OPTUM360®

EXPERT

2018

ICD-10-CM Expert for Physicians

The complete official code set
Codes valid October 1, 2017 through September 30, 2018

D1405275

Publisher's Notice

The *ICD-10-CM Expert for Physicians: The Complete Official Code Set* is designed to be an accurate and authoritative source regarding coding and every reasonable effort has been made to ensure accuracy and completeness of the content. However, Optum360 makes no guarantee, warranty, or representation that this publication is accurate, complete or without errors. It is understood that Optum360 is not rendering any legal or other professional services or advice in this publication and that Optum360 bears no liability for any results or consequences that may arise from the use of this book.

Acknowledgments

Lauri Gray, RHIT, CPC, AHIMA-approved ICD-10-CM/PCS Trainer, *Product Manager*
Karen Schmidt, BSN, *Technical Director*
Anita Schmidt, BS, RHIT, AHIMA-approved ICD-10-CM/PCS Trainer, *Clinical Technical Editor*
Leanne Patterson, CPC, *Clinical Technical Editor*
Anne Kenney, BA, MBA, CCA, CCS, *Clinical Technical Editor*
Karen Krawzik, RHIT, CCS, AHIMA-approved ICD-10-CM/PCS Trainer, *Clinical Technical Editor*
Peggy Willard, CCS, AHIMA-approved ICD-10-CM/PCS Trainer, *Clinical Technical Editor*
Dr. Vikas Kumar, BHMS, CPC, CPC-H, *Clinical Technical Editor*
Stacy Perry, *Manager, Desktop Publishing*
Lisa Singley, *Project Manager*
Tracy Betzler, *Senior Desktop Publishing Specialist*
Hope M. Dunn, *Senior Desktop Publishing Specialist*
Katie Russell, *Desktop Publishing Specialist*
Kate Holden, *Editor*

Our Commitment to Accuracy

Optum360 is committed to producing accurate and reliable materials.

To report corrections, please visit www.optum360coding.com/accuracy or email accuracy@optum.com. You can also reach customer service by calling 1.800.464.3649, option 1.

Anita Schmidt, BS, RHIT, AHIMA-approved ICD-10-CM/PCS Trainer

Ms. Schmidt has expertise in Level I Adult and Pediatric Trauma hospital coding, specializing in ICD-9-CM, ICD-10-CM/PCS, DRG, and CPT coding. Her experience includes analysis of medical record documentation, assignment of ICD-10-CM and PCS codes, DRG validation, as well as CPT code assignments for same-day surgery cases. She has conducted coding training and auditing, including DRG validation, conducted electronic health record training, and worked with clinical documentation specialists to identify documentation needs and potential areas for physician education. Most recently she has been developing content for resource and educational products related to ICD-10-CM and ICD-10-PCS. Ms. Schmidt is an AHIMA-approved ICD-10-CM/PCS trainer, and is an active member of the American Health Information Management Association (AHIMA) and the Minnesota Health Information Management Association (MHIMA).

Leanne Patterson, CPC

Ms. Patterson has more than 10 years of experience in the health care profession. She has an extensive background in professional component coding, with expertise in E/M coding and auditing, and HIPAA compliance. Her experience includes general surgery coding, serving as director of compliance, conducting chart-to-claim audits and physician education. She has been responsible for coding and denial management in large multispecialty physician practices, and most recently served as a practice manager where she supervised implementation of a new EHR system. Ms. Patterson is credentialed by the American Academy of Professional Coders (AAPC) as a Certified Professional Coder (CPC).

Contents

Contents

Preface

ICD-10-CM Official Preface

This FY 2018 update of the International Statistical Classification of Diseases and Related Health Problems, 10th revision, Clinical Modification (ICD-10-CM) is being published by the United States government in recognition of its responsibility to promulgate this classification throughout the United States for morbidity coding. The International Statistical Classification of Diseases and Related Health Problems, 10th Revision (ICD-10), published by the World Health Organization (WHO), is the foundation of ICD-10-CM. ICD-10 continues to be the classification used in cause-of-death coding in the United States. The ICD-10-CM is comparable with the ICD-10. The WHO Collaborating Center for the Family of International Classifications in North America, housed at the Centers for Disease Control and Prevention's National Center for Health Statistics (NCHS), has responsibility for the implementation of ICD and other WHO-FIC classifications and serves as a liaison with the WHO, fulfilling international obligations for comparable classifications and the national health data needs of the United States. The historical background of ICD and ICD-10 can be found in the Introduction to the International Classification of Diseases and Related Health Problems (ICD-10), 2010, World Health Organization, Geneva, Switzerland.

ICD-10-CM is the United States' clinical modification of the World Health Organization's ICD-10. The term "clinical" is used to emphasize the modification's intent: to serve as a useful tool in the area of classification of morbidity data for indexing of health records, medical care review, and ambulatory and other health care programs, as well as for basic health statistics. To describe the clinical picture of the patient the codes must be more precise than those needed only for statistical groupings and trend analysis.

Characteristics of ICD-10-CM

ICD-10-CM far exceeds its predecessors in the number of concepts and codes provided. The disease classification has been expanded to include health-related conditions and to provide greater specificity at the sixth and seventh character level. The sixth and seventh characters are not optional and are intended for use in recording the information documented in the clinical record.

ICD-10-CM extensions, interpretations, modifications, addenda, or errata other than those approved by the Centers for Disease Control and Prevention are not to be considered official and should not be utilized. Continuous maintenance of the ICD-10-CM is the responsibility of the aforementioned agencies. However, because the ICD-10-CM represents the best in contemporary thinking of clinicians, nosologists, epidemiologists, and statisticians from both public and private sectors, when future modifications are considered, advice will be sought from all stakeholders.

All official authorized addenda since the last complete update (October 1, 2017) have been included in this revision. For more detailed information please see the complete official authorized addenda to ICD-10-CM, including the "ICD-10-CM Official Guidelines for Coding and Reporting," and a description of the ICD-10-CM updating and maintenance process.

What's New for 2018

Official Updates

The National Center for Health Statistics (NCHS), a section of the Centers for Disease Control and Prevention (CDC), is the agency charged with maintaining and updating ICD-10-CM. The 2018 official addendum was posted to the Centers for Medicare and Medicaid Services (CMS) website on June 13, 2017, identifying the changes to the ICD-10-CM code set for fiscal 2018. A summary of changes is provided below:

- 360 new codes added

- 226 code descriptions revised

- 34 codes changed from valid to invalid

Note: Validity changes are the result of new codes being added to the classification, changing a previously valid code to an invalid code, creating a new subcategory.

A04.7	Enterocolitis due to Clostridium difficile
C96.2	Malignant mast cell tumor
D47.0	Histiocytic and mast cell tumors of uncertain behavior
E85.8	Other amyloidosis
H54.0	Blindness, both eyes
H54.11	Blindness, right eye, low vision left eye
H54.12	Blindness, left eye, low vision right eye
H54.2	Low vision, both eyes
H54.41	Blindness, right eye, normal vision left eye
H54.42	Blindness, left eye, normal vision right eye
H54.51	Low vision, right eye, normal vision left eye
H54.52	Low vision, left eye, normal vision right eye
I27.2	Other secondary pulmonary hypertension
K06.0	Gingival recession
K56.5	Intestinal adhesions [bands] with obstruction (postprocedural) (postinfection)
K56.60	Unspecified intestinal obstruction
K56.69	Other intestinal obstruction
K91.3	Postprocedural intestinal obstruction
M48.06	Spinal stenosis, lumbar region
N63	Unspecified lump in breast
O00.10	Tubal pregnancy without intrauterine pregnancy
O00.11	Tubal pregnancy with intrauterine pregnancy
O00.20	Ovarian pregnancy without intrauterine pregnancy
O00.21	Ovarian pregnancy with intrauterine pregnancy
P29.3	Persistent fetal circulation
P83.8	Other specified conditions of integument specific to newborn
P91.8	Other specified disturbances of cerebral status of newborn
Q53.11	Abdominal testis, unilateral
Q53.21	Abdominal testis, bilateral
T07	Unspecified multiple injuries
T14.8	Other injury of unspecified body region
T14.90	Injury, unspecified
T14.91	Suicide attempt
Z36	Encounter for antenatal screening of mother

- 122 codes deleted from the classification

S06.1X7D	Traumatic cerebral edema with loss of consciousness of any duration with death due to brain injury prior to regaining consciousness, subsequent encounter
S06.1X7S	Traumatic cerebral edema with loss of consciousness of any duration with death due to brain injury prior to regaining consciousness, sequela
S06.1X8D	Traumatic cerebral edema with loss of consciousness of any duration with death due to other cause prior to regaining consciousness, subsequent encounter
S06.1X8S	Traumatic cerebral edema with loss of consciousness of any duration with death due to other cause prior to regaining consciousness, sequela
S06.2X7D	Diffuse traumatic brain injury with loss of consciousness of any duration with death due to brain injury prior to regaining consciousness, subsequent encounter
S06.2X7S	Diffuse traumatic brain injury with loss of consciousness of any duration with death due to brain injury prior to regaining consciousness, sequela
S06.2X8D	Diffuse traumatic brain injury with loss of consciousness of any duration with death due to other cause prior to regaining consciousness, subsequent encounter
S06.2X8S	Diffuse traumatic brain injury with loss of consciousness of any duration with death due to other cause prior to regaining consciousness, sequela
S06.307D	Unspecified focal traumatic brain injury with loss of consciousness of any duration with death due to brain injury prior to regaining consciousness, subsequent encounter
S06.307S	Unspecified focal traumatic brain injury with loss of consciousness of any duration with death due to brain injury prior to regaining consciousness, sequela
S06.308D	Unspecified focal traumatic brain injury with loss of consciousness of any duration with death due to other cause prior to regaining consciousness, subsequent encounter
S06.308S	Unspecified focal traumatic brain injury with loss of consciousness of any duration with death due to other cause prior to regaining consciousness, sequela
S06.317D	Contusion and laceration of right cerebrum with loss of consciousness of any duration with death due to brain injury prior to regaining consciousness, subsequent encounter
S06.317S	Contusion and laceration of right cerebrum with loss of consciousness of any duration with death due to brain injury prior to regaining consciousness, sequela
S06.318D	Contusion and laceration of right cerebrum with loss of consciousness of any duration with death due to other cause prior to regaining consciousness, subsequent encounter
S06.318S	Contusion and laceration of right cerebrum with loss of consciousness of any duration with death due to other cause prior to regaining consciousness, sequela
S06.327D	Contusion and laceration of left cerebrum with loss of consciousness of any duration with death due to brain injury prior to regaining consciousness, subsequent encounter
S06.327S	Contusion and laceration of left cerebrum with loss of consciousness of any duration with death due to brain injury prior to regaining consciousness, sequela
S06.328D	Contusion and laceration of left cerebrum with loss of consciousness of any duration with death due to other cause prior to regaining consciousness, subsequent encounter
S06.328S	Contusion and laceration of left cerebrum with loss of consciousness of any duration with death due to other cause prior to regaining consciousness, sequela
S06.337D	Contusion and laceration of cerebrum, unspecified, with loss of consciousness of any duration with death due to brain injury prior to regaining consciousness, subsequent encounter
S06.337S	Contusion and laceration of cerebrum, unspecified, with loss of consciousness of any duration with death due to brain injury prior to regaining consciousness, sequela
S06.338D	Contusion and laceration of cerebrum, unspecified, with loss of consciousness of any duration with death due to other cause prior to regaining consciousness, subsequent encounter
S06.338S	Contusion and laceration of cerebrum, unspecified, with loss of consciousness of any duration with death due to other cause prior to regaining consciousness, sequela
S06.347D	Traumatic hemorrhage of right cerebrum with loss of consciousness of any duration with death due to brain injury prior to regaining consciousness, subsequent encounter

S06.347S Traumatic hemorrhage of right cerebrum with loss of consciousness of any duration with death due to brain injury prior to regaining consciousness, sequela

S06.348D Traumatic hemorrhage of right cerebrum with loss of consciousness of any duration with death due to other cause prior to regaining consciousness, subsequent encounter

S06.348S Traumatic hemorrhage of right cerebrum with loss of consciousness of any duration with death due to other cause prior to regaining consciousness, sequela

S06.357D Traumatic hemorrhage of left cerebrum with loss of consciousness of any duration with death due to brain injury prior to regaining consciousness, subsequent encounter

S06.357S Traumatic hemorrhage of left cerebrum with loss of consciousness of any duration with death due to brain injury prior to regaining consciousness, sequela

S06.358D Traumatic hemorrhage of left cerebrum with loss of consciousness of any duration with death due to other cause prior to regaining consciousness, subsequent encounter

S06.358S Traumatic hemorrhage of left cerebrum with loss of consciousness of any duration with death due to other cause prior to regaining consciousness, sequela

S06.367D Traumatic hemorrhage of cerebrum, unspecified, with loss of consciousness of any duration with death due to brain injury prior to regaining consciousness, subsequent encounter

S06.367S Traumatic hemorrhage of cerebrum, unspecified, with loss of consciousness of any duration with death due to brain injury prior to regaining consciousness, sequela

S06.368D Traumatic hemorrhage of cerebrum, unspecified, with loss of consciousness of any duration with death due to other cause prior to regaining consciousness, subsequent encounter

S06.368S Traumatic hemorrhage of cerebrum, unspecified, with loss of consciousness of any duration with death due to other cause prior to regaining consciousness, sequela

S06.377D Contusion, laceration, and hemorrhage of cerebellum with loss of consciousness of any duration with death due to brain injury prior to regaining consciousness, subsequent encounter

S06.377S Contusion, laceration, and hemorrhage of cerebellum with loss of consciousness of any duration with death due to brain injury prior to regaining consciousness, sequela

S06.378D Contusion, laceration, and hemorrhage of cerebellum with loss of consciousness of any duration with death due to other cause prior to regaining consciousness, subsequent encounter

S06.378S Contusion, laceration, and hemorrhage of cerebellum with loss of consciousness of any duration with death due to other cause prior to regaining consciousness, sequela

S06.387D Contusion, laceration, and hemorrhage of brainstem with loss of consciousness of any duration with death due to brain injury prior to regaining consciousness, subsequent encounter

S06.387S Contusion, laceration, and hemorrhage of brainstem with loss of consciousness of any duration with death due to brain injury prior to regaining consciousness, sequela

S06.388D Contusion, laceration, and hemorrhage of brainstem with loss of consciousness of any duration with death due to other cause prior to regaining consciousness, subsequent encounter

S06.388S Contusion, laceration, and hemorrhage of brainstem with loss of consciousness of any duration with death due to other cause prior to regaining consciousness, sequela

S06.4X7D Epidural hemorrhage with loss of consciousness of any duration with death due to brain injury prior to regaining consciousness, subsequent encounter

S06.4X7S Epidural hemorrhage with loss of consciousness of any duration with death due to brain injury prior to regaining consciousness, sequela

S06.4X8D Epidural hemorrhage with loss of consciousness of any duration with death due to other causes prior to regaining consciousness, subsequent encounter

S06.4X8S Epidural hemorrhage with loss of consciousness of any duration with death due to other causes prior to regaining consciousness, sequela

S06.5X7D Traumatic subdural hemorrhage with loss of consciousness of any duration with death due to brain injury before regaining consciousness, subsequent encounter

S06.5X7S Traumatic subdural hemorrhage with loss of consciousness of any duration with death due to brain injury before regaining consciousness, sequela

S06.5X8D Traumatic subdural hemorrhage with loss of consciousness of any duration with death due to other cause before regaining consciousness, subsequent encounter

S06.5X8S Traumatic subdural hemorrhage with loss of consciousness of any duration with death due to other cause before regaining consciousness, sequela

S06.6X7D Traumatic subarachnoid hemorrhage with loss of consciousness of any duration with death due to brain injury prior to regaining consciousness, subsequent encounter

S06.6X7S Traumatic subarachnoid hemorrhage with loss of consciousness of any duration with death due to brain injury prior to regaining consciousness, sequela

S06.6X8D Traumatic subarachnoid hemorrhage with loss of consciousness of any duration with death due to other cause prior to regaining consciousness, subsequent encounter

S06.6X8S Traumatic subarachnoid hemorrhage with loss of consciousness of any duration with death due to other cause prior to regaining consciousness, sequela

S06.817D Injury of right internal carotid artery, intracranial portion, not elsewhere classified with loss of consciousness of any duration with death due to brain injury prior to regaining consciousness, subsequent encounter

S06.817S Injury of right internal carotid artery, intracranial portion, not elsewhere classified with loss of consciousness of any duration with death due to brain injury prior to regaining consciousness, sequela

S06.818D Injury of right internal carotid artery, intracranial portion, not elsewhere classified with loss of consciousness of any duration with death due to other cause prior to regaining consciousness, subsequent encounter

S06.818S Injury of right internal carotid artery, intracranial portion, not elsewhere classified with loss of consciousness of any duration with death due to other cause prior to regaining consciousness, sequela

S06.827D Injury of left internal carotid artery, intracranial portion, not elsewhere classified with loss of consciousness of any duration with death due to brain injury prior to regaining consciousness, subsequent encounter

S06.827S Injury of left internal carotid artery, intracranial portion, not elsewhere classified with loss of consciousness of any duration with death due to brain injury prior to regaining consciousness, sequela

S06.828D Injury of left internal carotid artery, intracranial portion, not elsewhere classified with loss of consciousness of any duration with death due to other cause prior to regaining consciousness, subsequent encounter

S06.828S Injury of left internal carotid artery, intracranial portion, not elsewhere classified with loss of consciousness of any duration with death due to other cause prior to regaining consciousness, sequela

S06.897D Other specified intracranial injury with loss of consciousness of any duration with death due to brain injury prior to regaining consciousness, subsequent encounter

S06.897S Other specified intracranial injury with loss of consciousness of any duration with death due to brain injury prior to regaining consciousness, sequela

S06.898D Other specified intracranial injury with loss of consciousness of any duration with death due to other cause prior to regaining consciousness, subsequent encounter

S06.898S Other specified intracranial injury with loss of consciousness of any duration with death due to other cause prior to regaining consciousness, sequela

S06.9X7D Unspecified intracranial injury with loss of consciousness of any duration with death due to brain injury prior to regaining consciousness, subsequent encounter

S06.9X7S   Unspecified intracranial injury with loss of consciousness of any duration with death due to brain injury prior to regaining consciousness, sequela

S06.9X8D   Unspecified intracranial injury with loss of consciousness of any duration with death due to other cause prior to regaining consciousness, subsequent encounter

S06.9X8S   Unspecified intracranial injury with loss of consciousness of any duration with death due to other cause prior to regaining consciousness, sequela

S63.13   Subluxation and dislocation of proximal interphalangeal joint of thumb

S63.131   Subluxation of proximal interphalangeal joint of right thumb

S63.131A   Subluxation of proximal interphalangeal joint of right thumb, initial encounter

S63.131D   Subluxation of proximal interphalangeal joint of right thumb, subsequent encounter

S63.131S   Subluxation of proximal interphalangeal joint of right thumb, sequela

S63.132   Subluxation of proximal interphalangeal joint of left thumb

S63.132A   Subluxation of proximal interphalangeal joint of left thumb, initial encounter

S63.132D   Subluxation of proximal interphalangeal joint of left thumb, subsequent encounter

S63.132S   Subluxation of proximal interphalangeal joint of left thumb, sequela

S63.133   Subluxation of proximal interphalangeal joint of unspecified thumb

S63.133A   Subluxation of proximal interphalangeal joint of unspecified thumb, initial encounter

S63.133D   Subluxation of proximal interphalangeal joint of unspecified thumb, subsequent encounter

S63.133S   Subluxation of proximal interphalangeal joint of unspecified thumb, sequela

S63.134   Dislocation of proximal interphalangeal joint of right thumb

S63.134A   Dislocation of proximal interphalangeal joint of right thumb, initial encounter

S63.134D   Dislocation of proximal interphalangeal joint of right thumb, subsequent encounter

S63.134S   Dislocation of proximal interphalangeal joint of right thumb, sequela

S63.135   Dislocation of proximal interphalangeal joint of left thumb

S63.135A   Dislocation of proximal interphalangeal joint of left thumb, initial encounter

S63.135D   Dislocation of proximal interphalangeal joint of left thumb, subsequent encounter

S63.135S   Dislocation of proximal interphalangeal joint of left thumb, sequela

S63.136   Dislocation of proximal interphalangeal joint of unspecified thumb

S63.136A   Dislocation of proximal interphalangeal joint of unspecified thumb, initial encounter

S63.136D   Dislocation of proximal interphalangeal joint of unspecified thumb, subsequent encounter

S63.136S   Dislocation of proximal interphalangeal joint of unspecified thumb, sequela

S63.14   Subluxation and dislocation of distal interphalangeal joint of thumb

S63.141   Subluxation of distal interphalangeal joint of right thumb

S63.141A   Subluxation of distal interphalangeal joint of right thumb, initial encounter

S63.141D   Subluxation of distal interphalangeal joint of right thumb, subsequent encounter

S63.141S   Subluxation of distal interphalangeal joint of right thumb, sequela

S63.142   Subluxation of distal interphalangeal joint of left thumb

S63.142A   Subluxation of distal interphalangeal joint of left thumb, initial encounter

S63.142D   Subluxation of distal interphalangeal joint of left thumb, subsequent encounter

S63.142S   Subluxation of distal interphalangeal joint of left thumb, sequela

S63.143   Subluxation of distal interphalangeal joint of unspecified thumb

S63.143A   Subluxation of distal interphalangeal joint of unspecified thumb, initial encounter

S63.143D   Subluxation of distal interphalangeal joint of unspecified thumb, subsequent encounter

S63.143S   Subluxation of distal interphalangeal joint of unspecified thumb, sequela

S63.144   Dislocation of distal interphalangeal joint of right thumb

S63.144A   Dislocation of distal interphalangeal joint of right thumb, initial encounter

S63.144D   Dislocation of distal interphalangeal joint of right thumb, subsequent encounter

S63.144S   Dislocation of distal interphalangeal joint of right thumb, sequela

S63.145   Dislocation of distal interphalangeal joint of left thumb

S63.145A   Dislocation of distal interphalangeal joint of left thumb, initial encounter

S63.145D   Dislocation of distal interphalangeal joint of left thumb, subsequent encounter

S63.145S   Dislocation of distal interphalangeal joint of left thumb, sequela

S63.146   Dislocation of distal interphalangeal joint of unspecified thumb

S63.146A   Dislocation of distal interphalangeal joint of unspecified thumb, initial encounter

S63.146D   Dislocation of distal interphalangeal joint of unspecified thumb, subsequent encounter

S63.146S   Dislocation of distal interphalangeal joint of unspecified thumb, sequela

Proprietary Updates

The following proprietary features have also been added:

- 150+ new definitions that describe, in lay terms, a specific condition or disease process

- 50+ new illustrations

- Updated *AHA Coding Clinic* references through second quarter 2017

- Updated pharmacology list

- New HCC icon identifying CMS hierarchical condition category (CMS-HCC) codes

- New appendix outlining the Medicare Advantage risk-adjustment model

- Updated coding examples in the chapter-specific guideline sections that are specific to the physician setting

Introduction

History of ICD-10-CM

The ICD-10-CM classification system was developed by the National Center for Health Statistics (NCHS) as a clinical modification to the ICD-10 system developed by the World Health Organization (WHO), primarily as a unique system for use in the United States for morbidity and mortality reporting. Although ICD-10 replaced ICD-9 for use in coding and classifying mortality data from death certificates beginning January 1, 1999, ICD-10-CM implementation was postponed many years until legislation to replace ICD-9-CM, volumes 1 and 2, with ICD-10-CM was approved.

ICD-10 is the copyrighted product of the World Health Organization (WHO), which has authorized the development of a clinical modification (CM) of ICD-10 for use in the United States. However, all modifications to the ICD-10 must conform to WHO conventions for ICD. The development of ICD-10-CM included comprehensive evaluation by a Technical Advisory Panel and extensive consultation with physician groups, clinical coders, and other industry experts.

The ICD-10-CM draft and crosswalk between ICD-9-CM and ICD-10-CM were made available on the Centers for Medicare and Medicaid Services (CMS) website for public comment. The initial public comment period extended from December 1997 through February 1998. A field test for ICD-10-CM was conducted in the summer of 2003 jointly by the American Hospital Association (AHA) and the American Health Information Management Association (AHIMA). Public comments and suggestions were reviewed and additional modifications to ICD-10-CM were made. Revisions were made to ICD-10-CM based on the established update process for ICD-10-CM (the ICD-10-CM Coordination and Maintenance Committee) and the World Health Organization's ICD-10 (the Update and Revision Committee).

These revisions to ICD-10-CM have included:

- Information relevant to ambulatory and managed care encounters
- Expanded injury codes
- Creation of combination diagnosis/symptom codes to reduce the number of codes needed to fully describe a condition
- The addition of 6th and 7th character classifications
- Incorporation of common 4th and 5th character classifications
- Classifications specific to laterality
- Classification refinement for increased data granularity

This new structure allows for further expansion than was possible with the ICD-9-CM classification system.

The Department of Health and Human Services (HHS) published the final rule regarding the adoption of both ICD-10-CM and ICD-10-PCS in the January 16, 2009, *Federal Register* (45 CFR part 162 [CMS—0013—F]). The initial compliance date for implementation of ICD-10-CM and ICD-10-PCS as a replacement for ICD-9-CM was set at October 1, 2013. On April 17, 2012, the Department of Health and Human Services (HHS) released a notice to postpone the date by which certain health care entities have to comply with International Classification of Diseases, 10th Revision diagnosis and procedure codes (ICD-10). The compliance date for implementation of ICD-10-CM and ICD-10-PCS as a replacement for ICD-9-CM was changed to October 1, 2014. On April 1, 2014, Congress enacted the Protecting Access to Medicare Act of 2014, which contained a provision to delay the implementation of ICD-10-CM/PCS by at least one year, prohibiting the Department of Health and Human Services (HHS) from adopting the ICD-10-CM/PCS code sets as the mandatory standard until October 1, 2015. Eventually, the ICD-10-CM/PCS code sets were implemented in their entirety on October 1, 2015, and volumes 1 and 2 of ICD-9-CM were retired.

ICD-10-CM: The Complete Official Code Set

ICD-10-CM for Physicians: The Complete Official Code Set 2018 edition includes many of the enhancements described below in direct response to requests from our subscribers.

As you review the content, you will find the following:

- Optum360 Exclusive feature — Check Placeholder Alert symbol, indicating the need for one or more "filler" X character assignments in the 5th and/or 6th character position, in order to appropriately assign a required character in the 7th character position

- Optum360 Exclusive feature — Key word differentiation by the use of a green font that highlights the differentiating terms in similar code descriptions in a given category

- Optum360 Exclusive color coding, symbols, and footnotes that alert coders to coding and reimbursement issues, including the majority of the Medicare code edits

- Optum360 Exclusive feature — Exclusive *following* references and Check Additional Character symbol in the indexes. The *following* references (designed and used exclusively by Optum360) help coders locate those alphanumeric codes that are out of sequence in the tabular section.

- Optum360 Exclusive feature — Exclusive shaded guides in the index that help users easily follow the indent levels for the subterms under a main term

- Illustrations throughout the tabular list and at the back of the book that feature anatomy and terminology included in the ICD-10-CM classification system

- Optum360 Exclusive feature — Detailed Muscle/Tendon tables that correspond to codes in chapters 13 and 19

- The complete ICD-10-CM Official Guidelines for Coding and Reporting, published by the U.S. Department of Health and Human Services and approved by the cooperating parties (American Health Information Management Association, National Center for Health Statistics, Centers for Medicare and Medicaid Services, American Hospital Association)

- Optum360 Exclusive feature — Official chapter-specific guidelines with coding examples at the beginning of each chapter

- All the official ICD-10-CM codes, indexes, notes, footnotes, and symbols

- Icons and definitions to differentiate between the two types of Excludes notes

- Check 4th, 5th, 6th, and 7th character symbols that identify codes that require the addition of a 4th, 5th, 6th, or 7th character for code specificity and validity

- Color coding and symbol legend at the bottom of each page

Please review "How to Use *ICD-10-CM Expert for Physicians*" in this section to learn about the features that will help you assign and report correct codes, ensuring appropriate reimbursement.

How to Use ICD-10-CM Expert for Physicians 2018

This International Classification of Diseases, 10th Revision, Clinical Modification (ICD-10-CM) is being published by the United States Government in recognition of its responsibility to promulgate this classification throughout the United States for morbidity coding. This code book represents an adaptation of ICD-10 that was created specifically for use in the United States. Revisions to ICD-10-CM will be made based on the established update process for ICD-10-CM (the ICD-10-CM Coordination and Maintenance Committee) and the World Health Organization's ICD-10 (the Update and Revision Committee).

Use of Official Sources

The *ICD-10-CM Expert for Physicians* contains the official U.S. Department of Health and Human Services, Tenth Revision, Clinical Modification, ICD-10-CM codes, effective for the current year.

Much of the color coding and many of the symbols that identify coding and reimbursement issues are derived from official federal government sources, including the Integrated Outpatient Code Editor (IOCE), version 18.2.

For the most current IOCE documents please refer to the following: https://www.cms.gov/Medicare/Coding/OutpatientCodeEdit/OCEQtrReleaseSpecs.html.

Steps to Correct Coding

1. Before beginning to use this code book, review section I.A., "Conventions for the ICD-10-CM," and section I.B., "General Coding Guidelines," of the ICD-10-CM Official Guidelines for Coding and Reporting.

2. Look up the main term in the alphabetic index and scan the subterm entries as appropriate. Review continued lines and additional subterms that may appear in the next column or on the next page.

3. Note all parenthetical terms (nonessential modifiers) that help in code selection but do not affect code assignment. Shaded vertical guidelines in the index are provided to help determine the indentation level for each subterm in relation to the main terms.

4. Pay close attention to the following instructions in the index:
   - "See," "see also," and "see category" cross-references
   - "With"/"without" notes
   - "Omit code" notes
   - "Due to" subterms
   - Other instructions found in note boxes, such as "code by site"
   - *Following* references and Check Additional Character symbol in the indexes. The *following* references (designed and used exclusively by Optum360) help coders locate those alphanumeric codes that are out of sequence in the tabular section.

5. Do not code from the alphabetic index without verifying the accuracy of the code in the tabular list. Locate the code in the alphanumerically arranged tabular list.

6. To determine the appropriateness of the code selection and proper coding, read all instructional material:
   - "Includes" and both types of "Excludes" notes
   - "Use additional code" and "code first underlying disease" instructions

   - "Code also"
   - 4th, 5th, and 6th character requirements and 7th character extension requirements
   - Age and sex symbols

7. Consult the official ICD-10-CM guidelines, which govern the use of specific codes. These guidelines provide both general and chapter-specific coding guidance.

8. Confirm and assign the correct code.

Organization

This book is organized in the following manner:

Introduction

The introductory material in this book includes the ICD-10-CM Official Preface, the history of ICD-10-CM as well as an overview of the classification system.

Official ICD-10-CM Conventions and Guidelines

This section provides an explanation of the conventions and guidelines regulating the appropriate assignment and reporting of ICD-10-CM codes. This coding guidance is presented by the National Center for Health Statistics (NCHS), a governmental agency of the Centers for Disease Control and Prevention (CDC), within the United States Department of Health and Human Services (DHHS).

Alphabetic Index to Diseases

The Alphabetic Index to Diseases is arranged in alphabetic order by disease — by specific illness, injury, eponym, abbreviation, or other descriptive diagnostic term. The Index also lists diagnostic terms for other reasons for encounters with health care professionals.

Neoplasm Table

The Neoplasm Table provides the proper code based upon histology of the neoplasm and site.

Table of Drugs and Chemicals

The Table of Drugs and Chemicals lists the drug and the specific codes that identify the drug and the intent. No additional external cause of injury and poisoning code is assigned in ICD-10-CM.

Index to External Causes

The Alphabetic Index to External Causes of Injuries is arranged in alphabetic order by main term indicating the event.

Tabular List of Diseases

ICD-10-CM codes and descriptors are arranged numerically within the tabular list of diseases within 21 separate chapters according to body system or nature of injury and disease. Classifications that were previously considered supplemental to ICD-9-CM (e.g., V codes and E codes) are incorporated into the tabular listing of ICD-10-CM as individual chapters. Chapters 20, "External Causes of Morbidity," and 21, "Factors Influencing Health Status and Contact with Health Services," include chapter-specific guidelines.

Appendixes

The additional resources described below have been included as appendixes for the *ICD-10-CM Expert for Physicians*. These resources further instruct the professional coder on the appropriate application of the ICD-10-CM code set.

Appendix A: 10 Steps to Correct Coding

This step-by-step tutorial walks the coder through the process of locating the correct code in the alphabetic index and verifying it in the tabular section while following applicable conventions and guidelines. Detailed examples are provided and explained along with advice for proper sequencing.

Appendix B: Valid 3-character ICD-10-CM Codes

The user may consult this table to confirm that no further specificity, such as the use of 4th, 5th, 6th, or 7th characters or placeholders (X), is necessary. All ICD-10-CM codes that are valid at the three-character level are listed.

Appendix C: Pharmacology List 2018

This reference is a comprehensive but not all-inclusive list of pharmacological agents used to treat acute and/or chronic conditions. Drugs are listed in alphabetical order by their brand and/or generic names along with their drug action and indications for which they may commonly be prescribed. Some drugs have also been mapped to their appropriate Z code for long-term drug use.

Appendix D: Z Codes for Long-Term Drug Use with Associated Drugs

This resource correlates Z codes that are used to identify current long-term drug use with a list of drugs that are typically categorized to that class of drug.

Note: These tables are not all-inclusive but list some of the more commonly used drugs.

Appendix E: Z Codes Only as Principal/First-Listed Diagnosis

Chapter 21, "Factors Influencing Health Status and Contact with Health Services," provides codes to deal with encounters for circumstances other than a disease or injury. Many of these codes may be reported *only* as the principal/first-listed diagnosis. This resource lists all of these codes in one table for quick and easy reference to ensure accurate reporting.

Appendix F: Centers for Medicare & Medicaid Services Hierarchical Condition Categories (CMS-HCC)

This resource provides the framework behind the Centers for Medicare and Medicaid Services' (CMS) Medicare Advantage (MA) program, a risk-adjustment model developed as a means of compensating health care plans with large numbers of Medicare Part C beneficiaries. It includes a brief synopsis of the evolution of the program from its inception; insight into the various elements needed to predict risk, including the principles used to develop the hierarchical condition categories (HCCs), which make up one of the fundamental components of the risk-adjustment model. This appendix also outlines the audit process used to ensure the accuracy of payments made to MA plans.

Illustrations

This section includes illustrations of normal anatomy with ICD-10-CM specific terminology.

Overview of ICD-10-CM Official Conventions

This is an overview of the ICD-10-CM official conventions, which are general rules for using the classification system, independent of the guidelines. The official conventions and instructions of the classification, which take precedence over the guidelines, are incorporated within the alphabetic index and tabular list as instructional notes and are applicable regardless of the health care setting. For the full version of the official conventions, see the ICD-10-CM Official Guidelines for Coding and Reporting, section I.A., which is included in this book.

Format

ICD-10-CM is divided into two main parts: the index, an alphabetical list of terms and their corresponding code, and the tabular list, a sequential, alphanumeric list of codes divided into chapters based on body system or condition. The index contains the Index to Diseases and Injuries (main index) and the Index to External Causes of Injury. Also included in the main index is the Neoplasm Table and a Table of Drugs and Chemicals.

The tabular list contains categories, subcategories, and valid codes. ICD-10-CM is an alphanumeric classification system. The 1st character of a three-character category is a letter. The 2nd and 3rd characters may be numbers or alpha characters. A three-character category without further subclassification is equivalent to a valid three-character code. Subcategories are either four or five characters. Subcategory characters include either letters or numbers. Codes may be three, four, five, six, or seven characters in length, in which each level of subdivision after a category is a subcategory. The final level of subdivision is a valid code. The final character in a code may be either a letter or a number.

The ICD-10-CM uses the letter "X" as a placeholder. A placeholder "X" is used as a 5th character placeholder at certain six-character codes to allow for future expansion, without disturbing the 6th character structure. For instance, an initial encounter for accidental poisoning by penicillin is coded to T36.0X1A. The "X" in the 5th character position is a placeholder, or filler character.

Similarly, certain categories have applicable 7th character extensions. In these cases, the 7th character extension is required for all codes within the category, or as otherwise instructed in the tabular list notations. 7th character extensions must always be the last character in the data field. If a code is not a full six characters in length, a dummy placeholder "X" must be used to fill in the empty characters when a 7th character extension is required.

Punctuation

[ ]   In the tabular list, brackets are used to enclose synonyms, alternative wording, or explanatory phrases. In the index, brackets are used to identify manifestation codes.

( )   Parentheses are used in both the index and tabular list to enclose nonessential modifiers; supplementary words that may be present or absent in the statement of a disease or procedure without affecting the code number to which it is assigned.

:   Colons are used in the tabular list after an incomplete term that needs one or more of the modifiers following the colon to make it assignable to a given category.

Abbreviations

NEC

The abbreviation NEC, "Not elsewhere classifiable" represents "other specified" in the ICD-10-CM. An index entry that states NEC directs the coder to an "other specified" code in the tabular list. Codes titled "Other" or "Other specified" in the tabular list (usually a code with a 4th or 6th character 8 and 5th character 9) are for use when the information in the medical record provides detail for which a specific code does not exist.

NOS

The abbreviation NOS, "Not otherwise specified," in the tabular list may be interpreted as "unspecified." Codes in the tabular list with "Unspecified" in the title (usually a code with a 4th or 6th character 9 and 5th character Ø) are for use when the information in the medical record is insufficient to assign a more specific code.

Typeface

Boldface

Boldface type is used for main term entries in the alphabetic index, and all codes and descriptions in the tabular list.

General Notes

The following conventions and notes appear only in the tabular list of diseases:

Includes Notes

The word INCLUDES appears immediately under certain categories to further define, clarify, or give examples of the content of a code category.

Inclusion Terms

Lists of inclusion terms are included under certain codes. These terms indicate some of the conditions for which that code number may be used. Inclusion terms may be synonyms with the code title, or, in the case of "other specified" codes, the terms may also provide a list of various conditions included within a classification code. The inclusion terms are not exhaustive. The index may provide additional terms that may also be assigned to a given code.

Excludes Notes

ICD-10-CM has two types of excludes notes. Each note has a different definition for use. However, they are similar in that they both indicate that codes excluded from each other are independent of each other.

Excludes 1

An EXCLUDES 1 note is a "pure" excludes. It means "NOT CODED HERE!" An Excludes 1 note indicates mutually exclusive codes: two conditions that cannot be reported together. For example, a congenital form of a disease may not be reported with the acquired form of the same condition. The code excluded should never be reported with the applicable codes listed above the excludes notation.

An exception to the Excludes 1 definition is when the two conditions are unrelated to each other. If it is not clear whether the two conditions involving an Excludes 1 note are related or not, query the provider. For example, code F45.8 Other somatoform disorders, has an Excludes 1 note for "sleep related teeth grinding (G47.63)" because "teeth grinding" is an inclusion term under F45.8. Only one of these two codes should be assigned for teeth grinding. However psychogenic dysmenorrhea is also an inclusion term under F45.8, and a patient could have both this condition and sleep-related teeth grinding. In this case, the two conditions are clearly unrelated to each other, so it would be appropriate to report F45.8 and G47.63 together.

Excludes 2

An EXCLUDES 2 note means "NOT INCLUDED HERE." An Excludes 2 note indicates that although the excluded condition is not part of the condition it is excluded from, a patient may have both conditions at the same time. Therefore, when an Excludes 2 note appears under a code, it may be acceptable to use both the code and the excluded code together if supported by the medical documentation.

Note

NOTE The term "NOTE" appears as an icon and precedes the instructional information. These notes function as alerts to highlight coding instructions within the text.

Default Codes

In the index, the default code is the code listed next to the main term. The default code represents the condition most commonly associated with the main term. This code may be assigned when documentation does not facilitate reporting a more specific code. Alternatively, it may provide an unspecified code for the condition.

Syndromes

Follow the alphabetic index guidance when coding syndromes. In the absence of index guidance, assign codes for the documented manifestations of the syndrome.

And

When the term "and" is used in a narrative statement or code title it may be interpreted as "and/or."

With

The word "with" or "in" should be interpreted to mean "associated with" or "due to" when it appears in a code title, the Alphabetic Index, or an instructional note in the Tabular List. The classification presumes a causal relationship between the two conditions linked by these terms in the Alphabetic Index or Tabular List. These conditions should be coded as related even in the absence of provider documentation explicitly linking them, unless the documentation clearly states the conditions are unrelated or when another guideline exists that specifically requires a documented linkage between two conditions (e.g., sepsis guideline for "acute organ dysfunction that is not clearly associated with the sepsis"). For conditions not specifically linked by these relational terms in the classification or when a guideline requires that a linkage between two conditions be explicitly documented, provider documentation must link the conditions in order to code them as related.

The word "with" in the Alphabetic Index is sequenced immediately following the main term, not in alphabetical order.

See and See Also

When the instruction "See" follows a main term in the alphabetic index, it indicates that another term must be referenced in order to locate the correct code. The instructional note "See also" simply provides alternative terms that may be useful in determining the correct code but is not necessary to follow if the main term supplies the appropriate code.

Instructional Notes Used in the Tabular List

In the tabular section, the following instructional notes appear in red type for emphasis:

Code First/Use additional code:

These instructional notes provide sequencing instruction. They may appear independently of each other or to designate certain etiology/manifestation paired codes. These instructions signal the coder that an additional code should be reported to provide a more complete picture of that diagnosis.

In etiology/manifestation coding, ICD-10-CM requires the underlying condition to be sequenced first, followed by the manifestation. In these situations, codes with "In diseases classified elsewhere" in the code description are never permitted as a first-listed or principal diagnosis code and must be sequenced following the underlying condition code.

Code Also:

A "code also" note alerts the coder that more than one code may be required to fully describe the condition. The sequencing depends on the circumstances of the encounter. Factors that may determine sequencing include severity and reason for the encounter.

Code Assignment and Clinical Criteria

Diagnosis code assignment must be based on the provider's diagnostic statement that the condition exists and is not based on clinical criteria the provider used to establish the diagnosis. Conflicting documentation must be queried.

Additional Annotations

Code-Level Notations

The tabular section of ICD-10-CM has various colors, symbols, and other tabular annotations that may help in code selection, provide clinical or coding information, or alert the coder to reimbursement issues affected by the diagnosis code assignment. Some codes may have more than one annotation. For quick reference to the meanings of the colors and symbols, look at the color/symbol legend at the bottom of each page in the tabular list.

Italics

Italicized type is used for all exclusion notes and to identify manifestation codes, those codes that should not be reported as first-listed (principal) diagnoses.

Color Coding/Symbols

New Code

This ● icon identifies the codes that are new to the classification system for the current year. The new code icon is to the left of the code.

Revised Code Title

This ▲ icon to the left of a code alerts the user to a change in that code's title. This change may be as simple as adding or removing punctuation, which may or may not change the intent of the code, to adding or removing specific terms from a code description that completely alter the circumstances in which the code would be used.

Revised Text

The revised text ▶◀ "bow ties" alert the user to changes in parenthetical notes for the current year. Revised text may include the following:

- A change in a current parenthetical description

- A change in the code(s) associated with a current parenthetical note

- A change in how a current parenthetical note is classified (e.g., an Excludes 1 note that changed to an Excludes 2 note)

- Addition of a new parenthetical note(s) to a code

Deleted Text

Strikethrough on code description(s) and/or code note(s) indicates a deletion from the classification for the current year. For example:

✓4ᵗʰ **N25 Disorders resulting from impaired renal tubular function**
     EXCLUDES 1   ~~metabolic disorders classifiable to E70-E88~~

The strikethrough over the Excludes 1 note indicates that this note was deleted from the classification and is no longer applicable to codes in category N25.

✓7ᵗʰ ~~S63.131   Subluxation of proximal interphalangeal joint of right thumb~~

The strikethrough over the code and the code description indicates that all codes in subcategory S63.131 (S63.131A, S63.131D, and S63.131S) have been deleted from the classification.

Additional Characters Required

✓4ᵗʰ This symbol indicates that the code requires a 4th character.

✓5ᵗʰ This symbol indicates that the code requires a 5th character.

✓6ᵗʰ This symbol indicates that the code requires a 6th character.

✓7ᵗʰ This symbol indicates that the code requires a 7th character.

✓x7ᵗʰ This symbol indicates that the code requires a 7th character following the placeholder "X." Codes with fewer than six characters

that require a 7th character must contain placeholder "X" to fill in the empty character(s).

Key Word

Green font is used throughout the Tabular List of Diseases to differentiate the key words that appear in similar code descriptions in a given category or subcategory.

For example, refer to the list of codes below from category C7A:

C7A.020   Malignant carcinoid tumor of the appendix

C7A.021   Malignant carcinoid tumor of the cecum

C7A.022   Malignant carcinoid tumor of the ascending colon

C7A.023   Malignant carcinoid tumor of the transverse colon

C7A.024   Malignant carcinoid tumor of the descending colon

C7A.025   Malignant carcinoid tumor of the sigmoid colon

C7A.026   Malignant carcinoid tumor of the rectum

C7A.029   Malignant carcinoid tumor of the large intestine, unspecified portion

The portion of the code description that appears in green font in the tabular list assists the coder in quickly identifying the key terms and in identifying the correct code. This convention is especially useful when the codes describe laterality, such as the following codes from subcategory H40.22:

H40.221   Chronic angle-closure glaucoma, right eye

H40.222   Chronic angle-closure glaucoma, left eye

H40.223   Chronic angle-closure glaucoma, bilateral

H40.229   Chronic angle-closure glaucoma, unspecified eye

The key word convention is used only in those categories in which there are multiple codes with very similar descriptions with only a few words that differentiate them.

Medicare Code Edits

Medicare Administrative Contractors and many payers use Medicare code edits to check the coding accuracy on claims. The coding edit information in this manual reflects those edits used for outpatient institutional providers, which also include hospitals that are subject to the outpatient prospective payment system (OPPS). These edits have been updated to reflect changes in the Integrated Outpatient Code Editor (IOCE), version 18.2.

Manifestation Code

These codes appear in italic type, with a ***blue color bar*** over the title. A manifestation code cannot be reported as a first-listed or principal diagnosis. By definition, a manifestation code represents a demonstration of some aspect of an underlying disease, which is separately classifiable. In the alphabetic index, these codes are listed as the secondary code in brackets. The underlying disease code is listed first.

Age and Sex Edit

The age and sex edits below are used to detect inconsistencies between the patient's age and/or sex and the patient's diagnosis. The following edit symbols appear in the tabular list to the right of the code description.

Newborn Age: 0   Ⓝ

These diagnoses are intended for newborns and neonates and the patient's age must be 0 years.

Pediatric Age: 0-17   P

> These diagnoses are intended for children and the patient's age must be between 0 and 17 years.

Maternity Age: 12-55   M

> These diagnoses are intended for childbearing patients between the age of 12 and 55 years.

Adult Age: 15-124   A

> These diagnoses are intended for patients between the age of 15 and 124 years.

Male diagnosis only   ♂

Female diagnosis only   ♀

Medicare Advantage Risk Adjustment Edits

Medicare Advantage plans provided as part of the Medicare Part C program use a risk-adjustment model to plan for future healthcare costs of Medicare Part C participants. The risk-adjustment model measures disease burden by assigning certain ICD-10-CM diagnosis codes to hierarchical condition categories (HCC). The HCC information in this manual has been updated to reflect the CMS-HCC model category for v22 of the CMS-HCC risk-adjustment software.

HCC   HCC

This symbol indicates that the condition is considered a CMS-HCC diagnosis. All HCC conditions that are appropriately documented are used in the risk-adjustment model for Medicare Advantage to provide a means of comparing quality of care across Medicare Part C participants as well as predict future healthcare costs.

The HCC icon appears to the right of the code description.

Other Code-Level Notations

Unspecified Code   ▽

Use these codes when neither the diagnostic statement nor the documentation provides enough information to assign a more specific diagnosis code. These codes may be stated as "Unspecified" or "Not otherwise specified (NOS)."

Note: Do not assign these codes when a more specific diagnosis has been determined.

PDx Symbol   PDx

This symbol identifies a Z code that generally is for use as a first-listed (or principal) diagnosis only but may be used as an additional diagnosis if the patient has more than one encounter on the same day or there is more than one reason for the encounter.

The instructions for Z code use contained in the ICD-10-CM official coding guidelines identify those Z codes that can be used only as a PDx. All other Z codes may either be SDx or PDx, depending upon circumstances of the encounter, by meeting the definition of first-listed or principal diagnosis, and by following any specific Z code guidelines in section I.C.21 a-c. The responsibility of those assigning the Z codes as PDx is to make sure the circumstances of the encounter meet the definition of first-listed or principal diagnosis, follow all coding instructions, and follow the Z code specific guidelines. Optum360 does not include any SDx edit since there is no official source for it and the Z code use is determined by circumstances of the encounter.

Note: Please note that the symbols indicating the Z code "principal or first-listed only" designation and the Z codes that may be principal or first-listed diagnoses included in the official coding guidelines [section I.C.21.c.16] are consistent with reporting guidelines for health care encounters *excluding acute care inpatient admissions*. These Z code edits are often in conflict with the inpatient prospective payment system (IPPS) edits. For example, code Z34.9Ø Encounter for supervision of normal pregnancy, unspecified, unspecified trimester, may be an appropriate primary reason for an outpatient encounter. However, supervision for a normal pregnancy is not an acceptable principal diagnosis or reason for an inpatient admission and will have an unacceptable principal diagnosis edit under the inpatient prospective payment system (IPPS).

AHA:

This symbol precedes official citations from AHA's *Coding Clinic for ICD-10-CM/PCS*. Similar to the parenthetical notes, AHA references are placed in a hierarchical pattern at the chapter, code block, category, subcategory, or valid code level. This means that the information found in the reference applies to one or more codes depending on where the citation is placed.

The citations appear in purple type and are listed with the most current citation first. *Coding Clinic* citations included in this edition have been updated through second quarter 2017.

DEF:

This symbol precedes a definition of a condition or disease.

The definition appears in purple type directly under the code.

TIP:

This symbol precedes coding advice that is not readily available within the ICD-10-CM classification. It may relate official coding guidelines, indexing nuances, or advice from *AHA's Coding Clinic for ICD-10-CM/PCS*.

The tip appears in purple type directly under the code.

Footnotes

All footnotes are identified by a numerical superscript that appears to the upper left of the code. For example:

> [1] ✓x7ᵗʰ **M48.5Ø**   **Collapsed vertebra, not elsewhere classified, site unspecified**   HCC

The footnote 1 indicates "HCC with 7th character indicating initial encounter." This means that a collapsed vertebra would be considered an HCC only when the 7th character represents an initial encounter, such as 7th character A, B, or C, depending on the category.

The following list identifies the meaning of each footnote number in the Tabular List of Diseases:

1   These codes are considered an HCC when reported with a 7th character indicating an initial encounter (7th character A, B, or C).

2   These codes are considered an HCC when reported with a 7th character indicating an initial encounter (7th character A or B) OR sequela.

3   These codes are considered an HCC when reported with a 7th character indicating sequela.

Chapter-Level Notations

Chapter-Specific Guidelines with Coding Examples

Each chapter begins with the Official Guidelines for Coding and Reporting specific to that chapter, where provided. Coding examples specific to outpatient care settings have been provided to illustrate the coding and/or sequencing guidance in these guidelines.

Muscle and Tendon Table

ICD-10-CM categorizes certain muscles and tendons in the upper and lower extremities by their action (e.g., extension or flexion) as well as their anatomical location. The Muscle/Tendon table is provided at the beginning of chapter 13 and chapter 19 to help users when code selection depends on the action of the muscle and/or tendon.

Note: This table is not all-inclusive, and proper code assignment should be based on the provider's documentation.

Index Notations

▽ Subterms under main terms may continue to next column or page. This warning statement is a reminder to always check for additional subterms and information that may continue onto the next page or column before making a final selection.

Following References

The index includes *following* references to assist in locating "out-of-sequence" codes in the tabular list. "Out-of-sequence" codes contain an alphabetic character (letter) in the 3rd or 4th character position. These codes are placed according to the classification rules — the placement of the codes according to condition — not according to alphabetic or numeric sequencing rules.

Examples:

Carcinoma (malignant) (*see also,* Neoplasm, by site, malignant)
   neuroendocrine (*see also* Tumor, neuroendocrine)
      high grade, any site C7A.1 (*following* C75)
      poorly differentiated, any site C7A.1 (*following* C75)

In the tabular rubric, C7A is included after rubric C75 and before C76.

Gout, chronic (*see also* Gout, gouty) M1A.9
   drug-induced M1A.20 (*following* M08)
      ankle M1A.27-(*following* M08)
      elbow M1A.22-(*following* M08)

In the tabular rubric, M1A is included after rubric M08 and before M10.

ICD-10-CM Official Guidelines for Coding and Reporting

Narrative changes appear in **bold** text

Items <u>underlined</u> have been moved within the guidelines since the FY 2017 version

Italics are used to indicate revisions to heading changes

The Centers for Medicare and Medicaid Services (CMS) and the National Center for Health Statistics (NCHS), two departments within the U.S. Federal Government's Department of Health and Human Services (DHHS) provide the following guidelines for coding and reporting using the International Classification of Diseases, 10th Revision, Clinical Modification (ICD-10-CM). These guidelines should be used as a companion document to the official version of the ICD-10-CM as published on the NCHS website. The ICD-10-CM is a morbidity classification published by the United States for classifying diagnoses and reason for visits in all health care settings. The ICD-10-CM is based on the ICD-10, the statistical classification of disease published by the World Health Organization (WHO).

These guidelines have been approved by the four organizations that make up the Cooperating Parties for the ICD-10-CM: the American Hospital Association (AHA), the American Health Information Management Association (AHIMA), CMS, and NCHS.

These guidelines are a set of rules that have been developed to accompany and complement the official conventions and instructions provided within the ICD-10-CM itself. The instructions and conventions of the classification take precedence over guidelines. These guidelines are based on the coding and sequencing instructions in the Tabular List and Alphabetic Index of ICD-10-CM, but provide additional instruction. Adherence to these guidelines when assigning ICD-10-CM diagnosis codes is required under the Health Insurance Portability and Accountability Act (HIPAA). The diagnosis codes (Tabular List and Alphabetic Index) have been adopted under HIPAA for all healthcare settings. A joint effort between the healthcare provider and the coder is essential to achieve complete and accurate documentation, code assignment, and reporting of diagnoses and procedures. These guidelines have been developed to assist both the healthcare provider and the coder in identifying those diagnoses that are to be reported. The importance of consistent, complete documentation in the medical record cannot be overemphasized. Without such documentation accurate coding cannot be achieved. The entire record should be reviewed to determine the specific reason for the encounter and the conditions treated.

The term encounter is used for all settings, including hospital admissions. In the context of these guidelines, the term provider is used throughout the guidelines to mean physician or any qualified health care practitioner who is legally accountable for establishing the patient's diagnosis. Only this set of guidelines, approved by the Cooperating Parties, is official.

The guidelines are organized into sections. Section I includes the structure and conventions of the classification and general guidelines that apply to the entire classification, and chapter-specific guidelines that correspond to the chapters as they are arranged in the classification. Section II includes guidelines for selection of principal diagnosis for non-outpatient settings. Section III includes guidelines for reporting additional diagnoses in non-outpatient settings. Section IV is for outpatient coding and reporting. It is necessary to review all sections of the guidelines to fully understand all of the rules and instructions needed to code properly.

Section I. Conventions, general coding guidelines and chapter specific guidelines

The conventions, general guidelines and chapter-specific guidelines are applicable to all health care settings unless otherwise indicated. The conventions and instructions of the classification take precedence over guidelines.

A. Conventions for the ICD-10-CM

The conventions for the ICD-10-CM are the general rules for use of the classification independent of the guidelines. These conventions are incorporated within the Alphabetic Index and Tabular List of the ICD-10-CM as instructional notes.

1. **The Alphabetic Index and Tabular List**

   The ICD-10-CM is divided into the Alphabetic Index, an alphabetical list of terms and their corresponding code, and the Tabular List, a structured list of codes divided into chapters based on body system or condition. The Alphabetic Index consists of the following parts: the Index of Diseases and Injury, the Index of External Causes of Injury, the Table of Neoplasms and the Table of Drugs and Chemicals.

   See Section I.C2. General guidelines

   See Section I.C.19. Adverse effects, poisoning, underdosing and toxic effects

2. **Format and Structure:**

   The ICD-10-CM Tabular List contains categories, subcategories and codes. Characters for categories, subcategories and codes may be either a letter or a number. All categories are 3 characters. A three-character category that has no further subdivision is equivalent to a code. Subcategories are either 4 or 5 characters. Codes may be 3, 4, 5, 6 or 7 characters. That is, each level of subdivision after a category is a subcategory. The final level of subdivision is a code. Codes that have applicable 7th characters are still referred to as codes, not subcategories. A code that has an applicable 7th character is considered invalid without the 7th character.

   The ICD-10-CM uses an indented format for ease in reference.

3. **Use of codes for reporting purposes**

   For reporting purposes only codes are permissible, not categories or subcategories, and any applicable 7th character is required.

4. **Placeholder character**

   The ICD-10-CM utilizes a placeholder character "X". The "X" is used as a placeholder at certain codes to allow for future expansion. An example of this is at the poisoning, adverse effect and underdosing codes, categories T36-T50.

   Where a placeholder exists, the X must be used in order for the code to be considered a valid code.

5. **7th Characters**

   Certain ICD-10-CM categories have applicable 7th characters. The applicable 7th character is required for all codes within the category, or as the notes in the Tabular List instruct. The 7th character must always be the 7th character in the data field. If a code that requires a 7th character is not 6 characters, a placeholder X must be used to fill in the empty characters.

6. **Abbreviations**

   a. **Alphabetic Index abbreviations**

      NEC "Not elsewhere classifiable"

      This abbreviation in the Alphabetic Index represents "other specified." When a specific code is not available for a condition, the Alphabetic Index directs the coder to the "other specified" code in the Tabular List.

      NOS "Not otherwise specified"

      This abbreviation is the equivalent of unspecified.

   b. **Tabular List abbreviations**

      NEC "Not elsewhere classifiable"

      This abbreviation in the Tabular List represents "other specified". When a specific code is not available for a condition, the Tabular List includes an NEC entry under a code to identify the code as the "other specified" code.

      NOS "Not otherwise specified"

      This abbreviation is the equivalent of unspecified.

7. **Punctuation**

   [ ]   Brackets are used in the Tabular List to enclose synonyms, alternative wording or explanatory phrases. Brackets are used in the Alphabetic Index to identify manifestation codes.

   ( )   Parentheses are used in both the Alphabetic Index and Tabular List to enclose supplementary words that may be present or absent in the statement of a disease or procedure without affecting the code number to which it is assigned. The terms within the parentheses are referred to as nonessential modifiers. The nonessential modifiers in the Alphabetic Index to Diseases apply to subterms following a main term except when a nonessential modifier and a subentry are mutually exclusive, the subentry takes precedence. For example, in the ICD-10-CM Alphabetic Index under the main term Enteritis, "acute" is a nonessential modifier and "chronic" is a subentry. In this case, the nonessential modifier "acute" does not apply to the subentry "chronic".

   :   Colons are used in the Tabular List after an incomplete term which needs one or more of the modifiers following the colon to make it assignable to a given category.

8. **Use of "and".**

   See Section I.A.14. Use of the term "And"

9. **Other and Unspecified codes**

   a. **"Other" codes**

      Codes titled "other" or "other specified" are for use when the information in the medical record provides detail for which a specific code does not exist. Alphabetic Index entries with NEC in the line designate "other" codes in the Tabular List. These Alphabetic Index entries represent specific disease entities for which no specific code exists so the term is included within an "other" code.

   b. **"Unspecified" codes**

      Codes titled "unspecified" are for use when the information in the medical record is insufficient to assign a more specific code. For those categories for which an unspecified code is not provided, the "other specified" code may represent both other and unspecified.

      See Section I.B.18 Use of Signs/Symptom/Unspecified Codes

10. **Includes Notes**

    This note appears immediately under a three character code title to further define, or give examples of, the content of the category.

11. **Inclusion terms**

    List of terms is included under some codes. These terms are the conditions for which that code is to be used. The terms may be synonyms of the code title, or, in the case of "other specified" codes, the terms are a list of the various conditions assigned to that code. The inclusion terms are not necessarily exhaustive. Additional terms found only in the Alphabetic Index may also be assigned to a code.

12. **Excludes Notes**

    The ICD-10-CM has two types of excludes notes. Each type of note has a different definition for use but they are all similar in that they indicate that codes excluded from each other are independent of each other.

    a. **Excludes1**

       A type 1 Excludes note is a pure excludes note. It means "NOT CODED HERE!" An Excludes1 note indicates that the code excluded should never be used at the same time as the code above the Excludes1 note. An Excludes1 is used when two conditions cannot occur together, such as a congenital form versus an acquired form of the same condition.

       An exception to the Excludes1 definition is the circumstance when the two conditions are unrelated to each other. If it is not clear whether the two conditions involving an Excludes1 note are related or not, query the provider. For example, code F45.8, Other somatoform disorders, has an Excludes1 note for "sleep related teeth grinding (G47.63)," because "teeth grinding" is an inclusion term under F45.8. Only one of these two codes should be assigned for teeth grinding. However psychogenic dysmenorrhea is also an inclusion term under F45.8, and a patient could have both this condition and sleep related teeth grinding. In this case, the two conditions are clearly unrelated to each other, and so it would be appropriate to report F45.8 and G47.63 together.

b. **Excludes2**

A type 2 Excludes note represents "Not included here." An excludes2 note indicates that the condition excluded is not part of the condition represented by the code, but a patient may have both conditions at the same time. When an Excludes2 note appears under a code, it is acceptable to use both the code and the excluded code together, when appropriate.

13. **Etiology/manifestation convention ("code first", "use additional code" and "in diseases classified elsewhere" notes)**

Certain conditions have both an underlying etiology and multiple body system manifestations due to the underlying etiology. For such conditions, the ICD-10-CM has a coding convention that requires the underlying condition be sequenced first, if applicable, followed by the manifestation. Wherever such a combination exists, there is a "use additional code" note at the etiology code, and a "code first" note at the manifestation code. These instructional notes indicate the proper sequencing order of the codes, etiology followed by manifestation.

In most cases the manifestation codes will have in the code title, "in diseases classified elsewhere." Codes with this title are a component of the etiology/ manifestation convention. The code title indicates that it is a manifestation code. "In diseases classified elsewhere" codes are never permitted to be used as first-listed or principal diagnosis codes. They must be used in conjunction with an underlying condition code and they must be listed following the underlying condition. See category F02, Dementia in other diseases classified elsewhere, for an example of this convention.

There are manifestation codes that do not have "in diseases classified elsewhere" in the title. For such codes, there is a "use additional code" note at the etiology code and a "code first" note at the manifestation code, and the rules for sequencing apply.

In addition to the notes in the Tabular List, these conditions also have a specific Alphabetic Index entry structure. In the Alphabetic Index both conditions are listed together with the etiology code first followed by the manifestation codes in brackets. The code in brackets is always to be sequenced second.

An example of the etiology/manifestation convention is dementia in Parkinson's disease. In the Alphabetic Index, code G20 is listed first, followed by code F02.80 or F02.81 in brackets. Code G20 represents the underlying etiology, Parkinson's disease, and must be sequenced first, whereas code F02.80 and F02.81 represent the manifestation of dementia in diseases classified elsewhere, with or without behavioral disturbance.

"Code first" and "Use additional code" notes are also used as sequencing rules in the classification for certain codes that are not part of an etiology/ manifestation combination.

See Section I.B.7. Multiple coding for a single condition.

14. **"And"**

The word "and" should be interpreted to mean either "and" or "or" when it appears in a title.

For example, cases of "tuberculosis of bones", "tuberculosis of joints" and "tuberculosis of bones and joints" are classified to subcategory A18.0, Tuberculosis of bones and joints.

15. **"With"**

The word "with" **or "in"** should be interpreted to mean "associated with" or "due to" when it appears in a code title, the Alphabetic Index, or an instructional note in the Tabular List. The classification presumes a causal relationship between the two conditions linked by these terms in the Alphabetic Index or Tabular List. These conditions should be coded as related even in the absence of provider documentation explicitly linking them, unless the documentation clearly states the conditions are unrelated **or when another guideline exists that specifically requires a documented linkage between two conditions (e.g., sepsis guideline for "acute organ dysfunction that is not clearly associated with the sepsis").**

For conditions not specifically linked by these relational terms in the classification **or when a guideline requires that a linkage between two conditions be explicitly documented,** provider documentation must link the conditions in order to code them as related.

The word "with" in the Alphabetic Index is sequenced immediately following the main term, not in alphabetical order.

16. **"See" and "See Also"**

The "see" instruction following a main term in the Alphabetic Index indicates that another term should be referenced. It is necessary to go to the main term referenced with the "see" note to locate the correct code.

A "see also" instruction following a main term in the Alphabetic Index instructs that there is another main term that may also be referenced that may provide additional Alphabetic Index entries that may be useful. It is not necessary to follow the "see also" note when the original main term provides the necessary code.

17. **"Code also" note**

A "code also" note instructs that two codes may be required to fully describe a condition, but this note does not provide sequencing direction. **The sequencing depends on the circumstances of the encounter.**

18. **Default codes**

A code listed next to a main term in the ICD-10-CM Alphabetic Index is referred to as a default code. The default code represents that condition that is most commonly associated with the main term, or is the unspecified code for the condition. If a condition is documented in a medical record (for example, appendicitis) without any additional information, such as acute or chronic, the default code should be assigned.

19. **Code assignment and Clinical Criteria**

The assignment of a diagnosis code is based on the provider's diagnostic statement that the condition exists. The provider's statement that the patient has a particular condition is sufficient. Code assignment is not based on clinical criteria used by the provider to establish the diagnosis.

B. General Coding Guidelines

1. **Locating a code in the ICD-10-CM**

To select a code in the classification that corresponds to a diagnosis or reason for visit documented in a medical record, first locate the term in the Alphabetic Index, and then verify the code in the Tabular List. Read and be guided by instructional notations that appear in both the Alphabetic Index and the Tabular List.

It is essential to use both the Alphabetic Index and Tabular List when locating and assigning a code. The Alphabetic Index does not always provide the full code. Selection of the full code, including laterality and any applicable 7th character can only be done in the Tabular List. A dash (-) at the end of an Alphabetic Index entry indicates that additional characters are required. Even if a dash is not included at the Alphabetic Index entry, it is necessary to refer to the Tabular List to verify that no 7th character is required.

2. **Level of Detail in Coding**

Diagnosis codes are to be used and reported at their highest number of characters available.

ICD-10-CM diagnosis codes are composed of codes with 3, 4, 5, 6 or 7 characters. Codes with three characters are included in ICD-10-CM as the heading of a category of codes that may be further subdivided by the use of fourth and/or fifth characters and/or sixth characters, which provide greater detail.

A three-character code is to be used only if it is not further subdivided. A code is invalid if it has not been coded to the full number of characters required for that code, including the 7th character, if applicable.

3. **Code or codes from A00.0 through T88.9, Z00-Z99.8**

The appropriate code or codes from A00.0 through T88.9, Z00-Z99.8 must be used to identify diagnoses, symptoms, conditions, problems, complaints or other reason(s) for the encounter/visit.

4. **Signs and symptoms**

Codes that describe symptoms and signs, as opposed to diagnoses, are acceptable for reporting purposes when a related definitive diagnosis has not been established (confirmed) by the provider. Chapter 18 of ICD-10-CM, Symptoms, Signs, and Abnormal Clinical and Laboratory Findings, Not Elsewhere Classified (codes R00.0 - R99) contains many, but not all, codes for symptoms.

See Section I.B.18 Use of Signs/Symptom/Unspecified Codes

5. **Conditions that are an integral part of a disease process**

Signs and symptoms that are associated routinely with a disease process should not be assigned as additional codes, unless otherwise instructed by the classification.

6. Conditions that are not an integral part of a disease process

Additional signs and symptoms that may not be associated routinely with a disease process should be coded when present.

7. Multiple coding for a single condition

In addition to the etiology/manifestation convention that requires two codes to fully describe a single condition that affects multiple body systems, there are other single conditions that also require more than one code. "Use additional code" notes are found in the Tabular List at codes that are not part of an etiology/manifestation pair where a secondary code is useful to fully describe a condition. The sequencing rule is the same as the etiology/manifestation pair, "use additional code" indicates that a secondary code should be added, **if known.**

For example, for bacterial infections that are not included in chapter 1, a secondary code from category B95, Streptococcus, Staphylococcus, and Enterococcus, as the cause of diseases classified elsewhere, or B96, Other bacterial agents as the cause of diseases classified elsewhere, may be required to identify the bacterial organism causing the infection. A "use additional code" note will normally be found at the infectious disease code, indicating a need for the organism code to be added as a secondary code.

"Code first" notes are also under certain codes that are not specifically manifestation codes but may be due to an underlying cause. When there is a "code first" note and an underlying condition is present, the underlying condition should be sequenced first, **if known.**

"Code, if applicable, any causal condition first" notes indicate that this code may be assigned as a principal diagnosis when the causal condition is unknown or not applicable. If a causal condition is known, then the code for that condition should be sequenced as the principal or first-listed diagnosis.

Multiple codes may be needed for sequela, complication codes and obstetric codes to more fully describe a condition. See the specific guidelines for these conditions for further instruction.

8. Acute and Chronic Conditions

If the same condition is described as both acute (subacute) and chronic, and separate subentries exist in the Alphabetic Index at the same indentation level, code both and sequence the acute (subacute) code first.

9. Combination Code

A combination code is a single code used to classify:

Two diagnoses, or

A diagnosis with an associated secondary process (manifestation)

A diagnosis with an associated complication

Combination codes are identified by referring to subterm entries in the Alphabetic Index and by reading the inclusion and exclusion notes in the Tabular List.

Assign only the combination code when that code fully identifies the diagnostic conditions involved or when the Alphabetic Index so directs. Multiple coding should not be used when the classification provides a combination code that clearly identifies all of the elements documented in the diagnosis. When the combination code lacks necessary specificity in describing the manifestation or complication, an additional code should be used as a secondary code.

10. Sequela (Late Effects)

A sequela is the residual effect (condition produced) after the acute phase of an illness or injury has terminated. There is no time limit on when a sequela code can be used. The residual may be apparent early, such as in cerebral infarction, or it may occur months or years later, such as that due to a previous injury. Examples of sequela include: scar formation resulting from a burn, deviated septum due to a nasal fracture, and infertility due to tubal occlusion from old tuberculosis. Coding of sequela generally requires two codes sequenced in the following order: the condition or nature of the sequela is sequenced first. The sequela code is sequenced second.

An exception to the above guidelines are those instances where the code for the sequela is followed by a manifestation code identified in the Tabular List and title, or the sequela code has been expanded (at the fourth, fifth or sixth character levels) to include the manifestation(s). The code for the acute phase of an illness or injury that led to the sequela is never used with a code for the late effect.

See Section I.C.9. Sequelae of cerebrovascular disease

See Section I.C.15. Sequelae of complication of pregnancy, childbirth and the puerperium

See Section I.C.19. Application of 7th characters for Chapter 19

11. Impending or Threatened Condition

Code any condition described at the time of discharge as "impending" or "threatened" as follows:

If it did occur, code as confirmed diagnosis.

If it did not occur, reference the Alphabetic Index to determine if the condition has a subentry term for "impending" or "threatened" and also reference main term entries for "Impending" and for "Threatened."

If the subterms are listed, assign the given code.

If the subterms are not listed, code the existing underlying condition(s) and not the condition described as impending or threatened.

12. Reporting Same Diagnosis Code more than Once

Each unique ICD-10-CM diagnosis code may be reported only once for an encounter. This applies to bilateral conditions when there are no distinct codes identifying laterality or two different conditions classified to the same ICD-10-CM diagnosis code.

13. Laterality

Some ICD-10-CM codes indicate laterality, specifying whether the condition occurs on the left, right or is bilateral. If no bilateral code is provided and the condition is bilateral, assign separate codes for both the left and right side. If the side is not identified in the medical record, assign the code for the unspecified side.

When a patient has a bilateral condition and each side is treated during separate encounters, assign the "bilateral" code (as the condition still exists on both sides), including for the encounter to treat the first side. For the second encounter for treatment after one side has previously been treated and the condition no longer exists on that side, assign the appropriate unilateral code for the side where the condition still exists (e.g., cataract surgery performed on each eye in separate encounters). The bilateral code would not be assigned for the subsequent encounter, as the patient no longer has the condition in the previously-treated site. If the treatment on the first side did not completely resolve the condition, then the bilateral code would still be appropriate.

14. Documentation for BMI, Depth of Non-pressure ulcers, Pressure Ulcer Stages, Coma Scale, and NIH Stroke Scale

For the Body Mass Index (BMI**)**, depth of non-pressure chronic ulcers, pressure ulcer stage, coma scale, and NIH stroke scale (NIHSS) codes, code assignment may be based on medical record documentation from clinicians who are not the patient's provider (i.e., physician or other qualified healthcare practitioner legally accountable for establishing the patient's diagnosis), since this information is typically documented by other clinicians involved in the care of the patient (e.g., a dietitian often documents the BMI, a nurse often documents the pressure ulcer stages, and an emergency medical technician often documents the coma scale). However, the associated diagnosis (such as overweight, obesity, acute stroke, or pressure ulcer) must be documented by the patient's provider. If there is conflicting medical record documentation, either from the same clinician or different clinicians, the patient's attending provider should be queried for clarification.

The BMI, coma scale, and NIHSS codes should only be reported as secondary diagnoses.

15. Syndromes

Follow the Alphabetic Index guidance when coding syndromes. In the absence of Alphabetic Index guidance, assign codes for the documented manifestations of the syndrome. Additional codes for manifestations that are not an integral part of the disease process may also be assigned when the condition does not have a unique code.

16. Documentation of Complications of Care

Code assignment is based on the provider's documentation of the relationship between the condition and the care or procedure, unless otherwise instructed by the classification. The guideline extends to any complications of care, regardless of the chapter the code is located in. It is important to note that not all conditions that occur during or following medical care or surgery are classified as complications. There must be a cause-and-effect relationship between the care provided and the condition, and an indication in the documentation that it is a complication. Query the provider for clarification, if the complication is not clearly documented.

17. Borderline Diagnosis

If the provider documents a "borderline" diagnosis at the time of discharge, the diagnosis is coded as confirmed, unless the classification provides a specific entry (e.g., borderline diabetes). If a borderline condition has a specific index entry in ICD-10-CM, it should be coded as such. Since borderline conditions are not uncertain diagnoses, no distinction is made between the care setting (inpatient versus outpatient). Whenever the documentation is unclear regarding a borderline condition, coders are encouraged to query for clarification.

18. Use of Sign/Symptom/Unspecified Codes

Sign/symptom and "unspecified" codes have acceptable, even necessary, uses. While specific diagnosis codes should be reported when they are supported by the available medical record documentation and clinical knowledge of the patient's health condition, there are instances when signs/symptoms or unspecified codes are the best choices for accurately reflecting the healthcare encounter. Each healthcare encounter should be coded to the level of certainty known for that encounter.

If a definitive diagnosis has not been established by the end of the encounter, it is appropriate to report codes for sign(s) and/or symptom(s) in lieu of a definitive diagnosis. When sufficient clinical information isn't known or available about a particular health condition to assign a more specific code, it is acceptable to report the appropriate "unspecified" code (e.g., a diagnosis of pneumonia has been determined, but not the specific type). Unspecified codes should be reported when they are the codes that most accurately reflect what is known about the patient's condition at the time of that particular encounter. It would be inappropriate to select a specific code that is not supported by the medical record documentation or conduct medically unnecessary diagnostic testing in order to determine a more specific code.

C. Chapter-Specific Coding Guidelines

In addition to general coding guidelines, there are guidelines for specific diagnoses and/or conditions in the classification. Unless otherwise indicated, these guidelines apply to all health care settings. Please refer to Section II for guidelines on the selection of principal diagnosis.

1. Chapter 1: Certain Infectious and Parasitic Diseases (A00-B99)

a. Human Immunodeficiency Virus (HIV) Infections

1) Code only confirmed cases

Code only confirmed cases of HIV infection/illness. This is an exception to the hospital inpatient guideline Section II, H.

In this context, "confirmation" does not require documentation of positive serology or culture for HIV; the provider's diagnostic statement that the patient is HIV positive, or has an HIV-related illness is sufficient.

2) Selection and sequencing of HIV codes

(a) Patient admitted for HIV-related condition

If a patient is admitted for an HIV-related condition, the principal diagnosis should be B20, Human immunodeficiency virus [HIV] disease followed by additional diagnosis codes for all reported HIV-related conditions.

(b) Patient with HIV disease admitted for unrelated condition

If a patient with HIV disease is admitted for an unrelated condition (such as a traumatic injury), the code for the unrelated condition (e.g., the nature of injury code) should be the principal diagnosis. Other diagnoses would be B20 followed by additional diagnosis codes for all reported HIV-related conditions.

(c) Whether the patient is newly diagnosed

Whether the patient is newly diagnosed or has had previous admissions/encounters for HIV conditions is irrelevant to the sequencing decision.

(d) Asymptomatic human immunodeficiency virus

Z21, Asymptomatic human immunodeficiency virus [HIV] infection status, is to be applied when the patient without any documentation of symptoms is listed as being "HIV positive," "known HIV," "HIV test positive," or similar terminology. Do not use this code if the term "AIDS" is used

or if the patient is treated for any HIV-related illness or is described as having any condition(s) resulting from his/her HIV positive status; use B20 in these cases.

(e) Patients with inconclusive HIV serology

Patients with inconclusive HIV serology, but no definitive diagnosis or manifestations of the illness, may be assigned code R75, Inconclusive laboratory evidence of human immunodeficiency virus [HIV].

(f) Previously diagnosed HIV-related illness

Patients with any known prior diagnosis of an HIV-related illness should be coded to B20. Once a patient has developed an HIV-related illness, the patient should always be assigned code B20 on every subsequent admission/encounter. Patients previously diagnosed with any HIV illness (B20) should never be assigned to R75 or Z21, Asymptomatic human immunodeficiency virus [HIV] infection status.

(g) HIV Infection in Pregnancy, Childbirth and the Puerperium

During pregnancy, childbirth or the puerperium, a patient admitted (or presenting for a health care encounter) because of an HIV-related illness should receive a principal diagnosis code of O98.7-, Human immunodeficiency [HIV] disease complicating pregnancy, childbirth and the puerperium, followed by B20 and the code(s) for the HIV-related illness(es). Codes from Chapter 15 always take sequencing priority.

Patients with asymptomatic HIV infection status admitted (or presenting for a health care encounter) during pregnancy, childbirth, or the puerperium should receive codes of O98.7- and Z21.

(h) Encounters for testing for HIV

If a patient is being seen to determine his/her HIV status, use code Z11.4, Encounter for screening for human immunodeficiency virus [HIV]. Use additional codes for any associated high risk behavior.

If a patient with signs or symptoms is being seen for HIV testing, code the signs and symptoms. An additional counseling code Z71.7, Human immunodeficiency virus [HIV] counseling, may be used if counseling is provided during the encounter for the test.

When a patient returns to be informed of his/her HIV test results and the test result is negative, use code Z71.7, Human immunodeficiency virus [HIV] counseling.

If the results are positive, see previous guidelines and assign codes as appropriate.

b. Infectious agents as the cause of diseases classified to other chapters

Certain infections are classified in chapters other than Chapter 1 and no organism is identified as part of the infection code. In these instances, it is necessary to use an additional code from Chapter 1 to identify the organism. A code from category B95, Streptococcus, Staphylococcus, and Enterococcus as the cause of diseases classified to other chapters, B96, Other bacterial agents as the cause of diseases classified to other chapters, or B97, Viral agents as the cause of diseases classified to other chapters, is to be used as an additional code to identify the organism. An instructional note will be found at the infection code advising that an additional organism code is required.

c. Infections resistant to antibiotics

Many bacterial infections are resistant to current antibiotics. It is necessary to identify all infections documented as antibiotic resistant. Assign a code from category Z16, Resistance to antimicrobial drugs, following the infection code only if the infection code does not identify drug resistance.

d. Sepsis, Severe Sepsis, and Septic Shock

1) Coding of Sepsis and Severe Sepsis

(a) Sepsis

For a diagnosis of sepsis, assign the appropriate code for the underlying systemic infection. If the type of infection or causal organism is not further specified, assign code A41.9, Sepsis, unspecified organism.

A code from subcategory R65.2, Severe sepsis, should not be assigned unless severe sepsis or an associated acute organ dysfunction is documented.

(i) Negative or inconclusive blood cultures and sepsis

Negative or inconclusive blood cultures do not preclude a diagnosis of sepsis in patients with clinical evidence of the condition; however, the provider should be queried.

(ii) Urosepsis

The term urosepsis is a nonspecific term. It is not to be considered synonymous with sepsis. It has no default code in the Alphabetic Index. Should a provider use this term, he/she must be queried for clarification.

(iii) Sepsis with organ dysfunction

If a patient has sepsis and associated acute organ dysfunction or multiple organ dysfunction (MOD), follow the instructions for coding severe sepsis.

(iv) Acute organ dysfunction that is not clearly associated with the sepsis

If a patient has sepsis and an acute organ dysfunction, but the medical record documentation indicates that the acute organ dysfunction is related to a medical condition other than the sepsis, do not assign a code from subcategory R65.2, Severe sepsis. An acute organ dysfunction must be associated with the sepsis in order to assign the severe sepsis code. If the documentation is not clear as to whether an acute organ dysfunction is related to the sepsis or another medical condition, query the provider.

(b) Severe sepsis

The coding of severe sepsis requires a minimum of 2 codes: first a code for the underlying systemic infection, followed by a code from subcategory R65.2, Severe sepsis. If the causal organism is not documented, assign code A41.9, Sepsis, unspecified organism, for the infection. Additional code(s) for the associated acute organ dysfunction are also required.

Due to the complex nature of severe sepsis, some cases may require querying the provider prior to assignment of the codes.

2) Septic shock

(a) Septic shock generally refers to circulatory failure associated with severe sepsis, and therefore, it represents a type of acute organ dysfunction.

For cases of septic shock, the code for the systemic infection should be sequenced first, followed by code R65.21, Severe sepsis with septic shock or code T81.12, Postprocedural septic shock. Any additional codes for the other acute organ dysfunctions should also be assigned. As noted in the sequencing instructions in the Tabular List, the code for septic shock cannot be assigned as a principal diagnosis.

3) Sequencing of severe sepsis

If severe sepsis is present on admission, and meets the definition of principal diagnosis, the underlying systemic infection should be assigned as principal diagnosis followed by the appropriate code from subcategory R65.2 as required by the sequencing rules in the Tabular List. A code from subcategory R65.2 can never be assigned as a principal diagnosis.

When severe sepsis develops during an encounter (it was not present on admission), the underlying systemic infection and the appropriate code from subcategory R65.2 should be assigned as secondary diagnoses.

Severe sepsis may be present on admission, but the diagnosis may not be confirmed until sometime after admission. If the documentation is not clear whether severe sepsis was present on admission, the provider should be queried.

4) Sepsis and severe sepsis with a localized infection

If the reason for admission is both sepsis or severe sepsis and a localized infection, such as pneumonia or cellulitis, a code(s) for the underlying systemic infection should be assigned first and the code for the localized infection should be assigned as a secondary diagnosis. If the patient has severe sepsis, a code from subcategory R65.2 should also be assigned as a secondary diagnosis. If the patient is admitted with a localized infection, such as pneumonia, and sepsis/severe sepsis doesn't develop until after admission, the localized infection should be assigned first, followed by the appropriate sepsis/severe sepsis codes.

5) Sepsis due to a postprocedural infection

(a) Documentation of causal relationship

As with all postprocedural complications, code assignment is based on the provider's documentation of the relationship between the infection and the procedure.

(b) Sepsis due to a postprocedural infection

For such cases, the postprocedural infection code, such as T80.2, Infections following infusion, transfusion, and therapeutic injection, T81.4, Infection following a procedure, T88.0, Infection following immunization, or O86.0, Infection of obstetric surgical wound, should be coded first, followed by the code for the specific infection. If the patient has severe sepsis, the appropriate code from subcategory R65.2 should also be assigned with the additional code(s) for any acute organ dysfunction.

(c) Postprocedural infection and postprocedural septic shock

In cases where a postprocedural infection has occurred and has resulted in severe sepsis the code for the precipitating complication such as code T81.4, Infection following a procedure, or O86.0, Infection of obstetrical surgical wound should be coded first followed by code R65.20, Severe sepsis without septic shock. A code for the systemic infection should also be assigned.

If a postprocedural infection has resulted in postprocedural septic shock, the code for the precipitating complication such as code T81.4, Infection following a procedure, or O86.0, Infection of obstetrical surgical wound should be coded first followed by code T81.12-, Postprocedural septic shock. A code for the systemic infection should also be assigned.

6) Sepsis and severe sepsis associated with a noninfectious process (condition)

In some cases a noninfectious process (condition), such as trauma, may lead to an infection which can result in sepsis or severe sepsis. If sepsis or severe sepsis is documented as associated with a noninfectious condition, such as a burn or serious injury, and this condition meets the definition for principal diagnosis, the code for the noninfectious condition should be sequenced first, followed by the code for the resulting infection. If severe sepsis is present, a code from subcategory R65.2 should also be assigned with any associated organ dysfunction(s) codes. It is not necessary to assign a code from subcategory R65.1, Systemic inflammatory response syndrome (SIRS) of non-infectious origin, for these cases.

If the infection meets the definition of principal diagnosis, it should be sequenced before the non-infectious condition. When both the associated non-infectious condition and the infection meet the definition of principal diagnosis, either may be assigned as principal diagnosis.

Only one code from category R65, Symptoms and signs specifically associated with systemic inflammation and infection, should be assigned. Therefore, when a non-infectious condition leads to an infection resulting in severe sepsis, assign the appropriate code from subcategory R65.2, Severe sepsis. Do not additionally assign a code from subcategory R65.1, Systemic inflammatory response syndrome (SIRS) of non-infectious origin.

See Section I.C.18. SIRS due to non-infectious process

7) Sepsis and septic shock complicating abortion, pregnancy, childbirth, and the puerperium

See Section I.C.15. Sepsis and septic shock complicating abortion, pregnancy, childbirth and the puerperium

8) Newborn sepsis

See Section I.C.16. f. Bacterial sepsis of Newborn

e. Methicillin Resistant Staphylococcus aureus (MRSA) Conditions

1) Selection and sequencing of MRSA codes

(a) Combination codes for MRSA infection

When a patient is diagnosed with an infection that is due to methicillin resistant *Staphylococcus aureus* (MRSA), and that infection has a combination code that includes the causal organism (e.g., sepsis, pneumonia) assign the appropriate combination code for the condition (e.g., code A41.02, Sepsis due to Methicillin resistant Staphylococcus aureus or code J15.212, Pneumonia due to Methicillin resistant Staphylococcus aureus). Do not assign code B95.62, Methicillin resistant Staphylococcus aureus infection as the cause of diseases classified elsewhere, as an additional code, because the combination code includes the type of infection and the MRSA organism. Do not assign a code from subcategory Z16.11, Resistance to penicillins, as an additional diagnosis.

See Section C.1. for instructions on coding and sequencing of sepsis and severe sepsis.

(b) Other codes for MRSA infection

When there is documentation of a current infection (e.g., wound infection, stitch abscess, urinary tract infection) due to MRSA, and that infection does not have a combination code that includes the causal organism, assign the appropriate code to identify the condition along with code B95.62, Methicillin resistant Staphylococcus aureus infection as the cause of diseases classified elsewhere for the MRSA infection. Do not assign a code from subcategory Z16.11, Resistance to penicillins.

(c) Methicillin susceptible Staphylococcus aureus (MSSA) and MRSA colonization

The condition or state of being colonized or carrying MSSA or MRSA is called colonization or carriage, while an individual person is described as being colonized or being a carrier. Colonization means that MSSA or MSRA is present on or in the body without necessarily causing illness. A positive MRSA colonization test might be documented by the provider as "MRSA screen positive" or "MRSA nasal swab positive".

Assign code Z22.322, Carrier or suspected carrier of Methicillin resistant Staphylococcus aureus, for patients documented as having MRSA colonization. Assign code Z22.321, Carrier or suspected carrier of Methicillin susceptible Staphylococcus aureus, for patient documented as having MSSA colonization. Colonization is not necessarily indicative of a disease process or as the cause of a specific condition the patient may have unless documented as such by the provider.

(d) MRSA colonization and infection

If a patient is documented as having both MRSA colonization and infection during a hospital admission, code Z22.322, Carrier or suspected carrier of Methicillin resistant Staphylococcus aureus, and a code for the MRSA infection may both be assigned.

f. Zika virus infections

1) Code only confirmed cases

Code only a confirmed diagnosis of Zika virus (A92.5, Zika virus disease) as documented by the provider. This is an exception to the hospital inpatient guideline Section II, H. In this context, "confirmation" does not require documentation of the type of test performed; the physician's diagnostic statement that the condition is confirmed is sufficient. This code should be assigned regardless of the stated mode of transmission.

If the provider documents "suspected", "possible" or "probable" Zika, do not assign code A92.5. Assign a code(s) explaining the reason for encounter (such as fever, rash, or joint pain) or Z20.828, Contact with and (suspected) exposure to other viral communicable diseases.

2. Chapter 2: Neoplasms (C00-D49)
General guidelines

Chapter 2 of the ICD-10-CM contains the codes for most benign and all malignant neoplasms. Certain benign neoplasms, such as prostatic adenomas, may be found in the specific body system chapters. To properly code a neoplasm it is necessary to determine from the record if the neoplasm is benign, in-situ, malignant, or of uncertain histologic behavior. If malignant, any secondary (metastatic) sites should also be determined.

Primary malignant neoplasms overlapping site boundaries

A primary malignant neoplasm that overlaps two or more contiguous (next to each other) sites should be classified to the subcategory/code .8 ('overlapping lesion'), unless the combination is specifically indexed elsewhere. For multiple neoplasms of the same site that are not contiguous such as tumors in different quadrants of the same breast, codes for each site should be assigned.

Malignant neoplasm of ectopic tissue

Malignant neoplasms of ectopic tissue are to be coded to the site of origin mentioned, e.g., ectopic pancreatic malignant neoplasms involving the stomach are coded to **malignant neoplasm of** pancreas, unspecified (C25.9).

The neoplasm table in the Alphabetic Index should be referenced first. However, if the histological term is documented, that term should be referenced first, rather than going immediately to the Neoplasm Table, in order to determine which column in the Neoplasm Table is appropriate. For example, if the documentation indicates "adenoma," refer to the term in the Alphabetic Index to review the entries under this term and the instructional note to "see also neoplasm, by site, benign." The table provides the proper code based on the type of neoplasm and the site. It is important to select the proper column in the table that corresponds to the type of neoplasm. The Tabular List should then be referenced to verify that the correct code has been selected from the table and that a more specific site code does not exist.

See Section I.C.21. Factors influencing health status and contact with health services, Status, for information regarding Z15.0, codes for genetic susceptibility to cancer.

a. Treatment directed at the malignancy

If the treatment is directed at the malignancy, designate the malignancy as the principal diagnosis.

The only exception to this guideline is if a patient admission/encounter is solely for the administration of chemotherapy, immunotherapy or **external beam** radiation therapy, assign the appropriate Z51.-- code as the first-listed or principal diagnosis, and the diagnosis or problem for which the service is being performed as a secondary diagnosis.

b. Treatment of secondary site

When a patient is admitted because of a primary neoplasm with metastasis and treatment is directed toward the secondary site only, the secondary neoplasm is designated as the principal diagnosis even though the primary malignancy is still present.

c. Coding and sequencing of complications

Coding and sequencing of complications associated with the malignancies or with the therapy thereof are subject to the following guidelines:

1) Anemia associated with malignancy

When admission/encounter is for management of an anemia associated with the malignancy, and the treatment is only for anemia, the appropriate code for the malignancy is sequenced as the principal or first-listed diagnosis followed by the appropriate code for the anemia (such as code D63.0, Anemia in neoplastic disease).

2) Anemia associated with chemotherapy, immunotherapy and radiation therapy

When the admission/encounter is for management of an anemia associated with an adverse effect of the administration of chemotherapy or immunotherapy and the only treatment is for the anemia, the anemia code is sequenced first followed by the appropriate codes for the neoplasm and the adverse effect (T45.1X5-, Adverse effect of antineoplastic and immunosuppressive drugs).

When the admission/encounter is for management of an anemia associated with an adverse effect of radiotherapy, the anemia code should be sequenced first, followed by the appropriate neoplasm code and code Y84.2, Radiological procedure and radiotherapy as the cause of abnormal reaction of the patient, or of later complication, without mention of misadventure at the time of the procedure.

3) Management of dehydration due to the malignancy
When the admission/encounter is for management of dehydration due to the malignancy and only the dehydration is being treated (intravenous rehydration), the dehydration is sequenced first, followed by the code(s) for the malignancy.

4) Treatment of a complication resulting from a surgical procedure
When the admission/encounter is for treatment of a complication resulting from a surgical procedure, designate the complication as the principal or first-listed diagnosis if treatment is directed at resolving the complication.

d. Primary malignancy previously excised
When a primary malignancy has been previously excised or eradicated from its site and there is no further treatment directed to that site and there is no evidence of any existing primary malignancy, a code from category Z85, Personal history of malignant neoplasm, should be used to indicate the former site of the malignancy. Any mention of extension, invasion, or metastasis to another site is coded as a secondary malignant neoplasm to that site. The secondary site may be the principal or first-listed with the Z85 code used as a secondary code.

e. Admissions/Encounters involving chemotherapy, immunotherapy and radiation therapy

1) Episode of care involves surgical removal of neoplasm
When an episode of care involves the surgical removal of a neoplasm, primary or secondary site, followed by adjunct chemotherapy or radiation treatment during the same episode of care, the code for the neoplasm should be assigned as principal or first-listed diagnosis**.**

2) Patient admission/encounter solely for administration of chemotherapy, immunotherapy and radiation therapy
If a patient admission/encounter is solely for the administration of chemotherapy, immunotherapy or **external beam** radiation therapy assign code Z51.0, Encounter for antineoplastic radiation therapy, or Z51.11, Encounter for antineoplastic chemotherapy, or Z51.12, Encounter for antineoplastic immunotherapy as the first-listed or principal diagnosis. If a patient receives more than one of these therapies during the same admission more than one of these codes may be assigned, in any sequence.

The malignancy for which the therapy is being administered should be assigned as a secondary diagnosis.

If a patient admission/encounter is for the insertion or implantation of radioactive elements (e.g., brachytherapy) the appropriate code for the malignancy is sequenced as the principal or first-listed diagnosis. Code Z51.0 should not be assigned.

3) Patient admitted for radiation therapy, chemotherapy or immunotherapy and develops complications
When a patient is admitted for the purpose of **external beam** radiotherapy, immunotherapy or chemotherapy and develops complications such as uncontrolled nausea and vomiting or dehydration, the principal or first-listed diagnosis is Z51.0, Encounter for antineoplastic radiation therapy, or Z51.11, Encounter for antineoplastic chemotherapy, or Z51.12, Encounter for antineoplastic immunotherapy followed by any codes for the complications.

When a patient is admitted for the purpose of insertion or implantation of radioactive elements (e.g., brachytherapy) and develops complications such as uncontrolled nausea and vomiting or dehydration, the principal or first-listed diagnosis is the appropriate code for the malignancy followed by any codes for the complications.

f. Admission/encounter to determine extent of malignancy
When the reason for admission/encounter is to determine the extent of the malignancy, or for a procedure such as paracentesis or thoracentesis, the primary malignancy or appropriate metastatic site is designated as the principal or first-listed diagnosis, even though chemotherapy or radiotherapy is administered.

g. Symptoms, signs, and abnormal findings listed in Chapter 18 associated with neoplasms
Symptoms, signs, and ill-defined conditions listed in Chapter 18 characteristic of, or associated with, an existing primary or

secondary site malignancy cannot be used to replace the malignancy as principal or first-listed diagnosis, regardless of the number of admissions or encounters for treatment and care of the neoplasm.
See section I.C.21. Factors influencing health status and contact with health services, Encounter for prophylactic organ removal.

h. Admission/encounter for pain control/management
See Section I.C.6. for information on coding admission/encounter for pain control/management.

i. Malignancy in two or more noncontiguous sites
A patient may have more than one malignant tumor in the same organ. These tumors may represent different primaries or metastatic disease, depending on the site. Should the documentation be unclear, the provider should be queried as to the status of each tumor so that the correct codes can be assigned.

j. Disseminated malignant neoplasm, unspecified
Code C80.0, Disseminated malignant neoplasm, unspecified, is for use only in those cases where the patient has advanced metastatic disease and no known primary or secondary sites are specified. It should not be used in place of assigning codes for the primary site and all known secondary sites.

k. Malignant neoplasm without specification of site
Code C80.1, Malignant (primary) neoplasm, unspecified, equates to Cancer, unspecified. This code should only be used when no determination can be made as to the primary site of a malignancy. This code should rarely be used in the inpatient setting.

l. Sequencing of neoplasm codes

1) Encounter for treatment of primary malignancy
If the reason for the encounter is for treatment of a primary malignancy, assign the malignancy as the principal/first-listed diagnosis. The primary site is to be sequenced first, followed by any metastatic sites.

2) Encounter for treatment of secondary malignancy
When an encounter is for a primary malignancy with metastasis and treatment is directed toward the metastatic (secondary) site(s) only, the metastatic site(s) is designated as the principal/first-listed diagnosis. The primary malignancy is coded as an additional code.

3) Malignant neoplasm in a pregnant patient
When a pregnant woman has a malignant neoplasm, a code from subcategory O9A.1-, Malignant neoplasm complicating pregnancy, childbirth, and the puerperium, should be sequenced first, followed by the appropriate code from Chapter 2 to indicate the type of neoplasm.

4) Encounter for complication associated with a neoplasm
When an encounter is for management of a complication associated with a neoplasm, such as dehydration, and the treatment is only for the complication, the complication is coded first, followed by the appropriate code(s) for the neoplasm.

The exception to this guideline is anemia. When the admission/encounter is for management of an anemia associated with the malignancy, and the treatment is only for anemia, the appropriate code for the malignancy is sequenced as the principal or first-listed diagnosis followed by code D63.0, Anemia in neoplastic disease.

5) Complication from surgical procedure for treatment of a neoplasm
When an encounter is for treatment of a complication resulting from a surgical procedure performed for the treatment of the neoplasm, designate the complication as the principal/first-listed diagnosis. See guideline regarding the coding of a current malignancy versus personal history to determine if the code for the neoplasm should also be assigned.

6) Pathologic fracture due to a neoplasm
When an encounter is for a pathological fracture due to a neoplasm, and the focus of treatment is the fracture, a code from subcategory M84.5, Pathological fracture in neoplastic disease, should be sequenced first, followed by the code for the neoplasm.

If the focus of treatment is the neoplasm with an associated pathological fracture, the neoplasm code should be sequenced first, followed by a code from M84.5 for the pathological fracture.

m. Current malignancy versus personal history of malignancy
When a primary malignancy has been excised but further treatment, such as an additional surgery for the malignancy, radiation therapy or chemotherapy is directed to that site, the primary malignancy code should be used until treatment is completed.

When a primary malignancy has been previously excised or eradicated from its site, there is no further treatment (of the malignancy) directed to that site, and there is no evidence of any existing primary malignancy, a code from category Z85, Personal history of malignant neoplasm, should be used to indicate the former site of the malignancy.

See Section I.C.21. Factors influencing health status and contact with health services, History (of)

n. Leukemia, Multiple Myeloma, and Malignant Plasma Cell Neoplasms in remission versus personal history
The categories for leukemia, and category C90, Multiple myeloma and malignant plasma cell neoplasms, have codes indicating whether or not the leukemia has achieved remission. There are also codes Z85.6, Personal history of leukemia, and Z85.79, Personal history of other malignant neoplasms of lymphoid, hematopoietic and related tissues. If the documentation is unclear as to whether the leukemia has achieved remission, the provider should be queried.

See Section I.C.21. Factors influencing health status and contact with health services, History (of)

o. Aftercare following surgery for neoplasm
See Section I.C.21. Factors influencing health status and contact with health services, Aftercare

p. Follow-up care for completed treatment of a malignancy
See Section I.C.21. Factors influencing health status and contact with health services, Follow-up

q. Prophylactic organ removal for prevention of malignancy
See Section I.C. 21, Factors influencing health status and contact with health services, Prophylactic organ removal

r. Malignant neoplasm associated with transplanted organ
A malignant neoplasm of a transplanted organ should be coded as a transplant complication. Assign first the appropriate code from category T86.-, Complications of transplanted organs and tissue, followed by code C80.2, Malignant neoplasm associated with transplanted organ. Use an additional code for the specific malignancy.

3. Chapter 3: Disease of the blood and blood-forming organs and certain disorders involving the immune mechanism (D50-D89)
Reserved for future guideline expansion

4. Chapter 4: Endocrine, Nutritional, and Metabolic Diseases (E00-E89)
a. Diabetes mellitus
The diabetes mellitus codes are combination codes that include the type of diabetes mellitus, the body system affected, and the complications affecting that body system. As many codes within a particular category as are necessary to describe all of the complications of the disease may be used. They should be sequenced based on the reason for a particular encounter. Assign as many codes from categories E08 – E13 as needed to identify all of the associated conditions that the patient has.

1) Type of diabetes
The age of a patient is not the sole determining factor, though most type 1 diabetics develop the condition before reaching puberty. For this reason type 1 diabetes mellitus is also referred to as juvenile diabetes.

2) Type of diabetes mellitus not documented
If the type of diabetes mellitus is not documented in the medical record the default is E11.-, Type 2 diabetes mellitus.

3) Diabetes mellitus and the use of insulin and oral hypoglycemics
If the documentation in a medical record does not indicate the type of diabetes but does indicate that the patient uses insulin, code E11-, Type 2 diabetes mellitus, should be assigned. **An additional code should be assigned from category Z79 to** identify the long-term (current) use of insulin or oral hypoglycemic drugs. If the patient is treated with both oral medications and insulin, only the code for long-term (current) use of insulin should be assigned. Code Z79.4 should not be assigned if insulin is given temporarily to bring a type 2 patient's blood sugar under control during an encounter.

4) Diabetes mellitus in pregnancy and gestational diabetes
See Section I.C.15. Diabetes mellitus in pregnancy.

See Section I.C.15. Gestational (pregnancy induced) diabetes

5) Complications due to insulin pump malfunction
(a) Underdose of insulin due to insulin pump failure
An underdose of insulin due to an insulin pump failure should be assigned to a code from subcategory T85.6, Mechanical complication of other specified internal and external prosthetic devices, implants and grafts, that specifies the type of pump malfunction, as the principal or first-listed code, followed by code T38.3X6-, Underdosing of insulin and oral hypoglycemic [antidiabetic] drugs. Additional codes for the type of diabetes mellitus and any associated complications due to the underdosing should also be assigned.

(b) Overdose of insulin due to insulin pump failure
The principal or first-listed code for an encounter due to an insulin pump malfunction resulting in an overdose of insulin, should also be T85.6-, Mechanical complication of other specified internal and external prosthetic devices, implants and grafts, followed by code T38.3X1-, Poisoning by insulin and oral hypoglycemic [antidiabetic] drugs, accidental (unintentional).

6) Secondary diabetes mellitus
Codes under categories E08, Diabetes mellitus due to underlying condition, E09, Drug or chemical induced diabetes mellitus, and E13, Other specified diabetes mellitus, identify complications/manifestations associated with secondary diabetes mellitus. Secondary diabetes is always caused by another condition or event (e.g., cystic fibrosis, malignant neoplasm of pancreas, pancreatectomy, adverse effect of drug, or poisoning).

(a) Secondary diabetes mellitus and the use of insulin or *oral* hypoglycemic drugs
For patients with secondary diabetes mellitus who routinely use insulin or oral hypoglycemic drugs, an additional code from category Z79 should be assigned to identify the long-term (current) use of insulin or oral hypoglycemic drugs. If the patient is treated with both oral medications and insulin, only the code for long-term (current) use of insulin should be assigned. Code Z79.4 should not be assigned if insulin is given temporarily to bring a type 2 patient's blood sugar under control during an encounter.

(b) Assigning and sequencing secondary diabetes codes and its causes
The sequencing of the secondary diabetes codes in relationship to codes for the cause of the diabetes is based on the Tabular List instructions for categories E08, E09 and E13.

(i) Secondary diabetes mellitus due to pancreatectomy
For postpancreatectomy diabetes mellitus (lack of insulin due to the surgical removal of all or part of the pancreas), assign code E89.1, Postprocedural hypoinsulinemia. Assign a code from category E13 and a code from subcategory Z90.41, Acquired absence of pancreas, as additional codes.

(ii) Secondary diabetes due to drugs
Secondary diabetes may be caused by an adverse effect of correctly administered medications, poisoning or sequela of poisoning.
See section I.C.19.e for coding of adverse effects and poisoning, and section I.C.20 for external cause code reporting.

5. **Chapter 5: Mental, Behavioral and Neurodevelopmental disorders (F01 – F99)**
   a. **Pain disorders related to psychological factors**
      Assign code F45.41, for pain that is exclusively related to psychological disorders. As indicated by the Excludes 1 note under category G89, a code from category G89 should not be assigned with code F45.41.

      Code F45.42, Pain disorders with related psychological factors, should be used with a code from category G89, Pain, not elsewhere classified, if there is documentation of a psychological component for a patient with acute or chronic pain.

      See Section I.C.6. Pain

   b. **Mental and behavioral disorders due to psychoactive substance use**
      1) **In Remission**
         Selection of codes for "in remission" for categories F10-F19, Mental and behavioral disorders due to psychoactive substance use (categories F10-F19 with **-11,** -.21) requires the provider's clinical judgment. The appropriate codes for "in remission" are assigned only on the basis of provider documentation (as defined in the Official Guidelines for Coding and Reporting), **unless otherwise instructed by the classification.**

         Mild substance use disorders in early or sustained remission are classified to the appropriate codes for substance abuse in remission, and moderate or severe substance use disorders in early or sustained remission are classified to the appropriate codes for substance dependence in remission.

      2) **Psychoactive Substance Use, Abuse and Dependence**
         When the provider documentation refers to use, abuse and dependence of the same substance (e.g. alcohol, opioid, cannabis, etc.), only one code should be assigned to identify the pattern of use based on the following hierarchy:
         - If both use and abuse are documented, assign only the code for abuse
         - If both abuse and dependence are documented, assign only the code for dependence
         - If use, abuse and dependence are all documented, assign only the code for dependence
         - If both use and dependence are documented, assign only the code for dependence.

      3) **Psychoactive Substance Use** *Disorders*
         As with all other diagnoses, the codes for psychoactive substance use **disorders** (F10.9-, F11.9-, F12.9-, F13.9-, F14.9-, F15.9-, F16.9-) should only be assigned based on provider documentation and when they meet the definition of a reportable diagnosis (see Section III, Reporting Additional Diagnoses). The codes are to be used only when the psychoactive substance use is associated with a **physical,** mental or behavioral disorder, and such a relationship is documented by the provider.

6. **Chapter 6: Diseases of the Nervous System (G00-G99)**
   a. **Dominant/nondominant side**
      Codes from category G81, Hemiplegia and hemiparesis, and subcategories G83.1, Monoplegia of lower limb, G83.2, Monoplegia of upper limb, and G83.3, Monoplegia, unspecified, identify whether the dominant or nondominant side is affected. Should the affected side be documented, but not specified as dominant or nondominant, and the classification system does not indicate a default, code selection is as follows:
      - For ambidextrous patients, the default should be dominant.
      - If the left side is affected, the default is non-dominant.
      - If the right side is affected, the default is dominant.

   b. **Pain - Category G89**
      1) **General coding information**
         Codes in category G89, Pain, not elsewhere classified, may be used in conjunction with codes from other categories and chapters to provide more detail about acute or chronic pain and neoplasm-related pain, unless otherwise indicated below.

         If the pain is not specified as acute or chronic, post-thoracotomy, postprocedural, or neoplasm-related, do not assign codes from category G89.

A code from category G89 should not be assigned if the underlying (definitive) diagnosis is known, unless the reason for the encounter is pain control/ management and not management of the underlying condition.

When an admission or encounter is for a procedure aimed at treating the underlying condition (e.g., spinal fusion, kyphoplasty), a code for the underlying condition (e.g., vertebral fracture, spinal stenosis) should be assigned as the principal diagnosis. No code from category G89 should be assigned.

(a) **Category G89 Codes as Principal or First-Listed Diagnosis**
   Category G89 codes are acceptable as principal diagnosis or the first-listed code:
   - When pain control or pain management is the reason for the admission/encounter (e.g., a patient with displaced intervertebral disc, nerve impingement and severe back pain presents for injection of steroid into the spinal canal). The underlying cause of the pain should be reported as an additional diagnosis, if known.
   - When a patient is admitted for the insertion of a neurostimulator for pain control, assign the appropriate pain code as the principal or first-listed diagnosis. When an admission or encounter is for a procedure aimed at treating the underlying condition and a neurostimulator is inserted for pain control during the same admission/encounter, a code for the underlying condition should be assigned as the principal diagnosis and the appropriate pain code should be assigned as a secondary diagnosis.

(b) **Use of Category G89 Codes in Conjunction with Site Specific Pain Codes**
   (i) **Assigning Category G89 and Site-Specific Pain Codes**
       Codes from category G89 may be used in conjunction with codes that identify the site of pain (including codes from chapter 18) if the category G89 code provides additional information. For example, if the code describes the site of the pain, but does not fully describe whether the pain is acute or chronic, then both codes should be assigned.
   (ii) **Sequencing of Category G89 Codes with Site-Specific Pain Codes**
       The sequencing of category G89 codes with site-specific pain codes (including chapter 18 codes), is dependent on the circumstances of the encounter/admission as follows:
       - If the encounter is for pain control or pain management, assign the code from category G89 followed by the code identifying the specific site of pain (e.g., encounter for pain management for acute neck pain from trauma is assigned code G89.11, Acute pain due to trauma, followed by code M54.2, Cervicalgia, to identify the site of pain).
       - If the encounter is for any other reason except pain control or pain management, and a related definitive diagnosis has not been established (confirmed) by the provider, assign the code for the specific site of pain first, followed by the appropriate code from category G89.

2) **Pain due to devices, implants and grafts**
   See Section I.C.19. Pain due to medical devices

3) **Postoperative Pain**
   The provider's documentation should be used to guide the coding of postoperative pain, as well as *Section III. Reporting Additional Diagnoses and Section IV. Diagnostic Coding and Reporting in the Outpatient Setting.*

   The default for post-thoracotomy and other postoperative pain not specified as acute or chronic is the code for the acute form.

   Routine or expected postoperative pain immediately after surgery should not be coded.

(a) Postoperative pain not associated with specific postoperative complication
Postoperative pain not associated with a specific postoperative complication is assigned to the appropriate postoperative pain code in category G89.

(b) Postoperative pain associated with specific postoperative complication
Postoperative pain associated with a specific postoperative complication (such as painful wire sutures) is assigned to the appropriate code(s) found in Chapter 19, Injury, poisoning, and certain other consequences of external causes. If appropriate, use additional code(s) from category G89 to identify acute or chronic pain (G89.18 or G89.28).

4) Chronic pain
Chronic pain is classified to subcategory G89.2. There is no time frame defining when pain becomes chronic pain. The provider's documentation should be used to guide use of these codes.

5) Neoplasm Related Pain
Code G89.3 is assigned to pain documented as being related, associated or due to cancer, primary or secondary malignancy, or tumor. This code is assigned regardless of whether the pain is acute or chronic.

This code may be assigned as the principal or first-listed code when the stated reason for the admission/encounter is documented as pain control/pain management. The underlying neoplasm should be reported as an additional diagnosis.

When the reason for the admission/encounter is management of the neoplasm and the pain associated with the neoplasm is also documented, code G89.3 may be assigned as an additional diagnosis. It is not necessary to assign an additional code for the site of the pain.

See Section I.C.2 for instructions on the sequencing of neoplasms for all other stated reasons for the admission/encounter (except for pain control/pain management).

6) Chronic pain syndrome
Central pain syndrome (G89.0) and chronic pain syndrome (G89.4) are different than the term "chronic pain," and therefore codes should only be used when the provider has specifically documented this condition.

See Section I.C.5. Pain disorders related to psychological factors

7. Chapter 7: Diseases of the Eye and Adnexa (H00-H59)
a. Glaucoma

1) Assigning Glaucoma Codes
Assign as many codes from category H40, Glaucoma, as needed to identify the type of glaucoma, the affected eye, and the glaucoma stage.

2) Bilateral glaucoma with same type and stage
When a patient has bilateral glaucoma and both eyes are documented as being the same type and stage, and there is a code for bilateral glaucoma, report only the code for the type of glaucoma, bilateral, with the seventh character for the stage.

When a patient has bilateral glaucoma and both eyes are documented as being the same type and stage, and the classification does not provide a code for bilateral glaucoma (i.e. subcategories H40.10, H40.11 and H40.20) report only one code for the type of glaucoma with the appropriate seventh character for the stage.

3) Bilateral glaucoma stage with different types or stages
When a patient has bilateral glaucoma and each eye is documented as having a different type or stage, and the classification distinguishes laterality, assign the appropriate code for each eye rather than the code for bilateral glaucoma.

When a patient has bilateral glaucoma and each eye is documented as having a different type, and the classification does not distinguish laterality (i.e. subcategories H40.10, H40.11 and H40.20), assign one code for each type of glaucoma with the appropriate seventh character for the stage.

When a patient has bilateral glaucoma and each eye is documented as having the same type, but different stage, and the classification does not distinguish laterality (i.e. subcategories H40.10, H40.11 and H40.20), assign a code for

the type of glaucoma for each eye with the seventh character for the specific glaucoma stage documented for each eye.

4) Patient admitted with glaucoma and stage evolves during the admission
If a patient is admitted with glaucoma and the stage progresses during the admission, assign the code for highest stage documented.

5) Indeterminate stage glaucoma
Assignment of the seventh character "4" for "indeterminate stage" should be based on the clinical documentation. The seventh character "4" is used for glaucomas whose stage cannot be clinically determined. This seventh character should not be confused with the seventh character "0", unspecified, which should be assigned when there is no documentation regarding the stage of the glaucoma.

b. Blindness
If "blindness" or "low vision" of both eyes is documented but the visual impairment category is not documented, assign code H54.3, Unqualified visual loss, both eyes. If "blindness" or "low vision" in one eye is documented but the visual impairment category is not documented, assign a code from H54.6-, Unqualified visual loss, one eye. If "blindness" or "visual loss" is documented without any information about whether one or both eyes are affected, assign code H54.7, Unspecified visual loss.

8. Chapter 8: Diseases of the Ear and Mastoid Process (H60-H95)
Reserved for future guideline expansion

9. Chapter 9: Diseases of the Circulatory System (I00-I99)
a. Hypertension
The classification presumes a causal relationship between hypertension and heart involvement and between hypertension and kidney involvement, as the two conditions are linked by the term "with" in the Alphabetic Index. These conditions should be coded as related even in the absence of provider documentation explicitly linking them, unless the documentation clearly states the conditions are unrelated.

For hypertension and conditions not specifically linked by relational terms such as "with," "associated with" or "due to" in the classification, provider documentation must link the conditions in order to code them as related.

1) Hypertension with Heart Disease
Hypertension with heart conditions classified to I50.- or I51.4-I51.9, are assigned to a code from category I11, Hypertensive heart disease. Use additional code(s) from category I50, Heart failure, to identify the type(s) of heart failure in those patients with heart failure.

The same heart conditions (I50.-, I51.4-I51.9) with hypertension are coded separately if the provider has specifically documented a different cause. Sequence according to the circumstances of the admission/encounter.

2) Hypertensive Chronic Kidney Disease
Assign codes from category I12, Hypertensive chronic kidney disease, when both hypertension and a condition classifiable to category N18, Chronic kidney disease (CKD), are present. CKD should not be coded as hypertensive if the physician has specifically documented a different cause.

The appropriate code from category N18 should be used as a secondary code with a code from category I12 to identify the stage of chronic kidney disease.

See Section I.C.14. Chronic kidney disease.

If a patient has hypertensive chronic kidney disease and acute renal failure, an additional code for the acute renal failure is required.

3) Hypertensive Heart and Chronic Kidney Disease
Assign codes from combination category I13, Hypertensive heart and chronic kidney disease, when there is hypertension with both heart and kidney involvement. If heart failure is present, assign an additional code from category I50 to identify the type of heart failure.

The appropriate code from category N18, Chronic kidney disease, should be used as a secondary code with a code from category I13 to identify the stage of chronic kidney disease.

See Section I.C.14. Chronic kidney disease.

The codes in category I13, Hypertensive heart and chronic kidney disease, are combination codes that include hypertension, heart disease and chronic kidney disease. The Includes note at I13 specifies that the conditions included at I11 and I12 are included together in I13. If a patient has hypertension, heart disease and chronic kidney disease, then a code from I13 should be used, not individual codes for hypertension, heart disease and chronic kidney disease, or codes from I11 or I12.

For patients with both acute renal failure and chronic kidney disease, an additional code for acute renal failure is required.

4) Hypertensive Cerebrovascular Disease
For hypertensive cerebrovascular disease, first assign the appropriate code from categories I60-I69, followed by the appropriate hypertension code.

5) Hypertensive Retinopathy
Subcategory H35.0, Background retinopathy and retinal vascular changes, should be used with a code from category I10- I15, Hypertensive disease to include the systemic hypertension. The sequencing is based on the reason for the encounter.

6) Hypertension, Secondary
Secondary hypertension is due to an underlying condition. Two codes are required: one to identify the underlying etiology and one from category I15 to identify the hypertension. Sequencing of codes is determined by the reason for admission/encounter.

7) Hypertension, Transient
Assign code R03.0, Elevated blood pressure reading without diagnosis of hypertension, unless patient has an established diagnosis of hypertension. Assign code O13.-, Gestational [pregnancy-induced] hypertension without significant proteinuria, or O14.-, Pre-eclampsia, for transient hypertension of pregnancy.

8) Hypertension, Controlled
This diagnostic statement usually refers to an existing state of hypertension under control by therapy. Assign the appropriate code from categories I10-I15, Hypertensive diseases.

9) Hypertension, Uncontrolled
Uncontrolled hypertension may refer to untreated hypertension or hypertension not responding to current therapeutic regimen. In either case, assign the appropriate code from categories I10-I15, Hypertensive diseases.

10) Hypertensive Crisis
Assign a code from category I16, Hypertensive crisis, for documented hypertensive urgency, hypertensive emergency or unspecified hypertensive crisis. Code also any identified hypertensive disease (I10-I15). The sequencing is based on the reason for the encounter.

10) Pulmonary Hypertension
Pulmonary hypertension is classified to category I27, Other pulmonary heart diseases. For secondary pulmonary hypertension (I27.1, I27.2-), code also any associated conditions or adverse effects of drugs or toxins. The sequencing is based on the reason for the encounter.

b. Atherosclerotic Coronary Artery Disease and Angina
ICD-10-CM has combination codes for atherosclerotic heart disease with angina pectoris. The subcategories for these codes are I25.11, Atherosclerotic heart disease of native coronary artery with angina pectoris and I25.7, Atherosclerosis of coronary artery bypass graft(s) and coronary artery of transplanted heart with angina pectoris.

When using one of these combination codes it is not necessary to use an additional code for angina pectoris. A causal relationship can be assumed in a patient with both atherosclerosis and angina pectoris, unless the documentation indicates the angina is due to something other than the atherosclerosis.

If a patient with coronary artery disease is admitted due to an acute myocardial infarction (AMI), the AMI should be sequenced before the coronary artery disease.

See Section I.C.9. Acute myocardial infarction (AMI)

c. Intraoperative and Postprocedural Cerebrovascular Accident
Medical record documentation should clearly specify the cause-and-effect relationship between the medical intervention and the cerebrovascular accident in order to assign a code for intraoperative or postprocedural cerebrovascular accident.

Proper code assignment depends on whether it was an infarction or hemorrhage and whether it occurred intraoperatively or postoperatively. If it was a cerebral hemorrhage, code assignment depends on the type of procedure performed.

d. Sequelae of Cerebrovascular Disease
1) Category I69, Sequelae of Cerebrovascular disease
Category I69 is used to indicate conditions classifiable to categories I60-I67 as the causes of sequela (neurologic deficits), themselves classified elsewhere. These "late effects" include neurologic deficits that persist after initial onset of conditions classifiable to categories I60-I67. The neurologic deficits caused by cerebrovascular disease may be present from the onset or may arise at any time after the onset of the condition classifiable to categories I60-I67.

Codes from category I69, Sequelae of cerebrovascular disease, that specify hemiplegia, hemiparesis and monoplegia identify whether the dominant or nondominant side is affected. Should the affected side be documented, but not specified as dominant or nondominant, and the classification system does not indicate a default, code selection is as follows:

- For ambidextrous patients, the default should be dominant.
- If the left side is affected, the default is non-dominant.
- If the right side is affected, the default is dominant.

2) Codes from category I69 with codes from I60-I67
Codes from category I69 may be assigned on a health care record with codes from I60-I67, if the patient has a current cerebrovascular disease and deficits from an old cerebrovascular disease.

3) Codes from category I69 and Personal history of transient ischemic attack (TIA) and cerebral infarction (Z86.73)
Codes from category I69 should not be assigned if the patient does not have neurologic deficits.

See Section I.C.21. 4. History (of) for use of personal history codes

e. Acute myocardial infarction (AMI)
1) Type 1 ST elevation myocardial infarction (STEMI) and non-ST elevation myocardial infarction (NSTEMI)
The ICD-10-CM codes for **type 1** acute myocardial infarction (AMI) identify the site, such as anterolateral wall or true posterior wall. Subcategories I21.0-I21.2 and code I21.3 are used for **type 1** ST elevation myocardial infarction (STEMI). Code I21.4, Non-ST elevation (NSTEMI) myocardial infarction, is used for **type 1** non ST elevation myocardial infarction (NSTEMI) and nontransmural MIs.

If **a type 1** NSTEMI evolves to STEMI, assign the STEMI code. If **a type 1** STEMI converts to NSTEMI due to thrombolytic therapy, it is still coded as STEMI.

For encounters occurring while the myocardial infarction is equal to, or less than, four weeks old, including transfers to another acute setting or a postacute setting, and the myocardial infarction meets the definition for "other diagnoses" (see Section III, Reporting Additional Diagnoses), codes from category I21 may continue to be reported. For encounters after the 4 week time frame and the patient is still receiving care related to the myocardial infarction, the appropriate aftercare code should be assigned, rather than a code from category I21. For old or healed myocardial infarctions not requiring further care, code I25.2, Old myocardial infarction, may be assigned.

2) Acute myocardial infarction, unspecified
Code **I21.9, Acute myocardial infarction, unspecified,** is the default for unspecified acute myocardial infarction **or unspecified type.** If only **type 1** STEMI or transmural MI without the site is documented, assign code I21.3, **ST elevation (STEMI) myocardial infarction of unspecified site.**

3) AMI documented as nontransmural or subendocardial but site provided
If an AMI is documented as nontransmural or subendocardial, but the site is provided, it is still coded as a subendocardial AMI.

See Section I.C.21.3 for information on coding status post administration of tPA in a different facility within the last 24 hours.

4) **Subsequent acute myocardial infarction**

A code from category I22, Subsequent ST elevation (STEMI) and non-ST elevation (NSTEMI) myocardial infarction, is to be used when a patient who has suffered **a type 1 or unspecified** AMI has a new AMI within the 4 week time frame of the initial AMI. A code from category I22 must be used in conjunction with a code from category I21. The sequencing of the I22 and I21 codes depends on the circumstances of the encounter.

Do not assign code I22 for subsequent myocardial infarctions other than type 1 or unspecified. For subsequent type 2 AMI assign only code I21.A1. For subsequent type 4 or type 5 AMI, assign only code I21.A9.

5) **Other Types of Myocardial Infarction**

The ICD-10-CM provides codes for different types of myocardial infarction. Type 1 myocardial infarctions are assigned to codes I21.0-I21.4.

Type 2 myocardial infarction, and myocardial infarction due to demand ischemia or secondary to ischemic balance, is assigned to code I21.A1, Myocardial infarction type 2 with a code for the underlying cause. Do not assign code I24.8, Other forms of acute ischemic heart disease for the demand ischemia. Sequencing of type 2 AMI or the underlying cause is dependent on the circumstances of admission. When a type 2 AMI code is described as NSTEMI or STEMI, only assign code I21.A1. Codes I21.01-I21.4 should only be assigned for type 1 AMIs.

Acute myocardial infarctions type 3, 4a, 4b, 4c and 5 are assigned to code I21.A9, Other myocardial infarction type.

The "Code also" and "Code first" notes should be followed related to complications, and for coding of postprocedural myocardial infarctions during or following cardiac surgery.

10. **Chapter 10: Diseases of the Respiratory System (J00-J99)**
    a. **Chronic Obstructive Pulmonary Disease [COPD] and Asthma**
       1) **Acute exacerbation of chronic obstructive bronchitis and asthma**

          The codes in categories J44 and J45 distinguish between uncomplicated cases and those in acute exacerbation. An acute exacerbation is a worsening or a decompensation of a chronic condition. An acute exacerbation is not equivalent to an infection superimposed on a chronic condition, though an exacerbation may be triggered by an infection.

    b. **Acute Respiratory Failure**
       1) **Acute respiratory failure as principal diagnosis**

          A code from subcategory J96.0, Acute respiratory failure, or subcategory J96.2, Acute and chronic respiratory failure, may be assigned as a principal diagnosis when it is the condition established after study to be chiefly responsible for occasioning the admission to the hospital, and the selection is supported by the Alphabetic Index and Tabular List. However, chapter-specific coding guidelines (such as obstetrics, poisoning, HIV, newborn) that provide sequencing direction take precedence.

       2) **Acute respiratory failure as secondary diagnosis**

          Respiratory failure may be listed as a secondary diagnosis if it occurs after admission, or if it is present on admission, but does not meet the definition of principal diagnosis.

       3) **Sequencing of acute respiratory failure and another acute condition**

          When a patient is admitted with respiratory failure and another acute condition, (e.g., myocardial infarction, cerebrovascular accident, aspiration pneumonia), the principal diagnosis will not be the same in every situation. This applies whether the other acute condition is a respiratory or nonrespiratory condition. Selection of the principal diagnosis will be dependent on the circumstances of admission. If both the respiratory failure and the other acute condition are equally responsible for occasioning the admission to the hospital, and there are no chapter-specific sequencing rules, the guideline regarding two or more diagnoses that equally meet the definition for principal diagnosis *(Section II, C.)* may be applied in these situations.

If the documentation is not clear as to whether acute respiratory failure and another condition are equally responsible for occasioning the admission, query the provider for clarification.

c. **Influenza due to certain identified influenza viruses**

Code only confirmed cases of influenza due to certain identified influenza viruses (category J09), and due to other identified influenza virus (category J10). This is an exception to the hospital inpatient guideline Section II, H. (Uncertain Diagnosis).

In this context, "confirmation" does not require documentation of positive laboratory testing specific for avian or other novel influenza A or other identified influenza virus. However, coding should be based on the provider's diagnostic statement that the patient has avian influenza, or other novel influenza A, for category J09, or has another particular identified strain of influenza, such as H1N1 or H3N2, but not identified as novel or variant, for category J10.

If the provider records "suspected" or "possible" or "probable" avian influenza, or novel influenza, or other identified influenza, then the appropriate influenza code from category J11, Influenza due to unidentified influenza virus, should be assigned. A code from category J09, Influenza due to certain identified influenza viruses, should not be assigned nor should a code from category J10, Influenza due to other identified influenza virus.

d. **Ventilator associated Pneumonia**
   1) **Documentation of Ventilator associated Pneumonia**

      As with all procedural or postprocedural complications, code assignment is based on the provider's documentation of the relationship between the condition and the procedure.

      Code J95.851, Ventilator associated pneumonia, should be assigned only when the provider has documented ventilator associated pneumonia (VAP). An additional code to identify the organism (e.g., Pseudomonas aeruginosa, code B96.5) should also be assigned. Do not assign an additional code from categories J12-J18 to identify the type of pneumonia.

      Code J95.851 should not be assigned for cases where the patient has pneumonia and is on a mechanical ventilator and the provider has not specifically stated that the pneumonia is ventilator-associated pneumonia. If the documentation is unclear as to whether the patient has a pneumonia that is a complication attributable to the mechanical ventilator, query the provider.

   2) **Ventilator associated Pneumonia Develops after Admission**

      A patient may be admitted with one type of pneumonia (e.g., code J13, Pneumonia due to Streptococcus pneumonia) and subsequently develop VAP. In this instance, the principal diagnosis would be the appropriate code from categories J12-J18 for the pneumonia diagnosed at the time of admission. Code J95.851, Ventilator associated pneumonia, would be assigned as an additional diagnosis when the provider has also documented the presence of ventilator associated pneumonia.

11. **Chapter 11: Diseases of the Digestive System (K00-K95)**
    Reserved for future guideline expansion

12. **Chapter 12: Diseases of the Skin and Subcutaneous Tissue (L00-L99)**
    a. **Pressure ulcer stage codes**
       1) **Pressure ulcer stages**

          Codes from category L89, Pressure ulcer, identify the site of the pressure ulcer as well as the stage of the ulcer.

          The ICD-10-CM classifies pressure ulcer stages based on severity, which is designated by stages 1-4, unspecified stage and unstageable.

          Assign as many codes from category L89 as needed to identify all the pressure ulcers the patient has, if applicable.

       2) **Unstageable pressure ulcers**

          Assignment of the code for unstageable pressure ulcer (L89.--0) should be based on the clinical documentation. These codes are used for pressure ulcers whose stage cannot be clinically determined (e.g., the ulcer is covered by eschar or has been treated with a skin or muscle graft) and pressure ulcers that are documented as deep tissue injury but not documented as due to trauma. This code should not be confused with the codes for unspecified stage (L89.--9). When there is no documentation regarding the stage of the pressure ulcer, assign the appropriate code for unspecified stage (L89.--9).

3) **Documented pressure ulcer stage**
Assignment of the pressure ulcer stage code should be guided by clinical documentation of the stage or documentation of the terms found in the Alphabetic Index. For clinical terms describing the stage that are not found in the Alphabetic Index, and there is no documentation of the stage, the provider should be queried.

4) **Patients admitted with pressure ulcers documented as healed**
No code is assigned if the documentation states that the pressure ulcer is completely healed.

5) **Patients admitted with pressure ulcers documented as healing**
Pressure ulcers described as healing should be assigned the appropriate pressure ulcer stage code based on the documentation in the medical record. If the documentation does not provide information about the stage of the healing pressure ulcer, assign the appropriate code for unspecified stage.

If the documentation is unclear as to whether the patient has a current (new) pressure ulcer or if the patient is being treated for a healing pressure ulcer, query the provider.

For ulcers that were present on admission but healed at the time of discharge, assign the code for the site and stage of the pressure ulcer at the time of admission.

6) **Patient admitted with pressure ulcer evolving into another stage during the admission**
If a patient is admitted **to an inpatient hospital** with a pressure ulcer at one stage and it progresses to a higher stage, two separate codes should be assigned: one code for the site and stage of the ulcer on admission and a second code for the same ulcer site and the highest stage reported during the stay.

b. **Non-Pressure Chronic Ulcers**

1) **Patients admitted with non-pressure ulcers documented as healed**
No code is assigned if the documentation states that the non-pressure ulcer is completely healed.

2) **Patients admitted with non-pressure ulcers documented as healing**
Non-pressure ulcers described as healing should be assigned the appropriate non-pressure ulcer code based on the documentation in the medical record. If the documentation does not provide information about the severity of the healing non-pressure ulcer, assign the appropriate code for unspecified severity.

If the documentation is unclear as to whether the patient has a current (new) non-pressure ulcer or if the patient is being treated for a healing non-pressure ulcer, query the provider.

For ulcers that were present on admission but healed at the time of discharge, assign the code for the site and severity of the non-pressure ulcer at the time of admission.

3) **Patient admitted with non-pressure ulcer that progresses to another severity level during the admission**
If a patient is admitted to an inpatient hospital with a non-pressure ulcer at one severity level and it progresses to a higher severity level, two separate codes should be assigned: one code for the site and severity level of the ulcer on admission and a second code for the same ulcer site and the highest severity level reported during the stay.

13. **Chapter 13: Diseases of the Musculoskeletal System and Connective Tissue (M00-M99)**
a. **Site and laterality**
Most of the codes within Chapter 13 have site and laterality designations. The site represents the bone, joint or the muscle involved. For some conditions where more than one bone, joint or muscle is usually involved, such as osteoarthritis, there is a "multiple sites" code available. For categories where no multiple site code is provided and more than one bone, joint or muscle is involved,

multiple codes should be used to indicate the different sites involved.

1) **Bone versus joint**
For certain conditions, the bone may be affected at the upper or lower end, (e.g., avascular necrosis of bone, M87, Osteoporosis, M80, M81). Though the portion of the bone affected may be at the joint, the site designation will be the bone, not the joint.

b. **Acute traumatic versus chronic or recurrent musculoskeletal conditions**
Many musculoskeletal conditions are a result of previous injury or trauma to a site, or are recurrent conditions. Bone, joint or muscle conditions that are the result of a healed injury are usually found in chapter 13. Recurrent bone, joint or muscle conditions are also usually found in chapter 13. Any current, acute injury should be coded to the appropriate injury code from chapter 19. Chronic or recurrent conditions should generally be coded with a code from chapter 13. If it is difficult to determine from the documentation in the record which code is best to describe a condition, query the provider.

c. **Coding of Pathologic Fractures**
7th character A is for use as long as the patient is receiving active treatment for the fracture. While the patient may be seen by a new or different provider over the course of treatment for a pathological fracture, assignment of the 7th character is based on whether the patient is undergoing active treatment and not whether the provider is seeing the patient for the first time.

7th character D is to be used for encounters after the patient has completed active treatment **for the fracture and is receiving routine care for the fracture during the healing or recovery phase.** The other 7th characters, listed under each subcategory in the Tabular List, are to be used for subsequent encounters for treatment of problems associated with the healing, such as malunions, nonunions, and sequelae.

Care for complications of surgical treatment for fracture repairs during the healing or recovery phase should be coded with the appropriate complication codes.

See Section I.C.19. Coding of traumatic fractures.

d. **Osteoporosis**
Osteoporosis is a systemic condition, meaning that all bones of the musculoskeletal system are affected. Therefore, site is not a component of the codes under category M81, Osteoporosis without current pathological fracture. The site codes under category M80, Osteoporosis with current pathological fracture, identify the site of the fracture, not the osteoporosis.

1) **Osteoporosis without pathological fracture**
Category M81, Osteoporosis without current pathological fracture, is for use for patients with osteoporosis who do not currently have a pathologic fracture due to the osteoporosis, even if they have had a fracture in the past. For patients with a history of osteoporosis fractures, status code Z87.310, Personal history of (healed) osteoporosis fracture, should follow the code from M81.

2) **Osteoporosis with current pathological fracture**
Category M80, Osteoporosis with current pathological fracture, is for patients who have a current pathologic fracture at the time of an encounter. The codes under M80 identify the site of the fracture. A code from category M80, not a traumatic fracture code, should be used for any patient with known osteoporosis who suffers a fracture, even if the patient had a minor fall or trauma, if that fall or trauma would not usually break a normal, healthy bone.

14. **Chapter 14: Diseases of Genitourinary System (N00-N99)**
a. **Chronic kidney disease**
1) **Stages of chronic kidney disease (CKD)**
The ICD-10-CM classifies CKD based on severity. The severity of CKD is designated by stages 1-5. Stage 2, code N18.2, equates to mild CKD; stage 3, code N18.3, equates to moderate CKD; and stage 4, code N18.4, equates to severe CKD. Code N18.6, End stage renal disease (ESRD), is assigned when the provider has documented end-stage-renal disease (ESRD).

If both a stage of CKD and ESRD are documented, assign code N18.6 only.

2) Chronic kidney disease and kidney transplant status
Patients who have undergone kidney transplant may still have some form of chronic kidney disease (CKD) because the kidney transplant may not fully restore kidney function. Therefore, the presence of CKD alone does not constitute a transplant complication. Assign the appropriate N18 code for the patient's stage of CKD and code Z94.0, Kidney transplant status. If a transplant complication such as failure or rejection or other transplant complication is documented, see section I.C.19.g for information on coding complications of a kidney transplant. If the documentation is unclear as to whether the patient has a complication of the transplant, query the provider.

3) Chronic kidney disease with other conditions
Patients with CKD may also suffer from other serious conditions, most commonly diabetes mellitus and hypertension. The sequencing of the CKD code in relationship to codes for other contributing conditions is based on the conventions in the Tabular List.

See I.C.9. Hypertensive chronic kidney disease.

See I.C.19. Chronic kidney disease and kidney transplant complications.

15. Chapter 15: Pregnancy, Childbirth, and the Puerperium (O00-O9A)
a. General Rules for Obstetric Cases
1) Codes from chapter 15 and sequencing priority
Obstetric cases require codes from chapter 15, codes in the range O00-O9A, Pregnancy, Childbirth, and the Puerperium. Chapter 15 codes have sequencing priority over codes from other chapters. Additional codes from other chapters may be used in conjunction with chapter 15 codes to further specify conditions. Should the provider document that the pregnancy is incidental to the encounter, then code Z33.1, Pregnant state, incidental, should be used in place of any chapter 15 codes. It is the provider's responsibility to state that the condition being treated is not affecting the pregnancy.

2) Chapter 15 codes used only on the maternal record
Chapter 15 codes are to be used only on the maternal record, never on the record of the newborn.

3) Final character for trimester
The majority of codes in Chapter 15 have a final character indicating the trimester of pregnancy. The timeframes for the trimesters are indicated at the beginning of the chapter. If trimester is not a component of a code, it is because the condition always occurs in a specific trimester, or the concept of trimester of pregnancy is not applicable. Certain codes have characters for only certain trimesters because the condition does not occur in all trimesters, but it may occur in more than just one.

Assignment of the final character for trimester should be based on the provider's documentation of the trimester (or number of weeks) for the current admission/encounter. This applies to the assignment of trimester for pre-existing conditions as well as those that develop during or are due to the pregnancy. The provider's documentation of the number of weeks may be used to assign the appropriate code identifying the trimester.

Whenever delivery occurs during the current admission, and there is an "in childbirth" option for the obstetric complication being coded, the "in childbirth" code should be assigned.

4) Selection of trimester for inpatient admissions that encompass more than one trimester
In instances when a patient is admitted to a hospital for complications of pregnancy during one trimester and remains in the hospital into a subsequent trimester, the trimester character for the antepartum complication code should be assigned on the basis of the trimester when the complication developed, not the trimester of the discharge. If the condition developed prior to the current admission/encounter or represents a pre-existing condition, the trimester character for the trimester at the time of the admission/encounter should be assigned.

5) Unspecified trimester
Each category that includes codes for trimester has a code for "unspecified trimester." The "unspecified trimester" code should rarely be used, such as when the documentation in the record is insufficient to determine the trimester and it is not possible to obtain clarification.

6) 7th character for Fetus Identification
Where applicable, a 7th character is to be assigned for certain categories (O31, O32, O33.3 - O33.6, O35, O36, O40, O41, O60.1, O60.2, O64, and O69) to identify the fetus for which the complication code applies.

Assign 7th character "0":

- For single gestations
- When the documentation in the record is insufficient to determine the fetus affected and it is not possible to obtain clarification.
- When it is not possible to clinically determine which fetus is affected.

b. Selection of OB Principal or First-listed Diagnosis
1) Routine outpatient prenatal visits
For routine outpatient prenatal visits when no complications are present, a code from category Z34, Encounter for supervision of normal pregnancy, should be used as the first-listed diagnosis. These codes should not be used in conjunction with chapter 15 codes.

2) Supervision of High-Risk Pregnancy
Codes from category O09, Supervision of high-risk pregnancy, are intended for use only during the prenatal period. For complications during the labor or delivery episode as a result of a high-risk pregnancy, assign the applicable complication codes from Chapter 15. If there are no complications during the labor or delivery episode, assign code O80, Encounter for full-term uncomplicated delivery.

For routine prenatal outpatient visits for patients with high-risk pregnancies, a code from category O09, Supervision of high-risk pregnancy, should be used as the first-listed diagnosis. Secondary chapter 15 codes may be used in conjunction with these codes if appropriate.

3) Episodes when no delivery occurs
In episodes when no delivery occurs, the principal diagnosis should correspond to the principal complication of the pregnancy which necessitated the encounter. Should more than one complication exist, all of which are treated or monitored, any of the complications codes may be sequenced first.

4) When a delivery occurs
When an obstetric patient is admitted and delivers during that admission, the condition that prompted the admission should be sequenced as the principal diagnosis. If multiple conditions prompted the admission, sequence the one most related to the delivery as the principal diagnosis. A code for any complication of the delivery should be assigned as an additional diagnosis. In cases of cesarean delivery, if the patient was admitted with a condition that resulted in the performance of a cesarean procedure, that condition should be selected as the principal diagnosis. If the reason for the admission was unrelated to the condition resulting in the cesarean delivery, the condition related to the reason for the admission should be selected as the principal diagnosis.

5) Outcome of delivery
A code from category Z37, Outcome of delivery, should be included on every maternal record when a delivery has occurred. These codes are not to be used on subsequent records or on the newborn record.

c. Pre-existing conditions versus conditions due to the pregnancy
Certain categories in Chapter 15 distinguish between conditions of the mother that existed prior to pregnancy (pre-existing) and those that are a direct result of pregnancy. When assigning codes from Chapter 15, it is important to assess if a condition was pre-existing prior to pregnancy or developed during or due to the pregnancy in order to assign the correct code.

Categories that do not distinguish between pre-existing and pregnancy-related conditions may be used for either. It is acceptable to use codes specifically for the puerperium with codes complicating pregnancy and childbirth if a condition arises postpartum during the delivery encounter.

d. Pre-existing hypertension in pregnancy
Category O10, Pre-existing hypertension complicating pregnancy, childbirth and the puerperium, includes codes for hypertensive heart and hypertensive chronic kidney disease. When assigning one of the O10 codes that includes hypertensive heart disease or hypertensive chronic kidney disease, it is necessary to add a secondary code from the appropriate hypertension category to specify the type of heart failure or chronic kidney disease.

See Section I.C.9. Hypertension.

e. Fetal Conditions Affecting the Management of the Mother
1) Codes from categories O35 and O36
Codes from categories O35, Maternal care for known or suspected fetal abnormality and damage, and O36, Maternal care for other fetal problems, are assigned only when the fetal condition is actually responsible for modifying the management of the mother, i.e., by requiring diagnostic studies, additional observation, special care, or termination of pregnancy. The fact that the fetal condition exists does not justify assigning a code from this series to the mother's record.

2) In utero surgery
In cases when surgery is performed on the fetus, a diagnosis code from category O35, Maternal care for known or suspected fetal abnormality and damage, should be assigned identifying the fetal condition. Assign the appropriate procedure code for the procedure performed.

No code from Chapter 16, the perinatal codes, should be used on the mother's record to identify fetal conditions. Surgery performed in utero on a fetus is still to be coded as an obstetric encounter.

f. HIV Infection in Pregnancy, Childbirth and the Puerperium
During pregnancy, childbirth or the puerperium, a patient admitted because of an HIV-related illness should receive a principal diagnosis from subcategory O98.7-, Human immunodeficiency [HIV] disease complicating pregnancy, childbirth and the puerperium, followed by the code(s) for the HIV-related illness(es).

Patients with asymptomatic HIV infection status admitted during pregnancy, childbirth, or the puerperium should receive codes of O98.7- and Z21, Asymptomatic human immunodeficiency virus [HIV] infection status.

g. Diabetes mellitus in pregnancy
Diabetes mellitus is a significant complicating factor in pregnancy. Pregnant women who are diabetic should be assigned a code from category O24, Diabetes mellitus in pregnancy, childbirth, and the puerperium, first, followed by the appropriate diabetes code(s) (E08-E13) from Chapter 4.

h. Long term use of insulin and oral hypoglycemics
See section I.C.4.a.3 for information on the long term use of insulin and oral hypoglycemic.

i. Gestational (pregnancy induced) diabetes
Gestational (pregnancy induced) diabetes can occur during the second and third trimester of pregnancy in women who were not diabetic prior to pregnancy. Gestational diabetes can cause complications in the pregnancy similar to those of pre-existing diabetes mellitus. It also puts the woman at greater risk of developing diabetes after the pregnancy. Codes for gestational diabetes are in subcategory O24.4, Gestational diabetes mellitus. No other code from category O24, Diabetes mellitus in pregnancy, childbirth, and the puerperium, should be used with a code from O24.4.

The codes under subcategory O24.4 include diet controlled, insulin controlled, and controlled by oral hypoglycemic drugs. If a patient with gestational diabetes is treated with both diet and insulin, only the code for insulin-controlled is required. If a patient with gestational diabetes is treated with both diet and oral hypoglycemic medications, only the code for "controlled by oral hypoglycemic drugs" is required. Code Z79.4, Long-term (current) use of insulin or code Z79.84, Long-term (current) use of oral hypoglycemic drugs, should not be assigned with codes from subcategory O24.4.

An abnormal glucose tolerance in pregnancy is assigned a code from subcategory O99.81, Abnormal glucose complicating pregnancy, childbirth, and the puerperium.

j. Sepsis and septic shock complicating abortion, pregnancy, childbirth and the puerperium
When assigning a chapter 15 code for sepsis complicating abortion, pregnancy, childbirth, and the puerperium, a code for the specific type of infection should be assigned as an additional diagnosis. If severe sepsis is present, a code from subcategory R65.2, Severe sepsis, and code(s) for associated organ dysfunction(s) should also be assigned as additional diagnoses.

k. Puerperal sepsis
Code O85, Puerperal sepsis, should be assigned with a secondary code to identify the causal organism (e.g., for a bacterial infection, assign a code from category B95-B96, Bacterial infections in conditions classified elsewhere). A code from category A40, Streptococcal sepsis, or A41, Other sepsis, should not be used for puerperal sepsis. If applicable, use additional codes to identify severe sepsis (R65.2-) and any associated acute organ dysfunction.

l. Alcohol and tobacco use during pregnancy, childbirth and the puerperium
1) Alcohol use during pregnancy, childbirth and the puerperium
Codes under subcategory O99.31, Alcohol use complicating pregnancy, childbirth, and the puerperium, should be assigned for any pregnancy case when a mother uses alcohol during the pregnancy or postpartum. A secondary code from category F10, Alcohol related disorders, should also be assigned to identify manifestations of the alcohol use.

2) Tobacco use during pregnancy, childbirth and the puerperium
Codes under subcategory O99.33, Smoking (tobacco) complicating pregnancy, childbirth, and the puerperium, should be assigned for any pregnancy case when a mother uses any type of tobacco product during the pregnancy or postpartum. A secondary code from category F17, Nicotine dependence, should also be assigned to identify the type of nicotine dependence.

m. Poisoning, toxic effects, adverse effects and underdosing in a pregnant patient
A code from subcategory O9A.2, Injury, poisoning and certain other consequences of external causes complicating pregnancy, childbirth, and the puerperium, should be sequenced first, followed by the appropriate injury, poisoning, toxic effect, adverse effect or underdosing code, and then the additional code(s) that specifies the condition caused by the poisoning, toxic effect, adverse effect or underdosing.

See Section I.C.19. Adverse effects, poisoning, underdosing and toxic effects.

n. Normal Delivery, Code O80
1) Encounter for full term uncomplicated delivery
Code O80 should be assigned when a woman is admitted for a full-term normal delivery and delivers a single, healthy infant without any complications antepartum, during the delivery, or postpartum during the delivery episode. Code O80 is always a principal diagnosis. It is not to be used if any other code from chapter 15 is needed to describe a current complication of the antenatal, delivery, or perinatal period. Additional codes from other chapters may be used with code O80 if they are not related to or are in any way complicating the pregnancy.

2) Uncomplicated delivery with resolved antepartum complication
Code O80 may be used if the patient had a complication at some point during the pregnancy, but the complication is not present at the time of the admission for delivery.

3) Outcome of delivery for O80
Z37.0, Single live birth, is the only outcome of delivery code appropriate for use with O80.

o. The Peripartum and Postpartum Periods
1) Peripartum and Postpartum periods
The postpartum period begins immediately after delivery and continues for six weeks following delivery. The peripartum period is defined as the last month of pregnancy to five months postpartum.

2) Peripartum and postpartum complication

A postpartum complication is any complication occurring within the six-week period.

3) Pregnancy-related complications after 6 week period

Chapter 15 codes may also be used to describe pregnancy-related complications after the peripartum or postpartum period if the provider documents that a condition is pregnancy related.

4) Admission for routine postpartum care following delivery outside hospital

When the mother delivers outside the hospital prior to admission and is admitted for routine postpartum care and no complications are noted, code Z39.0, Encounter for care and examination of mother immediately after delivery, should be assigned as the principal diagnosis.

5) Pregnancy associated cardiomyopathy

Pregnancy associated cardiomyopathy, code O90.3, is unique in that it may be diagnosed in the third trimester of pregnancy but may continue to progress months after delivery. For this reason, it is referred to as peripartum cardiomyopathy. Code O90.3 is only for use when the cardiomyopathy develops as a result of pregnancy in a woman who did not have pre-existing heart disease.

p. Code O94, Sequelae of complication of pregnancy, childbirth, and the puerperium

1) Code O94

Code O94, Sequelae of complication of pregnancy, childbirth, and the puerperium, is for use in those cases when an initial complication of a pregnancy develops a sequelae requiring care or treatment at a future date.

2) After the initial postpartum period

This code may be used at any time after the initial postpartum period.

3) Sequencing of Code O94

This code, like all sequela codes, is to be sequenced following the code describing the sequelae of the complication.

q. Termination of Pregnancy and Spontaneous abortions

1) Abortion with Liveborn Fetus

When an attempted termination of pregnancy results in a liveborn fetus, assign code Z33.2, Encounter for elective termination of pregnancy and a code from category Z37, Outcome of Delivery.

2) Retained Products of Conception following an abortion

Subsequent encounters for retained products of conception following a spontaneous abortion or elective termination of pregnancy, **without complications** are assigned O03.**4, Incomplete spontaneous,** abortion **without complication,** or codes O07.4, Failed attempted termination of pregnancy without complication. This advice is appropriate even when the patient was discharged previously with a discharge diagnosis of complete abortion. **If the patient has a specific complication associated with the spontaneous abortion or elective termination of pregnancy in addition to retained products of conception, assign the appropriate complication in category O03 or O07 instead of code O03.4 or O07.4**

3) Complications leading to abortion

Codes from Chapter 15 may be used as additional codes to identify any documented complications of the pregnancy in conjunction with codes in categories in **O04,** O07 and O08.

r. Abuse in a pregnant patient

For suspected or confirmed cases of abuse of a pregnant patient, a code(s) from subcategories O9A.3, Physical abuse complicating pregnancy, childbirth, and the puerperium, O9A.4, Sexual abuse complicating pregnancy, childbirth, and the puerperium, and O9A.5, Psychological abuse complicating pregnancy, childbirth, and the puerperium, should be sequenced first, followed by the appropriate codes (if applicable) to identify any associated current injury due to physical abuse, sexual abuse, and the perpetrator of abuse.

See Section I.C.19. Adult and child abuse, neglect and other maltreatment.

16. Chapter 16: Certain Conditions Originating in the Perinatal Period (P00-P96)

For coding and reporting purposes the perinatal period is defined as before birth through the 28th day following birth. The following guidelines are provided for reporting purposes.

a. General Perinatal Rules

1) Use of Chapter 16 Codes

Codes in this chapter are never for use on the maternal record. Codes from Chapter 15, the obstetric chapter, are never permitted on the newborn record. Chapter 16 codes may be used throughout the life of the patient if the condition is still present.

2) Principal Diagnosis for Birth Record

When coding the birth episode in a newborn record, assign a code from category Z38, Liveborn infants according to place of birth and type of delivery, as the principal diagnosis. A code from category Z38 is assigned only once, to a newborn at the time of birth. If a newborn is transferred to another institution, a code from category Z38 should not be used at the receiving hospital.

A code from category Z38 is used only on the newborn record, not on the mother's record.

3) Use of Codes from other Chapters with Codes from Chapter 16

Codes from other chapters may be used with codes from chapter 16 if the codes from the other chapters provide more specific detail. Codes for signs and symptoms may be assigned when a definitive diagnosis has not been established. If the reason for the encounter is a perinatal condition, the code from chapter 16 should be sequenced first.

4) Use of Chapter 16 Codes after the Perinatal Period

Should a condition originate in the perinatal period, and continue throughout the life of the patient, the perinatal code should continue to be used regardless of the patient's age.

5) Birth process or community acquired conditions

If a newborn has a condition that may be either due to the birth process or community acquired and the documentation does not indicate which it is, the default is due to the birth process and the code from Chapter 16 should be used. If the condition is community-acquired, a code from Chapter 16 should not be assigned.

6) Code all clinically significant conditions

All clinically significant conditions noted on routine newborn examination should be coded. A condition is clinically significant if it requires:

- clinical evaluation; or
- therapeutic treatment; or
- diagnostic procedures; or
- extended length of hospital stay; or
- increased nursing care and/or monitoring; or
- has implications for future health care needs

Note: The perinatal guidelines listed above are the same as the general coding guidelines for "additional diagnoses", except for the final point regarding implications for future health care needs. Codes should be assigned for conditions that have been specified by the provider as having implications for future health care needs.

b. Observation and Evaluation of Newborns for Suspected Conditions not Found

1) Use of Z05 codes

Assign a code from category Z05, Observation and evaluation of newborns and infants for suspected conditions ruled out, to identify those instances when a healthy newborn is evaluated for a suspected condition that is determined after study not to be present. Do not use a code from category Z05 when the patient has identified signs or symptoms of a suspected problem; in such cases code the sign or symptom.

2) Z05 on Other than the Birth Record

A code from category Z05 may also be assigned as a principal or first-listed code for readmissions or encounters when the code from category Z38 code no longer applies. Codes from category

ZØ5 are for use only for healthy newborns and infants for which no condition after study is found to be present.

3) ZØ5 on a birth record

A code from category ZØ5 is to be used as a secondary code after the code from category Z38, Liveborn infants according to place of birth and type of delivery.

c. Coding Additional Perinatal Diagnoses

1) Assigning codes for conditions that require treatment

Assign codes for conditions that require treatment or further investigation, prolong the length of stay, or require resource utilization.

2) Codes for conditions specified as having implications for future health care needs

Assign codes for conditions that have been specified by the provider as having implications for future health care needs.

Note: This guideline should not be used for adult patients.

d. Prematurity and Fetal Growth Retardation

Providers utilize different criteria in determining prematurity. A code for prematurity should not be assigned unless it is documented. Assignment of codes in categories PØ5, Disorders of newborn related to slow fetal growth and fetal malnutrition, and PØ7, Disorders of newborn related to short gestation and low birth weight, not elsewhere classified, should be based on the recorded birth weight and estimated gestational age.

When both birth weight and gestational age are available, two codes from category PØ7 should be assigned, with the code for birth weight sequenced before the code for gestational age.

e. Low birth weight and immaturity status

Codes from category PØ7, Disorders of newborn related to short gestation and low birth weight, not elsewhere classified, are for use for a child or adult who was premature or had a low birth weight as a newborn and this is affecting the patient's current health status.

See Section I.C.21. Factors influencing health status and contact with health services, Status.

f. Bacterial Sepsis of Newborn

Category P36, Bacterial sepsis of newborn, includes congenital sepsis. If a perinate is documented as having sepsis without documentation of congenital or community acquired, the default is congenital and a code from category P36 should be assigned. If the P36 code includes the causal organism, an additional code from category B95, Streptococcus, Staphylococcus, and Enterococcus as the cause of diseases classified elsewhere, or B96, Other bacterial agents as the cause of diseases classified elsewhere, should not be assigned. If the P36 code does not include the causal organism, assign an additional code from category B96. If applicable, use additional codes to identify severe sepsis (R65.2-) and any associated acute organ dysfunction.

g. Stillbirth

Code P95, Stillbirth, is only for use in institutions that maintain separate records for stillbirths. No other code should be used with P95. Code P95 should not be used on the mother's record.

17. Chapter 17: Congenital malformations, deformations, and chromosomal abnormalities (QØØ-Q99)

Assign an appropriate code(s) from categories QØØ-Q99, Congenital malformations, deformations, and chromosomal abnormalities when a malformation/deformation or chromosomal abnormality is documented. A malformation/deformation/or chromosomal abnormality may be the principal/first-listed diagnosis on a record or a secondary diagnosis.

When a malformation/deformation or chromosomal abnormality does not have a unique code assignment, assign additional code(s) for any manifestations that may be present.

When the code assignment specifically identifies the malformation/deformation or chromosomal abnormality, manifestations that are an inherent component of the anomaly should not be coded separately. Additional codes should be assigned for manifestations that are not an inherent component.

Codes from Chapter 17 may be used throughout the life of the patient. If a congenital malformation or deformity has been corrected, a personal history code should be used to identify the history of the malformation or deformity. Although present at birth, malformation/deformation/or chromosomal abnormality may not be identified until later in life.

Whenever the condition is diagnosed by the physician, it is appropriate to assign a code from codes QØØ-Q99. For the birth admission, the appropriate code from category Z38, Liveborn infants, according to place of birth and type of delivery, should be sequenced as the principal diagnosis, followed by any congenital anomaly codes, QØØ-Q99.

18. Chapter 18: Symptoms, signs, and abnormal clinical and laboratory findings, not elsewhere classified (RØØ-R99)

Chapter 18 includes symptoms, signs, abnormal results of clinical or other investigative procedures, and ill-defined conditions regarding which no diagnosis classifiable elsewhere is recorded. Signs and symptoms that point to a specific diagnosis have been assigned to a category in other chapters of the classification.

a. Use of symptom codes

Codes that describe symptoms and signs are acceptable for reporting purposes when a related definitive diagnosis has not been established (confirmed) by the provider.

b. Use of a symptom code with a definitive diagnosis code

Codes for signs and symptoms may be reported in addition to a related definitive diagnosis when the sign or symptom is not routinely associated with that diagnosis, such as the various signs and symptoms associated with complex syndromes. The definitive diagnosis code should be sequenced before the symptom code.

Signs or symptoms that are associated routinely with a disease process should not be assigned as additional codes, unless otherwise instructed by the classification.

c. Combination codes that include symptoms

ICD-10-CM contains a number of combination codes that identify both the definitive diagnosis and common symptoms of that diagnosis.

When using one of these combination codes, an additional code should not be assigned for the symptom.

d. Repeated falls

Code R29.6, Repeated falls, is for use for encounters when a patient has recently fallen and the reason for the fall is being investigated.

Code Z91.81, History of falling, is for use when a patient has fallen in the past and is at risk for future falls. When appropriate, both codes R29.6 and Z91.81 may be assigned together.

e. Coma scale

The coma scale codes (R4Ø.2-) can be used in conjunction with traumatic brain injury codes, acute cerebrovascular disease or sequelae of cerebrovascular disease codes. These codes are primarily for use by trauma registries, but they may be used in any setting where this information is collected. The coma scale may also be used to assess the status of the central nervous system for other non-trauma conditions, such as monitoring patients in the intensive care unit regardless of medical condition. The coma scale codes should be sequenced after the diagnosis code(s).

These codes, one from each subcategory, are needed to complete the scale. The 7th character indicates when the scale was recorded. The 7th character should match for all three codes.

At a minimum, report the initial score documented on presentation at your facility. This may be a score from the emergency medicine technician (EMT) or in the emergency department. If desired, a facility may choose to capture multiple coma scale scores.

Assign code R4Ø.24, Glasgow coma scale, total score, when only the total score is documented in the medical record and not the individual score(s).

f. Functional quadriplegia

GUIDELINE HAS BEEN DELETED EFFECTIVE OCTOBER 1, 2017

g. SIRS due to Non-Infectious Process

The systemic inflammatory response syndrome (SIRS) can develop as a result of certain non-infectious disease processes, such as trauma, malignant neoplasm, or pancreatitis. When SIRS is documented with a noninfectious condition, and no subsequent infection is documented, the code for the underlying condition, such as an injury, should be assigned, followed by code R65.1Ø, Systemic inflammatory response syndrome (SIRS) of non-infectious origin without acute organ dysfunction, or code R65.11, Systemic inflammatory response syndrome (SIRS) of non-infectious origin with acute organ dysfunction. If an associated acute organ dysfunction is documented, the appropriate code(s) for the specific type of organ dysfunction(s) should be assigned in addition to code

R65.11. If acute organ dysfunction is documented, but it cannot be determined if the acute organ dysfunction is associated with SIRS or due to another condition (e.g., directly due to the trauma), the provider should be queried.

h. Death NOS
Code R99, Ill-defined and unknown cause of mortality, is only for use in the very limited circumstance when a patient who has already died is brought into an emergency department or other healthcare facility and is pronounced dead upon arrival. It does not represent the discharge disposition of death.

i. NIHSS Stroke Scale
The NIH stroke scale (NIHSS) codes (R29.7- -) can be used in conjunction with acute stroke codes (I63) to identify the patient's neurological status and the severity of the stroke. The stroke scale codes should be sequenced after the acute stroke diagnosis code(s).

At a minimum, report the initial score documented. If desired, a facility may choose to capture multiple stroke scale scores.

See Section I.B.14. for information concerning the medical record documentation that may be used for assignment of the NIHSS codes.

19. Chapter 19: Injury, poisoning, and certain other consequences of external causes (S00-T88)
a. Application of 7th Characters in Chapter 19
Most categories in chapter 19 have a 7th character requirement for each applicable code. Most categories in this chapter have three 7th character values (with the exception of fractures): A, initial encounter, D, subsequent encounter and S, sequela. Categories for traumatic fractures have additional 7th character values. While the patient may be seen by a new or different provider over the course of treatment for an injury, assignment of the 7th character is based on whether the patient is undergoing active treatment and not whether the provider is seeing the patient for the first time.

For complication codes, active treatment refers to treatment for the condition described by the code, even though it may be related to an earlier precipitating problem. For example, code T84.50XA, Infection and inflammatory reaction due to unspecified internal joint prosthesis, initial encounter, is used when active treatment is provided for the infection, even though the condition relates to the prosthetic device, implant or graft that was placed at a previous encounter.

7th character "A", initial encounter is used for each encounter where the patient is receiving active treatment for the condition.

7th character "D" subsequent encounter is used for encounters after the patient has completed active treatment of the condition and is receiving routine care for the condition during the healing or recovery phase.

The aftercare Z codes should not be used for aftercare for conditions such as injuries or poisonings, where 7th characters are provided to identify subsequent care. For example, for aftercare of an injury, assign the acute injury code with the 7th character "D" (subsequent encounter).

7th character "S", sequela, is for use for complications or conditions that arise as a direct result of a condition, such as scar formation after a burn. The scars are sequelae of the burn. When using 7th character "S", it is necessary to use both the injury code that precipitated the sequela and the code for the sequela itself. The "S" is added only to the injury code, not the sequela code. The 7th character "S" identifies the injury responsible for the sequela. The specific type of sequela (e.g. scar) is sequenced first, followed by the injury code.

See Section I.B.10 Sequelae, (Late Effects)

b. Coding of Injuries
When coding injuries, assign separate codes for each injury unless a combination code is provided, in which case the combination code is assigned. **Codes from category** T07, Unspecified multiple injuries should not be assigned in the inpatient setting unless information for a more specific code is not available. Traumatic injury codes (S00-T14.9) are not to be used for normal, healing surgical wounds or to identify complications of surgical wounds.

The code for the most serious injury, as determined by the provider and the focus of treatment, is sequenced first.

1) Superficial injuries
Superficial injuries such as abrasions or contusions are not coded when associated with more severe injuries of the same site.

2) Primary injury with damage to nerves/blood vessels
When a primary injury results in minor damage to peripheral nerves or blood vessels, the primary injury is sequenced first with additional code(s) for injuries to nerves and spinal cord (such as category S04), and/or injury to blood vessels (such as category S15). When the primary injury is to the blood vessels or nerves, that injury should be sequenced first.

c. Coding of Traumatic Fractures
The principles of multiple coding of injuries should be followed in coding fractures. Fractures of specified sites are coded individually by site in accordance with both the provisions within categories S02, S12, S22, S32, S42, S49, S52, S59, S62, S72, S79, S82, S89, S92 and the level of detail furnished by medical record content.

A fracture not indicated as open or closed should be coded to closed. A fracture not indicated whether displaced or not displaced should be coded to displaced.

More specific guidelines are as follows:

1) Initial vs. Subsequent Encounter for Fractures
Traumatic fractures are coded using the appropriate 7th character for initial encounter (A, B, C) for each encounter where the patient is receiving active treatment for the fracture. The appropriate 7th character for initial encounter should also be assigned for a patient who delayed seeking treatment for the fracture or nonunion.

Fractures are coded using the appropriate 7th character for subsequent care for encounters after the patient has completed active treatment of the fracture and is receiving routine care for the fracture during the healing or recovery phase.

Care for complications of surgical treatment for fracture repairs during the healing or recovery phase should be coded with the appropriate complication codes.

Care of complications of fractures, such as malunion and nonunion, should be reported with the appropriate 7th character for subsequent care with nonunion (K, M, N,) or subsequent care with malunion (P, Q, R).

Malunion/nonunion: The appropriate 7th character for initial encounter should also be assigned for a patient who delayed seeking treatment for the fracture or nonunion.

The open fracture designations in the assignment of the 7th character for fractures of the forearm, femur and lower leg, including ankle are based on the Gustilo open fracture classification. When the Gustilo classification type is not specified for an open fracture, the 7th character for open fracture type I or II should be assigned (B, E, H, M, Q).

A code from category M80, not a traumatic fracture code, should be used for any patient with known osteoporosis who suffers a fracture, even if the patient had a minor fall or trauma, if that fall or trauma would not usually break a normal, healthy bone.

See Section I.C.13. Osteoporosis.

The aftercare Z codes should not be used for aftercare for traumatic fractures. For aftercare of a traumatic fracture, assign the acute fracture code with the appropriate 7th character.

2) Multiple fractures sequencing
Multiple fractures are sequenced in accordance with the severity of the fracture.

d. Coding of Burns and Corrosions
The ICD-10-CM makes a distinction between burns and corrosions. The burn codes are for thermal burns, except sunburns, that come from a heat source, such as a fire or hot appliance. The burn codes are also for burns resulting from electricity and radiation. Corrosions are burns due to chemicals. The guidelines are the same for burns and corrosions.

Current burns (T20-T25) are classified by depth, extent and by agent (X code). Burns are classified by depth as first degree (erythema), second degree (blistering), and third degree (full-thickness involvement). Burns of the eye and internal organs (T26-T28) are classified by site, but not by degree.

1) **Sequencing of burn and related condition codes**
Sequence first the code that reflects the highest degree of burn when more than one burn is present.

   a. When the reason for the admission or encounter is for treatment of external multiple burns, sequence first the code that reflects the burn of the highest degree.

   b. When a patient has both internal and external burns, the circumstances of admission govern the selection of the principal diagnosis or first-listed diagnosis.

   c. When a patient is admitted for burn injuries and other related conditions such as smoke inhalation and/or respiratory failure, the circumstances of admission govern the selection of the principal or first-listed diagnosis.

2) **Burns of the same local site**
Classify burns of the same local site (three-character category level, T20-T28) but of different degrees to the subcategory identifying the highest degree recorded in the diagnosis.

3) **Non-healing burns**
Non-healing burns are coded as acute burns.

Necrosis of burned skin should be coded as a non-healed burn.

4) **Infected Burn**
For any documented infected burn site, use an additional code for the infection.

5) **Assign separate codes for each burn site**
When coding burns, assign separate codes for each burn site. Category T30, Burn and corrosion, body region unspecified is extremely vague and should rarely be used.

6) **Burns and Corrosions Classified According to Extent of Body Surface Involved**
Assign codes from category T31, Burns classified according to extent of body surface involved, or T32, Corrosions classified according to extent of body surface involved, when the site of the burn is not specified or when there is a need for additional data. It is advisable to use category T31 as additional coding when needed to provide data for evaluating burn mortality, such as that needed by burn units. It is also advisable to use category T31 as an additional code for reporting purposes when there is mention of a third-degree burn involving 20 percent or more of the body surface.

Categories T31 and T32 are based on the classic "rule of nines" in estimating body surface involved: head and neck are assigned nine percent, each arm nine percent, each leg 18 percent, the anterior trunk 18 percent, posterior trunk 18 percent, and genitalia one percent. Providers may change these percentage assignments where necessary to accommodate infants and children who have proportionately larger heads than adults, and patients who have large buttocks, thighs, or abdomen that involve burns.

7) **Encounters for treatment of sequela of burns**
Encounters for the treatment of the late effects of burns or corrosions (i.e., scars or joint contractures) should be coded with a burn or corrosion code with the 7th character "S" for sequela.

8) **Sequelae with a late effect code and current burn**
When appropriate, both a code for a current burn or corrosion with 7th character "A" or "D" and a burn or corrosion code with 7th character "S" may be assigned on the same record (when both a current burn and sequelae of an old burn exist). Burns and corrosions do not heal at the same rate and a current healing wound may still exist with sequela of a healed burn or corrosion.

See Section I.B.10 Sequela (Late Effects)

9) **Use of an external cause code with burns and corrosions**
An external cause code should be used with burns and corrosions to identify the source and intent of the burn, as well as the place where it occurred.

e. **Adverse Effects, Poisoning, Underdosing and Toxic Effects**
Codes in categories T36-T65 are combination codes that include the substance that was taken as well as the intent. No additional external cause code is required for poisonings, toxic effects, adverse effects and underdosing codes.

1) **Do not code directly from the Table of Drugs**
Do not code directly from the Table of Drugs and Chemicals. Always refer back to the Tabular List.

2) **Use as many codes as necessary to describe**
Use as many codes as necessary to describe completely all drugs, medicinal or biological substances.

3) **If the same code would describe the causative agent**
If the same code would describe the causative agent for more than one adverse reaction, poisoning, toxic effect or underdosing, assign the code only once.

4) **If two or more drugs, medicinal or biological substances**
If two or more drugs, medicinal or biological substances are reported, code each individually unless a combination code is listed in the Table of Drugs and Chemicals.

5) **The occurrence of drug toxicity is classified in ICD-10-CM as follows:**

   (a) Adverse Effect
When coding an adverse effect of a drug that has been correctly prescribed and properly administered, assign the appropriate code for the nature of the adverse effect followed by the appropriate code for the adverse effect of the drug (T36-T50). The code for the drug should have a 5th or 6th character "5" (for example T36.0X5-) Examples of the nature of an adverse effect are tachycardia, delirium, gastrointestinal hemorrhaging, vomiting, hypokalemia, hepatitis, renal failure, or respiratory failure.

   (b) Poisoning
When coding a poisoning or reaction to the improper use of a medication (e.g., overdose, wrong substance given or taken in error, wrong route of administration), first assign the appropriate code from categories T36-T50. The poisoning codes have an associated intent as their 5th or 6th character (accidental, intentional self-harm, assault and undetermined. If the intent of the poisoning is unknown or unspecified, code the intent as accidental intent. The undetermined intent is only for use if the documentation in the record specifies that the intent cannot be determined. Use additional code(s) for all manifestations of poisonings.

If there is also a diagnosis of abuse or dependence of the substance, the abuse or dependence is assigned as an additional code.

Examples of poisoning include:

   (i) Error was made in drug prescription
Errors made in drug prescription or in the administration of the drug by provider, nurse, patient, or other person.

   (ii) Overdose of a drug intentionally taken
If an overdose of a drug was intentionally taken or administered and resulted in drug toxicity, it would be coded as a poisoning.

   (iii) Nonprescribed drug taken with correctly prescribed and properly administered drug
If a nonprescribed drug or medicinal agent was taken in combination with a correctly prescribed and properly administered drug, any drug toxicity or other reaction resulting from the interaction of the two drugs would be classified as a poisoning.

   (iv) Interaction of drug(s) and alcohol
When a reaction results from the interaction of a drug(s) and alcohol, this would be classified as poisoning.

See Section I.C.4. if poisoning is the result of insulin pump malfunctions.

   (c) Underdosing
Underdosing refers to taking less of a medication than is prescribed by a provider or a manufacturer's instruction. For underdosing, assign the code from categories T36-T50 (fifth or sixth character "6").

Codes for underdosing should never be assigned as principal or first-listed codes. If a patient has a relapse or exacerbation of the medical condition for which the drug is prescribed because of the reduction in dose, then the medical condition itself should be coded.

Noncompliance (Z91.12-, Z91.13-) or complication of care (Y63.6-Y63.9) codes are to be used with an underdosing code to indicate intent, if known.

(d) Toxic Effects

When a harmful substance is ingested or comes in contact with a person, this is classified as a toxic effect. The toxic effect codes are in categories T51-T65.

Toxic effect codes have an associated intent: accidental, intentional self-harm, assault and undetermined.

f. Adult and child abuse, neglect and other maltreatment

Sequence first the appropriate code from categories T74, Adult and child abuse, neglect and other maltreatment, confirmed) or T76, Adult and child abuse, neglect and other maltreatment, suspected) for abuse, neglect and other maltreatment, followed by any accompanying mental health or injury code(s).

If the documentation in the medical record states abuse or neglect it is coded as confirmed (T74.-). It is coded as suspected if it is documented as suspected (T76.-).

For cases of confirmed abuse or neglect an external cause code from the assault section (X92-Y09) should be added to identify the cause of any physical injuries. A perpetrator code (Y07) should be added when the perpetrator of the abuse is known. For suspected cases of abuse or neglect, do not report external cause or perpetrator code.

If a suspected case of abuse, neglect or mistreatment is ruled out during an encounter code Z04.71, Encounter for examination and observation following alleged physical adult abuse, ruled out, or code Z04.72, Encounter for examination and observation following alleged child physical abuse, ruled out, should be used, not a code from T76.

If a suspected case of alleged rape or sexual abuse is ruled out during an encounter code Z04.41, Encounter for examination and observation following alleged adult rape or code Z04.42, Encounter for examination and observation following alleged child rape, should be used, not a code from T76.

See Section I.C.15. Abuse in a pregnant patient.

g. Complications of care

1) General guidelines for complications of care

(a) Documentation of complications of care

See Section I.B.16. for information on documentation of complications of care.

2) Pain due to medical devices

Pain associated with devices, implants or grafts left in a surgical site (for example painful hip prosthesis) is assigned to the appropriate code(s) found in Chapter 19, Injury, poisoning, and certain other consequences of external causes. Specific codes for pain due to medical devices are found in the T code section of the ICD-10-CM. Use additional code(s) from category G89 to identify acute or chronic pain due to presence of the device, implant or graft (G89.18 or G89.28).

3) Transplant complications

(a) Transplant complications other than kidney

Codes under category T86, Complications of transplanted organs and tissues, are for use for both complications and rejection of transplanted organs. A transplant complication code is only assigned if the complication affects the function of the transplanted organ. Two codes are required to fully describe a transplant complication: the appropriate code from category T86 and a secondary code that identifies the complication.

Pre-existing conditions or conditions that develop after the transplant are not coded as complications unless they affect the function of the transplanted organs.

See I.C.21. for transplant organ removal status

See I.C.2. for malignant neoplasm associated with transplanted organ.

(b) Kidney transplant complications

Patients who have undergone kidney transplant may still have some form of chronic kidney disease (CKD) because the kidney transplant may not fully restore kidney function.

Code T86.1- should be assigned for documented complications of a kidney transplant, such as transplant failure or rejection or other transplant complication. Code T86.1- should not be assigned for post kidney transplant patients who have chronic kidney (CKD) unless a transplant complication such as transplant failure or rejection is documented. If the documentation is unclear as to whether the patient has a complication of the transplant, query the provider.

Conditions that affect the function of the transplanted kidney, other than CKD, should be assigned a code from subcategory T86.1, Complications of transplanted organ, Kidney, and a secondary code that identifies the complication.

For patients with CKD following a kidney transplant, but who do not have a complication such as failure or rejection, *see section I.C.14. Chronic kidney disease and kidney transplant status.*

4) Complication codes that include the external cause

As with certain other T codes, some of the complications of care codes have the external cause included in the code. The code includes the nature of the complication as well as the type of procedure that caused the complication. No external cause code indicating the type of procedure is necessary for these codes.

5) Complications of care codes within the body system chapters

Intraoperative and postprocedural complication codes are found within the body system chapters with codes specific to the organs and structures of that body system. These codes should be sequenced first, followed by a code(s) for the specific complication, if applicable.

20. Chapter 20: External Causes of Morbidity (V00-Y99)

The external causes of morbidity codes should never be sequenced as the first-listed or principal diagnosis.

External cause codes are intended to provide data for injury research and evaluation of injury prevention strategies. These codes capture how the injury or health condition happened (cause), the intent (unintentional or accidental; or intentional, such as suicide or assault), the place where the event occurred the activity of the patient at the time of the event, and the person's status (e.g., civilian, military).

There is no national requirement for mandatory ICD-10-CM external cause code reporting. Unless a provider is subject to a state-based external cause code reporting mandate or these codes are required by a particular payer, reporting of ICD-10-CM codes in Chapter 20, External Causes of Morbidity, is not required. In the absence of a mandatory reporting requirement, providers are encouraged to voluntarily report external cause codes, as they provide valuable data for injury research and evaluation of injury prevention strategies.

a. General External Cause Coding Guidelines

1) Used with any code in the range of A00.0-T88.9 Z00-Z99

An external cause code may be used with any code in the range of A00.0-T88.9, Z00-Z99, classification that **represent**s a health condition due to an external cause. Though they are most applicable to injuries, they are also valid for use with such things as infections or diseases due to an external source, and other health conditions, such as a heart attack that occurs during strenuous physical activity.

2) External cause code used for length of treatment

Assign the external cause code, with the appropriate 7th character (initial encounter, subsequent encounter or sequela) for each encounter for which the injury or condition is being treated.

Most categories in chapter 20 have a 7th character requirement for each applicable code. Most categories in this chapter have three 7th character values: A, initial encounter, D, subsequent encounter and S, sequela. While the patient may be seen by a new or different provider over the course of treatment for an injury or condition, assignment of the 7th character for external cause should match the 7th character of the code assigned for the associated injury or condition for the encounter.

3) **Use the full range of external cause codes**
Use the full range of external cause codes to completely describe the cause, the intent, the place of occurrence, and if applicable, the activity of the patient at the time of the event, and the patient's status, for all injuries, and other health conditions due to an external cause.

4) **Assign as many external cause codes as necessary**
Assign as many external cause codes as necessary to fully explain each cause. If only one external code can be recorded, assign the code most related to the principal diagnosis.

5) **The selection of the appropriate external cause code**
The selection of the appropriate external cause code is guided by the Alphabetic Index of External Causes and by Inclusion and Exclusion notes in the Tabular List.

6) **External cause code can never be a principal diagnosis**
An external cause code can never be a principal (first-listed) diagnosis.

7) **Combination external cause codes**
Certain of the external cause codes are combination codes that identify sequential events that result in an injury, such as a fall which results in striking against an object. The injury may be due to either event or both. The combination external cause code used should correspond to the sequence of events regardless of which caused the most serious injury.

8) **No external cause code needed in certain circumstances**
No external cause code from Chapter 20 is needed if the external cause and intent are included in a code from another chapter (e.g. T36.0X1- Poisoning by penicillins, accidental (unintentional)).

b. **Place of Occurrence Guideline**
Codes from category Y92, Place of occurrence of the external cause, are secondary codes for use after other external cause codes to identify the location of the patient at the time of injury or other condition.

Generally, a place of occurrence code is assigned only once, at the initial encounter for treatment. However, in the rare instance that a new injury occurs during hospitalization, an additional place of occurrence code may be assigned. No 7th characters are used for Y92.

Do not use place of occurrence code Y92.9 if the place is not stated or is not applicable.

c. **Activity Code**
Assign a code from category Y93, Activity code, to describe the activity of the patient at the time the injury or other health condition occurred.

An activity code is used only once, at the initial encounter for treatment. Only one code from Y93 should be recorded on a medical record.

The activity codes are not applicable to poisonings, adverse effects, misadventures or sequela.

Do not assign Y93.9, Unspecified activity, if the activity is not stated.

A code from category Y93 is appropriate for use with external cause and intent codes if identifying the activity provides additional information about the event.

d. **Place of Occurrence, Activity, and Status Codes Used with other External Cause Code**
When applicable, place of occurrence, activity, and external cause status codes are sequenced after the main external cause code(s). Regardless of the number of external cause codes assigned, generally there should be only one place of occurrence code, one activity code, and one external cause status code assigned to an encounter. However, in the rare instance that a new injury occurs during hospitalization, an additional place of occurrence code may be assigned.

e. **If the Reporting Format Limits the Number of External Cause Codes**
If the reporting format limits the number of external cause codes that can be used in reporting clinical data, report the code for the cause/intent most related to the principal diagnosis. If the format permits capture of additional external cause codes, the cause/intent, including medical misadventures, of the additional events should be reported rather than the codes for place, activity, or external status.

f. **Multiple External Cause Coding Guidelines**
More than one external cause code is required to fully describe the external cause of an illness or injury. The assignment of external cause codes should be sequenced in the following priority:

If two or more events cause separate injuries, an external cause code should be assigned for each cause. The first-listed external cause code will be selected in the following order:

External codes for child and adult abuse take priority over all other external cause codes.

See Section I.C.19., Child and Adult abuse guidelines.

External cause codes for terrorism events take priority over all other external cause codes except child and adult abuse.

External cause codes for cataclysmic events take priority over all other external cause codes except child and adult abuse and terrorism.

External cause codes for transport accidents take priority over all other external cause codes except cataclysmic events, child and adult abuse and terrorism.

Activity and external cause status codes are assigned following all causal (intent) external cause codes.

The first-listed external cause code should correspond to the cause of the most serious diagnosis due to an assault, accident, or self-harm, following the order of hierarchy listed above.

g. **Child and Adult Abuse Guideline**
Adult and child abuse, neglect and maltreatment are classified as assault. Any of the assault codes may be used to indicate the external cause of any injury resulting from the confirmed abuse.

For confirmed cases of abuse, neglect and maltreatment, when the perpetrator is known, a code from Y07, Perpetrator of maltreatment and neglect, should accompany any other assault codes.

See Section I.C.19. Adult and child abuse, neglect and other maltreatment

h. **Unknown or Undetermined Intent Guideline**
If the intent (accident, self-harm, assault) of the cause of an injury or other condition is unknown or unspecified, code the intent as accidental intent. All transport accident categories assume accidental intent.

1) **Use of undetermined intent**
External cause codes for events of undetermined intent are only for use if the documentation in the record specifies that the intent cannot be determined.

i. **Sequelae (Late Effects) of External Cause Guidelines**
1) **Sequelae external cause codes**
Sequela are reported using the external cause code with the 7th character "S" for sequela. These codes should be used with any report of a late effect or sequela resulting from a previous injury.

See Section I.B.10 Sequela (Late Effects)

2) **Sequela external cause code with a related current injury**
A sequela external cause code should never be used with a related current nature of injury code.

3) **Use of sequela external cause codes for subsequent visits**
Use a late effect external cause code for subsequent visits when a late effect of the initial injury is being treated. Do not use a late effect external cause code for subsequent visits for follow-up care (e.g., to assess healing, to receive rehabilitative therapy) of the injury when no late effect of the injury has been documented.

j. **Terrorism Guidelines**
1) **Cause of injury identified by the Federal Government (FBI) as terrorism**
When the cause of an injury is identified by the Federal Government (FBI) as terrorism, the first-listed external cause code should be a code from category Y38, Terrorism. The definition of terrorism employed by the FBI is found at the inclusion note at the beginning of category Y38. Use additional code for place of occurrence (Y92.-). More than one Y38 code

may be assigned if the injury is the result of more than one mechanism of terrorism.

   2)   Cause of an injury is suspected to be the result of terrorism
   When the cause of an injury is suspected to be the result of terrorism a code from category Y38 should not be assigned. Suspected cases should be classified as assault.

   3)   Code Y38.9, Terrorism, secondary effects
   Assign code Y38.9, Terrorism, secondary effects, for conditions occurring subsequent to the terrorist event. This code should not be assigned for conditions that are due to the initial terrorist act.

   It is acceptable to assign code Y38.9 with another code from Y38 if there is an injury due to the initial terrorist event and an injury that is a subsequent result of the terrorist event.

k.   External cause status
   A code from category Y99, External cause status, should be assigned whenever any other external cause code is assigned for an encounter, including an Activity code, except for the events noted below. Assign a code from category Y99, External cause status, to indicate the work status of the person at the time the event occurred. The status code indicates whether the event occurred during military activity, whether a non-military person was at work, whether an individual including a student or volunteer was involved in a non-work activity at the time of the causal event.

   A code from Y99, External cause status, should be assigned, when applicable, with other external cause codes, such as transport accidents and falls. The external cause status codes are not applicable to poisonings, adverse effects, misadventures or late effects.

   Do not assign a code from category Y99 if no other external cause codes (cause, activity) are applicable for the encounter.

   An external cause status code is used only once, at the initial encounter for treatment. Only one code from Y99 should be recorded on a medical record.

   Do not assign code Y99.9, Unspecified external cause status, if the status is not stated.

21. Chapter 21: Factors influencing health status and contact with health services (Z00-Z99)
   Note: The chapter specific guidelines provide additional information about the use of Z codes for specified encounters.

a.   Use of Z codes in any healthcare setting
   Z codes are for use in any healthcare setting. Z codes may be used as either a first-listed (principal diagnosis code in the inpatient setting) or secondary code, depending on the circumstances of the encounter. Certain Z codes may only be used as first-listed or principal diagnosis.

b.   Z Codes indicate a reason for an encounter
   Z codes are not procedure codes. A corresponding procedure code must accompany a Z code to describe any procedure performed.

c.   Categories of Z Codes
   1)   Contact/Exposure
   Category Z20 indicates contact with, and suspected exposure to, communicable diseases. These codes are for patients who do not show any sign or symptom of a disease but are suspected to have been exposed to it by close personal contact with an infected individual or are in an area where a disease is epidemic.

   Category Z77, Other contact with and (suspected) exposures hazardous to health, indicates contact with and suspected exposures hazardous to health.

   Contact/exposure codes may be used as a first-listed code to explain an encounter for testing, or, more commonly, as a secondary code to identify a potential risk.

   2)   Inoculations and vaccinations
   Code Z23 is for encounters for inoculations and vaccinations. It indicates that a patient is being seen to receive a prophylactic inoculation against a disease. Procedure codes are required to identify the actual administration of the injection and the type(s) of immunizations given. Code Z23 may be used as a secondary code if the inoculation is given as a routine part of preventive health care, such as a well-baby visit.

3)   Status
   Status codes indicate that a patient is either a carrier of a disease or has the sequelae or residual of a past disease or condition. This includes such things as the presence of prosthetic or mechanical devices resulting from past treatment. A status code is informative, because the status may affect the course of treatment and its outcome. A status code is distinct from a history code. The history code indicates that the patient no longer has the condition.

   A status code should not be used with a diagnosis code from one of the body system chapters, if the diagnosis code includes the information provided by the status code. For example, code Z94.1, Heart transplant status, should not be used with a code from subcategory T86.2, Complications of heart transplant. The status code does not provide additional information. The complication code indicates that the patient is a heart transplant patient.

   For encounters for weaning from a mechanical ventilator, assign a code from subcategory J96.1, Chronic respiratory failure, followed by code Z99.11, Dependence on respirator [ventilator] status.

   The status Z codes/categories are:

   Z14   Genetic carrier

   Genetic carrier status indicates that a person carries a gene, associated with a particular disease, which may be passed to offspring who may develop that disease. The person does not have the disease and is not at risk of developing the disease.

   Z15   Genetic susceptibility to disease

   Genetic susceptibility indicates that a person has a gene that increases the risk of that person developing the disease.

   Codes from category Z15 should not be used as principal or first-listed codes. If the patient has the condition to which he/she is susceptible, and that condition is the reason for the encounter, the code for the current condition should be sequenced first. If the patient is being seen for follow-up after completed treatment for this condition, and the condition no longer exists, a follow-up code should be sequenced first, followed by the appropriate personal history and genetic susceptibility codes. If the purpose of the encounter is genetic counseling associated with procreative management, code Z31.5, Encounter for genetic counseling, should be assigned as the first-listed code, followed by a code from category Z15. Additional codes should be assigned for any applicable family or personal history.

   Z16   Resistance to antimicrobial drugs

   This code indicates that a patient has a condition that is resistant to antimicrobial drug treatment. Sequence the infection code first.

   Z17   Estrogen receptor status

   Z18   Retained foreign body fragments

   Z19   Hormone sensitivity malignancy status

   Z21   Asymptomatic HIV infection status

   This code indicates that a patient has tested positive for HIV but has manifested no signs or symptoms of the disease.

   Z22   Carrier of infectious disease

   Carrier status indicates that a person harbors the specific organisms of a disease without manifest symptoms and is capable of transmitting the infection.

   Z28.3   Underimmunization status

   Z33.1   Pregnant state, incidental

   This code is a secondary code only for use when the pregnancy is in no way complicating the reason for visit. Otherwise, a code from the obstetric chapter is required.

   Z66   Do not resuscitate

This code may be used when it is documented by the provider that a patient is on do not resuscitate status at any time during the stay.

Z67 Blood type

Z68 Body mass index (BMI)

As with all other secondary diagnosis codes, the BMI codes should only be assigned when they meet the definition of a reportable diagnosis (see Section III, Reporting Additional Diagnoses).

Z74.01 Bed confinement status

Z76.82 Awaiting organ transplant status

Z78 Other specified health status

Code Z78.1, Physical restraint status, may be used when it is documented by the provider that a patient has been put in restraints during the current encounter. Please note that this code should not be reported when it is documented by the provider that a patient is temporarily restrained during a procedure.

Z79 Long-term (current) drug therapy

Codes from this category indicate a patient's continuous use of a prescribed drug (including such things as aspirin therapy) for the long-term treatment of a condition or for prophylactic use. It is not for use for patients who have addictions to drugs. This subcategory is not for use of medications for detoxification or maintenance programs to prevent withdrawal symptoms in patients with drug dependence (e.g., methadone maintenance for opiate dependence). Assign the appropriate code for the drug dependence instead.

Assign a code from Z79 if the patient is receiving a medication for an extended period as a prophylactic measure (such as for the prevention of deep vein thrombosis) or as treatment of a chronic condition (such as arthritis) or a disease requiring a lengthy course of treatment (such as cancer). Do not assign a code from category Z79 for medication being administered for a brief period of time to treat an acute illness or injury (such as a course of antibiotics to treat acute bronchitis).

Z88 Allergy status to drugs, medicaments and biological substances

Except: Z88.9, Allergy status to unspecified drugs, medicaments and biological substances status

Z89 Acquired absence of limb

Z90 Acquired absence of organs, not elsewhere classified

Z91.0- Allergy status, other than to drugs and biological substances

Z92.82 Status post administration of tPA (rtPA) in a different facility within the last 24 hours prior to admission to a current facility

Assign code Z92.82, Status post administration of tPA (rtPA) in a different facility within the last 24 hours prior to admission to current facility, as a secondary diagnosis when a patient is received by transfer into a facility and documentation indicates they were administered tissue plasminogen activator (tPA) within the last 24 hours prior to admission to the current facility.

This guideline applies even if the patient is still receiving the tPA at the time they are received into the current facility.

The appropriate code for the condition for which the tPA was administered (such as cerebrovascular disease or myocardial infarction) should be assigned first.

Code Z92.82 is only applicable to the receiving facility record and not to the transferring facility record.

Z93 Artificial opening status

Z94 Transplanted organ and tissue status

Z95 Presence of cardiac and vascular implants and grafts

Z96 Presence of other functional implants

Z97 Presence of other devices

Z98 Other postprocedural states

Assign code Z98.85, Transplanted organ removal status, to indicate that a transplanted organ has been previously removed. This code should not be assigned for the encounter in which the transplanted organ is removed. The complication necessitating removal of the transplant organ should be assigned for that encounter.

See section I.C19. for information on the coding of organ transplant complications.

Z99 Dependence on enabling machines and devices, not elsewhere classified

Note: Categories Z89-Z90 and Z93-Z99 are for use only if there are no complications or malfunctions of the organ or tissue replaced, the amputation site or the equipment on which the patient is dependent.

4) **History (of)**

There are two types of history Z codes, personal and family. Personal history codes explain a patient's past medical condition that no longer exists and is not receiving any treatment, but that has the potential for recurrence, and therefore may require continued monitoring.

Family history codes are for use when a patient has a family member(s) who has had a particular disease that causes the patient to be at higher risk of also contracting the disease.

Personal history codes may be used in conjunction with follow-up codes and family history codes may be used in conjunction with screening codes to explain the need for a test or procedure. History codes are also acceptable on any medical record regardless of the reason for visit. A history of an illness, even if no longer present, is important information that may alter the type of treatment ordered.

The history Z code categories are:

Z80 Family history of primary malignant neoplasm

Z81 Family history of mental and behavioral disorders

Z82 Family history of certain disabilities and chronic diseases (leading to disablement)

Z83 Family history of other specific disorders

Z84 Family history of other conditions

Z85 Personal history of malignant neoplasm

Z86 Personal history of certain other diseases

Z87 Personal history of other diseases and conditions

Z91.4- Personal history of psychological trauma, not elsewhere classified

Z91.5 Personal history of self-harm

Z91.81 History of falling

Z91.82 Personal history of military deployment

Z92 Personal history of medical treatment

Except: Z92.0, Personal history of contraception

Except: Z92.82, Status post administration of tPA (rtPA) in a different facility within the last 24 hours prior to admission to a current facility

5) **Screening**

Screening is the testing for disease or disease precursors in seemingly well individuals so that early detection and treatment can be provided for those who test positive for the disease (e.g., screening mammogram).

The testing of a person to rule out or confirm a suspected diagnosis because the patient has some sign or symptom is a diagnostic examination, not a screening. In these cases, the sign or symptom is used to explain the reason for the test.

A screening code may be a first-listed code if the reason for the visit is specifically the screening exam. It may also be used as an additional code if the screening is done during an office visit for other health problems. A screening code is not necessary if the screening is inherent to a routine examination, such as a pap smear done during a routine pelvic examination.

Should a condition be discovered during the screening then the code for the condition may be assigned as an additional diagnosis.

The Z code indicates that a screening exam is planned. A procedure code is required to confirm that the screening was performed.

The screening Z codes/categories:

Z11   Encounter for screening for infectious and parasitic diseases

Z12   Encounter for screening for malignant neoplasms

Z13   Encounter for screening for other diseases and disorders

       Except: Z13.9, Encounter for screening, unspecified

Z36   Encounter for antenatal screening for mother

6) Observation

There are three observation Z code categories. They are for use in very limited circumstances when a person is being observed for a suspected condition that is ruled out. The observation codes are not for use if an injury or illness or any signs or symptoms related to the suspected condition are present. In such cases the diagnosis/symptom code is used with the corresponding external cause code.

The observation codes are to be used as principal diagnosis only. The only exception to this is when the principal diagnosis is required to be a code from category Z38, Liveborn infants according to place of birth and type of delivery. Then a code from category Z05, Encounter for observation and evaluation of newborn for suspected diseases and conditions ruled out, is sequenced after the Z38 code. Additional codes may be used in addition to the observation code, but only if they are unrelated to the suspected condition being observed.

Codes from subcategory Z03.7, Encounter for suspected maternal and fetal conditions ruled out, may either be used as a first-listed or as an additional code assignment depending on the case. They are for use in very limited circumstances on a maternal record when an encounter is for a suspected maternal or fetal condition that is ruled out during that encounter (for example, a maternal or fetal condition may be suspected due to an abnormal test result). These codes should not be used when the condition is confirmed. In those cases, the confirmed condition should be coded. In addition, these codes are not for use if an illness or any signs or symptoms related to the suspected condition or problem are present. In such cases the diagnosis/symptom code is used.

Additional codes may be used in addition to the code from subcategory Z03.7, but only if they are unrelated to the suspected condition being evaluated.

Codes from subcategory Z03.7 may not be used for encounters for antenatal screening of mother. See Section I.C.21. Screening.

For encounters for suspected fetal condition that are inconclusive following testing and evaluation, assign the appropriate code from category O35, O36, O40 or O41.

The observation Z code categories:

Z03   Encounter for medical observation for suspected diseases and conditions ruled out

Z04   Encounter for examination and observation for other reasons

       Except: Z04.9, Encounter for examination and observation for unspecified reason

Z05   Encounter for observation and evaluation of newborn for suspected diseases and conditions ruled out

7) Aftercare

Aftercare visit codes cover situations when the initial treatment of a disease has been performed and the patient requires continued care during the healing or recovery phase, or for the long-term consequences of the disease. The aftercare Z code should not be used if treatment is directed at a current, acute disease. The diagnosis code is to be used in these cases. Exceptions to this rule are codes Z51.0, Encounter for antineoplastic radiation therapy, and codes from subcategory Z51.1, Encounter for antineoplastic chemotherapy and immunotherapy. These codes are to be first-listed, followed by the diagnosis code when a patient's encounter is solely to receive radiation therapy, chemotherapy, or immunotherapy for the treatment of a neoplasm. If the reason for the encounter is more than one type of antineoplastic therapy, code Z51.0 and a code from subcategory Z51.1 may be assigned together, in which case one of these codes would be reported as a secondary diagnosis.

The aftercare Z codes should also not be used for aftercare for injuries. For aftercare of an injury, assign the acute injury code with the appropriate 7th character (for subsequent encounter).

The aftercare codes are generally first-listed to explain the specific reason for the encounter. An aftercare code may be used as an additional code when some type of aftercare is provided in addition to the reason for admission and no diagnosis code is applicable. An example of this would be the closure of a colostomy during an encounter for treatment of another condition.

Aftercare codes should be used in conjunction with other aftercare codes or diagnosis codes to provide better detail on the specifics of an aftercare encounter visit, unless otherwise directed by the classification. Should a patient receive multiple types of antineoplastic therapy during the same encounter, code Z51.0, Encounter for antineoplastic radiation therapy, and codes from subcategory Z51.1, Encounter for antineoplastic chemotherapy and immunotherapy, may be used together on a record. The sequencing of multiple aftercare codes depends on the circumstances of the encounter.

Certain aftercare Z code categories need a secondary diagnosis code to describe the resolving condition or sequelae. For others, the condition is included in the code title.

Additional Z code aftercare category terms include fitting and adjustment, and attention to artificial openings.

Status Z codes may be used with aftercare Z codes to indicate the nature of the aftercare. For example code Z95.1, Presence of aortocoronary bypass graft, may be used with code Z48.812, Encounter for surgical aftercare following surgery on the circulatory system, to indicate the surgery for which the aftercare is being performed. A status code should not be used when the aftercare code indicates the type of status, such as using Z43.0, Encounter for attention to tracheostomy, with Z93.0, Tracheostomy status.

The aftercare Z category/codes:

Z42   Encounter for plastic and reconstructive surgery following medical procedure or healed injury

Z43   Encounter for attention to artificial openings

Z44   Encounter for fitting and adjustment of external prosthetic device

Z45   Encounter for adjustment and management of implanted device

Z46   Encounter for fitting and adjustment of other devices

Z47   Orthopedic aftercare

Z48   Encounter for other postprocedural aftercare

Z49   Encounter for care involving renal dialysis

Z51   Encounter for other aftercare and medical care

8) Follow-up

The follow-up codes are used to explain continuing surveillance following completed treatment of a disease, condition, or injury. They imply that the condition has been fully treated and no longer exists. They should not be confused with aftercare codes, or injury codes with a 7th character for subsequent encounter, that explain ongoing care of a healing condition or its sequelae. Follow-up codes may be used in conjunction with history codes to provide the full picture of the healed condition and its treatment. The follow-up code is sequenced first, followed by the history code.

A follow-up code may be used to explain multiple visits. Should a condition be found to have recurred on the follow-up visit, then the diagnosis code for the condition should be assigned in place of the follow-up code.

The follow-up Z code categories:

Z08   Encounter for follow-up examination after completed treatment for malignant neoplasm

Z09   Encounter for follow-up examination after completed treatment for conditions other than malignant neoplasm

Z39   Encounter for maternal postpartum care and examination

9) Donor

Codes in category Z52, Donors of organs and tissues, are used for living individuals who are donating blood or other body tissue. These codes are only for individuals donating for others, not for self-donations. They are not used to identify cadaveric donations.

10) Counseling

Counseling Z codes are used when a patient or family member receives assistance in the aftermath of an illness or injury, or when support is required in coping with family or social problems.

The counseling Z codes/categories:

Z30.0-   Encounter for general counseling and advice on contraception

Z31.5   Encounter for **procreative** genetic counseling

Z31.6-   Encounter for general counseling and advice on procreation

Z32.2   Encounter for childbirth instruction

Z32.3   Encounter for childcare instruction

Z69   Encounter for mental health services for victim and perpetrator of abuse

Z70   Counseling related to sexual attitude, behavior and orientation

Z71   Persons encountering health services for other counseling and medical advice, not elsewhere classified

Z76.81 Expectant mother prebirth pediatrician visit

11) Encounters for Obstetrical and Reproductive Services

See Section I.C.15. Pregnancy, Childbirth, and the Puerperium, for further instruction on the use of these codes.

Z codes for pregnancy are for use in those circumstances when none of the problems or complications included in the codes from the Obstetrics chapter exist (a routine prenatal visit or postpartum care). Codes in category Z34, Encounter for supervision of normal pregnancy, are always first-listed and are not to be used with any other code from the OB chapter.

Codes in category Z3A, Weeks of gestation, may be assigned to provide additional information about the pregnancy. Category Z3A codes should not be assigned for pregnancies with abortive outcomes (categories O00-O08), elective termination of pregnancy (code **Z33.2**), nor for postpartum conditions, as category Z3A is not applicable to these conditions. The date of the admission should be used to determine weeks of gestation for inpatient admissions that encompass more than one gestational week.

The outcome of delivery, category Z37, should be included on all maternal delivery records. It is always a secondary code. Codes in category Z37 should not be used on the newborn record.

Z codes for family planning (contraceptive) or procreative management and counseling should be included on an obstetric record either during the pregnancy or the postpartum stage, if applicable.

Z codes/categories for obstetrical and reproductive services:

Z30   Encounter for contraceptive management

Z31   Encounter for procreative management

Z32.2   Encounter for childbirth instruction

Z32.3   Encounter for childcare instruction

Z33   Pregnant state

Z34   Encounter for supervision of normal pregnancy

Z36   Encounter for antenatal screening of mother

Z3A   Weeks of gestation

Z37   Outcome of delivery

Z39   Encounter for maternal postpartum care and examination

Z76.81 Expectant mother prebirth pediatrician visit

12) Newborns and Infants

See Section I.C.16. Newborn (Perinatal) Guidelines, for further instruction on the use of these codes.

Newborn Z codes/categories:

Z76.1   Encounter for health supervision and care of foundling

Z00.1-   Encounter for routine child health examination

Z38'   Liveborn infants according to place of birth and type of delivery

13) Routine and administrative examinations

The Z codes allow for the description of encounters for routine examinations, such as, a general check-up, or, examinations for administrative purposes, such as, a pre-employment physical. The codes are not to be used if the examination is for diagnosis of a suspected condition or for treatment purposes. In such cases the diagnosis code is used. During a routine exam, should a diagnosis or condition be discovered, it should be coded as an additional code. Pre-existing and chronic conditions and history codes may also be included as additional codes as long as the examination is for administrative purposes and not focused on any particular condition.

Some of the codes for routine health examinations distinguish between "with" and "without" abnormal findings. Code assignment depends on the information that is known at the time the encounter is being coded. For example, if no abnormal findings were found during the examination, but the encounter is being coded before test results are back, it is acceptable to assign the code for "without abnormal findings." When assigning a code for "with abnormal findings," additional code(s) should be assigned to identify the specific abnormal finding(s).

Pre-operative examination and pre-procedural laboratory examination Z codes are for use only in those situations when a patient is being cleared for a procedure or surgery and no treatment is given.

The Z codes/categories for routine and administrative examinations:

Z00   Encounter for general examination without complaint, suspected or reported diagnosis

Z01   Encounter for other special examination without complaint, suspected or reported diagnosis

Z02   Encounter for administrative examination

     Except: Z02.9, Encounter for administrative examinations, unspecified

Z32.0-   Encounter for pregnancy test

14) Miscellaneous Z codes

The miscellaneous Z codes capture a number of other health care encounters that do not fall into one of the other categories.

Certain of these codes identify the reason for the encounter; others are for use as additional codes that provide useful information on circumstances that may affect a patient's care and treatment.

Prophylactic Organ Removal

For encounters specifically for prophylactic removal of an organ (such as prophylactic removal of breasts due to a genetic susceptibility to cancer or a family history of cancer), the principal or first-listed code should be a code from category Z40, Encounter for prophylactic surgery, followed by the appropriate codes to identify the associated risk factor (such as genetic susceptibility or family history).

If the patient has a malignancy of one site and is having prophylactic removal at another site to prevent either a new primary malignancy or metastatic disease, a code for the malignancy should also be assigned in addition to a code from subcategory Z40.0, Encounter for prophylactic surgery for risk factors related to malignant neoplasms. A Z40.0 code should not be assigned if the patient is having organ removal for treatment of a malignancy, such as the removal of the testes for the treatment of prostate cancer.

Miscellaneous Z codes/categories:

Z28   Immunization not carried out

    Except: Z28.3, Underimmunization status

Z29   Encounter for other prophylactic measures

Z40   Encounter for prophylactic surgery

Z41   Encounter for procedures for purposes other than remedying health state

    Except: Z41.9, Encounter for procedure for purposes other than remedying health state, unspecified

Z53   Persons encountering health services for specific procedures and treatment, not carried out

Z55   Problems related to education and literacy

Z56   Problems related to employment and unemployment

Z57   Occupational exposure to risk factors

Z58   Problems related to physical environment

Z59   Problems related to housing and economic circumstances

Z60   Problems related to social environment

Z62   Problems related to upbringing

Z63   Other problems related to primary support group, including family circumstances

Z64   Problems related to certain psychosocial circumstances

Z65   Problems related to other psychosocial circumstances

Z72   Problems related to lifestyle

    Note: These codes should be assigned only when the documentation specifies that the patient has an associated problem

Z73   Problems related to life management difficulty

Z74   Problems related to care provider dependency

    Except: Z74.01, Bed confinement status

Z75   Problems related to medical facilities and other health care

Z76.0   Encounter for issue of repeat prescription

Z76.3   Healthy person accompanying sick person

Z76.4   Other boarder to healthcare facility

Z76.5   Malingerer [conscious simulation]

Z91.1-   Patient's noncompliance with medical treatment and regimen

Z91.83   Wandering in diseases classified elsewhere

Z91.84-Oral health risk factors

Z91.89   Other specified personal risk factors, not elsewhere classified

15) Nonspecific Z codes

Certain Z codes are so non-specific, or potentially redundant with other codes in the classification, that there can be little justification for their use in the inpatient setting. Their use in the outpatient setting should be limited to those instances when there is no further documentation to permit more precise coding. Otherwise, any sign or symptom or any other reason for visit that is captured in another code should be used.

Nonspecific Z codes/categories:

Z02.9   Encounter for administrative examinations, unspecified

Z04.9   Encounter for examination and observation for unspecified reason

Z13.9   Encounter for screening, unspecified

Z41.9   Encounter for procedure for purposes other than remedying health state, unspecified

Z52.9   Donor of unspecified organ or tissue

Z86.59   Personal history of other mental and behavioral disorders

Z88.9   Allergy status to unspecified drugs, medicaments and biological substances status

Z92.0   Personal history of contraception

16) Z Codes That May Only be Principal/First-Listed Diagnosis

The following Z codes/categories may only be reported as the principal/first-listed diagnosis, except when there are multiple encounters on the same day and the medical records for the encounters are combined:

Z00   Encounter for general examination without complaint, suspected or reported diagnosis

    Except: Z00.6

Z01   Encounter for other special examination without complaint, suspected or reported diagnosis

Z02   Encounter for administrative examination

Z03   Encounter for medical observation for suspected diseases and conditions ruled out

Z04   Encounter for examination and observation for other reasons

Z33.2   Encounter for elective termination of pregnancy

Z31.81   Encounter for male factor infertility in female patient

Z31.83   Encounter for assisted reproductive fertility procedure cycle

Z31.84   Encounter for fertility preservation procedure

Z34   Encounter for supervision of normal pregnancy

Z39   Encounter for maternal postpartum care and examination

Z38   Liveborn infants according to place of birth and type of delivery

Z40   Encounter for prophylactic surgery

Z42   Encounter for plastic and reconstructive surgery following medical procedure or healed injury

Z51.0   Encounter for antineoplastic radiation therapy

Z51.1-   Encounter for antineoplastic chemotherapy and immunotherapy

Z52   Donors of organs and tissues

    Except: Z52.9, Donor of unspecified organ or tissue

Z76.1   Encounter for health supervision and care of foundling

Z76.2   Encounter for health supervision and care of other healthy infant and child

Z99.12   Encounter for respirator [ventilator] dependence during power failure

Section II. Selection of Principal Diagnosis

The circumstances of inpatient admission always govern the selection of principal diagnosis. The principal diagnosis is defined in the Uniform Hospital Discharge Data Set (UHDDS) as "that condition established after study to be chiefly responsible for occasioning the admission of the patient to the hospital for care."

The UHDDS definitions are used by hospitals to report inpatient data elements in a standardized manner. These data elements and their definitions can be found in the July 31, 1985, Federal Register (Vol. 50, No, 147), pp. 31038-40.

Since that time the application of the UHDDS definitions has been expanded to include all non-outpatient settings (acute care, short term, long term care and psychiatric hospitals; home health agencies; rehab facilities; nursing homes, etc). The UHDDS definitions also apply to hospice services (all levels of care).

In determining principal diagnosis, coding conventions in the ICD-10-CM, the Tabular List and Alphabetic Index take precedence over these official coding guidelines.

(See Section I.A., Conventions for the ICD-10-CM)

The importance of consistent, complete documentation in the medical record cannot be overemphasized. Without such documentation the application of all coding guidelines is a difficult, if not impossible, task.

A. Codes for symptoms, signs, and ill-defined conditions
Codes for symptoms, signs, and ill-defined conditions from Chapter 18 are not to be used as principal diagnosis when a related definitive diagnosis has been established.

B. Two or more interrelated conditions, each potentially meeting the definition for principal diagnosis.
When there are two or more interrelated conditions (such as diseases in the same ICD-10-CM chapter or manifestations characteristically associated with a certain disease) potentially meeting the definition of principal diagnosis, either condition may be sequenced first, unless the circumstances of the admission, the therapy provided, the Tabular List, or the Alphabetic Index indicate otherwise.

C. Two or more diagnoses that equally meet the definition for principal diagnosis
In the unusual instance when two or more diagnoses equally meet the criteria for principal diagnosis as determined by the circumstances of admission, diagnostic workup and/or therapy provided, and the Alphabetic Index, Tabular List, or another coding guidelines does not provide sequencing direction, any one of the diagnoses may be sequenced first.

D. Two or more comparative or contrasting conditions
In those rare instances when two or more contrasting or comparative diagnoses are documented as "either/or" (or similar terminology), they are coded as if the diagnoses were confirmed and the diagnoses are sequenced according to the circumstances of the admission. If no further determination can be made as to which diagnosis should be principal, either diagnosis may be sequenced first.

E. A symptom(s) followed by contrasting/comparative diagnoses
GUIDELINE HAS BEEN DELETED EFFECTIVE OCTOBER 1, 2014

F. Original treatment plan not carried out
Sequence as the principal diagnosis the condition, which after study occasioned the admission to the hospital, even though treatment may not have been carried out due to unforeseen circumstances.

G. Complications of surgery and other medical care
When the admission is for treatment of a complication resulting from surgery or other medical care, the complication code is sequenced as the principal diagnosis. If the complication is classified to the T80-T88 series and the code lacks the necessary specificity in describing the complication, an additional code for the specific complication should be assigned.

H. Uncertain Diagnosis
If the diagnosis documented at the time of discharge is qualified as "probable", "suspected", "likely", "questionable", "possible", or "still to be ruled out", or other similar terms indicating uncertainty, code the condition as if it existed or was established. The bases for these guidelines are the diagnostic workup, arrangements for further workup or observation, and initial therapeutic approach that correspond most closely with the established diagnosis.

Note: This guideline is applicable only to inpatient admissions to short-term, acute, long-term care and psychiatric hospitals.

I. Admission from Observation Unit
1. Admission Following Medical Observation
When a patient is admitted to an observation unit for a medical condition, which either worsens or does not improve, and is subsequently admitted as an inpatient of the same hospital for this same medical condition, the principal diagnosis would be the medical condition which led to the hospital admission.

2. Admission Following Post-Operative Observation
When a patient is admitted to an observation unit to monitor a condition (or complication) that develops following outpatient surgery, and then is subsequently admitted as an inpatient of the same hospital, hospitals should apply the Uniform Hospital Discharge Data Set (UHDDS) definition of principal diagnosis as "that condition established after study to be chiefly responsible for occasioning the admission of the patient to the hospital for care."

J. Admission from Outpatient Surgery
When a patient receives surgery in the hospital's outpatient surgery department and is subsequently admitted for continuing inpatient care at the same hospital, the following guidelines should be followed in selecting the principal diagnosis for the inpatient admission:
- If the reason for the inpatient admission is a complication, assign the complication as the principal diagnosis.
- If no complication, or other condition, is documented as the reason for the inpatient admission, assign the reason for the outpatient surgery as the principal diagnosis.
- If the reason for the inpatient admission is another condition unrelated to the surgery, assign the unrelated condition as the principal diagnosis.

K. Admissions/Encounters for Rehabilitation
When the purpose for the admission/encounter is rehabilitation, sequence first the code for the condition for which the service is being performed. For example, for an admission/encounter for rehabilitation for right-sided dominant hemiplegia following a cerebrovascular infarction, report code I69.351, Hemiplegia and hemiparesis following cerebral infarction affecting right dominant side, as the first-listed or principal diagnosis.

If the condition for which the rehabilitation service is no longer present, report the appropriate aftercare code **as the first-listed or principal diagnosis, unless the rehabilitation service is being provided following an injury. For rehabilitation services following active treatment of an injury, assign the injury code with the appropriate seventh character for subsequent encounter** as the first-listed or principal diagnosis. For example, if a patient with severe degenerative osteoarthritis of the hip, underwent hip replacement and the current encounter/admission is for rehabilitation, report code Z47.1, Aftercare following joint replacement surgery, as the first-listed or principal diagnosis. **If the patient requires rehabilitation post hip replacement for right intertrochanteric femur fracture, report code S72.141D, Displaced intertrochanteric fracture of right femur, subsequent encounter for closed fracture with routine healing, as the first-listed or principal diagnosis.**

See Section I.C.21.c.7, Factors influencing health states and contact with health services, Aftercare.

See Section I.C.19.a for additional information about the use of 7th characters for injury codes.

Section III. Reporting Additional Diagnoses
GENERAL RULES FOR OTHER (ADDITIONAL) DIAGNOSES

For reporting purposes the definition for "other diagnoses" is interpreted as additional conditions that affect patient care in terms of requiring:

> clinical evaluation; or
> therapeutic treatment; or
> diagnostic procedures; or
> extended length of hospital stay; or
> increased nursing care and/or monitoring.

The UHDDS item #11-b defines Other Diagnoses as "all conditions that coexist at the time of admission, that develop subsequently, or that affect the treatment received and/or the length of stay. Diagnoses that relate to an earlier episode which have no bearing on the current hospital stay are to be excluded." UHDDS definitions apply to inpatients in acute care, short-term, long term care and psychiatric hospital setting. The UHDDS definitions are used by acute care short-term hospitals to report inpatient data elements in a standardized manner. These data elements and their definitions can be found in the July 31, 1985, Federal Register (Vol. 50, No, 147), pp. 31038-40.

Since that time the application of the UHDDS definitions has been expanded to include all non-outpatient settings (acute care, short term, long term care and psychiatric hospitals; home health agencies; rehab facilities; nursing homes, etc). The UHDDS definitions also apply to hospice services (all levels of care).

The following guidelines are to be applied in designating "other diagnoses" when neither the Alphabetic Index nor the Tabular List in ICD-10-CM provide direction. The listing of the diagnoses in the patient record is the responsibility of the attending provider.

A. Previous conditions
If the provider has included a diagnosis in the final diagnostic statement, such as the discharge summary or the face sheet, it should ordinarily be coded. Some providers include in the diagnostic statement resolved conditions or diagnoses and status-post procedures from previous admission that have no bearing on the current stay. Such conditions are not to be reported and are coded only if required by hospital policy.

However, history codes (categories Z80-Z87) may be used as secondary codes if the historical condition or family history has an impact on current care or influences treatment.

B. Abnormal findings

Abnormal findings (laboratory, x-ray, pathologic, and other diagnostic results) are not coded and reported unless the provider indicates their clinical significance. If the findings are outside the normal range and the attending provider has ordered other tests to evaluate the condition or prescribed treatment, it is appropriate to ask the provider whether the abnormal finding should be added.

Please note: This differs from the coding practices in the outpatient setting for coding encounters for diagnostic tests that have been interpreted by a provider.

C. Uncertain Diagnosis

If the diagnosis documented at the time of discharge is qualified as "probable", "suspected", "likely", "questionable", "possible", or "still to be ruled out" or other similar terms indicating uncertainty, code the condition as if it existed or was established. The bases for these guidelines are the diagnostic workup, arrangements for further workup or observation, and initial therapeutic approach that correspond most closely with the established diagnosis.

Note: This guideline is applicable only to inpatient admissions to short-term, acute, long-term care and psychiatric hospitals.

Section IV.Diagnostic Coding and Reporting Guidelines for Outpatient Services

These coding guidelines for outpatient diagnoses have been approved for use by hospitals/ providers in coding and reporting hospital-based outpatient services and provider-based office visits. Guidelines in Section I, Conventions, general coding guidelines and chapter-specific guidelines, should also be applied for outpatient services and office visits.

Information about the use of certain abbreviations, punctuation, symbols, and other conventions used in the ICD-10-CM Tabular List (code numbers and titles), can be found in Section IA of these guidelines, under "Conventions Used in the Tabular List." Section I.B. contains general guidelines that apply to the entire classification. Section I.C. contains chapter-specific guidelines that correspond to the chapters as they are arranged in the classification. Information about the correct sequence to use in finding a code is also described in Section I.

The terms encounter and visit are often used interchangeably in describing outpatient service contacts and, therefore, appear together in these guidelines without distinguishing one from the other.

Though the conventions and general guidelines apply to all settings, coding guidelines for outpatient and provider reporting of diagnoses will vary in a number of instances from those for inpatient diagnoses, recognizing that:

The Uniform Hospital Discharge Data Set (UHDDS) definition of principal diagnosis does not apply to hospital-based outpatient services and provider-based office visits.

Coding guidelines for inconclusive diagnoses (probable, suspected, rule out, etc.) were developed for inpatient reporting and do not apply to outpatients.

A. Selection of first-listed condition

In the outpatient setting, the term first-listed diagnosis is used in lieu of principal diagnosis.

In determining the first-listed diagnosis the coding conventions of ICD-10-CM, as well as the general and disease specific guidelines take precedence over the outpatient guidelines.

Diagnoses often are not established at the time of the initial encounter/visit. It may take two or more visits before the diagnosis is confirmed.

The most critical rule involves beginning the search for the correct code assignment through the Alphabetic Index. Never begin searching initially in the Tabular List as this will lead to coding errors.

1. Outpatient Surgery

When a patient presents for outpatient surgery (same day surgery), code the reason for the surgery as the first-listed diagnosis (reason for the encounter), even if the surgery is not performed due to a contraindication.

2. Observation Stay

When a patient is admitted for observation for a medical condition, assign a code for the medical condition as the first-listed diagnosis.

When a patient presents for outpatient surgery and develops complications requiring admission to observation, code the reason for the surgery as the first reported diagnosis (reason for the encounter), followed by codes for the complications as secondary diagnoses.

B. Codes from A00.0 through T88.9, Z00-Z99

The appropriate code(s) from A00.0 through T88.9, Z00-Z99 must be used to identify diagnoses, symptoms, conditions, problems, complaints, or other reason(s) for the encounter/visit.

C. Accurate reporting of ICD-10-CM diagnosis codes

For accurate reporting of ICD-10-CM diagnosis codes, the documentation should describe the patient's condition, using terminology which includes specific diagnoses as well as symptoms, problems, or reasons for the encounter. There are ICD-10-CM codes to describe all of these.

D. Codes that describe symptoms and signs

Codes that describe symptoms and signs, as opposed to diagnoses, are acceptable for reporting purposes when a diagnosis has not been established (confirmed) by the provider. Chapter 18 of ICD-10-CM, Symptoms, Signs, and Abnormal Clinical and Laboratory Findings Not Elsewhere Classified (codes R00-R99) contain many, but not all codes for symptoms.

E. Encounters for circumstances other than a disease or injury

ICD-10-CM provides codes to deal with encounters for circumstances other than a disease or injury. The Factors Influencing Health Status and Contact with Health Services codes (Z00-Z99) are provided to deal with occasions when circumstances other than a disease or injury are recorded as diagnosis or problems.

See Section I.C.21. Factors influencing health status and contact with health services.

F. Level of Detail in Coding

1. ICD-10-CM codes with 3, 4, 5, 6 or 7 characters

ICD-10-CM is composed of codes with 3, 4, 5, 6 or 7 characters. Codes with three characters are included in ICD-10-CM as the heading of a category of codes that may be further subdivided by the use of fourth, fifth, sixth or seventh characters to provide greater specificity.

2. Use of full number of characters required for a code

A three-character code is to be used only if it is not further subdivided. A code is invalid if it has not been coded to the full number of characters required for that code, including the 7th character, if applicable.

G. ICD-10-CM code for the diagnosis, condition, problem, or other reason for encounter/visit

List first the ICD-10-CM code for the diagnosis, condition, problem, or other reason for encounter/visit shown in the medical record to be chiefly responsible for the services provided. List additional codes that describe any coexisting conditions. In some cases the first-listed diagnosis may be a symptom when a diagnosis has not been established (confirmed) by the physician.

H. Uncertain diagnosis

Do not code diagnoses documented as "probable", "suspected," "questionable," "rule out," or "working diagnosis" or other similar terms indicating uncertainty. Rather, code the condition(s) to the highest degree of certainty for that encounter/visit, such as symptoms, signs, abnormal test results, or other reason for the visit.

Please note: This differs from the coding practices used by short-term, acute care, long-term care and psychiatric hospitals.

I. Chronic diseases

Chronic diseases treated on an ongoing basis may be coded and reported as many times as the patient receives treatment and care for the condition(s)

J. Code all documented conditions that coexist

Code all documented conditions that coexist at the time of the encounter/visit, and require or affect patient care treatment or management. Do not code conditions that were previously treated and no longer exist. However, history codes (categories Z80-Z87) may be used as secondary codes if the historical condition or family history has an impact on current care or influences treatment.

K. Patients receiving diagnostic services only

For patients receiving diagnostic services only during an encounter/visit, sequence first the diagnosis, condition, problem, or other reason for encounter/visit shown in the medical record to be chiefly responsible for the outpatient services provided during the encounter/visit. Codes for other diagnoses (e.g., chronic conditions) may be sequenced as additional diagnoses.

For encounters for routine laboratory/radiology testing in the absence of any signs, symptoms, or associated diagnosis, assign Z01.89, Encounter for other specified special examinations. If routine testing is performed during the same encounter as a test to evaluate a sign, symptom, or diagnosis, it is appropriate to assign both the Z code and the code describing the reason for the non-routine test.

For outpatient encounters for diagnostic tests that have been interpreted by a physician, and the final report is available at the time of coding, code any confirmed or definitive diagnosis(es) documented in the interpretation. Do not code related signs and symptoms as additional diagnoses.

Please note: This differs from the coding practice in the hospital inpatient setting regarding abnormal findings on test results.

L. Patients receiving therapeutic services only

For patients receiving therapeutic services only during an encounter/visit, sequence first the diagnosis, condition, problem, or other reason for encounter/visit shown in the medical record to be chiefly responsible for the outpatient services provided during the encounter/visit. Codes for other diagnoses (e.g., chronic conditions) may be sequenced as additional diagnoses.

The only exception to this rule is that when the primary reason for the admission/encounter is chemotherapy or radiation therapy, the appropriate Z code for the service is listed first, and the diagnosis or problem for which the service is being performed listed second.

M. Patients receiving preoperative evaluations only

For patients receiving preoperative evaluations only, sequence first a code from subcategory Z01.81, Encounter for pre-procedural examinations, to describe the pre-op consultations. Assign a code for the condition to describe the reason for the surgery as an additional diagnosis. Code also any findings related to the pre-op evaluation.

N. Ambulatory surgery

For ambulatory surgery, code the diagnosis for which the surgery was performed. If the postoperative diagnosis is known to be different from the preoperative diagnosis at the time the diagnosis is confirmed, select the postoperative diagnosis for coding, since it is the most definitive.

O. Routine outpatient prenatal visits

See Section I.C.15. Routine outpatient prenatal visits.

P. Encounters for general medical examinations with abnormal findings

The subcategories for encounters for general medical examinations, **Z00.0- and encounter for routine child health examination, Z00.12-,** provide codes for with and without abnormal findings. Should a general medical examination result in an abnormal finding, the code for general medical examination with abnormal finding should be assigned as the first-listed diagnosis. An examination with abnormal findings refers to a condition/diagnosis that is newly identified or a change in severity of a chronic condition (such as uncontrolled hypertension, or an acute exacerbation of chronic obstructive pulmonary disease) during a routine physical examination. A secondary code for the abnormal finding should also be coded.

Q. Encounters for routine health screenings

See Section I.C.21. Factors influencing health status and contact with health services, Screening

Appendix I. Present on Admission Reporting Guidelines

Introduction

These guidelines are to be used as a supplement to the *ICD-10-CM Official Guidelines for Coding and Reporting* to facilitate the assignment of the Present on Admission (POA) indicator for each diagnosis and external cause of injury code reported on claim forms (UB-04 and 837 Institutional).

These guidelines are not intended to replace any guidelines in the main body of the *ICD-10-CM Official Guidelines for Coding and Reporting*. The POA guidelines are not intended to provide guidance on when a condition should be coded, but rather, how to apply the POA indicator to the final set of diagnosis codes that have been assigned in accordance with Sections I, II, and III of the official coding guidelines. Subsequent to the assignment of the ICD-10-CM codes, the POA indicator should then be assigned to those conditions that have been coded.

As stated in the Introduction to the ICD-10-CM Official Guidelines for Coding and Reporting, a joint effort between the healthcare provider and the coder is essential to achieve complete and accurate documentation, code assignment, and reporting of diagnoses and procedures. The importance of consistent, complete documentation in the medical record cannot be overemphasized. Medical record documentation from any provider involved in the care and treatment of the patient may be used to support the determination of whether a condition was present on admission or not. In the context of the official coding guidelines, the term "provider" means a physician or any qualified healthcare practitioner who is legally accountable for establishing the patient's diagnosis.

These guidelines are not a substitute for the provider's clinical judgment as to the determination of whether a condition was/was not present on admission. The provider should be queried regarding issues related to the linking of signs/symptoms, timing of test results, and the timing of findings.

Please see the CDC website for the detailed list of ICD-10-CM codes that do not require the use of a POA indicator (https://www.cdc.gov/nchs/icd/icd10cm.htm) (https://www.cms.gov/Medicare/Coding/ICD10/2018-ICD-10-CM-and-GEMs. html). The **codes and categories** on this exempt list **are** for circumstances regarding the healthcare encounter or factors influencing health status that do not represent a current disease or injury or **that describe conditions that** are always present on admission.

General Reporting Requirements

All claims involving inpatient admissions to general acute care hospitals or other facilities that are subject to a law or regulation mandating collection of present on admission information.

Present on admission is defined as present at the time the order for inpatient admission occurs -- conditions that develop during an outpatient encounter, including emergency department, observation, or outpatient surgery, are considered as present on admission.

POA indicator is assigned to principal and secondary diagnoses (as defined in Section II of the Official Guidelines for Coding and Reporting) and the external cause of injury codes.

Issues related to inconsistent, missing, conflicting or unclear documentation must still be resolved by the provider.

If a condition would not be coded and reported based on UHDDS definitions and current official coding guidelines, then the POA indicator would not be reported.

Reporting Options

    Y - Yes

    N - No

    U - Unknown

    W – Clinically undetermined

Unreported/Not used – (Exempt from POA reporting)

Reporting Definitions

    Y = present at the time of inpatient admission

    N = not present at the time of inpatient admission

    U = documentation is insufficient to determine if condition is present on admission

    W = provider is unable to clinically determine whether condition was present on admission or not

Timeframe for POA Identification and Documentation

There is no required timeframe as to when a provider (per the definition of "provider" used in these guidelines) must identify or document a condition to be present on admission. In some clinical situations, it may not be possible for a provider to make a definitive diagnosis (or a condition may not be recognized or reported by the patient) for a period of time after admission. In some cases it may be several days before the provider arrives at a definitive diagnosis. This does not mean that the condition was not present on admission. Determination of whether the condition was present on admission or not will be based on the applicable POA guideline as identified in this document, or on the provider's best clinical judgment.

If at the time of code assignment the documentation is unclear as to whether a condition was present on admission or not, it is appropriate to query the provider for clarification.

Assigning the POA Indicator

Condition is on the "Exempt from Reporting" list

Leave the "present on admission" field blank if the condition is on the list of ICD-10-CM codes for which this field is not applicable. This is the only circumstance in which the field may be left blank.

POA Explicitly Documented

Assign Y for any condition the provider explicitly documents as being present on admission.

Assign N for any condition the provider explicitly documents as not present at the time of admission.

Conditions diagnosed prior to inpatient admission

Assign "Y" for conditions that were diagnosed prior to admission (example: hypertension, diabetes mellitus, asthma)

Conditions diagnosed during the admission but clearly present before admission

Assign "Y" for conditions diagnosed during the admission that were clearly present but not diagnosed until after admission occurred.

Diagnoses subsequently confirmed after admission are considered present on admission if at the time of admission they are documented as suspected, possible, rule out, differential diagnosis, or constitute an underlying cause of a symptom that is present at the time of admission.

Condition develops during outpatient encounter prior to inpatient admission

Assign Y for any condition that develops during an outpatient encounter prior to a written order for inpatient admission.

Documentation does not indicate whether condition was present on admission

Assign "U" when the medical record documentation is unclear as to whether the condition was present on admission. "U" should not be routinely assigned and used only in very limited circumstances. Coders are encouraged to query the providers when the documentation is unclear.

Documentation states that it cannot be determined whether the condition was or was not present on admission

Assign "W" when the medical record documentation indicates that it cannot be clinically determined whether or not the condition was present on admission.

Chronic condition with acute exacerbation during the admission

If a single code identifies both the chronic condition and the acute exacerbation, see POA guidelines pertaining to codes that contain multiple clinical concepts.

If a single code only identifies the chronic condition and not the acute exacerbation (e.g., acute exacerbation of chronic leukemia), assign "Y."

Conditions documented as possible, probable, suspected, or rule out at the time of discharge

If the final diagnosis contains a possible, probable, suspected, or rule out diagnosis, and this diagnosis was based on signs, symptoms or clinical findings suspected at the time of inpatient admission, assign "Y."

If the final diagnosis contains a possible, probable, suspected, or rule out diagnosis, and this diagnosis was based on signs, symptoms or clinical findings that were not present on admission, assign "N".

Conditions documented as impending or threatened at the time of discharge

If the final diagnosis contains an impending or threatened diagnosis, and this diagnosis is based on symptoms or clinical findings that were present on admission, assign "Y".

If the final diagnosis contains an impending or threatened diagnosis, and this diagnosis is based on symptoms or clinical findings that were not present on admission, assign "N".

Acute and Chronic Conditions

Assign "Y" for acute conditions that are present at time of admission and N for acute conditions that are not present at time of admission.

Assign "Y" for chronic conditions, even though the condition may not be diagnosed until after admission.

If a single code identifies both an acute and chronic condition, see the POA guidelines for codes that contain multiple clinical concepts.

Codes That Contain Multiple Clinical Concepts

Assign "N" if at least one of the clinical concepts included in the code was not present on admission (e.g., COPD with acute exacerbation and the exacerbation was not present on admission; gastric ulcer that does not start bleeding until after admission; asthma patient develops status asthmaticus after admission).

Assign "Y" if all of the clinical concepts included in the code were present on admission (e.g., duodenal ulcer that perforates prior to admission).

For infection codes that include the causal organism, assign "Y" if the infection (or signs of the infection) were present on admission, even though the culture results may not be known until after admission (e.g., patient is admitted with pneumonia and the provider documents Pseudomonas as the causal organism a few days later).

Same Diagnosis Code for Two or More Conditions

When the same ICD-10-CM diagnosis code applies to two or more conditions during the same encounter (e.g. two separate conditions classified to the same ICD-10-CM diagnosis code):

Assign "Y" if all conditions represented by the single ICD-10-CM code were present on admission (e.g. bilateral unspecified age-related cataracts).

Assign "N" if any of the conditions represented by the single ICD-10-CM code was not present on admission (e.g. traumatic secondary and recurrent hemorrhage and seroma is assigned to a single code T79.2, but only one of the conditions was present on admission).

Obstetrical conditions

Whether or not the patient delivers during the current hospitalization does not affect assignment of the POA indicator. The determining factor for POA assignment is whether the pregnancy complication or obstetrical condition described by the code was present at the time of admission or not.

If the pregnancy complication or obstetrical condition was present on admission (e.g., patient admitted in preterm labor), assign "Y".

If the pregnancy complication or obstetrical condition was not present on admission (e.g., 2nd degree laceration during delivery, postpartum hemorrhage that occurred during current hospitalization, fetal distress develops after admission), assign "N".

If the obstetrical code includes more than one diagnosis and any of the diagnoses identified by the code were not present on admission assign "N". (e.g., Category O11, Pre-existing hypertension with pre-eclampsia)

Perinatal conditions

Newborns are not considered to be admitted until after birth. Therefore, any condition present at birth or that developed in utero is considered present at admission and should be assigned "Y". This includes conditions that occur during delivery (e.g., injury during delivery, meconium aspiration, exposure to streptococcus B in the vaginal canal).

Congenital conditions and anomalies

Assign "Y" for congenital conditions and anomalies except for categories Q00-Q99, Congenital anomalies, which are on the exempt list. Congenital conditions are always considered present on admission.

External cause of injury codes

Assign "Y" for any external cause code representing an external cause of morbidity that occurred prior to inpatient admission (e.g., patient fell out of bed at home, patient fell out of bed in emergency room prior to admission)

Assign "N" for any external cause code representing an external cause of morbidity that occurred during inpatient hospitalization (e.g., patient fell out of hospital bed during hospital stay, patient experienced an adverse reaction to a medication administered after inpatient admission)

ICD-10-CM Index to Diseases and Injuries

A

Aarskog's syndrome Q87.1
Abandonment — *see* Maltreatment
Abasia (-astasia) (hysterical) F44.4
Abderhalden-Kaufmann-Lignac syndrome (cystinosis) E72.04
Abdomen, abdominal (*see also* condition)
  acute R10.0
  angina K55.1
  muscle deficiency syndrome Q79.4
Abdominalgia — *see* Pain, abdominal
Abduction contracture, hip or other joint — *see* Contraction, joint
Aberrant (congenital) (*see also* Malposition, congenital)
  adrenal gland Q89.1
  artery (peripheral) Q27.8
    basilar NEC Q28.1
    cerebral Q28.3
    coronary Q24.5
    digestive system Q27.8
    eye Q15.8
    lower limb Q27.8
    precerebral Q28.1
    pulmonary Q25.79
    renal Q27.2
    retina Q14.1
    specified site NEC Q27.8
    subclavian Q27.8
    upper limb Q27.8
    vertebral Q28.1
  breast Q83.8
  endocrine gland NEC Q89.2
  hepatic duct Q44.5
  pancreas Q45.3
  parathyroid gland Q89.2
  pituitary gland Q89.2
  sebaceous glands, mucous membrane, mouth, congenital Q38.6
  spleen Q89.09
  subclavian artery Q27.8
  thymus (gland) Q89.2
  thyroid gland Q89.2
  vein (peripheral) NEC Q27.8
    cerebral Q28.3
    digestive system Q27.8
    lower limb Q27.8
    precerebral Q28.1
    specified site NEC Q27.8
    upper limb Q27.8
Aberration
  distantial — *see* Disturbance, visual
  mental F99
Abetalipoproteinemia E78.6
Abiotrophy R68.89
Ablatio, ablation
  retinae — *see* Detachment, retina
Ablepharia, ablepharon Q10.3
Abnormal, abnormality, abnormalities (*see also* Anomaly)
  acid-base balance (mixed) E87.4
  albumin R77.0
  alphafetoprotein R77.2
  alveolar ridge K08.9
  anatomical relationship Q89.9
  apertures, congenital, diaphragm Q79.1
  auditory perception H93.29- ☑
    diplacusis — *see* Diplacusis
    hyperacusis — *see* Hyperacusis
    recruitment — *see* Recruitment, auditory
    threshold shift — *see* Shift, auditory threshold
  autosomes Q99.9
    fragile site Q95.5
  basal metabolic rate R94.8
  biosynthesis, testicular androgen E29.1
  bleeding time R79.1
  blood level (of)
    cobalt R79.0
    copper R79.0
    iron R79.0
    lithium R78.89
    magnesium R79.0

Abnormal, abnormality, abnormalities — *continued*
  blood level — *continued*
    mineral NEC R79.0
    zinc R79.0
  blood pressure
    elevated R03.0
    low reading (nonspecific) R03.1
  blood sugar R73.09
  blood-gas level R79.81
  bowel sounds R19.15
    absent R19.11
    hyperactive R19.12
  brain scan R94.02
  breathing R06.9
  caloric test R94.138
  cerebrospinal fluid R83.9
    cytology R83.6
    drug level R83.2
    enzyme level R83.0
    hormones R83.1
    immunology R83.4
    microbiology R83.5
    nonmedicinal level R83.3
    specified type NEC R83.8
  chemistry, blood R79.9
    C-reactive protein R79.82
    drugs — *see* Findings, abnormal, in blood
    gas level R79.81
    minerals R79.0
    pancytopenia D61.818
    PTT R79.1
    specified NEC R79.89
    toxins — *see* Findings, abnormal, in blood
  chest sounds (friction) (rales) R09.89
  chromosome, chromosomal Q99.9
    with more than three X chromosomes, female Q97.1
    analysis result R89.8
      bronchial washings R84.8
      cerebrospinal fluid R83.8
      cervix uteri NEC R87.89
      nasal secretions R84.8
      nipple discharge R89.9
      peritoneal fluid R85.89
      pleural fluid R84.8
      prostatic secretions R86.8
      saliva R85.89
      seminal fluid R86.8
      sputum R84.8
      synovial fluid R89.8
      throat scrapings R84.8
      vagina R87.89
      vulva R87.89
      wound secretions R89.8
    dicentric replacement Q93.2
    ring replacement Q93.2
    sex Q99.8
      female phenotype Q97.9
        specified NEC Q97.8
      male phenotype Q98.9
        specified NEC Q98.8
      structural male Q98.6
    specified NEC Q99.8
  clinical findings NEC R68.89
  coagulation D68.9
    newborn, transient P61.6
    profile R79.1
    time R79.1
  communication — *see* Fistula
  conjunctiva, vascular H11.41- ☑
  coronary artery Q24.5
  cortisol-binding globulin E27.8
  course, eustachian tube Q17.8
  creatinine clearance R94.4
  cytology
    anus R85.619
      atypical squamous cells cannot exclude high grade squamous intraepithelial lesion (ASC-H) R85.611
      atypical squamous cells of undetermined significance (ASC-US) R85.610
      cytologic evidence of malignancy R85.614

Abnormal, abnormality, abnormalities — *continued*
  cytology — *continued*
    anus — *continued*
      high grade squamous intraepithelial lesion (HGSIL) R85.613
      human papillomavirus (HPV) DNA test
        high risk positive R85.81
        low risk postive R85.82
      inadequate smear R85.615
      low grade squamous intraepithelial lesion (LGSIL) R85.612
      satisfactory anal smear but lacking transformation zone R85.616
      specified NEC R85.618
      unsatisfactory smear R85.615
    female genital organs — *see* Abnormal, Papanicolaou (smear)
  dark adaptation curve H53.61
  dentofacial NEC — *see* Anomaly, dentofacial
  development, developmental Q89.9
    central nervous system Q07.9
  diagnostic imaging
    abdomen, abdominal region NEC R93.5
    biliary tract R93.2
    bladder R93.41
    breast R92.8
    central nervous system NEC R90.89
    cerebrovascular NEC R90.89
    coronary circulation R93.1
    digestive tract NEC R93.3
    gastrointestinal (tract) R93.3
    genitourinary organs R93.8
    head R93.0
    heart R93.1
    intrathoracic organ NEC R93.8
    kidney R93.42- ☑
    limbs R93.6
    liver R93.2
    lung (field) R91.8
    musculoskeletal system NEC R93.7
    renal pelvis R93.41
    retroperitoneum R93.5
    site specified NEC R93.8
    skin and subcutaneous tissue R93.8
    skull R93.0
    ureter R93.41
    urinary organs specified NEC R93.49
  direction, teeth, fully erupted M26.30
  ear ossicles, acquired NEC H74.39- ☑
    ankylosis — *see* Ankylosis, ear ossicles
    discontinuity — *see* Discontinuity, ossicles, ear
    partial loss — *see* Loss, ossicles, ear (partial)
  Ebstein Q22.5
  echocardiogram R93.1
  echoencephalogram R90.81
  echogram — *see* Abnormal, diagnostic imaging
  electrocardiogram [ECG] [EKG] R94.31
  electroencephalogram [EEG] R94.01
  electrolyte — *see* Imbalance, electrolyte
  electromyogram [EMG] R94.131
  electro-oculogram [EOG] R94.110
  electrophysiological intracardiac studies R94.39
  electroretinogram [ERG] R94.111
  erythrocytes
    congenital, with perinatal jaundice D58.9
  feces (color) (contents) (mucus) R19.5
  finding — *see* Findings, abnormal, without diagnosis
  fluid
    amniotic — *see* Abnormal, specimen, specified
    cerebrospinal — *see* Abnormal, cerebrospinal fluid
    peritoneal — *see* Abnormal, specimen, digestive organs
    pleural — *see* Abnormal, specimen, respiratory organs
    synovial — *see* Abnormal, specimen, specified
    thorax (bronchial washings) (pleural fluid) — *see* Abnormal, specimen, respiratory organs
    vaginal — *see* Abnormal, specimen, female genital organs
  form
    teeth K00.2
    uterus — *see* Anomaly, uterus

Abnormal, abnormality, abnormalities — *continued*
 function studies
  auditory R94.120
  bladder R94.8
  brain R94.09
  cardiovascular R94.30
  ear R94.128
  endocrine NEC R94.7
  eye NEC R94.118
  kidney R94.4
  liver R94.5
  nervous system
   central NEC R94.09
   peripheral NEC R94.138
  pancreas R94.8
  placenta R94.8
  pulmonary R94.2
  special senses NEC R94.128
  spleen R94.8
  thyroid R94.6
  vestibular R94.121
 gait — *see* Gait
  hysterical F44.4
 gastrin secretion E16.4
 globulin R77.1
  cortisol-binding E27.8
  thyroid-binding E07.89
 glomerular, minor (*see also* N00-N07 with fourth
   character .0) N05.0
 glucagon secretion E16.3
 glucose tolerance (test) (non-fasting) R73.09
 gravitational (G) forces or states (effect of) T75.81 ☑
 hair (color) (shaft) L67.9
  specified NEC L67.8
 hard tissue formation in pulp (dental) K04.3
 head movement R25.0
 heart
  rate R00.9
   specified NEC R00.8
  shadow R93.1
  sounds NEC R01.2
 hemoglobin (disease) (*see also* Disease, hemoglobin)
   D58.2
  trait — *see* Trait, hemoglobin, abnormal
 histology NEC R89.7
 immunological findings R89.4
  in serum R76.9
   specified NEC R76.8
 increase in appetite R63.2
 involuntary movement — *see* Abnormal, movement,
   involuntary
 jaw closure M26.51
 karyotype R89.8
 kidney function test R94.4
 knee jerk R29.2
 leukocyte (cell) (differential) NEC D72.9
 liver function test R94.5
 loss of
  height R29.890
  weight R63.4
 mammogram NEC R92.8
  calcification (calculus) R92.1
  microcalcification R92.0
 Mantoux test R76.11
 movement (disorder) (*see also* Disorder, movement)
  head R25.0
  involuntary R25.9
   fasciculation R25.3
   of head R25.0
   spasm R25.2
   specified type NEC R25.8
   tremor R25.1
 myoglobin (Aberdeen) (Annapolis) R89.7
 neonatal screening P09
 oculomotor study R94.113
 palmar creases Q82.8
 Papanicolaou (smear)
  anus R85.619
   atypical squamous cells cannot exclude high
     grade squamous intraepithelial lesion
     (ASC-H) R85.611
   atypical squamous cells of undetermined signif-
     icance (ASC-US) R85.610
   cytologic evidence of malignancy R85.614
   high grade squamous intraepithelial lesion
     (HGSIL) R85.613
   human papillomavirus (HPV) DNA test
    high risk positive R85.81

Abnormal, abnormality, abnormalities — *continued*
 Papanicolaou — *continued*
  anus — *continued*
   human papillomavirus DNA test — *contin-
     ued*
    low risk positive R85.82
   inadequate smear R85.615
   low grade squamous intraepithelial lesion
     (LGSIL) R85.612
   satisfactory anal smear but lacking transforma-
     tion zone R85.616
   specified NEC R85.618
   unsatisfactory smear R85.615
  bronchial washings R84.6
  cerebrospinal fluid R83.6
  cervix R87.619
   atypical squamous cells cannot exclude high
     grade squamous intraepithelial lesion
     (ASC-H) R87.611
   atypical squamous cells of undetermined signif-
     icance (ASC-US) R87.610
   cytologic evidence of malignancy R87.614
   high grade squamous intraepithelial lesion
     (HGSIL) R87.613
   inadequate smear R87.615
   low grade squamous intraepithelial lesion
     (LGSIL) R87.612
   non-atypical endometrial cells R87.618
   satisfactory cervical smear but lacking transfor-
     mation zone R87.616
   specified NEC R87.618
   thin preparaton R87.619
   unsatisfactory smear R87.615
  nasal secretions R84.6
  nipple discharge R89.6
  peritoneal fluid R85.69
  pleural fluid R84.6
  prostatic secretions R86.6
  saliva R85.69
  seminal fluid R86.6
  sites NEC R89.6
  sputum R84.6
  synovial fluid R89.6
  throat scrapings R84.6
  vagina R87.629
   atypical squamous cells cannot exclude high
     grade squamous intraepithelial lesion
     (ASC-H) R87.621
   atypical squamous cells of undetermined signif-
     icance (ASC-US) R87.620
   cytologic evidence of malignancy R87.624
   high grade squamous intraepithelial lesion
     (HGSIL) R87.623
   inadequate smear R87.625
   low grade squamous intraepithelial lesion
     (LGSIL) R87.622
   specified NEC R87.628
   thin preparation R87.629
   unsatisfactory smear R87.625
  vulva R87.69
  wound secretions R89.6
 partial thromboplastin time (PTT) R79.1
 pelvis (bony) — *see* Deformity, pelvis
 percussion, chest (tympany) R09.89
 periods (grossly) — *see* Menstruation
 phonocardiogram R94.39
 plantar reflex R29.2
 plasma
  protein R77.9
   specified NEC R77.8
  viscosity R70.1
 pleural (folds) Q34.0
 posture R29.3
 product of conception O02.9
  specified type NEC O02.89
 prothrombin time (PT) R79.1
 pulmonary
  artery, congenital Q25.79
  function, newborn P28.89
  test results R94.2
 pulsations in neck R00.2
 pupillary H21.56- ☑
  function (reaction) (reflex) — *see* Anomaly, pupil,
    function
 radiological examination — *see* Abnormal, diagnostic
   imaging
 red blood cell(s) (morphology) (volume) R71.8
 reflex — *see* Reflex

Abnormal, abnormality, abnormalities — *continued*
 renal function test R94.4
 response to nerve stimulation R94.130
 retinal correspondence H53.31
 retinal function study R94.111
 rhythm, heart (*see also* Arrhythmia)
 saliva — *see* Abnormal, specimen, digestive organs
 scan
  kidney R94.4
  liver R93.2
  thyroid R94.6
 secretion
  gastrin E16.4
  glucagon E16.3
 semen, seminal fluid — *see* Abnormal, specimen, male
   genital organs
 serum level (of)
  acid phosphatase R74.8
  alkaline phosphatase R74.8
  amylase R74.8
  enzymes R74.9
   specified NEC R74.8
  lipase R74.8
  triacylglycerol lipase R74.8
 shape
  gravid uterus — *see* Anomaly, uterus
 sinus venosus Q21.1
 size, tooth, teeth K00.2
 spacing, tooth, teeth, fully erupted M26.30
 specimen
  digestive organs (peritoneal fluid) (saliva) R85.9
   cytology R85.69
   drug level R85.2
   enzyme level R85.0
   histology R85.7
   hormones R85.1
   immunology R85.4
   microbiology R85.5
   nonmedicinal level R85.3
   specified type NEC R85.89
  female genital organs (secretions) (smears) R87.9
   cytology R87.69
    cervix R87.619
     human papillomavirus (HPV) DNA test
      high risk positive R87.810
      low risk positive R87.820
     inadequate (unsatisfactory) smear
       R87.615
     non-atypical endometrial cells R87.618
     specified NEC R87.618
    vagina R87.629
     human papillomavirus (HPV) DNA test
      high risk positive R87.811
      low risk positive R87.821
     inadequate (unsatisfactory) smear
       R87.625
    vulva R87.69
   drug level R87.2
   enzyme level R87.0
   histological R87.7
   hormones R87.1
   immunology R87.4
   microbiology R87.5
   nonmedicinal level R87.3
   specified type NEC R87.89
  male genital organs (prostatic secretions) (semen)
    R86.9
   cytology R86.6
   drug level R86.2
   enzyme level R86.0
   histological R86.7
   hormones R86.1
   immunology R86.4
   microbiology R86.5
   nonmedicinal level R86.3
   specified type NEC R86.8
  nipple discharge — *see* Abnormal, specimen,
    specified
  respiratory organs (bronchial washings) (nasal se-
    cretions) (pleural fluid) (sputum) R84.9
   cytology R84.6
   drug level R84.2
   enzyme level R84.0
   histology R84.7
   hormones R84.1
   immunology R84.4
   microbiology R84.5
   nonmedicinal level R84.3

Abnormal, abnormality, abnormalities — *continued*
  specimen — *continued*
    respiratory organs — *continued*
      specified type NEC R84.8
    specified organ, system and tissue NOS R89.9
      cytology R89.6
      drug level R89.2
      enzyme level R89.0
      histology R89.7
      hormones R89.1
      immunology R89.4
      microbiology R89.5
      nonmedicinal level R89.3
      specified type NEC R89.8
    synovial fluid — *see* Abnormal, specimen, specified
    thorax (bronchial washings) (pleural fluids) — *see* Abnormal, specimen, respiratory organs
    vagina (secretion) (smear) R87.629
    vulva (secretion) (smear) R87.69
    wound secretion — *see* Abnormal, specimen, specified
  spermatozoa — *see* Abnormal, specimen, male genital organs
  sputum (amount) (color) (odor) R09.3
  stool (color) (contents) (mucus) R19.5
    bloody K92.1
    guaiac positive R19.5
  synchondrosis Q78.8
  thermography (*see also* Abnormal, diagnostic imaging) R93.8
  thyroid-binding globulin E07.89
  tooth, teeth (form) (size) K00.2
  toxicology (findings) R78.9
  transport protein E88.09
  tumor marker NEC R97.8
  ultrasound results — *see* Abnormal, diagnostic imaging
  umbilical cord complicating delivery O69.9 ☑
  urination NEC R39.198
  urine (constituents) R82.90
    bile R82.2
    cytological examination R82.8
    drugs R82.5
    fat R82.0
    glucose R81
    heavy metals R82.6
    hemoglobin R82.3
    histological examination R82.8
    ketones R82.4
    microbiological examination (culture) R82.79
    myoglobin R82.1
    positive culture R82.79
    protein — *see* Proteinuria
    specified substance NEC R82.99
      chromoabnormality NEC R82.91
    substances nonmedical R82.6
  uterine hemorrhage — *see* Hemorrhage, uterus
  vectorcardiogram R94.39
  visually evoked potential (VEP) R94.112
  white blood cells D72.9
    specified NEC D72.89
  X-ray examination — *see* Abnormal, diagnostic imaging
Abnormity (any organ or part) — *see* Anomaly
Abocclusion M26.29
  hemolytic disease (newborn) P55.1
  incompatibility reaction ABO — *see* Complication(s), transfusion, incompatibility reaction, ABO
Abolition, language R48.8
Aborter, habitual or recurrent — *see* Loss (of), pregnancy, recurrent
Abortion (complete) (spontaneous) O03.9
  with
    retained products of conception — *see* Abortion, incomplete
  attempted (elective) (failed) O07.4
    complicated by O07.30
      afibrinogenemia O07.1
      cardiac arrest O07.36
      chemical damage of pelvic organ(s) O07.34
      circulatory collapse O07.31
      cystitis O07.38
      defibrination syndrome O07.1
      electrolyte imbalance O07.33
      embolism (air) (amniotic fluid) (blood clot) (fat) (pulmonary) (septic) (soap) O07.2
      endometritis O07.0

Abortion — *continued*
  attempted — *continued*
    complicated by — *continued*
      genital tract and pelvic infection O07.0
      hemolysis O07.1
      hemorrhage (delayed) (excessive) O07.1
      infection
        genital tract or pelvic O07.0
        urinary tract tract O07.38
      intravascular coagulation O07.1
      laceration of pelvic organ(s) O07.34
      metabolic disorder O07.33
      oliguria O07.32
      oophoritis O07.0
      parametritis O07.0
      pelvic peritonitis O07.0
      perforation of pelvic organ(s) O07.34
      renal failure or shutdown O07.32
      salpingitis or salpingo-oophoritis O07.0
      sepsis O07.37
      shock O07.31
      specified condition NEC O07.39
      tubular necrosis (renal) O07.32
      uremia O07.32
      urinary tract infection O07.38
      venous complication NEC O07.35
        embolism (air) (amniotic fluid) (blood clot) (fat) (pulmonary) (septic) (soap) O07.2
  complicated (by) (following) O03.80
    afibrinogenemia O03.6
    cardiac arrest O03.86
    chemical damage of pelvic organ(s) O03.84
    circulatory collapse O03.81
    cystitis O03.88
    defibrination syndrome O03.6
    electrolyte imbalance O03.83
    embolism (air) (amniotic fluid) (blood clot) (fat) (pulmonary) (septic) (soap) O03.7
    endometritis O03.5
    genital tract and pelvic infection O03.5
    hemolysis O03.6
    hemorrhage (delayed) (excessive) O03.6
    infection
      genital tract or pelvic O03.5
      urinary tract O03.88
    intravascular coagulation O03.6
    laceration of pelvic organ(s) O03.84
    metabolic disorder O03.83
    oliguria O03.82
    oophoritis O03.5
    parametritis O03.5
    pelvic peritonitis O03.5
    perforation of pelvic organ(s) O03.84
    renal failure or shutdown O03.82
    salpingitis or salpingo-oophoritis O03.5
    sepsis O03.87
    shock O03.81
    specified condition NEC O03.89
    tubular necrosis (renal) O03.82
    uremia O03.82
    urinary tract infection O03.88
    venous complication NEC O03.85
      embolism (air) (amniotic fluid) (blood clot) (fat) (pulmonary) (septic) (soap) O03.7
  failed — *see* Abortion, attempted
  habitual or recurrent N96
    with current abortion — *see* categories O03-O04
    without current pregnancy N96
    care in current pregnancy O26.2- ☑
  incomplete (spontaneous) O03.4
    complicated (by) (following) O03.30
      afibrinogenemia O03.1
      cardiac arrest O03.36
      chemical damage of pelvic organ(s) O03.34
      circulatory collapse O03.31
      cystitis O03.38
      defibrination syndrome O03.1
      electrolyte imbalance O03.33
      embolism (air) (amniotic fluid) (blood clot) (fat) (pulmonary) (septic) (soap) O03.2
      endometritis O03.0
      genital tract and pelvic infection O03.0
      hemolysis O03.1
      hemorrhage (delayed) (excessive) O03.1
      infection
        genital tract or pelvic O03.0
        urinary tract O03.38
      intravascular coagulation O03.1
      laceration of pelvic organ(s) O03.34

Abortion — *continued*
  incomplete — *continued*
    complicated — *continued*
      metabolic disorder O03.33
      oliguria O03.32
      oophoritis O03.0
      parametritis O03.0
      pelvic peritonitis O03.0
      perforation of pelvic organ(s) O03.34
      renal failure or shutdown O03.32
      salpingitis or salpingo-oophoritis O03.0
      sepsis O03.37
      shock O03.31
      specified condition NEC O03.39
      tubular necrosis (renal) O03.32
      uremia O03.32
      urinary infection O03.38
      venous complication NEC O03.35
        embolism (air) (amniotic fluid) (blood clot) (fat) (pulmonary) (septic) (soap) O03.2
  induced (encounter for) Z33.2
    complicated by O04.80
      afibrinogenemia O04.6
      cardiac arrest O04.86
      chemical damage of pelvic organ(s) O04.84
      circulatory collapse O04.81
      cystitis O04.88
      defibrination syndrome O04.6
      electrolyte imbalance O04.83
      embolism (air) (amniotic fluid) (blood clot) (fat) (pulmonary) (septic) (soap) O04.7
      endometritis O04.5
      genital tract and pelvic infection O04.5
      hemolysis O04.6
      hemorrhage (delayed) (excessive) O04.6
      infection
        genital tract or pelvic O04.5
        urinary tract O04.88
      intravascular coagulation O04.6
      laceration of pelvic organ(s) O04.84
      metabolic disorder O04.83
      oliguria O04.82
      oophoritis O04.5
      parametritis O04.5
      pelvic peritonitis O04.5
      perforation of pelvic organ(s) O04.84
      renal failure or shutdown O04.82
      salpingitis or salpingo-oophoritis O04.5
      sepsis O04.87
      shock O04.81
      specified condition NEC O04.89
      tubular necrosis (renal) O04.82
      uremia O04.82
      urinary tract infection O04.88
      venous complication NEC O04.85
        embolism (air) (amniotic fluid) (blood clot) (fat) (pulmonary) (septic) (soap) O04.7
  missed O02.1
  spontaneous — *see* Abortion (complete) (spontaneous)
    threatened O20.0
  threatened (spontaneous) O20.0
  tubal O00.10- ☑
    with intrauterine pregnancy O00.11- ☑
Abortus fever A23.1
Aboulomania F60.7
Abrami's disease D59.8
Abramov-Fiedler myocarditis (acute isolated myocarditis) I40.1
Abrasion T14.8 ☑
  abdomen, abdominal (wall) S30.811 ☑
  alveolar process S00.512 ☑
  ankle S90.51- ☑
  antecubital space — *see* Abrasion, elbow
  anus S30.817 ☑
  arm (upper) S40.81- ☑
  auditory canal — *see* Abrasion, ear
  auricle — *see* Abrasion, ear
  axilla — *see* Abrasion, arm
  back, lower S30.810 ☑
  breast S20.11- ☑
  brow S00.81 ☑
  buttock S30.810 ☑
  calf — *see* Abrasion, leg
  canthus — *see* Abrasion, eyelid
  cheek S00.81 ☑
    internal S00.512 ☑
  chest wall — *see* Abrasion, thorax

Abrasion — *continued*
- chin S00.81 ☑
- clitoris S30.814 ☑
- cornea S05.0- ☑
- costal region — *see* Abrasion, thorax
- dental K03.1
- digit(s)
  - foot — *see* Abrasion, toe
  - hand — *see* Abrasion, finger
- ear S00.41- ☑
- elbow S50.31- ☑
- epididymis S30.813 ☑
- epigastric region S30.811 ☑
- epiglottis S10.11 ☑
- esophagus (thoracic) S27.818 ☑
  - cervical S10.11 ☑
- eyebrow — *see* Abrasion, eyelid
- eyelid S00.21- ☑
- face S00.81 ☑
- finger(s) S60.41- ☑
  - index S60.41- ☑
  - little S60.41- ☑
  - middle S60.41- ☑
  - ring S60.41- ☑
- flank S30.811 ☑
- foot (except toe(s) alone) S90.81- ☑
  - toe — *see* Abrasion, toe
- forearm S50.81- ☑
  - elbow only — *see* Abrasion, elbow
- forehead S00.81 ☑
- genital organs, external
  - female S30.816 ☑
  - male S30.815 ☑
- groin S30.811 ☑
- gum S00.512 ☑
- hand S60.51- ☑
- head S00.91 ☑
  - ear — *see* Abrasion, ear
  - eyelid — *see* Abrasion, eyelid
  - lip S00.511 ☑
  - nose S00.31 ☑
  - oral cavity S00.512 ☑
  - scalp S00.01 ☑
  - specified site NEC S00.81 ☑
- heel — *see* Abrasion, foot
- hip S70.21- ☑
- inguinal region S30.811 ☑
- interscapular region S20.419 ☑
- jaw S00.81 ☑
- knee S80.21- ☑
- labium (majus) (minus) S30.814 ☑
- larynx S10.11 ☑
- leg (lower) S80.81- ☑
  - knee — *see* Abrasion, knee
  - upper — *see* Abrasion, thigh
- lip S00.511 ☑
- lower back S30.810 ☑
- lumbar region S30.810 ☑
- malar region S00.81 ☑
- mammary — *see* Abrasion, breast
- mastoid region S00.81 ☑
- mouth S00.512 ☑
- nail
  - finger — *see* Abrasion, finger
  - toe — *see* Abrasion, toe
- nape S10.81 ☑
- nasal S00.31 ☑
- neck S10.91 ☑
  - specified site NEC S10.81 ☑
  - throat S10.11 ☑
- nose S00.31 ☑
- occipital region S00.01 ☑
- oral cavity S00.512 ☑
- orbital region — *see* Abrasion, eyelid
- palate S00.512 ☑
- palm — *see* Abrasion, hand
- parietal region S00.01 ☑
- pelvis S30.810 ☑
- penis S30.812 ☑
- perineum
  - female S30.814 ☑
  - male S30.810 ☑
- periocular area — *see* Abrasion, eyelid
- phalanges
  - finger — *see* Abrasion, finger
  - toe — *see* Abrasion, toe

Abrasion — *continued*
- pharynx S10.11 ☑
- pinna — *see* Abrasion, ear
- popliteal space — *see* Abrasion, knee
- prepuce S30.812 ☑
- pubic region S30.810 ☑
- pudendum
  - female S30.816 ☑
  - male S30.815 ☑
- sacral region S30.810 ☑
- scalp S00.01 ☑
- scapular region — *see* Abrasion, shoulder
- scrotum S30.813 ☑
- shin — *see* Abrasion, leg
- shoulder S40.21- ☑
- skin NEC T14.8 ☑
- sternal region S20.319 ☑
- submaxillary region S00.81 ☑
- submental region S00.81 ☑
- subungual
  - finger(s) — *see* Abrasion, finger
  - toe(s) — *see* Abrasion, toe
- supraclavicular fossa S10.81 ☑
- supraorbital S00.81 ☑
- temple S00.81 ☑
- temporal region S00.81 ☑
- testis S30.813 ☑
- thigh S70.31- ☑
- thorax, thoracic (wall) S20.91 ☑
  - back S20.41- ☑
  - front S20.31- ☑
- throat S10.11 ☑
- thumb S60.31- ☑
- toe(s) (lesser) S90.416 ☑
  - great S90.41- ☑
- tongue S00.512 ☑
- tooth, teeth (dentifrice) (habitual) (hard tissues) (occupational) (ritual) (traditional) K03.1
- trachea S10.11 ☑
- tunica vaginalis S30.813 ☑
- tympanum, tympanic membrane — *see* Abrasion, ear
- uvula S00.512 ☑
- vagina S30.814 ☑
- vocal cords S10.11 ☑
- vulva S30.814 ☑
- wrist S60.81- ☑

Abrism — *see* Poisoning, food, noxious, plant

Abruptio placentae O45.9- ☑
- with
  - afibrinogenemia O45.01- ☑
  - coagulation defect O45.00- ☑
    - specified NEC O45.09- ☑
  - disseminated intravascular coagulation O45.02- ☑
  - hypofibrinogenemia O45.01- ☑
- specified NEC O45.8- ☑

Abruption, placenta — *see* Abruptio placentae

Abscess (connective tissue) (embolic) (fistulous) (infective) (metastatic) (multiple) (pernicious) (pyogenic) (septic) L02.91
- with
  - diverticular disease (intestine) K57.80
    - with bleeding K57.81
    - large intestine K57.20
      - with
        - bleeding K57.21
        - small intestine K57.40
          - with bleeding K57.41
    - small intestine K57.00
      - with
        - bleeding K57.01
        - large intestine K57.40
          - with bleeding K57.41
  - lymphangitis — *code by* site under Abscess
- abdomen, abdominal
  - cavity K65.1
  - wall L02.211
- abdominopelvic K65.1
- accessory sinus — *see* Sinusitis
- adrenal (capsule) (gland) E27.8
- alveolar K04.7
  - with sinus K04.6
- amebic A06.4
  - brain (and liver or lung abscess) A06.6
  - genitourinary tract A06.82
  - liver (without mention of brain or lung abscess) A06.4

Abscess — *continued*
- amebic — *continued*
  - lung (and liver) (without mention of brain abscess) A06.5
    - specified site NEC A06.89
    - spleen A06.89
- anerobic A48.0
- ankle — *see* Abscess, lower limb
- anorectal K61.2
- antecubital space — *see* Abscess, upper limb
- antrum (chronic) (Highmore) — *see* Sinusitis, maxillary
- anus K61.0
- apical (tooth) K04.7
  - with sinus (alveolar) K04.6
- appendix K35.3
- areola (acute) (chronic) (nonpuerperal) N61.1
  - puerperal, postpartum or gestational — *see* Infection, nipple
- arm (any part) — *see* Abscess, upper limb
- artery (wall) I77.89
- atheromatous I77.2
- auricle, ear — *see* Abscess, ear, external
- axilla (region) L02.41- ☑
  - lymph gland or node L04.2
- back (any part, except buttock) L02.212
- Bartholin's gland N75.1
  - with
    - abortion — *see* Abortion, by type complicated by, sepsis
    - ectopic or molar pregnancy O08.0
    - following ectopic or molar pregnancy O08.0
- Bezold's — *see* Mastoiditis, acute
- bilharziasis B65.1
- bladder (wall) — *see* Cystitis, specified type NEC
- bone (subperiosteal) (*see also* Osteomyelitis, specified type NEC)
  - accessory sinus (chronic) — *see* Sinusitis
  - chronic or old — *see* Osteomyelitis, chronic
  - jaw (lower) (upper) M27.2
  - mastoid — *see* Mastoiditis, acute, subperiosteal
  - petrous — *see* Petrositis
  - spinal (tuberculous) A18.01
    - nontuberculous — *see* Osteomyelitis, vertebra
- bowel K63.0
- brain (any part) (cystic) (otogenic) G06.0
  - amebic (with abscess of any other site) A06.6
  - gonococcal A54.82
  - pheomycotic (chromomycotic) B43.1
  - tuberculous A17.81
- breast (acute) (chronic) (nonpuerperal) N61.1
  - newborn P39.0
  - puerperal, postpartum, gestational — *see* Mastitis, obstetric, purulent
- broad ligament N73.2
  - acute N73.0
  - chronic N73.1
- Brodie's (localized) (chronic) M86.8X- ☑
- bronchi J98.09
- buccal cavity K12.2
- bulbourethral gland N34.0
- bursa M71.00
  - ankle M71.07- ☑
  - elbow M71.02- ☑
  - foot M71.07- ☑
  - hand M71.04- ☑
  - hip M71.05- ☑
  - knee M71.06- ☑
  - multiple sites M71.09
  - pharyngeal J39.1
  - shoulder M71.01- ☑
  - specified site NEC M71.08
  - wrist M71.03- ☑
- buttock L02.31
- canthus — *see* Blepharoconjunctivitis
- cartilage — *see* Disorder, cartilage, specified type NEC
- cecum K35.3
- cerebellum, cerebellar G06.0
  - sequelae G09
- cerebral (embolic) G06.0
  - sequelae G09
- cervical (meaning neck) L02.11
  - lymph gland or node L04.0
- cervix (stump) (uteri) — *see* Cervicitis
- cheek (external) L02.01
  - inner K12.2
- chest J86.9
  - with fistula J86.0
  - wall L02.213

Abscess — continued
  chin L02.01
  choroid — see Inflammation, chorioretinal
  circumtonsillar J36
  cold (lung) (tuberculous) (see also Tuberculosis, abscess, lung)
    articular — see Tuberculosis, joint
  colon (wall) K63.0
  colostomy K94.02
  conjunctiva — see Conjunctivitis, acute
  cornea H16.31- ☑
  corpus
    cavernosum N48.21
    luteum — see Oophoritis
  Cowper's gland N34.0
  cranium G06.0
  cul-de-sac (Douglas') (posterior) — see Peritonitis, pelvic, female
  cutaneous — see Abscess, by site
  dental K04.7
    with sinus (alveolar) K04.6
  dentoalveolar K04.7
    with sinus K04.6
  diaphragm, diaphragmatic K65.1
  Douglas' cul-de-sac or pouch — see Peritonitis, pelvic, female
  Dubois A50.59
  ear (middle) (see also Otitis, media, suppurative)
    acute — see Otitis, media, suppurative, acute
    external H60.0- ☑
  entamebic — see Abscess, amebic
  enterostomy K94.12
  epididymis N45.4
  epidural G06.2
    brain G06.0
    spinal cord G06.1
  epiglottis J38.7
  epiploon, epiploic K65.1
  erysipelatous — see Erysipelas
  esophagus K20.8
  ethmoid (bone) (chronic) (sinus) J32.2
  external auditory canal — see Abscess, ear, external
  extradural G06.2
    brain G06.0
      sequelae G09
    spinal cord G06.1
  extraperitoneal K68.19
  eye — see Endophthalmitis, purulent
  eyelid H00.03- ☑
  face (any part, except ear, eye and nose) L02.01
  fallopian tube — see Salpingitis
  fascia M72.8
  fauces J39.1
  fecal K63.0
  femoral (region) — see Abscess, lower limb
  filaria, filarial — see Infestation, filarial
  finger (any) (see also Abscess, hand)
    nail — see Cellulitis, finger
  foot L02.61- ☑
  forehead L02.01
  frontal sinus (chronic) J32.1
  gallbladder K81.0
  genital organ or tract
    female (external) N76.4
    male N49.9
      multiple sites N49.8
      specified NEC N49.8
  gestational mammary O91.11- ☑
  gestational subareolar O91.11- ☑
  gingival — see Peridontitis, aggressive, localized
  gland, glandular (lymph) (acute) — see Lymphadenitis, acute
  gluteal (region) L02.31
  gonorrheal — see Gonococcus
  groin L02.214
  gum — see Peridontitis, aggressive, localized
  hand L02.51- ☑
  head NEC L02.811
    face (any part, except ear, eye and nose) L02.01
  heart — see Carditis
  heel — see Abscess, foot
  helminthic — see Infestation, helminth
  hepatic (cholangitic) (hematogenic) (lymphogenic) (pylephlebitic) K75.0
    amebic A06.4
  hip (region) — see Abscess, lower limb
  ileocecal K35.3
  ileostomy (bud) K94.12

Abscess — continued
  iliac (region) L02.214
    fossa K35.3
  infraclavicular (fossa) — see Abscess, upper limb
  inguinal (region) L02.214
    lymph gland or node L04.1
  intestine, intestinal NEC K63.0
    rectal K61.1
  intra-abdominal (see also Abscess, peritoneum) K65.1
    postprocedural T81.4 ☑
      retroperitoneal K68.11
  intracranial G06.0
  intramammary — see Abscess, breast
  intraorbital — see Abscess, orbit
  intraperitoneal K65.1
  intrasphincteric (anus) K61.4
  intraspinal G06.1
  intratonsillar J36
  ischiorectal (fossa) K61.3
  jaw (bone) (lower) (upper) M27.2
  joint — see Arthritis, pyogenic or pyemic
    spine (tuberculous) A18.01
      nontuberculous — see Spondylopathy, infective
  kidney N15.1
    with calculus N20.0
      with hydronephrosis N13.6
    puerperal (postpartum) O86.21
  knee (see also Abscess, lower limb)
    joint M00.9
  labium (majus) (minus) N76.4
  lacrimal
    caruncle — see Inflammation, lacrimal, passages, acute
    gland — see Dacryoadenitis
    passages (duct) (sac) — see Inflammation, lacrimal, passages, acute
  lacunar N34.0
  larynx J38.7
  lateral (alveolar) K04.7
    with sinus K04.6
  leg (any part) — see Abscess, lower limb
  lens H27.8
  lingual K14.0
    tonsil J36
  lip K13.0
  Littre's gland N34.0
  liver (cholangitic) (hematogenic) (lymphogenic) (pylephlebitic) (pyogenic) K75.0
    amebic (due to Entamoeba histolytica) (dysenteric) (tropical) A06.4
      with
        brain abscess (and liver or lung abscess) A06.6
        lung abscess A06.5
  loin (region) L02.211
  lower limb L02.41- ☑
  lumbar (tuberculous) A18.01
    nontuberculous L02.212
  lung (miliary) (putrid) J85.2
    with pneumonia J85.1
      due to specified organism (see Pneumonia, in (due to))
    amebic (with liver abscess) A06.5
      with
        brain abscess A06.6
        pneumonia A06.5
  lymph, lymphatic, gland or node (acute) (see also Lymphadenitis, acute)
    mesentery I88.0
  malar M27.2
  mammary gland — see Abscess, breast
  marginal, anus K61.0
  mastoid — see Mastoiditis, acute
  maxilla, maxillary M27.2
    molar (tooth) K04.7
      with sinus K04.6
    premolar K04.7
    sinus (chronic) J32.0
  mediastinum J85.3
  meibomian gland — see Hordeolum
  meninges G06.2
  mesentery, mesenteric K65.1
  mesosalpinx — see Salpingitis
  mons pubis L02.215
  mouth (floor) K12.2
  muscle — see Myositis, infective
  myocardium I40.0

Abscess — continued
  nabothian (follicle) — see Cervicitis
  nasal J32.9
  nasopharyngeal J39.1
  navel L02.216
    newborn P38.9
      with mild hemorrhage P38.1
      without hemorrhage P38.9
  neck (region) L02.11
    lymph gland or node L04.0
  nephritic — see Abscess, kidney
  nipple N61.1
    associated with
      lactation — see Pregnancy, complicated by
      pregnancy — see Pregnancy, complicated by
  nose (external) (fossa) (septum) J34.0
    sinus (chronic) — see Sinusitis
  omentum K65.1
  operative wound T81.4 ☑
  orbit, orbital — see Cellulitis, orbit
  otogenic G06.0
  ovary, ovarian (corpus luteum) — see Oophoritis
  oviduct — see Oophoritis
  palate (soft) K12.2
    hard M27.2
  palmar (space) — see Abscess, hand
  pancreas (duct) — see Pancreatitis, acute
  parafrenal N48.21
  parametric, parametrium N73.2
    acute N73.0
    chronic N73.1
  paranephric N15.1
  parapancreatic — see Pancreatitis, acute
  parapharyngeal J39.0
  pararectal K61.1
  parasinus — see Sinusitis
  parauterine (see also Disease, pelvis, inflammatory) N73.2
  paravaginal — see Vaginitis
  parietal region (scalp) L02.811
  parodontal — see Peridontitis, aggressive, localized
  parotid (duct) (gland) K11.3
    region K12.2
  pectoral (region) L02.213
  pelvis, pelvic
    female — see Disease, pelvis, inflammatory
    male, peritoneal K65.1
  penis N48.21
    gonococcal (accessory gland) (periurethral) A54.1
  perianal K61.0
  periapical K04.7
    with sinus (alveolar) K04.6
  periappendicular K35.3
  pericardial I30.1
  pericecal K35.3
  pericemental — see Peridontitis, aggressive, localized
  pericholecystic — see Cholecystitis, acute
  pericoronal — see Peridontitis, aggressive, localized
  peridental — see Peridontitis, aggressive, localized
  perimetric (see also Disease, pelvis, inflammatory) N73.2
  perinephric, perinephritic — see Abscess, kidney
  perineum, perineal (superficial) L02.215
    urethra N34.0
  periodontal (parietal) — see Peridontitis, aggressive, localized
    apical K04.7
  periosteum, periosteal (see also Osteomyelitis, specified type NEC)
    with osteomyelitis (see also Osteomyelitis, specified type NEC)
      acute — see Osteomyelitis, acute
      chronic — see Osteomyelitis, chronic
  peripharyngeal J39.0
  peripleuritic J86.9
    with fistula J86.0
  periprostatic N41.2
  perirectal K61.1
  perirenal (tissue) — see Abscess, kidney
  perisinuous (nose) — see Sinusitis
  peritoneum, peritoneal (perforated) (ruptured) K65.1
    with appendicitis K35.3
    pelvic
      female — see Peritonitis, pelvic, female
      male K65.1
    postoperative T81.4 ☑
    puerperal, postpartum, childbirth O85
    tuberculous A18.31

Abscess — *continued*
peritonsillar J36
perityphlic K35.3
periureteral N28.89
periurethral N34.0
gonococcal (accessory gland) (periurethral) A54.1
periuterine (*see also* Disease, pelvis, inflammatory) N73.2
perivesical — *see* Cystitis, specified type NEC
petrous bone — *see* Petrositis
phagedenic NOS L02.91
chancroid A57
pharynx, pharyngeal (lateral) J39.1
pilonidal L05.01
pituitary (gland) E23.6
pleura J86.9
with fistula J86.0
popliteal — *see* Abscess, lower limb
postcecal K35.3
postlaryngeal J38.7
postnasal J34.0
postoperative (any site) T81.4 ☑
retroperitoneal K68.11
postpharyngeal J39.0
posttonsillar J36
post-typhoid A01.09
pouch of Douglas — *see* Peritonitis, pelvic, female
premammary — *see* Abscess, breast
prepatellar — *see* Abscess, lower limb
prostate N41.2
gonococcal (acute) (chronic) A54.22
psoas muscle K68.12
puerperal — *code by* site under Puerperal, abscess
pulmonary — *see* Abscess, lung
pulp, pulpal (dental) K04.01
irreversible K04.02
reversible K04.01
rectovaginal septum K63.0
rectovesical — *see* Cystitis, specified type NEC
rectum K61.1
renal — *see* Abscess, kidney
retina — *see* Inflammation, chorioretinal
retrobulbar — *see* Abscess, orbit
retrocecal K65.1
retrolaryngeal J38.7
retromammary — *see* Abscess, breast
retroperitoneal NEC K68.19
postprocedural K68.11
retropharyngeal J39.0
retrouterine — *see* Peritonitis, pelvic, female
retrovesical — *see* Cystitis, specified type NEC
root, tooth K04.7
with sinus (alveolar) K04.6
round ligament (*see also* Disease, pelvis, inflammatory) N73.2
rupture (spontaneous) NOS L02.91
sacrum (tuberculous) A18.01
nontuberculous M46.28
salivary (duct) (gland) K11.3
scalp (any part) L02.811
scapular — *see* Osteomyelitis, specified type NEC
sclera — *see* Scleritis
scrofulous (tuberculous) A18.2
scrotum N49.2
seminal vesicle N49.0
septal, dental K04.7
with sinus (alveolar) K04.6
serous — *see* Periostitis
shoulder (region) — *see* Abscess, upper limb
sigmoid K63.0
sinus (accessory) (chronic) (nasal) (*see also* Sinusitis)
intracranial venous (any) G06.0
Skene's duct or gland N34.0
skin — *see* Abscess, by site
specified site NEC L02.818
spermatic cord N49.1
sphenoidal (sinus) (chronic) J32.3
spinal cord (any part) (staphylococcal) G06.1
tuberculous A17.81
spine (column) (tuberculous) A18.01
epidural G06.1
nontuberculous — *see* Osteomyelitis, vertebra
spleen D73.3
amebic A06.89
stitch T81.4 ☑
subarachnoid G06.2
brain G06.0
spinal cord G06.1

Abscess — *continued*
subareolar — *see* Abscess, breast
subcecal K35.3
subcutaneous (*see also* Abscess, by site)
pheomycotic (chromomycotic) B43.2
subdiaphragmatic K65.1
subdural G06.2
brain G06.0
sequelae G09
spinal cord G06.1
subgaleal L02.811
subhepatic K65.1
sublingual K12.2
gland K11.3
submammary — *see* Abscess, breast
submandibular (region) (space) (triangle) K12.2
gland K11.3
submaxillary (region) L02.01
gland K11.3
submental L02.01
gland K11.3
subperiosteal — *see* Osteomyelitis, specified type NEC
subphrenic K65.1
postoperative T81.4 ☑
suburethral N34.0
sudoriparous L75.8
supraclavicular (fossa) — *see* Abscess, upper limb
suprapelvic, acute N73.0
suprarenal (capsule) (gland) E27.8
sweat gland L74.8
tear duct — *see* Inflammation, lacrimal, passages, acute
temple L02.01
temporal region L02.01
temporosphenoidal G06.0
tendon (sheath) M65.00
ankle M65.07- ☑
foot M65.07- ☑
forearm M65.03- ☑
hand M65.04- ☑
lower leg M65.06- ☑
pelvic region M65.05- ☑
shoulder region M65.01- ☑
specified site NEC M65.08
thigh M65.05- ☑
upper arm M65.02- ☑
testis N45.4
thigh — *see* Abscess, lower limb
thorax J86.9
with fistula J86.0
throat J39.1
thumb (*see also* Abscess, hand)
nail — *see* Cellulitis, finger
thymus (gland) E32.1
thyroid (gland) E06.0
toe (any) (*see also* Abscess, foot)
nail — *see* Cellulitis, toe
tongue (staphylococcal) K14.0
tonsil(s) (lingual) J36
tonsillopharyngeal J36
tooth, teeth (root) K04.7
with sinus (alveolar) K04.6
supporting structures NEC — *see* Peridontitis, aggressive, localized
trachea J39.8
trunk L02.219
abdominal wall L02.211
back L02.212
chest wall L02.213
groin L02.214
perineum L02.215
umbilicus L02.216
tubal — *see* Salpingitis
tuberculous — *see* Tuberculosis, abscess
tubo-ovarian — *see* Salpingo-oophoritis
tunica vaginalis N49.1
umbilicus L02.216
upper
limb L02.41- ☑
respiratory J39.8
urethral (gland) N34.0
urinary N34.0
uterus, uterine (wall) (*see also* Endometritis)
ligament (*see also* Disease, pelvis, inflammatory) N73.2
neck — *see* Cervicitis
uvula K12.2
vagina (wall) — *see* Vaginitis

Abscess — *continued*
vaginorectal — *see* Vaginitis
vas deferens N49.1
vermiform appendix K35.3
vertebra (column) (tuberculous) A18.01
nontuberculous — *see* Osteomyelitis, vertebra
vesical — *see* Cystitis, specified type NEC
vesico-uterine pouch — *see* Peritonitis, pelvic, female
vitreous (humor) — *see* Endophthalmitis, purulent
vocal cord J38.3
von Bezold's — *see* Mastoiditis, acute
vulva N76.4
vulvovaginal gland N75.1
web space — *see* Abscess, hand
wound T81.4 ☑
wrist — *see* Abscess, upper limb
Absence (of) (organ or part) (complete or partial)
adrenal (gland) (congenital) Q89.1
acquired E89.6
albumin in blood E88.09
alimentary tract (congenital) Q45.8
upper Q40.8
alveolar process (acquired) — *see* Anomaly, alveolar
ankle (acquired) Z89.44- ☑
anus (congenital) Q42.3
with fistula Q42.2
aorta (congenital) Q25.41
appendix, congenital Q42.8
arm (acquired) Z89.20- ☑
above elbow Z89.22- ☑
congenital (with hand present) — *see* Agenesis, arm, with hand present
and hand — *see* Agenesis, forearm, and hand
below elbow Z89.21- ☑
congenital (with hand present) — *see* Agenesis, arm, with hand present
and hand — *see* Agenesis, forearm, and hand
congenital — *see* Defect, reduction, upper limb
shoulder (following explantation of shoulder joint prosthesis) (joint) (with or without presence of antibiotic-impregnated cement spacer) Z89.23- ☑
congenital (with hand present) — *see* Agenesis, arm, with hand present
artery (congenital) (peripheral) Q27.8
brain Q28.3
coronary Q24.5
pulmonary Q25.79
specified NEC Q27.8
umbilical Q27.0
atrial septum (congenital) Q21.1
auditory canal (congenital) (external) Q16.1
auricle (ear), congenital Q16.0
bile, biliary duct, congenital Q44.5
bladder (acquired) Z90.6
congenital Q64.5
bowel sounds R19.11
brain Q00.0
part of Q04.3
breast(s) (and nipple(s)) (acquired) Z90.1- ☑
congenital Q83.8
broad ligament Q50.6
bronchus (congenital) Q32.4
canaliculus lacrimalis, congenital Q10.4
cerebellum (vermis) Q04.3
cervix (acquired) (with uterus) Z90.710
with remaining uterus Z90.712
congenital Q51.5
chin, congenital Q18.8
cilia (congenital) Q10.3
acquired — *see* Madarosis
clitoris (congenital) Q52.6
coccyx, congenital Q76.49
cold sense R20.8
congenital
lumen — *see* Atresia
organ or site NEC — *see* Agenesis
septum — *see* Imperfect, closure
corpus callosum Q04.0
cricoid cartilage, congenital Q31.8
diaphragm (with hernia), congenital Q79.1
digestive organ(s) or tract, congenital Q45.8
acquired NEC Z90.49
upper Q40.8
ductus arteriosus Q28.8
duodenum (acquired) Z90.49

Absence — *continued*
  duodenum — *continued*
    congenital Q41.0
  ear, congenital Q16.9
    acquired H93.8- ☑
    auricle Q16.0
    external Q16.0
    inner Q16.5
    lobe, lobule Q17.8
    middle, except ossicles Q16.4
      ossicles Q16.3
    ossicles Q16.3
  ejaculatory duct (congenital) Q55.4
  endocrine gland (congenital) NEC Q89.2
    acquired E89.89
  epididymis (congenital) Q55.4
    acquired Z90.79
  epiglottis, congenital Q31.8
  esophagus (congenital) Q39.8
    acquired (partial) Z90.49
  eustachian tube (congenital) Q16.2
  extremity (acquired) Z89.9
    congenital Q73.0
    knee (following explanation of knee joint prosthe-
      sis) (joint) (with or without presence of an-
      tibiotic-impregnated cement spacer)
      Z89.52- ☑
    lower (above knee) Z89.619
      below knee Z89.51- ☑
    upper — *see* Absence, arm
  eye (acquired) Z90.01
    congenital Q11.1
    muscle (congenital) Q10.3
  eyeball (acquired) Z90.01
  eyelid (fold) (congenital) Q10.3
    acquired Z90.01
  face, specified part NEC Q18.8
  fallopian tube(s) (acquired) Z90.79
    congenital Q50.6
  family member (causing problem in home) NEC (*see
    also* Disruption, family) Z63.32
  femur, congenital — *see* Defect, reduction, lower limb,
    longitudinal, femur
  fibrinogen (congenital) D68.2
    acquired D65
  finger(s) (acquired) Z89.02- ☑
    congenital — *see* Agenesis, hand
  foot (acquired) Z89.43- ☑
    congenital — *see* Agenesis, foot
  forearm (acquired) — *see* Absence, arm, below elbow
  gallbladder (acquired) Z90.49
    congenital Q44.0
  gamma globulin in blood D80.1
    hereditary D80.0
  genital organs
    acquired (female) (male) Z90.79
    female, congenital Q52.8
      external Q52.71
      internal NEC Q52.8
    male, congenital Q55.8
  genitourinary organs, congenital NEC
    female Q52.8
    male Q55.8
  globe (acquired) Z90.01
    congenital Q11.1
  glottis, congenital Q31.8
  hand and wrist (acquired) Z89.11- ☑
    congenital — *see* Agenesis, hand
  head, part (acquired) NEC Z90.09
  heat sense R20.8
  hip (following explanation of hip joint prosthesis)
    (joint) (with or without presence of antibiotic-
    impregnated cement spacer) Z89.62- ☑
  hymen (congenital) Q52.4
  ileum (acquired) Z90.49
    congenital Q41.2
  immunoglobulin, isolated NEC D80.3
    IgA D80.2
    IgG D80.3
    IgM D80.4
  incus (acquired) — *see* Loss, ossicles, ear
    congenital Q16.3
  inner ear, congenital Q16.5
  intestine (acquired) (small) Z90.49
    congenital Q41.9
      specified NEC Q41.8
    large Z90.49
      congenital Q42.9

Absence — *continued*
  intestine — *continued*
    large — *continued*
      congenital — *continued*
        specified NEC Q42.8
  iris, congenital Q13.1
  jejunum (acquired) Z90.49
    congenital Q41.1
  joint
    acquired
      hip (following explanation of hip joint prosthe-
        sis) (with or without presence of antibiot-
        ic-impregnated cement spacer)
        Z89.62- ☑
      knee (following explanation of knee joint
        prosthesis) (with or without presence of
        antibiotic-impregnated cement spacer)
        Z89.52- ☑
      shoulder (following explanation of shoulder
        joint prosthesis) (with or without pres-
        ence of antibiotic-impregnated cement
        spacer) Z89.23- ☑
    congenital NEC Q74.8
  kidney(s) (acquired) Z90.5
    congenital Q60.2
      bilateral Q60.1
      unilateral Q60.0
  knee (following explanation of knee joint prosthesis)
    (joint) (with or without presence of antibiotic-
    impregnated cement spacer) Z89.52- ☑
  labyrinth, membranous Q16.5
  larynx (congenital) Q31.8
    acquired Z90.02
  leg (acquired) (above knee) Z89.61- ☑
    below knee (acquired) Z89.51- ☑
    congenital — *see* Defect, reduction, lower limb
  lens (acquired) (*see also* Aphakia)
    congenital Q12.3
    post cataract extraction Z98.4- ☑
  limb (acquired) — *see* Absence, extremity
  lip Q38.6
  liver (congenital) Q44.7
  lung (fissure) (lobe) (bilateral) (unilateral) (congenital)
    Q33.3
    acquired (any part) Z90.2
  menstruation — *see* Amenorrhea
  muscle (congenital) (pectoral) Q79.8
    ocular Q10.3
  neck, part Q18.8
  neutrophil — *see* Agranulocytosis
  nipple(s) (with breast(s)) (acquired) Z90.1- ☑
    congenital Q83.2
  nose (congenital) Q30.1
    acquired Z90.09
  organ
    of Corti, congenital Q16.5
    or site, congenital NEC Q89.8
      acquired NEC Z90.89
  osseous meatus (ear) Q16.4
  ovary (acquired)
    bilateral Z90.722
    congenital
      bilateral Q50.02
      unilateral Q50.01
    unilateral Z90.721
  oviduct (acquired)
    bilateral Z90.722
    congenital Q50.6
    unilateral Z90.721
  pancreas (congenital) Q45.0
    acquired Z90.410
      complete Z90.410
      partial Z90.411
      total Z90.410
  parathyroid gland (acquired) E89.2
    congenital Q89.2
  patella, congenital Q74.1
  penis (congenital) Q55.5
    acquired Z90.79
  pericardium (congenital) Q24.8
  pituitary gland (congenital) Q89.2
    acquired E89.3
  prostate (acquired) Z90.79
    congenital Q55.4
  pulmonary valve Q22.0
  punctum lacrimale (congenital) Q10.4
  radius, congenital — *see* Defect, reduction, upper limb,
    longitudinal, radius

Absence — *continued*
  rectum (congenital) Q42.1
    with fistula Q42.0
    acquired Z90.49
  respiratory organ NOS Q34.9
  rib (acquired) Z90.89
    congenital Q76.6
  sacrum, congenital Q76.49
  salivary gland(s), congenital Q38.4
  scrotum, congenital Q55.29
  seminal vesicles (congenital) Q55.4
    acquired Z90.79
  septum
    atrial (congenital) Q21.1
    between aorta and pulmonary artery Q21.4
    ventricular (congenital) Q20.4
  sex chromosome
    female phenotype Q97.8
    male phenotype Q98.8
  skull bone (congenital) Q75.8
    with
      anencephaly Q00.0
      encephalocele — *see* Encephalocele
      hydrocephalus Q03.9
        with spina bifida — *see* Spina bifida, by site,
          with hydrocephalus
      microcephaly Q02
  spermatic cord, congenital Q55.4
  spine, congenital Q76.49
  spleen (congenital) Q89.01
    acquired Z90.81
  sternum, congenital Q76.7
  stomach (acquired) (partial) Z90.3
    congenital Q40.2
  superior vena cava, congenital Q26.8
  teeth, tooth (congenital) K00.0
    acquired (complete) K08.109
      class I K08.101
      class II K08.102
      class III K08.103
      class IV K08.104
      due to
        caries K08.139
          class I K08.131
          class II K08.132
          class III K08.133
          class IV K08.134
        periodontal disease K08.129
          class I K08.121
          class II K08.122
          class III K08.123
          class IV K08.124
        specified NEC K08.199
          class I K08.191
          class II K08.192
          class III K08.193
          class IV K08.194
        trauma K08.119
          class I K08.111
          class II K08.112
          class III K08.113
          class IV K08.114
    partial K08.409
      class I K08.401
      class II K08.402
      class III K08.403
      class IV K08.404
      due to
        caries K08.439
          class I K08.431
          class II K08.432
          class III K08.433
          class IV K08.434
        periodontal disease K08.429
          class I K08.421
          class II K08.422
          class III K08.423
          class IV K08.424
        specified NEC K08.499
          class I K08.491
          class II K08.492
          class III K08.493
          class IV K08.494
        trauma K08.419
          class I K08.411
          class II K08.412
          class III K08.413
          class IV K08.414
  tendon (congenital) Q79.8

Absence — continued
 testis (congenital) Q55.0
  acquired Z90.79
 thumb (acquired) Z89.01- ☑
  congenital — see Agenesis, hand
 thymus gland Q89.2
 thyroid (gland) (acquired) E89.0
  cartilage, congenital Q31.8
  congenital E03.1
 toe(s) (acquired) Z89.42- ☑
  with foot — see Absence, foot and ankle
  congenital — see Agenesis, foot
  great Z89.41- ☑
 tongue, congenital Q38.3
 trachea (cartilage), congenital Q32.1
 transverse aortic arch, congenital Q25.49
 tricuspid valve Q22.4
 umbilical artery, congenital Q27.0
 upper arm and forearm with hand present, congenital
   — see Agenesis, arm, with hand present
 ureter (congenital) Q62.4
  acquired Z90.6
 urethra, congenital Q64.5
 uterus (acquired) Z90.710
  with cervix Z90.710
  with remaining cervical stump Z90.711
  congenital Q51.0
 uvula, congenital Q38.5
 vagina, congenital Q52.0
 vas deferens (congenital) Q55.4
  acquired Z90.79
 vein (peripheral) congenital NEC Q27.8
  cerebral Q28.3
  digestive system Q27.8
  great Q26.8
  lower limb Q27.8
  portal Q26.5
  precerebral Q28.1
  specified site NEC Q27.8
  upper limb Q27.8
 vena cava (inferior) (superior), congenital Q26.8
 ventricular septum Q20.4
 vertebra, congenital Q76.49
 vulva, congenital Q52.71
 wrist (acquired) Z89.12- ☑
Absorbent system disease I87.8
Absorption
 carbohydrate, disturbance K90.49
 chemical — see Table of Drugs and Chemicals
  through placenta (newborn) P04.9
   environmental substance P04.6
   nutritional substance P04.5
   obstetric anesthetic or analgesic drug P04.0
 drug NEC — see Table of Drugs and Chemicals
  addictive
   through placenta (newborn) P04.49
    cocaine P04.41
  medicinal
   through placenta (newborn) P04.1
  through placenta (newborn) P04.1
   obstetric anesthetic or analgesic drug P04.0
 fat, disturbance K90.49
  pancreatic K90.3
 noxious substance — see Table of Drugs and Chemicals
 protein, disturbance K90.49
 starch, disturbance K90.49
 toxic substance — see Table of Drugs and Chemicals
 uremic — see Uremia
Abstinence symptoms, syndrome
 alcohol F10.239
  with delirium F10.231
 cocaine F14.23
 neonatal P96.1
 nicotine — see Dependence, drug, nicotine, with,
   withdrawal
 opioid F11.93
  with dependence F11.23
 psychoactive NEC F19.939
  with
   delirium F19.931
   dependence F19.239
    with
     delirium F19.231
     perceptual disturbance F19.232
    uncomplicated F19.230
   perceptual disturbance F19.932
  uncomplicated F19.930

Abstinence symptoms, syndrome — continued
 sedative F13.939
  with
   delirium F13.931
   dependence F13.239
    with
     delirium F13.231
     perceptual disturbance F13.232
    uncomplicated F13.230
   perceptual disturbance F13.932
  uncomplicated F13.930
 stimulant NEC F15.93
  with dependence F15.23
Abulia R68.89
Abulomania F60.7
Abuse
 adult — see Maltreatment, adult
  as reason for
   couple seeking advice (including offender)
    Z63.0
 alcohol (non-dependent) F10.10
  with
   anxiety disorder F10.180
   intoxication F10.129
    with delirium F10.121
    uncomplicated F10.120
   mood disorder F10.14
   other specified disorder F10.188
   psychosis F10.159
    delusions F10.150
    hallucinations F10.151
   sexual dysfunction F10.181
   sleep disorder F10.182
   unspecified disorder F10.19
  counseling and surveillance Z71.41
  in remission (early) (sustained) F10.11
 amphetamine (or related substance) — see Abuse,
   drug, stimulant NEC
 analgesics (non-prescribed) (over the counter) F55.8
 antacids F55.0
 antidepressants — see Abuse, drug, psychoactive NEC
 anxiolytic — see Abuse, drug, sedative
 barbiturates — see Abuse, drug, sedative
 caffeine — see Abuse, drug, stimulant NEC
 cannabis, cannabinoids — see Abuse, drug, cannabis
 child — see Maltreatment, child
 cocaine — see Abuse, drug, cocaine
 drug NEC (non-dependent) F19.10
  with sleep disorder F19.182
  amphetamine type — see Abuse, drug, stimulant
    NEC
  analgesics (non-prescribed) (over the counter)
    F55.8
  antacids F55.0
  antidepressants — see Abuse, drug, psychoactive
    NEC
  anxiolytics — see Abuse, drug, sedative
  barbiturates — see Abuse, drug, sedative
  caffeine — see Abuse, drug, stimulant NEC
  cannabis F12.10
   with
    anxiety disorder F12.180
    intoxication F12.129
     with
      delirium F12.121
      perceptual disturbance F12.122
     uncomplicated F12.120
    other specified disorder F12.188
    psychosis F12.159
     delusions F12.150
     hallucinations F12.151
    unspecified disorder F12.19
   in remission (early) (sustained) F12.11
  cocaine F14.10
   with
    anxiety disorder F14.180
    intoxication F14.129
     with
      delirium F14.121
      perceptual disturbance F14.122
     uncomplicated F14.120
    mood disorder F14.14
    other specified disorder F14.188
    psychosis F14.159
     delusions F14.150
     hallucinations F14.151
    sexual dysfunction F14.181
    sleep disorder F14.182

Abuse — continued
 drug — continued
  cocaine — continued
   with — continued
    unspecified disorder F14.19
   in remission (early) (sustained) F14.11
  counseling and surveillance Z71.51
  hallucinogen F16.10
   with
    anxiety disorder F16.180
    flashbacks F16.183
    intoxication F16.129
     with
      delirium F16.121
      perceptual disturbance F16.122
     uncomplicated F16.120
    mood disorder F16.14
    other specified disorder F16.188
    perception disorder, persisting F16.183
    psychosis F16.159
     delusions F16.150
     hallucinations F16.151
    unspecified disorder F16.19
   in remission (early) (sustained) F16.11
  hashish — see Abuse, drug, cannabis
  herbal or folk remedies F55.1
  hormones F55.3
  hypnotics — see Abuse, drug, sedative
  in remission (early) (sustained) F19.11
  inhalant F18.10
   with
    anxiety disorder F18.180
    dementia, persisting F18.17
    intoxication F18.129
     with delirium F18.121
     uncomplicated F18.120
    mood disorder F18.14
    other specified disorder F18.188
    psychosis F18.159
     delusions F18.150
     hallucinations F18.151
    unspecified disorder F18.19
   in remission (early) (sustained) F18.11
  laxatives F55.2
  LSD — see Abuse, drug, hallucinogen
  marihuana — see Abuse, drug, cannabis
  morphine type (opioids) — see Abuse, drug, opioid
  opioid F11.10
   with
    intoxication F11.129
     with
      delirium F11.121
      perceptual disturbance F11.122
     uncomplicated F11.120
    mood disorder F11.14
    other specified disorder F11.188
    psychosis F11.159
     delusions F11.150
     hallucinations F11.151
    sexual dysfunction F11.181
    sleep disorder F11.182
    unspecified disorder F11.19
   in remission (early) (sustained) F11.11
  PCP (phencyclidine) (or related substance) — see
    Abuse, drug, hallucinogen
  psychoactive NEC F19.10
   with
    amnestic disorder F19.16
    anxiety disorder F19.180
    dementia F19.17
    intoxication F19.129
     with
      delirium F19.121
      perceptual disturbance F19.122
     uncomplicated F19.120
    mood disorder F19.14
    other specified disorder F19.188
    psychosis F19.159
     delusions F19.150
     hallucinations F19.151
    sexual dysfunction F19.181
    sleep disorder F19.182
    unspecified disorder F19.19
  sedative, hypnotic or anxiolytic F13.10
   with
    anxiety disorder F13.180
    intoxication F13.129
     with delirium F13.121
     uncomplicated F13.120

Abuse — *continued*
  drug — *continued*
    sedative, hypnotic or anxiolytic — *continued*
      with — *continued*
        mood disorder F13.14
        other specified disorder F13.188
        psychosis F13.159
          delusions F13.150
          hallucinations F13.151
        sexual dysfunction F13.181
        sleep disorder F13.182
        unspecified disorder F13.19
      in remission (early) (sustained) F13.11
    solvent — *see* Abuse, drug, inhalant
    steroids F55.3
    stimulant NEC F15.10
      with
        anxiety disorder F15.180
        intoxication F15.129
          with
            delirium F15.121
            perceptual disturbance F15.122
          uncomplicated F15.120
        mood disorder F15.14
        other specified disorder F15.188
        psychosis F15.159
          delusions F15.150
          hallucinations F15.151
        sexual dysfunction F15.181
        sleep disorder F15.182
        unspecified disorder F15.19
      in remission (early) (sustained) F15.11
    tranquilizers — *see* Abuse, drug, sedative
    vitamins F55.4
  hallucinogens — *see* Abuse, drug, hallucinogen
  hashish — *see* Abuse, drug, cannabis
  herbal or folk remedies F55.1
  hormones F55.3
  hypnotic — *see* Abuse, drug, sedative
  inhalant — *see* Abuse, drug, inhalant
  laxatives F55.2
  LSD — *see* Abuse, drug, hallucinogen
  marihuana — *see* Abuse, drug, cannabis
  morphine type (opioids) — *see* Abuse, drug, opioid
  non-psychoactive substance NEC F55.8
    antacids F55.0
    folk remedies F55.1
    herbal remedies F55.1
    hormones F55.3
    laxatives F55.2
    steroids F55.3
    vitamins F55.4
  opioids — *see* Abuse, drug, opioid
  PCP (phencyclidine) (or related substance) — *see* Abuse, drug, hallucinogen
  physical (adult) (child) — *see* Maltreatment
  psychoactive substance — *see* Abuse, drug, psychoactive NEC
  psychological (adult) (child) — *see* Maltreatment
  sedative — *see* Abuse, drug, sedative
  sexual — *see* Maltreatment
  solvent — *see* Abuse, drug, inhalant
  steroids F55.3
  vitamins F55.4
Acalculia R48.8
  developmental F81.2
Acanthamebiasis (with) B60.10
  conjunctiva B60.12
  keratoconjunctivitis B60.13
  meningoencephalitis B60.11
  other specified B60.19
Acanthocephaliasis B83.8
Acanthocheilonemiasis B74.4
Acanthocytosis E78.6
Acantholysis L11.9
Acanthosis (acquired) (nigricans) L83
  benign Q82.8
  congenital Q82.8
  seborrheic L82.1
    inflamed L82.0
  tongue K14.3
Acapnia E87.3
Acarbia E87.2
Acardia, acardius Q89.8
Acardiacus amorphus Q89.8
Acardiotrophia I51.4
Acariasis B88.0
  scabies B86

Acarodermatitis (urticarioides) B88.0
Acarophobia F40.218
Acatalasemia, acatalasia E80.3
Acathisia (drug induced) G25.71
Accelerated atrioventricular conduction I45.6
Accentuation of personality traits (type A) Z73.1
Accessory (congenital)
  adrenal gland Q89.1
  anus Q43.4
  appendix Q43.4
  atrioventricular conduction I45.6
  auditory ossicles Q16.3
  auricle (ear) Q17.0
  biliary duct or passage Q44.5
  bladder Q64.79
  blood vessels NEC Q27.9
    coronary Q24.5
  bone NEC Q79.8
  breast tissue, axilla Q83.1
  carpal bones Q74.0
  cecum Q43.4
  chromosome(s) NEC (nonsex) Q92.9
    with complex rearrangements NEC Q92.5
      seen only at prometaphase Q92.8
    13 — *see* Trisomy, 13
    18 — *see* Trisomy, 18
    21 — *see* Trisomy, 21
    partial Q92.9
    sex
      female phenotype Q97.8
  coronary artery Q24.5
  cusp(s), heart valve NEC Q24.8
    pulmonary Q22.3
  cystic duct Q44.5
  digit(s) Q69.9
  ear (auricle) (lobe) Q17.0
  endocrine gland NEC Q89.2
  eye muscle Q10.3
  eyelid Q10.3
  face bone(s) Q75.8
  fallopian tube (fimbria) (ostium) Q50.6
  finger(s) Q69.0
  foreskin N47.8
  frontonasal process Q75.8
  gallbladder Q44.1
  genital organ(s)
    female Q52.8
      external Q52.79
      internal NEC Q52.8
    male Q55.8
  genitourinary organs NEC Q89.8
    female Q52.8
    male Q55.8
  hallux Q69.2
  heart Q24.8
    valve NEC Q24.8
      pulmonary Q22.3
  hepatic ducts Q44.5
  hymen Q52.4
  intestine (large) (small) Q43.4
  kidney Q63.0
  lacrimal canal Q10.6
  leaflet, heart valve NEC Q24.8
  ligament, broad Q50.6
  liver Q44.7
    duct Q44.5
  lobule (ear) Q17.0
  lung (lobe) Q33.1
  muscle Q79.8
  navicular of carpus Q74.0
  nervous system, part NEC Q07.8
  nipple Q83.3
  nose Q30.8
  organ or site not listed — *see* Anomaly, by site
  ovary Q50.31
  oviduct Q50.6
  pancreas Q45.3
  parathyroid gland Q89.2
  parotid gland (and duct) Q38.4
  pituitary gland Q89.2
  preauricular appendage Q17.0
  prepuce N47.8
  renal arteries (multiple) Q27.2
  rib Q76.6
    cervical Q76.5
  roots (teeth) K00.2
  salivary gland Q38.4
  sesamoid bones Q74.8

Accessory — *continued*
  sesamoid bones — *continued*
    foot Q74.2
    hand Q74.0
  skin tags Q82.8
  spleen Q89.09
  sternum Q76.7
  submaxillary gland Q38.4
  tarsal bones Q74.2
  teeth, tooth K00.1
  tendon Q79.8
  thumb Q69.1
  thymus gland Q89.2
  thyroid gland Q89.2
  toes Q69.2
  tongue Q38.3
  tooth, teeth K00.1
  tragus Q17.0
  ureter Q62.5
  urethra Q64.79
  urinary organ or tract NEC Q64.8
  uterus Q51.2
  vagina Q52.10
  valve, heart NEC Q24.8
    pulmonary Q22.3
  vertebra Q76.49
  vocal cords Q31.8
  vulva Q52.79
Accident
  birth — *see* Birth, injury
  cardiac — *see* Infarct, myocardium
  cerebral I63.9
  cerebrovascular (embolic) (ischemic) (thrombotic) I63.9
    aborted I63.9
    hemorrhagic — *see* Hemorrhage, intracranial, intracerebral
    old (without sequelae) Z86.73
      with sequelae (of) — *see* Sequelae, infarction, cerebral
  coronary — *see* Infarct, myocardium
  craniovascular I63.9
  vascular, brain I63.9
Accidental — *see* condition
Accommodation (disorder) (*see also* condition)
  hysterical paralysis of F44.89
  insufficiency of H52.4
  paresis — *see* Paresis, of accommodation
  spasm — *see* Spasm, of accommodation
Accouchement — *see* Delivery
Accreta placenta O43.21- ☑
Accretio cordis (nonrheumatic) I31.0
Accretions, tooth, teeth K03.6
Acculturation difficulty Z60.3
Accumulation secretion, prostate N42.89
Acephalia, acephalism, acephalus, acephaly Q00.0
Acephalobrachia monster Q89.8
Acephalochirus monster Q89.8
Acephalogaster Q89.8
Acephalostomus monster Q89.8
Acephalothorax Q89.8
Acerophobia F40.298
Acetonemia R79.89
  in Type 1 diabetes E10.10
    with coma E10.11
Acetonuria R82.4
Achalasia (cardia) (esophagus) K22.0
  congenital Q39.5
  pylorus Q40.0
  sphincteral NEC K59.8
Ache(s) — *see* Pain
Acheilia Q38.6
Achillobursitis — *see* Tendinitis, Achilles
Achillodynia — *see* Tendinitis, Achilles
Achlorhydria, achlorhydric (neurogenic) K31.83
  anemia D50.8
  diarrhea K31.83
  psychogenic F45.8
  secondary to vagotomy K91.1
Achluophobia F40.228
Acholia K82.8
Acholuric jaundice (familial) (splenomegalic) (*see also* Spherocytosis)
  acquired D59.8
Achondrogenesis Q77.0
Achondroplasia (osteosclerosis congenita) Q77.4
Achroma, cutis L80

Achromat (ism), achromatopsia (acquired) (congenital) H53.51
Achromia, congenital — see Albinism
Achromia parasitica B36.0
Achylia gastrica K31.89
 psychogenic F45.8
Acid
 burn — see Corrosion
 deficiency
  amide nicotinic E52
  ascorbic E54
  folic E53.8
  nicotinic E52
  pantothenic E53.8
 intoxication E87.2
 peptic disease K30
 phosphatase deficiency E83.39
 stomach K30
  psychogenic F45.8
Acidemia E87.2
 argininosuccinic E72.22
 isovaleric E71.110
 metabolic (newborn) P19.9
  first noted before onset of labor P19.0
  first noted during labor P19.1
  noted at birth P19.2
 methylmalonic E71.120
 pipecolic E72.3
 propionic E71.121
Acidity, gastric (high) K30
 psychogenic F45.8
Acidocytopenia — see Agranulocytosis
Acidocytosis D72.1
Acidopenia — see Agranulocytosis
Acidosis (lactic) (respiratory) E87.2
 in Type 1 diabetes E10.10
  with coma E10.11
 kidney, tubular N25.89
 lactic E87.2
 metabolic NEC E87.2
  with respiratory acidosis E87.4
  late, of newborn P74.0
 mixed metabolic and respiratory, newborn P84
 newborn P84
 renal (hyperchloremic) (tubular) N25.89
 respiratory E87.2
  complicated by
   metabolic
    acidosis E87.4
    alkalosis E87.4
Aciduria
 argininosuccinic E72.22
 glutaric (type I) E72.3
  type II E71.313
  type III E71.5- ☑
 orotic (congenital) (hereditary) (pyrimidine deficiency) E79.8
  anemia D53.0
Acladiosis (skin) B36.0
Aclasis, diaphyseal Q78.6
Acleistocardia Q21.1
Aclusion — see Anomaly, dentofacial, malocclusion
Acne L70.9
 artificialis L70.8
 atrophica L70.2
 cachecticorum (Hebra) L70.8
 conglobata L70.1
 cystic L70.0
 decalvans L66.2
 excoriée (des jeunes filles) L70.5
 frontalis L70.2
 indurata L70.0
 infantile L70.4
 keloid L73.0
 lupoid L70.2
 necrotic, necrotica (miliaris) L70.2
 neonatal L70.4
 nodular L70.0
 occupational L70.8
 picker's L70.5
 pustular L70.0
 rodens L70.2
 rosacea L71.9
 specified NEC L70.8
 tropica L70.3
 varioliformis L70.2
 vulgaris L70.0
Acnitis (primary) A18.4

Acosta's disease T70.29 ☑
Acoustic — see condition
Acousticophobia F40.298
Acquired (see also condition)
 immunodeficiency syndrome (AIDS) B20
Acrania Q00.0
Acroangiodermatitis I78.9
Acroasphyxia, chronic I73.89
Acrobystitis N47.7
Acrocephalopolysyndactyly Q87.0
Acrocephalosyndactyly Q87.0
Acrocephaly Q75.0
Acrochondrohyperplasia — see Syndrome, Marfan's
Acrocyanosis I73.8 ☑
 newborn P28.2
  meaning transient blue hands and feet — omit code
Acrodermatitis L30.8
 atrophicans (chronica) L90.4
 continua (Hallopeau) L40.2
 enteropathica (hereditary) E83.2
 Hallopeau's L40.2
 infantile papular L44.4
 perstans L40.2
 pustulosa continua L40.2
 recalcitrant pustular L40.2
Acrodynia — see Poisoning, mercury
Acromegaly, acromegalia E22.0
Acromelalgia I73.81
Acromicria, acromikria Q79.8
Acronyx L60.0
Acropachy, thyroid — see Thyrotoxicosis
Acroparesthesia (simple) (vasomotor) I73.89
Acropathy, thyroid — see Thyrotoxicosis
Acrophobia F40.241
Acroposthitis N47.7
Acroscleriasis, acroscleroderma, acrosclerosis — see Sclerosis, systemic
Acrosphacelus I96
Acrospiroma, eccrine — see Neoplasm, skin, benign
Acrostealgia — see Osteochondropathy
Acrotrophodynia — see Immersion
ACTH ectopic syndrome E24.3
Actinic — see condition
Actinobacillosis, actinobacillus A28.8
 mallei A24.0
 muris A25.1
Actinomyces israelii (infection) — see Actinomycosis
Actinomycetoma (foot) B47.1
Actinomycosis, actinomycotic A42.9
 with pneumonia A42.0
 abdominal A42.1
 cervicofacial A42.2
 cutaneous A42.89
 gastrointestinal A42.1
 pulmonary A42.0
 sepsis A42.7
 specified site NEC A42.89
Actinoneuritis G62.82
Action, heart
 disorder I49.9
 irregular I49.9
  psychogenic F45.8
Activated protein C resistance D68.51
Activation
 mast cell (disorder) (syndrome) D89.40
  idiopathic D89.42
  monoclonal D89.41
  secondary D89.43
  specified type NEC D89.49
Active — see condition
Acute (see also condition)
 abdomen R10.0
 gallbladder — see Cholecystitis, acute
Acyanotic heart disease (congenital) Q24.9
Acystia Q64.5
Adair-Dighton syndrome (brittle bones and blue sclera, deafness) Q78.0
Adamantinoblastoma — see Ameloblastoma
Adamantinoma (see also Cyst, calcifying odontogenic)
 long bones C40.90
  lower limb C40.2- ☑
  upper limb C40.0- ☑
 malignant C41.1
  jaw (bone) (lower) C41.1
   upper C41.0
 tibial C40.2- ☑

Adamantoblastoma — see Ameloblastoma
Adams-Stokes (-Morgagni) disease or syndrome I45.9
Adaption reaction — see Disorder, adjustment
Addiction (see also Dependence) F19.20
 alcohol, alcoholic (ethyl) (methyl) (wood) (without remission) F10.20
  with remission F10.21
 drug — see Dependence, drug
 ethyl alcohol (without remission) F10.20
  with remission F10.21
 heroin — see Dependence, drug, opioid
 methyl alcohol (without remission) F10.20
  with remission F10.21
 methylated spirit (without remission) F10.20
  with remission F10.21
 morphine (-like substances) — see Dependence, drug, opioid
 nicotine — see Dependence, drug, nicotine
 opium and opioids — see Dependence, drug, opioid
 tobacco — see Dependence, drug, nicotine
Addison-Biermer anemia (pernicious) D51.0
Addisonian crisis E27.2
Addison's
 anemia (pernicious) D51.0
 disease (bronze) or syndrome E27.1
  tuberculous A18.7
 keloid L94.0
Addison-Schilder complex E71.528
Additional (see also Accessory)
 chromosome(s) Q99.8
  21 — see Trisomy, 21
 sex — see Abnormal, chromosome, sex
Adduction contracture, hip or other joint — see Contraction, joint
Adenitis (see also Lymphadenitis)
 acute, unspecified site L04.9
 axillary I88.9
  acute L04.2
  chronic or subacute I88.1
 Bartholin's gland N75.8
 bulbourethral gland — see Urethritis
 cervical I88.9
  acute L04.0
  chronic or subacute I88.1
 chancroid (Hemophilus ducreyi) A57
 chronic, unspecified site I88.1
 Cowper's gland — see Urethritis
 due to Pasteurella multocida (P. septica) A28.0
 epidemic, acute B27.09
 gangrenous L04.9
 gonorrheal NEC A54.89
 groin I88.9
  acute L04.1
  chronic or subacute I88.1
 infectious (acute) (epidemic) B27.09
 inguinal I88.9
  acute L04.1
  chronic or subacute I88.1
 lymph gland or node, except mesenteric I88.9
  acute — see Lymphadenitis, acute
  chronic or subacute I88.1
 mesenteric (acute) (chronic) (nonspecific) (subacute) I88.0
 parotid gland (suppurative) — see Sialoadenitis
 salivary gland (any) (suppurative) — see Sialoadenitis
 scrofulous (tuberculous) A18.2
 Skene's duct or gland — see Urethritis
 strumous, tuberculous A18.2
 subacute, unspecified site I88.1
 sublingual gland (suppurative) — see Sialoadenitis
 submandibular gland (suppurative) — see Sialoadenitis
 submaxillary gland (suppurative) — see Sialoadenitis
 tuberculous — see Tuberculosis, lymph gland
 urethral gland — see Urethritis
 Wharton's duct (suppurative) — see Sialoadenitis
Adenoacanthoma — see Neoplasm, malignant, by site
Adenoameloblastoma — see Cyst, calcifying odontogenic
Adenocarcinoid (tumor) — see Neoplasm, malignant, by site
Adenocarcinoma (see also Neoplasm, malignant, by site)
 acidophil
  specified site — see Neoplasm, malignant, by site
  unspecified site C75.1
 adrenal cortical C74.0- ☑
 alveolar — see Neoplasm, lung, malignant

☑ **Additional Character Required** — Refer to the Tabular List for Character Selection   ▽ **Subterms under main terms may continue to next column or page**

Adenocarcinoma — *continued*
  apocrine
    breast — *see* Neoplasm, breast, malignant
    in situ
      breast D05.8- ☑
      specified site NEC — *see* Neoplasm, skin, in situ
      unspecified site D04.9
    specified site NEC — *see* Neoplasm, skin, malignant
    unspecified site C44.99
  basal cell
    specified site — *see* Neoplasm, skin, malignant
    unspecified site C08.9
  basophil
    specified site — *see* Neoplasm, malignant, by site
    unspecified site C75.1
  bile duct type C22.1
    liver C22.1
    specified site NEC — *see* Neoplasm, malignant, by
      site
    unspecified site C22.1
  bronchiolar — *see* Neoplasm, lung, malignant
  bronchioloalveolar — *see* Neoplasm, lung, malignant
  ceruminous C44.29- ☑
  cervix, in situ (*see also* Carcinoma, cervix uteri, in situ)
    D06.9
  chromophobe
    specified site — *see* Neoplasm, malignant, by site
    unspecified site C75.1
  diffuse type
    specified site — *see* Neoplasm, malignant, by site
    unspecified site C16.9
  duct
    infiltrating
      with Paget's disease — *see* Neoplasm, breast,
        malignant
      specified site — *see* Neoplasm, malignant, by
        site
      unspecified site (female) C50.91- ☑
        male C50.92- ☑
    specified site — *see* Neoplasm, malignant, by site
    unspecified site
      female C56.9
      male C61
  eosinophil
    specified site — *see* Neoplasm, malignant, by site
    unspecified site C75.1
  follicular
    with papillary C73
    moderately differentiated C73
    specified site — *see* Neoplasm, malignant, by site
    trabecular C73
    unspecified site C73
    well differentiated C73
  Hurthle cell C73
  in
    adenomatous
      polyposis coli C18.9
  infiltrating duct
    with Paget's disease — *see* Neoplasm, breast, ma-
      lignant
    specified site — *see* Neoplasm, by site, malignant
    unspecified site (female) C50.91- ☑
      male C50.92- ☑
  inflammatory
    specified site — *see* Neoplasm, by site, malignant
    unspecified site (female) C50.91- ☑
      male C50.92- ☑
  intestinal type
    specified site — *see* Neoplasm, by site, malignant
    unspecified site C16.9
  intracystic papillary
  intraductal
    breast D05.1- ☑
    noninfiltrating
      breast D05.1- ☑
      papillary
        with invasion
          specified site — *see* Neoplasm, by site,
            malignant
          unspecified site (female) C50.91- ☑
            male C50.92- ☑
        breast D05.1- ☑
        specified site NEC — *see* Neoplasm, in situ,
          by site
        unspecified site D05.1- ☑
      specified site NEC — *see* Neoplasm, in situ, by
        site

Adenocarcinoma — *continued*
  intraductal — *continued*
    noninfiltrating — *continued*
      unspecified site D05.1- ☑
    papillary
      with invasion
        specified site — *see* Neoplasm, malignant,
          by site
        unspecified site (female) C50.91- ☑
          male C50.92- ☑
      breast D05.1- ☑
    specified site — *see* Neoplasm, in situ, by site
    unspecified site D05.1- ☑
  specified site NEC — *see* Neoplasm, in situ, by site
  unspecified site D05.1- ☑
  islet cell
    with exocrine, mixed
      specified site — *see* Neoplasm, malignant, by
        site
      unspecified site C25.9
    pancreas C25.4
    specified site NEC — *see* Neoplasm, malignant, by
      site
    unspecified site C25.4
  lobular
    in situ
      breast D05.0- ☑
      specified site NEC — *see* Neoplasm, in situ, by
        site
      unspecified site D05.0- ☑
    specified site — *see* Neoplasm, malignant, by site
    unspecified site (female) C50.91- ☑
      male C50.92- ☑
  mucoid (*see also* Neoplasm, malignant, by site)
    cell
      specified site — *see* Neoplasm, malignant, by
        site
      unspecified site C75.1
  nonencapsulated sclerosing C73
  papillary
    with follicular C73
    follicular variant C73
    intraductal (noninfiltrating)
      with invasion
        specified site — *see* Neoplasm, malignant,
          by site
        unspecified site (female) C50.91- ☑
          male C50.92- ☑
      breast D05.1- ☑
      specified site NEC — *see* Neoplasm, in situ, by
        site
      unspecified site D05.1- ☑
    serous
      specified site — *see* Neoplasm, malignant, by
        site
      unspecified site C56.9
  papillocystic
    specified site — *see* Neoplasm, malignant, by site
    unspecified site C56.9
  pseudomucinous
    specified site — *see* Neoplasm, malignant, by site
    unspecified site C56.9
  renal cell C64- ☑
  sebaceous — *see* Neoplasm, skin, malignant
  serous (*see also* Neoplasm, malignant, by site)
    papillary
      specified site — *see* Neoplasm, malignant, by
        site
      unspecified site C56.9
  sweat gland — *see* Neoplasm, skin, malignant
  water-clear cell C75.0
Adenocarcinoma-in-situ (*see also* Neoplasm, in situ, by
  site)
  breast D05.9- ☑
Adenofibroma
  clear cell — *see* Neoplasm, benign, by site
  endometrioid D27.9
    borderline malignancy D39.10
    malignant C56- ☑
  mucinous
    specified site — *see* Neoplasm, benign, by site
    unspecified site D27.9
  papillary
    specified site — *see* Neoplasm, benign, by site
    unspecified site D27.9
  prostate — *see* Enlargement, enlarged, prostate

Adenofibroma — *continued*
  serous
    specified site — *see* Neoplasm, benign, by site
    unspecified site D27.9
  specified site — *see* Neoplasm, benign, by site
  unspecified site D27.9
Adenofibrosis
  breast — *see* Fibroadenosis, breast
  endometrioid N80.0
Adenoiditis (chronic) J35.02
  with tonsillitis J35.03
  acute J03.90
    recurrent J03.91
    specified organism NEC J03.80
      recurrent J03.81
    staphylococcal J03.80
      recurrent J03.81
    streptococcal J03.00
      recurrent J03.01
Adenoids — *see* condition
Adenolipoma — *see* Neoplasm, benign, by site
Adenolipomatosis, Launois-Bensaude E88.89
Adenolymphoma
  specified site — *see* Neoplasm, benign, by site
  unspecified site D11.9
Adenoma (*see also* Neoplasm, benign, by site)
  acidophil
    specified site — *see* Neoplasm, benign, by site
    unspecified site D35.2
  acidophil-basophil, mixed
    specified site — *see* Neoplasm, benign, by site
    unspecified site D35.2
  adrenal (cortical) D35.00
    clear cell D35.00
    compact cell D35.00
    glomerulosa cell D35.00
    heavily pigmented variant D35.00
    mixed cell D35.00
  alpha-cell
    pancreas D13.7
    specified site NEC — *see* Neoplasm, benign, by site
    unspecified site D13.7
  alveolar D14.30
  apocrine
    breast D24- ☑
    specified site NEC — *see* Neoplasm, skin, benign,
      by site
    unspecified site D23.9
  basal cell D11.9
  basophil
    specified site — *see* Neoplasm, benign, by site
    unspecified site D35.2
  basophil-acidophil, mixed
    specified site — *see* Neoplasm, benign, by site
    unspecified site D35.2
  beta-cell
    pancreas D13.7
    specified site NEC — *see* Neoplasm, benign, by site
    unspecified site D13.7
  bile duct D13.4
    common D13.5
    extrahepatic D13.5
    intrahepatic D13.4
    specified site NEC — *see* Neoplasm, benign, by site
    unspecified site D13.4
  black D35.00
  bronchial D38.1
    cylindroid type — *see* Neoplasm, lung, malignant
  ceruminous D23.2- ☑
  chief cell D35.1
  chromophobe
    specified site — *see* Neoplasm, benign, by site
    unspecified site D35.2
  colloid
    specified site — *see* Neoplasm, benign, by site
    unspecified site D34
  duct
  eccrine, papillary — *see* Neoplasm, skin, benign
  endocrine, multiple
    single specified site — *see* Neoplasm, uncertain
      behavior, by site
    two or more specified sites D44- ☑
    unspecified site D44.9
  endometrioid (*see also* Neoplasm, benign)
    borderline malignancy — *see* Neoplasm, uncertain
      behavior, by site
  eosinophil
    specified site — *see* Neoplasm, benign, by site

Adenoma — *continued*
eosinophil — *continued*
unspecified site D35.2
fetal
specified site — *see* Neoplasm, benign, by site
unspecified site D34
follicular
specified site — *see* Neoplasm, benign, by site
unspecified site D34
hepatocellular D13.4
Hurthle cell D34
islet cell
pancreas D13.7
specified site NEC — *see* Neoplasm, benign, by site
unspecified site D13.7
liver cell D13.4
macrofollicular
specified site — *see* Neoplasm, benign, by site
unspecified site D34
malignant, malignum — *see* Neoplasm, malignant, by site
microcystic
pancreas D13.6
specified site NEC — *see* Neoplasm, benign, by site
unspecified site D13.6
microfollicular
specified site — *see* Neoplasm, benign, by site
unspecified site D34
mucoid cell
specified site — *see* Neoplasm, benign, by site
unspecified site D35.2
multiple endocrine
single specified site — *see* Neoplasm, uncertain behavior, by site
two or more specified sites D44- ☑
unspecified site D44.9
nipple D24- ☑
papillary (*see also* Neoplasm, benign, by site)
eccrine — *see* Neoplasm, skin, benign, by site
Pick's tubular
specified site — *see* Neoplasm, benign, by site
unspecified site
female D27.9
male D29.20
pleomorphic
carcinoma in — *see* Neoplasm, salivary gland, malignant
specified site — *see* Neoplasm, malignant, by site
unspecified site C08.9
polypoid (*see also* Neoplasm, benign)
adenocarcinoma in — *see* Neoplasm, malignant, by site
adenocarcinoma in situ — *see* Neoplasm, in situ, by site
prostate — *see* Neoplasm, benign, prostate
rete cell D29.20
sebaceous — *see* Neoplasm, skin, benign
Sertoli cell
specified site — *see* Neoplasm, benign, by site
unspecified site
female D27.9
male D29.20
skin appendage — *see* Neoplasm, skin, benign
sudoriferous gland — *see* Neoplasm, skin, benign
sweat gland — *see* Neoplasm, skin, benign
testicular
specified site — *see* Neoplasm, benign, by site
unspecified site
female D27.9
male D29.20
tubular (*see also* Neoplasm, benign, by site)
adenocarcinoma in — *see* Neoplasm, malignant, by site
adenocarcinoma in situ — *see* Neoplasm, in situ, by site
Pick's
specified site — *see* Neoplasm, benign, by site
unspecified site
female D27.9
male D29.20
tubulovillous (*see also* Neoplasm, benign, by site)
adenocarcinoma in — *see* Neoplasm, malignant, by site
adenocarcinoma in situ — *see* Neoplasm, in situ, by site
villous — *see* Neoplasm, uncertain behavior, by site

Adenoma — *continued*
villous — *see* Neoplasm, uncertain behavior, by site
— *continued*
adenocarcinoma in — *see* Neoplasm, malignant, by site
adenocarcinoma in situ — *see* Neoplasm, in situ, by site
water-clear cell D35.1
Adenomatosis
endocrine (multiple) E31.20
single specified site — *see* Neoplasm, uncertain behavior, by site
erosive of nipple D24- ☑
pluriendocrine — *see* Adenomatosis, endocrine
pulmonary D38.1
malignant — *see* Neoplasm, lung, malignant
specified site — *see* Neoplasm, benign, by site
unspecified site D12.6
Adenomatous
goiter (nontoxic) E04.9
with hyperthyroidism — *see* Hyperthyroidism, with, goiter, nodular
toxic — *see* Hyperthyroidism, with, goiter, nodular
Adenomyoma (*see also* Neoplasm, benign, by site)
prostate — *see* Enlarged, prostate
Adenomyometritis N80.0
Adenomyosis N80.0
Adenopathy (lymph gland) R59.9
generalized R59.1
inguinal R59.0
localized R59.0
mediastinal R59.0
mesentery R59.0
syphilitic (secondary) A51.49
tracheobronchial R59.0
tuberculous A15.4
primary (progressive) A15.7
tuberculous (*see also* Tuberculosis, lymph gland)
tracheobronchial A15.4
primary (progressive) A15.7
Adenosalpingitis — *see* Salpingitis
Adenosarcoma — *see* Neoplasm, malignant, by site
Adenosclerosis I88.8
Adenosis (sclerosing) breast — *see* Fibroadenosis, breast
Adenovirus, as cause of disease classified elsewhere B97.0
Adentia (complete) (partial) — *see* Absence, teeth
Adherent (*see also* Adhesions)
labia (minora) N90.89
pericardium (nonrheumatic) I31.0
rheumatic I09.2
placenta (with hemorrhage) O72.0
without hemorrhage O73.0
prepuce, newborn N47.0
scar (skin) L90.5
tendon in scar L90.5
Adhesions, adhesive (postinfective) K66.0
with intestinal obstruction K56.50
complete K56.52
incomplete K56.51
partial K56.51
abdominal (wall) — *see* Adhesions, peritoneum
appendix K38.8
bile duct (common) (hepatic) K83.8
bladder (sphincter) N32.89
bowel — *see* Adhesions, peritoneum
cardiac I31.0
rheumatic I09.2
cecum — *see* Adhesions, peritoneum
cervicovaginal N88.1
congenital Q52.8
postpartal O90.89
old N88.1
cervix N88.1
ciliary body NEC — *see* Adhesions, iris
clitoris N90.89
colon — *see* Adhesions, peritoneum
common duct K83.8
congenital (*see also* Anomaly, by site)
fingers — *see* Syndactylism, complex, fingers
omental, anomalous Q43.3
peritoneal Q43.3
tongue (to gum or roof of mouth) Q38.3
conjunctiva (acquired) H11.21- ☑
congenital Q15.8
cystic duct K82.8
diaphragm — *see* Adhesions, peritoneum
due to foreign body — *see* Foreign body

Adhesions, adhesive — *continued*
duodenum — *see* Adhesions, peritoneum
ear
middle H74.1- ☑
epididymis N50.89
epidural — *see* Adhesions, meninges
epiglottis J38.7
eyelid H02.59
female pelvis N73.6
gallbladder K82.8
globe H44.89
heart I31.0
rheumatic I09.2
ileocecal (coil) — *see* Adhesions, peritoneum
ileum — *see* Adhesions, peritoneum
intestine (*see also* Adhesions, peritoneum)
with obstruction K56.50
complete K56.52
incomplete K56.51
partial K56.51
intra-abdominal — *see* Adhesions, peritoneum
iris H21.50- ☑
anterior H21.51- ☑
goniosynechiae H21.52- ☑
posterior H21.54- ☑
to corneal graft T85.898 ☑
joint — *see* Ankylosis
knee M23.8X ☑
temporomandibular M26.61- ☑
labium (majus) (minus), congenital Q52.5
liver — *see* Adhesions, peritoneum
lung J98.4
mediastinum J98.59
meninges (cerebral) (spinal) G96.12
congenital Q07.8
tuberculous (cerebral) (spinal) A17.0
mesenteric — *see* Adhesions, peritoneum
nasal (septum) (to turbinates) J34.89
ocular muscle — *see* Strabismus, mechanical
omentum — *see* Adhesions, peritoneum
ovary N73.6
congenital (to cecum, kidney or omentum) Q50.39
paraovarian N73.6
pelvic (peritoneal)
female N73.6
postprocedural N99.4
male — *see* Adhesions, peritoneum
postpartal (old) N73.6
tuberculous A18.17
penis to scrotum (congenital) Q55.8
periappendiceal (*see also* Adhesions, peritoneum)
pericardium (nonrheumatic) I31.0
focal I31.8
rheumatic I09.2
tuberculous A18.84
pericholecystic K82.8
perigastric — *see* Adhesions, peritoneum
periovarian N73.6
periprostatic N42.89
perirectal — *see* Adhesions, peritoneum
perirenal N28.89
peritoneum, peritoneal (postinfective)
with obstruction (intestinal) K56.50
complete K56.52
incomplete K56.51
partial K56.51
congenital Q43.3
pelvic, female N73.6
postprocedural N99.4
postpartal, pelvic N73.6
postprocedural K66.0
to uterus N73.6
peritubal N73.6
periureteral N28.89
periuterine N73.6
perivesical N32.89
perivesicular (seminal vesicle) N50.89
pleura, pleuritic J94.8
tuberculous NEC A15.6
pleuropericardial J94.8
postoperative (gastrointestinal tract) K66.0
with obstruction (*see also* Obstruction, intestine, postoperative) K91.30
due to foreign body accidentally left in wound — *see* Foreign body, accidentally left during a procedure
pelvic peritoneal N99.4
urethra — *see* Stricture, urethra, postprocedural

Adhesions, adhesive — *continued*
　postoperative — *continued*
　　vagina N99.2
　postpartal, old (vulva or perineum) N90.89
　preputial, prepuce N47.5
　pulmonary J98.4
　pylorus — *see* Adhesions, peritoneum
　sciatic nerve — *see* Lesion, nerve, sciatic
　seminal vesicle N50.89
　shoulder (joint) — *see* Capsulitis, adhesive
　sigmoid flexure — *see* Adhesions, peritoneum
　spermatic cord (acquired) N50.89
　　congenital Q55.4
　spinal canal G96.12
　stomach — *see* Adhesions, peritoneum
　subscapular — *see* Capsulitis, adhesive
　temporomandibular M26.61- ☑
　tendinitis (*see also* Tenosynovitis, specified type NEC)
　　shoulder — *see* Capsulitis, adhesive
　testis N44.8
　tongue, congenital (to gum or roof of mouth) Q38.3
　　acquired K14.8
　trachea J39.8
　tubo-ovarian N73.6
　tunica vaginalis N44.8
　uterus N73.6
　　internal N85.6
　　to abdominal wall N73.6
　vagina (chronic) N89.5
　　postoperative N99.2
　vitreomacular H43.82- ☑
　vitreous H43.89
　vulva N90.89
Adiaspiromycosis B48.8
Adie (-Holmes) pupil or syndrome — *see* Anomaly,
　pupil, function, tonic pupil
Adiponecrosis neonatorum P83.88
Adiposis (*see also* Obesity)
　cerebralis E23.6
　dolorosa E88.2
Adiposity (*see also* Obesity)
　heart — *see* Degeneration, myocardial
　localized E65
Adiposogenital dystrophy E23.6
Adjustment
　disorder — *see* Disorder, adjustment
　implanted device — *see* Encounter (for), adjustment
　　(of)
　prosthesis, external — *see* Fitting
　reaction — *see* Disorder, adjustment
Administration of tPA (rtPA) in a different facility within
　the last 24 hours prior to admission to current facil-
　ity Z92.82
Admission (for) (*see also* Encounter (for))
　adjustment (of)
　　artificial
　　　arm Z44.00- ☑
　　　　complete Z44.01- ☑
　　　　partial Z44.02- ☑
　　　eye Z44.2 ☑
　　　leg Z44.10- ☑
　　　　complete Z44.11- ☑
　　　　partial Z44.12- ☑
　　　brain neuropacemaker Z46.2
　　　　implanted Z45.42
　　　breast
　　　　implant Z45.81 ☑
　　　　prosthesis (external) Z44.3 ☑
　　　colostomy belt Z46.89
　　　contact lenses Z46.0
　　　cystostomy device Z46.6
　　　dental prosthesis Z46.3
　　　device NEC
　　　　abdominal Z46.89
　　　　implanted Z45.89
　　　　　cardiac Z45.09
　　　　　　defibrillator (with synchronous cardiac
　　　　　　　pacemaker) Z45.02
　　　　　　pacemaker (cardiac resynchronization
　　　　　　　therapy (CRT-P)) Z45.018
　　　　　　　pulse generator Z45.010
　　　　　　resynchronization therapy defibrillator
　　　　　　　(CRT-D) Z45.02
　　　　　hearing device Z45.328
　　　　　　bone conduction Z45.320
　　　　　　cochlear Z45.321
　　　　　infusion pump Z45.1
　　　　　nervous system Z45.49

Admission — *continued*
　adjustment — *continued*
　　device — *continued*
　　　implanted — *continued*
　　　　nervous system — *continued*
　　　　　CSF drainage Z45.41
　　　　　hearing device — *see* Admission, adjust-
　　　　　　ment, device, implanted, hearing
　　　　　　device
　　　　　neuropacemaker Z45.42
　　　　　visual substitution Z45.31
　　　　specified NEC Z45.89
　　　　vascular access Z45.2
　　　　visual substitution Z45.31
　　　nervous system Z46.2
　　　　implanted — *see* Admission, adjustment,
　　　　　device, implanted, nervous system
　　　orthodontic Z46.4
　　　prosthetic Z44.9
　　　　arm — *see* Admission, adjustment, artificial,
　　　　　arm
　　　　breast Z44.3 ☑
　　　　dental Z46.3
　　　　eye Z44.2 ☑
　　　　leg — *see* Admission, adjustment, artificial,
　　　　　leg
　　　　specified type NEC Z44.8
　　　substitution
　　　　auditory Z46.2
　　　　　implanted — *see* Admission, adjust-
　　　　　　ment, device, implanted, hearing
　　　　　　device
　　　　nervous system Z46.2
　　　　　implanted — *see* Admission, adjust-
　　　　　　ment, device, implanted, nervous
　　　　　　system
　　　　visual Z46.2
　　　　　implanted Z45.31
　　　urinary Z46.6
　　hearing aid Z46.1
　　　implanted — *see* Admission, adjustment, de-
　　　　vice, implanted, hearing device
　　ileostomy device Z46.89
　　intestinal appliance or device NEC Z46.89
　　neuropacemaker (brain) (peripheral nerve) (spinal
　　　cord) Z46.2
　　　implanted Z45.42
　　orthodontic device Z46.4
　　orthopedic (brace) (cast) (device) (shoes) Z46.89
　　pacemaker (cardiac resynchronization therapy
　　　(CRT-P))
　　　cardiac Z45.018
　　　　pulse generator Z45.010
　　　nervous system Z46.2
　　　　implanted Z45.42
　　portacath (port-a-cath) Z45.2
　　prosthesis Z44.9
　　　arm — *see* Admission, adjustment, artificial,
　　　　arm
　　　breast Z44.3 ☑
　　　dental Z46.3
　　　eye Z44.2 ☑
　　　leg — *see* Admission, adjustment, artificial, leg
　　　specified NEC Z44.8
　　spectacles Z46.0
　aftercare (*see also* Aftercare) Z51.89
　　postpartum
　　　immediately after delivery Z39.0
　　　routine follow-up Z39.2
　　radiation therapy (antineoplastic) Z51.0
　attention to artificial opening (of) Z43.9
　　artificial vagina Z43.7
　　colostomy Z43.3
　　cystostomy Z43.5
　　enterostomy Z43.4
　　gastrostomy Z43.1
　　ileostomy Z43.2
　　jejunostomy Z43.4
　　nephrostomy Z43.6
　　specified site NEC Z43.8
　　　intestinal tract Z43.4
　　　urinary tract Z43.6
　　tracheostomy Z43.0
　　ureterostomy Z43.6
　　urethrostomy Z43.6
　breast augmentation or reduction Z41.1
　breast reconstruction following mastectomy Z42.1

Admission — *continued*
　change of
　　dressing (nonsurgical) Z48.00
　　neuropacemaker device (brain) (peripheral nerve)
　　　(spinal cord) Z46.2
　　　implanted Z45.42
　　surgical dressing Z48.01
　circumcision, ritual or routine (in absence of diagnosis)
　　Z41.2
　clinical research investigation (control) (normal com-
　　parison) (participant) Z00.6
　contraceptive management Z30.9
　cosmetic surgery NEC Z41.1
　counseling (*see also* Counseling)
　　dietary Z71.3
　　gestational carrier Z31.7
　　HIV Z71.7
　　human immunodeficiency virus Z71.7
　　nonattending third party Z71.0
　　procreative management NEC Z31.69
　delivery, full-term, uncomplicated O80
　　cesarean, without indication O82
　desensitization to allergens Z51.6
　dietary surveillance and counseling Z71.3
　ear piercing Z41.3
　examination at health care facility (adult) (*see also*
　　Examination) Z00.00
　　with abnormal findings Z00.01
　　clinical research investigation (control) (normal
　　　comparison) (participant) Z00.6
　　dental Z01.20
　　　with abnormal findings Z01.21
　　donor (potential) Z00.5
　　ear Z01.10
　　　with abnormal findings NEC Z01.118
　　eye Z01.00
　　　with abnormal findings Z01.01
　　general, specified reason NEC Z00.8
　　hearing Z01.10
　　　with abnormal findings NEC Z01.118
　　postpartum checkup Z39.2
　　psychiatric (general) Z00.8
　　　requested by authority Z04.6
　　vision Z01.00
　　　with abnormal findings Z01.01
　fitting (of)
　　artificial
　　　arm — *see* Admission, adjustment, artificial,
　　　　arm
　　　eye Z44.2 ☑
　　　leg — *see* Admission, adjustment, artificial, leg
　　brain neuropacemaker Z46.2
　　　implanted Z45.42
　　breast prosthesis (external) Z44.3 ☑
　　colostomy belt Z46.89
　　contact lenses Z46.0
　　cystostomy device Z46.6
　　dental prosthesis Z46.3
　　dentures Z46.3
　　device NEC
　　　abdominal Z46.89
　　　nervous system Z46.2
　　　　implanted — *see* Admission, adjustment,
　　　　　device, implanted, nervous system
　　　orthodontic Z46.4
　　　prosthetic Z44.9
　　　　breast Z44.3 ☑
　　　　dental Z46.3
　　　　eye Z44.2 ☑
　　　substitution
　　　　auditory Z46.2
　　　　　implanted — *see* Admission, adjust-
　　　　　　ment, device, implanted, hearing
　　　　　　device
　　　　nervous system Z46.2
　　　　　implanted — *see* Admission, adjust-
　　　　　　ment, device, implanted, nervous
　　　　　　system
　　　　visual Z46.2
　　　　　implanted Z45.31
　　hearing aid Z46.1
　　ileostomy device Z46.89
　　intestinal appliance or device NEC Z46.89
　　neuropacemaker (brain) (peripheral nerve) (spinal
　　　cord) Z46.2
　　　implanted Z45.42
　　orthodontic device Z46.4
　　orthopedic device (brace) (cast) (shoes) Z46.89

Admission — *continued*
  fitting — *continued*
    prosthesis Z44.9
      arm — *see* Admission, adjustment, artificial, arm
      breast Z44.3 ☑
      dental Z46.3
      eye Z44.2 ☑
      leg — *see* Admission, adjustment, artificial, leg
        specified type NEC Z44.8
    spectacles Z46.0
  follow-up examination Z09
  intrauterine device management Z30.431
    initial prescription Z30.014
  mental health evaluation Z00.8
    requested by authority Z04.6
  observation — *see* Observation
  Papanicolaou smear, cervix Z12.4
    for suspected malignant neoplasm Z12.4
  plastic and reconstructive surgery following medical procedure or healed injury NEC Z42.8
  plastic surgery, cosmetic NEC Z41.1
  postpartum observation
    immediately after delivery Z39.0
    routine follow-up Z39.2
  poststerilization (for restoration) Z31.0
    aftercare Z31.42
  procreative management Z31.9
  prophylactic (measure) — (*see also* Encounter, prophylactic measures)
    organ removal Z40.00
      breast Z40.01
      fallopian tube(s) Z40.03
        with ovary(s) Z40.02
      ovary(s) Z40.02
      specified organ NEC Z40.09
      testes Z40.09
    vaccination Z23
  psychiatric examination (general) Z00.8
    requested by authority Z04.6
  radiation therapy (antineoplastic) Z51.0
  reconstructive surgery following medical procedure or healed injury NEC Z42.8
  removal of
    cystostomy catheter Z43.5
    drains Z48.03
    dressing (nonsurgical) Z48.00
    implantable subdermal contraceptive Z30.46
    intrauterine contraceptive device Z30.432
    neuropacemaker (brain) (peripheral nerve) (spinal cord) Z46.2
      implanted Z45.42
    staples Z48.02
    surgical dressing Z48.01
    sutures Z48.02
    ureteral stent Z46.6
  respirator [ventilator] use during power failure Z99.12
  restoration of organ continuity (poststerilization) Z31.0
    aftercare Z31.42
  sensitivity test (*see also* Test, skin)
    allergy NEC Z01.82
    Mantoux Z11.1
  tuboplasty following previous sterilization Z31.0
    aftercare Z31.42
  vasoplasty following previous sterilization Z31.0
    aftercare Z31.42
  vision examination Z01.00
    with abnormal findings Z01.01
  waiting period for admission to other facility Z75.1
Adnexitis (suppurative) — *see* Salpingo-oophoritis
Adolescent X-linked adrenoleukodystrophy E71.521
Adrenal (gland) — *see* condition
Adrenalism, tuberculous A18.7
Adrenalitis, adrenitis E27.8
  autoimmune E27.1
  meningococcal, hemorrhagic A39.1
Adrenarche, premature E27.0
Adrenocortical syndrome — *see* Cushing's, syndrome
Adrenogenital syndrome E25.9
  acquired E25.8
  congenital E25.0
  salt loss E25.0
Adrenogenitalism, congenital E25.0
Adrenoleukodystrophy E71.529
  neonatal E71.511
  X-linked E71.529
    Addison only phenotype E71.528
    Addison-Schilder E71.528

Adrenoleukodystrophy — *continued*
  X-linked — *continued*
    adolescent E71.521
    adrenomyeloneuropathy E71.522
    childhood cerebral E71.520
    other specified E71.528
Adrenomyeloneuropathy E71.522
Adventitious bursa — *see* Bursopathy, specified type NEC
Adverse effect — *see* Table of Drugs and Chemicals, categories T36-T50, with 6th character 5
Advice — *see* Counseling
Adynamia (episodica) (hereditary) (periodic) G72.3
Aeration lung imperfect, newborn — *see* Atelectasis
Aerobullosis T70.3 ☑
Aerocele — *see* Embolism, air
Aerodermectasia
  subcutaneous (traumatic) T79.7 ☑
Aerodontalgia T70.29 ☑
Aeroembolism T70.3 ☑
Aerogenes capsulatus infection A48.0
Aero-otitis media T70.0 ☑
Aerophagy, aerophagia (psychogenic) F45.8
Aerophobia F40.228
Aerosinusitis T70.1 ☑
Aerotitis T70.0 ☑
Affection — *see* Disease
Afibrinogenemia (*see also* Defect, coagulation) D68.8
  acquired D65
  congenital D68.2
  following ectopic or molar pregnancy O08.1
  in abortion — *see* Abortion, by type, complicated by, afibrinogenemia
  puerperal O72.3
African
  sleeping sickness B56.9
  tick fever A68.1
  trypanosomiasis B56.9
    gambian B56.0
    rhodesian B56.1
Aftercare (*see also* Care) Z51.89
  following surgery (for) (on)
    amputation Z47.81
    attention to
      drains Z48.03
      dressings (nonsurgical) Z48.00
        surgical Z48.01
      sutures Z48.02
    circulatory system Z48.812
    delayed (planned) wound closure Z48.1
    digestive system Z48.815
    explantation of joint prosthesis (staged procedure)
      hip Z47.32
      knee Z47.33
      shoulder Z47.31
    genitourinary system Z48.816
    joint replacement Z47.1
    neoplasm Z48.3
    nervous system Z48.811
    oral cavity Z48.814
    organ transplant
      bone marrow Z48.290
      heart Z48.21
      heart-lung Z48.280
      kidney Z48.22
      liver Z48.23
      lung Z48.24
      multiple organs NEC Z48.288
      specified NEC Z48.298
    orthopedic NEC Z47.89
    planned wound closure Z48.1
    removal of internal fixation device Z47.2
    respiratory system Z48.813
    scoliosis Z47.82
    sense organs Z48.810
    skin and subcutaneous tissue Z48.817
    specified body system
      circulatory Z48.812
      digestive Z48.815
      genitourinary Z48.816
      nervous Z48.811
      oral cavity Z48.814
      respiratory Z48.813
      sense organs Z48.810
      skin and subcutaneous tissue Z48.817
      teeth Z48.814
    specified NEC Z48.89
    spinal Z47.89

Aftercare — *continued*
  following surgery — *continued*
    teeth Z48.814
  fracture — *code to* fracture with seventh character D
  involving
    removal of
      drains Z48.03
      dressings (nonsurgical) Z48.00
      staples Z48.02
      surgical dressings Z48.01
      sutures Z48.02
    neuropacemaker (brain) (peripheral nerve) (spinal cord) Z46.2
      implanted Z45.42
  orthopedic NEC Z47.89
  postprocedural — *see* Aftercare, following surgery
After-cataract — *see* Cataract, secondary
Agalactia (primary) O92.3
  elective, secondary or therapeutic O92.5
Agammaglobulinemia (acquired (secondary) (nonfamilial) D80.1
  with
    immunoglobulin-bearing B-lymphocytes D80.1
    lymphopenia D81.9
  autosomal recessive (Swiss type) D80.0
  Bruton's X-linked D80.0
  common variable (CVAgamma) D80.1
  congenital sex-linked D80.0
  hereditary D80.0
  lymphopenic D81.9
  Swiss type (autosomal recessive) D80.0
  X-linked (with growth hormone deficiency) (Bruton) D80.0
Aganglionosis (bowel) (colon) Q43.1
Age (old) — *see* Senility
Agenesis
  adrenal (gland) Q89.1
  alimentary tract (complete) (partial) NEC Q45.8
    upper Q40.8
  anus, anal (canal) Q42.3
    with fistula Q42.2
  aorta Q25.41
  appendix Q42.8
  arm (complete) Q71.0- ☑
    with hand present Q71.1- ☑
  artery (peripheral) Q27.9
    brain Q28.3
    coronary Q24.5
    pulmonary Q25.79
    specified NEC Q27.8
    umbilical Q27.0
  auditory (canal) (external) Q16.1
  auricle (ear) Q16.0
  bile duct or passage Q44.5
  bladder Q64.5
  bone Q79.9
  brain Q00.0
    part of Q04.3
  breast (with nipple present) Q83.8
    with absent nipple Q83.0
  bronchus Q32.4
  canaliculus lacrimalis Q10.4
  carpus — *see* Agenesis, hand
  cartilage Q79.9
  cecum Q42.8
  cerebellum Q04.3
  cervix Q51.5
  chin Q18.8
  cilia Q10.3
  circulatory system, part NOS Q28.9
  clavicle Q74.0
  clitoris Q52.6
  coccyx Q76.49
  colon Q42.9
    specified NEC Q42.8
  corpus callosum Q04.0
  cricoid cartilage Q31.8
  diaphragm (with hernia) Q79.1
  digestive organ(s) or tract (complete) (partial) NEC Q45.8
    upper Q40.8
  ductus arteriosus Q28.8
  duodenum Q41.0
  ear Q16.9
    auricle Q16.0
    lobe Q17.8
  ejaculatory duct Q55.4
  endocrine (gland) NEC Q89.2

Agenesis — *continued*
  epiglottis Q31.8
  esophagus Q39.8
  eustachian tube Q16.2
  eye Q11.1
    adnexa Q15.8
  eyelid (fold) Q10.3
  face
    bones NEC Q75.8
    specified part NEC Q18.8
  fallopian tube Q50.6
  femur — *see* Defect, reduction, lower limb, longitudinal, femur
  fibula — *see* Defect, reduction, lower limb, longitudinal, fibula
  finger (complete) (partial) — *see* Agenesis, hand
  foot (and toes) (complete) (partial) Q72.3- ☑
  forearm (with hand present) — *see* Agenesis, arm, with hand present
    and hand Q71.2- ☑
  gallbladder Q44.0
  gastric Q40.2
  genitalia, genital (organ(s))
    female Q52.8
      external Q52.71
      internal NEC Q52.8
    male Q55.8
  glottis Q31.8
  hair Q84.0
  hand (and fingers) (complete) (partial) Q71.3- ☑
  heart Q24.8
    valve NEC Q24.8
      pulmonary Q22.0
  hepatic Q44.7
  humerus — *see* Defect, reduction, upper limb
  hymen Q52.4
  ileum Q41.2
  incus Q16.3
  intestine (small) Q41.9
    large Q42.9
      specified NEC Q42.8
  iris (dilator fibers) Q13.1
  jaw M26.09
  jejunum Q41.1
  kidney(s) (partial) Q60.2
    bilateral Q60.1
    unilateral Q60.0
  labium (majus) (minus) Q52.71
  labyrinth, membranous Q16.5
  lacrimal apparatus Q10.4
  larynx Q31.8
  leg (complete) Q72.0- ☑
    with foot present Q72.1- ☑
      lower leg (with foot present) — *see* Agenesis, leg, with foot present
        and foot Q72.2- ☑
  lens Q12.3
  limb (complete) Q73.0
    lower — *see* Agenesis, leg
    upper — *see* Agenesis, arm
  lip Q38.0
  liver Q44.7
  lung (fissure) (lobe) (bilateral) (unilateral) Q33.3
  mandible, maxilla M26.09
  metacarpus — *see* Agenesis, hand
  metatarsus — *see* Agenesis, foot
  muscle Q79.8
    eyelid Q10.3
    ocular Q15.8
  musculoskeletal system NEC Q79.8
  nail(s) Q84.3
  neck, part Q18.8
  nerve Q07.8
  nervous system, part NEC Q07.8
  nipple Q83.2
  nose Q30.1
  nuclear Q07.8
  organ
    of Corti Q16.5
    or site not listed — *see* Anomaly, by site
  osseous meatus (ear) Q16.1
  ovary
    bilateral Q50.02
    unilateral Q50.01
  oviduct Q50.6
  pancreas Q45.0
  parathyroid (gland) Q89.2
  parotid gland(s) Q38.4

Agenesis — *continued*
  patella Q74.1
  pelvic girdle (complete) (partial) Q74.2
  penis Q55.5
  pericardium Q24.8
  pituitary (gland) Q89.2
  prostate Q55.4
  punctum lacrimale Q10.4
  radioulnar — *see* Defect, reduction, upper limb
  radius — *see* Defect, reduction, upper limb, longitudinal, radius
  rectum Q42.1
    with fistula Q42.0
  renal Q60.2
    bilateral Q60.1
    unilateral Q60.0
  respiratory organ NEC Q34.8
  rib Q76.6
  roof of orbit Q75.8
  round ligament Q52.8
  sacrum Q76.49
  salivary gland Q38.4
  scapula Q74.0
  scrotum Q55.29
  seminal vesicles Q55.4
  septum
    atrial Q21.1
    between aorta and pulmonary artery Q21.4
    ventricular Q20.4
  shoulder girdle (complete) (partial) Q74.0
  skull (bone) Q75.8
    with
      anencephaly Q00.0
      encephalocele — *see* Encephalocele
      hydrocephalus Q03.9
        with spina bifida — *see* Spina bifida, by site, with hydrocephalus
      microcephaly Q02
  spermatic cord Q55.4
  spinal cord Q06.0
  spine Q76.49
  spleen Q89.01
  sternum Q76.7
  stomach Q40.2
  submaxillary gland(s) (congenital) Q38.4
  tarsus — *see* Agenesis, foot
  tendon Q79.8
  testicle Q55.0
  thymus (gland) Q89.2
  thyroid (gland) E03.1
    cartilage Q31.8
  tibia — *see* Defect, reduction, lower limb, longitudinal, tibia
  tibiofibular — *see* Defect, reduction, lower limb, specified type NEC
  toe (and foot) (complete) (partial) — *see* Agenesis, foot
  tongue Q38.3
  trachea (cartilage) Q32.1
  ulna — *see* Defect, reduction, upper limb, longitudinal, ulna
  upper limb — *see* Agenesis, arm
  ureter Q62.4
  urethra Q64.5
  urinary tract NEC Q64.8
  uterus Q51.0
  uvula Q38.5
  vagina Q52.0
  vas deferens Q55.4
  vein(s) (peripheral) Q27.9
    brain Q28.3
    great NEC Q26.8
    portal Q26.5
  vena cava (inferior) (superior) Q26.8
  vermis of cerebellum Q04.3
  vertebra Q76.49
  vulva Q52.71
Ageusia R43.2
Agitated — *see* condition
Agitation R45.1
Aglossia (congenital) Q38.3
Aglossia-adactylia syndrome Q87.0
Aglycogenosis E74.00
Agnosia (body image) (other senses) (tactile) R48.1
  developmental F88
  verbal R48.1
    auditory R48.1
      developmental F80.2

Agnosia — *continued*
  verbal — *continued*
    developmental F80.2
  visual (object) R48.3
Agoraphobia F40.00
  with panic disorder F40.01
  without panic disorder F40.02
Agrammatism R48.8
Agranulocytopenia — *see* Agranulocytosis
Agranulocytosis (chronic) (cyclical) (genetic) (infantile) (periodic) (pernicious) (*see also* Neutropenia) D70.9
  congenital D70.0
  cytoreductive cancer chemotherapy sequela D70.1
  drug-induced D70.2
    due to cytoreductive cancer chemotherapy D70.1
  due to infection D70.3
  secondary D70.4
    drug-induced D70.2
      due to cytoreductive cancer chemotherapy D70.1
Agraphia (absolute) R48.8
  with alexia R48.0
  developmental F81.81
Ague (dumb) — *see* Malaria
Agyria Q04.3
Ahumada-del Castillo syndrome E23.0
Aichomophobia F40.298
AIDS (related complex) B20
Ailment heart — *see* Disease, heart
Ailurophobia F40.218
AIN — *see* Neoplasia, intraepithelial, anal
Ainhum (disease) L94.6
AIPHI (acute idiopathic pulmonary hemorrhage in infants (over 28 days old)) R04.81
Air
  anterior mediastinum J98.2
  compressed, disease T70.3 ☑
  conditioner lung or pneumonitis J67.7
  embolism (artery) (cerebral) (any site) T79.0 ☑
    with ectopic or molar pregnancy O08.2
    due to implanted device NEC — *see* Complications, by site and type, specified NEC
    following
      abortion — *see* Abortion by type, complicated by, embolism
      ectopic or molar pregnancy O08.2
    infusion, therapeutic injection or transfusion T80.0 ☑
    in pregnancy, childbirth or puerperium — *see* Embolism, obstetric
    traumatic T79.0 ☑
  hunger, psychogenic F45.8
  rarefied, effects of — *see* Effect, adverse, high altitude
  sickness T75.3 ☑
Airplane sickness T75.3 ☑
Akathisia (drug-induced) (treatment-induced) G25.71
  neuroleptic induced (acute) G25.71
  tardive G25.71
Akinesia R29.898
Akinetic mutism R41.89
Akureyri's disease G93.3
Alactasia, congenital E73.0
Alagille's syndrome Q44.7
Alastrim B03
Albers-Schönberg syndrome Q78.2
Albert's syndrome — *see* Tendinitis, Achilles
Albinism, albino E70.30
  with hematologic abnormality E70.339
    Chédiak-Higashi syndrome E70.330
    Hermansky-Pudlak syndrome E70.331
    other specified E70.338
  I E70.320
  II E70.321
  ocular E70.319
    autosomal recessive E70.311
    other specified E70.318
    X-linked E70.310
  oculocutaneous E70.329
    other specified E70.328
    tyrosinase (ty) negative E70.320
    tyrosinase (ty) positive E70.321
  other specified E70.39
Albinismus E70.30
Albright (-McCune)(-Sternberg) syndrome Q78.1
Albuminous — *see* condition
Albuminuria, albuminuric (acute) (chronic) (subacute) (*see also* Proteinuria) R80.9

Albuminuria, albuminuric — *continued*
  complicating pregnancy — *see* Proteinuria, gestational
    with
      gestational hypertension — *see* Pre-eclampsia
      pre-existing hypertension — *see* Hypertension, complicating pregnancy, pre-existing, with, pre-eclampsia
  gestational — *see* Proteinuria, gestational
    with
      gestational hypertension — *see* Pre-eclampsia
      pre-existing hypertension — *see* Hypertension, complicating pregnancy, pre-existing, with, pre-eclampsia
  orthostatic R80.2
  postural R80.2
  pre-eclamptic — *see* Pre-eclampsia
  scarlatinal A38.8
Albuminurophobia F40.298
Alcaptonuria E70.29
Alcohol, alcoholic, alcohol-induced
  addiction (without remission) F10.20
    with remission F10.21
  amnestic disorder, persisting F10.96
    with dependence F10.26
  anxiety disorder F10.980
  bipolar and related disorder F10.94
  brain syndrome, chronic F10.97
    with dependence F10.27
  cardiopathy I42.6
  counseling and surveillance Z71.41
    family member Z71.42
  delirium (acute) (tremens) (withdrawal) F10.231
    with intoxication F10.921
      in
        abuse F10.121
        dependence F10.221
  dementia F10.97
    with dependence F10.27
  depressive disorder F10.94
  deterioration F10.97
    with dependence F10.27
  hallucinosis (acute) F10.951
    in
      abuse F10.151
      dependence F10.251
  insanity F10.959
  intoxication (acute) (without dependence) F10.129
    with
      delirium F10.121
      dependence F10.229
        with delirium F10.221
        uncomplicated F10.220
      uncomplicated F10.120
  jealousy F10.988
  Korsakoff's, Korsakov's, Korsakow's F10.26
  liver K70.9
    acute — *see* Disease, liver, alcoholic, hepatitis
  major neurocognitive disorder, amnestic-confabulatory type F10.96
  major neurocognitive disorder, nonamnestic-confabulatory type F10.97
  mania (acute) (chronic) F10.959
  mild neurocognitive disorder F10.988
  paranoia, paranoid (type) psychosis F10.950
  pellagra E52
  poisoning, accidental (acute) NEC — *see* Table of Drugs and Chemicals, alcohol, poisoning
  psychosis — *see* Psychosis, alcoholic
  psychotic disorder F10.959
  sexual dysfunction F10.981
  sleep disorder F10.982
  withdrawal (without convulsions) F10.239
    with delirium F10.231
Alcoholism (chronic) (without remission) F10.20
  with
    psychosis — *see* Psychosis, alcoholic
    remission F10.21
  Korsakov's F10.96
    with dependence F10.26
Alder (-Reilly) **anomaly or syndrome** (leukocyte granulation) D72.0
Aldosteronism E26.9
  familial (type I) E26.02
  glucocorticoid-remediable E26.02
  primary (due to (bilateral) adrenal hyperplasia) E26.09
  primary NEC E26.09
  secondary E26.1
  specified NEC E26.89

Aldosteronoma D44.10
Aldrich (-Wiskott) **syndrome** (eczema-thrombocytopenia) D82.0
Alektorophobia F40.218
Aleppo boil B55.1
Aleukemic — *see* condition
Aleukia
  congenital D70.0
  hemorrhagica D61.9
    congenital D61.09
  splenica D73.1
Alexia R48.0
  developmental F81.0
  secondary to organic lesion R48.0
Algoneurodystrophy M89.00
  ankle M89.07- ☑
  foot M89.07- ☑
  forearm M89.03- ☑
  hand M89.04- ☑
  lower leg M89.06- ☑
  multiple sites M89.0- ☑
  shoulder M89.01- ☑
  specified site NEC M89.08
  thigh M89.05- ☑
  upper arm M89.02- ☑
Algophobia F40.298
Alienation, mental — *see* Psychosis
Alkalemia E87.3
Alkalosis E87.3
  metabolic E87.3
    with respiratory acidosis E87.4
  respiratory E87.3
Alkaptonuria E70.29
Allen-Masters syndrome N83.8
Allergy, allergic (reaction) (to) T78.40 ☑
  air-borne substance NEC (rhinitis) J30.89
  alveolitis (extrinsic) J67.9
    due to
      Aspergillus clavatus J67.4
      Cryptostroma corticale J67.6
      organisms (fungal, thermophilic actinomycete) growing in ventilation (air conditioning) systems J67.7
    specified type NEC J67.8
  anaphylactic reaction or shock T78.2 ☑
  angioneurotic edema T78.3 ☑
  animal (dander) (epidermal) (hair) (rhinitis) J30.81
  bee sting (anaphylactic shock) — *see* Toxicity, venom, arthropod, bee
  biological — *see* Allergy, drug
  colitis (*see also* Colitis, allergic) K52.29
  dander (animal) (rhinitis) J30.81
  dandruff (rhinitis) J30.81
  dental restorative material (existing) K08.55
  dermatitis — *see* Dermatitis, contact, allergic
  diathesis — *see* History, allergy
  drug, medicament & biological (any) (external) (internal) T78.40 ☑
    correct substance properly administered — *see* Table of Drugs and Chemicals, by drug, adverse effect
    wrong substance given or taken NEC (by accident) — *see* Table of Drugs and Chemicals, by drug, poisoning
  due to pollen J30.1
  dust (house) (stock) (rhinitis) J30.89
    with asthma — *see* Asthma, allergic extrinsic
  eczema — *see* Dermatitis, contact, allergic
  epidermal (animal) (rhinitis) J30.81
  feathers (rhinitis) J30.89
  food (any) (ingested) NEC T78.1 ☑
    anaphylactic shock — *see* Shock, anaphylactic, due to food
    dermatitis — *see* Dermatitis, due to, food
    dietary counseling and surveillance Z71.3
    in contact with skin L23.6
    rhinitis J30.5
    status (without reaction) Z91.018
      eggs Z91.012
      milk products Z91.011
      peanuts Z91.010
      seafood Z91.013
      specified NEC Z91.018
    gastrointestinal — *see also* specific type of allergic reaction
      meaning colitis (*see also* Colitis, allergic) K52.29

Allergy, allergic — *continued*
  gastrointestinal — *see also* specific type of allergic reaction — *continued*
    meaning gastroenteritis (*see also* Gastroenteritis, allergic) K52.29
    meaning other adverse food reaction not elsewhere classified T78.1 ☑
  grain J30.1
  grass (hay fever) (pollen) J30.1
    asthma — *see* Asthma, allergic extrinsic
  hair (animal) (rhinitis) J30.81
  history (of) — *see* History, allergy
  horse serum — *see* Allergy, serum
  inhalant (rhinitis) J30.89
    pollen J30.1
  kapok (rhinitis) J30.89
  medicine — *see* Allergy, drug
  milk protein (*see also* Allergy, food) Z91.011
    anaphylactic reaction T78.07 ☑
    dermatitis L27.2
    enterocolitis syndrome K52.21
    enteropathy K52.22
    gastroenteritis K52.29
    gastroesophageal reflux (*see also* Reaction, adverse, food) K21.9
      with esophagitis K21.0
    proctocolitis K52.82
  nasal, seasonal due to pollen J30.1
  pneumonia J82
  pollen (any) (hay fever) J30.1
    asthma — *see* Asthma, allergic extrinsic
  primrose J30.1
  primula J30.1
  proctocolitis K52.82
  purpura D69.0
  ragweed (hay fever) (pollen) J30.1
    asthma — *see* Asthma, allergic extrinsic
  rose (pollen) J30.1
  seasonal NEC J30.2
  Senecio jacobae (pollen) J30.1
  serum (*see also* Reaction, serum) T80.69 ☑
    anaphylactic shock T80.59 ☑
  shock (anaphylactic) T78.2 ☑
    due to
      administration of blood and blood products T80.51 ☑
      adverse effect of correct medicinal substance properly administered T88.6 ☑
      immunization T80.52 ☑
      serum NEC T80.59 ☑
      vaccination T80.52 ☑
  specific NEC T78.49 ☑
  tree (any) (hay fever) (pollen) J30.1
    asthma — *see* Asthma, allergic extrinsic
  upper respiratory J30.9
  urticaria L50.0
  vaccine — *see* Allergy, serum
  wheat — *see* Allergy, food
Allescheriasis B48.2
Alligator skin disease Q80.9
Allocheiria, allochiria R20.8
Almeida's disease — *see* Paracoccidioidomycosis
Alopecia (hereditaria) (seborrheica) L65.9
  androgenic L64.9
    drug-induced L64.0
    specified NEC L64.8
  areata L63.9
    ophiasis L63.2
    specified NEC L63.8
    totalis L63.0
    universalis L63.1
  cicatricial L66.9
    specified NEC L66.8
  circumscripta L63.9
  congenital, congenitalis Q84.0
  due to cytotoxic drugs NEC L65.8
  mucinosa L65.2
  postinfective NEC L65.8
  postpartum L65.0
  premature L64.8
  specific (syphilitic) A51.32
  specified NEC L65.8
  syphilitic (secondary) A51.32
  totalis (capitis) L63.0
  universalis (entire body) L63.1
  X-ray L58.1
Alpers' disease G31.81
Alpine sickness T70.29 ☑

Alport syndrome Q87.81
ALTE (apparent life threatening event) **in newborn and infant** R68.13
Alteration (of), **Altered**
  awareness
    transient R40.4
    unintended under general anesthesia, during procedure T88.53 ☑
  mental status R41.82
  pattern of family relationships affecting child Z62.898
  sensation
    following
      cerebrovascular disease I69.998
        cerebral infarction I69.398
        intracerebral hemorrhage I69.198
        nontraumatic intracranial hemorrhage NEC I69.298
        specified disease NEC I69.898
        subarachnoid hemorrhage I69.098
Alternating — *see* condition
Altitude, high (effects) — *see* Effect, adverse, high altitude
Aluminosis (of lung) J63.0
Alveolitis
  allergic (extrinsic) — *see* Pneumonitis, hypersensitivity due to
    Aspergillus clavatus J67.4
    Cryptostroma corticale J67.6
  fibrosing (cryptogenic) (idiopathic) J84.112
  jaw M27.3
  sicca dolorosa M27.3
Alveolus, alveolar — *see* condition
Alymphocytosis D72.810
  thymic (with immunodeficiency) D82.1
Alymphoplasia, thymic D82.1
Alzheimer's disease or sclerosis — *see* Disease, Alzheimer's
Amastia (with nipple present) Q83.8
  with absent nipple Q83.0
Amathophobia F40.228
Amaurosis (acquired) (congenital) (*see also* Blindness)
  fugax G45.3
  hysterical F44.6
  Leber's congenital H35.50
  uremic — *see* Uremia
Amaurotic idiocy (infantile) (juvenile) (late) E75.4
Amaxophobia F40.248
Ambiguous genitalia Q56.4
Amblyopia (congenital) (ex anopsia) (partial) (suppression) H53.00- ☑
  anisometropic — *see* Amblyopia, refractive
  deprivation H53.01- ☑
  hysterical F44.6
  nocturnal (*see also* Blindness, night)
    vitamin A deficiency E50.5
  refractive H53.02- ☑
  strabismic H53.03- ☑
  suspect H53.04- ☑
  tobacco H53.8
  toxic NEC H53.8
  uremic — *see* Uremia
Ameba, amebic (histolytica) (*see also* Amebiasis)
  abscess (liver) A06.4
Amebiasis A06.9
  with abscess — *see* Abscess, amebic
  acute A06.0
  chronic (intestine) A06.1
    with abscess — *see* Abscess, amebic
  cutaneous A06.7
  cutis A06.7
  cystitis A06.81
  genitourinary tract NEC A06.82
  hepatic — *see* Abscess, liver, amebic
  intestine A06.0
  nondysenteric colitis A06.2
  skin A06.7
  specified site NEC A06.89
Ameboma (of intestine) A06.3
Amelia Q73.0
  lower limb — *see* Agenesis, leg
  upper limb — *see* Agenesis, arm
Ameloblastoma (*see also* Cyst, calcifying odontogenic)
  long bones C40.9-
    lower limb C40.2- ☑
    upper limb C40.0- ☑
  malignant C41.1
    jaw (bone) (lower) C41.1

Ameloblastoma — *continued*
  malignant — *continued*
    jaw — *continued*
      upper C41.0
  tibial C40.2- ☑
Amelogenesis imperfecta K00.5
  nonhereditaria (segmentalis) K00.4
Amenorrhea N91.2
  hyperhormonal E28.8
  primary N91.0
  secondary N91.1
Amentia — *see* Disability, intellectual
  Meynert's (nonalcoholic) F04
American
  leishmaniasis B55.2
  mountain tick fever A93.2
Ametropia — *see* Disorder, refraction
AMH (asymptomatic microscopic hematuria) R31.21
Amianthosis J61
Amimia R48.8
Amino-acid disorder E72.9
  anemia D53.0
Aminoacidopathy E72.9
Aminoaciduria E72.9
Amnesia R41.3
  anterograde R41.1
  auditory R48.8
  dissociative F44.0
    with dissociative fugue F44.1
  hysterical F44.0
  postictal in epilepsy — *see* Epilepsy
  psychogenic F44.0
  retrograde R41.2
  transient global G45.4
Amnes(t)ic syndrome (post-traumatic) F04
  induced by
    alcohol F10.96
      with dependence F10.26
    psychoactive NEC F19.96
      with
        abuse F19.16
        dependence F19.26
    sedative F13.96
      with dependence F13.26
Amnion, amniotic — *see* condition
Amnionitis — *see* Pregnancy, complicated by
Amok F68.8
Amoral traits F60.89
Amphetamine (or other stimulant) -**induced**
  anxiety disorder F15.980
  bipolar and related disorder F15.94
  delirium F15.921
  depressive disorder F15.94
  obsessive-compulsive and related disorder F15.988
  psychotic disorder F15.959
  sexual dysfunction F15.981
  sleep disorder F15.982
  stimulant withdrawal F15.23
Ampulla
  lower esophagus K22.8
  phrenic K22.8
Amputation (*see also* Absence, by site, acquired)
  neuroma (postoperative) (traumatic) — *see* Complications, amputation stump, neuroma
  stump (surgical)
    abnormal, painful, or with complication (late) — *see* Complications, amputation stump
    healed or old NOS Z89.9
  traumatic (complete) (partial)
    arm (upper) (complete) S48.91- ☑
      at
        elbow S58.01- ☑
          partial S58.02- ☑
        shoulder joint (complete) S48.01- ☑
          partial S48.02- ☑
      between
        elbow and wrist (complete) S58.11- ☑
          partial S58.12- ☑
        shoulder and elbow (complete) S48.11- ☑
          partial S48.12- ☑
      partial S48.92- ☑
    breast (complete) S28.21- ☑
      partial S28.22- ☑
    clitoris (complete) S38.211 ☑
      partial S38.212 ☑
    ear (complete) S08.11- ☑
      partial S08.12- ☑

Amputation — *continued*
  traumatic — *continued*
    finger (complete) (metacarpophalangeal)
      S68.11- ☑
      index S68.11- ☑
      little S68.11- ☑
      middle S68.11- ☑
      partial S68.12- ☑
        index S68.12- ☑
        little S68.12- ☑
        middle S68.12- ☑
        ring S68.12- ☑
      ring S68.11- ☑
      thumb — *see* Amputation, traumatic, thumb
      transphalangeal (complete) S68.61- ☑
        index S68.61- ☑
        little S68.61- ☑
        middle S68.61- ☑
        partial S68.62- ☑
          index S68.62- ☑
          little S68.62- ☑
          middle S68.62- ☑
          ring S68.62- ☑
        ring S68.61- ☑
    foot (complete) S98.91- ☑
      at ankle level S98.01- ☑
        partial S98.02- ☑
      midfoot S98.31- ☑
        partial S98.32- ☑
      partial S98.92- ☑
    forearm (complete) S58.91- ☑
      at elbow level (complete) S58.01- ☑
        partial S58.02- ☑
      between elbow and wrist (complete) S58.11- ☑
        partial S58.12- ☑
      partial S58.92- ☑
    genital organ(s) (external)
      female (complete) S38.211 ☑
        partial S38.212 ☑
      male
        penis (complete) S38.221 ☑
          partial S38.222 ☑
        scrotum (complete) S38.231 ☑
          partial S38.232 ☑
        testes (complete) S38.231 ☑
          partial S38.232 ☑
    hand (complete) (wrist level) S68.41- ☑
      finger(s) alone — *see* Amputation, traumatic, finger
      partial S68.42- ☑
      thumb alone — *see* Amputation, traumatic, thumb
      transmetacarpal (complete) S68.71- ☑
        partial S68.72- ☑
    head
      ear — *see* Amputation, traumatic, ear
      nose (partial) S08.812 ☑
        complete S08.811 ☑
      part S08.89 ☑
      scalp S08.0 ☑
    hip (and thigh) (complete) S78.91- ☑
      at hip joint (complete) S78.01- ☑
        partial S78.02- ☑
      between hip and knee (complete) S78.11- ☑
        partial S78.12- ☑
      partial S78.92- ☑
    labium (majus) (minus) (complete) S38.21- ☑
      partial S38.21- ☑
    leg (lower) S88.91- ☑
      at knee level S88.01- ☑
        partial S88.02- ☑
      between knee and ankle (complete) S88.11- ☑
        partial S88.12- ☑
      partial S88.92- ☑
    nose (partial) S08.812 ☑
      complete S08.811 ☑
    penis (complete) S38.221 ☑
      partial S38.222 ☑
    scrotum (complete) S38.231 ☑
      partial S38.232 ☑
    shoulder — *see* Amputation, traumatic, arm
      at shoulder joint — *see* Amputation, traumatic, arm, at shoulder joint
    testes (complete) S38.231 ☑
      partial S38.232 ☑
    thigh — *see* Amputation, traumatic, hip

Amputation — continued
traumatic — continued
thorax, part of S28.1 ☑
breast — see Amputation, traumatic, breast
thumb (complete) (metacarpophalangeal)
S68.01- ☑
partial S68.02- ☑
transphalangeal (complete) S68.51- ☑
partial S68.52- ☑
toe (lesser) S98.13- ☑
great S98.11- ☑
partial S98.12- ☑
more than one S98.21- ☑
partial S98.22- ☑
partial S98.14- ☑
vulva (complete) S38.211 ☑
partial S38.212 ☑
Amputee (bilateral) (old) Z89.9
Amsterdam dwarfism Q87.1
Amusia R48.8
developmental F80.89
Amyelencephalus, amyelencephaly Q00.0
Amyelia Q06.0
Amygdalitis — see Tonsillitis
Amygdalolith J35.8
Amyloid heart (disease) E85.4 [I43]
Amyloidosis (generalized) (primary) E85.9
with lung involvement E85.4 [J99]
familial E85.2
genetic E85.2
heart E85.4 [I43]
hemodialysis-associated E85.3
light chain (AL) E85.81
liver E85.4 [K77]
localized E85.4
neuropathic heredofamilial E85.1
non-neuropathic heredofamilial E85.0
organ limited E85.4
Portuguese E85.1
pulmonary E85.4 [J99]
secondary systemic E85.3
senile systemic (SSA) E85.82
skin (lichen) (macular) E85.4 [L99]
specified NEC E85.89
subglottic E85.4 [J99]
wild-type transthyretin-related (ATTR) E85.82
Amylopectinosis (brancher enzyme deficiency) E74.03
Amylophagia — see Pica
Amyoplasia congenita Q79.8
Amyotonia M62.89
congenita G70.2
Amyotrophia, amyotrophy, amyotrophic G71.8
congenita Q79.8
diabetic — see Diabetes, amyotrophy
lateral sclerosis G12.21
neuralgic G54.5
spinal progressive G12.25
Anacidity, gastric K31.83
psychogenic F45.8
Anaerosis of newborn P28.89
Analbuminemia E88.09
Analgesia — see Anesthesia
Analphalipoproteinemia E78.6
Anaphylactic
purpura D69.0
shock or reaction — see Shock, anaphylactic
Anaphylactoid shock or reaction — see Shock, anaphylactic
Anaphylactoid syndrome of pregnancy O88.01- ☑
Anaphylaxis — see Shock, anaphylactic
Anaplasia cervix (see also Dysplasia, cervix) N87.9
Anaplasmosis, human A77.49
Anarthria R47.1
Anasarca R60.1
cardiac — see Failure, heart, congestive
lung J18.2
newborn P83.2
nutritional E43
pulmonary J18.2
renal N04.9
Anastomosis
aneurysmal — see Aneurysm
arteriovenous ruptured brain I60.8
intestinal K63.89
complicated NEC K91.89
involving urinary tract N99.89
retinal and choroidal vessels (congenital) Q14.8

Anatomical narrow angle H40.03- ☑
Ancylostoma, ancylostomiasis (braziliense) (caninum) (ceylanicum) (duodenale) B76.0
Necator americanus B76.1
Andersen's disease (glycogen storage) E74.09
Anderson-Fabry disease E75.21
Andes disease T70.29 ☑
Andrews' disease (bacterid) L08.89
Androblastoma
benign
specified site — see Neoplasm, benign, by site
unspecified site
female D27.9
male D29.20
malignant
specified site — see Neoplasm, malignant, by site
unspecified site
female C56.9
male C62.90
specified site — see Neoplasm, uncertain behavior, by site
tubular
with lipid storage
specified site — see Neoplasm, benign, by site
unspecified site
female D27.9
male D29.20
specified site — see Neoplasm, benign, by site
unspecified site
female D27.9
male D29.20
unspecified site
female D39.10
male D40.10
Androgen insensitivity syndrome (see also Syndrome, androgen insensitivity) E34.50
Androgen resistance syndrome (see also Syndrome, androgen insensitivity) E34.50
Android pelvis Q74.2
with disproportion (fetopelvic) O33.3 ☑
causing obstructed labor O65.3
Androphobia F40.290
Anectasis, pulmonary (newborn) — see Atelectasis
Anemia (essential) (general) (hemoglobin deficiency) (infantile) (primary) (profound) D64.9
with (due to) (in)
disorder of
anaerobic glycolysis D55.2
pentose phosphate pathway D55.1
koilonychia D50.9
achlorhydric D50.8
achrestic D53.1
Addison (-Biermer) (pernicious) D51.0
agranulocytic — see Agranulocytosis
amino-acid-deficiency D53.0
aplastic D61.9
congenital D61.09
drug-induced D61.1
due to
drugs D61.1
external agents NEC D61.2
infection D61.2
radiation D61.2
idiopathic D61.3
red cell (pure) D60.9
chronic D60.0
congenital D61.01
specified type NEC D60.8
transient D60.1
specified type NEC D61.89
toxic D61.2
aregenerative
congenital D61.09
asiderotic D50.9
atypical (primary) D64.9
Baghdad spring D55.0
Balantidium coli A07.0
Biermer's (pernicious) D51.0
blood loss (chronic) D50.0
acute D62
bothriocephalus B70.0 [D63.8]
brickmaker's B76.9 [D63.8]
cerebral I67.89
childhood D58.9
chlorotic D50.8
chronic
blood loss D50.0
hemolytic D58.9

Anemia — continued
chronic — continued
hemolytic — continued
idiopathic D59.9
simple D53.9
chronica congenita aregenerativa D61.09
combined system disease NEC D51.0 [G32.0]
due to dietary vitamin B12 deficiency D51.3 [G32.0]
complicating pregnancy, childbirth or puerperium — see Pregnancy, complicated by (management affected by), anemia
congenital P61.4
aplastic D61.09
due to isoimmunization NOS P55.9
dyserythropoietic, dyshematopoietic D64.4
following fetal blood loss P61.3
Heinz body D58.2
hereditary hemolytic NOS D58.9
pernicious D51.0
spherocytic D58.0
Cooley's (erythroblastic) D56.1
cytogenic D51.0
deficiency D53.9
6-PGD D55.1
2, 3 diphosphoglycurate mutase D55.2
2, 3 PG D55.2
6 phosphogluconate dehydrogenase D55.1
amino-acid D53.0
combined B12 and folate D53.1
enzyme D55.9
drug-induced (hemolytic) D59.2
glucose-6-phosphate dehydrogenase (G6PD) D55.0
glycolytic D55.2
nucleotide metabolism D55.3
related to hexose monophosphate (HMP) shunt pathway NEC D55.1
specified type NEC D55.8
erythrocytic glutathione D55.1
folate D52.9
dietary D52.0
drug-induced D52.1
folic acid D52.9
dietary D52.0
drug-induced D52.1
G SH D55.1
G6PD D55.0
GGS-R D55.1
glucose-6-phosphate dehydrogenase D55.0
glutathione reductase D55.1
glyceraldehyde phosphate dehydrogenase D55.2
hexokinase D55.2
iron D50.9
secondary to blood loss (chronic) D50.0
nutritional D53.9
with
poor iron absorption D50.8
specified deficiency NEC D53.8
phosphofructo-aldolase D55.2
phosphoglycerate kinase D55.2
PK D55.2
protein D53.0
pyruvate kinase D55.2
transcobalamin II D51.2
triose-phosphate isomerase D55.2
vitamin B12 NOS D51.9
dietary D51.3
due to
intrinsic factor deficiency D51.0
selective vitamin B12 malabsorption with proteinuria D51.1
pernicious D51.0
specified type NEC D51.8
Diamond-Blackfan (congenital hypoplastic) D61.01
dibothriocephalus B70.0 [D63.8]
dimorphic D53.1
diphasic D53.1
Diphyllobothrium (Dibothriocephalus) B70.0 [D63.8]
due to (in) (with)
antineoplastic chemotherapy D64.81
blood loss (chronic) D50.0
acute D62
chemotherapy, antineoplastic D64.81
chronic disease classified elsewhere NEC D63.8
chronic kidney disease D63.1
deficiency
amino-acid D53.0
copper D53.8
folate (folic acid) D52.9

☑ Additional Character Required — Refer to the Tabular List for Character Selection   ▽ Subterms under main terms may continue to next column or page

Anemia — continued
  due to — continued
    deficiency — continued
      folate — continued
        dietary D52.0
        drug-induced D52.1
      molybdenum D53.8
      protein D53.0
      zinc D53.8
    dietary vitamin B12 deficiency D51.3
    disorder of
      glutathione metabolism D55.1
      nucleotide metabolism D55.3
    drug — see Anemia, by type (see also Table of Drugs and Chemicals)
    end stage renal disease D63.1
    enzyme disorder D55.9
    fetal blood loss P61.3
    fish tapeworm (D.latum) infestation B70.0 [D63.8]
    hemorrhage (chronic) D50.0
      acute D62
    impaired absorption D50.9
    loss of blood (chronic) D50.0
      acute D62
    myxedema E03.9 [D63.8]
    Necator americanus B76.1 [D63.8]
    prematurity P61.2
    selective vitamin B12 malabsorption with proteinuria D51.1
    transcobalamin II deficiency D51.2
  Dyke-Young type (secondary) (symptomatic) D59.1
  dyserythropoietic (congenital) D64.4
  dyshematopoietic (congenital) D64.4
  Egyptian B76.9 [D63.8]
  elliptocytosis — see Elliptocytosis
  enzyme-deficiency, drug-induced D59.2
  epidemic (see also Ancylostomiasis) B76.9 [D63.8]
  erythroblastic
    familial D56.1
    newborn (see also Disease, hemolytic) P55.9
    of childhood D56.1
  erythrocytic glutathione deficiency D55.1
  erythropoietin-resistant anemia (EPO resistant anemia) D63.1
  Faber's (achlorhydric anemia) D50.9
  factitious (self-induced blood letting) D50.0
  familial erythroblastic D56.1
  Fanconi's (congenital pancytopenia) D61.09
  favism D55.0
  fish tapeworm (D. latum) infestation B70.0 [D63.8]
  folate (folic acid) deficiency D52.9
  glucose-6-phosphate dehydrogenase (G6PD) deficiency D55.0
  glutathione-reductase deficiency D55.1
  goat's milk D52.0
  granulocytic — see Agranulocytosis
  Heinz body, congenital D58.2
  hemolytic D58.9
    acquired D59.9
      with hemoglobinuria NEC D59.6
      autoimmune NEC D59.1
      infectious D59.4
      specified type NEC D59.8
      toxic D59.4
    acute D59.9
      due to enzyme deficiency specified type NEC D55.8
      Lederer's D59.1
    autoimmune D59.1
      drug-induced D59.0
    chronic D58.9
      idiopathic D59.9
    cold type (secondary) (symptomatic) D59.1
    congenital (spherocytic) — see Spherocytosis
    due to
      cardiac conditions D59.4
      drugs (nonautoimmune) D59.2
        autoimmune D59.0
      enzyme disorder D55.9
        drug-induced D59.2
      presence of shunt or other internal prosthetic device D59.4
    familial D58.9
    hereditary D58.9
      due to enzyme disorder D55.9
        specified type NEC D55.8
      specified type NEC D58.8
    idiopathic (chronic) D59.9
    mechanical D59.4

Anemia — continued
  hemolytic — continued
    microangiopathic D59.4
    nonautoimmune D59.4
      drug-induced D59.2
    nonspherocytic
      congenital or hereditary NEC D55.8
        glucose-6-phosphate dehydrogenase deficiency D55.0
        pyruvate kinase deficiency D55.2
        type
          I D55.1
          II D55.2
      type
        I D55.1
        II D55.2
    secondary D59.4
      autoimmune D59.1
    specified (hereditary) type NEC D58.8
    Stransky-Regala type (see also Hemoglobinopathy) D58.8
    symptomatic D59.4
      autoimmune D59.1
    toxic D59.4
    warm type (secondary) (symptomatic) D59.1
  hemorrhagic (chronic) D50.0
    acute D62
  Herrick's D57.1
  hexokinase deficiency D55.2
  hookworm B76.9 [D63.8]
  hypochromic (idiopathic) (microcytic) (normoblastic) D50.9
    due to blood loss (chronic) D50.0
      acute D62
    familial sex-linked D64.0
    pyridoxine-responsive D64.3
    sideroblastic, sex-linked D64.0
  hypoplasia, red blood cells D61.9
    congenital or familial D61.01
  hypoplastic (idiopathic) D61.9
    congenital or familial (of childhood) D61.01
  hypoproliferative (refractive) D61.9
  idiopathic D64.9
    aplastic D61.3
    hemolytic, chronic D59.9
  in (due to) (with)
    chronic kidney disease D63.1
    end stage renal disease D63.1
    failure, kidney (renal) D63.1
    neoplastic disease (see also Neoplasm) D63.0
  intertropical (see also Ancylostomiasis) D63.8
  iron deficiency D50.9
    secondary to blood loss (chronic) D50.0
      acute D62
    specified type NEC D50.8
  Joseph-Diamond-Blackfan (congenital hypoplastic) D61.01
  Lederer's (hemolytic) D59.1
  leukoerythroblastic D61.82
  macrocytic D53.9
    nutritional D52.0
    tropical D52.8
  malarial (see also Malaria) B54 [D63.8]
  malignant (progressive) D51.0
  malnutrition D53.9
  marsh (see also Malaria) B54 [D63.8]
  Mediterranean (with other hemoglobinopathy) D56.9
  megaloblastic D53.1
    combined B12 and folate deficiency D53.1
    hereditary D51.1
    nutritional D52.0
    orotic aciduria D53.0
    refractory D53.1
    specified type NEC D53.1
  megalocytic D53.1
  microcytic (hypochromic) D50.9
    due to blood loss (chronic) D50.0
      acute D62
    familial D56.8
  microdrepanocytosis D57.40
  microelliptopoikilocytic (Rietti-Greppi- Micheli) D56.9
  miner's B76.9 [D63.8]
  myelodysplastic D46.9
  myelofibrosis D75.81
  myelogenous D64.89
  myelopathic D64.89
  myelophthisic D61.82
  myeloproliferative D47.Z9 (following D47.4)
  newborn P61.4

Anemia — continued
  newborn — continued
    due to
      ABO (antibodies, isoimmunization, maternal/fetal incompatibility) P55.1
      Rh (antibodies, isoimmunization, maternal/fetal incompatibility) P55.0
    following fetal blood loss P61.3
    posthemorrhagic (fetal) P61.3
  nonspherocytic hemolytic — see Anemia, hemolytic, nonspherocytic
  normocytic (infectional) D64.9
    due to blood loss (chronic) D50.0
      acute D62
    myelophthisic D61.82
  nutritional (deficiency) D53.9
    with
      poor iron absorption D50.8
      specified deficiency NEC D53.8
    megaloblastic D52.0
  of prematurity P61.2
  orotaciduric (congenital) (hereditary) D53.0
  osteosclerotic D64.89
  ovalocytosis (hereditary) — see Elliptocytosis
  paludal (see also Malaria) B54 [D63.8]
  pernicious (congenital) (malignant) (progressive) D51.0
  pleochromic D64.89
    of sprue D52.8
  posthemorrhagic (chronic) D50.0
    acute D62
    newborn P61.3
  postoperative (postprocedural)
    due to (acute) blood loss D62
      chronic blood loss D50.0
    specified NEC D64.9
  postpartum O90.81
  pressure D64.89
  progressive D64.9
    malignant D51.0
    pernicious D51.0
  protein-deficiency D53.0
  pseudoleukemica infantum D64.89
  pure red cell D60.9
    congenital D61.01
  pyridoxine-responsive D64.3
  pyruvate kinase deficiency D55.2
  refractory D46.4
    with
      excess of blasts D46.20
        1 (RAEB 1) D46.21
        2 (RAEB 2) D46.22
        in transformation (RAEB T) — see Leukemia, acute myeloblastic
      hemochromatosis D46.1
      sideroblasts (ring) (RARS) D46.1
    without ring sideroblasts, so stated D46.0
    without sideroblasts without excess of blasts D46.0
    megaloblastic D53.1
    sideroblastic D46.1
    sideropenic D50.9
  Rietti-Greppi-Micheli D56.9
  scorbutic D53.2
  secondary to
    blood loss (chronic) D50.0
      acute D62
    hemorrhage (chronic) D50.0
      acute D62
  semiplastic D61.89
  sickle-cell — see Disease, sickle-cell
  sideroblastic D64.3
    hereditary D64.0
    hypochromic, sex-linked D64.0
    pyridoxine-responsive NEC D64.3
    refractory D46.1
    secondary (due to)
      disease D64.1
      drugs and toxins D64.2
    specified type NEC D64.3
  sideropenic (refractory) D50.9
    due to blood loss (chronic) D50.0
      acute D62
  simple chronic D53.9
  specified type NEC D64.89
  spherocytic (hereditary) — see Spherocytosis
  splenic D64.89
  splenomegalic D64.89
  stomatocytosis D58.8
  syphilitic (acquired) (late) A52.79 [D63.8]
  target cell D64.89

Anemia — continued
  thalassemia D56.9
  thrombocytopenic — see Thrombocytopenia
  toxic D61.2
  tropical B76.9 [D63.8]
    macrocytic D52.8
  tuberculous A18.89 [D63.8]
  vegan D51.3
  vitamin
    B6-responsive D64.3
    B12 deficiency (dietary) pernicious D51.0
  von Jaksch's D64.89
  Witts' (achlorhydric anemia) D50.8
Anemophobia F40.228
Anencephalus, anencephaly Q00.0
Anergasia — see Psychosis, organic
Anesthesia, anesthetic R20.0
  complication or reaction NEC (see also Complications, anesthesia) T88.59 ☑
    due to
      correct substance properly administered — see Table of Drugs and Chemicals, by drug, adverse effect
      overdose or wrong substance given — see Table of Drugs and Chemicals, by drug, poisoning
      unintended awareness under general anesthesia during procedure T88.53 ☑
        personal history of Z92.84
  cornea H18.81- ☑
  dissociative F44.6
  functional (hysterical) F44.6
  hyperesthetic, thalamic G89.0
  hysterical F44.6
  local skin lesion R20.0
  sexual (psychogenic) F52.1
  shock (due to) T88.2 ☑
  skin R20.0
  testicular N50.9
Anetoderma (maculosum) (of) L90.8
  Jadassohn-Pellizzari L90.2
  Schweniger-Buzzi L90.1
Aneurin deficiency E51.9
Aneurysm (anastomotic) (artery) (cirsoid) (diffuse) (false) (fusiform) (multiple) (saccular) I72.9
  abdominal (aorta) I71.4
    ruptured I71.3
    syphilitic A52.01
  aorta, aortic (nonsyphilitic) I71.9
    abdominal I71.4
      ruptured I71.3
    arch I71.2
      ruptured I71.1
    arteriosclerotic I71.9
      ruptured I71.8
    ascending I71.2
      ruptured I71.1
    congenital Q25.43
    descending I71.9
      abdominal I71.4
        ruptured I71.3
      ruptured I71.8
      thoracic I71.2
        ruptured I71.1
    root Q25.43
    ruptured I71.8
    sinus, congenital Q25.43
    syphilitic A52.01
    thoracic I71.2
      ruptured I71.1
    thoracoabdominal I71.6
      ruptured I71.5
    thorax, thoracic (arch) I71.2
      ruptured I71.1
    transverse I71.2
      ruptured I71.1
    valve (heart) (see also Endocarditis, aortic) I35.8
  arteriosclerotic I72.9
    cerebral I67.1
      ruptured — see Hemorrhage, intracranial, subarachnoid
  arteriovenous (congenital) (see also Malformation, arteriovenous)
    acquired I77.0
      brain I67.1
      coronary I25.41
      pulmonary I28.0
    brain Q28.2

Aneurysm — continued
  arteriovenous (see also Malformation, arteriovenous) — continued
    brain — continued
      ruptured I60.8
    peripheral — see Malformation, arteriovenous, peripheral
    precerebral vessels Q28.0
    specified site NEC (see also Malformation, arteriovenous)
      acquired I77.0
  basal — see Aneurysm, brain
  basilar (trunk) I72.5
  berry (congenital) (nonruptured) I67.1
    ruptured I60.7
  brain I67.1
    arteriosclerotic I67.1
      ruptured — see Hemorrhage, intracranial, subarachnoid
    arteriovenous (congenital) (nonruptured) Q28.2
      acquired I67.1
        ruptured I60.8
      ruptured I60.8
    berry (congenital) (nonruptured) I67.1
      ruptured (see also Hemorrhage, intracranial, subarachnoid) I60.7
    congenital Q28.3
      ruptured I60.7
    meninges I67.1
      ruptured I60.8
    miliary (congenital) (nonruptured) I67.1
      ruptured (see also Hemorrhage, intracranial, subarachnoid) I60.7
    mycotic I33.0
    ruptured — see Hemorrhage, intracranial, subarachnoid
    syphilitic (hemorrhage) A52.05
  cardiac (false) (see also Aneurysm, heart) I25.3
  carotid artery (common) (external) I72.0
    internal (intracranial) I67.1
      extracranial portion I72.0
      ruptured into brain I60.0- ☑
    syphilitic A52.09
      intracranial A52.05
  cavernous sinus I67.1
    arteriovenous (congenital) (nonruptured) Q28.3
      ruptured I60.8
  celiac I72.8
  central nervous system, syphilitic A52.05
  cerebral — see Aneurysm, brain
  chest — see Aneurysm, thorax
  circle of Willis I67.1
    congenital Q28.3
      ruptured I60.6
    ruptured I60.6
  common iliac artery I72.3
  congenital (peripheral) Q27.8
    aorta (root) (sinus) Q25.43
    brain Q28.3
      ruptured I60.7
    coronary Q24.5
    digestive system Q27.8
    lower limb Q27.8
    pulmonary Q25.79
    retina Q14.1
    specified site NEC Q27.8
    upper limb Q27.8
  conjunctiva — see Abnormality, conjunctiva, vascular
  conus arteriosus — see Aneurysm, heart
  coronary (arteriosclerotic) (artery) I25.41
    arteriovenous, congenital Q24.5
    congenital Q24.5
    ruptured — see Infarct, myocardium
    syphilitic A52.06
    vein I25.89
  cylindroid (aorta) I71.9
    ruptured I71.8
    syphilitic A52.01
  ductus arteriosus Q25.0
  endocardial, infective (any valve) I33.0
  femoral (artery) (ruptured) I72.4
  gastroduodenal I72.8
  gastroepiploic I72.8
  heart (wall) (chronic or with a stated duration of over 4 weeks) I25.3
    valve — see Endocarditis
  hepatic I72.8
  iliac (common) (artery) (ruptured) I72.3

Aneurysm — continued
  infective I72.9
    endocardial (any valve) I33.0
  innominate (nonsyphilitic) I72.8
    syphilitic A52.09
  interauricular septum — see Aneurysm, heart
  interventricular septum — see Aneurysm, heart
  intrathoracic (nonsyphilitic) I71.2
    ruptured I71.1
    syphilitic A52.01
  lower limb I72.4
  lung (pulmonary artery) I28.1
  mediastinal (nonsyphilitic) I72.8
    syphilitic A52.09
  miliary (congenital) I67.1
    ruptured — see Hemorrhage, intracerebral, subarachnoid, intracranial
  mitral (heart) (valve) I34.8
  mural — see Aneurysm, heart
  mycotic I72.9
    endocardial (any valve) I33.0
    ruptured, brain — see Hemorrhage, intracerebral, subarachnoid
  myocardium — see Aneurysm, heart
  neck I72.0
  pancreaticoduodenal I72.8
  patent ductus arteriosus Q25.0
  peripheral NEC I72.8
    congenital Q27.8
      digestive system Q27.8
      lower limb Q27.8
      specified site NEC Q27.8
      upper limb Q27.8
  popliteal (artery) (ruptured) I72.4
  precerebral
    congenital (nonruptured) Q28.1
    specified site, NEC I72.5
  pulmonary I28.1
    arteriovenous Q25.72
      acquired I28.0
    syphilitic A52.09
    valve (heart) — see Endocarditis, pulmonary
  racemose (peripheral) I72.9
    congenital — see Aneurysm, congenital
  radial I72.1
  Rasmussen NEC A15.0
  renal (artery) I72.2
  retina (see also Disorder, retina, microaneurysms)
    congenital Q14.1
    diabetic — see Diabetes, microaneurysms, retinal
  sinus of Valsalva Q25.49
  specified NEC I72.8
  spinal (cord) I72.8
    syphilitic (hemorrhage) A52.09
  splenic I72.8
  subclavian (artery) (ruptured) I72.8
    syphilitic A52.09
  superior mesenteric I72.8
  syphilitic (aorta) A52.01
    central nervous system A52.05
    congenital (late) A50.54 [I79.0]
    spine, spinal A52.09
  thoracoabdominal (aorta) I71.6
    ruptured I71.5
    syphilitic A52.01
  thorax, thoracic (aorta) (arch) (nonsyphilitic) I71.2
    ruptured I71.1
    syphilitic A52.01
  traumatic (complication) (early), specified site — see Injury, blood vessel
  tricuspid (heart) (valve) I07.8
  ulnar I72.1
  upper limb (ruptured) I72.1
  valve, valvular — see Endocarditis
  venous (see also Varix) I86.8
    congenital Q27.8
      digestive system Q27.8
      lower limb Q27.8
      specified site NEC Q27.8
      upper limb Q27.8
  ventricle — see Aneurysm, heart
  vertebral artery I72.6
  visceral NEC I72.8
Angelman syndrome Q93.5
Anger R45.4
Angiectasis, angiectopia I99.8
Angiitis I77.6
  allergic granulomatous M30.1

Angiitis — *continued*
　hypersensitivity M31.Ø
　necrotizing M31.9
　　specified NEC M31.8
　nervous system, granulomatous I67.7
Angina (attack) (cardiac) (chest) (heart) (pectoris) (syndrome) (vasomotor) I20.9
　with
　　atherosclerotic heart disease — *see* Arteriosclerosis, coronary (artery),
　　　documented spasm I20.1
　abdominal K55.1
　accelerated — *see* Angina, unstable
　agranulocytic — *see* Agranulocytosis
　angiospastic — *see* Angina, with documented spasm
　aphthous B08.5
　crescendo — *see* Angina, unstable
　croupous J05.0
　cruris I73.9
　de novo effort — *see* Angina, unstable
　diphtheritic, membranous A36.0
　equivalent I20.8
　exudative, chronic J37.0
　following acute myocardial infarction I23.7
　gangrenous diphtheritic A36.0
　intestinal K55.1
　Ludovici K12.2
　Ludwig's K12.2
　malignant diphtheritic A36.0
　membranous J05.0
　　diphtheritic A36.0
　　Vincent's A69.1
　mesenteric K55.1
　monocytic — *see* Mononucleosis, infectious
　of effort — *see* Angina, specified NEC
　phlegmonous J36
　　diphtheritic A36.0
　post-infarctional I23.7
　pre-infarctional — *see* Angina, unstable
　Prinzmetal — *see* Angina, with documented spasm
　progressive — *see* Angina, unstable
　pseudomembranous A69.1
　pultaceous, diphtheritic A36.0
　spasm-induced — *see* Angina, with documented spasm
　specified NEC I20.8
　stable I20.8
　stenocardia — *see* Angina, specified NEC
　stridulous, diphtheritic A36.2
　tonsil J36
　trachealis J05.0
　unstable I20.0
　variant — *see* Angina, with documented spasm
　Vincent's A69.1
　worsening effort — *see* Angina, unstable
Angioblastoma — *see* Neoplasm, connective tissue, uncertain behavior
Angiocholecystitis — *see* Cholecystitis, acute
Angiocholitis (*see also* Cholecystitis, acute) K83.0
Angiodysgenesis spinalis G95.19
Angiodysplasia (cecum) (colon) K55.20
　with bleeding K55.21
　duodenum (and stomach) K31.819
　　with bleeding K31.811
　stomach (and duodenum) K31.819
　　with bleeding K31.811
Angioedema (allergic) (any site) (with urticaria) T78.3 ☑
　hereditary D84.1
Angioendothelioma — *see* Neoplasm, uncertain behavior, by site
　benign D18.00
　　intra-abdominal D18.03
　　intracranial D18.02
　　skin D18.01
　　specified site NEC D18.09
　bone — *see* Neoplasm, bone, malignant
　Ewing's — *see* Neoplasm, bone, malignant
Angioendotheliomatosis C85.8- ☑
Angiofibroma (*see also* Neoplasm, benign, by site)
　juvenile
　　specified site — *see* Neoplasm, benign, by site
　　unspecified site D10.6
Angiohemophilia (A) (B) D68.0
Angioid streaks (choroid) (macula) (retina) H35.33
Angiokeratoma — *see* Neoplasm, skin, benign
　corporis diffusum E75.21
Angioleiomyoma — *see* Neoplasm, connective tissue, benign

Angiolipoma (*see also* Lipoma)
　infiltrating — *see* Lipoma
Angioma (*see also* Hemangioma, by site)
　capillary I78.1
　hemorrhagicum hereditaria I78.0
　intra-abdominal D18.03
　intracranial D18.02
　malignant — *see* Neoplasm, connective tissue, malignant
　plexiform D18.00
　　intra-abdominal D18.03
　　intracranial D18.02
　　skin D18.01
　　specified site NEC D18.09
　senile I78.1
　serpiginosum L81.7
　skin D18.01
　specified site NEC D18.09
　spider I78.1
　stellate I78.1
　venous Q28.3
Angiomatosis Q82.8
　bacillary A79.89
　encephalotrigeminal Q85.8
　hemorrhagic familial I78.0
　hereditary familial I78.0
　liver K76.4
Angiomyolipoma — *see* Lipoma
Angiomyoliposarcoma — *see* Neoplasm, connective tissue, malignant
Angiomyoma — *see* Neoplasm, connective tissue, benign
Angiomyosarcoma — *see* Neoplasm, connective tissue, malignant
Angiomyxoma — *see* Neoplasm, connective tissue, uncertain behavior
Angioneurosis F45.8
Angioneurotic edema (allergic) (any site) (with urticaria) T78.3 ☑
　hereditary D84.1
Angiopathia, angiopathy I99.9
　cerebral I67.9
　　amyloid E85.4 [I68.0]
　diabetic (peripheral) — *see* Diabetes, angiopathy
　peripheral I73.9
　　diabetic — *see* Diabetes, angiopathy
　　specified type NEC I73.89
　retinae syphilitica A52.05
　retinalis (juvenilis)
　　diabetic — *see* Diabetes, retinopathy
　　proliferative — *see* Retinopathy, proliferative
Angiosarcoma (*see also* Neoplasm, connective tissue, malignant)
　liver C22.3
Angiosclerosis — *see* Arteriosclerosis
Angiospasm (peripheral) (traumatic) (vessel) I73.9
　brachial plexus G54.0
　cerebral G45.9
　cervical plexus G54.2
　nerve
　　arm — *see* Mononeuropathy, upper limb
　　　axillary G54.0
　　　median — *see* Lesion, nerve, median
　　　ulnar — *see* Lesion, nerve, ulnar
　　axillary G54.0
　　leg — *see* Mononeuropathy, lower limb
　　median — *see* Lesion, nerve, median
　　plantar — *see* Lesion, nerve, plantar
　　ulnar — *see* Lesion, nerve, ulnar
Angiospastic disease or edema I73.9
Angiostrongyliasis
　due to
　　Parastrongylus
　　　cantonensis B83.2
　　　costaricensis B81.3
　intestinal B81.3
Anguillulosis — *see* Strongyloidiasis
Angulation
　cecum — *see* Obstruction, intestine
　coccyx (acquired) (*see also* subcategory) M43.8 ☑
　　congenital NEC Q76.49
　femur (acquired) (*see also* Deformity, limb, specified type NEC, thigh)
　　congenital Q74.2
　intestine (large) (small) — *see* Obstruction, intestine
　sacrum (acquired) (*see also* subcategory) M43.8 ☑
　　congenital NEC Q76.49
　sigmoid (flexure) — *see* Obstruction, intestine

Angulation — *continued*
　spine — *see* Dorsopathy, deforming, specified NEC
　tibia (acquired) (*see also* Deformity, limb, specified type NEC, lower leg)
　　congenital Q74.2
　ureter N13.5
　　with infection N13.6
　wrist (acquired) (*see also* Deformity, limb, specified type NEC, forearm)
　　congenital Q74.0
Angulus infectiosus (lips) K13.0
Anhedonia R45.84
　sexual F52.0
Anhidrosis L74.4
Anhydration E86.0
Anhydremia E86.0
Anidrosis L74.4
Aniridia (congenital) Q13.1
Anisakiasis (infection) (infestation) B81.0
Anisakis larvae infestation B81.0
Aniseikonia H52.32
Anisocoria (pupil) H57.02
　congenital Q13.2
Anisocytosis R71.8
Anisometropia (congenital) H52.31
Ankle — *see* condition
Ankyloblepharon (eyelid) (acquired) (*see also* Blepharophimosis)
　filiforme (adnatum) (congenital) Q10.3
　total Q10.3
Ankyloglossia Q38.1
Ankylosis (fibrous) (osseous) (joint) M24.60
　ankle M24.67- ☑
　arthrodesis status Z98.1
　cricoarytenoid (cartilage) (joint) (larynx) J38.7
　dental K03.5
　ear ossicles H74.31- ☑
　elbow M24.62- ☑
　foot M24.67- ☑
　hand M24.64- ☑
　hip M24.65- ☑
　incostapedial joint (infectional) — *see* Ankylosis, ear ossicles
　jaw (temporomandibular) M26.61- ☑
　knee M24.66- ☑
　lumbosacral (joint) M43.27
　postoperative (status) Z98.1
　produced by surgical fusion, status Z98.1
　sacro-iliac (joint) M43.28
　shoulder M24.61- ☑
　spine (joint) (*see also* Fusion, spine)
　　spondylitic — *see* Spondylitis, ankylosing
　surgical Z98.1
　temporomandibular M26.61- ☑
　tooth, teeth (hard tissues) K03.5
　wrist M24.63- ☑
Ankylostoma — *see* Ancylostoma
Ankylostomiasis — *see* Ancylostomiasis
Ankylurethria — *see* Stricture, urethra
Annular (*see also* condition)
　detachment, cervix N88.8
　organ or site, congenital NEC — *see* Distortion
　pancreas (congenital) Q45.1
Anodontia (complete) (partial) (vera) K00.0
　acquired K08.10 ☑
Anomaly, anomalous (congenital) (unspecified type) Q89.9
　abdominal wall NEC Q79.59
　acoustic nerve Q07.8
　adrenal (gland) Q89.1
　Alder (-Reilly) (leukocyte granulation) D72.0
　alimentary tract Q45.9
　　upper Q40.9
　alveolar M26.70
　　hyperplasia M26.79
　　　mandibular M26.72
　　　maxillary M26.71
　　hypoplasia M26.79
　　　mandibular M26.74
　　　maxillary M26.73
　　ridge (process) M26.79
　　specified NEC M26.79
　ankle (joint) Q74.2
　anus Q43.9
　aorta (arch) NEC Q25.40
　　coarctation (preductal) (postductal) Q25.1
　aortic cusp or valve Q23.9

Anomaly, anomalous — *continued*
  appendix Q43.8
  apple peel syndrome Q41.1
  aqueduct of Sylvius Q03.0
    with spina bifida — *see* Spina bifida, with hydro-
        cephalus
  arm Q74.0
  arteriovenous NEC
    coronary Q24.5
    gastrointestinal Q27.33
      acquired — *see* Angiodysplasia
  artery (peripheral) Q27.9
    basilar NEC Q28.1
    cerebral Q28.3
    coronary Q24.5
    digestive system Q27.8
    eye Q15.8
    great Q25.9
      specified NEC Q25.8
    lower limb Q27.8
    peripheral Q27.9
      specified NEC Q27.8
    pulmonary NEC Q25.79
    renal Q27.2
    retina Q14.1
    specified site NEC Q27.8
    subclavian Q27.8
      origin Q25.48
    umbilical Q27.0
    upper limb Q27.8
    vertebral NEC Q28.1
  aryteno-epiglottic folds Q31.8
  atrial
    bands or folds Q20.8
    septa Q21.1
  atrioventricular
    excitation I45.6
    septum Q21.0
  auditory canal Q17.8
  auricle
    ear Q17.8
      causing impairment of hearing Q16.9
    heart Q20.8
  Axenfeld's Q15.0
  back Q89.9
  band
    atrial Q20.8
    heart Q24.8
    ventricular Q24.8
  Bartholin's duct Q38.4
  biliary duct or passage Q44.5
  bladder Q64.70
    absence Q64.5
    diverticulum Q64.6
    exstrophy Q64.10
      cloacal Q64.12
      extroversion Q64.19
      specified type NEC Q64.19
      supravesical fissure Q64.11
    neck obstruction Q64.31
    specified type NEC Q64.79
  bone Q79.9
    arm Q74.0
    face Q75.9
    leg Q74.2
    pelvic girdle Q74.2
    shoulder girdle Q74.0
    skull Q75.9
      with
        anencephaly Q00.0
        encephalocele — *see* Encephalocele
        hydrocephalus Q03.9
          with spina bifida — *see* Spina bifida, by
            site, with hydrocephalus
        microcephaly Q02
  brain (multiple) Q04.9
    vessel Q28.3
  breast Q83.9
  broad ligament Q50.6
  bronchus Q32.4
  bulbus cordis Q21.9
  bursa Q79.9
  canal of Nuck Q52.4
  canthus Q10.3
  capillary Q27.9
  cardiac Q24.9
    chambers Q20.9
      specified NEC Q20.8
    septal closure Q21.9

Anomaly, anomalous — *continued*
  cardiac — *continued*
    septal closure — *continued*
      specified NEC Q21.8
    valve NEC Q24.8
      pulmonary Q22.3
  cardiovascular system Q28.8
  carpus Q74.0
  caruncle, lacrimal Q10.6
  cascade stomach Q40.2
  cauda equina Q06.3
  cecum Q43.9
  cerebral Q04.9
    vessels Q28.3
  cervix Q51.9
  Chédiak-Higashi (-Steinbrinck) (congenital gigantism
    of peroxidase granules) E70.330
  cheek Q18.9
  chest wall Q67.8
    bones Q76.9
  chin Q18.9
  chordae tendineae Q24.8
  choroid Q14.3
    plexus Q07.8
  chromosomes, chromosomal Q99.9
    D (1) — *see* condition, chromosome 13
    E (3) — *see* condition, chromosome 18
    G — *see* condition, chromosome 21
    sex
      female phenotype Q97.8
      gonadal dysgenesis (pure) Q99.1
      Klinefelter's Q98.4
      male phenotype Q98.9
      Turner's Q96.9
    specified NEC Q99.8
  cilia Q10.3
  circulatory system Q28.9
  clavicle Q74.0
  clitoris Q52.6
  coccyx Q76.49
  colon Q43.9
  common duct Q44.5
  communication
    coronary artery Q24.5
    left ventricle with right atrium Q21.0
  concha (ear) Q17.3
  connection
    portal vein Q26.5
    pulmonary venous Q26.4
      partial Q26.3
      total Q26.2
    renal artery with kidney Q27.2
  cornea (shape) Q13.4
  coronary artery or vein Q24.5
  cranium — *see* Anomaly, skull
  cricoid cartilage Q31.8
  cystic duct Q44.5
  dental
    alveolar — *see* Anomaly, alveolar
    arch relationship M26.20
      specified NEC M26.29
  dentofacial M26.9
    alveolar — *see* Anomaly, alveolar
    dental arch relationship M26.20
      specified NEC M26.29
    functional M26.50
      specified NEC M26.59
    jaw size M26.00
      macrogenia M26.05
      mandibular
        hyperplasia M26.03
        hypoplasia M26.04
      maxillary
        hyperplasia M26.01
        hypoplasia M26.02
      microgenia M26.06
      specified type NEC M26.09
    jaw-cranial base relationship M26.10
      asymmetry M26.12
      maxillary M26.11
      specified type NEC M26.19
    malocclusion M26.4
      dental arch relationship NEC M26.29
      jaw size — *see* Anomaly, dentofacial, jaw size
      jaw-cranial base relationship — *see* Anomaly,
        dentofacial, jaw-cranial base relationship
    specified type NEC M26.89
    temporomandibular joint M26.60- ☑

Anomaly, anomalous — *continued*
  dentofacial — *continued*
    temporomandibular joint — *continued*
      adhesions M26.61- ☑
      ankylosis M26.61- ☑
      arthralgia M26.62- ☑
      articular disc M26.63- ☑
      specified type NEC M26.69
    tooth position, fully erupted M26.30
      specified NEC M26.39
  dermatoglyphic Q82.8
  diaphragm (apertures) NEC Q79.1
  digestive organ(s) or tract Q45.9
    lower Q43.9
    upper Q40.9
  distance, interarch (excessive) (inadequate) M26.25
  distribution, coronary artery Q24.5
  ductus
    arteriosus Q25.0
    botalli Q25.0
  duodenum Q43.9
  dura (brain) Q04.9
    spinal cord Q06.9
  ear (external) Q17.9
    causing impairment of hearing Q16.9
    inner Q16.5
    middle (causing impairment of hearing) Q16.4
    ossicles Q16.3
  Ebstein's (heart) (tricuspid valve) Q22.5
  ectodermal Q82.9
  Eisenmenger's (ventricular septal defect) Q21.8
  ejaculatory duct Q55.4
  elbow Q74.0
  endocrine gland NEC Q89.2
  epididymis Q55.4
  epiglottis Q31.8
  esophagus Q39.9
  eustachian tube Q17.8
  eye Q15.9
    anterior segment Q13.9
      specified NEC Q13.89
    posterior segment Q14.9
      specified NEC Q14.8
    ptosis (eyelid) Q10.0
    specified NEC Q15.8
  eyebrow Q18.8
  eyelid Q10.3
    ptosis Q10.0
  face Q18.9
    bone(s) Q75.9
  fallopian tube Q50.6
  fascia Q79.9
  femur NEC Q74.2
  fibula NEC Q74.2
  finger Q74.0
  fixation, intestine Q43.3
  flexion (joint) NOS Q74.9
    hip or thigh Q65.89
  foot NEC Q74.2
    varus (congenital) Q66.3
  foramen
    Botalli Q21.1
    ovale Q21.1
  forearm Q74.0
  forehead Q75.8
  form, teeth K00.2
  fovea centralis Q14.1
  frontal bone — *see* Anomaly, skull
  gallbladder (position) (shape) (size) Q44.1
  Gartner's duct Q52.4
  gastrointestinal tract Q45.9
  genitalia, genital organ(s) or system
    female Q52.9
      external Q52.70
      internal NOS Q52.9
    male Q55.9
      hydrocele P83.5
      specified NEC Q55.8
  genitourinary NEC
    female Q52.9
    male Q55.9
  Gerbode Q21.0
  glottis Q31.8
  granulation or granulocyte, genetic (constitutional)
    (leukocyte) D72.0
  gum Q38.6
  gyri Q07.9
  hair Q84.2
  hand Q74.0

Anomaly, anomalous — *continued*
- hard tissue formation in pulp K04.3
- head — *see* Anomaly, skull
- heart Q24.9
  - auricle Q20.8
  - bands or folds Q24.8
  - fibroelastosis cordis I42.4
  - obstructive NEC Q22.6
  - patent ductus arteriosus (Botalli) Q25.0
  - septum Q21.9
    - auricular Q21.1
    - interatrial Q21.1
    - interventricular Q21.0
      - with pulmonary stenosis or atresia, dextra-position of aorta and hypertrophy of right ventricle Q21.3
    - specified NEC Q21.8
    - ventricular Q21.0
      - with pulmonary stenosis or atresia, dextra-position of aorta and hypertrophy of right ventricle Q21.3
  - tetralogy of Fallot Q21.3
  - valve NEC Q24.8
    - aortic
      - bicuspid valve Q23.1
      - insufficiency Q23.1
      - stenosis Q23.0
        - subaortic Q24.4
    - mitral
      - insufficiency Q23.3
      - stenosis Q23.2
    - pulmonary Q22.3
      - atresia Q22.0
      - insufficiency Q22.2
      - stenosis Q22.1
        - infundibular Q24.3
        - subvalvular Q24.3
    - tricuspid
      - atresia Q22.4
      - stenosis Q22.4
  - ventricle Q20.8
- heel NEC Q74.2
- Hegglin's D72.0
- hemianencephaly Q00.0
- hemicephaly Q00.0
- hemicrania Q00.0
- hepatic duct Q44.5
- hip NEC Q74.2
- hourglass stomach Q40.2
- humerus Q74.0
- hydatid of Morgagni
  - female Q50.5
  - male (epididymal) Q55.4
    - testicular Q55.29
- hymen Q52.4
- hypersegmentation of neutrophils, hereditary D72.0
- hypophyseal Q89.2
- ileocecal (coil) (valve) Q43.9
- ileum Q43.9
- ilium NEC Q74.2
- integument Q84.9
  - specified NEC Q84.8
- interarch distance (excessive) (inadequate) M26.25
- intervertebral cartilage or disc Q76.49
- intestine (large) (small) Q43.9
  - with anomalous adhesions, fixation or malrotation Q43.3
- iris Q13.2
- ischium NEC Q74.2
- jaw — *see* Anomaly, dentofacial
  - alveolar — *see* Anomaly, alveolar
- jaw-cranial base relationship — *see* Anomaly, dento-facial, jaw-cranial base relationship
- jejunum Q43.8
- joint Q74.9
  - specified NEC Q74.8
- Jordan's D72.0
- kidney(s) (calyx) (pelvis) Q63.9
  - artery Q27.2
  - specified NEC Q63.8
- Klippel-Feil (brevicollis) Q76.1
- knee Q74.1
- labium (majus) (minus) Q52.70
- labyrinth, membranous Q16.5
- lacrimal apparatus or duct Q10.6
- larynx, laryngeal (muscle) Q31.9
  - web (bed) Q31.0
- lens Q12.9
- leukocytes, genetic D72.0

Anomaly, anomalous — *continued*
- leukocytes, genetic — *continued*
  - granulation (constitutional) D72.0
- lid (fold) Q10.3
- ligament Q79.9
  - broad Q50.6
  - round Q52.8
- limb Q74.9
  - lower NEC Q74.2
    - reduction deformity — *see* Defect, reduction, lower limb
  - upper Q74.0
- lip Q38.0
- liver Q44.7
  - duct Q44.5
- lower limb NEC Q74.2
- lumbosacral (joint) (region) Q76.49
  - kyphosis — *see* Kyphosis, congenital
  - lordosis — *see* Lordosis, congenital
- lung (fissure) (lobe) Q33.9
- mandible — *see* Anomaly, dentofacial
- maxilla — *see* Anomaly, dentofacial
- May (-Hegglin) D72.0
- meatus urinarius NEC Q64.79
- meningeal bands or folds Q07.9
  - constriction of Q07.8
  - spinal Q06.9
- meninges Q07.9
  - cerebral Q04.8
  - spinal Q06.9
- meningocele Q05.9
- mesentery Q45.9
- metacarpus Q74.0
- metatarsus NEC Q74.2
- middle ear Q16.4
  - ossicles Q16.3
- mitral (leaflets) (valve) Q23.9
  - insufficiency Q23.3
  - specified NEC Q23.8
  - stenosis Q23.2
- mouth Q38.6
- Müllerian (*see also* Anomaly, by site)
  - uterus NEC Q51.818
- multiple NEC Q89.7
- muscle Q79.9
  - eyelid Q10.3
- musculoskeletal system, except limbs Q79.9
- myocardium Q24.8
- nail Q84.6
- narrowness, eyelid Q10.3
- nasal sinus (wall) Q30.8
- neck (any part) Q18.9
- nerve Q07.9
  - acoustic Q07.8
  - optic Q07.8
- nervous system (central) Q07.9
- nipple Q83.9
- nose, nasal (bones) (cartilage) (septum) (sinus) Q30.9
  - specified NEC Q30.8
- ocular muscle Q15.8
- omphalomesenteric duct Q43.0
- opening, pulmonary veins Q26.4
- optic
  - disc Q14.2
  - nerve Q07.8
- opticociliary vessels Q13.2
- orbit (eye) Q10.7
- organ Q89.9
  - of Corti Q16.5
- origin
  - artery
    - innominate Q25.8
    - pulmonary Q25.79
    - renal Q27.2
    - subclavian Q25.48
- osseous meatus (ear) Q16.1
- ovary Q50.39
- oviduct Q50.6
- palate (hard) (soft) NEC Q38.5
- pancreas or pancreatic duct Q45.3
- papillary muscles Q24.8
- parathyroid gland Q89.2
- paraurethral ducts Q64.79
- parotid (gland) Q38.4
- patella Q74.1
- Pelger-Huët (hereditary hyposegmentation) D72.0
- pelvic girdle NEC Q74.2
- pelvis (bony) NEC Q74.2
  - rachitic E64.3

Anomaly, anomalous — *continued*
- penis (glans) Q55.69
- pericardium Q24.8
- peripheral vascular system Q27.9
- Peter's Q13.4
- pharynx Q38.8
- pigmentation L81.9
  - congenital Q82.8
- pituitary (gland) Q89.2
- pleural (folds) Q34.0
- portal vein Q26.5
  - connection Q26.5
- position, tooth, teeth, fully erupted M26.30
  - specified NEC M26.39
- precerebral vessel Q28.1
- prepuce Q55.69
- prostate Q55.4
- pulmonary Q33.9
  - artery NEC Q25.79
  - valve Q22.3
    - atresia Q22.0
    - insufficiency Q22.2
    - specified type NEC Q22.3
    - stenosis Q22.1
      - infundibular Q24.3
      - subvalvular Q24.3
  - venous connection Q26.4
    - partial Q26.3
    - total Q26.2
- pupil Q13.2
  - function H57.00
    - anisocoria H57.02
    - Argyll Robertson pupil H57.01
    - miosis H57.03
    - mydriasis H57.04
    - specified type NEC H57.09
    - tonic pupil H57.05- ☑
- pylorus Q40.3
- radius Q74.0
- rectum Q43.9
- reduction (extremity) (limb)
  - femur (longitudinal) — *see* Defect, reduction, lower limb, longitudinal, femur
  - fibula (longitudinal) — *see* Defect, reduction, lower limb, longitudinal, fibula
  - lower limb — *see* Defect, reduction, lower limb
  - radius (longitudinal) — *see* Defect, reduction, upper limb, longitudinal, radius
  - tibia (longitudinal) — *see* Defect, reduction, lower limb, longitudinal, tibia
  - ulna (longitudinal) — *see* Defect, reduction, upper limb, longitudinal, ulna
  - upper limb — *see* Defect, reduction, upper limb
- refraction — *see* Disorder, refraction
- renal Q63.9
  - artery Q27.2
  - pelvis Q63.9
    - specified NEC Q63.8
- respiratory system Q34.9
  - specified NEC Q34.8
- retina Q14.1
- rib Q76.6
  - cervical Q76.5
- Rieger's Q13.81
- rotation — *see* Malrotation
  - hip or thigh Q65.89
- round ligament Q52.8
- sacroiliac (joint) NEC Q74.2
- sacrum NEC Q76.49
  - kyphosis — *see* Kyphosis, congenital
  - lordosis — *see* Lordosis, congenital
- saddle nose, syphilitic A50.57
- salivary duct or gland Q38.4
- scapula Q74.0
- scrotum — *see* Malformation, testis and scrotum
- sebaceous gland Q82.9
- seminal vesicles Q55.4
- sense organs NEC Q07.8
- sex chromosomes NEC (*see also* Anomaly, chromosomes)
  - female phenotype Q97.8
  - male phenotype Q98.9
- shoulder (girdle) (joint) Q74.0
- sigmoid (flexure) Q43.9
- simian crease Q82.8
- sinus of Valsalva Q25.49
- skeleton generalized Q78.9
- skin (appendage) Q82.9

Anomaly, anomalous — *continued*
  skull Q75.9
    with
      anencephaly Q00.0
      encephalocele — *see* Encephalocele
      hydrocephalus Q03.9
        with spina bifida — *see* Spina bifida, by site,
          with hydrocephalus
      microcephaly Q02
  specified organ or site NEC Q89.8
  spermatic cord Q55.4
  spine, spinal NEC Q76.49
    column NEC Q76.49
      kyphosis — *see* Kyphosis, congenital
      lordosis — *see* Lordosis, congenital
    cord Q06.9
    nerve root Q07.8
  spleen Q89.09
    agenesis Q89.01
  stenonian duct Q38.4
  sternum NEC Q76.7
  stomach Q40.3
  submaxillary gland Q38.4
  tarsus NEC Q74.2
  tendon Q79.9
  testis — *see* Malformation, testis and scrotum
  thigh NEC Q74.2
  thorax (wall) Q67.8
    bony Q76.9
  throat Q38.8
  thumb Q74.0
  thymus gland Q89.2
  thyroid (gland) Q89.2
    cartilage Q31.8
  tibia NEC Q74.2
    saber A50.56
  toe Q74.2
  tongue Q38.3
  tooth, teeth K00.9
    eruption K00.6
    position, fully erupted M26.30
    spacing, fully erupted M26.30
  trachea (cartilage) Q32.1
  tragus Q17.9
  tricuspid (leaflet) (valve) Q22.9
    atresia or stenosis Q22.4
    Ebstein's Q22.5
  Uhl's (hypoplasia of myocardium, right ventricle) Q24.8
  ulna Q74.0
  umbilical artery Q27.0
  union
    cricoid cartilage and thyroid cartilage Q31.8
    thyroid cartilage and hyoid bone Q31.8
    trachea with larynx Q31.8
  upper limb Q74.0
  urachus Q64.4
  ureter Q62.8
    obstructive NEC Q62.39
      cecoureterocele Q62.32
      orthotopic ureterocele Q62.31
  urethra Q64.70
    absence Q64.5
    double Q64.74
    fistula to rectum Q64.73
    obstructive Q64.39
      stricture Q64.32
    prolapse Q64.71
    specified type NEC Q64.79
  urinary tract Q64.9
  uterus Q51.9
    with only one functioning horn Q51.4
  uvula Q38.5
  vagina Q52.4
  valleculae Q31.8
  valve (heart) NEC Q24.8
    coronary sinus Q24.5
    inferior vena cava Q24.8
    pulmonary Q22.3
    sinus coronario Q24.5
    venae cavae inferioris Q24.8
  vas deferens Q55.4
  vascular Q27.9
    brain Q28.3
    ring Q25.45
  vein(s) (peripheral) Q27.9
    brain Q28.3
    cerebral Q28.3
    coronary Q24.5
    developmental Q28.3

Anomaly, anomalous — *continued*
  vein(s) — *continued*
    great Q26.9
      specified NEC Q26.8
  vena cava (inferior) (superior) Q26.9
  venous — *see* Anomaly, vein(s)
  venous return Q26.8
  ventricular
    bands or folds Q24.8
    septa Q21.0
  vertebra Q76.49
    kyphosis — *see* Kyphosis, congenital
    lordosis — *see* Lordosis, congenital
  vesicourethral orifice Q64.79
  vessel(s) Q27.9
    optic papilla Q14.2
    precerebral Q28.1
  vitelline duct Q43.0
  vitreous body or humor Q14.0
  vulva Q52.70
  wrist (joint) Q74.0
Anomia R48.8
Anonychia (congenital) Q84.3
  acquired L60.8
Anophthalmos, anophthalmus (congenital) (globe)
  Q11.1
  acquired Z90.01
Anopia, anopsia H53.46- ☑
  quadrant H53.46- ☑
Anorchia, anorchism, anorchidism Q55.0
Anorexia R63.0
  hysterical F44.89
  nervosa F50.00
    atypical F50.9
    binge-eating type F50.2
      with purging F50.02
    restricting type F50.01
Anorgasmy, psychogenic (female) F52.31
  male F52.32
Anosmia R43.0
  hysterical F44.6
  postinfectional J39.8
Anosognosia R41.89
Anosteoplasia Q78.9
Anovulatory cycle N97.0
Anoxemia R09.02
  newborn P84
Anoxia (pathological) R09.02
  altitude T70.29 ☑
  cerebral G93.1
    complicating
      anesthesia (general) (local) or other sedation
        T88.59 ☑
      in labor and delivery O74.3
      in pregnancy O29.21- ☑
      postpartum, puerperal O89.2
      delivery (cesarean) (instrumental) O75.4
    during a procedure G97.81
    newborn P84
    resulting from a procedure G97.82
  due to
    drowning T75.1 ☑
    high altitude T70.29 ☑
  heart — *see* Insufficiency, coronary
  intrauterine P84
  myocardial — *see* Insufficiency, coronary
  newborn P84
  spinal cord G95.11
  systemic (by suffocation) (low content in atmosphere)
    — *see* Asphyxia, traumatic
Anteflexion — *see* Anteversion
Antenatal
  care (normal pregnancy) Z34.90
  screening (encounter for) of mother (*see also* En-
    counter, antenatal screening) Z36.9
Antepartum — *see* condition
Anterior — *see* condition
Antero-occlusion M26.220
Anteversion
  cervix — *see* Anteversion, uterus
  femur (neck), congenital Q65.89
  uterus, uterine (cervix) (postinfectional) (postpartal,
    old) N85.4
    congenital Q51.818
    in pregnancy or childbirth — *see* Pregnancy,
      complicated by
Anthophobia F40.228
Anthracosilicosis J60

Anthracosis (lung) (occupational) J60
  lingua K14.3
Anthrax A22.9
  with pneumonia A22.1
  cerebral A22.8
  colitis A22.2
  cutaneous A22.0
  gastrointestinal A22.2
  inhalation A22.1
  intestinal A22.2
  meningitis A22.8
  pulmonary A22.1
  respiratory A22.1
  sepsis A22.7
  specified manifestation NEC A22.8
Anthropoid pelvis Q74.2
  with disproportion (fetopelvic) O33.0
Anthropophobia F40.10
  generalized F40.11
Antibodies, maternal (blood group) — *see* Isoimmunization, affecting management of pregnancy
  anti-D — *see* Isoimmunization, affecting management
    of pregnancy, Rh
  newborn P55.0
Antibody
  anticardiolipin R76.0
    with
      hemorrhagic disorder D68.312
      hypercoagulable state D68.61
  antiphosphatidylglycerol R76.0
    with
      hemorrhagic disorder D68.312
      hypercoagulable state D68.61
  antiphosphatidylinositol R76.0
    with
      hemorrhagic disorder D68.312
      hypercoagulable state D68.61
  antiphosphatidylserine R76.0
    with
      hemorrhagic disorder D68.312
      hypercoagulable state D68.61
  antiphospholipid R76.0
    with
      hemorrhagic disorder D68.312
      hypercoagulable state D68.61
Anticardiolipin syndrome D68.61
Anticoagulant, circulating (intrinsic) (*see also* Disorder,
  hemorrhagic) D68.318
  drug-induced (extrinsic) (*see also* Disorder, hemorrhag-
    ic) D68.32
  iatrogenic D68.32
Antidiuretic hormone syndrome E22.2
Antimonial cholera — *see* Poisoning, antimony
Antiphospholipid
  antibody
    with hemorrhagic disorder D68.312
    syndrome D68.61
Antisocial personality F60.2
Antithrombinemia — *see* Circulating anticoagulants
Antithromboplastinemia D68.318
Antithromboplastinogenemia D68.318
Antitoxin complication or reaction — *see* Complications, vaccination
Antlophobia F40.228
Antritis J32.0
  maxilla J32.0
    acute J01.00
      recurrent J01.01
  stomach K29.60
    with bleeding K29.61
Antrum, antral — *see* condition
Anuria R34
  calculous (impacted) (recurrent) (*see also* Calculus,
    urinary) N20.9
  following
    abortion — *see* Abortion by type complicated by,
      renal failure
    ectopic or molar pregnancy O08.4
  newborn P96.0
  postprocedural N99.0
  postrenal N13.8
  traumatic (following crushing) T79.5 ☑
Anus, anal — *see* condition
Anusitis K62.89
Anxiety F41.9
  depression F41.8
  episodic paroxysmal F41.0
  generalized F41.1

Anxiety — *continued*
  hysteria F41.8
  neurosis F41.1
  panic type F41.0
  reaction F41.1
  separation, abnormal (of childhood) F93.0
  specified NEC F41.8
  state F41.1
Aorta, aortic — *see* condition
Aortectasia — *see* Ectasia, aorta
  with aneurysm — *see* Aneurysm, aorta
Aortitis (nonsyphilitic) (calcific) I77.6
  arteriosclerotic I70.0
  Doehle-Heller A52.02
  luetic A52.02
  rheumatic — *see* Endocarditis, acute, rheumatic
  specific (syphilitic) A52.02
  syphilitic A52.02
    congenital A50.54 [I79.1]
Apathetic thyroid storm — *see* Thyrotoxicosis
Apathy R45.3
Apeirophobia F40.228
Apepsia K30
  psychogenic F45.8
Aperistalsis, esophagus K22.0
Apertognathia M26.29
Apert's syndrome Q87.0
Aphagia R13.0
  psychogenic F50.9
Aphakia (acquired) (postoperative) H27.0- ☑
  congenital Q12.3
Aphasia (amnestic) (global) (nominal) (semantic) (syntactic) R47.01
  acquired, with epilepsy (Landau-Kleffner syndrome) — *see* Epilepsy, specified NEC
  auditory (developmental) F80.2
  developmental (receptive type) F80.2
    expressive type F80.1
    Wernicke's F80.2
  following
    cerebrovascular disease I69.920
      cerebral infarction I69.320
      intracerebral hemorrhage I69.120
      nontraumatic intracranial hemorrhage NEC I69.220
      specified disease NEC I69.820
      subarachnoid hemorrhage I69.020
  primary progressive G31.01 [F02.80]
    with behavioral disturbance G31.01 [F02.81]
  progressive isolated G31.01 [F02.80]
    with behavioral disturbance G31.01 [F02.81]
  sensory F80.2
  syphilis, tertiary A52.19
  Wernicke's (developmental) F80.2
Aphonia (organic) R49.1
  hysterical F44.4
  psychogenic F44.4
Aphthae, aphthous (*see also* condition)
  Bednar's K12.0
  cachectic K14.0
  epizootic B08.8
  fever B08.8
  oral (recurrent) K12.0
  stomatitis (major) (minor) K12.0
  thrush B37.0
  ulcer (oral) (recurrent) K12.0
    genital organ(s) NEC
      female N76.6
      male N50.89
    larynx J38.7
Apical — *see* condition
Apiphobia F40.218
Aplasia (*see also* Agenesis)
  abdominal muscle syndrome Q79.4
  alveolar process (acquired) — *see* Anomaly, alveolar
    congenital Q38.6
  aorta (congenital) Q25.41
  axialis extracorticalis (congenita) E75.29
  bone marrow (myeloid) D61.9
    congenital D61.01
  brain Q00.0
    part of Q04.3
  bronchus Q32.4
  cementum K00.4
  cerebellum Q04.3
  cervix (congenital) Q51.5
  congenital pure red cell D61.01
  corpus callosum Q04.0

Aplasia — *continued*
  cutis congenita Q84.8
  erythrocyte congenital D61.01
  extracortical axial E75.29
  eye Q11.1
  fovea centralis (congenital) Q14.1
  gallbladder, congenital Q44.0
  iris Q13.1
  labyrinth, membranous Q16.5
  limb (congenital) Q73.8
    lower — *see* Defect, reduction, lower limb
    upper — *see* Agenesis, arm
  lung, congenital (bilateral) (unilateral) Q33.3
  pancreas Q45.0
  parathyroid-thymic D82.1
  Pelizaeus-Merzbacher E75.29
  penis Q55.5
  prostate Q55.4
  red cell (with thymoma) D60.9
    acquired D60.9
      due to drugs D60.9
    adult D60.9
    chronic D60.0
    congenital D61.01
    constitutional D61.01
    due to drugs D60.9
    hereditary D61.01
    of infants D61.01
    primary D61.01
    pure D61.01
      due to drugs D60.9
    specified type NEC D60.8
    transient D60.1
  round ligament Q52.8
  skin Q84.8
  spermatic cord Q55.4
  spleen Q89.01
  testicle Q55.0
  thymic, with immunodeficiency D82.1
  thyroid (congenital) (with myxedema) E03.1
  uterus Q51.0
  ventral horn cell Q06.1
Apnea, apneic (of) (spells) R06.81
  newborn NEC P28.4
    obstructive P28.4
    sleep (central) (obstructive) (primary) P28.3
  prematurity P28.4
  sleep G47.30
    central (primary) G47.31
      idiopathic G47.31
      in conditions classified elsewhere G47.37
    obstructive (adult) (pediatric) G47.33
      hypopnea G47.33
    primary central G47.31
    specified NEC G47.39
Apneumatosis, newborn P28.0
Apocrine metaplasia (breast) — *see* Dysplasia, mammary, specified type NEC
Apophysitis (bone) (*see also* Osteochondropathy)
  calcaneus M92.8
  juvenile M92.9
Apoplectiform convulsions (cerebral ischemia) I67.82
Apoplexia, apoplexy, apoplectic
  adrenal A39.1
  heart (auricle) (ventricle) — *see* Infarct, myocardium
  heat T67.0 ☑
  hemorrhagic (stroke) — *see* Hemorrhage, intracranial
  meninges, hemorrhagic — *see* Hemorrhage, intracranial, subarachnoid
  uremic N18.9 [I68.8]
Appearance
  bizarre R46.1
  specified NEC R46.89
  very low level of personal hygiene R46.0
Appendage
  epididymal (organ of Morgagni) Q55.4
  intestine (epiploic) Q43.8
  preauricular Q17.0
  testicular (organ of Morgagni) Q55.29
Appendicitis (pneumococcal) (retrocecal) K37
  with
    perforation or rupture K35.2
    peritoneal abscess K35.3
    peritonitis NEC K35.3
      generalized (with perforation or rupture) K35.2
      localized (with perforation or rupture) K35.3
  acute (catarrhal) (fulminating) (gangrenous) (obstructive) (retrocecal) (suppurative) K35.80

Appendicitis — *continued*
  acute — *continued*
    with
      peritoneal abscess K35.3
      peritonitis NEC K35.3
        generalized (with perforation or rupture) K35.2
        localized (with perforation or rupture) K35.3
    specified NEC K35.89
  amebic A06.89
  chronic (recurrent) K36
  exacerbation — *see* Appendicitis, acute
  gangrenous — *see* Appendicitis, acute
  healed (obliterative) K36
  interval K36
  neurogenic K36
  obstructive K36
  recurrent K36
  relapsing K36
  subacute (adhesive) K36
  subsiding K36
  suppurative — *see* Appendicitis, acute
  tuberculous A18.32
Appendicopathia oxyurica B80
Appendix, appendicular (*see also* condition)
  epididymis Q55.4
  Morgagni
    female Q50.5
    male (epididymal) Q55.4
      testicular Q55.29
  testis Q55.29
Appetite
  depraved — *see* Pica
  excessive R63.2
  lack or loss (*see also* Anorexia) R63.0
    nonorganic origin F50.89
    psychogenic F50.89
  perverted (hysterical) — *see* Pica
Apple peel syndrome Q41.1
Apprehension state F41.1
Apprehensiveness, abnormal F41.9
Approximal wear K03.0
Apraxia (classic) (ideational) (ideokinetic) (ideomotor) (motor) (verbal) R48.2
  following
    cerebrovascular disease I69.990
      cerebral infarction I69.390
      intracerebral hemorrhage I69.190
      nontraumatic intracranial hemorrhage NEC I69.290
      specified disease NEC I69.890
      subarachnoid hemorrhage I69.090
  oculomotor, congenital H51.8
Aptyalism K11.7
Apudoma — *see* Neoplasm, uncertain behavior, by site
Aqueous misdirection H40.83- ☑
Arabicum elephantiasis — *see* Infestation, filarial
Arachnitis — *see* Meningitis
Arachnodactyly — *see* Syndrome, Marfan's
Arachnoiditis (acute) (adhesive) (basal) (brain) (cerebrospinal) — *see* Meningitis
Arachnophobia F40.210
Arboencephalitis, Australian A83.4
Arborization block (heart) I45.5
ARC (AIDS-related complex) B20
Arch
  aortic Q25.49
  bovine Q25.49
Arches — *see* condition
Arcuate uterus Q51.810
Arcuatus uterus Q51.810
Arcus (cornea) senilis — *see* Degeneration, cornea, senile
Arc-welder's lung J63.4
Areflexia R29.2
Areola — *see* condition
Argentaffinoma (*see also* Neoplasm, uncertain behavior, by site)
  malignant — *see* Neoplasm, malignant, by site
  syndrome E34.0
Argininemia E72.21
Arginosuccinic aciduria E72.22
Argyll Robertson phenomenon, pupil or syndrome (syphilitic) A52.19
  atypical H57.09
  nonsyphilitic H57.09
Argyria, argyriasis ☑
  conjunctival H11.13- ☑

▽ Subterms under main terms may continue to next column or page   ☑ Additional Character Required — Refer to the Tabular List for Character Selection   25

Anxiety — Argyria, argyriasis

Argyria, argyriasis — continued
  from drug or medicament — see Table of Drugs and
    Chemicals, by substance
Argyrosis, conjunctival H11.13- ☑
Arhinencephaly Q04.1
Ariboflavinosis E53.0
Arm — see condition
Arnold-Chiari disease, obstruction or syndrome (type
  II) Q07.00
  with
    hydrocephalus Q07.02
      with spina bifida Q07.03
    spina bifida Q07.01
      with hydrocephalus Q07.03
  type III — see Encephalocele
  type IV Q04.8
Aromatic amino-acid metabolism disorder E70.9
  specified NEC E70.8
Arousals, confusional G47.51
Arrest, arrested
  cardiac I46.9
    complicating
      abortion — see Abortion, by type, complicated
        by, cardiac arrest
      anesthesia (general) (local) or other sedation
        — see Table of Drugs and Chemicals, by
        drug
        in labor and delivery O74.2
        in pregnancy O29.11- ☑
        postpartum, puerperal O89.1
      delivery (cesarean) (instrumental) O75.4
    due to
      cardiac condition I46.2
      specified condition NEC I46.8
    intraoperative I97.71- ☑
    newborn P29.81
    personal history, successfully resuscitated Z86.74
    postprocedural I97.12- ☑
      obstetric procedure O75.4
  cardiorespiratory — see Arrest, cardiac
  circulatory — see Arrest, cardiac
  deep transverse O64.0 ☑
  development or growth
    bone — see Disorder, bone, development or
      growth
    child R62.50
    tracheal rings Q32.1
  epiphyseal
    complete
      femur M89.15- ☑
      humerus M89.12- ☑
      tibia M89.16- ☑
      ulna M89.13- ☑
      forearm M89.13- ☑
        specified NEC M89.13- ☑
        ulna — see Arrest, epiphyseal, by type, ulna
      lower leg M89.16- ☑
        specified NEC M89.168
        tibia — see Arrest, epiphyseal, by type, tibia
    partial
      femur M89.15- ☑
      humerus M89.12- ☑
      tibia M89.16- ☑
      ulna M89.13- ☑
    specified NEC M89.18
  granulopoiesis — see Agranulocytosis
  growth plate — see Arrest, epiphyseal
  heart — see Arrest, cardiac
  legal, anxiety concerning Z65.3
  physeal — see Arrest, epiphyseal
  respiratory R09.2
    newborn P28.81
  sinus I45.5
  spermatogenesis (complete) — see Azoospermia
    incomplete — see Oligospermia
  transverse (deep) O64.0 ☑
Arrhenoblastoma
  benign
    specified site — see Neoplasm, benign, by site
    unspecified site
      female D27.9
      male D29.20
  malignant
    specified site — see Neoplasm, malignant, by site
    unspecified site
      female C56.9
      male C62.90

Arrhenoblastoma — continued
  specified site — see Neoplasm, uncertain behavior,
    by site
  unspecified site
    female D39.10
    male D40.10
Arrhythmia (auricle) (cardiac) (juvenile) (nodal) (reflex)
  (sinus) (supraventricular) (transitory) (ventricle) I49.9
  block I45.9
  extrasystolic I49.49
  newborn
    bradycardia P29.12
    occurring before birth P03.819
      before onset of labor P03.810
      during labor P03.811
    tachycardia P29.11
  psychogenic F45.8
  specified NEC I49.8
  vagal R55
  ventricular re-entry I47.0
Arrillaga-Ayerza syndrome (pulmonary sclerosis with
  pulmonary hypertension) I27.0
Arsenical pigmentation L81.8
  from drug or medicament — see Table of Drugs and
    Chemicals
Arsenism — see Poisoning, arsenic
Arterial — see condition
Arteriofibrosis — see Arteriosclerosis
Arteriolar sclerosis — see Arteriosclerosis
Arteriolith — see Arteriosclerosis
Arteriolitis I77.6
  necrotizing, kidney I77.5
  renal — see Hypertension, kidney
Arteriolosclerosis — see Arteriosclerosis
Arterionephrosclerosis — see Hypertension, kidney
Arteriopathy I77.9
Arteriosclerosis, arteriosclerotic (diffuse) (obliterans)
  (of) (senile) (with calcification) I70.90
  aorta I70.0
  arteries of extremities — see Arteriosclerosis, extrem-
    ities
  brain I67.2
  bypass graft
    coronary — see Arteriosclerosis, coronary, bypass
      graft
    extremities — see Arteriosclerosis, extremities,
      bypass graft
  cardiac — see Disease, heart, ischemic, atherosclerotic
  cardiopathy — see Disease, heart, ischemic,
    atherosclerotic
  cardiorenal — see Hypertension, cardiorenal
  cardiovascular — see Disease, heart, ischemic,
    atherosclerotic
  carotid (see also Occlusion, artery, carotid) I65.2- ☑
  central nervous system I67.2
  cerebral I67.2
  cerebrovascular I67.2
  coronary (artery) I25.10
    bypass graft I25.810
      with
        angina pectoris I25.709
          with documented spasm I25.701
          specified type NEC I25.708
          unstable I25.700
        ischemic chest pain I25.709
      autologous artery I25.810
        with
          angina pectoris I25.729
            with documented spasm I25.721
            specified type I25.728
            unstable I25.720
          ischemic chest pain I25.729
      autologous vein I25.810
        with
          angina pectoris I25.719
            with documented spasm I25.711
            specified type I25.718
            unstable I25.710
          ischemic chest pain I25.719
      nonautologous biological I25.810
        with
          angina pectoris I25.739
            with documented spasm I25.731
            specified type I25.738
            unstable I25.730
          ischemic chest pain I25.739
      specified type NEC I25.810

Arteriosclerosis, arteriosclerotic — continued
  coronary — continued
    bypass graft — continued
      specified type — continued
        with
          angina pectoris I25.799
            with documented spasm I25.791
            specified type I25.798
            unstable I25.790
          ischemic chest pain I25.799
    due to
      calcified coronary lesion (severely) I25.84
      lipid rich plaque I25.83
    native vessel
      with
        angina pectoris I25.119
          with documented spasm I25.111
          specified type NEC I25.118
          unstable I25.110
        ischemic chest pain I25.119
    transplanted heart I25.811
      bypass graft I25.812
        with
          angina pectoris I25.769
           with documented spasm I25.761
           specified type I25.768
           unstable I25.760
         ischemic chest pain I25.769
      native coronary artery I25.811
        with
          angina pectoris I25.759
           with documented spasm I25.751
           specified type I25.758
           unstable I25.750
         ischemic chest pain I25.759
  extremities (native arteries) I70.209
    bypass graft I70.309
      autologous vein graft I70.409
        leg I70.409
          with
            gangrene (and intermittent claudica-
              tion, rest pain and ulcer)
              I70.469
            intermittent claudication I70.419
            rest pain (and intermittent claudica-
              tion) I70.429
        bilateral I70.403
          with
            gangrene (and intermittent clau-
              dication, rest pain and ul-
              cer) I70.463
            intermittent claudication I70.463
            rest pain (and intermittent claudi-
              cation) I70.423
            specified type NEC I70.493
        left I70.402
          with
            gangrene (and intermittent clau-
              dication, rest pain and ul-
              cer) I70.462
            intermittent claudication I70.412
            rest pain (and intermittent claudi-
              cation) I70.422
            ulceration (and intermittent
              claudication and rest pain)
              I70.449
              ankle I70.443
              calf I70.442
              foot site NEC I70.445
              heel I70.444
              lower leg NEC I70.448
              midfoot I70.444
              thigh I70.441
            specified type NEC I70.492
        right I70.401
          with
            gangrene (and intermittent clau-
              dication, rest pain and ul-
              cer) I70.461
            intermittent claudication I70.411
            rest pain (and intermittent claudi-
              cation) I70.421
            ulceration (and intermittent
              claudication and rest pain)
              I70.439
              ankle I70.433
              calf I70.432
              foot site NEC I70.435
              heel I70.434

☑ Additional Character Required — Refer to the Tabular List for Character Selection   ▽ Subterms under main terms may continue to next column or page

Arteriosclerosis, arteriosclerotic — *continued*
  extremities — *continued*
    bypass graft — *continued*
      autologous vein graft — *continued*
        leg — *continued*
          right — *continued*
            with — *continued*
              ulceration — *continued*
                lower leg NEC I70.438
                midfoot I70.434
                thigh I70.431
              specified type NEC I70.491
          specified type NEC I70.499
          specified NEC I70.408
            with
              gangrene (and intermittent claudication, rest pain and ulcer) I70.468
              intermittent claudication I70.418
              rest pain (and intermittent claudication) I70.428
              ulceration (and intermittent claudication and rest pain) I70.45
              specified type NEC I70.498
        leg I70.309
          with
            gangrene (and intermittent claudication, rest pain and ulcer) I70.369
            intermittent claudication I70.319
            rest pain (and intermittent claudication) I70.329
            bilateral I70.303
              with
                gangrene (and intermittent claudication, rest pain and ulcer) I70.363
                intermittent claudication I70.313
                rest pain (and intermittent claudication) I70.323
              specified type NEC I70.393
            left I70.302
              with
                gangrene (and intermittent claudication, rest pain and ulcer) I70.362
                intermittent claudication I70.312
                rest pain (and intermittent claudication) I70.322
                ulceration (and intermittent claudication and rest pain) I70.349
                  ankle I70.343
                  calf I70.342
                  foot site NEC I70.345
                  heel I70.344
                  lower leg NEC I70.348
                  midfoot I70.344
                  thigh I70.341
              specified type NEC I70.392
            right I70.301
              with
                gangrene (and intermittent claudication, rest pain and ulcer) I70.361
                intermittent claudication I70.311
                rest pain (and intermittent claudication) I70.321
                ulceration (and intermittent claudication and rest pain) I70.339
                  ankle I70.333
                  calf I70.332
                  foot site NEC I70.335
                  heel I70.334
                  lower leg NEC I70.338
                  midfoot I70.334
                  thigh I70.331
              specified type NEC I70.391
          specified type NEC I70.399
      nonautologous biological graft I70.509
        leg I70.509
          with
            gangrene (and intermittent claudication, rest pain and ulcer) I70.569
            intermittent claudication I70.519
            rest pain (and intermittent claudication) I70.529
            bilateral I70.503

Arteriosclerosis, arteriosclerotic — *continued*
  extremities — *continued*
    bypass graft — *continued*
      nonautologous biological graft — *continued*
        leg — *continued*
          bilateral — *continued*
            with
              gangrene (and intermittent claudication, rest pain and ulcer) I70.563
              intermittent claudication I70.513
              rest pain (and intermittent claudication) I70.523
            specified type NEC I70.593
          left I70.502
            with
              gangrene (and intermittent claudication, rest pain and ulcer) I70.562
              intermittent claudication I70.512
              rest pain (and intermittent claudication) I70.522
              ulceration (and intermittent claudication and rest pain) I70.549
                ankle I70.543
                calf I70.542
                foot site NEC I70.545
                heel I70.544
                lower leg NEC I70.548
                midfoot I70.544
                thigh I70.541
            specified type NEC I70.592
          right I70.501
            with
              gangrene (and intermittent claudication, rest pain and ulcer) I70.561
              intermittent claudication I70.511
              rest pain (and intermittent claudication) I70.521
              ulceration (and intermittent claudication and rest pain) I70.539
                ankle I70.533
                calf I70.532
                foot site NEC I70.535
                heel I70.534
                lower leg NEC I70.538
                midfoot I70.534
                thigh I70.531
            specified type NEC I70.591
          specified type NEC I70.599
          specified NEC I70.508
            with
              gangrene (and intermittent claudication, rest pain and ulcer) I70.568
              intermittent claudication I70.518
              rest pain (and intermittent claudication) I70.528
              ulceration (and intermittent claudication and rest pain) I70.55
            specified type NEC I70.598
      nonbiological graft I70.609
        leg I70.609
          with
            gangrene (and intermittent claudication, rest pain and ulcer) I70.669
            intermittent claudication I70.619
            rest pain (and intermittent claudication) I70.629
          bilateral I70.603
            with
              gangrene (and intermittent claudication, rest pain and ulcer) I70.663
              intermittent claudication I70.613
              rest pain (and intermittent claudication) I70.623
            specified type NEC I70.693
          left I70.602
            with
              gangrene (and intermittent claudication, rest pain and ulcer) I70.662
              intermittent claudication I70.612

Arteriosclerosis, arteriosclerotic — *continued*
  extremities — *continued*
    bypass graft — *continued*
      nonbiological graft — *continued*
        leg — *continued*
          left — *continued*
            with — *continued*
              rest pain (and intermittent claudication) I70.622
              ulceration (and intermittent claudication and rest pain) I70.649
                ankle I70.643
                calf I70.642
                foot site NEC I70.645
                heel I70.644
                lower leg NEC I70.648
                midfoot I70.644
                thigh I70.641
            specified type NEC I70.692
          right I70.601
            with
              gangrene (and intermittent claudication, rest pain and ulcer) I70.661
              intermittent claudication I70.611
              rest pain (and intermittent claudication) I70.621
              ulceration (and intermittent claudication and rest pain) I70.639
                ankle I70.633
                calf I70.632
                foot site NEC I70.635
                heel I70.634
                lower leg NEC I70.638
                midfoot I70.634
                thigh I70.631
            specified type NEC I70.691
          specified NEC I70.608
            with
              gangrene (and intermittent claudication, rest pain and ulcer) I70.668
              intermittent claudication I70.618
              rest pain (and intermittent claudication) I70.628
              ulceration (and intermittent claudication and rest pain) I70.65
            specified type NEC I70.698
      specified graft NEC I70.709
        leg I70.709
          with
            gangrene (and intermittent claudication, rest pain and ulcer) I70.769
            intermittent claudication I70.719
            rest pain (and intermittent claudication) I70.729
          bilateral I70.703
            with
              gangrene (and intermittent claudication, rest pain and ulcer) I70.763
              intermittent claudication I70.713
              rest pain (and intermittent claudication) I70.723
            specified type NEC I70.793
          left I70.702
            with
              gangrene (and intermittent claudication, rest pain and ulcer) I70.762
              intermittent claudication I70.712
              rest pain (and intermittent claudication) I70.722
              ulceration (and intermittent claudication and rest pain) I70.749
                ankle I70.743
                calf I70.742
                foot site NEC I70.745
                heel I70.744
                lower leg NEC I70.748
                midfoot I70.744
                thigh I70.741
            specified type NEC I70.792
          right I70.701

Arteriosclerosis, arteriosclerotic — *continued*
  extremities — *continued*
    bypass graft — *continued*
      specified graft — *continued*
        leg — *continued*
          right — *continued*
            with
              gangrene (and intermittent claudication, rest pain and ulcer) I70.761
              intermittent claudication I70.711
              rest pain (and intermittent claudication) I70.721
              ulceration (and intermittent claudication and rest pain) I70.739
                ankle I70.733
                calf I70.732
                foot site NEC I70.735
                heel I70.734
                lower leg NEC I70.738
                midfoot I70.734
                thigh I70.731
            specified type NEC I70.791
        specified type NEC I70.799
      specified NEC I70.708
        with
          gangrene (and intermittent claudication, rest pain and ulcer) I70.768
          intermittent claudication I70.718
          rest pain (and intermittent claudication) I70.728
          ulceration (and intermittent claudication and rest pain) I70.75
        specified type NEC I70.798
    specified NEC I70.308
      with
        gangrene (and intermittent claudication, rest pain and ulcer) I70.368
        intermittent claudication I70.318
        rest pain (and intermittent claudication) I70.328
        ulceration (and intermittent claudication and rest pain) I70.35
      specifiec type NEC I70.398
  leg I70.209
    with
      gangrene (and intermittent claudication, rest pain and ulcer) I70.269
      intermittent claudication I70.219
      rest pain (and intermittent claudication) I70.229
    bilateral I70.203
      with
        gangrene (and intermittent claudication, rest pain and ulcer) I70.263
        intermittent claudication I70.213
        rest pain (and intermittent claudication) I70.223
      specified type NEC I70.293
    left I70.202
      with
        gangrene (and intermittent claudication, rest pain and ulcer) I70.262
        intermittent claudication I70.212
        rest pain (and intermittent claudication) I70.222
        ulceration (and intermittent claudication and rest pain) I70.249
          ankle I70.243
          calf I70.242
          foot site NEC I70.245
          heel I70.244
          lower leg NEC I70.248
          midfoot I70.244
          thigh I70.241
      specified type NEC I70.292
    right I70.201
      with
        gangrene (and intermittent claudication, rest pain and ulcer) I70.261
        intermittent claudication I70.211
        rest pain (and intermittent claudication) I70.221
        ulceration (and intermittent claudication and rest pain) I70.239
          ankle I70.233
          calf I70.232

Arteriosclerosis, arteriosclerotic — *continued*
  extremities — *continued*
    leg — *continued*
      right — *continued*
        with — *continued*
          ulceration — *continued*
            foot site NEC I70.235
            heel I70.234
            lower leg NEC I70.238
            midfoot I70.234
            thigh I70.231
          specified type NEC I70.291
        specified type NEC I70.299
    specified site NEC I70.208
      with
        gangrene (and intermittent claudication, rest pain and ulcer) I70.268
        intermittent claudication I70.218
        rest pain (and intermittent claudication) I70.228
        ulceration (and intermittent claudication and rest pain) I70.25
      specified type NEC I70.298
  generalized I70.91
  heart (disease) — *see* Arteriosclerosis, coronary (artery),
  kidney — *see* Hypertension, kidney
  medial — *see* Arteriosclerosis, extremities
  mesenteric (artery) K55.1
  Mönckeberg's — *see* Arteriosclerosis, extremities
  myocarditis I51.4
  peripheral (of extremities) — *see* Arteriosclerosis, extremities
  pulmonary (idiopathic) I27.0
  renal (arterioles) (*see also* Hypertension, kidney)
    artery I70.1
  retina (vascular) I70.8 [H35.0-] ☑
  specified artery NEC I70.8
  spinal (cord) G95.19
  vertebral (artery) I67.2
Arteriospasm I73.9
Arteriovenous — *see* condition
Arteritis I77.6
  allergic M31.0
  aorta (nonsyphilitic) I77.6
    syphilitic A52.02
  aortic arch M31.4
  brachiocephalic M31.4
  brain I67.7
    syphilitic A52.04
  cerebral I67.7
    in systemic lupus erythematosus M32.19
    listerial A32.89
    syphilitic A52.04
    tuberculous A18.89
  coronary (artery) I25.89
    rheumatic I01.8
      chronic I09.89
    syphilitic A52.06
  cranial (left) (right), giant cell M31.6
  deformans — *see* Arteriosclerosis
  giant cell NEC M31.6
    with polymyalgia rheumatica M31.5
  necrosing or necrotizing M31.9
    specified NEC M31.8
  nodosa M30.0
  obliterans — *see* Arteriosclerosis
  pulmonary I28.8
  rheumatic — *see* Fever, rheumatic
  senile — *see* Arteriosclerosis
  suppurative I77.2
  syphilitic (general) A52.09
    brain A52.04
    coronary A52.06
    spinal A52.09
  temporal, giant cell M31.6
  young female aortic arch syndrome M31.4
Artery, arterial (*see also* condition)
  abscess I77.89
  single umbilical Q27.0
Arthralgia (allergic) (*see also* Pain, joint)
  in caisson disease T70.3 ☑
  temporomandibular M26.62- ☑
Arthritis, arthritic (acute) (chronic) (nonpyogenic) (subacute) M19.90
  allergic — *see* Arthritis, specified form NEC
  ankylosing (crippling) (spine) (*see also* Spondylitis, ankylosing)

Arthritis, arthritic — *continued*
  ankylosing (*see also* Spondylitis, ankylosing) — *continued*
    sites other than spine — *see* Arthritis, specified form NEC
  atrophic — *see* Osteoarthritis
    spine — *see* Spondylitis, ankylosing
  back — *see* Spondylopathy, inflammatory
  blennorrhagic (gonococcal) A54.42
  Charcot's — *see* Arthropathy, neuropathic
    diabetic — *see* Diabetes, arthropathy, neuropathic
    syringomyelic G95.0
  chylous (filarial) (*see also* category M01) B74.9
  climacteric (any site) NEC — *see* Arthritis, specified form NEC
  crystal (-induced) — *see* Arthritis, in, crystals
  deformans — *see* Osteoarthritis
  degenerative — *see* Osteoarthritis
  due to or associated with
    acromegaly E22.0
    brucellosis — *see* Brucellosis
    caisson disease T70.3 ☑
    diabetes — *see* Diabetes, arthropathy
    dracontiasis (*see also* category M01) B72
    enteritis NEC
      regional — *see* Enteritis, regional
    erysipelas (*see also* category M01) A46
    erythema
      epidemic A25.1
      nodosum L52
    filariasis NOS B74.9
    glanders A24.0
    helminthiasis (*see also* category M01) B83.9
    hemophilia D66 [M36.2]
    Henoch- (Schönlein) purpura D69.0 [M36.4]
    human parvovirus (*see also* category M01) B97.6
    infectious disease NEC M01 ☑
    leprosy (see also category M01) (*see also* Leprosy) A30.9
    Lyme disease A69.23
    mycobacteria (*see also* category M01) A31.8
    parasitic disease NEC (*see also* category M01) B89
    paratyphoid fever (see also category M01) (*see also* Fever, paratyphoid) A01.4
    rat bite fever (*see also* category M01) A25.1
    regional enteritis — *see* Enteritis, regional
    respiratory disorder NOS J98.9
    serum sickness (*see also* Reaction, serum) T80.69 ☑
    syringomyelia G95.0
    typhoid fever A01.04
  epidemic erythema A25.1
  febrile — *see* Fever, rheumatic
  gonococcal A54.42
  gouty (acute) — *see* Gout
  in (due to)
    acromegaly (*see also* subcategory M14.8-) E22.0
    amyloidosis (*see also* subcategory M14.8-) E85.4
    bacterial disease (*see also* subcategory M01) A49.9
    Behçet's syndrome M35.2
    caisson disease (*see also* subcategory M14.8-) T70.3 ☑
    coliform bacilli (Escherichia coli) — *see* Arthritis, in, pyogenic organism NEC
    crystals M11.9
      dicalcium phosphate — *see* Arthritis, in, crystals, specified type NEC
      hydroxyapatite M11.0- ☑
      pyrophosphate — *see* Arthritis, in, crystals, specified type NEC
      specified type NEC M11.80
        ankle M11.87- ☑
        elbow M11.82- ☑
        foot joint M11.87- ☑
        hand joint M11.84- ☑
        hip M11.85- ☑
        knee M11.86- ☑
        multiple sites M11.8- ☑
        shoulder M11.81- ☑
        vertebrae M11.88
        wrist M11.83- ☑
    dermatoarthritis, lipoid E78.81
    dracontiasis (dracunculiasis) (*see also* category M01) B72
    endocrine disorder NEC (*see also* subcategory M14.8-) E34.9
    enteritis, infectious NEC (*see also* category M01) A09

☑ **Additional Character Required** — Refer to the Tabular List for Character Selection   ⚐ Subterms under main terms may continue to next column or page

Arthritis, arthritic — continued
in — continued
enteritis, infectious (see also category M01) — continued
specified organism NEC (see also category M01) A08.8
erythema
multiforme (see also subcategory M14.8-) L51.9
nodosum (see also subcategory M14.8-) L52
gout — see Gout
helminthiasis NEC (see also category M01) B83.9
hemochromatosis (see also subcategory M14.8-) E83.118
hemoglobinopathy NEC D58.2 [M36.3]
hemophilia NEC D66 [M36.2]
Hemophilus influenzae M00.8- [B96.3]
Henoch (-Schönlein) purpura D69.0 [M36.4]
hyperparathyroidism NEC (see also subcategory M14.8-) E21.3
hypersensitivity reaction NEC T78.49 [M36.4]
hypogammaglobulinemia (see also subcategory M14.8-) D80.1
hypothyroidism NEC (see also subcategory M14.8-) E03.9
infection — see Arthritis, pyogenic or pyemic
spine — see Spondylopathy, infective
infectious disease NEC M01
leprosy (see also category M01) A30.9
leukemia NEC C95.9- [M36.1]
lipoid dermatoarthritis E78.81
Lyme disease A69.23
Mediterranean fever, familial (see also subcategory M14.8-) M04.1
Meningococcus A39.83
metabolic disorder NEC (see also subcategory M14.8-) E88.9
multiple myelomatosis C90.0- [M36.1]
mumps B26.85
mycosis NEC (see also category M01) B49
myelomatosis (multiple) C90.0- [M36.1]
neurological disorder NEC G98.0
ochronosis (see also subcategory M14.8-) E70.29
O'nyong-nyong (see also category M01) A92.1
parasitic disease NEC (see also category M01) B89
paratyphoid fever (see also category M01) A01.4
Pseudomonas — see Arthritis, pyogenic, bacterial NEC
psoriasis L40.50
pyogenic organism NEC — see Arthritis, pyogenic, bacterial NEC
Reiter's disease — see Reiter's disease
respiratory disorder NEC (see also subcategory M14.8-) J98.9
reticulosis, malignant (see also subcategory M14.8-) C86.0
rubella B06.82
Salmonella (arizonae) (cholerae-suis) (enteritidis) (typhimurium) A02.23
sarcoidosis D86.86
specified bacteria NEC — see Arthritis, pyogenic, bacterial NEC
sporotrichosis B42.82
syringomyelia G95.0
thalassemia NEC D56.9 [M36.3]
tuberculosis — see Tuberculosis, arthritis
typhoid fever A01.04
urethritis, Reiter's — see Reiter's disease
viral disease NEC (see also category M01) B34.9
infectious or infective (see also Arthritis, pyogenic or pyemic)
spine — see Spondylopathy, infective
juvenile M08.90
with systemic onset — see Still's disease
ankle M08.97-
elbow M08.92-
foot joint M08.97-
hand joint M08.94-
hip M08.95-
knee M08.96-
multiple site M08.99
pauciarticular M08.40
ankle M08.47-
elbow M08.42-
foot joint M08.47-
hand joint M08.44-
hip M08.45-
knee M08.46-

Arthritis, arthritic — continued
juvenile — continued
pauciarticular — continued
shoulder M08.41-
vertebrae M08.48
wrist M08.43-
psoriatic L40.54
rheumatoid — see Arthritis, rheumatoid, juvenile
shoulder M08.91-
specified type NEC M08.80
ankle M08.87-
elbow M08.82-
foot joint M08.87-
hand joint M08.84-
hip M08.85-
knee M08.86-
multiple site M08.89
shoulder M08.81-
specified joint NEC M08.88
vertebrae M08.88
wrist M08.83-
wrist M08.93-
meaning osteoarthritis — see Osteoarthritis
meningococcal A39.83
menopausal (any site) NEC — see Arthritis, specified form NEC
mutilans (psoriatic) L40.52
mycotic NEC (see also category M01) B49
neuropathic (Charcot) — see Arthropathy, neuropathic
diabetic — see Diabetes, arthropathy, neuropathic
nonsyphilitic NEC G98.0
syringomyelic G95.0
ochronotic (see also subcategory M14.8-) E70.29
palindromic (any site) — see Rheumatism, palindromic
pneumococcal M00.10
ankle M00.17-
elbow M00.12-
foot joint — see Arthritis, pneumococcal, ankle
hand joint M00.14-
hip M00.15-
knee M00.16-
multiple site M00.19
shoulder M00.11-
vertebra M00.18
wrist M00.13-
postdysenteric — see Arthropathy, postdysenteric
postmeningococcal A39.84
postrheumatic, chronic — see Arthropathy, postrheumatic, chronic
primary progressive (see also Arthritis, specified form NEC)
spine — see Spondylitis, ankylosing
psoriatic L40.50
purulent (any site except spine) — see Arthritis, pyogenic or pyemic
spine — see Spondylopathy, infective
pyogenic or pyemic (any site except spine) M00.9
bacterial NEC M00.80
ankle M00.87-
elbow M00.82-
foot joint — see Arthritis, pyogenic, bacterial NEC, ankle
hand joint M00.84-
hip M00.85-
knee M00.86-
multiple site M00.89
shoulder M00.81-
vertebra M00.88
wrist M00.83-
pneumococcal — see Arthritis, pneumococcal
spine — see Spondylopathy, infective
staphylococcal — see Arthritis, staphylococcal
streptococcal — see Arthritis, streptococcal NEC
pneumococcal — see Arthritis, pneumococcal
reactive — see Reiter's disease
rheumatic (see also Arthritis, rheumatoid)
acute or subacute — see Fever, rheumatic
rheumatoid M06.9
with
carditis — see Rheumatoid, carditis
endocarditis — see Rheumatoid, carditis
heart involvement NEC — see Rheumatoid, carditis
lung involvement — see Rheumatoid, lung
myocarditis — see Rheumatoid, carditis
myopathy — see Rheumatoid, myopathy
pericarditis — see Rheumatoid, carditis

Arthritis, arthritic — continued
rheumatoid — continued
with — continued
polyneuropathy — see Rheumatoid, polyneuropathy
rheumatoid factor — see Arthritis, rheumatoid, seropositive
splenoadenomegaly and leukopenia — see Felty's syndrome
vasculitis — see Rheumatoid, vasculitis
visceral involvement NEC — see Rheumatoid, arthritis, with involvement of organs NEC
juvenile (with or without rheumatoid factor) M08.00
ankle M08.07-
elbow M08.02-
foot joint M08.07-
hand joint M08.04-
hip M08.05-
knee M08.06-
multiple site M08.09
shoulder M08.01-
vertebra M08.08
wrist M08.03-
seronegative M06.00
ankle M06.07-
elbow M06.02-
foot joint M06.07-
hand joint M06.04-
hip M06.05-
knee M06.06-
multiple site M06.09
shoulder M06.01-
vertebra M06.08
wrist M06.03-
seropositive M05.9
without organ involvement M05.70
ankle M05.77-
elbow M05.72-
foot joint M05.77-
hand joint M05.74-
hip M05.75-
knee M05.76-
multiple sites M05.79
shoulder M05.71-
vertebra — see Spondylitis, ankylosing
wrist M05.73-
specified NEC M05.80
ankle M05.87-
elbow M05.82-
foot joint M05.87-
hand joint M05.84-
hip M05.85-
knee M05.86-
multiple sites M05.89
shoulder M05.81-
vertebra — see Spondylitis, ankylosing
wrist M05.83-
specified type NEC M06.80
ankle M06.87-
elbow M06.82-
foot joint M06.87-
hand joint M06.84-
hip M06.85-
knee M06.86-
multiple site M06.89
shoulder M06.81-
vertebra M06.88
wrist M06.83-
spine — see Spondylitis, ankylosing
rubella B06.82
scorbutic (see also subcategory M14.8-) E54
senile or senescent — see Osteoarthritis
septic (any site except spine) — see Arthritis, pyogenic or pyemic
spine — see Spondylopathy, infective
serum (nontherapeutic) (therapeutic) — see Arthropathy, postimmunization
specified form NEC M13.80
ankle M13.87-
elbow M13.82-
foot joint M13.87-
hand joint M13.84-
hip M13.85-
knee M13.86-
multiple site M13.89

Arthritis, arthritic — continued
  specified form — continued
    shoulder M13.81- ☑
    specified joint NEC M13.88
    wrist M13.83- ☑
  spine (see also Spondylopathy, inflammatory)
    infectious or infective NEC — see Spondylopathy, infective
    Marie-Strümpell — see Spondylitis, ankylosing
    pyogenic — see Spondylopathy, infective
    rheumatoid — see Spondylitis, ankylosing
    traumatic (old) — see Spondylopathy, traumatic
    tuberculous A18.01
  staphylococcal M00.00
    ankle M00.07- ☑
    elbow M00.02- ☑
    foot joint — see Arthritis, staphylococcal, ankle
    hand joint M00.04- ☑
    hip M00.05- ☑
    knee M00.06- ☑
    multiple site M00.09
    shoulder M00.01- ☑
    vertebra M00.08
    wrist M00.03- ☑
  streptococcal NEC M00.20
    ankle M00.27- ☑
    elbow M00.22- ☑
    foot joint — see Arthritis, streptococcal, ankle
    hand joint M00.24- ☑
    hip M00.25- ☑
    knee M00.26- ☑
    multiple site M00.29
    shoulder M00.21- ☑
    vertebra M00.28
    wrist M00.23- ☑
  suppurative — see Arthritis, pyogenic or pyemic
  syphilitic (late) A52.16
    congenital A50.55 [M12.80]
  syphilitica deformans (Charcot) A52.16
  temporomandibular M26.69
  toxic of menopause (any site) — see Arthritis, specified form NEC
  transient — see Arthropathy, specified form NEC
  traumatic (chronic) — see Arthropathy, traumatic
  tuberculous A18.02
    spine A18.01
  uratic — see Gout
  urethritica (Reiter's) — see Reiter's disease
  vertebral — see Spondylopathy, inflammatory
  villous (any site) — see Arthropathy, specified form NEC
Arthrocele — see Effusion, joint
Arthrodesis status Z98.1
Arthrodynia (see also Pain, joint)
Arthrodysplasia Q74.9
Arthrofibrosis, joint — see Ankylosis
Arthrogryposis (congenital) Q68.8
  multiplex congenita Q74.3
Arthrokatadysis M24.7
Arthropathy (see also Arthritis) M12.9
  Charcot's — see Arthropathy, neuropathic
    diabetic — see Diabetes, arthropathy, neuropathic
    syringomyelic G95.0
  cricoarytenoid J38.7
  crystal (-induced) — see Arthritis, in, crystals
  diabetic NEC — see Diabetes, arthropathy
  distal interphalangeal, psoriatic L40.51
  enteropathic M07.60
    ankle M07.67- ☑
    elbow M07.62- ☑
    foot joint M07.67- ☑
    hand joint M07.64- ☑
    hip M07.65- ☑
    knee M07.66- ☑
    multiple site M07.69
    shoulder M07.61- ☑
    vertebra M07.68
    wrist M07.63- ☑
  following intestinal bypass M02.00
    ankle M02.07- ☑
    elbow M02.02- ☑
    foot joint M02.07- ☑
    hand joint M02.04- ☑
    hip M02.05- ☑
    knee M02.06- ☑
    multiple site M02.09
    shoulder M02.01- ☑

Arthropathy — continued
  following intestinal bypass — continued
    vertebra M02.08
    wrist M02.03- ☑
  gouty (see also Gout)
    in (due to)
      Lesch-Nyhan syndrome E79.1 [M14.8-] ☑
      sickle-cell disorders D57- ☑ [M14.8-] ☑
  hemophilic NEC D66 [M36.2]
    in (due to)
      hyperparathyroidism NEC E21.3 [M14.8-] ☑
      metabolic disease NOS E88.9 [M14.8-] ☑
  in (due to)
    acromegaly E22.0 [M14.8-] ☑
    amyloidosis E85.4 [M14.8-] ☑
    blood disorder NOS D75.9 [M36.3]
    diabetes — see Diabetes, arthropathy
    endocrine disease NOS E34.9 [M14.8-] ☑
    erythema
      multiforme L51.9 [M14.8-] ☑
      nodosum L52 [M14.8-] ☑
    hemochromatosis E83.118 [M14.8-] ☑
    hemoglobinopathy NEC D58.2 [M36.3]
    hemophilia NEC D66 [M36.2]
    Henoch-Schönlein purpura D69.0 [M36.4]
    hyperthyroidism E05.90 [M14.8-] ☑
    hypothyroidism E03.9 [M14.8-] ☑
    infective endocarditis I33.0 [M12.80]
    leukemia NEC C95.9- ☑ [M36.1]
    malignant histiocytosis C96.A [M36.1]
    metabolic disease NOS E88.9 [M14.8-] ☑
    multiple myeloma C90.0- ☑ [M36.1]
    neoplastic disease NOS (see also Neoplasm) D49.9 [M36.1]
    nutritional deficiency (see also subcategory M14.8-) E63.9
    psoriasis NOS L40.50
    sarcoidosis D86.86
    syphilis (late) A52.77
      congenital A50.55 [M12.80]
    thyrotoxicosis (see also subcategory M14.8-) E05.90
    ulcerative colitis K51.90 [M07.60]
    viral hepatitis (postinfectious) NEC B19.9 [M12.80]
    Whipple's disease (see also subcategory M14.8-) K90.81
  Jaccoud — see Arthropathy, postrheumatic, chronic
  juvenile — see Arthritis, juvenile
    psoriatic L40.54
  mutilans (psoriatic) L40.52
  neuropathic (Charcot) M14.60
    ankle M14.67- ☑
    diabetic — see Diabetes, arthropathy, neuropathic
    elbow M14.62- ☑
    foot joint M14.67- ☑
    hand joint M14.64- ☑
    hip M14.65- ☑
    knee M14.66- ☑
    multiple site M14.69
    nonsyphilitic NEC G98.0
    shoulder M14.61- ☑
    syringomyelic G95.0
    vertebra M14.68
    wrist M14.63- ☑
  osteopulmonary — see Osteoarthropathy, hypertrophic, specified NEC
  postdysenteric M02.10
    ankle M02.17- ☑
    elbow M02.12- ☑
    foot joint M02.17- ☑
    hand joint M02.14- ☑
    hip M02.15- ☑
    knee M02.16- ☑
    multiple site M02.19
    shoulder M02.11- ☑
    vertebra M02.18
    wrist M02.13- ☑
  postimmunization M02.20
    ankle M02.27- ☑
    elbow M02.22- ☑
    foot joint M02.27- ☑
    hand joint M02.24- ☑
    hip M02.25- ☑
    knee M02.26- ☑
    multiple site M02.29
    shoulder M02.21- ☑
    vertebra M02.28
    wrist M02.23- ☑

Arthropathy — continued
  postinfectious NEC B99 ☑ [M12.80]
    in (due to)
      enteritis due to Yersinia enterocolitica A04.6 [M12.80]
      syphilis A52.77
      viral hepatitis NEC B19.9 [M12.80]
  postrheumatic, chronic (Jaccoud) M12.00
    ankle M12.07- ☑
    elbow M12.02- ☑
    foot joint M12.07- ☑
    hand joint M12.04- ☑
    hip M12.05- ☑
    knee M12.06- ☑
    multiple site M12.09
    shoulder M12.01- ☑
    specified joint NEC M12.08
    vertebrae M12.08
    wrist M12.03- ☑
  psoriatic NEC L40.59
    interphalangeal, distal L40.51
  reactive M02.9
    in (due to)
      infective endocarditis I33.0 [M02.9]
      specified type NEC M02.80
        ankle M02.87- ☑
        elbow M02.82- ☑
        foot joint M02.87- ☑
        hand joint M02.84- ☑
        hip M02.85- ☑
        knee M02.86- ☑
        multiple site M02.89
        shoulder M02.81- ☑
        vertebra M02.88
        wrist M02.83- ☑
  specified form NEC M12.80
    ankle M12.87- ☑
    elbow M12.82- ☑
    foot joint M12.87- ☑
    hand joint M12.84- ☑
    hip M12.85- ☑
    knee M12.86- ☑
    multiple site M12.89
    shoulder M12.81- ☑
    specified joint NEC M12.88
    vertebrae M12.88
    wrist M12.83- ☑
  syringomyelic G95.0
  tabes dorsalis A52.16
  tabetic A52.16
  transient — see Arthropathy, specified form NEC
  traumatic M12.50
    ankle M12.57- ☑
    elbow M12.52- ☑
    foot joint M12.57- ☑
    hand joint M12.54- ☑
    hip M12.55- ☑
    knee M12.56- ☑
    multiple site M12.59
    shoulder M12.51- ☑
    specified joint NEC M12.58
    vertebrae M12.58
    wrist M12.53- ☑
Arthropyosis — see Arthritis, pyogenic or pyemic
Arthrosis (deformans) (degenerative) (localized) (see also Osteoarthritis) M19.90
  spine — see Spondylosis
Arthus' phenomenon or reaction T78.41 ☑
  due to
    drug — see Table of Drugs and Chemicals, by drug
Articular — see condition
Articulation, reverse (teeth) M26.24
Artificial
  insemination complication — see Complications, artificial, fertilization
  opening status (functioning) (without complication) Z93.9
    anus (colostomy) Z93.3
    colostomy Z93.3
    cystostomy Z93.50
      appendico-vesicostomy Z93.52
      cutaneous Z93.51
      specified NEC Z93.59
    enterostomy Z93.4
    gastrostomy Z93.1
    ileostomy Z93.2
    intestinal tract NEC Z93.4

☑ Additional Character Required — Refer to the Tabular List for Character Selection   ▽ Subterms under main terms may continue to next column or page

Artificial — *continued*
  opening status — *continued*
    jejunostomy Z93.4
    nephrostomy Z93.6
    specified site NEC Z93.8
    tracheostomy Z93.0
    ureterostomy Z93.6
    urethrostomy Z93.6
    urinary tract NEC Z93.6
    vagina Z93.8
    vagina status Z93.8
Arytenoid — *see* condition
Asbestosis (occupational) J61
Ascariasis B77.9
  with
    complications NEC B77.89
    intestinal complications B77.0
    pneumonia, pneumonitis B77.81
Ascaridosis, ascariadiasis — *see* Ascariasis
Ascaris (infection) (infestation) (lumbricoides) — *see* Ascariasis
Ascending — *see* condition
ASC-H (atypical squamous cells cannot exclude high grade squamous intraepithelial lesion on cytologic smear)
  anus R85.611
  cervix R87.611
  vagina R87.621
Aschoff's bodies — *see* Myocarditis, rheumatic
Ascites (abdominal) R18.8
  cardiac (*see also* Failure, heart, right) I50.810
  chylous (nonfilarial) I89.8
    filarial — *see* Infestation, filarial
  due to
    cirrhosis, alcoholic K70.31
    hepatitis
      alcoholic K70.11
      chronic active K71.51
    S. japonicum B65.2
  heart (*see also* Failure, heart, right) I50.810
  malignant R18.0
  pseudochylous R18.8
  syphilitic A52.74
  tuberculous A18.31
ASC-US (atypical squamous cells of undetermined significance on cytologic smear)
  anus R85.610
  cervix R87.610
  vagina R87.620
Aseptic — *see* condition
Asherman's syndrome N85.6
Asialia K11.7
Asiatic cholera — *see* Cholera
Asimultagnosia (simultanagnosia) R48.3
Askin's tumor — *see* Neoplasm, connective tissue, malignant
Asocial personality F60.2
Asomatognosia R41.4
Aspartylglucosaminuria E77.1
Asperger's disease or syndrome F84.5
Aspergilloma — *see* Aspergillosis
Aspergillosis (with pneumonia) B44.9
  bronchopulmonary, allergic B44.81
  disseminated B44.7
  generalized B44.7
  pulmonary NEC B44.1
    allergic B44.81
    invasive B44.0
  specified NEC B44.89
  tonsillar B44.2
Aspergillus (flavus) (fumigatus) (infection) (terreus) — *see* Aspergillosis
Aspermatogenesis — *see* Azoospermia
Aspermia (testis) — *see* Azoospermia
Asphyxia, asphyxiation (by) R09.01
  antenatal P84
  birth P84
  bunny bag — *see* Asphyxia, due to, mechanical threat to breathing, trapped in bed clothes
  crushing S28.0 ☑
  drowning T75.1 ☑
  gas, fumes, or vapor — *see* Table of Drugs and Chemicals
  inhalation — *see* Inhalation
  intrauterine P84
  local I73.00
    with gangrene I73.01

Asphyxia, asphyxiation — *continued*
  mucus (*see also* Foreign body, respiratory tract, causing asphyxia)
    newborn P84
  pathological R09.01
  postnatal P84
    mechanical — *see* Asphyxia, due to, mechanical threat to breathing
  prenatal P84
  reticularis R23.1
  strangulation — *see* Asphyxia, due to, mechanical threat to breathing
  submersion T75.1 ☑
  traumatic T71.9 ☑
    due to
      crushed chest S28.0 ☑
      foreign body (in) — *see* Foreign body, respiratory tract, causing asphyxia
      low oxygen content of ambient air T71.20 ☑
        due to
          being trapped in
            low oxygen environment T71.29 ☑
            in car trunk T71.221 ☑
              circumstances undetermined T71.224 ☑
              done with intent to harm by another person T71.223 ☑
                self T71.222 ☑
            in refrigerator T71.231 ☑
              circumstances undetermined T71.234 ☑
              done with intent to harm by another person T71.233 ☑
                self T71.232 ☑
        cave-in T71.21 ☑
      mechanical threat to breathing (accidental) T71.191 ☑
        circumstances undetermined T71.194 ☑
        done with intent to harm by
          another person T71.193 ☑
          self T71.192 ☑
        hanging T71.161 ☑
          circumstances undetermined T71.164 ☑
          done with intent to harm by
            another person T71.163 ☑
            self T71.162 ☑
        plastic bag T71.121 ☑
          circumstances undetermined T71.124 ☑
          done with intent to harm by
            another person T71.123 ☑
            self T71.122 ☑
      smothering
        in furniture T71.151 ☑
          circumstances undetermined T71.154 ☑
          done with intent to harm by
            another person T71.153 ☑
            self T71.152 ☑
        under
          another person's body T71.141 ☑
            circumstances undetermined T71.144 ☑
            done with intent to harm T71.143 ☑
          pillow T71.111 ☑
            circumstances undetermined T71.114 ☑
            done with intent to harm by
              another person T71.113 ☑
              self T71.112 ☑
        trapped in bed clothes T71.131 ☑
          circumstances undetermined T71.134 ☑
          done with intent to harm by
            another person T71.133 ☑
            self T71.132 ☑
  vomiting, vomitus — *see* Foreign body, respiratory tract, causing asphyxia
Aspiration
  amniotic (clear) fluid (newborn) P24.10
    with
      pneumonia (pneumonitis) P24.11
      respiratory symptoms P24.11
  blood
    newborn (without respiratory symptoms) P24.20
      with
        pneumonia (pneumonitis) P24.21
        respiratory symptoms P24.21

Aspiration — *continued*
  blood — *continued*
    specified age NEC — *see* Foreign body, respiratory tract
  bronchitis J69.0
  food or foreign body (with asphyxiation) — *see* Asphyxia, food
  liquor (amnii) (newborn) P24.10
    with
      pneumonia (pneumonitis) P24.11
      respiratory symptoms P24.11
  meconium (newborn) (without respiratory symptoms) P24.00
    with
      pneumonitis (pneumonitis) P24.01
      respiratory symptoms P24.01
  milk (newborn) (without respiratory symptoms) P24.30
    with
      pneumonia (pneumonitis) P24.31
      respiratory symptoms P24.31
    specified age NEC — *see* Foreign body, respiratory tract
  mucus (*see also* Foreign body, by site, causing asphyxia)
    newborn P24.10
      with
        pneumonia (pneumonitis) P24.11
        respiratory symptoms P24.11
    neonatal P24.9
      specific NEC (without respiratory symptoms) P24.80
        with
          pneumonia (pneumonitis) P24.81
          respiratory symptoms P24.81
    newborn P24.9
      specific NEC (without respiratory symptoms) P24.80
        with
          pneumonia (pneumonitis) P24.81
          respiratory symptoms P24.81
  pneumonia J69.0
  pneumonitis J69.0
  syndrome of newborn — *see* Aspiration, by substance, with pneumonia
  vernix caseosa (newborn) P24.80
    with
      pneumonia (pneumonitis) P24.81
      respiratory symptoms P24.81
  vomitus (*see also* Foreign body, respiratory tract)
    newborn (without respiratory symptoms) P24.30
      with
        pneumonia (pneumonitis) P24.31
        respiratory symptoms P24.31
Asplenia (congenital) Q89.01
  postsurgical Z90.81
Assam fever B55.0
Assault, sexual — *see* Maltreatment
Assmann's focus NEC A15.0
Astasia (-abasia) (hysterical) F44.4
Asteatosis cutis L85.3
Astereognosia, astereognosis R48.1
Asterixis R27.8
  in liver disease K71.3
Asteroid hyalitis — *see* Deposit, crystalline
Asthenia, asthenic R53.1
  cardiac (*see also* Failure, heart) I50.9
    psychogenic F45.8
  cardiovascular (*see also* Failure, heart) I50.9
    psychogenic F45.8
  heart (*see also* Failure, heart) I50.9
    psychogenic F45.8
  hysterical F44.4
  myocardial (*see also* Failure, heart) I50.9
    psychogenic F45.8
  nervous F48.8
  neurocirculatory F45.8
  neurotic F48.8
  psychogenic F48.8
  psychoneurotic F48.8
  psychophysiologic F48.8
  reaction (psychophysiologic) F48.8
  senile R54
Asthenopia (*see also* Discomfort, visual)
  hysterical F44.6
  psychogenic F44.6
Asthenospermia — *see* Abnormal, specimen, male genital organs
Asthma, asthmatic (bronchial) (catarrh) (spasmodic) J45.909

Asthma, asthmatic — *continued*
with
  chronic obstructive bronchitis J44.9
    with
      acute lower respiratory infection J44.0
      exacerbation (acute) J44.1
  chronic obstructive pulmonary disease J44.9
    with
      acute lower respiratory infection J44.0
      exacerbation (acute) J44.1
  exacerbation (acute) J45.901
  hay fever — *see* Asthma, allergic extrinsic
  rhinitis, allergic — *see* Asthma, allergic extrinsic
  status asthmaticus J45.902
allergic extrinsic J45.909
  with
    exacerbation (acute) J45.901
    status asthmaticus J45.902
atopic — *see* Asthma, allergic extrinsic
cardiac — *see* Failure, ventricular, left
cardiobronchial I50.1
childhood J45.909
  with
    exacerbation (acute) J45.901
    status asthmaticus J45.902
chronic obstructive J44.9
  with
    acute lower respiratory infection J44.0
    exacerbation (acute) J44.1
collier's J60
cough variant J45.991
detergent J69.8
due to
  detergent J69.8
  inhalation of fumes J68.3
eosinophilic J82
extrinsic, allergic — *see* Asthma, allergic extrinsic
grinder's J62.8
hay — *see* Asthma, allergic extrinsic
heart I50.1
idiosyncratic — *see* Asthma, nonallergic
intermittent (mild) J45.20
  with
    exacerbation (acute) J45.21
    status asthmaticus J45.22
intrinsic, nonallergic — *see* Asthma, nonallergic
Kopp's E32.8
late-onset J45.909
  with
    exacerbation (acute) J45.901
    status asthmaticus J45.902
mild intermittent J45.20
  with
    exacerbation (acute) J45.21
    status asthmaticus J45.22
mild persistent J45.30
  with
    exacerbation (acute) J45.31
    status asthmaticus J45.32
Millar's (laryngismus stridulus) J38.5
miner's J60
mixed J45.909
  with
    exacerbation (acute) J45.901
    status asthmaticus J45.902
moderate persistent J45.40
  with
    exacerbation (acute) J45.41
    status asthmaticus J45.42
nervous — *see* Asthma, nonallergic
nonallergic (intrinsic) J45.909
  with
    exacerbation (acute) J45.901
    status asthmaticus J45.902
persistent
  mild J45.30
    with
      exacerbation (acute) J45.31
      status asthmaticus J45.32
  moderate J45.40
    with
      exacerbation (acute) J45.41
      status asthmaticus J45.42
  severe J45.50
    with
      exacerbation (acute) J45.51
      status asthmaticus J45.52
platinum J45.998

Asthma, asthmatic — *continued*
pneumoconiotic NEC J64
potter's J62.8
predominantly allergic J45.909
psychogenic F54
pulmonary eosinophilic J82
red cedar J67.8
Rostan's I50.1
sandblaster's J62.8
sequoiosis J67.8
severe persistent J45.50
  with
    exacerbation (acute) J45.51
    status asthmaticus J45.52
specified NEC J45.998
stonemason's J62.8
thymic E32.8
tuberculous — *see* Tuberculosis, pulmonary
Wichmann's (laryngismus stridulus) J38.5
wood J67.8
Astigmatism (compound) (congenital) H52.20- ☑
irregular H52.21- ☑
regular H52.22- ☑
Astraphobia F40.220
Astroblastoma
specified site — *see* Neoplasm, malignant, by site
unspecified site C71.9
Astrocytoma (cystic)
anaplastic
  specified site — *see* Neoplasm, malignant, by site
  unspecified site C71.9
fibrillary
  specified site — *see* Neoplasm, malignant, by site
  unspecified site C71.9
fibrous
  specified site — *see* Neoplasm, malignant, by site
  unspecified site C71.9
gemistocytic
  specified site — *see* Neoplasm, malignant, by site
  unspecified site C71.9
juvenile
  specified site — *see* Neoplasm, malignant, by site
  unspecified site C71.9
pilocytic
  specified site — *see* Neoplasm, malignant, by site
  unspecified site C71.9
piloid
  specified site — *see* Neoplasm, malignant, by site
  unspecified site C71.9
protoplasmic
  specified site — *see* Neoplasm, malignant, by site
  unspecified site C71.9
specified site NEC — *see* Neoplasm, malignant, by site
subependymal D43.2
  giant cell
    specified site — *see* Neoplasm, uncertain behavior, by site
    unspecified site D43.2
  specified site — *see* Neoplasm, uncertain behavior, by site
  unspecified site D43.2
unspecified site C71.9
Astroglioma
specified site — *see* Neoplasm, malignant, by site
unspecified site C71.9
Asymbolia R48.8
Asymmetry (*see also* Distortion)
between native and reconstructed breast N65.1
face Q67.0
jaw (lower) — *see* Anomaly, dentofacial, jaw-cranial base relationship, asymmetry
Asynergia, asynergy R27.8
ventricular I51.89
Asystole (heart) — *see* Arrest, cardiac
At risk
for
  dental caries Z91.849
    high Z91.843
    low Z91.841
    moderate Z91.842
  falling Z91.81
Ataxia, ataxy, ataxic R27.0
acute R27.8
brain (hereditary) G11.9
cerebellar (hereditary) G11.9
  with defective DNA repair G11.3
  alcoholic G31.2
  early-onset G11.1

Ataxia, ataxy, ataxic — *continued*
cerebellar — *continued*
  in
    alcoholism G31.2
    myxedema E03.9 [G13.2]
    neoplastic disease (*see also* Neoplasm) D49.9 [G32.81]
    specified disease NEC G32.81
  late-onset (Marie's) G11.2
cerebral (hereditary) G11.9
congenital nonprogressive G11.0
family, familial — *see* Ataxia, hereditary
following
  cerebrovascular disease I69.993
    cerebral infarction I69.393
    intracerebral hemorrhage I69.193
    nontraumatic intracranial hemorrhage NEC I69.293
    specified disease NEC I69.893
    subarachnoid hemorrhage I69.093
Friedreich's (heredofamilial) (cerebellar) (spinal) G11.1
gait R26.0
  hysterical F44.4
general R27.8
gluten M35.9 [G32.81]
  with celiac disease K90.0 [G32.81]
hereditary G11.9
  with neuropathy G60.2
  cerebellar — *see* Ataxia, cerebellar
  spastic G11.4
  specified NEC G11.8
  spinal (Friedreich's) G11.1
heredofamilial — *see* Ataxia, hereditary
Hunt's G11.1
hysterical F44.4
locomotor (progressive) (syphilitic) (partial) (spastic) A52.11
  diabetic — *see* Diabetes, ataxia
Marie's (cerebellar) (heredofamilial) (late-onset) G11.2
nonorganic origin F44.4
nonprogressive, congenital G11.0
psychogenic F44.4
Roussy-Lévy G60.0
Sanger-Brown's (hereditary) G11.2
spastic hereditary G11.4
spinal
  hereditary (Friedreich's) G11.1
  progressive (syphilitic) A52.11
spinocerebellar, X-linked recessive G11.1
telangiectasia (Louis-Bar) G11.3
Ataxia-telangiectasia (Louis-Bar) G11.3
Atelectasis (massive) (partial) (pressure) (pulmonary) J98.11
newborn P28.10
  due to resorption P28.11
  partial P28.19
  primary P28.0
  secondary P28.19
primary (newborn) P28.0
tuberculous — *see* Tuberculosis, pulmonary
Atelocardia Q24.9
Atelomyelia Q06.1
Atheroembolism
of
  extremities
    lower I75.02- ☑
    upper I75.01- ☑
  kidney I75.81
  specified NEC I75.89
Atheroma, atheromatous (*see also* Arteriosclerosis) I70.90
aorta, aortic I70.0
  valve (*see also* Endocarditis, aortic) I35.8
aorto-iliac I70.0
artery — *see* Arteriosclerosis
basilar (artery) I67.2
carotid (artery) (common) (internal) I67.2
cerebral (arteries) I67.2
coronary (artery) I25.10
  with angina pectoris — *see* Arteriosclerosis, coronary (artery),
degeneration — *see* Arteriosclerosis
heart, cardiac — *see* Disease, heart, ischemic, atherosclerotic
mitral (valve) I34.8
myocardium, myocardial — *see* Disease, heart, ischemic, atherosclerotic

Atheroma, atheromatous — *continued*
  pulmonary valve (heart) (*see also* Endocarditis, pulmonary) I37.8
  tricuspid (heart) (valve) I36.8
  valve, valvular — *see* Endocarditis
  vertebral (artery) I67.2
Atheromatosis — *see* Arteriosclerosis
Atherosclerosis (*see also* Arteriosclerosis)
  coronary
    artery I25.10
      with angina pectoris — *see* Arteriosclerosis, coronary (artery),
      due to
        calcified coronary lesion (severely) I25.84
        lipid rich plaque I25.83
    transplanted heart I25.811
      bypass graft I25.812
        with angina pectoris — *see* Arteriosclerosis, coronary (artery),
      native coronary artery I25.811
        with angina pectoris — *see* Arteriosclerosis, coronary (artery),
Athetosis (acquired) R25.8
  bilateral (congenital) G80.3
  congenital (bilateral) (double) G80.3
  double (congenital) G80.3
  unilateral R25.8
Athlete's
  foot B35.3
  heart I51.7
Athrepsia E41
Athyrea (acquired) (*see also* Hypothyroidism)
  congenital E03.1
Atonia, atony, atonic
  bladder (sphincter) (neurogenic) N31.2
  capillary I78.8
  cecum K59.8
    psychogenic F45.8
  colon — *see* Atony, intestine
  congenital P94.2
  esophagus K22.8
  intestine K59.8
    psychogenic F45.8
  stomach K31.89
    neurotic or psychogenic F45.8
  uterus (during labor) O62.2
    with hemorrhage (postpartum) O72.1
    postpartum (with hemorrhage) O72.1
      without hemorrhage O75.89
Atopy — *see* History, allergy
Atransferrinemia, congenital E88.09
Atresia, atretic
  alimentary organ or tract NEC Q45.8
    upper Q40.8
  ani, anus, anal (canal) Q42.3
    with fistula Q42.2
  aorta (ring) Q25.29
  aortic (orifice) (valve) Q23.0
    arch Q25.21
    congenital with hypoplasia of ascending aorta and defective development of left ventricle (with mitral stenosis) Q23.4
    in hypoplastic left heart syndrome Q23.4
  aqueduct of Sylvius Q03.0
    with spina bifida — *see* Spina bifida, with hydrocephalus
  artery NEC Q27.8
    cerebral Q28.3
    coronary Q24.5
    digestive system Q27.8
    eye Q15.8
    lower limb Q27.8
    pulmonary Q25.5
    specified site NEC Q27.8
    umbilical Q27.0
    upper limb Q27.8
  auditory canal (external) Q16.1
  bile duct (common) (congenital) (hepatic) Q44.2
    acquired — *see* Obstruction, bile duct
  bladder (neck) Q64.39
    obstruction Q64.31
  bronchus Q32.4
  cecum Q42.8
  cervix (acquired) N88.2
    congenital Q51.828
    in pregnancy or childbirth — *see* Anomaly, cervix, in pregnancy or childbirth
      causing obstructed labor O65.5

Atresia, atretic — *continued*
  choana Q30.0
  colon Q42.9
    specified NEC Q42.8
  common duct Q44.2
  cricoid cartilage Q31.8
  cystic duct Q44.2
    acquired K82.8
      with obstruction K82.0
  digestive organs NEC Q45.8
  duodenum Q41.0
  ear canal Q16.1
  ejaculatory duct Q55.4
  epiglottis Q31.8
  esophagus Q39.0
    with tracheoesophageal fistula Q39.1
  eustachian tube Q17.8
  fallopian tube (congenital) Q50.6
    acquired N97.1
  follicular cyst N83.0- ☑
  foramen of
    Luschka Q03.1
      with spina bifida — *see* Spina bifida, with hydrocephalus
    Magendie Q03.1
      with spina bifida — *see* Spina bifida, with hydrocephalus
  gallbladder Q44.1
  genital organ
    external
      female Q52.79
      male Q55.8
    internal
      female Q52.8
      male Q55.8
  glottis Q31.8
  gullet Q39.0
    with tracheoesophageal fistula Q39.1
  heart valve NEC Q24.8
    pulmonary Q22.0
    tricuspid Q22.4
  hymen Q52.3
    acquired (postinfective) N89.6
  ileum Q41.2
  intestine (small) Q41.9
    large Q42.9
      specified NEC Q42.8
  iris, filtration angle Q15.0
  jejunum Q41.1
  lacrimal apparatus Q10.4
  larynx Q31.8
  meatus urinarius Q64.33
  mitral valve Q23.2
    in hypoplastic left heart syndrome Q23.4
  nares (anterior) (posterior) Q30.0
  nasopharynx Q34.8
  nose, nostril Q30.0
    acquired J34.89
  organ or site NEC Q89.8
  osseous meatus (ear) Q16.1
  oviduct (congenital) Q50.6
    acquired N97.1
  parotid duct Q38.4
    acquired K11.8
  pulmonary (artery) Q25.5
    valve Q22.0
  pulmonic Q22.0
  pupil Q13.2
  rectum Q42.1
    with fistula Q42.0
  salivary duct Q38.4
    acquired K11.8
  sublingual duct Q38.4
    acquired K11.8
  submandibular duct Q38.4
    acquired K11.8
  submaxillary duct Q38.4
    acquired K11.8
  thyroid cartilage Q31.8
  trachea Q32.1
  tricuspid valve Q22.4
  ureter Q62.10
    pelvic junction Q62.11
    vesical orifice Q62.12
  ureteropelvic junction Q62.11
  ureterovesical orifice Q62.12
  urethra (valvular) Q64.39
    stricture Q64.32
  urinary tract NEC Q64.8

Atresia, atretic — *continued*
  uterus Q51.818
    acquired N85.8
  vagina (congenital) Q52.4
    acquired (postinfectional) (senile) N89.5
  vas deferens Q55.3
  vascular NEC Q27.8
    cerebral Q28.3
    digestive system Q27.8
    lower limb Q27.8
    specified site NEC Q27.8
    upper limb Q27.8
  vein NEC Q27.8
    digestive system Q27.8
    great Q26.8
    lower limb Q27.8
    portal Q26.5
    pulmonary Q26.4
      partial Q26.3
      total Q26.2
    specified site NEC Q27.8
    upper limb Q27.8
  vena cava (inferior) (superior) Q26.8
  vesicourethral orifice Q64.31
  vulva Q52.79
    acquired N90.5
Atrichia, atrichosis — *see* Alopecia
Atrophia (*see also* Atrophy)
  cutis senilis L90.8
    due to radiation L57.8
  gyrata of choroid and retina H31.23
  senilis R54
    dermatological L90.8
      due to radiation (nonionizing) (solar) L57.8
  unguium L60.3
    congenita Q84.6
Atrophie blanche (en plaque) (de Milian) L95.0
Atrophoderma, atrophodermia (of) L90.9
  diffusum (idiopathic) L90.4
  maculatum L90.8
    et striatum L90.8
      due to syphilis A52.79
    syphilitic A51.39
  neuriticum L90.8
  Pasini and Pierini L90.3
  pigmentosum Q82.1
  reticulatum symmetricum faciei L66.4
  senile L90.8
    due to radiation (nonionizing) (solar) L57.8
  vermiculata (cheeks) L66.4
Atrophy, atrophic (of)
  adrenal (capsule) (gland) E27.49
    primary (autoimmune) E27.1
  alveolar process or ridge (edentulous) K08.20
  anal sphincter (disuse) N81.84
  appendix K38.8
  arteriosclerotic — *see* Arteriosclerosis
  bile duct (common) (hepatic) K83.8
  bladder N32.89
    neurogenic N31.8
  blanche (en plaque) (of Milian) L95.0
  bone (senile) NEC (*see also* Disorder, bone, specified type NEC)
    due to
      tabes dorsalis (neurogenic) A52.11
  brain (cortex) (progressive) G31.9
    frontotemporal circumscribed G31.01 [F02.80]
      with behavioral disturbance G31.01 [F02.81]
    senile NEC G31.1
  breast N64.2
    obstetric — *see* Disorder, breast, specified type NEC
  buccal cavity K13.79
  cardiac — *see* Degeneration, myocardial
  cartilage (infectional) (joint) — *see* Disorder, cartilage, specified NEC
  cerebellar — *see* Atrophy, brain
  cerebral — *see* Atrophy, brain
  cervix (mucosa) (senile) (uteri) N88.8
    menopausal N95.8
  Charcot-Marie-Tooth G60.0
  choroid (central) (macular) (myopic) (retina) H31.10- ☑
    diffuse secondary H31.12- ☑
    gyrate H31.23
    senile H31.11- ☑
  ciliary body — *see* Atrophy, iris
  conjunctiva (senile) H11.89
  corpus cavernosum N48.89

Atrophy, atrophic — *continued*
- cortical — *see* Atrophy, brain
- cystic duct K82.8
- Déjérine-Thomas G23.8
- disuse NEC — *see* Atrophy, muscle
- Duchenne-Aran G12.21
- ear H93.8- ☑
- edentulous alveolar ridge K08.20
- endometrium (senile) N85.8
  - cervix N88.8
- enteric K63.89
- epididymis N50.89
- eyeball — *see* Disorder, globe, degenerated condition, atrophy
- eyelid (senile) — *see* Disorder, eyelid, degenerative
- facial (skin) L90.9
- fallopian tube (senile) N83.32- ☑
  - with ovary N83.33- ☑
- fascioscapulohumeral (Landouzy- Déjérine) G71.0
- fatty, thymus (gland) E32.8
- gallbladder K82.8
- gastric K29.40
  - with bleeding K29.41
- gastrointestinal K63.89
- glandular I89.8
- globe H44.52- ☑
- gum — *see* Recession, gingival
- hair L67.8
- heart (brown) — *see* Degeneration, myocardial
- hemifacial Q67.4
  - Romberg G51.8
- infantile E41
  - paralysis, acute — *see* Poliomyelitis, paralytic
- intestine K63.89
- iris (essential) (progressive) H21.26- ☑
  - specified NEC H21.29
- kidney (senile) (terminal) (*see also* Sclerosis, renal) N26.1
  - congenital or infantile Q60.5
    - bilateral Q60.4
    - unilateral Q60.3
  - hydronephrotic — *see* Hydronephrosis
- lacrimal gland (primary) H04.14- ☑
  - secondary H04.15- ☑
- Landouzy-Déjérine G71.0
- laryngitis, infective J37.0
- larynx J38.7
- Leber's optic (hereditary) H47.22
- lip K13.0
- liver (yellow) K72.90
  - with coma K72.91
  - acute, subacute K72.00
    - with coma K72.01
  - chronic K72.10
    - with coma K72.11
- lung (senile) J98.4
- macular (dermatological) L90.8
  - syphilitic, skin A51.39
    - striated A52.79
- mandible (edentulous) K08.20
  - minimal K08.21
  - moderate K08.22
  - severe K08.23
- maxilla K08.20
  - minimal K08.24
  - moderate K08.25
  - severe K08.26
- muscle, muscular (diffuse) (general) (idiopathic) (primary) M62.50
  - ankle M62.57- ☑
  - Duchenne-Aran G12.21
  - foot M62.57- ☑
  - forearm M62.53- ☑
  - hand M62.54- ☑
  - infantile spinal G12.0
  - lower leg M62.56- ☑
  - multiple sites M62.59
  - myelopathic — *see* Atrophy, muscle, spinal
  - myotonic G71.11
  - neuritic G58.9
  - neuropathic (peroneal) (progressive) G60.0
  - pelvic (disuse) N81.84
  - peroneal G60.0
  - progressive (bulbar) G12.21
    - adult G12.1
    - infantile (spinal) G12.0
    - spinal G12.25
      - adult G12.1

Atrophy, atrophic — *continued*
- muscle, muscular — *continued*
  - progressive — *continued*
    - spinal — *continued*
      - infantile G12.0
  - pseudohypertrophic G71.0
  - shoulder region M62.51- ☑
  - specified site NEC M62.58
  - spinal G12.9
    - adult form G12.1
    - Aran-Duchenne G12.21
    - childhood form, type II G12.1
    - distal G12.1
    - hereditary NEC G12.1
    - infantile, type I (Werdnig-Hoffmann) G12.0
    - juvenile form, type III (Kugelberg- Welander) G12.1
    - progressive G12.25
    - scapuloperoneal form G12.1
    - specified NEC G12.8
  - syphilitic A52.78
  - thigh M62.55- ☑
  - upper arm M62.52- ☑
- myocardium — *see* Degeneration, myocardial
- myometrium (senile) N85.8
  - cervix N88.8
- myopathic NEC — *see* Atrophy, muscle
- myotonia G71.11
- nail L60.3
- nasopharynx J31.1
- nerve (*see also* Disorder, nerve)
  - abducens — *see* Strabismus, paralytic, sixth nerve
  - accessory G52.8
  - acoustic or auditory H93.3 ☑
  - cranial G52.9
    - eighth (auditory) H93.3 ☑
    - eleventh (accessory) G52.8
    - fifth (trigeminal) G50.8
    - first (olfactory) G52.0
    - fourth (trochlear) — *see* Strabismus, paralytic, fourth nerve
    - second (optic) H47.20
    - sixth (abducens) — *see* Strabismus, paralytic, sixth nerve
    - tenth (pneumogastric) (vagus) G52.2
    - third (oculomotor) — *see* Strabismus, paralytic, third nerve
    - twelfth (hypoglossal) G52.3
  - hypoglossal G52.3
  - oculomotor — *see* Strabismus, paralytic, third nerve
  - olfactory G52.0
  - optic (papillomacular bundle)
    - syphilitic (late) A52.15
      - congenital A50.44
  - pneumogastric G52.2
  - trigeminal G50.8
  - trochlear — *see* Strabismus, paralytic, fourth nerve
  - vagus (pneumogastric) G52.2
- neurogenic, bone, tabetic A52.11
- nutritional E41
- old age R54
- olivopontocerebellar G23.8
- optic (nerve) H47.20
  - glaucomatous H47.23- ☑
  - hereditary H47.22
  - primary H47.21- ☑
  - specified type NEC H47.29- ☑
  - syphilitic (late) A52.15
    - congenital A50.44
- orbit H05.31- ☑
- ovary (senile) N83.31- ☑
  - with fallopian tube N83.33- ☑
- oviduct (senile) — *see* Atrophy, fallopian tube
- palsy, diffuse (progressive) G12.22
- pancreas (duct) (senile) K86.89
- parotid gland K11.0
- pelvic muscle N81.84
- penis N48.89
- pharynx J39.2
- pluriglandular E31.8
  - autoimmune E31.0
- polyarthritis M15.9
- prostate N42.89
- pseudohypertrophic (muscle) G71.0
- renal (*see also* Sclerosis, renal) N26.1
- retina, retinal (postinfectional) H35.89
- rhinitis J31.0

Atrophy, atrophic — *continued*
- salivary gland K11.0
- scar L90.5
- sclerosis, lobar (of brain) G31.09 [F02.80]
  - with behavioral disturbance G31.09 [F02.81]
- scrotum N50.89
- seminal vesicle N50.89
- senile R54
  - due to radiation (nonionizing) (solar) L57.8
- skin (patches) (spots) L90.9
  - degenerative (senile) L90.8
  - due to radiation (nonionizing) (solar) L57.8
  - senile L90.8
- spermatic cord N50.89
- spinal (acute) (cord) G95.89
  - muscular — *see* Atrophy, muscle, spinal
  - paralysis G12.20
    - acute — *see* Poliomyelitis, paralytic
    - meaning progressive muscular atrophy G12.21
- spine (column) — *see* Spondylopathy, specified NEC
- spleen (senile) D73.0
- stomach K29.40
  - with bleeding K29.41
- striate (skin) L90.6
  - syphilitic A52.79
- subcutaneous L90.9
- sublingual gland K11.0
- submandibular gland K11.0
- submaxillary gland K11.0
- Sudeck's — *see* Algoneurodystrophy
- suprarenal (capsule) (gland) E27.49
  - primary E27.1
- systemic affecting central nervous system in
  - myxedema E03.9 [G13.2]
  - neoplastic disease (*see also* Neoplasm) D49.9 [G13.1]
  - specified disease NEC G13.8
- tarso-orbital fascia, congenital Q10.3
- testis N50.0
- thenar, partial — *see* Syndrome, carpal tunnel
- thymus (fatty) E32.8
- thyroid (gland) (acquired) E03.4
  - with cretinism E03.1
  - congenital (with myxedema) E03.1
- tongue (senile) K14.8
  - papillae K14.4
- trachea J39.8
- tunica vaginalis N50.89
- turbinate J34.89
- tympanic membrane (nonflaccid) H73.82- ☑
  - flaccid H73.81- ☑
- upper respiratory tract J39.8
- uterus, uterine (senile) N85.8
  - cervix N88.8
  - due to radiation (intended effect) N85.8
    - adverse effect or misadventure N99.89
- vagina (senile) N95.2
- vas deferens N50.89
- vascular I99.8
- vertebra (senile) — *see* Spondylopathy, specified NEC
- vulva (senile) N90.5
- Werdnig-Hoffmann G12.0
- yellow — *see* Failure, hepatic

Attack, attacks
- with alteration of consciousness (with automatisms) — *see* Epilepsy, localization-related, symptomatic, with complex partial seizures
- without alteration of consciousness — *see* Epilepsy, localization-related, symptomatic, with simple partial seizures
- Adams-Stokes I45.9
- akinetic — *see* Epilepsy, generalized, specified NEC
- angina — *see* Angina
- atonic — *see* Epilepsy, generalized, specified NEC
- benign shuddering G25.83
- cataleptic — *see* Catalepsy
- coronary — *see* Infarct, myocardium
- cyanotic, newborn P28.2
- drop NEC R55
- epileptic — *see* Epilepsy
- heart — *see* infarct, myocardium
- hysterical F44.9
- jacksonian — *see* Epilepsy, localization-related, symptomatic, with simple partial seizures
- myocardial, myocardial — *see* Infarct, myocardium
- myoclonic — *see* Epilepsy, generalized, specified NEC
- panic F41.0

ICD-10-CM 2018   **Band**

Index

Attack, attacks — *continued*
 psychomotor — *see* Epilepsy, localization-related,
  symptomatic, with complex partial seizures
 salaam — *see* Epilepsy, spasms
 schizophreniform, brief F23
 shuddering, benign G25.83
 Stokes-Adams I45.9
 syncope R55
 transient ischemic (TIA) G45.9
  specified NEC G45.8
 unconsciousness R55
  hysterical F44.89
 vasomotor R55
 vasovagal (paroxysmal) (idiopathic) R55
Attention (to)
 artificial
  opening (of) Z43.9
   digestive tract NEC Z43.4
    colon Z43.3
    ilium Z43.2
    stomach Z43.1
   specified NEC Z43.8
   trachea Z43.0
   urinary tract NEC Z43.6
    cystostomy Z43.5
    nephrostomy Z43.6
    ureterostomy Z43.6
    urethrostomy Z43.6
   vagina Z43.7
 colostomy Z43.3
 cystostomy Z43.5
 deficit disorder or syndrome F98.8
  with hyperactivity — *see* Disorder, attention-deficit
   hyperactivity
 gastrostomy Z43.1
 ileostomy Z43.2
 jejunostomy Z43.4
 nephrostomy Z43.6
 surgical dressings Z48.01
 sutures Z48.02
 tracheostomy Z43.0
 ureterostomy Z43.6
 urethrostomy Z43.6
Attrition
 gum — *see* Recession, gingival
 tooth, teeth (excessive) (hard tissues) K03.0
Atypical, atypism (*see also* condition)
 cells (on cytological smear) (endocervical) (endometrial) (glandular)
  cervix R87.619
  vagina R87.629
 cervical N87.9
 endometrium N85.9
  hyperplasia N85.00
 parenting situation Z62.9
Auditory — *see* condition
Aujeszky's disease B33.8
Aurantiasis, cutis E67.1
Auricle, auricular (*see also* condition)
 cervical Q18.2
Auriculotemporal syndrome G50.8
Austin Flint murmur (aortic insufficiency) I35.1
Australian
 Q fever A78
 X disease A83.4
Autism, autistic (childhood) (infantile) F84.0
 atypical F84.9
 spectrum disorder F84.0
Autodigestion R68.89
Autoerythrocyte sensitization (syndrome) D69.2
Autographism L50.3
Autoimmune
 disease (systemic) M35.9
 inhibitors to clotting factors D68.311
 lymphoproliferative syndrome [ALPS] D89.82
 thyroiditis E06.3
Autointoxication R68.89
Automatism G93.89
 with temporal sclerosis G93.81
 epileptic — *see* Epilepsy, localization-related, symptomatic, with complex partial seizures
 paroxysmal, idiopathic — *see* Epilepsy, localization-
  related, symptomatic, with complex partial
  seizures
Autonomic, autonomous
 bladder (neurogenic) N31.2
 hysteria seizure F44.5
Autosensitivity, erythrocyte D69.2

Autosensitization, cutaneous L30.2
Autosome — *see* condition by chromosome involved
Autotopagnosia R48.1
Autotoxemia R68.89
Autumn — *see* condition
Avellis' syndrome G46.8
Aversion
 oral R63.3
  newborn P92.- ☑
  nonorganic origin F98.2 ☑
 sexual F52.1
Aviator's
 disease or sickness — *see* Effect, adverse, high altitude
 ear T70.0 ☑
Avitaminosis (multiple) (*see also* Deficiency, vitamin)
  E56.9
 B E53.9
  with
   beriberi E51.11
   pellagra E52
 B2 E53.0
 B6 E53.1
 B12 E53.8
 D E55.9
  with rickets E55.0
 G E53.0
 K E56.1
 nicotinic acid E52
AVNRT (atrioventricular nodal re-entrant tachycardia)
  I47.1
AVRT (atrioventricular nodal re-entrant tachycardia) I47.1
Avulsion (traumatic)
 blood vessel — *see* Injury, blood vessel
 bone — *see* Fracture, by site
 cartilage (*see also* Dislocation, by site)
  symphyseal (inner), complicating delivery O71.6
 external site other than limb — *see* Wound, open, by
  site
 eye S05.7- ☑
 head (intracranial)
  external site NEC S08.89 ☑
  scalp S08.0 ☑
 internal organ or site — *see* Injury, by site
 joint (*see also* Dislocation, by site)
  capsule — *see* Sprain, by site
 kidney S37.06- ☑
 ligament — *see* Sprain, by site
 limb (*see also* Amputation, traumatic, by site)
  skin and subcutaneous tissue — *see* Wound, open,
   by site
 muscle — *see* Injury, muscle
 nerve (root) — *see* Injury, nerve
 scalp S08.0 ☑
 skin and subcutaneous tissue — *see* Wound, open, by
  site
 spleen S36.032 ☑
 symphyseal cartilage (inner), complicating delivery
  O71.6
 tendon — *see* Injury, muscle
 tooth S03.2 ☑
Awareness of heart beat R00.2
Axenfeld's
 anomaly or syndrome Q15.0
 degeneration (calcareous) Q13.4
Axilla, axillary (*see also* condition)
 breast Q83.1
Axonotmesis — *see* Injury, nerve
Ayerza's disease or syndrome (pulmonary artery sclerosis with pulmonary hypertension) I27.0
Azoospermia (organic) N46.01
 due to
  drug therapy N46.021
  efferent duct obstruction N46.023
  infection N46.022
  radiation N46.024
  specified cause NEC N46.029
  systemic disease N46.025
Azotemia R79.89
 meaning uremia N19
Aztec ear Q17.3
Azygos
 continuation inferior vena cava Q26.8
 lobe (lung) Q33.1

B

Baastrup's disease — *see* Kissing spine

Babesiosis B60.0
Babington's disease (familial hemorrhagic telangiectasia) I78.0
Babinski's syndrome A52.79
Baby
 crying constantly R68.11
 floppy (syndrome) P94.2
Bacillary — *see* condition
Bacilluria R82.71
Bacillus (*see also* Infection, bacillus)
 abortus infection A23.1
 anthracis infection A22.9
 coli infection (*see also* Escherichia coli) B96.20
 Flexner's A03.1
 mallei infection A24.0
 Shiga's A03.0
 suipestifer infection — *see* Infection, salmonella
Back — *see* condition
Backache (postural) M54.9
 sacroiliac M53.3
 specified NEC M54.89
Backflow — *see* Reflux
Backward reading (dyslexia) F81.0
Bacteremia R78.81
 with sepsis — *see* Sepsis
Bactericholia — *see* Cholecystitis, acute
Bacterid, bacteride (pustular) L40.3
Bacterium, bacteria, bacterial
 agent NEC, as cause of disease classified elsewhere
  B96.89
 in blood — *see* Bacteremia
 in urine — *see* Bacteriuria
Bacteriuria, bacteruria R82.71
 asymptomatic R82.71
Bacteroides
 fragilis, as cause of disease classified elsewhere B96.6
Bad
 heart — *see* Disease, heart
 trip
  due to drug abuse — *see* Abuse, drug, hallucinogen
  due to drug dependence — *see* Dependence, drug,
   hallucinogen
Baelz's disease (cheilitis glandularis apostematosa) K13.0
Baerensprung's disease (eczema marginatum) B35.6
Bagasse disease or pneumonitis J67.1
Bagassosis J67.1
Baker's cyst — *see* Cyst, Baker's
Bakwin-Krida syndrome (metaphyseal dysplasia) Q78.5
Balancing side interference M26.56
Balanitis (circinata) (erosiva) (gangrenosa) (phagedenic)
  (vulgaris) N48.1
 amebic A06.82
 candidal B37.42
 due to Haemophilus ducreyi A57
 gonococcal (acute) (chronic) A54.09
 xerotica obliterans N48.0
Balanoposthitis N47.6
 gonococcal (acute) (chronic) A54.09
 ulcerative (specific) A63.8
Balanorrhagia — *see* Balanitis
Balantidiasis, balantidiosis A07.0
Bald tongue K14.4
Baldness (*see also* Alopecia)
 male-pattern — *see* Alopecia, androgenic
Balkan grippe A78
Balloon disease — *see* Effect, adverse, high altitude
Balo's disease (concentric sclerosis) G37.5
Bamberger-Marie disease — *see* Osteoarthropathy,
  hypertrophic, specified type NEC
Bancroft's filariasis B74.0
Band(s)
 adhesive — *see* Adhesions, peritoneum
 anomalous or congenital (*see also* Anomaly, by site)
  heart (atrial) (ventricular) Q24.8
  intestine Q43.3
  omentum Q43.3
 cervix N88.1
 constricting, congenital Q79.8
 gallbladder (congenital) Q44.1
 intestinal (adhesive) — *see* Adhesions, peritoneum
 obstructive
  intestine K56.50
   complete K56.52
   incomplete K56.51
   partial K56.51
  peritoneum K56.50

▼ Subterms under main terms may continue to next column or page   ☑ Additional Character Required — Refer to the Tabular List for Character Selection   **35**

Band(s) — *continued*
  obstructive — *continued*
    peritoneum — *continued*
      complete K56.52
      incomplete K56.51
      partial K56.51
    periappendiceal, congenital Q43.3
    peritoneal (adhesive) — *see* Adhesions, peritoneum
    uterus N73.6
      internal N85.6
    vagina N89.5
Bandemia D72.825
Bandl's ring (contraction), complicating delivery O62.4
Bangkok hemorrhagic fever A91
Bang's disease (brucella abortus) A23.1
Bankruptcy, anxiety concerning Z59.8
Bannister's disease T78.3 ☑
  hereditary D84.1
Banti's disease or syndrome (with cirrhosis) (with portal hypertension) K76.6
Bar, median, prostate — *see* Enlargement, enlarged, prostate
Barcoo disease or rot — *see* Ulcer, skin
Barlow's disease E54
Barodontalgia T70.29 ☑
Baron Münchausen syndrome — *see* Disorder, factitious
Barosinusitis T70.1 ☑
Barotitis T70.0 ☑
Barotrauma T70.29 ☑
  odontalgia T70.29 ☑
  otitic T70.0 ☑
  sinus T70.1 ☑
Barraquer (-Simons) **disease or syndrome** (progressive lipodystrophy) E88.1
Barré-Guillain disease or syndrome G61.0
Barrel chest M95.4
Barré-Liéou syndrome (posterior cervical sympathetic) M53.0
Barrett's
  disease — *see* Barrett's, esophagus
  esophagus K22.70
    with dysplasia K22.719
      high grade K22.711
      low grade K22.710
    without dysplasia K22.70
  syndrome — *see* Barrett's, esophagus
  ulcer K22.10
    with bleeding K22.11
    without bleeding K22.10
Bársony (-Polgár) (-Teschendorf) **syndrome** (corkscrew esophagus) K22.4
Barth syndrome E78.71
Bartholinitis (suppurating) N75.8
  gonococcal (acute) (chronic) (with abscess) A54.1
Bartonellosis A44.9
  cutaneous A44.1
  mucocutaneous A44.1
  specified NEC A44.8
  systemic A44.0
Barton's fracture S52.56- ☑
Bartter's syndrome E26.81
Basal — *see* condition
Basan's (hidrotic) ectodermal dysplasia Q82.4
Baseball finger — *see* Dislocation, finger
Basedow's disease (exophthalmic goiter) — *see* Hyperthyroidism, with, goiter
Basic — *see* condition
Basilar — *see* condition
Bason's (hidrotic) ectodermal dysplasia Q82.4
Basopenia — *see* Agranulocytosis
Basophilia D72.824
Basophilism (cortico-adrenal) (Cushing's) (pituitary) E24.0
Bassen-Kornzweig disease or syndrome E78.6
Bat ear Q17.5
Bateman's
  disease B08.1
  purpura (senile) D69.2
Bathing cramp T75.1 ☑
Bathophobia F40.248
Batten (-Mayou) **disease** E75.4
  retina E75.4 [H36]
Batten-Steinert syndrome G71.11
Battered — *see* Maltreatment
Battey Mycobacterium infection A31.0
Battle exhaustion F43.0

Battledore placenta O43.19- ☑
Baumgarten-Cruveilhier cirrhosis, disease or syndrome K74.69
Bauxite fibrosis (of lung) J63.1
Bayle's disease (general paresis) A52.17
Bazin's disease (primary) (tuberculous) A18.4
Beach ear — *see* Swimmer's, ear
Beaded hair (congenital) Q84.1
Béal conjunctivitis or syndrome B30.2
Beard's disease (neurasthenia) F48.8
Beat(s)
  atrial, premature I49.1
  ectopic I49.49
  elbow — *see* Bursitis, elbow
  escaped, heart I49.49
  hand — *see* Bursitis, hand
  knee — *see* Bursitis, knee
  premature I49.40
    atrial I49.1
    auricular I49.1
    supraventricular I49.1
Beau's
  disease or syndrome — *see* Degeneration, myocardial
  lines (transverse furrows on fingernails) L60.4
Bechterev's syndrome — *see* Spondylitis, ankylosing
Becker's
  cardiomyopathy I42.8
  disease
    idiopathic mural endomyocardial disease I42.3
    myotonia congenita, recessive form G71.12
  dystrophy G71.0
  pigmented hairy nevus D22.5
Beck's syndrome (anterior spinal artery occlusion) I65.8
Beckwith-Wiedemann syndrome Q87.3
Bed confinement status Z74.01
Bed sore — *see* Ulcer, pressure, by site
Bedbug bite(s) — *see* Bite(s), by site, superficial, insect
Bedclothes, asphyxiation or suffocation by — *see* Asphyxia, traumatic, due to, mechanical, trapped
Bednar's
  aphthae K12.0
  tumor — *see* Neoplasm, malignant, by site
Bedridden Z74.01
Bedsore — *see* Ulcer, pressure, by site
Bedwetting — *see* Enuresis
Bee sting (with allergic or anaphylactic shock) — *see* Toxicity, venom, arthropod, bee
Beer drinker's heart (disease) I42.6
Begbie's disease (exophthalmic goiter) — *see* Hyperthyroidism, with, goiter
Behavior
  antisocial
    adult Z72.811
    child or adolescent Z72.810
  disorder, disturbance — *see* Disorder, conduct
  disruptive — *see* Disorder, conduct
  drug seeking Z76.5
  inexplicable R46.2
  marked evasiveness R46.5
  obsessive-compulsive R46.81
  overactivity R46.3
  poor responsiveness R46.4
  self-damaging (life-style) Z72.89
  sleep-incompatible Z72.821
  slowness R46.4
  specified NEC R46.89
  strange (and inexplicable) R46.2
  suspiciousness R46.5
  type A pattern Z73.1
  undue concern or preoccupation with stressful events R46.6
  verbosity and circumstantial detail obscuring reason for contact R46.7
Behçet's disease or syndrome M35.2
Behr's disease — *see* Degeneration, macula
Beigel's disease or morbus (white piedra) B36.2
Bejel A65
Bekhterev's syndrome — *see* Spondylitis, ankylosing
Belching — *see* Eructation
Bell's
  mania F30.8
  palsy, paralysis G51.0
    infant or newborn P11.3
  spasm G51.3
Bence Jones albuminuria or proteinuria NEC R80.3
Bends T70.3 ☑
Benedikt's paralysis or syndrome G46.3

Benign (*see also* condition)
  prostatic hyperplasia — *see* Hyperplasia, prostate
Bennett's fracture (displaced) S62.21- ☑
Benson's disease — *see* Deposit, crystalline
Bent
  back (hysterical) F44.4
  nose M95.0
    congenital Q67.4
Bereavement (uncomplicated) Z63.4
Bergeron's disease (hysterical chorea) F44.4
Berger's disease — *see* Nephropathy, IgA
Beriberi (dry) E51.11
  heart (disease) E51.12
  polyneuropathy E51.11
  wet E51.12
    involving circulatory system E51.11
Berlin's disease or edema (traumatic) S05.8X- ☑
Berlock (berloque) **dermatitis** L56.2
Bernard-Horner syndrome G90.2
Bernard-Soulier disease or thrombopathia D69.1
Bernhardt (-Roth) **disease** — *see* Mononeuropathy, lower limb, meralgia paresthetica
Bernheim's syndrome — *see* Failure, heart, right
Bertielliasis B71.8
Berylliosis (lung) J63.2
Besnier-Boeck (-Schaumann) **disease** — *see* Sarcoidosis
Besnier's
  lupus pernio D86.3
  prurigo L20.0
Bestiality F65.89
Best's disease H35.50
Betalipoproteinemia, broad or floating E78.2
Beta-mercaptolactate-cysteine disulfiduria E72.09
Betting and gambling Z72.6
  pathological (compulsive) F63.0
Bezoar T18.9 ☑
  intestine T18.3 ☑
  stomach T18.2 ☑
Bezold's abscess — *see* Mastoiditis, acute
Bianchi's syndrome R48.8
Bicornate or bicornis uterus Q51.3
  in pregnancy or childbirth O34.00
    causing obstructed labor O65.5
Bicuspid aortic valve Q23.1
Biedl-Bardet syndrome Q87.89
Bielschowsky (-Jansky) disease E75.4
Biermer's (pernicious) anemia or disease D51.0
Biett's disease L93.0
Bifid (congenital)
  apex, heart Q24.8
  clitoris Q52.6
  kidney Q63.8
  nose Q30.2
  patella Q74.1
  scrotum Q55.29
  toe NEC Q74.2
  tongue Q38.3
  ureter Q62.8
  uterus Q51.3
  uvula Q35.7
Biforis uterus (suprasimplex) Q51.3
Bifurcation (congenital)
  gallbladder Q44.1
  kidney pelvis Q63.8
  renal pelvis Q63.8
  rib Q76.6
  tongue, congenital Q38.3
  trachea Q32.1
  ureter Q62.8
  urethra Q64.74
  vertebra Q76.49
Big spleen syndrome D73.1
Bigeminal pulse R00.8
Bilateral — *see* condition
Bile
  duct — *see* condition
  pigments in urine R82.2
Bilharziasis (*see also* Schistosomiasis)
  chyluria B65.0
  cutaneous B65.3
  galacturia B65.0
  hematochyluria B65.0
  intestinal B65.1
  lipemia B65.9
  lipuria B65.0
  oriental B65.2
  piarhemia B65.9

☑ **Additional Character Required** — Refer to the Tabular List for Character Selection   ▽ **Subterms under main terms may continue to next column or page**

Bilharziasis — *continued*
  pulmonary NOS B65.9 [J99]
    pneumonia B65.9 [J17]
  tropical hematuria B65.0
  vesical B65.0
Biliary — *see* condition
Bilirubin metabolism disorder E80.7
  specified NEC E80.6
Bilirubinemia, familial nonhemolytic E80.4
Bilirubinuria R82.2
Biliuria R82.2
Bilocular stomach K31.2
Binswanger's disease I67.3
Biparta, bipartite
  carpal scaphoid Q74.0
  patella Q74.1
  vagina Q52.10
Bird
  face Q75.8
  fancier's disease or lung J67.2
Birth
  complications in mother — *see* Delivery, complicated
  compression during NOS P15.9
  defect — *see* Anomaly
  immature (less than 37 completed weeks) — *see*
    Preterm, newborn
    extremely (less than 28 completed weeks) — *see*
      Immaturity, extreme
  inattention, at or after — *see* Maltreatment, child, ne-
    glect
  injury NOS P15.9
    basal ganglia P11.1
    brachial plexus NEC P14.3
    brain (compression) (pressure) P11.2
    central nervous system NOS P11.9
    cerebellum P11.1
    cerebral hemorrhage P10.1
    external genitalia P15.5
    eye P15.3
    face P15.4
    fracture
      bone P13.9
        specified NEC P13.8
      clavicle P13.4
      femur P13.2
      humerus P13.3
      long bone, except femur P13.3
      radius and ulna P13.3
      skull P13.0
      spine P11.5
      tibia and fibula P13.3
    intracranial P11.2
      laceration or hemorrhage P10.9
        specified NEC P10.8
    intraventricular hemorrhage P10.2
    laceration
      brain P10.1
      by scalpel P15.8
      peripheral nerve P14.9
    liver P15.0
    meninges
      brain P11.1
      spinal cord P11.5
    nerve
      brachial plexus P14.3
      cranial NEC (except facial) P11.4
      facial P11.3
      peripheral P14.9
      phrenic (paralysis) P14.2
    paralysis
      facial nerve P11.3
      spinal P11.5
    penis P15.5
    rupture
      spinal cord P11.5
    scalp P12.9
    scalpel wound P15.8
    scrotum P15.5
    skull NEC P13.1
      fracture P13.0
    specified type NEC P15.8
    spinal cord P11.5
    spine P11.5
    spleen P15.1
    sternomastoid (hematoma) P15.2
    subarachnoid hemorrhage P10.3
    subcutaneous fat necrosis P15.6
    subdural hemorrhage P10.0

Birth — *continued*
  injury — *continued*
    tentorial tear P10.4
    testes P15.5
    vulva P15.5
  lack of care, at or after — *see* Maltreatment, child, ne-
    glect
  neglect, at or after — *see* Maltreatment, child, neglect
  palsy or paralysis, newborn, NOS (birth injury) P14.9
  premature (infant) — *see* Preterm, newborn
  shock, newborn P96.89
  trauma — *see* Birth, injury
  weight
    4000 grams to 4499 grams P08.1
    4500 grams or more P08.0
    low (2499 grams or less) — *see* Low, birthweight
      extremely (999 grams or less) — *see* Low,
        birthweight, extreme
Birthmark Q82.5
Birt-Hogg-Dube syndrome Q87.89
Bisalbuminemia E88.09
Biskra's button B55.1
Bite(s) (animal) (human)
  abdomen, abdominal
    wall S31.159 ☑
      with penetration into peritoneal cavity
        S31.659 ☑
      epigastric region S31.152 ☑
        with penetration into peritoneal cavity
          S31.652 ☑
      left
        lower quadrant S31.154 ☑
          with penetration into peritoneal cavity
            S31.654 ☑
        upper quadrant S31.151 ☑
          with penetration into peritoneal cavity
            S31.651 ☑
      periumbilic region S31.155 ☑
        with penetration into peritoneal cavity
          S31.655 ☑
      right
        lower quadrant S31.153 ☑
          with penetration into peritoneal cavity
            S31.653 ☑
        upper quadrant S31.150 ☑
          with penetration into peritoneal cavity
            S31.650 ☑
      superficial NEC S30.871 ☑
        insect S30.861 ☑
  alveolar (process) — *see* Bite, oral cavity
  amphibian (venomous) — *see* Venom, bite, amphibian
  animal (*see also* Bite, by site)
    venomous — *see* Venom
  ankle S91.05- ☑
    superficial NEC S90.57- ☑
      insect S90.56- ☑
  antecubital space — *see* Bite, elbow
  anus S31.835 ☑
    superficial NEC S30.877 ☑
      insect S30.867 ☑
  arm (upper) S41.15- ☑
    lower — *see* Bite, forearm
    superficial NEC S40.87- ☑
      insect S40.86- ☑
  arthropod NEC — *see* Venom, bite, arthropod
  auditory canal (external) (meatus) — *see* Bite, ear
  auricle, ear — *see* Bite, ear
  axilla — *see* Bite, arm
  back (*see also* Bite, thorax, back)
    lower S31.050 ☑
      with penetration into retroperitoneal space
        S31.051 ☑
      superficial NEC S30.870 ☑
        insect S30.860 ☑
  bedbug — *see* Bite(s), by site, superficial, insect
  breast S21.05- ☑
    superficial NEC S20.17- ☑
      insect S20.16- ☑
  brow — *see* Bite, head, specified site NEC
  buttock S31.805 ☑
    left S31.825 ☑
    right S31.815 ☑
    superficial NEC S30.870 ☑
      insect S30.860 ☑
  calf — *see* Bite, leg
  canaliculus lacrimalis — *see* Bite, eyelid

Bite(s) — *continued*
  canthus, eye — *see* Bite, eyelid
  centipede — *see* Toxicity, venom, arthropod, cen-
    tipede
  cheek (external) S01.45- ☑
    internal — *see* Bite, oral cavity
    superficial NEC S00.87 ☑
      insect S00.86 ☑
  chest wall — *see* Bite, thorax
  chigger B88.0
  chin — *see* Bite, head, specified site NEC
  clitoris — *see* Bite, vulva
  costal region — *see* Bite, thorax
  digit(s)
    hand — *see* Bite, finger
    toe — *see* Bite, toe
  ear (canal) (external) S01.35- ☑
    superficial NEC S00.47- ☑
      insect S00.46- ☑
  elbow S51.05- ☑
    superficial NEC S50.37- ☑
      insect S50.36- ☑
  epididymis — *see* Bite, testis
  epigastric region — *see* Bite, abdomen
  epiglottis — *see* Bite, neck, specified site NEC
  esophagus, cervical S11.25 ☑
    superficial NEC S10.17 ☑
      insect S10.16 ☑
  eyebrow — *see* Bite, eyelid
  eyelid S01.15- ☑
    superficial NEC S00.27- ☑
      insect S00.26- ☑
  face NEC — *see* Bite, head, specified site NEC
  finger(s) S61.259 ☑
    with
      damage to nail S61.359 ☑
    index S61.258 ☑
      with
        damage to nail S61.358 ☑
      left S61.251 ☑
        with
          damage to nail S61.351 ☑
      right S61.250 ☑
        with
          damage to nail S61.350 ☑
      superficial NEC S60.478 ☑
        insect S60.46- ☑
    little S61.25- ☑
      with
        damage to nail S61.35- ☑
      superficial NEC S60.47- ☑
        insect S60.46- ☑
    middle S61.25- ☑
      with
        damage to nail S61.35- ☑
      superficial NEC S60.47- ☑
        insect S60.46- ☑
    ring S61.25- ☑
      with
        damage to nail S61.35- ☑
      superficial NEC S60.47- ☑
        insect S60.46- ☑
    superficial NEC S60.479 ☑
      insect S60.469 ☑
    thumb — *see* Bite, thumb
  flank — *see* Bite, abdomen, wall
  flea — *see* Bite, by site, superficial, insect
  foot (except toe(s) alone) S91.35- ☑
    superficial NEC S90.87- ☑
      insect S90.86- ☑
    toe — *see* Bite, toe
  forearm S51.85- ☑
    elbow only — *see* Bite, elbow
    superficial NEC S50.87- ☑
      insect S50.86- ☑
  forehead — *see* Bite, head, specified site NEC
  genital organs, external
    female S31.552 ☑
      superficial NEC S30.876 ☑
        insect S30.866 ☑
      vagina and vulva — *see* Bite, vulva
    male S31.551 ☑
      penis — *see* Bite, penis
      scrotum — *see* Bite, scrotum
      superficial NEC S30.875 ☑
        insect S30.865 ☑

Bite(s) — *continued*
  genital organs, external — *continued*
    male — *continued*
      testes — *see* Bite, testis
  groin — *see* Bite, abdomen, wall
  gum — *see* Bite, oral cavity
  hand S61.45- ☑
    finger — *see* Bite, finger
    superficial NEC S60.57- ☑
      insect S60.56- ☑
    thumb — *see* Bite, thumb
  head S01.95 ☑
    cheek — *see* Bite, cheek
    ear — *see* Bite, ear
    eyelid — *see* Bite, eyelid
    lip — *see* Bite, lip
    nose — *see* Bite, nose
    oral cavity — *see* Bite, oral cavity
    scalp — *see* Bite, scalp
    specified site NEC S01.85 ☑
      superficial NEC S00.87 ☑
        insect S00.86 ☑
    superficial NEC S00.97 ☑
      insect S00.96 ☑
    temporomandibular area — *see* Bite, cheek
  heel — *see* Bite, foot
  hip S71.05- ☑
    superficial NEC S70.27- ☑
      insect S70.26- ☑
  hymen S31.45 ☑
  hypochondrium — *see* Bite, abdomen, wall
  hypogastric region — *see* Bite, abdomen, wall
  inguinal region — *see* Bite, abdomen, wall
  insect — *see* Bite, by site, superficial, insect
  instep — *see* Bite, foot
  interscapular region — *see* Bite, thorax, back
  jaw — *see* Bite, head, specified site NEC
  knee S81.05- ☑
    superficial NEC S80.27- ☑
      insect S80.26- ☑
  labium (majus) (minus) — *see* Bite, vulva
  lacrimal duct — *see* Bite, eyelid
  larynx S11.015 ☑
    superficial NEC S10.17 ☑
      insect S10.16 ☑
  leg (lower) S81.85- ☑
    ankle — *see* Bite, ankle
    foot — *see* Bite, foot
    knee — *see* Bite, knee
    superficial NEC S80.87- ☑
      insect S80.86- ☑
    toe — *see* Bite, toe
    upper — *see* Bite, thigh
  lip S01.551 ☑
    superficial NEC S00.571 ☑
      insect S00.561 ☑
  lizard (venomous) — *see* Venom, bite, reptile
  loin — *see* Bite, abdomen, wall
  lower back — *see* Bite, back, lower
  lumbar region — *see* Bite, back, lower
  malar region — *see* Bite, head, specified site NEC
  mammary — *see* Bite, breast
  marine animals (venomous) — *see* Toxicity, venom, marine animal
  mastoid region — *see* Bite, head, specified site NEC
  mouth — *see* Bite, oral cavity
  nail
    finger — *see* Bite, finger
    toe — *see* Bite, toe
  nape — *see* Bite, neck, specified site NEC
  nasal (septum) (sinus) — *see* Bite, nose
  nasopharynx — *see* Bite, head, specified site NEC
  neck S11.95 ☑
    involving
      cervical esophagus — *see* Bite, esophagus, cervical
      larynx — *see* Bite, larynx
      pharynx — *see* Bite, pharynx
      thyroid gland S11.15 ☑
      trachea — *see* Bite, trachea
    specified site NEC S11.85 ☑
      superficial NEC S10.87 ☑
        insect S10.86 ☑
    superficial NEC S10.97 ☑
      insect S10.96 ☑
    throat S11.85 ☑

Bite(s) — *continued*
  neck — *continued*
    throat — *continued*
      superficial NEC S10.17 ☑
        insect S10.16 ☑
  nose (septum) (sinus) S01.25 ☑
    superficial NEC S00.37 ☑
      insect S00.36 ☑
  occipital region — *see* Bite, scalp
  oral cavity S01.552 ☑
    superficial NEC S00.572 ☑
      insect S00.562 ☑
  orbital region — *see* Bite, eyelid
  palate — *see* Bite, oral cavity
  palm — *see* Bite, hand
  parietal region — *see* Bite, scalp
  pelvis S31.050 ☑
    with penetration into retroperitoneal space S31.051 ☑
    superficial NEC S30.870 ☑
      insect S30.860 ☑
  penis S31.25 ☑
    superficial NEC S30.872 ☑
      insect S30.862 ☑
  perineum
    female — *see* Bite, vulva
    male — *see* Bite, pelvis
  periocular area (with or without lacrimal passages) — *see* Bite, eyelid
  phalanges
    finger — *see* Bite, finger
    toe — *see* Bite, toe
  pharynx S11.25 ☑
    superficial NEC S10.17 ☑
      insect S10.16 ☑
  pinna — *see* Bite, ear
  poisonous — *see* Venom
  popliteal space — *see* Bite, knee
  prepuce — *see* Bite, penis
  pubic region — *see* Bite, abdomen, wall
  rectovaginal septum — *see* Bite, vulva
  red bug B88.0
  reptile NEC (*see also* Venom, bite, reptile)
    nonvenomous — *see* Bite, by site
    snake — *see* Venom, bite, snake
  sacral region — *see* Bite, back, lower
  sacroiliac region — *see* Bite, back, lower
  salivary gland — *see* Bite, oral cavity
  scalp S01.05 ☑
    superficial NEC S00.07 ☑
      insect S00.06 ☑
  scapular region — *see* Bite, shoulder
  scrotum S31.35 ☑
    superficial NEC S30.873 ☑
      insect S30.863 ☑
  sea-snake (venomous) — *see* Toxicity, venom, snake, sea snake
  shin — *see* Bite, leg
  shoulder S41.05- ☑
    superficial NEC S40.27- ☑
      insect S40.26- ☑
  snake (*see also* Venom, bite, snake)
    nonvenomous — *see* Bite, by site
  spermatic cord — *see* Bite, testis
  spider (venomous) — *see* Toxicity, venom, spider
    nonvenomous — *see* Bite, by site, superficial, insect
  sternal region — *see* Bite, thorax, front
  submaxillary region — *see* Bite, head, specified site NEC
  submental region — *see* Bite, head, specified site NEC
  subungual
    finger(s) — *see* Bite, finger
    toe — *see* Bite, toe
  superficial — *see* Bite, by site, superficial
  supraclavicular fossa S11.85 ☑
  supraorbital — *see* Bite, head, specified site NEC
  temple, temporal region — *see* Bite, head, specified site NEC
  temporomandibular area — *see* Bite, cheek
  testis S31.35 ☑
    superficial NEC S30.873 ☑
      insect S30.863 ☑
  thigh S71.15- ☑
    superficial NEC S70.37- ☑
      insect S70.36- ☑
  thorax, thoracic (wall) S21.95 ☑

Bite(s) — *continued*
  thorax, thoracic — *continued*
    back S21.25- ☑
      with penetration into thoracic cavity S21.45- ☑
    breast — *see* Bite, breast
    front S21.15- ☑
      with penetration into thoracic cavity S21.35- ☑
    superficial NEC S20.97 ☑
      back S20.47- ☑
      front S20.37- ☑
      insect S20.96 ☑
        back S20.46- ☑
        front S20.36- ☑
  throat — *see* Bite, neck, throat
  thumb S61.05- ☑
    with
      damage to nail S61.15- ☑
    superficial NEC S60.37- ☑
      insect S60.36- ☑
  thyroid S11.15
    superficial NEC S10.87 ☑
      insect S10.86 ☑
  toe(s) S91.15- ☑
    with
      damage to nail S91.25- ☑
    great S91.15- ☑
      with
        damage to nail S91.25- ☑
    lesser S91.15- ☑
      with
        damage to nail S91.25- ☑
    superficial NEC S90.47- ☑
      great S90.47- ☑
      insect S90.46- ☑
        great S90.46- ☑
  tongue S01.552 ☑
  trachea S11.025 ☑
    superficial NEC S10.17 ☑
      insect S10.16 ☑
  tunica vaginalis — *see* Bite, testis
  tympanum, tympanic membrane — *see* Bite, ear
  umbilical region S31.155 ☑
  uvula — *see* Bite, oral cavity
  vagina — *see* Bite, vulva
  venomous — *see* Venom
  vocal cords S11.035 ☑
    superficial NEC S10.17 ☑
      insect S10.16 ☑
  vulva S31.45 ☑
    superficial NEC S30.874 ☑
      insect S30.864 ☑
  wrist S61.55- ☑
    superficial NEC S60.87- ☑
      insect S60.86- ☑
Biting, cheek or lip K13.1
Biventricular failure (heart) I50.82
Björck (-Thorson) **syndrome** (malignant carcinoid) E34.0
Black
  death A20.9
  eye S00.1- ☑
  hairy tongue K14.3
  heel (foot) S90.3- ☑
  lung (disease) J60
  palm (hand) S60.22- ☑
Blackfan-Diamond anemia or syndrome (congenital hypoplastic anemia) D61.01
Blackhead L70.0
Blackout R55
Bladder — *see* condition
Blast (air) (hydraulic) (immersion) (underwater)
  blindness S05.8X- ☑
  injury
    abdomen or thorax — *see* Injury, by site
    ear (acoustic nerve trauma) — *see* Injury, nerve, acoustic, specified type NEC
    syndrome NEC T70.8
Blastoma — *see* Neoplasm, malignant, by site
  pulmonary — *see* Neoplasm, lung, malignant
Blastomycosis, blastomycotic B40.9
  Brazilian — *see* Paracoccidioidomycosis
  cutaneous B40.3
  disseminated B40.7
  European — *see* Cryptococcosis
  generalized B40.7
  keloidal B48.0
  North American B40.9

Blastomycosis, blastomycotic — *continued*
  primary pulmonary B40.0
  pulmonary B40.2
    acute B40.0
    chronic B40.1
  skin B40.3
  South American — *see* Paracoccidioidomycosis
  specified NEC B40.89
Bleb(s) R23.8
  emphysematous (lung) (solitary) J43.9
  endophthalmitis H59.43
  filtering (vitreous), after glaucoma surgery Z98.83
  inflamed (infected), postprocedural H59.40
    stage 1 H59.41
    stage 2 H59.42
    stage 3 H59.43
  lung (ruptured) J43.9
    congenital — *see* Atelectasis
    newborn P25.8
  subpleural (emphysematous) J43.9
Blebitis, postprocedural H59.40
  stage 1 H59.41
  stage 2 H59.42
  stage 3 H59.43
Bleeder (familial) (hereditary) — *see* Hemophilia
Bleeding (*see also* Hemorrhage)
  anal K62.5
  anovulatory N97.0
  atonic, following delivery O72.1
  capillary I78.8
    puerperal O72.2
  contact (postcoital) N93.0
  due to uterine subinvolution N85.3
  ear — *see* Otorrhagia
  excessive, associated with menopausal onset N92.4
  familial — *see* Defect, coagulation
  following intercourse N93.0
  gastrointestinal K92.2
  hemorrhoids — *see* Hemorrhoids
  intermenstrual (regular) N92.3
    irregular N92.1
  intraoperative — *see* Complication, intraoperative,
    hemorrhage
  irregular N92.6
  menopausal N92.4
  newborn, intraventricular — *see* Newborn, affected
    by, hemorrhage, intraventricular
  nipple N64.59
  nose R04.0
  ovulation N92.3
  postclimacteric N95.0
  postcoital N93.0
  postmenopausal N95.0
  postoperative — *see* Complication, postprocedural,
    hemorrhage
  preclimacteric N92.4
  pre-pubertal vaginal N93.1
  puberty (excessive, with onset of menstrual periods)
    N92.2
  rectum, rectal K62.5
    newborn P54.2
  tendencies — *see* Defect, coagulation
  throat R04.1
  tooth socket (post-extraction) K91.840
  umbilical stump P51.9
  uterus, uterine NEC N93.9
    climacteric N92.4
    dysfunctional or functional N93.8
    menopausal N92.4
    preclimacteric or premenopausal N92.4
    unrelated to menstrual cycle N93.9
  vagina, vaginal (abnormal) N93.9
    dysfunctional or functional N93.8
    newborn P54.6
    pre-pubertal N93.1
  vicarious N94.89
Blennorrhagia, blennorrhagic — *see* Gonorrhea
Blennorrhea (acute) (chronic) (*see also* Gonorrhea)
  inclusion (neonatal) (newborn) P39.1
  lower genitourinary tract (gonococcal) A54.00
  neonatorum (gonococcal ophthalmia) A54.31
Blepharelosis — *see* Entropion
Blepharitis (angularis) (ciliaris) (eyelid) (marginal)
  (nonulcerative) H01.009
  herpes zoster B02.39
  left H01.006
    lower H01.005
    upper H01.004

Blepharitis — *continued*
  right H01.003
    lower H01.002
    upper H01.001
  squamous H01.029
    left H01.026
      lower H01.025
      upper H01.024
    right H01.023
      lower H01.022
      upper H01.021
  ulcerative H01.019
    left H01.016
      lower H01.015
      upper H01.014
    right H01.013
      lower H01.012
      upper H01.011
Blepharochalasis H02.30
  congenital Q10.0
  left H02.36
    lower H02.35
    upper H02.34
  right H02.33
    lower H02.32
    upper H02.31
Blepharoclonus H02.59
Blepharoconjunctivitis H10.50- ☑
  angular H10.52- ☑
  contact H10.53- ☑
  ligneous H10.51- ☑
Blepharophimosis (eyelid) H02.529
  congenital Q10.3
  left H02.526
    lower H02.525
    upper H02.524
  right H02.523
    lower H02.522
    upper H02.521
Blepharoptosis H02.40- ☑
  congenital Q10.0
  mechanical H02.41- ☑
  myogenic H02.42- ☑
  neurogenic H02.43- ☑
  paralytic H02.43- ☑
Blepharopyorrhea, gonococcal A54.39
Blepharospasm G24.5
  drug induced G24.01
Blighted ovum O02.0
Blind (*see also* Blindness)
  bronchus (congenital) Q32.4
  loop syndrome K90.2
    congenital Q43.8
  sac, fallopian tube (congenital) Q50.6
  spot, enlarged — *see* Defect, visual field, localized,
    scotoma, blind spot area
  tract or tube, congenital NEC — *see* Atresia, by site
Blindness (acquired) (congenital) (both eyes) H54.0X- ☑
  blast S05.8X- ☑
  color — *see* Deficiency, color vision
  concussion S05.8X- ☑
  cortical H47.619
    left brain H47.612
    right brain H47.611
  day H53.11
  due to injury (current episode) S05.9- ☑
    sequelae — *code to* injury with seventh character
      S
  eclipse (total) — *see* Retinopathy, solar
  emotional (hysterical) F44.6
  face H53.16
  hysterical F44.6
  legal (both eyes) (USA definition) H54.8
  mind R48.8
  night H53.60
    abnormal dark adaptation curve H53.61
    acquired H53.62
    congenital H53.63
    specified type NEC H53.69
    vitamin A deficiency E50.5
  one eye (other eye normal) H54.40
    left (normal vision on right) H54.42- ☑
      low vision on right H54.12- ☑
    low vision, other eye H54.10
    right (normal vision on left) H54.41- ☑
      low vision on left H54.11- ☑
  psychic R48.8
  river B73.01

Blindness — *continued*
  snow — *see* Photokeratitis
  sun, solar — *see* Retinopathy, solar
  transient — *see* Disturbance, vision, subjective, loss,
    transient
  traumatic (current episode) S05.9- ☑
  word (developmental) F81.0
    acquired R48.0
    secondary to organic lesion R48.0
Blister (nonthermal)
  abdominal wall S30.821 ☑
  alveolar process S00.522 ☑
  ankle S90.52- ☑
  antecubital space — *see* Blister, elbow
  anus S30.827 ☑
  arm (upper) S40.82- ☑
  auditory canal — *see* Blister, ear
  auricle — *see* Blister, ear
  axilla — *see* Blister, arm
  back, lower S30.820 ☑
  beetle dermatitis L24.89
  breast S20.12- ☑
  brow S00.82 ☑
  calf — *see* Blister, leg
  canthus — *see* Blister, eyelid
  cheek S00.82 ☑
    internal S00.522 ☑
  chest wall — *see* Blister, thorax
  chin S00.82 ☑
  costal region — *see* Blister, thorax
  digit(s)
    foot — *see* Blister, toe
    hand — *see* Blister, finger
  due to burn — *see* Burn, by site, second degree
  ear S00.42- ☑
  elbow S50.32- ☑
  epiglottis S10.12 ☑
  esophagus, cervical S10.12 ☑
  eyebrow — *see* Blister, eyelid
  eyelid S00.22- ☑
  face S00.82 ☑
  fever B00.1
  finger(s) S60.429 ☑
    index S60.42- ☑
    little S60.42- ☑
    middle S60.42- ☑
    ring S60.42- ☑
  foot (except toe(s) alone) S90.82- ☑
    toe — *see* Blister, toe
  forearm S50.82- ☑
    elbow only — *see* Blister, elbow
  forehead S00.82 ☑
  fracture — *omit code*
  genital organ
    female S30.826 ☑
    male S30.825 ☑
  gum S00.522 ☑
  hand S60.52- ☑
  head S00.92 ☑
    ear — *see* Blister, ear
    eyelid — *see* Blister, eyelid
    lip S00.521 ☑
    nose S00.32 ☑
    oral cavity S00.522 ☑
    scalp S00.02 ☑
    specified site NEC S00.82 ☑
  heel — *see* Blister, foot
  hip S70.22- ☑
  interscapular region S20.429 ☑
  jaw S00.82 ☑
  knee S80.22- ☑
  larynx S10.12 ☑
  leg (lower) S80.82- ☑
    knee — *see* Blister, knee
    upper — *see* Blister, thigh
  lip S00.521 ☑
  malar region S00.82 ☑
  mammary — *see* Blister, breast
  mastoid region S00.82 ☑
  mouth S00.522 ☑
  multiple, skin, nontraumatic R23.8
  nail
    finger — *see* Blister, finger
    toe — *see* Blister, toe
  nasal S00.32 ☑
  neck S10.92 ☑

Blister — *continued*
neck — *continued*
specified site NEC S10.82 ☑
throat S10.12 ☑
nose S00.32 ☑
occipital region S00.02 ☑
oral cavity S00.522 ☑
orbital region — *see* Blister, eyelid
palate S00.522 ☑
palm — *see* Blister, hand
parietal region S00.02 ☑
pelvis S30.820 ☑
penis S30.822 ☑
periocular area — *see* Blister, eyelid
phalanges
finger — *see* Blister, finger
toe — *see* Blister, toe
pharynx S10.12 ☑
pinna — *see* Blister, ear
popliteal space — *see* Blister, knee
scalp S00.02 ☑
scapular region — *see* Blister, shoulder
scrotum S30.823 ☑
shin — *see* Blister, leg
shoulder S40.22- ☑
sternal region S20.329 ☑
submaxillary region S00.82 ☑
submental region S00.82 ☑
subungual
finger(s) — *see* Blister, finger
toe(s) — *see* Blister, toe
supraclavicular fossa S10.82 ☑
supraorbital S00.82 ☑
temple S00.82 ☑
temporal region S00.82 ☑
testis S30.823 ☑
thermal — *see* Burn, second degree, by site
thigh S70.32- ☑
thorax, thoracic (wall) S20.92 ☑
back S20.42- ☑
front S20.32- ☑
throat S10.12 ☑
thumb S60.32- ☑
toe(s) S90.42- ☑
great S90.42- ☑
tongue S00.522 ☑
trachea S10.12 ☑
tympanum, tympanic membrane — *see* Blister, ear
upper arm — *see* Blister, arm (upper)
uvula S00.522 ☑
vagina S30.824 ☑
vocal cords S10.12 ☑
vulva S30.824 ☑
wrist S60.82- ☑
Bloating R14.0
Bloch-Sulzberger disease or syndrome Q82.3
Block, blocked
alveolocapillary J84.10
arborization (heart) I45.5
arrhythmic I45.9
atrioventricular (incomplete) (partial) I44.30
with atrioventricular dissociation I44.2
complete I44.2
congenital Q24.6
congenital Q24.6
first degree I44.0
second degree (types I and II) I44.1
specified NEC I44.39
third degree I44.2
types I and II I44.1
auriculoventricular — *see* Block, atrioventricular
bifascicular (cardiac) I45.2
bundle-branch (complete) (false) (incomplete) I45.4
bilateral I45.2
left I44.7
with right bundle branch block I45.2
hemiblock I44.60
anterior I44.4
posterior I44.5
incomplete I44.7
with right bundle branch block I45.2
right I45.10
with
left bundle branch block I45.2
left fascicular block I45.2
specified NEC I45.19
Wilson's type I45.19

Block, blocked — *continued*
cardiac I45.9
conduction I45.9
complete I44.2
fascicular (left) I44.60
anterior I44.4
posterior I44.5
right I45.0
specified NEC I44.69
foramen Magendie (acquired) G91.1
congenital Q03.1
with spina bifida — *see* Spina bifida, by site, with hydrocephalus
heart I45.9
bundle branch I45.4
bilateral I45.2
complete (atrioventricular) I44.2
congenital Q24.6
first degree (atrioventricular) I44.0
second degree (atrioventricular) I44.1
specified type NEC I45.5
third degree (atrioventricular) I44.2
hepatic vein I82.0
intraventricular (nonspecific) I45.4
bundle branch
bilateral I45.2
kidney N28.9
postcystoscopic or postprocedural N99.0
Mobitz (types I and II) I44.1
myocardial — *see* Block, heart
nodal I45.5
organ or site, congenital NEC — *see* Atresia, by site
portal (vein) I81
second degree (types I and II) I44.1
sinoatrial I45.5
sinoauricular I45.5
third degree I44.2
trifascicular I45.3
tubal N97.1
vein NOS I82.90
Wenckebach (types I and II) I44.1
Blockage — *see* Obstruction
Blocq's disease F44.4
Blood
constituents, abnormal R78.9
disease D75.9
donor — *see* Donor, blood
dyscrasia D75.9
with
abortion — *see* Abortion, by type, complicated by, hemorrhage
ectopic pregnancy O08.1
molar pregnancy O08.1
following ectopic or molar pregnancy O08.1
newborn P61.9
puerperal, postpartum O72.3
flukes NEC — *see* Schistosomiasis
in
feces K92.1
occult R19.5
urine — *see* Hematuria
mole O02.0
occult in feces R19.5
pressure
decreased, due to shock following injury T79.4 ☑
examination only Z01.30
fluctuating I99.8
high — *see* Hypertension
borderline R03.0
incidental reading, without diagnosis of hypertension R03.0
low (*see also* Hypotension)
incidental reading, without diagnosis of hypotension R03.1
spitting — *see* Hemoptysis
staining cornea — *see* Pigmentation, cornea, stromal
transfusion
reaction or complication — *see* Complications, transfusion
type
A (Rh positive) Z67.10
Rh negative Z67.11
AB (Rh positive) Z67.30
Rh negative Z67.31
B (Rh positive) Z67.20
Rh negative Z67.21
O (Rh positive) Z67.40
Rh negative Z67.41

Blood — *continued*
type — *continued*
Rh (positive) Z67.90
negative Z67.91
vessel rupture — *see* Hemorrhage
vomiting — *see* Hematemesis
Blood-forming organs, disease D75.9
Bloodgood's disease — *see* Mastopathy, cystic
Bloom (-Machacek)(-Torre) **syndrome** Q82.8
Blount's disease or osteochondrosis — *see* Osteochondrosis, juvenile, tibia
Blue
baby Q24.9
diaper syndrome E72.09
dome cyst (breast) — *see* Cyst, breast
dot cataract Q12.0
nevus D22.9
sclera Q13.5
with fragility of bone and deafness Q78.0
toe syndrome I75.02- ☑
Blueness — *see* Cyanosis
Blues, postpartal O90.6
baby O90.6
Blurring, visual H53.8
Blushing (abnormal) (excessive) R23.2
BMI — *see* Body, mass index
Boarder, hospital NEC Z76.4
accompanying sick person Z76.3
healthy infant or child Z76.2
foundling Z76.1
Bochart's impetigo L01.02
Bodechtel-Guttman disease (subacute sclerosing panencephalitis) A81.1
Boder-Sedgwick syndrome (ataxia-telangiectasia) G11.3
Body, bodies
Aschoff's — *see* Myocarditis, rheumatic
asteroid, vitreous — *see* Deposit, crystalline
cytoid (retina) — *see* Occlusion, artery, retina
drusen (degenerative) (macula) (retinal) (*see also* Degeneration, macula, drusen)
optic disc — *see* Drusen, optic disc
foreign — *see* Foreign body
loose
joint, except knee — *see* Loose, body, joint
knee M23.4- ☑
sheath, tendon — *see* Disorder, tendon, specified type NEC
mass index (BMI)
adult
19.9 or less Z68.1
20.0-20.9 Z68.20
21.0-21.9 Z68.21
22.0-22.9 Z68.22
23.0-23.9 Z68.23
24.0-24.9 Z68.24
25.0-25.9 Z68.25
26.0-26.9 Z68.26
27.0-27.9 Z68.27
28.0-28.9 Z68.28
29.0-29.9 Z68.29
30.0-30.9 Z68.30
31.0-31.9 Z68.31
32.0-32.9 Z68.32
33.0-33.9 Z68.33
34.0-34.9 Z68.34
35.0-35.9 Z68.35
36.0-36.9 Z68.36
37.0-37.9 Z68.37
38.0-38.9 Z68.38
39.0-39.9 Z68.39
40.0-44.9 Z68.41
45.0-49.9 Z68.42
50.0-59.9 Z68.43
60.0-69.9 Z68.44
70 and over Z68.45
pediatric
5th percentile to less than 85th percentile for age Z68.52
85th percentile to less than 95th percentile for age Z68.53
less than fifth percentile for age Z68.51
greater than or equal to ninety-fifth percentile for age Z68.54
Mooser's A75.2
rice (*see also* Loose, body, joint)
knee M23.4- ☑
rocking F98.4

☑ Additional Character Required — Refer to the Tabular List for Character Selection ▽ Subterms under main terms may continue to next column or page

Boeck's
  disease or sarcoid — *see* Sarcoidosis
  lupoid (miliary) D86.3
Boerhaave's syndrome (spontaneous esophageal rupture) K22.3
Boggy
  cervix N88.8
  uterus N85.8
Boil (*see also* Furuncle, by site)
  Aleppo B55.1
  Baghdad B55.1
  Delhi B55.1
  lacrimal
    gland — *see* Dacryoadenitis
    passages (duct) (sac) — *see* Inflammation, lacrimal, passages, acute
  Natal B55.1
  orbit, orbital — *see* Abscess, orbit
  tropical B55.1
Bold hives — *see* Urticaria
Bombé, iris — *see* Membrane, pupillary
Bone — *see* condition
Bonnevie-Ullrich syndrome (*see also* Turner's syndrome) Q87.1
Bonnier's syndrome H81.8 ☑
Bonvale dam fever T73.3 ☑
Bony block of joint — *see* Ankylosis
BOOP (bronchiolitis obliterans organized pneumonia) J84.89
Borderline
  diabetes mellitus R73.03
  hypertension R03.0
  osteopenia M85.8- ☑
  pelvis, with obstruction during labor O65.1
  personality F60.3
Borna disease A83.9
Bornholm disease B33.0
Boston exanthem A88.0
Botalli, ductus (patent) (persistent) Q25.0
Bothriocephalus latus infestation B70.0
Botulism (foodborne intoxication) A05.1
  infant A48.51
  non-foodborne A48.52
  wound A48.52
Bouba — *see* Yaws
Bouchard's nodes (with arthropathy) M15.2
Bouffée délirante F23
Bouillaud's disease or syndrome (rheumatic heart disease) I01.9
Bourneville's disease Q85.1
Boutonniere deformity (finger) — *see* Deformity, finger, boutonniere
Bouveret (-Hoffmann) **syndrome** (paroxysmal tachycardia) I47.9
Bovine heart — *see* Hypertrophy, cardiac
Bowel — *see* condition
Bowen's
  dermatosis (precancerous) — *see* Neoplasm, skin, in situ
  disease — *see* Neoplasm, skin, in situ
  epithelioma — *see* Neoplasm, skin, in situ
  type
    epidermoid carcinoma-in-situ — *see* Neoplasm, skin, in situ
    intraepidermal squamous cell carcinoma — *see* Neoplasm, skin, in situ
Bowing
  femur (*see also* Deformity, limb, specified type NEC, thigh)
    congenital Q68.3
  fibula (*see also* Deformity, limb, specified type NEC, lower leg)
    congenital Q68.4
  forearm — *see* Deformity, limb, specified type NEC, forearm
  leg(s), long bones, congenital Q68.5
  radius — *see* Deformity, limb, specified type NEC, forearm
  tibia (*see also* Deformity, limb, specified type NEC, lower leg)
    congenital Q68.4
Bowleg(s) (acquired) M21.16- ☑
  congenital Q68.5
  rachitic E64.3
Boyd's dysentery A03.2
Brachial — *see* condition
Brachycardia R00.1

Brachycephaly Q75.0
Bradley's disease A08.19
Bradyarrhythmia, cardiac I49.8
Bradycardia (sinoatrial) (sinus) (vagal) R00.1
  neonatal P29.12
  reflex G90.09
  tachycardia syndrome I49.5
Bradykinesia R25.8
Bradypnea R06.89
Bradytachycardia I49.5
Brailsford's disease or osteochondrosis — *see* Osteochondrosis, juvenile, radius
Brain (*see also* condition)
  death G93.82
  syndrome — *see* Syndrome, brain
Branched-chain amino-acid disorder E71.2
Branchial — *see* condition
  cartilage, congenital Q18.2
Branchiogenic remnant (in neck) Q18.0
Brandt's syndrome (acrodermatitis enteropathica) E83.2
Brash (water) R12
Bravais-jacksonian epilepsy — *see* Epilepsy, localization-related, symptomatic, with simple partial seizures
Braxton Hicks contractions — *see* False, labor
Brazilian leishmaniasis B55.2
BRBPR K62.5
Break, retina (without detachment) H33.30- ☑
  with retinal detachment — *see* Detachment, retina
  horseshoe tear H33.31- ☑
  multiple H33.33- ☑
  round hole H33.32- ☑
Breakdown
  device, graft or implant (*see also* Complications, by site and type, mechanical) T85.618 ☑
    arterial graft NEC — *see* Complication, cardiovascular device, mechanical, vascular
    breast (implant) T85.41 ☑
    catheter NEC T85.618 ☑
      cystostomy T83.010 ☑
      dialysis (renal) T82.41 ☑
        intraperitoneal T85.611 ☑
      Hopkins T83.018 ☑
      ileostomy T83.018 ☑
      infusion NEC T82.514 ☑
        cranial T85.610- ☑
        epidural T85.610 ☑
        intrathecal T85.610 ☑
        spinal T85.610 ☑
        subarachnoid T85.610 ☑
        subdural T85.610 ☑
      nephrostomy T83.012 ☑
      urethral indwelling T83.011 ☑
      urinary NEC T83.018 ☑
      urostomy T83.018 ☑
    electronic (electrode) (pulse generator) (stimulator)
      bone T84.310 ☑
      cardiac T82.119 ☑
        electrode T82.110 ☑
        pulse generator T82.111 ☑
        specified type NEC T82.118 ☑
      nervous system — *see* Complication, prosthetic device, mechanical, electronic nervous system stimulator
      urinary — *see* Complication, genitourinary, device, urinary, mechanical
    fixation, internal (orthopedic) NEC — *see* Complication, fixation device, mechanical
    gastrointestinal — *see* Complications, prosthetic device, mechanical, gastrointestinal device
    genital NEC T83.418 ☑
      intrauterine contraceptive device T83.31 ☑
      penile prosthesis (cylinder) (implanted) (pump) (resevoir) T83.410 ☑
      testicular prosthesis T83.411 ☑
    heart NEC — *see* Complication, cardiovascular device, mechanical
    intrathecal infusion pump T85.615 ☑
    joint prosthesis — *see* Complications..., joint prosthesis,internal, mechanical, by site
    nervous system, specified device NEC T85.615 ☑
    ocular NEC — *see* Complications, prosthetic device, mechanical, ocular device
    orthopedic NEC — *see* Complication, orthopedic, device, mechanical
    specified NEC T85.618 ☑

Breakdown — *continued*
  device, graft or implant (*see also* Complications, by site and type, mechanical) — *continued*
    subcutaneous device pocket
      nervous system prosthetic device, implant, or graft T85.890 ☑
      other internal prosthetic device, implant, or graft T85.898 ☑
    sutures, permanent T85.612 ☑
      used in bone repair — *see* Complications, fixation device, internal (orthopedic), mechanical
    urinary NEC T83.118 ☑
      graft T83.21 ☑
      sphincter, implanted T83.111 ☑
      stent (ileal conduit) (nephroureteral) T83.113 ☑
        ureteral indwelling T83.112 ☑
    vascular NEC — *see* Complication, cardiovascular device, mechanical
    ventricular intracranial shunt T85.01 ☑
  nervous F48.8
  perineum O90.1
  respirator J95.850
    specified NEC J95.859
  ventilator J95.850
    specified NEC J95.859
Breast (*see also* condition)
  buds E30.1
    in newborn P96.89
  dense R92.2
  nodule (*see also* Lump, breast) N63.0
Breath
  foul R19.6
  holder, child R06.89
  holding spell R06.89
  shortness R06.02
Breathing
  labored — *see* Hyperventilation
  mouth R06.5
    causing malocclusion M26.5 ☑
  periodic R06.3
    high altitude G47.32
Breathlessness R06.81
Breda's disease — *see* Yaws
Breech presentation (mother) O32.1 ☑
  causing obstructed labor O64.1 ☑
  footling O32.8 ☑
    causing obstructed labor O64.8 ☑
  incomplete O32.8 ☑
    causing obstructed labor O64.8 ☑
Breisky's disease N90.4
Brennemann's syndrome I88.0
Brenner
  tumor (benign) D27.9
    borderline malignancy D39.1- ☑
    malignant C56 ☑
    proliferating D39.1- ☑
Bretonneau's disease or angina A36.0
Breus' mole O02.0
Brevicollis Q76.49
Brickmakers' anemia B76.9 [D63.8]
Bridge, myocardial Q24.5
Bright red blood per rectum (BRBPR) K62.5
Bright's disease (*see also* Nephritis)
  arteriosclerotic — *see* Hypertension, kidney
Brill (-Zinsser) **disease** (recrudescent typhus) A75.1
  flea-borne A75.2
  louse-borne A75.1
Brill-Symmers' disease C82.90
Brion-Kayser disease — *see* Fever, parathyroid
Briquet's disorder or syndrome F45.0
Brissaud's
  infantilism or dwarfism E23.0
  motor-verbal tic F95.2
Brittle
  bones disease Q78.0
  nails L60.3
    congenital Q84.6
Broad (*see also* condition)
  beta disease E78.2
  ligament laceration syndrome N83.8
Broad- or floating-betalipoproteinemia E78.2
Brock's syndrome (atelectasis due to enlarged lymph nodes) J98.19
Brocq-Duhring disease (dermatitis herpetiformis) L13.0
Brodie's abscess or disease M86.8X- ☑

Broken
arches (see also Deformity, limb, flat foot)
arm (meaning upper limb) — see Fracture, arm
back — see Fracture, vertebra
bone — see Fracture
implant or internal device — see Complications, by
    site and type, mechanical
leg (meaning lower limb) — see Fracture, leg
nose S02.2 ☑
tooth, teeth — see Fracture, tooth
Bromhidrosis, bromidrosis L75.0
Bromidism, bromism G92
chronic (dependence) F13.20
due to
    correct substance properly administered — see
        Table of Drugs and Chemicals, by drug, ad-
        verse effect
    overdose or wrong substance given or taken —
        see Table of Drugs and Chemicals, by drug,
        poisoning
Bromidrosiphobia F40.298
Bronchi, bronchial — see condition
Bronchiectasis (cylindrical) (diffuse) (fusiform) (localized)
    (saccular) J47.9
with
    acute
        bronchitis J47.0
        lower respiratory infection J47.0
        exacerbation (acute) J47.1
congenital Q33.4
tuberculous NEC — see Tuberculosis, pulmonary
Bronchiolectasis — see Bronchiectasis
Bronchiolitis (acute) (infective) (subacute) J21.9
with
    bronchospasm or obstruction J21.9
    influenza, flu or grippe — see Influenza, with, res-
        piratory manifestations NEC
chemical (chronic) J68.4
    acute J68.0
chronic (fibrosing) (obliterative) J44.9
due to
    external agent — see Bronchitis, acute, due to
    human metapneumovirus J21.1
    respiratory syncytial virus J21.0
    specified organism NEC J21.8
fibrosa obliterans J44.9
influenzal — see Influenza, with, respiratory manifes-
    tations NEC
obliterans J42
    with organizing pneumonia (BOOP) J84.89
obliterative (chronic) (subacute) J44.9
    due to chemicals, gases, fumes or vapors (inhala-
        tion) J68.4
    due to fumes or vapors J68.4
respiratory, interstitial lung disease J84.115
Bronchitis (diffuse) (fibrinous) (hypostatic) (infective)
    (membranous) J40
with
    influenza, flu or grippe — see Influenza, with, res-
        piratory manifestations NEC
    obstruction (airway) (lung) J44.9
    tracheitis (15 years of age and above) J40
        acute or subacute J20.9
        chronic J42
        under 15 years of age J20.9
acute or subacute (with bronchospasm or obstruction)
    J20.9
    with
        bronchiectasis J47.0
        chronic obstructive pulmonary disease J44.0
    chemical (due to gases, fumes or vapors) J68.0
    due to
        fumes or vapors J68.0
        Haemophilus influenzae J20.1
        Mycoplasma pneumoniae J20.0
        radiation J70.0
        specified organism NEC J20.8
        Streptococcus J20.2
        virus
            coxsackie J20.3
            echovirus J20.7
            parainfluenzae J20.4
            respiratory syncytial J20.5
            rhinovirus J20.6
    viral NEC J20.8
allergic (acute) J45.909
    with
        exacerbation (acute) J45.901

Bronchitis — continued
allergic — continued
    with — continued
        status asthmaticus J45.902
arachidic T17.528 ☑
aspiration (due to fumes or vapors) J68.0
asthmatic J45.9 ☑
    chronic J44.9
        with
            acute lower respiratory infection J44.0
            exacerbation (acute) J44.1
capillary — see Pneumonia, broncho
caseous (tuberculous) A15.5
Castellani's A69.8
catarrhal (15 years of age and above) J40
    acute — see Bronchitis, acute
    chronic J41.0
    under 15 years of age J20.9
chemical (acute) (subacute) J68.0
    chronic J68.4
    due to fumes or vapors J68.0
        chronic J68.4
chronic J42
    with
        airways obstruction J44.9
        tracheitis (chronic) J42
    asthmatic (obstructive) J44.9
    catarrhal J41.0
    chemical (due to fumes or vapors) J68.4
    due to
        chemicals, gases, fumes or vapors (inhalation)
            J68.4
        radiation J70.1
        tobacco smoking J41.0
    emphysematous J44.9
    mucopurulent J41.1
    non-obstructive J41.0
    obliterans J44.9
    obstructive J44.9
    purulent J41.1
    simple J41.0
croupous — see Bronchitis, acute
due to gases, fumes or vapors (chemical) J68.0
emphysematous (obstructive) J44.9
exudative — see Bronchitis, acute
fetid J41.1
grippal — see Influenza, with, respiratory manifesta-
    tions NEC
in those under 15 years age — see Bronchitis, acute
    chronic — see Bronchitis, chronic
influenzal — see Influenza, with, respiratory manifes-
    tations NEC
mixed simple and mucopurulent J41.8
moulder's J62.8
mucopurulent (chronic) (recurrent) J41.1
    acute or subacute J20.9
    simple (mixed) J41.8
obliterans (chronic) J44.9
obstructive (chronic) (diffuse) J44.9
pituitous J41.1
pneumococcal, acute or subacute J20.2
pseudomembranous, acute or subacute — see Bron-
    chitis, acute
purulent (chronic) (recurrent) J41.1
    acute or subacute — see Bronchitis, acute
putrid J41.1
senile (chronic) J42
simple and mucopurulent (mixed) J41.8
smokers' J41.0
spirochetal NEC A69.8
subacute — see Bronchitis, acute
suppurative (chronic) J41.1
    acute or subacute — see Bronchitis, acute
tuberculous A15.5
under 15 years of age — see Bronchitis, acute
    chronic — see Bronchitis, chronic
viral NEC, acute or subacute (see also Bronchitis, acute)
    J20.8
Bronchoalveolitis J18.0
Bronchoaspergillosis B44.1
Bronchocele meaning goiter E04.0
Broncholithiasis J98.09
    tuberculous NEC A15.5
Bronchomalacia J98.09
    congenital Q32.2
Bronchomycosis NOS B49 [J99]
    candidal B37.1
Bronchopleuropneumonia — see Pneumonia, broncho

Bronchopneumonia — see Pneumonia, broncho
Bronchopneumonitis — see Pneumonia, broncho
Bronchopulmonary — see condition
Bronchopulmonitis — see Pneumonia, broncho
Bronchorrhagia (see Hemoptysis)
Bronchorrhea J98.09
acute J98.9
chronic (infective) (purulent) J42
Bronchospasm (acute) J98.01
with
    bronchiolitis, acute J21.9
    bronchitis, acute (conditions in J20) — see Bronchi-
        tis, acute
due to external agent — see condition, respiratory,
    acute, due to
exercise induced J45.990
Bronchospirochetosis A69.8
Castellani A69.8
Bronchostenosis J98.09
Bronchus — see condition
Brontophobia F40.220
Bronze baby syndrome P83.88
Brooke's tumor — see Neoplasm, skin, benign
Brown enamel of teeth (hereditary) K00.5
Brown's sheath syndrome H50.61- ☑
Brown-Séquard disease, paralysis or syndrome
    G83.81
Bruce sepsis A23.0
Brucellosis (infection) A23.9
abortus A23.1
canis A23.3
dermatitis A23.9
melitensis A23.0
mixed A23.8
sepsis A23.9
    melitensis A23.0
    specified NEC A23.8
suis A23.2
Bruck-de Lange disease Q87.1
Bruck's disease — see Deformity, limb
BRUE (brief resolved unexplained event) R68.13
Brugsch's syndrome Q82.8
Bruise (skin surface intact) (see also Contusion)
with
    open wound — see Wound, open
internal organ — see Injury, by site
newborn P54.5
scalp, due to birth injury, newborn P12.3
umbilical cord O69.5 ☑
Bruit (arterial) R09.89
cardiac R01.1
Brush burn — see Abrasion, by site
Bruton's X-linked agammaglobulinemia D80.0
Bruxism
psychogenic F45.8
sleep related G47.63
Bubbly lung syndrome P27.0
Bubo I88.8
blennorrhagic (gonococcal) A54.89
chancroidal A57
climatic A55
due to Haemophilus ducreyi A57
gonococcal A54.89
indolent (nonspecific) I88.8
inguinal (nonspecific) I88.8
    chancroidal A57
    climatic A55
    due to H. ducreyi A57
    infective I88.8
scrofulous (tuberculous) A18.2
soft chancre A57
suppurating — see Lymphadenitis, acute
syphilitic (primary) A51.0
    congenital A50.07
tropical A55
virulent (chancroidal) A57
Bubonic plague A20.0
Bubonocele — see Hernia, inguinal
Buccal — see condition
Buchanan's disease or osteochondrosis M91.0
Buchem's syndrome (hyperostosis corticalis) M85.2
Bucket-handle fracture or tear (semilunar cartilage)
    — see Tear, meniscus
Budd-Chiari syndrome (hepatic vein thrombosis) I82.0
Budgerigar fancier's disease or lung J67.2
Buds
breast E30.1

Buds — *continued*
  breast — *continued*
    in newborn P96.89
Buerger's disease (thromboangiitis obliterans) I73.1
Bulbar — *see* condition
Bulbus cordis (left ventricle) (persistent) Q21.8
Bulimia (nervosa) F50.2
  atypical F50.9
  normal weight F50.9
Bulky
  stools R19.5
  uterus N85.2
Bulla (e) R23.8
  lung (emphysematous) (solitary) J43.9
    newborn P25.8
Bullet wound (*see also* Wound, open)
  fracture — *code as* Fracture, by site
  internal organ — *see* Injury, by site
Bundle
  branch block (complete) (false) (incomplete) — *see* Block, bundle-branch
  of His — *see* condition
Bunion M21.61- ☑
  tailor's M21.62- ☑
Bunionette M21.62- ☑
Buphthalmia, buphthalmos (congenital) Q15.0
Burdwan fever B55.0
Bürger-Grütz disease or syndrome E78.3
Buried
  penis (congenital) Q55.64
    acquired N48.83
  roots K08.3
Burke's syndrome K86.89
Burkitt
  cell leukemia C91.0- ☑
  lymphoma (malignant) C83.7- ☑
    small noncleaved, diffuse C83.7- ☑
    spleen C83.77
    undifferentiated C83.7- ☑
  tumor C83.7- ☑
  type
    acute lymphoblastic leukemia C91.0- ☑
    undifferentiated C83.7- ☑
Burn (electricity) (flame) (hot gas, liquid or hot object) (radiation) (steam) (thermal) T30.0
  abdomen, abdominal (muscle) (wall) T21.02 ☑
    first degree T21.12 ☑
    second degree T21.22 ☑
    third degree T21.32 ☑
  above elbow T22.039 ☑
    first degree T22.139 ☑
    left T22.032 ☑
      first degree T22.132 ☑
      second degree T22.232 ☑
      third degree T22.332 ☑
    right T22.031 ☑
      first degree T22.131 ☑
      second degree T22.231 ☑
      third degree T22.331 ☑
    second degree T22.239 ☑
    third degree T22.339 ☑
  acid (caustic) (external) (internal) — *see* Corrosion, by site
  alimentary tract NEC T28.2 ☑
    esophagus T28.1 ☑
    mouth T28.0 ☑
    pharynx T28.0 ☑
  alkaline (caustic) (external) (internal) — *see* Corrosion, by site
  ankle T25.019 ☑
    first degree T25.119 ☑
    left T25.012 ☑
      first degree T25.112 ☑
      second degree T25.212 ☑
      third degree T25.312 ☑
    multiple with foot — *see* Burn, lower, limb, multiple, ankle and foot
    right T25.011 ☑
      first degree T25.111 ☑
      second degree T25.211 ☑
      third degree T25.311 ☑
    second degree T25.219 ☑
    third degree T25.319 ☑
  anus — *see* Burn, buttock
  arm (lower) (upper) — *see* Burn, upper, limb
  axilla T22.049 ☑

Burn — *continued*
  axilla — *continued*
    first degree T22.149 ☑
    left T22.042 ☑
      first degree T22.142 ☑
      second degree T22.242 ☑
      third degree T22.342 ☑
    right T22.041 ☑
      first degree T22.141 ☑
      second degree T22.241 ☑
      third degree T22.341 ☑
    second degree T22.249 ☑
    third degree T22.349 ☑
  back (lower) T21.04 ☑
    first degree T21.14 ☑
    second degree T21.24 ☑
    third degree T21.34 ☑
    upper T21.03 ☑
      first degree T21.13 ☑
      second degree T21.23 ☑
      third degree T21.33 ☑
  blisters — *code as* Burn, second degree, by site
  breast(s) — *see* Burn, chest wall
  buttock(s) T21.05 ☑
    first degree T21.15 ☑
    second degree T21.25 ☑
    third degree T21.35 ☑
  calf T24.039 ☑
    first degree T24.139 ☑
    left T24.032 ☑
      first degree T24.132 ☑
      second degree T24.232 ☑
      third degree T24.332 ☑
    right T24.031 ☑
      first degree T24.131 ☑
      second degree T24.231 ☑
      third degree T24.331 ☑
    second degree T24.239 ☑
    third degree T24.339 ☑
  canthus (eye) — *see* Burn, eyelid
  caustic acid or alkaline — *see* Corrosion, by site
  cervix T28.3 ☑
  cheek T20.06 ☑
    first degree T20.16 ☑
    second degree T20.26 ☑
    third degree T20.36 ☑
  chemical (acids) (alkalines) (caustics) (external) (internal) — *see* Corrosion, by site
  chest wall T21.01 ☑
    first degree T21.11 ☑
    second degree T21.21 ☑
    third degree T21.31 ☑
  chin T20.03 ☑
    first degree T20.13 ☑
    second degree T20.23 ☑
    third degree T20.33 ☑
  colon T28.2 ☑
  conjunctiva (and cornea) — *see* Burn, cornea
  cornea (and conjunctiva) T26.1- ☑
    chemical — *see* Corrosion, cornea
  corrosion (external) (internal) — *see* Corrosion, by site
  deep necrosis of underlying tissue — *code as* Burn, third degree, by site
  dorsum of hand T23.069 ☑
    first degree T23.169 ☑
    left T23.062 ☑
      first degree T23.162 ☑
      second degree T23.262 ☑
      third degree T23.362 ☑
    right T23.061 ☑
      first degree T23.161 ☑
      second degree T23.261 ☑
      third degree T23.361 ☑
    second degree T23.269 ☑
    third degree T23.369 ☑
  due to ingested chemical agent — *see* Corrosion, by site
  ear (auricle) (external) (canal) T20.01 ☑
    first degree T20.11 ☑
    second degree T20.21 ☑
    third degree T20.31 ☑
  elbow T22.029 ☑
    first degree T22.129 ☑
    left T22.022 ☑
      first degree T22.122 ☑
      second degree T22.222 ☑

Burn — *continued*
  elbow — *continued*
    left — *continued*
      third degree T22.322 ☑
    right T22.021 ☑
      first degree T22.121 ☑
      second degree T22.221 ☑
      third degree T22.321 ☑
    second degree T22.229 ☑
    third degree T22.329 ☑
  epidermal loss — *code as* Burn, second degree, by site
  erythema, erythematous — *code as* Burn, first degree, by site
  esophagus T28.1 ☑
  extent (percentage of body surface)
    less than 10 percent T31.0
    10-19 percent T31.10
      with 0-9 percent third degree burns T31.10
      with 10-19 percent third degree burns T31.11
    20-29 percent T31.20
      with 0-9 percent third degree burns T31.20
      with 10-19 percent third degree burns T31.21
      with 20-29 percent third degree burns T31.22
    30-39 percent T31.30
      with 0-9 percent third degree burns T31.30
      with 10-19 percent third degree burns T31.31
      with 20-29 percent third degree burns T31.32
      with 30-39 percent third degree burns T31.33
    40-49 percent T31.40
      with 0-9 percent third degree burns T31.40
      with 10-19 percent third degree burns T31.41
      with 20-29 percent third degree burns T31.42
      with 30-39 percent third degree burns T31.43
      with 40-49 percent third degree burns T31.44
    50-59 percent T31.50
      with 0-9 percent third degree burns T31.50
      with 10-19 percent third degree burns T31.51
      with 20-29 percent third degree burns T31.52
      with 30-39 percent third degree burns T31.53
      with 40-49 percent third degree burns T31.54
      with 50-59 percent third degree burns T31.55
    60-69 percent T31.60
      with 0-9 percent third degree burns T31.60
      with 10-19 percent third degree burns T31.61
      with 20-29 percent third degree burns T31.62
      with 30-39 percent third degree burns T31.63
      with 40-49 percent third degree burns T31.64
      with 50-59 percent third degree burns T31.65
      with 60-69 percent third degree burns T31.66
    70-79 percent T31.70
      with 0-9 percent third degree burns T31.70
      with 10-19 percent third degree burns T31.71
      with 20-29 percent third degree burns T31.72
      with 30-39 percent third degree burns T31.73
      with 40-49 percent third degree burns T31.74
      with 50-59 percent third degree burns T31.75
      with 60-69 percent third degree burns T31.76
      with 70-79 percent third degree burns T31.77
    80-89 percent T31.80
      with 0-9 percent third degree burns T31.80
      with 10-19 percent third degree burns T31.81
      with 20-29 percent third degree burns T31.82
      with 30-39 percent third degree burns T31.83
      with 40-49 percent third degree burns T31.84
      with 50-59 percent third degree burns T31.85
      with 60-69 percent third degree burns T31.86
      with 70-79 percent third degree burns T31.87
      with 80-89 percent third degree burns T31.88
    90 percent or more T31.90
      with 0-9 percent third degree burns T31.90
      with 10-19 percent third degree burns T31.91
      with 20-29 percent third degree burns T31.92
      with 30-39 percent third degree burns T31.93
      with 40-49 percent third degree burns T31.94
      with 50-59 percent third degree burns T31.95
      with 60-69 percent third degree burns T31.96
      with 70-79 percent third degree burns T31.97
      with 80-89 percent third degree burns T31.98
      with 90 percent or more third degree burns T31.99
  extremity — *see* Burn, limb
  eye(s) and adnexa T26.4- ☑
    with resulting rupture and destruction of eyeball T26.2- ☑
    conjunctival sac — *see* Burn, cornea
    cornea — *see* Burn, cornea
    lid — *see* Burn, eyelid
    periocular area — *see* Burn, eyelid

▼ Subterms under main terms may continue to next column or page   ☑ Additional Character Required — Refer to the Tabular List for Character Selection   43

Buds — Burn

Burn — *continued*
eye(s) and adnexa — *continued*
    specified site NEC T26.3- ☑
eyeball — *see* Burn, eye
eyelid(s) T26.0-
  chemical — *see* Corrosion, eyelid
face — *see* Burn, head
finger T23.029 ☑
  first degree T23.129 ☑
  left T23.022 ☑
    first degree T23.122 ☑
    second degree T23.222 ☑
    third degree T23.322 ☑
  multiple sites (without thumb) T23.039 ☑
    with thumb T23.049 ☑
      first degree T23.149 ☑
      left T23.042 ☑
        first degree T23.142 ☑
        second degree T23.242 ☑
        third degree T23.342 ☑
      right T23.041 ☑
        first degree T23.141 ☑
        second degree T23.241 ☑
        third degree T23.341 ☑
      second degree T23.249 ☑
      third degree T23.349 ☑
    first degree T23.139 ☑
    left T23.032 ☑
      first degree T23.132 ☑
      second degree T23.232 ☑
      third degree T23.332 ☑
    right T23.031 ☑
      first degree T23.131 ☑
      second degree T23.231 ☑
      third degree T23.331 ☑
    second degree T23.239 ☑
    third degree T23.339 ☑
  right T23.021 ☑
    first degree T23.121 ☑
    second degree T23.221 ☑
    third degree T23.321 ☑
  second degree T23.229 ☑
  third degree T23.329 ☑
flank — *see* Burn, abdominal wall
foot T25.029 ☑
  first degree T25.129 ☑
  left T25.022 ☑
    first degree T25.122 ☑
    second degree T25.222 ☑
    third degree T25.322 ☑
  multiple with ankle — *see* Burn, lower, limb, multiple, ankle and foot
  right T25.021 ☑
    first degree T25.121 ☑
    second degree T25.221 ☑
    third degree T25.321 ☑
  second degree T25.229 ☑
  third degree T25.329 ☑
forearm T22.019 ☑
  first degree T22.119 ☑
  left T22.012 ☑
    first degree T22.112 ☑
    second degree T22.212 ☑
    third degree T22.312 ☑
  right T22.011 ☑
    first degree T22.111 ☑
    second degree T22.211 ☑
    third degree T22.311 ☑
  second degree T22.219 ☑
  third degree T22.319 ☑
forehead T20.06 ☑
  first degree T20.16 ☑
  second degree T20.26 ☑
  third degree T20.36 ☑
fourth degree — *code as* Burn, third degree, by site
friction — *see* Burn, by site
from swallowing caustic or corrosive substance NEC — *see* Corrosion, by site
full thickness skin loss — *code as* Burn, third degree, by site
gastrointestinal tract NEC T28.2 ☑
  from swallowing caustic or corrosive substance T28.7 ☑
genital organs
  external
    female T21.07 ☑

Burn — *continued*
genital organs — *continued*
  external — *continued*
    female — *continued*
      first degree T21.17 ☑
      second degree T21.27 ☑
      third degree T21.37 ☑
    male T21.06 ☑
      first degree T21.16 ☑
      second degree T21.26 ☑
      third degree T21.36 ☑
  internal T28.3 ☑
    from caustic or corrosive substance T28.8 ☑
groin — *see* Burn, abdominal wall
hand(s) T23.009 ☑
  back — *see* Burn, dorsum of hand
  finger — *see* Burn, finger
  first degree T23.109 ☑
  left T23.002 ☑
    first degree T23.102 ☑
    second degree T23.202 ☑
    third degree T23.302 ☑
  multiple sites with wrist T23.099 ☑
    first degree T23.199 ☑
    left T23.092 ☑
      first degree T23.192 ☑
      second degree T23.292 ☑
      third degree T23.392 ☑
    right T23.091 ☑
      first degree T23.191 ☑
      second degree T23.291 ☑
      third degree T23.391 ☑
    second degree T23.299 ☑
    third degree T23.399 ☑
  palm — *see* Burn, palm
  right T23.001 ☑
    first degree T23.101 ☑
    second degree T23.201 ☑
    third degree T23.301 ☑
  second degree T23.209 ☑
  third degree T23.309 ☑
  thumb — *see* Burn, thumb
head (and face) (and neck) T20.00 ☑
  cheek — *see* Burn, cheek
  chin — *see* Burn, chin
  ear — *see* Burn, ear
  eye(s) only — *see* Burn, eye
  first degree T20.10 ☑
  forehead — *see* Burn, forehead
  lip — *see* Burn, lip
  multiple sites T20.09 ☑
    first degree T20.19 ☑
    second degree T20.29 ☑
    third degree T20.39 ☑
  neck — *see* Burn, neck
  nose — *see* Burn, nose
  scalp — *see* Burn, scalp
  second degree T20.20 ☑
  third degree T20.30 ☑
hip(s) — *see* Burn, thigh
inhalation — *see* Burn, respiratory tract
  caustic or corrosive substance (fumes) — *see* Corrosion, respiratory tract
internal organ(s) T28.40 ☑
  alimentary tract T28.2 ☑
    esophagus T28.1 ☑
  eardrum T28.41 ☑
  esophagus T28.1 ☑
    from caustic or corrosive substance (swallowing) NEC — *see* Corrosion, by site
  genitourinary T28.3 ☑
  mouth T28.0 ☑
  pharynx T28.0 ☑
  respiratory tract — *see* Burn, respiratory tract
  specified organ NEC T28.49 ☑
interscapular region — *see* Burn, back, upper
intestine (large) (small) T28.2 ☑
knee T24.029 ☑
  first degree T24.129 ☑
  left T24.022 ☑
    first degree T24.122 ☑
    second degree T24.222 ☑
    third degree T24.322 ☑
  right T24.021 ☑
    first degree T24.121 ☑
    second degree T24.221 ☑

Burn — *continued*
knee — *continued*
  right — *continued*
    third degree T24.321 ☑
  second degree T24.229 ☑
  third degree T24.329 ☑
labium (majus) (minus) — *see* Burn, genital organs, external, female
lacrimal apparatus, duct, gland or sac — *see* Burn, eye, specified site NEC
larynx T27.0 ☑
  with lung T27.1 ☑
leg(s) (lower) (upper) — *see* Burn, lower, limb
lightning — *see* Burn, by site
limb(s)
  lower (except ankle or foot alone) — *see* Burn, lower, limb
  upper — *see* Burn, upper limb
lip(s) T20.02 ☑
  first degree T20.12 ☑
  second degree T20.22 ☑
  third degree T20.32 ☑
lower
  back — *see* Burn, back
  limb T24.009 ☑
    ankle — *see* Burn, ankle
    calf — *see* Burn, calf
    first degree T24.109 ☑
    foot — *see* Burn, foot
    hip — *see* Burn, thigh
    knee — *see* Burn, knee
    left T24.002 ☑
      first degree T24.102 ☑
      second degree T24.202 ☑
      third degree T24.302 ☑
    multiple sites, except ankle and foot T24.099 ☑
      ankle and foot T25.099 ☑
        first degree T25.199 ☑
        left T25.092 ☑
          first degree T25.192 ☑
          second degree T25.292 ☑
          third degree T25.392 ☑
        right T25.091 ☑
          first degree T25.191 ☑
          second degree T25.291 ☑
          third degree T25.391 ☑
        second degree T25.299 ☑
        third degree T25.399 ☑
      first degree T24.199 ☑
      left T24.092 ☑
        first degree T24.192 ☑
        second degree T24.292 ☑
        third degree T24.392 ☑
      right T24.091 ☑
        first degree T24.191 ☑
        second degree T24.291 ☑
        third degree T24.391 ☑
      second degree T24.299 ☑
      third degree T24.399 ☑
    right T24.001 ☑
      first degree T24.101 ☑
      second degree T24.201 ☑
      third degree T24.301 ☑
    second degree T24.209 ☑
    thigh — *see* Burn, thigh
    third degree T24.309 ☑
    toe — *see* Burn, toe
lung (with larynx and trachea) T27.1 ☑
mouth T28.0 ☑
neck T20.07 ☑
  first degree T20.17 ☑
  second degree T20.27 ☑
  third degree T20.37 ☑
nose (septum) T20.04 ☑
  first degree T20.14 ☑
  second degree T20.24 ☑
  third degree T20.34 ☑
ocular adnexa — *see* Burn, eye
orbit region — *see* Burn, eyelid
palm T23.059 ☑
  first degree T23.159 ☑
  left T23.052 ☑
    first degree T23.152 ☑
    second degree T23.252 ☑
    third degree T23.352 ☑
  right T23.051 ☑

Burn — *continued*
  palm — *continued*
    right — *continued*
      first degree T23.151 ☑
      second degree T23.251 ☑
      third degree T23.351 ☑
    second degree T23.259 ☑
    third degree T23.359 ☑
  partial thickness — *code as* Burn, unspecified degree, by site
  pelvis — *see* Burn, trunk
  penis — *see* Burn, genital organs, external, male
  perineum
    female — *see* Burn, genital organs, external, female
    male — *see* Burn, genital organs, external, male
  periocular area — *see* Burn, eyelid
  pharynx T28.0 ☑
  rectum T28.2 ☑
  respiratory tract T27.3 ☑
    larynx — *see* Burn, larynx
    specified part NEC T27.2 ☑
    trachea — *see* Burn, trachea
  sac, lacrimal — *see* Burn, eye, specified site NEC
  scalp T20.05 ☑
    first degree T20.15 ☑
    second degree T20.25 ☑
    third degree T20.35 ☑
  scapular region T22.069 ☑
    first degree T22.169 ☑
    left T22.062 ☑
      first degree T22.162 ☑
      second degree T22.262 ☑
      third degree T22.362 ☑
    right T22.061 ☑
      first degree T22.161 ☑
      second degree T22.261 ☑
      third degree T22.361 ☑
    second degree T22.269 ☑
    third degree T22.369 ☑
  sclera — *see* Burn, eye, specified site NEC
  scrotum — *see* Burn, genital organs, external, male
  shoulder T22.059 ☑
    first degree T22.159 ☑
    left T22.052 ☑
      first degree T22.152 ☑
      second degree T22.252 ☑
      third degree T22.352 ☑
    right T22.051 ☑
      first degree T22.151 ☑
      second degree T22.251 ☑
      third degree T22.351 ☑
    second degree T22.259 ☑
    third degree T22.359 ☑
  stomach T28.2 ☑
  temple — *see* Burn, head
  testis — *see* Burn, genital organs, external, male
  thigh T24.019 ☑
    first degree T24.119 ☑
    left T24.012 ☑
      first degree T24.112 ☑
      second degree T24.212 ☑
      third degree T24.312 ☑
    right T24.011 ☑
      first degree T24.111 ☑
      second degree T24.211 ☑
      third degree T24.311 ☑
    second degree T24.219 ☑
    third degree T24.319 ☑
  thorax (external) — *see* Burn, trunk
  throat (meaning pharynx) T28.0 ☑
  thumb(s) T23.019 ☑
    first degree T23.119 ☑
    left T23.012 ☑
      first degree T23.112 ☑
      second degree T23.212 ☑
      third degree T23.312 ☑
    multiple sites with fingers T23.049 ☑
      first degree T23.149 ☑
      left T23.042 ☑
        first degree T23.142 ☑
        second degree T23.242 ☑
        third degree T23.342 ☑
      right T23.041 ☑
        first degree T23.141 ☑
        second degree T23.241 ☑
        third degree T23.341 ☑

Burn — *continued*
  thumb(s) — *continued*
    multiple sites with fingers — *continued*
      second degree T23.249 ☑
      third degree T23.349 ☑
    right T23.011 ☑
      first degree T23.111 ☑
      second degree T23.211 ☑
      third degree T23.311 ☑
    second degree T23.219 ☑
    third degree T23.319 ☑
  toe T25.039 ☑
    first degree T25.139 ☑
    left T25.032 ☑
      first degree T25.132 ☑
      second degree T25.232 ☑
      third degree T25.332 ☑
    right T25.031 ☑
      first degree T25.131 ☑
      second degree T25.231 ☑
      third degree T25.331 ☑
    second degree T25.239 ☑
    third degree T25.339 ☑
  tongue T28.0 ☑
  tonsil(s) T28.0 ☑
  trachea T27.0 ☑
    with lung T27.1 ☑
  trunk T21.00 ☑
    abdominal wall — *see* Burn, abdominal wall
    anus — *see* Burn, buttock
    axilla — *see* Burn, upper limb
    back — *see* Burn, back
    breast — *see* Burn, chest wall
    buttock — *see* Burn, buttock
    chest wall — *see* Burn, chest wall
    first degree T21.10 ☑
    flank — *see* Burn, abdominal wall
    genital
      female — *see* Burn, genital organs, external, female
      male — *see* Burn, genital organs, external, male
    groin — *see* Burn, abdominal wall
    interscapular region — *see* Burn, back, upper
    labia — *see* Burn, genital organs, external, female
    lower back — *see* Burn, back
    penis — *see* Burn, genital organs, external, male
    perineum
      female — *see* Burn, genital organs, external, female
      male — *see* Burn, genital organs, external, male
    scapula region — *see* Burn, scapular region
    scrotum — *see* Burn, genital organs, external, male
    second degree T21.20 ☑
    specified site NEC T21.09 ☑
      first degree T21.19 ☑
      second degree T21.29 ☑
      third degree T21.39 ☑
    testes — *see* Burn, genital organs, external, male
    third degree T21.30 ☑
    upper back — *see* Burn, back, upper
    vulva — *see* Burn, genital organs, external, female
  unspecified site with extent of body surface involved specified
    less than 10 percent T31.0
    10-19 percent (0-9 percent third degree) T31.10
      with 10-19 percent third degree T31.11
    20-29 percent (0-9 percent third degree) T31.20
      with
        10-19 percent third degree T31.21
        20-29 percent third degree T31.22
    30-39 percent (0-9 percent third degree) T31.30
      with
        10-19 percent third degree T31.31
        20-29 percent third degree T31.32
        30-39 percent third degree T31.33
    40-49 percent (0-9 percent third degree) T31.40
      with
        10-19 percent third degree T31.41
        20-29 percent third degree T31.42
        30-39 percent third degree T31.43
        40-49 percent third degree T31.44
    50-59 percent (0-9 percent third degree) T31.50
      with
        10-19 percent third degree T31.51
        20-29 percent third degree T31.52
        30-39 percent third degree T31.53
        40-49 percent third degree T31.54

Burn — *continued*
  unspecified site with extent of body surface involved specified — *continued*
    50-59 percent — *continued*
      with — *continued*
        50-59 percent third degree T31.55
    60-69 percent (0-9 percent third degree) T31.60
      with
        10-19 percent third degree T31.61
        20-29 percent third degree T31.62
        30-39 percent third degree T31.63
        40-49 percent third degree T31.64
        50-59 percent third degree T31.65
        60-69 percent third degree T31.66
    70-79 percent (0-9 percent third degree) T31.70
      with
        10-19 percent third degree T31.71
        20-29 percent third degree T31.72
        30-39 percent third degree T31.73
        40-49 percent third degree T31.74
        50-59 percent third degree T31.75
        60-69 percent third degree T31.76
        70-79 percent third degree T31.77
    80-89 percent (0-9 percent third degree) T31.80
      with
        10-19 percent third degree T31.81
        20-29 percent third degree T31.82
        30-39 percent third degree T31.83
        40-49 percent third degree T31.84
        50-59 percent third degree T31.85
        60-69 percent third degree T31.86
        70-79 percent third degree T31.87
        80-89 percent third degree T31.88
    90 percent or more (0-9 percent third degree) T31.90
      with
        10-19 percent third degree T31.91
        20-29 percent third degree T31.92
        30-39 percent third degree T31.93
        40-49 percent third degree T31.94
        50-59 percent third degree T31.95
        60-69 percent third degree T31.96
        70-79 percent third degree T31.97
        80-89 percent third degree T31.98
        90-99 percent third degree T31.99
  upper limb T22.00 ☑
    above elbow — *see* Burn, above elbow
    axilla — *see* Burn, axilla
    elbow — *see* Burn, elbow
    first degree T22.10 ☑
    forearm — *see* Burn, forearm
    hand — *see* Burn, hand
    interscapular region — *see* Burn, back, upper
    multiple sites T22.099 ☑
      first degree T22.199 ☑
      left T22.092 ☑
        first degree T22.192 ☑
        second degree T22.292 ☑
        third degree T22.392 ☑
      right T22.091 ☑
        first degree T22.191 ☑
        second degree T22.291 ☑
        third degree T22.391 ☑
      second degree T22.299 ☑
      third degree T22.399 ☑
    scapular region — *see* Burn, scapular region
    second degree T22.20 ☑
    shoulder — *see* Burn, shoulder
    third degree T22.30 ☑
    wrist — *see* Burn, wrist
  uterus T28.3 ☑
  vagina T28.3 ☑
  vulva — *see* Burn, genital organs, external, female
  wrist T23.079 ☑
    first degree T23.179 ☑
    left T23.072 ☑
      first degree T23.172 ☑
      second degree T23.272 ☑
      third degree T23.372 ☑
    multiple sites with hand T23.099 ☑
      first degree T23.199 ☑
      left T23.092 ☑
        first degree T23.192 ☑
        second degree T23.292 ☑
        third degree T23.392 ☑
      right T23.091 ☑
        first degree T23.191 ☑

Burn — continued
  wrist — continued
    multiple sites with hand — continued
      right — continued
        second degree T23.291 ☑
          third degree T23.391 ☑
        second degree T23.299 ☑
        third degree T23.399 ☑
      right T23.071 ☑
        first degree T23.171 ☑
        second degree T23.271 ☑
        third degree T23.371 ☑
      second degree T23.279 ☑
      third degree T23.379 ☑
Burnett's syndrome E83.52
Burning
  feet syndrome E53.9
  sensation R20.8
  tongue K14.6
Burn-out (state) Z73.0
Burns' disease or osteochondrosis — see Osteochondrosis, juvenile, ulna
Bursa — see condition
Bursitis M71.9
  Achilles — see Tendinitis, Achilles
  adhesive — see Bursitis, specified NEC
  ankle — see Enthesopathy, lower limb, ankle, specified type NEC
  calcaneal — see Enthesopathy, foot, specified type NEC
  collateral ligament, tibial — see Bursitis, tibial collateral
  due to use, overuse, pressure (see also Disorder, soft tissue, due to use, specified type NEC)
    specified NEC — see Disorder, soft tissue, due to use, specified NEC
  Duplay's M75.0
  elbow NEC M70.3- ☑
    olecranon M70.2- ☑
  finger — see Disorder, soft tissue, due to use, specified type NEC, hand
  foot — see Enthesopathy, foot, specified type NEC
  gonococcal A54.49
  gouty — see Gout
  hand M70.1- ☑
  hip NEC M70.7- ☑
    trochanteric M70.6- ☑
  infective NEC M71.10
    abscess — see Abscess, bursa
    ankle M71.17- ☑
    elbow M71.12- ☑
    foot M71.17- ☑
    hand M71.14- ☑
    hip M71.15- ☑
    knee M71.16- ☑
    multiple sites M71.19
    shoulder M71.11- ☑
    specified site NEC M71.18
    wrist M71.13- ☑
  ischial — see Bursitis, hip
  knee NEC M70.5- ☑
    prepatellar M70.4- ☑
  occupational NEC (see also Disorder, soft tissue, due to, use)
  olecranon — see Bursitis, elbow, olecranon
  pharyngeal J39.1
  popliteal — see Bursitis, knee
  prepatellar M70.4- ☑
  radiohumeral M77.8
  rheumatoid M06.20
    ankle M06.27- ☑
    elbow M06.22- ☑
    foot joint M06.27- ☑
    hand joint M06.24- ☑
    hip M06.25- ☑
    knee M06.26- ☑
    multiple site M06.29
    shoulder M06.21- ☑
    vertebra M06.28
    wrist M06.23- ☑
  scapulohumeral — see Bursitis, shoulder
  semimembranous muscle (knee) — see Bursitis, knee
  shoulder M75.5- ☑
    adhesive — see Capsulitis, adhesive
  specified NEC M71.50
    ankle M71.57- ☑

Bursitis — continued
  specified — continued
    due to use, overuse or pressure — see Disorder, soft tissue, due to, use
    elbow M71.52- ☑
    foot M71.57- ☑
    hand M71.54- ☑
    hip M71.55- ☑
    knee M71.56- ☑
    shoulder — see Bursitis, shoulder
    specified site NEC M71.58
    tibial collateral M76.4- ☑
    wrist M71.53- ☑
  subacromial — see Bursitis, shoulder
  subcoracoid — see Bursitis, shoulder
  subdeltoid — see Bursitis, shoulder
  syphilitic A52.78
  Thornwaldt, Tornwaldt J39.2
  tibial collateral M76.4- ☑
  toe — see Enthesopathy, foot, specified type NEC
  trochanteric (area) — see Bursitis, hip, trochanteric
  wrist — see Bursitis, hand
Bursopathy M71.9
  specified type NEC M71.80
    ankle M71.87- ☑
    elbow M71.82- ☑
    foot M71.87- ☑
    hand M71.84- ☑
    hip M71.85- ☑
    knee M71.86- ☑
    multiple sites M71.89
    shoulder M71.81- ☑
    specified site NEC M71.88
    wrist M71.83- ☑
Burst stitches or sutures (complication of surgery) T81.31
  external operation wound T81.31 ☑
  internal operation wound T81.32 ☑
Buruli ulcer A31.1
Bury's disease L95.1
Buschke's
  disease B45.3
  scleredema — see Sclerosis, systemic
Busse-Buschke disease B45.3
Buttock — see condition
Button
  Biskra B55.1
  Delhi B55.1
  oriental B55.1
Buttonhole deformity (finger) — see Deformity, finger, boutonniere
Bwamba fever A92.8
Byssinosis J66.0
Bywaters' syndrome T79.5 ☑

C

Cachexia R64
  cancerous R64
  cardiac — see Disease, heart
  dehydration E86.0
  due to malnutrition R64
  exophthalmic — see Hyperthyroidism
  heart — see Disease, heart
  hypophyseal E23.0
  hypopituitary E23.0
  lead — see Poisoning, lead
  malignant R64
  marsh — see Malaria
  nervous F48.8
  old age R54
  paludal — see Malaria
  pituitary E23.0
  renal N28.9
  saturnine — see Poisoning, lead
  senile R54
  Simmonds' E23.0
  splenica D73.0
  strumipriva E03.4
  tuberculous NEC — see Tuberculosis
Café, au lait spots L81.3
Caffeine-induced
  anxiety disorder F15.980
  sleep disorder F15.982
Caffey's syndrome Q78.8
Caisson disease T70.3 ☑
Cake kidney Q63.1

Caked breast (puerperal, postpartum) O92.79
Calabar swelling B74.3
Calcaneal spur — see Spur, bone, calcaneal
Calcaneo-apophysitis M92.8
Calcareous — see condition
Calcicosis J62.8
Calciferol (vitamin D) deficiency E55.9
  with rickets E55.0
Calcification
  adrenal (capsule) (gland) E27.49
    tuberculous E35 [B90.8]
  aorta I70.0
  artery (annular) — see Arteriosclerosis
  auricle (ear) — see Disorder, pinna, specified type NEC
  basal ganglia G23.8
  bladder N32.89
    due to Schistosoma hematobium B65.0
  brain (cortex) — see Calcification, cerebral
  bronchus J98.09
  bursa M71.40
    ankle M71.47- ☑
    elbow M71.42- ☑
    foot M71.47- ☑
    hand M71.44- ☑
    hip M71.45- ☑
    knee M71.46- ☑
    multiple sites M71.49
    shoulder M75.3- ☑
    specified site NEC M71.48
    wrist M71.43- ☑
  cardiac — see Degeneration, myocardial
  cerebral (cortex) G93.89
    artery I67.2
  cervix (uteri) N88.8
  choroid plexus G93.89
  conjunctiva — see Concretion, conjunctiva
  corpora cavernosa (penis) N48.89
  cortex (brain) — see Calcification, cerebral
  dental pulp (nodular) K04.2
  dentinal papilla K00.4
  fallopian tube N83.8
  falx cerebri G96.19
  gallbladder K82.8
  general E83.59
  heart (see also Degeneration, myocardial)
    valve — see Endocarditis
  idiopathic infantile arterial (IIAC) Q28.8
  intervertebral cartilage or disc (postinfective) — see Disorder, disc, specified NEC
  intracranial — see Calcification, cerebral
  joint — see Disorder, joint, specified type NEC
  kidney N28.89
    tuberculous N29 [B90.1]
  larynx (senile) J38.7
  lens — see Cataract, specified NEC
  lung (active) (postinfectional) J98.4
    tuberculous B90.9
  lymph gland or node (postinfectional) I89.8
    tuberculous (see also Tuberculosis, lymph gland) B90.8
  mammographic R92.1
  massive (paraplegic) — see Myositis, ossificans, in, quadriplegia
  medial — see Arteriosclerosis, extremities
  meninges (cerebral) (spinal) G96.19
  metastatic E83.59
  Mönckeberg's — see Arteriosclerosis, extremities
  muscle M61.9
    due to burns — see Myositis, ossificans, in, burns
    paralytic — see Myositis, ossificans, in, quadriplegia
    specified type NEC M61.40
      ankle M61.47- ☑
      foot M61.47- ☑
      forearm M61.43- ☑
      hand M61.44- ☑
      lower leg M61.46- ☑
      multiple sites M61.49
      pelvic region M61.45- ☑
      shoulder region M61.41- ☑
      specified site NEC M61.48
      thigh M61.45- ☑
      upper arm M61.42- ☑
  myocardium, myocardial — see Degeneration, myocardial
  ovary N83.8
  pancreas K86.89
  penis N48.89

Calcification — *continued*
  periarticular — *see* Disorder, joint, specified type NEC
  pericardium (*see also* Pericarditis) I31.1
  pineal gland E34.8
  pleura J94.8
    postinfectional J94.8
    tuberculous NEC B90.9
  pulpal (dental) (nodular) K04.2
  sclera H15.89
  spleen D73.89
  subcutaneous L94.2
  suprarenal (capsule) (gland) E27.49
  tendon (sheath) (*see also* Tenosynovitis, specified type NEC)
    with bursitis, synovitis or tenosynovitis — *see* Tendinitis, calcific
  trachea J39.8
  ureter N28.89
  uterus N85.8
  vitreous — *see* Deposit, crystalline
Calcified — *see* Calcification
Calcinosis (interstitial) (tumoral) (universalis) E83.59
  with Raynaud's phenomenon, esophageal dysfunction, sclerodactyly, telangiectasia (CREST syndrome) M34.1
  circumscripta (skin) L94.2
  cutis L94.2
Calciphylaxis (*see also* Calcification, by site) E83.59
Calcium
  deposits — *see* Calcification, by site
  metabolism disorder E83.50
  salts or soaps in vitreous — *see* Deposit, crystalline
Calciuria R82.99
Calculi — *see* Calculus
Calculosis, intrahepatic — *see* Calculus, bile duct
Calculus, calculi, calculous
  ampulla of Vater — *see* Calculus, bile duct
  anuria (impacted) (recurrent) (*see also* Calculus, urinary) N20.9
  appendix K38.1
  bile duct (common) (hepatic) K80.50
    with
      calculus of gallbladder — *see* Calculus, gallbladder and bile duct
      cholangitis K80.30
        with
          cholecystitis — *see* Calculus, bile duct, with cholecystitis
          obstruction K80.31
        acute K80.32
          with
            chronic cholangitis K80.36
              with obstruction K80.37
            obstruction K80.33
        chronic K80.34
          with
            acute cholangitis K80.36
              with obstruction K80.37
            obstruction K80.35
      cholecystitis (with cholangitis) K80.40
        with obstruction K80.41
        acute K80.42
          with
            chronic cholecystitis K80.46
              with obstruction K80.47
            obstruction K80.43
        chronic K80.44
          with
            acute cholecystitis K80.46
              with obstruction K80.47
            obstruction K80.45
  biliary (*see also* Calculus, gallbladder)
    specified NEC K80.80
      with obstruction K80.81
  bilirubin, multiple — *see* Calculus, gallbladder
  bladder (encysted) (impacted) (urinary) (diverticulum) N21.0
  bronchus J98.09
  calyx (kidney) (renal) — *see* Calculus, kidney
  cholesterol (pure) (solitary) — *see* Calculus, gallbladder
  common duct (bile) — *see* Calculus, bile duct
  conjunctiva — *see* Concretion, conjunctiva
  cystic N21.0
    duct — *see* Calculus, gallbladder
  dental (subgingival) (supragingival) K03.6
  diverticulum
    bladder N21.0
    kidney N20.0

Calculus, calculi, calculous — *continued*
  epididymis N50.89
  gallbladder K80.20
    with
      bile duct calculus — *see* Calculus, gallbladder and bile duct
      cholecystitis K80.10
        with obstruction K80.11
        acute K80.00
          with
            chronic cholecystitis K80.12
              with obstruction K80.13
            obstruction K80.01
        chronic K80.10
          with
            acute cholecystitis K80.12
              with obstruction K80.13
            obstruction K80.11
      specified NEC K80.18
        with obstruction K80.19
    obstruction K80.21
  gallbladder and bile duct K80.70
    with
      cholecystitis K80.60
        with obstruction K80.61
        acute K80.62
          with
            chronic cholecystitis K80.66
              with obstruction K80.67
            obstruction K80.63
        chronic K80.64
          with
            acute cholecystitis K80.66
              with obstruction K80.67
            obstruction K80.65
    obstruction K80.71
  hepatic (duct) — *see* Calculus, bile duct
  ileal conduit N21.8
  intestinal (impaction) (obstruction) K56.49
  kidney (impacted) (multiple) (pelvis) (recurrent) (staghorn) N20.0
    with calculus, ureter N20.2
    congenital Q63.8
  lacrimal passages — *see* Dacryolith
  liver (impacted) — *see* Calculus, bile duct
  lung J98.4
  mammographic R92.1
  nephritic (impacted) (recurrent) — *see* Calculus, kidney
  nose J34.89
  pancreas (duct) K86.89
  parotid duct or gland K11.5
  pelvis, encysted — *see* Calculus, kidney
  prostate N42.0
  pulmonary J98.4
  pyelitis (impacted) (recurrent) N20.0
    with hydronephrosis N13.2
  pyelonephritis (impacted) (recurrent) N20 ☑
    with hydronephrosis N13.2
  renal (impacted) (recurrent) — *see* Calculus, kidney
  salivary (duct) (gland) K11.5
  seminal vesicle N50.89
  staghorn — *see* Calculus, kidney
  Stensen's duct K11.5
  stomach K31.89
  sublingual duct or gland K11.5
    congenital Q38.4
  submandibular duct, gland or region K11.5
  submaxillary duct, gland or region K11.5
  suburethral N21.8
  tonsil J35.8
  tooth, teeth (subgingival) (supragingival) K03.6
  tunica vaginalis N50.89
  ureter (impacted) (recurrent) N20.1
    with calculus, kidney N20.2
      with hydronephrosis N13.2
        with infection N13.6
  urethra (impacted) N21.1
  urinary (duct) (impacted) (passage) (tract) N20.9
    with hydronephrosis N13.2
      with infection N13.6
    in (due to)
    lower N21.9
      specified NEC N21.8
  vagina N89.8
  vesical (impacted) N21.0
  Wharton's duct K11.5
  xanthine E79.8 [N22]
Calicectasis N28.89

Caliectasis N28.89
California
  disease B38.9
  encephalitis A83.5
Caligo cornea — *see* Opacity, cornea, central
Callositas, callosity (infected) L84
Callus (infected) L84
  bone — *see* Osteophyte
  excessive, following fracture — *code as* Sequelae of fracture
CALME (childhood asymmetric labium majus enlargement) N90.61
Calorie deficiency or malnutrition (*see also* Malnutrition) E46
Calvé-Perthes disease — *see* Legg-Calvé-Perthes disease
Calvé's disease — *see* Osteochondrosis, juvenile, spine
Calvities — *see* Alopecia, androgenic
Cameroon fever — *see* Malaria
Camptocormia (hysterical) F44.4
Camurati-Engelmann syndrome Q78.3
Canal (*see also* condition)
  atrioventricular common Q21.2
Canaliculitis (lacrimal) (acute) (subacute) H04.33- ☑
  Actinomyces A42.89
  chronic H04.42- ☑
Canavan's disease E75.29
Canceled procedure (surgical) Z53.9
  because of
    contraindication Z53.09
      smoking Z53.01
    left against medical advice (AMA) Z53.21
    patient's decision Z53.20
      for reasons of belief or group pressure Z53.1
      specified reason NEC Z53.29
    specified reason NEC Z53.8
Cancer (*see also* Neoplasm, by site, malignant)
  bile duct type liver C22.1
  blood — *see* Leukemia
  breast (*see also* Neoplasm, breast, malignant) C50.91- ☑
  hepatocellular C22.0
  lung (*see also* Neoplasm, lung, malignant) C34.90
  ovarian (*see also* Neoplasm ovary, malignant) C56.9
  unspecified site (primary) C80.1
Cancer (o)**phobia** F45.29
Cancerous — *see* Neoplasm, malignant, by site
Cancrum oris A69.0
Candidiasis, candidal B37.9
  balanitis B37.42
  bronchitis B37.1
  cheilitis B37.83
  congenital P37.5
  cystitis B37.41
  disseminated B37.7
  endocarditis B37.6
  enteritis B37.82
  esophagitis B37.81
  intertrigo B37.2
  lung B37.1
  meningitis B37.5
  mouth B37.0
  nails B37.2
  neonatal P37.5
  onychia B37.2
  oral B37.0
  osteomyelitis B37.89
  otitis externa B37.84
  paronychia B37.2
  perionyxis B37.2
  pneumonia B37.1
  proctitis B37.82
  pulmonary B37.1
  pyelonephritis B37.49
  sepsis B37.7
  skin B37.2
  specified site NEC B37.89
  stomatitis B37.0
  systemic B37.7
  urethritis B37.41
  urogenital site NEC B37.49
  vagina B37.3
  vulva B37.3
  vulvovaginitis B37.3
Candidid L30.2
Candidosis — *see* Candidiasis
Candiru infection or infestation B88.8
Canities (premature) L67.1

⚐ Subterms under main terms may continue to next column or page   ☑ Additional Character Required — Refer to the Tabular List for Character Selection   47

Calcification — Canities

Canities — *continued*
congenital Q84.2
Canker (mouth) (sore) K12.0
rash A38.9
Cannabinosis J66.2
Cannabis induced
anxiety disorder F12.980
psychotic disorder F12.959
sleep disorder F12.988
Canton fever A75.9
Cantrell's syndrome Q87.89
Capillariasis (intestinal) B81.1
hepatic B83.8
Capillary — *see* condition
Caplan's syndrome — *see* Rheumatoid, lung
Capsule — *see* condition
Capsulitis (joint) (*see also* Enthesopathy)
adhesive (shoulder) M75.0- ☑
hepatic K65.8
labyrinthine — *see* Otosclerosis, specified NEC
thyroid E06.9
Caput
crepitus Q75.8
medusae I86.8
succedaneum P12.81
Car sickness T75.3 ☑
Carapata (disease) A68.0
Carate — *see* Pinta
Carbon lung J60
Carbuncle L02.93
abdominal wall L02.231
anus K61.0
auditory canal, external — *see* Abscess, ear, external
auricle ear — *see* Abscess, ear, external
axilla L02.43- ☑
back (any part) L02.232
breast N61.1
buttock L02.33
cheek (external) L02.03
chest wall L02.233
chin L02.03
corpus cavernosum N48.21
ear (any part) (external) (middle) — *see* Abscess, ear, external
external auditory canal — *see* Abscess, ear, external
eyelid — *see* Abscess, eyelid
face NEC L02.03
femoral (region) — *see* Carbuncle, lower limb
finger — *see* Carbuncle, hand
flank L02.231
foot L02.63- ☑
forehead L02.03
genital — *see* Abscess, genital
gluteal (region) L02.33
groin L02.234
hand L02.53- ☑
head NEC L02.831
heel — *see* Carbuncle, foot
hip — *see* Carbuncle, lower limb
kidney — *see* Abscess, kidney
knee — *see* Carbuncle, lower limb
labium (majus) (minus) N76.4
lacrimal
gland — *see* Dacryoadenitis
passages (duct) (sac) — *see* Inflammation, lacrimal, passages, acute
leg — *see* Carbuncle, lower limb
lower limb L02.43- ☑
malignant A22.0
navel L02.236
neck L02.13
nose (external) (septum) J34.0
orbit, orbital — *see* Abscess, orbit
palmar (space) — *see* Carbuncle, hand
partes posteriores L02.33
pectoral region L02.233
penis N48.21
perineum L02.235
pinna — *see* Abscess, ear, external
popliteal — *see* Carbuncle, lower limb
scalp L02.831
seminal vesicle N49.0
shoulder — *see* Carbuncle, upper limb
specified site NEC L02.838
temple (region) L02.03
thumb — *see* Carbuncle, hand
toe — *see* Carbuncle, foot

Carbuncle — *continued*
trunk L02.239
abdominal wall L02.231
back L02.232
chest wall L02.233
groin L02.234
perineum L02.235
umbilicus L02.236
umbilicus L02.236
upper limb L02.43- ☑
urethra N34.0
vulva N76.4
Carbunculus — *see* Carbuncle
Carcinoid (tumor) — *see* Tumor, carcinoid
Carcinoidosis E34.0
Carcinoma (malignant) (*see also* Neoplasm, by site, malignant)
acidophil
specified site — *see* Neoplasm, malignant, by site
unspecified site C75.1
acidophil-basophil, mixed
specified site — *see* Neoplasm, malignant, by site
unspecified site C75.1
adnexal (skin) — *see* Neoplasm, skin, malignant
adrenal cortical C74.0- ☑
alveolar — *see* Neoplasm, lung, malignant
cell — *see* Neoplasm, lung, malignant
ameloblastic C41.1
upper jaw (bone) C41.0
apocrine
breast — *see* Neoplasm, breast, malignant
specified site NEC — *see* Neoplasm, skin, malignant
unspecified site C44.99
basal cell (pigmented) (*see also* Neoplasm, skin, malignant) C44.91
fibro-epithelial — *see* Neoplasm, skin, malignant
morphea — *see* Neoplasm, skin, malignant
multicentric — *see* Neoplasm, skin, malignant
basaloid
basal-squamous cell, mixed — *see* Neoplasm, skin, malignant
basophil
specified site — *see* Neoplasm, malignant, by site
unspecified site C75.1
basophil-acidophil, mixed
specified site — *see* Neoplasm, malignant, by site
unspecified site C75.1
basosquamous — *see* Neoplasm, skin, malignant
bile duct
with hepatocellular, mixed C22.0
liver C22.1
specified site NEC — *see* Neoplasm, malignant, by site
unspecified site C22.1
branchial or branchiogenic C10.4
bronchial or bronchogenic — *see* Neoplasm, lung, malignant
bronchiolar — *see* Neoplasm, lung, malignant
bronchioloalveolar — *see* Neoplasm, lung, malignant
C cell
specified site — *see* Neoplasm, malignant, by site
unspecified site C73
ceruminous C44.29- ☑
cervix uteri
in situ D06.9
endocervix D06.0
exocervix D06.1
specified site NEC D06.7
chorionic
specified site — *see* Neoplasm, malignant, by site
unspecified site
female C58
male C62.90
chromophobe
specified site — *see* Neoplasm, malignant, by site
unspecified site C75.1
cloacogenic
specified site — *see* Neoplasm, malignant, by site
unspecified site C21.2
diffuse type
specified site — *see* Neoplasm, malignant, by site
unspecified site C16.9
duct (cell)
with Paget's disease — *see* Neoplasm, breast, malignant

Carcinoma — *continued*
duct — *continued*
infiltrating
with lobular carcinoma (in situ)
specified site — *see* Neoplasm, malignant, by site
unspecified site (female) C50.91- ☑
male C50.92- ☑
specified site — *see* Neoplasm, malignant, by site
unspecified site (female) C50.91- ☑
male C50.92- ☑
ductal
with lobular
specified site — *see* Neoplasm, malignant, by site
unspecified site (female) C50.91- ☑
male C50.92- ☑
ductular, infiltrating
specified site — *see* Neoplasm, malignant, by site
unspecified site (female) C50.91- ☑
male C50.92- ☑
embryonal
liver C22.7
endometrioid
specified site — *see* Neoplasm, malignant, by site
unspecified site
female C56.9
male C61
eosinophil
specified site — *see* Neoplasm, malignant, by site
unspecified site C75.1
epidermoid (*see also* Neoplasm, skin, malignant)
in situ, Bowen's type — *see* Neoplasm, skin, in situ
fibroepithelial, basal cell — *see* Neoplasm, skin, malignant
follicular
with papillary (mixed) C73
moderately differentiated C73
pure follicle C73
specified site — *see* Neoplasm, malignant, by site
trabecular C73
unspecified site C73
well differentiated C73
generalized, with unspecified primary site C80.0
glycogen-rich — *see* Neoplasm, breast, malignant
granulosa cell C56- ☑
hepatic cell C22.0
hepatocellular C22.0
with bile duct, mixed C22.0
fibrolamellar C22.0
hepatocholangiolitic C22.0
Hurthle cell C73
in
adenomatous
polyposis coli C18.9
pleomorphic adenoma — *see* Neoplasm, salivary glands, malignant
situ — *see* Carcinoma-in-situ
infiltrating
duct
with lobular
specified site — *see* Neoplasm, malignant, by site
unspecified site (female) C50.91- ☑
male C50.92- ☑
with Paget's disease — *see* Neoplasm, breast, malignant
specified site — *see* Neoplasm, malignant
unspecified site (female) C50.91- ☑
male C50.92- ☑
ductular
specified site — *see* Neoplasm, malignant
unspecified site (female) C50.91- ☑
male C50.92- ☑
lobular
specified site — *see* Neoplasm, malignant
unspecified site (female) C50.91- ☑
male C50.92- ☑
inflammatory
specified site — *see* Neoplasm, malignant
unspecified site (female) C50.91- ☑
male C50.92- ☑
intestinal type
specified site — *see* Neoplasm, malignant, by site
unspecified site C16.9

Canities — Carcinoma

48

☑ **Additional Character Required** — Refer to the Tabular List for Character Selection   ⬇ **Subterms under main terms may continue to next column or page**

Carcinoma — *continued*
  intracystic
    noninfiltrating — *see* Neoplasm, in situ, by site
  intraductal (noninfiltrating)
    with Paget's disease — *see* Neoplasm, breast, malignant
    breast D05.1- ☑
    papillary
      with invasion
        specified site — *see* Neoplasm, malignant, by site
        unspecified site (female) C50.91- ☑
          male C50.92- ☑
      breast D05.1- ☑
      specified site NEC — *see* Neoplasm, in situ, by site
      unspecified site (female) D05.1- ☑
    specified site NEC — *see* Neoplasm, in situ, by site
    unspecified site (female) D05.1- ☑
  intraepidermal — *see* Neoplasm, in situ
    squamous cell, Bowen's type — *see* Neoplasm, skin, in situ
  intraepithelial — *see* Neoplasm, in situ, by site
    squamous cell — *see* Neoplasm, in situ, by site
  intraosseous C41.1
    upper jaw (bone) C41.0
  islet cell
    with exocrine, mixed
      specified site — *see* Neoplasm, malignant, by site
      unspecified site C25.9
    pancreas C25.4
    specified site NEC — *see* Neoplasm, malignant, by site
    unspecified site C25.4
  juvenile, breast — *see* Neoplasm, breast, malignant
  large cell
    small cell
      specified site — *see* Neoplasm, malignant, by site
      unspecified site C34.90
  Leydig cell (testis)
    specified site — *see* Neoplasm, malignant, by site
    unspecified site
      female C56.9
      male C62.90
  lipid-rich (female) C50.91- ☑
    male C50.92- ☑
  liver cell C22.0
  liver NEC C22.7
  lobular (infiltrating)
    with intraductal
      specified site — *see* Neoplasm, malignant, by site
      unspecified site (female) C50.91- ☑
        male C50.92- ☑
    noninfiltrating
      breast D05.0- ☑
      specified site NEC — *see* Neoplasm, in situ, by site
      unspecified site D05.0- ☑
    specified site — *see* Neoplasm, malignant, by site
    unspecified site (female) C50.91- ☑
      male C50.92- ☑
  medullary
    with
      amyloid stroma
        specified site — *see* Neoplasm, malignant, by site
        unspecified site C73
      lymphoid stroma
        specified site — *see* Neoplasm, malignant, by site
        unspecified site (female) C50.91- ☑
          male C50.92- ☑
  Merkel cell C4A.9 (*following* C43)
    anal margin C4A.51 (*following* C43)
    anal skin C4A.51 (*following* C43)
    canthus C4A.1- ☑ (*following* C43)
    ear and external auricular canal C4A.2- ☑ (*following* C43)
    external auricular canal C4A.2- ☑ (*following* C43)
    eyelid, including canthus C4A.1- ☑ (*following* C43)
    face C4A.30 (*following* C43)
      specified NEC C4A.39 (*following* C43)
    hip C4A.7- ☑ (*following* C43)
    lip C4A.0 (*following* C43)

Carcinoma — *continued*
  Merkel cell — *continued*
    lower limb, including hip C4A.7- ☑ (*following* C43)
    neck C4A.4 (*following* C43)
    nodal presentation C7B.1 (*following* C75)
    nose C4A.31 (*following* C43)
    overlapping sites C4A.8 (*following* C43)
    perianal skin C4A.51 (*following* C43)
    scalp C4A.4 (*following* C43)
    secondary C7B.1 (*following* C75)
    shoulder C4A.6- ☑ (*following* C43)
    skin of breast C4A.52 (*following* C43)
    trunk NEC C4A.59 (*following* C43)
    upper limb, including shoulder C4A.6- ☑ (*following* C43)
    visceral metastatic C7B.1 (*following* C75)
  metastatic — *see* Neoplasm, secondary, by site
  metatypical — *see* Neoplasm, skin, malignant
  morphea, basal cell — *see* Neoplasm, skin, malignant
  mucoid
    cell
      specified site — *see* Neoplasm, malignant, by site
      unspecified site C75.1
  neuroendocrine (*see also* Tumor, neuroendocrine)
    high grade, any site C7A.1 (*following* C75)
    poorly differentiated, any site C7A.1 (*following* C75)
  nonencapsulated sclerosing C73
  noninfiltrating
    intracystic — *see* Neoplasm, in situ, by site
    intraductal
      breast D05.1- ☑
      papillary
        breast D05.1- ☑
        specified site NEC — *see* Neoplasm, in situ, by site
        unspecified site D05.1- ☑
      specified site — *see* Neoplasm, in situ, by site
      unspecified site D05.1- ☑
    lobular
      breast D05.0- ☑
      specified site NEC — *see* Neoplasm, in situ, by site
      unspecified site (female) D05.0- ☑
  oat cell
    specified site — *see* Neoplasm, malignant, by site
    unspecified site C34.90
  odontogenic C41.1
    upper jaw (bone) C41.0
  papillary
    with follicular (mixed) C73
    follicular variant C73
    intraductal (noninfiltrating)
      with invasion
        specified site — *see* Neoplasm, malignant, by site
        unspecified site (female) C50.91- ☑
          male C50.92- ☑
      breast D05.1- ☑
      specified site NEC — *see* Neoplasm, in situ, by site
      unspecified site D05.1- ☑
    serous
      specified site — *see* Neoplasm, malignant, by site
    surface
      specified site — *see* Neoplasm, malignant, by site
      unspecified site C56.9
    unspecified site C56.9
  papillocystic
    specified site — *see* Neoplasm, malignant, by site
    unspecified site C56.9
  parafollicular cell
    specified site — *see* Neoplasm, malignant, by site
    unspecified site C73
  pilomatrix — *see* Neoplasm, skin, malignant
  pseudomucinous
    specified site — *see* Neoplasm, malignant, by site
    unspecified site C56.9
  renal cell C64- ☑
  Schmincke — *see* Neoplasm, nasopharynx, malignant
  Schneiderian
    specified site — *see* Neoplasm, malignant, by site
    unspecified site C30.0
  sebaceous — *see* Neoplasm, skin, malignant

Carcinoma — *continued*
  secondary (*see also* Neoplasm, secondary, by site)
    Merkel cell C7B.1 (*following* C75)
  secretory, breast — *see* Neoplasm, breast, malignant
  serous
    papillary
      specified site — *see* Neoplasm, malignant, by site
      unspecified site C56.9
    surface, papillary
      specified site — *see* Neoplasm, malignant, by site
      unspecified site C56.9
  Sertoli cell
    specified site — *see* Neoplasm, malignant, by site
    unspecified site C62.90
      female C56.9
      male C62.90
  skin appendage — *see* Neoplasm, skin, malignant
  small cell
    fusiform cell
      specified site — *see* Neoplasm, malignant, by site
      unspecified site C34.90
    intermediate cell
      specified site — *see* Neoplasm, malignant, by site
      unspecified site C34.90
    large cell
      specified site — *see* Neoplasm, malignant, by site
      unspecified site C34.90
  solid
    with amyloid stroma
      specified site — *see* Neoplasm, malignant, by site
      unspecified site C73
    microinvasive
      specified site — *see* Neoplasm, malignant, by site
      unspecified site C53.9
  sweat gland — *see* Neoplasm, skin, malignant
  theca cell C56.- ☑
  thymic C37
    unspecified site (primary) C80.1
  water-clear cell C75.0
Carcinoma-in-situ (*see also* Neoplasm, in situ, by site)
  breast NOS D05.9- ☑
    specified type NEC D05.8- ☑
  epidermoid (*see also* Neoplasm, in situ, by site)
    with questionable stromal invasion
      cervix D06.9
      specified site NEC — *see* Neoplasm, in situ, by site
      unspecified site D06.9
    Bowen's type — *see* Neoplasm, skin, in situ
  intraductal
    breast D05.1- ☑
    specified site NEC — *see* Neoplasm, in situ, by site
    unspecified site D05.1- ☑
  lobular
    with
      infiltrating duct
        breast (female) C50.91- ☑
          male C50.92- ☑
        specified site NEC — *see* Neoplasm, malignant
        unspecified site (female) C50.91- ☑
          male C50.92- ☑
      intraductal
        breast D05.8- ☑
        specified site NEC — *see* Neoplasm, in situ, by site
        unspecified site (female) D05.8- ☑
    breast D05.0- ☑
    specified site NEC — *see* Neoplasm, in situ, by site
    unspecified site D05.0- ☑
  squamous cell (*see also* Neoplasm, in situ, by site)
    with questionable stromal invasion
      cervix D06.9
      specified site NEC — *see* Neoplasm, in situ, by site
      unspecified site D06.9
Carcinomaphobia F45.29
Carcinomatosis C80.0
  peritonei C78.6

Carcinomatosis — *continued*
  unspecified site (primary) (secondary) C80.0
Carcinosarcoma — *see* Neoplasm, malignant, by site
  embryonal — *see* Neoplasm, malignant, by site
Cardia, cardial — *see* condition
Cardiac (*see also* condition)
  death, sudden — *see* Arrest, cardiac
  pacemaker
    in situ Z95.0
    management or adjustment Z45.018
  tamponade I31.4
Cardialgia — *see* Pain, precordial
Cardiectasis — *see* Hypertrophy, cardiac
Cardiochalasia K21.9
Cardiomalacia I51.5
Cardiomegalia glycogenica diffusa E74.02 [I43]
Cardiomegaly (*see also* Hypertrophy, cardiac)
  congenital Q24.8
  glycogen E74.02 [I43]
  idiopathic I51.7
Cardiomyolipsis I51.5
Cardiomyopathy (familial) (idiopathic) I42.9
  alcoholic I42.6
  amyloid E85.4 [I43]
    transthyretin-related (ATTR) familial E85.4
  arteriosclerotic — *see* Disease, heart, ischemic, atherosclerotic
  beriberi E51.12
  cobalt-beer I42.6
  congenital I42.4
  congestive I42.0
  constrictive NOS I42.5
  dilated I42.0
  due to
    alcohol I42.6
    beriberi E51.12
    cardiac glycogenosis E74.02 [I43]
    drugs I42.7
    external agents NEC I42.7
    Friedreich's ataxia G11.1
    myotonia atrophica G71.11 [I43]
    progressive muscular dystrophy G71.0 [I43]
  glycogen storage E74.02 [I43]
  hypertensive — *see* Hypertension, heart
  hypertrophic (nonobstructive) I42.2
    obstructive I42.1
      congenital Q24.8
  in
    Chagas' disease (chronic) B57.2
      acute B57.0
    sarcoidosis D86.85
  ischemic I25.5
  metabolic E88.9 [I43]
    thyrotoxic E05.90 [I43]
      with thyroid storm E05.91 [I43]
  newborn I42.8
    congenital I42.4
  nutritional E63.9 [I43]
    beriberi E51.12
  obscure of Africa I42.8
  peripartum O90.3
  postpartum O90.3
  restrictive NEC I42.5
  rheumatic I09.0
  secondary I42.9
  stress induced I51.81
  takotsubo I51.81
  thyrotoxic E05.90 [I43]
    with thyroid storm E05.91 [I43]
  toxic NEC I42.7
  transthyretin-related (ATTR) familial amyloid E85.4
  tuberculous A18.84
  viral B33.24
Cardionephritis — *see* Hypertension, cardiorenal
Cardionephropathy — *see* Hypertension, cardiorenal
Cardionephrosis — *see* Hypertension, cardiorenal
Cardiopathia nigra I27.0
Cardiopathy (*see also* Disease, heart) I51.9
  idiopathic I42.9
  mucopolysaccharidosis E76.3 [I52]
Cardiopericarditis — *see* Pericarditis
Cardiophobia F45.29
Cardiorenal — *see* condition
Cardiorrhexis — *see* Infarct, myocardium
Cardiosclerosis — *see* Disease, heart, ischemic, atherosclerotic
Cardiosis — *see* Disease, heart
Cardiospasm (esophagus) (reflex) (stomach) K22.0

Cardiospasm — *continued*
  congenital Q39.5
    with megaesophagus Q39.5
Cardiostenosis — *see* Disease, heart
Cardiosymphysis I31.0
Cardiovascular — *see* condition
Carditis (acute) (bacterial) (chronic) (subacute) I51.89
  meningococcal A39.50
  rheumatic — *see* Disease, heart, rheumatic
  rheumatoid — *see* Rheumatoid, carditis
  viral B33.20
Care (of) (for) (following)
  child (routine) Z76.2
  family member (handicapped) (sick)
    creating problem for family Z63.6
    provided away from home for holiday relief Z75.5
    unavailable, due to
      absence (person rendering care) (sufferer) Z74.2
      inability (any reason) of person rendering care Z74.2
  foundling Z76.1
  holiday relief Z75.5
  improper — *see* Maltreatment
  lack of (at or after birth) (infant) — *see* Maltreatment, child, neglect
  lactating mother Z39.1
  palliative Z51.5
  postpartum
    immediately after delivery Z39.0
    routine follow-up Z39.2
  respite Z75.5
  unavailable, due to
    absence of person rendering care Z74.2
    inability (any reason) of person rendering care Z74.2
  well-baby Z76.2
Caries
  bone NEC A18.03
  dental (dentino enamel junction) (early childhood) (of dentine) (pre-eruptive) (recurrent) (to the pulp) K02.9
    arrested (coronal) (root) K02.3
    chewing surface
      limited to enamel K02.51
      penetrating into dentin K02.52
      penetrating into pulp K02.53
    coronal surface
      chewing surface
        limited to enamel K02.51
        penetrating into dentin K02.52
        penetrating into pulp K02.53
      pit and fissure surface
        limited to enamel K02.51
        penetrating into dentin K02.52
        penetrating into pulp K02.53
      smooth surface
        limited to enamel K02.61
        penetrating into dentin K02.62
        penetrating into pulp K02.63
    pit and fissure surface
      limited to enamel K02.51
      penetrating into dentin K02.52
      penetrating into pulp K02.53
    primary, cervical origin K02.52
    root K02.7
    smooth surface
      limited to enamel K02.61
      penetrating into dentin K02.62
      penetrating into pulp K02.63
  external meatus — *see* Disorder, ear, external, specified type NEC
  hip (tuberculous) A18.02
  initial (tooth)
    chewing surface K02.51
    pit and fissure surface K02.51
    smooth surface K02.61
  knee (tuberculous) A18.02
  labyrinth H83.8 ☑
  limb NEC (tuberculous) A18.03
  mastoid process (chronic) — *see* Mastoiditis, chronic
    tuberculous A18.03
  middle ear H74.8 ☑
  nose (tuberculous) A18.03
  orbit (tuberculous) A18.03
  ossicles, ear — *see* Abnormal, ear ossicles
  petrous bone — *see* Petrositis
  root (dental) (tooth) K02.7
  sacrum (tuberculous) A18.01

Caries — *continued*
  spine, spinal (column) (tuberculous) A18.01
  syphilitic A52.77
    congenital (early) A50.02 [M90.80]
  tooth, teeth — *see* Caries, dental
  tuberculous A18.03
  vertebra (column) (tuberculous) A18.01
Carious teeth — *see* Caries, dental
Carneous mole O02.0
Carnitine insufficiency E71.40
Carotid body or sinus syndrome G90.01
Carotidynia G90.01
Carotinemia (dietary) E67.1
Carotinosis (cutis) (skin) E67.1
Carpal tunnel syndrome — *see* Syndrome, carpal tunnel
Carpenter's syndrome Q87.0
Carpopedal spasm — *see* Tetany
Carr-Barr-Plunkett syndrome Q97.1
Carrier (suspected) of
  amebiasis Z22.1
  bacterial disease NEC Z22.39
    diphtheria Z22.2
    intestinal infectious NEC Z22.1
      typhoid Z22.0
    meningococcal Z22.31
    sexually transmitted Z22.4
    specified NEC Z22.39
    staphylococcal (Methicillin susceptible) Z22.321
      Methicillin resistant Z22.322
    streptococcal Z22.338
      group B Z22.330
        complicating pregnancy or delivery O99.82- ☑
  typhoid Z22.0
  cholera Z22.1
  diphtheria Z22.2
  gastrointestinal pathogens NEC Z22.1
  genetic Z14.8
    cystic fibrosis Z14.1
    hemophilia A (asymptomatic) Z14.01
      symptomatic Z14.02
  gestational, pregnant Z33.1
  gonorrhea Z22.4
  HAA (hepatitis Australian-antigen) B18.8
  HB (c)(s)-AG B18.1
  hepatitis (viral) B18.9
    Australia-antigen (HAA) B18.8
    B surface antigen (HBsAg) B18.1
      with acute delta- (super)infection B17.0
    C B18.2
    specified NEC B18.8
  human T-cell lymphotropic virus type-1 (HTLV-1) infection Z22.6
  infectious organism Z22.9
    specified NEC Z22.8
  meningococci Z22.31
  Salmonella typhosa Z22.0
  serum hepatitis — *see* Carrier, hepatitis
  staphylococci (Methicillin susceptible) Z22.321
    Methicillin resistant Z22.322
  streptococci Z22.338
    group B Z22.330
      complicating pregnancy or delivery O99.82- ☑
  syphilis Z22.4
  typhoid Z22.0
  venereal disease NEC Z22.4
Carrion's disease A44.0
Carter's relapsing fever (Asiatic) A68.1
Cartilage — *see* condition
Caruncle (inflamed)
  conjunctiva (acute) — *see* Conjunctivitis, acute
  labium (majus) (minus) N90.89
  lacrimal — *see* Inflammation, lacrimal, passages
  myrtiform N89.8
  urethral (benign) N36.2
Cascade stomach K31.2
Caseation lymphatic gland (tuberculous) A18.2
Cassidy (-Scholte) syndrome (malignant carcinoid) E34.0
Castellani's disease A69.8
Castration, traumatic, male S38.231 ☑
Casts in urine R82.99
Cat
  cry syndrome Q93.4
  ear Q17.3
  eye syndrome Q92.8
Catabolism, senile R54
Catalepsy (hysterical) F44.2
  schizophrenic F20.2

☑ **Additional Character Required** — Refer to the Tabular List for Character Selection   ⬚ Subterms under main terms may continue to next column or page

Cataplexy (idiopathic) — *see* Narcolepsy
Cataract (cortical) (immature) (incipient) H26.9
  with
    neovascularization — *see* Cataract, complicated
  age-related — *see* Cataract, senile
  anterior
    and posterior axial embryonal Q12.0
    pyramidal Q12.0
  associated with
    galactosemia E74.21 [H28]
    myotonic disorders G71.19 [H28]
  blue Q12.0
  central Q12.0
  cerulean Q12.0
  complicated H26.20
    with
      neovascularization H26.21- ☑
      ocular disorder H26.22- ☑
    glaucomatous flecks H26.23- ☑
  congenital Q12.0
  coraliform Q12.0
  coronary Q12.0
  crystalline Q12.0
  diabetic — *see* Diabetes, cataract
  drug-induced H26.3- ☑
  due to
    ocular disorder — *see* Cataract, complicated
    radiation H26.8
  electric H26.8
  extraction status Z98.4- ☑
  glass-blower's H26.8
  heat ray H26.8
  heterochromic — *see* Cataract, complicated
  hypermature — *see* Cataract, senile, morgagnian type
  in (due to)
    chronic iridocyclitis — *see* Cataract, complicated
    diabetes — *see* Diabetes, cataract
    endocrine disease E34.9 [H28]
    eye disease — *see* Cataract, complicated
    hypoparathyroidism E20.9 [H28]
    malnutrition-dehydration E46 [H28]
    metabolic disease E88.9 [H28]
    myotonic disorders G71.19 [H28]
    nutritional disease E63.9 [H28]
  infantile — *see* Cataract, presenile
  irradiational — *see* Cataract, specified NEC
  juvenile — *see* Cataract, presenile
  malnutrition-dehydration E46 [H28]
  morgagnian — *see* Cataract, senile, morgagnian type
  myotonic G71.19 [H28]
  myxedema E03.9 [H28]
  nuclear
    embryonal Q12.0
    sclerosis — *see* Cataract, senile, nuclear
  presenile H26.00- ☑
    combined forms H26.06- ☑
    cortical H26.01- ☑
    lamellar — *see* Cataract, presenile, cortical
    nuclear H26.03- ☑
    specified NEC H26.09
    subcapsular polar (anterior) H26.04- ☑
      posterior H26.05- ☑
    zonular — *see* Cataract, presenile, cortical
  secondary H26.40
    Soemmering's ring H26.41- ☑
    specified NEC H26.49- ☑
    to eye disease — *see* Cataract, complicated
  senile H25.9
    brunescens — *see* Cataract, senile, nuclear
    combined forms H25.81- ☑
    coronary — *see* Cataract, senile, incipient
    cortical H25.01- ☑
    hypermature — *see* Cataract, senile, morgagnian
      type
    incipient (mature) (total) H25.09- ☑
      cortical — *see* Cataract, senile, cortical
      subcapsular — *see* Cataract, senile, subcapsular
    morgagnian type (hypermature) H25.2- ☑
    nuclear (sclerosis) H25.1- ☑
    polar subcapsular (anterior) (posterior) — *see*
      Cataract, senile, incipient
    punctate — *see* Cataract, senile, incipient
    specified NEC H25.89
    subcapsular polar (anterior) H25.03- ☑
      posterior H25.04- ☑
  snowflake — *see* Diabetes, cataract
  specified NEC H26.8

Cataract — *continued*
  toxic — *see* Cataract, drug-induced
  traumatic H26.10- ☑
    localized H26.11- ☑
    partially resolved H26.12- ☑
    total H26.13- ☑
  zonular (perinuclear) Q12.0
Cataracta (*see also* Cataract)
  brunescens — *see* Cataract, senile, nuclear
  centralis pulverulenta Q12.0
  cerulea Q12.0
  complicata — *see* Cataract, complicated
  congenita Q12.0
  coralliformis Q12.0
  coronaria Q12.0
  diabetic — *see* Diabetes, cataract
  membranacea
    accreta — *see* Cataract, secondary
    congenita Q12.0
  nigra — *see* Cataract, senile, nuclear
  sunflower — *see* Cataract, complicated
Catarrh, catarrhal (acute) (febrile) (infectious) (inflammation) (*see also* condition) J00
  bronchial — *see* Bronchitis
  chest — *see* Bronchitis
  chronic J31.0
  due to congenital syphilis A50.03
  enteric — *see* Enteritis
  eustachian H68.009
  fauces — *see* Pharyngitis
  gastrointestinal — *see* Enteritis
  gingivitis K05.00
    nonplaque induced K05.01
    plaque induced K05.00
  hay — *see* Fever, hay
  intestinal — *see* Enteritis
  larynx, chronic J37.0
  liver B15.9
    with hepatic coma B15.0
  lung — *see* Bronchitis
  middle ear, chronic — *see* Otitis, media, nonsuppura-
    tive, chronic, serous
  mouth K12.1
  nasal (chronic) — *see* Rhinitis
  nasobronchial J31.1
  nasopharyngeal (chronic) J31.1
    acute J00
  pulmonary — *see* Bronchitis
  spring (eye) (vernal) — *see* Conjunctivitis, acute, atopic
  summer (hay) — *see* Fever, hay
  throat J31.2
  tubotympanal (*see also* Otitis, media, nonsuppurative)
    chronic — *see* Otitis, media, nonsuppurative,
      chronic, serous
Catatonia (schizophrenic) F20.2
Catatonic
  disorder due to known physiologic condition F06.1
  schizophrenia F20.2
  stupor R40.1
Cat-scratch (*see also* Abrasion)
  disease or fever A28.1
Cauda equina — *see* condition
Cauliflower ear M95.1- ☑
Causalgia (upper limb) G56.4- ☑
  lower limb G57.7- ☑
Cause
  external, general effects T75.89 ☑
Caustic burn — *see* Corrosion, by site
Cavare's disease (familial periodic paralysis) G72.3
Cave-in, injury
  crushing (severe) — *see* Crush
  suffocation — *see* Asphyxia, traumatic, due to low
    oxygen, due to cave-in
Cavernitis (penis) N48.29
Cavernositis N48.29
Cavernous — *see* condition
Cavitation of lung (*see also* Tuberculosis, pulmonary)
  nontuberculous J98.4
Cavities, dental — *see* Caries, dental
Cavity
  lung — *see* Cavitation of lung
  optic papilla Q14.2
  pulmonary — *see* Cavitation of lung
Cavovarus foot, congenital Q66.1
Cavus foot (congenital) Q66.7
  acquired — *see* Deformity, limb, foot, specified NEC
Cazenave's disease L10.2

Cecitis K52.9
  with perforation, peritonitis, or rupture K65.8
Cecum — *see* condition
Celiac
  artery compression syndrome I77.4
  disease (with steatorrhea) K90.0
  infantilism K90.0
Cell(s), **cellular** (*see also* condition)
  in urine R82.99
Cellulitis (diffuse) (phlegmonous) (septic) (suppurative)
  L03.90
  abdominal wall L03.311
  anaerobic A48.0
  ankle — *see* Cellulitis, lower limb
  anus K61.0
  arm — *see* Cellulitis, upper limb
  auricle (ear) — *see* Cellulitis, ear
  axilla L03.11- ☑
  back (any part) L03.312
  breast (acute) (nonpuerperal) (subacute) N61.0
    nipple N61.0
  broad ligament
    acute N73.0
  buttock L03.317
  cervical (meaning neck) L03.221
  cervix (uteri) — *see* Cervicitis
  cheek (external) L03.211
    internal K12.2
  chest wall L03.313
  chronic L03.90
  clostridial A48.0
  corpus cavernosum N48.22
  digit
    finger — *see* Cellulitis, finger
    toe — *see* Cellulitis, toe
  Douglas' cul-de-sac or pouch
    acute N73.0
  drainage site (following operation) T81.4 ☑
  ear (external) H60.1- ☑
  eosinophilic (granulomatous) L98.3
  erysipelatous — *see* Erysipelas
  external auditory canal — *see* Cellulitis, ear
  eyelid — *see* Abscess, eyelid
  face NEC L03.211
  finger (intrathecal) (periosteal) (subcutaneous) (subcu-
    ticular) L03.01- ☑
  foot — *see* Cellulitis, lower limb
  gangrenous — *see* Gangrene
  genital organ NEC
    female (external) N76.4
    male N49.9
      multiple sites N49.8
      specified NEC N49.8
  gluteal (region) L03.317
  gonococcal A54.89
  groin L03.314
  hand — *see* Cellulitis, upper limb
  head NEC L03.811
    face (any part, except ear, eye and nose) L03.211
  heel — *see* Cellulitis, lower limb
  hip — *see* Cellulitis, lower limb
  jaw (region) L03.211
  knee — *see* Cellulitis, lower limb
  labium (majus) (minus) — *see* Vulvitis
  lacrimal passages — *see* Inflammation, lacrimal, pas-
    sages
  larynx J38.7
  leg — *see* Cellulitis, lower limb
  lip K13.0
  lower limb L03.11- ☑
    toe — *see* Cellulitis, toe
  mouth (floor) K12.2
  multiple sites, so stated L03.90
  nasopharynx J39.1
  navel L03.316
    newborn P38.9
      with mild hemorrhage P38.1
      without hemorrhage P38.9
  neck (region) L03.221
  nipple (acute) (nonpuerperal) (subacute) N61.0
  nose (septum) (external) J34.0
  orbit, orbital H05.01- ☑
  palate (soft) K12.2
  pectoral (region) L03.313
  pelvis, pelvic (chronic)
    female (*see also* Disease, pelvis, inflammatory)
      N73.2
      acute N73.0

Cellulitis — *continued*
  pelvis, pelvic — *continued*
    following ectopic or molar pregnancy O08.0
      male K65.0
  penis N48.22
  perineal, perineum L03.315
  periorbital L03.213
  perirectal K61.1
  peritonsillar J36
  periurethral N34.0
  periuterine (*see also* Disease, pelvis, inflammatory) N73.2
    acute N73.0
  pharynx J39.1
  preseptal L03.213
  rectum K61.1
  retroperitoneal K68.9
  round ligament
    acute N73.0
  scalp (any part) L03.811
  scrotum N49.2
  seminal vesicle N49.0
  shoulder — *see* Cellulitis, upper limb
  specified site NEC L03.818
  submandibular (region) (space) (triangle) K12.2
    gland K11.3
  submaxillary (region) K12.2
    gland K11.3
  thigh — *see* Cellulitis, lower limb
  thumb (intrathecal) (periosteal) (subcutaneous) (subcuticular) — *see* Cellulitis, finger
  toe (intrathecal) (periosteal) (subcutaneous) (subcuticular) L03.03- ☑
  tonsil J36
  trunk L03.319
    abdominal wall L03.311
    back (any part) L03.312
    buttock L03.317
    chest wall L03.313
    groin L03.314
    perineal, perineum L03.315
    umbilicus L03.316
  tuberculous (primary) A18.4
  umbilicus L03.316
  upper limb L03.11- ☑
    axilla — *see* Cellulitis, axilla
    finger — *see* Cellulitis, finger
    thumb — *see* Cellulitis, finger
  vaccinal T88.0 ☑
  vocal cord J38.3
  vulva — *see* Vulvitis
  wrist — *see* Cellulitis, upper limb
Cementoblastoma, benign — *see* Cyst, calcifying odontogenic
Cementoma — *see* Cyst, calcifying odontogenic
Cementoperiostitis — *see* Periodontitis
Cementosis K03.4
Central auditory processing disorder H93.25
Central pain syndrome G89.0
Cephalematocele, cephal (o)hematocele
  newborn P52.8
    birth injury P10.8
  traumatic — *see* Hematoma, brain
Cephalematoma, cephalhematoma (calcified)
  newborn (birth injury) P12.0
  traumatic — *see* Hematoma, brain
Cephalgia, cephalalgia (*see also* Headache)
  histamine G44.009
    intractable G44.001
    not intractable G44.009
  trigeminal autonomic (TAC) NEC G44.099
    intractable G44.091
    not intractable G44.099
Cephalic — *see* condition
Cephalitis — *see* Encephalitis
Cephalocele — *see* Encephalocele
Cephalomenia N94.89
Cephalopelvic — *see* condition
Cerclage (with cervical incompetence) in pregnancy — *see* Incompetence, cervix, in pregnancy
Cerebellitis — *see* Encephalitis
Cerebellum, cerebellar — *see* condition
Cerebral — *see* condition
Cerebritis — *see* Encephalitis
Cerebro-hepato-renal syndrome Q87.89
Cerebromalacia — *see* Softening, brain
  sequelae of cerebrovascular disease I69.398
Cerebroside lipidosis E75.22

Cerebrospasticity (congenital) G80.1
Cerebrospinal — *see* condition
Cerebrum — *see* condition
Ceroid-lipofuscinosis, neuronal E75.4
Cerumen (accumulation) (impacted) H61.2- ☑
Cervical (*see also* condition)
  auricle Q18.2
  dysplasia in pregnancy — *see* Abnormal, cervix, in pregnancy or childbirth
  erosion in pregnancy — *see* Abnormal, cervix, in pregnancy or childbirth
  fibrosis in pregnancy — *see* Abnormal, cervix, in pregnancy or childbirth
  fusion syndrome Q76.1
  rib Q76.5
  shortening (complicating pregnancy) O26.87- ☑
Cervicalgia M54.2
Cervicitis (acute) (chronic) (nonvenereal) (senile (atrophic)) (subacute) (with ulceration) N72
  with
    abortion — *see* Abortion, by type complicated by genital tract and pelvic infection
    ectopic pregnancy O08.0
    molar pregnancy O08.0
  chlamydial A56.09
  gonococcal A54.03
  herpesviral A60.03
  puerperal (postpartum) O86.11
  syphilitic A52.76
  trichomonal A59.09
  tuberculous A18.16
Cervicocolpitis (emphysematosa) (see also Cervicitis) N72
Cervix — *see* condition
Cesarean delivery, previous, affecting management of pregnancy O34.219
  classical (vertical) scar O34.212
  low transverse scar O34.211
Céstan (-Chenais) paralysis or syndrome G46.3
Céstan-Raymond syndrome I65.8
Cestode infestation B71.9
  specified type NEC B71.8
Cestodiasis B71.9
Chabert's disease A22.9
Chacaleh E53.8
Chafing L30.4
Chagas' (-Mazza) disease (chronic) B57.2
  with
    cardiovascular involvement NEC B57.2
    digestive system involvement B57.30
      megacolon B57.32
      megaesophagus B57.31
      other specified B57.39
    megacolon B57.32
    megaesophagus B57.31
    myocarditis B57.2
    nervous system involvement B57.40
      meningitis B57.41
      meningoencephalitis B57.42
      other specified B57.49
    specified organ involvement NEC B57.5
  acute (with) B57.1
    cardiovascular NEC B57.0
    myocarditis B57.0
Chagres fever B50.9
Chairridden Z74.09
Chalasia (cardiac sphincter) K21.9
Chalazion H00.19
  left H00.16
    lower H00.15
    upper H00.14
  right H00.13
    lower H00.12
    upper H00.11
Chalcosis (*see also* Disorder, globe, degenerative, chalcosis)
  cornea — *see* Deposit, cornea
  crystalline lens — *see* Cataract, complicated
  retina H35.89
Chalicosis (pulmonum) J62.8
Chancre (any genital site) (hard) (hunterian) (mixed) (primary) (seronegative) (seropositive) (syphilitic) A51.0
  congenital A50.07
  conjunctiva NEC A51.2
  Ducrey's A57
  extragenital A51.2
  eyelid A51.2

Chancre — *continued*
  lip A51.2
  nipple A51.2
  Nisbet's A57
  of
    carate A67.0
    pinta A67.0
    yaws A66.0
  palate, soft A51.2
  phagedenic A57
  simple A57
  soft A57
    bubo A57
    palate A51.2
  urethra A51.0
  yaws A66.0
Chancroid (anus) (genital) (penis) (perineum) (rectum) (urethra) (vulva) A57
Chandler's disease (osteochondritis dissecans, hip) — *see* Osteochondritis, dissecans, hip
Change(s) (in) (of) (*see also* Removal)
  arteriosclerotic — *see* Arteriosclerosis
  bone (*see also* Disorder, bone)
    diabetic — *see* Diabetes, bone change
  bowel habit R19.4
  cardiorenal (vascular) — *see* Hypertension, cardiorenal
  cardiovascular — *see* Disease, cardiovascular
  circulatory I99.9
  cognitive (mild) (organic) R41.89
  color, tooth, teeth
    during formation K00.8
    posteruptive K03.7
  contraceptive device Z30.433
  corneal membrane H18.30
    Bowman's membrane fold or rupture H18.31- ☑
    Descemet's membrane
      fold H18.32- ☑
      rupture H18.33- ☑
  coronary — *see* Disease, heart, ischemic
  degenerative, spine or vertebra — *see* Spondylosis
  dental pulp, regressive K04.2
  dressing (nonsurgical) Z48.00
    surgical Z48.01
  heart — *see* Disease, heart
  hip joint — *see* Derangement, joint, hip
  hyperplastic larynx J38.7
  hypertrophic
    nasal sinus J34.89
    turbinate, nasal J34.3
    upper respiratory tract J39.8
  indwelling catheter Z46.6
  inflammatory (*see also* Inflammation)
    sacroiliac M46.1
  job, anxiety concerning Z56.1
  joint — *see* Derangement, joint
  life — *see* Menopause
  mental status R41.82
  minimal (glomerular) (*see also* N00-N07 with fourth character .0) N05.0
  myocardium, myocardial — *see* Degeneration, myocardial
  of life — *see* Menopause
  pacemaker Z45.018
    pulse generator Z45.010
  personality (enduring) F68.8
    due to (secondary to)
      general medical condition F07.0
    secondary (nonspecific) F60.89
  regressive, dental pulp K04.2
  renal — *see* Disease, renal
  retina H35.9
    myopic (*see also* Myopia, degenerative) H44.2- ☑
  sacroiliac joint M53.3
  senile (*see also* condition) R54
  sensory R20.8
  skin R23.9
    acute, due to ultraviolet radiation L56.9
      specified NEC L56.8
    chronic, due to nonionizing radiation L57.9
      specified NEC L57.8
    cyanosis R23.0
    flushing R23.2
    pallor R23.1
    petechiae R23.3
    specified change NEC R23.8
    swelling — *see* Mass, localized
    texture R23.4

Change(s) — *continued*
  trophic
    arm — *see* Mononeuropathy, upper limb
    leg — *see* Mononeuropathy, lower limb
  vascular I99.9
  vasomotor I73.9
  voice R49.9
    psychogenic F44.4
    specified NEC R49.8
Changing sleep-work schedule, affecting sleep
  G47.26
Changuinola fever A93.1
Chapping skin T69.8 ☑
Charcot-Marie-Tooth disease, paralysis or syndrome
  G60.0
Charcot's
  arthropathy — *see* Arthropathy, neuropathic
  cirrhosis K74.3
  disease (tabetic arthropathy) A52.16
  joint (disease) (tabetic) A52.16
    diabetic — *see* Diabetes, with, arthropathy
    syringomyelic G95.0
  syndrome (intermittent claudication) I73.9
CHARGE association Q89.8
Charley-horse (quadriceps) M62.831
  traumatic (quadriceps) S76.11- ☑
Charlouis' disease — *see* Yaws
Cheadle's disease E54
Checking (of)
  cardiac pacemaker (battery) (electrode(s)) Z45.018
    pulse generator Z45.010
  implantable subdermal contraceptive Z30.46
  intrauterine contraceptive device Z30.431
  wound Z48.0- ☑
    due to injury — code to Injury, by site, using appro-
      priate seventh character for subsequent en-
      counter
Check-up — *see* Examination
Chédiak-Higashi (-Steinbrinck) **syndrome** (congenital
  gigantism of peroxidase granules) E70.330
Cheek — *see* condition
Cheese itch B88.0
Cheese-washer's lung J67.8
Cheese-worker's lung J67.8
Cheilitis (acute) (angular) (catarrhal) (chronic) (exfoliative)
  (gangrenous) (glandular) (infectional) (suppurative)
  (ulcerative) (vesicular) K13.0
  actinic (due to sun) L56.8
    other than from sun L59.8
  candidal B37.83
Cheilodynia K13.0
Cheiloschisis — *see* Cleft, lip
Cheilosis (angular) K13.0
  with pellagra E52
  due to
    vitamin B2 (riboflavin) deficiency E53.0
Cheiromegaly M79.89
Cheiropompholyx L30.1
Cheloid — *see* Keloid
Chemical burn — *see* Corrosion, by site
Chemodectoma — *see* Paraganglioma, nonchromaffin
Chemosis, conjunctiva — *see* Edema, conjunctiva
Chemotherapy (session) (for)
  cancer Z51.11
  neoplasm Z51.11
Cherubism M27.8
Chest — *see* condition
Cheyne-Stokes breathing (respiration) R06.3
Chiari's
  disease or syndrome (hepatic vein thrombosis) I82.0
  malformation
    type I G93.5
    type II — *see* Spina bifida
    net Q24.8
Chicago disease B40.9
Chickenpox — *see* Varicella
Chiclero ulcer or sore B55.1
Chigger (infestation) B88.0
Chignon (disease) B36.8
  newborn (from vacuum extraction) (birth injury) P12.1
Chilaiditi's syndrome (subphrenic displacement, colon)
  Q43.3
Chilblain(s) (lupus) T69.1 ☑
Child
  custody dispute Z65.3
Childbirth — *see* Delivery

Childhood
  cerebral X-linked adrenoleukodystrophy E71.520
  period of rapid growth Z00.2
Chill(s) R68.83
  with fever R50.9
  without fever R68.83
  congestive in malarial regions B54
Chilomastigiasis A07.8
Chimera 46,XX/46,XY Q99.0
Chin — *see* condition
Chinese dysentery A03.9
Chionophobia F40.228
Chitral fever A93.1
Chlamydia, chlamydial A74.9
  cervicitis A56.09
  conjunctivitis A74.0
  cystitis A56.01
  endometritis A56.11
  epididymitis A56.19
  female
    pelvic inflammatory disease A56.11
    pelviperitonitis A56.11
  orchitis A56.19
  peritonitis A74.81
  pharyngitis A56.4
  proctitis A56.3
  psittaci (infection) A70
  salpingitis A56.11
  sexually-transmitted infection NEC A56.8
  specified NEC A74.89
  urethritis A56.01
  vulvovaginitis A56.02
Chlamydiosis — *see* Chlamydia
Chloasma (skin) (idiopathic) (symptomatic) L81.1
  eyelid H02.719
    hyperthyroid E05.90 [H02.719]
      with thyroid storm E05.91 [H02.719]
    left H02.716
      lower H02.715
      upper H02.714
    right H02.713
      lower H02.712
      upper H02.711
Chloroma C92.3- ☑
Chlorosis D50.9
  Egyptian B76.9 [D63.8]
  miner's B76.9 [D63.8]
Chlorotic anemia D50.8
Chocolate cyst (ovary) N80.1
Choked
  disc or disk — *see* Papilledema
  on food, phlegm, or vomitus NOS — *see* Foreign body,
    by site
  while vomiting NOS — *see* Foreign body, by site
Chokes (resulting from bends) T70.3 ☑
Choking sensation R09.89
Cholangiectasis K83.8
Cholangiocarcinoma
  with hepatocellular carcinoma, combined C22.0
  liver C22.1
  specified site NEC — *see* Neoplasm, malignant, by site
  unspecified site C22.1
Cholangiohepatitis K83.8
  due to fluke infestation B66.1
Cholangiohepatoma C22.0
Cholangiolitis (acute) (chronic) (extrahepatic) (gangrenous) (intrahepatic) K83.0
  paratyphoidal — *see* Fever, paratyphoid
  typhoidal A01.09
Cholangioma D13.4
  malignant — *see* Cholangiocarcinoma
Cholangitis (ascending) (primary) (recurrent) (sclerosing)
  (secondary) (stenosing) (suppurative) K83.0
  with calculus, bile duct — *see* Calculus, bile duct, with
    cholangitis
  chronic nonsuppurative destructive K74.3
Cholecystectasia K82.8
Cholecystitis K81.9
  with
    calculus, stones in
      bile duct (common) (hepatic) — *see* Calculus,
        bile duct, with cholecystitis
      cystic duct — *see* Calculus, gallbladder, with
        cholecystitis
      gallbladder — *see* Calculus, gallbladder, with
        cholecystitis
      choledocholithiasis — *see* Calculus, bile duct, with
        cholecystitis

Cholecystitis — *continued*
  with — *continued*
    cholelithiasis — *see* Calculus, gallbladder, with
      cholecystitis
  acute (emphysematous) (gangrenous) (suppurative)
    K81.0
    with
      calculus, stones in
        cystic duct — *see* Calculus, gallbladder, with
          cholecystitis, acute
        gallbladder — *see* Calculus, gallbladder,
          with cholecystitis, acute
      choledocholithiasis — *see* Calculus, bile duct,
        with cholecystitis, acute
      cholelithiasis — *see* Calculus, gallbladder, with
        cholecystitis, acute
      chronic cholecystitis K81.2
        with gallbladder calculus K80.12
          with obstruction K80.13
  chronic K81.1
    with acute cholecystitis K81.2
      with gallbladder calculus K80.12
        with obstruction K80.13
  emphysematous (acute) — *see* Cholecystitis, acute
  gangrenous — *see* Cholecystitis, acute
  paratyphoidal, current A01.4
  suppurative — *see* Cholecystitis, acute
  typhoidal A01.09
Cholecystolithiasis — *see* Calculus, gallbladder
Choledochitis (suppurative) K83.0
Choledocholith — *see* Calculus, bile duct
Choledocholithiasis (common duct) (hepatic duct) —
  see Calculus, bile duct
  cystic — *see* Calculus, gallbladder
  typhoidal A01.09
Cholelithiasis (cystic duct) (gallbladder) (impacted)
  (multiple) — *see* Calculus, gallbladder
  bile duct (common) (hepatic) — *see* Calculus, bile duct
  hepatic duct — *see* Calculus, bile duct
  specified NEC K80.80
    with obstruction K80.81
Cholemia (*see also* Jaundice)
  familial (simple) (congenital) E80.4
  Gilbert's E80.4
Choleperitoneum, choleperitonitis K65.3
Cholera (Asiatic) (epidemic) (malignant) A00.9
  antimonial — *see* Poisoning, antimony
  classical A00.0
  due to Vibrio cholerae 01 A00.9
    biovar cholerae A00.0
    biovar eltor A00.1
    el tor A00.1
  el tor A00.1
Cholerine — *see* Cholera
Cholestasis NEC K83.1
  with hepatocyte injury K71.0
  due to total parenteral nutrition (TPN) K76.89
  pure K71.0
Cholesteatoma (ear) (middle) (with reaction) H71.9- ☑
  attic H71.0- ☑
  external ear (canal) H60.4- ☑
  mastoid H71.2- ☑
  postmastoidectomy cavity (recurrent) — *see* Compli-
    cations, postmastoidectomy, recurrent
    cholesteatoma
  recurrent (postmastoidectomy) — *see* Complications,
    postmastoidectomy, recurrent cholesteatoma
  tympanum H71.1- ☑
Cholesteatosis, diffuse H71.3- ☑
Cholesteremia E78.00
Cholesterin in vitreous — *see* Deposit, crystalline
Cholesterol
  deposit
    retina H35.89
    vitreous — *see* Deposit, crystalline
  elevated (high) E78.00
    with elevated (high) triglycerides E78.2
    screening for Z13.220
  imbibition of gallbladder K82.4
Cholesterolemia (essential) (pure) E78.00
  familial E78.01
  hereditary E78.01
Cholesterolosis, cholesterosis (gallbladder) K82.4
  cerebrotendinous E75.5
Cholocolic fistula K82.3
Choluria R82.2
Chondritis M94.8X9

Chondritis — *continued*
- aurical H61.03- ☑
- costal (Tietze's) M94.0
- external ear H61.03- ☑
- patella, posttraumatic — *see* Chondromalacia, patella
- pinna H61.03- ☑
- purulent M94.8X- ☑
- tuberculous NEC A18.02
  - intervertebral A18.01

Chondroblastoma (*see also* Neoplasm, bone, benign)
- malignant — *see* Neoplasm, bone, malignant

Chondrocalcinosis M11.20
- ankle M11.27- ☑
- elbow M11.22- ☑
- familial M11.10
  - ankle M11.17- ☑
  - elbow M11.12- ☑
  - foot joint M11.17- ☑
  - hand joint M11.14- ☑
  - hip M11.15- ☑
  - knee M11.16- ☑
  - multiple site M11.19
  - shoulder M11.11- ☑
  - vertebrae M11.18
  - wrist M11.13- ☑
- foot joint M11.27- ☑
- hand joint M11.24- ☑
- hip M11.25- ☑
- knee M11.26- ☑
- multiple site M11.29
- shoulder M11.21- ☑
- specified type NEC M11.20
  - ankle M11.27- ☑
  - elbow M11.22- ☑
  - foot joint M11.27- ☑
  - hand joint M11.24- ☑
  - hip M11.25- ☑
  - knee M11.26- ☑
  - multiple site M11.29
  - shoulder M11.21- ☑
  - vertebrae M11.28
  - wrist M11.23- ☑
- vertebrae M11.28
- wrist M11.23- ☑

Chondrodermatitis nodularis helicis or anthelicis — *see* Perichondritis, ear

Chondrodysplasia Q78.9
- with hemangioma Q78.4
- calcificans congenita Q77.3
- fetalis Q77.4
- metaphyseal (Jansen's) (McKusick's) (Schmid's) Q78.8
- punctata Q77.3

Chondrodystrophy, chondrodystrophia (familial) (fetalis) (hypoplastic) Q78.9
- calcificans congenita Q77.3
- myotonic (congenital) G71.13
- punctata Q77.3

Chondroectodermal dysplasia Q77.6

Chondrogenesis imperfecta Q77.4

Chondrolysis M94.35- ☑

Chondroma (*see also* Neoplasm, cartilage, benign)
- juxtacortical — *see* Neoplasm, bone, benign
- periosteal — *see* Neoplasm, bone, benign

Chondromalacia (systemic) M94.20
- acromioclavicular joint M94.21- ☑
- ankle M94.27- ☑
- elbow M94.22- ☑
- foot joint M94.27- ☑
- glenohumeral joint M94.21- ☑
- hand joint M94.24- ☑
- hip M94.25- ☑
- knee M94.26- ☑
  - patella M22.4- ☑
- multiple sites M94.29
- patella M22.4- ☑
- rib M94.28
- sacroiliac joint M94.259
- shoulder M94.21- ☑
- sternoclavicular joint M94.21- ☑
- vertebral joint M94.28
- wrist M94.23- ☑

Chondromatosis (*see also* Neoplasm, cartilage, uncertain behavior)
- internal Q78.4

Chondromyxosarcoma — *see* Neoplasm, cartilage, malignant

Chondro-osteodysplasia (Morquio-Brailsford type) E76.219

Chondro-osteodystrophy E76.29

Chondro-osteoma — *see* Neoplasm, bone, benign

Chondropathia tuberosa M94.0

Chondrosarcoma — *see* Neoplasm, cartilage, malignant
- juxtacortical — *see* Neoplasm, bone, malignant
- mesenchymal — *see* Neoplasm, connective tissue, malignant
- myxoid — *see* Neoplasm, cartilage, malignant

Chordee (nonvenereal) N48.89
- congenital Q54.4
- gonococcal A54.09

Chorditis (fibrinous) (nodosa) (tuberosa) J38.2

Chordoma — *see* Neoplasm, vertebral (column), malignant

Chorea (chronic) (gravis) (posthemiplegic) (senile) (spasmodic) G25.5
- with
  - heart involvement I02.0
    - active or acute (conditions in I01-) I02.0
    - rheumatic I02.9
      - with valvular disorder I02.0
    - rheumatic heart disease (chronic) (inactive)(quiescent) — *code to* rheumatic heart condition involved
- drug-induced G25.4
- habit F95.8
- hereditary G10
- Huntington's G10
- hysterical F44.4
- minor I02.9
  - with heart involvement I02.0
- progressive G25.5
  - hereditary G10
- rheumatic (chronic) I02.9
  - with heart involvement I02.0
- Sydenham's I02.9
  - with heart involvement — *see* Chorea, with rheumatic heart disease
- nonrheumatic G25.5

Choreoathetosis (paroxysmal) G25.5

Chorioadenoma (destruens) D39.2

Chorioamnionitis O41.12- ☑

Chorioangioma D26.7

Choriocarcinoma — *see* Neoplasm, malignant, by site
- combined with
  - embryonal carcinoma — *see* Neoplasm, malignant, by site
  - other germ cell elements — *see* Neoplasm, malignant, by site
  - teratoma — *see* Neoplasm, malignant, by site
- specified site — *see* Neoplasm, malignant, by site
- unspecified site
  - female C58
  - male C62.90

Chorioencephalitis (acute) (lymphocytic) (serous) A87.2

Chorioepithelioma — *see* Choriocarcinoma

Choriomeningitis (acute) (lymphocytic) (serous) A87.2

Chorionepithelioma — *see* Choriocarcinoma

Chorioretinitis (*see also* Inflammation, chorioretinal)
- disseminated (*see also* Inflammation, chorioretinal, disseminated)
  - in neurosyphilis A52.19
- Egyptian B76.9 [D63.8]
- focal (*see also* Inflammation, chorioretinal, focal)
- histoplasmic B39.9 [H32]
- in (due to)
  - histoplasmosis B39.9 [H32]
  - syphilis (secondary) A51.43
    - late A52.71
  - toxoplasmosis (acquired) B58.01
    - congenital (active) P37.1 [H32]
  - tuberculosis A18.53
- juxtapapillary, juxtapapillaris — *see* Inflammation, chorioretinal, focal, juxtapapillary
- leprous A30.9 [H32]
- miner's B76.9 [D63.8]
- progressive myopia (degeneration) (*see also* Myopia, degenerative) H44.2- ☑
- syphilitic (secondary) A51.43
  - congenital (early) A50.01 [H32]
    - late A50.32
  - late A52.71
- tuberculous A18.53

Chorioretinopathy, central serous H35.71- ☑

Choroid — *see* condition

Choroideremia H31.21

Choroiditis — *see* Chorioretinitis

Choroidopathy — *see* Disorder, choroid

Choroidoretinitis — *see* Chorioretinitis

Choroidoretinopathy, central serous — *see* Chorioretinopathy, central serous

Christian-Weber disease M35.6

Christmas disease D67

Chromaffinoma (*see also* Neoplasm, benign, by site)
- malignant — *see* Neoplasm, malignant, by site

Chromatopsia — *see* Deficiency, color vision

Chromhidrosis, chromidrosis L75.1

Chromoblastomycosis — *see* Chromomycosis

Chromoconversion R82.91

Chromomycosis B43.9
- brain abscess B43.1
- cerebral B43.1
- cutaneous B43.0
- skin B43.0
- specified NEC B43.8
- subcutaneous abscess or cyst B43.2

Chromophytosis B36.0

Chromosome — *see* Anomaly, by chromosome involved
- D (1) — *see* Anomaly, chromosome 13
- E (3) — *see* Anomaly, chromosome 18
- G — *see* Anomaly, chromosome 21

Chromotrichomycosis B36.8

Chronic — *see* condition
- fracture — *see* Fracture, pathological

Churg-Strauss syndrome M30.1

Chyle cyst, mesentery I89.8

Chylocele (nonfilarial) I89.8
- filarial (*see also* Infestation, filarial) B74.9 [N51]
- tunica vaginalis N50.89
  - filarial (*see also* Infestation, filarial) B74.9 [N51]

Chylomicronemia (fasting) (with hyperprebetalipoproteinemia) E78.3

Chylopericardium I31.3
- acute I30.9

Chylothorax (nonfilarial) I89.8
- filarial (*see also* Infestation, filarial) B74.9 [J91.8]

Chylous — *see* condition

Chyluria (nonfilarial) R82.0
- due to
  - bilharziasis B65.0
  - Brugia (malayi) B74.1
    - timori B74.2
  - schistosomiasis (bilharziasis) B65.0
  - Wuchereria (bancrofti) B74.0
- filarial — *see* Infestation, filarial

Cicatricial (deformity) — *see* Cicatrix

Cicatrix (adherent) (contracted) (painful) (vicious) (*see also* Scar) L90.5
- adenoid (and tonsil) J35.8
- alveolar process M26.79
- anus K62.89
- auricle — *see* Disorder, pinna, specified type NEC
- bile duct (common) (hepatic) K83.8
- bladder N32.89
- bone — *see* Disorder, bone, specified type NEC
- brain G93.89
- cervix (postoperative) (postpartal) N88.1
- common duct K83.8
- cornea H17.9
  - tuberculous A18.59
- duodenum (bulb), obstructive K31.5
- esophagus K22.2
- eyelid — *see* Disorder, eyelid function
- hypopharynx J39.2
- lacrimal passages — *see* Obstruction, lacrimal
- larynx J38.7
- lung J98.4
- middle ear H74.8 ☑
- mouth K13.79
- muscle M62.89
  - with contracture — *see* Contraction, muscle NEC
- nasopharynx J39.2
- palate (soft) K13.79
- penis N48.89
- pharynx J39.2
- prostate N42.89
- rectum K62.89
- retina — *see* Scar, chorioretinal
- semilunar cartilage — *see* Derangement, meniscus
- seminal vesicle N50.89
- skin L90.5
  - infected L08.89
  - postinfective L90.5

Cicatrix — *continued*
- skin — *continued*
  - tuberculous B90.8
  - specified site NEC L90.5
  - throat J39.2
  - tongue K14.8
  - tonsil (and adenoid) J35.8
  - trachea J39.8
  - tuberculous NEC B90.9
  - urethra N36.8
  - uterus N85.8
  - vagina N89.8
    - postoperative N99.2
  - vocal cord J38.3
  - wrist, constricting (annular) L90.5

CIDP (chronic inflammatory demyelinating polyneuropathy) G61.81

CIN — *see* Neoplasia, intraepithelial, cervix

CINCA (chronic infantile neurological, cutaneous and articular syndrome) M04.2

Cinchonism — *see* Deafness, ototoxic
- correct substance properly administered — *see* Table of Drugs and Chemicals, by drug, adverse effect
- overdose or wrong substance given or taken — *see* Table of Drugs and Chemicals, by drug, poisoning

Circle of Willis — *see* condition

Circular — *see* condition

Circulating anticoagulants (*see also* Disorder, hemorrhagic) D68.318
- due to drugs (*see also* Disorder, hemorrhagic) D68.32
- following childbirth O72.3

Circulation
- collateral, any site I99.8
- defective (lower extremity) I99.9
  - congenital Q28.9
- embryonic Q28.9
- failure (peripheral) R57.9
  - newborn P29.89
- fetal, persistent P29.38
- heart, incomplete Q28.9

Circulatory system — *see* condition

Circulus senilis (cornea) — *see* Degeneration, cornea, senile

Circumcision (in absence of medical indication) (ritual) (routine) Z41.2

Circumscribed — *see* condition

Circumvallate placenta O43.11- ☑

Cirrhosis, cirrhotic (hepatic) (liver) K74.60
- alcoholic K70.30
  - with ascites K70.31
- atrophic — *see* Cirrhosis, liver
- Baumgarten-Cruveilhier K74.69
- biliary (cholangiolitic) (cholangitic) (hypertrophic) (obstructive) (pericholangiolitic) K74.5
  - due to
    - Clonorchiasis B66.1
    - flukes B66.3
  - primary K74.3
  - secondary K74.4
- cardiac (of liver) K76.1
- Charcot's K74.3
- cholangiolitic, cholangitic, cholostatic (primary) K74.3
- congestive K76.1
- Cruveilhier-Baumgarten K74.69
- cryptogenic (liver) K74.69
- due to
  - hepatolenticular degeneration E83.01
  - Wilson's disease E83.01
  - xanthomatosis E78.2
- fatty K76.0
  - alcoholic K70.0
- Hanot's (hypertrophic) K74.3
- hepatic — *see* Cirrhosis, liver
- hypertrophic K74.3
- Indian childhood K74.69
- kidney — *see* Sclerosis, renal
- Laennec's K70.30
  - with ascites K70.31
  - alcoholic K70.30
    - with ascites K70.31
  - nonalcoholic K74.69
- liver K74.60
  - alcoholic K70.30
    - with ascites K70.31
    - fatty K70.0
  - congenital P78.81
  - syphilitic A52.74

Cirrhosis, cirrhotic — *continued*
- lung (chronic) J84.10
- macronodular K74.69
  - alcoholic K70.30
    - with ascites K70.31
- micronodular K74.69
  - alcoholic K70.30
    - with ascites K70.31
- mixed type K74.69
- monolobular K74.3
- nephritis — *see* Sclerosis, renal
- nutritional K74.69
  - alcoholic K70.30
    - with ascites K70.31
- obstructive — *see* Cirrhosis, biliary
- ovarian N83.8
- pancreas (duct) K86.89
- pigmentary E83.110
- portal K74.69
  - alcoholic K70.30
    - with ascites K70.31
- postnecrotic K74.69
  - alcoholic K70.30
    - with ascites K70.31
- pulmonary J84.10
- renal — *see* Sclerosis, renal
- spleen D73.2
- stasis K76.1
- Todd's K74.3
- unilobar K74.3
- xanthomatous (biliary) K74.5
  - due to xanthomatosis (familial) (metabolic) (primary) E78.2

Cistern, subarachnoid R93.0

Citrullinemia E72.23

Citrullinuria E72.23

Civatte's disease or poikiloderma L57.3

Clam digger's itch B65.3

Clammy skin R23.1

Clap — *see* Gonorrhea

Clarke-Hadfield syndrome (pancreatic infantilism) K86.89

Clark's paralysis G80.9

Clastothrix L67.8

Claude Bernard-Horner syndrome G90.2
- traumatic — *see* Injury, nerve, cervical sympathetic

Claude's disease or syndrome G46.3

Claudicatio venosa intermittens I87.8

Claudication (intermittent) I73.9
- cerebral (artery) G45.9
- spinal cord (arteriosclerotic) G95.19
  - syphilitic A52.09
- venous (axillary) I87.8

Claustrophobia F40.240

Clavus (infected) L84

Clawfoot (congenital) Q66.89
- acquired — *see* Deformity, limb, clawfoot

Clawhand (acquired) (*see also* Deformity, limb, clawhand)
- congenital Q68.1

Clawtoe (congenital) Q66.89
- acquired — *see* Deformity, toe, specified NEC

Clay eating — *see* Pica

Cleansing of artificial opening — *see* Attention to, artificial, opening

Cleft (congenital) — *see also* Imperfect, closure
- alveolar process M26.79
- branchial (persistent) Q18.2
  - cyst Q18.0
    - fistula Q18.0
    - sinus Q18.0
- cricoid cartilage, posterior Q31.8
- cyst Q18.0
  - fistula Q18.0
  - sinus Q18.0
- foot Q72.7 ☑
- hand Q71.6 ☑
- lip (unilateral) Q36.9
  - with cleft palate Q37.9
    - hard Q37.1
      - with soft Q37.5
    - soft Q37.3
      - with hard Q37.5
  - bilateral Q36.0
    - with cleft palate Q37.8
      - hard Q37.0
        - with soft Q37.4
      - soft Q37.2
        - with hard Q37.4

Cleft — *continued*
- lip — *continued*
  - median Q36.1
  - nose Q30.2
- palate Q35.9
  - with cleft lip (unilateral) Q37.9
    - bilateral Q37.8
  - hard Q35.1
    - with
      - cleft lip (unilateral) Q37.1
        - bilateral Q37.0
      - soft Q35.5
        - with cleft lip (unilateral) Q37.5
          - bilateral Q37.4
  - medial Q35.5
    - soft Q35.3
      - with
        - cleft lip (unilateral) Q37.3
          - bilateral Q37.2
        - hard Q35.5
          - with cleft lip (unilateral) Q37.5
            - bilateral Q37.4
  - penis Q55.69
  - scrotum Q55.29
  - thyroid cartilage Q31.8
  - uvula Q35.7

Cleidocranial dysostosis Q74.0

Cleptomania F63.2

Clicking hip (newborn) R29.4

Climacteric (female) (*see also* Menopause)
- arthritis (any site) NEC — *see* Arthritis, specified form NEC
- depression (single episode) F32.89
  - recurrent episode F33.8
- male (symptoms) (syndrome) NEC N50.89
- melancholia (single episode) F32.89
  - recurrent episode F33.8
- paranoid state F22
- polyarthritis NEC — *see* Arthritis, specified form NEC
- symptoms (female) N95.1

Clinical research investigation (clinical trial) (control subject) (normal comparison) (participant) Z00.6

Clitoris — *see* condition

Cloaca (persistent) Q43.7

Clonorchiasis, clonorchis infection (liver) B66.1

Clonus R25.8

Closed bite M26.29

Clostridium (C.) **perfringens, as cause of disease classified elsewhere** B96.7

Closure
- congenital, nose Q30.0
- cranial sutures, premature Q75.0
- defective or imperfect NEC — *see* Imperfect, closure
- fistula, delayed — *see* Fistula
- foramen ovale, imperfect Q21.1
- hymen N89.6
- interauricular septum, defective Q21.1
- interventricular septum, defective Q21.0
- lacrimal duct (*see also* Stenosis, lacrimal, duct)
  - congenital Q10.5
- nose (congenital) Q30.0
  - acquired M95.0
- of artificial opening — *see* Attention to, artificial, opening
- vagina N89.5
- valve — *see* Endocarditis
- vulva N90.5

Clot (blood) (*see also* Embolism)
- artery (obstruction) (occlusion) — *see* Embolism
- bladder N32.89
- brain (intradural or extradural) — *see* Occlusion, artery, cerebral
- circulation I74.9
- heart (*see also* Infarct, myocardium)
  - not resulting in infarction I51.3
- vein — *see* Thrombosis

Clouded state R40.1
- epileptic — *see* Epilepsy, specified NEC
- paroxysmal — *see* Epilepsy, specified NEC

Cloudy antrum, antra J32.0

Clouston's (hidrotic) **ectodermal dysplasia** Q82.4

Clubbed nail pachydermoperiostosis M89.40 [L62]

Clubbing of finger(s) (nails) R68.3

Clubfinger R68.3
- congenital Q68.1

Clubfoot (congenital) Q66.89
- acquired — *see* Deformity, limb, clubfoot
- equinovarus Q66.0

⬚ Subterms under main terms may continue to next column or page   ☑ Additional Character Required — Refer to the Tabular List for Character Selection   **55**

Cicatrix — Clubfoot

Index

Clubfoot — Collapse

Clubfoot — continued
  paralytic — see Deformity, limb, clubfoot
Clubhand (congenital) (radial) Q71.4- ☑
  acquired — see Deformity, limb, clubhand
Clubnail R68.3
  congenital Q84.6
Clump, kidney Q63.1
Clumsiness, clumsy child syndrome F82
Cluttering F80.81
Clutton's joints A50.51 [M12.80]
Coagulation, intravascular (diffuse) (disseminated)
  (see also Defibrination syndrome)
  complicating abortion — see Abortion, by type, com-
    plicated by, intravascular coagulation
  following ectopic or molar pregnancy O08.1
Coagulopathy (see also Defect, coagulation)
  consumption D65
  intravascular D65
    newborn P60
Coalition
  calcaneo-scaphoid Q66.89
  tarsal Q66.89
Coalminer's
  elbow — see Bursitis, elbow, olecranon
  lung or pneumoconiosis J60
Coalworker's lung or pneumoconiosis J60
Coarctation
  aorta (preductal) (postductal) Q25.1
  pulmonary artery Q25.71
Coated tongue K14.3
Coats' disease (exudative retinopathy) — see
  Retinopathy, exudative
Cocaine-induced
  anxiety disorder F14.980
  bipolar and related disorder F14.94
  depressive disorder F14.94
  obsessive-compulsive and related disorder F14.988
  psychotic disorder F14.959
  sexual dysfunction F14.981
  sleep disorder F14.982
Cocainism — see Disorder, cocaine use
Coccidioidomycosis B38.9
  cutaneous B38.3
  disseminated B38.7
  generalized B38.7
  meninges B38.4
  prostate B38.81
  pulmonary B38.2
    acute B38.0
    chronic B38.1
  skin B38.3
  specified NEC B38.89
Coccidioidosis — see Coccidioidomycosis
Coccidiosis (intestinal) A07.3
Coccydynia, coccygodynia M53.3
Coccyx — see condition
Cochin-China diarrhea K90.1
Cockayne's syndrome Q87.1
Cocked up toe — see Deformity, toe, specified NEC
Cock's peculiar tumor L72.3
Codman's tumor — see Neoplasm, bone, benign
Coenurosis B71.8
Coffee-worker's lung J67.8
Cogan's syndrome H16.32- ☑
  oculomotor apraxia H51.8
Coitus, painful (female) N94.10
  male N53.12
  psychogenic F52.6
Cold J00
  with influenza, flu, or grippe — see Influenza, with,
    respiratory manifestations NEC
  agglutinin disease or hemoglobinuria (chronic) D59.1
  bronchial — see Bronchitis
  chest — see Bronchitis
  common (head) J00
  effects of T69.9 ☑
    specified effect NEC T69.8 ☑
  excessive, effects of T69.9 ☑
    specified effect NEC T69.8 ☑
  exhaustion from T69.8 ☑
  exposure to T69.9 ☑
    specified effect NEC T69.8 ☑
  head J00
  injury syndrome (newborn) P80.0
  on lung — see Bronchitis
  rose J30.1
  sensitivity, auto-immune D59.1

Cold — continued
  symptoms J00
  virus J00
Coldsore B00.1
Colibacillosis A49.8
  as the cause of other disease (see also Escherichia coli)
    B96.20
  generalized A41.50
Colic (bilious) (infantile) (intestinal) (recurrent) (spasmodic) R10.83
  abdomen R10.83
    psychogenic F45.8
  appendix, appendicular K38.8
  bile duct — see Calculus, bile duct
  biliary — see Calculus, bile duct
  common duct — see Calculus, bile duct
  cystic duct — see Calculus, gallbladder
  Devonshire NEC — see Poisoning, lead
  gallbladder — see Calculus, gallbladder
  gallstone — see Calculus, gallbladder
    gallbladder or cystic duct — see Calculus, gallblad-
      der
  hepatic (duct) — see Calculus, bile duct
  hysterical F45.8
  kidney N23
  lead NEC — see Poisoning, lead
  mucous K58.9
    with diarrhea K58.0
    psychogenic F54
  nephritic N23
  painter's NEC — see Poisoning, lead
  pancreas K86.89
  psychogenic F45.8
  renal N23
  saturnine NEC — see Poisoning, lead
  ureter N23
  urethral N36.8
    due to calculus N21.1
  uterus NEC N94.89
    menstrual — see Dysmenorrhea
  worm NOS B83.9
Colicystitis — see Cystitis
Colitis (acute) (catarrhal) (chronic) (noninfective) (hemorrhagic) (see also Enteritis) K52.9
  allergic K52.29
    with
      food protein-induced enterocolitis syndrome
        K52.21
      proctocolitis K52.82
  amebic (acute) (see also Amebiasis) A06.0
    nondysenteric A06.2
  anthrax A22.2
  bacillary — see Infection, Shigella
  balantidial A07.0
  Clostridium difficile
    not specified as recurrent A04.72
    recurrent A04.71
  coccidial A07.3
  collagenous K52.831
  cystica superficialis K52.89
  dietary counseling and surveillance (for) Z71.3
  dietetic (see also Colitis, allergic) K52.29
  drug-induced K52.1
  due to radiation K52.0
  eosinophilic K52.82
  food hypersensitivity (see also Colitis, allergic) K52.29
  giardial A07.1
  granulomatous — see Enteritis, regional, large intes-
    tine
  indeterminate, so stated K52.3
  infectious — see Enteritis, infectious
  ischemic K55.9
    acute (subacute) (see also Ischemia, intestine,
      acute) K55.039
    chronic K55.1
    due to mesenteric artery insufficiency K55.1
    fulminant (acute) (see also Ischemia, intestine,
      acute) K55.039
  left sided K51.50
    with
      abscess K51.514
      complication K51.519
        specified NEC K51.518
      fistula K51.513
      obstruction K51.512
      rectal bleeding K51.511
  lymphocytic K52.832

Colitis — continued
  membranous
    psychogenic F54
  microscopic K52.839
    specified NEC K52.838
  mucous — see Syndrome, irritable, bowel
    psychogenic F54
  noninfective K52.9
    specified NEC K52.89
  polyposa — see Polyp, colon, inflammatory
  protozoal A07.9
  pseudomembranous
    not specified as recurrent A04.72
    recurrent A04.71
  pseudomucinous — see Syndrome, irritable, bowel
  regional — see Enteritis, regional, large intestine
    infectious A09
  segmental — see Enteritis, regional, large intestine
  septic — see Enteritis, infectious
  spastic K58.9
    with diarrhea K58.0
    psychogenic F54
  staphylococcal A04.8
    foodborne A05.0
  subacute ischemic (see also Ischemia, intestine, acute)
    K55.039
  thromboulcerative (see also Ischemia, intestine, acute)
    K55.039
  toxic NEC K52.1
    due to Clostridium difficile
      not specified as recurrent A04.72
      recurrent A04.71
  transmural — see Enteritis, regional, large intestine
  trichomonal A07.8
  tuberculous (ulcerative) A18.32
  ulcerative (chronic) K51.90
    with
      complication K51.919
        abscess K51.914
        fistula K51.913
        obstruction K51.912
        rectal bleeding K51.911
        specified complication NEC K51.918
    enterocolitis — see Enterocolitis, ulcerative
    ileocolitis — see Ileocolitis, ulcerative
    mucosal proctocolitis — see Proctocolitis, mucosal
    proctitis — see Proctitis, ulcerative
    pseudopolyposis — see Polyp, colon, inflammatory
    psychogenic F54
    rectosigmoiditis — see Rectosigmoiditis, ulcerative
    specified type NEC K51.80
      with
        complication K51.819
          abscess K51.814
          fistula K51.813
          obstruction K51.812
          rectal bleeding K51.811
          specified complication NEC K51.818
Collagenosis, collagen disease (nonvascular) (vascular)
  M35.9
  cardiovascular I42.8
  reactive perforating L87.1
  specified NEC M35.8
Collapse R55
  adrenal E27.2
  cardiorespiratory R57.0
  cardiovascular R57.0
    newborn P29.89
  circulatory (peripheral) R57.9
    during or after labor and delivery O75.1
    following ectopic or molar pregnancy O08.3
    newborn P29.89
  during or
    after labor and delivery O75.1
    resulting from a procedure, not elsewhere classified
      T81.10 ☑
  external ear canal — see Stenosis, external ear canal
  general R55
  heart — see Disease, heart
  heat T67.1 ☑
  hysterical F44.89
  labyrinth, membranous (congenital) Q16.5
  lung (massive) (see also Atelectasis) J98.19
    pressure due to anesthesia (general) (local) or
      other sedation T88.2 ☑
      during labor and delivery O74.1
      in pregnancy O29.02- ☑
      postpartum, puerperal O89.09

56

☑ Additional Character Required — Refer to the Tabular List for Character Selection   ▽ Subterms under main terms may continue to next column or page

Collapse — *continued*
- myocardial — *see* Disease, heart
- nervous F48.8
- neurocirculatory F45.8
- nose M95.0
- postoperative T81.10 ☑
- pulmonary (*see also* Atelectasis) J98.19
  - newborn — *see* Atelectasis
- trachea J39.8
- tracheobronchial J98.09
- valvular — *see* Endocarditis
- vascular (peripheral) R57.9
  - during or after labor and delivery O75.1
  - following ectopic or molar pregnancy O08.3
  - newborn P29.89
- vertebra M48.50- ☑
  - cervical region M48.52- ☑
  - cervicothoracic region M48.53- ☑
  - in (due to)
    - metastasis — *see* Collapse, vertebra, in, specified disease NEC
    - osteoporosis (*see also* Osteoporosis) M80.88 ☑
      - cervical region M80.88 ☑
      - cervicothoracic region M80.88 ☑
      - lumbar region M80.88 ☑
      - lumbosacral region M80.88 ☑
      - multiple sites M80.88 ☑
      - occipito-atlanto-axial region M80.88 ☑
      - sacrococcygeal region M80.88 ☑
      - thoracic region M80.88 ☑
      - thoracolumbar region M80.88 ☑
    - specified disease NEC M48.50- ☑
      - cervical region M48.52- ☑
      - cervicothoracic region M48.53- ☑
      - lumbar region M48.56- ☑
      - lumbosacral region M48.57- ☑
      - occipito-atlanto-axial region M48.51- ☑
      - sacrococcygeal region M48.58- ☑
      - thoracic region M48.54- ☑
      - thoracolumbar region M48.55- ☑
  - lumbar region M48.56- ☑
  - lumbosacral region M48.57- ☑
  - occipito-atlanto-axial region M48.51- ☑
  - sacrococcygeal region M48.58- ☑
  - thoracic region M48.54- ☑
  - thoracolumbar region M48.55- ☑

Collateral (*see also* condition)
- circulation (venous) I87.8
- dilation, veins I87.8

Colles' fracture S52.53- ☑

Collet (-Sicard) syndrome G52.7

Collier's asthma or lung J60

Collodion baby Q80.2

Colloid nodule (of thyroid) (cystic) E04.1

Coloboma (iris) Q13.0
- eyelid Q10.3
- fundus Q14.8
- lens Q12.2
- optic disc (congenital) Q14.2
  - acquired H47.31- ☑

Coloenteritis — *see* Enteritis

Colon — *see* condition

Colonization
- MRSA (Methicillin resistant Staphylococcus aureus) Z22.322
- MSSA (Methicillin susceptible Staphylococcus aureus) Z22.321
- status — *see* Carrier (suspected) of

Coloptosis K63.4

Color blindness — *see* Deficiency, color vision

Colostomy
- attention to Z43.3
- fitting or adjustment Z46.89
- malfunctioning K94.03
- status Z93.3

Colpitis (acute) — *see* Vaginitis

Colpocele N81.5

Colpocystitis — *see* Vaginitis

Colpospasm N94.2

Column, spinal, vertebral — *see* condition

Coma R40.20
- with
  - motor response (none) R40.231 ☑
    - abnormal extensor posturing to pain or noxious stimuli (< 2 years of age) R40.232 ☑
    - abnormal flexure posturing to pain or noxious stimuli (0-5 years of age) R40.233 ☑

Coma — *continued*
- with — *continued*
  - motor response — *continued*
    - extensor posturing to pain or noxious stimuli (2-5 years of age) R40.232 ☑
    - flexion/decorticate posturing (< 2 years of age) R40.233 ☑
    - localizes pain (2-5 years of age) R40.235 ☑
    - normal or spontaneous movement (< 2 years of age) R40.236 ☑
    - obeys commands (2-5 years of age) R40.236 ☑
    - withdraws from pain or noxious stimuli (0-5 years of age) R40.234 ☑
    - withdraws to touch (< 2 years of age) R40.235 ☑
  - opening of eyes (never) R40.211 ☑
    - in response to
      - pain R40.212 ☑
      - sound R40.213 ☑
    - spontaneous R40.214 ☑
  - verbal response (none) R40.221 ☑
    - confused conversation R40.224 ☑
    - cooing or babbling or crying appropriately (< 2 years of age) R40.225 ☑
    - inappropriate crying or screaming (< 2 years of age) R40.223 ☑
    - inappropriate words (2-5 years of age) R40.224 ☑
    - incomprehensible sounds (2-5 years of age) R40.222 ☑
    - incomprehensible words R40.222 ☑
    - irritable cries (< 2 years of age) R40.224 ☑
    - moans/grunts to pain; restless (< 2 years old) R40.222 ☑
    - oriented R40.225 ☑
    - screaming (2-5 years of age) R40.223 ☑
    - uses appropriate words (2-5 years of age) R40.225 ☑
- eclamptic — *see* Eclampsia
- epileptic — *see* Epilepsy
- Glasgow, scale score — *see* Glasgow coma scale
- hepatic — *see* Failure, hepatic, by type, with coma
- hyperglycemic (diabetic) — *see* Diabetes, by type, with hyperosmolarity, with coma
- hyperosmolar (diabetic) — *see* Diabetes, by type, with hyperosmolarity, with coma
- hypoglycemic (diabetic) — *see* Diabetes, by type, with hypoglycemia, with coma
  - nondiabetic E15
- in diabetes — *see* Diabetes, coma
- insulin-induced — *see* Coma, hypoglycemic
- ketoacidotic (diabetic) — *see* Diabetes, by type, with ketoacidosis, with coma
- myxedematous E03.5
- newborn P91.5
- persistent vegetative state R40.3
- specified NEC, without documented Glasgow coma scale score, or with partial Glasgow coma scale score reported R40.244 ☑

Comatose — *see* Coma

Combat fatigue F43.0

Combined — *see* condition

Comedo, comedones (giant) L70.0

Comedocarcinoma (*see also* Neoplasm, breast, malignant)
- noninfiltrating
  - breast D05.8- ☑
  - specified site — *see* Neoplasm, in situ, by site
  - unspecified site D05.8- ☑

Comedomastitis — *see* Ectasia, mammary duct

Comminuted fracture — *code as* Fracture, closed

Common
- arterial trunk Q20.0
- atrioventricular canal Q21.2
- atrium Q21.1
- cold (head) J00
- truncus (arteriosus) Q20.0
- variable immunodeficiency — *see* Immunodeficiency, common variable
- ventricle Q20.4

Commotio, commotion (current)
- brain — *see* Injury, intracranial, concussion
- cerebri — *see* Injury, intracranial, concussion
- retinae S05.8X- ☑
- spinal cord — *see* Injury, spinal cord, by region
- spinalis — *see* Injury, spinal cord, by region

Communication
- between
  - base of aorta and pulmonary artery Q21.4
  - left ventricle and right atrium Q20.5
  - pericardial sac and pleural sac Q34.8
  - pulmonary artery and pulmonary vein, congenital Q25.72
- congenital between uterus and digestive or urinary tract Q51.7

Compartment syndrome (deep) (posterior) (traumatic) T79.A0 ☑ (*following* T79.7)
- abdomen T79.A3 ☑ (*following* T79.7)
- lower extremity (hip, buttock, thigh, leg, foot, toes) T79.A2 ☑ (*following* T79.7)
- nontraumatic
  - abdomen M79.A3 (*following* M79.7)
  - lower extremity (hip, buttock, thigh, leg, foot, toes) M79.A2- ☑ (*following* M79.7)
  - specified site NEC M79.A9 (*following* M79.7)
  - upper extremity (shoulder, arm, forearm, wrist, hand, fingers) M79.A1- ☑ (*following* M79.7)
- specified site NEC T79.A9 ☑ (*following* T79.7)
- upper extremity (shoulder, arm, forearm, wrist, hand, fingers) T79.A1- ☑ (*following* T79.7)

Compensation
- failure — *see* Disease, heart
- neurosis, psychoneurosis — *see* Disorder, factitious

Complaint (*see also* Disease)
- bowel, functional K59.9
  - psychogenic F45.8
- intestine, functional K59.9
  - psychogenic F45.8
- kidney — *see* Disease, renal
- miners' J60

Complete — *see* condition

Complex
- Addison-Schilder E71.528
- cardiorenal — *see* Hypertension, cardiorenal
- Costen's M26.69
- disseminated mycobacterium avium- intracellulare (DMAC) A31.2
- Eisenmenger's (ventricular septal defect) I27.83
- hypersexual F52.8
- jumped process, spine — *see* Dislocation, vertebra
- primary, tuberculous A15.7
- Schilder-Addison E71.528
- subluxation (vertebral) M99.19
  - abdomen M99.19
  - acromioclavicular M99.17
  - cervical region M99.11
  - cervicothoracic M99.11
  - costochondral M99.18
  - costovertebral M99.18
  - head region M99.10
  - hip M99.15
  - lower extremity M99.16
  - lumbar region M99.13
  - lumbosacral M99.13
  - occipitocervical M99.10
  - pelvic region M99.15
  - pubic M99.15
  - rib cage M99.18
  - sacral region M99.14
  - sacrococcygeal M99.14
  - sacroiliac M99.14
  - specified NEC M99.19
  - sternochondral M99.18
  - sternoclavicular M99.17
  - thoracic region M99.12
  - thoracolumbar M99.12
  - upper extremity M99.17
- Taussig-Bing (transposition, aorta and overriding pulmonary artery) Q20.1

Complication(s) (from) (of)
- accidental puncture or laceration during a procedure (of) — *see* Complications, intraoperative (intraprocedural), puncture or laceration
- amputation stump (surgical) (late) NEC T87.9
  - dehiscence T87.81
  - infection or inflammation T87.40
    - lower limb T87.4- ☑
    - upper limb T87.4- ☑
  - necrosis T87.50
    - lower limb T87.5- ☑
    - upper limb T87.5- ☑
  - neuroma T87.30
    - lower limb T87.3- ☑
    - upper limb T87.3- ☑

Complication(s) — *continued*
  amputation stump — *continued*
    specified type NEC T87.89
  anastomosis (and bypass) (*see also* Complications, prosthetic device or implant)
    intestinal (internal) NEC K91.89
      involving urinary tract N99.89
    urinary tract (involving intestinal tract) N99.89
    vascular — *see* Complications, cardiovascular device or implant
  anesthesia, anesthetic (*see also* Anesthesia, complication) T88.59 ✓
    brain, postpartum, puerperal O89.2
    cardiac
      in
        labor and delivery O74.2
        pregnancy O29.19- ✓
      postpartum, puerperal O89.1
    central nervous system
      in
        labor and delivery O74.3
        pregnancy O29.29- ✓
      postpartum, puerperal O89.2
    difficult or failed intubation T88.4 ✓
      in pregnancy O29.6- ✓
    failed sedation (conscious) (moderate) during procedure T88.52 ✓
    general, unintended awareness during procedure T88.53 ✓
    hyperthermia, malignant T88.3 ✓
    hypothermia T88.51 ✓
    intubation failure T88.4 ✓
    malignant hyperthermia T88.3 ✓
    pulmonary
      in
        labor and delivery O74.1
        pregnancy NEC O29.09- ✓
      postpartum, puerperal O89.09
    shock T88.2 ✓
    spinal and epidural
      in
        labor and delivery NEC O74.6
          headache O74.5
        pregnancy NEC O29.5X- ✓
      postpartum, puerperal NEC O89.5
        headache O89.4
    unintended awareness under general anesthesia during procedure T88.53 ✓
  anti-reflux device — *see* Complications, esophageal anti-reflux device
  aortic (bifurcation) graft — *see* Complications, graft, vascular
  aortocoronary (bypass) graft — *see* Complications, coronary artery (bypass) graft
  aortofemoral (bypass) graft — *see* Complications, extremity artery (bypass) graft
  arteriovenous
    fistula, surgically created T82.9 ✓
      embolism T82.818 ✓
      fibrosis T82.828 ✓
      hemorrhage T82.838 ✓
      infection or inflammation T82.7 ✓
      mechanical
        breakdown T82.510 ✓
        displacement T82.520 ✓
        leakage T82.530 ✓
        malposition T82.520 ✓
        obstruction T82.590 ✓
        perforation T82.590 ✓
        protrusion T82.590 ✓
      pain T82.848 ✓
      specified type NEC T82.898 ✓
      stenosis T82.858 ✓
      thrombosis T82.868 ✓
    shunt, surgically created T82.9 ✓
      embolism T82.818 ✓
      fibrosis T82.828 ✓
      hemorrhage T82.838 ✓
      infection or inflammation T82.7 ✓
      mechanical
        breakdown T82.511 ✓
        displacement T82.521 ✓
        leakage T82.531 ✓
        malposition T82.521 ✓
        obstruction T82.591 ✓
        perforation T82.591 ✓
        protrusion T82.591 ✓

Complication(s) — *continued*
  arteriovenous — *continued*
    shunt, surgically created — *continued*
      pain T82.848 ✓
      specified type NEC T82.898 ✓
      stenosis T82.858 ✓
      thrombosis T82.868 ✓
  arthroplasty — *see* Complications, joint prosthesis
  artificial
    fertilization or insemination N98.9
      attempted introduction (of)
        embryo in embryo transfer N98.3
        ovum following in vitro fertilization N98.2
      hyperstimulation of ovaries N98.1
      infection N98.0
      specified NEC N98.8
    heart T82.9 ✓
      embolism T82.817 ✓
      fibrosis T82.827 ✓
      hemorrhage T82.837 ✓
      infection or inflammation T82.7 ✓
      mechanical
        breakdown T82.512 ✓
        displacement T82.522 ✓
        leakage T82.532 ✓
        malposition T82.522 ✓
        obstruction T82.592 ✓
        perforation T82.592 ✓
        protrusion T82.592 ✓
      pain T82.847 ✓
      specified type NEC T82.897 ✓
      stenosis T82.857 ✓
      thrombosis T82.867 ✓
    opening
      cecostomy — *see* Complications, colostomy
      colostomy — *see* Complications, colostomy
      cystostomy — *see* Complications, cystostomy
      enterostomy — *see* Complications, enterostomy
      gastrostomy — *see* Complications, gastrostomy
      ileostomy — *see* Complications, enterostomy
      jejunostomy — *see* Complications, enterostomy
      nephrostomy — *see* Complications, stoma, urinary tract
      tracheostomy — *see* Complications, tracheostomy
      ureterostomy — *see* Complications, stoma, urinary tract
      urethrostomy — *see* Complications, stoma, urinary tract
  balloon implant or device
    gastrointestinal T85.9 ✓
      embolism T85.818 ✓
      fibrosis T85.828 ✓
      hemorrhage T85.838 ✓
      infection and inflammation T85.79 ✓
      pain T85.848 ✓
      specified type NEC T85.898 ✓
      stenosis T85.858 ✓
      thrombosis T85.868 ✓
    vascular (counterpulsation) T82.9 ✓
      embolism T82.818 ✓
      fibrosis T82.828 ✓
      hemorrhage T82.838 ✓
      infection or inflammation T82.7 ✓
      mechanical
        breakdown T82.513 ✓
        displacement T82.523 ✓
        leakage T82.533 ✓
        malposition T82.523 ✓
        obstruction T82.593 ✓
        perforation T82.593 ✓
        protrusion T82.593 ✓
      pain T82.848 ✓
      specified type NEC T82.898 ✓
      stenosis T82.858 ✓
      thrombosis T82.868 ✓
  bariatric procedure
    gastric band procedure K95.09
      infection K95.01
    specified procedure NEC K95.89
      infection K95.81
  bile duct implant (prosthetic) T85.9 ✓
    embolism T85.818 ✓
    fibrosis T85.828 ✓
    hemorrhage T85.838 ✓

Complication(s) — *continued*
  bile duct implant — *continued*
    infection and inflammation T85.79 ✓
    mechanical
      breakdown T85.510 ✓
      displacement T85.520 ✓
      malfunction T85.510 ✓
      malposition T85.520 ✓
      obstruction T85.590 ✓
      perforation T85.590 ✓
      protrusion T85.590 ✓
      specified NEC T85.590 ✓
    pain T85.848 ✓
    specified type NEC T85.898 ✓
    stenosis T85.858 ✓
    thrombosis T85.868 ✓
  bladder device (auxiliary) — *see* Complications, genitourinary, device or implant, urinary system
  bleeding (postoperative) — *see* Complication, postoperative, hemorrhage
    intraoperative — *see* Complication, intraoperative, hemorrhage
  blood vessel graft — *see* Complications, graft, vascular
  bone
    device NEC T84.9 ✓
      embolism T84.81 ✓
      fibrosis T84.82 ✓
      hemorrhage T84.83 ✓
      infection or inflammation T84.7 ✓
      mechanical
        breakdown T84.318 ✓
        displacement T84.328 ✓
        malposition T84.328 ✓
        obstruction T84.398 ✓
        perforation T84.398 ✓
        protrusion T84.398 ✓
      pain T84.84 ✓
      specified type NEC T84.89 ✓
      stenosis T84.85 ✓
      thrombosis T84.86 ✓
    graft — *see* Complications, graft, bone
    growth stimulator (electrode) — *see* Complications, electronic stimulator device, bone
    marrow transplant — *see* Complications, transplant, bone, marrow
  brain neurostimulator (electrode) — *see* Complications, electronic stimulator device, brain
  breast implant (prosthetic) T85.9 ✓
    capsular contracture T85.44 ✓
    embolism T85.818 ✓
    fibrosis T85.828 ✓
    hemorrhage T85.838 ✓
    infection and inflammation T85.79 ✓
    mechanical
      breakdown T85.41 ✓
      displacement T85.42 ✓
      leakage T85.43 ✓
      malposition T85.42 ✓
      obstruction T85.49 ✓
      perforation T85.49 ✓
      protrusion T85.49 ✓
      specified NEC T85.49 ✓
    pain T85.848 ✓
    specified type NEC T85.898 ✓
    stenosis T85.858 ✓
    thrombosis T85.868 ✓
  bypass (*see also* Complications, prosthetic device or implant)
    aortocoronary — *see* Complications, coronary artery (bypass) graft
    arterial (*see also* Complications, graft, vascular)
      extremity — *see* Complications, extremity artery (bypass) graft
  cardiac (*see also* Disease, heart)
    device, implant or graft T82.9 ✓
      embolism T82.817 ✓
      fibrosis T82.827 ✓
      hemorrhage T82.837 ✓
      infection or inflammation T82.7 ✓
        valve prosthesis T82.6 ✓
      mechanical
        breakdown T82.519 ✓
          specified device NEC T82.518 ✓
        displacement T82.529 ✓
          specified device NEC T82.528 ✓
        leakage T82.539 ✓

✓ **Additional Character Required** — Refer to the Tabular List for Character Selection   Subterms under main terms may continue to next column or page

Complication(s) — *continued*
  cardiac (*see also* Disease, heart) — *continued*
    device, implant or graft — *continued*
      mechanical — *continued*
        leakage — *continued*
          specified device NEC T82.538 ☑
        malposition T82.529 ☑
          specified device NEC T82.528 ☑
        obstruction T82.599 ☑
          specified device NEC T82.598 ☑
        perforation T82.599 ☑
          specified device NEC T82.598 ☑
        protrusion T82.599 ☑
          specified device NEC T82.598 ☑
      pain T82.847 ☑
      specified type NEC T82.897 ☑
      stenosis T82.857 ☑
      thrombosis T82.867 ☑
  cardiovascular device, graft or implant T82.9 ☑
    aortic graft — *see* Complications, graft, vascular
    arteriovenous
      fistula, artificial — *see* Complication, arteriovenous, fistula, surgically created
      shunt — *see* Complication, arteriovenous, shunt, surgically created
    artificial heart — *see* Complication, artificial, heart
    balloon (counterpulsation) device — *see* Complication, balloon implant, vascular
    carotid artery graft — *see* Complications, graft, vascular
    coronary bypass graft — *see* Complication, coronary artery (bypass) graft
    dialysis catheter (vascular) — *see* Complication, catheter, dialysis
    electronic T82.9 ☑
      electrode T82.9 ☑
        embolism T82.817 ☑
        fibrosis T82.827 ☑
        hemorrhage T82.837 ☑
        infection T82.7 ☑
        mechanical
          breakdown T82.110 ☑
          displacement T82.120 ☑
          leakage T82.190 ☑
          obstruction T82.190 ☑
          perforation T82.190 ☑
          protrusion T82.190 ☑
          specified type NEC T82.190 ☑
        pain T82.847 ☑
        specified NEC T82.897 ☑
        stenosis T82.857 ☑
        thrombosis T82.867 ☑
      embolism T82.817 ☑
      fibrosis T82.827 ☑
      hemorrhage T82.837 ☑
      infection T82.7 ☑
      mechanical
        breakdown T82.119 ☑
        displacement T82.129 ☑
        leakage T82.199 ☑
        obstruction T82.199 ☑
        perforation T82.199 ☑
        protrusion T82.199 ☑
        specified type NEC T82.199 ☑
      pain T82.847 ☑
      pulse generator T82.9 ☑
        embolism T82.817 ☑
        fibrosis T82.827 ☑
        hemorrhage T82.837 ☑
        infection T82.7 ☑
        mechanical
          breakdown T82.111 ☑
          displacement T82.121 ☑
          leakage T82.191 ☑
          obstruction T82.191 ☑
          perforation T82.191 ☑
          protrusion T82.191 ☑
          specified type NEC T82.191 ☑
        pain T82.847 ☑
        specified NEC T82.897 ☑
        stenosis T82.857 ☑
        thrombosis T82.867 ☑
      specified condition NEC T82.897 ☑
      specified device NEC T82.9 ☑
        embolism T82.817 ☑
        fibrosis T82.827 ☑

Complication(s) — *continued*
  cardiovascular device, graft or implant — *continued*
    electronic — *continued*
      specified device — *continued*
        hemorrhage T82.837 ☑
        infection T82.7 ☑
        mechanical
          breakdown T82.118 ☑
          displacement T82.128 ☑
          leakage T82.198 ☑
          obstruction T82.198 ☑
          perforation T82.198 ☑
          protrusion T82.198 ☑
          specified type NEC T82.198 ☑
        pain T82.847 ☑
        specified NEC T82.897 ☑
        stenosis T82.857 ☑
        thrombosis T82.867 ☑
      stenosis T82.857 ☑
      thrombosis T82.867 ☑
    extremity artery graft — *see* Complication, extremity artery (bypass) graft
    femoral artery graft — *see* Complication, extremity artery (bypass) graft
    heart
      transplant — *see* Complication, transplant, heart
      valve — *see* Complication, prosthetic device, heart valve
        graft — *see* Complication, heart, valve, graft
    heart-lung transplant — *see* Complication, transplant, heart, with lung
    infection or inflammation T82.7 ☑
    umbrella device — *see* Complication, umbrella device, vascular
    vascular graft (or anastomosis) — *see* Complication, graft, vascular
  carotid artery (bypass) graft — *see* Complications, graft, vascular
  catheter (device) NEC (*see also* Complications, prosthetic device or implant)
    cranial infusion
      infection and inflammation T85.735 ☑
      mechanical
        breakdown T85.610 ☑
        displacement T85.620 ☑
        leakage T85.630 ☑
        malfunction T85.690 ☑
        malposition T85.620 ☑
        obstruction T85.690 ☑
        perforation T85.690 ☑
        protrusion T85.690 ☑
        specified NEC T85.690 ☑
    cystostomy T83.9 ☑
      embolism T83.81 ☑
      fibrosis T83.82 ☑
      hemorrhage T83.83 ☑
      infection and inflammation T83.510 ☑
      mechanical
        breakdown T83.010 ☑
        displacement T83.020 ☑
        leakage T83.030 ☑
        malposition T83.020 ☑
        obstruction T83.090 ☑
        perforation T83.090 ☑
        protrusion T83.090 ☑
        specified NEC T83.090 ☑
      pain T83.84 ☑
      specified type NEC T83.89 ☑
      stenosis T83.85 ☑
      thrombosis T83.86 ☑
    dialysis (vascular) T82.9 ☑
      embolism T82.818 ☑
      fibrosis T82.828 ☑
      hemorrhage T82.838 ☑
      infection and inflammation T82.7 ☑
      intraperitoneal — *see* Complications, catheter, intraperitoneal
      mechanical
        breakdown T82.41 ☑
        displacement T82.42 ☑
        leakage T82.43 ☑
        malposition T82.42 ☑
        obstruction T82.49 ☑
        perforation T82.49 ☑

Complication(s) — *continued*
  catheter (*see also* Complications, prosthetic device or implant) — *continued*
    dialysis — *continued*
      mechanical — *continued*
        protrusion T82.49 ☑
      pain T82.848 ☑
      specified type NEC T82.898 ☑
      stenosis T82.858 ☑
      thrombosis T82.868 ☑
    epidural infusion T85.9 ☑
      embolism T85.810 ☑
      fibrosis T85.820 ☑
      hemorrhage T85.830 ☑
      infection and inflammation T85.735 ☑
      mechanical
        breakdown T85.610 ☑
        displacement T85.620 ☑
        leakage T85.630 ☑
        malfunction T85.610 ☑
        malposition T85.620 ☑
        obstruction T85.690 ☑
        perforation T85.690 ☑
        protrusion T85.690 ☑
        specified NEC T85.690 ☑
      pain T85.840 ☑
      specified type NEC T85.890 ☑
      stenosis T85.850 ☑
      thrombosis T85.860 ☑
    intraperitoneal dialysis T85.9 ☑
      embolism T85.818 ☑
      fibrosis T85.828 ☑
      hemorrhage T85.838 ☑
      infection and inflammation T85.71 ☑
      mechanical
        breakdown T85.611 ☑
        displacement T85.621 ☑
        leakage T85.631 ☑
        malfunction T85.611 ☑
        malposition T85.621 ☑
        obstruction T85.691 ☑
        perforation T85.691 ☑
        protrusion T85.691 ☑
        specified NEC T85.691 ☑
      pain T85.848 ☑
      specified type NEC T85.898 ☑
      stenosis T85.858 ☑
      thrombosis T85.868 ☑
    intrathecal infusion
      infection and inflammation T85.735 ☑
      mechanical
        breakdown T85.610 ☑
        displacement T85.620 ☑
        leakage T85.630 ☑
        malfunction T85.690 ☑
        malposition T85.620 ☑
        obstruction T85.690 ☑
        perforation T85.690 ☑
        protrusion T85.690 ☑
        specified NEC T85.690 ☑
    intravenous infusion T82.9 ☑
      embolism T82.818 ☑
      fibrosis T82.828 ☑
      hemorrhage T82.838 ☑
      infection or inflammation T82.7 ☑
      mechanical
        breakdown T82.514 ☑
        displacement T82.524 ☑
        leakage T82.534 ☑
        malposition T82.524 ☑
        obstruction T82.594 ☑
        perforation T82.594 ☑
        protrusion T82.594 ☑
      pain T82.848 ☑
      specified type NEC T82.898 ☑
      stenosis T82.858 ☑
      thrombosis T82.868 ☑
    spinal infusion
      infection and inflammation T85.735 ☑
      mechanical
        breakdown T85.610 ☑
        displacement T85.620 ☑
        leakage T85.630 ☑
        malfunction T85.690 ☑
        malposition T85.620 ☑
        obstruction T85.690 ☑

Complication(s) — *continued*
catheter (*see also* Complications, prosthetic device or implant) — *continued*
  spinal infusion — *continued*
    mechanical — *continued*
      perforation T85.690 ☑
      protrusion T85.690 ☑
      specified NEC T85.690 ☑
    subarachnoid infusion
      infection and inflammation T85.735 ☑
      mechanical
        breakdown T85.610 ☑
        displacement T85.620 ☑
        leakage T85.630 ☑
        malfunction T85.690 ☑
        malposition T85.620 ☑
        obstruction T85.690 ☑
        perforation T85.690 ☑
        protrusion T85.690 ☑
        specified NEC T85.690 ☑
    subdural infusion T85.9 ☑
      embolism T85.810 ☑
      fibrosis T85.820 ☑
      hemorrhage T85.830 ☑
      infection and inflammation T85.735 ☑
      mechanical
        breakdown T85.610 ☑
        displacement T85.620 ☑
        leakage T85.630 ☑
        malfunction T85.610 ☑
        malposition T85.620 ☑
        obstruction T85.690 ☑
        perforation T85.690 ☑
        protrusion T85.690 ☑
        specified NEC T85.690 ☑
      pain T85.840 ☑
      specified type NEC T85.890 ☑
      stenosis T85.850 ☑
      thrombosis T85.860 ☑
  urethral T83.9 ☑
    displacement T83.028 ☑
    embolism T83.81 ☑
    fibrosis T83.82 ☑
    hemorrhage T83.83 ☑
    indwelling
      breakdown T83.011 ☑
      displacement T83.021 ☑
      infection and inflammation T83.511 ☑
      leakage T83.031 ☑
      specified complication NEC T83.091 ☑
    infection and inflammation T83.511 ☑
    leakage T83.038 ☑
    malposition T83.028 ☑
    mechanical
      breakdown T83.011 ☑
    obstruction (mechanical) T83.091 ☑
    pain T83.84 ☑
    perforation T83.091 ☑
    protrusion T83.091 ☑
    specified type NEC T83.091 ☑
    stenosis T83.85 ☑
    thrombosis T83.86 ☑
  urinary NEC
    breakdown T83.018 ☑
    displacement T83.028 ☑
    infection and inflammation T83.518 ☑
    leakage T83.038 ☑
    specified complication NEC T83.098 ☑
cecostomy (stoma) — *see* Complications, colostomy
cesarean delivery wound NEC O90.89
  disruption O90.0
  hematoma O90.2
  infection (following delivery) O86.0
chemotherapy (antineoplastic) NEC T88.7 ☑
chin implant (prosthetic) — *see* Complication, prosthetic device or implant, specified NEC
circulatory system I99.8
  intraoperative I97.88
  postprocedural I97.89
    following cardiac surgery (*see also* Infarct, myocardium, associated with revascularization procedure) I97.19- ☑
      postcardiotomy syndrome I97.0
    hypertension I97.3
    lymphedema after mastectomy I97.2
    postcardiotomy syndrome I97.0

Complication(s) — *continued*
circulatory system — *continued*
  postprocedural — *continued*
    specified NEC I97.89
colostomy (stoma) K94.00
  hemorrhage K94.01
  infection K94.02
  malfunction K94.03
  mechanical K94.03
  specified complication NEC K94.09
contraceptive device, intrauterine — *see* Complications, intrauterine, contraceptive device
cord (umbilical) — *see* Complications, umbilical cord
corneal graft — *see* Complications, graft, cornea
coronary artery (bypass) graft T82.9 ☑
  atherosclerosis — *see* Arteriosclerosis, coronary (artery),
  embolism T82.818 ☑
  fibrosis T82.828 ☑
  hemorrhage T82.838 ☑
  infection and inflammation T82.7 ☑
  mechanical
    breakdown T82.211 ☑
    displacement T82.212 ☑
    leakage T82.213 ☑
    malposition T82.212 ☑
    obstruction T82.218 ☑
    perforation T82.218 ☑
    protrusion T82.218 ☑
    specified NEC T82.218 ☑
  pain T82.848 ☑
  specified type NEC T82.898 ☑
  stenosis T82.858 ☑
  thrombosis T82.868 ☑
counterpulsation device (balloon), intra- aortic — *see* Complications, balloon implant, vascular
cystostomy (stoma) N99.518
  catheter — *see* Complications, catheter, cystostomy
  hemorrhage N99.510
  infection N99.511
  malfunction N99.512
  specified type NEC N99.518
delivery (*see also* Complications, obstetric) O75.9
  procedure (instrumental) (manual) (surgical) O75.4
  specified NEC O75.89
dialysis (peritoneal) (renal) (*see also* Complications, infusion)
  catheter (vascular) — *see* Complication, catheter, dialysis
    peritoneal, intraperitoneal — *see* Complications, catheter, intraperitoneal
dorsal column (spinal) neurostimulator — *see* Complications, electronic stimulator device, spinal cord
drug NEC T88.7 ☑
ear procedure (*see also* Disorder, ear)
  intraoperative H95.88
    hematoma — *see* Complications, intraoperative, hemorrhage (hematoma) (of), ear
    hemorrhage — *see* Complications, intraoperative, hemorrhage (hematoma) (of), ear
    laceration — *see* Complications, intraoperative, puncture or laceration..., ear
    specified NEC H95.88
  postoperative H95.89
    external ear canal stenosis H95.81- ☑
    hematoma — *see* Complications, postprocedural, hematoma (of), ear
    hemorrhage — *see* Complications, postprocedural, hemorrhage (of), ear
    postmastoidectomy — *see* Complications, postmastoidectomy
    seroma — *see* Complications, postprocedural, seroma (of), mastoid process
    specified NEC H95.89
ectopic pregnancy O08.9
  damage to pelvic organs O08.6
  embolism O08.2
  genital infection O08.0
  hemorrhage (delayed) (excessive) O08.1
  metabolic disorder O08.5
  renal failure O08.4
  shock O08.3
  specified type NEC O08.0
  venous complication NEC O08.7

Complication(s) — *continued*
electronic stimulator device
  bladder (urinary) — *see* Complications, electronic stimulator device, urinary
  bone T84.9 ☑
    breakdown T84.310 ☑
    displacement T84.320 ☑
    embolism T84.81 ☑
    fibrosis T84.82 ☑
    hemorrhage T84.83 ☑
    infection or inflammation T84.7 ☑
    malfunction T84.310 ☑
    malposition T84.320 ☑
    mechanical NEC T84.390 ☑
    obstruction T84.390 ☑
    pain T84.84 ☑
    perforation T84.390 ☑
    protrusion T84.390 ☑
    specified type NEC T84.89 ☑
    stenosis T84.85 ☑
    thrombosis T84.86 ☑
  brain T85.9 ☑
    embolism T85.810 ☑
    fibrosis T85.820 ☑
    hemorrhage T85.830 ☑
    infection and inflammation T85.731 ☑
    mechanical
      breakdown T85.110 ☑
      displacement T85.120 ☑
      leakage T85.190 ☑
      malposition T85.120 ☑
      obstruction T85.190 ☑
      perforation T85.190 ☑
      protrusion T85.190 ☑
      specified NEC T85.190 ☑
    pain T85.840 ☑
    specified type NEC T85.890 ☑
    stenosis T85.850 ☑
    thrombosis T85.860 ☑
  cardiac (defibrillator) (pacemaker) — *see* Complications, cardiovascular device or implant, electronic
  generator (brain) (gastric) (peripheral) (sacral) (spinal)
    breakdown T85.113 ☑
    displacement T85.123 ☑
    leakage T85.193 ☑
    malposition T85.123 ☑
    obstruction T85.193 ☑
    perforation T85.193 ☑
    protrusion T85.193 ☑
    specified type NEC T85.193 ☑
  muscle T84.9 ☑
    breakdown T84.418 ☑
    displacement T84.428 ☑
    embolism T84.81 ☑
    fibrosis T84.82 ☑
    hemorrhage T84.83 ☑
    infection or inflammation T84.7 ☑
    mechanical NEC T84.498 ☑
    pain T84.84 ☑
    specified type NEC T84.89 ☑
    stenosis T84.85 ☑
    thrombosis T84.86 ☑
  nervous system T85.9 ☑
    brain — *see* Complications, electronic stimulator device, brain
    cranial nerve — *see* Complications, electronic stimulator device, peripheral nerve
    embolism T85.810 ☑
    fibrosis T85.820 ☑
    gastric nerve — *see* Complications, electronic stimulator device, peripheral nerve
    hemorrhage T85.830 ☑
    infection and inflammation T85.738 ☑
    mechanical
      breakdown T85.118 ☑
      displacement T85.128 ☑
      leakage T85.199 ☑
      malposition T85.128 ☑
      obstruction T85.199 ☑
      perforation T85.199 ☑
      protrusion T85.199 ☑
      specified NEC T85.199 ☑
    pain T85.840 ☑

Complication(s) — *continued*
  electronic stimulator device — *continued*
    nervous system — *continued*
      peripheral nerve — *see* Complications, electron-
        ic stimulator device, peripheral nerve
      sacral nerve — *see* Complications, electronic
        stimulator device, peripheral nerve
      specified type NEC T85.890 ☑
      spinal cord — *see* Complications, electronic
        stimulator device, spinal cord
      stenosis T85.850 ☑
      thrombosis T85.860 ☑
      vagal nerve — *see* Complications, electronic
        stimulator device, peripheral nerve
    peripheral nerve T85.9 ☑
      embolism T85.810 ☑
      fibrosis T85.820 ☑
      hemorrhage T85.830 ☑
      infection and inflammation T85.732 ☑
      mechanical
        breakdown T85.111 ☑
        displacement T85.121 ☑
        leakage T85.191 ☑
        malposition T85.121 ☑
        obstruction T85.191 ☑
        perforation T85.191 ☑
        protrusion T85.191 ☑
        specified NEC T85.191 ☑
      pain T85.840 ☑
      specified type NEC T85.890 ☑
      stenosis T85.850 ☑
      thrombosis T85.860 ☑
    spinal cord T85.9 ☑
      embolism T85.810 ☑
      fibrosis T85.820 ☑
      hemorrhage T85.830 ☑
      infection and inflammation T85.733 ☑
      mechanical
        breakdown T85.112 ☑
        displacement T85.122 ☑
        leakage T85.192 ☑
        malposition T85.122 ☑
        obstruction T85.192 ☑
        perforation T85.192 ☑
        protrusion T85.192 ☑
        specified NEC T85.192 ☑
      pain T85.840 ☑
      specified type NEC T85.890 ☑
      stenosis T85.850 ☑
      thrombosis T85.860 ☑
    urinary T83.9 ☑
      embolism T83.81 ☑
      fibrosis T83.82 ☑
      hemorrhage T83.83 ☑
      infection and inflammation T83.598 ☑
      mechanical
        breakdown T83.110 ☑
        displacement T83.120 ☑
        malposition T83.120 ☑
        perforation T83.190 ☑
        protrusion T83.190 ☑
        specified NEC T83.190 ☑
      pain T83.84 ☑
      specified type NEC T83.89 ☑
      stenosis T83.85 ☑
      thrombosis T83.86 ☑
  electroshock therapy T88.9 ☑
    specified NEC T88.8 ☑
  endocrine E34.9
    postprocedural
      adrenal hypofunction E89.6
      hypoinsulinemia E89.1
      hypoparathyroidism E89.2
      hypopituitarism E89.3
      hypothyroidism E89.0
      ovarian failure E89.40
        asymptomatic E89.40
        symptomatic E89.41
      specified NEC E89.89
      testicular hypofunction E89.5
  endodontic treatment NEC M27.59
  enterostomy (stoma) K94.10
    hemorrhage K94.11
    infection K94.12
    malfunction K94.13
    mechanical K94.13

Complication(s) — *continued*
  enterostomy — *continued*
    specified complication NEC K94.19
  episiotomy, disruption O90.1
  esophageal anti-reflux device T85.9 ☑
    embolism T85.818 ☑
    fibrosis T85.828 ☑
    hemorrhage T85.838 ☑
    infection and inflammation T85.79 ☑
    mechanical
      breakdown T85.511 ☑
      displacement T85.521 ☑
      malfunction T85.511 ☑
      malposition T85.521 ☑
      obstruction T85.591 ☑
      perforation T85.591 ☑
      protrusion T85.591 ☑
      specified NEC T85.591 ☑
    pain T85.848 ☑
    specified type NEC T85.898 ☑
    stenosis T85.858 ☑
    thrombosis T85.868 ☑
  esophagostomy K94.30
    hemorrhage K94.31
    infection K94.32
    malfunction K94.33
    mechanical K94.33
    specified complication NEC K94.39
  extracorporeal circulation T80.90 ☑
  extremity artery (bypass) graft T82.9 ☑
    arteriosclerosis — *see* Arteriosclerosis, extremities,
      bypass graft
    embolism T82.818 ☑
    fibrosis T82.828 ☑
    hemorrhage T82.838 ☑
    infection and inflammation T82.7 ☑
    mechanical
      breakdown T82.318 ☑
        femoral artery T82.312 ☑
      displacement T82.328 ☑
        femoral artery T82.322 ☑
      leakage T82.338 ☑
        femoral artery T82.332 ☑
      malposition T82.328 ☑
        femoral artery T82.322 ☑
      obstruction T82.398 ☑
        femoral artery T82.392 ☑
      perforation T82.398 ☑
        femoral artery T82.392 ☑
      protrusion T82.398 ☑
        femoral artery T82.392 ☑
    pain T82.848 ☑
    specified type NEC T82.898 ☑
    stenosis T82.858 ☑
    thrombosis T82.868 ☑
  eye H57.9
    corneal graft — *see* Complications, graft, cornea
    implant (prosthetic) T85.9 ☑
      embolism T85.818 ☑
      fibrosis T85.828 ☑
      hemorrhage T85.838 ☑
      infection and inflammation T85.79 ☑
      mechanical
        breakdown T85.318 ☑
        displacement T85.328 ☑
        leakage T85.398 ☑
        malposition T85.328 ☑
        obstruction T85.398 ☑
        perforation T85.398 ☑
        protrusion T85.398 ☑
        specified NEC T85.398 ☑
      pain T85.848 ☑
      specified type NEC T85.898 ☑
      stenosis T85.858 ☑
      thrombosis T85.868 ☑
    intraocular lens — *see* Complications, intraocular
      lens
    orbital prosthesis — *see* Complications, orbital
      prosthesis
  female genital N94.9
    device, implant or graft NEC — *see* Complications,
      genitourinary, device or implant, genital tract
  femoral artery (bypass) graft — *see* Complication, ex-
    tremity artery (bypass) graft
  fixation device, internal (orthopedic) T84.9 ☑
    infection and inflammation T84.60 ☑

Complication(s) — *continued*
  fixation device, internal — *continued*
    infection and inflammation — *continued*
      arm T84.61- ☑
        humerus T84.61- ☑
        radius T84.61- ☑
        ulna T84.61- ☑
      leg T84.629 ☑
        femur T84.62- ☑
        fibula T84.62- ☑
        tibia T84.62- ☑
      specified site NEC T84.89 ☑
      spine T84.63 ☑
    mechanical
      breakdown
        limb T84.119 ☑
          carpal T84.210 ☑
          femur T84.11- ☑
          fibula T84.11- ☑
          humerus T84.11- ☑
          metacarpal T84.210 ☑
          metatarsal T84.213 ☑
          phalanx
            foot T84.213 ☑
            hand T84.210 ☑
          radius T84.11- ☑
          tarsal T84.213 ☑
          tibia T84.11- ☑
          ulna T84.11- ☑
        specified bone NEC T84.218 ☑
        spine T84.216 ☑
      displacement
        limb T84.129 ☑
          carpal T84.220 ☑
          femur T84.12- ☑
          fibula T84.12- ☑
          humerus T84.12- ☑
          metacarpal T84.220 ☑
          metatarsal T84.223 ☑
          phalanx
            foot T84.223 ☑
            hand T84.220 ☑
          radius T84.12- ☑
          tarsal T84.223 ☑
          tibia T84.12- ☑
          ulna T84.12- ☑
        specified bone NEC T84.228 ☑
        spine T84.226 ☑
      malposition — *see* Complications, fixation de-
        vice, internal, mechanical, displacement
      obstruction — *see* Complications, fixation de-
        vice, internal, mechanical, specified type
        NEC
      perforation — *see* Complications, fixation de-
        vice, internal, mechanical, specified type
        NEC
      protrusion — *see* Complications, fixation de-
        vice, internal, mechanical, specified type
        NEC
      specified type NEC
        limb T84.199 ☑
          carpal T84.290 ☑
          femur T84.19- ☑
          fibula T84.19- ☑
          humerus T84.19- ☑
          metacarpal T84.290 ☑
          metatarsal T84.293 ☑
          phalanx
            foot T84.293 ☑
            hand T84.290 ☑
          radius T84.19- ☑
          tarsal T84.293 ☑
          tibia T84.19- ☑
          ulna T84.19- ☑
        specified bone NEC T84.298 ☑
        vertebra T84.296 ☑
    specified type NEC T84.89 ☑
      embolism T84.81 ☑
      fibrosis T84.82 ☑
      hemorrhage T84.83 ☑
      pain T84.84 ☑
      specified complication NEC T84.89 ☑
      stenosis T84.85 ☑
      thrombosis T84.86 ☑
  following
    acute myocardial infarction NEC I23.8

Complication — *continued*
following — *continued*
acute myocardial infarction — *continued*
aneurysm (false) (of cardiac wall) (of heart wall)
(ruptured) I23.3
angina I23.7
atrial
septal defect I23.1
thrombosis I23.6
cardiac wall rupture I23.3
chordae tendinae rupture I23.4
defect
septal
atrial (heart) I23.1
ventricular (heart) I23.2
hemopericardium I23.0
papillary muscle rupture I23.5
rupture
cardiac wall I23.3
with hemopericardium I23.0
chordae tendineae I23.4
papillary muscle I23.5
specified NEC I23.8
thrombosis
atrium I23.6
auricular appendage I23.6
ventricle (heart) I23.6
ventricular
septal defect I23.2
thrombosis I23.6
ectopic or molar pregnancy O08.9
cardiac arrest O08.81
sepsis O08.82
specified type NEC O08.89
urinary tract infection O08.83
termination of pregnancy — *see* Abortion
gastrointestinal K92.9
bile duct prosthesis — *see* Complications, bile duct
implant
esophageal anti-reflux device — *see* Complications,
esophageal anti-reflux device
postoperative
colostomy — *see* Complications, colostomy
dumping syndrome K91.1
enterostomy — *see* Complications, enterostomy
gastrostomy — *see* Complications, gastrostomy
malabsorption NEC K91.2
obstruction (*see also* Obstruction, intestine,
postoperative) K91.30
postcholecystectomy syndrome K91.5
specified NEC K91.89
vomiting after GI surgery K91.0
prosthetic device or implant
bile duct prosthesis — *see* Complications, bile
duct implant
esophageal anti-reflux device — *see* Complications, esophageal anti-reflux device
specified type NEC
embolism T85.818 ☑
fibrosis T85.828 ☑
hemorrhage T85.838 ☑
mechanical
breakdown T85.518 ☑
displacement T85.528 ☑
malfunction T85.518 ☑
malposition T85.528 ☑
obstruction T85.598 ☑
perforation T85.598 ☑
protrusion T85.598 ☑
specified NEC T85.598 ☑
pain T85.848 ☑
specified complication NEC T85.898 ☑
stenosis T85.858 ☑
thrombosis T85.868 ☑
gastrostomy (stoma) K94.20
hemorrhage K94.21
infection K94.22
malfunction K94.23
mechanical K94.23
specified complication NEC K94.29
genitourinary
device or implant T83.9 ☑
genital tract T83.9 ☑
infection or inflammation T83.69 ☑
intrauterine contraceptive device — *see*
Complications, intrauterine, contraceptive device

Complication(s) — *continued*
genitourinary — *continued*
device or implant — *continued*
genital tract — *continued*
mechanical — *see* Complications, by device,
mechanical
mesh — *see* Complications, mesh
penile prosthesis — *see* Complications,
prosthetic device, penile
specified type NEC T83.89 ☑
embolism T83.81 ☑
fibrosis T83.82 ☑
hemorrhage T83.83 ☑
pain T83.84 ☑
specified complication NEC T83.89 ☑
stenosis T83.85 ☑
thrombosis T83.86 ☑
vaginal mesh — *see* Complications, mesh
urinary system T83.9 ☑
cystostomy catheter — *see* Complication,
catheter, cystostomy
electronic stimulator — *see* Complications,
electronic stimulator device, urinary
indwelling urethral catheter — *see* Complications, catheter, urethral, indwelling
infection or inflammation T83.598 ☑
indwelling urethral catheter T83.511 ☑
kidney transplant — *see* Complication,
transplant, kidney
organ graft — *see* Complication, graft, urinary organ
specified type NEC T83.89 ☑
embolism T83.81 ☑
fibrosis T83.82 ☑
hemorrhage T83.83 ☑
mechanical T83.198 ☑
breakdown T83.118 ☑
displacement T83.128 ☑
malfunction T83.118 ☑
malposition T83.128 ☑
obstruction T83.198 ☑
perforation T83.198 ☑
protrusion T83.198 ☑
specified NEC T83.198 ☑
sphincter implant — *see* Complications,
implant, urinary sphincter
sphincter, implanted T83.191 ☑
stent (ileal conduit) (nephroureteral)
T83.193 ☑
pain T83.84 ☑
specified complication NEC T83.89 ☑
stenosis T83.85 ☑
thrombosis T83.86 ☑
ureteral indwelling T83.192 ☑
postprocedural
pelvic peritoneal adhesions N99.4
renal failure N99.0
specified NEC N99.89
stoma — *see* Complications, stoma, urinary
tract
urethral stricture — *see* Stricture, urethra,
postprocedural
vaginal
adhesions N99.2
vault prolapse N99.3
graft (bypass) (patch) (*see also* Complications, prosthetic device or implant)
aorta — *see* Complications, graft, vascular
arterial — *see* Complication, graft, vascular
bone T86.839
failure T86.831
infection T86.832
mechanical T84.318 ☑
breakdown T84.318 ☑
displacement T84.328 ☑
protrusion T84.398 ☑
specified type NEC T84.398 ☑
rejection T86.830
specified type NEC T86.838
carotid artery — *see* Complications, graft, vascular
cornea T86.849
failure T86.841
infection T86.842
mechanical T85.398 ☑
breakdown T85.318 ☑
displacement T85.328 ☑
protrusion T85.398 ☑

Complication(s) — *continued*
graft (*see also* Complications, prosthetic device or implant) — *continued*
cornea — *continued*
mechanical — *continued*
specified type NEC T85.398 ☑
rejection T86.840
retroprosthetic membrane T85.398 ☑
specified type NEC T86.848
femoral artery (bypass) — *see* Complication, extremity artery (bypass) graft
genital organ or tract — *see* Complications, genitourinary, device or implant, genital tract
muscle T84.9 ☑
breakdown T84.410 ☑
displacement T84.420 ☑
embolism T84.81 ☑
fibrosis T84.82 ☑
hemorrhage T84.83 ☑
infection and inflammation T84.7 ☑
mechanical NEC T84.490 ☑
pain T84.84 ☑
specified type NEC T84.89 ☑
stenosis T84.85 ☑
thrombosis T84.86 ☑
nerve — *see* Complication, prosthetic device or
implant, specified NEC
skin — *see* Complications, prosthetic device or
implant, skin graft
tendon T84.9 ☑
breakdown T84.410 ☑
displacement T84.420 ☑
embolism T84.81 ☑
fibrosis T84.82 ☑
hemorrhage T84.83 ☑
infection and inflammation T84.7 ☑
mechanical NEC T84.490 ☑
pain T84.84 ☑
specified type NEC T84.89 ☑
stenosis T84.85 ☑
thrombosis T84.86 ☑
urinary organ T83.9 ☑
embolism T83.81 ☑
fibrosis T83.82 ☑
hemorrhage T83.83 ☑
infection and inflammation T83.598 ☑
indwelling urethral catheter T83.511 ☑
mechanical
breakdown T83.21 ☑
displacement T83.22 ☑
erosion T83.24 ☑
exposure T83.25 ☑
leakage T83.23 ☑
malposition T83.22 ☑
obstruction T83.29 ☑
perforation T83.29 ☑
protrusion T83.29 ☑
specified NEC T83.29 ☑
pain T83.84 ☑
specified type NEC T83.89 ☑
stenosis T83.85 ☑
thrombosis T83.86 ☑
vascular T82.9 ☑
embolism T82.818 ☑
femoral artery — *see* Complication, extremity
artery (bypass) graft
fibrosis T82.828 ☑
hemorrhage T82.838 ☑
mechanical
breakdown T82.319 ☑
aorta (bifurcation) T82.310 ☑
carotid artery T82.311 ☑
specified vessel NEC T82.318 ☑
displacement T82.329 ☑
aorta (bifurcation) T82.320 ☑
carotid artery T82.321 ☑
specified vessel NEC T82.328 ☑
leakage T82.339 ☑
aorta (bifurcation) T82.330 ☑
carotid artery T82.331 ☑
specified vessel NEC T82.338 ☑
malposition T82.329 ☑
aorta (bifurcation) T82.320 ☑
carotid artery T82.321 ☑
specified vessel NEC T82.328 ☑
obstruction T82.399 ☑

Complication(s) — *continued*
 graft (*see also* Complications, prosthetic device or implant) — *continued*
  vascular — *continued*
   mechanical — *continued*
    obstruction — *continued*
     aorta (bifurcation) T82.390 ☑
     carotid artery T82.391 ☑
     specified vessel NEC T82.398 ☑
    perforation T82.399 ☑
     aorta (bifurcation) T82.390 ☑
     carotid artery T82.391 ☑
     specified vessel NEC T82.398 ☑
    protrusion T82.399 ☑
     aorta (bifurcation) T82.390 ☑
     carotid artery T82.391 ☑
     specified vessel NEC T82.398 ☑
   pain T82.848 ☑
   specified complication NEC T82.898 ☑
   stenosis T82.858 ☑
   thrombosis T82.868 ☑
 heart I51.9
  assist device
   infection and inflammation T82.7 ☑
  following acute myocardial infarction — *see* Complications, following, acute myocardial infarction
  postoperative — *see* Complications, circulatory system
  transplant — *see* Complication, transplant, heart and lung(s) — *see* Complications, transplant, heart, with lung
  valve
   graft (biological) T82.9 ☑
    embolism T82.817 ☑
    fibrosis T82.827 ☑
    hemorrhage T82.837 ☑
    infection and inflammation T82.7 ☑
    mechanical T82.228 ☑
     breakdown T82.221 ☑
     displacement T82.222 ☑
     leakage T82.223 ☑
     malposition T82.222 ☑
     obstruction T82.228 ☑
     perforation T82.228 ☑
     protrusion T82.228 ☑
    pain T82.847 ☑
    specified type NEC T82.897 ☑
    stenosis T82.857 ☑
    thrombosis T82.867 ☑
   prosthesis T82.9 ☑
    embolism T82.817 ☑
    fibrosis T82.827 ☑
    hemorrhage T82.837 ☑
    infection or inflammation T82.6 ☑
    mechanical T82.09 ☑
     breakdown T82.01 ☑
     displacement T82.02 ☑
     leakage T82.03 ☑
     malposition T82.02 ☑
     obstruction T82.09 ☑
     perforation T82.09 ☑
     protrusion T82.09 ☑
    pain T82.847 ☑
    specified type NEC T82.897 ☑
     mechanical T82.09 ☑
    stenosis T82.857 ☑
    thrombosis T82.867 ☑
 hematoma
  intraoperative — *see* Complication, intraoperative, hemorrhage
  postprocedural — *see* Complication, postprocedural, hematoma
 hemodialysis — *see* Complications, dialysis
 hemorrhage
  intraoperative — *see* Complication, intraoperative, hemorrhage
  postprocedural — *see* Complication, postprocedural, hemorrhage
 ileostomy (stoma) — *see* Complications, enterostomy
 immunization (procedure) — *see* Complications, vaccination
 implant (*see also* Complications, by site and type)
  urinary sphincter T83.9 ☑
   embolism T83.81 ☑
   fibrosis T83.82 ☑

Complication(s) — *continued*
 implant (*see also* Complications, by site and type) — *continued*
  urinary sphincter — *continued*
   hemorrhage T83.83 ☑
   infection and inflammation T83.591 ☑
   mechanical
    breakdown T83.111 ☑
    displacement T83.121 ☑
    leakage T83.191 ☑
    malposition T83.121 ☑
    obstruction T83.191 ☑
    perforation T83.191 ☑
    protrusion T83.191 ☑
    specified NEC T83.191 ☑
   pain T83.84 ☑
   specified type NEC T83.89 ☑
   stenosis T83.85 ☑
   thrombosis T83.86 ☑
 infusion (procedure) T80.90 ☑
  air embolism T80.0 ☑
  blood — *see* Complications, transfusion
  catheter — *see* Complications, catheter
  infection T80.29 ☑
  pump — *see* Complications, cardiovascular, device or implant
  sepsis T80.29 ☑
  serum reaction (*see also* Reaction, serum) T80.69 ☑
   anaphylactic shock (*see also* Shock, anaphylactic) T80.59 ☑
  specified type NEC T80.89 ☑
 inhalation therapy NEC T81.81 ☑
 injection (procedure) T80.90 ☑
  drug reaction — *see* Reaction, drug
  infection T80.29 ☑
  sepsis T80.29 ☑
  serum (prophylactic) (therapeutic) — *see* Complications, vaccination
  specified type NEC T80.89 ☑
  vaccine (any) — *see* Complications, vaccination
 inoculation (any) — *see* Complications, vaccination
 insulin pump
  infection and inflammation T85.72 ☑
  mechanical
   breakdown T85.614 ☑
   displacement T85.624 ☑
   leakage T85.633 ☑
   malposition T85.624 ☑
   obstruction T85.694 ☑
   perforation T85.694 ☑
   protrusion T85.694 ☑
   specified NEC T85.694 ☑
 intestinal pouch NEC K91.858
 intraocular lens (prosthetic) T85.9 ☑
  embolism T85.818 ☑
  fibrosis T85.828 ☑
  hemorrhage T85.838 ☑
  infection and inflammation T85.79 ☑
  mechanical
   breakdown T85.21 ☑
   displacement T85.22 ☑
   malposition T85.22 ☑
   obstruction T85.29 ☑
   perforation T85.29 ☑
   protrusion T85.29 ☑
   specified NEC T85.29 ☑
  pain T85.848 ☑
  specified type NEC T85.898 ☑
  stenosis T85.858 ☑
  thrombosis T85.868 ☑
 intraoperative (intraprocedural)
  cardiac arrest (*see also* Infarct, myocardium, associated with revascularization procedure)
   during cardiac surgery I97.710
   during other surgery I97.711
  cardiac functional disturbance NEC (*see also* Infarct, myocardium, associated with revascularization procedure)
   during cardiac surgery I97.790
   during other surgery I97.791
  hemorrhage (hematoma) (of)
   circulatory system organ or structure
    during cardiac bypass I97.411
    during cardiac catheterization I97.410
    during other circulatory system procedure I97.418

Complication(s) — *continued*
 intraoperative — *continued*
  hemorrhage — *continued*
   circulatory system organ or structure — *continued*
    during other procedure I97.42
   digestive system organ
    during procedure on digestive system K91.61
    during procedure on other organ K91.62
   ear
    during procedure on ear and mastoid process H95.21
    during procedure on other organ H95.22
   endocrine system organ or structure
    during procedure on endocrine system organ or structure E36.01
    during procedure on other organ E36.02
   eye and adnexa
    during ophthalmic procedure H59.11- ☑
    during other procedure H59.12- ☑
   genitourinary organ or structure
    during procedure on genitourinary organ or structure N99.61
    during procedure on other organ N99.62
   mastoid process
    during procedure on ear and mastoid process H95.21
    during procedure on other organ H95.22
   musculoskeletal structure
    during musculoskeletal surgery M96.810
    during non-orthopedic surgery M96.811
    during orthopedic surgery M96.810
   nervous system
    during a nervous system procedure G97.31
    during other procedure G97.32
   respiratory system
    during other procedure J95.62
    during procedure on respiratory system organ or structure J95.61
   skin and subcutaneous tissue
    during a dermatologic procedure L76.01
    during a procedure on other organ L76.02
   spleen
    during a procedure on other organ D78.02
    during a procedure on the spleen D78.01
  puncture or laceration (accidental) (unintentional) (of)
   brain
    during a nervous system procedure G97.48
    during other procedure G97.49
   circulatory system organ or structure
    during circulatory system procedure I97.51
    during other procedure I97.52
   digestive system
    during procedure on digestive system K91.71
    during procedure on other organ K91.72
   ear
    during procedure on ear and mastoid process H95.31
    during procedure on other organ H95.32
   endocrine system organ or structure
    during procedure on endocrine system organ or structure E36.11
    during procedure on other organ E36.12
   eye and adnexa
    during ophthalmic procedure H59.21- ☑
    during other procedure H59.22- ☑
   genitourinary organ or structure
    during procedure on genitourinary organ or structure N99.71
    during procedure on other organ N99.72
   mastoid process
    during procedure on ear and mastoid process H95.31
    during procedure on other organ H95.32
   musculoskeletal structure
    during musculoskeletal surgery M96.820
    during non-orthopedic surgery M96.821
    during orthopedic surgery M96.820
   nervous system
    during a nervous system procedure G97.48
    during other procedure G97.49
   respiratory system
    during other procedure J95.72
    during procedure on respiratory system organ or structure J95.71

Complication — Complication

▼ Subterms under main terms may continue to next column or page   ☑ Additional Character Required — Refer to the Tabular List for Character Selection   63

Complication(s) — *continued*
  intraoperative — *continued*
    puncture or laceration — *continued*
      skin and subcutaneous tissue
        during a dermatologic procedure L76.11
        during a procedure on other organ L76.12
      spleen
        during a procedure on other organ D78.12
        during a procedure on the spleen D78.11
    specified NEC
      circulatory system I97.88
      digestive system K91.81
      ear H95.88
      endocrine system E36.8
      eye and adnexa H59.88
      genitourinary system N99.81
      mastoid process H95.88
      musculoskeletal structure M96.89
      nervous system G97.81
      respiratory system J95.88
      skin and subcutaneous tissue L76.81
      spleen D78.81
  intraperitoneal catheter (dialysis) (infusion) — *see*
      Complications, catheter, intraperitoneal
  intrathecal infusion pump
    infection and inflammation T85.738 ☑
    mechanical
      breakdown T85.615 ☑
      displacement T85.625 ☑
      leakage T85.635 ☑
      malfunction T85.695 ☑
      malposition T85.625 ☑
      obstruction T85.695 ☑
      perforation T85.695 ☑
      protrusion T85.695 ☑
      specified NEC T85.695 ☑
  intrauterine
    contraceptive device
      embolism T83.81 ☑
      fibrosis T83.82 ☑
      hemorrhage T83.83 ☑
      infection and inflammation T83.69 ☑
      mechanical
        breakdown T83.31 ☑
        displacement T83.32 ☑
        malposition T83.32 ☑
        obstruction T83.39 ☑
        perforation T83.39 ☑
        protrusion T83.39 ☑
        specified NEC T83.39 ☑
      pain T83.84 ☑
      specified type NEC T83.89 ☑
      stenosis T83.85 ☑
      thrombosis T83.86 ☑
    procedure (fetal), to newborn P96.5
  jejunostomy (stoma) — *see* Complications, enterostomy
  joint prosthesis, internal T84.9 ☑
    breakage (fracture) T84.01- ☑
    dislocation T84.02- ☑
    fracture T84.01- ☑
    infection or inflammation T84.50 ☑
      hip T84.5- ☑
      knee T84.5- ☑
      specified joint NEC T84.59 ☑
    instability T84.02- ☑
    malposition — *see* Complications, joint prosthesis,
        mechanical, displacement
    mechanical
      breakage, broken T84.01- ☑
      dislocation T84.02- ☑
      fracture T84.01- ☑
      instability T84.02- ☑
      leakage — *see* Complications, joint prosthesis,
          mechanical, specified NEC
      loosening T84.039 ☑
        hip T84.03- ☑
        knee T84.03- ☑
        specified joint NEC T84.038 ☑
      obstruction — *see* Complications, joint prosthesis, mechanical, specified NEC
      perforation — *see* Complications, joint prosthesis, mechanical, specified NEC
      osteolysis T84.059 ☑
        hip T84.05- ☑
        knee T84.05- ☑
        other specified joint T84.058 ☑

Complication(s) — *continued*
  joint prosthesis, internal — *continued*
    mechanical — *continued*
      protrusion — *see* Complications, joint prosthesis, mechanical, specified NEC
      specified complication NEC T84.099 ☑
        hip T84.09- ☑
        knee T84.09- ☑
        other specified joint T84.098 ☑
      subluxation T84.02- ☑
      wear of articular bearing surface T84.069 ☑
        hip T84.06- ☑
        knee T84.06- ☑
        other specified joint T84.068 ☑
    specified joint NEC T84.89 ☑
      embolism T84.81 ☑
      fibrosis T84.82 ☑
      hemorrhage T84.83 ☑
      pain T84.84 ☑
      specified complication NEC T84.89 ☑
      stenosis T84.85 ☑
      thrombosis T84.86 ☑
    subluxation T84.02- ☑
  kidney transplant — *see* Complications, transplant, kidney
  labor O75.9
    specified NEC O75.89
  liver transplant (immune or nonimmune) — *see*
      Complications, transplant, liver
  lumbar puncture G97.1
    cerebrospinal fluid leak G97.0
    headache or reaction G97.1
  lung transplant — *see* Complications, transplant, lung
    and heart — *see* Complications, transplant, lung, with heart
  male genital N50.9
    device, implant or graft — *see* Complications, genitourinary, device or implant, genital tract
    postprocedural or postoperative — *see* Complications, genitourinary, postprocedural
    specified NEC N99.89
  mastoid (process) procedure
    intraoperative H95.88
      hematoma — *see* Complications, intraoperative, hemorrhage (hematoma) (of), mastoid process
      hemorrhage — *see* Complications, intraoperative, hemorrhage (hematoma) (of), mastoid process
      laceration — *see* Complications, intraoperative, puncture or laceration, mastoid process
      specified NEC H95.88
    postmastoidectomy — *see* Complications, postmastoidectomy
    postoperative H95.89
      external ear canal stenosis H95.81 ☑
      hematoma — *see* Complications, postprocedural, hematoma (of), mastoid process
      hemorrhage — *see* Complications, postprocedural, hemorrhage (of), mastoid process
      postmastoidectomy — *see* Complications, postmastoidectomy
      seroma — *see* Complications, postprocedural, seroma (of), mastoid process
      specified NEC H95.89
    mastoidectomy cavity — *see* Complications, postmastoidectomy
  mechanical — *see* Complications, by site and type, mechanical
  medical procedures (*see also* Complication(s), intraoperative) T88.9 ☑
  metabolic E88.9
    postoperative E89.89
      specified NEC E89.89
  molar pregnancy NOS O08.9
    damage to pelvic organs O08.6
    embolism O08.2
    genital infection O08.0
    hemorrhage (delayed) (excessive) O08.1
    metabolic disorder O08.5
    renal failure O08.4
    shock O08.3
    specified type NEC O08.0
    venous complication NEC O08.7

Complication(s) — *continued*
  musculoskeletal system (*see also* Complication, intraoperative (intraprocedural), by site)
    device, implant or graft NEC — *see* Complications, orthopedic, device or implant
      internal fixation (nail) (plate) (rod) — *see* Complications, fixation device, internal
      joint prosthesis — *see* Complications, joint prosthesis
    post radiation M96.89
      kyphosis M96.2
      scoliosis M96.5
      specified complication NEC M96.89
    postoperative (postprocedural) M96.89
      with osteoporosis — *see* Osteoporosis
      fracture following insertion of device — *see* Fracture, following insertion of orthopedic implant, joint prosthesis or bone plate
      joint instability after prosthesis removal M96.89
      lordosis M96.4
      postlaminectomy syndrome NEC M96.1
        kyphosis M96.3
      pseudarthrosis M96.0
      specified complication NEC M96.89
  nephrostomy (stoma) — *see* Complications, stoma, urinary tract, external NEC
  nervous system G98.8
    central G96.9
    device, implant or graft (*see also* Complication, prosthetic device or implant, specified NEC)
      electronic stimulator (electrode(s)) — *see* Complications, electronic stimulator device
      specified NEC
        infection and inflammation T85.738 ☑
        mechanical T85.695 ☑
          breakdown T85.615 ☑
          displacement T85.625 ☑
          leakage T85.635 ☑
          malfunction T85.695 ☑
          malposition T85.625 ☑
          obstruction T85.695 ☑
          perforation T85.695 ☑
          protrusion T85.695 ☑
          specified NEC T85.695 ☑
      ventricular shunt — *see* Complications, ventricular shunt
    electronic stimulator (electrode(s)) — *see* Complications, electronic stimulator device
    postprocedural G97.82
      intracranial hypotension G97.2
      specified NEC G97.82
      spinal fluid leak G97.0
  newborn, due to intrauterine (fetal) procedure P96.5
  nonabsorbable (permanent) sutures — *see* Complication, sutures, permanent
  obstetric O75.9
    procedure (instrumental) (manual) (surgical)
      specified NEC O75.4
    specified NEC O75.89
    surgical wound NEC O90.89
      hematoma O90.2
      infection O86.0
  ocular lens implant — *see* Complications, intraocular lens
  ophthalmologic
    postprocedural bleb — *see* Blebitis
  orbital prosthesis T85.9 ☑
    embolism T85.818 ☑
    fibrosis T85.828 ☑
    hemorrhage T85.838 ☑
    infection and inflammation T85.79 ☑
    mechanical
      breakdown T85.31- ☑
      displacement T85.32- ☑
      malposition T85.32- ☑
      obstruction T85.39- ☑
      perforation T85.39- ☑
      protrusion T85.39- ☑
      specified NEC T85.39- ☑
    pain T85.848 ☑
    specified type NEC T85.898 ☑
    stenosis T85.858 ☑
    thrombosis T85.868 ☑
  organ or tissue transplant (partial) (total) — *see* Complications, transplant

Complication(s) — *continued*
orthopedic (*see also* Disorder, soft tissue)
  device or implant T84.9 ☑
    bone
      device or implant — *see* Complication, bone, device NEC
      graft — *see* Complication, graft, bone
    breakdown T84.418 ☑
    displacement T84.428 ☑
    electronic bone stimulator — *see* Complications, electronic stimulator device, bone
    embolism T84.81 ☑
    fibrosis T84.82 ☑
    fixation device — *see* Complication, fixation device, internal
    hemorrhage T84.83 ☑
    infection or inflammation T84.7 ☑
    joint prosthesis — *see* Complication, joint prosthesis, internal
    malfunction T84.418 ☑
    malposition T84.428 ☑
    mechanical NEC T84.498 ☑
    muscle graft — *see* Complications, graft, muscle
    obstruction T84.498 ☑
    pain T84.84 ☑
    perforation T84.498 ☑
    protrusion T84.498 ☑
    specified complication NEC T84.89 ☑
    stenosis T84.85 ☑
    tendon graft — *see* Complications, graft, tendon
    thrombosis T84.86 ☑
  fracture (following insertion of device) — *see* Fracture, following insertion of orthopedic implant, joint prosthesis or bone plate
  postprocedural M96.89
    fracture — *see* Fracture, following insertion of orthopedic implant, joint prosthesis or bone plate
    postlaminectomy syndrome NEC M96.1
      kyphosis M96.3
      lordosis M96.4
    postradiation
      kyphosis M96.2
      scoliosis M96.5
    pseudarthrosis post-fusion M96.0
    specified type NEC M96.89
pacemaker (cardiac) — *see* Complications, cardiovascular device or implant, electronic
pancreas transplant — *see* Complications, transplant, pancreas
penile prosthesis (implant) — *see* Complications, prosthetic device, penile
perfusion NEC T80.90 ☑
perineal repair (obstetrical) NEC O90.89
  disruption O90.1
  hematoma O90.2
  infection (following delivery) O86.0
phototherapy T88.9 ☑
  specified NEC T88.8 ☑
postmastoidectomy NEC H95.19- ☑
  cyst, mucosal H95.13- ☑
  granulation H95.12- ☑
  inflammation, chronic H95.11- ☑
  recurrent cholesteatoma H95.0- ☑
postoperative — *see* Complications, postprocedural
  circulatory — *see* Complications, circulatory system
  ear — *see* Complications, ear
  endocrine — *see* Complications, endocrine
  eye — *see* Complications, eye
  lumbar puncture G97.1
    cerebrospinal fluid leak G97.0
  nervous system (central) (peripheral) — *see* Complications, nervous system
  respiratory system — *see* Complications, respiratory system
postprocedural (*see also* Complications, surgical procedure)
  cardiac arrest (*see also* Infarct, myocardium, associated with revascularization procedure)
    following cardiac surgery I97.120
    following other surgery I97.121
  cardiac functional disturbance NEC (*see also* Infarct, myocardium, associated with revascularization procedure)
    following cardiac surgery I97.190

Complication(s) — *continued*
postprocedural (*see also* Complications, surgical procedure) — *continued*
  cardiac functional disturbance (*see also* Infarct, myocardium, associated with revascularization procedure) — *continued*
    following other surgery I97.191
  cardiac insufficiency
    following cardiac surgery I97.110
    following other surgery I97.111
  chorioretinal scars following retinal surgery H59.81-
  following cataract surgery
    cataract (lens) fragments H59.02- ☑
    cystoid macular edema H59.03- ☑
    specified NEC H59.09- ☑
    vitreous (touch) syndrome H59.01- ☑
  heart failure
    following cardiac surgery I97.130
    following other surgery I97.131
  hematoma (of)
    circulatory system organ or structure
      following cardiac bypass I97.631
      following cardiac catheterization I97.630
      following other circulatory system procedure I97.638
      following other procedure I97.621
    digestive system
      following procedure on digestive system K91.870
      following procedure on other organ K91.871
    ear
      following other procedure H95.52
      following procedure on ear and mastoid process H95.51
    endocrine system
      following endocrine system procedure E89.820
      following other procedure E89.821
    eye and adnexa
      following ophthalmic procedure H59.33- ☑
      following other procedure H59.34- ☑
    genitourinary organ or structure
      following procedure on genitourinary organ or structure N99.840
      following procedure on other organ N99.841
    mastoid process
      following other procedure H95.52
      following procedure on ear and mastoid process H95.51
    musculoskeletal structure
      following musculoskeletal surgery M96.840
      following non-orthopedic surgery M96.841
      following orthopedic surgery M96.840
    nervous system
      following nervous system procedure G97.61
      following other procedure G97.62
    respiratory system
      following other procedure J95.861
      following procedure on respiratory system organ or structure J95.860
    skin and subcutaneous tissue
      following dermatologic procedure L76.31
      following procedure on other organ L76.32
    spleen
      following procedure on other organ D78.32
      following procedure on the spleen D78.31
  hemorrhage (of)
    circulatory system organ or structure
      following cardiac bypass I97.611
      following cardiac catheterization I97.610
      following other circulatory system procedure I97.618
      following other procedure I97.620
    digestive system
      following procedure on digestive system K91.840
      following procedure on other organ K91.841
    ear
      following other procedure H95.42
      following procedure on ear and mastoid process H95.41
    endocrine system
      following endocrine system procedure E89.810
      following other procedure E89.811

Complication(s) — *continued*
postprocedural (*see also* Complications, surgical procedure) — *continued*
  hemorrhage — *continued*
    eye and adnexa
      following ophthalmic procedure H59.31- ☑
      following other procedure H59.32- ☑
    genitourinary organ or structure
      following procedure on genitourinary organ or structure N99.820
      following procedure on other organ N99.821
    mastoid process
      following other procedure H95.42
      following procedure on ear and mastoid process H95.41
    musculoskeletal structure
      following musculoskeletal surgery M96.830
      following non-orthopedic surgery M96.831
      following orthopedic surgery M96.830
    nervous system
      following nervous system procedure G97.51
      following other procedure G97.52
    respiratory system
      following a respiratory system procedure J95.830
      following other procedure J95.831
    skin and subcutaneous tissue
      following a procedure on other organ L76.22
      following dermatologic procedure L76.21
    spleen
      following procedure on other organ D78.22
      following procedure on the spleen D78.21
  seroma (of)
    circulatory system organ or structure
      following cardiac bypass I97.641
      following cardiac catheterization I97.640
      following other circulatory system procedure I97.648
      following other procedure I97.622
    digestive system
      following procedure on digestive system K91.872
      following procedure on other organ K91.873
    ear
      following other procedure H95.54
      following procedure on ear and mastoid process H95.53
    endocrine system
      following endocrine system procedure E89.822
      following other procedure E89.823
    eye and adnexa
      following ophthalmic procedure H59.35- ☑
      following other procedure H59.36- ☑
    genitourinary organ or structure
      following procedure on genitourinary organ or structure N99.842
      following procedure on other organ N99.843
    mastoid process
      following other procedure H95.54
      following procedure on ear and mastoid process H95.53
    musculoskeletal structure
      following musculoskeletal surgery M96.842
      following non-orthopedic surgery M96.843
      following orthopedic surgery M96.842
    nervous system
      following nervous system procedure G97.63
      following other procedure G97.64
    respiratory system
      following other procedure J95.863
      following procedure on respiratory system organ or structure J95.862
    skin and subcutaneous tissue
      following dermatologic procedure L76.33
      following procedure on other organ L76.34
    spleen
      following procedure on other organ D78.34
      following procedure on the spleen D78.33
  specified NEC
    circulatory system I97.89
    digestive K91.89
    ear H95.89
    endocrine E89.89
    eye and adnexa H59.89
    genitourinary N99.89

Complication(s) — *continued*
 postprocedural (*see also* Complications, surgical procedure) — *continued*
  specified — *continued*
   mastoid process H95.89
   metabolic E89.89
   musculoskeletal structure M96.89
   nervous system G97.82
   respiratory system J95.89
   skin and subcutaneous tissue L76.82
   spleen D78.89
 pregnancy NEC — *see* Pregnancy, complicated by
 prosthetic device or implant T85.9 ☑
  bile duct — *see* Complications, bile duct implant
  breast — *see* Complications, breast implant
  bulking agent
   ureteral
    erosion T83.714 ☑
    exposure T83.724 ☑
   urethral
    erosion T83.713 ☑
    exposure T83.723 ☑
  cardiac and vascular NEC — *see* Complications, cardiovascular device or implant
  corneal transplant — *see* Complications, graft, cornea
  electronic nervous system stimulator — *see* Complications, electronic stimulator device
  epidural infusion catheter — *see* Complications, catheter, epidural
  esophageal anti-reflux device — *see* Complications, esophageal anti-reflux device
  genital organ or tract — *see* Complications, genitourinary, device or implant, genital tract
  specified NEC T83.79- ☑
  heart valve — *see* Complications, heart, valve, prosthesis
  infection or inflammation T85.79 ☑
   intestine transplant T86.892
   liver transplant T86.43
   lung transplant T86.812
   pancreas transplant T86.892
   skin graft T86.822
  intraocular lens — *see* Complications, intraocular lens
  intraperitoneal (dialysis) catheter — *see* Complications, catheter, intraperitoneal
  joint — *see* Complications, joint prosthesis, internal
  mechanical NEC T85.698 ☑
   dialysis catheter (vascular) (*see also* Complication, catheter, dialysis, mechanical)
    peritoneal — *see* Complications, catheter, intraperitoneal, mechanical
   gastrointestinal device T85.598 ☑
   ocular device T85.398 ☑
   subdural (infusion) catheter T85.690 ☑
   suture, permanent T85.692 ☑
    that for bone repair — *see* Complications, fixation device, internal (orthopedic), mechanical
   ventricular shunt
    breakdown T85.01 ☑
    displacement T85.02 ☑
    leakage T85.03 ☑
    malposition T85.02 ☑
    obstruction T85.09 ☑
    perforation T85.09 ☑
    protrusion T85.09 ☑
    specified NEC T85.09 ☑
  mesh
   erosion (to surrounding organ or tissue) T83.718 ☑
    urethral (into pelvic floor muscles) T83.712 ☑
    vaginal (into pelvic floor muscles) T83.711 ☑
   exposure (into surrounding organ or tissue) T83.728 ☑
    urethral (through urethral wall) T83.722 ☑
    vaginal (into vagina) (through vaginal wall) T83.721 ☑
  orbital — *see* Complications, orbital prosthesis
  penile T83.9 ☑
   embolism T83.81 ☑
   fibrosis T83.82 ☑
   hemorrhage T83.83 ☑
   infection and inflammation T83.61 ☑

Complication(s) — *continued*
 prosthetic device or implant — *continued*
  penile — *continued*
   mechanical
    breakdown T83.410 ☑
    displacement T83.420 ☑
    leakage T83.490 ☑
    malposition T83.420 ☑
    obstruction T83.490 ☑
    perforation T83.490 ☑
    protrusion T83.490 ☑
    specified NEC T83.490 ☑
   pain T83.84
   specified type NEC T83.89 ☑
   stenosis T83.85 ☑
   thrombosis T83.86 ☑
  prosthetic materials NEC
   erosion (to surrounding organ or tissue) T83.718 ☑
   exposure (into surrounding organ or tissue) T83.728 ☑
  skin graft T86.829
   artificial skin or decellularized allodermis
    embolism T85.818 ☑
    fibrosis T85.828 ☑
    hemorrhage T85.838 ☑
    infection and inflammation T85.79 ☑
    mechanical
     breakdown T85.613 ☑
     displacement T85.623 ☑
     malfunction T85.613 ☑
     malposition T85.623 ☑
     obstruction T85.693 ☑
     perforation T85.693 ☑
     protrusion T85.693 ☑
     specified NEC T85.693 ☑
    pain T85.848 ☑
    specified type NEC T85.898 ☑
    stenosis T85.858 ☑
    thrombosis T85.868 ☑
   failure T86.821
   infection T86.822
   rejection T86.820
   specified NEC T86.828
  sling
   urethral (female) (male)
    erosion T83.712 ☑
    exposure T83.722 ☑
  specified NEC T85.9 ☑
   embolism T85.818 ☑
   fibrosis T85.828 ☑
   hemorrhage T85.838 ☑
   infection and inflammation T85.79 ☑
   mechanical
    breakdown T85.618 ☑
    displacement T85.628 ☑
    leakage T85.638 ☑
    malfunction T85.618 ☑
    malposition T85.628 ☑
    obstruction T85.698 ☑
    perforation T85.698 ☑
    protrusion T85.698 ☑
    specified NEC T85.698 ☑
   pain T85.848 ☑
   specified type NEC T85.898 ☑
   stenosis T85.858 ☑
   thrombosis T85.868 ☑
  subdural infusion catheter — *see* Complications, catheter, subdural
  sutures — *see* Complications, sutures
  urinary organ or tract NEC — *see* Complications, genitourinary, device or implant, urinary system
  vascular — *see* Complications, cardiovascular device or implant
  ventricular shunt — *see* Complications, ventricular shunt (device)
 puerperium — *see* Puerperal
 puncture, spinal G97.1
  cerebrospinal fluid leak G97.0
  headache or reaction G97.1
 pyelogram N99.89
 radiation
  kyphosis M96.2
  scoliosis M96.5

Complication(s) — *continued*
 reattached
  extremity (infection) (rejection)
   lower T87.1X- ☑
   upper T87.0X- ☑
  specified body part NEC T87.2
 reconstructed breast
  asymmetry between native and reconstructed breast N65.1
  deformity N65.0
  disproportion between native and reconstructed breast N65.1
  excess tissue N65.0
  misshappen N65.0
 reimplant NEC (*see also* Complications, prosthetic device or implant)
  limb (infection) (rejection) — *see* Complications, reattached, extremity
  organ (partial) (total) — *see* Complications, transplant
  prosthetic device NEC — *see* Complications, prosthetic device
 renal N28.9
  allograft — *see* Complications, transplant, kidney
  dialysis — *see* Complications, dialysis
 respirator
  mechanical J95.850
  specified NEC J95.859
 respiratory system J98.9
  device, implant or graft — *see* Complication, prosthetic device or implant, specified NEC
  lung transplant — *see* Complications, prosthetic device or implant, lung transplant
  postoperative J95.89
   air leak J95.812
   Mendelson's syndrome (chemical pneumonitis) J95.4
   pneumothorax J95.811
   pulmonary insufficiency (acute) (after nonthoracic surgery) J95.2
    chronic J95.3
    following thoracic surgery J95.1
   respiratory failure (acute) J95.821
    acute and chronic J95.822
   specified NEC J95.89
   subglottic stenosis J95.5
   tracheostomy complication — *see* Complications, tracheostomy
  therapy T81.89 ☑
 sedation during labor and delivery O74.9
  cardiac O74.2
  central nervous system O74.3
  pulmonary NEC O74.1
 shunt (*see also* Complications, prosthetic device or implant)
  arteriovenous — *see* Complications, arteriovenous, shunt
  ventricular (communicating) — *see* Complications, ventricular shunt
 skin
  graft T86.829
   failure T86.821
   infection T86.822
   rejection T86.820
   specified type NEC T86.828
 spinal
  anesthesia — *see* Complications, anesthesia, spinal
  catheter (epidural) (subdural) — *see* Complications, catheter
  puncture or tap G97.1
   cerebrospinal fluid leak G97.0
   headache or reaction G97.1
 stent
  bile duct — *see* Complications, bile duct prosthesis
  ureteral indwelling
   breakdown T83.112 ☑
   displacement T83.122 ☑
   leakage T83.192 ☑
   malposition T83.122 ☑
   obstruction T83.192 ☑
   perforation T83.192 ☑
   protrusion T83.192 ☑
   specified NEC T83.192 ☑
  urinary NEC (ileal conduit) (nephroureteral) T83.193 ☑
   embolism T83.81 ☑
   fibrosis T83.82 ☑
   hemorrhage T83.83 ☑

Complication(s) — *continued*
  stent — *continued*
    urinary — *continued*
      infection and inflammation T83.593 ☑
      mechanical
        breakdown T83.113 ☑
        displacement T83.123 ☑
        leakage T83.193 ☑
        malposition T83.123 ☑
        obstruction T83.193 ☑
        perforation T83.193 ☑
        protrusion T83.193 ☑
        specified NEC T83.193 ☑
      pain T83.84 ☑
      specified type NEC T83.89 ☑
      stenosis T83.85 ☑
      thrombosis T83.86 ☑
    vascular
      end stent stenosis — *see* Restenosis, stent
      in stent stenosis — *see* Restenosis, stent
  stoma
    digestive tract
      colostomy — *see* Complications, colostomy
      enterostomy — *see* Complications, enterostomy
      esophagostomy — *see* Complications, esophagostomy
      gastrostomy — *see* Complications, gastrostomy
    urinary tract N99.528
      continent N99.538
        hemorrhage N99.530
        herniation N99.533
        infection N99.531
        malfunction N99.532
        specified type NEC N99.538
        stenosis N99.534
      cystostomy — *see* Complications, cystostomy
      external NOS N99.528
      hemorrhage N99.520
      herniation N99.523
      incontinent N99.528
        hemorrhage N99.520
        herniation N99.523
        infection N99.521
        malfunction N99.522
        specified type NEC N99.528
        stenosis N99.524
      infection N99.521
      malfunction N99.522
      specified type NEC N99.528
      stenosis N99.524
  stomach banding — *see* Complication(s), bariatric procedure
  stomach stapling — *see* Complication(s), bariatric procedure
  surgical material, nonabsorbable — *see* Complication, suture, permanent
  surgical procedure (on) T81.9 ☑
    amputation stump (late) — *see* Complications, amputation stump
    cardiac — *see* Complications, circulatory system
    cholesteatoma, recurrent — *see* Complications, postmastoidectomy, recurrent cholesteatoma
    circulatory (early) — *see* Complications, circulatory system
    digestive system — *see* Complications, gastrointestinal
    dumping syndrome (postgastrectomy) K91.1
    ear — *see* Complications, ear
    elephantiasis or lymphedema I97.89
      postmastectomy I97.2
    emphysema (surgical) T81.82 ☑
    endocrine — *see* Complications, endocrine
    eye — *see* Complications, eye
    fistula (persistent postoperative) T81.83 ☑
    foreign body inadvertently left in wound (sponge) (suture) (swab) — *see* Foreign body, accidentally left during a procedure
    gastrointestinal — *see* Complications, gastrointestinal
    genitourinary NEC N99.89
    hematoma
      intraoperative — *see* Complication, intraoperative, hemorrhage
      postprocedural — *see* Complication, postprocedural, hematoma

Complication(s) — *continued*
  surgical procedure — *continued*
    hemorrhage
      intraoperative — *see* Complication, intraoperative, hemorrhage
      postprocedural — *see* Complication, postprocedural, hemorrhage
    hepatic failure K91.82
    hyperglycemia (postpancreatectomy) E89.1
    hypoinsulinemia (postpancreatectomy) E89.1
    hypoparathyroidism (postparathyroidectomy) E89.2
    hypopituitarism (posthypophysectomy) E89.3
    hypothyroidism (post-thyroidectomy) E89.0
    intestinal obstruction (*see also* Obstruction, intestine, postoperative) K91.30
    intracranial hypotension following ventricular shunting (ventriculostomy) G97.2
    lymphedema I97.89
      postmastectomy I97.2
    malabsorption (postsurgical) NEC K91.2
      osteoporosis — *see* Osteoporosis, postsurgical malabsorption
    mastoidectomy cavity NEC — *see* Complications, postmastoidectomy
    metabolic E89.89
      specified NEC E89.89
    musculoskeletal — *see* Complications, musculoskeletal system
    nervous system (central) (peripheral) — *see* Complications, nervous system
    ovarian failure E89.40
      asymptomatic E89.40
      symptomatic E89.41
    peripheral vascular — *see* Complications, surgical procedure, vascular
    postcardiotomy syndrome I97.0
    postcholecystectomy syndrome K91.5
    postcommissurotomy syndrome I97.0
    postgastrectomy dumping syndrome K91.1
    postlaminectomy syndrome NEC M96.1
      kyphosis M96.3
    postmastectomy lymphedema syndrome I97.2
    postmastoidectomy cholesteatoma — *see* Complications, postmastoidectomy, recurrent cholesteatoma
    postvagotomy syndrome K91.1
    postvalvulotomy syndrome I97.0
    pulmonary insufficiency (acute) J95.2
      chronic J95.3
      following thoracic surgery J95.1
    reattached body part — *see* Complications, reattached
    respiratory — *see* Complications, respiratory system
    shock (hypovolemic) T81.19 ☑
    spleen (postoperative) D78.89
      intraoperative D78.81
    stitch abscess T81.4 ☑
    subglottic stenosis (postsurgical) J95.5
    testicular hypofunction E89.5
    transplant — *see* Complications, organ or tissue transplant
    urinary NEC N99.89
    vaginal vault prolapse (posthysterectomy) N99.3
    vascular (peripheral)
      artery T81.719 ☑
        mesenteric T81.710 ☑
        renal T81.711 ☑
        specified NEC T81.718 ☑
      vein T81.72 ☑
    wound infection T81.4 ☑
  suture, permanent (wire) NEC T85.9 ☑
    with repair of bone — *see* Complications, fixation device, internal
    embolism T85.818 ☑
    fibrosis T85.828 ☑
    hemorrhage T85.838 ☑
    infection and inflammation T85.79 ☑
    mechanical
      breakdown T85.612 ☑
      displacement T85.622 ☑
      malfunction T85.612 ☑
      malposition T85.622 ☑
      obstruction T85.692 ☑
      perforation T85.692 ☑
      protrusion T85.692 ☑

Complication(s) — *continued*
  suture, permanent — *continued*
    mechanical — *continued*
      specified NEC T85.692 ☑
    pain T85.848 ☑
    specified type NEC T85.898 ☑
    stenosis T85.858 ☑
    thrombosis T85.868 ☑
  tracheostomy J95.00
    granuloma J95.09
    hemorrhage J95.01
    infection J95.02
    malfunction J95.03
    mechanical J95.03
    obstruction J95.03
    specified type NEC J95.09
    tracheo-esophageal fistula J95.04
  transfusion (blood) (lymphocytes) (plasma) T80.92 ☑
    air emblism T80.0 ☑
    circulatory overload E87.71
    febrile nonhemolytic transfusion reaction R50.84
    hemochromatosis E83.111
    hemolysis T80.89 ☑
    hemolytic reaction (antigen unspecified) T80.919 ☑
    incompatibility reaction (antigen unspecified) T80.919 ☑
      ABO T80.30 ☑
        delayed serologic (DSTR) T80.39 ☑
        hemolytic transfusion reaction (HTR) (unspecified time after transfusion) T80.319 ☑
          acute (AHTR) (less than 24 hours after transfusion) T80.310 ☑
          delayed (DHTR) (24 hours or more after transfusion) T80.311 ☑
        specified NEC T80.39 ☑
      acute (antigen unspecified) T80.910 ☑
      delayed (antigen unspecified) T80.911 ☑
      delayed serologic (DSTR) T80.89 ☑
      non-ABO (minor antigens (Duffy) (Kell) (Kidd) (Lewis) (M) (N) (P) (S)) T80.A0 ☑ (*following* T80.4)
        delayed serologic (DSTR) T80.A9 ☑ (*following* T80.4)
        hemolytic transfusion reaction (HTR) (unspecified time after transfusion) T80.A19 ☑ (*following* T80.4)
          acute (AHTR) (less than 24 hours after transfusion) T80.A10 ☑ (*following* T80.4)
          delayed (DHTR) (24 hours or more after transfusion) T80.A11 ☑ (*following* T80.4)
        specified NEC T80.A9 ☑ (*following* T80.4)
      Rh (antigens (C) (c) (D) (E) (e)) (factor) T80.40 ☑
        delayed serologic (DSTR) T80.49 ☑
        hemolytic transfusion reaction (HTR) (unspecified time after transfusion) T80.419 ☑
          acute (AHTR) (less than 24 hours after transfusion) T80.410 ☑
          delayed (DHTR) (24 hours or more after transfusion) T80.411 ☑
        specified NEC T80.49 ☑
    infection T80.29 ☑
      acute T80.22- ☑
    reaction NEC T80.89 ☑
    sepsis T80.29 ☑
    shock T80.89 ☑
  transplant T86.90
    bone T86.839
      failure T86.831
      infection T86.832
      rejection T86.830
      specified type NEC T86.838
    bone marrow T86.00
      failure T86.02
      infection T86.03
      rejection T86.01
      specified type NEC T86.09
    cornea T86.849
      failure T86.841
      infection T86.842
      rejection T86.840
      specified type NEC T86.848
    failure T86.92

Complication(s) — *continued*
transplant — *continued*
heart T86.20
with lung T86.30
cardiac allograft vasculopathy T86.290
failure T86.32
infection T86.33
rejection T86.31
specified type NEC T86.39
failure T86.22
infection T86.23
rejection T86.21
specified type NEC T86.298
infection T86.93
intestine T86.859
failure T86.851
infection T86.852
rejection T86.850
specified type NEC T86.858
kidney T86.10
failure T86.12
infection T86.13
rejection T86.11
specified type NEC T86.19
liver T86.40
failure T86.42
infection T86.43
rejection T86.41
specified type NEC T86.49
lung T86.819
with heart T86.30
failure T86.32
infection T86.33
rejection T86.31
specified type NEC T86.39
failure T86.811
infection T86.812
rejection T86.810
specified type NEC T86.818
malignant neoplasm C80.2
pancreas T86.899
failure T86.891
infection T86.892
rejection T86.890
specified type NEC T86.898
peripheral blood stem cells T86.5
post-transplant lymphoproliferative disorder
(PTLD) D47.Z1 (*following* D47.4)
rejection T86.91
skin T86.829
failure T86.821
infection T86.822
rejection T86.820
specified type NEC T86.828
specified
tissue T86.899
failure T86.891
infection T86.892
rejection T86.890
specified type NEC T86.898
type NEC T86.99
stem cell (from peripheral blood) (from umbilical
cord) T86.5
umbilical cord stem cells T86.5
trauma (early) T79.9 ☑
specified NEC T79.8 ☑
ultrasound therapy NEC T88.9 ☑
umbilical cord NEC
complicating delivery O69.9 ☑
specified NEC O69.89 ☑
umbrella device, vascular T82.9 ☑
embolism T82.818 ☑
fibrosis T82.828 ☑
hemorrhage T82.838 ☑
infection or inflammation T82.7 ☑
mechanical
breakdown T82.515 ☑
displacement T82.525 ☑
leakage T82.535 ☑
malposition T82.525 ☑
obstruction T82.595 ☑
perforation T82.595 ☑
protrusion T82.595 ☑
pain T82.848 ☑
specified type NEC T82.898 ☑
stenosis T82.858 ☑
thrombosis T82.868 ☑

Complication(s) — *continued*
urethral catheter — *see* Complications, catheter, urethral, indwelling
vaccination T88.1 ☑
anaphylaxis NEC T80.52 ☑
arthropathy — *see* Arthropathy, postimmunization
cellulitis T88.0 ☑
encephalitis or encephalomyelitis G04.02
infection (general) (local) NEC T88.0 ☑
meningitis G03.8
myelitis G04.02
protein sickness T80.62 ☑
rash T88.1 ☑
reaction (allergic) T88.1 ☑
serum T80.62 ☑
sepsis T88.0 ☑
serum intoxication, sickness, rash, or other serum
reaction NEC T80.62 ☑
anaphylactic shock T80.52 ☑
shock (allergic) (anaphylactic) T80.52 ☑
vaccinia (generalized) (localized) T88.1 ☑
vas deferens device or implant — *see* Complications,
genitourinary, device or implant, genital tract
vascular I99.9
device or implant T82.9 ☑
embolism T82.818 ☑
fibrosis T82.828 ☑
hemorrhage T82.838 ☑
infection or inflammation T82.7 ☑
mechanical
breakdown T82.519 ☑
specified device NEC T82.518 ☑
displacement T82.529 ☑
specified device NEC T82.528 ☑
leakage T82.539 ☑
specified device NEC T82.538 ☑
malposition T82.529 ☑
specified device NEC T82.528 ☑
obstruction T82.599 ☑
specified device NEC T82.598 ☑
perforation T82.599 ☑
specified device NEC T82.598 ☑
protrusion T82.599 ☑
specified device NEC T82.598 ☑
pain T82.848 ☑
specified type NEC T82.898 ☑
stenosis T82.858 ☑
thrombosis T82.868 ☑
dialysis catheter — *see* Complication, catheter,
dialysis
following infusion, therapeutic injection or transfusion T80.1 ☑
graft T82.9 ☑
embolism T82.818 ☑
fibrosis T82.828 ☑
hemorrhage T82.838 ☑
mechanical
breakdown T82.319 ☑
aorta (bifurcation) T82.310 ☑
carotid artery T82.311 ☑
specified vessel NEC T82.318 ☑
displacement T82.329 ☑
aorta (bifurcation) T82.320 ☑
carotid artery T82.321 ☑
specified vessel NEC T82.328 ☑
leakage T82.339 ☑
aorta (bifurcation) T82.330 ☑
carotid artery T82.331 ☑
specified vessel NEC T82.338 ☑
malposition T82.329 ☑
aorta (bifurcation) T82.320 ☑
carotid artery T82.321 ☑
specified vessel NEC T82.328 ☑
obstruction T82.399 ☑
aorta (bifurcation) T82.390 ☑
carotid artery T82.391 ☑
specified vessel NEC T82.398 ☑
perforation T82.399 ☑
aorta (bifurcation) T82.390 ☑
carotid artery T82.391 ☑
specified vessel NEC T82.398 ☑
protrusion T82.399 ☑
aorta (bifurcation) T82.390 ☑
carotid artery T82.391 ☑
specified vessel NEC T82.398 ☑
pain T82.848 ☑

Complication(s) — *continued*
vascular — *continued*
graft — *continued*
specified complication NEC T82.898 ☑
stenosis T82.858 ☑
thrombosis T82.868 ☑
postoperative — *see* Complications, postoperative,
circulatory
vena cava device (filter) (sieve) (umbrella) — *see*
Complications, umbrella device, vascular
ventilation therapy NEC T81.81 ☑
ventilator
mechanical J95.850
specified NEC J95.859
ventricular (communicating) shunt (device) T85.9 ☑
embolism T85.810 ☑
fibrosis T85.820 ☑
hemorrhage T85.830 ☑
infection and inflammation T85.730 ☑
mechanical
breakdown T85.01 ☑
displacement T85.02 ☑
leakage T85.03 ☑
malposition T85.02 ☑
obstruction T85.09 ☑
perforation T85.09 ☑
protrusion T85.09 ☑
specified NEC T85.09 ☑
pain T85.840 ☑
specified type NEC T85.890 ☑
stenosis T85.850 ☑
thrombosis T85.860 ☑
wire suture, permanent (implanted) — *see* Complications, suture, permanent
Compressed air disease T70.3 ☑
Compression
with injury — *code by* Nature of injury
artery I77.1
celiac, syndrome I77.4
brachial plexus G54.0
brain (stem) G93.5
due to
contusion (diffuse) — *see* Injury, intracranial,
diffuse
focal — *see* Injury, intracranial, focal
injury NEC — *see* Injury, intracranial, diffuse
traumatic — *see* Injury, intracranial, diffuse
bronchus J98.09
cauda equina G83.4
celiac (artery) (axis) I77.4
cerebral — *see* Compression, brain
cervical plexus G54.2
cord
spinal — *see* Compression, spinal
umbilical — *see* Compression, umbilical cord
cranial nerve G52.9
eighth H93.3 ☑
eleventh G52.8
fifth G50.8
first G52.0
fourth — *see* Strabismus, paralytic, fourth nerve
ninth G52.1
second — *see* Disorder, nerve, optic
seventh G51.8
sixth — *see* Strabismus, paralytic, sixth nerve
tenth G52.2
third — *see* Strabismus, paralytic, third nerve
twelfth G52.3
diver's squeeze T70.3 ☑
during birth (newborn) P15.9
esophagus K22.2
eustachian tube — *see* Obstruction, eustachian tube,
cartilaginous
facies Q67.1
fracture
nontraumatic NOS — *see* Collapse, vertebra
pathological — *see* Fracture, pathological
traumatic — *see* Fracture, traumatic
heart — *see* Disease, heart
intestine — *see* Obstruction, intestine
laryngeal nerve, recurrent G52.2
with paralysis of vocal cords and larynx J38.00
bilateral J38.02
unilateral J38.01
lumbosacral plexus G54.1
lung J98.4
lymphatic vessel I89.0

☑ **Additional Character Required — Refer to the Tabular List for Character Selection** ▽ **Subterms under main terms may continue to next column or page**

Compression — *continued*
  medulla — *see also* Compression, brain
  nerve (*see also* Disorder, nerve) G58.9
    arm NEC — *see* Mononeuropathy, upper limb
    axillary G54.0
    cranial — *see* Compression, cranial nerve
    leg NEC — *see* Mononeuropathy, lower limb
    median (in carpal tunnel) — *see* Syndrome, carpal tunnel
    optic — *see* Disorder, nerve, optic
    plantar — *see* Lesion, nerve, plantar
    posterior tibial (in tarsal tunnel) — *see* Syndrome, tarsal tunnel
    root or plexus NOS (in) G54.9
      intervertebral disc disorder NEC — *see* Disorder, disc, with, radiculopathy
      with myelopathy — *see* Disorder, disc, with, myelopathy
      neoplastic disease (*see also* Neoplasm) D49.9 [G55]
      spondylosis — *see* Spondylosis, with radiculopathy
    sciatic (acute) — *see* Lesion, nerve, sciatic
    sympathetic G90.8
    traumatic — *see* Injury, nerve
    ulnar — *see* Lesion, nerve, ulnar
    upper extremity NEC — *see* Mononeuropathy, upper limb
  spinal (cord) G95.20
    by displacement of intervertebral disc NEC (*see also* Disorder, disc, with, myelopathy)
    nerve root NOS G54.9
      due to displacement of intervertebral disc NEC — *see* Disorder, disc, with, radiculopathy
      with myelopathy — *see* Disorder, disc, with, myelopathy
    specified NEC G95.29
    spondylogenic (cervical) (lumbar, lumbosacral) (thoracic) — *see* Spondylosis, with myelopathy NEC
      anterior — *see* Syndrome, anterior, spinal artery, compression
    traumatic — *see* Injury, spinal cord, by region
  subcostal nerve (syndrome) — *see* Mononeuropathy, upper limb, specified NEC
  sympathetic nerve NEC G90.8
  syndrome T79.5 ☑
  trachea J39.8
  ulnar nerve (by scar tissue) — *see* Lesion, nerve, ulnar
  umbilical cord
    complicating delivery O69.2 ☑
      cord around neck O69.1 ☑
      prolapse O69.0 ☑
      specified NEC O69.2 ☑
  ureter N13.5
  vein I87.1
  vena cava (inferior) (superior) I87.1
Compulsion, compulsive
  gambling F63.0
  neurosis F42.8
  personality F60.5
  states F42.8
  swearing F42.8
    in Gilles de la Tourette's syndrome F95.2
  tics and spasms F95.9
Concato's disease (pericardial polyserositis) A19.9
  nontubercular I31.1
  pleural — *see* Pleurisy, with effusion
Concavity chest wall M95.4
Concealed penis Q55.69
Concern (normal) **about sick person in family** Z63.6
Concrescence (teeth) K00.2
Concretio cordis I31.1
  rheumatic I09.2
Concretion (*see also* Calculus)
  appendicular K38.1
  canaliculus — *see* Dacryolith
  clitoris N90.89
  conjunctiva H11.12- ☑
  eyelid — *see* Disorder, eyelid, specified type NEC
  lacrimal passages — *see* Dacryolith
  prepuce (male) N47.8
  salivary gland (any) K11.5
  seminal vesicle N50.89
  tonsil J35.8
Concussion (brain) (cerebral) (current) S06.0X9 ☑

Concussion — *continued*
  with
    loss of consciousness of 30 minutes or less S06.0X1 ☑
    loss of consciousness of unspecified duration S06.0X9 ☑
    without loss of consciousness S06.0X0 ☑
  blast (air) (hydraulic) (immersion) (underwater)
    abdomen or thorax — *see* Injury, blast, by site
    ear with acoustic nerve injury — *see* Injury, nerve, acoustic, specified type NEC
  cauda equina S34.3 ☑
  conus medullaris S34.02 ☑
  ocular S05.8X- ☑
  spinal (cord)
    cervical S14.0 ☑
    lumbar S34.01 ☑
    sacral S34.02 ☑
    thoracic S24.0 ☑
  syndrome F07.81
Condition — *see* Disease
Conditions arising in the perinatal period — *see* Newborn, affected by
Conduct disorder — *see* Disorder, conduct
Condyloma A63.0
  acuminatum A63.0
  gonorrheal A54.09
  latum A51.31
  syphilitic A51.31
    congenital A50.07
  venereal, syphilitic A51.31
Conflagration (*see also* Burn)
  asphyxia (by inhalation of gases, fumes or vapors) (*see also* Table of Drugs and Chemicals) T59.9- ☑
Conflict (with) (*see also* Discord)
  family Z73.9
  marital Z63.0
    involving divorce or estrangement Z63.5
  parent-child Z62.820
    parent-adopted child Z62.821
    parent-biological child Z62.820
    parent-foster child Z62.822
  social role NEC Z73.5
Confluent — *see* condition
Confusion, confused R41.0
  epileptic F05
  mental state (psychogenic) F44.89
  psychogenic F44.89
  reactive (from emotional stress, psychological trauma) F44.89
Confusional arousals G47.51
Congelation T69.9
Congenital (*see also* condition)
  aortic septum Q25.49
  intrinsic factor deficiency D51.0
  malformation — *see* Anomaly
Congestion, congestive
  bladder N32.89
  bowel K63.89
  brain G93.89
  breast N64.59
  bronchial J98.09
  catarrhal J31.0
  chest R09.89
  chill, malarial — *see* Malaria
  circulatory NEC I99.8
  duodenum K31.89
  eye — *see* Hyperemia, conjunctiva
  facial, due to birth injury P15.4
  general R68.89
  glottis J37.0
  heart — *see* Failure, heart, congestive
  hepatic K76.1
  hypostatic (lung) — *see* Edema, lung
  intestine K63.89
  kidney N28.89
  labyrinth H83.8 ☑
  larynx J37.0
  liver K76.1
  lung R09.89
    active or acute — *see* Pneumonia
  malaria, malarial — *see* Malaria
  nasal R09.81
  nose R09.81
  orbit, orbital (*see also* Exophthalmos)
    inflammatory (chronic) — *see* Inflammation, orbit
  ovary N83.8

Congestion, congestive — *continued*
  pancreas K86.89
  pelvic, female N94.89
  pleural J94.8
  prostate (active) N42.1
  pulmonary — *see* Congestion, lung
  renal N28.89
  retina H35.81
  seminal vesicle N50.1
  spinal cord G95.19
  spleen (chronic) D73.2
  stomach K31.89
  trachea — *see* Tracheitis
  urethra N36.8
  uterus N85.8
    with subinvolution N85.3
  venous (passive) I87.8
  viscera R68.89
Congestive — *see* Congestion
Conical
  cervix (hypertrophic elongation) N88.4
  cornea — *see* Keratoconus
  teeth K00.2
Conjoined twins Q89.4
Conjugal maladjustment Z63.0
  involving divorce or estrangement Z63.5
Conjunctiva — *see* condition
Conjunctivitis (staphylococcal) (streptococcal) NOS H10.9
  Acanthamoeba B60.12
  acute H10.3- ☑
    atopic H10.1- ☑
    chemical (*see also* Corrosion, cornea) H10.21- ☑
    mucopurulent H10.02- ☑
      follicular H10.01- ☑
    pseudomembranous H10.22- ☑
    serous except viral H10.23- ☑
    viral — *see* Conjunctivitis, viral
    toxic H10.21- ☑
  adenoviral (acute) (follicular) B30.1
  allergic (acute) — *see* Conjunctivitis, acute, atopic
    chronic H10.45
      vernal H10.44
  anaphylactic — *see* Conjunctivitis, acute, atopic
  Apollo B30.3
  atopic (acute) — *see* Conjunctivitis, acute, atopic
  Béal's B30.2
  blennorrhagic (gonococcal) (neonatorum) A54.31
  chemical (acute) (*see also* Corrosion, cornea) H10.21- ☑
  chlamydial A74.0
    due to trachoma A71.1
    neonatal P39.1
  chronic (nodosa) (petrificans) (phlyctenular) H10.40- ☑
    allergic H10.45
      vernal H10.44
    follicular H10.43- ☑
    giant papillary H10.41- ☑
    simple H10.42- ☑
    vernal H10.44
  coxsackievirus 24 B30.3
  diphtheritic A36.86
  due to
    dust — *see* Conjunctivitis, acute, atopic
    filariasis B74.9
    mucocutaneous leishmaniasis B55.2
  enterovirus type 70 (hemorrhagic) B30.3
  epidemic (viral) B30.9
    hemorrhagic B30.3
  gonococcal (neonatorum) A54.31
  granular (trachomatous) A71.1
    sequelae (late effect) B94.0
  hemorrhagic (acute) (epidemic) B30.3
  herpes zoster B02.31
  in (due to)
    Acanthamoeba B60.12
    adenovirus (acute) (follicular) B30.1
    Chlamydia A74.0
    coxsackievirus 24 B30.3
    diphtheria A36.86
    enterovirus type 70 (hemorrhagic) B30.3
    filariasis B74.9
    gonococci A54.31
    herpes (simplex) virus B00.53
      zoster B02.31
    infectious disease NEC B99 ☑
    meningococci A39.89
    mucocutaneous leishmaniasis B55.2

Contact — continued
communicable disease Z20.9
  bacterial NEC Z20.818
  specified NEC Z20.89
  viral NEC Z20.828
cyanobacteria bloom Z77.121
dyes Z77.098
Escherichia coli (E. coli) Z20.01
fiberglass — see Table of Drugs and Chemicals, fiber-
    glass
German measles Z20.4
gonorrhea Z20.2
hazardous metals NEC Z77.018
hazardous substances NEC Z77.29
hazards in the physical environment NEC Z77.128
hazards to health NEC Z77.9
HIV Z20.6
HTLV-III/LAV Z20.6
human immunodeficiency virus (HIV) Z20.6
infection Z20.9
  specified NEC Z20.89
infestation (parasitic) NEC Z20.7
intestinal infectious disease NEC Z20.09
  Escherichia coli (E. coli) Z20.01
lead Z77.011
meningococcus Z20.811
mold (toxic) Z77.120
nickel dust Z77.018
noise Z77.122
parasitic disease Z20.7
pediculosis Z20.7
pfiesteria piscicida Z77.121
poliomyelitis Z20.89
pollution
  air Z77.110
  environmental NEC Z77.118
  soil Z77.112
  water Z77.111
polycyclic aromatic hydrocarbons Z77.028
rabies Z20.3
radiation, naturally occurring NEC Z77.123
radon Z77.123
red tide (Florida) Z77.121
rubella Z20.4
sexually-transmitted disease Z20.2
smallpox (laboratory) Z20.89
syphilis Z20.2
tuberculosis Z20.1
uranium Z77.012
varicella Z20.820
venereal disease Z20.2
viral disease NEC Z20.828
viral hepatitis Z20.5
water pollution Z77.111

Contamination, food — see Intoxication, foodborne

Contraception, contraceptive
advice Z30.09
counseling Z30.09
device (intrauterine) (in situ) Z97.5
  causing menorrhagia T83.83 ☑
  checking Z30.431
  complications — see Complications, intrauterine,
    contraceptive device
  in place Z97.5
  initial prescription Z30.014
  reinsertion Z30.433
  removal Z30.432
  replacement Z30.433
emergency (postcoital) Z30.012
initial prescription Z30.019
  barrier Z30.018
  diaphragm Z30.018
  injectable Z30.013
  intrauterine device Z30.014
  pills Z30.011
  postcoital (emergency) Z30.012
  specified type NEC Z30.018
  subdermal implantable Z30.017
  transdermal patch hormonal Z30.016
  vaginal ring hormonal Z30.015
maintenance Z30.40
  barrier Z30.49
  diaphragm Z30.49
  examination Z30.8
  injectable Z30.42
  intrauterine device Z30.431
  pills Z30.41
  specified type NEC Z30.49
  subdermal implantable Z30.46

Contraception, contraceptive — continued
maintenance — continued
  transdermal patch hormonal Z30.45
  vaginal ring hormonal Z30.44
management Z30.9
  specified NEC Z30.8
postcoital (emergency) Z30.012
prescription Z30.019
  repeat Z30.40
sterilization Z30.2
surveillance (drug) — see Contraception, maintenance

Contraction(s), contracture, contracted
Achilles tendon (see also Short, tendon, Achilles)
  congenital Q66.89
amputation stump (surgical) (flexion) (late) (next
    proximal joint) T87.89
anus K59.8
bile duct (common) (hepatic) K83.8
bladder N32.89
  neck or sphincter N32.0
bowel, cecum, colon or intestine, any part — see Ob-
    struction, intestine
Braxton Hicks — see False, labor
breast implant, capsular T85.44 ☑
bronchial J98.09
burn (old) — see Cicatrix
cervix — see Stricture, cervix
cicatricial — see Cicatrix
conjunctiva, trachomatous, active A71.1
  sequelae (late effect) B94.0
Dupuytren's M72.0
eyelid — see Disorder, eyelid function
fascia (lata) (postural) M72.8
  Dupuytren's M72.0
  palmar M72.0
  plantar M72.2
finger NEC (see also Deformity, finger)
  congenital Q68.1
  joint — see Contraction, joint, hand
flaccid — see Contraction, paralytic
gallbladder K82.0
heart valve — see Endocarditis
hip — see Contraction, joint, hip
hourglass
  bladder N32.89
    congenital Q64.79
  gallbladder K82.0
    congenital Q44.1
  stomach K31.89
    congenital Q40.2
    psychogenic F45.8
  uterus (complicating delivery) O62.4
hysterical F44.4
internal os — see Stricture, cervix
joint (abduction) (acquired) (adduction) (flexion) (ro-
    tation) M24.50
  ankle M24.57- ☑
  congenital NEC Q68.8
    hip Q65.89
  elbow M24.52- ☑
  foot joint M24.57- ☑
  hand joint M24.54- ☑
  hip M24.55- ☑
    congenital Q65.89
  hysterical F44.4
  knee M24.56- ☑
  shoulder M24.51- ☑
  wrist M24.53- ☑
kidney (granular) (secondary) N26.9
  congenital Q63.8
  hydronephritic — see Hydronephrosis
  Page N26.2
  pyelonephritic — see Pyelitis, chronic
  tuberculous A18.11
ligament (see also Disorder, ligament)
  congenital Q79.8
muscle (postinfective) (postural) NEC M62.40
  with contracture of joint — see Contraction, joint
  ankle M62.47- ☑
  congenital Q79.8
    sternocleidomastoid Q68.0
  extraocular — see Strabismus
  eye (extrinsic) — see Strabismus
  foot M62.47- ☑
  forearm M62.43- ☑
  hand M62.44- ☑
  hysterical F44.4

Contraction(s), contracture, contracted — continued
muscle — continued
  ischemic (Volkmann's) T79.6 ☑
  lower leg M62.46- ☑
  multiple sites M62.49
  pelvic region M62.45- ☑
  posttraumatic — see Strabismus, paralytic
  psychogenic F45.8
    conversion reaction F44.4
  shoulder region M62.41- ☑
  specified site NEC M62.48
  thigh M62.45- ☑
  upper arm M62.42- ☑
neck — see Torticollis
ocular muscle — see Strabismus
organ or site, congenital NEC — see Atresia, by site
outlet (pelvis) — see Contraction, pelvis
palmar fascia M72.0
paralytic
  joint — see Contraction, joint
  muscle (see also Contraction, muscle NEC)
    ocular — see Strabismus, paralytic
pelvis (acquired) (general) M95.5
  with disproportion (fetopelvic) O33.1
    causing obstructed labor O65.1
    inlet O33.2
    mid-cavity O33.3 ☑
    outlet O33.3 ☑
plantar fascia M72.2
premature
  atrium I49.1
  auriculoventricular I49.49
  heart I49.49
  junctional I49.2
  supraventricular I49.1
  ventricular I49.3
prostate N42.89
pylorus NEC (see also Pylorospasm)
  psychogenic F45.8
rectum, rectal (sphincter) K59.8
ring (Bandl's) (complicating delivery) O62.4
scar — see Cicatrix
spine — see Dorsopathy, deforming
sternocleidomastoid (muscle), congenital Q68.0
stomach K31.89
  hourglass K31.89
    congenital Q40.2
    psychogenic F45.8
  psychogenic F45.8
tendon (sheath) M62.40
  with contracture of joint — see Contraction, joint
  Achilles — see Short, tendon, Achilles
  ankle M62.47- ☑
    Achilles — see Short, tendon, Achilles
  foot M62.47- ☑
  forearm M62.43- ☑
  hand M62.44- ☑
  lower leg M62.46- ☑
  multiple sites M62.49
  neck M62.48
  pelvic region M62.45- ☑
  shoulder region M62.41- ☑
  specified site NEC M62.48
  thigh M62.45- ☑
  thorax M62.48
  trunk M62.48
  upper arm M62.42- ☑
toe — see Deformity, toe, specified NEC
ureterovesical orifice (postinfectional) N13.5
  with infection N13.6
urethra (see also Stricture, urethra)
  orifice N32.0
uterus N85.8
  abnormal NEC O62.9
  clonic (complicating delivery) O62.4
  dyscoordinate (complicating delivery) O62.4
  hourglass (complicating delivery) O62.4
  hypertonic O62.4
  hypotonic NEC O62.2
  inadequate
    primary O62.0
    secondary O62.1
  incoordinate (complicating delivery) O62.4
  poor O62.2
  tetanic (complicating delivery) O62.4
vagina (outlet) N89.5
vesical N32.89

Contraction(s), contracture, contracted — *continued*
- vesical — *continued*
  - neck or urethral orifice N32.0
- visual field — *see* Defect, visual field, generalized
- Volkmann's (ischemic) T79.6 ☑

Contusion (skin surface intact) T14.8 ☑
- abdomen, abdominal (muscle) (wall) S30.1 ☑
- adnexa, eye NEC S05.8X- ☑
- adrenal gland S37.812 ☑
- alveolar process S00.532 ☑
- ankle S90.0- ☑
- antecubital space — *see* Contusion, forearm
- anus S30.3 ☑
- arm (upper) S40.02- ☑
  - lower (with elbow) — *see* Contusion, forearm
- auditory canal — *see* Contusion, ear
- auricle — *see* Contusion, ear
- axilla — *see* Contusion, arm, upper
- back (*see also* Contusion, thorax, back)
  - lower S30.0 ☑
- bile duct S36.13 ☑
- bladder S37.22 ☑
- bone NEC T14.8 ☑
- brain (diffuse) — *see* Injury, intracranial, diffuse
  - focal — *see* Injury, intracranial, focal
- brainstem S06.38- ☑
- breast S20.0- ☑
- broad ligament S37.892 ☑
- brow S00.83 ☑
- buttock S30.0 ☑
- canthus, eye S00.1- ☑
- cauda equina S34.3 ☑
- cerebellar, traumatic S06.37- ☑
- cerebral S06.33- ☑
  - left side S06.32- ☑
  - right side S06.31- ☑
- cheek S00.83 ☑
  - internal S00.532 ☑
- chest (wall) — *see* Contusion, thorax
- chin S00.83 ☑
- clitoris S30.23 ☑
- colon — *see* Injury, intestine, large, contusion
- common bile duct S36.13 ☑
- conjunctiva S05.1- ☑
  - with foreign body (in conjunctival sac) — *see* Foreign body, conjunctival sac
- conus medullaris (spine) S34.139 ☑
- cornea — *see* Contusion, eyeball
  - with foreign body — *see* Foreign body, cornea
- corpus cavernosum S30.21 ☑
- cortex (brain) (cerebral) — *see* Injury, intracranial, diffuse
  - focal — *see* Injury, intracranial, focal
- costal region — *see* Contusion, thorax
- cystic duct S36.13 ☑
- diaphragm S27.802 ☑
- duodenum S36.420 ☑
- ear S00.43- ☑
- elbow S50.0- ☑
  - with forearm — *see* Contusion, forearm
- epididymis S30.22 ☑
- epigastric region S30.1 ☑
- epiglottis S10.0 ☑
- esophagus (thoracic) S27.812 ☑
  - cervical S10.0 ☑
- eyeball S05.1- ☑
- eyebrow S00.1- ☑
- eyelid (and periocular area) S00.1- ☑
- face NEC S00.83 ☑
- fallopian tube S37.529 ☑
  - bilateral S37.522 ☑
  - unilateral S37.521 ☑
- femoral triangle S30.1 ☑
- finger(s) S60.00 ☑
  - with damage to nail (matrix) S60.10 ☑
    - index S60.02- ☑
      - with damage to nail S60.12- ☑
    - little S60.05- ☑
      - with damage to nail S60.15- ☑
    - middle S60.03- ☑
      - with damage to nail S60.13- ☑
    - ring S60.04- ☑
      - with damage to nail S60.14- ☑
    - thumb — *see* Contusion, thumb
- flank S30.1 ☑

Contusion — *continued*
- foot (except toe(s) alone) S90.3- ☑
  - toe — *see* Contusion, toe
- forearm S50.1- ☑
  - elbow only — *see* Contusion, elbow
- forehead S00.83 ☑
- gallbladder S36.122 ☑
- genital organs, external
  - female S30.202 ☑
  - male S30.201 ☑
- globe (eye) — *see* Contusion, eyeball
- groin S30.1 ☑
- gum S00.532 ☑
- hand S60.22- ☑
  - finger(s) — *see* Contusion, finger
  - wrist — *see* Contusion, wrist
- head S00.93 ☑
  - ear — *see* Contusion, ear
  - eyelid — *see* Contusion, eyelid
  - lip S00.531 ☑
  - nose S00.33 ☑
  - oral cavity S00.532 ☑
  - scalp S00.03 ☑
  - specified part NEC S00.83 ☑
- heart (*see also* Injury, heart) S26.91 ☑
- heel — *see* Contusion, foot
- hepatic duct S36.13 ☑
- hip S70.0- ☑
- ileum S36.428 ☑
- iliac region S30.1 ☑
- inguinal region S30.1 ☑
- interscapular region S20.229 ☑
- intra-abdominal organ S36.92 ☑
  - colon — *see* Injury, intestine, large, contusion
  - liver S36.112 ☑
  - pancreas — *see* Contusion, pancreas
  - rectum S36.62 ☑
  - small intestine — *see* Injury, intestine, small, contusion
  - specified organ NEC S36.892 ☑
  - spleen — *see* Contusion, spleen
  - stomach S36.32 ☑
- iris (eye) — *see* Contusion, eyeball
- jaw S00.83 ☑
- jejunum S36.428 ☑
- kidney S37.01- ☑
  - major (greater than 2 cm) S37.02- ☑
  - minor (less than 2 cm) S37.01- ☑
- knee S80.0- ☑
- labium (majus) (minus) S30.23 ☑
- lacrimal apparatus, gland or sac S05.8X- ☑
- larynx S10.0 ☑
- leg (lower) S80.1- ☑
  - knee — *see* Contusion, knee
- lens — *see* Contusion, eyeball
- lip S00.531 ☑
- liver S36.112 ☑
- lower back S30.0 ☑
- lumbar region S30.0 ☑
- lung S27.329 ☑
  - bilateral S27.322 ☑
  - unilateral S27.321 ☑
- malar region S00.83 ☑
- mastoid region S00.83 ☑
- membrane, brain — *see* Injury, intracranial, diffuse
  - focal — *see* Injury, intracranial, focal
- mesentery S36.892 ☑
- mesosalpinx S37.892 ☑
- mouth S00.532 ☑
- muscle — *see* Contusion, by site
- nail
  - finger — *see* Contusion, finger, with damage to nail
  - toe — *see* Contusion, toe, with damage to nail
- nasal S00.33 ☑
- neck S10.93 ☑
  - specified site NEC S10.83 ☑
  - throat S10.0 ☑
- nerve — *see* Injury, nerve
- newborn P54.5
- nose S00.33 ☑
- occipital
  - lobe (brain) — *see* Injury, intracranial, diffuse
    - focal — *see* Injury, intracranial, focal
  - region (scalp) S00.03 ☑
- orbit (region) (tissues) S05.1- ☑

Contusion — *continued*
- ovary S37.429 ☑
  - bilateral S37.422 ☑
  - unilateral S37.421 ☑
- palate S00.532 ☑
- pancreas S36.229 ☑
  - body S36.221 ☑
  - head S36.220 ☑
  - tail S36.222 ☑
- parietal
  - lobe (brain) — *see* Injury, intracranial, diffuse
    - focal — *see* Injury, intracranial, focal
  - region (scalp) S00.03 ☑
- pelvic organ S37.92 ☑
  - adrenal gland S37.812 ☑
  - bladder S37.22 ☑
  - fallopian tube — *see* Contusion, fallopian tube
  - kidney — *see* Contusion, kidney
  - ovary — *see* Contusion, ovary
  - prostate S37.822 ☑
  - specified organ NEC S37.892 ☑
  - ureter S37.12 ☑
  - urethra S37.32 ☑
  - uterus S37.62 ☑
- pelvis S30.0 ☑
- penis S30.21 ☑
- perineum
  - female S30.23 ☑
  - male S30.0 ☑
- periocular area S00.1- ☑
- peritoneum S36.81 ☑
- periurethral tissue — *see* Contusion, urethra
- pharynx S10.0 ☑
- pinna — *see* Contusion, ear
- popliteal space — *see* Contusion, knee
- prepuce S30.21 ☑
- prostate S37.822 ☑
- pubic region S30.1 ☑
- pudendum
  - female S30.202 ☑
  - male S30.201 ☑
- quadriceps femoris — *see* Contusion, thigh
- rectum S36.62 ☑
- retroperitoneum S36.892 ☑
- round ligament S37.892 ☑
- sacral region S30.0 ☑
- scalp S00.03 ☑
  - due to birth injury P12.3
- scapular region — *see* Contusion, shoulder
- sclera — *see* Contusion, eyeball
- scrotum S30.22 ☑
- seminal vesicle S37.892 ☑
- shoulder S40.01- ☑
- skin NEC T14.8 ☑
- small intestine — *see* Injury, intestine, small, contusion
- spermatic cord S30.22 ☑
- spinal cord — *see* Injury, spinal cord, by region
  - cauda equina S34.3 ☑
  - conus medullaris S34.139 ☑
- spleen S36.029 ☑
  - major S36.021 ☑
  - minor S36.020 ☑
- sternal region S20.219 ☑
- stomach S36.32 ☑
- subconjunctival S05.1- ☑
- subcutaneous NEC T14.8 ☑
- submaxillary region S00.83 ☑
- submental region S00.83 ☑
- subperiosteal NEC T14.8 ☑
- subungual
  - finger — *see* Contusion, finger, with damage to nail
  - toe — *see* Contusion, toe, with damage to nail
- supraclavicular fossa S10.83 ☑
- supraorbital S00.83 ☑
- suprarenal gland S37.812 ☑
- temple (region) S00.83 ☑
- temporal
  - lobe (brain) — *see* Injury, intracranial, diffuse
    - focal — *see* Injury, intracranial, focal
  - region S00.83 ☑
- testis S30.22 ☑
- thigh S70.1- ☑
- thorax (wall) S20.20 ☑
  - back S20.22- ☑
  - front S20.21- ☑

Contusion — *continued*
  throat S10.0 ☑
  thumb S60.01- ☑
    with damage to nail S60.11- ☑
  toe(s) (lesser) S90.12- ☑
    with damage to nail S90.22- ☑
    great S90.11- ☑
      with damage to nail S90.21- ☑
  tongue S00.532 ☑
  trachea (cervical) S10.0 ☑
    thoracic S27.52 ☑
  tunica vaginalis S30.22 ☑
  tympanum, tympanic membrane — *see* Contusion, ear
  ureter S37.12 ☑
  urethra S37.32 ☑
  urinary organ NEC S37.892 ☑
  uterus S37.62 ☑
  uvula S00.532 ☑
  vagina S30.23 ☑
  vas deferens S37.892 ☑
  vesical S37.22 ☑
  vocal cord(s) S10.0 ☑
  vulva S30.23 ☑
  wrist S60.21- ☑
Conus (congenital) (any type) Q14.8
  cornea — *see* Keratoconus
  medullaris syndrome G95.81
Conversion hysteria, neurosis or reaction F44.9
Converter, tuberculosis (test reaction) R76.11
Conviction (legal), **anxiety concerning** Z65.0
  with imprisonment Z65.1
Convulsions (idiopathic) (*see also* Seizure(s)) R56.9
  apoplectiform (cerebral ischemia) I67.82
  dissociative F44.5
  epileptic — *see* Epilepsy
  epileptiform, epileptoid — *see* Seizure, epileptiform
  ether (anesthetic) — *see* Table of Drugs and Chemicals, by drug
  febrile R56.00
    with status epilepticus G40.901
    complex R56.01
      with status epilepticus G40.901
    simple R56.00
  hysterical F44.5
  infantile P90
    epilepsy — *see* Epilepsy
  jacksonian — *see* Epilepsy, localization-related, symptomatic, with simple partial seizures
  myoclonic G25.3
  newborn P90
  obstetrical (nephritic) (uremic) — *see* Eclampsia
  paretic A52.17
  post traumatic R56.1
  psychomotor — *see* Epilepsy, localization-related, symptomatic, with complex partial seizures
  recurrent R56.9
  reflex R25.8
  scarlatinal A38.8
  tetanus, tetanic — *see* Tetanus
  thymic E32.8
Convulsive (*see also* Convulsions)
Cooley's anemia D56.1
Coolie itch B76.9
Cooper's
  disease — *see* Mastopathy, cystic
  hernia — *see* Hernia, abdomen, specified site NEC
Copra itch B88.0
Coprophagy F50.89
Coprophobia F40.298
Coproporphyria, hereditary E80.29
Cor
  biloculare Q20.8
  bovis, bovinum — *see* Hypertrophy, cardiac
  pulmonale (chronic) I27.81
    acute I26.09
  triatriatum, triatrium Q24.2
  triloculare Q20.8
    biatrium Q20.4
    biventriculare Q21.1
Corbus' disease (gangrenous balanitis) N48.1
Cord (*see also* condition)
  around neck
    complicating delivery O69.81 ☑
      with compression O69.1 ☑
  bladder G95.89
    tabetic A52.19

Cordis ectopia Q24.8
Corditis (spermatic) N49.1
Corectopia Q13.2
Cori's disease (glycogen storage) E74.03
Corkhandler's disease or lung J67.3
Corkscrew esophagus K22.4
Corkworker's disease or lung J67.3
Corn (infected) L84
Cornea (*see also* condition)
  donor Z52.5
  plana Q13.4
Cornelia de Lange syndrome Q87.1
Cornu cutaneum L85.8
Cornual gestation or pregnancy O00.80
  with intrauterine pregnancy O00.81
Coronary (artery) — *see* condition
Coronavirus, as cause of disease classified elsewhere B97.29
  SARS-associated B97.21
Corpora (*see also* condition)
  amylacea, prostate N42.89
  cavernosa — *see* condition
Corpulence — *see* Obesity
Corpus — *see* condition
Corrected transposition Q20.5
Corrosion (injury) (acid) (caustic) (chemical) (lime) (external) (internal) T30.4
  abdomen, abdominal (muscle) (wall) T21.42 ☑
    first degree T21.52 ☑
    second degree T21.62 ☑
    third degree T21.72 ☑
  above elbow T22.439 ☑
    first degree T22.539 ☑
    left T22.432 ☑
      first degree T22.532 ☑
      second degree T22.632 ☑
      third degree T22.732 ☑
    right T22.431 ☑
      first degree T22.531 ☑
      second degree T22.631 ☑
      third degree T22.731 ☑
    second degree T22.639 ☑
    third degree T22.739 ☑
  alimentary tract NEC T28.7 ☑
  ankle T25.419 ☑
    first degree T25.519 ☑
    left T25.412 ☑
      first degree T25.512 ☑
      second degree T25.612 ☑
      third degree T25.712 ☑
    multiple with foot — *see* Corrosion, lower, limb, multiple, ankle and foot
    right T25.411 ☑
      first degree T25.511 ☑
      second degree T25.611 ☑
      third degree T25.711 ☑
    second degree T25.619 ☑
    third degree T25.719 ☑
  anus — *see* Corrosion, buttock
  arm(s) (meaning upper limb(s)) — *see* Corrosion, upper limb
  axilla T22.449 ☑
    first degree T22.549 ☑
    left T22.442 ☑
      first degree T22.542 ☑
      second degree T22.642 ☑
      third degree T22.742 ☑
    right T22.441 ☑
      first degree T22.541 ☑
      second degree T22.641 ☑
      third degree T22.741 ☑
    second degree T22.649 ☑
    third degree T22.749 ☑
  back (lower) T21.44 ☑
    first degree T21.54 ☑
    second degree T21.64 ☑
    third degree T21.74 ☑
    upper T21.43 ☑
      first degree T21.53 ☑
      second degree T21.63 ☑
      third degree T21.73 ☑
  blisters — *code as* Corrosion, second degree, by site
  breast(s) — *see* Corrosion, chest wall
  buttock(s) T21.45 ☑
    first degree T21.55 ☑
    second degree T21.65 ☑

Corrosion — *continued*
  buttock(s) — *continued*
    third degree T21.75 ☑
  calf T24.439 ☑
    first degree T24.539 ☑
    left T24.432 ☑
      first degree T24.532 ☑
      second degree T24.632 ☑
      third degree T24.732 ☑
    right T24.431 ☑
      first degree T24.531 ☑
      second degree T24.631 ☑
      third degree T24.731 ☑
    second degree T24.639 ☑
    third degree T24.739 ☑
  canthus (eye) — *see* Corrosion, eyelid
  cervix T28.8 ☑
  cheek T20.46 ☑
    first degree T20.56 ☑
    second degree T20.66 ☑
    third degree T20.76 ☑
  chest wall T21.41 ☑
    first degree T21.51 ☑
    second degree T21.61 ☑
    third degree T21.71 ☑
  chin T20.43 ☑
    first degree T20.53 ☑
    second degree T20.63 ☑
    third degree T20.73 ☑
  colon T28.7 ☑
  conjunctiva (and cornea) — *see* Corrosion, cornea
  cornea (and conjunctiva) T26.6- ☑
  deep necrosis of underlying tissue — *code as* Corrosion, third degree, by site
  dorsum of hand T23.469 ☑
    first degree T23.569 ☑
    left T23.462 ☑
      first degree T23.562 ☑
      second degree T23.662 ☑
      third degree T23.762 ☑
    right T23.461 ☑
      first degree T23.561 ☑
      second degree T23.661 ☑
      third degree T23.761 ☑
    second degree T23.669 ☑
    third degree T23.769 ☑
  ear (auricle) (external) (canal) T20.41 ☑
    drum T28.91 ☑
    first degree T20.51 ☑
    second degree T20.61 ☑
    third degree T20.71 ☑
  elbow T22.429 ☑
    first degree T22.529 ☑
    left T22.422 ☑
      first degree T22.522 ☑
      second degree T22.622 ☑
      third degree T22.722 ☑
    right T22.421 ☑
      first degree T22.521 ☑
      second degree T22.621 ☑
      third degree T22.721 ☑
    second degree T22.629 ☑
    third degree T22.729 ☑
  entire body — *see* Corrosion, multiple body regions
  epidermal loss — *code as* Corrosion, second degree, by site
  epiglottis T27.4 ☑
  erythema, erythematous — *code as* Corrosion, first degree, by site
  esophagus T28.6 ☑
  extent (percentage of body surface)
    less than 10 percent T32.0
    10-19 percent (0-9 percent third degree) T32.10
      with 10-19 percent third degree T32.11
    20-29 percent (0-9 percent third degree) T32.20
      with
        10-19 percent third degree T32.21
        20-29 percent third degree T32.22
    30-39 percent (0-9 percent third degree) T32.30
      with
        10-19 percent third degree T32.31
        20-29 percent third degree T32.32
        30-39 percent third degree T32.33
    40-49 percent (0-9 percent third degree) T32.40
      with
        10-19 percent third degree T32.41

⬚ Subterms under main terms may continue to next column or page   ☑ Additional Character Required — Refer to the Tabular List for Character Selection   73

Contusion — Corrosion

Corrosion — *continued*
  extent — *continued*
    40-49 percent — *continued*
      with — *continued*
        20-29 percent third degree T32.42
        30-39 percent third degree T32.43
        40-49 percent third degree T32.44
    50-59 percent (0-9 percent third degree) T32.50
      with
        10-19 percent third degree T32.51
        20-29 percent third degree T32.52
        30-39 percent third degree T32.53
        40-49 percent third degree T32.54
        50-59 percent third degree T32.55
    60-69 percent (0-9 percent third degree) T32.60
      with
        10-19 percent third degree T32.61
        20-29 percent third degree T32.62
        30-39 percent third degree T32.63
        40-49 percent third degree T32.64
        50-59 percent third degree T32.65
        60-69 percent third degree T32.66
    70-79 percent (0-9 percent third degree) T32.70
      with
        10-19 percent third degree T32.71
        20-29 percent third degree T32.72
        30-39 percent third degree T32.73
        40-49 percent third degree T32.74
        50-59 percent third degree T32.75
        60-69 percent third degree T32.76
        70-79 percent third degree T32.77
    80-89 percent (0-9 percent third degree) T32.80
      with
        10-19 percent third degree T32.81
        20-29 percent third degree T32.82
        30-39 percent third degree T32.83
        40-49 percent third degree T32.84
        50-59 percent third degree T32.85
        60-69 percent third degree T32.86
        70-79 percent third degree T32.87
        80-89 percent third degree T32.88
    90 percent or more (0-9 percent third degree) T32.90
      with
        10-19 percent third degree T32.91
        20-29 percent third degree T32.92
        30-39 percent third degree T32.93
        40-49 percent third degree T32.94
        50-59 percent third degree T32.95
        60-69 percent third degree T32.96
        70-79 percent third degree T32.97
        80-89 percent third degree T32.98
        90-99 percent third degree T32.99
  extremity — *see* Corrosion, limb
  eye(s) and adnexa T26.9- ✓
    with resulting rupture and destruction of eyeball T26.7- ✓
    conjunctival sac — *see* Corrosion, cornea
    cornea — *see* Corrosion, cornea
    lid — *see* Corrosion, eyelid
    periocular area — *see* Corrosion eyelid
    specified site NEC T26.8- ✓
  eyeball — *see* Corrosion, eye
  eyelid(s) T26.5- ✓
  face — *see* Corrosion, head
  finger T23.429 ✓
    first degree T23.529 ✓
    left T23.422 ✓
      first degree T23.522 ✓
      second degree T23.622 ✓
      third degree T23.722 ✓
    multiple sites (without thumb) T23.439 ✓
      with thumb T23.449 ✓
        first degree T23.549 ✓
        left T23.442 ✓
          first degree T23.542 ✓
          second degree T23.642 ✓
          third degree T23.742 ✓
        right T23.441 ✓
          first degree T23.541 ✓
          second degree T23.641 ✓
          third degree T23.741 ✓
        second degree T23.649 ✓
        third degree T23.749 ✓
      first degree T23.539 ✓
      left T23.432 ✓
        first degree T23.532 ✓

Corrosion — *continued*
  finger — *continued*
    multiple sites — *continued*
      left — *continued*
        second degree T23.632 ✓
        third degree T23.732 ✓
      right T23.431 ✓
        first degree T23.531 ✓
        second degree T23.631 ✓
        third degree T23.731 ✓
      second degree T23.639 ✓
      third degree T23.739 ✓
    right T23.421 ✓
      first degree T23.521 ✓
      second degree T23.621 ✓
      third degree T23.721 ✓
    second degree T23.629 ✓
    third degree T23.729 ✓
  flank — *see* Corrosion, abdomen
  foot T25.429 ✓
    first degree T25.529 ✓
    left T25.422 ✓
      first degree T25.522 ✓
      second degree T25.622 ✓
      third degree T25.722 ✓
    multiple with ankle — *see* Corrosion, lower, limb, multiple, ankle and foot
    right T25.421 ✓
      first degree T25.521 ✓
      second degree T25.621 ✓
      third degree T25.721 ✓
    second degree T25.629 ✓
    third degree T25.729 ✓
  forearm T22.419 ✓
    first degree T22.519 ✓
    left T22.412 ✓
      first degree T22.512 ✓
      second degree T22.612 ✓
      third degree T22.712 ✓
    right T22.411 ✓
      first degree T22.511 ✓
      second degree T22.611 ✓
      third degree T22.711 ✓
    second degree T22.619 ✓
    third degree T22.719 ✓
  forehead T20.46 ✓
    first degree T20.56 ✓
    second degree T20.66 ✓
    third degree T20.76 ✓
  fourth degree — *code as* Corrosion, third degree, by site
  full thickness skin loss — *code as* Corrosion, third degree, by site
  gastrointestinal tract NEC T28.7 ✓
  genital organs
    external
      female T21.47 ✓
        first degree T21.57 ✓
        second degree T21.67 ✓
        third degree T21.77 ✓
      male T21.46 ✓
        first degree T21.56 ✓
        second degree T21.66 ✓
        third degree T21.76 ✓
    internal T28.8 ✓
  groin — *see* Corrosion, abdominal wall
  hand(s) T23.409 ✓
    back — *see* Corrosion, dorsum of hand
    finger — *see* Corrosion, finger
    first degree T23.509 ✓
    left T23.402 ✓
      first degree T23.502 ✓
      second degree T23.602 ✓
      third degree T23.702 ✓
    multiple sites with wrist T23.499 ✓
      first degree T23.599 ✓
      left T23.492 ✓
        first degree T23.592 ✓
        second degree T23.692 ✓
        third degree T23.792 ✓
      right T23.491 ✓
        first degree T23.591 ✓
        second degree T23.691 ✓
        third degree T23.791 ✓
      second degree T23.699 ✓
      third degree T23.799 ✓

Corrosion — *continued*
  hand(s) — *continued*
    palm — *see* Corrosion, palm
      right T23.401 ✓
        first degree T23.501 ✓
        second degree T23.601 ✓
        third degree T23.701 ✓
      second degree T23.609 ✓
      third degree T23.709 ✓
    thumb — *see* Corrosion, thumb
  head (and face) (and neck) T20.40 ✓
    cheek — *see* Corrosion, cheek
    chin — *see* Corrosion, chin
    ear — *see* Corrosion, ear
    eye(s) only — *see* Corrosion, eye
    first degree T20.50 ✓
    forehead — *see* Corrosion, forehead
    lip — *see* Corrosion, lip
    multiple sites T20.49 ✓
      first degree T20.59 ✓
      second degree T20.69 ✓
      third degree T20.79 ✓
    neck — *see* Corrosion, neck
    nose — *see* Corrosion, nose
    scalp — *see* Corrosion, scalp
    second degree T20.60 ✓
    third degree T20.70 ✓
  hip(s) — *see* Corrosion, lower, limb
  inhalation — *see* Corrosion, respiratory tract
  internal organ(s) (*see also* Corrosion, by site) T28.90 ✓
    alimentary tract T28.7 ✓
      esophagus T28.6 ✓
    esophagus T28.6 ✓
    genitourinary T28.8 ✓
    mouth T28.5 ✓
    pharynx T28.5 ✓
    specified organ NEC T28.99 ✓
  interscapular region — *see* Corrosion, back, upper
  intestine (large) (small) T28.7 ✓
  knee T24.429 ✓
    first degree T24.529 ✓
    left T24.422 ✓
      first degree T24.522 ✓
      second degree T24.622 ✓
      third degree T24.722 ✓
    right T24.421 ✓
      first degree T24.521 ✓
      second degree T24.621 ✓
      third degree T24.721 ✓
    second degree T24.629 ✓
    third degree T24.729 ✓
  labium (majus) (minus) — *see* Corrosion, genital organs, external, female
  lacrimal apparatus, duct, gland or sac — *see* Corrosion, eye, specified site NEC
  larynx T27.4 ✓
    with lung T27.5 ✓
  leg(s) (meaning lower limb(s)) — *see* Corrosion, lower limb
  limb(s)
    lower — *see* Corrosion, lower, limb
    upper — *see* Corrosion, upper limb
  lip(s) T20.42 ✓
    first degree T20.52 ✓
    second degree T20.62 ✓
    third degree T20.72 ✓
  lower
    back — *see* Corrosion, back
    limb T24.409 ✓
      ankle — *see* Corrosion, ankle
      calf — *see* Corrosion, calf
      first degree T24.509 ✓
      foot — *see* Corrosion, foot
      knee — *see* Corrosion, knee
      left T24.402 ✓
        first degree T24.502 ✓
        second degree T24.602 ✓
        third degree T24.702 ✓
      multiple sites, except ankle and foot T24.499 ✓
        ankle and foot T25.499 ✓
          first degree T25.599 ✓
          left T25.492 ✓
            first degree T25.592 ✓
            second degree T25.692 ✓
            third degree T25.792 ✓
          right T25.491 ✓

Corrosion — *continued*
- lower — *continued*
  - limb — *continued*
    - multiple sites, except ankle and foot — *continued*
      - ankle and foot — *continued*
        - right — *continued*
          - first degree T25.591 ✓
          - second degree T25.691 ✓
          - third degree T25.791 ✓
        - second degree T25.699 ✓
        - third degree T25.799 ✓
      - first degree T24.599 ✓
      - left T24.492 ✓
        - first degree T24.592 ✓
        - second degree T24.692 ✓
        - third degree T24.792 ✓
      - right T24.491 ✓
        - first degree T24.591 ✓
        - second degree T24.691 ✓
        - third degree T24.791 ✓
      - second degree T24.699 ✓
      - third degree T24.799 ✓
    - right T24.401 ✓
      - first degree T24.501 ✓
      - second degree T24.601 ✓
      - third degree T24.701 ✓
    - thigh — *see* Corrosion, thigh
    - third degree T24.709 ✓
- lung (with larynx and trachea) T27.5 ✓
- mouth T28.5 ✓
- neck T20.47 ✓
  - first degree T20.57 ✓
  - second degree T20.67 ✓
  - third degree T20.77 ✓
- nose (septum) T20.44 ✓
  - first degree T20.54 ✓
  - second degree T20.64 ✓
  - third degree T20.74 ✓
- ocular adnexa — *see* Corrosion, eye
- orbit region — *see* Corrosion, eyelid
- palm T23.459 ✓
  - first degree T23.559 ✓
  - left T23.452 ✓
    - first degree T23.552 ✓
    - second degree T23.652 ✓
    - third degree T23.752 ✓
  - right T23.451 ✓
    - first degree T23.551 ✓
    - second degree T23.651 ✓
    - third degree T23.751 ✓
  - second degree T23.659 ✓
  - third degree T23.759 ✓
- partial thickness — *code as* Corrosion, unspecified degree, by site
- pelvis — *see* Corrosion, trunk
- penis — *see* Corrosion, genital organs, external, male
- perineum
  - female — *see* Corrosion, genital organs, external, female
  - male — *see* Corrosion, genital organs, external, male
- periocular area — *see* Corrosion, eyelid
- pharynx T28.5 ✓
- rectum T28.7 ✓
- respiratory tract T27.7 ✓
  - larynx — *see* Corrosion, larynx
  - specified part NEC T27.6 ✓
  - trachea — *see* Corrosion, larynx
- sac, lacrimal — *see* Corrosion, eye, specified site NEC
- scalp T20.45 ✓
  - first degree T20.55 ✓
  - second degree T20.65 ✓
  - third degree T20.75 ✓
- scapular region T22.469 ✓
  - first degree T22.569 ✓
  - left T22.462 ✓
    - first degree T22.562 ✓
    - second degree T22.662 ✓
    - third degree T22.762 ✓
  - right T22.461 ✓
    - first degree T22.561 ✓
    - second degree T22.661 ✓
    - third degree T22.761 ✓
  - second degree T22.669 ✓

Corrosion — *continued*
- scapular region — *continued*
  - third degree T22.769 ✓
- sclera — *see* Corrosion, eye, specified site NEC
- scrotum — *see* Corrosion, genital organs, external, male
- shoulder T22.459 ✓
  - first degree T22.559 ✓
  - left T22.452 ✓
    - first degree T22.552 ✓
    - second degree T22.652 ✓
    - third degree T22.752 ✓
  - right T22.451 ✓
    - first degree T22.551 ✓
    - second degree T22.651 ✓
    - third degree T22.751 ✓
  - second degree T22.659 ✓
  - third degree T22.759 ✓
- stomach T28.7 ✓
- temple — *see* Corrosion, head
- testis — *see* Corrosion, genital organs, external, male
- thigh T24.419 ✓
  - first degree T24.519 ✓
  - left T24.412 ✓
    - first degree T24.512 ✓
    - second degree T24.612 ✓
    - third degree T24.712 ✓
  - right T24.411 ✓
    - first degree T24.511 ✓
    - second degree T24.611 ✓
    - third degree T24.711 ✓
  - second degree T24.619 ✓
  - third degree T24.719 ✓
- thorax (external) — *see* Corrosion, trunk
- throat (meaning pharynx) T28.5 ✓
- thumb(s) T23.419 ✓
  - first degree T23.519 ✓
  - left T23.412 ✓
    - first degree T23.512 ✓
    - second degree T23.612 ✓
    - third degree T23.712 ✓
  - multiple sites with fingers T23.449 ✓
    - first degree T23.549 ✓
    - left T23.442 ✓
      - first degree T23.542 ✓
      - second degree T23.642 ✓
      - third degree T23.742 ✓
    - right T23.441 ✓
      - first degree T23.541 ✓
      - second degree T23.641 ✓
      - third degree T23.741 ✓
    - second degree T23.649 ✓
    - third degree T23.749 ✓
  - right T23.411 ✓
    - first degree T23.511 ✓
    - second degree T23.611 ✓
    - third degree T23.711 ✓
  - second degree T23.619 ✓
  - third degree T23.719 ✓
- toe T25.439 ✓
  - first degree T25.539 ✓
  - left T25.432 ✓
    - first degree T25.532 ✓
    - second degree T25.632 ✓
    - third degree T25.732 ✓
  - right T25.431 ✓
    - first degree T25.531 ✓
    - second degree T25.631 ✓
    - third degree T25.731 ✓
  - second degree T25.639 ✓
  - third degree T25.739 ✓
- tongue T28.5 ✓
- tonsil(s) T28.5 ✓
- total body — *see* Corrosion, multiple body regions
- trachea T27.4 ✓
  - with lung T27.5 ✓
- trunk T21.40 ✓
  - abdominal wall — *see* Corrosion, abdominal wall
  - anus — *see* Corrosion, buttock
  - axilla — *see* Corrosion, upper limb
  - back — *see* Corrosion, back
  - breast — *see* Corrosion, chest wall
  - buttock — *see* Corrosion, buttock
  - chest wall — *see* Corrosion, chest wall
  - first degree T21.50 ✓
  - flank — *see* Corrosion, abdominal wall

Corrosion — *continued*
- trunk — *continued*
  - genital
    - female — *see* Corrosion, genital organs, external, female
    - male — *see* Corrosion, genital organs, external, male
  - groin — *see* Corrosion, abdominal wall
  - interscapular region — *see* Corrosion, back, upper
  - labia — *see* Corrosion, genital organs, external, female
  - lower back — *see* Corrosion, back
  - penis — *see* Corrosion, genital organs, external, male
  - perineum
    - female — *see* Corrosion, genital organs, external, female
    - male — *see* Corrosion, genital organs, external, male
  - scapular region — *see* Corrosion, upper limb
  - scrotum — *see* Corrosion, genital organs, external, male
  - second degree T21.60 ✓
  - shoulder — *see* Corrosion, upper limb
  - specified site NEC T21.49 ✓
    - first degree T21.59 ✓
    - second degree T21.69 ✓
    - third degree T21.79 ✓
  - testes — *see* Corrosion, genital organs, external, male
  - third degree T21.70 ✓
  - upper back — *see* Corrosion, back, upper
  - vagina T28.8 ✓
  - vulva — *see* Corrosion, genital organs, external, female
- unspecified site with extent of body surface involved specified
  - less than 10 percent T32.0
  - 10-19 percent (0-9 percent third degree) T32.10
    - with 10-19 percent third degree T32.11
  - 20-29 percent (0-9 percent third degree) T32.20
    - with
      - 10-19 percent third degree T32.21
      - 20-29 percent third degree T32.22
  - 30-39 percent (0-9 percent third degree) T32.30
    - with
      - 10-19 percent third degree T32.31
      - 20-29 percent third degree T32.32
      - 30-39 percent third degree T32.33
  - 40-49 percent (0-9 percent third degree) T32.40
    - with
      - 10-19 percent third degree T32.41
      - 20-29 percent third degree T32.42
      - 30-39 percent third degree T32.43
      - 40-49 percent third degree T32.44
  - 50-59 percent (0-9 percent third degree) T32.50
    - with
      - 10-19 percent third degree T32.51
      - 20-29 percent third degree T32.52
      - 30-39 percent third degree T32.53
      - 40-49 percent third degree T32.54
      - 50-59 percent third degree T32.55
  - 60-69 percent (0-9 percent third degree) T32.60
    - with
      - 10-19 percent third degree T32.61
      - 20-29 percent third degree T32.62
      - 30-39 percent third degree T32.63
      - 40-49 percent third degree T32.64
      - 50-59 percent third degree T32.65
      - 60-69 percent third degree T32.66
  - 70-79 percent (0-9 percent third degree) T32.70
    - with
      - 10-19 percent third degree T32.71
      - 20-29 percent third degree T32.72
      - 30-39 percent third degree T32.73
      - 40-49 percent third degree T32.74
      - 50-59 percent third degree T32.75
      - 60-69 percent third degree T32.76
      - 70-79 percent third degree T32.77
  - 80-89 percent (0-9 percent third degree) T32.80
    - with
      - 10-19 percent third degree T32.81
      - 20-29 percent third degree T32.82
      - 30-39 percent third degree T32.83
      - 40-49 percent third degree T32.84
      - 50-59 percent third degree T32.85
      - 60-69 percent third degree T32.86
      - 70-79 percent third degree T32.87

⬥ Subterms under main terms may continue to next column or page   ✓ Additional Character Required — Refer to the Tabular List for Character Selection   **75**

Corrosion — Corrosion

Corrosion — *continued*
  unspecified site with extent of body surface involved
        specified — *continued*
      80-89 percent — *continued*
        with — *continued*
            80-89 percent third degree T32.88
      90 percent or more (0-9 percent third degree)
        T32.90
        with
            10-19 percent third degree T32.91
            20-29 percent third degree T32.92
            30-39 percent third degree T32.93
            40-49 percent third degree T32.94
            50-59 percent third degree T32.95
            60-69 percent third degree T32.96
            70-79 percent third degree T32.97
            80-89 percent third degree T32.98
            90-99 percent third degree T32.99
  upper limb (axilla) (scapular region) T22.40 ☑
    above elbow — *see* Corrosion, above elbow
    axilla — *see* Corrosion, axilla
    elbow — *see* Corrosion, elbow
    first degree T22.50 ☑
    forearm — *see* Corrosion, forearm
    hand — *see* Corrosion, hand
    interscapular region — *see* Corrosion, back, upper
    multiple sites T22.499 ☑
      first degree T22.599 ☑
      left T22.492 ☑
        first degree T22.592 ☑
        second degree T22.692 ☑
        third degree T22.792 ☑
      right T22.491 ☑
        first degree T22.591 ☑
        second degree T22.691 ☑
        third degree T22.791 ☑
      second degree T22.699 ☑
      third degree T22.799 ☑
    scapular region — *see* Corrosion, scapular region
    second degree T22.60 ☑
    shoulder — *see* Corrosion, shoulder
    third degree T22.70 ☑
    wrist — *see* Corrosion, hand
  uterus T28.8 ☑
  vagina T28.8 ☑
  vulva — *see* Corrosion, genital organs, external, female
  wrist T23.479 ☑
    first degree T23.579 ☑
    left T23.472 ☑
      first degree T23.572 ☑
      second degree T23.672 ☑
      third degree T23.772 ☑
    multiple sites with hand T23.499 ☑
      first degree T23.599 ☑
      left T23.492 ☑
        first degree T23.592 ☑
        second degree T23.692 ☑
        third degree T23.792 ☑
      right T23.491 ☑
        first degree T23.591 ☑
        second degree T23.691 ☑
        third degree T23.791 ☑
      second degree T23.699 ☑
      third degree T23.799 ☑
    right T23.471 ☑
      first degree T23.571 ☑
      second degree T23.671 ☑
      third degree T23.771 ☑
    second degree T23.679 ☑
    third degree T23.779 ☑
Corrosive burn — *see* Corrosion
Corsican fever — *see* Malaria
Cortical — *see* condition
Cortico-adrenal — *see* condition
Coryza (acute) J00
  with grippe or influenza — *see* Influenza, with, respiratory manifestations NEC
  syphilitic
    congenital (chronic) A50.05
Costen's syndrome or complex M26.69
Costiveness — *see* Constipation
Costochondritis M94.0
Cot death R99
Cotard's syndrome F22
Cotia virus B08.8
Cotton wool spots (retinal) H35.81

Cotungo's disease — *see* Sciatica
Cough (affected) (chronic) (epidemic) (nervous) R05
  with hemorrhage — *see* Hemoptysis
  bronchial R05
    with grippe or influenza — *see* Influenza, with, respiratory manifestations NEC
  functional F45.8
  hysterical F45.8
  laryngeal, spasmodic R05
  psychogenic F45.8
  smokers' J41.0
  tea taster's B49
Counseling (for) Z71.9
  abuse NEC
    perpetrator Z69.82
    victim Z69.81
  alcohol abuser Z71.41
    family Z71.42
  child abuse
    nonparental
      perpetrator Z69.021
      victim Z69.020
    parental
      perpetrator Z69.011
      victim Z69.010
  consanguinity Z71.89
  contraceptive Z30.09
  dietary Z71.3
  drug abuser Z71.51
    family member Z71.52
  exercise Z71.82
  family Z71.89
  fertility preservation (prior to cancer therapy) (prior to removal of gonads) Z31.62
  for non-attending third party Z71.0
    related to sexual behavior or orientation Z70.2
  genetic
    nonprocreative Z71.83
    procreative NEC Z31.5
  gestational carrier Z31.7
  health (advice) (education) (instruction) — *see* Counseling, medical
  human immunodeficiency virus (HIV) Z71.7
  impotence Z70.1
  insulin pump use Z46.81
  medical (for) Z71.9
    boarding school resident Z59.3
    consanguinity Z71.89
    feared complaint and no disease found Z71.1
    human immunodeficiency virus (HIV) Z71.7
    institutional resident Z59.3
    on behalf of another Z71.0
      related to sexual behavior or orientation Z70.2
    person living alone Z60.2
    specified reason NEC Z71.89
  natural family planning
    procreative Z31.61
    to avoid pregnancy Z30.02
  perpetrator (of)
    abuse NEC Z69.82
    child abuse
      non-parental Z69.021
      parental Z69.011
    rape NEC Z69.82
    spousal abuse Z69.12
  procreative NEC Z31.69
    fertility preservation (prior to cancer therapy) (prior to removal of gonads) Z31.62
    using natural family planning Z31.61
  promiscuity Z70.1
  rape victim Z69.81
  religious Z71.81
  sex, sexual (related to) Z70.9
    attitude(s) Z70.0
    behavior or orientation Z70.1
    combined concerns Z70.3
    non-responsiveness Z70.1
    on behalf of third party Z70.2
    specified reason NEC Z70.8
  specified reason NEC Z71.89
  spiritual Z71.81
  spousal abuse (perpetrator) Z69.12
    victim Z69.11
  substance abuse Z71.89
    alcohol Z71.41
    drug Z71.51
    tobacco Z71.6
  tobacco use Z71.6

Counseling — *continued*
  use (of)
    insulin pump Z46.81
  victim (of)
    abuse Z69.81
    child abuse
      by parent Z69.010
      non-parental Z69.020
    rape NEC Z69.81
Coupled rhythm R00.8
Couvelaire syndrome or uterus (complicating delivery) O45.8X- ☑
Cowperitis — *see* Urethritis
Cowper's gland — *see* condition
Cowpox B08.010
  due to vaccination T88.1 ☑
Coxa
  magna M91.4- ☑
  plana M91.2- ☑
  valga (acquired) (*see also* Deformity, limb, specified type NEC, thigh)
    congenital Q65.81
    sequelae (late effect) of rickets E64.3
  vara (acquired) (*see also* Deformity, limb, specified type NEC, thigh)
    congenital Q65.82
    sequelae (late effect) of rickets E64.3
Coxalgia, coxalgic (nontuberculous) (*see also* Pain, joint, hip)
  tuberculous A18.02
Coxitis — *see* Monoarthritis, hip
Coxsackie (virus) (infection) B34.1
  as cause of disease classified elsewhere B97.11
  carditis B33.20
  central nervous system NEC A88.8
  endocarditis B33.21
  enteritis A08.39
  meningitis (aseptic) A87.0
  myocarditis B33.22
  pericarditis B33.23
  pharyngitis B08.5
  pleurodynia B33.0
  specific disease NEC B33.8
Crabs, meaning pubic lice B85.3
Crack baby P04.41
Cracked nipple N64.0
  associated with
    lactation O92.13
    pregnancy O92.11- ☑
    puerperium O92.12
Cracked tooth K03.81
Cradle cap L21.0
Craft neurosis F48.8
Cramp(s) R25.2
  abdominal — *see* Pain, abdominal
  bathing T75.1 ☑
  colic R10.83
    psychogenic F45.8
  due to immersion T75.1 ☑
  fireman T67.2 ☑
  heat T67.2 ☑
  immersion T75.1 ☑
  intestinal — *see* Pain, abdominal
    psychogenic F45.8
  leg, sleep related G47.62
  limb (lower) (upper) NEC R25.2
    sleep related G47.62
  linotypist's F48.8
    organic G25.89
  muscle (limb) (general) R25.2
    due to immersion T75.1 ☑
    psychogenic F45.8
  occupational (hand) F48.8
    organic G25.89
  salt-depletion E87.1
  sleep related, leg G47.62
  stoker's T67.2 ☑
  swimmer's T75.1 ☑
  telegrapher's F48.8
    organic G25.89
  typist's F48.8
    organic G25.89
  uterus N94.89
    menstrual — *see* Dysmenorrhea
  writer's F48.8
    organic G25.89
Cranial — *see* condition

Craniocleidodysostosis Q74.0
Craniofenestria (skull) Q75.8
Craniolacunia (skull) Q75.8
Craniopagus Q89.4
Craniopathy, metabolic M85.2
Craniopharyngeal — see condition
Craniopharyngioma D44.4
Craniorachischisis (totalis) Q00.1
Cranioschisis Q75.8
Craniostenosis Q75.0
Craniosynostosis Q75.0
Craniotabes (cause unknown) M83.8
  neonatal P96.3
  rachitic E64.3
  syphilitic A50.56
Cranium — see condition
Craw-craw — see Onchocerciasis
Creaking joint — see Derangement, joint, specified type
    NEC
Creeping
  eruption B76.9
  palsy or paralysis G12.22
Crenated tongue K14.8
Creotoxism A05.9
Crepitus
  caput Q75.8
  joint — see Derangement, joint, specified type NEC
Crescent or conus choroid, congenital Q14.3
CREST syndrome M34.1
Cretin, cretinism (congenital) (endemic) (nongoitrous)
    (sporadic) E00.9
  pelvis
    with disproportion (fetopelvic) O33.0
      causing obstructed labor O65.0
  type
    hypothyroid E00.1
    mixed E00.2
    myxedematous E00.1
    neurological E00.0
Creutzfeldt-Jakob disease or syndrome (with demen-
    tia) A81.00
  familial A81.09
  iatrogenic A81.09
  specified NEC A81.09
  sporadic A81.09
  variant (vCJD) A81.01
Crib death R99
Cribriform hymen Q52.3
Cri-du-chat syndrome Q93.4
Crigler-Najjar disease or syndrome E80.5
Crime, victim of Z65.4
Crimean hemorrhagic fever A98.0
Criminalism F60.2
Crisis
  abdomen R10.0
  acute reaction F43.0
  addisonian E27.2
  adrenal (cortical) E27.2
  celiac K90.0
  Dietl's N13.8
  emotional (see also Disorder, adjustment)
    acute reaction to stress F43.0
    specific to childhood and adolescence F93.8
  glaucomatocyclitic — see Glaucoma, secondary, in-
    flammation
  heart — see Failure, heart
  nitritoid I95.2
    correct substance properly administered — see
      Table of Drugs and Chemicals, by drug, ad-
      verse effect
    overdose or wrong substance given or taken —
      see Table of Drugs and Chemicals, by drug,
      poisoning
  oculogyric H51.8
    psychogenic F45.8
  Pel's (tabetic) A52.11
  psychosexual identity F64.2
  renal N28.0
  sickle-cell D57.00
    with
      acute chest syndrome D57.01
      splenic sequestration D57.02
  state (acute reaction) F43.0
  tabetic A52.11
  thyroid — see Thyrotoxicosis with thyroid storm
  thyrotoxic — see Thyrotoxicosis with thyroid storm
Crocq's disease (acrocyanosis) I73.89

Crohn's disease — see Enteritis, regional
Crooked septum, nasal J34.2
Cross syndrome E70.328
Crossbite (anterior) (posterior) M26.24
Cross-eye — see Strabismus, convergent concomitant
Croup, croupous (catarrhal) (infectious) (inflammatory)
    (nondiphtheritic) J05.0
  bronchial J20.9
  diphtheritic A36.2
  false J38.5
  spasmodic J38.5
    diphtheritic A36.2
  stridulous J38.5
    diphtheritic A36.2
Crouzon's disease Q75.1
Crowding, tooth, teeth, fully erupted M26.31
CRST syndrome M34.1
Cruchet's disease A85.8
Cruelty in children (see also Disorder, conduct)
Crural ulcer — see Ulcer, lower limb
Crush, crushed, crushing T14.8 ☑
  abdomen S38.1 ☑
  ankle S97.0- ☑
  arm (upper) (and shoulder) S47.- ☑
  axilla — see Crush, arm
  back, lower S38.1 ☑
  buttock S38.1 ☑
  cheek S07.0 ☑
  chest S28.0 ☑
  cranium S07.1 ☑
  ear S07.0 ☑
  elbow S57.0- ☑
  extremity
    lower
      ankle — see Crush, ankle
      below knee — see Crush, leg
      foot — see Crush, foot
      hip — see Crush, hip
      knee — see Crush, knee
      thigh — see Crush, thigh
      toe — see Crush, toe
    upper
      below elbow S67.9- ☑
      elbow — see Crush, elbow
      finger — see Crush, finger
      forearm — see Crush, forearm
      hand — see Crush, hand
      thumb — see Crush, thumb
      upper arm — see Crush, arm
      wrist — see Crush, wrist
  face S07.0 ☑
  finger(s) S67.1- ☑
    with hand (and wrist) — see Crush, hand, specified
      site NEC
    index S67.19- ☑
    little S67.19- ☑
    middle S67.19- ☑
    ring S67.19- ☑
    thumb — see Crush, thumb
  foot S97.8- ☑
    toe — see Crush, toe
  forearm S57.8- ☑
  genitalia, external
    female S38.002 ☑
      vagina S38.03 ☑
      vulva S38.03 ☑
    male S38.001 ☑
      penis S38.01 ☑
      scrotum S38.02 ☑
      testis S38.02 ☑
  hand (except fingers alone) S67.2- ☑
    with wrist S67.4- ☑
  head S07.9 ☑
    specified NEC S07.8 ☑
  heel — see Crush, foot
  hip S77.0- ☑
    with thigh S77.2- ☑
  internal organ (abdomen, chest, or pelvis) NEC
    T14.8 ☑
  knee S87.0- ☑
  labium (majus) (minus) S38.03 ☑
  larynx S17.0 ☑
  leg (lower) S87.8- ☑
    knee — see Crush, knee
  lip S07.0 ☑

Crush, crushed, crushing — continued
  lower
    back S38.1 ☑
    leg — see Crush, leg
  neck S17.9 ☑
  nerve — see Injury, nerve
  nose S07.0 ☑
  pelvis S38.1 ☑
  penis S38.01 ☑
  scalp S07.8 ☑
  scapular region — see Crush, arm
  scrotum S38.02 ☑
  severe, unspecified site T14.8 ☑
  shoulder (and upper arm) — see Crush, arm
  skull S07.1 ☑
  syndrome (complication of trauma) T79.5 ☑
  testis S38.02 ☑
  thigh S77.1- ☑
    with hip S77.2- ☑
  throat S17.8 ☑
  thumb S67.0- ☑
    with hand (and wrist) — see Crush, hand, specified
      site NEC
  toe(s) S97.10- ☑
    great S97.11- ☑
    lesser S97.12- ☑
  trachea S17.0 ☑
  vagina S38.03 ☑
  vulva S38.03 ☑
  wrist S67.3- ☑
    with hand S67.4- ☑
Crusta lactea L21.0
Crusts R23.4
Crutch paralysis — see Injury, brachial plexus
**Cruveilhier-Baumgarten cirrhosis, disease or syn-
    drome** K74.69
Cruveilhier's atrophy or disease G12.8
Crying (constant) (continuous) (excessive)
  child, adolescent, or adult R45.83
  infant (baby) (newborn) R68.11
Cryofibrinogenemia D89.2
Cryoglobulinemia (essential) (idiopathic) (mixed) (pri-
    mary) (purpura) (secondary) (vasculitis) D89.1
  with lung involvement D89.1 [J99]
Cryptitis (anal) (rectal) K62.89
Cryptococcosis, cryptococcus (infection) (neoformans)
    B45.9
  bone B45.3
  cerebral B45.1
  cutaneous B45.2
  disseminated B45.7
  generalized B45.7
  meningitis B45.1
  meningocerebralis B45.1
  osseous B45.3
  pulmonary B45.0
  skin B45.2
  specified NEC B45.8
Cryptopapillitis (anus) K62.89
Cryptophthalmos Q11.2
  syndrome Q87.0
Cryptorchid, cryptorchism, cryptorchidism Q53.9
  bilateral Q53.20
    abdominal Q53.211
    perineal Q53.22
  unilateral Q53.10
    abdominal Q53.111
    perineal Q53.12
Cryptosporidiosis A07.2
  hepatobiliary B88.8
  respiratory B88.8
Cryptostromosis J67.6
Crystalluria R82.99
Cubitus
  congenital Q68.8
  valgus (acquired) M21.0- ☑
    congenital Q68.8
    sequelae (late effect) of rickets E64.3
  varus (acquired) M21.1- ☑
    congenital Q68.8
    sequelae (late effect) of rickets E64.3
Cultural deprivation or shock Z60.3
Curling esophagus K22.4
Curling's ulcer — see Ulcer, peptic, acute
Curschmann (-Batten) (-Steinert) **disease or syndrome**
    G71.11
Curse, Ondine's — see Apnea, sleep

Curvature
- organ or site, congenital NEC — *see* Distortion
- penis (lateral) Q55.61
- Pott's (spinal) A18.01
- radius, idiopathic, progressive (congenital) Q74.0
- spine (acquired) (angular) (idiopathic) (incorrect) (postural) — *see* Dorsopathy, deforming
    - congenital Q67.5
    - due to or associated with
        - Charcot-Marie-Tooth disease (*see also* subcategory M49.8) G60.0
        - osteitis
            - deformans M88.88
            - fibrosa cystica (*see also* subcategory M49.8) E21.0
        - tuberculosis (Pott's curvature) A18.01
    - sequelae (late effect) of rickets E64.3
    - tuberculous A18.01

Cushingoid due to steroid therapy E24.2
- correct substance properly administered — *see* Table of Drugs and Chemicals, by drug, adverse effect
- overdose or wrong substance given or taken — *see* Table of Drugs and Chemicals, by drug, poisoning

Cushing's
- syndrome or disease E24.9
    - drug-induced E24.2
    - iatrogenic E24.2
    - pituitary-dependent E24.0
    - specified NEC E24.8
- ulcer — *see* Ulcer, peptic, acute

Cusp, Carabelli — *omit code*

Cut (external) (*see also* Laceration)
- muscle — *see* Injury, muscle

Cutaneous (*see also* condition)
- hemorrhage R23.3
- larva migrans B76.9

Cutis (*see also* condition)
- hyperelastica Q82.8
    - acquired L57.4
- laxa (hyperelastica) — *see* Dermatolysis
- marmorata R23.8
- osteosis L94.2
- pendula — *see* Dermatolysis
- rhomboidalis nuchae L57.2
- verticis gyrata Q82.8
    - acquired L91.8

Cyanosis R23.0
- due to
    - patent foramen botalli Q21.1
    - persistent foramen ovale Q21.1
- enterogenous D74.8
- paroxysmal digital — *see* Raynaud's disease
    - with gangrene I73.01
- retina, retinal H35.89

Cyanotic heart disease I24.9
- congenital Q24.9

Cycle
- anovulatory N97.0
- menstrual, irregular N92.6

Cyclencephaly Q04.9

Cyclical vomiting (*see also* Vomiting, cyclical) G43.A0 (*following* G43.7)
- psychogenic F50.89

Cyclitis (*see also* Iridocyclitis) H20.9
- chronic — *see* Iridocyclitis, chronic
- Fuchs' heterochromic H20.81- ☑
- granulomatous — *see* Iridocyclitis, chronic
- lens-induced — *see* Iridocyclitis, lens-induced
- posterior H30.2- ☑

Cycloid personality F34.0

Cyclophoria H50.54

Cyclopia, cyclops Q87.0

Cyclopism Q87.0

Cyclosporiasis A07.4

Cyclothymia F34.0

Cyclothymic personality F34.0

Cyclotropia H50.41- ☑

Cylindroma (*see also* Neoplasm, malignant, by site)
- eccrine dermal — *see* Neoplasm, skin, benign
- skin — *see* Neoplasm, skin, benign

Cylindruria R82.99

Cynanche
- diphtheritic A36.2
- tonsillaris J36

Cynophobia F40.218

Cynorexia R63.2

Cyphosis — *see* Kyphosis

Cyprus fever — *see* Brucellosis

Cyst (colloid) (mucous) (simple) (retention)
- adenoid (infected) J35.8
- adrenal gland E27.8
    - congenital Q89.1
- air, lung J98.4
- allantoic Q64.4
- alveolar process (jaw bone) M27.40
- amnion, amniotic O41.8X- ☑
- aneurysmal M27.49
- anterior
    - chamber (eye) — *see* Cyst, iris
    - nasopalatine K09.1
- antrum J34.1
- anus K62.89
- apical (tooth) (periodontal) K04.8
- appendix K38.8
- arachnoid, brain (acquired) G93.0
    - congenital Q04.6
- arytenoid J38.7
- Baker's M71.2- ☑
    - ruptured M66.0
    - tuberculous A18.02
- Bartholin's gland N75.0
- bile duct (common) (hepatic) K83.5
- bladder (multiple) (trigone) N32.89
- blue dome (breast) — *see* Cyst, breast
- bone (local) NEC M85.60
    - aneurysmal M85.50
        - ankle M85.57- ☑
        - foot M85.57- ☑
        - forearm M85.53- ☑
        - hand M85.54- ☑
        - jaw M27.49
        - lower leg M85.56- ☑
        - multiple site M85.59
        - neck M85.58
        - rib M85.58
        - shoulder M85.51- ☑
        - skull M85.58
        - specified site NEC M85.58
        - thigh M85.55- ☑
        - toe M85.57- ☑
        - upper arm M85.52- ☑
        - vertebra M85.58
    - solitary M85.40
        - ankle M85.47- ☑
        - fibula M85.46- ☑
        - foot M85.47- ☑
        - hand M85.44- ☑
        - humerus M85.42- ☑
        - jaw M27.49
        - neck M85.48
        - pelvis M85.45- ☑
        - radius M85.43- ☑
        - rib M85.48
        - shoulder M85.41- ☑
        - skull M85.48
        - specified site NEC M85.48
        - tibia M85.46- ☑
        - toe M85.47- ☑
        - ulna M85.43- ☑
        - vertebra M85.48
    - specified type NEC M85.60
        - ankle M85.67- ☑
        - foot M85.67- ☑
        - forearm M85.63- ☑
        - hand M85.64- ☑
        - jaw M27.40
            - developmental (nonodontogenic) K09.1
            - odontogenic K09.0
            - latent M27.0
        - lower leg M85.66- ☑
        - multiple site M85.69
        - neck M85.68
        - rib M85.68
        - shoulder M85.61- ☑
        - skull M85.68
        - specified site NEC M85.68
        - thigh M85.65- ☑
        - toe M85.67- ☑
        - upper arm M85.62- ☑
        - vertebra M85.68
- brain (acquired) G93.0
    - congenital Q04.6
    - hydatid B67.99 [G94]

Cyst — *continued*
- brain — *continued*
    - third ventricle (colloid), congenital Q04.6
- branchial (cleft) Q18.0
- branchiogenic Q18.0
- breast (benign) (blue dome) (pedunculated) (solitary) N60.0- ☑
    - involution — *see* Dysplasia, mammary, specified type NEC
    - sebaceous — *see* Dysplasia, mammary, specified type NEC
- broad ligament (benign) N83.8
- bronchogenic (mediastinal) (sequestration) J98.4
    - congenital Q33.0
- buccal K09.8
- bulbourethral gland N36.8
- bursa, bursal NEC M71.30
    - with rupture — *see* Rupture, synovium
    - ankle M71.37- ☑
    - elbow M71.32- ☑
    - foot M71.37- ☑
    - hand M71.34- ☑
    - hip M71.35- ☑
    - multiple sites M71.39
    - pharyngeal J39.2
    - popliteal space — *see* Cyst, Baker's
    - shoulder M71.31- ☑
    - specified site NEC M71.38
    - wrist M71.33- ☑
- calcifying odontogenic D16.5
    - upper jaw (bone) (maxilla) D16.4
- canal of Nuck (female) N94.89
    - congenital Q52.4
- canthus — *see* Cyst, conjunctiva
- carcinomatous — *see* Neoplasm, malignant, by site
- cauda equina G95.89
- cavum septi pellucidi — *see* Cyst, brain
- celomic (pericardium) Q24.8
- cerebellopontine (angle) — *see* Cyst, brain
- cerebellum — *see* Cyst, brain
- cerebral — *see* Cyst, brain
- cervical lateral Q18.0
- cervix NEC N88.8
    - embryonic Q51.6
    - nabothian N88.8
- chiasmal optic NEC — *see* Disorder, optic, chiasm
- chocolate (ovary) N80.1
- choledochus, congenital Q44.4
- chorion O41.8X- ☑
- choroid plexus G93.0
- ciliary body — *see* Cyst, iris
- clitoris N90.7
- colon K63.89
- common (bile) duct K83.5
- congenital NEC Q89.8
    - adrenal gland Q89.1
    - epiglottis Q31.8
    - esophagus Q39.8
    - fallopian tube Q50.4
    - kidney Q61.00
        - more than one (multiple) Q61.02
            - specified as polycystic Q61.3
                - adult type Q61.2
                - infantile type NEC Q61.19
                    - collecting duct dilation Q61.11
        - solitary Q61.01
    - larynx Q31.8
    - liver Q44.6
    - lung Q33.0
    - mediastinum Q34.1
    - ovary Q50.1
    - oviduct Q50.4
    - periurethral (tissue) Q64.79
    - prepuce Q55.69
    - salivary gland (any) Q38.4
    - sublingual Q38.6
    - submaxillary gland Q38.6
    - thymus (gland) Q89.2
    - tongue Q38.3
    - ureterovesical orifice Q62.8
    - vulva Q52.79
- conjunctiva H11.44- ☑
- cornea H18.89- ☑
- corpora quadrigemina G93.0
- corpus
    - albicans N83.29- ☑
    - luteum (hemorrhagic) (ruptured) N83.1- ☑
- Cowper's gland (benign) (infected) N36.8

Cyst — *continued*
　cranial meninges G93.0
　craniobuccal pouch E23.6
　craniopharyngeal pouch E23.6
　cystic duct K82.8
　Cysticercus — *see* Cysticercosis
　Dandy-Walker Q03.1
　　with spina bifida — *see* Spina bifida
　dental (root) K04.8
　　developmental K09.0
　　eruption K09.0
　　primordial K09.0
　dentigerous (mandible) (maxilla) K09.0
　dermoid — *see* Neoplasm, benign, by site
　　with malignant transformation C56.- ☑
　　implantation
　　　external area or site (skin) NEC L72.0
　　　iris — *see* Cyst, iris, implantation
　　　vagina N89.8
　　　vulva N90.7
　　mouth K09.8
　　oral soft tissue K09.8
　　sacrococcygeal — *see* Cyst, pilonidal
　developmental K09.1
　　odontogenic K09.0
　　oral region (nonodontogenic) K09.1
　　ovary, ovarian Q50.1
　dura (cerebral) G93.0
　　spinal G96.19
　ear (external) Q18.1
　echinococcal — *see* Echinococcus
　embryonic
　　cervix uteri Q51.6
　　fallopian tube Q50.4
　　vagina Q52.4
　endometrium, endometrial (uterus) N85.8
　　ectopic — *see* Endometriosis
　enterogenous Q43.8
　epidermal, epidermoid (inclusion) (*see also* Cyst, skin)
　　　L72.0
　　mouth K09.8
　　oral soft tissue K09.8
　epididymis N50.3
　epiglottis J38.7
　epiphysis cerebri E34.8
　epithelial (inclusion) L72.0
　epoophoron Q50.5
　eruption K09.0
　esophagus K22.8
　ethmoid sinus J34.1
　external female genital organs NEC N90.7
　eyelid (sebaceous) H02.829
　　infected — *see* Hordeolum
　　left H02.826
　　　lower H02.825
　　　upper H02.824
　　right H02.823
　　　lower H02.822
　　　upper H02.821
　eye NEC H57.8
　　congenital Q15.8
　fallopian tube N83.8
　　congenital Q50.4
　fimbrial (twisted) Q50.4
　fissural (oral region) K09.1
　follicle (graafian) (hemorrhagic) N83.0- ☑
　　nabothian N88.8
　follicular (atretic) (hemorrhagic) (ovarian) N83.0- ☑
　　dentigerous K09.0
　　odontogenic K09.0
　　skin L72.9
　　　specified NEC L72.8
　frontal sinus J34.1
　gallbladder K82.8
　ganglion — *see* Ganglion
　Gartner's duct Q52.4
　gingiva K09.0
　gland of Moll — *see* Cyst, eyelid
　globulomaxillary K09.1
　graafian follicle (hemorrhagic) N83.0- ☑
　granulosal lutein (hemorrhagic) N83.1- ☑
　hemangiomatous D18.00
　　intra-abdominal D18.03
　　intracranial D18.02
　　skin D18.01
　　specified site NEC D18.09
　hemorrhagic M27.49
　hydatid (*see also* Echinococcus) B67.90

Cyst — *continued*
　hydatid (*see also* Echinococcus) — *continued*
　　brain B67.99 [G94]
　　liver (*see also* Cyst, liver, hydatid) B67.8
　　lung NEC B67.99 [J99]
　　Morgagni
　　　female Q50.5
　　　male (epididymal) Q55.4
　　　　testicular Q55.29
　　specified site NEC B67.99
　hymen N89.8
　　embryonic Q52.4
　hypopharynx J39.2
　hypophysis, hypophyseal (duct) (recurrent) E23.6
　　cerebri E23.6
　implantation (dermoid)
　　external area or site (skin) NEC L72.0
　　iris — *see* Cyst, iris, implantation
　　vagina N89.8
　　vulva N90.7
　incisive canal K09.1
　inclusion (epidermal) (epithelial) (epidermoid) (squa-
　　　mous) L72.0
　　not of skin — *code under* Cyst, by site
　intestine (large) (small) K63.89
　intracranial — *see* Cyst, brain
　intraligamentous (*see also* Disorder, ligament)
　　knee — *see* Derangement, knee
　intrasellar E23.6
　iris H21.309
　　exudative H21.31- ☑
　　idiopathic H21.30- ☑
　　implantation H21.32- ☑
　　parasitic H21.33- ☑
　　pars plana (primary) H21.34- ☑
　　　exudative H21.35- ☑
　jaw (bone) M27.40
　　aneurysmal M27.49
　　developmental (odontogenic) K09.0
　　fissural K09.1
　　hemorrhagic M27.49
　　traumatic M27.49
　joint NEC — *see* Disorder, joint, specified type NEC
　kidney (acquired) N28.1
　　calyceal — *see* Hydronephrosis
　　congenital Q61.00
　　　more than one (multiple) Q61.02
　　　　specified as polycystic Q61.3
　　　　　adult type (autosomal dominant) Q61.2
　　　　　infantile type (autosomal recessive) NEC
　　　　　　Q61.19
　　　　　　collecting duct dilation Q61.11
　　pyelogenic — *see* Hydronephrosis
　　simple N28.1
　　solitary (single) Q61.01
　　　acquired N28.1
　labium (majus) (minus) N90.7
　　sebaceous N90.7
　lacrimal (*see also* Disorder, lacrimal system, specified
　　　NEC)
　　gland H04.13- ☑
　　passages or sac — *see* Disorder, lacrimal system,
　　　specified NEC
　larynx J38.7
　lateral periodontal K09.0
　lens H27.8
　　congenital Q12.8
　lip (gland) K13.0
　liver (idiopathic) (simple) K76.89
　　congenital Q44.6
　　hydatid B67.8
　　　granulosus B67.0
　　　multilocularis B67.5
　lung J98.4
　　congenital Q33.0
　　giant bullous J43.9
　lutein N83.1- ☑
　lymphangiomatous D18.1
　lymphoepithelial, oral soft tissue K09.8
　macula — *see* Degeneration, macula, hole
　malignant — *see* Neoplasm, malignant, by site
　mammary gland — *see* Cyst, breast
　mandible M27.40
　　dentigerous K09.0
　　radicular K04.8
　maxilla M27.40
　　dentigerous K09.0
　　radicular K04.8

Cyst — *continued*
　medial, face and neck Q18.8
　median
　　anterior maxillary K09.1
　　palatal K09.1
　mediastinum, congenital Q34.1
　meibomian (gland) — *see* Chalazion
　　infected — *see* Hordeolum
　membrane, brain G93.0
　meninges (cerebral) G93.0
　　spinal G96.19
　meniscus, knee — *see* Derangement, knee, meniscus,
　　　cystic
　mesentery, mesenteric K66.8
　　chyle I89.8
　mesonephric duct
　　female Q50.5
　　male Q55.4
　milk N64.89
　Morgagni (hydatid)
　　female Q50.5
　　male (epididymal) Q55.4
　　　testicular Q55.29
　mouth K09.8
　Müllerian duct Q50.4
　　appendix testis Q55.29
　　cervix Q51.6
　　fallopian tube Q50.4
　　female Q50.4
　　male Q55.29
　　prostatic utricle Q55.4
　　vagina (embryonal) Q52.4
　multilocular (ovary) D39.10
　　benign — *see* Neoplasm, benign, by site
　myometrium N85.8
　nabothian (follicle) (ruptured) N88.8
　nasoalveolar K09.1
　nasolabial K09.1
　nasopalatine (anterior) (duct) K09.1
　nasopharynx J39.2
　neoplastic — *see* Neoplasm, uncertain behavior, by
　　　site
　　benign — *see* Neoplasm, benign, by site
　nervous system NEC G96.8
　neuroenteric (congenital) Q06.8
　nipple — *see* Cyst, breast
　nose (turbinates) J34.1
　　sinus J34.1
　odontogenic, developmental K09.0
　omentum (lesser) K66.8
　　congenital Q45.8
　ora serrata — *see* Cyst, retina, ora serrata
　oral
　　region K09.9
　　　developmental (nonodontogenic) K09.1
　　　specified NEC K09.8
　　soft tissue K09.9
　　　specified NEC K09.8
　orbit H05.81- ☑
　ovary, ovarian (twisted) N83.20- ☑
　　adherent N83.20- ☑
　　chocolate N80.1
　　corpus
　　　albicans N83.29- ☑
　　　luteum (hemorrhagic) N83.1- ☑
　　dermoid D27.9
　　developmental Q50.1
　　due to failure of involution NEC N83.20- ☑
　　endometrial N80.1
　　follicular (graafian) (hemorrhagic) N83.0- ☑
　　hemorrhagic N83.20- ☑
　　in pregnancy or childbirth O34.8- ☑
　　　with obstructed labor O65.5
　　multilocular D39.10
　　pseudomucinous D27.9
　　retention N83.29- ☑
　　serous N83.20- ☑
　　specified NEC N83.29- ☑
　　theca lutein (hemorrhagic) N83.1- ☑
　　tuberculous A18.18
　oviduct N83.8
　palate (median) (fissural) K09.1
　palatine papilla (jaw) K09.1
　pancreas, pancreatic (hemorrhagic) (true) K86.2
　　congenital Q45.2
　　false K86.3
　paralabral
　　hip M24.85- ☑

🔻 **Subterms under main terms may continue to next column or page**　　☑ **Additional Character Required — Refer to the Tabular List for Character Selection**　　79

Cyst — Cyst

Cyst — *continued*
paralabral — *continued*
  shoulder S43.43- ☑
paramesonephric duct Q50.4
  female Q50.4
  male Q55.29
paranephric N28.1
paraphysis, cerebri, congenital Q04.6
parasitic B89
parathyroid (gland) E21.4
paratubal N83.8
paraurethral duct N36.8
paroophoron Q50.5
parotid gland K11.6
parovarian Q50.5
pelvis, female N94.89
  in pregnancy or childbirth O34.8- ☑
    causing obstructed labor O65.5
penis (sebaceous) N48.89
periapical K04.8
pericardial (congenital) Q24.8
  acquired (secondary) I31.8
pericoronal K09.0
periodontal K04.8
  lateral K09.0
peripelvic (lymphatic) N28.1
peritoneum K66.8
  chylous I89.8
periventricular, acquired, newborn P91.1
pharynx (wall) J39.2
pilar L72.11
pilonidal (infected) (rectum) L05.91
  with abscess L05.01
  malignant C44.59- ☑
pituitary (duct) (gland) E23.6
placenta O43.19- ☑
pleura J94.8
popliteal — *see* Cyst, Baker's
porencephalic Q04.6
  acquired G93.0
postanal (infected) — *see* Cyst, pilonidal
postmastoidectomy cavity (mucosal) — *see* Complications, postmastoidectomy, cyst
preauricular Q18.1
prepuce N47.4
  congenital Q55.69
primordial (jaw) K09.0
prostate N42.83
pseudomucinous (ovary) D27.9
pupillary, miotic H21.27- ☑
radicular (residual) K04.8
radiculodental K04.8
ranular K11.8
Rathke's pouch E23.6
rectum (epithelium) (mucous) K62.89
renal — *see* Cyst, kidney
residual (radicular) K04.8
retention (ovary) N83.29- ☑
  salivary gland K11.6
retina H33.19- ☑
  ora serrata H33.11- ☑
  parasitic H33.12- ☑
retroperitoneal K68.9
sacrococcygeal (dermoid) — *see* Cyst, pilonidal
salivary gland or duct (mucous extravasation or retention) K11.6
Sampson's N80.1
sclera H15.89
scrotum L72.9
  sebaceous L72.3
sebaceous (duct) (gland) L72.3
  breast — *see* Dysplasia, mammary, specified type NEC
  eyelid — *see* Cyst, eyelid
  genital organ NEC
    female N94.89
    male N50.89
  scrotum L72.3
semilunar cartilage (knee) (multiple) — *see* Derangement, knee, meniscus, cystic
seminal vesicle N50.89
serous (ovary) N83.20- ☑
sinus (accessory) (nasal) J34.1
Skene's gland N36.8
skin L72.9
  breast — *see* Dysplasia, mammary, specified type NEC
  epidermal, epidermoid L72.0

Cyst — *continued*
skin — *continued*
  epithelial L72.0
  eyelid — *see* Cyst, eyelid
  genital organ NEC
    female N90.7
    male N50.89
  inclusion L72.0
  scrotum L72.9
  sebaceous L72.3
  sweat gland or duct L74.8
solitary
  bone — *see* Cyst, bone, solitary
  jaw M27.40
  kidney N28.1
spermatic cord N50.89
sphenoid sinus J34.1
spinal meninges G96.19
spleen NEC D73.4
  congenital Q89.09
  hydatid (*see also* Echinococcus) B67.99 [D77]
Stafne's M27.0
subarachnoid intrasellar R93.0
subcutaneous, pheomycotic (chromomycotic) B43.2
subdural (cerebral) G93.0
  spinal cord G96.19
sublingual gland K11.6
submandibular gland K11.6
submaxillary gland K11.6
suburethral N36.8
suprarenal gland E27.8
suprasellar — *see* Cyst, brain
sweat gland or duct L74.8
synovial (*see also* Cyst, bursa)
  ruptured — *see* Rupture, synovium
tarsal — *see* Chalazion
tendon (sheath) — *see* Disorder, tendon, specified type NEC
testis N44.2
  tunica albuginea N44.1
theca lutein (ovary) N83.1- ☑
Thornwaldt's J39.2
thymus (gland) E32.8
thyroglossal duct (infected) (persistent) Q89.2
thyroid (gland) E04.1
thyrolingual duct (infected) (persistent) Q89.2
tongue K14.8
tonsil J35.8
tooth — *see* Cyst, dental
Tornwaldt's J39.2
trichilemmal (proliferating) L72.12
trichodermal L72.12
tubal (fallopian) N83.8
  inflammatory — *see* Salpingitis, chronic
tubo-ovarian N83.8
  inflammatory N70.13
tunica
  albuginea testis N44.1
  vaginalis N50.89
turbinate (nose) J34.1
Tyson's gland N48.89
urachus, congenital Q64.4
ureter N28.89
ureterovesical orifice N28.89
urethra, urethral (gland) N36.8
uterine ligament N83.8
uterus (body) (corpus) (recurrent) N85.8
  embryonic Q51.818
    cervix Q51.6
vagina, vaginal (implantation) (inclusion) (squamous cell) (wall) N89.8
  embryonic Q52.4
vallecula, vallecular (epiglottis) J38.7
vesical (orifice) N32.89
vitreous body H43.89
vulva (implantation) (inclusion) N90.7
  congenital Q52.79
  sebaceous gland N90.7
vulvovaginal gland N90.7
wolffian
  female Q50.5
  male Q55.4
Cystadenocarcinoma — *see* Neoplasm, malignant, by site
bile duct C22.1
endometrioid — *see* Neoplasm, malignant, by site
  specified site — *see* Neoplasm, malignant, by site

Cystadenocarcinoma — *continued*
endometrioid — *see* Neoplasm, malignant, by site — *continued*
  unspecified site
    female C56.9
    male C61
mucinous
  papillary
    specified site — *see* Neoplasm, malignant, by site
    unspecified site C56.9
  specified site — *see* Neoplasm, malignant, by site
  unspecified site C56.9
papillary
  mucinous
    specified site — *see* Neoplasm, malignant, by site
    unspecified site C56.9
  pseudomucinous
    specified site — *see* Neoplasm, malignant, by site
    unspecified site C56.9
  serous
    specified site — *see* Neoplasm, malignant, by site
    unspecified site C56.9
  specified site — *see* Neoplasm, malignant, by site
  unspecified site C56.9
pseudomucinous
  papillary
    specified site — *see* Neoplasm, malignant, by site
    unspecified site C56.9
  specified site — *see* Neoplasm, malignant, by site
  unspecified site C56.9
serous
  papillary
    specified site — *see* Neoplasm, malignant, by site
    unspecified site C56.9
  specified site — *see* Neoplasm, malignant, by site
  unspecified site C56.9
Cystadenofibroma
clear cell — *see* Neoplasm, benign, by site
endometrioid D27.9
  borderline malignancy D39.1- ☑
  malignant C56.- ☑
mucinous
  specified site — *see* Neoplasm, benign, by site
  unspecified site D27.9
serous
  specified site — *see* Neoplasm, benign, by site
  unspecified site D27.9
specified site — *see* Neoplasm, benign, by site
unspecified site D27.9
Cystadenoma (*see also* Neoplasm, benign, by site)
bile duct D13.4
endometrioid — *see* Neoplasm, benign, by site
  borderline malignancy — *see* Neoplasm, uncertain behavior, by site
malignant — *see* Neoplasm, malignant, by site
mucinous
  borderline malignancy
    ovary C56.- ☑
    specified site NEC — *see* Neoplasm, uncertain behavior, by site
    unspecified site C56.9
  papillary
    borderline malignancy
      ovary C56.- ☑
      specified site NEC — *see* Neoplasm, uncertain behavior, by site
      unspecified site C56.9
    specified site — *see* Neoplasm, benign, by site
    unspecified site D27.9
  specified site — *see* Neoplasm, benign, by site
  unspecified site D27.9
papillary
  borderline malignancy
    ovary C56.- ☑
    specified site NEC — *see* Neoplasm, uncertain behavior, by site
    unspecified site C56.9
  lymphomatosum
    specified site — *see* Neoplasm, benign, by site
    unspecified site D11.9

☑ **Additional Character Required** — **Refer to the Tabular List for Character Selection**

▽ **Subterms under main terms may continue to next column or page**

Cyst — Cystadenoma

Cystadenoma — *continued*
  papillary — *continued*
    mucinous
      borderline malignancy
        ovary C56.- ☑
        specified site NEC — *see* Neoplasm, uncertain behavior, by site
        unspecified site C56.9
      specified site — *see* Neoplasm, benign, by site
      unspecified site D27.9
    pseudomucinous
      borderline malignancy
        ovary C56.- ☑
        specified site NEC — *see* Neoplasm, uncertain behavior, by site
        unspecified site C56.9
      specified site — *see* Neoplasm, benign, by site
      unspecified site D27.9
    serous
      borderline malignancy
        ovary C56.- ☑
        specified site NEC — *see* Neoplasm, uncertain behavior, by site
        unspecified site C56.9
      specified site — *see* Neoplasm, benign, by site
      unspecified site D27.9
    specified site — *see* Neoplasm, benign, by site
    unspecified site D27.9
  pseudomucinous
    borderline malignancy
      ovary C56.- ☑
      specified site NEC — *see* Neoplasm, uncertain behavior, by site
      unspecified site C56.9
    papillary
      borderline malignancy
        ovary C56.- ☑
        specified site NEC — *see* Neoplasm, uncertain behavior, by site
        unspecified site C56.9
      specified site — *see* Neoplasm, benign, by site
      unspecified site D27.9
    specified site — *see* Neoplasm, benign, by site
    unspecified site D27.9
  serous
    borderline malignancy
      ovary C56.- ☑
      specified site NEC — *see* Neoplasm, uncertain behavior, by site
      unspecified site C56.9
    papillary
      borderline malignancy
        ovary C56.- ☑
        specified site NEC — *see* Neoplasm, uncertain behavior, by site
        unspecified site C56.9
      specified site — *see* Neoplasm, benign, by site
      unspecified site D27.9
    specified site — *see* Neoplasm, benign, by site
    unspecified site D27.9
Cystathionine synthase deficiency E72.11
Cystathioninemia E72.19
Cystathioninuria E72.19
Cystic (*see also* condition)
  breast (chronic) — *see* Mastopathy, cystic
  corpora lutea (hemorrhagic) N83.1- ☑
  duct — *see* condition
  eyeball (congenital) Q11.0
  fibrosis — *see* Fibrosis, cystic
  kidney (congenital) Q61.9

Cystic — *continued*
  kidney — *continued*
    adult type Q61.2
    infantile type NEC Q61.19
      collecting duct dilatation Q61.11
    medullary Q61.5
  liver, congenital Q44.6
  lung disease J98.4
    congenital Q33.0
  mastitis, chronic — *see* Mastopathy, cystic
  medullary, kidney Q61.5
  meniscus — *see* Derangement, knee, meniscus, cystic
  ovary N83.20- ☑
Cysticercosis, cysticerciasis B69.9
  with
    epileptiform fits B69.0
    myositis B69.81
  brain B69.0
  central nervous system B69.0
  cerebral B69.0
  ocular B69.1
  specified NEC B69.89
Cysticercus cellulose infestation — *see* Cysticercosis
Cystinosis (malignant) E72.04
Cystinuria E72.01
Cystitis (exudative) (hemorrhagic) (septic) (suppurative) N30.90
  with
    fibrosis — *see* Cystitis, chronic, interstitial
    hematuria N30.91
    leukoplakia — *see* Cystitis, chronic, interstitial
    malakoplakia — *see* Cystitis, chronic, interstitial
    metaplasia — *see* Cystitis, chronic, interstitial
    prostatitis N41.3
  acute N30.00
    with hematuria N30.01
    of trigone N30.30
      with hematuria N30.31
  allergic — *see* Cystitis, specified type NEC
  amebic A06.81
  bilharzial B65.9 [N33]
  blennorrhagic (gonococcal) A54.01
  bullous — *see* Cystitis, specified type NEC
  calculous N21.0
  chlamydial A56.01
  chronic N30.20
    with hematuria N30.21
    interstitial N30.10
      with hematuria N30.11
    of trigone N30.30
      with hematuria N30.31
    specified NEC N30.20
      with hematuria N30.21
  cystic (a) — *see* Cystitis, specified type NEC
  diphtheritic A36.85
  echinococcal
    granulosus B67.39
    multilocularis B67.69
  emphysematous — *see* Cystitis, specified type NEC
  encysted — *see* Cystitis, specified type NEC
  eosinophilic — *see* Cystitis, specified type NEC
  follicular — *see* Cystitis, of trigone
  gangrenous — *see* Cystitis, specified type NEC
  glandularis — *see* Cystitis, specified type NEC
  gonococcal A54.01
  incrusted — *see* Cystitis, specified type NEC
  interstitial (chronic) — *see* Cystitis, chronic, interstitial
  irradiation N30.40
    with hematuria N30.41
  irritation — *see* Cystitis, specified type NEC

Cystitis — *continued*
  malignant — *see* Cystitis, specified type NEC
  of trigone N30.30
    with hematuria N30.31
  panmural — *see* Cystitis, chronic, interstitial
  polyposa — *see* Cystitis, specified type NEC
  prostatic N41.3
  puerperal (postpartum) O86.22
  radiation — *see* Cystitis, irradiation
  specified type NEC N30.80
    with hematuria N30.81
  subacute — *see* Cystitis, chronic
  submucous — *see* Cystitis, chronic, interstitial
  syphilitic (late) A52.76
  trichomonal A59.03
  tuberculous A18.12
  ulcerative — *see* Cystitis, chronic, interstitial
Cystocele (-urethrocele)
  female N81.10
    with prolapse of uterus — *see* Prolapse, uterus
    lateral N81.12
    midline N81.11
    paravaginal N81.12
  in pregnancy or childbirth O34.8- ☑
    causing obstructed labor O65.5
  male N32.89
Cystolithiasis N21.0
Cystoma (*see also* Neoplasm, benign, by site)
  endometrial, ovary N80.1
  mucinous
    specified site — *see* Neoplasm, benign, by site
    unspecified site D27.9
  serous
    specified site — *see* Neoplasm, benign, by site
    unspecified site D27.9
  simple (ovary) N83.29- ☑
Cystoplegia N31.2
Cystoptosis N32.89
Cystopyelitis — *see* Pyelonephritis
Cystorrhagia N32.89
Cystosarcoma phyllodes D48.6- ☑
  benign D24- ☑
  malignant — *see* Neoplasm, breast, malignant
Cystostomy
  attention to Z43.5
  complication — *see* Complications, cystostomy
  status Z93.50
    appendico-vesicostomy Z93.52
    cutaneous Z93.51
    specified NEC Z93.59
Cystourethritis — *see* Urethritis
Cystourethrocele (*see also* Cystocele)
  female N81.10
    with uterine prolapse — *see* Prolapse, uterus
    lateral N81.12
    midline N81.11
    paravaginal N81.12
  male N32.89
Cytomegalic inclusion disease
  congenital P35.1
Cytomegalovirus infection B25.9
Cytomycosis (reticuloendothelial) B39.4
Cytopenia D75.9
  refractory
    with multilineage dysplasia D46.A (*following* D46.2)
      and ring sideroblasts (RCMD RS) D46.B (*following* D46.2)
Czerny's disease (periodic hydrarthrosis of the knee) — *see* Effusion, joint, knee

Subterms under main terms may continue to next column or page   ☑ Additional Character Required — Refer to the Tabular List for Character Selection   81

Cystadenoma — Czerny's disease

D

Da Costa's syndrome F45.8
Daae (-Finsen) **disease** (epidemic pleurodynia) B33.0
Dabney's grip B33.0
Dacryoadenitis, dacryadenitis H04.00- ☑
  acute H04.01- ☑
  chronic H04.02- ☑
Dacryocystitis H04.30- ☑
  acute H04.32- ☑
  chronic H04.41- ☑
  neonatal P39.1
  phlegmonous H04.31- ☑
  syphilitic A52.71
    congenital (early) A50.01
  trachomatous, active A71.1
    sequelae (late effect) B94.0
Dacryocystoblenorrhea — see Inflammation, lacrimal, passages, chronic
Dacryocystocele — see Disorder, lacrimal system, changes
Dacryolith, dacryolithiasis H04.51- ☑
Dacryoma — see Disorder, lacrimal system, changes
Dacryopericystitis — see Dacryocystitis
Dacryops H04.11- ☑
Dacryostenosis (see also Stenosis, lacrimal)
  congenital Q10.5
Dactylitis
  bone — see Osteomyelitis
  sickle-cell D57.00
    Hb C D57.219
    Hb SS D57.00
    specified NEC D57.819
  skin L08.9
  syphilitic A52.77
  tuberculous A18.03
Dactylolysis spontanea (ainhum) L94.6
Dactylosymphysis Q70.9
  fingers — see Syndactylism, complex, fingers
  toes — see Syndactylism, complex, toes
Damage
  arteriosclerotic — see Arteriosclerosis
  brain (nontraumatic) G93.9
    anoxic, hypoxic G93.1
      resulting from a procedure G97.82
    child NEC G80.9
    due to birth injury P11.2
  cardiorenal (vascular) — see Hypertension, cardiorenal
  cerebral NEC — see Damage, brain
  coccyx, complicating delivery O71.6
  coronary — see Disease, heart, ischemic
  eye, birth injury P15.3
  liver (nontraumatic) K76.9
    alcoholic K70.9
    due to drugs — see Disease, liver, toxic
    toxic — see Disease, liver, toxic
  medication T88.7 ☑
  pelvic
    joint or ligament, during delivery O71.6
    organ NEC
      during delivery O71.5
      following ectopic or molar pregnancy O08.6
  renal — see Disease, renal
  subendocardium, subendocardial — see Degeneration, myocardial
  vascular I99.9
Dana-Putnam syndrome (subacute combined sclerosis with pernicious anemia) — see Degeneration, combined
Danbolt (-Cross) **syndrome** (acrodermatitis enteropathica) E83.2
Dandruff L21.0
Dandy-Walker syndrome Q03.1
  with spina bifida — see Spina bifida
Danlos' syndrome Q79.6
Darier (-White) **disease** (congenital) Q82.8
  meaning erythema annulare centrifugum L53.1
Darier-Roussy sarcoid D86.3
Darling's disease or histoplasmosis B39.4
Darwin's tubercle Q17.8
Dawson's (inclusion body) **encephalitis** A81.1

De Beurmann (-Gougerot) **disease** B42.1
De la Tourette's syndrome F95.2
De Lange's syndrome Q87.1
De Morgan's spots (senile angiomas) I78.1
De Quervain's
  disease (tendon sheath) M65.4
  syndrome E34.51
  thyroiditis (subacute granulomatous thyroiditis) E06.1
De Toni-Fanconi (-Debré) **syndrome** E72.09
  with cystinosis E72.04
Dead
  fetus, retained (mother) O36.4 ☑
    early pregnancy O02.1
  labyrinth H83.2 ☑
  ovum, retained O02.0
Deaf nonspeaking NEC H91.3
Deafmutism (acquired) (congenital) NEC H91.3
  hysterical F44.6
  syphilitic, congenital (see also subcategory) H94.8 A50.09
Deafness (acquired) (complete) (hereditary) (partial) H91.9-
  with blue sclera and fragility of bone Q78.0
  auditory fatigue — see Deafness, specified type NEC
  aviation T70.0 ☑
    nerve injury — see Injury, nerve, acoustic, specified type NEC
  boilermaker's H83.3 ☑
  central — see Deafness, sensorineural
  conductive H90.2
    and sensorineural
      mixed H90.8
        bilateral H90.6
    bilateral H90.0
    unilateral H90.1- ☑
      with restricted hearing on the contralateral side H90.A- ☑
  congenital H90.5
    with blue sclera and fragility of bone Q78.0
  due to toxic agents — see Deafness, ototoxic
  emotional (hysterical) F44.6
  functional (hysterical) F44.6
  high frequency H91.9- ☑
  hysterical F44.6
  low frequency H91.9- ☑
  mental R48.8
  mixed conductive and sensorineural H90.8
    bilateral H90.6
    unilateral H90.7- ☑
  nerve — see Deafness, sensorineural
  neural — see Deafness, sensorineural
  noise-induced (see also subcategory) H83.3 ☑
    nerve injury — see Injury, nerve, acoustic, specified type NEC
  nonspeaking H91.3
  ototoxic H91.0 ☑
  perceptive — see Deafness, sensorineural
  psychogenic (hysterical) F44.6
  sensorineural H90.5
    and conductive
      bilateral H90.6
      mixed H90.8
        bilateral H90.6
    bilateral H90.3
    unilateral H90.4- ☑
      with restricted hearing on the contralateral side H90.A- ☑
  sensory — see Deafness, sensorineural
  specified type NEC H91.8 ☑
  sudden (idiopathic) H91.2- ☑
  syphilitic A52.15
  transient ischemic H93.01- ☑
  traumatic — see Injury, nerve, acoustic, specified type NEC
  word (developmental) H93.25
Death (cause unknown) (of) (unexplained) (unspecified cause) R99
  brain G93.82
  cardiac (sudden) (with successful resuscitation) — code to underlying disease
    family history of Z82.41
    personal history of Z86.74

Death — continued
  family member (assumed) Z63.4
Debility (chronic) (general) (nervous) R53.81
  congenital or neonatal NOS P96.9
  nervous R53.81
  old age R54
  senile R54
Débove's disease (splenomegaly) R16.1
Decalcification
  bone — see Osteoporosis
  teeth K03.89
Decapsulation, kidney N28.89
Decay
  dental — see Caries, dental
  senile R54
  tooth, teeth — see Caries, dental
Deciduitis (acute)
  following ectopic or molar pregnancy O08.0
Decline (general) — see Debility
  cognitive, age-associated R41.81
Decompensation
  cardiac (acute) (chronic) — see Disease, heart
  cardiovascular — see Disease, cardiovascular
  heart — see Disease, heart
  hepatic — see Failure, hepatic
  myocardial (acute) (chronic) — see Disease, heart
  respiratory J98.8
Decompression sickness T70.3 ☑
Decrease (d)
  absolute neutrophile count — see Neutropenia
  blood
    platelets — see Thrombocytopenia
    pressure R03.1
      due to shock following
        injury T79.4 ☑
        operation T81.19 ☑
  estrogen E28.39
    postablative E89.40
      asymptomatic E89.40
      symptomatic E89.41
  fragility of erythrocytes D58.8
  function
    lipase (pancreatic) K90.3
    ovary in hypopituitarism E23.0
    parenchyma of pancreas K86.89
    pituitary (gland) (anterior) (lobe) E23.0
      posterior (lobe) E23.0
  functional activity R68.89
  glucose R73.09
  hematocrit R71.0
  hemoglobin R71.0
  leukocytes D72.819
    specified NEC D72.818
  libido R68.82
  lymphocytes D72.810
  platelets D69.6
  respiration, due to shock following injury T79.4 ☑
  sexual desire R68.82
  tear secretion NEC — see Syndrome, dry eye
  tolerance
    fat K90.49
    glucose R73.09
    pancreatic K90.3
    salt and water E87.8
  vision NEC H54.7
  white blood cell count D72.819
    specified NEC D72.818
Decubitus (ulcer) — see Ulcer, pressure, by site
  cervix N86
Deepening acetabulum — see Derangement, joint, specified type NEC, hip
Defect, defective Q89.9
  3-beta-hydroxysteroid dehydrogenase E25.0
  11-hydroxylase E25.0
  21-hydroxylase E25.0
  abdominal wall, congenital Q79.59
  antibody immunodeficiency D80.9
  aorticopulmonary septum Q21.4
  atrial septal (ostium secundum type) Q21.1
    following acute myocardial infarction (current complication) I23.1
    ostium primum type Q21.2

Defect, defective — *continued*
  atrioventricular
    canal Q21.2
    septum Q21.2
  auricular septal Q21.1
  bilirubin excretion NEC E80.6
  biosynthesis, androgen (testicular) E29.1
  bulbar septum Q21.0
  catalase E80.3
  cell membrane receptor complex (CR3) D71
  circulation I99.9
    congenital Q28.9
    newborn Q28.9
  coagulation (factor) (*see also* Deficiency, factor) D68.9
    with
      ectopic pregnancy O08.1
      molar pregnancy O08.1
    acquired D68.4
    antepartum with hemorrhage — *see* Hemorrhage,
      antepartum, with coagulation defect
    due to
      liver disease D68.4
      vitamin K deficiency D68.4
    hereditary NEC D68.2
    intrapartum O67.0
    newborn, transient P61.6
    postpartum O99.13
      with hemorrhage O72.3
    specified type NEC D68.8
  complement system D84.1
  conduction (heart) I45.9
    bone — *see* Deafness, conductive
  congenital, organ or site not listed — *see* Anomaly,
    by site
  coronary sinus Q21.1
  cushion, endocardial Q21.2
  degradation, glycoprotein E77.1
  dental bridge, crown, fillings — *see* Defect, dental
    restoration
  dental restoration K08.50
    specified NEC K08.59
  dentin (hereditary) K00.5
  Descemet's membrane, congenital Q13.89
  developmental (*see also* Anomaly)
    cauda equina Q06.3
  diaphragm
    with elevation, eventration or hernia — *see* Hernia,
      diaphragm
    congenital Q79.1
      with hernia Q79.0
      gross (with hernia) Q79.0
  ectodermal, congenital Q82.9
  Eisenmenger's Q21.8
  enzyme
    catalase E80.3
    peroxidase E80.3
  esophagus, congenital Q39.9
  extensor retinaculum M62.89
  fibrin polymerization D68.2
  filling
    bladder R93.41
    kidney R93.42- ☑
    renal pelvis R93.41
    stomach R93.3
    ureter R93.41
    urinary organs, specified NEC R93.49
  Gerbode Q21.0
  glycoprotein degradation E77.1
  Hageman (factor) D68.2
  hearing — *see* Deafness
  high grade F70
  interatrial septal Q21.1
  interauricular septal Q21.1
  interventricular septal Q21.0
    with dextroposition of aorta, pulmonary stenosis
      and hypertrophy of right ventricle Q21.3
    in tetralogy of Fallot Q21.3
  learning (specific) — *see* Disorder, learning
  lymphocyte function antigen-1 (LFA-1) D84.0
  lysosomal enzyme, post-translational modification
    E77.0
  major osseous M89.70
    ankle M89.77- ☑
    carpus M89.74- ☑
    clavicle M89.71- ☑
    femur M89.75- ☑
    fibula M89.76- ☑
    fingers M89.74- ☑

Defect, defective — *continued*
  major osseous — *continued*
    foot M89.77- ☑
    forearm M89.73- ☑
    hand M89.74- ☑
    humerus M89.72- ☑
    lower leg M89.76- ☑
    metacarpus M89.74- ☑
    metatarsus M89.77- ☑
    multiple sites M89.79
    pelvic region M89.75- ☑
    pelvis M89.75- ☑
    radius M89.73- ☑
    scapula M89.71- ☑
    shoulder region M89.71- ☑
    specified NEC M89.78
    tarsus M89.77- ☑
    thigh M89.75- ☑
    tibia M89.76- ☑
    toes M89.77- ☑
    ulna M89.73- ☑
  mental — *see* Disability, intellectual
  modification, lysosomal enzymes, post-translational
    E77.0
  obstructive, congenital
    renal pelvis Q62.39
    ureter Q62.39
      atresia — *see* Atresia, ureter
      cecoureterocele Q62.32
      megaureter Q62.2
      orthotopic ureterocele Q62.31
  osseous, major M89.70
    ankle M89.77- ☑
    carpus M89.74- ☑
    clavicle M89.71- ☑
    femur M89.75- ☑
    fibula M89.76- ☑
    fingers M89.74- ☑
    foot M89.77- ☑
    forearm M89.73- ☑
    hand M89.74- ☑
    humerus M89.72- ☑
    lower leg M89.76- ☑
    metacarpus M89.74- ☑
    metatarsus M89.77- ☑
    multiple sites M89.9
    pelvic region M89.75- ☑
    pelvis M89.75- ☑
    radius M89.73- ☑
    scapula M89.71- ☑
    shoulder region M89.71- ☑
    specified NEC M89.78
    tarsus M89.77- ☑
    thigh M89.75- ☑
    tibia M89.76- ☑
    toes M89.77- ☑
    ulna M89.73- ☑
  osteochondral NEC (*see also* Deformity) M95.8
  ostium
    primum Q21.2
    secundum Q21.1
  peroxidase E80.3
  placental blood supply — *see* Insufficiency, placental
  platelets, qualitative D69.1
    constitutional D68.0
  postural NEC, spine — *see* Dorsopathy, deforming
  reduction
    limb Q73.8
      lower Q72.9- ☑
        absence — *see* Agenesis, leg
          foot — *see* Agenesis, foot
        longitudinal
          femur Q72.4- ☑
          fibula Q72.6- ☑
          tibia Q72.5- ☑
        specified type NEC Q72.89- ☑
        split foot Q72.7- ☑
      specified type NEC Q73.8
      upper Q71.9- ☑
        absence — *see* Agenesis, arm
          forearm — *see* Agenesis, forearm
          hand — *see* Agenesis, hand
        lobster-claw hand Q71.6- ☑
        longitudinal
          radius Q71.4- ☑
          ulna Q71.5- ☑

Defect, defective — *continued*
  reduction — *continued*
    limb — *continued*
      upper — *continued*
        specified type NEC Q71.89- ☑
  renal pelvis Q63.8
    obstructive Q62.39
  respiratory system, congenital Q34.9
  restoration, dental K08.50
    specified NEC K08.59
  retinal nerve bundle fibers H35.89
  septal (heart) NOS Q21.9
    acquired (atrial) (auricular) (old) I51.0
    atrial Q21.1
      concurrent with acute myocardial infarction —
        see Infarct, myocardium
      following acute myocardial infarction (current
        complication) I23.1
    ventricular (*see also* Defect, ventricular septal)
      Q21.0
  sinus venosus Q21.1
  speech R47.9
    developmental F80.9
    specified NEC R47.89
  Taussig-Bing (aortic transposition and overriding pul-
    monary artery) Q20.1
  teeth, wedge K03.1
  vascular (local) I99.9
    congenital Q27.9
  ventricular septal Q21.0
    concurrent with acute myocardial infarction — *see*
      Infarct, myocardium
    following acute myocardial infarction (current
      complication) I23.2
    in tetralogy of Fallot Q21.3
  vision NEC H54.7
  visual field H53.40
    bilateral
      heteronymous H53.47
      homonymous H53.46- ☑
    generalized contraction H53.48- ☑
    localized
      arcuate H53.43- ☑
      scotoma (central area) H53.41- ☑
        blind spot area H53.42- ☑
      sector H53.43- ☑
      specified type NEC H53.45- ☑
  voice R49.9
    specified NEC R49.8
  wedge, tooth, teeth (abrasion) K03.1
Deferentitis N49.1
  gonorrheal (acute) (chronic) A54.23
Defibrination (syndrome) D65
  antepartum — *see* Hemorrhage, antepartum, with
    coagulation defect, disseminated intravascular
    coagulation
  following ectopic or molar pregnancy O08.1
  intrapartum O67.0
  newborn P60
  postpartum O72.3
Deficiency, deficient
  3-beta hydroxysteroid dehydrogenase E25.0
  5-alpha reductase (with male pseudo-
    hermaphroditism) E29.1
  11-hydroxylase E25.0
  21-hydroxylase E25.0
  abdominal muscle syndrome Q79.4
  AC globulin (congenital) (hereditary) D68.2
    acquired D68.4
  accelerator globulin (Ac G) (blood) D68.2
  acid phosphatase E83.39
  activating factor (blood) D68.2
  adenosine deaminase (ADA) D81.3
  aldolase (hereditary) E74.19
  alpha-1-antitrypsin E88.01
  amino-acids E72.9
  anemia — *see* Anemia
  aneurin E51.9
  antibody with
    hyperimmunoglobulinemia D80.6
    near-normal immunoglobins D80.6
  antidiuretic hormone E23.2
  anti-hemophilic
    factor (A) D66
      B D67
      C D68.1
    globulin (AHG) NEC D66
  antithrombin (antithrombin III) D68.59

Deficiency, deficient — continued
ascorbic acid E54
attention (disorder) (syndrome) F98.8
  with hyperactivity — see Disorder, attention-deficit
    hyperactivity
autoprothrombin
  C D68.2
  I D68.2
  II D67
beta-glucuronidase E76.29
biotin E53.8
biotin-dependent carboxylase D81.819
biotinidase D81.810
brancher enzyme (amylopectinosis) E74.03
C1 esterase inhibitor (C1-INH) D84.1
calciferol E55.9
  with
    adult osteomalacia M83.8
    rickets — see Rickets
calcium (dietary) E58
calorie, severe E43
  with marasmus E41
    and kwashiorkor E42
cardiac — see Insufficiency, myocardial
carnitine E71.40
  due to
    hemodialysis E71.43
    inborn errors of metabolism E71.42
    Valproic acid therapy E71.43
  iatrogenic E71.43
  muscle palmityltransferase E71.314
  primary E71.41
  secondary E71.448
carotene E50.9
central nervous system G96.8
ceruloplasmin (Wilson) E83.01
choline E53.8
Christmas factor D67
chromium E61.4
clotting (blood) (see also Deficiency, coagulation factor) D68.9
clotting factor NEC (hereditary) (see also Deficiency, factor) D68.2
coagulation NOS D68.9
  with
    ectopic pregnancy O08.1
    molar pregnancy O08.1
  acquired (any) D68.4
  antepartum hemorrhage — see Hemorrhage, antepartum, with coagulation defect
  clotting factor NEC (see also Deficiency, factor) D68.2
  due to
    hyperprothrombinemia D68.4
    liver disease D68.4
    vitamin K deficiency D68.4
  newborn, transient P61.6
  postpartum O72.3
  specified NEC D68.8
cognitive F09
color vision H53.50
  achromatopsia H53.51
  acquired H53.52
  deuteranomaly H53.53
  protanomaly H53.54
  specified type NEC H53.59
  tritanomaly H53.55
combined glucocorticoid and mineralocorticoid E27.49
contact factor D68.2
copper (nutritional) E61.0
corticoadrenal E27.40
  primary E27.1
craniofacial axis Q75.0
cyanocobalamin E53.8
debrancher enzyme (limit dextrinosis) E74.03
dehydrogenase
  long chain/very long chain acyl CoA E71.310
  medium chain acyl CoA E71.311
  short chain acyl CoA E71.312
diet E63.9
dihydropyrimidine dehydrogenase (DPD) E88.89
disaccharidase E73.9
edema — see Malnutrition, severe
endocrine E34.9
energy-supply — see Malnutrition
enzymes, circulating NEC E88.09
ergosterol E55.9

Deficiency, deficient — continued
ergosterol — continued
  with
    adult osteomalacia M83.8
    rickets — see Rickets
essential fatty acid (EFA) E63.0
factor (see also Deficiency, coagulation)
  Hageman D68.2
  I (congenital) (hereditary) D68.2
  II (congenital) (hereditary) D68.2
  IX (congenital) (functional) (hereditary) (with functional defect) D67
  multiple (congenital) D68.8
    acquired D68.4
  V (congenital) (hereditary) D68.2
  VII (congenital) (hereditary) D68.2
  VIII (congenital) (functional) (hereditary) (with functional defect) D66
    with vascular defect D68.0
  X (congenital) (hereditary) D68.2
  XI (congenital) (hereditary) D68.1
  XII (congenital) (hereditary) D68.2
  XIII (congenital) (hereditary) D68.2
femoral, proximal focal (congenital) — see Defect, reduction, lower limb, longitudinal, femur
fibrinase D68.2
fibrinogen (congenital) (hereditary) D68.2
  acquired D65
fibrin-stabilizing factor (congenital) (hereditary) D68.2
  acquired D68.4
folate E53.8
folic acid E53.8
foreskin N47.3
fructokinase E74.11
fructose 1,6-diphosphatase E74.19
fructose-1-phosphate aldolase E74.19
galactokinase E74.29
galactose-1-phosphate uridyl transferase E74.29
gammaglobulin in blood D80.1
  hereditary D80.0
glass factor D68.2
glucocorticoid E27.49
  mineralocorticoid E27.49
glucose-6-phosphatase E74.01
glucose-6-phosphate dehydrogenase anemia D55.0
glucuronyl transferase E80.5
glycogen synthetase E74.09
gonadotropin (isolated) E23.0
growth hormone (idiopathic) (isolated) E23.0
Hageman factor D68.2
hemoglobin D64.9
hepatophosphorylase E74.09
homogentisate 1,2-dioxygenase E70.29
hormone
  anterior pituitary (partial) NEC E23.0
    growth E23.0
  growth (isolated) E23.0
  pituitary E23.0
  testicular E29.1
hypoxanthine- (guanine)-phosphoribosyltransferase (HG- PRT) (total H-PRT) E79.1
immunity D84.9
  cell-mediated D84.8
    with thrombocytopenia and eczema D82.0
  combined D81.9
  humoral D80.9
  IgA (secretory) D80.2
  IgG D80.3
  IgM D80.4
immuno — see Immunodeficiency
immunoglobulin, selective
  A (IgA) D80.2
  G (IgG) (subclasses) D80.3
  M (IgM) D80.4
inositol (B complex) E53.8
intrinsic
  factor (congenital) D51.0
  sphincter N36.42
    with urethral hypermobility N36.43
iodine E61.8
  congenital syndrome — see Syndrome, iodine-deficiency, congenital
iron E61.1
  anemia D50.9
kalium E87.6
kappa-light chain D80.8
labile factor (congenital) (hereditary) D68.2
  acquired D68.4

Deficiency, deficient — continued
lacrimal fluid (acquired) (see also Syndrome, dry eye)
  congenital Q10.6
lactase
  congenital E73.0
  secondary E73.1
Laki-Lorand factor D68.2
lecithin cholesterol acyltransferase E78.6
lipocaic K86.89
lipoprotein (familial) (high density) E78.6
liver phosphorylase E74.09
lysosomal alpha-1, 4 glucosidase E74.02
magnesium E61.2
major histocompatibility complex
  class I D81.6
  class II D81.7
manganese E61.3
menadione (vitamin K) E56.1
  newborn P53
mental (familial) (hereditary) — see Disability, intellectual
methylenetetrahydrofolate reductase (MTHFR) E72.12
mevalonate kinase M04.1
mineralocorticoid E27.49
  with glucocorticoid E27.49
mineral NEC E61.8
molybdenum (nutritional) E61.5
moral F60.2
multiple nutrient elements E61.7
muscle
  carnitine (palmityltransferase) E71.314
  phosphofructokinase E74.09
myoadenylate deaminase E79.2
myocardial — see Insufficiency, myocardial
myophosphorylase E74.04
NADH diaphorase or reductase (congenital) D74.0
NADH-methemoglobin reductase (congenital) D74.0
natrium E87.1
niacin (amide) (-tryptophan) E52
nicotinamide E52
nicotinic acid E52
number of teeth — see Anodontia
nutrient element E61.9
  multiple E61.7
  specified NEC E61.8
nutrition, nutritional E63.9
  sequelae — see Sequelae, nutritional deficiency
  specified NEC E63.8
of interleukin 1 receptor antagonist [DIRA] M04.8
ornithine transcarbamylase E72.4
ovarian E28.39
oxygen — see Anoxia
pantothenic acid E53.8
parathyroid (gland) E20.9
perineum (female) N81.89
phenylalanine hydroxylase E70.1
phosphoenolpyruvate carboxykinase E74.4
phosphofructokinase E74.19
phosphomannomutase E74.8
phosphomannose isomerase E74.8
phosphomannosyl mutase E74.8
phosphorylase kinase, liver E74.09
pituitary hormone (isolated) E23.0
plasma thromboplastin
  antecedent (PTA) D68.1
  component (PTC) D67
platelet NEC D69.1
  constitutional D68.0
polyglandular E31.8
  autoimmune E31.0
potassium (K) E87.6
prepuce N47.3
proaccelerin (congenital) (hereditary) D68.2
  acquired D68.4
proconvertin factor (congenital) (hereditary) D68.2
  acquired D68.4
protein (see also Malnutrition) E46
  anemia D53.0
  C D68.59
  S D68.59
prothrombin (congenital) (hereditary) D68.2
  acquired D68.4
Prower factor D68.2
pseudocholinesterase E88.09
PTA (plasma thromboplastin antecedent) D68.1
PTC (plasma thromboplastin component) D67
purine nucleoside phosphorylase (PNP) D81.5

Deficiency, deficient — *continued*
  pyracin (alpha) (beta) E53.1
  pyridoxal E53.1
  pyridoxamine E53.1
  pyridoxine (derivatives) E53.1
  pyruvate
    carboxylase E74.4
    dehydrogenase E74.4
  riboflavin (vitamin B2) E53.0
  salt E87.1
  secretion
    ovary E28.39
    salivary gland (any) K11.7
    urine R34
  selenium (dietary) E59
  serum antitrypsin, familial E88.01
  short stature homeobox gene (SHOX)
    with
      dyschondrosteosis Q78.8
      short stature (idiopathic) E34.3
      Turner's syndrome Q96.9
  sodium (Na) E87.1
  SPCA (factor VII) D68.2
  sphincter, intrinsic N36.42
    with urethral hypermobility N36.43
  stable factor (congenital) (hereditary) D68.2
    acquired D68.4
  Stuart-Prower (factor X) D68.2
  sucrase E74.39
  sulfatase E75.29
  sulfite oxidase E72.19
  thiamin, thiaminic (chloride) E51.9
    beriberi (dry) E51.11
      wet E51.12
  thrombokinase D68.2
    newborn P53
  thyroid (gland) — *see* Hypothyroidism
  tocopherol E56.0
  tooth bud K00.0
  transcobalamine II (anemia) D51.2
  vanadium E61.6
  vascular I99.9
  vasopressin E23.2
  vertical ridge K06.8
  viosterol — *see* Deficiency, calciferol
  vitamin (multiple) NOS E56.9
    A E50.9
      with
        Bitot's spot (corneal) E50.1
        follicular keratosis E50.8
        keratomalacia E50.4
        manifestations NEC E50.8
        night blindness E50.5
        scar of cornea, xerophthalmic E50.6
        xeroderma E50.8
        xerophthalmia E50.7
        xerosis
          conjunctival E50.0
            and Bitot's spot E50.1
          cornea E50.2
            and ulceration E50.3
      sequelae E64.1
    B (complex) NOS E53.9
      with
        beriberi (dry) E51.11
          wet E51.12
        pellagra E52
    B1 NOS E51.9
      beriberi (dry) E51.11
        with circulatory system manifestations
          E51.11
        wet E51.12
    B2 (riboflavin) E53.0
    B6 E53.1
    B12 E53.8
    C E54
      sequelae E64.2
    D E55.9
      with
        adult osteomalacia M83.8
        rickets — *see* Rickets
      25-hydroxylase E83.32
    E E56.0
    folic acid E53.8
    G E53.0
    group B E53.9
      specified NEC E53.8
    H (biotin) E53.8
    K E56.1

Deficiency, deficient — *continued*
  vitamin — *continued*
    K — *continued*
      of newborn P53
    nicotinic E52
    P E56.8
    PP (pellagra-preventing) E52
    specified NEC E56.8
    thiamin E51.9
      beriberi — *see* Beriberi
  zinc, dietary E60
Deficit (*see also* Deficiency)
  attention and concentration R41.840
    disorder — *see* Attention, deficit
    following
      cerebral infarction I69.310
      cerebrovascular disease I69.910
        specified disease NEC I69.810
      nontraumatic
        intracerebral hemorrhage I69.110
        specified intracranial hemorrhage NEC
          I69.210
        subarachnoid hemorrhage I69.010
  cognitive
    communication R41.841
    emotional
      following
        cerebral infarction I69.315
        cerebrovascular disease I69.915
          specified disease NEC I69.815
        nontraumatic
          intracerebral hemorrhage I69.115
          specified intracranial hemorrhage NEC
            I69.215
          subarachnoid hemorrhage I69.015
    following
      cerebral infarction I69.319
      cerebrovascular disease I69.919
        specified disease NEC I69.819
      nontraumatic
        intracerebral hemorrhage I69.119
        specified intracranial hemorrhage NEC
          I69.219
        subarachnoid hemorrhage I69.019
    social
      following
        cerebral infarction I69.315
        cerebrovascular disease I69.915
          specified disease NEC I69.815
        nontraumatic
          intracerebral hemorrhage I69.115
          specified intracranial hemorrhage NEC
            I69.215
          subarachnoid hemorrhage I69.015
  cognitive NEC R41.89
    following
      cerebral infarction I69.318
      cerebrovascular disease I69.918
        specified disease NEC I69.818
      nontraumatic
        intracerebral hemorrhage I69.118
        specified intracranial hemorrhage NEC
          I69.218
        subarachnoid hemorrhage I69.018
  concentration R41.840
  executive function R41.844
    following
      cerebral infarction I69.314
      cerebrovascular disease I69.914
        specified disease NEC I69.814
      nontraumatic
        intracerebral hemorrhage I69.114
        specified intracranial hemorrhage NEC
          I69.214
        subarachnoid hemorrhage I69.014
  frontal lobe R41.844
    following
      cerebral infarction I69.314
      cerebrovascular disease I69.914
        specified disease NEC I69.814
      nontraumatic
        intracerebral hemorrhage I69.114
        specified intracranial hemorrhage NEC
          I69.214
        subarachnoid hemorrhage I69.014
  memory
    following
      cerebral infarction I69.311
      cerebrovascular disease I69.911

Deficit — *continued*
  memory — *continued*
    following — *continued*
      cerebrovascular disease — *continued*
        specified disease NEC I69.811
      nontraumatic
        intracerebral hemorrhage I69.111
        specified intracranial hemorrhage NEC
          I69.211
        subarachnoid hemorrhage I69.011
  neurologic NEC R29.818
    ischemic
      reversible (RIND) I63.9
        prolonged (PRIND) I63.9
  oxygen R09.02
  prolonged reversible ischemic neurologic (PRIND) I63.9
  psychomotor R41.843
    following
      cerebral infarction I69.313
      cerebrovascular disease I69.913
        specified disease NEC I69.813
      nontraumatic
        intracerebral hemorrhage I69.113
        specified intracranial hemorrhage NEC
          I69.213
        subarachnoid hemorrhage I69.013
  visuospatial R41.842
    following
      cerebral infarction I69.312
      cerebrovascular disease I69.912
        specified disease NEC I69.812
      nontraumatic
        intracerebral hemorrhage I69.112
        specified intracranial hemorrhage NEC
          I69.212
        subarachnoid hemorrhage I69.012
Deflection
  radius — *see* Deformity, limb, specified type NEC,
    forearm
  septum (acquired) (nasal) (nose) J34.2
  spine — *see* Curvature, spine
  turbinate (nose) J34.2
Defluvium
  capillorum — *see* Alopecia
  ciliorum — *see* Madarosis
  unguium L60.8
Deformity Q89.9
  abdomen, congenital Q89.9
  abdominal wall
    acquired M95.8
    congenital Q79.59
  acquired (unspecified site) M95.9
  adrenal gland Q89.1
  alimentary tract, congenital Q45.9
    upper Q40.9
  ankle (joint) (acquired) (*see also* Deformity, limb, lower
    leg)
    abduction — *see* Contraction, joint, ankle
    congenital Q68.8
    contraction — *see* Contraction, joint, ankle
    specified type NEC — *see* Deformity, limb, foot,
      specified NEC
  anus (acquired) K62.89
    congenital Q43.9
  aorta (arch) (congenital) Q25.40
    acquired I77.89
  aortic
    arch, acquired I77.89
    cusp or valve (congenital) Q23.8
      acquired (*see also* Endocarditis, aortic) I35.8
  arm (acquired) (upper) (*see also* Deformity, limb, upper
    arm)
    congenital Q68.8
    forearm — *see* Deformity, limb, forearm
  artery (congenital) (peripheral) NOS Q27.9
    acquired I77.89
    coronary (acquired) I25.9
      congenital Q24.5
    umbilical Q27.0
  atrial septal Q21.1
  auditory canal (external) (congenital) (*see also* Malfor-
    mation, ear, external)
    acquired — *see* Disorder, ear, external, specified
      type NEC
  auricle
    ear (congenital) (*see also* Malformation, ear, exter-
      nal)
      acquired — *see* Disorder, pinna, deformity

Deformity — *continued*
- back — *see* Dorsopathy, deforming
- bile duct (common) (congenital) (hepatic) Q44.5
  - acquired K83.8
- biliary duct or passage (congenital) Q44.5
  - acquired K83.8
- bladder (neck) (trigone) (sphincter) (acquired) N32.89
  - congenital Q64.79
- bone (acquired) NOS M95.9
  - congenital Q79.9
  - turbinate M95.0
- brain (congenital) Q04.9
  - acquired G93.89
  - reduction Q04.3
- breast (acquired) N64.89
  - congenital Q83.9
  - reconstructed N65.0
- bronchus (congenital) Q32.4
  - acquired NEC J98.09
- bursa, congenital Q79.9
- canaliculi (lacrimalis) (acquired) (*see also* Disorder, lacrimal system, changes)
  - congenital Q10.6
- canthus, acquired — *see* Disorder, eyelid, specified type NEC
- capillary (acquired) I78.8
- caruncle, lacrimal (acquired) (*see also* Disorder, lacrimal system, changes)
  - congenital Q10.6
- cascade, stomach K31.2
- cecum (congenital) Q43.9
  - acquired K63.89
- cerebral, acquired G93.89
  - congenital Q04.9
- cervix (uterus) (acquired) NEC N88.8
  - congenital Q51.9
- cheek (acquired) M95.2
  - congenital Q18.9
- chest (acquired) (wall) M95.4
  - congenital Q67.8
  - sequelae (late effect) of rickets E64.3
- chin (acquired) M95.2
  - congenital Q18.9
- choroid (congenital) Q14.3
  - acquired H31.8
  - plexus Q07.8
    - acquired G96.19
- cicatricial — *see* Cicatrix
- cilia, acquired — *see* Disorder, eyelid, specified type NEC
- clavicle (acquired) M95.8
  - congenital Q68.8
- clitoris (congenital) Q52.6
  - acquired N90.89
- clubfoot — *see* Clubfoot
- coccyx (acquired) — *see* subcategory M43.8 ☑
- colon (congenital) Q43.9
  - acquired K63.89
- concha (ear), congenital (*see also* Malformation, ear, external)
  - acquired — *see* Disorder, pinna, deformity
- cornea (acquired) H18.70
  - congenital Q13.4
  - descemetocele — *see* Descemetocele
  - ectasia — *see* Ectasia, cornea
  - specified NEC H18.79- ☑
  - staphyloma — *see* Staphyloma, cornea
- coronary artery (acquired) I25.9
  - congenital Q24.5
- cranium (acquired) — *see* Deformity, skull
- cricoid cartilage (congenital) Q31.8
  - acquired J38.7
- cystic duct (congenital) Q44.5
  - acquired K82.8
- Dandy-Walker Q03.1
  - with spina bifida — *see* Spina bifida
- diaphragm (congenital) Q79.1
  - acquired J98.6
- digestive organ NOS Q45.9
- ductus arteriosus Q25.0
- duodenal bulb K31.89
- duodenum (congenital) Q43.9
  - acquired K31.89
- dura — *see* Deformity, meninges
- ear (acquired) (*see also* Disorder, pinna, deformity)
  - congenital (external) Q17.9
    - internal Q16.5

Deformity — *continued*
- ear (*see also* Disorder, pinna, deformity) — *continued*
  - congenital — *continued*
    - middle Q16.4
      - ossicles Q16.3
    - ossicles Q16.3
- ectodermal (congenital) NEC Q84.9
- ejaculatory duct (congenital) Q55.4
  - acquired N50.89
- elbow (joint) (acquired) (*see also* Deformity, limb, upper arm)
  - congenital Q68.8
  - contraction — *see* Contraction, joint, elbow
- endocrine gland NEC Q89.2
- epididymis (congenital) Q55.4
  - acquired N50.89
- epiglottis (congenital) Q31.8
  - acquired J38.7
- esophagus (congenital) Q39.9
  - acquired K22.8
- eustachian tube (congenital) NEC Q17.8
- eye, congenital Q15.9
- eyebrow (congenital) Q18.8
- eyelid (acquired) (*see also* Disorder, eyelid, specified type NEC)
  - congenital Q10.3
- face (acquired) M95.2
  - congenital Q18.9
- fallopian tube, acquired N83.8
- femur (acquired) — *see* Deformity, limb, specified type NEC, thigh
- fetal
  - with fetopelvic disproportion O33.7 ☑
  - causing obstructed labor O66.3
- finger (acquired) M20.00- ☑
  - boutonniere M20.02- ☑
  - congenital Q68.1
  - flexion contracture — *see* Contraction, joint, hand
  - mallet finger M20.01- ☑
  - specified NEC M20.09- ☑
  - swan-neck M20.03- ☑
- flexion (joint) (acquired) (*see also* Deformity, limb, flexion) M21.20
  - congenital NOS Q74.9
  - hip Q65.89
- foot (acquired) (*see also* Deformity, limb, lower leg)
  - cavovarus (congenital) Q66.1
  - congenital NOS Q66.9
    - specified type NEC Q66.89
  - specified type NEC — *see* Deformity, limb, foot, specified NEC
  - valgus (congenital) Q66.6
    - acquired — *see* Deformity, valgus, ankle
  - varus (congenital) NEC Q66.3
    - acquired — *see* Deformity, varus, ankle
- forearm (acquired) (*see also* Deformity, limb, forearm)
  - congenital Q68.8
- forehead (acquired) M95.2
  - congenital Q75.8
- frontal bone (acquired) M95.2
  - congenital Q75.8
- gallbladder (congenital) Q44.1
  - acquired K82.8
- gastrointestinal tract (congenital) NOS Q45.9
  - acquired K63.89
- genitalia, genital organ(s) or system NEC
  - female (congenital) Q52.9
    - acquired N94.89
    - external Q52.70
  - male (congenital) Q55.9
    - acquired N50.89
- globe (eye) (congenital) Q15.8
  - acquired H44.89
- gum, acquired NEC K06.8
- hand (acquired) — *see* Deformity, limb, hand
  - congenital Q68.1
- head (acquired) M95.2
  - congenital Q75.8
- heart (congenital) Q24.9
  - septum Q21.9
    - auricular Q21.1
    - ventricular Q21.0
  - valve (congenital) NEC Q24.8
    - acquired — *see* Endocarditis
- heel (acquired) — *see* Deformity, foot
- hepatic duct (congenital) Q44.5
  - acquired K83.8

Deformity — *continued*
- hip (joint) (acquired) (*see also* Deformity, limb, thigh)
  - congenital Q65.9
  - due to (previous) juvenile osteochondrosis — *see* Coxa, plana
  - flexion — *see* Contraction, joint, hip
- hourglass — *see* Contraction, hourglass
- humerus (acquired) M21.82- ☑
  - congenital Q74.0
- hypophyseal (congenital) Q89.2
- ileocecal (coil) (valve) (acquired) K63.89
  - congenital Q43.9
- ileum (congenital) Q43.9
  - acquired K63.89
- ilium (acquired) M95.5
  - congenital Q74.2
- integument (congenital) Q84.9
- intervertebral cartilage or disc (acquired) — *see* Disorder, disc, specified NEC
- intestine (large) (small) (congenital) NOS Q43.9
  - acquired K63.89
- intrinsic minus or plus (hand) — *see* Deformity, limb, specified type NEC, forearm
- iris (acquired) H21.89
  - congenital Q13.2
- ischium (acquired) M95.5
  - congenital Q74.2
- jaw (acquired) (congenital) M26.9
- joint (acquired) NEC M21.90
  - congenital Q68.8
  - elbow M21.92- ☑
  - hand M21.94- ☑
  - hip M21.95- ☑
  - knee M21.96- ☑
  - shoulder M21.92- ☑
  - wrist M21.93- ☑
- kidney(s) (calyx) (pelvis) (congenital) Q63.9
  - acquired N28.89
  - artery (congenital) Q27.2
    - acquired I77.89
- Klippel-Feil (brevicollis) Q76.1
- knee (acquired) NEC (*see also* Deformity, limb, lower leg)
  - congenital Q68.2
- labium (majus) (minus) (congenital) Q52.79
  - acquired N90.89
- lacrimal passages or duct (congenital) NEC Q10.6
  - acquired — *see* Disorder, lacrimal system, changes
- larynx (muscle) (congenital) Q31.8
  - acquired J38.7
  - web (glottic) Q31.0
- leg (upper) (acquired) NEC (*see also* Deformity, limb, thigh)
  - congenital Q68.8
  - lower leg — *see* Deformity, limb, lower leg
- lens (acquired) H27.8
  - congenital Q12.9
- lid (fold) (acquired) (*see also* Disorder, eyelid, specified type NEC)
  - congenital Q10.3
- ligament (acquired) — *see* Disorder, ligament
  - congenital Q79.9
- limb (acquired) M21.90
  - clawfoot M21.53- ☑
  - clawhand M21.51- ☑
  - clubfoot M21.54- ☑
  - clubhand M21.52- ☑
  - congenital, except reduction deformity Q74.9
  - flat foot M21.4- ☑
  - flexion M21.20
    - ankle M21.27- ☑
    - elbow M21.22- ☑
    - finger M21.24- ☑
    - hip M21.25- ☑
    - knee M21.26- ☑
    - shoulder M21.21- ☑
    - toe M21.27- ☑
    - wrist M21.23- ☑
  - foot
    - claw — *see* Deformity, limb, clawfoot
    - club — *see* Deformity, limb, clubfoot
    - drop M21.37- ☑
    - flat — *see* Deformity, limb, flat foot
    - specified NEC M21.6X- ☑
  - forearm M21.93- ☑
  - hand M21.94- ☑
  - lower leg M21.96- ☑

Deformity — *continued*
limb — *continued*
specified type NEC M21.80
forearm M21.83- ☑
lower leg M21.86- ☑
thigh M21.85- ☑
upper arm M21.82- ☑
thigh M21.95- ☑
unequal length M21.70
short site is
femur M21.75- ☑
fibula M21.76- ☑
humerus M21.72- ☑
radius M21.73- ☑
tibia M21.76- ☑
ulna M21.73- ☑
upper arm M21.92- ☑
valgus — *see* Deformity, valgus
varus — *see* Deformity, varus
wrist drop M21.33- ☑
lip (acquired) NEC K13.0
congenital Q38.0
liver (congenital) Q44.7
acquired K76.89
lumbosacral (congenital) (joint) (region) Q76.49
acquired — *see* subcategory M43.8 ☑
kyphosis — *see* Kyphosis, congenital
lordosis — *see* Lordosis, congenital
lung (congenital) Q33.9
acquired J98.4
lymphatic system, congenital Q89.9
Madelung's (radius) Q74.0
mandible (acquired) (congenital) M26.9
maxilla (acquired) (congenital) M26.9
meninges or membrane (congenital) Q07.9
cerebral Q04.8
acquired G96.19
spinal cord (congenital) G96.19
acquired G96.19
metacarpus (acquired) — *see* Deformity, limb, forearm
congenital Q74.0
metatarsus (acquired) — *see* Deformity, foot
congenital Q66.9
middle ear (congenital) Q16.4
ossicles Q16.3
mitral (leaflets) (valve) I05.8
parachute Q23.2
stenosis, congenital Q23.2
mouth (acquired) K13.79
congenital Q38.6
multiple, congenital NEC Q89.7
muscle (acquired) M62.89
congenital Q79.9
sternocleidomastoid Q68.0
musculoskeletal system (acquired) M95.9
congenital Q79.9
specified NEC M95.8
nail (acquired) L60.8
congenital Q84.6
nasal — *see* Deformity, nose
neck (acquired) M95.3
congenital Q18.9
sternocleidomastoid Q68.0
nervous system (congenital) Q07.9
nipple (congenital) Q83.9
acquired N64.89
nose (acquired) (cartilage) M95.0
bone (turbinate) M95.0
congenital Q30.9
bent or squashed Q67.4
saddle M95.0
syphilitic A50.57
septum (acquired) J34.2
congenital Q30.8
sinus (wall) (congenital) Q30.8
acquired M95.0
syphilitic (congenital) A50.57
late A52.73
ocular muscle (congenital) Q10.3
acquired — *see* Strabismus, mechanical
opticociliary vessels (congenital) Q13.2
orbit (eye) (acquired) H05.30
atrophy — *see* Atrophy, orbit
congenital Q10.7
due to
bone disease NEC H05.32- ☑
trauma or surgery H05.33- ☑
enlargement — *see* Enlargement, orbit

Deformity — *continued*
orbit — *continued*
exostosis — *see* Exostosis, orbit
organ of Corti (congenital) Q16.5
ovary (congenital) Q50.39
acquired N83.8
oviduct, acquired N83.8
palate (congenital) Q38.5
acquired M27.8
cleft (congenital) — *see* Cleft, palate
pancreas (congenital) Q45.3
acquired K86.89
parathyroid (gland) Q89.2
parotid (gland) (congenital) Q38.4
acquired K11.8
patella (acquired) — *see* Disorder, patella, specified NEC
pelvis, pelvic (acquired) (bony) M95.5
with disproportion (fetopelvic) O33.0
causing obstructed labor O65.0
congenital Q74.2
rachitic sequelae (late effect) E64.3
penis (glans) (congenital) Q55.69
acquired N48.89
pericardium (congenital) Q24.8
acquired — *see* Pericarditis
pharynx (congenital) Q38.8
acquired J39.2
pinna, acquired (*see also* Disorder, pinna, deformity)
congenital Q17.9
pituitary (congenital) Q89.2
posture — *see* Dorsopathy, deforming
prepuce (congenital) Q55.69
acquired N47.8
prostate (congenital) Q55.4
acquired N42.89
pupil (congenital) Q13.2
acquired — *see* Abnormality, pupillary
pylorus (congenital) Q40.3
acquired K31.89
rachitic (acquired), old or healed E64.3
radius (acquired) (*see also* Deformity, limb, forearm)
congenital Q68.8
rectum (congenital) Q43.9
acquired K62.89
reduction (extremity) (limb), congenital (*see also* condition and site) Q73.8
brain Q04.3
lower — *see* Defect, reduction, lower limb
upper — *see* Defect, reduction, upper limb
renal — *see* Deformity, kidney
respiratory system (congenital) Q34.9
rib (acquired) M95.4
congenital Q76.6
cervical Q76.5
rotation (joint) (acquired) — *see* Deformity, limb, specified site NEC
congenital Q74.9
hip — *see* Deformity, limb, specified type NEC, thigh
congenital Q65.89
sacroiliac joint (congenital) — *see* subcategory Q74.2
acquired — *see* subcategory M43.8 ☑
sacrum (acquired) — *see* subcategory M43.8 ☑
saddle
back — *see* Lordosis
nose M95.0
syphilitic A50.57
salivary gland or duct (congenital) Q38.4
acquired K11.8
scapula (acquired) M95.8
congenital Q68.8
scrotum (congenital) (*see also* Malformation, testis and scrotum)
acquired N50.89
seminal vesicles (congenital) Q55.4
acquired N50.89
septum, nasal (acquired) J34.2
shoulder (joint) (acquired) — *see* Deformity, limb, upper arm
congenital Q74.0
contraction — *see* Contraction, joint, shoulder
sigmoid (flexure) (congenital) Q43.9
acquired K63.89
skin (congenital) Q82.9
skull (acquired) M95.2
congenital Q75.8

Deformity — *continued*
skull — *continued*
congenital — *continued*
with
anencephaly Q00.0
encephalocele — *see* Encephalocele
hydrocephalus Q03.9
with spina bifida — *see* Spina bifida, by site, with hydrocephalus
microcephaly Q02
soft parts, organs or tissues (of pelvis)
in pregnancy or childbirth NEC O34.8- ☑
causing obstructed labor O65.5
spermatic cord (congenital) Q55.4
acquired N50.89
torsion — *see* Torsion, spermatic cord
spinal — *see* Dorsopathy, deforming
column (acquired) — *see* Dorsopathy, deforming
congenital Q67.5
cord (congenital) Q06.9
acquired G95.89
nerve root (congenital) Q07.9
spine (acquired) (*see also* Dorsopathy, deforming)
congenital Q67.5
rachitic E64.3
specified NEC — *see* Dorsopathy, deforming, specified NEC
spleen
acquired D73.89
congenital Q89.09
Sprengel's (congenital) Q74.0
sternocleidomastoid (muscle), congenital Q68.0
sternum (acquired) M95.4
congenital NEC Q76.7
stomach (congenital) Q40.3
acquired K31.89
submandibular gland (congenital) Q38.4
submaxillary gland (congenital) Q38.4
acquired K11.8
talipes — *see* Talipes
testis (congenital) (*see also* Malformation, testis and scrotum)
acquired N44.8
torsion — *see* Torsion, testis
thigh (acquired) (*see also* Deformity, limb, thigh)
congenital NEC Q68.8
thorax (acquired) (wall) M95.4
congenital Q67.8
sequelae of rickets E64.3
thumb (acquired) (*see also* Deformity, finger)
congenital NEC Q68.1
thymus (tissue) Q89.2
thyroid (gland) (congenital) Q89.2
cartilage Q31.8
acquired J38.7
tibia (acquired) (*see also* Deformity, limb, specified type NEC, lower leg)
congenital NEC Q68.8
saber (syphilitic) A50.56
toe (acquired) M20.6- ☑
congenital Q66.9
hallux rigidus M20.2- ☑
hallux valgus M20.1- ☑
hallux varus M20.3- ☑
hammer toe M20.4- ☑
specified NEC M20.5X- ☑
tongue (congenital) Q38.3
acquired K14.8
tooth, teeth K00.2
trachea (rings) (congenital) Q32.1
acquired J39.8
transverse aortic arch (congenital) Q25.49
tricuspid (leaflets) (valve) I07.8
atresia or stenosis Q22.4
Ebstein's Q22.5
trunk (acquired) M95.8
congenital Q89.9
ulna (acquired) (*see also* Deformity, limb, forearm)
congenital NEC Q68.8
urachus, congenital Q64.4
ureter (opening) (congenital) Q62.8
acquired N28.89
urethra (congenital) Q64.79
acquired N36.8
urinary tract (congenital) Q64.9
urachus Q64.4
uterus (congenital) Q51.9
acquired N85.8

Deformity — *continued*
  uvula (congenital) Q38.5
  vagina (acquired) N89.8
    congenital Q52.4
  valgus NEC M21.00
    ankle M21.07- ☑
    elbow M21.02- ☑
    hip M21.05- ☑
    knee M21.06- ☑
  valve, valvular (congenital) (heart) Q24.8
    acquired — *see* Endocarditis
  varus NEC M21.10
    ankle M21.17- ☑
    elbow M21.12- ☑
    hip M21.15 ☑
    knee M21.16- ☑
    tibia — *see* Osteochondrosis, juvenile, tibia
  vas deferens (congenital) Q55.4
    acquired N50.89
  vein (congenital) Q27.9
    great Q26.9
  vertebra — *see* Dorsopathy, deforming
  vertical talus (congenital) Q66.80
    left foot Q66.82
    right foot Q66.81
  vesicourethral orifice (acquired) N32.89
    congenital NEC Q64.79
  vessels of optic papilla (congenital) Q14.2
  visual field (contraction) — *see* Defect, visual field
  vitreous body, acquired H43.89
  vulva (congenital) Q52.79
    acquired N90.89
  wrist (joint) (acquired) (*see also* Deformity, limb, forearm)
    congenital Q68.8
    contraction — *see* Contraction, joint, wrist

Degeneration, degenerative
  adrenal (capsule) (fatty) (gland) (hyaline) (infectional) E27.8
  amyloid (*see also* Amyloidosis) E85.9
  anterior cornua, spinal cord G12.29
  anterior labral S43.49- ☑
  aorta, aortic I70.0
    fatty I77.89
  aortic valve (heart) — *see* Endocarditis, aortic
  arteriovascular — *see* Arteriosclerosis
  artery, arterial (atheromatous) (calcareous) (*see also* Arteriosclerosis)
    cerebral, amyloid E85.4 [I68.0]
    medial — *see* Arteriosclerosis, extremities
  articular cartilage NEC — *see* Derangement, joint, articular cartilage, by site
  atheromatous — *see* Arteriosclerosis
  basal nuclei or ganglia G23.9
    specified NEC G23.8
  bone NEC — *see* Disorder, bone, specified type NEC
  brachial plexus G54.0
  brain (cortical) (progressive) G31.9
    alcoholic G31.2
    arteriosclerotic I67.2
    childhood G31.9
      specified NEC G31.89
    cystic G31.89
      congenital Q04.6
    in
      alcoholism G31.2
      beriberi E51.2
      cerebrovascular disease I67.9
      congenital hydrocephalus Q03.9
        with spina bifida (*see also* Spina bifida)
      Fabry-Anderson disease E75.21
      Gaucher's disease E75.22
      Hunter's syndrome E76.1
      lipidosis
        cerebral E75.4
        generalized E75.6
      mucopolysaccharidosis — *see* Mucopolysaccharidosis
      myxedema E03.9 [G32.89]
      neoplastic disease (*see also* Neoplasm) D49.6 [G32.89]
      Niemann-Pick disease E75.249 [G32.89]
      sphingolipidosis E75.3 [G32.89]
      vitamin B12 deficiency E53.8 [G32.89]
    senile NEC G31.1
  breast N64.89
  Bruch's membrane — *see* Degeneration, choroid
  capillaries (fatty) I78.8

Degeneration, degenerative — *continued*
  capillaries — *continued*
    amyloid E85.89 [I79.8]
  cardiac (*see also* Degeneration, myocardial)
    valve, valvular — *see* Endocarditis
  cardiorenal — *see* Hypertension, cardiorenal
  cardiovascular (*see also* Disease, cardiovascular)
    renal — *see* Hypertension, cardiorenal
  cerebellar NOS G31.9
    alcoholic G31.2
    primary (hereditary) (sporadic) G11.9
  cerebral — *see* Degeneration, brain
  cerebrovascular I67.9
    due to hypertension I67.4
  cervical plexus G54.2
  cervix N88.8
    due to radiation (intended effect) N88.8
      adverse effect or misadventure N99.89
  chamber angle H21.21- ☑
  changes, spine or vertebra — *see* Spondylosis
  chorioretinal (*see also* Degeneration, choroid)
    hereditary H31.20
  choroid (colloid) (drusen) H31.10- ☑
    atrophy — *see* Atrophy, choroidal
    hereditary — *see* Dystrophy, choroidal, hereditary
  ciliary body H21.22- ☑
  cochlear — *see* subcategory H83.8 ☑
  combined (spinal cord) (subacute) E53.8 [G32.0]
    with anemia (pernicious) D51.0 [G32.0]
      due to dietary vitamin B12 deficiency D51.3 [G32.0]
    in (due to)
      vitamin B12 deficiency E53.8 [G32.0]
        anemia D51.9 [G32.0]
  conjunctiva H11.10
    concretions — *see* Concretion, conjunctiva
    deposits — *see* Deposit, conjunctiva
    pigmentations — *see* Pigmentation, conjunctiva
    pinguecula — *see* Pinguecula
    xerosis — *see* Xerosis, conjunctiva
  cornea H18.40
    calcerous H18.43
      band keratopathy H18.42- ☑
    familial, hereditary — *see* Dystrophy, cornea
    hyaline (of old scars) H18.49
    keratomalacia — *see* Keratomalacia
    nodular H18.45- ☑
    peripheral H18.46- ☑
    senile H18.41- ☑
    specified type NEC H18.49
  cortical (cerebellar) (parenchymatous) G31.89
    alcoholic G31.2
    diffuse, due to arteriopathy I67.2
  corticobasal G31.85
  cutis L98.8
    amyloid E85.4 [L99]
  dental pulp K04.2
  disc disease — *see* Degeneration, intervertebral disc NEC
  dorsolateral (spinal cord) — *see* Degeneration, combined
  extrapyramidal G25.9
  eye, macular (*see also* Degeneration, macula)
    congenital or hereditary — *see* Dystrophy, retina
  facet joints — *see* Spondylosis
  fatty
    liver NEC K76.0
      alcoholic K70.0
  grey matter (brain) (Alpers') G31.81
  heart (*see also* Degeneration, myocardial)
    amyloid E85.4 [I43]
    atheromatous — *see* Disease, heart, ischemic, atherosclerotic
    ischemic — *see* Disease, heart, ischemic
  hepatolenticular (Wilson's) E83.01
  hepatorenal K76.7
  hyaline (diffuse) (generalized)
    localized — *see* Degeneration, by site
  infrapatellar fat pad M79.4
  intervertebral disc NOS
    with
      myelopathy — *see* Disorder, disc, with, myelopathy
      radiculitis or radiculopathy — *see* Disorder, disc, with, radiculopathy
    cervical, cervicothoracic — *see* Disorder, disc, cervical, degeneration

Degeneration, degenerative — *continued*
  intervertebral disc — *continued*
    cervical, cervicothoracic — *see* Disorder, disc, cervical, degeneration — *continued*
      with
        myelopathy — *see* Disorder, disc, cervical, with myelopathy
        neuritis, radiculitis or radiculopathy — *see* Disorder, disc, cervical, with neuritis
    lumbar region M51.36
      with
        myelopathy M51.06
        neuritis, radiculitis, radiculopathy or sciatica M51.16
    lumbosacral region M51.37
      with
        neuritis, radiculitis, radiculopathy or sciatica M51.17
    sacrococcygeal region M53.3
    thoracic region M51.34
      with
        myelopathy M51.04
        neuritis, radiculitis, radiculopathy M51.14
    thoracolumbar region M51.35
      with
        myelopathy M51.05
        neuritis, radiculitis, radiculopathy M51.15
  intestine, amyloid E85.4
  iris (pigmentary) H21.23- ☑
  ischemic — *see* Ischemia
  joint disease — *see* Osteoarthritis
  kidney N28.89
    amyloid E85.4 [N29]
    cystic, congenital Q61.9
    fatty N28.89
    polycystic Q61.3
      adult type (autosomal dominant) Q61.2
      infantile type (autosomal recessive) NEC Q61.19
        collecting duct dilatation Q61.11
  Kuhnt-Junius (*see also* Degeneration, macula) H35.32- ☑
  lens — *see* Cataract
  lenticular (familial) (progressive) (Wilson's) (with cirrhosis of liver) E83.01
  liver (diffuse) NEC K76.89
    amyloid E85.4 [K77]
    cystic K76.89
      congenital Q44.6
    fatty NEC K76.0
      alcoholic K70.0
    hypertrophic K76.89
    parenchymatous, acute or subacute K72.00
      with coma K72.01
    pigmentary K76.89
    toxic (acute) K71.9
  lung J98.4
  lymph gland I89.8
    hyaline I89.8
  macula, macular (acquired) (age-related) (senile) H35.30
    angioid streaks H35.33
    atrophic age-related H35.31- ☑
    congenital or hereditary — *see* Dystrophy, retina
    cystoid H35.35- ☑
    drusen H35.36- ☑
    dry age-related H35.31- ☑
    exudative H35.32- ☑
    hole H35.34- ☑
    nonexudative H35.31- ☑
    puckering H35.37- ☑
    toxic H35.38- ☑
    wet age-related H35.32- ☑
  membranous labyrinth, congenital (causing impairment of hearing) Q16.5
  meniscus — *see* Derangement, meniscus
  mitral — *see* Insufficiency, mitral
  Mönckeberg's — *see* Arteriosclerosis, extremities
  motor centers, senile G31.1
  multi-system G90.3
  mural — *see* Degeneration, myocardial
  muscle (fatty) (fibrous) (hyaline) (progressive) M62.89
    heart — *see* Degeneration, myocardial
  myelin, central nervous system G37.9
  myocardial, myocardium (fatty) (hyaline) (senile) I51.5
    with rheumatic fever (conditions in I00) I09.0
      active, acute or subacute I01.2
        with chorea I02.0
      inactive or quiescent (with chorea) I09.0

Degeneration, degenerative — *continued*
  myocardial, myocardium — *continued*
    hypertensive — *see* Hypertension, heart
    rheumatic — *see* Degeneration, myocardial, with
      rheumatic fever
    syphilitic A52.06
  nasal sinus (mucosa) J32.9
    frontal J32.1
    maxillary J32.0
  nerve — *see* Disorder, nerve
  nervous system G31.9
    alcoholic G31.2
    amyloid E85.4 [G99.8]
    autonomic G90.9
    fatty G31.89
    specified NEC G31.89
  nipple N64.89
  olivopontocerebellar (hereditary) (familial) G23.8
  osseous labyrinth — *see* subcategory H83.8 ☑
  ovary N83.8
    cystic N83.20- ☑
    microcystic N83.20- ☑
  pallidal pigmentary (progressive) G23.0
  pancreas K86.89
    tuberculous A18.83
  penis N48.89
  pigmentary (diffuse) (general)
    localized — *see* Degeneration, by site
    pallidal (progressive) G23.0
  pineal gland E34.8
  pituitary (gland) E23.6
  popliteal fat pad M79.4
  posterolateral (spinal cord) — *see* Degeneration,
    combined
  pulmonary valve (heart) I37.8
  pulp (tooth) K04.2
  pupillary margin H21.24- ☑
  renal — *see* Degeneration, kidney
  retina H35.9
    hereditary (cerebroretinal) (congenital) (juvenile)
      (macula) (peripheral) (pigmentary) — *see*
      Dystrophy, retina
    Kuhnt-Junius (*see also* Degeneration, macula)
      H35.32- ☑
    macula (cystic) (exudative) (hole) (nonexudative)
      (pseudohole) (senile) (toxic) — *see* Degener-
      ation, macula
    peripheral H35.40
      lattice H35.41- ☑
      microcystoid H35.42- ☑
      paving stone H35.43- ☑
      secondary
        pigmentary H35.45- ☑
        vitreoretinal H35.46- ☑
      senile reticular H35.44- ☑
    pigmentary (primary) (*see also* Dystrophy, retina)
      secondary — *see* Degeneration, retina, periph-
      eral, secondary
    posterior pole — *see* Degeneration, macula
  saccule, congenital (causing impairment of hearing)
    Q16.5
  senile R54
    brain G31.1
    cardiac, heart or myocardium — *see* Degeneration,
      myocardial
    motor centers G31.1
    vascular — *see* Arteriosclerosis
  sinus (cystic) (*see also* Sinusitis)
    polypoid J33.1
  skin L98.8
    amyloid E85.4 [L99]
    colloid L98.8
  spinal (cord) G31.89
    amyloid E85.4 [G32.89]
    combined (subacute) — *see* Degeneration, com-
      bined
    dorsolateral — *see* Degeneration, combined
    familial NEC G31.89
    fatty G31.89
    funicular — *see* Degeneration, combined
    posterolateral — *see* Degeneration, combined
    subacute combined — *see* Degeneration, com-
      bined
    tuberculous A17.81
  spleen D73.0
    amyloid E85.4 [D77]
  stomach K31.89
  striatonigral G23.2

Degeneration, degenerative — *continued*
  suprarenal (capsule) (gland) E27.8
  synovial membrane (pulpy) — *see* Disorder, synovium,
    specified type NEC
  tapetoretinal — *see* Dystrophy, retina
  thymus (gland) E32.8
    fatty E32.8
  thyroid (gland) E07.89
  tricuspid (heart) (valve) I07.9
  tuberculous NEC — *see* Tuberculosis
  turbinate J34.89
  uterus (cystic) N85.8
  vascular (senile) — *see* Arteriosclerosis
    hypertensive — *see* Hypertension
  vitreoretinal, secondary — *see* Degeneration, retina,
    peripheral, secondary, vitreoretinal
  vitreous (body) H43.81- ☑
  Wallerian — *see* Disorder, nerve
  Wilson's hepatolenticular E83.01
Deglutition
  paralysis R13.0
    hysterical F44.4
  pneumonia J69.0
Degos' disease I77.89
Dehiscence (of)
  amputation stump T87.81
  cesarean wound O90.0
  closure of
    cornea T81.31 ☑
    craniotomy T81.32 ☑
    fascia (muscular) (superficial) T81.32 ☑
    internal organ or tissue T81.32 ☑
    laceration (external) (internal) T81.33 ☑
    ligament T81.32 ☑
    mucosa T81.31 ☑
    muscle or muscle flap T81.32 ☑
    ribs or rib cage T81.32 ☑
    skin and subcutaneous tissue (full-thickness) (su-
      perficial) T81.31 ☑
    skull T81.32 ☑
    sternum (sternotomy) T81.32 ☑
    tendon T81.32 ☑
    traumatic laceration (external) (internal) T81.33 ☑
  episiotomy O90.1
  operation wound NEC T81.31 ☑
    external operation wound (superficial) T81.31 ☑
    internal operation wound (deep) T81.32 ☑
  perineal wound (postpartum) O90.1
  traumatic injury wound repair T81.33 ☑
  wound T81.30 ☑
    traumatic repair T81.33 ☑
Dehydration E86.0
  newborn P74.1
Déjérine-Roussy syndrome G89.0
Déjérine-Sottas disease or neuropathy (hypertrophic)
  G60.0
Déjérine-Thomas atrophy G23.8
Delay, delayed
  any plane in pelvis
    complicating delivery O66.9
  birth or delivery NOS O63.9
  closure, ductus arteriosus (Botalli) P29.38
  coagulation — *see* Defect, coagulation
  conduction (cardiac) (ventricular) I45.9
  delivery, second twin, triplet, etc O63.2
  development R62.50
    global F88
    intellectual (specific) F81.9
    language F80.9
      due to hearing loss F80.4
    learning F81.9
    pervasive F84.9
    physiological R62.50
      specified stage NEC R62.0
    reading F81.0
    sexual E30.0
    speech F80.9
      due to hearing loss F80.4
    spelling F81.81
  ejaculation F52.32
  gastric emptying K30
  menarche E30.0
  menstruation (cause unknown) N91.0
  milestone R62.0
  passage of meconium (newborn) P76.0
  primary respiration P28.9
  puberty (constitutional) E30.0

Delay, delayed — *continued*
  separation of umbilical cord P96.82
  sexual maturation, female E30.0
  sleep phase syndrome G47.21
  union, fracture — *see* Fracture, by site
  vaccination Z28.9
Deletion(s)
  autosome Q93.9
    identified by fluorescence in situ hybridization
      (FISH) Q93.89
    identified by in situ hybridization (ISH) Q93.89
  chromosome
    with complex rearrangements NEC Q93.7
    part of NEC Q93.5
    seen only at prometaphase Q93.89
    short arm
      22q11.2 Q93.81
      4 Q93.3
      5p Q93.4
    specified NEC Q93.89
  long arm chromosome 18 or 21 Q93.89
    with complex rearrangements NEC Q93.7
  microdeletions NEC Q93.88
Delhi boil or button B55.1
Delinquency (juvenile) (neurotic) F91.8
  group Z72.810
Delinquent immunization status Z28.3
Delirium, delirious (acute or subacute) (not alcohol- or
  drug-induced) (with dementia) R41.0
  alcoholic (acute) (tremens) (withdrawal) F10.921
    with
      in
        abuse F10.121
        dependence F10.221
  due to (secondary to)
    alcohol
      intoxication F10.921
        in
          abuse F10.121
          dependence F10.221
      withdrawal F10.231
    amphetamine intoxication F15.921
      in
        abuse F15.121
        dependence F15.221
    anxiolytic
      intoxication F13.921
        in
          abuse F13.121
          dependence F13.221
      withdrawal F13.231
    cannabis intoxication (acute) F12.921
      in
        abuse F12.121
        dependence F12.221
    cocaine intoxication (acute) F14.921
      in
        abuse F14.121
        dependence F14.221
    general medical condition F05
    hallucinogen intoxication F16.921
      in
        abuse F16.121
        dependence F16.221
    hypnotic
      intoxication F13.921
        in
          abuse F13.121
          dependence F13.221
      withdrawal F13.231
    inhalant intoxication (acute) F18.921
      in
        abuse F18.121
        dependence F18.221
    multiple etiologies F05
    opioid intoxication (acute) F11.921
      in
        abuse F11.121
        dependence F11.221
    other (or unknown) substance F19.921
    phencyclidine intoxication (acute) F16.921
      in
        abuse F16.121
        dependence F16.221
    psychoactive substance NEC intoxication (acute)
      F19.921
      in
        abuse F19.121
        dependence F19.221

Delirium, delirious — *continued*
 due to — *continued*
  sedative
   intoxication F13.921
    in
     abuse F13.121
     dependence F13.221
    withdrawal F13.231
  unknown etiology F05
  exhaustion F43.0
  hysterical F44.89
  postprocedural (postoperative) F05
  puerperal F05
  thyroid — *see* Thyrotoxicosis with thyroid storm
  traumatic — *see* Injury, intracranial
  tremens (alcohol-induced) F10.231
   sedative-induced F13.231
Delivery (childbirth) (labor)
 arrested active phase O62.1
 cesarean (for)
  without indication O82
  abnormal
   pelvis (bony) (deformity) (major) NEC with dis-
     proportion (fetopelvic) O33.0
    with obstructed labor O65.0
   presentation or position O32.9 ☑
  abruptio placentae (*see also* Abruptio placentae)
    O45.9- ☑
  acromion presentation O32.2 ☑
  atony, uterus O62.2
  breech presentation O32.1 ☑
   incomplete O32.8 ☑
  brow presentation O32.3 ☑
  cephalopelvic disproportion O33.9
  cerclage O34.3- ☑
  chin presentation O32.3 ☑
  cicatrix of cervix O34.4- ☑
  contracted pelvis (general)
   inlet O33.2
   outlet O33.3 ☑
  cord presentation or prolapse O69.0 ☑
  cystocele O34.8- ☑
  deformity (acquired) (congenital)
   pelvic organs or tissues NEC O34.8- ☑
   pelvis (bony) NEC O33.0
  disproportion NOS O33.9
  eclampsia — *see* Eclampsia
  face presentation O32.3 ☑
  failed
   forceps O66.5
   induction of labor O61.9
    instrumental O61.1
    mechanical O61.1
    medical O61.0
    specified NEC O61.8
    surgical O61.1
   trial of labor NOS O66.40
    following previous cesarean delivery O66.41
   vacuum extraction O66.5
   ventouse O66.5
  fetal-maternal hemorrhage O43.01- ☑
  hemorrhage (intrapartum) O67.9
   with coagulation defect O67.0
   specified cause NEC O67.8
  high head at term O32.4 ☑
  hydrocephalic fetus O33.6 ☑
  incarceration of uterus O34.51- ☑
  incoordinate uterine action O62.4
  increased size, fetus O33.5 ☑
  inertia, uterus O62.2
   primary O62.0
   secondary O62.1
  lateroversion, uterus O34.59- ☑
  mal lie O32.9 ☑
  malposition
   fetus O32.9 ☑
   pelvic organs or tissues NEC O34.8- ☑
   uterus NEC O34.59- ☑
  malpresentation NOS O32.9 ☑
  oblique presentation O32.2 ☑
  occurring after 37 completed weeks of gestation
    but before 39 completed weeks gestation
    due to (spontaneous) onset of labor O75.82
  oversize fetus O33.5 ☑
  pelvic tumor NEC O34.8- ☑
  placenta previa O44.0- ☑
   complete O44.0- ☑

Delivery — *continued*
 cesarean — *continued*
  placenta previa — *continued*
   complete — *continued*
    with hemorrhage O44.1- ☑
  placental insufficiency O36.51- ☑
  planned, occurring after 37 completed weeks of
    gestation but before 39 completed weeks
    gestation due to (spontaneous) onset of la-
    bor O75.82
  polyp, cervix O34.4- ☑
   causing obstructed labor O65.5
  poor dilatation, cervix O62.0
  pre-eclampsia O14.94
   mild O14.04
   moderate O14.04
   severe O14.14
    with hemolysis, elevated liver enzymes and
      low platelet count (HELLP) O14.24
  previous
   cesarean delivery O34.219
    classical (vertical) scar O34.212
    low transverse scar O34.211
   surgery (to)
    cervix O34.4- ☑
    gynecological NEC O34.8- ☑
    rectum O34.7- ☑
    uterus O34.29
    vagina O34.6- ☑
  prolapse
   arm or hand O32.2 ☑
   uterus O34.52- ☑
  prolonged labor NOS O63.9
  rectocele O34.8- ☑
  retroversion
   uterus O34.53- ☑
  rigid
   cervix O34.4- ☑
   pelvic floor O34.8- ☑
   perineum O34.7- ☑
   vagina O34.6- ☑
   vulva O34.7- ☑
  sacculation, pregnant uterus O34.59- ☑
  scar(s)
   cervix O34.4- ☑
   cesarean delivery O34.219
    classical (vertical) O34.212
    low transverse O34.211
   transmural uterine O34.29
   uterus O34.29
  Shirodkar suture in situ O34.3- ☑
  shoulder presentation O32.2 ☑
  stenosis or stricture, cervix O34.4- ☑
  streptococcus group B (GBS) carrier state O99.824
  transmural uterine scar O34.29
  transverse presentation or lie O32.2 ☑
  tumor, pelvic organs or tissues NEC O34.8- ☑
   cervix O34.4- ☑
  umbilical cord presentation or prolapse O69.0 ☑
 completely normal case O80
 complicated O75.9
  by
   abnormal, abnormality (of)
    forces of labor O62.9
     specified type NEC O62.8
    glucose O99.814
    uterine contractions NOS O62.9
   abruptio placentae (*see also* Abruptio placen-
     tae) O45.9- ☑
   abuse
    physical O9A.32 (*following* O99)
    psychological O9A.52 (*following* O99)
    sexual O9A.42 (*following* O99)
   adherent placenta O72.0
    without hemorrhage O73.0
   alcohol use O99.314
   anemia (pre-existing) O99.02
   anesthetic death O74.8
   annular detachment of cervix O71.3
   atony, uterus O62.2
   attempted vacuum extraction and forceps
     O66.5
   Bandl's ring O62.4
   bariatric surgery status O99.844
   biliary tract disorder O26.62
   bleeding — *see* Delivery, complicated by,
     hemorrhage
   blood disorder NEC O99.12

Delivery — *continued*
 complicated — *continued*
  by — *continued*
   cervical dystocia (hypotonic) O62.2
    primary O62.0
    secondary O62.1
   circulatory system disorder O99.42
   compression of cord (umbilical) NEC O69.2 ☑
   condition NEC O99.89
   contraction, contracted ring O62.4
   cord (umbilical)
    around neck
     with compression O69.1 ☑
     without compression O69.81 ☑
    bruising O69.5 ☑
    complication O69.9 ☑
     specified NEC O69.89 ☑
    compression NEC O69.2 ☑
    entanglement O69.2 ☑
     without compression O69.82 ☑
    hematoma O69.5 ☑
    presentation O69.0 ☑
    prolapse O69.0 ☑
    short O69.3 ☑
    thrombosis (vessels) O69.5 ☑
    vascular lesion O69.5 ☑
   Couvelaire uterus O45.8X- ☑
   damage to (injury to) NEC
    perineum O71.82
    periurethral tissue O71.82
    vulva O71.82
   delay following rupture of membranes (sponta-
     neous) — *see* Pregnancy, complicated
     by, premature rupture of membranes
   depressed fetal heart tones O76
   diabetes O24.92
    gestational O24.429
     diet controlled O24.420
     insulin controlled O24.424
     oral drug controlled (antidiabetic) (hypo-
       glycemic) O24.425
    pre-existing O24.32
     specified NEC O24.82
     type 1 O24.02
     type 2 O24.12
   diastasis recti (abdominis) O71.89
   dilatation
    bladder O66.8
    cervix incomplete, poor or slow O62.0
   disease NEC O99.89
   disruptio uteri — *see* Delivery, complicated by,
     rupture, uterus
   drug use O99.324
   dysfunction, uterus NOS O62.9
    hypertonic O62.4
    hypotonic O62.2
     primary O62.0
     secondary O62.1
    incoordinate O62.4
   eclampsia O15.1
   embolism (pulmonary) — *see* Embolism, obstet-
     ric
   endocrine, nutritional or metabolic disease NEC
     O99.284
   failed
    attempted vaginal birth after previous ce-
      sarean delivery O66.41
    induction of labor O61.9
     instrumental O61.1
     mechanical O61.1
     medical O61.0
     specified NEC O61.8
     surgical O61.1
    trial of labor O66.40
   female genital mutilation O65.5
   fetal
    abnormal acid-base balance O68
    acidemia O68
    acidosis O68
    alkalosis O68
    death, early O02.1
    deformity O66.3
    heart rate or rhythm (abnormal) (non-reas-
      suring) O76
    hypoxia O77.8
    stress O77.9
     due to drug administration O77.1
     electrocardiographic evidence of O77.8

Delivery — continued
  complicated — continued
    by — continued
      fetal — continued
        stress — continued
          specified NEC O77.8
          ultrasound evidence of O77.8
      fever during labor O75.2
      gastric banding status O99.844
      gastric bypass status O99.844
      gastrointestinal disease NEC O99.62
      gestational
        diabetes O24.429
          diet controlled O24.420
          insulin (and diet) controlled O24.424
          oral drug controlled (antidiabetic) (hypo-glycemic) O24.425
        edema O12.04
          with proteinuria O12.24
        proteinuria O12.14
      gonorrhea O98.22
      hematoma O71.7
        ischial spine O71.7
        pelvic O71.7
        vagina O71.7
        vulva or perineum O71.7
      hemorrhage (uterine) O67.9
        associated with
          afibrinogenemia O67.0
          coagulation defect O67.0
          hyperfibrinolysis O67.0
          hypofibrinogenemia O67.0
        due to
          low implantation of placenta O44.5- ☑
          low-lying placenta O44.5- ☑
          placenta previa O44.1- ☑
            marginal O44.3- ☑
            partial O44.3- ☑
          premature separation of placenta (nor-mally implanted) (see also Abrup-tio placentae) O45.9- ☑
          retained placenta O72.0
          uterine leiomyoma O67.8
        placenta NEC O67.8
        postpartum NEC (atonic) (immediate) O72.1
          with retained or trapped placenta O72.0
          delayed O72.2
          secondary O72.2
          third stage O72.0
      hourglass contraction, uterus O62.4
      hypertension, hypertensive (pre-existing) — see Hypertension, complicated by, child-birth (labor)
      hypotension O26.5- ☑
      incomplete dilatation (cervix) O62.0
      incoordinate uterus contractions O62.4
      inertia, uterus O62.2
        during latent phase of labor O62.0
        primary O62.0
        secondary O62.1
      infection (maternal) O98.92
        carrier state NEC O99.834
        gonorrhea O98.22
        human immunodeficiency virus (HIV) O98.72
        sexually transmitted NEC O98.32
        specified NEC O98.82
        syphilis O98.12
        tuberculosis O98.02
        viral hepatitis O98.42
        viral NEC O98.52
      injury (to mother) (see also Delivery, complicat-ed, by, damage to) O71.9
        nonobstetric O9A.22 (following O99)
          caused by abuse — see Delivery, compli-cated by, abuse
      intrauterine fetal death, early O02.1
      inversion, uterus O71.2
      laceration (perineal) O70.9
        anus (sphincter) O70.4
          with third degree laceration (see also Delivery, complicated, by, lacera-tion, perineum, third degree) O70.20
            with mucosa O70.3
          without third degree laceration O70.2 ☑
        bladder (urinary) O71.5
        bowel O71.5

Delivery — continued
  complicated — continued
    by — continued
      laceration — continued
        cervix (uteri) O71.3
        fourchette O70.0
        hymen O70.0
        labia O70.0
        pelvic
          floor O70.1
          organ NEC O71.5
        perineum, perineal O70.9
          first degree O70.0
          fourth degree O70.3
          muscles O70.1
          second degree O70.1
          skin O70.0
          slight O70.0
          third degree O70.20
            with
              less than 50% of external anal sphincter (EAS) thickness torn (IIIa) O70.21
              both external anal sphincter (EAS) and internal anal sphincter (IAS) torn (IIIc) O70.23
              more than 50% external anal sphincter (EAS) thickness torn (IIIb) O70.22
            IIIa O70.21
            IIIb O70.22
            IIIc O70.23
        peritoneum (pelvic) O71.5
        rectovaginal (septum) (without perineal laceration) O71.4
          with perineum (see also Delivery, compli-cated, by, laceration, perineum, third degree) O70.20
          with anal or rectal mucosa O70.3
        specified NEC O71.89
        sphincter ani — see Delivery, complicated, by, laceration, anus (sphincter)
        urethra O71.5
        uterus O71.81
          before labor O71.81
        vagina, vaginal (deep) (high) (without per-ineal laceration) O71.4
          with perineum O70.0
          muscles, with perineum O70.1
        vulva O70.0
      liver disorder O26.62
      malignancy O9A.12 (following O99)
      malnutrition O25.2
      malposition, malpresentation
        without obstruction (see also Delivery, complicated by, obstruction) O32.9 ☑
          breech O32.1 ☑
          compound O32.6 ☑
          face (brow) (chin) O32.3 ☑
          footling O32.8 ☑
          high head O32.4 ☑
          oblique O32.2 ☑
          specified NEC O32.8 ☑
          transverse O32.2 ☑
          unstable lie O32.0 ☑
        placenta O44.0- ☑
          with hemorrhage O44.1- ☑
        uterus or cervix O65.5
      meconium in amniotic fluid O77.0
      mental disorder NEC O99.344
      metrorrhexis — see Delivery, complicated by, rupture, uterus
      nervous system disorder O99.354
      obesity (pre-existing) O99.214
      obesity surgery status O99.844
      obstetric trauma O71.9
        specified NEC O71.89
      obstructed labor
        due to
          breech (complete) (frank) presentation O64.1 ☑
            incomplete O64.8 ☑
          brow presenation O64.3 ☑
          buttock presentation O64.1 ☑
          chin presentation O64.2 ☑
          compound presentation O64.5 ☑
          contracted pelvis O65.1
          deep transverse arrest O64.0 ☑

Delivery — continued
  complicated — continued
    by — continued
      obstructed labor — continued
        due to — continued
          deformed pelvis O65.0
          dystocia (fetal) O66.9
            due to
              conjoined twins O66.3
              fetal
                abnormality NEC O66.3
                ascites O66.3
                hydrops O66.3
                meningomyelocele O66.3
                sacral teratoma O66.3
                tumor O66.3
             hydrocephalic fetus O66.3
            shoulder O66.0
          face presentation O64.2 ☑
          fetopelvic disproportion O65.4
          footling presentation O64.8 ☑
          impacted shoulders O66.0
          incomplete rotation of fetal head O64.0 ☑
          large fetus O66.2
          locked twins O66.1
          malposition O64.9 ☑
            specified NEC O64.8 ☑
          malpresentation O64.9 ☑
            specified NEC O64.8 ☑
          multiple fetuses NEC O66.6
          pelvic
            abnormality (maternal) O65.9
              organ O65.5
              specified NEC O65.8
            contraction
              inlet O65.2
              mid-cavity O65.3
              outlet O65.3
          persistent (position)
            occipitoiliac O64.0 ☑
            occipitoposterior O64.0 ☑
            occipitosacral O64.0 ☑
            occipitotransverse O64.0 ☑
          prolapsed arm O64.4 ☑
          shoulder presentation O64.4 ☑
        specified NEC O66.8
      pathological retraction ring, uterus O62.4
      penetration, pregnant uterus by instrument O71.1
      perforation — see Delivery, complicated by, laceration
      placenta, placental
        ablatio (see also Abruptio placentae) O45.9- ☑
        abnormality O43.9- ☑
          specified NEC O43.89- ☑
        abruptio (see also Abruptio placentae) O45.9- ☑
        accreta O43.21- ☑
        adherent (with hemorrhage) O72.0
          without hemorrhage O73.0
        detachment (premature) (see also Abruptio placentae) O45.9- ☑
        disorder O43.9- ☑
          specified NEC O43.89- ☑
        hemorrhage NEC O67.8
        increta O43.22- ☑
        low (implantation) (lying) O44.4- ☑
          with hemorrhage O44.5- ☑
        malformation O43.10- ☑
        malposition O44.0- ☑
          without hemorrhage O44.1- ☑
        percreta O43.23- ☑
        previa (central) (complete) (lateral) (total) O44.0- ☑
          with hemorrhage O44.1- ☑
          marginal O44.2- ☑
            with hemorrhage O44.3- ☑
          partial O44.2- ☑
            with hemorrhage O44.3- ☑
        retained (with hemorrhage) O72.0
          without hemorrhage O73.0
        separation (premature) O45.9- ☑
          specified NEC O45.8X- ☑
        vicious insertion O44.1- ☑
      precipitate labor O62.3

Delivery — *continued*
  complicated — *continued*
    by — *continued*
      premature rupture, membranes (*see also* Pregnancy, complicated by, premature rupture of membranes) O42.90
      prolapse
        arm or hand O32.2 ☑
        cord (umbilical) O69.0 ☑
        foot or leg O32.8 ☑
        uterus O34.52- ☑
      prolonged labor O63.9
        first stage O63.0
        second stage O63.1
      protozoal disease (maternal) O98.62
      respiratory disease NEC O99.52
      retained membranes or portions of placenta O72.2
        without hemorrhage O73.1
      retarded birth O63.9
      retention of secundines (with hemorrhage) O72.0
        without hemorrhage O73.0
        partial O72.2
          without hemorrhage O73.1
      rupture
        bladder (urinary) O71.5
        cervix O71.3
        pelvic organ NEC O71.5
        urethra O71.5
        uterus (during or after labor) O71.1
          before labor O71.0- ☑
      separation, pubic bone (symphysis pubis) O71.6
      shock O75.1
      shoulder presentation O64.4 ☑
      skin disorder NEC O99.72
      spasm, cervix O62.4
      stenosis or stricture, cervix O65.5
      streptococcus group B (GBS) carrier state O99.824
      subluxation of symphysis (pubis) O26.72
      syphilis (maternal) O98.12
      tear — *see* Delivery, complicated by, laceration
      tetanic uterus O62.4
      trauma (obstetrical) (*see also* Delivery, complicated, by, damage to) O71.9
        non-obstetric O9A.22 (*following* O99)
        periurethral O71.82
        specified NEC O71.89
      tuberculosis (maternal) O98.02
      tumor, pelvic organs or tissues NEC O65.5
      umbilical cord around neck
        with compression O69.1 ☑
        without compression O69.81 ☑
      uterine inertia O62.2
        during latent phase of labor O62.0
        primary O62.0
        secondary O62.1
      vasa previa O69.4 ☑
      velamentous insertion of cord O43.12- ☑
    specified complication NEC O75.89
  delayed NOS O63.9
    following rupture of membranes
      artificial O75.5
    second twin, triplet, etc. O63.2
  forceps, low following failed vacuum extraction O66.5
  missed (at or near term) O36.4 ☑
  normal O80
  obstructed — *see* Delivery, complicated by, obstructed labor
  precipitate O62.3
  preterm (*see also* Pregnancy, complicated by, preterm labor) O60.10 ☑
  spontaneous O80
  term pregnancy NOS O80
  uncomplicated O80
  vaginal, following previous cesarean delivery O34.219
    classical (vertical) scar O34.212
    low transverse scar O34.211
Delusions (paranoid) — *see* Disorder, delusional
Dementia (degenerative (primary)) (old age) (persisting) F03.90
  with
    aggressive behavior F03.91
    behavioral disturbance F03.91
    combative behavior F03.91
    Lewy bodies G31.83 [F02.80]
      with behavioral disturbance G31.83 [F02.81]

Dementia — *continued*
  with — *continued*
    Parkinsonism G31.83 [F02.80]
      with behavioral disturbance G31.83 [F02.81]
    Parkinson's disease G20 [F02.80]
      with behavioral disturbance G20 [F02.81]
    violent behavior F03.91
  alcoholic F10.97
    with dependence F10.27
  Alzheimer's type — *see* Disease, Alzheimer's
  arteriosclerotic — *see* Dementia, vascular
  atypical, Alzheimer's type — *see* Disease, Alzheimer's, specified NEC
  congenital — *see* Disability, intellectual
  frontal (lobe) G31.09 [F02.80]
    with behavioral disturbance G31.09 [F02.81]
  frontotemporal G31.09 [F02.80]
    with behavioral disturbance G31.09 [F02.81]
    specified NEC G31.09 [F02.80]
      with behavioral disturbance G31.09 [F02.81]
  Huntington's disease or chorea G10
    with dementia G10 [F02.80]
  in (due to)
    with behavioral disturbance G31.83 [F02.81]
    alcohol F10.97
      with dependence F10.27
    Alzheimer's disease — *see* Disease, Alzheimer's
    arteriosclerotic brain disease — *see* Dementia, vascular
    cerebral lipidoses E75.- ☑ [F02.80]
      with behavioral disturbance E75.- ☑ [F02.81]
    Creutzfeldt-Jakob disease (*see also* Creutzfeldt-Jakob disease or syndrome (with dementia)) A81.00
    epilepsy G40.- ☑ [F02.80]
      with behavioral disturbance G40.- ☑ [F02.81]
    hepatolenticular degeneration E83.01 [F02.80]
      with behavioral disturbance E83.01 [F02.81]
    human immunodeficiency virus (HIV) disease B20 [F02.80]
      with behavioral disturbance B20 [F02.81]
    Huntington's disease or chorea G10 [F02.80]
      with behavioral disturbance G10 [F02.81]
    hypercalcemia E83.52 [F02.80]
      with behavioral disturbance E83.52 [F02.81]
    hypothyroidism, acquired E03.9 [F02.80]
      with behavioral disturbance E03.9 [F02.81]
      due to iodine deficiency E01.8 [F02.80]
        with behavioral disturbance E01.8 [F02.81]
    inhalants F18.97
      with dependence F18.27
    multiple
      etiologies F03 ☑
      sclerosis G35 [F02.80]
        with behavioral disturbance G35 [F02.81]
    neurosyphilis A52.17 [F02.80]
      with behavioral disturbance A52.17 [F02.81]
      juvenile A50.49 [F02.80]
        with behavioral disturbance A50.49 [F02.81]
    niacin deficiency E52 [F02.80]
      with behavioral disturbance E52 [F02.81]
    paralysis agitans G20 [F02.80]
      with behavioral disturbance G20 [F02.81]
    Parkinson's disease G20 [F02.80]
    pellagra E52 [F02.80]
      with behavioral disturbance E52 [F02.81]
    Pick's G31.01 [F02.80]
      with behavioral disturbance G31.01 [F02.81]
    polyarteritis nodosa M30.0 [F02.80]
      with behavioral disturbance M30.0 [F02.81]
    psychoactive drug F19.97
      with dependence F19.27
      inhalants F18.97
        with dependence F18.27
      sedatives, hypnotics or anxiolytics F13.97
        with dependence F13.27
    sedatives, hypnotics or anxiolytics F13.97
      with dependence F13.27
    systemic lupus erythematosus M32.- ☑ [F02.80]
      with behavioral disturbance M32.- ☑ [F02.81]
    trypanosomiasis
      African B56.9 [F02.80]
        with behavioral disturbance B56.9 [F02.81]
    unknown etiology F03 ☑
    vitamin B12 deficiency E53.8 [F02.80]
      with behavioral disturbance E53.8 [F02.81]
    volatile solvents F18.97
      with dependence F18.27

Dementia — *continued*
  infantile, infantilis F84.3
  Lewy body G31.83 [F02.80]
    with behavioral disturbance G31.83 [F02.81]
  multi-infarct — *see* Dementia, vascular
  paralytica, paralytic (syphilitic) A52.17 [F02.80]
    with behavioral disturbance A52.17 [F02.81]
    juvenilis A50.45
  paretic A52.17
  praecox — *see* Schizophrenia
  presenile F03 ☑
    Alzheimer's type — *see* Disease, Alzheimer's, early onset
  primary degenerative F03 ☑
  progressive, syphilitic A52.17
  senile F03 ☑
    with acute confusional state F05
    Alzheimer's type — *see* Disease, Alzheimer's, late onset
    depressed or paranoid type F03 ☑
  vascular (acute onset) (mixed) (multi-infarct) (subcortical) F01.50
    with behavioral disturbance F01.51
Demineralization, bone — *see* Osteoporosis
Demodex folliculorum (infestation) B88.0
Demophobia F40.248
Demoralization R45.3
Demyelination, demyelinization
  central nervous system G37.9
    specified NEC G37.8
  corpus callosum (central) G37.1
  disseminated, acute G36.9
    specified NEC G36.8
  global G35
  in optic neuritis G36.0
Dengue (classical) (fever) A90
  hemorrhagic A91
  sandfly A93.1
Dennie-Marfan syphilitic syndrome A50.45
Dens evaginatus, in dente or invaginatus K00.2
Dense breasts R92.2
Density
  increased, bone (disseminated) (generalized) (spotted) — *see* Disorder, bone, density and structure, specified type NEC
  lung (nodular) J98.4
Dental (*see also* condition)
  examination Z01.20
    with abnormal findings Z01.21
  restoration
    aesthetically inadequate or displeasing K08.56
    defective K08.50
      specified NEC K08.59
    failure of marginal integrity K08.51
    failure of periodontal anatomical integrity K08.54
Dentia praecox K00.6
Denticles (pulp) K04.2
Dentigerous cyst K09.0
Dentin
  irregular (in pulp) K04.3
  opalescent K00.5
  secondary (in pulp) K04.3
  sensitive K03.89
Dentinogenesis imperfecta K00.5
Dentinoma — *see* Cyst, calcifying odontogenic
Dentition (syndrome) K00.7
  delayed K00.6
  difficult K00.7
  precocious K00.6
  premature K00.6
  retarded K00.6
Dependence (on) (syndrome) F19.20
  with remission F19.21
  alcohol (ethyl) (methyl) (without remission) F10.20
    with
      amnestic disorder, persisting F10.26
      anxiety disorder F10.280
      dementia, persisting F10.27
      intoxication F10.229
        with delirium F10.221
        uncomplicated F10.220
      mood disorder F10.24
      psychotic disorder F10.259
        with
          delusions F10.250
          hallucinations F10.251
      remission F10.21
      sexual dysfunction F10.281

☑ **Additional Character Required** — Refer to the Tabular List for Character Selection   ▽ Subterms under main terms may continue to next column or page

Dependence — continued
  alcohol — continued
    with — continued
      sleep disorder F10.282
      specified disorder NEC F10.288
      withdrawal F10.239
        with
          delirium F10.231
          perceptual disturbance F10.232
        uncomplicated F10.230
    counseling and surveillance Z71.41
  amobarbital — see Dependence, drug, sedative
  amphetamine(s) (type) — see Dependence, drug, stimulant NEC
  amytal (sodium) — see Dependence, drug, sedative
  analgesic NEC F55.8
  anesthetic (agent) (gas) (general) (local) NEC — see Dependence, drug, psychoactive NEC
  anxiolytic NEC — see Dependence, drug, sedative
  barbital(s) — see Dependence, drug, sedative
  barbiturate(s) (compounds) (drugs classifiable to T42) — see Dependence, drug, sedative
  benzedrine — see Dependence, drug, stimulant NEC
  bhang — see Dependence, drug, cannabis
  bromide(s) NEC — see Dependence, drug, sedative
  caffeine — see Dependence, drug, stimulant NEC
  cannabis (sativa) (indica) (resin) (derivatives) (type) — see Dependence, drug, cannabis
  chloral (betaine) (hydrate) — see Dependence, drug, sedative
  chlordiazepoxide — see Dependence, drug, sedative
  coca (leaf) (derivatives) — see Dependence, drug, cocaine
  cocaine — see Dependence, drug, cocaine
  codeine — see Dependence, drug, opioid
  combinations of drugs F19.20
  dagga — see Dependence, drug, cannabis
  demerol — see Dependence, drug, opioid
  dexamphetamine — see Dependence, drug, stimulant NEC
  dexedrine — see Dependence, drug, stimulant NEC
  dextromethorphan — see Dependence, drug, opioid
  dextromoramide — see Dependence, drug, opioid
  dextro-nor-pseudo-ephedrine — see Dependence, drug, stimulant NEC
  dextrorphan — see Dependence, drug, opioid
  diazepam — see Dependence, drug, sedative
  dilaudid — see Dependence, drug, opioid
  D-lysergic acid diethylamide — see Dependence, drug, hallucinogen
  drug NEC F19.20
    with sleep disorder F19.282
    cannabis F12.20
      with
        anxiety disorder F12.280
        intoxication F12.229
          with
            delirium F12.221
            perceptual disturbance F12.222
          uncomplicated F12.220
        other specified disorder F12.288
        psychosis F12.259
          delusions F12.250
          hallucinations F12.251
        unspecified disorder F12.29
      in remission F12.21
    cocaine F14.20
      with
        anxiety disorder F14.280
        intoxication F14.229
          with
            delirium F14.221
            perceptual disturbance F14.222
          uncomplicated F14.220
        mood disorder F14.24
        other specified disorder F14.288
        psychosis F14.259
          delusions F14.250
          hallucinations F14.251
        sexual dysfunction F14.281
        sleep disorder F14.282
        unspecified disorder F14.29
        withdrawal F14.23
      in remission F14.21
      withdrawal symptoms in newborn P96.1
    counseling and surveillance Z71.51
    hallucinogen F16.20

Dependence — continued
  drug — continued
    hallucinogen — continued
      with
        anxiety disorder F16.280
        flashbacks F16.283
        intoxication F16.229
          with delirium F16.221
          uncomplicated F16.220
        mood disorder F16.24
        other specified disorder F16.288
        perception disorder, persisting F16.283
        psychosis F16.259
          delusions F16.250
          hallucinations F16.251
        unspecified disorder F16.29
      in remission F16.21
    in remission F19.21
    inhalant F18.20
      with
        anxiety disorder F18.280
        dementia, persisting F18.27
        intoxication F18.229
          with delirium F18.221
          uncomplicated F18.220
        mood disorder F18.24
        other specified disorder F18.288
        psychosis F18.259
          delusions F18.250
          hallucinations F18.251
        unspecified disorder F18.29
      in remission F18.21
    nicotine F17.200
      with disorder F17.209
        in remission F17.201
        specified disorder NEC F17.208
        withdrawal F17.203
      chewing tobacco F17.220
        with disorder F17.229
          in remission F17.221
          specified disorder NEC F17.228
          withdrawal F17.223
      cigarettes F17.210
        with disorder F17.219
          in remission F17.211
          specified disorder NEC F17.218
          withdrawal F17.213
      specified product NEC F17.290
        with disorder F17.299
          remission F17.291
          specified disorder NEC F17.298
          withdrawal F17.293
    opioid F11.20
      with
        intoxication F11.229
          with
            delirium F11.221
            perceptual disturbance F11.222
          uncomplicated F11.220
        mood disorder F11.24
        other specified disorder F11.288
        psychosis F11.259
          delusions F11.250
          hallucinations F11.251
        sexual dysfunction F11.281
        sleep disorder F11.282
        unspecified disorder F11.29
        withdrawal F11.23
      in remission F11.21
    psychoactive NEC F19.20
      with
        amnestic disorder F19.26
        anxiety disorder F19.280
        dementia F19.27
        intoxication F19.229
          with
            delirium F19.221
            perceptual disturbance F19.222
          uncomplicated F19.220
        mood disorder F19.24
        other specified disorder F19.288
        psychosis F19.259
          delusions F19.250
          hallucinations F19.251
        sexual dysfunction F19.281
        sleep disorder F19.282
        unspecified disorder F19.29
        withdrawal F19.239

Dependence — continued
  drug — continued
    psychoactive — continued
      with — continued
        withdrawal — continued
          with
            delirium F19.231
            perceptual disturbance F19.232
          uncomplicated F19.230
    sedative, hypnotic or anxiolytic F13.20
      with
        amnestic disorder F13.26
        anxiety disorder F13.280
        dementia, persisting F13.27
        intoxication F13.229
          with delirium F13.221
          uncomplicated F13.220
        mood disorder F13.24
        other specified disorder F13.288
        psychosis F13.259
          delusions F13.250
          hallucinations F13.251
        sexual dysfunction F13.281
        sleep disorder F13.282
        unspecified disorder F13.29
        withdrawal F13.239
          with
            delirium F13.231
            perceptual disturbance F13.232
          uncomplicated F13.230
      in remission F13.21
    stimulant NEC F15.20
      with
        anxiety disorder F15.280
        intoxication F15.229
          with
            delirium F15.221
            perceptual disturbance F15.222
          uncomplicated F15.220
        mood disorder F15.24
        other specified disorder F15.288
        psychosis F15.259
          delusions F15.250
          hallucinations F15.251
        sexual dysfunction F15.281
        sleep disorder F15.282
        unspecified disorder F15.29
        withdrawal F15.23
      in remission F15.21
  ethyl
    alcohol (without remission) F10.20
      with remission F10.21
    bromide — see Dependence, drug, sedative
    carbamate F19.20
    chloride F19.20
    morphine — see Dependence, drug, opioid
  ganja — see Dependence, drug, cannabis
  glue (airplane) (sniffing) — see Dependence, drug, inhalant
  glutethimide — see Dependence, drug, sedative
  hallucinogenics — see Dependence, drug, hallucinogen
  hashish — see Dependence, drug, cannabis
  hemp — see Dependence, drug, cannabis
  heroin (salt) (any) — see Dependence, drug, opioid
  hypnotic NEC — see Dependence, drug, sedative
  Indian hemp — see Dependence, drug, cannabis
  inhalants — see Dependence, drug, inhalant
  khat — see Dependence, drug, stimulant NEC
  laudanum — see Dependence, drug, opioid
  LSD (-25) (derivatives) — see Dependence, drug, hallucinogen
  luminal — see Dependence, drug, sedative
  lysergic acid — see Dependence, drug, hallucinogen
  maconha — see Dependence, drug, cannabis
  marihuana — see Dependence, drug, cannabis
  meprobamate — see Dependence, drug, sedative
  mescaline — see Dependence, drug, hallucinogen
  methadone — see Dependence, drug, opioid
  methamphetamine(s) — see Dependence, drug, stimulant NEC
  methaqualone — see Dependence, drug, sedative
  methyl
    alcohol (without remission) F10.20
      with remission F10.21
    bromide — see Dependence, drug, sedative
    morphine — see Dependence, drug, opioid

Index

Dependence — Derangement

Dependence — *continued*
  methyl — *continued*
    phenidate — *see* Dependence, drug, stimulant NEC
    sulfonal — *see* Dependence, drug, sedative
  morphine (sulfate) (sulfite) (type) — *see* Dependence, drug, opioid
  narcotic (drug) NEC — *see* Dependence, drug, opioid
  nembutal — *see* Dependence, drug, sedative
  neraval — *see* Dependence, drug, sedative
  neravan — *see* Dependence, drug, sedative
  neurobarb — *see* Dependence, drug, sedative
  nicotine — *see* Dependence, drug, nicotine
  nitrous oxide F19.20
  nonbarbiturate sedatives and tranquilizers with similar effect — *see* Dependence, drug, sedative
  on
    artificial heart (fully implantable) (mechanical) Z95.812
    aspirator Z99.0
    care provider (because of) Z74.9
      impaired mobility Z74.09
      need for
        assistance with personal care Z74.1
        continuous supervision Z74.3
        no other household member able to render care Z74.2
      specified reason NEC Z74.8
    machine Z99.89
      enabling NEC Z99.89
      specified type NEC Z99.89
    renal dialysis (hemodialysis) (peritoneal) Z99.2
    respirator Z99.11
    ventilator Z99.11
    wheelchair Z99.3
  opiate — *see* Dependence, drug, opioid
  opioids — *see* Dependence, drug, opioid
  opium (alkaloids) (derivatives) (tincture) — *see* Dependence, drug, opioid
  oxygen (long-term) (supplemental) Z99.81
  paraldehyde — *see* Dependence, drug, sedative
  paregoric — *see* Dependence, drug, opioid
  PCP (phencyclidine) (or related substance) — *see* Dependence, drug, hallucinogen
  pentobarbital — *see* Dependence, drug, sedative
  pentobarbitone (sodium) — *see* Dependence, drug, sedative
  pentothal — *see* Dependence, drug, sedative
  peyote — *see* Dependence, drug, hallucinogen
  phencyclidine (PCP) (or related substance) — *see* Dependence, drug, hallucinogen
  phenmetrazine — *see* Dependence, drug, stimulant NEC
  phenobarbital — *see* Dependence, drug, sedative
  polysubstance F19.20
  psilocibin, psilocin, psilocyn, psilocyline — *see* Dependence, drug, hallucinogen
  psychostimulant NEC — *see* Dependence, drug, stimulant NEC
  secobarbital — *see* Dependence, drug, sedative
  seconal — *see* Dependence, drug, sedative
  sedative NEC — *see* Dependence, drug, sedative
  specified drug NEC — *see* Dependence, drug
  stimulant NEC — *see* Dependence, drug, stimulant NEC
  substance NEC — *see* Dependence, drug
  supplemental oxygen Z99.81
  tobacco — *see* Dependence, drug, nicotine
    counseling and surveillance Z71.6
  tranquilizer NEC — *see* Dependence, drug, sedative
  vitamin B6 E53.1
  volatile solvents — *see* Dependence, drug, inhalant

Dependency
  care-provider Z74.9
  passive F60.7
  reactions (persistent) F60.7

Depersonalization (in neurotic state) (neurotic) (syndrome) F48.1

Depletion
  extracellular fluid E86.9
  plasma E86.1
  potassium E87.6
    nephropathy N25.89
  salt or sodium E87.1
    causing heat exhaustion or prostration T67.4 ☑
    nephropathy N28.9
  volume NOS E86.9

Deployment (current) (military) status Z56.82
  in theater or in support of military war, peacekeeping and humanitarian operations Z56.82
  personal history of Z91.82
    military war, peacekeeping and humanitarian deployment (current or past conflict) Z91.82
  returned from Z91.82

Depolarization, premature I49.40
  atrial I49.1
  junctional I49.2
  specified NEC I49.49
  ventricular I49.3

Deposit
  bone in Boeck's sarcoid D86.89
  calcareous, calcium — *see* Calcification
  cholesterol
    retina H35.89
    vitreous (body) (humor) — *see* Deposit, crystalline
  conjunctiva H11.11- ☑
  cornea H18.00- ☑
    argentous H18.02- ☑
    due to metabolic disorder H18.03- ☑
    Kayser-Fleischer ring H18.04- ☑
    pigmentation — *see* Pigmentation, cornea
  crystalline, vitreous (body) (humor) H43.2- ☑
  hemosiderin in old scars of cornea — *see* Pigmentation, cornea, stromal
  metallic in lens — *see* Cataract, specified NEC
  skin R23.8
  tooth, teeth (betel) (black) (green) (materia alba) (orange) (tobacco) K03.6
  urate, kidney — *see* Calculus, kidney

Depraved appetite — *see* Pica

Depressed
  HDL cholesterol E78.6

Depression (acute) (mental) F32.9
  agitated (single episode) F32.2
  anaclitic — *see* Disorder, adjustment
  anxiety F41.8
    persistent F34.1
  arches (*see also* Deformity, limb, flat foot)
  atypical (single episode) F32.89
    recurrent episode F33.8
  basal metabolic rate R94.8
  bone marrow D75.89
  central nervous system R09.2
  cerebral R29.818
    newborn P91.4
  cerebrovascular I67.9
  chest wall M95.4
  climacteric (single episode) F32.89
    recurrent episode F33.8
  endogenous (without psychotic symptoms) F33.2
    with psychotic symptoms F33.3
  functional activity R68.89
  hysterical F44.89
  involutional (single episode) F32.89
    recurrent episode F33.8
  major F32.9
    with psychotic symptoms F32.3
    recurrent — *see* Disorder, depressive, recurrent
  manic-depressive — *see* Disorder, depressive, recurrent
  masked (single episode) F32.89
  medullary G93.89
  menopausal (single episode) F32.89
    recurrent episode F33.8
  metatarsus — *see* Depression, arches
  monopolar F33.9
  nervous F34.1
  neurotic F34.1
  nose M95.0
  postnatal F53
  postpartum F53
  post-psychotic of schizophrenia F32.89
  post-schizophrenic F32.89
  psychogenic (reactive) (single episode) F32.9
  psychoneurotic F34.1
  psychotic (single episode) F32.3
    recurrent F33.3
  reactive (psychogenic) (single episode) F32.9
    psychotic (single episode) F32.3
  recurrent — *see* Disorder, depressive, recurrent
  respiratory center G93.89
  seasonal — *see* Disorder, depressive, recurrent
  senile F03 ☑
  severe, single episode F32.2
  situational F43.21

Depression — *continued*
  skull Q67.4
  specified NEC (single episode) F32.89
  sternum M95.4
  visual field — *see* Defect, visual field
  vital (recurrent) (without psychotic symptoms) F33.2
    with psychotic symptoms F33.3
    single episode F32.2

Deprivation
  cultural Z60.3
  effects NOS T73.9 ☑
    specified NEC T73.8 ☑
  emotional NEC Z65.8
    affecting infant or child — *see* Maltreatment, child, psychological
  food T73.0 ☑
  protein — *see* Malnutrition
  sleep Z72.820
  social Z60.4
    affecting infant or child — *see* Maltreatment, child, psychological
  specified NEC T73.8 ☑
  vitamins — *see* Deficiency, vitamin
  water T73.1 ☑

Derangement
  ankle (internal) — *see* Derangement, joint, ankle
  cartilage (articular) NEC — *see* Derangement, joint, articular cartilage, by site
    recurrent — *see* Dislocation, recurrent
  cruciate ligament, anterior, current injury — *see* Sprain, knee, cruciate, anterior
  elbow (internal) — *see* Derangement, joint, elbow
  hip (joint) (internal) (old) — *see* Derangement, joint, hip
  joint (internal) M24.9
    ankylosis — *see* Ankylosis
    articular cartilage M24.10
      ankle M24.17- ☑
      elbow M24.12- ☑
      foot M24.17- ☑
      hand M24.14- ☑
      hip M24.15- ☑
      knee NEC M23.9- ☑
      loose body — *see* Loose, body
      shoulder M24.11- ☑
      wrist M24.13- ☑
    contracture — *see* Contraction, joint
    current injury (*see also* Dislocation)
      knee, meniscus or cartilage — *see* Tear, meniscus
    dislocation
      pathological — *see* Dislocation, pathological
      recurrent — *see* Dislocation, recurrent
    knee — *see* Derangement, knee
    ligament — *see* Disorder, ligament
    loose body — *see* Loose, body
    recurrent — *see* Dislocation, recurrent
    specified type NEC M24.80
      ankle M24.87- ☑
      elbow M24.82- ☑
      foot joint M24.87- ☑
      hand joint M24.84- ☑
      hip M24.85- ☑
      shoulder M24.81- ☑
      wrist M24.83- ☑
    temporomandibular M26.69
  knee (recurrent) M23.9- ☑
    ligament disruption, spontaneous M23.60- ☑
      anterior cruciate M23.61- ☑
      capsular M23.67- ☑
      instability, chronic M23.5- ☑
      lateral collateral M23.64- ☑
      medial collateral M23.63- ☑
      posterior cruciate M23.62- ☑
    loose body M23.4- ☑
    meniscus M23.30- ☑
      cystic M23.00- ☑
        lateral M23.002
          anterior horn M23.04- ☑
          posterior horn M23.05- ☑
          specified NEC M23.06- ☑
        medial M23.005
          anterior horn M23.01- ☑
          posterior horn M23.02- ☑
          specified NEC M23.03- ☑

Derangement — continued
  knee — continued
    meniscus — continued
      degenerate — see Derangement, knee, meniscus, specified NEC
      detached — see Derangement, knee, meniscus, specified NEC
      due to old tear or injury M23.20- ☑
        lateral M23.20- ☑
          anterior horn M23.24- ☑
          posterior horn M23.25- ☑
          specified NEC M23.26- ☑
        medial M23.20- ☑
          anterior horn M23.21- ☑
          posterior horn M23.22- ☑
          specified NEC M23.23- ☑
      retained — see Derangement, knee, meniscus, specified NEC
      specified NEC M23.30- ☑
        lateral M23.30- ☑
          anterior horn M23.34- ☑
          posterior horn M23.35- ☑
          specified NEC M23.36- ☑
        medial M23.30- ☑
          anterior horn M23.31- ☑
          posterior horn M23.32- ☑
          specified NEC M23.33- ☑
      old M23.8X- ☑
      specified NEC — see subcategory M23.8 ☑
    low back NEC — see Dorsopathy, specified NEC
    meniscus — see Derangement, knee, meniscus
    mental — see Psychosis
    patella, specified NEC — see Disorder, patella, derangement NEC
    semilunar cartilage (knee) — see Derangement, knee, meniscus, specified NEC
    shoulder (internal) — see Derangement, joint, shoulder
Dercum's disease E88.2
Derealization (neurotic) F48.1
Dermal — see condition
Dermaphytid — see Dermatophytosis
Dermatitis (eczematous) L30.9
  ab igne L59.0
  acarine B88.0
  actinic (due to sun) L57.8
    other than from sun L59.8
  allergic — see Dermatitis, contact, allergic
  ambustionis, due to burn or scald — see Burn
  amebic A06.7
  ammonia L22
  arsenical (ingested) L27.8
  artefacta L98.1
    psychogenic F54
  atopic L20.9
    psychogenic F54
    specified NEC L20.89
  autoimmune progesterone L30.8
  berlock, berloque L56.2
  blastomycotic B40.3
  blister beetle L24.89
  bullous, bullosa L13.9
    mucosynechial, atrophic L12.1
    seasonal L30.8
    specified NEC L13.8
  calorica L59.0
    due to burn or scald — see Burn
  caterpillar L24.89
  cercarial B65.3
  combustionis L59.0
    due to burn or scald — see Burn
  congelationis T69.1 ☑
  contact (occupational) L25.9
    allergic L23.9
      due to
        adhesives L23.1
        cement L23.5
        chemical products NEC L23.5
        chromium L23.0
        cosmetics L23.2
        dander (cat) (dog) L23.81
        drugs in contact with skin L23.3
        dyes L23.4
        food in contact with skin L23.6
        hair (cat) (dog) L23.81
        insecticide L23.5
        metals L23.0

Dermatitis — continued
  contact — continued
    allergic — continued
      due to — continued
        nickel L23.0
        plants, non-food L23.7
        plastic L23.5
        rubber L23.5
        specified agent NEC L23.89
    due to
      cement L25.3
      chemical products NEC L25.3
      cosmetics L25.0
      dander (cat) (dog) L23.81
      drugs in contact with skin L25.1
      dyes L25.2
      food in contact with skin L25.4
      hair (cat) (dog) L23.81
      plants, non-food L25.5
      specified agent NEC L25.8
    irritant L24.9
      due to
        cement L24.5
        chemical products NEC L24.5
        cosmetics L24.3
        detergents L24.0
        drugs in contact with skin L24.4
        food in contact with skin L24.6
        oils and greases L24.1
        plants, non-food L24.7
        solvents L24.2
        specified agent NEC L24.89
  contusiformis L52
  diabetic — see E08-E13 with .620
  diaper L22
  diphtheritica A36.3
  dry skin L85.3
  due to
    acetone (contact) (irritant) L24.2
    acids (contact) (irritant) L24.5
    adhesive(s) (allergic) (contact) (plaster) L23.1
      irritant L24.5
    alcohol (irritant) (skin contact) (substances in category T51) L24.2
      taken internally L27.8
    alkalis (contact) (irritant) L24.5
    arsenic (ingested) L27.8
    carbon disulfide (contact) (irritant) L24.2
    caustics (contact) (irritant) L24.5
    cement (contact) L25.3
    cereal (ingested) L27.2
    chemical(s) NEC L25.3
      taken internally L27.8
    chlorocompounds L24.2
    chromium (contact) (irritant) L24.81
    coffee (ingested) L27.2
    cold weather L30.8
    cosmetics (contact) L25.0
      allergic L23.2
      irritant L24.3
    cyclohexanes L24.2
    dander (cat) (dog) L23.81
    Demodex species B88.0
    Dermanyssus gallinae B88.0
    detergents (contact) (irritant) L24.0
    dichromate L24.81
    drugs and medicaments (generalized) (internal use) L27.0
      external — see Dermatitis, due to, drugs, in contact with skin
      in contact with skin L25.1
        allergic L23.3
        irritant L24.4
      localized skin eruption L27.1
      specified substance — see Table of Drugs and Chemicals
    dyes (contact) L25.2
      allergic L23.4
      irritant L24.89
    epidermophytosis — see Dermatophytosis
    esters L24.2
    external irritant NEC L24.9
    fish (ingested) L27.2
    flour (ingested) L27.2
    food (ingested) L27.2
      in contact with skin L25.4
    fruit (ingested) L27.2
    furs (allergic) (contact) L23.81
    glues — see Dermatitis, due to, adhesives

Dermatitis — continued
  due to — continued
    glycols L24.2
    greases NEC (contact) (irritant) L24.1
    hair (cat) (dog) L23.81
    hot
      objects and materials — see Burn
      weather or places L59.0
    hydrocarbons L24.2
    infrared rays L59.8
    ingestion, ingested substance L27.9
      chemical NEC L27.8
      drugs and medicaments — see Dermatitis, due to, drugs
      food L27.2
      specified NEC L27.8
    insecticide in contact with skin L24.5
    internal agent L27.9
      drugs and medicaments (generalized) — see Dermatitis, due to, drugs
      food L27.2
    irradiation — see Dermatitis, due to, radioactive substance
    ketones L24.2
    lacquer tree (allergic) (contact) L23.7
    light (sun) NEC L57.8
      acute L56.8
      other L59.8
    Liponyssoides sanguineus B88.0
    low temperature L30.8
    meat (ingested) L27.2
    metals, metal salts (contact) (irritant) L24.81
    milk (ingested) L27.2
    nickel (contact) (irritant) L24.81
    nylon (contact) (irritant) L24.5
    oils NEC (contact) (irritant) L24.1
    paint solvent (contact) (irritant) L24.2
    petroleum products (contact) (irritant) (substances in T52.0) L24.2
    plants NEC (contact) L25.5
      allergic L23.7
      irritant L24.7
    plasters (adhesive) (any) (allergic) (contact) L23.1
      irritant L24.5
    plastic (contact) L25.3
    preservatives (contact) — see Dermatitis, due to, chemical, in contact with skin
    primrose (allergic) (contact) L23.7
    primula (allergic) (contact) L23.7
    radiation L59.8
      nonionizing (chronic exposure) L57.8
      sun NEC L57.8
        acute L56.8
    radioactive substance L58.9
      acute L58.0
      chronic L58.1
    radium L58.9
      acute L58.0
      chronic L58.1
    ragweed (allergic) (contact) L23.7
    Rhus (allergic) (contact) (diversiloba) (radicans) (toxicodendron) (venenata) (verniciflua) L23.7
    rubber (contact) L24.5
    Senecio jacobaea (allergic) (contact) L23.7
    solvents (contact) (irritant) (substances in category T52) L24.2
    specified agent NEC (contact) L25.8
      allergic L23.89
      irritant L24.89
    sunshine NEC L57.8
      acute L56.8
    tetrachlorethylene (contact) (irritant) L24.2
    toluene (contact) (irritant) L24.2
    turpentine (contact) L24.2
    ultraviolet rays (sun NEC) (chronic exposure) L57.8
      acute L56.8
    vaccine or vaccination L27.0
      specified substance — see Table of Drugs and Chemicals
    varicose veins — see Varix, leg, with, inflammation
    X-rays L58.9
      acute L58.0
      chronic L58.1
  dyshydrotic L30.1
  dysmenorrheica N94.6
  escharotica — see Burn
  exfoliative, exfoliativa (generalized) L26

Dermatitis — continued
exfoliative, exfoliativa — continued
  neonatorum L00
eyelid (see also Dermatosis, eyelid)
  allergic H01.119
    left H01.116
      lower H01.115
      upper H01.114
    right H01.113
      lower H01.112
      upper H01.111
  contact — see Dermatitis, eyelid, allergic
  due to
    Demodex species B88.0
    herpes (zoster) B02.39
      simplex B00.59
  eczematous H01.139
    left H01.136
      lower H01.135
      upper H01.134
    right H01.133
      lower H01.132
      upper H01.131
facta, factitia, factitial L98.1
  psychogenic F54
flexural NEC L20.82
friction L30.4
fungus B36.9
  specified type NEC B36.8
gangrenosa, gangrenous infantum L08.0
harvest mite B88.0
heat L59.0
herpesviral, vesicular (ear) (lip) B00.1
herpetiformis (bullous) (erythematous) (pustular)
  (vesicular) L13.0
  juvenile L12.2
  senile L12.0
hiemalis L30.8
hypostatic, hypostatica — see Varix, leg, with, inflammation
infectious eczematoid L30.3
infective L30.3
irritant — see Dermatitis, contact, irritant
Jacquet's (diaper dermatitis) L22
Leptus B88.0
lichenified NEC L28.0
medicamentosa (generalized) (internal use) — see
  Dermatitis, due to drugs
mite B88.0
multiformis L13.0
  juvenile L12.2
napkin L22
neurotica L13.0
nummular L30.0
papillaris capillitii L73.0
pellagrous E52
perioral L71.0
photocontact L56.2
polymorpha dolorosa L13.0
pruriginosa L13.0
pruritic NEC L30.8
psychogenic F54
purulent L08.0
pustular
  contagious B08.02
  subcorneal L13.1
pyococcal L08.0
pyogenica L08.0
repens L40.2
Ritter's (exfoliativa) L00
Schamberg's L81.7
schistosome B65.3
seasonal bullous L30.8
seborrheic L21.9
  infantile L21.1
  specified NEC L21.8
sensitization NOS L23.9
septic L08.0
solare L57.8
specified NEC L30.8
stasis I87.2
  with
    varicose ulcer — see Varix, leg, with ulcer, with
      inflammation
    varicose veins — see Varix, leg, with, inflamma-
      tion
  due to postthrombotic syndrome — see Syndrome,
    postthrombotic

Dermatitis — continued
suppurative L08.0
traumatic NEC L30.4
trophoneurotica L13.0
ultraviolet (sun) (chronic exposure) L57.8
  acute L56.8
varicose — see Varix, leg, with, inflammation
vegetans L10.1
verrucosa B43.0
vesicular, herpesviral B00.1
Dermatoarthritis, lipoid E78.81
Dermatochalasis, eyelid H02.839
  left H02.836
    lower H02.835
    upper H02.834
  right H02.833
    lower H02.832
    upper H02.831
Dermatofibroma (lenticulare) — see Neoplasm, skin,
  benign
  protuberans — see Neoplasm, skin, uncertain behavior
Dermatofibrosarcoma (pigmented) (protuberans) —
  see Neoplasm, skin, malignant
Dermatographia L50.3
Dermatolysis (exfoliativa) (congenital) Q82.8
  acquired L57.4
  eyelids — see Blepharochalasis
  palpebrarum — see Blepharochalasis
  senile L57.4
Dermatomegaly NEC Q82.8
Dermatomucosomyositis M33.10
  with
    myopathy M33.12
    respiratory involvement M33.11
    specified organ involvement NEC M33.19
Dermatomycosis B36.9
  furfuracea B36.0
  specified type NEC B36.8
Dermatomyositis (acute) (chronic) (see also Dermatopolymyositis)
  adult (see also Dermatomyositis, specified NEC) M33.10
  in (due to) neoplastic disease (see also Neoplasm)
    D49.9 [M36.0]
  juvenile M33.00
    with
      myopathy M33.02
      respiratory involvement M33.01
      specified organ involvement NEC M33.09
    without myopathy M33.03
  specified NEC M33.10
    with
      myopathy M33.12
      respiratory involvement M33.11
      specified organ involvement NEC M33.19
    without myopathy M33.13
Dermatoneuritis of children — see Poisoning, mercury
Dermatophilosis A48.8
Dermatophytid L30.2
Dermatophytide — see Dermatophytosis
Dermatophytosis (epidermophyton) (infection) (Microsporum) (tinea) (Trichophyton) B35.9
  beard B35.0
  body B35.4
  capitis B35.0
  corporis B35.4
  deep-seated B35.8
  disseminated B35.8
  foot B35.3
  granulomatous B35.8
  groin B35.6
  hand B35.2
  nail B35.1
  perianal (area) B35.6
  scalp B35.0
  specified NEC B35.8
Dermatopolymyositis M33.90
  with
    myopathy M33.92
    respiratory involvement M33.91
    specified organ involvement NEC M33.99
  without myopathy M33.93
  in neoplastic disease (see also Neoplasm)
    D49.9 [M36.0]
  juvenile M33.00
    with
      myopathy M33.02
      respiratory involvement M33.01
      specified organ involvement NEC M33.09

Dermatopolymyositis — continued
  specified NEC M33.10
    myopathy M33.12
    respiratory involvement M33.11
    specified organ involvement NEC M33.19
Dermatopolyneuritis — see Poisoning, mercury
Dermatorrhexis Q79.6
  acquired L57.4
Dermatosclerosis (see also Scleroderma)
  localized L94.0
Dermatosis L98.9
  Andrews' L98.89
  Bowen's — see Neoplasm, skin, in situ
  bullous L13.9
    specified NEC L13.8
  exfoliativa L26
  eyelid (noninfectious)
    dermatitis — see Dermatitis, eyelid
    discoid lupus erythematosus — see Lupus, erythe-
      matosus, eyelid
    xeroderma — see Xeroderma, acquired, eyelid
  factitial L98.1
  febrile neutrophilic L98.2
  gonococcal A54.89
  herpetiformis L13.0
    juvenile L12.2
  linear IgA L13.8
  menstrual NEC L98.8
  neutrophilic, febrile L98.2
  occupational — see Dermatitis, contact
  papulosa nigra L82.1
  pigmentary L81.9
    progressive L81.7
    Schamberg's L81.7
  psychogenic F54
  purpuric, pigmented L81.7
  pustular, subcorneal L13.1
  transient acantholytic L11.1
Dermographia, dermographism L50.3
Dermoid (cyst) (see also Neoplasm, benign, by site)
  with malignant transformation C56- ☑
  due to radiation (nonionizing) L57.8
Dermopathy
  infiltrative with thyrotoxicosis — see Thyrotoxicosis
  nephrogenic fibrosing L90.8
Dermophytosis — see Dermatophytosis
Descemetocele H18.73- ☑
Descemet's membrane — see condition
Descending — see condition
Descensus uteri — see Prolapse, uterus
Desert
  rheumatism B38.0
  sore — see Ulcer, skin
Desertion (newborn) — see Maltreatment
Desmoid (extra-abdominal) (tumor) — see Neoplasm,
  connective tissue, uncertain behavior
  abdominal D48.1
Despondency F32.9
Desquamation, skin R23.4
Destruction, destructive (see also Damage)
  articular facet (see also Derangement, joint, specified
    type NEC)
    knee M23.8X- ☑
    vertebra — see Spondylosis
  bone (see also Disorder, bone, specified type NEC)
    syphilitic A52.77
  joint (see also Derangement, joint, specified type NEC)
    sacroiliac M53.3
  rectal sphincter K62.89
  septum (nasal) J34.89
  tuberculous NEC — see Tuberculosis
  tympanum, tympanic membrane (nontraumatic) —
    see Disorder, tympanic membrane, specified
    NEC
  vertebral disc — see Degeneration, intervertebral disc
Destructiveness (see also Disorder, conduct)
  adjustment reaction — see Disorder, adjustment
Desultory labor O62.2
Detachment
  cartilage — see Sprain
  cervix, annular N88.8
    complicating delivery O71.3
  choroid (old) (postinfectional) (simple) (spontaneous)
    H31.40- ☑
    hemorrhagic H31.41- ☑
    serous H31.42- ☑
  ligament — see Sprain

Detachment — *continued*
  meniscus (knee) (*see also* Derangement, knee, menis-
    cus, specified NEC)
    current injury — *see* Tear, meniscus
    due to old tear or injury — *see* Derangement, knee,
      meniscus, due to old tear
  retina (without retinal break) (serous) H33.2- ☑
    with retinal:
      break H33.00- ☑
        giant H33.03- ☑
        multiple H33.02- ☑
        single H33.01- ☑
      dialysis H33.04- ☑
    pigment epithelium — *see* Degeneration, retina,
      separation of layers, pigment epithelium
      detachment
    rhegmatogenous — *see* Detachment, retina, with
      retinal, break
    specified NEC H33.8
    total H33.05- ☑
    traction H33.4- ☑
  vitreous (body) H43.81 ☑
Detergent asthma J69.8
Deterioration
  epileptic F06.8
  general physical R53.81
  heart, cardiac — *see* Degeneration, myocardial
  mental — *see* Psychosis
  myocardial, myocardium — *see* Degeneration, myocar-
    dial
  senile (simple) R54
Deuteranomaly (anomalous trichromat) H53.53
Deuteranopia (complete) (incomplete) H53.53
Development
  abnormal, bone Q79.9
  arrested R62.50
    bone — *see* Arrest, development or growth, bone
    child R62.50
    due to malnutrition E45
  defective, congenital (*see also* Anomaly, by site)
    cauda equina Q06.3
    left ventricle Q24.8
      in hypoplastic left heart syndrome Q23.4
    valve Q24.8
      pulmonary Q22.3
  delayed (*see also* Delay, development) R62.50
    arithmetical skills F81.2
    language (skills) (expressive) F80.1
    learning skill F81.9
    mixed skills F88
    motor coordination F82
    reading F81.0
    specified learning skill NEC F81.89
    speech F80.9
    spelling F81.81
    written expression F81.81
  imperfect, congenital (*see also* Anomaly, by site)
    heart Q24.9
    lungs Q33.6
  incomplete
    bronchial tree Q32.4
    organ or site not listed — *see* Hypoplasia, by site
    respiratory system Q34.9
  sexual, precocious NEC E30.1
  tardy, mental (*see also* Disability, intellectual) F79
Developmental — *see* condition
  testing, infant or child — *see* Examination, child
Devergie's disease (pityriasis rubra pilaris) L44.0
Deviation (in)
  conjugate palsy (eye) (spastic) H51.0
  esophagus (acquired) K22.8
  eye, skew H51.8
  midline (jaw) (teeth) (dental arch) M26.29
    specified site NEC — *see* Malposition
  nasal septum J34.2
    congenital Q67.4
  opening and closing of the mandible M26.53
  organ or site, congenital NEC — *see* Malposition,
    congenital
  septum (nasal) (acquired) J34.2
    congenital Q67.4
  sexual F65.9
    bestiality F65.89
    erotomania F52.8
    exhibitionism F65.2
    fetishism, fetishistic F65.0
      transvestism F65.1
    frotteurism F65.81

Deviation — *continued*
  sexual — *continued*
    masochism F65.51
    multiple F65.89
    necrophilia F65.89
    nymphomania F52.8
    pederosis F65.4
    pedophilia F65.4
    sadism, sadomasochism F65.52
    satyriasis F52.8
    specified type NEC F65.89
    transvestism F64.1
    voyeurism F65.3
  teeth, midline M26.29
  trachea J39.8
  ureter, congenital Q62.61
Device
  cerebral ventricle (communicating) in situ Z98.2
  contraceptive — *see* Contraceptive, device
  drainage, cerebrospinal fluid, in situ Z98.2
Devic's disease G36.0
Devil's
  grip B33.0
  pinches (purpura simplex) D69.2
Devitalized tooth K04.99
Devonshire colic — *see* Poisoning, lead
Dextraposition, aorta Q20.3
  in tetralogy of Fallot Q21.3
Dextrinosis, limit (debrancher enzyme deficiency)
  E74.03
Dextrocardia (true) Q24.0
  with
    complete transposition of viscera Q89.3
    situs inversus Q89.3
Dextrotransposition, aorta Q20.3
d-glycericacidemia E72.59
Dhat syndrome F48.8
Dhobi itch B35.6
Di George's syndrome D82.1
Di Guglielmo's disease C94.0- ☑
Diabetes, diabetic (mellitus) (sugar) E11.9
  with
    amyotrophy E11.44
    arthropathy NEC E11.618
    autonomic (poly)neuropathy E11.43
    cataract E11.36
    Charcot's joints E11.610
    chronic kidney disease E11.22
    circulatory complication NEC E11.59
    complication E11.8
      specified NEC E11.69
    dermatitis E11.620
    foot ulcer E11.621
    gangrene E11.52
    gastroparalysis E11.43
    gastroparesis E11.43
    glomerulonephrosis, intracapillary E11.21
    glomerulosclerosis, intercapillary E11.21
    hyperglycemia E11.65
    hyperosmolarity E11.00
      with coma E11.01
    hypoglycemia E11.649
      with coma E11.641
    ketoacidosis E11.10
      with coma E11.11
    kidney complications NEC E11.29
    Kimmelstiel-Wilson disease E11.21
    loss of protective sensation (LOPS) — *see* Diabetes,
      by type, with neuropathy
    mononeuropathy E11.41
    myasthenia E11.44
    necrobiosis lipoidica E11.620
    nephropathy E11.21
    neuralgia E11.42
    neurologic complication NEC E11.49
    neuropathic arthropathy E11.610
    neuropathy E11.40
    ophthalmic complication NEC E11.39
    oral complication NEC E11.638
    osteomyelitis E11.69
    periodontal disease E11.630
    peripheral angiopathy E11.51
      with gangrene E11.52
    polyneuropathy E11.42
    renal complication NEC E11.29
    renal tubular degeneration E11.29
    retinopathy E11.319
      with macular edema E11.311

Diabetes, diabetic — *continued*
  with — *continued*
    retinopathy — *continued*
      with macular edema — *continued*
        resolved following treatment E11.37 ☑
      nonproliferative E11.329 ☑
        with macular edema E11.321 ☑
        mild E11.329 ☑
          with macular edema E11.321 ☑
        moderate E11.339 ☑
          with macular edema E11.331 ☑
        severe E11.349 ☑
          with macular edema E11.341 ☑
      proliferative E11.359 ☑
        with
          combined traction retinal detachment
            and rhegmatogenous retinal de-
            tachment E11.354 ☑
          macular edema E11.351 ☑
          stable proliferative diabetic retinopathy
            E11.355 ☑
          traction retinal detachment involving
            the macula E11.352 ☑
          traction retinal detachment not involv-
            ing the macula E11.353 ☑
  skin complication NEC E11.628
  skin ulcer NEC E11.622
  brittle — *see* Diabetes, type 1
  bronzed E83.110
  complicating pregnancy — *see* Pregnancy, complicat-
    ed by, diabetes
  dietary counseling and surveillance Z71.3
  due to
    autoimmune process — *see* Diabetes, type 1
    immune mediated pancreatic islet beta-cell destruc-
      tion — *see* Diabetes, type 1
  due to drug or chemical E09.9
    with
      amyotrophy E09.44
      arthropathy NEC E09.618
      autonomic (poly)neuropathy E09.43
      cataract E09.36
      Charcot's joints E09.610
      chronic kidney disease E09.22
      circulatory complication NEC E09.59
      complication E09.8
        specified NEC E09.69
      dermatitis E09.620
      foot ulcer E09.621
      gangrene E09.52
      gastroparalysis E09.43
      gastroparesis E09.43
      glomerulonephrosis, intracapillary E09.21
      glomerulosclerosis, intercapillary E09.21
      hyperglycemia E09.65
      hyperosmolarity E09.00
        with coma E09.01
      hypoglycemia E09.649
        with coma E09.641
      ketoacidosis E09.10
        with coma E09.11
      kidney complications NEC E09.29
      Kimmelstiel-Wilson disease E09.21
      mononeuropathy E09.41
      myasthenia E09.44
      necrobiosis lipoidica E09.620
      nephropathy E09.21
      neuralgia E09.42
      neurologic complication NEC E09.49
      neuropathic arthropathy E09.610
      neuropathy E09.40
      ophthalmic complication NEC E09.39
      oral complication NEC E09.638
      periodontal disease E09.630
      peripheral angiopathy E09.51
        with gangrene E09.52
      polyneuropathy E09.42
      renal complication NEC E09.29
      renal tubular degeneration E09.29
      retinopathy E09.319
        with macular edema E09.311
        nonproliferative E09.329 ☑
          with macular edema E09.321 ☑
          mild E09.329 ☑
            with macular edema E09.321 ☑
          moderate E09.339 ☑
            with macular edema E09.331 ☑
          severe E09.349 ☑

Diabetes, diabetic — *continued*
  due to drug or chemical — *continued*
    with — *continued*
      retinopathy — *continued*
        nonproliferative — *continued*
          severe — *continued*
            with macular edema E09.341 ☑
        proliferative E09.359 ☑
          with
            combined traction retinal detachment and rhegmatogenous retinal detachment E09.354 ☑
            macular edema E09.351 ☑
            stable proliferative diabetic retinopathy E09.355 ☑
            traction retinal detachment involving the macula E09.352 ☑
            traction retinal detachment not involving the macula E09.353 ☑
        resolved following treatment E09.37 ☑
      skin complication NEC E09.628
      skin ulcer NEC E09.622
  due to underlying condition E08.9
    with
      amyotrophy E08.44
      arthropathy NEC E08.618
      autonomic (poly)neuropathy E08.43
      cataract E08.36
      Charcot's joints E08.610
      chronic kidney disease E08.22
      circulatory complication NEC E08.59
      complication E08.8
        specified NEC E08.69
      dermatitis E08.620
      foot ulcer E08.621
      gangrene E08.52
      gastroparalysis E08.43
      gastroparesis E08.43
      glomerulonephrosis, intracapillary E08.21
      glomerulosclerosis, intercapillary E08.21
      hyperglycemia E08.65
      hyperosmolarity E08.00
        with coma E08.01
      hypoglycemia E08.649
        with coma E08.641
      ketoacidosis E08.10
        with coma E08.11
      kidney complications NEC E08.29
      Kimmelstein-WIlson disease E08.21
      mononeuropathy E08.41
      myasthenia E08.44
      necrobiosis lipoidica E08.620
      nephropathy E08.21
      neuralgia E08.42
      neurologic complication NEC E08.49
      neuropathic arthropathy E08.610
      neuropathy E08.40
      ophthalmic complication NEC E08.39
      oral complication NEC E08.638
      periodontal disease E08.630
      peripheral angiopathy E08.51
        with gangrene E08.52
      polyneuropathy E08.42
      renal complication NEC E08.29
      renal tubular degeneration E08.29
      retinopathy E08.319
        with macular edema E08.311
        nonproliferative E08.329 ☑
          with macular edema E08.321 ☑
          mild E08.329 ☑
            with macular edema E08.321 ☑
          moderate E08.339 ☑
            with macular edema E08.331 ☑
          severe E08.349 ☑
            with macular edema E08.341 ☑
        proliferative E08.359 ☑
          with
            combined traction retinal detachment and rhegmatogenous retinal detachment E08.354 ☑
            macular edema E08.351 ☑
            stable proliferative diabetic retinopathy E08.355 ☑
            traction retinal detachment involving the macula E08.352 ☑
            traction retinal detachment not involving the macula E08.353 ☑
        resolved following treatment E08.37 ☑

Diabetes, diabetic — *continued*
  due to underlying condition — *continued*
    with — *continued*
      skin complication NEC E08.628
      skin ulcer NEC E08.622
  gestational (in pregnancy) O24.419
    affecting newborn P70.0
    diet controlled O24.410
    in childbirth O24.429
      diet controlled O24.420
      insulin (and diet) controlled O24.424
      oral drug controlled (antidiabetic) (hypoglycemic) O24.425
    insulin (and diet) controlled O24.414
    oral drug controlled (antidiabetic) (hypoglycemic) O24.415
    puerperal O24.439
      diet controlled O24.430
      insulin (and diet) controlled O24.434
      oral drug controlled (antidiabetic) (hypoglycemic) O24.435
  hepatogenous E13.9
  idiopathic — *see* Diabetes, type 1
  inadequately controlled — *code to* Diabetes, by type, with hyperglycemia
  insipidus E23.2
    nephrogenic N25.1
    pituitary E23.2
    vasopressin resistant N25.1
  insulin dependent — *code to* type of diabetes
  juvenile-onset — *see* Diabetes, type 1
  ketosis-prone — *see* Diabetes, type 1
  latent R73.03
  neonatal (transient) P70.2
  non-insulin dependent — *code to* type of diabetes
  out of control — *code to* Diabetes, by type, with hyperglycemia
  phosphate E83.39
  poorly controlled — *code to* Diabetes, by type, with hyperglycemia
  postpancreatectomy — *see* Diabetes, specified type NEC
  postprocedural — *see* Diabetes, specified type NEC
  secondary diabetes mellitus NEC — *see* Diabetes, specified type NEC
  specified type NEC E13.9
    with
      amyotrophy E13.44
      arthropathy NEC E13.618
      autonomic (poly)neuropathy E13.43
      cataract E13.36
      Charcot's joints E13.610
      chronic kidney disease E13.22
      circulatory complication NEC E13.59
      complication E13.8
        specified NEC E13.69
      dermatitis E13.620
      foot ulcer E13.621
      gangrene E13.52
      gastroparalysis E13.43
      gastroparesis E13.43
      glomerulonephrosis, intracapillary E13.21
      glomerulosclerosis, intercapillary E13.21
      hyperglycemia E13.65
      hyperosmolarity E13.00
        with coma E13.01
      hypoglycemia E13.649
        with coma E13.641
      ketoacidosis E13.10
        with coma E13.11
      kidney complications NEC E13.29
      Kimmelsteil-Wilson disease E13.21
      mononeuropathy E13.41
      myasthenia E13.44
      necrobiosis lipoidica E13.620
      nephropathy E13.21
      neuralgia E13.42
      neurologic complication NEC E13.49
      neuropathic arthropathy E13.610
      neuropathy E13.40
      ophthalmic complication NEC E13.39
      oral complication NEC E13.638
      periodontal disease E13.630
      peripheral angiopathy E13.51
        with gangrene E13.52
      polyneuropathy E13.42
      renal complication NEC E13.29
      renal tubular degeneration E13.29

Diabetes, diabetic — *continued*
  specified type — *continued*
    with — *continued*
      retinopathy E13.319
        with macular edema E13.311
        nonproliferative E13.329 ☑
          with macular edema E13.321 ☑
          mild E13.329 ☑
            with macular edema E13.321 ☑
          moderate E13.339 ☑
            with macular edema E13.331 ☑
          severe E13.349 ☑
            with macular edema E13.341 ☑
        proliferative E13.359 ☑
          with
            combined traction retinal detachment and rhegmatogenous retinal detachment E13.354 ☑
            macular edema E13.351 ☑
            stable proliferative diabetic retinopathy E13.355 ☑
            traction retinal detachment involving the macula E13.352 ☑
            traction retinal detachment not involving the macula E13.353 ☑
        resolved following treatment E13.37 ☑
      skin complication NEC E13.628
      skin ulcer NEC E13.622
  steroid-induced — *see* Diabetes, due to, drug or chemical
  type 1 E10.9
    with
      amyotrophy E10.44
      arthropathy NEC E10.618
      autonomic (poly)neuropathy E10.43
      cataract E10.36
      Charcot's joints E10.610
      chronic kidney disease E10.22
      circulatory complication NEC E10.59
      complication E10.8
        specified NEC E10.69
      dermatitis E10.620
      foot ulcer E10.621
      gangrene E10.52
      gastroparalysis E10.43
      gastroparesis E10.43
      glomerulonephrosis, intracapillary E10.21
      glomerulosclerosis, intercapillary E10.21
      hyperglycemia E10.65
      hypoglycemia E10.649
        with coma E10.641
      ketoacidosis E10.10
        with coma E10.11
      kidney complications NEC E10.29
      Kimmelsteil-Wilson disease E10.21
      mononeuropathy E10.41
      myasthenia E10.44
      necrobiosis lipoidica E10.620
      nephropathy E10.21
      neuralgia E10.42
      neurologic complication NEC E10.49
      neuropathic arthropathy E10.610
      neuropathy E10.40
      ophthalmic complication NEC E10.39
      oral complication NEC E10.638
      osteomyelitis E10.69
      periodontal disease E10.630
      peripheral angiopathy E10.51
        with gangrene E10.52
      polyneuropathy E10.42
      renal complication NEC E10.29
      renal tubular degeneration E10.29
      retinopathy E10.319
        with macular edema E10.311
        nonproliferative E10.329 ☑
          with macular edema E10.321 ☑
          mild E10.329 ☑
            with macular edema E10.321 ☑
          moderate E10.339 ☑
            with macular edema E10.331 ☑
          severe E10.349 ☑
            with macular edema E10.341 ☑
        proliferative E10.359 ☑
          with
            combined traction retinal detachment and rhegmatogenous retinal detachment E10.354 ☑
            macular edema E10.351 ☑

☑ **Additional Character Required — Refer to the Tabular List for Character Selection**   ▽ **Subterms under main terms may continue to next column or page**

Diabetes, diabetic — *continued*
  type 1 — *continued*
    with — *continued*
      retinopathy — *continued*
        proliferative — *continued*
          with — *continued*
            stable proliferative diabetic
              retinopathy E10.355 ☑
            traction retinal detachment involving
              the macula E10.352 ☑
            traction retinal detachment not in-
              volving the macula E10.353 ☑
          resolved following treatment E10.37 ☑
        skin complication NEC E10.628
        skin ulcer NEC E10.622
  type 2 E11.9
    with
      amyotrophy E11.44
      arthropathy NEC E11.618
      autonomic (poly)neuropathy E11.43
      cataract E11.36
      Charcot's joints E11.610
      chronic kidney disease E11.22
      circulatory complication NEC E11.59
      complication E11.8
        specified NEC E11.69
      dermatitis E11.620
      foot ulcer E11.621
      gangrene E11.52
      gastroparalysis E11.43
      gastroparesis E11.43
      glomerulonephrosis, intracapillary E11.21
      glomerulosclerosis, intercapillary E11.21
      hyperglycemia E11.65
      hyperosmolarity E11.00
        with coma E11.01
      hypoglycemia E11.649
        with coma E11.641
      ketoacidosis E11.10
        with coma E11.11
      kidney complications NEC E11.29
      Kimmelstiel-Wilson disease E11.21
      mononeuropathy E11.41
      myasthenia E11.44
      necrobiosis lipoidica E11.620
      nephropathy E11.21
      neuralgia E11.42
      neurologic complication NEC E11.49
      neuropathic arthropathy E11.610
      neuropathy E11.40
      ophthalmic complication NEC E11.39
      oral complication NEC E11.638
      osteomyelitis E11.69
      periodontal disease E11.630
      peripheral angiopathy E11.51
        with gangrene E11.52
      polyneuropathy E11.42
      renal complication NEC E11.29
      renal tubular degeneration E11.29
      retinopathy E11.319
        with macular edema E11.311
        nonproliferative E11.329 ☑
          with macular edema E11.321 ☑
          mild E11.329 ☑
            with macular edema E11.321 ☑
          moderate E11.339 ☑
            with macular edema E11.331 ☑
          severe E11.349 ☑
            with macular edema E11.341 ☑
        proliferative E11.359 ☑
          with
            combined traction retinal detach-
              ment and rhegmatogenous
              retinal detachment E11.354 ☑
            macular edema E11.351 ☑
            stable proliferative diabetic
              retinopathy E11.355 ☑
            traction retinal detachment involving
              the macula E11.352 ☑
            traction retinal detachment not in-
              volving the macula E11.353 ☑
          resolved following treatment E11.37 ☑
        skin complication NEC E11.628
        skin ulcer NEC E11.622
  uncontrolled
    meaning
      hyperglycemia — *see* Diabetes, by type, with,
        hyperglycemia

Diabetes, diabetic — *continued*
  uncontrolled — *continued*
    meaning — *continued*
      hypoglycemia — *see* Diabetes, by type, with,
        hypoglycemia
Diacyclothrombopathia D69.1
Diagnosis deferred R69
Dialysis (intermittent) (treatment)
  noncompliance (with) Z91.15
  renal (hemodialysis) (peritoneal), status Z99.2
  retina, retinal — *see* Detachment, retina, with retinal,
    dialysis
Diamond-Blackfan anemia (congenital hypoplastic)
    D61.01
Diamond-Gardener syndrome (autoerythrocyte sensi-
    tization) D69.2
Diaper rash L22
Diaphoresis (excessive) R61
Diaphragm — *see* condition
Diaphragmalgia R07.1
Diaphragmatitis, diaphragmitis J98.6
Diaphysial aclasis Q78.6
Diaphysitis — *see* Osteomyelitis, specified type NEC
Diarrhea, diarrheal (disease) (infantile) (inflammatory)
    R19.7
  achlorhydric K31.83
  allergic K52.29
    due to
      colitis — *see* Colitis, allergic
      enteritis — *see* Enteritis, allergic
  amebic (*see also* Amebiasis) A06.0
    with abscess — *see* Abscess, amebic
    acute A06.0
    chronic A06.1
    nondysenteric A06.2
  bacillary — *see* Dysentery, bacillary
  balantidial A07.0
  cachectic NEC K52.89
  Chilomastix A07.8
  choleriformis A00.1
  chronic (noninfectious) K52.9
  coccidial A07.3
  Cochin-China K90.1
    strongyloidiasis B78.0
  Dientamoeba A07.8
  dietetic (*see also* Diarrhea, allergic) K52.29
  drug-induced K52.1
  due to
    bacteria A04.9
      specified NEC A04.8
    Campylobacter A04.5
    Capillaria philippinensis B81.1
    Clostridium difficile
      not specified as recurrent A04.72
      recurrent A04.71
    Clostridium perfringens (C) (F) A04.8
    Cryptosporidium A07.2
    drugs K52.1
    Escherichia coli A04.4
      enteroaggregative A04.4
      enterohemorrhagic A04.3
      enteroinvasive A04.2
      enteropathogenic A04.0
      enterotoxigenic A04.1
      specified NEC A04.4
    food hypersensitivity (*see also* Diarrhea, allergic)
      K52.29
    Necator americanus B76.1
    S. japonicum B65.2
    specified organism NEC A08.8
      bacterial A04.8
      viral A08.39
    Staphylococcus A04.8
    Trichuris trichiuria B79
    virus — *see* Enteritis, viral
    Yersinia enterocolitica A04.6
  dysenteric A09
  endemic A09
  epidemic A09
  flagellate A07.9
  Flexner's (ulcerative) A03.1
  functional K59.1
    following gastrointestinal surgery K91.89
    psychogenic F45.8
  Giardia lamblia A07.1
  giardial A07.1
  hill K90.1
  infectious A09

Diarrhea, diarrheal — *continued*
  malarial — *see* Malaria
  mite B88.0
  mycotic NEC B49
  neonatal (noninfectious) P78.3
  nervous F45.8
  neurogenic K59.1
  noninfectious K52.9
  postgastrectomy K91.1
  postvagotomy K91.1
  protozoal A07.9
    specified NEC A07.8
  psychogenic F45.8
  specified
    bacterium NEC A04.8
    virus NEC A08.39
  strongyloidiasis B78.0
  toxic K52.1
  trichomonal A07.8
  tropical K90.1
  tuberculous A18.32
  viral — *see* Enteritis, viral
Diastasis
  cranial bones M84.88
    congenital NEC Q75.8
  joint (traumatic) — *see* Dislocation
  muscle M62.00
    ankle M62.07- ☑
    congenital Q79.8
    foot M62.07- ☑
    forearm M62.03- ☑
    hand M62.04- ☑
    lower leg M62.06- ☑
    pelvic region M62.05- ☑
    shoulder region M62.01- ☑
    specified site NEC M62.08
    thigh M62.05- ☑
    upper arm M62.02- ☑
  recti (abdomen)
    complicating delivery O71.89
    congenital Q79.59
Diastema, tooth, teeth, fully erupted M26.32
Diastematomyelia Q06.2
Diataxia, cerebral G80.4
Diathesis
  allergic — *see* History, allergy
  bleeding (familial) D69.9
  cystine (familial) E72.00
  gouty — *see* Gout
  hemorrhagic (familial) D69.9
    newborn NEC P53
  spasmophilic R29.0
Diaz's disease or osteochondrosis (juvenile) (talus) —
    see Osteochondrosis, juvenile, tarsus
Dibothriocephalus, dibothriocephaliasis (latus) (in-
    fection) (infestation) B70.0
  larval B70.1
Dicephalus, dicephaly Q89.4
Dichotomy, teeth K00.2
Dichromat, dichromatopsia (congenital) — *see* Defi-
    ciency, color vision
Dichuchwa A65
Dicroceliasis B66.2
Didelphia, didelphys — *see* Double uterus
Didymytis N45.1
  with orchitis N45.3
Dietary
  inadequacy or deficiency E63.9
  surveillance and counseling Z71.3
Dietl's crisis N13.8
Dieulafoy lesion (hemorrhagic)
  duodenum K31.82
  esophagus K22.8
  intestine (colon) K63.81
  stomach K31.82
Difficult, difficulty (in)
  acculturation Z60.3
  feeding R63.3
    newborn P92.9
      breast P92.5
      specified NEC P92.8
    nonorganic (infant or child) F98.29
  intubation, in anesthesia T88.4 ☑
  mechanical, gastroduodenal stoma K91.89
    causing obstruction (*see also* Obstruction, intestine,
      postoperative) K91.30
  micturition
    need to immediately re-void R39.191

Difficult, difficulty — *continued*
  micturition — *continued*
    position dependent R39.192
    specified NEC R39.198
  reading (developmental) F81.0
    secondary to emotional disorders F93.9
  spelling (specific) F81.81
    with reading disorder F81.89
    due to inadequate teaching Z55.8
  swallowing — *see* Dysphagia
  walking R26.2
  work
    conditions NEC Z56.5
    schedule Z56.3
Diffuse — *see* condition
Digestive — *see* condition
Dihydropyrimidine dehydrogenase disease (DPD) E88.89
Diktyoma — *see* Neoplasm, malignant, by site
Dilaceration, tooth K00.4
Dilatation
  anus K59.8
    venule — *see* Hemorrhoids
  aorta (focal) (general) — *see* Ectasia, aorta
    with aneuysm — *see* Aneurysm, aorta
    congenital Q25.44
  artery — *see* Aneurysm
  bladder (sphincter) N32.89
    congenital Q64.79
  blood vessel I99.8
  bronchial J47.9
    with
      exacerbation (acute) J47.1
      lower respiratory infection J47.0
  calyx (due to obstruction) — *see* Hydronephrosis
  capillaries I78.8
  cardiac (acute) (chronic) (*see also* Hypertrophy, cardiac)
    congenital Q24.8
      valve NEC Q24.8
        pulmonary Q22.3
    valve — *see* Endocarditis
  cavum septi pellucidi Q06.8
  cervix (uteri) (*see also* Incompetency, cervix)
    incomplete, poor, slow complicating delivery O62.0
  colon K59.39
    congenital Q43.1
    psychogenic F45.8
    toxic K59.31
  common duct (acquired) K83.8
    congenital Q44.5
  cystic duct (acquired) K82.8
    congenital Q44.5
  duct, mammary — *see* Ectasia, mammary duct
  duodenum K59.8
  esophagus K22.8
    congenital Q39.5
    due to achalasia K22.0
  eustachian tube, congenital Q17.8
  gallbladder K82.8
  gastric — *see* Dilatation, stomach
  heart (acute) (chronic) (*see also* Hypertrophy, cardiac)
    congenital Q24.8
    valve — *see* Endocarditis
  ileum K59.8
    psychogenic F45.8
  jejunum K59.8
    psychogenic F45.8
  kidney (calyx) (collecting structures) (cystic) (parenchyma) (pelvis) (idiopathic) N28.89
  lacrimal passages or duct — *see* Disorder, lacrimal system, changes
  lymphatic vessel I89.0
  mammary duct — *see* Ectasia, mammary duct
  Meckel's diverticulum (congenital) Q43.0
    malignant — *see* Table of Neoplasms, small intestine, malignant
  myocardium (acute) (chronic) — *see* Hypertrophy, cardiac
  organ or site, congenital NEC — *see* Distortion
  pancreatic duct K86.89
  pericardium — *see* Pericarditis
  pharynx J39.2
  prostate N42.89
  pulmonary
    artery (idiopathic) I28.8
    valve, congenital Q22.3
  pupil H57.04
  rectum K59.39

Dilatation — *continued*
  saccule, congenital Q16.5
  salivary gland (duct) K11.8
  sphincter ani K62.89
  stomach K31.89
    acute K31.0
    psychogenic F45.8
  submaxillary duct K11.8
  trachea, congenital Q32.1
  ureter (idiopathic) N28.82
    congenital Q62.2
    due to obstruction N13.4
  urethra (acquired) N36.8
  vasomotor I73.9
  vein I86.8
  ventricular, ventricle (acute) (chronic) (*see also* Hypertrophy, cardiac)
    cerebral, congenital Q04.8
  venule NEC I86.8
  vesical orifice N32.89
Dilated, dilation — *see* Dilatation
Diminished, diminution
  hearing (acuity) — *see* Deafness
  sense or sensation (cold) (heat) (tactile) (vibratory) R20.8
  vision NEC H54.7
  vital capacity R94.2
Diminuta taenia B71.0
Dimitri-Sturge-Weber disease Q85.8
Dimple
  congenital sacral Q82.6
  parasacral Q82.6
  pilonidal or postanal — *see* Cyst, pilonidal
Dioctophyme renalis (infection) (infestation) B83.8
Dipetalonemiasis B74.4
Diphallus Q55.69
Diphtheria, diphtheritic (gangrenous) (hemorrhagic) A36.9
  carrier (suspected) Z22.2
  cutaneous A36.3
  faucial A36.0
  infection of wound A36.3
  laryngeal A36.2
  myocarditis A36.81
  nasal, anterior A36.89
  nasopharyngeal A36.1
  neurological complication A36.89
  pharyngeal A36.0
  specified site NEC A36.89
  tonsillar A36.0
Diphyllobothriasis (intestine) B70.0
  larval B70.1
Diplacusis H93.22- ☑
Diplegia (upper limbs) G83.0
  congenital (cerebral) G80.8
  facial G51.0
  lower limbs G82.20
  spastic G80.1
Diplococcus, diplococcal — *see* condition
Diplopia H53.2
Dipsomania F10.20
  with
    psychosis — *see* Psychosis, alcoholic
    remission F10.21
Dipylidiasis B71.1
DIRA (deficiency of interleukin 1 receptor antagonist) M04.8
Direction, teeth, abnormal, fully erupted M26.30
Dirofilariasis B74.8
Dirt-eating child F98.3
Disability, disabilities
  heart — *see* Disease, heart
  intellectual F79
    with
      autistic features F84.9
    mild (I.Q. 50-69) F70
    moderate (I.Q. 35-49) F71
    profound (I.Q. under 20) F73
    severe (I.Q. 20-34) F72
    specified level NEC F78
  knowledge acquisition F81.9
  learning F81.9
  limiting activities Z73.6
  spelling, specific F81.81
Disappearance of family member Z63.4
Disarticulation — *see* Amputation
  meaning traumatic amputation — *see* Amputation, traumatic

Discharge (from)
  abnormal finding in — *see* Abnormal, specimen
  breast (female) (male) N64.52
  diencephalic autonomic idiopathic — *see* Epilepsy, specified NEC
  ear (*see also* Otorrhea)
    blood — *see* Otorrhagia
  excessive urine R35.8
  nipple N64.52
  penile R36.9
  postnasal R09.82
  prison, anxiety concerning Z65.2
  urethral R36.9
    without blood R36.0
    hematospermia R36.1
  vaginal N89.8
Discitis, diskitis M46.40
  cervical region M46.42
  cervicothoracic region M46.43
  lumbar region M46.46
  lumbosacral region M46.47
  multiple sites M46.49
  occipito-atlanto-axial region M46.41
  pyogenic — *see* Infection, intervertebral disc, pyogenic
  sacrococcygeal region M46.48
  thoracic region M46.44
  thoracolumbar region M46.45
Discoid
  meniscus (congenital) Q68.6
  semilunar cartilage (congenital) — *see* Derangement, knee, meniscus, specified NEC
Discoloration
  nails L60.8
  teeth (posteruptive) K03.7
    during formation K00.8
Discomfort
  chest R07.89
  visual H53.14- ☑
Discontinuity, ossicles, ear H74.2- ☑
Discord (with)
  boss Z56.4
  classmates Z55.4
  counselor Z64.4
  employer Z56.4
  family Z63.8
  fellow employees Z56.4
  in-laws Z63.1
  landlord Z59.2
  lodgers Z59.2
  neighbors Z59.2
  probation officer Z64.4
  social worker Z64.4
  teachers Z55.4
  workmates Z56.4
Discordant connection
  atrioventricular (congenital) Q20.5
  ventriculoarterial Q20.3
Discrepancy
  centric occlusion maximum intercuspation M26.55
  leg length (acquired) — *see* Deformity, limb, unequal length
    congenital — *see* Defect, reduction, lower limb
  uterine size date O26.84- ☑
Discrimination
  ethnic Z60.5
  political Z60.5
  racial Z60.5
  religious Z60.5
  sex Z60.5
Disease, diseased (*see also* Syndrome)
  absorbent system I87.8
  acid-peptic K30
  Acosta's T70.29 ☑
  Adams-Stokes (-Morgagni) (syncope with heart block) I45.9
  Addison's anemia (pernicious) D51.0
  adenoids (and tonsils) J35.9
  adrenal (capsule) (cortex) (gland) (medullary) E27.9
    hyperfunction E27.0
    specified NEC E27.8
  ainhum L94.6
  airway
    obstructive, chronic J44.9
      due to
        cotton dust J66.0
        specific organic dusts NEC J66.8
    reactive — *see* Asthma
  akamushi (scrub typhus) A75.3

☑ Additional Character Required — Refer to the Tabular List for Character Selection   ▽ Subterms under main terms may continue to next column or page

Disease, diseased — *continued*
- Albers-Schönberg (marble bones) Q78.2
- Albert's — *see* Tendinitis, Achilles
- alimentary canal K63.9
- alligator-skin Q80.9
  - acquired L85.0
- alpha heavy chain C88.3
- alpine T70.29 ☑
- altitude T70.20 ☑
- alveolar ridge
  - edentulous K06.9
    - specified NEC K06.8
- alveoli, teeth K08.9
- Alzheimer's G30.9 [F02.80]
  - with behavioral disturbance G30.9 [F02.81]
  - early onset G30.0 [F02.80]
    - with behavioral disturbance G30.0 [F02.81]
  - late onset G30.1 [F02.80]
    - with behavioral disturbance G30.1 [F02.81]
  - specified NEC G30.8 [F02.80]
    - with behavioral disturbance G30.8 [F02.81]
- amyloid — *see* Amyloidosis
- Andersen's (glycogenosis IV) E74.09
- Andes T70.29 ☑
- Andrews' (bacterid) L08.89
- angiospastic I73.9
  - cerebral G45.9
  - vein I87.8
- anterior
  - chamber H21.9
  - horn cell G12.29
- antiglomerular basement membrane (anti- GBM) antibody M31.0
  - tubulo-interstitial nephritis N12
- antral — *see* Sinusitis, maxillary
- anus K62.9
  - specified NEC K62.89
- aorta (nonsyphilitic) I77.9
  - syphilitic NEC A52.02
- aortic (heart) (valve) I35.9
  - rheumatic I06.9
- Apollo B30.3
- aponeuroses — *see* Enthesopathy
- appendix K38.9
  - specified NEC K38.8
- aqueous (chamber) H21.9
- Arnold-Chiari — *see* Arnold-Chiari disease
- arterial I77.9
  - occlusive — *see* Occlusion, by site
    - due to stricture or stenosis I77.1
- arteriocardiorenal — *see* Hypertension, cardiorenal
- arteriolar (generalized) (obliterative) I77.9
- arteriorenal — *see* Hypertension, kidney
- arteriosclerotic (*see also* Arteriosclerosis)
  - cardiovascular — *see* Disease, heart, ischemic, atherosclerotic
  - coronary (artery) — *see* Disease, heart, ischemic, atherosclerotic
  - heart — *see* Disease, heart, ischemic, atherosclerotic
- artery I77.9
  - cerebral I67.9
  - coronary I25.10
    - with angina pectoris — *see* Arteriosclerosis, coronary (artery)
- arthropod-borne NOS (viral) A94
  - specified type NEC A93.8
- atticoantral, chronic H66.20
  - left H66.22
    - with right H66.23
  - right H66.21
    - with left H66.23
- auditory canal — *see* Disorder, ear, external
- auricle, ear NEC — *see* Disorder, pinna
- Australian X A83.4
- autoimmune (systemic) NOS M35.9
  - hemolytic (cold type) (warm type) D59.1
    - drug-induced D59.0
  - thyroid E06.3
- aviator's — *see* Effect, adverse, high altitude
- Ayerza's (pulmonary artery sclerosis with pulmonary hypertension) I27.0
- Babington's (familial hemorrhagic telangiectasia) I78.0
- bacterial A49.9
  - specified NEC A48.8
  - zoonotic A28.9
    - specified type NEC A28.8
- Baelz's (cheilitis glandularis apostematosa) K13.0

Disease, diseased — *continued*
- bagasse J67.1
- balloon — *see* Effect, adverse, high altitude
- Bang's (brucella abortus) A23.1
- Bannister's T78.3 ☑
- barometer makers' — *see* Poisoning, mercury
- Barraquer (-Simons') (progressive lipodystrophy) E88.1
- Barrett's — *see* Barrett's, esophagus
- Bartholin's gland N75.9
- basal ganglia G25.9
  - degenerative G23.9
    - specified NEC G23.8
  - specified NEC G25.89
- Basedow's (exophthalmic goiter) — *see* Hyperthyroidism, with, goiter (diffuse)
- Bateman's B08.1
- Batten-Steinert G71.11
- Battey A31.0
- Beard's (neurasthenia) F48.8
- Becker
  - idiopathic mural endomyocardial I42.3
  - myotonia congenita G71.12
- Begbie's (exophthalmic goiter) — *see* Hyperthyroidism, with, goiter (diffuse)
- behavioral, organic F07.9
- Beigel's (white piedra) B36.2
- Benson's — *see* Deposit, crystalline
- Bernard-Soulier (thrombopathy) D69.1
- Bernhardt (-Roth) — *see* Mononeuropathy, lower limb, meralgia paresthetica
- Biermer's (pernicious anemia) D51.0
- bile duct (common) (hepatic) K83.9
  - with calculus, stones — *see* Calculus, bile duct
  - specified NEC K83.8
- biliary (tract) K83.9
  - specified NEC K83.8
- Billroth's — *see* Spina bifida
- bird fancier's J67.2
- black lung J60
- bladder N32.9
  - in (due to)
    - schistosomiasis (bilharziasis) B65.0 [N33]
  - specified NEC N32.89
- bleeder's D66
- blood D75.9
  - forming organs D75.9
  - vessel I99.9
- Bloodgood's — *see* Mastopathy, cystic
- Bodechtel-Guttmann (subacute sclerosing panencephalitis) A81.1
- bone (*see also* Disorder, bone)
  - aluminum M83.4
  - fibrocystic NEC
    - jaw M27.49
- bone-marrow D75.9
- Borna A83.9
- Bornholm (epidemic pleurodynia) B33.0
- Bouchard's (myopathic dilatation of the stomach) K31.0
- Bouillaud's (rheumatic heart disease) I01.9
- Bourneville (-Brissaud) (tuberous sclerosis) Q85.1
- Bouveret (-Hoffmann) (paroxysmal tachycardia) I47.9
- bowel K63.9
  - functional K59.9
    - psychogenic F45.8
- brain G93.9
  - arterial, artery I67.9
  - arteriosclerotic I67.2
  - congenital Q04.9
  - degenerative — *see* Degeneration, brain
  - inflammatory — *see* Encephalitis
  - organic G93.9
    - arteriosclerotic I67.2
  - parasitic NEC B71.9 [G94]
  - senile NEC G31.1
  - specified NEC G93.89
- breast (*see also* Disorder, breast) N64.9
  - cystic (chronic) — *see* Mastopathy, cystic
  - fibrocystic — *see* Mastopathy, cystic
  - Paget's
    - female, unspecified side C50.91- ☑
    - male, unspecified side C50.92- ☑
  - specified NEC N64.89
- Breda's — *see* Yaws
- Bretonneau's (diphtheritic malignant angina) A36.0
- Bright's — *see* Nephritis
  - arteriosclerotic — *see* Hypertension, kidney
- Brill's (recrudescent typhus) A75.1

Disease, diseased — *continued*
- Brill-Zinsser (recrudescent typhus) A75.1
- Brion-Kayser — *see* Fever, paratyphoid
- broad
  - beta E78.2
  - ligament (noninflammatory) N83.9
    - inflammatory — *see* Disease, pelvis, inflammatory
    - specified NEC N83.8
- Brocq-Duhring (dermatitis herpetiformis) L13.0
- Brocq's
  - meaning
    - dermatitis herpetiformis L13.0
    - prurigo L28.2
- bronchopulmonary J98.4
- bronchus NEC J98.09
- bronze Addison's E27.1
  - tuberculous A18.7
- budgerigar fancier's J67.2
- Buerger's (thromboangiitis obliterans) I73.1
- bullous L13.9
  - chronic of childhood L12.2
  - specified NEC L13.8
- Bürger-Grütz (essential familial hyperlipemia) E78.3
- bursa — *see* Bursopathy
- caisson T70.3 ☑
- California — *see* Coccidioidomycosis
- capillaries I78.9
  - specified NEC I78.8
- Carapata A68.0
- cardiac — *see* Disease, heart
- cardiopulmonary, chronic I27.9
- cardiorenal (hepatic) (hypertensive) (vascular) — *see* Hypertension, cardiorenal
- cardiovascular (atherosclerotic) I25.10
  - with angina pectoris — *see* Arteriosclerosis, coronary (artery),
  - congenital Q28.9
  - hypertensive — *see* Hypertension, heart
  - newborn P29.9
    - specified NEC P29.89
  - renal (hypertensive) — *see* Hypertension, cardiorenal
  - syphilitic (asymptomatic) A52.00
- cartilage — *see* Disorder, cartilage
- Castellani's A69.8
- Castleman (unicentric) (multicentric) D47.Z2
  - HHV-8-associated (*see also* Herpesvirus, human, 8) D47.Z2
- cat-scratch A28.1
- Cavare's (familial periodic paralysis) G72.3
- cecum K63.9
- celiac (adult) (infantile) (with steatorrhea) K90.0
- cellular tissue L98.9
- central core G71.2
- cerebellar, cerebellum — *see* Disease, brain
- cerebral (*see also* Disease, brain)
  - degenerative — *see* Degeneration, brain
- cerebrospinal G96.9
- cerebrovascular I67.9
  - acute I67.89
    - embolic I63.4- ☑
    - thrombotic I63.3- ☑
  - arteriosclerotic I67.2
  - specified NEC I67.89
- cervix (uteri) (noninflammatory) N88.9
  - inflammatory — *see* Cervicitis
  - specified NEC N88.8
- Chabert's A22.9
- Chandler's (osteochondritis dissecans, hip) — *see* Osteochondritis, dissecans, hip
- Charlouis — *see* Yaws
- Chédiak-Steinbrinck (-Higashi) (congenital gigantism of peroxidase granules) E70.330
- chest J98.9
- Chiari's (hepatic vein thrombosis) I82.0
- Chicago B40.9
- Chignon B36.8
- chigo, chigoe B88.1
- childhood granulomatous D71
- Chinese liver fluke B66.1
- chlamydial A74.9
  - specified NEC A74.89
- cholecystic K82.9
- choroid H31.9
  - specified NEC H31.8
- Christmas D67
- chronic bullous of childhood L12.2

Disease, diseased — *continued*
chylomicron retention E78.3
ciliary body H21.9
  specified NEC H21.89
circulatory (system) NEC I99.8
  newborn P29.9
  syphilitic A52.00
    congenital A50.54
coagulation factor deficiency (congenital) — *see* Defect, coagulation
coccidioidal — *see* Coccidioidomycosis
cold
  agglutinin or hemoglobinuria D59.1
    paroxysmal D59.6
  hemagglutinin (chronic) D59.1
collagen NOS (nonvascular) (vascular) M35.9
  specified NEC M35.8
colon K63.9
  functional K59.9
    congenital Q43.2
  ischemic (*see also* Ischemia, intestine, acute) K55.039
colonic inflammatory bowel, unclassified (IBDU) K52.3
combined system — *see* Degeneration, combined
compressed air T70.3 ☑
Concato's (pericardial polyserositis) A19.9
  nontubercular I31.1
  pleural — *see* Pleurisy, with effusion
conjunctiva H11.9
  chlamydial A74.0
  specified NEC H11.89
  viral B30.9
    specified NEC B30.8
connective tissue, systemic (diffuse) M35.9
  in (due to)
    hypogammaglobulinemia D80.1 [M36.8]
    ochronosis E70.29 [M36.8]
  specified NEC M35.8
Conor and Bruch's (boutonneuse fever) A77.1
Cooper's — *see* Mastopathy, cystic
Cori's (glycogenosis III) E74.03
corkhandler's or corkworker's J67.3
cornea H18.9
  specified NEC H18.89- ☑
coronary (artery) — *see* Disease, heart, ischemic, atherosclerotic
  congenital Q24.5
  ostial, syphilitic (aortic) (mitral) (pulmonary) A52.03
corpus cavernosum N48.9
  specified NEC N48.89
Cotugno's — *see* Sciatica
coxsackie (virus) NEC B34.1
cranial nerve NOS G52.9
Creutzfeldt-Jakob — *see* Creutzfeldt-Jakob disease or syndrome
Crocq's (acrocyanosis) I73.89
Crohn's — *see* Enteritis, regional
Curschmann G71.11
cystic
  breast (chronic) — *see* Mastopathy, cystic
  kidney, congenital Q61.9
  liver, congenital Q44.6
  lung J98.4
    congenital Q33.0
cytomegalic inclusion (generalized) B25.9
  with pneumonia B25.0
  congenital P35.1
cytomegaloviral B25.9
  specified NEC B25.8
Czerny's (periodic hydrarthrosis of the knee) — *see* Effusion, joint, knee
Daae (-Finsen) (epidemic pleurodynia) B33.0
Darling's — *see* Histoplasmosis capsulati
de Quervain's (tendon sheath) M65.4
  thyroid (subacute granulomatous thyroiditis) E06.1
Débove's (splenomegaly) R16.1
deer fly — *see* Tularemia
Degos' I77.89
demyelinating, demyelinizating (nervous system) G37.9
  multiple sclerosis G35
  specified NEC G37.8
dense deposit (*see also* N00-N07 with fourth character .6) N05.6
deposition, hydroxyapatite — *see* Disease, hydroxyapatite deposition
Devergie's (pityriasis rubra pilaris) L44.0
Devic's G36.0

diaphorase deficiency D74.0
diaphragm J98.6
diarrheal, infectious NEC A09
digestive system K92.9
  specified NEC K92.89
disc, degenerative — *see* Degeneration, intervertebral disc
discogenic (*see also* Displacement, intervertebral disc NEC)
  with myelopathy — *see* Disorder, disc, with, myelopathy
diverticular — *see* Diverticula
Dubois (thymus) A50.59 [E35]
Duchenne-Griesinger G71.0
Duchenne's
  muscular dystrophy G71.0
  pseudohypertrophy, muscles G71.0
ductless glands E34.9
Duhring's (dermatitis herpetiformis) L13.0
duodenum K31.9
  specified NEC K31.89
Dupré's (meningism) R29.1
Dupuytren's (muscle contracture) M72.0
Durand-Nicholas-Favre (climatic bubo) A55
Duroziez's (congenital mitral stenosis) Q23.2
ear — *see* Disorder, ear
Eberth's — *see* Fever, typhoid
Ebola (virus) A98.4
Ebstein's heart Q22.5
Echinococcus — *see* Echinococcus
echovirus NEC B34.1
Eddowes' (brittle bones and blue sclera) Q78.0
edentulous (alveolar) ridge K06.9
  specified NEC K06.8
Edsall's T67.2 ☑
Eichstedt's (pityriasis versicolor) B36.0
Eisenmenger's (irreversible) I27.83
Ellis-van Creveld (chondroectodermal dysplasia) Q77.6
end stage renal (ESRD) N18.6
  due to hypertension I12.0
endocrine glands or system NEC E34.9
endomyocardial (eosinophilic) I42.3
English (rickets) E55.0
enteroviral, enterovirus NEC B34.1
  central nervous system NEC A88.8
epidemic B99.9
  specified NEC B99.8
epididymis N50.9
Erb (-Landouzy) G71.0
Erdheim-Chester (ECD) E88.89
esophagus K22.9
  functional K22.4
  psychogenic F45.8
  specified NEC K22.8
Eulenburg's (congenital paramyotonia) G71.19
eustachian tube — *see* Disorder, eustachian tube
external
  auditory canal — *see* Disorder, ear, external
  ear — *see* Disorder, ear, external
extrapyramidal G25.9
  specified NEC G25.89
eye H57.9
  anterior chamber H21.9
  inflammatory NEC H57.8
  muscle (external) — *see* Strabismus
  specified NEC H57.8
  syphilitic — *see* Oculopathy, syphilitic
eyeball H44.9
  specified NEC H44.89
eyelid — *see* Disorder, eyelid
  specified NEC — *see* Disorder, eyelid, specified type NEC
eyeworm of Africa B74.3
facial nerve (seventh) G51.9
  newborn (birth injury) P11.3
Fahr (of brain) G23.8
Fahr Volhard (of kidney) I12.- ☑
fallopian tube (noninflammatory) N83.9
  inflammatory — *see* Salpingo-oophoritis
  specified NEC N83.8
familial periodic paralysis G72.3
Fanconi's (congenital pancytopenia) D61.09
fascia NEC (*see also* Disorder, muscle)
  inflammatory — *see* Myositis
  specified NEC M62.89
Fauchard's (periodontitis) — *see* Periodontitis
Favre-Durand-Nicolas (climatic bubo) A55

Disease, diseased — *continued*
Fede's K14.0
Feer's — *see* Poisoning, mercury
female pelvic inflammatory (*see also* Disease, pelvis, inflammatory) N73.9
  syphilitic (secondary) A51.42
  tuberculous A18.17
Fernels' (aortic aneurysm) I71.9
fibrocaseous of lung — *see* Tuberculosis, pulmonary
fibrocystic — *see* Fibrocystic disease
Fiedler's (leptospiral jaundice) A27.0
fifth B08.3
file-cutter's — *see* Poisoning, lead
fish-skin Q80.9
  acquired L85.0
Flajani (-Basedow) (exophthalmic goiter) — *see* Hyperthyroidism, with, goiter (diffuse)
flax-dresser's J66.1
fluke — *see* Infestation, fluke
foot and mouth B08.8
foot process N04.9
Forbes' (glycogenosis III) E74.03
Fordyce-Fox (apocrine miliaria) L75.2
Fordyce's (ectopic sebaceous glands) (mouth) Q38.6
Forestier's (rhizomelic pseudopolyarthritis) M35.3
  meaning ankylosing hyperostosis — *see* Hyperostosis, ankylosing
Fothergill's
  neuralgia — *see* Neuralgia, trigeminal
  scarlatina anginosa A38.9
Fournier (gangrene) N49.3
  female N76.89
fourth B08.8
Fox (-Fordyce) (apocrine miliaria) L75.2
Francis' — *see* Tularemia
Franklin C88.2
Frei's (climatic bubo) A55
Friedreich's
  combined systemic or ataxia G11.1
  myoclonia G25.3
frontal sinus — *see* Sinusitis, frontal
fungus NEC B49
Gaisböck's (polycythemia hypertonica) D75.1
gallbladder K82.9
  calculus — *see* Calculus, gallbladder
  cholecystitis — *see* Cholecystitis
  cholesterolosis K82.4
  fistula — *see* Fistula, gallbladder
  hydrops K82.1
  obstruction — *see* Obstruction, gallbladder
  perforation K82.2
  specified NEC K82.8
gamma heavy chain C88.2
Gamna's (siderotic splenomegaly) D73.2
Gamstorp's (adynamia episodica hereditaria) G72.3
Gandy-Nanta (siderotic splenomegaly) D73.2
ganister J62.8
gastric — *see* Disease, stomach
gastroesophageal reflux (GERD) K21.9
  with esophagitis K21.0
gastrointestinal (tract) K92.9
  amyloid E85.4
  functional K59.9
    psychogenic F45.8
  specified NEC K92.89
Gee (-Herter) (-Heubner) (-Thaysen) (nontropical sprue) K90.0
genital organs
  female N94.9
  male N50.9
Gerhardt's (erythromelalgia) I73.81
Gibert's (pityriasis rosea) L42
Gierke's (glycogenosis I) E74.01
Gilles de la Tourette's (motor-verbal tic) F95.2
gingiva K06.9
  plaque induced K05.00
  specified NEC K06.8
gland (lymph) I89.9
Glanzmann's (hereditary hemorrhagic thrombasthenia) D69.1
glass-blower's (cataract) — *see* Cataract, specified NEC
  salivary gland hypertrophy K11.1
Glisson's — *see* Rickets
globe H44.9
  specified NEC H44.89
glomerular (*see also* Glomerulonephritis)
  with edema — *see* Nephrosis
  acute — *see* Nephritis, acute

Disease, diseased — *continued*
  glomerular (*see also* Glomerulonephritis) — *continued*
    chronic — *see* Nephritis, chronic
    minimal change N05.0
    rapidly progressive N01.9
  glycogen storage E74.00
    Andersen's E74.09
    Cori's E74.03
    Forbes' E74.03
    generalized E74.00
    glucose-6-phosphatase deficiency E74.01
    heart E74.02 [I43]
    hepatorenal E74.09
    Hers' E74.09
    liver and kidney E74.09
    McArdle's E74.04
    muscle phosphofructokinase E74.09
    myocardium E74.02 [I43]
    Pompe's E74.02
    Tauri's E74.09
    type 0 E74.09
    type I E74.01
    type II E74.02
    type III E74.03
    type IV E74.09
    type V E74.04
    type VI-XI E74.09
    Von Gierke's E74.01
  Goldstein's (familial hemorrhagic telangiectasia) I78.0
  gonococcal NOS A54.9
  graft-versus-host (GVH) D89.813
    acute D89.810
    acute on chronic D89.812
    chronic D89.811
  grainhandler's J67.8
  granulomatous (childhood) (chronic) D71
  Graves' (exophthalmic goiter) — *see* Hyperthyroidism, with, goiter (diffuse)
  Griesinger's — *see* Ancylostomiasis
  Grisel's M43.6
  Gruby's (tinea tonsurans) B35.0
  Guillain-Barré G61.0
  Guinon's (motor-verbal tic) F95.2
  gum K06.9
  gynecological N94.9
  H (Hartnup's) E72.02
  Haff — *see* Poisoning, mercury
  Hageman (congenital factor XII deficiency) D68.2
  hair (color) (shaft) L67.9
    follicles L73.9
      specified NEC L73.8
  Hamman's (spontaneous mediastinal emphysema) J98.2
  hand, foot and mouth B08.4
  Hansen's — *see* Leprosy
  Hantavirus, with pulmonary manifestations B33.4
    with renal manifestations A98.5
  Harada's H30.81- ☑
  Hartnup (pellagra-cerebellar ataxia-renal aminoaciduria) E72.02
  Hart's (pellagra-cerebellar ataxia-renal aminoaciduria) E72.02
  Hashimoto's (struma lymphomatosa) E06.3
  Hb — *see* Disease, hemoglobin
  heart (organic) I51.9
    with
      pulmonary edema (acute) (*see also* Failure, ventricular, left) I50.1
      rheumatic fever (conditions in I00)
        active I01.9
          with chorea I02.0
          specified NEC I01.8
        inactive or quiescent (with chorea) I09.9
          specified NEC I09.89
    amyloid E85.4 [I43]
    aortic (valve) I35.9
    arteriosclerotic or sclerotic (senile) — *see* Disease, heart, ischemic, atherosclerotic
    artery, arterial — *see* Disease, heart, ischemic, atherosclerotic
    beer drinkers' I42.6
    beriberi (wet) E51.12
    black I27.0
    congenital Q24.9
      cyanotic Q24.9
      specified NEC Q24.8
    coronary — *see* Disease, heart, ischemic

Disease, diseased — *continued*
  heart — *continued*
    cryptogenic I51.9
    fibroid — *see* Myocarditis
    functional I51.89
      psychogenic F45.8
    glycogen storage E74.02 [I43]
    gonococcal A54.83
    hypertensive — *see* Hypertension, heart
    hyperthyroid (*see also* Hyperthyroidism)
      E05.90 [I43]
      with thyroid storm E05.91 [I43]
    ischemic (chronic or with a stated duration of over 4 weeks) I25.9
      atherosclerotic (of) I25.10
        with angina pectoris — *see* Arteriosclerosis, coronary (artery)
        coronary artery bypass graft — *see* Arteriosclerosis, coronary (artery), cardiomyopathy I25.5
      diagnosed on ECG or other special investigation, but currently presenting no symptoms I25.6
      silent I25.6
      specified form NEC I25.89
    kyphoscoliotic I27.1
    meningococcal A39.50
      endocarditis A39.51
      myocarditis A39.52
      pericarditis A39.53
    mitral I05.9
      specified NEC I05.8
    muscular — *see* Degeneration, myocardial
    psychogenic (functional) F45.8
    pulmonary (chronic) I27.9
      in schistosomiasis B65.9 [I52]
      specified NEC I27.89
    rheumatic (chronic) (inactive) (old) (quiescent) (with chorea) I09.9
      active or acute I01.9
        with chorea (acute) (rheumatic) (Sydenham's) I02.0
      specified NEC I09.89
    senile — *see* Myocarditis
    syphilitic A52.06
      aortic A52.03
        aneurysm A52.01
      congenital A50.54 [I52]
    thyrotoxic (*see also* Thyrotoxicosis) E05.90 [I43]
      with thyroid storm E05.91 [I43]
    valve, valvular (obstructive) (regurgitant) (*see also* Endocarditis)
      congenital NEC Q24.8
      pulmonary Q22.3
    vascular — *see* Disease, cardiovascular
  heavy chain NEC C88.2
    alpha C88.3
    gamma C88.2
    mu C88.2
  Hebra's
    pityriasis
      maculata et circinata L42
      rubra pilaris L44.0
    prurigo L28.2
  hematopoietic organs D75.9
  hemoglobin or Hb
    abnormal (mixed) NEC D58.2
      with thalassemia D56.9
    AS genotype D57.3
    Bart's D56.0
    C (Hb-C) D58.2
      with other abnormal hemoglobin NEC D58.2
      elliptocytosis D58.1
      Hb-S D57.2- ☑
      sickle-cell D57.2- ☑
      thalassemia D56.8
    Constant Spring D58.2
    D (Hb-D) D58.2
    E (Hb-E) D58.2
    E-beta thalassemia D56.5
    elliptocytosis D58.1
    H (Hb-H) (thalassemia) D56.0
      with other abnormal hemoglobin NEC D56.9
      Constant Spring D56.0
    I thalassemia D56.9
    M D74.0
    S or SS D57.1
    SC D57.2- ☑

Disease, diseased — *continued*
  hemoglobin or Hb — *continued*
    SD D57.8- ☑
    SE D57.8- ☑
    spherocytosis D58.0
    unstable, hemolytic D58.2
  hemolytic (newborn) P55.9
    autoimmune (cold type) (warm type) D59.1
    drug-induced D59.0
    due to or with
      incompatibility
        ABO (blood group) P55.1
        blood (group) (Duffy) (K(ell)) (Kidd) (Lewis) (M) (S) NEC P55.8
        Rh (blood group) (factor) P55.0
        Rh negative mother P55.0
    specified type NEC P55.8
    unstable hemoglobin D58.2
  hemorrhagic D69.9
    newborn P53
  Henoch (-Schönlein) (purpura nervosa) D69.0
  hepatic — *see* Disease, liver
  hepatolenticular E83.01
  heredodegenerative NEC
    spinal cord G95.89
  herpesviral, disseminated B00.7
  Hers' (glycogenosis VI) E74.09
  Herter (-Gee) (-Heubner) (nontropical sprue) K90.0
  Heubner-Herter (nontropical sprue) K90.0
  high fetal gene or hemoglobin thalassemia D56.9
  Hildenbrand's — *see* Typhus
  hip (joint) M25.9
    congenital Q65.89
    suppurative M00.9
    tuberculous A18.02
  His (-Werner) (trench fever) A79.0
  Hodgson's I71.2
    ruptured I71.1
  Holla — *see* Spherocytosis
  hookworm B76.9
    specified NEC B76.8
  host-versus-graft D89.813
    acute D89.810
    acute on chronic D89.812
    chronic D89.811
  human immunodeficiency virus (HIV) B20
  Huntington's G10
    with dementia G10 [F02.80]
  Hutchinson's (cheiropompholyx) — *see* Hutchinson's disease
  hyaline (diffuse) (generalized)
    membrane (lung) (newborn) P22.0
    adult J80
  hydatid — *see* Echinococcus
  hydroxyapatite deposition M11.00
    ankle M11.07- ☑
    elbow M11.02- ☑
    foot joint M11.07- ☑
    hand joint M11.04- ☑
    hip M11.05- ☑
    knee M11.06- ☑
    multiple site M11.09
    shoulder M11.01- ☑
    vertebra M11.08
    wrist M11.03- ☑
  hyperkinetic — *see* Hyperkinesia
  hypertensive — *see* Hypertension
  hypophysis E23.7
  Iceland G93.3
  I-cell E77.0
  immune D89.9
  immunoproliferative (malignant) C88.9
    small intestinal C88.3
    specified NEC C88.8
  inclusion B25.9
    salivary gland B25.9
  infectious, infective B99.9
    congenital P37.9
      specified NEC P37.8
      viral P35.9
        specified type NEC P35.8
    specified NEC B99.8
  inflammatory
    penis N48.29
      abscess N48.21
      cellulitis N48.22
    prepuce N47.7
      balanoposthitis N47.6

Disease, diseased — *continued*
  inflammatory — *continued*
    tubo-ovarian — *see* Salpingo-oophoritis
  intervertebral disc (*see also* Disorder, disc)
    with myelopathy — *see* Disorder, disc, with, myelopathy
    cervical, cervicothoracic — *see* Disorder, disc, cervical
      with
        myelopathy — *see* Disorder, disc, cervical, with myelopathy
        neuritis, radiculitis or radiculopathy — *see* Disorder, disc, cervical, with neuritis
        specified NEC — *see* Disorder, disc, cervical, specified type NEC
    lumbar (with)
      myelopathy M51.06
      neuritis, radiculitis, radiculopathy or sciatica M51.16
      specified NEC M51.86
    lumbosacral (with)
      neuritis, radiculitis, radiculopathy or sciatica M51.17
      specified NEC M51.87
    specified NEC — *see* Disorder, disc, specified NEC
    thoracic (with)
      myelopathy M51.04
      neuritis, radiculitis or radiculopathy M51.14
      specified NEC M51.84
    thoracolumbar (with)
      myelopathy M51.05
      neuritis, radiculitis or radiculopathy M51.15
      specified NEC M51.85
  intestine K63.9
    functional K59.9
      psychogenic F45.8
      specified NEC K59.8
    organic K63.9
    protozoal A07.9
    specified NEC K63.89
  iris H21.9
    specified NEC H21.89
  iron metabolism or storage E83.10
  island (scrub typhus) A75.3
  itai-itai — *see* Poisoning, cadmium
  Jakob-Creutzfeldt — *see* Creutzfeldt-Jakob disease or syndrome
  jaw M27.9
    fibrocystic M27.49
    specified NEC M27.8
  jigger B88.1
  joint (*see also* Disorder, joint)
    Charcot's — *see* Arthropathy, neuropathic (Charcot)
    degenerative — *see* Osteoarthritis
      multiple M15.9
      spine — *see* Spondylosis
    hypertrophic — *see* Osteoarthritis
    sacroiliac M53.3
    specified NEC — *see* Disorder, joint, specified type NEC
    spine NEC — *see* Dorsopathy
    suppurative — *see* Arthritis, pyogenic or pyemic
  Jourdain's (acute gingivitis) K05.00
    nonplaque induced K05.01
    plaque induced K05.00
  Kaschin-Beck (endemic polyarthritis) M12.10
    ankle M12.17- ☑
    elbow M12.12- ☑
    foot joint M12.17- ☑
    hand joint M12.14- ☑
    hip M12.15- ☑
    knee M12.16- ☑
    multiple site M12.19
    shoulder M12.11- ☑
    vertebra M12.18
    wrist M12.13- ☑
  Katayama B65.2
  Kedani (scrub typhus) A75.3
  Keshan E59
  kidney (functional) (pelvis) N28.9
    chronic N18.9
      hypertensive — *see* Hypertension, kidney
      stage 1 N18.1
      stage 2 (mild) N18.2
      stage 3 (moderate) N18.3
      stage 4 (severe) N18.4
      stage 5 N18.5

Disease, diseased — *continued*
  kidney — *continued*
    complicating pregnancy — *see* Pregnancy, complicated by, renal disease
    cystic (congenital) Q61.9
    fibrocystic (congenital) Q61.8
    hypertensive — *see* Hypertension, kidney
    in (due to)
      schistosomiasis (bilharziasis) B65.9 [N29]
    multicystic Q61.4
    polycystic Q61.3
      adult type Q61.2
      childhood type NEC Q61.19
        collecting duct dilatation Q61.11
  Kimmelstiel (-Wilson) (intercapillary polycystic (congenital) glomerulosclerosis) — *see* E08-E13 with .21
  Kinnier Wilson's (hepatolenticular degeneration) E83.01
  kissing — *see* Mononucleosis, infectious
  Klebs' (*see also* Glomerulonephritis) N05- ☑
  Klippel-Feil (brevicollis) Q76.1
  Köhler-Pellegrini-Stieda (calcification, knee joint) — *see* Bursitis, tibial collateral
  Kok Q89.8
  König's (osteochondritis dissecans) — *see* Osteochondritis, dissecans
  Korsakoff's (nonalcoholic) F04
    alcoholic F10.96
      with dependence F10.26
  Kostmann's (infantile genetic agranulocytosis) D70.0
  kuru A81.81
  Kyasanur Forest A98.2
  labyrinth, ear — *see* Disorder, ear, inner
  lacrimal system — *see* Disorder, lacrimal system
  Lafora's — *see* Epilepsy, generalized, idiopathic
  Lancereaux-Mathieu (leptospiral jaundice) A27.0
  Landry's G61.0
  Larrey-Weil (leptospiral jaundice) A27.0
  larynx J38.7
  legionnaires' A48.1
    nonpneumonic A48.2
  Lenegre's I44.2
  lens H27.9
    specified NEC H27.8
  Lev's (acquired complete heart block) I44.2
  Lewy body (dementia) G31.83 [F02.80]
    with behavioral disturbance G31.83 [F02.81]
  Lichtheim's (subacute combined sclerosis with pernicious anemia) D51.0
  Lightwood's (renal tubular acidosis) N25.89
  Lignac's (cystinosis) E72.04
  lip K13.0
  lipid-storage E75.6
    specified NEC E75.5
  Lipschütz's N76.6
  liver (chronic) (organic) K76.9
    alcoholic (chronic) K70.9
      acute — *see* Disease, liver, alcoholic, hepatitis
      cirrhosis K70.30
        with ascites K70.31
      failure K70.40
        with coma K70.41
      fatty liver K70.0
      fibrosis K70.2
      hepatitis K70.10
        with ascites K70.11
      sclerosis K70.2
    cystic, congenital Q44.6
    drug-induced (idiosyncratic) (toxic) (predictable) (unpredictable) — *see* Disease, liver, toxic
    end stage K72.90
      due to hepatitis — *see* Hepatitis
    fatty, nonalcoholic (NAFLD) K76.0
      alcoholic K70.0
    fibrocystic (congenital) Q44.6
    fluke
      Chinese B66.1
      oriental B66.1
      sheep B66.3
    gestational alloimmune (GALD) P78.84
    glycogen storage E74.09 [K77]
    in (due to)
      schistosomiasis (bilharziasis) B65.9 [K77]
    inflammatory K75.9
      alcoholic K70.1 ☑
      specified NEC K75.89
    polycystic (congenital) Q44.6

Disease, diseased — *continued*
  liver — *continued*
    toxic K71.9
      with
        cholestasis K71.0
        cirrhosis (liver) K71.7
        fibrosis (liver) K71.7
        focal nodular hyperplasia K71.8
        hepatic granuloma K71.8
        hepatic necrosis K71.10
          with coma K71.11
        hepatitis NEC K71.6
          acute K71.2
          chronic
            active K71.50
              with ascites K71.51
            lobular K71.4
            persistent K71.3
          lupoid K71.50
            with ascites K71.51
        peliosis hepatis K71.8
        veno-occlusive disease (VOD) of liver K71.8
    veno-occlusive K76.5
  Lobo's (keloid blastomycosis) B48.0
  Lobstein's (brittle bones and blue sclera) Q78.0
  Ludwig's (submaxillary cellulitis) K12.2
  lumbosacral region M53.87
  lung J98.4
    black J60
    congenital Q33.9
    cystic J98.4
      congenital Q33.0
    fibroid (chronic) — *see* Fibrosis, lung
    fluke B66.4
      oriental B66.4
    in
      amyloidosis E85.4 [J99]
      sarcoidosis D86.0
      Sjögren's syndrome M35.02
      systemic
        lupus erythematosus M32.13
        sclerosis M34.81
    interstitial J84.9
      of childhood, specified NEC J84.848
      respiratory bronchiolitis J84.115
      specified NEC J84.89
    obstructive (chronic) J44.9
      with
        acute
          bronchitis J44.0
          exacerbation NEC J44.1
          lower respiratory infection J44.0
        alveolitis, allergic J67.9
        asthma J44.9
        bronchiectasis J47.9
          with
            exacerbation (acute) J47.1
            lower respiratory infection J47.0
        bronchitis J44.9
          with
            exacerbation (acute) J44.1
            lower respiratory infection J44.0
        emphysema J43.9
        hypersensitivity pneumonitis J67.9
      decompensated J44.1
        with
          exacerbation (acute) J44.1
    polycystic J98.4
      congenital Q33.0
    rheumatoid (diffuse) (interstitial) — *see* Rheumatoid, lung
  Lutembacher's (atrial septal defect with mitral stenosis) Q21.1
  Lyme A69.20
  lymphatic (gland) (system) (channel) (vessel) I89.9
  lymphoproliferative D47.9
    specified NEC D47.Z9 (*following* D47.4)
    T-gamma D47.Z9 (*following* D47.4)
    X-linked D82.3
  Magitot's M27.2
  malarial — *see* Malaria
  malignant (*see also* Neoplasm, malignant, by site)
  Manson's B65.1
  maple bark J67.6
  maple-syrup-urine E71.0
  Marburg (virus) A98.3
  Marion's (bladder neck obstruction) N32.0
  Marsh's (exophthalmic goiter) — *see* Hyperthyroidism, with, goiter (diffuse)

☑ Additional Character Required — Refer to the Tabular List for Character Selection   🔻 Subterms under main terms may continue to next column or page

Disease, diseased — *continued*
- mastoid (process) — *see* Disorder, ear, middle
- Mathieu's (leptospiral jaundice) A27.0
- Maxcy's A75.2
- McArdle (-Schmid-Pearson) (glycogenosis V) E74.04
- mediastinum J98.59
- medullary center (idiopathic) (respiratory) G93.89
- Meige's (chronic hereditary edema) Q82.0
- meningococcal — *see* Infection, meningococcal
- mental F99
  - organic F09
- mesenchymal M35.9
- mesenteric embolic (*see also* Ischemia, intestine, acute) K55.039
- metabolic, metabolism E88.9
  - bilirubin E80.7
- metal-polisher's J62.8
- metastatic (*see also* Neoplasm, secondary, by site) C79.9
- microvascular - code to condition
- microvillus
  - atrophy Q43.8
  - inclusion (MVD) Q43.8
- middle ear — *see* Disorder, ear, middle
- Mikulicz' (dryness of mouth, absent or decreased lacrimation) K11.8
- Milroy's (chronic hereditary edema) Q82.0
- Minamata — *see* Poisoning, mercury
- minicore G71.2
- Minor's G95.19
- Minot's (hemorrhagic disease, newborn) P53
- Minot-von Willebrand-Jürgens (angiohemophilia) D68.0
- Mitchell's (erythromelalgia) I73.81
- mitral (valve) I05.9
  - nonrheumatic I34.9
- mixed connective tissue M35.1
- moldy hay J67.0
- Monge's T70.29 ☑
- Morgagni-Adams-Stokes (syncope with heart block) I45.9
- Morgagni's (syndrome) (hyperostosis frontalis interna) M85.2
- Morton's (with metatarsalgia) — *see* Lesion, nerve, plantar
- Morvan's G60.8
- motor neuron (bulbar) (mixed type) (spinal) G12.20
  - amyotrophic lateral sclerosis G12.21
  - familial G12.24
  - progressive bulbar palsy G12.22
  - specified NEC G12.29
- moyamoya I67.5
- mu heavy chain disease C88.2
- multicore G71.2
- muscle (*see also* Disorder, muscle)
  - inflammatory — *see* Myositis
  - ocular (external) — *see* Strabismus
- musculoskeletal system, soft tissue — *see also* Disorder, soft tissue
  - specified NEC — *see* Disorder, soft tissue, specified type NEC
- mushroom workers' J67.5
- mycotic B49
- myelodysplastic, not classified C94.6
- myeloproliferative, not classified C94.6
  - chronic D47.1
- myocardium, myocardial (*see also* Degeneration, myocardial) I51.5
  - primary (idiopathic) I42.9
- myoneural G70.9
- Naegeli's D69.1
- nails L60.9
  - specified NEC L60.8
- Nairobi (sheep virus) A93.8
- nasal J34.9
- nemaline body G71.2
- nerve — *see* Disorder, nerve
- nervous system G98.8
  - autonomic G90.9
  - central G96.9
    - specified NEC G96.8
  - congenital Q07.9
  - parasympathetic G90.9
  - specified NEC G98.8
  - sympathetic G90.9
  - vegetative G90.9
- neuromuscular system G70.9
- Newcastle B30.8

Disease, diseased — *continued*
- Nicolas (-Durand)-Favre (climatic bubo) A55
- nipple N64.9
  - Paget's C50.01- ☑
    - female C50.01- ☑
    - male C50.02- ☑
- Nishimoto (-Takeuchi) I67.5
- nonarthropod-borne NOS (viral) B34.9
  - enterovirus NEC B34.1
- nonautoimmune hemolytic D59.4
  - drug-induced D59.2
- Nonne-Milroy-Meige (chronic hereditary edema) Q82.0
- nose J34.9
- nucleus pulposus — *see* Disorder, disc
- nutritional E63.9
- oast-house-urine E72.19
  - ocular
    - herpesviral B00.50
    - zoster B02.30
- obliterative vascular I77.1
- Ohara's — *see* Tularemia
- Opitz's (congestive splenomegaly) D73.2
- Oppenheim-Urbach (necrobiosis lipoidica diabeticorum) — *see* E08-E13 with .620
- optic nerve NEC — *see* Disorder, nerve, optic
- orbit — *see* Disorder, orbit
- Oriental liver fluke B66.1
- Oriental lung fluke B66.4
- Ormond's N13.5
- Oropouche virus A93.0
- Osler-Rendu (familial hemorrhagic telangiectasia) I78.0
- osteofibrocystic E21.0
- Otto's M24.7
- outer ear — *see* Disorder, ear, external
- ovary (noninflammatory) N83.9
  - cystic N83.20- ☑
  - inflammatory — *see* Salpingo-oophoritis
  - polycystic E28.2
  - specified NEC N83.8
- Owren's (congenital) — *see* Defect, coagulation
- pancreas K86.9
  - cystic K86.2
  - fibrocystic E84.9
  - specified NEC K86.89
- panvalvular I08.9
  - specified NEC I08.8
- parametrium (noninflammatory) N83.9
- parasitic B89
  - cerebral NEC B71.9 [G94]
  - intestinal NOS B82.9
  - mouth B37.0
  - skin NOS B88.9
  - specified type — *see* Infestation
  - tongue B37.0
- parathyroid (gland) E21.5
  - specified NEC E21.4
- Parkinson's G20
- parodontal K05.6
- Parrot's (syphilitic osteochondritis) A50.02
- Parry's (exophthalmic goiter) — *see* Hyperthyroidism, with, goiter (diffuse)
- Parson's (exophthalmic goiter) — *see* Hyperthyroidism, with, goiter (diffuse)
- Paxton's (white piedra) B36.2
- pearl-worker's — *see* Osteomyelitis, specified type NEC
- Pellegrini-Stieda (calcification, knee joint) — *see* Bursitis, tibial collateral
- pelvis, pelvic
  - female NOS N94.9
    - specified NEC N94.89
  - gonococcal (acute) (chronic) A54.24
  - inflammatory (female) N73.9
    - acute N73.0
    - chlamydial A56.11
    - chronic N73.1
    - specified NEC N73.8
    - syphilitic (secondary) A51.42
      - late A52.76
    - tuberculous A18.17
  - organ, female N94.9
  - peritoneum, female NEC N94.89
- penis N48.9
  - inflammatory N48.29
    - abscess N48.21
    - cellulitis N48.22
  - specified NEC N48.89
- periapical tissues NOS K04.90

Disease, diseased — *continued*
- periodontal K05.6
  - specified NEC K05.5
- periosteum — *see* Disorder, bone, specified type NEC
- peripheral
  - arterial I73.9
  - autonomic nervous system G90.9
  - nerves — *see* Polyneuropathy
  - vascular NOS I73.9
- peritoneum K66.9
  - pelvic, female NEC N94.89
  - specified NEC K66.8
- persistent mucosal (middle ear) H66.20
  - left H66.22
    - with right H66.23
  - right H66.21
    - with left H66.23
- Petit's — *see* Hernia, abdomen, specified site NEC
- pharynx J39.2
  - specified NEC J39.2
- Phocas' — *see* Mastopathy, cystic
- photochromogenic (acid-fast bacilli) (pulmonary) A31.0
  - nonpulmonary A31.9
- Pick's G31.01 [F02.80]
  - with behavioral disturbance G31.01 [F02.81]
    - brain G31.01 [F02.80]
      - with behavioral disturbance G31.01 [F02.81]
  - of pericardium (pericardial pseudocirrhosis of liver) I31.1
- pigeon fancier's J67.2
- pineal gland E34.8
- pink — *see* Poisoning, mercury
- Pinkus' (lichen nitidus) L44.1
- pinworm B80
- Piry virus A93.8
- pituitary (gland) E23.7
- pituitary-snuff-taker's J67.8
- pleura (cavity) J94.9
  - specified NEC J94.8
- pneumatic drill (hammer) T75.21 ☑
- Pollitzer's (hidradenitis suppurativa) L73.2
- polycystic
  - kidney or renal Q61.3
    - adult type Q61.2
    - childhood type NEC Q61.19
      - collecting duct dilatation Q61.11
  - liver or hepatic Q44.6
  - lung or pulmonary J98.4
    - congenital Q33.0
  - ovary, ovaries E28.2
  - spleen Q89.09
- polyethylene T84.05- ☑
- Pompe's (glycogenosis II) E74.02
- Posadas-Wernicke B38.9
- Potain's (pulmonary edema) — *see* Edema, lung
- prepuce N47.8
  - inflammatory N47.7
    - balanoposthitis N47.6
- Pringle's (tuberous sclerosis) Q85.1
- prion, central nervous system A81.9
  - specified NEC A81.89
- prostate N42.9
  - specified NEC N42.89
- protozoal B64
  - acanthamebiasis — *see* Acanthamebiasis
  - African trypanosomiasis — *see* African trypanosomiasis
  - babesiosis B60.0
  - Chagas disease — *see* Chagas disease
  - intestine, intestinal A07.9
  - leishmaniasis — *see* Leishmaniasis
  - malaria — *see* Malaria
  - naegleriasis B60.2
  - pneumocystosis B59
  - specified organism NEC B60.8
  - toxoplasmosis — *see* Toxoplasmosis
- pseudo-Hurler's E77.0
- psychiatric F99
- psychotic — *see* Psychosis
- Puente's (simple glandular cheilitis) K13.0
- puerperal (*see also* Puerperal) O90.89
- pulmonary (*see also* Disease, lung)
  - artery I28.9
  - chronic obstructive J44.9
    - with
      - acute bronchitis J44.0
      - exacerbation (acute) J44.1

Disease, diseased — *continued*
 pulmonary (*see also* Disease, lung) — *continued*
  chronic obstructive — *continued*
   with — *continued*
    lower respiratory infection (acute) J44.0
    decompensated J44.1
     with
      exacerbation (acute) J44.1
  heart I27.9
   specified NEC I27.89
  hypertensive (vascular) (*see also* Hypertension, pulmonary) I27.20
   primary (idiopathic) I27.0
   NEC I27.2 ☑
  valve I37.9
   rheumatic I09.89
 pulp (dental) NOS K04.90
 pulseless M31.4
 Putnam's (subacute combined sclerosis with pernicious anemia) D51.0
 Pyle (-Cohn) (metaphyseal dysplasia) Q78.5
 ragpicker's or ragsorter's A22.1
 Raynaud's — *see* Raynaud's disease
 reactive airway — *see* Asthma
 Reclus' (cystic) — *see* Mastopathy, cystic
 rectum K62.9
  specified NEC K62.89
 Refsum's (heredopathia atactica polyneuritiformis) G60.1
 renal (functional) (pelvis) (*see also* Disease, kidney) N28.9
  with
   edema — *see* Nephrosis
   glomerular lesion — *see* Glomerulonephritis
    with edema — *see* Nephrosis
   interstitial nephritis N12
  acute N28.9
  chronic (*see also* Disease, kidney, chronic) N18.9
  cystic, congenital Q61.9
  diabetic — *see* E08-E13 with .22
  end-stage (failure) N18.6
   due to hypertension I12.0
  fibrocystic (congenital) Q61.8
  hypertensive — *see* Hypertension, kidney
  lupus M32.14
  phosphate-losing (tubular) N25.0
  polycystic (congenital) Q61.3
   adult type Q61.2
   childhood type NEC Q61.19
    collecting duct dilatation Q61.11
  rapidly progressive N01.9
  subacute N01.9
 Rendu-Osler-Weber (familial hemorrhagic telangiectasia) I78.0
 renovascular (arteriosclerotic) — *see* Hypertension, kidney
 respiratory (tract) J98.9
  acute or subacute NOS J06.9
   due to
    chemicals, gases, fumes or vapors (inhalation) J68.3
    external agent J70.9
     specified NEC J70.8
    radiation J70.0
    smoke inhalation J70.5
   noninfectious J39.8
  chronic NOS J98.9
   due to
    chemicals, gases, fumes or vapors J68.4
    external agent J70.9
     specified NEC J70.8
    radiation J70.1
   newborn P27.9
    specified NEC P27.8
  due to
   chemicals, gases, fumes or vapors J68.9
    acute or subacute NEC J68.3
    chronic J68.4
   external agent J70.9
    specified NEC J70.8
  newborn P28.9
   specified type NEC P28.89
  upper J39.9
   acute or subacute J06.9
   noninfectious NEC J39.8
   specified NEC J39.8
   streptococcal J06.9
 retina, retinal H35.9

Disease, diseased — *continued*
 retina, retinal — *continued*
  Batten's or Batten-Mayou E75.4 [H36]
  specified NEC H35.89
 rheumatoid — *see* Arthritis, rheumatoid
 rickettsial NOS A79.9
  specified type NEC A79.89
 Riga (-Fede) (cachectic aphthae) K14.0
 Riggs' (compound periodontitis) — *see* Periodontitis
 Ritter's L00
 Rivalta's (cervicofacial actinomycosis) A42.2
 Robles' (onchocerciasis) B73.01
 Roger's (congenital interventricular septal defect) Q21.0
 Rosenthal's (factor XI deficiency) D68.1
 Ross River B33.1
 Rossbach's (hyperchlorhydria) K30
 Rotes Quérol — *see* Hyperostosis, ankylosing
 Roth (-Bernhardt) — *see* Mononeuropathy, lower limb, meralgia paresthetica
 Runeberg's (progressive pernicious anemia) D51.0
 sacroiliac NEC M53.3
 salivary gland or duct K11.9
  inclusion B25.9
  specified NEC K11.8
  virus B25.9
 sandworm B76.9
 Schimmelbusch's — *see* Mastopathy, cystic
 Schmorl's — *see* Schmorl's disease or nodes
 Schönlein (-Henoch) (purpura rheumatica) D69.0
 Schottmüller's — *see* Fever, paratyphoid
 Schultz's (agranulocytosis) — *see* Agranulocytosis
 Schwalbe-Ziehen-Oppenheim G24.1
 Schwartz-Jampel G71.13
 sclera H15.9
  specified NEC H15.89
 scrofulous (tuberculous) A18.2
 scrotum N50.9
 sebaceous glands L73.9
 semilunar cartilage, cystic (*see also* Derangement, knee, meniscus, cystic)
 seminal vesicle N50.9
 serum NEC (*see also* Reaction, serum) T80.69 ☑
 sexually transmitted A64
  anogenital
   herpesviral infection — *see* Herpes, anogenital warts A63.0
   chancroid A57
   chlamydial infection — *see* Chlamydia
   gonorrhea — *see* Gonorrhea
   granuloma inguinale A58
   specified organism NEC A63.8
   syphilis — *see* Syphilis
   trichomoniasis — *see* Trichomoniasis
 Sézary C84.1- ☑
 shimamushi (scrub typhus) A75.3
 shipyard B30.0
 sickle-cell D57.1
  with crisis (vasoocclusive pain) D57.00
   with
    acute chest syndrome D57.01
    splenic sequestration D57.02
  elliptocytosis D57.8- ☑
  Hb-C D57.20
   with crisis (vasoocclusive pain) D57.219
    with
     acute chest syndrome D57.211
     splenic sequestration D57.212
   without crisis D57.20
  Hb-SD D57.80
   with crisis D57.819
    with
     acute chest syndrome D57.811
     splenic sequestration D57.812
  Hb-SE D57.80
   with crisis D57.819
    with
     acute chest syndrome D57.811
     splenic sequestration D57.812
  specified NEC D57.80
   with crisis D57.819
    with
     acute chest syndrome D57.811
     splenic sequestration D57.812
  spherocytosis D57.80
   with crisis D57.819
    with
     acute chest syndrome D57.811

Disease, diseased — *continued*
 sickle-cell — *continued*
  spherocytosis — *continued*
   with crisis — *continued*
    with — *continued*
     splenic sequestration D57.812
   thalassemia D57.40
    with crisis (vasoocclusive pain) D57.419
     with
      acute chest syndrome D57.411
      splenic sequestration D57.412
    without crisis D57.40
 silo-filler's J68.8
  bronchitis J68.0
  pneumonitis J68.0
  pulmonary edema J68.1
 simian B B00.4
 Simons' (progressive lipodystrophy) E88.1
 sin nombre virus B33.4
 sinus — *see* Sinusitis
 Sirkari's B55.0
 sixth B08.20
  due to human herpesvirus 6 B08.21
  due to human herpesvirus 7 B08.22
 skin L98.9
  due to metabolic disorder NEC E88.9 [L99]
  specified NEC L98.8
 slim (HIV) B20
 small vessel I73.9
 Sneddon-Wilkinson (subcorneal pustular dermatosis) L13.1
 South African creeping B88.0
 spinal (cord) G95.9
  congenital Q06.9
  specified NEC G95.89
 spine (*see also* Spondylopathy)
  joint — *see* Dorsopathy
  tuberculous A18.01
 spinocerebellar (hereditary) G11.9
  specified NEC G11.8
 spleen D73.9
  amyloid E85.4 [D77]
  organic D73.9
  polycystic Q89.09
  postinfectional D73.89
 sponge-diver's — *see* Toxicity, venom, marine animal, sea anemone
 Startle Q89.8
 Steinert's G71.11
 Sticker's (erythema infectiosum) B08.3
 Stieda's (calcification, knee joint) — *see* Bursitis, tibial collateral
 Stokes' (exophthalmic goiter) — *see* Hyperthyroidism, with, goiter (diffuse)
 Stokes-Adams (syncope with heart block) I45.9
 stomach K31.9
  functional, psychogenic F45.8
  specified NEC K31.89
 stonemason's J62.8
 storage
  glycogen — *see* Disease, glycogen storage
  mucopolysaccharide — *see* Mucopolysaccharidosis
 striatopallidal system NEC G25.89
 Stuart-Prower (congenital factor X deficiency) D68.2
 Stuart's (congenital factor X deficiency) D68.2
 subcutaneous tissue — *see* Disease, skin
 supporting structures of teeth K08.9
  specified NEC K08.89
 suprarenal (capsule) (gland) E27.9
  hyperfunction E27.0
  specified NEC E27.8
 sweat glands L74.9
  specified NEC L74.8
 Sweeley-Klionsky E75.21
 Swift (-Feer) — *see* Poisoning, mercury
 swimming-pool granuloma A31.1
 Sylvest's (epidemic pleurodynia) B33.0
 sympathetic nervous system G90.9
 synovium — *see* Disorder, synovium
 syphilitic — *see* Syphilis
 systemic tissue mast cell C96.20
 tanapox (virus) B08.71
 Tangier E78.6
 Tarral-Besnier (pityriasis rubra pilaris) L44.0
 Tauri's E74.09
 tear duct — *see* Disorder, lacrimal system
 tendon, tendinous (*see also* Disorder, tendon)
  nodular — *see* Trigger finger

Disease, diseased — *continued*
  terminal vessel I73.9
  testis N50.9
  thalassemia Hb-S — *see* Disease, sickle-cell, tha-
      lassemia
  Thaysen-Gee (nontropical sprue) K90.0
  Thomsen G71.12
  throat J39.2
      septic J02.0
  thromboembolic — *see* Embolism
  thymus (gland) E32.9
      specified NEC E32.8
  thyroid (gland) E07.9
      heart (*see also* Hyperthyroidism) E05.90 [I43]
          with thyroid storm E05.91 [I43]
      specified NEC E07.89
  Tietze's M94.0
  tongue K14.9
      specified NEC K14.8
  tonsils, tonsillar (and adenoids) J35.9
  tooth, teeth K08.9
      hard tissues K03.9
          specified NEC K03.89
      pulp NEC K04.99
      specified NEC K08.89
  Tourette's F95.2
  trachea NEC J39.8
  tricuspid I07.9
      nonrheumatic I36.9
  triglyceride-storage E75.5
  trophoblastic — *see* Mole, hydatidiform
  tsutsugamushi A75.3
  tube (fallopian) (noninflammatory) N83.9
      inflammatory — *see* Salpingitis
      specified NEC N83.8
  tuberculous NEC — *see* Tuberculosis
  tubo-ovarian (noninflammatory) N83.9
      inflammatory — *see* Salpingo-oophoritis
      specified NEC N83.8
  tubotympanic, chronic — *see* Otitis, media, suppura-
      tive, chronic, tubotympanic
  tubulo-interstitial N15.9
      specified NEC N15.8
  tympanum — *see* Disorder, tympanic membrane
  Uhl's Q24.8
  Underwood's (sclerema neonatorum) P83.0
  Unverricht (-Lundborg) — *see* Epilepsy, generalized,
      idiopathic
  Urbach-Oppenheim (necrobiosis lipoidica diabetico-
      rum) — *see* E08-E13 with .620
  ureter N28.9
      in (due to)
          schistosomiasis (bilharziasis) B65.0 [N29]
  urethra N36.9
      specified NEC N36.8
  urinary (tract) N39.9
      bladder N32.9
          specified NEC N32.89
      specified NEC N39.8
  uterus (noninflammatory) N85.9
      infective — *see* Endometritis
      inflammatory — *see* Endometritis
      specified NEC N85.8
  uveal tract (anterior) H21.9
      posterior H31.9
  vagabond's B85.1
  vagina, vaginal (noninflammatory) N89.9
      inflammatory NEC N76.89
      specified NEC N89.8
  valve, valvular I38
      multiple I08.9
      specified NEC I08.8
  van Creveld-von Gierke (glycogenosis I) E74.01
  vas deferens N50.9
  vascular I99.9
      arteriosclerotic — *see* Arteriosclerosis
      ciliary body NEC — *see* Disorder, iris, vascular
      hypertensive — *see* Hypertension
      iris NEC — *see* Disorder, iris, vascular
      obliterative I77.1
          peripheral I73.9
      occlusive I99.8
      peripheral (occlusive) I73.9
          in diabetes mellitus — *see* E08-E13 with .51
  vasomotor I73.9
  vasospastic I73.9
  vein I87.9
  venereal (*see also* Disease, sexually transmitted) A64

Disease, diseased — *continued*
  venereal (*see also* Disease, sexually transmitted) —
      continued
      chlamydial NEC A56.8
          anus A56.3
          genitourinary NOS A56.2
          pharynx A56.4
          rectum A56.3
      fifth A55
      sixth A55
      specified nature or type NEC A63.8
  vertebra, vertebral (*see also* Spondylopathy)
      disc — *see* Disorder, disc
  vibration — *see* Vibration, adverse effects
  viral, virus (*see also* Disease, by type of virus) B34.9
      arbovirus NOS A94
      arthropod-borne NOS A94
      congenital P35.9
          specified NEC P35.8
      Hanta (with renal manifestations) (Dobrava) (Pu-
          umala) (Seoul) A98.5
          with pulmonary manifestations (Andes) (Bayou)
              (Bermejo) (Black Creek Canal) (Choclo)
              (Juquitiba) (Laguna negra) (Lechiguanas)
              (New York) (Oran) (Sin nombre) B33.4
      Hantaan (Korean hemorrhagic fever) A98.5
      human immunodeficiency (HIV) B20
      Kunjin A83.4
      nonarthropod-borne NOS B34.9
      Powassan A84.8
      Rocio (encephalitis) A83.6
      Sin nombre (Hantavirus) (cardio)-pulmonary syn-
          drome) B33.4
      Tahyna B33.8
      vesicular stomatitis A93.8
  vitreous H43.9
      specified NEC H43.89
  vocal cord J38.3
  Volkmann's, acquired T79.6 ☑
  von Eulenburg's (congenital paramyotonia) G71.19
  von Gierke's (glycogenosis I) E74.01
  von Graefe's — *see* Strabismus, paralytic, ophthalmo-
      plegia, progressive
  von Willebrand (-Jürgens) (angiohemophilia) D68.0
  Vrolik's (osteogenesis imperfecta) Q78.0
  vulva (noninflammatory) N90.9
      inflammatory NEC N76.89
      specified NEC N90.89
  Wallgren's (obstruction of splenic vein with collateral
      circulation) I87.8
  Wassilieff's (leptospiral jaundice) A27.0
  wasting NEC R64
      due to malnutrition E41
  Waterhouse-Friderichsen A39.1
  Wegner's (syphilitic osteochondritis) A50.02
  Weil's (leptospiral jaundice of lung) A27.0
  Weir Mitchell's (erythromelalgia) I73.81
  Werdnig-Hoffmann G12.0
  Wermer's E31.21
  Werner-His (trench fever) A79.0
  Werner-Schultz (neutropenic splenomegaly) D73.81
  Wernicke-Posadas B38.9
  whipworm B79
  white blood cells D72.9
      specified NEC D72.89
  white matter R90.82
  white-spot, meaning lichen sclerosus et atrophicus
      L90.0
      penis N48.0
      vulva N90.4
  Wilkie's K55.1
  Wilkinson-Sneddon (subcorneal pustular dermatosis)
      L13.1
  Willis' — *see* Diabetes
  Wilson's (hepatolenticular degeneration) E83.01
  woolsorter's A22.1
  yaba monkey tumor B08.72
  yaba pox (virus) B08.72
  Zika virus A92.5
  zoonotic, bacterial A28.9
      specified type NEC A28.8
Disfigurement (due to scar) L90.5
Disgerminoma — *see* Dysgerminoma
DISH (diffuse idiopathic skeletal hyperostosis) — *see*
      Hyperostosis, ankylosing
Disinsertion, retina — *see* Detachment, retina
Dislocatable hip, congenital Q65.6

Dislocation (articular)
  with fracture — *see* Fracture
  acromioclavicular (joint) S43.10- ☑
      with displacement
          100%-200% S43.12- ☑
          more than 200% S43.13- ☑
      inferior S43.14- ☑
      posterior S43.15- ☑
  ankle S93.0- ☑
  astragalus — *see* Dislocation, ankle
  atlantoaxial S13.121 ☑
  atlantooccipital S13.111 ☑
  atloidooccipital S13.111 ☑
  breast bone S23.29 ☑
  capsule, joint — *code by* site under Dislocation
  carpal (bone) — *see* Dislocation, wrist
  carpometacarpal (joint) NEC S63.05- ☑
      thumb S63.04- ☑
  cartilage (joint) — *code by* site under Dislocation
  cervical spine (vertebra) — *see* Dislocation, vertebra,
      cervical
  chronic — *see* Dislocation, recurrent
  clavicle — *see* Dislocation, acromioclavicular joint
  coccyx S33.2 ☑
  congenital NEC Q68.8
  coracoid — *see* Dislocation, shoulder
  costal cartilage S23.29 ☑
  costochondral S23.29 ☑
  cricoarytenoid articulation S13.29 ☑
  cricothyroid articulation S13.29 ☑
  dorsal vertebra — *see* Dislocation, vertebra, thoracic
  ear ossicle — *see* Discontinuity, ossicles, ear
  elbow S53.10- ☑
      congenital Q68.8
      pathological — *see* Dislocation, pathological NEC,
          elbow
      radial head alone — *see* Dislocation, radial head
      recurrent — *see* Dislocation, recurrent, elbow
      traumatic S53.10- ☑
          anterior S53.11- ☑
          lateral S53.14- ☑
          medial S53.13- ☑
          posterior S53.12- ☑
          specified type NEC S53.19- ☑
  eye, nontraumatic — *see* Luxation, globe
  eyeball, nontraumatic — *see* Luxation, globe
  femur
      distal end — *see* Dislocation, knee
      proximal end — *see* Dislocation, hip
  fibula
      distal end — *see* Dislocation, ankle
      proximal end — *see* Dislocation, knee
  finger S63.25- ☑
      index S63.25- ☑
      interphalangeal S63.27- ☑
          distal S63.29- ☑
              index S63.29- ☑
              little S63.29- ☑
              middle S63.29- ☑
              ring S63.29- ☑
          index S63.27- ☑
          little S63.27- ☑
          middle S63.27- ☑
          proximal S63.28- ☑
              index S63.28- ☑
              little S63.28- ☑
              middle S63.28- ☑
              ring S63.28- ☑
          ring S63.27- ☑
      little S63.25- ☑
      metacarpophalangeal S63.26- ☑
          index S63.26- ☑
          little S63.26- ☑
          middle S63.26- ☑
          ring S63.26- ☑
      middle S63.25- ☑
      recurrent — *see* Dislocation, recurrent, finger
      ring S63.25- ☑
      thumb — *see* Dislocation, thumb
  foot S93.30- ☑
      recurrent — *see* Dislocation, recurrent, foot
      specified site NEC S93.33- ☑
      tarsal joint S93.31- ☑
      tarsometatarsal joint S93.32- ☑
      toe — *see* Dislocation, toe
  fracture — *see* Fracture

Dislocation — continued
glenohumeral (joint) — see Dislocation, shoulder
glenoid — see Dislocation, shoulder
habitual — see Dislocation, recurrent
hip S73.00- ☑
  anterior S73.03- ☑
    obturator S73.02- ☑
  central S73.04- ☑
  congenital (total) Q65.2
    bilateral Q65.1
    partial Q65.5
      bilateral Q65.4
      unilateral Q65.3- ☑
    unilateral Q65.0- ☑
  developmental M24.85- ☑
  pathological — see Dislocation, pathological NEC, hip
  posterior S73.01- ☑
  recurrent — see Dislocation, recurrent, hip
humerus, proximal end — see Dislocation, shoulder
incomplete — see Subluxation, by site
incus — see Discontinuity, ossicles, ear
infracoracoid — see Dislocation, shoulder
innominate (pubic junction) (sacral junction) S33.39 ☑
  acetabulum — see Dislocation, hip
interphalangeal (joint(s))
  finger S63.279 ☑
    distal S63.29- ☑
      index S63.29- ☑
      little S63.29- ☑
      middle S63.29- ☑
      ring S63.29- ☑
    index S63.27- ☑
    little S63.27- ☑
    middle S63.27- ☑
    proximal S63.28- ☑
      index S63.28- ☑
      little S63.28- ☑
      middle S63.28- ☑
      ring S63.28- ☑
    ring S63.27- ☑
  foot or toe — see Dislocation, toe
  thumb S63.12- ☑
    distal joint S63.14- ☑
    proximal joint S63.13- ☑
jaw (cartilage) (meniscus) S03.0- ☑
joint prosthesis — see Complications, joint prosthesis, mechanical, displacement, by site
knee S83.106 ☑
  cap — see Dislocation, patella
  congenital Q68.2
  old M23.8X- ☑
  patella — see Dislocation, patella
  pathological — see Dislocation, pathological NEC, knee
  proximal tibia
    anteriorly S83.11- ☑
    laterally S83.14- ☑
    medially S83.13- ☑
    posteriorly S83.12- ☑
  recurrent (see also Derangement, knee, specified NEC)
  specified type NEC S83.19- ☑
lacrimal gland H04.16- ☑
lens (complete) H27.10
  anterior H27.12- ☑
  congenital Q12.1
  ocular implant — see Complications, intraocular lens
  partial H27.11- ☑
  posterior H27.13- ☑
  traumatic S05.8X- ☑
ligament — code by site under Dislocation
lumbar (vertebra) — see Dislocation, vertebra, lumbar
lumbosacral (vertebra) (see also Dislocation, vertebra, lumbar)
  congenital Q76.49
mandible S03.0- ☑
meniscus (knee) — see Tear, meniscus
  other sites - code by site under Dislocation
metacarpal (bone)
  distal end — see Dislocation, finger
  proximal end S63.06- ☑
metacarpophalangeal (joint)
  finger S63.26- ☑
    index S63.26- ☑

Dislocation — continued
metacarpophalangeal — continued
  finger — continued
    little S63.26- ☑
    middle S63.26- ☑
    ring S63.26- ☑
    thumb S63.11- ☑
metatarsal (bone) — see Dislocation, foot
metatarsophalangeal (joint(s)) — see Dislocation, toe
midcarpal (joint) S63.03- ☑
midtarsal (joint) — see Dislocation, foot
neck S13.20
  specified site NEC S13.29 ☑
  vertebra — see Dislocation, vertebra, cervical
nose (septal cartilage) S03.1 ☑
occipitoatloid S13.111 ☑
old — see Derangement, joint, specified type NEC
ossicles, ear — see Discontinuity, ossicles, ear
partial — see Subluxation, by site
patella S83.006 ☑
  congenital Q74.1
  lateral S83.01- ☑
  recurrent (nontraumatic) M22.0- ☑
    incomplete M22.1- ☑
  specified type NEC S83.09- ☑
pathological NEC M24.30
  ankle M24.37- ☑
  elbow M24.32- ☑
  foot joint M24.37- ☑
  hand joint M24.34- ☑
  hip M24.35- ☑
  knee M24.36- ☑
  lumbosacral joint — see subcategory M53.2 ☑
  pelvic region — see Dislocation, pathological, hip
  sacroiliac — see subcategory M53.2 ☑
  shoulder M24.31- ☑
  wrist M24.33- ☑
pelvis NEC S33.30 ☑
  specified NEC S33.39 ☑
phalanx
  finger or hand — see Dislocation, finger
  foot or toe — see Dislocation, toe
prosthesis, internal — see Complications, prosthetic device, by site, mechanical
radial head S53.006 ☑
  anterior S53.01- ☑
  posterior S53.02- ☑
  specified type NEC S53.09- ☑
radiocarpal (joint) S63.02- ☑
radiohumeral (joint) — see Dislocation, radial head
radioulnar (joint)
  distal S63.01- ☑
  proximal — see Dislocation, elbow
radius
  distal end — see Dislocation, wrist
  proximal end — see Dislocation, radial head
recurrent M24.40
  ankle M24.47- ☑
  elbow M24.42- ☑
  finger M24.44- ☑
  foot joint M24.47- ☑
  hand joint M24.44- ☑
  hip M24.45- ☑
  knee M24.46- ☑
    patella — see Dislocation, patella, recurrent
  patella — see Dislocation, patella, recurrent
  sacroiliac — see subcategory M53.2 ☑
  shoulder M24.41- ☑
  toe M24.47- ☑
  vertebra (see also subcategory) M43.5 ☑
    atlantoaxial M43.4
      with myelopathy M43.3
  wrist M24.43- ☑
rib (cartilage) S23.29 ☑
sacrococcygeal S33.2 ☑
sacroiliac (joint) (ligament) S33.2 ☑
  congenital Q74.2
  recurrent — see subcategory M53.2 ☑
sacrum S33.2 ☑
scaphoid (bone) (hand) (wrist) — see Dislocation, wrist
  foot — see Dislocation, foot
scapula — see Dislocation, shoulder, girdle, scapula
semilunar cartilage, knee — see Tear, meniscus
septal cartilage (nose) S03.1 ☑
septum (nasal) (old) J34.2

Dislocation — continued
sesamoid bone — code by site under Dislocation
shoulder (blade) (ligament) (joint) (traumatic) S43.006 ☑
  acromioclavicular — see Dislocation, acromioclavicular
  chronic — see Dislocation, recurrent, shoulder
  congenital Q68.8
  girdle S43.30- ☑
    scapula S43.31- ☑
    specified site NEC S43.39- ☑
  humerus S43.00- ☑
    anterior S43.01- ☑
    inferior S43.03- ☑
    posterior S43.02- ☑
  pathological — see Dislocation, pathological NEC, shoulder
  recurrent — see Dislocation, recurrent, shoulder
  specified type NEC S43.08- ☑
spine
  cervical — see Dislocation, vertebra, cervical
  congenital Q76.49
  due to birth trauma P11.5
  lumbar — see Dislocation, vertebra, lumbar
  thoracic — see Dislocation, vertebra, thoracic
spontaneous — see Dislocation, pathological
sternoclavicular (joint) S43.206 ☑
  anterior S43.21- ☑
  posterior S43.22- ☑
sternum S23.29 ☑
subglenoid — see Dislocation, shoulder
symphysis pubis S33.4 ☑
talus — see Dislocation, ankle
tarsal (bone(s)) (joint(s)) — see Dislocation, foot
tarsometatarsal (joint(s)) — see Dislocation, foot
temporomandibular (joint) S03.0- ☑
thigh, proximal end — see Dislocation, hip
thorax S23.20 ☑
  specified site NEC S23.29 ☑
  vertebra — see Dislocation, vertebra
thumb S63.10- ☑
  interphalangeal joint — see Dislocation, interphalangeal (joint), thumb
  metacarpophalangeal joint — see Dislocation, metacarpophalangeal (joint), thumb
thyroid cartilage S13.29 ☑
tibia
  distal end — see Dislocation, ankle
  proximal end — see Dislocation, knee
tibiofibular (joint)
  distal — see Dislocation, ankle
  superior — see Dislocation, knee
toe(s) S93.106 ☑
  great S93.10- ☑
    interphalangeal joint S93.11- ☑
    metatarsophalangeal joint S93.12- ☑
  interphalangeal joint S93.119 ☑
  lesser S93.106 ☑
    interphalangeal joint S93.11- ☑
    metatarsophalangeal joint S93.12- ☑
  metatarsophalangeal joint S93.12- ☑
tooth S03.2 ☑
trachea S23.29 ☑
ulna
  distal end S63.07- ☑
  proximal end — see Dislocation, elbow
ulnohumeral (joint) — see Dislocation, elbow
vertebra (articular process) (body) (traumatic)
  cervical S13.101 ☑
    atlantoaxial joint S13.121 ☑
    atlantooccipital joint S13.111 ☑
    atloidooccipital joint S13.111 ☑
    joint between
      C0 and C1 S13.111 ☑
      C1 and C2 S13.121 ☑
      C2 and C3 S13.131 ☑
      C3 and C4 S13.141 ☑
      C4 and C5 S13.151 ☑
      C5 and C6 S13.161 ☑
      C6 and C7 S13.171 ☑
      C7 and T1 S13.181 ☑
    occipitoatloid joint S13.111 ☑
  congenital Q76.49
  lumbar S33.101 ☑
    joint between
      L1 and L2 S33.111 ☑

☑ Additional Character Required — Refer to the Tabular List for Character Selection   ▽ Subterms under main terms may continue to next column or page

Dislocation — continued
  vertebra — continued
    lumbar — continued
      joint between — continued
        L2 and L3 S33.121 ☑
        L3 and L4 S33.131 ☑
        L4 and L5 S33.141 ☑
    nontraumatic — see Displacement, intervertebral disc
    partial — see Subluxation, by site
    recurrent NEC — see subcategory M43.5 ☑
    thoracic S23.101 ☑
      joint between
        T1 and T2 S23.111 ☑
        T2 and T3 S23.121 ☑
        T3 and T4 S23.123 ☑
        T4 and T5 S23.131 ☑
        T5 and T6 S23.133 ☑
        T6 and T7 S23.141 ☑
        T7 and T8 S23.143 ☑
        T8 and T9 S23.151 ☑
        T9 and T10 S23.153 ☑
        T10 and T11 S23.161 ☑
        T11 and T12 S23.163 ☑
        T12 and L1 S23.171 ☑
  wrist (carpal bone) S63.006 ☑
    carpometacarpal joint — see Dislocation, carpometacarpal (joint)
    distal radioulnar joint — see Dislocation, radioulnar (joint), distal
    metacarpal bone, proximal — see Dislocation, metacarpal (bone), proximal end
    midcarpal — see Dislocation, midcarpal (joint)
    radiocarpal joint — see Dislocation, radiocarpal (joint)
    recurrent — see Dislocation, recurrent, wrist
    specified site NEC S63.09- ☑
    ulna — see Dislocation, ulna, distal end
  xiphoid cartilage S23.29 ☑

Disorder (of) (see also Disease)
  acantholytic L11.9
    specified NEC L11.8
  acute
    psychotic — see Psychosis, acute
    stress F43.0
  adjustment (grief) F43.20
    with
      anxiety F43.22
        with depressed mood F43.23
      conduct disturbance F43.24
        with emotional disturbance F43.25
      depressed mood F43.21
        with anxiety F43.23
      other specified symptom F43.29
  adrenal (capsule) (gland) (medullary) E27.9
    specified NEC E27.8
  adrenogenital E25.9
    drug-induced E25.8
    iatrogenic E25.8
    idiopathic E25.8
  adult personality (and behavior) F69
    specified NEC F68.8
  affective (mood) — see Disorder, mood
  aggressive, unsocialized F91.1
  alcohol use
    mild F10.10
      with
        alcohol intoxication F10.129
          delirium F10.121
        alcohol-induced
          anxiety disorder F10.180
          bipolar and related disorder F10.14
          depressive disorder F10.14
          psychotic disorder F10.159
          sexual dysfunction F10.181
          sleep disorder F10.182
      in remission (early) (sustained) F10.11
    moderate or severe F10.20
      with
        alcohol intoxication F10.229
          delirium F10.221
        alcohol-induced
          anxiety disorder F10.280
          bipolar and related disorder F10.24
          depressive disorder F10.24
          major neurocognitive disorder, amnestic-confabulatory type F10.26

Disorder — continued
  alcohol use — continued
    moderate or severe — continued
      with
        alcohol-induced — continued
          major neurocognitive disorder, non-amnestic-confabulatory type F10.27
          mild neurocognitive disorder F10.288
          psychotic disorder F10.259
          sexual dysfunction F10.281
          sleep disorder F10.282
      in remission (early) (sustained) F10.21
  alcohol-related F10.99
    with
      amnestic disorder, persisting F10.96
      anxiety disorder F10.980
      dementia, persisting F10.97
      intoxication F10.929
        with delirium F10.921
        uncomplicated F10.920
      mood disorder F10.94
      other specified F10.988
      psychotic disorder F10.959
        with
          delusions F10.950
          hallucinations F10.951
      sexual dysfunction F10.981
      sleep disorder F10.982
  allergic — see Allergy
  alveolar NEC J84.09
  amino-acid
    cystathioninuria E72.19
    cystinosis E72.04
    cystinuria E72.01
    glycinuria E72.09
    homocystinuria E72.11
    metabolism — see Disturbance, metabolism, amino-acid
    specified NEC E72.8
    neonatal, transitory P74.8
    renal transport NEC E72.09
    transport NEC E72.09
  amnesic, amnestic
    alcohol-induced F10.96
      with dependence F10.26
    due to (secondary to) general medical condition F04
    psychoactive NEC-induced F19.96
      with
        abuse F19.16
        dependence F19.26
    sedative, hypnotic or anxiolytic-induced F13.96
      with dependence F13.26
  amphetamine (or other stimulant) use
    mild
      with
        amphetamine, cocaine, or other stimulant intoxication
          with perceptual disturbances F15.122
          without perceptual disturbances F15.129
        amphetamine (or other stimulant) -induced
          anxiety disorder F15.180
          bipolar and related disorder F15.14
          depressive disorder F15.14
          obsessive-compulsive and related disorder F15.188
          psychotic disorder F15.159
          sexual dysfunction F15.181
        intoxication delirium F15.121
    moderate or severe
      with
        amphetamine, cocaine, or other stimulant intoxication
          with perceptual disturbances F15.222
          without perceptual disturbances F15.229
        amphetamine (or other stimulant) -induced
          anxiety disorder F15.280
          bipolar and related disorder F15.24
          depressive disorder F15.24
          obsessive-compulsive and related disorder F15.288
          psychotic disorder F15.259
          sexual dysfunction F15.281
        intoxication delirium F15.221
  amphetamine-type substance use
    mild F15.10
      in remission (early) (sustained) F15.11
    moderate F15.20

Disorder — continued
  amphetamine-type substance use — continued
    moderate — continued
      in remission (early) (sustained) F15.21
    severe F15.20
      in remission (early) (sustained) F15.21
  anaerobic glycolysis with anemia D55.2
  anxiety F41.9
    due to (secondary to)
      alcohol F10.980
        in
          abuse F10.180
          dependence F10.280
      amphetamine F15.980
        in
          abuse F15.180
          dependence F15.280
      anxiolytic F13.980
        in
          abuse F13.180
          dependence F13.280
      caffeine F15.980
        in
          abuse F15.180
          dependence F15.280
      cannabis F12.980
        in
          abuse F12.180
          dependence F12.280
      cocaine F14.980
        in
          abuse F14.180
          dependence F14.180
      general medical condition F06.4
      hallucinogen F16.980
        in
          abuse F16.180
          dependence F16.280
      hypnotic F13.980
        in
          abuse F13.180
          dependence F13.280
      inhalant F18.980
        in
          abuse F18.180
          dependence F18.280
      phencyclidine F16.980
        in
          abuse F16.180
          dependence F16.280
      psychoactive substance NEC F19.980
        in
          abuse F19.180
          dependence F19.280
      sedative F13.980
        in
          abuse F13.180
          dependence F13.280
      volatile solvents F18.980
        in
          abuse F18.180
          dependence F18.280
    generalized F41.1
    illness F45.21
    mixed
      with depression (mild) F41.8
      specified NEC F41.3
    organic F06.4
    phobic F40.9
      of childhood F40.8
    specified NEC F41.8
  aortic valve — see Endocarditis, aortic
  aromatic amino-acid metabolism E70.9
    specified NEC E70.8
  arteriole NEC I77.89
  artery NEC I77.89
  articulation — see Disorder, joint
  attachment (childhood)
    disinhibited F94.2
    reactive F94.1
  attention-deficit hyperactivity (adolescent) (adult) (child) F90.9
    combined
      presentation F90.2
      type F90.2
    hyperactive
      impulsive presentation F90.1
      type F90.1

Index

Disorder — *continued*
  attention-deficit hyperactivity — *continued*
    inattentive
      presentation F90.0
      type F90.0
    specified type NEC F90.8
  attention-deficit without hyperactivity (adolescent) (adult) (child) F98.8
  auditory processing (central) H93.25
  autism spectrum F84.0
  autistic F84.0
  autoimmune D89.89
  autonomic nervous system G90.9
    specified NEC G90.8
  avoidant
    child or adolescent F40.10
    restrictive food intake F50.82
  balance
    acid-base E87.8
      mixed E87.4
    electrolyte E87.8
    fluid NEC E87.8
  behavioral (disruptive) — *see* Disorder, conduct
  beta-amino-acid metabolism E72.8
  bile acid and cholesterol metabolism E78.70
    Barth syndrome E78.71
    other specified E78.79
    Smith-Lemli-Opitz syndrome E78.72
  bilirubin excretion E80.6
  binge eating F50.81
  binocular
    movement H51.9
      convergence
        excess H51.12
        insufficiency H51.11
      internuclear ophthalmoplegia — *see* Ophthalmoplegia, internuclear
      palsy of conjugate gaze H51.0
      specified type NEC H51.8
    vision NEC — *see* Disorder, vision, binocular
  bipolar (I) (type I) F31.9
    and related due to a known physiological condition
      with
        manic features F06.33
        manic- or hypomanic-like episodes F06.33
        mixed features F06.34
    current (or most recent) episode
      depressed F31.9
        with psychotic features F31.5
        without psychotic features F31.30
          mild F31.31
          moderate F31.32
          severe (without psychotic features) F31.4
            with psychotic features F31.5
      hypomanic F31.0
      manic F31.9
        with psychotic features F31.2
        without psychotic features F31.10
          mild F31.11
          moderate F31.12
          severe (without psychotic features) F31.13
            with psychotic features F31.2
      mixed F31.60
        mild F31.61
        moderate F31.62
        severe (without psychotic features) F31.63
          with psychotic features F31.64
      severe depression (without psychotic features) F31.4
        with psychotic features F31.5
    in remission (currently) F31.70
      in full remission
        most recent episode
          depressed F31.76
          hypomanic F31.72
          manic F31.74
          mixed F31.78
      in partial remission
        most recent episode
          depressed F31.75
          hypomanic F31.71
          manic F31.73
          mixed F31.77
    organic F06.30
    single manic episode F30.9
      mild F30.11
      moderate F30.12
      severe (without psychotic symptoms) F30.13

Disorder — *continued*
  bipolar — *continued*
    single manic episode — *continued*
      severe — *continued*
        with psychotic symptoms F30.2
      specified NEC F31.89
  bipolar II (type 2) F31.81
  bladder N32.9
    functional NEC N31.9
    in schistosomiasis B65.0 [N33]
    specified NEC N32.89
  bleeding D68.9
  blood D75.9
    in congenital early syphilis A50.09 [D77]
  body dysmorphic F45.22
  bone M89.9
    continuity M84.9
      specified type NEC M84.80
        ankle M84.87- ☑
        fibula M84.86- ☑
        foot M84.87- ☑
        hand M84.84- ☑
        humerus M84.82- ☑
        neck M84.88
        pelvis M84.88
        radius M84.83- ☑
        rib M84.88
        shoulder M84.81- ☑
        skull M84.88
        thigh M84.85- ☑
        tibia M84.86- ☑
        ulna M84.83- ☑
        vertebra M84.88
    density and structure M85.9
      cyst (*see also* Cyst, bone, specified type NEC)
        aneurysmal — *see* Cyst, bone, aneurysmal
        solitary — *see* Cyst, bone, solitary
      diffuse idiopathic skeletal hyperostosis — *see* Hyperostosis, ankylosing
      fibrous dysplasia (monostotic) — *see* Dysplasia, fibrous, bone
      fluorosis — *see* Fluorosis, skeletal
      hyperostosis of skull M85.2
      osteitis condensans — *see* Osteitis, condensans
      specified type NEC M85.8- ☑
        ankle M85.87- ☑
        foot M85.87- ☑
        forearm M85.83- ☑
        hand M85.84- ☑
        lower leg M85.86- ☑
        multiple sites M85.89
        neck M85.88
        rib M85.88
        shoulder M85.81- ☑
        skull M85.88
        thigh M85.85- ☑
        upper arm M85.82- ☑
        vertebra M85.88
    development and growth NEC M89.20
      carpus M89.24- ☑
      clavicle M89.21- ☑
      femur M89.25- ☑
      fibula M89.26- ☑
      finger M89.24- ☑
      humerus M89.22- ☑
      ilium M89.259
      ischium M89.259
      metacarpus M89.24- ☑
      metatarsus M89.27- ☑
      multiple sites M89.29
      neck M89.28
      radius M89.23- ☑
      rib M89.28
      scapula M89.21- ☑
      skull M89.28
      tarsus M89.27- ☑
      tibia M89.26- ☑
      toe M89.27- ☑
      ulna M89.23- ☑
      vertebra M89.28
      specified type NEC M89.8X- ☑
  brachial plexus G54.0
  branched-chain amino-acid metabolism E71.2
    specified NEC E71.19
  breast N64.9
    agalactia — *see* Agalactia

Disorder — *continued*
  breast — *continued*
    associated with
      lactation O92.70
        specified NEC O92.79
      pregnancy O92.20
        specified NEC O92.29
      puerperium O92.20
        specified NEC O92.29
    cracked nipple — *see* Cracked nipple
    galactorrhea — *see* Galactorrhea
    hypogalactia O92.4
    lactation disorder NEC O92.79
    mastitis — *see* Mastitis
    nipple infection — *see* Infection, nipple
    retracted nipple — *see* Retraction, nipple
    specified type NEC N64.89
  Briquet's F45.0
  bullous, in diseases classified elsewhere L14
  caffeine use
    mild
      with
        caffeine-induced
          anxiety disorder F15.180
          sleep disorder F15.182
    moderate or severe
      with
        caffeine-induced
          anxiety disorder F15.280
          sleep disorder F15.282
  cannabis use
    mild F12.10
      with
        cannabis intoxication delirium F12.121
          with perceptual disturbances F12.122
          without perceptual disturbances F12.129
        cannabis-induced
          anxiety disorder F12.180
          psychotic disorder F12.159
          sleep disorder F12.188
      in remission (early) (sustained) F12.11
    moderate or severe F12.20
      with
        cannabis intoxication
          with perceptual disturbances F12.222
          without perceptual disturbances F12.229
        cannabis-induced
          anxiety disorder F12.280
          psychotic disorder F12.259
          sleep disorder F12.288
        delirium F12.221
      in remission (early) (sustained) F12.21
  carbohydrate
    absorption, intestinal NEC E74.39
    metabolism (congenital) E74.9
      specified NEC E74.8
  cardiac, functional I51.89
  carnitine metabolism E71.40
  cartilage M94.9
    articular NEC — *see* Derangement, joint, articular cartilage
    chondrocalcinosis — *see* Chondrocalcinosis
    specified type NEC M94.8X- ☑
      articular — *see* Derangement, joint, articular cartilage
      multiple sites M94.8X0
  catatonia (due to known physiological condition) (with another mental disorder) F06.1
  catatonic
    due to (secondary to) known physiological condition F06.1
    organic F06.1
  central auditory processing H93.25
  cervical
    region NEC M53.82
    root (nerve) NEC G54.2
  character NOS F60.9
  childhood disintegrative NEC F84.3
  cholesterol and bile acid metabolism E78.70
    Barth syndrome E78.71
    other specified E78.79
    Smith-Lemli-Opitz syndrome E78.72
  choroid H31.9
    atrophy — *see* Atrophy, choroid
    degeneration — *see* Degeneration, choroid
    detachment — *see* Detachment, choroid
    dystrophy — *see* Dystrophy, choroid
    hemorrhage — *see* Hemorrhage, choroid

  ☑ Additional Character Required — Refer to the Tabular List for Character Selection   Subterms under main terms may continue to next column or page

Disorder — *continued*
  choroid — *continued*
    rupture — *see* Rupture, choroid
    scar — *see* Scar, chorioretinal
    solar retinopathy — *see* Retinopathy, solar
    specified type NEC H31.8
  ciliary body — *see* Disorder, iris
    degeneration — *see* Degeneration, ciliary body
  coagulation (factor) (*see also* Defect, coagulation)
    D68.9
    newborn, transient P61.6
  cocaine use
    mild F14.10
      with
        amphetamine, cocaine, or other stimulant
          intoxication
            with perceptual disturbances F14.122
            without perceptual disturbances F14.129
        cocaine intoxication delirium F14.121
        cocaine-induced
          anxiety disorder F14.180
          bipolar and related disorder F14.14
          depressive disorder F14.14
          obsessive-compulsive and related disor-
            der F14.188
          psychotic disorder F14.159
          sexual dysfunction F14.181
          sleep disorder F14.182
      in remission (early) (sustained) F14.11
    moderate or severe F14.20
      with
        amphetamine, cocaine, or other stimulant
          intoxication
            with perceptual disturbances F14.222
            without perceptual disturbances F14.229
        cocaine intoxication delirium F14.221
        cocaine-induced
          anxiety disorder F14.280
          bipolar and related disorder F14.24
          depressive disorder F14.24
          obsessive-compulsive and related disor-
            der F14.288
          psychotic disorder F14.259
          sexual dysfunction F14.281
          sleep disorder F14.282
      in remission (early) (sustained) F14.21
  coccyx NEC M53.3
  cognitive F09
    due to (secondary to) general medical condition
      F09
    persisting R41.89
      due to
        alcohol F10.97
          with dependence F10.27
        anxiolytics F13.97
          with dependence F13.27
        hypnotics F13.97
          with dependence F13.27
        sedatives F13.97
          with dependence F13.27
        specified substance NEC F19.97
          with
            abuse F19.17
            dependence F19.27
  communication F80.9
    social pragmatic F80.82
  conduct (childhood) F91.9
    adjustment reaction — *see* Disorder, adjustment
    adolescent onset type F91.2
    childhood onset type F91.1
    compulsive F63.9
    confined to family context F91.0
    depressive F91.8
    group type F91.2
    hyperkinetic — *see* Disorder, attention-deficit hy-
      peractivity
    oppositional defiance F91.3
    socialized F91.2
    solitary aggressive type F91.1
    specified NEC F91.8
    unsocialized (aggressive) F91.1
  conduction, heart I45.9
  congenital glycosylation (CDG) E74.8
  conjunctiva H11.9
    infection — *see* Conjunctivitis
  connective tissue, localized L94.9
    specified NEC L94.8

Disorder — *continued*
  conversion (functional neurological symptom disorder)
    with
      abnormal movement F44.4
      anesthesia or sensory loss F44.6
      attacks or seizures F44.5
      mixed symptoms F44.7
      special sensory symptoms F44.6
      speech symptoms F44.4
      swallowing symptoms F44.4
      weakness or paralysis F44.4
  convulsive (secondary) — *see* Convulsions
  cornea H18.9
    deformity — *see* Deformity, cornea
    degeneration — *see* Degeneration, cornea
    deposits — *see* Deposit, cornea
    due to contact lens H18.82- ☑
      specified as edema — *see* Edema, cornea
    edema — *see* Edema, cornea
    keratitis — *see* Keratitis
    keratoconjunctivitis — *see* Keratoconjunctivitis
    membrane change — *see* Change, corneal mem-
      brane
    neovascularization — *see* Neovascularization,
      cornea
    scar — *see* Opacity, cornea
    specified type NEC H18.89- ☑
    ulcer — *see* Ulcer, cornea
  corpus cavernosum N48.9
  cranial nerve — *see* Disorder, nerve, cranial
  cyclothymic F34.0
  defiant oppositional F91.3
  delusional (persistent) (systematized) F22
    induced F24
  depersonalization F48.1
  depressive F32.9
    due to known physiological condition
      with
        depressive features F06.31
        major depressive-like episode F06.32
        mixed features F06.34
    major F32.9
      with psychotic symptoms F32.3
      in remission (full) F32.5
        partial F32.4
      recurrent F33.9
        with psychotic features F33.3
      single episode F32.9
        mild F32.0
        moderate F32.1
        severe (without psychotic symptoms) F32.2
          with psychotic symptoms F32.3
    organic F06.31
    persistent F34.1
    recurrent F33.9
      current episode
        mild F33.0
        moderate F33.1
        severe (without psychotic symptoms) F33.2
          with psychotic symptoms F33.3
      in remission F33.40
        full F33.42
        partial F33.41
      specified NEC F33.8
    single episode — *see* Episode, depressive
    specified NEC F32.89
  developmental F89
    arithmetical skills F81.2
    coordination (motor) F82
    expressive writing F81.81
    language F80.9
      expressive F80.1
      mixed receptive and expressive F80.2
      receptive type F80.2
      specified NEC F80.89
    learning F81.9
      arithmetical F81.2
      reading F81.0
    mixed F88
    motor coordination or function F82
    pervasive F84.9
      specified NEC F84.8
    phonological F80.0
    reading F81.0
    scholastic skills (*see also* Disorder, learning)
      mixed F81.89
    specified NEC F88
    speech F80.9

Disorder — *continued*
  developmental — *continued*
    speech — *continued*
      articulation F80.0
      specified NEC F80.89
    written expression F81.81
  diaphragm J98.6
  digestive (system) K92.9
    newborn P78.9
      specified NEC P78.89
    postprocedural — *see* Complication, gastrointesti-
      nal
    psychogenic F45.8
  disc (intervertebral) M51.9
    with
      myelopathy
        cervical region M50.00
        cervicothoracic region M50.03
        high cervical region M50.01
        lumbar region M51.06
        mid-cervical region M50.020
        sacrococcygeal region M53.3
        thoracic region M51.04
        thoracolumbar region M51.05
      radiculopathy
        cervical region M50.10
        cervicothoracic region M50.13
        high cervical region M50.11
        lumbar region M51.16
        lumbosacral region M51.17
        mid-cervical region M50.120
        sacrococcygeal region M53.3
        thoracic region M51.14
        thoracolumbar region M51.15
    cervical M50.90
      with
        myelopathy M50.00
          C2-C3 M50.01
          C3-C4 M50.01
          C4-C5 M50.021
          C5-C6 M50.022
          C6-C7 M50.023
          C7-T1 M50.03
          cervicothoracic region M50.03
          high cervical region M50.01
          mid-cervical region M50.020
        neuritis, radiculitis or radiculopathy M50.10
          C2-C3 M50.11
          C3-C4 M50.11
          C4-C5 M50.121
          C5-C6 M50.122
          C6-C7 M50.123
          C7-T1 M50.13
          cervicothoracic region M50.13
          high cervical region M50.11
          mid-cervical region M50.120
      C2-C3 M50.91
      C3-C4 M50.91
      C4-C5 M50.921
      C5-C6 M50.922
      C6-C7 M50.923
      C7-T1 M50.93
      cervicothoracic region M50.93
      degeneration M50.30
        C2-C3 M50.31
        C3-C4 M50.31
        C4-C5 M50.321
        C5-C6 M50.322
        C6-C7 M50.323
        C7-T1 M50.33
        cervicothoracic region M50.33
        high cervical region M50.31
        mid-cervical region M50.320
      displacement M50.20
        C2-C3 M50.21
        C3-C4 M50.21
        C4-C5 M50.221
        C5-C6 M50.222
        C6-C7 M50.223
        C7-T1 M50.23
        cervicothoracic region M50.23
        high cervical region M50.21
        mid-cervical region M50.220
      high cervical region M50.91
      mid-cervical region M50.920
      specified type NEC M50.80
        C2-C3 M50.81
        C3-C4 M50.81
        C4-C5 M50.821

▽ **Subterms under main terms may continue to next column or page**   ☑ **Additional Character Required** — Refer to the Tabular List for Character Selection   **111**

Disorder — Disorder

Disorder — continued
    disc — continued
        cervical — continued
            specified type — continued
                C5-C6 M50.822
                C6-C7 M50.823
                C7-T1 M50.83
                cervicothoracic region M50.83
                high cervical region M50.81
                mid-cervical region M50.820
            specified NEC
                lumbar region M51.86
                lumbosacral region M51.87
                sacrococcygeal region M53.3
                thoracic region M51.84
                thoracolumbar region M51.85
    disinhibited attachment (childhood) F94.2
    disintegrative, childhood NEC F84.3
    disruptive F91.9
        mood dysregulation F34.81
        specified NEC F91.8
    disruptive behavior — see Disorder, conduct
    dissocial personality F60.2
    dissociative F44.9
        affecting
            motor function F44.4
                and sensation F44.7
            sensation F44.6
                and motor function F44.7
        brief reactive F43.0
        due to (secondary to) general medical condition
            F06.8
        mixed F44.7
        organic F06.8
        other specified NEC F44.89
    double heterozygous sickling — see Disease, sickle-
        cell
    dream anxiety F51.5
    drug induced hemorrhagic D68.32
    drug related F19.99
        abuse — see Abuse, drug
        dependence — see Dependence, drug
    dysmorphic body F45.22
    dysthymic F34.1
    ear H93.9- ☑
        bleeding — see Otorrhagia
        deafness — see Deafness
        degenerative H93.09- ☑
        discharge — see Otorrhea
        external H61.9- ☑
            auditory canal stenosis — see Stenosis, external
                ear canal
            exostosis — see Exostosis, external ear canal
            impacted cerumen — see Impaction, cerumen
            otitis — see Otitis, externa
            perichondritis — see Perichondritis, ear
            pinna — see Disorder, pinna
            specified type NEC H61.89- ☑
        inner H83.9- ☑
            vestibular dysfunction — see Disorder,
                vestibular function
        middle H74.9- ☑
            adhesive H74.1- ☑
            ossicle — see Abnormal, ear ossicles
            polyp — see Polyp, ear (middle)
            specified NEC, in diseases classified elsewhere
                H75.8- ☑
        postprocedural — see Complications, ear, proce-
            dure
        specified NEC, in diseases classified elsewhere
            H94.8- ☑
    eating (adult) (psychogenic) F50.9
        anorexia — see Anorexia
        binge F50.81
        bulimia F50.2
        child F98.29
            pica F98.3
            rumination disorder F98.21
        pica F50.89
            childhood F98.3
    electrolyte (balance) NEC E87.8
        with
            abortion — see Abortion by type complicated
                by specified condition NEC
            ectopic pregnancy O08.5
            molar pregnancy O08.5
        acidosis (metabolic) (respiratory) E87.2
        alkalosis (metabolic) (respiratory) E87.3

Disorder — continued
    elimination, transepidermal L87.9
        specified NEC L87.8
    emotional (persistent) F34.9
        of childhood F93.9
            specified NEC F93.8
    endocrine E34.9
        postprocedural E89.89
            specified NEC E89.89
    erectile (male) (organic) (see also Dysfunction, sexual,
        male, erectile) N52.9
        nonorganic F52.21
    erythematous — see Erythema
    esophagus K22.9
        functional K22.4
        psychogenic F45.8
    eustachian tube H69.9- ☑
        infection — see Salpingitis, eustachian
        obstruction — see Obstruction, eustachian tube
        patulous — see Patulous, eustachian tube
        specified NEC H69.8- ☑
    exhibitionistic F65.2
    extrapyramidal G25.9
        in deseases classified elsewhere — see category
            G26
        specified type NEC G25.89
    eye H57.9
        postprocedural — see Complication, postprocedu-
            ral, eye
    eyelid H02.9
        cyst — see Cyst, eyelid
        degenerative H02.70
            chloasma — see Chloasma, eyelid
            madarosis — see Madarosis
            specified type NEC H02.79
            vitiligo — see Vitiligo, eyelid
            xanthelasma — see Xanthelasma
        dermatochalasis — see Dermatochalasis
        edema — see Edema, eyelid
        elephantiasis — see Elephantiasis, eyelid
        foreign body, retained — see Foreign body, re-
            tained, eyelid
        function H02.59
            abnormal innervation syndrome — see Syn-
                drome, abnormal innervation
            blepharochalasis — see Blepharochalasis
            blepharoclonus — see Blepharoclonus
            blepharophimosis — see Blepharophimosis
            blepharoptosis — see Blepharoptosis
            lagophthalmos — see Lagophthalmos
            lid retraction — see Retraction, lid
        hypertrichosis — see Hypertrichosis, eyelid
        specified type NEC H02.89
        vascular H02.879
            left H02.876
                lower H02.875
                upper H02.874
            right H02.873
                lower H02.872
                upper H02.871
    factitious F68.10
        with predominantly
            physical symptoms F68.12
                with psychological symptoms F68.13
            psychological symptoms F68.11
                with physical symptoms F68.13
    factor, coagulation — see Defect, coagulation
    fatty acid
        metabolism E71.30
            specified NEC E71.39
        oxidation
            LCAD E71.310
            MCAD E71.311
            SCAD E71.312
            specified deficiency NEC E71.318
    feeding (infant or child) (see also Disorder, eating)
        R63.3
        or eating disorder F50.9
        specified NEC F50.9
    feigned (with obvious motivation) Z76.5
        without obvious motivation — see Disorder, facti-
            tious
    female
        hypoactive sexual desire F52.0
        orgasmic F52.31
        sexual interest/arousal F52.22
    fetishistic F65.0
    fibroblastic M72.9

Disorder — continued
    fibroblastic — continued
        specified NEC M72.8
    fluency
        adult onset F98.5
        childhood onset F80.81
        following
            cerebral infarction I69.323
            cerebrovascular disease I69.923
                specified disease NEC I69.823
            intracerebral hemorrhage I69.123
            nontraumatic intracranial hemorrhage NEC
                I69.223
            subarachnoid hemorrhage I69.023
        in conditions classified elsewhere R47.82
    fluid balance E87.8
    follicular (skin) L73.9
        specified NEC L73.8
    frotteuristic F65.81
    fructose metabolism E74.10
        essential fructosuria E74.11
        fructokinase deficiency E74.11
        fructose-1, 6-diphosphatase deficiency E74.19
        hereditary fructose intolerance E74.12
        other specified E74.19
    functional polymorphonuclear neutrophils D71
    gallbladder, biliary tract and pancreas in diseases
        classified elsewhere K87
    gambling F63.0
    gamma-glutamyl cycle E72.8
    gastric (functional) K31.9
        motility K30
        psychogenic F45.8
        secretion K30
    gastrointestinal (functional) NOS K92.9
        newborn P78.9
        psychogenic F45.8
    gender-identity or -role F64.9
        childhood F64.2
        effect on relationship F66
        of adolescence or adulthood F64.0
            nontranssexual F64.8
        specified NEC F64.8
        uncertainty F66
    genito-pelvic pain penetration F52.6
    genitourinary system
        female N94.9
        male N50.9
        psychogenic F45.8
    globe H44.9
        degenerated condition H44.50
            absolute glaucoma H44.51- ☑
            atrophy H44.52- ☑
            leucocoria H44.53- ☑
        degenerative H44.30
            chalcosis H44.31- ☑
            myopia (see also Myopia, degenerative)
                H44.2- ☑
            siderosis H44.32- ☑
            specified type NEC H44.39- ☑
        endophthalmitis — see Endophthalmitis
        foreign body, retained — see Foreign body, intraoc-
            ular, old, retained
        hemophthalmos — see Hemophthalmos
        hypotony H44.40
            due to
                ocular fistula H44.42- ☑
                specified disorder NEC H44.43- ☑
            flat anterior chamber H44.41- ☑
            primary H44.44- ☑
        luxation — see Luxation, globe
        specified type NEC H44.89
    glomerular (in) N05.9
        amyloidosis E85.4 [N08]
        cryoglobulinemia D89.1 [N08]
        disseminated intravascular coagulation D65 [N08]
        Fabry's disease E75.21 [N08]
        familial lecithin cholesterol acyltransferase deficien-
            cy E78.6 [N08]
        Goodpasture's syndrome M31.0
        hemolytic-uremic syndrome D59.3
        Henoch (-Schönlein) purpura D69.0 [N08]
        malariae malaria B52.0
        microscopic polyangiitis M31.7 [N08]
        multiple myeloma C90.0- ☑ [N08]
        mumps B26.83
        schistosomiasis B65.9 [N08]
        sepsis NEC A41.- ☑ [N08]

☑ Additional Character Required — Refer to the Tabular List for Character Selection   ▽ Subterms under main terms may continue to next column or page

Disorder — *continued*
  glomerular — *continued*
    sepsis — *continued*
      streptococcal A40.- ☑ [NØ8]
      sickle-cell disorders D57.- ☑ [NØ8]
      strongyloidiasis B78.9 [NØ8]
      subacute bacterial endocarditis I33.Ø [NØ8]
      syphilis A52.75
      systemic lupus erythematosus M32.14
      thrombotic thrombocytopenic purpura
        M31.1 [NØ8]
      Waldenström macroglobulinemia C88.Ø [NØ8]
      Wegener's granulomatosis M31.31
  gluconeogenesis E74.4
  glucosaminoglycan metabolism — *see* Disorder,
    metabolism, glucosaminoglycan
  glycine metabolism E72.5Ø
    d-glycericacidemia E72.59
    hyperhydroxyprolinemia E72.59
    hyperoxaluria E72.53
    hyperprolinemia E72.59
    non-ketotic hyperglycinemia E72.51
    oxalosis E72.53
    oxaluria E72.53
    sarcosinemia E72.59
    trimethylaminuria E72.52
  glycoprotein metabolism E77.9
    specified NEC E77.8
  habit (and impulse) F63.9
    involving sexual behavior NEC F65.9
    specified NEC F63.89
  hallucinogen use
    mild F16.1Ø
      with
        hallucinogen intoxication delirium F16.121
        hallucinogen-induced
          anxiety disorder F16.18Ø
          bipolar and related disorder F16.14
          depressive disorder F16.14
          psychotic disorder F16.159
        other hallucinogen intoxication F16.129
      in remission (early) (sustained) F16.11
    moderate or severe F16.2Ø
      with
        hallucinogen intoxication delirium F16.221
        hallucinogen-induced
          anxiety disorder F16.28Ø
          bipolar and related disorder F16.24
          depressive disorder F16.24
          psychotic disorder F16.259
        other hallucinogen intoxication F16.229
      in remission (early) (sustained) F16.21
  heart action I49.9
  hematological D75.9
    newborn (transient) P61.9
      specified NEC P61.8
  hematopoietic organs D75.9
  hemorrhagic NEC D69.9
    drug-induced D68.32
    due to
      extrinsic circulating anticoagulants D68.32
      increase in
        anti-IIa D68.32
        anti-Xa D68.32
      intrinsic
        circulating anticoagulants D68.318
        increase in
          anti-IXa D68.318
          antithrombin D68.318
          anti-VIIIa D68.318
          anti-XIa D68.318
    following childbirth O72.3
  hemostasis — *see* Defect, coagulation
  histidine metabolism E7Ø.4Ø
    histidinemia E7Ø.41
    other specified E7Ø.49
  hoarding F42.3
  hyperkinetic — *see* Disorder, attention-deficit hyper-
    activity
  hyperleucine-isoleucinemia E71.19
  hypervalinemia E71.19
  hypoactive sexual desire F52.Ø
  hypochondriacal F45.2Ø
    body dysmorphic F45.22
    neurosis F45.21
    other specified F45.29
  identity
    dissociative F44.81
    illness anxiety F45.21

Disorder — *continued*
  identity — *continued*
    of childhood F93.8
  immune mechanism (immunity) D89.9
    specified type NEC D89.89
  impaired renal tubular function N25.9
    specified NEC N25.89
  impulse (control) F63.9
  inflammatory
    pelvic, in diseases classified elsewhere — *see* cate-
      gory N74
    penis N48.29
      abscess N48.21
      cellulitis N48.22
  inhalant use
    mild F18.1Ø
      with
        inhalant intoxication F18.129
        inhalant intoxication delirium F18.121
        inhalant-induced
          anxiety disorder F18.18Ø
          depressive disorder F18.14
          major neurocognitive disorder F18.17
          mild neurocognitive disorder F18.188
          psychotic disorder F18.159
      in remission (early) (sustained) F18.11
    moderate or severe F18.2Ø
      with
        inhalant intoxication F18.229
        inhalant intoxication delirium F18.221
        inhalant-induced
          anxiety disorder F18.28Ø
          depressive disorder F18.24
          major neurocognitive disorder F18.27
          mild neurocognitive disorder F18.288
          psychotic disorder F18.259
      in remission (early) (sustained) F18.21
  integument, newborn P83.9
    specified NEC P83.88
  intermittent explosive F63.81
  internal secretion pancreas — *see* Increased, secretion,
    pancreas, endocrine
  intestine, intestinal
    carbohydrate absorption NEC E74.39
    postoperative K91.2
    functional NEC K59.9
      postoperative K91.89
    psychogenic F45.8
    vascular K55.9
      chronic K55.1
      specified NEC K55.8
  intraoperative (intraprocedural) — *see* Complications,
    intraoperative
  involuntary emotional expression (IEED) FØ7.89
  iris H21.9
    adhesions — *see* Adhesions, iris
    atrophy — *see* Atrophy, iris
    chamber angle recession — *see* Recession, cham-
      ber angle
    cyst — *see* Cyst, iris
    degeneration — *see* Degeneration, iris
    in diseases classified elsewhere H22
    iridodialysis — *see* Iridodialysis
    iridoschisis — *see* Iridoschisis
    miotic pupillary cyst — *see* Cyst, pupillary
    pupillary
      abnormality — *see* Abnormality, pupillary
      membrane — *see* Membrane, pupillary
    specified type NEC H21.89
    vascular NEC H21.1X- ☑
  iron metabolism E83.1Ø
    specified NEC E83.19
  isovaleric acidemia E71.11Ø
  jaw, developmental M27.Ø
    temporomandibular (*see also* Anomaly, dentofacial,
      temporomandibular joint) M26.6Ø- ☑
  joint M25.9
    derangement — *see* Derangement, joint
    effusion — *see* Effusion, joint
    fistula — *see* Fistula, joint
    hemarthrosis — *see* Hemarthrosis
    instability — *see* Instability, joint
    osteophyte — *see* Osteophyte
    pain — *see* Pain, joint
    psychogenic F45.8
    specified type NEC M25.8Ø
      ankle M25.87- ☑
      elbow M25.82- ☑

Disorder — *continued*
  joint — *continued*
    specified type — *continued*
      foot joint M25.87- ☑
      hand joint M25.84- ☑
      hip M25.85- ☑
      knee M25.86- ☑
      shoulder M25.81- ☑
      wrist M25.83- ☑
    stiffness — *see* Stiffness, joint
  ketone metabolism E71.32
  kidney N28.9
    functional (tubular) N25.9
    in
      schistosomiasis B65.9 [N29]
    tubular function N25.9
    specified NEC N25.89
  lacrimal system HØ4.9
    changes HØ4.69
      fistula — *see* Fistula, lacrimal
    gland HØ4.19
      atrophy — *see* Atrophy, lacrimal gland
      cyst — *see* Cyst, lacrimal, gland
      dacryops — *see* Dacryops
      dislocation — *see* Dislocation, lacrimal gland
      dry eye syndrome — *see* Syndrome, dry eye
      infection — *see* Dacryoadenitis
      granuloma — *see* Granuloma, lacrimal
      inflammation — *see* Inflammation, lacrimal
      obstruction — *see* Obstruction, lacrimal
      specified NEC HØ4.89
  lactation NEC O92.79
  language (developmental) F8Ø.9
    expressive F8Ø.1
    mixed receptive and expressive F8Ø.2
    receptive F8Ø.2
  late luteal phase dysphoric N94.89
  learning (specific) F81.9
    acalculia R48.8
    alexia R48.Ø
    mathematics F81.2
    reading F81.Ø
    specified
      with impairment in
        mathematics F81.2
        reading F81.Ø
        written expression F81.81
    specified NEC F81.89
    spelling F81.81
    written expression F81.81
  lens H27.9
    aphakia — *see* Aphakia
    cataract — *see* Cataract
    dislocation — *see* Dislocation, lens
    specified type NEC H27.8
  ligament M24.2Ø
    ankle M24.27- ☑
    attachment, spine — *see* Enthesopathy, spinal
    elbow M24.22- ☑
    foot joint M24.27- ☑
    hand joint M24.24- ☑
    hip M24.25- ☑
    knee — *see* Derangement, knee, specified NEC
    shoulder M24.21- ☑
    vertebra M24.28
    wrist M24.23- ☑
  ligamentous attachments (*see also* Enthesopathy)
    spine — *see* Enthesopathy, spinal
  lipid
    metabolism, congenital E78.9
    storage E75.6
      specified NEC E75.5
  lipoprotein
    deficiency (familial) E78.6
    metabolism E78.9
      specified NEC E78.89
  liver K76.9
    malarial B54 [K77]
  low back (*see also* Dorsopathy, specified NEC)
  lumbosacral
    plexus G54.1
    root (nerve) NEC G54.4
  lung, interstitial, drug-induced J7Ø.4
    acute J7Ø.2
    chronic J7Ø.3
  lymphoproliferative, post-transplant (PTLD) D47.Z1
    (*following* D47.4)
  lysine and hydroxylysine metabolism E72.3

☟ Subterms under main terms may continue to next column or page   ☑ Additional Character Required — Refer to the Tabular List for Character Selection   113

Disorder — Disorder

Disorder — *continued*
  major neurocognitive — *see* Dementia, in (due to)
  male
    erectile (organic) (*see also* Dysfunction, sexual, male, erectile) N52.9
      nonorganic F52.21
    hypoactive sexual desire F52.0
    orgasmic F52.32
  manic F30.9
    organic F06.33
  mast cell activation — *see* Activation, mast cell
  mastoid (*see also* Disorder, ear, middle)
    postprocedural — *see* Complications, ear, procedure
  meniscus — *see* Derangement, knee, meniscus
  menopausal N95.9
    specified NEC N95.8
  menstrual N92.6
    psychogenic F45.8
    specified NEC N92.5
  mental (or behavioral) (nonpsychotic) F99
    due to (secondary to)
      amphetamine
        due to drug abuse — *see* Abuse, drug, stimulant
        due to drug dependence — *see* Dependence, drug, stimulant
      brain disease, damage and dysfunction F09
      caffeine use
        due to drug abuse — *see* Abuse, drug, stimulant
        due to drug dependence — *see* Dependence, drug, stimulant
      cannabis use
        due to drug abuse — *see* Abuse, drug, cannabis
        due to drug dependence — *see* Dependence, drug, cannabis
      general medical condition F09
      sedative or hypnotic use
        due to drug abuse — *see* Abuse, drug, sedative
        due to drug dependence — *see* Dependence, drug, sedative
      tobacco (nicotine) use — *see* Dependence, drug, nicotine
    following organic brain damage F07.9
      frontal lobe syndrome F07.0
      personality change F07.0
      postconcussional syndrome F07.81
      specified NEC F07.89
    infancy, childhood or adolescence F98.9
    neurotic — *see* Neurosis
    organic or symptomatic F09
    presenile, psychotic F03 ☑
    problem NEC
    psychoneurotic — *see* Neurosis
    psychotic — *see* Psychosis
    puerperal F53
    senile, psychotic NEC F03 ☑
  metabolic, amino acid, transitory, newborn P74.8
  metabolism NOS E88.9
    amino-acid E72.9
      aromatic E70.9
        albinism — *see* Albinism
        histidine E70.40
          histidinemia E70.41
          other specified E70.49
        hyperphenylalaninemia E70.1
          classical phenylketonuria E70.0
        other specified E70.8
        tryptophan E70.5
        tyrosine E70.20
          hypertyrosinemia E70.21
          other specified E70.29
      branched chain E71.2
        3-methylglutaconic aciduria E71.111
        hyperleucine-isoleucinemia E71.19
        hypervalinemia E71.19
        isovaleric acidemia E71.110
        maple syrup urine disease E71.0
        methylmalonic acidemia E71.120
        organic aciduria NEC E71.118
        other specified E71.19
        proprionate NEC E71.128
        proprionic acidemia E71.121
      glycine E72.50
        d-glycericacidemia E72.59

Disorder — *continued*
  metabolism — *continued*
    amino-acid — *continued*
      glycine — *continued*
        hyperhydroxyprolinemia E72.59
        hyperoxaluria E72.53
        hyperprolinemia E72.59
        non-ketotic hyperglycinemia E72.51
        other specified E72.59
        sarcosinemia E72.59
        trimethylaminuria E72.52
      hydroxylysine E72.3
      lysine E72.3
      ornithine E72.4
      other specified E72.8
        beta-amino acid E72.8
        gamma-glutamyl cycle E72.8
      straight-chain E72.8
      sulfur-bearing E72.10
        homocystinuria E72.11
        methylenetetrahydrofolate reductase deficiency E72.12
        other specified E72.19
    bile acid and cholesterol metabolism E78.70
    bilirubin E80.7
      specified NEC E80.6
    calcium E83.50
      hypercalcemia E83.52
      hypocalcemia E83.51
      other specified E83.59
    carbohydrate E74.9
      specified NEC E74.8
    cholesterol and bile acid metabolism E78.70
    congenital E88.9
    copper E83.00
      specified type NEC E83.09
      Wilson's disease E83.01
    cystinuria E72.01
    fructose E74.10
    galactose E74.20
    glucosaminoglycan E76.9
      mucopolysaccharidosis — *see* Mucopolysaccharidosis
      specified NEC E76.8
    glutamine E72.8
    glycine E72.50
    glycogen storage (hepatorenal) E74.09
    glycoprotein E77.9
      specified NEC E77.8
    glycosaminoglycan E76.9
      specified NEC E76.8
    in labor and delivery O75.89
    iron E83.10
    isoleucine E71.19
    leucine E71.19
    lipoid E78.9
    lipoprotein E78.9
      specified NEC E78.89
    magnesium E83.40
      hypermagnesemia E83.41
      hypomagnesemia E83.42
      other specified E83.49
    mineral E83.9
      specified NEC E83.89
    mitochondrial E88.40
      MELAS syndrome E88.41
      MERRF syndrome (myoclonic epilepsy associated with ragged-red fibers) E88.42
      other specified E88.49
    ornithine E72.4
    phosphatases E83.30
    phosphorus E83.30
      acid phosphatase deficiency E83.39
      hypophosphatasia E83.39
      hypophosphatemia E83.39
        familial E83.31
      other specified E83.39
      pseudovitamin D deficiency E83.32
    plasma protein NEC E88.09
    porphyrin — *see* Porphyria
    postprocedural E89.89
      specified NEC E89.89
    purine E79.9
      specified NEC E79.8
    pyrimidine E79.9
      specified NEC E79.8
    pyruvate E74.4
    serine E72.8
    sodium E87.8

Disorder — *continued*
  metabolism — *continued*
    specified NEC E88.89
    threonine E72.8
    valine E71.19
    zinc E83.2
  methylmalonic acidemia E71.120
  micturition NEC (*see also* Difficulty, micturition) R39.198
    feeling of incomplete emptying R39.14
    hesitancy R39.11
    poor stream R39.12
    psychogenic F45.8
    split stream R39.13
    straining R39.16
    urgency R39.15
  mild neurocognitive G31.84
  mitochondrial metabolism E88.40
  mitral (valve) — *see* Endocarditis, mitral
  mixed
    anxiety and depressive F41.8
    of scholastic skills (developmental) F81.89
    receptive expressive language F80.2
  mood F39
    bipolar — *see* Disorder, bipolar
    depressive — *see* Disorder, depressive
    due to (secondary to)
      alcohol F10.94
      amphetamine F15.94
        in
          abuse F15.14
          dependence F15.24
      anxiolytic F13.94
        in
          abuse F13.14
          dependence F13.24
      cocaine F14.94
        in
          abuse F14.14
          dependence F14.24
      general medical condition F06.30
      hallucinogen F16.94
        in
          abuse F16.14
          dependence F16.24
      hypnotic F13.94
        in
          abuse F13.14
          dependence F13.24
      inhalant F18.94
        in
          abuse F18.14
          dependence F18.24
      opioid F11.94
        in
          abuse F11.14
          dependence F11.24
      phencyclidine (PCP) F16.94
        in
          abuse F16.14
          dependence F16.24
      physiological condition F06.30
        with
          depressive features F06.31
          major depressive-like episode F06.32
          manic features F06.33
          mixed features F06.34
      psychoactive substance NEC F19.94
        in
          abuse F19.14
          dependence F19.24
      sedative F13.94
        in
          abuse F13.14
          dependence F13.24
      volatile solvents F18.94
        in
          abuse F18.14
          dependence F18.24
    manic episode F30.9
      with psychotic symptoms F30.2
      without psychotic symptoms F30.10
        mild F30.11
        moderate F30.12
        severe F30.13
      in remission (full) F30.4
        partial F30.3
      specified type NEC F30.8
    organic F06.30

☑ **Additional Character Required** — Refer to the Tabular List for Character Selection   ▽ Subterms under main terms may continue to next column or page

Disorder — continued
  mood — continued
    organic — continued
      right hemisphere F07.89
    persistent F34.9
      cyclothymia F34.0
      dysthymia F34.1
      specified type NEC F34.89
    recurrent F39
    right hemisphere organic F07.89
  movement G25.9
    drug-induced G25.70
      akathisia G25.71
      specified NEC G25.79
    hysterical F44.4
    in diseases classified elsewhere — see category G26
    periodic limb G47.61
      sleep related G47.61
    sleep related NEC G47.69
    specified NEC G25.89
    stereotyped F98.4
    treatment-induced G25.9
  multiple personality F44.81
  muscle M62.9
    attachment, spine — see Enthesopathy, spinal
    in trichinellosis — see Trichinellosis, with muscle disorder
    psychogenic F45.8
    specified type NEC M62.89
    tone, newborn P94.9
      specified NEC P94.8
  muscular
    attachments (see also Enthesopathy)
      spine — see Enthesopathy, spinal
    urethra N36.44
  musculoskeletal system, soft tissue — see Disorder, soft tissue
    postprocedural M96.89
    psychogenic F45.8
  myoneural G70.9
    due to lead G70.1
    specified NEC G70.89
    toxic G70.1
  myotonic NEC G71.19
  nail, in diseases classified elsewhere L62
  neck region NEC — see Dorsopathy, specified NEC
  neonatal onset multisystemic inflammatory (NOMID) M04.2
  nerve G58.9
    abducent NEC — see Strabismus, paralytic, sixth nerve
    accessory G52.8
    acoustic — see subcategory H93.3 ☑
    auditory — see subcategory H93.3 ☑
    auriculotemporal G50.8
    axillary G54.0
    cerebral — see Disorder, nerve, cranial
    cranial G52.9
      eighth — see subcategory H93.3 ☑
      eleventh G52.8
      fifth G50.9
      first G52.0
      fourth NEC — see Strabismus, paralytic, fourth nerve
      multiple G52.7
      ninth G52.1
      second NEC — see Disorder, nerve, optic
      seventh NEC G51.8
      sixth NEC — see Strabismus, paralytic, sixth nerve
      specified NEC G52.8
      tenth G52.2
      third NEC — see Strabismus, paralytic, third nerve
      twelfth G52.3
    entrapment — see Neuropathy, entrapment
    facial G51.9
      specified NEC G51.8
    femoral — see Lesion, nerve, femoral
    glossopharyngeal NEC G52.1
    hypoglossal G52.3
    intercostal G58.0
    lateral
      cutaneous of thigh — see Mononeuropathy, lower limb, meralgia paresthetica
      popliteal — see Lesion, nerve, popliteal
      lower limb — see Mononeuropathy, lower limb

Disorder — continued
  nerve — continued
    medial popliteal — see Lesion, nerve, popliteal, medial
    median NEC — see Lesion, nerve, median
    multiple G58.7
    oculomotor NEC — see Strabismus, paralytic, third nerve
    olfactory G52.0
    optic NEC H47.09- ☑
      hemorrhage into sheath — see Hemorrhage, optic nerve
      ischemic H47.01- ☑
    peroneal — see Lesion, nerve, popliteal
    phrenic G58.8
    plantar — see Lesion, nerve, plantar
    pneumogastric G52.2
    posterior tibial — see Syndrome, tarsal tunnel
    radial — see Lesion, nerve, radial
    recurrent laryngeal G52.2
    root G54.9
      cervical G54.2
      lumbosacral G54.1
      specified NEC G54.8
      thoracic G54.3
    sciatic NEC — see Lesion, nerve, sciatic
    specified NEC G58.8
      lower limb — see Mononeuropathy, lower limb, specified NEC
      upper limb — see Mononeuropathy, upper limb, specified NEC
    sympathetic G90.9
    tibial — see Lesion, nerve, popliteal, medial
    trigeminal G50.9
      specified NEC G50.8
    trochlear NEC — see Strabismus, paralytic, fourth nerve
    ulnar — see Lesion, nerve, ulnar
    upper limb — see Mononeuropathy, upper limb
    vagus G52.2
  nervous system G98.8
    autonomic (peripheral) G90.9
      specified NEC G90.8
    central G96.9
      specified NEC G96.8
    parasympathetic G90.9
    specified NEC G98.8
    sympathetic G90.9
    vegetative G90.9
  neurocognitive R41.9
    major
      with
        aggressive behavior F01.51
        combative behavior F01.51
        violent behavior F01.51
      without behavioral disturbance F01.50
      due to vascular disease, with behavioral disturbance F01.51
      in (due to) (other diseases classified elsewhere) (see also Dementia, in (due to)) F02.80
        with
          aggressive behavior F02.81
          combative behavior F02.81
          violent behavior F02.81
    mild G31.84
  neurodevelopmental F89
    specified NEC F88
  neurohypophysis NEC E23.3
  neurological NEC R29.818
  neuromuscular G70.9
    hereditary NEC G71.9
    specified NEC G70.89
    toxic G70.1
  neurotic F48.9
    specified NEC F48.8
  neutrophil, polymorphonuclear D71
  nicotine use — see Dependence, drug, nicotine
  nightmare F51.5
  non-rapid eye movement sleep arousal
    sleep terror type F51.4
    sleepwalking type F51.3
  nose J34.9
    specified NEC J34.89
  obsessive-compulsive F42.9
    and related disorder due to a known physiological condition F06.8
  odontogenesis NOS K00.9

Disorder — continued
  opioid use
    with
      opioid-induced psychotic disorder F11.959
        with
          delusions F11.950
          hallucinations F11.951
    due to drug abuse — see Abuse, drug, opioid
    due to drug dependence — see Dependence, drug, opioid
    mild F11.10
      with
        opioid intoxication
          with perceptual disturbances F11.122
          without perceptual disturbances F11.129
          delirium F11.121
        opioid-induced
          anxiety disorder F11.188
          depressive disorder F11.14
          sexual dysfunction F11.181
      in remission (early) (sustained) F11.11
    moderate or severe F11.20
      with
        opioid intoxication
          with perceptual disturbances F11.222
          without perceptual disturbances F11.229
          delirium F11.221
        opioid-induced
          anxiety disorder F11.288
          anxiety disorder F11.988
          depressive disorder F11.24
          depressive disorder F11.94
          sexual dysfunction F11.281
          sexual dysfunction F11.981
      in remission (early) (sustained) F11.21
  oppositional defiant F91.3
  optic
    chiasm H47.49
      due to
        inflammatory disorder H47.41
        neoplasm H47.42
        vascular disorder H47.43
    disc H47.39- ☑
      coloboma — see Coloboma, optic disc
      drusen — see Drusen, optic disc
      pseudopapilledema — see Pseudopapilledema
    radiations — see Disorder, visual, pathway
    tracts — see Disorder, visual, pathway
  orbit H05.9
    cyst — see Cyst, orbit
    deformity — see Deformity, orbit
    edema — see Edema, orbit
    enophthalmos — see Enophthalmos
    exophthalmos — see Exophthalmos
    hemorrhage — see Hemorrhage, orbit
    inflammation — see Inflammation, orbit
    myopathy — see Myopathy, extraocular muscles
    retained foreign body — see Foreign body, orbit, old
    specified type NEC H05.89
  organic
    anxiety F06.4
    catatonic F06.1
    delusional F06.2
    dissociative F06.8
    emotionally labile (asthenic) F06.8
    mood (affective) F06.30
    schizophrenia-like F06.2
  orgasmic (female) F52.31
    male F52.32
  ornithine metabolism E72.4
  overanxious F41.1
    of childhood F93.8
  pain
    with related psychological factors F45.42
    exclusively related to psychological factors F45.41
    genito-pelvic penetration disorder F52.6
  pancreatic internal secretion E16.9
    specified NEC E16.8
  panic F41.0
    with agoraphobia F40.01
  papulosquamous L44.9
    in diseases classified elsewhere L45
    specified NEC L44.8
  paranoid F22
    induced F24
    shared F24
  paraphilic F65.9

▽ Subterms under main terms may continue to next column or page   ☑ Additional Character Required — Refer to the Tabular List for Character Selection   **115**

Disorder — Disorder

Disorder — continued
  paraphilic — continued
    specified NEC F65.89
  parathyroid (gland) E21.5
    specified NEC E21.4
  parietoalveolar NEC J84.09
  paroxysmal, mixed R56.9
  patella M22.9- ☑
    chondromalacia — see Chondromalacia, patella
    derangement NEC M22.3X- ☑
    recurrent
      dislocation — see Dislocation, patella, recurrent
      subluxation — see Dislocation, patella, recurrent, incomplete
    specified NEC M22.8X- ☑
  patellofemoral M22.2X- ☑
  pedophilic F65.4
  pentose phosphate pathway with anemia D55.1
  perception, due to hallucinogens F16.983
    in
      abuse F16.183
      dependence F16.283
  peripheral nervous system NEC G64
  peroxisomal E71.50
    biogenesis
      neonatal adrenoleukodystrophy E71.511
      specified disorder NEC E71.518
      Zellweger syndrome E71.510
    rhizomelic chondrodysplasia punctata E71.540
    specified form NEC E71.548
      group 1 E71.518
      group 2 E71.53
      group 3 E71.542
    X-linked adrenoleukodystrophy E71.529
      adolescent E71.521
      adrenomyeloneuropathy E71.522
      childhood E71.520
      specified form NEC E71.528
    Zellweger-like syndrome E71.541
  persistent
    (somatoform) pain F45.41
    affective (mood) F34.9
  personality (see also Personality) F60.9
    affective F34.0
    aggressive F60.3
    amoral F60.2
    anankastic F60.5
    antisocial F60.2
    anxious F60.6
    asocial F60.2
    asthenic F60.7
    avoidant F60.6
    borderline F60.3
    change (secondary) due to general medical condition F07.0
    compulsive F60.5
    cyclothymic F34.0
    dependent (passive) F60.7
    depressive F34.1
    dissocial F60.2
    emotional instability F60.3
    expansive paranoid F60.0
    explosive F60.3
    following organic brain damage F07.9
    histrionic F60.4
    hyperthymic F34.0
    hypothymic F34.1
    hysterical F60.4
    immature F60.89
    inadequate F60.7
    labile F60.3
    mixed (nonspecific) F60.89
    moral deficiency F60.2
    narcissistic F60.81
    negativistic F60.89
    obsessional F60.5
    obsessive (-compulsive) F60.5
    organic F07.9
    overconscientious F60.5
    paranoid F60.0
    passive (-dependent) F60.7
    passive-aggressive F60.89
    pathological NEC F60.9
    pseudosocial F60.2
    psychopathic F60.2
    schizoid F60.1
    schizotypal F21
    self-defeating F60.7

Disorder — continued
  personality (see also Personality) — continued
    specified NEC F60.89
    type A F60.5
    unstable (emotional) F60.3
  pervasive, developmental F84.9
  phencyclidine use
    mild F16.10
      with
        phencyclidine intoxication F16.129
        phencyclidine intoxication delirium F16.121
        phencyclidine-induced
          anxiety disorder F16.180
          bipolar and related disorder F16.14
          depressive disorder F16.14
          psychotic disorder F16.159
      in remission (early) (sustained) F16.11
    moderate or severe F16.20
      with
        phencyclidine intoxication F16.229
        phencyclidine intoxication delirium F16.221
        phencyclidine-induced
          anxiety disorder F16.280
          bipolar and related disorder F16.14
          depressive disorder F16.24
          psychotic disorder F16.259
      in remission (early) (sustained) F16.21
  phobic anxiety, childhood F40.8
  phosphate-losing tubular N25.0
  pigmentation L81.9
    choroid, congenital Q14.3
    diminished melanin formation L81.6
    iron L81.8
    specified NEC L81.8
  pinna (noninfective) H61.10- ☑
    deformity, acquired H61.11- ☑
    hematoma H61.12- ☑
    perichondritis — see Perichondritis, ear
    specified type NEC H61.19- ☑
  pituitary gland E23.7
    iatrogenic (postprocedural) E89.3
    specified NEC E23.6
  platelets D69.1
  plexus G54.9
    specified NEC G54.8
  polymorphonuclear neutrophils D71
  porphyrin metabolism — see Porphyria
  postconcussional F07.81
  posthallucinogen perception F16.983
    in
      abuse F16.183
      dependence F16.283
  postmenopausal N95.9
    specified NEC N95.8
  postprocedural (postoperative) — see Complications, postprocedural
  post-transplant lymphoproliferative D47.Z1 (following D47.4)
  post-traumatic stress (PTSD) F43.10
    acute F43.11
    chronic F43.12
  premenstrual dysphoric (PMDD) F32.81
  prepuce N47.8
  propionic acidemia E71.121
  prostate N42.9
    specified NEC N42.89
  psychogenic NOS (see also condition) F45.9
    anxiety F41.8
    appetite F50.9
    asthenic F48.8
    cardiovascular (system) F45.8
    compulsive F42.8
    cutaneous F54
    depressive F32.9
    digestive (system) F45.8
    dysmenorrheic F45.8
    dyspneic F45.8
    endocrine (system) F54
    eye NEC F45.8
    feeding — see Disorder, eating
    functional NEC F45.8
    gastric F45.8
    gastrointestinal (system) F45.8
    genitourinary (system) F45.8
    heart (function) (rhythm) F45.8
    hyperventilatory F45.8
    hypochondriacal — see Disorder, hypochondriacal
    intestinal F45.8

Disorder — continued
  psychogenic (see also condition) — continued
    joint F45.8
    learning F81.9
    limb F45.8
    lymphatic (system) F45.8
    menstrual F45.8
    micturition F45.8
    monoplegic NEC F44.4
    motor F44.4
    muscle F45.8
    musculoskeletal F45.8
    neurocirculatory F45.8
    obsessive F42.8
    occupational F48.8
    organ or part of body NEC F45.8
    paralytic NEC F44.4
    phobic F40.9
    physical NEC F45.8
    rectal F45.8
    respiratory (system) F45.8
    rheumatic F45.8
    sexual (function) F52.9
    skin (allergic) (eczematous) F54
    sleep F51.9
    specified part of body NEC F45.8
    stomach F45.8
  psychological F99
    associated with
      disease classified elsewhere F54
      sexual
        development F66
        relationship F66
      uncertainty about gender identity F64.9
  psychomotor NEC F44.4
    hysterical F44.4
  psychoneurotic (see also Neurosis)
    mixed NEC F48.8
  psychophysiologic — see Disorder, somatoform
  psychosexual F65.9
    development F66
    identity of childhood F64.2
  psychosomatic NOS — see Disorder, somatoform
    multiple F45.0
    undifferentiated F45.1
  psychotic — see Psychosis
    transient (acute) F23
  puberty E30.9
    specified NEC E30.8
  pulmonary (valve) — see Endocarditis, pulmonary
  purine metabolism E79.9
  pyrimidine metabolism E79.9
  pyruvate metabolism E74.4
  reactive attachment (childhood) F94.1
  reading R48.0
    developmental (specific) F81.0
  receptive language F80.2
  receptor, hormonal, peripheral (see also Syndrome, androgen insensitivity) E34.50
  recurrent brief depressive F33.8
  reflex R29.2
  refraction H52.7
    aniseikonia H52.32
    anisometropia H52.31
    astigmatism — see Astigmatism
    hypermetropia — see Hypermetropia
    myopia — see Myopia
    presbyopia H52.4
    specified NEC H52.6
  relationship F68.8
    due to sexual orientation F66
  REM sleep behavior G47.52
  renal function, impaired (tubular) N25.9
  resonance R49.9
    specified NEC R49.8
  respiratory function, impaired (see also Failure, respiration)
    postprocedural — see Complication, postoperative, respiratory system
    psychogenic F45.8
  retina H35.9
    angioid streaks H35.33
    changes in vascular appearance H35.01- ☑
    degeneration — see Degeneration, retina
    dystrophy (hereditary) — see Dystrophy, retina
    edema H35.81
    hemorrhage — see Hemorrhage, retina
    ischemia H35.82

Disorder — continued
  retina — continued
    macular degeneration — see Degeneration, macula
    microaneurysms H35.04- ☑
    microvascular abnormality NEC H35.09
    neovascularization — see Neovascularization, retina
    retinopathy — see Retinopathy
    separation of layers H35.70
      central serous chorioretinopathy H35.71- ☑
      pigment epithelium detachment (serous) H35.72- ☑
        hemorrhagic H35.73- ☑
    specified type NEC H35.89
    telangiectasis — see Telangiectasis, retina
    vasculitis — see Vasculitis, retina
  retroperitoneal K68.9
  right hemisphere organic affective F07.89
  rumination (infant or child) F98.21
  sacrum, sacrococcygeal NEC M53.3
  schizoaffective F25.9
    bipolar type F25.0
    depressive type F25.1
    manic type F25.0
    mixed type F25.0
    specified NEC F25.8
  schizoid of childhood F84.5
  schizophrenia spectrum and other psychotic disorder F29
    specified NEC F28
  schizophreniform F20.81
    brief F23
  schizotypal (personality) F21
  secretion, thyrocalcitonin E07.0
  sedative, hypnotic, or anxiolytic use
    mild F13.10
      with
        sedative, hypnotic, or anxiolytic intoxication F13.129
        sedative, hypnotic, or anxiolytic intoxication delirium F13.121
        sedative, hypnotic, or anxiolytic-induced
          anxiety disorder F13.180
          bipolar and related disorder F13.14
          depressive disorder F13.14
          psychotic disorder F13.159
          sexual dysfunction F13.181
      in remission (early) (sustained) F13.11
    moderate or severe F13.20
      with
        sedative, hypnotic, or anxiolytic intoxication F13.229
        sedative, hypnotic, or anxiolytic intoxication delirium F13.221
        sedative, hypnotic, or anxiolytic-induced
          anxiety disorder F13.280
          bipolar and related disorder F13.24
          depressive disorder F13.24
          major neurocognitive disorder F13.27
          mild neurocognitive disorder F13.288
          psychotic disorder F13.259
          sexual dysfunction F13.281
      in remission (early) (sustained) F13.21
  seizure (see also Epilepsy) G40.909
    intractable G40.919
      with status epilepticus G40.911
  semantic pragmatic F80.89
    with autism F84.0
  sense of smell R43.1
    psychogenic F45.8
  separation anxiety, of childhood F93.0
  sexual
    aversion F52.1
    function, psychogenic F52.9
    interest/arousal, female F52.22
    masochism F65.51
    maturation F66
    nonorganic F52.9
    preference (see also Deviation, sexual) F65.9
      fetishistic transvestism F65.1
    relationship F66
    sadism F65.52
  shyness, of childhood and adolescence F40.10
  sibling rivalry F93.8
  sickle-cell (sickling) (homozygous) — see Disease, sickle-cell
    heterozygous D57.3
    specified type NEC D57.8- ☑

Disorder — continued
  sickle-cell — see Disease, sickle-cell — continued
    trait D57.3
  sinus (nasal) J34.9
    specified NEC J34.89
  skin L98.9
    atrophic L90.9
      specified NEC L90.8
    granulomatous L92.9
      specified NEC L92.8
    hypertrophic L91.9
      specified NEC L91.8
    infiltrative NEC L98.6
    newborn P83.9
      specified NEC P83.88
    picking F42.4
    psychogenic (allergic) (eczematous) F54
  sleep G47.9
    breathing-related — see Apnea, sleep
    circadian rhythm G47.20
      advance sleep phase type G47.22
      delayed sleep phase type G47.21
      due to
        alcohol
          abuse F10.182
          dependence F10.282
          use F10.982
        amphetamines
          abuse F15.182
          dependence F15.282
          use F15.982
        caffeine
          abuse F15.182
          dependence F15.282
          use F15.982
        cocaine
          abuse F14.182
          dependence F14.282
          use F14.982
        drug NEC
          abuse F19.182
          dependence F19.282
          use F19.982
        opioid
          abuse F11.182
          dependence F11.282
          use F11.982
        psychoactive substance NEC
          abuse F19.182
          dependence F19.282
          use F19.982
        sedative, hypnotic, or anxiolytic
          abuse F13.182
          dependence F13.282
          use F13.982
        stimulant NEC
          abuse F15.182
          dependence F15.282
          use F15.982
      free running type G47.24
      in conditions classified elsewhere G47.27
      irregular sleep wake type G47.23
      jet lag type G47.25
      non-24-hour sleep-wake type G47.24
      shift work type G47.26
      specified NEC G47.29
    due to
      alcohol
        abuse F10.182
        dependence F10.282
        use F10.982
      amphetamine
        abuse F15.182
        dependence F15.282
        use F15.982
      anxiolytic
        abuse F13.182
        dependence F13.282
        use F13.982
      caffeine
        abuse F15.182
        dependence F15.282
        use F15.982
      cocaine
        abuse F14.182
        dependence F14.282
        use F14.982
      drug NEC
        abuse F19.182

Disorder — continued
  sleep — continued
    due to — continued
      drug — continued
        dependence F19.282
        use F19.982
      hypnotic
        abuse F13.182
        dependence F13.282
        use F13.982
      opioid
        abuse F11.182
        dependence F11.282
        use F11.982
      psychoactive substance NEC
        abuse F19.182
        dependence F19.282
        use F19.982
      sedative
        abuse F13.182
        dependence F13.282
        use F13.982
      stimulant NEC
        abuse F15.182
        dependence F15.282
        use F15.982
    emotional F51.9
    excessive somnolence — see Hypersomnia
    hypersomnia type — see Hypersomnia
    initiating or maintaining — see Insomnia
    nightmares F51.5
    nonorganic F51.9
      specified NEC F51.8
    parasomnia type G47.50
    specified NEC G47.8
    terrors F51.4
    walking F51.3
  sleep-wake pattern or schedule (see also Disorder, sleep, circadian rhythm) G47.9
    specified NEC G47.8
  social
    anxiety (of childhood) F40.10
      generalized F40.11
    functioning in childhood F94.9
      specified NEC F94.8
    pragmatic F80.82
  soft tissue M79.9
    ankle M79.9
    due to use, overuse and pressure M70.90
      ankle M70.97- ☑
      bursitis — see Bursitis
      foot M70.97- ☑
      forearm M70.93- ☑
      hand M70.94- ☑
      lower leg M70.96- ☑
      multiple sites M70.99
      pelvic region M70.95- ☑
      shoulder region M70.91- ☑
      specified site NEC M70.98
      specified type NEC M70.80
        ankle M70.87- ☑
        foot M70.87- ☑
        forearm M70.83- ☑
        hand M70.84- ☑
        lower leg M70.86- ☑
        multiple sites M70.89
        pelvic region M70.85- ☑
        shoulder region M70.81- ☑
        specified site NEC M70.88
        thigh M70.85- ☑
        upper arm M70.82- ☑
      thigh M70.95- ☑
      upper arm M70.92- ☑
    foot M79.9
    forearm M79.9
    hand M79.9
    lower leg M79.9
    multiple sites M79.9
    occupational — see Disorder, soft tissue, due to use, overuse and pressure
    pelvic region M79.9
    shoulder region M79.9
    specified type NEC M79.89
    thigh M79.9
    upper arm M79.9
  somatic symptom F45.1
  somatization F45.0
  somatoform F45.9

▽ Subterms under main terms may continue to next column or page   ☑ Additional Character Required — Refer to the Tabular List for Character Selection   117

Disorder — Disorder

Disorder — *continued*
  somatoform — *continued*
    pain (persistent) F45.41
    somatization (multiple) (long-lasting) F45.0
    specified NEC F45.8
    undifferentiated F45.1
  somnolence, excessive — *see* Hypersomnia
  specific
    arithmetical F81.2
    developmental, of motor F82
    reading F81.0
    speech and language F80.9
    spelling F81.81
    written expression F81.81
  speech R47.9
    articulation (functional) (specific) F80.0
    developmental F80.9
    specified NEC R47.89
  speech-sound F80.0
  spelling (specific) F81.81
  spine (*see also* Dorsopathy)
    ligamentous or muscular attachments, peripheral — *see* Enthesopathy, spinal
    specified NEC — *see* Dorsopathy, specified NEC
  stereotyped, habit or movement F98.4
  stimulant use (other) (unspecified)
    mild F15.10
      in remission (early) (sustained) F15.11
    moderate or severe F15.20
      in remission (early) (sustained) F15.21
  stomach (functional) — *see* Disorder, gastric
  stress F43.9
    acute F43.0
    post-traumatic F43.10
      acute F43.11
      chronic F43.12
  substance use (other) (unknown)
    mild F19.10
      with substance-induced
        anxiety disorder F19.180
        bipolar and related disorder F19.14
        depressive disorder F19.14
        major neurocognitive disorder F19.17
        mild neurocognitive disorder F19.188
        obsessive-compulsive and related disorder F19.188
        sexual dysfunction F19.181
      substance intoxication F19.129
      substance intoxication delirium F19.121
    moderate or severe F19.20
      with substance-induced
        anxiety disorder F19.280
        bipolar and related disorder F19.24
        depressive disorder F19.24
        major neurocognitive disorder F19.27
        mild neurocognitive disorder F19.288
        obsessive-compulsive and related disorder F19.288
        sexual dysfunction F19.281
      in remission (early) (sustained) F19.21
      substance intoxication F19.229
      substance intoxication delirium F19.221
  sulfur-bearing amino-acid metabolism E72.10
  sweat gland (eccrine) L74.9
    apocrine L75.9
      specified NEC L75.8
    specified NEC L74.8
  synovium M67.90
    acromioclavicular M67.91- ☑
    ankle M67.97- ☑
    elbow M67.92- ☑
    foot M67.97- ☑
    forearm M67.93- ☑
    hand M67.94- ☑
    hip M67.95- ☑
    knee M67.96- ☑
    multiple sites M67.99
    rupture — *see* Rupture, synovium
    shoulder M67.91- ☑
    specified type NEC M67.80
      acromioclavicular M67.81- ☑
      ankle M67.87- ☑
      elbow M67.82- ☑
      foot M67.87- ☑
      hand M67.84- ☑
      hip M67.85- ☑
      knee M67.86- ☑
      multiple sites M67.89

Disorder — *continued*
  synovium — *continued*
    specified type — *continued*
      wrist M67.83- ☑
    synovitis — *see* Synovitis
    upper arm M67.92- ☑
    wrist M67.93- ☑
  temperature regulation, newborn P81.9
    specified NEC P81.8
  temporomandibular joint M26.60- ☑
  tendon M67.90
    acromioclavicular M67.91- ☑
    ankle M67.97- ☑
    contracture — *see* Contracture, tendon
    elbow M67.92- ☑
    foot M67.97- ☑
    forearm M67.93- ☑
    hand M67.94- ☑
    hip M67.95- ☑
    knee M67.96- ☑
    multiple sites M67.99
    rupture — *see* Rupture, tendon
    shoulder M67.91- ☑
    specified type NEC M67.80
      acromioclavicular M67.81- ☑
      ankle M67.87- ☑
      elbow M67.82- ☑
      foot M67.87- ☑
      hand M67.84- ☑
      hip M67.85- ☑
      knee M67.86- ☑
      multiple sites M67.89
      trunk M67.88
      wrist M67.83- ☑
    synovitis — *see* Synovitis
    tendinitis — *see* Tendinitis
    tenosynovitis — *see* Tenosynovitis
    trunk M67.98
    upper arm M67.92- ☑
    wrist M67.93- ☑
  thoracic root (nerve) NEC G54.3
  thyrocalcitonin hypersecretion E07.0
  thyroid (gland) E07.9
    function NEC, neonatal, transitory P72.2
    iodine-deficiency related E01.8
    specified NEC E07.89
  tic — *see* Tic
  tobacco use
    chewing tobacco (mild) (moderate) (severe)
      in remission (early) (sustained) F17.221
    cigarettes (mild) (moderate) (severe)
      in remission (early) (sustained) F17.211
    mild Z72.0
      in remission (early) (sustained) F17.201
    moderate F17.200
      in remission (early) (sustained) F17.201
    severe F17.200
      in remission (early) (sustained) F17.201
    specified product NEC (mild) (moderate) (severe)
      in remission (early) (sustained) F17.291
  tooth K08.9
    development K00.9
      specified NEC K00.8
    eruption K00.6
  Tourette's F95.2
  trance and possession F44.89
  transvestic F65.1
  trauma and stressor-related F43.9
    other specified F43.8
  tricuspid (valve) — *see* Endocarditis, tricuspid
  tryptophan metabolism E70.5
  tubular, phosphate-losing N25.0
  tubulo-interstitial (in)
    brucellosis A23.9 [N16]
    cystinosis E72.04
    diphtheria A36.84
    glycogen storage disease E74.00 [N16]
    leukemia NEC C95.9- ☑ [N16]
    lymphoma NEC C85.9- ☑ [N16]
    mixed cryoglobulinemia D89.1 [N16]
    multiple myeloma C90.0- ☑ [N16]
    Salmonella infection A02.25
    sarcoidosis D86.84
    sepsis A41.9 [N16]
      streptococcal A40.9 [N16]
    systemic lupus erythematosus M32.15
    toxoplasmosis B58.83

Disorder — *continued*
  tubulo-interstitial — *continued*
    transplant rejection T86.91 [N16]
    Wilson's disease E83.01 [N16]
  tubulo-renal function, impaired N25.9
    specified NEC N25.89
  tympanic membrane H73.9- ☑
    atrophy — *see* Atrophy, tympanic membrane
    infection — *see* Myringitis
    perforation — *see* Perforation, tympanum
    specified NEC H73.89- ☑
  unsocialized aggressive F91.1
  urea cycle metabolism E72.20
    argininemia E72.21
    argininosuccinic aciduria E72.22
    citrullinemia E72.23
    ornithine transcarbamylase deficiency E72.4
    other specified E72.29
  ureter (in) N28.9
    schistosomiasis B65.0 [N29]
    tuberculosis A18.11
  urethra N36.9
    specified NEC N36.8
  urinary system N39.9
    specified NEC N39.8
  valve, heart
    aortic — *see* Endocarditis, aortic
    mitral — *see* Endocarditis, mitral
    pulmonary — *see* Endocarditis, pulmonary
    rheumatic
      aortic — *see* Endocarditis, aortic, rheumatic
      mitral — *see* Endocarditis, mitral
      pulmonary — *see* Endocarditis, pulmonary, rheumatic
      tricuspid — *see* Endocarditis, tricuspid
    tricuspid — *see* Endocarditis, tricuspid
  vestibular function H81.9- ☑
    specified NEC — *see* subcategory H81.8 ☑
      in diseases classified elsewhere H82.- ☑
    vertigo — *see* Vertigo
  vision, binocular H53.30
    abnormal retinal correspondence H53.31
    diplopia H53.2
    fusion with defective stereopsis H53.32
    simultaneous perception H53.33
    suppression H53.34
  visual
    cortex
      blindness H47.619
        left brain H47.612
        right brain H47.611
      due to
        inflammatory disorder H47.629
          left brain H47.622
          right brain H47.621
        neoplasm H47.639
          left brain H47.632
          right brain H47.631
        vascular disorder H47.649
          left brain H47.642
          right brain H47.641
    pathway H47.9
      due to
        inflammatory disorder H47.51- ☑
        neoplasm H47.52- ☑
        vascular disorder H47.53- ☑
      optic chiasm — *see* Disorder, optic, chiasm
  vitreous body H43.9
    crystalline deposits — *see* Deposit, crystalline
    degeneration — *see* Degeneration, vitreous
    hemorrhage — *see* Hemorrhage, vitreous
    opacities — *see* Opacity, vitreous
    prolapse — *see* Prolapse, vitreous
    specified type NEC H43.89
  voice R49.9
    specified type NEC R49.8
  volatile solvent use
    due to drug abuse — *see* Abuse, drug, inhalant
    due to drug dependence — *see* Dependence, drug, inhalant
  voyeuristic F65.3
  white blood cells D72.9
    specified NEC D72.89
  withdrawing, child or adolescent F40.10
Disorientation R41.0
Displacement, displaced
  acquired traumatic of bone, cartilage, joint, tendon NEC — *see* Dislocation

Displacement, displaced — *continued*
  adrenal gland (congenital) Q89.1
  appendix, retrocecal (congenital) Q43.8
  auricle (congenital) Q17.4
  bladder (acquired) N32.89
    congenital Q64.19
  brachial plexus (congenital) Q07.8
  brain stem, caudal (congenital) Q04.8
  canaliculus (lacrimalis), congenital Q10.6
  cardia through esophageal hiatus (congenital) Q40.1
  cerebellum, caudal (congenital) Q04.8
  cervix — *see* Malposition, uterus
  colon (congenital) Q43.3
  device, implant or graft (*see also* Complications, by
      site and type, mechanical) T85.628 ☑
    arterial graft NEC — *see* Complication, cardiovas-
        cular device, mechanical, vascular
    breast (implant) T85.42 ☑
    catheter NEC T85.628 ☑
      dialysis (renal) T82.42 ☑
        intraperitoneal T85.621 ☑
      infusion NEC T82.524 ☑
        spinal (epidural) (subdural) T85.620 ☑
      urinary
        cystostomy T83.020 ☑
        Hopkins T83.028 ☑
        ileostomy T83.028 ☑
        indwelling T83.021 ☑
        nephrostomy T83.022 ☑
        specified NEC T83.028 ☑
        urostomy T83.028 ☑
    electronic (electrode) (pulse generator) (stimulator)
        — *see* Complication, electronic stimulator
    fixation, internal (orthopedic) NEC — *see* Compli-
        cation, fixation device, mechanical
    gastrointestinal — *see* Complications, prosthetic
        device, mechanical, gastrointestinal device
    genital NEC T83.428 ☑
      intrauterine contraceptive device (string)
          T83.32 ☑
      penile prosthesis (cylinder) (implanted) (pump)
          (reservoir) T83.420 ☑
      testicular prosthesis T83.421 ☑
    heart NEC — *see* Complication, cardiovascular de-
        vice, mechanical
    joint prosthesis — *see* Complications, joint prosthe-
        sis, mechanical
    ocular — *see* Complications, prosthetic device,
        mechanical, ocular device
    orthopedic NEC — *see* Complication, orthopedic,
        device or graft, mechanical
    specified NEC T85.628 ☑
    urinary NEC T83.128 ☑
      graft T83.22 ☑
      sphincter, implanted T83.121 ☑
      stent (ileal conduit) (nephroureteral) T83.123 ☑
        ureteral indwelling T83.122 ☑
    vascular NEC — *see* Complication, cardiovascular
        device, mechanical
    ventricular intracranial shunt T85.02 ☑
  electronic stimulator
    bone T84.320 ☑
    cardiac — *see* Complications, cardiac device, elec-
        tronic
    nervous system — *see* Complication, prosthetic
        device, mechanical, electronic nervous sys-
        tem stimulator
    urinary — *see* Complications, electronic stimulator,
        urinary
  esophageal mucosa into cardia of stomach, congenital
      Q39.8
  esophagus (acquired) K22.8
    congenital Q39.8
  eyeball (acquired) (lateral) (old) — *see* Displacement,
      globe
    congenital Q15.8
    current — *see* Avulsion, eye
  fallopian tube (acquired) N83.4- ☑
    congenital Q50.6
    opening (congenital) Q50.6
  gallbladder (congenital) Q44.1
  gastric mucosa (congenital) Q40.2
  globe (acquired) (old) (lateral) H05.21- ☑
    current — *see* Avulsion, eye
  heart (congenital) Q24.8
    acquired I51.89
  hymen (upward) (congenital) Q52.4

Displacement, displaced — *continued*
  intervertebral disc NEC
    with myelopathy — *see* Disorder, disc, with,
        myelopathy
    cervical, cervicothoracic (with) M50.20
      myelopathy — *see* Disorder, disc, cervical, with
          myelopathy
      neuritis, radiculitis or radiculopathy — *see* Dis-
          order, disc, cervical, with neuritis
    due to trauma — *see* Dislocation, vertebra
    lumbar region M51.26
      with
        myelopathy M51.06
        neuritis, radiculitis, radiculopathy or sciatica
            M51.16
    lumbosacral region M51.27
      with
        neuritis, radiculitis, radiculopathy or sciatica
            M51.17
    sacrococcygeal region M53.3
    thoracic region M51.24
      with
        myelopathy M51.04
        neuritis, radiculitis, radiculopathy M51.14
    thoracolumbar region M51.25
      with
        myelopathy M51.05
        neuritis, radiculitis, radiculopathy M51.15
  intrauterine device (string) T83.32 ☑
  kidney (acquired) N28.83
    congenital Q63.2
  lachrymal, lacrimal apparatus or duct (congenital)
      Q10.6
  lens, congenital Q12.1
  macula (congenital) Q14.1
  Meckel's diverticulum Q43.0
    malignant — *see* Table of Neoplasms, small intes-
        tine, malignant
  nail (congenital) Q84.6
    acquired L60.8
  opening of Wharton's duct in mouth Q38.4
  organ or site, congenital NEC — *see* Malposition,
      congenital
  ovary (acquired) N83.4- ☑
    congenital Q50.39
    free in peritoneal cavity (congenital) Q50.39
    into hernial sac N83.4- ☑
  oviduct (acquired) N83.4- ☑
    congenital Q50.6
  parathyroid (gland) E21.4
  parotid gland (congenital) Q38.4
  punctum lacrimale (congenital) Q10.6
  sacro-iliac (joint) (congenital) Q74.2
    current injury S33.2 ☑
    old — *see* subcategory M53.2 ☑
  salivary gland (any) (congenital) Q38.4
  spleen (congenital) Q89.09
  stomach, congenital Q40.2
  sublingual duct Q38.4
  tongue (downward) (congenital) Q38.3
  tooth, teeth, fully erupted M26.30
    horizontal M26.33
    vertical M26.34
  trachea (congenital) Q32.1
  ureter or ureteric opening or orifice (congenital)
      Q62.62
  uterine opening of oviducts or fallopian tubes Q50.6
  uterus, uterine — *see* Malposition, uterus
  ventricular septum Q21.0
    with rudimentary ventricle Q20.4
Disproportion
  between native and reconstructed breast N65.1
  fiber-type G71.2
Disruptio uteri — *see* Rupture, uterus
Disruption (of)
  ciliary body NEC H21.89
  closure of
    cornea T81.31 ☑
    craniotomy T81.32 ☑
    fascia (muscular) (superficial) T81.32 ☑
    internal organ or tissue T81.32 ☑
    laceration (external) (internal) T81.33 ☑
    ligament T81.32 ☑
    mucosa T81.31 ☑
    muscle or muscle flap T81.32 ☑
    ribs or rib cage T81.32 ☑
    skin and subcutaneous tissue (full-thickness) (su-
        perficial) T81.31 ☑

Disruption — *continued*
  closure of — *continued*
    skull T81.32 ☑
    sternum (sternotomy) T81.32 ☑
    tendon T81.32 ☑
    traumatic laceration (external) (internal) T81.33 ☑
  family Z63.8
    due to
      absence of family member due to military de-
          ployment Z63.31
      absence of family member NEC Z63.32
      alcoholism and drug addiction in family Z63.72
      bereavement Z63.4
      death (assumed) or disappearance of family
          member Z63.4
      divorce or separation Z63.5
      drug addiction in family Z63.72
      return of family member from military deploy-
          ment (current or past conflict) Z63.71
      stressful life events NEC Z63.79
  iris NEC H21.89
  ligament(s) (*see also* Sprain)
    knee
      current injury — *see* Dislocation, knee
      old (chronic) — *see* Derangement, knee, insta-
          bility
      spontaneous NEC — *see* Derangement, knee,
          disruption ligament
  ossicular chain — *see* Discontinuity, ossicles, ear
  pelvic ring (stable) S32.810 ☑
    unstable S32.811 ☑
  traumatic injury wound repair T81.33 ☑
  wound T81.30 ☑
    episiotomy O90.1
    operation T81.31 ☑
      cesarean O90.0
      external operation wound (superficial)
          T81.31 ☑
      internal operation wound (deep) T81.32 ☑
    perineal (obstetric) O90.1
    traumatic injury repair T81.33 ☑
Dissatisfaction with
  employment Z56.9
  school environment Z55.4
Dissecting — *see* condition
Dissection
  aorta I71.00
    abdominal I71.02
    thoracic I71.01
    thoracoabdominal I71.03
  artery I77.70
    basilar (trunk) I77.75
    carotid I77.71
    cerebral (nonruptured) I67.0
      ruptured — *see* Hemorrhage, intracranial,
          subarachnoid
    coronary I25.42
    extremity
      lower I77.77
      upper I77.76
    iliac I77.72
    precerebral
      congenital (nonruptured) Q28.1
      specified site NEC I77.75
    renal I77.73
    specified NEC I77.79
    vertebral I77.74
  precerebral artery, congenital (nonruptured) Q28.1
    Heartland A93.8
  traumatic — *see* Wound, open, by site
  vascular I99.8
  wound — *see* Wound, open
Disseminated — *see* condition
Dissociation
  auriculoventricular or atrioventricular (AV) (any de-
      gree) (isorhythmic) I45.89
    with heart block I44.2
  interference I45.89
Dissociative reaction, state F44.9
Dissolution, vertebra — *see* Osteoporosis
Distension, distention
  abdomen R14.0
  bladder N32.89
  cecum K63.89
  colon K63.89
  gallbladder K82.8
  intestine K63.89
  kidney N28.89

Distension, distention — *continued*
  liver K76.89
  seminal vesicle N50.89
  stomach K31.89
    acute K31.0
    psychogenic F45.8
  ureter — *see* Dilatation, ureter
  uterus N85.8
Distoma hepaticum infestation B66.3
Distomiasis B66.9
  bile passages B66.3
  hemic B65.9
  hepatic B66.3
    due to Clonorchis sinensis B66.1
  intestinal B66.5
  liver B66.3
    due to Clonorchis sinensis B66.1
  lung B66.4
  pulmonary B66.4
Distomolar (fourth molar) K00.1
Disto-occlusion (Division I) (Division II) M26.212
Distortion(s) (congenital)
  adrenal (gland) Q89.1
  arm NEC Q68.8
  bile duct or passage Q44.5
  bladder Q64.79
  brain Q04.9
  cervix (uteri) Q51.9
  chest (wall) Q67.8
    bones Q76.8
  clavicle Q74.0
  clitoris Q52.6
  coccyx Q76.49
  common duct Q44.5
  coronary Q24.5
  cystic duct Q44.5
  ear (auricle) (external) Q17.3
    inner Q16.5
    middle Q16.4
      ossicles Q16.3
  endocrine NEC Q89.2
  eustachian tube Q17.8
  eye (adnexa) Q15.8
  face bone(s) NEC Q75.8
  fallopian tube Q50.6
  femur NEC Q68.8
  fibula NEC Q68.8
  finger(s) Q68.1
  foot Q66.9
  genitalia, genital organ(s)
    female Q52.8
      external Q52.79
      internal NEC Q52.8
  gyri Q04.8
  hand bone(s) Q68.1
  heart (auricle) (ventricle) Q24.8
    valve (cusp) Q24.8
  hepatic duct Q44.5
  humerus NEC Q68.8
  hymen Q52.4
  intrafamilial communications Z63.8
  jaw NEC M26.89
  labium (majus) (minus) Q52.79
  leg NEC Q68.8
  lens Q12.8
  liver Q44.7
  lumbar spine Q76.49
    with disproportion O33.8
      causing obstructed labor O65.0
  lumbosacral (joint) (region) Q76.49
    kyphosis — *see* Kyphosis, congenital
    lordosis — *see* Lordosis, congenital
  nerve Q07.8
  nose Q30.8
  organ
    of Corti Q16.5
    or site not listed — *see* Anomaly, by site
  ossicles, ear Q16.3
  oviduct Q50.6
  pancreas Q45.3
  parathyroid (gland) Q89.2
  pituitary (gland) Q89.2
  radius NEC Q68.8
  sacroiliac joint Q74.2
  sacrum Q76.49
  scapula Q74.0
  shoulder girdle Q74.0
  skull bone(s) NEC Q75.8

Distortion(s) — *continued*
  skull bone(s) — *continued*
    with
      anencephalus Q00.0
      encephalocele — *see* Encephalocele
      hydrocephalus Q03.9
        with spina bifida — *see* Spina bifida, with hydrocephalus
      microcephaly Q02
  spinal cord Q06.8
  spine Q76.49
    kyphosis — *see* Kyphosis, congenital
    lordosis — *see* Lordosis, congenital
  spleen Q89.09
  sternum NEC Q76.7
  thorax (wall) Q67.8
    bony Q76.8
  thymus (gland) Q89.2
  thyroid (gland) Q89.2
  tibia NEC Q68.8
  toe(s) Q66.9
  tongue Q38.3
  trachea (cartilage) Q32.1
  ulna NEC Q68.8
  ureter Q62.8
  urethra Q64.79
    causing obstruction Q64.39
  uterus Q51.9
  vagina Q52.4
  vertebra Q76.49
    kyphosis — *see* Kyphosis, congenital
    lordosis — *see* Lordosis, congenital
  visual (*see also* Disturbance, vision)
    shape and size H53.15
  vulva Q52.79
  wrist (bones) (joint) Q68.8
Distress
  abdomen — *see* Pain, abdominal
  acute respiratory R06.03
    syndrome (adult) (child) J80
  epigastric R10.13
  fetal P84
    complicating pregnancy — *see* Stress, fetal
  gastrointestinal (functional) K30
    psychogenic F45.8
  intestinal (functional) NOS K59.9
    psychogenic F45.8
  maternal, during labor and delivery O75.0
  relationship, with spouse or intimate partner Z63.0
  respiratory (adult) (child) R06.03
    newborn P22.9
      specified NEC P22.8
    orthopnea R06.01
    psychogenic F45.8
    shortness of breath R06.02
    specified type NEC R06.09
Distribution vessel, atypical Q27.9
  coronary artery Q24.5
  precerebral Q28.1
Districhiasis L68.8
Disturbance(s) (*see also* Disease)
  absorption K90.9
    calcium E58
    carbohydrate K90.49
    fat K90.49
      pancreatic K90.3
    protein K90.49
    starch K90.49
    vitamin — *see* Deficiency, vitamin
  acid-base equilibrium E87.8
    mixed E87.4
  activity and attention (with hyperkinesis) — *see* Disorder, attention-deficit hyperactivity
  amino acid transport E72.00
  assimilation, food K90.9
  auditory nerve, except deafness — *see* subcategory H93.3 ☑
  behavior — *see* Disorder, conduct
  blood clotting (mechanism) (*see also* Defect, coagulation) D68.9
  cerebral
    nerve — *see* Disorder, nerve, cranial
    status, newborn P91.9
      specified NEC P91.88
  circulatory I99.9
  conduct (*see also* Disorder, conduct) F91.9
    adjustment reaction — *see* Disorder, adjustment
    compulsive F63.9

Disturbance(s) — *continued*
  conduct (*see also* Disorder, conduct) — *continued*
    disruptive F91.9
    hyperkinetic — *see* Disorder, attention-deficit hyperactivity
    socialized F91.2
    specified NEC F91.8
    unsocialized F91.1
  coordination R27.8
  cranial nerve — *see* Disorder, nerve, cranial
  deep sensibility — *see* Disturbance, sensation
  digestive K30
    psychogenic F45.8
  electrolyte (*see also* Imbalance, electrolyte)
    newborn, transitory P74.4
      hyperammonemia P74.6
      potassium balance P74.3
      sodium balance P74.2
      specified type NEC P74.4
  emotions specific to childhood and adolescence F93.9
    with
      anxiety and fearfulness NEC F93.8
      elective mutism F94.0
      oppositional disorder F91.3
      sensitivity (withdrawal) F40.10
      shyness F40.10
      social withdrawal F40.10
    involving relationship problems F93.8
    mixed F93.8
    specified NEC F93.8
  endocrine (gland) E34.9
    neonatal, transitory P72.9
      specified NEC P72.8
  equilibrium R42
  fructose metabolism E74.10
  gait — *see* Gait
    hysterical F44.4
    psychogenic F44.4
  gastrointestinal (functional) K30
    psychogenic F45.8
  habit, child F98.9
  hearing, except deafness and tinnitus — *see* Abnormal, auditory perception
  heart, functional (conditions in I44-I50)
    due to presence of (cardiac) prosthesis I97.19- ☑
    postoperative I97.89
      cardiac surgery (*see also* Infarct, myocardium, associated with revascularization procedure) I97.19- ☑
  hormones E34.9
  innervation uterus (parasympathetic) (sympathetic) N85.8
  keratinization NEC
    gingiva K05.10
      nonplaque induced K05.11
      plaque induced K05.10
    lip K13.0
    oral (mucosa) (soft tissue) K13.29
    tongue K13.29
  learning (specific) — *see* Disorder, learning
  memory — *see* Amnesia
    mild, following organic brain damage F06.8
  mental F99
    associated with diseases classified elsewhere F54
  metabolism E88.9
    with
      abortion — *see* Abortion, by type with other specified complication
      ectopic pregnancy O08.5
      molar pregnancy O08.5
    amino-acid E72.9
      aromatic E70.9
      branched-chain E71.2
      straight-chain E72.8
      sulfur-bearing E72.10
    ammonia E72.20
    arginine E72.21
    arginosuccinic acid E72.22
    carbohydrate E74.9
    cholesterol E78.9
    citrulline E72.23
    cystathionine E72.19
    general E88.9
    glutamine E72.8
    histidine E70.40
    homocystine E72.19
    hydroxylysine E72.3
    in labor or delivery O75.89

Disturbance(s) — *continued*
metabolism — *continued*
iron E83.10
lipoid E78.9
lysine E72.3
methionine E72.19
neonatal, transitory P74.9
calcium and magnesium P71.9
specified type NEC P71.8
carbohydrate metabolism P70.9
specified type NEC P70.8
specified NEC P74.8
ornithine E72.4
phosphate E83.39
sodium NEC E87.8
threonine E72.8
tryptophan E70.5
tyrosine E70.20
urea cycle E72.20
motor R29.2
nervous, functional R45.0
neuromuscular mechanism (eye), due to syphilis
A52.15
nutritional E63.9
nail L60.3
ocular motion H51.9
psychogenic F45.8
oculogyric H51.8
psychogenic F45.8
oculomotor H51.9
psychogenic F45.8
olfactory nerve R43.1
optic nerve NEC — *see* Disorder, nerve, optic
oral epithelium, including tongue NEC K13.29
perceptual due to
alcohol withdrawal F10.232
amphetamine intoxication F15.922
in
abuse F15.122
dependence F15.222
anxiolytic withdrawal F13.232
cannabis intoxication (acute) F12.922
in
abuse F12.122
dependence F12.222
cocaine intoxication (acute) F14.922
in
abuse F14.122
dependence F14.222
hypnotic withdrawal F13.232
opioid intoxication (acute) F11.922
in
abuse F11.122
dependence F11.222
phencyclidine intoxication (acute) F16.122
sedative withdrawal F13.232
personality (pattern) (trait) (*see also* Disorder, personality) F60.9
following organic brain damage F07.9
polyglandular E31.9
specified NEC E31.8
potassium balance, newborn P74.3
psychogenic F45.9
psychomotor F44.4
psychophysical visual H53.16
pupillary — *see* Anomaly, pupil, function
reflex R29.2
rhythm, heart I49.9
salivary secretion K11.7
sensation (cold) (heat) (localization) (tactile discrimination) (texture) (vibratory) NEC R20.9
hysterical F44.6
skin R20.9
anesthesia R20.0
hyperesthesia R20.3
hypoesthesia R20.1
paresthesia R20.2
specified type NEC R20.8
smell R43.9
and taste (mixed) R43.8
anosmia R43.0
parosmia R43.1
specified NEC R43.8
taste R43.9
and smell (mixed) R43.8
parageusia R43.2
specified NEC R43.8
sensory — *see* Disturbance, sensation

Disturbance(s) — *continued*
situational (transient) (*see also* Disorder, adjustment)
acute F43.0
sleep G47.9
nonorganic origin F51.9
smell — *see* Disturbance, sensation, smell
sociopathic F60.2
sodium balance, newborn P74.2
speech R47.9
developmental F80.9
specified NEC R47.89
stomach (functional) K31.9
sympathetic (nerve) G90.9
taste — *see* Disturbance, sensation, taste
temperature
regulation, newborn P81.9
specified NEC P81.8
sense R20.8
hysterical F44.6
tooth
eruption K00.6
formation K00.4
structure, hereditary NEC K00.5
touch — *see* Disturbance, sensation
vascular I99.9
arteriosclerotic — *see* Arteriosclerosis
vasomotor I73.9
vasospastic I73.9
vision, visual H53.9
following
cerebral infarction I69.398
cerebrovascular disease I69.998
specified NEC I69.898
intracerebral hemorrhage I69.198
nontraumatic intracranial hemorrhage NEC I69.298
specified disease NEC I69.898
subarachnoid hemorrhage I69.098
psychophysical H53.16
specified NEC H53.8
subjective H53.10
day blindness H53.11
discomfort H53.14- ☑
distortions of shape and size H53.15
loss
sudden H53.13- ☑
transient H53.12- ☑
specified type NEC H53.19
voice R49.9
psychogenic F44.4
specified NEC R49.8
Diuresis R35.8
Diver's palsy, paralysis or squeeze T70.3 ☑
Diverticulitis (acute) K57.92
bladder — *see* Cystitis
ileum — *see* Diverticulitis, intestine, small
intestine K57.92
with
abscess, perforation or peritonitis K57.80
with bleeding K57.81
bleeding K57.93
congenital Q43.8
large K57.32
with
abscess, perforation or peritonitis K57.20
with bleeding K57.21
bleeding K57.33
small intestine K57.52
with
abscess, perforation or peritonitis K57.40
with bleeding K57.41
bleeding K57.53
small K57.12
with
abscess, perforation or peritonitis K57.00
with bleeding K57.01
bleeding K57.13
large intestine K57.52
with
abscess, perforation or peritonitis K57.40
with bleeding K57.41
bleeding K57.53
Diverticulosis K57.90
with bleeding K57.91
large intestine K57.30

Diverticulosis — *continued*
large intestine — *continued*
with
bleeding K57.31
small intestine K57.50
with bleeding K57.51
small intestine K57.10
with
bleeding K57.11
large intestine K57.50
with bleeding K57.51
Diverticulum, diverticula (multiple) K57.90
appendix (noninflammatory) K38.2
bladder (sphincter) N32.3
congenital Q64.6
bronchus (congenital) Q32.4
acquired J98.09
calyx, calyceal (kidney) N28.89
cardia (stomach) K31.4
cecum — *see* Diverticulosis, intestine, large
congenital Q43.8
colon — *see* Diverticulosis, intestine, large
congenital Q43.8
duodenum — *see* Diverticulosis, intestine, small
congenital Q43.8
epiphrenic (esophagus) K22.5
esophagus (congenital) Q39.6
acquired (epiphrenic) (pulsion) (traction) K22.5
eustachian tube — *see* Disorder, eustachian tube, specified NEC
fallopian tube N83.8
gastric K31.4
heart (congenital) Q24.8
ileum — *see* Diverticulosis, intestine, small
jejunum — *see* Diverticulosis, intestine, small
kidney (pelvis) (calyces) N28.89
with calculus — *see* Calculus, kidney
Meckel's (displaced) (hypertrophic) Q43.0
malignant — *see* Table of Neoplasms, small intestine, malignant
midthoracic K22.5
organ or site, congenital NEC — *see* Distortion
pericardium (congenital) (cyst) Q24.8
acquired I31.8
pharyngoesophageal (congenital) Q39.6
acquired K22.5
pharynx (congenital) Q38.7
rectosigmoid — *see* Diverticulosis, intestine, large
congenital Q43.8
rectum — *see* Diverticulosis, intestine, large
Rokitansky's K22.5
seminal vesicle N50.89
sigmoid — *see* Diverticulosis, intestine, large
congenital Q43.8
stomach (acquired) K31.4
congenital Q40.2
trachea (acquired) J39.8
ureter (acquired) N28.89
congenital Q62.8
ureterovesical orifice N28.89
urethra (acquired) N36.1
congenital Q64.79
ventricle, left (congenital) Q24.8
vesical N32.3
congenital Q64.6
Zenker's (esophagus) K22.5
Division
cervix uteri (acquired) N88.8
glans penis Q55.69
labia minora (congenital) Q52.79
ligament (partial or complete) (current) (*see also* Sprain)
with open wound — *see* Wound, open
muscle (partial or complete) (current) (*see also* Injury, muscle)
with open wound — *see* Wound, open
nerve (traumatic) — *see* Injury, nerve
spinal cord — *see* Injury, spinal cord, by region
vein I87.8
Divorce, causing family disruption Z63.5
Dix-Hallpike neurolabyrinthitis — *see* Neuronitis, vestibular
Dizziness R42
hysterical F44.89
psychogenic F45.8
DMAC (disseminated mycobacterium avium- intracellulare complex) A31.2
DNR (do not resuscitate) Z66

Doan-Wiseman syndrome (primary splenic neutropenia) — see Agranulocytosis
Doehle-Heller aortitis A52.02
Dog bite — see Bite
Dohle body panmyelopathic syndrome D72.0
Dolichocephaly Q67.2
Dolichocolon Q43.8
Dolichostenomelia — see Syndrome, Marfan's
Donohue's syndrome E34.8
Donor (organ or tissue) Z52.9
  blood (whole) Z52.000
    autologous Z52.010
    specified component (lymphocytes) (platelets) NEC Z52.008
      autologous Z52.018
      specified donor NEC Z52.098
    specified donor NEC Z52.090
    stem cells Z52.001
      autologous Z52.011
      specified donor NEC Z52.091
  bone Z52.20
    autologous Z52.21
    marrow Z52.3
    specified type NEC Z52.29
  cornea Z52.5
  egg (Oocyte) Z52.819
    age 35 and over Z52.812
      anonymous recipient Z52.812
      designated recipient Z52.813
    under age 35 Z52.810
      anonymous recipient Z52.810
      designated recipient Z52.811
  kidney Z52.4
  liver Z52.6
  lung Z52.89
  lymphocyte — see Donor, blood, specified components NEC
  Oocyte — see Donor, egg
  platelets Z52.008
  potential, examination of Z00.5
  semen Z52.89
  skin Z52.10
    autologous Z52.11
    specified type NEC Z52.19
  specified organ or tissue NEC Z52.89
  sperm Z52.89
Donovanosis A58
Dorsalgia M54.9
  psychogenic F45.41
  specified NEC M54.89
Dorsopathy M53.9
  deforming M43.9
    specified NEC — see subcategory M43.8 ☑
  specified NEC M53.80
    cervical region M53.82
    cervicothoracic region M53.83
    lumbar region M53.86
    lumbosacral region M53.87
    occipito-atlanto-axial region M53.81
    sacrococcygeal region M53.88
    thoracic region M53.84
    thoracolumbar region M53.85
Double
  albumin E88.09
  aortic arch Q25.45
  auditory canal Q17.8
  auricle (heart) Q20.8
  bladder Q64.79
  cervix Q51.820
    with doubling of uterus (and vagina) Q51.10
      with obstruction Q51.11
  inlet ventricle Q20.4
  kidney with double pelvis (renal) Q63.0
  meatus urinarius Q64.75
  monster Q89.4
  outlet
    left ventricle Q20.2
    right ventricle Q20.1
  pelvis (renal) with double ureter Q62.5
  tongue Q38.3
  ureter (one or both sides) Q62.5
    with double pelvis (renal) Q62.5
  urethra Q64.74
  urinary meatus Q64.75
  uterus Q51.2
    with
      doubling of cervix (and vagina) Q51.10
        with obstruction Q51.11

Double — continued
  uterus — continued
    in pregnancy or childbirth O34.59- ☑
      causing obstructed labor O65.5
  vagina Q52.10
    with doubling of uterus (and cervix) Q51.10
      with obstruction Q51.11
  vision H53.2
  vulva Q52.79
Douglas' pouch, cul-de-sac — see condition
Down syndrome Q90.9
  meiotic nondisjunction Q90.0
  mitotic nondisjunction Q90.1
  mosaicism Q90.1
  translocation Q90.2
DPD (dihydropyrimidine dehydrogenase deficiency) E88.89
Dracontiasis B72
Dracunculiasis, dracunculosis B72
Dream state, hysterical F44.89
Drepanocytic anemia — see Disease, sickle-cell
Dresbach's syndrome (elliptocytosis) D58.1
Dreschlera (hawaiiensis) (infection) B43.8
Dressler's syndrome I24.1
Drift, ulnar — see Deformity, limb, specified type NEC, forearm
Drinking (alcohol)
  excessive, to excess NEC (without dependence) F10.10
    habitual (continual) (without remission) F10.20
      with remission F10.21
Drip, postnasal (chronic) R09.82
  due to
    allergic rhinitis — see Rhinitis, allergic
    common cold J00
    gastroesophageal reflux — see Reflux, gastroesophageal
    nasopharyngitis — see Nasopharyngitis
    other known condition — code to condition
    sinusitis — see Sinusitis
Droop
  facial R29.810
    cerebrovascular disease I69.992
      cerebral infarction I69.392
      intracerebral hemorrhage I69.192
      nontraumatic intracranial hemorrhage NEC I69.292
      specified disease NEC I69.892
      subarachnoid hemorrhage I69.092
Drop (in)
  attack NEC R55
  finger — see Deformity, finger
  foot — see Deformity, limb, foot, drop
  hematocrit (precipitous) R71.0
  hemoglobin R71.0
  toe — see Deformity, toe, specified NEC
  wrist — see Deformity, limb, wrist drop
Dropped heart beats I45.9
Dropsy, dropsical (see also Hydrops)
  abdomen R18.8
  brain — see Hydrocephalus
  cardiac, heart — see Failure, heart, congestive
  gangrenous — see Gangrene
  heart — see Failure, heart, congestive
  kidney — see Nephrosis
  lung — see Edema, lung
  newborn due to isoimmunization P56.0
  pericardium — see Pericarditis
Drowned, drowning (near) T75.1 ☑
Drowsiness R40.0
Drug
  abuse counseling and surveillance Z71.51
  addiction — see Dependence
  dependence — see Dependence
  habit — see Dependence
  harmful use — see Abuse, drug
  induced fever R50.2
  overdose — see Table of Drugs and Chemicals, by drug, poisoning
  poisoning — see Table of Drugs and Chemicals, by drug, poisoning
  resistant organism infection (see also Resistant, organism, to, drug) Z16.30
  therapy
    long term (current) (prophylactic) — see Therapy, drug long-term (current) (prophylactic)

Drug — continued
  therapy — continued
    short term — omit code
  wrong substance given or taken in error — see Table of Drugs and Chemicals, by drug, poisoning
Drunkenness (without dependence) F10.129
  acute in alcoholism F10.229
  chronic (without remission) F10.20
    with remission F10.21
  pathological (without dependence) F10.129
    with dependence F10.229
  sleep F51.9
Drusen
  macula (degenerative) (retina) — see Degeneration, macula, drusen
  optic disc H47.32- ☑
Dry, dryness (see also condition)
  larynx J38.7
  mouth R68.2
    due to dehydration E86.0
  nose J34.89
  socket (teeth) M27.3
  throat J39.2
DSAP L56.5
Duane's syndrome H50.81- ☑
Dubin-Johnson disease or syndrome E80.6
Dubois' disease (thymus gland) A50.59 [E35]
Dubowitz' syndrome Q87.1
Duchenne-Aran muscular atrophy G12.21
Duchenne-Griesinger disease G71.0
Duchenne's
  disease or syndrome
    motor neuron disease G12.22
    muscular dystrophy G71.0
  locomotor ataxia (syphilitic) A52.11
  paralysis
    birth injury P14.0
    due to or associated with
      motor neuron disease G12.22
      muscular dystrophy G71.0
Ducrey's chancre A57
Duct, ductus — see condition
Duhring's disease (dermatitis herpetiformis) L13.0
Dullness, cardiac (decreased) (increased) R01.2
Dumb ague — see Malaria
Dumbness — see Aphasia
Dumdum fever B55.0
Dumping syndrome (postgastrectomy) K91.1
Duodenitis (nonspecific) (peptic) K29.80
  with bleeding K29.81
Duodenocholangitis — see Cholangitis
Duodenum, duodenal — see condition
Duplay's bursitis or periarthritis — see Tendinitis, calcific, shoulder
Duplication, duplex (see also Accessory)
  alimentary tract Q45.8
  anus Q43.4
  appendix (and cecum) Q43.4
  biliary duct (any) Q44.5
  bladder Q64.79
  cecum (and appendix) Q43.4
  cervix Q51.820
  chromosome NEC
    with complex rearrangements NEC Q92.5
    seen only at prometaphase Q92.8
  cystic duct Q44.5
  digestive organs Q45.8
  esophagus Q39.8
  frontonasal process Q75.8
  intestine (large) (small) Q43.4
  kidney Q63.0
  liver Q44.7
  pancreas Q45.3
  penis Q55.69
  respiratory organs NEC Q34.8
  salivary duct Q38.4
  spinal cord (incomplete) Q06.2
  stomach Q40.2
Dupré's disease (meningism) R29.1
Dupuytren's contraction or disease M72.0
Durand-Nicolas-Favre disease A55
Durotomy (inadvertent) (incidental) G97.41
Duroziez's disease (congenital mitral stenosis) Q23.2
Dutton's relapsing fever (West African) A68.1
Dwarfism E34.3
  achondroplastic Q77.4
  congenital E34.3
  constitutional E34.3

Dwarfism — *continued*
  hypochondroplastic Q77.4
  hypophyseal E23.0
  infantile E34.3
  Laron-type E34.3
  Lorain (-Levi) type E23.0
  metatropic Q77.8
  nephrotic-glycosuric (with hypophosphatemic rickets) E72.09
  nutritional E45
  pancreatic K86.89
  pituitary E23.0
  renal N25.0
  thanatophoric Q77.1
Dyke-Young anemia (secondary) (symptomatic) D59.1
Dysacusis — *see* Abnormal, auditory perception
Dysadrenocortism E27.9
  hyperfunction E27.0
Dysarthria R47.1
  following
    cerebral infarction I69.322
    cerebrovascular disease I69.922
      specified disease NEC I69.822
    intracerebral hemorrhage I69.122
    nontraumatic intracranial hemorrhage NEC I69.222
    subarachnoid hemorrhage I69.022
Dysautonomia (familial) G90.1
Dysbarism T70.3 ☑
Dysbasia R26.2
  angiosclerotica intermittens I73.9
  hysterical F44.4
  lordotica (progressiva) G24.1
  nonorganic origin F44.4
  psychogenic F44.4
Dysbetalipoproteinemia (familial) E78.2
Dyscalculia R48.8
  developmental F81.2
Dyschezia K59.00
Dyschondroplasia (with hemangiomata) Q78.4
Dyschromia (skin) L81.9
Dyscollagenosis M35.9
Dyscranio-pygo-phalangy Q87.0
Dyscrasia
  blood (with) D75.9
    antepartum hemorrhage — *see* Hemorrhage, antepartum, with coagulation defect
    intrapartum hemorrhage O67.0
    newborn P61.9
      specified type NEC P61.8
    puerperal, postpartum O72.3
  polyglandular, pluriglandular E31.9
Dysendocrinism E34.9
Dysentery, dysenteric (catarrhal) (diarrhea) (epidemic) (hemorrhagic) (infectious) (sporadic) (tropical) A09
  abscess, liver A06.4
  amebic (*see also* Amebiasis) A06.0
    with abscess — *see* Abscess, amebic
    acute A06.0
    chronic A06.1
  arthritis (*see also* category M01) A09
    bacillary (*see also* category M01) A03.9
  bacillary A03.9
    arthritis (*see also* category M01) A03.9
    Boyd A03.2
    Flexner A03.1
    Schmitz (-Stutzer) A03.0
    Shiga (-Kruse) A03.0
    Shigella A03.9
      boydii A03.2
      dysenteriae A03.0
      flexneri A03.1
      group A A03.0
      group B A03.1
      group C A03.2
      group D A03.3
      sonnei A03.3
      specified type NEC A03.8
    Sonne A03.3
    specified type NEC A03.8
  balantidial A07.0
  Balantidium coli A07.0
  Boyd's A03.2
  candidal B37.82
  Chilomastix A07.8
  Chinese A03.9
  coccidial A07.3
  Dientamoeba (fragilis) A07.8
  Embadomonas A07.8

Dysentery, dysenteric — *continued*
  Entamoeba, entambic — *see* Dysentery, amebic
  Flexner-Boyd A03.2
  Flexner's A03.1
  Giardia lamblia A07.1
  Hiss-Russell A03.1
  Lamblia A07.1
  leishmanial B55.0
  malarial — *see* Malaria
  metazoal B82.0
  monilial B37.82
  protozoal A07.9
  Salmonella A02.0
  schistosomal B65.1
  Schmitz (-Stutzer) A03.0
  Shiga (-Kruse) A03.0
  Shigella NOS — *see* Dysentery, bacillary
  Sonne A03.3
  strongyloidiasis B78.0
  trichomonal A07.8
  viral (*see also* Enteritis, viral) A08.4
Dysequilibrium R42
Dysesthesia R20.8
  hysterical F44.6
Dysfibrinogenemia (congenital) D68.2
Dysfunction
  adrenal E27.9
    hyperfunction E27.0
  autonomic
    due to alcohol G31.2
    somatoform F45.8
  bladder N31.9
    neurogenic NOS — *see* Dysfunction, bladder, neuromuscular
    neuromuscular NOS N31.9
      atonic (motor) (sensory) N31.2
      autonomous N31.2
      flaccid N31.2
      nonreflex N31.2
      reflex N31.1
      specified NEC N31.8
      uninhibited N31.0
  bleeding, uterus N93.8
  cerebral G93.89
  colon K59.9
    psychogenic F45.8
  colostomy K94.03
  cystic duct K82.8
  cystostomy (stoma) — *see* Complications, cystostomy
  ejaculatory N53.19
    anejaculatory orgasm N53.13
    painful N53.12
    premature F52.4
    retarded N53.11
  endocrine NOS E34.9
  endometrium N85.8
  enterostomy K94.13
  erectile — *see* Dysfunction, sexual, male, erectile
  gallbladder K82.8
  gastrostomy (stoma) K94.23
  gland, glandular NOS E34.9
  heart I51.89
  hemoglobin D75.89
  hepatic K76.89
  hypophysis E23.7
  hypothalamic NEC E23.3
  ileostomy (stoma) K94.13
  jejunostomy (stoma) K94.13
  kidney — *see* Disease, renal
  labyrinthine — *see* subcategory H83.2 ☑
  left ventricular, following sudden emotional stress I51.81
  liver K76.89
  male — *see* Dysfunction, sexual, male
  orgasmic (female) F52.31
    male F52.32
  ovary E28.9
    specified NEC E28.8
  papillary muscle I51.89
  parathyroid E21.4
  physiological NEC R68.89
    psychogenic F59
  pineal gland E34.8
  pituitary (gland) E23.3
  platelets D69.1
  polyglandular E31.9
    specified NEC E31.8
  psychophysiologic F59

Dysfunction — *continued*
  psychosexual F52.9
    with
      dyspareunia F52.6
      premature ejaculation F52.4
      vaginismus F52.5
  pylorus K31.9
  rectum K59.9
    psychogenic F45.8
  reflex (sympathetic) — *see* Syndrome, pain, complex regional I
  segmental — *see* Dysfunction, somatic
  senile R54
  sexual (due to) R37
    alcohol F10.981
    amphetamine F15.981
      in
        abuse F15.181
        dependence F15.281
    anxiolytic F13.981
      in
        abuse F13.181
        dependence F13.281
    cocaine F14.981
      in
        abuse F14.181
        dependence F14.281
    excessive sexual drive F52.8
    failure of genital response (male) F52.21
      female F52.22
    female N94.9
      aversion F52.1
      dyspareunia N94.10
        psychogenic F52.6
      frigidity F52.22
      nymphomania F52.8
      orgasmic F52.31
      psychogenic F52.9
        aversion F52.1
        dyspareunia F52.6
        frigidity F52.22
        nymphomania F52.8
        orgasmic F52.31
        vaginismus F52.5
      vaginismus N94.2
        psychogenic F52.5
    hypnotic F13.981
      in
        abuse F13.181
        dependence F13.281
    inhibited orgasm (female) F52.31
      male F52.32
    lack
      of sexual enjoyment F52.1
      or loss of sexual desire F52.0
    male N53.9
      anejaculatory orgasm N53.13
      ejaculatory N53.19
        painful N53.12
        premature F52.4
        retarded N53.11
      erectile N52.9
        drug induced N52.2
        due to
          disease classified elsewhere N52.1
          drug N52.2
          postoperative (postprocedural) N52.39
            following
              cryotherapy N52.37
              interstitial seed therapy N52.36
              prostate ablative therapy N52.37
              prostatectomy N52.34
                radical N52.31
              radiation therapy N52.35
              radical cystectomy N52.32
              ultrasound ablative therapy N52.37
              urethral surgery N52.33
        psychogenic F52.21
        specified cause NEC N52.8
        vasculogenic
          arterial insufficiency N52.01
            with corporo-venous occlusive N52.03
          corporo-venous occlusive N52.02
            with arterial insufficiency N52.03
      impotence — *see* Dysfunction, sexual, male, erectile
      psychogenic F52.9
        aversion F52.1

Dysfunction — continued
  sexual — continued
    male — continued
      psychogenic — continued
        erectile F52.21
        orgasmic F52.32
        premature ejaculation F52.4
        satyriasis F52.8
        specified type NEC F52.8
      specified type NEC N53.8
    nonorganic F52.9
      specified NEC F52.8
    opioid F11.981
      in
        abuse F11.181
        dependence F11.281
    orgasmic dysfunction (female) F52.31
      male F52.32
    premature ejaculation F52.4
    psychoactive substances NEC F19.981
      in
        abuse F19.181
        dependence F19.281
    psychogenic F52.9
    sedative F13.981
      in
        abuse F13.181
        dependence F13.281
    sexual aversion F52.1
    vaginismus (nonorganic) (psychogenic) F52.5
  sinoatrial node I49.5
  somatic M99.09
    abdomen M99.09
    acromioclavicular M99.07
    cervical region M99.01
    cervicothoracic M99.01
    costochondral M99.08
    costovertebral M99.08
    head region M99.00
    hip M99.05
    lower extremity M99.06
    lumbar region M99.03
    lumbosacral M99.03
    occipitocervical M99.00
    pelvic region M99.05
    pubic M99.05
    rib cage M99.08
    sacral region M99.04
    sacrococcygeal M99.04
    sacroiliac M99.04
    specified NEC M99.09
    sternochondral M99.08
    sternoclavicular M99.07
    thoracic region M99.02
    thoracolumbar M99.02
    upper extremity M99.07
  somatoform autonomic F45.8
  stomach K31.89
    psychogenic F45.8
  suprarenal E27.9
    hyperfunction E27.0
  symbolic R48.9
    specified type NEC R48.8
  temporomandibular (joint) M26.69
    joint-pain syndrome M26.62- ☑
  testicular (endocrine) E29.9
    specified NEC E29.8
  thymus E32.9
  thyroid E07.9
  ureterostomy (stoma) — see Complications, stoma,
    urinary tract
  urethrostomy (stoma) — see Complications, stoma,
    urinary tract
  uterus, complicating delivery O62.9
    hypertonic O62.4
    hypotonic O62.2
      primary O62.0
      secondary O62.1
  ventricular I51.9
    with congestive heart failure (see also Failure,
      heart) I50.9
    left, reversible, following sudden emotional stress
      I51.81

Dysgenesis
  gonadal (due to chromosomal anomaly) Q96.9
    pure Q99.1
  renal Q60.5
    bilateral Q60.4
    unilateral Q60.3

Dysgenesis — continued
  reticular D72.0
  tidal platelet D69.3
Dysgerminoma
  specified site — see Neoplasm, malignant, by site
  unspecified site
    female C56.9
    male C62.90
Dysgeusia R43.2
Dysgraphia R27.8
Dyshidrosis, dysidrosis L30.1
Dyskaryotic cervical smear R87.619
Dyskeratosis L85.8
  cervix — see Dysplasia, cervix
  congenital Q82.8
  uterus NEC N85.8
Dyskinesia G24.9
  biliary (cystic duct or gallbladder) K82.8
  drug induced
    orofacial G24.01
  esophagus K22.4
  hysterical F44.4
  intestinal K59.8
  nonorganic origin F44.4
  orofacial (idiopathic) G24.4
    drug induced G24.01
  psychogenic F44.4
  subacute, drug induced G24.01
  tardive G24.01
    neuroleptic induced G24.01
  trachea J39.8
  tracheobronchial J98.09
Dyslalia (developmental) F80.0
Dyslexia R48.0
  developmental F81.0
Dyslipidemia E78.5
  depressed HDL cholesterol E78.6
  elevated fasting triglycerides E78.1
Dysmaturity (see also Light for dates)
  pulmonary (newborn) (Wilson-Mikity) P27.0
Dysmenorrhea (essential) (exfoliative) N94.6
  congestive (syndrome) N94.6
  primary N94.4
  psychogenic F45.8
  secondary N94.5
Dysmetabolic syndrome X E88.81
Dysmetria R27.8
Dysmorphism (due to)
  alcohol Q86.0
  exogenous cause NEC Q86.8
  hydantoin Q86.1
  warfarin Q86.2
Dysmorphophobia (nondelusional) F45.22
  delusional F22
Dysnomia R47.01
Dysorexia R63.0
  psychogenic F50.89
Dysostosis
  cleidocranial, cleidocranialis Q74.0
  craniofacial Q75.1
  Fairbank's (idiopathic familial generalized osteophyto-
    sis) Q78.9
  mandibulofacial (incomplete) Q75.4
  multiplex E76.01
  oculomandibular Q75.5
Dyspareunia (female) N94.10
  deep N94.12
  male N53.12
  nonorganic F52.6
  psychogenic F52.6
  secondary N94.19
  specified NEC N94.19
  superficial (introital) N94.11
Dyspepsia R10.13
  atonic K30
  functional (allergic) (congenital) (gastrointestinal)
    (occupational) (reflex) K30
  intestinal K59.8
  nervous F45.8
  neurotic F45.8
  psychogenic F45.8
Dysphagia R13.10
  cervical R13.19
  following
    cerebral infarction I69.391
    cerebrovascular disease I69.991
      specified NEC I69.891
    intracerebral hemorrhage I69.191

Dysphagia — continued
  following — continued
    nontraumatic intracranial hemorrhage NEC I69.291
    specified disease NEC I69.891
    subarachnoid hemorrhage I69.091
  functional (hysterical) F45.8
  hysterical F45.8
  nervous (hysterical) F45.8
  neurogenic R13.19
  oral phase R13.11
  oropharyngeal phase R13.12
  pharyngeal phase R13.13
  pharyngoesophageal phase R13.14
  psychogenic F45.8
  sideropenic D50.1
  spastica K22.4
  specified NEC R13.19
Dysphagocytosis, congenital D71
Dysphasia R47.02
  developmental
    expressive type F80.1
    receptive type F80.2
  following
    cerebrovascular disease I69.921
      cerebral infarction I69.321
      intracerebral hemorrhage I69.121
      nontraumatic intracranial hemorrhage NEC
        I69.221
      specified disease NEC I69.821
      subarachnoid hemorrhage I69.021
Dysphonia R49.0
  functional F44.4
  hysterical F44.4
  psychogenic F44.4
  spastica J38.3
Dysphoria
  gender F64.9
    in
      adolescence and adulthood F64.0
      children F64.2
    specified NEC F64.8
  postpartal O90.6
Dyspituitarism E23.3
Dysplasia (see also Anomaly)
  acetabular, congenital Q65.89
  alveolar capillary, with vein misalignment J84.843
  anus (histologically confirmed) (mild) (moderate)
    K62.82
    severe D01.3
  arrhythmogenic right ventricular I42.8
  arterial, fibromuscular I77.3
  asphyxiating thoracic (congenital) Q77.2
  brain Q07.9
  bronchopulmonary, perinatal P27.1
  cervix (uteri) N87.9
    mild N87.0
    moderate N87.1
    severe D06.9
  chondroectodermal Q77.6
  colon D12.6
  craniometaphyseal Q78.8
  dentinal K00.5
  diaphyseal, progressive Q78.3
  dystrophic Q77.5
  ectodermal (anhidrotic) (congenital) (hereditary) Q82.4
    hydrotic Q82.8
  epithelial, uterine cervix — see Dysplasia, cervix
  eye (congenital) Q11.2
  fibrous
    bone NEC (monostotic) M85.00
      ankle M85.07- ☑
      foot M85.07- ☑
      forearm M85.03- ☑
      hand M85.04- ☑
      lower leg M85.06- ☑
      multiple site M85.09
      neck M85.08
      rib M85.08
      shoulder M85.01- ☑
      skull M85.08
      specified site NEC M85.08
      thigh M85.05- ☑
      toe M85.07- ☑
      upper arm M85.02- ☑
      vertebra M85.08
    diaphyseal, progressive Q78.3
  jaw M27.8
  polyostotic Q78.1

Dysplasia — *continued*
  florid osseous (*see also* Cyst, calcifying odontogenic)
  high grade, focal D12.6
  hip, congenital Q65.89
  joint, congenital Q74.8
  kidney Q61.4
    multicystic Q61.4
  leg Q74.2
  lung, congenital (not associated with short gestation) Q33.6
  mammary (gland) (benign) N60.9- ☑
    cyst (solitary) — *see* Cyst, breast
    cystic — *see* Mastopathy, cystic
    duct ectasia — *see* Ectasia, mammary duct
    fibroadenosis — *see* Fibroadenosis, breast
    fibrosclerosis — *see* Fibrosclerosis, breast
    specified type NEC N60.8- ☑
  metaphyseal Q78.5
  muscle Q79.8
  oculodentodigital Q87.0
  periapical (cemental) (cemento-osseous) — *see* Cyst, calcifying odontogenic
  periosteum — *see* Disorder, bone, specified type NEC
  polyostotic fibrous Q78.1
  prostate (*see also* Neoplasia, intraepithelial, prostate) N42.30
    severe D07.5
    specified NEC N42.39
  renal Q61.4
    multicystic Q61.4
  retinal, congenital Q14.1
  right ventricular, arrhythmogenic I42.8
  septo-optic Q04.4
  skin L98.8
  spinal cord Q06.1
  spondyloepiphyseal Q77.7
  thymic, with immunodeficiency D82.1
  vagina N89.3
    mild N89.0
    moderate N89.1
    severe NEC D07.2
  vulva N90.3
    mild N90.0
    moderate N90.1
    severe NEC D07.1
Dyspnea (nocturnal) (paroxysmal) R06.00
  asthmatic (bronchial) J45.909
    with
      bronchitis J45.909
        with
          exacerbation (acute) J45.901
          status asthmaticus J45.902
        chronic J44.9
      exacerbation (acute) J45.901
      status asthmaticus J45.902
    cardiac — *see* Failure, ventricular, left
  cardiac — *see* Failure, ventricular, left
  functional F45.8
  hyperventilation R06.4
  hysterical F45.8
  newborn P28.89
  orthopnea R06.01
  psychogenic F45.8
  shortness of breath R06.02
  specified type NEC R06.09
Dyspraxia R27.8
  developmental (syndrome) F82
Dysproteinemia E88.09
Dysreflexia, autonomic G90.4
Dysrhythmia
  cardiac I49.9
    newborn
      bradycardia P29.12
      occurring before birth P03.819
        before onset of labor P03.810
        during labor P03.811
      tachycardia P29.11
    postoperative I97.89
  cerebral or cortical — *see* Epilepsy
Dyssomnia — *see* Disorder, sleep
Dyssynergia
  biliary K83.8
  bladder sphincter N36.44
  cerebellaris myoclonica (Hunt's ataxia) G11.1
Dysthymia F34.1
Dysthyroidism E07.9
Dystocia O66.9
  affecting newborn P03.1

Dystocia — *continued*
  cervical (hypotonic) O62.2
    affecting newborn P03.6
    primary O62.0
    secondary O62.1
  contraction ring O62.4
  fetal O66.9
    abnormality NEC O66.3
    conjoined twins O66.3
    oversize O66.2
  maternal O66.9
  positional O64.9 ☑
  shoulder (girdle) O66.0
    causing obstructed labor O66.0
  uterine NEC O62.4
Dystonia G24.9
  deformans progressiva G24.1
  drug induced NEC G24.09
    acute G24.02
    specified NEC G24.09
  familial G24.1
  idiopathic G24.1
    familial G24.1
    nonfamilial G24.2
    orofacial G24.4
  lenticularis G24.8
  musculorum deformans G24.1
  neuroleptic induced (acute) G24.02
  orofacial (idiopathic) G24.4
  oromandibular G24.4
    due to drug G24.01
  specified NEC G24.8
  torsion (familial) (idiopathic) G24.1
    acquired G24.8
    genetic G24.1
    symptomatic (nonfamilial) G24.2
Dystonic movements R25.8
Dystrophy, dystrophia
  adiposogenital E23.6
  Becker's type G71.0
  cervical sympathetic G90.2
  choroid (hereditary) H31.20
    central areolar H31.22
    choroideremia H31.21
    gyrate atrophy H31.23
    specified type NEC H31.29
  cornea (hereditary) H18.50
    endothelial H18.51
    epithelial H18.52
    granular H18.53
    lattice H18.54
    macular H18.55
    specified type NEC H18.59
  Duchenne's type G71.0
  due to malnutrition E45
  Erb's G71.0
  Fuchs' H18.51
  Gower's muscular G71.0
  hair L67.8
  infantile neuraxonal G31.89
  Landouzy-Déjérine G71.0
  Leyden-Möbius G71.0
  muscular G71.0
    benign (Becker type) G71.0
    congenital (hereditary) (progressive) (with specific morphological abnormalities of the muscle fiber) G71.0
      myotonic G71.11
    distal G71.0
    Duchenne type G71.0
    Emery-Dreifuss G71.0
    Erb type G71.0
    facioscapulohumeral G71.0
    Gower's G71.0
    hereditary (progressive) G71.0
    Landouzy-Déjérine type G71.0
    limb-girdle G71.0
    myotonic G71.11
    progressive (hereditary) G71.0
      Charcot-Marie (-Tooth) type G60.0
    pseudohypertrophic (infantile) G71.0
    severe (Duchenne type) G71.0
  myocardium, myocardial — *see* Degeneration, myocardial
  nail L60.3
    congenital Q84.6
  nutritional E45
  ocular G71.0
  oculocerebrorenal E72.03

Dystrophy, dystrophia — *continued*
  oculopharyngeal G71.0
  ovarian N83.8
  polyglandular E31.8
  reflex (neuromuscular) (sympathetic) — *see* Syndrome, pain, complex regional I
  retinal (hereditary) H35.50
    in
      lipid storage disorders E75.6 [H36]
      systemic lipidoses E75.6 [H36]
    involving
      pigment epithelium H35.54
      sensory area H35.53
    pigmentary H35.52
    vitreoretinal H35.51
  Salzmann's nodular — *see* Degeneration, cornea, nodular
  scapuloperoneal G71.0
  skin NEC L98.8
  sympathetic (reflex) — *see* Syndrome, pain, complex regional I
    cervical G90.2
  tapetoretinal H35.54
  thoracic, asphyxiating Q77.2
  unguium L60.3
    congenital Q84.6
  vitreoretinal H35.51
  vulva N90.4
  yellow (liver) — *see* Failure, hepatic
Dysuria R30.0
  psychogenic F45.8

E

Eales' disease H35.06- ☑
Ear (*see also* condition)
  piercing Z41.3
  tropical NEC B36.9 [H62.40]
    in
      aspergillosis B44.89
      candidiasis B37.84
      moniliasis B37.84
  wax (impacted) H61.20
    left H61.22
      with right H61.23
    right H61.21
      with left H61.23
Earache — *see* subcategory H92.0 ☑
Early satiety R68.81
Eaton-Lambert syndrome — *see* Syndrome, Lambert-Eaton
Eberth's disease (typhoid fever) A01.00
Ebola virus disease A98.4
Ebstein's anomaly or syndrome (heart) Q22.5
Eccentro-osteochondrodysplasia E76.29
Ecchondroma — *see* Neoplasm, bone, benign
Ecchondrosis D48.0
Ecchymosis R58
  conjunctiva — *see* Hemorrhage, conjunctiva
  eye (traumatic) — *see* Contusion, eyeball
  eyelid (traumatic) — *see* Contusion, eyelid
  newborn P54.5
  spontaneous R23.3
  traumatic — *see* Contusion
Echinococciasis — *see* Echinococcus
Echinococcosis — *see* Echinococcus
Echinococcus (infection) B67.90
  granulosus B67.4
    bone B67.2
    liver B67.0
    lung B67.1
    multiple sites B67.32
    specified site NEC B67.39
    thyroid B67.31
  liver NOS B67.8
    granulosus B67.0
    multilocularis B67.5
  lung NEC B67.99
    granulosus B67.1
    multilocularis B67.69
  multilocularis B67.7
    liver B67.5
    multiple sites B67.61
    specified site NEC B67.69
  specified site NEC B67.99
    granulosus B67.39
    multilocularis B67.69
  thyroid NEC B67.99

⑯ **Subterms under main terms may continue to next column or page**   ☑ **Additional Character Required** — Refer to the Tabular List for Character Selection   **125**

Dysplasia — Echinococcus

Index

Echinococcus — Edema, edematous

Echinococcus — *continued*
  thyroid — *continued*
    granulosus B67.31
    multilocularis B67.69 [E35]
Echinorhynchiasis B83.8
Echinostomiasis B66.8
Echolalia R48.8
Echovirus, as cause of disease classified elsewhere B97.12
Eclampsia, eclamptic (coma) (convulsions) (delirium) (with hypertension) NEC O15.9
  complicating
    labor and delivery O15.1
    postpartum O15.2
    pregnancy O15.0- ☑
    puerperium O15.2
Economic circumstances affecting care Z59.9
Economo's disease A85.8
Ectasia, ectasis
  annuloaortic I35.8
  aorta I77.819
    with aneurysm — *see* Aneurysm, aorta
    abdominal I77.811
    thoracic I77.810
    thoracoabdominal I77.812
  breast — *see* Ectasia, mammary duct
  capillary I78.8
  cornea H18.71- ☑
  gastric antral vascular (GAVE) K31.819
    with hemorrhage K31.811
    without hemorrhage K31.819
  mammary duct N60.4- ☑
  salivary gland (duct) K11.8
  sclera — *see* Sclerectasia
Ecthyma L08.0
  contagiosum B08.02
  gangrenosum L08.0
  infectiosum B08.02
Ectocardia Q24.8
Ectodermal dysplasia (anhidrotic) Q82.4
Ectodermosis erosiva pluriorificialis L51.1
Ectopic, ectopia (congenital)
  abdominal viscera Q45.8
    due to defect in anterior abdominal wall Q79.59
  ACTH syndrome E24.3
  adrenal gland Q89.1
  anus Q43.5
  atrial beats I49.1
  beats I49.49
    atrial I49.1
    ventricular I49.3
  bladder Q64.10
  bone and cartilage in lung Q33.5
  brain Q04.8
  breast tissue Q83.8
  cardiac Q24.8
  cerebral Q04.8
  cordis Q24.8
  endometrium — *see* Endometriosis
  gastric mucosa Q40.2
  gestation — *see* Pregnancy, by site
  heart Q24.8
  hormone secretion NEC E34.2
  kidney (crossed) (pelvis) Q63.2
  lens, lentis Q12.1
  mole — *see* Pregnancy, by site
  organ or site NEC — *see* Malposition, congenital
  pancreas Q45.3
  pregnancy — *see* Pregnancy, ectopic
  pupil — *see* Abnormality, pupillary
  renal Q63.2
  sebaceous glands of mouth Q38.6
  spleen Q89.09
  testis Q53.00
    bilateral Q53.02
    unilateral Q53.01
  thyroid Q89.2
  tissue in lung Q33.5
  ureter Q62.63
  ventricular beats I49.3
  vesicae Q64.10
Ectromelia Q73.8
  lower limb — *see* Defect, reduction, limb, lower, specified type NEC
  upper limb — *see* Defect, reduction, limb, upper, specified type NEC
Ectropion H02.109
  cervix N86

Ectropion — *continued*
  cervix — *continued*
    with cervicitis N72
  congenital Q10.1
  eyelid (paralytic) H02.109
    cicatricial H02.119
      left H02.116
        lower H02.115
        upper H02.114
      right H02.113
        lower H02.112
        upper H02.111
    congenital Q10.1
    left H02.106
      lower H02.105
      upper H02.104
    mechanical H02.129
      left H02.126
        lower H02.125
        upper H02.124
      right H02.123
        lower H02.122
        upper H02.121
    right H02.103
      lower H02.102
      upper H02.101
    senile H02.139
      left H02.136
        lower H02.135
        upper H02.134
      right H02.133
        lower H02.132
        upper H02.131
    spastic H02.149
      left H02.146
        lower H02.145
        upper H02.144
      right H02.143
        lower H02.142
        upper H02.141
  iris H21.89
  lip (acquired) K13.0
    congenital Q38.0
  urethra N36.8
  uvea H21.89
Eczema (acute) (chronic) (erythematous) (fissum) (rubrum) (squamous) (*see also* Dermatitis) L30.9
  contact — *see* Dermatitis, contact
  dyshydrotic L30.1
  external ear — *see* Otitis, externa, acute, eczematoid
  flexural L20.82
  herpeticum B00.0
  hypertrophicum L28.0
  hypostatic — *see* Varix, leg, with, inflammation
  impetiginous L01.1
  infantile (due to any substance) L20.83
    intertriginous L21.1
    seborrheic L21.1
  intertriginous NEC L30.4
    infantile L21.1
  intrinsic (allergic) L20.84
  lichenified NEC L28.0
  marginatum (hebrae) B35.6
  pustular L30.3
  stasis I87.2
    with varicose veins — *see* Varix, leg, with, inflammation
  vaccination, vaccinatum T88.1 ☑
  varicose — *see* Varix, leg, with, inflammation
Eczematid L30.2
Eddowes (-Spurway) **syndrome** Q78.0
Edema, edematous (infectious) (pitting) (toxic) R60.9
  with nephritis — *see* Nephrosis
  allergic T78.3 ☑
  amputation stump (surgical) (sequelae (late effect)) T87.89
  angioneurotic (allergic) (any site) (with urticaria) T78.3 ☑
    hereditary D84.1
  angiospastic I73.9
  Berlin's (traumatic) S05.8X- ☑
  brain (cytotoxic) (vasogenic) G93.6
    due to birth injury P11.0
    newborn (anoxia or hypoxia) P52.4
      birth injury P11.0
    traumatic — *see* Injury, intracranial, cerebral edema
  cardiac — *see* Failure, heart, congestive
  cardiovascular — *see* Failure, heart, congestive

Edema, edematous — *continued*
  cerebral — *see* Edema, brain
  cerebrospinal — *see* Edema, brain
  cervix (uteri) (acute) N88.8
    puerperal, postpartum O90.89
  chronic hereditary Q82.0
  circumscribed, acute T78.3 ☑
    hereditary D84.1
  conjunctiva H11.42- ☑
  cornea H18.2- ☑
    idiopathic H18.22- ☑
    secondary H18.23- ☑
      due to contact lens H18.21- ☑
  due to
    lymphatic obstruction I89.0
    salt retention E87.0
  epiglottis — *see* Edema, glottis
  essential, acute T78.3 ☑
    hereditary D84.1
  extremities, lower — *see* Edema, legs
  eyelid NEC H02.849
    left H02.846
      lower H02.845
      upper H02.844
    right H02.843
      lower H02.842
      upper H02.841
  familial, hereditary Q82.0
  famine — *see* Malnutrition, severe
  generalized R60.1
  glottis, glottic, glottidis (obstructive) (passive) J38.4
    allergic T78.3 ☑
      hereditary D84.1
  heart — *see* Failure, heart, congestive
  heat T67.7 ☑
  hereditary Q82.0
  inanition — *see* Malnutrition, severe
  intracranial G93.6
  iris H21.89
  joint — *see* Effusion, joint
  larynx — *see* Edema, glottis
  legs R60.0
    due to venous obstruction I87.1
    hereditary Q82.0
  localized R60.0
    due to venous obstruction I87.1
  lower limbs — *see* Edema, legs
  lung J81.1
    with heart condition or failure — *see* Failure, ventricular, left
    acute J81.0
      chemical (acute) J68.1
        chronic J68.1
    chronic J81.1
      due to
        chemicals, gases, fumes or vapors (inhalation) J68.1
        external agent J70.9
          specified NEC J70.8
        radiation J70.1
    due to
      chemicals, fumes or vapors (inhalation) J68.1
      external agent J70.9
        specified NEC J70.8
      high altitude T70.29 ☑
      near drowning T75.1 ☑
      radiation J70.0
    meaning failure, left ventricle I50.1
  lymphatic I89.0
    due to mastectomy I97.2
  macula H35.81
    cystoid, following cataract surgery — *see* Complications, postprocedural, following cataract surgery
    diabetic — *see* Diabetes, by type, with, retinopathy, with macular edema
  malignant — *see* Gangrene, gas
  Milroy's Q82.0
  nasopharynx J39.2
  newborn P83.30
    hydrops fetalis — *see* Hydrops, fetalis
    specified NEC P83.39
  nutritional (*see also* Malnutrition, severe)
    with dyspigmentation, skin and hair E40
  optic disc or nerve — *see* Papilledema
  orbit H05.22- ☑
  pancreas K86.89
  papilla, optic — *see* Papilledema

Edema, edematous — continued
penis N48.89
periodic T78.3 ☑
hereditary D84.1
pharynx J39.2
pulmonary — see Edema, lung
Quincke's T78.3 ☑
hereditary D84.1
renal — see Nephrosis
retina H35.81
diabetic — see Diabetes, by type, with, retinopathy, with macular edema
salt E87.0
scrotum N50.89
seminal vesicle N50.89
spermatic cord N50.89
spinal (cord) (vascular) (nontraumatic) G95.19
starvation — see Malnutrition, severe
stasis — see Hypertension, venous, (chronic)
subglottic — see Edema, glottis
supraglottic — see Edema, glottis
testis N44.8
tunica vaginalis N50.89
vas deferens N50.89
vulva (acute) N90.89
Edentulism — see Absence, teeth, acquired
Edsall's disease T67.2 ☑
Educational handicap Z55.9
specified NEC Z55.8
Edward's syndrome — see Trisomy, 18
Effect(s) (of) (from) — see Effect, adverse NEC
Effect, adverse
abnormal gravitational (G) forces or states T75.81 ☑
abuse — see Maltreatment
air pressure T70.9 ☑
specified NEC T70.8 ☑
altitude (high) — see Effect, adverse, high altitude
anesthesia (see also Anesthesia) T88.59 ☑
in labor and delivery O74.9
local, toxic
in labor and delivery O74.4
in pregnancy NEC O29.3- ☑
postpartum, puerperal O89.3
postpartum, puerperal O89.9
specified NEC T88.59 ☑
in labor and delivery O74.8
postpartum, puerperal O89.8
spinal and epidural T88.59 ☑
headache T88.59 ☑
in labor and delivery O74.5
postpartum, puerperal O89.4
specified NEC
in labor and delivery O74.6
postpartum, puerperal O89.5
antitoxin — see Complications, vaccination
atmospheric pressure T70.9 ☑
due to explosion T70.8 ☑
high T70.3 ☑
low — see Effect, adverse, high altitude
specified effect NEC T70.8 ☑
biological, correct substance properly administered — see Effect, adverse, drug
blood (derivatives) (serum) (transfusion) — see Complications, transfusion
chemical substance — see Table of Drugs and Chemicals
cold (temperature) (weather) T69.9 ☑
chilblains T69.1 ☑
frostbite — see Frostbite
specified effect NEC T69.8 ☑
drugs and medicaments T88.7 ☑
specified drug — see Table of Drugs and Chemicals, by drug, adverse effect
specified effect — code to condition
electric current, electricity (shock) T75.4 ☑
burn — see Burn
exertion (excessive) T73.3 ☑
exposure — see Exposure
external cause NEC T75.89 ☑
foodstuffs T78.1 ☑
allergic reaction — see Allergy, food
causing anaphylaxis — see Shock, anaphylactic, due to food
noxious — see Poisoning, food, noxious
gases, fumes, or vapors T59.9- ☑
specified agent — see Table of Drugs and Chemicals

Effect, adverse — continued
glue (airplane) sniffing
due to drug abuse — see Abuse, drug, inhalant
due to drug dependence — see Dependence, drug, inhalant
heat — see Heat
high altitude NEC T70.29 ☑
anoxia T70.29 ☑
on
ears T70.0 ☑
sinuses T70.1 ☑
polycythemia D75.1
high pressure fluids T70.4 ☑
hot weather — see Heat
hunger T73.0 ☑
immersion, foot — see Immersion
immunization — see Complications, vaccination
immunological agents — see Complications, vaccination
infrared (radiation) (rays) NOS T66 ☑
dermatitis or eczema L59.8
infusion — see Complications, infusion
lack of care of infants — see Maltreatment, child
lightning — see Lightning
medical care T88.9 ☑
specified NEC T88.8 ☑
medicinal substance, correct, properly administered — see Effect, adverse, drug
motion T75.3 ☑
noise, on inner ear — see subcategory H83.3 ☑
overheated places — see Heat
psychosocial, of work environment Z56.5
radiation (diagnostic) (infrared) (natural source) (therapeutic) (ultraviolet) (X-ray) NOS T66 ☑
dermatitis or eczema — see Dermatitis, due to, radiation
fibrosis of lung J70.1
pneumonitis J70.0
pulmonary manifestations
acute J70.0
chronic J70.1
skin L59.9
radioactive substance NOS
dermatitis or eczema — see Radiodermatitis
reduced temperature T69.9 ☑
immersion foot or hand — see Immersion
specified effect NEC T69.8 ☑
serum NEC (see also Reaction, serum) T80.69 ☑
specified NEC T78.8 ☑
external cause NEC T75.89 ☑
strangulation — see Asphyxia, traumatic
submersion T75.1 ☑
thirst T73.1 ☑
toxic — see Toxicity
transfusion — see Complications, transfusion
ultraviolet (radiation) (rays) NOS T66 ☑
burn — see Burn
dermatitis or eczema — see Dermatitis, due to, ultraviolet rays
acute L56.8
vaccine (any) — see Complications, vaccination
vibration — see Vibration, adverse effects
water pressure NEC T70.9 ☑
specified NEC T70.8 ☑
weightlessness T75.82 ☑
whole blood — see Complications, transfusion
work environment Z56.5
Effects, late — see Sequelae
Effluvium
anagen L65.1
telogen L65.0
Effort syndrome (psychogenic) F45.8
Effusion
amniotic fluid — see Pregnancy, complicated by, premature rupture of membranes
brain (serous) G93.6
bronchial — see Bronchitis
cerebral G93.6
cerebrospinal (see also Meningitis)
vessel G93.6
chest — see Effusion, pleura
chylous, chyliform (pleura) J94.0
intracranial G93.6
joint M25.40
ankle M25.47- ☑
elbow M25.42- ☑
foot joint M25.47- ☑

Effusion — continued
joint — continued
hand joint M25.44- ☑
hip M25.45- ☑
knee M25.46- ☑
shoulder M25.41- ☑
specified joint NEC M25.48
wrist M25.43- ☑
malignant pleural J91.0
meninges — see Meningitis
pericardium, pericardial (noninflammatory) I31.3
acute — see Pericarditis, acute
peritoneal (chronic) R18.8
pleura, pleurisy, pleuritic, pleuropericardial J90
chylous, chyliform J94.0
due to systemic lupus erythematosis M32.13
in conditions classified elsewhere J91.8
influenzal — see Influenza, with, respiratory manifestations NEC
malignant J91.0
newborn P28.89
tuberculous NEC A15.6
primary (progressive) A15.7
spinal — see Meningitis
thorax, thoracic — see Effusion, pleura
Egg shell nails L60.3
congenital Q84.6
Egyptian splenomegaly B65.1
Ehlers-Danlos syndrome Q79.6
Ehrlichiosis A77.40
due to
E. chafeensis A77.41
E. sennetsu A79.81
specified organism NEC A77.49
Eichstedt's disease B36.0
Eisenmenger's
complex or syndrome I27.83
defect Q21.8
Ejaculation
delayed F52.32
painful N53.12
premature F52.4
retarded N53.11
retrograde N53.14
semen, painful N53.12
psychogenic F52.6
Ekbom's syndrome (restless legs) G25.81
Ekman's syndrome (brittle bones and blue sclera) Q78.0
Elastic skin Q82.8
acquired L57.4
Elastofibroma — see Neoplasm, connective tissue, benign
Elastoma (juvenile) Q82.8
Miescher's L87.2
Elastomyofibrosis I42.4
Elastosis
actinic, solar L57.8
atrophicans (senile) L57.4
perforans serpiginosa L87.2
senilis L57.4
Elbow — see condition
Electric current, electricity, effects (concussion) (fatal) (nonfatal) (shock) T75.4 ☑
burn — see Burn
Electric feet syndrome E53.8
Electrocution T75.4 ☑
from electroshock gun (taser) T75.4 ☑
Electrolyte imbalance E87.8
with
abortion — see Abortion by type, complicated by, electrolyte imbalance
ectopic pregnancy O08.5
molar pregnancy O08.5
Elephantiasis (nonfilarial) I89.0
arabicum — see Infestation, filarial
bancroftian B74.0
congenital (any site) (hereditary) Q82.0
due to
Brugia (malayi) B74.1
timori B74.2
mastectomy I97.2
Wuchereria (bancrofti) B74.0
eyelid H02.859
left H02.856
lower H02.855
upper H02.854
right H02.853
lower H02.852

Subterms under main terms may continue to next column or page   ☑ Additional Character Required — Refer to the Tabular List for Character Selection   **127**

Edema, edematous — Elephantiasis

Elephantiasis — *continued*
  eyelid — *continued*
    right — *continued*
      upper H02.851
  filarial, filariensis — *see* Infestation, filarial
  glandular I89.0
  graecorum A30.9
  lymphangiectatic I89.0
  lymphatic vessel I89.0
    due to mastectomy I97.2
  scrotum (nonfilarial) I89.0
  streptococcal I89.0
  surgical I97.89
    postmastectomy I97.2
  telangiectodes I89.0
  vulva (nonfilarial) N90.89

Elevated, elevation
  antibody titer R76.0
  basal metabolic rate R94.8
  blood pressure (*see also* Hypertension)
    reading (incidental) (isolated) (nonspecific), no diagnosis of hypertension R03.0
  blood sugar R73.9
  body temperature (of unknown origin) R50.9
  cancer antigen 125 [CA 125] R97.1
  carcinoembryonic antigen [CEA] R97.0
  cholesterol E78.00
    with high triglycerides E78.2
  conjugate, eye H51.0
  C-reactive protein (CRP) R79.82
  diaphragm, congenital Q79.1
  erythrocyte sedimentation rate R70.0
  fasting glucose R73.01
  fasting triglycerides E78.1
  finding on laboratory examination — *see* Findings, abnormal, inconclusive, without diagnosis, by type of exam
  GFR (glomerular filtration rate) — *see* Findings, abnormal, inconclusive, without diagnosis, by type of exam
  glucose tolerance (oral) R73.02
  immunoglobulin level R76.8
  indoleacetic acid R82.5
  lactic acid dehydrogenase (LDH) level R74.0
  leukocytes D72.829
  lipoprotein a level E78.8 ☑
  liver function
    study R94.5
    test R79.89
      alkaline phosphatase R74.8
      aminotransferase R74.0
      bilirubin R17
      hepatic enzyme R74.8
      lactate dehydrogenase R74.0
  lymphocytes D72.820
  prostate specific antigen [PSA] R97.20
  Rh titer — *see* Complication(s), transfusion, incompatibility reaction, Rh (factor)
  scapula, congenital Q74.0
  sedimentation rate R70.0
  SGOT R74.0
  SGPT R74.0
  transaminase level R74.0
  triglycerides E78.1
    with high cholesterol E78.2
  tumor associated antigens [TAA] NEC R97.8
  tumor specific antigens [TSA] NEC R97.8
  urine level of
    17-ketosteroids R82.5
    catecholamine R82.5
    indoleacetic acid R82.5
    steroids R82.5
    vanillylmandelic acid (VMA) R82.5
  venous pressure I87.8
  white blood cell count D72.829
    specified NEC D72.828

Elliptocytosis (congenital) (hereditary) D58.1
  Hb C (disease) D58.1
  hemoglobin disease D58.1
  sickle-cell (disease) D57.8- ☑
    trait D57.3

Ellison-Zollinger syndrome E16.4
Ellis-van Creveld syndrome (chondroectodermal dysplasia) Q77.6
Elongated, elongation (congenital) (*see also* Distortion)
  bone Q79.9
  cervix (uteri) Q51.828
    acquired N88.4

Elongated, elongation — *continued*
  cervix — *continued*
    hypertrophic N88.4
  colon Q43.8
  common bile duct Q44.5
  cystic duct Q44.5
  frenulum, penis Q55.69
  labia minora (acquired) N90.69
  ligamentum patellae Q74.1
  petiolus (epiglottidis) Q31.8
  tooth, teeth K00.2
  uvula Q38.6

Eltor cholera A00.1
Emaciation (due to malnutrition) E41
Embadomoniasis A07.8
Embedded tooth, teeth K01.0
  root only K08.3
Embolic — *see* condition
Embolism (multiple) (paradoxical) I74.9
  air (any site) (traumatic) T79.0 ☑
    following
      abortion — *see* Abortion by type complicated by embolism
      ectopic pregnancy O08.2
      infusion, therapeutic injection or transfusion T80.0 ☑
      molar pregnancy O08.2
      procedure NEC
        artery T81.719 ☑
          mesenteric T81.710 ☑
          renal T81.711 ☑
          specified NEC T81.718 ☑
        vein T81.72 ☑
    in pregnancy, childbirth or puerperium — *see* Embolism, obstetric
  amniotic fluid (pulmonary) (*see also* Embolism, obstetric)
    following
      abortion — *see* Abortion by type complicated by embolism
      ectopic pregnancy O08.2
      molar pregnancy O08.2
  aorta, aortic I74.10
    abdominal I74.09
      saddle I74.01
    bifurcation I74.09
    saddle I74.01
    thoracic I74.11
  artery I74.9
    auditory, internal I65.8
    basilar — *see* Occlusion, artery, basilar
    carotid (common) (internal) — *see* Occlusion, artery, carotid
    cerebellar (anterior inferior) (posterior inferior) (superior) I66.3
    cerebral — *see* Occlusion, artery, cerebral
    choroidal (anterior) I65.8
    communicating posterior I65.8
    coronary (*see also* Infarct, myocardium)
      not resulting in infarction I24.0
    extremity I74.4
      lower I74.3
      upper I74.2
    hypophyseal I65.8
    iliac I74.5
    limb I74.4
      lower I74.3
      upper I74.2
    mesenteric (with gangrene) (*see also* Ischemia, intestine, acute) K55.059
    ophthalmic — *see* Occlusion, artery, retina
    peripheral I74.4
    pontine I65.8
    precerebral — *see* Occlusion, artery, precerebral
    pulmonary — *see* Embolism, pulmonary
    renal N28.0
    retinal — *see* Occlusion, artery, retina
    septic I76
    specified NEC I74.8
    vertebral — *see* Occlusion, artery, vertebral
  basilar (artery) I65.1
  blood clot
    following
      abortion — *see* Abortion by type complicated by embolism
      ectopic or molar pregnancy O08.2
    in pregnancy, childbirth or puerperium — *see* Embolism, obstetric

Embolism — *continued*
  brain (*see also* Occlusion, artery, cerebral)
    following
      abortion — *see* Abortion by type complicated by embolism
      ectopic or molar pregnancy O08.2
      puerperal, postpartum, childbirth — *see* Embolism, obstetric
  capillary I78.8
  cardiac (*see also* Infarct, myocardium)
    not resulting in infarction I51.3
  carotid (artery) (common) (internal) — *see* Occlusion, artery, carotid
  cavernous sinus (venous) — *see* Embolism, intracranial venous sinus
  cerebral — *see* Occlusion, artery, cerebral
  cholesterol — *see* Atheroembolism
  coronary (artery or vein) (systemic) — Occlusion, coronary
  due to device, implant or graft (*see also* Complications, by site and type, specified NEC)
    arterial graft NEC T82.818 ☑
    breast (implant) T85.818 ☑
    catheter NEC T85.818 ☑
      dialysis (renal) T82.818 ☑
        intraperitoneal T85.818 ☑
      infusion NEC T82.818 ☑
        spinal (epidural) (subdural) T85.810 ☑
      urinary (indwelling) T83.81 ☑
    electronic (electrode) (pulse generator) (stimulator)
      bone T84.81 ☑
      cardiac T82.817 ☑
      nervous system (brain) (peripheral nerve) (spinal) T85.810 ☑
      urinary T83.81 ☑
    fixation, internal (orthopedic) NEC T84.81 ☑
    gastrointestinal (bile duct) (esophagus) T85.818 ☑
    genital NEC T83.81 ☑
    heart (graft) (valve) T82.817 ☑
    joint prosthesis T84.81 ☑
    ocular (corneal graft) (orbital implant) T85.818 ☑
    orthopedic (bone graft) NEC T86.838
    specified NEC T85.818 ☑
    urinary (graft) NEC T83.81 ☑
    vascular NEC T82.818 ☑
    ventricular intracranial shunt T85.810 ☑
  extremities
    lower — *see* Embolism, vein, lower extremity
      arterial I74.3
    upper I74.2
  eye H34.9
  fat (cerebral) (pulmonary) (systemic) T79.1 ☑
    complicating delivery — *see* Embolism, obstetric
    following
      abortion — *see* Abortion by type complicated by embolism
      ectopic or molar pregnancy O08.2
  following
    abortion — *see* Abortion by type complicated by embolism
    ectopic or molar pregnancy O08.2
    infusion, therapeutic injection or transfusion
      air T80.0 ☑
  heart (fatty) (*see also* Infarct, myocardium)
    not resulting in infarction I51.3
  hepatic (vein) I82.0
  in pregnancy, childbirth or puerperium — *see* Embolism, obstetric
  intestine (artery) (vein) (with gangrene) (*see also* Ischemia, intestine, acute) K55.039
  intracranial (*see also* Occlusion, artery, cerebral)
    venous sinus (any) G08
      nonpyogenic I67.6
  intraspinal venous sinuses or veins G08
    nonpyogenic G95.19
  kidney (artery) N28.0
  lateral sinus (venous) — *see* Embolism, intracranial, venous sinus
  leg — *see* Embolism, vein, lower extremity
    arterial I74.3
  longitudinal sinus (venous) — *see* Embolism, intracranial, venous sinus
  lung (massive) — *see* Embolism, pulmonary
  meninges I66.8
  mesenteric (artery) (vein) (with gangrene) (*see also* Ischemia, intestine, acute) K55.059

☑ **Additional Character Required** — Refer to the Tabular List for Character Selection ⬇ **Subterms under main terms may continue to next column or page**

Embolism — *continued*
  obstetric (in) (pulmonary)
    childbirth O88.22
      air O88.02
      amniotic fluid O88.12
      blood clot O88.22
      fat O88.82
      pyemic O88.32
      septic O88.32
      specified type NEC O88.82
    pregnancy O88.21- ☑
      air O88.0́1- ☑
      amniotic fluid O88.11- ☑
      blood clot O88.21- ☑
      fat O88.81- ☑
      pyemic O88.31- ☑
      septic O88.31- ☑
      specified type NEC O88.81- ☑
    puerperal O88.23
      air O88.03
      amniotic fluid O88.13
      blood clot O88.23
      fat O88.83
      pyemic O88.33
      septic O88.33
      specified type NEC O88.83
  ophthalmic — *see* Occlusion, artery, retina
  penis N48.81
  peripheral artery NOS I74.4
  pituitary E23.6
  popliteal (artery) I74.3
  portal (vein) I81
  postoperative, postprocedural
    artery T81.719 ☑
      mesenteric T81.710 ☑
      renal T81.711 ☑
      specified NEC T81.718 ☑
    vein T81.72 ☑
  precerebral artery — *see* Occlusion, artery, precerebral
  puerperal — *see* Embolism, obstetric
  pulmonary (acute) (artery) (vein) I26.99
    with acute cor pulmonale I26.09
    chronic I27.82
    following
      abortion — *see* Abortion by type complicated
        by embolism
      ectopic or molar pregnancy O08.2
    healed or old Z86.711
    in pregnancy, childbirth or puerperium — *see*
      Embolism, obstetric
    personal history of Z86.711
    saddle I26.92
      with acute cor pulmonale I26.02
    septic I26.90
      with acute cor pulmonale I26.01
  pyemic (multiple) I76
    following
      abortion — *see* Abortion by type complicated
        by embolism
      ectopic or molar pregnancy O08.2
    Hemophilus influenzae A41.3
    pneumococcal A40.3
      with pneumonia J13
    puerperal, postpartum, childbirth (any organism)
      — *see* Embolism, obstetric
    specified organism NEC A41.89
    staphylococcal A41.2
    streptococcal A40.9
  renal (artery) N28.0
    vein I82.3
  retina, retinal — *see* Occlusion, artery, retina
  saddle
    abdominal aorta I74.01
    pulmonary artery I26.92
      with acute cor pulmonale I26.02
  septic (arterial) I76
    complicating abortion — *see* Abortion, by type,
      complicated by, embolism
  sinus — *see* Embolism, intracranial, venous sinus
  soap complicating abortion — *see* Abortion, by type,
    complicated by, embolism
  spinal cord G95.19
    pyogenic origin G06.1
  spleen, splenic (artery) I74.8
  upper extremity I74.2
  vein (acute) I82.90
    antecubital I82.61- ☑
      chronic I82.71- ☑

Embolism — *continued*
  vein — *continued*
    axillary I82.A1- ☑ (*following* I82.7)
      chronic I82.A2- ☑ (*following* I82.7)
    basilic I82.61- ☑
      chronic I82.71- ☑
    brachial I82.62- ☑
      chronic I82.72- ☑
    brachiocephalic (innominate) I82.290
      chronic I82.291
    cephalic I82.61- ☑
      chronic I82.71- ☑
    chronic I82.91
    deep (DVT) I82.40- ☑
      calf I82.4Z- ☑
        chronic I82.5Z- ☑
      lower leg I82.4Z- ☑
        chronic I82.5Z- ☑
      thigh I82.4Y- ☑
        chronic I82.5Y- ☑
      upper leg I82.4Y ☑
        chronic I82.5Y-
    femoral I82.41- ☑
      chronic I82.51- ☑
    iliac (iliofemoral) I82.42- ☑
      chronic I82.52- ☑
    innominate I82.290
      chronic I82.291
    internal jugular I82.C1- ☑ (*following* I82.7)
      chronic I82.C2- ☑ (*following* I82.7)
    lower extremity
      deep I82.40- ☑
        chronic I82.50- ☑
        specified NEC I82.49- ☑
          chronic NEC I82.59- ☑
      distal
        deep I82.4Z- ☑
      proximal
        deep I82.4Y- ☑
          chronic I82.5Y- ☑
      superficial I82.81- ☑
    popliteal I82.43- ☑
      chronic I82.53- ☑
    radial I82.62- ☑
      chronic I82.72- ☑
    renal I82.3
    saphenous (greater) (lesser) I82.81- ☑
    specified NEC I82.890
      chronic NEC I82.891
    subclavian I82.B1- ☑ (*following* I82.7)
      chronic I82.B2- ☑ (*following* I82.7)
    thoracic NEC I82.290
      chronic I82.291
    tibial I82.44- ☑
      chronic I82.54- ☑
    ulnar I82.62- ☑
      chronic I82.72- ☑
    upper extremity I82.60- ☑
      chronic I82.70- ☑
      deep I82.62- ☑
        chronic I82.72- ☑
      superficial I82.61- ☑
        chronic I82.71- ☑
    vena cava
      inferior (acute) I82.220
        chronic I82.221
      superior (acute) I82.210
        chronic I82.211
    venous sinus G08
    vessels of brain — *see* Occlusion, artery, cerebral
Embolus — *see* Embolism
Embryoma (*see also* Neoplasm, uncertain behavior, by
    site)
  benign — *see* Neoplasm, benign, by site
  kidney C64.- ☑
  liver C22.0
  malignant (*see also* Neoplasm, malignant, by site)
    kidney C64.- ☑
    liver C22.0
    testis C62.9- ☑
      descended (scrotal) C62.1- ☑
      undescended C62.0- ☑
  testis C62.9- ☑
    descended (scrotal) C62.1- ☑
    undescended C62.0- ☑

Embryonic
  circulation Q28.9
  heart Q28.9
  vas deferens Q55.4
Embryopathia NOS Q89.9
Embryotoxon Q13.4
Emesis — *see* Vomiting
Emotional lability R45.86
Emotionality, pathological F60.3
Emotogenic disease — *see* Disorder, psychogenic
Emphysema (atrophic) (bullous) (chronic) (interlobular)
    (lung) (obstructive) (pulmonary) (senile) (vesicular)
    J43.9
  cellular tissue (traumatic) T79.7 ☑
    surgical T81.82 ☑
  centrilobular J43.2
  compensatory J98.3
  congenital (interstitial) P25.0
  conjunctiva H11.89
  connective tissue (traumatic) T79.7 ☑
    surgical T81.82 ☑
  due to chemicals, gases, fumes or vapors J68.4
  eyelid(s) — *see* Disorder, eyelid, specified type NEC
    surgical T81.82 ☑
    traumatic T79.7 ☑
  interstitial J98.2
    congenital P25.0
    perinatal period P25.0
  laminated tissue T79.7 ☑
    surgical T81.82 ☑
  mediastinal J98.2
    newborn P25.2
  orbit, orbital — *see* Disorder, orbit, specified type NEC
  panacinar J43.1
  panlobular J43.1
  specified NEC J43.8
  subcutaneous (traumatic) T79.7 ☑
    nontraumatic J98.2
    postprocedural T81.82 ☑
    surgical T81.82 ☑
  surgical T81.82 ☑
  thymus (gland) (congenital) E32.8
  traumatic (subcutaneous) T79.7 ☑
  unilateral J43.0
Empty nest syndrome Z60.0
Empyema (acute) (chest) (double) (pleura) (supradi-
    aphragmatic) (thorax) J86.9
  with fistula J86.0
  accessory sinus (chronic) — *see* Sinusitis
  antrum (chronic) — *see* Sinusitis, maxillary
  brain (any part) — *see* Abscess, brain
  ethmoidal (chronic) (sinus) — *see* Sinusitis, ethmoidal
  extradural — *see* Abscess, extradural
  frontal (chronic) (sinus) — *see* Sinusitis, frontal
  gallbladder K81.0
  mastoid (process) (acute) — *see* Mastoiditis, acute
  maxilla, maxillary M27.2
    sinus (chronic) — *see* Sinusitis, maxillary
  nasal sinus (chronic) — *see* Sinusitis
  sinus (accessory) (chronic) (nasal) — *see* Sinusitis
  sphenoidal (sinus) (chronic) — *see* Sinusitis, sphe-
    noidal
  subarachnoid — *see* Abscess, extradural
  subdural — *see* Abscess, subdural
  tuberculous A15.6
  ureter — *see* Ureteritis
  ventricular — *see* Abscess, brain
En coup de sabre lesion L94.1
Enamel pearls K00.2
Enameloma K00.2
Enanthema, viral B09
Encephalitis (chronic) (hemorrhagic) (idiopathic)
    (nonepidemic) (spurious) (subacute) G04.90
  acute (*see also* Encephalitis, viral) A86
    disseminated G04.00
      infectious G04.01
      noninfectious G04.81
      postimmunization (postvaccination) G04.02
      postinfectious G04.01
    inclusion body A85.8
    necrotizing hemorrhagic G04.30
      postimmunization G04.32
      postinfectious G04.31
      specified NEC G04.39
  arboviral, arbovirus NEC A85.2
  arthropod-borne NEC (viral) A85.2
  Australian A83.4

Encephalitis — continued
California (virus) A83.5
Central European (tick-borne) A84.1
Czechoslovakian A84.1
Dawson's (inclusion body) A81.1
diffuse sclerosing A81.1
disseminated, acute G04.00
due to
cat scratch disease A28.1
human immunodeficiency virus (HIV) disease
B20 [G05.3]
malaria — see Malaria
rickettsiosis — see Rickettsiosis
smallpox inoculation G04.02
typhus — see Typhus
Eastern equine A83.2
endemic (viral) A86
epidemic NEC (viral) A86
equine (acute) (infectious) (viral) A83.9
Eastern A83.2
Venezuelan A92.2
Western A83.1
Far Eastern (tick-borne) A84.0
following vaccination or other immunization procedure G04.02
herpes zoster B02.0
herpesviral B00.4
due to herpesvirus 6 B10.01
due to herpesvirus 7 B10.09
specified NEC B10.09
Ilheus (virus) A83.8
in (due to)
actinomycosis A42.82
adenovirus A85.1
African trypanosomiasis B56.9 [G05.3]
Chagas' disease (chronic) B57.42
cytomegalovirus B25.8
enterovirus A85.0
herpes (simplex) virus B00.4
due to herpesvirus 6 B10.01
due to herpesvirus 7 B10.09
specified NEC B10.09
infectious disease NEC B99 ☑ [G05.3]
influenza — see Influenza, with, encephalopathy
listeriosis A32.12
measles B05.0
mumps B26.2
naegleriasis B60.2
parasitic disease NEC B89 [G05.3]
poliovirus A80.9 [G05.3]
rubella B06.01
syphilis
congenital A50.42
late A52.14
systemic lupus erythematosus M32.19
toxoplasmosis (acquired) B58.2
congenital P37.1
tuberculosis A17.82
zoster B02.0
inclusion body A81.1
infectious (acute) (virus) NEC A86
Japanese (B type) A83.0
La Crosse A83.5
lead — see Poisoning, lead
lethargica (acute) (infectious) A85.8
louping ill A84.8
lupus erythematosus, systemic M32.19
lymphatica A87.2
Mengo A85.8
meningococcal A39.81
Murray Valley A83.4
otitic NEC H66.40 [G05.3]
parasitic NOS B71.9
periaxial G37.0
periaxialis (concentrica) (diffuse) G37.5
postchickenpox B01.11
postexanthematous NEC B09
postimmunization G04.02
postinfectious NEC G04.01
postmeasles B05.0
postvaccinal G04.02
postvaricella B01.11
postviral NEC A86
Powassan A84.8
Rasmussen G04.81
Rio Bravo A85.8
Russian
autumnal A83.0
spring-summer (taiga) A84.0

Encephalitis — continued
saturnine — see Poisoning, lead
specified NEC G04.81
St. Louis A83.3
subacute sclerosing A81.1
summer A83.0
suppurative G04.81
tick-borne A84.9
Torula, torular (cryptococcal) B45.1
toxic NEC G92
trichinosis B75 [G05.3]
type
B A83.0
C A83.3
van Bogaert's A81.1
Venezuelan equine A92.2
Vienna A85.8
viral, virus A86
arthropod-borne NEC A85.2
mosquito-borne A83.9
Australian X disease A83.4
California virus A83.5
Eastern equine A83.2
Japanese (B type) A83.0
Murray Valley A83.4
specified NEC A83.8
St. Louis A83.3
type B A83.0
type C A83.3
Western equine A83.1
tick-borne A84.9
biundulant A84.1
central European A84.1
Czechoslovakian A84.1
diphasic meningoencephalitis A84.1
Far Eastern A84.0
Russian spring-summer (taiga) A84.0
specified NEC A84.8
specified type NEC A85.8
Western equine A83.1
Encephalocele Q01.9
frontal Q01.0
nasofrontal Q01.1
occipital Q01.2
specified NEC Q01.8
Encephalocystocele — see Encephalocele
Encephaloduroarteriomyosynangiosis (EDAMS) I67.5
Encephalomalacia (brain) (cerebellar) (cerebral) — see
Softening, brain
Encephalomeningitis — see Meningoencephalitis
Encephalomeningocele — see Encephalocele
Encephalomeningomyelitis — see Meningoencephalitis
Encephalomyelitis (see also Encephalitis) G04.90
acute disseminated G04.00
infectious G04.01
noninfectious G04.81
postimmunization G04.02
postinfectious G04.01
acute necrotizing hemorrhagic G04.30
postimmunization G04.32
postinfectious G04.31
specified NEC G04.39
benign myalgic G93.3
equine A83.9
Eastern A83.2
Venezuelan A92.2
Western A83.1
in diseases classified elsewhere G05.3
myalgic, benign G93.3
postchickenpox B01.11
postinfectious NEC G04.01
postmeasles B05.0
postvaccinal G04.02
postvaricella B01.11
rubella B06.01
specified NEC G04.81
Venezuelan equine A92.2
Encephalomyelocele — see Encephalocele
Encephalomyelomeningitis — see Meningoencephalitis
Encephalomyelopathy G96.9
Encephalomyeloradiculitis (acute) G61.0
Encephalomyeloradiculoneuritis (acute) (Guillain-
Barré) G61.0
Encephalomyeloradiculopathy G96.9
Encephalopathia hyperbilirubinemica, newborn
P57.9

Encephalopathia hyperbilirubinemica, newborn —
continued
due to isoimmunization (conditions in P55) P57.0
Encephalopathy (acute) G93.40
acute necrotizing hemorrhagic G04.30
postimmunization G04.32
postinfectious G04.31
specified NEC G04.39
alcoholic G31.2
anoxic — see Damage, brain, anoxic
arteriosclerotic I67.2
centrolobar progressive (Schilder) G37.0
congenital Q07.9
degenerative, in specified disease NEC G32.89
demyelinating callosal G37.1
due to
drugs (see also Table of Drugs and Chemicals) G92
hepatic — see Failure, hepatic
hyperbilirubinemic, newborn P57.9
due to isoimmunization (conditions in P55) P57.0
hypertensive I67.4
hypoglycemic E16.2
hypoxic — see Damage, brain, anoxic
hypoxic ischemic P91.60
mild P91.61
moderate P91.62
severe P91.63
in (due to) (with)
birth injury P11.1
hyperinsulinism E16.1 [G94]
influenza — see Influenza, with, encephalopathy
lack of vitamin (see also Deficiency, vitamin)
E56.9 [G32.89]
neoplastic disease (see also Neoplasm)
D49.9 [G13.1]
serum (see also Reaction, serum) T80.69 ☑
syphilis A52.17
trauma (postconcussional) F07.81
current injury — see Injury, intracranial
vaccination G04.02
lead — see Poisoning, lead
metabolic G93.41
drug induced G92
toxic G92
myoclonic, early, symptomatic — see Epilepsy, generalized, specified NEC
necrotizing, subacute (Leigh) G31.82
neonatal P91.819
in diseases classified elsewhere P91.811
pellagrous E52 [G32.89]
portosystemic — see Failure, hepatic
postcontusional F07.81
current injury — see Injury, intracranial, diffuse
posthypoglycemic (coma) E16.1 [G94]
postradiation G93.89
saturnine — see Poisoning, lead
septic G93.41
specified NEC G93.49
spongioform, subacute (viral) A81.09
toxic G92
metabolic G92
traumatic (postconcussional) F07.81
current injury — see Injury, intracranial
vitamin B deficiency NEC E53.9 [G32.89]
vitamin B1 E51.2
Wernicke's E51.2
Encephalorrhagia — see Hemorrhage, intracranial, intracerebral
Encephalosis, posttraumatic F07.81
Enchondroma (see also Neoplasm, bone, benign)
Enchondromatosis (cartilaginous) (multiple) Q78.4
Encopresis R15.9
functional F98.1
nonorganic origin F98.1
psychogenic F98.1
Encounter (with health service) (for) Z76.89
adjustment and management (of)
breast implant Z45.81 ☑
implanted device NEC Z45.89
myringotomy device (stent) (tube) Z45.82
administrative purpose only Z02.9
examination for
adoption Z02.82
armed forces Z02.3
disability determination Z02.71
driving license Z02.4
employment Z02.1
insurance Z02.6

☑ **Additional Character Required** — Refer to the Tabular List for Character Selection   ▽ **Subterms under main terms may continue to next column or page**

Encounter — *continued*
  administrative purpose only — *continued*
    examination for — *continued*
      medical certificate NEC Z02.79
      paternity testing Z02.81
      residential institution admission Z02.2
      school admission Z02.0
      sports Z02.5
      specified reason NEC Z02.89
  aftercare — *see* Aftercare
  antenatal screening Z36.9
    cervical length Z36.86
    chromosomal anomalies Z36.0
    congenital cardiac abnormalities Z36.83
    elevated maternal serum alphafetoprotein Z36.1
    fetal growth retardation Z36.4
    fetal lung maturity Z36.84
    fetal macrosomia Z36.88
    hydrops fetalis Z36.81
    intrauterine growth restriction (IUGR) /small-for-
      dates Z36.4
    isoimmunization Z36.5
    large-for-dates Z36.88
    malformations Z36.3
    non-visualized anatomy on a previous scan Z36.2
    nuchal translucency Z36.82
    raised alphafetoprotein level Z36.1
    risk of pre-term labor Z36.86
    specified follow-up NEC Z36.2
    specified genetic defects NEC Z36.8A
    specified type NEC Z36.89
    Streptococcus B Z36.85
    suspected anomaly Z36.3
    uncertain dates Z36.87
  assisted reproductive fertility procedure cycle Z31.83
  blood typing Z01.83
    Rh typing Z01.83
  breast augmentation or reduction Z41.1
  breast implant exchange (different material) (different
    size) Z45.81 ☑
  breast reconstruction following mastectomy Z42.1
  check-up — *see* Examination
  chemotherapy for neoplasm Z51.11
  colonoscopy, screening Z12.11
  counseling — *see* Counseling
  delivery, full-term, uncomplicated O80
    cesarean, without indication O82
  desensitization to allergens Z51.6
  ear piercing Z41.3
  examination — *see* Examination
  expectant parent(s) (adoptive) pre-birth pediatrician
    visit Z76.81
  fertility preservation procedure (prior to cancer thera-
    py) (prior to removal of gonads) Z31.84
  fitting (of) — *see* Fitting (and adjustment) (of)
  genetic
    counseling
      nonprocreative Z71.83
      procreative Z31.5
    testing — *see* Test, genetic
  hearing conservation and treatment Z01.12
  immunotherapy for neoplasm Z51.12
  in vitro fertilization cycle Z31.83
  instruction (in)
    child care (postpartal) (prenatal) Z32.3
    childbirth Z32.2
    natural family planning
      procreative Z31.61
      to avoid pregnancy Z30.02
  insulin pump titration Z46.81
  joint prosthesis insertion following prior explantation
    of joint prosthesis (staged procedure)
    hip Z47.32
    knee Z47.33
    shoulder Z47.31
  laboratory (as part of a general medical examination)
    Z00.00
    with abnormal findings Z00.01
  mental health services (for)
    abuse NEC
      perpetrator Z69.82
      victim Z69.81
    child abuse
      nonparental
        perpetrator Z69.021
        victim Z69.020
      parental
        perpetrator Z69.011

Encounter — *continued*
  mental health services — *continued*
    child abuse — *continued*
      parental — *continued*
        victim Z69.010
    child neglect
      nonparental
        perpetrator Z69.021
        victim Z69.020
      parental
        perpetrator Z69.011
        victim Z69.010
    child psychological abuse
      nonparental
        perpetrator Z69.021
        victim Z69.020
      parental
        perpetrator Z69.011
        victim Z69.010
    child sexual abuse
      nonparental
        perpetrator Z69.021
        victim Z69.020
      parental
        perpetrator Z69.011
        victim Z69.010
    non-spousal adult abuse (perpetrator) (victim)
      Z69.81
    spousal or partner
      abuse
        perpetrator Z69.12
        victim Z69.11
      neglect
        perpetrator Z69.12
        victim Z69.11
      psychological abuse
        perpetrator Z69.12
        victim Z69.11
      violence
        perpetrator (physical) (sexual) Z69.12
        victim (physical) Z69.11
          sexual Z69.81
  observation (for) (ruled out)
    exposure to (suspected)
      anthrax Z03.810
      biological agent NEC Z03.818
  pediatrician visit, by expectant parent(s) (adoptive)
    Z76.81
  placental sample (taken vaginally) (*see also* Encounter,
    antenatal screening) Z36.9
  plastic and reconstructive surgery following medical
    procedure or healed injury NEC Z42.8
  pregnancy
    supervision of — *see* Pregnancy, supervision of
    test Z32.00
      result negative Z32.02
      result positive Z32.01
  procreative management and counseling for gestation-
    al carrier Z31.7
  prophylactic measures Z29.9
    antivenin Z29.12
    fluoride administration Z29.3
    immunotherapy for respiratory syncytial virus (RSV)
      Z29.11
    rabies immune globin Z29.14
    Rho (D) immune globulin Z29.13
    specified NEC Z29.8
  radiation therapy (antineoplastic) Z51.0
  radiological (as part of a general medical examination)
    Z00.00
    with abnormal findings Z00.01
  reconstructive surgery following medical procedure
    or healed injury NEC Z42.8
  removal (of) (*see also* Removal)
    artificial
      arm Z44.00- ☑
        complete Z44.01- ☑
        partial Z44.02- ☑
      eye Z44.2- ☑
      leg Z44.10- ☑
        complete Z44.11- ☑
        partial Z44.12- ☑
    breast implant Z45.81 ☑
      tissue expander (without synchronous insertion
        of permanent implant) Z45.81 ☑
    device Z46.9
      specified NEC Z46.89

Encounter — *continued*
  removal (*see also* Removal) — *continued*
    external
      fixation device — *code to* fracture with seventh
        character D
      prosthesis, prosthetic device Z44.9
        breast Z44.3- ☑
        specified NEC Z44.8
    implanted device NEC Z45.89
    insulin pump Z46.81
    internal fixation device Z47.2
    myringotomy device (stent) (tube) Z45.82
    nervous system device NEC Z46.2
      brain neuropacemaker Z46.2
      visual substitution device Z46.2
        implanted Z45.31
    non-vascular catheter Z46.82
    orthodontic device Z46.4
    stent
      ureteral Z46.6
    urinary device Z46.6
  repeat cervical smear to confirm findings of recent
    normal smear following initial abnormal smear
    Z01.42
  respirator [ventilator] use during power failure Z99.12
  Rh typing Z01.83
  screening — *see* Screening
  specified NEC Z76.89
  sterilization Z30.2
  suspected condition, ruled out
    amniotic cavity and membrane Z03.71
    cervical shortening Z03.75
    fetal anomaly Z03.73
    fetal growth Z03.74
    maternal and fetal conditions NEC Z03.79
    oligohydramnios Z03.71
    placental problem Z03.72
    polyhydramnios Z03.71
  suspected exposure (to), ruled out
    anthrax Z03.810
    biological agents NEC Z03.818
  termination of pregnancy, elective Z33.2
  testing — *see* Test
  therapeutic drug level monitoring Z51.81
  titration, insulin pump Z46.81
  to determine fetal viability of pregnancy O36.80 ☑
  training
    insulin pump Z46.81
  X-ray of chest (as part of a general medical examina-
    tion) Z00.00
    with abnormal findings Z00.01
Encystment — *see* Cyst
Endarteritis (bacterial, subacute) (infective) I77.6
  brain I67.7
  cerebral or cerebrospinal I67.7
  deformans — *see* Arteriosclerosis
  embolic — *see* Embolism
  obliterans (*see also* Arteriosclerosis)
    pulmonary I28.8
  pulmonary I28.8
  retina — *see* Vasculitis, retina
  senile — *see* Arteriosclerosis
  syphilitic A52.09
    brain or cerebral A52.04
    congenital A50.54 [I79.8]
  tuberculous A18.89
Endemic — *see* condition
Endocarditis (chronic) (marantic) (nonbacterial)
    (thrombotic) (valvular) I38
  with rheumatic fever (conditions in I00)
    active — *see* Endocarditis, acute, rheumatic
    inactive or quiescent (with chorea) I09.1
  acute or subacute I33.9
    infective I33.0
    rheumatic (aortic) (mitral) (pulmonary) (tricuspid)
      I01.1
      with chorea (acute) (rheumatic) (Sydenham's)
        I02.0
  aortic (heart) (nonrheumatic) (valve) I35.8
    with
      mitral disease I08.0
        with tricuspid (valve) disease I08.3
        active or acute I01.1
          with chorea (acute) (rheumatic) (Syden-
            ham's) I02.0
      rheumatic fever (conditions in I00)
        active — *see* Endocarditis, acute, rheumatic
        inactive or quiescent (with chorea) I06.9

Endocarditis — *continued*
  aortic — *continued*
    with — *continued*
      tricuspid (valve) disease I08.2
        with mitral (valve) disease I08.3
    acute or subacute I33.9
    arteriosclerotic I35.8
    rheumatic I06.9
      with mitral disease I08.0
        with tricuspid (valve) disease I08.3
          active or acute I01.1
            with chorea (acute) (rheumatic) (Sydenham's) I02.0
        active or acute I01.1
          with chorea (acute) (rheumatic) (Sydenham's) I02.0
      specified NEC I06.8
    specified cause NEC I35.8
    syphilitic A52.03
  arteriosclerotic I38
  atypical verrucous (Libman-Sacks) M32.11
  bacterial (acute) (any valve) (subacute) I33.0
  candidal B37.6
  congenital Q24.8
  constrictive I33.0
  Coxiella burnetii A78 [I39]
  Coxsackie B33.21
  due to
    prosthetic cardiac valve T82.6 ☑
    Q fever A78 [I39]
    Serratia marcescens I33.0
    typhoid (fever) A01.02
  gonococcal A54.83
  infectious or infective (acute) (any valve) (subacute) I33.0
  lenta (acute) (any valve) (subacute) I33.0
  Libman-Sacks M32.11
  listerial A32.82
  Löffler's I42.3
  malignant (acute) (any valve) (subacute) I33.0
  meningococcal A39.51
  mitral (chronic) (double) (fibroid) (heart) (inactive) (valve) (with chorea) I05.9
    with
      aortic (valve) disease I08.0
        with tricuspid (valve) disease I08.3
          active or acute I01.1
            with chorea (acute) (rheumatic) (Sydenham's) I02.0
      rheumatic fever (conditions in I00)
        active — *see* Endocarditis, acute, rheumatic
        inactive or quiescent (with chorea) I05.9
      tricuspid (valve) disease I08.1
        with aortic (valve) disease I08.3
          active or acute I01.1
            with chorea (acute) (rheumatic) (Sydenham's) I02.0
          bacterial I33.0
      arteriosclerotic I34.8
      nonrheumatic I34.8
        acute or subacute I33.9
    specified NEC I05.8
  monilial B37.6
  multiple valves I08.9
    specified disorders I08.8
  mycotic (acute) (any valve) (subacute) I33.0
  pneumococcal (acute) (any valve) (subacute) I33.0
  pulmonary (chronic) (heart) (valve) I37.8
    with rheumatic fever (conditions in I00)
      active — *see* Endocarditis, acute, rheumatic
      inactive or quiescent (with chorea) I09.89
        with aortic, mitral or tricuspid disease I08.8
    acute or subacute I33.9
      rheumatic I01.1
        with chorea (acute) (rheumatic) (Sydenham's) I02.0
    arteriosclerotic I37.8
    congenital Q22.2
    rheumatic (chronic) (inactive) (with chorea) I09.89
      active or acute I01.1
        with chorea (acute) (rheumatic) (Sydenham's) I02.0
    syphilitic A52.03
  purulent (acute) (any valve) (subacute) I33.0
  Q fever A78 [I39]
  rheumatic (chronic) (inactive) (with chorea) I09.1
    active or acute (aortic) (mitral) (pulmonary) (tricuspid) I01.1

Endocarditis — *continued*
  rheumatic — *continued*
    active or acute — *continued*
      with chorea (acute) (rheumatic) (Sydenham's) I02.0
  rheumatoid — *see* Rheumatoid, carditis
  septic (acute) (any valve) (subacute) I33.0
  streptococcal (acute) (any valve) (subacute) I33.0
  subacute — *see* Endocarditis, acute
  suppurative (acute) (any valve) (subacute) I33.0
  syphilitic A52.03
  toxic I33.9
  tricuspid (chronic) (heart) (inactive) (rheumatic) (valve) (with chorea) I07.9
    with
      aortic (valve) disease I08.2
        mitral (valve) disease I08.3
      mitral (valve) disease I08.1
        aortic (valve) disease I08.3
      rheumatic fever (conditions in I00)
        active — *see* Endocarditis, acute, rheumatic
        inactive or quiescent (with chorea) I07.8
    active or acute I01.1
      with chorea (acute) (rheumatic) (Sydenham's) I02.0
    arteriosclerotic I36.8
    nonrheumatic I36.8
      acute or subacute I33.9
    specified cause, except rheumatic I36.8
  tuberculous — *see* Tuberculosis, endocarditis
  typhoid A01.02
  ulcerative (acute) (any valve) (subacute) I33.0
  vegetative (acute) (any valve) (subacute) I33.0
  verrucous (atypical) (nonbacterial) (nonrheumatic) M32.11
Endocardium, endocardial (*see also* condition)
  cushion defect Q21.2
Endocervicitis (*see also* Cervicitis)
  due to intrauterine (contraceptive) device T83.69 ☑
  hyperplastic N72
Endocrine — *see* condition
Endocrinopathy, pluriglandular E31.9
Endodontic
  overfill M27.52
  underfill M27.53
Endodontitis K04.01
  irreversible K04.02
  reversible K04.01
Endomastoiditis — *see* Mastoiditis
Endometrioma N80.9
Endometriosis N80.9
  appendix N80.5
  bladder N80.8
  bowel N80.5
  broad ligament N80.3
  cervix N80.0
  colon N80.5
  cul-de-sac (Douglas') N80.3
  exocervix N80.0
  fallopian tube N80.2
  female genital organ NEC N80.8
  gallbladder N80.8
  in scar of skin N80.6
  internal N80.0
  intestine N80.5
  lung N80.8
  myometrium N80.0
  ovary N80.1
  parametrium N80.3
  pelvic peritoneum N80.3
  peritoneal (pelvic) N80.3
  rectovaginal septum N80.4
  rectum N80.5
  round ligament N80.3
  skin (scar) N80.6
  specified site NEC N80.8
  stromal D39.0
  thorax N80.8
  umbilicus N80.8
  uterus (internal) N80.0
  vagina N80.4
  vulva N80.8
Endometritis (decidual) (nonspecific) (purulent) (senile) (atrophic) (suppurative) N71.9
  with ectopic pregnancy O08.0
  acute N71.0
  blenorrhagic (gonococcal) (acute) (chronic) A54.24

Endometritis — *continued*
  cervix, cervical (with erosion or ectropion) (*see also* Cervicitis)
    hyperplastic N72
  chlamydial A56.11
  chronic N71.1
  following
    abortion — *see* Abortion by type complicated by genital infection
    ectopic or molar pregnancy O08.0
  gonococcal, gonorrheal (acute) (chronic) A54.24
  hyperplastic (*see also* Hyperplasia, endometrial) N85.00
    cervix N72
  puerperal, postpartum, childbirth O86.12
  subacute N71.0
  tuberculous A18.17
Endometrium — *see* condition
Endomyocardiopathy, South African I42.3
Endomyocarditis — *see* Endocarditis
Endomyofibrosis I42.3
Endomyometritis — *see* Endometritis
Endopericarditis — *see* Endocarditis
Endoperineuritis — *see* Disorder, nerve
Endophlebitis — *see* Phlebitis
Endophthalmia — *see* Endophthalmitis, purulent
Endophthalmitis (acute) (infective) (metastatic) (subacute) H44.009
  bleb associated (*see also* Bleb, inflamed (infected), postprocedural H59.4 ☑
  gonorrhea A54.39
  in (due to)
    cysticercosis B69.1
    onchocerciasis B73.01
    toxocariasis B83.0
  panuveitis — *see* Panuveitis
  parasitic H44.12- ☑
  purulent H44.00- ☑
    panophthalmitis — *see* Panophthalmitis
    vitreous abscess H44.02- ☑
  specified NEC H44.19
  sympathetic — *see* Uveitis, sympathetic
Endosalpingioma D28.2
Endosalpingiosis N94.89
Endosteitis — *see* Osteomyelitis
Endothelioma, bone — *see* Neoplasm, bone, malignant
Endotheliosis (hemorrhagic infectional) D69.8
Endotoxemia — code to condition
Endotrachelitis — *see* Cervicitis
Engelmann (-Camurati) **syndrome** Q78.3
English disease — *see* Rickets
Engman's disease L30.3
Engorgement
  breast N64.59
    newborn P83.4
    puerperal, postpartum O92.79
  lung (passive) — *see* Edema, lung
  pulmonary (passive) — *see* Edema, lung
  stomach K31.89
  venous, retina — *see* Occlusion, retina, vein, engorgement
Enlargement, enlarged (*see also* Hypertrophy)
  adenoids J35.2
    with tonsils J35.3
  alveolar ridge K08.89
    congenital — *see* Anomaly, alveolar
  apertures of diaphragm (congenital) Q79.1
  gingival K06.1
  heart, cardiac — *see* Hypertrophy, cardiac
  labium majus, childhood asymmetric (CALME) N90.61
  lacrimal gland, chronic H04.03- ☑
  liver — *see* Hypertrophy, liver
  lymph gland or node R59.9
    generalized R59.1
    localized R59.0
  orbit H05.34- ☑
  organ or site, congenital NEC — *see* Anomaly, by site
  parathyroid (gland) E21.0
  pituitary fossa R93.0
  prostate N40.0
    with lower urinary tract symptoms (LUTS) N40.1
    without lower urinary tract symtpoms (LUTS) N40.0
  sella turcica R93.0
  spleen — *see* Splenomegaly
  thymus (gland) (congenital) E32.0
  thyroid (gland) — *see* Goiter
  tongue K14.8
  tonsils J35.1

Enlargement, enlarged — *continued*
  tonsils — *continued*
    with adenoids J35.3
  uterus N85.2
  vestibular aqueduct Q16.5
Enophthalmos H05.40- ☑
  due to
    orbital tissue atrophy H05.41- ☑
    trauma or surgery H05.42- ☑
Enostosis M27.8
Entamebic, entamebiasis — *see* Amebiasis
Entanglement
  umbilical cord(s) O69.82 ☑
    with compression O69.2 ☑
    without compression O69.82 ☑
    around neck (with compression) O69.81 ☑
      with compression O69.1 ☑
      without compression O69.81 ☑
    of twins in monoamniotic sac O69.2 ☑
Enteralgia — *see* Pain, abdominal
Enteric — *see* condition
Enteritis (acute) (diarrheal) (hemorrhagic) (noninfective) K52.9
  adenovirus A08.2
  aertrycke infection A02.0
  allergic K52.29
    with
      eosinophilic gastritis or gastroenteritis K52.81
      food protein-induced enterocolitis syndrome K52.21
      food protein-induced enteropathy K52.22
  amebic (acute) A06.0
    with abscess — *see* Abscess, amebic
    chronic A06.1
      with abscess — *see* Abscess, amebic
      nondysenteric A06.2
    nondysenteric A06.2
  astrovirus A08.32
  bacillary NOS A03.9
  bacterial A04.9
    specified NEC A04.8
  calicivirus A08.31
  candidal B37.82
  Chilomastix A07.8
  choleriformis A00.1
  chronic (noninfectious) K52.9
    ulcerative — *see* Colitis, ulcerative
  cicatrizing (chronic) — *see* Enteritis, regional, small intestine
  Clostridium
    botulinum (food poisoning) A05.1
    difficile
      not specified as recurrent A04.72
      recurrent A04.71
  coccidial A07.3
  coxsackie virus A08.39
  dietetic (*see also* Enteritis, allergic) K52.29
  drug-induced K52.1
  due to
    astrovirus A08.32
    calicivirus A08.31
    coxsackie virus A08.39
    drugs K52.1
    echovirus A08.39
    enterovirus NEC A08.39
    food hypersensitivity (*see also* Enteritis, allergic) K52.29
    infectious organism (bacterial) (viral) — *see* Enteritis, infectious
    torovirus A08.39
    Yersinia enterocolitica A04.6
  echovirus A08.39
  eltor A00.1
  enterovirus NEC A08.39
  eosinophilic K52.81
  epidemic (infectious) A09
  fulminant (*see also* Ischemia, intestine, acute) K55.019
  gangrenous — *see* Enteritis, infectious
  giardial A07.1
  infectious NOS A09
    due to
      adenovirus A08.2
      Aerobacter aerogenes A04.8
      Arizona (bacillus) A02.0
      bacteria NOS A04.9
        specified NEC A04.8
      Campylobacter A04.5

Enteritis — *continued*
  infectious — *continued*
    due to — *continued*
      Clostridium difficile
        not specified as recurrent A04.72
        recurrent A04.71
      Clostridium perfringens A04.8
      Enterobacter aerogenes A04.8
      enterovirus A08.39
      Escherichia coli A04.4
        enteroaggregative A04.4
        enterohemorrhagic A04.3
        enteroinvasive A04.2
        enteropathogenic A04.0
        enterotoxigenic A04.1
        specified NEC A04.4
      specified
        bacteria NEC A04.8
        virus NEC A08.39
      Staphylococcus A04.8
      virus NEC A08.4
        specified type NEC A08.39
      Yersinia enterocolitica A04.6
    specified organism NEC A08.8
  influenzal — *see* Influenza, with, digestive manifestations
  ischemic K55.9
    acute (*see also* Ischemia, intestine, acute) K55.019
    chronic K55.1
  microsporidial A07.8
  mucomembranous, myxomembranous — *see* Syndrome, irritable bowel
  mucous — *see* Syndrome, irritable bowel
  necroticans A05.2
  necrotizing of newborn — *see* Enterocolitis, necrotizing, in newborn
  neurogenic — *see* Syndrome, irritable bowel
  newborn necrotizing — *see* Enterocolitis, necrotizing, in newborn
  noninfectious K52.9
  norovirus A08.11
  parasitic NEC B82.9
  paratyphoid (fever) — *see* Fever, paratyphoid
  protozoal A07.9
    specified NEC A07.8
  radiation K52.0
  regional (of) K50.90
    with
      complication K50.919
        abscess K50.914
        fistula K50.913
        intestinal obstruction K50.912
        rectal bleeding K50.911
        specified complication NEC K50.918
    colon — *see* Enteritis, regional, large intestine
    duodenum — *see* Enteritis, regional, small intestine
    ileum — *see* Enteritis, regional, small intestine
    jejunum — *see* Enteritis, regional, small intestine
    large bowel — *see* Enteritis, regional, large intestine
    large intestine (colon) (rectum) K50.10
      with
        complication K50.119
          abscess K50.114
          fistula K50.113
          intestinal obstruction K50.112
          rectal bleeding K50.111
          small intestine (duodenum) (ileum) (jejunum) involvement K50.80
            with
              complication K50.819
                abscess K50.814
                fistula K50.813
                intestinal obstruction K50.812
                rectal bleeding K50.811
                specified complication NEC K50.818
        specified complication NEC K50.118
    rectum — *see* Enteritis, regional, large intestine
    small intestine (duodenum) (ileum) (jejunum) K50.00
      with
        complication K50.019
          abscess K50.014
          fistula K50.013
          intestinal obstruction K50.012
          large intestine (colon) (rectum) involvement K50.80

Enteritis — *continued*
  regional — *continued*
    small intestine — *continued*
      with — *continued*
        complication — *continued*
          large intestine involvement — *continued*
            with
              complication K50.819
                abscess K50.814
                fistula K50.813
                intestinal obstruction K50.812
                rectal bleeding K50.811
                specified complication NEC K50.818
          rectal bleeding K50.011
          specified complication NEC K50.018
  rotaviral A08.0
  Salmonella, salmonellosis (arizonae) (cholerae-suis) (enteritidis) (typhimurium) A02.0
  segmental — *see* Enteritis, regional
  septic A09
  Shigella — *see* Infection, Shigella
  small round structured NEC A08.19
  spasmodic, spastic — *see* Syndrome, irritable bowel
  staphylococcal A04.8
    due to food A05.0
  torovirus A08.39
  toxic NEC K52.1
    due to Clostridium difficile
      not specified as recurrent A04.72
      recurrent A04.71
  trichomonal A07.8
  tuberculous A18.32
  typhosa A01.00
  ulcerative (chronic) — *see* Colitis, ulcerative
  viral A08.4
    adenovirus A08.2
    enterovirus A08.39
    Rotavirus A08.0
    small round structured NEC A08.19
    specified NEC A08.39
    virus specified NEC A08.39
Enterobiasis B80
Enterobius vermicularis (infection) (infestation) B80
Enterocele (*see also* Hernia, abdomen)
  pelvic, pelvis (acquired) (congenital) N81.5
  vagina, vaginal (acquired) (congenital) NEC N81.5
Enterocolitis (*see also* Enteritis) K52.9
  due to Clostridium difficile
    not specified as recurrent A04.72
    recurrent A04.71
  fulminant ischemic (*see also* Ischemia, intestine, acute) K55.059
  granulomatous — *see* Enteritis, regional
  hemorrhagic (acute) (*see also* Ischemia, intestine, acute) K55.059
    chronic K55.1
  infectious NEC A09
  ischemic K55.9
  necrotizing K55.30
    with
      perforation K55.33
      pneumatosis K55.32
        and perforation K55.33
    without pneumatosis or perforation K55.31
    due to Clostridium difficile
      not specified as recurrent A04.72
      recurrent A04.71
    in newborn P77.9
      stage 1 (without pneumatosis, without perforation) P77.1
      stage 2 (with pneumatosis, without perforation) P77.2
      stage 3 (with pneumatosis, with perforation) P77.3
    in non-newborn K55.30
      stage 1 (without pneumatosis, without perforation) K55.31
      stage 2 (with pneumatosis, without perforation) K55.32
      stage 3 (with pneumatosis, with perforation) K55.33
  noninfectious K52.9
    newborn — *see* Enterocolitis, necrotizing, in newborn
  pseudomembranous (newborn)
    not specified as recurrent A04.72

Enterocolitis — continued
pseudomembranous — continued
recurrent A04.71
radiation K52.0
newborn — see Enterocolitis, necrotizing, in newborn
ulcerative (chronic) — see Pancolitis, ulcerative (chronic)
Enterogastritis — see Enteritis
Enteropathy K63.9
celiac-gluten-sensitive K90.0
non-celiac K90.41
food protein-induced enterocolitis K52.22
hemorrhagic, terminal (see also Ischemia, intestine, acute) K55.059
protein-losing K90.49
Enteroperitonitis — see Peritonitis
Enteroptosis K63.4
Enterorrhagia K92.2
Enterospasm (see also Syndrome, irritable, bowel)
psychogenic F45.8
Enterostenosis (see also Obstruction, intestine, specified NEC) K56.699
Enterostomy
complication — see Complication, enterostomy
status Z93.4
Enterovirus, as cause of disease classified elsewhere B97.10
coxsackievirus B97.11
echovirus B97.12
other specified B97.19
Enthesopathy (peripheral) M77.9
Achilles tendinitis — see Tendinitis, Achilles
ankle and tarsus M77.9
specified type NEC — see Enthesopathy, foot, specified type NEC
anterior tibial syndrome M76.81- ☑
calcaneal spur — see Spur, bone, calcaneal
elbow region M77.9
lateral epicondylitis — see Epicondylitis, lateral
medial epicondylitis — see Epicondylitis, medial
foot NEC M77.9
metatarsalgia — see Metatarsalgia
specified type NEC M77.5- ☑
forearm M77.9
gluteal tendinitis — see Tendinitis, gluteal
hand M77.9
hip — see Enthesopathy, lower limb, specified type NEC
iliac crest spur — see Spur, bone, iliac crest
iliotibial band syndrome — see Syndrome, iliotibial band
knee — see Enthesopathy, lower limb, lower leg, specified type NEC
lateral epicondylitis — see Epicondylitis, lateral
lower limb (excluding foot) M76.9
Achilles tendinitis — see Tendinitis, Achilles
anterior tibial syndrome M76.81- ☑
gluteal tendinitis — see Tendinitis, gluteal
iliac crest spur — see Spur, bone, iliac crest
iliotibial band syndrome — see Syndrome, iliotibial band
patellar tendinitis — see Tendinitis, patellar
pelvic region — see Enthesopathy, lower limb, specified type NEC
peroneal tendinitis — see Tendinitis, peroneal
posterior tibial syndrome M76.82- ☑
psoas tendinitis — see Tendinitis, psoas
shoulder M77.9
specified type NEC M76.89- ☑
tibial collateral bursitis — see Bursitis, tibial collateral
medial epicondylitis — see Epicondylitis, medial
metatarsalgia — see Metatarsalgia
multiple sites M77.9
patellar tendinitis — see Tendinitis, patellar
pelvis M77.9
periarthritis of wrist — see Periarthritis, wrist
peroneal tendinitis — see Tendinitis, peroneal
posterior tibial syndrome M76.82- ☑
psoas tendinitis — see Tendinitis, psoas
shoulder region — see Lesion, shoulder
specified site NEC M77.9
specified type NEC M77.8
spinal M46.00
cervical region M46.02
cervicothoracic region M46.03

Enthesopathy — continued
spinal — continued
lumbar region M46.06
lumbosacral region M46.07
multiple sites M46.09
occipito-atlanto-axial region M46.01
sacrococcygeal region M46.08
thoracic region M46.04
thoracolumbar region M46.05
tibial collateral bursitis — see Bursitis, tibial collateral
upper arm M77.9
wrist and carpus NEC M77.8
calcaneal spur — see Spur, bone, calcaneal
periarthritis of wrist — see Periarthritis, wrist
Entomophobia F40.218
Entomophthoromycosis B46.8
Entrance, air into vein — see Embolism, air
Entrapment, nerve — see Neuropathy, entrapment
Entropion (eyelid) (paralytic) H02.009
cicatricial H02.019
left H02.016
lower H02.015
upper H02.014
right H02.013
lower H02.012
upper H02.011
congenital Q10.2
left H02.006
lower H02.005
upper H02.004
mechanical H02.029
left H02.026
lower H02.025
upper H02.024
right H02.023
lower H02.022
upper H02.021
right H02.003
lower H02.002
upper H02.001
senile H02.039
left H02.036
lower H02.035
upper H02.034
right H02.033
lower H02.032
upper H02.031
spastic H02.049
left H02.046
lower H02.045
upper H02.044
right H02.043
lower H02.042
upper H02.041
Enucleated eye (traumatic, current) S05.7- ☑
Enuresis R32
functional F98.0
habit disturbance F98.0
nocturnal N39.44
psychogenic F98.0
nonorganic origin F98.0
psychogenic F98.0
Eosinopenia — see Agranulocytosis
Eosinophilia (allergic) (hereditary) (idiopathic) (secondary) D72.1
with
angiolymphoid hyperplasia (ALHE) D18.01
infiltrative J82
Löffler's J82
peritoneal — see Peritonitis, eosinophilic
pulmonary NEC J82
tropical (pulmonary) J82
Eosinophilia-myalgia syndrome M35.8
Ependymitis (acute) (cerebral) (chronic) (granular) — see Encephalomyelitis
Ependymoblastoma
specified site — see Neoplasm, malignant, by site
unspecified site C71.9
Ependymoma (epithelial) (malignant)
anaplastic
specified site — see Neoplasm, malignant, by site
unspecified site C71.9
benign
specified site — see Neoplasm, benign, by site
unspecified site D33.2
myxopapillary D43.2
specified site — see Neoplasm, uncertain behavior, by site

Ependymoma — continued
myxopapillary — continued
unspecified site D43.2
papillary D43.2
specified site — see Neoplasm, uncertain behavior, by site
unspecified site D43.2
specified site — see Neoplasm, malignant, by site
unspecified site C71.9
Ependymopathy G93.89
Ephelis, ephelides L81.2
Epiblepharon (congenital) Q10.3
Epicanthus, epicanthic fold (eyelid) (congenital) Q10.3
Epicondylitis (elbow)
lateral M77.1- ☑
medial M77.0- ☑
Epicystitis — see Cystitis
Epidemic — see condition
Epidermidalization, cervix — see Dysplasia, cervix
Epidermis, epidermal — see condition
Epidermodysplasia verruciformis B07.8
Epidermolysis
bullosa (congenital) Q81.9
acquired L12.30
drug-induced L12.31
specified cause NEC L12.35
dystrophica Q81.2
letalis Q81.1
simplex Q81.0
specified NEC Q81.8
necroticans combustiformis L51.2
due to drug — see Table of Drugs and Chemicals, by drug
Epidermophytid — see Dermatophytosis
Epidermophytosis (infected) — see Dermatophytosis
Epididymis — see condition
Epididymitis (acute) (nonvenereal) (recurrent) (residual) N45.1
with orchitis N45.3
blennorrhagic (gonococcal) A54.23
caseous (tuberculous) A18.15
chlamydial A56.19
filarial (see also Infestation, filarial) B74.9 [N51]
gonococcal A54.23
syphilitic A52.76
tuberculous A18.15
Epididymo-orchitis (see also Epididymitis) N45.3
Epidural — see condition
Epigastrium, epigastric — see condition
Epigastrocele — see Hernia, ventral
Epiglottis — see condition
Epiglottitis, epiglottiditis (acute) J05.10
with obstruction J05.11
chronic J37.0
Epignathus Q89.4
Epilepsia partialis continua (see also Kozhevnikof's epilepsy) G40.1- ☑
Epilepsy, epileptic, epilepsia (attack) (cerebral) (convulsion) (fit) (seizure) G40.909

> Note: the following terms are to be considered equivalent to intractable: pharmacoresistant (pharmacologically resistant), treatment resistant, refractory (medically) and poorly controlled

with
complex partial seizures — see Epilepsy, localization-related, symptomatic, with complex partial seizures
grand mal seizures on awakening — see Epilepsy, generalized, specified NEC
myoclonic absences — see Epilepsy, generalized, specified NEC
myoclonic-astatic seizures — see Epilepsy, generalized, specified NEC
simple partial seizures — see Epilepsy, localization-related, symptomatic, with simple partial seizures
akinetic — see Epilepsy, generalized, specified NEC
benign childhood with centrotemporal EEG spikes — see Epilepsy, localization-related, idiopathic
benign myoclonic in infancy G40.80- ☑
Bravais-jacksonian — see Epilepsy, localization-related, symptomatic, with simple partial seizures
childhood
with occipital EEG paroxysms — see Epilepsy, localization-related, idiopathic
absence G40.A09 (following G40.3)

Epilepsy, epileptic, epilepsia — *continued*
  childhood — *continued*
    absence — *continued*
      intractable G40.A19 (*following* G40.3)
        with status epilepticus G40.A11 (*following* G40.3)
        without status epilepticus G40.A19 (*following* G40.3)
      not intractable G40.A09 (*following* G40.3)
        with status epilepticus G40.A01 (*following* G40.3)
        without status epilepticus G40.A09 (*following* G40.3)
  climacteric — *see* Epilepsy, specified NEC
  cysticercosis B69.0
  deterioration (mental) F06.8
  due to syphilis A52.19
  focal — *see* Epilepsy, localization-related, symptomatic, with simple partial seizures
  generalized
    idiopathic G40.309
      intractable G40.319
        with status epilepticus G40.311
        without status epilepticus G40.319
      not intractable G40.309
        with status epilepticus G40.301
        without status epilepticus G40.309
    specified NEC G40.409
      intractable G40.419
        with status epilepticus G40.411
        without status epilepticus G40.419
      not intractable G40.409
        with status epilepticus G40.401
        without status epilepticus G40.409
  impulsive petit mal — *see* Epilepsy, juvenile myoclonic
  intractable G40.919
    with status epilepticus G40.911
    without status epilepticus G40.919
  juvenile absence G40.A09 (*following* G40.3)
    intractable G40.A19 (*following* G40.3)
      with status epilepticus G40.A11 (*following* G40.3)
      without status epilepticus G40.A19 (*following* G40.3)
    not intractable G40.A09 (*following* G40.3)
      with status epilepticus G40.A01 (*following* G40.3)
      without status epilepticus G40.A09 (*following* G40.3)
  juvenile myoclonic G40.B09 (*following* G40.3)
    intractable G40.B19 (*following* G40.3)
      with status epilepticus G40.B11 (*following* G40.3)
      without status epilepticus G40.B19 (*following* G40.3)
    not intractable G40.B09 (*following* G40.3)
      with status epilepticus G40.B01 (*following* G40.3)
      without status epilepticus G40.B09 (*following* G40.3)
  localization-related (focal) (partial)
    idiopathic G40.009
      with seizures of localized onset G40.009
        intractable G40.019
          with status epilepticus G40.011
          without status epilepticus G40.019
        not intractable G40.009
          with status epilepticus G40.001
          without status epilepticus G40.009
    symptomatic
      with complex partial seizures G40.209
        intractable G40.219
          with status epilepticus G40.211
          without status epilepticus G40.219
        not intractable G40.209
          with status epilepticus G40.201
          without status epilepticus G40.209
      with simple partial seizures G40.109
        intractable G40.119
          with status epilepticus G40.111
          without status epilepticus G40.119
        not intractable G40.109
          with status epilepticus G40.101
          without status epilepticus G40.109
  myoclonus, myoclonic — *see* Epilepsy, generalized, specified NEC
  progressive — *see* Epilepsy, generalized, idiopathic
  not intractable G40.909
    with status epilepticus G40.901

Epilepsy, epileptic, epilepsia — *continued*
  not intractable — *continued*
    without status epilepticus G40.909
  on awakening — *see* Epilepsy, generalized, specified NEC
  parasitic NOS B71.9 [G94]
  partialis continua (*see also* Kozhevnikof's epilepsy) G40.1- ☑
  peripheral — *see* Epilepsy, specified NEC
  procursiva — *see* Epilepsy, localization-related, symptomatic, with simple partial seizures
  progressive (familial) myoclonic — *see* Epilepsy, generalized, idiopathic
  reflex — *see* Epilepsy, specified NEC
  related to
    alcohol G40.509
      not intractable G40.509
        with status epilepticus G40.501
        without status epliepticus G40.509
    drugs G40.509
      not intractable G40.509
        with status epilepticus G40.501
        without status epliepticus G40.509
    external causes G40.509
      not intractable G40.509
        with status epilepticus G40.501
        without status epliepticus G40.509
    hormonal changes G40.509
      not intractable G40.509
        with status epilepticus G40.501
        without status epliepticus G40.509
    sleep deprivation G40.509
      not intractable G40.509
        with status epilepticus G40.501
        without status epliepticus G40.509
    stress G40.509
      not intractable G40.509
        with status epilepticus G40.501
        without status epliepticus G40.509
  somatomotor — *see* Epilepsy, localization-related, symptomatic, with simple partial seizures
  somatosensory — *see* Epilepsy, localization-related, symptomatic, with simple partial seizures
  spasms G40.822
    intractable G40.824
      with status epilepticus G40.823
      without status epilepticus G40.824
    not intractable G40.822
      with status epilepticus G40.821
      without status epilepticus G40.822
  specified NEC G40.802
    intractable G40.804
      with status epilepticus G40.803
      without status epilepticus G40.804
    not intractable G40.802
      with status epilepticus G40.801
      without status epilepticus G40.802
  syndromes
    generalized
      idiopathic G40.309
        intractable G40.319
          with status epilepticus G40.311
          without status epilepticus G40.319
        not intractable G40.309
          with status epilepticus G40.301
          without status epilepticus G40.309
      specified NEC G40.409
        intractable G40.419
          with status epilepticus G40.411
          without status epilepticus G40.419
        not intractable G40.409
          with status epilepticus G40.401
          without status epilepticus G40.409
    localization-related (focal) (partial)
      idiopathic G40.009
        with seizures of localized onset G40.009
          intractable G40.019
            with status epilepticus G40.011
            without status epilepticus G40.019
          not intractable G40.009
            with status epilepticus G40.001
            without status epilepticus G40.009
      symptomatic
        with complex partial seizures G40.209
          intractable G40.219
            with status epilepticus G40.211
            without status epilepticus G40.219
          not intractable G40.209

Epilepsy, epileptic, epilepsia — *continued*
  syndromes — *continued*
    localization-related — *continued*
      symptomatic — *continued*
        with complex partial seizures — *continued*
          not intractable — *continued*
            with status epilepticus G40.201
            without status epilepticus G40.209
        with simple partial seizures G40.109
          intractable G40.119
            with status epilepticus G40.111
            without status epilepticus G40.119
          not intractable G40.109
            with status epilepticus G40.101
            without status epilepticus G40.109
    specified NEC G40.802
      intractable G40.804
        with status epilepticus G40.803
        without status epilepticus G40.804
      not intractable G40.802
        with status epilepticus G40.801
        without status epilepticus G40.802
  tonic (-clonic) — *see* Epilepsy, generalized, specified NEC
  twilight F05
  uncinate (gyrus) — *see* Epilepsy, localization-related, symptomatic, with complex partial seizures
  Unverricht (-Lundborg) (familial myoclonic) — *see* Epilepsy, generalized, idiopathic
  visceral — *see* Epilepsy, specified NEC
  visual — *see* Epilepsy, specified NEC
Epiloia Q85.1
Epimenorrhea N92.0
Epipharyngitis — *see* Nasopharyngitis
Epiphora H04.20- ☑
  due to
    excess lacrimation H04.21- ☑
    insufficient drainage H04.22- ☑
Epiphyseal arrest — *see* Arrest, epiphyseal
Epiphyseolysis, epiphysiolysis — *see* Osteochondropathy
Epiphysitis (*see also* Osteochondropathy)
  juvenile M92.9
  syphilitic (congenital) A50.02
Epiplocele — *see* Hernia, abdomen
Epiploitis — *see* Peritonitis
Epiplosarcomphalocele — *see* Hernia, umbilicus
Episcleritis (suppurative) H15.10- ☑
  in (due to)
    syphilis A52.71
    tuberculosis A18.51
  nodular H15.12- ☑
  periodica fugax H15.11- ☑
    angioneurotic — *see* Edema, angioneurotic
  syphilitic (late) A52.71
  tuberculous A18.51
Episode
  affective, mixed F39
  depersonalization (in neurotic state) F48.1
  depressive F32.9
    major F32.9
      mild F32.0
      moderate F32.1
      severe (without psychotic symptoms) F32.2
        with psychotic symptoms F32.3
    recurrent F33.9
      brief F33.8
    specified NEC F32.89
  hypomanic F30.8
  manic F30.9
    with
      psychotic symptoms F30.2
      remission (full) F30.4
        partial F30.3
    without psychotic symptoms F30.10
      mild F30.11
      moderate F30.12
      severe (without psychotic symptoms) F30.13
        with psychotic symptoms F30.2
    other specified F30.8
    recurrent F31.89
  psychotic F23
    organic F06.8
  schizophrenic (acute) NEC, brief F23
Epispadias (female) (male) Q64.0
Episplenitis D73.89
Epistaxis (multiple) R04.0

Epistaxis — *continued*
  hereditary I78.0
  vicarious menstruation N94.89
Epithelioma (malignant) (*see also* Neoplasm, malignant, by site)
  adenoides cysticum — *see* Neoplasm, skin, benign
  basal cell — *see* Neoplasm, skin, malignant
  benign — *see* Neoplasm, benign, by site
  Bowen's — *see* Neoplasm, skin, in situ
  calcifying, of Malherbe — *see* Neoplasm, skin, benign
  external site — *see* Neoplasm, skin, malignant
  intraepidermal, Jadassohn — *see* Neoplasm, skin, benign
  squamous cell — *see* Neoplasm, malignant, by site
Epitheliomatosis pigmented Q82.1
Epitheliopathy, multifocal placoid pigment H30.14- ☑
Epithelium, epithelial — *see* condition
Epituberculosis (with atelectasis) (allergic) A15.7
Eponychia Q84.6
Epstein's
  nephrosis or syndrome — *see* Nephrosis
  pearl K09.8
Epulis (gingiva) (fibrous) (giant cell) K06.8
Equinia A24.0
Equinovarus (congenital) (talipes) Q66.0
  acquired — *see* Deformity, limb, clubfoot
Equivalent
  convulsive (abdominal) — *see* Epilepsy, specified NEC
  epileptic (psychic) — *see* Epilepsy, localization-related, symptomatic, with complex partial seizures
Erb (-Duchenne) **paralysis** (birth injury) (newborn) P14.0
Erb-Goldflam disease or syndrome G70.00
  with exacerbation (acute) G70.01
  in crisis G70.01
Erb's
  disease G71.0
  palsy, paralysis (brachial) (birth) (newborn) P14.0
   spinal (spastic) syphilitic A52.17
  pseudohypertrophic muscular dystrophy G71.0
Erdheim's syndrome (acromegalic macrospondylitis) E22.0
Erection, painful (persistent) — *see* Priapism
Ergosterol deficiency (vitamin D) E55.9
  with
   adult osteomalacia M83.8
   rickets — *see* Rickets
Ergotism (*see also* Poisoning, food, noxious, plant)
  from ergot used as drug (migraine therapy) — *see* Table of Drugs and Chemicals
Erosio interdigitalis blastomycetica B37.2
Erosion
  artery I77.2
   without rupture I77.89
  bone — *see* Disorder, bone, density and structure, specified NEC
  bronchus J98.09
  cartilage (joint) — *see* Disorder, cartilage, specified type NEC
  cervix (uteri) (acquired) (chronic) (congenital) N86
   with cervicitis N72
  cornea (nontraumatic) — *see* Ulcer, cornea
   recurrent H18.83- ☑
   traumatic — *see* Abrasion, cornea
  dental (idiopathic) (occupational) (due to diet, drugs or vomiting) K03.2
  duodenum, postpyloric — *see* Ulcer, duodenum
  esophagus K22.10
   with bleeding K22.11
  gastric — *see* Ulcer, stomach
  gastrojejunal — *see* Ulcer, gastrojejunal
  implanted mesh — *see* Complications, mesh
  intestine K63.3
  lymphatic vessel I89.8
  pylorus, pyloric (ulcer) — *see* Ulcer, stomach
  spine, aneurysmal A52.09
  stomach — *see* Ulcer, stomach
  subcutaneous device pocket
   nervous system prosthetic device, implant, or graft T85.890 ☑
   other internal prosthetic device, implant, or graft T85.898 ☑
  teeth (idiopathic) (occupational) (due to diet, drugs or vomiting) K03.2
  urethra N36.8
  uterus N85.8
Erotomania F52.8

Error
  metabolism, inborn — *see* Disorder, metabolism
  refractive — *see* Disorder, refraction
Eructation R14.2
  nervous or psychogenic F45.8
Eruption
  creeping B76.9
  drug (generalized) (taken internally) L27.0
   fixed L27.1
   in contact with skin — *see* Dermatitis, due to drugs
   localized L27.1
  Hutchinson, summer L56.4
  Kaposi's varicelliform B00.0
  napkin L22
  polymorphous light (sun) L56.4
  recalcitrant pustular L13.8
  ringed R23.8
  skin (nonspecific) R21
   creeping (meaning hookworm) B76.9
   due to inoculation/vaccination (generalized) (*see also* Dermatitis, due to, vaccine) L27.0
    localized L27.1
   erysipeloid A26.0
   feigned L98.1
   Kaposi's varicelliform B00.0
   lichenoid L28.0
   meaning dermatitis — *see* Dermatitis
   toxic NEC L53.0
  tooth, teeth, abnormal (incomplete) (late) (premature) (sequence) K00.6
  vesicular R23.8
Erysipelas (gangrenous) (infantile) (newborn) (phlegmonous) (suppurative) A46
  external ear A46 [H62.40]
  puerperal, postpartum O86.89
Erysipeloid A26.9
  cutaneous (Rosenbach's) A26.0
  disseminated A26.8
  sepsis A26.7
  specified NEC A26.8
Erythema, erythematous (infectional) (inflammation) L53.9
  ab igne L59.0
  annulare (centrifugum) (rheumaticum) L53.1
  arthriticum epidemicum A25.1
  brucellum — *see* Brucellosis
  chronic figurate NEC L53.3
  chronicum migrans (Borrelia burgdorferi) A69.20
  diaper L22
  due to
   chemical NEC L53.0
    in contact with skin L24.5
   drug (internal use) — *see* Dermatitis, due to, drugs
  elevatum diutinum L95.1
  endemic E52
  epidemic, arthritic A25.1
  figuratum perstans L53.3
  gluteal L22
  heat — *code by site under* Burn, first degree
  ichthyosiforme congenitum bullous Q80.3
  in diseases classified elsewhere L54
  induratum (nontuberculous) L52
   tuberculous A18.4
  infectiosum B08.3
  intertrigo L30.4
  iris L51.9
  marginatum L53.2
   in (due to) acute rheumatic fever I00
  medicamentosum — *see* Dermatitis, due to, drugs
  migrans A26.0
   chronicum A69.20
   tongue K14.1
  multiforme (major) (minor) L51.9
   bullous, bullosum L51.1
   conjunctiva L51.1
   nonbullous L51.0
   pemphigoides L12.0
   specified NEC L51.8
  napkin L22
  neonatorum P83.88
   toxic P83.1
  nodosum L52
   tuberculous A18.4
  palmar L53.8
  pernio T69.1 ☑
  rash, newborn P83.88
  scarlatiniform (recurrent) (exfoliative) L53.8
  solare L55.0

Erythema, erythematous — *continued*
  specified NEC L53.8
  toxic, toxicum NEC L53.0
   newborn P83.1
  tuberculous (primary) A18.4
Erythematous, erythematosus — *see* condition
Erythermalgia (primary) I73.81
Erythralgia I73.81
Erythrasma L08.1
Erythredema (polyneuropathy) — *see* Poisoning, mercury
Erythremia (acute) C94.0- ☑
  chronic D45
  secondary D75.1
Erythroblastopenia (*see also* Aplasia, red cell) D60.9
  congenital D61.01
Erythroblastophthisis D61.09
Erythroblastosis (fetalis) (newborn) P55.9
  due to
   ABO (antibodies) (incompatibility) (isoimmunization) P55.1
   Rh (antibodies) (incompatibility) (isoimmunization) P55.0
Erythrocyanosis (crurum) I73.89
Erythrocythemia — *see* Erythremia
Erythrocytosis (megalosplenic) (secondary) D75.1
  familial D75.0
  oval, hereditary — *see* Elliptocytosis
  secondary D75.1
  stress D75.1
Erythroderma (secondary) (*see also* Erythema) L53.9
  bullous ichthyosiform, congenital Q80.3
  desquamativum L21.1
  ichthyosiform, congenital (bullous) Q80.3
  neonatorum P83.88
  psoriaticum L40.8
Erythrodysesthesia, palmar plantar (PPE) L27.1
Erythrogenesis imperfecta D61.09
Erythroleukemia C94.0- ☑
Erythromelalgia I73.81
Erythrophagocytosis D75.89
Erythrophobia F40.298
Erythroplakia, oral epithelium, and tongue K13.29
Erythroplasia (Queyrat) D07.4
  specified site — *see* Neoplasm, skin, in situ
  unspecified site D07.4
Escherichia coli (E. coli), **as cause of disease classified elsewhere** B96.20
  non-O157 Shiga toxin-producing (with known O group) B96.22
  non-Shiga toxin-producing B96.29
  O157 B96.21
  O157 with confirmation of Shiga toxin when H antigen is unknown, or is not H7 B96.21
  O157:H- (nonmotile) with confirmation of Shiga toxin B96.21
  O157:H7 with or without confirmation of Shiga toxin-production B96.21
  Shiga toxin-producing (with unspecified O group) (STEC) B96.23
  specified NEC B96.29
Esophagismus K22.4
Esophagitis (acute) (alkaline) (chemical) (chronic) (infectional) (necrotic) (peptic) (postoperative) K20.9
  candidal B37.81
  due to gastrointestinal reflux disease K21.0
  eosinophilic K20.0
  reflux K21.0
  specified NEC K20.8
  tuberculous A18.83
  ulcerative K22.10
   with bleeding K22.11
Esophagocele K22.5
Esophagomalacia K22.8
Esophagospasm K22.4
Esophagostenosis K22.2
Esophagostomiasis B81.8
Esophagotracheal — *see* condition
Esophagus — *see* condition
Esophoria H50.51
  convergence, excess H51.12
  divergence, insufficiency H51.8
Esotropia — *see* Strabismus, convergent concomitant
Espundia B55.2
Essential — *see* condition
Esthesioneuroblastoma C30.0
Esthesioneurocytoma C30.0

Esthesioneuroepithelioma C30.0
Esthiomene A55
Estivo-autumnal malaria (fever) B50.9
Estrangement (marital) Z63.5
  parent-child NEC Z62.890
Estriasis — *see* Myiasis
Ethanolism — *see* Alcoholism
Etherism — *see* Dependence, drug, inhalant
Ethmoid, ethmoidal — *see* condition
Ethmoiditis (chronic) (nonpurulent) (purulent) (*see also* Sinusitis, ethmoidal)
  influenzal — *see* Influenza, with, respiratory manifestations NEC
  Woakes' J33.1
Ethylism — *see* Alcoholism
Eulenburg's disease (congenital paramyotonia) G71.19
Eumycetoma B47.0
Eunuchoidism E29.1
  hypogonadotropic E23.0
European blastomycosis — *see* Cryptococcosis
Eustachian — *see* condition
Evaluation (for) (of)
  development state
    adolescent Z00.3
    period of
      delayed growth in childhood Z00.70
        with abnormal findings Z00.71
      rapid growth in childhood Z00.2
      puberty Z00.3
  growth and developmental state (period of rapid growth) Z00.2
    delayed growth Z00.70
      with abnormal findings Z00.71
  mental health (status) Z00.8
    requested by authority Z04.6
  period of
    delayed growth in childhood Z00.70
      with abnormal findings Z00.71
    rapid growth in childhood Z00.2
  suspected condition — *see* Observation
Evans syndrome D69.41
Event
  apparent life threatening in newborn and infant (ALTE) R68.13
  brief resolved unexplained event (BRUE) R68.13
Eventration (*see also* Hernia, ventral)
  colon into chest — *see* Hernia, diaphragm
  diaphragm (congenital) Q79.1
Eversion
  bladder N32.89
  cervix (uteri) N86
    with cervicitis N72
  foot NEC (*see also* Deformity, valgus, ankle)
    congenital Q66.6
  punctum lacrimale (postinfectional) (senile) H04.52- ☑
  ureter (meatus) N28.89
  urethra (meatus) N36.8
  uterus N81.4
Evidence
  cytologic
    of malignancy on anal smear R85.614
    of malignancy on cervical smear R87.614
    of malignancy on vaginal smear R87.624
Evisceration
  birth injury P15.8
  traumatic NEC
    eye — *see* Enucleated eye
Evulsion — *see* Avulsion
Ewing's sarcoma or tumor — *see* Neoplasm, bone, malignant
Examination (for) (following) (general) (of) (routine) Z00.00
  with abnormal findings Z00.01
  abuse, physical (alleged), ruled out
    adult Z04.71
    child Z04.72
  adolescent (development state) Z00.3
  alleged rape or sexual assault (victim), ruled out
    adult Z04.41
    child Z04.42
  allergy Z01.82
  annual (adult) (periodic) (physical) Z00.00
    with abnormal findings Z00.01
    gynecological Z01.419
      with abnormal findings Z01.411
  antibody response Z01.84
  blood — *see* Examination, laboratory
  blood pressure Z01.30

Examination — *continued*
  blood pressure — *continued*
    with abnormal findings Z01.31
  cancer staging — *see* Neoplasm, malignant, by site
  cervical Papanicolaou smear Z12.4
    as part of routine gynecological examination Z01.419
    with abnormal findings Z01.411
  child (over 28 days old) Z00.129
    with abnormal findings Z00.121
    under 28 days old — *see* Newborn, examination
  clinical research control or normal comparison (control) (participant) Z00.6
  contraceptive (drug) maintenance (routine) Z30.8
    device (intrauterine) Z30.431
  dental Z01.20
    with abnormal findings Z01.21
  developmental — *see* Examination, child
  donor (potential) Z00.5
  ear Z01.10
    with abnormal findings NEC Z01.118
  eye Z01.00
    with abnormal findings Z01.01
  following
    accident NEC Z04.3
      transport Z04.1
      work Z04.2
    assault, alleged, ruled out
      adult Z04.71
      child Z04.72
    motor vehicle accident Z04.1
    treatment (for) Z09
      combined NEC Z09
        fracture Z09
        malignant neoplasm Z08
      malignant neoplasm Z08
      mental disorder Z09
      specified condition NEC Z09
  follow-up (routine) (following) Z09
    chemotherapy NEC Z09
      malignant neoplasm Z08
    fracture Z09
    malignant neoplasm Z08
    postpartum Z39.2
    psychotherapy Z09
    radiotherapy NEC Z09
      malignant neoplasm Z08
    surgery NEC Z09
      malignant neoplasm Z08
  gynecological Z01.419
    with abnormal findings Z01.411
    for contraceptive maintenance Z30.8
  health — *see* Examination, medical
  hearing Z01.10
    with abnormal findings NEC Z01.118
    following failed hearing screening Z01.110
  immunity status testing Z01.84
  laboratory (as part of a general medical examination) Z00.00
    with abnormal findings Z00.01
    preprocedural Z01.812
  lactating mother Z39.1
  medical (adult) (for) (of) Z00.00
    with abnormal findings Z00.01
    administrative purpose only Z02.9
      specified NEC Z02.89
    admission to
      armed forces Z02.3
      old age home Z02.2
      prison Z02.89
      residential institution Z02.2
      school Z02.0
        following illness or medical treatment Z02.0
      summer camp Z02.89
    adoption Z02.82
    blood alcohol or drug level Z02.83
    camp (summer) Z02.89
    clinical research, normal subject (control) (participant) Z00.6
    control subject in clinical research (normal comparison) (participant) Z00.6
    donor (potential) Z00.5
    driving license Z02.4
    general (adult) Z00.00
      with abnormal findings Z00.01
    immigration Z02.89
    insurance purposes Z02.6
    marriage Z02.89
    medicolegal reasons NEC Z04.8

Examination — *continued*
  medical — *continued*
    naturalization Z02.89
    participation in sport Z02.5
    paternity testing Z02.81
    population survey Z00.8
    pre-employment Z02.1
    pre-operative — *see* Examination, pre-procedural
    pre-procedural
      cardiovascular Z01.810
      respiratory Z01.811
      specified NEC Z01.818
    preschool children
      for admission to school Z02.0
    prisoners
      for entrance into prison Z02.89
    recruitment for armed forces Z02.3
    specified NEC Z00.8
    sport competition Z02.5
  medicolegal reason NEC Z04.8
  newborn — *see* Newborn, examination
  pelvic (annual) (periodic) Z01.419
    with abnormal findings Z01.411
  period of rapid growth in childhood Z00.2
  periodic (adult) (annual) (routine) Z00.00
    with abnormal findings Z00.01
  physical (adult) (*see also* Examination, medical) Z00.00
    sports Z02.5
  postpartum
    immediately after delivery Z39.0
    routine follow-up Z39.2
  pre-chemotherapy (antineoplastic) Z01.818
  prenatal (normal pregnancy) (*see also* Pregnancy, normal) Z34.9- ☑
  pre-procedural (pre-operative)
    cardiovascular Z01.810
    laboratory Z01.812
    respiratory Z01.811
    specified NEC Z01.818
  prior to chemotherapy (antineoplastic) Z01.818
  psychiatric NEC Z00.8
    follow-up not needing further care Z09
    requested by authority Z04.6
  radiological (as part of a general medical examination) Z00.00
    with abnormal findings Z00.01
  repeat cervical smear to confirm findings of recent normal smear following initial abnormal smear Z01.42
  skin (hypersensitivity) Z01.82
  special (*see also* Examination, by type) Z01.89
    specified type NEC Z01.89
  specified type or reason NEC Z04.8
  teeth Z01.20
    with abnormal findings Z01.21
  urine — *see* Examination, laboratory
  vision Z01.00
    with abnormal findings Z01.01
Exanthem, exanthema (*see also* Rash)
  with enteroviral vesicular stomatitis B08.4
  Boston A88.0
  epidemic with meningitis A88.0 [G02]
  subitum B08.20
    due to human herpesvirus 6 B08.21
    due to human herpesvirus 7 B08.22
  viral, virus B09
    specified type NEC B08.8
Excess, excessive, excessively
  alcohol level in blood R78.0
  androgen (ovarian) E28.1
  attrition, tooth, teeth K03.0
  carotene, carotin (dietary) E67.1
  cold, effects of T69.9 ☑
    specified effect NEC T69.8 ☑
  convergence H51.12
  crying
    in child, adolescent, or adult R45.83
    in infant R68.11
  development, breast N62
  divergence H51.8
  drinking (alcohol) NEC (without dependence) F10.10
    habitual (continual) (without remission) F10.20
  eating R63.2
  estrogen E28.0
  fat (*see also* Obesity)
    in heart — *see* Degeneration, myocardial
    localized E65
  foreskin N47.8

Excess, excessive, excessively — *continued*
gas R14.0
glucagon E16.3
heat — *see* Heat
intermaxillary vertical dimension of fully erupted teeth M26.37
interocclusal distance of fully erupted teeth M26.37
kalium E87.5
large
  colon K59.39
    congenital Q43.8
  infant P08.0
  organ or site, congenital NEC — *see* Anomaly, by site
long
  organ or site, congenital NEC — *see* Anomaly, by site
menstruation (with regular cycle) N92.0
  with irregular cycle N92.1
napping Z72.821
natrium E87.0
number of teeth K00.1
nutrient (dietary) NEC R63.2
potassium (K) E87.5
salivation K11.7
secretion (*see also* Hypersecretion)
  milk O92.6
  sputum R09.3
  sweat R61
sexual drive F52.8
short
  organ or site, congenital NEC — *see* Anomaly, by site
  umbilical cord in labor or delivery O69.3 ☑
skin L98.7
  and subcutaneous tissue L98.7
  eyelid (acquired) — *see* Blepharochalasis
    congenital Q10.3
sodium (Na) E87.0
spacing of fully erupted teeth M26.32
sputum R09.3
sweating R61
thirst R63.1
  due to deprivation of water T73.1 ☑
tuberosity of jaw M26.07
vitamin
  A (dietary) E67.0
    administered as drug (prolonged intake) — *see* Table of Drugs and Chemicals, vitamins, adverse effect
    overdose or wrong substance given or taken — *see* Table of Drugs and Chemicals, vitamins, poisoning
  D (dietary) E67.3
    administered as drug (prolonged intake) — *see* Table of Drugs and Chemicals, vitamins, adverse effect
    overdose or wrong substance given or taken — *see* Table of Drugs and Chemicals, vitamins, poisoning
weight
  gain R63.5
  loss R63.4
Excitability, abnormal, under minor stress (personality disorder) F60.3
Excitation
anomalous atrioventricular I45.6
psychogenic F30.8
reactive (from emotional stress, psychological trauma) F30.8
Excitement
hypomanic F30.8
manic F30.9
mental, reactive (from emotional stress, psychological trauma) F30.8
state, reactive (from emotional stress, psychological trauma) F30.8
Excoriation (traumatic) (*see also* Abrasion)
neurotic L98.1
skin picking disorder F42.4
Exfoliation
due to erythematous conditions according to extent of body surface involved L49.0
  less than 10 percent of body surface L49.0
  10-19 percent of body surface L49.1
  20-29 percent of body surface L49.2
  30-39 percent of body surface L49.3
  40-49 percent of body surface L49.4

Exfoliation — *continued*
due to erythematous conditions according to extent of body surface involved — *continued*
  50-59 percent of body surface L49.5
  60-69 percent of body surface L49.6
  70-79 percent of body surface L49.7
  80-89 percent of body surface L49.8
  90-99 percent of body surface L49.9
teeth, due to systemic causes K08.0
Exfoliative — *see* condition
Exhaustion, exhaustive (physical NEC) R53.83
battle F43.0
cardiac — *see* Failure, heart
delirium F43.0
due to
  cold T69.8 ☑
  excessive exertion T73.3 ☑
  exposure T73.2 ☑
  neurasthenia F48.8
heart — *see* Failure, heart
heat (*see also* Heat, exhaustion) T67.5 ☑
  due to
    salt depletion T67.4 ☑
    water depletion T67.3 ☑
maternal, complicating delivery O75.81
mental F48.8
myocardium, myocardial — *see* Failure, heart
nervous F48.8
old age R54
psychogenic F48.8
psychosis F43.0
senile R54
vital NEC Z73.0
Exhibitionism F65.2
Exocervicitis — *see* Cervicitis
Exomphalos Q79.2
meaning hernia — *see* Hernia, umbilicus
Exophoria H50.52
convergence, insufficiency H51.11
divergence, excess H51.8
Exophthalmos H05.2- ☑
congenital Q15.8
constant NEC H05.24- ☑
displacement, globe — *see* Displacement, globe
due to thyrotoxicosis (hyperthyroidism) — *see* Hyperthyroidism, with, goiter (diffuse)
dysthyroid — *see* Hyperthyroidism, with, goiter (diffuse)
goiter — *see* Hyperthyroidism, with, goiter (diffuse)
intermittent NEC H05.25- ☑
malignant — *see* Hyperthyroidism, with, goiter (diffuse)
orbital
  edema — *see* Edema, orbit
  hemorrhage — *see* Hemorrhage, orbit
pulsating NEC H05.26- ☑
thyrotoxic, thyrotropic — *see* Hyperthyroidism, with, goiter (diffuse)
Exostosis (*see also* Disorder, bone)
cartilaginous — *see* Neoplasm, bone, benign
congenital (multiple) Q78.6
external ear canal H61.81- ☑
gonococcal A54.49
jaw (bone) M27.8
multiple, congenital Q78.6
orbit H05.35- ☑
osteocartilaginous — *see* Neoplasm, bone, benign
syphilitic A52.77
Exotropia — *see* Strabismus, divergent concomitant
Explanation of
investigation finding Z71.2
medication Z71.89
Exposure (to) (*see also* Contact, with) T75.89 ☑
acariasis Z20.7
AIDS virus Z20.6
air pollution Z77.110
algae and algae toxins Z77.121
algae bloom Z77.121
anthrax Z20.810
aromatic amines Z77.020
aromatic (hazardous) compounds NEC Z77.028
aromatic dyes NOS Z77.028
arsenic Z77.010
asbestos Z77.090
bacterial disease NEC Z20.818
benzene Z77.021
blue-green algae bloom Z77.121

Exposure — *continued*
body fluids (potentially hazardous) Z77.21
brown tide Z77.121
chemicals (chiefly nonmedicinal) (hazardous) NEC Z77.098
cholera Z20.09
chromium compounds Z77.018
cold, effects of T69.9 ☑
  specified effect NEC T69.8 ☑
communicable disease Z20.9
  bacterial NEC Z20.818
  specified NEC Z20.89
  viral NEC Z20.828
cyanobacteria bloom Z77.121
disaster Z65.5
discrimination Z60.5
dyes Z77.098
effects of T73.9 ☑
environmental tobacco smoke (acute) (chronic) Z77.22
Escherichia coli (E. coli) Z20.01
exhaustion due to T73.2 ☑
fiberglass — *see* Table of Drugs and Chemicals, fiberglass
German measles Z20.4
gonorrhea Z20.2
hazardous metals NEC Z77.018
hazardous substances NEC Z77.29
hazards in the physical environment NEC Z77.128
hazards to health NEC Z77.9
human immunodeficiency virus (HIV) Z20.6
human T-lymphotropic virus type-1 (HTLV-1) Z20.89
implanted
  mesh — *see* Complications, mesh
  prosthetic materials NEC — *see* Complications, prosthetic materials NEC
infestation (parasitic) NEC Z20.7
intestinal infectious disease NEC Z20.09
  Escherichia coli (E. coli) Z20.01
lead Z77.011
meningococcus Z20.811
mold (toxic) Z77.120
nickel dust Z77.018
noise Z77.122
occupational
  air contaminants NEC Z57.39
  dust Z57.2
  environmental tobacco smoke Z57.31
  extreme temperature Z57.6
  noise Z57.0
  radiation Z57.1
  risk factors Z57.9
    specified NEC Z57.8
  toxic agents (gases) (liquids) (solids) (vapors) in agriculture Z57.4
  toxic agents (gases) (liquids) (solids) (vapors) in industry NEC Z57.5
  vibration Z57.7
parasitic disease NEC Z20.7
pediculosis Z20.7
persecution Z60.5
pfiesteria piscicida Z77.121
poliomyelitis Z20.89
pollution
  air Z77.110
  environmental NEC Z77.118
  soil Z77.112
  water Z77.111
polycyclic aromatic hydrocarbons Z77.028
prenatal (drugs) (toxic chemicals) — *see* Newborn, affected by, noxious substances transmitted via placenta or breast milk
rabies Z20.3
radiation, naturally occurring NEC Z77.123
radon Z77.123
red tide (Florida) Z77.121
rubella Z20.4
second hand tobacco smoke (acute) (chronic) Z77.22
  in the perinatal period P96.81
sexually-transmitted disease Z20.2
smallpox (laboratory) Z20.89
syphilis Z20.2
terrorism Z65.4
torture Z65.4
tuberculosis Z20.1
uranium Z77.012
varicella Z20.820
venereal disease Z20.2
viral disease NEC Z20.828

Exposure — *continued*
  war Z65.5
  water pollution Z77.111
Exsanguination — *see* Hemorrhage
Exstrophy
  abdominal contents Q45.8
  bladder Q64.10
    cloacal Q64.12
    specified type NEC Q64.19
    supravesical fissure Q64.11
Extensive — *see* condition
Extra (*see also* Accessory)
  marker chromosomes (normal individual) Q92.61
    in abnormal individual Q92.62
  rib Q76.6
    cervical Q76.5
Extrasystoles (supraventricular) I49.49
  atrial I49.1
  auricular I49.1
  junctional I49.2
  ventricular I49.3
Extrauterine gestation or pregnancy — *see* Pregnancy, by site
Extravasation
  blood R58
  chyle into mesentery I89.8
  pelvicalyceal N13.8
  pyelosinus N13.8
  urine (from ureter) R39.0
  vesicant agent
    antineoplastic chemotherapy T80.810 ☑
    other agent NEC T80.818 ☑
Extremity — *see* condition, limb
Extrophy — *see* Exstrophy
Extroversion
  bladder Q64.19
  uterus N81.4
    complicating delivery O71.2
    postpartal (old) N81.4
Extruded tooth (teeth) M26.34
Extrusion
  breast implant (prosthetic) T85.42 ☑
  eye implant (globe) (ball) T85.328 ☑
  intervertebral disc — *see* Displacement, intervertebral disc
  ocular lens implant (prosthetic) — *see* Complications, intraocular lens
  vitreous — *see* Prolapse, vitreous
Exudate
  pleural — *see* Effusion, pleura
  retina H35.89
Exudative — *see* condition
Eye, eyeball, eyelid — *see* condition
Eyestrain — *see* Disturbance, vision, subjective
Eyeworm disease of Africa B74.3

F

Faber's syndrome (achlorhydric anemia) D50.9
Fabry (-Anderson) **disease** E75.21
Faciocephalalgia, autonomic (*see also* Neuropathy, peripheral, autonomic) G90.09
Factor(s)
  psychic, associated with diseases classified elsewhere F54
  psychological
    affecting physical conditions F54
    or behavioral
      affecting general medical condition F54
      associated with disorders or diseases classified elsewhere F54
Fahr disease (of brain) G23.8
Fahr Volhard disease (of kidney) I12.- ☑
Failure, failed
  abortion — *see* Abortion, attempted
  aortic (valve) I35.8
    rheumatic I06.8
  attempted abortion — *see* Abortion, attempted
  biventricular I50.82
    due to left heart failure I50.814
  bone marrow — *see* Anemia, aplastic
  cardiac — *see* Failure, heart
  cardiorenal (chronic) (*see also* Failure, renal, and Failure, heart) I50.9
    hypertensive I13.2
  cardiorespiratory (*see also* Failure, heart) R09.2
  cardiovascular (chronic) — *see* Failure, heart

Failure, failed — *continued*
  cerebrovascular I67.9
  cervical dilatation in labor O62.0
  circulation, circulatory (peripheral) R57.9
    newborn P29.89
  compensation — *see* Disease, heart
  compliance with medical treatment or regimen — *see* Noncompliance
  congestive — *see* Failure, heart, congestive
  dental implant (endosseous) M27.69
    due to
      failure of dental prosthesis M27.63
      lack of attached gingiva M27.62
      occlusal trauma (poor prosthetic design) M27.62
      parafunctional habits M27.62
      periodontal infection (peri-implantitis) M27.62
      poor oral hygiene M27.62
    osseointegration M27.61
      due to
        complications of systemic disease M27.61
        poor bone quality M27.61
      iatrogenic M27.61
    post-osseointegration
      biological M27.62
      due to complications of systemic disease M27.62
      iatrogenic M27.62
      mechanical M27.63
    pre-integration M27.61
    pre-osseointegration M27.61
    specified NEC M27.69
  descent of head (at term) of pregnancy (mother) O32.4 ☑
  endosseous dental implant — *see* Failure, dental implant
  engagement of head (term of pregnancy) (mother) O32.4 ☑
  erection (penile) (*see also* Dysfunction, sexual, male, erectile) N52.9
    nonorganic F52.21
  examination(s), anxiety concerning Z55.2
  expansion terminal respiratory units (newborn) (primary) P28.0
  forceps NOS (with subsequent cesarean delivery) O66.5
  gain weight (child over 28 days old) R62.51
    adult R62.7
    newborn P92.6
  genital response (male) F52.21
    female F52.22
  heart (acute) (senile) (sudden) I50.9
    with
      acute pulmonary edema — *see* Failure, ventricular, left
      decompensation (*see also* Failure, heart, by type as diastolic or systolic, acute and chronic) I50.9
      dilatation — *see* Disease, heart
      normal ejection fraction — *see* Failure, heart, diastolic
      preserved ejection fraction — *see* Failure, heart, diastolic
      reduced ejection fraction — *see* Failure, heart, systolic
    arteriosclerotic I70.90
    biventricular I50.82
      due to left heart failure I50.814
    combined left-right sided I50.82
      due to left heart failure I50.814
    compensated (*see also* Failure, heart, by type as diastolic or systolic, chronic) I50.9
    complicating
      anesthesia (general) (local) or other sedation
        in labor and delivery O74.2
        in pregnancy O29.12- ☑
        postpartum, puerperal O89.1
      delivery (cesarean) (instrumental) O75.4
    congestive I50.9
      with rheumatic fever (conditions in I00)
        active I01.8
        inactive or quiescent (with chorea) I09.81
      newborn P29.0
      rheumatic (chronic) (inactive) (with chorea) I09.81
        active or acute I01.8
          with chorea I02.0
    decompensated (*see also* Failure, heart, by type as diastolic or systolic, acute and chronic) I50.9

Failure, failed — *continued*
  heart — *continued*
    degenerative — *see* Degeneration, myocardial
    diastolic (congestive) (left ventricular) I50.30
      acute (congestive) I50.31
        and (on) chronic (congestive) I50.33
      chronic (congestive) I50.32
        and (on) acute (congestive) I50.33
      combined with systolic (congestive) I50.40
        acute (congestive) I50.41
          and (on) chronic (congestive) I50.43
        chronic (congestive) I50.42
          and (on) acute (congestive) I50.43
    due to presence of cardiac prosthesis I97.13- ☑
    end stage (*see also* Failure, heart, by type as diastolic or systolic, chronic) I50.84
    following cardiac surgery I97.13- ☑
    high output NOS I50.83
    hypertensive — *see* Hypertension, heart
    left (ventricular) (*see also* Failure, ventricular, left)
      combined diastolic and systolic — *see* Failure, heart, diastolic, combined with systolic
      diastolic — *see* Failure, heart, diastolic
      systolic — *see* Failure, heart, systolic
    low output (syndrome) NOS I50.9
    newborn P29.0
    organic — *see* Disease, heart
    peripartum O90.3
    postprocedural I97.13- ☑
    rheumatic (chronic) (inactive) I09.9
    right (isolated) (ventricular) I50.810
      acute I50.811
        and (on) chronic I50.813
      chronic I50.812
        and acute I50.813
      secondary to left heart failure I50.814
    specified NEC I50.89

> Note: heart failure stages A, B, C, and D are based on the American College of Cardiology and American Heart Association stages of heart failure, which complement and should not be confused with the New York Heart Association Classification of Heart Failure, into Class I, Class II, Class III, and Class IV

    stage A Z91.89
    stage B (*see also* Failure, heart, by type as diastolic or systolic) I50.9
    stage C (*see also* Failure, heart, by type as diastolic or systolic) I50.9
    stage D (*see also* Failure, heart, by type as diastolic or systolic, chronic) I50.84
    systolic (congestive) (left ventricular) I50.20
      acute (congestive) I50.21
        and (on) chronic (congestive) I50.23
      chronic (congestive) I50.22
        and (on) acute (congestive) I50.23
      combined with diastolic (congestive) I50.40
        acute (congestive) I50.41
          and (on) chronic (congestive) I50.43
        chronic (congestive) I50.42
          and (on) acute (congestive) I50.43
    thyrotoxic (*see also* Thyrotoxicosis) E05.90 [I43]
      with
        high output (*see also* Thyrotoxicosis) I50.83
        thyroid storm E05.91 [I43]
          high output (*see also* Thyrotoxicosis) I50.83
    valvular — *see* Endocarditis
  hepatic K72.90
    with coma K72.91
    acute or subacute K72.00
      with coma K72.01
      due to drugs K71.10
        with coma K71.11
    alcoholic (acute) (chronic) (subacute) K70.40
      with coma K70.41
    chronic K72.10
      with coma K72.11
      due to drugs (acute) (subacute) (chronic) K71.10
        with coma K71.11
    due to drugs (acute) (subacute) (chronic) K71.10
      with coma K71.11
    postprocedural K91.82
  hepatorenal K76.7
  induction (of labor) O61.9
    abortion — *see* Abortion, attempted
    by
      oxytocic drugs O61.0

Failure, failed — *continued*
- induction — *continued*
  - by — *continued*
    - prostaglandins O61.0
  - instrumental O61.1
  - mechanical O61.1
  - medical O61.0
  - specified NEC O61.8
  - surgical O61.1
- intubation during anesthesia T88.4 ☑
  - in pregnancy O29.6- ☑
  - labor and delivery O74.7
  - postpartum, puerperal O89.6
- involution, thymus (gland) E32.0
- kidney (*see also* Disease, kidney, chronic) N19
  - acute (*see also* Failure, renal, acute) N17.9
- lactation (complete) O92.3
  - partial O92.4
- Leydig's cell, adult E29.1
- liver — *see* Failure, hepatic
- menstruation at puberty N91.0
- mitral I05.8
- myocardial, myocardium (*see also* Failure, heart) I50.9
  - chronic (*see also* Failure, heart, congestive) I50.9
  - congestive (*see also* Failure, heart, congestive) I50.9
- orgasm (female) (psychogenic) F52.31
  - male F52.32
- ovarian (primary) E28.39
  - iatrogenic E89.40
    - asymptomatic E89.40
    - symptomatic E89.41
  - postprocedural (postablative) (postirradiation) (postsurgical) E89.40
    - asymptomatic E89.40
    - symptomatic E89.41
- ovulation causing infertility N97.0
- polyglandular, autoimmune E31.0
- prosthetic joint implant — *see* Complications, joint prosthesis, mechanical, breakdown, by site
- renal N19
  - with
    - tubular necrosis (acute) N17.0
  - acute N17.9
    - with
      - cortical necrosis N17.1
      - medullary necrosis N17.2
      - tubular necrosis N17.0
    - specified NEC N17.8
  - chronic N18.9
    - hypertensive — *see* Hypertension, kidney
  - congenital P96.0
  - end stage (chronic) N18.6
    - due to hypertension I12.0
  - following
    - abortion — *see* Abortion by type complicated by specified condition NEC
    - crushing T79.5 ☑
    - ectopic or molar pregnancy O08.4
    - labor and delivery O90.4
  - hypertensive — *see* Hypertension, kidney
  - postprocedural N99.0
- respiration, respiratory J96.90
  - with
    - hypercapnia J96.92
    - hypercarbia J96.02
    - hypoxia J96.91
  - acute J96.00
    - with
      - hypercapnia J96.02
      - hypercarbia J96.02
      - hypoxia J96.01
  - acute and (on) chronic J96.20
    - with
      - hypercapnia J96.22
      - hypercarbia J96.22
      - hypoxia J96.21
  - center G93.89
  - chronic J96.10
    - with
      - hypercapnia J96.12
      - hypercarbia J96.12
      - hypoxia J96.11
  - newborn P28.5
  - postprocedural (acute) J95.821
    - acute and chronic J95.822
- rotation
  - cecum Q43.3
  - colon Q43.3

Failure, failed — *continued*
- rotation — *continued*
  - intestine Q43.3
  - kidney Q63.2
- sedation (conscious) (moderate) during procedure T88.52 ☑
  - history of Z92.83
- segmentation (*see also* Fusion)
  - fingers — *see* Syndactylism, complex, fingers
  - vertebra Q76.49
    - with scoliosis Q76.3
- seminiferous tubule, adult E29.1
- senile (general) R54
- sexual arousal (male) F52.21
  - female F52.22
- testicular endocrine function E29.1
- to thrive (child over 28 days old) R62.51
  - adult R62.7
  - newborn P92.6
- transplant T86.92
  - bone T86.831
    - marrow T86.02
  - cornea T86.841
  - heart T86.22
    - with lung(s) T86.32
  - intestine T86.851
  - kidney T86.12
  - liver T86.42
  - lung(s) T86.811
    - with heart T86.32
  - pancreas T86.891
  - skin (allograft) (autograft) T86.821
  - specified organ or tissue NEC T86.891
  - stem cell (peripheral blood) (umbilical cord) T86.5
- trial of labor (with subsequent cesarean delivery) O66.40
  - following previous cesarean delivery O66.41
- tubal ligation N99.89
- urinary — *see* Disease, kidney, chronic
- vacuum extraction NOS (with subsequent cesarean delivery) O66.5
- vasectomy N99.89
- ventouse NOS (with subsequent cesarean delivery) O66.5
- ventricular (*see also* Failure, heart) I50.9
  - left (*see also* Failure, heart, left) I50.1
    - with rheumatic fever (conditions in I00)
      - active I01.8
        - with chorea I02.0
      - inactive or quiescent (with chorea) I09.81
      - rheumatic (chronic) (inactive) (with chorea) I09.81
        - active or acute I01.8
          - with chorea I02.0
  - right — *see* Failure, heart, right
- vital centers, newborn P91.88

Fainting (fit) R55
Fallen arches — *see* Deformity, limb, flat foot
Falling, falls (repeated) R29.6
- any organ or part — *see* Prolapse
Fallopian
- insufflation Z31.41
- tube — *see* condition
Fallot's
- pentalogy Q21.8
- tetrad or tetralogy Q21.3
- triad or trilogy Q22.3
False (*see also* condition)
- croup J38.5
- joint — *see* Nonunion, fracture
- labor (pains) O47.9
  - at or after 37 completed weeks of gestation O47.1
  - before 37 completed weeks of gestation O47.0- ☑
- passage, urethra (prostatic) N36.5
- pregnancy F45.8
Family, familial (*see also* condition)
- disruption Z63.8
  - involving divorce or separation Z63.5
- Li-Fraumeni (syndrome) Z15.01
- planning advice Z30.09
- problem Z63.9
  - specified NEC Z63.8
- retinoblastoma C69.2- ☑
Famine (effects of) T73.0 ☑
- edema — *see* Malnutrition, severe
Fanconi (-de Toni)(-Debré) **syndrome** E72.09
- with cystinosis E72.04
Fanconi's anemia (congenital pancytopenia) D61.09

Farber's disease or syndrome E75.29
Farcy A24.0
Farmer's
- lung J67.0
- skin L57.8
Farsightedness — *see* Hypermetropia
Fascia — *see* condition
Fasciculation R25.3
Fasciitis M72.9
- diffuse (eosinophilic) M35.4
- infective M72.8
  - necrotizing M72.6
- necrotizing M72.6
- nodular M72.4
- perirenal (with ureteral obstruction) N13.5
  - with infection N13.6
- plantar M72.2
- specified NEC M72.8
- traumatic (old) M72.8
  - current — *code by* site under Sprain
Fascioliasis B66.3
Fasciolopsis, fasciolopsiasis (intestinal) B66.5
Fascioscapulohumeral myopathy G71.0
Fast pulse R00.0
Fat
- embolism — *see* Embolism, fat
- excessive (*see also* Obesity)
  - in heart — *see* Degeneration, myocardial
- in stool R19.5
- localized (pad) E65
  - heart — *see* Degeneration, myocardial
  - knee M79.4
  - retropatellar M79.4
- necrosis
  - breast N64.1
  - mesentery K65.4
  - omentum K65.4
- pad E65
  - knee M79.4
Fatigue R53.83
- auditory deafness — *see* Deafness
- chronic R53.82
- combat F43.0
- general R53.83
  - psychogenic F48.8
- heat (transient) T67.6 ☑
- muscle M62.89
- myocardium — *see* Failure, heart
- neoplasm-related R53.0
- nervous, neurosis F48.8
- operational F48.8
- psychogenic (general) F48.8
- senile R54
- voice R49.8
Fatness — *see* Obesity
Fatty (*see also* condition)
- apron E65
- degeneration — *see* Degeneration, fatty
- heart (enlarged) — *see* Degeneration, myocardial
- liver NEC K76.0
  - alcoholic K70.0
  - nonalcoholic K76.0
- necrosis — *see* Degeneration, fatty
Fauces — *see* condition
Fauchard's disease (periodontitis) — *see* Periodontitis
Faucitis J02.9
Favism (anemia) D55.0
Favus — *see* Dermatophytosis
Fazio-Londe disease or syndrome G12.1
Fear complex or reaction F40.9
Fear of — *see* Phobia
Feared complaint unfounded Z71.1
Febris, febrile (*see also* Fever)
- flava (*see also* Fever, yellow) A95.9
- melitensis A23.0
- pestis — *see* Plague
- recurrens — *see* Fever, relapsing
- rubra A38.9
Fecal
- incontinence R15.9
- smearing R15.1
- soiling R15.1
- urgency R15.2
Fecalith (impaction) K56.41
- appendix K38.1
- congenital P76.8
Fede's disease K14.0

Feeble rapid pulse due to shock following injury
  T79.4 ☑
Feeble-minded F70
Feeding
  difficulties R63.3
  problem R63.3
    newborn P92.9
      specified NEC P92.8
    nonorganic (adult) — see Disorder, eating
Feeling (of)
  foreign body in throat R09.89
Feer's disease — see Poisoning, mercury
Feet — see condition
Feigned illness Z76.5
Feil-Klippel syndrome (brevicollis) Q76.1
Feinmesser's (hidrotic) **ectodermal dysplasia** Q82.4
Felinophobia F40.218
Felon (see also Cellulitis, digit)
  with lymphangitis — see Lymphangitis, acute, digit
Felty's syndrome M05.00
  ankle M05.07- ☑
  elbow M05.02- ☑
  foot joint M05.07- ☑
  hand joint M05.04- ☑
  hip M05.05- ☑
  knee M05.06- ☑
  multiple site M05.09
  shoulder M05.01- ☑
  vertebra — see Spondylitis, ankylosing
  wrist M05.03- ☑
Female genital cutting status — see Female genital
    mutilation status (FGM)
Female genital mutilation status (FGM) N90.810
  specified NEC N90.818
  type I (clitorectomy status) N90.811
  type II (clitorectomy with excision of labia minora status) N90.812
  type III (infibulation status) N90.813
  type IV N90.818
Femur, femoral — see condition
Fenestration, fenestrated (see also Imperfect, closure)
  aortico-pulmonary Q21.4
  cusps, heart valve NEC Q24.8
    pulmonary Q22.3
  pulmonic cusps Q22.3
Fernell's disease (aortic aneurysm) I71.9
Fertile eunuch syndrome E23.0
Fetid
  breath R19.6
  sweat L75.0
Fetishism F65.0
  transvestic F65.1
Fetus, fetal (see also condition)
  alcohol syndrome (dysmorphic) Q86.0
  compressus O31.0- ☑
  hydantoin syndrome Q86.1
  lung tissue P28.0
  papyraceous O31.0- ☑
Fever (inanition) (of unknown origin) (persistent) (with chills) (with rigor) R50.9
  abortus A23.1
  Aden (dengue) A90
  African tick-borne A68.1
  American
    mountain (tick) A93.2
    spotted A77.0
  aphthous B08.8
  arbovirus, arboviral A94
    hemorrhagic A94
    specified NEC A93.8
  Argentinian hemorrhagic A96.0
  Assam B55.0
  Australian Q A78
  Bangkok hemorrhagic A91
  Barmah forest A92.8
  Bartonella A44.0
  bilious, hemoglobinuric B50.8
  blackwater B50.8
  blister B00.1
  Bolivian hemorrhagic A96.1
  Bonvale dam T73.3 ☑
  boutonneuse A77.1
  brain — see Encephalitis
  Brazilian purpuric A48.4
  breakbone A90
  Bullis A77.0
  Bunyamwera A92.8

Fever — continued
  Burdwan B55.0
  Bwamba A92.8
  Cameroon — see Malaria
  Canton A75.9
  catarrhal (acute) J00
    chronic J31.0
  cat-scratch A28.1
  Central Asian hemorrhagic A98.0
  cerebral — see Encephalitis
  cerebrospinal meningococcal A39.0
  Chagres B50.9
  Chandipura A92.8
  Changuinola A93.1
  Charcot's (biliary) (hepatic) (intermittent) — see Calculus, bile duct
  Chikungunya (viral) (hemorrhagic) A92.0
  Chitral A93.1
  Colombo — see Fever, paratyphoid
  Colorado tick (virus) A93.2
  congestive (remittent) — see Malaria
  Congo virus A98.0
  continued malarial B50.9
  Corsican — see Malaria
  Crimean-Congo hemorrhagic A98.0
  Cyprus — see Brucellosis
  dandy A90
  deer fly — see Tularemia
  dengue (virus) A90
    hemorrhagic A91
    sandfly A93.1
  desert B38.0
  drug induced R50.2
  due to
    conditions classified elsewhere R50.81
    heat T67.0 ☑
  enteric A01.00
  enteroviral exanthematous (Boston exanthem) A88.0
  ephemeral (of unknown origin) R50.9
  epidemic hemorrhagic A98.5
  erysipelatous — see Erysipelas
  estivo-autumnal (malarial) B50.9
  famine A75.0
  five day A79.0
  following delivery O86.4
  Fort Bragg A27.89
  gastroenteric A01.00
  gastromalarial — see Malaria
  Gibraltar — see Brucellosis
  glandular — see Mononucleosis, infectious
  Guama (viral) A92.8
  Haverhill A25.1
  hay (allergic) J30.1
    with asthma (bronchial) J45.909
      with
        exacerbation (acute) J45.901
        status asthmaticus J45.902
    due to
      allergen other than pollen J30.89
      pollen, any plant or tree J30.1
  heat (effects) T67.0 ☑
  hematuric, bilious B50.8
  hemoglobinuric (malarial) (bilious) B50.8
  hemorrhagic (arthropod-borne) NOS A94
    with renal syndrome A98.5
    arenaviral A96.9
      specified NEC A96.8
    Argentinian A96.0
    Bangkok A91
    Bolivian A96.1
    Central Asian A98.0
    Chikungunya A92.0
    Crimean-Congo A98.0
    dengue (virus) A91
    epidemic A98.5
    Junin (virus) A96.0
    Korean A98.5
    Kyasanur forest A98.2
    Machupo (virus) A96.1
    mite-borne A93.8
    mosquito-borne A92.8
    Omsk A98.1
    Philippine A91
    Russian A98.5
    Singapore A91
    Southeast Asia A91
    Thailand A91
    tick-borne NEC A93.8

Fever — continued
  hemorrhagic — continued
    viral A99
      specified NEC A98.8
  hepatic — see Cholecystitis
  herpetic — see Herpes
  icterohemorrhagic A27.0
  Indiana A93.8
  infective B99.9
    specified NEC B99.8
  intermittent (bilious) (see also Malaria)
    of unknown origin R50.9
    pernicious B50.9
  iodide R50.2
  Japanese river A75.3
  jungle (see also Malaria)
    yellow A95.0
  Junin (virus) hemorrhagic A96.0
  Katayama B65.2
  kedani A75.3
  Kenya (tick) A77.1
  Kew Garden A79.1
  Korean hemorrhagic A98.5
  Lassa A96.2
  Lone Star A77.0
  Machupo (virus) hemorrhagic A96.1
  malaria, malarial — see Malaria
  Malta A23.9
  Marseilles A77.1
  marsh — see Malaria
  Mayaro (viral) A92.8
  Mediterranean (see also Brucellosis) A23.9
    familial M04.1
    tick A77.1
  meningeal — see Meningitis
  Meuse A79.0
  Mexican A75.2
  mianeh A68.1
  miasmatic — see Malaria
  mosquito-borne (viral) A92.9
    hemorrhagic A92.8
  mountain (see also Brucellosis)
    meaning Rocky Mountain spotted fever A77.0
    tick (American) (Colorado) (viral) A93.2
  Mucambo (viral) A92.8
  mud A27.9
  Neapolitan — see Brucellosis
  neutropenic D70.9
  newborn P81.9
    environmental P81.0
  Nine-Mile A78
  non-exanthematous tick A93.2
  North Asian tick-borne A77.2
  Omsk hemorrhagic A98.1
  O'nyong-nyong (viral) A92.1
  Oropouche (viral) A93.0
  Oroya A44.0
  paludal — see Malaria
  Panama (malarial) B50.9
  Pappataci A93.1
  paratyphoid A01.4
    A A01.1
    B A01.2
    C A01.3
  parrot A70
  periodic (Mediterranean) M04.1
  persistent (of unknown origin) R50.9
  petechial A39.0
  pharyngoconjunctival B30.2
  Philippine hemorrhagic A91
  phlebotomus A93.1
  Piry (virus) A93.8
  Pixuna (viral) A92.8
  Plasmodium ovale B53.0
  polioviral (nonparalytic) A80.4
  Pontiac A48.2
  postimmunization R50.83
  postoperative R50.82
    due to infection T81.4 ☑
  posttransfusion R50.84
  postvaccination R50.83
  presenting with conditions classified elsewhere R50.81
  pretibial A27.89
  puerperal O86.4
  Q A78
  quadrilateral A78
  quartan (malaria) B52.9
  Queensland (coastal) (tick) A77.3

Fever — *continued*
quintan A79.Ø
rabbit — *see* Tularemia
rat-bite A25.9
   due to
      Spirillum A25.Ø
      Streptobacillus moniliformis A25.1
recurrent — *see* Fever, relapsing
relapsing (Borrelia) A68.9
   Carter's (Asiatic) A68.1
   Dutton's (West African) A68.1
   Koch's A68.9
   louse-borne A68.Ø
   Novy's
      louse-borne A68.Ø
      tick-borne A68.1
   Obermeyer's (European) A68.Ø
   tick-borne A68.1
remittent (bilious) (congestive) (gastric) — *see* Malaria
rheumatic (active) (acute) (chronic) (subacute) IØØ
   with central nervous system involvement IØ2.9
   active with heart involvement — *see* category
      IØ1 ☑
   inactive or quiescent with
      cardiac hypertrophy IØ9.89
      carditis IØ9.9
      endocarditis IØ9.1
         aortic (valve) IØ6.9
            with mitral (valve) disease IØ8.Ø
         mitral (valve) IØ5.9
            with aortic (valve) disease IØ8.Ø
         pulmonary (valve) IØ9.89
         tricuspid (valve) IØ7.8
      heart disease NEC IØ9.89
      heart failure (congestive) (conditions in I5Ø.) IØ9.81
      left ventricular failure (conditions in I5Ø.1-I5Ø.4-) IØ9.81
      myocarditis, myocardial degeneration (conditions in I51.4) IØ9.Ø
      pancarditis IØ9.9
      pericarditis IØ9.2
Rift Valley (viral) A92.4
Rocky Mountain spotted A77.Ø
rose J3Ø.1
Ross River B33.1
Russian hemorrhagic A98.5
San Joaquin (Valley) B38.Ø
sandfly A93.1
Sao Paulo A77.Ø
scarlet A38.9
seven day (leptospirosis) (autumnal) (Japanese) A27.89
   dengue A9Ø
shin-bone A79.Ø
Singapore hemorrhagic A91
solar A9Ø
Songo A98.5
sore BØØ.1
South African tick-bite A68.1
Southeast Asia hemorrhagic A91
spinal — *see* Meningitis
spirillary A25.Ø
splenic — *see* Anthrax
spotted A77.9
   American A77.Ø
   Brazilian A77.Ø
   cerebrospinal meningitis A39.Ø
   Colombian A77.Ø
   due to Rickettsia
      australis A77.3
      conorii A77.1
      rickettsii A77.Ø
      sibirica A77.2
      specified type NEC A77.8
   Ehrlichiosis A77.4Ø
      due to
         E. chafeensis A77.41
         specified organism NEC A77.49
   Rocky Mountain A77.Ø
steroid R5Ø.2
streptobacillary A25.1
subtertian B5Ø.9
Sumatran mite A75.3
sun A9Ø
swamp A27.9
swine AØ2.8
sylvatic, yellow A95.Ø
Tahyna B33.8

Fever — *continued*
tertian — *see* Malaria, tertian
Thailand hemorrhagic A91
thermic T67.Ø ☑
three-day A93.1
tick
   American mountain A93.2
   Colorado A93.2
   Kemerovo A93.8
   Mediterranean A77.1
   mountain A93.2
   nonexanthematous A93.2
   Quaranfil A93.8
tick-bite NEC A93.8
tick-borne (hemorrhagic) NEC A93.8
trench A79.Ø
tsutsugamushi A75.3
typhogastric AØ1.ØØ
typhoid (abortive) (hemorrhagic) (intermittent) (malignant) AØ1.ØØ
   complicated by
      arthritis AØ1.Ø4
      heart involvement AØ1.Ø2
      meningitis AØ1.Ø1
      osteomyelitis AØ1.Ø5
      pneumonia AØ1.Ø3
      specified NEC AØ1.Ø9
typhomalarial — *see* Malaria
typhus — *see* Typhus (fever)
undulant — *see* Brucellosis
unknown origin R5Ø.9
uveoparotid D86.89
valley B38.Ø
Venezuelan equine A92.2
vesicular stomatitis A93.8
viral hemorrhagic — *see* Fever, hemorrhagic, by type of virus
Volhynian A79.Ø
Wesselsbron (viral) A92.8
West
   African B5Ø.8
   Nile (viral) A92.3Ø
      with
         complications NEC A92.39
         cranial nerve disorders A92.32
         encephalitis A92.31
         encephalomyelitis A92.31
         neurologic manifestation NEC A92.32
         optic neuritis A92.32
         polyradiculitis A92.32
Whitmore's — *see* Melioidosis
Wolhynian A79.Ø
worm B83.9
yellow A95.9
   jungle A95.Ø
   sylvatic A95.Ø
   urban A95.1
Zika virus A92.5
Fibrillation
atrial or auricular (established) I48.91
   chronic I48.2
   paroxysmal I48.Ø
   permanent I48.2
   persistent I48.1
cardiac I49.8
heart I49.8
muscular M62.89
ventricular I49.Ø1
Fibrin
ball or bodies, pleural (sac) J94.1
chamber, anterior (eye) (gelatinous exudate) — *see* Iridocyclitis, acute
Fibrinogenolysis — *see* Fibrinolysis
Fibrinogenopenia D68.8
acquired D65
congenital D68.2
Fibrinolysis (hemorrhagic) (acquired) D65
antepartum hemorrhage — *see* Hemorrhage, antepartum, with coagulation defect
following
   abortion — *see* Abortion by type complicated by hemorrhage
   ectopic or molar pregnancy OØ8.1
intrapartum O67.Ø
newborn, transient P6Ø
postpartum O72.3
Fibrinopenia (hereditary) D68.2
acquired D68.4

Fibrinopurulent — *see* condition
Fibrinous — *see* condition
Fibroadenoma
cellular intracanalicular D24- ☑
giant D24- ☑
intracanalicular
   cellular D24- ☑
   giant D24- ☑
   specified site — *see* Neoplasm, benign, by site
   unspecified site D24- ☑
juvenile D24- ☑
pericanalicular
   specified site — *see* Neoplasm, benign, by site
   unspecified site D24- ☑
phyllodes D24- ☑
prostate D29.1
specified site NEC — *see* Neoplasm, benign, by site
unspecified site D24- ☑
Fibroadenosis, breast (chronic) (cystic) (diffuse) (periodic) (segmental) N6Ø.2- ☑
Fibroangioma (*see also* Neoplasm, benign, by site)
juvenile
   specified site — *see* Neoplasm, benign, by site
   unspecified site D1Ø.6
Fibrochondrosarcoma — *see* Neoplasm, cartilage, malignant
Fibrocystic
disease (*see also* Fibrosis, cystic)
   breast — *see* Mastopathy, cystic
   jaw M27.49
   kidney (congenital) Q61.8
   liver Q44.6
   pancreas E84.9
kidney (congenital) Q61.8
Fibrodysplasia ossificans progressiva — *see* Myositis, ossificans, progressiva
Fibroelastosis (cordis) (endocardial) (endomyocardial) I42.4
Fibroid (tumor) (*see also* Neoplasm, connective tissue, benign)
disease, lung (chronic) — *see* Fibrosis, lung
heart (disease) — *see* Myocarditis
in pregnancy or childbirth O34.1- ☑
   causing obstructed labor O65.5
induration, lung (chronic) — *see* Fibrosis, lung
lung — *see* Fibrosis, lung
pneumonia (chronic) — *see* Fibrosis, lung
uterus (*see also* Leiomyoma, uterus) D25.9
Fibrolipoma — *see* Lipoma
Fibroliposarcoma — *see* Neoplasm, connective tissue, malignant
Fibroma (*see also* Neoplasm, connective tissue, benign)
ameloblastic — *see* Cyst, calcifying odontogenic
bone (nonossifying) — *see* Disorder, bone, specified type NEC
   ossifying — *see* Neoplasm, bone, benign
cementifying — *see* Neoplasm, bone, benign
chondromyxoid — *see* Neoplasm, bone, benign
desmoplastic — *see* Neoplasm, connective tissue, uncertain behavior
durum — *see* Neoplasm, connective tissue, benign
fascial — *see* Neoplasm, connective tissue, benign
invasive — *see* Neoplasm, connective tissue, uncertain behavior
molle — *see* Lipoma
myxoid — *see* Neoplasm, connective tissue, benign
nasopharynx, nasopharyngeal (juvenile) D1Ø.6
nonosteogenic (nonossifying) — *see* Dysplasia, fibrous
odontogenic (central) — *see* Cyst, calcifying odontogenic
ossifying — *see* Neoplasm, bone, benign
periosteal — *see* Neoplasm, bone, benign
soft — *see* Lipoma
Fibromatosis M72.9
abdominal — *see* Neoplasm, connective tissue, uncertain behavior
aggressive — *see* Neoplasm, connective tissue, uncertain behavior
congenital generalized — *see* Neoplasm, connective tissue, uncertain behavior
Dupuytren's M72.Ø
gingival KØ6.1
palmar (fascial) M72.Ø
plantar (fascial) M72.2
pseudosarcomatous (proliferative) (subcutaneous) M72.4
retroperitoneal D48.3

☑ **Additional Character Required** — Refer to the Tabular List for Character Selection ▽ Subterms under main terms may continue to next column or page

Fibromatosis — *continued*
  specified NEC M72.8
Fibromyalgia M79.7
Fibromyoma (*see also* Neoplasm, connective tissue, benign)
  uterus (corpus) (*see also* Leiomyoma, uterus)
    in pregnancy or childbirth — *see* Fibroid, in pregnancy or childbirth
      causing obstructed labor O65.5
Fibromyositis M79.7
Fibromyxolipoma D17.9
Fibromyxoma — *see* Neoplasm, connective tissue, benign
Fibromyxosarcoma — *see* Neoplasm, connective tissue, malignant
Fibro-odontoma, ameloblastic — *see* Cyst, calcifying odontogenic
Fibro-osteoma — *see* Neoplasm, bone, benign
Fibroplasia, retrolental H35.17- ☑
Fibropurulent — *see* condition
Fibrosarcoma (*see also* Neoplasm, connective tissue, malignant)
  ameloblastic C41.1
    upper jaw (bone) C41.0
  congenital — *see* Neoplasm, connective tissue, malignant
  fascial — *see* Neoplasm, connective tissue, malignant
  infantile — *see* Neoplasm, connective tissue, malignant
  odontogenic C41.1
    upper jaw (bone) C41.0
  periosteal — *see* Neoplasm, bone, malignant
Fibrosclerosis
  breast N60.3- ☑
  multifocal M35.5
  penis (corpora cavernosa) N48.6
Fibrosis, fibrotic
  adrenal (gland) E27.8
  amnion O41.8X- ☑
  anal papillae K62.89
  arteriocapillary — *see* Arteriosclerosis
  bladder N32.89
    interstitial — *see* Cystitis, chronic, interstitial
    localized submucosal — *see* Cystitis, chronic, interstitial
    panmural — *see* Cystitis, chronic, interstitial
  breast — *see* Fibrosclerosis, breast
  capillary (*see also* Arteriosclerosis) I70.90
    lung (chronic) — *see* Fibrosis, lung
  cardiac — *see* Myocarditis
  cervix N88.8
  chorion O41.8X- ☑
  corpus cavernosum (sclerosing) N48.6
  cystic (of pancreas) E84.9
    with
      distal intestinal obstruction syndrome E84.19
      fecal impaction E84.19
      intestinal manifestations NEC E84.19
      pulmonary manifestations E84.0
      specified manifestations NEC E84.8
    due to device, implant or graft (*see also* Complications, by site and type, specified NEC) T85.828 ☑
      arterial graft NEC T82.828 ☑
      breast (implant) T85.828 ☑
      catheter NEC T85.828 ☑
        dialysis (renal) T82.828 ☑
          intraperitoneal T85.828 ☑
        infusion NEC T82.828 ☑
          spinal (epidural) (subdural) T85.820 ☑
        urinary (indwelling) T83.82 ☑
      electronic (electrode) (pulse generator) (stimulator)
        bone T84.82 ☑
        cardiac T82.827 ☑
        nervous system (brain) (peripheral nerve) (spinal) T85.820 ☑
        urinary T83.82 ☑
      fixation, internal (orthopedic) NEC T84.82 ☑
      gastrointestinal (bile duct) (esophagus) T85.828 ☑
      genital NEC T83.82 ☑
      heart NEC T82.827 ☑
      joint prosthesis T84.82 ☑
      ocular (corneal graft) (orbital implant) NEC T85.828 ☑
      orthopedic NEC T84.82 ☑
      specified NEC T85.828 ☑
      urinary NEC T83.82 ☑
      vascular NEC T82.828 ☑

Fibrosis, fibrotic — *continued*
  due to device, implant or graft (*see also* Complications, by site and type, specified) — *continued*
    ventricular intracranial shunt T85.820 ☑
  ejaculatory duct N50.89
  endocardium — *see* Endocarditis
  endomyocardial (tropical) I42.3
  epididymis N50.89
  eye muscle — *see* Strabismus, mechanical
  heart — *see* Myocarditis
  hepatic — *see* Fibrosis, liver
  hepatolienal (portal hypertension) K76.6
  hepatosplenic (portal hypertension) K76.6
  infrapatellar fat pad M79.4
  intrascrotal N50.89
  kidney N26.9
  liver K74.0
    with sclerosis K74.2
    alcoholic K70.2
  lung (atrophic) (chronic) (confluent) (massive) (perialveolar) (peribronchial) J84.10
    with
      anthracosilicosis J60
      anthracosis J60
      asbestosis J61
      bagassosis J67.1
      bauxite J63.1
      berylliosis J63.2
      byssinosis J66.0
      calcicosis J62.8
      chalicosis J62.8
      dust reticulation J64
      farmer's lung J67.0
      ganister disease J62.8
      graphite J63.3
      pneumoconiosis NOS J64
      siderosis J63.4
      silicosis J62.8
    capillary J84.10
    congenital P27.8
    diffuse (idiopathic) J84.10
      chemicals, gases, fumes or vapors (inhalation) J68.4
      interstitial J84.10
        acute J84.114
        talc J62.0
    following radiation J70.1
    idiopathic J84.112
    postinflammatory J84.10
    silicotic J62.8
    tuberculous — *see* Tuberculosis, pulmonary
  lymphatic gland I89.8
  median bar — *see* Hyperplasia, prostate
  mediastinum (idiopathic) J98.59
  meninges G96.19
  myocardium, myocardial — *see* Myocarditis
  ovary N83.8
  oviduct N83.8
  pancreas K86.89
  penis NEC N48.6
  pericardium I31.0
  perineum, in pregnancy or childbirth O34.7- ☑
    causing obstructed labor O65.5
  pleura J94.1
  popliteal fat pad M79.4
  prostate (chronic) — *see* Hyperplasia, prostate
  pulmonary (*see also* Fibrosis, lung) J84.10
    congenital P27.8
    idiopathic J84.112
  rectal sphincter K62.89
  retroperitoneal, idiopathic (with ureteral obstruction) N13.5
    with infection N13.6
  sclerosing mesenteric (idiopathic) K65.4
  scrotum N50.89
  seminal vesicle N50.89
  senile R54
  skin L90.5
  spermatic cord N50.89
  spleen D73.89
    in schistosomiasis (bilharziasis) B65.9 [D77]
  subepidermal nodular — *see* Neoplasm, skin, benign
  submucous (oral) (tongue) K13.5
  testis N44.8
    chronic, due to syphilis A52.76
  thymus (gland) E32.8
  tongue, submucous K13.5
  tunica vaginalis N50.89

Fibrosis, fibrotic — *continued*
  uterus (non-neoplastic) N85.8
  vagina N89.8
  valve, heart — *see* Endocarditis
  vas deferens N50.89
  vein I87.8
Fibrositis (periarticular) M79.7
  nodular, chronic (Jaccoud's) (rheumatoid) — *see* Arthropathy, postrheumatic, chronic
Fibrothorax J94.1
Fibrotic — *see* Fibrosis
Fibrous — *see* condition
Fibroxanthoma (*see also* Neoplasm, connective tissue, benign)
  atypical — *see* Neoplasm, connective tissue, uncertain behavior
  malignant — *see* Neoplasm, connective tissue, malignant
Fibroxanthosarcoma — *see* Neoplasm, connective tissue, malignant
Fiedler's
  disease (icterohemorrhagic leptospirosis) A27.0
  myocarditis (acute) I40.1
Fifth disease B08.3
  venereal A55
Filaria, filarial, filariasis — *see* Infestation, filarial
Filatov's disease — *see* Mononucleosis, infectious
File-cutter's disease — *see* Poisoning, lead
Filling defect
  biliary tract R93.2
  bladder R93.41
  duodenum R93.3
  gallbladder R93.2
  gastrointestinal tract R93.3
  intestine R93.3
  kidney R93.42- ☑
  stomach R93.3
  ureter R93.41
  urinary organs, specified NEC R93.49
Fimbrial cyst Q50.4
Financial problem affecting care NOS Z59.9
  bankruptcy Z59.8
  foreclosure on loan Z59.8
Findings, abnormal, inconclusive, without diagnosis
  (*see also* Abnormal)
  17-ketosteroids, elevated R82.5
  acetonuria R82.4
  alcohol in blood R78.0
  anisocytosis R71.8
  antenatal screening of mother O28.9
    biochemical O28.1
    chromosomal O28.5
    cytological O28.2
    genetic O28.5
    hematological O28.0
    radiological O28.4
    specified NEC O28.8
    ultrasonic O28.3
  antibody titer, elevated R76.0
  anticardiolipin antibody R76.0
  antiphosphatidylglycerol antibody R76.0
  antiphosphatidylinositol antibody R76.0
  antiphosphatidylserine antibody R76.0
  antiphospholipid antibody R76.0
  bacteriuria R82.71
  bicarbonate E87.8
  bile in urine R82.2
  blood sugar R73.09
    high R73.9
    low (transient) E16.2
  body fluid or substance, specified NEC R88.8
  casts, urine R82.99
  catecholamines R82.5
  cells, urine R82.99
  chloride E87.8
  cholesterol E78.9
    high E78.00
      with high triglycerides E78.2
  chyluria R82.0
  cloudy
    dialysis effluent R88.0
    urine R82.90
  creatinine clearance R94.4
  crystals, urine R82.99
  culture
    blood R78.81
      positive — *see* Positive, culture
  echocardiogram R93.1

☑ **Additional Character Required** — Refer to the Tabular List for Character Selection   Subterms under main terms may continue to next column or page

Fistula — *continued*
- enterouterine N82.4
  - congenital Q51.7
- enterovaginal N82.4
  - congenital Q52.2
  - large intestine N82.3
  - small intestine N82.2
- enterovesical N32.1
- epididymis N50.89
  - tuberculous A18.15
- esophagobronchial J86.0
  - congenital Q39.2
    - with atresia of esophagus Q39.1
- esophagocutaneous K22.8
- esophagopleural-cutaneous J86.0
- esophagotracheal J86.0
  - congenital Q39.2
    - with atresia of esophagus Q39.1
- esophagus K22.8
  - congenital Q39.2
    - with atresia of esophagus Q39.1
- ethmoid — *see* Sinusitis, ethmoidal
- eyeball (cornea) (sclera) — *see* Disorder, globe, hypotony
- eyelid H01.8
- fallopian tube, external N82.5
- fecal K63.2
  - congenital Q43.6
- from periapical abscess K04.6
- frontal sinus — *see* Sinusitis, frontal
- gallbladder K82.3
  - with calculus, cholelithiasis, stones — *see* Calculus, gallbladder
- gastric K31.6
- gastrocolic K31.6
  - congenital Q40.2
  - tuberculous A18.32
- gastroenterocolic K31.6
- gastroesophageal K31.6
- gastrojejunal K31.6
- gastrojejunocolic K31.6
- genital tract (female) N82.9
  - specified NEC N82.8
  - to intestine NEC N82.4
  - to skin N82.5
- hepatic artery-portal vein, congenital Q26.6
- hepatopleural J86.0
- hepatopulmonary J86.0
- ileorectal or ileosigmoidal K63.2
- ileovaginal N82.2
- ileovesical N32.1
- ileum K63.2
- in ano K60.3
  - tuberculous A18.32
- inner ear (labyrinth) — *see* subcategory H83.1 ☑
- intestine NEC K63.2
- intestinocolonic (abdominal) K63.2
- intestinoureteral N28.89
- intestinouterine N82.4
- intestinovaginal N82.4
  - large intestine N82.3
  - small intestine N82.2
- intestinovesical N32.1
- ischiorectal (fossa) K61.3
- jejunum K63.2
- joint M25.10
  - ankle M25.17- ☑
  - elbow M25.12- ☑
  - foot joint M25.17- ☑
  - hand joint M25.14- ☑
  - hip M25.15- ☑
  - knee M25.16- ☑
  - shoulder M25.11- ☑
  - specified joint NEC M25.18
  - tuberculous — *see* Tuberculosis, joint
  - vertebrae M25.18
  - wrist M25.13- ☑
- kidney N28.89
- labium (majus) (minus) N82.8
- labyrinth — *see* subcategory H83.1 ☑
- lacrimal (gland) (sac) H04.61- ☑
- lacrimonasal duct — *see* Fistula, lacrimal
- laryngotracheal, congenital Q34.8
- larynx J38.7
- lip K13.0
  - congenital Q38.0
- lumbar, tuberculous A18.01
- lung J86.0

Fistula — *continued*
- lymphatic I89.8
- mammary (gland) N61.0
- mastoid (process) (region) — *see* Mastoiditis, chronic
- maxillary J32.0
- medial, face and neck Q18.8
- mediastinal J86.0
- mediastinobronchial J86.0
- mediastinocutaneous J86.0
- middle ear — *see* subcategory H74.8 ☑
- mouth K12.2
- nasal J34.89
  - sinus — *see* Sinusitis
- nasopharynx J39.2
- nipple N64.0
- nose J34.89
- oral (cutaneous) K12.2
  - maxillary J32.0
  - nasal (with cleft palate) — *see* Cleft, palate
- orbit, orbital — *see* Disorder, orbit, specified type NEC
- oroantral J32.0
- oviduct, external N82.5
- palate (hard) M27.8
- pancreatic K86.89
- pancreaticoduodenal K86.89
- parotid (gland) K11.4
  - region K12.2
- penis N48.89
- perianal K60.3
- pericardium (pleura) (sac) — *see* Pericarditis
- pericecal K63.2
- perineorectal K60.4
- perineosigmoidal K63.2
- perineum, perineal (with urethral involvement) NEC N36.0
  - tuberculous A18.13
  - ureter N28.89
- perirectal K60.4
  - tuberculous A18.32
- peritoneum K65.9
- pharyngoesophageal J39.2
- pharynx J39.2
  - branchial cleft (congenital) Q18.0
- pilonidal (infected) (rectum) — *see* Sinus, pilonidal
- pleura, pleural, pleurocutaneous, pleuroperitoneal J86.0
  - tuberculous NEC A15.6
- pleuropericardial I31.8
- portal vein-hepatic artery, congenital Q26.6
- postauricular H70.81- ☑
- postoperative, persistent T81.83 ☑
  - specified site — *see* Fistula, by site
- preauricular (congenital) Q18.1
- prostate N42.89
- pulmonary J86.0
  - arteriovenous I28.0
    - congenital Q25.72
  - tuberculous — *see* Tuberculosis, pulmonary
- pulmonoperitoneal J86.0
- rectolabial N82.4
- rectosigmoid (intercommunicating) K63.2
- rectoureteral N28.89
- rectourethral N36.0
  - congenital Q64.73
- rectouterine N82.4
  - congenital Q51.7
- rectovaginal N82.3
  - congenital Q52.2
  - tuberculous A18.18
- rectovesical N32.1
  - congenital Q64.79
- rectovesicovaginal N82.3
- rectovulval N82.4
  - congenital Q52.79
- rectum (to skin) K60.4
  - congenital Q43.6
    - with absence, atresia and stenosis Q42.0
  - tuberculous A18.32
- renal N28.89
- retroauricular — *see* Fistula, postauricular
- salivary duct or gland (any) K11.4
  - congenital Q38.4
- scrotum (urinary) N50.89
  - tuberculous A18.15
- semicircular canals — *see* subcategory H83.1 ☑
- sigmoid K63.2
  - to bladder N32.1
- sinus — *see* Sinusitis

Fistula — *continued*
- skin L98.8
  - to genital tract (female) N82.5
- splenocolic D73.89
- stercoral K63.2
- stomach K31.6
- sublingual gland K11.4
- submandibular gland K11.4
- submaxillary (gland) K11.4
  - region K12.2
- thoracic J86.0
  - duct I89.8
- thoracoabdominal J86.0
- thoracogastric J86.0
- thoracointestinal J86.0
- thorax J86.0
- thyroglossal duct Q89.2
- thyroid E07.89
- trachea, congenital (external) (internal) Q32.1
- tracheoesophageal J86.0
  - congenital Q39.2
    - with atresia of esophagus Q39.1
  - following tracheostomy J95.04
- traumatic arteriovenous — *see* Injury, blood vessel, by site
- tuberculous — *code by* site under Tuberculosis
- typhoid A01.09
- umbilicourinary Q64.8
- urachus, congenital Q64.4
- ureter (persistent) N28.89
- ureteroabdominal N28.89
- ureterorectal N28.89
- ureterosigmoido-abdominal N28.89
- ureterovaginal N82.1
- ureterovesical N32.2
- urethra N36.0
  - congenital Q64.79
  - tuberculous A18.13
- urethroperineal N36.0
- urethroperineovesical N32.2
- urethrorectal N36.0
  - congenital Q64.73
- urethroscrotal N50.89
- urethrovaginal N82.1
- urethrovesical N32.2
- urinary (tract) (persistent) (recurrent) N36.0
- uteroabdominal N82.5
  - congenital Q51.7
- uteroenteric, uterointestinal N82.4
  - congenital Q51.7
- uterorectal N82.4
  - congenital Q51.7
- uteroureteric N82.1
- uterourethral Q51.7
- uterovaginal N82.8
- uterovesical N82.1
  - congenital Q51.7
- uterus N82.8
- vagina (postpartal) (wall) N82.8
- vaginocutaneous (postpartal) N82.5
- vaginointestinal NEC N82.4
  - large intestine N82.3
  - small intestine N82.2
- vaginoperineal N82.5
- vasocutaneous, congenital Q55.7
- vesical NEC N32.2
- vesicoabdominal N32.2
- vesicocervicovaginal N82.1
- vesicocolic N32.1
- vesicocutaneous N32.2
- vesicoenteric N32.1
- vesicointestinal N32.1
- vesicometrorectal N82.4
- vesicoperineal N32.2
- vesicorectal N32.1
  - congenital Q64.79
- vesicosigmoidal N32.1
- vesicosigmoidovaginal N82.3
- vesicoureteral N32.2
- vesicoureterovaginal N82.1
- vesicourethral N32.2
- vesicourethrorectal N32.1
- vesicouterine N82.1
  - congenital Q51.7
- vesicovaginal N82.0
- vulvorectal N82.4
  - congenital Q52.79

Fit R56.9
- epileptic — *see* Epilepsy

Fit — *continued*
  fainting R55
  hysterical F44.5
  newborn P90
Fitting (and adjustment) (of)
  artificial
    arm — *see* Admission, adjustment, artificial, arm
    breast Z44.3 ☑
    eye Z44.2 ☑
    leg — *see* Admission, adjustment, artificial, leg
  automatic implantable cardiac defibrillator (with synchronous cardiac pacemaker) Z45.02
  brain neuropacemaker Z46.2
    implanted Z45.42
  cardiac defibrillator — *see* Fitting (and adjustment) (of), automatic implantable cardiac defibrillator
  catheter, non-vascular Z46.82
  colostomy belt Z46.89
  contact lenses Z46.0
  CRT-D (resynchronization therapy defibrillator) Z45.02
  CRT-P (cardiac resynchronization therapy pacemaker) Z45.018
    pulse generator Z45.010
  cystostomy device Z46.6
  defibrillator, cardiac — *see* Fitting (and adjustment) (of), automatic implantable cardiac defibrillator
  dentures Z46.3
  device NOS Z46.9
    abdominal Z46.89
    gastrointestinal NEC Z46.59
    implanted NEC Z45.89
    nervous system Z46.2
      implanted — *see* Admission, adjustment, device, implanted, nervous system
    orthodontic Z46.4
    orthoptic Z46.0
    orthotic Z46.89
    prosthetic (external) Z44.9
      breast Z44.3 ☑
      dental Z46.3
      eye Z44.2 ☑
      specified NEC Z44.8
    specified NEC Z46.89
    substitution
      auditory Z46.2
        implanted — *see* Admission, adjustment, device, implanted, hearing device
      nervous system Z46.2
        implanted — *see* Admission, adjustment, device, implanted, nervous system
      visual Z46.2
        implanted Z45.31
    urinary Z46.6
  gastric lap band Z46.51
  gastrointestinal appliance NEC Z46.59
  glasses (reading) Z46.0
  hearing aid Z46.1
  ileostomy device Z46.89
  insulin pump Z46.81
  intestinal appliance NEC Z46.89
  myringotomy device (stent) (tube) Z45.82
  neuropacemaker Z46.2
    implanted Z45.42
  non-vascular catheter Z46.82
  orthodontic device Z46.4
  orthopedic device (brace) (cast) (corset) (shoes) Z46.89
  pacemaker (cardiac) (cardiac resynchronization therapy (CRT-P)) Z45.018
    nervous system (brain) (peripheral nerve) (spinal cord) Z46.2
      implanted Z45.42
    pulse generator Z45.010
  portacath (port-a-cath) Z45.2
  prosthesis (external) Z44.9
    arm — *see* Admission, adjustment, artificial, arm
    breast Z44.3 ☑
    dental Z46.3
    eye Z44.2 ☑
    leg — *see* Admission, adjustment, artificial, leg
    specified NEC Z44.8
  spectacles Z46.0
  wheelchair Z46.89
Fitzhugh-Curtis syndrome
  due to
    Chlamydia trachomatis A74.81
    Neisseria gonorrhorea (gonococcal peritonitis) A54.85

Fitz's syndrome (acute hemorrhagic pancreatitis) (*see also* Pancreatitis, acute) K85.80
Fixation
  joint — *see* Ankylosis
  larynx J38.7
  stapes — *see* Ankylosis, ear ossicles
    deafness — *see* Deafness, conductive
  uterus (acquired) — *see* Malposition, uterus
  vocal cord J38.3
Flabby ridge K06.8
Flaccid (*see also* condition)
  palate, congenital Q38.5
Flail
  chest S22.5 ☑
    newborn (birth injury) P13.8
  joint (paralytic) M25.20
    ankle M25.27- ☑
    elbow M25.22- ☑
    foot joint M25.27- ☑
    hand joint M25.24- ☑
    hip M25.25- ☑
    knee M25.26- ☑
    shoulder M25.21- ☑
    specified joint NEC M25.28
    wrist M25.23- ☑
Flajani's disease — *see* Hyperthyroidism, with, goiter (diffuse)
Flap, liver K71.3
Flashbacks (residual to hallucinogen use) F16.283
Flat
  chamber (eye) — *see* Disorder, globe, hypotony, flat anterior chamber
  chest, congenital Q67.8
  foot (acquired) (fixed type) (painful) (postural) (*see also* Deformity, limb, flat foot)
    congenital (rigid) (spastic) (everted) Q66.5- ☑
    rachitic sequelae (late effect) E64.3
  organ or site, congenital NEC — *see* Anomaly, by site
  pelvis M95.5
    with disproportion (fetopelvic) O33.0
      causing obstructed labor O65.0
    congenital Q74.2
Flatau-Schilder disease G37.0
Flatback syndrome M40.30
  lumbar region M40.36
  lumbosacral region M40.37
  thoracolumbar region M40.35
Flattening
  head, femur M89.8X5
  hip — *see* Coxa, plana
  lip (congenital) Q18.8
  nose (congenital) Q67.4
    acquired M95.0
Flatulence R14.3
  psychogenic F45.8
Flatus R14.3
  vaginalis N89.8
Flax-dresser's disease J66.1
Flea bite — *see* Injury, bite, by site, superficial, insect
Flecks, glaucomatous (subcapsular) — *see* Cataract, complicated
Fleischer (-Kayser) **ring** (cornea) H18.04- ☑
Fleshy mole O02.0
Flexibilitas cerea — *see* Catalepsy
Flexion
  amputation stump (surgical) T87.89
  cervix — *see* Malposition, uterus
  contracture, joint — *see* Contraction, joint
  deformity, joint (*see also* Deformity, limb, flexion) M21.20
    hip, congenital Q65.89
  uterus (*see also* Malposition, uterus)
    lateral — *see* Lateroversion, uterus
Flexner-Boyd dysentery A03.2
Flexner's dysentery A03.1
Flexure — *see* Flexion
Flint murmur (aortic insufficiency) I35.1
Floater, vitreous — *see* Opacity, vitreous
Floating
  cartilage (joint) (*see also* Loose, body, joint)
    knee — *see* Derangement, knee, loose body
  gallbladder, congenital Q44.1
  kidney N28.89
    congenital Q63.8
  spleen D73.89
Flooding N92.0
Floor — *see* condition

Floppy
  baby syndrome (nonspecific) P94.2
  iris syndrome (intraoperative) (IFIS) H21.81
  nonrheumatic mitral valve syndrome I34.1
Flu (*see also* Influenza)
  avian (*see also* Influenza, due to, identified novel influenza A virus) J09.X2
  bird (*see also* Influenza, due to, identified novel influenza A virus) J09.X2
  intestinal NEC A08.4
  swine (viruses that normally cause infections in pigs) (*see also* Influenza, due to, identified novel influenza A virus) J09.X2
Fluctuating blood pressure I99.8
Fluid
  abdomen R18.8
  chest J94.8
  heart — *see* Failure, heart, congestive
  joint — *see* Effusion, joint
  loss (acute) E86.9
  lung — *see* Edema, lung
  overload E87.70
    specified NEC E87.79
  peritoneal cavity R18.8
  pleural cavity J94.8
  retention R60.9
Flukes NEC (*see also* Infestation, fluke)
  blood NEC — *see* Schistosomiasis
  liver B66.3
Fluor (vaginalis) N89.8
  trichomonal or due to Trichomonas (vaginalis) A59.00
Fluorosis
  dental K00.3
  skeletal M85.10
    ankle M85.17- ☑
    foot M85.17- ☑
    forearm M85.13- ☑
    hand M85.14- ☑
    lower leg M85.16- ☑
    multiple site M85.19
    neck M85.18
    rib M85.18
    shoulder M85.11- ☑
    skull M85.18
    specified site NEC M85.18
    thigh M85.15- ☑
    toe M85.17- ☑
    upper arm M85.12- ☑
    vertebra M85.18
Flush syndrome E34.0
Flushing R23.2
  menopausal N95.1
Flutter
  atrial or auricular I48.92
    atypical I48.4
    type I I48.3
    type II I48.4
    typical I48.3
  heart I49.8
    atrial or auricular I48.92
      atypical I48.4
      type I I48.3
      type II I48.4
      typical I48.3
    ventricular I49.02
  ventricular I49.02
FNHTR (febrile nonhemolytic transfusion reaction) R50.84
Fochier's abscess — *code by* site under Abscess
Focus, Assmann's — *see* Tuberculosis, pulmonary
Fogo selvagem L10.3
Foix-Alajouanine syndrome G95.19
Fold, folds (anomalous) (*see also* Anomaly, by site)
  Descemet's membrane — *see* Change, corneal membrane, Descemet's, fold
  epicanthic Q10.3
  heart Q24.8
Folie à deux F24
Follicle
  cervix (nabothian) (ruptured) N88.8
  graafian, ruptured, with hemorrhage N83.0- ☑
  nabothian N88.8
Follicular — *see* condition
Folliculitis (superficial) L73.9
  abscedens et suffodiens L66.3
  cyst N83.0- ☑
  decalvans L66.2
  deep — *see* Furuncle, by site

☑ **Additional Character Required** — Refer to the Tabular List for Character Selection

▽ **Subterms under main terms may continue to next column or page**

Folliculitis — *continued*
  gonococcal (acute) (chronic) A54.01
  keloid, keloidalis L73.0
  pustular L01.02
  ulerythematosa reticulata L66.4
Folliculome lipidique
  specified site — *see* Neoplasm, benign, by site
  unspecified site
    female D27.9
    male D29.20
Følling's disease E70.0
Follow-up — *see* Examination, follow-up
Fong's syndrome (hereditary osteo-onychodysplasia)
  Q87.2
Food
  allergy L27.2
  asphyxia (from aspiration or inhalation) — *see* Foreign
    body, by site
  choked on — *see* Foreign body, by site
  deprivation T73.0 ☑
    specified kind of food NEC E63.8
  intoxication — *see* Poisoning, food
  lack of T73.0 ☑
  poisoning — *see* Poisoning, food
  rejection NEC — *see* Disorder, eating
  strangulation or suffocation — *see* Foreign body, by
    site
  toxemia — *see* Poisoning, food
Foot — *see* condition
Foramen ovale (nonclosure) (patent) (persistent) Q21.1
Forbes' glycogen storage disease E74.03
Fordyce-Fox disease L75.2
Fordyce's disease (mouth) Q38.6
Forearm — *see* condition
Foreign body
  with
    laceration — *see* Laceration, by site, with foreign
      body
    puncture wound — *see* Puncture, by site, with
      foreign body
  accidentally left following a procedure T81.509 ☑
    aspiration T81.506 ☑
      resulting in
        adhesions T81.516 ☑
        obstruction T81.526 ☑
        perforation T81.536 ☑
        specified complication NEC T81.596 ☑
    cardiac catheterization T81.505 ☑
      resulting in
        acute reaction T81.60 ☑
          aseptic peritonitis T81.61 ☑
          specified NEC T81.69 ☑
        adhesions T81.515 ☑
        obstruction T81.525 ☑
        perforation T81.535 ☑
        specified complication NEC T81.595 ☑
    causing
      acute reaction T81.60 ☑
        aseptic peritonitis T81.61 ☑
        specified complication NEC T81.69 ☑
      adhesions T81.519 ☑
      aseptic peritonitis T81.61 ☑
      obstruction T81.529 ☑
      perforation T81.539 ☑
      specified complication NEC T81.599 ☑
    endoscopy T81.504 ☑
      resulting in
        adhesions T81.514 ☑
        obstruction T81.524 ☑
        perforation T81.534 ☑
        specified complication NEC T81.594 ☑
    immunization T81.503 ☑
      resulting in
        adhesions T81.513 ☑
        obstruction T81.523 ☑
        perforation T81.533 ☑
        specified complication NEC T81.593 ☑
    infusion T81.501 ☑
      resulting in
        adhesions T81.511 ☑
        obstruction T81.521 ☑
        perforation T81.531 ☑
        specified complication NEC T81.591 ☑
    injection T81.503 ☑
      resulting in
        adhesions T81.513 ☑

Foreign body — *continued*
  accidentally left following a procedure — *contin-*
    ued
    injection — *continued*
      resulting in — *continued*
        obstruction T81.523 ☑
        perforation T81.533 ☑
        specified complication NEC T81.593 ☑
    kidney dialysis T81.502 ☑
      resulting in
        adhesions T81.512 ☑
        obstruction T81.522 ☑
        perforation T81.532 ☑
        specified complication NEC T81.592 ☑
    packing removal T81.507 ☑
      resulting in
        acute reaction T81.60 ☑
          aseptic peritonitis T81.61 ☑
          specified NEC T81.69 ☑
        adhesions T81.517 ☑
        obstruction T81.527 ☑
        perforation T81.537 ☑
        specified complication NEC T81.597 ☑
    puncture T81.506 ☑
      resulting in
        adhesions T81.516 ☑
        obstruction T81.526 ☑
        perforation T81.536 ☑
        specified complication NEC T81.596 ☑
    specified procedure NEC T81.508 ☑
      resulting in
        acute reaction T81.60 ☑
          aseptic peritonitis T81.61 ☑
          specified NEC T81.69 ☑
        adhesions T81.518 ☑
        obstruction T81.528 ☑
        perforation T81.538 ☑
        specified complication NEC T81.598 ☑
    surgical operation T81.500 ☑
      resulting in
        acute reaction T81.60 ☑
          aseptic peritonitis T81.61 ☑
          specified NEC T81.69 ☑
        adhesions T81.510 ☑
        obstruction T81.520 ☑
        perforation T81.530 ☑
        specified complication NEC T81.590 ☑
    transfusion T81.501 ☑
      resulting in
        adhesions T81.511 ☑
        obstruction T81.521 ☑
        perforation T81.531 ☑
        specified complication NEC T81.591 ☑
  alimentary tract T18.9 ☑
    anus T18.5 ☑
    colon T18.4 ☑
    esophagus — *see* Foreign body, esophagus
    mouth T18.0 ☑
    multiple sites T18.8 ☑
    rectosigmoid (junction) T18.5 ☑
    rectum T18.5 ☑
    small intestine T18.3 ☑
    specified site NEC T18.8 ☑
    stomach T18.2 ☑
  anterior chamber (eye) S05.5- ☑
  auditory canal — *see* Foreign body, entering through
    orifice, ear
  bronchus T17.508 ☑
    causing
      asphyxiation T17.500 ☑
        food (bone) (seed) T17.520 ☑
        gastric contents (vomitus) T17.510 ☑
        specified type NEC T17.590 ☑
      injury NEC T17.508 ☑
        food (bone) (seed) T17.528 ☑
        gastric contents (vomitus) T17.518 ☑
        specified type NEC T17.598 ☑
  canthus — *see* Foreign body, conjunctival sac
  ciliary body (eye) S05.5- ☑
  conjunctival sac T15.1- ☑
  cornea T15.0- ☑
  entering through orifice
    accessory sinus T17.0 ☑
    alimentary canal T18.9 ☑
      multiple parts T18.8 ☑
      specified part NEC T18.8 ☑

Foreign body — *continued*
  entering through orifice — *continued*
    alveolar process T18.0 ☑
    antrum (Highmore's) T17.0 ☑
    anus T18.5 ☑
    appendix T18.4 ☑
    auditory canal — *see* Foreign body, entering
      through orifice, ear
    auricle — *see* Foreign body, entering through ori-
      fice, ear
    bladder T19.1 ☑
    bronchioles — *see* Foreign body, respiratory tract,
      specified site NEC
    bronchus (main) — *see* Foreign body, bronchus
    buccal cavity T18.0 ☑
    canthus (inner) — *see* Foreign body, conjunctival
      sac
    cecum T18.4 ☑
    cervix (canal) (uteri) T19.3 ☑
    colon T18.4 ☑
    conjunctival sac — *see* Foreign body, conjunctival
      sac
    cornea — *see* Foreign body, cornea
    digestive organ or tract NOS T18.9 ☑
      multiple parts T18.8 ☑
      specified part NEC T18.8 ☑
    duodenum T18.3 ☑
    ear (external) T16.- ☑
    esophagus — *see* Foreign body, esophagus
    eye (external) NOS T15.9- ☑
      conjunctival sac — *see* Foreign body, conjunc-
        tival sac
      cornea — *see* Foreign body, cornea
      specified part NEC T15.8- ☑
    eyeball (*see also* Foreign body, entering through
      orifice, eye, specified part NEC)
      with penetrating wound — *see* Puncture, eye-
        ball
    eyelid (*see also* Foreign body, conjunctival sac)
      with
        laceration — *see* Laceration, eyelid, with
          foreign body
        puncture — *see* Puncture, eyelid, with for-
          eign body
        superficial injury — *see* Foreign body, super-
          ficial, eyelid
    gastrointestinal tract T18.9 ☑
      multiple parts T18.8 ☑
      specified part NEC T18.8 ☑
    genitourinary tract T19.9 ☑
      multiple parts T19.8 ☑
      specified part NEC T19.8 ☑
    globe — *see* Foreign body, entering through ori-
      fice, eyeball
    gum T18.0 ☑
    Highmore's antrum T17.0 ☑
    hypopharynx — *see* Foreign body, pharynx
    ileum T18.3 ☑
    intestine (small) T18.3 ☑
      large T18.4 ☑
    lacrimal apparatus (punctum) — *see* Foreign body,
      entering through orifice, eye, specified part
      NEC
    large intestine T18.4 ☑
    larynx — *see* Foreign body, larynx
    lung — *see* Foreign body, respiratory tract, speci-
      fied site NEC
    maxillary sinus T17.0 ☑
    mouth T18.0 ☑
    nasal sinus T17.0 ☑
    nasopharynx — *see* Foreign body, pharynx
    nose (passage) T17.1 ☑
    nostril T17.1 ☑
    oral cavity T18.0 ☑
    palate T18.0 ☑
    penis T19.4 ☑
    pharynx — *see* Foreign body, pharynx
    piriform sinus — *see* Foreign body, pharynx
    rectosigmoid (junction) T18.5 ☑
    rectum T18.5 ☑
    respiratory tract — *see* Foreign body, respiratory
      tract
    sinus (accessory) (frontal) (maxillary) (nasal)
      T17.0 ☑
      piriform — *see* Foreign body, pharynx
    small intestine T18.3 ☑

Foreign body — *continued*
  entering through orifice — *continued*
    stomach T18.2 ☑
    suffocation by — *see* Foreign body, by site
    tear ducts or glands — *see* Foreign body, entering
      through orifice, eye, specified part NEC
    throat — *see* Foreign body, pharynx
    tongue T18.0 ☑
    tonsil, tonsillar (fossa) — *see* Foreign body, pharynx
    trachea — *see* Foreign body, trachea
    ureter T19.8 ☑
    urethra T19.0 ☑
    uterus (any part) T19.3 ☑
    vagina T19.2 ☑
    vulva T19.2 ☑
  esophagus T18.108 ☑
    causing
      injury NEC T18.108 ☑
        food (bone) (seed) T18.128 ☑
        gastric contents (vomitus) T18.118 ☑
        specified type NEC T18.198 ☑
      tracheal compression T18.100 ☑
        food (bone) (seed) T18.120 ☑
        gastric contents (vomitus) T18.110 ☑
        specified type NEC T18.190 ☑
  feeling of, in throat R09.89
  fragment — *see* Retained, foreign body fragments
    (type of)
  genitourinary tract T19.9 ☑
    bladder T19.1 ☑
    multiple parts T19.8 ☑
    penis T19.4 ☑
    specified site NEC T19.8 ☑
    urethra T19.0 ☑
    uterus T19.3 ☑
      IUD Z97.5
    vagina T19.2 ☑
      contraceptive device Z97.5
    vulva T19.2 ☑
  granuloma (old) (soft tissue) (*see also* Granuloma,
    foreign body)
    skin L92.3
  in
    laceration — *see* Laceration, by site, with foreign
      body
    puncture wound — *see* Puncture, by site, with
      foreign body
    soft tissue (residual) M79.5
  inadvertently left in operation wound — *see* Foreign
    body, accidentally left during a procedure
  ingestion, ingested NOS T18.9 ☑
  inhalation or inspiration — *see* Foreign body, by site
  internal organ, not entering through a natural orifice
    — code as specific injury with foreign body
  intraocular S05.5- ☑
    old, retained (nonmagnetic) H44.70- ☑
      anterior chamber H44.71- ☑
      ciliary body H44.72- ☑
      iris H44.72- ☑
      lens H44.73- ☑
      magnetic H44.60- ☑
        anterior chamber H44.61- ☑
        ciliary body H44.62- ☑
        iris H44.62- ☑
        lens H44.63- ☑
        posterior wall H44.64- ☑
        specified site NEC H44.69- ☑
        vitreous body H44.65- ☑
      posterior wall H44.74- ☑
      specified site NEC H44.79- ☑
      vitreous body H44.75- ☑
  iris — *see* Foreign body, intraocular
  lacrimal punctum — *see* Foreign body, entering
    through orifice, eye, specified part NEC
  larynx T17.308 ☑
    causing
      asphyxiation T17.300 ☑
        food (bone) (seed) T17.320 ☑
        gastric contents (vomitus) T17.310 ☑
        specified type NEC T17.390 ☑
      injury NEC T17.308 ☑
        food (bone) (seed) T17.328 ☑
        gastric contents (vomitus) T17.318 ☑
        specified type NEC T17.398 ☑
  lens — *see* Foreign body, intraocular
  ocular muscle S05.4- ☑

Foreign body — *continued*
  ocular muscle — *continued*
    old, retained — *see* Foreign body, orbit, old
  old or residual
    soft tissue (residual) M79.5
  operation wound, left accidentally — *see* Foreign
    body, accidentally left during a procedure
  orbit S05.4- ☑
    old, retained H05.5- ☑
  pharynx T17.208 ☑
    causing
      asphyxiation T17.200 ☑
        food (bone) (seed) T17.220 ☑
        gastric contents (vomitus) T17.210 ☑
        specified type NEC T17.290 ☑
      injury NEC T17.208 ☑
        food (bone) (seed) T17.228 ☑
        gastric contents (vomitus) T17.218 ☑
        specified type NEC T17.298 ☑
  respiratory tract T17.908 ☑
    bronchioles — *see* Foreign body, respiratory tract,
      specified site NEC
    bronchus — *see* Foreign body, bronchus
    causing
      asphyxiation T17.900 ☑
        food (bone) (seed) T17.920 ☑
        gastric contents (vomitus) T17.910 ☑
        specified type NEC T17.990 ☑
      injury NEC T17.908 ☑
        food (bone) (seed) T17.928 ☑
        gastric contents (vomitus) T17.918 ☑
        specified type NEC T17.998 ☑
    larynx — *see* Foreign body, larynx
    lung — *see* Foreign body, respiratory tract, speci-
      fied site NEC
    multiple parts — *see* Foreign body, respiratory
      tract, specified site NEC
    nasal sinus T17.0 ☑
    nasopharynx — *see* Foreign body, pharynx
    nose T17.1 ☑
    nostril T17.1 ☑
    pharynx — *see* Foreign body, pharynx
    specified site NEC T17.808 ☑
      causing
        asphyxiation T17.800 ☑
          food (bone) (seed) T17.820 ☑
          gastric contents (vomitus) T17.810 ☑
          specified type NEC T17.890 ☑
        injury NEC T17.808 ☑
          food (bone) (seed) T17.828 ☑
          gastric contents (vomitus) T17.818 ☑
          specified type NEC T17.898 ☑
    throat — *see* Foreign body, pharynx
    trachea — *see* Foreign body, trachea
  retained (old) (nonmagnetic) (in)
    anterior chamber (eye) — *see* Foreign body, intraoc-
      ular, old, retained, anterior chamber
      magnetic — *see* Foreign body, intraocular, old,
        retained, magnetic, anterior chamber
    ciliary body — *see* Foreign body, intraocular, old,
      retained, ciliary body
      magnetic — *see* Foreign body, intraocular, old,
        retained, magnetic, ciliary body
    eyelid H02.819
      left H02.816
        lower H02.815
        upper H02.814
      right H02.813
        lower H02.812
        upper H02.811
    fragments — *see* Retained, foreign body fragments
      (type of)
    globe — *see* Foreign body, intraocular, old, re-
      tained
      magnetic — *see* Foreign body, intraocular, old,
        retained, magnetic
    intraocular — *see* Foreign body, intraocular, old,
      retained
      magnetic — *see* Foreign body, intraocular, old,
        retained, magnetic
    iris — *see* Foreign body, intraocular, old, retained,
      iris
      magnetic — *see* Foreign body, intraocular, old,
        retained, magnetic, iris
    lens — *see* Foreign body, intraocular, old, retained,
      lens

Foreign body — *continued*
  retained — *continued*
    lens — *see* Foreign body, intraocular, old, retained,
      lens — *continued*
      magnetic — *see* Foreign body, intraocular, old,
        retained, magnetic, lens
    muscle — *see* Foreign body, retained, soft tissue
    orbit — *see* Foreign body, orbit, old
    posterior wall of globe — *see* Foreign body, intraoc-
      ular, old, retained, posterior wall
      magnetic — *see* Foreign body, intraocular, old,
        retained, magnetic, posterior wall
    retrobulbar — *see* Foreign body, orbit, old,
      retrobulbar
    soft tissue M79.5
    vitreous — *see* Foreign body, intraocular, old, re-
      tained, vitreous body
      magnetic — *see* Foreign body, intraocular, old,
        retained, magnetic, vitreous body
  retina S05.5- ☑
  superficial, without open wound
    abdomen, abdominal (wall) S30.851 ☑
    alveolar process S00.552 ☑
    ankle S90.55- ☑
    antecubital space — *see* Foreign body, superficial,
      forearm
    anus S30.857 ☑
    arm (upper) S40.85- ☑
    auditory canal — *see* Foreign body, superficial, ear
    auricle — *see* Foreign body, superficial, ear
    axilla — *see* Foreign body, superficial, arm
    back, lower S30.850 ☑
    breast S20.15- ☑
    brow S00.85 ☑
    buttock S30.850 ☑
    calf — *see* Foreign body, superficial, leg
    canthus — *see* Foreign body, superficial, eyelid
    cheek S00.85 ☑
      internal S00.552 ☑
    chest wall — *see* Foreign body, superficial, thorax
    chin S00.85 ☑
    clitoris S30.854 ☑
    costal region — *see* Foreign body, superficial,
      thorax
    digit(s)
      foot — *see* Foreign body, superficial, toe
      hand — *see* Foreign body, superficial, finger
    ear S00.45- ☑
    elbow S50.35- ☑
    epididymis S30.853 ☑
    epigastric region S30.851 ☑
    epiglottis S10.15 ☑
    esophagus, cervical S10.15 ☑
    eyebrow — *see* Foreign body, superficial, eyelid
    eyelid S00.25- ☑
    face S00.85 ☑
    finger(s) S60.459 ☑
      index S60.45- ☑
      little S60.45- ☑
      middle S60.45- ☑
      ring S60.45- ☑
    flank S30.851 ☑
    foot (except toe(s) alone) S90.85- ☑
      toe — *see* Foreign body, superficial, toe
    forearm S50.85- ☑
      elbow only — *see* Foreign body, superficial, el-
      bow
    forehead S00.85 ☑
    genital organs, external
      female S30.856 ☑
      male S30.855 ☑
    groin S30.851 ☑
    gum S00.552 ☑
    hand S60.55- ☑
    head S00.95 ☑
      ear — *see* Foreign body, superficial, ear
      eyelid — *see* Foreign body, superficial, eyelid
      lip S00.551 ☑
      nose S00.35 ☑
      oral cavity S00.552 ☑
      scalp S00.05 ☑
      specified site NEC S00.85 ☑
    heel — *see* Foreign body, superficial, foot
    hip S70.25- ☑
    inguinal region S30.851 ☑
    interscapular region S20.459 ☑

Foreign body — *continued*
  superficial, without open wound — *continued*
    jaw S00.85 ☑
    knee S80.25- ☑
    labium (majus) (minus) S30.854 ☑
    larynx S10.15 ☑
    leg (lower) S80.85- ☑
      knee — *see* Foreign body, superficial, knee
      upper — *see* Foreign body, superficial, thigh
    lip S00.551 ☑
    lower back S30.850 ☑
    lumbar region S30.850 ☑
    malar region S00.85 ☑
    mammary — *see* Foreign body, superficial, breast
    mastoid region S00.85 ☑
    mouth S00.552 ☑
    nail
      finger — *see* Foreign body, superficial, finger
      toe — *see* Foreign body, superficial, toe
    nape S10.85 ☑
    nasal S00.35 ☑
    neck S10.95 ☑
      specified site NEC S10.85 ☑
      throat S10.15 ☑
    nose S00.35 ☑
    occipital region S00.05 ☑
    oral cavity S00.552 ☑
    orbital region — *see* Foreign body, superficial, eyelid
    palate S00.552 ☑
    palm — *see* Foreign body, superficial, hand
    parietal region S00.05 ☑
    pelvis S30.850 ☑
    penis S30.852 ☑
    perineum
      female S30.854 ☑
      male S30.850 ☑
    periocular area — *see* Foreign body, superficial, eyelid
    phalanges
      finger — *see* Foreign body, superficial, finger
      toe — *see* Foreign body, superficial, toe
    pharynx S10.15 ☑
    pinna — *see* Foreign body, superficial, ear
    popliteal space — *see* Foreign body, superficial, knee
    prepuce S30.852 ☑
    pubic region S30.850 ☑
    pudendum
      female S30.856 ☑
      male S30.855 ☑
    sacral region S30.850 ☑
    scalp S00.05 ☑
    scapular region — *see* Foreign body, superficial, shoulder
    scrotum S30.853 ☑
    shin — *see* Foreign body, superficial, leg
    shoulder S40.25- ☑
    sternal region S20.359 ☑
    submaxillary region S00.85 ☑
    submental region S00.85 ☑
    subungual
      finger(s) — *see* Foreign body, superficial, finger
      toe(s) — *see* Foreign body, superficial, toe
    supraclavicular fossa S10.85 ☑
    supraorbital S00.85 ☑
    temple S00.85 ☑
    temporal region S00.85 ☑
    testis S30.853 ☑
    thigh S70.35- ☑
    thorax, thoracic (wall) S20.95 ☑
      back S20.45- ☑
      front S20.35- ☑
    throat S10.15 ☑
    thumb S60.35- ☑
    toe(s) (lesser) S90.456 ☑
      great S90.45- ☑
    tongue S00.552 ☑
    trachea S10.15 ☑
    tunica vaginalis S30.853 ☑
    tympanum, tympanic membrane — *see* Foreign body, superficial, ear
    uvula S00.552 ☑
    vagina S30.854 ☑
    vocal cords S10.15 ☑
    vulva S30.854 ☑

Foreign body — *continued*
  superficial, without open wound — *continued*
    wrist S60.85- ☑
    swallowed T18.9 ☑
    trachea T17.408 ☑
      causing
        asphyxiation T17.400 ☑
          food (bone) (seed) T17.420 ☑
          gastric contents (vomitus) T17.410 ☑
          specified type NEC T17.490 ☑
        injury NEC T17.408 ☑
          food (bone) (seed) T17.428 ☑
          gastric contents (vomitus) T17.418 ☑
          specified type NEC T17.498 ☑
    type of fragment — *see* Retained, foreign body fragments (type of)
    vitreous (humor) S05.5- ☑
Forestier's disease (rhizomelic pseudopolyarthritis) M35.3
  meaning ankylosing hyperostosis — *see* Hyperostosis, ankylosing
Formation
  hyalin in cornea — *see* Degeneration, cornea
  sequestrum in bone (due to infection) — *see* Osteomyelitis, chronic
  valve
    colon, congenital Q43.8
    ureter (congenital) Q62.39
Formication R20.2
Fort Bragg fever A27.89
Fossa (*see also* condition)
  pyriform — *see* condition
Foster-Kennedy syndrome H47.14- ☑
Fothergill's
  disease (trigeminal neuralgia) (*see also* Neuralgia, trigeminal)
  scarlatina anginosa A38.9
Foul breath R19.6
Foundling Z76.1
Fournier disease or gangrene N49.3
  female N76.89
Fourth
  cranial nerve — *see* condition
  molar K00.1
Foville's (peduncular) **disease or syndrome** G46.3
Fox (-Fordyce) disease (apocrine miliaria) L75.2
Fracture, burst — *see* Fracture, traumatic, by site
Fracture, chronic — *see* Fracture, pathological, by site
Fracture, insufficiency — *see* Fracture, pathological, by site
Fracture, nontraumatic, NEC
  atypical
    femur M84.750- ☑
      complete
        oblique M84.759 ☑
          left side M84.758 ☑
          right side M84.757 ☑
        transverse M84.756 ☑
          left side M84.755 ☑
          right side M84.754 ☑
      incomplete M84.753 ☑
        left side M84.752 ☑
        right side M84.751 ☑
Fracture, pathological (pathologic) (*see also* Fracture, traumatic) M84.40 ☑
  ankle M84.47- ☑
  carpus M84.44- ☑
  clavicle M84.41- ☑
  compression (not due to trauma) (*see also* Collapse, vertebra) M48.50- ☑
  dental implant M27.63
  dental restorative material K08.539
    with loss of material K08.531
    without loss of material K08.530
  due to
    neoplastic disease NEC (*see also* Neoplasm) M84.50
      ankle M84.57- ☑
      carpus M84.54- ☑
      clavicle M84.51- ☑
      femur M84.55- ☑
      fibula M84.56- ☑
      finger M84.54- ☑
      hip M84.559 ☑
      humerus M84.52- ☑
      ilium M84.550 ☑

Fracture, pathological — *continued*
  due to — *continued*
    neoplastic disease (*see also* Neoplasm) — *continued*
      ischium M84.550 ☑
      metacarpus M84.54- ☑
      metatarsus M84.57- ☑
      neck M84.58 ☑
      pelvis M84.550 ☑
      radius M84.53- ☑
      rib M84.58 ☑
      scapula M84.51- ☑
      skull M84.58 ☑
      specified site NEC M84.58 ☑
      tarsus M84.57- ☑
      tibia M84.56- ☑
      toe M84.57- ☑
      ulna M84.53- ☑
      vertebra M84.58 ☑
    osteoporosis M80.00 ☑
      disuse — *see* Osteoporosis, specified type NEC, with pathological fracture
      drug-induced — *see* Osteoporosis, drug-induced, with pathological fracture
      idiopathic — *see* Osteoporosis, specified type NEC, with pathological fracture
      postmenopausal — *see* Osteoporosis, postmenopausal, with pathological fracture
      postoophorectomy — *see* Osteoporosis, postoophorectomy, with pathological fracture
      postsurgical malabsorption — *see* Osteoporosis, specified type NEC, with pathological fracture
      specified cause NEC — *see* Osteoporosis, specified type NEC, with pathological fracture
    specified disease NEC M84.60 ☑
      ankle M84.67- ☑
      carpus M84.64- ☑
      clavicle M84.61- ☑
      femur M84.65- ☑
      fibula M84.66- ☑
      finger M84.64- ☑
      hip M84.65- ☑
      humerus M84.62- ☑
      ilium M84.650 ☑
      ischium M84.650 ☑
      metacarpus M84.64- ☑
      metatarsus M84.67- ☑
      neck M84.68 ☑
      radius M84.63- ☑
      rib M84.68 ☑
      scapula M84.61- ☑
      skull M84.68 ☑
      tarsus M84.67- ☑
      tibia M84.66- ☑
      toe M84.67- ☑
      ulna M84.63- ☑
      vertebra M84.68 ☑
  femur M84.45- ☑
  fibula M84.46- ☑
  finger M84.44- ☑
  hip M84.459 ☑
  humerus M84.42- ☑
  ilium M84.454 ☑
  ischium M84.454 ☑
  joint prosthesis — *see* Complications, joint prosthesis, mechanical, breakdown, by site
    periprosthetic — *see* Fracture, pathological, periprosthetic
  metacarpus M84.44- ☑
  metatarsus M84.47- ☑
  neck M84.48 ☑
  pelvis M84.454 ☑
  periprosthetic M97.9 ☑
    ankle M97.2- ☑
    elbow M97.4- ☑
    finger M97.8 ☑
    hip M97.0- ☑
    knee M97.1- ☑
    other specified joint M97.8 ☑
    shoulder M97.3- ☑
    spinal joint M97.8 ☑
    toe joint M97.8 ☑
    wrist joint M97.8 ☑
  radius M84.43- ☑

Fracture, pathological — *continued*
  restorative material (dental) K08.539
    with loss of material K08.531
    without loss of material K08.530
  rib M84.48 ☑
  scapula M84.41- ☑
  skull M84.48 ☑
  tarsus M84.47- ☑
  tibia M84.46- ☑
  toe M84.47- ☑
  ulna M84.43- ☑
  vertebra M84.48 ☑
Fracture, traumatic (abduction) (adduction) (separation)
  (*see also* Fracture, pathological) T14.8 ☑
  acetabulum S32.40- ☑
    column
      anterior (displaced) (iliopubic) S32.43- ☑
        nondisplaced S32.436 ☑
      posterior (displaced) (ilioischial) S32.443 ☑
        nondisplaced S32.44- ☑
    dome (displaced) S32.48- ☑
      nondisplaced S32.48 ☑
    specified NEC S32.49- ☑
    transverse (displaced) S32.45- ☑
      with associated posterior wall fracture (displaced) S32.46- ☑
        nondisplaced S32.46- ☑
      nondisplaced S32.45- ☑
    wall
      anterior (displaced) S32.41- ☑
        nondisplaced S32.41- ☑
      medial (displaced) S32.47- ☑
        nondisplaced S32.47- ☑
      posterior (displaced) S32.42- ☑
        with associated transverse fracture (displaced) S32.46- ☑
          nondisplaced S32.46- ☑
        nondisplaced S32.42- ☑
  acromion — *see* Fracture, scapula, acromial process
  ankle S82.899 ☑
    bimalleolar (displaced) S82.84- ☑
      nondisplaced S82.84- ☑
    lateral malleolus only (displaced) S82.6- ☑
      nondisplaced S82.6- ☑
    medial malleolus (displaced) S82.5- ☑
      associated with Maisonneuve's fracture — *see* Fracture, Maisonneuve's
      nondisplaced S82.5- ☑
    talus — *see* Fracture, tarsal, talus
    trimalleolar (displaced) S82.85- ☑
      nondisplaced S82.85- ☑
  arm (upper) (*see also* Fracture, humerus, shaft)
    humerus — *see* Fracture, humerus
    radius — *see* Fracture, radius
    ulna — *see* Fracture, ulna
  astragalus — *see* Fracture, tarsal, talus
  atlas — *see* Fracture, neck, cervical vertebra, first
  axis — *see* Fracture, neck, cervical vertebra, second
  back — *see* Fracture, vertebra
  Barton's — *see* Barton's fracture
  base of skull — *see* Fracture, skull, base
  basicervical (basal) (femoral) S72.0 ☑
  Bennett's — *see* Bennett's fracture
  bimalleolar — *see* Fracture, ankle, bimalleolar
  blow-out S02.3- ☑
  bone NEC T14.8 ☑
    birth injury P13.9
    following insertion of orthopedic implant, joint prosthesis or bone plate — *see* Fracture, following insertion of orthopedic implant, joint prosthesis or bone plate
    in (due to) neoplastic disease NEC — *see* Fracture, pathological, due to, neoplastic disease
    pathological (cause unknown) — *see* Fracture, pathological
  breast bone — *see* Fracture, sternum
  bucket handle (semilunar cartilage) — *see* Tear, meniscus
  burst — *see* Fracture, traumatic, by site
  calcaneus — *see* Fracture, tarsal, calcaneus
  carpal bone(s) S62.10- ☑
    capitate (displaced) S62.13- ☑
      nondisplaced S62.13- ☑
    cuneiform — *see* Fracture, carpal bone, triquetrum
    hamate (body) (displaced) S62.143 ☑
      hook process (displaced) S62.15- ☑

Fracture, traumatic — *continued*
  carpal bone(s) — *continued*
    hamate — *continued*
      hook process — *continued*
        nondisplaced S62.15- ☑
      nondisplaced S62.14- ☑
    larger multangular — *see* Fracture, carpal bones, trapezium
    lunate (displaced) S62.12- ☑
      nondisplaced S62.12- ☑
    navicular S62.00- ☑
      distal pole (displaced) S62.01- ☑
        nondisplaced S62.01- ☑
      middle third (displaced) S62.02- ☑
        nondisplaced S62.02- ☑
      proximal third (displaced) S62.03- ☑
        nondisplaced S62.03- ☑
      volar tuberosity — *see* Fracture, carpal bones, navicular, distal pole
    os magnum — *see* Fracture, carpal bones, capitate
    pisiform (displaced) S62.16- ☑
      nondisplaced S62.16- ☑
    semilunar — *see* Fracture, carpal bones, lunate
    smaller multangular — *see* Fracture, carpal bones, trapezoid
    trapezium (displaced) S62.17- ☑
      nondisplaced S62.17- ☑
    trapezoid (displaced) S62.18- ☑
      nondisplaced S62.18- ☑
    triquetrum (displaced) S62.11- ☑
      nondisplaced S62.11- ☑
    unciform — *see* Fracture, carpal bones, hamate
  cervical — *see* Fracture, vertebra, cervical
  clavicle S42.00- ☑
    acromial end (displaced) S42.03- ☑
      nondisplaced S42.03- ☑
    birth injury P13.4
    lateral end — *see* Fracture, clavicle, acromial end
    shaft (displaced) S42.02- ☑
      nondisplaced S42.02- ☑
    sternal end (anterior) (displaced) S42.01- ☑
      nondisplaced S42.01- ☑
      posterior S42.01- ☑
  coccyx S32.2 ☑
  collapsed — *see* Collapse, vertebra
  collar bone — *see* Fracture, clavicle
  Colles' — *see* Colles' fracture
  coronoid process — *see* Fracture, ulna, upper end, coronoid process
  corpus cavernosum penis S39.840 ☑
  costochondral cartilage S23.41 ☑
  costochondral, costosternal junction — *see* Fracture, rib
  cranium — *see* Fracture, skull
  cricoid cartilage S12.8 ☑
  cuboid (ankle) — *see* Fracture, tarsal, cuboid
  cuneiform
    foot — *see* Fracture, tarsal, cuneiform
    wrist — *see* Fracture, carpal, triquetrum
  delayed union — *see* Delay, union, fracture
  dental restorative material K08.539
    with loss of material K08.531
    without loss of material K08.530
  due to
    birth injury — *see* Birth, injury, fracture
    osteoporosis — *see* Osteoporosis, with fracture
  Dupuytren's — *see* Fracture, ankle, lateral malleolus
  elbow S42.40- ☑
  ethmoid (bone) (sinus) — *see* Fracture, skull, base
  face bone S02.92 ☑
  fatigue (*see also* Fracture, stress)
    vertebra M48.40 ☑
      cervical region M48.42 ☑
      cervicothoracic region M48.43 ☑
      lumbar region M48.46 ☑
      lumbosacral region M48.47 ☑
      occipito-atlanto-axial region M48.41 ☑
      sacrococcygeal region M48.48 ☑
      thoracic region M48.44 ☑
      thoracolumbar region M48.45 ☑
  femur, femoral S72.9- ☑
    basicervical (basal) S72.0 ☑
    birth injury P13.2
    capital epiphyseal S79.01- ☑
    condyles, epicondyles — *see* Fracture, femur, lower end

Fracture, traumatic — *continued*
  femur, femoral — *continued*
    distal end — *see* Fracture, femur, lower end
    epiphysis
      head — *see* Fracture, femur, upper end, epiphysis
      lower — *see* Fracture, femur, lower end, epiphysis
      upper — *see* Fracture, femur, upper end, epiphysis
    following insertion of implant, prosthesis or plate M96.66- ☑
    head — *see* Fracture, femur, upper end, head
    intertrochanteric — *see* Fracture, femur, trochanteric
    intratrochanteric — *see* Fracture, femur, trochanteric
    lower end S72.40- ☑
      condyle (displaced) S72.41- ☑
        lateral (displaced) S72.42- ☑
          nondisplaced S72.42- ☑
        medial (displaced) S72.43- ☑
          nondisplaced S72.43- ☑
        nondisplaced S72.41- ☑
      epiphysis (displaced) S72.44- ☑
        nondisplaced S72.44- ☑
      physeal S79.10- ☑
        Salter-Harris
          Type I S79.11- ☑
          Type II S79.12- ☑
          Type III S79.13- ☑
          Type IV S79.14- ☑
        specified NEC S79.19- ☑
      specified NEC S72.49- ☑
      supracondylar (displaced) S72.45- ☑
        with intracondylar extension (displaced) S72.46- ☑
          nondisplaced S72.46- ☑
        nondisplaced S72.45- ☑
      torus S72.47- ☑
    neck — *see* Fracture, femur, upper end, neck
    pertrochanteric — *see* Fracture, femur, trochanteric
    shaft (lower third) (middle third) (upper third) S72.30- ☑
      comminuted (displaced) S72.35- ☑
        nondisplaced S72.35- ☑
      oblique (displaced) S72.33- ☑
        nondisplaced S72.33- ☑
      segmental (displaced) S72.36- ☑
        nondisplaced S72.36- ☑
      specified NEC S72.39- ☑
      spiral (displaced) S72.34- ☑
        nondisplaced S72.34- ☑
      transverse (displaced) S72.32- ☑
        nondisplaced S72.32- ☑
    specified site NEC — *see* subcategory S72.8
    subcapital (displaced) S72.01- ☑
    subtrochanteric (region) (section) (displaced) S72.2- ☑
      nondisplaced S72.2- ☑
    transcervical — *see* Fracture, femur, upper end, neck
    transtrochanteric — *see* Fracture, femur, trochanteric
    trochanteric S72.10- ☑
      apophyseal (displaced) S72.13- ☑
        nondisplaced S72.13- ☑
      greater trochanter (displaced) S72.11- ☑
        nondisplaced S72.11- ☑
      intertrochanteric (displaced) S72.14- ☑
        nondisplaced S72.14- ☑
      lesser trochanter (displaced) S72.12- ☑
        nondisplaced S72.12- ☑
    upper end S72.00- ☑
      apophyseal (displaced) S72.13- ☑
        nondisplaced S72.13- ☑
      cervicotrochanteric — *see* Fracture, femur, upper end, neck, base
      epiphysis (displaced) S72.02- ☑
        nondisplaced S72.02- ☑
      head S72.05- ☑
        articular (displaced) S72.06- ☑
          nondisplaced S72.06- ☑
        specified NEC S72.09- ☑
      intertrochanteric (displaced) S72.14- ☑

Fracture, traumatic — *continued*
  femur, femoral — *continued*
    upper end — *continued*
      intertrochanteric — *continued*
        nondisplaced S72.14- ☑
      intracapsular S72.01- ☑
      midcervical (displaced) S72.03- ☑
        nondisplaced S72.03- ☑
      neck S72.00- ☑
        base (displaced) S72.04- ☑
          nondisplaced S72.04- ☑
        specified NEC S72.09- ☑
      pertrochanteric — *see* Fracture, femur, upper end, trochanteric
      physeal S79.00- ☑
        Salter-Harris type I S79.01- ☑
        specified NEC S79.09- ☑
      subcapital (displaced) S72.01- ☑
      subtrochanteric (displaced) S72.2- ☑
        nondisplaced S72.2- ☑
      transcervical — *see* Fracture, femur, upper end, midcervical
      trochanteric S72.10- ☑
        greater (displaced) S72.11- ☑
          nondisplaced S72.11- ☑
        lesser (displaced) S72.12- ☑
          nondisplaced S72.12- ☑
  fibula (shaft) (styloid) S82.40- ☑
    comminuted (displaced) S82.45- ☑
      nondisplaced S82.45- ☑
    following insertion of implant, prosthesis or plate M96.67- ☑
    involving ankle or malleolus — *see* Fracture, fibula, lateral malleolus
    lateral malleolus (displaced) S82.6- ☑
      nondisplaced S82.6- ☑
    lower end
      physeal S89.30- ☑
        Salter-Harris
          Type I S89.31- ☑
          Type II S89.32- ☑
        specified NEC S89.39- ☑
      specified NEC S82.83- ☑
      torus S82.82- ☑
    oblique (displaced) S82.43- ☑
      nondisplaced S82.43- ☑
    segmental (displaced) S82.46- ☑
      nondisplaced S82.46- ☑
    specified NEC S82.49- ☑
    spiral (displaced) S82.44- ☑
      nondisplaced S82.44- ☑
    transverse (displaced) S82.42- ☑
      nondisplaced S82.42- ☑
    upper end
      physeal S89.20- ☑
        Salter-Harris
          Type I S89.21- ☑
          Type II S89.22- ☑
        specified NEC S89.29- ☑
      specified NEC S82.83- ☑
      torus S82.81- ☑
  finger (except thumb) S62.60- ☑
    distal phalanx (displaced) S62.63- ☑
      nondisplaced S62.66- ☑
    index S62.60- ☑
      distal phalanx (displaced) S62.63- ☑
        nondisplaced S62.66- ☑
      medial phalanx (displaced) S62.62- ☑
        nondisplaced S62.65- ☑
      proximal phalanx (displaced) S62.61- ☑
        nondisplaced S62.64- ☑
    little S62.60- ☑
      distal phalanx (displaced) S62.63- ☑
        nondisplaced S62.66- ☑
      medial phalanx (displaced) S62.62- ☑
        nondisplaced S62.65- ☑
      proximal phalanx (displaced) S62.61- ☑
        nondisplaced S62.64- ☑
    medial phalanx (displaced) S62.62- ☑
      nondisplaced S62.65- ☑
    middle S62.60- ☑
      distal phalanx (displaced) S62.63- ☑
        nondisplaced S62.66- ☑
      medial phalanx (displaced) S62.62- ☑
        nondisplaced S62.65- ☑
      proximal phalanx (displaced) S62.61- ☑

Fracture, traumatic — *continued*
  finger — *continued*
    middle — *continued*
      proximal phalanx — *continued*
        nondisplaced S62.64- ☑
    proximal phalanx (displaced) S62.61- ☑
      nondisplaced S62.64- ☑
    ring S62.60- ☑
      distal phalanx (displaced) S62.63- ☑
        nondisplaced S62.66- ☑
      medial phalanx (displaced) S62.62- ☑
        nondisplaced S62.65- ☑
      proximal phalanx (displaced) S62.61- ☑
        nondisplaced S62.64- ☑
    thumb — *see* Fracture, thumb
  following insertion (intraoperative) (postoperative) of orthopedic implant, joint prosthesis or bone plate M96.69
    femur M96.66- ☑
    fibula M96.67- ☑
    humerus M96.62- ☑
    pelvis M96.65
    radius M96.63- ☑
    specified bone NEC M96.69
    tibia M96.67- ☑
    ulna M96.63- ☑
  foot S92.90- ☑
    astragalus — *see* Fracture, tarsal, talus
    calcaneus — *see* Fracture, tarsal, calcaneus
    cuboid — *see* Fracture, tarsal, cuboid
    cuneiform — *see* Fracture, tarsal, cuneiform
    metatarsal — *see* Fracture, metatarsal
    navicular — *see* Fracture, tarsal, navicular
    sesamoid S92.81- ☑
    specified NEC S92.81- ☑
    talus — *see* Fracture, tarsal, talus
    tarsal — *see* Fracture, tarsal
    toe — *see* Fracture, toe
  forearm S52.9- ☑
    radius — *see* Fracture, radius
    ulna — *see* Fracture, ulna
  fossa (anterior) (middle) (posterior) S02.19 ☑
  frontal (bone) (skull) S02.0 ☑
    sinus S02.19 ☑
  glenoid (cavity) (scapula) — *see* Fracture, scapula, glenoid cavity
  greenstick — *see* Fracture, by site
  hallux — *see* Fracture, toe, great
  hand S62.9- ☑
    carpal — *see* Fracture, carpal bone
    finger (except thumb) — *see* Fracture, finger
    metacarpal — *see* Fracture, metacarpal
    navicular (scaphoid) (hand) — *see* Fracture, carpal bone, navicular
    thumb — *see* Fracture, thumb
  healed or old
    with complications — *code by* Nature of the complication
  heel bone — *see* Fracture, tarsal, calcaneus
  Hill-Sachs S42.29- ☑
  hip — *see* Fracture, femur, neck
  humerus S42.30- ☑
    anatomical neck — *see* Fracture, humerus, upper end
    articular process — *see* Fracture, humerus, lower end
    capitellum — *see* Fracture, humerus, lower end, condyle, lateral
    distal end — *see* Fracture, humerus, lower end
    epiphysis
      lower — *see* Fracture, humerus, lower end, physeal
      upper — *see* Fracture, humerus, upper end, physeal
    external condyle — *see* Fracture, humerus, lower end, condyle, lateral
    following insertion of implant, prosthesis or plate M96.62- ☑
    great tuberosity — *see* Fracture, humerus, upper end, greater tuberosity
    intercondylar — *see* Fracture, humerus, lower end
    internal epicondyle — *see* Fracture, humerus, lower end, epicondyle, medial
    lesser tuberosity — *see* Fracture, humerus, upper end, lesser tuberosity
    lower end S42.40- ☑

Fracture, traumatic — *continued*
  humerus — *continued*
    lower end — *continued*
      condyle
        lateral (displaced) S42.45- ☑
          nondisplaced S42.45- ☑
        medial (displaced) S42.46- ☑
          nondisplaced S42.46- ☑
      epicondyle
        lateral (displaced) S42.43- ☑
          nondisplaced S42.43- ☑
        medial (displaced) S42.44- ☑
          incarcerated S42.44- ☑
          nondisplaced S42.44- ☑
      physeal S49.10- ☑
        Salter-Harris
          Type I S49.11- ☑
          Type II S49.12- ☑
          Type III S49.13- ☑
          Type IV S49.14- ☑
        specified NEC S49.19- ☑
      specified NEC (displaced) S42.49- ☑
        nondisplaced S42.49- ☑
      supracondylar (simple) (displaced) S42.41- ☑
        with intercondylar fracture — *see* Fracture, humerus, lower end
        comminuted (displaced) S42.42- ☑
          nondisplaced S42.42- ☑
          nondisplaced S42.41- ☑
      torus S42.48- ☑
      transcondylar (displaced) S42.47- ☑
        nondisplaced S42.47- ☑
    proximal end — *see* Fracture, humerus, upper end
    shaft S42.30- ☑
      comminuted (displaced) S42.35- ☑
        nondisplaced S42.35- ☑
      greenstick S42.31- ☑
      oblique (displaced) S42.33- ☑
        nondisplaced S42.33- ☑
      segmental (displaced) S42.36- ☑
        nondisplaced S42.36- ☑
      specified NEC S42.39- ☑
      spiral (displaced) S42.34- ☑
        nondisplaced S42.34- ☑
      transverse (displaced) S42.32- ☑
        nondisplaced S42.32- ☑
    supracondylar — *see* Fracture, humerus, lower end
    surgical neck — *see* Fracture, humerus, upper end, surgical neck
    trochlea — *see* Fracture, humerus, lower end, condyle, medial
    tuberosity — *see* Fracture, humerus, upper end
    upper end S42.20- ☑
      anatomical neck — *see* Fracture, humerus, upper end, specified NEC
      articular head — *see* Fracture, humerus, upper end, specified NEC
      epiphysis — *see* Fracture, humerus, upper end, physeal
      greater tuberosity (displaced) S42.25- ☑
        nondisplaced S42.25- ☑
      lesser tuberosity (displaced) S42.26- ☑
        nondisplaced S42.26- ☑
      physeal S49.00- ☑
        Salter-Harris
          Type I S49.01- ☑
          Type II S49.02- ☑
          Type III S49.03- ☑
          Type IV S49.04- ☑
        specified NEC S49.09- ☑
      specified NEC (displaced) S42.29- ☑
        nondisplaced S42.29- ☑
      surgical neck (displaced) S42.21- ☑
        four-part S42.24- ☑
        nondisplaced S42.21- ☑
        three-part S42.23- ☑
        two-part (displaced) S42.22- ☑
          nondisplaced S42.22- ☑
      torus S42.27- ☑
      transepiphyseal — *see* Fracture, humerus, upper end, physeal
  hyoid bone S12.8 ☑
  ilium S32.30- ☑
    with disruption of pelvic ring — *see* Disruption, pelvic ring
    avulsion (displaced) S32.31- ☑

Fracture, traumatic — *continued*
  ilium — *continued*
    avulsion — *continued*
      nondisplaced S32.31- ☑
    specified NEC S32.39- ☑
  impaction, impacted — *code as* Fracture, by site
  innominate bone — *see* Fracture, ilium
  instep — *see* Fracture, foot
  ischium S32.60- ☑
    with disruption of pelvic ring — *see* Disruption, pelvic ring
    avulsion (displaced) S32.61- ☑
      nondisplaced S32.61- ☑
    specified NEC S32.69- ☑
  jaw (bone) (lower) — *see* Fracture, mandible
    upper — *see* Fracture, maxilla
  joint prosthesis — *see* Complications, joint prosthesis, mechanical, breakdown, by site
    periprosthetic — *see* Fracture, traumatic, periprosthetic
  knee cap — *see* Fracture, patella
  larynx S12.8 ☑
  late effects — *see* Sequelae, fracture
  leg (lower) S82.9- ☑
    ankle — *see* Fracture, ankle
    femur — *see* Fracture, femur
    fibula — *see* Fracture, fibula
    malleolus — *see* Fracture, ankle
    patella — *see* Fracture, patella
    specified site NEC S82.89- ☑
    tibia — *see* Fracture, tibia
  lumbar spine — *see* Fracture, vertebra, lumbar
  lumbosacral spine S32.9 ☑
  Maisonneuve's (displaced) S82.86- ☑
    nondisplaced S82.86- ☑
  malar bone (*see also* Fracture, maxilla) S02.400 ☑
    left side S02.40B ☑
    right side S02.40A ☑
  malleolus — *see* Fracture, ankle
  malunion — *see* Fracture, by site
  mandible (lower jaw (bone)) S02.609 ☑
    alveolus S02.67- ☑
    angle (of jaw) S02.65- ☑
    body, unspecified S02.600 ☑
      left side S02.602 ☑
      right side S02.601 ☑
    condylar process S02.61- ☑
    coronoid process S02.63- ☑
    ramus, unspecified S02.64- ☑
    specified site NEC S02.69 ☑
    subcondylar process S02.62- ☑
    symphysis S02.66 ☑
  manubrium (sterni) S22.21 ☑
    dissociation from sternum S22.23 ☑
  march — *see* Fracture, traumatic, stress, by site
  maxilla, maxillary (bone) (sinus) (superior) (upper jaw) S02.401 ☑
    alveolus S02.42 ☑
    inferior — *see* Fracture, mandible
    LeFort I S02.411 ☑
    LeFort II S02.412 ☑
    LeFort III S02.413 ☑
    left side S02.40D ☑
    right side S02.40C ☑
  metacarpal S62.309 ☑
    base (displaced) S62.319 ☑
      nondisplaced S62.349 ☑
    fifth S62.30- ☑
      base (displaced) S62.31- ☑
        nondisplaced S62.34- ☑
      neck (displaced) S62.33- ☑
        nondisplaced S62.36- ☑
      shaft (displaced) S62.32- ☑
        nondisplaced S62.35- ☑
      specified NEC S62.398 ☑
    first S62.20- ☑
      base NEC (displaced) S62.23- ☑
        nondisplaced S62.23- ☑
      Bennett's — *see* Bennett's fracture
      neck (displaced) S62.25- ☑
        nondisplaced S62.25- ☑
      shaft (displaced) S62.24- ☑
        nondisplaced S62.24- ☑
      specified NEC S62.29- ☑
    fourth S62.30- ☑
      base (displaced) S62.31- ☑

Fracture, traumatic — *continued*
  metacarpal — *continued*
    fourth — *continued*
      base — *continued*
        nondisplaced S62.34- ☑
      neck (displaced) S62.33- ☑
        nondisplaced S62.36- ☑
      shaft (displaced) S62.32- ☑
        nondisplaced S62.35- ☑
      specified NEC S62.39- ☑
    neck (displaced) S62.33- ☑
      nondisplaced S62.36- ☑
    Rolando's — *see* Rolando's fracture
    second S62.30- ☑
      base (displaced) S62.31- ☑
        nondisplaced S62.34- ☑
      neck (displaced) S62.33- ☑
        nondisplaced S62.36- ☑
      shaft (displaced) S62.32- ☑
        nondisplaced S62.35- ☑
      specified NEC S62.39- ☑
    shaft (displaced) S62.32- ☑
      nondisplaced S62.35- ☑
    specified NEC S62.399 ☑
    third S62.30- ☑
      base (displaced) S62.31- ☑
        nondisplaced S62.34- ☑
      neck (displaced) S62.33- ☑
        nondisplaced S62.36- ☑
      shaft (displaced) S62.32- ☑
        nondisplaced S62.35- ☑
      specified NEC S62.39- ☑
  metastatic — *see* Fracture, pathological, due to, neoplastic disease (*see also* Neoplasm)
  metatarsal bone S92.30- ☑
    fifth (displaced) S92.35- ☑
      nondisplaced S92.35- ☑
    first (displaced) S92.31- ☑
      nondisplaced S92.31- ☑
    fourth (displaced) S92.34- ☑
      nondisplaced S92.34- ☑
    physeal S99.10- ☑
      Salter-Harris
        Type I S99.11- ☑
        Type II S99.12- ☑
        Type III S99.13- ☑
        Type IV S99.14- ☑
      specified NEC S99.19- ☑
    second (displaced) S92.32- ☑
      nondisplaced S92.32- ☑
    third (displaced) S92.33- ☑
      nondisplaced S92.33- ☑
  Monteggia's — *see* Monteggia's fracture
  multiple
    hand (and wrist) NEC — *see* Fracture, by site
    ribs — *see* Fracture, rib, multiple
  nasal (bone(s)) S02.2 ☑
  navicular (scaphoid) (foot) (*see also* Fracture, tarsal, navicular)
    hand — *see* Fracture, carpal, navicular
  neck S12.9 ☑
    cervical vertebra S12.9 ☑
      fifth (displaced) S12.400 ☑
        nondisplaced S12.401 ☑
        specified type NEC (displaced) S12.490 ☑
          nondisplaced S12.491 ☑
      first (displaced) S12.000 ☑
        burst (stable) S12.01 ☑
          unstable S12.02 ☑
        lateral mass (displaced) S12.040 ☑
          nondisplaced S12.041 ☑
        nondisplaced S12.001 ☑
        posterior arch (displaced) S12.030 ☑
          nondisplaced S12.031 ☑
        specified type NEC (displaced) S12.090 ☑
          nondisplaced S12.091 ☑
      fourth (displaced) S12.300 ☑
        nondisplaced S12.301 ☑
        specified type NEC (displaced) S12.390 ☑
          nondisplaced S12.391 ☑
      second (displaced) S12.100 ☑
        dens (anterior) (displaced) (type II) S12.110 ☑
          nondisplaced S12.112 ☑
          posterior S12.111 ☑

Fracture, traumatic — *continued*
  neck — *continued*
    cervical vertebra — *continued*
      second — *continued*
        dens — *continued*
          specified type NEC (displaced) S12.120 ☑
          nondisplaced S12.121 ☑
        nondisplaced S12.101 ☑
        specified type NEC (displaced) S12.190 ☑
          nondisplaced S12.191 ☑
      seventh (displaced) S12.600 ☑
        nondisplaced S12.601 ☑
        specified type NEC (displaced) S12.690 ☑
          nondisplaced S12.691 ☑
      sixth (displaced) S12.500 ☑
        nondisplaced S12.501 ☑
        specified type NEC (displaced) S12.590 ☑
          nondisplaced S12.591 ☑
      third (displaced) S12.200 ☑
        nondisplaced S12.201 ☑
        specified type NEC (displaced) S12.290 ☑
          nondisplaced S12.291 ☑
    hyoid bone S12.8 ☑
    larynx S12.8 ☑
    specified site NEC S12.8 ☑
    thyroid cartilage S12.8 ☑
    trachea S12.8 ☑
  neoplastic NEC — *see* Fracture, pathological, due to, neoplastic disease
  neural arch — *see* Fracture, vertebra
  newborn — *see* Birth, injury, fracture
  nontraumatic — *see* Fracture, pathological
  nonunion — *see* Nonunion, fracture
  nose, nasal (bone) (septum) S02.2 ☑
  occiput — *see* Fracture, skull, base, occiput
  odontoid process — *see* Fracture, neck, cervical vertebra, second
  olecranon (process) (ulna) — *see* Fracture, ulna, upper end, olecranon process
  orbit, orbital (bone) (region) S02.8- ☑
    floor (blow-out) S02.3- ☑
    roof S02.19 ☑
  os
    calcis — *see* Fracture, tarsal, calcaneus
    magnum — *see* Fracture, carpal, capitate
    pubis — *see* Fracture, pubis
  palate S02.8- ☑
  parietal bone (skull) S02.0 ☑
  patella S82.00- ☑
    comminuted (displaced) S82.04- ☑
      nondisplaced S82.04- ☑
    longitudinal (displaced) S82.02- ☑
      nondisplaced S82.02- ☑
    osteochondral (displaced) S82.01- ☑
      nondisplaced S82.01- ☑
    specified NEC S82.09- ☑
    transverse (displaced) S82.03- ☑
      nondisplaced S82.03- ☑
  pedicle (of vertebral arch) — *see* Fracture, vertebra
  pelvis, pelvic (bone) S32.9 ☑
    acetabulum — *see* Fracture, acetabulum
    circle — *see* Disruption, pelvic ring
    following insertion of implant, prosthesis or plate M96.65
    ilium — *see* Fracture, ilium
    ischium — *see* Fracture, ischium
    multiple
      with disruption of pelvic ring (circle) — *see* Disruption, pelvic ring
      without disruption of pelvic ring (circle) S32.82 ☑
    pubis — *see* Fracture, pubis
    sacrum — *see* Fracture, sacrum
    specified site NEC S32.89 ☑
  periprosthetic, around internal prosthetic joint M97.9
    ankle M97.2- ☑
    elbow M97.4- ☑
    finger M97.8 ☑
    hip M97.0- ☑
    knee M97.1- ☑
    shoulder M97.3- ☑
    specified joint NEC M97.8 ☑
    spine M97.8 ☑
    toe M97.8 ☑

Fracture, traumatic — *continued*
  periprosthetic, around internal prosthetic joint —
        continued
    wrist M97.8 ☑
  phalanx
    foot — *see* Fracture, toe
    hand — *see* Fracture, finger
  pisiform — *see* Fracture, carpal, pisiform
  pond — *see* Fracture, skull
  prosthetic device, internal — *see* Complications,
        prosthetic device, by site, mechanical
  pubis S32.50- ☑
    with disruption of pelvic ring — *see* Disruption,
          pelvic ring
    specified site NEC S32.59- ☑
    superior rim S32.51- ☑
  radius S52.9- ☑
    distal end — *see* Fracture, radius, lower end
    following insertion of implant, prosthesis or plate
          M96.63- ☑
    head — *see* Fracture, radius, upper end, head
    lower end S52.50- ☑
      Barton's — *see* Barton's fracture
      Colles' — *see* Colles' fracture
      extraarticular NEC S52.55- ☑
      intraarticular NEC S52.57- ☑
      physeal S59.20- ☑
        Salter-Harris
          Type I S59.21- ☑
          Type II S59.22- ☑
          Type III S59.23- ☑
          Type IV S59.24- ☑
        specified NEC S59.29- ☑
      Smith's — *see* Smith's fracture
      specified NEC S52.59- ☑
      styloid process (displaced) S52.51- ☑
        nondisplaced S52.51- ☑
      torus S52.52- ☑
    neck — *see* Fracture, radius, upper end
    proximal end — *see* Fracture, radius, upper end
    shaft S52.30- ☑
      bent bone S52.38- ☑
      comminuted (displaced) S52.35- ☑
        nondisplaced S52.35- ☑
      Galeazzi's — *see* Galeazzi's fracture
      greenstick S52.31- ☑
      oblique (displaced) S52.33- ☑
        nondisplaced S52.33- ☑
      segmental (displaced) S52.36- ☑
        nondisplaced S52.36- ☑
      specified NEC S52.39- ☑
      spiral (displaced) S52.34- ☑
        nondisplaced S52.34- ☑
      transverse (displaced) S52.32- ☑
        nondisplaced S52.32- ☑
    upper end S52.10- ☑
      head (displaced) S52.12- ☑
        nondisplaced S52.12- ☑
      neck (displaced) S52.13- ☑
        nondisplaced S52.13- ☑
      physeal S59.10- ☑
        Salter-Harris
          Type I S59.11- ☑
          Type II S59.12- ☑
          Type III S59.13- ☑
          Type IV S59.14- ☑
        specified NEC S59.19- ☑
      specified NEC S52.18- ☑
      torus S52.11- ☑
  ramus
    inferior or superior, pubis — *see* Fracture, pubis
    mandible — *see* Fracture, mandible
  restorative material (dental) K08.539
    with loss of material K08.531
    without loss of material K08.530
  rib S22.3- ☑
    with flail chest — *see* Flail, chest
    multiple S22.4- ☑
      with flail chest — *see* Flail, chest
  root, tooth — *see* Fracture, tooth
  sacrum S32.10 ☑
    specified NEC S32.19 ☑
    Type
      1 S32.14 ☑
      2 S32.15 ☑
      3 S32.16 ☑

Fracture, traumatic — *continued*
  sacrum — *continued*
    Type — *continued*
      4 S32.17 ☑
    Zone
      I S32.119 ☑
        displaced (minimally) S32.111 ☑
          severely S32.112 ☑
        nondisplaced S32.110 ☑
      II S32.129 ☑
        displaced (minimally) S32.121 ☑
          severely S32.122 ☑
        nondisplaced S32.120 ☑
      III S32.139 ☑
        displaced (minimally) S32.131 ☑
          severely S32.132 ☑
        nondisplaced S32.130 ☑
  scaphoid (hand) (*see also* Fracture, carpal, navicular)
    foot — *see* Fracture, tarsal, navicular
  scapula S42.10- ☑
    acromial process (displaced) S42.12- ☑
      nondisplaced S42.12- ☑
    body (displaced) S42.11- ☑
      nondisplaced S42.11- ☑
    coracoid process (displaced) S42.13- ☑
      nondisplaced S42.13- ☑
    glenoid cavity (displaced) S42.14- ☑
      nondisplaced S42.14- ☑
    neck (displaced) S42.15- ☑
      nondisplaced S42.15- ☑
    specified NEC S42.19- ☑
  semilunar bone, wrist — *see* Fracture, carpal, lunate
  sequelae — *see* Sequelae, fracture
  sesamoid bone
    foot S92.81- ☑
    hand — *see* Fracture, carpal
    other — *see* Fracture, traumatic, by site
  shepherd's — *see* Fracture, tarsal, talus
  shoulder (girdle) S42.9- ☑
    blade — *see* Fracture, scapula
  sinus (ethmoid) (frontal) S02.19 ☑
  skull S02.91 ☑
    base S02.10- ☑
      occiput S02.119 ☑
        condyle S02.113 ☑
          specified NEC S02.118 ☑
            left side S02.11H ☑
            right side S02.11G ☑
          type I S02.110 ☑
            left side S02.11B ☑
            right side S02.11A ☑
          type II S02.111 ☑
            left side S02.11D ☑
            right side S02.11C ☑
          type III S02.112 ☑
            left side S02.11F ☑
            right side S02.11E ☑
      specified NEC S02.19 ☑
    birth injury P13.0
    frontal bone S02.0 ☑
    parietal bone S02.0 ☑
    specified site NEC S02.8- ☑
    temporal bone S02.19 ☑
    vault S02.0 ☑
  Smith's — *see* Smith's fracture
  sphenoid (bone) (sinus) S02.19 ☑
  spine — *see* Fracture, vertebra
  spinous process — *see* Fracture, vertebra
  spontaneous (cause unknown) — *see* Fracture,
        pathological
  stave (of thumb) — *see* Fracture, metacarpal, first
  sternum S22.20 ☑
    with flail chest — *see* Flail, chest
    body S22.22 ☑
    manubrium S22.21 ☑
    xiphoid (process) S22.24 ☑
  stress M84.30 ☑
    ankle M84.37- ☑
    carpus M84.34- ☑
    clavicle M84.31- ☑
    femoral neck M84.359 ☑
    femur M84.35- ☑
    fibula M84.36- ☑
    finger M84.34- ☑
    hip M84.359 ☑
    humerus M84.32- ☑

Fracture, traumatic — *continued*
  stress — *continued*
    ilium M84.350 ☑
    ischium M84.350 ☑
    metacarpus M84.34- ☑
    metatarsus M84.37- ☑
    neck — *see* Fracture, fatigue, vertebra
    pelvis M84.350 ☑
    radius M84.33- ☑
    rib M84.38 ☑
    scapula M84.31- ☑
    skull M84.38 ☑
    tarsus M84.37- ☑
    tibia M84.36- ☑
    toe M84.37- ☑
    ulna M84.33- ☑
    vertebra — *see* Fracture, fatigue, vertebra
  supracondylar, elbow — *see* Fracture, humerus, lower
        end, supracondylar
  symphysis pubis — *see* Fracture, pubis
  talus (ankle bone) — *see* Fracture, tarsal, talus
  tarsal bone(s) S92.20- ☑
    astragalus — *see* Fracture, tarsal, talus
    calcaneus S92.00- ☑
      anterior process (displaced) S92.02- ☑
        nondisplaced S92.02- ☑
      body (displaced) S92.01- ☑
        nondisplaced S92.01- ☑
      extraarticular NEC (displaced) S92.05- ☑
        nondisplaced S92.05- ☑
      intraarticular (displaced) S92.06- ☑
        nondisplaced S92.06- ☑
      physeal S99.00- ☑
        Salter-Harris
          Type I S99.01- ☑
          Type II S99.02- ☑
          Type III S99.03- ☑
          Type IV S99.04- ☑
        specified NEC S99.09- ☑
      tuberosity (displaced) S92.04- ☑
        avulsion (displaced) S92.03- ☑
          nondisplaced S92.03- ☑
        nondisplaced S92.04- ☑
    cuboid (displaced) S92.21- ☑
      nondisplaced S92.21- ☑
    cuneiform
      intermediate (displaced) S92.23- ☑
        nondisplaced S92.23- ☑
      lateral (displaced) S92.22- ☑
        nondisplaced S92.22- ☑
      medial (displaced) S92.24- ☑
        nondisplaced S92.24- ☑
    navicular (displaced) S92.25- ☑
      nondisplaced S92.25- ☑
    scaphoid — *see* Fracture, tarsal, navicular
    talus S92.10- ☑
      avulsion (displaced) S92.15- ☑
        nondisplaced S92.15- ☑
      body (displaced) S92.12- ☑
        nondisplaced S92.12- ☑
      dome (displaced) S92.14- ☑
        nondisplaced S92.14- ☑
      head (displaced) S92.12- ☑
        nondisplaced S92.12- ☑
      lateral process (displaced) S92.14- ☑
        nondisplaced S92.14- ☑
      neck (displaced) S92.11- ☑
        nondisplaced S92.11- ☑
      posterior process (displaced) S92.13- ☑
        nondisplaced S92.13- ☑
      specified NEC S92.19- ☑
  temporal bone (styloid) S02.19 ☑
  thorax (bony) S22.9 ☑
    with flail chest — *see* Flail, chest
    rib S22.3- ☑
      multiple S22.4- ☑
        with flail chest — *see* Flail, chest
    sternum S22.20 ☑
      body S22.22 ☑
      manubrium S22.21 ☑
      xiphoid process S22.24 ☑
    vertebra (displaced) S22.009 ☑
      burst (stable) S22.001 ☑
        unstable S22.002 ☑
      eighth S22.069 ☑
        burst (stable) S22.061 ☑

Fracture, traumatic — Fracture, traumatic

Fracture, traumatic — *continued*
  thorax — *continued*
    vertebra — *continued*
      eighth — *continued*
        burst — *continued*
          unstable S22.062 ☑
        specified type NEC S22.068 ☑
        wedge compression S22.060 ☑
      eleventh S22.089 ☑
        burst (stable) S22.081 ☑
          unstable S22.082 ☑
        specified type NEC S22.088 ☑
        wedge compression S22.080 ☑
      fifth S22.059 ☑
        burst (stable) S22.051 ☑
          unstable S22.052 ☑
        specified type NEC S22.058 ☑
        wedge compression S22.050 ☑
      first S22.019 ☑
        burst (stable) S22.011 ☑
          unstable S22.012 ☑
        specified type NEC S22.018 ☑
        wedge compression S22.010 ☑
      fourth S22.049 ☑
        burst (stable) S22.041 ☑
          unstable S22.042 ☑
        specified type NEC S22.048 ☑
        wedge compression S22.040 ☑
      ninth S22.079 ☑
        burst (stable) S22.071 ☑
          unstable S22.072 ☑
        specified type NEC S22.078 ☑
        wedge compression S22.070 ☑
      nondisplaced S22.001 ☑
      second S22.029 ☑
        burst (stable) S22.021 ☑
          unstable S22.022 ☑
        specified type NEC S22.028 ☑
        wedge compression S22.020 ☑
      seventh S22.069 ☑
        burst (stable) S22.061 ☑
          unstable S22.062 ☑
        specified type NEC S22.068 ☑
        wedge compression S22.060 ☑
      sixth S22.059 ☑
        burst (stable) S22.051 ☑
          unstable S22.052 ☑
        specified type NEC S22.058 ☑
        wedge compression S22.050 ☑
      specified type NEC S22.008 ☑
      tenth S22.079 ☑
        burst (stable) S22.071 ☑
          unstable S22.072 ☑
        specified type NEC S22.078 ☑
        wedge compression S22.070 ☑
      third S22.039 ☑
        burst (stable) S22.031 ☑
          unstable S22.032 ☑
        specified type NEC S22.038 ☑
        wedge compression S22.030 ☑
      twelfth S22.089 ☑
        burst (stable) S22.081 ☑
          unstable S22.082 ☑
        specified type NEC S22.088 ☑
        wedge compression S22.080 ☑
      wedge compression S22.000 ☑
  thumb S62.50- ☑
    distal phalanx (displaced) S62.52- ☑
      nondisplaced S62.52- ☑
    proximal phalanx (displaced) S62.51- ☑
      nondisplaced S62.51- ☑
  thyroid cartilage S12.8 ☑
  tibia (shaft) S82.20- ☑
    comminuted (displaced) S82.25- ☑
      nondisplaced S82.25- ☑
    condyles — *see* Fracture, tibia, upper end
    distal end — *see* Fracture, tibia, lower end
    epiphysis
      lower — *see* Fracture, tibia, lower end
      upper — *see* Fracture, tibia, upper end
    following insertion of implant, prosthesis or plate
      M96.67- ☑
    head (involving knee joint) — *see* Fracture, tibia,
      upper end
    intercondyloid eminence — *see* Fracture, tibia,
      upper end

Fracture, traumatic — *continued*
  tibia — *continued*
    involving ankle or malleolus — *see* Fracture, ankle,
      medial malleolus
    lower end S82.30- ☑
      physeal S89.10- ☑
        Salter-Harris
          Type I S89.11- ☑
          Type II S89.12- ☑
          Type III S89.13- ☑
          Type IV S89.14- ☑
        specified NEC S89.19- ☑
      pilon (displaced) S82.87- ☑
        nondisplaced S82.87- ☑
      specified NEC S82.39- ☑
      torus S82.31- ☑
    malleolus — *see* Fracture, ankle, medial malleolus
    oblique (displaced) S82.23- ☑
      nondisplaced S82.23- ☑
    pilon — *see* Fracture, tibia, lower end, pilon
    proximal end — *see* Fracture, tibia, upper end
    segmental (displaced) S82.26- ☑
      nondisplaced S82.26- ☑
    specified NEC S82.29- ☑
    spine — *see* Fracture, tibia, upper end, spine
    spiral (displaced) S82.24- ☑
      nondisplaced S82.24- ☑
    transverse (displaced) S82.22- ☑
      nondisplaced S82.22- ☑
    tuberosity — *see* Fracture, tibia, upper end,
      tuberosity
    upper end S82.10- ☑
      bicondylar (displaced) S82.14- ☑
        nondisplaced S82.14- ☑
      lateral condyle (displaced) S82.12- ☑
        nondisplaced S82.12- ☑
      medial condyle (displaced) S82.13- ☑
        nondisplaced S82.13- ☑
      physeal S89.00- ☑
        Salter-Harris
          Type I S89.01- ☑
          Type II S89.02- ☑
          Type III S89.03- ☑
          Type IV S89.04- ☑
        specified NEC S89.09- ☑
      plateau — *see* Fracture, tibia, upper end, bi-
        condylar
      specified NEC S82.19- ☑
      spine (displaced) S82.11- ☑
        nondisplaced S82.11- ☑
      torus S82.16- ☑
      tuberosity (displaced) S82.15- ☑
        nondisplaced S82.15- ☑
  toe S92.91- ☑
    great (displaced) S92.40- ☑
      distal phalanx (displaced) S92.42- ☑
        nondisplaced S92.42- ☑
      nondisplaced S92.40- ☑
      proximal phalanx (displaced) S92.41- ☑
        nondisplaced S92.41- ☑
      specified NEC S92.49- ☑
    lesser (displaced) S92.50- ☑
      distal phalanx (displaced) S92.53- ☑
        nondisplaced S92.53- ☑
      medial phalanx (displaced) S92.52- ☑
        nondisplaced S92.52- ☑
      nondisplaced S92.50- ☑
      proximal phalanx (displaced) S92.51- ☑
        nondisplaced S92.51- ☑
      specified NEC S92.59- ☑
    physeal
      phalanx S99.20- ☑
        Salter-Harris
          Type I S99.21- ☑
          Type II S99.22- ☑
          Type III S99.23- ☑
          Type IV S99.24- ☑
        specified NEC S99.29- ☑
  tooth (root) S02.5 ☑
  trachea (cartilage) S12.8 ☑
  transverse process — *see* Fracture, vertebra
  trapezium or trapezoid bone — *see* Fracture, carpal
  trimalleolar — *see* Fracture, ankle, trimalleolar
  triquetrum (cuneiform of carpus) — *see* Fracture,
    carpal, triquetrum
  trochanter — *see* Fracture, femur, trochanteric

Fracture, traumatic — *continued*
  tuberosity (external) — *see* Fracture, traumatic, by site
  ulna (shaft) S52.20- ☑
    bent bone S52.28- ☑
    coronoid process — *see* Fracture, ulna, upper end,
      coronoid process
    distal end — *see* Fracture, ulna, lower end
    following insertion of implant, prosthesis or plate
      M96.63- ☑
    head S52.60- ☑
    lower end S52.60- ☑
      physeal S59.00- ☑
        Salter-Harris
          Type I S59.01- ☑
          Type II S59.02- ☑
          Type III S59.03- ☑
          Type IV S59.04- ☑
        specified NEC S59.09- ☑
      specified NEC S52.69- ☑
      styloid process (displaced) S52.61- ☑
        nondisplaced S52.61- ☑
      torus S52.62- ☑
    proximal end — *see* Fracture, ulna, upper end
    shaft S52.20- ☑
      comminuted (displaced) S52.25- ☑
        nondisplaced S52.25- ☑
      greenstick S52.21- ☑
      Monteggia's — *see* Monteggia's fracture
      oblique (displaced) S52.23- ☑
        nondisplaced S52.23- ☑
      segmental (displaced) S52.26- ☑
        nondisplaced S52.26- ☑
      specified NEC S52.29- ☑
      spiral (displaced) S52.24- ☑
        nondisplaced S52.24- ☑
      transverse (displaced) S52.22- ☑
        nondisplaced S52.22- ☑
    upper end S52.00- ☑
      coronoid process (displaced) S52.04- ☑
        nondisplaced S52.04- ☑
      olecranon process (displaced) S52.02- ☑
        with intraarticular extension S52.03- ☑
        nondisplaced S52.02- ☑
          with intraarticular extension S52.03- ☑
      specified NEC S52.09- ☑
      torus S52.01- ☑
  unciform — *see* Fracture, carpal, hamate
  vault of skull S02.0 ☑
  vertebra, vertebral (arch) (body) (column) (neural arch)
    (pedicle) (spinous process) (transverse process)
    atlas — *see* Fracture, neck, cervical vertebra, first
    axis — *see* Fracture, neck, cervical vertebra, second
    cervical (teardrop) S12.9 ☑
      axis — *see* Fracture, neck, cervical vertebra,
        second
      first (atlas) — *see* Fracture, neck, cervical verte-
        bra, first
      second (axis) — *see* Fracture, neck, cervical
        vertebra, second
    chronic M84.48 ☑
    coccyx S32.2 ☑
    dorsal — *see* Fracture, thorax, vertebra
    lumbar S32.009 ☑
      burst (stable) S32.001 ☑
        unstable S32.002 ☑
      fifth S32.059 ☑
        burst (stable) S32.051 ☑
          unstable S32.052 ☑
        specified type NEC S32.058 ☑
        wedge compression S32.050 ☑
      first S32.019 ☑
        burst (stable) S32.011 ☑
          unstable S32.012 ☑
        specified type NEC S32.018 ☑
        wedge compression S32.010 ☑
      fourth S32.049 ☑
        burst (stable) S32.041 ☑
          unstable S32.042 ☑
        specified type NEC S32.048 ☑
        wedge compression S32.040 ☑
      second S32.029 ☑
        burst (stable) S32.021 ☑
          unstable S32.022 ☑
        specified type NEC S32.028 ☑
        wedge compression S32.020 ☑
      specified type NEC S32.008 ☑

Fracture, traumatic — *continued*
  vertebra, vertebral — *continued*
    lumbar — *continued*
      third S32.039 ☑
        burst (stable) S32.031 ☑
          unstable S32.032 ☑
        specified type NEC S32.038 ☑
        wedge compression S32.030 ☑
      wedge compression S32.000 ☑
      metastatic — *see* Collapse, vertebra, in, specified
        disease NEC (*see also* Neoplasm)
    newborn (birth injury) P11.5
    sacrum S32.10 ☑
      specified NEC S32.19 ☑
      Type
        1 S32.14 ☑
        2 S32.15 ☑
        3 S32.16 ☑
        4 S32.17 ☑
      Zone
        I S32.119 ☑
          displaced (minimally) S32.111 ☑
            severely S32.112 ☑
          nondisplaced S32.110 ☑
        II S32.129 ☑
          displaced (minimally) S32.121 ☑
            severely S32.122 ☑
          nondisplaced S32.120 ☑
        III S32.139 ☑
          displaced (minimally) S32.131 ☑
            severely S32.132 ☑
          nondisplaced S32.130 ☑
    thoracic — *see* Fracture, thorax, vertebra
  vertex S02.0 ☑
  vomer (bone) S02.2 ☑
  wrist S62.10- ☑
    carpal — *see* Fracture, carpal bone
    navicular (scaphoid) (hand) — *see* Fracture, carpal,
      navicular
  xiphisternum, xiphoid (process) S22.24 ☑
  zygoma S02.402 ☑
    left side S02.40F ☑
    right side S02.40E ☑
Fragile, fragility
  autosomal site Q95.5
  bone, congenital (with blue sclera) Q78.0
  capillary (hereditary) D69.8
  hair L67.8
  nails L60.3
  non-sex chromosome site Q95.5
  X chromosome Q99.2
Fragilitas
  crinium L67.8
  ossium (with blue sclerae) (hereditary) Q78.0
  unguium L60.3
    congenital Q84.6
Fragments, cataract (lens), **following cataract surgery**
  H59.02- ☑
  retained foreign body — *see* Retained, foreign body
    fragments (type of)
Frailty (frail) R54
  mental R41.81
Frambesia, frambesial (tropica) (*see also* Yaws)
  initial lesion or ulcer A66.0
  primary A66.0
Frambeside
  gummatous A66.4
  of early yaws A66.2
Frambesioma A66.1
Franceschetti-Klein (-Wildervanck) **disease or syndrome** Q75.4
Francis' disease — *see* Tularemia
Franklin disease C88.2
Frank's essential thrombocytopenia D69.3
Fraser's syndrome Q87.0
Freckle(s) L81.2
  malignant melanoma in — *see* Melanoma
  melanotic (Hutchinson's) — *see* Melanoma, in situ
  retinal D49.81
Frederickson's hyperlipoproteinemia, type
  I and V E78.3
  IIA E78.00
  IIB and III E78.2
  IV E78.1
Freeman Sheldon syndrome Q87.0
Freezing (*see also* Effect, adverse, cold) T69.9 ☑

Freiberg's disease (infraction of metatarsal head or osteochondrosis) — *see* Osteochondrosis, juvenile, metatarsus
Frei's disease A55
Fremitus, friction, cardiac R01.2
Frenum, frenulum
  external os Q51.828
  tongue (shortening) (congenital) Q38.1
Frequency micturition (nocturnal) R35.0
  psychogenic F45.8
Frey's syndrome
  auriculotemporal G50.8
  hyperhidrosis L74.52
Friction
  burn — *see* Burn, by site
  fremitus, cardiac R01.2
  precordial R01.2
  sounds, chest R09.89
Friderichsen-Waterhouse syndrome or disease A39.1
Friedländer's B (bacillus) **NEC** (*see also* condition) A49.8
Friedreich's
  ataxia G11.1
  combined systemic disease G11.1
  facial hemihypertrophy Q67.4
  sclerosis (cerebellum) (spinal cord) G11.1
Frigidity F52.22
Fröhlich's syndrome E23.6
Frontal (*see also* condition)
  lobe syndrome F07.0
Frostbite (superficial) T33.90 ☑
  with
    partial thickness skin loss — *see* Frostbite (superficial), by site
    tissue necrosis T34.90 ☑
  abdominal wall T33.3
    with tissue necrosis T34.3 ☑
  ankle T33.81- ☑
    with tissue necrosis T34.81- ☑
  arm T33.4- ☑
    with tissue necrosis T34.4- ☑
    finger(s) — *see* Frostbite, finger
    hand — *see* Frostbite, hand
    wrist — *see* Frostbite, wrist
  ear T33.01- ☑
    with tissue necrosis T34.01- ☑
  face T33.09 ☑
    with tissue necrosis T34.09 ☑
  finger T33.53- ☑
    with tissue necrosis T34.53- ☑
  foot T33.82- ☑
    with tissue necrosis T34.82- ☑
  hand T33.52- ☑
    with tissue necrosis T34.52- ☑
  head T33.09 ☑
    with tissue necrosis T34.09 ☑
    ear — *see* Frostbite, ear
    nose — *see* Frostbite, nose
  hip (and thigh) T33.6- ☑
    with tissue necrosis T34.6- ☑
  knee T33.7- ☑
    with tissue necrosis T34.7- ☑
  leg T33.9- ☑
    with tissue necrosis T34.9- ☑
    ankle — *see* Frostbite, ankle
    foot — *see* Frostbite, foot
    knee — *see* Frostbite, knee
    lower T33.7- ☑
      with tissue necrosis T34.7- ☑
    thigh — *see* Frostbite, hip
    toe — *see* Frostbite, toe
  limb
    lower T33.99 ☑
      with tissue necrosis T34.99 ☑
    upper — *see* Frostbite, arm
  neck T33.1 ☑
    with tissue necrosis T34.1 ☑
  nose T33.02 ☑
    with tissue necrosis T34.02 ☑
  pelvis T33.3 ☑
    with tissue necrosis T34.3 ☑
  specified site NEC T33.99 ☑
    with tissue necrosis T34.99 ☑
  thigh — *see* Frostbite, hip
  thorax T33.2 ☑
    with tissue necrosis T34.2 ☑
  toes T33.83- ☑

Frostbite — *continued*
  toes — *continued*
    with tissue necrosis T34.83- ☑
  trunk T33.99
    with tissue necrosis T34.99 ☑
  wrist T33.51- ☑
    with tissue necrosis T34.51- ☑
Frotteurism F65.81
Frozen (*see also* Effect, adverse, cold) T69.9 ☑
  pelvis (female) N94.89
    male K66.8
  shoulder — *see* Capsulitis, adhesive
Fructokinase deficiency E74.11
Fructose 1,6 diphosphatase deficiency E74.19
Fructosemia (benign) (essential) E74.12
Fructosuria (benign) (essential) E74.11
Fuchs'
  black spot (myopic) (*see also* Myopia, degenerative) H44.2- ☑
  dystrophy (corneal endothelium) H18.51
  heterochromic cyclitis — *see* Cyclitis, Fuchs' heterochromic
Fucosidosis E77.1
Fugue R68.89
  dissociative F44.1
  hysterical (dissociative) F44.1
  postictal in epilepsy — *see* Epilepsy
  reaction to exceptional stress (transient) F43.0
Fulminant, fulminating — *see* condition
Functional (*see also* condition)
  bleeding (uterus) N93.8
Functioning, intellectual, borderline R41.83
Fundus — *see* condition
Fungemia NOS B49
Fungus, fungous
  cerebral G93.89
  disease NOS B49
  infection — *see* Infection, fungus
Funiculitis (acute) (chronic) (endemic) N49.1
  gonococcal (acute) (chronic) A54.23
  tuberculous A18.15
Funnel
  breast (acquired) M95.4
    congenital Q67.6
    sequelae (late effect) of rickets E64.3
  chest (acquired) M95.4
    congenital Q67.6
    sequelae (late effect) of rickets E64.3
  pelvis (acquired) M95.5
    with disproportion (fetopelvic) O33.3 ☑
      causing obstructed labor O65.3
    congenital Q74.2
FUO (fever of unknown origin) R50.9
Furfur L21.0
  microsporon B36.0
Furrier's lung J67.8
Furrowed K14.5
  nail(s) (transverse) L60.4
    congenital Q84.6
  tongue K14.5
    congenital Q38.3
Furuncle L02.92
  abdominal wall L02.221
  ankle — *see* Furuncle, lower limb
  antecubital space — *see* Furuncle, upper limb
  anus K61.0
  arm — *see* Furuncle, upper limb
  auditory canal, external — *see* Abscess, ear, external
  auricle (ear) — *see* Abscess, ear, external
  axilla (region) L02.42- ☑
  back (any part) L02.222
  breast N61.1
  buttock L02.32
  cheek (external) L02.02
  chest wall L02.223
  chin L02.02
  corpus cavernosum N48.21
  ear, external — *see* Abscess, ear, external
  external auditory canal — *see* Abscess, ear, external
  eyelid — *see* Abscess, eyelid
  face L02.02
  femoral (region) — *see* Furuncle, lower limb
  finger — *see* Furuncle, hand
  flank L02.221
  foot L02.62- ☑
  forehead L02.02
  gluteal (region) L02.32

▽ Subterms under main terms may continue to next column or page   ☑ Additional Character Required — Refer to the Tabular List for Character Selection   155

Fracture, traumatic — Furuncle

Furuncle — *continued*
  groin L02.224
  hand L02.52- ☑
  head L02.821
    face L02.02
  hip — *see* Furuncle, lower limb
  kidney — *see* Abscess, kidney
  knee — *see* Furuncle, lower limb
  labium (majus) (minus) N76.4
  lacrimal
    gland — *see* Dacryoadenitis
    passages (duct) (sac) — *see* Inflammation, lacrimal, passages, acute
  leg (any part) — *see* Furuncle, lower limb
  lower limb L02.42- ☑
  malignant A22.0
  mouth K12.2
  navel L02.226
  neck L02.12
  nose J34.0
  orbit, orbital — *see* Abscess, orbit
  palmar (space) — *see* Furuncle, hand
  partes posteriores L02.32
  pectoral region L02.223
  penis N48.21
  perineum L02.225
  pinna — *see* Abscess, ear, external
  popliteal — *see* Furuncle, lower limb
  prepatellar — *see* Furuncle, lower limb
  scalp L02.821
  seminal vesicle N49.0
  shoulder — *see* Furuncle, upper limb
  specified site NEC L02.828
  submandibular K12.2
  temple (region) L02.02
  thumb — *see* Furuncle, hand
  toe — *see* Furuncle, foot
  trunk L02.229
    abdominal wall L02.221
    back L02.222

Furuncle — *continued*
  trunk — *continued*
    chest wall L02.223
    groin L02.224
    perineum L02.225
    umbilicus L02.226
  umbilicus L02.226
  upper limb L02.42- ☑
  vulva N76.4
Furunculosis — *see* Furuncle
Fused — *see* Fusion, fused
Fusion, fused (congenital)
  astragaloscaphoid Q74.2
  atria Q21.1
  auditory canal Q16.1
  auricles, heart Q21.1
  binocular with defective stereopsis H53.32
  bone Q79.8
  cervical spine M43.22
  choanal Q30.0
  commissure, mitral valve Q23.2
  cusps, heart valve NEC Q24.8
    mitral Q23.2
    pulmonary Q22.1
    tricuspid Q22.4
  ear ossicles Q16.3
  fingers Q70.0 ☑
  hymen Q52.3
  joint (acquired) (*see also* Ankylosis)
    congenital Q74.8
  kidneys (incomplete) Q63.1
  labium (majus) (minus) Q52.5
  larynx and trachea Q34.8
  limb, congenital Q74.8
    lower Q74.2
    upper Q74.0
  lobes, lung Q33.8
  lumbosacral (acquired) M43.27
    arthrodesis status Z98.1
    congenital Q76.49

Fusion, fused — *continued*
  lumbosacral — *continued*
    postprocedural status Z98.1
  nares, nose, nasal, nostril(s) Q30.0
  organ or site not listed — *see* Anomaly, by site
  ossicles Q79.9
    auditory Q16.3
  pulmonic cusps Q22.1
  ribs Q76.6
  sacroiliac (joint) (acquired) M43.28
    arthrodesis status Z98.1
    congenital Q74.2
    postprocedural status Z98.1
  spine (acquired) NEC M43.20
    arthrodesis status Z98.1
    cervical region M43.22
    cervicothoracic region M43.23
    congenital Q76.49
    lumbar M43.26
    lumbosacral region M43.27
    occipito-atlanto-axial region M43.21
    postoperative status Z98.1
    sacrococcygeal region M43.28
    thoracic region M43.24
    thoracolumbar region M43.25
  sublingual duct with submaxillary duct at opening in mouth Q38.4
  testes Q55.1
  toes Q70.2- ☑
  tooth, teeth K00.2
  trachea and esophagus Q39.8
  twins Q89.4
  vagina Q52.4
  ventricles, heart Q21.0
  vertebra (arch) — *see* Fusion, spine
  vulva Q52.5
Fusospirillosis (mouth) (tongue) (tonsil) A69.1
Fussy baby R68.12

Furuncle — Fussy baby

G

Gain in weight (abnormal) (excessive) (*see also* Weight, gain)
Gaisböck's disease (polycythemia hypertonica) D75.1
Gait abnormality R26.9
  ataxic R26.0
  falling R29.6
  hysterical (ataxic) (staggering) F44.4
  paralytic R26.1
  spastic R26.1
  specified type NEC R26.89
  staggering R26.0
  unsteadiness R26.81
  walking difficulty NEC R26.2
Galactocele (breast) N64.89
  puerperal, postpartum O92.79
Galactokinase deficiency E74.29
Galactophoritis N61.0
  gestational, puerperal, postpartum O91.2- ☑
Galactorrhea O92.6
  not associated with childbirth N64.3
Galactosemia (classic) (congenital) E74.21
Galactosuria E74.29
Galacturia R82.0
  schistosomiasis (bilharziasis) B65.0
GALD (gestational alloimmune liver disease) P78.84
Galeazzi's fracture S52.37- ☑
Galen's vein — *see* condition
Galeophobia F40.218
Gall duct — *see* condition
Gallbladder (*see also* condition)
  acute K81.0
Gallop rhythm R00.8
Gallstone (colic) (cystic duct) (gallbladder) (impacted) (multiple) (*see also* Calculus, gallbladder)
  with
    cholecystitis — *see* Calculus, gallbladder, with cholecystitis
  bile duct (common) (hepatic) — *see* Calculus, bile duct
  causing intestinal obstruction K56.3
  specified NEC K80.80
    with obstruction K80.81
Gambling Z72.6
  pathological (compulsive) F63.0
Gammopathy (of undetermined significance [MGUS]) D47.2
  associated with lymphoplasmacytic dyscrasia D47.2
  monoclonal D47.2
  polyclonal D89.0
Gamna's disease (siderotic splenomegaly) D73.1
Gamophobia F40.298
Gampsodactylia (congenital) Q66.7
Gamstorp's disease (adynamia episodica hereditaria) G72.3
Gandy-Nanta disease (siderotic splenomegaly) D73.1
Gang
  membership offenses Z72.810
Gangliocytoma D36.10
Ganglioglioma — *see* Neoplasm, uncertain behavior, by site
Ganglion (compound) (diffuse) (joint) (tendon (sheath)) M67.40
  ankle M67.47- ☑
  foot M67.47- ☑
  forearm M67.43- ☑
  hand M67.44- ☑
  lower leg M67.46- ☑
  multiple sites M67.49
  of yaws (early) (late) A66.6
  pelvic region M67.45- ☑
  periosteal — *see* Periostitis
  shoulder region M67.41- ☑
  specified site NEC M67.48
  thigh region M67.45- ☑
  tuberculous A18.09
  upper arm M67.42- ☑
  wrist M67.43- ☑
Ganglioneuroblastoma — *see* Neoplasm, nerve, malignant
Ganglioneuroma D36.10
  malignant — *see* Neoplasm, nerve, malignant
Ganglioneuromatosis D36.10
Ganglionitis
  fifth nerve — *see* Neuralgia, trigeminal
  gasserian (postherpetic) (postzoster) B02.21

Ganglionitis — *continued*
  geniculate G51.1
    newborn (birth injury) P11.3
    postherpetic, postzoster B02.21
  herpes zoster B02.21
  postherpetic geniculate B02.21
Gangliosidosis E75.10
  GM1 E75.19
  GM2 E75.00
    other specified E75.09
    Sandhoff disease E75.01
    Tay-Sachs disease E75.02
  GM3 E75.19
  mucolipidosis IV E75.11
Gangosa A66.5
Gangrene, gangrenous (connective tissue) (dropsical) (dry) (moist) (skin) (ulcer) (*see also* Necrosis) I96
  with diabetes (mellitus) — *see* Diabetes, gangrene
  abdomen (wall) I96
  alveolar M27.3
  appendix K35.80
    with
      perforation or rupture K35.2
      peritoneal abscess K35.3
      peritonitis NEC K35.3
        generalized (with perforation or rupture) K35.2
        localized (with perforation or rupture) K35.3
  arteriosclerotic (general) (senile) — *see* Arteriosclerosis, extremities, with, gangrene
  auricle I96
  Bacillus welchii A48.0
  bladder (infectious) — *see* Cystitis, specified type NEC
  bowel, cecum, or colon — *see* Gangrene, intestine
  Clostridium perfringens or welchii A48.0
  cornea H18.89- ☑
  corpora cavernosa N48.29
    noninfective N48.89
  cutaneous, spreading I96
  decubital — *see* Ulcer, pressure, by site
  diabetic (any site) — *see* Diabetes, gangrene
  emphysematous — *see* Gangrene, gas
  epidemic — *see* Poisoning, food, noxious, plant
  epididymis (infectional) N45.1
  erysipelas — *see* Erysipelas
  extremity (lower) (upper) I96
  Fournier N49.3
    female N76.89
  fusospirochetal A69.0
  gallbladder — *see* Cholecystitis, acute
  gas (bacillus) A48.0
    following
      abortion — *see* Abortion by type complicated by infection
      ectopic or molar pregnancy O08.0
  glossitis K14.0
  hernia — *see* Hernia, by site, with gangrene
  intestine, intestinal (hemorrhagic) (massive) (*see also* Infarct, intestine) K55.069
    with
      mesenteric embolism (*see also* Infarct, intestine) K55.069
      obstruction — *see* Obstruction, intestine
  laryngitis J04.0
  limb (lower) (upper) I96
  lung J85.0
    spirochetal A69.8
  lymphangitis I89.1
  Meleney's (synergistic) — *see* Ulcer, skin
  mesentery (*see also* Infarct, intestine) K55.069
    with
      embolism (*see also* Infarct, intestine) K55.069
      intestinal obstruction — *see* Obstruction, intestine
  mouth A69.0
  ovary — *see* Oophoritis
  pancreas — *see* Pancreatitis, acute
  penis N48.29
    noninfective N48.89
  perineum I96
  pharynx (*see also* Pharyngitis)
    Vincent's A69.1
  presenile I73.1
  progressive synergistic — *see* Ulcer, skin
  pulmonary J85.0
  pulpal (dental) K04.1
  quinsy J36
  Raynaud's (symmetric gangrene) I73.01

Gangrene, gangrenous — *continued*
  retropharyngeal J39.2
  scrotum N49.3
    noninfective N50.89
  senile (atherosclerotic) — *see* Arteriosclerosis, extremities, with, gangrene
  spermatic cord N49.1
    noninfective N50.89
  spine I96
  spirochetal NEC A69.8
  spreading cutaneous I96
  stomatitis A69.0
  symmetrical I73.01
  testis (infectional) N45.2
    noninfective N44.8
  throat (*see also* Pharyngitis)
    diphtheritic A36.0
    Vincent's A69.1
  thyroid (gland) E07.89
  tooth (pulp) K04.1
  tuberculous NEC — *see* Tuberculosis
  tunica vaginalis N49.1
    noninfective N50.89
  umbilicus I96
  uterus — *see* Endometritis
  uvulitis K12.2
  vas deferens N49.1
    noninfective N50.89
  vulva N76.89
Ganister disease J62.8
Ganser's syndrome (hysterical) F44.89
Gardner-Diamond syndrome (autoerythrocyte sensitization) D69.2
Gargoylism E76.01
Garré's disease, osteitis (sclerosing), osteomyelitis — *see* Osteomyelitis, specified type NEC
Garrod's pad, knuckle M72.1
Gartner's duct
  cyst Q52.4
  persistent Q50.6
Gas R14.3
  asphyxiation, inhalation, poisoning, suffocation NEC — *see* Table of Drugs and Chemicals
  excessive R14.0
  gangrene A48.0
    following
      abortion — *see* Abortion by type complicated by infection
      ectopic or molar pregnancy O08.0
  on stomach R14.0
  pains R14.1
Gastralgia (*see also* Pain, abdominal)
Gastrectasis K31.0
  psychogenic F45.8
Gastric — *see* condition
Gastrinoma
  malignant
    pancreas C25.4
    specified site NEC — *see* Neoplasm, malignant, by site
    unspecified site C25.4
  specified site — *see* Neoplasm, uncertain behavior
  unspecified site D37.9
Gastritis (simple) K29.70
  with bleeding K29.71
  acute (erosive) K29.00
    with bleeding K29.01
  alcoholic K29.20
    with bleeding K29.21
  allergic K29.60
    with bleeding K29.61
  atrophic (chronic) K29.40
    with bleeding K29.41
  chronic (antral) (fundal) K29.50
    with bleeding K29.51
    atrophic K29.40
      with bleeding K29.41
    superficial K29.30
      with bleeding K29.31
  dietary counseling and surveillance Z71.3
  due to diet deficiency E63.9
  eosinophilic K52.81
  giant hypertrophic K29.60
    with bleeding K29.61
  granulomatous K29.60
    with bleeding K29.61
  hypertrophic (mucosa) K29.60
    with bleeding K29.61

Gastritis — *continued*
nervous F54
spastic K29.60
with bleeding K29.61
specified NEC K29.60
with bleeding K29.61
superficial chronic K29.30
with bleeding K29.31
tuberculous A18.83
viral NEC A08.4
Gastrocarcinoma — *see* Neoplasm, malignant, stomach
Gastrocolic — *see* condition
Gastrodisciasis, gastrodiscoidiasis B66.8
Gastroduodenitis K29.90
with bleeding K29.91
virus, viral A08.4
specified type NEC A08.39
Gastrodynia — *see* Pain, abdominal
Gastroenteritis (acute) (chronic) (noninfectious) (*see also* Enteritis) K52.9
allergic K52.29
with
eosinophilic gastritis or gastroenteritis K52.81
food protein-induced enterocolitis syndrome K52.21
food protein-induced enteropathy K52.22
dietetic (*see also* Gastroenteritis, allergic) K52.29
drug-induced K52.1
due to
Cryptosporidium A07.2
drugs K52.1
food poisoning — *see* Intoxication, foodborne
radiation K52.0
eosinophilic K52.81
epidemic (infectious) A09
food hypersensitivity (*see also* Gastroenteritis, allergic) K52.29
infectious — *see* Enteritis, infectious
influenzal — *see* Influenza, with gastroenteritis
noninfectious K52.9
specified NEC K52.89
rotaviral A08.0
Salmonella A02.0
toxic K52.1
viral NEC A08.4
acute infectious A08.39
type Norwalk A08.11
infantile (acute) A08.39
Norwalk agent A08.11
rotaviral A08.0
severe of infants A08.39
specified type NEC A08.39
Gastroenteropathy (*see also* Gastroenteritis) K52.9
acute, due to Norovirus A08.11
acute, due to Norwalk agent A08.11
infectious A09
Gastroenteroptosis K63.4
Gastroesophageal laceration- hemorrhage syndrome K22.6
Gastrointestinal — *see* condition
Gastrojejunal — *see* condition
Gastrojejunitis (*see also* Enteritis) K52.9
Gastrojejunocolic — *see* condition
Gastroliths K31.89
Gastromalacia K31.89
Gastroparalysis K31.84
diabetic — *see* Diabetes, gastroparalysis
Gastroparesis K31.84
diabetic — *see* Diabetes, by type, with gastroparesis
Gastropathy K31.9
congestive portal K31.89
erythematous K29.70
exudative K90.89
portal hypertensive K31.89
Gastroptosis K31.89
Gastrorrhagia K92.2
psychogenic F45.8
Gastroschisis (congenital) Q79.3
Gastrospasm (neurogenic) (reflex) K31.89
neurotic F45.8
psychogenic F45.8
Gastrostaxis — *see* Gastritis, with bleeding
Gastrostenosis K31.89
Gastrostomy
attention to Z43.1
status Z93.1
Gastrosuccorrhea (continuous) (intermittent) K31.89
neurotic F45.8

Gastrosuccorrhea — *continued*
psychogenic F45.8
Gatophobia F40.218
Gaucher's disease or splenomegaly (adult) (infantile) E75.22
Gee (-Herter)(-Thaysen) **disease** (nontropical sprue) K90.0
Gélineau's syndrome G47.419
with cataplexy G47.411
Gemination, tooth, teeth K00.2
Gemistocytoma
specified site — *see* Neoplasm, malignant, by site
unspecified site C71.9
General, generalized — *see* condition
Genetic
carrier (status)
cystic fibrosis Z14.1
hemophilia A (asymptomatic) Z14.01
symptomatic Z14.02
specified NEC Z14.8
susceptibility to disease NEC Z15.89
malignant neoplasm Z15.09
breast Z15.01
endometrium Z15.04
ovary Z15.02
prostate Z15.03
specified NEC Z15.09
multiple endocrine neoplasia Z15.81
Genital — *see* condition
Genito-anorectal syndrome A55
Genitourinary system — *see* condition
Genu
congenital Q74.1
extrorsum (acquired) (*see also* Deformity, varus, knee) Q74.1
congenital Q74.1
sequelae (late effect) of rickets E64.3
introrsum (acquired) (*see also* Deformity, valgus, knee) Q74.1
congenital Q74.1
sequelae (late effect) of rickets E64.3
rachitic (old) E64.3
recurvatum (acquired) (*see also* Deformity, limb, specified type NEC, lower leg)
congenital Q68.2
sequelae (late effect) of rickets E64.3
valgum (acquired) (knock-knee) M21.06- ☑
congenital Q74.1
sequelae (late effect) of rickets E64.3
varum (acquired) (bowleg) M21.16- ☑
congenital Q74.1
sequelae (late effect) of rickets E64.3
Geographic tongue K14.1
Geophagia — *see* Pica
Geotrichosis B48.3
stomatitis B48.3
Gephyrophobia F40.242
GERD (gastroesophageal reflux disease) K21.9
Gerhardt's
disease (erythromelalgia) I73.81
syndrome (vocal cord paralysis) J38.00
bilateral J38.02
unilateral J38.01
German measles (*see also* Rubella)
exposure to Z20.4
Germinoblastoma (diffuse) C85.9- ☑
follicular C82.9- ☑
Germinoma — *see* Neoplasm, malignant, by site
Gerontoxon — *see* Degeneration, cornea, senile
Gerstmann's syndrome R48.8
developmental F81.2
Gerstmann-Sträussler-Scheinker syndrome (GSS) A81.82
Gestation (period) (*see also* Pregnancy)
ectopic — *see* Pregnancy, by site
multiple O30.9- ☑
greater than quadruplets — *see* Pregnancy, multiple (gestation), specified NEC
specified NEC — *see* Pregnancy, multiple (gestation), specified NEC
Gestational
mammary abscess O91.11- ☑
purulent mastitis O91.11- ☑
subareolar abscess O91.11- ☑
Ghon tubercle, primary infection A15.7
Ghost
teeth K00.4
vessels (cornea) H16.41- ☑
Ghoul hand A66.3

Gianotti-Crosti disease L44.4
Giant
cell
epulis K06.8
peripheral granuloma K06.8
esophagus, congenital Q39.5
kidney, congenital Q63.3
urticaria T78.3 ☑
hereditary D84.1
Giardiasis A07.1
Gibert's disease or pityriasis L42
Giddiness R42
hysterical F44.89
psychogenic F45.8
Gierke's disease (glycogenosis I) E74.01
Gigantism (cerebral) (hypophyseal) (pituitary) E22.0
constitutional E34.4
Gilbert's disease or syndrome E80.4
Gilchrist's disease B40.9
Gilford-Hutchinson disease E34.8
Gilles de la Tourette's disease or syndrome (motor-verbal tic) F95.2
Gingivitis K05.10
acute (catarrhal) K05.00
necrotizing A69.1
nonplaque induced K05.01
plaque induced K05.00
chronic (desquamative) (hyperplastic) (simple marginal) (pregnancy associated) (ulcerative) K05.10
nonplaque induced K05.11
plaque induced K05.10
expulsiva — *see* Periodontitis
necrotizing ulcerative (acute) A69.1
pellagrous E52
acute necrotizing A69.1
Vincent's A69.1
Gingivoglossitis K14.0
Gingivopericementitis — *see* Periodontitis
Gingivosis — *see* Gingivitis, chronic
Gingivostomatitis K05.10
herpesviral B00.2
necrotizing ulcerative (acute) A69.1
Gland, glandular — *see* condition
Glanders A24.0
Glanzmann (-Naegeli) **disease or thrombasthenia** D69.1
Glasgow coma scale
total score
3-8 R40.243 ☑
9-12 R40.242 ☑
13-15 R40.241 ☑
Glass-blower's disease (cataract) — *see* Cataract, specified NEC
Glaucoma H40.9
with
increased episcleral venous pressure H40.81- ☑
pseudoexfoliation of lens — *see* Glaucoma, open angle, primary, capsular
absolute H44.51- ☑
angle-closure (primary) H40.20- ☑
acute (attack) (crisis) H40.21- ☑
chronic H40.22- ☑
intermittent H40.23- ☑
residual stage H40.24- ☑
borderline H40.00- ☑
capsular (with pseudoexfoliation of lens) — *see* Glaucoma, open angle, primary, capsular
childhood Q15.0
closed angle — *see* Glaucoma, angle-closure
congenital Q15.0
corticosteroid-induced — *see* Glaucoma, secondary, drugs
hypersecretion H40.82- ☑
in (due to)
amyloidosis E85.4 [H42]
aniridia Q13.1 [H42]
concussion of globe — *see* Glaucoma, secondary, trauma
dislocation of lens — *see* Glaucoma, secondary
disorder of lens NEC — *see* Glaucoma, secondary
drugs — *see* Glaucoma, secondary, drugs
endocrine disease NOS E34.9 [H42]
eye
inflammation — *see* Glaucoma, secondary, inflammation
trauma — *see* Glaucoma, secondary, trauma

Glaucoma — *continued*
  in — *continued*
    hypermature cataract — *see* Glaucoma, secondary
    iridocyclitis — *see* Glaucoma, secondary, inflammation
    lens disorder — *see* Glaucoma, secondary
    Lowe's syndrome E72.03 [H42]
    metabolic disease NOS E88.9 [H42]
    ocular disorders NEC — *see* Glaucoma, secondary
    onchocerciasis B73.02
    pupillary block — *see* Glaucoma, secondary
    retinal vein occlusion — *see* Glaucoma, secondary
    Rieger's anomaly Q13.81 [H42]
    rubeosis of iris — *see* Glaucoma, secondary
    tumor of globe — *see* Glaucoma, secondary
  infantile Q15.0
  low tension — *see* Glaucoma, open angle, primary, low-tension
  malignant H40.83- ☑
  narrow angle — *see* Glaucoma, angle-closure
  newborn Q15.0
  noncongestive (chronic) — *see* Glaucoma, open angle
  nonobstructive — *see* Glaucoma, open angle
  obstructive (*see also* Glaucoma, angle-closure)
    due to lens changes — *see* Glaucoma, secondary
  open angle H40.10- ☑
    primary H40.11- ☑
      capsular (with pseudoexfoliation of lens) H40.14- ☑
      low-tension H40.12- ☑
      pigmentary H40.13- ☑
      residual stage H40.15- ☑
  phacolytic — *see* Glaucoma, secondary
  pigmentary — *see* Glaucoma, open angle, primary, pigmentary
  postinfectious — *see* Glaucoma, secondary, inflammation
  secondary (to) H40.5- ☑
    drugs H40.6- ☑
    inflammation H40.4- ☑
    trauma H40.3- ☑
  simple (chronic) H40.11- ☑
  simplex H40.11- ☑
  specified type NEC H40.89
  suspect H40.00- ☑
  syphilitic A52.71
  traumatic (*see also* Glaucoma, secondary, trauma)
    newborn (birth injury) P15.3
  tuberculous A18.59
Glaucomatous flecks (subcapsular) — *see* Cataract, complicated
Glazed tongue K14.4
Gleet (gonococcal) A54.01
Glénard's disease K63.4
Glioblastoma (multiforme)
  with sarcomatous component
    specified site — *see* Neoplasm, malignant, by site
    unspecified site C71.9
  giant cell
    specified site — *see* Neoplasm, malignant, by site
    unspecified site C71.9
  specified site — *see* Neoplasm, malignant, by site
  unspecified site C71.9
Glioma (malignant)
  astrocytic
    specified site — *see* Neoplasm, malignant, by site
    unspecified site C71.9
  mixed
    specified site — *see* Neoplasm, malignant, by site
    unspecified site C71.9
  nose Q30.8
  specified site NEC — *see* Neoplasm, malignant, by site
  subependymal D43.2
    specified site — *see* Neoplasm, uncertain behavior, by site
    unspecified site D43.2
  unspecified site C71.9
Gliomatosis cerebri C71.0
Glioneuroma — *see* Neoplasm, uncertain behavior, by site
Gliosarcoma
  specified site — *see* Neoplasm, malignant, by site
  unspecified site C71.9
Gliosis (cerebral) G93.89
  spinal G95.89
Glisson's disease — *see* Rickets
Globinuria R82.3

Globus (hystericus) F45.8
Glomangioma D18.00
  intra-abdominal D18.03
  intracranial D18.02
  skin D18.01
  specified site NEC D18.09
Glomangiomyoma D18.00
  intra-abdominal D18.03
  intracranial D18.02
  skin D18.01
  specified site NEC D18.09
Glomangiosarcoma — *see* Neoplasm, connective tissue, malignant
Glomerular
  disease in syphilis A52.75
  nephritis — *see* Glomerulonephritis
Glomerulitis — *see* Glomerulonephritis
Glomerulonephritis (*see also* Nephritis) N05.9
  with
    edema — *see* Nephrosis
    minimal change N05.0
    minor glomerular abnormality N05.0
  acute N00.9
  chronic N03.9
  crescentic (diffuse) NEC (*see also* N00-N07 with fourth character .7) N05.7
  dense deposit (*see also* N00-N07 with fourth character .6) N05.6
  diffuse
    crescentic (*see also* N00-N07 with fourth character .7) N05.7
    endocapillary proliferative (*see also* N00-N07 with fourth character .4) N05.4
    membranous (*see also* N00-N07 with fourth character .2) N05.2
    mesangial proliferative (*see also* N00-N07 with fourth character .3) N05.3
    mesangiocapillary (*see also* N00-N07 with fourth character .5) N05.5
    sclerosing N18.9
  endocapillary proliferative (diffuse) NEC (*see also* N00-N07 with fourth character .4) N05.4
  extracapillary NEC (*see also* N00-N07 with fourth character .7) N05.7
  focal (and segmental) (*see also* N00-N07 with fourth character .1) N05.1
  hypocomplementemic — *see* Glomerulonephritis, membranoproliferative
  IgA — *see* Nephropathy, IgA
  immune complex (circulating) NEC N05.8
  in (due to)
    amyloidosis E85.4 [N08]
    bilharziasis B65.9 [N08]
    cryoglobulinemia D89.1 [N08]
    defibrination syndrome D65 [N08]
    diabetes mellitus — *see* Diabetes, glomerulosclerosis
    disseminated intravascular coagulation D65 [N08]
    Fabry (-Anderson) disease E75.21 [N08]
    Goodpasture's syndrome M31.0
    hemolytic-uremic syndrome D59.3
    Henoch (-Schönlein) purpura D69.0 [N08]
    lecithin cholesterol acyltransferase deficiency E78.6 [N08]
    microscopic polyangiitis M31.7 [N08]
    multiple myeloma C90.0- ☑ [N08]
    Plasmodium malariae B52.0
    schistosomiasis B65.9 [N08]
    sepsis A41.9 [N08]
      streptococcal A40- ☑ [N08]
    sickle-cell disorders D57.- ☑ [N08]
    strongyloidiasis B78.9 [N08]
    subacute bacterial endocarditis I33.0 [N08]
    syphilis (late) congenital A50.59 [N08]
    systemic lupus erythematosus M32.14
    thrombotic thrombocytopenic purpura M31.1 [N08]
    typhoid fever A01.09
    Waldenström macroglobulinemia C88.0 [N08]
    Wegener's granulomatosis M31.31
  latent or quiescent N03.9
  lobular, lobulonodular — *see* Glomerulonephritis, membranoproliferative
  membranoproliferative (diffuse)(type 1 or 3) (*see also* N00-N07 with fourth character .5) N05.5
    dense deposit (type 2) NEC (*see also* N00-N07 with fourth character .6) N05.6

Glomerulonephritis — *continued*
  membranous (diffuse) NEC (*see also* N00-N07 with fourth character .2) N05.2
  mesangial
    IgA/IgG — *see* Nephropathy, IgA
    proliferative (diffuse) NEC (*see also* N00-N07 with fourth character .3) N05.3
  mesangiocapillary (diffuse) NEC (*see also* N00-N07 with fourth character .5) N05.5
  necrotic, necrotizing NEC (*see also* N00- N07 with fourth character .8) N05.8
  nodular — *see* Glomerulonephritis, membranoproliferative
  poststreptococcal NEC N05.9
    acute N00.9
    chronic N03.9
    rapidly progressive N01.9
  proliferative NEC (*see also* N00-N07 with fourth character .8) N05.8
    diffuse (lupus) M32.14
  rapidly progressive N01.9
  sclerosing, diffuse N18.9
  specified pathology NEC (*see also* N00- N07 with fourth character .8) N05.8
  subacute N01.9
Glomerulopathy — *see* Glomerulonephritis
Glomerulosclerosis (*see also* Sclerosis, renal)
  intercapillary (nodular) (with diabetes) — *see* Diabetes, glomerulosclerosis
  intracapillary — *see* Diabetes, glomerulosclerosis
Glossagra K14.6
Glossalgia K14.6
Glossitis (chronic superficial) (gangrenous) (Moeller's) K14.0
  areata exfoliativa K14.1
  atrophic K14.4
  benign migratory K14.1
  cortical superficial, sclerotic K14.0
  Hunter's D51.0
  interstitial, sclerous K14.0
  median rhomboid K14.2
  pellagrous E52
  superficial, chronic K14.0
Glossocele K14.8
Glossodynia K14.6
  exfoliativa K14.4
Glossoncus K14.8
Glossopathy K14.9
Glossophytia K14.3
Glossoplegia K14.8
Glossoptosis K14.8
Glossopyrosis K14.6
Glossotrichia K14.3
Glossy skin L90.8
Glottis — *see* condition
Glottitis (*see also* Laryngitis) J04.0
Glucagonoma
  pancreas
    benign D13.7
    malignant C25.4
    uncertain behavior D37.8
  specified site NEC
    benign — *see* Neoplasm, benign, by site
    malignant — *see* Neoplasm, malignant, by site
    uncertain behavior — *see* Neoplasm, uncertain behavior, by site
  unspecified site
    benign D13.7
    malignant C25.4
    uncertain behavior D37.8
Glucoglycinuria E72.51
Glucose-galactose malabsorption E74.39
Glue
  ear — *see* Otitis, media, nonsuppurative, chronic, mucoid
  sniffing (airplane) — *see* Abuse, drug, inhalant
    dependence — *see* Dependence, drug, inhalant
Glutaric aciduria E72.3
Glycinemia E72.51
Glycinuria (renal) (with ketosis) E72.09
Glycogen
  infiltration — *see* Disease, glycogen storage
  storage disease — *see* Disease, glycogen storage
Glycogenosis (diffuse) (generalized) (*see also* Disease, glycogen storage)
  cardiac E74.02 [I43]

Index

Glycogenosis — *continued*
  diabetic, secondary — *see* Diabetes, glycogenosis, secondary
  pulmonary interstitial J84.842
Glycopenia E16.2
Glycosuria R81
  renal E74.8
Gnathostoma spinigerum (infection) (infestation), **gnathostomiasis** (wandering swelling) B83.1
Goiter (plunging) (substernal) E04.9
  with
    hyperthyroidism (recurrent) — *see* Hyperthyroidism, with, goiter
    thyrotoxicosis — *see* Hyperthyroidism, with, goiter
  adenomatous — *see* Goiter, nodular
  cancerous C73
  congenital (nontoxic) E03.0
    diffuse E03.0
    parenchymatous E03.0
    transitory, with normal functioning P72.0
  cystic E04.2
    due to iodine-deficiency E01.1
  due to
    enzyme defect in synthesis of thyroid hormone E07.1
    iodine-deficiency (endemic) E01.2
  dyshormonogenetic (familial) E07.1
  endemic (iodine-deficiency) E01.2
    diffuse E01.0
    multinodular E01.1
  exophthalmic — *see* Hyperthyroidism, with, goiter
  iodine-deficiency (endemic) E01.2
    diffuse E01.0
    multinodular E01.1
    nodular E01.1
  lingual Q89.2
  lymphadenoid E06.3
  malignant C73
  multinodular (cystic) (nontoxic) E04.2
    toxic or with hyperthyroidism E05.20
      with thyroid storm E05.21
  neonatal NEC P72.0
  nodular (nontoxic) (due to) E04.9
    with
      hyperthyroidism E05.20
        with thyroid storm E05.21
      thyrotoxicosis E05.20
        with thyroid storm E05.21
    endemic E01.1
    iodine-deficiency E01.1
    sporadic E04.9
    toxic E05.20
      with thyroid storm E05.21
  nontoxic E04.9
    diffuse (colloid) E04.0
    multinodular E04.2
    simple E04.0
    specified NEC E04.8
    uninodular E04.1
  simple E04.0
  toxic — *see* Hyperthyroidism, with, goiter
  uninodular (nontoxic) E04.1
    toxic or with hyperthyroidism E05.10
      with thyroid storm E05.11
Goiter-deafness syndrome E07.1
Goldberg syndrome Q89.8
Goldberg-Maxwell syndrome E34.51
Goldblatt's hypertension or kidney I70.1
Goldenhar (-Gorlin) **syndrome** Q87.0
Goldflam-Erb disease or syndrome G70.00
  with exacerbation (acute) G70.01
  in crisis G70.01
Goldscheider's disease Q81.8
Goldstein's disease (familial hemorrhagic telangiectasia) I78.0
Golfer's elbow — *see* Epicondylitis, medial
Gonadoblastoma
  specified site — *see* Neoplasm, uncertain behavior, by site
  unspecified site
    female D39.10
    male D40.10
Gonecystitis — *see* Vesiculitis
Gongylonemiasis B83.8
Goniosynechiae — *see* Adhesions, iris, goniosynechiae
Gonococcemia A54.86
Gonococcus, gonococcal (disease) (infection) (*see also* condition) A54.9

Gonococcus, gonococcal — *continued*
  anus A54.6
  bursa, bursitis A54.49
  conjunctiva, conjunctivitis (neonatorum) A54.31
  endocardium A54.83
  eye A54.30
    conjunctivitis A54.31
    iridocyclitis A54.32
    keratitis A54.33
    newborn A54.31
    other specified A54.39
  fallopian tubes (acute) (chronic) A54.24
  genitourinary (organ) (system) (tract) (acute)
    lower A54.00
      with abscess (accessory gland) (periurethral) A54.1
    upper (*see also* condition) A54.29
  heart A54.83
  iridocyclitis A54.32
  joint A54.42
  lymphatic (gland) (node) A54.89
  meninges, meningitis A54.81
  musculoskeletal A54.40
    arthritis A54.42
    osteomyelitis A54.43
    other specified A54.49
    spondylopathy A54.41
  pelviperitonitis A54.24
  pelvis (acute) (chronic) A54.24
  pharynx A54.5
  proctitis A54.6
  pyosalpinx (acute) (chronic) A54.24
  rectum A54.6
  skin A54.89
  specified site NEC A54.89
  tendon sheath A54.49
  throat A54.5
  urethra (acute) (chronic) A54.01
    with abscess (accessory gland) (periurethral) A54.1
  vulva (acute) (chronic) A54.02
Gonocytoma
  specified site — *see* Neoplasm, uncertain behavior, by site
  unspecified site
    female D39.10
    male D40.10
Gonorrhea (acute) (chronic) A54.9
  Bartholin's gland (acute) (chronic) (purulent) A54.02
    with abscess (accessory gland) (periurethral) A54.1
  bladder A54.01
  cervix A54.03
  conjunctiva, conjunctivitis (neonatorum) A54.31
  contact Z20.2
  Cowper's gland (with abscess) A54.1
  exposure to Z20.2
  fallopian tube (acute) (chronic) A54.24
  kidney (acute) (chronic) A54.21
  lower genitourinary tract A54.00
    with abscess (accessory gland) (periurethral) A54.1
  ovary (acute) (chronic) A54.24
  pelvis (acute) (chronic) A54.24
    female pelvic inflammatory disease A54.24
  penis A54.09
  prostate (acute) (chronic) A54.22
  seminal vesicle (acute) (chronic) A54.23
  specified site not listed (*see also* Gonococcus) A54.89
  spermatic cord (acute) (chronic) A54.23
  urethra A54.01
    with abscess (accessory gland) (periurethral) A54.1
  vagina A54.02
  vas deferens (acute) (chronic) A54.23
  vulva A54.02
Goodall's disease A08.19
Goodpasture's syndrome M31.0
Gopalan's syndrome (burning feet) E53.0
Gorlin-Chaudry-Moss syndrome Q87.0
Gottron's papules L94.4
Gougerot-Blum syndrome (pigmented purpuric lichenoid dermatitis) L81.7
Gougerot-Carteaud disease or syndrome (confluent reticulate papillomatosis) L83
Gougerot's syndrome (trisymptomatic) L81.7
Gouley's syndrome (constrictive pericarditis) I31.1
Goundou A66.6
Gout, chronic (*see also* Gout, gouty) M1A.9 ☑ (*following* M08)
  drug-induced M1A.20 ☑ (*following* M08)
    ankle M1A.27- ☑ (*following* M08)

Gout, chronic — *continued*
  drug-induced — *continued*
    elbow M1A.22- ☑ (*following* M08)
    foot joint M1A.27- ☑ (*following* M08)
    hand joint M1A.24- ☑ (*following* M08)
    hip M1A.25- ☑ (*following* M08)
    knee M1A.26- ☑ (*following* M08)
    multiple site M1A.29- ☑ (*following* M08)
    shoulder M1A.21- ☑ (*following* M08)
    vertebrae M1A.28 ☑ (*following* M08)
    wrist M1A.23- ☑ (*following* M08)
  idiopathic M1A.00 ☑ (*following* M08)
    ankle M1A.07- ☑ (*following* M08)
    elbow M1A.02- ☑ (*following* M08)
    foot joint M1A.07- ☑ (*following* M08)
    hand joint M1A.04- ☑ (*following* M08)
    hip M1A.05- ☑ (*following* M08)
    knee M1A.06- ☑ (*following* M08)
    multiple site M1A.09 ☑ (*following* M08)
    shoulder M1A.01- ☑ (*following* M08)
    vertebrae M1A.08 ☑ (*following* M08)
    wrist M1A.03- ☑ (*following* M08)
  in (due to) renal impairment M1A.30 ☑ (*following* M08)
    ankle M1A.37- ☑ (*following* M08)
    elbow M1A.32- ☑ (*following* M08)
    foot joint M1A.37- ☑ (*following* M08)
    hand joint M1A.34- ☑ (*following* M08)
    hip M1A.35- ☑ (*following* M08)
    knee M1A.36- ☑ (*following* M08)
    multiple site M1A.39 ☑ (*following* M08)
    shoulder M1A.31- ☑ (*following* M08)
    vertebrae M1A.38 ☑ (*following* M08)
    wrist M1A.33- ☑ (*following* M08)
  lead-induced M1A.10 ☑ (*following* M08)
    ankle M1A.17- ☑ (*following* M08)
    elbow M1A.12- ☑ (*following* M08)
    foot joint M1A.17- ☑ (*following* M08)
    hand joint M1A.14- ☑ (*following* M08)
    hip M1A.15- ☑ (*following* M08)
    knee M1A.16- ☑ (*following* M08)
    multiple site M1A.19 ☑ (*following* M08)
    shoulder M1A.11- ☑ (*following* M08)
    vertebrae M1A.18 ☑ (*following* M08)
    wrist M1A.13- ☑ (*following* M08)
  primary — *see* Gout, chronic, idiopathic
  saturnine — *see* Gout, chronic, lead-induced
  secondary NEC M1A.40 ☑ (*following* M08)
    ankle M1A.47- ☑ (*following* M08)
    elbow M1A.42- ☑ (*following* M08)
    foot joint M1A.47- ☑ (*following* M08)
    hand joint M1A.44- ☑ (*following* M08)
    hip M1A.45- ☑ (*following* M08)
    knee M1A.46- ☑ (*following* M08)
    multiple site M1A.49 ☑ (*following* M08)
    shoulder M1A.41- ☑ (*following* M08)
    vertebrae M1A.48 ☑ (*following* M08)
    wrist M1A.43- ☑ (*following* M08)
  syphilitic (*see also* subcategory M14.8-) A52.77
  tophi M1A.9 ☑ (*following* M08)
Gout, gouty (acute) (attack) (flare) (*see also* Gout, chronic) M10.9
  drug-induced M10.20
    ankle M10.27- ☑
    elbow M10.22- ☑
    foot joint M10.27- ☑
    hand joint M10.24- ☑
    hip M10.25- ☑
    knee M10.26- ☑
    multiple site M10.29
    shoulder M10.21- ☑
    vertebrae M10.28
    wrist M10.23- ☑
  idiopathic M10.00
    ankle M10.07- ☑
    elbow M10.02- ☑
    foot joint M10.07- ☑
    hand joint M10.04- ☑
    hip M10.05- ☑
    knee M10.06- ☑
    multiple site M10.09
    shoulder M10.01- ☑
    vertebrae M10.08
    wrist M10.03- ☑
  in (due to) renal impairment M10.30
    ankle M10.37- ☑

Glycogenosis — Gout, gouty

Gout, gouty — continued
  in renal impairment — continued
    elbow M10.32- ☑
    foot joint M10.37- ☑
    hand joint M10.34- ☑
    hip M10.35- ☑
    knee M10.36- ☑
    multiple site M10.39
    shoulder M10.31- ☑
    vertebrae M10.38
    wrist M10.33- ☑
  lead-induced M10.10
    ankle M10.17- ☑
    elbow M10.12- ☑
    foot joint M10.17- ☑
    hand joint M10.14- ☑
    hip M10.15- ☑
    knee M10.16- ☑
    multiple site M10.19
    shoulder M10.11- ☑
    vertebrae M10.18
    wrist M10.13- ☑
  primary — see Gout, idiopathic
  saturnine — see Gout, lead-induced
  secondary NEC M10.40
    ankle M10.47- ☑
    elbow M10.42- ☑
    foot joint M10.47- ☑
    hand joint M10.44- ☑
    hip M10.45- ☑
    knee M10.46- ☑
    multiple site M10.49
    shoulder M10.41- ☑
    vertebrae M10.48
    wrist M10.43- ☑
  syphilitic (see also subcategory M14.8-) A52.77
  tophi — see Gout, chronic
Gower's
  muscular dystrophy G71.0
  syndrome (vasovagal attack) R55
Gradenigo's syndrome — see Otitis, media, suppurative, acute
Graefe's disease — see Strabismus, paralytic, ophthalmoplegia, progressive
Graft-versus-host disease D89.813
  acute D89.810
  acute on chronic D89.812
  chronic D89.811
Grain mite (itch) B88.0
Grainhandler's disease or lung J67.8
Grand mal — see Epilepsy, generalized, specified NEC
Grand multipara status only (not pregnant) Z64.1
  pregnant — see Pregnancy, complicated by, grand multiparity
Granite worker's lung J62.8
Granular (see also condition)
  inflammation, pharynx J31.2
  kidney (contracting) — see Sclerosis, renal
  liver K74.69
Granulation tissue (abnormal) (excessive) L92.9
  postmastoidectomy cavity — see Complications, postmastoidectomy, granulation
Granulocytopenia (primary) (malignant) — see Agranulocytosis
Granuloma L92.9
  abdomen K66.8
    from residual foreign body L92.3
    pyogenicum L98.0
  actinic L57.5
  annulare (perforating) L92.0
  apical K04.5
  aural — see Otitis, externa, specified NEC
  beryllium (skin) L92.3
  bone
    eosinophilic C96.6
    from residual foreign body — see Osteomyelitis, specified type NEC
    lung C96.6
  brain (any site) G06.0
    schistosomiasis B65.9 [G07]
  canaliculus lacrimalis — see Granuloma, lacrimal
  candidal (cutaneous) B37.2
  cerebral (any site) G06.0
  coccidioidal (primary) (progressive) B38.7
    lung B38.1
    meninges B38.4
  colon K63.89

Granuloma — continued
  conjunctiva H11.22- ☑
  dental K04.5
  ear, middle — see Cholesteatoma
  eosinophilic C96.6
    bone C96.6
    lung C96.6
    oral mucosa K13.4
    skin L92.2
  eyelid H01.8
  facial (e) L92.2
  foreign body (in soft tissue) NEC M60.20
    ankle M60.27- ☑
    foot M60.27- ☑
    forearm M60.23- ☑
    hand M60.24- ☑
    in operation wound — see Foreign body, accidentally left during a procedure
    lower leg M60.26- ☑
    pelvic region M60.25- ☑
    shoulder region M60.21- ☑
    skin L92.3
    specified site NEC M60.28
    subcutaneous tissue L92.3
    thigh M60.25- ☑
    upper arm M60.22- ☑
  gangraenescens M31.2
  genito-inguinale A58
  giant cell (central) (reparative) (jaw) M27.1
    gingiva (peripheral) K06.8
  gland (lymph) I88.8
  hepatic NEC K75.3
    in (due to)
      berylliosis J63.2 [K77]
      sarcoidosis D86.89
  Hodgkin C81.9 ☑
  ileum K63.89
  infectious B99.9
    specified NEC B99.8
  inguinale (Donovan) (venereal) A58
  intestine NEC K63.89
  intracranial (any site) G06.0
  intraspinal (any part) G06.1
  iridocyclitis — see Iridocyclitis, chronic
  jaw (bone) (central) M27.1
    reparative giant cell M27.1
  kidney (see also Infection, kidney) N15.8
  lacrimal H04.81- ☑
  larynx J38.7
  lethal midline (faciale(e)) M31.2
  liver NEC — see Granuloma, hepatic
  lung (infectious) (see also Fibrosis, lung)
    coccidioidal B38.1
    eosinophilic C96.6
  Majocchi's B35.8
  malignant (facial(e)) M31.2
  mandible (central) M27.1
  midline (lethal) M31.2
  monilial (cutaneous) B37.2
  nasal sinus — see Sinusitis
  operation wound T81.89 ☑
    foreign body — see Foreign body, accidentally left during a procedure
    stitch T81.89 ☑
    talc — see Foreign body, accidentally left during a procedure
  oral mucosa K13.4
  orbit, orbital H05.11- ☑
  paracoccidioidal B41.8
  penis, venereal A58
  periapical K04.5
  peritoneum K66.8
    due to ova of helminths NOS (see also Helminthiasis) B83.9 [K67]
  postmastoidectomy cavity — see Complications, postmastoidectomy, recurrent cholesteatoma
  prostate N42.89
  pudendi (ulcerating) A58
  pulp, internal (tooth) K03.3
  pyogenic, pyogenicum (of) (skin) L98.0
    gingiva K06.8
    maxillary alveolar ridge K04.5
    oral mucosa K13.4
  rectum K62.89
  reticulohistiocytic D76.3
  rubrum nasi L74.8
  Schistosoma — see Schistosomiasis
  septic (skin) L98.0

Granuloma — continued
  silica (skin) L92.3
  sinus (accessory) (infective) (nasal) — see Sinusitis
  skin L92.9
    from residual foreign body L92.3
    pyogenicum L98.0
  spine
    syphilitic (epidural) A52.19
    tuberculous A18.01
  stitch (postoperative) T81.89 ☑
  suppurative (skin) L98.0
  swimming pool A31.1
  talc (see also Granuloma, foreign body)
    in operation wound — see Foreign body, accidentally left during a procedure
  telangiectaticum (skin) L98.0
  tracheostomy J95.09
  trichophyticum B35.8
  tropicum A66.4
  umbilical P83.81
  umbilicus P83.81
  urethra N36.8
  uveitis — see Iridocyclitis, chronic
  vagina A58
  venereum A58
  vocal cord J38.3
Granulomatosis L92.9
  lymphoid C83.8- ☑
  miliary (listerial) A32.89
  necrotizing, respiratory M31.30
  progressive septic D71
  specified NEC L92.8
  Wegener's M31.30
    with renal involvement M31.31
Granulomatous tissue (abnormal) (excessive) L92.9
Granulosis rubra nasi L74.8
Graphite fibrosis (of lung) J63.3
Graphospasm F48.8
  organic G25.89
Grating scapula M89.8X1
Gravel (urinary) — see Calculus, urinary
Graves' disease — see Hyperthyroidism, with, goiter
Gravis — see condition
Grawitz tumor C64.- ☑
Gray syndrome (newborn) P93.0
Grayness, hair (premature) L67.1
  congenital Q84.2
Green sickness D50.8
Greenfield's disease
  meaning
    concentric sclerosis (encephalitis periaxialis concentrica) G37.5
    metachromatic leukodystrophy E75.25
Greenstick fracture — code as Fracture, by site
Grey syndrome (newborn) P93.0
Grief F43.21
  prolonged F43.29
  reaction (see also Disorder, adjustment) F43.20
Griesinger's disease B76.9
Grinder's lung or pneumoconiosis J62.8
Grinding, teeth
  psychogenic F45.8
  sleep related G47.63
Grip
  Dabney's B33.0
  devil's B33.0
Grippe, grippal (see also Influenza)
  Balkan A78
  summer, of Italy A93.1
Grisel's disease M43.6
Groin — see condition
Grooved tongue K14.5
Ground itch B76.9
Grover's disease or syndrome L11.1
Growing pains, children R29.898
Growth (fungoid) (neoplastic) (new) (see also Neoplasm)
  adenoid (vegetative) J35.8
  benign — see Neoplasm, benign, by site
  malignant — see Neoplasm, malignant, by site
  rapid, childhood Z00.2
  secondary — see Neoplasm, secondary, by site
Gruby's disease B35.0
Gubler-Millard paralysis or syndrome G46.3
Guerin-Stern syndrome Q74.3
Guidance, insufficient anterior (occlusal) M26.54
Guillain-Barré disease or syndrome G61.0
  sequelae G65.0

Guinea worms (infection) (infestation) B72
Guinon's disease (motor-verbal tic) F95.2
Gull's disease E03.4
Gum — *see* condition
Gumboil K04.7
  with sinus K04.6
Gumma (syphilitic) A52.79
  artery A52.09
    cerebral A52.04
  bone A52.77
    of yaws (late) A66.6
  brain A52.19
  cauda equina A52.19
  central nervous system A52.3
  ciliary body A52.71
  congenital A50.59
  eyelid A52.71
  heart A52.06
  intracranial A52.19
  iris A52.71
  kidney A52.75
  larynx A52.73
  leptomeninges A52.19
  liver A52.74
  meninges A52.19
  myocardium A52.06
  nasopharynx A52.73
  neurosyphilitic A52.3
  nose A52.73
  orbit A52.71
  palate (soft) A52.79
  penis A52.76
  pericardium A52.06
  pharynx A52.73
  pituitary A52.79
  scrofulous (tuberculous) A18.4
  skin A52.79
  specified site NEC A52.79
  spinal cord A52.19
  tongue A52.79
  tonsil A52.73
  trachea A52.73
  tuberculous A18.4
  ulcerative due to yaws A66.4
  ureter A52.75
  yaws A66.4
    bone A66.6
Gunn's syndrome Q07.8
Gunshot wound (*see also* Wound, open)
  fracture — *code as* Fracture, by site
  internal organs — *see* Injury, by site
Gynandrism Q56.0
Gynandroblastoma
  specified site — *see* Neoplasm, uncertain behavior,
    by site
  unspecified site
    female D39.10
    male D40.10
Gynecological examination (periodic) (routine) Z01.419
  with abnormal findings Z01.411
Gynecomastia N62
Gynephobia F40.291
Gyrate scalp Q82.8

H

H (Hartnup's) **disease** E72.02
Haas' disease or osteochondrosis (juvenile) (head of
  humerus) — *see* Osteochondrosis, juvenile,
  humerus
Habit, habituation
  bad sleep Z72.821
  chorea F95.8
  disturbance, child F98.9
  drug — *see* Dependence, drug
  irregular sleep Z72.821
  laxative F55.2
  spasm — *see* Tic
  tic — *see* Tic
Haemophilus (H.) **influenzae, as cause of disease
  classified elsewhere** B96.3
Haff disease — *see* Poisoning, mercury
Hageman's factor defect, deficiency or disease D68.2
Haglund's disease or osteochondrosis (juvenile) (os
  tibiale externum) — *see* Osteochondrosis, juvenile,
  tarsus
Hailey-Hailey disease Q82.8

Hair (*see also* condition)
  plucking F63.3
    in stereotyped movement disorder F98.4
  tourniquet syndrome (*see also* Constriction, external,
    by site)
    finger S60.44- ☑
    penis S30.842 ☑
    thumb S60.34- ☑
    toe S90.44- ☑
Hairball in stomach T18.2 ☑
Hair-pulling, pathological (compulsive) F63.3
Hairy black tongue K14.3
Half vertebra Q76.49
Halitosis R19.6
Hallerman-Streiff syndrome Q87.0
Hallervorden-Spatz disease G23.0
Hallopeau's acrodermatitis or disease L40.2
Hallucination R44.3
  auditory R44.0
  gustatory R44.2
  olfactory R44.2
  specified NEC R44.2
  tactile R44.2
  visual R44.1
Hallucinosis (chronic) F28
  alcoholic (acute) F10.951
    in
      abuse F10.151
      dependence F10.251
  drug-induced F19.951
    cannabis F12.951
    cocaine F14.951
    hallucinogen F16.151
    in
      abuse F19.151
        cannabis F12.151
        cocaine F14.151
        hallucinogen F16.151
        inhalant F18.151
        opioid F11.151
        sedative, anxiolytic or hypnotic F13.151
        stimulant NEC F15.151
      dependence F19.251
        cannabis F12.251
        cocaine F14.251
        hallucinogen F16.251
        inhalant F18.251
        opioid F11.251
        sedative, anxiolytic or hypnotic F13.251
        stimulant NEC F15.251
    inhalant F18.951
    opioid F11.951
    sedative, anxiolytic or hypnotic F13.951
    stimulant NEC F15.951
  organic F06.0
Hallux
  deformity (acquired) NEC M20.5X- ☑
  limitus M20.5X- ☑
  malleus (acquired) NEC M20.3- ☑
  rigidus (acquired) M20.2- ☑
    congenital Q74.2
    sequelae (late effect) of rickets E64.3
  valgus (acquired) M20.1- ☑
    congenital Q66.6
  varus (acquired) M20.3- ☑
    congenital Q66.3
Halo, visual H53.19
Hamartoma, hamartoblastoma Q85.9
  epithelial (gingival), odontogenic, central or peripheral
    — *see* Cyst, calcifying odontogenic
Hamartosis Q85.9
Hamman-Rich syndrome J84.114
Hammer toe (acquired) NEC (*see also* Deformity, toe,
  hammer toe)
  congenital Q66.89
  sequelae (late effect) of rickets E64.3
Hand — *see* condition
Hand-foot syndrome L27.1
Handicap, handicapped
  educational Z55.9
  specified NEC Z55.8
Hand-Schüller-Christian disease or syndrome C96.5
Hanging (asphyxia) (strangulation) (suffocation) — *see*
  Asphyxia, traumatic, due to mechanical threat
Hangnail (*see also* Cellulitis, digit)
  with lymphangitis — *see* Lymphangitis, acute, digit
Hangover (alcohol) F10.129

Hanhart's syndrome Q87.0
Hanot-Chauffard (-Troisier) **syndrome** E83.19
Hanot's cirrhosis or disease K74.3
Hansen's disease — *see* Leprosy
Hantaan virus disease (Korean hemorrhagic fever) A98.5
Hantavirus disease (with renal manifestations) (Dobra-
  va) (Puumala) (Seoul) A98.5
  with pulmonary manifestations (Andes) (Bayou)
    (Bermejo) (Black Creek Canal) (Choclo) (Juquiti-
    ba) (Laguna negra) (Lechiguanas) (New York)
    (Oran) (Sin nombre) B33.4
Happy puppet syndrome Q93.5
Harada's disease or syndrome H30.81- ☑
Hardening
  artery — *see* Arteriosclerosis
  brain G93.89
Harelip (complete) (incomplete) — *see* Cleft, lip
Harlequin (newborn) Q80.4
Harley's disease D59.6
Harmful use (of)
  alcohol F10.10
  anxiolytics — *see* Abuse, drug, sedative
  cannabinoids — *see* Abuse, drug, cannabis
  cocaine — *see* Abuse, drug, cocaine
  drug — *see* Abuse, drug
  hallucinogens — *see* Abuse, drug, hallucinogen
  hypnotics — *see* Abuse, drug, sedative
  opioids — *see* Abuse, drug, opioid
  PCP (phencyclidine) — *see* Abuse, drug, hallucinogen
  sedatives — *see* Abuse, drug, sedative
  stimulants NEC — *see* Abuse, drug, stimulant
Harris' lines — *see* Arrest, epiphyseal
Hartnup's disease E72.02
Harvester's lung J67.0
Harvesting ovum for in vitro fertilization Z31.83
Hashimoto's disease or thyroiditis E06.3
Hashitoxicosis (transient) E06.3
Hassal-Henle bodies or warts (cornea) H18.49
Haut mal — *see* Epilepsy, generalized, specified NEC
Haverhill fever A25.1
Hay fever (*see also* Fever, hay) J30.1
Hayem-Widal syndrome D59.8
Haygarth's nodes M15.8
Haymaker's lung J67.0
Hb (abnormal)
  Bart's disease D56.0
  disease — *see* Disease, hemoglobin
  trait — *see* Trait
Head — *see* condition
Headache R51
  allergic NEC G44.89
  associated with sexual activity G44.82
  chronic daily R51
  cluster G44.009
    chronic G44.029
      intractable G44.021
      not intractable G44.029
    episodic G44.019
      intractable G44.011
      not intractable G44.019
    intractable G44.001
    not intractable G44.009
  cough (primary) G44.83
  daily chronic R51
  drug-induced NEC G44.40
    intractable G44.41
    not intractable G44.40
  exertional (primary) G44.84
  histamine G44.009
    intractable G44.001
    not intractable G44.009
  hypnic G44.81
  lumbar puncture G97.1
  medication overuse G44.40
    intractable G44.41
    not intractable G44.40
  menstrual — *see* Migraine, menstrual
  migraine (type) (*see also* Migraine) G43.909
  nasal septum R51
  neuralgiform, short lasting unilateral, with conjunctival
    injection and tearing (SUNCT) G44.059
    intractable G44.051
    not intractable G44.059
  new daily persistent (NDPH) G44.52
  orgasmic G44.82
  periodic syndromes in adults and children G43.C0
    (*following* G43.7)

Headache — *continued*
  periodic syndromes in adults and children — *continued*
    with refractory migraine G43.C1 (*following* G43.7)
    without refractory migraine G43.C0 (*following* G43.7)
    intractable G43.C1 (*following* G43.7)
    not intractable G43.C0 (*following* G43.7)
  postspinal puncture G97.1
  post-traumatic G44.309
    acute G44.319
      intractable G44.311
      not intractable G44.319
    chronic G44.329
      intractable G44.321
      not intractable G44.329
    intractable G44.301
    not intractable G44.309
  pre-menstrual — *see* Migraine, menstrual
  preorgasmic G44.82
  primary
    cough G44.83
    exertional G44.84
    stabbing G44.85
    thunderclap G44.53
  rebound G44.40
    intractable G44.41
    not intractable G44.40
  short lasting unilateral neuralgiform, with conjunctival injection and tearing (SUNCT) G44.059
    intractable G44.051
    not intractable G44.059
  specified syndrome NEC G44.89
  spinal and epidural anesthesia - induced T88.59 ☑
    in labor and delivery O74.5
    in pregnancy O29.4- ☑
    postpartum, puerperal O89.4
  spinal fluid loss (from puncture) G97.1
  stabbing (primary) G44.85
  tension (-type) G44.209
    chronic G44.229
      intractable G44.221
      not intractable G44.229
    episodic G44.219
      intractable G44.211
      not intractable G44.219
    intractable G44.201
    not intractable G44.209
  thunderclap (primary) G44.53
  vascular NEC G44.1
Healthy
  infant
    accompanying sick mother Z76.3
    receiving care Z76.2
  person accompanying sick person Z76.3
Hearing examination Z01.10
  with abnormal findings NEC Z01.118
  following failed hearing screening Z01.110
  for hearing conservation and treatment Z01.12
Heart — *see* condition
Heart beat
  abnormality R00.9
    specified NEC R00.8
  awareness R00.2
  rapid R00.0
  slow R00.1
Heartburn R12
  psychogenic F45.8
Heartland virus disease A93.8
Heat (effects) T67.9 ☑
  apoplexy T67.0 ☑
  burn (*see also* Burn) L55.9
  collapse T67.1 ☑
  cramps T67.2 ☑
  dermatitis or eczema L59.0
  edema T67.7 ☑
  erythema — *code by site under* Burn, first degree
  excessive T67.9 ☑
    specified effect NEC T67.8 ☑
  exhaustion T67.5 ☑
    anhydrotic T67.3 ☑
    due to
      salt (and water) depletion T67.4 ☑
      water depletion T67.3 ☑
        with salt depletion T67.4 ☑
  fatigue (transient) T67.6 ☑
  fever T67.0 ☑
  hyperpyrexia T67.0 ☑

Heat — *continued*
  prickly L74.0
  prostration — *see* Heat, exhaustion
  pyrexia T67.0 ☑
  rash L74.0
  specified effect NEC T67.8 ☑
  stroke T67.0 ☑
  sunburn — *see* Sunburn
  syncope T67.1 ☑
Heavy-for-dates NEC (infant) (4000g to 4499g) P08.1
  exceptionally (4500g or more) P08.0
Hebephrenia, hebephrenic (schizophrenia) F20.1
Heberden's disease or nodes (with arthropathy) M15.1
Hebra's
  pityriasis L26
  prurigo L28.2
Heel — *see* condition
Heerfordt's disease D86.89
Hegglin's anomaly or syndrome D72.0
Heilmeyer-Schoner disease D45
Heine-Medin disease A80.9
Heinz body anemia, congenital D58.2
Heliophobia F40.228
Heller's disease or syndrome F84.3
HELLP syndrome (hemolysis, elevated liver enzymes and low platelet count) O14.2- ☑
  complicating
    childbirth O14.24
    puerperium O14.25
Helminthiasis (*see also* Infestation, helminth)
  Ancylostoma B76.0
  intestinal B82.0
    mixed types (types classifiable to more than one of the titles B65.0-B81.3 and B81.8) B81.4
    specified type NEC B81.8
  mixed types (intestinal) (types classifiable to more than one of the titles B65.0-B81.3 and B81.8) B81.4
  Necator (americanus) B76.1
  specified type NEC B83.8
Heloma L84
Hemangioblastoma — *see* Neoplasm, connective tissue, uncertain behavior
  malignant — *see* Neoplasm, connective tissue, malignant
Hemangioendothelioma (*see also* Neoplasm, uncertain behavior, by site)
  benign D18.00
    intra-abdominal D18.03
    intracranial D18.02
    skin D18.01
    specified site NEC D18.09
  bone (diffuse) — *see* Neoplasm, bone, malignant
  epithelioid (*see also* Neoplasm, uncertain behavior, by site)
    malignant — *see* Neoplasm, malignant, by site
  malignant — *see* Neoplasm, connective tissue, malignant
Hemangiofibroma — *see* Neoplasm, benign, by site
Hemangiolipoma — *see* Lipoma
Hemangioma D18.00
  arteriovenous D18.00
    intra-abdominal D18.03
    intracranial D18.02
    skin D18.01
    specified site NEC D18.09
  capillary D18.00
    intra-abdominal D18.03
    intracranial D18.02
    skin D18.01
    specified site NEC D18.09
  cavernous D18.00
    intra-abdominal D18.03
    intracranial D18.02
    skin D18.01
    specified site NEC D18.09
  epithelioid D18.00
    intra-abdominal D18.03
    intracranial D18.02
    skin D18.01
    specified site NEC D18.09
  histiocytoid D18.00
    intra-abdominal D18.03
    intracranial D18.02
    skin D18.01
    specified site NEC D18.09
  infantile D18.00
    intra-abdominal D18.03

Hemangioma — *continued*
  infantile — *continued*
    intracranial D18.02
    skin D18.01
    specified site NEC D18.09
  intra-abdominal D18.03
  intracranial D18.02
  intramuscular D18.00
    intra-abdominal D18.03
    intracranial D18.02
    skin D18.01
    specified site NEC D18.09
  intrathoracic structures D18.09
  juvenile D18.00
  malignant — *see* Neoplasm,connective tissue, malignant
  plexiform D18.00
    intra-abdominal D18.03
    intracranial D18.02
    skin D18.01
    specified site NEC D18.09
  racemose D18.00
    intra-abdominal D18.03
    intracranial D18.02
    skin D18.01
    specified site NEC D18.09
  sclerosing — *see* Neoplasm, skin, benign
  simplex D18.00
    intra-abdominal D18.03
    intracranial D18.02
    skin D18.01
    specified site NEC D18.09
  skin D18.01
  specified site NEC D18.09
  venous D18.00
    intra-abdominal D18.03
    intracranial D18.02
    skin D18.01
    specified site NEC D18.09
  verrucous keratotic D18.00
    intra-abdominal D18.03
    intracranial D18.02
    skin D18.01
    specified site NEC D18.09
Hemangiomatosis (systemic) I78.8
  involving single site — *see* Hemangioma
Hemangiopericytoma (*see also* Neoplasm, connective tissue, uncertain behavior)
  benign — *see* Neoplasm, connective tissue, benign
  malignant — *see* Neoplasm, connective tissue, malignant
Hemangiosarcoma — *see* Neoplasm, connective tissue, malignant
Hemarthrosis (nontraumatic) M25.00
  ankle M25.07- ☑
  elbow M25.02- ☑
  foot joint M25.07- ☑
  hand joint M25.04- ☑
  hip M25.05- ☑
  in hemophilic arthropathy — *see* Arthropathy, hemophilic
  knee M25.06- ☑
  shoulder M25.01- ☑
  specified joint NEC M25.08
  traumatic — *see* Sprain, by site
  vertebrae M25.08
  wrist M25.03- ☑
Hematemesis K92.0
  with ulcer — *code by site under* Ulcer, with hemorrhage K27.4
  newborn, neonatal P54.0
    due to swallowed maternal blood P78.2
Hematidrosis L74.8
Hematinuria (*see also* Hemoglobinuria)
  malarial B50.8
Hematobilia K83.8
Hematocele
  female NEC N94.89
    with ectopic pregnancy O00.90
      with intrauterine pregnancy O00.91
    ovary N83.8
  male N50.1
Hematochezia (*see also* Melena) K92.1
Hematochyluria (*see also* Infestation, filarial)
  schistosomiasis (bilharziasis) B65.0
Hematocolpos (with hematometra or hematosalpinx) N89.7
Hematocornea — *see* Pigmentation, cornea, stromal

Index

Headache — Hematocornea

Hematogenous — see condition
Hematoma (traumatic) (skin surface intact) (see also Contusion)
  with
    injury of internal organs — see Injury, by site
    open wound — see Wound, open
  amputation stump (surgical) (late) T87.89
  aorta, dissecting I71.00
    abdominal I71.02
    thoracic I71.01
    thoracoabdominal I71.03
  aortic intramural — see Dissection, aorta
  arterial (complicating trauma) — see Injury, blood vessel, by site
  auricle — see Contusion, ear
    nontraumatic — see Disorder, pinna, hematoma
  birth injury NEC P15.8
  brain (traumatic)
    with
      cerebral laceration or contusion (diffuse) — see Injury, intracranial, diffuse
        focal — see Injury, intracranial, focal
    cerebellar, traumatic S06.37- ☑
    intracerebral, traumatic — see Injury, intracranial, intracerebral hemorrhage
    newborn NEC P52.4
      birth injury P10.1
    nontraumatic — see Hemorrhage, intracranial
    subarachnoid, arachnoid, traumatic — see Injury, intracranial, subarachnoid hemorrhage
    subdural, traumatic — see Injury, intracranial, subdural hemorrhage
  breast (nontraumatic) N64.89
  broad ligament (nontraumatic) N83.7
    traumatic S37.892 ☑
  cerebellar, traumatic S06.37- ☑
  cerebral — see Hematoma, brain
  cerebrum S06.36- ☑
    left S06.35- ☑
    right S06.34- ☑
  cesarean delivery wound O90.2
  complicating delivery (perineal) (pelvic) (vagina) (vulva) O71.7
  corpus cavernosum (nontraumatic) N48.89
  epididymis (nontraumatic) N50.1
  epidural (traumatic) — see Injury, intracranial, epidural hemorrhage
    spinal — see Injury, spinal cord, by region
  episiotomy O90.2
  face, birth injury P15.4
  genital organ NEC (nontraumatic)
    female (nonobstetric) N94.89
      traumatic S30.202 ☑
    male N50.1
      traumatic S30.201 ☑
  internal organs — see Injury, by site
  intracerebral, traumatic — see Injury, intracranial, intracerebral hemorrhage
  intraoperative — see Complications, intraoperative, hemorrhage
  labia (nontraumatic) (nonobstetric) N90.89
  liver (subcapsular) (nontraumatic) K76.89
    birth injury P15.0
  mediastinum — see Injury, intrathoracic
  mesosalpinx (nontraumatic) N83.7
    traumatic S37.898 ☑
  muscle — code by site under Contusion
  nontraumatic
    muscle M79.81
    soft tissue M79.81
  obstetrical surgical wound O90.2
  orbit, orbital (nontraumatic) (see also Hemorrhage, orbit)
    traumatic — see Contusion, orbit
  pelvis (female) (nontraumatic) (nonobstetric) N94.89
    obstetric O71.7
    traumatic — see Injury, by site
  penis (nontraumatic) N48.89
    birth injury P15.5
  perianal (nontraumatic) K64.5
  perineal S30.23 ☑
    complicating delivery O71.7
  perirenal — see Injury, kidney
  pinna — see Contusion, ear
    nontraumatic — see Disorder, pinna, hematoma
  placenta O43.89- ☑

Hematoma — continued
  postoperative (postprocedural) — see Complication, postprocedural, hematoma
  retroperitoneal (nontraumatic) K66.1
    traumatic S36.892 ☑
  scrotum, superficial S30.22 ☑
    birth injury P15.5
  seminal vesicle (nontraumatic) N50.1
    traumatic S37.892 ☑
  spermatic cord (traumatic) S37.892 ☑
    nontraumatic N50.1
  spinal (cord) (meninges) (see also Injury, spinal cord, by region)
    newborn (birth injury) P11.5
  spleen D73.5
    intraoperative — see Complications, intraoperative, hemorrhage, spleen
    postprocedural (postoperative) — see Complications, postprocedural, hemorrhage, spleen
  sternocleidomastoid, birth injury P15.2
  sternomastoid, birth injury P15.2
  subarachnoid (traumatic) — see Injury, intracranial, subarachnoid hemorrhage
    newborn (nontraumatic) P52.5
      due to birth injury P10.3
    nontraumatic — see Hemorrhage, intracranial, subarachnoid
  subdural (traumatic) — see Injury, intracranial, subdural hemorrhage
    newborn (localized) P52.8
      birth injury P10.0
    nontraumatic — see Hemorrhage, intracranial, subdural
  superficial, newborn P54.5
  testis (nontraumatic) N50.1
    birth injury P15.5
  tunica vaginalis (nontraumatic) N50.1
  umbilical cord, complicating delivery O69.5 ☑
  uterine ligament (broad) (nontraumatic) N83.7
    traumatic S37.892 ☑
  vagina (ruptured) (nontraumatic) N89.8
    complicating delivery O71.7
  vas deferens (nontraumatic) N50.1
    traumatic S37.892 ☑
  vitreous — see Hemorrhage, vitreous
  vulva (nontraumatic) (nonobstetric) N90.89
    complicating delivery O71.7
    newborn (birth injury) P15.5
Hematometra N85.7
  with hematocolpos N89.7
Hematomyelia (central) G95.19
  newborn (birth injury) P11.5
  traumatic T14.8 ☑
Hematomyelitis G04.90
Hematoperitoneum — see Hemoperitoneum
Hematophobia F40.230
Hematopneumothorax (see Hemothorax)
Hematopoiesis, cyclic D70.4
Hematoporphyria — see Porphyria
Hematorachis, hematorrhachis G95.19
  newborn (birth injury) P11.5
Hematosalpinx N83.6
  with
    hematocolpos N89.7
    hematometra N85.7
      with hematocolpos N89.7
  infectional — see Salpingitis
Hematospermia R36.1
Hematothorax (see Hemothorax)
Hematuria R31.9
  benign (familial) (of childhood) (see also Hematuria, idiopathic)
    essential microscopic R31.1
  due to sulphonamide, sulfonamide — see Table of Drugs and Chemicals, by drug
  endemic (see also Schistosomiasis) B65.0
  gross R31.0
  idiopathic N02.9
    with glomerular lesion
      crescentic (diffuse) glomerulonephritis N02.7
      dense deposit disease N02.6
      endocapillary proliferative glomerulonephritis N02.4
      focal and segmental hyalinosis or sclerosis N02.1
      membranoproliferative (diffuse) N02.5
      membranous (diffuse) N02.2
      mesangial proliferative (diffuse) N02.3

Hematuria — continued
  idiopathic — continued
    with glomerular lesion — continued
      mesangiocapillary (diffuse) N02.5
      minor abnormality N02.0
      proliferative NEC N02.8
      specified pathology NEC N02.8
  intermittent — see Hematuria, idiopathic
  malarial B50.8
  microscopic NEC (with symptoms) R31.29
    asymptomatic R31.21
    benign essential R31.1
  paroxysmal (see also Hematuria, idiopathic)
    nocturnal D59.5
  persistent — see Hematuria, idiopathic
  recurrent — see Hematuria, idiopathic
  tropical (see also Schistosomiasis) B65.0
  tuberculous A18.13
Hemeralopia (day blindness) H53.11
  vitamin A deficiency E50.5
Hemi-akinesia R41.4
Hemianalgesia R20.0
Hemianencephaly Q00.0
Hemianesthesia R20.0
Hemianopia, hemianopsia (heteronymous) H53.47
  homonymous H53.46- ☑
  syphilitic A52.71
Hemiathetosis R25.8
Hemiatrophy R68.89
  cerebellar G31.9
  face, facial, progressive (Romberg) G51.8
  tongue K14.8
Hemiballism (us) G25.5
Hemicardia Q24.8
Hemicephalus, hemicephaly Q00.0
Hemichorea G25.5
Hemicolitis, left — see Colitis, left sided
Hemicrania
  congenital malformation Q00.0
  continua G44.51
  meaning migraine (see also Migraine) G43.909
  paroxysmal G44.039
    chronic G44.049
      intractable G44.041
      not intractable G44.049
    episodic G44.039
      intractable G44.031
      not intractable G44.039
    intractable G44.031
    not intractable G44.039
Hemidystrophy — see Hemiatrophy
Hemiectromelia Q73.8
Hemihypalgesia R20.8
Hemihypesthesia R20.1
Hemi-inattention R41.4
Hemimelia Q73.8
  lower limb — see Defect, reduction, lower limb, specified type NEC
  upper limb — see Defect, reduction, upper limb, specified type NEC
Hemiparalysis — see Hemiplegia
Hemiparesis — see Hemiplegia
Hemiparesthesia R20.2
Hemiparkinsonism G20
Hemiplegia G81.9- ☑
  alternans facialis G83.89
  ascending NEC G81.90
    spinal G95.89
  congenital (cerebral) G80.8
    spastic G80.2
  embolic (current episode) I63.4- ☑
  flaccid G81.0- ☑
  following
    cerebrovascular disease I69.959
      cerebral infarction I69.35- ☑
      intracerebral hemorrhage I69.15- ☑
      nontraumatic intracranial hemorrhage NEC I69.25- ☑
      specified disease NEC I69.85- ☑
      stroke NOS I69.35- ☑
      subarachnoid hemorrhage I69.05- ☑
  hysterical F44.4
  newborn NEC P91.88
    birth injury P11.9
  spastic G81.1- ☑
    congenital G80.2
  thrombotic (current episode) I63.3- ☑

Hemisection, spinal cord — see Injury, spinal cord, by region
Hemispasm (facial) R25.2
Hemisporosis B48.8
Hemitremor R25.1
Hemivertebra Q76.49
  failure of segmentation with scoliosis Q76.3
  fusion with scoliosis Q76.3
Hemochromatosis E83.119
  with refractory anemia D46.1
  due to repeated red blood cell transfusion E83.111
  hereditary (primary) E83.110
  neonatal P78.84
  primary E83.110
  specified NEC E83.118
Hemoglobin (see also condition)
  abnormal (disease) — see Disease, hemoglobin
  AS genotype D57.3
  Constant Spring D58.2
  E-beta thalassemia D56.5
  fetal, hereditary persistence (HPFH) D56.4
  H Constant Spring D56.0
  low NOS D64.9
  S (Hb S), heterozygous D57.3
Hemoglobinemia D59.9
  due to blood transfusion T80.89 ☑
  paroxysmal D59.6
    nocturnal D59.5
Hemoglobinopathy (mixed) D58.2
  with thalassemia D56.8
  sickle-cell D57.1
    with thalassemia D57.40
      with crisis (vasoocclusive pain) D57.419
        with
          acute chest syndrome D57.411
          splenic sequestration D57.412
      without crisis D57.40
Hemoglobinuria R82.3
  with anemia, hemolytic, acquired (chronic) NEC D59.6
  cold (agglutinin) (paroxysmal) (with Raynaud's syndrome) D59.6
  due to exertion or hemolysis NEC D59.6
  intermittent D59.6
  malarial B50.8
  march D59.6
  nocturnal (paroxysmal) D59.5
  paroxysmal (cold) D59.6
    nocturnal D59.5
Hemolymphangioma D18.1
Hemolysis
  intravascular
    with
      abortion — see Abortion, by type, complicated by, hemorrhage
      ectopic or molar pregnancy O08.1
      hemorrhage
        antepartum — see Hemorrhage, antepartum, with coagulation defect
        intrapartum (see also Hemorrhage, complicating, delivery) O67.0
      postpartum O72.3
  neonatal (excessive) P58.9
    specified NEC P58.8
Hemolytic — see condition
Hemopericardium I31.2
  following acute myocardial infarction (current complication) I23.0
  newborn P54.8
  traumatic — see Injury, heart, with hemopericardium
Hemoperitoneum K66.1
  infectional K65.9
  traumatic S36.899 ☑
    with open wound — see Wound, open, with penetration into peritoneal cavity
Hemophilia (classical) (familial) (hereditary) D66
  A D66
  acquired D68.311
  autoimmune D68.311
  B D67
  C D68.1
  calcipriva (see also Defect, coagulation) D68.4
  nonfamilial (see also Defect, coagulation) D68.4
  secondary D68.311
  vascular D68.0
Hemophthalmos H44.81- ☑
Hemopneumothorax (see also Hemothorax)
  traumatic S27.2 ☑
Hemoptysis R04.2

Hemoptysis — continued
  newborn P26.9
  tuberculous — see Tuberculosis, pulmonary
Hemorrhage, hemorrhagic (concealed) R58
  abdomen R58
  accidental antepartum — see Hemorrhage, antepartum
  acute idiopathic pulmonary, in infants R04.81
  adenoid J35.8
  adrenal (capsule) (gland) E27.49
    medulla E27.8
    newborn P54.4
  after delivery — see Hemorrhage, postpartum
  alveolar
    lung, newborn P26.8
    process K08.89
  alveolus K08.89
  amputation stump (surgical) T87.89
  anemia (chronic) D50.0
    acute D62
  antepartum (with) O46.90
    with coagulation defect O46.00- ☑
      afibrinogenemia O46.01- ☑
      disseminated intravascular coagulation O46.02- ☑
      hypofibrinogenemia O46.01- ☑
      specified defect NEC O46.09- ☑
    before 20 weeks gestation O20.9
      specified type NEC O20.8
      threatened abortion O20.0
    due to
      abruptio placenta (see also Abruptio placentae) O45.9- ☑
      leiomyoma, uterus — see Hemorrhage, antepartum, specified cause NEC
      placenta previa O44.1- ☑
    specified cause NEC — see subcategory O46.8X- ☑
  anus (sphincter) K62.5
  apoplexy (stroke) — see Hemorrhage, intracranial, intracerebral
  arachnoid — see Hemorrhage, intracranial, subarachnoid
  artery R58
    brain — see Hemorrhage, intracranial, intracerebral
  basilar (ganglion) I61.0
  bladder N32.89
  bowel K92.2
    newborn P54.3
  brain (miliary) (nontraumatic) — see Hemorrhage, intracranial, intracerebral
    due to
      birth injury P10.1
      syphilis A52.05
    epidural or extradural (traumatic) — see Injury, intracranial, epidural hemorrhage
    newborn P52.4
      birth injury P10.1
    subarachnoid — see Hemorrhage, intracranial, subarachnoid
    subdural — see Hemorrhage, intracranial, subdural
  brainstem (nontraumatic) I61.3
    traumatic S06.38- ☑
  breast N64.59
  bronchial tube — see Hemorrhage, lung
  bronchopulmonary — see Hemorrhage, lung
  bronchus — see Hemorrhage, lung
  bulbar I61.5
  capillary I78.8
    primary D69.8
  cecum K92.2
  cerebellar, cerebellum (nontraumatic) I61.4
    newborn P52.6
    traumatic S06.37- ☑
  cerebral, cerebrum (see also Hemorrhage, intracranial, intracerebral)
    lobe I61.1
    newborn (anoxic) P52.4
      birth injury P10.1
  cerebromeningeal I61.8
  cerebrospinal — see Hemorrhage, intracranial, intracerebral
  cervix (uteri) (stump) NEC N88.8
  chamber, anterior (eye) — see Hyphema
  childbirth — see Hemorrhage, complicating, delivery
  choroid H31.30- ☑
    expulsive H31.31- ☑
  ciliary body — see Hyphema
  cochlea — see subcategory H83.8 ☑

Hemorrhage, hemorrhagic — continued
  colon K92.2
  complicating
    abortion — see Abortion, by type, complicated by, hemorrhage
    delivery O67.9
      associated with coagulation defect (afibrinogenemia) (DIC) (hyperfibrinolysis) O67.0
      specified cause NEC O67.8
    surgical procedure — see Hemorrhage, intraoperative
  conjunctiva H11.3- ☑
    newborn P54.8
  cord, newborn (stump) P51.9
  corpus luteum (ruptured) cyst N83.1- ☑
  cortical (brain) I61.1
  cranial — see Hemorrhage, intracranial
  cutaneous R23.3
    due to autosensitivity, erythrocyte D69.2
    newborn P54.5
  delayed
    following ectopic or molar pregnancy O08.1
    postpartum O72.2
  diathesis (familial) D69.9
  disease D69.9
    newborn P53
    specified type NEC D69.8
  due to or associated with
    afibrinogenemia or other coagulation defect (conditions in categories D65- D69)
      antepartum — see Hemorrhage, antepartum, with coagulation defect
      intrapartum O67.0
    dental implant M27.61
    device, implant or graft (see also Complications, by site and type, specified NEC) T85.838 ☑
      arterial graft NEC T82.838 ☑
      breast T85.838 ☑
      catheter NEC T85.838 ☑
        dialysis (renal) T82.838 ☑
          intraperitoneal T85.838 ☑
        infusion NEC T82.838 ☑
          spinal (epidural) (subdural) T85.830 ☑
        urinary (indwelling) T83.83 ☑
      electronic (electrode) (pulse generator) (stimulator)
        bone T84.83 ☑
        cardiac T82.837 ☑
        nervous system (brain) (peripheral nerve) (spinal) T85.830 ☑
        urinary T83.83 ☑
      fixation, internal (orthopedic) NEC T84.83 ☑
      gastrointestinal (bile duct) (esophagus) T85.838 ☑
      genital NEC T83.83 ☑
      heart NEC T82.837 ☑
      joint prosthesis T84.83 ☑
      ocular (corneal graft) (orbital implant) NEC T85.838 ☑
      orthopedic NEC T84.83 ☑
        bone graft T86.838
      specified NEC T85.838 ☑
      urinary NEC T83.83 ☑
      vascular NEC T82.838 ☑
      ventricular intracranial shunt T85.830 ☑
  duodenum, duodenal K92.2
    ulcer — see Ulcer, duodenum, with hemorrhage
  dura mater — see Hemorrhage, intracranial, subdural
  endotracheal — see Hemorrhage, lung
  epicranial subaponeurotic (massive), birth injury P12.2
  epidural (traumatic) (see also Injury, intracranial, epidural hemorrhage)
    nontraumatic I62.1
  esophagus K22.8
    varix I85.01
      secondary I85.11
  excessive, following ectopic gestation (subsequent episode) O08.1
  extradural (traumatic) — see Injury, intracranial, epidural hemorrhage
    birth injury P10.8
    newborn (anoxic) (nontraumatic) P52.8
    nontraumatic I62.1
  eye NEC H57.8
    fundus — see Hemorrhage, retina
    lid — see Disorder, eyelid, specified type NEC
  fallopian tube N83.6

Hemorrhage, hemorrhagic — *continued*
fibrinogenolysis — *see* Fibrinolysis
fibrinolytic (acquired) — *see* Fibrinolysis
from
  ear (nontraumatic) — *see* Otorrhagia
  tracheostomy stoma J95.01
fundus, eye — *see* Hemorrhage, retina
funis — *see* Hemorrhage, umbilicus, cord
gastric — *see* Hemorrhage, stomach
gastroenteric K92.2
  newborn P54.3
gastrointestinal (tract) K92.2
  newborn P54.3
genital organ, male N50.1
genitourinary (tract) NOS R31.9
gingiva K06.8
globe (eye) — *see* Hemophthalmos
graafian follicle cyst (ruptured) N83.0- ☑
gum K06.8
heart I51.89
hypopharyngeal (throat) R04.1
intermenstrual (regular) N92.3
  irregular N92.1
internal (organs) NEC R58
  capsule I61.0
  ear — *see* subcategory H83.8 ☑
  newborn P54.8
intestine K92.2
  newborn P54.3
intra-abdominal R58
intra-alveolar (lung), newborn P26.8
intracerebral (nontraumatic) — *see* Hemorrhage, intracranial, intracerebral
intracranial (nontraumatic) I62.9
  birth injury P10.9
  epidural, nontraumatic I62.1
  extradural, nontraumatic I62.1
  intracerebral (nontraumatic) (in) I61.9
    brain stem I61.3
    cerebellum I61.4
    hemisphere I61.2
      cortical (superficial) I61.1
      subcortical (deep) I61.0
    intraoperative
      during a nervous system procedure G97.31
      during other procedure G97.32
    intraventricular I61.5
    multiple localized I61.6
    newborn P52.4
      birth injury P10.1
    postprocedural
      following a nervous system procedure G97.51
      following other procedure G97.52
    specified NEC I61.8
    superficial I61.1
    traumatic (diffuse) — *see* Injury, intracranial, diffuse
      focal — *see* Injury, intracranial, focal
  newborn P52.9
    specified NEC P52.8
  subarachnoid (nontraumatic) (from) I60.9
    intracranial (cerebral) artery I60.7
      anterior communicating I60.2
      basilar I60.4
      carotid siphon and bifurcation I60.0- ☑
      communicating I60.7
        anterior I60.2
        posterior I60.3- ☑
      middle cerebral I60.1- ☑
      posterior communicating I60.3- ☑
      specified artery NEC I60.6
      vertebral I60.5- ☑
    newborn P52.5
      birth injury P10.3
    specified NEC I60.8
    traumatic S06.6X- ☑
  subdural (nontraumatic) I62.00
    acute I62.01
    birth injury P10.0
    chronic I62.03
    newborn (anoxic) (hypoxic) P52.8
      birth injury P10.0
    spinal G95.19
    subacute I62.02
    traumatic — *see* Injury, intracranial, subdural hemorrhage

Hemorrhage, hemorrhagic — *continued*
intracranial — *continued*
  traumatic — *see* Injury, intracranial, focal brain injury
intramedullary NEC G95.19
intraocular — *see* Hemophthalmos
intraoperative, intraprocedural — *see* Complication, hemorrhage (hematoma), intraoperative (intraprocedural), by site
intrapartum — *see* Hemorrhage, complicating, delivery
intrapelvic
  female N94.89
  male K66.1
intraperitoneal K66.1
intrapontine I61.3
intraprocedural — *see* Complication, hemorrhage (hematoma), intraoperative (intraprocedural), by site
intrauterine N85.7
  complicating delivery (*see also* Hemorrhage, complicating, delivery) O67.9
  postpartum — *see* Hemorrhage, postpartum
intraventricular I61.5
  newborn (nontraumatic) (*see also* Newborn, affected by, hemorrhage) P52.3
    due to birth injury P10.2
    grade
      1 P52.0
      2 P52.1
      3 P52.21
      4 P52.22
intravesical N32.89
iris (postinfectional) (postinflammatory) (toxic) — *see* Hyphema
joint (nontraumatic) — *see* Hemarthrosis
kidney N28.89
knee (joint) (nontraumatic) — *see* Hemarthrosis, knee
labyrinth — *see* subcategory H83.8 ☑
lenticular striate artery I61.0
ligature, vessel — *see* Hemorrhage, postoperative
liver K76.89
lung R04.89
  newborn P26.9
    massive P26.1
    specified NEC P26.8
  tuberculous — *see* Tuberculosis, pulmonary
massive umbilical, newborn P51.0
mediastinum — *see* Hemorrhage, lung
medulla I61.3
membrane (brain) I60.8
  spinal cord — *see* Hemorrhage, spinal cord
meninges, meningeal (brain) (middle) I60.8
  spinal cord — *see* Hemorrhage, spinal cord
mesentery K66.1
metritis — *see* Endometritis
mouth K13.79
mucous membrane NEC R58
  newborn P54.8
muscle M62.89
nail (subungual) L60.8
nasal turbinate R04.0
  newborn P54.8
navel, newborn P51.9
newborn P54.9
  specified NEC P54.8
nipple N64.59
nose R04.0
  newborn P54.8
omentum K66.1
optic nerve (sheath) H47.02- ☑
orbit, orbital H05.23- ☑
ovary NEC N83.8
oviduct N83.6
pancreas K86.89
parathyroid (gland) (spontaneous) E21.4
parturition — *see* Hemorrhage, complicating, delivery
penis N48.89
pericardium, pericarditis I31.2
peritoneum, peritoneal K66.1
peritonsillar tissue J35.8
  due to infection J36
petechial R23.3
  due to autosensitivity, erythrocyte D69.2
pituitary (gland) E23.6
pleura — *see* Hemorrhage, lung
polioencephalitis, superior E51.2
polymyositis — *see* Polymyositis

Hemorrhage, hemorrhagic — *continued*
pons, pontine I61.3
posterior fossa (nontraumatic) I61.8
  newborn P52.6
postmenopausal N95.0
postnasal R04.0
postoperative — *see* Complications, postprocedural, hemorrhage, by site
postpartum NEC (following delivery of placenta) O72.1
  delayed or secondary O72.2
  retained placenta O72.0
  third stage O72.0
pregnancy — *see* Hemorrhage, antepartum
preretinal — *see* Hemorrhage, retina
prostate N42.1
puerperal — *see* Hemorrhage, postpartum
  delayed or secondary O72.2
pulmonary R04.89
  newborn P26.9
    massive P26.1
    specified NEC P26.8
  tuberculous — *see* Tuberculosis, pulmonary
purpura (primary) D69.3
rectum (sphincter) K62.5
  newborn P54.2
recurring, following initial hemorrhage at time of injury T79.2 ☑
renal N28.89
respiratory passage or tract R04.9
  specified NEC R04.89
retina, retinal (vessels) H35.6- ☑
  diabetic — *see* Diabetes, retinal, hemorrhage
retroperitoneal R58
scalp R58
scrotum N50.1
secondary (nontraumatic) R58
  following initial hemorrhage at time of injury T79.2 ☑
seminal vesicle N50.1
skin R23.3
  newborn P54.5
slipped umbilical ligature P51.8
spermatic cord N50.1
spinal (cord) G95.19
  newborn (birth injury) P11.5
spleen D73.5
  intraoperative — *see* Complications, intraoperative, hemorrhage, spleen
  postprocedural — *see* Complications, postprocedural, hemorrhage, spleen
stomach K92.2
  newborn P54.3
  ulcer — *see* Ulcer, stomach, with hemorrhage
subarachnoid (nontraumatic) — *see* Hemorrhage, intracranial, subarachnoid
subconjunctival (*see also* Hemorrhage, conjunctiva)
  birth injury P15.3
subcortical (brain) I61.0
subcutaneous R23.3
subdiaphragmatic R58
subdural (acute) (nontraumatic) — *see* Hemorrhage, intracranial, subdural
subependymal
  newborn P52.0
    with intraventricular extension P52.1
      and intracerebral extension P52.22
subgaleal P12.2
subhyaloid — *see* Hemorrhage, retina
subperiosteal — *see* Disorder, bone, specified type NEC
subretinal — *see* Hemorrhage, retina
subtentorial — *see* Hemorrhage, intracranial, subdural
subungual L60.8
suprarenal (capsule) (gland) E27.49
  newborn P54.4
tentorium (traumatic) NEC — *see* Hemorrhage, brain
  newborn (birth injury) P10.4
testis N50.1
third stage (postpartum) O72.0
thorax — *see* Hemorrhage, lung
throat R04.1
thymus (gland) E32.8
thyroid (cyst) (gland) E07.89
tongue K14.8
tonsil J35.8
trachea — *see* Hemorrhage, lung
tracheobronchial R04.89
  newborn P26.0

☑ **Additional Character Required** — Refer to the Tabular List for Character Selection   ▽ **Subterms under main terms may continue to next column or page**

Hemorrhage, hemorrhagic — *continued*
  traumatic — *code to* specific injury
    cerebellar — *see* Hemorrhage, brain
    intracranial — *see* Hemorrhage, brain
    recurring or secondary (following initial hemorrhage at time of injury) T79.2 ☑
  tuberculous NEC (*see also* Tuberculosis, pulmonary) A15.0
  tunica vaginalis N50.1
  ulcer — *code by* site under Ulcer, with hemorrhage K27.4
  umbilicus, umbilical
    cord
      after birth, newborn P51.9
      complicating delivery O69.5 ☑
    newborn P51.9
      massive P51.0
      slipped ligature P51.8
    stump P51.9
  urethra (idiopathic) N36.8
  uterus, uterine (abnormal) N93.9
    climacteric N92.4
    complicating delivery — *see* Hemorrhage, complicating, delivery
    dysfunctional or functional N93.8
    intermenstrual (regular) N92.3
      irregular N92.1
    postmenopausal N95.0
    postpartum — *see* Hemorrhage, postpartum
    preclimacteric or premenopausal N92.4
    prepubertal N93.8
    pubertal N92.2
  vagina (abnormal) N93.9
    newborn P54.6
  vas deferens N50.1
  vasa previa O69.4 ☑
  ventricular I61.5
  vesical N32.89
  viscera NEC R58
    newborn P54.8
  vitreous (humor) (intraocular) H43.1- ☑
  vulva N90.89
Hemorrhoids (bleeding) (without mention of degree) K64.9
  1st degree (grade/stage I) (without prolapse outside of anal canal) K64.0
  2nd degree (grade/stage II) (that prolapse with straining but retract spontaneously) K64.1
  3rd degree (grade/stage III) (that prolapse with straining and require manual replacement back inside anal canal) K64.2
  4th degree (grade/stage IV) (with prolapsed tissue that cannot be manually replaced) K64.3
  complicating
    pregnancy O22.4 ☑
    puerperium O87.2
  external K64.4
    with
      thrombosis K64.5
  internal (without mention of degree) K64.8
  prolapsed K64.8
  skin tags
    anus K64.4
    residual K64.4
  specified NEC K64.8
  strangulated (*see also* Hemorrhoids, by degree) K64.8
  thrombosed (*see also* Hemorrhoids, by degree) K64.5
  ulcerated (*see also* Hemorrhoids, by degree) K64.8
Hemosalpinx N83.6
  with
    hematocolpos N89.7
    hematometra N85.7
      with hematocolpos N89.7
Hemosiderosis (dietary) E83.19
  pulmonary, idiopathic E83.1- ☑ [J84.03]
  transfusion T80.89 ☑
Hemothorax (bacterial) (nontuberculous) J94.2
  newborn P54.8
  traumatic S27.1 ☑
    with pneumothorax S27.2 ☑
  tuberculous NEC A15.6
Henoch (-Schönlein) **disease or syndrome** (purpura) D69.0
Henpue, henpuye A66.6
Hepar lobatum (syphilitic) A52.74
Hepatalgia K76.89
Hepatitis K75.9
  acute B17.9

Hepatitis — *continued*
  acute — *continued*
    with coma K72.01
    with hepatic failure — *see* Failure, hepatic
    alcoholic — *see* Hepatitis, alcoholic
    infectious B17.9
    non-viral K72.0 ☑
    viral B17.9
  alcoholic (acute) (chronic) K70.10
    with ascites K70.11
  amebic — *see* Abscess, liver, amebic
  anicteric, (viral) — *see* Hepatitis, viral
  antigen-associated (HAA) — *see* Hepatitis, B
  Australia-antigen (positive) — *see* Hepatitis, B
  autoimmune K75.4
  B B19.10
    with hepatic coma B19.11
    acute B16.9
      with
        delta-agent (coinfection) (without hepatic coma) B16.1
          with hepatic coma B16.0
        hepatic coma (without delta-agent coinfection) B16.2
    chronic B18.1
      with delta-agent B18.0
  bacterial NEC K75.89
  C (viral) B19.20
    with hepatic coma B19.21
    acute B17.10
      with hepatic coma B17.11
    chronic B18.2
  catarrhal (acute) B15.9
    with hepatic coma B15.0
  cholangiolitic K75.89
  cholestatic K75.89
  chronic K73.9
    active NEC K73.2
    lobular NEC K73.1
    persistent NEC K73.0
    specified NEC K73.8
  cytomegaloviral B25.1
  due to ethanol (acute) (chronic) — *see* Hepatitis, alcoholic
  epidemic B15.9
    with hepatic coma B15.0
  fulminant NEC (viral) — *see* Hepatitis, viral
  granulomatous NEC K75.3
  herpesviral B00.81
  history of
    B Z86.19
    C Z86.19
  homologous serum — *see* Hepatitis, viral, type B
  in (due to)
    mumps B26.81
    toxoplasmosis (acquired) B58.1
      congenital (active) P37.1 [K77]
  infectious, infective B15.9
    acute (subacute) B17.9
    chronic B18.9
  inoculation — *see* Hepatitis, viral, type B
  interstitial (chronic) K74.69
  lupoid NEC K75.4
  malignant NEC (with hepatic failure) K72.90
    with coma K72.91
  neonatal (idiopathic) (toxic) P59.29
  neonatal giant cell P59.29
  newborn P59.29
  non-viral K72.0 ☑
  postimmunization — *see* Hepatitis, viral, type B
  post-transfusion — *see* Hepatitis, viral, type B
  reactive, nonspecific K75.2
  serum — *see* Hepatitis, viral, type B
  specified type NEC
    with hepatic failure — *see* Failure, hepatic
  syphilitic (late) A52.74
    congenital (early) A50.08 [K77]
      late A50.59 [K77]
    secondary A51.45
  toxic (*see also* Disease, liver, toxic) K71.6
  tuberculous A18.83
  viral, virus B19.9
    with hepatic coma B19.0
    acute B17.9
    chronic B18.9
      specified NEC B18.8
      type
        B B18.1

Hepatitis — *continued*
  viral, virus — *continued*
    chronic — *continued*
      type — *continued*
        B — *continued*
          with delta-agent B18.0
        C B18.2
    congenital P35.3
    coxsackie B33.8 [K77]
    cytomegalic inclusion B25.1
    in remission, any type — *code to* Hepatitis, chronic, by type
    non-A, non-B B17.8
    specified type NEC (with or without coma) B17.8
    type
      A B15.9
        with hepatic coma B15.0
      B B19.10
        with hepatic coma B19.11
        acute B16.9
          with
            delta-agent (coinfection) (without hepatic coma) B16.1
              with hepatic coma B16.0
            hepatic coma (without delta-agent coinfection) B16.2
        chronic B18.1
          with delta-agent B18.0
      C B19.20
        with hepatic coma B19.21
        acute B17.10
          with hepatic coma B17.11
        chronic B18.2
      E B17.2
    non-A, non-B B17.8
Hepatization lung (acute) — *see* Pneumonia, lobar
Hepatoblastoma C22.2
Hepatocarcinoma C22.0
Hepatocholangiocarcinoma C22.0
Hepatocholangioma, benign D13.4
Hepatocholangitis K75.89
Hepatolenticular degeneration E83.01
Hepatoma (malignant) C22.0
  benign D13.4
  embryonal C22.0
Hepatomegaly (*see also* Hypertrophy, liver)
  with splenomegaly R16.2
  congenital Q44.7
  in mononucleosis
    gammaherpesviral B27.09
    infectious specified NEC B27.89
Hepatoptosis K76.89
Hepatorenal syndrome following labor and delivery O90.4
Hepatosis K76.89
Hepatosplenomegaly R16.2
  hyperlipemic (Bürger-Grütz type) E78.3 [K77]
Hereditary — *see* condition
Heredodegeneration, macular — *see* Dystrophy, retina
Heredopathia atactica polyneuritiformis G60.1
Heredosyphilis — *see* Syphilis, congenital
Herlitz' syndrome Q81.1
Hermansky-Pudlak syndrome E70.331
Hermaphrodite, hermaphroditism (true) Q56.0
  46,XX with streak gonads Q99.1
  46,XX/46,XY Q99.0
  46,XY with streak gonads Q99.1
  chimera 46,XX/46,XY Q99.0
Hernia, hernial (acquired) (recurrent) K46.9
  with
    gangrene — *see* Hernia, by site, with, gangrene
    incarceration — *see* Hernia, by site, with, obstruction
    irreducible — *see* Hernia, by site, with, obstruction
    obstruction — *see* Hernia, by site, with, obstruction
    strangulation — *see* Hernia, by site, with, obstruction
  abdomen, abdominal K46.9
    with
      gangrene (and obstruction) K46.1
      obstruction K46.0
    femoral — *see* Hernia, femoral
    incisional — *see* Hernia, incisional
    inguinal — *see* Hernia, inguinal
    specified site NEC K45.8
      with
        gangrene (and obstruction) K45.1
        obstruction K45.0

Hernia, hernial — *continued*
  abdomen, abdominal — *continued*
    umbilical — *see* Hernia, umbilical
    wall — *see* Hernia, ventral
  appendix — *see* Hernia, abdomen
  bladder (mucosa) (sphincter)
    congenital (female) (male) Q79.51
    female — *see* Cystocele
    male N32.89
  brain, congenital — *see* Encephalocele
  cartilage, vertebra — *see* Displacement, intervertebral
      disc
  cerebral, congenital (*see also* Encephalocele)
    endaural Q01.8
  ciliary body (traumatic) S05.2- ☑
  colon — *see* Hernia, abdomen
  Cooper's — *see* Hernia, abdomen, specified site NEC
  crural — *see* Hernia, femoral
  diaphragm, diaphragmatic K44.9
    with
      gangrene (and obstruction) K44.1
      obstruction K44.0
    congenital Q79.0
  direct (inguinal) — *see* Hernia, inguinal
  diverticulum, intestine — *see* Hernia, abdomen
  double (inguinal) — *see* Hernia, inguinal, bilateral
  due to adhesions (with obstruction) K56.50
  epigastric (*see also* Hernia, ventral) K43.9
  esophageal hiatus — *see* Hernia, hiatal
  external (inguinal) — *see* Hernia, inguinal
  fallopian tube N83.4- ☑
  fascia M62.89
  femoral K41.90
    with
      gangrene (and obstruction) K41.40
        not specified as recurrent K41.40
        recurrent K41.41
      obstruction K41.30
        not specified as recurrent K41.30
        recurrent K41.31
    bilateral K41.20
      with
        gangrene (and obstruction) K41.10
          not specified as recurrent K41.10
          recurrent K41.11
        obstruction K41.00
          not specified as recurrent K41.00
          recurrent K41.01
      not specified as recurrent K41.20
      recurrent K41.21
    not specified as recurrent K41.90
    recurrent K41.91
    unilateral K41.90
      with
        gangrene (and obstruction) K41.40
          not specified as recurrent K41.40
          recurrent K41.41
        obstruction K41.30
          not specified as recurrent K41.30
          recurrent K41.31
      not specified as recurrent K41.90
      recurrent K41.91
  foramen magnum G93.5
    congenital Q01.8
  funicular (umbilical) (*see also* Hernia, umbilicus)
    spermatic (cord) — *see* Hernia, inguinal
  gastrointestinal tract — *see* Hernia, abdomen
  Hesselbach's — *see* Hernia, femoral, specified site NEC
  hiatal (esophageal) (sliding) K44.9
    with
      gangrene (and obstruction) K44.1
      obstruction K44.0
    congenital Q40.1
  hypogastric — *see* Hernia, ventral
  incarcerated (*see also* Hernia, by site, with obstruction)
    with gangrene — *see* Hernia, by site, with gan-
        grene
  incisional K43.2
    with
      gangrene (and obstruction) K43.1
      obstruction K43.0
  indirect (inguinal) — *see* Hernia, inguinal
  inguinal (direct) (external) (funicular) (indirect) (inter-
      nal) (oblique) (scrotal) (sliding) K40.90
    with
      gangrene (and obstruction) K40.40
        not specified as recurrent K40.40
        recurrent K40.41

Hernia, hernial — *continued*
  inguinal — *continued*
    with — *continued*
      obstruction K40.30
        not specified as recurrent K40.30
        recurrent K40.31
    bilateral K40.20
      with
        gangrene (and obstruction) K40.10
          not specified as recurrent K40.10
          recurrent K40.11
        obstruction K40.00
          not specified as recurrent K40.00
          recurrent K40.01
      not specified as recurrent K40.20
      recurrent K40.21
    not specified as recurrent K40.90
    recurrent K40.91
    unilateral K40.90
      with
        gangrene (and obstruction) K40.40
          not specified as recurrent K40.40
          recurrent K40.41
        obstruction K40.30
          not specified as recurrent K40.30
          recurrent K40.31
      not specified as recurrent K40.90
      recurrent K40.91
  internal (*see also* Hernia, abdomen)
    inguinal — *see* Hernia, inguinal
  interstitial — *see* Hernia, abdomen
  intervertebral cartilage or disc — *see* Displacement,
      intervertebral disc
  intestine, intestinal — *see* Hernia, by site
  intra-abdominal — *see* Hernia, abdomen
  iris (traumatic) S05.2- ☑
  irreducible (*see also* Hernia, by site, with obstruction)
    with gangrene — *see* Hernia, by site, with gan-
        grene
  ischiatic — *see* Hernia, abdomen, specified site NEC
  ischiorectal — *see* Hernia, abdomen, specified site
      NEC
  lens (traumatic) S05.2- ☑
  linea (alba) (semilunaris) — *see* Hernia, ventral
  Littre's — *see* Hernia, abdomen
  lumbar — *see* Hernia, abdomen, specified site NEC
  lung (subcutaneous) J98.4
  mediastinum J98.59
  mesenteric (internal) — *see* Hernia, abdomen
  midline — *see* Hernia, ventral
  muscle (sheath) M62.89
  nucleus pulposus — *see* Displacement, intervertebral
      disc
  oblique (inguinal) — *see* Hernia, inguinal
  obstructive (*see also* Hernia, by site, with obstruction)
    with gangrene — *see* Hernia, by site, with gan-
        grene
  obturator — *see* Hernia, abdomen, specified site NEC
  omental — *see* Hernia, abdomen
  ovary N83.4- ☑
  oviduct N83.4- ☑
  paraesophageal (*see also* Hernia, diaphragm)
    congenital Q40.1
  parastomal K43.5
    with
      gangrene (and obstruction) K43.4
      obstruction K43.3
  paraumbilical — *see* Hernia, umbilicus
  perineal — *see* Hernia, abdomen, specified site NEC
  Petit's — *see* Hernia, abdomen, specified site NEC
  postoperative — *see* Hernia, incisional
  pregnant uterus — *see* Abnormal, uterus in pregnancy
      or childbirth
  prevesical N32.89
  properitoneal — *see* Hernia, abdomen, specified site
      NEC
  pudendal — *see* Hernia, abdomen, specified site NEC
  rectovaginal N81.6
  retroperitoneal — *see* Hernia, abdomen, specified site
      NEC
  Richter's — *see* Hernia, abdomen, with obstruction
  Rieux's, Riex's — *see* Hernia, abdomen, specified site
      NEC
  sac condition (adhesion) (dropsy) (inflammation)
      (laceration) (suppuration) — *code by site under*
      Hernia
  sciatic — *see* Hernia, abdomen, specified site NEC

Hernia, hernial — *continued*
  scrotum, scrotal — *see* Hernia, inguinal
  sliding (inguinal) (*see also* Hernia, inguinal)
    hiatus — *see* Hernia, hiatal
  spigelian — *see* Hernia, ventral
  spinal — *see* Spina bifida
  strangulated (*see also* Hernia, by site, with obstruction)
    with gangrene — *see* Hernia, by site, with gan-
        grene
  subxiphoid — *see* Hernia, ventral
  supra-umbilicus — *see* Hernia, ventral
  tendon — *see* Disorder, tendon, specified type NEC
  Treitz's (fossa) — *see* Hernia, abdomen, specified site
      NEC
  tunica vaginalis Q55.29
  umbilicus, umbilical K42.9
    with
      gangrene (and obstruction) K42.1
      obstruction K42.0
  ureter N28.89
  urethra, congenital Q64.79
  urinary meatus, congenital Q64.79
  uterus N81.4
    pregnant — *see* Abnormal, uterus in pregnancy or
        childbirth
  vaginal (anterior) (wall) — *see* Cystocele
  Velpeau's — *see* Hernia, femoral
  ventral K43.9
    with
      gangrene (and obstruction) K43.7
      obstruction K43.6
    incisional K43.2
      with
        gangrene (and obstruction) K43.1
        obstruction K43.0
      recurrent — *see* Hernia, incisional
    specified NEC K43.9
      with
        gangrene (and obstruction) K43.7
        obstruction K43.6
  vesical
    congenital (female) (male) Q79.51
    female — *see* Cystocele
    male N32.89
  vitreous (into wound) S05.2- ☑
    into anterior chamber — *see* Prolapse, vitreous
Herniation (*see also* Hernia)
  brain (stem) G93.5
  cerebral G93.5
  mediastinum J98.59
  nucleus pulposus — *see* Displacement, intervertebral
      disc
Herpangina B08.5
Herpes, herpesvirus, herpetic B00.9
  anogenital A60.9
    perianal skin A60.1
    rectum A60.1
    urogenital tract A60.00
      cervix A60.03
      male genital organ NEC A60.02
      penis A60.01
      specified site NEC A60.09
      vagina A60.04
      vulva A60.04
  blepharitis (zoster) B02.39
    simplex B00.59
  circinatus B35.4
    bullosus L12.0
  conjunctivitis (simplex) B00.53
    zoster B02.31
  cornea B02.33
  encephalitis B00.4
    due to herpesvirus 6 B10.01
    due to herpesvirus 7 B10.09
    specified NEC B10.09
  eye (zoster) B02.30
    simplex B00.50
  eyelid (zoster) B02.39
    simplex B00.59
  facialis B00.1
  febrilis B00.1
  geniculate ganglionitis B02.21
  genital, genitalis A60.00
    female A60.09
    male A60.02
  gestational, gestationis O26.4- ☑
  gingivostomatitis B00.2
  human B00.9

☑ Additional Character Required — Refer to the Tabular List for Character Selection   ▽ Subterms under main terms may continue to next column or page

Herpes, herpesvirus, herpetic — continued
  human — continued
    1 — see Herpes, simplex
    2 — see Herpes, simplex
    3 — see Varicella
    4 — see Mononucleosis, Epstein-Barr (virus)
    5 — see Disease, cytomegalic inclusion (generalized)
    6
      encephalitis B10.01
      specified NEC B10.81
    7
      encephalitis B10.09
      specified NEC B10.82
    8 B10.89
    infection NEC B10.89
      Kaposi's sarcoma associated B10.89
    iridocyclitis (simplex) B00.51
      zoster B02.32
    iris (vesicular erythema multiforme) L51.9
    iritis (simplex) B00.51
    Kaposi's sarcoma associated B10.89
    keratitis (simplex) (dendritic) (disciform) (interstitial) B00.52
      zoster (interstitial) B02.33
    keratoconjunctivitis (simplex) B00.52
      zoster B02.33
    labialis B00.1
    lip B00.1
    meningitis (simplex) B00.3
      zoster B02.1
    ophthalmicus (zoster) NEC B02.30
      simplex B00.50
    penis A60.01
    perianal skin A60.1
    pharyngitis, pharyngotonsillitis B00.2
    rectum A60.1
    scrotum A60.02
    sepsis B00.7
    simplex B00.9
      complicated NEC B00.89
      congenital P35.2
      conjunctivitis B00.53
      external ear B00.1
      eyelid B00.59
      hepatitis B00.81
      keratitis (interstitial) B00.52
      myelitis B00.82
      specified complication NEC B00.89
      visceral B00.89
    stomatitis B00.2
    tonsurans B35.0
    visceral B00.89
    vulva A60.04
    whitlow B00.89
    zoster (see also condition) B02.9
      auricularis B02.21
      complicated NEC B02.8
      conjunctivitis B02.31
      disseminated B02.7
      encephalitis B02.0
      eye (lid) B02.39
      geniculate ganglionitis B02.21
      keratitis (interstitial) B02.33
      meningitis B02.1
      myelitis B02.24
      neuritis, neuralgia B02.29
      ophthalmicus NEC B02.30
      oticus B02.21
      polyneuropathy B02.23
      specified complication NEC B02.8
      trigeminal neuralgia B02.22
Herpesvirus (human) — see Herpes
Herpetophobia F40.218
Herrick's anemia — see Disease, sickle-cell
Hers' disease E74.09
Herter-Gee syndrome K90.0
Herxheimer's reaction R68.89
Hesitancy
  of micturition R39.11
  urinary R39.11
Hesselbach's hernia — see Hernia, femoral, specified site NEC
Heterochromia (congenital) Q13.2
  cataract — see Cataract, complicated
  cyclitis (Fuchs) — see Cyclitis, Fuchs' heterochromic
  hair L67.1
  iritis — see Cyclitis, Fuchs' heterochromic

Heterochromia — continued
  retained metallic foreign body (nonmagnetic) — see Foreign body, intraocular, old, retained
    magnetic — see Foreign body, intraocular, old, retained, magnetic
  uveitis — see Cyclitis, Fuchs' heterochromic
Heterophoria — see Strabismus, heterophoria
Heterophyes, heterophyiasis (small intestine) B66.8
Heterotopia, heterotopic (see also Malposition, congenital)
  cerebralis Q04.8
Heterotropia — see Strabismus
Heubner-Herter disease K90.0
Hexadactylism Q69.9
HGSIL (cytology finding) (high grade squamous intraepithelial lesion on cytologic smear) (Pap smear finding)
  anus R85.613
  cervix R87.613
    biopsy (histology) finding — see Neoplasia, intraepithelial, cervix, grade II or grade III
  vagina R87.623
    biopsy (histology) finding — see Neoplasia, intraepithelial, cervix, grade II or grade III
Hibernoma — see Lipoma
Hiccup, hiccough R06.6
  epidemic B33.0
  psychogenic F45.8
Hidden penis (congenital) Q55.64
  acquired N48.83
Hidradenitis (axillaris) (suppurative) L73.2
Hidradenoma (nodular) (see also Neoplasm, skin, benign)
  clear cell — see Neoplasm, skin, benign
  papillary — see Neoplasm, skin, benign
Hidrocystoma — see Neoplasm, skin, benign
High
  altitude effects T70.20 ☑
    anoxia T70.29 ☑
    on
      ears T70.0 ☑
      sinuses T70.1 ☑
    polycythemia D75.1
  arch
    foot Q66.7
    palate, congenital Q38.5
  arterial tension — see Hypertension
  basal metabolic rate R94.8
  blood pressure (see also Hypertension)
    borderline R03.0
    reading (incidental) (isolated) (nonspecific), without diagnosis of hypertension R03.0
  cholesterol E78.00
    with high triglycerides E78.2
  diaphragm (congenital) Q79.1
  expressed emotional level within family Z63.8
  head at term O32.4 ☑
  palate, congenital Q38.5
  risk
    infant NEC Z76.2
    sexual behavior (heterosexual) Z72.51
      bisexual Z72.53
      homosexual Z72.52
  scrotal testis, testes
    bilateral Q53.23
    unilateral Q53.13
  temperature (of unknown origin) R50.9
  thoracic rib Q76.6
  triglycerides E78.1
    with high cholesterol E78.2
Hildenbrand's disease A75.0
Hilum — see condition
Hip — see condition
Hippel's disease Q85.8
Hippophobia F40.218
Hippus H57.09
Hirschsprung's disease or megacolon Q43.1
Hirsutism, hirsuties L68.0
Hirudiniasis
  external B88.3
  internal B83.4
Hiss-Russell dysentery A03.1
Histidinemia, histidinuria E70.41
Histiocytoma (see also Neoplasm, skin, benign)
  fibrous (see also Neoplasm, skin, benign)
    atypical — see Neoplasm, connective tissue, uncertain behavior

Histiocytoma — continued
  fibrous (see also Neoplasm, skin, benign) — continued
    malignant — see Neoplasm, connective tissue, malignant
Histiocytosis D76.3
  acute differentiated progressive C96.0
  Langerhans' cell NEC C96.6
    multifocal X
      multisystemic (disseminated) C96.0
      unisystemic C96.5
    pulmonary, adult (adult PLCH) J84.82
    unifocal (X) C96.6
  lipid, lipoid D76.3
    essential E75.29
  malignant C96.A (following C96.6)
  mononuclear phagocytes NEC D76.1
    Langerhans' cells C96.6
  non-Langerhans cell D76.3
  polyostotic sclerosing D76.3
  sinus, with massive lymphadenopathy D76.3
  syndrome NEC D76.3
  X NEC C96.6
    acute (progressive) C96.0
    chronic C96.6
    multifocal C96.5
    multisystemic C96.0
    unifocal C96.6
Histoplasmosis B39.9
  with pneumonia NEC B39.2
  African B39.5
  American — see Histoplasmosis, capsulati
  capsulati B39.4
    disseminated B39.3
    generalized B39.3
    pulmonary B39.2
      acute B39.0
      chronic B39.1
  Darling's B39.4
  duboisii B39.5
  lung NEC B39.2
History
  family (of) (see also History, personal (of))
    alcohol abuse Z81.1
    allergy NEC Z84.89
    anemia Z83.2
    arthritis Z82.61
    asthma Z82.5
    blindness Z82.1
    cardiac death (sudden) Z82.41
    carrier of genetic disease Z84.81
    chromosomal anomaly Z82.79
    chronic
      disabling disease NEC Z82.8
      lower respiratory disease Z82.5
    colonic polyps Z83.71
    congenital malformations and deformations Z82.79
      polycystic kidney Z82.71
    consanguinity Z84.3
    deafness Z82.2
    diabetes mellitus Z83.3
    disability NEC Z82.8
    disease or disorder (of)
      allergic NEC Z84.89
      behavioral NEC Z81.8
      blood and blood-forming organs Z83.2
      cardiovascular NEC Z82.49
      chronic disabling NEC Z82.8
      digestive Z83.79
      ear NEC Z83.52
      endocrine NEC Z83.49
      eye NEC Z83.518
        glaucoma Z83.511
      familial hypercholesterolemia Z83.42
      genitourinary NEC Z84.2
      glaucoma Z83.511
      hematological Z83.2
      immune mechanism Z83.2
      infectious NEC Z83.1
      ischemic heart Z82.49
      kidney Z84.1
      mental NEC Z81.8
      metabolic Z83.49
      musculoskeletal NEC Z82.69
      neurological NEC Z82.0
      nutritional Z83.49
      parasitic NEC Z83.1
      psychiatric NEC Z81.8
      respiratory NEC Z83.6

History — *continued*
  family (*see also* History, personal) — *continued*
    disease or disorder — *continued*
      skin and subcutaneous tissue NEC Z84.0
      specified NEC Z84.89
    drug abuse NEC Z81.3
    epilepsy Z82.0
    familial hypercholesterolemia Z83.42
    genetic disease carrier Z84.81
    glaucoma Z83.511
    hearing loss Z82.2
    human immunodeficiency virus (HIV) infection
      Z83.0
    Huntington's chorea Z82.0
    intellectual disability Z81.0
    leukemia Z80.6
    malignant neoplasm (of) NOS Z80.9
      bladder Z80.52
      breast Z80.3
      bronchus Z80.1
      digestive organ Z80.0
      gastrointestinal tract Z80.0
      genital organ Z80.49
        ovary Z80.41
        prostate Z80.42
        specified organ NEC Z80.49
        testis Z80.43
      hematopoietic NEC Z80.7
      intrathoracic organ NEC Z80.2
      kidney Z80.51
      lung Z80.1
      lymphatic NEC Z80.7
      ovary Z80.41
      prostate Z80.42
      respiratory organ NEC Z80.2
      specified site NEC Z80.8
      testis Z80.43
      trachea Z80.1
      urinary organ or tract Z80.59
        bladder Z80.52
        kidney Z80.51
    mental
      disorder NEC Z81.8
    multiple endocrine neoplasia (MEN) syndrome
      Z83.41
    osteoporosis Z82.62
    polycystic kidney Z82.71
    polyps (colon) Z83.71
    psychiatric disorder Z81.8
    psychoactive substance abuse NEC Z81.3
    respiratory condition NEC Z83.6
      asthma and other lower respiratory conditions
        Z82.5
    self-harmful behavior Z81.8
    SIDS (sudden infant death syndrome) Z84.82
    skin condition Z84.0
    specified condition NEC Z84.89
    stroke (cerebrovascular) Z82.3
    substance abuse NEC Z81.4
      alcohol Z81.1
      drug NEC Z81.3
      psychoactive NEC Z81.3
      tobacco Z81.2
    sudden
      cardiac death Z82.41
      infant death syndrome (SIDS) Z84.82
    tobacco abuse Z81.2
    violence, violent behavior Z81.8
    visual loss Z82.1
  personal (of) (*see also* History, family (of))
    abuse
      adult Z91.419
        physical and sexual Z91.410
        psychological Z91.411
      childhood Z62.819
        physical Z62.810
        psychological Z62.811
        sexual Z62.810
    alcohol dependence F10.21
    allergy (to) Z88.9
      analgesic agent NEC Z88.6
      anesthetic Z88.4
      antibiotic agent NEC Z88.1
      anti-infective agent NEC Z88.3
      contrast media Z91.041
      drugs, medicaments and biological substances
        Z88.9
        specified NEC Z88.8
      food Z91.018

History — *continued*
  personal (*see also* History, family) — *continued*
    allergy — *continued*
      food — *continued*
        additives Z91.02
        eggs Z91.012
        milk products Z91.011
        peanuts Z91.010
        seafood Z91.013
        specified food NEC Z91.018
      insect Z91.038
        bee Z91.030
      latex Z91.040
      medicinal agents Z88.9
        specified NEC Z88.8
      narcotic agent NEC Z88.5
      nonmedicinal agents Z91.048
      penicillin Z88.0
      serum Z88.7
      specified NEC Z91.09
      sulfonamides Z88.2
      vaccine Z88.7
    anaphylactic shock Z87.892
    anaphylaxis Z87.892
    behavioral disorders Z86.59
    benign carcinoid tumor Z86.012
    benign neoplasm Z86.018
      brain Z86.011
      carcinoid Z86.012
      colonic polyps Z86.010
    brain injury (traumatic) Z87.820
    breast implant removal Z98.86
    calculi, renal Z87.442
    cancer — *see* History, personal (of), malignant
      neoplasm (of)
    cardiac arrest (death), successfully resuscitated
      Z86.74
    cerebral infarction without residual deficit Z86.73
    cervical dysplasia Z87.410
    chemotherapy for neoplastic condition Z92.21
    childhood abuse — *see* History, personal (of),
      abuse
    cleft lip (corrected) Z87.730
    cleft palate (corrected) Z87.730
    collapsed vertebra (healed) Z87.311
      due to osteoporosis Z87.310
    combat and operational stress reaction Z86.51
    congenital malformation (corrected) Z87.798
      circulatory system (corrected) Z87.74
      digestive system (corrected) NEC Z87.738
      ear (corrected) Z87.721
      eye (corrected) Z87.720
      face and neck (corrected) Z87.790
      genitourinary system (corrected) NEC Z87.718
      heart (corrected) Z87.74
      integument (corrected) Z87.76
      limb(s) (corrected) Z87.76
      musculoskeletal system (corrected) Z87.76
      neck (corrected) Z87.790
      nervous system (corrected) NEC Z87.728
      respiratory system (corrected) Z87.75
      sense organs (corrected) NEC Z87.728
      specified NEC Z87.798
    contraception Z92.0
    deployment (military) Z91.82
    diabetic foot ulcer Z86.31
    disease or disorder (of) Z87.898
      anaphylaxis Z87.892
      blood and blood-forming organs Z86.2
      circulatory system Z86.79
        specified condition NEC Z86.79
      connective tissue Z87.39
      digestive system Z87.19
        colonic polyp Z86.010
        peptic ulcer disease Z87.11
        specified condition NEC Z87.19
      ear Z86.69
      endocrine Z86.39
        diabetic foot ulcer Z86.31
        gestational diabetes Z86.32
        specified type NEC Z86.39
      eye Z86.69
      genital (track) system NEC
        female Z87.42
        male Z87.438
      hematological Z86.2
      Hodgkin Z85.71
      immune mechanism Z86.2
      infectious Z86.19

History — *continued*
  personal (*see also* History, family) — *continued*
    disease or disorder — *continued*
      infectious — *continued*
        malaria Z86.13
        Methicillin resistant Staphylococcus aureus
          (MRSA) Z86.14
        poliomyelitis Z86.12
        specified NEC Z86.19
        tuberculosis Z86.11
      mental NEC Z86.59
      metabolic Z86.39
        diabetic foot ulcer Z86.31
        gestational diabetes Z86.32
        specified type NEC Z86.39
      musculoskeletal NEC Z87.39
      nervous system Z86.69
      nutritional Z86.39
      parasitic Z86.19
      respiratory system NEC Z87.09
      sense organs Z86.69
      skin Z87.2
      specified site or type NEC Z87.898
      subcutaneous tissue Z87.2
      trophoblastic Z87.59
      urinary system NEC Z87.448
    drug dependence — *see* Dependence, drug, by
      type, in remission
    drug therapy
      antineoplastic chemotherapy Z92.21
      estrogen Z92.23
      immunosupression Z92.25
      inhaled steroids Z92.240
      monoclonal drug Z92.22
      specified NEC Z92.29
      steroid Z92.241
      systemic steroids Z92.241
    dysplasia
      cervical (mild) (moderate) Z87.410
        severe (grade III) Z86.001
      prostatic Z87.430
      vaginal (mild) (moderate) Z87.411
        severe (grade III) Z86.008
      vulvar (mild) (moderate) Z87.412
        severe (grade III) Z86.008
    embolism (venous) Z86.718
      pulmonary Z86.711
    encephalitis Z86.61
    estrogen therapy Z92.23
    extracorporeal membrane oxygenation (ECMO)
      Z92.81
    failed conscious sedation Z92.83
    failed moderate sedation Z92.83
    fall, falling Z91.81
    fracture (healed)
      fatigue Z87.312
      fragility Z87.310
      osteoporosis Z87.310
      pathological NEC Z87.311
      stress Z87.312
      traumatic Z87.81
    gestational diabetes Z86.32
    hepatitis
      B Z86.19
      C Z86.19
    Hodgkin disease Z85.71
    hyperthermia, malignant Z88.4
    hypospadias (corrected) Z87.710
    hysterectomy Z90.710
    immunosupression therapy Z92.25
    in situ neoplasm
      breast Z86.000
      cervix uteri Z86.001
      specified NEC Z86.008
    in utero procedure during pregnancy Z98.870
    in utero procedure while a fetus Z98.871
    infection NEC Z86.19
      central nervous system Z86.61
      Methicillin resistant Staphylococcus aureus
        (MRSA) Z86.14
      urinary (recurrent) (tract) Z87.440
    injury NEC Z87.828
    irradiation Z92.3
    kidney stones Z87.442
    leukemia Z85.6
    lymphoma (non-Hodgkin) Z85.72
    malignant melanoma (skin) Z85.820
    malignant neoplasm (of) Z85.9
      accessory sinuses Z85.22

☑ Additional Character Required — Refer to the Tabular List for Character Selection   ▽ Subterms under main terms may continue to next column or page

History — continued
  personal (see also History, family) — continued
    malignant neoplasm — continued
      anus NEC Z85.048
        carcinoid Z85.040
      bladder Z85.51
      bone Z85.830
      brain Z85.841
      breast Z85.3
      bronchus NEC Z85.118
        carcinoid Z85.110
      carcinoid — see History, personal (of), malig-
        nant neoplasm, by site, carcinioid
      cervix Z85.41
      colon NEC Z85.038
        carcinoid Z85.030
      digestive organ Z85.00
        specified NEC Z85.09
      endocrine gland NEC Z85.858
      epididymis Z85.48
      esophagus Z85.01
      eye Z85.840
      gastrointestinal tract — see History, malignant
        neoplasm, digestive organ
      genital organ
        female Z85.40
          specified NEC Z85.44
        male Z85.45
          specified NEC Z85.49
      hematopoietic NEC Z85.79
      intrathoracic organ Z85.20
      kidney NEC Z85.528
        carcinoid Z85.520
      large intestine NEC Z85.038
        carcinoid Z85.030
      larynx Z85.21
      liver Z85.05
      lung NEC Z85.118
        carcinoid Z85.110
      mediastinum Z85.29
      Merkel cell Z85.821
      middle ear Z85.22
      nasal cavities Z85.22
      nervous system NEC Z85.848
      oral cavity Z85.819
        specified site NEC Z85.818
      ovary Z85.43
      pancreas Z85.07
      pelvis Z85.53
      pharynx Z85.819
        specified site NEC Z85.818
      pleura Z85.29
      prostate Z85.46
      rectosigmoid junction NEC Z85.048
        carcinoid Z85.040
      rectum NEC Z85.048
        carcinoid Z85.040
      respiratory organ Z85.20
      sinuses, accessory Z85.22
      skin NEC Z85.828
        melanoma Z85.820
        Merkel cell Z85.821
      small intestine NEC Z85.068
        carcinoid Z85.060
      soft tissue Z85.831
      specified site NEC Z85.89
      stomach NEC Z85.028
        carcinoid Z85.020
      testis Z85.47
      thymus NEC Z85.238
        carcinoid Z85.230
      thyroid Z85.850
      tongue Z85.810
      trachea Z85.12
      urinary organ or tract Z85.50
        specified NEC Z85.59
      uterus Z85.42
    maltreatment Z91.89
    medical treatment NEC Z92.89
    melanoma (malignant) (skin) Z85.820
    meningitis Z86.61
    mental disorder Z86.59
    Merkel cell carcinoma (skin) Z85.821
    Methicillin resistant Staphylococcus aureus (MRSA)
      Z86.14
    military deployment Z91.82
    military war, peacekeeping and humanitarian de-
      ployment (current or past conflict) Z91.82
    myocardial infarction (old) I25.2

History — continued
  personal (see also History, family) — continued
    neglect (in)
      adult Z91.412
      childhood Z62.812
    neoplasm
      benign Z86.018
        brain Z86.011
        colon polyp Z86.010
      in situ
        breast Z86.000
        cervix uteri Z86.001
        specified NEC Z86.008
      malignant — see History of, malignant neo-
        plasm
      uncertain behavior Z86.03
    nephrotic syndrome Z87.441
    nicotine dependence Z87.891
    noncompliance with medical treatment or regimen
      — see Noncompliance
    nutritional deficiency Z86.39
    obstetric complications Z87.59
      childbirth Z87.59
      pregnancy Z87.59
      pre-term labor Z87.51
      puerperium Z87.59
    osteoporosis fractures Z87.31 ☑
    parasuicide (attempt) Z91.5
    physical trauma NEC Z87.828
      self-harm or suicide attempt Z91.5
    pneumonia (recurrent) Z87.01
    poisoning NEC Z91.89
      self-harm or suicide attempt Z91.5
    poor personal hygiene Z91.89
    preterm labor Z87.51
    procedure during pregnancy Z98.870
    procedure while a fetus Z98.871
    prolonged reversible ischemic neurologic deficit
      (PRIND) Z86.73
    prostatic dysplasia Z87.430
    psychological
      abuse
        adult Z91.411
        child Z62.811
      trauma, specified NEC Z91.49
    radiation therapy Z92.3
    removal
      implant
        breast Z98.86
    renal calculi Z87.442
    respiratory condition NEC Z87.09
    retained foreign body fully removed Z87.821
    risk factors NEC Z91.89
    self-harm Z91.5
    self-poisoning attempt Z91.5
    sex reassignment Z87.890
    sleep-wake cycle problem Z72.821
    specified NEC Z87.898
    steroid therapy (systemic) Z92.241
      inhaled Z92.240
    stroke without residual deficits Z86.73
    substance abuse NEC F10-F19
    sudden cardiac arrest Z86.74
    sudden cardiac death successfully resuscitated
      Z86.74
    suicide attempt Z91.5
    surgery NEC Z98.890
      with uterine scar Z98.891
      sex reassignment Z87.890
      transplant — see Transplant
    thrombophlebitis Z86.72
    thrombosis (venous) Z86.718
      pulmonary Z86.711
    tobacco dependence Z87.891
    transient ischemic attack (TIA) without residual
      deficits Z86.73
    trauma (physical) NEC Z87.828
      psychological NEC Z91.49
      self-harm Z91.5
    traumatic brain injury Z87.820
    unhealthy sleep-wake cycle Z72.821
    unintended awareness under general anesthesia
      Z92.84
    urinary calculi Z87.442
    urinary (recurrent) (tract) infection(s) Z87.440
    uterine scar from previous surgery Z98.891
    vaginal dysplasia Z87.411
    venous thrombosis or embolism Z86.718
      pulmonary Z86.711

History — continued
  personal (see also History, family) — continued
    vulvar dysplasia Z87.412
His-Werner disease A79.0
HIV (see also Human, immunodeficiency virus) B20
  laboratory evidence (nonconclusive) R75
  nonconclusive test (in infants) R75
  positive, seropositive Z21
Hives (bold) — see Urticaria
Hoarseness R49.0
Hobo Z59.0
Hodgkin disease — see Lymphoma, Hodgkin
Hodgson's disease I71.2
  ruptured I71.1
Hoffa-Kastert disease E88.89
Hoffa's disease E88.89
Hoffmann-Bouveret syndrome I47.9
Hoffmann's syndrome E03.9 [G73.7]
Hole (round)
  macula H35.34- ☑
  retina (without detachment) — see Break, retina,
    round hole
    with detachment — see Detachment, retina, with
      retinal, break
Holiday relief care Z75.5
Hollenhorst's plaque — see Occlusion, artery, retina
Hollow foot (congenital) Q66.7
  acquired — see Deformity, limb, foot, specified NEC
Holoprosencephaly Q04.2
Holt-Oram syndrome Q87.2
Homelessness Z59.0
Homesickness — see Disorder, adjustment
Homocystinemia, homocystinuria E72.11
Homogentisate 1,2-dioxygenase deficiency E70.29
Homologous serum hepatitis (prophylactic) (therapeu-
  tic) — see Hepatitis, viral, type B
Honeycomb lung J98.4
  congenital Q33.0
Hooded
  clitoris Q52.6
  penis Q55.69
Hookworm (anemia) (disease) (infection) (infestation)
  B76.9
  specified NEC B76.8
Hordeolum (eyelid) (externum) (recurrent) H00.019
  internum H00.029
    left H00.026
      lower H00.025
      upper H00.024
    right H00.023
      lower H00.022
      upper H00.021
  left H00.016
    lower H00.015
    upper H00.014
  right H00.013
    lower H00.012
    upper H00.011
Horn
  cutaneous L85.8
  nail L60.2
    congenital Q84.6
Horner (-Claude Bernard) **syndrome** G90.2
  traumatic — see Injury, nerve, cervical sympathetic
Horseshoe kidney (congenital) Q63.1
Horton's headache or neuralgia G44.099
  intractable G44.091
  not intractable G44.099
Hospital hopper syndrome — see Disorder, factitious
Hospitalism in children — see Disorder, adjustment
Hostility R45.5
  towards child Z62.3
Hot flashes
  menopausal N95.1
Hourglass (contracture) (see also Contraction, hourglass)
  stomach K31.89
    congenital Q40.2
    stricture K31.2
Household, housing circumstance affecting care
  Z59.9
  specified NEC Z59.8
Housemaid's knee — see Bursitis, prepatellar
Hudson (-Stähli) **line** (cornea) — see Pigmentation,
  cornea, anterior
Human
  bite (open wound) (see also Bite)
    intact skin surface — see Bite, superficial

Human — *continued*
  herpesvirus — *see* Herpes
  immunodeficiency virus (HIV) disease (infection) B20
    asymptomatic status Z21
    contact Z20.6
    counseling Z71.7
    dementia B20 [F02.80]
      with behavioral disturbance B20 [F02.81]
    exposure to Z20.6
    laboratory evidence R75
    type-2 (HIV 2) as cause of disease classified else-
        where B97.35
  papillomavirus (HPV)
    DNA test positive
      high risk
        cervix R87.810
        vagina R87.811
      low risk
        cervix R87.820
        vagina R87.821
    screening for Z11.51
  T-cell lymphotropic virus
    type-1 (HTLV-I) infection B33.3
      as cause of disease classified elsewhere B97.33
      carrier Z22.6
    type-2 (HTLV-II) as cause of disease classified else-
        where B97.34
Humidifier lung or pneumonitis J67.7
Humiliation (experience) **in childhood** Z62.898
Humpback (acquired) — *see* Kyphosis
Hunchback (acquired) — *see* Kyphosis
Hunger T73.0 ☑
  air, psychogenic F45.8
Hungry bone syndrome E83.81
Hunner's ulcer — *see* Cystitis, chronic, interstitial
Hunter's
  glossitis D51.0
  syndrome E76.1
Huntington's disease or chorea G10
  with dementia G10 [F02.80]
    with behavioral disturbance G10 [F02.81]
Hunt's
  disease or syndrome (herpetic geniculate ganglionitis)
      B02.21
    dyssynergia cerebellaris myoclonica G11.1
  neuralgia B02.21
Hurler (-Scheie) **disease or syndrome** E76.02
Hurst's disease G36.1
Hurthle cell
  adenocarcinoma C73
  adenoma D34
  carcinoma C73
  tumor D34
Hutchinson-Boeck disease or syndrome — *see* Sar-
    coidosis
Hutchinson-Gilford disease or syndrome E34.8
Hutchinson's
  disease, meaning
    angioma serpiginosum L81.7
    pompholyx (cheiropompholyx) L30.1
    prurigo estivalis L56.4
    summer eruption or summer prurigo L56.4
  melanotic freckle — *see* Melanoma, in situ
    malignant melanoma in — *see* Melanoma
  teeth or incisors (congenital syphilis) A50.52
  triad (congenital syphilis) A50.53
Hyalin plaque, sclera, senile H15.89
Hyaline membrane (disease) (lung) (pulmonary) (new-
    born) P22.0
Hyalinosis
  cutis (et mucosae) E78.89
  focal and segmental (glomerular) (*see also* N00-N07
    with fourth character .1) N05.1
Hyalitis, hyalosis, asteroid (*see also* Deposit, crystalline)
  syphilitic (late) A52.71
Hydatid
  cyst or tumor — *see* Echinococcus
  mole — *see* Hydatidiform mole
  Morgagni
    female Q50.5
    male (epididymal) Q55.4
    testicular Q55.29
Hydatidiform mole (benign) (complicating pregnancy)
    (delivered) (undelivered) O01.9
  classical O01.0
  complete O01.0
  incomplete O01.1
  invasive D39.2

Hydatidiform mole — *continued*
  malignant D39.2
  partial O01.1
Hydatidosis — *see* Echinococcus
Hydradenitis (axillaris) (suppurative) L73.2
Hydradenoma — *see* Hidradenoma
Hydramnios O40.- ☑
Hydrancephaly, hydranencephaly Q04.3
  with spina bifida — *see* Spina bifida, with hydro-
      cephalus
Hydrargyrism NEC — *see* Poisoning, mercury
Hydrarthrosis (*see also* Effusion, joint)
  gonococcal A54.42
  intermittent M12.40
    ankle M12.47- ☑
    elbow M12.42- ☑
    foot joint M12.47- ☑
    hand joint M12.44- ☑
    hip M12.45- ☑
    knee M12.46- ☑
    multiple site M12.49
    shoulder M12.41- ☑
    specified joint NEC M12.48
    wrist M12.43- ☑
  of yaws (early) (late) (*see also* subcategory M14.8-)
      A66.6
  syphilitic (late) A52.77
    congenital A50.55 [M12.80]
Hydremia D64.89
Hydrencephalocele (congenital) — *see* Encephalocele
Hydrencephalomeningocele (congenital) — *see* En-
    cephalocele
Hydroa R23.8
  aestivale L56.4
  vacciniforme L56.4
Hydroadenitis (axillaris) (suppurative) L73.2
Hydrocalycosis — *see* Hydronephrosis
Hydrocele (spermatic cord) (testis) (tunica vaginalis)
    N43.3
  canal of Nuck N94.89
  communicating N43.2
    congenital P83.5
  congenital P83.5
  encysted N43.0
  female NEC N94.89
  infected N43.1
  newborn P83.5
  round ligament N94.89
  specified NEC N43.2
  spinalis — *see* Spina bifida
  vulva N90.89
Hydrocephalus (acquired) (external) (internal) (malig-
    nant) (recurrent) G91.9
  aqueduct Sylvius stricture Q03.0
  causing disproportion O33.6 ☑
    with obstructed labor O66.3
  communicating G91.0
  congenital (external) (internal) Q03.9
    with spina bifida Q05.4
      cervical Q05.0
      dorsal Q05.1
      lumbar Q05.2
      lumbosacral Q05.2
      sacral Q05.3
      thoracic Q05.1
      thoracolumbar Q05.1
    specified NEC Q03.8
  due to toxoplasmosis (congenital) P37.1
  foramen Magendie block (acquired) G91.1
    congenital (*see also* Hydrocephalus, congenital)
        Q03.1
  in (due to)
    infectious disease NEC B89 [G91.4]
    neoplastic disease NEC (*see also* Neoplasm) G91.4
    parasitic disease B89 [G91.4]
  newborn Q03.9
    with spina bifida — *see* Spina bifida, with hydro-
        cephalus
  noncommunicating G91.1
  normal pressure G91.2
    secondary G91.0
  obstructive G91.1
  otitic G93.2
  post-traumatic NEC G91.3
  secondary G91.4
    post-traumatic G91.3
  specified NEC G91.8
  syphilitic, congenital A50.49

Hydrocolpos (congenital) N89.8
Hydrocystoma — *see* Neoplasm, skin, benign
Hydroencephalocele (congenital) — *see* Encephalocele
Hydroencephalomeningocele (congenital) — *see* En-
    cephalocele
Hydrohematopneumothorax — *see* Hemothorax
Hydromeningitis — *see* Meningitis
Hydromeningocele (spinal) (*see also* Spina bifida)
  cranial — *see* Encephalocele
Hydrometra N85.8
Hydrometrocolpos N89.8
Hydromicrocephaly Q02
Hydromphalos (since birth) Q45.8
Hydromyelia Q06.4
Hydromyelocele — *see* Spina bifida
Hydronephrosis (atrophic) (early) (functionless) (inter-
    mittent) (primary) (secondary) NEC N13.30
  with
    infection N13.6
    obstruction (by) (of)
      renal calculus N13.2
        with infection N13.6
      ureteral NEC N13.1
        with infection N13.6
        calculus N13.2
          with infection N13.6
      ureteropelvic junction (congenital) Q62.11
        acquired N13.0
          with infection N13.6
      ureteral stricture NEC N13.1
        with infection N13.6
  congenital Q62.0
    due to acquired occlusion of ureteropelvic junction
        N13.0
  specified type NEC N13.39
  tuberculous A18.11
Hydropericarditis — *see* Pericarditis
Hydropericardium — *see* Pericarditis
Hydroperitoneum R18.8
Hydrophobia — *see* Rabies
Hydrophthalmos Q15.0
Hydropneumohemothorax — *see* Hemothorax
Hydropneumopericarditis — *see* Pericarditis
Hydropneumopericardium — *see* Pericarditis
Hydropneumothorax J94.8
  traumatic — *see* Injury, intrathoracic, lung
  tuberculous NEC A15.6
Hydrops R60.9
  abdominis R18.8
  articulorum intermittens — *see* Hydrarthrosis, inter-
      mittent
  cardiac — *see* Failure, heart, congestive
  causing obstructed labor (mother) O66.3
  endolymphatic H81.0- ☑
  fetal — *see* Pregnancy, complicated by, hydrops, fetalis
  fetalis P83.2
    due to
      ABO isoimmunization P56.0
      alpha thalassemia D56.0
      hemolytic disease P56.90
        specified NEC P56.99
      isoimmunization (ABO) (Rh) P56.0
      other specified nonhemolytic disease NEC P83.2
      Rh incompatibility P56.0
    during pregnancy — *see* Pregnancy, complicated
        by, hydrops, fetalis
  gallbladder K82.1
  joint — *see* Effusion, joint
  labyrinth H81.0- ☑
  newborn (idiopathic) P83.2
    due to
      ABO isoimmunization P56.0
      alpha thalassemia D56.0
      hemolytic disease P56.90
        specified NEC P56.99
      isoimmunization (ABO) (Rh) P56.0
      Rh incompatibility P56.0
  nutritional — *see* Malnutrition, severe
  pericardium — *see* Pericarditis
  pleura — *see* Hydrothorax
  spermatic cord — *see* Hydrocele
Hydropyonephrosis N13.6
Hydrorachis Q06.4
Hydrorrhea (nasal) J34.89
  pregnancy — *see* Rupture, membranes, premature
Hydrosadenitis (axillaris) (suppurative) L73.2
Hydrosalpinx (fallopian tube) (follicularis) N70.11

☑ Additional Character Required — Refer to the Tabular List for Character Selection   ▽ Subterms under main terms may continue to next column or page

Hydrothorax (double) (pleura) J94.8
　chylous (nonfilarial) I89.8
　　filarial (see also Infestation, filarial) B74.9 [J91.8]
　traumatic — see Injury, intrathoracic
　tuberculous NEC (non primary) A15.6
Hydroureter (see also Hydronephrosis) N13.4
　with infection N13.6
　congenital Q62.39
Hydroureteronephrosis — see Hydronephrosis
Hydrourethra N36.8
Hydroxykynureninuria E70.8
Hydroxylysinemia E72.3
Hydroxyprolinemia E72.59
Hygiene, sleep
　abuse Z72.821
　inadequate Z72.821
　poor Z72.821
Hygroma (congenital) (cystic) D18.1
　praepatellare, prepatellar — see Bursitis, prepatellar
　subdural I62.03
Hymen — see condition
Hymenolepis, hymenolepiasis (diminuta) (infection) (infestation) (nana) B71.0
Hypalgesia R20.8
Hyperacidity (gastric) K31.89
　psychogenic F45.8
Hyperactive, hyperactivity F90.9
　basal cell, uterine cervix — see Dysplasia, cervix
　bowel sounds R19.12
　cervix epithelial (basal) — see Dysplasia, cervix
　child F90.9
　　attention deficit — see Disorder, attention-deficit hyperactivity
　detrusor muscle N32.81
　gastrointestinal K31.89
　　psychogenic F45.8
　nasal mucous membrane J34.3
　stomach K31.89
　thyroid (gland) — see Hyperthyroidism
Hyperacusis H93.23- ☑
Hyperadrenalism E27.5
Hyperadrenocorticism E24.9
　congenital E25.0
　iatrogenic E24.2
　　correct substance properly administered — see Table of Drugs and Chemicals, by drug, adverse effect
　　overdose or wrong substance given or taken — see Table of Drugs and Chemicals, by drug, poisoning
　not associated with Cushing's syndrome E27.0
　pituitary-dependent E24.0
Hyperaldosteronism E26.9
　familial (type I) E26.02
　glucocorticoid-remediable E26.02
　primary (due to (bilateral) adrenal hyperplasia) E26.09
　primary NEC E26.09
　secondary E26.1
　specified NEC E26.89
Hyperalgesia R20.8
Hyperalimentation R63.2
　carotene, carotin E67.1
　specified NEC E67.8
　vitamin
　　A E67.0
　　D E67.3
Hyperaminoaciduria
　arginine E72.21
　cystine E72.01
　lysine E72.3
　ornithine E72.4
Hyperammonemia (congenital) E72.20
Hyperazotemia — see Uremia
Hyperbetalipoproteinemia (familial) E78.00
　with prebetalipoproteinemia E78.2
Hyperbilirubinemia
　constitutional E80.6
　familial conjugated E80.6
　neonatal (transient) — see Jaundice, newborn
Hypercalcemia, hypocalciuric, familial E83.52
Hypercalciuria, idiopathic E83.52
Hypercapnia R06.89
　newborn P84
Hypercarotenemia, hypercarotinemia (dietary) E67.1
Hypercementosis K03.4
Hyperchloremia E87.8
Hyperchlorhydria K31.89

Hyperchlorhydria — continued
　neurotic F45.8
　psychogenic F45.8
Hypercholesterinemia — see Hypercholesterolemia
Hypercholesterolemia (essential) (primary) (pure) E78.00
　with hyperglyceridemia, endogenous E78.2
　dietary counseling and surveillance Z71.3
　familial E78.01
　hereditary E78.01
Hyperchylia gastrica, psychogenic F45.8
Hyperchylomicronemia (familial) (primary) E78.3
　with hyperbetalipoproteinemia E78.3
Hypercoagulable (state) D68.59
　activated protein C resistance D68.51
　antithrombin (III) deficiency D68.59
　factor V Leiden mutation D68.51
　primary NEC D68.59
　protein C deficiency D68.59
　protein S deficiency D68.59
　prothrombin gene mutation D68.52
　secondary D68.69
　specified NEC D68.69
Hypercoagulation (state) D68.59
Hypercorticalism, pituitary-dependent E24.0
Hypercorticosolism — see Cushing's, syndrome
Hypercorticosteronism E24.2
　correct substance properly administered — see Table of Drugs and Chemicals, by drug, adverse effect
　overdose or wrong substance given or taken — see Table of Drugs and Chemicals, by drug, poisoning
Hypercortisonism E24.2
　correct substance properly administered — see Table of Drugs and Chemicals, by drug, adverse effect
　overdose or wrong substance given or taken — see Table of Drugs and Chemicals, by drug, poisoning
Hyperekplexia Q89.8
Hyperelectrolytemia E87.8
Hyperemesis R11.10
　with nausea R11.2
　gravidarum (mild) O21.0
　　with
　　　carbohydrate depletion O21.1
　　　dehydration O21.1
　　　electrolyte imbalance O21.1
　　　metabolic disturbance O21.1
　　severe (with metabolic disturbance) O21.1
　projectile R11.12
　psychogenic F45.8
Hyperemia (acute) (passive) R68.89
　anal mucosa K62.89
　bladder N32.89
　cerebral I67.89
　conjunctiva H11.43- ☑
　ear internal, acute — see subcategory H83.0 ☑
　enteric K59.8
　eye — see Hyperemia, conjunctiva
　eyelid (active) (passive) — see Disorder, eyelid, specified type NEC
　intestine K59.8
　iris — see Disorder, iris, vascular
　kidney N28.89
　labyrinth — see subcategory H83.0 ☑
　liver (active) K76.89
　lung (passive) — see Edema, lung
　pulmonary (passive) — see Edema, lung
　renal N28.89
　retina H35.89
　stomach K31.89
Hyperesthesia (body surface) R20.3
　larynx (reflex) J38.7
　　hysterical F44.89
　pharynx (reflex) J39.2
　　hysterical F44.89
Hyperestrogenism (drug-induced) (iatrogenic) E28.0
Hyperexplexia Q89.8
Hyperfibrinolysis — see Fibrinolysis
Hyperfructosemia E74.19
Hyperfunction
　adrenal cortex, not associated with Cushing's syndrome E27.0
　medulla E27.5
　　adrenomedullary E27.5
　virilism E25.9
　　congenital E25.0
　ovarian E28.8

Hyperfunction — continued
　pancreas K86.89
　parathyroid (gland) E21.3
　pituitary (gland) (anterior) E22.9
　　specified NEC E22.8
　polyglandular E31.1
　testicular E29.0
Hypergammaglobulinemia D89.2
　polyclonal D89.0
　Waldenström D89.0
Hypergastrinemia E16.4
Hyperglobulinemia R77.1
Hyperglycemia, hyperglycemic (transient) R73.9
　coma — see Diabetes, by type, with coma
　postpancreatectomy E89.1
Hyperglyceridemia (endogenous) (essential) (familial) (hereditary) (pure) E78.1
　mixed E78.3
Hyperglycinemia (non-ketotic) E72.51
Hypergonadism
　ovarian E28.8
　testicular (primary) (infantile) E29.0
Hyperheparinemia D68.32
Hyperhidrosis, hyperidrosis R61
　focal
　　primary L74.519
　　　axilla L74.510
　　　face L74.511
　　　palms L74.512
　　　soles L74.513
　　secondary L74.52
　generalized R61
　localized
　　primary L74.519
　　　axilla L74.510
　　　face L74.511
　　　palms L74.512
　　　soles L74.513
　　secondary L74.52
　psychogenic F45.8
　secondary R61
　　focal L74.52
Hyperhistidinemia E70.41
Hyperhomocysteinemia E72.11
Hyperhydroxyprolinemia E72.59
Hyperinsulinism (functional) E16.1
　with
　　coma (hypoglycemic) E15
　　encephalopathy E16.1 [G94]
　ectopic E16.1
　therapeutic misadventure (from administration of insulin) — see subcategory T38.3 ☑
Hyperkalemia E87.5
Hyperkeratosis (see also Keratosis) L85.9
　cervix N88.0
　due to yaws (early) (late) (palmar or plantar) A66.3
　follicularis Q82.8
　　penetrans (in cutem) L87.0
　palmoplantaris climacterica L85.1
　pinta A67.1
　senile (with pruritus) L57.0
　universalis congenita Q80.8
　vocal cord J38.3
　vulva N90.4
Hyperkinesia, hyperkinetic (disease) (reaction) (syndrome) (childhood) (adolescence) (see also Disorder, attention-deficit hyperactivity)
　heart I51.89
Hyperleucine-isoleucinemia E71.19
Hyperlipemia, hyperlipidemia E78.5
　combined E78.2
　　familial E78.4
　group
　　A E78.00
　　B E78.1
　　C E78.2
　　D E78.3
　mixed E78.2
　specified NEC E78.4
Hyperlipidosis E75.6
　hereditary NEC E75.5
Hyperlipoproteinemia E78.5
　Fredrickson's type
　　I E78.3
　　IIa E78.00
　　IIb E78.2
　　III E78.2
　　IV E78.1

Hyperlipoproteinemia — *continued*
  Fredrickson's type — *continued*
    V E78.3
    low-density-lipoprotein-type (LDL) E78.00
    very-low-density-lipoprotein-type (VLDL) E78.1
Hyperlucent lung, unilateral J43.0
Hyperlysinemia E72.3
Hypermagnesemia E83.41
  neonatal P71.8
Hypermenorrhea N92.0
Hypermethioninemia E72.19
Hypermetropia (congenital) H52.0- ☑
Hypermobility, hypermotility
  cecum — *see* Syndrome, irritable bowel
  coccyx — *see* subcategory M53.2 ☑
  colon — *see* Syndrome, irritable bowel
    psychogenic F45.8
  ileum K58.9
  intestine (*see also* Syndrome, irritable bowel) K58.9
    psychogenic F45.8
  meniscus (knee) — *see* Derangement, knee, meniscus
  scapula — *see* Instability, joint, shoulder
  stomach K31.89
    psychogenic F45.8
  syndrome M35.7
  urethra N36.41
    with intrinsic sphincter deficiency N36.43
Hypernasality R49.21
Hypernatremia E87.0
Hypernephroma C64.- ☑
Hyperopia — *see* Hypermetropia
Hyperorexia nervosa F50.2
Hyperornithinemia E72.4
Hyperosmia R43.1
Hyperosmolality E87.0
Hyperostosis (monomelic) (*see also* Disorder, bone, density and structure, specified NEC)
  ankylosing (spine) M48.10
    cervical region M48.12
    cervicothoracic region M48.13
    lumbar region M48.16
    lumbosacral region M48.17
    multiple sites M48.19
    occipito-atlanto-axial region M48.11
    sacrococcygeal region M48.18
    thoracic region M48.14
    thoracolumbar region M48.15
  cortical (skull) M85.2
    infantile M89.8X- ☑
  frontal, internal of skull M85.2
  interna frontalis M85.2
  skeletal, diffuse idiopathic — *see* Hyperostosis, ankylosing
  skull M85.2
    congenital Q75.8
  vertebral, ankylosing — *see* Hyperostosis, ankylosing
Hyperovarism E28.8
Hyperoxaluria (primary) E72.53
Hyperparathyroidism E21.3
  primary E21.0
  secondary (renal) N25.81
    non-renal E21.1
  specified NEC E21.2
  tertiary E21.2
Hyperpathia R20.8
Hyperperistalsis R19.2
  psychogenic F45.8
Hyperpermeability, capillary I78.8
Hyperphagia R63.2
Hyperphenylalaninemia NEC E70.1
Hyperphoria (alternating) H50.53
Hyperphosphatemia E83.39
Hyperpiesis, hyperpiesia — *see* Hypertension
Hyperpigmentation (*see also* Pigmentation)
  melanin NEC L81.4
  postinflammatory L81.0
Hyperpinealism E34.8
Hyperpituitarism E22.9
Hyperplasia, hyperplastic
  adenoids J35.2
  adrenal (capsule) (cortex) (gland) E27.8
    with
      sexual precocity (male) E25.9
        congenital E25.0
      virilism, adrenal E25.9
        congenital E25.0
      virilization (female) E25.9

Hyperplasia, hyperplastic — *continued*
  adrenal — *continued*
    with — *continued*
      virilization — *continued*
        congenital E25.0
    congenital E25.0
    salt-losing E25.0
  adrenomedullary E27.5
  angiolymphoid, eosinophilia (ALHE) D18.01
  appendix (lymphoid) K38.0
  artery, fibromuscular I77.3
  bone (*see also* Hypertrophy, bone)
    marrow D75.89
  breast (*see also* Hypertrophy, breast)
    ductal (atypical) N60.9- ☑
  C-cell, thyroid E07.0
  cementation (tooth) (teeth) K03.4
  cervical gland R59.0
  cervix (uteri) (basal cell) (endometrium) (polypoid) (*see also* Dysplasia, cervix)
    congenital Q51.828
  clitoris, congenital Q52.6
  denture K06.2
  endocervicitis N72
  endometrium, endometrial (adenomatous) (benign) (cystic) (glandular) (glandular-cystic) (polypoid) N85.00
    with atypia N85.02
    cervix — *see* Dysplasia, cervix
    complex (without atypia) N85.01
    simple (without atypia) N85.01
  epithelial L85.9
    focal, oral, including tongue K13.29
    nipple N62
    skin L85.9
    tongue K13.29
    vaginal wall N89.3
  erythroid D75.89
  fibromuscular of artery (carotid) (renal) I77.3
  genital
    female NEC N94.89
    male N50.89
  gingiva K06.1
  glandularis cystica uteri (interstitialis) (*see also* Hyperplasia, endometrial) N85.00
  gum K06.1
  hymen, congenital Q52.4
  irritative, edentulous (alveolar) K06.2
  jaw M26.09
    alveolar M26.79
    lower M26.03
      alveolar M26.72
    upper M26.01
      alveolar M26.71
  kidney (congenital) Q63.3
  labia N90.69
    epithelial N90.3
  liver (congenital) Q44.7
    nodular, focal K76.89
  lymph gland or node R59.9
  mandible, mandibular M26.03
    alveolar M26.72
    unilateral condylar M27.8
  maxilla, maxillary M26.01
    alveolar M26.71
  myometrium, myometrial N85.2
  neuroendocrine cell, of infancy J84.841
  nose
    lymphoid J34.89
    polypoid J33.9
  oral mucosa (irritative) K13.6
  organ or site, congenital NEC — *see* Anomaly, by site
  ovary N83.8
  palate, papillary (irritative) K13.6
  pancreatic islet cells E16.9
    alpha E16.8
      with excess
        gastrin E16.4
        glucagon E16.3
    beta E16.1
  parathyroid (gland) E21.0
  pharynx (lymphoid) J39.2
  prostate (adenofibromatous) (nodular) N40.0
    with lower urinary tract symptoms (LUTS) N40.1
    without lower urinary tract symptoms (LUTS) N40.0
  renal artery I77.89
  reticulo-endothelial (cell) D75.89
  salivary gland (any) K11.1

Hyperplasia, hyperplastic — *continued*
  Schimmelbusch's — *see* Mastopathy, cystic
  suprarenal capsule (gland) E27.8
  thymus (gland) (persistent) E32.0
  thyroid (gland) — *see* Goiter
  tonsils (faucial) (infective) (lingual) (lymphoid) J35.1
    with adenoids J35.3
  unilateral condylar M27.8
  uterus, uterine N85.2
    endometrium (glandular) (*see also* Hyperplasia, endometrial) N85.00
  vulva N90.69
    epithelial N90.3
Hyperpnea — *see* Hyperventilation
Hyperpotassemia E87.5
Hyperprebetalipoproteinemia (familial) E78.1
Hyperprolactinemia E22.1
Hyperprolinemia (type I) (type II) E72.59
Hyperproteinemia E88.09
Hyperprothrombinemia, causing coagulation factor deficiency D68.4
Hyperpyrexia R50.9
  heat (effects) T67.0 ☑
  malignant, due to anesthetic T88.3 ☑
  rheumatic — *see* Fever, rheumatic
  unknown origin R50.9
Hyper-reflexia R29.2
Hypersalivation K11.7
Hypersecretion
  ACTH (not associated with Cushing's syndrome) E27.0
    pituitary E24.0
  adrenaline E27.5
  adrenomedullary E27.5
  androgen (testicular) E29.0
    ovarian (drug-induced) (iatrogenic) E28.1
  calcitonin E07.0
  catecholamine E27.5
  corticoadrenal E24.9
  cortisol E24.9
  epinephrine E27.5
  estrogen E28.0
  gastric K31.89
    psychogenic F45.8
  gastrin E16.4
  glucagon E16.3
  hormone(s)
    ACTH (not associated with Cushing's syndrome) E27.0
      pituitary E24.0
    antidiuretic E22.2
    growth E22.0
    intestinal NEC E34.1
    ovarian androgen E28.1
    pituitary E22.9
    testicular E29.0
    thyroid stimulating E05.80
      with thyroid storm E05.81
  insulin — *see* Hyperinsulinism
  lacrimal glands — *see* Epiphora
  medulloadrenal E27.5
  milk O92.6
  ovarian androgens E28.1
  salivary gland (any) K11.7
  thyrocalcitonin E07.0
  upper respiratory J39.8
Hypersegmentation, leukocytic, hereditary D72.0
Hypersensitive, hypersensitiveness, hypersensitivity (*see also* Allergy)
  carotid sinus G90.01
  colon — *see* Irritable, colon
  drug T88.7 ☑
  gastrointestinal K52.29
    immediate K52.29
    psychogenic F45.8
  labyrinth — *see* subcategory H83.2 ☑
  pain R20.8
  pneumonitis — *see* Pneumonitis, allergic
  reaction T78.40 ☑
    upper respiratory tract NEC J39.3
Hypersomnia (organic) G47.10
  due to
    alcohol
      abuse F10.182
      dependence F10.282
      use F10.982
    amphetamines
      abuse F15.182
      dependence F15.282

Hypersomnia — *continued*
  due to — *continued*
    amphetamines — *continued*
      use F15.982
    caffeine
      abuse F15.182
      dependence F15.282
      use F15.982
    cocaine
      abuse F14.182
      dependence F14.282
      use F14.982
    drug NEC
      abuse F19.182
      dependence F19.282
      use F19.982
    medical condition G47.14
    mental disorder F51.13
    opioid
      abuse F11.182
      dependence F11.282
      use F11.982
    psychoactive substance NEC
      abuse F19.182
      dependence F19.282
      use F19.982
    sedative, hypnotic, or anxiolytic
      abuse F13.182
      dependence F13.282
      use F13.982
    stimulant NEC
      abuse F15.182
      dependence F15.282
      use F15.982
  idiopathic G47.11
    with long sleep time G47.11
    without long sleep time G47.12
  menstrual related G47.13
  nonorganic origin F51.11
    specified NEC F51.19
  not due to a substance or known physiological condi-
    tion F51.11
    specified NEC F51.19
  primary F51.11
  recurrent G47.13
  specified NEC G47.19
Hypersplenia, hypersplenism D73.1
Hyperstimulation, ovaries (associated with induced
  ovulation) N98.1
Hypersusceptibility — *see* Allergy
Hypertelorism (ocular) (orbital) Q75.2
Hypertension, hypertensive (accelerated) (benign)
  (essential) (idiopathic) (malignant) (systemic) I10
  with
    heart failure (congestive) I11.0
    heart involvement (conditions in I50.-, I51.4- I51.9
      due to hypertension) — *see* Hypertension,
      heart
    kidney involvement — *see* Hypertension, kidney
  benign, intracranial G93.2
  borderline R03.0
  cardiorenal (disease) I13.10
    with heart failure I13.0
      with stage 1 through stage 4 chronic kidney
        disease I13.0
      with stage 5 or end stage renal disease I13.2
    without heart failure I13.10
      with stage 1 through stage 4 chronic kidney
        disease I13.10
      with stage 5 or end stage renal disease I13.11
  cardiovascular
    disease (arteriosclerotic) (sclerotic) — *see* Hyper-
      tension, heart
    renal (disease) — *see* Hypertension, cardiorenal
  chronic venous — *see* Hypertension, venous (chronic)
  complicating
    childbirth (labor) O16.4
      pre-existing O10.92
        with
          heart disease O10.12
            with renal disease O10.32
          pre-eclampsia O11.4
          renal disease O10.22
            with heart disease O10.32
        essential O10.02
      secondary O10.42
    pregnancy O16.- ☑
      with edema (*see also* Pre-eclampsia) O14.9- ☑

Hypertension, hypertensive — *continued*
  complicating — *continued*
    pregnancy — *continued*
      gestational (pregnancy induced) (without pro-
        teinuria) O13.- ☑
        with proteinuria O14.9- ☑
          mild pre-eclampsia O14.0- ☑
          moderate pre-eclampsia O14.0- ☑
          severe pre-eclampsia O14.1- ☑
            with hemolysis, elevated liver en-
              zymes and low platelet count
              (HELLP) O14.2- ☑
      pre-existing O10.91- ☑
        with
          heart disease O10.11- ☑
            with renal disease O10.31- ☑
          pre-eclampsia — *see* category O11
          renal disease O10.21- ☑
            with heart disease O10.31- ☑
        essential O10.01- ☑
        secondary O10.41- ☑
      transient O13- ☑
    puerperium, pre-existing O16.5
      pre-existing
        with
          heart disease O10.13
            with renal disease O10.33
          pre-eclampsia O11.5
          renal disease O10.23
            with heart disease O10.33
        essential O10.03
      pregnancy-induced O13.9
      secondary O10.43
  crisis I16.9
  due to
    endocrine disorders I15.2
    pheochromocytoma I15.2
    renal disorders NEC I15.1
      arterial I15.0
    renovascular disorders I15.0
    specified disease NEC I15.8
  emergency I16.1
  encephalopathy I67.4
  gestational (without significant proteinuria) (pregnan-
    cy-induced) (transient) O13.- ☑
    with significant proteinuria — *see* Pre-eclampsia
    complicating
      delivery O13.4
      puerperium O13.5
  Goldblatt's I70.1
  heart (disease) (conditions in I51.4-I51.9 due to hyper-
    tension) I11.9
    with
      heart failure (congestive) I11.0
      kidney disease (chronic) — *see* Hypertension,
        cardiorenal
  intracranial (benign) G93.2
  kidney I12.9
    with
      heart disease — *see* Hypertension, cardiorenal
      stage 1 through stage 4 chronic kidney disease
        I12.9
      stage 5 chronic kidney disease (CKD) or end
        stage renal disease (ESRD) I12.0
  lesser circulation I27.0
  maternal O16- ☑
  newborn P29.2
    pulmonary (persistent) P29.30
  ocular H40.05- ☑
  pancreatic duct — *code to* underlying condition
    with chronic pancreatitis K86.1
  portal (due to chronic liver disease) (idiopathic) K76.6
    gastropathy K31.89
    in (due to) schistosomiasis (bilharziasis) B65.9 [K77]
  postoperative I97.3
  psychogenic F45.8
  pulmonary I27.20
    with
      cor pulmonale (chronic) I27.29
        acute I26.09
      right heart ventricular strain/failure I27.29
        acute I26.09
      right to left shunt related to congenital heart
        disease I27.83
      unclear multifactorial mechanisms I27.29
    arterial (associated) (drug-induced) (toxin-induced)
      I27.21
    chronic thromboembolic I27.24

Hypertension, hypertensive — *continued*
  pulmonary — *continued*
    due to
      hematologic disorders I27.29
      left heart disease I27.22
      lung diseases and hypoxia I27.23
      metabolic disorders I27.29
      specified systemic disorders I27.29
    group 1 (associated) (drug-induced) (toxin-in-
      duced) I27.21
    group 2 I27.22
    group 3 I27.23
    group 4 I27.24
    group 5 I27.29
    of newborn (persistent) P29.30
    primary (idiopathic) I27.0
    secondary
      arterial I27.21
      specified NEC I27.29
  renal — *see* Hypertension, kidney
  renovascular I15.0
  secondary NEC I15.9
    due to
      endocrine disorders I15.2
      pheochromocytoma I15.2
      renal disorders NEC I15.1
        arterial I15.0
      renovascular disorders I15.0
    specified NEC I15.8
  transient, of pregnancy O13- ☑
  urgency I16.0
  venous (chronic)
    due to
      deep vein thrombosis — *see* Syndrome, post-
        thrombotic
    idiopathic I87.309
      with
        inflammation I87.32- ☑
          with ulcer I87.33- ☑
        specified complication NEC I87.39- ☑
        ulcer I87.31- ☑
          with inflammation I87.33- ☑
      asymptomatic I87.30- ☑
Hypertensive urgency — *see* Hypertension
Hyperthecosis ovary E28.8
Hyperthermia (of unknown origin) (*see also* Hyperpyrexia)
  malignant, due to anesthesia T88.3 ☑
  newborn P81.9
    environmental P81.0
Hyperthyroid (recurrent) — *see* Hyperthyroidism
Hyperthyroidism (latent) (pre-adult) (recurrent) E05.90
  with
    goiter (diffuse) E05.00
      with thyroid storm E05.01
      nodular (multinodular) E05.20
        with thyroid storm E05.21
        uninodular E05.10
          with thyroid storm E05.11
    storm E05.91
  due to ectopic thyroid tissue E05.30
    with thyroid storm E05.31
  neonatal, transitory P72.1
  specified NEC E05.80
    with thyroid storm E05.81
Hypertony, hypertonia, hypertonicity
  bladder N31.8
  congenital P94.1
  stomach K31.89
    psychogenic F45.8
  uterus, uterine (contractions) (complicating delivery)
    O62.4
Hypertrichosis L68.9
  congenital Q84.2
  eyelid H02.869
    left H02.866
      lower H02.865
      upper H02.864
    right H02.863
      lower H02.862
      upper H02.861
  lanuginosa Q84.2
    acquired L68.1
  localized L68.2
  specified NEC L68.8
Hypertriglyceridemia, essential E78.1

Index

Hypertrophy, hypertrophic

adenofibromatous, prostate — see Enlargement, enlarged, prostate
adenoids (infective) J35.2
    with tonsils J35.3
adrenal cortex E27.8
alveolar process or ridge — see Anomaly, alveolar
anal papillae K62.89
anal papillae K62.89
artery I77.89
    congenital NEC Q27.8
        digestive system Q27.8
        lower limb Q27.8
        specified site NEC Q27.8
        upper limb Q27.8
auricular — see Hypertrophy, cardiac
Bartholin's gland N75.8
bile duct (common) (hepatic) K83.8
bladder (sphincter) (trigone) N32.89
bone M89.3Ø
    carpus M89.34- ☑
    clavicle M89.31- ☑
    femur M89.35- ☑
    fibula M89.36- ☑
    finger M89.34- ☑
    humerus M89.32- ☑
    ilium M89.359
    ischium M89.359
    metacarpus M89.34- ☑
    metatarsus M89.37- ☑
    multiple sites M89.39
    neck M89.38
    radius M89.33- ☑
    rib M89.38
    scapula M89.31- ☑
    skull M89.38
    tarsus M89.37- ☑
    tibia M89.36- ☑
    toe M89.37- ☑
    ulna M89.33- ☑
    vertebra M89.38
brain G93.89
breast N62
    cystic — see Mastopathy, cystic
    newborn P83.4
    pubertal, massive N62
    puerperal, postpartum — see Disorder, breast, specified type NEC
    senile (parenchymatous) N62
cardiac (chronic) (idiopathic) I51.7
    with rheumatic fever (conditions in IØØ)
        active IØ1.8
        inactive or quiescent (with chorea) IØ9.89
    congenital NEC Q24.8
    fatty — see Degeneration, myocardial
    hypertensive — see Hypertension, heart
    rheumatic (with chorea) IØ9.89
        active or acute IØ1.8
            with chorea IØ2.Ø
    valve — see Endocarditis
cartilage — see Disorder, cartilage, specified type NEC
cecum — see Megacolon
cervix (uteri) N88.8
    congenital Q51.828
    elongation N88.4
clitoris (cirrhotic) N9Ø.89
    congenital Q52.6
colon (see also Megacolon)
    congenital Q43.2
conjunctiva, lymphoid H11.89
corpora cavernosa N48.89
cystic duct K82.8
duodenum K31.89
endometrium (glandular) (see also Hyperplasia, endometrial) N85.ØØ
    cervix N88.8
epididymis N5Ø.89
esophageal hiatus (congenital) Q79.1
    with hernia — see Hernia, hiatal
eyelid — see Disorder, eyelid, specified type NEC
fat pad E65
    knee (infrapatellar) (popliteal) (prepatellar) (retropatellar) M79.4
foot (congenital) Q74.2
frenulum, frenum (tongue) K14.8
    lip K13.Ø
gallbladder K82.8
gastric mucosa K29.6Ø
    with bleeding K29.61

Hypertrophy, hypertrophic — continued

gland, glandular R59.9
    generalized R59.1
    localized R59.Ø
gum (mucous membrane) KØ6.1
heart (idiopathic) (see also Hypertrophy, cardiac)
    valve (see also Endocarditis) I38
hemifacial Q67.4
hepatic — see Hypertrophy, liver
hiatus (esophageal) Q79.1
hilus gland R59.Ø
hymen, congenital Q52.4
ileum K63.89
intestine NEC K63.89
jejunum K63.89
kidney (compensatory) N28.81
    congenital Q63.3
labium (majus) (minus) N9Ø.6Ø
ligament — see Disorder, ligament
lingual tonsil (infective) J35.1
    with adenoids J35.3
lip K13.Ø
    congenital Q18.6
liver R16.Ø
    acute K76.89
    cirrhotic — see Cirrhosis, liver
    congenital Q44.7
    fatty — see Fatty, liver
lymph, lymphatic gland R59.9
    generalized R59.1
    localized R59.Ø
    tuberculous — see Tuberculosis, lymph gland
mammary gland — see Hypertrophy, breast
Meckel's diverticulum (congenital) Q43.Ø
    malignant — see Table of Neoplasms, small intestine, malignant
median bar — see Hyperplasia, prostate
meibomian gland — see Chalazion
meniscus, knee, congenital Q74.1
metatarsal head — see Hypertrophy, bone, metatarsus
metatarsus — see Hypertrophy, bone, metatarsus
mucous membrane
    alveolar ridge KØ6.2
    gum KØ6.1
    nose (turbinate) J34.3
muscle M62.89
muscular coat, artery I77.89
myocardium (see also Hypertrophy, cardiac)
    idiopathic I42.2
myometrium N85.2
nail L6Ø.2
    congenital Q84.5
nasal J34.89
    alae J34.89
    bone J34.89
    cartilage J34.89
    mucous membrane (septum) J34.3
    sinus J34.89
    turbinate J34.3
nasopharynx, lymphoid (infectional) (tissue) (wall) J35.2
nipple N62
organ or site, congenital NEC — see Anomaly, by site
ovary N83.8
palate (hard) M27.8
    soft K13.79
pancreas, congenital Q45.3
parathyroid (gland) E21.Ø
parotid gland K11.1
penis N48.89
pharyngeal tonsil J35.2
pharynx J39.2
    lymphoid (infectional) (tissue) (wall) J35.2
pituitary (anterior) (fossa) (gland) E23.6
prepuce (congenital) N47.8
    female N9Ø.89
prostate — see Enlargement, enlarged, prostate
    congenital Q55.4
pseudomuscular G71.Ø
pylorus (adult) (muscle) (sphincter) K31.1
    congenital or infantile Q4Ø.Ø
rectal, rectum (sphincter) K62.89
rhinitis (turbinate) J31.Ø
salivary gland (any) K11.1
    congenital Q38.4
scaphoid (tarsal) — see Hypertrophy, bone, tarsus
scar L91.Ø
scrotum N5Ø.89

Hypertrophy, hypertrophic — continued

seminal vesicle N5Ø.89
sigmoid — see Megacolon
skin L91.9
    specified NEC L91.8
spermatic cord N5Ø.89
spleen — see Splenomegaly
spondylitis — see Spondylosis
stomach K31.89
sublingual gland K11.1
submandibular gland K11.1
suprarenal cortex (gland) E27.8
synovial NEC M67.2Ø
    acromioclavicular M67.21- ☑
    ankle M67.27- ☑
    elbow M67.22- ☑
    foot M67.27- ☑
    hand M67.24- ☑
    hip M67.25- ☑
    knee M67.26- ☑
    multiple sites M67.29
    specified site NEC M67.28
    wrist M67.23- ☑
tendon — see Disorder, tendon, specified type NEC
testis N44.8
    congenital Q55.29
thymic, thymus (gland) (congenital) E32.Ø
thyroid (gland) — see Goiter
toe (congenital) Q74.2
    acquired (see also Deformity, toe, specified NEC)
tongue K14.8
    congenital Q38.2
    papillae (foliate) K14.3
tonsils (faucial) (infective) (lingual) (lymphoid) J35.1
    with adenoids J35.3
tunica vaginalis N5Ø.89
ureter N28.89
urethra N36.8
uterus N85.2
    neck (with elongation) N88.4
    puerperal O9Ø.89
uvula K13.79
vagina N89.8
vas deferens N5Ø.89
vein I87.8
ventricle, ventricular (heart) (see also Hypertrophy, cardiac)
    congenital Q24.8
    in tetralogy of Fallot Q21.3
verumontanum N36.8
vocal cord J38.3
vulva N9Ø.6Ø
    stasis (nonfilarial) N9Ø.69

Hypertropia H5Ø.2- ☑
Hypertyrosinemia E7Ø.21
Hyperuricemia (asymptomatic) E79.Ø
Hypervalinemia E71.19
Hyperventilation (tetany) RØ6.4
    hysterical F45.8
    psychogenic F45.8
    syndrome F45.8
Hypervitaminosis (dietary) NEC E67.8
    A E67.Ø
        administered as drug (prolonged intake) — see Table of Drugs and Chemicals, vitamins, adverse effect
        overdose or wrong substance given or taken — see Table of Drugs and Chemicals, vitamins, poisoning
    B6 E67.2
    D E67.3
        administered as drug (prolonged intake) — see Table of Drugs and Chemicals, vitamins, adverse effect
        overdose or wrong substance given or taken — see Table of Drugs and Chemicals, vitamins, poisoning
    K E67.8
        administered as drug (prolonged intake) — see Table of Drugs and Chemicals, vitamins, adverse effect
        overdose or wrong substance given or taken — see Table of Drugs and Chemicals, vitamins, poisoning
Hypervolemia E87.7Ø
    specified NEC E87.79
Hypesthesia R2Ø.1
    cornea — see Anesthesia, cornea

Hypertrophy, hypertrophic — Hypesthesia

Hyphema H21.0- ☑
  traumatic S05.1- ☑
Hypoacidity, gastric K31.89
  psychogenic F45.8
Hypoadrenalism, hypoadrenia E27.40
  primary E27.1
  tuberculous A18.7
Hypoadrenocorticism E27.40
  pituitary E23.0
  primary E27.1
Hypoalbuminemia E88.09
Hypoaldosteronism E27.40
Hypoalphalipoproteinemia E78.6
Hypobarism T70.29 ☑
Hypobaropathy T70.29 ☑
Hypobetalipoproteinemia (familial) E78.6
Hypocalcemia E83.51
  dietary E58
  neonatal P71.1
    due to cow's milk P71.0
  phosphate-loading (newborn) P71.1
Hypochloremia E87.8
Hypochlorhydria K31.89
  neurotic F45.8
  psychogenic F45.8
Hypochondria, hypochondriac, hypochondriasis (reaction) F45.21
  sleep F51.03
Hypochondrogenesis Q77.0
Hypochondroplasia Q77.4
Hypochromasia, blood cells D50.8
Hypodontia — see Anodontia
Hypoeosinophilia D72.89
Hypoesthesia R20.1
Hypofibrinogenemia D68.8
  acquired D65
  congenital (hereditary) D68.2
Hypofunction
  adrenocortical E27.40
    drug-induced E27.3
    postprocedural E89.6
    primary E27.1
  adrenomedullary, postprocedural E89.6
  cerebral R29.818
  corticoadrenal NEC E27.40
  intestinal K59.8
  labyrinth — see subcategory H83.2 ☑
  ovary E28.39
  pituitary (gland) (anterior) E23.0
  testicular E29.1
    postprocedural (postsurgical) (postirradiation) (iatrogenic) E89.5
Hypogalactia O92.4
Hypogammaglobulinemia (see also Agammaglobulinemia) D80.1
  hereditary D80.0
  nonfamilial D80.1
  transient, of infancy D80.7
Hypogenitalism (congenital) — see Hypogonadism
Hypoglossia Q38.3
Hypoglycemia (spontaneous) E16.2
  coma E15
    diabetic — see Diabetes, by type, with hypoglycemia, with coma
  diabetic — see Diabetes, hypoglycemia
  dietary counseling and surveillance Z71.3
  drug-induced E16.0
    with coma (nondiabetic) E15
  due to insulin E16.0
    with coma (nondiabetic) E15
    therapeutic misadventure — see subcategory T38.3 ☑
  functional, nonhyperinsulinemic E16.1
  iatrogenic E16.0
    with coma (nondiabetic) E15
  in infant of diabetic mother P70.1
    gestational diabetes P70.0
  infantile E16.1
  leucine-induced E71.19
  neonatal (transitory) P70.4
    iatrogenic P70.3
  reactive (not drug-induced) E16.1
  transitory neonatal P70.4
Hypogonadism
  female E28.39
  hypogonadotropic E23.0
  male E29.1
  ovarian (primary) E28.39

Hypogonadism — continued
  pituitary E23.0
  testicular (primary) E29.1
Hypohidrosis, hypoidrosis L74.4
Hypoinsulinemia, postprocedural E89.1
Hypokalemia E87.6
Hypoleukocytosis — see Agranulocytosis
Hypolipoproteinemia (alpha) (beta) E78.6
Hypomagnesemia E83.42
  neonatal P71.2
Hypomania, hypomanic reaction F30.8
Hypomenorrhea — see Oligomenorrhea
Hypometabolism R63.8
Hypomotility
  gastrointestinal (tract) K31.89
    psychogenic F45.8
  intestine K59.8
    psychogenic F45.8
  stomach K31.89
    psychogenic F45.8
Hyponasality R49.22
Hyponatremia E87.1
Hypo-osmolality E87.1
Hypo-ovarianism, hypo-ovarism E28.39
Hypoparathyroidism E20.9
  familial E20.8
  idiopathic E20.0
  neonatal, transitory P71.4
  postprocedural E89.2
  specified NEC E20.8
Hypoperfusion (in)
  newborn P96.89
Hypopharyngitis — see Laryngopharyngitis
Hypophoria H50.53
Hypophosphatemia, hypophosphatasia (acquired) (congenital) (renal) E83.39
  familial E83.31
Hypophyseal, hypophysis (see also condition)
  dwarfism E23.0
  gigantism E22.0
Hypopiesis — see Hypotension
Hypopinealism E34.8
Hypopituitarism (juvenile) E23.0
  drug-induced E23.1
  due to
    hypophysectomy E89.3
    radiotherapy E89.3
  iatrogenic NEC E23.1
  postirradiation E89.3
  postpartum O99.285
  postprocedural E89.3
Hypoplasia, hypoplastic
  adrenal (gland), congenital Q89.1
  alimentary tract, congenital Q45.8
    upper Q40.8
  anus, anal (canal) Q42.3
    with fistula Q42.2
  aorta, aortic Q25.42
    ascending, in hypoplastic left heart syndrome Q23.4
    valve Q23.1
      in hypoplastic left heart syndrome Q23.4
  areola, congenital Q83.8
  arm (congenital) — see Defect, reduction, upper limb
  artery (peripheral) Q27.8
    brain (congenital) Q28.3
    coronary Q24.5
    digestive system Q27.8
    lower limb Q27.8
    pulmonary Q25.79
      functional, unilateral J43.0
    retinal (congenital) Q14.1
    specified site NEC Q27.8
    umbilical Q27.0
    upper limb Q27.8
  auditory canal Q17.8
    causing impairment of hearing Q16.9
  biliary duct or passage Q44.5
  bone NOS Q79.9
    face Q75.8
    marrow D61.9
      megakaryocytic D69.49
    skull — see Hypoplasia, skull
  brain Q02
    gyri Q04.3
    part of Q04.3
  breast (areola) N64.82
  bronchus Q32.4

Hypoplasia, hypoplastic — continued
  cardiac Q24.8
  carpus — see Defect, reduction, upper limb, specified type NEC
  cartilage hair Q78.8
  cecum Q42.8
  cementum K00.4
  cephalic Q02
  cerebellum Q04.3
  cervix (uteri), congenital Q51.821
  clavicle (congenital) Q74.0
  coccyx Q76.49
  colon Q42.9
    specified NEC Q42.8
  corpus callosum Q04.0
  cricoid cartilage Q31.2
  digestive organ(s) or tract NEC Q45.8
    upper (congenital) Q40.8
  ear (auricle) (lobe) Q17.2
    middle Q16.4
  enamel of teeth (neonatal) (postnatal) (prenatal) K00.4
  endocrine (gland) NEC Q89.2
  endometrium N85.8
  epididymis (congenital) Q55.4
  epiglottis Q31.2
  erythroid, congenital D61.01
  esophagus (congenital) Q39.8
  eustachian tube Q17.8
  eye Q11.2
  eyelid (congenital) Q10.3
  face Q18.8
    bone(s) Q75.8
  femur (congenital) — see Defect, reduction, lower limb, specified type NEC
  fibula (congenital) — see Defect, reduction, lower limb, specified type NEC
  finger (congenital) — see Defect, reduction, upper limb, specified type NEC
  focal dermal Q82.8
  foot — see Defect, reduction, lower limb, specified type NEC
  gallbladder Q44.0
  genitalia, genital organ(s)
    female, congenital Q52.8
      external Q52.79
      internal NEC Q52.8
    in adiposogenital dystrophy E23.6
  glottis Q31.2
  hair Q84.2
  hand (congenital) — see Defect, reduction, upper limb, specified type NEC
  heart Q24.8
  humerus (congenital) — see Defect, reduction, upper limb, specified type NEC
  intestine (small) Q41.9
    large Q42.9
      specified NEC Q42.8
  jaw M26.09
    alveolar M26.79
    lower M26.04
      alveolar M26.74
    upper M26.02
      alveolar M26.73
  kidney(s) Q60.5
    bilateral Q60.4
    unilateral Q60.3
  labium (majus) (minus), congenital Q52.79
  larynx Q31.2
  left heart syndrome Q23.4
  leg (congenital) — see Defect, reduction, lower limb
  limb Q73.8
    lower (congenital) — see Defect, reduction, lower limb
    upper (congenital) — see Defect, reduction, upper limb
  liver Q44.7
  lung (lobe) (not associated with short gestation) Q33.6
    associated with immaturity, low birth weight, prematurity, or short gestation P28.0
  mammary (areola), congenital Q83.8
  mandible, mandibular M26.04
    alveolar M26.74
    unilateral condylar M27.8
  maxillary M26.02
    alveolar M26.73
  medullary D61.9
  megakaryocytic D69.49

IIAC (idiopathic infantile arterial calcification) Q28.8
Ileitis (chronic) (noninfectious) (see also Enteritis) K52.9
  backwash — see Pancolitis, ulcerative (chronic)
  infectious A09
  regional (ulcerative) — see Enteritis, regional, small
    intestine
  segmental — see Enteritis, regional
  terminal (ulcerative) — see Enteritis, regional, small
    intestine
Ileocolitis (see also Enteritis) K52.9
  infectious A09
  regional — see Enteritis, regional
  ulcerative K51.0- ☑
Ileostomy
  attention to Z43.2
  malfunctioning K94.13
  status Z93.2
    with complication — see Complications, enterostomy
Ileotyphus — see Typhoid
Ileum — see condition
Ileus (bowel) (colon) (inhibitory) (intestine) K56.7
  adynamic K56.0
  due to gallstone (in intestine) K56.3
  duodenal (chronic) K31.5
  gallstone K56.3
  mechanical NEC (see also Obstruction, intestine, specified NEC) K56.699
  meconium P76.0
    in cystic fibrosis E84.11
    meaning meconium plug (without cystic fibrosis) P76.0
  myxedema K59.8
  neurogenic K56.0
    Hirschsprung's disease or megacolon Q43.1
  newborn
    due to meconium P76.0
      in cystic fibrosis E84.11
      meaning meconium plug (without cystic fibrosis) P76.0
    transitory P76.1
  obstructive (see also Obstruction, intestine, specified NEC) K56.699
  paralytic K56.0
  postoperative K91.89
Iliac — see condition
Iliotibial band syndrome M76.3- ☑
Illiteracy Z55.0
Illness (see also Disease) R69
  manic-depressive — see Disorder, bipolar
Imbalance R26.89
  autonomic G90.8
  constituents of food intake E63.1
  electrolyte E87.8
    with
      abortion — see Abortion by type, complicated by, electrolyte imbalance
      molar pregnancy O08.5
    due to hyperemesis gravidarum O21.1
    following ectopic or molar pregnancy O08.5
    neonatal, transitory NEC P74.4
      potassium P74.3
      sodium P74.2
  endocrine E34.9
  eye muscle NOS H50.9
  hormone E34.9
  hysterical F44.4
  labyrinth — see subcategory H83.2 ☑
  posture R29.3
  protein-energy — see Malnutrition
  sympathetic G90.8
Imbecile, imbecility (I.Q. 35-49) F71
Imbedding, intrauterine device T83.39 ☑
Imbibition, cholesterol (gallbladder) K82.4
Imbrication, teeth,, fully erupted M26.30
Imerslund (-Gräsbeck) **syndrome** D51.1
Immature (see also Immaturity)
  birth (less than 37 completed weeks) — see Preterm, newborn
    extremely (less than 28 completed weeks) — see Immaturity, extreme
  personality F60.89
Immaturity (less than 37 completed weeks) (see also Preterm, newborn)
  extreme of newborn (less than 28 completed weeks of gestation) (less than 196 completed days of gestation) (unspecified weeks of gestation) P07.20

Immaturity — continued
  extreme of newborn — continued
    gestational age
      less than 23 completed weeks P07.21
      23 completed weeks (23 weeks, 0 days through 23 weeks, 6 days) P07.22
      24 completed weeks (24 weeks, 0 days through 24 weeks, 6 days) P07.23
      25 completed weeks (25 weeks, 0 days through 25 weeks, 6 days) P07.24
      26 completed weeks (26 weeks, 0 days through 26 weeks, 6 days) P07.25
      27 completed weeks (27 weeks, 0 days through 27 weeks, 6 days) P07.26
  fetus or infant light-for-dates — see Light-for-dates
  lung, newborn P28.0
  organ or site NEC — see Hypoplasia
  pulmonary, newborn P28.0
  reaction F60.89
  sexual (female) (male), after puberty E30.0
Immersion T75.1 ☑
  foot T69.02- ☑
  hand T69.01- ☑
Immobile, immobility
  complete, due to severe physical disability or frailty R53.2
  intestine K59.8
  syndrome (paraplegic) M62.3
Immune reconstitution (inflammatory) syndrome [IRIS] D89.3
Immunization (see also Vaccination)
  ABO — see Incompatibility, ABO
    in newborn P55.1
  complication — see Complications, vaccination
  encounter for Z23
  not done (not carried out) Z28.9
    because (of)
      acute illness of patient Z28.01
      allergy to vaccine (or component) Z28.04
      caregiver refusal Z28.82
      chronic illness of patient Z28.02
      contraindication NEC Z28.09
      group pressure Z28.1
      guardian refusal Z28.82
      immune compromised state of patient Z28.03
      parent refusal Z28.82
      patient had disease being vaccinated against Z28.81
      patient refusal Z28.21
      patient's belief Z28.1
      religious beliefs of patient Z28.1
      specified reason NEC Z28.89
        of patient Z28.29
      unspecified patient reason Z28.20
  Rh factor
    affecting management of pregnancy NEC O36.09- ☑
    anti-D antibody O36.01- ☑
  from transfusion — see Complication(s), transfusion, incompatibility reaction, Rh (factor)
Immunocytoma C83.0- ☑
Immunodeficiency D84.9
  with
    adenosine-deaminase deficiency D81.3
    antibody defects D80.9
      specified type NEC D80.8
    hyperimmunoglobulinemia D80.6
    increased immunoglobulin M (IgM) D80.5
    major defect D82.9
      specified type NEC D82.8
    partial albinism D82.8
    short-limbed stature D82.2
    thrombocytopenia and eczema D82.0
  antibody with
    hyperimmunoglobulinemia D80.6
    near-normal immunoglobulins D80.6
  autosomal recessive, Swiss type D80.0
  combined D81.9
    biotin-dependent carboxylase D81.819
      biotinidase D81.810
      holocarboxylase synthetase D81.818
      specified type NEC D81.818
    severe (SCID) D81.9
      with
        low or normal B-cell numbers D81.2
        low T- and B-cell numbers D81.1
        reticular dysgenesis D81.0
  specified type NEC D81.89

Immunodeficiency — continued
  common variable D83.9
    with
      abnormalities of B-cell numbers and function D83.0
      autoantibodies to B- or T-cells D83.2
      immunoregulatory T-cell disorders D83.1
      specified type NEC D83.8
  following hereditary defective response to Epstein-Barr virus (EBV) D82.3
  selective, immunoglobulin
    A (IgA) D80.2
    G (IgG) (subclasses) D80.3
    M (IgM) D80.4
  severe combined (SCID) D81.9
  specified type NEC D84.8
  X-linked, with increased IgM D80.5
Immunotherapy (encounter for)
  antineoplastic Z51.12
Impaction, impacted
  bowel, colon, rectum (see also Impaction, fecal) K56.49
    by gallstone K56.3
  calculus — see Calculus
  cerumen (ear) (external) H61.2- ☑
  cuspid — see Impaction, tooth
  dental (same or adjacent tooth) K01.1
  fecal, feces K56.41
  fracture — see Fracture, by site
  gallbladder — see Calculus, gallbladder
  gallstone(s) — see Calculus, gallbladder
    bile duct (common) (hepatic) — see Calculus, bile duct
    cystic duct — see Calculus, gallbladder
    in intestine, with obstruction (any part) K56.3
  intestine (calculous) NEC (see also Impaction, fecal) K56.49
    gallstone, with ileus K56.3
  intrauterine device (IUD) T83.39 ☑
  molar — see Impaction, tooth
  shoulder, causing obstructed labor O66.0
  tooth, teeth K01.1
  turbinate J34.89
Impaired, impairment (function)
  auditory discrimination — see Abnormal, auditory perception
  cognitive, mild, so stated G31.84
  dual sensory Z73.82
  fasting glucose R73.01
  glucose tolerance (oral) R73.02
  hearing — see Deafness
  heart — see Disease, heart
  kidney N28.9
    disorder resulting from N25.9
      specified NEC N25.89
  liver K72.90
    with coma K72.91
  mastication K08.89
  mild cognitive, so stated G31.84
  mobility
    ear ossicles — see Ankylosis, ear ossicles
    requiring care provider Z74.09
  myocardium, myocardial — see Insufficiency, myocardial
  rectal sphincter R19.8
  renal (acute) (chronic) N28.9
    disorder resulting from N25.9
      specified NEC N25.89
  vision NEC H54.7
    both eyes H54.3
Impediment, speech R47.9
  psychogenic (childhood) F98.8
  slurring R47.81
  specified NEC R47.89
Impending
  coronary syndrome I20.0
  delirium tremens F10.239
  myocardial infarction I20.0
Imperception auditory (acquired) (see also Deafness)
  congenital H93.25
Imperfect
  aeration, lung (newborn) NEC — see Atelectasis
  closure (congenital)
    alimentary tract NEC Q45.8
      lower Q43.8
      upper Q40.8
    atrioventricular ostium Q21.2
    atrium (secundum) Q21.1
    branchial cleft NOS Q18.2

Imperfect — *continued*
- closure — *continued*
  - branchial cleft — *continued*
    - cyst Q18.0
    - fistula Q18.0
    - sinus Q18.0
  - choroid Q14.3
  - cricoid cartilage Q31.8
  - cusps, heart valve NEC Q24.8
    - pulmonary Q22.3
  - ductus
    - arteriosus Q25.0
    - Botalli Q25.0
  - ear drum (causing impairment of hearing) Q16.4
  - esophagus with communication to bronchus or trachea Q39.1
  - eyelid Q10.3
  - foramen
    - botalli Q21.1
    - ovale Q21.1
  - genitalia, genital organ(s) or system
    - female Q52.8
      - external Q52.79
      - internal NEC Q52.8
    - male Q55.8
  - glottis Q31.8
  - interatrial ostium or septum Q21.1
  - interauricular ostium or septum Q21.1
  - interventricular ostium or septum Q21.0
  - larynx Q31.8
  - lip — *see* Cleft, lip
  - nasal septum Q30.3
  - nose Q30.2
  - omphalomesenteric duct Q43.0
  - optic nerve entry Q14.2
  - organ or site not listed — *see* Anomaly, by site
  - ostium
    - interatrial Q21.1
    - interauricular Q21.1
    - interventricular Q21.0
  - palate — *see* Cleft, palate
  - preauricular sinus Q18.1
  - retina Q14.1
  - roof of orbit Q75.8
  - sclera Q13.5
  - septum
    - aorticopulmonary Q21.4
    - atrial (secundum) Q21.1
    - between aorta and pulmonary artery Q21.4
    - heart Q21.9
    - interatrial (secundum) Q21.1
    - interauricular (secundum) Q21.1
    - interventricular Q21.0
      - in tetralogy of Fallot Q21.3
    - nasal Q30.3
    - ventricular Q21.0
      - with pulmonary stenosis or atresia, dextraposition of aorta, and hypertrophy of right ventricle Q21.3
      - in tetralogy of Fallot Q21.3
  - skull Q75.0
    - with
      - anencephaly Q00.0
      - encephalocele — *see* Encephalocele
      - hydrocephalus Q03.9
        - with spina bifida — *see* Spina bifida, by site, with hydrocephalus
      - microcephaly Q02
  - spine (with meningocele) — *see* Spina bifida
  - trachea Q32.1
  - tympanic membrane (causing impairment of hearing) Q16.4
  - uterus Q51.818
  - vitelline duct Q43.0
- erection — *see* Dysfunction, sexual, male, erectile
- fusion — *see* Imperfect, closure
- inflation, lung (newborn) — *see* Atelectasis
- posture R29.3
- rotation, intestine Q43.3
- septum, ventricular Q21.0

Imperfectly descended testis — *see* Cryptorchid
Imperforate (congenital) (*see also* Atresia)
- anus Q42.3
  - with fistula Q42.2
- cervix (uteri) Q51.828
- esophagus Q39.0
  - with tracheoesophageal fistula Q39.1
- hymen Q52.3

Imperforate — *continued*
- jejunum Q41.1
- pharynx Q38.8
- rectum Q42.1
  - with fistula Q42.0
- urethra Q64.39
- vagina Q52.4
Impervious (congenital) (*see also* Atresia)
- anus Q42.3
  - with fistula Q42.2
- bile duct Q44.2
- esophagus Q39.0
  - with tracheoesophageal fistula Q39.1
- intestine (small) Q41.9
  - large Q42.9
    - specified NEC Q42.8
- rectum Q42.1
  - with fistula Q42.0
- ureter — *see* Atresia, ureter
- urethra Q64.39
Impetiginization of dermatoses L01.1
Impetigo (any organism) (any site) (circinate) (contagiosa) (simplex) (vulgaris) L01.00
- Bockhart's L01.02
- bullous, bullosa L01.03
- external ear L01.00 [H62.40]
- follicularis L01.02
- furfuracea L30.5
- herpetiformis L40.1
  - nonobstetrical L40.1
- neonatorum L01.03
- nonbullous L01.01
- specified type NEC L01.09
- ulcerative L01.09
Impingement (on teeth)
- soft tissue
  - anterior M26.81
  - posterior M26.82
Implant, endometrial N80.9
Implantation
- anomalous — *see* Anomaly, by site
  - ureter Q62.63
- cyst
  - external area or site (skin) NEC L72.0
  - iris — *see* Cyst, iris, implantation
  - vagina N89.8
  - vulva N90.7
- dermoid (cyst) — *see* Implantation, cyst
Impotence (sexual) N52.9
- counseling Z70.1
- organic origin (*see also* Dysfunction, sexual, male, erectile) N52.9
- psychogenic F52.21
Impression, basilar Q75.8
Imprisonment, anxiety concerning Z65.1
Improper care (child) (newborn) — *see* Maltreatment
Improperly tied umbilical cord (causing hemorrhage) P51.8
Impulsiveness (impulsive) R45.87
Inability to swallow — *see* Aphagia
Inaccessible, inaccessibility
- health care NEC Z75.3
  - due to
    - waiting period Z75.2
      - for admission to facility elsewhere Z75.1
  - other helping agencies Z75.4
Inactive — *see* condition
Inadequate, inadequacy
- aesthetics of dental restoration K08.56
- biologic, constitutional, functional, or social F60.7
- development
  - child R62.50
  - genitalia
    - after puberty NEC E30.0
    - congenital
      - female Q52.8
        - external Q52.79
        - internal Q52.8
      - male Q55.8
  - lungs Q33.6
    - associated with short gestation P28.0
  - organ or site not listed — *see* Anomaly, by site
- diet (causing nutritional deficiency) E63.9
- eating habits Z72.4
- environment, household Z59.1
- family support Z63.8
- food (supply) NEC Z59.4
  - hunger effects T73.0 ☑

Inadequate, inadequacy — *continued*
- functional F60.7
- household care, due to
  - family member
    - handicapped or ill Z74.2
    - on vacation Z75.5
    - temporarily away from home Z74.2
  - technical defects in home Z59.1
  - temporary absence from home of person rendering care Z74.2
- housing (heating) (space) Z59.1
- income (financial) Z59.6
- intrafamilial communication Z63.8
- material resources Z59.9
- mental — *see* Disability, intellectual
- parental supervision or control of child Z62.0
- personality F60.7
- pulmonary
  - function R06.89
    - newborn P28.5
  - ventilation, newborn P28.5
- sample of cytologic smear
  - anus R85.615
  - cervix R87.615
  - vagina R87.625
- social F60.7
  - insurance Z59.7
  - skills NEC Z73.4
- supervision of child by parent Z62.0
- teaching affecting education Z55.8
- welfare support Z59.7
Inanition R64
- with edema — *see* Malnutrition, severe
- due to
  - deprivation of food T73.0 ☑
  - malnutrition — *see* Malnutrition
- fever R50.9
Inappropriate
- change in quantitative human chorionic gonadotropin (hCG) in early pregnancy O02.81
- diet or eating habits Z72.4
- level of quantitative human chorionic gonadotropin (hCG) for gestational age in early pregnancy O02.81
- secretion
  - antidiuretic hormone (ADH) (excessive) E22.2
    - deficiency E23.2
  - pituitary (posterior) E22.2
Inattention at or after birth — *see* Neglect
Incarceration, incarcerated
- enterocele K46.0
  - gangrenous K46.1
- epiplocele K46.0
  - gangrenous K46.1
- exomphalos K42.0
  - gangrenous K42.1
- hernia (*see also* Hernia, by site, with obstruction)
  - with gangrene — *see* Hernia, by site, with gangrene
- iris, in wound — *see* Injury, eye, laceration, with prolapse
- lens, in wound — *see* Injury, eye, laceration, with prolapse
- omphalocele K42.0
- prison, anxiety concerning Z65.1
- rupture — *see* Hernia, by site
- sarcoepiplocele K46.0
  - gangrenous K46.1
- sarcoepiplomphalocele K42.0
  - with gangrene K42.1
- uterus N85.8
  - gravid O34.51- ☑
    - causing obstructed labor O65.5
Incised wound
- external — *see* Laceration
- internal organs — *see* Injury, by site
Incision, incisional
- hernia K43.2
  - with
    - gangrene (and obstruction) K43.1
    - obstruction K43.0
  - surgical, complication — *see* Complications, surgical procedure
  - traumatic
    - external — *see* Laceration
    - internal organs — *see* Injury, by site
Inclusion
- azurophilic leukocytic D72.0

Inclusion — *continued*
  blennorrhea (neonatal) (newborn) P39.1
  gallbladder in liver (congenital) Q44.1
Incompatibility
  ABO
    affecting management of pregnancy O36.11- ☑
      anti-A sensitization O36.11- ☑
      anti-B sensitization O36.19- ☑
      specified NEC O36.19- ☑
    infusion or transfusion reaction — *see* Complication(s), transfusion, incompatibility reaction, ABO
    newborn P55.1
  blood (group) (Duffy) (K(ell)) (Kidd) (Lewis) (M) (S) NEC
    affecting management of pregnancy O36.11- ☑
      anti-A sensitization O36.11- ☑
      anti-B sensitization O36.19- ☑
    infusion or transfusion reaction T80.89 ☑
    newborn P55.8
  divorce or estrangement Z63.5
  Rh (blood group) (factor) Z31.82
    affecting management of pregnancy NEC O36.09- ☑
      anti-D antibody O36.01- ☑
    infusion or transfusion reaction — *see* Complication(s), transfusion, incompatibility reaction, Rh (factor)
    newborn P55.0
  rhesus — *see* Incompatibility, Rh
Incompetency, incompetent, incompetence
  annular
    aortic (valve) — *see* Insufficiency, aortic
    mitral (valve) I34.0
    pulmonary valve (heart) I37.1
  aortic (valve) — *see* Insufficiency, aortic
  cardiac valve — *see* Endocarditis
  cervix, cervical (os) N88.3
    in pregnancy O34.3- ☑
  chronotropic I45.89
    with
      autonomic dysfunction G90.8
      ischemic heart disease I25.89
      left ventricular dysfunction I51.89
      sinus node dysfunction I49.8
  esophagogastric (junction) (sphincter) K22.0
  mitral (valve) — *see* Insufficiency, mitral
  pelvic fundus N81.89
  pubocervical tissue N81.82
  pulmonary valve (heart) I37.1
    congenital Q22.3
  rectovaginal tissue N81.83
  tricuspid (annular) (valve) — *see* Insufficiency, tricuspid
  valvular — *see* Endocarditis
    congenital Q24.8
  vein, venous (saphenous) (varicose) — *see* Varix, leg
Incomplete (*see also* condition)
  bladder, emptying R33.9
  defecation R15.0
  expansion lungs (newborn) NEC — *see* Atelectasis
  rotation, intestine Q43.3
Inconclusive
  diagnostic imaging due to excess body fat of patient R93.9
  findings on diagnostic imaging of breast NEC R92.8
  mammogram (due to dense breasts) R92.2
Incontinence R32
  anal sphincter R15.9
  coital N39.491
  feces R15.9
    nonorganic origin F98.1
  insensible (urinary) N39.42
  overflow N39.490
  postural (urinary) N39.492
  psychogenic F45.8
  rectal R15.9
  reflex N39.498
  stress (female) (male) N39.3
    and urge N39.46
  urethral sphincter R32
  urge N39.41
    and stress (female) (male) N39.46
  urine (urinary) R32
    continuous N39.45
    due to cognitive impairment, or severe physical disability or immobility R39.81
    functional R39.81
    insensible N39.42
    mixed (stress and urge) N39.46

Incontinence — *continued*
  urine — *continued*
    nocturnal N39.44
    nonorganic origin F98.0
    overflow N39.490
    post dribbling N39.43
    postural N39.492
    reflex N39.498
    specified NEC N39.498
    stress (female) (male) N39.3
      and urge N39.46
    total N39.498
    unaware N39.42
    urge N39.41
      and stress (female) (male) N39.46
Incontinentia pigmenti Q82.3
Incoordinate, incoordination
  esophageal-pharyngeal (newborn) — *see* Dysphagia
  muscular R27.8
  uterus (action) (contractions) (complicating delivery) O62.4
Increase, increased
  abnormal, in development R63.8
  androgens (ovarian) E28.1
  anticoagulants (antithrombin) (anti-VIIIa) (anti-IXa) (anti-Xa) (anti-XIa) — *see* Circulating anticoagulants
  cold sense R20.8
  estrogen E28.0
  function
    adrenal
      cortex — *see* Cushing's, syndrome
      medulla E27.5
    pituitary (gland) (anterior) (lobe) E22.9
      posterior E22.2
  heat sense R20.8
  intracranial pressure (benign) G93.2
  permeability, capillaries I78.8
  pressure, intracranial G93.2
  secretion
    gastrin E16.4
    glucagon E16.3
    pancreas, endocrine E16.9
      growth hormone-releasing hormone E16.8
      pancreatic polypeptide E16.8
      somatostatin E16.8
      vasoactive-intestinal polypeptide E16.8
  sphericity, lens Q12.4
  splenic activity D73.1
  venous pressure I87.8
    portal K76.6
Increta placenta O43.22- ☑
Incrustation, cornea, foreign body (lead)(zinc) — *see* Foreign body, cornea
Incyclophoria H50.54
Incyclotropia — *see* Cyclotropia
Indeterminate sex Q56.4
India rubber skin Q82.8
Indigestion (acid) (bilious) (functional) K30
  catarrhal K31.89
  due to decomposed food NOS A05.9
  nervous F45.8
  psychogenic F45.8
Indirect — *see* condition
Induratio penis plastica N48.6
Induration, indurated
  brain G93.89
  breast (fibrous) N64.51
    puerperal, postpartum O92.29
  broad ligament N83.8
  chancre
    anus A51.1
    congenital A50.07
    extragenital NEC A51.2
  corpora cavernosa (penis) (plastic) N48.6
  liver (chronic) K76.89
  lung (black) (chronic) (fibroid) (*see also* Fibrosis, lung) J84.10
    essential brown J84.03
  penile (plastic) N48.6
  phlebitic — *see* Phlebitis
  skin R23.4
Inebriety (without dependence) — *see* Alcohol, intoxication
Inefficiency, kidney N28.9
Inelasticity, skin R23.4
Inequality, leg (length) (acquired) (*see also* Deformity, limb, unequal length)
  congenital — *see* Defect, reduction, lower limb

Inequality, leg — *continued*
  lower leg — *see* Deformity, limb, unequal length
Inertia
  bladder (neurogenic) N31.2
  stomach K31.89
    psychogenic F45.8
  uterus, uterine during labor O62.2
    during latent phase of labor O62.0
    primary O62.0
    secondary O62.1
  vesical (neurogenic) N31.2
Infancy, infantile, infantilism (*see also* condition)
  celiac K90.0
  genitalia, genitals (after puberty) E30.0
  Herter's (nontropical sprue) K90.0
  intestinal K90.0
  Lorain E23.0
  pancreatic K86.89
  pelvis M95.5
    with disproportion (fetopelvic) O33.1
      causing obstructed labor O65.1
  pituitary E23.0
  renal N25.0
  uterus — *see* Infantile, genitalia
Infant(s) (*see also* Infancy)
  excessive crying R68.11
  irritable child R68.12
  lack of care — *see* Neglect
  liveborn (singleton) Z38.2
    born in hospital Z38.00
      by cesarean Z38.01
    born outside hospital Z38.1
    multiple NEC Z38.8
      born in hospital Z38.68
        by cesarean Z38.69
      born outside hospital Z38.7
    quadruplet Z38.8
      born in hospital Z38.63
        by cesarean Z38.64
      born outside hospital Z38.7
    quintuplet Z38.8
      born in hospital Z38.65
        by cesarean Z38.66
      born outside hospital Z38.7
    triplet Z38.8
      born in hospital Z38.61
        by cesarean Z38.62
      born outside hospital Z38.7
    twin Z38.5
      born in hospital Z38.30
        by cesarean Z38.31
      born outside hospital Z38.4
  of diabetic mother (syndrome of) P70.1
    gestational diabetes P70.0
Infantile (*see also* condition)
  genitalia, genitals E30.0
  os, uterine E30.0
  penis E30.0
  testis E29.1
  uterus E30.0
Infantilism — *see* Infancy
Infarct, infarction
  adrenal (capsule) (gland) E27.49
  appendices epiploicae (*see also* Infarct, intestine) K55.069
  bowel (*see also* Infarct, intestine) K55.069
  brain (stem) — *see* Infarct, cerebral
  breast N64.89
  brewer's (kidney) N28.0
  cardiac — *see* Infarct, myocardium
  cerebellar — *see* Infarct, cerebral
  cerebral (*see also* Occlusion, artery cerebral or precerebral, with infarction) I63.9
    aborted I63.9
    cortical I63.9
    due to
      cerebral venous thrombosis, nonpyogenic I63.6
      embolism
        cerebral arteries I63.4- ☑
        precerebral arteries I63.1- ☑
      occlusion NEC
        cerebral arteries I63.5- ☑
        precerebral arteries I63.2- ☑
      stenosis NEC
        cerebral arteries I63.5- ☑
        precerebral arteries I63.2- ☑

Infarct, infarction — *continued*
cerebral (*see also* Occlusion, artery cerebral or precerebral, with infarction) — *continued*
  due to — *continued*
    thrombosis
      cerebral artery I63.3- ☑
      precerebral artery I63.0- ☑
    intraoperative
      during cardiac surgery I97.810
      during other surgery I97.811
    postprocedural
      following cardiac surgery I97.820
      following other surgery I97.821
    specified NEC I63.8
  colon (acute) (agnogenic) (embolic) (hemorrhagic) (nonocclusive) (nonthrombotic) (occlusive) (segmental) (thrombotic) (with gangrene) (*see also* Infarct, intestine) K55.049
  coronary artery — *see* Infarct, myocardium
  embolic — *see* Embolism
  fallopian tube N83.8
  gallbladder K82.8
  heart — *see* Infarct, myocardium
  hepatic K76.3
  hypophysis (anterior lobe) E23.6
  impending (myocardium) I20.0
  intestine (acute) (agnogenic) (embolic) (hemorrhagic) (nonocclusive) (nonthrombotic) (occlusive) (thrombotic) (with gangrene) K55.069
    diffuse K55.062
    focal K55.061
    large K55.049
      diffuse K55.042
      focal K55.041
    small K55.029
      diffuse K55.022
      focal K55.021
  kidney N28.0
  liver K76.3
  lung (embolic) (thrombotic) — *see* Embolism, pulmonary
  lymph node I89.8
  mesentery, mesenteric (embolic) (thrombotic) (with gangrene) (*see also* Infarct, intestine) K55.069
  muscle (ischemic) M62.20
    ankle M62.27- ☑
    foot M62.27- ☑
    forearm M62.23- ☑
    hand M62.24- ☑
    lower leg M62.26- ☑
    pelvic region M62.25- ☑
    shoulder region M62.21- ☑
    specified site NEC M62.28
    thigh M62.25- ☑
    upper arm M62.22- ☑
  myocardium, myocardial (acute) (with stated duration of 4 weeks or less) I21.9
    associated with revascularization procedure I21.A9
    diagnosed on ECG, but presenting no symptoms I25.2
    due to
      demand ischemia I21.A1
      ischemic imbalance I21.A1
    healed or old I25.2
    intraoperative (*see also* Infarct, myocardium, associated with revascularization procedure)
      during cardiac surgery I97.790
      during other surgery I97.791
    non-Q wave I21.4
    non-ST elevation (NSTEMI) I21.4
      subsequent I22.2
    nontransmural I21.4
    past (diagnosed on ECG or other investigation, but currently presenting no symptoms) I25.2
    postprocedural (*see also* Infarct, myocardium, associated with revascularization procedure)
      following cardiac surgery (*see also* Infarct, myocardium, type 4 or type 5) I97.190
      following other surgery I97.191
    Q wave (see also, Infarct, myocardium, by site) I21.3
    secondary to
      demand ischemia I21.A1
      ischemic imbalance I21.A1
    ST elevation (STEMI) I21.3
      anterior (anteroapical) (anterolateral) (anteroseptal) (Q wave) (wall) I21.09
        subsequent I22.0

Infarct, infarction — *continued*
myocardium, myocardial — *continued*
  ST elevation — *continued*
    inferior (diaphragmatic) (inferolateral) (inferoposterior) (wall) NEC I21.19
      subsequent I22.1
    inferoposterior transmural (Q wave) I21.11
    involving
      coronary artery of anterior wall NEC I21.09
      coronary artery of inferior wall NEC I21.19
      diagonal coronary artery I21.02
      left anterior descending coronary artery I21.02
      left circumflex coronary artery I21.21
      left main coronary artery I21.01
      oblique marginal coronary artery I21.21
      right coronary artery I21.11
    lateral (apical-lateral) (basal-lateral) (high) I21.29
      subsequent I22.8
    posterior (posterobasal) (posterolateral) (posteroseptal) (true) I21.29
      subsequent I22.8
    septal I21.29
      subsequent I22.8
    specified NEC I21.29
      subsequent I22.8
    subsequent I22.9
  subsequent (recurrent) (reinfarction) I22.9
    anterior (anteroapical) (anterolateral) (anteroseptal) (wall) I22.0
    diaphragmatic (wall) I22.1
    inferior (diaphragmatic) (inferolateral) (inferoposterior) (wall) I22.1
    lateral (apical-lateral) (basal-lateral) (high) I22.8
    non-ST elevation (NSTEMI) I22.2
    posterior (posterobasal) (posterolateral) (posteroseptal) (true) I22.8
    septal I22.8
    specified NEC I22.8
    ST elevation I22.9
      anterior (anteroapical) (anterolateral) (anteroseptal) (wall) I22.0
      inferior (diaphragmatic) (inferolateral) (inferoposterior) (wall) I22.1
      specified NEC I22.8
    subendocardial I22.2
    transmural I22.9
      anterior (anteroapical) (anterolateral) (anteroseptal) (wall) I22.0
      diaphragmatic (wall) I22.1
      inferior (diaphragmatic) (inferolateral) (inferoposterior) (wall) I22.1
      lateral (apical-lateral) (basal-lateral) (high) I22.8
      posterior (posterobasal) (posterolateral) (posteroseptal) (true) I22.8
      specified NEC I22.8
    type 1 (*see also* Infarction, myocardial, subsequent, by site, or by ST elevation or non-ST elevation) I22.9
    type 2 I21.A1
    type 3 I21.A9
    type 4 I21.A9
    type 5 I21.A9
  syphilitic A52.06
  transmural I21.9
    anterior (anteroapical) (anterolateral) (anteroseptal) (Q wave) (wall) NEC I21.09
    inferior (diaphragmatic) (inferolateral) (inferoposterior) (Q wave) (wall) NEC I21.19
    inferoposterior (Q wave) I21.11
    lateral (apical-lateral) (basal-lateral) (high) NEC I21.29
    posterior (posterobasal) (posterolateral) (posteroseptal) (true) NEC I21.29
    septal NEC I21.29
    specified NEC I21.29
  type 1 (*see also* Infarction, myocardial, by site, or by ST elevation or non-ST elevation) I21.9
  type 2 I21.A1
  type 3 I21.A9
  type 4 (a) (b) (c) I21.A9
  type 5 I21.A9
  nontransmural I21.4
omentum (*see also* Infarct, intestine) K55.069
ovary N83.8
pancreas K86.89
papillary muscle — *see* Infarct, myocardium

Infarct, infarction — *continued*
parathyroid gland E21.4
pituitary (gland) E23.6
placenta O43.81- ☑
prostate N42.89
pulmonary (artery) (vein) (hemorrhagic) — *see* Embolism, pulmonary
renal (embolic) (thrombotic) N28.0
retina, retinal (artery) — *see* Occlusion, artery, retina
spinal (cord) (acute) (embolic) (nonembolic) G95.11
spleen D73.5
  embolic or thrombotic I74.8
subendocardial (acute) (nontransmural) I21.4
suprarenal (capsule) (gland) E27.49
testis N50.1
thrombotic (*see also* Thrombosis)
  artery, arterial — *see* Embolism
thyroid (gland) E07.89
ventricle (heart) — *see* Infarct, myocardium
Infecting — *see* condition
Infection, infected, infective (opportunistic) B99.9
  with
    drug resistant organism — *see* Resistance (to), drug (*see also* specific organism)
    lymphangitis — *see* Lymphangitis
    organ dysfunction (acute) R65.20
      with septic shock R65.21
  abscess (skin) — *code by* site under Abscess
  Absidia — *see* Mucormycosis
  Acanthamoeba — *see* Acanthamebiasis
  Acanthocheilonema (perstans) (streptocerca) B74.4
  accessory sinus (chronic) — *see* Sinusitis
  achorion — *see* Dermatophytosis
  Acremonium falciforme B47.0
  acromioclavicular M00.9
  Actinobacillus (actinomycetem-comitans) A28.8
    mallei A24.0
    muris A25.1
  Actinomadura B47.1
  Actinomyces (israelii) (*see also* Actinomycosis) A42.9
  Actinomycetales — *see* Actinomycosis
  actinomycotic NOS — *see* Actinomycosis
  adenoid (and tonsil) J03.90
    chronic J35.02
  adenovirus NEC
    as cause of disease classified elsewhere B97.0
    unspecified nature or site B34.0
  aerogenes capsulatus A48.0
  aertrycke — *see* Infection, salmonella
  alimentary canal NOS — *see* Enteritis, infectious
  Allescheria boydii B48.2
  Alternaria B48.8
  alveolus, alveolar (process) K04.7
  Ameba, amebic (histolytica) — *see* Amebiasis
  amniotic fluid, sac or cavity O41.10- ☑
    chorioamnionitis O41.12- ☑
    placentitis O41.14- ☑
  amputation stump (surgical) — *see* Complication, amputation stump, infection
  Ancylostoma (duodenalis) B76.0
  Anisakiasis, Anisakis larvae B81.0
  anthrax — *see* Anthrax
  antrum (chronic) — *see* Sinusitis, maxillary
  anus, anal (papillae) (sphincter) K62.89
  arbovirus (arbor virus) A94
    specified type NEC A93.8
  artificial insemination N98.0
  Ascaris lumbricoides — *see* Ascariasis
  Ascomycetes B47.0
  Aspergillus (flavus) (fumigatus) (terreus) — *see* Aspergillosis
  atypical
    acid-fast (bacilli) — *see* Mycobacterium, atypical
    mycobacteria — *see* Mycobacterium, atypical
    virus A81.9
      specified type NEC A81.89
  auditory meatus (external) — *see* Otitis, externa, infective
  auricle (ear) — *see* Otitis, externa, infective
  axillary gland (lymph) L04.2
  Bacillus A49.9
    abortus A23.1
    anthracis — *see* Anthrax
    Ducrey's (any location) A57
    Flexner's A03.1
    Friedländer's NEC A49.8
    gas (gangrene) A48.0
    mallei A24.0

Infection, infected, infective — *continued*
  Bacillus — *continued*
    melitensis A23.0
    paratyphoid, paratyphosus A01.4
      A A01.1
      B A01.2
      C A01.3
    Shiga (-Kruse) A03.0
    suipestifer — *see* Infection, salmonella
    swimming pool A31.1
    typhosa A01.00
    welchii — *see* Gangrene, gas
  bacterial NOS A49.9
    as cause of disease classified elsewhere B96.89
      Bacteroides fragilis [B. fragilis] B96.6
      Clostridium perfringens [C. perfringens] B96.7
      Enterobacter sakazakii B96.89
      Enterococcus B95.2
      Escherichia coli [E. coli] (*see also* Escherichia coli) B96.20
      Helicobacter pylori [H.pylori] B96.81
      Hemophilus influenzae [H. influenzae] B96.3
      Klebsiella pneumoniae [K. pneumoniae] B96.1
      Mycoplasma pneumoniae [M. pneumoniae] B96.0
      Proteus (mirabilis) (morganii) B96.4
      Pseudomonas (aeruginosa) (mallei) (pseudomallei) B96.5
      Staphylococcus B95.8
        aureus (methicillin susceptible) (MSSA) B95.61
          methicillin resistant (MRSA) B95.62
        specified NEC B95.7
      Streptococcus B95.5
        group A B95.0
        group B B95.1
        pneumoniae B95.3
        specified NEC B95.4
      Vibrio vulnificus B96.82
    specified NEC A48.8
  Bacterium
    paratyphosum A01.4
      A A01.1
      B A01.2
      C A01.3
    typhosum A01.00
  Bacteroides NEC A49.8
    fragilis, as cause of disease classified elsewhere B96.6
  Balantidium coli A07.0
  Bartholin's gland N75.8
  Basidiobolus B46.8
  bile duct (common) (hepatic) — *see* Cholangitis
  bladder — *see* Cystitis
  Blastomyces, blastomycotic (*see also* Blastomycosis)
    brasiliensis — *see* Paracoccidioidomycosis
    dermatitidis — *see* Blastomycosis
    European — *see* Cryptococcosis
    Loboi B48.0
    North American B40.9
    South American — *see* Paracoccidioidomycosis
  bleb, postprocedure — *see* Blebitis
  bone — *see* Osteomyelitis
  Bordetella — *see* Whooping cough
  Borrelia bergdorfi A69.20
  brain (*see also* Encephalitis) G04.90
    membranes — *see* Meningitis
    septic G06.0
      meninges — *see* Meningitis, bacterial
  branchial cyst Q18.0
  breast — *see* Mastitis
  bronchus — *see* Bronchitis
  Brucella A23.9
    abortus A23.1
    canis A23.3
    melitensis A23.0
    mixed A23.8
    specified NEC A23.8
    suis A23.2
  Brugia (malayi) B74.1
    timori B74.2
  bursa — *see* Bursitis, infective
  buttocks (skin) L08.9
  Campylobacter, intestinal A04.5
    as cause of disease classified elsewhere B96.81
  Candida (albicans) (tropicalis) — *see* Candidiasis
  candiru B88.8
  Capillaria (intestinal) B81.1

Infection, infected, infective — *continued*
  Capillaria — *continued*
    hepatica B83.8
    philippinensis B81.1
  cartilage — *see* Disorder, cartilage, specified type NEC
  cat liver fluke B66.0
  catheter-related bloodstream (CRBSI) T80.211 ☑
  cellulitis — *code by* site under Cellulitis
  central line-associated T80.219 ☑
    bloodstream (CLABSI) T80.211 ☑
    specified NEC T80.218 ☑
  Cephalosporium falciforme B47.0
  cerebrospinal — *see* Meningitis
  cervical gland (lymph) L04.0
  cervix — *see* Cervicitis
  cesarean delivery wound (puerperal) O86.0
  cestodes — *see* Infestation, cestodes
  chest J22
  Chilomastix (intestinal) A07.8
  Chlamydia, chlamydial A74.9
    anus A56.3
    genitourinary tract A56.2
      lower A56.00
      specified NEC A56.19
    lymphogranuloma A55
    pharynx A56.4
    psittaci A70
    rectum A56.3
    sexually transmitted NEC A56.8
  cholera — *see* Cholera
  Cladosporium
    bantianum (brain abscess) B43.1
    carrionii B43.0
    castellanii B36.1
    trichoides (brain abscess) B43.1
    werneckii B36.1
  Clonorchis (sinensis) (liver) B66.1
  Clostridium NEC
    bifermentans A48.0
    botulinum (food poisoning) A05.1
      infant A48.51
      wound A48.52
    difficile
      as cause of disease classified elsewhere B96.89
      foodborne (disease)
        not specified as recurrent A04.72
        recurrent A04.71
      gas gangrene A48.0
      necrotizing enterocolitis
        not specified as recurrent A04.72
        recurrent A04.71
      sepsis A41.4
    gas-forming NEC A48.0
    histolyticum A48.0
    novyi, causing gas gangrene A48.0
    oedematiens A48.0
    perfringens
      as cause of disease classified elsewhere B96.7
      due to food A05.2
      foodborne (disease) A05.2
      gas gangrene A48.0
      sepsis A41.4
    septicum, causing gas gangrene A48.0
    sordellii, causing gas gangrene A48.0
    welchii
      as cause of disease classified elsewhere B96.7
      foodborne (disease) A05.2
      gas gangrene A48.0
      necrotizing enteritis A05.2
      sepsis A41.4
  Coccidioides (immitis) — *see* Coccidioidomycosis
  colon — *see* Enteritis, infectious
  colostomy K94.02
  common duct — *see* Cholangitis
  congenital P39.9
    Candida (albicans) P37.5
    cytomegalovirus P35.1
    hepatitis, viral P35.3
    herpes simplex P35.2
    infectious or parasitic disease P37.9
      specified NEC P37.8
    listeriosis (disseminated) P37.2
    malaria NEC P37.4
      falciparum P37.3
    Plasmodium falciparum P37.3
    poliomyelitis P35.8
    rubella P35.0
    skin P39.4

Infection, infected, infective — *continued*
  congenital — *continued*
    toxoplasmosis (acute) (subacute) (chronic) P37.1
    tuberculosis P37.0
    urinary (tract) P39.3
    vaccinia P35.8
    virus P35.9
      specified type NEC P35.8
  Conidiobolus B46.8
  coronavirus NEC B34.2
    as cause of disease classified elsewhere B97.29
    severe acute respiratory syndrome (SARS associated) B97.21
  corpus luteum — *see* Salpingo-oophoritis
  Corynebacterium diphtheriae — *see* Diphtheria
  cotia virus B08.8
  Coxiella burnetii A78
  coxsackie — *see* Coxsackie
  Cryptococcus neoformans — *see* Cryptococcosis
  Cryptosporidium A07.2
  Cunninghamella — *see* Mucormycosis
  cyst — *see* Cyst
  cystic duct (*see also* Cholecystitis) K81.9
  Cysticercus cellulosae — *see* Cysticercosis
  cytomegalovirus, cytomegaloviral B25.9
    congenital P35.1
    maternal, maternal care for (suspected) damage to fetus O35.3 ☑
    mononucleosis B27.10
      with
        complication NEC B27.19
        meningitis B27.12
        polyneuropathy B27.11
  delta-agent (acute), in hepatitis B carrier B17.0
  dental (pulpal origin) K04.7
  Deuteromycetes B47.0
  Dicrocoelium dendriticum B66.2
  Dipetalonema (perstans) (streptocerca) B74.4
  diphtherial — *see* Diphtheria
  Diphyllobothrium (adult) (latum) (pacificum) B70.0
    larval B70.1
  Diplogonoporus (grandis) B71.8
  Dipylidium caninum B67.4
  Dirofilaria B74.8
  Dracunculus medinensis B72
  Drechslera (hawaiiensis) B43.8
  Ducrey Haemophilus (any location) A57
  due to or resulting from
    artificial insemination N98.0
    central venous catheter T80.219 ☑
      bloodstream T80.211 ☑
      exit or insertion site T80.212 ☑
      localized T80.212 ☑
      port or reservoir T80.212 ☑
      specified NEC T80.218 ☑
      tunnel T80.212 ☑
    device, implant or graft (*see also* Complications, by site and type, infection or inflammation) T85.79 ☑
      arterial graft NEC T82.7 ☑
      breast (implant) T85.79 ☑
      catheter NEC T85.79 ☑
        dialysis (renal) T82.7 ☑
          intraperitoneal T85.71 ☑
        infusion NEC T82.7 ☑
          cranial T85.735 ☑
          intrathecal T85.735 ☑
          spinal (epidural) (subdural) T85.735 ☑
          subarachnoid T85.735 ☑
        urinary T83.518 ☑
          cystostomy T83.510 ☑
          Hopkins T83.518 ☑
          ileostomy T83.518 ☑
          nephrostomy T83.512 ☑
          specified NEC T83.518 ☑
          urethral indwelling T83.511 ☑
          urostomy T83.518 ☑
      electronic (electrode) (pulse generator) (stimulator)
        bone T84.7 ☑
        cardiac T82.7 ☑
        nervous system T85.738 ☑
          brain T85.731 ☑
          cranial nerve T85.732 ☑
          gastric nerve T85.732 ☑
          generator pocket T85.734 ☑
          neurostimulator generator T85.734 ☑

Infection, infected, infective — *continued*
  due to or resulting from — *continued*
    device, implant or graft (*see also* Complications, by site and type, infection or inflammation) — *continued*
      electronic — *continued*
        nervous system — *continued*
          peripheral nerve T85.732 ☑
          sacral nerve T85.732 ☑
          spinal cord T85.733 ☑
          vagal nerve T85.732 ☑
          urinary (indwelling) T83.51
      fixation, internal (orthopedic) NEC — *see* Complication, fixation device, infection
      gastrointestinal (bile duct) (esophagus) T85.79
        neurostimulator electrode (lead) T85.732 ☑
      genital NEC T83.69 ☑
      heart NEC T82.7 ☑
        valve (prosthesis) T82.6 ☑
          graft T82.7 ☑
      joint prosthesis — *see* Complication, joint prosthesis, infection
      ocular (corneal graft) (orbital implant) NEC T85.79
      orthopedic NEC T84.7 ☑
      penile (cylinder) (pump) (resevoir) T83.61 ☑
      specified NEC T85.79 ☑
      testicular T83.62 ☑
      urinary NEC T83.598 ☑
        ileal conduit stent T83.593 ☑
        implanted neurostimulation T83.590 ☑
        implanted sphincter T83.591 ☑
        indwelling ureteral stent T83.592 ☑
        nephroureteral stent T83.593 ☑
        specified stent NEC T83.593 ☑
      vascular NEC T82.7 ☑
      ventricular intracranial (communicating) shunt T85.730 ☑
    Hickman catheter T80.219 ☑
      bloodstream T80.211 ☑
      localized T80.212 ☑
      specified NEC T80.218 ☑
    immunization or vaccination T88.0 ☑
    infusion, injection or transfusion NEC T80.29 ☑
    injury NEC — *code by* site under Wound, open
    peripherally inserted central catheter (PICC) T80.219 ☑
      bloodstream T80.211 ☑
      localized T80.212 ☑
      specified NEC T80.218 ☑
    portacath (port-a-cath) T80.219 ☑
      bloodstream T80.211 ☑
      localized T80.212 ☑
      specified NEC T80.218 ☑
    pulmonary artery catheter — *see* Infection, due to or resulting from, central venous catheter
    surgery T81.4 ☑
    Swan Ganz catheter — *see* Infection, due to or resulting from, central venous catheter
    triple lumen catheter T80.219 ☑
      bloodstream T80.211 ☑
      localized T80.212 ☑
      specified NEC T80.218 ☑
    umbilical venous catheter T80.219 ☑
      bloodstream T80.211 ☑
      localized T80.212 ☑
      specified NEC T80.218 ☑
  during labor NEC O75.3
  ear (middle) (*see also* Otitis media)
    external — *see* Otitis, externa, infective
    inner — *see* subcategory H83.0 ☑
  Eberthella typhosa A01.00
  Echinococcus — *see* Echinococcus
  echovirus
    as cause of disease classified elsewhere B97.12
    unspecified nature or site B34.1
  endocardium I33.0
  endocervix — *see* Cervicitis
  Entamoeba — *see* Amebiasis
  enteric — *see* Enteritis, infectious
  Enterobacter sakazakii B96.89
  Enterobius vermicularis B80
  enterostomy K94.12
  enterovirus B34.1
    as cause of disease classified elsewhere B97.10

Infection, infected, infective — *continued*
  enterovirus — *continued*
    as cause of disease classified elsewhere — *continued*
      coxsackievirus B97.11
      echovirus B97.12
      specified NEC B97.19
  Entomophthora B46.8
  Epidermophyton — *see* Dermatophytosis
  epididymis — *see* Epididymitis
  episiotomy (puerperal) O86.0
  Erysipelothrix (insidiosa) (rhusiopathiae) — *see* Erysipeloid
  erythema infectiosum B08.3
  Escherichia (E.) coli NEC A49.8
    as cause of disease classified elsewhere (*see also* Escherichia coli) B96.20
    congenital P39.8
      sepsis P36.4
    generalized A41.51
    intestinal — *see* Enteritis, infectious, due to, Escherichia coli
  ethmoidal (chronic) (sinus) — *see* Sinusitis, ethmoidal
  eustachian tube (ear) — *see* Salpingitis, eustachian
  external auditory canal (meatus) NEC — *see* Otitis, externa, infective
  eye (purulent) — *see* Endophthalmitis, purulent
  eyelid — *see* Inflammation, eyelid
  fallopian tube — *see* Salpingo-oophoritis
  Fasciola (gigantica) (hepatica) (indica) B66.3
  Fasciolopsis (buski) B66.5
  filarial — *see* Infestation, filarial
  finger (skin) L08.9
    nail L03.01- ☑
      fungus B35.1
  fish tapeworm B70.0
    larval B70.1
  flagellate, intestinal A07.9
  fluke — *see* Infestation, fluke
  focal
    teeth (pulpal origin) K04.7
    tonsils J35.01
  Fonsecaea (compactum) (pedrosoi) B43.0
  food — *see* Intoxication, foodborne
  foot (skin) L08.9
    dermatophytic fungus B35.3
  Francisella tularensis — *see* Tularemia
  frontal (sinus) (chronic) — *see* Sinusitis, frontal
  fungus NOS B49
    beard B35.0
    dermatophytic — *see* Dermatophytosis
    foot B35.3
    groin B35.6
    hand B35.2
    nail B35.1
    pathogenic to compromised host only B48.8
    perianal (area) B35.6
    scalp B35.0
    skin B36.9
      foot B35.3
      hand B35.2
      toenails B35.1
  Fusarium B48.8
  gallbladder — *see* Cholecystitis
  gas bacillus — *see* Gangrene, gas
  gastrointestinal — *see* Enteritis, infectious
  generalized NEC — *see* Sepsis
  generator pocket, implanted electronic neurostimulator T85.734 ☑
  genital organ or tract
    female — *see* Disease, pelvis, inflammatory
    male N49.9
      multiple sites N49.8
      specified NEC N49.8
  Ghon tubercle, primary A15.7
  Giardia lamblia A07.1
  gingiva (chronic) K05.10
    acute K05.00
      nonplaque induced K05.01
      plaque induced K05.00
    nonplaque induced K05.11
    plaque induced K05.10
  glanders A24.0
  glenosporopsis B48.0
  Gnathostoma (spinigerum) B83.1
  Gongylonema B83.8
  gonococcal — *see* Gonococcus
  gram-negative bacilli NOS A49.9

Infection, infected, infective — *continued*
  guinea worm B72
  gum (chronic) K05.10
    acute K05.00
      nonplaque induced K05.01
      plaque induced K05.00
    nonplaque induced K05.11
    plaque induced K05.10
  Haemophilus — *see* Infection, Hemophilus
  heart — *see* Carditis
  Helicobacter pylori A04.8
    as cause of disease classified elsewhere B96.81
  helminths B83.9
    intestinal B82.0
      mixed (types classifiable to more than one of the titles B65.0-B81.3 and B81.8) B81.4
      specified type NEC B81.8
    specified type NEC B83.8
  Hemophilus
    aegyptius, systemic A48.4
    ducrey (any location) A57
    generalized A41.3
    influenzae NEC A49.2
      as cause of disease classified elsewhere B96.3
  herpes (simplex) (*see also* Herpes)
    congenital P35.2
    disseminated B00.7
    zoster B02.9
  herpesvirus, herpesviral — *see* Herpes
  Heterophyes (heterophyes) B66.8
  hip (joint) NEC M00.9
    due to internal joint prosthesis
      left T84.52 ☑
      right T84.51 ☑
    skin NEC L08.9
  Histoplasma — *see* Histoplasmosis
    American B39.4
    capsulatum B39.4
  hookworm B76.9
  human
    papilloma virus A63.0
    T-cell lymphotropic virus type-1 (HTLV-1) B33.3
  hydrocele N43.0
  Hymenolepis B71.0
  hypopharynx — *see* Pharyngitis
  inguinal (lymph) glands L04.1
    due to soft chancre A57
  intervertebral disc, pyogenic M46.30
    cervical region M46.32
    cervicothoracic region M46.33
    lumbar region M46.36
    lumbosacral region M46.37
    multiple sites M46.39
    occipito-atlanto-axial region M46.31
    sacrococcygeal region M46.38
    thoracic region M46.34
    thoracolumbar region M46.35
  intestine, intestinal — *see* Enteritis, infectious
    specified NEC A08.8
  intra-amniotic affecting newborn NEC P39.2
  Isospora belli or hominis A07.3
  Japanese B encephalitis A83.0
  jaw (bone) (lower) (upper) M27.2
  joint NEC M00.9
    due to internal joint prosthesis T84.50 ☑
  kidney (cortex) (hematogenous) N15.9
    with calculus N20.0
      with hydronephrosis N13.6
    following ectopic gestation O08.83
    pelvis and ureter (cystic) N28.85
    puerperal (postpartum) O86.21
    specified NEC N15.8
  Klebsiella (K.) pneumoniae NEC A49.8
    as cause of disease classified elsewhere B96.1
  knee (joint) NEC M00.9
    due to internal joint prosthesis
      left T84.54 ☑
      right T84.53 ☑
    joint M00.9
    skin L08.9
  Koch's — *see* Tuberculosis
  labia (majora) (minora) (acute) — *see* Vulvitis
  lacrimal
    gland — *see* Dacryoadenitis
    passages (duct) (sac) — *see* Inflammation, lacrimal, passages
  lancet fluke B66.2
  larynx NEC J38.7

Infection, infected, infective — *continued*
- leg (skin) NOS L08.9
- Legionella pneumophila A48.1
  - nonpneumonic A48.2
- Leishmania (*see also* Leishmaniasis)
  - aethiopica B55.1
  - braziliensis B55.2
  - chagasi B55.0
  - donovani B55.0
  - infantum B55.0
  - major B55.1
  - mexicana B55.1
  - tropica B55.1
- lentivirus, as cause of disease classified elsewhere B97.31
- Leptosphaeria senegalensis B47.0
- Leptospira interrogans A27.9
  - autumnalis A27.89
  - canicola A27.89
  - hebdomadis A27.89
  - icterohaemorrhagiae A27.0
  - pomona A27.89
  - specified type NEC A27.89
- leptospirochetal NEC — *see* Leptospirosis
- Listeria monocytogenes (*see also* Listeriosis)
  - congenital P37.2
- Loa loa B74.3
  - with conjunctival infestation B74.3
  - eyelid B74.3
- Loboa loboi B48.0
- local, skin (staphylococcal) (streptococcal) L08.9
  - abscess — *code by* site under Abscess
  - cellulitis — *code by* site under Cellulitis
  - specified NEC L08.89
  - ulcer — *see* Ulcer, skin
- Loefflerella mallei A24.0
- lung (*see also* Pneumonia) J18.9
  - atypical Mycobacterium A31.0
  - spirochetal A69.8
  - tuberculous — *see* Tuberculosis, pulmonary
  - virus — *see* Pneumonia, viral
- lymph gland (*see also* Lymphadenitis, acute)
  - mesenteric I88.0
- lymphoid tissue, base of tongue or posterior pharynx, NEC (chronic) J35.03
- Madurella (grisea) (mycetomii) B47.0
- major
  - following ectopic or molar pregnancy O08.0
  - puerperal, postpartum, childbirth O85
- Malassezia furfur B36.0
- Malleomyces
  - mallei A24.0
  - pseudomallei (whitmori) — *see* Melioidosis
- mammary gland N61.0
- Mansonella (ozzardi) (perstans) (streptocerca) B74.4
- mastoid — *see* Mastoiditis
- maxilla, maxillary M27.2
  - sinus (chronic) — *see* Sinusitis, maxillary
- mediastinum J98.51
- Medina (worm) B72
- meibomian cyst or gland — *see* Hordeolum
- meninges — *see* Meningitis, bacterial
- meningococcal (*see also* condition) A39.9
  - adrenals A39.1
  - brain A39.81
  - cerebrospinal A39.0
  - conjunctiva A39.89
  - endocardium A39.51
  - heart A39.50
    - endocardium A39.51
    - myocardium A39.52
    - pericardium A39.53
  - joint A39.83
  - meninges A39.0
  - meningococcemia A39.4
    - acute A39.2
    - chronic A39.3
  - myocardium A39.52
  - pericardium A39.53
  - retrobulbar neuritis A39.82
  - specified site NEC A39.89
- mesenteric lymph nodes or glands NEC I88.0
- Metagonimus B66.8
- metatarsophalangeal M00.9
- methicillin
  - resistant Staphylococcus aureus (MRSA) A49.02
  - susceptible Staphylococcus aureus (MSSA) A49.01
- Microsporum, microsporic — *see* Dermatophytosis

Infection, infected, infective — *continued*
- mixed flora (bacterial) NEC A49.8
- Monilia — *see* Candidiasis
- Monosporium apiospermum B48.2
- mouth, parasitic B37.0
- Mucor — *see* Mucormycosis
- muscle NEC — *see* Myositis, infective
- mycelium NOS B49
- mycetoma B47.9
  - actinomycotic NEC B47.1
  - mycotic NEC B47.0
- Mycobacterium, mycobacterial — *see* Mycobacterium
- Mycoplasma NEC A49.3
  - pneumoniae, as cause of disease classified elsewhere B96.0
- mycotic NOS B49
  - pathogenic to compromised host only B48.8
  - skin NOS B36.9
- myocardium NEC I40.0
- nail (chronic)
  - with lymphangitis — *see* Lymphangitis, acute, digit
  - finger L03.01- ☑
    - fungus B35.1
  - ingrowing L60.0
  - toe L03.03- ☑
    - fungus B35.1
- nasal sinus (chronic) — *see* Sinusitis
- nasopharynx — *see* Nasopharyngitis
- navel L08.82
- Necator americanus B76.1
- Neisseria — *see* Gonococcus
- Neotestudina rosatii B47.0
- newborn P39.9
  - intra-amniotic NEC P39.2
  - skin P39.4
  - specified type NEC P39.8
- nipple N61.0
  - associated with
    - lactation O91.03
    - pregnancy O91.01- ☑
    - puerperium O91.02
- Nocardia — *see* Nocardiosis
- obstetrical surgical wound (puerperal) O86.0
- Oesophagostomum (apiostomum) B81.8
- Oestrus ovis — *see* Myiasis
- Oidium albicans B37.9
- Onchocerca (volvulus) — *see* Onchocerciasis
- oncovirus, as cause of disease classified elsewhere B97.32
- operation wound T81.4 ☑
- Opisthorchis (felineus) (viverrini) B66.0
- orbit, orbital — *see* Inflammation, orbit
- orthopoxvirus NEC B08.09
- ovary — *see* Salpingo-oophoritis
- Oxyuris vermicularis B80
- pancreas (acute) — *see* Pancreatitis, acute
  - abscess — *see* Pancreatitis, acute
  - specified NEC (*see also* Pancreatitis, acute) K85.80
- papillomavirus, as cause of disease classified elsewhere B97.7
- papovavirus NEC B34.4
- Paracoccidioides brasiliensis — *see* Paracoccidioidomycosis
- Paragonimus (westermani) B66.4
- parainfluenza virus B34.8
- parameningococcus NOS A39.9
- parapoxvirus B08.60
  - specified NEC B08.69
- parasitic B89
- Parastrongylus
  - cantonensis B83.2
  - costaricensis B81.3
  - paratyphoid A01.4
    - Type A A01.1
    - Type B A01.2
    - Type C A01.3
- paraurethral ducts N34.2
- parotid gland — *see* Sialoadenitis
- parvovirus NEC B34.3
  - as cause of disease classified elsewhere B97.6
- Pasteurella NEC A28.0
  - multocida A28.0
  - pestis — *see* Plague
  - pseudotuberculosis A28.0
  - septica (cat bite) (dog bite) A28.0
  - tularensis — *see* Tularemia
- pelvic, female — *see* Disease, pelvis, inflammatory

Infection, infected, infective — *continued*
- Penicillium (marneffei) B48.4
- penis (glans) (retention) NEC N48.29
- periapical K04.5
- peridental, periodontal K05.20
  - generalized — *see* Peridontitis, aggressive, generalized
  - localized — *see* Peridontitis, aggressive, localized
- perinatal period P39.9
  - specified type NEC P39.8
- perineal repair (puerperal) O86.0
- periorbital — *see* Inflammation, orbit
- perirectal K62.89
- perirenal — *see* Infection, kidney
- peritoneal — *see* Peritonitis
- periureteral N28.89
- Petriellidium boydii B48.2
- pharynx (*see also* Pharyngitis)
  - coxsackievirus B08.5
  - posterior, lymphoid (chronic) J35.03
- Phialophora
  - gougerotii (subcutaneous abscess or cyst) B43.2
  - jeanselmei (subcutaneous abscess or cyst) B43.2
  - verrucosa (skin) B43.0
- Piedraia hortae B36.3
- pinta A67.9
  - intermediate A67.1
  - late A67.2
  - mixed A67.3
  - primary A67.0
- pinworm B80
- pityrosporum furfur B36.0
- pleuro-pneumonia-like organism (PPLO) NEC A49.3
  - as cause of disease classified elsewhere B96.0
- pneumococcus, pneumococcal NEC A49.1
  - as cause of disease classified elsewhere B95.3
  - generalized (purulent) A40.3
    - with pneumonia J13
- Pneumocystis carinii (pneumonia) B59
- Pneumocystis jiroveci (pneumonia) B59
- port or reservoir T80.212 ☑
- postoperative T81.4 ☑
- postoperative wound T81.4 ☑
- postprocedural T81.4 ☑
- postvaccinal T88.0 ☑
- prepuce NEC N47.7
  - with penile inflammation N47.6
- prion — *see* Disease, prion, central nervous system
- prostate (capsule) — *see* Prostatitis
- Proteus (mirabilis) (morganii) (vulgaris) NEC A49.8
  - as cause of disease classified elsewhere B96.4
- protozoal NEC B64
  - intestinal A07.9
    - specified NEC A07.8
  - specified NEC B60.8
- Pseudoallescheria boydii B48.2
- Pseudomonas NEC A49.8
  - as cause of disease classified elsewhere B96.5
  - mallei A24.0
  - pneumonia J15.1
  - pseudomallei — *see* Melioidosis
- puerperal O86.4
  - genitourinary tract NEC O86.89
  - major or generalized O85
  - minor O86.4
  - specified NEC O86.89
- pulmonary — *see* Infection, lung
- purulent — *see* Abscess
- Pyrenochaeta romeroi B47.0
- Q fever A78
- rectum (sphincter) K62.89
- renal (*see also* Infection, kidney)
  - pelvis and ureter (cystic) N28.85
- reovirus, as cause of disease classified elsewhere B97.5
- respiratory (tract) NEC J98.8
  - acute J22
  - chronic J98.8
  - influenzal (upper) (acute) — *see* Influenza, with, respiratory manifestations NEC
  - lower (acute) J22
    - chronic — *see* Bronchitis, chronic
  - rhinovirus J00
  - syncytial virus, as cause of disease classified elsewhere B97.4
  - upper (acute) NOS J06.9
    - chronic J39.8
    - streptococcal J06.9
    - viral NOS J06.9

Infection, infected, infective — *continued*
- resulting from
  - presence of internal prosthesis, implant, graft — *see* Complications, by site and type, infection
- retortamoniasis A07.8
- retroperitoneal NEC K68.9
- retrovirus B33.3
  - as cause of disease classified elsewhere B97.30
    - human
      - immunodeficiency, type 2 (HIV 2) B97.35
        - T-cell lymphotropic
          - type I (HTLV-I) B97.33
          - type II (HTLV-II) B97.34
    - lentivirus B97.31
    - oncovirus B97.32
    - specified NEC B97.39
- Rhinosporidium (seeberi) B48.1
- rhinovirus
  - as cause of disease classified elsewhere B97.89
  - unspecified nature or site B34.8
- Rhizopus — *see* Mucormycosis
- rickettsial NOS A79.9
- roundworm (large) NEC B82.0
  - Ascariasis (*see also* Ascariasis) B77.9
- rubella — *see* Rubella
- Saccharomyces — *see* Candidiasis
- salivary duct or gland (any) — *see* Sialoadenitis
- Salmonella (aertrycke) (arizonae) (callinarum) (cholerae-suis) (enteritidis) (suipestifer) (typhimurium) A02.9
  - with
    - (gastro)enteritis A02.0
    - sepsis A02.1
    - specified manifestation NEC A02.8
  - due to food (poisoning) A02.9
  - hirschfeldii A01.3
  - localized A02.20
    - arthritis A02.23
    - meningitis A02.21
    - osteomyelitis A02.24
    - pneumonia A02.22
    - pyelonephritis A02.25
    - specified NEC A02.29
  - paratyphi A01.4
    - A A01.1
    - B A01.2
    - C A01.3
  - schottmuelleri A01.2
  - typhi, typhosa — *see* Typhoid
- Sarcocystis A07.8
- scabies B86
- Schistosoma — *see* Infestation, Schistosoma
- scrotum (acute) NEC N49.2
- seminal vesicle — *see* Vesiculitis
- septic
  - localized, skin — *see* Abscess
- sheep liver fluke B66.3
- Shigella A03.9
  - boydii A03.2
  - dysenteriae A03.0
  - flexneri A03.1
  - group
    - A A03.0
    - B A03.1
    - C A03.2
    - D A03.3
  - Schmitz (-Stutzer) A03.0
  - schmitzii A03.0
  - shigae A03.0
  - sonnei A03.3
  - specified NEC A03.8
- shoulder (joint) NEC M00.9
  - due to internal joint prosthesis T84.59 ☑
  - skin NEC L08.9
- sinus (accessory) (chronic) (nasal) (*see also* Sinusitis)
  - pilonidal — *see* Sinus, pilonidal
  - skin NEC L08.89
- Skene's duct or gland — *see* Urethritis
- skin (local) (staphylococcal) (streptococcal) L08.9
  - abscess — *code by* site under Abscess
  - cellulitis — *code by* site under Cellulitis
  - due to fungus B36.9
    - specified type NEC B36.8
  - mycotic B36.9
    - specified type NEC B36.8
  - newborn P39.4
  - ulcer — *see* Ulcer, skin
- slow virus A81.9

Infection, infected, infective — *continued*
- slow virus — *continued*
  - specified NEC A81.89
- Sparganum (mansoni) (proliferum) (baxteri) B70.1
- specific (*see also* Syphilis)
  - to perinatal period — *see* Infection, congenital
- specified NEC B99.8
- spermatic cord NEC N49.1
- sphenoidal (sinus) — *see* Sinusitis, sphenoidal
- spinal cord NOS (*see also* Myelitis) G04.91
  - abscess G06.1
  - meninges — *see* Meningitis
  - streptococcal G04.89
- Spirillum A25.0
- spirochetal NOS A69.9
  - lung A69.8
  - specified NEC A69.8
- Spirometra larvae B70.1
- spleen D73.89
- Sporotrichum, Sporothrix (schenckii) — *see* Sporotrichosis
- staphylococcal, unspecified site
  - as cause of disease classified elsewhere B95.8
    - aureus (methicillin susceptible) (MSSA) B95.61
      - methicillin resistant (MRSA) B95.62
    - specified NEC B95.7
  - aureus (methicillin susceptible) (MSSA) A49.01
    - methicillin resistant (MRSA) A49.02
  - food poisoning A05.0
  - generalized (purulent) A41.2
  - pneumonia — *see* Pneumonia, staphylococcal
- Stellantchasmus falcatus B66.8
- streptobacillus moniliformis A25.1
- streptococcal NEC A49.1
  - as cause of disease classified elsewhere B95.5
    - B genitourinary complicating
      - childbirth O98.82
      - pregnancy O98.81- ☑
      - puerperium O98.83
    - congenital
      - sepsis P36.10
        - group B P36.0
        - specified NEC P36.19
    - generalized (purulent) A40.9
- Streptomyces B47.1
- Strongyloides (stercoralis) — *see* Strongyloidiasis
- stump (amputation) (surgical) — *see* Complication, amputation stump, infection
- subcutaneous tissue, local L08.9
- suipestifer — *see* Infection, salmonella
- swimming pool bacillus A31.1
- Taenia — *see* Infestation, Taenia
- Taeniarhynchus saginatus B68.1
- tapeworm — *see* Infestation, tapeworm
- tendon (sheath) — *see* Tenosynovitis, infective NEC
- Ternidens diminutus B81.8
- testis — *see* Orchitis
- threadworm B80
- throat — *see* Pharyngitis
- thyroglossal duct K14.8
- toe (skin) L08.9
  - cellulitis L03.03- ☑
    - fungus B35.1
  - nail L03.03- ☑
    - fungus B35.1
- tongue NEC K14.0
  - parasitic B37.0
- tonsil (and adenoid) (faucial) (lingual) (pharyngeal) — *see* Tonsillitis
- tooth, teeth K04.7
  - periapical K04.7
  - peridental, periodontal K05.20
    - generalized — *see* Peridontitis, aggressive, generalized
    - localized — *see* Peridontitis, aggressive, localized
  - pulp K04.01
    - irreversible K04.02
    - reversible K04.01
  - socket M27.3
- TORCH — *see* Infection, congenital
  - without active infection P00.2
- Torula histolytica — *see* Cryptococcosis
- Toxocara (canis) (cati) (felis) B83.0
- Toxoplasma gondii — *see* Toxoplasma
- trachea, chronic J42
- trematode NEC — *see* Infestation, fluke
- trench fever A79.0

Infection, infected, infective — *continued*
- Treponema pallidum — *see* Syphilis
- Trichinella (spiralis) B75
- Trichomonas A59.9
  - cervix A59.09
  - intestine A07.8
  - prostate A59.02
  - specified site NEC A59.8
  - urethra A59.03
  - urogenitalis A59.00
  - vagina A59.01
  - vulva A59.01
- Trichophyton, trichophytic — *see* Dermatophytosis
- Trichosporon (beigelii) cutaneum B36.2
- Trichostrongylus B81.2
- Trichuris (trichiura) B79
- Trombicula (irritans) B88.0
- Trypanosoma
  - brucei
    - gambiense B56.0
    - rhodesiense B56.1
  - cruzi — *see* Chagas' disease
- tubal — *see* Salpingo-oophoritis
- tuberculous NEC — *see* Tuberculosis
- tubo-ovarian — *see* Salpingo-oophoritis
- tunica vaginalis N49.1
- tunnel T80.212 ☑
- tympanic membrane NEC — *see* Myringitis
- typhoid (abortive) (ambulant) (bacillus) — *see* Typhoid
- typhus A75.9
  - flea-borne A75.2
  - mite-borne A75.3
  - recrudescent A75.1
  - tick-borne A77.9
    - African A77.1
    - North Asian A77.2
- umbilicus L08.82
- ureter N28.86
- urethra — *see* Urethritis
- urinary (tract) N39.0
  - bladder — *see* Cystitis
  - complicating
    - pregnancy O23.4- ☑
      - specified type NEC O23.3- ☑
  - kidney — *see* Infection, kidney
  - newborn P39.3
  - puerperal (postpartum) O86.20
  - tuberculous A18.13
  - urethra — *see* Urethritis
- uterus, uterine — *see* Endometritis
- vaccination T88.0 ☑
- vaccinia not from vaccination B08.011
- vagina (acute) — *see* Vaginitis
- varicella B01.9
- varicose veins — *see* Varix
- vas deferens NEC N49.1
- vesical — *see* Cystitis
- Vibrio
  - cholerae A00.0
    - El Tor A00.1
  - parahaemolyticus (food poisoning) A05.3
  - vulnificus
    - as cause of disease classified elsewhere B96.82
    - foodborne intoxication A05.5
- Vincent's (gum) (mouth) (tonsil) A69.1
- virus, viral NOS B34.9
  - adenovirus
    - as cause of disease classified elsewhere B97.0
    - unspecified nature or site B34.0
  - arborvirus, arbovirus arthropod-borne A94
  - as cause of disease classified elsewhere B97.89
    - adenovirus B97.0
    - coronavirus B97.29
      - SARS-associated B97.21
    - coxsackievirus B97.11
    - echovirus B97.12
    - enterovirus B97.10
      - coxsackievirus B97.11
      - echovirus B97.12
      - specified NEC B97.19
    - human
      - immunodeficiency, type 2 (HIV 2) B97.35
      - metapneumovirus B97.81
      - T-cell lymphotropic,
        - type I (HTLV-I) B97.33
        - type II (HTLV-II) B97.34
    - papillomavirus B97.7
    - parvovirus B97.6

Infection, infected, infective — *continued*
  virus, viral — *continued*
    as cause of disease classified elsewhere — *continued*
      reovirus B97.5
      respiratory syncytial B97.4
      retrovirus B97.30
        human
          immunodeficiency, type 2 (HIV 2) B97.35
          T-cell lymphotropic,
            type I (HTLV-I) B97.33
            type II (HTLV-II) B97.34
        lentivirus B97.31
        oncovirus B97.32
        specified NEC B97.39
      specified NEC B97.89
  central nervous system A89
    atypical A81.9
      specified NEC A81.89
    enterovirus NEC A88.8
      meningitis A87.0
    slow virus A81.9
      specified NEC A81.89
    specified NEC A88.8
  chest J98.8
  cotia B08.8
  coxsackie (*see also* Infection, coxsackie) B34.1
    as cause of disease classified elsewhere B97.11
  ECHO
    as cause of disease classified elsewhere B97.12
    unspecified nature or site B34.1
  encephalitis, tick-borne A84.9
  enterovirus, as cause of disease classified elsewhere
      B97.10
    coxsackievirus B97.11
    echovirus B97.12
    specified NEC B97.19
  exanthem NOS B09
  human metapneumovirus as cause of disease
      classified elsewhere B97.81
  human papilloma as cause of disease classified
      elsewhere B97.7
  intestine — *see* Enteritis, viral
  respiratory syncytial
    as cause of disease classified elsewhere B97.4
    bronchopneumonia J12.1
    common cold syndrome J00
    nasopharyngitis (acute) J00
  rhinovirus
    as cause of disease classified elsewhere B97.89
    unspecified nature or site B34.8
  slow A81.9
    specified NEC A81.89
  specified type NEC B33.8
    as cause of disease classified elsewhere B97.89
    unspecified nature or site B34.8
  unspecified nature or site B34.9
  West Nile — *see* Virus, West Nile
vulva (acute) — *see* Vulvitis
West Nile — *see* Virus, West Nile
whipworm B79
worms B83.9
  specified type NEC B83.8
Wuchereria (bancrofti) B74.0
  malayi B74.1
yatapoxvirus B08.70
  specified NEC B08.79
yeast (*see also* Candidiasis) B37.9
yellow fever — *see* Fever, yellow
Yersinia
  enterocolitica (intestinal) A04.6
  pestis — *see* Plague
  pseudotuberculosis A28.2
Zeis' gland — *see* Hordeolum
Zika virus A92.5
zoonotic bacterial NOS A28.9
Zopfia senegalensis B47.0
Infective, infectious — *see* condition
Infertility
  female N97.9
    age-related N97.8
    associated with
      anovulation N97.0
      cervical (mucus) disease or anomaly N88.3
      congenital anomaly
        cervix N88.3
        fallopian tube N97.1
        uterus N97.2

Infertility — *continued*
  female — *continued*
    associated with — *continued*
      congenital anomaly — *continued*
        vagina N97.8
      dysmucorrhea N88.3
      fallopian tube disease or anomaly N97.1
      pituitary-hypothalamic origin E23.0
      specified origin NEC N97.8
      Stein-Leventhal syndrome E28.2
      uterine disease or anomaly N97.2
      vaginal disease or anomaly N97.8
    due to
      cervical anomaly N88.3
      fallopian tube anomaly N97.1
      ovarian failure E28.39
      Stein-Leventhal syndrome E28.2
      uterine anomaly N97.2
      vaginal anomaly N97.8
    nonimplantation N97.2
    origin
      cervical N88.3
      tubal (block) (occlusion) (stenosis) N97.1
      uterine N97.2
      vaginal N97.8
  male N46.9
    azoospermia N46.01
      extratesticular cause N46.029
        drug therapy N46.021
        efferent duct obstruction N46.023
        infection N46.022
        radiation N46.024
        specified cause NEC N46.029
        systemic disease N46.025
    oligospermia N46.11
      extratesticular cause N46.129
        drug therapy N46.121
        efferent duct obstruction N46.123
        infection N46.122
        radiation N46.124
        specified cause NEC N46.129
        systemic disease N46.125
    specified type NEC N46.8
Infestation B88.9
  Acanthocheilonema (perstans) (streptocerca) B74.4
  Acariasis B88.0
    demodex folliculorum B88.0
    sarcoptes scabiei B86
    trombiculae B88.0
  Agamofilaria streptocerca B74.4
  Ancylostoma, ankylostoma (braziliense) (caninum)
      (ceylanicum) (duodenale) B76.0
    americanum B76.1
    new world B76.1
  Anisakis larvae, anisakiasis B81.0
  arthropod NEC B88.2
  Ascaris lumbricoides — *see* Ascariasis
  Balantidium coli A07.0
  beef tapeworm B68.1
  Bothriocephalus (latus) B70.0
    larval B70.1
  broad tapeworm B70.0
    larval B70.1
  Brugia (malayi) B74.1
    timori B74.2
  candiru B88.8
  Capillaria
    hepatica B83.8
    philippinensis B81.1
  cat liver fluke B66.0
  cestodes B71.9
    diphyllobothrium — *see* Infestation, diphyllobothrium
    dipylidiasis B71.1
    hymenolepiasis B71.0
    specified type NEC B71.8
  chigger B88.0
  chigo, chigoe B88.1
  Clonorchis (sinensis) (liver) B66.1
  coccidial A07.3
  crab-lice B85.3
  Cysticercus cellulosae — *see* Cysticercosis
  Demodex (folliculorum) B88.0
  Dermanyssus gallinae B88.0
  Dermatobia (hominis) — *see* Myiasis
  Dibothriocephalus (latus) B70.0
    larval B70.1
  Dicrocoelium dendriticum B66.2

Infestation — *continued*
  Diphyllobothrium (adult) (latum) (intestinal) (pacificum) B70.0
    larval B70.1
  Diplogonoporus (grandis) B71.8
  Dipylidium caninum B67.4
  Distoma hepaticum B66.3
  dog tapeworm B67.4
  Dracunculus medinensis B72
  dragon worm B72
  dwarf tapeworm B71.0
  Echinococcus — *see* Echinococcus
  Echinostomum ilocanum B66.8
  Entamoeba (histolytica) — *see* Infection, Ameba
  Enterobius vermicularis B80
  eyelid
    in (due to)
      leishmaniasis B55.1
      loiasis B74.3
      onchocerciasis B73.09
      phthiriasis B85.3
    parasitic NOS B89
  eyeworm B74.3
  Fasciola (gigantica) (hepatica) (indica) B66.3
  Fasciolopsis (buski) (intestine) B66.5
  filarial B74.9
    bancroftian B74.0
    conjunctiva B74.9
    due to
      Acanthocheilonema (perstans) (streptocerca)
          B74.4
      Brugia (malayi) B74.1
        timori B74.2
      Dracunculus medinensis B72
      guinea worm B72
      loa loa B74.3
      Mansonella (ozzardi) (perstans) (streptocerca)
          B74.4
      Onchocerca volvulus B73.00
        eye B73.00
        eyelid B73.09
      Wuchereria (bancrofti) B74.0
    Malayan B74.1
    ozzardi B74.4
    specified type NEC B74.8
  fish tapeworm B70.0
    larval B70.1
  fluke B66.9
    blood NOS — *see* Schistosomiasis
    cat liver B66.0
    intestinal B66.5
    lancet B66.2
    liver (sheep) B66.3
      cat B66.0
      Chinese B66.1
      due to clonorchiasis B66.1
      oriental B66.1
    lung (oriental) B66.4
    sheep liver B66.3
    specified type NEC B66.8
  fly larvae — *see* Myiasis
  Gasterophilus (intestinalis) — *see* Myiasis
  Gastrodiscoides hominis B66.8
  Giardia lamblia A07.1
  Gnathostoma (spinigerum) B83.1
  Gongylonema B83.8
  guinea worm B72
  helminth B83.9
    angiostrongyliasis B83.2
      intestinal B81.3
    gnathostomiasis B83.1
    hirudiniasis, internal B83.4
    intestinal B82.0
      angiostrongyliasis B81.3
      anisakiasis B81.0
      ascariasis — *see* Ascariasis
      capillariasis B81.1
      cysticercosis — *see* Cysticercosis
      diphyllobothriasis — *see* Infestation, diphyllobothriasis
      dracunculiasis B72
      echinococcus — *see* Echinococcosis
      enterobiasis B80
      filariasis — *see* Infestation, filarial
      fluke — *see* Infestation, fluke
      hookworm — *see* Infestation, hookworm
      mixed (types classifiable to more than one of
          the titles B65.0-B81.3 and B81.8) B81.4

Infestation — *continued*
    helminth — *continued*
        intestinal — *continued*
            onchocerciasis — *see* Onchocerciasis
            schistosomiasis — *see* Infestation, schistosoma
            specified
                cestode NEC — *see* Infestation, cestode
                    type NEC B81.8
                strongyloidiasis — *see* Strongyloidiasis
                taenia — *see* Infestation, taenia
                trichinellosis B75
                trichostrongyliasis B81.2
                trichuriasis B79
            specified type NEC B83.8
            syngamiasis B83.3
            visceral larva migrans B83.0
        Heterophyes (heterophyes) B66.8
        hookworm B76.9
            ancylostomiasis B76.0
            necatoriasis B76.1
            specified type NEC B76.8
        Hymenolepis (diminuta) (nana) B71.0
        intestinal NEC B82.9
        leeches (aquatic) (land) — *see* Hirudiniasis
        Leishmania — *see* Leishmaniasis
        lice, louse — *see* Infestation, Pediculus
        Linguatula B88.8
        Liponyssoides sanguineus B88.0
        Loa loa B74.3
            conjunctival B74.3
            eyelid B74.3
        louse — *see* Infestation, Pediculus
        maggots — *see* Myiasis
        Mansonella (ozzardi) (perstans) (streptocerca) B74.4
        Medina (worm) B72
        Metagonimus (yokogawai) B66.8
        microfilaria streptocerca — *see* Onchocerciasis
            eye B73.00
            eyelid B73.09
        mites B88.9
            scabic B86
        Monilia (albicans) — *see* Candidiasis
        mouth B37.0
        Necator americanus B76.1
        nematode NEC (intestinal) B82.0
            Ancylostoma B76.0
            conjunctiva NEC B83.9
            Enterobius vermicularis B80
            Gnathostoma spinigerum B83.1
            physaloptera B80
            specified NEC B81.8
            trichostrongylus B81.2
            trichuris (trichuria) B79
        Oesophagostomum (apiostomum) B81.8
        Oestrus ovis (see also Myiasis) B87.9
        Onchocerca (volvulus) — *see* Onchocerciasis
        Opisthorchis (felineus) (viverrini) B66.0
        orbit, parasitic NOS B89
        Oxyuris vermicularis B80
        Paragonimus (westermani) B66.4
        parasite, parasitic B89
            eyelid B89
            intestinal NOS B82.9
            mouth B37.0
            skin B88.9
            tongue B37.0
        Parastrongylus
            cantonensis B83.2
            costaricensis B81.3
        Pediculus B85.2
            body B85.1
            capitis (humanus) (any site) B85.0
            corporis (humanus) (any site) B85.1
            head B85.0
            mixed (classifiable to more than one of the titles
                B85.0 - B85.3) B85.4
            pubis (any site) B85.3
        Pentastoma B88.8
        Phthirus (pubis) (any site) B85.3
            with any infestation classifiable to B85.0 - B85.2
                B85.4
        pinworm B80
        pork tapeworm (adult) B68.0
        protozoal NEC B64
            intestinal A07.9
                specified NEC A07.8
            specified NEC B60.8
        pubic, louse B85.3

Infestation — *continued*
    rat tapeworm B71.0
    red bug B88.0
    roundworm (large) NEC B82.0
        Ascariasis (see also Ascariasis) B77.9
    sandflea B88.1
    Sarcoptes scabiei B86
    scabies B86
    Schistosoma B65.9
        bovis B65.8
        cercariae B65.3
        haematobium B65.0
        intercalatum B65.8
        japonicum B65.2
        mansoni B65.1
        mattheei B65.8
        mekongi B65.8
        specified type NEC B65.8
        spindale B65.8
    screw worms — *see* Myiasis
    skin NOS B88.9
    Sparganum (mansoni) (proliferum) (baxteri) B70.1
        larval B70.1
    specified type NEC B88.8
    Spirometra larvae B70.1
    Stellantchasmus falcatus B66.8
    Strongyloides stercoralis — *see* Strongyloidiasis
    Taenia B68.9
        diminuta B71.0
        echinococcus — *see* Echinococcus
        mediocanellata B68.1
        nana B71.0
        saginata B68.1
        solium (intestinal form) B68.0
            larval form — *see* Cysticercosis
    Taeniarhynchus saginatus B68.1
    tapeworm B71.9
        beef B68.1
        broad B70.0
            larval B70.1
        dog B67.4
        dwarf B71.0
        fish B70.0
            larval B70.1
        pork B68.0
        rat B71.0
    Ternidens diminutus B81.8
    Tetranychus molestissimus B88.0
    threadworm B80
    tongue B37.0
    Toxocara (canis) (cati) (felis) B83.0
    trematode(s) NEC — *see* Infestation, fluke
    Trichinella (spiralis) B75
    Trichocephalus B79
    Trichomonas — *see* Trichomoniasis
    Trichostrongylus B81.2
    Trichuris (trichiura) B79
    Trombicula (irritans) B88.0
    Tunga penetrans B88.1
    Uncinaria americana B76.1
    Vandellia cirrhosa B88.8
    whipworm B79
    worms B83.9
        intestinal B82.0
    Wuchereria (bancrofti) B74.0

Infiltrate, infiltration
    amyloid (generalized) (localized) — *see* Amyloidosis
    calcareous NEC R89.7
        localized — *see* Degeneration, by site
    calcium salt R89.7
    cardiac
        fatty — *see* Degeneration, myocardial
        glycogenic E74.02 [I43]
    corneal — *see* Edema, cornea
    eyelid — *see* Inflammation, eyelid
    glycogen, glycogenic — *see* Disease, glycogen storage
    heart, cardiac
        fatty — *see* Degeneration, myocardial
        glycogenic E74.02 [I43]
    inflammatory in vitreous H43.89
    kidney N28.89
    leukemic — *see* Leukemia
    liver K76.89
        fatty — *see* Fatty, liver NEC
        glycogen (see also Disease, glycogen storage)
            E74.03 [K77]
    lung R91.8
        eosinophilic J82

Infiltrate, infiltration — *continued*
    lymphatic (see also Leukemia, lymphatic) C91.9- ☑
        gland I88.9
    muscle, fatty M62.89
    myocardium, myocardial
        fatty — *see* Degeneration, myocardial
        glycogenic E74.02 [I43]
    on chest x-ray R91.8
    pulmonary R91.8
        with eosinophilia J82
    skin (lymphocytic) L98.6
    thymus (gland) (fatty) E32.8
    urine R39.0
    vesicant agent
        antineoplastic chemotherapy T80.810 ☑
        other agent NEC T80.818 ☑
    vitreous body H43.89
Infirmity R68.89
    senile R54
Inflammation, inflamed, inflammatory (with exudation)
    abducent (nerve) — *see* Strabismus, paralytic, sixth
        nerve
    accessory sinus (chronic) — *see* Sinusitis
    adrenal (gland) E27.8
    alveoli, teeth M27.3
        scorbutic E54
    anal canal, anus K62.89
    antrum (chronic) — *see* Sinusitis, maxillary
    appendix — *see* Appendicitis
    arachnoid — *see* Meningitis
    areola N61.0
        puerperal, postpartum or gestational — *see* Infection, nipple
    areolar tissue NOS L08.9
    artery — *see* Arteritis
    auditory meatus (external) — *see* Otitis, externa
    Bartholin's gland N75.8
    bile duct (common) (hepatic) or passage — *see* Cholangitis
    bladder — *see* Cystitis
    bone — *see* Osteomyelitis
    brain (see also Encephalitis)
        membrane — *see* Meningitis
    breast N61.0
        puerperal, postpartum, gestational — *see* Mastitis, obstetric
    broad ligament — *see* Disease, pelvis, inflammatory
    bronchi — *see* Bronchitis
    catarrhal J00
    cecum — *see* Appendicitis
    cerebral (see also Encephalitis)
        membrane — *see* Meningitis
    cerebrospinal
        meningococcal A39.0
    cervix (uteri) — *see* Cervicitis
    chest J98.8
    chorioretinal H30.9- ☑
        cyclitis — *see* Cyclitis
        disseminated H30.10- ☑
            generalized H30.13- ☑
            peripheral H30.12- ☑
            posterior pole H30.11- ☑
        epitheliopathy — *see* Epitheliopathy
        focal H30.00- ☑
            juxtapapillary H30.01- ☑
            macular H30.04- ☑
            paramacular — *see* Inflammation, chorioretinal, focal, macular
            peripheral H30.03- ☑
            posterior pole H30.02- ☑
        specified type NEC H30.89- ☑
    choroid — *see* Inflammation, chorioretinal
    chronic, postmastoidectomy cavity — *see* Complications, postmastoidectomy, inflammation
    colon — *see* Enteritis
    connective tissue (diffuse) NEC — *see* Disorder, soft tissue, specified type NEC
    cornea — *see* Keratitis
    corpora cavernosa N48.29
    cranial nerve — *see* Disorder, nerve, cranial
    Douglas' cul-de-sac or pouch (chronic) N73.0
    due to device, implant or graft (see also Complications, by site and type, infection or inflammation)
        arterial graft T82.7 ☑
        breast (implant) T85.79 ☑
        catheter T85.79 ☑

Inflammation, inflamed, inflammatory —
continued
due to device, implant or graft (*see also* Complications, by site and type, infection or inflammation) — *continued*
catheter — *continued*
dialysis (renal) T82.7 ☑
intraperitoneal T85.71 ☑
infusion T82.7 ☑
cranial T85.735 ☑
intrathecal T85.735 ☑
spinal (epidural) (subdural) T85.735 ☑
subarachnoid T85.735 ☑
urinary T83.518 ☑
cystostomy T83.510 ☑
Hopkins T83.518 ☑
ileostomy T83.518 ☑
nephrostomy T83.512 ☑
specified NEC T83.518 ☑
urethral indwelling T83.511 ☑
urostomy T83.518 ☑
electronic (electrode) (pulse generator) (stimulator)
bone T84.7 ☑
cardiac T82.7 ☑
nervous system T85.738 ☑
brain T85.731 ☑
cranial nerve T85.732 ☑
gastric nerve T85.732 ☑
neurostimulator generator T85.734 ☑
peripheral nerve T85.732 ☑
sacral nerve T85.732 ☑
spinal cord T85.733 ☑
vagal nerve T85.732 ☑
urinary T83.590 ☑
fixation, internal (orthopedic) NEC — *see* Complication, fixation device, infection
gastrointestinal (bile duct) (esophagus) T85.79 ☑
neurostimulator electrode (lead) T85.732 ☑
genital NEC T83.69 ☑
heart NEC T82.7 ☑
valve (prosthesis) T82.6 ☑
graft T82.7 ☑
joint prosthesis — *see* Complication, joint prosthesis, infection
ocular (corneal graft) (orbital implant) NEC T85.79 ☑
orthopedic NEC T84.7 ☑
penile (cylinder) (pump) (resevoir) T83.61 ☑
specified NEC T85.79 ☑
testicular T83.62 ☑
urinary NEC T83.598 ☑
ileal conduit stent T83.593 ☑
implanted neurostimulation T83.590 ☑
implanted sphincter T83.591 ☑
indwelling ureteral stent T83.592 ☑
nephroureteral stent T83.593 ☑
specified stent NEC T83.593 ☑
vascular NEC T82.7 ☑
ventricular intracranial (communicating) shunt T85.730 ☑
duodenum K29.80
with bleeding K29.81
dura mater — *see* Meningitis
ear (middle) (*see also* Otitis, media)
external — *see* Otitis, externa
inner — *see* subcategory H83.0 ☑
epididymis — *see* Epididymitis
esophagus K20.9
ethmoidal (sinus) (chronic) — *see* Sinusitis, ethmoidal
eustachian tube (catarrhal) — *see* Salpingitis, eustachian
eyelid H01.9
abscess — *see* Abscess, eyelid
blepharitis — *see* Blepharitis
chalazion — *see* Chalazion
dermatosis (noninfectious) — *see* Dermatosis, eyelid
hordeolum — *see* Hordeolum
specified NEC H01.8
fallopian tube — *see* Salpingo-oophoritis
fascia — *see* Myositis
follicular, pharynx J31.2
frontal (sinus) (chronic) — *see* Sinusitis, frontal
gallbladder — *see* Cholecystitis
gastric — *see* Gastritis
gastrointestinal — *see* Enteritis

Inflammation, inflamed, inflammatory —
continued
genital organ (internal) (diffuse)
female — *see* Disease, pelvis, inflammatory
male N49.9
multiple sites N49.8
specified NEC N49.8
gland (lymph) — *see* Lymphadenitis
glottis — *see* Laryngitis
granular, pharynx J31.2
gum K05.10
nonplaque induced K05.11
plaque induced K05.10
heart — *see* Carditis
hepatic duct — *see* Cholangitis
ileoanal (internal) pouch K91.850
ileum (*see also* Enteritis)
regional or terminal — *see* Enteritis, regional
intestinal pouch K91.850
intestine (any part) — *see* Enteritis
jaw (acute) (bone) (chronic) (lower) (suppurative) (upper) M27.2
joint NEC — *see* Arthritis
sacroiliac M46.1
kidney — *see* Nephritis
knee (joint) M13.169
tuberculous A18.02
labium (majus) (minus) — *see* Vulvitis
lacrimal
gland — *see* Dacryoadenitis
passages (duct) (sac) (*see also* Dacryocystitis)
canaliculitis — *see* Canaliculitis, lacrimal
larynx — *see* Laryngitis
leg NOS L08.9
lip K13.0
liver (capsule) (*see also* Hepatitis)
chronic K73.9
suppurative K75.0
lung (acute) (*see also* Pneumonia)
chronic J98.4
lymph gland or node — *see* Lymphadenitis
lymphatic vessel — *see* Lymphangitis
maxilla, maxillary M27.2
sinus (chronic) — *see* Sinusitis, maxillary
membranes of brain or spinal cord — *see* Meningitis
meninges — *see* Meningitis
mouth K12.1
muscle — *see* Myositis
myocardium — *see* Myocarditis
nasal sinus (chronic) — *see* Sinusitis
nasopharynx — *see* Nasopharyngitis
navel L08.82
nerve NEC — *see* Neuralgia
nipple N61.0
puerperal, postpartum or gestational — *see* Infection, nipple
nose — *see* Rhinitis
oculomotor (nerve) — *see* Strabismus, paralytic, third nerve
optic nerve — *see* Neuritis, optic
orbit (chronic) H05.10
acute H05.00
abscess — *see* Abscess, orbit
cellulitis — *see* Cellulitis, orbit
osteomyelitis — *see* Osteomyelitis, orbit
periostitis — *see* Periostitis, orbital
tenonitis — *see* Tenonitis, eye
granuloma — *see* Granuloma, orbit
myositis — *see* Myositis, orbital
ovary — *see* Salpingo-oophoritis
oviduct — *see* Salpingo-oophoritis
pancreas (acute) — *see* Pancreatitis
parametrium N73.0
parotid region L08.9
pelvis, female — *see* Disease, pelvis, inflammatory
penis (corpora cavernosa) N48.29
perianal K62.89
pericardium — *see* Pericarditis
perineum (female) (male) L08.9
perirectal K62.89
peritoneum — *see* Peritonitis
periuterine — *see* Disease, pelvis, inflammatory
perivesical — *see* Cystitis
petrous bone (acute) (chronic) — *see* Petrositis
pharynx (acute) — *see* Pharyngitis
pia mater — *see* Meningitis
pleura — *see* Pleurisy

Inflammation, inflamed, inflammatory —
continued
polyp, colon (*see also* Polyp, colon, inflammatory) K51.40
prostate (*see also* Prostatitis)
specified type NEC N41.8
rectosigmoid — *see* Rectosigmoiditis
rectum (*see also* Proctitis) K62.89
respiratory, upper (*see also* Infection, respiratory, upper) J06.9
acute, due to radiation J70.0
chronic, due to external agent — *see* condition, respiratory, chronic, due to
due to
chemicals, gases, fumes or vapors (inhalation) J68.2
radiation J70.1
retina — *see* Chorioretinitis
retrocecal — *see* Appendicitis
retroperitoneal — *see* Peritonitis
salivary duct or gland (any) (suppurative) — *see* Sialoadenitis
scorbutic, alveoli, teeth E54
scrotum N49.2
seminal vesicle — *see* Vesiculitis
sigmoid — *see* Enteritis
sinus — *see* Sinusitis
Skene's duct or gland — *see* Urethritis
skin L08.9
spermatic cord N49.1
sphenoidal (sinus) — *see* Sinusitis, sphenoidal
spinal
cord — *see* Encephalitis
membrane — *see* Meningitis
nerve — *see* Disorder, nerve
spine — *see* Spondylopathy, inflammatory
spleen (capsule) D73.89
stomach — *see* Gastritis
subcutaneous tissue L08.9
suprarenal (gland) E27.8
synovial — *see* Tenosynovitis
tendon (sheath) NEC — *see* Tenosynovitis
testis — *see* Orchitis
throat (acute) — *see* Pharyngitis
thymus (gland) E32.8
thyroid (gland) — *see* Thyroiditis
tongue K14.0
tonsil — *see* Tonsillitis
trachea — *see* Tracheitis
trochlear (nerve) — *see* Strabismus, paralytic, fourth nerve
tubal — *see* Salpingo-oophoritis
tuberculous NEC — *see* Tuberculosis
tubo-ovarian — *see* Salpingo-oophoritis
tunica vaginalis N49.1
tympanic membrane — *see* Tympanitis
umbilicus, umbilical L08.82
uterine ligament — *see* Disease, pelvis, inflammatory
uterus (catarrhal) — *see* Endometritis
uveal tract (anterior) NOS (*see also* Iridocyclitis)
posterior — *see* Chorioretinitis
vagina — *see* Vaginitis
vas deferens N49.1
vein (*see also* Phlebitis)
intracranial or intraspinal (septic) G08
thrombotic I80.9
leg — *see* Phlebitis, leg
lower extremity — *see* Phlebitis, leg
vocal cord J38.3
vulva — *see* Vulvitis
Wharton's duct (suppurative) — *see* Sialoadenitis
Inflation, lung, imperfect (newborn) — *see* Atelectasis
Influenza (bronchial) (epidemic) (respiratory (upper)) (unidentified influenza virus) J11.1
with
digestive manifestations J11.2
encephalopathy J11.81
enteritis J11.2
gastroenteritis J11.2
gastrointestinal manifestations J11.2
laryngitis J11.1
myocarditis J11.82
otitis media J11.83
pharyngitis J11.1
pneumonia J11.00
specified type J11.08
respiratory manifestations NEC J11.1

Influenza — *continued*
  with — *continued*
    specified manifestation NEC J11.89
  A/H5N1 (*see also* Influenza, due to, identified novel influenza A virus) J09.X2
  avian (*see also* Influenza, due to, identified novel influenza A virus) J09.X2
  bird (*see also* Influenza, due to, identified novel influenza A virus) J09.X2
  due to
    avian (*see also* Influenza, due to, identified novel influenza A virus) J09.X2
    identified influenza virus NEC J10.1
      with
        digestive manifestations J10.2
        encephalopathy J10.81
        enteritis J10.2
        gastroenteritis J10.2
        gastrointestinal manifestations J10.2
        laryngitis J10.1
        myocarditis J10.82
        otitis media J10.83
        pharyngitis J10.1
        pneumonia (unspecified type) J10.00
          with same identified influenza virus J10.01
          specified type NEC J10.08
        respiratory manifestations NEC J10.1
        specified manifestation NEC J10.89
    identified novel influenza A virus J09.X2
      with
        digestive manifestations J09.X3
        encephalopathy J09.X9
        enteritis J09.X3
        gastroenteritis J09.X3
        gastrointestinal manifestations J09.X3
        laryngitis J09.X2
        myocarditis J09.X9
        otitis media J09.X9
        pharyngitis J09.X2
        pneumonia J09.X1
        respiratory manifestations NEC J09.X2
        specified manifestation NEC J09.X9
        upper respiratory symptoms J09.X2
    novel (2009) H1N1 influenza (*see also* Influenza, due to, identified influenza virus NEC) J10.1
    novel influenza A/H1N1 (*see also* Influenza, due to, identified influenza virus NEC) J10.1
    of other animal origin, not bird or swine (*see also* Influenza, due to, identified novel influenza A virus) J09.X2
    swine (viruses that normally cause infections in pigs) (*see also* Influenza, due to, identified novel influenza A virus) J09.X2
Influenzal — *see* Influenza
Influenza-like disease — *see* Influenza
Infraction, Freiberg's (metatarsal head) — *see* Osteochondrosis, juvenile, metatarsus
Infraeruption of tooth (teeth) M26.34
Infusion complication, misadventure, or reaction — *see* Complications, infusion
Ingestion
  chemical — *see* Table of Drugs and Chemicals, by substance, poisoning
  drug or medicament
    correct substance properly administered — *see* Table of Drugs and Chemicals, by drug, adverse effect
    overdose or wrong substance given or taken — *see* Table of Drugs and Chemicals, by drug, poisoning
  foreign body — *see* Foreign body, alimentary tract
  tularemia A21.3
Ingrowing
  hair (beard) L73.1
  nail (finger) (toe) L60.0
Inguinal (*see also* condition)
  testicle Q53.9
    bilateral Q53.212
    unilateral Q53.112
Inhalant-induced
  anxiety disorder F18.980
  depressive disorder F18.94
  major neurocognitive disorder F18.97
  mild neurocognitive disorder F18.988
  psychotic disorder F18.959
Inhalation
  anthrax A22.1

Inhalation — *continued*
  flame T27.3 ☑
  food or foreign body — *see* Foreign body, by site
  gases, fumes, or vapors NEC T59.9-
    specified agent — *see* Table of Drugs and Chemicals, by substance
  liquid or vomitus — *see* Asphyxia
  meconium (newborn) P24.00
    with
      with respiratory symptoms P24.01
      pneumonia (pneumonitis) P24.01
  mucus — *see* Asphyxia, mucus
  oil or gasoline (causing suffocation) — *see* Foreign body, by site
  smoke J70.5
    due to chemicals, gases, fumes and vapors J68.9
  steam — *see* Toxicity, vapors
  stomach contents or secretions — *see* Foreign body, by site
    due to anesthesia (general) (local) or other sedation T88.59 ☑
      in labor and delivery O74.0
      in pregnancy O29.01- ☑
      postpartum, puerperal O89.01
Inhibition, orgasm
  female F52.31
  male F52.32
Inhibitor, systemic lupus erythematosus (presence of) D68.62
Iniencephalus, iniencephaly Q00.2
Injection, traumatic jet (air) (industrial) (water) (paint or dye) T70.4 ☑
Injury (*see also* specified injury type) T14.90 ☑
  abdomen, abdominal S39.91 ☑
    blood vessel — *see* Injury, blood vessel, abdomen
    cavity — *see* Injury, intra-abdominal
    contusion S30.1 ☑
    internal — *see* Injury, intra-abdominal
    intra-abdominal organ — *see* Injury, intra-abdominal
    nerve — *see* Injury, nerve, abdomen
    open — *see* Wound, open, abdomen
    specified NEC S39.81 ☑
    superficial — *see* Injury, superficial, abdomen
  Achilles tendon S86.00- ☑
    laceration S86.02- ☑
    specified type NEC S86.09- ☑
    strain S86.01- ☑
  acoustic, resulting in deafness — *see* Injury, nerve, acoustic
  adrenal (gland) S37.819 ☑
    contusion S37.812 ☑
    laceration S37.813 ☑
    specified type NEC S37.818 ☑
  alveolar (process) S09.93 ☑
  ankle S99.91- ☑
    contusion — *see* Contusion, ankle
    dislocation — *see* Dislocation, ankle
    fracture — *see* Fracture, ankle
    nerve — *see* Injury, nerve, ankle
    open — *see* Wound, open, ankle
    specified type NEC S99.81- ☑
    sprain — *see* Sprain, ankle
    superficial — *see* Injury, superficial, ankle
  anterior chamber, eye — *see* Injury, eye, specified site NEC
  anus — *see* Injury, abdomen
  aorta (thoracic) S25.00 ☑
    abdominal S35.00 ☑
      laceration (minor) (superficial) S35.01 ☑
        major S35.02 ☑
      specified type NEC S35.09 ☑
    laceration (minor) (superficial) S25.01 ☑
      major S25.02 ☑
    specified type NEC S25.09 ☑
  arm (upper) S49.9- ☑
    blood vessel — *see* Injury, blood vessel, arm
    contusion — *see* Contusion, arm, upper
    fracture — *see* Fracture, humerus
    lower — *see* Injury, forearm
    muscle — *see* Injury, muscle, shoulder
    nerve — *see* Injury, nerve, arm
    open — *see* Wound, open, arm
    specified type NEC S49.8- ☑
    superficial — *see* Injury, superficial, arm

Injury — *continued*
  artery (complicating trauma) (*see also* Injury, blood vessel, by site)
    cerebral or meningeal — *see* Injury, intracranial
  auditory canal (external) (meatus) S09.91 ☑
  auricle, auris, ear S09.91 ☑
  axilla — *see* Injury, shoulder
  back — *see* Injury, back, lower
  bile duct S36.13 ☑
  birth (*see also* Birth, injury) P15.9
  bladder (sphincter) S37.20 ☑
    at delivery O71.5
    contusion S37.22 ☑
    laceration S37.23 ☑
    obstetrical trauma O71.5
    specified type NEC S37.29 ☑
  blast (air) (hydraulic) (immersion) (underwater) NEC T14.8 ☑
    acoustic nerve trauma — *see* Injury, nerve, acoustic
    bladder — *see* Injury, bladder
    brain — *see* Concussion
    colon — *see* Injury, intestine, large
    ear (primary) S09.31- ☑
      secondary S09.39- ☑
    generalized T70.8 ☑
    lung — *see* Injury, intrathoracic, lung
    multiple body organs T70.8 ☑
    peritoneum S36.81 ☑
    rectum S36.61 ☑
    retroperitoneum S36.898 ☑
    small intestine S36.419 ☑
      duodenum S36.410 ☑
      specified site NEC S36.418 ☑
    specified
      intra-abdominal organ NEC S36.898 ☑
      pelvic organ NEC S37.899 ☑
  blood vessel NEC T14.8 ☑
    abdomen S35.9 ☑
      aorta — *see* Injury, aorta, abdominal
      celiac artery — *see* Injury, blood vessel, celiac artery
      iliac vessel — *see* Injury, blood vessel, iliac
      laceration S35.91 ☑
      mesenteric vessel — *see* Injury, mesenteric
      portal vein — *see* Injury, blood vessel, portal vein
      renal vessel — *see* Injury, blood vessel, renal
      specified vessel NEC S35.8X- ☑
      splenic vessel — *see* Injury, blood vessel, splenic
      vena cava — *see* Injury, vena cava, inferior
    ankle — *see* Injury, blood vessel, foot
    aorta (abdominal) (thoracic) — *see* Injury, aorta
    arm (upper) NEC S45.90- ☑
      forearm — *see* Injury, blood vessel, forearm
      laceration S45.91- ☑
      specified
        site NEC S45.80- ☑
          laceration S45.81- ☑
          specified type NEC S45.89- ☑
        type NEC S45.99- ☑
      superficial vein S45.30- ☑
        laceration S45.31- ☑
        specified type NEC S45.39- ☑
    axillary
      artery S45.00- ☑
        laceration S45.01- ☑
        specified type NEC S45.09- ☑
      vein S45.20- ☑
        laceration S45.21- ☑
        specified type NEC S45.29- ☑
    azygos vein — *see* Injury, blood vessel, thoracic, specified site NEC
    brachial
      artery S45.10- ☑
        laceration S45.11- ☑
        specified type NEC S45.19- ☑
      vein S45.20- ☑
        laceration S45.219 ☑
        specified type NEC S45.29- ☑
    carotid artery (common) (external) (internal, extracranial) S15.00- ☑
      internal, intracranial S06.8- ☑
        laceration (minor) (superficial) S15.01- ☑
          major S15.02- ☑
        specified type NEC S15.09- ☑

Injury — *continued*
　blood vessel — *continued*
　　celiac artery S35.219 ☑
　　　branch S35.299 ☑
　　　　laceration (minor) (superficial) S35.291 ☑
　　　　　major S35.292 ☑
　　　　specified NEC S35.298 ☑
　　　laceration (minor) (superficial) S35.211 ☑
　　　　major S35.212 ☑
　　　specified type NEC S35.218 ☑
　　cerebral — *see* Injury, intracranial
　　deep plantar — *see* Injury, blood vessel, plantar
　　　artery
　　digital (hand) — *see* Injury, blood vessel, finger
　　dorsal
　　　artery (foot) S95.00- ☑
　　　　laceration S95.01- ☑
　　　　specified type NEC S95.09- ☑
　　　vein (foot) S95.20- ☑
　　　　laceration S95.21- ☑
　　　　specified type NEC S95.29- ☑
　　due to accidental laceration during procedure —
　　　see Laceration, accidental complicating
　　　surgery
　　extremity — *see* Injury, blood vessel, limb
　　femoral
　　　artery (common) (superficial) S75.00- ☑
　　　　laceration (minor) (superficial) S75.01- ☑
　　　　　major S75.02- ☑
　　　　specified type NEC S75.09- ☑
　　　vein (hip level) (thigh level) S75.10- ☑
　　　　laceration (minor) (superficial) S75.11- ☑
　　　　　major S75.12- ☑
　　　　specified type NEC S75.19- ☑
　　finger S65.50- ☑
　　　index S65.50- ☑
　　　　laceration S65.51- ☑
　　　　specified type NEC S65.59- ☑
　　　laceration S65.51- ☑
　　　little S65.50- ☑
　　　　laceration S65.51- ☑
　　　　specified type NEC S65.59- ☑
　　　middle S65.50- ☑
　　　　laceration S65.51- ☑
　　　　specified type NEC S65.59- ☑
　　　specified type NEC S65.59- ☑
　　　thumb — *see* Injury, blood vessel, thumb
　　foot S95.90- ☑
　　　dorsal
　　　　artery — *see* Injury, blood vessel, dorsal,
　　　　　artery
　　　　vein — *see* Injury, blood vessel, dorsal, vein
　　　laceration S95.91- ☑
　　　plantar artery — *see* Injury, blood vessel, plan-
　　　　tar artery
　　　specified
　　　　site NEC S95.80- ☑
　　　　　laceration S95.81- ☑
　　　　　specified type NEC S95.89- ☑
　　　　specified type NEC S95.99- ☑
　　forearm S55.90- ☑
　　　laceration S55.91- ☑
　　　radial artery — *see* Injury, blood vessel, radial
　　　　artery
　　　specified
　　　　site NEC S55.80- ☑
　　　　　laceration S55.81- ☑
　　　　　specified type NEC S55.89- ☑
　　　　type NEC S55.99- ☑
　　　ulnar artery — *see* Injury, blood vessel, ulnar
　　　　artery
　　　vein S55.20- ☑
　　　　laceration S55.21- ☑
　　　　specified type NEC S55.29- ☑
　　gastric
　　　artery — *see* Injury, mesenteric, artery, branch
　　　vein — *see* Injury, blood vessel, abdomen
　　gastroduodenal artery — *see* Injury, mesenteric,
　　　artery, branch
　　greater saphenous vein (lower leg level) S85.30- ☑
　　　hip (and thigh) level S75.20- ☑
　　　　laceration (minor) (superficial) S75.21- ☑
　　　　　major S75.22- ☑
　　　　specified type NEC S75.29- ☑
　　　laceration S85.31- ☑
　　　specified type NEC S85.39- ☑

Injury — *continued*
　blood vessel — *continued*
　　hand (level) S65.90- ☑
　　　finger — *see* Injury, blood vessel, finger
　　　laceration S65.91- ☑
　　　palmar arch — *see* Injury, blood vessel, palmar
　　　　arch
　　　radial artery — *see* Injury, blood vessel, radial
　　　　artery, hand
　　　specified
　　　　site NEC S65.80- ☑
　　　　　laceration S65.81- ☑
　　　　　specified type NEC S65.89- ☑
　　　　type NEC S65.99- ☑
　　　thumb — *see* Injury, blood vessel, thumb
　　　ulnar artery — *see* Injury, blood vessel, ulnar
　　　　artery, hand
　　head S09.0 ☑
　　　intracranial — *see* Injury, intracranial
　　　multiple S09.0 ☑
　　hepatic
　　　artery — *see* Injury, mesenteric, artery
　　　vein — *see* Injury, vena cava, inferior
　　hip S75.90- ☑
　　　femoral artery — *see* Injury, blood vessel,
　　　　femoral, artery
　　　femoral vein — *see* Injury, blood vessel,
　　　　femoral, vein
　　　greater saphenous vein — *see* Injury, blood
　　　　vessel, greater saphenous, hip level
　　　laceration S75.91- ☑
　　　specified
　　　　site NEC S75.80- ☑
　　　　　laceration S75.81- ☑
　　　　　specified type NEC S75.89- ☑
　　　　type NEC S75.99- ☑
　　hypogastric (artery) (vein) — *see* Injury, blood
　　　vessel, iliac
　　iliac S35.5- ☑
　　　artery S35.51- ☑
　　　specified vessel NEC S35.5- ☑
　　　uterine vessel — *see* Injury, blood vessel, uter-
　　　　ine
　　　vein S35.51- ☑
　　innominate — *see* Injury, blood vessel, thoracic,
　　　innominate
　　intercostal (artery) (vein) — *see* Injury, blood vessel,
　　　thoracic, intercostal
　　jugular vein (external) S15.20- ☑
　　　internal S15.30- ☑
　　　　laceration (minor) (superficial) S15.31- ☑
　　　　　major S15.32- ☑
　　　　specified type NEC S15.39- ☑
　　　laceration (minor) (superficial) S15.21- ☑
　　　　major S15.22- ☑
　　　specified type NEC S15.29- ☑
　　leg (level) (lower) S85.90- ☑
　　　greater saphenous — *see* Injury, blood vessel,
　　　　greater saphenous
　　　laceration S85.91- ☑
　　　lesser saphenous — *see* Injury, blood vessel,
　　　　lesser saphenous
　　　peroneal artery — *see* Injury, blood vessel,
　　　　peroneal artery
　　　popliteal
　　　　artery — *see* Injury, blood vessel, popliteal,
　　　　　artery
　　　　vein — *see* Injury, blood vessel, popliteal,
　　　　　vein
　　　specified
　　　　site NEC S85.80- ☑
　　　　　laceration S85.81- ☑
　　　　　specified type NEC S85.89- ☑
　　　　type NEC S85.99- ☑
　　　thigh — *see* Injury, blood vessel, hip
　　　tibial artery — *see* Injury, blood vessel, tibial
　　　　artery
　　lesser saphenous vein (lower leg level) S85.40- ☑
　　　laceration S85.41- ☑
　　　specified type NEC S85.49- ☑
　　limb
　　　lower — *see* Injury, blood vessel, leg
　　　upper — *see* Injury, blood vessel, arm
　　lower back — *see* Injury, blood vessel, abdomen
　　　specified NEC — *see* Injury, blood vessel, ab-
　　　　domen, specified, site NEC

Injury — *continued*
　blood vessel — *continued*
　　mammary (artery) (vein) — *see* Injury, blood vessel,
　　　thoracic, specified site NEC
　　mesenteric (inferior) (superior)
　　　artery — *see* Injury, mesenteric, artery
　　　vein — *see* Injury, blood vessel, mesenteric,
　　　　vein
　　neck S15.9 ☑
　　　specified site NEC S15.8 ☑
　　ovarian (artery) (vein) — *see* subcategory S35.8 ☑
　　palmar arch (superficial) S65.20- ☑
　　　deep S65.30- ☑
　　　　laceration S65.31- ☑
　　　　specified type NEC S65.39- ☑
　　　laceration S65.21- ☑
　　　specified type NEC S65.29- ☑
　　pelvis — *see* Injury, blood vessel, abdomen
　　　specified NEC — *see* Injury, blood vessel, ab-
　　　　domen, specified, site NEC
　　peroneal artery S85.20- ☑
　　　laceration S85.21- ☑
　　　specified type NEC S85.29- ☑
　　plantar artery (deep) (foot) S95.10- ☑
　　　laceration S95.11- ☑
　　　specified type NEC S95.19- ☑
　　popliteal
　　　artery S85.00- ☑
　　　　laceration S85.01- ☑
　　　　specified type NEC S85.09- ☑
　　　vein S85.50- ☑
　　　　laceration S85.51- ☑
　　　　specified type NEC S85.59- ☑
　　portal vein S35.319 ☑
　　　laceration S35.311 ☑
　　　specified type NEC S35.318 ☑
　　precerebral — *see* Injury, blood vessel, neck
　　pulmonary (artery) (vein) — *see* Injury, blood ves-
　　　sel, thoracic, pulmonary
　　radial artery (forearm level) S55.10- ☑
　　　hand and wrist (level) S65.10- ☑
　　　　laceration S65.11- ☑
　　　　specified type NEC S65.19- ☑
　　　laceration S55.11- ☑
　　　specified type NEC S55.19- ☑
　　renal
　　　artery S35.40- ☑
　　　　laceration S35.41- ☑
　　　　specified NEC S35.49- ☑
　　　vein S35.40- ☑
　　　　laceration S35.41- ☑
　　　　specified NEC S35.49- ☑
　　saphenous vein (greater) (lower leg level) — *see*
　　　Injury, blood vessel, greater saphenous
　　　hip and thigh level — *see* Injury, blood vessel,
　　　　greater saphenous, hip level
　　　lesser — *see* Injury, blood vessel, lesser saphe-
　　　　nous
　　shoulder
　　　specified NEC — *see* Injury, blood vessel, arm,
　　　　specified site NEC
　　　superficial vein — *see* Injury, blood vessel, arm,
　　　　superficial vein
　　specified NEC T14.8 ☑
　　splenic
　　　artery — *see* Injury, blood vessel, celiac artery,
　　　　branch
　　　vein S35.329 ☑
　　　　laceration S35.321 ☑
　　　　specified NEC S35.328 ☑
　　subclavian — *see* Injury, blood vessel, thoracic, in-
　　　nominate
　　thigh — *see* Injury, blood vessel, hip
　　thoracic S25.90 ☑
　　　aorta S25.00 ☑
　　　　laceration (minor) (superficial) S25.01 ☑
　　　　　major S25.02 ☑
　　　　specified type NEC S25.09 ☑
　　　azygos vein — *see* Injury, blood vessel, thoracic,
　　　　specified, site NEC
　　　innominate
　　　　artery S25.10- ☑
　　　　　laceration (minor) (superficial)
　　　　　　S25.11- ☑
　　　　　　major S25.12- ☑
　　　　　specified type NEC S25.19- ☑

Injury — *continued*
- blood vessel — *continued*
  - thoracic — *continued*
    - innominate — *continued*
      - vein S25.30- ☑
        - laceration (minor) (superficial) S25.31- ☑
          - major S25.32- ☑
        - specified type NEC S25.39- ☑
    - intercostal S25.50- ☑
      - laceration S25.51- ☑
      - specified type NEC S25.59- ☑
    - laceration S25.91 ☑
    - mammary vessel — *see* Injury, blood vessel, thoracic, specified, site NEC
    - pulmonary S25.40- ☑
      - laceration (minor) (superficial) S25.41- ☑
        - major S25.42- ☑
      - specified type NEC S25.49- ☑
    - specified
      - site NEC S25.80- ☑
        - laceration S25.81 ☑
        - specified type NEC S25.89 ☑
      - type NEC S25.99 ☑
    - subclavian — *see* Injury, blood vessel, thoracic, innominate
    - vena cava (superior) S25.20 ☑
      - laceration (minor) (superficial) S25.21 ☑
        - major S25.22 ☑
      - specified type NEC S25.29 ☑
  - thumb S65.40- ☑
    - laceration S65.41- ☑
    - specified type NEC S65.49- ☑
  - tibial artery S85.10- ☑
    - anterior S85.13- ☑
      - laceration S85.14- ☑
      - specified injury NEC S85.15- ☑
    - laceration S85.11- ☑
    - posterior S85.16- ☑
      - laceration S85.17- ☑
      - specified injury NEC S85.18- ☑
    - specified injury NEC S85.12- ☑
  - ulnar artery (forearm level) S55.00- ☑
    - hand and wrist (level) S65.00- ☑
      - laceration S65.01- ☑
      - specified type NEC S65.09- ☑
    - laceration S55.01- ☑
    - specified type NEC S55.09- ☑
  - upper arm (level) — *see* Injury, blood vessel, arm
    - superficial vein — *see* Injury, blood vessel, arm, superficial vein
  - uterine S35.5- ☑
    - artery S35.53- ☑
    - vein S35.53- ☑
  - vena cava — *see* Injury, vena cava
  - vertebral artery S15.10- ☑
    - laceration (minor) (superficial) S15.11- ☑
      - major S15.12- ☑
    - specified type NEC S15.19- ☑
  - wrist (level) — *see* Injury, blood vessel, hand
- brachial plexus S14.3 ☑
  - newborn P14.3
- brain (traumatic) S06.9- ☑
  - diffuse (axonal) S06.2X- ☑
  - focal S06.30- ☑
- brainstem S06.38- ☑
- breast NOS S29.9 ☑
- broad ligament — *see* Injury, pelvic organ, specified site NEC
- bronchus, bronchi — *see* Injury, intrathoracic, bronchus
- brow S09.90 ☑
- buttock S39.92 ☑
- canthus, eye S05.90 ☑
- cardiac plexus — *see* Injury, nerve, thorax, sympathetic
- cauda equina S34.3 ☑
- cavernous sinus — *see* Injury, intracranial
- cecum — *see* Injury, colon
- celiac ganglion or plexus — *see* Injury, nerve, lumbosacral, sympathetic
- cerebellum — *see* Injury, intracranial
- cerebral — *see* Injury, intracranial
- cervix (uteri) — *see* Injury, uterus
- cheek (wall) S09.93 ☑
- chest — *see* Injury, thorax

Injury — *continued*
- childbirth (newborn) (*see also* Birth, injury)
  - maternal NEC O71.9
- chin S09.93 ☑
- choroid (eye) — *see* Injury, eye, specified site NEC
- clitoris S39.94 ☑
- coccyx (*see also* Injury, back, lower)
  - complicating delivery O71.6
- colon — *see* Injury, intestine, large
- common bile duct — *see* Injury, liver
- conjunctiva (superficial) — *see* Injury, eye, conjunctiva
- conus medullaris — *see* Injury, spinal, sacral
- cord
  - spermatic (pelvic region) S37.898 ☑
    - scrotal region S39.848 ☑
  - spinal — *see* Injury, spinal cord, by region
- cornea — *see* Injury, eye, specified site NEC
  - abrasion — *see* Injury, eye, cornea, abrasion
- cortex (cerebral) (*see also* Injury, intracranial)
  - visual — *see* Injury, nerve, optic
- costal region NEC S29.9 ☑
- costochondral NEC S29.9 ☑
- cranial
  - cavity — *see* Injury, intracranial
  - nerve — *see* Injury, nerve, cranial
- crushing — *see* Crush
- cutaneous sensory nerve
- cystic duct — *see* Injury, liver
- deep tissue — *see* Contusion, by site
  - meaning pressure ulcer — *see* Ulcer, pressure, unstageable, by site
- delivery (newborn) P15.9
  - maternal NEC O71.9
- Descemet's membrane — *see* Injury, eyeball, penetrating
- diaphragm — *see* Injury, intrathoracic, diaphragm
- duodenum — *see* Injury, intestine, small, duodenum
- ear (auricle) (external) (canal) S09.91 ☑
  - abrasion — *see* Abrasion, ear
  - bite — *see* Bite, ear
  - blister — *see* Blister, ear
  - bruise — *see* Contusion, ear
  - contusion — *see* Contusion, ear
  - external constriction — *see* Constriction, external, ear
  - hematoma — *see* Hematoma, ear
  - inner — *see* Injury, ear, middle
  - laceration — *see* Laceration, ear
  - middle S09.30- ☑
    - blast — *see* Injury, blast, ear
    - specified NEC S09.39- ☑
  - puncture — *see* Puncture, ear
  - superficial — *see* Injury, superficial, ear
- eighth cranial nerve (acoustic or auditory) — *see* Injury, nerve, acoustic
- elbow S59.90- ☑
  - contusion — *see* Contusion, elbow
  - dislocation — *see* Dislocation, elbow
  - fracture — *see* Fracture, ulna, upper end
  - open — *see* Wound, open, elbow
  - specified NEC S59.80- ☑
  - sprain — *see* Sprain, elbow
  - superficial — *see* Injury, superficial, elbow
- eleventh cranial nerve (accessory) — *see* Injury, nerve, accessory
- epididymis S39.94 ☑
- epigastric region S39.91 ☑
- epiglottis NEC S19.89 ☑
- esophageal plexus — *see* Injury, nerve, thorax, sympathetic
- esophagus (thoracic part) (*see also* Injury, intrathoracic, esophagus)
  - cervical NEC S19.85 ☑
- eustachian tube S09.30 ☑
- eye S05.9- ☑
  - avulsion S05.7- ☑
  - ball — *see* Injury, eyeball
  - conjunctiva S05.0- ☑
  - cornea
    - abrasion S05.0- ☑
  - laceration S05.3- ☑
    - with prolapse S05.2- ☑
  - lacrimal apparatus S05.8X- ☑
  - orbit penetration S05.4- ☑
  - specified site NEC S05.8X- ☑
- eyeball S05.8X- ☑

Injury — *continued*
- eyeball — *continued*
  - contusion S05.1- ☑
  - penetrating S05.6- ☑
    - with
      - foreign body S05.5- ☑
      - prolapse or loss of intraocular tissue S05.2- ☑
      - without prolapse or loss of intraocular tissue S05.3- ☑
    - specified type NEC S05.8- ☑
- eyebrow S09.93 ☑
- eyelid S09.93 ☑
  - abrasion — *see* Abrasion, eyelid
  - contusion — *see* Contusion, eyelid
  - open — *see* Wound, open, eyelid
- face S09.93 ☑
- fallopian tube S37.509 ☑
  - bilateral S37.502 ☑
    - blast injury S37.512 ☑
    - contusion S37.522 ☑
    - laceration S37.532 ☑
    - specified type NEC S37.592 ☑
  - blast injury (primary) S37.519 ☑
    - bilateral S37.512 ☑
    - secondary — *see* Injury, fallopian tube, specified type NEC
    - unilateral S37.511 ☑
  - contusion S37.529 ☑
    - bilateral S37.522 ☑
    - unilateral S37.521 ☑
  - laceration S37.539 ☑
    - bilateral S37.532 ☑
    - unilateral S37.531 ☑
  - specified type NEC S37.599 ☑
    - bilateral S37.592 ☑
    - unilateral S37.591 ☑
  - unilateral S37.501 ☑
    - blast injury S37.511 ☑
    - contusion S37.521 ☑
    - laceration S37.531 ☑
    - specified type NEC S37.591 ☑
- fascia — *see* Injury, muscle
- fifth cranial nerve (trigeminal) — *see* Injury, nerve, trigeminal
- finger (nail) S69.9- ☑
  - blood vessel — *see* Injury, blood vessel, finger
  - contusion — *see* Contusion, finger
  - dislocation — *see* Dislocation, finger
  - fracture — *see* Fracture, finger
  - muscle — *see* Injury, muscle, finger
  - nerve — *see* Injury, nerve, digital, finger
  - open — *see* Wound, open, finger
  - specified NEC S69.8- ☑
  - sprain — *see* Sprain, finger
  - superficial — *see* Injury, superficial, finger
- first cranial nerve (olfactory) — *see* Injury, nerve, olfactory
- flank — *see* Injury, abdomen
- foot S99.92- ☑
  - blood vessel — *see* Injury, blood vessel, foot
  - contusion — *see* Contusion, foot
  - dislocation — *see* Dislocation, foot
  - fracture — *see* Fracture, foot
  - muscle — *see* Injury, muscle, foot
  - open — *see* Wound, open, foot
  - specified type NEC S99.82- ☑
  - sprain — *see* Sprain, foot
  - superficial — *see* Injury, superficial, foot
- forceps NOS P15.9
- forearm S59.91- ☑
  - blood vessel — *see* Injury, blood vessel, forearm
  - contusion — *see* Contusion, forearm
  - fracture — *see* Fracture, forearm
  - muscle — *see* Injury, muscle, forearm
  - nerve — *see* Injury, nerve, forearm
  - open — *see* Wound, open, forearm
  - specified NEC S59.81- ☑
  - superficial — *see* Injury, superficial, forearm
- forehead S09.90 ☑
- fourth cranial nerve (trochlear) — *see* Injury, nerve, trochlear
- gallbladder S36.129 ☑
  - contusion S36.122 ☑
  - laceration S36.123 ☑
  - specified NEC S36.128 ☑

☑ **Additional Character Required** — Refer to the Tabular List for Character Selection   ▽ **Subterms under main terms may continue to next column or page**

Injury — continued
- ganglion
  - celiac, coeliac — see Injury, nerve, lumbosacral, sympathetic
  - gasserian — see Injury, nerve, trigeminal
  - stellate — see Injury, nerve, thorax, sympathetic
  - thoracic sympathetic — see Injury, nerve, thorax, sympathetic
- gasserian ganglion — see Injury, nerve, trigeminal
- gastric artery — see Injury, blood vessel, celiac artery, branch
- gastroduodenal artery — see Injury, blood vessel, celiac artery, branch
- gastrointestinal tract — see Injury, intra-abdominal
  - with open wound into abdominal cavity — see Wound, open, with penetration into peritoneal cavity
  - colon — see Injury, intestine, large
  - rectum — see Injury, intestine, large, rectum
    - with open wound into abdominal cavity S36.61 ☑
  - small intestine — see Injury, intestine, small
  - specified site NEC — see Injury, intra-abdominal, specified, site NEC
  - stomach — see Injury, stomach
- genital organ(s)
  - external S39.94 ☑
    - specified NEC S39.848 ☑
  - internal S37.90 ☑
    - fallopian tube — see Injury, fallopian tube
    - ovary — see Injury, ovary
    - prostate — see Injury, prostate
    - seminal vesicle — see Injury, pelvis, organ, specified site NEC
    - uterus — see Injury, uterus
    - vas deferens — see Injury, pelvis, organ, specified site NEC
  - obstetrical trauma O71.9
- gland
  - lacrimal laceration — see Injury, eye, specified site NEC
  - salivary S09.93 ☑
  - thyroid NEC S19.84 ☑
- globe (eye) S05.90 ☑
  - specified NEC S05.8X- ☑
- groin — see Injury, abdomen
- gum S09.90 ☑
- hand S69.9- ☑
  - blood vessel — see Injury, blood vessel, hand
  - contusion — see Contusion, hand
  - fracture — see Fracture, hand
  - muscle — see Injury, muscle, hand
  - nerve — see Injury, nerve, hand
  - open — see Wound, open, hand
  - specified NEC S69.8- ☑
  - sprain — see Sprain, hand
  - superficial — see Injury, superficial, hand
- head S09.90 ☑
  - with loss of consciousness S06.9- ☑
  - specified NEC S09.8 ☑
- heart S26.90 ☑
  - with hemopericardium S26.00 ☑
    - contusion S26.01 ☑
    - laceration (mild) S26.020 ☑
      - major S26.022 ☑
      - moderate S26.021 ☑
    - specified type NEC S26.09 ☑
  - without hemopericardium S26.10 ☑
    - contusion S26.11 ☑
    - laceration S26.12 ☑
    - specified type NEC S26.19 ☑
  - contusion S26.91 ☑
  - laceration S26.92 ☑
  - specified type NEC S26.99 ☑
- heel — see Injury, foot
- hepatic
  - artery — see Injury, blood vessel, celiac artery, branch
  - duct — see Injury, liver
  - vein — see Injury, vena cava, inferior
- hip S79.91- ☑
  - blood vessel — see Injury, blood vessel, hip
  - contusion — see Contusion, hip
  - dislocation — see Dislocation, hip
  - fracture — see Fracture, femur, neck
  - muscle — see Injury, muscle, hip

Injury — continued
- hip — continued
  - nerve — see Injury, nerve, hip
  - open — see Wound, open, hip
  - specified NEC S79.81- ☑
  - sprain — see Sprain, hip
  - superficial — see Injury, superficial, hip
- hymen S39.94 ☑
- hypogastric
  - blood vessel — see Injury, blood vessel, iliac
  - plexus — see Injury, nerve, lumbosacral, sympathetic
- ileum — see Injury, intestine, small
- iliac region S39.91 ☑
- instrumental (during surgery) — see Laceration, accidental complicating surgery
  - birth injury — see Birth, injury
  - nonsurgical — see Injury, by site
  - obstetrical O71.9
    - bladder O71.5
    - cervix O71.3
    - high vaginal O71.4
    - perineal NOS O70.9
    - urethra O71.5
    - uterus O71.5
      - with rupture or perforation O71.1
- internal T14.8 ☑
  - aorta — see Injury, aorta
  - bladder (sphincter) — see Injury, bladder
    - with
      - ectopic or molar pregnancy O08.6
      - following ectopic or molar pregnancy O08.6
      - obstetrical trauma O71.5
  - bronchus, bronchi — see Injury, intrathoracic, bronchus
  - cecum — see Injury, intestine, large
  - cervix (uteri) (see also Injury, uterus)
    - with ectopic or molar pregnancy O08.6
    - following ectopic or molar pregnancy O08.6
    - obstetrical trauma O71.3
  - chest — see Injury, intrathoracic
  - gastrointestinal tract — see Injury, intra-abdominal
  - heart — see Injury, heart
  - intestine NEC — see Injury, intestine
  - intrauterine — see Injury, uterus
  - mesentery — see Injury, intra-abdominal, specified, site NEC
  - pelvis, pelvic (organ) S37.90 ☑
    - following ectopic or molar pregnancy (subsequent episode) O08.6
    - obstetrical trauma NEC O71.5
      - rupture or perforation O71.1
    - specified NEC S39.83 ☑
  - rectum — see Injury, intestine, large, rectum
  - stomach — see Injury, stomach
  - ureter — see Injury, ureter
  - urethra (sphincter) following ectopic or molar pregnancy O08.6
  - uterus — see Injury, uterus
- interscapular area — see Injury, thorax
- intestine
  - large S36.509 ☑
    - ascending (right) S36.500 ☑
      - blast injury (primary) S36.510 ☑
        - secondary S36.590 ☑
      - contusion S36.520 ☑
      - laceration S36.530 ☑
      - specified type NEC S36.590 ☑
    - blast injury (primary) S36.519 ☑
      - ascending (right) S36.510 ☑
      - descending (left) S36.512 ☑
      - rectum S36.61 ☑
      - sigmoid S36.513 ☑
      - specified site NEC S36.518 ☑
      - transverse S36.511 ☑
    - contusion S36.529 ☑
      - ascending (right) S36.520 ☑
      - descending (left) S36.522 ☑
      - rectum S36.62 ☑
      - sigmoid S36.523 ☑
      - specified site NEC S36.528 ☑
      - transverse S36.521 ☑
    - descending (left) S36.502 ☑
      - blast injury (primary) S36.512 ☑
        - secondary S36.592 ☑
      - contusion S36.522 ☑
      - laceration S36.532 ☑

Injury — continued
- intestine — continued
  - large — continued
    - descending — continued
      - specified type NEC S36.592 ☑
    - laceration S36.539 ☑
      - ascending (right) S36.530 ☑
      - descending (left) S36.532 ☑
      - rectum S36.63 ☑
      - sigmoid S36.533 ☑
      - specified site NEC S36.538 ☑
      - transverse S36.531 ☑
    - rectum S36.60 ☑
      - blast injury (primary) S36.61 ☑
        - secondary S36.69 ☑
      - contusion S36.62 ☑
      - laceration S36.63 ☑
      - specified type NEC S36.69 ☑
    - sigmoid S36.503 ☑
      - blast injury (primary) S36.513 ☑
        - secondary S36.593 ☑
      - contusion S36.523 ☑
      - laceration S36.533 ☑
      - specified type NEC S36.593 ☑
    - specified
      - site NEC S36.508 ☑
        - blast injury (primary) S36.518 ☑
          - secondary S36.598 ☑
        - contusion S36.528 ☑
        - laceration S36.538 ☑
        - specified type NEC S36.598 ☑
      - type NEC S36.599 ☑
        - ascending (right) S36.590 ☑
        - descending (left) S36.592 ☑
        - rectum S36.69 ☑
        - sigmoid S36.593 ☑
        - specified site NEC S36.598 ☑
        - transverse S36.591 ☑
    - transverse S36.501 ☑
      - blast injury (primary) S36.511 ☑
        - secondary S36.591 ☑
      - contusion S36.521 ☑
      - laceration S36.531 ☑
      - specified type NEC S36.591 ☑
  - small S36.409 ☑
    - blast injury (primary) S36.419 ☑
      - duodenum S36.410 ☑
      - secondary S36.499 ☑
        - duodenum S36.490 ☑
        - specified site NEC S36.498 ☑
      - specified site NEC S36.418 ☑
    - contusion S36.429 ☑
      - duodenum S36.420 ☑
      - specified site NEC S36.428 ☑
    - duodenum S36.400 ☑
      - blast injury (primary) S36.410 ☑
        - secondary S36.490 ☑
      - contusion S36.420 ☑
      - laceration S36.430 ☑
      - specified NEC S36.490 ☑
    - laceration S36.439 ☑
      - duodenum S36.430 ☑
      - specified site NEC S36.438 ☑
    - specified
      - site NEC S36.408 ☑
      - type NEC S36.499 ☑
        - duodenum S36.490 ☑
        - specified site NEC S36.498 ☑
- intra-abdominal S36.90 ☑
  - adrenal gland — see Injury, adrenal gland
  - bladder — see Injury, bladder
  - colon — see Injury, intestine, large
  - contusion S36.92 ☑
  - fallopian tube — see Injury, fallopian tube
  - gallbladder — see Injury, gallbladder
  - intestine — see Injury, intestine
  - kidney — see Injury, kidney
  - laceration S36.93 ☑
  - liver — see Injury, liver
  - ovary — see Injury, ovary
  - pancreas — see Injury, pancreas
  - pelvic NOS S37.90 ☑
  - peritoneum — see Injury, intra-abdominal, specified, site NEC
  - prostate — see Injury, prostate
  - rectum — see Injury, intestine, large, rectum

Injury — *continued*
- intra-abdominal — *continued*
  - retroperitoneum — *see* Injury, intra-abdominal, specified, site NEC
  - seminal vesicle — *see* Injury, pelvis, organ, specified site NEC
  - small intestine — *see* Injury, intestine, small
  - specified
    - pelvic S37.90 ☑
      - specified
        - site NEC S37.899 ☑
          - specified type NEC S37.898 ☑
        - type NEC S37.99 ☑
    - site NEC S36.899 ☑
      - contusion S36.892 ☑
      - laceration S36.893 ☑
      - specified type NEC S36.898 ☑
    - type NEC S36.99 ☑
  - spleen — *see* Injury, spleen
  - stomach — *see* Injury, stomach
  - ureter — *see* Injury, ureter
  - urethra — *see* Injury, urethra
  - uterus — *see* Injury, uterus
  - vas deferens — *see* Injury, pelvis, organ, specified site NEC
- intracranial (traumatic) S06.9- ☑
  - cerebellar hemorrhage, traumatic — *see* Injury, intracranial, focal
  - cerebral edema, traumatic S06.1X- ☑
    - diffuse S06.1X- ☑
    - focal S06.1X- ☑
  - diffuse (axonal) S06.2X- ☑
  - epidural hemorrhage (traumatic) S06.4X- ☑
  - focal brain injury S06.30- ☑
    - contusion — *see* Contusion, cerebral
    - laceration — *see* Laceration, cerebral
    - intracerebral hemorrhage, traumatic S06.36- ☑
      - left side S06.35- ☑
      - right side S06.34- ☑
  - subarachnoid hemorrhage, traumatic S06.6X- ☑
  - subdural hemorrhage, traumatic S06.5X- ☑
- intraocular — *see* Injury, eyeball, penetrating
- intrathoracic S27.9 ☑
  - bronchus S27.409 ☑
    - bilateral S27.402 ☑
    - blast injury (primary) S27.419 ☑
      - bilateral S27.412 ☑
      - secondary — *see* Injury, intrathoracic, bronchus, specified type NEC
      - unilateral S27.411 ☑
    - contusion S27.429 ☑
      - bilateral S27.422 ☑
      - unilateral S27.421 ☑
    - laceration S27.439 ☑
      - bilateral S27.432 ☑
      - unilateral S27.431 ☑
    - specified type NEC S27.499 ☑
      - bilateral S27.492 ☑
      - unilateral S27.491 ☑
    - unilateral S27.401 ☑
  - diaphragm S27.809 ☑
    - contusion S27.802 ☑
    - laceration S27.803 ☑
    - specified type NEC S27.808 ☑
  - esophagus (thoracic) S27.819 ☑
    - contusion S27.812 ☑
    - laceration S27.813 ☑
    - specified type NEC S27.818 ☑
  - heart — *see* Injury, heart
  - hemopneumothorax S27.2 ☑
  - hemothorax S27.1 ☑
  - lung S27.309 ☑
    - aspiration J69.0
    - bilateral S27.302 ☑
    - blast injury (primary) S27.319 ☑
      - bilateral S27.312 ☑
      - secondary — *see* Injury, intrathoracic, lung, specified type NEC
      - unilateral S27.311 ☑
    - contusion S27.329 ☑
      - bilateral S27.322 ☑
      - unilateral S27.321 ☑
    - laceration S27.339 ☑
      - bilateral S27.332 ☑
      - unilateral S27.331 ☑
    - specified type NEC S27.399 ☑

Injury — *continued*
- intrathoracic — *continued*
  - lung — *continued*
    - specified type — *continued*
      - bilateral S27.392 ☑
      - unilateral S27.391 ☑
    - unilateral S27.301 ☑
  - pleura S27.60 ☑
    - laceration S27.63 ☑
    - specified type NEC S27.69 ☑
  - pneumothorax S27.0 ☑
  - specified organ NEC S27.899 ☑
    - contusion S27.892 ☑
    - laceration S27.893 ☑
    - specified type NEC S27.898 ☑
  - thoracic duct — *see* Injury, intrathoracic, specified organ NEC
  - thymus gland — *see* Injury, intrathoracic, specified organ NEC
  - trachea, thoracic S27.50 ☑
    - blast (primary) S27.51 ☑
    - contusion S27.52 ☑
    - laceration S27.53 ☑
    - specified type NEC S27.59 ☑
- iris — *see* Injury, eye, specified site NEC
  - penetrating — *see* Injury, eyeball, penetrating
- jaw S09.93 ☑
- jejunum — *see* Injury, intestine, small
- joint NOS T14.8 ☑
  - old or residual — *see* Disorder, joint, specified type NEC
- kidney S37.00- ☑
  - acute (nontraumatic) N17.9
  - contusion — *see* Contusion, kidney
  - laceration — *see* Laceration, kidney
  - specified NEC S37.09- ☑
- knee S89.9- ☑
  - contusion — *see* Contusion, knee
  - dislocation — *see* Dislocation, knee
  - meniscus (lateral) (medial) — *see* Sprain, knee, specified site NEC
    - old injury or tear — *see* Derangement, knee, meniscus, due to old injury
  - open — *see* Wound, open, knee
  - specified NEC S89.8- ☑
  - sprain — *see* Sprain, knee
  - superficial — *see* Injury, superficial, knee
- labium (majus) (minus) S39.94 ☑
- labyrinth, ear S09.30- ☑
- lacrimal apparatus, duct, gland, or sac — *see* Injury, eye, specified site NEC
- larynx NEC S19.81 ☑
- leg (lower) S89.9- ☑
  - blood vessel — *see* Injury, blood vessel, leg
  - contusion — *see* Contusion, leg
  - fracture — *see* Fracture, leg
  - muscle — *see* Injury, muscle, leg
  - nerve — *see* Injury, nerve, leg
  - open — *see* Wound, open, leg
  - specified NEC S89.8- ☑
  - superficial — *see* Injury, superficial, leg
- lens, eye — *see* Injury, eye, specified site NEC
  - penetrating — *see* Injury, eyeball, penetrating
- limb NEC T14.8 ☑
- lip S09.93 ☑
- liver S36.119 ☑
  - contusion S36.112 ☑
  - laceration S36.113 ☑
    - major (stellate) S36.116 ☑
    - minor S36.114 ☑
    - moderate S36.115 ☑
  - specified NEC S36.118 ☑
- lower back S39.92 ☑
  - specified NEC S39.82 ☑
- lumbar, lumbosacral (region) S39.92 ☑
  - plexus — *see* Injury, lumbosacral plexus
- lumbosacral plexus S34.4 ☑
- lung (*see also* Injury, intrathoracic, lung)
  - aspiration J69.0
  - transfusion-related (TRALI) J95.84
- lymphatic thoracic duct — *see* Injury, intrathoracic, specified organ NEC
- malar region S09.93 ☑
- mastoid region S09.90 ☑
- maxilla S09.93 ☑

Injury — *continued*
- mediastinum — *see* Injury, intrathoracic, specified organ NEC
- membrane, brain — *see* Injury, intracranial
- meningeal artery — *see* Injury, intracranial, subdural hemorrhage
- meninges (cerebral) — *see* Injury, intracranial
- mesenteric
  - artery
    - branch S35.299 ☑
      - laceration (minor) (superficial) S35.291 ☑
        - major S35.292 ☑
      - specified NEC S35.298 ☑
    - inferior S35.239 ☑
      - laceration (minor) (superficial) S35.231 ☑
        - major S35.232 ☑
      - specified NEC S35.238 ☑
    - superior S35.229 ☑
      - laceration (minor) (superficial) S35.221 ☑
        - major S35.222 ☑
      - specified NEC S35.228 ☑
  - plexus (inferior) (superior) — *see* Injury, nerve, lumbosacral, sympathetic
  - vein
    - inferior S35.349 ☑
      - laceration S35.341 ☑
      - specified NEC S35.348 ☑
    - superior S35.339 ☑
      - laceration S35.331 ☑
      - specified NEC S35.338 ☑
- mesentery — *see* Injury, intra-abdominal, specified site NEC
- mesosalpinx — *see* Injury, pelvic organ, specified site NEC
- middle ear S09.30- ☑
- midthoracic region NOS S29.9 ☑
- mouth S09.93 ☑
- multiple NOS T07 ☑
- muscle (and fascia) (and tendon)
  - abdomen S39.001 ☑
    - laceration S39.021 ☑
    - specified type NEC S39.091 ☑
    - strain S39.011 ☑
  - abductor
    - thumb, forearm level — *see* Injury, muscle, thumb, abductor
  - adductor
    - thigh S76.20- ☑
      - laceration S76.22- ☑
      - specified type NEC S76.29- ☑
      - strain S76.21- ☑
  - ankle — *see* Injury, muscle, foot
  - anterior muscle group, at leg level (lower) S86.20- ☑
    - laceration S86.22- ☑
    - specified type NEC S86.29- ☑
    - strain S86.21- ☑
  - arm (upper) — *see* Injury, muscle, shoulder
  - biceps (parts NEC) S46.20- ☑
    - laceration S46.22- ☑
    - long head S46.10- ☑
      - laceration S46.12- ☑
      - specified type NEC S46.19- ☑
      - strain S46.11- ☑
    - specified type NEC S46.29- ☑
    - strain S46.21- ☑
  - extensor
    - finger(s) (other than thumb) — *see* Injury, muscle, finger by site, extensor
    - forearm level, specified NEC — *see* Injury, muscle, forearm, extensor
    - thumb — *see* Injury, muscle, thumb, extensor
    - toe (large) (ankle level) (foot level) — *see* Injury, muscle, toe, extensor
  - finger
    - extensor (forearm level) S56.40- ☑
      - hand level S66.309 ☑
        - laceration S66.329 ☑
        - specified type NEC S66.399 ☑
        - strain S66.319 ☑
      - laceration S56.429 ☑
      - specified type NEC S56.499 ☑
      - strain S56.419 ☑
    - flexor (forearm level) S56.10- ☑
      - hand level S66.109 ☑
        - laceration S66.129 ☑

☑ **Additional Character Required** — Refer to the Tabular List for Character Selection   ▽ **Subterms under main terms may continue to next column or page**

Injury — *continued*
  muscle — *continued*
    finger — *continued*
      flexor — *continued*
        hand level — *continued*
          specified type NEC S66.199 ☑
          strain S66.119 ☑
        laceration S56.129 ☑
        specified type NEC S56.199 ☑
        strain S56.119 ☑
      index
        extensor (forearm level)
          hand level S66.308 ☑
            laceration S66.32- ☑
            specified type NEC S66.39- ☑
            strain S66.31- ☑
          specified type NEC S56.492- ☑
        flexor (forearm level)
          hand level S66.108 ☑
            laceration S66.12- ☑
            specified type NEC S66.19- ☑
            strain S66.11- ☑
          specified type NEC S56.19- ☑
          strain S56.11- ☑
        intrinsic S66.50- ☑
          laceration S66.52- ☑
          specified type NEC S66.59- ☑
          strain S66.51- ☑
      intrinsic S66.509 ☑
        laceration S66.529 ☑
        specified type NEC S66.599 ☑
        strain S66.519 ☑
      little
        extensor (forearm level)
          hand level S66.30- ☑
            laceration S66.32- ☑
            specified type NEC S66.39- ☑
            strain S66.31- ☑
          laceration S56.42- ☑
          specified type NEC S56.49- ☑
          strain S56.41- ☑
        flexor (forearm level)
          hand level S66.10- ☑
            laceration S66.12- ☑
            specified type NEC S66.19- ☑
            strain S66.11- ☑
          laceration S56.12- ☑
          specified type NEC S56.19- ☑
          strain S56.11- ☑
        intrinsic S66.50- ☑
          laceration S66.52- ☑
          specified type NEC S66.59- ☑
          strain S66.51- ☑
      middle
        extensor (forearm level)
          hand level S66.30- ☑
            laceration S66.32- ☑
            specified type NEC S66.39- ☑
            strain S66.31- ☑
          laceration S56.42- ☑
          specified type NEC S56.49- ☑
          strain S56.41- ☑
        flexor (forearm level)
          hand level S66.10- ☑
            laceration S66.12- ☑
            specified type NEC S66.19- ☑
            strain S66.11- ☑
          laceration S56.12- ☑
          specified type NEC S56.19- ☑
          strain S56.11- ☑
        intrinsic S66.50- ☑
          laceration S66.52- ☑
          specified type NEC S66.59- ☑
          strain S66.51- ☑
      ring
        extensor (forearm level)
          hand level S66.30- ☑
            laceration S66.32- ☑
            specified type NEC S66.39- ☑
            strain S66.31- ☑
          laceration S56.42- ☑
          specified type NEC S56.49- ☑
          strain S56.41- ☑
        flexor (forearm level)
          hand level S66.10- ☑
            laceration S66.12- ☑

Injury — *continued*
  muscle — *continued*
    finger — *continued*
      ring — *continued*
        flexor — *continued*
          hand level — *continued*
            specified type NEC S66.19- ☑
            strain S66.11- ☑
          laceration S56.12- ☑
          specified type NEC S56.19- ☑
          strain S56.11- ☑
        intrinsic S66.50- ☑
          laceration S66.52- ☑
          specified type NEC S66.59- ☑
          strain S66.51- ☑
    flexor
      finger(s) (other than thumb) — *see* Injury,
        muscle, finger
      forearm level, specified NEC — *see* Injury,
        muscle, forearm, flexor
      thumb — *see* Injury, muscle, thumb, flexor
      toe (long) (ankle level) (foot level) — *see* Injury,
        muscle, toe, flexor
    foot S96.90- ☑
      intrinsic S96.20- ☑
        laceration S96.22- ☑
        specified type NEC S96.29- ☑
        strain S96.21- ☑
      laceration S96.92- ☑
      long extensor, toe — *see* Injury, muscle, toe,
        extensor
      long flexor, toe — *see* Injury, muscle, toe, flexor
      specified
        site NEC S96.80- ☑
          laceration S96.82- ☑
          specified type NEC S96.89- ☑
          strain S96.81- ☑
        type S96.99- ☑
      strain S96.91- ☑
    forearm (level) S56.90- ☑
      extensor S56.50- ☑
        laceration S56.52- ☑
        specified type NEC S56.59- ☑
        strain S56.51- ☑
      flexor S56.20- ☑
        laceration S56.22- ☑
        specified type NEC S56.29- ☑
        strain S56.21- ☑
      laceration S56.92- ☑
      specified
        site NEC S56.80- ☑
          laceration S56.82- ☑
          strain S56.81- ☑
          type NEC S56.89- ☑
      strain S56.91- ☑
    hand (level) S66.90- ☑
      laceration S66.92- ☑
      specified
        site NEC S66.80- ☑
          laceration S66.82- ☑
          specified type NEC S66.89- ☑
          strain S66.81- ☑
          type NEC S66.99- ☑
      strain S66.91- ☑
    head S09.10 ☑
      laceration S09.12 ☑
      specified type NEC S09.19 ☑
      strain S09.11 ☑
    hip NEC S76.00- ☑
      laceration S76.02- ☑
      specified type NEC S76.09- ☑
      strain S76.01- ☑
    intrinsic
      ankle and foot level — *see* Injury, muscle, foot,
        intrinsic
      finger (other than thumb) — *see* Injury, muscle,
        finger by site, intrinsic
      foot (level) — *see* Injury, muscle, foot, intrinsic
      thumb — *see* Injury, muscle, thumb, intrinsic
    leg (level) (lower) S86.90- ☑
      Achilles tendon — *see* Injury, Achilles tendon
      anterior muscle group — *see* Injury, muscle,
        anterior muscle group
      laceration S86.92- ☑
      peroneal muscle group — *see* Injury, muscle,
        peroneal muscle group

Injury — *continued*
  muscle — *continued*
    leg — *continued*
      posterior muscle group — *see* Injury, muscle,
        posterior muscle group, leg level
      specified
        site NEC S86.80- ☑
          laceration S86.82- ☑
          specified type NEC S86.89- ☑
          strain S86.81- ☑
        type NEC S86.99- ☑
      strain S86.91- ☑
    long
      extensor toe, at ankle and foot level — *see* In-
        jury, muscle, toe, extensor
      flexor, toe, at ankle and foot level — *see* Injury,
        muscle, toe, flexor
      head, biceps — *see* Injury, muscle, biceps, long
        head
    lower back S39.002 ☑
      laceration S39.022 ☑
      specified type NEC S39.092 ☑
      strain S39.012 ☑
    neck (level) S16.9 ☑
      laceration S16.2 ☑
      specified type NEC S16.8 ☑
      strain S16.1 ☑
    pelvis S39.003 ☑
      laceration S39.023 ☑
      specified type NEC S39.093 ☑
      strain S39.013 ☑
    peroneal muscle group, at leg level (lower)
      S86.30- ☑
      laceration S86.32- ☑
      specified type NEC S86.39- ☑
      strain S86.31- ☑
    posterior muscle (group)
      leg level (lower) S86.10- ☑
        laceration S86.12- ☑
        specified type NEC S86.19- ☑
        strain S86.11- ☑
      thigh level S76.30- ☑
        laceration S76.32- ☑
        specified type NEC S76.39- ☑
        strain S76.31- ☑
    quadriceps (thigh) S76.10- ☑
      laceration S76.12- ☑
      specified type NEC S76.19- ☑
      strain S76.11- ☑
    shoulder S46.90- ☑
      laceration S46.92- ☑
      rotator cuff — *see* Injury, rotator cuff
      specified site NEC S46.80- ☑
        laceration S46.82- ☑
        specified type NEC S46.89- ☑
        strain S46.81- ☑
      specified type NEC S46.99- ☑
      strain S46.91- ☑
    thigh NEC (level) S76.90- ☑
      adductor — *see* Injury, muscle, adductor, thigh
      laceration S76.92- ☑
      posterior muscle (group) — *see* Injury, muscle,
        posterior muscle, thigh level
      quadriceps — *see* Injury, muscle, quadriceps
      specified
        site NEC S76.80- ☑
          laceration S76.82- ☑
          specified type NEC S76.89- ☑
          strain S76.81- ☑
        type NEC S76.99- ☑
      strain S76.91- ☑
    thorax (level) S29.009 ☑
      back wall S29.002 ☑
      front wall S29.001 ☑
      laceration S29.029 ☑
        back wall S29.022 ☑
        front wall S29.021 ☑
      specified type NEC S29.099 ☑
        back wall S29.092 ☑
        front wall S29.091 ☑
      strain S29.019 ☑
        back wall S29.012 ☑
        front wall S29.011 ☑
    thumb
      abductor (forearm level) S56.30- ☑
        laceration S56.32- ☑

Injury — *continued*
  muscle — *continued*
    thumb — *continued*
      abductor — *continued*
        specified type NEC S56.39- ☑
        strain S56.31- ☑
      extensor (forearm level) S56.30- ☑
        hand level S66.20- ☑
          laceration S66.22- ☑
          specified type NEC S66.29- ☑
          strain S66.21- ☑
        laceration S56.32- ☑
        specified type NEC S56.39- ☑
        strain S56.31- ☑
      flexor (forearm level) S56.00- ☑
        hand level S66.00- ☑
          laceration S66.02- ☑
          specified type NEC S66.09- ☑
          strain S66.01- ☑
        laceration S56.02- ☑
        specified type NEC S56.09- ☑
        strain S56.01- ☑
        wrist level — *see* Injury, muscle, thumb, flexor, hand level
      intrinsic S66.40- ☑
        laceration S66.42- ☑
        specified type NEC S66.49- ☑
        strain S66.41- ☑
    toe (*see also* Injury, muscle, foot)
      extensor, long S96.10- ☑
        laceration S96.12- ☑
        specified type NEC S96.19- ☑
        strain S96.11- ☑
      flexor, long S96.00- ☑
        laceration S96.02- ☑
        specified type NEC S96.09- ☑
        strain S96.01- ☑
    triceps S46.30- ☑
      laceration S46.32- ☑
      specified type NEC S46.39- ☑
      strain S46.31- ☑
    wrist (and hand) level — *see* Injury, muscle, hand
  musculocutaneous nerve — *see* Injury, nerve, musculocutaneous
  myocardium — *see* Injury, heart
  nape — *see* Injury, neck
  nasal (septum) (sinus) S09.92 ☑
  nasopharynx S09.92 ☑
  neck S19.9 ☑
    specified NEC S19.80 ☑
    specified site NEC S19.89 ☑
  nerve NEC T14.8 ☑
    abdomen S34.9 ☑
      peripheral S34.6 ☑
      specified site NEC S34.8 ☑
    abducens S04.4- ☑
      contusion S04.4- ☑
      laceration S04.4- ☑
      specified type NEC S04.4- ☑
    abducent — *see* Injury, nerve, abducens
    accessory S04.7- ☑
      contusion S04.7- ☑
      laceration S04.7- ☑
      specified type NEC S04.7- ☑
    acoustic S04.6- ☑
      contusion S04.6- ☑
      laceration S04.6- ☑
      specified type NEC S04.6- ☑
    ankle S94.9- ☑
      cutaneous sensory S94.3- ☑
      specified site NEC — *see* subcategory S94.8 ☑
    anterior crural, femoral — *see* Injury, nerve, femoral
    arm (upper) S44.9- ☑
      axillary — *see* Injury, nerve, axillary
      cutaneous — *see* Injury, nerve, cutaneous, arm
      median — *see* Injury, nerve, median, upper arm
      musculocutaneous — *see* Injury, nerve, musculocutaneous
      radial — *see* Injury, nerve, radial, upper arm
      specified site NEC — *see* subcategory S44.8 ☑
      ulnar — *see* Injury, nerve, ulnar, arm
    auditory — *see* Injury, nerve, acoustic
    axillary S44.3- ☑
    brachial plexus — *see* Injury, brachial plexus
    cervical sympathetic S14.5 ☑
    cranial S04.9 ☑

Injury — *continued*
  nerve — *continued*
    cranial — *continued*
      contusion S04.9 ☑
      eighth (acoustic or auditory) — *see* Injury, nerve, acoustic
      eleventh (accessory) — *see* Injury, nerve, accessory
      fifth (trigeminal) — *see* Injury, nerve, trigeminal
      first (olfactory) — *see* Injury, nerve, olfactory
      fourth (trochlear) — *see* Injury, nerve, trochlear
      laceration S04.9 ☑
      ninth (glossopharyngeal) — *see* Injury, nerve, glossopharyngeal
      second (optic) — *see* Injury, nerve, optic
      seventh (facial) — *see* Injury, nerve, facial
      sixth (abducent) — *see* Injury, nerve, abducens
      specified
        nerve NEC S04.89- ☑
          contusion S04.89- ☑
          laceration S04.89- ☑
          specified type NEC S04.89- ☑
        type NEC S04.9 ☑
      tenth (pneumogastric or vagus) — *see* Injury, nerve, vagus
      third (oculomotor) — *see* Injury, nerve, oculomotor
      twelfth (hypoglossal) — *see* Injury, nerve, hypoglossal
    cutaneous sensory
      ankle (level) S94.3- ☑
      arm (upper) (level) S44.5- ☑
      foot (level) — *see* Injury, nerve, cutaneous sensory, ankle
      forearm (level) S54.3- ☑
      hip (level) S74.2- ☑
      leg (lower level) S84.2- ☑
      shoulder (level) — *see* Injury, nerve, cutaneous sensory, arm
      thigh (level) — *see* Injury, nerve, cutaneous sensory, hip
    deep peroneal — *see* Injury, nerve, peroneal, foot
    digital
      finger S64.4- ☑
        index S64.49- ☑
        little S64.49- ☑
        middle S64.49- ☑
        ring S64.49- ☑
        thumb S64.3- ☑
      toe — *see* Injury, nerve, ankle, specified site NEC
    eighth cranial (acoustic or auditory) — *see* Injury, nerve, acoustic
    eleventh cranial (accessory) — *see* Injury, nerve, accessory
    facial S04.5- ☑
      contusion S04.5- ☑
      laceration S04.5- ☑
      newborn P11.3
      specified type NEC S04.5- ☑
    femoral (hip level) (thigh level) S74.1- ☑
    fifth cranial (trigeminal) — *see* Injury, nerve, trigeminal
    finger (digital) — *see* Injury, nerve, digital, finger
    first cranial (olfactory) — *see* Injury, nerve, olfactory
    foot S94.9- ☑
      cutaneous sensory S94.3- ☑
      deep peroneal S94.2- ☑
      lateral plantar S94.0- ☑
      medial plantar S94.1- ☑
      specified site NEC — *see* subcategory S94.8 ☑
    forearm (level) S54.9- ☑
      cutaneous sensory — *see* Injury, nerve, cutaneous sensory, forearm
      median — *see* Injury, nerve, median
      radial — *see* Injury, nerve, radial
      specified site NEC — *see* subcategory S54.8 ☑
      ulnar — *see* Injury, nerve, ulnar
    fourth cranial (trochlear) — *see* Injury, nerve, trochlear
    glossopharyngeal S04.89- ☑
      specified type NEC S04.89- ☑
    hand S64.9- ☑
      median — *see* Injury, nerve, median, hand
      radial — *see* Injury, nerve, radial, hand
      specified NEC — *see* subcategory S64.8 ☑

Injury — *continued*
  nerve — *continued*
    hand — *continued*
      ulnar — *see* Injury, nerve, ulnar, hand
    hip (level) S74.9- ☑
      cutaneous sensory — *see* Injury, nerve, cutaneous sensory, hip
      femoral — *see* Injury, nerve, femoral
      sciatic — *see* Injury, nerve, sciatic
      specified site NEC — *see* subcategory S74.8 ☑
    hypoglossal S04.89- ☑
      specified type NEC S04.89- ☑
    lateral plantar S94.0- ☑
    leg (lower) S84.9- ☑
      cutaneous sensory — *see* Injury, nerve, cutaneous sensory, leg
      peroneal — *see* Injury, nerve, peroneal
      specified site NEC — *see* subcategory S84.8 ☑
      tibial — *see* Injury, nerve, tibial
      upper — *see* Injury, nerve, thigh
    lower
      back — *see* Injury, nerve, abdomen, specified site NEC
        peripheral — *see* Injury, nerve, abdomen, peripheral
      limb — *see* Injury, nerve, leg
    lumbar plexus — *see* Injury, nerve, lumbosacral, sympathetic
    lumbar spinal — *see* Injury, nerve, spinal, lumbar
    lumbosacral
      plexus — *see* Injury, nerve, lumbosacral, sympathetic
      sympathetic S34.5 ☑
    medial plantar S94.1- ☑
    median (forearm level) S54.1- ☑
      hand (level) S64.1- ☑
      upper arm (level) S44.1- ☑
      wrist (level) — *see* Injury, nerve, median, hand
    musculocutaneous S44.4- ☑
    musculospiral (upper arm level) — *see* Injury, nerve, radial, upper arm
    neck S14.9 ☑
      peripheral S14.4 ☑
      specified site NEC S14.8 ☑
      sympathetic S14.5 ☑
    ninth cranial (glossopharyngeal) — *see* Injury, nerve, glossopharyngeal
    oculomotor S04.1- ☑
      contusion S04.1- ☑
      laceration S04.1- ☑
      specified type NEC S04.1- ☑
    olfactory S04.81- ☑
      specified type NEC S04.81- ☑
    optic S04.01- ☑
      contusion S04.01- ☑
      laceration S04.01- ☑
      specified type NEC S04.01- ☑
    pelvic girdle — *see* Injury, nerve, hip
    pelvis — *see* Injury, nerve, abdomen, specified site NEC
      peripheral — *see* Injury, nerve, abdomen, peripheral
    peripheral NEC T14.8 ☑
      abdomen — *see* Injury, nerve, abdomen, peripheral
      lower back — *see* Injury, nerve, abdomen, peripheral
      neck — *see* Injury, nerve, neck, peripheral
      pelvis — *see* Injury, nerve, abdomen, peripheral
      specified NEC T14.8 ☑
    peroneal (lower leg level) S84.1- ☑
      foot S94.2- ☑
    plexus
      brachial — *see* Injury, brachial plexus
      celiac, coeliac — *see* Injury, nerve, lumbosacral, sympathetic
      mesenteric, inferior — *see* Injury, nerve, lumbosacral, sympathetic
      sacral — *see* Injury, lumbosacral plexus
      spinal
        brachial — *see* Injury, brachial plexus
        lumbosacral — *see* Injury, lumbosacral plexus
    pneumogastric — *see* Injury, nerve, vagus
    radial (forearm level) S54.2- ☑
      hand (level) S64.2- ☑

☑ Additional Character Required — Refer to the Tabular List for Character Selection   ▽ Subterms under main terms may continue to next column or page

Injury — *continued*
 nerve — *continued*
  radial — *continued*
   upper arm (level) S44.2- ☑
   wrist (level) — *see* Injury, nerve, radial, hand
  root — *see* Injury, nerve, spinal, root
  sacral plexus — *see* Injury, lumbosacral plexus
  sacral spinal — *see* Injury, nerve, spinal, sacral
  sciatic (hip level) (thigh level) S74.0- ☑
  second cranial (optic) — *see* Injury, nerve, optic
  seventh cranial (facial) — *see* Injury, nerve, facial
  shoulder — *see* Injury, nerve, arm
  sixth cranial (abducent) — *see* Injury, nerve, abducens
  spinal
   plexus — *see* Injury, nerve, plexus, spinal
   root
    cervical S14.2 ☑
    dorsal S24.2 ☑
    lumbar S34.21 ☑
    sacral S34.22 ☑
    thoracic — *see* Injury, nerve, spinal, root, dorsal
  splanchnic — *see* Injury, nerve, lumbosacral, sympathetic
  sympathetic NEC — *see* Injury, nerve, lumbosacral, sympathetic
   cervical — *see* Injury, nerve, cervical sympathetic
  tenth cranial (pneumogastric or vagus) — *see* Injury, nerve, vagus
  thigh (level) — *see* Injury, nerve, hip
   cutaneous sensory — *see* Injury, nerve, cutaneous sensory, hip
   femoral — *see* Injury, nerve, femoral
   sciatic — *see* Injury, nerve, sciatic
   specified NEC — *see* Injury, nerve, hip
  third cranial (oculomotor) — *see* Injury, nerve, oculomotor
  thorax S24.9 ☑
   peripheral S24.3 ☑
   specified site NEC S24.8 ☑
   sympathetic S24.4 ☑
  thumb, digital — *see* Injury, nerve, digital, thumb
  tibial (lower leg level) (posterior) S84.0- ☑
  toe — *see* Injury, nerve, ankle
  trigeminal S04.3- ☑
   contusion S04.3- ☑
   laceration S04.3- ☑
   specified type NEC S04.3- ☑
  trochlear S04.2- ☑
   contusion S04.2- ☑
   laceration S04.2- ☑
   specified type NEC S04.2- ☑
  twelfth cranial (hypoglossal) — *see* Injury, nerve, hypoglossal
  ulnar (forearm level) S54.0- ☑
   arm (upper) (level) S44.0- ☑
   hand (level) S64.0- ☑
   wrist (level) — *see* Injury, nerve, ulnar, hand
  vagus S04.89- ☑
   specified type NEC S04.89- ☑
  wrist (level) — *see* Injury, nerve, hand
 ninth cranial nerve (glossopharyngeal) — *see* Injury, nerve, glossopharyngeal
 nose (septum) S09.92 ☑
 obstetrical O71.9
  specified NEC O71.89
 occipital (region) (scalp) S09.90 ☑
  lobe — *see* Injury, intracranial
 optic chiasm S04.02 ☑
 optic radiation S04.03- ☑
 optic tract and pathways S04.03- ☑
 orbit, orbital (region) — *see* Injury, eye
  penetrating (with foreign body) — *see* Injury, eye, orbit, penetrating
  specified NEC — *see* Injury, eye, specified site NEC
 ovary, ovarian S37.409 ☑
  bilateral S37.402 ☑
   contusion S37.422 ☑
   laceration S37.432 ☑
   specified type NEC S37.492 ☑
  blood vessel — *see* Injury, blood vessel, ovarian
  contusion S37.429 ☑
   bilateral S37.422 ☑
   unilateral S37.421 ☑

Injury — *continued*
 ovary, ovarian — *continued*
  laceration S37.439 ☑
   bilateral S37.432 ☑
   unilateral S37.431 ☑
  specified type NEC S37.499 ☑
   bilateral S37.492 ☑
   unilateral S37.491 ☑
  unilateral S37.401 ☑
   contusion S37.421 ☑
   laceration S37.431 ☑
   specified type NEC S37.491 ☑
 palate (hard) (soft) S09.93 ☑
 pancreas S36.209 ☑
  body S36.201 ☑
   contusion S36.221 ☑
   laceration S36.231 ☑
    major S36.261 ☑
    minor S36.241 ☑
    moderate S36.251 ☑
   specified type NEC S36.291 ☑
  contusion S36.229 ☑
  head S36.200 ☑
   contusion S36.220 ☑
   laceration S36.230 ☑
    major S36.260 ☑
    minor S36.240 ☑
    moderate S36.250 ☑
   specified type NEC S36.290 ☑
  laceration S36.239 ☑
   major S36.269 ☑
   minor S36.249 ☑
   moderate S36.259 ☑
  specified type NEC S36.299 ☑
  tail S36.202 ☑
   contusion S36.222 ☑
   laceration S36.232 ☑
    major S36.262 ☑
    minor S36.242 ☑
    moderate S36.252 ☑
   specified type NEC S36.292 ☑
 parietal (region) (scalp) S09.90 ☑
  lobe — *see* Injury, intracranial
 patellar ligament (tendon) S76.10- ☑
  laceration S76.12- ☑
  specified NEC S76.19- ☑
  strain S76.11- ☑
 pelvis, pelvic (floor) S39.93 ☑
  complicating delivery O70.1
  joint or ligament, complicating delivery O71.6
  organ S37.90 ☑
   with ectopic or molar pregnancy O08.6
   complication of abortion — *see* Abortion
   contusion S37.92 ☑
   following ectopic or molar pregnancy O08.6
   laceration S37.93 ☑
   obstetrical trauma NEC O71.5
   specified
    site NEC S37.899 ☑
     contusion S37.892 ☑
     laceration S37.893 ☑
     specified type NEC S37.898 ☑
    type NEC S37.99 ☑
  specified NEC S39.83 ☑
 penis S39.94 ☑
 perineum S39.94 ☑
 peritoneum S36.81 ☑
  laceration S36.893 ☑
 periurethral tissue — *see* Injury, urethra
  complicating delivery O71.82
 phalanges
  foot — *see* Injury, foot
  hand — *see* Injury, hand
 pharynx NEC S19.85 ☑
 pleura — *see* Injury, intrathoracic, pleura
 plexus
  brachial — *see* Injury, brachial plexus
  cardiac — *see* Injury, nerve, thorax, sympathetic
  celiac, coeliac — *see* Injury, nerve, lumbosacral, sympathetic
  esophageal — *see* Injury, nerve, thorax, sympathetic
  hypogastric — *see* Injury, nerve, lumbosacral, sympathetic
  lumbar, lumbosacral — *see* Injury, lumbosacral plexus

Injury — *continued*
 plexus — *continued*
  mesenteric — *see* Injury, nerve, lumbosacral, sympathetic
  pulmonary — *see* Injury, nerve, thorax, sympathetic
 postcardiac surgery (syndrome) I97.0
 prepuce S39.94 ☑
 prostate S37.829 ☑
  contusion S37.822 ☑
  laceration S37.823 ☑
  specified type NEC S37.828 ☑
 pubic region S39.94 ☑
 pudendum S39.94 ☑
 pulmonary plexus — *see* Injury, nerve, thorax, sympathetic
 rectovaginal septum NEC S39.83 ☑
 rectum — *see* Injury, intestine, large, rectum
 retina — *see* Injury, eye, specified site NEC
  penetrating — *see* Injury, eyeball, penetrating
 retroperitoneal — *see* Injury, intra-abdominal, specified site NEC
 rotator cuff (muscle(s)) (tendon(s)) S46.00- ☑
  laceration S46.02- ☑
  specified type NEC S46.09- ☑
  strain S46.01- ☑
 round ligament — *see* Injury, pelvic organ, specified site NEC
 sacral plexus — *see* Injury, lumbosacral plexus
 salivary duct or gland S09.93 ☑
 scalp S09.90 ☑
  newborn (birth injury) P12.9
   due to monitoring (electrode) (sampling incision) P12.4
   specified NEC P12.89
    caput succedaneum P12.81
 scapular region — *see* Injury, shoulder
 sclera — *see* Injury, eye, specified site NEC
  penetrating — *see* Injury, eyeball, penetrating
 scrotum S39.94 ☑
 second cranial nerve (optic) — *see* Injury, nerve, optic
 seminal vesicle — *see* Injury, pelvic organ, specified site NEC
 seventh cranial nerve (facial) — *see* Injury, nerve, facial
 shoulder S49.9- ☑
  blood vessel — *see* Injury, blood vessel, arm
  contusion — *see* Contusion, shoulder
  dislocation — *see* Dislocation, shoulder
  fracture — *see* Fracture, shoulder
  muscle — *see* Injury, muscle, shoulder
  nerve — *see* Injury, nerve, shoulder
  open — *see* Wound, open, shoulder
  specified type NEC S49.8- ☑
  sprain — *see* Sprain, shoulder girdle
  superficial — *see* Injury, superficial, shoulder
 sinus
  cavernous — *see* Injury, intracranial
  nasal S09.92 ☑
 sixth cranial nerve (abducent) — *see* Injury, nerve, abducens
 skeleton, birth injury P13.9
  specified part NEC P13.8
 skin NEC T14.8 ☑
  surface intact — *see* Injury, superficial
 skull NEC S09.90 ☑
 specified NEC T14.8 ☑
 spermatic cord (pelvic region) S37.898 ☑
  scrotal region S39.848 ☑
 spinal (cord)
  cervical (neck) S14.109 ☑
   anterior cord syndrome S14.139 ☑
    C1 level S14.131 ☑
    C2 level S14.132 ☑
    C3 level S14.133 ☑
    C4 level S14.134 ☑
    C5 level S14.135 ☑
    C6 level S14.136 ☑
    C7 level S14.137 ☑
    C8 level S14.138 ☑
   Brown-Séquard syndrome S14.149 ☑
    C1 level S14.141 ☑
    C2 level S14.142 ☑
    C3 level S14.143 ☑
    C4 level S14.144 ☑
    C5 level S14.145 ☑
    C6 level S14.146 ☑

Injury — *continued*
  spinal — *continued*
    cervical — *continued*
      Brown-Séquard syndrome — *continued*
        C7 level S14.147 ☑
        C8 level S14.148 ☑
      C1 level S14.101 ☑
      C2 level S14.102 ☑
      C3 level S14.103 ☑
      C4 level S14.104 ☑
      C5 level S14.105 ☑
      C6 level S14.106 ☑
      C7 level S14.107 ☑
      C8 level S14.108 ☑
      central cord syndrome S14.129 ☑
        C1 level S14.121 ☑
        C2 level S14.122 ☑
        C3 level S14.123 ☑
        C4 level S14.124 ☑
        C5 level S14.125 ☑
        C6 level S14.126 ☑
        C7 level S14.127 ☑
        C8 level S14.128 ☑
      complete lesion S14.119 ☑
        C1 level S14.111 ☑
        C2 level S14.112 ☑
        C3 level S14.113 ☑
        C4 level S14.114 ☑
        C5 level S14.115 ☑
        C6 level S14.116 ☑
        C7 level S14.117 ☑
        C8 level S14.118 ☑
      concussion S14.0 ☑
      edema S14.0 ☑
      incomplete lesion specified NEC S14.159 ☑
        C1 level S14.151 ☑
        C2 level S14.152 ☑
        C3 level S14.153 ☑
        C4 level S14.154 ☑
        C5 level S14.155 ☑
        C6 level S14.156 ☑
        C7 level S14.157 ☑
        C8 level S14.158 ☑
      posterior cord syndrome S14.159 ☑
        C1 level S14.151 ☑
        C2 level S14.152 ☑
        C3 level S14.153 ☑
        C4 level S14.154 ☑
        C5 level S14.155 ☑
        C6 level S14.156 ☑
        C7 level S14.157 ☑
        C8 level S14.158 ☑
    dorsal — *see* Injury, spinal, thoracic
    lumbar S34.109 ☑
      complete lesion S34.119 ☑
        L1 level S34.111 ☑
        L2 level S34.112 ☑
        L3 level S34.113 ☑
        L4 level S34.114 ☑
        L5 level S34.115 ☑
      concussion S34.01 ☑
      edema S34.01 ☑
      incomplete lesion S34.129 ☑
        L1 level S34.121 ☑
        L2 level S34.122 ☑
        L3 level S34.123 ☑
        L4 level S34.124 ☑
        L5 level S34.125 ☑
      L1 level S34.101 ☑
      L2 level S34.102 ☑
      L3 level S34.103 ☑
      L4 level S34.104 ☑
      L5 level S34.105 ☑
    nerve root NEC
      cervical — *see* Injury, nerve, spinal, root, cervical
      dorsal — *see* Injury, nerve, spinal, root, dorsal
      lumbar S34.21 ☑
      sacral S34.22 ☑
      thoracic — *see* Injury, nerve, spinal, root, dorsal
    plexus
      brachial — *see* Injury, brachial plexus
      lumbosacral — *see* Injury, lumbosacral plexus
    sacral S34.139 ☑
      complete lesion S34.131 ☑
      incomplete lesion S34.132 ☑

Injury — *continued*
  spinal — *continued*
    thoracic S24.109 ☑
      anterior cord syndrome S24.139 ☑
        T1 level S24.131 ☑
        T2-T6 level S24.132 ☑
        T7-T10 level S24.133 ☑
        T11-T12 level S24.134 ☑
      Brown-Séquard syndrome S24.149 ☑
        T1 level S24.141 ☑
        T2-T6 level S24.142 ☑
        T7-T10 level S24.143 ☑
        T11-T12 level S24.144 ☑
      complete lesion S24.119 ☑
        T1 level S24.111 ☑
        T2-T6 level S24.112 ☑
        T7-T10 level S24.113 ☑
        T11-T12 level S24.114 ☑
      concussion S24.0 ☑
      edema S24.0 ☑
      incomplete lesion specified NEC S24.159 ☑
        T1 level S24.151 ☑
        T2-T6 level S24.152 ☑
        T7-T10 level S24.153 ☑
        T11-T12 level S24.154 ☑
      posterior cord syndrome S24.159 ☑
        T1 level S24.151 ☑
        T2-T6 level S24.152 ☑
        T7-T10 level S24.153 ☑
        T11-T12 level S24.154 ☑
      T1 level S24.101 ☑
      T2-T6 level S24.102 ☑
      T7-T10 level S24.103 ☑
      T11-T12 level S24.104 ☑
    splanchnic nerve — *see* Injury, nerve, lumbosacral, sympathetic
    spleen S36.00 ☑
      contusion S36.029 ☑
        major S36.021 ☑
        minor S36.020 ☑
      laceration S36.039 ☑
        major (massive) (stellate) S36.032 ☑
        moderate S36.031 ☑
        superficial (capsular) (minor) S36.030 ☑
      specified type NEC S36.09 ☑
    splenic artery — *see* Injury, blood vessel, celiac artery, branch
    stellate ganglion — *see* Injury, nerve, thorax, sympathetic
    sternal region S29.9 ☑
    stomach S36.30 ☑
      contusion S36.32 ☑
      laceration S36.33 ☑
      specified type NEC S36.39 ☑
    subconjunctival — *see* Injury, eye, conjunctiva
    subcutaneous NEC T14.8 ☑
    submaxillary region S09.93 ☑
    submental region S09.93 ☑
    subungual
      fingers — *see* Injury, hand
      toes — *see* Injury, foot
    superficial NEC T14.8 ☑
      abdomen, abdominal (wall) S30.92 ☑
        abrasion S30.811 ☑
        bite S30.871 ☑
          insect S30.861 ☑
        contusion S30.1 ☑
        external constriction S30.841 ☑
        foreign body S30.851 ☑
      abrasion — *see* Abrasion, by site
      adnexa, eye NEC — *see* Injury, eye, specified site NEC
      alveolar process — *see* Injury, superficial, oral cavity
      ankle S90.91- ☑
        abrasion — *see* Abrasion, ankle
        bite — *see* Bite, ankle
        blister — *see* Blister, ankle
        contusion — *see* Contusion, ankle
        external constriction — *see* Constriction, external, ankle
        foreign body — *see* Foreign body, superficial, ankle
      anus S30.98 ☑
      arm (upper) S40.92- ☑
        abrasion — *see* Abrasion, arm

Injury — *continued*
  superficial — *continued*
    arm — *continued*
      bite — *see* Bite, superficial, arm
      blister — *see* Blister, arm (upper)
      contusion — *see* Contusion, arm
      external constriction — *see* Constriction, external, arm
      foreign body — *see* Foreign body, superficial, arm
    auditory canal (external) (meatus) — *see* Injury, superficial, ear
    auricle — *see* Injury, superficial, ear
    axilla — *see* Injury, superficial, arm
    back (*see also* Injury, superficial, thorax, back)
      lower S30.91
        abrasion S30.810 ☑
        contusion S30.0 ☑
        external constriction S30.840 ☑
        superficial
          bite NEC S30.870 ☑
            insect S30.860 ☑
          foreign body S30.850 ☑
    bite NEC — *see* Bite, superficial NEC, by site
    blister — *see* Blister, by site
    breast S20.10- ☑
      abrasion — *see* Abrasion, breast
      bite — *see* Bite, superficial, breast
      contusion — *see* Contusion, breast
      external constriction — *see* Constriction, external, breast
      foreign body — *see* Foreign body, superficial, breast
    brow — *see* Injury, superficial, head, specified NEC
    buttock S30.91 ☑
    calf — *see* Injury, superficial, leg
    canthus, eye — *see* Injury, superficial, periocular area
    cheek (external) — *see* Injury, superficial, head, specified NEC
      internal — *see* Injury, superficial, oral cavity
    chest wall — *see* Injury, superficial, thorax
    chin — *see* Injury, superficial, head NEC
    clitoris S30.95 ☑
    conjunctiva — *see* Injury, eye, conjunctiva
      with foreign body (in conjunctival sac) — *see* Foreign body, conjunctival sac
    contusion — *see* Contusion, by site
    costal region — *see* Injury, superficial, thorax
    digit(s)
      hand — *see* Injury, superficial, finger
    ear (auricle) (canal) (external) S00.40- ☑
      abrasion — *see* Abrasion, ear
      bite — *see* Bite, superficial, ear
      contusion — *see* Contusion, ear
      external constriction — *see* Constriction, external, ear
      foreign body — *see* Foreign body, superficial, ear
    elbow S50.90- ☑
      abrasion — *see* Abrasion, elbow
      bite — *see* Bite, superficial, elbow
      blister — *see* Blister, elbow
      contusion — *see* Contusion, elbow
      external constriction — *see* Constriction, external, elbow
      foreign body — *see* Foreign body, superficial, elbow
    epididymis S30.94 ☑
    epigastric region S30.92 ☑
    epiglottis — *see* Injury, superficial, throat
    esophagus
      cervical — *see* Injury, superficial, throat
    external constriction — *see* Constriction, external, by site
    extremity NEC T14.8 ☑
    eyeball NEC — *see* Injury, eye, specified site NEC
    eyebrow — *see* Injury, superficial, periocular area
    eyelid S00.20- ☑
      abrasion — *see* Abrasion, eyelid
      bite — *see* Bite, superficial, eyelid
      contusion — *see* Contusion, eyelid
      external constriction — *see* Constriction, external, eyelid
      foreign body — *see* Foreign body, superficial, eyelid

☑ **Additional Character Required** — Refer to the Tabular List for Character Selection   ▽ **Subterms under main terms may continue to next column or page**

Injury — *continued*
  superficial — *continued*
    face NEC — *see* Injury, superficial, head, specified NEC
    finger(s) S60.949 ☑
      abrasion — *see* Abrasion, finger
      bite — *see* Bite, superficial, finger
      blister — *see* Blister, finger
      contusion — *see* Contusion, finger
      external constriction — *see* Constriction, external, finger
      foreign body — *see* Foreign body, superficial, finger
      index S60.94- ☑
      insect bite — *see* Bite, by site, superficial, insect
      little S60.94- ☑
      middle S60.94- ☑
      ring S60.94- ☑
    flank S30.92 ☑
    foot S90.92- ☑
      abrasion — *see* Abrasion, foot
      bite — *see* Bite, foot
      blister — *see* Blister, foot
      contusion — *see* Contusion, foot
      external constriction — *see* Constriction, external, foot
      foreign body — *see* Foreign body, superficial, foot
    forearm S50.91- ☑
      abrasion — *see* Abrasion, forearm
      bite — *see* Bite, forearm, superficial
      blister — *see* Blister, forearm
      contusion — *see* Contusion, forearm
      elbow only — *see* Injury, superficial, elbow
      external constriction — *see* Constriction, external, forearm
      foreign body — *see* Foreign body, superficial, forearm
    forehead — *see* Injury, superficial, head NEC
    foreign body — *see* Foreign body, superficial
    genital organs, external
      female S30.97 ☑
      male S30.96 ☑
    globe (eye) — *see* Injury, eye, specified site NEC
    groin S30.92 ☑
    gum — *see* Injury, superficial, oral cavity
    hand S60.92- ☑
      abrasion — *see* Abrasion, hand
      bite — *see* Bite, superficial, hand
      contusion — *see* Contusion, hand
      external constriction — *see* Constriction, external, hand
      foreign body — *see* Foreign body, superficial, hand
    head S00.90 ☑
      ear — *see* Injury, superficial, ear
      eyelid — *see* Injury, superficial, eyelid
      nose S00.30 ☑
      oral cavity S00.502 ☑
      scalp S00.00 ☑
      specified site NEC S00.80 ☑
    heel — *see* Injury, superficial, foot
    hip S70.91- ☑
      abrasion — *see* Abrasion, hip
      bite — *see* Bite, superficial, hip
      blister — *see* Blister, hip
      contusion — *see* Contusion, hip
      external constriction — *see* Constriction, external, hip
      foreign body — *see* Foreign body, superficial, hip
    iliac region — *see* Injury, superficial, abdomen
    inguinal region — *see* Injury, superficial, abdomen
    insect bite — *see* Bite, by site, superficial, insect
    interscapular region — *see* Injury, superficial, thorax, back
    jaw — *see* Injury, superficial, head, specified NEC
    knee S80.91- ☑
      abrasion — *see* Abrasion, knee
      bite — *see* Bite, superficial, knee
      blister — *see* Blister, knee
      contusion — *see* Contusion, knee
      external constriction — *see* Constriction, external, knee
      foreign body — *see* Foreign body, superficial, knee

Injury — *continued*
  superficial — *continued*
    labium (majus) (minus) S30.95 ☑
    lacrimal (apparatus) (gland) (sac) — *see* Injury, eye, specified site NEC
    larynx — *see* Injury, superficial, throat
    leg (lower) S80.92- ☑
      abrasion — *see* Abrasion, leg
      bite — *see* Bite, superficial, leg
      contusion — *see* Contusion, leg
      external constriction — *see* Constriction, external, leg
      foreign body — *see* Foreign body, superficial, leg
      knee — *see* Injury, superficial, knee
    limb NEC T14.8 ☑
    lip S00.501 ☑
    lower back S30.91 ☑
    lumbar region S30.91 ☑
    malar region — *see* Injury, superficial, head, specified NEC
    mammary — *see* Injury, superficial, breast
    mastoid region — *see* Injury, superficial, head, specified NEC
    mouth — *see* Injury, superficial, oral cavity
    muscle NEC T14.8 ☑
    nail NEC T14.8 ☑
      finger — *see* Injury, superficial, finger
      toe — *see* Injury, superficial, toe
    nasal (septum) — *see* Injury, superficial, nose
    neck S10.90 ☑
      specified site NEC S10.80 ☑
    nose (septum) S00.30 ☑
    occipital region — *see* Injury, superficial, scalp
    oral cavity S00.502 ☑
    orbital region — *see* Injury, superficial, periocular area
    palate — *see* Injury, superficial, oral cavity
    palm — *see* Injury, superficial, hand
    parietal region — *see* Injury, superficial, scalp
    pelvis S30.91 ☑
      girdle — *see* Injury, superficial, hip
    penis S30.93 ☑
    perineum
      female S30.95 ☑
      male S30.91 ☑
    periocular area S00.20- ☑
      abrasion — *see* Abrasion, eyelid
      bite — *see* Bite, superficial, eyelid
      contusion — *see* Contusion, eyelid
      external constriction — *see* Constriction, external, eyelid
      foreign body — *see* Foreign body, superficial, eyelid
    phalanges
      finger — *see* Injury, superficial, finger
      toe — *see* Injury, superficial, toe
    pharynx — *see* Injury, superficial, throat
    pinna — *see* Injury, superficial, ear
    popliteal space — *see* Injury, superficial, knee
    prepuce S30.93 ☑
    pubic region S30.91 ☑
    pudendum
      female S30.97 ☑
      male S30.96 ☑
    sacral region S30.91 ☑
    scalp S00.00 ☑
    scapular region — *see* Injury, superficial, shoulder
    sclera — *see* Injury, eye, specified site NEC
    scrotum S30.94 ☑
    shin — *see* Injury, superficial, leg
    shoulder S40.91- ☑
      abrasion — *see* Abrasion, shoulder
      bite — *see* Bite, superficial, shoulder
      blister — *see* Blister, shoulder
      contusion — *see* Contusion, shoulder
      external constriction — *see* Constriction, external, shoulder
      foreign body — *see* Foreign body, superficial, shoulder
    skin NEC T14.8 ☑
    sternal region — *see* Injury, superficial, thorax, front
    subconjunctival — *see* Injury, eye, specified site NEC
    subcutaneous NEC T14.8 ☑

Injury — *continued*
  superficial — *continued*
    submaxillary region — *see* Injury, superficial, head, specified NEC
    submental region — *see* Injury, superficial, head, specified NEC
    subungual
      finger(s) — *see* Injury, superficial, finger
      toe(s) — *see* Injury, superficial, toe
    supraclavicular fossa — *see* Injury, superficial, neck
    supraorbital — *see* Injury, superficial, head, specified NEC
    temple — *see* Injury, superficial, head, specified NEC
    temporal region — *see* Injury, superficial, head, specified NEC
    testis S30.94 ☑
    thigh S70.92- ☑
      abrasion — *see* Abrasion, thigh
      bite — *see* Bite, superficial, thigh
      blister — *see* Blister, thigh
      contusion — *see* Contusion, thigh
      external constriction — *see* Constriction, external, thigh
      foreign body — *see* Foreign body, superficial, thigh
    thorax, thoracic (wall) S20.90 ☑
      abrasion — *see* Abrasion, thorax
      back S20.40- ☑
      bite — *see* Bite, thorax, superficial
      blister — *see* Blister, thorax
      contusion — *see* Contusion, thorax
      external constriction — *see* Constriction, external, thorax
      foreign body — *see* Foreign body, superficial, thorax
      front S20.30- ☑
    throat S10.10 ☑
      abrasion S10.11 ☑
      bite S10.17 ☑
        insect S10.16 ☑
      blister S10.12 ☑
      contusion S10.0 ☑
      external constriction S10.14 ☑
      foreign body S10.15 ☑
    thumb S60.93- ☑
      abrasion — *see* Abrasion, thumb
      bite — *see* Bite, superficial, thumb
      blister — *see* Blister, thumb
      contusion — *see* Contusion, thumb
      external constriction — *see* Constriction, external, thumb
      foreign body — *see* Foreign body, superficial, thumb
      insect bite — *see* Bite, by site, superficial, insect
      specified type NEC S60.39 ☑
    toe(s) S90.93- ☑
      abrasion — *see* Abrasion, toe
      bite — *see* Bite, toe
      blister — *see* Blister, toe
      contusion — *see* Contusion, toe
      external constriction — *see* Constriction, external, toe
      foreign body — *see* Foreign body, superficial, toe
      great S90.93- ☑
    tongue — *see* Injury, superficial, oral cavity
    tooth, teeth — *see* Injury, superficial, oral cavity
    trachea S10.10 ☑
    tunica vaginalis S30.94 ☑
    tympanum, tympanic membrane — *see* Injury, superficial, ear
    uvula — *see* Injury, superficial, oral cavity
    vagina S30.95 ☑
    vocal cords — *see* Injury, superficial, throat
    vulva S30.95 ☑
    wrist S60.91- ☑
  supraclavicular region — *see* Injury, neck
  supraorbital S09.93 ☑
  suprarenal gland (multiple) — *see* Injury, adrenal
  surgical complication (external or internal site) — *see* Laceration, accidental complicating surgery
  temple S09.90 ☑
  temporal region S09.90 ☑
  tendon (*see also* Injury, muscle, by site)
    abdomen — *see* Injury, muscle, abdomen

Injury — continued
tendon (see also Injury, muscle, by site) — continued
Achilles — see Injury, Achilles tendon
lower back — see Injury, muscle, lower back
pelvic organs — see Injury, muscle, pelvis
tenth cranial nerve (pneumogastric or vagus) — see Injury, nerve, vagus
testis S39.94 ✓
thigh S79.92- ✓
blood vessel — see Injury, blood vessel, hip
contusion — see Contusion, thigh
fracture — see Fracture, femur
muscle — see Injury, muscle, thigh
nerve — see Injury, nerve, thigh
open — see Wound, open, thigh
specified NEC S79.82- ✓
superficial — see Injury, superficial, thigh
third cranial nerve (oculomotor) — see Injury, nerve, oculomotor
thorax, thoracic S29.9 ✓
blood vessel — see Injury, blood vessel, thorax
cavity — see Injury, intrathoracic
dislocation — see Dislocation, thorax
external (wall) S29.9 ✓
contusion — see Contusion, thorax
nerve — see Injury, nerve, thorax
open — see Wound, open, thorax
specified NEC S29.8 ✓
sprain — see Sprain, thorax
superficial — see Injury, superficial, thorax
fracture — see Fracture, thorax
internal — see Injury, intrathoracic
intrathoracic organ — see Injury, intrathoracic
sympathetic ganglion — see Injury, nerve, thorax, sympathetic
throat (see also Injury, neck) S19.9 ✓
thumb S69.9- ✓
blood vessel — see Injury, blood vessel, thumb
contusion — see Contusion, thumb
dislocation — see Dislocation, thumb
fracture — see Fracture, thumb
muscle — see Injury, muscle, thumb
nerve — see Injury, nerve, digital, thumb
open — see Wound, open, thumb
specified NEC S69.8- ✓
sprain — see Sprain, thumb
superficial — see Injury, superficial, thumb
thymus (gland) — see Injury, intrathoracic, specified organ NEC
thyroid (gland) NEC S19.84 ✓
toe S99.92- ✓
contusion — see Contusion, toe
dislocation — see Dislocation, toe
fracture — see Fracture, toe
muscle — see Injury, muscle, toe
open — see Wound, open, toe
specified type NEC S99.82- ✓
sprain — see Sprain, toe
superficial — see Injury, superficial, toe
tongue S09.93 ✓
tonsil S09.93 ✓
tooth S09.93 ✓
trachea (cervical) NEC S19.82 ✓
thoracic — see Injury, intrathoracic, trachea, thoracic
transfusion-related acute lung (TRALI) J95.84
tunica vaginalis S39.94 ✓
twelfth cranial nerve (hypoglossal) — see Injury, nerve, hypoglossal
ureter S37.10 ✓
contusion S37.12 ✓
laceration S37.13 ✓
specified type NEC S37.19 ✓
urethra (sphincter) S37.30 ✓
at delivery O71.5
contusion S37.32 ✓
laceration S37.33 ✓
specified type NEC S37.39 ✓
urinary organ S37.90 ✓
contusion S37.92 ✓
laceration S37.93 ✓
specified
site NEC S37.899 ✓
contusion S37.892 ✓
laceration S37.893 ✓

Injury — continued
urinary organ — continued
specified — continued
site — continued
specified type NEC S37.898 ✓
type NEC S37.99 ✓
uterus, uterine S37.60 ✓
with ectopic or molar pregnancy O08.6
blood vessel — see Injury, blood vessel, iliac
contusion S37.62 ✓
laceration S37.63 ✓
cervix at delivery O71.3
rupture associated with obstetrics — see Rupture, uterus
specified type NEC S37.69 ✓
uvula S09.93 ✓
vagina S39.93 ✓
abrasion S30.814 ✓
bite S31.45 ✓
insect S30.864 ✓
superficial NEC S30.874 ✓
contusion S30.23 ✓
crush S38.03 ✓
during delivery — see Laceration, vagina, during delivery
external constriction S30.844 ✓
insect bite S30.864 ✓
laceration S31.41 ✓
with foreign body S31.42 ✓
open wound S31.40 ✓
puncture S31.43 ✓
with foreign body S31.44 ✓
superficial S30.95 ✓
foreign body S30.854 ✓
vas deferens — see Injury, pelvic organ, specified site NEC
vascular NEC T14.8 ✓
vein — see Injury, blood vessel
vena cava (superior) S25.20 ✓
inferior S35.10 ✓
laceration (minor) (superficial) S35.11 ✓
major S35.12 ✓
specified type NEC S35.19 ✓
laceration (minor) (superficial) S25.21 ✓
major S25.22 ✓
specified type NEC S25.29 ✓
vesical (sphincter) — see Injury, bladder
visual cortex S04.04- ✓
vitreous (humor) S05.90 ✓
specified NEC S05.8X- ✓
vocal cord NEC S19.83 ✓
vulva S39.94 ✓
abrasion S30.814 ✓
bite S31.45 ✓
insect S30.864 ✓
superficial NEC S30.874 ✓
contusion S30.23 ✓
crush S38.03 ✓
during delivery — see Laceration, perineum, female, during delivery
external constriction S30.844 ✓
insect bite S30.864 ✓
laceration S31.41 ✓
with foreign body S31.42 ✓
open wound S31.40 ✓
puncture S31.43 ✓
with foreign body S31.44 ✓
superficial S30.95 ✓
foreign body S30.854 ✓
whiplash (cervical spine) S13.4 ✓
wrist S69.9- ✓
blood vessel — see Injury, blood vessel, hand
contusion — see Contusion, wrist
dislocation — see Dislocation, wrist
fracture — see Fracture, wrist
muscle — see Injury, muscle, hand
nerve — see Injury, nerve, hand
open — see Wound, open, wrist
specified NEC S69.8- ✓
sprain — see Sprain, wrist
superficial — see Injury, superficial, wrist
Inoculation (see also Vaccination)
complication or reaction — see Complications, vaccination
Insanity, insane (see also Psychosis)
adolescent — see Schizophrenia

Insanity, insane — continued
confusional F28
acute or subacute F05
delusional F22
senile F03 ✓
Insect
bite — see Bite, by site, superficial, insect
venomous, poisoning NEC (by) — see Venom, arthropod
Insensitivity
adrenocorticotropin hormone (ACTH) E27.49
androgen E34.50
complete E34.51
partial E34.52
Insertion
cord (umbilical) lateral or velamentous O43.12- ✓
intrauterine contraceptive device (encounter for) — see Intrauterine contraceptive device
Insolation (sunstroke) T67.0 ✓
Insomnia (organic) G47.00
without objective findings F51.02
adjustment F51.02
adjustment disorder F51.02
behavioral, of childhood Z73.819
combined type Z73.812
limit setting type Z73.811
sleep-onset association type Z73.810
childhood Z73.819
chronic F51.04
somatized tension F51.04
conditioned F51.04
due to
alcohol
abuse F10.182
dependence F10.282
use F10.982
amphetamines
abuse F15.182
dependence F15.282
use F15.982
anxiety disorder F51.05
caffeine
abuse F15.182
dependence F15.282
use F15.982
cocaine
abuse F14.182
dependence F14.282
use F14.982
depression F51.05
drug NEC
abuse F19.182
dependence F19.282
use F19.982
medical condition G47.01
mental disorder NEC F51.05
opioid
abuse F11.182
dependence F11.282
use F11.982
psychoactive substance NEC
abuse F19.182
dependence F19.182
use F19.982
sedative, hypnotic, or anxiolytic
abuse F13.182
dependence F13.282
use F13.982
stimulant NEC
abuse F15.182
dependence F15.282
use F15.982
fatal familial (FFI) A81.83
idiopathic F51.01
learned F51.3
nonorganic origin F51.01
not due to a substance or known physiological condition F51.01
specified NEC F51.09
paradoxical F51.03
primary F51.01
psychiatric F51.05
psychophysiologic F51.04
related to psychopathology F51.05
short-term F51.02
specified NEC G47.09
stress-related F51.02
transient F51.02

✓ **Additional Character Required** — Refer to the Tabular List for Character Selection   ▽ **Subterms under main terms may continue to next column or page**

Inspiration
  food or foreign body — *see* Foreign body, by site
  mucus — *see* Asphyxia, mucus
Inspissated bile syndrome (newborn) P59.1
Instability
  emotional (excessive) F60.3
  joint (post-traumatic) M25.30
    ankle M25.37- ☑
    due to old ligament injury — *see* Disorder, liga-
      ment
    elbow M25.32- ☑
    flail — *see* Flail, joint
    foot M25.37- ☑
    hand M25.34- ☑
    hip M25.35- ☑
    knee M25.36- ☑
    lumbosacral — *see* subcategory M53.2 ☑
    prosthesis — *see* Complications, joint prosthesis,
      mechanical, displacement, by site
    sacroiliac — *see* subcategory M53.2 ☑
    secondary to
      old ligament injury — *see* Disorder, ligament
      removal of joint prosthesis M96.89
    shoulder (region) M25.31- ☑
    spine — *see* subcategory M53.2 ☑
    wrist M25.33- ☑
  knee (chronic) M23.5- ☑
  lumbosacral — *see* subcategory M53.2 ☑
  nervous F48.8
  personality (emotional) F60.3
  spine — *see* Instability, joint, spine
  vasomotor R55
Institutional syndrome (childhood) F94.2
Institutionalization, affecting child Z62.22
  disinhibited attachment F94.2
Insufficiency, insufficient
  accommodation, old age H52.4
  adrenal (gland) E27.40
    primary E27.1
  adrenocortical E27.40
    drug-induced E27.3
    iatrogenic E27.3
    primary E27.1
  anatomic crown height K08.89
  anterior (occlusal) guidance M26.54
  anus K62.89
  aortic (valve) I35.1
    with
      mitral (valve) disease I08.0
        with tricuspid (valve) disease I08.3
      stenosis I35.2
      tricuspid (valve) disease I08.2
        with mitral (valve) disease I08.3
    congenital Q23.1
    rheumatic I06.1
      with
        mitral (valve) disease I08.0
          with tricuspid (valve) disease I08.3
        stenosis I06.2
          with mitral (valve) disease I08.0
            with tricuspid (valve) disease I08.3
        tricuspid (valve) disease I08.2
          with mitral (valve) disease I08.3
    specified cause NEC I35.1
    syphilitic A52.03
  arterial I77.1
    basilar G45.0
    carotid (hemispheric) G45.1
    cerebral I67.81
    coronary (acute or subacute) I24.8
    mesenteric K55.1
    peripheral I73.9
    precerebral (multiple) (bilateral) G45.2
    vertebral G45.0
  arteriovenous I99.8
  biliary K83.8
  cardiac (*see also* Insufficiency, myocardial)
    due to presence of (cardiac) prosthesis I97.11- ☑
      postprocedural I97.11- ☑
  cardiorenal, hypertensive I13.2
  cardiovascular — *see* Disease, cardiovascular
  cerebrovascular (acute) I67.81
    with transient focal neurological signs and symp-
      toms G45.8
  circulatory NEC I99.8
    newborn P29.89
  clinical crown length K08.89
  convergence H51.11

Insufficiency, insufficient — *continued*
  coronary (acute or subacute) I24.8
    chronic or with a stated duration of over 4 weeks
      I25.89
  corticoadrenal E27.40
    primary E27.1
  dietary E63.9
  divergence H51.8
  food T73.0 ☑
  gastroesophageal K22.8
  gonadal
    ovary E28.39
    testis E29.1
  heart (*see also* Insufficiency, myocardial)
    newborn P29.0
    valve — *see* Endocarditis
  hepatic — *see* Failure, hepatic
  idiopathic autonomic G90.09
  interocclusal distance of fully erupted teeth (ridge)
    M26.36
  kidney N28.9
    acute N28.9
    chronic N18.9
  lacrimal (secretion) H04.12- ☑
    passages — *see* Stenosis, lacrimal
  liver — *see* Failure, hepatic
  lung — *see* Insufficiency, pulmonary
  mental (congenital) — *see* Disability, intellectual
  mesenteric K55.1
  mitral (valve) I34.0
    with
      aortic valve disease I08.0
        with tricuspid (valve) disease I08.3
      obstruction or stenosis I05.2
        with aortic valve disease I08.0
      tricuspid (valve) disease I08.1
        with aortic (valve) disease I08.3
    congenital Q23.3
    rheumatic I05.1
      with
        aortic valve disease I08.0
          with tricuspid (valve) disease I08.3
        obstruction or stenosis I05.2
          with aortic valve disease I08.0
            with tricuspid (valve) disease I08.3
        tricuspid (valve) disease I08.1
          with aortic (valve) disease I08.3
      active or acute I01.1
        with chorea, rheumatic (Sydenham's) I02.0
    specified cause, except rheumatic I34.0
  muscle (*see also* Disease, muscle)
    heart — *see* Insufficiency, myocardial
    ocular NEC H50.9
  myocardial, myocardium (with arteriosclerosis) (*see
    also* Failure, heart) I50.9
    with
      rheumatic fever (conditions in I00) I09.0
        active, acute or subacute I01.2
          with chorea I02.0
        inactive or quiescent (with chorea) I09.0
    congenital Q24.8
    hypertensive — *see* Hypertension, heart
    newborn P29.0
    rheumatic I09.0
      active, acute, or subacute I01.2
    syphilitic A52.06
  nourishment T73.0 ☑
  pancreatic K86.89
    exocrine K86.81
  parathyroid (gland) E20.9
  peripheral vascular (arterial) I73.9
  pituitary E23.0
  placental (mother) O36.51- ☑
  platelets D69.6
  prenatal care affecting management of pregnancy
    O09.3- ☑
  progressive pluriglandular E31.0
  pulmonary J98.4
    acute, following surgery (nonthoracic) J95.2
      thoracic J95.1
    chronic, following surgery J95.3
    following
      shock J98.4
      trauma J98.4
    newborn P28.5
    valve I37.1
      with stenosis I37.2
      congenital Q22.2

Insufficiency, insufficient — *continued*
  pulmonary — *continued*
    valve — *continued*
      rheumatic I09.89
        with aortic, mitral or tricuspid (valve) disease
          I08.8
  pyloric K31.89
  renal (acute) N28.9
    chronic N18.9
  respiratory R06.89
    newborn P28.5
  rotation — *see* Malrotation
  sleep syndrome F51.12
  social insurance Z59.7
  suprarenal E27.40
    primary E27.1
  tarso-orbital fascia, congenital Q10.3
  testis E29.1
  thyroid (gland) (acquired) E03.9
    congenital E03.1
  tricuspid (valve) (rheumatic) I07.1
    with
      aortic (valve) disease I08.2
        with mitral (valve) disease I08.3
      mitral (valve) disease I08.1
        with aortic (valve) disease I08.3
      obstruction or stenosis I07.2
        with aortic (valve) disease I08.2
          with mitral (valve) disease I08.3
    congenital Q22.8
    nonrheumatic I36.1
      with stenosis I36.2
  urethral sphincter R32
  valve, valvular (heart) I38
    aortic — *see* Insufficiency, aortic (valve)
    congenital Q24.8
    mitral — *see* Insufficiency, mitral (valve)
    pulmonary — *see* Insufficiency, pulmonary, valve
    tricuspid — *see* Insufficiency, tricuspid (valve)
  vascular I99.8
    intestine K55.9
      acute (*see also* Ischemia, intestine, acute)
        K55.059
    mesenteric K55.1
    peripheral I73.9
    renal — *see* Hypertension, kidney
  velopharyngeal
    acquired K13.79
    congenital Q38.8
  venous (chronic) (peripheral) I87.2
  ventricular — *see* Insufficiency, myocardial
  welfare support Z59.7
Insufflation, fallopian Z31.41
Insular — *see* condition
Insulinoma
  pancreas
    benign D13.7
    malignant C25.4
    uncertain behavior D37.8
  specified site
    benign — *see* Neoplasm, by site, benign
    malignant — *see* Neoplasm, by site, malignant
    uncertain behavior — *see* Neoplasm, by site, uncer-
      tain behavior
  unspecified site
    benign D13.7
    malignant C25.4
    uncertain behavior D37.8
Insuloma — *see* Insulinoma
Interference
  balancing side M26.56
  non-working side M26.56
Intermenstrual — *see* condition
Intermittent — *see* condition
Internal — *see* condition
Interrogation
  cardiac defibrillator (automatic) (implantable) Z45.02
  cardiac pacemaker Z45.018
  cardiac (event) (loop) recorder Z45.09
  infusion pump (implanted) (intrathecal) Z45.1
  neurostimulator Z46.2
Interruption
  aortic arch Q25.21
  bundle of His I44.30
  phase-shift, sleep cycle — *see* Disorder, sleep, circadian
    rhythm
  sleep phase-shift, or 24 hour sleep-wake cycle — *see*
    Disorder, sleep, circadian rhythm

▼ Subterms under main terms may continue to next column or page   ☑ Additional Character Required — Refer to the Tabular List for Character Selection

Interstitial — *see* condition
Intertrigo L30.4
  labialis K13.0
Intervertebral disc — *see* condition
Intestine, intestinal — *see* condition
Intolerance
  carbohydrate K90.49
  disaccharide, hereditary E73.0
  fat NEC K90.49
    pancreatic K90.3
  food K90.49
    dietary counseling and surveillance Z71.3
  fructose E74.10
    hereditary E74.12
  glucose (-galactose) E74.39
  gluten K90.41
  lactose E73.9
    specified NEC E73.8
  lysine E72.3
  milk NEC K90.49
    lactose E73.9
  protein K90.49
  starch NEC K90.49
  sucrose (-isomaltose) E74.31
Intoxicated NEC (without dependence) — *see* Alcohol, intoxication
Intoxication
  acid E87.2
  alcoholic (acute) (without dependence) — *see* Alcohol, intoxication
  alimentary canal K52.1
  amphetamine (without dependence) — *see* Abuse, drug, stimulant, with intoxication
    with dependence — *see* Dependence, drug, stimulant, with intoxication
  anxiolytic (acute) (without dependence) — *see* Abuse, drug, sedative, with intoxication
    with dependence — *see* Dependence, drug, sedative, with intoxication
  caffeine F15.929
    with dependence — *see* Dependence, drug, stimulant, with intoxication
  cannabinoids (acute) (without dependence) — *see* Use, cannabis, with intoxication
    with
      abuse — *see* Abuse, drug, cannabis, with intoxication
      dependence — *see* Dependence, drug, cannabis, with intoxication
  chemical — *see* Table of Drugs and Chemicals
    via placenta or breast milk — *see* - Absorption, chemical, through placenta
  cocaine (acute) (without dependence) — *see* Abuse, drug, cocaine, with intoxication
    with dependence — *see* Dependence, drug, cocaine, with intoxication
  drug
    acute (without dependence) — *see* Abuse, drug, by type with intoxication
      with dependence — *see* Dependence, drug, by type with intoxication
    addictive
      via placenta or breast milk — *see* Absorption, drug, addictive, through placenta
    newborn P93.8
      gray baby syndrome P93.0
    overdose or wrong substance given or taken — *see* Table of Drugs and Chemicals, by drug, poisoning
  enteric K52.1
  foodborne A05.9
    bacterial A05.9
    classical (Clostridium botulinum) A05.1
    due to
      Bacillus cereus A05.4
      bacterium A05.9
        specified NEC A05.8
      Clostridium
        botulinum A05.1
        perfringens A05.2
        welchii A05.2
      Salmonella A02.9
        with
          (gastro)enteritis A02.0
          localized infection(s) A02.20
            arthritis A02.23
            meningitis A02.21
            osteomyelitis A02.24

Intoxication — *continued*
  foodborne — *continued*
    due to — *continued*
      Salmonella — *continued*
        with — *continued*
          localized infection(s) — *continued*
            pneumonia A02.22
            pyelonephritis A02.25
            specified NEC A02.29
          sepsis A02.1
          specified manifestation NEC A02.8
      Staphylococcus A05.0
      Vibrio
        parahaemolyticus A05.3
        vulnificus A05.5
    enterotoxin, staphylococcal A05.0
    noxious — *see* Poisoning, food, noxious
  gastrointestinal K52.1
  hallucinogenic (without dependence) — *see* Abuse, drug, hallucinogen, with intoxication
    with dependence — *see* Dependence, drug, hallucinogen, with intoxication
  hypnotic (acute) (without dependence) — *see* Abuse, drug, sedative, with intoxication
    with dependence — *see* Dependence, drug, sedative, with intoxication
  inhalant (acute) (without dependence) — *see* Abuse, drug, inhalant, with intoxication
    with dependence — *see* Dependence, drug, inhalant, with intoxication
  meaning
    inebriation — *see* category F10 ☑
    poisoning — *see* Table of Drugs and Chemicals
  methyl alcohol (acute) (without dependence) — *see* Alcohol, intoxication
  opioid (acute) (without dependence) — *see* Abuse, drug, opioid, with intoxication
    with dependence — *see* Dependence, drug, opioid, with intoxication
  pathologic NEC (without dependence) — *see* Alcohol, intoxication
  phencyclidine (without dependence) — *see* Abuse, drug, hallucinogen, with intoxication
    with dependence — *see* Dependence, drug, hallucinogen, with intoxication
  potassium (K) E87.5
  psychoactive substance NEC (without dependence) — *see* Abuse, drug, psychoactive NEC, with intoxication
    with dependence — *see* Dependence, drug, psychoactive NEC, with intoxication
  sedative (acute) (without dependence) — *see* Abuse, drug, sedative, with intoxication
    with dependence — *see* Dependence, drug, sedative, with intoxication
  serum (*see also* Reaction, serum) T80.69 ☑
  uremic — *see* Uremia
  volatile solvents (acute) (without dependence) — *see* Abuse, drug, inhalant, with intoxication
    with dependence — *see* Dependence, drug, inhalant, with intoxication
  water E87.79
Intraabdominal testis, testes
  bilateral Q53.211
  unilateral Q53.111
Intracranial — *see* condition
Intrahepatic gallbladder Q44.1
Intraligamentous — *see* condition
Intrathoracic (*see also* condition)
  kidney Q63.2
Intrauterine contraceptive device
  checking Z30.431
  in situ Z97.5
  insertion Z30.430
    immediately following removal Z30.433
  management Z30.431
  reinsertion Z30.433
  removal Z30.432
  replacement Z30.433
  retention in pregnancy O26.3- ☑
Intraventricular — *see* condition
Intrinsic deformity — *see* Deformity
Intubation, difficult or failed T88.4 ☑
Intumescence, lens (eye) (cataract) — *see* Cataract
Intussusception (bowel) (colon) (enteric) (ileocecal) (ileocolic) (intestine) (rectum) K56.1
  appendix K38.8
  congenital Q43.8

Intussusception — *continued*
  ureter (with obstruction) N13.5
Invagination (bowel, colon, intestine or rectum) K56.1
Inversion
  albumin-globulin (A-G) ratio E88.09
  bladder N32.89
  cecum — *see* Intussusception
  cervix N88.8
  chromosome in normal individual Q95.1
  circadian rhythm — *see* Disorder, sleep, circadian rhythm
  nipple N64.59
    congenital Q83.8
    gestational — *see* Retraction, nipple
    puerperal, postpartum — *see* Retraction, nipple
  nyctohemeral rhythm — *see* Disorder, sleep, circadian rhythm
  optic papilla Q14.2
  organ or site, congenital NEC — *see* Anomaly, by site
  sleep rhythm — *see* Disorder, sleep, circadian rhythm
  testis (congenital) Q55.29
  uterus (chronic) (postinfectional) (postpartal, old) N85.5
    postpartum O71.2
  vagina (posthysterectomy) N99.3
  ventricular Q20.5
Investigation (*see also* Examination) Z04.9
  clinical research subject (control) (normal comparison) (participant) Z00.6
Involuntary movement, abnormal R25.9
Involution, involutional (*see also* condition)
  breast, cystic — *see* Dysplasia, mammary, specified type NEC
  depression (single episode) F32.89
    recurrent episode F33.9
  melancholia (single episode) F32.89
    recurrent episode F33.8
  ovary, senile — *see* Atrophy, ovary
  thymus failure E32.8
I.Q.
  under 20 F73
  20-34 F72
  35-49 F71
  50-69 F70
IRDS (type I) P22.0
  type II P22.1
Irideremia Q13.1
Iridis rubeosis — *see* Disorder, iris, vascular
Iridochoroiditis (panuveitis) — *see* Panuveitis
Iridocyclitis H20.9
  acute H20.0-
    hypopyon H20.05- ☑
    primary H20.01- ☑
    recurrent H20.02- ☑
    secondary (noninfectious) H20.04- ☑
      infectious H20.03- ☑
  chronic H20.1- ☑
  due to allergy — *see* Iridocyclitis, acute, secondary
  endogenous — *see* Iridocyclitis, acute, primary
  Fuchs' — *see* Cyclitis, Fuchs' heterochromic
  gonococcal A54.32
  granulomatous — *see* Iridocyclitis, chronic
  herpes, herpetic (simplex) B00.51
    zoster B02.32
  hypopyon — *see* Iridocyclitis, acute, hypopyon
  in (due to)
    ankylosing spondylitis M45.9
    gonococcal infection A54.32
    herpes (simplex) virus B00.51
      zoster B02.32
    infectious disease NOS B99 ☑
    parasitic disease NOS B89 [H22]
    sarcoidosis D86.83
    syphilis A51.43
    tuberculosis A18.54
    zoster B02.32
  lens-induced H20.2- ☑
  nongranulomatous — *see* Iridocyclitis, acute
  recurrent — *see* Iridocyclitis, acute, recurrent
  rheumatic — *see* Iridocyclitis, chronic
  subacute — *see* Iridocyclitis, acute
  sympathetic — *see* Uveitis, sympathetic
  syphilitic (secondary) A51.43
  tuberculous (chronic) A18.54
  Vogt-Koyanagi H20.82- ☑
Iridocyclochoroiditis (panuveitis) — *see* Panuveitis
Iridodialysis H21.53- ☑

Iridodonesis H21.89
Iridoplegia (complete) (partial) (reflex) H57.09
Iridoschisis H21.25- ☑
Iris (see also condition)
  bombé — see Membrane, pupillary
Iritis (see also Iridocyclitis)
  chronic — see Iridocyclitis, chronic
  diabetic — see E08-E13 with .39
  due to
    herpes simplex B00.51
    leprosy A30.9 [H22]
  gonococcal A54.32
  gouty (see also Gout, by type) M10.9 [H22]
  granulomatous — see Iridocyclitis, chronic
  lens induced — see Iridocyclitis, lens-induced
  papulosa (syphilitic) A52.71
  rheumatic — see Iridocyclitis, chronic
  syphilitic (secondary) A51.43
    congenital (early) A50.01
    late A52.71
  tuberculous A18.54
Iron — see condition
Iron-miner's lung J63.4
Irradiated enamel (tooth, teeth) K03.89
Irradiation effects, adverse T66 ☑
Irreducible, irreducibility — see condition
Irregular, irregularity
  action, heart I49.9
  alveolar process K08.89
  bleeding N92.6
  breathing R06.89
  contour of cornea (acquired) — see Deformity, cornea
    congenital Q13.4
  contour, reconstructed breast N65.0
  dentin (in pulp) K04.3
  eye movements H55.89
    nystagmus — see Nystagmus
    saccadic H55.81
  labor O62.2
  menstruation (cause unknown) N92.6
  periods N92.6
  prostate N42.9
  pupil — see Abnormality, pupillary
  reconstructed breast N65.0
  respiratory R06.89
  septum (nasal) J34.2
  shape, organ or site, congenital NEC — see Distortion
  sleep-wake pattern (rhythm) G47.23
Irritable, irritability R45.4
  bladder N32.89
  bowel (syndrome) K58.9
    with
      constipation K58.1
      diarrhea K58.0
    mixed K58.2
    psychogenic F45.8
    specified NEC K58.8
  bronchial — see Bronchitis
  cerebral, in newborn P91.3
  colon (see also Irritable, bowel) K58.9
    with diarrhea K58.0
    psychogenic F45.8
  duodenum K59.8
  heart (psychogenic) F45.8
  hip — see Derangement, joint, specified type NEC, hip
  ileum K59.8
  infant R68.12
  jejunum K59.8
  rectum K59.8
  stomach K31.89
    psychogenic F45.8
  sympathetic G90.8
  urethra N36.8
Irritation
  anus K62.89
  axillary nerve G54.0
  bladder N32.89
  brachial plexus G54.0
  bronchial — see Bronchitis
  cervical plexus G54.2
  cervix — see Cervicitis
  choroid, sympathetic — see Endophthalmitis
  cranial nerve — see Disorder, nerve, cranial
  gastric K31.89
    psychogenic F45.8
  globe, sympathetic — see Uveitis, sympathetic
  labyrinth — see subcategory H83.2 ☑
  lumbosacral plexus G54.1

Irritation — continued
  meninges (traumatic) — see Injury, intracranial
    nontraumatic — see Meningismus
  nerve — see Disorder, nerve
  nervous R45.0
  penis N48.89
  perineum NEC L29.3
  peripheral autonomic nervous system G90.8
  peritoneum — see Peritonitis
  pharynx J39.2
  plantar nerve — see Lesion, nerve, plantar
  spinal (cord) (traumatic) (see also Injury, spinal cord, by region)
    nerve G58.9
      root NEC — see Radiculopathy
    nontraumatic — see Myelopathy
  stomach K31.89
    psychogenic F45.8
  sympathetic nerve NEC G90.8
  ulnar nerve — see Lesion, nerve, ulnar
  vagina N89.8
Ischemia, ischemic I99.8
  bowel (transient)
    acute (see also Ischemia, intestine, acute) K55.059
    chronic K55.1
    due to mesenteric artery insufficiency K55.1
  brain — see Ischemia, cerebral
  cardiac (see Disease, heart, ischemic)
  cardiomyopathy I25.5
  cerebral (chronic) (generalized) I67.82
    arteriosclerotic I67.2
    intermittent G45.9
    newborn P91.0
    recurrent focal G45.8
    transient G45.9
  colon chronic (due to mesenteric artery insufficiency) K55.1
  coronary — see Disease, heart, ischemic
  demand (coronary) (see also Angina) I24.8
    with myocardial infarction I21.A1
    resulting in myocardial infarction I21.A1
  heart (chronic or with a stated duration of over 4 weeks) I25.9
    acute or with a stated duration of 4 weeks or less I24.9
    subacute I24.9
  infarction, muscle — see Infarct, muscle
  intestine (large) (small) (transient) K55.9
    acute K55.059
      diffuse K55.052
      focal K55.051
      large K55.039
        diffuse K55.032
        focal K55.031
      small K55.019
        diffuse K55.012
        focal K55.011
    chronic K55.1
    due to mesenteric artery insufficiency K55.1
  kidney N28.0
  mesenteric, acute (see also Ischemia, intestine, acute) K55.059
  muscle, traumatic T79.6 ☑
  myocardium, myocardial (chronic or with a stated duration of over 4 weeks) I25.9
    acute, without myocardial infarction I51.3
    silent (asymptomatic) I25.6
    transient of newborn P29.4
  renal N28.0
  retina, retinal — see Occlusion, artery, retina
  small bowel
    acute K55.019
      diffuse K55.012
      focal K55.011
    chronic K55.1
    due to mesenteric artery insufficiency K55.1
  spinal cord G95.11
  subendocardial — see Insufficiency, coronary
  supply (coronary) (see also Angina) I25.9
    due to vasospasm I20.1
Ischial spine — see condition
Ischialgia — see Sciatica
Ischiopagus Q89.4
Ischium, ischial — see condition
Ischuria R34
Iselin's disease or osteochondrosis — see Osteochondrosis, juvenile, metatarsus

Islands of
  parotid tissue in
    lymph nodes Q38.6
    neck structures Q38.6
  submaxillary glands in
    fascia Q38.6
    lymph nodes Q38.6
    neck muscles Q38.6
Islet cell tumor, pancreas D13.7
Isoimmunization NEC (see also Incompatibility)
  affecting management of pregnancy (ABO) (with hydrops fetalis) O36.11- ☑
    anti-A sensitization O36.11- ☑
    anti-B sensitization O36.19- ☑
    anti-c sensitization O36.09- ☑
    anti-C sensitization O36.09- ☑
    anti-e sensitization O36.09- ☑
    anti-E sensitization O36.09- ☑
    Rh NEC O36.09- ☑
      anti-D antibody O36.01- ☑
    specified NEC O36.19- ☑
  newborn P55.9
    with
      hydrops fetalis P56.0
      kernicterus P57.0
    ABO (blood groups) P55.1
    Rhesus (Rh) factor P55.0
    specified type NEC P55.8
Isolation, isolated
  dwelling Z59.8
  family Z63.79
  social Z60.4
Isoleucinosis E71.19
Isomerism atrial appendages (with asplenia or polysplenia) Q20.6
Isosporiasis, isosporosis A07.3
Isovaleric acidemia E71.110
Issue of
  medical certificate Z02.79
    for disability determination Z02.71
  repeat prescription (appliance) (glasses) (medicinal substance, medicament, medicine) Z76.0
    contraception — see Contraception
Itch, itching (see also Pruritus)
  baker's L23.6
  barber's B35.0
  bricklayer's L24.5
  cheese B88.0
  clam digger's B65.3
  coolie B76.9
  copra B88.0
  dew B76.9
  dhobi B35.6
  filarial — see Infestation, filarial
  grain B88.0
  grocer's B88.0
  ground B76.9
  harvest B88.0
  jock B35.6
  Malabar B35.5
    beard B35.0
    foot B35.3
    scalp B35.0
  meaning scabies B86
  Norwegian B86
  perianal L29.0
  poultrymen's B88.0
  sarcoptic B86
  scabies B86
  scrub B88.0
  straw B88.0
  swimmer's B65.3
  water B76.9
  winter L29.8
Ivemark's syndrome (asplenia with congenital heart disease) Q89.01
Ivory bones Q78.2
Ixodiasis NEC B88.8

J

Jaccoud's syndrome — see Arthropathy, postrheumatic, chronic
Jackson's
  membrane Q43.3
  paralysis or syndrome G83.89
  veil Q43.3
Jacquet's dermatitis (diaper dermatitis) L22

Jadassohn-Pellizari's disease or anetoderma L90.2
Jadassohn's
  blue nevus — *see* Nevus
  intraepidermal epithelioma — *see* Neoplasm, skin, benign
Jaffe-Lichtenstein (-Uehlinger) **syndrome** — *see* Dysplasia, fibrous, bone NEC
Jakob-Creutzfeldt disease or syndrome — *see* Creutzfeldt-Jakob disease or syndrome
Jaksch-Luzet disease D64.89
Jamaican
  neuropathy G92
  paraplegic tropical ataxic-spastic syndrome G92
Janet's disease F48.8
Janiceps Q89.4
Jansky-Bielschowsky amaurotic idiocy E75.4
Japanese
  B-type encephalitis A83.0
  river fever A75.3
Jaundice (yellow) R17
  acholuric (familial) (splenomegalic) (*see also* Spherocytosis)
    acquired D59.8
  breast-milk (inhibitor) P59.3
  catarrhal (acute) B15.9
    with hepatic coma B15.0
  cholestatic (benign) R17
  due to or associated with
    delayed conjugation P59.8
      associated with (due to) preterm delivery P59.0
    preterm delivery P59.0
  epidemic (catarrhal) B15.9
    with hepatic coma B15.0
    leptospiral A27.0
    spirochetal A27.0
  familial nonhemolytic (congenital) (Gilbert) E80.4
    Crigler-Najjar E80.5
  febrile (acute) B15.9
    with hepatic coma B15.0
    leptospiral A27.0
    spirochetal A27.0
  hematogenous D59.9
  hemolytic (acquired) D59.9
    congenital — *see* Spherocytosis
  hemorrhagic (acute) (leptospiral) (spirochetal) A27.0
  infectious (acute) (subacute) B15.9
    with hepatic coma B15.0
    leptospiral A27.0
    spirochetal A27.0
  leptospiral (hemorrhagic) A27.0
  malignant (without coma) K72.90
    with coma K72.91
  neonatal — *see* Jaundice, newborn
  newborn P59.9
    due to or associated with
      ABO
        antibodies P55.1
        incompatibility, maternal/fetal P55.1
        isoimmunization P55.1
      absence or deficiency of enzyme system for bilirubin conjugation (congenital) P59.8
      bleeding P58.1
      breast milk inhibitors to conjugation P59.3
        associated with preterm delivery P59.0
      bruising P58.0
      Crigler-Najjar syndrome E80.5
      delayed conjugation P59.8
        associated with preterm delivery P59.0
      drugs or toxins
        given to newborn P58.42
        transmitted from mother P58.41
      excessive hemolysis P58.9
        due to
          bleeding P58.1
          bruising P58.0
          drugs or toxins
            given to newborn P58.42
            transmitted from mother P58.41
          infection P58.2
          polycythemia P58.3
          swallowed maternal blood P58.5
        specified type NEC P58.8
      galactosemia E74.21
      Gilbert syndrome E80.4
      hemolytic disease P55.9
        ABO isoimmunization P55.1
        Rh isoimmunization P55.0
        specified NEC P55.8

Jaundice — *continued*
  newborn — *continued*
    due to or associated with — *continued*
      hepatocellular damage P59.20
        specified NEC P59.29
      hereditary hemolytic anemia P58.8
      hypothyroidism, congenital E03.1
      incompatibility, maternal/fetal NOS P55.9
      infection P58.2
      inspissated bile syndrome P59.1
      isoimmunization NOS P55.9
      mucoviscidosis E84.9
      polycythemia P58.3
      preterm delivery P59.0
      Rh
        antibodies P55.0
        incompatibility, maternal/fetal P55.0
        isoimmunization P55.0
      specified cause NEC P59.8
      swallowed maternal blood P58.5
    spherocytosis (congenital) D58.0
  nonhemolytic congenital familial (Gilbert) E80.4
  nuclear, newborn (*see also* Kernicterus of newborn) P57.9
  obstructive (*see also* Obstruction, bile duct) K83.1
  post-immunization — *see* Hepatitis, viral, type, B
  post-transfusion — *see* Hepatitis, viral, type, B
  regurgitation (*see also* Obstruction, bile duct) K83.1
  serum (homologous) (prophylactic) (therapeutic) — *see* Hepatitis, viral, type, B
  spirochetal (hemorrhagic) A27.0
  symptomatic R17
    newborn P59.9
Jaw — *see* condition
Jaw-winking phenomenon or syndrome Q07.8
Jealousy
  alcoholic F10.988
  childhood F93.8
  sibling F93.8
Jejunitis — *see* Enteritis
Jejunostomy status Z93.4
Jejunum, jejunal — *see* condition
Jensen's disease — *see* Inflammation, chorioretinal, focal, juxtapapillary
Jerks, myoclonic G25.3
Jervell-Lange-Nielsen syndrome I45.81
Jeune's disease Q77.2
Jigger disease B88.1
Job's syndrome (chronic granulomatous disease) D71
Joint (*see also* condition)
  mice — *see* Loose, body, joint
    knee M23.4-
Jordan's anomaly or syndrome D72.0
Joseph-Diamond-Blackfan anemia (congenital hypoplastic) D61.01
Jungle yellow fever A95.0
Jüngling's disease — *see* Sarcoidosis
Juvenile — *see* condition

K

Kahler's disease C90.0- ☑
Kakke E51.11
Kala-azar B55.0
Kallmann's syndrome E23.0
Kanner's syndrome (autism) — *see* Psychosis, childhood
Kaposi's
  dermatosis (xeroderma pigmentosum) Q82.1
  lichen ruber L44.0
    acuminatus L44.0
  sarcoma
    colon C46.4
    connective tissue C46.1
    gastrointestinal organ C46.4
    lung C46.5- ☑
    lymph node (multiple) C46.3
    palate (hard) (soft) C46.2
    rectum C46.4
    skin (multiple sites) C46.0
    specified site NEC C46.7
    stomach C46.4
    unspecified site C46.9
  varicelliform eruption B00.0
    vaccinia T88.1 ☑
Kartagener's syndrome or triad (sinusitis, bronchiectasis, situs inversus) Q89.3

Karyotype
  with abnormality except iso (Xq) Q96.2
  45,X Q96.0
  46,X
    iso (Xq) Q96.1
  46,XX Q98.3
    with streak gonads Q50.32
    hermaphrodite (true) Q99.1
    male Q98.3
  46,XY
    with streak gonads Q56.1
    female Q97.3
    hermaphrodite (true) Q99.1
  47,XXX Q97.0
  47,XXY Q98.0
  47,XYY Q98.5
Kaschin-Beck disease — *see* Disease, Kaschin-Beck
Katayama's disease or fever B65.2
Kawasaki's syndrome M30.3
Kayser-Fleischer ring (cornea) (pseudosclerosis) H18.04-
Kaznelson's syndrome (congenital hypoplastic anemia) D61.01
Kearns-Sayre syndrome H49.81- ☑
Kedani fever A75.3
Kelis L91.0
Kelly (-Patterson) **syndrome** (sideropenic dysphagia) D50.1
Keloid, cheloid L91.0
  acne L73.0
  Addison's L94.0
  cornea — *see* Opacity, cornea
  Hawkin's L91.0
  scar L91.0
Keloma L91.0
Kenya fever A77.1
Keratectasia (*see also* Ectasia, cornea)
  congenital Q13.4
Keratinization of alveolar ridge mucosa
  excessive K13.23
  minimal K13.22
Keratinized residual ridge mucosa
  excessive K13.23
  minimal K13.22
Keratitis (nodular) (nonulcerative) (simple) (zonular) H16.9
  with ulceration (central) (marginal) (perforated) (ring) — *see* Ulcer, cornea
  actinic — *see* Photokeratitis
  arborescens (herpes simplex) B00.52
  areolar H16.11- ☑
  bullosa H16.8
  deep H16.309
    specified type NEC H16.399
  dendritic (a) (herpes simplex) B00.52
  disciform (is) (herpes simplex) B00.52
    varicella B01.81
  filamentary H16.12- ☑
  gonococcal (congenital or prenatal) A54.33
  herpes, herpetic (simplex) B00.52
    zoster B02.33
  in (due to)
    acanthamebiasis B60.13
    adenovirus B30.0
    exanthema (*see also* Exanthem) B09
    herpes (simplex) virus B00.52
    measles B05.81
    syphilis A50.31
    tuberculosis A18.52
    zoster B02.33
  interstitial (nonsyphilitic) H16.30- ☑
    diffuse H16.32- ☑
    herpes, herpetic (simplex) B00.52
      zoster B02.33
    sclerosing H16.33- ☑
    specified type NEC H16.39- ☑
    syphilitic (congenital) (late) A50.31
    tuberculous A18.52
  macular H16.11- ☑
  nummular H16.11- ☑
  oyster shuckers' H16.8
  parenchymatous — *see* Keratitis, interstitial
  petrificans H16.8
  postmeasles B05.81
  punctata
    leprosa A30.9 [H16.14-] ☑
    syphilitic (profunda) A50.31
  punctate H16.14- ☑

Keratitis — *continued*
   purulent H16.8
   rosacea L71.8
   sclerosing H16.33- ☑
   specified type NEC H16.8
   stellate H16.11- ☑
   striate H16.11- ☑
   superficial H16.10- ☑
     with conjunctivitis — *see* Keratoconjunctivitis
     due to light — *see* Photokeratitis
   suppurative H16.8
   syphilitic (congenital) (prenatal) A50.31
   trachomatous A71.1
     sequelae B94.0
   tuberculous A18.52
   vesicular H16.8
   xerotic (*see also* Keratomalacia) H16.8
     vitamin A deficiency E50.4
Keratoacanthoma L85.8
Keratocele — *see* Descemetocele
Keratoconjunctivitis H16.20- ☑
   Acanthamoeba B60.13
   adenoviral B30.0
   epidemic B30.0
   exposure H16.21- ☑
   herpes, herpetic (simplex) B00.52
     zoster B02.33
   in exanthema (*see also* Exanthem) B09
   infectious B30.0
   lagophthalmic — *see* Keratoconjunctivitis, specified
     type NEC
   neurotrophic H16.23- ☑
   phlyctenular H16.25- ☑
   postmeasles B05.81
   shipyard B30.0
   sicca (Sjogren's) M35.0- ☑
     not Sjogren's H16.22- ☑
   specified type NEC H16.29- ☑
   tuberculous (phlyctenular) A18.52
   vernal H16.26- ☑
Keratoconus H18.60- ☑
   congenital Q13.4
   stable H18.61- ☑
   unstable H18.62- ☑
Keratocyst (dental) (odontogenic) — *see* Cyst, calcifying
   odontogenic
Keratoderma, keratodermia (congenital) (palmaris et
   plantaris) (symmetrical) Q82.8
   acquired L85.1
     in diseases classified elsewhere L86
   climactericum L85.1
   gonococcal A54.89
   gonorrheal A54.89
   punctata L85.2
   Reiter's — *see* Reiter's disease
Keratodermatocele — *see* Descemetocele
Keratoglobus H18.79 ☑
   congenital Q15.8
     with glaucoma Q15.0
Keratohemia — *see* Pigmentation, cornea, stromal
Keratoiritis (*see also* Iridocyclitis)
   syphilitic A50.39
   tuberculous A18.54
Keratoma L57.0
   palmaris and plantaris hereditarium Q82.8
   senile L57.0
Keratomalacia H18.44- ☑
   vitamin A deficiency E50.4
Keratomegaly Q13.4
Keratomycosis B49
   nigrans, nigricans (palmaris) B36.1
Keratopathy H18.9
   band H18.42- ☑
   bullous (aphakic), following cataract surgery
     H59.01- ☑
     bullous H18.1- ☑
Keratoscleritis, tuberculous A18.52
Keratosis L57.0
   actinic L57.0
   arsenical L85.8
   congenital, specified NEC Q80.8
   female genital NEC N94.89
   follicularis Q82.8
     acquired L11.0
     congenita Q82.8
     et parafollicularis in cutem penetrans L87.0
     spinulosa (decalvans) Q82.8

Keratosis — *continued*
   follicularis — *continued*
     vitamin A deficiency E50.8
   gonococcal A54.89
   male genital (external) N50.89
   nigricans L83
   obturans, external ear (canal) — *see* Cholesteatoma,
     external ear
   palmaris et plantaris (inherited) (symmetrical) Q82.8
     acquired L85.1
   penile N48.89
   pharynx J39.2
   pilaris, acquired L85.8
   punctata (palmaris et plantaris) L85.2
   scrotal N50.89
   seborrheic L82.1
     inflamed L82.0
   senile L57.0
   solar L57.0
   tonsillaris J35.8
   vagina N89.4
   vegetans Q82.8
   vitamin A deficiency E50.8
   vocal cord J38.3
Kerato-uveitis — *see* Iridocyclitis
Kerion (celsi) B35.0
Kernicterus of newborn (not due to isoimmunization)
   P57.9
   due to isoimmunization (conditions in P55.0-P55.9)
     P57.0
   specified type NEC P57.8
Kerunoparalysis T75.09 ☑
Keshan disease E59
Ketoacidosis E87.2
   diabetic — *see* Diabetes, by type, with ketoacidosis
Ketonuria R82.4
Ketosis NEC E88.89
   diabetic — *see* Diabetes, by type, with with ketoacido-
     sis
Kew Garden fever A79.1
Kidney — *see* condition
Kienböck's disease (*see also* Osteochondrosis, juvenile,
   hand, carpal lunate)
   adult M93.1
Kimmelstiel (-Wilson) **disease** — *see* Diabetes, Kimmelstiel (-Wilson) disease
Kink, kinking
   artery I77.1
   hair (acquired) L67.8
   ileum or intestine — *see* Obstruction, intestine
   Lane's — *see* Obstruction, intestine
   organ or site, congenital NEC — *see* Anomaly, by site
   ureter (pelvic junction) N13.5
     with
       hydronephrosis N13.1
         with infection N13.6
       pyelonephritis (chronic) N11.1
     congenital Q62.39
   vein(s) I87.8
     caval I87.1
     peripheral I87.1
Kinnier Wilson's disease (hepatolenticular degeneration) E83.01
Kissing spine M48.20
   cervical region M48.22
   cervicothoracic region M48.23
   lumbar region M48.26
   lumbosacral region M48.27
   occipito-atlanto-axial region M48.21
   thoracic region M48.24
   thoracolumbar region M48.25
Klatskin's tumor C22.1
Klauder's disease A26.8
Klebs' disease (*see also* Glomerulonephritis) N05- ☑
Klebsiella (K.) **pneumoniae, as cause of disease
   classified elsewhere** B96.1
Klein (e)-**Levin syndrome** G47.13
Kleptomania F63.2
Klinefelter's syndrome Q98.4
   karyotype 47,XXY Q98.0
   male with more than two X chromosomes Q98.1
Klippel-Feil deficiency, disease, or syndrome (brevi-
   collis) Q76.1
Klippel's disease I67.2
Klippel-Trenaunay (-Weber) **syndrome** Q87.2
Klumpke (-Déjerine) **palsy, paralysis** (birth) (newborn)
   P14.1
Knee — *see* condition

Knock knee (acquired) M21.06- ☑
   congenital Q74.1
Knot(s)
   intestinal, syndrome (volvulus) K56.2
   surfer S89.8- ☑
   umbilical cord (true) O69.2 ☑
Knotting (of)
   hair L67.8
   intestine K56.2
Knuckle pad (Garrod's) M72.1
Koch's
   infection — *see* Tuberculosis
   relapsing fever A68.9
Koch-Weeks' conjunctivitis — *see* Conjunctivitis, acute,
   mucopurulent
Köebner's syndrome Q81.8
Köenig's disease (osteochondritis dissecans) — *see* Osteochondritis, dissecans
Köhler-Pellegrini-Steida disease or syndrome (calcification, knee joint) — *see* Bursitis, tibial collateral
Köhler's disease
   patellar — *see* Osteochondrosis, juvenile, patella
   tarsal navicular — *see* Osteochondrosis, juvenile, tarsus
Koilonychia L60.3
   congenital Q84.6
Kojevnikov's, epilepsy — *see* Kozhevnikof's epilepsy
Koplik's spots B05.9
Kopp's asthma E32.8
Korsakoff's (Wernicke) **disease, psychosis or syn-
   drome** (alcoholic) F10.96
   with dependence F10.26
   drug-induced
     due to drug abuse — *see* Abuse, drug, by type,
       with amnestic disorder
     due to drug dependence — *see* Dependence, drug,
       by type, with amnestic disorder
   nonalcoholic F04
Korsakov's disease, psychosis or syndrome — *see*
   Korsakoff's disease
Korsakow's disease, psychosis or syndrome — *see*
   Korsakoff's disease
Kostmann's disease or syndrome (infantile genetic
   agranulocytosis) — *see* Agranulocytosis
Kozhevnikof's epilepsy G40.109
   intractable G40.119
     with status epilepticus G40.111
     without status epilepticus G40.119
   not intractable G40.109
     with status epilepticus G40.101
     without status epilepticus G40.109
Krabbe's
   disease E75.23
   syndrome, congenital muscle hypoplasia Q79.8
Kraepelin-Morel disease — *see* Schizophrenia
Kraft-Weber-Dimitri disease Q85.8
Kraurosis
   ani K62.89
   penis N48.0
   vagina N89.8
   vulva N90.4
Kreotoxism A05.9
Krukenberg's
   spindle — *see* Pigmentation, cornea, posterior
   tumor C79.6- ☑
Kufs' disease E75.4
Kugelberg-Welander disease G12.1
Kuhnt-Junius degeneration (*see also* Degeneration,
   macula) H35.32- ☑
Kümmell's disease or spondylitis — *see* Spondylopa-
   thy, traumatic
Kupffer cell sarcoma C22.3
Kuru A81.81
Kussmaul's
   disease M30.0
   respiration E87.2
     in diabetic acidosis — *see* Diabetes, by type, with
       ketoacidosis
Kwashiorkor E40
   marasmic, marasmus type E42
Kyasanur Forest disease A98.2
Kyphoscoliosis, kyphoscoliotic (acquired) (*see also*
   Scoliosis) M41.9
   congenital Q67.5
   heart (disease) I27.1
   sequelae of rickets E64.3
   tuberculous A18.01
Kyphosis, kyphotic (acquired) M40.209

Kyphosis, kyphotic — *continued*
  cervical region M40.202
  cervicothoracic region M40.203
  congenital Q76.419
    cervical region Q76.412
    cervicothoracic region Q76.413
    occipito-atlanto-axial region Q76.411
    thoracic region Q76.414
    thoracolumbar region Q76.415
  Morquio-Brailsford type (spinal) (*see also* subcategory M49.8) E76.219
  postlaminectomy M96.3
  postradiation therapy M96.2
  postural (adolescent) M40.00
    cervicothoracic region M40.03
    thoracic region M40.04
    thoracolumbar region M40.05
  secondary NEC M40.10
    cervical region M40.12
    cervicothoracic region M40.13
    thoracic region M40.14
    thoracolumbar region M40.15
  sequelae of rickets E64.3
  specified type NEC M40.299
    cervical region M40.292
    cervicothoracic region M40.293
    thoracic region M40.294
    thoracolumbar region M40.295
  syphilitic, congenital A50.56
  thoracic region M40.204
  thoracolumbar region M40.205
  tuberculous A18.01
Kyrle disease L87.0

L

Labia, labium — *see* condition
Labile
  blood pressure R09.89
  vasomotor system I73.9
Labioglossal paralysis G12.29
Labium leporinum — *see* Cleft, lip
Labor — *see* Delivery
Labored breathing — *see* Hyperventilation
Labyrinthitis (circumscribed) (destructive) (diffuse) (inner ear) (latent) (purulent) (suppurative) (*see also* sub-category) H83.0 ☑
  syphilitic A52.79
Laceration
  with abortion — *see* Abortion, by type, complicated by laceration of pelvic organs
  abdomen, abdominal
    wall S31.119 ☑
      with
        foreign body S31.129 ☑
        penetration into peritoneal cavity S31.619 ☑
          with foreign body S31.629 ☑
      epigastric region S31.112 ☑
        with
          foreign body S31.122 ☑
          penetration into peritoneal cavity S31.612 ☑
            with foreign body S31.622 ☑
      left
        lower quadrant S31.114 ☑
          with
            foreign body S31.124 ☑
            penetration into peritoneal cavity S31.614 ☑
              with foreign body S31.624 ☑
        upper quadrant S31.111 ☑
          with
            foreign body S31.121 ☑
            penetration into peritoneal cavity S31.611 ☑
              with foreign body S31.621 ☑
      periumbilic region S31.115 ☑
        with
          foreign body S31.125 ☑
          penetration into peritoneal cavity S31.615 ☑
            with foreign body S31.625 ☑
      right
        lower quadrant S31.113 ☑
          with
            foreign body S31.123 ☑

Laceration — *continued*
  abdomen, abdominal — *continued*
    wall — *continued*
      right — *continued*
        lower quadrant — *continued*
          with — *continued*
            penetration into peritoneal cavity S31.613 ☑
              with foreign body S31.623 ☑
        upper quadrant S31.110 ☑
          with
            foreign body S31.120 ☑
            penetration into peritoneal cavity S31.610 ☑
              with foreign body S31.620 ☑
    accidental, complicating surgery — *see* Complications, surgical, accidental puncture or laceration
  Achilles tendon S86.02- ☑
  adrenal gland S37.813 ☑
  alveolar (process) — *see* Laceration, oral cavity
  ankle S91.01- ☑
    with
      foreign body S91.02- ☑
  antecubital space — *see* Laceration, elbow
  anus (sphincter) S31.831 ☑
    with
      ectopic or molar pregnancy O08.6
      foreign body S31.832 ☑
    complicating delivery — *see* Delivery, complicated, by, laceration, anus (sphincter)
    following ectopic or molar pregnancy O08.6
    nontraumatic, nonpuerperal — *see* Fissure, anus
  arm (upper) S41.11- ☑
    with foreign body S41.12- ☑
    lower — *see* Laceration, forearm
  auditory canal (external) (meatus) — *see* Laceration, ear
  auricle, ear — *see* Laceration, ear
  axilla — *see* Laceration, arm
  back (*see also* Laceration, thorax, back)
    lower S31.010 ☑
      with
        foreign body S31.020 ☑
          with penetration into retroperitoneal space S31.021 ☑
        penetration into retroperitoneal space S31.011 ☑
  bile duct S36.13 ☑
  bladder S37.23 ☑
    with ectopic or molar pregnancy O08.6
    following ectopic or molar pregnancy O08.6
    obstetrical trauma O71.5
  blood vessel — *see* Injury, blood vessel
  bowel (*see also* Laceration, intestine)
    with ectopic or molar pregnancy O08.6
    complicating abortion — *see* Abortion, by type, complicated by, specified condition NEC
    following ectopic or molar pregnancy O08.6
    obstetrical trauma O71.5
  brain (any part) (cortex) (diffuse) (membrane) (*see also* Injury, intracranial, diffuse)
    during birth P10.8
      with hemorrhage P10.1
    focal — *see* Injury, intracranial, focal brain injury
  brainstem S06.38- ☑
  breast S21.01- ☑
    with foreign body S21.02- ☑
  broad ligament S37.893 ☑
    with ectopic or molar pregnancy O08.6
    following ectopic or molar pregnancy O08.6
    laceration syndrome N83.8
    obstetrical trauma O71.6
    syndrome (laceration) N83.8
  buttock S31.801 ☑
    with foreign body S31.802 ☑
    left S31.821 ☑
      with foreign body S31.822 ☑
    right S31.811 ☑
      with foreign body S31.812 ☑
  calf — *see* Laceration, leg
  canaliculus lacrimalis — *see* Laceration, eyelid
  canthus, eye — *see* Laceration, eyelid
  capsule, joint — *see* Sprain
  causing eversion of cervix uteri (old) N86
  central (perineal), complicating delivery O70.9
  cerebellum, traumatic S06.37- ☑
  cerebral S06.33- ☑

Laceration — *continued*
  cerebral — *continued*
    during birth P10.8
      with hemorrhage P10.1
    left side S06.32- ☑
    right side S06.31- ☑
  cervix (uteri)
    with ectopic or molar pregnancy O08.6
    following ectopic or molar pregnancy O08.6
    nonpuerperal, nontraumatic N88.1
    obstetrical trauma (current) O71.3
    old (postpartal) N88.1
    traumatic S37.63 ☑
  cheek (external) S01.41- ☑
    with foreign body S01.42- ☑
    internal — *see* Laceration, oral cavity
  chest wall — *see* Laceration, thorax
  chin — *see* Laceration, head, specified site NEC
  chordae tendinae NEC I51.1
    concurrent with acute myocardial infarction — *see* Infarct, myocardium
    following acute myocardial infarction (current complication) I23.4
  clitoris — *see* Laceration, vulva
  colon — *see* Laceration, intestine, large, colon
  common bile duct S36.13 ☑
  cortex (cerebral) — *see* Injury, intracranial, diffuse
  costal region — *see* Laceration, thorax
  cystic duct S36.13 ☑
  diaphragm S27.803 ☑
  digit(s)
    foot — *see* Laceration, toe
    hand — *see* Laceration, finger
  duodenum S36.430 ☑
  ear (canal) (external) S01.31- ☑
    with foreign body S01.32- ☑
    drum S09.2- ☑
  elbow S51.01- ☑
    with
      foreign body S51.02- ☑
  epididymis — *see* Laceration, testis
  epigastric region — *see* Laceration, abdomen, wall, epigastric region
  esophagus K22.8
    traumatic
      cervical S11.21 ☑
        with foreign body S11.22 ☑
      thoracic S27.813 ☑
  eye (ball) S05.3- ☑
    with prolapse or loss of intraocular tissue S05.2- ☑
    penetrating S05.6- ☑
  eyebrow — *see* Laceration, eyelid
  eyelid S01.11- ☑
    with foreign body S01.12- ☑
  face NEC — *see* Laceration, head, specified site NEC
  fallopian tube S37.539 ☑
    bilateral S37.532 ☑
    unilateral S37.531 ☑
  finger(s) S61.219 ☑
    with
      damage to nail S61.319 ☑
        with
          foreign body S61.329 ☑
      foreign body S61.229 ☑
    index S61.218 ☑
      with
        damage to nail S61.318 ☑
          with
            foreign body S61.328 ☑
        foreign body S61.228 ☑
      left S61.211 ☑
        with
          damage to nail S61.311 ☑
            with
              foreign body S61.321 ☑
          foreign body S61.221 ☑
      right S61.210 ☑
        with
          damage to nail S61.310 ☑
            with
              foreign body S61.320 ☑
          foreign body S61.220 ☑
    little S61.218 ☑
      with
        damage to nail S61.318 ☑
          with
            foreign body S61.328 ☑

Laceration — *continued*
finger(s) — *continued*
  little — *continued*
    with — *continued*
      foreign body S61.228 ☑
    left S61.217 ☑
      with
        damage to nail S61.317 ☑
          with
            foreign body S61.327 ☑
        foreign body S61.227 ☑
    right S61.216 ☑
      with
        damage to nail S61.316 ☑
          with
            foreign body S61.326 ☑
        foreign body S61.226 ☑
  middle S61.218 ☑
    with
      damage to nail S61.318 ☑
        with
          foreign body S61.328 ☑
      foreign body S61.228 ☑
    left S61.213 ☑
      with
        damage to nail S61.313 ☑
          with
            foreign body S61.323 ☑
        foreign body S61.223 ☑
    right S61.212 ☑
      with
        damage to nail S61.312 ☑
          with
            foreign body S61.322 ☑
        foreign body S61.222 ☑
  ring S61.218 ☑
    with
      damage to nail S61.318 ☑
        with
          foreign body S61.328 ☑
      foreign body S61.228 ☑
    left S61.215 ☑
      with
        damage to nail S61.315 ☑
          with
            foreign body S61.325 ☑
        foreign body S61.225 ☑
    right S61.214 ☑
      with
        damage to nail S61.314 ☑
          with
            foreign body S61.324 ☑
        foreign body S61.224 ☑
flank S31.119 ☑
  with foreign body S31.129 ☑
foot (except toe(s) alone) S91.319 ☑
  with foreign body S91.329 ☑
  left S91.312 ☑
    with foreign body S91.322 ☑
  right S91.311 ☑
    with foreign body S91.321 ☑
  toe — *see* Laceration, toe
forearm S51.819 ☑
  with
    foreign body S51.829 ☑
  elbow only — *see* Laceration, elbow
  left S51.812 ☑
    with
      foreign body S51.822 ☑
  right S51.811 ☑
    with
      foreign body S51.821 ☑
forehead S01.81 ☑
  with foreign body S01.82 ☑
fourchette O70.0
  with ectopic or molar pregnancy O08.6
  complicating delivery O70.0
  following ectopic or molar pregnancy O08.6
gallbladder S36.123 ☑
genital organs, external
  female S31.512 ☑
    with foreign body S31.522 ☑
    vagina — *see* Laceration, vagina
    vulva — *see* Laceration, vulva
  male S31.511 ☑
    with foreign body S31.521 ☑

Laceration — *continued*
genital organs, external — *continued*
  male — *continued*
    penis — *see* Laceration, penis
    scrotum — *see* Laceration, scrotum
    testis — *see* Laceration, testis
groin — *see* Laceration, abdomen, wall
gum — *see* Laceration, oral cavity
hand S61.419 ☑
  with
    foreign body S61.429 ☑
  finger — *see* Laceration, finger
  left S61.412 ☑
    with
      foreign body S61.422 ☑
  right S61.411 ☑
    with
      foreign body S61.421 ☑
  thumb — *see* Laceration, thumb
head S01.91 ☑
  with foreign body S01.92 ☑
  cheek — *see* Laceration, cheek
  ear — *see* Laceration, ear
  eyelid — *see* Laceration, eyelid
  lip — *see* Laceration, lip
  nose — *see* Laceration, nose
  oral cavity — *see* Laceration, oral cavity
  scalp S01.01 ☑
    with foreign body S01.02 ☑
  specified site NEC S01.81 ☑
    with foreign body S01.82 ☑
  temporomandibular area — *see* Laceration, cheek
heart — *see* Injury, heart, laceration
heel — *see* Laceration, foot
hepatic duct S36.13 ☑
hip S71.019 ☑
  with foreign body S71.029 ☑
  left S71.012 ☑
    with foreign body S71.022 ☑
  right S71.011 ☑
    with foreign body S71.021 ☑
hymen — *see* Laceration, vagina
hypochondrium — *see* Laceration, abdomen, wall
hypogastric region — *see* Laceration, abdomen, wall
ileum S36.438 ☑
inguinal region — *see* Laceration, abdomen, wall
instep — *see* Laceration, foot
internal organ — *see* Injury, by site
interscapular region — *see* Laceration, thorax, back
intestine
  large
    colon S36.539 ☑
      ascending S36.530 ☑
      descending S36.532 ☑
      sigmoid S36.533 ☑
      specified site NEC S36.538 ☑
    rectum S36.63 ☑
      transverse S36.531 ☑
    small S36.439 ☑
      duodenum S36.430 ☑
      specified site NEC S36.438 ☑
intra-abdominal organ S36.93 ☑
  intestine — *see* Laceration, intestine
  liver — *see* Laceration, liver
  pancreas — *see* Laceration, pancreas
  peritoneum S36.81 ☑
  specified site NEC S36.893 ☑
  spleen — *see* Laceration, spleen
  stomach — *see* Laceration, stomach
intracranial NEC (*see also* Injury, intracranial, diffuse)
  birth injury P10.9
jaw — *see* Laceration, head, specified site NEC
jejunum S36.438 ☑
joint capsule — *see* Sprain, by site
kidney S37.03- ☑
  major (greater than 3 cm) (massive) (stellate) S37.06- ☑
  minor (less than 1 cm) S37.04- ☑
  moderate (1 to 3 cm) S37.05- ☑
    multiple S37.06- ☑
knee S81.01- ☑
  with foreign body S81.02- ☑
labium (majus) (minus) — *see* Laceration, vulva
lacrimal duct — *see* Laceration, eyelid
large intestine — *see* Laceration, intestine, large
larynx S11.011 ☑

Laceration — *continued*
larynx — *continued*
  with foreign body S11.012 ☑
leg (lower) S81.819 ☑
  with foreign body S81.829 ☑
  foot — *see* Laceration, foot
  knee — *see* Laceration, knee
  left S81.812 ☑
    with foreign body S81.822 ☑
  right S81.811 ☑
    with foreign body S81.821 ☑
  upper — *see* Laceration, thigh
ligament — *see* Sprain
lip S01.511 ☑
  with foreign body S01.521 ☑
liver S36.113 ☑
  major (stellate) S36.116 ☑
  minor S36.114 ☑
  moderate S36.115 ☑
loin — *see* Laceration, abdomen, wall
lower back — *see* Laceration, back, lower
lumbar region — *see* Laceration, back, lower
lung S27.339 ☑
  bilateral S27.332 ☑
  unilateral S27.331 ☑
malar region — *see* Laceration, head, specified site NEC
mammary — *see* Laceration, breast
mastoid region — *see* Laceration, head, specified site NEC
meninges — *see* Injury, intracranial, diffuse
meniscus — *see* Tear, meniscus
mesentery S36.893 ☑
mesosalpinx S37.893 ☑
mouth — *see* Laceration, oral cavity
muscle — *see* Injury, muscle, by site, laceration
nail
  finger — *see* Laceration, finger, with damage to nail
  toe — *see* Laceration, toe, with damage to nail
nasal (septum) (sinus) — *see* Laceration, nose
nasopharynx — *see* Laceration, head, specified site NEC
neck S11.91 ☑
  with foreign body S11.92 ☑
  involving
    cervical esophagus S11.21 ☑
      with foreign body S11.22 ☑
    larynx — *see* Laceration, larynx
    pharynx — *see* Laceration, pharynx
    thyroid gland — *see* Laceration, thyroid gland
    trachea — *see* Laceration, trachea
  specified site NEC S11.81 ☑
    with foreign body S11.82 ☑
nerve — *see* Injury, nerve
nose (septum) (sinus) S01.21 ☑
  with foreign body S01.22 ☑
ocular NOS S05.3- ☑
  adnexa NOS S01.11- ☑
oral cavity S01.512 ☑
  with foreign body S01.522 ☑
orbit (eye) — *see* Wound, open, ocular, orbit
ovary S37.439 ☑
  bilateral S37.432 ☑
  unilateral S37.431 ☑
palate — *see* Laceration, oral cavity
palm — *see* Laceration, hand
pancreas S36.239 ☑
pelvic S31.010 ☑
  with
    foreign body S31.020 ☑
      penetration into retroperitoneal cavity S31.021 ☑
    penetration into retroperitoneal cavity S31.011 ☑
  floor (*see also* Laceration, back, lower)
    with ectopic or molar pregnancy O08.6
    complicating delivery O70.1
    following ectopic or molar pregnancy O08.6
    old (postpartal) N81.89
  organ S37.93 ☑
penis S31.21 ☑
  with foreign body S31.22 ☑
perineum
  female S31.41 ☑

Laceration — *continued*
  perineum — *continued*
    female — *continued*
      with
        ectopic or molar pregnancy O08.6
        foreign body S31.42 ☑
      during delivery O70.9
        first degree O70.0
        fourth degree O70.3
        second degree O70.1
        third degree (*see also* Delivery, complicated, by, laceration, perineum, third degree) O70.20
      old (postpartal) N81.89
      postpartal N81.89
      secondary (postpartal) O90.1
    male S31.119 ☑
      with foreign body S31.129 ☑
  periocular area (with or without lacrimal passages) — *see* Laceration, eyelid
  peritoneum S36.893 ☑
  periumbilic region — *see* Laceration, abdomen, wall, periumbilic
  periurethral tissue — *see* Laceration, urethra
  phalanges
    finger — *see* Laceration, finger
    toe — *see* Laceration, toe
  pharynx S11.21 ☑
    with foreign body S11.22 ☑
  pinna — *see* Laceration, ear
  popliteal space — *see* Laceration, knee
  prepuce — *see* Laceration, penis
  prostate S37.823 ☑
  pubic region S31.119 ☑
    with foreign body S31.129 ☑
  pudendum — *see* Laceration, genital organs, external
  rectovaginal septum — *see* Laceration, vagina
  rectum S36.63 ☑
  retroperitoneum S36.893 ☑
  round ligament S37.893 ☑
  sacral region — *see* Laceration, back, lower
  sacroiliac region — *see* Laceration, back, lower
  salivary gland — *see* Laceration, oral cavity
  scalp S01.01 ☑
    with foreign body S01.02 ☑
  scapular region — *see* Laceration, shoulder
  scrotum S31.31 ☑
    with foreign body S31.32 ☑
  seminal vesicle S37.893 ☑
  shin — *see* Laceration, leg
  shoulder S41.019 ☑
    with foreign body S41.029 ☑
    left S41.012 ☑
      with foreign body S41.022 ☑
    right S41.011 ☑
      with foreign body S41.021 ☑
  small intestine — *see* Laceration, intestine, small
  spermatic cord — *see* Laceration, testis
  spinal cord (meninges) (*see also* Injury, spinal cord, by region)
    due to injury at birth P11.5
    newborn (birth injury) P11.5
  spleen S36.039 ☑
    major (massive) (stellate) S36.032 ☑
    moderate S36.031 ☑
    superficial (minor) S36.030 ☑
  sternal region — *see* Laceration, thorax, front
  stomach S36.33 ☑
  submaxillary region — *see* Laceration, head, specified site NEC
  submental region — *see* Laceration, head, specified site NEC
  subungual
    finger(s) — *see* Laceration, finger, with damage to nail
    toe(s) — *see* Laceration, toe, with damage to nail
  suprarenal gland — *see* Laceration, adrenal gland
  temple, temporal region — *see* Laceration, head, specified site NEC
  temporomandibular area — *see* Laceration, cheek
  tendon — *see* Injury, muscle, by site, laceration
    Achilles S86.02- ☑
  tentorium cerebelli — *see* Injury, intracranial, diffuse
  testis S31.31 ☑
    with foreign body S31.32 ☑
  thigh S71.11- ☑
    with foreign body S71.12- ☑

Laceration — *continued*
  thorax, thoracic (wall) S21.91 ☑
    with foreign body S21.92 ☑
    back S21.22- ☑
      with penetration into thoracic cavity S21.42- ☑
    front S21.12- ☑
      with penetration into thoracic cavity S21.32- ☑
    back S21.21- ☑
      with
        foreign body S21.22- ☑
          with penetration into thoracic cavity S21.42- ☑
        penetration into thoracic cavity S21.41- ☑
    breast — *see* Laceration, breast
    front S21.11- ☑
      with
        foreign body S21.12- ☑
          with penetration into thoracic cavity S21.32- ☑
        penetration into thoracic cavity S21.31- ☑
  thumb S61.019 ☑
    with
      damage to nail S61.119 ☑
        with
          foreign body S61.129 ☑
      foreign body S61.029 ☑
    left S61.012 ☑
      with
        damage to nail S61.112 ☑
          with
            foreign body S61.122 ☑
        foreign body S61.022 ☑
    right S61.011 ☑
      with
        damage to nail S61.111 ☑
          with
            foreign body S61.121 ☑
        foreign body S61.021 ☑
  thyroid gland S11.11 ☑
    with foreign body S11.12 ☑
  toe(s) S91.119 ☑
    with
      damage to nail S91.219 ☑
        with
          foreign body S91.229 ☑
      foreign body S91.129 ☑
    great S91.113 ☑
      with
        damage to nail S91.213 ☑
          with
            foreign body S91.223 ☑
        foreign body S91.123 ☑
      left S91.112 ☑
        with
          damage to nail S91.212 ☑
            with
              foreign body S91.222 ☑
          foreign body S91.122 ☑
      right S91.111 ☑
        with
          damage to nail S91.211 ☑
            with
              foreign body S91.221 ☑
          foreign body S91.121 ☑
    lesser S91.116 ☑
      with
        damage to nail S91.216 ☑
          with
            foreign body S91.226 ☑
        foreign body S91.126 ☑
      left S91.115 ☑
        with
          damage to nail S91.215 ☑
            with
              foreign body S91.225 ☑
          foreign body S91.125 ☑
      right S91.114 ☑
        with
          damage to nail S91.214 ☑
            with
              foreign body S91.224 ☑
          foreign body S91.124 ☑
  tongue — *see* Laceration, oral cavity
  trachea S11.021 ☑

Laceration — *continued*
  trachea — *continued*
    with foreign body S11.022 ☑
  tunica vaginalis — *see* Laceration, testis
  tympanum, tympanic membrane — *see* Laceration, ear, drum
  umbilical region S31.115 ☑
    with foreign body S31.125 ☑
  ureter S37.13 ☑
  urethra S37.33 ☑
    with or following ectopic or molar pregnancy O08.6
    obstetrical trauma O71.5
  urinary organ NEC S37.893 ☑
  uterus S37.63 ☑
    with ectopic or molar pregnancy O08.6
    following ectopic or molar pregnancy O08.6
    nonpuerperal, nontraumatic N85.8
    obstetrical trauma NEC O71.81
    old (postpartal) N85.8
  uvula — *see* Laceration, oral cavity
  vagina S31.41 ☑
    with
      ectopic or molar pregnancy O08.6
      foreign body S31.42 ☑
    during delivery O71.4
      with perineal laceration — *see* Laceration, perineum, female, during delivery
    following ectopic or molar pregnancy O08.6
    nonpuerperal, nontraumatic N89.8
    old (postpartal) N89.8
  vas deferens S37.893 ☑
  vesical — *see* Laceration, bladder
  vocal cords S11.031 ☑
    with foreign body S11.032 ☑
  vulva S31.41 ☑
    with
      ectopic or molar pregnancy O08.6
      foreign body S31.42 ☑
    complicating delivery O70.0
    following ectopic or molar pregnancy O08.6
    nonpuerperal, nontraumatic N90.89
    old (postpartal) N90.89
  wrist S61.519 ☑
    with
      foreign body S61.529 ☑
    left S61.512 ☑
      with
        foreign body S61.522 ☑
    right S61.511 ☑
      with
        foreign body S61.521 ☑

Lack of
  achievement in school Z55.3
  adequate
    food Z59.4
    intermaxillary vertical dimension of fully erupted teeth M26.36
    sleep Z72.820
  appetite (see Anorexia) R63.0
  awareness R41.9
  care
    in home Z74.2
    of infant (at or after birth) T76.02 ☑
      confirmed T74.02 ☑
  cognitive functions R41.9
  coordination R27.9
    ataxia R27.0
    specified type NEC R27.8
  development (physiological) R62.50
    failure to thrive (child over 28 days old) R62.51
      adult R62.7
      newborn P92.6
    short stature R62.52
    specified type NEC R62.59
  energy R53.83
  financial resources Z59.6
  food T73.0 ☑
  growth R62.52
  heating Z59.1
  housing (permanent) (temporary) Z59.0
    adequate Z59.1
  learning experiences in childhood Z62.898
  leisure time (affecting life-style) Z73.2
  material resources Z59.9
  memory (*see also* Amnesia)
    mild, following organic brain damage F06.8
  ovulation N97.0
  parental supervision or control of child Z62.0

Lack of — *continued*
  person able to render necessary care Z74.2
  physical exercise Z72.3
  play experience in childhood Z62.898
  posterior occlusal support M26.57
  relaxation (affecting life-style) Z73.2
  sexual
    desire F52.0
    enjoyment F52.1
  shelter Z59.0
  sleep (adequate) Z72.820
  supervision of child by parent Z62.0
  support, posterior occlusal M26.57
  water T73.1 ☑
Lacrimal — *see* condition
Lacrimation, abnormal — *see* Epiphora
Lacrimonasal duct — *see* condition
Lactation, lactating (breast) (puerperal, postpartum)
  associated
    cracked nipple O92.13
    retracted nipple O92.03
  defective O92.4
  disorder NEC O92.79
  excessive O92.6
  failed (complete) O92.3
    partial O92.4
  mastitis NEC — *see* Mastitis, obstetric
  mother (care and/or examination) Z39.1
  nonpuerperal N64.3
Lacticemia, excessive E87.2
Lacunar skull Q75.8
Laennec's cirrhosis K70.30
  with ascites K70.31
  nonalcoholic K74.69
Lafora's disease — *see* Epilepsy, generalized, idiopathic
Lag, lid (nervous) — *see* Retraction, lid
Lagophthalmos (eyelid) (nervous) H02.209
  cicatricial H02.219
    left H02.216
      lower H02.215
      upper H02.214
    right H02.213
      lower H02.212
      upper H02.211
  keratoconjunctivitis — *see* Keratoconjunctivitis
  left H02.206
    lower H02.205
    upper H02.204
  mechanical H02.229
    left H02.226
      lower H02.225
      upper H02.224
    right H02.223
      lower H02.222
      upper H02.221
  paralytic H02.239
    left H02.236
      lower H02.235
      upper H02.234
    right H02.233
      lower H02.232
      upper H02.231
  right H02.203
    lower H02.202
    upper H02.201
Laki-Lorand factor deficiency — *see* Defect, coagulation, specified type NEC
Lalling F80.0
Lambert-Eaton syndrome — *see* Syndrome, Lambert-Eaton
Lambliasis, lambliosis A07.1
Landau-Kleffner syndrome — *see* Epilepsy, specified NEC
Landouzy-Déjérine dystrophy or facioscapulohumeral atrophy G71.0
Landouzy's disease (icterohemorrhagic leptospirosis) A27.0
Landry-Guillain-Barré, syndrome or paralysis G61.0
Landry's disease or paralysis G61.0
Lane's
  band Q43.3
  kink — *see* Obstruction, intestine
  syndrome K90.2
Langdon Down syndrome — *see* Trisomy, 21
Lapsed immunization schedule status Z28.3
Large
  baby (regardless of gestational age) (4000g to 4499g) P08.1

Large — *continued*
  ear, congenital Q17.1
  physiological cup Q14.2
  stature R68.89
Large-for-dates NEC (infant) (4000g to 4499g) P08.1
  affecting management of pregnancy O36.6- ☑
  exceptionally (4500g or more) P08.0
Larsen-Johansson disease orosteochondrosis — *see* Osteochondrosis, juvenile, patella
Larsen's syndrome (flattened facies and multiple congenital dislocations) Q74.8
Larva migrans
  cutaneous B76.9
    Ancylostoma B76.0
  visceral B83.0
Laryngeal — *see* condition
Laryngismus (stridulus) J38.5
  congenital P28.89
  diphtheritic A36.2
Laryngitis (acute) (edematous) (fibrinous) (infective) (infiltrative) (malignant) (membranous) (phlegmonous) (pneumococcal) (pseudomembranous) (septic) (subglottic) (suppurative) (ulcerative) J04.0
  with
    influenza, flu, or grippe — *see* Influenza, with, laryngitis
    tracheitis (acute) — *see* Laryngotracheitis
  atrophic J37.0
  catarrhal J37.0
  chronic J37.0
    with tracheitis (chronic) J37.1
  diphtheritic A36.2
  due to external agent — *see* Inflammation, respiratory, upper, due to
  H. influenzae J04.0
  Hemophilus influenzae J04.0
  hypertrophic J37.0
  influenzal — *see* Influenza, with, respiratory manifestations NEC
  obstructive J05.0
  sicca J37.0
  spasmodic J05.0
    acute J04.0
  streptococcal J04.0
  stridulous J05.0
  syphilitic (late) A52.73
    congenital A50.59 [J99]
    early A50.03 [J99]
  tuberculous A15.5
  Vincent's A69.1
Laryngocele (congenital) (ventricular) Q31.3
Laryngofissure J38.7
  congenital Q31.8
Laryngomalacia (congenital) Q31.5
Laryngopharyngitis (acute) J06.0
  chronic J37.0
  due to external agent — *see* Inflammation, respiratory, upper, due to
Laryngoplegia J38.00
  bilateral J38.02
  unilateral J38.01
Laryngoptosis J38.7
Laryngospasm J38.5
Laryngostenosis J38.6
Laryngotracheitis (acute) (Infectional) (infective) (viral) J04.2
  atrophic J37.1
  catarrhal J37.1
  chronic J37.1
  diphtheritic A36.2
  due to external agent — *see* Inflammation, respiratory, upper, due to
  Hemophilus influenzae J04.2
  hypertrophic J37.1
  influenzal — *see* Influenza, with, respiratory manifestations NEC
  pachydermic J38.7
  sicca J37.1
  spasmodic J38.5
    acute J05.0
  streptococcal J04.2
  stridulous J38.5
  syphilitic (late) A52.73
    congenital A50.59 [J99]
    early A50.03 [J99]
  tuberculous A15.5
  Vincent's A69.1
Laryngotracheobronchitis — *see* Bronchitis

Larynx, laryngeal — *see* condition
Lassa fever A96.2
Lassitude — *see* Weakness
Late
  talker R62.0
  walker R62.0
Late effect(s) — *see* Sequelae
Latent — *see* condition
Laterocession — *see* Lateroversion
Lateroflexion — *see* Lateroversion
Lateroversion
  cervix — *see* Lateroversion, uterus
  uterus, uterine (cervix) (postinfectional) (postpartal, old) N85.4
    congenital Q51.818
    in pregnancy or childbirth O34.59- ☑
Lathyrism — *see* Poisoning, food, noxious, plant
Launois' syndrome (pituitary gigantism) E22.0
Launois-Bensaude adenolipomatosis E88.89
Laurence-Moon (-Bardet)-**Biedl syndrome** Q87.89
Lax, laxity (*see also* Relaxation)
  ligament (ous) (*see also* Disorder, ligament)
    familial M35.7
    knee — *see* Derangement, knee
  skin (acquired) L57.4
    congenital Q82.8
Laxative habit F55.2
Lazy leukocyte syndrome D70.8
Lead miner's lung J63.6
Leak, leakage
  air NEC J93.82
    postprocedural J95.812
  amniotic fluid — *see* Rupture, membranes, premature
  blood (microscopic), fetal, into maternal circulation
    affecting management of pregnancy — *see* Pregnancy, complicated by
  cerebrospinal fluid G96.0
    from spinal (lumbar) puncture G97.0
  device, implant or graft (*see also* Complications, by site and type, mechanical)
    arterial graft NEC — *see* Complication, cardiovascular device, mechanical, vascular
    breast (implant) T85.43 ☑
    catheter NEC T85.638 ☑
      dialysis (renal) T82.43 ☑
        intraperitoneal T85.631 ☑
      infusion NEC T82.534 ☑
        spinal (epidural) (subdural) T85.630 ☑
      urinary T83.038 ☑
        cystostomy T83.030 ☑
        Hopkins T83.038 ☑
        ileostomy T83.038 ☑
        indwelling T83.031 ☑
        nephrostomy T83.032 ☑
        specified T83.038 ☑
        urostomy T83.038 ☑
    gastrointestinal — *see* Complications, prosthetic device, mechanical, gastrointestinal device
    genital NEC T83.498 ☑
      penile prosthesis (cylinder) (implanted) (pump) (reservoir) T83.490 ☑
      testicular prosthesis T83.491 ☑
    heart NEC — *see* Complication, cardiovascular device, mechanical
    joint prosthesis — *see* Complications, joint prosthesis, mechanical, specified NEC, by site
    ocular NEC — *see* Complications, prosthetic device, mechanical, ocular device
    orthopedic NEC — *see* Complication, orthopedic, device, mechanical
    persistent air J93.82
    specified NEC T85.638 ☑
    urinary NEC (*see also* Complication, genitourinary, device, urinary, mechanical)
      graft T83.23 ☑
    vascular NEC — *see* Complication, cardiovascular device, mechanical
    ventricular intracranial shunt T85.03 ☑
  urine — *see* Incontinence
Leaky heart — *see* Endocarditis
Learning defect (specific) F81.9
Leather bottle stomach C16.9
Leber's
  congenital amaurosis H35.50
  optic atrophy (hereditary) H47.22
Lederer's anemia D59.1
Leeches (external) — *see* Hirudiniasis

Leg — *see* condition

Legg (-Calvé)-**Perthes disease, syndrome or osteochondrosis** M91.1- ☑

Legionellosis A48.1
  nonpneumonic A48.2

Legionnaires'
  disease A48.1
    nonpneumonic A48.2
  pneumonia A48.1

Leigh's disease G31.82

Leiner's disease L21.1

Leiofibromyoma — *see* Leiomyoma

Leiomyoblastoma — *see* Neoplasm, connective tissue, benign

Leiomyofibroma (*see also* Neoplasm, connective tissue, benign)
  uterus (cervix) (corpus) D25.9

Leiomyoma (*see also* Neoplasm, connective tissue, benign)
  bizarre — *see* Neoplasm, connective tissue, benign
  cellular — *see* Neoplasm, connective tissue, benign
  epithelioid — *see* Neoplasm, connective tissue, benign
  uterus (cervix) (corpus) D25.9
    intramural D25.1
    submucous D25.0
    subserosal D25.2
  vascular — *see* Neoplasm, connective tissue, benign

Leiomyoma, leiomyomatosis (intravascular) — *see* Neoplasm, connective tissue, uncertain behavior

Leiomyosarcoma (*see also* Neoplasm, connective tissue, malignant)
  epithelioid — *see* Neoplasm, connective tissue, malignant
  myxoid — *see* Neoplasm, connective tissue, malignant

Leishmaniasis B55.9
  American (mucocutaneous) B55.2
    cutaneous B55.1
  Asian Desert B55.1
  Brazilian B55.2
  cutaneous (any type) B55.1
  dermal (*see also* Leishmaniasis, cutaneous)
    post-kala-azar B55.0
  eyelid B55.1
  infantile B55.0
  Mediterranean B55.0
  mucocutaneous (American) (New World) B55.2
  naso-oral B55.2
  nasopharyngeal B55.2
  old world B55.1
  tegumentaria diffusa B55.1
  visceral B55.0

Leishmanoid, dermal (*see also* Leishmaniasis, cutaneous)
  post-kala-azar B55.0

Lenegre's disease I44.2

Lengthening, leg — *see* Deformity, limb, unequal length

Lennert's lymphoma — *see* Lymphoma, Lennert's

Lennox-Gastaut syndrome G40.812
  intractable G40.814
    with status epilepticus G40.813
    without status epilepticus G40.814
  not intractable G40.812
    with status epilepticus G40.811
    without status epilepticus G40.812

Lens — *see* condition

Lenticonus (anterior) (posterior) (congenital) Q12.8

Lenticular degeneration, progressive E83.01

Lentiglobus (posterior) (congenital) Q12.8

Lentigo (congenital) L81.4
  maligna (*see also* Melanoma, in situ)
    melanoma — *see* Melanoma

Lentivirus, as cause of disease classified elsewhere B97.31

Leontiasis
  ossium M85.2
  syphilitic (late) A52.78
    congenital A50.59

Lepothrix A48.8

Lepra — *see* Leprosy

Leprechaunism E34.8

Leprosy A30.- ☑
  with muscle disorder A30.9 [M63.80]
    ankle A30.9 [M63.87-] ☑
    foot A30.9 [M63.87-] ☑
    forearm A30.9 [M63.83-] ☑
    hand A30.9 [M63.84-] ☑
    lower leg A30.9 [M63.86-] ☑

Leprosy — *continued*
  with muscle disorder — *continued*
    multiple sites A30.9 [M63.89]
    pelvic region A30.9 [M63.85-] ☑
    shoulder region A30.9 [M63.81-] ☑
    specified site NEC A30.9 [M63.88]
    thigh A30.9 [M63.85-] ☑
    upper arm A30.9 [M63.82-] ☑
  anesthetic A30.9
  BB A30.3
  BL A30.4
  borderline (infiltrated) (neuritic) A30.3
    lepromatous A30.4
    tuberculoid A30.2
  BT A30.2
  dimorphous (infiltrated) (neuritic) A30.3
  I A30.0
  indeterminate (macular) (neuritic) A30.0
  lepromatous (diffuse) (infiltrated) (macular) (neuritic) (nodular) A30.5
  LL A30.5
  macular (early) (neuritic) (simple) A30.9
  maculoanesthetic A30.9
  mixed A30.3
  neural A30.9
  nodular A30.5
  primary neuritic A30.3
  specified type NEC A30.8
  TT A30.1
  tuberculoid (major) (minor) A30.1

Leptocytosis, hereditary D56.9

Leptomeningitis (chronic) (circumscribed) (hemorrhagic) (nonsuppurative) — *see* Meningitis

Leptomeningopathy G96.19

Leptospiral — *see* condition

Leptospirochetal — *see* condition

Leptospirosis A27.9
  canicola A27.89
  due to Leptospira interrogans serovar icterohaemorrhagiae A27.0
  icterohemorrhagica A27.0
  pomona A27.89
  Weil's disease A27.0

Leptus dermatitis B88.0

Leriche's syndrome (aortic bifurcation occlusion) I74.09

Leri's pleonosteosis Q78.8

Leri-Weill syndrome Q77.8

Lermoyez' syndrome — *see* Vertigo, peripheral NEC

Lesch-Nyhan syndrome E79.1

Leser-Trélat disease L82.1
  inflamed L82.0

Lesion(s) (nontraumatic)
  abducens nerve — *see* Strabismus, paralytic, sixth nerve
  alveolar process K08.9
  angiocentric immunoproliferative D47.Z9 (*following* D47.4)
  anorectal K62.9
  aortic (valve) I35.9
  auditory nerve — *see* subcategory H93.3 ☑
  basal ganglion G25.9
  bile duct — *see* Disease, bile duct
  biomechanical M99.9
    specified type NEC M99.89
      abdomen M99.89
      acromioclavicular M99.87
      cervical region M99.81
      cervicothoracic M99.81
      costochondral M99.88
      costovertebral M99.88
      head region M99.80
      hip M99.85
      lower extremity M99.86
      lumbar region M99.83
      lumbosacral M99.83
      occipitocervical M99.80
      pelvic region M99.85
      pubic M99.85
      rib cage M99.88
      sacral region M99.84
      sacrococcygeal M99.84
      sacroiliac M99.84
      specified NEC M99.89
      sternochondral M99.88
      sternoclavicular M99.87
      thoracic region M99.82
      thoracolumbar M99.82
      upper extremity M99.87

Lesion(s) — *continued*
  bladder N32.9
  bone — *see* Disorder, bone
  brachial plexus G54.0
  brain G93.9
    congenital Q04.9
    vascular I67.9
      degenerative I67.9
      hypertensive I67.4
  buccal cavity K13.79
  calcified — *see* Calcification
  canthus — *see* Disorder, eyelid
  carate — *see* Pinta, lesions
  cardia K31.9
  cardiac (*see also* Disease, heart) I51.9
    congenital Q24.9
    valvular — *see* Endocarditis
  cauda equina G83.4
  cecum K63.9
  cerebral — *see* Lesion, brain
  cerebrovascular I67.9
    degenerative I67.9
    hypertensive I67.4
  cervical (nerve) root NEC G54.2
  chiasmal — *see* Disorder, optic, chiasm
  chorda tympani G51.8
  coin, lung R91.1
  colon K63.9
  combined periodontic - endodontic K05.5
  congenital — *see* Anomaly, by site
  conjunctiva H11.9
  conus medullaris — *see* Injury, conus medullaris
  coronary artery — *see* Ischemia, heart
  cranial nerve G52.9
    eighth — *see* Disorder, ear
    eleventh G52.9
    fifth G50.9
    first G52.0
    fourth — *see* Strabismus, paralytic, fourth nerve
    seventh G51.9
    sixth — *see* Strabismus, paralytic, sixth nerve
    tenth G52.2
    twelfth G52.3
  cystic — *see* Cyst
  degenerative — *see* Degeneration
  duodenum K31.9
  edentulous (alveolar) ridge, associated with trauma, due to traumatic occlusion K06.2
  en coup de sabre L94.1
  eyelid — *see* Disorder, eyelid
  gasserian ganglion G50.8
  gastric K31.9
  gastroduodenal K31.9
  gastrointestinal K63.9
  gingiva, associated with trauma K06.2
  glomerular
    focal and segmental (*see also* N00-N07 with fourth character .1) N05.1
    minimal change (*see also* N00-N07 with fourth character .0) N05.0
  heart (organic) — *see* Disease, heart
  hyperchromic, due to pinta (carate) A67.1
  hyperkeratotic — *see* Hyperkeratosis
  hypothalamic E23.7
  ileocecal K63.9
  ileum K63.9
  iliohypogastric nerve G57.8- ☑
  inflammatory — *see* Inflammation
  intestine K63.9
  intracerebral — *see* Lesion, brain
  intrachiasmal (optic) — *see* Disorder, optic, chiasm
  intracranial, space-occupying R90.0
  joint — *see* Disorder, joint
    sacroiliac (old) M53.3
  keratotic — *see* Keratosis
  kidney — *see* Disease, renal
  laryngeal nerve (recurrent) G52.2
  lip K13.0
  liver K76.9
  lumbosacral
    plexus G54.1
    root (nerve) NEC G54.4
  lung (coin) R91.1
  maxillary sinus J32.0
  mitral I05.9
  Morel-Lavallée — *see* Hematoma, by site
  motor cortex NEC G93.89
  mouth K13.79

☑ Additional Character Required — Refer to the Tabular List for Character Selection   ▽ Subterms under main terms may continue to next column or page

Lesion(s) — *continued*
　nerve G58.9
　　femoral G57.2- ☑
　　median G56.1- ☑
　　　carpal tunnel syndrome — *see* Syndrome, carpal tunnel
　　plantar G57.6- ☑
　　popliteal (lateral) G57.3- ☑
　　　medial G57.4- ☑
　　radial G56.3- ☑
　　sciatic G57.0- ☑
　　spinal — *see* Injury, nerve, spinal
　　ulnar G56.2- ☑
　nervous system, congenital Q07.9
　nonallopathic — *see* Lesion, biomechanical
　nose (internal) J34.89
　obstructive — *see* Obstruction
　obturator nerve G57.8- ☑
　oral mucosa K13.70
　organ or site NEC — *see* Disease, by site
　osteolytic — *see* Osteolysis
　peptic K27.9
　periodontal, due to traumatic occlusion K05.5
　pharynx J39.2
　pigment, pigmented (skin) L81.9
　pinta — *see* Pinta, lesions
　polypoid — *see* Polyp
　prechiasmal (optic) — *see* Disorder, optic, chiasm
　primary (*see also* Syphilis, primary) A51.0
　　carate A67.0
　　pinta A67.0
　　yaws A66.0
　pulmonary J98.4
　　valve I37.9
　pylorus K31.9
　rectosigmoid K63.9
　retina, retinal H35.9
　sacroiliac (joint) (old) M53.3
　salivary gland K11.9
　　benign lymphoepithelial K11.8
　saphenous nerve G57.8- ☑
　sciatic nerve G57.0- ☑
　secondary — *see* Syphilis, secondary
　shoulder (region) M75.9- ☑
　　specified NEC M75.8- ☑
　sigmoid K63.9
　sinus (accessory) (nasal) J34.89
　skin L98.9
　　suppurative L08.0
　SLAP S43.43- ☑
　spinal cord G95.9
　　congenital Q06.9
　spleen D73.89
　stomach K31.9
　superior glenoid labrum S43.43- ☑
　syphilitic — *see* Syphilis
　tertiary — *see* Syphilis, tertiary
　thoracic root (nerve) NEC G54.3
　tonsillar fossa J35.9
　tooth, teeth K08.9
　　white spot
　　　chewing surface K02.51
　　　pit and fissure surface K02.51
　　　smooth surface K02.61
　traumatic — *see* specific type of injury by site
　tricuspid (valve) I07.9
　　nonrheumatic I36.9
　trigeminal nerve G50.9
　ulcerated or ulcerative — *see* Ulcer, skin
　uterus N85.9
　vagus nerve G52.2
　valvular — *see* Endocarditis
　vascular I99.9
　　affecting central nervous system I67.9
　　following trauma NEC T14.8
　　umbilical cord, complicating delivery O69.5 ☑
　warty — *see* Verruca
　white spot (tooth)
　　chewing surface K02.51
　　pit and fissure surface K02.51
　　smooth surface K02.61
Lethargic — *see* condition
Lethargy R53.83
Letterer-Siwe's disease C96.0
Leukemia, leukemic C95.9- ☑
　acute basophilic C94.8- ☑
　acute bilineal C95.0- ☑

Leukemia, leukemic — *continued*
　acute erythroid C94.0- ☑
　acute lymphoblastic C91.0- ☑
　acute megakaryoblastic C94.2- ☑
　acute megakaryocytic C94.2- ☑
　acute mixed lineage C95.0- ☑
　acute monoblastic (monoblastic/monocytic) C93.0- ☑
　acute monocytic (monoblastic/monocytic) C93.0- ☑
　acute myeloblastic (minimal differentiation) (with maturation) C92.0- ☑
　acute myeloid
　　with
　　　11q23-abnormality C92.6- ☑
　　　dysplasia of remaining hematopoesis and/or myelodysplastic disease in its history C92.A- ☑ (*following* C92.6)
　　　multilineage dysplasia C92.A- ☑ (*following* C92.6)
　　　variation of MLL-gene C92.6- ☑
　　M6 (a)(b) C94.0- ☑
　　M7 C94.2- ☑
　acute myelomonocytic C92.5- ☑
　acute promyelocytic C92.4- ☑
　adult T-cell (HTLV-1-associated) (acute variant) (chronic variant) (lymphomatoid variant) (smouldering variant) C91.5- ☑
　aggressive NK-cell C94.8- ☑
　AML (1/ETO) (M0) (M1) (M2) (without a FAB classification) C92.0- ☑
　AML M3 C92.4- ☑
　AML M4 (Eo with inv(16) or t(16;16)) C92.5- ☑
　AML M5 C93.0- ☑
　AML M5a C93.0- ☑
　AML M5b C93.0- ☑
　AML M6 with t (15;17) and variants C92.4- ☑
　atypical chronic myeloid, BCR/ABL-negative C92.2- ☑
　biphenotypic acute C95.0- ☑
　blast cell C95.0- ☑
　Burkitt-type, mature B-cell C91.A- ☑ (*following* C91.6)
　chronic lymphocytic, of B-cell type C91.1- ☑
　chronic monocytic C93.1- ☑
　chronic myelogenous (Philadelphia chromosome (Ph1) positive) (t(9;22)) (q34;q11) (with crisis of blast cells) C92.1- ☑
　chronic myeloid, BCR/ABL-positive C92.1- ☑
　　atypical, BCR/ABL-negative C92.2- ☑
　chronic myelomonocytic C93.1- ☑
　chronic neutrophilic D47.1
　CMML (-1) (-2) (with eosinophilia) C93.1- ☑
　granulocytic (*see also* Category C92) C92.9- ☑
　hairy cell C91.4- ☑
　juvenile myelomonocytic C93.3- ☑
　lymphoid C91.9- ☑
　　specified NEC C91.Z- ☑ (*following* C91.6)
　mast cell C94.3- ☑
　mature B-cell, Burkitt-type C91.A- ☑ (*following* C91.6)
　monocytic (subacute) C93.9- ☑
　　specified NEC C93.Z- ☑ (*following* C93.3)
　myelogenous (*see also* Category C92) C92.9- ☑
　myeloid C92.9- ☑
　　specified NEC C92.Z- ☑ (*following* C92.6)
　plasma cell C90.1- ☑
　plasmacytic C90.1- ☑
　prolymphocytic
　　of B-cell type C91.3- ☑
　　of T-cell type C91.6- ☑
　specified NEC C94.8- ☑
　stem cell, of unclear lineage C95.0- ☑
　subacute lymphocytic C91.9- ☑
　T-cell large granular lymphocytic C91.Z- ☑ (*following* C91.6)
　unspecified cell type C95.9- ☑
　　acute C95.0- ☑
　　chronic C95.1- ☑
Leukemoid reaction (*see also* Reaction, leukemoid) D72.823
Leukoaraiosis (hypertensive) I67.81
Leukoariosis — *see* Leukoaraiosis
Leukocoria — *see* Disorder, globe, degenerated condition, leucocoria
Leukocytopenia D72.819
Leukocytosis D72.829
　eosinophilic D72.1
Leukoderma, leukodermia NEC L81.5
　syphilitic A51.39
　　late A52.79

Leukodystrophy E75.29
Leukoedema, oral epithelium K13.29
Leukoencephalitis G04.81
　acute (subacute) hemorrhagic G36.1
　　postimmunization or postvaccinal G04.02
　postinfectious G04.01
　subacute sclerosing A81.1
　van Bogaert's (sclerosing) A81.1
Leukoencephalopathy (*see also* Encephalopathy) G93.49
　Binswanger's I67.3
　heroin vapor G92
　metachromatic E75.25
　multifocal (progressive) A81.2
　postimmunization and postvaccinal G04.02
　progressive multifocal A81.2
　reversible, posterior G93.6
　van Bogaert's (sclerosing) A81.1
　vascular, progressive I67.3
Leukoerythroblastosis D75.9
Leukokeratosis (*see also* Leukoplakia)
　mouth K13.21
　nicotina palati K13.24
　oral mucosa K13.21
　tongue K13.21
　vocal cord J38.3
Leukokraurosis vulva (e) N90.4
Leukoma (cornea) (*see also* Opacity, cornea)
　adherent H17.0- ☑
　interfering with central vision — *see* Opacity, cornea, central
Leukomalacia, cerebral, newborn P91.2
　periventricular P91.2
Leukomelanopathy, hereditary D72.0
Leukonychia (punctata) (striata) L60.8
　congenital Q84.4
Leukopathia unguium L60.8
　congenital Q84.4
Leukopenia D72.819
　basophilic D72.818
　chemotherapy (cancer) induced D70.1
　congenital D70.0
　cyclic D70.0
　drug induced NEC D70.2
　　due to cytoreductive cancer chemotherapy D70.1
　eosinophilic D72.818
　familial D70.0
　infantile genetic D70.0
　malignant D70.9
　periodic D70.0
　transitory neonatal P61.5
Leukopenic — *see* condition
Leukoplakia
　anus K62.89
　bladder (postinfectional) N32.89
　buccal K13.21
　cervix (uteri) N88.0
　esophagus K22.8
　gingiva K13.21
　hairy (oral mucosa) (tongue) K13.3
　kidney (pelvis) N28.89
　larynx J38.7
　lip K13.21
　mouth K13.21
　oral epithelium, including tongue (mucosa) K13.21
　palate K13.21
　pelvis (kidney) N28.89
　penis (infectional) N48.0
　rectum K62.89
　syphilitic (late) A52.79
　tongue K13.21
　ureter (postinfectional) N28.89
　urethra (postinfectional) N36.8
　uterus N85.8
　vagina N89.4
　vocal cord J38.3
　vulva N90.4
Leukorrhea N89.8
　due to Trichomonas (vaginalis) A59.00
　trichomonal A59.00
Leukosarcoma C85.9- ☑
Levocardia (isolated) Q24.1
　with situs inversus Q89.3
Levotransposition Q20.5
Lev's disease or syndrome (acquired complete heart block) I44.2
Levulosuria — *see* Fructosuria
Levurid L30.2

Lewy body (ies) (dementia) (disease) G31.83
Leyden-Moebius dystrophy G71.0
Leydig cell
  carcinoma
    specified site — *see* Neoplasm, malignant, by site
    unspecified site
      female C56.9
      male C62.9- ☑
  tumor
    benign
      specified site — *see* Neoplasm, benign, by site
      unspecified site
        female D27.- ☑
        male D29.2- ☑
    malignant
      specified site — *see* Neoplasm, malignant, by site
      unspecified site
        female C56.- ☑
        male C62.9- ☑
    specified site — *see* Neoplasm, uncertain behavior, by site
    unspecified site
      female D39.1- ☑
      male D40.1- ☑
Leydig-Sertoli cell tumor
  specified site — *see* Neoplasm, benign, by site
  unspecified site
    female D27.- ☑
    male D29.2- ☑
LGSIL (Low grade squamous intraepithelial lesion on cytologic smear of)
  anus R85.612
  cervix R87.612
  vagina R87.622
Liar, pathologic F60.2
Libido
  decreased R68.82
Libman-Sacks disease M32.11
Lice (infestation) B85.2
  body (Pediculus corporis) B85.1
  crab B85.3
  head (Pediculus capitis) B85.0
  mixed (classifiable to more than one of the titles B85.0-B85.3) B85.4
  pubic (Phthirus pubis) B85.3
Lichen L28.0
  albus L90.0
    penis N48.0
    vulva N90.4
  amyloidosis E85.4 [L99]
  atrophicus L90.0
    penis N48.0
    vulva N90.4
  congenital Q82.8
  myxedematosus L98.5
  nitidus L44.1
  pilaris Q82.8
    acquired L85.8
  planopilaris L66.1
  planus (chronicus) L43.9
    annularis L43.8
    bullous L43.1
    follicular L66.1
    hypertrophic L43.0
    moniliformis L44.3
    of Wilson L43.9
    specified NEC L43.8
    subacute (active) L43.3
    tropicus L43.3
  ruber
    acuminatus L44.0
    moniliformis L44.3
    planus L43.9
  sclerosus (et atrophicus) L90.0
    penis N48.0
    vulva N90.4
  scrofulosus (primary) (tuberculous) A18.4
  simplex (chronicus) (circumscriptus) L28.0
  striatus L44.2
  urticatus L28.2
Lichenification L28.0
Lichenoides tuberculosis (primary) A18.4
Lichtheim's disease or syndrome — *see* Degeneration, combined
Lien migrans D73.89
Ligament — *see* condition

Light
  for gestational age — *see* Light for dates
  headedness R42
Light-for-dates (infant) P05.00
  with weight of
    1000-1249 grams P05.04
    1250-1499 grams P05.05
    1500-1749 grams P05.06
    1750-1999 grams P05.07
    2000-2499 grams P05.08
    2500 grams and over P05.09
    499 grams or less P05.01
    500-749 grams P05.02
    750-999 grams P05.03
  affecting management of pregnancy O36.59- ☑
  and small-for-dates — *see* Small for dates
  specified NEC P05.09
Lightning (effects) (stroke) (struck by) T75.00 ☑
  burn — *see* Burn
  foot E53.8
  shock T75.01 ☑
  specified effect NEC T75.09 ☑
Lightwood-Albright syndrome N25.89
Lightwood's disease or syndrome (renal tubular acidosis) N25.89
Lignac (-de Toni) (-Fanconi) (-Debré) **disease or syndrome** E72.09
  with cystinosis E72.04
Ligneous thyroiditis E06.5
Likoff's syndrome I20.8
Limb — *see* condition
Limbic epilepsy personality syndrome F07.0
Limitation, limited
  activities due to disability Z73.6
  cardiac reserve — *see* Disease, heart
  eye muscle duction, traumatic — *see* Strabismus, mechanical
  mandibular range of motion M26.52
Lindau (-von Hippel) **disease** Q85.8
Line(s)
  Beau's L60.4
  Harris' — *see* Arrest, epiphyseal
  Hudson's (cornea) — *see* Pigmentation, cornea, anterior
  Stähli's (cornea) — *see* Pigmentation, cornea, anterior
Linea corneae senilis — *see* Change, cornea, senile
Lingua
  geographica K14.1
  nigra (villosa) K14.3
  plicata K14.5
  tylosis K13.29
Lingual — *see* condition
Linguatulosis B88.8
Linitis (gastric) **plastica** C16.9
Lip — *see* condition
Lipedema — *see* Edema
Lipemia (*see also* Hyperlipidemia)
  retina, retinalis E78.3
Lipidosis E75.6
  cerebral (infantile) (juvenile) (late) E75.4
  cerebroretinal E75.4
  cerebroside E75.22
  cholesterol (cerebral) E75.5
  glycolipid E75.21
  hepatosplenomegalic E78.3
  sphingomyelin — *see* Niemann-Pick disease or syndrome
  sulfatide E75.29
Lipoadenoma — *see* Neoplasm, benign, by site
Lipoblastoma — *see* Lipoma
Lipoblastomatosis — *see* Lipoma
Lipochondrodystrophy E76.01
Lipochrome histiocytosis (familial) D71
Lipodermatosclerosis — *see* Varix, leg, with, inflammation
  ulcerated — *see* Varix, leg, with, ulcer, with inflammation by site
Lipodystrophia progressiva E88.1
Lipodystrophy (progressive) E88.1
  insulin E88.1
  intestinal K90.81
  mesenteric K65.4
Lipofibroma — *see* Lipoma
Lipofuscinosis, neuronal (with ceroidosis) E75.4
Lipogranuloma, sclerosing L92.8
Lipogranulomatosis E78.89
Lipoid (*see also* condition)

Lipoid — *continued*
  histiocytosis D76.3
    essential E75.29
  nephrosis N04.9
  proteinosis of Urbach E78.89
Lipoidemia — *see* Hyperlipidemia
Lipoidosis — *see* Lipidosis
Lipoma D17.9
  fetal D17.9
    fat cell D17.9
  infiltrating D17.9
  intramuscular D17.9
  pleomorphic D17.9
  site classification
    arms (skin) (subcutaneous) D17.2- ☑
    connective tissue D17.30
      intra-abdominal D17.5
      intrathoracic D17.4
      peritoneum D17.79
      retroperitoneum D17.79
      specified site NEC D17.39
      spermatic cord D17.6
    face (skin) (subcutaneous) D17.0
    genitourinary organ NEC D17.72
    head (skin) (subcutaneous) D17.0
    intra-abdominal D17.5
    intrathoracic D17.4
    kidney D17.71
    legs (skin) (subcutaneous) D17.2- ☑
    neck (skin) (subcutaneous) D17.0
    peritoneum D17.79
    retroperitoneum D17.79
    skin D17.30
      specified site NEC D17.39
    specified site NEC D17.79
    spermatic cord D17.6
    subcutaneous D17.30
      specified site NEC D17.39
    trunk (skin) (subcutaneous) D17.1
    unspecified D17.9
  spindle cell D17.9
Lipomatosis E88.2
  dolorosa (Dercum) E88.2
  fetal — *see* Lipoma
  Launois-Bensaude E88.89
Lipomyoma — *see* Lipoma
Lipomyxoma — *see* Lipoma
Lipomyxosarcoma — *see* Neoplasm, connective tissue, malignant
Lipoprotein metabolism disorder E78.9
Lipoproteinemia E78.5
  broad-beta E78.2
  floating-beta E78.2
  hyper-pre-beta E78.1
Liposarcoma (*see also* Neoplasm, connective tissue, malignant)
  dedifferentiated — *see* Neoplasm, connective tissue, malignant
  differentiated type — *see* Neoplasm, connective tissue, malignant
  embryonal — *see* Neoplasm, connective tissue, malignant
  mixed type — *see* Neoplasm, connective tissue, malignant
  myxoid — *see* Neoplasm, connective tissue, malignant
  pleomorphic — *see* Neoplasm, connective tissue, malignant
  round cell — *see* Neoplasm, connective tissue, malignant
  well differentiated type — *see* Neoplasm, connective tissue, malignant
Liposynovitis prepatellaris E88.89
Lipping, cervix N86
Lipschütz disease or ulcer N76.6
Lipuria R82.0
  schistosomiasis (bilharziasis) B65.0
Lisping F80.0
Lissauer's paralysis A52.17
Lissencephalia, lissencephaly Q04.3
Listeriosis, listerellosis A32.9
  congenital (disseminated) P37.2
  cutaneous A32.0
  neonatal, newborn (disseminated) P37.2
  oculoglandular A32.81
  specified NEC A32.89
Lithemia E79.0
Lithiasis — *see* Calculus
Lithosis J62.8

Lithuria R82.99
Litigation, anxiety concerning Z65.3
Little leaguer's elbow — *see* Epicondylitis, medial
Little's disease G80.9
Littre's
  gland — *see* condition
  hernia — *see* Hernia, abdomen
Littritis — *see* Urethritis
Livedo (annularis) (racemosa) (reticularis) R23.1
Liver — *see* condition
Living alone (problems with) Z60.2
  with handicapped person Z74.2
Lloyd's syndrome — *see* Adenomatosis, endocrine
Loa loa, loaiasis, loasis B74.3
Lobar — *see* condition
Lobomycosis B48.0
Lobo's disease B48.0
Lobotomy syndrome F07.0
Lobstein (-Ekman) **disease or syndrome** Q78.0
Lobster-claw hand Q71.6- ☑
Lobulation (congenital) (*see also* Anomaly, by site)
  kidney, Q63.1
  liver, abnormal Q44.7
  spleen Q89.09
Lobule, lobular — *see* condition
Local, localized — *see* condition
Locked twins causing obstructed labor O66.1
Locked-in state G83.5
Locking
  joint — *see* Derangement, joint, specified type NEC
    knee — *see* Derangement, knee
Lockjaw — *see* Tetanus
Löffler's
  endocarditis I42.3
  eosinophilia J82
  pneumonia J82
  syndrome (eosinophilic pneumonitis) J82
Loiasis (with conjunctival infestation) (eyelid) B74.3
Lone Star fever A77.0
Long
  labor O63.9
    first stage O63.0
    second stage O63.1
  QT syndrome I45.81
Longitudinal stripes or grooves, nails L60.8
  congenital Q84.6
Long-term (current) (prophylactic) **drug therapy** (use of)
  agents affecting estrogen receptors and estrogen levels NEC Z79.818
  anastrozole (Arimidex) Z79.811
  antibiotics Z79.2
    short-term use — *omit code*
  anticoagulants Z79.01
  anti-inflammatory, non-steroidal (NSAID) Z79.1
  antiplatelet Z79.02
  antithrombotics Z79.02
  aromatase inhibitors Z79.811
  aspirin Z79.82
  birth control pill or patch Z79.3
  bisphosphonates Z79.83
  contraceptive, oral Z79.3
  drug, specified NEC Z79.899
  estrogen receptor downregulators Z79.818
  Evista Z79.810
  exemestane (Aromasin) Z79.811
  Fareston Z79.810
  fulvestrant (Faslodex) Z79.818
  gonadotropin-releasing hormone (GnRH) agonist Z79.818
  goserelin acetate (Zoladex) Z79.818
  hormone replacement Z79.890
  insulin Z79.4
  letrozole (Femara) Z79.811
  leuprolide acetate (leuprorelin) (Lupron) Z79.818
  megestrol acetate (Megace) Z79.818
  methadone for pain management Z79.891
  Nolvadex Z79.810
  non-steroidal anti-inflammatories (NSAID) Z79.1
  opiate analgesic Z79.891
  oral
    antidiabetic Z79.84
    contraceptive Z79.3
    hypoglycemic Z79.84
  raloxifene (Evista) Z79.810
  selective estrogen receptor modulators (SERMs) Z79.810

Long-term (current) (prophylactic) **drug therapy** — *continued*
  steroids
    inhaled Z79.51
    systemic Z79.52
  tamoxifen (Nolvadex) Z79.810
  toremifene (Fareston) Z79.810
Loop
  intestine — *see* Volvulus
  vascular on papilla (optic) Q14.2
Loose (*see also* condition)
  body
    joint M24.00
      ankle M24.07- ☑
      elbow M24.02- ☑
      hand M24.04- ☑
      hip M24.05- ☑
      knee M23.4- ☑
      shoulder (region) M24.01- ☑
      specified site NEC M24.08
      toe M24.07- ☑
      vertebra M24.08
      wrist M24.03- ☑
    knee M23.4- ☑
    sheath, tendon — *see* Disorder, tendon, specified type NEC
  cartilage — *see* Loose, body, joint
  skin and subcutaneous tissue (following bariatric surgery weight loss) (following dietary weight loss) L98.7
  tooth, teeth K08.89
Loosening
  aseptic
    joint prosthesis — *see* Complications, joint prosthesis, mechanical, loosening, by site
    epiphysis — *see* Osteochondropathy
  mechanical
    joint prosthesis — *see* Complications, joint prosthesis, mechanical, loosening, by site
Looser-Milkman (-Debray) **syndrome** M83.8
Lop ear (deformity) Q17.3
Lorain (-Levi) **short stature syndrome** E23.0
Lordosis M40.50
  acquired — *see* Lordosis, specified type NEC
  congenital Q76.429
    lumbar region Q76.426
    lumbosacral region Q76.427
    sacral region Q76.428
    sacrococcygeal region Q76.428
    thoracolumbar region Q76.425
  lumbar region M40.56
  lumbosacral region M40.57
  postsurgical M96.4
  postural — *see* Lordosis, specified type NEC
  rachitic (late effect) (sequelae) E64.3
  sequelae of rickets E64.3
  specified type NEC M40.40
    lumbar region M40.46
    lumbosacral region M40.47
    thoracolumbar region M40.45
  thoracolumbar region M40.55
  tuberculous A18.01
Loss (of)
  appetite (*see also* Anorexia) R63.0
    hysterical F50.89
    nonorganic origin F50.89
    psychogenic F50.89
  blood — *see* Hemorrhage
  bone —*see* Loss, substance of, bone
  consciousness, transient R55
    traumatic — *see* Injury, intracranial
  control, sphincter, rectum R15.9
    nonorganic origin F98.1
  elasticity, skin R23.4
  family (member) in childhood Z62.898
  fluid (acute) E86.9
  function of labyrinth — *see* subcategory H83.2 ☑
  hair, nonscarring — *see* Alopecia
  hearing (*see also* Deafness)
    central NOS H90.5
    conductive H90.2
      bilateral H90.0
      unilateral
        with
          restricted hearing on the contralateral side H90.A1- ☑
          unrestricted hearing on the contralateral side H90.1- ☑

Loss — *continued*
  hearing (*see also* Deafness) — *continued*
    mixed conductive and sensorineural hearing loss H90.8
      bilateral H90.6
      unilateral
        with
          restricted hearing on the contralateral side H90.A3- ☑
          unrestricted hearing on the contralateral side H90.7- ☑
    neural NOS H90.5
    perceptive NOS H90.5
    sensorineural NOS H90.5
      bilateral H90.3
      unilateral
        with
          restricted hearing onthe contralateral side H90.A2- ☑
          unrestricted hearing on the contralateral side H90.4- ☑
    sensory NOS H90.5
  height R29.890
  limb or member, traumatic, current — *see* Amputation, traumatic
  love relationship in childhood Z62.898
  memory (*see also* Amnesia)
    mild, following organic brain damage F06.8
  mind — *see* Psychosis
  occlusal vertical dimension of fully erupted teeth M26.37
  organ or part — *see* Absence, by site, acquired
  ossicles, ear (partial) H74.32- ☑
  parent in childhood Z63.4
  pregnancy, recurrent N96
    without current pregnancy N96
    care in current pregnancy O26.2- ☑
  recurrent pregnancy — *see* Loss, pregnancy, recurrent
  self-esteem, in childhood Z62.898
  sense of
    smell — *see* Disturbance, sensation, smell
    taste — *see* Disturbance, sensation, taste
    touch R20.8
  sensory R44.9
    dissociative F44.6
  sexual desire F52.0
  sight (acquired) (complete) (congenital) — *see* Blindness
  substance of
    bone — *see* Disorder, bone, density and structure, specified NEC
      horizontal alveolar K06.3
    cartilage — *see* Disorder, cartilage, specified type NEC
      auricle (ear) — *see* Disorder, pinna, specified type NEC
    vitreous (humor) H15.89
  tooth, teeth — *see* Absence, teeth, acquired
  vision, visual H54.7
    both eyes H54.3
    one eye H54.60
      left (normal vision on right) H54.62
      right (normal vision on left) H54.61
    specified as blindness — *see* Blindness
    subjective
      sudden H53.13- ☑
      transient H53.12- ☑
  vitreous — *see* Prolapse, vitreous
  voice — *see* Aphonia
  weight (abnormal) (cause unknown) R63.4
Louis-Bar syndrome (ataxia-telangiectasia) G11.3
Louping ill (encephalitis) A84.8
Louse, lousiness — *see* Lice
Low
  achiever, school Z55.3
  back syndrome M54.5
  basal metabolic rate R94.8
  birthweight (2499 grams or less) P07.10
    with weight of
      1000-1249 grams P07.14
      1250-1499 grams P07.15
      1500-1749 grams P07.16
      1750-1999 grams P07.17
      2000-2499 grams P07.18
    extreme (999 grams or less) P07.00
      with weight of
        499 grams or less P07.01
        500-749 grams P07.02

Low — continued
  birthweight — continued
    extreme — continued
      with weight of — continued
        750-999 grams P07.03
    for gestational age — see Light for dates
  blood pressure (see also Hypotension)
    reading (incidental) (isolated) (nonspecific) R03.1
  cardiac reserve — see Disease, heart
  function (see also Hypofunction)
    kidney N28.9
  hematocrit D64.9
  hemoglobin D64.9
  income Z59.6
  level of literacy Z55.0
  lying
    kidney N28.89
    organ or site, congenital — see Malposition, congenital
  output syndrome (cardiac) — see Failure, heart
  platelets (blood) — see Thrombocytopenia
  reserve, kidney N28.89
  salt syndrome E87.1
  self esteem R45.81
  set ears Q17.4
  vision H54.2X- ☑
    one eye (other eye normal) H54.50
      left (normal vision on right) H54.52A- ☑
      other eye blind — see Blindness
      right (normal vision on left) H54.511- ☑
Low-density-lipoprotein-type (LDL) **hyperlipoproteinemia** E78.00
Lowe's syndrome E72.03
Lown-Ganong-Levine syndrome I45.6
LSD reaction (acute) (without dependence) F16.90
  with dependence F16.20
L-shaped kidney Q63.8
Ludwig's angina or disease K12.2
Lues (venerea), **luetic** — see Syphilis
Luetscher's syndrome (dehydration) E86.0
Lumbago, lumbalgia M54.5
  with sciatica M54.4- ☑
    due to intervertebral disc disorder M51.17
    due to displacement, intervertebral disc M51.27
      with sciatica M51.17
Lumbar — see condition
Lumbarization, vertebra, congenital Q76.49
Lumbermen's itch B88.0
Lump (see also Mass)
  breast N63.0
    axillary tail
      left N63.32
      right N63.31
    left
      lower inner quadrant N63.24
      lower outer quadrant N63.23
      unspecified quadrant N63.20
      upper inner quadrant N63.22
      upper outer quadrant N63.21
    right
      lower inner quadrant N63.14
      lower outer quadrant N63.13
      unspecified quadrant N63.10
      upper inner quadrant N63.12
      upper outer quadrant N63.11
    subareolar
      left N63.42
      right N63.41
Lunacy — see Psychosis
Lung — see condition
Lupoid (miliary) **of Boeck** D86.3
Lupus
  anticoagulant D68.62
    with
      hemorrhagic disorder D68.312
      hypercoagulable state D68.62
    finding without diagnosis R76.0
  discoid (local) L93.0
  erythematosus (discoid) (local) L93.0
    disseminated — see Lupus, erythematosus, systemic
    eyelid H01.129
      left H01.126
        lower H01.125
        upper H01.124
      right H01.123
        lower H01.122
        upper H01.121

Lupus — continued
  erythematosus — continued
    profundus L93.2
    specified NEC L93.2
    subacute cutaneous L93.1
    systemic M32.9
      with organ or system involvement M32.10
        endocarditis M32.11
        lung M32.13
        pericarditis M32.12
        renal (glomerular) M32.14
          tubulo-interstitial M32.15
        specified organ or system NEC M32.19
      drug-induced M32.0
      inhibitor (presence of) D68.62
        with
          hemorrhagic disorder D68.312
          hypercoagulable state D68.62
        finding without diagnosis R76.0
      specified NEC M32.8
  exedens A18.4
  hydralazine M32.0
    correct substance properly administered — see Table of Drugs and Chemicals, by drug, adverse effect
    overdose or wrong substance given or taken — see Table of Drugs and Chemicals, by drug, poisoning
  nephritis (chronic) M32.14
  nontuberculous, not disseminated L93.0
  panniculitis L93.2
  pernio (Besnier) D86.3
  systemic — see Lupus, erythematosus, systemic
  tuberculous A18.4
    eyelid A18.4
  vulgaris A18.4
    eyelid A18.4
Luteinoma D27.- ☑
Lutembacher's disease or syndrome (atrial septal defect with mitral stenosis) Q21.1
Luteoma D27.- ☑
Lutz (-Splendore-de Almeida) **disease** — see Paracoccidioidomycosis
Luxation (see also Dislocation)
  eyeball (nontraumatic) — see Luxation, globe
    birth injury P15.3
  globe, nontraumatic H44.82- ☑
  lacrimal gland — see Dislocation, lacrimal gland
  lens (old) (partial) (spontaneous)
    congenital Q12.1
    syphilitic A50.39
Lycanthropy F22
Lyell's syndrome L51.2
  due to drug L51.2
    correct substance properly administered — see Table of Drugs and Chemicals, by drug, adverse effect
    overdose or wrong substance given or taken — see Table of Drugs and Chemicals, by drug, poisoning
Lyme disease A69.20
Lymph
  gland or node — see condition
  scrotum — see Infestation, filarial
Lymphadenitis I88.9
  with ectopic or molar pregnancy O08.0
  acute L04.9
    axilla L04.2
    face L04.0
    head L04.0
    hip L04.3
    limb
      lower L04.3
      upper L04.2
    neck L04.0
    shoulder L04.2
    specified site NEC L04.8
    trunk L04.1
  anthracosis (occupational) J60
  any site, except mesenteric I88.9
    chronic I88.1
    subacute I88.1
  breast
    gestational — see Mastitis, obstetric
    puerperal, postpartum (nonpurulent) O91.22
  chancroidal (congenital) A57
  chronic I88.1
    mesenteric I88.0

Lymphadenitis — continued
  due to
    Brugia (malayi) B74.1
      timori B74.2
    chlamydial lymphogranuloma A55
    diphtheria (toxin) A36.89
    lymphogranuloma venereum A55
    Wuchereria bancrofti B74.0
  following ectopic or molar pregnancy O08.0
  gonorrheal A54.89
  infective — see Lymphadenitis, acute
  mesenteric (acute) (chronic) (nonspecific) (subacute) I88.0
    due to Salmonella typhi A01.09
    tuberculous A18.39
  mycobacterial A31.8
  purulent — see Lymphadenitis, acute
  pyogenic — see Lymphadenitis, acute
  regional, nonbacterial I88.8
  septic — see Lymphadenitis, acute
  subacute, unspecified site I88.1
  suppurative — see Lymphadenitis, acute
  syphilitic (early) (secondary) A51.49
    late A52.79
  tuberculous — see Tuberculosis, lymph gland
  venereal (chlamydial) A55
Lymphadenoid goiter E06.3
Lymphadenopathy (generalized) R59.1
  angioimmunoblastic, with dysproteinemia (AILD) C86.5
  due to toxoplasmosis (acquired) B58.89
    congenital (acute) (subacute) (chronic) P37.1
  localized R59.0
  syphilitic (early) (secondary) A51.49
Lymphadenosis R59.1
Lymphangiectasis I89.0
  conjunctiva H11.89
  postinfectional I89.0
  scrotum I89.0
Lymphangiectatic elephantiasis, nonfilarial I89.0
Lymphangioendothelioma D18.1
  malignant — see Neoplasm, connective tissue, malignant
Lymphangioleiomyomatosis J84.81
Lymphangioma D18.1
  capillary D18.1
  cavernous D18.1
  cystic D18.1
  malignant — see Neoplasm, connective tissue, malignant
Lymphangiomyoma D18.1
Lymphangiomyomatosis J84.81
Lymphangiosarcoma — see Neoplasm, connective tissue, malignant
Lymphangitis I89.1
  with
    abscess — code by site under Abscess
    cellulitis — code by site under Cellulitis
    ectopic or molar pregnancy O08.0
  acute L03.91
    abdominal wall L03.321
    ankle — see Lymphangitis, acute, lower limb
    arm — see Lymphangitis, acute, upper limb
    auricle (ear) — see Lymphangitis, acute, ear
    axilla L03.12- ☑
    back (any part) L03.322
    buttock L03.327
    cervical (meaning neck) L03.222
    cheek (external) L03.212
    chest wall L03.323
    digit
      finger — see Lymphangitis, acute, finger
      toe — see Lymphangitis, acute, toe
    ear (external) H60.1- ☑
    external auditory canal — see Lymphangitis, acute, ear
    eyelid — see Abscess, eyelid
    face NEC L03.212
    finger (intrathecal) (periosteal) (subcutaneous) (subcuticular) L03.02- ☑
    foot — see Lymphangitis, acute, lower limb
    gluteal (region) L03.327
    groin L03.324
    hand — see Lymphangitis, acute, upper limb
    head NEC L03.891
      face (any part, except ear, eye and nose) L03.212
    heel — see Lymphangitis, acute, lower limb

Lymphangitis — *continued*
- acute — *continued*
    - hip — *see* Lymphangitis, acute, lower limb
    - jaw (region) L03.212
    - knee — *see* Lymphangitis, acute, lower limb
    - leg — *see* Lymphangitis, acute, lower limb
    - lower limb L03.12- ☑
        - toe — *see* Lymphangitis, acute, toe
    - navel L03.326
    - neck (region) L03.222
    - orbit, orbital — *see* Cellulitis, orbit
    - pectoral (region) L03.323
    - perineal, perineum L03.325
    - scalp (any part) L03.891
    - shoulder — *see* Lymphangitis, acute, upper limb
    - specified site NEC L03.898
    - thigh — *see* Lymphangitis, acute, lower limb
    - thumb (intrathecal) (periosteal) (subcutaneous) (subcuticular) — *see* Lymphangitis, acute, finger
    - toe (intrathecal) (periosteal) (subcutaneous) (subcuticular) L03.04- ☑
    - trunk L03.329
        - abdominal wall L03.321
        - back (any part) L03.322
        - buttock L03.327
        - chest wall L03.323
        - groin L03.324
        - perineal, perineum L03.325
        - umbilicus L03.326
    - umbilicus L03.326
    - upper limb L03.12- ☑
        - axilla — *see* Lymphangitis, acute, axilla
        - finger — *see* Lymphangitis, acute, finger
        - thumb — *see* Lymphangitis, acute, finger
        - wrist — *see* Lymphangitis, acute, upper limb
- breast
    - gestational — *see* Mastitis, obstetric
- chancroidal A57
- chronic (any site) I89.1
- due to
    - Brugia (malayi) B74.1
        - timori B74.2
    - Wuchereria bancrofti B74.0
- following ectopic or molar pregnancy O08.89
- penis
    - acute N48.29
    - gonococcal (acute) (chronic) A54.09
- puerperal, postpartum, childbirth O86.89
- strumous, tuberculous A18.2
- subacute (any site) I89.1
- tuberculous — *see* Tuberculosis, lymph gland

Lymphatic (vessel) — *see* condition
Lymphatism E32.8
Lymphectasia I89.0
Lymphedema (acquired) (*see also* Elephantiasis)
- congenital Q82.0
- hereditary (chronic) (idiopathic) Q82.0
- postmastectomy I97.2
- praecox I89.0
- secondary I89.0
- surgical NEC I97.89
    - postmastectomy (syndrome) I97.2

Lymphoblastic — *see* condition
Lymphoblastoma (diffuse) — *see* Lymphoma, lymphoblastic (diffuse)
- giant follicular — *see* Lymphoma, lymphoblastic (diffuse)
- macrofollicular — *see* Lymphoma, lymphoblastic (diffuse)

Lymphocele I89.8
Lymphocytic
- chorioencephalitis (acute) (serous) A87.2
- choriomeningitis (acute) (serous) A87.2
- meningoencephalitis A87.2

Lymphocytoma, benign cutis L98.8
Lymphocytopenia D72.810
Lymphocytosis (symptomatic) D72.820
- infectious (acute) B33.8

Lymphoepithelioma — *see* Neoplasm, malignant, by site
Lymphogranuloma (malignant) (*see also* Lymphoma, Hodgkin)
- chlamydial A55
- inguinale A55
- venereum (any site) (chlamydial) (with stricture of rectum) A55

Lymphogranulomatosis (malignant) (*see also* Lymphoma, Hodgkin)
- benign (Boeck's sarcoid) (Schaumann's) D86.1
Lymphohistiocytosis, hemophagocytic (familial) D76.1
Lymphoid — *see* condition
Lymphoma (of) (malignant) C85.90
- adult T-cell (HTLV-1-associated) (acute variant) (chronic variant) (lymphomatoid variant) (smouldering variant) C91.5-
- anaplastic large cell
    - ALK-negative C84.7- ☑
    - ALK-positive C84.6- ☑
    - CD30-positive C84.6- ☑
        - primary cutaneous C86.6
- angioimmunoblastic T-cell C86.5
- BALT C88.4
- B-cell C85.1- ☑
- blastic NK-cell C86.4
- blastic plasmacytoid dendritic cell neoplasm (BPDCN) C86.4
- B-precursor C83.5- ☑
- bronchial-associated lymphoid tissue [BALT-lymphoma] C88.4
- Burkitt (atypical) C83.7- ☑
- Burkitt-like C83.7- ☑
- centrocytic C83.1- ☑
- cutaneous follicle center C82.6- ☑
- cutaneous T-cell C84.A- ☑ (*following* C84.7)
- diffuse follicle center C82.5- ☑
- diffuse large cell C83.3- ☑
    - anaplastic C83.3- ☑
    - B-cell C83.3- ☑
    - CD30-positive C83.3- ☑
    - centroblastic C83.3- ☑
    - immunoblastic C83.3- ☑
    - plasmablastic C83.3- ☑
    - subtype not specified C83.3- ☑
    - T-cell rich C83.3- ☑
- enteropathy-type (associated) (intestinal) T-cell C86.2
- extranodal marginal zone B-cell lymphoma of mucosa-associated lymphoid tissue [MALT-lymphoma] C88.4
- extranodal NK/T-cell, nasal type C86.0
- follicular C82.9- ☑
    - grade
        - I C82.0- ☑
        - II C82.1- ☑
        - III C82.2- ☑
        - IIIa C82.3- ☑
        - IIIb C82.4- ☑
    - specified NEC C82.8- ☑
- hepatosplenic T-cell (alpha-beta) (gamma-delta) C86.1
- histiocytic C85.9- ☑
    - true C96.A (*following* C96.6)
- Hodgkin C81.9 ☑
    - lymphocyte depleted (classical) C81.3- ☑
    - lymphocyte-rich (classical) C81.4- ☑
    - mixed cellularity (classical) C81.2- ☑
    - nodular
        - lymphocyte predominant C81.0- ☑
        - sclerosis (classical) C81.1- ☑
    - nodular sclerosis (classical) C81.1- ☑
    - specified NEC (classical) C81.7- ☑
- intravascular large B-cell C83.8- ☑
- Lennert's C84.4- ☑
- lymphoblastic (diffuse) C83.5- ☑
- lymphoblastic B-cell C83.5- ☑
- lymphoblastic T-cell C83.5- ☑
- lymphoepithelioid C84.4- ☑
- lymphoplasmacytic C83.0- ☑
    - with IgM-production C88.0
- MALT C88.4
- mantle cell C83.1- ☑
- mature T-cell NEC C84.4- ☑
- mature T/NK-cell C84.9- ☑
    - specified NEC C84.Z- ☑ (*following* C84.7)
- mediastinal (thymic) large B-cell C85.2- ☑
- Mediterranean C88.3
- mucosa-associated lymphoid tissue [MALT-lymphoma] C88.4
- NK/T cell C84.9- ☑
- nodal marginal zone C83.0- ☑
- non-follicular (diffuse) C83.9- ☑
    - specified NEC C83.8- ☑
- non-Hodgkin (*see also* Lymphoma, by type) C85.9- ☑
    - specified NEC C85.8- ☑

Lymphoma — *continued*
- non-leukemic variant of B-CLL C83.0- ☑
- peripheral T-cell, not classified C84.4- ☑
- primary cutaneous
    - anaplastic large cell C86.6
    - CD30-positive large T-cell C86.6
- primary effusion B-cell C83.8- ☑
- SALT C88.4
- skin-associated lymphoid tissue [SALT-lymphoma] C88.4
- small cell B-cell C83.0- ☑
- splenic marginal zone C83.0- ☑
- subcutaneous panniculitis-like T-cell C86.3
- T-precursor C83.5- ☑
- true histiocytic C96.A (*following* C96.6)

Lymphomatosis — *see* Lymphoma
Lymphopathia venereum, veneris A55
Lymphopenia D72.810
Lymphoplasmacytic leukemia — *see* Leukemia, chronic lymphocytic, B-cell type
Lymphoproliferation, X-linked disease D82.3
Lymphoreticulosis, benign (of inoculation) A28.1
Lymphorrhea I89.8
Lymphosarcoma (diffuse) (*see also* Lymphoma) C85.9- ☑
Lymphostasis I89.8
Lypemania — *see* Melancholia
Lysine and hydroxylysine metabolism disorder E72.3
Lyssa — *see* Rabies

M

Macacus ear Q17.3
Maceration, wet feet, tropical (syndrome) T69.02- ☑
MacLeod's syndrome J43.0
Macrocephalia, macrocephaly Q75.3
Macrocheilia, macrochilia (congenital) Q18.6
Macrocolon (*see also* Megacolon) Q43.1
Macrocornea Q15.8
- with glaucoma Q15.0
Macrocytic — *see* condition
Macrocytosis D75.89
Macrodactylia, macrodactylism (fingers) (thumbs) Q74.0
- toes Q74.2
Macrodontia K00.2
Macrogenia M26.05
Macrogenitosomia (adrenal) (male) (praecox) E25.9
- congenital E25.0
Macroglobulinemia (idiopathic) (primary) C88.0
- monoclonal (essential) D47.2
- Waldenström C88.0
Macroglossia (congenital) Q38.2
- acquired K14.8
Macrognathia, macrognathism (congenital) (mandibular) (maxillary) M26.09
Macrogyria (congenital) Q04.8
Macrohydrocephalus — *see* Hydrocephalus
Macromastia — *see* Hypertrophy, breast
Macrophthalmos Q11.3
- in congenital glaucoma Q15.0
Macropsia H53.15
Macrosigmoid K59.39
- congenital Q43.2
Macrospondylitis , acromegalic E22.0
Macrostomia (congenital) Q18.4
Macrotia (external ear) (congenital) Q17.1
Macula
- cornea, corneal — *see* Opacity, cornea
- degeneration (atrophic) (exudative) (senile) (*see also* Degeneration, macula)
    - hereditary — *see* Dystrophy, retina
Maculae ceruleae B85.1
Maculopathy, toxic — *see* Degeneration, macula, toxic
Madarosis (eyelid) H02.729
- left H02.726
    - lower H02.725
    - upper H02.724
- right H02.729
    - lower H02.722
    - upper H02.721
Madelung's
- deformity (radius) Q74.0
- disease
    - radial deformity Q74.0
    - symmetrical lipomas, neck E88.89
Madness — *see* Psychosis

Madura
foot B47.9
  actinomycotic B47.1
  mycotic B47.0
Maduromycosis B47.0
Maffucci's syndrome Q78.4
Magnesium metabolism disorder — *see* Disorder, metabolism, magnesium
Main en griffe (acquired) (*see also* Deformity, limb, clawhand)
congenital Q74.0
Maintenance (encounter for)
antineoplastic chemotherapy Z51.11
antineoplastic radiation therapy Z51.0
methadone F11.20
Majocchi's
disease L81.7
granuloma B35.8
Major — *see* condition
Mal de los pintos — *see* Pinta
Mal de mer T75.3 ☑
Malabar itch (any site) B35.5
Malabsorption K90.9
calcium K90.89
carbohydrate K90.49
disaccharide E73.9
fat K90.49
galactose E74.20
glucose (-galactose) E74.39
intestinal K90.9
  specified NEC K90.89
isomaltose E74.31
lactose E73.9
methionine E72.19
monosaccharide E74.39
postgastrectomy K91.2
postsurgical K91.2
protein K90.49
starch K90.49
sucrose E74.39
syndrome K90.9
  postsurgical K91.2
Malacia, bone (adult) M83.9
juvenile — *see* Rickets
Malacoplakia
bladder N32.89
pelvis (kidney) N28.89
ureter N28.89
urethra N36.8
Malacosteon, juvenile — *see* Rickets
Maladaptation — *see* Maladjustment
Maladie de Roger Q21.0
Maladjustment
conjugal Z63.0
  involving divorce or estrangement Z63.5
educational Z55.4
family Z63.9
marital Z63.0
  involving divorce or estrangement Z63.5
occupational NEC Z56.89
simple, adult — *see* Disorder, adjustment
situational — *see* Disorder, adjustment
social Z60.9
  due to
    acculturation difficulty Z60.3
    discrimination and persecution (perceived) Z60.5
    exclusion and isolation Z60.4
    life-cycle (phase of life) transition Z60.0
    rejection Z60.4
    specified reason NEC Z60.8
Malaise R53.81
Malakoplakia — *see* Malacoplakia
Malaria, malarial (fever) B54
with
  blackwater fever B50.8
    hemoglobinuric (bilious) B50.8
  hemoglobinuria B50.8
accidentally induced (therapeutically) — *code by* type under Malaria
algid B50.9
cerebral B50.0 [G94]
clinically diagnosed (without parasitological confirmation) B54
congenital NEC P37.4
  falciparum P37.3
congestion, congestive B54
continued (fever) B50.9

Malaria, malarial — *continued*
estivo-autumnal B50.9
falciparum B50.9
  with complications NEC B50.8
    cerebral B50.0 [G94]
  severe B50.8
hemorrhagic B54
malariae B52.9
with
  complications NEC B52.8
  glomerular disorder B52.0
malignant (tertian) — *see* Malaria, falciparum
mixed infections — *code to* first listed type in B50-B53
ovale B53.0
parasitologically confirmed NEC B53.8
pernicious, acute — *see* Malaria, falciparum
Plasmodium (P.)
  falciparum NEC — *see* Malaria, falciparum
  malariae NEC B52.9
    with Plasmodium
      falciparum (and or vivax) — *see* Malaria, falciparum
      vivax (*see also* Malaria, vivax)
        and falciparum — *see* Malaria, falciparum
  ovale B53.0
    with Plasmodium malariae (*see also* Malaria, malariae)
      and vivax (*see also* Malaria, vivax)
        and falciparum — *see* Malaria, falciparum
  simian B53.1
    with Plasmodium malariae (*see also* Malaria, malariae)
      and vivax (*see also* Malaria, vivax)
        and falciparum — *see* Malaria, falciparum
  vivax NEC B51.9
    with Plasmodium falciparum — *see* Malaria, falciparum
quartan — *see* Malaria, malariae
quotidian — *see* Malaria, falciparum
recurrent B54
remittent B54
specified type NEC (parasitologically confirmed) B53.8
spleen B54
subtertian (fever) — *see* Malaria, falciparum
tertian (benign) (*see also* Malaria, vivax)
  malignant B50.9
tropical B50.9
typhoid B54
vivax B51.9
with
  complications NEC B51.8
  ruptured spleen B51.0
Malassez's disease (cystic) N50.89
Malassimilation K90.9
Maldescent, testis Q53.9
bilateral Q53.20
  abdominal Q53.211
  perineal Q53.22
unilateral Q53.10
  abdominal Q53.111
  perineal Q53.12
Maldevelopment (*see also* Anomaly)
brain Q07.9
colon Q43.9
hip Q74.2
  congenital dislocation Q65.2
    bilateral Q65.1
    unilateral Q65.0- ☑
mastoid process Q75.8
middle ear Q16.4
  except ossicles Q16.4
  ossicles Q16.3
ossicles Q16.3
spine Q76.49
toe Q74.2
Male type pelvis Q74.2
with disproportion (fetopelvic) O33.3 ☑
  causing obstructed labor O65.3
Malformation (congenital) (*see also* Anomaly)
adrenal gland Q89.1
affecting multiple systems with skeletal changes NEC Q87.5
alimentary tract Q45.9
  specified type NEC Q45.8
  upper Q40.9

Malformation — *continued*
alimentary tract — *continued*
  upper — *continued*
    specified type NEC Q40.8
aorta Q25.40
  absence Q25.41
  aneurysm, congenital Q25.43
  aplasia Q25.41
  atresia Q25.29
    aortic arch Q25.21
  coarctation (preductal) (postductal) Q25.1
  dilatation, congenital Q25.44
  hypoplasia Q25.42
  patent ductus arteriosus Q25.0
  specified type NEC Q25.49
  stenosis Q25.1
    supravalvular Q25.3
aortic valve Q23.9
  specified NEC Q23.8
arteriovenous, aneurysmatic (congenital) Q27.30
  brain Q28.2
  cerebral Q28.2
  peripheral Q27.30
    digestive system Q27.33
    lower limb Q27.32
    other specified site Q27.39
    renal vessel Q27.34
    upper limb Q27.31
  precerebral vessels (nonruptured) Q28.0
auricle
  ear (congenital) Q17.3
    acquired H61.119
      left H61.112
        with right H61.113
      right H61.111
        with left H61.113
bile duct Q44.5
bladder Q64.79
  aplasia Q64.5
  diverticulum Q64.6
  exstrophy — *see* Exstrophy, bladder
  neck obstruction Q64.31
bone Q79.9
  face Q75.9
    specified type NEC Q75.8
  skull Q75.9
    specified type NEC Q75.8
brain (multiple) Q04.9
  arteriovenous Q28.2
  specified type NEC Q04.8
branchial cleft Q18.2
breast Q83.9
  specified type NEC Q83.8
broad ligament Q50.6
bronchus Q32.4
bursa Q79.9
cardiac
  chambers Q20.9
    specified type NEC Q20.8
  septum Q21.9
    specified type NEC Q21.8
cerebral Q04.9
  vessels Q28.3
cervix uteri Q51.9
  specified type NEC Q51.828
Chiari
  Type I G93.5
  Type II Q07.01
choroid (congenital) Q14.3
  plexus Q07.8
circulatory system Q28.9
cochlea Q16.5
cornea Q13.4
coronary vessels Q24.5
corpus callosum (congenital) Q04.0
diaphragm Q79.1
digestive system NEC, specified type NEC Q45.8
dura Q07.9
  brain Q04.9
  spinal Q06.9
ear Q17.9
  causing impairment of hearing Q16.9
  external Q17.9
    accessory auricle Q17.0
    causing impairment of hearing Q16.9
      absence of
        auditory canal Q16.1
        auricle Q16.0
    macrotia Q17.1

▽ Subterms under main terms may continue to next column or page

Malformation — *continued*
- ear — *continued*
  - external — *continued*
    - microtia Q17.2
    - misplacement Q17.4
    - misshapen NEC Q17.3
    - prominence Q17.5
    - specified type NEC Q17.8
  - inner Q16.5
  - middle Q16.4
    - absence of eustachian tube Q16.2
    - ossicles (fusion) Q16.3
  - ossicles Q16.3
  - specified type NEC Q17.8
- epididymis Q55.4
- esophagus Q39.9
  - specified type NEC Q39.8
- eye Q15.9
  - lid Q10.3
  - specified NEC Q15.8
- fallopian tube Q50.6
- genital organ — *see* Anomaly, genitalia
- great
  - artery Q25.9
    - aorta — *see* Malformation, aorta
    - pulmonary artery — *see* Malformation, pulmonary, artery
    - specified type NEC Q25.8
  - vein Q26.9
    - anomalous
      - portal venous connection Q26.5
      - pulmonary venous connection Q26.4
        - partial Q26.3
        - total Q26.2
    - persistent left superior vena cava Q26.1
    - portal vein-hepatic artery fistula Q26.6
    - specified type NEC Q26.8
    - vena cava stenosis, congenital Q26.0
- gum Q38.6
- hair Q84.2
- heart Q24.9
  - specified type NEC Q24.8
- integument Q84.9
  - specified type NEC Q84.8
- internal ear Q16.5
- intestine Q43.9
  - specified type NEC Q43.8
- iris Q13.2
- joint Q74.9
  - ankle Q74.2
  - lumbosacral Q76.49
  - sacroiliac Q74.2
  - specified type NEC Q74.8
- kidney Q63.9
  - accessory Q63.0
  - giant Q63.3
  - horseshoe Q63.1
  - hydronephrosis Q62.0
  - malposition Q63.2
  - specified type NEC Q63.8
- lacrimal apparatus Q10.6
- lingual Q38.3
- lip Q38.0
- liver Q44.7
- lung Q33.9
- meninges or membrane (congenital) Q07.9
  - cerebral Q04.8
  - spinal (cord) Q06.9
- middle ear Q16.4
  - ossicles Q16.3
- mitral valve Q23.9
  - specified NEC Q23.8
- Mondini's (congenital) (malformation, cochlea) Q16.5
- mouth (congenital) Q38.6
- multiple types NEC Q89.7
- musculoskeletal system Q79.9
- myocardium Q24.8
- nail Q84.6
- nervous system (central) Q07.9
- nose Q30.9
  - specified type NEC Q30.8
- optic disc Q14.2
- orbit Q10.7
- ovary Q50.39
- palate Q38.5
- parathyroid gland Q89.2
- pelvic organs or tissues NEC
  - in pregnancy or childbirth O34.8- ☑
    - causing obstructed labor O65.5

Malformation — *continued*
- penis Q55.69
  - aplasia Q55.5
  - curvature (lateral) Q55.61
  - hypoplasia Q55.62
- pericardium Q24.8
- peripheral vascular system Q27.9
  - specified type NEC Q27.8
- pharynx Q38.8
- precerebral vessels Q28.1
- prostate Q55.4
- pulmonary
  - arteriovenous Q25.72
  - artery Q25.9
    - atresia Q25.5
    - specified type NEC Q25.79
    - stenosis Q25.6
  - valve Q22.3
- renal artery Q27.2
- respiratory system Q34.9
- retina Q14.1
- scrotum — *see* Malformation, testis and scrotum
- seminal vesicles Q55.4
- sense organs NEC Q07.9
- skin Q82.9
- specified NEC Q89.8
- spinal
  - cord Q06.9
  - nerve root Q07.8
- spine Q76.49
  - kyphosis — *see* Kyphosis, congenital
  - lordosis — *see* Lordosis, congenital
- spleen Q89.09
- stomach Q40.3
  - specified type NEC Q40.2
- teeth, tooth K00.9
- tendon Q79.9
- testis and scrotum Q55.20
  - aplasia Q55.0
  - hypoplasia Q55.1
  - polyorchism Q55.21
  - retractile testis Q55.22
  - scrotal transposition Q55.23
  - specified NEC Q55.29
- thorax, bony Q76.9
- throat Q38.8
- thyroid gland Q89.2
- tongue (congenital) Q38.3
  - hypertrophy Q38.2
  - tie Q38.1
- trachea Q32.1
- tricuspid valve Q22.9
  - specified type NEC Q22.8
- umbilical cord NEC (complicating delivery) O69.89 ☑
- umbilicus Q89.9
- ureter Q62.8
  - agenesis Q62.4
  - duplication Q62.5
  - malposition — *see* Malposition, congenital, ureter
  - obstructive defect — *see* Defect, obstructive, ureter
  - vesico-uretero-renal reflux Q62.7
- urethra Q64.79
  - aplasia Q64.5
  - duplication Q64.74
  - posterior valves Q64.2
  - prolapse Q64.71
  - stricture Q64.32
- urinary system Q64.9
- uterus Q51.9
  - specified type NEC Q51.818
- vagina Q52.4
- vas deferens Q55.4
  - atresia Q55.3
- vascular system, peripheral Q27.9
- venous — *see* Anomaly, vein(s)
- vulva Q52.70

Malfunction (*see also* Dysfunction)
- cardiac electronic device T82.119 ☑
  - electrode T82.110 ☑
  - pulse generator T82.111 ☑
  - specified type NEC T82.118 ☑
- catheter device NEC T85.618 ☑
  - cystostomy T83.010 ☑
  - dialysis (renal) (vascular) T82.41 ☑
    - intraperitoneal T85.611 ☑
  - infusion NEC T82.514 ☑
    - cranial T85.610 ☑
    - epidural T85.610 ☑

Malfunction — *continued*
- catheter device — *continued*
  - infusion — *continued*
    - intrathecal T85.610 ☑
    - spinal T85.610 ☑
    - subarachnoid T85.610 ☑
    - subdural T85.610 ☑
  - urinary (*see also* Breakdown, device, catheter) T83.018 ☑
- colostomy K94.03
  - valve K94.03
- cystostomy (stoma) N99.512
  - catheter T83.010 ☑
- enteric stoma K94.13
- enterostomy K94.13
- esophagostomy K94.33
- gastroenteric K31.89
- gastrostomy K94.23
- ileostomy K94.13
  - valve K94.13
- intrathecal infusion pump T85.615 ☑
- jejunostomy K94.13
- nervous system device, implant or graft, specified NEC T85.615 ☑
- pacemaker — *see* Malfunction, cardiac electronic device
- prosthetic device, internal — *see* Complications, prosthetic device, by site, mechanical
- tracheostomy J95.03
- urinary device NEC — *see* Complication, genitourinary, device, urinary, mechanical
- valve
  - colostomy K94.03
  - heart T82.09 ☑
  - ileostomy K94.13
- vascular graft or shunt NEC — *see* Complication, cardiovascular device, mechanical, vascular
- ventricular (communicating shunt) T85.01 ☑

Malherbe's tumor — *see* Neoplasm, skin, benign
Malibu disease L98.8
Malignancy (*see also* Neoplasm, malignant, by site)
- unspecified site (primary) C80.1
Malignant — *see* condition
Malingerer, malingering Z76.5
Mallet finger (acquired) — *see* Deformity, finger, mallet finger
- congenital Q74.0
- sequelae of rickets E64.3
Malleus A24.0
Mallory's bodies R89.7
Mallory-Weiss syndrome K22.6
Malnutrition E46
- degree
  - first E44.1
    - mild (protein) E44.1
    - moderate (protein) E44.0
  - second E44.0
  - severe (protein-energy) E43
    - intermediate form E42
      - with
        - kwashiorkor (and marasmus) E42
        - marasmus E41
  - third E43
- following gastrointestinal surgery K91.2
- intrauterine
  - light-for-dates — *see* Light for dates
  - small-for-dates — *see* Small for dates
- lack of care, or neglect (child) (infant) T76.02 ☑
  - confirmed T74.02 ☑
- malignant E40
- protein E46
  - calorie E46
    - mild E44.1
    - moderate E44.0
    - severe E43
      - intermediate form E42
        - with
          - kwashiorkor (and marasmus) E42
          - marasmus E41
  - energy E46
    - mild E44.1
    - moderate E44.0
    - severe E43
      - intermediate form E42
        - with
          - kwashiorkor (and marasmus) E42
          - marasmus E41
- severe (protein-energy) E43

⬇ Subterms under main terms may continue to next column or page   ☑ Additional Character Required — Refer to the Tabular List for Character Selection   **217**

Malformation — Malnutrition

Malnutrition — *continued*
  severe — *continued*
    with
      kwashiorkor (and marasmus) E42
      marasmus E41
Malocclusion (teeth) M26.4
  Angle's M26.219
    class I M26.211
    class II M26.212
    class III M26.213
  due to
    abnormal swallowing M26.59
    mouth breathing M26.59
    tongue, lip or finger habits M26.59
  temporomandibular (joint) M26.69
Malposition
  cervix — *see* Malposition, uterus
  congenital
    adrenal (gland) Q89.1
    alimentary tract Q45.8
      lower Q43.8
      upper Q40.8
    aorta Q25.49
    appendix Q43.8
    arterial trunk Q20.0
    artery (peripheral) Q27.8
      coronary Q24.5
      digestive system Q27.8
      lower limb Q27.8
      pulmonary Q25.79
      specified site NEC Q27.8
      upper limb Q27.8
    auditory canal Q17.8
      causing impairment of hearing Q16.9
    auricle (ear) Q17.4
      causing impairment of hearing Q16.9
      cervical Q18.2
    biliary duct or passage Q44.5
    bladder (mucosa) — *see* Exstrophy, bladder
    brachial plexus Q07.8
    brain tissue Q04.8
    breast Q83.8
    bronchus Q32.4
    cecum Q43.8
    clavicle Q74.0
    colon Q43.8
    digestive organ or tract NEC Q45.8
      lower Q43.8
      upper Q40.8
    ear (auricle) (external) Q17.4
      ossicles Q16.3
    endocrine (gland) NEC Q89.2
    epiglottis Q31.8
    eustachian tube Q17.8
    eye Q15.8
    facial features Q18.8
    fallopian tube Q50.6
    finger(s) Q68.1
      supernumerary Q69.0
    foot Q66.9
    gallbladder Q44.1
    gastrointestinal tract Q45.8
    genitalia, genital organ(s) or tract
      female Q52.8
        external Q52.79
        internal NEC Q52.8
      male Q55.8
    glottis Q31.8
    hand Q68.1
    heart Q24.8
      dextrocardia Q24.0
        with complete transposition of viscera Q89.3
    hepatic duct Q44.5
    hip (joint) Q65.89
    intestine (large) (small) Q43.8
      with anomalous adhesions, fixation or malrotation Q43.3
    joint NEC Q68.8
    kidney Q63.2
    larynx Q31.8
    limb Q68.8
      lower Q68.8
      upper Q68.8
    liver Q44.7
    lung (lobe) Q33.8
    nail(s) Q84.6
    nerve Q07.8
    nervous system NEC Q07.8
    nose, nasal (septum) Q30.8

Malposition — *continued*
  congenital — *continued*
    organ or site not listed — *see* Anomaly, by site
    ovary Q50.39
    pancreas Q45.3
    parathyroid (gland) Q89.2
    patella Q74.1
    peripheral vascular system Q27.8
    pituitary (gland) Q89.2
    respiratory organ or system NEC Q34.8
    rib (cage) Q76.6
      supernumerary in cervical region Q76.5
    scapula Q74.0
    shoulder Q74.0
    spinal cord Q06.8
    spleen Q89.09
    sternum NEC Q76.7
    stomach Q40.2
    symphysis pubis Q74.2
    thymus (gland) Q89.2
    thyroid (gland) (tissue) Q89.2
      cartilage Q31.8
    toe(s) Q66.9
      supernumerary Q69.2
    tongue Q38.3
    trachea Q32.1
    ureter Q62.60
      deviation Q62.61
      displacement Q62.62
      ectopia Q62.63
      specified type NEC Q62.69
    uterus Q51.818
    vein(s) (peripheral) Q27.8
      great Q26.8
    vena cava (inferior) (superior) Q26.8
  device, implant or graft (*see also* Complications, by site and type, mechanical) T85.628 ☑
    arterial graft NEC — *see* Complication, cardiovascular device, mechanical, vascular
    breast (implant) T85.42 ☑
    catheter NEC T85.628 ☑
      cystostomy T83.020 ☑
      dialysis (renal) T82.42 ☑
        intraperitoneal T85.621 ☑
      infusion NEC T82.524 ☑
        spinal (epidural) (subdural) T85.620 ☑
      urinary (*see also* Displacement, device, catheter, urinary) T83.028 ☑
    electronic (electrode) (pulse generator) (stimulator)
      bone T84.320 ☑
      cardiac T82.129 ☑
        electrode T82.120 ☑
        pulse generator T82.121 ☑
        specified type NEC T82.128 ☑
      nervous system — *see* Complication, prosthetic device, mechanical, electronic nervous system stimulator
      urinary — *see* Complication, genitourinary, device, urinary, mechanical
    fixation, internal (orthopedic) NEC — *see* Complication, fixation device, mechanical
    gastrointestinal — *see* Complications, prosthetic device, mechanical, gastrointestinal device
    genital NEC T83.428 ☑
      intrauterine contraceptive device (string) T83.32 ☑
      penile prosthesis (cylinder) (implanted) (pump) (reservoir) T83.420 ☑
      testicular prosthesis T83.421 ☑
    heart NEC — *see* Complication, cardiovascular device, mechanical
    joint prosthesis — *see* Complication, joint prosthesis, mechanical
    ocular NEC — *see* Complications, prosthetic device, mechanical, ocular device
    orthopedic NEC — *see* Complication, orthopedic, device, mechanical
    specified NEC T85.628 ☑
    urinary NEC (*see also* Complication, genitourinary, device, urinary, mechanical)
      graft T83.22 ☑
    vascular NEC — *see* Complication, cardiovascular device, mechanical
    ventricular intracranial shunt T85.02 ☑
  fetus — *see* Pregnancy, complicated by (management affected by), presentation, fetal
  gallbladder K82.8

Malposition — *continued*
  gastrointestinal tract, congenital Q45.8
  heart, congenital NEC Q24.8
  joint prosthesis — *see* Complications, joint prosthesis, mechanical, displacement, by site
  stomach K31.89
    congenital Q40.2
  tooth, teeth, fully erupted M26.30
  uterus (acute) (acquired) (adherent) (asymptomatic) (postinfectional) (postpartal, old) N85.4
    anteflexion or anteversion N85.4
      congenital Q51.818
    flexion N85.4
      lateral — *see* Lateroversion, uterus
    inversion N85.5
    lateral (flexion) (version) — *see* Lateroversion, uterus
      in pregnancy or childbirth — *see* subcategory O34.5 ☑
    retroflexion or retroversion — *see* Retroversion, uterus
Malposture R29.3
Malrotation
  cecum Q43.3
  colon Q43.3
  intestine Q43.3
  kidney Q63.2
Malta fever — *see* Brucellosis
Maltreatment
  adult
    abandonment
      confirmed T74.01 ☑
      suspected T76.01 ☑
    confirmed T74.91 ☑
    history of Z91.419
    neglect
      confirmed T74.01 ☑
      suspected T76.01 ☑
    physical abuse
      confirmed T74.11 ☑
      suspected T76.11 ☑
    psychological abuse
      confirmed T74.31 ☑
      history of Z91.411
      suspected T76.31 ☑
    sexual abuse
      confirmed T74.21 ☑
      suspected T76.21 ☑
    suspected T76.91 ☑
  child
    abandonment
      confirmed T74.02 ☑
      suspected T76.02 ☑
    confirmed T74.92 ☑
    history of — *see* History, personal (of), abuse
    neglect
      confirmed T74.02 ☑
      history of — *see* History, personal (of), abuse
      suspected T76.02 ☑
    physical abuse
      confirmed T74.12 ☑
      history of — *see* History, personal (of), abuse
      suspected T76.12 ☑
    psychological abuse
      confirmed T74.32 ☑
      history of — *see* History, personal (of), abuse
      suspected T76.32 ☑
    sexual abuse
      confirmed T74.22 ☑
      history of — *see* History, personal (of), abuse
      suspected T76.22 ☑
    suspected T76.92 ☑
  personal history of Z91.89
Maltworker's lung J67.4
Malunion, fracture — *see* Fracture, by site
Mammillitis N61.0
  puerperal, postpartum O91.02
Mammitis — *see* Mastitis
Mammogram (examination) Z12.39
  routine Z12.31
Mammoplasia N62
Management (of)
  bone conduction hearing device (implanted) Z45.320
  cardiac pacemaker NEC Z45.018
  cerebrospinal fluid drainage device Z45.41
  cochlear device (implanted) Z45.321
  contraceptive Z30.9

Management — *continued*
  contraceptive — *continued*
    specified NEC Z30.8
    implanted device Z45.9
      specified NEC Z45.89
    infusion pump Z45.1
    procreative Z31.9
      male factor infertility in female Z31.81
      specified NEC Z31.89
    prosthesis (external) (*see also* Fitting) Z44.9
      implanted Z45.9
        specified NEC Z45.89
    renal dialysis catheter Z49.01
    vascular access device Z45.2
Mangled — *see* specified injury by site
Mania (monopolar) (*see also* Disorder, mood, manic episode)
  with psychotic symptoms F30.2
  without psychotic symptoms F30.10
    mild F30.11
    moderate F30.12
    severe F30.13
  Bell's F30.8
  chronic (recurrent) F31.89
  hysterical F44.89
  puerperal F30.8
  recurrent F31.89
Manic depression F31.9
Manic-depressive insanity, psychosis, or syndrome — *see* Disorder, bipolar
Mannosidosis E77.1
Mansonelliasis, mansonellosis B74.4
Manson's
  disease B65.1
  schistosomiasis B65.1
Manual — *see* condition
Maple-bark-stripper's lung (disease) J67.6
Maple-syrup-urine disease E71.0
Marable's syndrome (celiac artery compression) I77.4
Marasmus E41
  due to malnutrition E41
  intestinal E41
  nutritional E41
  senile R54
  tuberculous NEC — *see* Tuberculosis
Marble
  bones Q78.2
  skin R23.8
Marburg virus disease A98.3
March
  fracture — *see* Fracture, traumatic, stress, by site
  hemoglobinuria D59.6
Marchesani (-Weill) **syndrome** Q87.0
Marchiafava (-Bignami) **syndrome or disease** G37.1
Marchiafava-Micheli syndrome D59.5
Marcus Gunn's syndrome Q07.8
Marfan's syndrome — *see* Syndrome, Marfan's
Marie-Bamberger disease — *see* Osteoarthropathy, hypertrophic, specified NEC
Marie-Charcot-Tooth neuropathic muscular atrophy G60.0
Marie's
  cerebellar ataxia (late-onset) G11.2
  disease or syndrome (acromegaly) E22.0
Marie-Strümpell arthritis, disease or spondylitis — *see* Spondylitis, ankylosing
Marion's disease (bladder neck obstruction) N32.0
Marital conflict Z63.0
Mark
  port wine Q82.5
  raspberry Q82.5
  strawberry Q82.5
  stretch L90.6
  tattoo L81.8
Marker heterochromatin — *see* Extra, marker chromosomes
Maroteaux-Lamy syndrome (mild) (severe) E76.29
Marrow (bone)
  arrest D61.9
  poor function D75.89
Marseilles fever A77.1
Marsh fever — *see* Malaria
Marshall's (hidrotic) **ectodermal dysplasia** Q82.4
Marsh's disease (exophthalmic goiter) E05.00
  with storm E05.01
Masculinization (female) **with adrenal hyperplasia** E25.9

Masculinization (female) **with adrenal hyperplasia** — *continued*
  congenital E25.0
Masculinovoblastoma D27.- ☑
Masochism (sexual) F65.51
Mason's lung J62.8
Mass
  abdominal R19.00
    epigastric R19.06
    generalized R19.07
    left lower quadrant R19.04
    left upper quadrant R19.02
    periumbilic R19.05
    right lower quadrant R19.03
    right upper quadrant R19.01
    specified site NEC R19.09
  breast (*see also* Lump, breast) N63.0
  chest R22.2
  cystic — *see* Cyst
  ear H93.8- ☑
  head R22.0
  intra-abdominal (diffuse) (generalized) — *see* Mass, abdominal
  kidney N28.89
  liver R16.0
  localized (skin) R22.9
    chest R22.2
    head R22.0
    limb
      lower R22.4- ☑
      upper R22.3- ☑
    neck R22.1
    trunk R22.2
  lung R91.8
  malignant — *see* Neoplasm, malignant, by site
  neck R22.1
  pelvic (diffuse) (generalized) — *see* Mass, abdominal
  specified organ NEC — *see* Disease, by site
  splenic R16.1
  substernal thyroid — *see* Goiter
  superficial (localized) R22.9
  umbilical (diffuse) (generalized) R19.09
Massive — *see* condition
Mast cell
  disease, systemic tissue D47.02
  leukemia C94.3- ☑
  neoplasm
    malignant C96.20
      specified type NEC C96.29
    of uncertain behavior NEC D47.09
  sarcoma C96.22
  tumor D47.09
Mastalgia N64.4
Masters-Allen syndrome N83.8
Mastitis (acute) (diffuse) (nonpuerperal) (subacute) N61.0
  with abscess N61.1
  without abscess N61.0
  chronic (cystic) — *see* Mastopathy, cystic
  cystic (Schimmelbusch's type) — *see* Mastopathy, cystic
  fibrocystic — *see* Mastopathy, cystic
  infective N61.0
    newborn P39.0
  interstitial, gestational or puerperal — *see* Mastitis, obstetric
  neonatal (noninfective) P83.4
    infective P39.0
  obstetric (interstitial) (nonpurulent)
    associated with
      lactation O91.23
      pregnancy O91.21- ☑
      puerperium O91.22
    purulent
      associated with
        lactation O91.13
        pregnancy O91.11- ☑
        puerperium O91.12
  periductal — *see* Ectasia, mammary duct
  phlegmonous — *see* Mastopathy, cystic
  plasma cell — *see* Ectasia, mammary duct
Mastocytoma (extracutaneous) D47.09
  malignant C96.29
  solitary D47.01
Mastocytosis D47.09
  aggressive systemic C96.21
  cutaneous (diffuse) (maculopapular) D47.01
    congenital Q82.2
    of neonatal onset Q82.2

Mastocytosis — *continued*
  cutaneous — *continued*
    of newborn onset Q82.2
  indolent systemic D47.02
  isolated bone marrow D47.02
  malignant C96.29
  systemic (indolent) (smoldering)
    with an associated hematological non-mast cell lineage disease (SM-AHNMD) D47.02
Mastodynia N64.4
Mastoid — *see* condition
Mastoidalgia — *see* subcategory H92.0 ☑
Mastoiditis (coalescent) (hemorrhagic) (suppurative) H70.9- ☑
  acute, subacute H70.00- ☑
    complicated NEC H70.09- ☑
    subperiosteal H70.01- ☑
  chronic (necrotic) (recurrent) H70.1- ☑
  in (due to)
    infectious disease NEC B99 ☑ [H75.0-] ☑
    parasitic disease NEC B89 [H75.0-] ☑
    tuberculosis A18.03
  petrositis — *see* Petrositis
  postauricular fistula — *see* Fistula, postauricular
  specified NEC H70.89- ☑
  tuberculous A18.03
Mastopathy, mastopathia N64.9
  chronica cystica — *see* Mastopathy, cystic
  cystic (chronic) (diffuse) N60.1- ☑
    with epithelial proliferation N60.3- ☑
  diffuse cystic — *see* Mastopathy, cystic
  estrogenic, oestrogenica N64.89
  ovarian origin N64.89
Mastoplasia, mastoplastia N62
Masturbation (excessive) F98.8
Maternal care (for) — *see* Pregnancy (complicated by) (management affected by)
Matheiu's disease (leptospiral jaundice) A27.0
Mauclaire's disease or osteochondrosis — *see* Osteochondrosis, juvenile, hand, metacarpal
Maxcy's disease A75.2
Maxilla, maxillary — *see* condition
May (-Hegglin) **anomaly or syndrome** D72.0
McArdle (-Schmid)(-Pearson) **disease** (glycogen storage) E74.04
McCune-Albright syndrome Q78.1
McQuarrie's syndrome (idiopathic familial hypoglycemia) E16.2
Meadow's syndrome Q86.1
Measles (black) (hemorrhagic) (suppressed) B05.9
  with
    complications NEC B05.89
    encephalitis B05.0
    intestinal complications B05.4
    keratitis (keratoconjunctivitis) B05.81
    meningitis B05.1
    otitis media B05.3
    pneumonia B05.2
  French — *see* Rubella
  German — *see* Rubella
  Liberty — *see* Rubella
Meatitis, urethral — *see* Urethritis
Meatus, meatal — *see* condition
Meat-wrappers' asthma J68.9
Meckel-Gruber syndrome Q61.9
Meckel's diverticulitis, diverticulum (displaced) (hypertrophic) Q43.0
  malignant — *see* Table of Neoplasms, small intestine, malignant
Meconium
  ileus, newborn P76.0
    in cystic fibrosis E84.11
    meaning meconium plug (without cystic fibrosis) P76.0
  obstruction, newborn P76.0
    due to fecaliths P76.0
    in mucoviscidosis E84.11
  peritonitis P78.0
  plug syndrome (newborn) NEC P76.0
Median (*see also* condition)
  arcuate ligament syndrome I77.4
  bar (prostate) (vesical orifice) — *see* Hyperplasia, prostate
  rhomboid glossitis K14.2
Mediastinal shift R93.8
Mediastinitis (acute) (chronic) J98.51
  syphilitic A52.73

Mediastinitis — *continued*
  tuberculous A15.8
Mediastinopericarditis (*see also* Pericarditis)
  acute I30.9
  adhesive I31.0
  chronic I31.8
    rheumatic I09.2
Mediastinum, mediastinal — *see* condition
Medicine poisoning — *see* Table of Drugs and Chemicals, by drug, poisoning
Mediterranean
  fever — *see* Brucellosis
    familial M04.1
    tick A77.1
  kala-azar B55.0
  leishmaniasis B55.0
  tick fever A77.1
Medulla — *see* condition
Medullary cystic kidney Q61.5
Medullated fibers
  optic (nerve) Q14.8
  retina Q14.1
Medulloblastoma
  desmoplastic C71.6
  specified site — *see* Neoplasm, malignant, by site
  unspecified site C71.6
Medulloepithelioma (*see also* Neoplasm, malignant, by site)
  teratoid — *see* Neoplasm, malignant, by site
Medullomyoblastoma
  specified site — *see* Neoplasm, malignant, by site
  unspecified site C71.6
Meekeren-Ehlers-Danlos syndrome Q79.6
Megacolon (acquired) (functional) (not Hirschsprung's disease) (in) K59.39
  Chagas' disease B57.32
  congenital, congenitum (aganglionic) Q43.1
  Hirschsprung's (disease) Q43.1
  toxic NEC K59.31
    due to Clostridium difficile
      not specified as recurrent A04.72
      recurrent A04.71
Megaesophagus (functional) K22.0
  congenital Q39.5
  in (due to) Chagas' disease B57.31
Megalencephaly Q04.5
Megalerythema (epidemic) B08.3
Megaloappendix Q43.8
Megalocephalus, megalocephaly NEC Q75.3
Megalocornea Q15.8
  with glaucoma Q15.0
Megalocytic anemia D53.1
Megalodactylia (fingers) (thumbs) (congenital) Q74.0
  toes Q74.2
Megaloduodenum Q43.8
Megaloesophagus (functional) K22.0
  congenital Q39.5
Megalogastria (acquired) K31.89
  congenital Q40.2
Megalophthalmos Q11.3
Megalopsia H53.15
Megalosplenia — *see* Splenomegaly
Megaloureter N28.82
  congenital Q62.2
Megarectum K62.89
Megasigmoid K59.39
  congenital Q43.2
Megaureter N28.82
  congenital Q62.2
Megavitamin-B6 syndrome E67.2
Megrim — *see* Migraine
Meibomian
  cyst, infected — *see* Hordeolum
  gland — *see* condition
  sty, stye — *see* Hordeolum
Meibomitis — *see* Hordeolum
Meige-Milroy disease (chronic hereditary edema) Q82.0
Meige's syndrome Q82.0
Melalgia, nutritional E53.8
Melancholia F32.9
  climacteric (single episode) F32.89
    recurrent episode F33.8
  hypochondriac F45.29
  intermittent (single episode) F32.89
    recurrent episode F33.8
  involutional (single episode) F32.89
    recurrent episode F33.8

Melancholia — *continued*
  menopausal (single episode) F32.89
    recurrent episode F33.8
  puerperal F32.89
  reactive (emotional stress or trauma) F32.3
  recurrent F33.9
  senile F03 ☑
  stuporous (single episode) F32.89
    recurrent episode F33.8
Melanemia R79.89
Melanoameloblastoma — *see* Neoplasm, bone, benign
Melanoblastoma — *see* Melanoma
Melanocarcinoma — *see* Melanoma
Melanocytoma, eyeball D31.9- ☑
Melanocytosis, neurocutaneous Q82.8
Melanoderma, melanodermia L81.4
Melanodontia, infantile K03.89
Melanodontoclasia K03.89
Melanoepithelioma — *see* Melanoma
Melanoma (malignant) C43.9
  acral lentiginous, malignant — *see* Melanoma, skin, by site
  amelanotic — *see* Melanoma, skin, by site
  balloon cell — *see* Melanoma, skin, by site
  benign — *see* Nevus
  desmoplastic, malignant — *see* Melanoma, skin, by site
  epithelioid cell — *see* Melanoma, skin, by site
    with spindle cell, mixed — *see* Melanoma, skin, by site
  in
    giant pigmented nevus — *see* Melanoma, skin, by site
    Hutchinson's melanotic freckle — *see* Melanoma, skin, by site
    junctional nevus — *see* Melanoma, skin, by site
    precancerous melanosis — *see* Melanoma, skin, by site
  in situ D03.9
    abdominal wall D03.59
    ala nasi D03.39
    ankle D03.7- ☑
    anus, anal (margin) (skin) D03.51
    arm D03.6- ☑
    auditory canal D03.2- ☑
    auricle (ear) D03.2- ☑
    axilla, axillary fold D03.59
    back D03.59
    breast D03.52
    brow D03.39
    buttock D03.59
    canthus (eye) D03.1- ☑
    cheek (external) D03.39
    chest wall D03.59
    chin D03.39
    choroid D03.8
    conjunctiva D03.8
    ear (external) D03.2- ☑
    external meatus (ear) D03.2- ☑
    eye D03.8
    eyebrow D03.39
    eyelid (lower) (upper) D03.1- ☑
    face D03.30
      specified NEC D03.39
    female genital organ (external) NEC D03.8
    finger D03.6- ☑
    flank D03.59
    foot D03.7- ☑
    forearm D03.6- ☑
    forehead D03.39
    foreskin D03.8
    gluteal region D03.59
    groin D03.59
    hand D03.6- ☑
    heel D03.7- ☑
    helix D03.2- ☑
    hip D03.7- ☑
    interscapular region D03.59
    iris D03.8
    jaw D03.39
    knee D03.7- ☑
    labium (majus) (minus) D03.8
    lacrimal gland D03.8
    leg D03.7- ☑
    lip (lower) (upper) D03.0
    lower limb NEC D03.7- ☑

Melanoma — *continued*
  in situ — *continued*
    male genital organ (external) NEC D03.8
    nail D03.9
      finger D03.6- ☑
      toe D03.7- ☑
    neck D03.4
    nose (external) D03.39
    orbit D03.8
    penis D03.8
    perianal skin D03.51
    perineum D03.51
    pinna D03.2- ☑
    popliteal fossa or space D03.7- ☑
    prepuce D03.8
    pudendum D03.8
    retina D03.8
    retrobulbar D03.8
    scalp D03.4
    scrotum D03.8
    shoulder D03.6- ☑
    specified site NEC D03.8
    submammary fold D03.52
    temple D03.39
    thigh D03.7- ☑
    toe D03.7- ☑
    trunk NEC D03.59
    umbilicus D03.59
    upper limb NEC D03.6- ☑
    vulva D03.8
  juvenile — *see* Nevus
  malignant, of soft parts except skin — *see* Neoplasm, connective tissue, malignant
  metastatic
    breast C79.81
    genital organ C79.82
    specified site NEC C79.89
  neurotropic, malignant — *see* Melanoma, skin, by site
  nodular — *see* Melanoma, skin, by site
  regressing, malignant — *see* Melanoma, skin, by site
  skin C43.9
    abdominal wall C43.59
    ala nasi C43.31
    ankle C43.7- ☑
    anus, anal (skin) C43.51
    arm C43.6- ☑
    auditory canal (external) C43.2- ☑
    auricle (ear) C43.2- ☑
    auricular canal (external) C43.2- ☑
    axilla, axillary fold C43.59
    back C43.59
    breast (female) (male) C43.52
    brow C43.39
    buttock C43.59
    canthus (eye) C43.1- ☑
    cheek (external) C43.39
    chest wall C43.59
    chin C43.39
    ear (external) C43.2- ☑
    elbow C43.6- ☑
    external meatus (ear) C43.2- ☑
    eyebrow C43.39
    eyelid (lower) (upper) C43.1- ☑
    face C43.30
      specified NEC C43.39
    female genital organ (external) NEC C51.9
    finger C43.6- ☑
    flank C43.59
    foot C43.7- ☑
    forearm C43.6- ☑
    forehead C43.39
    foreskin C60.0
    glabella C43.39
    gluteal region C43.59
    groin C43.59
    hand C43.6- ☑
    heel C43.7- ☑
    helix C43.2- ☑
    hip C43.7- ☑
    interscapular region C43.59
    jaw (external) C43.39
    knee C43.7- ☑
    labium C51.9
      majus C51.0
      minus C51.1
    leg C43.7- ☑
    lip (lower) (upper) C43.0

☑ **Additional Character Required** — Refer to the Tabular List for Character Selection   ⬇ Subterms under main terms may continue to next column or page

Index

Melanoma — *continued*
  skin — *continued*
    lower limb NEC C43.7- ☑
    male genital organ (external) NEC C63.9
    nail
      finger C43.6- ☑
      toe C43.7- ☑
    nasolabial groove C43.39
    nates C43.59
    neck C43.4
    nose (external) C43.31
    overlapping site C43.8
    palpebra C43.1- ☑
    penis C60.9
    perianal skin C43.51
    perineum C43.51
    pinna C43.2- ☑
    popliteal fossa or space C43.7- ☑
    prepuce C60.0
    pudendum C51.9
    scalp C43.4
    scrotum C63.2
    shoulder C43.6- ☑
    skin NEC C43.9
    submammary fold C43.52
    temple C43.39
    thigh C43.7- ☑
    toe C43.7- ☑
    trunk NEC C43.59
    umbilicus C43.59
    upper limb NEC C43.6- ☑
    vulva C51.9
      overlapping sites C51.8
  spindle cell
    with epithelioid, mixed — *see* Melanoma, skin, by site
    type A C69.4- ☑
    type B C69.4- ☑
  superficial spreading — *see* Melanoma, skin, by site
Melanosarcoma (*see also* Melanoma)
  epithelioid cell — *see* Melanoma
Melanosis L81.4
  addisonian E27.1
    tuberculous A18.7
  adrenal E27.1
  colon K63.89
  conjunctiva — *see* Pigmentation, conjunctiva
    congenital Q13.89
  cornea (presenile) (senile) (*see also* Pigmentation, cornea)
    congenital Q13.4
  eye NEC H57.8
    congenital Q15.8
  lenticularis progressiva Q82.1
  liver K76.89
  precancerous (*see also* Melanoma, in situ)
    malignant melanoma in — *see* Melanoma
  Riehl's L81.4
  sclera H15.89
    congenital Q13.89
  suprarenal E27.1
  tar L81.4
  toxic L81.4
Melanuria R82.99
MELAS syndrome E88.41
Melasma L81.1
  adrenal (gland) E27.1
  suprarenal (gland) E27.1
Melena K92.1
  with ulcer — *code by* site under Ulcer, with hemorrhage K27.4
  due to swallowed maternal blood P78.2
  newborn, neonatal P54.1
    due to swallowed maternal blood P78.2
Meleney's
  gangrene (cutaneous) — *see* Ulcer, skin
  ulcer (chronic undermining) — *see* Ulcer, skin
Melioidosis A24.9
  acute A24.1
  chronic A24.2
  fulminating A24.1
  pneumonia A24.1
  pulmonary (chronic) A24.2
    acute A24.1
    subacute A24.2
  sepsis A24.1
  specified NEC A24.3
  subacute A24.2

Melitensis, febris A23.0
Melkersson (-Rosenthal) **syndrome** G51.2
Mellitus, diabetes — *see* Diabetes
Melorheostosis (bone) — *see* Disorder, bone, density and structure, specified NEC
Meloschisis Q18.4
Melotia Q17.4
Membrana
  capsularis lentis posterior Q13.89
  epipapillaris Q14.2
Membranacea placenta O43.19- ☑
Membranaceous uterus N85.8
Membrane(s), membranous (*see also* condition)
  cyclitic — *see* Membrane, pupillary
  folds, congenital — *see* Web
  Jackson's Q43.3
  over face of newborn P28.9
  premature rupture — *see* Rupture, membranes, premature
  pupillary H21.4- ☑
    persistent Q13.89
  retained (with hemorrhage) (complicating delivery) O72.2
    without hemorrhage O73.1
  secondary cataract — *see* Cataract, secondary
  unruptured (causing asphyxia) — *see* Asphyxia, newborn
  vitreous — *see* Opacity, vitreous, membranes and strands
Membranitis — *see* Chorioamnionitis
Memory disturbance, lack or loss (*see also* Amnesia)
  mild, following organic brain damage F06.8
Menadione deficiency E56.1
Menarche
  delayed E30.0
  precocious E30.1
Mendacity, pathologic F60.2
Mendelson's syndrome (due to anesthesia) J95.4
  in labor and delivery O74.0
  in pregnancy O29.01- ☑
  obstetric O74.0
  postpartum, puerperal O89.01
Ménétrier's disease or syndrome K29.60
  with bleeding K29.61
Ménière's disease, syndrome or vertigo H81.0- ☑
Meninges, meningeal — *see* condition
Meningioma (*see also* Neoplasm, meninges, benign)
  angioblastic — *see* Neoplasm, meninges, benign
  angiomatous — *see* Neoplasm, meninges, benign
  endotheliomatous — *see* Neoplasm, meninges, benign
  fibroblastic — *see* Neoplasm, meninges, benign
  fibrous — *see* Neoplasm, meninges, benign
  hemangioblastic — *see* Neoplasm, meninges, benign
  hemangiopericytic — *see* Neoplasm, meninges, benign
  malignant — *see* Neoplasm, meninges, malignant
  meningiothelial — *see* Neoplasm, meninges, benign
  meningotheliomatous — *see* Neoplasm, meninges, benign
  mixed — *see* Neoplasm, meninges, benign
  multiple — *see* Neoplasm, meninges, uncertain behavior
  papillary — *see* Neoplasm, meninges, uncertain behavior
  psammomatous — *see* Neoplasm, meninges, benign
  syncytial — *see* Neoplasm, meninges, benign
  transitional — *see* Neoplasm, meninges, benign
Meningiomatosis (diffuse) — *see* Neoplasm, meninges, uncertain behavior
Meningism — *see* Meningismus
Meningismus (infectional) (pneumococcal) R29.1
  due to serum or vaccine R29.1
  influenzal — *see* Influenza, with, manifestations NEC
Meningitis (basal) (basic) (brain) (cerebral) (cervical) (congestive) (diffuse) (hemorrhagic) (infantile) (membranous) (metastatic) (nonspecific) (pontine) (progressive) (simple) (spinal) (subacute) (sympathetic) (toxic) G03.9
  abacterial G03.0
  actinomycotic A42.81
  adenoviral A87.1
  arbovirus A87.8
  aseptic (acute) G03.0
  bacterial G00.9
    Escherichia coli (E. coli) G00.8
    Friedländer (bacillus) G00.8
    gram-negative G00.9

Meningitis — *continued*
  bacterial — *continued*
    H. influenzae G00.0
    Klebsiella G00.8
    pneumococcal G00.1
    specified organism NEC G00.8
    staphylococcal G00.3
    streptococcal (acute) G00.2
  benign recurrent (Mollaret) G03.2
  candidal B37.5
  caseous (tuberculous) A17.0
  cerebrospinal A39.0
  chronic NEC G03.1
  clear cerebrospinal fluid NEC G03.0
  coxsackievirus A87.0
  cryptococcal B45.1
  diplococcal (gram positive) A39.0
  echovirus A87.0
  enteroviral A87.0
  eosinophilic B83.2
  epidemic NEC A39.0
  Escherichia coli (E. coli) G00.8
  fibrinopurulent G00.9
    specified organism NEC G00.8
  Friedländer (bacillus) G00.8
  gonococcal A54.81
  gram-negative cocci G00.9
  gram-positive cocci G00.9
  H. influenzae G00.0
  Haemophilus (influenzae) G00.0
  in (due to)
    adenovirus A87.1
    African trypanosomiasis B56.9 [G02]
    anthrax A22.8
    bacterial disease NEC A48.8 [G01]
    Chagas' disease (chronic) B57.41
    chickenpox B01.0
    coccidioidomycosis B38.4
    Diplococcus pneumoniae G00.1
    enterovirus A87.0
    herpes (simplex) virus B00.3
      zoster B02.1
    infectious mononucleosis B27.92
    leptospirosis A27.81
    Listeria monocytogenes A32.11
    Lyme disease A69.21
    measles B05.1
    mumps (virus) B26.1
    neurosyphilis (late) A52.13
    parasitic disease NEC B89 [G02]
    poliovirus A80.9 [G02]
    preventive immunization, inoculation or vaccination G03.8
    rubella B06.02
    Salmonella infection A02.21
    specified cause NEC G03.8
    Streptococcal pneumoniae G00.1
    typhoid fever A01.01
    varicella B01.0
    viral disease NEC A87.8
    whooping cough A37.90
    zoster B02.1
  infectious G00.9
  influenzal (H. influenzae) G00.0
  Klebsiella G00.8
  leptospiral (aseptic) A27.81
  lymphocytic (acute) (benign) (serous) A87.2
  meningococcal A39.0
  Mima polymorpha G00.8
  Mollaret (benign recurrent) G03.2
  monilial B37.5
  mycotic NEC B49 [G02]
  Neisseria A39.0
  nonbacterial G03.0
  nonpyogenic NEC G03.0
  ossificans G96.19
  pneumococcal streptococcus pneumoniae G00.1
  poliovirus A80.9 [G02]
  postmeasles B05.1
  purulent G00.9
    specified organism NEC G00.8
  pyogenic G00.9
    specified organism NEC G00.8
  Salmonella (arizonae) (Cholerae-Suis) (enteritidis) (typhimurium) A02.21
  septic G00.9
    specified organism NEC G00.8
  serosa circumscripta NEC G03.0
  serous NEC G93.2

Melanoma — Meningitis

Meningitis — *continued*
  specified organism NEC G00.8
  sporotrichosis B42.81
  staphylococcal G00.3
  sterile G03.0
  Streptococcal (acute) G00.2
    pneumoniae G00.1
  suppurative G00.9
    specified organism NEC G00.8
  syphilitic (late) (tertiary) A52.13
    acute A51.41
    congenital A50.41
    secondary A51.41
  Torula histolytica (cryptococcal) B45.1
  traumatic (complication of injury) T79.8 ☑
  tuberculous A17.0
  typhoid A01.01
  viral NEC A87.9
  Yersinia pestis A20.3
Meningocele (spinal) (*see also* Spina bifida)
  with hydrocephalus — *see* Spina bifida, by site, with
    hydrocephalus
  acquired (traumatic) G96.19
  cerebral — *see* Encephalocele
Meningocerebritis — *see* Meningoencephalitis
Meningococcemia A39.4
  acute A39.2
  chronic A39.3
Meningococcus, meningococcal (*see also* condition) A39.9
  adrenalitis, hemorrhagic A39.1
  carrier (suspected) of Z22.31
  meningitis (cerebrospinal) A39.0
Meningoencephalitis (*see also* Encephalitis) G04.90
  acute NEC (*see also* Encephalitis, viral) A86
  bacterial NEC G04.2
  California A83.5
  diphasic A84.1
  eosinophilic B83.2
  epidemic A39.81
  herpesviral, herpetic B00.4
    due to herpesvirus 6 B10.01
    due to herpesvirus 7 B10.09
    specified NEC B10.09
  in (due to)
    blastomycosis NEC B40.81
    diseases classified elsewhere G05.3
    free-living amebae B60.2
    H. influenzae G00.0
    Hemophilus influenzae (H .influenzae) G00.0
    herpes B00.4
      due to herpesvirus 6 B10.01
      due to herpesvirus 7 B10.09
      specified NEC B10.09
    Lyme disease A69.22
    mercury — *see* subcategory T56.1 ☑
    mumps B26.2
    Naegleria (amebae) (organisms) (fowleri) B60.2
    Parastrongylus cantonensis B83.2
    toxoplasmosis (acquired) B58.2
      congenital P37.1
  infectious (acute) (viral) A86
  influenzal (H. influenzae) G00.0
  Listeria monocytogenes A32.12
  lymphocytic (serous) A87.2
  mumps B26.2
  parasitic NEC B89 [G05.3]
  pneumococcal G04.2
  primary amebic B60.2
  specific (syphilitic) A52.14
  specified organism NEC G04.81
  staphylococcal G04.2
  streptococcal G04.2
  syphilitic A52.14
  toxic NEC G92
    due to mercury — *see* subcategory T56.1 ☑
  tuberculous A17.82
  virus NEC A86
Meningoencephalocele (*see also* Encephalocele)
  syphilitic A52.19
  congenital A50.49
Meningoencephalomyelitis (*see also* Meningoen-cephalitis)
  acute NEC (viral) A86
    disseminated G04.00
      postimmunization or postvaccination G04.02
      postinfectious G04.01

Meningoencephalomyelitis — *continued*
  due to
    actinomycosis A42.82
    Torula B45.1
    Toxoplasma or toxoplasmosis (acquired) B58.2
      congenital P37.1
  postimmunization or postvaccination G04.02
Meningoencephalomyelopathy G96.9
Meningoencephalopathy G96.9
Meningomyelitis (*see also* Meningoencephalitis)
  bacterial NEC G04.2
  blastomycotic NEC B40.81
  cryptococcal B45.1
  in diseases classified elsewhere G05.4
  meningococcal A39.81
  syphilitic A52.14
  tuberculous A17.82
Meningomyelocele (*see also* Spina bifida)
  syphilitic A52.19
Meningomyeloneuritis — *see* Meningoencephalitis
Meningoradiculitis — *see* Meningitis
Meningovascular — *see* condition
Menkes' disease or syndrome E83.09
  meaning maple-syrup-urine disease E71.0
Menometrorrhagia N92.1
Menopause, menopausal (asymptomatic) (state) Z78.0
  arthritis (any site) NEC — *see* Arthritis, specified form NEC
  bleeding N92.4
  depression (single episode) F32.89
    agitated (single episode) F32.2
      recurrent episode F33.9
    psychotic (single episode) F32.89
      recurrent episode F33.9
    recurrent episode F33.8
  melancholia (single episode) F32.89
    recurrent episode F33.8
  paranoid state F22
  premature E28.319
    asymptomatic E28.319
      postirradiation E89.40
      postsurgical E89.40
    symptomatic E28.310
      postirradiation E89.41
      postsurgical E89.41
  psychosis NEC F28
  symptomatic N95.1
  toxic polyarthritis NEC — *see* Arthritis, specified form NEC
Menorrhagia (primary) N92.0
  climacteric N92.4
    menopausal N92.4
  menopausal N92.4
  postclimacteric N95.0
  postmenopausal N95.0
  preclimacteric or premenopausal N92.4
  pubertal (menses retained) N92.2
Menostaxis N92.0
Menses, retention N94.89
Menstrual — *see* Menstruation
Menstruation
  absent — *see* Amenorrhea
  anovulatory N97.0
  cycle, irregular N92.6
  delayed N91.0
  disorder N93.9
    psychogenic F45.8
  during pregnancy O20.8
  excessive (with regular cycle) N92.0
    with irregular cycle N92.1
    at puberty N92.2
  frequent N92.0
  infrequent — *see* Oligomenorrhea
  irregular N92.6
    specified NEC N92.5
  latent N92.5
  membranous N92.5
  painful (*see also* Dysmenorrhea) N94.6
    primary N94.4
    psychogenic F45.8
    secondary N94.5
  passage of clots N92.0
  precocious E30.1
  protracted N92.5
  rare — *see* Oligomenorrhea
  retained N94.89
  retrograde N92.5
  scanty — *see* Oligomenorrhea

Menstruation — *continued*
  suppression N94.89
  vicarious (nasal) N94.89
Mental (*see also* condition)
  deficiency — *see* Disability, intellectual
  deterioration — *see* Psychosis
  disorder — *see* Disorder, mental
  exhaustion F48.8
  insufficiency (congenital) — *see* Disability, intellectual
  observation without need for further medical care Z03.89
  retardation — *see* Disability, intellectual
  subnormality — *see* Disability, intellectuall
  upset — *see* Disorder, mental
Meralgia paresthetica G57.1- ☑
Mercurial — *see* condition
Mercurialism — *see* subcategory T56.1 ☑
Merkel cell tumor — *see* Carcinoma, Merkel cell
Merocele — *see* Hernia, femoral
Meromelia
  lower limb — *see* Defect, reduction, lower limb
    intercalary
      femur — *see* Defect, reduction, lower limb, specified type NEC
        tibiofibular (complete) (incomplete) — *see* Defect, reduction, lower limb
  upper limb — *see* Defect, reduction, upper limb
    intercalary, humeral, radioulnar — *see* Agenesis, arm, with hand present
MERRF syndrome (myoclonic epilepsy associated with ragged-red fiber) E88.42
Merzbacher-Pelizaeus disease E75.29
Mesaortitis — *see* Aortitis
Mesarteritis — *see* Arteritis
Mesencephalitis — *see* Encephalitis
Mesenchymoma (*see also* Neoplasm, connective tissue, uncertain behavior)
  benign — *see* Neoplasm, connective tissue, benign
  malignant — *see* Neoplasm, connective tissue, malignant
Mesenteritis
  retractile K65.4
  sclerosing K65.4
Mesentery, mesenteric — *see* condition
Mesiodens, mesiodentes K00.1
Mesio-occlusion M26.213
Mesocolon — *see* condition
Mesonephroma (malignant) — *see* Neoplasm, malignant, by site
  benign — *see* Neoplasm, benign, by site
Mesophlebitis — *see* Phlebitis
Mesostromal dysgenesia Q13.89
Mesothelioma (malignant) C45.9
  benign
    mesentery D19.1
    mesocolon D19.1
    omentum D19.1
    peritoneum D19.1
    pleura D19.0
    specified site NEC D19.7
    unspecified site D19.9
  biphasic C45.9
    benign
      mesentery D19.1
      mesocolon D19.1
      omentum D19.1
      peritoneum D19.1
      pleura D19.0
      specified site NEC D19.7
      unspecified site D19.9
  cystic D48.4
  epithelioid C45.9
    benign
      mesentery D19.1
      mesocolon D19.1
      omentum D19.1
      peritoneum D19.1
      pleura D19.0
      specified site NEC D19.7
      unspecified site D19.9
  fibrous C45.9
    benign
      mesentery D19.1
      mesocolon D19.1
      omentum D19.1
      peritoneum D19.1
      pleura D19.0
      specified site NEC D19.7

Mesothelioma — *continued*
  fibrous — *continued*
    benign — *continued*
      unspecified site D19.9
    site classification
      liver C45.7
      lung C45.7
      mediastinum C45.7
      mesentery C45.1
      mesocolon C45.1
      omentum C45.1
      pericardium C45.2
      peritoneum C45.1
      pleura C45.0
        parietal C45.0
      retroperitoneum C45.7
      specified site NEC C45.7
      unspecified C45.9
Metabolic syndrome E88.81
Metagonimiasis B66.8
Metagonimus infestation (intestine) B66.8
Metal
  pigmentation L81.8
  polisher's disease J62.8
Metamorphopsia H53.15
Metaplasia
  apocrine (breast) — *see* Dysplasia, mammary, specified type NEC
  cervix (squamous) — *see* Dysplasia, cervix
  endometrium (squamous) (uterus) N85.8
  esophagus K22.7- ☑
  kidney (pelvis) (squamous) N28.89
  myelogenous D73.1
  myeloid (agnogenic) (megakaryocytic) D73.1
  spleen D73.1
  squamous cell, bladder N32.89
Metastasis, metastatic
  abscess — *see* Abscess
  calcification E83.59
  cancer
    from specified site — *see* Neoplasm, malignant, by site
    to specified site — *see* Neoplasm, secondary, by site
  deposits (in) — *see* Neoplasm, secondary, by site
  disease (*see also* Neoplasm, secondary, by site) C79.9
  spread (to) — *see* Neoplasm, secondary, by site
Metastrongyliasis B83.8
Metatarsalgia M77.4- ☑
  anterior G57.6- ☑
  Morton's G57.6- ☑
Metatarsus, metatarsal (*see also* condition)
  adductus, congenital Q66.22
  valgus (abductus), congenital Q66.6
  varus (congenital) Q66.22
    primus Q66.21
Methadone use — *see* Use, opioid
Methemoglobinemia D74.9
  acquired (with sulfhemoglobinemia) D74.8
  congenital D74.0
  enzymatic (congenital) D74.0
  Hb M disease D74.0
  hereditary D74.0
  toxic D74.8
Methemoglobinuria — *see* Hemoglobinuria
Methioninemia E72.19
Methylmalonic acidemia E71.120
Metritis (catarrhal) (hemorrhagic) (septic) (suppurative) (*see also* Endometritis)
  cervical — *see* Cervicitis
Metropathia hemorrhagica N93.8
Metroperitonitis — *see* Peritonitis, pelvic, female
Metrorrhagia N92.1
  climacteric N92.4
  menopausal N92.4
  postpartum NEC (atonic) (following delivery of placenta) O72.1
    delayed or secondary O72.2
  preclimacteric or premenopausal N92.4
  psychogenic F45.8
Metrorrhexis — *see* Rupture, uterus
Metrosalpingitis N70.91
Metrostaxis N93.8
Metrovaginitis — *see* Endometritis
Meyer-Schwickerath and Weyers syndrome Q87.0
Meynert's amentia (nonalcoholic) F04
  alcoholic F10.96

Meynert's amentia — *continued*
  alcoholic — *continued*
    with dependence F10.26
Mibelli's disease (porokeratosis) Q82.8
Mice, joint — *see* Loose, body, joint
  knee M23.4- ☑
Micrencephalon, micrencephaly Q02
Microalbuminuria R80.9
Microaneurysm, retinal (*see also* Disorder, retina, microaneurysms)
  diabetic — *see* E08-E13 with .31
Microangiopathy (peripheral) I73.9
  thrombotic M31.1
Microcalcifications, breast R92.0
Microcephalus, microcephalic, microcephaly Q02
  due to toxoplasmosis (congenital) P37.1
Microcheilia Q18.7
Microcolon (congenital) Q43.8
Microcornea (congenital) Q13.4
Microcytic — *see* condition
Microdeletions NEC Q93.88
Microdontia K00.2
Microdrepanocytosis D57.40
  with crisis (vasoocclusive pain) D57.419
    with
      acute chest syndrome D57.411
      splenic sequestration D57.412
Microembolism
  atherothrombotic — *see* Atheroembolism
  retinal — *see* Occlusion, artery, retina
Microencephalon Q02
Microfilaria streptocerca infestation — *see* Onchocerciasis
Microgastria (congenital) Q40.2
Microgenia M26.06
Microgenitalia, congenital
  female Q52.8
  male Q55.8
Microglioma — *see* Lymphoma, non-Hodgkin, specified NEC
Microglossia (congenital) Q38.3
Micrognathia, micrognathism (congenital) (mandibular) (maxillary) M26.09
Microgyria (congenital) Q04.3
Microinfarct of heart — *see* Insufficiency, coronary
Microlentia (congenital) Q12.8
Microlithiasis, alveolar, pulmonary J84.02
Micromastia N64.82
Micromyelia (congenital) Q06.8
Micropenis Q55.62
Microphakia (congenital) Q12.8
Microphthalmos, microphthalmia (congenital) Q11.2
  due to toxoplasmosis P37.1
Micropsia H53.15
Microscopic polyangiitis (polyarteritis) M31.7
Microsporidiosis B60.8
  intestinal A07.8
Microsporon furfur infestation B36.0
Microsporosis (*see also* Dermatophytosis)
  nigra B36.1
Microstomia (congenital) Q18.5
Microtia (congenital) (external ear) Q17.2
Microtropia H50.40
Microvillus inclusion disease (MVD) (MVID) Q43.8
Micturition
  disorder NEC (*see also* Difficulty, micturition) R39.198
    psychogenic F45.8
  frequency R35.0
    psychogenic F45.8
  hesitancy R39.11
  incomplete emptying R39.14
  nocturnal R35.1
  painful R30.9
    dysuria R30.0
    psychogenic F45.8
    tenesmus R30.1
  poor stream R39.12
  position dependent R39.192
  split stream R39.13
  straining R39.16
  urgency R39.15
Mid plane — *see* condition
Middle
  ear — *see* condition
  lobe (right) syndrome J98.19
Miescher's elastoma L87.2
Mietens' syndrome Q87.2

Migraine (idiopathic) G43.909
  with aura (acute-onset) (prolonged) (typical) (without headache) G43.109
    with refractory migraine G43.119
      with status migrainosus G43.111
      without status migrainosus G43.119
    without mention of refractory migraine G43.109
      with status migrainosus G43.101
      without status migrainosus G43.109
    intractable G43.119
      with status migrainosus G43.111
      without status migrainosus G43.119
    not intractable G43.109
      with status migrainosus G43.101
      without status migrainosus G43.109
    persistent G43.509
      with cerebral infarction G43.609
        with refractory migraine G43.619
          with status migrainosus G43.611
          without status migrainosus G43.619
        without refractory migraine G43.609
          with status migrainosus G43.601
          without status migrainosus G43.609
        intractable G43.619
          with status migrainosus G43.611
          without status migrainosus G43.619
        not intractable G43.609
          with status migrainosus G43.601
          without status migrainosus G43.609
      without cerebral infarction G43.509
        with refractory migraine G43.519
          with status migrainosus G43.511
          without status migrainosus G43.519
        without refractory migraine G43.509
          with status migrainosus G43.501
          without status migrainosus G43.509
        intractable G43.519
          with status migrainosus G43.511
          without status migrainosus G43.519
        not intractable G43.509
          with status migrainosus G43.501
          without status migrainosus G43.509
  with refractory migraine G43.919
    with status migrainosus G43.911
    without status migrainosus G43.919
  without aura G43.009
    with refractory migraine G43.019
      with status migrainosus G43.011
      without status migrainosus G43.019
    without mention of refractory migraine G43.009
      with status migrainosus G43.001
      without status migrainosus G43.009
    chronic G43.709
      with refractory migraine G43.719
        with status migrainosus G43.711
        without status migrainosus G43.719
      without refractory migraine G43.709
        with status migrainosus G43.701
        without status migrainosus G43.709
      intractable
        with status migrainosus G43.711
        without status migrainosus G43.719
      not intractable
        with status migrainosus G43.701
        without status migrainosus G43.709
    intractable
      with status migrainosus G43.011
      without status migrainosus G43.019
    not intractable
      with status migrainosus G43.001
      without status migrainosus G43.009
  without refractory migraine G43.909
    with status migrainosus G43.901
    without status migrainosus G43.919
  abdominal G43.D0 (*following* G43.7)
    with refractory migraine G43.D1 (*following* G43.7)
    without refractory migraine G43.D0 (*following* G43.7)
    intractable G43.D1 (*following* G43.7)
    not intractable G43.D0 (*following* G43.7)
  basilar — *see* Migraine, with aura
  classical — *see* Migraine, with aura
  common — *see* Migraine, without aura
  complicated G43.109
  equivalents — *see* Migraine, with aura
  familiar — *see* Migraine, hemiplegic
  hemiplegic G43.409
    with refractory migraine G43.419
      with status migrainosus G43.411

Migraine — *continued*
  hemiplegic — *continued*
    with refractory migraine — *continued*
      without status migrainosus G43.419
    without refractory migraine G43.409
      with status migrainosus G43.401
      without status migrainosus G43.409
    intractable G43.419
      with status migrainosus G43.411
      without status migrainosus G43.419
    not intractable G43.409
      with status migrainosus G43.401
      without status migrainosus G43.409
    intractable G43.919
      with status migrainosus G43.911
      without status migrainosus G43.919
  menstrual G43.829
    with refractory migraine G43.839
      with status migrainosus G43.831
      without status migrainosus G43.839
    without refractory migraine G43.829
      with status migrainosus G43.821
      without status migrainosus G43.829
    intractable G43.839
      with status migrainosus G43.831
      without status migrainosus G43.839
    not intractable 4G43.829
      with status migrainosus G43.821
      without status migrainosus G43.829
  menstrually related — *see* Migraine, menstrual
  not intractable G43.909
    with status migrainosus G43.901
    without status migrainosus G43.919
  ophthalmoplegic G43.B0 (*following* G43.7)
    with refractory migraine G43.B1 (*following* G43.7)
    without refractory migraine G43.B0 (*following* G43.7)
    intractable G43.B1 (*following* G43.7)
    not intractable G43.B0 (*following* G43.7)
  persistent aura (with, without) cerebral infarction — *see* Migraine, with aura, persistent
  preceded or accompanied by transient focal neurological phenomena — *see* Migraine, with aura
  pre-menstrual — *see* Migraine, menstrual
  pure menstrual — *see* Migraine, menstrual
  retinal — *see* Migraine, with aura
  specified NEC G43.809
    intractable G43.819
      with status migrainosus G43.811
      without status migrainosus G43.819
    not intractable G43.809
      with status migrainosus G43.801
      without status migrainosus G43.809
  sporadic — *see* Migraine, hemiplegic
  transformed — *see* Migraine, without aura, chronic
  triggered seizures — *see* Migraine, with aura
Migrant, social Z59.0
Migration, anxiety concerning Z60.3
Migratory, migrating (*see also* condition)
  person Z59.0
  testis Q55.29
Mikity-Wilson disease or syndrome P27.0
Mikulicz' disease or syndrome K11.8
Miliaria L74.3
  alba L74.1
  apocrine L75.2
  crystallina L74.1
  profunda L74.2
  rubra L74.0
  tropicalis L74.2
Miliary — *see* condition
Milium L72.0
  colloid L57.8
Milk
  crust L21.0
  excessive secretion O92.6
  poisoning — *see* Poisoning, food, noxious
  retention O92.79
  sickness — *see* Poisoning, food, noxious
  spots I31.0
Milk-alkali disease or syndrome E83.52
Milk-leg (deep vessels) (nonpuerperal) — *see* Embolism, vein, lower extremity
  complicating pregnancy O22.3- ☑
  puerperal, postpartum, childbirth O87.1
Milkman's disease or syndrome M83.8
Milky urine — *see* Chyluria
Millard-Gubler (-Foville) **paralysis or syndrome** G46.3

Millar's asthma J38.5
Miller Fisher syndrome G61.0
Mills' disease — *see* Hemiplegia
Millstone maker's pneumoconiosis J62.8
Milroy's disease (chronic hereditary edema) Q82.0
Minamata disease T56.1 ☑
Miners' asthma or lung J60
Minkowski-Chauffard syndrome — *see* Spherocytosis
Minor — *see* condition
Minor's disease (hematomyelia) G95.19
Minot's disease (hemorrhagic disease), newborn P53
Minot-von Willebrand-Jurgens disease or syndrome (angiohemophilia) D68.0
Minus (and plus) **hand** (intrinsic) — *see* Deformity, limb, specified type NEC, forearm
Miosis (pupil) H57.03
Mirizzi's syndrome (hepatic duct stenosis) K83.1
Mirror writing F81.0
Misadventure (of) (prophylactic) (therapeutic) (*see also* Complications) T88.9 ☑
  administration of insulin (by accident) — *see* subcategory T38.3 ☑
  infusion — *see* Complications, infusion
  local applications (of fomentations, plasters, etc.) T88.9 ☑
    burn or scald — *see* Burn
    specified NEC T88.8 ☑
  medical care (early) (late) T88.9 ☑
    adverse effect of drugs or chemicals — *see* Table of Drugs and Chemicals
    burn or scald — *see* Burn
    specified NEC T88.8 ☑
  specified NEC T88.8 ☑
  surgical procedure (early) (late) — *see* Complications, surgical procedure
  transfusion — *see* Complications, transfusion
  vaccination or other immunological procedure — *see* Complications, vaccination
Miscarriage O03.9
Misdirection, aqueous H40.83- ☑
Misperception, sleep state F51.02
Misplaced, misplacement
  ear Q17.4
  kidney (acquired) N28.89
    congenital Q63.2
  organ or site, congenital NEC — *see* Malposition, congenital
Missed
  abortion O02.1
  delivery O36.4 ☑
Missing (*see also* Absence)
  string of intrauterine contraceptive device T83.32- ☑
Misuse of drugs F19.99
Mitchell's disease (erythromelalgia) I73.81
Mite(s) (infestation) B88.9
  diarrhea B88.0
  grain (itch) B88.0
  hair follicle (itch) B88.0
  in sputum B88.0
Mitral — *see* condition
Mittelschmerz N94.0
Mixed — *see* condition
MMN (multifocal motor neuropathy) G61.82
MNGIE (Mitochondrial Neurogastrointestinal Encephalopathy) **syndrome** E88.49
Mobile, mobility
  cecum Q43.3
  excessive — *see* Hypermobility
  gallbladder, congenital Q44.1
  kidney N28.89
  organ or site, congenital NEC — *see* Malposition, congenital
Mobitz heart block (atrioventricular) I44.1
Moebius, Möbius
  disease (ophthalmoplegic migraine) — *see* Migraine, ophthalmoplegic
  syndrome Q87.0
    congenital oculofacial paralysis (with other anomalies) Q87.0
    ophthalmoplegic migraine — *see* Migraine, ophthalmoplegic
Moeller's glossitis K14.0
Mohr's syndrome (Types I and II) Q87.0
Mola destruens D39.2
Molar pregnancy O02.0
Molarization of premolars K00.2

Molding, head (during birth) — *omit code*
Mole (pigmented) (*see also* Nevus)
  blood O02.0
  Breus' O02.0
  cancerous — *see* Melanoma
  carneous O02.0
  destructive D39.2
  fleshy O02.0
  hydatid, hydatidiform (benign) (complicating pregnancy) (delivered) (undelivered) O01.9
    classical O01.0
    complete O01.0
    incomplete O01.1
    invasive D39.2
    malignant D39.2
    partial O01.1
  intrauterine O02.0
  invasive (hydatidiform) D39.2
  malignant
    meaning
      malignant hydatidiform mole D39.2
      melanoma — *see* Melanoma
  nonhydatidiform O02.0
  nonpigmented — *see* Nevus
  pregnancy NEC O02.0
  skin — *see* Nevus
  tubal O00.10- ☑
    with intrauterine pregnancy O00.11- ☑
  vesicular — *see* Mole, hydatidiform
Molimen, molimina (menstrual) N94.3
Molluscum contagiosum (epitheliale) B08.1
Mönckeberg's arteriosclerosis, disease, or sclerosis — *see* Arteriosclerosis, extremities
Mondini's malformation (cochlea) Q16.5
Mondor's disease I80.8
Monge's disease T70.29 ☑
Monilethrix (congenital) Q84.1
Moniliasis (*see also* Candidiasis) B37.9
  neonatal P37.5
Monitoring (encounter for)
  therapeutic drug level Z51.81
Monkey malaria B53.1
Monkeypox B04
Monoarthritis M13.10
  ankle M13.17- ☑
  elbow M13.12- ☑
  foot joint M13.17- ☑
  hand joint M13.14- ☑
  hip M13.15- ☑
  knee M13.16- ☑
  shoulder M13.11- ☑
  wrist M13.13- ☑
Monoblastic — *see* condition
Monochromat (ism), monochromatopsia (acquired) (congenital) H53.51
Monocytic — *see* condition
Monocytopenia D72.818
Monocytosis (symptomatic) D72.821
Monomania — *see* Psychosis
Mononeuritis G58.9
  cranial nerve — *see* Disorder, nerve, cranial
  femoral nerve G57.2- ☑
  lateral
    cutaneous nerve of thigh G57.1- ☑
    popliteal nerve G57.3- ☑
  lower limb G57.9- ☑
    specified NEC G57.8- ☑
  medial popliteal nerve G57.4- ☑
  median nerve G56.1- ☑
  multiplex G58.7
  plantar nerve G57.6- ☑
  posterior tibial nerve G57.5- ☑
  radial nerve G56.3- ☑
  sciatic nerve G57.0- ☑
  specified NEC G58.8
  tibial nerve G57.4- ☑
  ulnar nerve G56.2- ☑
  upper limb G56.9- ☑
    specified nerve NEC G56.8- ☑
  vestibular — *see* subcategory H93.3 ☑
Mononeuropathy G58.9
  carpal tunnel syndrome — *see* Syndrome, carpal tunnel
  diabetic NEC — *see* E08-E13 with .41
  femoral nerve — *see* Lesion, nerve, femoral
  ilioinguinal nerve G57.8- ☑
  in diseases classified elsewhere — *see* category G59

Mononeuropathy — *continued*
  intercostal G58.0
  lower limb G57.9- ☑
    causalgia — *see* Causalgia, lower limb
    femoral nerve — *see* Lesion, nerve, femoral
    meralgia paresthetica G57.1- ☑
    plantar nerve — *see* Lesion, nerve, plantar
    popliteal nerve — *see* Lesion, nerve, popliteal
    sciatic nerve — *see* Lesion, nerve, sciatic
    specified NEC G57.8- ☑
    tarsal tunnel syndrome — *see* Syndrome, tarsal tunnel
  median nerve — *see* Lesion, nerve, median
  multiplex G58.7
  obturator nerve G57.8- ☑
  popliteal nerve — *see* Lesion, nerve, popliteal
  radial nerve — *see* Lesion, nerve, radial
  saphenous nerve G57.8- ☑
  specified NEC G58.8
  tarsal tunnel syndrome — *see* Syndrome, tarsal tunnel
  tuberculous A17.83
  ulnar nerve — *see* Lesion, nerve, ulnar
  upper limb G56.9- ☑
    carpal tunnel syndrome — *see* Syndrome, carpal tunnel
    causalgia — *see* Causalgia
    median nerve — *see* Lesion, nerve, median
    radial nerve — *see* Lesion, nerve, radial
    specified site NEC G56.8- ☑
    ulnar nerve — *see* Lesion, nerve, ulnar
Mononucleosis, infectious B27.90
  with
    complication NEC B27.99
    meningitis B27.92
    polyneuropathy B27.91
  cytomegaloviral B27.10
    with
      complication NEC B27.19
      meningitis B27.12
      polyneuropathy B27.11
  Epstein-Barr (virus) B27.00
    with
      complication NEC B27.09
      meningitis B27.02
      polyneuropathy B27.01
  gammaherpesviral B27.00
    with
      complication NEC B27.09
      meningitis B27.02
      polyneuropathy B27.01
  specified NEC B27.80
    with
      complication NEC B27.89
      meningitis B27.82
      polyneuropathy B27.81
Monoplegia G83.3- ☑
  congenital (cerebral) G80.8
    spastic G80.1
  embolic (current episode) I63.4- ☑
  following
    cerebrovascular disease
      cerebral infarction
        lower limb I69.34- ☑
        upper limb I69.33- ☑
      intracerebral hemorrhage
        lower limb I69.14- ☑
        upper limb I69.13- ☑
      lower limb I69.94- ☑
      nontraumatic intracranial hemorrhage NEC
        lower limb I69.24- ☑
        upper limb I69.23- ☑
      specified disease NEC
        lower limb I69.84- ☑
        upper limb I69.83- ☑
      stroke NOS
        lower limb I69.34- ☑
        upper limb I69.33- ☑
      subarachnoid hemorrhage
        lower limb I69.04- ☑
        upper limb I69.03- ☑
      upper limb I69.93- ☑
  hysterical (transient) F44.4
  lower limb G83.1- ☑
  psychogenic (conversion reaction) F44.4
  thrombotic (current episode) I63.3- ☑
  transient R29.818
  upper limb G83.2- ☑

Monorchism, monorchidism Q55.0
Monosomy (*see also* Deletion, chromosome) Q93.9
  specified NEC Q93.89
  whole chromosome
    meiotic nondisjunction Q93.0
    mitotic nondisjunction Q93.1
    mosaicism Q93.1
  X Q96.9
Monster, monstrosity (single) Q89.7
  acephalic Q00.0
  twin Q89.4
Monteggia's fracture (-dislocation) S52.27- ☑
Mooren's ulcer (cornea) — *see* Ulcer, cornea, Mooren's
Moore's syndrome — *see* Epilepsy, specified NEC
Mooser-Neill reaction A75.2
Mooser's bodies A75.2
Morbidity not stated or unknown R69
Morbilli — *see* Measles
Morbus (*see also* Disease)
  angelicus, anglorum E55.0
  Beigel B36.2
  caducus — *see* Epilepsy
  celiacus K90.0
  comitialis — *see* Epilepsy
  cordis (*see also* Disease, heart) I51.9
    valvulorum — *see* Endocarditis
  coxae senilis M16.9
    tuberculous A18.02
  hemorrhagicus neonatorum P53
  maculosus neonatorum P54.5
Morel (-Stewart)(-Morgagni) **syndrome** M85.2
Morel-Kraepelin disease — *see* Schizophrenia
Morel-Moore syndrome M85.2
Morgagni's
  cyst, organ, hydatid, or appendage
    female Q50.5
    male (epididymal) Q55.4
      testicular Q55.29
  syndrome M85.2
Morgagni-Stewart-Morel syndrome M85.2
Morgagni-Stokes-Adams syndrome I45.9
Morgagni-Turner (-Albright) **syndrome** Q96.9
Moria F07.0
Moron (I.Q. 50-69) F70
Morphea L94.0
Morphinism (without remission) F11.20
  with remission F11.21
Morphinomania (without remission) F11.20
  with remission F11.21
Morquio (-Ullrich)(-Brailsford) **disease or syndrome** — *see* Mucopolysaccharidosis
Mortification (dry) (moist) — *see* Gangrene
Morton's metatarsalgia (neuralgia)(neuroma) (syndrome) G57.6- ☑
Morvan's disease or syndrome G60.8
Mosaicism, mosaic (autosomal) (chromosomal)
  45,X/46,XX Q96.3
  45,X/other cell lines NEC with abnormal sex chromosome Q96.4
  sex chromosome
    female Q97.8
    lines with various numbers of X chromosomes Q97.2
    male Q98.7
  XY Q96.3
Moschowitz' disease M31.1
Mother yaw A66.0
Motion sickness (from travel, any vehicle) (from roundabouts or swings) T75.3 ☑
Mottled, mottling, teeth (enamel) (endemic) (nonendemic) K00.3
Mounier-Kuhn syndrome Q32.4
  with bronchiectasis J47.9
    exacerbation (acute) J47.1
    lower respiratory infection J47.0
  acquired J98.09
    with bronchiectasis J47.9
      with
        exacerbation (acute) J47.1
        lower respiratory infection J47.0
Mountain
  sickness T70.29 ☑
    with polycythemia , acquired (acute) D75.1
  tick fever A93.2
Mouse, joint — *see* Loose, body, joint
  knee M23.4- ☑
Mouth — *see* condition

Movable
  coccyx — *see* subcategory M53.2 ☑
  kidney N28.89
    congenital Q63.8
  spleen D73.89
Movements, dystonic R25.8
Moyamoya disease I67.5
MRSA (Methicillin resistant Staphylococcus aureus)
  infection A49.02
    as the cause of diseases classified elsewhere B95.62
  sepsis A41.02
MSSA (Methicillin susceptible Staphylococcus aureus)
  infection A49.01
    as the cause of diseases classified elsewhere B95.61
  sepsis A41.01
Mucha-Habermann disease L41.0
Mucinosis (cutaneous) (focal) (papular) (skin) L98.5
  oral K13.79
Mucocele
  appendix K38.8
  buccal cavity K13.79
  gallbladder K82.1
  lacrimal sac, chronic H04.43- ☑
  nasal sinus J34.1
  nose J34.1
  salivary gland (any) K11.6
  sinus (accessory) (nasal) J34.1
  turbinate (bone) (middle) (nasal) J34.1
  uterus N85.8
Mucolipidosis
  I E77.1
  II, III E77.0
  IV E75.11
Mucopolysaccharidosis E76.3
  beta-gluduronidase deficiency E76.29
  cardiopathy E76.3 [I52]
  Hunter's syndrome E76.1
  Hurler's syndrome E76.01
  Hurler-Scheie syndrome E76.02
  Maroteaux-Lamy syndrome E76.29
  Morquio syndrome E76.219
    A E76.210
    B E76.211
    classic E76.210
  Sanfilippo syndrome E76.22
  Scheie's syndrome E76.03
  specified NEC E76.29
  type
    I
      Hurler's syndrome E76.01
      Hurler-Scheie syndrome E76.02
      Scheie's syndrome E76.03
    II E76.1
    III E76.22
    IV E76.219
    IVA E76.210
    IVB E76.211
    VI E76.29
    VII E76.29
Mucormycosis B46.5
  cutaneous B46.3
  disseminated B46.4
  gastrointestinal B46.2
  generalized B46.4
  pulmonary B46.0
  rhinocerebral B46.1
  skin B46.3
  subcutaneous B46.3
Mucositis (ulcerative) K12.30
  due to drugs NEC K12.32
  gastrointestinal K92.81
  mouth (oral) (oropharyngeal) K12.30
    due to antineoplastic therapy K12.31
    due to drugs NEC K12.32
    due to radiation K12.33
    specified NEC K12.39
    viral K12.39
  nasal J34.81
  oral cavity — *see* Mucositis, mouth
  oral soft tissues — *see* Mucositis, mouth
  vagina and vulva N76.81
Mucositis necroticans agranulocytica — *see* Agranulocytosis
Mucous (*see also* condition)
  patches (syphilitic) A51.39
    congenital A50.07
Mucoviscidosis E84.9
  with meconium obstruction E84.11

Mucus
asphyxia or suffocation — *see* Asphyxia, mucus
in stool R19.5
plug — *see* Asphyxia, mucus
Muguet B37.0
Mulberry molars (congenital syphilis) A50.52
Müllerian mixed tumor
specified site — *see* Neoplasm, malignant, by site
unspecified site C54.9
Multicystic kidney (development) Q61.4
Multiparity (grand) Z64.1
affecting management of pregnancy, labor and delivery (supervision only) O09.4- ☑
requiring contraceptive management — *see* Contraception
Multipartita placenta O43.19- ☑
Multiple, multiplex (*see also* condition)
digits (congenital) Q69.9
endocrine neoplasia — *see* Neoplasia, endocrine, multiple (MEN)
personality F44.81
Mumps B26.9
arthritis B26.85
complication NEC B26.89
encephalitis B26.2
hepatitis B26.81
meningitis (aseptic) B26.1
meningoencephalitis B26.2
myocarditis B26.82
oophoritis B26.89
orchitis B26.0
pancreatitis B26.3
polyneuropathy B26.84
Mumu (*see also* Infestation, filarial) B74.9 [N51]
Münchhausen's syndrome — *see* Disorder, factitious
Münchmeyer's syndrome — *see* Myositis, ossificans, progressiva
Mural — *see* condition
Murmur (cardiac) (heart) (organic) R01.1
abdominal R19.15
aortic (valve) — *see* Endocarditis, aortic
benign R01.0
diastolic — *see* Endocarditis
Flint I35.1
functional R01.0
Graham Steell I37.1
innocent R01.0
mitral (valve) — *see* Insufficiency, mitral
nonorganic R01.0
presystolic, mitral — *see* Insufficiency, mitral
pulmonic (valve) I37.8
systolic R01.1
tricuspid (valve) I07.9
valvular — *see* Endocarditis
Murri's disease (intermittent hemoglobinuria) D59.6
Muscle, muscular (*see also* condition)
carnitine (palmityltransferase) deficiency E71.314
Musculoneuralgia — *see* Neuralgia
Mushrooming hip — *see* Derangement, joint, specified NEC, hip
Mushroom-workers' (pickers') **disease or lung** J67.5
Mutation(s)
factor V Leiden D68.51
prothrombin gene D68.52
surfactant, of lung J84.83
Mutism (*see also* Aphasia)
deaf (acquired) (congenital) NEC H91.3
elective (adjustment reaction) (childhood) F94.0
hysterical F44.4
selective (childhood) F94.0
MVD (microvillus inclusion disease) Q43.8
MVID (microvillus inclusion disease) Q43.8
Myalgia M79.1
epidemic (cervical) B33.0
traumatic NEC T14.8 ☑
Myasthenia G70.9
congenital G70.2
cordis — *see* Failure, heart
developmental G70.2
gravis G70.00
with exacerbation (acute) G70.01
in crisis G70.01
neonatal, transient P94.0
pseudoparalytica G70.00
with exacerbation (acute) G70.01
in crisis G70.01
stomach, psychogenic F45.8

Myasthenia — *continued*
syndrome
in
diabetes mellitus — *see* E08-E13 with .44
neoplastic disease (*see also* Neoplasm) D49.9 [G73.3]
pernicious anemia D51.0 [G73.3]
thyrotoxicosis E05.90 [G73.3]
with thyroid storm E05.91 [G73.3]
Myasthenic M62.81
Mycelium infection B49
Mycetismus — *see* Poisoning, food, noxious, mushroom
Mycetoma B47.9
actinomycotic B47.1
bone (mycotic) B47.9 [M90.80]
eumycotic B47.0
foot B47.9
actinomycotic B47.1
mycotic B47.0
madurae NEC B47.9
mycotic B47.0
maduromycotic B47.0
mycotic B47.0
nocardial B47.1
Mycobacteriosis — *see* Mycobacterium
Mycobacterium, mycobacterial (infection) A31.9
anonymous A31.9
atypical A31.9
cutaneous A31.1
pulmonary A31.0
tuberculous — *see* Tuberculosis, pulmonary
specified site NEC A31.8
avium (intracellulare complex) A31.0
balnei A31.1
Battey A31.0
chelonei A31.8
cutaneous A31.1
extrapulmonary systemic A31.8
fortuitum A31.8
intracellulare (Battey bacillus) A31.0
kakaferifu A31.8
kansasii (yellow bacillus) A31.0
kasongo A31.8
leprae (*see also* Leprosy) A30.9
luciflavum A31.1
marinum (M. balnei) A31.1
nonspecific — *see* Mycobacterium, atypical
pulmonary (atypical) A31.0
tuberculous — *see* Tuberculosis, pulmonary
scrofulaceum A31.8
simiae A31.8
systemic, extrapulmonary A31.8
szulgai A31.8
terrae A31.8
triviale A31.8
tuberculosis (human, bovine) — *see* Tuberculosis
ulcerans A31.1
xenopi A31.8
Mycoplasma (M.) **pneumoniae, as cause of disease classified elsewhere** B96.0
Mycosis, mycotic B49
cutaneous NEC B36.9
ear B36.9
in
aspergillosis B44.89
candidiasis B37.84
moniliasis B37.84
fungoides (extranodal) (solid organ) C84.0- ☑
mouth B37.0
nails B35.1
opportunistic B48.8
skin NEC B36.9
specified NEC B48.8
stomatitis B37.0
vagina, vaginitis (candidal) B37.3
Mydriasis (pupil) H57.04
Myelatelia Q06.1
Myelinolysis, pontine, central G37.2
Myelitis (acute) (ascending) (childhood) (chronic) (descending) (diffuse) (disseminated) (idiopathic) (pressure) (progressive) (spinal cord) (subacute) (*see also* Encephalitis) G04.91
herpes simplex B00.82
herpes zoster B02.24
in diseases classified elsewhere G05.4
necrotizing, subacute G37.4
optic neuritis in G36.0
postchickenpox B01.12

Myelitis — *continued*
postherpetic B02.24
postimmunization G04.02
postinfectious NEC G04.89
postvaccinal G04.02
specified NEC G04.89
syphilitic (transverse) A52.14
toxic G92
transverse (in demyelinating diseases of central nervous system) G37.3
tuberculous A17.82
varicella B01.12
Myeloblastic — *see* condition
Myeloblastoma
granular cell (*see also* Neoplasm, connective tissue)
malignant — *see* Neoplasm, connective tissue, malignant
tongue D10.1
Myelocele — *see* Spina bifida
Myelocystocele — *see* Spina bifida
Myelocytic — *see* condition
Myelodysplasia D46.9
specified NEC D46.Z (*following* D46.4)
spinal cord (congenital) Q06.1
Myelodysplastic syndrome D46.9
with
5q deletion D46.C (*following* D46.2)
isolated del (5q) chromosomal abnormality D46.C (*following* D46.2)
specified NEC D46.Z (*following* D46.4)
Myeloencephalitis — *see* Encephalitis
Myelofibrosis D75.81
with myeloid metaplasia D47.4
acute C94.4- ☑
idiopathic (chronic) D47.4
primary D47.1
secondary D75.81
in myeloproliferative disease D47.4
Myelogenous — *see* condition
Myeloid — *see* condition
Myelokathexis D70.9
Myeloleukodystrophy E75.29
Myelolipoma — *see* Lipoma
Myeloma (multiple) C90.0- ☑
monostotic C90.3 ☑
plasma cell C90.0- ☑
plasma cell C90.0- ☑
solitary (*see also* Plasmacytoma, solitary) C90.3- ☑
Myelomalacia G95.89
Myelomatosis C90.0- ☑
Myelomeningitis — *see* Meningoencephalitis
Myelomeningocele (spinal cord) — *see* Spina bifida
Myelo-osteo-musculodysplasia hereditaria Q79.8
Myelopathic
anemia D64.89
muscle atrophy — *see* Atrophy, muscle, spinal
pain syndrome G89.0
Myelopathy (spinal cord) G95.9
drug-induced G95.89
in (due to)
degeneration or displacement, intervertebral disc NEC — *see* Disorder, disc, with, myelopathy
infection — *see* Encephalitis
intervertebral disc disorder (*see also* Disorder, disc, with, myelopathy)
mercury — *see* subcategory T56.1 ☑
neoplastic disease (*see also* Neoplasm) D49.9 [G99.2]
pernicious anemia D51.0 [G99.2]
spondylosis — *see* Spondylosis, with myelopathy NEC
necrotic (subacute) (vascular) G95.19
radiation-induced G95.89
spondylogenic NEC — *see* Spondylosis, with myelopathy NEC
toxic G95.89
transverse, acute G37.3
vascular G95.19
vitamin B12 E53.8 [G32.0]
Myelophthisis D61.82
Myeloradiculitis G04.91
Myeloradiculodysplasia (spinal) Q06.1
Myelosarcoma C92.3- ☑
Myelosclerosis D75.89
with myeloid metaplasia D47.4
disseminated, of nervous system G35
megakaryocytic D47.4

226

☑ Additional Character Required — Refer to the Tabular List for Character Selection   ▽ Subterms under main terms may continue to next column or page

Mucus — Myelosclerosis

Myelosclerosis — *continued*
- megakaryocytic — *continued*
  - with myeloid metaplasia D47.4

Myelosis
- acute C92.0- ☑
- aleukemic C92.9- ☑
- chronic D47.1
- erythremic (acute) C94.0- ☑
- megakaryocytic C94.2- ☑
- nonleukemic D72.828
- subacute C92.9- ☑

Myiasis (cavernous) B87.9
- aural B87.4
- creeping B87.0
- cutaneous B87.0
- dermal B87.0
- ear (external) (middle) B87.4
- eye B87.2
- genitourinary B87.81
- intestinal B87.82
- laryngeal B87.3
- nasopharyngeal B87.3
- ocular B87.2
- orbit B87.2
- skin B87.0
- specified site NEC B87.89
- traumatic B87.1
- wound B87.1

Myoadenoma, prostate — *see* Hyperplasia, prostate

Myoblastoma
- granular cell (*see also* Neoplasm, connective tissue, benign)
  - malignant — *see* Neoplasm, connective tissue, malignant
- tongue D10.1

Myocardial — *see* condition

Myocardiopathy (congestive) (constrictive) (familial) (hypertrophic nonobstructive) (idiopathic) (infiltrative) (obstructive) (primary) (restrictive) (sporadic) (*see also* Cardiomyopathy) I42.9
- alcoholic I42.6
- cobalt-beer I42.6
- glycogen storage E74.02 [I43]
- hypertrophic obstructive I42.1
- in (due to)
  - beriberi E51.12
  - cardiac glycogenosis E74.02 [I43]
  - Friedreich's ataxia G11.1 [I43]
  - myotonia atrophica G71.11 [I43]
  - progressive muscular dystrophy G71.0 [I43]
- obscure (African) I42.8
- secondary I42.9
- thyrotoxic E05.90 [I43]
  - with storm E05.91 [I43]
- toxic NEC I42.7

Myocarditis (with arteriosclerosis)(chronic)(fibroid) (interstitial) (old) (progressive) (senile) I51.4
- with
  - rheumatic fever (conditions in I00) I09.0
    - active — *see* Myocarditis, acute, rheumatic
    - inactive or quiescent (with chorea) I09.0
- active I40.9
  - rheumatic I01.2
    - with chorea (acute) (rheumatic) (Sydenham's) I02.0
- acute or subacute (interstitial) I40.9
  - due to
    - streptococcus (beta-hemolytic) I01.2
  - idiopathic I40.1
  - rheumatic I01.2
    - with chorea (acute) (rheumatic) (Sydenham's) I02.0
  - specified NEC I40.8
- aseptic of newborn B33.22
- bacterial (acute) I40.0
- Coxsackie (virus) B33.22
- diphtheritic A36.81
- eosinophilic I40.1
- epidemic of newborn (Coxsackie) B33.22
- Fiedler's (acute) (isolated) I40.1
- giant cell (acute) (subacute) I40.1
- gonococcal A54.83
- granulomatous (idiopathic) (isolated) (nonspecific) I40.1
- hypertensive — *see* Hypertension, heart
- idiopathic (granulomatous) I40.1
- in (due to)
  - diphtheria A36.81

Myocarditis — *continued*
- in — *continued*
  - epidemic louse-borne typhus A75.0 [I41]
  - Lyme disease A69.29
  - sarcoidosis D86.85
  - scarlet fever A38.1
  - toxoplasmosis (acquired) B58.81
  - typhoid A01.02
  - typhus NEC A75.9 [I41]
- infective I40.0
- influenzal — *see* Influenza, with, myocarditis
- isolated (acute) I40.1
- meningococcal A39.52
- mumps B26.82
- nonrheumatic, active I40.9
- parenchymatous I40.9
- pneumococcal I40.0
- rheumatic (chronic) (inactive) (with chorea) I09.0
  - active or acute I01.2
    - with chorea (acute) (rheumatic) (Sydenham's) I02.0
- rheumatoid — *see* Rheumatoid, carditis
- septic I40.0
- staphylococcal I40.0
- suppurative I40.0
- syphilitic (chronic) A52.06
- toxic I40.8
  - rheumatic — *see* Myocarditis, acute, rheumatic
- tuberculous A18.84
- typhoid A01.02
- valvular — *see* Endocarditis
- virus, viral I40.0
  - of newborn (Coxsackie) B33.22

Myocardium, myocardial — *see* condition

Myocardosis — *see* Cardiomyopathy

Myoclonus, myoclonic, myoclonia (familial) (essential) (multifocal) (simplex) G25.3
- drug-induced G25.3
- epilepsy (*see also* Epilepsy, generalized, specified NEC) G40.4- ☑
  - familial (progressive) G25.3
- epileptica G40.409
  - with status epilepticus G40.401
- facial G51.3
- familial progressive G25.3
- Friedreich's G25.3
- jerks G25.3
- massive G25.3
- palatal G25.3
- pharyngeal G25.3

Myocytolysis I51.5

Myodiastasis — *see* Diastasis, muscle

Myoendocarditis — *see* Endocarditis

Myoepithelioma — *see* Neoplasm, benign, by site

Myofasciitis (acute) — *see* Myositis

Myofibroma (*see also* Neoplasm, connective tissue, benign)
- uterus (cervix) (corpus) — *see* Leiomyoma

Myofibromatosis D48.1
- infantile Q89.8

Myofibrosis M62.89
- heart — *see* Myocarditis
- scapulohumeral — *see* Lesion, shoulder, specified NEC

Myofibrositis M79.7
- scapulohumeral — *see* Lesion, shoulder, specified NEC

Myoglobulinuria, myoglobinuria (primary) R82.1

Myokymia, facial G51.4

Myolipoma — *see* Lipoma

Myoma (*see also* Neoplasm, connective tissue, benign)
- malignant — *see* Neoplasm, connective tissue, malignant
- prostate D29.1
- uterus (cervix) (corpus) — *see* Leiomyoma

Myomalacia M62.89

Myometritis — *see* Endometritis

Myometrium — *see* condition

Myonecrosis, clostridial A48.0

Myopathy G72.9
- acute
  - necrotizing G72.81
    - quadriplegic G72.81
- alcoholic G72.1
- benign congenital G71.2
- central core G71.2
- centronuclear G71.2
- congenital (benign) G71.2
- critical illness G72.81
- distal G71.0

Myopathy — *continued*
- drug-induced G72.0
- endocrine NEC E34.9 [G73.7]
- extraocular muscles H05.82- ☑
- facioscapulohumeral G71.0
- hereditary G71.9
  - specified NEC G71.8
- immune NEC G72.49
- in (due to)
  - Addison's disease E27.1 [G73.7]
  - alcohol G72.1
  - amyloidosis E85.0 [G73.7]
  - cretinism E00.9 [G73.7]
  - Cushing's syndrome E24.9 [G73.7]
  - drugs G72.0
  - endocrine disease NEC E34.9 [G73.7]
  - giant cell arteritis M31.6 [G73.7]
  - glycogen storage disease E74.00 [G73.7]
  - hyperadrenocorticism E24.9 [G73.7]
  - hyperparathyroidism NEC E21.3 [G73.7]
  - hypoparathyroidism E20.9 [G73.7]
  - hypopituitarism E23.0 [G73.7]
  - hypothyroidism E03.9 [G73.7]
  - infectious disease NEC B99 ☑ [G73.7]
  - lipid storage disease E75.6 [G73.7]
  - metabolic disease NEC E88.9 [G73.7]
  - myxedema E03.9 [G73.7]
  - parasitic disease NEC B89 [G73.7]
  - polyarteritis nodosa M30.0 [G73.7]
  - rheumatoid arthritis — *see* Rheumatoid, myopathy
  - sarcoidosis D86.87
  - scleroderma M34.82
  - sicca syndrome M35.03
  - Sjögren's syndrome M35.03
  - systemic lupus erythematosus M32.19
  - thyrotoxicosis (hyperthyroidism) E05.90 [G73.7]
    - with thyroid storm E05.91 [G73.7]
  - toxic agent NEC G72.2
- inflammatory NEC G72.49
- intensive care (ICU) G72.81
- limb-girdle G71.0
- mitochondrial NEC G71.3
- myotubular G71.2
- mytonic, proximal (PROMM) G71.11
- nemaline G71.2
- ocular G71.0
- oculopharyngeal G71.0
- of critical illness G72.81
- primary G71.9
  - specified NEC G71.8
- progressive NEC G72.89
- proximal myotonic (PROMM) G71.11
- rod G71.2
- scapulohumeral G71.0
- specified NEC G72.89
- toxic G72.2

Myopericarditis (*see also* Pericarditis)
- chronic rheumatic I09.2

Myopia (axial) (congenital) H52.1- ☑
- degenerative (malignant) H44.20
  - with
    - choroidal neovascularization H44.2A- ☑
    - foveoschisis H44.2D- ☑
    - macular hole H44.2B- ☑
    - retinal detachment H44.2C- ☑
    - specified maculopathy NEC H44.2E- ☑
  - bilateral H44.23
  - left eye H44.22
  - right eye H44.21
- malignant (*see also* Myopia, degenerative) H44.2- ☑
- pernicious (*see also* Myopia, degenerative) H44.2- ☑
- progressive high (degenerative) (*see also* Myopia, degenerative) H44.2- ☑

Myosarcoma — *see* Neoplasm, connective tissue, malignant

Myosis (pupil) H57.03
- stromal (endolymphatic) D39.0

Myositis M60.9
- clostridial A48.0
- due to posture — *see* Myositis, specified type NEC
- epidemic B33.0
- fibrosa or fibrous (chronic), Volkmann's T79.6 ☑
- foreign body granuloma — *see* Granuloma, foreign body
- in (due to)
  - bilharziasis B65.9 [M63.8-] ☑
  - cysticercosis B69.81
  - leprosy A30.9 [M63.8-] ☑

Myositis — *continued*
  in — *continued*
    mycosis B49 [M63.8-] ☑
    sarcoidosis D86.87
    schistosomiasis B65.9 [M63.8-] ☑
    syphilis
      late A52.78
      secondary A51.49
    toxoplasmosis (acquired) B58.82
    trichinellosis B75 [M63.8-] ☑
    tuberculosis A18.09
  inclusion body [IBM] G72.41
  infective M60.009
    arm M60.002
      left M60.001
      right M60.000
    leg M60.005
      left M60.004
      right M60.003
    lower limb M60.005
      ankle M60.07- ☑
      foot M60.07- ☑
      lower leg M60.06- ☑
      thigh M60.05- ☑
      toe M60.07- ☑
    multiple sites M60.09
    specified site NEC M60.08
    upper limb M60.002
      finger M60.04- ☑
      forearm M60.03- ☑
      hand M60.04- ☑
      shoulder region M60.01- ☑
      upper arm M60.02- ☑
  interstitial M60.10
    ankle M60.17- ☑
    foot M60.17- ☑
    forearm M60.13- ☑
    hand M60.14- ☑
    lower leg M60.16- ☑
    multiple sites M60.19
    shoulder region M60.11- ☑
    specified site NEC M60.18
    thigh M60.15- ☑
    upper arm M60.12- ☑
  mycotic B49 [M63.8-] ☑
  orbital, chronic H05.12- ☑
  ossificans or ossifying (circumscripta) (*see also* Ossification, muscle, specified NEC)
    in (due to)
      burns M61.30
        ankle M61.37- ☑
        foot M61.37- ☑
        forearm M61.33- ☑
        hand M61.34- ☑
        lower leg M61.36- ☑
        multiple sites M61.39
        pelvic region M61.35- ☑

Myositis — *continued*
  ossificans or ossifying (*see also* Ossification, muscle, specified) — *continued*
    in — *continued*
      burns — *continued*
        shoulder region M61.31- ☑
        specified site NEC M61.38
        thigh M61.35- ☑
        upper arm M61.32- ☑
      quadriplegia or paraplegia M61.20
        ankle M61.27- ☑
        foot M61.27- ☑
        forearm M61.23- ☑
        hand M61.24- ☑
        lower leg M61.26- ☑
        multiple sites M61.29
        pelvic region M61.25- ☑
        shoulder region M61.21- ☑
        specified site NEC M61.28
        thigh M61.25- ☑
        upper arm M61.22- ☑
    progressiva M61.10
      ankle M61.17- ☑
      finger M61.14- ☑
      foot M61.17- ☑
      forearm M61.13- ☑
      hand M61.14- ☑
      lower leg M61.16- ☑
      multiple sites M61.19
      pelvic region M61.15- ☑
      shoulder region M61.11- ☑
      specified site NEC M61.18
      thigh M61.15- ☑
      toe M61.17- ☑
      upper arm M61.12- ☑
    traumatica M61.00
      ankle M61.07- ☑
      foot M61.07- ☑
      forearm M61.03- ☑
      hand M61.04- ☑
      lower leg M61.06- ☑
      multiple sites M61.09
      pelvic region M61.05- ☑
      shoulder region M61.01- ☑
      specified site NEC M61.08
      thigh M61.05- ☑
      upper arm M61.02- ☑
  purulent — *see* Myositis, infective
  specified type NEC M60.80
    ankle M60.87- ☑
    foot M60.87- ☑
    forearm M60.83- ☑
    hand M60.84- ☑
    lower leg M60.86- ☑
    multiple sites M60.89
    pelvic region M60.85- ☑
    shoulder region M60.81- ☑

Myositis — *continued*
  specified type — *continued*
    specified site NEC M60.88
    thigh M60.85- ☑
    upper arm M60.82- ☑
  suppurative — *see* Myositis, infective
  traumatic (old) — *see* Myositis, specified type NEC
Myospasia impulsiva F95.2
Myotonia (acquisita) (intermittens) M62.89
  atrophica G71.11
  chondrodystrophic G71.13
  congenita (acetazolamide responsive) (dominant) (recessive) G71.12
  drug-induced G71.14
  dystrophica G71.11
  fluctuans G71.19
  levior G71.12
  permanens G71.19
  symptomatic G71.19
Myotonic pupil — *see* Anomaly, pupil, function, tonic pupil
Myriapodiasis B88.2
Myringitis H73.2- ☑
  with otitis media — *see* Otitis, media
  acute H73.00- ☑
    bullous H73.01- ☑
    specified NEC H73.09- ☑
  bullous — *see* Myringitis, acute, bullous
  chronic H73.1- ☑
Mysophobia F40.228
Mytilotoxism — *see* Poisoning, fish
Myxadenitis labialis K13.0
Myxedema (adult) (idiocy) (infantile) (juvenile) (*see also* Hypothyroidism) E03.9
  circumscribed E05.90
    with storm E05.91
  coma E03.5
  congenital E00.1
  cutis L98.5
  localized (pretibial) E05.90
    with storm E05.91
  papular L98.5
Myxochondrosarcoma — *see* Neoplasm, cartilage, malignant
Myxofibroma — *see* Neoplasm, connective tissue, benign
  odontogenic — *see* Cyst, calcifying odontogenic
Myxofibrosarcoma — *see* Neoplasm, connective tissue, malignant
Myxolipoma D17.9
Myxoliposarcoma — *see* Neoplasm, connective tissue, malignant
Myxoma (*see also* Neoplasm, connective tissue, benign)
  nerve sheath — *see* Neoplasm, nerve, benign
  odontogenic — *see* Cyst, calcifying odontogenic
Myxosarcoma — *see* Neoplasm, connective tissue, malignant

N

Naegeli's
  disease Q82.8
  leukemia, monocytic C93.1- ☑
Naegleriasis (with meningoencephalitis) B60.2
Naffziger's syndrome G54.0
Naga sore — see Ulcer, skin
Nägele's pelvis M95.5
  with disproportion (fetopelvic) O33.0
    causing obstructed labor O65.0
Nail (see also condition)
  biting F98.8
  patella syndrome Q87.2
Nanism, nanosomia — see Dwarfism
Nanophyetiasis B66.8
Nanukayami A27.89
Napkin rash L22
Narcolepsy G47.419
  with cataplexy G47.411
  in conditions classified elsewhere G47.429
    with cataplexy G47.421
Narcosis R06.89
Narcotism — see Dependence
NARP (Neuropathy, Ataxia and Retinitis pigmentosa) syndrome E88.49
Narrow
  anterior chamber angle H40.03- ☑
  gingival width (of periodontal soft tissue) K05.5
  pelvis — see Contraction, pelvis
Narrowing (see also Stenosis)
  artery I77.1
    auditory, internal I65.8
    basilar — see Occlusion, artery, basilar
    carotid — see Occlusion, artery, carotid
    cerebellar — see Occlusion, artery, cerebellar
    cerebral — see Occlusion artery, cerebral
    choroidal — see Occlusion, artery, cerebral, specified NEC
    communicating posterior — see Occlusion, artery, cerebral, specified NEC
    coronary (see also Disease, heart, ischemic, atherosclerotic)
      congenital Q24.5
      syphilitic A50.54 [I52]
      due to syphilis NEC A52.06
    hypophyseal — see Occlusion, artery, cerebral, specified NEC
    pontine — see Occlusion, artery, cerebral, specified NEC
    precerebral — see Occlusion, artery, precerebral
    vertebral — see Occlusion, artery, vertebral
  auditory canal (external) — see Stenosis, external ear canal
  eustachian tube — see Obstruction, eustachian tube
  eyelid — see Disorder, eyelid function
  larynx J38.6
  mesenteric artery (see also Ischemia, intestine, acute) K55.059
  palate M26.89
  palpebral fissure — see Disorder, eyelid function
  ureter N13.5
    with infection N13.6
  urethra — see Stricture, urethra
Narrowness, abnormal, eyelid Q10.3
Nasal — see condition
Nasolachrymal, nasolacrimal — see condition
Nasopharyngeal (see also condition)
  pituitary gland Q89.2
  torticollis M43.6
Nasopharyngitis (acute) (infective) (streptococcal) (subacute) J00
  chronic (suppurative) (ulcerative) J31.1
Nasopharynx, nasopharyngeal — see condition
Natal tooth, teeth K00.6
Nausea (without vomiting) R11.0
  with vomiting R11.2
  gravidarum — see Hyperemesis, gravidarum
  marina T75.3 ☑
  navalis T75.3 ☑
Navel — see condition
Neapolitan fever — see Brucellosis
Near drowning T75.1 ☑
Nearsightedness — see Myopia
Near-syncope R55
Nebula, cornea — see Opacity, cornea

Necator americanus infestation B76.1
Necatoriasis B76.1
Neck — see condition
Necrobiosis R68.89
  lipoidica NEC L92.1
    with diabetes — see E08-E13 with .620
Necrolysis, toxic epidermal L51.2
  due to drug
    correct substance properly administered — see Table of Drugs and Chemicals, by drug, adverse effect
    overdose or wrong substance given or taken — see Table of Drugs and Chemicals, by drug, poisoning
Necrophilia F65.89
Necrosis, necrotic (ischemic) (see also Gangrene)
  adrenal (capsule) (gland) E27.49
  amputation stump (surgical) (late) T87.50
    arm T87.5- ☑
    leg T87.5- ☑
  antrum J32.0
  aorta (hyaline) (see also Aneurysm, aorta)
    cystic medial — see Dissection, aorta
  artery I77.5
  bladder (aseptic) (sphincter) N32.89
  bone (see also Osteonecrosis) M87.9
    aseptic or avascular — see Osteonecrosis
      idiopathic M87.00
    ethmoid J32.2
    jaw M27.2
    tuberculous — see Tuberculosis, bone
  brain I67.89
  breast (aseptic) (fat) (segmental) N64.1
  bronchus J98.09
  central nervous system NEC I67.89
  cerebellar I67.89
  cerebral I67.89
  colon (see also Infarct, intestine) K55.049
  cornea H18.89- ☑
  cortical (acute) (renal) N17.1
  cystic medial (aorta) — see Dissection, aorta
  dental pulp K04.1
  esophagus K22.8
  ethmoid (bone) J32.2
  eyelid — see Disorder, eyelid, degenerative
  fat, fatty (generalized) (see also Disorder, soft tissue, specified type NEC)
    abdominal wall K65.4
    breast (aseptic) (segmental) N64.1
    localized — see Degeneration, by site, fatty
    mesentery K65.4
    omentum K65.4
    pancreas K86.89
    peritoneum K65.4
    skin (subcutaneous), newborn P83.0
    subcutaneous, due to birth injury P15.6
  gallbladder — see Cholecystitis, acute
  heart — see Infarct, myocardium
  hip, aseptic or avascular — see Osteonecrosis, by type, femur
  intestine (acute) (hemorrhagic) (massive) (see also Infarct, intestine) K55.069
  jaw M27.2
  kidney (bilateral) N28.0
    acute N17.9
    cortical (acute) (bilateral) N17.1
      with ectopic or molar pregnancy O08.4
    medullary (bilateral) (in acute renal failure) (papillary) N17.2
    papillary (bilateral) (in acute renal failure) N17.2
    tubular N17.0
      with ectopic or molar pregnancy O08.4
      complicating
        abortion — see Abortion, by type, complicated by, tubular necrosis
        ectopic or molar pregnancy O08.4
        pregnancy — see Pregnancy, complicated by, diseases of, specified type or system NEC
      following ectopic or molar pregnancy O08.4
      traumatic T79.5 ☑
  larynx J38.7
  liver (with hepatic failure) (cell) — see Failure, hepatic hemorrhagic, central K76.2
  lung J85.0
  lymphatic gland — see Lymphadenitis, acute
  mammary gland (fat) (segmental) N64.1
  mastoid (chronic) — see Mastoiditis, chronic

Necrosis, necrotic — continued
  medullary (acute) (renal) N17.2
  mesentery (see also Infarct, intestine) K55.069
    fat K65.4
  mitral valve — see Insufficiency, mitral
  myocardium, myocardial — see Infarct, myocardium
  nose J34.0
  omentum (with mesenteric infarction) (see also Infarct, intestine) K55.069
    fat K65.4
  orbit, orbital — see Osteomyelitis, orbit
  ossicles, ear — see Abnormal, ear ossicles
  ovary N70.92
  pancreas (aseptic) (duct) (fat) K86.89
    acute (infective) — see Pancreatitis, acute
    infective — see Pancreatitis, acute
  papillary (acute) (renal) N17.2
  perineum N90.89
  peritoneum (with mesenteric infarction) (see also Infarct, intestine) K55.069
    fat K65.4
  pharynx J02.9
    in granulocytopenia — see Neutropenia
    Vincent's A69.1
  phosphorus — see subcategory T54.2 ☑
  pituitary (gland) E23.0
    postpartum O99.285
    Sheehan O99.285
  pressure — see Ulcer, pressure, by site
  pulmonary J85.0
  pulp (dental) K04.1
  radiation — see Necrosis, by site
  radium — see Necrosis, by site
  renal — see Necrosis, kidney
  sclera H15.89
  scrotum N50.89
  skin or subcutaneous tissue NEC I96
  spine, spinal (column) (see also Osteonecrosis, by type, vertebra)
    cord G95.19
  spleen D73.5
  stomach K31.89
  stomatitis (ulcerative) A69.0
  subcutaneous fat, newborn P83.88
  subendocardial (acute) I21.4
    chronic I25.89
  suprarenal (capsule) (gland) E27.49
  testis N50.89
  thymus (gland) E32.8
  tonsil J35.8
  trachea J39.8
  tuberculous NEC — see Tuberculosis
  tubular (acute) (anoxic) (renal) (toxic) N17.0
    postprocedural N99.0
  vagina N89.8
  vertebra (see also Osteonecrosis, by type, vertebra)
    tuberculous A18.01
  vulva N90.89
  X-ray — see Necrosis, by site
Necrospermia — see Infertility, male
Need (for)
  care provider because (of)
    assistance with personal care Z74.1
    continuous supervision required Z74.3
    impaired mobility Z74.09
    no other household member able to render care Z74.2
    specified reason NEC Z74.8
  immunization — see Vaccination
  vaccination — see Vaccination
Neglect
  adult
    confirmed T74.01 ☑
    history of Z91.412
    suspected T76.01 ☑
  child (childhood)
    confirmed T74.02 ☑
    history of Z62.812
    suspected T76.02 ☑
  emotional, in childhood Z62.898
  hemispatial R41.4
  left-sided R41.4
  sensory R41.4
  visuospatial R41.4
Neisserian infection NEC — see Gonococcus
Nelaton's syndrome G60.8
Nelson's syndrome E24.1
Nematodiasis (intestinal) B82.0

Nematodiasis — *continued*
  Ancylostoma B76.Ø
Neonatal (*see also* Newborn)
  acne L7Ø.4
  bradycardia P29.12
  screening, abnormal findings on PØ9
  tachycardia P29.11
  tooth, teeth KØØ.6
Neonatorum — *see* condition
Neoplasia
  endocrine, multiple (MEN) E31.2Ø
    type I E31.21
    type IIA E31.22
    type IIB E31.23
  intraepithelial (histologically confirmed)
    anal (AIN) (histologically confirmed) K62.82
      grade I K62.82
      grade II K62.82
      severe DØ1.3
    cervical glandular (histologically confirmed) DØ6.9
    cervix (uteri) (CIN) (histologically confirmed) N87.9
      glandular DØ6.9
      grade I N87.Ø
      grade II N87.1
      grade III (severe dysplasia) (*see also* Carcinoma, cervix uteri, in situ) DØ6.9
    prostate (histologically confirmed) (PIN) N42.31
      grade I N42.31
      grade II N42.31
      grade III (severe dysplasia) DØ7.5
    vagina (histologically confirmed) (VAIN) N89.3
      grade I N89.Ø
      grade II N89.1
      grade III (severe dysplasia) DØ7.2
    vulva (histologically confirmed) (VIN) N9Ø.3
      grade I N9Ø.Ø
      grade II N9Ø.1
      grade III (severe dysplasia) DØ7.1
Neoplasm, neoplastic (*see also* Table of Neoplasms)
  lipomatous, benign — *see* Lipoma
  malignant mast cell C96.2Ø
    specified type NEC C96.29
  mast cell, of uncertain behavior NEC D47.Ø9
Neovascularization
  ciliary body — *see* Disorder, iris, vascular
  cornea H16.4Ø- ☑
    deep H16.44- ☑
    ghost vessels — *see* Ghost, vessels
    localized H16.43- ☑
    pannus — *see* Pannus
  iris — *see* Disorder, iris, vascular
  retina H35.Ø5- ☑
Nephralgia N23
Nephritis, nephritic (albuminuric) (azotemic) (congenital) (disseminated) (epithelial) (familial) (focal) (granulomatous) (hemorrhagic) (infantile) (nonsuppurative, excretory) (uremic) NØ5.9
  with
    dense deposit disease NØ5.6
    diffuse
      crescentic glomerulonephritis NØ5.7
      endocapillary proliferative glomerulonephritis NØ5.4
      membranous glomerulonephritis NØ5.2
      mesangial proliferative glomerulonephritis NØ5.3
      mesangiocapillary glomerulonephritis NØ5.5
    edema — *see* Nephrosis
    focal and segmental glomerular lesions NØ5.1
    foot process disease NØ4.9
    glomerular lesion
      diffuse sclerosing NØ5.8
      hypocomplementemic — *see* Nephritis, membranoproliferative
      IgA — *see* Nephropathy, IgA
      lobular, lobulonodular — *see* Nephritis, membranoproliferative
      nodular — *see* Nephritis, membranoproliferative
    lesion of
      glomerulonephritis, proliferative NØ5.8
      renal necrosis NØ5.9
    minor glomerular abnormality NØ5.Ø
    specified morphological changes NEC NØ5.8
  acute NØØ.9
    with
      dense deposit disease NØØ.6

Nephritis, nephritic — *continued*
  acute — *continued*
    with — *continued*
      diffuse
        crescentic glomerulonephritis NØØ.7
        endocapillary proliferative glomerulonephritis NØØ.4
        membranous glomerulonephritis NØØ.2
        mesangial proliferative glomerulonephritis NØØ.3
        mesangiocapillary glomerulonephritis NØØ.5
      focal and segmental glomerular lesions NØØ.1
      minor glomerular abnormality NØØ.Ø
      specified morphological changes NEC NØØ.8
  amyloid E85.4 [NØ8]
  antiglomerular basement membrane (anti-GBM) antibody NEC
    in Goodpasture's syndrome M31.Ø
  antitubular basement membrane (tubulo-interstitial) NEC N12
    toxic — *see* Nephropathy, toxic
  arteriolar — *see* Hypertension, kidney
  arteriosclerotic — *see* Hypertension, kidney
  ascending — *see* Nephritis, tubulo-interstitial
  atrophic NØ3.9
  Balkan (endemic) N15.Ø
  calculous, calculus — *see* Calculus, kidney
  cardiac — *see* Hypertension, kidney
  cardiovascular — *see* Hypertension, kidney
  chronic NØ3.9
    with
      dense deposit disease NØ3.6
      diffuse
        crescentic glomerulonephritis NØ3.7
        endocapillary proliferative glomerulonephritis NØ3.4
        membranous glomerulonephritis NØ3.2
        mesangial proliferative glomerulonephritis NØ3.3
        mesangiocapillary glomerulonephritis NØ3.5
      focal and segmental glomerular lesions NØ3.1
      minor glomerular abnormality NØ3.Ø
      specified morphological changes NEC NØ3.8
    arteriosclerotic — *see* Hypertension, kidney
  cirrhotic N26.9
  complicating pregnancy O26.83- ☑
  croupous NØØ.9
  degenerative — *see* Nephrosis
  diffuse sclerosing NØ5.8
  due to
    diabetes mellitus — *see* EØ8-E13 with .21
    subacute bacterial endocarditis I33.Ø
    systemic lupus erythematosus (chronic) M32.14
    typhoid fever AØ1.Ø9
  gonococcal (acute) (chronic) A54.21
  hypocomplementemic — *see* Nephritis, membranoproliferative
  IgA — *see* Nephropathy, IgA
  immune complex (circulating) NEC NØ5.8
  infective — *see* Nephritis, tubulo-interstitial
  interstitial — *see* Nephritis, tubulo-interstitial
  lead N14.3
  membranoproliferative (diffuse) (type 1 or 3) (*see also* NØØ-NØ7 with fourth character .5) NØ5.5
    type 2 (*see also* NØØ-NØ7 with fourth character .6) NØ5.6
  minimal change NØ5.Ø
  necrotic, necrotizing NEC (*see also* NØØ-NØ7 with fourth character .8) NØ5.8
  nephrotic — *see* Nephrosis
  nodular — *see* Nephritis, membranoproliferative
  polycystic Q61.3
    adult type Q61.2
    autosomal
      dominant Q61.2
      recessive NEC Q61.19
    childhood type NEC Q61.19
    infantile type NEC Q61.19
  poststreptococcal NØ5.9
    acute NØØ.9
    chronic NØ3.9
    rapidly progressive NØ1.9
  proliferative NEC (*see also* NØØ-NØ7 with fourth character .8) NØ5.8
  purulent — *see* Nephritis, tubulo-interstitial
  rapidly progressive NØ1.9
    with
      dense deposit disease NØ1.6

Nephritis, nephritic — *continued*
  rapidly progressive — *continued*
    with — *continued*
      diffuse
        crescentic glomerulonephritis NØ1.7
        endocapillary proliferative glomerulonephritis NØ1.4
        membranous glomerulonephritis NØ1.2
        mesangial proliferative glomerulonephritis NØ1.3
        mesangiocapillary glomerulonephritis NØ1.5
      focal and segmental glomerular lesions NØ1.1
      minor glomerular abnormality NØ1.Ø
      specified morphological changes NEC NØ1.8
  salt losing or wasting NEC N28.89
  saturnine N14.3
  sclerosing, diffuse NØ5.8
  septic — *see* Nephritis, tubulo-interstitial
  specified pathology NEC (*see also* NØØ-NØ7 with fourth character .8) NØ5.8
  subacute NØ1.9
  suppurative — *see* Nephritis, tubulo-interstitial
  syphilitic (late) A52.75
    congenital A5Ø.59 [NØ8]
    early (secondary) A51.44
  toxic — *see* Nephropathy, toxic
  tubal, tubular — *see* Nephritis, tubulo-interstitial
  tuberculous A18.11
  tubulo-interstitial (in) N12
    acute (infectious) N1Ø
    chronic (infectious) N11.9
      nonobstructive N11.8
        reflux-associated N11.Ø
      obstructive N11.1
      specified NEC N11.8
    due to
      brucellosis A23.9 [N16]
      cryoglobulinemia D89.1 [N16]
      glycogen storage disease E74.ØØ [N16]
      Sjögren's syndrome M35.Ø4
  vascular — *see* Hypertension, kidney
  war NØØ.9
Nephroblastoma (epithelial) (mesenchymal) C64- ☑
Nephrocalcinosis E83.59 [N29]
Nephrocystitis, pustular — *see* Nephritis, tubulo-interstitial
Nephrolithiasis (congenital) (pelvis) (recurrent) (*see also* Calculus, kidney)
Nephroma C64- ☑
  mesoblastic D41.Ø- ☑
Nephronephritis — *see* Nephrosis
Nephronophthisis Q61.5
Nephropathia epidemica A98.5
Nephropathy (*see also* Nephritis) N28.9
  with
    edema — *see* Nephrosis
    glomerular lesion — *see* Glomerulonephritis
  amyloid, hereditary E85.Ø
  analgesic N14.Ø
    with medullary necrosis, acute N17.2
  Balkan (endemic) N15.Ø
  chemical — *see* Nephropathy, toxic
  diabetic — *see* EØ8-E13 with .21
  drug-induced N14.2
    specified NEC N14.1
  focal and segmental hyalinosis or sclerosis NØ2.1
  heavy metal-induced N14.3
  hereditary NEC NØ7.9
    with
      dense deposit disease NØ7.6
      diffuse
        crescentic glomerulonephritis NØ7.7
        endocapillary proliferative glomerulonephritis NØ7.4
        membranous glomerulonephritis NØ7.2
        mesangial proliferative glomerulonephritis NØ7.3
        mesangiocapillary glomerulonephritis NØ7.5
      focal and segmental glomerular lesions NØ7.1
      minor glomerular abnormality NØ7.Ø
      specified morphological changes NEC NØ7.8
  hypercalcemic N25.89
  hypertensive — *see* Hypertension, kidney
  hypokalemic (vacuolar) N25.89
  IgA NØ2.8
    with glomerular lesion NØ2.9
      focal and segmental hyalinosis or sclerosis NØ2.1

Nephropathy — *continued*
  IgA — *continued*
    with glomerular lesion — *continued*
      membranoproliferative (diffuse) N02.5
      membranous (diffuse) N02.2
      mesangial proliferative (diffuse) N02.3
      mesangiocapillary (diffuse) N02.5
      proliferative NEC N02.8
      specified pathology NEC N02.8
  lead N14.3
  membranoproliferative (diffuse) N02.5
  membranous (diffuse) N02.2
  mesangial (IgA/IgG) — *see* Nephropathy, IgA
    proliferative (diffuse) N02.3
  mesangiocapillary (diffuse) N02.5
  obstructive N13.8
  phenacetin N17.2
  phosphate-losing N25.0
  potassium depletion N25.89
  pregnancy-related O26.83- ☑
  proliferative NEC (*see also* N00-N07 with fourth character .8) N05.8
  protein-losing N25.89
  saturnine N14.3
  sickle-cell D57.- ☑ [N08]
  toxic NEC N14.4
    due to
      drugs N14.2
        analgesic N14.0
        specified NEC N14.1
      heavy metals N14.3
  vasomotor N17.0
  water-losing N25.89
Nephroptosis N28.83
Nephropyosis — *see* Abscess, kidney
Nephrorrhagia N28.89
Nephrosclerosis (arteriolar)(arteriosclerotic) (chronic) (hyaline) (*see also* Hypertension, kidney)
  hyperplastic — *see* Hypertension, kidney
  senile N26.9
Nephrosis, nephrotic (Epstein's) (syndrome) (congenital) N04.9
  with
    foot process disease N04.9
    glomerular lesion N04.1
    hypocomplementemic N04.5
  acute N04.9
  anoxic — *see* Nephrosis, tubular
  chemical — *see* Nephrosis, tubular
  cholemic K76.7
  diabetic — *see* E08-E13 with .21
  Finnish type (congenital) Q89.8
  hemoglobin N10
  hemoglobinuric — *see* Nephrosis, tubular
  in
    amyloidosis E85.4 [N08]
    diabetes mellitus — *see* E08-E13 with .21
    epidemic hemorrhagic fever A98.5
    malaria (malariae) B52.0
  ischemic — *see* Nephrosis, tubular
  lipoid N04.9
  lower nephron — *see* Nephrosis, tubular
  malarial (malariae) B52.0
  minimal change N04.0
  myoglobin N10
  necrotizing — *see* Nephrosis, tubular
  osmotic (sucrose) N25.89
  radiation N04.9
  syphilitic (late) A52.75
  toxic — *see* Nephrosis, tubular
  tubular (acute) N17.0
    postprocedural N99.0
    radiation N04.9
Nephrosonephritis, hemorrhagic (endemic) A98.5
Nephrostomy
  attention to Z43.6
  status Z93.6
Nerve (*see also* condition)
  injury — *see* Injury, nerve, by body site
Nerves R45.0
Nervous (*see also* condition) R45.0
  heart F45.8
  stomach F45.8
  tension R45.0
Nervousness R45.0
Nesidioblastoma
  pancreas D13.7
  specified site NEC — *see* Neoplasm, benign, by site

Nesidioblastoma — *continued*
  unspecified site D13.7
Nettleship's syndrome — *see* Urticaria pigmentosa
Neumann's disease or syndrome L10.1
Neuralgia, neuralgic (acute) M79.2
  accessory (nerve) G52.8
  acoustic (nerve) — *see* subcategory H93.3 ☑
  auditory (nerve) — *see* subcategory H93.3 ☑
  ciliary G44.009
    intractable G44.001
    not intractable G44.009
  cranial
    nerve (*see also* Disorder, nerve, cranial)
      fifth or trigeminal — *see* Neuralgia, trigeminal
      postherpetic, postzoster B02.29
  ear — *see* subcategory H92.0 ☑
  facialis vera G51.1
  Fothergill's — *see* Neuralgia, trigeminal
  glossopharyngeal (nerve) G52.1
  Horton's G44.099
    intractable G44.091
    not intractable G44.099
  Hunt's B02.21
  hypoglossal (nerve) G52.3
  infraorbital — *see* Neuralgia, trigeminal
  malarial — *see* Malaria
  migrainous G44.009
    intractable G44.001
    not intractable G44.009
  Morton's G57.6- ☑
  nerve, cranial — *see* Disorder, nerve, cranial
  nose G52.0
  occipital M54.81
  olfactory G52.0
  penis N48.9
  perineum R10.2
  postherpetic NEC B02.29
    trigeminal B02.22
  pubic region R10.2
  scrotum R10.2
  Sluder's G44.89
  specified nerve NEC G58.8
  spermatic cord R10.2
  sphenopalatine (ganglion) G90.09
  trifacial — *see* Neuralgia, trigeminal
  trigeminal G50.0
    postherpetic, postzoster B02.22
  vagus (nerve) G52.2
  writer's F48.8
    organic G25.89
Neurapraxia — *see* Injury, nerve
Neurasthenia F48.8
  cardiac F45.8
  gastric F45.8
  heart F45.8
Neurilemmoma (*see also* Neoplasm, nerve, benign)
  acoustic (nerve) D33.3
  malignant (*see also* Neoplasm, nerve, malignant)
    acoustic (nerve) C72.4- ☑
Neurilemmosarcoma — *see* Neoplasm, nerve, malignant
Neurinoma — *see* Neoplasm, nerve, benign
Neurinomatosis — *see* Neoplasm, nerve, uncertain behavior
Neuritis (rheumatoid) M79.2
  abducens (nerve) — *see* Strabismus, paralytic, sixth nerve
  accessory (nerve) G52.8
  acoustic (nerve) (*see also* subcategory) H93.3 ☑
    in (due to)
      infectious disease NEC B99 ☑ [H94.0-] ☑
      parasitic disease NEC B89 [H94.0-] ☑
    syphilitic A52.15
  alcoholic G62.1
    with psychosis — *see* Psychosis, alcoholic
  amyloid, any site E85.4 [G63]
  auditory (nerve) — *see* subcategory H93.3 ☑
  brachial — *see* Radiculopathy
    due to displacement, intervertebral disc — *see* Disorder, disc, cervical, with neuritis
  cranial nerve
    due to Lyme disease A69.22
    eighth or acoustic or auditory — *see* subcategory H93.3 ☑
    eleventh or accessory G52.8
    fifth or trigeminal G51.0
    first or olfactory G52.0

Neuritis — *continued*
  cranial nerve — *continued*
    fourth or trochlear — *see* Strabismus, paralytic, fourth nerve
    second or optic — *see* Neuritis, optic
    seventh or facial G51.8
      newborn (birth injury) P11.3
    sixth or abducent — *see* Strabismus, paralytic, sixth nerve
    tenth or vagus G52.2
    third or oculomotor — *see* Strabismus, paralytic, third nerve
    twelfth or hypoglossal G52.3
  Déjérine-Sottas G60.0
  diabetic (mononeuropathy) — *see* E08-E13 with .41
    polyneuropathy — *see* E08-E13 with .42
  due to
    beriberi E51.11
    displacement, prolapse or rupture, intervertebral disc — *see* Disorder, disc, with, radiculopathy
    herniation, nucleus pulposus M51.9 [G55]
  endemic E51.11
  facial G51.8
    newborn (birth injury) P11.3
  general — *see* Polyneuropathy
  geniculate ganglion G51.1
    due to herpes (zoster) B02.21
  gouty (*see also* Gout, by type) M10.9 [G63]
  hypoglossal (nerve) G52.3
  ilioinguinal (nerve) G57.9- ☑
  infectious (multiple) NEC G61.0
  interstitial hypertrophic progressive G60.0
  lumbar M54.16
  lumbosacral M54.17
  multiple (*see also* Polyneuropathy)
    endemic E51.11
    infective, acute G61.0
  multiplex endemica E51.11
  nerve root — *see* Radiculopathy
  oculomotor (nerve) — *see* Strabismus, paralytic, third nerve
  olfactory nerve G52.0
  optic (nerve) (hereditary) (sympathetic) H46.9
    with demyelination G36.0
    in myelitis G36.0
    nutritional H46.2
    papillitis — *see* Papillitis, optic
    retrobulbar H46.1- ☑
    specified type NEC H46.8
    toxic H46.3
  peripheral (nerve) G62.9
    multiple — *see* Polyneuropathy
    single — *see* Mononeuritis
  pneumogastric (nerve) G52.2
  postherpetic, postzoster B02.29
  progressive hypertrophic interstitial G60.0
  retrobulbar (*see also* Neuritis, optic, retrobulbar)
    in (due to)
      late syphilis A52.15
      meningococcal infection A39.82
    meningococcal A39.82
    syphilitic A52.15
  sciatic (nerve) (*see also* Sciatica)
    due to displacement of intervertebral disc — *see* Disorder, disc, with, radiculopathy
  serum (*see also* Reaction, serum) T80.69 ☑
  shoulder-girdle G54.5
  specified nerve NEC G58.8
  spinal (nerve) root — *see* Radiculopathy
  syphilitic A52.15
  thenar (median) G56.1- ☑
  thoracic M54.14
  toxic NEC G62.2
  trochlear (nerve) — *see* Strabismus, paralytic, fourth nerve
  vagus (nerve) G52.2
Neuroastrocytoma — *see* Neoplasm, uncertain behavior, by site
Neuroavitaminosis E56.9 [G99.8]
Neuroblastoma
  olfactory C30.0
  specified site — *see* Neoplasm, malignant, by site
  unspecified site C74.90
Neurochorioretinitis — *see* Chorioretinitis
Neurocirculatory asthenia F45.8
Neurocysticercosis B69.0
Neurocytoma — *see* Neoplasm, benign, by site

Neurodermatitis (circumscribed) (circumscripta) (local) L28.0
- atopic L20.81
- diffuse (Brocq) L20.81
- disseminated L20.81

Neuroencephalomyelopathy, optic G36.0

Neuroepithelioma (see also Neoplasm, malignant, by site)
- olfactory C30.0

Neurofibroma (see also Neoplasm, nerve, benign)
- melanotic — see Neoplasm, nerve, benign
- multiple — see Neurofibromatosis
- plexiform — see Neoplasm, nerve, benign

Neurofibromatosis (multiple) (nonmalignant) Q85.00
- acoustic Q85.02
- malignant — see Neoplasm, nerve, malignant
- specified NEC Q85.09
- type 1 (von Recklinghausen) Q85.01
- type 2 Q85.02

Neurofibrosarcoma — see Neoplasm, nerve, malignant

Neurogenic (see also condition)
- bladder (see also Dysfunction, bladder, neuromuscular) N31.9
  - cauda equina syndrome G83.4
- bowel NEC K59.2
- heart F45.8

Neuroglioma — see Neoplasm, uncertain behavior, by site

Neurolabyrinthitis (of Dix and Hallpike) — see Neuronitis, vestibular

Neurolathyrism — see Poisoning, food, noxious, plant

Neuroleprosy A30.9

Neuroma (see also Neoplasm, nerve, benign)
- acoustic (nerve) D33.3
- amputation (stump) (traumatic) (surgical complication) (late) T87.3- ☑
  - arm T87.3- ☑
  - leg T87.3- ☑
- digital (toe) G57.6- ☑
- interdigital G58.8
  - lower limb (toe) G57.8- ☑
  - upper limb G56.8- ☑
- intermetatarsal G57.8- ☑
- Morton's G57.6- ☑
- nonneoplastic
  - arm G56.9- ☑
  - leg G57.9- ☑
  - lower extremity G57.9- ☑
  - upper extremity G56.9- ☑
- optic (nerve) D33.3
- plantar G57.6- ☑
- plexiform — see Neoplasm, nerve, benign
- surgical (nonneoplastic)
  - arm G56.9- ☑
  - leg G57.9- ☑
  - lower extremity G57.9- ☑
  - upper extremity G56.9- ☑

Neuromyalgia — see Neuralgia

Neuromyasthenia (epidemic) (postinfectious) G93.3

Neuromyelitis G36.9
- ascending G61.0
- optica G36.0

Neuromyopathy G70.9
- paraneoplastic D49.9 [G13.0]

Neuromyotonia (Isaacs) G71.19

Neuronevus — see Nevus

Neuronitis G58.9
- ascending (acute) G57.2- ☑
- vestibular H81.2- ☑

Neuroparalytic — see condition

Neuropathy, neuropathic G62.9
- acute motor G62.81
- alcoholic G62.1
  - with psychosis — see Psychosis, alcoholic
- arm G56.9- ☑
- autonomic, peripheral — see Neuropathy, peripheral, autonomic
- axillary G56.9- ☑
- bladder N31.9
  - atonic (motor) (sensory) N31.2
  - autonomous N31.2
  - flaccid N31.2
  - nonreflex N31.2
  - reflex N31.1
  - uninhibited N31.0
- brachial plexus G54.0
- cervical plexus G54.2

Neuropathy, neuropathic — continued
- chronic
  - progressive segmentally demyelinating G62.89
  - relapsing demyelinating G62.89
- Déjérine-Sottas G60.0
- diabetic — see E08-E13 with .40
  - mononeuropathy — see E08-E13 with .41
  - polyneuropathy — see E08-E13 with .42
- entrapment G58.9
  - iliohypogastric nerve G57.8- ☑
  - ilioinguinal nerve G57.8- ☑
  - lateral cutaneous nerve of thigh G57.1- ☑
  - median nerve G56.0- ☑
  - obturator nerve G57.8- ☑
  - peroneal nerve G57.3- ☑
  - posterior tibial nerve G57.5- ☑
  - saphenous nerve G57.8- ☑
  - ulnar nerve G56.2- ☑
- facial nerve G51.9
- hereditary G60.9
  - motor and sensory (types I-IV) G60.0
  - sensory G60.8
  - specified NEC G60.8
- hypertrophic G60.0
  - Charcot-Marie-Tooth G60.0
  - Déjérine-Sottas G60.0
  - interstitial progressive G60.0
  - of infancy G60.0
  - Refsum G60.1
- idiopathic G60.9
  - progressive G60.3
  - specified NEC G60.8
- in association with hereditary ataxia G60.2
- intercostal G58.0
- ischemic — see Disorder, nerve
- Jamaica (ginger) G62.2
- leg NEC G57.9- ☑
- lower extremity G57.9- ☑
- lumbar plexus G54.1
- median nerve G56.1- ☑
- motor and sensory (see also Polyneuropathy)
  - hereditary (types I-IV) G60.0
- multifocal motor (MMN) G61.82
- multiple (acute) (chronic) — see Polyneuropathy
- optic (nerve) (see also Neuritis, optic)
  - ischemic H47.01- ☑
- paraneoplastic (sensorial) (Denny Brown) D49.9 [G13.0]
- peripheral (nerve) (see also Polyneuropathy) G62.9
  - autonomic G90.9
    - idiopathic G90.09
    - in (due to)
      - amyloidosis E85.4 [G99.0]
      - diabetes mellitus — see E08-E13 with .43
      - endocrine disease NEC E34.9 [G99.0]
      - gout M10.00 [G99.0]
      - hyperthyroidism E05.90 [G99.0]
        - with thyroid storm E05.91 [G99.0]
      - metabolic disease NEC E88.9 [G99.0]
  - idiopathic G60.9
    - progressive G60.3
  - in (due to)
    - antitetanus serum G62.0
    - arsenic G62.2
    - drugs NEC G62.0
    - lead G62.2
    - organophosphate compounds G62.2
    - toxic agent NEC G62.2
- plantar nerves G57.6- ☑
- progressive
  - hypertrophic interstitial G60.0
  - inflammatory G62.81
- radicular NEC — see Radiculopathy
- sacral plexus G54.1
- sciatic G57.0- ☑
- serum G61.1
- toxic NEC G62.2
- trigeminal sensory G50.8
- ulnar nerve G56.2- ☑
- uremic N18.9 [G63]
- vitamin B12 E53.8 [G63]
  - with anemia (pernicious) D51.0 [G63]
    - due to dietary deficiency D51.3 [G63]

Neurophthisis (see also Disorder, nerve)
- peripheral, diabetic — see E08-E13 with .42

Neuroretinitis — see Chorioretinitis

Neuroretinopathy, hereditary optic H47.22

Neurosarcoma — see Neoplasm, nerve, malignant

Neurosclerosis — see Disorder, nerve

Neurosis, neurotic F48.9
- anankastic F42.8
- anxiety (state) F41.1
  - panic type F41.0
- asthenic F48.8
- bladder F45.8
- cardiac (reflex) F45.8
- cardiovascular F45.8
- character F60.9
- colon F45.8
- compensation F68.1 ☑
- compulsive, compulsion F42.8
- conversion F44.9
- craft F48.8
- cutaneous F45.8
- depersonalization F48.1
- depressive (reaction) (type) F34.1
- environmental F48.8
- excoriation L98.1
- fatigue F48.8
- functional — see Disorder, somatoform
- gastric F45.8
- gastrointestinal F45.8
- heart F45.8
- hypochondriacal F45.21
- hysterical F44.9
- incoordination F45.8
  - larynx F45.8
  - vocal cord F45.8
- intestine F45.8
- larynx (sensory) F45.8
  - hysterical F44.4
- mixed NEC F48.8
- musculoskeletal F45.8
- obsessional F42.8
- obsessive-compulsive F42.8
- occupational F48.8
- ocular NEC F45.8
- organ — see Disorder, somatoform
- pharynx F45.8
- phobic F40.9
- posttraumatic (situational) F43.10
  - acute F43.11
  - chronic F43.12
- psychasthenic (type) F48.8
- railroad F48.8
- rectum F45.8
- respiratory F45.8
- rumination F45.8
- sexual F65.9
- situational F48.8
- social F40.10
  - generalized F40.11
- specified type NEC F48.8
- state F48.9
  - with depersonalization episode F48.1
- stomach F45.8
- traumatic F43.10
  - acute F43.11
  - chronic F43.12
- vasomotor F45.8
- visceral F45.8
- war F48.8

Neurospongioblastosis diffusa Q85.1

Neurosyphilis (arrested) (early) (gumma) (late) (latent) (recurrent) (relapse) A52.3
- with ataxia (cerebellar) (locomotor) (spastic) (spinal) A52.19
- aneurysm (cerebral) A52.05
- arachnoid (adhesive) A52.13
- arteritis (any artery) (cerebral) A52.04
- asymptomatic A52.2
- congenital A50.40
- dura (mater) A52.13
- general paresis A52.17
- hemorrhagic A52.05
- juvenile (asymptomatic) (meningeal) A50.40
- leptomeninges (aseptic) A52.13
- meningeal, meninges (adhesive) A52.13
- meningitis A52.13
- meningovascular (diffuse) A52.13
- optic atrophy A52.15
- parenchymatous (degenerative) A52.19
- paresis, paretic A52.17
  - juvenile A50.45
- remission in (sustained) A52.3
- serological (without symptoms) A52.2
- specified nature or site NEC A52.19
- tabes, tabetic (dorsalis) A52.11

☑ **Additional Character Required** — **Refer to the Tabular List for Character Selection**   ▽ **Subterms under main terms may continue to next column or page**

Neurosyphilis — *continued*
  tabes, tabetic — *continued*
    juvenile A50.45
    taboparesis A52.17
      juvenile A50.45
  thrombosis (cerebral) A52.05
  vascular (cerebral) NEC A52.05
Neurothekeoma — *see* Neoplasm, nerve, benign
Neurotic — *see* Neurosis
Neurotoxemia — *see* Toxemia
Neuroclusion M26.211
Neutropenia, neutropenic (chronic) (genetic) (idiopathic) (immune) (infantile) (malignant) (pernicious) (splenic) D70.9
  congenital (primary) D70.0
  cyclic D70.4
  cytoreductive cancer chemotherapy sequela D70.1
  drug-induced D70.2
    due to cytoreductive cancer chemotherapy D70.1
  due to infection D70.3
  fever D70.9
  neonatal, transitory (isoimmune) (maternal transfer) P61.5
  periodic D70.4
  secondary (cyclic) (periodic) (splenic) D70.4
    drug-induced D70.2
      due to cytoreductive cancer chemotherapy D70.1
  toxic D70.8
Neutrophilia, hereditary giant D72.0
Nevocarcinoma — *see* Melanoma
Nevus D22.9
  achromic — *see* Neoplasm, skin, benign
  amelanotic — *see* Neoplasm, skin, benign
  angiomatous D18.00
    intra-abdominal D18.03
    intracranial D18.02
    skin D18.01
    specified site NEC D18.09
  araneus I78.1
  balloon cell — *see* Neoplasm, skin, benign
  bathing trunk D48.5
  blue — *see* Neoplasm, skin, benign
    cellular — *see* Neoplasm, skin, benign
    giant — *see* Neoplasm, skin, benign
    Jadassohn's — *see* Neoplasm, skin, benign
    malignant — *see* Melanoma
  capillary D18.00
    intra-abdominal D18.03
    intracranial D18.02
    skin D18.01
    specified site NEC D18.09
  cavernous D18.00
    intra-abdominal D18.03
    intracranial D18.02
    skin D18.01
    specified site NEC D18.09
  cellular — *see* Neoplasm, skin, benign
    blue — *see* Neoplasm, skin, benign
  choroid D31.3- ☑
  comedonicus Q82.5
  conjunctiva D31.0- ☑
  dermal — *see* Neoplasm, skin, benign
    with epidermal nevus — *see* Neoplasm, skin, benign
  dysplastic — *see* Neoplasm, skin, benign
  eye D31.9- ☑
  flammeus Q82.5
  hemangiomatous D18.00
    intra-abdominal D18.03
    intracranial D18.02
    skin D18.01
    specified site NEC D18.09
  iris D31.4- ☑
  lacrimal gland D31.5- ☑
  lymphatic D18.1
  magnocellular
    specified site — *see* Neoplasm, benign, by site
    unspecified site D31.40
  malignant — *see* Melanoma
  meaning hemangioma D18.00
    intra-abdominal D18.03
    intracranial D18.02
    skin D18.01
    specified site NEC D18.09
  mouth (mucosa) D10.30
    specified site NEC D10.39
    white sponge Q38.6

Nevus — *continued*
  multiplex Q85.1
  non-neoplastic I78.1
  oral mucosa D10.30
    specified site NEC D10.39
    white sponge Q38.6
  orbit D31.6- ☑
  pigmented
    giant (*see also* Neoplasm, skin, uncertain behavior) D48.5
      malignant melanoma in — *see* Melanoma
  portwine Q82.5
  retina D31.2- ☑
  retrobulbar D31.6- ☑
  sanguineous Q82.5
  senile I78.1
  skin D22.9
    abdominal wall D22.5
    ala nasi D22.39
    ankle D22.7- ☑
    anus, anal D22.5
    arm D22.6- ☑
    auditory canal (external) D22.2- ☑
    auricle (ear) D22.2- ☑
    auricular canal (external) D22.2- ☑
    axilla, axillary fold D22.5
    back D22.5
    breast D22.5
    brow D22.39
    buttock D22.5
    canthus (eye) D22.1- ☑
    cheek (external) D22.39
    chest wall D22.5
    chin D22.39
    ear (external) D22.2- ☑
    external meatus (ear) D22.2- ☑
    eyebrow D22.39
    eyelid (lower) (upper) D22.1- ☑
    face D22.30
      specified NEC D22.39
    female genital organ (external) NEC D28.0
    finger D22.6- ☑
    flank D22.5
    foot D22.7- ☑
    forearm D22.6- ☑
    forehead D22.39
    foreskin D29.0
    genital organ (external) NEC
      female D28.0
      male D29.9
    gluteal region D22.5
    groin D22.5
    hand D22.6- ☑
    heel D22.7- ☑
    helix D22.2- ☑
    hip D22.7- ☑
    interscapular region D22.5
    jaw D22.39
    knee D22.7- ☑
    labium (majus) (minus) D28.0
    leg D22.7- ☑
    lip (lower) (upper) D22.0
    lower limb D22.7- ☑
    male genital organ (external) D29.9
    nail D22.9
      finger D22.6- ☑
      toe D22.7- ☑
    nasolabial groove D22.39
    nates D22.5
    neck D22.4
    nose (external) D22.39
    palpebra D22.1- ☑
    penis D29.0
    perianal skin D22.5
    perineum D22.5
    pinna D22.2- ☑
    popliteal fossa or space D22.7- ☑
    prepuce D29.0
    pudendum D28.0
    scalp D22.4
    scrotum D29.4
    shoulder D22.6- ☑
    submammary fold D22.5
    temple D22.39
    thigh D22.7- ☑
    toe D22.7- ☑
    trunk NEC D22.5

Nevus — *continued*
  skin — *continued*
    umbilicus D22.5
    upper limb D22.6- ☑
    vulva D28.0
  specified site NEC — *see* Neoplasm, by site, benign
  spider I78.1
  stellar I78.1
  strawberry Q82.5
  Sutton's benign D22.9
  unius lateris Q82.5
  Unna's Q82.5
  vascular Q82.5
  verrucous Q82.5
Newborn (infant) (liveborn) (singleton) Z38.2
  abstinence syndrome P96.1
  acne L70.4
  affected by
    abnormalities of membranes P02.9
      specified NEC P02.8
    abruptio placenta P02.1
    amino-acid metabolic disorder, transitory P74.8
    amniocentesis (while in utero) P00.6
    amnionitis P02.7
    apparent life threatening event (ALTE) R68.13
    bleeding (into)
      cerebral cortex P52.22
      germinal matrix P52.0
      ventricles P52.1
    breech delivery P03.0
    cardiac arrest P29.81
    cardiomyopathy I42.8
      congenital I42.4
    cerebral ischemia P91.0
    Cesarean delivery P03.4
    chemotherapy agents P04.1
    chorioamnionitis P02.7
    cocaine (crack) P04.41
    complications of labor and delivery P03.9
      specified NEC P03.89
    compression of umbilical cord NEC P02.5
    contracted pelvis P03.1
    delivery P03.9
      Cesarean P03.4
      forceps P03.2
      vacuum extractor P03.3
    entanglement (knot) in umbilical cord P02.5
    environmental chemicals P04.6
    fetal (intrauterine)
      growth retardation P05.9
      malnutrition not light or small for gestational age P05.2
    forceps delivery P03.2
    heart rate abnormalities
      bradycardia P29.12
      intrauterine P03.819
        before onset of labor P03.810
        during labor P03.811
      tachycardia P29.11
    hemorrhage (antepartum) P02.1
      cerebellar (nontraumatic) P52.6
      intracerebral (nontraumatic) P52.4
      intracranial (nontraumatic) P52.9
        specified NEC P52.8
      intraventricular (nontraumatic) P52.3
        grade 1 P52.0
        grade 2 P52.1
        grade 3 P52.21
        grade 4 P52.22
      posterior fossa (nontraumatic) P52.6
      subarachnoid (nontraumatic) P52.5
      subependymal P52.0
        with intracerebral extension P52.22
        with intraventricular extension P52.1
          with enlargment of ventricles P52.21
        without intraventricular extension P52.0
    hypoxic ischemic encephalopathy [HIE] P91.60
      mild P91.61
      moderate P91.62
      severe P91.63
    induction of labor P03.89
    intestinal perforation P78.0
    intrauterine (fetal) blood loss P50.9
      due to (from)
        cut end of co-twin cord P50.5
        hemorrhage into
          co-twin P50.3
          maternal circulation P50.4
          placenta P50.2

Newborn — continued
  affected by — continued
    intrauterine blood loss — continued
      due to — continued
        ruptured cord blood P50.1
        vasa previa P50.0
      specified NEC P50.8
    intrauterine (fetal) hemorrhage P50.9
    intrauterine (in utero) procedure P96.5
    malpresentation (malposition) NEC P03.1
    maternal (complication of) (use of)
      alcohol P04.3
      analgesia (maternal) P04.0
      anesthesia (maternal) P04.0
      blood loss P02.1
      circulatory disease P00.3
      condition P00.9
        specified NEC P00.89
      delivery P03.9
        Cesarean P03.4
        forceps P03.2
        vacuum extractor P03.3
      diabetes mellitus (pre-existing) P70.1
      disorder P00.9
        specified NEC P00.89
      drugs (addictive) (illegal) NEC P04.49
      ectopic pregnancy P01.4
      gestational diabetes P70.0
      hemorrhage P02.1
      hypertensive disorder P00.0
      incompetent cervix P01.0
      infectious disease P00.2
      injury P00.5
      labor and delivery P03.9
      malpresentation before labor P01.7
      maternal death P01.6
      medical procedure P00.7
      medication P04.1
      multiple pregnancy P01.5
      nutritional disorder P00.4
      oligohydramnios P01.2
      parasitic disease P00.2
      periodontal disease P00.81
      placenta previa P02.0
      polyhydramnios P01.3
      precipitate delivery P03.5
      pregnancy P01.9
        specified P01.8
      premature rupture of membranes P01.1
      renal disease P00.1
      respiratory disease P00.3
      surgical procedure P00.6
      urinary tract disease P00.1
      uterine contraction (abnormal) P03.6
    meconium peritonitis P78.0
    medication (legal) (maternal use) (prescribed) P04.1
    membrane abnormalities P02.9
      specified NEC P02.8
    membranitis P02.7
    methamphetamine(s) P04.49
    mixed metabolic and respiratory acidosis P84
    neonatal abstinence syndrome P96.1
    noxious substances transmitted via placenta or breast milk P04.9
      specified NEC P04.8
    nutritional supplements P04.5
    placenta previa P02.0
    placental
      abnormality (functional) (morphological) P02.20
        specified NEC P02.29
      dysfunction P02.29
      infarction P02.29
      insufficiency P02.29
      separation NEC P02.1
      transfusion syndromes P02.3
    placentitis P02.7
    precipitate delivery P03.5
    prolapsed cord P02.4
    respiratory arrest P28.81
    slow intrauterine growth P05.9
    tobacco P04.2
    twin to twin transplacental transfusion P02.3
    umbilical cord (tightly) around neck P02.5
    umbilical cord condition P02.60
      short cord P02.69
      specified NEC P02.69
    uterine contractions (abnormal) P03.6
    vasa previa P02.69

Newborn — continued
  affected by — continued
    vasa previa — continued
      from intrauterine blood loss P50.0
  apnea P28.4
    obstructive P28.4
    primary P28.3
    sleep (central) (obstructive) (primary) P28.3
  born in hospital Z38.00
    by cesarean Z38.01
  born outside hospital Z38.1
  breast buds P96.89
  breast engorgement P83.4
  check-up — see Newborn, examination
  convulsion P90
  dehydration P74.1
  examination
    8 to 28 days old Z00.111
    under 8 days old Z00.110
  fever P81.9
    environmentally-induced P81.0
  hyperbilirubinemia P59.9
    of prematurity P59.0
  hypernatremia P74.2
  hyponatremia P74.2
  infection P39.9
    candidal P37.5
    specified NEC P39.8
    urinary tract P39.3
  jaundice P59.9
    due to
      breast milk inhibitor P59.3
      hepatocellular damage P59.20
        specified NEC P59.29
      preterm delivery P59.0
    of prematurity P59.0
    specified NEC P59.8
  late metabolic acidosis P74.0
  mastitis P39.0
    infective P39.0
    noninfective P83.4
  multiple born NEC Z38.8
    born in hospital Z38.68
      by cesarean Z38.69
    born outside hospital Z38.7
  omphalitis P38.9
    with mild hemorrhage P38.1
    without hemorrhage P38.9
  post-term P08.21
  prolonged gestation (over 42 completed weeks) P08.22
  quadruplet Z38.8
    born in hospital Z38.63
      by cesarean Z38.64
    born outside hospital Z38.7
  quintuplet Z38.8
    born in hospital Z38.65
      by cesarean Z38.66
    born outside hospital Z38.7
  seizure P90
  sepsis (congenital) P36.9
    due to
      anaerobes NEC P36.5
      Escherichia coli P36.4
      Staphylococcus P36.30
        aureus P36.2
        specified NEC P36.39
      Streptococcus P36.10
        group B P36.0
        specified NEC P36.19
      specified NEC P36.8
  triplet Z38.8
    born in hospital Z38.61
      by cesarean Z38.62
    born outside hospital Z38.7
  twin Z38.5
    born in hospital Z38.30
      by cesarean Z38.31
    born outside hospital Z38.4
  vomiting P92.09
    bilious P92.01
  weight check Z00.111

Newcastle conjunctivitis or disease B30.8
Nezelof's syndrome (pure alymphocytosis) D81.4
Niacin (amide) **deficiency** E52
Nicolas (-Durand)-**Favre disease** A55
Nicotine — see Tobacco
Nicotinic acid deficiency E52

Niemann-Pick disease or syndrome E75.249
  specified NEC E75.248
  type
    A E75.240
    B E75.241
    C E75.242
    D E75.243
Night
  blindness — see Blindness, night
  sweats R61
  terrors (child) F51.4
Nightmares (REM sleep type) F51.5
NIHSS (National Institutes of Health Stroke Scale) **score** R29.7- ☑
Nipple — see condition
Nisbet's chancre A57
Nishimoto (-Takeuchi) **disease** I67.5
Nitritoid crisis or reaction — see Crisis, nitritoid
Nitrosohemoglobinemia D74.8
Njovera A65
Nocardiosis, nocardiasis A43.9
  cutaneous A43.1
  lung A43.0
  pneumonia A43.0
  pulmonary A43.0
  specified site NEC A43.8
Nocturia R35.1
  psychogenic F45.8
Nocturnal — see condition
Nodal rhythm I49.8
Node(s) (see also Nodule)
  Bouchard's (with arthropathy) M15.2
  Haygarth's M15.8
  Heberden's (with arthropathy) M15.1
  larynx J38.7
  lymph — see condition
  milker's B08.03
  Osler's I33.0
  Schmorl's — see Schmorl's disease
  singer's J38.2
  teacher's J38.2
  tuberculous — see Tuberculosis, lymph gland
  vocal cord J38.2
Nodule(s), **nodular**
  actinomycotic — see Actinomycosis
  breast NEC (see also Lump, breast) N63.0
  colloid (cystic), thyroid E04.1
  cutaneous — see Swelling, localized
  endometrial (stromal) D26.1
  Haygarth's M15.8
  inflammatory — see Inflammation
  juxta-articular
    syphilitic A52.77
    yaws A66.7
  larynx J38.7
  lung, solitary (subsegmental branch of the bronchial tree) R91.1
    multiple R91.8
  milker's B08.03
  prostate N40.2
    with lower urinary tract symptoms (LUTS) N40.3
    without lower urinary tract symtpoms (LUTS) N40.2
  pulmonary, solitary (subsegmental branch of the bronchial tree) R91.1
  retrocardiac R09.89
  rheumatoid M06.30
    ankle M06.37- ☑
    elbow M06.32- ☑
    foot joint M06.37- ☑
    hand joint M06.34- ☑
    hip M06.35- ☑
    knee M06.36- ☑
    multiple site M06.39
    shoulder M06.31- ☑
    vertebra M06.38
    wrist M06.33- ☑
  scrotum (inflammatory) N49.2
  singer's J38.2
  solitary, lung (subsegmental branch of the bronchial tree) R91.1
    multiple R91.8
  subcutaneous — see Swelling, localized
  teacher's J38.2
  thyroid (cold) (gland) (nontoxic) E04.1
    with thyrotoxicosis E05.20
      with thyroid storm E05.21
    toxic or with hyperthyroidism E05.20
      with thyroid storm E05.21

Nodule(s), nodular — *continued*
  vocal cord J38.2
Noma (gangrenous) (hospital) (infective) A69.Ø
  auricle I96
  mouth A69.Ø
  pudendi N76.89
  vulvae N76.89
Nomad, nomadism Z59.Ø
NOMID (neonatal onset multisystemic inflammatory
  disorder) MØ4.2
Nonadherence to medical treatment Z91.19
Nonautoimmune hemolytic anemia D59.4
  drug-induced D59.2
Nonclosure (*see also* Imperfect, closure)
  ductus arteriosus (Botallo's) Q25.Ø
  foramen
    botalli Q21.1
    ovale Q21.1
Noncompliance Z91.19
  with
    dialysis Z91.15
    dietary regimen Z91.11
    medical treatment Z91.19
    medication regimen NEC Z91.14
      underdosing (*see also* Table of Drugs and
        Chemicals, categories T36-T5Ø, with final
        character 6) Z91.14
        intentional NEC Z91.128
          due to financial hardship of patient
            Z91.12Ø
        unintentional NEC Z91.138
          due to patient's age related debility
            Z91.13Ø
    renal dialysis Z91.15
Nondescent (congenital) (*see also* Malposition, congenital)
  cecum Q43.3
  colon Q43.3
  testicle Q53.9
    bilateral Q53.2Ø
      abdominal Q53.211
      perineal Q53.22
    unilateral Q53.1Ø
      abdominal Q53.111
      perineal Q53.12
Nondevelopment
  brain QØ2
    part of QØ4.3
  heart Q24.8
  organ or site, congenital NEC — *see* Hypoplasia
Nonengagement
  head NEC O32.4 ☑
    in labor, causing obstructed labor O64.8 ☑
Nonexanthematous tick fever A93.2
Nonexpansion, lung (newborn) P28.Ø
Nonfunctioning
  cystic duct (*see also* Disease, gallbladder) K82.8
  gallbladder (*see also* Disease, gallbladder) K82.8
  kidney N28.9
  labyrinth — *see* subcategory H83.2 ☑
Non-Hodgkin lymphoma NEC — *see* Lymphoma, non-
  Hodgkin
Nonimplantation, ovum N97.2
Noninsufflation, fallopian tube N97.1
Non-ketotic hyperglycinemia E72.51
Nonne-Milroy syndrome Q82.Ø
Nonovulation N97.Ø
Non-palpable testicle(s)
  bilateral R39.84
  unilateral R39.83
Nonpatent fallopian tube N97.1
Nonpneumatization, lung NEC P28.Ø
Nonrotation — *see* Malrotation
Nonsecretion, urine — *see* Anuria
Nonunion
  fracture — *see* Fracture, by site
  joint, following fusion or arthrodesis M96.Ø
  organ or site, congenital NEC — *see* Imperfect, closure
  symphysis pubis, congenital Q74.2
Nonvisualization, gallbladder R93.2
Nonvital, nonvitalized tooth KØ4.99
Non-working side interference M26.56
Noonan's syndrome Q87.1
Normocytic anemia (infectional) due to blood loss
  (chronic) D5Ø.Ø
  acute D62
Norrie's disease (congenital) Q15.8

North American blastomycosis B4Ø.9
Norwegian itch B86
Nose, nasal — *see* condition
Nosebleed RØ4.Ø
Nose-picking F98.8
Nosomania F45.21
Nosophobia F45.22
Nostalgia F43.2Ø
Notch of iris Q13.2
Notching nose, congenital (tip) Q3Ø.2
Nothnagel's
  syndrome — *see* Strabismus, paralytic, third nerve
  vasomotor acroparesthesia I73.89
Novy's relapsing fever A68.9
  louse-borne A68.Ø
  tick-borne A68.1
Noxious
  foodstuffs, poisoning by — *see* Poisoning, food, nox-
    ious, plant
  substances transmitted through placenta or breast
    milk PØ4.9
Nucleus pulposus — *see* condition
Numbness R2Ø.Ø
Nuns' knee — *see* Bursitis, prepatellar
Nursemaid's elbow S53.Ø3- ☑
Nutcracker esophagus K22.4
Nutmeg liver K76.1
Nutrient element deficiency E61.9
  specified NEC E61.8
Nutrition deficient or insufficient (*see also* Malnutrition) E46
  due to
    insufficient food T73.Ø ☑
    lack of
      care (child) T76.Ø2 ☑
        adult T76.Ø1 ☑
      food T73.Ø ☑
Nutritional stunting E45
Nyctalopia (night blindness) — *see* Blindness, night
Nycturia R35.1
  psychogenic F45.8
Nymphomania F52.8
Nystagmus H55.ØØ
  benign paroxysmal — *see* Vertigo, benign paroxysmal
  central positional H81.4- ☑
  congenital H55.Ø1
  dissociated H55.Ø4
  latent H55.Ø2
  miners' H55.Ø9
  positional
    benign paroxysmal H81.4- ☑
    central H81.4- ☑
  specified form NEC H55.Ø9
  visual deprivation H55.Ø3

O

Obermeyer's relapsing fever (European) A68.Ø
Obesity E66.9
  with alveolar hypoventilation E66.2
  adrenal E27.8
  complicating
    childbirth O99.214
    pregnancy O99.21- ☑
    puerperium O99.215
  constitutional E66.8
  dietary counseling and surveillance Z71.3
  drug-induced E66.1
  due to
    drug E66.1
    excess calories E66.Ø9
      morbid E66.Ø1
      severe E66.Ø1
  endocrine E66.8
  endogenous E66.8
  exogenous E66.Ø9
  familial E66.8
  glandular E66.8
  hypothyroid — *see* Hypothyroidism
  hypoventilation syndrome (OHS) E66.2
  morbid E66.Ø1
    with
      alveolar hypoventilation E66.2
      obesity hypoventilation syndrome (OHS) E66.2
    due to excess calories E66.Ø1
  nutritional E66.Ø9
  pituitary E23.6

Obesity — *continued*
  severe E66.Ø1
  specified type NEC E66.8
Oblique — *see* condition
Obliteration
  appendix (lumen) K38.8
  artery I77.1
  bile duct (noncalculous) K83.1
  common duct (noncalculous) K83.1
  cystic duct — *see* Obstruction, gallbladder
  disease, arteriolar I77.1
  endometrium N85.8
  eye, anterior chamber — *see* Disorder, globe, hy-
    potony
  fallopian tube N97.1
  lymphatic vessel I89.Ø
    due to mastectomy I97.2
  organ or site, congenital NEC — *see* Atresia, by site
  ureter N13.5
    with infection N13.6
  urethra — *see* Stricture, urethra
  vein I87.8
  vestibule (oral) KØ8.89
Observation (following) (for) (without need for further
  medical care) ZØ4.9
  accident NEC ZØ4.3
    at work ZØ4.2
    transport ZØ4.1
  adverse effect of drug ZØ3.6
  alleged rape or sexual assault (victim), ruled out
    adult ZØ4.41
    child ZØ4.42
  criminal assault ZØ4.8
  development state
    adolescent ZØØ.3
    period of rapid growth in childhood ZØØ.2
    puberty ZØØ.3
  disease, specified NEC ZØ3.89
  following work accident ZØ4.2
  growth and development state — *see* Observation,
    development state
  injuries (accidental) NEC (*see also* Observation, acci-
    dent)
  newborn (for)
    suspected condition, related to exposure from the
      mother or birth process — *see* Newborn, af-
      fected by, maternal
      ruled out ZØ5.9
        cardiac ZØ5.Ø
        connective tissue ZØ5.73
        gastrointestinal ZØ5.5
        genetic ZØ5.41
        genitourinary ZØ5.6
        immunologic ZØ5.43
        infectious ZØ5.1
        metabolic ZØ5.42
        musculoskeletal ZØ5.72
        neurological ZØ5.2
        respiratory ZØ5.3
        skin and subcutaneous tissue ZØ5.71
        specified condition NEC ZØ5.8
  postpartum
    immediately after delivery Z39.Ø
    routine follow-up Z39.2
  pregnancy (normal) (without complication) Z34.9- ☑
    high risk OØ9.9- ☑
  suicide attempt, alleged NEC ZØ3.89
    self-poisoning ZØ3.6
  suspected, ruled out (*see also* Suspected condition,
    ruled out)
    abuse, physical
      adult ZØ4.71
      child ZØ4.72
    accident at work ZØ4.2
    adult battering victim ZØ4.71
    child battering victim ZØ4.72
    condition NEC ZØ3.89
      newborn (*see also* Observation, newborn (for),
        suspected condition, ruled out) ZØ5.9
    drug poisoning or adverse effect ZØ3.6
    exposure (to)
      anthrax ZØ3.81Ø
      biological agent NEC ZØ3.818
    inflicted injury NEC ZØ4.8
    suicide attempt, alleged ZØ3.89
      self-poisoning ZØ3.6
    toxic effects from ingested substance (drug) (poi-
      son) ZØ3.6

Observation — *continued*
  toxic effects from ingested substance (drug) (poison) Z03.6
Obsession, obsessional state F42.8
  mixed thoughts and acts F42.2
Obsessive-compulsive neurosis or reaction F42.8
Obstetric embolism, septic — *see* Embolism, obstetric, septic
Obstetrical trauma (complicating delivery) O71.9
  with or following ectopic or molar pregnancy O08.6
  specified type NEC O71.89
Obstipation — *see* Constipation
Obstruction, obstructed, obstructive
  airway J98.8
    with
      allergic alveolitis J67.9
      asthma J45.909
        with
          exacerbation (acute) J45.901
          status asthmaticus J45.902
      bronchiectasis J47.9
        with
          exacerbation (acute) J47.1
          lower respiratory infection J47.0
      bronchitis (chronic) J44.9
      emphysema J43.9
    chronic J44.9
      with
        allergic alveolitis — *see* Pneumonitis, hypersensitivity
        bronchiectasis J47.9
          with
            exacerbation (acute) J47.1
            lower respiratory infection J47.0
    due to
      foreign body — *see* Foreign body, by site, causing asphyxia
      inhalation of fumes or vapors J68.9
      laryngospasm J38.5
  ampulla of Vater K83.1
  aortic (heart) (valve) — *see* Stenosis, aortic
  aortoiliac I74.09
  aqueduct of Sylvius G91.1
    congenital Q03.0
      with spina bifida — *see* Spina bifida, by site, with hydrocephalus
  Arnold-Chiari — *see* Arnold-Chiari disease
  artery (*see also* Atherosclerosis, artery) I70.9 ☑
    basilar (complete) (partial) — *see* Occlusion, artery, basilar
    carotid (complete) (partial) — *see* Occlusion, artery, carotid
    cerebellar — *see* Occlusion, artery, cerebellar
    cerebral (anterior) (middle) (posterior) — *see* Occlusion, artery, cerebral
    precerebral — *see* Occlusion, artery, precerebral
    renal N28.0
    retinal NEC — *see* Occlusion, artery, retina
    stent — *see* Restenosis, stent
    vertebral (complete) (partial) — *see* Occlusion, artery, vertebral
  band (intestinal) (*see also* Obstruction, intestine, specified NEC) K56.699
  bile duct or passage (common) (hepatic) (noncalculous) K83.1
    with calculus K80.51
    congenital (causing jaundice) Q44.3
  biliary (duct) (tract) K83.1
    gallbladder K82.0
  bladder-neck (acquired) N32.0
    congenital Q64.31
    due to hyperplasia (hypertrophy) of prostate — *see* Hyperplasia, prostate
  bowel — *see* Obstruction, intestine
  bronchus J98.09
  canal, ear — *see* Stenosis, external ear canal
  cardia K22.2
  caval veins (inferior) (superior) I87.1
  cecum — *see* Obstruction, intestine
  circulatory I99.8
  colon — *see* Obstruction, intestine
  common duct (noncalculous) K83.1
  coronary (artery) — *see* Occlusion, coronary
  cystic duct (*see also* Obstruction, gallbladder)
    with calculus K80.21
  device, implant or graft (*see also* Complications, by site and type, mechanical) T85.698 ☑

Obstruction, obstructed, obstructive — *continued*
  device, implant or graft (*see also* Complications, by site and type, mechanical) — *continued*
    arterial graft NEC — *see* Complication, cardiovascular device, mechanical, vascular
    catheter NEC T85.628 ☑
      cystostomy T83.090 ☑
      dialysis (renal) T82.49 ☑
        intraperitoneal T85.691 ☑
      Hopkins T83.098 ☑
      ileostomy T83.098 ☑
      infusion NEC T82.594 ☑
        spinal (epidural) (subdural) T85.690 ☑
      nephrostomy T83.092 ☑
      urethral indwelling T83.091 ☑
      urinary T83.098 ☑
      urostomy T83.098 ☑
    due to infection T85.79 ☑
    gastrointestinal — *see* Complications, prosthetic device, mechanical, gastrointestinal device
    genital NEC T83.498 ☑
      intrauterine contraceptive device T83.39 ☑
      penile prosthesis (cylinder) (implanted) (pump) (resevoir) T83.490 ☑
      testicular prosthesis T83.491 ☑
    heart NEC — *see* Complication, cardiovascular device, mechanical
    joint prosthesis — *see* Complications, joint prosthesis, mechanical, specified NEC, by site
    orthopedic NEC — *see* Complication, orthopedic, device, mechanical
    specified NEC T85.628 ☑
    urinary NEC (*see also* Complication, genitourinary, device, urinary, mechanical)
      graft T83.29 ☑
    vascular NEC — *see* Complication, cardiovascular device, mechanical
    ventricular intracranial shunt T85.09 ☑
    due to foreign body accidentally left in operative wound T81.529 ☑
  duodenum K31.5
  ejaculatory duct N50.89
  esophagus K22.2
  eustachian tube (complete) (partial) H68.10- ☑
    cartilagenous (extrinsic) H68.13- ☑
      intrinsic H68.12- ☑
    osseous H68.11- ☑
  fallopian tube (bilateral) N97.1
  fecal K56.41
    with hernia — *see* Hernia, by site, with obstruction
  foramen of Monro (congenital) Q03.8
    with spina bifida — *see* Spina bifida, by site, with hydrocephalus
  foreign body — *see* Foreign body
  gallbladder K82.0
    with calculus, stones K80.21
    congenital Q44.1
  gastric outlet K31.1
  gastrointestinal — *see* Obstruction, intestine
  hepatic K76.89
    duct (noncalculous) K83.1
  ileum — *see* Obstruction, intestine
  iliofemoral (artery) I74.5
  intestine K56.609
    with
      adhesions (intestinal) (peritoneal) K56.50
        complete K56.52
        incomplete K56.51
        partial K56.51
    adynamic K56.0
    by gallstone K56.3
    complete K56.601
    congenital (small) Q41.9
      large Q42.9
        specified part NEC Q42.8
    incomplete K56.600
    neurogenic K56.0
      Hirschsprung's disease or megacolon Q43.1
    newborn P76.9
      due to
        fecaliths P76.8
        inspissated milk P76.2
        meconium (plug) P76.0
          in mucoviscidosis E84.11
      specified NEC P76.8
    partial K56.600
    postoperative K91.30

Obstruction, obstructed, obstructive — *continued*
  intestine — *continued*
    postoperative — *continued*
      complete K91.32
      incomplete K91.31
      partial K91.31
    reflex K56.0
    specified NEC K56.699
      complete K56.691
      incomplete K56.690
      partial K56.690
    volvulus K56.2
  intracardiac ball valve prosthesis T82.09 ☑
  jejunum — *see* Obstruction, intestine
  joint prosthesis — *see* Complications, joint prosthesis, mechanical, specified NEC, by site
  kidney (calices) N28.89
  labor — *see* Delivery
  lacrimal (passages) (duct)
    by
      dacryolith — *see* Dacryolith
      stenosis — *see* Stenosis, lacrimal
    congenital Q10.5
    neonatal H04.53- ☑
  lacrimonasal duct — *see* Obstruction, lacrimal
  lacteal, with steatorrhea K90.2
  laryngitis — *see* Laryngitis
  larynx NEC J38.6
    congenital Q31.8
  lung J98.4
    disease, chronic J44.9
  lymphatic I89.0
  meconium (plug)
    newborn P76.0
      due to fecaliths P76.0
      in mucoviscidosis E84.11
  mitral — *see* Stenosis, mitral
  nasal J34.89
  nasolacrimal duct (*see also* Obstruction, lacrimal)
    congenital Q10.5
  nasopharynx J39.2
  nose J34.89
  organ or site, congenital NEC — *see* Atresia, by site
  pancreatic duct K86.89
  parotid duct or gland K11.8
  pelviureteral junction N13.5
    with hydronephrosis N13.0
    congenital Q62.39
  pharynx J39.2
  portal (circulation) (vein) I81
  prostate (*see also* Hyperplasia, prostate)
    valve (urinary) N32.0
  pulmonary valve (heart) I37.0
  pyelonephritis (chronic) N11.1
  pylorus
    adult K31.1
    congenital or infantile Q40.0
  rectosigmoid — *see* Obstruction, intestine
  rectum K62.4
  renal N28.89
    outflow N13.8
    pelvis, congenital Q62.39
  respiratory J98.8
    chronic J44.9
  retinal (vessels) H34.9
  salivary duct (any) K11.8
    with calculus K11.5
  sigmoid — *see* Obstruction, intestine
  sinus (accessory) (nasal) J34.89
  Stensen's duct K11.8
  stomach NEC K31.89
    acute K31.0
    congenital Q40.2
    due to pylorospasm K31.3
  submandibular duct K11.8
  submaxillary gland K11.8
    with calculus K11.5
  thoracic duct I89.0
  thrombotic — *see* Thrombosis
  trachea J39.8
  tracheostomy airway J95.03
  tricuspid (valve) — *see* Stenosis, tricuspid
  upper respiratory, congenital Q34.8
  ureter (functional) (pelvic junction) NEC N13.5
    with
      hydronephrosis N13.1
        with infection N13.6
      pyelonephritis (chronic) N11.1

☑ **Additional Character Required** — Refer to the Tabular List for Character Selection   ▽ **Subterms under main terms may continue to next column or page**

Obstruction, obstructed, obstructive — *continued*
  ureter — *continued*
    congenital Q62.39
    due to calculus — *see* Calculus, ureter
  urethra NEC N36.8
    congenital Q64.39
  urinary (moderate) N13.9
    due to hyperplasia (hypertrophy) of prostate —
      see Hyperplasia, prostate
    organ or tract (lower) N13.9
    prostatic valve N32.0
    specified NEC N13.8
  uropathy N13.9
  uterus N85.8
  vagina N89.5
  valvular — *see* Endocarditis
  vein, venous I87.1
    caval (inferior) (superior) I87.1
    thrombotic — *see* Thrombosis
    vena cava (inferior) (superior) I87.1
  vesical NEC N32.0
  vesicourethral orifice N32.0
    congenital Q64.31
  vessel NEC I99.8
    stent — *see* Restenosis, stent
Obturator — *see* condition
Occlusal wear, teeth K03.0
Occlusio pupillae — *see* Membrane, pupillary
Occlusion, occluded
  anus K62.4
    congenital Q42.3
      with fistula Q42.2
  aortoiliac (chronic) I74.09
  aqueduct of Sylvius G91.1
    congenital Q03.0
      with spina bifida — *see* Spina bifida, by site,
        with hydrocephalus
  artery (*see also* Atherosclerosis, artery) I70.9 ☑
    auditory, internal I65.8
    basilar I65.1
      with
        infarction I63.22
          due to
            embolism I63.12
            thrombosis I63.02
    brain or cerebral I66.9
      with infarction (due to) I63.5- ☑
        embolism I63.4- ☑
        thrombosis I63.3- ☑
    carotid I65.2- ☑
      with
        infarction I63.23- ☑
          due to
            embolism I63.13- ☑
            thrombosis I63.03- ☑
    cerebellar (anterior inferior) (posterior inferior)
      (superior) I66.3
      with infarction I63.54- ☑
        due to
          embolism I63.44- ☑
          thrombosis I63.34- ☑
    cerebral I66.9
      with infarction I63.50
        due to
          embolism I63.40
            specified NEC I63.49
          thrombosis I63.30
            specified NEC I63.39
      anterior I66.1-
        with infarction I63.52- ☑
          due to
            embolism I63.42- ☑
            thrombosis I63.32- ☑
      middle I66.0- ☑
        with infarction I63.51- ☑
          due to
            embolism I63.41- ☑
            thrombosis I63.31- ☑
      posterior I66.2- ☑
        with infarction I63.53- ☑
          due to
            embolism I63.43- ☑
            thrombosis I63.33- ☑
      specified NEC I66.8
        with infarction I63.59
          due to
            embolism I63.4- ☑

Occlusion, occluded — *continued*
  artery (*see also* Atherosclerosis, artery) — *contin-ued*
    cerebral — *continued*
      specified — *continued*
        with infarction — *continued*
          due to — *continued*
            thrombosis I63.3- ☑
    choroidal (anterior) — *see* Occlusion, artery, pre-cerebral, specified NEC
    communicating posterior — *see* Occlusion, artery, precerebral, specified NEC
    complete
      coronary I25.82
      extremities I70.92
    coronary (acute) (thrombotic) (without myocardial infarction) I24.0
      with myocardial infarction — *see* Infarction, myocardium
      chronic total I25.82
      complete I25.82
      healed or old I25.2
      total (chronic) I25.82
    hypophyseal — *see* Occlusion, artery, precerebral, specified NEC
    iliac I74.5
    lower extremities due to stenosis or stricture I77.1
    mesenteric (embolic) (thrombotic) (*see also* Infarct, intestine) K55.069
    perforating — *see* Occlusion, artery, cerebral, specified NEC
    peripheral I77.9
      thrombotic or embolic I74.4
    pontine — *see* Occlusion, artery, precerebral, specified NEC
    precerebral I65.9
      with infarction I63.20
        due to
          embolism I63.10
            specified NEC I63.19
          thrombosis I63.00
            specified NEC I63.09
        specified NEC I63.29
      basilar — *see* Occlusion, artery, basilar
      carotid — *see* Occlusion, artery, carotid
      puerperal O88.23
      specified NEC I65.8
        with infarction I63.29
          due to
            embolism I63.19
            thrombosis I63.09
      vertebral — *see* Occlusion, artery, vertebral
    renal N28.0
    retinal
      branch H34.23- ☑
      central H34.1- ☑
      partial H34.21- ☑
      transient H34.0- ☑
    spinal — *see* Occlusion, artery, precerebral, verte-bral
    total (chronic)
      coronary I25.82
      extremities I70.92
    vertebral I65.0- ☑
      with
        infarction I63.21- ☑
          due to
            embolism I63.11- ☑
            thrombosis I63.01- ☑
  basilar artery — *see* Occlusion, artery, basilar
  bile duct (common) (hepatic) (noncalculous) K83.1
  bowel — *see* Obstruction, intestine
  carotid (artery) (common) (internal) — *see* Occlusion, artery, carotid
  centric (of teeth) M26.59
    maximum intercuspation discrepancy M26.55
  cerebellar (artery) — *see* Occlusion, artery, cerebellar
  cerebral (artery) — *see* Occlusion, artery, cerebral
  cerebrovascular (*see also* Occlusion, artery, cerebral)
    with infarction I63.5- ☑
  cervical canal — *see* Stricture, cervix
  cervix (uteri) — *see* Stricture, cervix
  choanal Q30.0
  choroidal (artery) — *see* Occlusion, artery, precerebral, specified NEC
  colon — *see* Obstruction, intestine
  communicating posterior artery — *see* Occlusion, artery, precerebral, specified NEC

Occlusion, occluded — *continued*
  coronary (artery) (vein) (thrombotic) (*see also* Infarct, myocardium)
    chronic total I25.82
    healed or old I25.2
    not resulting in infarction I24.0
    total (chronic) I25.82
  cystic duct — *see* Obstruction, gallbladder
  embolic — *see* Embolism
  fallopian tube N97.1
    congenital Q50.6
  gallbladder (*see also* Obstruction, gallbladder)
    congenital (causing jaundice) Q44.1
  gingiva, traumatic K06.2
  hymen N89.6
    congenital Q52.3
  hypophyseal (artery) — *see* Occlusion, artery, precere-bral, specified NEC
  iliac artery I74.5
  intestine — *see* Obstruction, intestine
  lacrimal passages — *see* Obstruction, lacrimal
  lung J98.4
  lymph or lymphatic channel I89.0
  mammary duct N64.89
  mesenteric artery (embolic) (thrombotic) (*see also* In-farct, intestine) K55.069
  nose J34.89
    congenital Q30.0
  organ or site, congenital NEC — *see* Atresia, by site
  oviduct N97.1
    congenital Q50.6
  peripheral arteries
    due to stricture or stenosis I77.1
    upper extremity I74.2
  pontine (artery) — *see* Occlusion, artery, precerebral, specified NEC
  posterior lingual, of mandibular teeth M26.29
  precerebral artery — *see* Occlusion, artery, precerebral
  punctum lacrimale — *see* Obstruction, lacrimal
  pupil — *see* Membrane, pupillary
  pylorus, adult (*see also* Stricture, pylorus) K31.1
  renal artery N28.0
  retina, retinal
    artery — *see* Occlusion, artery, retinal
    vein (central) H34.81- ☑
      engorgement H34.82- ☑
      tributary H34.83- ☑
    vessels H34.9
  spinal artery — *see* Occlusion, artery, precerebral, vertebral
  teeth (mandibular) (posterior lingual) M26.29
  thoracic duct I89.0
  thrombotic — *see* Thrombosis, artery
  traumatic
    edentulous (alveolar) ridge K06.2
    gingiva K06.2
    periodontal K05.5
  tubal N97.1
  ureter (complete) (partial) N13.5
    congenital Q62.10
  ureteropelvic junction N13.5
    congenital Q62.11
  ureterovesical orifice N13.5
    congenital Q62.12
  urethra — *see* Stricture, urethra
  uterus N85.8
  vagina N89.5
  vascular NEC I99.8
  vein — *see* Thrombosis
    retinal — *see* Occlusion, retinal, vein
  vena cava (inferior) (superior) — *see* Embolism, vena cava
  ventricle (brain) NEC G91.1
  vertebral (artery) — *see* Occlusion, artery, vertebral
  vessel (blood) I99.8
  vulva N90.5
Occult
  blood in feces (stools) R19.5
Occupational
  problems NEC Z56.89
Ochlophobia — *see* Agoraphobia
Ochronosis (endogenous) E70.29
Ocular muscle — *see* condition
Oculogyric crisis or disturbance H51.8
  psychogenic F45.8
Oculomotor syndrome H51.9
Oculopathy
  syphilitic NEC A52.71

Oculopathy — continued
  syphilitic — continued
    congenital
      early A50.01
      late A50.30
    early (secondary) A51.43
    late A52.71
Oddi's sphincter spasm K83.4
Odontalgia K08.89
Odontoameloblastoma — see Cyst, calcifying odontogenic
Odontoclasia K03.89
Odontodysplasia, regional K00.4
Odontogenesis imperfecta K00.5
Odontoma (ameloblastic) (complex) (compound) (fibroameloblastic) — see Cyst, calcifying odontogenic
Odontomyelitis (closed) (open) K04.01
  irreversible K04.02
  reversible K04.01
Odontorrhagia K08.89
Odontosarcoma, ameloblastic C41.1
  upper jaw (bone) C41.0
Oestriasis — see Myiasis
Oguchi's disease H53.63
Ohara's disease — see Tularemia
OHS (obesity hypoventilation syndrome) E66.2
Oidiomycosis — see Candidiasis
Oidium albicans infection — see Candidiasis
Old age (without mention of debility) R54
  dementia F03 ☑
Old (previous) **myocardial infarction** I25.2
Olfactory — see condition
Oligemia — see Anemia
Oligoastrocytoma
  specified site — see Neoplasm, malignant, by site
  unspecified site C71.9
Oligocythemia D64.9
Oligodendroblastoma
  specified site — see Neoplasm, malignant
  unspecified site C71.9
Oligodendroglioma
  anaplastic type
    specified site — see Neoplasm, malignant, by site
    unspecified site C71.9
  specified site — see Neoplasm, malignant, by site
  unspecified site C71.9
Oligodontia — see Anodontia
Oligoencephalon Q02
Oligohidrosis L74.4
Oligohydramnios O41.0- ☑
Oligohydrosis L74.4
Oligomenorrhea N91.5
  primary N91.3
  secondary N91.4
Oligophrenia (see also Disability, intellectual)
  phenylpyruvic E70.0
Oligospermia N46.11
  due to
    drug therapy N46.121
    efferent duct obstruction N46.123
    infection N46.122
    radiation N46.124
    specified cause NEC N46.129
    systemic disease N46.125
Oligotrichia — see Alopecia
Oliguria R34
  postprocedural N99.0
  with, complicating or following ectopic or molar pregnancy O08.4
Ollier's disease Q78.4
Omenotocele — see Hernia, abdomen, specified site NEC
Omentitis — see Peritonitis
Omentum, omental — see condition
Omphalitis (congenital) (newborn) P38.9
  with mild hemorrhage P38.1
  without hemorrhage P38.9
  not of newborn L08.82
  tetanus A33
Omphalocele Q79.2
Omphalomesenteric duct, persistent Q43.0
Omphalorrhagia, newborn P51.9
Omsk hemorrhagic fever A98.1
Onanism (excessive) F98.8
Onchocerciasis, onchocercosis B73.1
  with
    eye disease B73.00

Onchocerciasis, onchocercosis — continued
  with — continued
    eye disease — continued
      endophthalmitis B73.01
      eyelid B73.09
      glaucoma B73.02
      specified NEC B73.09
  eyelid B73.09
  eye NEC B73.00
Oncocytoma — see Neoplasm, benign, by site
Oncovirus, as cause of disease classified elsewhere B97.32
Ondine's curse — see Apnea, sleep
Oneirophrenia F23
Onychauxis L60.2
  congenital Q84.5
Onychia (see also Cellulitis, digit)
  with lymphangitis — see Lymphangitis, acute, digit
  candidal B37.2
  dermatophytic B35.1
Onychitis (see also Cellulitis, digit)
  with lymphangitis — see Lymphangitis, acute, digit
Onychocryptosis L60.0
Onychodystrophy L60.3
  congenital Q84.6
Onychogryphosis, onychogryposis L60.2
Onycholysis L60.1
Onychomadesis L60.8
Onychomalacia L60.3
Onychomycosis (finger) (toe) B35.1
Onycho-osteodysplasia Q87.2
Onychophagia F98.8
Onychophosis L60.8
Onychoptosis L60.8
Onychorrhexis L60.3
  congenital Q84.6
Onychoschizia L60.3
Onyxis (finger) (toe) L60.0
Onyxitis (see also Cellulitis, digit)
  with lymphangitis — see Lymphangitis, acute, digit
Oophoritis (cystic) (infectional) (interstitial) N70.92
  with salpingitis N70.93
  acute N70.02
    with salpingitis N70.03
  chronic N70.12
    with salpingitis N70.13
  complicating abortion — see Abortion, by type, complicated by, oophoritis
Oophorocele N83.4 ☑
Opacity, opacities
  cornea H17.- ☑
    central H17.1- ☑
    congenital Q13.3
    degenerative — see Degeneration, cornea
    hereditary — see Dystrophy, cornea
    inflammatory — see Keratitis
    minor H17.81- ☑
    peripheral H17.82- ☑
    sequelae of trachoma (healed) B94.0
    specified NEC H17.89
  enamel (teeth) (fluoride) (nonfluoride) K00.3
  lens — see Cataract
  snowball — see Deposit, crystalline
  vitreous (humor) NEC H43.39- ☑
    congenital Q14.0
    membranes and strands H43.31- ☑
Opalescent dentin (hereditary) K00.5
Open, opening
  abnormal, organ or site, congenital — see Imperfect, closure
  angle with
    borderline
      findings
        high risk H40.02- ☑
        low risk H40.01- ☑
      intraocular pressure H40.00- ☑
    cupping of discs H40.01- ☑
    glaucoma (primary) — see Glaucoma, open angle
  bite
    anterior M26.220
    posterior M26.221
  false — see Imperfect, closure
  margin on tooth restoration K08.51
  restoration margins of tooth K08.51
  wound — see Wound, open
Operational fatigue F48.8
Operative — see condition

Operculitis — see Periodontitis
Operculum — see Break, retina
Ophiasis L63.2
Ophthalmia (see also Conjunctivitis) H10.9
  actinic rays — see Photokeratitis
  allergic (acute) — see Conjunctivitis, acute, atopic
  blennorrhagic (gonococcal) (neonatorum) A54.31
  diphtheritic A36.86
  Egyptian A71.1
  electrica — see Photokeratitis
  gonococcal (neonatorum) A54.31
  metastatic — see Endophthalmitis, purulent
  migraine — see Migraine, ophthalmoplegic
  neonatorum, newborn P39.1
    gonococcal A54.31
  nodosa H16.24- ☑
  purulent — see Conjunctivitis, acute, mucopurulent
  spring — see Conjunctivitis, acute, atopic
  sympathetic — see Uveitis, sympathetic
Ophthalmitis — see Ophthalmia
Ophthalmocele (congenital) Q15.8
Ophthalmoneuromyelitis G36.0
Ophthalmoplegia (see also Strabismus, paralytic)
  anterior internuclear — see Ophthalmoplegia, internuclear
  ataxia-areflexia G61.0
  diabetic — see E08-E13 with .39
  exophthalmic E05.00
    with thyroid storm E05.01
  external H49.88- ☑
    progressive H49.4- ☑
      with pigmentary retinopathy — see Kearns-Sayre syndrome
    total H49.3- ☑
  internal (complete) (total) H52.51- ☑
  internuclear H51.2- ☑
  migraine — see Migraine, ophthalmoplegic
  Parinaud's H49.88- ☑
  progressive external — see Ophthalmoplegia, external, progressive
  supranuclear, progressive G23.1
  total (external) — see Ophthalmoplegia, external, total
Opioid(s)
  abuse — see Abuse, drug, opioids
  dependence — see Dependence, drug, opioids
  induced, without use disorder
    anxiety disorder F11.988
    delirium F11.921
    depressive disorder F11.94
    sexual dysfunction F11.981
    sleep disorder F11.982
Opisthognathism M26.09
Opisthorchiasis (felineus) (viverrini) B66.0
Opitz' disease D73.2
Opiumism — see Dependence, drug, opioid
Oppenheim's disease G70.2
Oppenheim-Urbach disease (necrobiosis lipoidica diabeticorum) — see E08-E13 with .620
Optic nerve — see condition
Orbit — see condition
Orchioblastoma C62.9- ☑
Orchitis (gangrenous) (nonspecific) (septic) (suppurative) N45.2
  blennorrhagic (gonococcal) (acute) (chronic) A54.23
  chlamydial A56.19
  filarial (see also Infestation, filarial) B74.9 [N51]
  gonococcal (acute) (chronic) A54.23
  mumps B26.0
  syphilitic A52.76
  tuberculous A18.15
Orf (virus disease) B08.02
Organic (see also condition)
  brain syndrome F09
  heart — see Disease, heart
  mental disorder F09
  psychosis F09
Orgasm
  anejaculatory N53.13
Oriental
  bilharziasis B65.2
  schistosomiasis B65.2
Orifice — see condition
Origin of both great vessels from right ventricle Q20.1
Ormond's disease (with ureteral obstruction) N13.5
  with infection N13.6
Ornithine metabolism disorder E72.4

☑ **Additional Character Required — Refer to the Tabular List for Character Selection**

▽ Subterms under main terms may continue to next column or page

Ornithinemia (Type I) (Type II) E72.4
Ornithosis A70
Orotaciduria, oroticaciduria (congenital) (hereditary) (pyrimidine deficiency) E79.8
  anemia D53.0
Orthodontics
  adjustment Z46.4
  fitting Z46.4
Orthopnea R06.01
Orthopoxvirus B08.09
  specified NEC B08.09
Os, uterus — *see* condition
Osgood-Schlatter disease or osteochondrosis — *see* Osteochondrosis, juvenile, tibia
Osler (-Weber)-**Rendu disease** I78.0
Osler's nodes I33.0
Osmidrosis L75.0
Osseous — *see* condition
Ossification
  artery — *see* Arteriosclerosis
  auricle (ear) — *see* Disorder, pinna, specified type NEC
  bronchial J98.09
  cardiac — *see* Degeneration, myocardial
  cartilage (senile) — *see* Disorder, cartilage, specified type NEC
  coronary (artery) — *see* Disease, heart, ischemic, atherosclerotic
  diaphragm J98.6
  ear, middle — *see* Otosclerosis
  falx cerebri G96.19
  fontanel, premature Q75.0
  heart (*see also* Degeneration, myocardial)
    valve — *see* Endocarditis
  larynx J38.7
  ligament — *see* Disorder, tendon, specified type NEC
    posterior longitudinal — *see* Spondylopathy, specified NEC
  meninges (cerebral) (spinal) G96.19
  multiple, eccentric centers — *see* Disorder, bone, development or growth
  muscle (*see also* Calcification, muscle)
    due to burns — *see* Myositis, ossificans, in, burns
    paralytic — *see* Myositis, ossificans, in, quadriplegia
    progressive — *see* Myositis, ossificans, progressiva
    specified NEC M61.50
      ankle M61.57- ☑
      foot M61.57- ☑
      forearm M61.53- ☑
      hand M61.54- ☑
      lower leg M61.56- ☑
      multiple sites M61.59
      pelvic region M61.55- ☑
      shoulder region M61.51- ☑
      specified site NEC M61.58
      thigh M61.55- ☑
      upper arm M61.52- ☑
    traumatic — *see* Myositis, ossificans, traumatica
  myocardium, myocardial — *see* Degeneration, myocardial
  penis N48.89
  periarticular — *see* Disorder, joint, specified type NEC
  pinna — *see* Disorder, pinna, specified type NEC
  rider's bone — *see* Ossification, muscle, specified NEC
  sclera H15.89
  subperiosteal, post-traumatic M89.8X- ☑
  tendon — *see* Disorder, tendon, specified type NEC
  trachea J39.8
  tympanic membrane — *see* Disorder, tympanic membrane, specified NEC
  vitreous (humor) — *see* Deposit, crystalline
Osteitis (*see also* Osteomyelitis)
  alveolar M27.3
  condensans M85.30
    ankle M85.37- ☑
    foot M85.37- ☑
    forearm M85.33- ☑
    hand M85.34- ☑
    lower leg M85.36- ☑
    multiple site M85.39
    neck M85.38
    rib M85.38
    shoulder M85.31- ☑
    skull M85.38
    specified site NEC M85.38
    thigh M85.35- ☑
    toe M85.37- ☑
    upper arm M85.32- ☑

Osteitis — *continued*
  condensans — *continued*
    vertebra M85.38
  deformans M88.9
    in (due to)
      malignant neoplasm of bone C41.9 [M90.60]
      neoplastic disease (*see also* Neoplasm) D49.9 [M90.60]
        carpus D49.9 [M90.64-] ☑
        clavicle D49.9 [M90.61-] ☑
        femur D49.9 [M90.65-] ☑
        fibula D49.9 [M90.66-] ☑
        finger D49.9 [M90.64-] ☑
        humerus D49.9 [M90.62-] ☑
        ilium D49.9 [M90.65-] ☑
        ischium D49.9 [M90.65-] ☑
        metacarpus D49.9 [M90.64-] ☑
        metatarsus D49.9 [M90.67-] ☑
        multiple sites D49.9 [M90.69]
        neck D49.9 [M90.68]
        radius D49.9 [M90.63-] ☑
        rib D49.9 [M90.68]
        scapula D49.9 [M90.61-] ☑
        skull D49.9 [M90.68]
        tarsus D49.9 [M90.67-] ☑
        tibia D49.9 [M90.66-] ☑
        toe D49.9 [M90.67-] ☑
        ulna D49.9 [M90.63-] ☑
        vertebra D49.9 [M90.68]
    skull M88.0
    specified NEC — *see* Paget's disease, bone, by site
    vertebra M88.1
  due to yaws A66.6
  fibrosa NEC — *see* Cyst, bone, by site
    circumscripta — *see* Dysplasia, fibrous, bone NEC
    cystica (generalisata) E21.0
    disseminata Q78.1
    osteoplastica E21.0
  fragilitans Q78.0
  Garr's (sclerosing) — *see* Osteomyelitis, specified type NEC
  jaw (acute) (chronic) (lower) (suppurative) (upper) M27.2
  parathyroid E21.0
  petrous bone (acute) (chronic) — *see* Petrositis
  sclerotic, nonsuppurative — *see* Osteomyelitis, specified type NEC
  tuberculosa A18.09
    cystica D86.89
    multiplex cystoides D86.89
Osteoarthritis M19.90
  ankle M19.07- ☑
  elbow M19.02- ☑
  foot joint M19.07- ☑
  generalized M15.9
    erosive M15.4
    primary M15.0
    specified NEC M15.8
  hand joint M19.04- ☑
    first carpometacarpal joint M18.9
  hip M16.1- ☑
    bilateral M16.0
    due to hip dysplasia (unilateral) M16.3- ☑
      bilateral M16.2
  interphalangeal
    distal (Heberden) M15.1
    proximal (Bouchard) M15.2
  knee M17.1- ☑
    bilateral M17.0
  post-traumatic NEC M19.92
    ankle M19.17- ☑
    elbow M19.12- ☑
    foot joint M19.17- ☑
    hand joint M19.14- ☑
      first carpometacarpal joint M18.3- ☑
        bilateral M18.2
    hip M16.5- ☑
      bilateral M16.4
    knee M17.3- ☑
      bilateral M17.2
    shoulder M19.11- ☑
    wrist M19.13- ☑
  primary M19.91
    ankle M19.07- ☑
    elbow M19.02- ☑
    foot joint M19.07- ☑
    hand joint M19.04- ☑

Osteoarthritis — *continued*
  primary — *continued*
    hand joint — *continued*
      first carpometacarpal joint M18.1- ☑
        bilateral M18.0
    hip M16.1- ☑
      bilateral M16.0
    knee M17.1- ☑
      bilateral M17.0
    shoulder M19.01- ☑
    spine — *see* Spondylosis
    wrist M19.03- ☑
  secondary M19.93
    ankle M19.27- ☑
    elbow M19.22- ☑
    foot joint M19.27- ☑
    hand joint M19.24- ☑
      first carpometacarpal joint M18.5- ☑
        bilateral M18.4
    hip M16.7
      bilateral M16.6
    knee M17.5
      bilateral M17.4
    multiple M15.3
    shoulder M19.21- ☑
    spine — *see* Spondylosis
    wrist M19.23- ☑
  shoulder M19.01- ☑
  spine — *see* Spondylosis
  wrist M19.03- ☑
Osteoarthropathy (hypertrophic) M19.90
  ankle — *see* Osteoarthritis, primary, ankle
  elbow — *see* Osteoarthritis, primary, elbow
  foot joint — *see* Osteoarthritis, primary, foot
  hand joint — *see* Osteoarthritis, primary, hand joint
  knee joint — *see* Osteoarthritis, primary, knee
  multiple site — *see* Osteoarthritis, primary, multiple joint
  pulmonary (*see also* Osteoarthropathy, specified type NEC)
    hypertrophic — *see* Osteoarthropathy, hypertrophic, specified type NEC
  secondary — *see* Osteoarthropathy, specified type NEC
  secondary hypertrophic — *see* Osteoarthropathy, specified type NEC
  shoulder — *see* Osteoarthritis, primary, shoulder
  specified joint NEC — *see* Osteoarthritis, primary, specified joint NEC
  specified type NEC M89.40
    carpus M89.44- ☑
    clavicle M89.41- ☑
    femur M89.45- ☑
    fibula M89.46- ☑
    finger M89.44- ☑
    humerus M89.42- ☑
    ilium M89.459
    ischium M89.459
    metacarpus M89.44- ☑
    metatarsus M89.47- ☑
    multiple sites M89.49
    neck M89.48
    radius M89.43- ☑
    rib M89.48
    scapula M89.41- ☑
    skull M89.48
    tarsus M89.47- ☑
    tibia M89.46- ☑
    toe M89.47- ☑
    ulna M89.43- ☑
    vertebra M89.48
  spine — *see* Spondylosis
  wrist — *see* Osteoarthritis, primary, wrist
Osteoarthrosis (degenerative) (hypertrophic) (joint) (*see also* Osteoarthritis)
  deformans alkaptonurica E70.29 [M36.8]
  erosive M15.4
  generalized M15.9
    primary M15.0
  polyarticular M15.9
  spine — *see* Spondylosis
Osteoblastoma — *see* Neoplasm, bone, benign
  aggressive — *see* Neoplasm, bone, uncertain behavior
Osteochondritis (*see also* Osteochondropathy, by site)
  Brailsford's — *see* Osteochondrosis, juvenile, radius
  dissecans M93.20
    ankle M93.27- ☑

Osteochondritis — continued
  dissecans — continued
    elbow M93.22- ☑
    foot M93.27- ☑
    hand M93.24- ☑
    hip M93.25- ☑
    knee M93.26- ☑
    multiple sites M93.29
    shoulder joint M93.21- ☑
    specified site NEC M93.28
    wrist M93.23- ☑
  juvenile M92.9
    patellar — see Osteochondrosis, juvenile, patella
  syphilitic (congenital) (early) A50.02 [M90.80]
    ankle A50.02 [M90.87-] ☑
    elbow A50.02 [M90.82-] ☑
    foot A50.02 [M90.87-] ☑
    forearm A50.02 [M90.83-] ☑
    hand A50.02 [M90.84-] ☑
    hip A50.02 [M90.85-] ☑
    knee A50.02 [M90.86-] ☑
    multiple sites A50.02 [M90.89]
    shoulder joint A50.02 [M90.81-] ☑
    specified site NEC A50.02 [M90.88]
Osteochondroarthrosis deformans endemica — see
  Disease, Kaschin-Beck
Osteochondrodysplasia Q78.9
  with defects of growth of tubular bones and spine
    Q77.9
    specified NEC Q77.8
  specified NEC Q78.8
Osteochondrodystrophy E78.9
Osteochondrolysis — see Osteochondritis, dissecans
Osteochondroma — see Neoplasm, bone, benign
Osteochondromatosis D48.0
  syndrome Q78.4
Osteochondromyxosarcoma — see Neoplasm, bone,
  malignant
Osteochondropathy M93.90
  ankle M93.97- ☑
  elbow M93.92- ☑
  foot M93.97- ☑
  hand M93.94- ☑
  hip M93.95- ☑
  Kienböck's disease of adults M93.1
  knee M93.96- ☑
  multiple joints M93.99
  osteochondritis dissecans — see Osteochondritis,
    dissecans
  osteochondrosis — see Osteochondrosis
  shoulder region M93.91- ☑
  slipped upper femoral epiphysis — see Slipped, epiph-
    ysis, upper femoral
  specified joint NEC M93.98
  specified type NEC M93.80
    ankle M93.87- ☑
    elbow M93.82- ☑
    foot M93.87- ☑
    hand M93.84- ☑
    hip M93.85- ☑
    knee M93.86- ☑
    multiple joints M93.89
    shoulder region M93.81- ☑
    specified joint NEC M93.88
    wrist M93.83- ☑
  syphilitic, congenital
    early A50.02 [M90.80]
    late A50.56 [M90.80]
  wrist M93.93- ☑
Osteochondrosarcoma — see Neoplasm, bone, malignant
Osteochondrosis (see also Osteochondropathy, by site)
  acetabulum (juvenile) M91.0
  adult — see Osteochondropathy, specified type NEC,
    by site
  astragalus (juvenile) — see Osteochondrosis, juvenile,
    tarsus
  Blount's — see Osteochondrosis, juvenile, tibia
  Buchanan's M91.0
  Burns' — see Osteochondrosis, juvenile, ulna
  calcaneus (juvenile) — see Osteochondrosis, juvenile,
    tarsus
  capitular epiphysis (femur) (juvenile) — see Legg-
    Calvé-Perthes disease
  carpal (juvenile) (lunate) (scaphoid) — see Osteochon-
    drosis, juvenile, hand, carpal lunate
    adult M93.1

Osteochondrosis — continued
  coxae juvenilis — see Legg-Calvé-Perthes disease
  deformans juvenilis, coxae — see Legg-Calvé-Perthes
    disease
  Diaz's — see Osteochondrosis, juvenile, tarsus
  dissecans (knee) (shoulder) — see Osteochondritis,
    dissecans
  femoral capital epiphysis (juvenile) — see Legg-Calvé-
    Perthes disease
  femur (head), juvenile — see Legg-Calvé-Perthes dis-
    ease
  fibula (juvenile) — see Osteochondrosis, juvenile,
    fibula
  foot NEC (juvenile) M92.8
  Freiberg's — see Osteochondrosis, juvenile, metatarsus
  Haas' (juvenile) — see Osteochondrosis, juvenile,
    humerus
  Haglund's — see Osteochondrosis, juvenile, tarsus
  hip (juvenile) — see Legg-Calvé-Perthes disease
  humerus (capitulum) (head) (juvenile) — see Osteo-
    chondrosis, juvenile, humerus
  ilium, iliac crest (juvenile) M91.0
  ischiopubic synchondrosis M91.0
  Iselin's — see Osteochondrosis, juvenile, metatarsus
  juvenile, juvenilis M92.9
    after congenital dislocation of hip reduction — see
      Osteochondrosis, juvenile, hip, specified NEC
    arm — see Osteochondrosis, juvenile, upper limb
      NEC
    capitular epiphysis (femur) — see Legg-Calvé-
      Perthes disease
    clavicle, sternal epiphysis — see Osteochondrosis,
      juvenile, upper limb NEC
    coxae — see Legg-Calvé-Perthes disease
    deformans M92.9
    fibula M92.5- ☑
    foot NEC M92.8
    hand M92.20- ☑
      carpal lunate M92.21- ☑
      metacarpal head M92.22- ☑
      specified site NEC M92.29- ☑
    head of femur — see Legg-Calvé-Perthes disease
    hip and pelvis M91.9- ☑
      coxa plana — see Coxa, plana
      femoral head — see Legg-Calvé-Perthes disease
      pelvis M91.0
      pseudocoxalgia — see Pseudocoxalgia
      specified NEC M91.8- ☑
    humerus M92.0- ☑
    limb
      lower NEC M92.8
      upper NEC — see Osteochondrosis, juvenile,
        upper limb NEC
    medial cuneiform bone — see Osteochondrosis,
      juvenile, tarsus
    metatarsus M92.7- ☑
    patella M92.4- ☑
    radius M92.1- ☑
    specified site NEC M92.8
    spine M42.00
      cervical region M42.02
      cervicothoracic region M42.03
      lumbar region M42.06
      lumbosacral region M42.07
      multiple sites M42.09
      occipito-atlanto-axial region M42.01
      sacrococcygeal region M42.08
      thoracic region M42.04
      thoracolumbar region M42.05
    tarsus M92.6- ☑
    tibia M92.5- ☑
    ulna M92.1- ☑
    upper limb NEC M92.3- ☑
    vertebra (body) (epiphyseal plates) (Calvé's)
      (Scheuermann's) — see Osteochondrosis,
      juvenile, spine
  Kienböck's — see Osteochondrosis, juvenile, hand,
    carpal lunate
    adult M93.1
  Köhler's
    patellar — see Osteochondrosis, juvenile, patella
    tarsal navicular — see Osteochondrosis, juvenile,
      tarsus
  Legg-Perthes (-Calvé)(-Waldenström) — see Legg-
    Calvé-Perthes disease
  limb
    lower NEC (juvenile) M92.8

Osteochondrosis — continued
  limb — continued
    upper NEC (juvenile) — see Osteochondrosis, juve-
      nile, upper limb NEC
  lunate bone (carpal) (juvenile) (see also Osteochondro-
    sis, juvenile, hand, carpal lunate)
    adult M93.1
  Mauclaire's — see Osteochondrosis, juvenile, hand,
    metacarpal
  metacarpal (head) (juvenile) — see Osteochondrosis,
    juvenile, hand, metacarpal
  metatarsus (fifth) (head) (juvenile) (second) — see
    Osteochondrosis, juvenile, metatarsus
  navicular (juvenile) — see Osteochondrosis, juvenile,
    tarsus
  os
    calcis (juvenile) — see Osteochondrosis, juvenile,
      tarsus
    tibiale externum (juvenile) — see Osteochondrosis,
      juvenile, tarsus
  Osgood-Schlatter — see Osteochondrosis, juvenile,
    tibia
  Panner's — see Osteochondrosis, juvenile, humerus
  patellar center (juvenile) (primary) (secondary) — see
    Osteochondrosis, juvenile, patella
  pelvis (juvenile) M91.0
  Pierson's M91.0
  radius (head) (juvenile) — see Osteochondrosis, juve-
    nile, radius
  Scheuermann's — see Osteochondrosis, juvenile, spine
  Sever's — see Osteochondrosis, juvenile, tarsus
  Sinding-Larsen — see Osteochondrosis, juvenile,
    patella
  spine M42.9
    adult M42.10
      cervical region M42.12
      cervicothoracic region M42.13
      lumbar region M42.16
      lumbosacral region M42.17
      multiple sites M42.19
      occipito-atlanto-axial region M42.11
      sacrococcygeal region M42.18
      thoracic region M42.14
      thoracolumbar region M42.15
    juvenile — see Osteochondrosis, juvenile, spine
  symphysis pubis (juvenile) M91.0
  syphilitic (congenital) A50.02
  talus (juvenile) — see Osteochondrosis, juvenile, tarsus
  tarsus (navicular) (juvenile) — see Osteochondrosis,
    juvenile, tarsus
  tibia (proximal) (tubercle) (juvenile) — see Osteochon-
    drosis, juvenile, tibia
  tuberculous — see Tuberculosis, bone
  ulna (lower) (juvenile) — see Osteochondrosis, juve-
    nile, ulna
  van Neck's M91.0
  vertebral — see Osteochondrosis, spine
Osteoclastoma D48.0
  malignant — see Neoplasm, bone, malignant
Osteodynia — see Disorder, bone, specified type NEC
Osteodystrophy Q78.9
  azotemic N25.0
  congenital Q78.9
  parathyroid, secondary E21.1
  renal N25.0
Osteofibroma — see Neoplasm, bone, benign
Osteofibrosarcoma — see Neoplasm, bone, malignant
Osteogenesis imperfecta Q78.0
Osteogenic — see condition
Osteolysis M89.50
  carpus M89.54- ☑
  clavicle M89.51- ☑
  femur M89.55- ☑
  fibula M89.56- ☑
  finger M89.54- ☑
  humerus M89.52- ☑
  ilium M89.559
  ischium M89.559
  joint prosthesis (periprosthetic) — see Complications,
    joint prosthesis, mechanical, periprosthetic, os-
    teolysis, by site
  metacarpus M89.54- ☑
  metatarsus M89.57- ☑
  multiple sites M89.59
  neck M89.58
  periprosthetic — see Complications, joint prosthesis,
    mechanical, periprosthetic, osteolysis, by site

Osteolysis — continued
　radius M89.53- ✓
　rib M89.58
　scapula M89.51- ✓
　skull M89.58
　tarsus M89.57- ✓
　tibia M89.56- ✓
　toe M89.57- ✓
　ulna M89.53- ✓
　vertebra M89.58
Osteoma (see also Neoplasm, bone, benign)
　osteoid (see also Neoplasm, bone, benign)
　　giant — see Neoplasm, bone, benign
Osteomalacia M83.9
　adult M83.9
　　drug-induced NEC M83.5
　　due to
　　　malabsorption (postsurgical) M83.2
　　　malnutrition M83.3
　　specified NEC M83.8
　aluminium-induced M83.4
　infantile — see Rickets
　juvenile — see Rickets
　oncogenic E83.89
　pelvis M83.8
　puerperal M83.0
　senile M83.1
　vitamin-D-resistant in adults E83.31 [M90.8-] ✓
　　carpus E83.31 [M90.84-] ✓
　　clavicle E83.31 [M90.81-] ✓
　　femur E83.31 [M90.85-] ✓
　　fibula E83.31 [M90.86-] ✓
　　finger E83.31 [M90.84-] ✓
　　humerus E83.31 [M90.82-] ✓
　　ilium E83.31 [M90.859]
　　ischium E83.31 [M90.859]
　　metacarpus E83.31 [M90.84-] ✓
　　metatarsus E83.31 [M90.87-] ✓
　　multiple sites E83.31 [M90.89]
　　neck E83.31 [M90.88]
　　radius E83.31 [M90.83-] ✓
　　rib E83.31 [M90.88]
　　scapula E83.31 [M90.819]
　　skull E83.31 [M90.88]
　　tarsus E83.31 [M90.879]
　　tibia E83.31 [M90.869]
　　toe E83.31 [M90.879]
　　ulna E83.31 [M90.839]
　　vertebra E83.31 [M90.88]
Osteomyelitis (general) (infective) (localized) (neonatal)
　　(purulent) (septic) (staphylococcal) (streptococcal)
　　(suppurative) (with periostitis) M86.9
　acute M86.10
　　carpus M86.14- ✓
　　clavicle M86.11- ✓
　　femur M86.15- ✓
　　fibula M86.16- ✓
　　finger M86.14- ✓
　　hematogenous M86.00
　　　carpus M86.04- ✓
　　　clavicle M86.01- ✓
　　　femur M86.05- ✓
　　　fibula M86.06- ✓
　　　finger M86.04- ✓
　　　humerus M86.02- ✓
　　　ilium M86.059
　　　ischium M86.059
　　　mandible M27.2
　　　metacarpus M86.04- ✓
　　　metatarsus M86.07- ✓
　　　multiple sites M86.09
　　　neck M86.08
　　　orbit H05.02- ✓
　　　petrous bone — see Petrositis
　　　radius M86.03- ✓
　　　rib M86.08
　　　scapula M86.01- ✓
　　　skull M86.08
　　　tarsus M86.07- ✓
　　　tibia M86.06- ✓
　　　toe M86.07- ✓
　　　ulna M86.03- ✓
　　　vertebra — see Osteomyelitis, vertebra
　　humerus M86.12- ✓
　　ilium M86.159
　　ischium M86.159
　　mandible M27.2

Osteomyelitis — continued
　acute — continued
　　metacarpus M86.14- ✓
　　metatarsus M86.17- ✓
　　multiple sites M86.19
　　neck M86.18
　　orbit H05.02- ✓
　　petrous bone — see Petrositis
　　radius M86.13- ✓
　　rib M86.18
　　scapula M86.11- ✓
　　skull M86.18
　　tarsus M86.17- ✓
　　tibia M86.16- ✓
　　toe M86.17- ✓
　　ulna M86.13- ✓
　　vertebra — see Osteomyelitis, vertebra
　chronic (or old) M86.60
　　with draining sinus M86.40
　　　carpus M86.44- ✓
　　　clavicle M86.41- ✓
　　　femur M86.45- ✓
　　　fibula M86.46- ✓
　　　finger M86.44- ✓
　　　humerus M86.42- ✓
　　　ilium M86.459
　　　ischium M86.459
　　　mandible M27.2
　　　metacarpus M86.44- ✓
　　　metatarsus M86.47- ✓
　　　multiple sites M86.49
　　　neck M86.48
　　　orbit H05.02- ✓
　　　petrous bone — see Petrositis
　　　radius M86.43- ✓
　　　rib M86.48
　　　scapula M86.41- ✓
　　　skull M86.48
　　　tarsus M86.47- ✓
　　　tibia M86.46- ✓
　　　toe M86.47- ✓
　　　ulna M86.43- ✓
　　　vertebra — see Osteomyelitis, vertebra
　　carpus M86.64- ✓
　　clavicle M86.61- ✓
　　femur M86.65- ✓
　　fibula M86.66- ✓
　　finger M86.64- ✓
　　hematogenous NEC M86.50
　　　carpus M86.54- ✓
　　　clavicle M86.51- ✓
　　　femur M86.55- ✓
　　　fibula M86.56- ✓
　　　finger M86.54- ✓
　　　humerus M86.52- ✓
　　　ilium M86.559
　　　ischium M86.559
　　　mandible M27.2
　　　metacarpus M86.54- ✓
　　　metatarsus M86.57- ✓
　　　multifocal M86.30
　　　　carpus M86.34- ✓
　　　　clavicle M86.31- ✓
　　　　femur M86.35- ✓
　　　　fibula M86.36- ✓
　　　　finger M86.34- ✓
　　　　humerus M86.32- ✓
　　　　ilium M86.359
　　　　ischium M86.359
　　　　metacarpus M86.34- ✓
　　　　metatarsus M86.37- ✓
　　　　multiple sites M86.39
　　　　neck M86.38
　　　　radius M86.33- ✓
　　　　rib M86.38
　　　　scapula M86.31- ✓
　　　　skull M86.38
　　　　tarsus M86.37- ✓
　　　　tibia M86.36- ✓
　　　　toe M86.37- ✓
　　　　ulna M86.33- ✓
　　　　vertebra — see Osteomyelitis, vertebra
　　　multiple sites M86.59
　　　neck M86.58
　　　orbit H05.02- ✓
　　　petrous bone — see Petrositis

Osteomyelitis — continued
　chronic — continued
　　hematogenous — continued
　　　radius M86.53- ✓
　　　rib M86.58
　　　scapula M86.51- ✓
　　　skull M86.58
　　　tarsus M86.57- ✓
　　　tibia M86.56- ✓
　　　toe M86.57- ✓
　　　ulna M86.53- ✓
　　　vertebra — see Osteomyelitis, vertebra
　　humerus M86.62- ✓
　　ilium M86.659
　　ischium M86.659
　　mandible M27.2
　　metacarpus M86.64- ✓
　　metatarsus M86.67- ✓
　　multifocal — see Osteomyelitis, chronic,
　　　　hematogenous, multifocal
　　multiple sites M86.69
　　neck M86.68
　　orbit H05.02- ✓
　　petrous bone — see Petrositis
　　radius M86.63- ✓
　　rib M86.68
　　scapula M86.61- ✓
　　skull M86.68
　　tarsus M86.67- ✓
　　tibia M86.66- ✓
　　toe M86.67- ✓
　　ulna M86.63- ✓
　　vertebra — see Osteomyelitis, vertebra
　echinococcal B67.2
　Garr's — see Osteomyelitis, specified type NEC
　in diabetes mellitus — see E08-E13 with .69
　jaw (acute) (chronic) (lower) (neonatal) (suppurative)
　　　(upper) M27.2
　nonsuppurating — see Osteomyelitis, specified type
　　　NEC
　orbit H05.02- ✓
　petrous bone — see Petrositis
　Salmonella (arizonae) (cholerae-suis) (enteritidis) (ty-
　　　phimurium) A02.24
　sclerosing, nonsuppurative — see Osteomyelitis,
　　　specified type NEC
　specified type NEC (see also subcategory) M86.8X- ✓
　　mandible M27.2
　　orbit H05.02- ✓
　　petrous bone — see Petrositis
　　vertebra — see Osteomyelitis, vertebra
　subacute M86.20
　　carpus M86.24- ✓
　　clavicle M86.21- ✓
　　femur M86.25- ✓
　　fibula M86.26- ✓
　　finger M86.24- ✓
　　humerus M86.22- ✓
　　mandible M27.2
　　metacarpus M86.24- ✓
　　metatarsus M86.27- ✓
　　multiple sites M86.29
　　neck M86.28
　　orbit H05.02- ✓
　　petrous bone — see Petrositis
　　radius M86.23- ✓
　　rib M86.28
　　scapula M86.21- ✓
　　skull M86.28
　　tarsus M86.27- ✓
　　tibia M86.26- ✓
　　toe M86.27- ✓
　　ulna M86.23- ✓
　　vertebra — see Osteomyelitis, vertebra
　syphilitic A52.77
　　congenital (early) A50.02 [M90.80]
　tuberculous — see Tuberculosis, bone
　typhoid A01.05
　vertebra M46.20
　　cervical region M46.22
　　cervicothoracic region M46.23
　　lumbar region M46.26
　　lumbosacral region M46.27
　　occipito-atlanto-axial region M46.21
　　sacrococcygeal region M46.28
　　thoracic region M46.24
　　thoracolumbar region M46.25

Osteomyelofibrosis D47.4
Osteomyelosclerosis D75.89
Osteonecrosis M87.9
  due to
    drugs — see Osteonecrosis, secondary, due to, drugs
    trauma — see Osteonecrosis, secondary, due to, trauma
  idiopathic aseptic M87.00
    ankle M87.07- ☑
    carpus M87.03- ☑
    clavicle M87.01- ☑
    femur M87.05- ☑
    fibula M87.06- ☑
    finger M87.04- ☑
    humerus M87.02- ☑
    ilium M87.050
    ischium M87.050
    metacarpus M87.04- ☑
    metatarsus M87.07- ☑
    multiple sites M87.09
    neck M87.08
    pelvis M87.050
    radius M87.03- ☑
    rib M87.08
    scapula M87.01- ☑
    skull M87.08
    tarsus M87.07- ☑
    tibia M87.06- ☑
    toe M87.07- ☑
    ulna M87.03- ☑
    vertebra M87.08
  secondary NEC M87.30
    carpus M87.33- ☑
    clavicle M87.31- ☑
    due to
      drugs M87.10
        carpus M87.13- ☑
        clavicle M87.11- ☑
        femur M87.15- ☑
        fibula M87.16- ☑
        finger M87.14- ☑
        humerus M87.12- ☑
        ilium M87.159
        ischium M87.159
        jaw M87.180
        metacarpus M87.14- ☑
        metatarsus M87.17- ☑
        multiple sites M87.19
        neck M87.18
        radius M87.13- ☑
        rib M87.18 ☑
        scapula M87.11- ☑
        skull M87.18 ☑
        tarsus M87.17- ☑
        tibia M87.16- ☑
        toe M87.17- ☑
        ulna M87.13- ☑
        vertebra M87.18 ☑
      hemoglobinopathy NEC D58.2 [M90.50]
        carpus D58.2 [M90.54-] ☑
        clavicle D58.2 [M90.51-] ☑
        femur D58.2 [M90.55-] ☑
        fibula D58.2 [M90.56-] ☑
        finger D58.2 [M90.54-] ☑
        humerus D58.2 [M90.52-] ☑
        ilium D58.2 [M90.55-] ☑
        ischium D58.2 [M90.55-] ☑
        metacarpus D58.2 [M90.54-] ☑
        metatarsus D58.2 [M90.57-] ☑
        multiple sites D58.2 [M90.58]
        neck D58.2 [M90.58]
        radius D58.2 [M90.53-] ☑
        rib D58.2 [M90.58]
        scapula D58.2 [M90.51-] ☑
        skull D58.2 [M90.58]
        tarsus D58.2 [M90.57-] ☑
        tibia D58.2 [M90.56-] ☑
        toe D58.2 [M90.57-] ☑
        ulna D58.2 [M90.53-] ☑
        vertebra D58.2 [M90.58]
      trauma (previous) M87.20
        carpus M87.23- ☑
        clavicle M87.21- ☑
        femur M87.25- ☑
        fibula M87.26- ☑

Osteonecrosis — continued
  secondary — continued
    due to — continued
      trauma — continued
        finger M87.24- ☑
        humerus M87.22- ☑
        ilium M87.25- ☑
        ischium M87.25- ☑
        metacarpus M87.24- ☑
        metatarsus M87.27- ☑
        multiple sites M87.29
        neck M87.28
        radius M87.23- ☑
        rib M87.28
        scapula M87.21- ☑
        skull M87.28
        tarsus M87.27- ☑
        tibia M87.26- ☑
        toe M87.27- ☑
        ulna M87.23- ☑
        vertebra M87.28
    femur M87.35- ☑
    fibula M87.36- ☑
    finger M87.34- ☑
    humerus M87.32- ☑
    ilium M87.350
    in
      caisson disease T70.3 ☑ [M90.50]
        carpus T70.3 ☑ [M90.54-] ☑
        clavicle T70.3 ☑ [M90.51-] ☑
        femur T70.3 ☑ [M90.55-] ☑
        fibula T70.3 ☑ [M90.56-] ☑
        finger T70.3 ☑ [M90.54-] ☑
        humerus T70.3 ☑ [M90.52-] ☑
        ilium T70.3 ☑ [M90.55-] ☑
        ischium T70.3 ☑ [M90.55-] ☑
        metacarpus T70.3 ☑ [M90.54-] ☑
        metatarsus T70.3 ☑ [M90.57-] ☑
        multiple sites T70.3 ☑ [M90.59]
        neck T70.3 ☑ [M90.58]
        radius T70.3 ☑ [M90.53-] ☑
        rib T70.3 ☑ [M90.58]
        scapula T70.3 ☑ [M90.51-] ☑
        skull T70.3 ☑ [M90.58]
        tarsus T70.3 ☑ [M90.57-] ☑
        tibia T70.3 ☑ [M90.56-] ☑
        toe T70.3 ☑ [M90.57-] ☑
        ulna T70.3 ☑ [M90.53-] ☑
        vertebra T70.3 ☑ [M90.58]
    ischium M87.350
    metacarpus M87.34- ☑
    metatarsus M87.37- ☑
    multiple site M87.39
    neck M87.38
    radius M87.33- ☑
    rib M87.38
    scapula M87.319
    skull M87.38
    tarsus M87.379
    tibia M87.366
    toe M87.379
    ulna M87.33- ☑
    vertebra M87.38
  specified type NEC M87.80
    carpus M87.83- ☑
    clavicle M87.81- ☑
    femur M87.85- ☑
    fibula M87.86- ☑
    finger M87.84- ☑
    humerus M87.82- ☑
    ilium M87.85- ☑
    ischium M87.85- ☑
    metacarpus M87.84- ☑
    metatarsus M87.87- ☑
    multiple sites M87.89
    neck M87.88
    radius M87.83- ☑
    rib M87.88
    scapula M87.81- ☑
    skull M87.88
    tarsus M87.87- ☑
    tibia M87.86- ☑
    toe M87.87- ☑
    ulna M87.83- ☑
    vertebra M87.88
Osteo-onycho-arthro-dysplasia Q87.2

Osteo-onychodysplasia, hereditary Q87.2
Osteopathia condensans disseminata Q78.8
Osteopathy (see also Osteomyelitis, Osteonecrosis, Osteoporosis)
  after poliomyelitis M89.60
    carpus M89.64- ☑
    clavicle M89.61- ☑
    femur M89.65- ☑
    fibula M89.66- ☑
    finger M89.64- ☑
    humerus M89.62- ☑
    ilium M89.659
    ischium M89.659
    metacarpus M89.64- ☑
    metatarsus M89.67- ☑
    multiple sites M89.69
    neck M89.68
    radius M89.63- ☑
    rib M89.68
    scapula M89.61- ☑
    skull M89.68
    tarsus M89.67- ☑
    tibia M89.66- ☑
    toe M89.67- ☑
    ulna M89.63- ☑
    vertebra M89.68
  in (due to)
    renal osteodystrophy N25.0
    specified diseases classified elsewhere — see subcategory M90.8 ☑
Osteopenia M85.8- ☑
  borderline M85.8- ☑
Osteoperiostitis — see Osteomyelitis, specified type NEC
Osteopetrosis (familial) Q78.2
Osteophyte M25.70
  ankle M25.77- ☑
  elbow M25.72- ☑
  foot joint M25.77- ☑
  hand joint M25.74- ☑
  hip M25.75- ☑
  knee M25.76- ☑
  shoulder M25.71- ☑
  spine M25.78
  vertebrae M25.78
  wrist M25.73- ☑
Osteopoikilosis Q78.8
Osteoporosis (female) (male) M81.0
  with current pathological fracture M80.00 ☑
  age-related M81.0
    with current pathologic fracture M80.00 ☑
      carpus M80.04- ☑
      clavicle M80.01- ☑
      fibula M80.06- ☑
      finger M80.04- ☑
      humerus M80.02- ☑
      ilium M80.05- ☑
      ischium M80.05- ☑
      metacarpus M80.04- ☑
      metatarsus M80.07- ☑
      pelvis M80.05- ☑
      radius M80.03- ☑
      scapula M80.01- ☑
      tarsus M80.07- ☑
      tibia M80.06- ☑
      toe M80.07- ☑
      ulna M80.03- ☑
      vertebra M80.08 ☑
  disuse M81.8
    with current pathological fracture M80.80 ☑
      carpus M80.84- ☑
      clavicle M80.81- ☑
      fibula M80.86- ☑
      finger M80.84- ☑
      humerus M80.82- ☑
      ilium M80.85- ☑
      ischium M80.85- ☑
      metacarpus M80.84- ☑
      metatarsus M80.87- ☑
      pelvis M80.85- ☑
      radius M80.83- ☑
      scapula M80.81- ☑
      tarsus M80.87- ☑
      tibia M80.86- ☑
      toe M80.87- ☑
      ulna M80.83- ☑

Osteoporosis — *continued*
  disuse — *continued*
    with current pathological fracture — *continued*
      vertebra M80.88 ☑
  drug-induced — *see* Osteoporosis, specified type NEC
  idiopathic — *see* Osteoporosis, specified type NEC
  involutional — *see* Osteoporosis, age-related
  Lequesne M81.6
  localized M81.6
  postmenopausal M81.0
    with pathological fracture M80.00 ☑
      carpus M80.04- ☑
      clavicle M80.01- ☑
      fibula M80.06- ☑
      finger M80.04- ☑
      humerus M80.02- ☑
      ilium M80.05- ☑
      ischium M80.05- ☑
      metacarpus M80.04- ☑
      metatarsus M80.07- ☑
      pelvis M80.05- ☑
      radius M80.03- ☑
      scapula M80.01- ☑
      tarsus M80.07- ☑
      tibia M80.06- ☑
      toe M80.07- ☑
      ulna M80.03- ☑
      vertebra M80.08 ☑
  postoophorectomy — *see* Osteoporosis, specified type NEC
  postsurgical malabsorption — *see* Osteoporosis, specified type NEC
  post-traumatic — *see* Osteoporosis, specified type NEC
  senile — *see* Osteoporosis, age-related
  specified type NEC M81.8
    with pathological fracture M80.80 ☑
      carpus M80.84- ☑
      clavicle M80.81- ☑
      fibula M80.86- ☑
      finger M80.84- ☑
      humerus M80.82- ☑
      ilium M80.85- ☑
      ischium M80.85- ☑
      metacarpus M80.84- ☑
      metatarsus M80.87- ☑
      pelvis M80.85- ☑
      radius M80.83- ☑
      scapula M80.81- ☑
      tarsus M80.87- ☑
      tibia M80.86- ☑
      toe M80.87- ☑
      ulna M80.83- ☑
      vertebra M80.88 ☑

Osteopsathyrosis (idiopathica) Q78.0
Osteoradionecrosis, jaw (acute) (chronic) (lower) (suppurative) (upper) M27.2
Osteosarcoma (any form) — *see* Neoplasm, bone, malignant
Osteosclerosis Q78.2
  acquired M85.8- ☑
  congenita Q77.4
  fragilitas (generalisata) Q78.2
  myelofibrosis D75.81
Osteosclerotic anemia D64.89
Osteosis
  cutis L94.2
  renal fibrocystic N25.0
Österreicher-Turner syndrome Q87.2
Ostium
  atrioventriculare commune Q21.2
  primum (arteriosum) (defect) (persistent) Q21.2
  secundum (arteriosum) (defect) (patent) (persistent) Q21.1
Ostrum-Furst syndrome Q75.8
Otalgia H92.0 ☑
Otitis (acute) H66.90
  with effusion (*see also* Otitis, media, nonsuppurative)
    purulent — *see* Otitis, media, suppurative
  adhesive — *see* subcategory H74.1 ☑
  chronic (*see also* Otitis, media, chronic)
    with effusion (*see also* Otitis, media, nonsuppurative, chronic)
  externa H60.9- ☑
    abscess — *see* Abscess, ear, external
    acute (noninfective) H60.50- ☑

Otitis — *continued*
  externa — *continued*
    acute — *continued*
      actinic H60.51- ☑
      chemical H60.52- ☑
      contact H60.53- ☑
      eczematoid H60.54- ☑
      infective — *see* Otitis, externa, infective
      reactive H60.55- ☑
      specified NEC H60.59- ☑
    cellulitis — *see* Cellulitis, ear
    chronic H60.6- ☑
    diffuse — *see* Otitis, externa, infective, diffuse
    hemorrhagic — *see* Otitis, externa, infective, hemorrhagic
    in (due to)
      aspergillosis B44.89
      candidiasis B37.84
      erysipelas A46 [H62.40]
      herpes (simplex) virus infection B00.1
        zoster B02.8
      impetigo L01.00 [H62.40]
      infectious disease NEC B99 [H62.4-] ☑
      mycosis NEC B36.9 [H62.40]
      parasitic disease NEC B89 [H62.40]
      viral disease NEC B34.9 [H62.40]
      zoster B02.8
    infective NEC H60.39- ☑
      abscess — *see* Abscess, ear, external
      cellulitis — *see* Cellulitis, ear
      diffuse H60.31- ☑
      hemorrhagic H60.32- ☑
      swimmer's ear — *see* Swimmer's, ear
    malignant H60.2- ☑
    mycotic NEC B36.9 [H62.40]
      in
        aspergillosis B44.89
        candidiasis B37.84
        moniliasis B37.84
    necrotizing — *see* Otitis, externa, malignant
    Pseudomonas aeruginosa — *see* Otitis, externa, malignant
    reactive — *see* Otitis, externa, acute, reactive
    specified NEC — *see* subcategory H60.8 ☑
    tropical NEC B36.9 [H62.40]
      in
        aspergillosis B44.89
        candidiasis B37.84
        moniliasis B37.84
  insidiosa — *see* Otosclerosis
  interna H83.0 ☑
  media (hemorrhagic) (staphylococcal) (streptococcal) H66.9- ☑
    with effusion (nonpurulent) — *see* Otitis, media, nonsuppurative
    acute, subacute H66.90
      allergic — *see* Otitis, media, nonsuppurative, acute, allergic
      exudative — *see* Otitis, media, suppurative, acute
      mucoid — *see* Otitis, media, nonsuppurative, acute
      necrotizing (*see also* Otitis, media, suppurative, acute)
        in
          measles B05.3
          scarlet fever A38.0
      nonsuppurative NEC — *see* Otitis, media, nonsuppurative, acute
      purulent — *see* Otitis, media, suppurative, acute
      sanguinous — *see* Otitis, media, nonsuppurative, acute
      secretory — *see* Otitis, media, nonsuppurative, acute, serous
      seromucinous — *see* Otitis, media, nonsuppurative, acute
      serous — *see* Otitis, media, nonsuppurative, acute, serous
      suppurative — *see* Otitis, media, suppurative, acute
    allergic — *see* Otitis, media, nonsuppurative
    catarrhal — *see* Otitis, media, nonsuppurative
    chronic H66.90
      with effusion (nonpurulent) — *see* Otitis, media, nonsuppurative, chronic

Otitis — *continued*
  media — *continued*
    chronic — *continued*
      allergic — *see* Otitis, media, nonsuppurative, chronic, allergic
      benign suppurative — *see* Otitis, media, suppurative, chronic, tubotympanic
      catarrhal — *see* Otitis, media, nonsuppurative, chronic, serous
      exudative — *see* Otitis, media, nonsuppurative, chronic
      mucinous — *see* Otitis, media, nonsuppurative, chronic, mucoid
      mucoid — *see* Otitis, media, nonsuppurative, chronic, mucoid
      nonsuppurative NEC — *see* Otitis, media, nonsuppurative, chronic
      purulent — *see* Otitis, media, suppurative, chronic
      secretory — *see* Otitis, media, nonsuppurative, chronic, mucoid
      seromucinous — *see* Otitis, media, nonsuppurative, chronic
      serous — *see* Otitis, media, nonsuppurative, chronic, serous
      suppurative — *see* Otitis, media, suppurative, chronic
      transudative — *see* Otitis, media, nonsuppurative, chronic, mucoid
    exudative — *see* Otitis, media, suppurative
    in (due to) (with)
      influenza — *see* Influenza, with, otitis media
      measles B05.3
      scarlet fever A38.0
      tuberculosis A18.6
      viral disease NEC B34.- ☑ [H67.-] ☑
    mucoid — *see* Otitis, media, nonsuppurative
    nonsuppurative H65.9- ☑
      acute or subacute NEC H65.19- ☑
        allergic H65.11- ☑
          recurrent H65.11- ☑
        recurrent H65.19- ☑
        secretory — *see* Otitis, media, nonsuppurative, serous
        serous H65.0- ☑
          recurrent H65.0- ☑
      chronic H65.49- ☑
        allergic H65.41- ☑
        mucoid H65.3- ☑
        serous H65.2- ☑
    postmeasles B05.3
    purulent — *see* Otitis, media, suppurative
    secretory — *see* Otitis, media, nonsuppurative
    seromucinous — *see* Otitis, media, nonsuppurative
    serous — *see* Otitis, media, nonsuppurative
    suppurative H66.4- ☑
      acute H66.00- ☑
        with rupture of ear drum H66.01- ☑
        recurrent H66.00- ☑
          with rupture of ear drum H66.01- ☑
      chronic (*see also* subcategory) H66.3 ☑
        atticoantral H66.2- ☑
        benign — *see* Otitis, media, suppurative, chronic, tubotympanic
        tubotympanic H66.1- ☑
    transudative — *see* Otitis, media, nonsuppurative
    tuberculous A18.6
Otocephaly Q18.2
Otolith syndrome — *see* subcategory H81.8 ☑
Otomycosis (diffuse) **NEC** B36.9 [H62.40]
  in
    aspergillosis B44.89
    candidiasis B37.84
    moniliasis B37.84
Otoporosis — *see* Otosclerosis
Otorrhagia (nontraumatic) H92.2- ☑
  traumatic — *code by* Type of injury
Otorrhea H92.1- ☑
  cerebrospinal G96.0
Otosclerosis (general) H80.9- ☑
  cochlear (endosteal) H80.2- ☑
  involving
    otic capsule — *see* Otosclerosis, cochlear
    oval window
      nonobliterative H80.0- ☑
      obliterative H80.1- ☑
    round window — *see* Otosclerosis, cochlear

⚑ Subterms under main terms may continue to next column or page   ☑ Additional Character Required — Refer to the Tabular List for Character Selection   243

Osteoporosis — Otosclerosis

Otosclerosis — *continued*
nonobliterative — *see* Otosclerosis, involving, oval window, nonobliterative
obliterative — *see* Otosclerosis, involving, oval window, obliterative
specified NEC H80.8- ☑
Otospongiosis — *see* Otosclerosis
Otto's disease or pelvis M24.7
Outcome of delivery Z37.9
multiple births Z37.9
all liveborn Z37.50
quadruplets Z37.52
quintuplets Z37.53
sextuplets Z37.54
specified number NEC Z37.59
triplets Z37.51
all stillborn Z37.7
some liveborn Z37.60
quadruplets Z37.62
quintuplets Z37.63
sextuplets Z37.64
specified number NEC Z37.69
triplets Z37.61
single NEC Z37.9
liveborn Z37.0
stillborn Z37.1
twins NEC Z37.9
both liveborn Z37.2
both stillborn Z37.4
one liveborn, one stillborn Z37.3
Outlet — *see* condition
Ovalocytosis (congenital) (hereditary) — *see* Elliptocytosis
Ovarian — *see* Condition
Ovariocele N83.4- ☑
Ovaritis (cystic) — *see* Oophoritis
Ovary, ovarian (*see also* condition)
resistant syndrome E28.39
vein syndrome N13.8
Overactive (*see also* Hyperfunction)
adrenal cortex NEC E27.0
bladder N32.81
hypothalamus E23.3
thyroid — *see* Hyperthyroidism
Overactivity R46.3
child — *see* Disorder, attention-deficit hyperactivity
Overbite (deep) (excessive) (horizontal) (vertical) M26.29
Overbreathing — *see* Hyperventilation
Overconscientious personality F60.5
Overdevelopment — *see* Hypertrophy
Overdistension — *see* Distension
Overdose, overdosage (drug) — *see* Table of Drugs and Chemicals, by drug, poisoning
Overeating R63.2
nonorganic origin F50.89
psychogenic F50.89
Overexertion (effects) (exhaustion) T73.3 ☑
Overexposure (effects) T73.9 ☑
exhaustion T73.2 ☑
Overfeeding — *see* Overeating
newborn P92.4
Overfill, endodontic M27.52
Overgrowth, bone — *see* Hypertrophy, bone
Overhanging of dental restorative material (unrepairable) K08.52
Overheated (places) (effects) — *see* Heat
Overjet (excessive horizontal) M26.23
Overlaid, overlying (suffocation) — *see* Asphyxia, traumatic, due to mechanical threat
Overlap, excessive horizontal (teeth) M26.23
Overlapping toe (acquired) (*see also* Deformity, toe, specified NEC)
congenital (fifth toe) Q66.89
Overload
circulatory, due to transfusion (blood) (blood components) (TACO) E87.71
fluid E87.70
due to transfusion (blood) (blood components) E87.71
specified NEC E87.79
iron, due to repeated red blood cell transfusions E83.111
potassium (K) E87.5
sodium (Na) E87.0
Overnutrition — *see* Hyperalimentation
Overproduction (*see also* Hypersecretion)
ACTH E27.0

Overproduction — *continued*
catecholamine E27.5
growth hormone E22.0
Overprotection, child by parent Z62.1
Overriding
aorta Q25.49
finger (acquired) — *see* Deformity, finger
congenital Q68.1
toe (acquired) (*see also* Deformity, toe, specified NEC)
congenital Q66.89
Overstrained R53.83
heart — *see* Hypertrophy, cardiac
Overuse, muscle NEC M70.8- ☑
Overweight E66.3
Overworked R53.83
Oviduct — *see* condition
Ovotestis Q56.0
Ovulation (cycle)
failure or lack of N97.0
pain N94.0
Ovum — *see* condition
Owren's disease or syndrome (parahemophilia) D68.2
Ox heart — *see* Hypertrophy, cardiac
Oxalosis E72.53
Oxaluria E72.53
Oxycephaly, oxycephalic Q75.0
syphilitic, congenital A50.02
Oxyuriasis B80
Oxyuris vermicularis (infestation) B80
Ozena J31.0

P

Pachyderma, pachydermia L85.9
larynx (verrucosa) J38.7
Pachydermatocele (congenital) Q82.8
Pachydermoperiostosis (*see also* Osteoarthropathy, hypertrophic, specified type NEC)
clubbed nail M89.40 [L62]
Pachygyria Q04.3
Pachymeningitis (adhesive) (basal) (brain) (cervical) (chronic)(circumscribed) (external) (fibrous) (hemorrhagic) (hypertrophic) (internal) (purulent) (spinal) (suppurative) — *see* Meningitis
Pachyonychia (congenital) Q84.5
Pacinian tumor — *see* Neoplasm, skin, benign
Pad, knuckle or Garrod's M72.1
Paget's disease
with infiltrating duct carcinoma — *see* Neoplasm, breast, malignant
bone M88.9
carpus M88.84- ☑
clavicle M88.81- ☑
femur M88.85- ☑
fibula M88.86- ☑
finger M88.84- ☑
humerus M88.82- ☑
ilium M88.85- ☑
in neoplastic disease — *see* Osteitis, deformans, in neoplastic disease
ischium M88.85- ☑
metacarpus M88.84- ☑
metatarsus M88.87- ☑
multiple sites M88.89
neck M88.88
radius M88.83- ☑
rib M88.88
scapula M88.81- ☑
skull M88.0
tarsus M88.87- ☑
tibia M88.86- ☑
toe M88.87- ☑
ulna M88.83- ☑
vertebra M88.88
breast (female) C50.01- ☑
male C50.02- ☑
extramammary (*see also* Neoplasm, skin, malignant)
anus C21.0
margin C44.590
skin C44.590
intraductal carcinoma — *see* Neoplasm, breast, malignant
malignant — *see* Neoplasm, skin, malignant
breast (female) C50.01- ☑
male C50.02- ☑
unspecified site (female) C50.01- ☑
male C50.02- ☑

Paget's disease — *continued*
mammary — *see* Paget's disease, breast
nipple — *see* Paget's disease, breast
osteitis deformans — *see* Paget's disease, bone
Paget-Schroetter syndrome I82.890
Pain(s) (*see also* Painful) R52
abdominal R10.9
colic R10.83
generalized R10.84
with acute abdomen R10.0
lower R10.30
left quadrant R10.32
pelvic or perineal R10.2
periumbilical R10.33
right quadrant R10.31
rebound — *see* Tenderness, abdominal, rebound
severe with abdominal rigidity R10.0
tenderness — *see* Tenderness, abdominal
upper R10.10
epigastric R10.13
left quadrant R10.12
right quadrant R10.11
acute R52
due to trauma G89.11
neoplasm related G89.3
postprocedural NEC G89.18
post-thoracotomy G89.12
specified by site — *code to* Pain, by site
adnexa (uteri) R10.2
anginoid — *see* Pain, precordial
anus K62.89
arm — *see* Pain, limb, upper
axillary (axilla) M79.62- ☑
back (postural) M54.9
bladder R39.89
associated with micturition — *see* Micturition, painful
chronic R39.82
bone — *see* Disorder, bone, specified type NEC
breast N64.4
broad ligament R10.2
cancer associated (acute) (chronic) G89.3
cecum — *see* Pain, abdominal
cervicobrachial M53.1
chest (central) R07.9
anterior wall R07.89
atypical R07.89
ischemic I20.9
musculoskeletal R07.89
non-cardiac R07.89
on breathing R07.1
pleurodynia R07.81
precordial R07.2
wall (anterior) R07.89
chronic G89.29
associated with significant psychosocial dysfunction G89.4
due to trauma G89.21
neoplasm related G89.3
postoperative NEC G89.28
postprocedural NEC G89.28
post-thoracotomy G89.22
specified NEC G89.29
coccyx M53.3
colon — *see* Pain, abdominal
coronary — *see* Angina
costochondral R07.1
diaphragm R07.1
due to cancer G89.3
due to device, implant or graft (*see also* Complications, by site and type, specified NEC) T85.848 ☑
arterial graft NEC T82.848 ☑
breast (implant) T85.848 ☑
catheter NEC T85.848 ☑
dialysis (renal) T82.848 ☑
intraperitoneal T85.848 ☑
infusion NEC T82.848 ☑
spinal (epidural) (subdural) T85.840 ☑
urinary (indwelling) T83.84 ☑
electronic (electrode) (pulse generator) (stimulator)
bone T85.840 ☑
cardiac T82.847 ☑
nervous system (brain) (peripheral nerve) (spinal) T85.84 ☑
urinary T83.84 ☑
fixation, internal (orthopedic) NEC T84.84 ☑
gastrointestinal (bile duct) (esophagus) T85.848 ☑
genital NEC T83.84 ☑

Pain(s) — *continued*
 due to device, implant or graft (*see also* Complications, by site and type, specified) — *continued*
  heart NEC T82.847 ☑
  infusion NEC T85.848 ☑
  joint prosthesis T84.84 ☑
  ocular (corneal graft) (orbital implant) NEC T85.848 ☑
  orthopedic NEC T84.84 ☑
  specified NEC T85.848 ☑
  urinary NEC T83.84 ☑
  vascular NEC T82.848 ☑
  ventricular intracranial shunt T85.840 ☑
 due to malignancy (primary) (secondary) G89.3
 ear — *see* subcategory H92.0 ☑
 epigastric, epigastrium R10.13
 eye — *see* Pain, ocular
 face, facial R51
  atypical G50.1
 female genital organs NEC N94.89
 finger — *see* Pain, limb, upper
 flank — *see* Pain, abdominal
 foot — *see* Pain, limb, lower
 gallbladder K82.9
 gas (intestinal) R14.1
 gastric — *see* Pain, abdominal
 generalized NOS R52
 genital organ
  female N94.89
  male N50.89
 groin — *see* Pain, abdominal, lower
 hand — *see* Pain, limb, upper
 head — *see* Headache
 heart — *see* Pain, precordial
 infra-orbital — *see* Neuralgia, trigeminal
 intercostal R07.82
 intermenstrual N94.0
 jaw R68.84
 joint M25.50
  ankle M25.57- ☑
  elbow M25.52- ☑
  finger M25.54- ☑
  foot M25.57- ☑
  hand M25.54- ☑
  hip M25.55- ☑
  knee M25.56- ☑
  shoulder M25.51- ☑
  toe M25.57- ☑
  wrist M25.53- ☑
 kidney N23
 laryngeal R07.0
 leg — *see* Pain, limb, lower
 limb M79.609
  lower M79.60- ☑
   foot M79.67- ☑
   lower leg M79.66- ☑
   thigh M79.65- ☑
   toe M79.67- ☑
  upper M79.60- ☑
   axilla M79.62- ☑
   finger M79.64- ☑
   forearm M79.63- ☑
   hand M79.64- ☑
   upper arm M79.62- ☑
 loin M54.5
 low back M54.5
 lumbar region M54.5
 mandibular R68.84
 mastoid — *see* subcategory H92.0 ☑
 maxilla R68.84
 menstrual (*see also* Dysmenorrhea) N94.6
 metacarpophalangeal (joint) — *see* Pain, joint, hand
 metatarsophalangeal (joint) — *see* Pain, joint, foot
 mouth K13.79
 muscle — *see* Myalgia
 musculoskeletal (*see also* Pain, by site) M79.1
 myofascial M79.1
 nasal J34.89
 nasopharynx J39.2
 neck NEC M54.2
 nerve NEC — *see* Neuralgia
 neuromuscular — *see* Neuralgia
 nose J34.89
 ocular H57.1- ☑
 ophthalmic — *see* Pain, ocular
 orbital region — *see* Pain, ocular
 ovary N94.89

Pain(s) — *continued*
 over heart — *see* Pain, precordial
 ovulation N94.0
 pelvic (female) R10.2
 penis N48.89
 pericardial — *see* Pain, precordial
 perineal, perineum R10.2
 pharynx J39.2
 pleura, pleural, pleuritic R07.81
 postoperative NOS G89.18
 postprocedural NOS G89.18
 post-thoracotomy G89.12
 precordial (region) R07.2
 premenstrual N94.3
 psychogenic (persistent) (any site) F45.41
 radicular (spinal) — *see* Radiculopathy
 rectum K62.89
 respiration R07.1
 retrosternal R07.2
 rheumatoid, muscular — *see* Myalgia
 rib R07.81
 root (spinal) — *see* Radiculopathy
 round ligament (stretch) R10.2
 sacroiliac M53.3
 sciatic — *see* Sciatica
 scrotum N50.82
 seminal vesicle N50.89
 shoulder M25.51- ☑
 spermatic cord N50.89
 spinal root — *see* Radiculopathy
 spine M54.9
  cervical M54.2
  low back M54.5
   with sciatica M54.4- ☑
  thoracic M54.6
 stomach — *see* Pain, abdominal
 substernal R07.2
 temporomandibular (joint) M26.62- ☑
 testis N50.81- ☑
 thoracic spine M54.6
  with radicular and visceral pain M54.14
 throat R07.0
 tibia — *see* Pain, limb, lower
 toe — *see* Pain, limb, lower
 tongue K14.6
 tooth K08.89
 trigeminal — *see* Neuralgia, trigeminal
 tumor associated G89.3
 ureter N23
 urinary (organ) (system) N23
 uterus NEC N94.89
 vagina R10.2
 vertebrogenic (syndrome) M54.89
 vesical R39.89
  associated with micturition — *see* Micturition, painful
 vulva R10.2
Painful (*see also* Pain)
 coitus
  female N94.10
  male N53.12
  psychogenic F52.6
 ejaculation (semen) N53.12
  psychogenic F52.6
 erection — *see* Priapism
 feet syndrome E53.8
 joint replacement (hip) (knee) T84.84 ☑
 menstruation — *see* Dysmenorrhea
  psychogenic F45.8
 micturition — *see* Micturition, painful
 respiration R07.1
 scar NEC L90.5
 wire sutures T81.89 ☑
Painter's colic — *see* subcategory T56.0 ☑
Palate — *see* condition
Palatoplegia K13.79
Palatoschisis — *see* Cleft, palate
Palilalia R48.8
Palliative care Z51.5
Pallor R23.1
 optic disc, temporal — *see* Atrophy, optic
Palmar (*see also* condition)
 fascia — *see* condition
Palpable
 cecum K63.89
 kidney N28.89
 ovary N83.8
 prostate N42.9

Palpable — *continued*
 spleen — *see* Splenomegaly
Palpitations (heart) R00.2
 psychogenic F45.8
Palsy (*see also* Paralysis) G83.9
 atrophic diffuse (progressive) G12.22
 Bell's (*see also* Palsy, facial)
  newborn P11.3
 brachial plexus NEC G54.0
  newborn (birth injury) P14.3
 brain — *see* Palsy, cerebral
 bulbar (progressive) (chronic) G12.22
  of childhood (Fazio-Londe) G12.1
  pseudo NEC G12.29
  supranuclear (progressive) G23.1
 cerebral (congenital) G80.9
  ataxic G80.4
  athetoid G80.3
  choreathetoid G80.3
  diplegic G80.8
   spastic G80.1
  dyskinetic G80.3
   athetoid G80.3
   choreathetoid G80.3
   distonic G80.3
  dystonic G80.3
  hemiplegic G80.8
   spastic G80.2
  mixed G80.8
  monoplegic G80.8
   spastic G80.1
  paraplegic G80.8
   spastic G80.1
  quadriplegic G80.8
   spastic G80.0
  spastic G80.1
   diplegic G80.1
   hemiplegic G80.2
   monoplegic G80.1
   quadriplegic G80.0
   specified NEC G80.1
   tetrapelgic G80.0
  specified NEC G80.8
  syphilitic A52.12
   congenital A50.49
  tetraplegic G80.8
   spastic G80.0
 cranial nerve (*see also* Disorder, nerve, cranial)
  multiple G52.7
   in
    infectious disease B99 ☑ [G53]
    neoplastic disease (*see also* Neoplasm) D49.9 [G53]
    parasitic disease B89 [G53]
    sarcoidosis D86.82
 creeping G12.22
 diver's T70.3 ☑
 Erb's P14.0
 facial G51.0
  newborn (birth injury) P11.3
 glossopharyngeal G52.1
 Klumpke (-Déjérine) P14.1
 lead — *see* subcategory T56.0 ☑
 median nerve (tardy) G56.1- ☑
 nerve G58.9
  specified NEC G58.8
 peroneal nerve (acute) (tardy) G57.3- ☑
 progressive supranuclear G23.1
 pseudobulbar NEC G12.29
 radial nerve (acute) G56.3- ☑
 seventh nerve (*see also* Palsy, facial)
  newborn P11.3
 shaking — *see* Parkinsonism
 spastic (cerebral) (spinal) G80.1
 ulnar nerve (tardy) G56.2- ☑
 wasting G12.29
Paludism — *see* Malaria
Panangiitis M30.0
Panaris, panaritium (*see also* Cellulitis, digit)
 with lymphangitis — *see* Lymphangitis, acute, digit
Panarteritis nodosa M30.0
 brain or cerebral I67.7
Pancake heart R93.1
 with cor pulmonale (chronic) I27.81
Pancarditis (acute) (chronic) I51.89
 rheumatic I09.89
  active or acute I01.8
Pancoast's syndrome or tumor C34.1- ☑

Pancolitis, ulcerative (chronic) K51.00
with
abscess K51.014
complication K51.019
fistula K51.013
obstruction K51.012
rectal bleeding K51.011
specified complication NEC K51.018
Pancreas, pancreatic — see condition
Pancreatitis (annular) (apoplectic) (calcareous) (edematous) (hemorrhagic) (malignant) (recurrent) (subacute) (suppurative) K85.90
with necrosis (uninfected) K85.91
infected K85.92
acute (without necrosis or infection) K85.90
with necrosis (uninfected) K85.91
infected K85.92
alcohol induced (without necrosis or infection) K85.20
with necrosis (uninfected) K85.21
infected K85.22
biliary (without necrosis or infection) K85.10
with necrosis (uninfected) K85.11
infected K85.12
drug induced (without necrosis or infection) K85.30
with necrosis (uninfected) K85.31
infected K85.32
gallstone (without necrosis or infection) K85.10
with necrosis (uninfected) K85.11
infected K85.12
idiopathic (without necrosis or infection) K85.00
with necrosis (uninfected) K85.01
infected K85.02
specified NEC (without necrosis or infection) K85.80
with necrosis (uninfected) K85.81
infected K85.82
chronic (infectious) K86.1
alcohol-induced K86.0
recurrent K86.1
relapsing K86.1
cystic (chronic) K86.1
cytomegaloviral B25.2
fibrous (chronic) K86.1
gallstone (without necrosis or infection) K85.10
with necrosis (uninfected) K85.11
infected K85.12
gangrenous — see Pancreatitis, acute
interstitial (chronic) K86.1
acute (see also Pancreatitis, acute) K85.80
mumps B26.3
recurrent (chronic) K86.1
relapsing, chronic K86.1
syphilitic A52.74
Pancreatoblastoma — see Neoplasm, pancreas, malignant
Pancreolithiasis K86.89
Pancytolysis D75.89
Pancytopenia (acquired) D61.818
with
malformations D61.09
myelodysplastic syndrome — see Syndrome, myelodysplastic
antineoplastic chemotherapy induced D61.810
congenital D61.09
drug-induced NEC D61.811
PANDAS (pediatric autoimmune neuropsychiatric disorders associated with streptococcal infections syndrome) D89.89
Panencephalitis, subacute, sclerosing A81.1
Panhematopenia D61.9
congenital D61.09
constitutional D61.09
splenic, primary D73.1
Panhemocytopenia D61.9
congenital D61.09
constitutional D61.09
Panhypogonadism E29.1
Panhypopituitarism E23.0
prepubertal E23.0
Panic (attack) (state) F41.0
reaction to exceptional stress (transient) F43.0
Panmyelopathy, familial, constitutional D61.09
Panmyelophthisis D61.82
congenital D61.09
Panmyelosis (acute) (with myelofibrosis) C94.4- ☑
Panner's disease — see Osteochondrosis, juvenile, humerus
Panneuritis endemica E51.11

Panniculitis (nodular) (nonsuppurative) M79.3
back M54.00
cervical region M54.02
cervicothoracic region M54.03
lumbar region M54.06
lumbosacral region M54.07
multiple sites M54.09
occipito-atlanto-axial region M54.01
sacrococcygeal region M54.08
thoracic region M54.04
thoracolumbar region M54.05
lupus L93.2
mesenteric K65.4
neck M54.02
cervicothoracic region M54.03
occipito-atlanto-axial region M54.01
relapsing M35.6
Panniculus adiposus (abdominal) E65
Pannus (allergic) (cornea) (degenerativus) (keratic) H16.42- ☑
abdominal (symptomatic) E65
trachomatosus, trachomatous (active) A71.1
Panophthalmitis H44.01- ☑
Pansinusitis (chronic) (hyperplastic) (nonpurulent) (purulent) J32.4
acute J01.40
recurrent J01.41
tuberculous A15.8
Panuveitis (sympathetic) H44.11- ☑
Panvalvular disease I08.9
specified NEC I08.8
PAPA (pyogenic arthritis, pyoderma gangrenosum, and acne syndrome) M04.8
Papanicolaou smear, cervix Z12.4
as part of routine gynecological examination Z01.419
with abnormal findings Z01.411
for suspected neoplasm Z12.4
nonspecific abnormal finding R87.619
routine Z01.419
with abnormal findings Z01.411
Papilledema (choked disc) H47.10
associated with
decreased ocular pressure H47.12
increased intracranial pressure H47.11
retinal disorder H47.13
Foster-Kennedy syndrome H47.14- ☑
Papillitis H46.00
anus K62.89
chronic lingual K14.4
necrotizing, kidney N17.2
optic H46.0- ☑
rectum K62.89
renal, necrotizing N17.2
tongue K14.0
Papilloma (see also Neoplasm, benign, by site)
acuminatum (female) (male) (anogenital) A63.0
basal cell L82.1
inflamed L82.0
benign pinta (primary) A67.0
bladder (urinary) (transitional cell) D41.4
choroid plexus (lateral ventricle) (third ventricle) D33.0
anaplastic C71.5
fourth ventricle D33.1
malignant C71.5
renal pelvis (transitional cell) D41.1- ☑
benign D30.1- ☑
Schneiderian
specified site — see Neoplasm, benign, by site
unspecified site D14.0
serous surface
borderline malignancy
specified site — see Neoplasm, uncertain behavior, by site
unspecified site D39.10
specified site — see Neoplasm, benign, by site
unspecified site D27.9
transitional (cell)
bladder (urinary) D41.4
inverted type — see Neoplasm, uncertain behavior, by site
renal pelvis D41.1- ☑
ureter D41.2- ☑
ureter (transitional cell) D41.2- ☑
benign D30.2- ☑
urothelial — see Neoplasm, uncertain behavior, by site
villous — see Neoplasm, uncertain behavior, by site

Papilloma — continued
villous — see Neoplasm, uncertain behavior, by site — continued
adenocarcinoma in — see Neoplasm, malignant, by site
in situ — see Neoplasm, in situ
yaws, plantar or palmar A66.1
Papillomata, multiple, of yaws A66.1
Papillomatosis (see also Neoplasm, benign, by site)
confluent and reticulated L83
cystic, breast — see Mastopathy, cystic
ductal, breast — see Mastopathy, cystic
intraductal (diffuse) — see Neoplasm, benign, by site
subareolar duct D24- ☑
Papillomavirus, as cause of disease classified elsewhere B97.7
Papillon-Léage and Psaume syndrome Q87.0
Papule(s) R23.8
carate (primary) A67.0
fibrous, of nose D22.39
Gottron's L94.4
pinta (primary) A67.0
Papulosis
lymphomatoid C86.6
malignant I77.89
Papyraceous fetus O31.0- ☑
Para-albuminemia E88.09
Paracephalus Q89.7
Parachute mitral valve Q23.2
Paracoccidioidomycosis B41.9
disseminated B41.7
generalized B41.7
mucocutaneous-lymphangitic B41.8
pulmonary B41.0
specified NEC B41.8
visceral B41.8
Paradentosis K05.4
Paraffinoma T88.8 ☑
Paraganglioma D44.7
adrenal D35.0- ☑
malignant C74.1- ☑
aortic body D44.7
malignant C75.5
carotid body D44.6
malignant C75.4
chromaffin (see also Neoplasm, benign, by site)
malignant — see Neoplasm, malignant, by site
extra-adrenal D44.7
malignant C75.5
specified site — see Neoplasm, malignant, by site
unspecified site C75.5
specified site — see Neoplasm, uncertain behavior, by site
unspecified site D44.7
gangliocytic D13.2
specified site — see Neoplasm, benign, by site
unspecified site D13.2
glomus jugulare D44.7
malignant C75.5
jugular D44.7
malignant C75.5
specified site — see Neoplasm, malignant, by site
unspecified site C75.5
nonchromaffin D44.7
malignant C75.5
specified site — see Neoplasm, malignant, by site
unspecified site C75.5
specified site — see Neoplasm, uncertain behavior, by site
unspecified site D44.7
parasympathetic D44.7
specified site — see Neoplasm, uncertain behavior, by site
unspecified site D44.7
specified site — see Neoplasm, uncertain behavior, by site
sympathetic D44.7
specified site — see Neoplasm, uncertain behavior, by site
unspecified site D44.7
unspecified site D44.7
Parageusia R43.2
psychogenic F45.8
Paragonimiasis B66.4

Paragranuloma, Hodgkin — *see* Lymphoma, Hodgkin,
   specified NEC
Parahemophilia (*see also* Defect, coagulation) D68.2
Parakeratosis R23.4
  variegata L41.0
Paralysis, paralytic (complete) (incomplete) G83.9
  with
     syphilis A52.17
  abducens, abducent (nerve) — *see* Strabismus, para-
    lytic, sixth nerve
  abductor, lower extremity G57.9- ☑
  accessory nerve G52.8
  accommodation (*see also* Paresis, of accommodation)
    hysterical F44.89
  acoustic nerve (except Deafness) H93.3 ☑
  agitans (*see also* Parkinsonism) G20
    arteriosclerotic G21.4
  alternating (oculomotor) G83.89
  amyotrophic G12.21
  ankle G57.9- ☑
  anus (sphincter) K62.89
  arm — *see* Monoplegia, upper limb
  ascending (spinal), acute G61.0
  association G12.29
  asthenic bulbar G70.00
    with exacerbation (acute) G70.01
    in crisis G70.01
  ataxic (hereditary) G11.9
    general (syphilitic) A52.17
  atrophic G58.9
    infantile, acute — *see* Poliomyelitis, paralytic
    progressive G12.22
    spinal (acute) — *see* Poliomyelitis, paralytic
  axillary G54.0
  Babinski-Nageotte's G83.89
  Bell's G51.0
    newborn P11.3
  Benedikt's G46.3
  birth injury P14.9
    spinal cord P11.5
  bladder (neurogenic) (sphincter) N31.2
  bowel, colon or intestine K56.0
  brachial plexus G54.0
    birth injury P14.3
    newborn (birth injury) P14.3
  brain G83.9
    diplegia G83.0
    triplegia G83.89
  bronchial J98.09
  Brown-Séquard G83.81
  bulbar (chronic) (progressive) G12.22
    infantile — *see* Poliomyelitis, paralytic
    poliomyelitic — *see* Poliomyelitis, paralytic
    pseudo G12.29
  bulbospinal G70.00
    with exacerbation (acute) G70.01
    in crisis G70.01
  cardiac (*see also* Failure, heart) I50.9
  cerebrocerebellar, diplegic G80.1
  cervical
    plexus G54.2
    sympathetic G90.09
  Céstan-Chenais G46.3
  Charcot-Marie-Tooth type G60.0
  Clark's G80.9
  colon K56.0
  compressed air T70.3 ☑
  compression
    arm G56.9- ☑
    leg G57.9- ☑
    lower extremity G57.9- ☑
    upper extremity G56.9- ☑
  congenital (cerebral) — *see* Palsy, cerebral
  conjugate movement (gaze) (of eye) H51.0
    cortical (nuclear) (supranuclear) H51.0
  cordis — *see* Failure, heart
  cranial or cerebral nerve G52.9
  creeping G12.22
  crossed leg G83.89
  crutch — *see* Injury, brachial plexus
  deglutition R13.0
    hysterical F44.4
  dementia A52.17
  descending (spinal) NEC G12.29
  diaphragm (flaccid) J98.6
    due to accidental dissection of phrenic nerve dur-
      ing procedure — *see* Puncture, accidental
      complicating surgery

Paralysis, paralytic — *continued*
  digestive organs NEC K59.8
  diplegic — *see* Diplegia
  divergence (nuclear) H51.8
  diver's T70.3 ☑
  Duchenne's
    birth injury P14.0
    due to or associated with
      motor neuron disease G12.22
      muscular dystrophy G71.0
  due to intracranial or spinal birth injury — *see* Palsy,
    cerebral
  embolic (current episode) I63.4- ☑
  Erb (-Duchenne) (birth) (newborn) P14.0
  Erb's syphilitic spastic spinal A52.17
  esophagus K22.8
  eye muscle (extrinsic) H49.9
    intrinsic (*see also* Paresis, of accommodation)
  facial (nerve) G51.0
    birth injury P11.3
    congenital P11.3
    following operation NEC — *see* Puncture, acciden-
      tal complicating surgery
    newborn (birth injury) P11.3
  familial (recurrent) (periodic) G72.3
    spastic G11.4
  fauces J39.2
  finger G56.9- ☑
  gait R26.1
  gastric nerve (nondiabetic) G52.2
  gaze, conjugate H51.0
  general (progressive) (syphilitic) A52.17
    juvenile A50.45
  glottis J38.00
    bilateral J38.02
    unilateral J38.01
  gluteal G54.1
  Gubler (-Millard) G46.3
  hand — *see* Monoplegia, upper limb
  heart — *see* Arrest, cardiac
  hemiplegic — *see* Hemiplegia
  hyperkalemic periodic (familial) G72.3
  hypoglossal (nerve) G52.3
  hypokalemic periodic G72.3
  hysterical F44.4
  ileus K56.0
  infantile (*see also* Poliomyelitis, paralytic) A80.30
    bulbar — *see* Poliomyelitis, paralytic
    cerebral — *see* Palsy, cerebral
    spastic — *see* Palsy, cerebral, spastic
  infective — *see* Poliomyelitis, paralytic
  inferior nuclear G83.9
  internuclear — *see* Ophthalmoplegia, internuclear
  intestine K56.0
  iris H57.09
    due to diphtheria (toxin) A36.89
  ischemic, Volkmann's (complicating trauma) T79.6 ☑
  Jackson's G83.89
  jake — *see* Poisoning, food, noxious, plant
  Jamaica ginger (jake) G62.2
  juvenile general A50.45
  Klumpke (-Déjérine) (birth) (newborn) P14.1
  labioglossal (laryngeal) (pharyngeal) G12.29
  Landry's G61.0
  laryngeal nerve (recurrent) (superior) (unilateral) J38.00
    bilateral J38.02
    unilateral J38.01
  larynx J38.00
    bilateral J38.02
    due to diphtheria (toxin) A36.2
    unilateral J38.01
  lateral G12.23
  lead T56.0 ☑
  left side — *see* Hemiplegia
  leg G83.1- ☑
    both — *see* Paraplegia
    crossed G83.89
    hysterical F44.4
    psychogenic F44.4
    transient or transitory R29.818
      traumatic NEC — *see* Injury, nerve, leg
  levator palpebrae superioris — *see* Blepharoptosis,
    paralytic
  limb — *see* Monoplegia
  lip K13.0
  Lissauer's A52.17
  lower limb — *see* Monoplegia, lower limb
    both — *see* Paraplegia

Paralysis, paralytic — *continued*
  lung J98.4
  median nerve G56.1- ☑
  medullary (tegmental) G83.89
  mesencephalic NEC G83.89
    tegmental G83.89
  middle alternating G83.89
  Millard-Gubler-Foville G46.3
  monoplegic — *see* Monoplegia
  motor G83.9
  muscle, muscular NEC G72.89
    due to nerve lesion G58.9
    eye (extrinsic) H49.9
      intrinsic — *see* Paresis, of accommodation
      oblique — *see* Strabismus, paralytic, fourth
        nerve
    iris sphincter H21.9
    ischemic (Volkmann's) (complicating trauma)
      T79.6 ☑
    progressive G12.21
    pseudohypertrophic G71.0
  musculocutaneous nerve G56.9- ☑
  musculospiral G56.9- ☑
  nerve (*see also* Disorder, nerve)
    abducent — *see* Strabismus, paralytic, sixth nerve
    accessory G52.8
    auditory (except Deafness) H93.3 ☑
    birth injury P14.9
    cranial or cerebral G52.9
    facial G51.0
      birth injury P11.3
      congenital P11.3
      newborn (birth injury) P11.3
    fourth or trochlear — *see* Strabismus, paralytic,
      fourth nerve
    newborn (birth injury) P14.9
    oculomotor — *see* Strabismus, paralytic, third
      nerve
    phrenic (birth injury) P14.2
    radial G56.3- ☑
    seventh or facial G51.0
      newborn (birth injury) P11.3
    sixth or abducent — *see* Strabismus, paralytic, sixth
      nerve
    syphilitic A52.15
    third or oculomotor — *see* Strabismus, paralytic,
      third nerve
    trigeminal G50.9
    trochlear — *see* Strabismus, paralytic, fourth nerve
    ulnar G56.2- ☑
  normokalemic periodic G72.3
  ocular H49.9
    alternating G83.89
  oculofacial, congenital (Moebius) Q87.0
  oculomotor (external bilateral) (nerve) — *see* Strabis-
    mus, paralytic, third nerve
  palate (soft) K13.79
  paratrigeminal G50.9
  periodic (familial) (hyperkalemic) (hypokalemic) (my-
    otonic) (normokalemic) (potassium sensitive)
    (secondary) G72.3
  peripheral autonomic nervous system — *see* Neuropa-
    thy, peripheral, autonomic
  peroneal (nerve) G57.3- ☑
  pharynx J39.2
  phrenic nerve G56.8- ☑
  plantar nerve(s) G57.6- ☑
  pneumogastric nerve G52.2
  poliomyelitis (current) — *see* Poliomyelitis, paralytic
  popliteal nerve G57.3- ☑
  postepileptic transitory G83.84
  progressive (atrophic) (bulbar) (spinal) G12.22
    general A52.17
    infantile acute — *see* Poliomyelitis, paralytic
    supranuclear G23.1
  pseudobulbar G12.29
  pseudohypertrophic (muscle) G71.0
  psychogenic F44.4
  quadriceps G57.9- ☑
  quadriplegic — *see* Tetraplegia
  radial nerve G56.3- ☑
  rectus muscle (eye) H49.9
  recurrent isolated sleep G47.53
  respiratory (muscle) (system) (tract) R06.81
    center NEC G93.89
    congenital P28.89
    newborn P28.89
  right side — *see* Hemiplegia

Paralysis, paralytic — *continued*
  saturnine T56.0 ☑
  sciatic nerve G57.0- ☑
  senile G83.9
  shaking — *see* Parkinsonism
  shoulder G56.9- ☑
  sleep, recurrent isolated G47.53
  spastic G83.9
    cerebral — *see* Palsy, cerebral, spastic
    congenital (cerebral) — *see* Palsy, cerebral, spastic
    familial G11.4
    hereditary G11.4
    quadriplegic G80.0
    syphilitic (spinal) A52.17
  sphincter, bladder — *see* Paralysis, bladder
  spinal (cord) G83.9
    accessory nerve G52.8
    acute — *see* Poliomyelitis, paralytic
    ascending acute G61.0
    atrophic (acute) (*see also* Poliomyelitis, paralytic)
      spastic, syphilitic A52.17
    congenital NEC — *see* Palsy, cerebral
    hereditary G95.89
    infantile — *see* Poliomyelitis, paralytic
    progressive G12.21
    sequelae NEC G83.89
  sternomastoid G52.8
  stomach K31.84
    diabetic — *see* Diabetes, by type, with gastroparesis
    nerve G52.2
      diabetic — *see* Diabetes, by type, with gastroparesis
  stroke — *see* Infarct, brain
  subcapsularis G56.8- ☑
  supranuclear (progressive) G23.1
  sympathetic G90.8
    cervical G90.09
    nervous system — *see* Neuropathy, peripheral, autonomic
  syndrome G83.9
    specified NEC G83.89
  syphilitic spastic spinal (Erb's) A52.17
  thigh G57.9- ☑
  throat J39.2
    diphtheritic A36.0
    muscle J39.2
  thrombotic (current episode) I63.3- ☑
  thumb G56.9- ☑
  tick — *see* Toxicity, venom, arthropod, specified NEC
  Todd's (postepileptic transitory paralysis) G83.84
  toe G57.6- ☑
  tongue K14.8
  transient R29.5
    arm or leg NEC R29.818
    traumatic NEC — *see* Injury, nerve
  trapezius G52.8
  traumatic, transient NEC — *see* Injury, nerve
  trembling — *see* Parkinsonism
  triceps brachii G56.9- ☑
  trigeminal nerve G50.9
  trochlear (nerve) — *see* Strabismus, paralytic, fourth nerve
  ulnar nerve G56.2- ☑
  upper limb — *see* Monoplegia, upper limb
  uremic N18.9 [G99.8]
  uveoparotitic D86.89
  uvula K13.79
    postdiphtheritic A36.0
  vagus nerve G52.2
  vasomotor NEC G90.8
  velum palati K13.79
  vesical — *see* Paralysis, bladder
  vestibular nerve (except Vertigo) H93.3 ☑
  vocal cords J38.00
    bilateral J38.02
    unilateral J38.01
  Volkmann's (complicating trauma) T79.6 ☑
  wasting G12.29
  Weber's G46.3
  wrist G56.9- ☑
Paramedial urethrovesical orifice Q64.79
Paramenia N92.6
Parametritis (*see also* Disease, pelvis, inflammatory) N73.2
  acute N73.0

Parametritis — *continued*
  complicating abortion — *see* Abortion, by type, complicated by, parametritis
Parametrium, parametric — *see* condition
Paramnesia — *see* Amnesia
Paramolar K00.1
Paramyloidosis E85.89
Paramyoclonus multiplex G25.3
Paramyotonia (congenita) G71.19
Parangi — *see* Yaws
Paranoia (querulans) F22
  senile F03 ☑
Paranoid
  dementia (senile) F03 ☑
    praecox — *see* Schizophrenia
  personality F60.0
  psychosis (climacteric) (involutional) (menopausal) F22
    psychogenic (acute) F23
    senile F03 ☑
  reaction (acute) F23
    chronic F22
  schizophrenia F20.0
  state (climacteric) (involutional) (menopausal) (simple) F22
    senile F03 ☑
  tendencies F60.0
  traits F60.0
  trends F60.0
  type, psychopathic personality F60.0
Paraparesis — *see* Paraplegia
Paraphasia R47.02
Paraphilia F65.9
Paraphimosis (congenital) N47.2
  chancroidal A57
Paraphrenia, paraphrenic (late) F22
  schizophrenia F20.0
Paraplegia (lower) G82.20
  ataxic — *see* Degeneration, combined, spinal cord
  complete G82.21
  congenital (cerebral) G80.8
    spastic G80.1
  familial spastic G11.4
  functional (hysterical) F44.4
  hereditary, spastic G11.4
  hysterical F44.4
  incomplete G82.22
  Pott's A18.01
  psychogenic F44.4
  spastic
    Erb's spinal, syphilitic A52.17
    hereditary G11.4
    tropical G04.1
  syphilitic (spastic) A52.17
  tropical spastic G04.1
Parapoxvirus B08.60
  specified NEC B08.69
Paraproteinemia D89.2
  benign (familial) D89.2
  monoclonal D47.2
  secondary to malignant disease D47.2
Parapsoriasis L41.9
  en plaques L41.4
  guttata L41.1
  large plaque L41.4
  retiform, retiformis L41.5
  small plaque L41.3
  specified NEC L41.8
  varioliformis (acuta) L41.0
Parasitic (*see also* condition)
  disease NEC B89
  stomatitis B37.0
  sycosis (beard) (scalp) B35.0
  twin Q89.4
Parasitism B89
  intestinal B82.9
  skin B88.9
  specified — *see* Infestation
Parasitophobia F40.218
Parasomnia G47.50
  due to
    alcohol
      abuse F10.182
      dependence F10.282
      use F10.982
    amphetamines
      abuse F15.182
      dependence F15.282

Parasomnia — *continued*
  due to — *continued*
    amphetamines — *continued*
      use F15.982
    caffeine
      abuse F15.182
      dependence F15.282
      use F15.982
    cocaine
      abuse F14.182
      dependence F14.282
      use F14.982
    drug NEC
      abuse F19.182
      dependence F19.282
      use F19.982
    opioid
      abuse F11.182
      dependence F11.282
      use F11.982
    psychoactive substance NEC
      abuse F19.182
      dependence F19.282
      use F19.982
    sedative, hypnotic, or anxiolytic
      abuse F13.182
      dependence F13.282
      use F13.982
    stimulant NEC
      abuse F15.182
      dependence F15.282
      use F15.982
  in conditions classified elsewhere G47.54
  nonorganic origin F51.8
  organic G47.50
  specified NEC G47.59
Paraspadias Q54.9
Paraspasmus facialis G51.8
Parasuicide (attempt)
  history of (personal) Z91.5
    in family Z81.8
Parathyroid gland — *see* condition
Parathyroid tetany E20.9
Paratrachoma A74.0
Paratyphilitis — *see* Appendicitis
Paratyphoid (fever) — *see* Fever, paratyphoid
Paratyphus — *see* Fever, paratyphoid
Paraurethral duct Q64.79
  nonorganic origin F51.5
Paraurethritis (*see also* Urethritis)
  gonococcal (acute) (chronic) (with abscess) A54.1
Paravaccinia NEC B08.04
Paravaginitis — *see* Vaginitis
Parencephalitis (*see also* Encephalitis)
  sequelae G09
Parent-child conflict — *see* Conflict, parent-child
  estrangement NEC Z62.890
Paresis (*see also* Paralysis)
  accommodation — *see* Paresis, of accommodation
  Bernhardt's G57.1- ☑
  bladder (sphincter) (*see also* Paralysis, bladder)
    tabetic A52.17
  bowel, colon or intestine K56.0
  extrinsic muscle, eye H49.9
  general (progressive) (syphilitic) A52.17
    juvenile A50.45
  heart — *see* Failure, heart
  insane (syphilitic) A52.17
  juvenile (general) A50.45
  of accommodation H52.52- ☑
  peripheral progressive (idiopathic) G60.3
  pseudohypertrophic G71.0
  senile G83.9
  syphilitic (general) A52.17
    congenital A50.45
  vesical NEC N31.2
Paresthesia (*see also* Disturbance, sensation, skin) R20.2
  Bernhardt G57.1- ☑
Paretic — *see* condition
Parinaud's
  conjunctivitis H10.89
  oculoglandular syndrome H10.89
  ophthalmoplegia H49.88- ☑
Parkinsonism (idiopathic) (primary) G20
  with neurogenic orthostatic hypotension (symptomatic) G90.3
  arteriosclerotic G21.4
  dementia G31.83 [F02.80]

Parkinsonism — *continued*
  dementia — *continued*
    with behavioral disturbance G31.83 [FØ2.81]
    due to
      drugs NEC G21.19
        neuroleptic G21.11
    medication-induced NEC G21.19
    neuroleptic induced G21.11
  postencephalitic G21.3
  secondary G21.9
    due to
      arteriosclerosis G21.4
      drugs NEC G21.19
        neuroleptic G21.11
      encephalitis G21.3
      external agents NEC G21.2
      syphilis A52.19
    specified NEC G21.8
  syphilitic A52.19
  treatment-induced NEC G21.19
  vascular G21.4
Parkinson's disease, syndrome or tremor — *see* Parkinsonism
Parodontitis — *see* Periodontitis
Parodontosis KØ5.4
Paronychia (*see also* Cellulitis, digit)
  with lymphangitis — *see* Lymphangitis, acute, digit
  candidal (chronic) B37.2
  tuberculous (primary) A18.4
Parorexia (psychogenic) F5Ø.89
Parosmia R43.1
  psychogenic F45.8
Parotid gland — *see* condition
Parotitis, parotiditis (allergic)(nonspecific toxic) (purulent) (septic) (suppurative) (*see also* Sialoadenitis)
  epidemic — *see* Mumps
  infectious — *see* Mumps
  postoperative K91.89
  surgical K91.89
Parrot fever A7Ø
Parrot's disease (early congenital syphilitic pseudoparalysis) A5Ø.Ø2
Parry-Romberg syndrome G51.8
Parry's disease or syndrome EØ5.ØØ
  with thyroid storm EØ5.Ø1
Pars planitis — *see* Cyclitis
Parsonage (-Aldren)-**Turner syndrome** G54.5
Parson's disease (exophthalmic goiter) EØ5.ØØ
  with thyroid storm EØ5.Ø1
Particolored infant Q82.8
Parturition — *see* Delivery
Parulis KØ4.7
  with sinus KØ4.6
Parvovirus, as cause of disease classified elsewhere B97.6
Pasini and Pierini's atrophoderma L9Ø.3
Passage
  false, urethra N36.5
  meconium (newborn) during delivery PØ3.82
  of sounds or bougies — *see* Attention to, artificial, opening
Passive — *see* condition
  smoking Z77.22
Pasteurella septica A28.Ø
Pasteurellosis — *see* Infection, Pasteurella
PAT (paroxysmal atrial tachycardia) I47.1
Patau's syndrome — *see* Trisomy, 13
Patches
  mucous (syphilitic) A51.39
    congenital A5Ø.Ø7
  smokers' (mouth) K13.24
Patellar — *see* condition
Patent (*see also* Imperfect, closure)
  canal of Nuck Q52.4
  cervix N88.3
  ductus arteriosus or Botallo's Q25.Ø
  foramen
    botalli Q21.1
    ovale Q21.1
  interauricular septum Q21.1
  interventricular septum Q21.Ø
  omphalomesenteric duct Q43.Ø
  os (uteri) — *see* Patent, cervix
  ostium secundum Q21.1
  urachus Q64.4
  vitelline duct Q43.Ø
Paterson (-Brown)(-Kelly) **syndrome or web** D5Ø.1

Pathologic, pathological (*see also* condition)
  asphyxia RØ9.Ø1
  fire-setting F63.1
  gambling F63.Ø
  ovum OØ2.Ø
  resorption, tooth KØ3.3
  stealing F63.2
Pathology (of) — *see* Disease
  periradicular, associated with previous endodontic treatment NEC M27.59
Pattern, sleep-wake, irregular G47.23
Patulous (*see also* Imperfect, closure (congenital))
  alimentary tract Q45.8
    lower Q43.8
    upper Q4Ø.8
  eustachian tube H69.Ø- ☑
Pause, sinoatrial I49.5
Paxton's disease B36.2
Pearl(s)
  enamel KØØ.2
  Epstein's KØ9.8
Pearl-worker's disease — *see* Osteomyelitis, specified type NEC
Pectenosis K62.4
Pectoral — *see* condition
Pectus
  carinatum (congenital) Q67.7
    acquired M95.4
    rachitic sequelae (late effect) E64.3
  excavatum (congenital) Q67.6
    acquired M95.4
    rachitic sequelae (late effect) E64.3
  recurvatum (congenital) Q67.6
Pedatrophia E41
Pederosis F65.4
Pediculosis (infestation) B85.2
  capitis (head-louse) (any site) B85.Ø
  corporis (body-louse) (any site) B85.1
  eyelid B85.Ø
  mixed (classifiable to more than one of the titles B85.Ø-B85.3) B85.4
  pubis (pubic louse) (any site) B85.3
  vestimenti B85.1
  vulvae B85.3
Pediculus (infestation) — *see* Pediculosis
Pedophilia F65.4
Peg-shaped teeth KØØ.2
Pelade — *see* Alopecia, areata
Pelger-Huët anomaly or syndrome D72.Ø
Peliosis (rheumatica) D69.Ø
  hepatis K76.4
    with toxic liver disease K71.8
Pelizaeus-Merzbacher disease E75.29
Pellagra (alcoholic) (with polyneuropathy) E52
Pellagra-cerebellar-ataxia-renal aminoaciduria syndrome E72.Ø2
Pellegrini (-Stieda) **disease or syndrome** — *see* Bursitis, tibial collateral
Pellizzi's syndrome E34.8
Pel's crisis A52.11
Pelvic (*see also* condition)
  examination (periodic) (routine) ZØ1.419
    with abnormal findings ZØ1.411
  kidney, congenital Q63.2
Pelviolithiasis — *see* Calculus, kidney
Pelviperitonitis (*see also* Peritonitis, pelvic)
  gonococcal A54.24
  puerperal O85
Pelvis — *see* condition or type
Pemphigoid L12.9
  benign, mucous membrane L12.1
  bullous L12.Ø
  cicatricial L12.1
  juvenile L12.2
  ocular L12.1
  specified NEC L12.8
Pemphigus L1Ø.9
  benign familial (chronic) Q82.8
  Brazilian L1Ø.3
  circinatus L13.Ø
  conjunctiva L12.1
  drug-induced L1Ø.5
  erythematosus L1Ø.4
  foliaceous L1Ø.2
  gangrenous — *see* Gangrene
  neonatorum LØ1.Ø3
  ocular L12.1
  paraneoplastic L1Ø.81

Pemphigus — *continued*
  specified NEC L1Ø.89
  syphilitic (congenital) A5Ø.Ø6
  vegetans L1Ø.1
  vulgaris L1Ø.Ø
  wildfire L1Ø.3
Pendred's syndrome EØ7.1
Pendulous
  abdomen, in pregnancy — *see* Pregnancy, complicated by, abnormal, pelvic organs or tissues NEC
  breast N64.89
Penetrating wound (*see also* Puncture)
  with internal injury — *see* Injury, by site
  eyeball — *see* Puncture, eyeball
  orbit (with or without foreign body) — *see* Puncture, orbit
  uterus by instrument with or following ectopic or molar pregnancy OØ8.6
Penicillosis B48.4
Penis — *see* condition
Penitis N48.29
Pentalogy of Fallot Q21.8
Pentasomy X syndrome Q97.1
Pentosuria (essential) E74.8
Percreta placenta - O43.23 ☑
Peregrinating patient — *see* Disorder, factitious
Perforation, perforated (nontraumatic) (of)
  accidental during procedure (blood vessel) (nerve) (organ) — *see* Complication, accidental puncture or laceration
  antrum — *see* Sinusitis, maxillary
  appendix K35.2
    with localized peritonitis K35.3
  atrial septum, multiple Q21.1
  attic, ear — *see* Perforation, tympanum, attic
  bile duct (common) (hepatic) K83.2
    cystic K82.2
  bladder (urinary)
    with or following ectopic or molar pregnancy OØ8.6
    obstetrical trauma O71.5
    traumatic S37.29 ☑
      at delivery O71.5
  bowel K63.1
    with or following ectopic or molar pregnancy OØ8.6
    newborn P78.Ø
    obstetrical trauma O71.5
    traumatic — *see* Laceration, intestine
  broad ligament N83.8
    with or following ectopic or molar pregnancy OØ8.6
    obstetrical trauma O71.6
  by
    device, implant or graft (*see also* Complications, by site and type, mechanical) T85.628 ☑
      arterial graft NEC — *see* Complication, cardiovascular device, mechanical, vascular
      breast (implant) T85.49 ☑
      catheter NEC T85.698 ☑
        cystostomy T83.Ø9Ø ☑
        dialysis (renal) T82.49 ☑
          intraperitoneal T85.691 ☑
        infusion NEC T82.594 ☑
          spinal (epidural) (subdural) T85.69Ø ☑
        urinary (*see also* Complications, catheter, urinary T83.Ø98 ☑
      electronic (electrode) (pulse generator) (stimulator)
        bone T84.39Ø ☑
        cardiac T82.199 ☑
          electrode T82.19Ø ☑
          pulse generator T82.191 ☑
          specified type NEC T82.198 ☑
        nervous system — *see* Complication, prosthetic device, mechanical, electronic nervous system stimulator
        urinary — *see* Complication, genitourinary, device, urinary, mechanical
      fixation, internal (orthopedic) NEC — *see* Complication, fixation device, mechanical
      gastrointestinal — *see* Complications, prosthetic device, mechanical, gastrointestinal device
      genital NEC T83.498 ☑
        intrauterine contraceptive device T83.39 ☑
        penile prosthesis T83.49Ø ☑
      heart NEC — *see* Complication, cardiovascular device, mechanical

---

Perforation, perforated — *continued*
  by — *continued*
    device, implant or graft (*see also* Complications, by site and type, mechanical) — *continued*
      joint prosthesis — *see* Complications, joint prosthesis, mechanical, specified NEC, by site
      ocular NEC — *see* Complications, prosthetic device, mechanical, ocular device
      orthopedic NEC — *see* Complication, orthopedic, device, mechanical
      specified NEC T85.628 ☑
      urinary NEC (*see also* Complication, genitourinary, device, urinary, mechanical)
        graft T83.29 ☑
      vascular NEC — *see* Complication, cardiovascular device, mechanical
      ventricular intracranial shunt T85.09 ☑
    foreign body left accidentally in operative wound T81.539 ☑
    instrument (any) during a procedure, accidental — *see* Puncture, accidental complicating surgery
  cecum K35.2
    with localized peritonitis K35.3
  cervix (uteri) N88.8
    with or following ectopic or molar pregnancy O08.6
    obstetrical trauma O71.3
  colon K63.1
    newborn P78.0
    obstetrical trauma O71.5
    traumatic — *see* Laceration, intestine, large
  common duct (bile) K83.2
  cornea (due to ulceration) — *see* Ulcer, cornea, perforated
  cystic duct K82.2
  diverticulum (intestine) K57.80
    with bleeding K57.81
    large intestine K57.20
      with
        bleeding K57.21
        small intestine K57.40
          with bleeding K57.41
    small intestine K57.00
      with
        bleeding K57.01
        large intestine K57.40
          with bleeding K57.41
  ear drum — *see* Perforation, tympanum
  esophagus K22.3
  ethmoidal sinus — *see* Sinusitis, ethmoidal
  frontal sinus — *see* Sinusitis, frontal
  gallbladder K82.2
  heart valve — *see* Endocarditis
  ileum K63.1
    newborn P78.0
    obstetrical trauma O71.5
    traumatic — *see* Laceration, intestine, small
  instrumental, surgical (accidental) (blood vessel) (nerve) (organ) — *see* Puncture, accidental complicating surgery
  intestine NEC K63.1
    with ectopic or molar pregnancy O08.6
    newborn P78.0
    obstetrical trauma O71.5
    traumatic — *see* Laceration, intestine
    ulcerative NEC K63.1
      newborn P78.0
  jejunum, jejunal K63.1
    obstetrical trauma O71.5
    traumatic — *see* Laceration, intestine, small
    ulcer — *see* Ulcer, gastrojejunal, with perforation
  joint prosthesis — *see* Complications, joint prosthesis, mechanical, specified NEC, by site
  mastoid (antrum) (cell) — *see* Disorder, mastoid, specified NEC
  maxillary sinus — *see* Sinusitis, maxillary
  membrana tympani — *see* Perforation, tympanum
  nasal
    septum J34.89
      congenital Q30.3
      syphilitic A52.73
    sinus J34.89
      congenital Q30.8
      due to sinusitis — *see* Sinusitis
  palate (*see also* Cleft, palate) Q35.9
    syphilitic A52.79
  palatine vault (*see also* Cleft, palate, hard) Q35.1

Perforation, perforated — *continued*
  palatine vault (*see also* Cleft, palate, hard) — *continued*
    syphilitic A52.79
    congenital A50.59
  pars flaccida (ear drum) — *see* Perforation, tympanum, attic
  pelvic
    floor S31.030 ☑
      with
        ectopic or molar pregnancy O08.6
        penetration into retroperitoneal space S31.031 ☑
        retained foreign body S31.040 ☑
          with penetration into retroperitoneal space S31.041 ☑
      following ectopic or molar pregnancy O08.6
      obstetrical trauma O70.1
    organ S37.99 ☑
      adrenal gland S37.818 ☑
      bladder — *see* Perforation, bladder
      fallopian tube S37.599 ☑
        bilateral S37.592 ☑
        unilateral S37.591 ☑
      kidney S37.09- ☑
      obstetrical trauma O71.5
      ovary S37.499 ☑
        bilateral S37.492 ☑
        unilateral S37.491 ☑
      prostate S37.828 ☑
      specified organ NEC S37.898 ☑
      ureter — *see* Perforation, ureter
      urethra — *see* Perforation, urethra
      uterus — *see* Perforation, uterus
  perineum — *see* Laceration, perineum
  pharynx J39.2
  rectum K63.1
    newborn P78.0
    obstetrical trauma O71.5
    traumatic S36.63 ☑
  root canal space due to endodontic treatment M27.51
  sigmoid K63.1
    newborn P78.0
    obstetrical trauma O71.5
    traumatic S36.533 ☑
  sinus (accessory) (chronic) (nasal) J34.89
  sphenoidal sinus — *see* Sinusitis, sphenoidal
  surgical (accidental) (by instrument) (blood vessel) (nerve) (organ) — *see* Puncture, accidental complicating surgery
  traumatic
    external — *see* Puncture
    eye — *see* Puncture, eyeball
    internal organ — *see* Injury, by site
  tympanum, tympanic (membrane) (persistent post-traumatic) (postinflammatory) H72.9- ☑
    attic H72.1- ☑
      multiple — *see* Perforation, tympanum, multiple
      total — *see* Perforation, tympanum, total
    central H72.0- ☑
      multiple — *see* Perforation, tympanum, multiple
      total — *see* Perforation, tympanum, total
    marginal NEC — *see* subcategory H72.2 ☑
    multiple H72.81- ☑
    pars flaccida — *see* Perforation, tympanum, attic
    total H72.82- ☑
    traumatic, current episode S09.2- ☑
  typhoid, gastrointestinal — *see* Typhoid
  ulcer — *see* Ulcer, by site, with perforation
  ureter N28.89
    traumatic S37.19 ☑
  urethra N36.8
    with ectopic or molar pregnancy O08.6
    following ectopic or molar pregnancy O08.6
    obstetrical trauma O71.5
    traumatic S37.39 ☑
      at delivery O71.5
  uterus
    with ectopic or molar pregnancy O08.6
    by intrauterine contraceptive device T83.39 ☑
    following ectopic or molar pregnancy O08.6
    obstetrical trauma O71.1
    traumatic S37.69 ☑
      obstetric O71.1
  uvula K13.79

Perforation, perforated — *continued*
  uvula — *continued*
    syphilitic A52.79
  vagina O71.4
    obstetrical trauma O71.4
    other trauma — *see* Puncture, vagina
Periadenitis mucosa necrotica recurrens K12.0
Periappendicitis (acute) — *see* Appendicitis
Periarteritis nodosa (disseminated) (infectious) (necrotizing) M30.0
Periarthritis (joint) (*see also* Enthesopathy)
  Duplay's M75.0- ☑
  gonococcal A54.42
  humeroscapularis — *see* Capsulitis, adhesive
  scapulohumeral — *see* Capsulitis, adhesive
  shoulder — *see* Capsulitis, adhesive
  wrist M77.2- ☑
Periarthrosis (angioneural) — *see* Enthesopathy
Pericapsulitis, adhesive (shoulder) — *see* Capsulitis, adhesive
Pericarditis (with decompensation) (with effusion) I31.9
  with rheumatic fever (conditions in I00)
    active — *see* Pericarditis, rheumatic
    inactive or quiescent I09.2
  acute (hemorrhagic) (nonrheumatic) (Sicca) I30.9
    with chorea (acute) (rheumatic) (Sydenham's) I02.0
    benign I30.8
    nonspecific I30.0
    rheumatic I01.0
      with chorea (acute) (Sydenham's) I02.0
  adhesive or adherent (chronic) (external) (internal) I31.0
    acute — *see* Pericarditis, acute
    rheumatic I09.2
  bacterial (acute) (subacute) (with serous or seropurulent effusion) I30.1
  calcareous I31.1
  cholesterol (chronic) I31.8
    acute I30.9
  chronic (nonrheumatic) I31.9
    rheumatic I09.2
  constrictive (chronic) I31.1
  coxsackie B33.23
  fibrinocaseous (tuberculous) A18.84
  fibrinopurulent I30.1
  fibrinous I30.8
  fibrous I31.0
  gonococcal A54.83
  idiopathic I30.0
  in systemic lupus erythematosus M32.12
  infective I30.1
  meningococcal A39.53
  neoplastic (chronic) I31.8
    acute I30.9
  obliterans, obliterating I31.0
  plastic I31.0
  pneumococcal I30.1
  postinfarction I24.1
  purulent I30.1
  rheumatic (active) (acute) (with effusion) (with pneumonia) I01.0
    with chorea (acute) (rheumatic) (Sydenham's) I02.0
    chronic or inactive (with chorea) I09.2
  rheumatoid — *see* Rheumatoid, carditis
  septic I30.1
  serofibrinous I30.8
  staphylococcal I30.1
  streptococcal I30.1
  suppurative I30.1
  syphilitic A52.06
  tuberculous A18.84
  uremic N18.9 [I32]
  viral I30.1
Pericardium, pericardial — *see* condition
Pericellulitis — *see* Cellulitis
Pericementitis (chronic) (suppurative) (*see also* Periodontitis)
  acute K05.20
    generalized — *see* Peridontitis, aggressive, generalized
    localized — *see* Peridontitis, aggressive, localized
Perichondritis
  auricle — *see* Perichondritis, ear
  bronchus J98.09
  ear (external) H61.00- ☑
    acute H61.01- ☑
    chronic H61.02- ☑
  external auditory canal — *see* Perichondritis, ear

Perichondritis — *continued*
  larynx J38.7
    syphilitic A52.73
    typhoid A01.09
  nose J34.89
  pinna — *see* Perichondritis, ear
  trachea J39.8
Periclasia K05.4
Pericoronitis — *see* Periodontitis
Pericystitis N30.90
  with hematuria N30.91
Peridiverticulitis (intestine) K57.92
  cecum — *see* Diverticulitis, intestine, large
  colon — *see* Diverticulitis, intestine, large
  duodenum — *see* Diverticulitis, intestine, small
  intestine — *see* Diverticulitis, intestine
  jejunum — *see* Diverticulitis, intestine, small
  rectosigmoid — *see* Diverticulitis, intestine, large
  rectum — *see* Diverticulitis, intestine, large
  sigmoid — *see* Diverticulitis, intestine, large
Periendocarditis — *see* Endocarditis
Periepididymitis N45.1
Perifolliculitis L01.02
  abscedens, caput, scalp L66.3
  capitis, abscedens (et suffodiens) L66.3
  superficial pustular L01.02
Perihepatitis K65.8
Perilabyrinthitis (acute) — *see* subcategory H83.0 ☑
Perimeningitis — *see* Meningitis
Perimetritis — *see* Endometritis
Perimetrosalpingitis — *see* Salpingo-oophoritis
Perineocele N81.81
Perinephric, perinephritic — *see* condition
Perinephritis (*see also* Infection, kidney)
  purulent — *see* Abscess, kidney
Perineum, perineal — *see* condition
Perineuritis NEC — *see* Neuralgia
Periodic — *see* condition
Periodontitis (chronic) (complex) (compound) (local)
  (simplex) K05.30
  acute K05.20
    generalized K05.229
      moderate K05.222
      severe K05.223
      slight K05.221
    localized K05.219
      moderate K05.212
      severe K05.213
      slight K05.211
  apical K04.5
    acute (pulpal origin) K04.4
  generalized K05.329
    moderate K05.322
    severe K05.323
    slight K05.321
  localized K05.319
    moderate K05.312
    severe K05.313
    slight K05.311
Periodontoclasia K05.4
Periodontosis (juvenile) K05.4
Periods (*see also* Menstruation)
  heavy N92.0
  irregular N92.6
  shortened intervals (irregular) N92.1
Perionychia (*see also* Cellulitis, digit)
  with lymphangitis — *see* Lymphangitis, acute, digit
Perioophoritis — *see* Salpingo-oophoritis
Periorchitis N45.2
Periosteum, periosteal — *see* condition
Periostitis (albuminosa) (circumscribed) (diffuse) (infective) (monomelic) (*see also* Osteomyelitis)
  alveolar M27.3
  alveolodental M27.3
  dental M27.3
  gonorrheal A54.43
  jaw (lower) (upper) M27.2
  orbit H05.03- ☑
  syphilitic A52.77
    congenital (early) A50.02 [M90.80]
    secondary A51.46
  tuberculous — *see* Tuberculosis, bone
  yaws (hypertrophic) (early) (late) A66.6 [M90.80]
Periostosis (hyperplastic) (*see also* Disorder, bone, specified type NEC)
  with osteomyelitis — *see* Osteomyelitis, specified type NEC

Peripartum
  cardiomyopathy O90.3
Periphlebitis — *see* Phlebitis
Periproctitis K62.89
Periprostatitis — *see* Prostatitis
Perirectal — *see* condition
Perirenal — *see* condition
Perisalpingitis — *see* Salpingo-oophoritis
Perisplenitis (infectional) D73.89
Peristalsis, visible or reversed R19.2
Peritendinitis — *see* Enthesopathy
Peritoneum, peritoneal — *see* condition
Peritonitis (adhesive) (bacterial) (fibrinous) (hemorrhagic) (idiopathic) (localized) (perforative) (primary) (with adhesions) (with effusion) K65.9
  with or following
    abscess K65.1
    appendicitis K35.3
      with perforation or rupture K35.2
      generalized K35.2
      localized K35.3
    diverticular disease (intestine) K57.80
      with bleeding K57.81
      ectopic or molar pregnancy O08.0
      large intestine K57.20
        with
          bleeding K57.21
          small intestine K57.40
            with bleeding K57.41
      small intestine K57.00
        with
          bleeding K57.01
          large intestine K57.40
            with bleeding K57.41
  acute (generalized) K65.0
  aseptic T81.61 ☑
  bile, biliary K65.3
  chemical T81.61 ☑
  chlamydial A74.81
  chronic proliferative K65.8
  complicating abortion — *see* Abortion, by type, complicated by, pelvic peritonitis
  congenital P78.1
  diaphragmatic K65.0
  diffuse K65.0
  diphtheritic A36.89
  disseminated K65.0
  due to
    bile K65.3
    foreign
      body or object accidentally left during a procedure (instrument) (sponge) (swab) T81.599 ☑
      substance accidentally left during a procedure (chemical) (powder) (talc) T81.61 ☑
    talc T81.61 ☑
    urine K65.8
  eosinophilic K65.8
    acute K65.0
  fibrocaseous (tuberculous) A18.31
  fibropurulent K65.0
  following ectopic or molar pregnancy O08.0
  general (ized) K65.0
  gonococcal A54.85
  meconium (newborn) P78.0
  neonatal P78.1
    meconium P78.0
  pancreatic K65.0
  paroxysmal, familial E85.0
    benign E85.0
  pelvic
    female N73.5
      acute N73.3
      chronic N73.4
        with adhesions N73.6
    male K65.0
  periodic, familial E85.0
  proliferative, chronic K65.8
  puerperal, postpartum, childbirth O85
  purulent K65.0
  septic K65.0
  specified NEC K65.8
  spontaneous bacterial K65.2
  subdiaphragmatic K65.0
  subphrenic K65.0
  suppurative K65.0
  syphilitic A52.74
    congenital (early) A50.08 [K67]

Peritonitis — *continued*
  talc T81.61 ☑
  tuberculous A18.31
  urine K65.8
Peritonsillar — *see* condition
Peritonsillitis J36
Perityphlitis K37
Periureteritis N28.89
Periurethral — *see* condition
Periurethritis (gangrenous) — *see* Urethritis
Periuterine — *see* condition
Perivaginitis — *see* Vaginitis
Perivasculitis, retinal H35.06- ☑
Perivasitis (chronic) N49.1
Perivesiculitis (seminal) — *see* Vesiculitis
Perlèche NEC K13.0
  due to
    candidiasis B37.83
    moniliasis B37.83
    riboflavin deficiency E53.0
    vitamin B2 (riboflavin) deficiency E53.0
Pernicious — *see* condition
Pernio, perniosis T69.1 ☑
Perpetrator (of abuse) — *see* Index to External Causes of Injury, Perpetrator
Persecution
  delusion F22
  social Z60.5
Perseveration (tonic) R48.8
Persistence, persistent (congenital)
  anal membrane Q42.3
    with fistula Q42.2
  arteria stapedia Q16.3
  atrioventricular canal Q21.2
  branchial cleft NOS Q18.2
    cyst Q18.0
    fistula Q18.0
    sinus Q18.0
  bulbus cordis in left ventricle Q21.8
  canal of Cloquet Q14.0
  capsule (opaque) Q12.8
  cilioretinal artery or vein Q14.8
  cloaca Q43.7
  communication — *see* Fistula, congenital
  convolutions
    aortic arch Q25.46
    fallopian tube Q50.6
    oviduct Q50.6
    uterine tube Q50.6
  double aortic arch Q25.45
  ductus arteriosus (Botalli) Q25.0
  fetal
    circulation P29.38
    form of cervix (uteri) Q51.828
    hemoglobin, hereditary (HPFH) D56.4
  foramen
    Botalli Q21.1
    ovale Q21.1
  Gartner's duct Q52.4
  hemoglobin, fetal (hereditary) (HPFH) D56.4
  hyaloid
    artery (generally incomplete) Q14.0
    system Q14.8
  hymen, in pregnancy or childbirth — *see* Pregnancy, complicated by, abnormal, vulva
  lanugo Q84.2
  left
    posterior cardinal vein Q26.8
    root with right arch of aorta Q25.49
    superior vena cava Q26.1
  Meckel's diverticulum Q43.0
    malignant — *see* Table of Neoplasms, small intestine, malignant
  mucosal disease (middle ear) — *see* Otitis, media, suppurative, chronic, tubotympanic
  nail(s), anomalous Q84.6
  omphalomesenteric duct Q43.0
  organ or site not listed — *see* Anomaly, by site
  ostium
    atrioventriculare commune Q21.2
    primum Q21.2
    secundum Q21.1
  ovarian rests in fallopian tube Q50.6
  pancreatic tissue in intestinal tract Q43.8
  primary (deciduous)
    teeth K00.6
    vitreous hyperplasia Q14.0
  pupillary membrane Q13.89

Persistence, persistent — *continued*
rhesus (Rh) titer — *see* Complication(s), transfusion, incompatibility reaction, Rh (factor)
right aortic arch Q25.47
sinus
  urogenitalis
    female Q52.8
    male Q55.8
  venosus with imperfect incorporation in right auricle Q26.8
thymus (gland) (hyperplasia) E32.0
thyroglossal duct Q89.2
thyrolingual duct Q89.2
truncus arteriosus or communis Q20.0
tunica vasculosa lentis Q12.2
umbilical sinus Q64.4
urachus Q64.4
vitelline duct Q43.0
Person (with)
admitted for clinical research, as a control subject (normal comparison) (participant) Z00.6
awaiting admission to adequate facility elsewhere Z75.1
concern (normal) about sick person in family Z63.6
consulting on behalf of another Z71.0
feigning illness Z76.5
living (in)
  without
    adequate housing (heating) (space) Z59.1
    housing (permanent) (temporary) Z59.0
    person able to render necessary care Z74.2
    shelter Z59.0
  alone Z60.2
  boarding school Z59.3
  residential institution Z59.3
on waiting list Z75.1
sick or handicapped in family Z63.6
Personality (disorder) F60.9
accentuation of traits (type A pattern) Z73.1
affective F34.0
aggressive F60.3
amoral F60.2
anacastic, anankastic F60.5
antisocial F60.2
anxious F60.6
asocial F60.2
asthenic F60.7
avoidant F60.6
borderline F60.3
change due to organic condition (enduring) F07.0
compulsive F60.5
cycloid F34.0
cyclothymic F34.0
dependent F60.7
depressive F34.1
dissocial F60.2
dual F44.81
eccentric F60.89
emotionally unstable F60.3
expansive paranoid F60.0
explosive F60.3
fanatic F60.0
haltlose type F60.89
histrionic F60.4
hyperthymic F34.0
hypothymic F34.1
hysterical F60.4
immature F60.89
inadequate F60.7
labile (emotional) F60.3
mixed (nonspecific) F60.89
morally defective F60.2
multiple F44.81
narcissistic F60.81
obsessional F60.5
obsessive (-compulsive) F60.5
organic F07.0
overconscientious F60.5
paranoid F60.0
passive (-dependent) F60.7
passive-aggressive F60.89
pathologic F60.9
pattern defect or disturbance F60.9
pseudopsychopathic (organic) F07.0
pseudoretarded (organic) F07.0
psychoinfantile F60.4
psychoneurotic NEC F60.89
psychopathic F60.2
querulant F60.0

Personality — *continued*
sadistic F60.89
schizoid F60.1
self-defeating F60.7
sensitive paranoid F60.0
sociopathic (amoral) (antisocial) (asocial) (dissocial) F60.2
specified NEC F60.89
type A Z73.1
unstable (emotional) F60.3
Perthes' disease — *see* Legg-Calvé-Perthes disease
Pertussis (*see also* Whooping cough) A37.90
Perversion, perverted
appetite F50.89
  psychogenic F50.89
function
  pituitary gland E23.2
    posterior lobe E22.2
sense of smell and taste R43.8
  psychogenic F45.8
sexual — *see* Deviation, sexual
Pervious, congenital (*see also* Imperfect, closure)
ductus arteriosus Q25.0
Pes (congenital) (*see also* Talipes)
acquired (*see also* Deformity, limb, foot, specified NEC)
  planus — *see* Deformity, limb, flat foot
adductus Q66.89
cavus Q66.7
deformity NEC, acquired — *see* Deformity, limb, foot, specified NEC
planus (acquired) (any degree) (*see also* Deformity, limb, flat foot)
  rachitic sequelae (late effect) E64.3
valgus Q66.6
Pest, pestis — *see* Plague
Petechia, petechiae R23.3
newborn P54.5
Petechial typhus A75.9
Peter's anomaly Q13.4
Petit mal seizure — *see* Epilepsy, generalized, specified NEC
Petit's hernia — *see* Hernia, abdomen, specified site NEC
Petrellidosis B48.2
Petrositis H70.20- ☑
acute H70.21- ☑
chronic H70.22- ☑
Peutz-Jeghers disease or syndrome Q85.8
Peyronie's disease N48.6
PFAPA (periodic fever, aphthous stomatitis, pharyngitis, and adenopathy syndrome) M04.8
Pfeiffer's disease — *see* Mononucleosis, infectious
Phagedena (dry) (moist) (sloughing) (*see also* Gangrene)
geometric L88
penis N48.29
tropical — *see* Ulcer, skin
vulva N76.6
Phagedenic — *see* condition
Phakoma H35.89
Phakomatosis (*see also* specific eponymous syndromes) Q85.9
Bourneville's Q85.1
specified NEC Q85.8
Phantom limb syndrome (without pain) G54.7
with pain G54.6
Pharyngeal pouch syndrome D82.1
Pharyngitis (acute) (catarrhal)(gangrenous) (infective) (malignant) (membranous) (phlegmonous) (pseudomembranous) (simple) (subacute) (suppurative) (ulcerative) (viral) J02.9
with influenza, flu, or grippe — *see* Influenza, with, pharyngitis
aphthous B08.5
atrophic J31.2
chlamydial A56.4
chronic (atrophic) (granular) (hypertrophic) J31.2
coxsackievirus B08.5
diphtheritic A36.0
enteroviral vesicular B08.5
follicular (chronic) J31.2
fusospirochetal A69.1
gonococcal A54.5
granular (chronic) J31.2
herpesviral B00.2
hypertrophic J31.2
infectional, chronic J31.2
influenzal — *see* Influenza, with, respiratory manifestations NEC

Pharyngitis — *continued*
lymphonodular, acute (enteroviral) B08.8
pneumococcal J02.8
purulent J02.9
putrid J02.9
septic J02.0
sicca J31.2
specified organism NEC J02.8
staphylococcal J02.8
streptococcal J02.0
syphilitic, congenital (early) A50.03
tuberculous A15.8
vesicular, enteroviral B08.5
viral NEC J02.8
Pharyngoconjunctivitis, viral B30.2
Pharyngolaryngitis (acute) J06.0
chronic J37.0
Pharyngoplegia J39.2
Pharyngotonsillitis, herpesviral B00.2
Pharyngotracheitis, chronic J42
Pharynx, pharyngeal — *see* condition
Phencyclidine-induced
anxiety disorder F16.980
bipolar and related disorder F16.94
depressive disorder F16.94
psychotic disorder F16.959
Phenomenon
Arthus' — *see* Arthus' phenomenon
jaw-winking Q07.8
lupus erythematosus (LE) cell M32.9
Raynaud's (secondary) I73.00
  with gangrene I73.01
vasomotor R55
vasospastic I73.9
vasovagal R55
Wenckebach's I44.1
Phenylketonuria E70.1
classical E70.0
maternal E70.1
Pheochromoblastoma
specified site — *see* Neoplasm, malignant, by site
unspecified site C74.10
Pheochromocytoma
malignant
  specified site — *see* Neoplasm, malignant, by site
  unspecified site C74.10
specified site — *see* Neoplasm, benign, by site
unspecified site D35.00
Pheohyphomycosis — *see* Chromomycosis
Pheomycosis — *see* Chromomycosis
Phimosis (congenital) (due to infection) N47.1
chancroidal A57
Phlebectasia (*see also* Varix)
congenital Q27.4
Phlebitis (infective) (pyemic) (septic) (suppurative) I80.9
antepartum — *see* Thrombophlebitis, antepartum
blue — *see* Phlebitis, leg, deep
breast, superficial I80.8
cavernous (venous) sinus — *see* Phlebitis, intracranial (venous) sinus
cerebral (venous) sinus — *see* Phlebitis, intracranial (venous) sinus
chest wall, superficial I80.8
cranial (venous) sinus — *see* Phlebitis, intracranial (venous) sinus
tuberculous A15.8
deep (vessels) — *see* Phlebitis, leg, deep
due to implanted device — *see* Complications, by site and type, specified NEC
during or resulting from a procedure T81.72 ☑
femoral vein (superficial) I80.1- ☑
femoropopliteal vein I80.0- ☑
gestational — *see* Phlebopathy, gestational
hepatic veins I80.8
iliofemoral — *see* Phlebitis, femoral vein
intracranial (venous) sinus (any) G08
  nonpyogenic I67.6
intraspinal venous sinuses and veins G08
  nonpyogenic G95.19
lateral (venous) sinus — *see* Phlebitis, intracranial (venous) sinus
leg I80.3
  antepartum — *see* Thrombophlebitis, antepartum
  deep (vessels) NEC I80.20- ☑
    iliac I80.21- ☑
    popliteal vein I80.22- ☑
    specified vessel NEC I80.29- ☑
    tibial vein I80.23- ☑

Phlebitis — *continued*
  leg — *continued*
    femoral vein (superficial) I80.1- ☑
    superficial (vessels) I80.0- ☑
  longitudinal sinus — *see* Phlebitis, intracranial (venous) sinus
  lower limb — *see* Phlebitis, leg
  migrans, migrating (superficial) I82.1
  pelvic
    with ectopic or molar pregnancy O08.0
    following ectopic or molar pregnancy O08.0
    puerperal, postpartum O87.1
  popliteal vein — *see* Phlebitis, leg, deep, popliteal
  portal (vein) K75.1
  postoperative T81.72 ☑
  pregnancy — *see* Thrombophlebitis, antepartum
  puerperal, postpartum, childbirth O87.0
    deep O87.1
    pelvic O87.1
    superficial O87.0
  retina — *see* Vasculitis, retina
  saphenous (accessory) (great) (long) (small) — *see* Phlebitis, leg, superficial
  sinus (meninges) — *see* Phlebitis, intracranial (venous) sinus
  specified site NEC I80.8
  syphilitic A52.09
  tibial vein — *see* Phlebitis, leg, deep, tibial
  ulcerative I80.9
    leg — *see* Phlebitis, leg
  umbilicus I80.8
  uterus (septic) — *see* Endometritis
  varicose (leg) (lower limb) — *see* Varix, leg, with, inflammation
Phlebofibrosis I87.8
Phleboliths I87.8
Phlebopathy,
  gestational O22.9- ☑
  puerperal O87.9
Phlebosclerosis I87.8
Phlebothrombosis (*see also* Thrombosis)
  antepartum — *see* Thrombophlebitis, antepartum
  pregnancy — *see* Thrombophlebitis, antepartum
  puerperal — *see* Thrombophlebitis, puerperal
Phlebotomus fever A93.1
Phlegmasia
  alba dolens O87.1
    nonpuerperal — *see* Phlebitis, femoral vein
  cerulea dolens — *see* Phlebitis, leg, deep
Phlegmon — *see* Abscess
Phlegmonous — *see* condition
Phlyctenulosis (allergic) (keratoconjunctivitis) (nontuberculous) (*see also* Keratoconjunctivitis)
  cornea — *see* Keratoconjunctivitis
  tuberculous A18.52
Phobia, phobic F40.9
  animal F40.218
    spiders F40.210
  examination F40.298
  reaction F40.9
  simple F40.298
  social F40.10
    generalized F40.11
  specific (isolated) F40.298
    animal F40.218
      spiders F40.210
    blood F40.230
    injection F40.231
    injury F40.233
    men F40.290
    natural environment F40.228
      thunderstorms F40.220
    situational F40.248
      bridges F40.242
      closed in spaces F40.240
      flying F40.243
      heights F40.241
    specified focus NEC F40.298
    transfusion F40.231
    women F40.291
  specified NEC F40.8
    medical care NEC F40.232
  state F40.9
Phocas' disease — *see* Mastopathy, cystic
Phocomelia Q73.1
  lower limb — *see* Agenesis, leg, with foot present
  upper limb — *see* Agenesis, arm, with hand present

Phoria H50.50
Phosphate-losing tubular disorder N25.0
Phosphatemia E83.39
Phosphaturia E83.39
Photodermatitis (sun) L56.8
  chronic L57.8
  due to drug L56.8
  light other than sun L59.8
Photokeratitis H16.13- ☑
Photophobia H53.14- ☑
Photophthalmia — *see* Photokeratitis
Photopsia H53.19
Photoretinitis — *see* Retinopathy, solar
Photosensitivity, photosensitization (sun) skin L56.8
  light other than sun L59.8
Phrenitis — *see* Encephalitis
Phrynoderma (vitamin A deficiency) E50.8
Phthiriasis (pubis) B85.3
  with any infestation classifiable to B85.0-B85.2 B85.4
Phthirus infestation — *see* Phthiriasis
Phthisis (*see also* Tuberculosis)
  bulbi (infectional) — *see* Disorder, globe, degenerated condition, atrophy
  eyeball (due to infection) — *see* Disorder, globe, degenerated condition, atrophy
Phycomycosis — *see* Zygomycosis
Physalopteriasis B81.8
Physical restraint status Z78.1
Phytobezoar T18.9 ☑
  intestine T18.3 ☑
  stomach T18.2 ☑
Pian — *see* Yaws
Pianoma A66.1
Pica F50.89
  in adults F50.89
  infant or child F98.3
Picking, nose F98.8
Pick-Niemann disease — *see* Niemann-Pick disease or syndrome
Pick's
  cerebral atrophy G31.01 [F02.80]
    with behavioral disturbance G31.01 [F02.81]
  disease or syndrome (brain) G31.01 [F02.80]
    with behavioral disturbance G31.01 [F02.81]
    brain G31.01 [F02.80]
      with behavioral disturbance G31.01 [F02.81]
    pericardium (pericardial pseudocirrhosis of liver) I31.1
  syndrome
    brain G31.01 [F02.80]
      with behavioral disturbance G31.01 [F02.81]
    of heart (pericardial pseudocirrhosis of liver) I31.1
Pickwickian syndrome E66.2
Piebaldism E70.39
Piedra (beard) (scalp) B36.8
  black B36.3
  white B36.2
Pierre Robin deformity or syndrome Q87.0
Pierson's disease or osteochondrosis M91.0
Pig-bel A05.2
Pigeon
  breast or chest (acquired) M95.4
    congenital Q67.7
    rachitic sequelae (late effect) E64.3
  breeder's disease or lung J67.2
  fancier's disease or lung J67.2
  toe — *see* Deformity, toe, specified NEC
Pigmentation (abnormal) (anomaly) L81.9
  conjunctiva H11.13- ☑
  cornea (anterior) H18.01- ☑
    posterior H18.05- ☑
    stromal H18.06- ☑
  diminished melanin formation NEC L81.6
  iron L81.8
  lids, congenital Q82.8
  limbus corneae — *see* Pigmentation, cornea
  metals L81.8
  optic papilla, congenital Q14.2
  retina, congenital (grouped) (nevoid) Q14.1
  scrotum, congenital Q82.8
  tattoo L81.8
Piles (*see also* Hemorrhoids) K64.9
Pili
  annulati or torti (congenital) Q84.1
  incarnati L73.1
Pill roller hand (intrinsic) — *see* Parkinsonism
Pilomatrixoma — *see* Neoplasm, skin, benign

Pilomatrixoma — *continued*
  malignant — *see* Neoplasm, skin, malignant
Pilonidal — *see* condition
Pimple R23.8
PIN — *see* Neoplasia, intraepithelial, prostate
Pinched nerve — *see* Neuropathy, entrapment
Pindborg tumor — *see* Cyst, calcifying odontogenic
Pineal body or gland — *see* condition
Pinealoblastoma C75.3
Pinealoma D44.5
  malignant C75.3
Pineoblastoma C75.3
Pineocytoma D44.5
Pinguecula H11.15- ☑
Pingueculitis H10.81- ☑
Pinhole meatus (*see also* Stricture, urethra) N35.9
Pink
  disease — *see* subcategory T56.1 ☑
  eye — *see* Conjunctivitis, acute, mucopurulent
Pinkus' disease (lichen nitidus) L44.1
Pinpoint
  meatus — *see* Stricture, urethra
  os (uteri) — *see* Stricture, cervix
Pins and needles R20.2
Pinta A67.9
  cardiovascular lesions A67.2
  chancre (primary) A67.0
  erythematous plaques A67.1
  hyperchromic lesions A67.1
  hyperkeratosis A67.1
  lesions A67.9
    cardiovascular A67.2
    hyperchromic A67.1
    intermediate A67.1
    late A67.2
    mixed A67.3
    primary A67.0
    skin (achromic) (cicatricial) (dyschromic) A67.2
      hyperchromic A67.1
      mixed (achromic and hyperchromic) A67.3
  papule (primary) A67.0
  skin lesions (achromic) (cicatricial) (dyschromic) A67.2
    hyperchromic A67.1
    mixed (achromic and hyperchromic) A67.3
  vitiligo A67.2
Pintids A67.1
Pinworm (disease) (infection) (infestation) B80
Piroplasmosis B60.0
Pistol wound — *see* Gunshot wound
Pitchers' elbow — *see* Derangement, joint, specified type NEC, elbow
Pithecoid pelvis Q74.2
  with disproportion (fetopelvic) O33.0
    causing obstructed labor O65.0
Pithiatism F48.8
Pitted — *see* Pitting
Pitting (*see also* Edema) R60.9
  lip R60.0
  nail L60.8
  teeth K00.4
Pituitary gland — *see* condition
Pituitary-snuff-taker's disease J67.8
Pityriasis (capitis) L21.0
  alba L30.5
  circinata (et maculata) L42
  furfuracea L21.0
  Hebra's L26
  lichenoides L41.0
    chronica L41.1
    et varioliformis (acuta) L41.0
  maculata (et circinata) L30.5
  nigra B36.1
  pilaris, Hebra's L44.0
  rosea L42
  rotunda L44.8
  rubra (Hebra) pilaris L44.0
  simplex L30.5
  specified type NEC L30.5
  streptogenes L30.5
  versicolor (scrotal) B36.0
Placenta, placental — *see* Pregnancy, complicated by (care of) (management affected by), specified condition
Placentitis O41.14- ☑
Plagiocephaly Q67.3
Plague A20.9
  abortive A20.8

▽ **Subterms under main terms may continue to next column or page**   ☑ **Additional Character Required — Refer to the Tabular List for Character Selection**   **253**

Phlebitis — Plague

Plague — *continued*
ambulatory A20.8
asymptomatic A20.8
bubonic A20.0
cellulocutaneous A20.1
cutaneobubonic A20.1
lymphatic gland A20.0
meningitis A20.3
pharyngeal A20.8
pneumonic (primary) (secondary) A20.2
pulmonary, pulmonic A20.2
septicemic A20.7
tonsillar A20.8
septicemic A20.7
Planning, family
contraception Z30.9
procreation Z31.69
Plaque(s)
artery, arterial — *see* Arteriosclerosis
calcareous — *see* Calcification
coronary, lipid rich I25.83
epicardial I31.8
erythematous, of pinta A67.1
Hollenhorst's — *see* Occlusion, artery, retina
lipid rich, coronary I25.83
pleural (without asbestos) J92.9
with asbestos J92.0
tongue K13.29
Plasmacytoma C90.3- ☑
extramedullary C90.2- ☑
medullary C90.0- ☑
solitary C90.3- ☑
Plasmacytopenia D72.818
Plasmacytosis D72.822
Plaster ulcer — *see* Ulcer, pressure, by site
Plateau iris syndrome (post-iridectomy) (postprocedural) (without glaucoma) H21.82
with glaucoma H40.22- ☑
Platybasia Q75.8
Platyonychia (congenital) Q84.6
acquired L60.8
Platypelloid pelvis M95.5
with disproportion (fetopelvic) O33.0
causing obstructed labor O65.0
congenital Q74.2
Platyspondylisis Q76.49
Plaut (-Vincent) **disease** (*see also* Vincent's) A69.1
Plethora R23.2
newborn P61.1
Pleura, pleural — *see* condition
Pleuralgia R07.81
Pleurisy (acute) (adhesive) (chronic) (costal) (diaphragmatic) (double) (dry) (fibrinous) (fibrous) (interlobar) (latent) (plastic) (primary) (residual) (sicca) (sterile) (subacute) (unresolved) R09.1
with
adherent pleura J86.0
effusion J90
chylous, chyliform J94.0
tuberculous (non primary) A15.6
primary (progressive) A15.7
tuberculosis — *see* Pleurisy, tuberculous (non primary)
encysted — *see* Pleurisy, with effusion
exudative — *see* Pleurisy, with effusion
fibrinopurulent, fibropurulent — *see* Pyothorax
hemorrhagic — *see* Hemothorax
pneumococcal J90
purulent — *see* Pyothorax
septic — *see* Pyothorax
serofibrinous — *see* Pleurisy, with effusion
seropurulent — *see* Pyothorax
serous — *see* Pleurisy, with effusion
staphylococcal J86.9
streptococcal J90
suppurative — *see* Pyothorax
traumatic (post) (current) — *see* Injury, intrathoracic, pleura
tuberculous (with effusion) (non primary) A15.6
primary (progressive) A15.7
Pleuritis sicca — *see* Pleurisy
Pleurobronchopneumonia — *see* Pneumonia, broncho-
Pleurodynia R07.81
epidemic B33.0
viral B33.0
Pleuropericarditis (*see also* Pericarditis)
acute I30.9

Pleuropneumonia (acute) (bilateral) (double) (septic) (*see also* Pneumonia) J18.8
chronic — *see* Fibrosis, lung
Pleuro-pneumonia-like-organism (PPLO), as cause of disease classified elsewhere B96.0
Pleurorrhea — *see* Pleurisy, with effusion
Plexitis, brachial G54.0
Plica
polonica B85.0
syndrome, knee M67.5- ☑
tonsil J35.8
Plicated tongue K14.5
Plug
bronchus NEC J98.09
meconium (newborn) NEC syndrome P76.0
mucus — *see* Asphyxia, mucus
Plumbism — *see* subcategory T56.0 ☑
Plummer's disease E05.20
with thyroid storm E05.21
Plummer-Vinson syndrome D50.1
Pluricarential syndrome of infancy E40
Plus (and minus) **hand** (intrinsic) — *see* Deformity, limb, specified type NEC, forearm
Pneumathemia — *see* Air, embolism
Pneumatic hammer (drill) syndrome T75.21 ☑
Pneumatocele (lung) J98.4
intracranial G93.89
tension J44.9
Pneumatosis
cystoides intestinalis K63.89
intestinalis K63.89
peritonei K66.8
Pneumaturia R39.89
Pneumoblastoma — *see* Neoplasm, lung, malignant
Pneumocephalus G93.89
Pneumococcemia A40.3
Pneumococcus, pneumococcal — *see* condition
Pneumoconiosis (due to) (inhalation of) J64
with tuberculosis (any type in A15) J65
aluminum J63.0
asbestos J61
bagasse, bagassosis J67.1
bauxite J63.1
beryllium J63.2
coal miners' (simple) J60
coalworkers' (simple) J60
collier's J60
cotton dust J66.0
diatomite (diatomaceous earth) J62.8
dust
inorganic NEC J63.6
lime J62.8
marble J62.8
organic NEC J66.8
fumes or vapors (from silo) J68.9
graphite J63.3
grinder's J62.8
kaolin J62.8
mica J62.8
millstone maker's J62.8
mineral fibers NEC J61
miner's J60
moldy hay J67.0
potter's J62.8
rheumatoid — *see* Rheumatoid, lung
sandblaster's J62.8
silica, silicate NEC J62.8
with carbon J60
stonemason's J62.8
talc (dust) J62.0
Pneumocystis carinii pneumonia B59
Pneumocystis jiroveci (pneumonia) B59
Pneumocystosis (with pneumonia) B59
Pneumohemopericardium I31.2
Pneumohemothorax J94.2
traumatic S27.2 ☑
Pneumohydropericardium — *see* Pericarditis
Pneumohydrothorax — *see* Hydrothorax
Pneumomediastinum J98.2
congenital or perinatal P25.2
Pneumomycosis B49 [J99]
Pneumonia (acute) (double) (migratory) (purulent) (septic) (unresolved) J18.9
with
influenza — *see* Influenza, with, pneumonia
lung abscess J85.1

Pneumonia — *continued*
with — *continued*
lung abscess — *continued*
due to specified organism — *see* Pneumonia, in (due to)
adenoviral J12.0
adynamic J18.2
alba A50.04
allergic (eosinophilic) J82
alveolar — *see* Pneumonia, lobar
anaerobes J15.8
anthrax A22.1
apex, apical — *see* Pneumonia, lobar
Ascaris B77.81
aspiration J69.0
due to
aspiration of microorganisms
bacterial J15.9
viral J12.9
food (regurgitated) J69.0
gastric secretions J69.0
milk (regurgitated) J69.0
oils, essences J69.1
solids, liquids NEC J69.8
vomitus J69.0
newborn P24.81
amniotic fluid (clear) P24.11
blood P24.21
food (regurgitated) P24.31
liquor (amnii) P24.11
meconium P24.01
milk P24.31
mucus P24.11
specified NEC P24.81
stomach contents P24.31
postprocedural J95.4
atypical NEC J18.9
bacillus J15.9
specified NEC J15.8
bacterial J15.9
specified NEC J15.8
Bacteroides (fragilis) (oralis) (melaninogenicus) J15.8
basal, basic, basilar — *see* Pneumonia, by type
bronchiolitis obliterans organized (BOOP) J84.89
broncho-, bronchial (confluent) (croupous) (diffuse) (disseminated) (hemorrhagic) (involving lobes) (lobar) (terminal) J18.0
allergic (eosinophilic) J82
aspiration — *see* Pneumonia, aspiration
bacterial J15.9
specified NEC J15.8
chronic — *see* Fibrosis, lung
diplococcal J13
Eaton's agent J15.7
Escherichia coli (E. coli) J15.5
Friedländer's bacillus J15.0
Hemophilus influenzae J14
hypostatic J18.2
inhalation (*see also* Pneumonia, aspiration)
due to fumes or vapors (chemical) J68.0
of oils or essences J69.1
Klebsiella (pneumoniae) J15.0
lipid, lipoid J69.1
endogenous J84.89
Mycoplasma (pneumoniae) J15.7
pleuro-pneumonia-like-organisms (PPLO) J15.7
pneumococcal J13
Proteus J15.6
Pseudomonas J15.1
Serratia marcescens J15.6
specified organism NEC J16.8
staphylococcal — *see* Pneumonia, staphylococcal
streptococcal NEC J15.4
group B J15.3
pneumoniae J13
viral, virus — *see* Pneumonia, viral
Butyrivibrio (fibriosolvens) J15.8
Candida B37.1
caseous — *see* Tuberculosis, pulmonary
catarrhal — *see* Pneumonia, broncho
chlamydial J16.0
congenital P23.1
cholesterol J84.89
cirrhotic (chronic) — *see* Fibrosis, lung
Clostridium (haemolyticum) (novyi) J15.8
confluent — *see* Pneumonia, broncho
congenital (infective) P23.9

Pneumonia — continued
congenital — continued
  due to
    bacterium NEC P23.6
    Chlamydia P23.1
    Escherichia coli P23.4
    Haemophilus influenzae P23.6
    infective organism NEC P23.8
    Klebsiella pneumoniae P23.6
    Mycoplasma P23.6
    Pseudomonas P23.5
    Staphylococcus P23.2
    Streptococcus (except group B) P23.6
      group B P23.3
    viral agent P23.0
  specified NEC P23.8
croupous — see Pneumonia, lobar
cryptogenic organizing J84.116
cytomegalic inclusion B25.0
cytomegaloviral B25.0
deglutition — see Pneumonia, aspiration
desquamative interstitial J84.117
diffuse — see Pneumonia, broncho
diplococcal, diplococcus (broncho-) (lobar) J13
disseminated (focal) — see Pneumonia, broncho
Eaton's agent J15.7
embolic, embolism — see Embolism, pulmonary
Enterobacter J15.6
eosinophilic J82
Escherichia coli (E. coli) J15.5
Eubacterium J15.8
fibrinous — see Pneumonia, lobar
fibroid, fibrous (chronic) — see Fibrosis, lung
Friedländer's bacillus J15.0
Fusobacterium (nucleatum) J15.8
gangrenous J85.0
giant cell (measles) B05.2
gonococcal A54.84
gram-negative bacteria NEC J15.6
  anaerobic J15.8
Hemophilus influenzae (broncho) (lobar) J14
human metapneumovirus J12.3
hypostatic (broncho) (lobar) J18.2
in (due to)
  actinomycosis A42.0
  adenovirus J12.0
  anthrax A22.1
  ascariasis B77.81
  aspergillosis B44.9
  Bacillus anthracis A22.1
  Bacterium anitratum J15.6
  candidiasis B37.1
  chickenpox B01.2
  Chlamydia J16.0
    neonatal P23.1
  coccidioidomycosis B38.2
    acute B38.0
    chronic B38.1
  cytomegalovirus disease B25.0
  Diplococcus (pneumoniae) J13
  Eaton's agent J15.7
  Enterobacter J15.6
  Escherichia coli (E. coli) J15.5
  Friedländer's bacillus J15.0
  fumes and vapors (chemical) (inhalation) J68.0
  gonorrhea A54.84
  Hemophilus influenzae (H. influenzae) J14
  Herellea J15.6
  histoplasmosis B39.2
    acute B39.0
    chronic B39.1
  human metapneumovirus J12.3
  Klebsiella (pneumoniae) J15.0
  measles B05.2
  Mycoplasma (pneumoniae) J15.7
  nocardiosis, nocardiasis A43.0
  ornithosis A70
  parainfluenza virus J12.2
  pleuro-pneumonia-like-organism (PPLO) J15.7
  pneumococcus J13
  pneumocystosis (Pneumocystis carinii) (Pneumo-
    cystis jiroveci) B59
  Proteus J15.6
  Pseudomonas NEC J15.1
    pseudomallei A24.1
  psittacosis A70
  Q fever A78
  respiratory syncytial virus J12.1

Pneumonia — continued
in — continued
  rheumatic fever I00 [J17]
  rubella B06.81
  Salmonella (infection) A02.22
    typhi A01.03
  schistosomiasis B65.9 [J17]
  Serratia marcescens J15.6
  specified
    bacterium NEC J15.8
    organism NEC J16.8
  spirochetal NEC A69.8
  Staphylococcus J15.20
    aureus (methicillin susceptible) (MSSA) J15.211
      methicillin resistant (MRSA) J15.212
    specified NEC J15.29
  Streptococcus J15.4
    group B J15.3
    pneumoniae J13
    specified NEC J15.4
  toxoplasmosis B58.3
  tularemia A21.2
  typhoid (fever) A01.03
  varicella B01.2
  virus — see Pneumonia, viral
  whooping cough A37.91
    due to
      Bordetella parapertussis A37.11
      Bordetella pertussis A37.01
      specified NEC A37.81
  Yersinia pestis A20.2
inhalation of food or vomit — see Pneumonia, aspiration
interstitial J84.9
  chronic J84.111
  desquamative J84.117
  due to
    collagen vascular disease J84.17
    known underlying cause J84.17
  idiopathic NOS J84.111
  in disease classified elsewhere J84.17
  lymphocytic (due to collagen vascular disease) (in
    diseases classified elsewhere) J84.17
  lymphoid J84.2
  non-specific J84.89
    due to
      collagen vascular disease J84.17
      known underlying cause J84.17
    idiopathic J84.113
    in diseases classified elsewhere J84.17
  plasma cell B59
  pseudomonas J15.1
  usual J84.112
    due to collagen vascular disease J84.17
    idiopathic J84.112
    in diseases classified elsewhere J84.17
Klebsiella (pneumoniae) J15.0
lipid, lipoid (exogenous) J69.1
  endogenous J84.89
lobar (disseminated) (double) (interstitial) J18.1
  bacterial J15.9
    specified NEC J15.8
  chronic — see Fibrosis, lung
  Escherichia coli (E. coli) J15.5
  Friedländer's bacillus J15.0
  Hemophilus influenzae J14
  hypostatic J18.2
  Klebsiella (pneumoniae) J15.0
  pneumococcal J13
  Proteus J15.6
  Pseudomonas J15.1
  specified organism NEC J16.8
  staphylococcal — see Pneumonia, staphylococcal
  streptococcal NEC J15.4
  Streptococcus pneumoniae J13
  viral, virus — see Pneumonia, viral
lobular — see Pneumonia, broncho
Löffler's J82
lymphoid interstitial J84.2
massive — see Pneumonia, lobar
meconium P24.01
MRSA (methicillin resistant Staphylococcus aureus)
  J15.212
MSSA (methicillin susceptible Staphylococcus aureus)
  J15.211
multilobar — see Pneumonia, by type
Mycoplasma (pneumoniae) J15.7
necrotic J85.0

Pneumonia — continued
neonatal P23.9
  aspiration — see Aspiration, by substance, with
    pneumonia
nitrogen dioxide J68.0
organizing J84.89
  due to
    collagen vascular disease J84.17
    known underlying cause J84.17
  in diseases classified elsewhere J84.17
orthostatic J18.2
parainfluenza virus J12.2
parenchymatous — see Fibrosis, lung
passive J18.2
patchy — see Pneumonia, broncho
Peptococcus J15.8
Peptostreptococcus J15.8
plasma cell (of infants) B59
pleurolobar — see Pneumonia, lobar
pleuro-pneumonia-like organism (PPLO) J15.7
pneumococcal (broncho) (lobar) J13
Pneumocystis (carinii) (jiroveci) B59
postinfectional NEC B99 ☑ [J17]
postmeasles B05.2
Proteus J15.6
Pseudomonas J15.1
psittacosis A70
radiation J70.0
respiratory syncytial virus J12.1
resulting from a procedure J95.89
rheumatic I00 [J17]
Salmonella (arizonae) (cholerae-suis) (enteritidis) (ty-
    phimurium) A02.22
  typhi A01.03
  typhoid fever A01.03
SARS-associated coronavirus J12.81
segmented, segmental — see Pneumonia, broncho-
Serratia marcescens J15.6
specified NEC J18.8
  bacterium NEC J15.8
  organism NEC J16.8
  virus NEC J12.89
spirochetal NEC A69.8
staphylococcal (broncho) (lobar) J15.20
  aureus (methicillin susceptible) (MSSA) J15.211
    methicillin resistant (MRSA) J15.212
  specified NEC J15.29
static, stasis J18.2
streptococcal NEC (broncho) (lobar) J15.4
  group
    A J15.4
    B J15.3
    specified NEC J15.4
Streptococcus pneumoniae J13
syphilitic, congenital (early) A50.04
traumatic (complication) (early) (secondary) T79.8 ☑
tuberculous (any) — see Tuberculosis, pulmonary
tularemic A21.2
varicella B01.2
Veillonella J15.8
ventilator associated J95.851
viral, virus (broncho) (interstitial) (lobar) J12.9
  adenoviral J12.0
  congenital P23.0
  human metapneumovirus J12.3
  parainfluenza J12.2
  respiratory syncytial J12.1
  SARS-associated coronavirus J12.81
  specified NEC J12.89
white (congenital) A50.04
Pneumonic — see condition
Pneumonitis (acute) (primary) (see also Pneumonia)
air-conditioner J67.7
allergic (due to) J67.9
  organic dust NEC J67.8
  red cedar dust J67.8
  sequoiosis J67.8
  wood dust J67.8
aspiration J69.0
  due to
    anesthesia J95.4
      during
        labor and delivery O74.0
        pregnancy O29.01- ☑
        puerperium O89.01
    fumes or gases J68.0
  obstetric O74.0

☜ Subterms under main terms may continue to next column or page   ☑ Additional Character Required — Refer to the Tabular List for Character Selection   255

Pneumonia — Pneumonitis

Pneumonitis — *continued*
  chemical (due to gases, fumes or vapors) (inhalation) J68.0
    due to anesthesia J95.4
  cholesterol J84.89
  chronic — *see* Fibrosis, lung
  congenital rubella P35.0
  crack (cocaine) J68.0
  due to
    beryllium J68.0
    cadmium J68.0
    crack (cocaine) J68.0
    detergent J69.8
    fluorocarbon-polymer J68.0
    food, vomit (aspiration) J69.0
    fumes or vapors J68.0
    gases, fumes or vapors (inhalation) J68.0
    inhalation
      blood J69.8
      essences J69.1
      food (regurgitated), milk, vomit J69.0
      oils, essences J69.1
      saliva J69.0
      solids, liquids NEC J69.8
    manganese J68.0
    nitrogen dioxide J68.0
    oils, essences J69.1
    solids, liquids NEC J69.8
    toxoplasmosis (acquired) B58.3
      congenital P37.1
    vanadium J68.0
    ventilator J95.851
  eosinophilic J82
  hypersensitivity J67.9
    air conditioner lung J67.7
    bagassosis J67.1
    bird fancier's lung J67.2
    farmer's lung J67.0
    maltworker's lung J67.4
    maple bark-stripper's lung J67.6
    mushroom worker's lung J67.5
    specified organic dust NEC J67.8
    suberosis J67.3
  interstitial (chronic) J84.89
    acute J84.114
    lymphoid J84.2
    non-specific J84.89
      idiopathic J84.113
  lymphoid, interstitial J84.2
  meconium P24.01
  postanesthetic J95.4
    correct substance properly administered — *see* Table of Drugs and Chemicals, by drug, adverse effect
    in labor and delivery O74.0
    in pregnancy O29.01- ☑
      obstetric O74.0
    overdose or wrong substance given or taken (by accident) — *see* Table of Drugs and Chemicals, by drug, poisoning
    postpartum, puerperal O89.01
  postoperative J95.4
    obstetric O74.0
  radiation J70.0
  rubella, congenital P35.0
  ventilation (air-conditioning) J67.7
  ventilator associated J95.851
  wood-dust J67.8
Pneumoconiosis — *see* Pneumoconiosis
Pneumoparotid K11.8
Pneumopathy NEC J98.4
  alveolar J84.09
  due to organic dust NEC J66.8
  parietoalveolar J84.09
Pneumopericarditis (*see also* Pericarditis)
  acute I30.9
Pneumopericardium (*see also* Pericarditis)
  congenital P25.3
  newborn P25.3
  traumatic (post) — *see* Injury, heart
Pneumophagia (psychogenic) F45.8
Pneumopleurisy, pneumopleuritis (*see also* Pneumonia) J18.8
Pneumopyopericardium I30.1
Pneumopyothorax — *see* Pyopneumothorax
  with fistula J86.0
Pneumorrhagia (*see also* Hemorrhage, lung)
  tuberculous — *see* Tuberculosis, pulmonary

Pneumothorax NOS J93.9
  acute J93.83
  chronic J93.81
  congenital P25.1
  perinatal period P25.1
  postprocedural J95.811
  specified NEC J93.83
  spontaneous NOS J93.83
    newborn P25.1
    primary J93.11
    secondary J93.12
    tension J93.0
  tense valvular, infectional J93.0
  tension (spontaneous) J93.0
  traumatic S27.0 ☑
    with hemothorax S27.2 ☑
  tuberculous — *see* Tuberculosis, pulmonary
Podagra (*see also* Gout) M10.9
Podencephalus Q01.9
Poikilocytosis R71.8
Poikiloderma L81.6
  Civatte's L57.3
  congenital Q82.8
  vasculare atrophicans L94.5
Poikilodermatomyositis M33.10
  with
    myopathy M33.12
    respiratory involvement M33.11
    specified organ involvement NEC M33.19
Pointed ear (congenital) Q17.3
Poison ivy, oak, sumac or other plant dermatitis (allergic) (contact) L23.7
Poisoning (acute) (*see also* Table of Drugs and Chemicals)
  algae and toxins T65.82- ☑
  Bacillus B (aertrycke) (cholerae (suis)) (paratyphosus) (suipestifer) A02.9
    botulinus A05.1
  bacterial toxins A05.9
  berries, noxious — *see* Poisoning, food, noxious, berries
  botulism A05.1
  ciguatera fish T61.0- ☑
  Clostridium botulinum A05.1
  death-cap (Amanita phalloides) (Amanita verna) — *see* Poisoning, food, noxious, mushrooms
  drug — *see* Table of Drugs and Chemicals, by drug, poisoning
  epidemic, fish (noxious) — *see* Poisoning, seafood
    bacterial A05.9
  fava bean D55.0
  fish (noxious) T61.9- ☑
    bacterial — *see* Intoxication, foodborne, by agent
    ciguatera fish — *see* Poisoning, ciguatera fish
    scombroid fish — *see* Poisoning, scombroid fish
    specified type NEC T61.77- ☑
  food (acute) (diseased) (infected) (noxious) NEC T62.9- ☑
    bacterial — *see* Intoxication, foodborne, by agent
    due to
      Bacillus (aertrycke) (choleraesuis) (paratyphosus) (suipestifer) A02.9
        botulinus A05.1
      Clostridium (perfringens) (Welchii) A05.2
      salmonella (aertrycke) (callinarum) (choleraesuis) (enteritidis) (paratyphi) (suipestifer) A02.9
        with
          gastroenteritis A02.0
          sepsis A02.1
      staphylococcus A05.0
      Vibrio
        parahaemolyticus A05.3
        vulnificus A05.5
    noxious or naturally toxic T62.9- ☑
      berries — *see* subcategory T62.1 ☑
      fish — *see* Poisoning, seafood
      mushrooms — *see* subcategory T62.0X ☑
      plants NEC — *see* subcategory T62.2X ☑
      seafood — *see* Poisoning, seafood
      specified NEC — *see* subcategory T62.8X ☑
  ichthyotoxism — *see* Poisoning, seafood
  kreotoxism, food A05.9
  latex T65.81- ☑
  lead T56.0- ☑
  mushroom — *see* Poisoning, food, noxious, mushroom
  mussels (*see also* Poisoning, shellfish)
    bacterial — *see* Intoxication, foodborne, by agent

Poisoning — *continued*
  nicotine (tobacco) T65.2- ☑
  noxious foodstuffs — *see* Poisoning, food, noxious
  plants, noxious — *see* Poisoning, food, noxious, plants NEC
  ptomaine — *see* Poisoning, food
  radiation J70.0
  Salmonella (arizonae) (cholerae-suis) (enteritidis) (typhimurium) A02.9
  scombroid fish T61.1- ☑
  seafood (noxious) T61.9- ☑
    bacterial — *see* Intoxication, foodborne, by agent
    fish — *see* Poisoning, fish
    shellfish — *see* Poisoning, shellfish
    specified NEC — *see* subcategory T61.8X ☑
  shellfish (amnesic) (azaspiracid) (diarrheic) (neurotoxic) (noxious) (paralytic) T61.78- ☑
    bacterial — *see* Intoxication, foodborne, by agent
    ciguatera mollusk — *see* Poisoning, ciguatera fish
  specified substance NEC T65.891 ☑
  Staphylococcus, food A05.0
  tobacco (nicotine) T65.2- ☑
  water E87.79
Poker spine — *see* Spondylitis, ankylosing
Poland syndrome Q79.8
Polioencephalitis (acute) (bulbar) A80.9
  inferior G12.22
  influenzal — *see* Influenza, with, encephalopathy
  superior hemorrhagic (acute) (Wernicke's) E51.2
  Wernicke's E51.2
Polioencephalomyelitis (acute) (anterior) A80.9
  with beriberi E51.2
Polioencephalopathy, superior hemorrhagic E51.2
  with
    beriberi E51.11
    pellagra E52
Poliomeningoencephalitis — *see* Meningoencephalitis
Poliomyelitis (acute) (anterior) (epidemic) A80.9
  with paralysis (bulbar) — *see* Poliomyelitis, paralytic
  abortive A80.4
  ascending (progressive) — *see* Poliomyelitis, paralytic
  bulbar (paralytic) — *see* Poliomyelitis, paralytic
  congenital P35.8
  nonepidemic A80.9
  nonparalytic A80.4
  paralytic A80.30
    specified NEC A80.39
    vaccine-associated A80.0
    wild virus
      imported A80.1
      indigenous A80.2
  spinal, acute A80.9
Poliosis (eyebrow) (eyelashes) L67.1
  circumscripta, acquired L67.1
Pollakiuria R35.0
  psychogenic F45.8
Pollinosis J30.1
Pollitzer's disease L73.2
Polyadenitis (*see also* Lymphadenitis)
  malignant A20.0
Polyalgia M79.89
Polyangiitis M30.0
  microscopic M31.7
  overlap syndrome M30.8
Polyarteritis
  microscopic M31.7
  nodosa M30.0
    with lung involvement M30.1
    juvenile M30.2
    related condition NEC M30.8
Polyarthralgia — *see* Pain, joint
Polyarthritis, polyarthropathy (*see also* Arthritis) M13.0
  due to or associated with other specified conditions — *see* Arthritis
  epidemic (Australian) (with exanthema) B33.1
  infective — *see* Arthritis, pyogenic or pyemic
  inflammatory M06.4
  juvenile (chronic) (seronegative) M08.3
  migratory — *see* Fever, rheumatic
  rheumatic, acute — *see* Fever, rheumatic
Polyarthrosis M15.9
  post-traumatic M15.3
  primary M15.0
  specified NEC M15.8
Polycarential syndrome of infancy E40
Polychondritis (atrophic) (chronic) (*see also* Disorder, cartilage, specified type NEC)
  relapsing M94.1

☑ **Additional Character Required** — **Refer to the Tabular List for Character Selection** ⬇ **Subterms under main terms may continue to next column or page**

Polycoria Q13.2
Polycystic (disease)
  degeneration, kidney Q61.3
    autosomal dominant (adult type) Q61.2
    autosomal recessive (infantile type)
      NEC Q61.19
  kidney Q61.3
    autosomal
      dominant Q61.2
      recessive NEC Q61.19
    autosomal dominant (adult type) Q61.2
    autosomal recessive (childhood type) NEC Q61.19
    infantile type NEC Q61.19
  liver Q44.6
  lung J98.4
    congenital Q33.0
  ovary, ovaries E28.2
  spleen Q89.09
Polycythemia (secondary) D75.1
  acquired D75.1
  benign (familial) D75.0
  due to
    donor twin P61.1
    erythropoietin D75.1
    fall in plasma volume D75.1
    high altitude D75.1
    maternal-fetal transfusion P61.1
    stress D75.1
  emotional D75.1
  erythropoietin D75.1
  familial (benign) D75.0
  Gaisböck's (hypertonica) D75.1
  high altitude D75.1
  hypertonica D75.1
  hypoxemic D75.1
  neonatorum P61.1
  nephrogenous D75.1
  relative D75.1
  secondary D75.1
  spurious D75.1
  stress D75.1
  vera D45
Polycytosis cryptogenica D75.1
Polydactylism, polydactyly Q69.9
  toes Q69.2
Polydipsia R63.1
Polydystrophy, pseudo-Hurler E77.0
Polyembryoma — *see* Neoplasm, malignant, by site
Polyglandular
  deficiency E31.0
  dyscrasia E31.9
  dysfunction E31.9
  syndrome E31.8
Polyhydramnios O40.- ☑
Polymastia Q83.1
Polymenorrhea N92.0
Polymyalgia M35.3
  arteritica, giant cell M31.5
  rheumatica M35.3
    with giant cell arteritis M31.5
Polymyositis (acute) (chronic) (hemorrhagic) M33.20
  with
    myopathy M33.22
    respiratory involvement M33.21
    skin involvement — *see* Dermatopolymyositis
    specified organ involvement NEC M33.29
  ossificans (generalisata) (progressiva) — *see* Myositis, ossificans, progressiva
Polyneuritis, polyneuritic (*see also* Polyneuropathy)
  acute (post-)infective G61.0
  alcoholic G62.1
  cranialis G52.7
  demyelinating, chronic inflammatory (CIDP) G61.81
  diabetic — *see* Diabetes, polyneuropathy
  diphtheritic A36.83
  due to lack of vitamin NEC E56.9 [G63]
  endemic E51.11
  erythredema — *see* subcategory T56.1 ☑
  febrile, acute G61.0
  hereditary ataxic G60.1
  idiopathic, acute G61.0
  infective (acute) G61.0
  inflammatory, chronic demyelinating (CIDP) G61.81
  nutritional E63.9 [G63]
  postinfective (acute) G61.0
  specified NEC G62.89
Polyneuropathy (peripheral) G62.9

Polyneuropathy — *continued*
  alcoholic G62.1
  amyloid (Portuguese) E85.1 [G63]
    transthyretin-related (ATTR) familial E85.1
  arsenical G62.2
  critical illness G62.81
  demyelinating, chronic inflammatory (CIDP) G61.81
  diabetic — *see* Diabetes, polyneuropathy
  drug-induced G62.0
  hereditary G60.9
    specified NEC G60.8
  idiopathic G60.9
    progressive G60.3
  in (due to)
    alcohol G62.1
      sequelae G65.2
    amyloidosis, familial (Portuguese) E85.1 [G63]
    antitetanus serum G61.1
    arsenic G62.2
      sequelae G65.2
    avitaminosis NEC E56.9 [G63]
    beriberi E51.11
    collagen vascular disease NEC M35.9 [G63]
    deficiency (of)
      B (-complex) vitamins E53.9 [G63]
      vitamin B6 E53.1 [G63]
    diabetes — *see* Diabetes, polyneuropathy
    diphtheria A36.83
    drug or medicament G62.0
      correct substance properly administered — *see* Table of Drugs and Chemicals, by drug, adverse effect
      overdose or wrong substance given or taken — *see* Table of Drugs and Chemicals, by drug, poisoning
    endocrine disease NEC E34.9 [G63]
    herpes zoster B02.23
    hypoglycemia E16.2 [G63]
    infectious
      disease NEC B99 ☑ [G63]
      mononucleosis B27.91
    lack of vitamin NEC E56.9 [G63]
    lead G62.2
      sequelae G65.2
    leprosy A30.9 [G63]
    Lyme disease A69.22
    metabolic disease NEC E88.9 [G63]
    microscopic polyangiitis M31.7 [G63]
    mumps B26.84
    neoplastic disease (*see also* Neoplasm) D49.9 [G63]
    nutritional deficiency NEC E63.9 [G63]
    organophosphate compounds G62.2
      sequelae G65.2
    parasitic disease NEC B89 [G63]
    pellagra E52 [G63]
    polyarteritis nodosa M30.0
    porphyria E80.20 [G63]
    radiation G62.82
    rheumatoid arthritis — *see* Rheumatoid, polyneuropathy
    sarcoidosis D86.89
    serum G61.1
    syphilis (late) A52.15
      congenital A50.43
    systemic
      connective tissue disorder M35.9 [G63]
      lupus erythematosus M32.19
    toxic agent NEC G62.2
      sequelae G65.2
  inflammatory G61.9
    chronic demyelinating (CIDP) G61.81
    sequelae G65.1
    specified NEC G61.89
  lead G62.2
    sequelae G65.2
  nutritional NEC E63.9 [G63]
  postherpetic (zoster) B02.23
  progressive G60.3
  radiation-induced G62.82
  sensory (hereditary) (idiopathic) G60.8
  specified NEC G62.89
  syphilitic (late) A52.15
    congenital A50.43
  transthyretin-related (ATTR) familial amyloid E85.1
    triorthocresyl phosphate G62.2
      sequelae G65.2
    tuberculosis A17.89
    uremia N18.9 [G63]

Polyneuropathy — *continued*
  transthyretin-related familial amyloid — *continued*
    vitamin B12 deficiency E53.8 [G63]
      with anemia (pernicious) D51.0 [G63]
      due to dietary deficiency D51.3 [G63]
    zoster B02.23
Polyopia H53.8
Polyorchism, polyorchidism Q55.21
Polyosteoarthritis (*see also* Osteoarthritis, generalized) M15.9
  post-traumatic M15.3
  specified NEC M15.8
Polyostotic fibrous dysplasia Q78.1
Polyotia Q17.0
Polyp, polypus
  accessory sinus J33.8
  adenocarcinoma in — *see* Neoplasm, malignant, by site
  adenocarcinoma in situ in — *see* Neoplasm, in situ, by site
  adenoid tissue J33.0
  adenomatous (*see also* Neoplasm, benign, by site)
    adenocarcinoma in — *see* Neoplasm, malignant, by site
    adenocarcinoma in situ in — *see* Neoplasm, in situ, by site
    carcinoma in — *see* Neoplasm, malignant, by site
    carcinoma in situ in — *see* Neoplasm, in situ, by site
    multiple — *see* Neoplasm, benign
      adenocarcinoma in — *see* Neoplasm, malignant, by site
      adenocarcinoma in situ in — *see* Neoplasm, in situ, by site
  antrum J33.8
  anus, anal (canal) K62.0
  Bartholin's gland N84.3
  bladder D41.4
  carcinoma in — *see* Neoplasm, malignant, by site
  carcinoma in situ in — *see* Neoplasm, in situ, by site
  cecum D12.0
  cervix (uteri) N84.1
    in pregnancy or childbirth — *see* Pregnancy, complicated by, abnormal, cervix
    mucous N84.1
    nonneoplastic N84.1
  choanal J33.0
  cholesterol K82.4
  clitoris N84.3
  colon K63.5
    adenomatous D12.6
    ascending D12.2
    cecum D12.0
    descending D12.4
    inflammatory K51.40
      with
        abscess K51.414
        complication K51.419
          specified NEC K51.418
        fistula K51.413
        intestinal obstruction K51.412
        rectal bleeding K51.411
    sigmoid D12.5
    transverse D12.3
  corpus uteri N84.0
  dental K04.01
    irreversible K04.02
    reversible K04.01
  duodenum K31.7
  ear (middle) H74.4- ☑
  endometrium N84.0
  ethmoidal (sinus) J33.8
  fallopian tube N84.8
  female genital tract N84.9
    specified NEC N84.8
  frontal (sinus) J33.8
  gallbladder K82.4
  gingiva, gum K06.8
  labia, labium (majus) (minus) N84.3
  larynx (mucous) J38.1
    adenomatous D14.1
  malignant — *see* Neoplasm, malignant, by site
  maxillary (sinus) J33.8
  middle ear — *see* Polyp, ear (middle)
  myometrium N84.0
  nares
    anterior J33.9
    posterior J33.0

☑ **Additional Character Required** — Refer to the Tabular List for Character Selection   ▽ Subterms under main terms may continue to next column or page

Precocious — *continued*
  puberty — *continued*
    central E22.8
  sexual development NEC E30.1
  thelarche E30.8
Precocity, sexual (constitutional) (cryptogenic) (female)
    (idiopathic) (male) E30.1
  with adrenal hyperplasia E25.9
    congenital E25.0
Precordial pain R07.2
Predeciduous teeth K00.2
Prediabetes, prediabetic R73.03
  complicating
    pregnancy — *see* Pregnancy, complicated by, dis-
      eases of, specified type or system NEC
    puerperium O99.89
Predislocation status of hip at birth Q65.6
Pre-eclampsia O14.9- ☑
  with pre-existing hypertension — *see* Hypertension,
      complicating pregnancy, pre-existing, with, pre-
      eclampsia
  complicating
    childbirth O14.94
    puerperium O14.95
  mild O14.0- ☑
    complicating
      childbirth O14.04
      puerperium O14.05
  moderate O14.0- ☑
    complicating
      childbirth O14.04
      puerperium O14.05
  severe O14.1- ☑
    with hemolysis, elevated liver enzymes and low
        platelet count (HELLP) O14.2- ☑
      complicating
        childbirth O14.24
        puerperium O14.25
    complicating
      childbirth O14.14
      puerperium O14.15
Pre-eruptive color change, teeth, tooth K00.8
Pre-excitation atrioventricular conduction I45.6
Preglaucoma H40.00- ☑
Pregnancy (single) (uterine) (*see also* Delivery and
    Puerperal)

> *Note: The Tabular must be reviewed for assign-*
> *ment of appropriate seventh character for multi-*
> *ple gestation codes in Chapter 15*

> *Note: The Tabular must be reviewed for assign-*
> *ment of the appropriate character indicating the*
> *trimester of the pregnancy*

  abdominal (ectopic) O00.00
    with intrauterine pregnancy O00.01
    with viable fetus O36.7- ☑
  ampullar O00.10- ☑
    with intrauterine pregnancy O00.11- ☑
  biochemical O02.81
  broad ligament O00.80
    with intrauterine pregnancy O00.81
  cervical O00.8
    with intrauterine pregnancy O00.81
  chemical O02.81
  complicated by (care of) (management affected by)
    abnormal, abnormality
      cervix O34.4- ☑
        causing obstructed labor O65.5
      cord (umbilical) O69.9 ☑
      fetal heart rate or rhythm O36.83- ☑
      findings on antenatal screening of mother
          O28.9
        biochemical O28.1
        chromosomal O28.5
        cytological O28.2
        genetic O28.5
        hematological O28.0
        radiological O28.4
        specified NEC O28.8
        ultrasonic O28.3
      glucose (tolerance) NEC O99.810
      pelvic organs O34.9- ☑
        specified NEC O34.8- ☑
          causing obstructed labor O65.5
      pelvis (bony) (major) NEC O33.0
      perineum O34.7- ☑

Pregnancy — *continued*
  complicated by — *continued*
    abnormal, abnormality — *continued*
      position
        placenta O44.0- ☑
          with hemorrhage O44.1- ☑
        uterus O34.59- ☑
      uterus O34.59- ☑
        causing obstructed labor O65.5
        congenital O34.0- ☑
      vagina O34.6- ☑
        causing obstructed labor O65.5
      vulva O34.7- ☑
        causing obstructed labor O65.5
    abruptio placentae — *see* Abruptio placentae
    abscess or cellulitis
      bladder O23.1- ☑
      breast O91.11- ☑
      genital organ or tract O23.9- ☑
    abuse
      physical O9A.31 ☑ (*following* O99)
      psychological O9A.51 ☑ (*following* O99)
      sexual O9A.41 ☑ (*following* O99)
    adverse effect anesthesia O29.9- ☑
      aspiration pneumonitis O29.01- ☑
      cardiac arrest O29.11- ☑
      cardiac complication NEC O29.19- ☑
      cardiac failure O29.12- ☑
      central nervous system complication NEC
          O29.29- ☑
      cerebral anoxia O29.21- ☑
      failed or difficult intubation O29.6- ☑
      inhalation of stomach contents or secretions
          NOS O29.01- ☑
      local, toxic reaction O29.3X ☑
      Mendelson's syndrome O29.01- ☑
      pressure collapse of lung O29.02- ☑
      pulmonary complications NEC O29.09- ☑
      specified NEC O29.8X- ☑
      spinal and epidural type NEC O29.5X ☑
        induced headache O29.4- ☑
    albuminuria (*see also* Proteinuria, gestational)
        O12.1- ☑
    alcohol use O99.31- ☑
    amnionitis O41.12- ☑
    anaphylactoid syndrome of pregnancy O88.01- ☑
    anemia (conditions in D50-D64) (pre-existing)
        O99.01- ☑
      complicating the puerperium O99.03
    antepartum hemorrhage O46.9- ☑
      with coagulation defect — *see* Hemorrhage,
          antepartum, with coagulation defect
      specified NEC O46.8X- ☑
    appendicitis O99.61- ☑
    atrophy (yellow) (acute) liver (subacute) O26.61- ☑
    bariatric surgery status O99.84- ☑
    bicornis or bicornuate uterus O34.0- ☑
    biliary tract problems O26.61- ☑
    breech presentation O32.1 ☑
    cardiovascular diseases (conditions in I00-I09, I20-
        I52, I70-I99) O99.41- ☑
    cerebrovascular disorders (conditions in I60-I69)
        O99.41- ☑
    cervical shortening O26.87- ☑
    cervicitis O23.51- ☑
    chloasma (gravidarum) O26.89- ☑
    cholecystitis O99.61- ☑
    cholestasis (intrahepatic) O26.61- ☑
    chorioamnionitis O41.12- ☑
    circulatory system disorder (conditions in I00-I09,
        I20-I99, O99.41-)
    compound presentation O32.6 ☑
    conjoined twins O30.02- ☑
    connective system disorders (conditions in M00-
        M99) O99.89
    contracted pelvis (general) O33.1
      inlet O33.2
      outlet O33.3
    convulsions (eclamptic) (uremic) (*see also* Eclamp-
        sia) O15.9
    cracked nipple O92.11- ☑
    cystitis O23.1- ☑
    cystocele O34.8- ☑
    death of fetus (near term) O36.4 ☑
      early pregnancy O02.1

Pregnancy — *continued*
  complicated by — *continued*
    death of fetus — *continued*
      of one fetus or more in multiple gestation
          O31.2- ☑
    deciduitis O41.14- ☑
    decreased fetal movement O36.81- ☑
    dental problems O99.61- ☑
    diabetes (mellitus) O24.91- ☑
      gestational (pregnancy induced) — *see* Dia-
          betes, gestational
      pre-existing O24.31- ☑
        specified NEC O24.81- ☑
        type 1 O24.01- ☑
        type 2 O24.11- ☑
    digestive system disorders (conditions in K00-K93)
        O99.61- ☑
    diseases of — *see* Pregnancy, complicated by,
        specified body system disease
      biliary tract O26.61- ☑
      blood NEC (conditions in D65-D77) O99.11- ☑
      liver O26.61- ☑
      specified NEC O99.89
    disorders of — *see* Pregnancy, complicated by,
        specified body system disorder
      amniotic fluid and membranes O41.9- ☑
        specified NEC O41.8X- ☑
      biliary tract O26.61- ☑
      ear and mastoid process (conditions in H60-
          H95) O99.89
      eye and adnexa (conditions in H00-H59) O99.89
      liver O26.61- ☑
      skin (conditions in L00-L99) O99.71- ☑
      specified NEC O99.89
    displacement, uterus NEC O34.59- ☑
      causing obstructed labor O65.5
    disproportion (due to) O33.9
      fetal (ascites) (hydrops) (meningomyelocele)
          (sacral teratoma) (tumor) deformities NEC
          O33.7
      generally contracted pelvis O33.1
      hydrocephalic fetus O33.6 ☑
      inlet contraction of pelvis O33.2
      mixed maternal and fetal origin O33.4
      specified NEC O33.8
    double uterus O34.0- ☑
      causing obstructed labor O65.5
    drug use (conditions in F11-F19) O99.32- ☑
    eclampsia, eclamptic (coma) (convulsions) (deliri-
        um) (nephritis) (uremia) (*see also* Eclampsia)
        O15.- ☑
    ectopic pregnancy — *see* Pregnancy, ectopic
    edema O12.0- ☑
      with
        gestational hypertension, mild (*see also* Pre-
            eclampsia) O14.0- ☑
        proteinuria O12.2- ☑
    effusion, amniotic fluid — *see* Pregnancy, compli-
        cated by, premature rupture of membranes
    elderly
      multigravida O09.52- ☑
      primigravida O09.51- ☑
    embolism (*see also* Embolism, obstetric, pregnancy)
        O88.- ☑
    endocrine diseases NEC O99.28- ☑
    endometritis O86.12
    excessive weight gain O26.0- ☑
    exhaustion O26.81- ☑
      during labor and delivery O75.81
    face presentation O32.3 ☑
    failed induction of labor O61.9
      instrumental O61.1
      mechanical O61.1
      medical O61.0
      specified NEC O61.8
      surgical O61.1
    failed or difficult intubation for anesthesia
        O29.6- ☑
    false labor (pains) O47.9
      at or after 37 completed weeks of pregnancy
          O47.1
      before 37 completed weeks of pregnancy
          O47.0- ☑
    fatigue O26.81- ☑
      during labor and delivery O75.81
    fatty metamorphosis of liver O26.61- ☑
    female genital mutilation O34.8- ☑ [N90.81-] ☑

Pregnancy — continued
  complicated by — continued
    fetal (maternal care for)
      abnormality or damage O35.9 ☑
        acid-base balance O68
        specified type NEC O35.8 ☑
      acidemia O68
      acidosis O68
      alkalosis O68
      anemia and thrombocytopenia O36.82- ☑
      anencephaly O35.0 ☑
      chromosomal abnormality (conditions in Q90-Q99) O35.1 ☑
      conjoined twins O30.02- ☑
      damage from
        amniocentesis O35.7 ☑
        biopsy procedures O35.7 ☑
        drug addiction O35.5 ☑
        hematological investigation O35.7 ☑
        intrauterine contraceptive device O35.7 ☑
        maternal
          alcohol addiction O35.4 ☑
          cytomegalovirus infection O35.3 ☑
          disease NEC O35.8 ☑
          drug addiction O35.5 ☑
          listeriosis O35.8 ☑
          rubella O35.3 ☑
          toxoplasmosis O35.8 ☑
          viral infection O35.3 ☑
        medical procedure NEC O35.7 ☑
        radiation O35.6 ☑
      death (near term) O36.4 ☑
        early pregnancy O02.1
      decreased movement O36.81- ☑
      disproportion due to deformity (fetal) O33.7 ☑
      excessive growth (large for dates) O36.6- ☑
      growth retardation O36.59- ☑
        light for dates O36.59- ☑
        small for dates O36.59- ☑
      heart rate irregularity (bradycardia) (decelerations) (tachycardia) O76
      hereditary disease O35.2 ☑
      hydrocephalus O35.0 ☑
      intrauterine death O36.4 ☑
      poor growth O36.59- ☑
        light for dates O36.59- ☑
        small for dates O36.59- ☑
      problem O36.9- ☑
        specified NEC O36.89- ☑
      reduction (elective) O31.3- ☑
      selective termination O31.3- ☑
      spina bifida O35.0 ☑
      thrombocytopenia O36.82- ☑
    fibroid (tumor) (uterus) O34.1- ☑
    fissure of nipple O92.11- ☑
    gallstones O99.61- ☑
    gastric banding status O99.84- ☑
    gastric bypass status O99.84- ☑
    genital herpes (asymptomatic) (history of) (inactive) O98.3- ☑
    genital tract infection O23.9- ☑
    glomerular diseases (conditions in N00-N07) O26.83- ☑
      with hypertension, pre-existing — see Hypertension, complicating, pregnancy, pre-existing, with, renal disease
    gonorrhea O98.21- ☑
    grand multiparity O09.4 ☑
    habitual aborter — see Pregnancy, complicated by, recurrent pregnancy loss
    HELLP syndrome (hemolysis, elevated liver enzymes and low platelet count) O14.2- ☑
    hemorrhage
      antepartum — see Hemorrhage, antepartum
      before 20 completed weeks gestation O20.9
        specified NEC O20.8
      due to premature separation, placenta (see also Abruptio placentae) O45.9- ☑
      early O20.9
        specified NEC O20.8
        threatened abortion O20.0
    hemorrhoids O22.4- ☑
    hepatitis (viral) O98.41- ☑
    herniation of uterus O34.59- ☑
    high
      head at term O32.4 ☑

Pregnancy — continued
  complicated by — continued
    high — continued
      risk — see Supervision (of) (for), high-risk
    history of in utero procedure during previous pregnancy O09.82- ☑
    HIV O98.71- ☑
    human immunodeficiency virus (HIV) disease O98.71- ☑
    hydatidiform mole (see also Mole, hydatidiform) O01.9
    hydramnios O40.- ☑
    hydrocephalic fetus (disproportion) O33.6 ☑
    hydrops
      amnii O40.- ☑
      fetalis O36.2- ☑
        associated with isoimmunization (see also Pregnancy, complicated by, isoimmunization) O36.11- ☑
    hydrorrhea O42.90
    hyperemesis (gravidarum) (mild) (see also Hyperemesis, gravidarum) O21.0
    hypertension — see Hypertension, complicating pregnancy
    hypertensive
      heart and renal disease, pre-existing — see Hypertension, complicating, pregnancy, pre-existing, with, heart disease, with renal disease
      heart disease, pre-existing — see Hypertension, complicating, pregnancy, pre-existing, with, heart disease
      renal disease, pre-existing — see Hypertension, complicating, pregnancy, pre-existing, with, renal disease
    hypotension O26.5- ☑
    immune disorders NEC (conditions in D80-D89) O99.11- ☑
    incarceration, uterus O34.51- ☑
    incompetent cervix O34.3- ☑
    inconclusive fetal viability O36.80 ☑
    infection(s) O98.91- ☑
      amniotic fluid or sac O41.10- ☑
      bladder O23.1- ☑
      carrier state NEC O99.830
        streptococcus B O99.820
      genital organ or tract O23.9- ☑
        specified NEC O23.59- ☑
      genitourinary tract O23.9- ☑
      gonorrhea O98.21- ☑
      hepatitis (viral) O98.41- ☑
      HIV O98.71- ☑
      human immunodeficiency virus (HIV) O98.71- ☑
      kidney O23.0- ☑
      nipple O91.01- ☑
      parasitic disease O98.91- ☑
        specified NEC O98.81- ☑
      protozoal disease O98.61- ☑
      sexually transmitted NEC O98.31- ☑
      specified type NEC O98.81- ☑
      syphilis O98.11- ☑
      tuberculosis O98.01- ☑
      urethra O23.2- ☑
      urinary (tract) O23.4- ☑
        specified NEC O23.3- ☑
      viral disease O98.51- ☑
    injury or poisoning (conditions in S00-T88) O9A.21- ☑ (following O99)
      due to abuse
        physical O9A.31- ☑ (following O99)
        psychological O9A.51- ☑ (following O99)
        sexual O9A.41- ☑ (following O99)
    insufficient
      prenatal care O09.3- ☑
      weight gain O26.1- ☑
    insulin resistance O26.89 ☑
    intrauterine fetal death (near term) O36.4 ☑
      early pregnancy O02.1
      multiple gestation (one fetus or more) O31.2- ☑
    isoimmunization O36.11- ☑
      anti-A sensitization O36.11- ☑
      anti-B sensitization O36.19- ☑
      Rh O36.09- ☑
        anti-D antibody O36.01- ☑

Pregnancy — continued
  complicated by — continued
    isoimmunization — continued
      specified NEC O36.19- ☑
    laceration of uterus NEC O71.81
    malformation
      placenta, placental (vessel) O43.10- ☑
        specified NEC O43.19- ☑
      uterus (congenital) O34.0- ☑
    malnutrition (conditions in E40-E46) O25.1- ☑
    maternal hypotension syndrome O26.5- ☑
    mental disorders (conditions in F01-F09, F20-F99) O99.34- ☑
      alcohol use O99.31- ☑
      drug use O99.32- ☑
      smoking O99.33- ☑
    mentum presentation O32.3 ☑
    metabolic disorders O99.28- ☑
    missed
      abortion O02.1
      delivery O36.4 ☑
    multiple gestations O30.9- ☑
      conjoined twins O30.02- ☑
      quadruplet — see Pregnancy, quadruplet
      specified complication NEC O31.8X- ☑
      specified number of multiples NEC — see Pregnancy, multiple (gestation), specified NEC
      triplet — see Pregnancy, triplet
      twin — see Pregnancy, twin
    musculoskeletal condition (conditions is M00-M99) O99.89
    necrosis, liver (conditions in K72) O26.61- ☑
    neoplasm
      benign
        cervix O34.4- ☑
        corpus uteri O34.1- ☑
        uterus O34.1- ☑
      malignant O9A.11- ☑ (following O99)
    nephropathy NEC O26.83- ☑
    nervous system condition (conditions in G00-G99) O99.35- ☑
    nutritional diseases NEC O99.28- ☑
    obesity (pre-existing) O99.21- ☑
    obesity surgery status O99.84- ☑
    oblique lie or presentation O32.2 ☑
    older mother — see Pregnancy, complicated by, elderly
    oligohydramnios O41.0- ☑
      with premature rupture of membranes (see also Pregnancy, complicated by, premature rupture of membranes) O42.- ☑
    onset (spontaneous) of labor after 37 completed weeks of gestation but before 39 completed weeks gestation, with delivery by (planned) cesarean section O75.82
    oophoritis O23.52- ☑
    overdose, drug (see also Table of Drugs and Chemicals, by drug, poisoning) O9A.21- ☑ (following O99)
    oversize fetus O33.5 ☑
    papyraceous fetus O31.0- ☑
    pelvic inflammatory disease O99.89
    periodontal disease O99.61- ☑
    peripheral neuritis O26.82- ☑
    peritoneal (pelvic) adhesions O99.89
    phlebitis O22.9- ☑
    phlebopathy O22.9- ☑
    phlebothrombosis (superficial) O22.2- ☑
      deep O22.3- ☑
    placenta accreta O43.21- ☑
    placenta increta O43.22- ☑
    placenta percreta O43.23- ☑
    placenta previa O44.0- ☑
      complete O44.0- ☑
        with hemorrhage O44.1- ☑
      marginal O44.2- ☑
        with hemorrhage O44.3- ☑
      partial O44.2- ☑
        with hemorrhage O44.3- ☑
    placental disorder O43.9- ☑
      specified NEC O43.89- ☑
    placental dysfunction O43.89- ☑
    placental infarction O43.81- ☑
    placental insufficiency O36.51- ☑

260

☑ Additional Character Required — Refer to the Tabular List for Character Selection   ▽ Subterms under main terms may continue to next column or page

Pregnancy — continued
  complicated by — continued
    placental transfusion syndromes
      fetomaternal O43.01- ☑
      fetus to fetus O43.02- ☑
      maternofetal O43.01- ☑
    placentitis O41.14- ☑
    pneumonia O99.51- ☑
    poisoning (see also Table of Drugs and Chemicals)
      O9A.21 ☑ (following O99)
    polyhydramnios O40- ☑
    polymorphic eruption of pregnancy O26.86
    poor obstetric history NEC O09.29- ☑
    postmaturity (post-term) (40 to 42 weeks) O48.0
      more than 42 completed weeks gestation
        (prolonged) O48.1
    pre-eclampsia O14.9- ☑
      mild O14.0- ☑
      moderate O14.0- ☑
      severe O14.1- ☑
        with hemolysis, elevated liver enzymes and
          low platelet count (HELLP) O14.2- ☑
    premature labor — see Pregnancy, complicated
      by, preterm labor
    premature rupture of membranes O42.90
      with onset of labor
        after 24 hours O42.10
          at or after 37 weeks gestation, onset of
            labor more than 24 hours follow-
            ing rupture O42.12
          pre-term (before 37 completed weeks
            of gestation) O42.11- ☑
        within 24 hours O42.00
          at or after 37 weeks gestation, onset of
            labor within 24 hours of rupture
            O42.02
          pre-term (before 37 completed weeks
            of gestation) O42.01- ☑
      at or after 37 weeks gestation, unspecified as
        to length of time between rupture and
        onset of labor O42.92
      full-term, unspecified as to length of time be-
        tween rupture and onset of labor O42.92
      pre-term (before 37 completed weeks of gesta-
        tion) O42.91- ☑
    premature separation of placenta (see also Abrup-
      tio placentae) O45.9- ☑
    presentation, fetal — see Delivery, complicated
      by, malposition
    preterm delivery O60.10 ☑
    preterm labor
      with delivery O60.10 ☑
        preterm O60.10 ☑
        term O60.20 ☑
      without delivery O60.00
        second trimester O60.02
        third trimester O60.03
      second trimester
        with preterm delivery
          second trimester O60.12 ☑
          third trimester O60.13 ☑
        with term delivery O60.22 ☑
        without delivery O60.02
      third trimester
        with term delivery O60.23 ☑
        with third trimester preterm delivery
          O60.14 ☑
        without delivery O60.03
    previous history of — see Pregnancy, supervision
      of, high-risk
    prolapse, uterus O34.52- ☑
    proteinuria (gestational) (see also Proteinuria,
      gestational) O12.1- ☑
      with edema O12.2- ☑
    pruritic urticarial papules and plaques of pregnancy
      (PUPPP) O26.86
    pruritus (neurogenic) O26.89- ☑
    psychosis or psychoneurosis (puerperal) F53
    ptyalism O26.89- ☑
    PUPPP (pruritic urticarial papules and plaques of
      pregnancy) O26.86
    pyelitis O23.0- ☑
    recurrent pregnancy loss O26.2- ☑
    renal disease or failure NEC O26.83- ☑
      with secondary hypertension, pre-existing —
        see Hypertension, complicating, pregnan-
        cy, pre-existing, secondary

Pregnancy — continued
  complicated by — continued
    renal disease or failure — continued
      hypertensive, pre-existing — see Hypertension,
        complicating, pregnancy, pre-existing,
        with, renal disease
    respiratory condition (conditions in J00-J99)
      O99.51- ☑
    retained, retention
      dead ovum O02.0
      intrauterine contraceptive device O26.3- ☑
    retroversion, uterus O34.53- ☑
    Rh immunization, incompatibility or sensitization
      NEC O36.09- ☑
      anti-D antibody O36.01- ☑
    rupture
      amnion (premature) (see also Pregnancy, com-
        plicated by, premature rupture of mem-
        branes) O42- ☑
      membranes (premature) (see also Pregnancy,
        complicated by, premature rupture of
        membranes) O42- ☑
      uterus (during labor) O71.1
        before onset of labor O71.0- ☑
    salivation (excessive) O26.89- ☑
    salpingitis O23.52- ☑
    salpingo-oophoritis O23.52- ☑
    sepsis (conditions in A40, A41) O98.81- ☑
    size date discrepancy (uterine) O26.84- ☑
    skin condition (conditions in L00-L99) O99.71- ☑
    smoking (tobacco) O99.33- ☑
    social problem O99.7- ☑
    specified condition NEC O26.89- ☑
    spotting O26.85- ☑
    streptococcus group B (GBS) carrier state O99.820
    subluxation of symphysis (pubis) O26.71- ☑
    syphilis (conditions in A50-A53) O98.11- ☑
    threatened
      abortion O20.0
      labor O47.9
        at or after 37 completed weeks of gestation
          O47.1
        before 37 completed weeks of gestation
          O47.0- ☑
    thrombophlebitis (superficial) O22.2- ☑
    thrombosis O22.9- ☑
      cerebral venous O22.5- ☑
      cerebrovenous sinus O22.5- ☑
      deep O22.3- ☑
    tobacco use disorder (smoking) O99.33- ☑
    torsion of uterus O34.59- ☑
    toxemia O14.9- ☑
    transverse lie or presentation O32.2 ☑
    tuberculosis (conditions in A15-A19) O98.01- ☑
    tumor (benign)
      cervix O34.4- ☑
      malignant O9A.11- ☑ (following O99)
      uterus O34.1- ☑
    unstable lie O32.0
    upper respiratory infection O99.51- ☑
    urethritis O23.2- ☑
    uterine size date discrepancy O26.84- ☑
    vaginitis or vulvitis O23.59- ☑
    varicose veins (lower extremities) O22.0- ☑
      genitals O22.1- ☑
      legs O22.0- ☑
      perineal O22.1- ☑
      vaginal or vulval O22.1- ☑
    venereal disease NEC (conditions in A63.8)
      O98.31- ☑
    venous disorders O22.9- ☑
      specified NEC O22.8X- ☑
    very young mother — see Pregnancy, complicated
      by, young mother
    viral diseases (conditions in A80-B09, B25-B34)
      O98.51- ☑
    vomiting O21.9
      due to diseases classified elsewhere O21.8
      hyperemesis gravidarum (mild) (see also Hyper-
        emesis, gravidarum) O21.0
      late (occurring after 20 weeks of gestation)
        O21.2
    young mother
      multigravida O09.62- ☑
      primigravida O09.61- ☑
  complicated NOS O26.9- ☑
  concealed O09.3- ☑

Pregnancy — continued
  continuing following
    elective fetal reduction of one or more fetus
      O31.3-
    intrauterine death of one or more fetus O31.2- ☑
    spontaneous abortion of one or more fetus
      O31.1- ☑
  cornual O00.80
    with intrauterine pregnancy O00.81
  ectopic (ruptured) O00.90
    with intrauterine pregnancy O00.91
    abdominal O00.00
      with
        intrauterine pregnancy O00.01
        viable fetus O36.7- ☑
    cervical O00.80
      with intrauterine pregnancy O00.81
    complicated (by) O08.9
      afibrinogenemia O08.1
      cardiac arrest O08.81
      chemical damage of pelvic organ(s) O08.6
      circulatory collapse O08.3
      defibrination syndrome O08.1
      electrolyte imbalance O08.5
      embolism (amniotic fluid) (blood clot) (pul-
        monary) (septic) O08.2
      endometritis O08.0
      genital tract and pelvic infection O08.0
      hemorrhage (delayed) (excessive) O08.1
      infection
        genital tract or pelvic O08.0
        kidney O08.83
        urinary tract O08.3
      intravascular coagulation O08.1
      laceration of pelvic organ(s) O08.6
      metabolic disorder O08.5
      oliguria O08.4
      oophoritis O08.0
      parametritis O08.0
      pelvic peritonitis O08.0
      perforation of pelvic organ(s) O08.6
      renal failure or shutdown O08.4
      salpingitis or salpingo-oophoritis O08.0
      sepsis O08.82
      shock O08.83
        septic O08.82
      specified condition NEC O08.89
      tubular necrosis (renal) O08.4
      uremia O08.4
      urinary infection O08.83
      venous complication NEC O08.7
        embolism O08.2
    cornual O00.80
      with intrauterine pregnancy O00.81
    intraligamentous O00.80
      with intrauterine pregnancy O00.81
    mural O00.80
      with intrauterine pregnancy O00.81
    ovarian O00.20- ☑
      with intrauterine pregnancy O00.21- ☑
    specified site NEC O00.80
      with intrauterine pregnancy O00.81
    tubal (ruptured) O00.10- ☑
      with intrauterine pregnancy O00.11- ☑
  examination (normal) Z34.9- ☑
    first Z34.0- ☑
    high-risk — see Pregnancy, supervision of, high-
      risk
    specified Z34.8- ☑
  extrauterine — see Pregnancy, ectopic
  fallopian O00.10- ☑
    with intrauterine pregnancy O00.11- ☑
  false F45.8
  gestational carrier Z33.3
  hidden O09.3- ☑
  high-risk — see Pregnancy, supervision of, high-risk
  incidental finding Z33.1
  interstitial O00.80
    with intrauterine pregnancy O00.81
  intraligamentous O00.80
    with intrauterine pregnancy O00.81
  intramural O00.80
    with intrauterine pregnancy O00.81
  intraperitoneal O00.00
    with intrauterine pregnancy O00.01
  isthmian O00.10- ☑
    with intrauterine pregnancy O00.11- ☑
  mesometric (mural) O00.80

Pregnancy — *continued*
  mesometric — *continued*
    with intrauterine pregnancy O00.81
  molar NEC O02.0
    complicated (by) O08.9
      afibrinogenemia O08.1
      cardiac arrest O08.81
      chemical damage of pelvic organ(s) O08.6
      circulatory collapse O08.3
      defibrination syndrome O08.1
      electrolyte imbalance O08.5
      embolism (amniotic fluid) (blood clot) (pulmonary) (septic) O08.2
      endometritis O08.0
      genital tract and pelvic infection O08.0
      hemorrhage (delayed) (excessive) O08.1
      infection
        genital tract or pelvic O08.0
        kidney O08.83
        urinary tract O08.83
      intravascular coagulation O08.1
      laceration of pelvic organ(s) O08.6
      metabolic disorder O08.5
      oliguria O08.4
      oophoritis O08.0
      parametritis O08.0
      pelvic peritonitis O08.0
      perforation of pelvic organ(s) O08.6
      renal failure or shutdown O08.4
      salpingitis or salpingo-oophoritis O08.0
      sepsis O08.82
      shock O08.3
        septic O08.82
      specified condition NEC O08.89
      tubular necrosis (renal) O08.4
      uremia O08.4
      urinary infection O08.83
      venous complication NEC O08.7
        embolism O08.2
    hydatidiform (*see also* Mole, hydatidiform) O01.9
  multiple (gestation) O30.9- ☑
    greater than quadruplets — *see* Pregnancy, multiple (gestation), specified NEC
    specified NEC O30.80- ☑
      with
        two or more monoamniotic fetuses O30.82- ☑
        two or more monochorionic fetuses O30.81- ☑
      two or more monoamniotic fetuses O30.82- ☑
      two or more monochorionic fetuses O30.81- ☑
      unable to determine number of placenta and number of amniotic sacs O30.89- ☑
      unspecified number of placenta and unspecified number of amniotic sacs O30.80- ☑
  mural O00.80
    with intrauterine pregnancy O00.81
  normal (supervision of) Z34.9- ☑
    first Z34.0- ☑
    high-risk — *see* Pregnancy, supervision of, high-risk
    specified Z34.8- ☑
  ovarian O00.20- ☑
    with intrauterine pregnancy O00.21- ☑
  postmature (40 to 42 weeks) O48.0
    more than 42 weeks gestation O48.1
  post-term (40 to 42 weeks) O48.0
  prenatal care only Z34.9- ☑
    first Z34.0- ☑
    high-risk — *see* Pregnancy, supervision of, high-risk
    specified Z34.8- ☑
  prolonged (more than 42 weeks gestation) O48.1
  quadruplet O30.20- ☑
    with
        two or more monoamniotic fetuses O30.22- ☑
        two or more monochorionic fetuses O30.21- ☑
      two or more monoamniotic fetuses O30.22- ☑
      two or more monochorionic fetuses O30.21- ☑
      unable to determine number of placenta and number of amniotic sacs O30.29- ☑
      unspecified number of placenta and unspecified number of amniotic sacs O30.20- ☑
  quintuplet — *see* Pregnancy, multiple (gestation), specified NEC
  sextuplet — *see* Pregnancy, multiple (gestation), specified NEC

Pregnancy — *continued*
  supervision of
    concealed pregnancy O09.3- ☑
    elderly mother
      multigravida O09.52- ☑
      primigravida O09.51- ☑
    hidden pregnancy O09.3- ☑
    high-risk O09.9- ☑
      due to (history of)
        ectopic pregnancy O09.1- ☑
        elderly — *see* Pregnancy, supervision, elderly mother
        grand multiparity O09.4 ☑
        in utero procedure during previous pregnancy O09.82- ☑
        in vitro fertilization O09.81- ☑
        infertility O09.0- ☑
        insufficient prenatal care O09.3- ☑
        molar pregnancy O09.A- ☑
        multiple previous pregnancies O09.4- ☑
        older mother — *see* Pregnancy, supervision of, elderly mother
        poor reproductive or obstetric history NEC O09.29- ☑
        pre-term labor O09.21- ☑
        previous
          neonatal death O09.29- ☑
        social problems O09.7- ☑
        specified NEC O09.89- ☑
        very young mother — *see* Pregnancy, supervision, young mother
      resulting from in vitro fertilization O09.81- ☑
    normal Z34.9- ☑
      first Z34.0- ☑
      specified NEC Z34.8- ☑
    young mother
      multigravida O09.62- ☑
      primigravida O09.61- ☑
  triplet O30.10- ☑
    with
        two or more monoamniotic fetuses O30.12- ☑
        two or more monochorionic fetuses O30.11- ☑
      two or more monoamniotic fetuses O30.12- ☑
      two or more monochorionic fetuses O30.11- ☑
      unable to determine number of placenta and number of amniotic sacs O30.19- ☑
      unspecified number of placenta and unspecified number of amniotic sacs O30.10- ☑
  tubal (with abortion) (with rupture) O00.10- ☑
    with intrauterine pregnancy O00.11- ☑
  twin O30.00- ☑
    conjoined O30.02- ☑
    dichorionic/diamniotic (two placenta, two amniotic sacs) O30.04- ☑
    monochorionic/diamniotic (one placenta, two amniotic sacs) O30.03- ☑
    monochorionic/monoamniotic (one placenta, one amniotic sac) O30.01- ☑
    unable to determine number of placenta and number of amniotic sacs O30.09- ☑
    unspecified number of placenta and unspecified number of amniotic sacs O30.00- ☑
  unwanted Z64.0
  weeks of gestation
    less than 8 weeks Z3A.01 (*following* Z36)
    8 weeks Z3A.08 (*following* Z36)
    9 weeks Z3A.09 (*following* Z36)
    10 weeks Z3A.10 (*following* Z36)
    11 weeks Z3A.11 (*following* Z36)
    12 weeks Z3A.12 (*following* Z36)
    13 weeks Z3A.13 (*following* Z36)
    14 weeks Z3A.14 (*following* Z36)
    15 weeks Z3A.15 (*following* Z36)
    16 weeks Z3A.16 (*following* Z36)
    17 weeks Z3A.17 (*following* Z36)
    18 weeks Z3A.18 (*following* Z36)
    19 weeks Z3A.19 (*following* Z36)
    20 weeks Z3A.20 (*following* Z36)
    21 weeks Z3A.21 (*following* Z36)
    22 weeks Z3A.22 (*following* Z36)
    23 weeks Z3A.23 (*following* Z36)
    24 weeks Z3A.24 (*following* Z36)
    25 weeks Z3A.25 (*following* Z36)
    26 weeks Z3A.26 (*following* Z36)
    27 weeks Z3A.27 (*following* Z36)
    28 weeks Z3A.28 (*following* Z36)
    29 weeks Z3A.29 (*following* Z36)

Pregnancy — *continued*
  weeks of gestation — *continued*
    30 weeks Z3A.30 (*following* Z36)
    31 weeks Z3A.31 (*following* Z36)
    32 weeks Z3A.32 (*following* Z36)
    33 weeks Z3A.33 (*following* Z36)
    34 weeks Z3A.34 (*following* Z36)
    35 weeks Z3A.35 (*following* Z36)
    36 weeks Z3A.36 (*following* Z36)
    37 weeks Z3A.37 (*following* Z36)
    38 weeks Z3A.38 (*following* Z36)
    39 weeks Z3A.39 (*following* Z36)
    40 weeks Z3A.40 (*following* Z36)
    41 weeks Z3A.41 (*following* Z36)
    42 weeks Z3A.42 (*following* Z36)
    greater than 42 weeks Z3A.49 (*following* Z36)
    not specified Z3A.00 (*following* Z36)
Preiser's disease — *see* Osteonecrosis, secondary, due to, trauma, metacarpus
Pre-kwashiorkor — *see* Malnutrition, severe
Preleukemia (syndrome) D46.9
Preluxation, hip, congenital Q65.6
Premature (*see also* condition)
  adrenarche E27.0
  aging E34.8
  beats I49.40
    atrial I49.1
    auricular I49.1
    supraventricular I49.1
  birth NEC — *see* Preterm, newborn
  closure, foramen ovale Q21.8
  contraction
    atrial I49.1
    atrioventricular I49.2
    auricular I49.1
    auriculoventricular I49.49
    heart (extrasystole) I49.49
    junctional I49.2
    ventricular I49.3
  delivery (*see also* Pregnancy, complicated by, preterm labor) O60.10 ☑
  ejaculation F52.4
  infant NEC — *see* Preterm, newborn
    light-for-dates — *see* Light for dates
  labor — *see* Pregnancy, complicated by, preterm labor
  lungs P28.0
  menopause E28.319
    asymptomatic E28.319
    symptomatic E28.310
  newborn
    less than 37 completed weeks — *see* Preterm, newborn
    extreme (less than 28 completed weeks) — *see* Immaturity, extreme
  puberty E30.1
  rupture membranes or amnion — *see* Pregnancy, complicated by, premature rupture of membranes
  senility E34.8
  thelarche E30.8
  ventricular systole I49.3
Prematurity NEC (less than 37 completed weeks) — *see* Preterm, newborn
  extreme (less than 28 completed weeks) — *see* Immaturity, extreme
Premenstrual
  dysphoric disorder (PMDD) F32.81
  tension (syndrome) N94.3
Premolarization, cuspids K00.2
Prenatal
  care, normal pregnancy — *see* Pregnancy, normal
  screening of mother (*see also* Encounter, antenatal screening) Z36.9
  teeth K00.6
Preparatory care for subsequent treatment NEC
  for dialysis Z49.01
    peritoneal Z49.02
Prepartum — *see* condition
Preponderance, left or right ventricular I51.7
Prepuce — *see* condition
PRES (posterior reversible encephalopathy syndrome) I67.83
Presbycardia R54
Presbycusis, presbyacusia H91.1- ☑
Presbyesophagus K22.8
Presbyophrenia F03 ☑
Presbyopia H52.4
Prescription of contraceptives (initial) Z30.019

Prescription of contraceptives — continued
  barrier Z30.018
    diaphragm Z30.018
  emergency (postcoital) Z30.012
  implantable subdermal Z30.017
  injectable Z30.013
  intrauterine contraceptive device Z30.014
  pills Z30.011
  postcoital (emergency) Z30.012
  repeat Z30.40
    barrier Z30.49
    diaphragm Z30.49
    implantable subdermal Z30.46
    injectable Z30.42
    pills Z30.41
    specified type NEC Z30.49
    transdermal patch hormonal Z30.45
    vaginal ring hormonal Z30.44
  specified type NEC Z30.018
    transdermal patch hormonal Z30.016
    vaginal ring hormonal Z30.015
Presence (of)
  ankle-joint implant (functional) (prosthesis) Z96.66- ☑
  aortocoronary (bypass) graft Z95.1
  arterial-venous shunt (dialysis) Z99.2
  artificial
    eye (globe) Z97.0
    heart (fully implantable) (mechanical) Z95.812
      valve Z95.2
    larynx Z96.3
    lens (intraocular) Z96.1
    limb (complete) (partial) Z97.1- ☑
      arm Z97.1- ☑
        bilateral Z97.15
      leg Z97.1- ☑
        bilateral Z97.16
  audiological implant (functional) Z96.29
  bladder implant (functional) Z96.0
  bone
    conduction hearing device Z96.29
    implant (functional) NEC Z96.7
    joint (prosthesis) — see Presence, joint implant
  cardiac
    defibrillator (functional) (with synchronous cardiac pacemaker) Z95.810
    implant or graft Z95.9
      specified type NEC Z95.818
    pacemaker Z95.0
    resynchronization therapy
      defibrillator Z95.810
      pacemaker Z95.0
  cardioverter-defibrillator (ICD) Z95.810
  cerebrospinal fluid drainage device Z98.2
  cochlear implant (functional) Z96.21
  contact lens (es) Z97.3
  coronary artery graft or prosthesis Z95.5
  CRT-D (cardiac resynchronization therapy defibrillator) Z95.810
  CRT-P (cardiac resynchronization therapy pacemaker) Z95.0
  CSF shunt Z98.2
  dental prosthesis device Z97.2
  dentures Z97.2
  device (external) NEC Z97.8
    cardiac NEC Z95.818
    heart assist Z95.811
    implanted (functional) Z96.9
      specified NEC Z96.89
    prosthetic Z97.8
  ear implant Z96.20
    cochlear implant Z96.21
    myringotomy tube Z96.22
    specified type NEC Z96.29
  elbow-joint implant (functional) (prosthesis) Z96.62- ☑
  endocrine implant (functional) NEC Z96.49
  eustachian tube stent or device (functional) Z96.29
  external hearing-aid or device Z97.4
  finger-joint implant (functional) (prosthetic) Z96.69- ☑
  functional implant Z96.9
    specified NEC Z96.89
  graft
    cardiac NEC Z95.818
    vascular NEC Z95.828
  hearing-aid or device (external) Z97.4
    implant (bone) (cochlear) (functional) Z96.21
  heart assist device Z95.811
  heart valve implant (functional) Z95.2

Presence — continued
  heart valve implant — continued
    prosthetic Z95.2
    specified type NEC Z95.4
    xenogenic Z95.3
  hip-joint implant (functional) (prosthesis) Z96.64- ☑
  ICD (cardioverter-defibrillator) Z95.810
  implanted device (artificial) (functional) (prosthetic) Z96.9
    automatic cardiac defibrillator (with synchronous cardiac pacemaker) Z95.810
    cardiac pacemaker Z95.0
    cochlear Z96.21
    dental Z96.5
    heart Z95.812
    heart valve Z95.2
      prosthetic Z95.2
      specified NEC Z95.4
      xenogenic Z95.3
    insulin pump Z96.41
    intraocular lens Z96.1
    joint Z96.60
      ankle Z96.66- ☑
      elbow Z96.62- ☑
      finger Z96.69- ☑
      hip Z96.64- ☑
      knee Z96.65- ☑
      shoulder Z96.61- ☑
      specified NEC Z96.698
      wrist Z96.63- ☑
    larynx Z96.3
    myringotomy tube Z96.22
    otological Z96.20
      cochlear Z96.21
      eustachian stent Z96.29
      myringotomy Z96.22
      specified NEC Z96.29
      stapes Z96.29
    skin Z96.81
    skull plate Z96.7
    specified NEC Z96.89
    urogenital Z96.0
  insulin pump (functional) Z96.41
  intestinal bypass or anastomosis Z98.0
  intraocular lens (functional) Z96.1
  intrauterine contraceptive device (IUD) Z97.5
  intravascular implant (functional) (prosthetic) NEC Z95.9
    coronary artery Z95.5
    defibrillator (with synchronous cardiac pacemaker) Z95.810
    peripheral vessel (with angioplasty) Z95.820
  joint implant (prosthetic) (any) Z96.60
    ankle — see Presence, ankle joint implant
    elbow — see Presence, elbow joint implant
    finger — see Presence, finger joint implant
    hip — see Presence, hip joint implant
    knee — see Presence, knee joint implant
    shoulder — see Presence, shoulder joint implant
    specified joint NEC Z96.698
    wrist — see Presence, wrist joint implant
  knee-joint implant (functional) (prosthesis) Z96.65- ☑
  laryngeal implant (functional) Z96.3
  mandibular implant (dental) Z96.5
  myringotomy tube(s) Z96.22
  orthopedic-joint implant (prosthetic) (any) — see Presence, joint implant
  otological implant (functional) Z96.29
  shoulder-joint implant (functional) (prosthesis) Z96.61- ☑
  skull-plate implant Z96.7
  spectacles Z97.3
  stapes implant (functional) Z96.29
  systemic lupus erythematosus [SLE] inhibitor D68.62
  tendon implant (functional) (graft) Z96.7
  tooth root(s) implant Z96.5
  ureteral stent Z96.0
  urethral stent Z96.0
  urogenital implant (functional) Z96.0
  vascular implant or device Z95.9
    access port device Z95.828
    specified type NEC Z95.828
  wrist-joint implant (functional) (prosthesis) Z96.63- ☑
Presenile (see also condition)
  dementia F03 ☑
  premature aging E34.8
Presentation, fetal — see Delivery, complicated by, malposition

Prespondylolisthesis (congenital) Q76.2
Pressure
  area, skin — see Ulcer, pressure, by site
  brachial plexus G54.0
  brain G93.5
    injury at birth NEC P11.1
  cerebral — see Pressure, brain
  chest R07.89
  cone, tentorial G93.5
  hyposystolic (see also Hypotension)
    incidental reading, without diagnosis of hypotension R03.1
  increased
    intracranial (benign) G93.2
      injury at birth P11.0
    intraocular H40.05- ☑
  lumbosacral plexus G54.1
  mediastinum J98.59
  necrosis (chronic) — see Ulcer, pressure, by site
  parental, inappropriate (excessive) Z62.6
  sore (chronic) — see Ulcer, pressure, by site
  spinal cord G95.20
  ulcer (chronic) — see Ulcer, pressure, by site
  venous, increased I87.8
Pre-syncope R55
Preterm
  delivery (see also Pregnancy, complicated by, preterm labor) O60.10 ☑
  labor — see Pregnancy, complicated by, preterm labor
  newborn (infant) P07.30
    gestational age
      28 completed weeks (28 weeks, 0 days through 28 weeks, 6 days) P07.31
      29 completed weeks (29 weeks, 0 days through 29 weeks, 6 days) P07.32
      30 completed weeks (30 weeks, 0 days through 30 weeks, 6 days) P07.33
      31 completed weeks (31 weeks, 0 days through 31 weeks, 6 days) P07.34
      32 completed weeks (32 weeks, 0 days through 32 weeks, 6 days) P07.35
      33 completed weeks (33 weeks, 0 days through 33 weeks, 6 days) P07.36
      34 completed weeks (34 weeks, 0 days through 34 weeks, 6 days) P07.37
      35 completed weeks (35 weeks, 0 days through 35 weeks, 6 days) P07.38
      36 completed weeks (36 weeks, 0 days through 36 weeks, 6 days) P07.39
Previa
  placenta (total) (without hemorrhage) O44.0- ☑
    with hemorrhage O44.1- ☑
    complete O44.0- ☑
      with hemorrhage O44.1- ☑
    low (see also Delivery, complicated, by, placenta, low) O44.4- ☑
      with hemorrhage O44.5- ☑
    marginal O44.2- ☑
      with hemorrhage O44.3- ☑
    partial O44.2- ☑
      with hemorrhage O44.3- ☑
  vasa O69.4 ☑
Priapism N48.30
  due to
    disease classified elsewhere N48.32
    drug N48.33
    specified cause NEC N48.39
    trauma N48.31
Prickling sensation (skin) R20.2
Prickly heat L74.0
Primary — see condition
Primigravida
  elderly, affecting management of pregnancy, labor and delivery (supervision only) — see Pregnancy, complicated by, elderly, primigravida
  older, affecting management of pregnancy, labor and delivery (supervision only) — see Pregnancy, complicated by, elderly, primigravida
  very young, affecting management of pregnancy, labor and delivery (supervision only) — see Pregnancy, complicated by, young mother, primigravida
Primipara
  elderly, affecting management of pregnancy, labor and delivery (supervision only) — see Pregnancy, complicated by, elderly, primigravida

Index

Primipara — Proctocele

Primipara — *continued*
  older, affecting management of pregnancy, labor and delivery (supervision only) — *see* Pregnancy, complicated by, elderly, primigravida
  very young, affecting management of pregnancy, labor and delivery (supervision only) — *see* Pregnancy, complicated by, young mother, primigravida
Primus varus (bilateral) Q66.2 ✓
PRIND (Prolonged reversible ischemic neurologic deficit) I63.9
Pringle's disease (tuberous sclerosis) Q85.1
Prinzmetal angina I20.1
Prizefighter ear — *see* Cauliflower ear
Problem (with) (related to)
  academic Z55.8
  acculturation Z60.3
  adjustment (to)
    change of job Z56.1
    life-cycle transition Z60.0
    pension Z60.0
    retirement Z60.0
  adopted child Z62.821
  alcoholism in family Z63.72
  atypical parenting situation Z62.9
  bankruptcy Z59.8
  behavioral (adult) F69
    drug seeking Z76.5
  birth of sibling affecting child Z62.898
  care (of)
    provider dependency Z74.9
      specified NEC Z74.8
    sick or handicapped person in family or household Z63.6
  child
    abuse (affecting the child) — *see* Maltreatment, child
    custody or support proceedings Z65.3
    in care of non-parental family member Z62.21
    in foster care Z62.21
    in welfare custody Z62.21
    living in orphanage or group home Z62.22
  child-rearing Z62.9
    specified NEC Z62.898
  communication (developmental) F80.9
  conflict or discord (with)
    boss Z56.4
    classmates Z55.4
    counselor Z64.4
    employer Z56.4
    family Z63.9
      specified NEC Z63.8
    probation officer Z64.4
    social worker Z64.4
    teachers Z55.4
    workmates Z56.4
  conviction in legal proceedings Z65.0
    with imprisonment Z65.1
  counselor Z64.4
  creditors Z59.8
  digestive K92.9
  drug addict in family Z63.72
  ear — *see* Disorder, ear
  economic Z59.9
    affecting care Z59.9
    specified NEC Z59.8
  education Z55.9
    specified NEC Z55.8
  employment Z56.9
    change of job Z56.1
    discord Z56.4
    environment Z56.5
    sexual harassment Z56.81
    specified NEC Z56.89
    stressful schedule Z56.3
    stress NEC Z56.6
    threat of job loss Z56.2
    unemployment Z56.0
  enuresis, child F98.0
  eye H57.9
  failed examinations (school) Z55.2
  falling Z91.81
  family (*see also* Disruption, family) Z63.9
    specified NEC Z63.8
  feeding (elderly) (infant) R63.3
    newborn P92.9
      breast P92.5
      overfeeding P92.4
      slow P92.2

Problem — *continued*
  feeding — *continued*
    newborn — *continued*
      specified NEC P92.8
      underfeeding P92.3
    nonorganic F50.89
  finance Z59.9
    specified NEC Z59.8
  foreclosure on loan Z59.8
  foster child Z62.822
  frightening experience(s) in childhood Z62.898
  genital NEC
    female N94.9
    male N50.9
  health care Z75.9
    specified NEC Z75.8
  hearing — *see* Deafness
  homelessness Z59.0
  housing Z59.9
    inadequate Z59.1
    isolated Z59.8
    specified NEC Z59.8
  identity (of childhood) F93.8
  illegitimate pregnancy (unwanted) Z64.0
  illiteracy Z55.0
  impaired mobility Z74.09
  imprisonment or incarceration Z65.1
  inadequate teaching affecting education Z55.8
  inappropriate (excessive) parental pressure Z62.6
  influencing health status NEC Z78.9
  in-law Z63.1
  institutionalization, affecting child Z62.22
  intrafamilial communication Z63.8
  jealousy, child F93.8
  landlord Z59.2
  language (developmental) F80.9
  learning (developmental) F81.9
  legal Z65.3
    conviction without imprisonment Z65.0
    imprisonment Z65.1
    release from prison Z65.2
  life-management Z73.9
    specified NEC Z73.89
  life-style Z72.9
    gambling Z72.6
    high-risk sexual behavior (heterosexual) Z72.51
      bisexual Z72.53
      homosexual Z72.52
    inappropriate eating habits Z72.4
    self-damaging behavior NEC Z72.89
    specified NEC Z72.89
    tobacco use Z72.0
  literacy Z55.9
    low level Z55.0
    specified NEC Z55.8
  living alone Z60.2
  lodgers Z59.2
  loss of love relationship in childhood Z62.898
  marital Z63.0
    involving
      divorce Z63.5
      estrangement Z63.5
      gender identity F66
  mastication K08.89
  medical
    care, within family Z63.6
    facilities Z75.9
      specified NEC Z75.8
  mental F48.9
  multiparity Z64.1
  negative life events in childhood Z62.9
    altered pattern of family relationships Z62.898
    frightening experience Z62.898
    loss of
      love relationship Z62.898
      self-esteem Z62.898
    physical abuse (alleged) — *see* Maltreatment, child
    removal from home Z62.29
    specified event NEC Z62.898
  neighbor Z59.2
  neurological NEC R29.818
  new step-parent affecting child Z62.898
  none (feared complaint unfounded) Z71.1
  occupational NEC Z56.89
  parent-child — *see* Conflict, parent-child
  personal hygiene Z91.89
  personality F69
  phase-of-life transition, adjustment Z60.0

Problem — *continued*
  presence of sick or disabled person in family or household Z63.79
    needing care Z63.6
  primary support group (family) Z63.9
    specified NEC Z63.8
  probation officer Z64.4
  psychiatric F99
  psychosexual (development) F66
  psychosocial Z65.9
    religious or spiritual Z65.8
    specified NEC Z65.8
  relationship Z63.9
    childhood F93.8
  release from prison Z65.2
    religious or spiritual Z65.8
  removal from home affecting child Z62.29
  seeking and accepting known hazardous and harmful
    behavioral or psychological interventions Z65.8
    chemical, nutritional or physical interventions Z65.8
  sexual function (nonorganic) F52.9
  sight H54.7
  sleep disorder, child F51.9
  smell — *see* Disturbance, sensation, smell
  social
    environment Z60.9
      specified NEC Z60.8
    exclusion and rejection Z60.4
    worker Z64.4
  speech R47.9
    developmental F80.9
    specified NEC R47.89
  swallowing — *see* Dysphagia
  taste — *see* Disturbance, sensation, taste
  tic, child F95.0
  underachievement in school Z55.3
  unemployment Z56.0
    threatened Z56.2
  unwanted pregnancy Z64.0
  upbringing Z62.9
    specified NEC Z62.898
  urinary N39.9
  voice production R47.89
  work schedule (stressful) Z56.3
Procedure (surgical)
  converted
    arthroscopic to open Z53.33
    laparoscopic to open Z53.31
    specified procedure NEC to open Z53.39
    thoracoscopic to open Z53.32
  for purpose other than remedying health state Z41.9
    specified NEC Z41.8
  not done Z53.9
    because of
      administrative reasons Z53.8
      contraindication Z53.09
        smoking Z53.01
      patient's decision Z53.20
        for reasons of belief or group pressure Z53.1
        left against medical advice (AMA) Z53.21
        specified reason NEC Z53.29
      specified reason NEC Z53.8
Procidentia (uteri) N81.3
Proctalgia K62.89
  fugax K59.4
  spasmodic K59.4
Proctitis K62.89
  amebic (acute) A06.0
  chlamydial A56.3
  gonococcal A54.6
  granulomatous — *see* Enteritis, regional, large intestine
  herpetic A60.1
  radiation K62.7
  tuberculous A18.32
  ulcerative (chronic) K51.20
    with
      complication K51.219
        abscess K51.214
        fistula K51.213
        obstruction K51.212
        rectal bleeding K51.211
        specified NEC K51.218
Proctocele
  female (without uterine prolapse) N81.6
    with uterine prolapse N81.2
      complete N81.3
  male K62.3

Proctocolitis
food protein-induced K52.82
food-induced eosinophilic K52.82
milk protein-induced K52.82
mucosal — see Rectosigmoiditis, ulcerative
Proctoptosis K62.3
Proctorrhagia K62.5
Proctosigmoiditis K63.89
ulcerative (chronic) — see Rectosigmoiditis, ulcerative
Proctospasm K59.4
psychogenic F45.8
Profichet's disease — see Disorder, soft tissue, specified type NEC
Progeria E34.8
Prognathism (mandibular) (maxillary) M26.19
Progonoma (melanotic) — see Neoplasm, benign, by site
Progressive — see condition
Prolactinoma
specified site — see Neoplasm, benign, by site
unspecified site D35.2
Prolapse, prolapsed
anus, anal (canal) (sphincter) K62.2
arm or hand O32.2 ☑
causing obstructed labor O64.4 ☑
bladder (mucosa) (sphincter) (acquired)
congenital Q79.4
female — see Cystocele
male N32.89
breast implant (prosthetic) T85.49 ☑
cecostomy K94.09
cecum K63.4
cervix, cervical (hypertrophied) N81.2
anterior lip, obstructing labor O65.5
congenital Q51.828
postpartal, old N81.2
stump N81.85
ciliary body (traumatic) — see Laceration, eye(ball), with prolapse or loss of interocular tissue
colon (pedunculated) K63.4
colostomy K94.09
disc (intervertebral) — see Displacement, intervertebral disc
eye implant (orbital) T85.398 ☑
lens (ocular) — see Complications, intraocular lens
fallopian tube N83.4- ☑
gastric (mucosa) K31.89
genital, female N81.9
specified NEC N81.89
globe, nontraumatic — see Luxation, globe
ileostomy bud K94.19
intervertebral disc — see Displacement, intervertebral disc
intestine (small) K63.4
iris (traumatic) — see Laceration, eye(ball), with prolapse or loss of interocular tissue
nontraumatic H21.89
kidney N28.83
congenital Q63.2
laryngeal muscles or ventricle J38.7
liver K76.89
meatus urinarius N36.8
mitral (valve) I34.1
ocular lens implant — see Complications, intraocular lens
organ or site, congenital NEC — see Malposition, congenital
ovary N83.4- ☑
pelvic floor, female N81.89
perineum, female N81.89
rectum (mucosa) (sphincter) K62.3
due to trichuris trichuria B79
spleen D73.89
stomach K31.89
umbilical cord
complicating delivery O69.0 ☑
urachus, congenital Q64.4
ureter N28.89
with obstruction N13.5
with infection N13.6
ureterovesical orifice N28.89
urethra (acquired) (infected) (mucosa) N36.8
congenital Q64.71
urinary meatus N36.8
congenital Q64.72
uterovaginal N81.4
complete N81.3
incomplete N81.2

Prolapse, prolapsed — continued
uterus (with prolapse of vagina) N81.4
complete N81.3
congenital Q51.818
first degree N81.2
in pregnancy or childbirth — see Pregnancy, complicated by, abnormal, uterus
incomplete N81.2
postpartal (old) N81.4
second degree N81.2
third degree N81.3
uveal (traumatic) — see Laceration, eye(ball), with prolapse or loss of interocular tissue
vagina (anterior) (wall) — see Cystocele
with prolapse of uterus N81.4
complete N81.3
incomplete N81.2
posterior wall N81.6
posthysterectomy N99.3
vitreous (humor) H43.0-
in wound — see Laceration, eye(ball), with prolapse or loss of interocular tissue
womb — see Prolapse, uterus
Prolapsus, female N81.9
specified NEC N81.89
Proliferation(s)
primary cutaneous CD30-positive large T-cell C86.6
prostate, atypical small acinar N42.32
Proliferative — see condition
Prolonged, prolongation (of)
bleeding (time) (idiopathic) R79.1
coagulation (time) R79.1
gestation (over 42 completed weeks)
mother O48.1
newborn P08.22
interval I44.0
labor O63.9
first stage O63.0
second stage O63.1
partial thromboplastin time (PTT) R79.1
pregnancy (more than 42 weeks gestation) O48.1
prothrombin time R79.1
QT interval I45.81
uterine contractions in labor O62.4
Prominence, prominent
auricle (congenital) (ear) Q17.5
ischial spine or sacral promontory
with disproportion (fetopelvic) O33.0
causing obstructed labor O65.0
nose (congenital) acquired M95.0
Promiscuity — see High, risk, sexual behavior
Pronation
ankle — see Deformity, limb, foot, specified NEC
foot (see also Deformity, limb, foot, specified NEC)
congenital Q74.2
Prophylactic
administration of
antibiotics, long-term Z79.2
short-term use — omit code
drug (see also Long-term (current) drug therapy (use of)) Z79.899
medication Z79.899
organ removal (for neoplasia management) Z40.00
breast Z40.01
fallopian tube(s) Z40.03
with ovary(s) Z40.02
ovary(s) Z40.02
specified site NEC Z40.09
surgery Z40.9
for risk factors related to malignant neoplasm — see Prophylactic, organ removal
specified NEC Z40.8
vaccination Z23
Propionic acidemia E71.121
Proptosis (ocular) (see also Exophthalmos)
thyroid — see Hyperthyroidism, with goiter
Prosecution, anxiety concerning Z65.3
Prosopagnosia R48.3
Prostadynia N42.81
Prostate, prostatic — see condition
Prostatism — see Hyperplasia, prostate
Prostatitis (congestive) (suppurative) (with cystitis) N41.9
acute N41.0
cavitary N41.8
chronic N41.1
diverticular N41.8
due to Trichomonas (vaginalis) A59.02
fibrous N41.1

Prostatitis — continued
gonococcal (acute) (chronic) A54.22
granulomatous N41.4
hypertrophic N41.1
subacute N41.1
trichomonal A59.02
tuberculous A18.14
Prostatocystitis N41.3
Prostatorrhea N42.89
Prostatosis N42.82
Prostration R53.83
heat (see also Heat, exhaustion)
anhydrotic T67.3 ☑
due to
salt (and water) depletion T67.4 ☑
water depletion T67.3 ☑
nervous F48.8
senile R54
Protanomaly (anomalous trichromat) H53.54
Protanopia (complete) (incomplete) H53.54
Protection (against) (from) — see Prophylactic
Protein
deficiency NEC — see Malnutrition
malnutrition — see Malnutrition
sickness (see also Reaction, serum) T80.69 ☑
Proteinemia R77.9
Proteinosis
alveolar (pulmonary) J84.01
lipid or lipoid (of Urbach) E78.89
Proteinuria R80.9
Bence Jones R80.3
complicating pregnancy — see Proteinuria, gestational
gestational
complicating
childbirth O12.14
pregnancy O12.1- ☑
with edema O12.2- ☑
puerperium O12.15
idiopathic R80.0
isolated R80.0
with glomerular lesion N06.9
dense deposit disease N06.6
diffuse
crescentic glomerulonephritis N06.7
endocapillary proliferative glomerulonephritis N06.4
mesangiocapillary glomerulonephritis N06.5
focal and segmental hyalinosis or sclerosis N06.1
membranous (diffuse) N06.2
mesangial proliferative (diffuse) N06.3
minimal change N06.0
specified pathology NEC N06.8
orthostatic R80.2
with glomerular lesion — see Proteinuria, isolated, with glomerular lesion
persistent R80.1
with glomerular lesion — see Proteinuria, isolated, with glomerular lesion
postural R80.2
with glomerular lesion — see Proteinuria, isolated, with glomerular lesion
pre-eclamptic — see Pre-eclampsia
puerperal O12.15
specified type NEC R80.8
Proteolysis, pathologic D65
Proteus (mirabilis) (morganii), **as cause of disease classified elsewhere** B96.4
Prothrombin gene mutation D68.52
Protoporphyria, erythropoietic E80.0
Protozoal (see also condition)
disease B64
specified NEC B60.8
Protrusion, protrusio
acetabuli M24.7
acetabulum (into pelvis) M24.7
device, implant or graft (see also Complications, by site and type, mechanical) T85.698 ☑
arterial graft NEC — see Complication, cardiovascular device, mechanical, vascular
breast (implant) T85.49 ☑
catheter NEC T85.698 ☑
cystostomy T83.090 ☑
dialysis (renal) T82.49 ☑
intraperitoneal T85.691 ☑
infusion NEC T82.594 ☑
spinal (epidural) (subdural) T85.690 ☑

Protrusion, protrusio — *continued*
  device, implant or graft (*see also* Complications, by site and type, mechanical) — *continued*
    catheter — *continued*
      urinary (*see also* Complications, catheter, urinary) T83.098 ☑
    electronic (electrode) (pulse generator) (stimulator) bone T84.390 ☑
      nervous system — *see* Complication, prosthetic device, mechanical, electronic nervous system stimulator
    fixation, internal (orthopedic) NEC — *see* Complication, fixation device, mechanical
    gastrointestinal — *see* Complications, prosthetic device, mechanical, gastrointestinal device
    genital NEC T83.498 ☑
      intrauterine contraceptive device T83.39 ☑
      penile prosthesis (cylinder) (implanted) (pump) (resevoir) T83.490 ☑
      testicular prosthesis T83.491 ☑
    heart NEC — *see* Complication, cardiovascular device, mechanical
    joint prosthesis — *see* Complications, joint prosthesis, mechanical, specified NEC, by site
    ocular NEC — *see* Complications, prosthetic device, mechanical, ocular device
    orthopedic NEC — *see* Complication, orthopedic, device, mechanical
    specified NEC T85.628 ☑
    urinary NEC (*see also* Complication, genitourinary, device, urinary, mechanical)
      graft T83.29 ☑
    vascular NEC — *see* Complication, cardiovascular device, mechanical
    ventricular intracranial shunt T85.09 ☑
  intervertebral disc — *see* Displacement, intervertebral disc
  joint prosthesis — *see* Complications, joint prosthesis, mechanical, specified NEC, by site
  nucleus pulposus — *see* Displacement, intervertebral disc
Prune belly (syndrome) Q79.4
Prurigo (ferox) (gravis) (Hebrae) (Hebra's) (mitis) (simplex) L28.2
  Besnier's L20.0
  estivalis L56.4
  nodularis L28.1
  psychogenic F45.8
Pruritus, pruritic (essential) L29.9
  ani, anus L29.0
    psychogenic F45.8
  anogenital L29.3
    psychogenic F45.8
  due to onchocerca volvulus B73.1
  gravidarum — *see* Pregnancy, complicated by, specified pregnancy-related condition NEC
  hiemalis L29.8
  neurogenic (any site) F45.8
  perianal L29.0
  psychogenic (any site) F45.8
  scroti, scrotum L29.1
    psychogenic F45.8
  senile, senilis L29.8
  specified NEC L29.8
    psychogenic F45.8
  Trichomonas A59.9
  vulva, vulvae L29.2
    psychogenic F45.8
Pseudarthrosis, pseudoarthrosis (bone) — *see* Nonunion, fracture
  clavicle, congenital Q74.0
  joint, following fusion or arthrodesis M96.0
Pseudoaneurysm — *see* Aneurysm
Pseudoangina (pectoris) — *see* Angina
Pseudoangioma I81
Pseudoarteriosus Q28.8
Pseudoarthrosis — *see* Pseudarthrosis
Pseudobulbar affect (PBA) F48.2
Pseudochromhidrosis L67.8
Pseudocirrhosis, liver, pericardial I31.1
Pseudocowpox B08.03
Pseudocoxalgia M91.3- ☑
Pseudocroup J38.5
Pseudo-Cushing's syndrome, alcohol-induced E24.4
Pseudocyesis F45.8
Pseudocyst
  lung J98.4

Pseudocyst — *continued*
  pancreas K86.3
  retina — *see* Cyst, retina
Pseudoelephantiasis neuroarthritica Q82.0
Pseudoexfoliation, capsule (lens) — *see* Cataract, specified NEC
Pseudofolliculitis barbae L73.1
Pseudoglioma H44.89
Pseudohemophilia (Bernuth's) (hereditary) (type B) D68.0
  Type A D69.8
  vascular D69.8
Pseudohermaphroditism Q56.3
  adrenal E25.8
  female Q56.2
    with adrenocortical disorder E25.8
    without adrenocortical disorder Q56.2
    adrenal (congenital) E25.0
    unspecified E25.9
  male Q56.1
    with
      5-alpha-reductase deficiency E29.1
      adrenocortical disorder E25.8
      androgen resistance E34.51
      cleft scrotum Q56.1
      feminizing testis E34.51
    without gonadal disorder Q56.1
    adrenal E25.8
    unspecified E25.9
Pseudo-Hurler's polydystrophy E77.0
Pseudohydrocephalus G93.2
Pseudohypertrophic muscular dystrophy (Erb's) G71.0
Pseudohypertrophy, muscle G71.0
Pseudohypoparathyroidism E20.1
Pseudoinsomnia F51.03
Pseudoleukemia, infantile D64.89
Pseudomembranous — *see* condition
Pseudomeningocele (cerebral) (infective) (post-traumatic) G96.19
  postprocedural (spinal) G97.82
Pseudomenses (newborn) P54.6
Pseudomenstruation (newborn) P54.6
Pseudomonas
  aeruginosa, as cause of disease classified elsewhere B96.5
  mallei infection A24.0
    as cause of disease classified elsewhere B96.5
  pseudomallei, as cause of disease classified elsewhere B96.5
Pseudomyotonia G71.19
Pseudomyxoma peritonei C78.6
Pseudoneuritis, optic (nerve) (disc) (papilla), **congenital** Q14.2
Pseudo-obstruction intestine (acute) (chronic) (idiopathic) (intermittent secondary) (primary) K59.8
Pseudopapilledema H47.33- ☑
  congenital Q14.2
Pseudoparalysis
  arm or leg R29.818
  atonic, congenital P94.2
Pseudopelade L66.0
Pseudophakia Z96.1
Pseudopolyarthritis, rhizomelic M35.3
Pseudopolycythemia D75.1
Pseudopseudohypoparathyroidism E20.1
Pseudopterygium H11.81- ☑
Pseudoptosis (eyelid) — *see* Blepharochalasis
Pseudopuberty, precocious
  female heterosexual E25.8
  male isosexual E25.8
Pseudorickets (renal) N25.0
Pseudorubella B08.20
Pseudosclerema, newborn P83.88
Pseudosclerosis (brain)
  Jakob's — *see* Creutzfeldt-Jakob disease or syndrome of Westphal (Strümpell) E83.01
  spastic — *see* Creutzfeldt-Jakob disease or syndrome
Pseudotetanus — *see* Convulsions
Pseudotetany R29.0
  hysterical F44.5
Pseudotruncus arteriosus Q25.49
Pseudotuberculosis A28.2
  enterocolitis A04.8
  pasteurella (infection) A28.0
Pseudotumor
  cerebri G93.2
  orbital H05.11 ☑

Pseudoxanthoma elasticum Q82.8
Psilosis (sprue) (tropical) K90.1
  nontropical K90.0
Psittacosis A70
Psoitis M60.88
Psoriasis L40.9
  arthropathic L40.50
    arthritis mutilans L40.52
    distal interphalangeal L40.51
    juvenile L40.54
    other specified L40.59
    spondylitis L40.53
  buccal K13.29
  flexural L40.8
  guttate L40.4
  mouth K13.29
  nummular L40.0
  plaque L40.0
  psychogenic F54
  pustular (generalized) L40.1
    palmaris et plantaris L40.3
  specified NEC L40.8
  vulgaris L40.0
Psychasthenia F48.8
Psychiatric disorder or problem F99
Psychogenic (*see also* condition)
  factors associated with physical conditions F54
Psychological and behavioral factors affecting medical condition F59
Psychoneurosis, psychoneurotic (*see also* Neurosis)
  anxiety (state) F41.1
  depersonalization F48.1
  hypochondriacal F45.21
  hysteria F44.9
  neurasthenic F48.8
  personality NEC F60.89
Psychopathy, psychopathic
  affectionless F94.2
  autistic F84.5
  constitution, post-traumatic F07.81
  personality — *see* Disorder, personality
  sexual — *see* Deviation, sexual
  state F60.2
Psychosexual identity disorder of childhood F64.2
Psychosis, psychotic F29
  acute (transient) F23
    hysterical F44.9
  affective — *see* Disorder, mood
  alcoholic F10.959
    with
      abuse F10.159
      anxiety disorder F10.980
        with
          abuse F10.180
          dependence F10.280
      delirium tremens F10.231
      delusions F10.950
        with
          abuse F10.150
          dependence F10.250
      dementia F10.97
        with dependence F10.27
      dependence F10.259
      hallucinosis F10.951
        with
          abuse F10.151
          dependence F10.251
      mood disorder F10.94
        with
          abuse F10.14
          dependence F10.24
      paranoia F10.950
        with
          abuse F10.150
          dependence F10.250
      persisting amnesia F10.96
        with dependence F10.26
    amnestic confabulatory F10.96
      with dependence F10.26
    delirium tremens F10.231
    Korsakoff's, Korsakov's, Korsakow's F10.26
    paranoid type F10.950
      with
        abuse F10.150
        dependence F10.250
  anergastic — *see* Psychosis, organic
  arteriosclerotic (simple type) (uncomplicated) F01.50
    with behavioral disturbance F01.51

☑ **Additional Character Required** — **Refer to the Tabular List for Character Selection**   ▽ **Subterms under main terms may continue to next column or page**

Psychosis, psychotic — *continued*
  childhood F84.0
    atypical F84.8
  climacteric — *see* Psychosis, involutional
  confusional F29
    acute or subacute F05
    reactive F23
  cycloid F23
  depressive — *see* Disorder, depressive
  disintegrative (childhood) F84.3
  drug-induced — *see* F11-F19 with .X59
    paranoid and hallucinatory states — *see* F11-F19
      with .X50 or .X51
  due to or associated with
    addiction, drug — *see* F11-F19 with .X59
    dependence
      alcohol F10.259
      drug — *see* F11-F19 with .X59
    epilepsy F06.8
    Huntington's chorea F06.8
    ischemia, cerebrovascular (generalized) F06.8
    multiple sclerosis F06.8
    physical disease F06.8
    presenile dementia F03 ☑
    senile dementia F03 ☑
    vascular disease (arteriosclerotic) (cerebral) F01.50
      with behavioral disturbance F01.51
  epileptic F06.8
  episode F23
    due to or associated with physical condition F06.8
  exhaustive F43.0
  hallucinatory, chronic F28
  hypomanic F30.8
  hysterical (acute) F44.9
  induced F24
  infantile F84.0
    atypical F84.8
  infective (acute) (subacute) F05
  involutional F28
    depressive — *see* Disorder, depressive
    melancholic — *see* Disorder, depressive
    paranoid (state) F22
  Korsakoff's, Korsakov's, Korsakow's (nonalcoholic) F04
    alcoholic F10.96
      in dependence F10.26
    induced by other psychoactive substance — *see*
      categories F11-F19 with .X5X
  mania, manic (single episode) F30.2
    recurrent type F31.89
  manic-depressive — *see* Disorder, bipolar
  menopausal — *see* Psychosis, involutional
  mixed schizophrenic and affective F25.8
  multi-infarct (cerebrovascular) F01.50
    with behavioral disturbance F01.51
  nonorganic F29
    specified NEC F28
  organic F09
    due to or associated with
      arteriosclerosis (cerebral) — *see* Psychosis, ar-
        teriosclerotic
      cerebrovascular disease, arteriosclerotic — *see*
        Psychosis, arteriosclerotic
      childbirth — *see* Psychosis, puerperal
      Creutzfeldt-Jakob disease or syndrome — *see*
        Creutzfeldt-Jakob disease or syndrome
      dependence, alcohol F10.259
      disease
        alcoholic liver F10.259
        brain, arteriosclerotic — *see* Psychosis, arte-
          riosclerotic
        cerebrovascular F01.50
          with behavioral disturbance F01.51
        Creutzfeldt-Jakob — *see* Creutzfeldt-Jakob
          disease or syndrome
        endocrine or metabolic F06.8
          acute or subacute F05
        liver, alcoholic F10.259
      epilepsy transient (acute) F05
      infection
        brain (intracranial) F06.8
          acute or subacute F05
      intoxication
        alcoholic (acute) F10.259
        drug F11-F19 with .X59
      ischemia, cerebrovascular (generalized) — *see*
        Psychosis, arteriosclerotic
      puerperium — *see* Psychosis, puerperal

Psychosis, psychotic — *continued*
  organic — *continued*
    due to or associated with — *continued*
      trauma, brain (birth) (from electric current)
        (surgical) F06.8
        acute or subacute F05
      infective F06.8
        acute or subacute F05
      post-traumatic F06.8
        acute or subacute F05
  paranoiac F22
  paranoid (climacteric) (involutional) (menopausal) F22
    psychogenic (acute) F23
    schizophrenic F20.0
    senile F03 ☑
  postpartum F53
  presbyophrenic (type) F03 ☑
  presenile F03 ☑
  psychogenic (paranoid) F23
    depressive F32.3
  puerperal F53
    specified type — *see* Psychosis, by type
  reactive (brief) (transient) (emotional stress) (psycho-
    logical trauma) F23
    depressive F32.3
      recurrent F33.3
    excitative type F30.8
  schizoaffective F25.9
    depressive type F25.1
    manic type F25.0
  schizophrenia, schizophrenic — *see* Schizophrenia
  schizophrenia-like, in epilepsy F06.2
  schizophreniform F20.81
    affective type F25.9
    brief F23
    confusional type F23
    mixed type F25.0
  senile NEC F03 ☑
    depressed or paranoid type F03 ☑
    simple deterioration F03 ☑
    specified type — *code to* condition
  shared F24
  situational (reactive) F23
  symbiotic (childhood) F84.3
  symptomatic F09
Psychosomatic — *see* Disorder, psychosomatic
Psychosyndrome, organic F07.9
**Psychotic episode due to or associated with physical
    condition** F06.8
Pterygium (eye) H11.00- ☑
  amyloid H11.01- ☑
  central H11.02- ☑
  colli Q18.3
  double H11.03- ☑
  peripheral
    progressive H11.05- ☑
    stationary H11.04- ☑
  recurrent H11.06- ☑
Ptilosis (eyelid) — *see* Madarosis
Ptomaine (poisoning) — *see* Poisoning, food
Ptosis (*see also* Blepharoptosis)
  adiposa (false) — *see* Blepharoptosis
  breast N64.81
  cecum K63.4
  colon K63.4
  congenital (eyelid) Q10.0
    specified site NEC — *see* Anomaly, by site
  eyelid — *see* Blepharoptosis
    congenital Q10.0
  gastric K31.89
  intestine K63.4
  kidney N28.83
  liver K76.89
  renal N28.83
  splanchnic K63.4
  spleen D73.89
  stomach K31.89
  viscera K63.4
PTP D69.51
Ptyalism (periodic) K11.7
  hysterical F45.8
  pregnancy — *see* Pregnancy, complicated by, specified
    pregnancy-related condition NEC
  psychogenic F45.8
Ptyalolithiasis K11.5
Pubarche, precocious E30.1
Pubertas praecox E30.1
Puberty (development state) Z00.3

Puberty — *continued*
  bleeding (excessive) N92.2
  delayed E30.0
  precocious (constitutional) (cryptogenic) (idiopathic)
    E30.1
    central E22.8
    due to
      ovarian hyperfunction E28.1
        estrogen E28.0
      testicular hyperfunction E29.0
  premature E30.1
    due to
      adrenal cortical hyperfunction E25.8
      pineal tumor E34.8
      pituitary (anterior) hyperfunction E22.8
Puckering, macula — *see* Degeneration, macula, puck-
    ering
Pudenda, pudendum — *see* condition
Puente's disease (simple glandular cheilitis) K13.0
Puerperal, puerperium (complicated by, complications)
  abnormal glucose (tolerance test) O99.815
  abscess
    areola O91.02
      associated with lactation O91.03
    Bartholin's gland O86.19
    breast O91.12
      associated with lactation O91.13
    cervix (uteri) O86.11
    genital organ NEC O86.19
    kidney O86.21
    mammary O91.12
      associated with lactation O91.13
    nipple O91.02
      associated with lactation O91.03
    peritoneum O85
    subareolar O91.12
      associated with lactation O91.13
    urinary tract — *see* Puerperal, infection, urinary
    uterus O86.12
    vagina (wall) O86.13
    vaginorectal O86.13
    vulvovaginal gland O86.13
  adnexitis O86.19
  afibrinogenemia, or other coagulation defect O72.3
  albuminuria (acute) (subacute) — *see* Proteinuria,
    gestational
  alcohol use O99.315
  anemia O90.81
    pre-existing (pre-pregnancy) O99.03
  anesthetic death O89.8
  apoplexy O99.43
  bariatric surgery status O99.845
  blood disorder NEC O99.13
  blood dyscrasia O72.3
  cardiomyopathy O90.3
  cerebrovascular disorder (conditions in I60-I69) O99.43
  cervicitis O86.11
  circulatory system disorder O99.43
  coagulopathy (any) O99.13
    with hemorrhage O72.3
  complications O90.9
    specified NEC O90.89
  convulsions — *see* Eclampsia
  cystitis O86.22
  cystopyelitis O86.29
  delirium NEC F05
  diabetes O24.93
    gestational — *see* Puerperal, gestational diabetes
    pre-existing O24.33
      specified NEC O24.83
      type 1 O24.03
      type 2 O24.13
  digestive system disorder O99.63
  disease O90.9
    breast NEC O92.29
    cerebrovascular (acute) O99.43
    nonobstetric NEC O99.89
    tubo-ovarian O86.19
    Valsuani's O99.03
  disorder O90.9
    biliary tract O26.63
    lactation O92.70
    liver O26.63
    nonobstetric NEC O99.89
  disruption
    cesarean wound O90.0
    episiotomy wound O90.1
    perineal laceration wound O90.1

Puerperal, puerperium — continued
- drug use O99.325
- eclampsia (with pre-existing hypertension) O15.2
- embolism (pulmonary) (blood clot) — see Embolism, obstetric, puerperal
- endocrine, nutritional or metabolic disease NEC O99.285
- endophlebitis — see Puerperal, phlebitis
- endotrachelitis O86.11
- failure
  - lactation (complete) O92.3
    - partial O92.4
  - renal, acute O90.4
- fever (of unknown origin) O86.4
  - septic O85
- fissure, nipple O92.12
  - associated with lactation O92.13
- fistula
  - breast (due to mastitis) O91.12
    - associated with lactation O91.13
  - nipple O91.02
    - associated with lactation O91.03
- galactophoritis O91.22
  - associated with lactation O91.23
- galactorrhea O92.6
- gastric banding status O99.845
- gastric bypass status O99.845
- gastrointestinal disease NEC O99.63
- gestational
  - diabetes O24.439
    - diet controlled O24.430
    - insulin (and diet) controlled O24.434
    - oral drug controlled (antidiabetic) (hypoglycemic) O24.435
  - edema O12.05
    - with proteinuria O12.25
  - proteinuria O12.15
- gonorrhea O98.23
- hematoma, subdural O99.43
- hemiplegia, cerebral O99.355
  - due to cerbrovascular disorder O99.43
- hemorrhage O72.1
  - brain O99.43
  - bulbar O99.43
  - cerebellar O99.43
  - cerebral O99.43
  - cortical O99.43
  - delayed or secondary O72.2
  - extradural O99.43
  - internal capsule O99.43
  - intracranial O99.43
  - intrapontine O99.43
  - meningeal O99.43
  - pontine O99.43
  - retained placenta O72.0
  - subarachnoid O99.43
  - subcortical O99.43
  - subdural O99.43
  - third stage O72.0
  - uterine, delayed O72.2
  - ventricular O99.43
- hemorrhoids O87.2
- hepatorenal syndrome O90.4
- hypertension — see Hypertension, complicating, puerperium
- hypertrophy, breast O92.29
- induration breast (fibrous) O92.29
- infection O86.4
  - cervix O86.11
  - generalized O85
  - genital tract NEC O86.19
    - obstetric surgical wound O86.0
  - kidney (bacillus coli) O86.21
  - maternal O98.93
    - carrier state NEC O99.835
    - gonorrhea O98.23
    - human immunodeficiency virus (HIV) O98.73
    - protozoal O98.63
    - sexually transmitted NEC O98.33
    - specified NEC O98.83
    - streptococcus group B (GBS) carrier state O99.825
    - syphilis O98.13
    - tuberculosis O98.03
    - viral hepatitis O98.43
    - viral NEC O98.53
  - nipple O91.02
    - associated with lactation O91.03
  - peritoneum O85

Puerperal, puerperium — continued
- infection — continued
  - renal O86.21
  - specified NEC O86.89
  - urinary (asymptomatic) (tract) NEC O86.20
    - bladder O86.22
    - kidney O86.21
    - specified site NEC O86.29
    - urethra O86.22
  - vagina O86.13
  - vein — see Puerperal, phlebitis
- ischemia, cerebral O99.43
- lymphangitis O86.89
  - breast O91.22
    - associated with lactation O91.23
- malignancy O9A.13 (following O99)
- malnutrition O25.3
- mammillitis O91.02
  - associated with lactation O91.03
- mammitis O91.22
  - associated with lactation O91.23
- mania F30.8
- mastitis O91.22
  - associated with lactation O91.23
  - purulent O91.12
    - associated with lactation O91.13
- melancholia — see Disorder, depressive
- mental disorder NEC O99.345
- metroperitonitis O85
- metrorrhagia — see Hemorrhage, postpartum
- metrosalpingitis O86.19
- metrovaginitis O86.13
- milk leg O87.1
- monoplegia, cerebral O99.43
- mood disturbance O90.6
- necrosis, liver (acute) (subacute) (conditions in subcategory K72.0) O26.63
  - with renal failure O90.4
- nervous system disorder O99.355
- obesity (pre-existing prior to pregnancy) O99.215
- obesity surgery status O99.845
- occlusion, precerebral artery O99.43
- paralysis
  - bladder (sphincter) O90.89
  - cerebral O99.43
- paralytic stroke O99.43
- parametritis O85
- paravaginitis O86.13
- pelviperitonitis O85
- perimetritis O86.12
- perimetrosalpingitis O86.19
- perinephritis O86.21
- periphlebitis — see Puerperal phlebitis
- peritoneal infection O85
- peritonitis (pelvic) O85
- perivaginitis O86.13
- phlebitis O87.0
  - deep O87.1
  - pelvic O87.1
  - superficial O87.0
- phlebothrombosis, deep O87.1
- phlegmasia alba dolens O87.1
- placental polyp O90.89
- pneumonia, embolic — see Embolism, obstetric, puerperal
- pre-eclampsia — see Pre-eclampsia
- psychosis F53
- pyelitis O86.29
- pyelocystitis O86.29
- pyelonephritis O86.21
- pyelonephrosis O86.21
- pyemia O85
- pyocystitis O86.29
- pyohemia O85
- pyometra O86.12
- pyonephritis O86.21
- pyosalpingitis O86.19
- pyrexia (of unknown origin) O86.4
- renal
  - disease NEC O90.89
  - failure O90.4
- respiratory disease NEC O99.53
- retention
  - decidua — see Retention, decidua
  - placenta O72.0
  - secundines — see Retention, secundines
- retrated nipple O92.02
- salpingo-ovaritis O86.19

Puerperal, puerperium — continued
- salpingoperitonitis O85
- secondary perineal tear O90.1
- sepsis (pelvic) O85
- sepsis O85
- septic thrombophlebitis O86.81
- skin disorder NEC O99.73
- specified condition NEC O99.89
- stroke O99.43
- subinvolution (uterus) O90.89
- subluxation of symphysis (pubis) O26.73
- suppuration — see Puerperal, abscess
- tetanus A34
- thelitis O91.02
  - associated with lactation O91.03
- thrombocytopenia O72.3
- thrombophlebitis (superficial) O87.0
  - deep O87.1
  - pelvic O87.1
  - septic O86.81
- thrombosis (venous) — see Thrombosis, puerperal
- thyroiditis O90.5
- toxemia (eclamptic) (pre-eclamptic) (with convulsions) O15.2
- trauma, non-obstetric O9A.23 (following O99)
  - caused by abuse (physical) (suspected) O9A.33 (following O99)
    - confirmed O9A.33 (following O99)
    - psychological (suspected) O9A.53 (following O99)
      - confirmed O9A.53 (following O99)
    - sexual (suspected) O9A.43 (following O99)
      - confirmed O9A.43 (following O99)
- uremia (due to renal failure) O90.4
- urethritis O86.22
- vaginitis O86.13
- varicose veins (legs) O87.4
  - vulva or perineum O87.8
- venous O87.9
- vulvitis O86.19
- vulvovaginitis O86.13
- white leg O87.1

Puerperium — see Puerperal

Pulmolithiasis J98.4

Pulmonary — see condition

Pulpitis (acute) (anachoretic) (chronic) (hyperplastic) (putrescent) (suppurative) (ulcerative) K04.01
- irreversible K04.02
- reversible K04.01

Pulpless tooth K04.99

Pulse
- alternating R00.8
- bigeminal R00.8
- fast R00.0
- feeble, rapid due to shock following injury T79.4 ☑
- rapid R00.0
- weak R09.89

Pulsus alternans or trigeminus R00.8

Punch drunk F07.81

Punctum lacrimale occlusion — see Obstruction, lacrimal

Puncture
- abdomen, abdominal
  - wall S31.139 ☑
    - with
      - foreign body S31.149 ☑
      - penetration into peritoneal cavity S31.639 ☑
        - with foreign body S31.649 ☑
    - epigastric region S31.132 ☑
      - with
        - foreign body S31.142 ☑
        - penetration into peritoneal cavity S31.632 ☑
          - with foreign body S31.642 ☑
    - left
      - lower quadrant S31.134 ☑
        - with
          - foreign body S31.144 ☑
          - penetration into peritoneal cavity S31.634 ☑
            - with foreign body S31.644 ☑
      - upper quadrant S31.131 ☑
        - with
          - foreign body S31.141 ☑
          - penetration into peritoneal cavity S31.631 ☑
            - with foreign body S31.641 ☑

☑ Additional Character Required — Refer to the Tabular List for Character Selection   ▽ Subterms under main terms may continue to next column or page

Puncture — *continued*
abdomen, abdominal — *continued*
wall — *continued*
periumbilic region S31.135 ☑
with
foreign body S31.145 ☑
penetration into peritoneal cavity
S31.635 ☑
with foreign body S31.645 ☑
right
lower quadrant S31.133 ☑
with
foreign body S31.143 ☑
penetration into peritoneal cavity
S31.633 ☑
with foreign body S31.643 ☑
upper quadrant S31.130 ☑
with
foreign body S31.140 ☑
penetration into peritoneal cavity
S31.630 ☑
with foreign body S31.640 ☑
accidental, complicating surgery — *see* Complication,
accidental puncture or laceration
alveolar (process) — *see* Puncture, oral cavity
ankle S91.039 ☑
with
foreign body S91.049 ☑
left S91.032 ☑
with
foreign body S91.042 ☑
right S91.031 ☑
with
foreign body S91.041 ☑
anus S31.833 ☑
with foreign body S31.834 ☑
arm (upper) S41.139 ☑
with foreign body S41.149 ☑
left S41.132 ☑
with foreign body S41.142 ☑
lower — *see* Puncture, forearm
right S41.131 ☑
with foreign body S41.141 ☑
auditory canal (external) (meatus) — *see* Puncture,
ear
auricle, ear — *see* Puncture, ear
axilla — *see* Puncture, arm
back (*see also* Puncture, thorax, back)
lower S31.030 ☑
with
foreign body S31.040 ☑
with penetration into retroperitoneal
space S31.041 ☑
penetration into retroperitoneal space
S31.031 ☑
bladder (traumatic) S37.29 ☑
nontraumatic N32.89
breast S21.039 ☑
with foreign body S21.049 ☑
left S21.032 ☑
with foreign body S21.042 ☑
right S21.031 ☑
with foreign body S21.041 ☑
buttock S31.803 ☑
with foreign body S31.804 ☑
left S31.823 ☑
with foreign body S31.824 ☑
right S31.813 ☑
with foreign body S31.814 ☑
by
device, implant or graft — *see* Complications, by
site and type, mechanical
foreign body left accidentally in operative wound
T81.539 ☑
instrument (any) during a procedure, accidental
— *see* Puncture, accidental complicating
surgery
calf — *see* Puncture, leg
canaliculus lacrimalis — *see* Puncture, eyelid
canthus, eye — *see* Puncture, eyelid
cervical esophagus S11.23 ☑
with foreign body S11.24 ☑
cheek (external) S01.439 ☑
with foreign body S01.449 ☑
internal — *see* Puncture, oral cavity
left S01.432 ☑

Puncture — *continued*
cheek — *continued*
left — *continued*
with foreign body S01.442 ☑
right S01.431 ☑
with foreign body S01.441 ☑
chest wall — *see* Puncture, thorax
chin — *see* Puncture, head, specified site NEC
clitoris — *see* Puncture, vulva
costal region — *see* Puncture, thorax
digit(s)
foot — *see* Puncture, toe
hand — *see* Puncture, finger
ear (canal) (external) S01.339 ☑
with foreign body S01.349 ☑
drum S09.2- ☑
left S01.332 ☑
with foreign body S01.342 ☑
right S01.331 ☑
with foreign body S01.341 ☑
elbow S51.039 ☑
with
foreign body S51.049 ☑
left S51.032 ☑
with
foreign body S51.042 ☑
right S51.031 ☑
with
foreign body S51.041 ☑
epididymis — *see* Puncture, testis
epigastric region — *see* Puncture, abdomen, wall,
epigastric
epiglottis S11.83 ☑
with foreign body S11.84 ☑
esophagus
cervical S11.23 ☑
with foreign body S11.24 ☑
thoracic S27.818 ☑
eyeball S05.6- ☑
with foreign body S05.5- ☑
eyebrow — *see* Puncture, eyelid
eyelid S01.13- ☑
with foreign body S01.14- ☑
left S01.132 ☑
with foreign body S01.142 ☑
right S01.131 ☑
with foreign body S01.141 ☑
face NEC — *see* Puncture, head, specified site NEC
finger(s) S61.239 ☑
with
damage to nail S61.339 ☑
with
foreign body S61.349 ☑
foreign body S61.249 ☑
index S61.238 ☑
with
damage to nail S61.338 ☑
with
foreign body S61.348 ☑
foreign body S61.248 ☑
left S61.231 ☑
with
damage to nail S61.331 ☑
with
foreign body S61.341 ☑
foreign body S61.241 ☑
right S61.230 ☑
with
damage to nail S61.330 ☑
with
foreign body S61.340 ☑
foreign body S61.240 ☑
little S61.238 ☑
with
damage to nail S61.338 ☑
with
foreign body S61.348 ☑
foreign body S61.248 ☑
left S61.237 ☑
with
damage to nail S61.337 ☑
with
foreign body S61.347 ☑
foreign body S61.247 ☑
right S61.236 ☑

Puncture — *continued*
finger(s) — *continued*
little — *continued*
right — *continued*
with
damage to nail S61.336 ☑
with
foreign body S61.346 ☑
foreign body S61.246 ☑
middle S61.238 ☑
with
damage to nail S61.338 ☑
with
foreign body S61.348 ☑
foreign body S61.248 ☑
left S61.233 ☑
with
damage to nail S61.333 ☑
with
foreign body S61.343 ☑
foreign body S61.243 ☑
right S61.232 ☑
with
damage to nail S61.332 ☑
with
foreign body S61.342 ☑
foreign body S61.242 ☑
ring S61.238 ☑
with
damage to nail S61.338 ☑
with
foreign body S61.348 ☑
foreign body S61.248 ☑
left S61.235 ☑
with
damage to nail S61.335 ☑
with
foreign body S61.345 ☑
foreign body S61.245 ☑
right S61.234 ☑
with
damage to nail S61.334 ☑
with
foreign body S61.344 ☑
foreign body S61.244 ☑
flank S31.139 ☑
with foreign body S31.149 ☑
foot (except toe(s) alone) S91.339 ☑
with foreign body S91.349 ☑
left S91.332 ☑
with foreign body S91.342 ☑
right S91.331 ☑
with foreign body S91.341 ☑
toe — *see* Puncture, toe
forearm S51.839 ☑
with
foreign body S51.849 ☑
elbow only — *see* Puncture, elbow
left S51.832 ☑
with
foreign body S51.842 ☑
right S51.831 ☑
with
foreign body S51.841 ☑
forehead — *see* Puncture, head, specified site NEC
genital organs, external
female S31.532 ☑
with foreign body S31.542 ☑
vagina — *see* Puncture, vagina
vulva — *see* Puncture, vulva
male S31.531 ☑
with foreign body S31.541 ☑
penis — *see* Puncture, penis
scrotum — *see* Puncture, scrotum
testis — *see* Puncture, testis
groin — *see* Puncture, abdomen, wall
gum — *see* Puncture, oral cavity
hand S61.439 ☑
with
foreign body S61.449 ☑
finger — *see* Puncture, finger
left S61.432 ☑
with
foreign body S61.442 ☑
right S61.431 ☑

Puncture — *continued*
  hand — *continued*
    right — *continued*
      with
        foreign body S61.441 ☑
    thumb — *see* Puncture, thumb
  head S01.93 ☑
    with foreign body S01.94 ☑
    cheek — *see* Puncture, cheek
    ear — *see* Puncture, ear
    eyelid — *see* Puncture, eyelid
    lip — *see* Puncture, oral cavity
    nose — *see* Puncture, nose
    oral cavity — *see* Puncture, oral cavity
    scalp S01.03 ☑
      with foreign body S01.04 ☑
    specified site NEC S01.83 ☑
      with foreign body S01.84 ☑
    temporomandibular area — *see* Puncture, cheek
  heart S26.99 ☑
    with hemopericardium S26.09 ☑
    without hemopericardium S26.19 ☑
  heel — *see* Puncture, foot
  hip S71.039 ☑
    with foreign body S71.049 ☑
    left S71.032 ☑
      with foreign body S71.042 ☑
    right S71.031 ☑
      with foreign body S71.041 ☑
  hymen — *see* Puncture, vagina
  hypochondrium — *see* Puncture, abdomen, wall
  hypogastric region — *see* Puncture, abdomen, wall
  inguinal region — *see* Puncture, abdomen, wall
  instep — *see* Puncture, foot
  internal organs — *see* Injury, by site
  interscapular region — *see* Puncture, thorax, back
  intestine
    large
      colon S36.599 ☑
        ascending S36.590 ☑
        descending S36.592 ☑
        sigmoid S36.593 ☑
        specified site NEC S36.598 ☑
        transverse S36.591 ☑
      rectum S36.69 ☑
    small S36.499 ☑
      duodenum S36.490 ☑
      specified site NEC S36.498 ☑
  intra-abdominal organ S36.99 ☑
    gallbladder S36.128 ☑
    intestine — *see* Puncture, intestine
    liver S36.118 ☑
    pancreas — *see* Puncture, pancreas
    peritoneum S36.81 ☑
    specified site NEC S36.898 ☑
    spleen S36.09 ☑
    stomach S36.39 ☑
  jaw — *see* Puncture, head, specified site NEC
  knee S81.039 ☑
    with foreign body S81.049 ☑
    left S81.032 ☑
      with foreign body S81.042 ☑
    right S81.031 ☑
      with foreign body S81.041 ☑
  labium (majus) (minus) — *see* Puncture, vulva
  lacrimal duct — *see* Puncture, eyelid
  larynx S11.013 ☑
    with foreign body S11.014 ☑
  leg (lower) S81.839 ☑
    with foreign body S81.849 ☑
    foot — *see* Puncture, foot
    knee — *see* Puncture, knee
    left S81.832 ☑
      with foreign body S81.842 ☑
    right S81.831 ☑
      with foreign body S81.841 ☑
    upper — *see* Puncture, thigh
  lip S01.531 ☑
    with foreign body S01.541 ☑
  loin — *see* Puncture, abdomen, wall
  lower back — *see* Puncture, back, lower
  lumbar region — *see* Puncture, back, lower
  malar region — *see* Puncture, head, specified site NEC
  mammary — *see* Puncture, breast
  mastoid region — *see* Puncture, head, specified site NEC

Puncture — *continued*
  mouth — *see* Puncture, oral cavity
  nail
    finger — *see* Puncture, finger, with damage to nail
    toe — *see* Puncture, toe, with damage to nail
  nasal (septum) (sinus) — *see* Puncture, nose
  nasopharynx — *see* Puncture, head, specified site NEC
  neck S11.93 ☑
    with foreign body S11.94 ☑
    involving
      cervical esophagus — *see* Puncture, cervical esophagus
      larynx — *see* Puncture, larynx
      pharynx — *see* Puncture, pharynx
      thyroid gland — *see* Puncture, thyroid gland
      trachea — *see* Puncture, trachea
    specified site NEC S11.83 ☑
      with foreign body S11.84 ☑
  nose (septum) (sinus) S01.23 ☑
    with foreign body S01.24 ☑
  ocular — *see* Puncture, eyeball
  oral cavity S01.532 ☑
    with foreign body S01.542 ☑
  orbit S05.4- ☑
  palate — *see* Puncture, oral cavity
  palm — *see* Puncture, hand
  pancreas S36.299 ☑
    body S36.291 ☑
    head S36.290 ☑
    tail S36.292 ☑
  pelvis — *see* Puncture, back, lower
  penis S31.23 ☑
    with foreign body S31.24 ☑
  perineum
    female S31.43 ☑
      with foreign body S31.44 ☑
    male S31.139 ☑
      with foreign body S31.149 ☑
  periocular area (with or without lacrimal passages) — *see* Puncture, eyelid
  phalanges
    finger — *see* Puncture, finger
    toe — *see* Puncture, toe
  pharynx S11.23 ☑
    with foreign body S11.24 ☑
  pinna — *see* Puncture, ear
  popliteal space — *see* Puncture, knee
  prepuce — *see* Puncture, penis
  pubic region S31.139 ☑
    with foreign body S31.149 ☑
  pudendum — *see* Puncture, genital organs, external
  rectovaginal septum — *see* Puncture, vagina
  sacral region — *see* Puncture, back, lower
  sacroiliac region — *see* Puncture, back, lower
  salivary gland — *see* Puncture, oral cavity
  scalp S01.03 ☑
    with foreign body S01.04 ☑
  scapular region — *see* Puncture, shoulder
  scrotum S31.33 ☑
    with foreign body S31.34 ☑
  shin — *see* Puncture, leg
  shoulder S41.039 ☑
    with foreign body S41.049 ☑
    left S41.032 ☑
      with foreign body S41.042 ☑
    right S41.031 ☑
      with foreign body S41.041 ☑
  spermatic cord — *see* Puncture, testis
  sternal region — *see* Puncture, thorax, front
  submaxillary region — *see* Puncture, head, specified site NEC
  submental region — *see* Puncture, head, specified site NEC
  subungual
    finger(s) — *see* Puncture, finger, with damage to nail
    toe — *see* Puncture, toe, with damage to nail
  supraclavicular fossa — *see* Puncture, neck, specified site NEC
  temple, temporal region — *see* Puncture, head, specified site NEC
  temporomandibular area — *see* Puncture, cheek
  testis S31.33 ☑
    with foreign body S31.34 ☑
  thigh S71.139 ☑
    with foreign body S71.149 ☑

Puncture — *continued*
  thigh — *continued*
    left S71.132 ☑
      with foreign body S71.142 ☑
    right S71.131 ☑
      with foreign body S71.141 ☑
  thorax, thoracic (wall) S21.93 ☑
    with foreign body S21.94 ☑
    back S21.23- ☑
      with
        foreign body S21.24- ☑
          with penetration S21.44 ☑
        penetration S21.43 ☑
    breast — *see* Puncture, breast
    front S21.13- ☑
      with
        foreign body S21.14- ☑
          with penetration S21.34 ☑
        penetration S21.33 ☑
  throat — *see* Puncture, neck
  thumb S61.039 ☑
    with
      damage to nail S61.139 ☑
        with
          foreign body S61.149 ☑
      foreign body S61.049 ☑
    left S61.032 ☑
      with
        damage to nail S61.132 ☑
          with
            foreign body S61.142 ☑
        foreign body S61.042 ☑
    right S61.031 ☑
      with
        damage to nail S61.131 ☑
          with
            foreign body S61.141 ☑
        foreign body S61.041 ☑
  thyroid gland S11.13 ☑
    with foreign body S11.14 ☑
  toe(s) S91.139 ☑
    with
      damage to nail S91.239 ☑
        with
          foreign body S91.249 ☑
      foreign body S91.149 ☑
    great S91.133 ☑
      with
        damage to nail S91.233 ☑
          with
            foreign body S91.243 ☑
        foreign body S91.143 ☑
      left S91.132 ☑
        with
          damage to nail S91.232 ☑
            with
              foreign body S91.242 ☑
          foreign body S91.142 ☑
      right S91.131 ☑
        with
          damage to nail S91.231 ☑
            with
              foreign body S91.241 ☑
          foreign body S91.141 ☑
    lesser S91.136 ☑
      with
        damage to nail S91.236 ☑
          with
            foreign body S91.246 ☑
        foreign body S91.146 ☑
      left S91.135 ☑
        with
          damage to nail S91.235 ☑
            with
              foreign body S91.245 ☑
          foreign body S91.145 ☑
      right S91.134 ☑
        with
          damage to nail S91.234 ☑
            with
              foreign body S91.244 ☑
          foreign body S91.144 ☑
  tongue — *see* Puncture, oral cavity
  trachea S11.023 ☑
    with foreign body S11.024 ☑
  tunica vaginalis — *see* Puncture, testis

Puncture — *continued*
  tympanum, tympanic membrane S09.2- ☑
  umbilical region S31.135 ☑
    with foreign body S31.145 ☑
  uvula — *see* Puncture, oral cavity
  vagina S31.43 ☑
    with foreign body S31.44 ☑
  vocal cords S11.033 ☑
    with foreign body S11.034 ☑
  vulva S31.43 ☑
    with foreign body S31.44 ☑
  wrist S61.539 ☑
    with
      foreign body S61.549 ☑
    left S61.532 ☑
      with
        foreign body S61.542 ☑
    right S61.531 ☑
      with
        foreign body S61.541 ☑
PUO (pyrexia of unknown origin) R50.9
Pupillary membrane (persistent) Q13.89
Pupillotonia — *see* Anomaly, pupil, function, tonic pupil
Purpura D69.2
  abdominal D69.0
  allergic D69.0
  anaphylactoid D69.0
  annularis telangiectodes L81.7
  arthritic D69.0
  autoerythrocyte sensitization D69.2
  autoimmune D69.0
  bacterial D69.0
  Bateman's (senile) D69.2
  capillary fragility (hereditary) (idiopathic) D69.8
  cryoglobulinemic D89.1
  Devil's pinches D69.2
  fibrinolytic — *see* Fibrinolysis
  fulminans, fulminous D65
  gangrenous D65
  hemorrhagic, hemorrhagica D69.3
    not due to thrombocytopenia D69.0
  Henoch (-Schönlein) (allergic) D69.0
  hypergammaglobulinemic (benign) (Waldenström) D89.0
  idiopathic (thrombocytopenic) D69.3
    nonthrombocytopenic D69.0
  immune thrombocytopenic D69.3
  infectious D69.0
  malignant D69.0
  neonatorum P54.5
  nervosa D69.0
  newborn P54.5
  nonthrombocytopenic D69.2
    hemorrhagic D69.0
    idiopathic D69.0
  nonthrombopenic D69.2
  peliosis rheumatica D69.0
  posttransfusion (post-transfusion) (from (fresh) whole blood or blood products) D69.51
  primary D69.49
  red cell membrane sensitivity D69.2
  rheumatica D69.0
  Schönlein (-Henoch) (allergic) D69.0
  scorbutic E54 [D77]
  senile D69.2
  simplex D69.2
  symptomatica D69.0
  telangiectasia annularis L81.7
  thrombocytopenic D69.49
    congenital D69.42
    hemorrhagic D69.3
    hereditary D69.42
    idiopathic D69.3
    immune D69.3
    neonatal, transitory P61.0
    thrombotic M31.1
  thrombohemolytic — *see* Fibrinolysis
  thrombolytic — *see* Fibrinolysis
  thrombopenic D69.49
  thrombotic, thrombocytopenic M31.1
  toxic D69.0
  vascular D69.0
  visceral symptoms D69.0
Purpuric spots R23.3
Purulent — *see* condition
Pus
  in
    stool R19.5

Pus — *continued*
  in — *continued*
    urine N39.0
    tube (rupture) — *see* Salpingo-oophoritis
Pustular rash L08.0
Pustule (nonmalignant) L08.9
  malignant A22.0
Pustulosis palmaris et plantaris L40.3
Putnam (-Dana) **disease or syndrome** — *see* Degeneration, combined
Putrescent pulp (dental) K04.1
Pyarthritis, pyarthrosis — *see* Arthritis, pyogenic or pyemic
  tuberculous — *see* Tuberculosis, joint
Pyelectasis — *see* Hydronephrosis
Pyelitis (congenital) (uremic) (*see also* Pyelonephritis)
  with
    calculus — *see* category N20 ☑
      with hydronephrosis N13.2
    contracted kidney N11.9
  acute N10
  chronic N11.9
    with calculus — *see* category N20 ☑
      with hydronephrosis N13.2
  cystica N28.84
  puerperal (postpartum) O86.21
  tuberculous A18.11
Pyelocystitis — *see* Pyelonephritis
Pyelonephritis (*see also* Nephritis, tubulo-interstitial)
  with
    calculus — *see* category N20 ☑
      with hydronephrosis N13.2
    contracted kidney N11.9
  acute N10
  calculous — *see* category N20 ☑
    with hydronephrosis N13.2
  chronic N11.9
    with calculus — *see* category N20 ☑
      with hydronephrosis N13.2
    associated with ureteral obstruction or stricture N11.1
    nonobstructive N11.8
      with reflux (vesicoureteral) N11.0
    obstructive N11.1
    specified NEC N11.8
  in (due to)
    brucellosis A23.9 [N16]
    cryoglobulinemia (mixed) D89.1 [N16]
    cystinosis E72.04
    diphtheria A36.84
    glycogen storage disease E74.09 [N16]
    leukemia NEC C95.9- ☑ [N16]
    lymphoma NEC C85.90 [N16]
    multiple myeloma C90.0- ☑ [N16]
    obstruction N11.1
    Salmonella infection A02.25
    sarcoidosis D86.84
    sepsis A41.9 [N16]
    Sjögren's disease M35.04
    toxoplasmosis B58.83
    transplant rejection T86.91 [N16]
    Wilson's disease E83.01 [N16]
  nonobstructive N12
    with reflux (vesicoureteral) N11.0
    chronic N11.8
  syphilitic A52.75
Pyelonephrosis (obstructive) N11.1
  chronic N11.9
Pyelophlebitis I80.8
Pyeloureteritis cystica N28.85
Pyemia, pyemic (fever) (infection) (purulent) (*see also* Sepsis)
  joint — *see* Arthritis, pyogenic or pyemic
  liver K75.1
  pneumococcal A40.3
  portal K75.1
  postvaccinal T88.0 ☑
  puerperal, postpartum, childbirth O85
  specified organism NEC A41.89
  tuberculous — *see* Tuberculosis, miliary
Pygopagus Q89.4
Pyknoepilepsy (idiopathic) — *see* Pyknolepsy
Pyknolepsy G40.A09 (following G40.3)
  intractable G40.A19 (following G40.3)
    with status epilepticus G40.A11 (following G40.3)
    without status epilepticus G40.A19 (following G40.3)
  not intractable G40.A09 (following G40.3)

Pyknolepsy — *continued*
  not intractable — *continued*
    with status epilepticus G40.A01 (following G40.3)
    without status epilepticus G40.A09 (following G40.3)
Pylephlebitis K75.1
Pyle's syndrome Q78.5
Pylethrombophlebitis K75.1
Pylethrombosis K75.1
Pyloritis K29.90
  with bleeding K29.91
Pylorospasm (reflex) **NEC** K31.3
  congenital or infantile Q40.0
  neurotic F45.8
  newborn Q40.0
  psychogenic F45.8
Pylorus, pyloric — *see* condition
Pyoarthrosis — *see* Arthritis, pyogenic or pyemic
Pyocele
  mastoid — *see* Mastoiditis, acute
  sinus (accessory) — *see* Sinusitis
  turbinate (bone) J32.9
  urethra (*see also* Urethritis) N34.0
Pyocolpos — *see* Vaginitis
Pyocystitis N30.80
  with hematuria N30.81
Pyoderma, pyodermia L08.0
  gangrenosum L88
  newborn P39.4
  phagedenic L88
  vegetans L08.81
Pyodermatitis L08.0
  vegetans L08.81
Pyogenic — *see* condition
Pyohydronephrosis N13.6
Pyometra, pyometrium, pyometritis — *see* Endometritis
Pyomyositis (tropical) — *see* Myositis, infective
Pyonephritis N12
Pyonephrosis N13.6
  tuberculous A18.11
Pyo-oophoritis — *see* Salpingo-oophoritis
Pyo-ovarium — *see* Salpingo-oophoritis
Pyopericarditis, pyopericardium I30.1
Pyophlebitis — *see* Phlebitis
Pyopneumopericardium I30.1
Pyopneumothorax (infective) J86.9
  with fistula J86.0
  tuberculous NEC A15.6
Pyosalpinx, pyosalpingitis (*see also* Salpingo-oophoritis)
Pyothorax J86.9
  with fistula J86.0
  tuberculous NEC A15.6
Pyoureter N28.89
  tuberculous A18.11
Pyramidopallidonigral syndrome G20
Pyrexia (of unknown origin) R50.9
  atmospheric T67.0 ☑
  during labor NEC O75.2
  heat T67.0 ☑
  newborn P81.9
    environmentally-induced P81.0
  persistent R50.9
  puerperal O86.4
Pyroglobulinemia NEC E88.09
Pyromania F63.1
Pyrosis R12
Pyuria (bacterial) N39.0

Q

Q fever A78
  with pneumonia A78
Quadricuspid aortic valve Q23.8
Quadrilateral fever A78
Quadriparesis — *see* Quadriplegia
  meaning muscle weakness M62.81
Quadriplegia G82.50
  complete
    C1-C4 level G82.51
    C5-C7 level G82.53
  congenital (cerebral) (spinal) G80.8
    spastic G80.0
  embolic (current episode) I63.4- ☑
  functional R53.2

Quadriplegia — continued
- incomplete
  - C1-C4 level G82.52
  - C5-C7 level G82.54
- thrombotic (current episode) I63.3- ☑
- traumatic — code to injury with seventh character S
  - current episode — see Injury, spinal (cord), cervical

Quadruplet, pregnancy — see Pregnancy, quadruplet

Quarrelsomeness F60.3

Queensland fever A77.3

Quervain's disease M65.4
- thyroid E06.1

Queyrat's erythroplasia D07.4
- penis D07.4
- specified site — see Neoplasm, skin, in situ
- unspecified site D07.4

Quincke's disease or edema T78.3 ☑
- hereditary D84.1

Quinsy (gangrenous) J36

Quintan fever A79.0

Quintuplet, pregnancy — see Pregnancy, quintuplet

R

Rabbit fever — see Tularemia

Rabies A82.9
- contact Z20.3
- exposure to Z20.3
- inoculation reaction — see Complications, vaccination
- sylvatic A82.0
- urban A82.1

Rachischisis — see Spina bifida

Rachitic (see also condition)
- deformities of spine (late effect) (sequelae) E64.3
- pelvis (late effect) (sequelae) E64.3
  - with disproportion (fetopelvic) O33.0
    - causing obstructed labor O65.0

Rachitis, rachitism (acute) (tarda) (see also Rickets)
- renalis N25.0
- sequelae E64.3

Radial nerve — see condition

Radiation
- burn — see Burn
- effects NOS T66 ☑
- sickness NOS T66 ☑
- therapy, encounter for Z51.0

Radiculitis (pressure) (vertebrogenic) — see Radiculopathy

Radiculomyelitis (see also Encephalitis)
- toxic, due to
  - Clostridium tetani A35
  - Corynebacterium diphtheriae A36.82

Radiculopathy M54.10
- cervical region M54.12
- cervicothoracic region M54.13
- due to
  - disc disorder
    - C3 M50.11
    - C4 M50.11
    - C5 M50.121
    - C6 M50.122
    - C7 M50.123
  - displacement of intervertebral disc — see Disorder, disc, with, radiculopathy
- leg M54.1- ☑
- lumbar region M54.16
- lumbosacral region M54.17
- occipito-atlanto-axial region M54.11
- postherpetic B02.29
- sacrococcygeal region M54.18
- syphilitic A52.11
- thoracic region (with visceral pain) M54.14
- thoracolumbar region M54.15

Radiodermal burns (acute, chronic, or occupational) — see Burn

Radiodermatitis L58.9
- acute L58.0
- chronic L58.1

Radiotherapy session Z51.0

RAEB (refractory anemia with excess blasts) D46.2- ☑

Rage, meaning rabies — see Rabies

Ragpicker's disease A22.1

Ragsorter's disease A22.1

Raillietiniasis B71.8

Railroad neurosis F48.8

Railway spine F48.8

Raised (see also Elevated)
- antibody titer R76.0

Rake teeth, tooth M26.39

Rales R09.89

Ramifying renal pelvis Q63.8

Ramsay-Hunt disease or syndrome (see also Hunt's disease) B02.21
- meaning dyssynergia cerebellaris myoclonica G11.1

Ranula K11.6
- congenital Q38.4

Rape
- adult
  - confirmed T74.21 ☑
  - suspected T76.21 ☑
- alleged, observation or examination, ruled out
  - adult Z04.41
  - child Z04.42
- child
  - confirmed T74.22 ☑
  - suspected T76.22 ☑

Rapid
- feeble pulse, due to shock, following injury T79.4 ☑
- heart (beat) R00.0
  - psychogenic F45.8
- second stage (delivery) O62.3
- time-zone change syndrome — see Disorder, sleep, circadian rhythm, psychogenic

Rarefaction, bone — see Disorder, bone, density and structure, specified NEC

Rash (toxic) R21
- canker A38.9
- diaper L22
- drug (internal use) L27.0
  - contact (see also Dermatitis, due to, drugs, external) L25.1
- following immunization T88.1 ☑
- food — see Dermatitis, due to, food
- heat L74.0
- napkin (psoriasiform) L22
- nettle — see Urticaria
- pustular L08.0
- rose R21
  - epidemic B06.9
- scarlet A38.9
- serum (see also Reaction, serum) T80.69 ☑
- wandering tongue K14.1

Rasmussen aneurysm — see Tuberculosis, pulmonary

Rasmussen encephalitis G04.81

Rat-bite fever A25.9
- due to Streptobacillus moniliformis A25.1
- spirochetal (morsus muris) A25.0

Rathke's pouch tumor D44.3

Raymond (-Céstan) **syndrome** I65.8

Raynaud's disease, phenomenon or syndrome (secondary) I73.00
- with gangrene (symmetric) I73.01

RDS (newborn) (type I) P22.0
- type II P22.1

Reaction (see also Disorder)
- adaptation — see Disorder, adjustment
- adjustment (anxiety) (conduct disorder) (depressiveness) (distress) — see Disorder, adjustment
  - with
    - mutism, elective (child) (adolescent) F94.0
- adverse
  - food (any) (ingested) NEC T78.1 ☑
    - anaphylactic — see Shock, anaphylactic, due to food
- affective — see Disorder, mood
- allergic — see Allergy
- anaphylactic — see Shock, anaphylactic
- anaphylactoid — see Shock, anaphylactic
- anesthesia — see Anesthesia, complication
- antitoxin (prophylactic) (therapeutic) — see Complications, vaccination
- anxiety F41.1
- Arthus — see Arthus' phenomenon
- asthenic F48.8
- combat and operational stress F43.0
- compulsive F42.8
- conversion F44.9
- crisis, acute F43.0
- deoxyribonuclease (DNA) (DNase) hypersensitivity D69.2
- depressive (single episode) F32.9
  - affective (single episode) F31.4
    - recurrent episode F33.9

Reaction — continued
- depressive — continued
  - neurotic F34.1
  - psychoneurotic F34.1
  - psychotic F32.3
  - recurrent — see Disorder, depressive, recurrent
- dissociative F44.9
- drug NEC T88.7 ☑
  - addictive — see Dependence, drug
    - transmitted via placenta or breast milk — see Absorption, drug, addictive, through placenta
  - allergic — see Allergy, drug
  - lichenoid L43.2
  - newborn P93.8
    - gray baby syndrome P93.0
  - overdose or poisoning (by accident) — see Table of Drugs and Chemicals, by drug, poisoning
  - photoallergic L56.1
  - phototoxic L56.0
  - withdrawal — see Dependence, by drug, with, withdrawal
    - infant of dependent mother P96.1
    - newborn P96.1
  - wrong substance given or taken (by accident) — see Table of Drugs and Chemicals, by drug, poisoning
- fear F40.9
  - child (abnormal) F93.8
- febrile nonhemolytic transfusion (FNHTR) R50.84
- fluid loss, cerebrospinal G97.1
- foreign
  - body NEC — see Granuloma, foreign body
    - in operative wound (inadvertently left) — see Foreign body, accidentally left during a procedure
  - substance accidentally left during a procedure (chemical) (powder) (talc) T81.60 ☑
    - aseptic peritonitis T81.61 ☑
    - body or object (instrument) (sponge) (swab) — see Foreign body, accidentally left during a procedure
    - specified reaction NEC T81.69 ☑
- grief — see Disorder, adjustment
- Herxheimer's R68.89
- hyperkinetic — see Hyperkinesia
- hypochondriacal F45.20
- hypoglycemic, due to insulin E16.0
  - with coma (diabetic) — see Diabetes, coma nondiabetic E15
  - therapeutic misadventure — see subcategory T38.3 ☑
- hypomanic F30.8
- hysterical F44.9
- immunization — see Complications, vaccination
- incompatibility
  - ABO blood group (infusion) (transfusion) — see Complication(s), transfusion, incompatibility reaction, ABO
  - delayed serologic T80.39 ☑
  - minor blood group (Duffy) (E) (K(ell)) (Kidd) (Lewis) (M) (N) (P) (S) T80.89 ☑
  - Rh (factor) (infusion) (transfusion) — see Complication(s), transfusion, incompatibility reaction, Rh (factor)
- inflammatory — see Infection
- infusion — see Complications, infusion
- inoculation (immune serum) — see Complications, vaccination
- insulin T38.3- ☑
- involutional psychotic — see Disorder, depressive
- leukemoid D72.823
  - basophilic D72.823
  - lymphocytic D72.823
  - monocytic D72.823
  - myelocytic D72.823
  - neutrophilic D72.823
- LSD (acute)
  - due to drug abuse — see Abuse, drug, hallucinogen
  - due to drug dependence — see Dependence, drug, hallucinogen
- lumbar puncture G97.1
- manic-depressive — see Disorder, bipolar
- neurasthenic F48.8
- neurogenic — see Neurosis
- neurotic F48.9
- neurotic-depressive F34.1

Reaction — *continued*
  nitritoid — *see* Crisis, nitritoid
  nonspecific
   to
    cell mediated immunity measurement of gamma interferon antigen response without active tuberculosis R76.12
    QuantiFERON-TB test (QFT) without active tuberculosis R76.12
    tuberculin test (*see also* Reaction, tuberculin skin test) R76.11
  obsessive-compulsive F42.8
  organic, acute or subacute — *see* Delirium
  paranoid (acute) F23
   chronic F22
   senile F03 ☑
  passive dependency F60.7
  phobic F40.9
  post-traumatic stress, uncomplicated Z73.3
  psychogenic F99
  psychoneurotic (*see also* Neurosis)
   compulsive F42.8
   depersonalization F48.1
   depressive F34.1
   hypochondriacal F45.20
   neurasthenic F48.8
   obsessive F42.8
  psychophysiologic — *see* Disorder, somatoform
  psychosomatic — *see* Disorder, somatoform
  psychotic — *see* Psychosis
  scarlet fever toxin — *see* Complications, vaccination
  schizophrenic F23
   acute (brief) (undifferentiated) F23
   latent F21
   undifferentiated (acute) (brief) F23
  serological for syphilis — *see* Serology for syphilis
  serum T80.69 ☑
   anaphylactic (immediate) (*see also* Shock, anaphylactic) T80.59 ☑
   specified reaction NEC
    due to
     administration of blood and blood products T80.61 ☑
     immunization T80.62 ☑
     serum specified NEC T80.69 ☑
     vaccination T80.62 ☑
  situational — *see* Disorder, adjustment
  somatization — *see* Disorder, somatoform
  spinal puncture G97.1
  stress (severe) F43.9
   acute (agitation) ("daze") (disorientation) (disturbance of consciousness) (flight reaction) (fugue) F43.0
   specified NEC F43.8
  surgical procedure — *see* Complications, surgical procedure
  tetanus antitoxin — *see* Complications, vaccination
  toxic, to local anesthesia T88.59 ☑
   in labor and delivery O74.4
   in pregnancy O29.3X- ☑
   postpartum, puerperal O89.3
  toxin-antitoxin — *see* Complications, vaccination
  transfusion (blood) (bone marrow) (lymphocytes) (allergic) — *see* Complications, transfusion
  tuberculin skin test, abnormal R76.11
  vaccination (any) — *see* Complications, vaccination
  withdrawing, child or adolescent F93.8
Reactive airway disease — *see* Asthma
Reactive depression — *see* Reaction, depressive
Rearrangement
  chromosomal
   balanced (in) Q95.9
    abnormal individual (autosomal) Q95.2
     non-sex (autosomal) chromosomes Q95.2
     sex/non-sex chromosomes Q95.3
    specified NEC Q95.8
Recalcitrant patient — *see* Noncompliance
Recanalization, thrombus — *see* Thrombosis
Recession, receding
  chamber angle (eye) H21.55- ☑
  chin M26.09
  gingival (postinfective) (postoperative)
   generalized K06.020
    minimal K06.021
    moderate K06.022
    severe K06.023
   localized K06.010
    minimal K06.011

Recession, receding — *continued*
  gingival — *continued*
   localized — *continued*
    moderate K06.012
    severe K06.013
Recklinghausen disease Q85.01
  bones E21.0
Reclus' disease (cystic) — *see* Mastopathy, cystic
Recrudescent typhus (fever) A75.1
Recruitment, auditory H93.21- ☑
Rectalgia K62.89
Rectitis K62.89
Rectocele
  female (without uterine prolapse) N81.6
   with uterine prolapse N81.4
    incomplete N81.2
  in pregnancy — *see* Pregnancy, complicated by, abnormal, pelvic organs or tissues NEC
  male K62.3
Rectosigmoid junction — *see* condition
Rectosigmoiditis K63.89
  ulcerative (chronic) K51.30
   with
    complication K51.319
     abscess K51.314
     fistula K51.313
     obstruction K51.312
     rectal bleeding K51.311
     specified NEC K51.318
Rectourethral — *see* condition
Rectovaginal — *see* condition
Rectovesical — *see* condition
Rectum, rectal — *see* condition
Recurrent — *see* condition
  pregnancy loss — *see* Loss (of), pregnancy, recurrent
Red bugs B88.0
Red tide (*see also* Table of Drugs and Chemicals)
  T65.82- ☑
Red-cedar lung or pneumonitis J67.8
Reduced
  mobility Z74.09
  ventilatory or vital capacity R94.2
Redundant, redundancy
  anus (congenital) Q43.8
  clitoris N90.89
  colon (congenital) Q43.8
  foreskin (congenital) N47.8
  intestine (congenital) Q43.8
  labia N90.69
  organ or site, congenital NEC — *see* Accessory
  panniculus (abdominal) E65
  prepuce (congenital) N47.8
  pylorus K31.89
  rectum (congenital) Q43.8
  scrotum N50.89
  sigmoid (congenital) Q43.8
  skin L98.7
   and subcutaneous tissue L98.7
   of face L57.4
    eyelids — *see* Blepharochalasis
  stomach K31.89
Reduplication — *see* Duplication
Reflex R29.2
  hyperactive gag J39.2
  pupillary, abnormal — *see* Anomaly, pupil, function
  vasoconstriction I73.9
  vasovagal R55
Reflux K21.9
  acid K21.9
  esophageal K21.9
   with esophagitis K21.0
   newborn P78.83
  gastroesophageal K21.9
   with esophagitis K21.0
  mitral — *see* Insufficiency, mitral
  ureteral — *see* Reflux, vesicoureteral
  vesicoureteral (with scarring) N13.70
   with
    nephropathy N13.729
     with hydroureter N13.739
      bilateral N13.732
      unilateral N13.731
     without hydroureter N13.729
      bilateral N13.722
      unilateral N13.721
    bilateral N13.722
    unilateral N13.721
    pyelonephritis (chronic) N11.0

Reflux — *continued*
  vesicoureteral — *continued*
   without nephropathy N13.71
   congenital Q62.7
Reforming, artificial openings — *see* Attention to, artificial, opening
Refractive error — *see* Disorder, refraction
Refsum's disease or syndrome G60.1
Refusal of
  food, psychogenic F50.89
  treatment (because of) Z53.20
   left against medical advice (AMA) Z53.21
   patient's decision NEC Z53.29
   reasons of belief or group pressure Z53.1
Regional — *see* condition
Regurgitation R11.10
  aortic (valve) — *see* Insufficiency, aortic
  food (*see also* Vomiting)
   with reswallowing — *see* Rumination
   newborn P92.1
  gastric contents — *see* Vomiting
  heart — *see* Endocarditis
  mitral (valve) — *see* Insufficiency, mitral
   congenital Q23.3
  myocardial — *see* Endocarditis
  pulmonary (valve) (heart) I37.1
   congenital Q22.2
   syphilitic A52.03
  tricuspid — *see* Insufficiency, tricuspid
  valve, valvular — *see* Endocarditis
   congenital Q24.8
  vesicoureteral — *see* Reflux, vesicoureteral
Reichmann's disease or syndrome K31.89
Reifenstein syndrome E34.52
Reinsertion
  implantable subdermal contraceptive Z30.46
  intrauterine contraceptive device Z30.433
Reiter's disease, syndrome, or urethritis M02.30
  ankle M02.37- ☑
  elbow M02.32- ☑
  foot joint M02.37- ☑
  hand joint M02.34- ☑
  hip M02.35- ☑
  knee M02.36- ☑
  multiple site M02.39
  shoulder M02.31- ☑
  vertebra M02.38
  wrist M02.33- ☑
Rejection
  food, psychogenic F50.89
  transplant T86.91
   bone T86.830
    marrow T86.01
   cornea T86.840
   heart T86.21
    with lung(s) T86.31
   intestine T86.850
   kidney T86.11
   liver T86.41
   lung(s) T86.810
    with heart T86.31
   organ (immune or nonimmune cause) T86.91
   pancreas T86.890
   skin (allograft) (autograft) T86.820
   specified NEC T86.890
   stem cell (peripheral blood) (umbilical cord) T86.5
Relapsing fever A68.9
  Carter's (Asiatic) A68.1
  Dutton's (West African) A68.1
  Koch's A68.9
  louse-borne (epidemic) A68.0
  Novy's (American) A68.1
  Obermeyers's (European) A68.0
  Spirillum A68.9
  tick-borne (endemic) A68.1
Relationship
  occlusal
   open anterior M26.220
   open posterior M26.221
Relaxation
  anus (sphincter) K62.89
   psychogenic F45.8
  arch (foot) (*see also* Deformity, limb, flat foot)
  back ligaments — *see* Instability, joint, spine
  bladder (sphincter) N31.2
  cardioesophageal K21.9
  cervix — *see* Incompetency, cervix
  diaphragm J98.6

Subterms under main terms may continue to next column or page   ☑ Additional Character Required — Refer to the Tabular List for Character Selection   273

Reaction — Relaxation

Relaxation — continued
  joint (capsule) (ligament) (paralytic) — see Flail, joint
    congenital NEC Q74.8
  lumbosacral (joint) — see subcategory M53.2 ☑
  pelvic floor N81.89
  perineum N81.89
  posture R29.3
  rectum (sphincter) K62.89
  sacroiliac (joint) — see subcategory M53.2 ☑
  scrotum N50.89
  urethra (sphincter) N36.44
  vesical N31.2
Release from prison, anxiety concerning Z65.2
Remains
  canal of Cloquet Q14.0
  capsule (opaque) Q14.8
Remittent fever (malarial) B54
Remnant
  canal of Cloquet Q14.0
  capsule (opaque) Q14.8
  cervix, cervical stump (acquired) (postoperative) N88.8
  cystic duct, postcholecystectomy K91.5
  fingernail L60.8
    congenital Q84.6
  meniscus, knee — see Derangement, knee, meniscus,
    specified NEC
  thyroglossal duct Q89.2
  tonsil J35.8
    infected (chronic) J35.01
  urachus Q64.4
Removal (from) (of)
  artificial
    arm Z44.00- ☑
      complete Z44.01- ☑
      partial Z44.02- ☑
    eye Z44.2- ☑
    leg Z44.10- ☑
      complete Z44.11- ☑
      partial Z44.12- ☑
  breast implant Z45.81 ☑
  cardiac pulse generator (battery) (end-of-life) Z45.010
  catheter (urinary) (indwelling) Z46.6
    from artificial opening — see Attention to, artificial,
      opening
    non-vascular Z46.82
    vascular NEC Z45.2
  device Z46.9
    contraceptive Z30.432
      implantable subdermal Z30.46
    implanted NEC Z45.89
    specified NEC Z46.89
  drains Z48.03
  dressing (nonsurgical) Z48.00
    surgical Z48.01
  external
    fixation device — code to fracture with seventh
      character D
    prosthesis, prosthetic device Z44.9
      breast Z44.3- ☑
      specified NEC Z44.8
  home in childhood (to foster home or institution)
    Z62.29
  ileostomy Z43.2
  insulin pump Z46.81
  myringotomy device (stent) (tube) Z45.82
  nervous system device NEC Z46.2
    brain neuropacemaker Z46.2
    visual substitution device Z46.2
      implanted Z45.31
  non-vascular catheter Z46.82
  organ, prophylactic (for neoplasia management) —
    see Prophylactic, organ removal
  orthodontic device Z46.4
  staples Z48.02
  stent
    ureteral Z46.6
  suture Z48.02
  urinary device Z46.6
  vascular access device or catheter Z45.2
Ren
  arcuatus Q63.1
  mobile, mobilis N28.89
    congenital Q63.8
  unguliformis Q63.1
Renal — see condition
Rendu-Osler-Weber disease or syndrome I78.0
Reninoma D41.0- ☑
Renon-Delille syndrome E23.3

Reovirus, as cause of disease classified elsewhere
  B97.5
Repeated falls NEC R29.6
Replaced chromosome by dicentric ring Q93.2
Replacement by artificial or mechanical device or
    prosthesis of
  bladder Z96.0
  blood vessel NEC Z95.828
  bone NEC Z96.7
  cochlea Z96.21
  coronary artery Z95.5
  eustachian tube Z96.29
  eye globe Z97.0
  heart Z95.812
    valve Z95.2
      prosthetic Z95.2
      specified NEC Z95.4
      xenogenic Z95.3
  intestine Z96.89
  joint Z96.60
    hip — see Presence, hip joint implant
    knee — see Presence, knee joint implant
    specified site NEC Z96.698
  larynx Z96.3
  lens Z96.1
  limb(s) — see Presence, artificial, limb
  mandible NEC (for tooth root implant(s)) Z96.5
  organ NEC Z96.89
  peripheral vessel NEC Z95.828
  stapes Z96.29
  teeth Z97.2
  tendon Z96.7
  tissue NEC Z96.89
  tooth root(s) Z96.5
  vessel NEC Z95.828
    coronary (artery) Z95.5
Request for expert evidence Z04.8
Reserve, decreased or low
  cardiac — see Disease, heart
  kidney N28.89
Residual (see also condition)
  ovary syndrome N99.83
  state, schizophrenic F20.5
  urine R39.198
Resistance, resistant (to)
  activated protein C D68.51
  complicating pregnancy O26.89 ☑
  insulin E88.81
  organism(s)
    to
      drug Z16.30
        aminoglycosides Z16.29
        amoxicillin Z16.11
        ampicillin Z16.11
        antibiotic(s) Z16.20
          multiple Z16.24
          specified NEC Z16.29
        antifungal Z16.32
        antimicrobial (single) Z16.30
          multiple Z16.35
          specified NEC Z16.39
        antimycobacterial (single) Z16.341
          multiple Z16.342
        antiparasitic Z16.31
        antiviral Z16.33
        beta lactam antibiotics Z16.10
          specified NEC Z16.19
        cephalosporins Z16.19
        extended beta lactamase (ESBL) Z16.12
        fluoroquinolones Z16.23
        macrolides Z16.29
        methicillin — see MRSA
        multiple drugs (MDRO)
          antibiotics Z16.24
          antimicrobial Z16.35
          antimycobacterials Z16.342
        penicillins Z16.11
        quinine (and related compounds) Z16.31
        quinolones Z16.23
        sulfonamides Z16.29
        tetracyclines Z16.29
        tuberculostatics (single) Z16.341
          multiple Z16.342
        vancomycin Z16.21
          related antibiotics Z16.22
      thyroid hormone E07.89
Resorption
  dental (roots) K03.3

Resorption — continued
  dental — continued
    alveoli M26.79
    teeth (external) (internal) (pathological) (roots) K03.3
Respiration
  Cheyne-Stokes R06.3
  decreased due to shock, following injury T79.4 ☑
  disorder of, psychogenic F45.8
  insufficient, or poor R06.89
    newborn P28.5
  painful R07.1
  sighing, psychogenic F45.8
Respiratory (see also condition)
  distress syndrome (newborn) (type I) P22.0
    type II P22.1
  syncytial virus, as cause of disease classified elsewhere
    B97.4
Respite care Z75.5
Response (drug)
  photoallergic L56.1
  phototoxic L56.0
Restenosis
  stent
    vascular
      end stent
        adjacent to stent — see Arteriosclerosis
        within the stent
          coronary T82.855 ☑
          peripheral T82.856 ☑
      in stent
        coronary vessel T82.855 ☑
        peripheral vessel T82.856 ☑
Restless legs (syndrome) G25.81
Restlessness R45.1
Restoration (of)
  dental
    aesthetically inadequate or displeasing K08.56
    defective K08.50
      specified NEC K08.59
    failure of marginal integrity K08.51
    failure of periodontal anatomical intergrity K08.54
  organ continuity from previous sterilization (tuboplas-
    ty) (vasoplasty) Z31.0
    aftercare Z31.42
  tooth (existing)
    contours biologically incompatible with oral health
      K08.54
    open margins K08.51
    overhanging K08.52
    poor aesthetic K08.56
    poor gingival margins K08.51
  unsatisfactory, of tooth K08.50
    specified NEC K08.59
Restorative material (dental)
  allergy to K08.55
  fractured K08.539
    with loss of material K08.531
    without loss of material K08.530
  unrepairable overhanging of K08.52
Restriction of housing space Z59.1
Rests, ovarian, in fallopian tube Q50.6
Restzustand (schizophrenic) F20.5
Retained (see also Retention)
  cholelithiasis following cholecystectomy K91.86
  foreign body fragments (type of) Z18.9
    acrylics Z18.2
    animal quill(s) or spines Z18.31
    cement Z18.83
    concrete Z18.83
    crystalline Z18.83
    depleted isotope Z18.09
    depleted uranium Z18.01
    diethylhexylphthalates Z18.2
    glass Z18.81
    isocyanate Z18.2
    magnetic metal Z18.11
    metal Z18.10
    nonmagnectic metal Z18.12
    nontherapeutic radioactive Z18.09
    organic NEC Z18.39
    plastic Z18.2
    quill(s) (animal) Z18.31
    radioactive (nontherapeutic) NEC Z18.09
    specified NEC Z18.89
    spine(s) (animal) Z18.31
    stone Z18.83
    tooth (teeth) Z18.32
    wood Z18.33

274

☑ Additional Character Required — Refer to the Tabular List for Character Selection   ▼ Subterms under main terms may continue to next column or page

Retained — *continued*
- fragments (type of) Z18.9
  - acrylics Z18.2
  - animal quill(s) or spines Z18.31
  - cement Z18.83
  - concrete Z18.83
  - crystalline Z18.83
  - depleted isotope Z18.09
  - depleted uranium Z18.01
  - diethylhexylphthalates Z18.2
  - glass Z18.81
  - isocyanate Z18.2
  - magnetic metal Z18.11
  - metal Z18.10
  - nonmagnectic metal Z18.12
  - nontherapeutic radioactive Z18.09
  - organic NEC Z18.39
  - plastic Z18.2
  - quill(s) (animal) Z18.31
  - radioactive (nontherapeutic) NEC Z18.09
  - specified NEC Z18.89
  - spine(s) (animal) Z18.31
  - stone Z18.83
  - tooth (teeth) Z18.32
  - wood Z18.33
- gallstones, following cholecystectomy K91.86

Retardation
- development, developmental, specific — *see* Disorder, developmental
- endochondral bone growth — *see* Disorder, bone, development or growth
- growth R62.50
  - due to malnutrition E45
- mental — *see* Disability, intellectual
- motor function, specific F82
- physical (child) R62.52
  - due to malnutrition E45
- reading (specific) F81.0
- spelling (specific) (without reading disorder) F81.81

Retching — *see* Vomiting

Retention (*see also* Retained)
- bladder — *see* Retention, urine
- carbon dioxide E87.2
- cholelithiasis following cholecystectomy K91.86
- cyst — *see* Cyst
- dead
  - fetus (at or near term) (mother) O36.4 ☑
    - early fetal death O02.1
  - ovum O02.0
- decidua (fragments) (following delivery) (with hemorrhage) O72.2
  - without hemorrhage O73.1
- deciduous tooth K00.6
- dental root K08.3
- fecal — *see* Constipation
- fetus
  - dead O36.4 ☑
    - early O02.1
- fluid R60.9
- foreign body (*see also* Foreign body, retained)
  - current trauma — *code as* Foreign body, by site or type
- gallstones, following cholecystectomy K91.86
- gastric K31.89
- intrauterine contraceptive device, in pregnancy — *see* Pregnancy, complicated by, retention, intrauterine device
- membranes (complicating delivery) (with hemorrhage) O72.2
  - with abortion — *see* Abortion, by type
  - without hemorrhage O73.1
- meniscus — *see* Derangement, meniscus
- menses N94.89
- milk (puerperal, postpartum) O92.79
- nitrogen, extrarenal R39.2
- ovary syndrome N99.83
- placenta (total) (with hemorrhage) O72.0
  - without hemorrhage O73.0
  - portions or fragments (with hemorrhage) O72.2
    - without hemorrhage O73.1
- products of conception
  - early pregnancy (dead fetus) O02.1
  - following
    - delivery (with hemorrhage) O72.2
      - without hemorrhage O73.1
- secundines (following delivery) (with hemorrhage) O72.0
  - without hemorrhage O73.0

Retention — *continued*
- secundines — *continued*
  - complicating puerperium (delayed hemorrhage) O72.2
  - partial O72.2
    - without hemorrhage O73.1
- smegma, clitoris N90.89
- urine R33.9
  - drug-induced R33.0
  - due to hyperplasia (hypertrophy) of prostate — *see* Hyperplasia, prostate
  - organic R33.8
    - drug-induced R33.0
  - psychogenic F45.8
  - specified NEC R33.8
- water (in tissues) — *see* Edema

Reticulation, dust — *see* Pneumoconiosis
Reticulocytosis R70.1
Reticuloendotheliosis
- acute infantile C96.0
- leukemic C91.4- ☑
- nonlipid C96.0

Reticulohistiocytoma (giant-cell) D76.3
Reticuloid, actinic L57.1
Reticulosis (skin)
- acute of infancy C96.0
- hemophagocytic, familial D76.1
- histiocytic medullary C96.A (*following* C96.6)
- lipomelanotic I89.8
- malignant (midline) C86.0
- polymorphic C83.8- ☑
- Sézary — *see* Sézary disease

Retina, retinal (*see also* condition)
- dark area D49.81

Retinitis (*see also* Inflammation, chorioretinal)
- albuminurica N18.9 [H32]
- diabetic — *see* Diabetes, retinitis
- disciformis — *see* Degeneration, macula
- focal — *see* Inflammation, chorioretinal, focal
- gravidarum — *see* Pregnancy, complicated by, specified pregnancy-related condition NEC
- juxtapapillaris — *see* Inflammation, chorioretinal, focal, juxtapapillary
- luetic — *see* Retinitis, syphilitic
- pigmentosa H35.52
- proliferans — *see* Disorder, globe, degenerative, specified type NEC
- proliferating — *see* Disorder, globe, degenerative, specified type NEC
- renal N18.9 [H32]
- syphilitic (early) (secondary) A51.43
  - central, recurrent A52.71
  - congenital (early) A50.01 [H32]
  - late A52.71
- tuberculous A18.53

Retinoblastoma C69.2- ☑
- differentiated C69.2- ☑
- undifferentiated C69.2- ☑

Retinochoroiditis (*see also* Inflammation, chorioretinal)
- disseminated — *see* Inflammation, chorioretinal, disseminated
  - syphilitic A52.71
- focal — *see* Inflammation, chorioretinal
- juxtapapillaris — *see* Inflammation, chorioretinal, focal, juxtapapillary

Retinopathy (background) H35.00
- arteriosclerotic I70.8 [H35.0-] ☑
- atherosclerotic I70.8 [H35.0-] ☑
- central serous — *see* Chorioretinopathy, central serous
- Coats H35.02- ☑
- diabetic — *see* Diabetes, retinopathy
- exudative H35.02- ☑
- hypertensive H35.03- ☑
- in (due to)
  - diabetes — *see* Diabetes, retinopathy
  - sickle-cell disorders D57.- ☑ [H36]
- of prematurity H35.10- ☑
  - stage 0 H35.11- ☑
  - stage 1 H35.12- ☑
  - stage 2 H35.13- ☑
  - stage 3 H35.14- ☑
  - stage 4 H35.15- ☑
  - stage 5 H35.16- ☑
- pigmentary, congenital — *see* Dystrophy, retina
- proliferative NEC H35.2- ☑
  - diabetic — *see* Diabetes, retinopathy, proliferative
  - sickle-cell D57.- ☑ [H36]

Retinopathy — *continued*
- solar H31.02- ☑
Retinoschisis H33.10- ☑
- congenital Q14.1
- specified type NEC H33.19- ☑
Retortamoniasis A07.8
Retractile testis Q55.22
Retraction
- cervix — *see* Retroversion, uterus
- drum (membrane) — *see* Disorder, tympanic membrane, specified NEC
- finger — *see* Deformity, finger
- lid H02.539
  - left H02.536
    - lower H02.535
    - upper H02.534
  - right H02.533
    - lower H02.532
    - upper H02.531
- lung J98.4
- mediastinum J98.59
- nipple N64.53
  - associated with
    - lactation O92.03
    - pregnancy O92.01- ☑
    - puerperium O92.02
  - congenital Q83.8
- palmar fascia M72.0
- pleura — *see* Pleurisy
- ring, uterus (Bandl's) (pathological) O62.4
- sternum (congenital) Q76.7
  - acquired M95.4
- uterus — *see* Retroversion, uterus
- valve (heart) — *see* Endocarditis
Retrobulbar — *see* condition
Retrocecal — *see* condition
Retrocession — *see* Retroversion
Retrodisplacement — *see* Retroversion
Retroflection, retroflexion — *see* Retroversion
Retrognathia, retrognathism (mandibular) (maxillary) M26.19
Retrograde menstruation N92.5
Retroperineal — *see* condition
Retroperitoneal — *see* condition
Retroperitonitis K68.9
Retropharyngeal — *see* condition
Retroplacental — *see* condition
Retroposition — *see* Retroversion
Retroprosthetic membrane T85.398 ☑
Retrosternal thyroid (congenital) Q89.2
Retroversion, retroverted
- cervix — *see* Retroversion, uterus
- female NEC — *see* Retroversion, uterus
- iris H21.89
- testis (congenital) Q55.29
- uterus (acquired) (acute) (any degree) (asymptomatic) (cervix) (postinfectional) (postpartal, old) N85.4
  - congenital Q51.818
  - in pregnancy O34.53- ☑
Retrovirus, as cause of disease classified elsewhere B97.30
- human
  - immunodeficiency, type 2 (HIV 2) B97.35
  - T-cell lymphotropic
    - type I (HTLV-I) B97.33
    - type II (HTLV-II) B97.34
- lentivirus B97.31
- oncovirus B97.32
- specified NEC B97.39
Retrusion, premaxilla (developmental) M26.09
Rett's disease or syndrome F84.2
Reverse peristalsis R19.2
Reye's syndrome G93.7
Rh (factor)
- hemolytic disease (newborn) P55.0
- incompatibility, immunization or sensitization
  - affecting management of pregnancy NEC O36.09- ☑
    - anti-D antibody O36.01- ☑
  - newborn P55.0
    - transfusion reaction — *see* Complication(s), transfusion, incompatibility reaction, Rh (factor)
- negative mother affecting newborn P55.0
- titer elevated — *see* Complication(s), transfusion, incompatibility reaction, Rh (factor)
- transfusion reaction — *see* Complication(s), transfusion, incompatibility reaction, Rh (factor)

Index

Rhabdomyolysis (idiopathic) NEC M62.82
  traumatic T79.6 ☑
Rhabdomyoma (see also Neoplasm, connective tissue, benign)
  adult — see Neoplasm, connective tissue, benign
  fetal — see Neoplasm, connective tissue, benign
  glycogenic — see Neoplasm, connective tissue, benign
Rhabdomyosarcoma (any type) — see Neoplasm, connective tissue, malignant
Rhabdosarcoma — see Rhabdomyosarcoma
Rhesus (factor) **incompatibility** — see Rh, incompatibility
Rheumatic (acute) (subacute) (chronic)
  adherent pericardium I09.2
  coronary arteritis I01.9
  degeneration, myocardium I09.0
  fever (acute) — see Fever, rheumatic
  heart — see Disease, heart, rheumatic
  myocardial degeneration — see Degeneration, myocardium
  myocarditis (chronic) (inactive) (with chorea) I09.0
    with chorea (acute) (rheumatic) (Sydenham's) I02.0
    active or acute I01.2
  pancarditis, acute I01.8
    with chorea (acute) (rheumatic) Sydenham's) I02.0
  pericarditis (active) (acute) (with effusion) (with pneumonia) I01.0
    with chorea (acute) (rheumatic) (Sydenham's) I02.0
    chronic or inactive I09.2
  pneumonia I00 [J17]
  torticollis M43.6
  typhoid fever A01.09
Rheumatism (articular) (neuralgic) (nonarticular) M79.0
  gout — see Arthritis, rheumatoid
  intercostal, meaning Tietze's disease M94.0
  palindromic (any site) M12.30
    ankle M12.37- ☑
    elbow M12.32- ☑
    foot joint M12.37- ☑
    hand joint M12.34- ☑
    hip M12.35- ☑
    knee M12.36- ☑
    multiple site M12.39
    shoulder M12.31- ☑
    specified joint NEC M12.38
    vertebrae M12.38
    wrist M12.33- ☑
  sciatic M54.4- ☑
Rheumatoid (see also condition)
  arthritis (see also Arthritis, rheumatoid)
    with involvement of organs NEC M05.60
      ankle M05.67- ☑
      elbow M05.62- ☑
      foot joint M05.67- ☑
      hand joint M05.64- ☑
      hip M05.65- ☑
      knee M05.66- ☑
      multiple site M05.69
      shoulder M05.61- ☑
      vertebra — see Spondylitis, ankylosing
      wrist M05.63- ☑
    seronegative — see Arthritis, rheumatoid, seronegative
    seropositive — see Arthritis, rheumatoid, seropositive
  carditis M05.30
    ankle M05.37- ☑
    elbow M05.32- ☑
    foot joint M05.37- ☑
    hand joint M05.34- ☑
    hip M05.35- ☑
    knee M05.36- ☑
    multiple site M05.39
    shoulder M05.31- ☑
    vertebra — see Spondylitis, ankylosing
    wrist M05.33- ☑
  endocarditis — see Rheumatoid, carditis
  lung (disease) M05.10
    ankle M05.17- ☑
    elbow M05.12- ☑
    foot joint M05.17- ☑
    hand joint M05.14- ☑
    hip M05.15- ☑
    knee M05.16- ☑
    multiple site M05.19
    shoulder M05.11- ☑
    vertebra — see Spondylitis, ankylosing

Rheumatoid — continued
  lung — continued
    wrist M05.13- ☑
  myocarditis — see Rheumatoid, carditis
  myopathy M05.40
    ankle M05.47- ☑
    elbow M05.42- ☑
    foot joint M05.47- ☑
    hand joint M05.44- ☑
    hip M05.45- ☑
    knee M05.46- ☑
    multiple site M05.49
    shoulder M05.41- ☑
    vertebra — see Spondylitis, ankylosing
    wrist M05.43- ☑
  pericarditis — see Rheumatoid, carditis
  polyarthritis — see Arthritis, rheumatoid
  polyneuropathy M05.50
    ankle M05.57- ☑
    elbow M05.52- ☑
    foot joint M05.57- ☑
    hand joint M05.54- ☑
    hip M05.55- ☑
    knee M05.56- ☑
    multiple site M05.59
    shoulder M05.51- ☑
    vertebra — see Spondylitis, ankylosing
    wrist M05.53- ☑
  vasculitis M05.20
    ankle M05.27- ☑
    elbow M05.22- ☑
    foot joint M05.27- ☑
    hand joint M05.24- ☑
    hip M05.25- ☑
    knee M05.26- ☑
    multiple site M05.29
    shoulder M05.21- ☑
    vertebra — see Spondylitis, ankylosing
    wrist M05.23- ☑
Rhinitis (atrophic) (catarrhal) (chronic) (croupous) (fibrinous) (granulomatous) (hyperplastic) (hypertrophic) (membranous) (obstructive) (purulent) (suppurative) (ulcerative) J31.0
  with
    sore throat — see Nasopharyngitis
  acute J00
  allergic J30.9
    with asthma J45.909
      with
        exacerbation (acute) J45.901
        status asthmaticus J45.902
    due to
      food J30.5
      pollen J30.1
    nonseasonal J30.89
    perennial J30.89
    seasonal NEC J30.2
    specified NEC J30.89
  infective J00
  pneumococcal J00
  syphilitic A52.73
    congenital A50.05 [J99]
  tuberculous A15.8
  vasomotor J30.0
Rhinoantritis (chronic) — see Sinusitis, maxillary
Rhinodacryolith — see Dacryolith
Rhinolith (nasal sinus) J34.89
Rhinomegaly J34.89
Rhinopharyngitis (acute) (subacute) (see also Nasopharyngitis)
  chronic J31.1
  destructive ulcerating A66.5
  mutilans A66.5
Rhinophyma L71.1
Rhinorrhea J34.89
  cerebrospinal (fluid) G96.0
  paroxysmal — see Rhinitis, allergic
  spasmodic — see Rhinitis, allergic
Rhinosalpingitis — see Salpingitis, eustachian
Rhinoscleroma A48.8
Rhinosporidiosis B48.1
Rhinovirus infection NEC B34.8
Rhizomelic chondrodysplasia punctata E71.540
Rhythm
  atrioventricular nodal I49.8
  disorder I49.9
    coronary sinus I49.8

Rhythm — continued
  disorder — continued
    ectopic I49.8
    nodal I49.8
    escape I49.9
    heart, abnormal I49.9
    idioventricular I44.2
    nodal I49.8
    sleep, inversion G47.2- ☑
      nonorganic origin — see Disorder, sleep, circadian rhythm, psychogenic
Rhytidosis facialis L98.8
Rib (see also condition)
  cervical Q76.5
Riboflavin deficiency E53.0
Rice bodies (see also Loose, body, joint)
  knee M23.4- ☑
Richter syndrome — see Leukemia, chronic lymphocytic, B-cell type
Richter's hernia — see Hernia, abdomen, with obstruction
Ricinism — see Poisoning, food, noxious, plant
Rickets (active) (acute) (adolescent) (chest wall) (congenital) (current) (infantile) (intestinal) E55.0
  adult — see Osteomalacia
  celiac K90.0
  hypophosphatemic with nephrotic-glycosuric dwarfism E72.09
  inactive E64.3
  kidney N25.0
  renal N25.0
  sequelae, any E64.3
  vitamin-D-resistant E83.31 [M90.80]
Rickettsial disease A79.9
  specified type NEC A79.89
Rickettsialpox (Rickettsia akari) A79.1
Rickettsiosis A79.9
  due to
    Ehrlichia sennetsu A79.81
    Rickettsia akari (rickettsialpox) A79.1
  specified type NEC A79.89
  tick-borne A77.9
  vesicular A79.1
Rider's bone — see Ossification, muscle, specified NEC
Ridge, alveolus (see also condition)
  flabby K06.8
Ridged ear, congenital Q17.3
Riedel's
  lobe, liver Q44.7
  struma, thyroiditis or disease E06.5
Rieger's anomaly or syndrome Q13.81
Riehl's melanosis L81.4
Rietti-Greppi-Micheli anemia D56.9
Rieux's hernia — see Hernia, abdomen, specified site NEC
Riga (-Fede) **disease** K14.0
Riggs' disease — see Periodontitis
Right aortic arch Q25.47
Right middle lobe syndrome J98.11
Rigid, rigidity (see also condition)
  abdominal R19.30
    with severe abdominal pain R10.0
    epigastric R19.36
    generalized R19.37
    left lower quadrant R19.34
    left upper quadrant R19.32
    periumbilic R19.35
    right lower quadrant R19.33
    right upper quadrant R19.31
  articular, multiple, congenital Q68.8
  cervix (uteri) in pregnancy — see Pregnancy, complicated by, abnormal, cervix
  hymen (acquired) (congenital) N89.6
  nuchal R29.1
  pelvic floor in pregnancy — see Pregnancy, complicated by, abnormal, pelvic organs or tissues NEC
  perineum or vulva in pregnancy — see Pregnancy, complicated by, abnormal, vulva
  spine — see Dorsopathy, specified NEC
  vagina in pregnancy — see Pregnancy, complicated by, abnormal, vagina
Rigors R68.89
  with fever R50.9
Riley-Day syndrome G90.1
RIND (reversible ischemic neurologic deficit) I63.9
Ring(s)
  aorta (vascular) Q25.45
  Bandl's O62.4

Ring(s) — *continued*
  contraction, complicating delivery O62.4
  esophageal, lower (muscular) K22.2
  Fleischer's (cornea) H18.04- ☑
  hymenal, tight (acquired) (congenital) N89.6
  Kayser-Fleischer (cornea) H18.04- ☑
  retraction, uterus, pathological O62.4
  Schatzki's (esophagus) (lower) K22.2
    congenital Q39.3
  Soemmerring's — *see* Cataract, secondary
  vascular (congenital) Q25.8
    aorta Q25.45
Ringed hair (congenital) Q84.1
Ringworm B35.9
  beard B35.0
  black dot B35.0
  body B35.4
  Burmese B35.5
  corporeal B35.4
  foot B35.3
  groin B35.6
  hand B35.2
  honeycomb B35.0
  nails B35.1
  perianal (area) B35.6
  scalp B35.0
  specified NEC B35.8
  Tokelau B35.5
Rise, venous pressure I87.8
Rising, PSA following treatment for malignant neoplasm of prostate R97.21
Risk
  for
    dental caries Z91.849
      high Z91.843
      low Z91.841
      moderate Z91.842
  suicidal
    meaning personal history of attempted suicide Z91.5
    meaning suicidal ideation — *see* Ideation, suicidal
Ritter's disease L00
Rivalry, sibling Z62.891
Rivalta's disease A42.2
River blindness B73.01
Robert's pelvis Q74.2
  with disproportion (fetopelvic) O33.0
    causing obstructed labor O65.0
Robin (-Pierre) **syndrome** Q87.0
Robinow-Silvermann-Smith syndrome Q87.1
Robinson's (hidrotic) **ectodermal dysplasia or syndrome** Q82.4
Robles' disease B73.01
Rocky Mountain (spotted) **fever** A77.0
Roetheln — *see* Rubella
Roger's disease Q21.0
Rokitansky-Aschoff sinuses (gallbladder) K82.8
Rolando's fracture (displaced) S62.22- ☑
  nondisplaced S62.22- ☑
Romano-Ward (prolonged QT interval) **syndrome** I45.81
Romberg's disease or syndrome G51.8
Roof, mouth — *see* condition
Rosacea L71.9
  acne L71.9
  keratitis L71.8
  specified NEC L71.8
Rosary, rachitic E55.0
Rose
  cold J30.1
  fever J30.1
  rash R21
    epidemic B06.9
Rosenbach's erysipeloid A26.0
Rosenthal's disease or syndrome D68.1
Roseola B09
  infantum B08.20
    due to human herpesvirus 6 B08.21
    due to human herpesvirus 7 B08.22
Ross River disease or fever B33.1
Rossbach's disease K31.89
  psychogenic F45.8
Rostan's asthma (cardiac) — *see* Failure, ventricular, left
Rotation
  anomalous, incomplete or insufficient, intestine Q43.3
  cecum (congenital) Q43.3
  colon (congenital) Q43.3

Rotation — *continued*
  spine, incomplete or insufficient — *see* Dorsopathy, deforming, specified NEC
  tooth, teeth, fully erupted M26.35
  vertebra, incomplete or insufficient — *see* Dorsopathy, deforming, specified NEC
Rotes Quérol disease or syndrome — *see* Hyperostosis, ankylosing
Roth (-Bernhardt) **disease or syndrome** — *see* Meralgia paraesthetica
Rothmund (-Thomson) **syndrome** Q82.8
Rotor's disease or syndrome E80.6
Round
  back (with wedging of vertebrae) — *see* Kyphosis
    sequelae (late effect) of rickets E64.3
  worms (large) (infestation) NEC B82.0
    Ascariasis (*see also* Ascariasis) B77.9
Roussy-Lévy syndrome G60.0
Rubella (German measles) B06.9
  complication NEC B06.09
    neurological B06.00
  congenital P35.0
  contact Z20.4
  exposure to Z20.4
  maternal
    care for (suspected) damage to fetus O35.3 ☑
    manifest rubella in infant P35.0
    suspected damage to fetus affecting management of pregnancy O35.3 ☑
  specified complications NEC B06.89
Rubeola (meaning measles) — *see* Measles
  meaning rubella — *see* Rubella
Rubeosis, iris — *see* Disorder, iris, vascular
Rubinstein-Taybi syndrome Q87.2
Rudimentary (congenital) (*see also* Agenesis)
  arm — *see* Defect, reduction, upper limb
  bone Q79.9
  cervix uteri Q51.828
  eye Q11.2
  lobule of ear Q17.3
  patella Q74.1
  respiratory organs in thoracopagus Q89.4
  tracheal bronchus Q32.4
  uterus Q51.818
    in male Q56.1
  vagina Q52.0
Ruled out condition — *see* Observation, suspected
Rumination R11.10
  with nausea R11.2
  disorder of infancy F98.21
  neurotic F42.8
  newborn P92.1
  obsessional F42.8
  psychogenic F42.8
Runeberg's disease D51.0
Runny nose R09.89
Rupia (syphilitic) A51.39
  congenital A50.06
  tertiary A52.79
Rupture, ruptured
  abscess (spontaneous) — *code by* site under Abscess
  aneurysm — *see* Aneurysm
  anus (sphincter) — *see* Laceration, anus
  aorta, aortic I71.8
    abdominal I71.3
    arch I71.1
    ascending I71.1
    descending I71.8
      abdominal I71.3
      thoracic I71.1
    syphilitic A52.01
    thoracoabdominal I71.5
    thorax, thoracic I71.1
    transverse I71.1
    traumatic — *see* Injury, aorta, laceration, major
    valve or cusp (*see also* Endocarditis, aortic) I35.8
  appendix (with peritonitis) K35.2
    with localized peritonitis K35.3
  arteriovenous fistula, brain I60.8
  artery I77.2
    brain — *see* Hemorrhage, intracranial, intracerebral
    coronary — *see* Infarct, myocardium
    heart — *see* Infarct, myocardium
    pulmonary I28.8
    traumatic (complication) — *see* Injury, blood vessel
  bile duct (common) (hepatic) K83.2
    cystic K82.2

Rupture, ruptured — *continued*
  bladder (sphincter) (nontraumatic) (spontaneous) N32.89
    following ectopic or molar pregnancy O08.6
    obstetrical trauma O71.5
    traumatic S37.29 ☑
  blood vessel (*see also* Hemorrhage)
    brain — *see* Hemorrhage, intracranial, intracerebral
    heart — *see* Infarct, myocardium
    traumatic (complication) — *see* Injury, blood vessel, laceration, major, by site
  bone — *see* Fracture
  bowel (nontraumatic) K63.1
  brain
    aneurysm (congenital) (*see also* Hemorrhage, intracranial, subarachnoid)
      syphilitic A52.05
    hemorrhagic — *see* Hemorrhage, intracranial, intracerebral
  capillaries I78.8
  cardiac (auricle) (ventricle) (wall) I23.3
    with hemopericardium I23.0
    infectional I40.9
    traumatic — *see* Injury, heart
  cartilage (articular) (current) (*see also* Sprain)
    knee S83.3- ☑
    semilunar — *see* Tear, meniscus
  cecum (with peritonitis) K65.0
    with peritoneal abscess K35.3
    traumatic S36.598 ☑
  celiac artery, traumatic — *see* Injury, blood vessel, celiac artery, laceration, major
  cerebral aneurysm (congenital) (*See* Hemorrhage, intracranial, subarachnoid)
  cervix (uteri)
    with ectopic or molar pregnancy O08.6
    following ectopic or molar pregnancy O08.6
    obstetrical trauma O71.3
    traumatic S37.69 ☑
  chordae tendineae NEC I51.1
    concurrent with acute myocardial infarction — *see* Infarct, myocardium
    following acute myocardial infarction (current complication) I23.4
  choroid (direct) (indirect) (traumatic) H31.32- ☑
  circle of Willis I60.6
  colon (nontraumatic) K63.1
    traumatic — *see* Injury, intestine, large
  cornea (traumatic) — *see* Injury, eye, laceration
  coronary (artery) (thrombotic) — *see* Infarct, myocardium
  corpus luteum (infected) (ovary) N83.1- ☑
  cyst — *see* Cyst
  cystic duct K82.2
  Descemet's membrane — *see* Change, corneal membrane, Descemet's, rupture
    traumatic — *see* Injury, eye, laceration
  diaphragm, traumatic — *see* Injury, intrathoracic, diaphragm
  disc — *see* Rupture, intervertebral disc
  diverticulum (intestine) K57.80
    with bleeding K57.81
    bladder N32.3
    large intestine K57.20
      with
        bleeding K57.21
        small intestine K57.40
          with bleeding K57.41
    small intestine K57.00
      with
        bleeding K57.01
        large intestine K57.40
          with bleeding K57.41
  duodenal stump K31.89
  ear drum (nontraumatic) (*see also* Perforation, tympanum)
    traumatic S09.2- ☑
    due to blast injury — *see* Injury, blast, ear
  esophagus K22.3
  eye (without prolapse or loss of intraocular tissue) — *see* Injury, eye, laceration
  fallopian tube NEC (nonobstetric) (nontraumatic) N83.8
    due to pregnancy O00.10- ☑
    with intrauterine pregnancy O00.11- ☑
  fontanel P13.1
  gallbladder K82.2
    traumatic S36.128 ☑

Rupture, ruptured — continued
  gastric (see also Rupture, stomach)
    vessel K92.2
  globe (eye) (traumatic) — see Injury, eye, laceration
  graafian follicle (hematoma) N83.0- ☑
  heart — see Rupture, cardiac
  hymen (nontraumatic) (nonintentional) N89.8
  internal organ, traumatic — see Injury, by site
  intervertebral disc — see Displacement, intervertebral
      disc
    traumatic — see Rupture, traumatic, intervertebral
        disc
  intestine NEC (nontraumatic) K63.1
    traumatic — see Injury, intestine
  iris (see also Abnormality, pupillary)
    traumatic — see Injury, eye, laceration
  joint capsule, traumatic — see Sprain
  kidney (traumatic) S37.06- ☑
    birth injury P15.8
    nontraumatic N28.89
  lacrimal duct (traumatic) — see Injury, eye, specified
      site NEC
  lens (cataract) (traumatic) — see Cataract, traumatic
  ligament, traumatic — see Rupture, traumatic, liga-
      ment, by site
  liver S36.116 ☑
    birth injury P15.0
  lymphatic vessel I89.8
  marginal sinus (placental) (with hemorrhage) — see
      Hemorrhage, antepartum, specified cause NEC
  membrana tympani (nontraumatic) — see Perforation,
      tympanum
  membranes (spontaneous)
    artificial
      delayed delivery following O75.5
      delayed delivery following — see Pregnancy,
          complicated by, premature rupture of
          membranes
  meningeal artery I60.8
  meniscus (knee) (see also Tear, meniscus)
    old — see Derangement, meniscus
    site other than knee — code as Sprain
  mesenteric artery, traumatic — see Injury, mesenteric,
      artery, laceration, major
  mesentery (nontraumatic) K66.8
    traumatic — see Injury, intra-abdominal, specified,
        site NEC
  mitral (valve) I34.8
  muscle (traumatic) (see also Strain)
    diastasis — see Diastasis, muscle
    nontraumatic M62.10
      ankle M62.17- ☑
      foot M62.17- ☑
      forearm M62.13- ☑
      hand M62.14- ☑
      lower leg M62.16- ☑
      pelvic region M62.15- ☑
      shoulder region M62.11- ☑
      specified site NEC M62.18
      thigh M62.15- ☑
      upper arm M62.12- ☑
    traumatic — see Strain, by site
  musculotendinous junction NEC, nontraumatic — see
      Rupture, tendon, spontaneous
  mycotic aneurysm causing cerebral hemorrhage —
      see Hemorrhage, intracranial, subarachnoid
  myocardium, myocardial — see Rupture, cardiac
    traumatic — see Injury, heart
  nontraumatic, meaning hernia — see Hernia
  obstructed — see Hernia, by site, obstructed
  operation wound — see Disruption, wound, operation
  ovary, ovarian N83.8
    corpus luteum cyst N83.1- ☑
    follicle (graafian) N83.0- ☑
  oviduct (nonobstetric) (nontraumatic) N83.8
    due to pregnancy O00.10- ☑
      with intrauterine pregnancy O00.11- ☑
  pancreas (nontraumatic) K86.89
    traumatic S36.299 ☑
  papillary muscle NEC I51.2
    following acute myocardial infarction (current
        complication) I23.5
  pelvic
    floor, complicating delivery O70.1
    organ NEC, obstetrical trauma O71.5
  perineum (nonobstetric) (nontraumatic) N90.89

Rupture, ruptured — continued
  perineum — continued
    complicating delivery — see Delivery, complicated,
        by, laceration, anus (sphincter)
  postoperative wound — see Disruption, wound, oper-
      ation
  prostate (traumatic) S37.828 ☑
  pulmonary
    artery I28.8
    valve (heart) I37.8
    vein I28.8
    vessel I28.8
  pus tube — see Salpingitis
  pyosalpinx — see Salpingitis
  rectum (nontraumatic) K63.1
    traumatic S36.69 ☑
  retina, retinal (traumatic) (without detachment) (see
      also Break, retina)
    with detachment — see Detachment, retina, with
        retinal, break
  rotator cuff (nontraumatic) M75.10- ☑
    complete M75.12- ☑
    incomplete M75.11- ☑
  sclera — see Injury, eye, laceration
  sigmoid (nontraumatic) K63.1
    traumatic S36.593 ☑
  spinal cord (see also Injury, spinal cord, by region)
    due to injury at birth P11.5
    newborn (birth injury) P11.5
  spleen (traumatic) S36.09 ☑
    birth injury P15.1
    congenital (birth injury) P15.1
    due to P. vivax malaria B51.0
    nontraumatic D73.5
    spontaneous D73.5
  splenic vein R58
    traumatic — see Injury, blood vessel, splenic vein
  stomach (nontraumatic) (spontaneous) K31.89
    traumatic S36.39 ☑
  supraspinatus (complete) (incomplete) (nontraumatic)
      — see Tear, rotator cuff
  symphysis pubis
    obstetric O71.6
    traumatic S33.4 ☑
  synovium (cyst) M66.10
    ankle M66.17- ☑
    elbow M66.12- ☑
    finger M66.14- ☑
    foot M66.17- ☑
    forearm M66.13- ☑
    hand M66.14- ☑
    pelvic region M66.15- ☑
    shoulder region M66.11- ☑
    specified site NEC M66.18
    thigh M66.15- ☑
    toe M66.17- ☑
    upper arm M66.12- ☑
    wrist M66.13- ☑
  tendon (traumatic) — see Strain
    nontraumatic (spontaneous) M66.9
      ankle M66.87- ☑
      extensor M66.20
        ankle M66.27- ☑
        foot M66.27- ☑
        forearm M66.23- ☑
        hand M66.24- ☑
        lower leg M66.26- ☑
        multiple sites M66.29
        pelvic region M66.25- ☑
        shoulder region M66.21- ☑
        specified site NEC M66.28
        thigh M66.25- ☑
        upper arm M66.22- ☑
      flexor M66.30
        ankle M66.37- ☑
        foot M66.37- ☑
        forearm M66.33- ☑
        hand M66.34- ☑
        lower leg M66.36- ☑
        multiple sites M66.39
        pelvic region M66.35- ☑
        shoulder region M66.31- ☑
        specified site NEC M66.38
        thigh M66.35- ☑
        upper arm M66.32- ☑
      foot M66.87- ☑
      forearm M66.83- ☑

Rupture, ruptured — continued
  tendon — see Strain — continued
    nontraumatic — continued
      hand M66.84- ☑
      lower leg M66.86- ☑
      multiple sites M66.89
      pelvic region M66.85- ☑
      shoulder region M66.81- ☑
      specified
        site NEC M66.88
        tendon M66.80
      thigh M66.85- ☑
      upper arm M66.82- ☑
  thoracic duct I89.8
  tonsil J35.8
  traumatic
    aorta — see Injury, aorta, laceration, major
    diaphragm — see Injury, intrathoracic, diaphragm
    external site — see Wound, open, by site
    eye — see Injury, eye, laceration
    internal organ — see Injury, by site
    intervertebral disc
      cervical S13.0 ☑
      lumbar S33.0 ☑
      thoracic S23.0 ☑
    kidney S37.06- ☑
    ligament (see also Sprain)
      ankle — see Sprain, ankle
      carpus — see Rupture, traumatic, ligament,
          wrist
      collateral (hand) — see Rupture, traumatic,
          ligament, finger, collateral
      finger (metacarpophalangeal) (interphalangeal)
          S63.40- ☑
        collateral S63.41- ☑
          index S63.41- ☑
          little S63.41- ☑
          middle S63.41- ☑
          ring S63.41- ☑
        index S63.40- ☑
        little S63.40- ☑
        middle S63.40- ☑
        palmar S63.42- ☑
          index S63.42- ☑
          little S63.42- ☑
          middle S63.42- ☑
          ring S63.42- ☑
        ring S63.40- ☑
        specified site NEC S63.499 ☑
          index S63.49- ☑
          little S63.49- ☑
          middle S63.49- ☑
          ring S63.49- ☑
        volar plate S63.43- ☑
          index S63.43- ☑
          little S63.43- ☑
          middle S63.43- ☑
          ring S63.43- ☑
      foot — see Sprain, foot
      radial collateral S53.2- ☑
      radiocarpal — see Rupture, traumatic, ligament,
          wrist, radiocarpal
      ulnar collateral S53.3- ☑
      ulnocarpal — see Rupture, traumatic, ligament,
          wrist, ulnocarpal
      wrist S63.30- ☑
        collateral S63.31- ☑
        radiocarpal S63.32- ☑
        specified site NEC S63.39- ☑
        ulnocarpal (palmar) S63.33- ☑
    liver S36.116 ☑
    membrana tympani — see Rupture, ear drum,
        traumatic
    muscle or tendon — see Strain
    myocardium — see Injury, heart
    pancreas S36.299 ☑
    rectum S36.69 ☑
    sigmoid S36.593 ☑
    spleen S36.09 ☑
    stomach S36.39 ☑
    symphysis pubis S33.4 ☑
    tympanum, tympanic (membrane) — see Rupture,
        ear drum, traumatic
    ureter S37.19 ☑
    uterus S37.69 ☑
    vagina — see Injury, vagina

Rupture, ruptured — continued

traumatic — continued

vena cava — see Injury, vena cava, laceration, major

tricuspid (heart) (valve) I07.8

tube, tubal (nonobstetric) (nontraumatic) N83.8

abscess — see Salpingitis

due to pregnancy O00.10-

with intrauterine pregnancy O00.11-

tympanum, tympanic (membrane) (nontraumatic) (see also Perforation, tympanic membrane) H72.9-

traumatic — see Rupture, ear drum, traumatic

umbilical cord, complicating delivery O69.89

ureter (traumatic) S37.19

nontraumatic N28.89

urethra (nontraumatic) N36.8

with ectopic or molar pregnancy O08.6

following ectopic or molar pregnancy O08.6

obstetrical trauma O71.5

traumatic S37.39

uterosacral ligament (nonobstetric) (nontraumatic) N83.8

uterus (traumatic) S37.69

before labor O71.0-

during or after labor O71.1

nonpuerperal, nontraumatic N85.8

pregnant (during labor) O71.1

before labor O71.0-

vagina — see Injury, vagina

valve, valvular (heart) — see Endocarditis

varicose vein — see Varix

varix — see Varix

vena cava R58

traumatic — see Injury, vena cava, laceration, major

vesical (urinary) N32.89

vessel (blood) R58

pulmonary I28.8

traumatic — see Injury, blood vessel

viscus R19.8

vulva complicating delivery O70.0

Russell-Silver syndrome Q87.1

Russian spring-summer type encephalitis A84.0

Rust's disease (tuberculous cervical spondylitis) A18.01

Ruvalcaba-Myhre-Smith syndrome E71.440

Rytand-Lipsitch syndrome I44.2

S

Saber, sabre shin or tibia (syphilitic) A50.56 [M90.8-]

Sac lacrimal — see condition

Saccharomyces infection B37.9

Saccharopinuria E72.3

Saccular — see condition

Sacculation

aorta (nonsyphilitic) — see Aneurysm, aorta

bladder N32.3

intralaryngeal (congenital) (ventricular) Q31.3

larynx (congenital) (ventricular) Q31.3

organ or site, congenital — see Distortion

pregnant uterus — see Pregnancy, complicated by, abnormal, uterus

ureter N28.89

urethra N36.1

vesical N32.3

Sachs' amaurotic familial idiocy or disease E75.02

Sachs-Tay disease E75.02

Sacks-Libman disease M32.11

Sacralgia M53.3

Sacralization Q76.49

Sacrodynia M53.3

Sacroiliac joint — see condition

Sacroiliitis NEC M46.1

Sacrum — see condition

Saddle

back — see Lordosis

embolus

abdominal aorta I74.01

pulmonary artery I26.92

with acute cor pulmonale I26.02

injury — code to condition

nose M95.0

due to syphilis A50.57

Sadism (sexual) F65.52

Sadness, postpartal O90.6

Sadomasochism F65.50

Saemisch's ulcer (cornea) — see Ulcer, cornea, central

Sagging

skin and subcutaneous tissue (following bariatric surgery weight loss) (following dietary weight loss) L98.7

Sahib disease B55.0

Sailors' skin L57.8

Saint

Anthony's fire — see Erysipelas

triad — see Hernia, diaphragm

Vitus' dance — see Chorea, Sydenham's

Salaam

attack(s) — see Epilepsy, spasms

tic R25.8

Salicylism

abuse F55.8

overdose or wrong substance given — see Table of Drugs and Chemicals, by drug, poisoning

Salivary duct or gland — see condition

Salivation, excessive K11.7

Salmonella — see Infection, Salmonella

Salmonellosis A02.0

Salpingitis (catarrhal) (fallopian tube) (nodular) (pseudofollicular) (purulent) (septic) N70.91

with oophoritis N70.93

acute N70.01

with oophoritis N70.03

chlamydial A56.11

chronic N70.11

with oophoritis N70.13

complicating abortion — see Abortion, by type, complicated by, salpingitis

ear — see Salpingitis, eustachian

eustachian (tube) H68.00-

acute H68.01-

chronic H68.02-

follicularis N70.11

with oophoritis N70.13

gonococcal (acute) (chronic) A54.24

interstitial, chronic N70.11

with oophoritis N70.13

isthmica nodosa N70.11

with oophoritis N70.13

specific (gonococcal) (acute) (chronic) A54.24

tuberculous (acute) (chronic) A18.17

venereal (gonococcal) (acute) (chronic) A54.24

Salpingocele N83.4-

Salpingo-oophoritis (catarrhal) (purulent) (ruptured) (septic) (suppurative) N70.93

acute N70.03

with ectopic or molar pregnancy O08.0

following ectopic or molar pregnancy O08.0

gonococcal A54.24

chronic N70.13

following ectopic or molar pregnancy O08.0

gonococcal (acute) (chronic) A54.24

puerperal O86.19

specific (gonococcal) (acute) (chronic) A54.24

subacute N70.03

tuberculous (acute) (chronic) A18.17

venereal (gonococcal) (acute) (chronic) A54.24

Salpingo-ovaritis — see Salpingo-oophoritis

Salpingoperitonitis — see Salpingo-oophoritis

Salzmann's nodular dystrophy — see Degeneration, cornea, nodular

Sampson's cyst or tumor N80.1

San Joaquin (Valley) **fever** B38.0

Sandblaster's asthma, lung or pneumoconiosis J62.8

Sander's disease (paranoia) F22

Sandfly fever A93.1

Sandhoff's disease E75.01

Sanfilippo (Type B) (Type C) (Type D) **syndrome** E76.22

Sanger-Brown ataxia G11.2

Sao Paulo fever or typhus A77.0

Saponification, mesenteric K65.8

Sarcocele (benign)

syphilitic A52.76

congenital A50.59

Sarcocystosis A07.8

Sarcoepiplocele — see Hernia

Sarcoepiplomphalocele Q79.2

Sarcoid (see also Sarcoidosis)

arthropathy D86.86

Boeck's D86.9

Darier-Roussy D86.3

iridocyclitis D86.83

meningitis D86.81

myocarditis D86.85

Sarcoid — continued

myositis D86.87

pyelonephritis D86.84

Spiegler-Fendt L08.89

Sarcoidosis D86.9

with

cranial nerve palsies D86.82

hepatic granuloma D86.89

polyarthritis D86.86

tubulo-interstitial nephropathy D86.84

combined sites NEC D86.89

lung D86.0

and lymph nodes D86.2

lymph nodes D86.1

and lung D86.2

meninges D86.81

skin D86.3

specified type NEC D86.89

Sarcoma (of) (see also Neoplasm, connective tissue, malignant)

alveolar soft part — see Neoplasm, connective tissue, malignant

ameloblastic C41.1

upper jaw (bone) C41.0

botryoid — see Neoplasm, connective tissue, malignant

botryoides — see Neoplasm, connective tissue, malignant

cerebellar C71.6

circumscribed (arachnoidal) C71.6

circumscribed (arachnoidal) cerebellar C71.6

clear cell (see also Neoplasm, connective tissue, malignant)

kidney C64.-

dendritic cells (accessory cells) C96.4

embryonal — see Neoplasm, connective tissue, malignant

endometrial (stromal) C54.1

isthmus C54.0

epithelioid (cell) — see Neoplasm, connective tissue, malignant

Ewing's — see Neoplasm, bone, malignant

follicular dendritic cell C96.4

germinoblastic (diffuse) — see Lymphoma, diffuse large cell

follicular — see Lymphoma, follicular, specified NEC

giant cell (except of bone) (see also Neoplasm, connective tissue, malignant)

bone — see Neoplasm, bone, malignant

glomoid — see Neoplasm, connective tissue, malignant

granulocytic C92.3-

hemangioendothelial — see Neoplasm, connective tissue, malignant

hemorrhagic, multiple — see Sarcoma, Kaposi's

histiocytic C96.A (following C96.6)

Hodgkin — see Lymphoma, Hodgkin

immunoblastic (diffuse) — see Lymphoma, diffuse large cell

interdigitating dendritic cell C96.4

Kaposi's

colon C46.4

connective tissue C46.1

gastrointestinal organ C46.4

lung C46.5-

lymph node(s) C46.3

palate (hard) (soft) C46.2

rectum C46.4

skin C46.0

specified site NEC C46.7

stomach C46.4

unspecified site C46.9

Kupffer cell C22.3

Langerhans cell C96.4

leptomeningeal — see Neoplasm, meninges, malignant

liver NEC C22.4

lymphangioendothelial — see Neoplasm, connective tissue, malignant

lymphoblastic — see Lymphoma, lymphoblastic (diffuse)

lymphocytic — see Lymphoma, small cell B-cell

mast cell C96.22

melanotic — see Melanoma

meningeal — see Neoplasm, meninges, malignant

meningothelial — see Neoplasm, meninges, malignant

◥ Subterms under main terms may continue to next column or page ☑ Additional Character Required — Refer to the Tabular List for Character Selection

279

Rupture, ruptured — Sarcoma

Index

Sarcoma — *continued*
- mesenchymal (*see also* Neoplasm, connective tissue, malignant)
  - mixed — *see* Neoplasm, connective tissue, malignant
  - mesothelial — *see* Mesothelioma
- monstrocellular
  - specified site — *see* Neoplasm, malignant, by site
  - unspecified site C71.9
- myeloid C92.3- ☑
- neurogenic — *see* Neoplasm, nerve, malignant
- odontogenic C41.1
  - upper jaw (bone) C41.0
- osteoblastic (*see also* Neoplasm, bone, malignant)
- osteogenic (*see also* Neoplasm, bone, malignant)
  - juxtacortical — *see* Neoplasm, bone, malignant
  - periosteal — *see* Neoplasm, bone, malignant
- periosteal (*see also* Neoplasm, bone, malignant)
  - osteogenic — *see* Neoplasm, bone, malignant
- pleomorphic cell — *see* Neoplasm, connective tissue, malignant
- reticulum cell (diffuse) — *see* Lymphoma, diffuse large cell
  - nodular — *see* Lymphoma, follicular
  - pleomorphic cell type — *see* Lymphoma, diffuse large cell
- rhabdoid — *see* Neoplasm, malignant, by site
- round cell — *see* Neoplasm, connective tissue, malignant
- small cell — *see* Neoplasm, connective tissue, malignant
- soft tissue — *see* Neoplasm, connective tissue, malignant
- spindle cell — *see* Neoplasm, connective tissue, malignant
- stromal (endometrial) C54.1
  - isthmus C54.0
- synovial (*see also* Neoplasm, connective tissue, malignant)
  - biphasic — *see* Neoplasm, connective tissue, malignant
  - epithelioid cell — *see* Neoplasm, connective tissue, malignant
  - spindle cell — *see* Neoplasm, connective tissue, malignant

Sarcomatosis
- meningeal — *see* Neoplasm, meninges, malignant
- specified site NEC — *see* Neoplasm, connective tissue, malignant
- unspecified site C80.1

Sarcopenia (age-related) M62.84
Sarcosinemia E72.59
Sarcosporidiosis (intestinal) A07.8
Satiety, early R68.81
Saturnine — *see* condition
Saturnism
- overdose or wrong substance given or taken — *see* Table of Drugs and Chemicals, by drug, poisoning

Satyriasis F52.8
Sauriasis — *see* Ichthyosis
SBE (subacute bacterial endocarditis) I33.0
Scabies (any site) B86
Scabs R23.4
Scaglietti-Dagnini syndrome E22.0
Scald — *see* Burn
Scalenus anticus (anterior) **syndrome** G54.0
Scales R23.4
Scaling, skin R23.4
Scalp — *see* condition
Scapegoating affecting child Z62.3
Scaphocephaly Q75.0
Scapulalgia M89.8X1
Scapulohumeral myopathy G71.0
Scar, scarring (*see also* Cicatrix) L90.5
- adherent L90.5
- atrophic L90.5
- cervix
  - in pregnancy or childbirth — *see* Pregnancy, complicated by, abnormal cervix
- cheloid L91.0
- chorioretinal H31.00- ☑
  - posterior pole macula H31.01- ☑
  - postsurgical H59.81- ☑
  - solar retinopathy H31.02- ☑
  - specified type NEC H31.09- ☑
- choroid — *see* Scar, chorioretinal

Scar, scarring — *continued*
- conjunctiva H11.24- ☑
- cornea H17.9
  - xerophthalmic (*see also* Opacity, cornea)
    - vitamin A deficiency E50.6
- duodenum, obstructive K31.5
- hypertrophic L91.0
- keloid L91.0
- labia N90.89
- lung (base) J98.4
- macula — *see* Scar, chorioretinal, posterior pole
- muscle M62.89
- myocardium, myocardial I25.2
- painful L90.5
- posterior pole (eye) — *see* Scar, chorioretinal, posterior pole
- retina — *see* Scar, chorioretinal
- trachea J39.8
- transmural uterine, in pregnancy O34.29
- uterus N85.8
  - in pregnancy O34.29
- vagina N89.8
  - postoperative N99.2
- vulva N90.89

Scarabiasis B88.2
Scarlatina (anginosa) (maligna) A38.9
- myocarditis (acute) A38.1
  - old — *see* Myocarditis
- otitis media A38.0
- ulcerosa A38.8

Scarlet fever (albuminuria) (angina) A38.9
Schamberg's disease (progressive pigmentary dermatosis) L81.7
Schatzki's ring (acquired) (esophagus) (lower) K22.2
- congenital Q39.3
Schaufenster krankheit I20.8
Schaumann's
- benign lymphogranulomatosis D86.1
- disease or syndrome — *see* Sarcoidosis
Scheie's syndrome E76.03
Schenck's disease B42.1
Scheuermann's disease or osteochondrosis — *see* Osteochondrosis, juvenile, spine
Schilder (-Flatau) **disease** G37.0
Schilling-type monocytic leukemia C93.0- ☑
Schimmelbusch's disease, cystic mastitis, or hyperplasia — *see* Mastopathy, cystic
Schistosoma infestation — *see* Infestation, Schistosoma
Schistosomiasis B65.9
- with muscle disorder B65.9 [M63.80]
  - ankle B65.9 [M63.87-] ☑
  - foot B65.9 [M63.87-] ☑
  - forearm B65.9 [M63.83-] ☑
  - hand B65.9 [M63.84-] ☑
  - lower leg B65.9 [M63.86-] ☑
  - multiple sites B65.9 [M63.89]
  - pelvic region B65.9 [M63.85-] ☑
  - shoulder region B65.9 [M63.81-] ☑
  - specified site NEC B65.9 [M63.88]
  - thigh B65.9 [M63.85-] ☑
  - upper arm B65.9 [M63.82-] ☑
- Asiatic B65.2
- bladder B65.0
- chestermani B65.8
- colon B65.1
- cutaneous B65.3
- due to
  - S. haematobium B65.0
  - S. japonicum B65.2
  - S. mansoni B65.1
  - S. mattheii B65.8
- Eastern B65.2
- genitourinary tract B65.0
- intestinal B65.1
- lung NEC B65.9 [J99]
  - pneumonia B65.9 [J17]
- Manson's (intestinal) B65.1
- oriental B65.2
- pulmonary NEC B65.9 [J99]
  - pneumonia B65.9
- Schistosoma
  - haematobium B65.0
  - japonicum B65.2
  - mansoni B65.1
- specified type NEC B65.8
- urinary B65.0
- vesical B65.0
Schizencephaly Q04.6

Schizoaffective psychosis F25.9
Schizodontia K00.2
Schizoid personality F60.1
Schizophrenia, schizophrenic F20.9
- acute (brief) (undifferentiated) F23
- atypical (form) F20.3
- borderline F21
- catalepsy F20.2
- catatonic (type) (excited) (withdrawn) F20.2
- cenesthopathic, cenesthesiopathic F20.89
- childhood type F84.5
- chronic undifferentiated F20.5
- cyclic F25.0
- disorganized (type) F20.1
- flexibilitas cerea F20.2
- hebephrenic (type) F20.1
- incipient F21
- latent F21
- negative type F20.5
- paranoid (type) F20.0
- paraphrenic F20.0
- post-psychotic depression F32.89
- prepsychotic F21
- prodromal F21
- pseudoneurotic F21
- pseudopsychopathic F21
- reaction F23
- residual (state) (type) F20.5
- restzustand F20.5
- schizoaffective (type) — *see* Psychosis, schizoaffective
- simple (type) F20.89
- simplex F20.89
- specified type NEC F20.89
- spectrum and other psychotic disorder F29
  - specified NEC F28
- stupor F20.2
- syndrome of childhood F84.5
- undifferentiated (type) F20.3
  - chronic F20.5
Schizothymia (persistent) F60.1
Schlatter-Osgood disease or osteochondrosis — *see* Osteochondrosis, juvenile, tibia
Schlatter's tibia — *see* Osteochondrosis, juvenile, tibia
Schmidt's syndrome (polyglandular, autoimmune) E31.0
Schmincke's carcinoma or tumor — *see* Neoplasm, nasopharynx, malignant
Schmitz (-Stutzer) **dysentery** A03.0
Schmorl's disease or nodes
- lumbar region M51.46
- lumbosacral region M51.47
- sacrococcygeal region M53.3
- thoracic region M51.44
- thoracolumbar region M51.45
Schneiderian
- papilloma — *see* Neoplasm, nasopharynx, benign
  - specified site — *see* Neoplasm, benign, by site
  - unspecified site D14.0
- specified site — *see* Neoplasm, malignant, by site
  - unspecified site C30.0
Scholte's syndrome (malignant carcinoid) E34.0
Scholz (-Bielchowsky-Henneberg) **disease or syndrome** E75.25
Schönlein (-Henoch) disease or purpura (primary) (rheumatic) D69.0
Schottmuller's disease A01.4
Schroeder's syndrome (endocrine hypertensive) E27.0
Schüller-Christian disease or syndrome C96.5
Schultze's type acroparesthesia, simple I73.89
Schultz's disease or syndrome — *see* Agranulocytosis
Schwalbe-Ziehen-Oppenheim disease G24.1
Schwannoma (*see also* Neoplasm, nerve, benign)
- malignant (*see also* Neoplasm, nerve, malignant)
  - with rhabdomyoblastic differentiation — *see* Neoplasm, nerve, malignant
- melanocytic — *see* Neoplasm, nerve, benign
- pigmented — *see* Neoplasm, nerve, benign
Schwannomatosis Q85.03
Schwartz (-Jampel) **syndrome** G71.13
Schwartz-Bartter syndrome E22.2
Schweniger-Buzzi anetoderma L90.1
Sciatic — *see* condition
Sciatica (infective)
- with lumbago M54.4- ☑
  - due to intervertebral disc disorder — *see* Disorder, disc, with, radiculopathy
- due to displacement of intervertebral disc (with lumbago) — *see* Disorder, disc, with, radiculopathy

Sciatica — *continued*
  wallet M54.3- ☑
Scimitar syndrome Q26.8
Sclera — *see* condition
Sclerectasia H15.84- ☑
Scleredema
  adultorum — *see* Sclerosis, systemic
  Buschke's — *see* Sclerosis, systemic
  newborn P83.8
Sclerema (adiposum) (edematosum) (neonatorum)
  (newborn) P83.0
  adultorum — *see* Sclerosis, systemic
Scleriasis — *see* Scleroderma
Scleritis H15.00- ☑
  with corneal involvement H15.04- ☑
  anterior H15.01- ☑
  brawny H15.02- ☑
  in (due to) zoster B02.34
  posterior H15.03- ☑
  specified type NEC H15.09- ☑
  syphilitic A52.71
  tuberculous (nodular) A18.51
Sclerochoroiditis H31.8
Scleroconjunctivitis — *see* Scleritis
Sclerocystic ovary syndrome E28.2
Sclerodactyly, sclerodactylia L94.3
Scleroderma, sclerodermia (acrosclerotic) (diffuse)
  (generalized) (progressive) (pulmonary) (*see also*
  Sclerosis, systemic) M34.9
  circumscribed L94.0
  linear L94.1
  localized L94.0
  newborn P83.88
  systemic M34.9
Sclerokeratitis H16.8
  tuberculous A18.52
Scleroma nasi A48.8
Scleromalacia (perforans) H15.05- ☑
Scleromyxedema L98.5
Sclérose en plaques G35
Sclerosis, sclerotic
  adrenal (gland) E27.8
  Alzheimer's — *see* Disease, Alzheimer's
  amyotrophic (lateral) G12.21
  aorta, aortic I70.0
    valve — *see* Endocarditis, aortic
  artery, arterial, arteriolar, arteriovascular — *see* Arteriosclerosis
  ascending multiple G35
  brain (generalized) (lobular) G37.9
    artery, arterial I67.2
    diffuse G37.0
    disseminated G35
    insular G35
    Krabbe's E75.23
    miliary G35
    multiple G35
    presenile (Alzheimer's) — *see* Disease, Alzheimer's,
      early onset
    senile (arteriosclerotic) I67.2
    stem, multiple G35
    tuberous Q85.1
  bulbar, multiple G35
  bundle of His I44.39
  cardiac — *see* Disease, heart, ischemic, atherosclerotic
  cardiorenal — *see* Hypertension, cardiorenal
  cardiovascular (*see also* Disease, cardiovascular)
    renal — *see* Hypertension, cardiorenal
  cerebellar — *see* Sclerosis, brain
  cerebral — *see* Sclerosis, brain
  cerebrospinal (disseminated) (multiple) G35
  cerebrovascular I67.2
  choroid — *see* Degeneration, choroid
  combined (spinal cord) (*see also* Degeneration, combined)
    multiple G35
  concentric (Balo) G37.5
  cornea — *see* Opacity, cornea
  coronary (artery) I25.10
    with angina pectoris — *see* Arteriosclerosis, coronary (artery),
  corpus cavernosum
    female N90.89
    male N48.6
  diffuse (brain) (spinal cord) G37.0
  disseminated G35
  dorsal G35

Sclerosis, sclerotic — *continued*
  dorsolateral (spinal cord) — *see* Degeneration, combined
  endometrium N85.5
  extrapyramidal G25.9
  eye, nuclear (senile) — *see* Cataract, senile, nuclear
  focal and segmental (glomerular) (*see also* N00-N07
    with fourth character .1) N05.1
  Friedreich's (spinal cord) G11.1
  funicular (spermatic cord) N50.89
  general (vascular) — *see* Arteriosclerosis
  gland (lymphatic) I89.8
  hepatic K74.1
    alcoholic K70.2
  hereditary
    cerebellar G11.9
    spinal (Friedreich's ataxia) G11.1
  hippocampal G93.81
  insular G35
  kidney — *see* Sclerosis, renal
  larynx J38.7
  lateral (amyotrophic) (descending) (spinal) G12.21
    primary G12.23
  lens, senile nuclear — *see* Cataract, senile, nuclear
  liver K74.1
    with fibrosis K74.2
      alcoholic K70.2
    alcoholic K70.2
    cardiac K76.1
  lung — *see* Fibrosis, lung
  mastoid — *see* Mastoiditis, chronic
  mesial temporal G93.81
  mitral I05.8
  Mönckeberg's (medial) — *see* Arteriosclerosis, extremities
  multiple (brain stem) (cerebral) (generalized) (spinal cord) G35
  myocardium, myocardial — *see* Disease, heart, ischemic, atherosclerotic
  nuclear (senile), eye — *see* Cataract, senile, nuclear
  ovary N83.8
  pancreas K86.89
  penis N48.6
  peripheral arteries — *see* Arteriosclerosis, extremities
  plaques G35
  pluriglandular E31.8
  polyglandular E31.8
  posterolateral (spinal cord) — *see* Degeneration, combined
  presenile (Alzheimer's) — *see* Disease, Alzheimer's, early onset
  primary, lateral G12.23
  progressive, systemic M34.0
  pulmonary — *see* Fibrosis, lung
    artery I27.0
    valve (heart) — *see* Endocarditis, pulmonary
  renal N26.9
    with
      cystine storage disease E72.09
      hypertensive heart disease (conditions in I11) — *see* Hypertension, cardiorenal
    arteriolar (hyaline) (hyperplastic) — *see* Hypertension, kidney
  retina (senile) (vascular) H35.00
  senile (vascular) — *see* Arteriosclerosis
  spinal (cord) (progressive) G95.89
    ascending G61.0
    combined (*see also* Degeneration, combined)
      multiple G35
      syphilitic A52.11
    disseminated G35
    dorsolateral — *see* Degeneration, combined
    hereditary (Friedreich's) (mixed form) G11.1
    lateral (amyotrophic) G12.23
    multiple G35
    posterior (syphilitic) A52.11
  stomach K31.89
  subendocardial, congenital I42.4
  systemic M34.9
    with
      lung involvement M34.81
      myopathy M34.82
      polyneuropathy M34.83
    drug-induced M34.2
    due to chemicals NEC M34.2
    progressive M34.0
    specified NEC M34.89
  temporal (mesial) G93.81

Sclerosis, sclerotic — *continued*
  tricuspid (heart) (valve) I07.8
  tuberous (brain) Q85.1
  tympanic membrane — *see* Disorder, tympanic membrane, specified NEC
  valve, valvular (heart) — *see* Endocarditis
  vascular — *see* Arteriosclerosis
  vein I87.8
Scoliosis (acquired) (postural) M41.9
  adolescent (idiopathic) — *see* Scoliosis, idiopathic, adolescent
  congenital Q67.5
    due to bony malformation Q76.3
    failure of segmentation (hemivertebra) Q76.3
    hemivertebra fusion Q76.3
    postural Q67.5
  idiopathic M41.20
    adolescent M41.129
      cervical region M41.122
      cervicothoracic region M41.123
      lumbar region M41.126
      lumbosacral region M41.127
      thoracic region M41.124
      thoracolumbar region M41.125
    cervical region M41.22
    cervicothoracic region M41.23
    infantile M41.00
      cervical region M41.02
      cervicothoracic region M41.03
      lumbar region M41.06
      lumbosacral region M41.07
      sacrococcygeal region M41.08
      thoracic region M41.04
      thoracolumbar region M41.05
    juvenile M41.119
      cervical region M41.112
      cervicothoracic region M41.113
      lumbar region M41.116
      lumbosacral region M41.117
      thoracic region M41.114
      thoracolumbar region M41.115
    lumbar region M41.26
    lumbosacral region M41.27
    thoracic region M41.24
    thoracolumbar region M41.25
  infantile — *see* Scoliosis, idiopathic, infantile
  neuromuscular M41.40
    cervical region M41.42
    cervicothoracic region M41.43
    lumbar region M41.46
    lumbosacral region M41.47
    occipito-atlanto-axial region M41.41
    thoracic region M41.44
    thoracolumbar region M41.45
  paralytic — *see* Scoliosis, neuromuscular
  postradiation therapy M96.5
  rachitic (late effect or sequelae) E64.3 [M49.80]
    cervical region E64.3 [M49.82]
    cervicothoracic region E64.3 [M49.83]
    lumbar region E64.3 [M49.86]
    lumbosacral region E64.3 [M49.87]
    multiple sites E64.3 [M49.89]
    occipito-atlanto-axial region E64.3 [M49.81]
    sacrococcygeal region E64.3 [M49.88]
    thoracic region E64.3 [M49.84]
    thoracolumbar region E64.3 [M49.85]
  sciatic M54.4- ☑
  secondary (to) NEC M41.50
    cerebral palsy, Friedreich's ataxia, poliomyelitis, neuromuscular disorders — *see* Scoliosis, neuromuscular
    cervical region M41.52
    cervicothoracic region M41.53
    lumbar region M41.56
    lumbosacral region M41.57
    thoracic region M41.54
    thoracolumbar region M41.55
  specified form NEC M41.80
    cervical region M41.82
    cervicothoracic region M41.83
    lumbar region M41.86
    lumbosacral region M41.87
    thoracic region M41.84
    thoracolumbar region M41.85
  thoracogenic M41.30
    thoracic region M41.34
    thoracolumbar region M41.35
  tuberculous A18.01

☑ Subterms under main terms may continue to next column or page   ☑ Additional Character Required — Refer to the Tabular List for Character Selection   281

Sciatica — Scoliosis

Scoliotic pelvis
  with disproportion (fetopelvic) O33.0
    causing obstructed labor O65.0
Scorbutus, scorbutic (*see also* Scurvy)
  anemia D53.2
Score, NIHSS (National Institutes of Health Stroke Scale)
  R29.7- ☑
Scotoma (arcuate) (Bjerrum) (central) (ring) (*see also*
  Defect, visual field, localized, scotoma)
  scintillating H53.19
Scratch — *see* Abrasion
Scratchy throat R09.89
Screening (for) Z13.9
  alcoholism Z13.89
  anemia Z13.0
  anomaly, congenital Z13.89
  antenatal, of mother (*see also* Encounter, antenatal
    screening) Z36.9
  arterial hypertension Z13.6
  arthropod-borne viral disease NEC Z11.59
  bacteriuria, asymptomatic Z13.89
  behavioral disorder Z13.89
  brain injury, traumatic Z13.850
  bronchitis, chronic Z13.83
  brucellosis Z11.2
  cardiovascular disorder Z13.6
  cataract Z13.5
  chlamydial diseases Z11.8
  cholera Z11.0
  chromosomal abnormalities (nonprocreative) NEC
    Z13.79
  colonoscopy Z12.11
  congenital
    dislocation of hip Z13.89
    eye disorder Z13.5
    malformation or deformation Z13.89
  contamination NEC Z13.88
  cystic fibrosis Z13.228
  dengue fever Z11.59
  dental disorder Z13.84
  depression Z13.89
  developmental handicap Z13.4
    in early childhood Z13.4
    infant Z13.4
  diabetes mellitus Z13.1
  diphtheria Z11.2
  disability, intellectual Z13.4
    infant Z13.4
  disease or disorder Z13.9
    bacterial NEC Z11.2
      intestinal infectious Z11.0
      respiratory tuberculosis Z11.1
    blood or blood-forming organ Z13.0
    cardiovascular Z13.6
    Chagas' Z11.6
    chlamydial Z11.8
    dental Z13.89
    developmental Z13.4
      in child Z13.4
      infant Z13.4
    digestive tract NEC Z13.818
      lower GI Z13.811
      upper GI Z13.810
    ear Z13.5
    endocrine Z13.29
    eye Z13.5
    genitourinary Z13.89
    heart Z13.6
    human immunodeficiency virus (HIV) infection
      Z11.4
    immunity Z13.0
    infection
      intestinal Z11.0
        specified NEC Z11.6
    infectious Z11.9
    mental Z13.89
    metabolic Z13.228
    neurological Z13.89
    nutritional Z13.21
      metabolic Z13.228
        lipoid disorders Z13.220
    protozoal Z11.6
      intestinal Z11.0
    respiratory Z13.83
    rheumatic Z13.828
    rickettsial Z11.8
    sexually-transmitted NEC Z11.3
      human immunodeficiency virus (HIV) Z11.4

Screening — *continued*
  disease or disorder — *continued*
    sickle-cell (trait) Z13.0
    skin Z13.89
    specified NEC Z13.89
    spirochetal Z11.8
    thyroid Z13.29
    vascular Z13.6
    venereal Z11.3
    viral NEC Z11.59
      human immunodeficiency virus (HIV) Z11.4
      intestinal Z11.0
  elevated titer Z13.89
  emphysema Z13.83
  encephalitis, viral (mosquito- or tick-borne) Z11.59
  exposure to contaminants (toxic) Z13.88
  fever
    dengue Z11.59
    hemorrhagic Z11.59
    yellow Z11.59
  filariasis Z11.6
  galactosemia Z13.228
  gastrointestinal condition Z13.818
  genetic (nonprocreative) - for procreative manage-
    ment — *see* Testing, genetic, for procreative
    management
    disease carrier status (nonprocreative) Z13.71
    specified NEC (nonprocreative) Z13.79
  genitourinary condition Z13.89
  glaucoma Z13.5
  gonorrhea Z11.3
  gout Z13.89
  helminthiasis (intestinal) Z11.6
  hematopoietic malignancy Z12.89
  hemoglobinopathies NEC Z13.0
  hemorrhagic fever Z11.59
  Hodgkin disease Z12.89
  human immunodeficiency virus (HIV) Z11.4
  human papillomavirus Z11.51
  hypertension Z13.6
  immunity disorders Z13.0
  infection
    mycotic Z11.8
    parasitic Z11.8
  ingestion of radioactive substance Z13.88
  intellectual disability Z13.4
    infant Z13.4
  intestinal
    helminthiasis Z11.6
    infectious disease Z11.0
  leishmaniasis Z11.6
  leprosy Z11.2
  leptospirosis Z11.8
  leukemia Z12.89
  lymphoma Z12.89
  malaria Z11.6
  malnutrition Z13.29
    metabolic Z13.228
    nutritional Z13.21
  measles Z11.59
  mental disorder Z13.89
  metabolic errors, inborn Z13.228
  multiphasic Z13.89
  musculoskeletal disorder Z13.828
    osteoporosis Z13.820
  mycoses Z11.8
  myocardial infarction (acute) Z13.6
  neoplasm (malignant) (of) Z12.9
    bladder Z12.6
    blood Z12.89
    breast Z12.39
      routine mammogram Z12.31
    cervix Z12.4
    colon Z12.11
    genitourinary organs NEC Z12.79
      bladder Z12.6
      cervix Z12.4
      ovary Z12.73
      prostate Z12.5
      testis Z12.71
      vagina Z12.72
    hematopoietic system Z12.89
    intestinal tract Z12.10
      colon Z12.11
      rectum Z12.12
      small intestine Z12.13
    lung Z12.2
    lymph (glands) Z12.89
    nervous system Z12.82

Screening — *continued*
  neoplasm — *continued*
    oral cavity Z12.81
    prostate Z12.5
    rectum Z12.12
    respiratory organs Z12.2
    skin Z12.83
    small intestine Z12.13
    specified site NEC Z12.89
    stomach Z12.0
  nephropathy Z13.89
  nervous system disorders NEC Z13.858
  neurological condition Z13.89
  osteoporosis Z13.820
  parasitic infestation Z11.9
    specified NEC Z11.8
  phenylketonuria Z13.228
  plague Z11.2
  poisoning (chemical) (heavy metal) Z13.88
  poliomyelitis Z11.59
  postnatal, chromosomal abnormalities Z13.89
  prenatal, of mother (*see also* Encounter, antenatal
    screening) Z36.9
  protozoal disease Z11.6
    intestinal Z11.0
  pulmonary tuberculosis Z11.1
  radiation exposure Z13.88
  respiratory condition Z13.83
  respiratory tuberculosis Z11.1
  rheumatoid arthritis Z13.828
  rubella Z11.59
  schistosomiasis Z11.6
  sexually-transmitted disease NEC Z11.3
    human immunodeficiency virus (HIV) Z11.4
  sickle-cell disease or trait Z13.0
  skin condition Z13.89
  sleeping sickness Z11.6
  special Z13.9
    specified NEC Z13.89
  syphilis Z11.3
  tetanus Z11.2
  trachoma Z11.8
  traumatic brain injury Z13.850
  trypanosomiasis Z11.6
  tuberculosis, respiratory Z11.1
  venereal disease Z11.3
  viral encephalitis (mosquito- or tick-borne) Z11.59
  whooping cough Z11.2
  worms, intestinal Z11.6
  yaws Z11.8
  yellow fever Z11.59
Scrofula, scrofulosis (tuberculosis of cervical lymph
  glands) A18.2
Scrofulide (primary) (tuberculous) A18.4
Scrofuloderma, scrofulodermia (any site) (primary)
  A18.4
Scrofulosus lichen (primary) (tuberculous) A18.4
Scrofulous — *see* condition
Scrotal tongue K14.5
Scrotum — *see* condition
Scurvy, scorbutic E54
  anemia D53.2
  gum E54
  infantile E54
  rickets E55.0 [M90.80]
Sealpox B08.62
Seasickness T75.3 ☑
Seatworm (infection) (infestation) B80
Sebaceous (*see also* condition)
  cyst — *see* Cyst, sebaceous
Seborrhea, seborrheic L21.9
  capillitii R23.8
  capitis L21.0
  dermatitis L21.9
    infantile L21.1
  eczema L21.9
    infantile L21.1
  sicca L21.0
Seckel's syndrome Q87.1
Seclusion, pupil — *see* Membrane, pupillary
Second hand tobacco smoke exposure (acute)
  (chronic) Z77.22
  in the perinatal period P96.81
Secondary
  dentin (in pulp) K04.3
  neoplasm, secondaries — *see* Table of Neoplasms,
    secondary

Secretion
- antidiuretic hormone, inappropriate E22.2
- catecholamine, by pheochromocytoma E27.5
- hormone
  - antidiuretic, inappropriate (syndrome) E22.2
  - by
    - carcinoid tumor E34.0
    - pheochromocytoma E27.5
  - ectopic NEC E34.2
- urinary
  - excessive R35.8
  - suppression R34

Section
- nerve, traumatic — see Injury, nerve

Sedative, hypnotic, or anxiolytic-induced
- anxiety disorder F13.980
- bipolar and related disorder F13.94
- delirium F13.921
- depressive disorder F13.94
- major neurocognitive disorder F13.97
- mild neurocognitive disorder F13.988
- psychotic disorder F13.959
- sexual dysfunction F13.981
- sleep disorder F13.982

Segmentation, incomplete (congenital) (see also Fusion)
- bone NEC Q78.8
- lumbosacral (joint) (vertebra) Q76.49

Seitelberger's syndrome (infantile neuraxonal dystrophy) G31.89

Seizure(s) (see also Convulsions) R56.9
- akinetic — see Epilepsy, generalized, specified NEC
- atonic — see Epilepsy, generalized, specified NEC
- autonomic (hysterical) F44.5
- convulsive — see Convulsions
- cortical (focal) (motor) — see Epilepsy, localization-related, symptomatic, with simple partial seizures
- disorder (see also Epilepsy) G40.909
- due to stroke — see Sequelae (of), disease, cerebrovascular, by type, specified NEC
- epileptic — see Epilepsy
- febrile (simple) R56.00
  - with status epilepticus G40.901
  - complex (atypical) (complicated) R56.01
    - with status epilepticus G40.901
- grand mal G40.409
  - intractable G40.419
    - with status epilepticus G40.411
    - without status epilepticus G40.419
  - not intractable G40.409
    - with status epilepticus G40.401
    - without status epilepticus G40.409
- heart — see Disease, heart
- hysterical F44.5
- intractable G40.919
  - with status epilepticus G40.911
- Jacksonian (focal) (motor type) (sensory type) — see Epilepsy, localization-related, symptomatic, with simple partial seizures
- newborn P90
- nonspecific epileptic
  - atonic — see Epilepsy, generalized, specified NEC
  - clonic — see Epilepsy, generalized, specified NEC
  - myoclonic — see Epilepsy, generalized, specified NEC
  - tonic — see Epilepsy, generalized, specified NEC
  - tonic-clonic — see Epilepsy, generalized, specified NEC
- partial, developing into secondarily generalized seizures
  - complex — see Epilepsy, localization-related, symptomatic, with complex partial seizures
  - simple — see Epilepsy, localization-related, symptomatic, with simple partial seizures
- petit mal G40.409
  - intractable G40.419
    - with status epilepticus G40.411
    - without status epilepticus G40.419
  - not intractable G40.409
    - with status epilepticus G40.401
    - without status epilepticus G40.409
- post traumatic R56.1
- recurrent G40.909
- specified NEC G40.89
- uncinate — see Epilepsy, localization-related, symptomatic, with complex partial seizures

Selenium deficiency, dietary E59

Self-damaging behavior (life-style) Z72.89
Self-harm (attempted)
- history (personal) Z91.5
  - in family Z81.8
Self-mutilation (attempted)
- history (personal) Z91.5
  - in family Z81.8
Self-poisoning
- history (personal) Z91.5
  - in family Z81.8
- observation following (alleged) attempt Z03.6
Semicoma R40.1
Seminal vesiculitis N49.0
Seminoma C62.9- ☑
- specified site — see Neoplasm, malignant, by site
Senear-Usher disease or syndrome L10.4
Senectus R54
Senescence (without mention of psychosis) R54
Senile, senility (see also condition) R41.81
- with
  - acute confusional state F05
  - mental changes NOS F03 ☑
  - psychosis NEC — see Psychosis, senile
- asthenia R54
- cervix (atrophic) N88.8
- debility R54
- endometrium (atrophic) N85.8
- fallopian tube (atrophic) — see Atrophy, fallopian tube
- heart (failure) R54
- ovary (atrophic) — see Atrophy, ovary
- premature E34.8
- vagina, vaginitis (atrophic) N95.2
- wart L82.1
Sensation
- burning (skin) R20.8
  - tongue K14.6
- loss of R20.8
- prickling (skin) R20.2
- tingling (skin) R20.2
Sense loss
- smell — see Disturbance, sensation, smell
- taste — see Disturbance, sensation, taste
- touch R20.8
Sensibility disturbance (cortical) (deep) (vibratory) R20.9
Sensitive, sensitivity (see also Allergy)
- carotid sinus G90.01
- child (excessive) F93.8
- cold, autoimmune D59.1
- dentin K03.89
- gluten (non-celiac) K90.41
- latex Z91.040
- methemoglobin D74.8
- tuberculin, without clinical or radiological symptoms R76.11
- visual
  - glare H53.71
  - impaired contrast H53.72
Sensitiver Beziehungswahn F22
Sensitization, auto-erythrocytic D69.2
Separation
- anxiety, abnormal (of childhood) F93.0
- apophysis, traumatic — code as Fracture, by site
- choroid — see Detachment, choroid
- epiphysis, epiphyseal
  - nontraumatic (see also Osteochondropathy, specified type NEC)
    - upper femoral — see Slipped, epiphysis, upper femoral
  - traumatic — code as Fracture, by site
- fracture — see Fracture
- infundibulum cardiac from right ventricle by a partition Q24.3
- joint (traumatic) (current) — code by site under Dislocation
- pubic bone, obstetrical trauma O71.6
- retina, retinal — see Detachment, retina
- symphysis pubis, obstetrical trauma O71.6
- tracheal ring, incomplete, congenital Q32.1
Sepsis (generalized) (unspecified organism) A41.9
- with
  - organ dysfunction (acute) (multiple) R65.20
    - with septic shock R65.21
- actinomycotic A42.7
- adrenal hemorrhage syndrome (meningococcal) A39.1
- anaerobic A41.4
- Bacillus anthracis A22.7
- Brucella (see also Brucellosis) A23.9

Sepsis — continued
- candidal B37.7
- cryptogenic A41.9
- due to device, implant or graft T85.79 ☑
  - arterial graft NEC T82.7 ☑
  - breast (implant) T85.79 ☑
  - catheter NEC T85.79 ☑
    - dialysis (renal) T82.7 ☑
      - intraperitoneal T85.71 ☑
    - infusion NEC T82.7 ☑
      - spinal (cranial) (epidural) (intrathecal) (spinal) (subarachnoid) (subdural) T85.735 ☑
    - urethral indwelling T83.511 ☑
    - urinary T83.518 ☑
  - ectopic or molar pregnancy O08.82
  - electronic (electrode) (pulse generator) (stimulator)
    - bone T84.7 ☑
    - cardiac T82.7 ☑
    - nervous system T85.738 ☑
      - brain T85.731 ☑
      - neurostimulator generator T85.734 ☑
      - peripheral nerve T85.732 ☑
      - spinal cord T85.733 ☑
    - urinary T83.590 ☑
  - fixation, internal (orthopedic) — see Complication, fixation device, infection
  - gastrointestinal (bile duct) (esophagus) T85.79 ☑
    - neurostimulator electrode (lead) T85.732 ☑
  - genital T83.69 ☑
  - heart NEC T82.7 ☑
    - valve (prosthesis) T82.6 ☑
    - graft T82.7 ☑
  - joint prosthesis — see Complication, joint prosthesis, infection
  - ocular (corneal graft) (orbital implant) T85.79 ☑
  - orthopedic NEC T84.7 ☑
    - fixation device, internal — see Complication, fixation device, infection
  - specified NEC T85.79 ☑
  - vascular T82.7 ☑
  - ventricular intracranial (communicating) shunt T85.730 ☑
- during labor O75.3
- Enterococcus A41.81
- Erysipelothrix (rhusiopathiae) (erysipeloid) A26.7
- Escherichia coli (E. coli) A41.5 ☑
- extraintestinal yersiniosis A28.2
- following
  - abortion (subsequent episode) O08.0
    - current episode — see Abortion
  - ectopic or molar pregnancy O08.82
  - immunization T88.0 ☑
  - infusion, therapeutic injection or transfusion NEC T80.29 ☑
- gangrenous A41.9
- gonococcal A54.86
- Gram-negative (organism) A41.5 ☑
  - anaerobic A41.4
- Haemophilus influenzae A41.3
- herpesviral B00.7
- intra-abdominal K65.1
- intraocular — see Endophthalmitis, purulent
- Listeria monocytogenes A32.7
- localized — code to specific localized infection
  - in operation wound T81.4 ☑
  - skin — see Abscess
- malleus A24.0
- melioidosis A24.1
- meningeal — see Meningitis
- meningococcal A39.4
  - acute A39.2
  - chronic A39.3
- MSSA (Methicillin susceptible Staphylococcus aureus) A41.01
- newborn P36.9
  - due to
    - anaerobes NEC P36.5
    - Escherichia coli P36.4
    - Staphylococcus P36.30
      - aureus P36.2
      - specified NEC P36.39
    - Streptococcus P36.10
      - group B P36.0
      - specified NEC P36.19
  - specified NEC P36.8
- Pasteurella multocida A28.0

Sepsis — continued
- pelvic, puerperal, postpartum, childbirth O85
- pneumococcal A40.3
- postprocedural T81.4 ☑
- puerperal, postpartum, childbirth (pelvic) O85
- Salmonella (arizonae) (cholerae-suis) (enteritidis) (typhimurium) A02.1
- severe R65.20
  - with septic shock R65.21
- Shigella (see also Dysentery, bacillary) A03.9
- skin, localized — see Abscess
- specified organism NEC A41.89
- Staphylococcus, staphylococcal A41.2
  - aureus (methicillin susceptible) (MSSA) A41.01
    - methicillin resistant (MRSA) A41.02
  - coagulase-negative A41.1
  - specified NEC A41.1
- Streptococcus, streptococcal A40.9
  - agalactiae A40.1
  - group
    - A A40.0
    - B A40.1
    - D A41.81
  - neonatal P36.10
    - group B P36.0
    - specified NEC P36.19
  - pneumoniae A40.3
  - pyogenes A40.0
  - specified NEC A40.8
- tracheostomy stoma J95.02
- tularemic A21.7
- umbilical, umbilical cord (newborn) — see Sepsis, newborn
- Yersinia pestis A20.7

Septate — see Septum

Septic — see condition
- arm — see Cellulitis, upper limb
  - with lymphangitis — see Lymphangitis, acute, upper limb
- embolus — see Embolism
- finger — see Cellulitis, digit
  - with lymphangitis — see Lymphangitis, acute, digit
- foot — see Cellulitis, lower limb
  - with lymphangitis — see Lymphangitis, acute, lower limb
- gallbladder (acute) K81.0
- hand — see Cellulitis, upper limb
  - with lymphangitis — see Lymphangitis, acute, upper limb
- joint — see Arthritis, pyogenic or pyemic
- leg — see Cellulitis, lower limb
  - with lymphangitis — see Lymphangitis, acute, lower limb
- nail (see also Cellulitis, digit)
  - with lymphangitis — see Lymphangitis, acute, digit
- sore (see also Abscess)
  - throat J02.0
    - streptococcal J02.0
- spleen (acute) D73.89
- teeth, tooth (pulpal origin) K04.4
- throat — see Pharyngitis
- thrombus — see Thrombosis
- toe — see Cellulitis, digit
  - with lymphangitis — see Lymphangitis, acute, digit
- tonsils, chronic J35.01
  - with adenoiditis J35.03
- uterus — see Endometritis

Septicemia A41.9
- meaning sepsis — see Sepsis

Septum, septate (congenital) (see also Anomaly, by site)
- anal Q42.3
  - with fistula Q42.2
- aqueduct of Sylvius Q03.0
  - with spina bifida — see Spina bifida, by site, with hydrocephalus
- uterus (complete) (partial) Q51.2
- vagina Q52.10
  - in pregnancy — see Pregnancy, complicated by, abnormal vagina
    - causing obstructed labor O65.5
  - longitudinal Q52.129
    - microperforate
      - left side Q52.124
      - right side Q52.123
    - nonobstruction Q52.120

Septum, septate — continued
- vagina — continued
  - longitudinal — continued
    - obstructing Q52.129
      - left side Q52.122
      - right side Q52.121
  - transverse Q52.11

Sequelae (of) (see also condition)
- abscess, intracranial or intraspinal (conditions in G06) G09
- amputation — code to injury with seventh character S
- burn and corrosion — code to injury with seventh character S
- calcium deficiency E64.8
- cerebrovascular disease — see Sequelae, disease, cerebrovascular
- childbirth O94
- contusion — code to injury with seventh character S
- corrosion — see Sequelae, burn and corrosion
- crushing injury — code to injury with seventh character S
- disease
  - cerebrovascular I69.90
    - alteration of sensation I69.998
    - aphasia I69.920
    - apraxia I69.990
    - ataxia I69.993
    - cognitive deficits I69.91 ☑
    - disturbance of vision I69.998
    - dysarthria I69.922
    - dysphagia I69.991
    - dysphasia I69.921
    - facial droop I69.992
    - facial weakness I69.992
    - fluency disorder I69.923
    - hemiplegia I69.95- ☑
    - hemorrhage
      - intracerebral — see Sequelae, hemorrhage, intracerebral
      - intracranial, nontraumatic NEC — see Sequelae, hemorrhage, intracranial, nontraumatic
      - subarachnoid — see Sequelae, hemorrhage, subarachnoid
    - language deficit I69.928
    - monoplegia
      - lower limb I69.94- ☑
      - upper limb I69.93- ☑
    - paralytic syndrome I69.96- ☑
    - specified effect NEC I69.998
    - specified type NEC I69.80
      - alteration of sensation I69.898
      - aphasia I69.820
      - apraxia I69.890
      - ataxia I69.893
      - cognitive deficits I69.81 ☑
      - disturbance of vision I69.898
      - dysarthria I69.822
      - dysphagia I69.891
      - dysphasia I69.821
      - facial droop I69.892
      - facial weakness I69.892
      - fluency disorder I69.823
      - hemiplegia I69.85- ☑
      - language deficit I69.828
      - monoplegia
        - lower limb I69.84- ☑
        - upper limb I69.83- ☑
      - paralytic syndrome I69.86- ☑
      - specified effect NEC I69.898
    - speech deficit I69.928
      - speech deficit I69.828
    - stroke NOS — see Sequelae, stroke NOS
- dislocation — code to injury with seventh character S
- encephalitis or encephalomyelitis (conditions in G04) G09
  - in infectious disease NEC B94.8
  - viral B94.1
- external cause — code to injury with seventh character S
- foreign body entering natural orifice — code to injury with seventh character S
- fracture — code to injury with seventh character S
- frostbite — code to injury with seventh character S
- Hansen's disease B92
- hemorrhage
  - intracerebral I69.10

Sequelae — continued
- hemorrhage — continued
  - intracerebral — continued
    - alteration of sensation I69.198
    - aphasia I69.120
    - apraxia I69.190
    - ataxia I69.193
    - cognitive deficits I69.11 ☑
    - disturbance of vision I69.198
    - dysarthria I69.122
    - dysphagia I69.191
    - dysphasia I69.121
    - facial droop I69.192
    - facial weakness I69.192
    - fluency disorder I69.123
    - hemiplegia I69.15- ☑
    - language deficit NEC I69.128
    - monoplegia
      - lower limb I69.14- ☑
      - upper limb I69.13- ☑
    - paralytic syndrome I69.16- ☑
    - specified effect NEC I69.198
    - speech deficit NEC I69.128
  - intracranial, nontraumatic NEC I69.20
    - alteration of sensation I69.298
    - aphasia I69.220
    - apraxia I69.290
    - ataxia I69.293
    - cognitive deficits I69.21 ☑
    - disturbance of vision I69.298
    - dysarthria I69.222
    - dysphagia I69.291
    - dysphasia I69.221
    - facial droop I69.292
    - facial weakness I69.292
    - fluency disorder I69.223
    - hemiplegia I69.25- ☑
    - language deficit NEC I69.228
    - monoplegia
      - lower limb I69.24- ☑
      - upper limb I69.23- ☑
    - paralytic syndrome I69.26- ☑
    - specified effect NEC I69.298
    - speech deficit NEC I69.228
  - subarachnoid I69.00
    - alteration of sensation I69.098
    - aphasia I69.020
    - apraxia I69.090
    - ataxia I69.093
    - cognitive deficits — see subcategory I69.01- ☑
    - disturbance of vision I69.098
    - dysarthria I69.022
    - dysphagia I69.091
    - dysphasia I69.021
    - facial droop I69.092
    - facial weakness I69.092
    - fluency disorder I69.023
    - hemiplegia I69.05- ☑
    - language deficit NEC I69.028
    - monoplegia
      - lower limb I69.04- ☑
      - upper limb I69.03- ☑
    - paralytic syndrome I69.06- ☑
    - specified effect NEC I69.098
    - speech deficit NEC I69.028
- hepatitis, viral B94.2
- hyperalimentation E68
- infarction
  - cerebral I69.30
    - alteration of sensation I69.398
    - aphasia I69.320
    - apraxia I69.390
    - ataxia I69.393
    - cognitive deficits I69.31 ☑
    - disturbance of vision I69.398
    - dysarthria I69.322
    - dysphagia I69.391
    - dysphasia I69.321
    - facial droop I69.392
    - facial weakness I69.392
    - fluency disorder I69.323
    - hemiplegia I69.35- ☑
    - language deficit NEC I69.328
    - monoplegia
      - lower limb I69.34- ☑
      - upper limb I69.33- ☑
    - paralytic syndrome I69.36- ☑
    - specified effect NEC I69.398

☑ **Additional Character Required** — Refer to the Tabular List for Character Selection   ▽ Subterms under main terms may continue to next column or page

Sequelae — continued
  infarction — continued
    cerebral — continued
      speech deficit NEC I69.328
  infection, pyogenic, intracranial or intraspinal G09
  infectious disease B94.9
    specified NEC B94.8
  injury — code to injury with seventh character S
  leprosy B92
  meningitis
    bacterial (conditions in G00) G09
    other or unspecified cause (conditions in G03) G09
  muscle (and tendon) injury — code to injury with
    seventh character S
  myelitis — see Sequelae, encephalitis
  niacin deficiency E64.8
  nutritional deficiency E64.9
    specified NEC E64.8
  obstetrical condition O94
  parasitic disease B94.9
  phlebitis or thrombophlebitis of intracranial or in-
    traspinal venous sinuses and veins (conditions
    in G08) G09
  poisoning — code to poisoning with seventh character
    S
    nonmedicinal substance — see Sequelae, toxic ef-
      fect, nonmedicinal substance
  poliomyelitis (acute) B91
  pregnancy O94
  protein-energy malnutrition E64.0
  puerperium O94
  rickets E64.3
  selenium deficiency E64.8
  sprain and strain — code to injury with seventh char-
    acter S
  stroke NOS I69.30
    alteration in sensation I69.398
    aphasia I69.320
    apraxia I69.390
    ataxia I69.393
    cognitive deficits I69.31 ☑
    disturbance of vision I69.398
    dysarthria I69.322
    dysphagia I69.391
    dysphasia I69.321
    facial droop I69.392
    facial weakness I69.392
    hemiplegia I69.35- ☑
    language deficit NEC I69.328
    monoplegia
      lower limb I69.34- ☑
      upper limb I69.33- ☑
    paralytic syndrome I69.36- ☑
    specified effect NEC I69.398
    speech deficit NEC I69.328
  tendon and muscle injury — code to injury with sev-
    enth character S
  thiamine deficiency E64.8
  trachoma B94.0
  tuberculosis B90.9
    bones and joints B90.2
    central nervous system B90.0
    genitourinary B90.1
    pulmonary (respiratory) B90.9
    specified organs NEC B90.8
  viral
    encephalitis B94.1
    hepatitis B94.2
  vitamin deficiency NEC E64.8
    A E64.1
    B E64.8
    C E64.2
  wound, open — code to injury with seventh character
    S
Sequestration (see also Sequestrum)
  disk — see Displacement, intervertebral disk
  lung, congenital Q33.2
Sequestrum
  bone — see Osteomyelitis, chronic
  dental M27.2
  jaw bone M27.2
  orbit — see Osteomyelitis, orbit
  sinus (accessory) (nasal) — see Sinusitis
Sequoiosis lung or pneumonitis J67.8

Serology for syphilis
  doubtful
    with signs or symptoms — code by site and stage
      under Syphilis
    follow-up of latent syphilis — see Syphilis, latent
  negative, with signs or symptoms — code by site and
    stage under Syphilis
  positive A53.0
    with signs or symptoms — code by site and stage
      under Syphilis
  reactivated A53.0
Seroma (see also Hematoma)
  postprocedural — see Complication, postprocedural,
    seroma
  traumatic, secondary and recurrent T79.2 ☑
Seropurulent — see condition
Serositis, multiple K65.8
  pericardial I31.1
  peritoneal K65.8
Serous — see condition
Sertoli cell
  adenoma
    specified site — see Neoplasm, benign, by site
    unspecified site
      female D27.9
      male D29.20
  carcinoma
    specified site — see Neoplasm, malignant, by site
    unspecified site (male) C62.9- ☑
      female C56.9
  tumor
    with lipid storage
      specified site — see Neoplasm, benign, by site
      unspecified site
        female D27.9
        male D29.20
    specified site — see Neoplasm, benign, by site
    unspecified site
      female D27.9
      male D29.20
Sertoli-Leydig cell tumor — see Neoplasm, benign, by
    site
  specified site — see Neoplasm, benign, by site
  unspecified site
    female D27.9
    male D29.20
Serum
  allergy, allergic reaction (see also Reaction, serum)
    T80.69 ☑
    shock (see also Shock, anaphylactic) T80.59 ☑
  arthritis (see also Reaction, serum) T80.69 ☑
  complication or reaction NEC (see also Reaction, serum)
    T80.69 ☑
  disease NEC (see also Reaction, serum) T80.69 ☑
  hepatitis (see also Hepatitis, viral, type B)
    carrier (suspected) of B18.1
  intoxication (see also Reaction, serum) T80.69 ☑
  neuritis (see also Reaction, serum) T80.69 ☑
  neuropathy G61.1
  poisoning NEC (see also Reaction, serum) T80.69 ☑
  rash NEC (see also Reaction, serum) T80.69 ☑
  reaction NEC (see also Reaction, serum) T80.69 ☑
  sickness NEC (see also Reaction, serum) T80.69 ☑
  urticaria (see also Reaction, serum) T80.69 ☑
Sesamoiditis M25.8- ☑
Severe sepsis R65.20
  with septic shock R65.21
Sever's disease or osteochondrosis — see Osteochon-
    drosis, juvenile, tarsus
Sex
  chromosome mosaics Q97.8
    lines with various numbers of X chromosomes
      Q97.2
  education Z70.8
  reassignment surgery status Z87.890
Sextuplet pregnancy — see Pregnancy, sextuplet
Sexual
  function, disorder of (psychogenic) F52.9
  immaturity (female) (male) E30.0
  impotence (psychogenic) organic origin NEC — see
    Dysfunction, sexual, male
  precocity (constitutional) (cryptogenic) (female) (idio-
    pathic) (male) E30.1
Sexuality, pathologic — see Deviation, sexual
Sézary disease C84.1- ☑
Shadow, lung R91.8
Shaking palsy or paralysis — see Parkinsonism

Shallowness, acetabulum — see Derangement, joint,
    specified type NEC, hip
Shaver's disease J63.1
Sheath (tendon) — see condition
Sheathing, retinal vessels H35.01- ☑
Shedding
  nail L60.8
  premature, primary (deciduous) teeth K00.6
Sheehan's disease or syndrome E23.0
Shelf, rectal K62.89
Shell teeth K00.5
Shellshock (current) F43.0
  lasting state — see Disorder, post-traumatic stress
Shield kidney Q63.1
Shift
  auditory threshold (temporary) H93.24- ☑
  mediastinal R93.8
Shifting sleep-work schedule (affecting sleep) G47.26
Shiga (-Kruse) **dysentery** A03.0
Shiga's bacillus A03.0
Shigella (dysentery) — see Dysentery, bacillary
Shigellosis A03.9
  Group A A03.0
  Group B A03.1
  Group C A03.2
  Group D A03.3
Shin splints S86.89- ☑
Shingles — see Herpes, zoster
Shipyard disease or eye B30.0
Shirodkar suture, in pregnancy — see Pregnancy,
    complicated by, incompetent cervix
Shock R57.9
  with ectopic or molar pregnancy O08.3
  adrenal (cortical) (Addisonian) E27.2
  adverse food reaction (anaphylactic) — see Shock,
    anaphylactic, due to food
  allergic — see Shock, anaphylactic
  anaphylactic T78.2 ☑
    chemical — see Table of Drugs and Chemicals
    due to drug or medicinal substance
      correct substance properly administered
        T88.6 ☑
      overdose or wrong substance given or taken
        (by accident) — see Table of Drugs and
        Chemicals, by drug, poisoning
    due to food (nonpoisonous) T78.00 ☑
      additives T78.06 ☑
      dairy products T78.07 ☑
      eggs T78.08 ☑
      fish T78.03 ☑
        shellfish T78.02 ☑
      fruit T78.04 ☑
      milk T78.07 ☑
      nuts T78.05 ☑
        multiple types T78.05 ☑
        peanuts T78.01 ☑
      peanuts T78.01 ☑
      seeds T78.05 ☑
      specified type NEC T78.09 ☑
      vegetable T78.04 ☑
    following sting(s) — see Venom
    immunization T80.52 ☑
    serum T80.59 ☑
      blood and blood products T80.51 ☑
      immunization T80.52 ☑
      specified NEC T80.59 ☑
      vaccination T80.52 ☑
  anaphylactoid — see Shock, anaphylactic
  anesthetic
    correct substance properly administered T88.2 ☑
    overdose or wrong substance given or taken —
      see Table of Drugs and Chemicals, by drug,
      poisoning
    specified anesthetic — see Table of Drugs and
      Chemicals, by drug, poisoning
  cardiogenic R57.0
  chemical substance — see Table of Drugs and Chemi-
    cals
  complicating ectopic or molar pregnancy O08.3
  culture — see Disorder, adjustment
  drug
    due to correct substance properly administered
      T88.6 ☑
    overdose or wrong substance given or taken (by
      accident) — see Table of Drugs and Chemi-
      cals, by drug, poisoning
  during or after labor and delivery O75.1

Shock — *continued*
electric T75.4 ☑
(taser) T75.4 ☑
endotoxic R65.21
postprocedural (resulting from a procedure, not elsewhere classified) T81.12 ☑
following
ectopic or molar pregnancy O08.3
injury (immediate) (delayed) T79.4 ☑
labor and delivery O75.1
food (anaphylactic) — *see* Shock, anaphylactic, due to food
from electroshock gun (taser) T75.4 ☑
gram-negative R65.21
postprocedural (resulting from a procedure, not elsewhere classified) T81.12 ☑
hematologic R57.8
hemorrhagic R57.8
surgery (intraoperative) (postoperative) T81.19 ☑
trauma T79.4 ☑
hypovolemic R57.1
surgical T81.19 ☑
traumatic T79.4 ☑
insulin E15
therapeutic misadventure — *see* subcategory T38.3 ☑
kidney N17.0
traumatic (following crushing) T79.5 ☑
lightning T75.01 ☑
liver K72.00
lung J80
obstetric O75.1
with ectopic or molar pregnancy O08.3
following ectopic or molar pregnancy O08.3
pleural (surgical) T81.19 ☑
due to trauma T79.4 ☑
postprocedural (postoperative) T81.10 ☑
with ectopic or molar pregnancy O08.3
cardiogenic T81.11 ☑
endotoxic T81.12 ☑
following ectopic or molar pregnancy O08.3
gram-negative T81.12 ☑
hypovolemic T81.19 ☑
septic T81.12 ☑
specified type NEC T81.19 ☑
psychic F43.0
septic (due to severe sepsis) R65.21
specified NEC R57.8
surgical T81.10 ☑
taser gun (taser) T75.4 ☑
therapeutic misadventure NEC T81.10 ☑
thyroxin
overdose or wrong substance given or taken — *see* Table of Drugs and Chemicals, by drug, poisoning
toxic, syndrome A48.3
transfusion — *see* Complications, transfusion
traumatic (immediate) (delayed) T79.4 ☑
Shoemaker's chest M95.4
Short, shortening, shortness
arm (acquired) (*see also* Deformity, limb, unequal length)
congenital Q71.81- ☑
forearm — *see* Deformity, limb, unequal length
bowel syndrome K91.2
breath R06.02
cervical (complicating pregnancy) O26.87- ☑
non-gravid uterus N88.3
common bile duct, congenital Q44.5
cord (umbilical), complicating delivery O69.3 ☑
cystic duct, congenital Q44.5
esophagus (congenital) Q39.8
femur (acquired) — *see* Deformity, limb, unequal length, femur
congenital — *see* Defect, reduction, lower limb, longitudinal, femur
frenum, frenulum, linguae (congenital) Q38.1
hip (acquired) (*see also* Deformity, limb, unequal length)
congenital Q65.89
leg (acquired) (*see also* Deformity, limb, unequal length)
congenital Q72.81- ☑
lower leg (*see also* Deformity, limb, unequal length)
limbed stature, with immunodeficiency D82.2
lower limb (acquired) (*see also* Deformity, limb, unequal length)

Short, shortening, shortness — *continued*
lower limb (*see also* Deformity, limb, unequal length) — *continued*
congenital Q72.81- ☑
organ or site, congenital NEC — *see* Distortion
palate, congenital Q38.5
radius (acquired) (*see also* Deformity, limb, unequal length)
congenital — *see* Defect, reduction, upper limb, longitudinal, radius
rib syndrome Q77.2
stature (child) (hereditary) (idiopathic) NEC R62.52
constitutional E34.3
due to endocrine disorder E34.3
Laron-type E34.3
tendon (*see also* Contraction, tendon)
with contracture of joint — *see* Contraction, joint
Achilles (acquired) M67.0- ☑
congenital Q66.89
congenital Q79.8
thigh (acquired) (*see also* Deformity, limb, unequal length, femur)
congenital — *see* Defect, reduction, lower limb, longitudinal, femur
tibialis anterior (tendon) — *see* Contraction, tendon
umbilical cord
complicating delivery O69.3 ☑
upper limb, congenital — *see* Defect, reduction, upper limb, specified type NEC
urethra N36.8
uvula, congenital Q38.5
vagina (congenital) Q52.4
Shortsightedness — *see* Myopia
Shoshin (acute fulminating beriberi) E51.11
Shoulder — *see* condition
Shovel-shaped incisors K00.2
Shower, thromboembolic — *see* Embolism
Shunt
arterial-venous (dialysis) Z99.2
arteriovenous, pulmonary (acquired) I28.0
congenital Q25.72
cerebral ventricle (communicating) in situ Z98.2
surgical, prosthetic, with complications — *see* Complications, cardiovascular, device or implant
Shutdown, renal N28.9
Shy-Drager syndrome G90.3
Sialadenitis, sialadenosis (any gland) (chronic) (periodic) (suppurative) — *see* Sialoadenitis
Sialectasia K11.8
Sialidosis E77.1
Sialitis, silitis (any gland) (chronic) (suppurative) — *see* Sialoadenitis
Sialoadenitis (any gland) (periodic) (suppurative) K11.20
acute K11.21
recurrent K11.22
chronic K11.23
Sialoadenopathy K11.9
Sialoangitis — *see* Sialoadenitis
Sialodochitis (fibrinosa) — *see* Sialoadenitis
Sialodocholithiasis K11.5
Sialolithiasis K11.5
Sialometaplasia, necrotizing K11.8
Sialorrhea (*see also* Ptyalism)
periodic — *see* Sialoadenitis
Sialosis K11.7
Siamese twin Q89.4
Sibling rivalry Z62.891
Sicard's syndrome G52.7
Sicca syndrome M35.00
with
keratoconjunctivitis M35.01
lung involvement M35.02
myopathy M35.03
renal tubulo-interstitial disorders M35.04
specified organ involvement NEC M35.09
Sick R69
or handicapped person in family Z63.79
needing care at home Z63.6
sinus (syndrome) I49.5
Sick-euthyroid syndrome E07.81
Sickle-cell
anemia — *see* Disease, sickle-cell
trait D57.3
Sicklemia (*see also* Disease, sickle-cell)
trait D57.3
Sickness
air (travel) T75.3 ☑

Sickness — *continued*
airplane T75.3 ☑
alpine T70.29 ☑
altitude T70.20 ☑
Andes T70.29 ☑
aviator's T70.29 ☑
balloon T70.29 ☑
car T75.3 ☑
compressed air T70.3 ☑
decompression T70.3 ☑
green D50.8
milk — *see* Poisoning, food, noxious
motion T75.3 ☑
mountain T70.29 ☑
acute D75.1
protein (*see also* Reaction, serum) T80.69 ☑
radiation T66 ☑
roundabout (motion) T75.3 ☑
sea T75.3 ☑
serum NEC (*see also* Reaction, serum) T80.69 ☑
sleeping (African) B56.9
by Trypanosoma B56.9
brucei
gambiense B56.0
rhodesiense B56.1
East African B56.1
Gambian B56.0
Rhodesian B56.1
West African B56.0
swing (motion) T75.3 ☑
train (railway) (travel) T75.3 ☑
travel (any vehicle) T75.3 ☑
Sideropenia — *see* Anemia, iron deficiency
Siderosilicosis J62.8
Siderosis (lung) J63.4
eye (globe) — *see* Disorder, globe, degenerative, siderosis
Siemens' syndrome (ectodermal dysplasia) Q82.8
Sighing R06.89
psychogenic F45.8
Sigmoid (*see also* condition)
flexure — *see* condition
kidney Q63.1
Sigmoiditis (*see also* Enteritis) K52.9
infectious A09
noninfectious K52.9
Silfversköld's syndrome Q78.9
Silicosiderosis J62.8
Silicosis, silicotic (simple) (complicated) J62.8
with tuberculosis J65
Silicotuberculosis J65
Silo-fillers' disease J68.8
bronchitis J68.0
pneumonitis J68.0
pulmonary edema J68.1
Silver's syndrome Q87.1
Simian malaria B53.1
Simmonds' cachexia or disease E23.0
Simons' disease or syndrome (progressive lipodystrophy) E88.1
Simple, simplex — *see* condition
Simulation, conscious (of illness) Z76.5
Simultanagnosia (asimultagnosia) R48.3
Sin Nombre virus disease (Hantavirus) (cardio)-pulmonary syndrome) B33.4
Sinding-Larsen disease or osteochondrosis — *see* Osteochondrosis, juvenile, patella
Singapore hemorrhagic fever A91
Singer's node or nodule J38.2
Single
atrium Q21.2
coronary artery Q24.5
umbilical artery Q27.0
ventricle Q20.4
Singultus R06.6
epidemicus B33.0
Sinus (*see also* Fistula)
abdominal K63.89
arrest I45.5
arrhythmia I49.8
bradycardia R00.1
branchial cleft (internal) (external) Q18.0
coccygeal — *see* Sinus, pilonidal
dental K04.6
dermal (congenital) Q06.8
with abscess Q06.8
coccygeal, pilonidal — *see* Sinus, coccygeal

☑ Additional Character Required — Refer to the Tabular List for Character Selection   ▽ Subterms under main terms may continue to next column or page

Index

Sinus — *continued*
  infected, skin NEC L08.89
  marginal, ruptured or bleeding — *see* Hemorrhage, antepartum, specified cause NEC
  medial, face and neck Q18.8
  pause I45.5
  pericranii Q01.9
  pilonidal (infected) (rectum) L05.92
    with abscess L05.02
  preauricular Q18.1
  rectovaginal N82.3
  Rokitansky-Aschoff (gallbladder) K82.8
  sacrococcygeal (dermoid) (infected) — *see* Sinus, pilonidal
  tachycardia R00.0
    paroxysmal I47.1
  tarsi syndrome M25.57- ☑
  testis N50.89
  tract (postinfective) — *see* Fistula
  urachus Q64.4
Sinusitis (accessory) (chronic) (hyperplastic) (nasal) (nonpurulent) (purulent) J32.9
  acute J01.90
    ethmoidal J01.20
      recurrent J01.21
    frontal J01.10
      recurrent J01.11
    involving more than one sinus, other than pansinusitis J01.80
      recurrent J01.81
    maxillary J01.00
      recurrent J01.01
    pansinusitis J01.40
      recurrent J01.41
    recurrent J01.91
    specified NEC J01.80
      recurrent J01.81
    sphenoidal J01.30
      recurrent J01.31
  allergic — *see* Rhinitis, allergic
  due to high altitude T70.1 ☑
  ethmoidal J32.2
    acute J01.20
      recurrent J01.21
  frontal J32.1
    acute J01.10
      recurrent J01.11
  influenzal — *see* Influenza, with, respiratory manifestations NEC
  involving more than one sinus but not pansinusitis J32.8
    acute J01.80
      recurrent J01.81
  maxillary J32.0
    acute J01.00
      recurrent J01.01
  sphenoidal J32.3
    acute J01.30
      recurrent J01.31
  tuberculous, any sinus A15.8
Sinusitis-bronchiectasis-situs inversus (syndrome) (triad) Q89.3
Sipple's syndrome E31.22
Sirenomelia (syndrome) Q87.2
Siriasis T67.0 ☑
Sirkari's disease B55.0
Siti A65
Situation, psychiatric F99
Situational
  disturbance (transient) — *see* Disorder, adjustment
    acute F43.0
  maladjustment — *see* Disorder, adjustment
  reaction — *see* Disorder, adjustment
    acute F43.0
Situs inversus or transversus (abdominalis) (thoracis) Q89.3
Sixth disease B08.20
  due to human herpesvirus 6 B08.21
  due to human herpesvirus 7 B08.22
Sjögren-Larsson syndrome Q87.1
Sjögren's syndrome or disease — *see* Sicca syndrome
Skeletal — *see* condition
Skene's gland — *see* condition
Skenitis — *see* Urethritis
Skerljevo A65
Skevas-Zerfus disease — *see* Toxicity, venom, marine animal, sea anemone
Skin (*see also* condition)

Skin — *continued*
  clammy R23.1
  donor — *see* Donor, skin
  hidebound M35.9
Slate-dressers' or slate-miners' lung J62.8
Sleep
  apnea — *see* Apnea, sleep
  deprivation Z72.820
  disorder or disturbance G47.9
    child F51.9
    nonorganic origin F51.9
    specified NEC G47.8
  disturbance G47.9
    nonorganic origin F51.9
  drunkenness F51.9
  rhythm inversion G47.2- ☑
  terrors F51.4
  walking F51.3
    hysterical F44.89
Sleep hygiene
  abuse Z72.821
  inadequate Z72.821
  poor Z72.821
Sleeping sickness — *see* Sickness, sleeping
Sleeplessness — *see* Insomnia
  menopausal N95.1
Sleep-wake schedule disorder G47.20
Slim disease (in HIV infection) B20
Slipped, slipping
  epiphysis (traumatic) (*see also* Osteochondropathy, specified type NEC)
    capital femoral (traumatic)
      acute (on chronic) S79.01- ☑
    current traumatic — *code as* Fracture, by site
    upper femoral (nontraumatic) M93.00- ☑
      acute M93.01- ☑
        on chronic M93.03- ☑
      chronic M93.02- ☑
  intervertebral disc — *see* Displacement, intervertebral disc
  ligature, umbilical P51.8
  patella — *see* Disorder, patella, derangement NEC
  rib M89.8X8
  sacroiliac joint — *see* subcategory M53.2 ☑
  tendon — *see* Disorder, tendon
  ulnar nerve, nontraumatic — *see* Lesion, nerve, ulnar
  vertebra NEC — *see* Spondylolisthesis
Slocumb's syndrome E27.0
Sloughing (multiple) (phagedena) (skin) (*see also* Gangrene)
  abscess — *see* Abscess
  appendix K38.8
  fascia — *see* Disorder, soft tissue, specified type NEC
  scrotum N50.89
  tendon — *see* Disorder, tendon
  transplanted organ — *see* Rejection, transplant
  ulcer — *see* Ulcer, skin
Slow
  feeding, newborn P92.2
  flow syndrome, coronary I20.8
  heart (beat) R00.1
Slowing, urinary stream R39.198
Sluder's neuralgia (syndrome) G44.89
Slurred, slurring speech R47.81
Small (ness)
  for gestational age — *see* Small for dates
  introitus, vagina N89.6
  kidney (unknown cause) N27.9
    bilateral N27.1
    unilateral N27.0
  ovary (congenital) Q50.39
  pelvis
    with disproportion (fetopelvic) O33.1
      causing obstructed labor O65.1
  uterus N85.8
  white kidney N03.9
Small-and-light-for-dates — *see* Small for dates
Small-for-dates (infant) P05.10
  with weight of
    499 grams or less P05.11
    500-749 grams P05.12
    750-999 grams P05.13
    1000-1249 grams P05.14
    1250-1499 grams P05.15
    1500-1749 grams P05.16
    1750-1999 grams P05.17
    2000-2499 grams P05.18

Small-for-dates — *continued*
  with weight of — *continued*
    2500 grams and over P05.19
  specified NEC P05.19
Smallpox B03
Smearing, fecal R15.1
Smith-Lemli-Opitz syndrome E78.72
Smith's fracture S52.54- ☑
Smoker — *see* Dependence, drug, nicotine
Smoker's
  bronchitis J41.0
  cough J41.0
  palate K13.24
  throat J31.2
  tongue K13.24
Smoking
  passive Z77.22
Smothering spells R06.81
Snaggle teeth, tooth M26.39
Snapping
  finger — *see* Trigger finger
  hip — *see* Derangement, joint, specified type NEC, hip
    involving the iliotiblial band M76.3- ☑
  knee — *see* Derangement, knee
    involving the iliotiblial band M76.3- ☑
Sneddon-Wilkinson disease or syndrome (sub-corneal pustular dermatosis) L13.1
Sneezing (intractable) R06.7
Sniffing
  cocaine
    abuse — *see* Abuse, drug, cocaine
    dependence — *see* Dependence, drug, cocaine
  gasoline
    abuse — *see* Abuse, drug, inhalant
    dependence — *see* Dependence, drug, inhalant
  glue (airplane)
    abuse — *see* Abuse, drug, inhalant
    drug dependence — *see* Dependence, drug, inhalant
Sniffles
  newborn P28.89
Snoring R06.83
Snow blindness — *see* Photokeratitis
Snuffles (non-syphilitic) R06.5
  newborn P28.89
  syphilitic (infant) A50.05 [J99]
Social
  exclusion Z60.4
    due to discrimination or persecution (perceived) Z60.5
  migrant Z59.0
    acculturation difficulty Z60.3
  rejection Z60.4
    due to discrimination or persecution Z60.5
  role conflict NEC Z73.5
  skills inadequacy NEC Z73.4
  transplantation Z60.3
Sodoku A25.0
Soemmerring's ring — *see* Cataract, secondary
Soft (*see also* condition)
  nails L60.3
Softening
  bone — *see* Osteomalacia
  brain (necrotic) (progressive) G93.89
    congenital Q04.8
    embolic I63.4- ☑
    hemorrhagic — *see* Hemorrhage, intracranial, intracerebral
    occlusive I63.5- ☑
    thrombotic I63.3- ☑
  cartilage M94.2- ☑
    patella M22.4- ☑
  cerebellar — *see* Softening, brain
  cerebral — *see* Softening, brain
  cerebrospinal — *see* Softening, brain
  myocardial, heart — *see* Degeneration, myocardial
  spinal cord G95.89
  stomach K31.89
Soldier's
  heart F45.8
  patches I31.0
Solitary
  cyst, kidney N28.1
  kidney, congenital Q60.0
Solvent abuse — *see* Abuse, drug, inhalant
  dependence — *see* Dependence, drug, inhalant

Somatization reaction, somatic reaction — *see* Disorder, somatoform
Somnambulism F51.3
  hysterical F44.89
Somnolence R40.0
  nonorganic origin F51.11
Sonne dysentery A03.3
Soor B37.0
Sore
  bed — *see* Ulcer, pressure, by site
  chiclero B55.1
  Delhi B55.1
  desert — *see* Ulcer, skin
  eye H57.1- ☑
  Lahore B55.1
  mouth K13.79
    canker K12.0
  muscle M79.1
  Naga — *see* Ulcer, skin
  of skin — *see* Ulcer, skin
  oriental B55.1
  pressure — *see* Ulcer, pressure, by site
  skin L98.9
  soft A57
  throat (acute) (*see also* Pharyngitis)
    with influenza, flu, or grippe — *see* Influenza, with, respiratory manifestations NEC
    chronic J31.2
    coxsackie (virus) B08.5
    diphtheritic A36.0
    herpesviral B00.2
    influenzal — *see* Influenza, with, respiratory manifestations NEC
    septic J02.0
    streptococcal (ulcerative) J02.0
    viral NEC J02.8
      coxsackie B08.5
  tropical — *see* Ulcer, skin
  veldt — *see* Ulcer, skin
Soto's syndrome (cerebral gigantism) Q87.3
South African cardiomyopathy syndrome I42.8
Southeast Asian hemorrhagic fever A91
Spacing
  abnormal, tooth, teeth, fully erupted M26.30
  excessive, tooth, fully erupted M26.32
Spade-like hand (congenital) Q68.1
Spading nail L60.8
  congenital Q84.6
Spanish collar N47.1
Sparganosis B70.1
Spasm(s), spastic, spasticity (*see also* condition) R25.2
  accommodation — *see* Spasm, of accommodation
  ampulla of Vater K83.4
  anus, ani (sphincter) (reflex) K59.4
    psychogenic F45.8
  artery I73.9
    cerebral G45.9
  Bell's G51.3
  bladder (sphincter, external or internal) N32.89
    psychogenic F45.8
  bronchus, bronchiole J98.01
  cardia K22.0
  cardiac I20.1
  carpopedal — *see* Tetany
  cerebral (arteries) (vascular) G45.9
  cervix, complicating delivery O62.4
  ciliary body (of accommodation) — *see* Spasm, of accommodation
  colon (*see also* Irritable, bowel) K58.9
    with diarrhea K58.0
    psychogenic F45.8
  common duct K83.8
  compulsive — *see* Tic
  conjugate H51.8
  coronary (artery) I20.1
  diaphragm (reflex) R06.6
    epidemic B33.0
    psychogenic F45.8
  duodenum K59.8
  epidemic diaphragmatic (transient) B33.0
  esophagus (diffuse) K22.4
    psychogenic F45.8
  facial G51.3
  fallopian tube N83.8
  gastrointestinal (tract) K31.89
    psychogenic F45.8
  glottis J38.5
    hysterical F44.4

Spasm(s), spastic, spasticity — *continued*
  glottis — *continued*
    psychogenic F45.8
      conversion reaction F44.4
    reflex through recurrent laryngeal nerve J38.5
  habit — *see* Tic
  heart I20.1
  hemifacial (clonic) G51.3
  hourglass — *see* Contraction, hourglass
  hysterical F44.4
  infantile — *see* Epilepsy, spasms
  inferior oblique, eye H51.8
  intestinal (*see also* Syndrome, irritable bowel) K58.9
    psychogenic F45.8
  larynx, laryngeal J38.5
    hysterical F44.4
    psychogenic F45.8
      conversion reaction F44.4
  levator palpebrae superioris — *see* Disorder, eyelid function
  muscle NEC M62.838
    back M62.830
  nerve, trigeminal G51.0
  nervous F45.8
  nodding F98.4
  occupational F48.8
  oculogyric H51.8
    psychogenic F45.8
  of accommodation H52.53- ☑
  ophthalmic artery — *see* Occlusion, artery, retina
  perineal, female N94.89
  peroneo-extensor (*see also* Deformity, limb, flat foot)
  pharynx (reflex) J39.2
    hysterical F45.8
    psychogenic F45.8
  psychogenic F45.8
  pylorus NEC K31.3
    adult hypertrophic K31.89
    congenital or infantile Q40.0
    psychogenic F45.8
  rectum (sphincter) K59.4
    psychogenic F45.8
  retinal (artery) — *see* Occlusion, artery, retina
  sigmoid (*see also* Syndrome, irritable bowel) K58.9
    psychogenic F45.8
  sphincter of Oddi K83.4
  stomach K31.89
    neurotic F45.8
  throat J39.2
    hysterical F45.8
    psychogenic F45.8
  tic F95.9
    chronic F95.1
    transient of childhood F95.0
  tongue K14.8
  torsion (progressive) G24.1
  trigeminal nerve — *see* Neuralgia, trigeminal
  ureter N13.5
  urethra (sphincter) N35.9
  uterus N85.8
    complicating labor O62.4
  vagina N94.2
    psychogenic F52.5
  vascular I73.9
  vasomotor I73.9
  vein NEC I87.8
  viscera — *see* Pain, abdominal
Spasmodic — *see* condition
Spasmophilia — *see* Tetany
Spasmus nutans F98.4
Spastic, spasticity (*see also* Spasm)
  child (cerebral) (congenital) (paralysis) G80.1
Speaker's throat R49.8
Specific, specified — *see* condition
Speech
  defect, disorder, disturbance, impediment R47.9
    psychogenic, in childhood and adolescence F98.8
    slurring R47.81
    specified NEC R47.89
Spencer's disease A08.19
Spens' syndrome (syncope with heart block) I45.9
Sperm counts (fertility testing) Z31.41
  postvasectomy Z30.8
    reversal Z31.42
Spermatic cord — *see* condition
Spermatocele N43.40
  congenital Q55.4
  multiple N43.42

Spermatocele — *continued*
  single N43.41
Spermatocystitis N49.0
Spermatocytoma C62.9- ☑
  specified site — *see* Neoplasm, malignant, by site
Spermatorrhea N50.89
Sphacelus — *see* Gangrene
Sphenoidal — *see* condition
Sphenoiditis (chronic) — *see* Sinusitis, sphenoidal
Sphenopalatine ganglion neuralgia G90.09
Sphericity, increased, lens (congenital) Q12.4
Spherocytosis (congenital) (familial) (hereditary) D58.0
  hemoglobin disease D58.0
  sickle-cell (disease) D57.8- ☑
Spherophakia Q12.4
Sphincter — *see* condition
Sphincteritis, sphincter of Oddi — *see* Cholangitis
Sphingolipidosis E75.3
  specified NEC E75.29
Sphingomyelinosis E75.3
Spicule tooth K00.2
Spider
  bite — *see* Toxicity, venom, spider
  fingers — *see* Syndrome, Marfan's
  nevus I78.1
  toes — *see* Syndrome, Marfan's
  vascular I78.1
Spiegler-Fendt
  benign lymphocytoma L98.8
  sarcoid L08.89
Spielmeyer-Vogt disease E75.4
Spina bifida (aperta) Q05.9
  with hydrocephalus NEC Q05.4
  cervical Q05.5
    with hydrocephalus Q05.0
  dorsal Q05.6
    with hydrocephalus Q05.1
  lumbar Q05.7
    with hydrocephalus Q05.2
  lumbosacral Q05.7
    with hydrocephalus Q05.2
  occulta Q76.0
  sacral Q05.8
    with hydrocephalus Q05.3
  thoracic Q05.6
    with hydrocephalus Q05.1
  thoracolumbar Q05.6
    with hydrocephalus Q05.1
Spindle, Krukenberg's — *see* Pigmentation, cornea, posterior
Spine, spinal — *see* condition
Spiradenoma (eccrine) — *see* Neoplasm, skin, benign
Spirillosis A25.0
Spirillum
  minus A25.0
  obermeieri infection A68.0
Spirochetal — *see* condition
Spirochetosis A69.9
  arthritic, arthritica A69.9
  bronchopulmonary A69.8
  icterohemorrhagic A27.0
  lung A69.8
Spirometrosis B70.1
Spitting blood — *see* Hemoptysis
Splanchnoptosis K63.4
Spleen, splenic — *see* condition
Splenectasis — *see* Splenomegaly
Splenitis (interstitial) (malignant) (nonspecific) D73.89
  malarial (*see also* Malaria) B54 [D77]
  tuberculous A18.85
Splenocele D73.89
Splenomegaly, splenomegalia (Bengal) (cryptogenic) (idiopathic) (tropical) R16.1
  with hepatomegaly R16.2
  cirrhotic D73.2
  congenital Q89.09
  congestive, chronic D73.2
  Egyptian B65.1
  Gaucher's E75.22
  malarial (*see also* Malaria) B54 [D77]
  neutropenic D73.81
  Niemann-Pick — *see* Niemann-Pick disease or syndrome
  siderotic D73.2
  syphilitic A52.79
    congenital (early) A50.08 [D77]
Splenopathy D73.9

Splenoptosis D73.89
Splenosis D73.89
Splinter — *see* Foreign body, superficial, by site
Split, splitting
  foot Q72.7- ☑
  hand Q71.6 ☑
  heart sounds R01.2
  lip, congenital — *see* Cleft, lip
  nails L60.3
  urinary stream R39.13
Spondylarthrosis — *see* Spondylosis
Spondylitis (chronic) (*see also* Spondylopathy, inflammatory)
  ankylopoietica — *see* Spondylitis, ankylosing
  ankylosing (chronic) M45.9
    with lung involvement M45.9 [J99]
    cervical region M45.2
    cervicothoracic region M45.3
    juvenile M08.1
    lumbar region M45.6
    lumbosacral region M45.7
    multiple sites M45.0
    occipito-atlanto-axial region M45.1
    sacrococcygeal region M45.8
    thoracic region M45.4
    thoracolumbar region M45.5
  atrophic (ligamentous) — *see* Spondylitis, ankylosing
  deformans (chronic) — *see* Spondylosis
  gonococcal A54.41
  gouty (*see also* Gout, by type, vertebrae) M10.08
  in (due to)
    brucellosis A23.9 [M49.80]
      cervical region A23.9 [M49.82]
      cervicothoracic region A23.9 [M49.83]
      lumbar region A23.9 [M49.86]
      lumbosacral region A23.9 [M49.87]
      multiple sites A23.9 [M49.89]
      occipito-atlanto-axial region A23.9 [M49.81]
      sacrococcygeal region A23.9 [M49.88]
      thoracic region A23.9 [M49.84]
      thoracolumbar region A23.9 [M49.85]
    enterobacteria (*see also* subcategory M49.8) A04.9
    tuberculosis A18.01
  infectious NEC — *see* Spondylopathy, infective
  juvenile ankylosing (chronic) M08.1
  Kümmell's — *see* Spondylopathy, traumatic
  Marie-Strümpell — *see* Spondylitis, ankylosing
  muscularis — *see* Spondylopathy, specified NEC
  psoriatic L40.53
  rheumatoid — *see* Spondylitis, ankylosing
  rhizomelica — *see* Spondylitis, ankylosing
  sacroiliac NEC M46.1
  senescent, senile — *see* Spondylosis
  traumatic (chronic) or post-traumatic — *see* Spondylopathy, traumatic
  tuberculous A18.01
  typhosa A01.05
Spondylolisthesis (acquired) (degenerative) M43.10
  with disproportion (fetopelvic) O33.0
    causing obstructed labor O65.0
  cervical region M43.12
  cervicothoracic region M43.13
  congenital Q76.2
  lumbar region M43.16
  lumbosacral region M43.17
  multiple sites M43.19
  occipito-atlanto-axial region M43.11
  sacrococcygeal region M43.18
  thoracic region M43.14
  thoracolumbar region M43.15
  traumatic (old) M43.10
    acute
      fifth cervical (displaced) S12.430 ☑
        nondisplaced S12.431 ☑
        specified type NEC (displaced) S12.450 ☑
          nondisplaced S12.451 ☑
        type III S12.44 ☑
      fourth cervical (displaced) S12.330 ☑
        nondisplaced S12.331 ☑
        specified type NEC (displaced) S12.350 ☑
          nondisplaced S12.351 ☑
        type III S12.34 ☑
      second cervical (displaced) S12.130 ☑
        nondisplaced S12.131 ☑
        specified type NEC (displaced) S12.150 ☑
          nondisplaced S12.151 ☑
        type III S12.14 ☑

Spondylolisthesis — *continued*
  traumatic — *continued*
    acute — *continued*
      seventh cervical (displaced) S12.630 ☑
        nondisplaced S12.631 ☑
        specified type NEC (displaced) S12.650 ☑
          nondisplaced S12.651 ☑
        type III S12.64 ☑
      sixth cervical (displaced) S12.530 ☑
        nondisplaced S12.531 ☑
        specified type NEC (displaced) S12.550 ☑
          nondisplaced S12.551 ☑
        type III S12.54 ☑
      third cervical (displaced) S12.230 ☑
        nondisplaced S12.231 ☑
        specified type NEC (displaced) S12.250 ☑
          nondisplaced S12.251 ☑
        type III S12.24 ☑
Spondylolysis (acquired) M43.00
  cervical region M43.02
  cervicothoracic region M43.03
  congenital Q76.2
  lumbar region M43.06
  lumbosacral region M43.07
    with disproportion (fetopelvic) O33.0
      causing obstructed labor O65.8
  multiple sites M43.09
  occipito-atlanto-axial region M43.01
  sacrococcygeal region M43.08
  thoracic region M43.04
  thoracolumbar region M43.05
Spondylopathy M48.9
  infective NEC M46.50
    cervical region M46.52
    cervicothoracic region M46.53
    lumbar region M46.56
    lumbosacral region M46.57
    multiple sites M46.59
    occipito-atlanto-axial region M46.51
    sacrococcygeal region M46.58
    thoracic region M46.54
    thoracolumbar region M46.55
  inflammatory M46.90
    cervical region M46.92
    cervicothoracic region M46.93
    lumbar region M46.96
    lumbosacral region M46.97
    multiple sites M46.99
    occipito-atlanto-axial region M46.91
    sacrococcygeal region M46.98
    specified type NEC M46.80
      cervical region M46.82
      cervicothoracic region M46.83
      lumbar region M46.86
      lumbosacral region M46.87
      multiple sites M46.89
      occipito-atlanto-axial region M46.81
      sacrococcygeal region M46.88
      thoracic region M46.84
      thoracolumbar region M46.85
    thoracic region M46.94
    thoracolumbar region M46.95
  neuropathic, in
    syringomyelia and syringobulbia G95.0
    tabes dorsalis A52.11
  specified NEC — *see* subcategory M48.8 ☑
  traumatic M48.30
    cervical region M48.32
    cervicothoracic region M48.33
    lumbar region M48.36
    lumbosacral region M48.37
    occipito-atlanto-axial region M48.31
    sacrococcygeal region M48.38
    thoracic region M48.34
    thoracolumbar region M48.35
Spondylosis M47.9
  with
    disproportion (fetopelvic) O33.0
      causing obstructed labor O65.0
    myelopathy NEC M47.10
      cervical region M47.12
      cervicothoracic region M47.13
      lumbar region M47.16
      occipito-atlanto-axial region M47.11
      thoracic region M47.14
      thoracolumbar region M47.15
    radiculopathy M47.20
      cervical region M47.22

Spondylosis — *continued*
  with — *continued*
    radiculopathy — *continued*
      cervicothoracic region M47.23
      lumbar region M47.26
      lumbosacral region M47.27
      occipito-atlanto-axial region M47.21
      sacrococcygeal region M47.28
      thoracic region M47.24
      thoracolumbar region M47.25
  without myelopathy or radiculopathy M47.819
    cervical region M47.812
    cervicothoracic region M47.813
    lumbar region M47.816
    lumbosacral region M47.817
    occipito-atlanto-axial region M47.811
    sacrococcygeal region M47.818
    thoracic region M47.814
    thoracolumbar region M47.815
  specified NEC M47.899
    cervical region M47.892
    cervicothoracic region M47.893
    lumbar region M47.896
    lumbosacral region M47.897
    occipito-atlanto-axial region M47.891
    sacrococcygeal region M47.898
    thoracic region M47.894
    thoracolumbar region M47.895
  traumatic — *see* Spondylopathy, traumatic
Sponge
  inadvertently left in operation wound — *see* Foreign body, accidentally left during a procedure
  kidney (medullary) Q61.5
Sponge-diver's disease — *see* Toxicity, venom, marine animal, sea anemone
Spongioblastoma (any type) — *see* Neoplasm, malignant, by site
  specified site — *see* Neoplasm, malignant, by site
  unspecified site C71.9
Spongioneuroblastoma — *see* Neoplasm, malignant, by site
Spontaneous (*see also* condition)
  fracture (cause unknown) — *see* Fracture, pathological
Spoon nail L60.3
  congenital Q84.6
Sporadic — *see* condition
Sporothrix schenckii infection — *see* Sporotrichosis
Sporotrichosis B42.9
  arthritis B42.82
  disseminated B42.7
  generalized B42.7
  lymphocutaneous (fixed) (progressive) B42.1
  pulmonary B42.0
  specified NEC B42.89
Spots, spotting (in) (of)
  Bitot's (*see also* Pigmentation, conjunctiva)
    in the young child E50.1
    vitamin A deficiency E50.1
  café, au lait L81.3
  Cayenne pepper I78.1
  cotton wool, retina — *see* Occlusion, artery, retina
  de Morgan's (senile angiomas) I78.1
  Fuchs' black (myopic) (*see also* Myopia, degenerative) H44.2- ☑
  intermenstrual (regular) N92.0
    irregular N92.1
  Koplik's B05.9
  liver L81.4
  pregnancy O26.85- ☑
  purpuric R23.3
  ruby I78.1
Spotted fever — *see* Fever, spotted N92.3
Sprain (joint) (ligament)
  acromioclavicular joint or ligament S43.5- ☑
  ankle S93.40- ☑
    calcaneofibular ligament S93.41- ☑
    deltoid ligament S93.42- ☑
    internal collateral ligament — *see* Sprain, ankle, specified ligament NEC
    specified ligament NEC S93.49- ☑
    talofibular ligament — *see* Sprain, ankle, specified ligament NEC
    tibiofibular ligament S93.43- ☑
  anterior longitudinal, cervical S13.4 ☑
  atlas, atlanto-axial, atlanto-occipital S13.4 ☑
  breast bone — *see* Sprain, sternum
  calcaneofibular — *see* Sprain, ankle
  carpal — *see* Sprain, wrist

Sprain — continued
  carpometacarpal — see Sprain, hand, specified site NEC
  cartilage
    costal S23.41 ☑
    semilunar (knee) — see Sprain, knee, specified site NEC
      with current tear — see Tear, meniscus
    thyroid region S13.5 ☑
    xiphoid — see Sprain, sternum
  cervical, cervicodorsal, cervicothoracic S13.4 ☑
  chondrosternal S23.421 ☑
  coracoclavicular S43.8- ☑
  coracohumeral S43.41- ☑
  coronary, knee — see Sprain, knee, specified site NEC
  costal cartilage S23.41 ☑
  cricoarytenoid articulation or ligament S13.5 ☑
  cricothyroid articulation S13.5 ☑
  cruciate, knee — see Sprain, knee, cruciate
  deltoid, ankle — see Sprain, ankle
  dorsal (spine) S23.3 ☑
  elbow S53.40- ☑
    radial collateral ligament S53.43- ☑
    radiohumeral S53.41- ☑
    rupture
      radial collateral ligament — see Rupture, traumatic, ligament, radial collateral
      ulnar collateral ligament — see Rupture, traumatic, ligament, ulnar collateral
    specified type NEC S53.49- ☑
    ulnar collateral ligament S53.44- ☑
    ulnohumeral S53.42- ☑
  femur, head — see Sprain, hip
  fibular collateral, knee — see Sprain, knee, collateral
  fibulocalcaneal — see Sprain, ankle
  finger(s) S63.61- ☑
    index S63.61- ☑
    interphalangeal (joint) S63.63- ☑
      index S63.63- ☑
      little S63.63- ☑
      middle S63.63- ☑
      ring S63.63- ☑
    little S63.61- ☑
    metacarpophalangeal (joint) S63.65- ☑
    middle S63.61- ☑
    ring S63.61- ☑
    specified site NEC S63.69- ☑
      index S63.69- ☑
      little S63.69- ☑
      middle S63.69- ☑
      ring S63.69- ☑
  foot S93.60- ☑
    specified ligament NEC S93.69- ☑
    tarsal ligament S93.61- ☑
    tarsometatarsal ligament S93.62- ☑
    toe — see Sprain, toe
  hand S63.9- ☑
    finger — see Sprain, finger
    specified site NEC — see subcategory S63.8 ☑
    thumb — see Sprain, thumb
  head S03.9 ☑
  hip S73.10- ☑
    iliofemoral ligament S73.11- ☑
    ischiocapsular (ligament) S73.12- ☑
    specified NEC S73.19- ☑
  iliofemoral — see Sprain, hip
  innominate
    acetabulum — see Sprain, hip
    sacral junction S33.6 ☑
  internal
    collateral, ankle — see Sprain, ankle
    semilunar cartilage — see Sprain, knee, specified site NEC
  interphalangeal
    finger — see Sprain, finger, interphalangeal (joint)
    toe — see Sprain, toe, interphalangeal joint
  ischiocapsular — see Sprain, hip
  ischiofemoral — see Sprain, hip
  jaw (articular disc) (cartilage) (meniscus) S03.4- ☑
    old M26.69
  knee S83.9- ☑
    collateral ligament S83.40- ☑
      lateral (fibular) S83.42- ☑
      medial (tibial) S83.41- ☑
    cruciate ligament S83.50- ☑
      anterior S83.51- ☑

Sprain — continued
  knee — continued
    cruciate ligament — continued
      posterior S83.52- ☑
    lateral (fibular) collateral ligament S83.42- ☑
    medial (tibial) collateral ligament S83.41- ☑
    patellar ligament S76.11- ☑
    specified site NEC S83.8X- ☑
    superior tibiofibular joint (ligament) S83.6- ☑
  lateral collateral, knee — see Sprain, knee, collateral
  lumbar (spine) S33.5 ☑
  lumbosacral S33.9 ☑
  mandible (articular disc) S03.4- ☑
    old M26.69
  medial collateral, knee — see Sprain, knee, collateral
  meniscus
    jaw S03.4- ☑
      old M26.69
    knee — see Sprain, knee, specified site NEC
      with current tear — see Tear, meniscus
        old — see Derangement, knee, meniscus, due to old tear
    mandible S03.4- ☑
      old M26.69
  metacarpal (distal) (proximal) — see Sprain, hand, specified site NEC
  metacarpophalangeal — see Sprain, finger, metacarpophalangeal (joint)
  metatarsophalangeal — see Sprain, toe, metatarsophalangeal joint
  midcarpal — see Sprain, hand, specified site NEC
  midtarsal — see Sprain, foot, specified site NEC
  neck S13.9 ☑
    anterior longitudinal cervical ligament S13.4 ☑
    atlanto-axial joint S13.4 ☑
    atlanto-occipital joint S13.4 ☑
    cervical spine S13.4 ☑
    cricoarytenoid ligament S13.5 ☑
    cricothyroid ligament S13.5 ☑
    specified site NEC S13.8 ☑
    thyroid region (cartilage) S13.5 ☑
  nose S03.8 ☑
  orbicular, hip — see Sprain, hip
  patella — see Sprain, knee, specified site NEC
  patellar ligament S76.11- ☑
  pelvis NEC S33.8 ☑
  phalanx
    finger — see Sprain, finger
    toe — see Sprain, toe
  pubofemoral — see Sprain, hip
  radiocarpal — see Sprain, wrist
  radiohumeral — see Sprain, elbow
  radius, collateral — see Rupture, traumatic, ligament, radial collateral
  rib (cage) S23.41 ☑
  rotator cuff (capsule) S43.42- ☑
  sacroiliac (region)
    chronic or old — see subcategory M53.2 ☑
    joint S33.6 ☑
  scaphoid (hand) — see Sprain, hand, specified site NEC
  scapula (r) — see Sprain, shoulder girdle, specified site NEC
  semilunar cartilage (knee) — see Sprain, knee, specified site NEC
    with current tear — see Tear, meniscus
      old — see Derangement, knee, meniscus, due to old tear
  shoulder joint S43.40- ☑
    acromioclavicular joint (ligament) — see Sprain, acromioclavicular joint
    blade — see Sprain, shoulder, girdle, specified site NEC
    coracoclavicular joint (ligament) — see Sprain, coracoclavicular joint
    coracohumeral ligament — see Sprain, coracohumeral joint
    girdle S43.9- ☑
      specified site NEC S43.8- ☑
    rotator cuff — see Sprain, rotator cuff
    specified site NEC S43.49- ☑
    sternoclavicular joint (ligament) — see Sprain, sternoclavicular joint
  spine
    cervical S13.4 ☑
    lumbar S33.5 ☑

Sprain — continued
  spine — continued
    thoracic S23.3 ☑
  sternoclavicular joint S43.6- ☑
  sternum S23.429 ☑
    chondrosternal joint S23.421 ☑
    specified site NEC S23.428 ☑
    sternoclavicular (joint) (ligament) S23.420 ☑
  symphysis
    jaw S03.4- ☑
      old M26.69
    mandibular S03.4- ☑
      old M26.69
  talofibular — see Sprain, ankle
  tarsal — see Sprain, foot, specified site NEC
  tarsometatarsal — see Sprain, foot, specified site NEC
  temporomandibular S03.4- ☑
    old M26.69
  thorax S23.9 ☑
    ribs S23.41 ☑
    specified site NEC S23.8 ☑
    spine S23.3 ☑
    sternum — see Sprain, sternum
  thumb S63.60- ☑
    interphalangeal (joint) S63.62- ☑
    metacarpophalangeal (joint) S63.64- ☑
    specified site NEC S63.68- ☑
  thyroid cartilage or region S13.5 ☑
  tibia (proximal end) — see Sprain, knee, specified site NEC
  tibial collateral, knee — see Sprain, knee, collateral
  tibiofibular
    distal — see Sprain, ankle
    superior — see Sprain, knee, specified site NEC
  toe(s) S93.50- ☑
    great S93.50- ☑
    interphalangeal joint S93.51- ☑
      great S93.51- ☑
      lesser S93.51- ☑
    lesser S93.50- ☑
    metatarsophalangeal joint S93.52- ☑
      great S93.52- ☑
      lesser S93.52- ☑
  ulna, collateral — see Rupture, traumatic, ligament, ulnar collateral
  ulnohumeral — see Sprain, elbow
  wrist S63.50- ☑
    carpal S63.51- ☑
    radiocarpal S63.52- ☑
    specified site NEC S63.59- ☑
  xiphoid cartilage — see Sprain, sternum
Sprengel's deformity (congenital) Q74.0
Sprue (tropical) K90.1
  celiac K90.0
  idiopathic K90.49
  meaning thrush B37.0
  nontropical K90.0
Spur, bone (see also Enthesopathy)
  calcaneal M77.3- ☑
  iliac crest M76.2- ☑
  nose (septum) J34.89
Spurway's syndrome Q78.0
Sputum
  abnormal (amount) (color) (odor) (purulent) R09.3
  blood-stained R04.2
  excessive (cause unknown) R09.3
Squamous (see also condition)
  epithelium in
    cervical canal (congenital) Q51.828
    uterine mucosa (congenital) Q51.818
Squashed nose M95.0
  congenital Q67.4
Squeeze, diver's T70.3 ☑
Squint (see also Strabismus)
  accommodative — see Strabismus, convergent concomitant
St. Hubert's disease A82.9
Stab (see also Laceration)
  internal organs — see Injury, by site
Stafne's cyst or cavity M27.0
Staggering gait R26.0
  hysterical F44.4
Staghorn calculus — see Calculus, kidney
Stähli's line (cornea) (pigment) — see Pigmentation, cornea, anterior

Stain, staining
meconium (newborn) P96.83
port wine Q82.5
tooth, teeth (hard tissues) (extrinsic) KØ3.6
  due to
    accretions KØ3.6
    deposits (betel) (black) (green) (materia alba)
      (orange) (soft) (tobacco) KØ3.6
    metals (copper) (silver) KØ3.7
    nicotine KØ3.6
    pulpal bleeding KØ3.7
    tobacco KØ3.6
  intrinsic KØØ.8

Stammering (see also Disorder, fluency) F80.81

Standstill
auricular I45.5
cardiac — see Arrest, cardiac
sinoatrial I45.5
ventricular — see Arrest, cardiac

Stannosis J63.5

Stanton's disease — see Melioidosis

Staphylitis (acute) (catarrhal) (chronic) (gangrenous) (membranous) (suppurative) (ulcerative) K12.2

Staphylococcal scalded skin syndrome LØØ

Staphylococcemia A41.2

Staphylococcus, staphylococcal (see also condition)
as cause of disease classified elsewhere B95.8
  aureus (methicillin susceptible) (MSSA) B95.61
    methicillin resistant (MRSA) B95.62
  specified NEC, as cause of disease classified elsewhere B95.7

Staphyloma (sclera)
cornea H18.72- ☑
equatorial H15.81- ☑
localized (anterior) H15.82- ☑
posticum H15.83- ☑
ring H15.85- ☑

Stargardt's disease — see Dystrophy, retina

Starvation (inanition) (due to lack of food) T73.Ø ☑
edema — see Malnutrition, severe

Stasis
bile (noncalculous) K83.1
bronchus J98.Ø9
  with infection — see Bronchitis
cardiac — see Failure, heart, congestive
cecum K59.8
colon K59.8
dermatitis I87.2
  with
    varicose ulcer — see Varix, leg, with ulcer, with inflammation
    varicose veins — see Varix, leg, with, inflammation
  due to postthrombotic syndrome — see Syndrome, postthrombotic
duodenal K31.5
eczema — see Varix, leg, with, inflammation
edema — see Hypertension, venous (chronic), idiopathic
foot T69.Ø- ☑
ileocecal coil K59.8
ileum K59.8
intestinal K59.8
jejunum K59.8
kidney N19
liver (cirrhotic) K76.1
lymphatic I89.8
pneumonia J18.2
pulmonary — see Edema, lung
rectal K59.8
renal N19
  tubular N17.Ø
ulcer — see Varix, leg, with, ulcer
  without varicose veins I87.2
urine — see Retention, urine
venous I87.8

State (of)
affective and paranoid, mixed, organic psychotic FØ6.8
agitated R45.1
  acute reaction to stress F43.Ø
anxiety (neurotic) F41.1
apprehension F41.1
burn-out Z73.Ø
climacteric, female Z78.Ø
  symptomatic N95.1
compulsive F42.8
  mixed with obsessional thoughts F42.2
confusional (psychogenic) F44.89

State — continued
confusional — continued
  acute (see also Delirium)
    with
      arteriosclerotic dementia FØ1.5Ø
        with behavioral disturbance FØ1.51
      senility or dementia FØ5
    alcoholic F1Ø.231
    epileptic FØ5
    reactive (from emotional stress, psychological trauma) F44.89
    subacute — see Delirium
convulsive — see Convulsions
crisis F43.Ø
depressive F32.9
  neurotic F34.1
dissociative F44.9
emotional shock (stress) R45.7
hypercoagulation — see Hypercoagulable
locked-in G83.5
menopausal Z78.Ø
  symptomatic N95.1
neurotic F48.9
  with depersonalization F48.1
obsessional F42.8
oneiroid (schizophrenia-like) F23
organic
  hallucinatory (nonalcoholic) FØ6.Ø
  paranoid (-hallucinatory) FØ6.2
panic F41.Ø
paranoid F22
  climacteric F22
  involutional F22
  menopausal F22
  organic FØ6.2
  senile FØ3 ☑
  simple F22
persistent vegetative R4Ø.3
phobic F4Ø.9
postleukotomy FØ7.Ø
pregnant
  gestational carrier Z33.3
  incidental Z33.1
psychogenic, twilight F44.89
psychopathic (constitutional) F6Ø.2
psychotic, organic (see also Psychosis, organic)
  mixed paranoid and affective FØ6.8
  senile or presenile FØ3 ☑
  transient NEC FØ6.8
    with
      depression FØ6.31
      hallucinations FØ6.Ø
residual schizophrenic F2Ø.5
restlessness R45.1
stress (emotional) R45.7
tension (mental) F48.9
  specified NEC F48.8
transient organic psychotic NEC FØ6.8
  depressive type FØ6.31
  hallucinatory type FØ6.Ø
twilight
  epileptic FØ5
  psychogenic F44.89
vegetative, persistent R4Ø.3
vital exhaustion Z73.Ø
withdrawal, — see Withdrawal, state

Status (post) (see also Presence (of))
absence, epileptic — see Epilepsy, by type, with status epilepticus
administration of tPA (rtPA) in a different facility within the last 24 hours prior to admission to current facility Z92.82
adrenalectomy (unilateral) (bilateral) E89.6
anastomosis Z98.Ø
anginosus I2Ø.9
angioplasty (peripheral) Z98.62
  with implant Z95.82Ø
  coronary artery Z98.61
    with implant Z95.5
aortocoronary bypass Z95.1
arthrodesis Z98.1
artificial opening (of) Z93.9
  gastrointestinal tract Z93.4
  specified NEC Z93.8
  urinary tract Z93.6
  vagina Z93.8
asthmaticus — see Asthma, by type, with status asthmaticus

Status — continued
awaiting organ transplant Z76.82
bariatric surgery Z98.84
bed confinement Z74.Ø1
bleb, filtering (vitreous), after glaucoma surgery Z98.83
breast implant Z98.82
  removal Z98.86
cataract extraction Z98.4- ☑
cholecystectomy Z9Ø.49
clitorectomy N9Ø.811
  with excision of labia minora N9Ø.812
colectomy (complete) (partial) Z9Ø.49
colonization — see Carrier (suspected) of
colostomy Z93.3
convulsivus idiopathicus — see Epilepsy, by type, with status epilepticus
coronary artery angioplasty — see Status, angioplasty, coronary artery
coronary artery bypass graft Z95.1
cystectomy (urinary bladder) Z9Ø.6
cystostomy Z93.5Ø
  appendico-vesicostomy Z93.52
  cutaneous Z93.51
  specified NEC Z93.59
delinquent immunization Z28.3
dental Z98.818
  crown Z98.811
  fillings Z98.811
  restoration Z98.811
  sealant Z98.81Ø
  specified NEC Z98.818
deployment (current) (military) Z56.82
dialysis (hemodialysis) (peritoneal) Z99.2
do not resuscitate (DNR) Z66
donor — see Donor
embedded fragments — see Retained, foreign body fragments (type of)
embedded splinter — see Retained, foreign body fragments (type of)
enterostomy Z93.4
epileptic, epilepticus (see also Epilepsy, by type, with status epilepticus) G4Ø.9Ø1
estrogen receptor
  negative Z17.1
  positive Z17.Ø
female genital cutting — see Female genital mutilation status
female genital mutilation — see Female genital mutilation status
filtering (vitreous) bleb after glaucoma surgery Z98.83
gastrectomy (complete) (partial) Z9Ø.3
gastric banding Z98.84
gastric bypass for obesity Z98.84
gastrostomy Z93.1
human immunodeficiency virus (HIV) infection, asymptomatic Z21
hysterectomy (complete) (total) Z9Ø.71Ø
  partial (with remaining cervial stump) Z9Ø.711
ileostomy Z93.2
implant
  breast Z98.82
infibulation N9Ø.813
intestinal bypass Z98.Ø
jejunostomy Z93.4
lapsed immunization schedule Z28.3
laryngectomy Z9Ø.Ø2
lymphaticus E32.8
malignancy
  castrate resistant prostate Z19.2
  hormone resistant Z19.2
  hormone sensitive Z19.1
marmoratus G8Ø.3
mastectomy (unilateral) (bilateral) Z9Ø.1- ☑
military deployment status (current) Z56.82
  in theater or in support of military war, peacekeeping and humanitarian operations Z56.82
nephrectomy (unilateral) (bilateral) Z9Ø.5
nephrostomy Z93.6
obesity surgery Z98.84
oophorectomy
  bilateral Z9Ø.722
  unilateral Z9Ø.721
organ replacement
  by artificial or mechanical device or prosthesis of
    artery Z95.828
    bladder Z96.Ø
    blood vessel Z95.828
    breast Z97.8

Status — *continued*
  organ replacement — *continued*
    by artificial or mechanical device or prosthesis of — *continued*
      eye globe Z97.0
      heart Z95.812
        valve Z95.2
      intestine Z97.8
      joint Z96.60
        hip — *see* Presence, hip joint implant
        knee — *see* Presence, knee joint implant
        specified site NEC Z96.698
      kidney Z97.8
      larynx Z96.3
      lens Z96.1
      limbs — *see* Presence, artificial, limb
      liver Z97.8
      lung Z97.8
      pancreas Z97.8
    by organ transplant (heterologous)(homologous) — *see* Transplant
  pacemaker
    brain Z96.89
    cardiac Z95.0
    specified NEC Z96.89
  pancreatectomy Z90.410
    complete Z90.410
    partial Z90.411
    total Z90.410
  physical restraint Z78.1
  pneumonectomy (complete) (partial) Z90.2
  pneumothorax, therapeutic Z98.3
  postcommotio cerebri F07.81
  postoperative (postprocedural) NEC Z98.890
    breast implant Z98.82
    dental Z98.818
      crown Z98.811
      fillings Z98.811
      restoration Z98.811
      sealant Z98.810
      specified NEC Z98.818
    pneumothorax, therapeutic Z98.3
    uterine scar Z98.891
  postpartum (routine follow-up) Z39.2
    care immediately after delivery Z39.0
  postsurgical (postprocedural) NEC Z98.890
    pneumothorax, therapeutic Z98.3
  pregnancy, incidental Z33.1
  prosthesis coronary angioplasty Z95.5
  pseudophakia Z96.1
  renal dialysis (hemodialysis) (peritoneal) Z99.2
  retained foreign body — *see* Retained, foreign body fragments (type of)
  reversed jejunal transposition (for bypass) Z98.0
  salpingo-oophorectomy
    bilateral Z90.722
    unilateral Z90.721
  sex reassignment surgery status Z87.890
  shunt
    arteriovenous (for dialysis) Z99.2
    cerebrospinal fluid Z98.2
    ventricular (communicating) (for drainage) Z98.2
  splenectomy Z90.81
  thymicolymphaticus E32.8
  thymicus E32.8
  thymolymphaticus E32.8
  thyroidectomy (hypothyroidism) E89.0
  tooth (teeth) extraction (*see also* Absence, teeth, acquired) K08.409
  tPA (rtPA) administration in a different facility within the last 24 hours prior to admission to current facility Z92.82
  tracheostomy Z93.0
  transplant — *see* Transplant
    organ removed Z98.85
  tubal ligation Z98.51
  underimmunization Z28.3
  ureterostomy Z93.6
  urethrostomy Z93.6
  vagina, artificial Z93.8
  vasectomy Z98.52
  wheelchair confinement Z99.3
Stealing
  child problem F91.8
    in company with others Z72.810
  pathological (compulsive) F63.2
Steam burn — *see* Burn
Steatocystoma multiplex L72.2

Steatohepatitis (nonalcoholic) (NASH) K75.81
Steatoma L72.3
  eyelid (cystic) — *see* Dermatosis, eyelid
    infected — *see* Hordeolum
Steatorrhea (chronic) K90.9
  with lacteal obstruction K90.2
  idiopathic (adult) (infantile) K90.9
  pancreatic K90.3
  primary K90.0
  tropical K90.1
Steatosis E88.89
  heart — *see* Degeneration, myocardial
  kidney N28.89
  liver NEC K76.0
Steele-Richardson-Olszewski disease or syndrome G23.1
Steinbrocker's syndrome G90.8
Steinert's disease G71.11
Stein-Leventhal syndrome E28.2
Stein's syndrome E28.2
STEMI (*see also* Infarct, myocardium, ST elevation) I21.3
Stenocardia I20.8
Stenocephaly Q75.8
Stenosis, stenotic (cicatricial) (*see also* Stricture)
  ampulla of Vater K83.1
  anus, anal (canal) (sphincter) K62.4
    and rectum K62.4
    congenital Q42.3
      with fistula Q42.2
  aorta (ascending) (supraventricular) (congenital) Q25.1
    arteriosclerotic I70.0
    calcified I70.0
    supravalvular Q25.3
  aortic (valve) I35.0
    with insufficiency I35.2
    congenital Q23.0
    rheumatic I06.0
      with
        incompetency, insufficiency or regurgitation I06.2
          with mitral (valve) disease I08.0
            with tricuspid (valve) disease I08.3
        mitral (valve) disease I08.0
          with tricuspid (valve) disease I08.3
        tricuspid (valve) disease I08.2
          with mitral (valve) disease I08.3
    specified cause NEC I35.0
    syphilitic A52.03
  aqueduct of Sylvius (congenital) Q03.0
    with spina bifida — *see* Spina bifida, by site, with hydrocephalus
    acquired G91.1
  artery NEC (*see also* Arteriosclerosis) I77.1
    celiac I77.4
    cerebral — *see* Occlusion, artery, cerebral
    extremities — *see* Arteriosclerosis, extremities
    precerebral — *see* Occlusion, artery, precerebral
    pulmonary (congenital) Q25.6
      acquired I28.8
    renal I70.1
    stent
      coronary T82.855 ☑
      peripheral T82.856 ☑
  bile duct (common) (hepatic) K83.1
    congenital Q44.3
  bladder-neck (acquired) N32.0
    congenital Q64.31
  brain G93.89
  bronchus J98.09
    congenital Q32.3
    syphilitic A52.72
  cardia (stomach) K22.2
    congenital Q39.3
  cardiovascular — *see* Disease, cardiovascular
  caudal M48.08
  cervix, cervical (canal) N88.2
    congenital Q51.828
    in pregnancy or childbirth — *see* Pregnancy, complicated by, abnormal cervix
  colon (*see also* Obstruction, intestine)
    congenital Q42.9
      specified NEC Q42.8
  colostomy K94.03
  common (bile) duct K83.1
    congenital Q44.3
  coronary (artery) — *see* Disease, heart, ischemic, atherosclerotic
  cystic duct — *see* Obstruction, gallbladder

Stenosis, stenotic — *continued*
  due to presence of device, implant or graft (*see also* Complications, by site and type, specified NEC) T85.858 ☑
    arterial graft NEC T82.858 ☑
    breast (implant) T85.858 ☑
    catheter T85.858 ☑
      dialysis (renal) T82.858 ☑
        intraperitoneal T85.858 ☑
      infusion NEC T82.858 ☑
        spinal (epidural) (subdural) T85.850 ☑
      urinary (indwelling) T83.85 ☑
    fixation, internal (orthopedic) NEC T84.85 ☑
    gastrointestinal (bile duct) (esophagus) T85.858 ☑
    genital NEC T83.85 ☑
    heart NEC T82.857 ☑
    joint prosthesis T84.85 ☑
    ocular (corneal graft) (orbital implant) NEC T85.858 ☑
    orthopedic NEC T84.85 ☑
    specified NEC T85.858 ☑
    urinary NEC T83.85 ☑
    vascular NEC T82.858 ☑
    ventricular intracranial shunt T85.850 ☑
  duodenum K31.5
    congenital Q41.0
  ejaculatory duct NEC N50.89
    stent
      vascular
        end stent
          adjacent to stent — *see* Arteriosclerosis
          within the stent
            coronary T82.855 ☑
            peripheral T82.856 ☑
        in stent
          coronary vessel T82.855 ☑
          peripheral vessel T82.856 ☑
  endocervical os — *see* Stenosis, cervix
  enterostomy K94.13
  esophagus K22.2
    congenital Q39.3
    syphilitic A52.79
      congenital A50.59 [K23]
  eustachian tube — *see* Obstruction, eustachian tube
  external ear canal (acquired) H61.30- ☑
    congenital Q16.1
    due to
      inflammation H61.32- ☑
      trauma H61.31- ☑
    postprocedural H95.81- ☑
    specified cause NEC H61.39- ☑
  gallbladder — *see* Obstruction, gallbladder
  glottis J38.6
  heart valve (congenital) Q24.8
    aortic Q23.0
    mitral Q23.2
    pulmonary Q22.1
    tricuspid Q22.4
  hepatic duct K83.1
  hymen N89.6
  hypertrophic subaortic (idiopathic) I42.1
  ileum (*see also* Obstruction, intestine, specified NEC) K56.699
    congenital Q41.2
  infundibulum cardia Q24.3
  intervertebral foramina (*see also* Lesion, biomechanical, specified NEC)
    connective tissue M99.79
      abdomen M99.79
      cervical region M99.71
      cervicothoracic M99.71
      head region M99.70
      lumbar region M99.73
      lumbosacral M99.73
      occipitocervical M99.70
      sacral region M99.74
      sacrococcygeal M99.74
      sacroiliac M99.74
      specified NEC M99.79
      thoracic region M99.72
      thoracolumbar M99.72
    disc M99.79
      abdomen M99.79
      cervical region M99.71
      cervicothoracic M99.71
      head region M99.70
      lower extremity M99.76

Stenosis, stenotic — continued
  intervertebral foramina (see also Lesion, biomechanical, specified) — continued
    disc — continued
      lumbar region M99.73
      lumbosacral M99.73
      occipitocervical M99.70
      pelvic M99.75
      rib cage M99.78
      sacral region M99.74
      sacrococcygeal M99.74
      sacroiliac M99.74
      specified NEC M99.79
      thoracic region M99.72
      thoracolumbar M99.72
      upper extremity M99.77
    osseous M99.69
      abdomen M99.69
      cervical region M99.61
      cervicothoracic M99.61
      head region M99.60
      lower extremity M99.66
      lumbar region M99.63
      lumbosacral M99.63
      occipitocervical M99.60
      pelvic M99.65
      rib cage M99.68
      sacral region M99.64
      sacrococcygeal M99.64
      sacroiliac M99.64
      specified NEC M99.69
      thoracic region M99.62
      thoracolumbar M99.62
      upper extremity M99.67
    subluxation — see Stenosis, intervertebral foramina, osseous
  intestine (see also Obstruction, intestine)
    congenital (small) Q41.9
      large Q42.9
        specified NEC Q42.8
      specified NEC Q41.8
  jejunum (see also Obstruction, intestine, specified NEC) K56.699
    congenital Q41.1
  lacrimal (passage)
    canaliculi H04.54- ☑
    congenital Q10.5
    duct H04.55- ☑
    punctum H04.56- ☑
    sac H04.57- ☑
  lacrimonasal duct — see Stenosis, lacrimal, duct
    congenital Q10.5
  larynx J38.6
    congenital NEC Q31.8
      subglottic Q31.1
    syphilitic A52.73
      congenital A50.59 [J99]
  mitral (chronic) (inactive) (valve) I05.0
    with
      aortic valve disease I08.0
      incompetency, insufficiency or regurgitation I05.2
    active or acute I01.1
      with rheumatic or Sydenham's chorea I02.0
    congenital Q23.2
    specified cause, except rheumatic I34.2
    syphilitic A52.03
  myocardium, myocardial (see also Degeneration, myocardial)
    hypertrophic subaortic (idiopathic) I42.1
  nares (anterior) (posterior) J34.89
    congenital Q30.0
  nasal duct (see also Stenosis, lacrimal, duct)
    congenital Q10.5
  nasolacrimal duct (see also Stenosis, lacrimal, duct)
    congenital Q10.5
  neural canal (see also Lesion, biomechanical, specified NEC)
    connective tissue M99.49
      abdomen M99.49
      cervical region M99.41
      cervicothoracic M99.41
      head region M99.40
      lower extremity M99.46
      lumbar region M99.43
      lumbosacral M99.43
      occipitocervical M99.40
      pelvic M99.45

Stenosis, stenotic — continued
  neural canal (see also Lesion, biomechanical, specified) — continued
    connective tissue — continued
      rib cage M99.48
      sacral region M99.44
      sacrococcygeal M99.44
      sacroiliac M99.44
      specified NEC M99.49
      thoracic region M99.42
      thoracolumbar M99.42
      upper extremity M99.47
    intervertebral disc M99.59
      abdomen M99.59
      cervical region M99.51
      cervicothoracic M99.51
      head region M99.50
      lower extremity M99.56
      lumbar region M99.53
      lumbosacral M99.53
      occipitocervical M99.50
      pelvic M99.55
      rib cage M99.58
      sacral region M99.54
      sacrococcygeal M99.54
      sacroiliac M99.54
      specified NEC M99.59
      thoracic region M99.52
      thoracolumbar M99.52
      upper extremity M99.57
    osseous M99.39
      abdomen M99.39
      cervical region M99.31
      cervicothoracic M99.31
      head region M99.30
      lower extremity M99.36
      lumbar region M99.33
      lumbosacral M99.33
      occipitocervical M99.30
      pelvic M99.35
      rib cage M99.38
      sacral region M99.34
      sacrococcygeal M99.34
      sacroiliac M99.34
      specified NEC M99.39
      thoracic region M99.32
      thoracolumbar M99.32
      upper extremity M99.37
    subluxation M99.29
      cervical region M99.21
      cervicothoracic M99.21
      head region M99.20
      lower extremity M99.26
      lumbar region M99.23
      lumbosacral M99.23
      occipitocervical M99.20
      pelvic M99.25
      rib cage M99.28
      sacral region M99.24
      sacrococcygeal M99.24
      sacroiliac M99.24
      specified NEC M99.29
      thoracic region M99.22
      thoracolumbar M99.22
      upper extremity M99.27
  organ or site, congenital NEC — see Atresia, by site
  papilla of Vater K83.1
  pulmonary (artery) (congenital) Q25.6
    with ventricular septal defect, transposition of aorta, and hypertrophy of right ventricle Q21.3
    acquired I28.8
    in tetralogy of Fallot Q21.3
    infundibular Q24.3
    subvalvular Q24.3
    supravalvular Q25.6
    valve I37.0
      with insufficiency I37.2
      congenital Q22.1
      rheumatic I09.89
        with aortic, mitral or tricuspid (valve) disease I08.8
    vein, acquired I28.8
    vessel NEC I28.8
  pulmonic (congenital) Q22.1
    infundibular Q24.3
    subvalvular Q24.3
  pylorus (hypertrophic) (acquired) K31.1
    adult K31.1

Stenosis, stenotic — continued
  pylorus — continued
    congenital Q40.0
    infantile Q40.0
  rectum (sphincter) — see Stricture, rectum
  renal artery I70.1
    congenital Q27.1
  salivary duct (any) K11.8
  sphincter of Oddi K83.1
  spinal M48.00
    cervical region M48.02
    cervicothoracic region M48.03
    lumbar region (NOS) (without neurogenic claudication) M48.061
      with neurogenic claudication M48.062
    lumbosacral region M48.07
    occipito-atlanto-axial region M48.01
    sacrococcygeal region M48.08
    thoracic region M48.04
    thoracolumbar region M48.05
  stomach, hourglass K31.2
  subaortic (congenital) Q24.4
    hypertrophic (idiopathic) I42.1
  subglottic J38.6
    congenital Q31.1
    postprocedural J95.5
  trachea J39.8
    congenital Q32.1
    syphilitic A52.73
    tuberculous NEC A15.5
  tracheostomy J95.03
  tricuspid (valve) I07.0
    with
      aortic (valve) disease I08.2
      incompetency, insufficiency or regurgitation I07.2
        with aortic (valve) disease I08.2
          with mitral (valve) disease I08.3
      mitral (valve) disease I08.1
        with aortic (valve) disease I08.3
    congenital Q22.4
    nonrheumatic I36.0
      with insufficiency I36.2
  tubal N97.1
  ureter — see Atresia, ureter
  ureteropelvic junction, congenital Q62.11
  ureterovesical orifice, congenital Q62.12
  urethra (valve) (see also Stricture, urethra)
    congenital Q64.32
  urinary meatus, congenital Q64.33
  vagina N89.5
    congenital Q52.4
    in pregnancy — see Pregnancy, complicated by, abnormal vagina
    causing obstructed labor O65.5
  valve (cardiac) (heart) (see also Endocarditis) I38
    congenital Q24.8
      aortic Q23.0
      mitral Q23.2
      pulmonary Q22.1
      tricuspid Q22.4
  vena cava (inferior) (superior) I87.1
    congenital Q26.0
  vesicourethral orifice Q64.31
  vulva N90.5
Stent jail T82.897 ☑
Stercolith (impaction) K56.41
    appendix K38.1
Stercoraceous, stercoral ulcer K63.3
    anus or rectum K62.6
Stereotypies NEC F98.4
Sterility — see Infertility
Sterilization — see Encounter (for), sterilization
Sternalgia — see Angina
Sternopagus Q89.4
Sternum bifidum Q76.7
Steroid
    effects (adverse) (adrenocortical) (iatrogenic)
      cushingoid E24.2
        correct substance properly administered — see Table of Drugs and Chemicals, by drug, adverse effect
        overdose or wrong substance given or taken — see Table of Drugs and Chemicals, by drug, poisoning
      diabetes — see subcategory E09 ☑

Steroid — *continued*
  effects — *continued*
    diabetes — *see subcategory* — *continued*
      correct substance properly administered — *see* Table of Drugs and Chemicals, by drug, adverse effect
      overdose or wrong substance given or taken — *see* Table of Drugs and Chemicals, by drug, poisoning
    fever R50.2
    insufficiency E27.3
      correct substance properly administered — *see* Table of Drugs and Chemicals, by drug, adverse effect
      overdose or wrong substance given or taken — *see* Table of Drugs and Chemicals, by drug, poisoning
    responder H40.04- ☑
Stevens-Johnson disease or syndrome L51.1
  toxic epidermal necrolysis overlap L51.3
Stewart-Morel syndrome M85.2
Sticker's disease B08.3
Sticky eye — *see* Conjunctivitis, acute, mucopurulent
Stieda's disease — *see* Bursitis, tibial collateral
Stiff neck — *see* Torticollis
Stiff-man syndrome G25.82
Stiffness, joint NEC M25.60
  ankle M25.67- ☑
  ankylosis — *see* Ankylosis, joint
  contracture — *see* Contraction, joint
  elbow M25.62- ☑
  foot M25.67- ☑
  hand M25.64- ☑
  hip M25.65- ☑
  knee M25.66- ☑
  shoulder M25.61- ☑
  wrist M25.63- ☑
Stigmata congenital syphilis A50.59
Stillbirth P95
Still-Felty syndrome — *see* Felty's syndrome
Still's disease or syndrome (juvenile) M08.20
  adult-onset M06.1
  ankle M08.27- ☑
  elbow M08.22- ☑
  foot joint M08.27- ☑
  hand joint M08.24- ☑
  hip M08.25- ☑
  knee M08.26- ☑
  multiple site M08.29
  shoulder M08.21- ☑
  vertebra M08.28
  wrist M08.23- ☑
Stimulation, ovary E28.1
Sting (venomous) (with allergic or anaphylactic shock) — *see* Table of Drugs and Chemicals, by animal or substance, poisoning
Stippled epiphyses Q78.8
Stitch
  abscess T81.4 ☑
  burst (in operation wound) — *see* Disruption, wound, operation
Stokes' disease E05.00
  with thyroid storm E05.01
Stokes-Adams disease or syndrome I45.9
Stokvis (-Talma) **disease** D74.8
Stoma malfunction
  colostomy K94.03
  enterostomy K94.13
  gastrostomy K94.23
  ileostomy K94.13
  tracheostomy J95.03
Stomach — *see* condition
Stomatitis (denture) (ulcerative) K12.1
  angular K13.0
    due to dietary or vitamin deficiency E53.0
  aphthous K12.0
  bovine B08.61
  candidal B37.0
  catarrhal K12.1
  diphtheritic A36.89
  due to
    dietary deficiency E53.0
    thrush B37.0
    vitamin deficiency
      B group NEC E53.9
      B2 (riboflavin) E53.0
  epidemic B08.8

Stomatitis — *continued*
  epizootic B08.8
  follicular K12.1
  gangrenous A69.0
  Geotrichum B48.3
  herpesviral, herpetic B00.2
  herpetiformis K12.0
  malignant K12.1
  membranous acute K12.1
  monilial B37.0
  mycotic B37.0
  necrotizing ulcerative A69.0
  parasitic B37.0
  septic K12.1
  spirochetal A69.1
  suppurative (acute) K12.2
  ulceromembranous A69.1
  vesicular K12.1
    with exanthem (enteroviral) B08.4
    virus disease A93.8
  Vincent's A69.1
Stomatocytosis D58.8
Stomatomycosis B37.0
Stomatorrhagia K13.79
Stone(s) (*see also* Calculus)
  bladder (diverticulum) N21.0
  cystine E72.09
  heart syndrome I50.1
  kidney N20.0
  prostate N42.0
  pulpal (dental) K04.2
  renal N20.0
  salivary gland or duct (any) K11.5
  urethra (impacted) N21.1
  urinary (duct) (impacted) (passage) N20.9
    bladder (diverticulum) N21.0
    lower tract N21.9
    specified NEC N21.8
  xanthine E79.8 [N22]
Stonecutter's lung J62.8
Stonemason's asthma, disease, lung or pneumoconiosis J62.8
Stoppage
  heart — *see* Arrest, cardiac
  urine — *see* Retention, urine
Storm, thyroid — *see* Thyrotoxicosis
Strabismus (congenital) (nonparalytic) H50.9
  concomitant H50.40
    convergent — *see* Strabismus, convergent concomitant
    divergent — *see* Strabismus, divergent concomitant
  convergent concomitant H50.00
    accommodative component H50.43
    alternating H50.05
      with
        A pattern H50.06
        specified nonconcomitances NEC H50.08
        V pattern H50.07
    monocular H50.01- ☑
      with
        A pattern H50.02- ☑
        specified nonconcomitances NEC H50.04- ☑
        V pattern H50.03- ☑
      intermittent H50.31- ☑
        alternating H50.32
  cyclotropia H50.41 ☑
  divergent concomitant H50.10
    alternating H50.15
      with
        A pattern H50.16
        specified noncomitances NEC H50.18
        V pattern H50.17
    monocular H50.11- ☑
      with
        A pattern H50.12- ☑
        specified nonconcomitances NEC H50.14- ☑
        V pattern H50.13- ☑
      intermittent H50.33 ☑
        alternating H50.34
  Duane's syndrome H50.81- ☑
  due to adhesions, scars H50.69
  heterophoria H50.50
    alternating H50.55
    cyclophoria H50.54
    esophoria H50.51
    exophoria H50.52
    vertical H50.53

Strabismus — *continued*
  heterotropia H50.40
    intermittent H50.30
  hypertropia H50.2- ☑
  hypotropia — *see* Hypertropia
  latent H50.50
  mechanical H50.60
    Brown's sheath syndrome H50.61- ☑
    specified type NEC H50.69
  monofixation syndrome H50.42
  paralytic H49.9
    abducens nerve H49.2- ☑
    fourth nerve H49.1- ☑
    Kearns-Sayre syndrome H49.81- ☑
    ophthalmoplegia (external)
      progressive H49.4- ☑
        with pigmentary retinopathy H49.81- ☑
      total H49.3- ☑
    sixth nerve H49.2- ☑
    specified type NEC H49.88- ☑
    third nerve H49.0- ☑
    trochlear nerve H49.1- ☑
  specified type NEC H50.89
  vertical H50.2- ☑
Strain
  back S39.012 ☑
  cervical S16.1 ☑
  eye NEC — *see* Disturbance, vision, subjective
  heart — *see* Disease, heart
  low back S39.012 ☑
  mental NOS Z73.3
    work-related Z56.6
  muscle (tendon) — *see* Injury, muscle, by site, strain
  neck S16.1 ☑
  physical NOS Z73.3
    work-related Z56.6
  postural (*see also* Disorder, soft tissue, due to use)
  psychological NEC Z73.3
  tendon — *see* Injury, muscle, by site, strain
Straining, on urination R39.16
Strand, vitreous — *see* Opacity, vitreous, membranes and strands
Strangulation, strangulated (*see also* Asphyxia, traumatic)
  appendix K38.8
  bladder-neck N32.0
  bowel or colon K56.2
  food or foreign body — *see* Foreign body, by site
  hemorrhoids — *see* Hemorrhoids, with complication
  hernia (*see also* Hernia, by site, with obstruction)
    with gangrene — *see* Hernia, by site, with gangrene
  intestine (large) (small) K56.2
    with hernia (*see also* Hernia, by site, with obstruction)
      with gangrene — *see* Hernia, by site, with gangrene
  mesentery K56.2
  mucus — *see* Asphyxia, mucus
  omentum K56.2
  organ or site, congenital NEC — *see* Atresia, by site
  ovary — *see* Torsion, ovary
  penis N48.89
    foreign body T19.4 ☑
  rupture — *see* Hernia, by site, with obstruction
  stomach due to hernia (*see also* Hernia, by site, with obstruction)
    with gangrene — *see* Hernia, by site, with gangrene
  vesicourethral orifice N32.0
Strangury R30.0
Straw itch B88.0
Strawberry
  gallbladder K82.4
  mark Q82.5
  tongue (red) (white) K14.3
Streak(s)
  macula, angioid H35.33
  ovarian Q50.32
Strephosymbolia F81.0
  secondary to organic lesion R48.8
Streptobacillary fever A25.1
Streptobacillosis A25.1
Streptobacillus moniliformis A25.1
Streptococcus, streptococcal (*see also* condition)
  as cause of disease classified elsewhere B95.5

Streptococcus, streptococcal — *continued*
  group
    A, as cause of disease classified elsewhere B95.0
    B, as cause of disease classified elsewhere B95.1
    D, as cause of disease classified elsewhere B95.2
  pneumoniae, as cause of disease classified elsewhere
    B95.3
  specified NEC, as cause of disease classified elsewhere
    B95.4
Streptomycosis B47.1
Streptotrichosis A48.8
Stress F43.9
  family — *see* Disruption, family
  fetal P84
    complicating pregnancy O77.9
      due to drug administration O77.1
  mental NEC Z73.3
    work-related Z56.6
  physical NEC Z73.3
    work-related Z56.6
  polycythemia D75.1
  reaction (*see also* Reaction, stress) F43.9
  work schedule Z56.3
Stretching, nerve — *see* Injury, nerve
Striae albicantes, atrophicae or distensae (cutis) L90.6
Stricture (*see also* Stenosis)
  ampulla of Vater K83.1
  anus (sphincter) K62.4
    congenital Q42.3
      with fistula Q42.2
    infantile Q42.3
      with fistula Q42.2
  aorta (ascending) (congenital) Q25.1
    arteriosclerotic I70.0
    calcified I70.0
    supravalvular, congenital Q25.3
  aortic (valve) — *see* Stenosis, aortic
  aqueduct of Sylvius (congenital) Q03.0
    with spina bifida — *see* Spina bifida, by site, with
      hydrocephalus
    acquired G91.1
  artery I77.1
    basilar — *see* Occlusion, artery, basilar
    carotid — *see* Occlusion, artery, carotid
    celiac I77.4
    congenital (peripheral) Q27.8
      cerebral Q28.3
      coronary Q24.5
      digestive system Q27.8
      lower limb Q27.8
      retinal Q14.1
      specified site NEC Q27.8
      umbilical Q27.0
      upper limb Q27.8
    coronary — *see* Disease, heart, ischemic,
      atherosclerotic
      congenital Q24.5
    precerebral — *see* Occlusion, artery, precerebral
    pulmonary (congenital) Q25.6
      acquired I28.8
    renal I70.1
    vertebral — *see* Occlusion, artery, vertebral
  auditory canal (external) (congenital)
    acquired — *see* Stenosis, external ear canal
  bile duct (common) (hepatic) K83.1
    congenital Q44.3
    postoperative K91.89
  bladder N32.89
    neck N32.0
  bowel — *see* Obstruction, intestine
  brain G93.89
  bronchus J98.09
    congenital Q32.3
    syphilitic A52.72
  cardia (stomach) K22.2
    congenital Q39.3
  cardiac (*see also* Disease, heart)
    orifice (stomach) K22.2
  cecum — *see* Obstruction, intestine
  cervix, cervical (canal) N88.2
    congenital Q51.828
    in pregnancy — *see* Pregnancy, complicated by,
      abnormal cervix
        causing obstructed labor O65.5
  colon (*see also* Obstruction, intestine)
    congenital Q42.9
      specified NEC Q42.8
  colostomy K94.03

Stricture — *continued*
  common (bile) (duct) K83.1
  coronary (artery) — *see* Disease, heart, ischemic,
    atherosclerotic
  cystic duct — *see* Obstruction, gallbladder
  digestive organs NEC, congenital Q45.8
  duodenum K31.5
    congenital Q41.0
  ear canal (external) (congenital) Q16.1
    acquired — *see* Stricture, auditory canal, acquired
  ejaculatory duct N50.89
  enterostomy K94.13
  esophagus K22.2
    congenital Q39.3
    syphilitic A52.79
      congenital A50.59 [K23]
  eustachian tube (*see also* Obstruction, eustachian tube)
    congenital Q17.8
  fallopian tube N97.1
    gonococcal A54.24
    tuberculous A18.17
  gallbladder — *see* Obstruction, gallbladder
  glottis J38.6
  heart (*see also* Disease, heart)
    valve (*see also* Endocarditis) I38
      aortic Q23.0
      mitral Q23.2
      pulmonary Q22.1
      tricuspid Q22.4
  hepatic duct K83.1
  hourglass, of stomach K31.2
  hymen N89.6
  hypopharynx J39.2
  ileum (*see also* Obstruction, intestine, specified NEC)
    K56.699
    congenital Q41.2
  intestine (*see also* Obstruction, intestine)
    congenital (small) Q41.9
      large Q42.9
        specified NEC Q42.8
      specified NEC Q41.8
    ischemic K55.1
  jejunum (*see also* Obstruction, intestine, specified NEC)
    K56.699
    congenital Q41.1
  lacrimal passages (*see also* Stenosis, lacrimal)
    congenital Q10.5
  larynx J38.6
    congenital NEC Q31.8
      subglottic Q31.1
    syphilitic A52.73
      congenital A50.59 [J99]
  meatus
    ear (congenital) Q16.1
      acquired — *see* Stricture, auditory canal, ac-
        quired
    osseous (ear) (congenital) Q16.1
      acquired — *see* Stricture, auditory canal, ac-
        quired
    urinarius (*see also* Stricture, urethra)
      congenital Q64.33
  mitral (valve) — *see* Stenosis, mitral
  myocardium, myocardial I51.5
    hypertrophic subaortic (idiopathic) I42.1
  nares (anterior) (posterior) J34.89
    congenital Q30.0
  nasal duct (*see also* Stenosis, lacrimal, duct)
    congenital Q10.5
  nasolacrimal duct (*see also* Stenosis, lacrimal, duct)
    congenital Q10.5
  nasopharynx J39.2
    syphilitic A52.73
  nose J34.89
    congenital Q30.0
  nostril (anterior) (posterior) J34.89
    congenital Q30.0
    syphilitic A52.73
      congenital A50.59 [J99]
  organ or site, congenital NEC — *see* Atresia, by site
  os uteri — *see* Stricture, cervix
  osseous meatus (ear) (congenital) Q16.1
    acquired — *see* Stricture, auditory canal, acquired
  oviduct — *see* Stricture, fallopian tube
  pelviureteric junction (congenital) Q62.11
    acquired, with hydronephrosis N13.0
  penis, by foreign body T19.4 ☑
  pharynx J39.2
  prostate N42.89

Stricture — *continued*
  pulmonary, pulmonic
    artery (congenital) Q25.6
      acquired I28.8
      noncongenital I28.8
    infundibulum (congenital) Q24.3
    valve I37.0
      congenital Q22.1
    vein, acquired I28.8
    vessel NEC I28.8
  punctum lacrimale (*see also* Stenosis, lacrimal, punc-
    tum)
    congenital Q10.5
  pylorus (hypertrophic) K31.1
    adult K31.1
    congenital Q40.0
    infantile Q40.0
  rectosigmoid (*see also* Obstruction, intestine, specified
    NEC) K56.699
  rectum (sphincter) K62.4
    congenital Q42.1
      with fistula Q42.0
    due to
      chlamydial lymphogranuloma A55
      irradiation K91.89
      lymphogranuloma venereum A55
    gonococcal A54.6
    inflammatory (chlamydial) A55
    syphilitic A52.74
    tuberculous A18.32
  renal artery I70.1
    congenital Q27.1
  salivary duct or gland (any) K11.8
  sigmoid (flexure) — *see* Obstruction, intestine
  spermatic cord N50.89
  stoma (following) (of)
    colostomy K94.03
    enterostomy K94.13
    gastrostomy K94.23
    ileostomy K94.13
    tracheostomy J95.03
  stomach K31.89
    congenital Q40.2
    hourglass K31.2
  subaortic Q24.4
    hypertrophic (acquired) (idiopathic) I42.1
  subglottic J38.6
  syphilitic NEC A52.79
  trachea J39.8
    congenital Q32.1
    syphilitic A52.73
    tuberculous NEC A15.5
  tracheostomy J95.03
  tricuspid (valve) — *see* Stenosis, tricuspid
  tunica vaginalis N50.89
  ureter (postoperative) N13.5
    with
      hydronephrosis N13.1
        with infection N13.6
      pyelonephritis (chronic) N11.1
    congenital — *see* Atresia, ureter
    tuberculous A18.11
  ureteropelvic junction (congenital) Q62.11
    acquired, with hydronephrosis N13.0
  ureterovesical orifice N13.5
    with infection N13.6
  urethra (organic) (spasmodic) N35.9
    associated with schistosomiasis B65.0 [N37]
    congenital Q64.39
      valvular (posterior) Q64.2
    due to
      infection — *see* Stricture, urethra, postinfective
      trauma — *see* Stricture, urethra, post-traumatic
    gonococcal, gonorrheal A54.01
    infective NEC — *see* Stricture, urethra, postinfective
    late effect (sequelae) of injury — *see* Stricture,
      urethra, post-traumatic
    postcatheterization — *see* Stricture, urethra, post-
      procedural
    postinfective NEC
      female N35.12
      male N35.119
        anterior urethra N35.114
        bulbous urethra N35.112
        meatal N35.111
        membranous urethra N35.113
    postobstetric N35.021

Stricture — continued
  urethra — continued
    postoperative — see Stricture, urethra, postprocedural
    postprocedural
      female N99.12
      male N99.114
        anterior bulbous urethra N99.113
        bulbous urethra N99.111
        fossa navicularis N99.115
        meatal N99.110
        membranous urethra N99.112
    post-traumatic
      female N35.028
        due to childbirth N35.021
      male N35.014
        anterior urethra N35.013
        bulbous urethra N35.011
        meatal N35.010
        membranous urethra N35.012
    sequela (late effect) of
      childbirth N35.021
      injury — see Stricture, urethra, post-traumatic
    specified cause NEC N35.8
    syphilitic A52.76
    traumatic — see Stricture, urethra, post-traumatic
    valvular (posterior), congenital Q64.2
  urinary meatus — see Stricture, urethra
  uterus, uterine (synechiae) N85.6
    os (external) (internal) — see Stricture, cervix
  vagina (outlet) — see Stenosis, vagina
  valve (cardiac) (heart) (see also Endocarditis)
    congenital
      aortic Q23.0
      mitral Q23.2
      pulmonary Q22.1
      tricuspid Q22.4
  vas deferens N50.89
    congenital Q55.4
  vein I87.1
  vena cava (inferior) (superior) NEC I87.1
    congenital Q26.0
  vesicourethral orifice N32.0
    congenital Q64.31
  vulva (acquired) N90.5
Stridor R06.1
  congenital (larynx) P28.89
Stridulous — see condition
Stroke (apoplectic) (brain) (embolic) (ischemic) (paralytic) (thrombotic) I63.9
  cryptogenic (see also Infarction, cerebral) I63.9
  epileptic — see Epilepsy
  heat T67.0 ☑
  in evolution I63.9
  intraoperative
    during cardiac surgery I97.810
    during other surgery I97.811
  lightning — see Lightning
  meaning
    cerebral hemorrhage — code to Hemorrhage, intracranial
    cerebral infarction — code to Infarction, cerebral
  postprocedural
    following cardiac surgery I97.820
    following other surgery I97.821
  unspecified (NOS) I63.9
Stromatosis, endometrial D39.0
Strongyloidiasis, strongyloidosis B78.9
  cutaneous B78.1
  disseminated B78.7
  intestinal B78.0
Strophulus pruriginosus L28.2
Struck by lightning — see Lightning
Struma (see also Goiter)
  Hashimoto E06.3
  lymphomatosa E06.3
  nodosa (simplex) E04.9
    endemic E01.2
      multinodular E01.1
    multinodular E04.2
      iodine-deficiency related E01.1
    toxic or with hyperthyroidism E05.20
      with thyroid storm E05.21
      multinodular E05.20
        with thyroid storm E05.21
      uninodular E05.10
        with thyroid storm E05.11
    toxicosa E05.20

Struma — continued
  nodosa — continued
    toxicosa — continued
      with thyroid storm E05.21
      multinodular E05.20
        with thyroid storm E05.21
      uninodular E05.10
        with thyroid storm E05.11
    uninodular E04.1
  ovarii D27.- ☑
  Riedel's E06.5
Strumipriva cachexia E03.4
Strümpell-Marie spine — see Spondylitis, ankylosing
Strümpell-Westphal pseudosclerosis E83.01
Stuart deficiency disease (factor X) D68.2
Stuart-Prower factor deficiency (factor X) D68.2
Student's elbow — see Bursitis, elbow, olecranon
Stump — see Amputation
Stunting, nutritional E45
Stupor (catatonic) R40.1
  depressive (single episode) F32.89
    recurrent episode F33.8
  dissociative F44.2
  manic F30.2
  manic-depressive F31.89
  psychogenic (aneric) F44.2
  reaction to exceptional stress (transient) F43.0
Sturge (-Weber) (-Dimitri) (-Kalischer) **disease or syndrome** Q85.8
Stuttering F80.81
  adult onset F98.5
  childhood onset F80.81
  following cerebrovascular disease — see Disorder, fluency. following cerebrovascular disease
  in conditions classified elsewhere R47.82
Sty, stye (external) (internal) (meibomian) (zeisian) — see Hordeolum
Subacidity, gastric K31.89
  psychogenic F45.8
Subacute — see condition
Subarachnoid — see condition
Subcortical — see condition
Subcostal syndrome, nerve compression — see Mononeuropathy, upper limb, specified site NEC
Subcutaneous, subcuticular — see condition
Subdural — see condition
Subendocardium — see condition
Subependymoma
  specified site — see Neoplasm, uncertain behavior, by site
  unspecified site D43.2
Suberosis J67.3
Subglossitis — see Glossitis
Subhemophilia D66
Subinvolution
  breast (postlactational) (postpuerperal) N64.89
  puerperal O90.89
  uterus (chronic) (nonpuerperal) N85.3
    puerperal O90.89
Sublingual — see condition
Sublinguitis — see Sialoadenitis
Subluxatable hip Q65.6
Subluxation (see also Dislocation)
  acromioclavicular S43.11- ☑
  ankle S93.0- ☑
  atlantoaxial, recurrent M43.4
    with myelopathy M43.3
  carpometacarpal (joint) NEC S63.05- ☑
    thumb S63.04- ☑
  complex, vertebral — see Complex, subluxation
  congenital (see also Malposition, congenital)
    hip — see Dislocation, hip, congenital, partial
    joint (excluding hip)
      lower limb Q68.8
      shoulder Q68.8
      upper limb Q68.8
  elbow (traumatic) S53.10- ☑
    anterior S53.11- ☑
    lateral S53.14- ☑
    medial S53.13- ☑
    posterior S53.12- ☑
    specified type NEC S53.19- ☑
  finger S63.20- ☑
    index S63.20- ☑
    interphalangeal S63.22- ☑
      distal S63.24- ☑
        index S63.24- ☑

Subluxation — continued
  finger — continued
    interphalangeal — continued
      distal — continued
        little S63.24- ☑
        middle S63.24- ☑
        ring S63.24- ☑
      index S63.22- ☑
      little S63.22- ☑
      middle S63.22- ☑
      proximal S63.23- ☑
        index S63.23- ☑
        little S63.23- ☑
        middle S63.23- ☑
        ring S63.23- ☑
      ring S63.22- ☑
    little S63.20- ☑
    metacarpophalangeal S63.21- ☑
      index S63.21- ☑
      little S63.21- ☑
      middle S63.21- ☑
      ring S63.21- ☑
    middle S63.20- ☑
    ring S63.20- ☑
  foot S93.30- ☑
    specified site NEC S93.33- ☑
    tarsal joint S93.31- ☑
    tarsometatarsal joint S93.32- ☑
    toe — see Subluxation, toe
  hip S73.00- ☑
    anterior S73.03- ☑
      obturator S73.02- ☑
    central S73.04- ☑
    posterior S73.01- ☑
  interphalangeal (joint)
    finger S63.22- ☑
      distal joint S63.24- ☑
        index S63.24- ☑
        little S63.24- ☑
        middle S63.24- ☑
        ring S63.24- ☑
      index S63.22- ☑
      little S63.22- ☑
      middle S63.22- ☑
      proximal joint S63.23- ☑
        index S63.23- ☑
        little S63.23- ☑
        middle S63.23- ☑
        ring S63.23- ☑
      ring S63.22- ☑
    thumb S63.12- ☑
      distal joint S63.14- ☑
      proximal joint S63.13- ☑
    toe S93.13- ☑
      great S93.13- ☑
      lesser S93.13- ☑
  joint prosthesis — see Complications, joint prosthesis, mechanical, displacement, by site
  knee S83.10- ☑
    cap — see Subluxation, patella
    patella — see Subluxation, patella
    proximal tibia
      anteriorly S83.11- ☑
      laterally S83.14- ☑
      medially S83.13- ☑
      posteriorly S83.12- ☑
    specified type NEC S83.19- ☑
  lens — see Dislocation, lens, partial
  ligament, traumatic — see Sprain, by site
  metacarpal (bone)
    proximal end S63.06- ☑
  metacarpophalangeal (joint)
    finger S63.21- ☑
      index S63.21- ☑
      little S63.21- ☑
      middle S63.21- ☑
      ring S63.21- ☑
    thumb S63.11- ☑
  metatarsophalangeal joint S93.14- ☑
    great toe S93.14- ☑
    lesser toe S93.14- ☑
  midcarpal (joint) S63.03- ☑
  patella S83.00- ☑
    lateral S83.01- ☑
    recurrent (nontraumatic) — see Dislocation, patella, recurrent, incomplete

☑ Additional Character Required — Refer to the Tabular List for Character Selection
  ▽ Subterms under main terms may continue to next column or page

Subluxation — *continued*
- patella — *continued*
  - specified type NEC S83.09- ☑
- pathological — *see* Dislocation, pathological
- radial head S53.00- ☑
  - anterior S53.01- ☑
  - nursemaid's elbow S53.03- ☑
  - posterior S53.02- ☑
  - specified type NEC S53.09- ☑
- radiocarpal (joint) S63.02- ☑
- radioulnar (joint)
  - distal S63.01- ☑
  - proximal — *see* Subluxation, elbow
- shoulder
  - congenital Q68.8
  - girdle S43.30- ☑
    - scapula S43.31- ☑
    - specified site NEC S43.39- ☑
  - traumatic S43.00- ☑
    - anterior S43.01- ☑
    - inferior S43.03- ☑
    - posterior S43.02- ☑
    - specified type NEC S43.08- ☑
- sternoclavicular (joint) S43.20- ☑
  - anterior S43.21- ☑
  - posterior S43.22- ☑
- symphysis (pubis)
- thumb S63.103 ☑
  - interphalangeal joint — *see* Subluxation, interphalangeal (joint), thumb
  - metacarpophalangeal joint — *see* Subluxation, metacarpophalangeal (joint), thumb
- toe(s) S93.10- ☑
  - great S93.10- ☑
    - interphalangeal joint S93.13- ☑
    - metatarsophalangeal joint S93.14- ☑
  - interphalangeal joint S93.13- ☑
  - lesser S93.10- ☑
    - interphalangeal joint S93.13- ☑
    - metatarsophalangeal joint S93.14- ☑
  - metatarsophalangeal joint S93.149 ☑
- ulna
  - distal end S63.07- ☑
  - proximal end — *see* Subluxation, elbow
- ulnohumeral joint — *see* Subluxation, elbow
- vertebral
  - recurrent NEC — *see* subcategory M43.5 ☑
  - traumatic
    - cervical S13.100 ☑
      - atlantoaxial joint S13.120 ☑
      - atlantooccipital joint S13.110 ☑
      - atloidooccipital joint S13.110 ☑
      - joint between
        - C0 and C1 S13.110 ☑
        - C1 and C2 S13.120 ☑
        - C2 and C3 S13.130 ☑
        - C3 and C4 S13.140 ☑
        - C4 and C5 S13.150 ☑
        - C5 and C6 S13.160 ☑
        - C6 and C7 S13.170 ☑
        - C7 and T1 S13.180 ☑
      - occipitoatloid joint S13.110 ☑
    - lumbar S33.100 ☑
      - joint between
        - L1 and L2 S33.110 ☑
        - L2 and L3 S33.120 ☑
        - L3 and L4 S33.130 ☑
        - L4 and L5 S33.140 ☑
    - thoracic S23.100 ☑
      - joint between
        - T1 and T2 S23.110 ☑
        - T2 and T3 S23.120 ☑
        - T3 and T4 S23.122 ☑
        - T4 and T5 S23.130 ☑
        - T5 and T6 S23.132 ☑
        - T6 and T7 S23.140 ☑
        - T7 and T8 S23.142 ☑
        - T8 and T9 S23.150 ☑
        - T9 and T10 S23.152 ☑
        - T10 and T11 S23.160 ☑
        - T11 and T12 S23.162 ☑
        - T12 and L1 S23.170 ☑
- wrist (carpal bone) S63.00- ☑
  - carpometacarpal joint — *see* Subluxation, carpometacarpal (joint)

Subluxation — *continued*
- wrist — *continued*
  - distal radioulnar joint — *see* Subluxation, radioulnar (joint), distal
  - metacarpal bone, proximal — *see* Subluxation, metacarpal (bone), proximal end
  - midcarpal — *see* Subluxation, midcarpal (joint)
  - radiocarpal joint — *see* Subluxation, radiocarpal (joint)
  - recurrent — *see* Dislocation, recurrent, wrist
  - specified site NEC S63.09- ☑
  - ulna — *see* Subluxation, ulna, distal end
Submaxillary — *see* condition
Submersion (fatal) (nonfatal) T75.1 ☑
Submucous — *see* condition
Subnormal, subnormality
- accommodation (old age) H52.4
- mental — *see* Disability, intellectual
- temperature (accidental) T68 ☑
Subphrenic — *see* condition
Subscapular nerve — *see* condition
Subseptus uterus Q51.2
Subsiding appendicitis K36
Substance (other psychoactive) **-induced**
- anxiety disorder F19.980
- bipolar and related disorder F19.94
- delirium F19.921
- depressive disorder F19.94
- major neurocognitive disorder F19.97
- mild neurocognitive disorder F19.988
- obsessive-compulsive and related disorder F19.988
- psychotic disorder F19.959
- sexual dysfunction F19.981
- sleep disorder F19.982
Substernal thyroid E04.9
- congenital Q89.2
Substitution disorder F44.9
Subtentorial — *see* condition
Subthyroidism (acquired) (*see also* Hypothyroidism)
- congenital E03.1
Succenturiate placenta O43.19- ☑
Sucking thumb, child (excessive) F98.8
Sudamen, sudamina L74.1
Sudanese kala-azar B55.0
Sudden
- hearing loss — *see* Deafness, sudden
- heart failure — *see* Failure, heart
Sudeck's atrophy, disease, or syndrome — *see* Algoneurodystrophy
Suffocation — *see* Asphyxia, traumatic
Sugar
- blood
  - high (transient) R73.9
  - low (transient) E16.2
- in urine R81
Suicide, suicidal (attempted) T14.91 ☑
- by poisoning — *see* Table of Drugs and Chemicals
- history of (personal) Z91.5
  - in family Z81.8
- ideation — *see* Ideation, suicidal
- risk
  - meaning personal history of attempted suicide Z91.5
  - meaning suicidal ideation — *see* Ideation, suicidal
- tendencies
  - meaning personal history of attempted suicide Z91.5
  - meaning suicidal ideation — *see* Ideation, suicidal
- trauma — *see* nature of injury by site
Suipestifer infection — *see* Infection, salmonella
Sulfhemoglobinemia, sulphemoglobinemia (acquired) (with methemoglobinemia) D74.8
Sumatran mite fever A75.3
Summer — *see* condition
Sunburn L55.9
- due to
  - tanning bed (acute) L56.8
    - chronic L57.8
  - ultraviolet radiation (acute) L56.8
    - chronic L57.8
- first degree L55.0
- second degree L55.1
- third degree L55.2
SUNCT (short lasting unilateral neuralgiform headache with conjunctival injection and tearing) G44.059
- intractable G44.051
- not intractable G44.059

Sundowning F05
Sunken acetabulum — *see* Derangement, joint, specified type NEC, hip
Sunstroke T67.0 ☑
Superfecundation — *see* Pregnancy, multiple
Superfetation — *see* Pregnancy, multiple
Superinvolution (uterus) N85.8
Supernumerary (congenital)
- aortic cusps Q23.8
- auditory ossicles Q16.3
- bone Q79.8
- breast Q83.1
- carpal bones Q74.0
- cusps, heart valve NEC Q24.8
  - aortic Q23.8
  - mitral Q23.2
  - pulmonary Q22.3
- digit(s) Q69.9
- ear (lobule) Q17.0
- fallopian tube Q50.6
- finger Q69.0
- hymen Q52.4
- kidney Q63.0
- lacrimonasal duct Q10.6
- lobule (ear) Q17.0
- mitral cusps Q23.2
- muscle Q79.8
- nipple(s) Q83.3
- organ or site not listed — *see* Accessory
- ossicles, auditory Q16.3
- ovary Q50.31
- oviduct Q50.6
- pulmonary, pulmonic cusps Q22.3
- rib Q76.6
  - cervical or first (syndrome) Q76.5
- roots (of teeth) K00.2
- spleen Q89.09
- tarsal bones Q74.2
- teeth K00.1
- testis Q55.29
- thumb Q69.1
- toe Q69.2
- uterus Q51.2
- vagina Q52.1 ☑
- vertebra Q76.49
Supervision (of)
- contraceptive — *see* Prescription, contraceptives
- dietary (for) Z71.3
  - allergy (food) Z71.3
  - colitis Z71.3
  - diabetes mellitus Z71.3
  - food allergy or intolerance Z71.3
  - gastritis Z71.3
  - hypercholesterolemia Z71.3
  - hypoglycemia Z71.3
  - intolerance (food) Z71.3
  - obesity Z71.3
  - specified NEC Z71.3
- healthy infant or child Z76.2
  - foundling Z76.1
- high-risk pregnancy — *see* Pregnancy, complicated by, high, risk
- lactation Z39.1
- pregnancy — *see* Pregnancy, supervision of
Supplemental teeth K00.1
Suppression
- binocular vision H53.34
- lactation O92.5
- menstruation N94.89
- ovarian secretion E28.39
- renal N28.9
- urine, urinary secretion R34
Suppuration, suppurative (*see also* condition)
- accessory sinus (chronic) — *see* Sinusitis
- adrenal gland
- antrum (chronic) — *see* Sinusitis, maxillary
- bladder — *see* Cystitis
- brain G06.0
  - sequelae G09
- breast N61.1
  - puerperal, postpartum or gestational — *see* Mastitis, obstetric, purulent
- dental periosteum M27.3
- ear (middle) (*see also* Otitis, media)
  - external NEC — *see* Otitis, externa, infective
  - internal — *see* subcategory H83.0 ☑
- ethmoidal (chronic) (sinus) — *see* Sinusitis, ethmoidal
- fallopian tube — *see* Salpingo-oophoritis

Suppuration, suppurative — continued
frontal (chronic) (sinus) — see Sinusitis, frontal
gallbladder (acute) K81.0
gum K05.20
generalized — see Peridontitis, aggressive, generalized
localized — see Peridontitis, aggressive, localized
intracranial G06.0
joint — see Arthritis, pyogenic or pyemic
labyrinthine — see subcategory H83.0 ☑
lung — see Abscess, lung
mammary gland N61.1
puerperal, postpartum O91.12
associated with lactation O91.13
maxilla, maxillary M27.2
sinus (chronic) — see Sinusitis, maxillary
muscle — see Myositis, infective
nasal sinus (chronic) — see Sinusitis
pancreas, acute (see also Pancreatitis, acute) K85.80
parotid gland — see Sialoadenitis
pelvis, pelvic
female — see Disease, pelvis, inflammatory
male K65.0
pericranial — see Osteomyelitis
salivary duct or gland (any) — see Sialoadenitis
sinus (accessory) (chronic) (nasal) — see Sinusitis
sphenoidal sinus (chronic) — see Sinusitis, sphenoidal
thymus (gland) E32.1
thyroid (gland) E06.0
tonsil — see Tonsillitis
uterus — see Endometritis
Supraeruption of tooth (teeth) M26.34
Supraglottitis J04.30
with obstruction J04.31
Suprarenal (gland) — see condition
Suprascapular nerve — see condition
Suprasellar — see condition
Surfer's knots or nodules S89.8- ☑
Surgical
emphysema T81.82 ☑
procedures, complication or misadventure — see Complications, surgical procedures
shock T81.10 ☑
Surveillance (of) (for) (see also Observation)
alcohol abuse Z71.41
contraceptive — see Prescription, contraceptives
dietary Z71.3
drug abuse Z71.51
Susceptibility to disease, genetic Z15.89
malignant neoplasm Z15.09
breast Z15.01
endometrium Z15.04
ovary Z15.02
prostate Z15.03
specified NEC Z15.09
multiple endocrine neoplasia Z15.81
Suspected condition, ruled out (see also Observation, suspected)
amniotic cavity and membrane Z03.71
cervical shortening Z03.75
fetal anomaly Z03.73
fetal growth Z03.74
maternal and fetal conditions NEC Z03.79
newborn (see also Observation, newborn, suspected condition ruled out) Z05.9
oligohydramnios Z03.71
placental problem Z03.72
polyhydramnios Z03.71
Suspended uterus
in pregnancy or childbirth — see Pregnancy, complicated by, abnormal uterus
Sutton's nevus D22.9
Suture
burst (in operation wound) T81.31 ☑
external operation wound T81.31 ☑
internal operation wound T81.32 ☑
inadvertently left in operation wound — see Foreign body, accidentally left during a procedure
removal Z48.02
Swab inadvertently left in operation wound — see Foreign body, accidentally left during a procedure
Swallowed, swallowing
difficulty — see Dysphagia
foreign body — see Foreign body, alimentary tract
Swan-neck deformity (finger) — see Deformity, finger, swan-neck
Swearing, compulsive F42.8

Swearing, compulsive — continued
in Gilles de la Tourette's syndrome F95.2
Sweat, sweats
fetid L75.0
night R61
Sweating, excessive R61
Sweeley-Klionsky disease E75.21
Sweet's disease or dermatosis L98.2
Swelling (of) R60.9
abdomen, abdominal (not referable to any particular organ) — see Mass, abdominal
ankle — see Effusion, joint, ankle
arm M79.89
forearm M79.89
breast (see also Lump, breast) N63.0
Calabar B74.3
cervical gland R59.0
chest, localized R22.2
ear H93.8- ☑
extremity (lower) (upper) — see Disorder, soft tissue, specified type NEC
finger M79.89
foot M79.89
glands R59.9
generalized R59.1
localized R59.0
hand M79.89
head (localized) R22.0
inflammatory — see Inflammation
intra-abdominal — see Mass, abdominal
joint — see Effusion, joint
leg M79.89
lower M79.89
limb — see Disorder, soft tissue, specified type NEC
localized (skin) R22.9
chest R22.2
head R22.0
limb
lower — see Mass, localized, limb, lower
upper — see Mass, localized, limb, upper
neck R22.1
trunk R22.2
neck (localized) R22.1
pelvic — see Mass, abdominal
scrotum N50.89
splenic — see Splenomegaly
testis N50.89
toe M79.89
umbilical R19.09
wandering, due to Gnathostoma (spinigerum) B83.1
white — see Tuberculosis, arthritis
Swift (-Feer) **disease**
overdose or wrong substance given or taken — see Table of Drugs and Chemicals, by drug, poisoning
Swimmer's
cramp T75.1 ☑
ear H60.33- ☑
itch B65.3
Swimming in the head R42
Swollen — see Swelling
Swyer syndrome Q99.1
Sycosis L73.8
barbae (not parasitic) L73.8
contagiosa (mycotic) B35.0
lupoides L73.8
mycotic B35.0
parasitic B35.0
vulgaris L73.8
Sydenham's chorea — see Chorea, Sydenham's
Sylvatic yellow fever A95.0
Sylvest's disease B33.0
Symblepharon H11.23- ☑
congenital Q10.3
Symond's syndrome G93.2
Sympathetic — see condition
Sympatheticotonia G90.8
Sympathicoblastoma
specified site — see Neoplasm, malignant, by site
unspecified site C74.90
Sympathogonioma — see Sympathicoblastoma
Symphalangy (fingers) (toes) Q70.9
Symptoms NEC R68.89
breast NEC N64.59
cold J00
development NEC R63.8
factitious, self-induced — see Disorder, factitious

Symptoms — continued
genital organs, female R10.2
involving
abdomen NEC R19.8
appearance NEC R46.89
awareness R41.9
altered mental status R41.82
amnesia — see Amnesia
borderline intellectual functioning R41.83
coma — see Coma
disorientation R41.0
neurologic neglect syndrome R41.4
senile cognitive decline R41.81
specified symptom NEC R41.89
behavior NEC R46.89
cardiovascular system NEC R09.89
chest NEC R09.89
circulatory system NEC R09.89
cognitive functions R41.9
altered mental status R41.82
amnesia — see Amnesia
borderline intellectual functioning R41.83
coma — see Coma
disorientation R41.0
neurologic neglect syndrome R41.4
senile cognitive decline R41.81
specified symptom NEC R41.89
development NEC R62.50
digestive system NEC R19.8
emotional state NEC R45.89
emotional lability R45.86
food and fluid intake R63.8
general perceptions and sensations R44.9
specified NEC R44.8
musculoskeletal system R29.91
specified NEC R29.898
nervous system R29.90
specified NEC R29.818
pelvis NEC R19.8
respiratory system NEC R09.89
skin and integument R23.9
urinary system R39.9
menopausal N95.1
metabolism NEC R63.8
neurotic F48.8
of infancy R68.19
pelvis NEC, female R10.2
skin and integument NEC R23.9
subcutaneous tissue NEC R23.9
viral cold J00
Sympus Q74.2
Syncephalus Q89.4
Synchondrosis
abnormal (congenital) Q78.8
ischiopubic M91.0
Synchysis (scintillans) (senile) (vitreous body) H43.89
Syncope (near) (pre-) R55
anginosa I20.8
bradycardia R00.1
cardiac R55
carotid sinus G90.01
due to spinal (lumbar) puncture G97.1
heart R55
heat T67.1 ☑
laryngeal R05
psychogenic F48.8
tussive R05
vasoconstriction R55
vasodepressor R55
vasomotor R55
vasovagal R55
Syndactylism, syndactyly Q70.9
complex (with synostosis)
fingers Q70.0- ☑
toes Q70.2- ☑
simple (without synostosis)
fingers Q70.1- ☑
toes Q70.3- ☑
Syndrome (see also Disease)
48,XXXX Q97.1
49,XXXXX Q97.1
5q minus NOS D46.C (following D46.2)
abdominal
acute R10.0
muscle deficiency Q79.4
abnormal innervation H02.519
left H02.516
lower H02.515

Syndrome — *continued*
    abnormal innervation — *continued*
        left — *continued*
            upper H02.514
        right H02.513
            lower H02.512
            upper H02.511
    abstinence, neonatal P96.1
    acid pulmonary aspiration, obstetric O74.0
    acquired immunodeficiency — *see* Human, immunod-
            eficiency virus (HIV) disease
    acute abdominal R10.0
    acute respiratory distress (adult) (child) J80-
        idiopathic J84.114
    Adair-Dighton Q78.0
    Adams-Stokes (-Morgagni) I45.9
    adiposogenital E23.6
    adrenal
        hemorrhage (meningococcal) A39.1
        meningococcic A39.1
    adrenocortical — *see* Cushing's, syndrome
    adrenogenital E25.9
        congenital, associated with enzyme deficiency
            E25.0
    afferent loop NEC K91.89
    Alagille's Q44.7
    alcohol withdrawal (without convulsions) — *see* De-
            pendence, alcohol, with, withdrawal
    Alder's D72.0
    Aldrich (-Wiskott) D82.0
    alien hand R41.4
    Alport Q87.81
    alveolar hypoventilation E66.2
    alveolocapillary block J84.10
    amnesic, amnestic (confabulatory) (due to) — *see*
            Disorder, amnesic
    amyostatic (Wilson's disease) E83.01
    androgen insensitivity E34.50
        complete E34.51
        partial E34.52
    androgen resistance (*see also* Syndrome, androgen
            insensitivity) E34.50
    Angelman Q93.5
    anginal — *see* Angina
    ankyloglossia superior Q38.1
    anterior
        chest wall R07.89
        cord G83.82
        spinal artery G95.19
            compression M47.019
                cervical region M47.012
                cervicothoracic region M47.013
                lumbar region M47.016
                occipito-atlanto-axial region M47.011
                thoracic region M47.014
                thoracolumbar region M47.015
        tibial M76.81- ☑
    antibody deficiency D80.9
        agammaglobulinemic D80.1
            hereditary D80.0
        congenital D80.0
        hypogammaglobulinemic D80.1
            hereditary D80.0
    anticardiolipin (-antibody) D68.61
    antidepressant discontinuation T43.205 ☑
    antiphospholipid (-antibody) D68.61
    aortic
        arch M31.4
        bifurcation I74.09
    aortomesenteric duodenum occlusion K31.5
    apical ballooning (transient left ventricular) I51.81
    arcuate ligament I77.4
    argentaffin, argintaffinoma E34.0
    Arnold-Chiari — *see* Arnold-Chiari disease
    Arrillaga-Ayerza I27.0
    arterial tortuosity Q87.82
    arteriovenous steal T82.898- ☑
    Asherman's N85.6
    aspiration, of newborn — *see* Aspiration, by substance,
            with pneumonia
        meconium P24.01
    ataxia-telangiectasia G11.3
    auriculotemporal G50.8
    autoerythrocyte sensitization (Gardner-Diamond)
            D69.2
    autoimmune lymphoproliferative [ALPS] D89.82
    autoimmune polyglandular E31.0
    autoinflammatory M04.9

Syndrome — *continued*
    autoinflammatory — *continued*
        specified type NEC M04.8
    autosomal — *see* Abnormal, autosomes
    Avellis' G46.8
    Ayerza (-Arrillaga) I27.0
    Babinski-Nageotte G83.89
    Bakwin-Krida Q78.5
    bare lymphocyte D81.6
    Barré-Guillain G61.0
    Barré-Liéou M53.0
    Barrett's — *see* Barrett's, esophagus
    Barsony-Polgar K22.4
    Bársony-Teschendorf K22.4
    Barth E78.71
    Bartter's E26.81
    basal cell nevus Q87.89
    Basedow's E05.00
        with thyroid storm E05.01
    basilar artery G45.0
    Batten-Steinert G71.11
    battered
        baby or child — *see* Maltreatment, child, physical
            abuse
        spouse — *see* Maltreatment, adult, physical abuse
    Beals Q87.40
    Beau's I51.5
    Beck's I65.8
    Benedikt's G46.3
    Béquez César (-Steinbrinck-Chédiak-Higashi) E70.330
    Bernhardt-Roth — *see* Meralgia paresthetica
    Bernheim's — *see* Failure, heart, right
    big spleen D73.1
    bilateral polycystic ovarian E28.2
    Bing-Horton's — *see* Horton's headache
    Birt-Hogg-Dube syndrome Q87.89
    Björck (-Thorsen) E34.0
    black
        lung J60
        widow spider bite — *see* Toxicity, venom, spider,
            black widow
    Blackfan-Diamond D61.01
    Blau M04.8
    blind loop K90.2
        congenital Q43.8
        postsurgical K91.2
    blue sclera Q78.0
    blue toe I75.02- ☑
    Boder-Sedgewick G11.3
    Boerhaave's K22.3
    Borjeson Forssman Lehmann Q89.8
    Bouillaud's I01.9
    Bourneville (-Pringle) Q85.1
    Bouveret (-Hoffman) I47.9
    brachial plexus G54.0
    bradycardia-tachycardia I49.5
    brain (nonpsychotic) F09
        with psychosis, psychotic reaction F09
        acute or subacute — *see* Delirium
        congenital — *see* Disability, intellectual
        organic F09
            post-traumatic (nonpsychotic) F07.81
                psychotic F09
            personality change F07.0
            postcontusional F07.81
            post-traumatic, nonpsychotic F07.81
            psycho-organic F09
            psychotic F06.8
    brain stem stroke G46.3
    Brandt's (acrodermatitis enteropathica) E83.2
    broad ligament laceration N83.8
    Brock's J98.11
    bronze baby P83.88
    Brown-Sequard G83.81
    Brugada I49.8
    bubbly lung P27.0
    Buchem's M85.2
    Budd-Chiari I82.0
    bulbar (progressive) G12.22
    Bürger-Grütz E78.3
    Burke's K86.89
    Burnett's (milk-alkali) E83.52
    burning feet E53.9
    Bywaters' T79.5 ☑
    Call-Fleming I67.841
    carbohydrate-deficient glycoprotein (CDGS) E77.8
    carcinogenic thrombophlebitis I82.1
    carcinoid E34.0

Syndrome — *continued*
    cardiac asthma I50.1
    cardiacos negros I27.0
    cardiofaciocutaneous Q87.89
    cardiopulmonary-obesity E66.2
    cardiorenal — *see* Hypertension, cardiorenal
    cardiorespiratory distress (idiopathic), newborn P22.0
    cardiovascular renal — *see* Hypertension, cardiorenal
    carotid
        artery (hemispheric) (internal) G45.1
        body G90.01
        sinus G90.01
    carpal tunnel G56.0- ☑
    Cassidy (-Scholte) E34.0
    cat cry Q93.4
    cat eye Q92.8
    cauda equina G83.4
    causalgia — *see* Causalgia
    celiac K90.0
        artery compression I77.4
        axis I77.4
    central pain G89.0
    cerebellar
        hereditary G11.9
        stroke G46.4
    cerebellomedullary malformation — *see* Spina bifida
    cerebral
        artery
            anterior G46.1
            middle G46.0
            posterior G46.2
        gigantism E22.0
    cervical (root) M53.1
        disc — *see* Disorder, disc, cervical, with neuritis
        fusion Q76.1
        posterior, sympathicus M53.0
        rib Q76.5
        sympathetic paralysis G90.2
    cervicobrachial (diffuse) M53.1
    cervicocranial M53.0
    cervicodorsal outlet G54.2
    cervicothoracic outlet G54.0
    Céstan (-Raymond) I65.8
    Charcot's (angina cruris) (intermittent claudication)
            I73.9
    Charcot-Weiss-Baker G90.09
    CHARGE Q89.8
    Chédiak-Higashi (-Steinbrinck) E70.330
    chest wall R07.1
    Chiari's (hepatic vein thrombosis) I82.0
    Chilaiditi's Q43.3
    child maltreatment — *see* Maltreatment, child
    chondrocostal junction M94.0
    chondroectodermal dysplasia Q77.6
    chromosome 4 short arm deletion Q93.3
    chromosome 5 short arm deletion Q93.4
    chronic
        infantile neurological, cutaneous and articular
            (CINCA) M04.2
        pain G89.4
            personality F68.8
    Clarke-Hadfield K86.89
    Clerambault's automatism G93.89
    Clouston's (hidrotic ectodermal dysplasia) Q82.4
    clumsiness, clumsy child F82
    cluster headache G44.009
        intractable G44.001
        not intractable G44.009
    Coffin-Lowry Q89.8
    cold injury (newborn) P80.0
    combined immunity deficiency D81.9
    compartment (deep) (posterior) (traumatic) T79.A0 ☑
            (*following* T79.7)
        abdomen T79.A3 ☑ (*following* T79.7)
        lower extremity (hip, buttock, thigh, leg, foot, toes)
            T79.A2 ☑ (*following* T79.7)
        nontraumatic
            abdomen M79.A3 (*following* M79.7)
            lower extremity (hip, buttock, thigh, leg, foot,
                toes) M79.A2- ☑ (*following* M79.7)
            specified site NEC M79.A9 (*following* M79.7)
            upper extremity (shoulder, arm, forearm, wrist,
                hand, fingers) M79.A1- ☑ (*following*
                M79.7)
        postprocedural — *see* Syndrome, compartment,
            nontraumatic
        specified site NEC T79.A9 ☑ (*following* T79.7)

Syndrome — *continued*
  compartment — *continued*
    upper extremity (shoulder, arm, forearm, wrist, hand, fingers) T79.A1 ☑ (*following* T79.7)
  complex regional pain — *see* Syndrome, pain, complex regional
  compression T79.5 ☑
    anterior spinal — *see* Syndrome, anterior, spinal artery, compression
    cauda equina G83.4
    celiac artery I77.4
    vertebral artery M47.029
      cervical region M47.022
      occipito-atlanto-axial region M47.021
  concussion F07.81
  congenital
    affecting multiple systems NEC Q87.89
    central alveolar hypoventilation G47.35
    facial diplegia Q87.0
    muscular hypertrophy-cerebral Q87.89
    oculo-auriculovertebral Q87.0
    oculofacial diplegia (Moebius) Q87.0
    rubella (manifest) P35.0
  congestion-fibrosis (pelvic), female N94.89
  congestive dysmenorrhea N94.6
  connective tissue M35.9
    overlap NEC M35.1
  Conn's E26.01
  conus medullaris G95.81
  cord
    anterior G83.82
    posterior G83.83
  coronary
    acute NEC I24.9
    insufficiency or intermediate I20.0
    slow flow I20.8
  Costen's (complex) M26.69
  costochondral junction M94.0
  costoclavicular G54.0
  costovertebral E22.0
  Cowden Q85.8
  craniovertebral M53.0
  Creutzfeldt-Jakob — *see* Creutzfeldt-Jakob disease or syndrome
  crib death R99
  cricopharyngeal — *see* Dysphagia
  cri-du-chat Q93.4
  croup J05.0
  CRPS I — *see* Syndrome, pain, complex regional I
  crush T79.5 ☑
  cryopyrin-associated perodic M04.2
  cryptophthalmos Q87.0
  cubital tunnel — *see* Lesion, nerve, ulnar
  Curschmann (-Batten) (-Steinert) G71.11
  Cushing's E24.9
    alcohol-induced E24.4
    drug-induced E24.2
    due to
      alcohol
      drugs E24.2
      ectopic ACTH E24.3
      overproduction of pituitary ACTH E24.0
      overdose or wrong substance given or taken — *see* Table of Drugs and Chemicals, by drug, poisoning
    pituitary-dependent E24.0
    specified type NEC E24.8
  cystic duct stump K91.5
  Dana-Putnam D51.0
  Danbolt (-Cross) (acrodermatitis enteropathica) E83.2
  Dandy-Walker Q03.1
    with spina bifida Q07.01
  Danlos' Q79.6
  De Quervain E34.51
  de Toni-Fanconi (-Debré) E72.09
    with cystinosis E72.04
  defibrination (*see also* Fibrinolysis)
    with
      antepartum hemorrhage — *see* Hemorrhage, antepartum, with coagulation defect
      intrapartum hemorrhage — *see* Hemorrhage, complicating, delivery
    newborn P60
    postpartum O72.3
  Degos' I77.89
  Déjérine-Roussy G89.0
  delayed sleep phase G47.21
  demyelinating G37.9

Syndrome — *continued*
  dependence — *see* F10-F19 with fourth character .2
  depersonalization (-derealization) F48.1
  di George's D82.1
  diabetes mellitus in newborn infant P70.2
  diabetes mellitus-hypertension-nephrosis — *see* Diabetes, nephrosis
  diabetes-nephrosis — *see* Diabetes, nephrosis
  diabetic amyotrophy — *see* Diabetes, amyotrophy
  dialysis associated steal T82.898- ☑
  Diamond-Blackfan D61.01
  Diamond-Gardener D69.2
  DIC (diffuse or disseminated intravascular coagulopathy) D65
  Dighton's Q78.0
  disequilibrium E87.8
  Döhle body-panmyelopathic D72.0
  dorsolateral medullary G46.4
  double athetosis G80.3
  Down (*see also* Down syndrome) Q90.9
  Dresbach's (elliptocytosis) D58.1
  Dressler's (postmyocardial infarction) I24.1
    postcardiotomy I97.0
  drug withdrawal, infant of dependent mother P96.1
  dry eye H04.12- ☑
  due to abnormality
    chromosomal Q99.9
      sex
        female phenotype Q97.9
        male phenotype Q98.9
      specified NEC Q99.8
  dumping (postgastrectomy) K91.1
    nonsurgical K31.89
  Dupré's (meningism) R29.1
  dysmetabolic X E88.81
  dyspraxia, developmental F82
  Eagle-Barrett Q79.4
  Eaton-Lambert — *see* Syndrome, Lambert-Eaton
  Ebstein's Q22.5
  ectopic ACTH E24.3
  eczema-thrombocytopenia D82.0
  Eddowes' Q78.0
  effort (psychogenic) F45.8
  Ehlers-Danlos Q79.6
  Eisenmenger's I27.83
  Ekman's Q78.0
  electric feet E53.8
  Ellis-van Creveld Q77.6
  empty nest Z60.0
  endocrine-hypertensive E27.0
  entrapment — *see* Neuropathy, entrapment
  eosinophilia-myalgia M35.8
  epileptic (*see also* Epilepsy, by type)
    absence G40.A09 (*following* G40.3)
      intractable G40.A19 (*following* G40.3)
        with status epilepticus G40.A11 (*following* G40.3)
        without status epilepticus G40.A19 (*following* G40.3)
      not intractable G40.A09 (*following* G40.3)
        with status epilepticus G40.A01 (*following* G40.3)
        without status epilepticus G40.A09 (*following* G40.3)
  Erdheim-Chester (ECD) E88.89
  Erdheim's E22.0
  erythrocyte fragmentation D59.4
  Evans D69.41
  exhaustion F48.8
  extrapyramidal G25.9
    specified NEC G25.89
  eye retraction — *see* Strabismus
  eyelid-malar-mandible Q87.0
  Faber's D50.9
  facial pain, paroxysmal G50.0
  Fallot's Q21.3
  familial cold autoinflammatory M04.2
  familial eczema-thrombocytopenia (Wiskott-Aldrich) D82.0
  Fanconi (-de Toni) (-Debré) E72.09
    with cystinosis E72.04
  Fanconi's (anemia) (congenital pancytopenia) D61.09
  fatigue
    chronic R53.82
    psychogenic F48.8
  faulty bowel habit K59.39
  Feil-Klippel (brevicollis) Q76.1
  Felty's — *see* Felty's syndrome

Syndrome — *continued*
  fertile eunuch E23.0
  fetal
    alcohol (dysmorphic) Q86.0
    hydantoin Q86.1
  Fiedler's I40.1
  first arch Q87.0
  fish odor E72.8
  Fisher's G61.0
  Fitzhugh-Curtis
    due to
      Chlamydia trachomatis A74.81
      Neisseria gonorrhorea (gonococcal peritonitis) A54.85
  Fitz's (*see also* Pancreatitis, acute) K85.80
  Flajani (-Basedow) E05.00
    with thyroid storm E05.01
  flatback — *see* Flatback syndrome
  floppy
    baby P94.2
    iris (intraoeprative) (IFIS) H21.81
    mitral valve I34.1
  flush E34.0
  Foix-Alajouanine G95.19
  Fong's Q87.2
  food protein-induced enterocolitis K52.21
  foramen magnum G93.5
  Foster-Kennedy H47.14- ☑
  Foville's (peduncular) G46.3
  fragile X Q99.2
  Franceschetti Q75.4
  Frey's
    auriculotemporal G50.8
    hyperhidrosis L74.52
  Friderichsen-Waterhouse A39.1
  Froin's G95.89
  frontal lobe F07.0
  Fukuhara E88.49
  functional
    bowel K59.9
    prepubertal castrate E29.1
  Gaisböck's D75.1
  ganglion (basal ganglia brain) G25.9
    geniculi G51.1
  Gardner-Diamond D69.2
  gastroesophageal
    junction K22.0
    laceration-hemorrhage K22.6
  gastrojejunal loop obstruction K91.89
  Gee-Herter-Heubner K90.0
  Gelineau's G47.419
    with cataplexy G47.411
  genito-anorectal A55
  Gerstmann-Sträussler-Scheinker (GSS) A81.82
  Gianotti-Crosti L44.4
  giant platelet (Bernard-Soulier) D69.1
  Gilles de la Tourette's F95.2
  goiter-deafness E07.1
  Goldberg Q89.8
  Goldberg-Maxwell E34.51
  Good's D83.8
  Gopalan' (burning feet) E53.8
  Gorlin's Q87.89
  Gougerot-Blum L81.7
  Gouley's I31.1
  Gower's R55
  gray or grey (newborn) P93.0
    platelet D69.1
  Gubler-Millard G46.3
  Guillain-Barré (-Strohl) G61.0
  gustatory sweating G50.8
  Hadfield-Clarke K86.89
  hair tourniquet — *see* Constriction, external, by site
  Hamman's J98.19
  hand-foot L27.1
  hand-shoulder G90.8
  hantavirus (cardio)-pulmonary (HPS) (HCPS) B33.4
  happy puppet Q93.5
  Harada's H30.81- ☑
  Hayem-Faber D50.9
  headache NEC G44.89
    complicated NEC G44.59
  Heberden's I20.8
  Hedinger's E34.0
  Hegglin's D72.0
  HELLP (hemolysis, elevated liver enzymes and low platelet count) O14.2- ☑
    complicating
      childbirth O14.24

Syndrome — *continued*
  HELLP — *continued*
    complicating — *continued*
      puerperium O14.25
  hemolytic-uremic D59.3
  hemophagocytic, infection-associated D76.2
  Henoch-Schönlein D69.0
  hepatic flexure K59.8
  hepatopulmonary K76.81
  hepatorenal K76.7
    following delivery O90.4
    postoperative or postprocedural K91.83
    postpartum, puerperal O90.4
  hepatourologic K76.7
  Herter (-Gee) (nontropical sprue) K90.0
  Heubner-Herter K90.0
  Heyd's K76.7
  Hilger's G90.09
  histamine-like (fish poisoning) — *see* Poisoning, fish
  histiocytic D76.3
  histiocytosis NEC D76.3
  HIV infection, acute B20
  Hoffmann-Werdnig G12.0
  Hollander-Simons E88.1
  Hoppe-Goldflam G70.00
    with exacerbation (acute) G70.01
    in crisis G70.01
  Horner's G90.2
  hungry bone E83.81
  hunterian glossitis D51.0
  Hutchinson's triad A50.53
  hyperabduction G54.0
  hyperammonemia-hyperornithinemia-homocitrulline-mia E72.4
  hypereosinophilic (idiopathic) D72.1
  hyperimmunoglobulin D M04.1
  hyperimmunoglobulin E (IgE) D82.4
  hyperkalemic E87.5
  hyperkinetic — *see* Hyperkinesia
  hypermobility M35.7
  hypernatremia E87.0
  hyperosmolarity E87.0
  hyperperfusion G97.82
  hypersplenic D73.1
  hypertransfusion, newborn P61.1
  hyperventilation F45.8
  hyperviscosity (of serum)
    polycythemic D75.1
    sclerothymic D58.8
  hypoglycemic (familial) (neonatal) E16.2
  hypokalemic E87.6
  hyponatremic E87.1
  hypopituitarism E23.0
  hypoplastic left-heart Q23.4
  hypopotassemia E87.6
  hyposmolality E87.1
  hypotension, maternal O26.5- ☑
  hypothenar hammer I73.89
  hypoventilation, obesity (OHS) E66.2
  ICF (intravascular coagulation-fibrinolysis) D65
  idiopathic
    cardiorespiratory distress, newborn P22.0
    nephrotic (infantile) N04.9
  iliotibial band M76.3- ☑
  immobility, immobilization (paraplegic) M62.3
  immune reconstitution D89.3
  immune reconstitution inflammatory [IRIS] D89.3
  immunity deficiency, combined D81.9
  immunodeficiency
    acquired — *see* Human, immunodeficiency virus (HIV) disease
    combined D81.9
  impending coronary I20.0
  impingement, shoulder M75.4- ☑
  inappropriate secretion of antidiuretic hormone E22.2
  infant
    gestational diabetes P70.0
    of diabetic mother P70.1
  infantilism (pituitary) E23.0
  inferior vena cava I87.1
  inspissated bile (newborn) P59.1
  institutional (childhood) F94.2
  insufficient sleep F51.12
  intermediate coronary (artery) I20.0
  interspinous ligament — *see* Spondylopathy, specified NEC
  intestinal
    carcinoid E34.0

Syndrome — *continued*
  intestinal — *continued*
    knot K56.2
  intravascular coagulation-fibrinolysis (ICF) D65
  iodine-deficiency, congenital E00.9
    type
      mixed E00.2
      myxedematous E00.1
      neurological E00.0
  IRDS (idiopathic respiratory distress, newborn) P22.0
  irritable
    bowel K58.9
      with
        constipation K58.1
        diarrhea K58.0
      mixed K58.2
      psychogenic F45.8
      specified NEC K58.8
    heart (psychogenic) F45.8
    weakness F48.8
  ischemic
    bowel (transient) K55.9
      chronic K55.1
      due to mesenteric artery insufficiency K55.1
    steal T82.898 ☑
  IVC (intravascular coagulopathy) D65
  Ivemark's Q89.01
  Jaccoud's — *see* Arthropathy, postrheumatic, chronic
  Jackson's G83.89
  Jakob-Creutzfeldt — *see* Creutzfeldt-Jakob disease or syndrome
  jaw-winking Q07.8
  Jervell-Lange-Nielsen I45.81
  jet lag G47.25
  Job's D71
  Joseph-Diamond-Blackfan D61.01
  jugular foramen G52.7
  Kabuki Q89.8
  Kanner's (autism) F84.0
  Kartagener's Q89.3
  Kelly's D50.1
  Kimmelstiel-Wilson — *see* Diabetes, specified type, with Kimmelstiel-Wilson disease
  Klein (e)-Levine G47.13
  Klippel-Feil (brevicollis) Q76.1
  Köhler-Pellegrini-Steida — *see* Bursitis, tibial collateral
  König's K59.8
  Korsakoff (-Wernicke) (nonalcoholic) F04
    alcoholic F10.26
  Kostmann's D70.0
  Krabbe's congenital muscle hypoplasia Q79.8
  labyrinthine — *see* subcategory H83.2 ☑
  lacunar NEC G46.7
  Lambert-Eaton G70.80
    in
      neoplastic disease G73.1
      specified disease NEC G70.81
  Landau-Kleffner — *see* Epilepsy, specified NEC
  Larsen's Q74.8
  lateral
    cutaneous nerve of thigh G57.1- ☑
    medullary G46.4
  Launois' E22.0
  lazy
    leukocyte D70.8
    posture M62.3
  Lemiere I80.8
  Lennox-Gastaut G40.812
    intractable G40.814
      with status epilepticus G40.813
      without status epilepticus G40.814
    not intractable G40.812
      with status epilepticus G40.811
      without status epilepticus G40.812
  lenticular, progressive E83.01
  Leopold-Levi's E05.90
  Lev's I44.2
  Lichtheim's D51.0
  Li-Fraumeni Z15.01
  Lightwood's N25.89
  Lignac (de Toni) (-Fanconi) (-Debré) E72.09
    with cystinosis E72.04
  Likoff's I20.8
  limbic epilepsy personality F07.0
  liver-kidney K76.7
  lobotomy F07.0
  Loffler's J82
  long arm 18 or 21 deletion Q93.89

Syndrome — *continued*
  long QT I45.81
  Louis-Barré G11.3
  low
    atmospheric pressure T70.29 ☑
    back M54.5
    output (cardiac) I50.9
  lower radicular, newborn (birth injury) P14.8
  Luetscher's (dehydration) E86.0
  Lupus anticoagulant D68.62
  Lutembacher's Q21.1
  macrophage activation D76.1
    due to infection D76.2
  magnesium-deficiency R29.0
  Majeed M04.8
  Mal de Debarquement R42
  malabsorption K90.9
    postsurgical K91.2
  malformation, congenital, due to
    alcohol Q86.0
    exogenous cause NEC Q86.8
    hydantoin Q86.1
    warfarin Q86.2
  malignant
    carcinoid E34.0
    neuroleptic G21.0
  Mallory-Weiss K22.6
  mandibulofacial dysostosis Q75.4
  manic-depressive — *see* Disorder, bipolar
  maple-syrup-urine E71.0
  Marable's I77.4
  Marfan's Q87.40
    with
      cardiovascular manifestations Q87.418
        aortic dilation Q87.410
      ocular manifestations Q87.42
      skeletal manifestations Q87.43
  Marie's (acromegaly) E22.0
  mast cell activation — *see* Activation, mast cell
  maternal hypotension — *see* Syndrome, hypotension, maternal
  May (-Hegglin) D72.0
  McArdle (-Schmidt) (-Pearson) E74.04
  McQuarrie's E16.2
  meconium plug (newborn) P76.0
  median arcuate ligament I77.4
  Meekeren-Ehlers-Danlos Q79.6
  megavitamin-B6 E67.2
  Meige G24.4
  MELAS E88.41
  Mendelson's O74.0
  MERRF (myoclonic epilepsy associated with ragged-red fibers) E88.42
  mesenteric
    artery (superior) K55.1
    vascular insufficiency K55.1
  metabolic E88.81
  metastatic carcinoid E34.0
  micrognathia-glossoptosis Q87.0
  midbrain NEC G93.89
  middle lobe (lung) J98.19
  middle radicular G54.0
  migraine (*see also* Migraine) G43.909
  Mikulicz' K11.8
  milk-alkali E83.52
  Millard-Gubler G46.3
  Miller-Dieker Q93.88
  Miller-Fisher G61.0
  Minkowski-Chauffard D58.0
  Mirizzi's K83.1
  MNGIE (Mitochondrial Neurogastrointestinal En-cephalopathy) E88.49
  Möbius, ophthalmoplegic migraine — *see* Migraine, ophthalmoplegic
  monofixation H50.42
  Morel-Moore M85.2
  Morel-Morgagni M85.2
  Morgagni (-Morel) (-Stewart) M85.2
  Morgagni-Adams-Stokes I45.9
  Mounier-Kuhn Q32.4
    with bronchiectasis J47.9
      with
        exacerbation (acute) J47.1
        lower respiratory infection J47.0
    acquired J98.09
      with bronchiectasis J47.9
        with
          exacerbation (acute) J47.1
          lower respiratory infection J47.0

Syndrome — continued
- Muckle-Wells M04.2
- mucocutaneous lymph node (acute febrile) (MCLS) M30.3
- multiple endocrine neoplasia (MEN) — see Neoplasia, endocrine, multiple (MEN)
- multiple operations — see Disorder, factitious
- myasthenic G70.9
  - in
    - diabetes mellitus — see Diabetes, amyotrophy
    - endocrine disease NEC E34.9 [G73.3]
    - neoplastic disease (see also Neoplasm) D49.9 [G73.3]
    - thyrotoxicosis (hyperthyroidism) E05.90 [G73.3]
      - with thyroid storm E05.91 [G73.3]
- myelodysplastic D46.9
  - with
    - 5q deletion D46.C (following D46.2)
    - isolated del (5q) chromosomal abnormality D46.C (following D46.2)
    - lesions, low grade D46.20
    - specified NEC D46.Z (following D46.4)
- myelopathic pain G89.0
- myeloproliferative (chronic) D47.1
- myofascial pain M79.1
- Naffziger's G54.0
- nail patella Q87.2
- NARP (Neuropathy, Ataxia and Retinitis pigmentosa) E88.49
- neonatal abstinence P96.1
- nephritic (see also Nephritis)
  - with edema — see Nephrosis
  - acute N00.9
  - chronic N03.9
  - rapidly progressive N01.9
- nephrotic (congenital) (see also Nephrosis) N04.9
  - with
    - dense deposit disease N04.6
    - diffuse
      - crescentic glomerulonephritis N04.7
      - endocapillary proliferative glomerulonephritis N04.4
      - membranous glomerulonephritis N04.2
      - mesangial proliferative glomerulonephritis N04.3
      - mesangiocapillary glomerulonephritis N04.5
    - focal and segmental glomerular lesions N04.1
    - minor glomerular abnormality N04.0
    - specified morphological changes NEC N04.8
  - diabetic — see Diabetes, nephrosis
- neurologic neglect R41.4
- Nezelof's D81.4
- Nonne-Milroy-Meige Q82.0
- Nothnagel's vasomotor acroparesthesia I73.89
- obesity hypoventilation (OHS) E66.2
- oculomotor H51.9
- ophthalmoplegia-cerebellar ataxia — see Strabismus, paralytic, third nerve
- oral allergy T78.1 ✓
- oral-facial-digital Q87.0
- organic
  - affective F06.30
  - amnesic (not alcohol- or drug-induced) F04
  - brain F09
  - depressive F06.31
  - hallucinosis F06.0
  - personality F07.0
- Ormond's N13.5
- oro-facial-digital Q87.0
- os trigonum Q68.8
- Osler-Weber-Rendu I78.0
- osteoporosis-osteomalacia M83.8
- Osterreicher-Turner Q87.2
- otolith — see subcategory H81.8 ✓
- oto-palatal-digital Q87.0
- outlet (thoracic) G54.0
- ovary
  - polycystic E28.2
  - resistant E28.39
  - sclerocystic E28.2
- Owren's D68.2
- Paget-Schroetter I82.890
- pain (see also Pain)
  - complex regional I G90.50
    - lower limb G90.52- ✓
    - specified site NEC G90.59
    - upper limb G90.51- ✓
  - complex regional II — see Causalgia

Syndrome — continued
- painful
  - bruising D69.2
  - feet E53.8
  - prostate N42.81
- paralysis agitans — see Parkinsonism
- paralytic G83.9
  - specified NEC G83.89
- Parinaud's H51.0
- parkinsonian — see Parkinsonism
- Parkinson's — see Parkinsonism
- paroxysmal facial pain G50.0
- Parry's E05.00
  - with thyroid storm E05.01
- Parsonage (-Aldren)-Turner G54.5
- patella clunk M25.86- ✓
- Paterson (-Brown) (-Kelly) D50.1
- pectoral girdle I77.89
- pectoralis minor I77.89
- pediatric autoimmune neuropsychiatric disorders associated with streptococcal infections (PANDAS) D89.89
- Pelger-Huet D72.0
- pellagra-cerebellar ataxia-renal aminoaciduria E72.02
- pellagroid E52
- Pellegrini-Stieda — see Bursitis, tibial collateral
- pelvic congestion-fibrosis, female N94.89
- penta X Q97.1
- peptic ulcer — see Ulcer, peptic
- perabduction I77.89
- periodic fever M04.1
- periodic fever, aphthous stomatitis, pharyngitis, and adenopathy [PFAPA] M04.8
- periodic headache, in adults and children — see Headache, periodic syndromes in adults and children
- periurethral fibrosis N13.5
- phantom limb (without pain) G54.7
  - with pain G54.6
- pharyngeal pouch D82.1
- Pick's — see Disease, Pick's
- Pickwickian E66.2
- PIE (pulmonary infiltration with eosinophilia) J82
- pigmentary pallidal degeneration (progressive) G23.0
- pineal E34.8
- pituitary E22.0
- placental transfusion — see Pregnancy, complicated by, placental transfusion syndromes
- plantar fascia M72.2
- plateau iris (post-iridectomy) (postprocedural) H21.82
- Plummer-Vinson D50.1
- pluricarential of infancy E40
- plurideficiency E40
- pluriglandular (compensatory) E31.8
  - autoimmune E31.0
- pneumatic hammer T75.21 ✓
- polyangiitis overlap M30.8
- polycarential of infancy E40
- polyglandular E31.8
  - autoimmune E31.0
- polysplenia Q89.09
- pontine NEC G93.89
- popliteal
  - artery entrapment I77.89
  - web Q87.89
- post chemoembolization — code to associated conditions
- postcardiac injury
  - postcardiotomy I97.0
  - postmyocardial infarction I24.1
- postcardiotomy I97.0
- postcholecystectomy K91.5
- postcommissurotomy I97.0
- postconcussional F07.81
- postcontusional F07.81
- postencephalitic F07.89
- posterior
  - cervical sympathetic M53.0
  - cord G83.83
  - fossa compression G93.5
  - reversible encephalopathy (PRES) I67.83
- postgastrectomy (dumping) K91.1
- postgastric surgery K91.1
- postinfarction I24.1
- postlaminectomy NEC M96.1
- postleukotomy F07.0
- postmastectomy lymphedema I97.2
- postmyocardial infarction I24.1

Syndrome — continued
- postoperative NEC T81.9 ✓
  - blind loop K90.2
- postpartum panhypopituitary (Sheehan) E23.0
- postpolio (myelitic) G14
- postthrombotic I87.009
  - with
    - inflammation I87.02- ✓
      - with ulcer I87.03- ✓
    - specified complication NEC I87.09- ✓
    - ulcer I87.01- ✓
      - with inflammation I87.03- ✓
  - asymptomatic I87.00- ✓
- postvagotomy K91.1
- postvalvulotomy I97.0
- postviral NEC G93.3
  - fatigue G93.3
- Potain's K31.0
- potassium intoxication E87.5
- precerebral artery (multiple) (bilateral) G45.2
- preinfarction I20.0
- preleukemic D46.9
- premature senility E34.8
- premenstrual dysphoric F32.89
- premenstrual tension N94.3
- Prinzmetal-Massumi R07.1
- prune belly Q79.4
- pseudo -Turner's Q87.1
- pseudocarpal tunnel (sublimis) — see Syndrome, carpal tunnel
- pseudoparalytica G70.00
  - with exacerbation (acute) G70.01
  - in crisis G70.01
- psycho-organic (nonpsychotic severity) F07.9
  - acute or subacute F05
  - depressive type F06.31
  - hallucinatory type F06.0
  - nonpsychotic severity F07.0
  - specified NEC F07.89
- pulmonary
  - arteriosclerosis I27.0
  - dysmaturity (Wilson-Mikity) P27.0
  - hypoperfusion (idiopathic) P22.0
  - renal (hemorrhagic) (Goodpasture's) M31.0
- pure
  - motor lacunar G46.5
  - sensory lacunar G46.6
- Putnam-Dana D51.0
- pyogenic arthritis, pyoderma gangrenosum, and acne [PAPA] M04.8
- pyramidopallidonigral G20
- pyriformis — see Lesion, nerve, sciatic
- QT interval prolongation I45.81
- radicular NEC — see Radiculopathy
  - upper limbs, newborn (birth injury) P14.3
- rapid time-zone change G47.25
- Rasmussen G04.81
- Raymond (-Céstan) I65.8
- Raynaud's I73.00
  - with gangrene I73.01
- RDS (respiratory distress syndrome, newborn) P22.0
- reactive airways dysfunction J68.3
- Refsum's G60.1
- Reifenstein E34.52
- renal glomerulohyalinosis-diabetic — see Diabetes, nephrosis
- Rendu-Osler-Weber I78.0
- residual ovary N99.83
- resistant ovary E28.39
- respiratory
  - distress
    - acute J80
      - adult J80
      - child J80
      - idiopathic J84.114
    - newborn (idiopathic) (type I) P22.0
      - type II P22.1
- restless legs G25.81
- retinoblastoma (familial) C69.2 ✓
- retroperitoneal fibrosis N13.5
- retroviral seroconversion (acute) Z21
- Reye's G93.7
- Richter — see Leukemia, chronic lymphocytic, B-cell type
- Ridley's I50.1
- right
  - heart, hypoplastic Q22.6

✓ Additional Character Required — Refer to the Tabular List for Character Selection

▼ Subterms under main terms may continue to next column or page

Syndrome — *continued*
   right — *continued*
      ventricular obstruction — *see* Failure, heart, con-
            gestive
   Romano-Ward (prolonged QT interval) I45.81
   rotator cuff, shoulder (*see also* Tear, rotator cuff)
         M75.10- ☑
   Rotes Quérol — *see* Hyperostosis, ankylosing
   Roth — *see* Meralgia paresthetica
   rubella (congenital) P35.0
   Ruvalcaba-Myhre-Smith E71.440
   Rytand-Lipsitch I44.2
   salt
      depletion E87.1
         due to heat NEC T67.8 ☑
            causing heat exhaustion or prostration
                  T67.4 ☑
      low E87.1
   salt-losing N28.89
   Scaglietti-Dagnini E22.0
   scalenus anticus (anterior) G54.0
   scapulocostal — *see* Mononeuropathy, upper limb,
         specified site NEC
   scapuloperoneal G71.0
   schizophrenic, of childhood NEC F84.5
   Schnitzler D47.2
   Scholte's E34.0
   Schroeder's E27.0
   Schüller-Christian C96.5
   Schwachman's — *see* Syndrome, Shwachman's
   Schwartz (-Jampel) G71.13
   Schwartz-Bartter E22.2
   scimitar Q26.8
   sclerocystic ovary E28.2
   Seitelberger's G31.89
   septicemic adrenal hemorrhage A39.1
   seroconversion, retroviral (acute) Z21
   serous meningitis G93.2
   severe acute respiratory (SARS) J12.81
   shaken infant T74.4 ☑
   shock (traumatic) T79.4 ☑
      kidney N17.0
         following crush injury T79.5 ☑
      toxic A48.3
   shock-lung J80
   Shone's — *code to* specific anomalies
   short
      bowel K91.2
      rib Q77.2
   shoulder-hand — *see* Algoneurodystrophy
   Shwachman's D70.4
   sicca — *see* Sicca syndrome
   sick
      cell E87.1
      sinus I49.5
   sick-euthyroid E07.81
   sideropenic D50.1
   Siemens' ectodermal dysplasia Q82.4
   Silfversköld's Q78.9
   Simons' E88.1
   sinus tarsi M25.57- ☑
   sinusitis-bronchiectasis-situs inversus Q89.3
   Sipple's E31.22
   sirenomelia Q87.2
   Slocumb's E27.0
   slow flow, coronary I20.8
   Sluder's G44.89
   Smith-Magenis Q93.88
   Sneddon-Wilkinson L13.1
   Sotos' Q87.3
   South African cardiomyopathy I42.8
   spasmodic
      upward movement, eyes H51.8
      winking F95.8
   Spen's I45.9
   splenic
      agenesis Q89.01
      flexure K59.8
      neutropenia D73.81
   Spurway's Q78.0
   staphylococcal scalded skin L00
   steal
      arteriovenous T82.898- ☑
      ischemic T82.898- ☑
      subclavian G45.8
   Stein-Leventhal E28.2
   Stein's E28.2
   Stevens-Johnson syndrome L51.1

Syndrome — *continued*
   Stevens-Johnson syndrome — *continued*
      toxic epidermal necrolysis overlap L51.3
   Stewart-Morel M85.2
   Stickler Q89.8
   stiff baby Q89.8
   stiff man G25.82
   Still-Felty — *see* Felty's syndrome
   Stokes (-Adams) I45.9
   stone heart I50.1
   straight back, congenital Q76.49
   subclavian steal G45.8
   subcoracoid-pectoralis minor G54.0
   subcostal nerve compression I77.89
   subphrenic interposition Q43.3
   superior
      cerebellar artery I63.8
      mesenteric artery K55.1
      semi-circular canal dehiscence H83.8X- ☑
      vena cava I87.1
   supine hypotensive (maternal) — *see* Syndrome, hy-
         potension, maternal
   suprarenal cortical E27.0
   supraspinatus (*see also* Tear, rotator cuff) M75.10- ☑
   Susac G93.49
   swallowed blood P78.2
   sweat retention L74.0
   Swyer Q99.1
   Symond's G93.2
   sympathetic
      cervical paralysis G90.2
      pelvic, female N94.89
   systemic inflammatory response (SIRS), of non-infec-
         tious origin (without organ dysfunction) R65.10
      with acute organ dysfunction R65.11
   tachycardia-bradycardia I49.5
   takotsubo I51.81
   TAR (thrombocytopenia with absent radius) Q87.2
   tarsal tunnel G57.5- ☑
   teething K00.7
   tegmental G93.89
   telangiectasic-pigmentation-cataract Q82.8
   temporal pyramidal apex — *see* Otitis, media, suppu-
         rative, acute
   temporomandibular joint-pain-dysfunction M26.62- ☑
   Terry's (*see also* Myopia, degenerative) H44.2- ☑
   testicular feminization (*see also* Syndrome, androgen
         insensitivity) E34.51
   thalamic pain (hyperesthetic) G89.0
   thoracic outlet (compression) G54.0
   Thorson-Björck E34.0
   thrombocytopenia with absent radius (TAR) Q87.2
   thyroid-adrenocortical insufficiency E31.0
   tibial
      anterior M76.81- ☑
      posterior M76.82- ☑
   Tietze's M94.0
   time-zone (rapid) G47.25
   Toni-Fanconi E72.09
      with cystinosis E72.04
   Touraine's Q79.8
   tourniquet — *see* Constriction, external, by site
   toxic shock A48.3
   transient left ventricular apical ballooning I51.81
   traumatic vasospastic T75.22 ☑
   Treacher Collins Q75.4
   triple X, female Q97.0
   trisomy Q92.9
      13 Q91.7
         meiotic nondisjunction Q91.4
         mitotic nondisjunction Q91.5
         mosaicism Q91.5
         translocation Q91.6
      18 Q91.3
         meiotic nondisjunction Q91.0
         mitotic nondisjunction Q91.1
         mosaicism Q91.1
         translocation Q91.2
      20 (q)(p) Q92.8
      21 Q90.9
         meiotic nondisjunction Q90.0
         mitotic nondisjunction Q90.1
         mosaicism Q90.1
         translocation Q90.2
      22 Q92.8
   tropical wet feet T69.0- ☑
   Trousseau's I82.1

Syndrome — *continued*
   tumor lysis (following antineoplastic chemotherapy)
         (spontaneous) NEC E88.3
   tumor necrosis factor receptor associated periodic
         (TRAPS) M04.1
   Twiddler's (due to)
      automatic implantable defibrillator T82.198 ☑
      cardiac pacemaker T82.198 ☑
   Unverricht (-Lundborg) — *see* Epilepsy, generalized,
         idiopathic
   upward gaze H51.8
   uremia, chronic (*see also* Disease, kidney, chronic)
         N18.9
   urethral N34.3
   urethro-oculo-articular — *see* Reiter's disease
   urohepatic K76.7
   vago-hypoglossal G52.7
   van Buchem's M85.2
   van der Hoeve's Q78.0
   vascular NEC in cerebrovascular disease G46.8
   vasoconstriction, reversible cerebrovascular I67.841
   vasomotor I73.9
   vasospastic (traumatic) T75.22 ☑
   vasovagal R55
   VATER Q87.2
   velo-cardio-facial Q93.81
   vena cava (inferior) (superior) (obstruction) I87.1
   vertebral
      artery G45.0
         compression — *see* Syndrome, anterior, spinal
               artery, compression
      steal G45.0
   vertebro-basilar artery G45.0
   vertebrogenic (pain) M54.89
   vertiginous — *see* Disorder, vestibular function
   Vinson-Plummer D50.1
   virus B34.9
   visceral larva migrans B83.0
   visual disorientation H53.8
   vitamin B6 deficiency E53.1
   vitreal corneal H59.01- ☑
   vitreous (touch) H59.01- ☑
   Vogt-Koyanagi H20.82- ☑
   Volkmann's T79.6 ☑
   von Schroetter's I82.890
   von Willebrand (-Jürgen) D68.0
   Waldenström-Kjellberg D50.1
   Wallenberg's G46.3
   water retention E87.79
   Waterhouse (-Friderichsen) A39.1
   Weber-Gubler G46.3
   Weber-Leyden G46.3
   Weber's G46.3
   Wegener's M31.30
      with
         kidney involvement M31.31
         lung involvement M31.30
            with kidney involvement M31.31
   Weingarten's (tropical eosinophilia) J82
   Weiss-Baker G90.09
   Werdnig-Hoffman G12.0
   Wermer's E31.21
   Werner's E34.8
   Wernicke-Korsakoff (nonalcoholic) F04
      alcoholic F10.26
   Westphal-Strümpell E83.01
   West's — *see* Epilepsy, spasms
   wet
      feet (maceration) (tropical) T69.0- ☑
      lung, newborn P22.1
   whiplash S13.4 ☑
   whistling face Q87.0
   Wilkie's K55.1
   Wilkinson-Sneddon L13.1
   Willebrand (-Jürgens) D68.0
   Wilson's (hepatolenticular degeneration) E83.01
   Wiskott-Aldrich D82.0
   withdrawal — *see* Withdrawal, state
      drug
         infant of dependent mother P96.1
         therapeutic use, newborn P96.2
   Woakes' (ethmoiditis) J33.1
   Wright's (hyperabduction) G54.0
   X I20.9
   XXXX Q97.1
   XXXXX Q97.1
   XXXXY Q98.1
   XXY Q98.0

Syndrome — *continued*
yellow nail L60.5
Zahorsky's B08.5
Zellweger syndrome E71.510
Zellweger-like syndrome E71.541
Synechia (anterior) (iris) (posterior) (pupil) (*see also* Adhesions, iris)
intra-uterine (traumatic) N85.6
Synesthesia R20.8
Syngamiasis, syngamosis B83.3
Synodontia K00.2
Synorchidism, synorchism Q55.1
Synostosis (congenital) Q78.8
astragalo-scaphoid Q74.2
radioulnar Q74.0
Synovial sarcoma — *see* Neoplasm, connective tissue, malignant
Synovioma (malignant) (*see also* Neoplasm, connective tissue, malignant)
benign — *see* Neoplasm, connective tissue, benign
Synoviosarcoma — *see* Neoplasm, connective tissue, malignant
Synovitis (*see also* Tenosynovitis) M65.9
crepitant
hand M70.0- ☑
wrist M70.03- ☑
gonococcal A54.49
gouty — *see* Gout
in (due to)
crystals M65.8- ☑
gonorrhea A54.49
syphilis (late) A52.78
use, overuse, pressure — *see* Disorder, soft tissue, due to use
infective NEC — *see* Tenosynovitis, infective NEC
specified NEC — *see* Tenosynovitis, specified type NEC
syphilitic A52.78
congenital (early) A50.02
toxic — *see* Synovitis, transient
transient M67.3- ☑
ankle M67.37- ☑
elbow M67.32- ☑
foot joint M67.37- ☑
hand joint M67.34- ☑
hip M67.35- ☑
knee M67.36- ☑
multiple site M67.39
pelvic region M67.35- ☑
shoulder M67.31- ☑
specified joint NEC M67.38
wrist M67.33- ☑
traumatic, current — *see* Sprain
tuberculous — *see* Tuberculosis, synovitis
villonodular (pigmented) M12.2- ☑
ankle M12.27- ☑
elbow M12.22- ☑
foot joint M12.27- ☑
hand joint M12.24- ☑
hip M12.25- ☑
knee M12.26- ☑
multiple site M12.29
pelvic region M12.25- ☑
shoulder M12.21- ☑
specified joint NEC M12.28
vertebrae M12.28
wrist M12.23- ☑
Syphilid A51.39
congenital A50.06
newborn A50.06
tubercular (late) A52.79
Syphilis, syphilitic (acquired) A53.9
abdomen (late) A52.79
acoustic nerve A52.15
adenopathy (secondary) A51.49
adrenal (gland) (with cortical hypofunction) A52.79
age under 2 years NOS (*see also* Syphilis, congenital, early)
acquired A51.9
alopecia (secondary) A51.32
anemia (late) A52.79 [D63.8]
aneurysm (aorta) (ruptured) A52.01
central nervous system A52.05
congenital A50.54 [I79.0]
anus (late) A52.74
primary A51.1
secondary A51.39
aorta (arch) (abdominal) (thoracic) A52.02

Syphilis, syphilitic — *continued*
aorta — *continued*
aneurysm A52.01
aortic (insufficiency) (regurgitation) (stenosis) A52.03
aneurysm A52.01
arachnoid (adhesive) (cerebral) (spinal) A52.13
asymptomatic — *see* Syphilis, latent
ataxia (locomotor) A52.11
atrophoderma maculatum A51.39
auricular fibrillation A52.06
bladder (late) A52.76
bone A52.77
secondary A51.46
brain A52.17
breast (late) A52.79
bronchus (late) A52.72
bubo (primary) A51.0
bulbar palsy A52.19
bursa (late) A52.78
cardiac decompensation A52.06
cardiovascular A52.00
central nervous system (late) (recurrent) (relapse) (tertiary) A52.3
with
ataxia A52.11
general paralysis A52.17
juvenile A50.45
paresis (general) A52.17
juvenile A50.45
tabes (dorsalis) A52.11
juvenile A50.45
taboparesis A52.17
juvenile A50.45
aneurysm A52.05
congenital A50.40
juvenile A50.40
remission in (sustained) A52.3
serology doubtful, negative, or positive A52.3
specified nature or site NEC A52.19
vascular A52.05
cerebral A52.17
meningovascular A52.13
nerves (multiple palsies) A52.15
sclerosis A52.17
thrombosis A52.05
cerebrospinal (tabetic type) A52.12
cerebrovascular A52.05
cervix (late) A52.76
chancre (multiple) A51.0
extragenital A51.2
Rollet's A51.0
Charcot's joint A52.16
chorioretinitis A51.43
congenital A50.01
late A52.71
prenatal A50.01
choroiditis — *see* Syphilitic chorioretinitis
choroidoretinitis — *see* Syphilitic chorioretinitis
ciliary body (secondary) A51.43
late A52.71
colon (late) A52.74
combined spinal sclerosis A52.11
condyloma (latum) A51.31
congenital A50.9
with
paresis (general) A50.45
tabes (dorsalis) A50.45
taboparesis A50.45
early, or less than 2 years after birth NEC A50.2
with manifestations — *see* Syphilis, congenital, early, symptomatic
latent (without manifestations) A50.1
negative spinal fluid test A50.1
serology positive A50.1
symptomatic A50.09
cutaneous A50.06
mucocutaneous A50.07
oculopathy A50.01
osteochondropathy A50.02
pharyngitis A50.03
pneumonia A50.04
rhinitis A50.05
visceral A50.08
chorioretinitis, choroiditis A50.01 [H32]
interstitial keratitis A50.31
juvenile neurosyphilis A50.45
late, or 2 years or more after birth NEC A50.7
chorioretinitis, choroiditis A50.32
interstitial keratitis A50.31

Syphilis, syphilitic — *continued*
congenital — *continued*
late, or 2 years or more after birth — *continued*
juvenile neurosyphilis A50.45
latent (without manifestations) A50.6
negative spinal fluid test A50.6
serology positive A50.6
symptomatic or with manifestations NEC A50.59
arthropathy A50.55
cardiovascular A50.54
Clutton's joints A50.51
Hutchinson's teeth A50.52
Hutchinson's triad A50.53
osteochondropathy A50.56
saddle nose A50.57
conjugal A53.9
tabes A52.11
conjunctiva (late) A52.71
contact Z20.2
cord bladder A52.19
cornea, late A52.71
coronary (artery) (sclerosis) A52.06
coryza, congenital A50.05
cranial nerve A52.15
multiple palsies A52.15
cutaneous — *see* Syphilis, skin
dacryocystitis (late) A52.71
degeneration, spinal cord A52.12
dementia paralytica A52.17
juvenilis A50.45
destruction of bone A52.77
dilatation, aorta A52.01
due to blood transfusion A53.9
dura mater A52.13
ear A52.79
inner A52.79
nerve (eighth) A52.15
neurorecurrence A52.15
early A51.9
cardiovascular A52.00
central nervous system A52.3
latent (without manifestations) (less than 2 years after infection) A51.5
negative spinal fluid test A51.5
serological relapse after treatment A51.5
serology positive A51.5
relapse (treated, untreated) A51.9
skin A51.39
symptomatic A51.9
extragenital chancre A51.2
primary, except extragenital chancre A51.0
secondary (*see also* Syphilis, secondary) A51.39
relapse (treated, untreated) A51.49
ulcer A51.39
eighth nerve (neuritis) A52.15
endemic A65
endocarditis A52.03
aortic A52.03
pulmonary A52.03
epididymis (late) A52.76
epiglottis (late) A52.73
epiphysitis (congenital) (early) A50.02
episcleritis (late) A52.71
esophagus A52.79
eustachian tube A52.73
exposure to Z20.2
eye A52.71
eyelid (late) (with gumma) A52.71
fallopian tube (late) A52.76
fracture A52.77
gallbladder (late) A52.74
gastric (polyposis) (late) A52.74
general A53.9
paralysis A52.17
juvenile A50.45
genital (primary) A51.0
glaucoma A52.71
gumma NEC A52.79
cardiovascular system A52.00
central nervous system A52.3
congenital A50.59
heart (block) (decompensation) (disease) (failure) A52.06 [I52]
valve NEC A52.03
hemianesthesia A52.19
hemianopsia A52.71
hemiparesis A52.17
hemiplegia A52.17

Subterms under main terms may continue to next column or page

Syphilis, syphilitic — *continued*
  hepatic artery A52.09
  hepatis A52.74
  hepatomegaly, congenital A50.08
  hereditaria tarda — *see* Syphilis, congenital, late
  hereditary — *see* Syphilis, congenital
  Hutchinson's teeth A50.52
  hyalitis A52.71
  inactive — *see* Syphilis, latent
  infantum — *see* Syphilis, congenital
  inherited — *see* Syphilis, congenital
  internal ear A52.79
  intestine (late) A52.74
  iris, iritis (secondary) A51.43
    late A52.71
  joint (late) A52.77
  keratitis (congenital) (interstitial) (late) A50.31
  kidney (late) A52.75
  lacrimal passages (late) A52.71
  larynx (late) A52.73
  late A52.9
    cardiovascular A52.00
    central nervous system A52.3
    kidney A52.75
    latent or 2 years or more after infection (without
      manifestations) A52.8
      negative spinal fluid test A52.8
      serology positive A52.8
    paresis A52.17
    specified site NEC A52.79
    symptomatic or with manifestations A52.79
    tabes A52.11
  latent A53.0
    with signs or symptoms — *code by* site and stage
      under Syphilis
    early, or less than 2 years after infection A51.5
    central nervous system A52.2
    date of infection unspecified A53.0
    follow-up of latent syphilis A53.0
      date of infection unspecified A53.0
      late, or 2 years or more after infection A52.8
    late, or 2 years or more after infection A52.8
    positive serology (only finding) A53.0
      early, or less than 2 years after infection A51.5
      date of infection unspecified A53.0
      late, or 2 years or more after infection A52.8
  lens (late) A52.71
  leukoderma A51.39
    late A52.79
  lienitis A52.79
  lip A51.39
    chancre (primary) A51.2
    late A52.79
  Lissauer's paralysis A52.17
  liver A52.74
  locomotor ataxia A52.11
  lung A52.72
  lymph gland (early) (secondary) A51.49
    late A52.79
  lymphadenitis (secondary) A51.49
  macular atrophy of skin A51.39
    striated A52.79
  mediastinum (late) A52.73
  meninges (adhesive) (brain) (spinal cord) A52.13
  meningitis A52.13
    acute (secondary) A51.41
    congenital A50.41
  meningoencephalitis A52.14
  meningovascular A52.13
    congenital A50.41
  mesarteritis A52.09
    brain A52.04
  middle ear A52.77
  mitral stenosis A52.03
  monoplegia A52.17
  mouth (secondary) A51.39
    late A52.79
  mucocutaneous (secondary) A51.39
    late A52.79
  mucous
    membrane (secondary) A51.39
      late A52.79
    patches A51.39
      congenital A50.07
  mulberry molars A50.52
  muscle A52.78
  myocardium A52.06
  nasal sinus (late) A52.73

Syphilis, syphilitic — *continued*
  neonatorum — *see* Syphilis, congenital
  nephrotic syndrome (secondary) A51.44
  nerve palsy (any cranial nerve) A52.15
    multiple A52.15
  nervous system, central A52.3
  neuritis A52.15
    acoustic A52.15
  neurorecidive of retina A52.19
  neuroretinitis A52.19
  newborn — *see* Syphilis, congenital
  nodular superficial (late) A52.79
  nonvenereal A65
  nose (late) A52.73
    saddle back deformity A50.57
  occlusive arterial disease A52.09
  oculopathy A52.71
  ophthalmic (late) A52.71
  optic nerve (atrophy) (neuritis) (papilla) A52.15
  orbit (late) A52.71
  organic A53.9
  osseous (late) A52.77
  osteochondritis (congenital) (early) A50.02 [M90.80]
  osteoporosis A52.77
  ovary (late) A52.76
  oviduct (late) A52.76
  palate (late) A52.79
  pancreas (late) A52.74
  paralysis A52.17
    general A52.17
      juvenile A50.45
  paresis (general) A52.17
    juvenile A50.45
  paresthesia A52.19
  Parkinson's disease or syndrome A52.19
  paroxysmal tachycardia A52.06
  pemphigus (congenital) A50.06
  penis (chancre) A51.0
    late A52.76
  pericardium A52.06
  perichondritis, larynx (late) A52.73
  periosteum (late) A52.77
    congenital (early) A50.02 [M90.80]
    early (secondary) A51.46
  peripheral nerve A52.79
  petrous bone (late) A52.77
  pharynx (late) A52.73
    secondary A51.39
  pituitary (gland) A52.79
  pleura (late) A52.73
  pneumonia, white A50.04
  pontine lesion A52.17
  portal vein A52.09
  primary A51.0
    anal A51.1
    and secondary — *see* Syphilis, secondary
    central nervous system A52.3
    extragenital chancre NEC A51.2
    fingers A51.2
    genital A51.0
    lip A51.2
    specified site NEC A51.2
    tonsils A51.2
  prostate (late) A52.76
  ptosis (eyelid) A52.71
  pulmonary (late) A52.72
    artery A52.09
  pyelonephritis (late) A52.75
  recently acquired, symptomatic A51.9
  rectum (late) A52.74
  respiratory tract (late) A52.73
  retina, late A52.71
  retrobulbar neuritis A52.15
  salpingitis A52.76
  sclera (late) A52.71
  sclerosis
    cerebral A52.17
    coronary A52.06
    multiple A52.11
  scotoma (central) A52.71
  scrotum (late) A52.76
  secondary (and primary) A51.49
    adenopathy A51.49
    anus A51.39
    bone A51.46
    chorioretinitis, choroiditis A51.43
    hepatitis A51.45
    liver A51.45
    lymphadenitis A51.49

Syphilis, syphilitic — *continued*
  secondary — *continued*
    meningitis (acute) A51.41
    mouth A51.39
    mucous membranes A51.39
    periosteum, periostitis A51.46
    pharynx A51.39
    relapse (treated, untreated) A51.49
    skin A51.39
    specified form NEC A51.49
    tonsil A51.39
    ulcer A51.39
    viscera NEC A51.49
    vulva A51.39
  seminal vesicle (late) A52.76
  seronegative with signs or symptoms — *code by* site
    and stage under Syphilis
  seropositive
    with signs or symptoms — *code by* site and stage
      under Syphilis
    follow-up of latent syphilis — *see* Syphilis, latent
    only finding — *see* Syphilis, latent
  seventh nerve (paralysis) A52.15
  sinus, sinusitis (late) A52.73
  skeletal system A52.77
  skin (with ulceration) (early) (secondary) A51.39
    late or tertiary A52.79
  small intestine A52.74
  spastic spinal paralysis A52.17
  spermatic cord (late) A52.76
  spinal (cord) A52.12
  spleen A52.79
  splenomegaly A52.79
  spondylitis A52.77
  staphyloma A52.71
  stigmata (congenital) A50.59
  stomach A52.74
  synovium A52.78
  tabes dorsalis (late) A52.11
    juvenile A50.45
  tabetic type A52.11
    juvenile A50.45
  taboparesis A52.17
    juvenile A50.45
  tachycardia A52.06
  tendon (late) A52.78
  tertiary A52.9
    with symptoms NEC A52.79
    cardiovascular A52.00
    central nervous system A52.3
    multiple NEC A52.79
    specified site NEC A52.79
  testis A52.76
  thorax A52.73
  throat A52.73
  thymus (gland) (late) A52.79
  thyroid (late) A52.79
  tongue (late) A52.79
  tonsil (lingual) (late) A52.73
    primary A51.2
    secondary A51.39
  trachea (late) A52.73
  tunica vaginalis (late) A52.76
  ulcer (any site) (early) (secondary) A51.39
    late A52.79
    perforating A52.79
      foot A52.11
  urethra (late) A52.76
  urogenital (late) A52.76
  uterus (late) A52.76
  uveal tract (secondary) A51.43
    late A52.71
  uveitis (secondary) A51.43
    late A52.71
  uvula (late) (perforated) A52.79
  vagina A51.0
    late A52.76
  valvulitis NEC A52.03
  vascular A52.00
    brain (cerebral) A52.05
  ventriculi A52.74
  vesicae urinariae (late) A52.76
  viscera (abdominal) (late) A52.74
    secondary A51.49
  vitreous (opacities) (late) A52.71
    hemorrhage A52.71
  vulva A51.0
    late A52.76
    secondary A51.39

Syphiloma A52.79
    cardiovascular system A52.00
    central nervous system A52.3
    circulatory system A52.00
    congenital A50.59
Syphilophobia F45.29
Syringadenoma (*see also* Neoplasm, skin, benign)
    papillary — *see* Neoplasm, skin, benign

Syringobulbia G95.0
Syringocystadenoma — *see* Neoplasm, skin, benign
    papillary — *see* Neoplasm, skin, benign
Syringoma (*see also* Neoplasm, skin, benign)
    chondroid — *see* Neoplasm, skin, benign
Syringomyelia G95.0
Syringomyelitis — *see* Encephalitis
Syringomyelocele — *see* Spina bifida

Syringopontia G95.0
System, systemic (*see also* condition)
    disease, combined — *see* Degeneration, combined
    inflammatory response syndrome (SIRS) of non-infectious origin (without organ dysfunction) R65.10
        with acute organ dysfunction R65.11
    lupus erythematosus M32.9
        inhibitor present D68.62

T

Tabacism, tabacosis, tabagism (see also Poisoning, tobacco)
  meaning dependence (without remission) F17.200
    with
      disorder F17.299
        in remission F17.211
        specified disorder NEC F17.298
        withdrawal F17.203
Tabardillo A75.9
  flea-borne A75.2
  louse-borne A75.0
Tabes, tabetic A52.10
  with
    central nervous system syphilis A52.10
    Charcot's joint A52.16
    cord bladder A52.19
    crisis, viscera (any) A52.19
    paralysis, general A52.17
    paresis (general) A52.17
    perforating ulcer (foot) A52.19
  arthropathy (Charcot) A52.16
  bladder A52.19
  bone A52.11
  cerebrospinal A52.12
  congenital A50.45
  conjugal A52.10
  dorsalis A52.11
    juvenile A50.49
  juvenile A50.49
  latent A52.19
  mesenterica A18.39
  paralysis, insane, general A52.17
  spasmodic A52.17
  syphilis (cerebrospinal) A52.12
Taboparalysis A52.17
Taboparesis (remission) A52.17
  juvenile A50.45
TAC (trigeminal autonomic cephalgia) **NEC** G44.099
  intractable G44.091
  not intractable G44.099
Tache noir S60.22- ☑
Tachyalimentation K91.2
Tachyarrhythmia, tachyrhythmia — see Tachycardia
Tachycardia R00.0
  atrial (paroxysmal) I47.1
  auricular I47.1
  AV nodal re-entry (re-entrant) I47.1
  junctional (paroxysmal) I47.1
  newborn P29.11
  nodal (paroxysmal) I47.1
  non-paroxysmal AV nodal I45.89
  paroxysmal (sustained) (nonsustained) I47.9
    with sinus bradycardia I49.5
    atrial (PAT) I47.1
    atrioventricular (AV) (re-entrant) I47.1
      psychogenic F54
    junctional I47.1
      ectopic I47.1
    nodal I47.1
    psychogenic (atrial) (supraventricular) (ventricular) F54
    supraventricular (sustained) I47.1
      psychogenic F54
    ventricular I47.2
      psychogenic F54
  psychogenic F45.8
  sick sinus I49.5
  sinoauricular NOS R00.0
    paroxysmal I47.1
  sinus [sinusal] NOS R00.0
    paroxysmal I47.1
  supraventricular I47.1
  ventricular (paroxysmal) (sustained) I47.2
    psychogenic F54
Tachygastria K31.89
Tachypnea R06.82
  hysterical F45.8
  newborn (idiopathic) (transitory) P22.1
  psychogenic F45.8
  transitory, of newborn P22.1
TACO (transfusion associated circulatory overload) E87.71
Taenia (infection) (infestation) B68.9
  diminuta B71.0
  echinococcal infestation B67.90
  mediocanellata B68.1

Taenia — continued
  nana B71.0
  saginata B68.1
  solium (intestinal form) B68.0
    larval form — see Cysticercosis
Taeniasis (intestine) — see Taenia
Tag (hypertrophied skin) (infected) L91.8
  adenoid J35.8
  anus K64.4
  hemorrhoidal K64.4
  hymen N89.8
  perineal N90.89
  preauricular Q17.0
  sentinel K64.4
  skin L91.8
    accessory (congenital) Q82.8
    anus K64.4
    congenital Q82.8
    preauricular Q17.0
  tonsil J35.8
  urethra, urethral N36.8
  vulva N90.89
Tahyna fever B33.8
Takahara's disease E80.3
Takayasu's disease or syndrome M31.4
Talcosis (pulmonary) J62.0
Talipes (congenital) Q66.89
  acquired, planus — see Deformity, limb, flat foot
  asymmetric Q66.89
  calcaneovalgus Q66.4
  calcaneovarus Q66.1
  calcaneus Q66.89
  cavus Q66.7
  equinovalgus Q66.6
  equinovarus Q66.0
  equinus Q66.89
  percavus Q66.7
  planovalgus Q66.6
  planus (acquired) (any degree) (see also Deformity, limb, flat foot)
    congenital Q66.5- ☑
    due to rickets (sequelae) E64.3
  valgus Q66.6
  varus Q66.3
Tall stature, constitutional E34.4
Talma's disease M62.89
Talon noir S90.3- ☑
  hand S60.22- ☑
  heel S90.3- ☑
  toe S90.1- ☑
Tamponade, heart I31.4
Tanapox (virus disease) B08.71
Tangier disease E78.6
Tantrum, child problem F91.8
Tapeworm (infection) (infestation) — see Infestation, tapeworm
Tapia's syndrome G52.7
TAR (thrombocytopenia with absent radius) **syndrome** Q87.2
Tarral-Besnier disease L44.0
Tarsal tunnel syndrome — see Syndrome, tarsal tunnel
Tarsalgia — see Pain, limb, lower
Tarsitis (eyelid) H01.8
  syphilitic A52.71
  tuberculous A18.4
Tartar (teeth) (dental calculus) K03.6
Tattoo (mark) L81.8
Tauri's disease E74.09
Taurodontism K00.2
Taussig-Bing syndrome Q20.1
Taybi's syndrome Q87.2
Tay-Sachs amaurotic familial idiocy or disease E75.02
TBI (traumatic brain injury) S06.9 ☑
Teacher's node or nodule J38.2
Tear, torn (traumatic) (see also Laceration)
  with abortion — see Abortion
  annular fibrosis M51.35
  anus, anal (sphincter) S31.831 ☑
    complicating delivery
      with third degree perineal laceration (see also Delivery, complicated, by, laceration, perineum, third degree) O70.20
        with mucosa O70.3
      without third degree perineal laceration O70.4
    nontraumatic (healed) (old) K62.81
  articular cartilage, old — see Derangement, joint, articular cartilage, by site

Tear, torn — continued
  bladder
    with ectopic or molar pregnancy O08.6
    following ectopic or molar pregnancy O08.6
    obstetrical O71.5
    traumatic — see Injury, bladder
  bowel
    with ectopic or molar pregnancy O08.6
    following ectopic or molar pregnancy O08.6
    obstetrical trauma O71.5
  broad ligament
    with ectopic or molar pregnancy O08.6
    following ectopic or molar pregnancy O08.6
    obstetrical trauma O71.6
  bucket handle (knee) (meniscus) — see Tear, meniscus
  capsule, joint — see Sprain
  cartilage (see also Sprain)
    articular, old — see Derangement, joint, articular cartilage, by site
  cervix
    with ectopic or molar pregnancy O08.6
    following ectopic or molar pregnancy O08.6
    obstetrical trauma (current) O71.3
    old N88.1
    traumatic — see Injury, uterus
  dural G97.41
    nontraumatic G96.11
  internal organ — see Injury, by site
  knee cartilage
    articular (current) S83.3- ☑
    old — see Derangement, knee, meniscus, due to old tear
  ligament — see Sprain
  meniscus (knee) (current injury) S83.209 ☑
    bucket-handle S83.20- ☑
    lateral
      bucket-handle S83.25- ☑
      complex S83.27- ☑
      peripheral S83.26- ☑
      specified type NEC S83.28- ☑
    medial
      bucket-handle S83.21- ☑
      complex S83.23- ☑
      peripheral S83.22- ☑
      specified type NEC S83.24- ☑
    old — see Derangement, knee, meniscus, due to old tear
    site other than knee — code as Sprain
    specified type NEC S83.20- ☑
  muscle — see Strain
  pelvic
    floor, complicating delivery O70.1
    organ NEC, obstetrical trauma O71.5
      with ectopic or molar pregnancy O08.6
      following ectopic or molar pregnancy O08.6
  perineal, secondary O90.1
  periurethral tissue, obstetrical trauma O71.82
    with ectopic or molar pregnancy O08.6
    following ectopic or molar pregnancy O08.6
  rectovaginal septum — see Laceration, vagina
  retina, retinal (without detachment) (horseshoe) (see also Break, retina, horseshoe)
    with detachment — see Detachment, retina, with retinal, break
  rotator cuff (nontraumatic) M75.10- ☑
    complete M75.12- ☑
    incomplete M75.11- ☑
    traumatic S46.01- ☑
      capsule S43.42- ☑
  semilunar cartilage, knee — see Tear, meniscus
  supraspinatus (complete) (incomplete) (nontraumatic) (see also Tear, rotator cuff) M75.10- ☑
  tendon — see Strain
  tentorial, at birth P10.4
  umbilical cord
    complicating delivery O69.89 ☑
  urethra
    with ectopic or molar pregnancy O08.6
    following ectopic or molar pregnancy O08.6
    obstetrical trauma O71.5
  uterus — see Injury, uterus
  vagina — see Laceration, vagina
  vessel, from catheter — see Puncture, accidental complicating surgery
  vulva, complicating delivery O70.0
Tear-stone — see Dacryolith

Teeth (see also condition)
  grinding
    psychogenic F45.8
    sleep related G47.63
Teething (syndrome) K00.7
Telangiectasia, telangiectasis (verrucous) I78.1
  ataxic (cerebellar) (Louis-Bar) G11.3
  familial I78.0
  hemorrhagic, hereditary (congenital) (senile) I78.0
  hereditary, hemorrhagic (congenital) (senile) I78.0
  juxtafoveal H35.07- ☑
  macular H35.07- ☑
  macularis eruptiva perstans D47.01
  parafoveal H35.07- ☑
  retinal (idiopathic) (juxtafoveal) (macular) (parafoveal) H35.07- ☑
  spider I78.1
Telephone scatologia F65.89
Telescoped bowel or intestine K56.1
  congenital Q43.8
Temperature
  body, high (of unknown origin) R50.9
  cold, trauma from T69.9 ☑
    newborn P80.0
    specified effect NEC T69.8 ☑
Temple — see condition
Temporal — see condition
Temporomandibular joint pain-dysfunction syndrome M26.62- ☑
Temporosphenoidal — see condition
Tendency
  bleeding — see Defect, coagulation
  suicide
    meaning personal history of attempted suicide Z91.5
    meaning suicidal ideation — see Ideation, suicidal
    to fall R29.6
Tenderness, abdominal R10.819
  epigastric R10.816
  generalized R10.817
  left lower quadrant R10.814
  left upper quadrant R10.812
  periumbilic R10.815
  rebound R10.829
    epigastric R10.826
    generalized R10.827
    left lower quadrant R10.824
    left upper quadrant R10.822
    periumbilic R10.825
    right lower quadrant R10.823
    right upper quadrant R10.821
  right lower quadrant R10.813
  right upper quadrant R10.811
Tendinitis, tendonitis (see also Enthesopathy)
  Achilles M76.6- ☑
  adhesive — see Tenosynovitis, specified type NEC
    shoulder — see Capsulitis, adhesive
  bicipital M75.2- ☑
  calcific M65.2- ☑
    ankle M65.27- ☑
    foot M65.27- ☑
    forearm M65.23- ☑
    hand M65.24- ☑
    lower leg M65.26- ☑
    multiple sites M65.29
    pelvic region M65.25- ☑
    shoulder M75.3- ☑
    specified site NEC M65.28
    thigh M65.25- ☑
    upper arm M65.22- ☑
  due to use, overuse, pressure (see also Disorder, soft tissue, due to use)
    specified NEC — see Disorder, soft tissue, due to use, specified NEC
  gluteal M76.0- ☑
  patellar M76.5- ☑
  peroneal M76.7- ☑
  psoas M76.1- ☑
  tibial (posterior) M76.82- ☑
    anterior M76.81- ☑
  trochanteric — see Bursitis, hip, trochanteric
Tendon — see condition
Tendosynovitis — see Tenosynovitis
Tenesmus (rectal) R19.8
  vesical R30.1
Tennis elbow — see Epicondylitis, lateral

Tenonitis (see also Tenosynovitis)
  eye (capsule) H05.04- ☑
Tenontosynovitis — see Tenosynovitis
Tenontothecitis — see Tenosynovitis
Tenophyte — see Disorder, synovium, specified type NEC
Tenosynovitis (see also Synovitis) M65.9
  adhesive — see Tenosynovitis, specified type NEC
    shoulder — see Capsulitis, adhesive
  bicipital (calcifying) — see Tendinitis, bicipital
  gonococcal A54.49
  in (due to)
    crystals M65.8- ☑
    gonorrhea A54.49
    syphilis (late) A52.78
    use, overuse, pressure (see also Disorder, soft tissue, due to use)
      specified NEC — see Disorder, soft tissue, due to use, specified NEC
  infective NEC M65.1- ☑
    ankle M65.17- ☑
    foot M65.17- ☑
    forearm M65.13- ☑
    hand M65.14- ☑
    lower leg M65.16- ☑
    multiple sites M65.19
    pelvic region M65.15- ☑
    shoulder region M65.11- ☑
    specified site NEC M65.18
    thigh M65.15- ☑
    upper arm M65.12- ☑
  radial styloid M65.4
  shoulder region M65.81- ☑
    adhesive — see Capsulitis, adhesive
  specified type NEC M65.88
    ankle M65.87- ☑
    foot M65.87- ☑
    forearm M65.83- ☑
    hand M65.84- ☑
    lower leg M65.86- ☑
    multiple sites M65.89
    pelvic region M65.85- ☑
    shoulder region M65.81- ☑
    specified site NEC M65.88
    thigh M65.85- ☑
    upper arm M65.82- ☑
  tuberculous — see Tuberculosis, tenosynovitis
Tenovaginitis — see Tenosynovitis
Tension
  arterial, high (see also Hypertension)
    without diagnosis of hypertension R03.0
  headache G44.209
    intractable G44.201
    not intractable G44.209
  nervous R45.0
  pneumothorax J93.0
  premenstrual N94.3
  state (mental) F48.9
Tentorium — see condition
Teratencephalus Q89.8
Teratism Q89.7
Teratoblastoma (malignant) — see Neoplasm, malignant, by site
Teratocarcinoma (see also Neoplasm, malignant, by site)
  liver C22.7
Teratoma (solid) (see also Neoplasm, uncertain behavior, by site)
  with embryonal carcinoma, mixed — see Neoplasm, malignant, by site
  with malignant transformation — see Neoplasm, malignant, by site
  adult (cystic) — see Neoplasm, benign, by site
  benign — see Neoplasm, benign, by site
  combined with choriocarcinoma — see Neoplasm, malignant, by site
  cystic (adult) — see Neoplasm, benign, by site
  differentiated — see Neoplasm, benign, by site
  embryonal (see also Neoplasm, malignant, by site)
    liver C22.7
  immature — see Neoplasm, malignant, by site
  liver C22.7
    adult, benign, cystic, differentiated type or mature D13.4
  malignant (see also Neoplasm, malignant, by site)
    anaplastic — see Neoplasm, malignant, by site
    intermediate — see Neoplasm, malignant, by site

Teratoma — continued
  malignant (see also Neoplasm, malignant, by site) — continued
    intermediate — see Neoplasm, malignant, by site — continued
      specified site — see Neoplasm, malignant, by site
      unspecified site C62.90
    undifferentiated — see Neoplasm, malignant, by site
  mature — see Neoplasm, uncertain behavior, by site
    malignant — see Neoplasm, by site, malignant, by site
  ovary D27.- ☑
    embryonal, immature or malignant C56- ☑
  solid — see Neoplasm, uncertain behavior, by site
  testis C62.9-
    adult, benign, cystic, differentiated type or mature D29.2- ☑
    scrotal C62.1- ☑
    undescended C62.0- ☑
Termination
  anomalous (see also Malposition, congenital)
    right pulmonary vein Q26.3
  pregnancy, elective Z33.2
Ternidens diminutus infestation B81.8
Ternidensiasis B81.8
Terror(s) night (child) F51.4
Terrorism, victim of Z65.4
Terry's syndrome (see also Myopia, degenerative) H44.2- ☑
Tertiary — see condition
Test, tests, testing (for)
  adequacy (for dialysis)
    hemodialysis Z49.31
    peritoneal Z49.32
  blood pressure Z01.30
    abnormal reading — see Blood, pressure
  blood typing Z01.83
    Rh typing Z01.83
  blood-alcohol Z04.8
    positive — see Findings, abnormal, in blood
  blood-drug Z04.8
    positive — see Findings, abnormal, in blood
  cardiac pulse generator (battery) Z45.010
  fertility Z31.41
  genetic
    disease carrier status for procreative management
      female Z31.430
      male Z31.440
    male partner of patient with recurrent pregnancy loss Z31.441
    procreative management NEC
      female Z31.438
      male Z31.448
  hearing Z01.10
    with abnormal findings NEC Z01.118
  HIV (human immunodeficiency virus)
    nonconclusive (in infants) R75
    positive Z21
    seropositive Z21
  immunity status Z01.84
  intelligence NEC Z01.89
  laboratory (as part of a general medical examination) Z00.00
    with abnormal finding Z00.01
    for medicolegal reason NEC Z04.8
  male partner of patient with recurrent pregnancy loss Z31.441
  Mantoux (for tuberculosis) Z11.1
    abnormal result R76.11
  pregnancy, positive first pregnancy — see Pregnancy, normal, first
  procreative Z31.49
    fertility Z31.41
  skin, diagnostic
    allergy Z01.82
      special screening examination — see Screening, by name of disease
    Mantoux Z11.1
    tuberculin Z11.1
  specified NEC Z01.89
  tuberculin Z11.1
    abnormal result R76.11
  vision Z01.00
    with abnormal findings Z01.01
  Wassermann Z11.3
    positive — see Serology for syphilis, positive

☑ **Additional Character Required** — Refer to the Tabular List for Character Selection   ▽ **Subterms under main terms may continue to next column or page**

Testicle, testicular, testis (*see also* condition)
  feminization syndrome (*see also* Syndrome, androgen
    insensitivity) E34.51
  migrans Q55.29
Tetanus, tetanic (cephalic) (convulsions) A35
  with
    abortion A34
    ectopic or molar pregnancy O08.0
  following ectopic or molar pregnancy O08.0
  inoculation reaction (due to serum) — *see* Complica-
    tions, vaccination
  neonatorum A33
  obstetrical A34
  puerperal, postpartum, childbirth A34
Tetany (due to) R29.0
  alkalosis E87.3
  associated with rickets E55.0
  convulsions R29.0
    hysterical F44.5
  functional (hysterical) F44.5
  hyperkinetic R29.0
    hysterical F44.5
  hyperpnea R06.4
    hysterical F44.5
    psychogenic F45.8
  hyperventilation (*see also* Hyperventilation) R06.4
    hysterical F44.5
  neonatal (without calcium or magnesium deficiency)
    P71.3
  parathyroid (gland) E20.9
  parathyroprival E89.2
  post- (para)thyroidectomy E89.2
  postoperative E89.2
  pseudotetany R29.0
  psychogenic (conversion reaction) F44.5
Tetralogy of Fallot Q21.3
Tetraplegia (chronic) (*see also* Quadriplegia) G82.50
Thailand hemorrhagic fever A91
Thalassanemia — *see* Thalassemia
Thalassemia (anemia) (disease) D56.9
  with other hemoglobinopathy D56.8
  alpha (major) (severe) (triple gene defect) D56.0
    minor D56.3
      silent carrier D56.3
      trait D56.3
  beta (severe) D56.1
    homozygous D56.1
    major D56.1
    minor D56.3
    trait D56.3
  delta-beta (homozygous) D56.2
    minor D56.3
    trait D56.3
  dominant D56.8
  hemoglobin
    C D56.8
    E-beta D56.5
  intermedia D56.1
  major D56.1
  minor D56.3
  mixed D56.8
  sickle-cell — *see* Disease, sickle-cell, thalassemia
  specified type NEC D56.8
  trait D56.3
  variants D56.8
Thanatophoric dwarfism or short stature Q77.1
Thaysen-Gee disease (nontropical sprue) K90.0
Thaysen's disease K90.0
Thecoma D27-
  luteinized D27- ☑
  malignant C56- ☑
Thelarche, premature E30.8
Thelaziasis B83.8
Thelitis N61.0
  puerperal, postpartum or gestational — *see* Infection,
    nipple
Therapeutic — *see* condition
Therapy
  drug, long-term (current) (prophylactic)
    agents affecting estrogen receptors and estrogen
      levels NEC Z79.818
    anastrozole (Arimidex) Z79.811
    antibiotics Z79.2
      short-term use — *omit code*
    anticoagulants Z79.01
    anti-inflammatory Z79.1
    antiplatelet Z79.02
    antithrombotics Z79.02

Therapy — *continued*
  drug, long-term — *continued*
    aromatase inhibitors Z79.811
    aspirin Z79.82
    birth control pill or patch Z79.3
    bisphosphonates Z79.83
    contraceptive, oral Z79.3
    drug, specified NEC Z79.899
    estrogen receptor downregulators Z79.818
    Evista Z79.810
    exemestane (Aromasin) Z79.811
    Fareston Z79.810
    fulvestrant (Faslodex) Z79.818
    gonadotropin-releasing hormone (GnRH) agonist
      Z79.818
    goserelin acetate (Zoladex) Z79.818
    hormone replacement Z79.890
    insulin Z79.4
    letrozole (Femara) Z79.811
    leuprolide acetate (leuprorelin) (Lupron) Z79.818
    megestrol acetate (Megace) Z79.818
    methadone
      for pain management Z79.891
      maintenance therapy F11.20
    Nolvadex Z79.810
    opiate analgesic Z79.891
    oral contraceptive Z79.3
    raloxifene (Evista) Z79.810
    selective estrogen receptor modulators (SERMs)
      Z79.810
    short term — *omit code*
    steroids
      inhaled Z79.51
      systemic Z79.52
    tamoxifen (Nolvadex) Z79.810
    toremifene (Fareston) Z79.810
Thermic — *see* condition
Thermography (abnormal) (*see also* Abnormal, diagnostic imaging) R93.8
  breast R92.8
Thermoplegia T67.0 ☑
Thesaurismosis, glycogen — *see* Disease, glycogen
  storage
Thiamin deficiency E51.9
  specified NEC E51.8
Thiaminic deficiency with beriberi E51.11
Thibierge-Weissenbach syndrome — *see* Sclerosis,
  systemic
Thickening
  bone — *see* Hypertrophy, bone
  breast N64.59
  endometrium R93.8
  epidermal L85.9
    specified NEC L85.8
  hymen N89.6
  larynx J38.7
  nail L60.2
    congenital Q84.5
  periosteal — *see* Hypertrophy, bone
  pleura J92.9
    with asbestos J92.0
  skin R23.4
  subepiglottic J38.7
  tongue K14.8
  valve, heart — *see* Endocarditis
Thigh — *see* condition
Thinning vertebra — *see* Spondylopathy, specified NEC
Thirst, excessive R63.1
  due to deprivation of water T73.1 ☑
Thomsen disease G71.12
Thoracic (*see also* condition)
  kidney Q63.2
  outlet syndrome G54.0
Thoracogastroschisis (congenital) Q79.8
Thoracopagus Q89.4
Thorax — *see* condition
Thorn's syndrome N28.89
Thorson-Björck syndrome E34.0
Threadworm (infection) (infestation) B80
Threatened
  abortion O20.0
    with subsequent abortion O03.9
  job loss, anxiety concerning Z56.2
  labor (without delivery) O47.9
    at or after 37 completed weeks of gestation O47.1
    before 37 completed weeks of gestation O47.0- ☑
  loss of job, anxiety concerning Z56.2
  miscarriage O20.0

Threatened — *continued*
  unemployment, anxiety concerning Z56.2
Three-day fever A93.1
Threshers' lung J67.0
Thrix annulata (congenital) Q84.1
Throat — *see* condition
Thrombasthenia (Glanzmann) (hemorrhagic) (heredi-
  tary) D69.1
Thromboangiitis I73.1
  obliterans (general) I73.1
    cerebral I67.89
    vessels
      brain I67.89
      spinal cord I67.89
Thromboarteritis — *see* Arteritis
Thromboasthenia (Glanzmann) (hemorrhagic) (heredi-
  tary) D69.1
Thrombocytasthenia (Glanzmann) D69.1
Thrombocythemia (essential) (hemorrhagic) (idiopathic)
  (primary) D47.3
Thrombocytopathy (dystrophic) (granulopenic) D69.1
Thrombocytopenia, thrombocytopenic D69.6
  with absent radius (TAR) Q87.2
  congenital D69.42
  dilutional D69.59
  due to
    (massive) blood transfusion D69.59
    drugs D69.59
    extracorporeal circulation of blood D69.59
    platelet alloimmunization D69.59
  essential D69.3
  heparin induced (HIT) D75.82
  hereditary D69.42
  idiopathic D69.3
  neonatal, transitory P61.0
    due to
      exchange transfusion P61.0
      idiopathic maternal thrombocytopenia P61.0
      isoimmunization P61.0
  primary NEC D69.49
    idiopathic D69.3
  puerperal, postpartum O72.3
  secondary D69.59
  transient neonatal P61.0
Thrombocytosis, essential D47.3
  primary D47.3
Thromboembolism — *see* Embolism
Thrombopathy (Bernard-Soulier) D69.1
  constitutional D68.0
  Willebrand-Jurgens D68.0
Thrombopenia — *see* Thrombocytopenia
Thrombophilia D68.59
  primary NEC D68.59
  secondary NEC D68.69
  specified NEC D68.69
Thrombophlebitis I80.9
  antepartum O22.2- ☑
    deep O22.3- ☑
    superficial O22.2- ☑
  cavernous (venous) sinus G08
    complicating pregnancy O22.5- ☑
    nonpyogenic I67.6
  cerebral (sinus) (vein) G08
    nonpyogenic I67.6
    sequelae G09
  due to implanted device — *see* Complications, by site
    and type, specified NEC
  during or resulting from a procedure NEC T81.72 ☑
  femoral vein (superficial) I80.1- ☑
  femoropopliteal vein I80.0- ☑
  hepatic (vein) I80.8
  idiopathic, recurrent I82.1
  iliofemoral I80.1- ☑
  intracranial venous sinus (any) G08
    nonpyogenic I67.6
    sequelae G09
  intraspinal venous sinuses and veins G08
    nonpyogenic G95.19
  lateral (venous) sinus G08
    nonpyogenic I67.6
  leg I80.3
    superficial I80.0- ☑
  longitudinal (venous) sinus G08
    nonpyogenic I67.6
  lower extremity I80.299
  migrans, migrating I82.1
  pelvic
    with ectopic or molar pregnancy O08.0

Index

Thrombophlebitis — *continued*
  pelvic — *continued*
    following ectopic or molar pregnancy O08.0
    puerperal O87.1
  popliteal vein — *see* Phlebitis, leg, deep, popliteal
  portal (vein) K75.1
  postoperative T81.72 ☑
  pregnancy — *see* Thrombophlebitis, antepartum
  puerperal, postpartum, childbirth O87.0
    deep O87.1
    pelvic O87.1
    septic O86.81
    superficial O87.0
  saphenous (greater) (lesser) I80.0- ☑
  sinus (intracranial) G08
    nonpyogenic I67.6
  specified site NEC I80.8
  tibial vein I80.23- ☑
Thrombosis, thrombotic (bland) (multiple) (progressive)
  (silent) (vessel) I82.90
  anal K64.5
  antepartum — *see* Thrombophlebitis, antepartum
  aorta, aortic I74.10
    abdominal I74.09
      saddle I74.01
    bifurcation I74.09
    saddle I74.01
    specified site NEC I74.19
    terminal I74.09
    thoracic I74.11
    valve — *see* Endocarditis, aortic
  apoplexy I63.3- ☑
  artery, arteries (postinfectional) I74.9
    auditory, internal — *see* Occlusion, artery, precerebral, specified NEC
    basilar — *see* Occlusion, artery, basilar
    carotid (common) (internal) — *see* Occlusion, artery, carotid
    cerebellar (anterior inferior) (posterior inferior) (superior) — *see* Occlusion, artery, cerebellar
    cerebral — *see* Occlusion, artery, cerebral
    choroidal (anterior) — *see* Occlusion, artery, precerebral, specified NEC
    communicating, posterior — *see* Occlusion, artery, precerebral, specified NEC
    coronary (*see also* Infarct, myocardium)
      not resulting in infarction I24.0
    hepatic I74.8
    hypophyseal — *see* Occlusion, artery, precerebral, specified NEC
    iliac I74.5
    limb I74.4
      lower I74.3
      upper I74.2
    meningeal, anterior or posterior — *see* Occlusion, artery, cerebral, specified NEC
    mesenteric (with gangrene) (*see also* Infarct, intestine) K55.069
    ophthalmic — *see* Occlusion, artery, retina
    pontine — *see* Occlusion, artery, precerebral, specified NEC
    precerebral — *see* Occlusion, artery, precerebral
    pulmonary (iatrogenic) — *see* Embolism, pulmonary
    renal N28.0
    retinal — *see* Occlusion, artery, retina
    spinal, anterior or posterior G95.11
    traumatic NEC T14.8 ☑
    vertebral — *see* Occlusion, artery, vertebral
  atrium, auricular (*see also* Infarct, myocardium)
    following acute myocardial infarction (current complication) I23.6
    not resulting in infarction I51.3
    old I51.3
  basilar (artery) — *see* Occlusion, artery, basilar
  brain (artery) (stem) (*see also* Occlusion, artery, cerebral)
    due to syphilis A52.05
    puerperal O99.43
    sinus — *see* Thrombosis, intracranial venous sinus
  capillary I78.8
  cardiac (*see also* Infarct, myocardium)
    not resulting in infarction I51.3
    old I51.3
    valve — *see* Endocarditis
  carotid (artery) (common) (internal) — *see* Occlusion, artery, carotid

Thrombosis, thrombotic — *continued*
  cavernous (venous) sinus — *see* Thrombosis, intracranial venous sinus
  cerebellar artery (anterior inferior) (posterior inferior) (superior) I66.3
  cerebral (artery) — *see* Occlusion, artery, cerebral
  cerebrovenous sinus (*see also* Thrombosis, intracranial venous sinus)
    puerperium O87.3
  chronic I82.91
  coronary (artery) (vein) (*see also* Infarct, myocardium)
    not resulting in infarction I24.0
  corpus cavernosum N48.89
  cortical I66.9
  deep — *see* Embolism, vein, lower extremity
  due to device, implant or graft (*see also* Complications, by site and type, specified NEC) T85.868 ☑
    arterial graft NEC T82.868 ☑
    breast (implant) T85.868 ☑
    catheter NEC T85.868 ☑
      dialysis (renal) T82.868 ☑
        intraperitoneal T85.868 ☑
      infusion NEC T82.868 ☑
        spinal (epidural) (subdural) T85.860 ☑
      urinary (indwelling) T83.86 ☑
    electronic (electrode) (pulse generator) (stimulator)
      bone T84.86 ☑
      cardiac T82.867 ☑
      nervous system (brain) (peripheral nerve) (spinal) T85.860 ☑
      urinary T83.86 ☑
    fixation, internal (orthopedic) NEC T84.86 ☑
    gastrointestinal (bile duct) (esophagus) T85.868 ☑
    genital NEC T83.86 ☑
    heart T82.867 ☑
    joint prosthesis T84.86 ☑
    ocular (corneal graft) (orbital implant) NEC T85.868 ☑
    orthopedic NEC T84.86 ☑
    specified NEC T85.868 ☑
    urinary NEC T83.86 ☑
    vascular NEC T82.868 ☑
    ventricular intracranial shunt T85.860 ☑
  during the puerperium — *see* Thrombosis, puerperal
  endocardial (*see also* Infarct, myocardium)
    not resulting in infarction I51.3
  eye — *see* Occlusion, retina
  genital organ
    female NEC N94.89
      pregnancy — *see* Thrombophlebitis, antepartum
    male N50.1
  gestational — *see* Phlebopathy, gestational
  heart (chamber) (*see also* Infarct, myocardium)
    not resulting in infarction I51.3
    old I51.3
  hepatic (vein) I82.0
    artery I74.8
  history (of) Z86.718
  intestine (with gangrene) (*see also* Infarct, intestine) K55.069
  intracardiac NEC (apical) (atrial) (auricular) (ventricular) (old) I51.3
  intracranial (arterial) I66.9
    venous sinus (any) G08
      nonpyogenic origin I67.6
      puerperium O87.3
  intramural (*see also* Infarct, myocardium)
    not resulting in infarction I51.3
    old I51.3
  intraspinal venous sinuses and veins G08
    nonpyogenic G95.19
  kidney (artery) N28.0
  lateral (venous) sinus — *see* Thrombosis, intracranial venous sinus
  leg — *see* Thrombosis, vein, lower extremity
    arterial I74.3
  liver (venous) I82.0
    artery I74.8
    portal vein I81
  longitudinal (venous) sinus — *see* Thrombosis, intracranial venous sinus
  lower limb — *see* Thrombosis, vein, lower extremity
  lung (iatrogenic) (postoperative) — *see* Embolism, pulmonary
  meninges (brain) (arterial) I66.8

Thrombosis, thrombotic — *continued*
  mesenteric (artery) (with gangrene) (*see also* Infarct, intestine) K55.069
    vein (inferior) (superior) I81
  mitral I34.8
  mural (*see also* Infarct, myocardium)
    due to syphilis A52.06
    not resulting in infarction I51.3
    old I51.3
  omentum (with gangrene) (*see also* Infarct, intestine) K55.069
  ophthalmic — *see* Occlusion, retina
  pampiniform plexus (male) N50.1
  parietal (*see also* Infarct, myocardium)
    not resulting in infarction I24.0
  penis, superficial vein N48.81
  perianal venous K64.5
  peripheral arteries I74.4
    upper I74.2
  personal history (of) Z86.718
  portal I81
    due to syphilis A52.09
  precerebral artery — *see* Occlusion, artery, precerebral
  puerperal, postpartum O87.0
    brain (artery) O99.43
      venous (sinus) O87.3
    cardiac O99.43
    cerebral (artery) O99.43
      venous (sinus) O87.3
    superficial O87.0
  pulmonary (artery) (iatrogenic) (postoperative) (vein) — *see* Embolism, pulmonary
  renal (artery) N28.0
    vein I82.3
  resulting from presence of device, implant or graft — *see* Complications, by site and type, specified NEC
  retina, retinal — *see* Occlusion, retina
  scrotum N50.1
  seminal vesicle N50.1
  sigmoid (venous) sinus — *see* Thrombosis, intracranial venous sinus
  sinus, intracranial (any) — *see* Thrombosis, intracranial venous sinus
  specified site NEC I82.890
    chronic I82.891
  spermatic cord N50.1
  spinal cord (arterial) G95.11
    due to syphilis A52.09
    pyogenic origin G06.1
  spleen, splenic D73.5
    artery I74.8
  testis N50.1
  traumatic NEC T14.8 ☑
  tricuspid I07.8
  tumor — *see* Neoplasm, unspecified behavior, by site
  tunica vaginalis N50.1
  umbilical cord (vessels), complicating delivery O69.5 ☑
  vas deferens N50.1
  vein (acute) I82.90
    antecubital I82.61- ☑
      chronic I82.71- ☑
    axillary I82.A1- ☑ (*following* I82.7)
      chronic I82.A2- ☑ (*following* I82.7)
    basilic I82.61- ☑
      chronic I82.71- ☑
    brachial I82.62- ☑
      chronic I82.72- ☑
    brachiocephalic (innominate) I82.290
      chronic I82.291
    cephalic I82.61- ☑
      chronic I82.71- ☑
    cerebral, nonpyogenic I67.6
    chronic I82.91
    deep (DVT) I82.40- ☑
      calf I82.4Z- ☑
        chronic I82.5Z- ☑
      lower leg I82.4Z- ☑
        chronic I82.5Z- ☑
      thigh I82.4Y- ☑
        chronic I82.5Y- ☑
      upper leg I82.4Y ☑
        chronic I82.5Y- ☑
    femoral I82.41- ☑
      chronic I82.51- ☑
    iliac (iliofemoral) I82.42- ☑
      chronic I82.52- ☑

Thrombosis, thrombotic — continued
  vein — continued
    innominate I82.290
      chronic I82.291
    internal jugular I82.C1- ☑ (following I82.7)
      chronic I82.C2- ☑ (following I82.7)
    lower extremity
      deep I82.40- ☑
        chronic I82.50- ☑
        specified NEC I82.49- ☑
          chronic NEC I82.59- ☑
      distal
        deep I82.4Z- ☑
      proximal
        deep I82.4Y- ☑
          chronic I82.5Y- ☑
      superficial I82.81- ☑
    perianal K64.5
    popliteal I82.43- ☑
      chronic I82.53- ☑
    radial I82.62- ☑
      chronic I82.72- ☑
    renal I82.3
    saphenous (greater) (lesser) I82.81- ☑
    specified NEC I82.890
      chronic NEC I82.891
    subclavian I82.B1- ☑ (following I82.7)
      chronic I82.B2- ☑ (following I82.7)
    thoracic NEC I82.290
      chronic I82.291
    tibial I82.44- ☑
      chronic I82.54- ☑
    ulnar I82.62- ☑
      chronic I82.72- ☑
    upper extremity I82.60- ☑
      chronic I82.70- ☑
      deep I82.62- ☑
        chronic I82.72- ☑
      superficial I82.61- ☑
        chronic I82.71- ☑
  vena cava
    inferior I82.220
      chronic I82.221
    superior I82.210
      chronic I82.211
  venous, perianal K64.5
  ventricle (see also Infarct, myocardium)
    following acute myocardial infarction (current complication) I23.6
    not resulting in infarction I24.0
    old I51.3
Thrombus — see Thrombosis
Thrush (see also Candidiasis)
  newborn P37.5
  oral B37.0
  vaginal B37.3
Thumb (see also condition)
  sucking (child problem) F98.8
Thymitis E32.8
Thymoma (benign) D15.0
  malignant C37
Thymus, thymic (gland) — see condition
Thyrocele — see Goiter
Thyroglossal (see also condition)
  cyst Q89.2
  duct, persistent Q89.2
Thyroid (gland) (body) (see also condition)
  hormone resistance E07.89
  lingual Q89.2
  nodule (cystic) (nontoxic) (single) E04.1
Thyroiditis E06.9
  acute (nonsuppurative) (pyogenic) (suppurative) E06.0
  autoimmune E06.3
  chronic (nonspecific) (sclerosing) E06.5
    with thyrotoxicosis, transient E06.2
    fibrous E06.5
    lymphadenoid E06.3
    lymphocytic E06.3
    lymphoid E06.3
  de Quervain's E06.1
  drug-induced E06.4
  fibrous (chronic) E06.5
  giant-cell (follicular) E06.1
  granulomatous (de Quervain) (subacute) E06.1
  Hashimoto's (struma lymphomatosa) E06.3
  iatrogenic E06.4
  ligneous E06.5

Thyroiditis — continued
  lymphocytic (chronic) E06.3
  lymphoid E06.3
  lymphomatous E06.3
  nonsuppurative E06.1
  postpartum, puerperal O90.5
  pseudotuberculous E06.1
  pyogenic E06.0
  radiation E06.4
  Riedel's E06.5
  subacute (granulomatous) E06.1
  suppurative E06.0
  tuberculous A18.81
  viral E06.1
  woody E06.5
Thyrolingual duct, persistent Q89.2
Thyromegaly E01.0
Thyrotoxic
  crisis — see Thyrotoxicosis
  heart disease or failure (see also Thyrotoxicosis) E05.90 [I43]
    with thyroid storm E05.91 [I43]
  storm — see Thyrotoxicosis
Thyrotoxicosis (recurrent) E05.90
  with
    goiter (diffuse) E05.00
      with thyroid storm E05.01
      adenomatous uninodular E05.10
        with thyroid storm E05.11
      multinodular E05.20
        with thyroid storm E05.21
      nodular E05.20
        with thyroid storm E05.21
      uninodular E05.10
        with thyroid storm E05.11
    infiltrative
      dermopathy E05.00
        with thyroid storm E05.01
      ophthalmopathy E05.00
        with thyroid storm E05.01
    single thyroid nodule E05.10
      with thyroid storm E05.11
    thyroid storm E05.91
  due to
    ectopic thyroid nodule or tissue E05.30
      with thyroid storm E05.31
    ingestion of (excessive) thyroid material E05.40
      with thyroid storm E05.41
    overproduction of thyroid-stimulating hormone E05.80
      with thyroid storm E05.81
    specified cause NEC E05.80
      with thyroid storm E05.81
  factitia E05.40
    with thyroid storm E05.41
  heart (see also Failure, heart, high-output) E05.90 [I43]
    with thyroid storm (see also Failure, heart, high-output) E05.91 [I43]
    failure (see also Failure, heart, high-output) E05.90 [I43]
  neonatal (transient) P72.1
  transient with chronic thyroiditis E06.2
Tibia vara — see Osteochondrosis, juvenile, tibia
Tic (disorder) F95.9
  breathing F95.8
  child problem F95.0
  compulsive F95.1
  de la Tourette F95.2
  degenerative (generalized) (localized) G25.69
    facial G25.69
  disorder
    chronic
      motor F95.1
      vocal F95.1
    combined vocal and multiple motor F95.2
    transient F95.0
  douloureux G50.0
    atypical G50.1
    postherpetic, postzoster B02.22
  drug-induced G25.61
  eyelid F95.8
  habit F95.9
    chronic F95.1
    transient of childhood F95.0
  lid, transient of childhood F95.0
  motor-verbal F95.2
  occupational F48.8
  orbicularis F95.8

Tic — continued
  orbicularis — continued
    transient of childhood F95.0
  organic origin G25.69
  postchoreic G25.69
  provisional F95.0
  psychogenic, compulsive F95.1
  salaam R25.8
  spasm (motor or vocal) F95.9
    chronic F95.1
    transient of childhood F95.0
  specified NEC F95.8
Tick-borne — see condition
Tietze's disease or syndrome M94.0
Tight, tightness
  anus K62.89
  chest R07.89
  fascia (lata) M62.89
  foreskin (congenital) N47.1
  hymen, hymenal ring N89.6
  introitus (acquired) (congenital) N89.6
  rectal sphincter K62.89
  tendon — see Short, tendon
  urethral sphincter N35.9
Tilting vertebra — see Dorsopathy, deforming, specified NEC
Timidity, child F93.8
Tinea (intersecta) (tarsi) B35.9
  amiantacea L44.8
  asbestina B35.0
  barbae B35.0
  beard B35.0
  black dot B35.0
  blanca B36.2
  capitis B35.0
  corporis B35.4
  cruris B35.6
  flava B36.0
  foot B35.3
  furfuracea B36.0
  imbricata (Tokelau) B35.5
  kerion B35.0
  manuum B35.2
  microsporic — see Dermatophytosis
  nigra B36.1
  nodosa — see Piedra
  pedis B35.3
  scalp B35.0
  specified NEC B35.8
  sycosis B35.0
  tonsurans B35.0
  trichophytic — see Dermatophytosis
  unguium B35.1
  versicolor B36.0
Tingling sensation (skin) R20.2
Tin-miner's lung J63.5
Tinnitus NOS H93.1- ☑
  audible H93.1- ☑
  aurium H93.1- ☑
  pulsatile H93.A- ☑
  subjective H93.1- ☑
Tipped tooth (teeth) M26.33
Tipping
  pelvis M95.5
    with disproportion (fetopelvic) O33.0
      causing obstructed labor O65.0
  tooth (teeth), fully erupted M26.33
Tiredness R53.83
Tissue — see condition
Tobacco (nicotine)
  abuse — see Tobacco, use
  dependence — see Dependence, drug, nicotine
  harmful use Z72.0
  heart — see Tobacco, toxic effect
  maternal use, affecting newborn P04.2
  toxic effect — see Table of Drugs and Chemicals, by substance, poisoning
    chewing tobacco — see Table of Drugs and Chemicals, by substance, poisoning
    cigarettes — see Table of Drugs and Chemicals, by substance, poisoning
  use Z72.0
    complicating
      childbirth O99.334
      pregnancy O99.33- ☑
      puerperium O99.335
    counseling and surveillance Z71.6
    history Z87.891

Tobacco — *continued*
  withdrawal state (*see also* Dependence, drug, nicotine) F17.203
Tocopherol deficiency E56.0
Todd's
  cirrhosis K74.3
  paralysis (postepileptic) (transitory) G83.84
Toe — *see* condition
Toilet, artificial opening — *see* Attention to, artificial, opening
Tokelau (ringworm) B35.5
Tollwut — *see* Rabies
Tommaselli's disease R31.9
  correct substance properly administered — *see* Table of Drugs and Chemicals, by drug, adverse effect
  overdose or wrong substance given or taken — *see* Table of Drugs and Chemicals, by drug, poisoning
Tongue (*see also* condition)
  tie Q38.1
Tonic pupil — *see* Anomaly, pupil, function, tonic pupil
Toni-Fanconi syndrome (cystinosis) E72.09
  with cystinosis E72.04
Tonsil — *see* condition
Tonsillitis (acute) (catarrhal) (croupous) (follicular) (gangrenous) (infective) (lacunar) (lingual) (malignant) (membranous) (parenchymatous) (phlegmonous) (pseudomembranous) (purulent) (septic) (subacute) (suppurative) (toxic) (ulcerative) (vesicular) (viral) J03.90
  chronic J35.01
    with adenoiditis J35.03
  diphtheritic A36.0
  hypertrophic J35.01
    with adenoiditis J35.03
  recurrent J03.91
  specified organism NEC J03.80
    recurrent J03.81
  staphylococcal J03.80
    recurrent J03.81
  streptococcal J03.00
    recurrent J03.01
  tuberculous A15.8
  Vincent's A69.1
Tooth, teeth — *see* condition
Toothache K08.89
Topagnosis R20.8
Tophi — *see* Gout, chronic
TORCH infection — *see* Infection, congenital
  without active infection P00.2
Torn — *see* Tear
Tornwaldt's cyst or disease J39.2
Torsion
  accessory tube — *see* Torsion, fallopian tube
  adnexa (female) — *see* Torsion, fallopian tube
  aorta, acquired I77.1
  appendix epididymis N44.04
  appendix testis N44.03
  bile duct (common) (hepatic) K83.8
    congenital Q44.5
  bowel, colon or intestine K56.2
  cervix — *see* Malposition, uterus
  cystic duct K82.8
  dystonia — *see* Dystonia, torsion
  epididymis (appendix) N44.04
  fallopian tube N83.52- ☑
    with ovary N83.53
  gallbladder K82.8
    congenital Q44.1
  hydatid of Morgagni
    female N83.52- ☑
    male N44.03
  kidney (pedicle) (leading to infarction) N28.0
  Meckel's diverticulum (congenital) Q43.0
    malignant — *see* Table of Neoplasms, small intestine, malignant
  mesentery K56.2
  omentum K56.2
  organ or site, congenital NEC — *see* Anomaly, by site
  ovary (pedicle) N83.51- ☑
    with fallopian tube N83.53
    congenital Q50.2
  oviduct — *see* Torsion, fallopian tube
  penis (acquired) N48.82
    congenital Q55.63
  spasm — *see* Dystonia, torsion
  spermatic cord N44.02
    extravaginal N44.01

Torsion — *continued*
  spermatic cord — *continued*
    intravaginal N44.02
  spleen D73.5
  testis, testicle N44.00
    appendix N44.03
  tibia — *see* Deformity, limb, specified type NEC, lower leg
  uterus — *see* Malposition, uterus
Torticollis (intermittent) (spastic) M43.6
  congenital (sternomastoid) Q68.0
  due to birth injury P15.8
  hysterical F44.4
  ocular R29.891
  psychogenic F45.8
    conversion reaction F44.4
  rheumatic M43.6
  rheumatoid M06.88
  spasmodic G24.3
  traumatic, current S13.4 ☑
Tortipelvis G24.1
Tortuous
  aortic arch Q25.46
  artery I77.1
  organ or site, congenital NEC — *see* Distortion
  retinal vessel, congenital Q14.1
  ureter N13.8
  urethra N36.8
  vein — *see* Varix
Torture, victim of Z65.4
Torula, torular (histolytica) (infection) — *see* Cryptococcosis
Torulosis — *see* Cryptococcosis
Torus (mandibularis) (palatinus) M27.0
  fracture — *see* Fracture, by site, torus
Touraine's syndrome Q79.8
Tourette's syndrome F95.2
Tourniquet syndrome — *see* Constriction, external, by site
Tower skull Q75.0
  with exophthalmos Q87.0
Toxemia R68.89
  bacterial — *see* Sepsis
  burn — *see* Burn
  eclamptic (with pre-existing hypertension) — *see* Eclampsia
  erysipelatous — *see* Erysipelas
  fatigue R68.89
  food — *see* Poisoning, food
  gastrointestinal K52.1
  intestinal K52.1
  kidney — *see* Uremia
  malarial — *see* Malaria
  myocardial — *see* Myocarditis, toxic
  of pregnancy — *see* Pre-eclampsia
  pre-eclamptic — *see* Pre-eclampsia
  small intestine K52.1
  staphylococcal, due to food A05.0
  stasis R68.89
  uremic — *see* Uremia
  urinary — *see* Uremia
Toxemica cerebropathia psychica (nonalcoholic) F04
  alcoholic — *see* Alcohol, amnestic disorder
Toxic (poisoning) (*see also* condition) T65.91 ☑
  effect — *see* Table of Drugs and Chemicals, by substance, poisoning
  shock syndrome A48.3
  thyroid (gland) — *see* Thyrotoxicosis
Toxicemia — *see* Toxemia
Toxicity — *see* Table of Drugs and Chemicals, by substance, poisoning
  fava bean D55.0
  food, noxious — *see* Poisoning, food
  from drug or nonmedicinal substance — *see* Table of Drugs and Chemicals, by drug
Toxicosis (*see also* Toxemia)
  capillary, hemorrhagic D69.0
Toxinfection, gastrointestinal K52.1
Toxocariasis B83.0
Toxoplasma, toxoplasmosis (acquired) B58.9
  with
    hepatitis B58.1
    meningoencephalitis B58.2
    ocular involvement B58.00
    other organ involvement B58.89
    pneumonia, pneumonitis B58.3
  congenital (acute) (subacute) (chronic) P37.1

Toxoplasma, toxoplasmosis — *continued*
  maternal, manifest toxoplasmosis in infant (acute) (subacute) (chronic) P37.1
tPA (rtPA) **administration in a different facility within the last 24 hours prior to admission to current facility** Z92.82
Trabeculation, bladder N32.89
Trachea — *see* condition
Tracheitis (catarrhal) (infantile) (membranous) (plastic) (septal) (suppurative) (viral) J04.10
  with
    bronchitis (15 years of age and above) J40
      acute or subacute — *see* Bronchitis, acute
      chronic J42
      tuberculous NEC A15.5
      under 15 years of age J20.9
    laryngitis (acute) J04.2
      chronic J37.1
      tuberculous NEC A15.5
  acute J04.10
    with obstruction J04.11
  chronic J42
    with
      bronchitis (chronic) J42
      laryngitis (chronic) J37.1
  diphtheritic (membranous) A36.89
  due to external agent — *see* Inflammation, respiratory, upper, due to
  syphilitic A52.73
  tuberculous A15.5
Trachelitis (nonvenereal) — *see* Cervicitis
Tracheobronchial — *see* condition
Tracheobronchitis (15 years of age and above) (*see also* Bronchitis)
  due to
    Bordetella bronchiseptica A37.80
      with pneumonia A37.81
    Francisella tularensis A21.8
Tracheobronchomegaly Q32.4
  with bronchiectasis J47.9
    with
      exacerbation (acute) J47.1
      lower respiratory infection J47.0
  acquired J98.09
    with bronchiectasis J47.9
      with
        exacerbation (acute) J47.1
        lower respiratory infection J47.0
Tracheobronchopneumonitis — *see* Pneumonia, broncho-
Tracheocele (external) (internal) J39.8
  congenital Q32.1
Tracheomalacia J39.8
  congenital Q32.0
Tracheopharyngitis (acute) J06.9
  chronic J42
  due to external agent — *see* Inflammation, respiratory, upper, due to
Tracheostenosis J39.8
Tracheostomy
  complication — *see* Complication, tracheostomy
  status Z93.0
    attention to Z43.0
    malfunctioning J95.03
Trachoma, trachomatous A71.9
  active (stage) A71.1
  contraction of conjunctiva A71.1
  dubium A71.0
  healed or sequelae B94.0
  initial (stage) A71.0
  pannus A71.1
  Türck's J37.0
Traction, vitreomacular H43.82- ☑
Train sickness T75.3 ☑
Trait(s)
  Hb-S D57.3
  hemoglobin
    abnormal NEC D58.2
      with thalassemia D56.3
    C — *see* Disease, hemoglobin C
    S (Hb-S) D57.3
  Lepore D56.3
  personality, accentuated Z73.1
  sickle-cell D57.3
    with elliptocytosis or spherocytosis D57.3
  type A personality Z73.1
Tramp Z59.0
Trance R41.89

312

☑ Additional Character Required — Refer to the Tabular List for Character Selection   ▽ Subterms under main terms may continue to next column or page

Trance — *continued*
  hysterical F44.89
Transaminasemia R74.0
Transection
  abdomen (partial) S38.3 ☑
  aorta (incomplete) (*see also* Injury, aorta)
    complete — *see* Injury, aorta, laceration, major
  carotid artery (incomplete) (*see also* Injury, blood vessel, carotid, laceration)
    complete — *see* Injury, blood vessel, carotid, laceration, major
  celiac artery (incomplete) S35.211 ☑
    branch (incomplete) S35.291 ☑
      complete S35.292 ☑
    complete S35.212 ☑
  innominate
    artery (incomplete) (*see also* Injury, blood vessel, thoracic, innominate, artery, laceration)
      complete — *see* Injury, blood vessel, thoracic, innominate, artery, laceration, major
    vein (incomplete) (*see also* Injury, blood vessel, thoracic, innominate, vein, laceration)
      complete — *see* Injury, blood vessel, thoracic, innominate, vein, laceration, major
  jugular vein (external) (incomplete) (*see also* Injury, blood vessel, jugular vein, laceration)
    complete — *see* Injury, blood vessel, jugular vein, laceration, major
    internal (incomplete) (*see also* Injury, blood vessel, jugular vein, internal, laceration)
      complete — *see* Injury, blood vessel, jugular vein, internal, laceration, major
  mesenteric artery (incomplete) (*see also* Injury, mesenteric, artery, laceration)
    complete — *see* Injury, mesenteric artery, laceration, major
  pulmonary vessel (incomplete) (*see also* Injury, blood vessel, thoracic, pulmonary, laceration)
    complete — *see* Injury, blood vessel, thoracic, pulmonary, laceration, major
  subclavian — *see* Transection, innominate
  vena cava (incomplete) (*see also* Injury, vena cava)
    complete — *see* Injury, vena cava, laceration, major
  vertebral artery (incomplete) (*see also* Injury, blood vessel, vertebral, laceration)
    complete — *see* Injury, blood vessel, vertebral, laceration, major
Transfusion
  associated (red blood cell) hemochromatosis E83.111
  blood
    ABO incompatible — *see* Complication(s), transfusion, incompatibility reaction, ABO
    minor blood group (Duffy) (E) (K(ell)) (Kidd) (Lewis) (M) (N) (P) (S) T80.89 ☑
    reaction or complication — *see* Complications, transfusion
  fetomaternal (mother) — *see* Pregnancy, complicated by, placenta, transfusion syndrome
  maternofetal (mother) — *see* Pregnancy, complicated by, placenta, transfusion syndrome
  placental (syndrome) (mother) — *see* Pregnancy, complicated by, placenta, transfusion syndrome
  reaction (adverse) — *see* Complications, transfusion
  related acute lung injury (TRALI) J95.84
  twin-to-twin — *see* Pregnancy, complicated by, placenta, transfusion syndrome, fetus to fetus
Transient (meaning homeless) (*see also* condition) Z59.0
Translocation
  balanced autosomal Q95.9
    in normal individual Q95.0
  chromosomes NEC Q99.8
    balanced and insertion in normal individual Q95.0
  Down syndrome Q90.2
  trisomy
    13 Q91.6
    18 Q91.2
    21 Q90.2
Translucency, iris — *see* Degeneration, iris
Transmission of chemical substances through the placenta — *see* Absorption, chemical, through placenta
Transparency, lung, unilateral J43.0
Transplant (ed) (status) Z94.9
  awaiting organ Z76.82
  bone Z94.6
    marrow Z94.81
  candidate Z76.82

Transplant — *continued*
  complication — *see* Complication, transplant
  cornea Z94.7
  heart Z94.1
    and lung(s) Z94.3
    valve Z95.2
      prosthetic Z95.2
      specified NEC Z95.4
      xenogenic Z95.3
  intestine Z94.82
  kidney Z94.0
  liver Z94.4
  lung(s) Z94.2
    and heart Z94.3
  organ (failure) (infection) (rejection) Z94.9
    removal status Z98.85
  pancreas Z94.83
  skin Z94.5
  social Z60.3
  specified organ or tissue NEC Z94.89
  stem cells Z94.84
  tissue Z94.9
Transplants, ovarian, endometrial N80.1
Transposed — *see* Transposition
Transposition (congenital) (*see also* Malposition, congenital)
  abdominal viscera Q89.3
  aorta (dextra) Q20.3
  appendix Q43.8
  colon Q43.8
  corrected Q20.5
  great vessels (complete) (partial) Q20.3
  heart Q24.0
    with complete transposition of viscera Q89.3
  intestine (large) (small) Q43.8
  reversed jejunal (for bypass) (status) Z98.0
  scrotum Q55.23
  stomach Q40.2
    with general transposition of viscera Q89.3
  tooth, teeth, fully erupted M26.30
  vessels, great (complete) (partial) Q20.3
  viscera (abdominal) (thoracic) Q89.3
Transsexualism F64.0
Transverse (*see also* condition)
  arrest (deep), in labor O64.0 ☑
  lie (mother) O32.2 ☑
    causing obstructed labor O64.8 ☑
Transvestism, transvestitism (dual-role) F64.1
  fetishistic F65.1
Trapped placenta (with hemorrhage) O72.0
  without hemorrhage O73.0
TRAPS (tumor necrosis factor receptor associated periodic syndrome) M04.1
Trauma, traumatism (*see also* Injury)
  acoustic — *see* subcategory H83.3 ☑
  birth — *see* Birth, injury
  complicating ectopic or molar pregnancy O08.6
  during delivery O71.9
  following ectopic or molar pregnancy O08.6
  obstetric O71.9
    specified NEC O71.89
  occlusal
    primary K08.81
    secondary K08.82
Traumatic (*see also* condition)
  brain injury S06.9 ☑
Treacher Collins syndrome Q75.4
Treitz's hernia — *see* Hernia, abdomen, specified site NEC
Trematode infestation — *see* Infestation, fluke
Trematodiasis — *see* Infestation, fluke
Trembling paralysis — *see* Parkinsonism
Tremor(s) R25.1
  drug induced G25.1
  essential (benign) G25.0
  familial G25.0
  hereditary G25.0
  hysterical F44.4
  intention G25.2
  medication induced postural G25.1
  mercurial — *see* subcategory T56.1 ☑
  Parkinson's — *see* Parkinsonism
  psychogenic (conversion reaction) F44.4
  senilis R54
  specified type NEC G25.2
Trench
  fever A79.0
  foot — *see* Immersion, foot

Trench — *continued*
  mouth A69.1
Treponema pallidum infection — *see* Syphilis
Treponematosis
  due to
    T. pallidum — *see* Syphilis
    T. pertenue — *see* Yaws
Triad
  Hutchinson's (congenital syphilis) A50.53
  Kartagener's Q89.3
  Saint's — *see* Hernia, diaphragm
Trichiasis (eyelid) H02.059
  with entropion — *see* Entropion
  left H02.056
    lower H02.055
    upper H02.054
  right H02.053
    lower H02.052
    upper H02.051
Trichinella spiralis (infection) (infestation) B75
Trichinellosis, trichiniasis, trichinelliasis, trichinosis B75
  with muscle disorder B75 [M63.80]
    ankle B75 [M63.87-] ☑
    foot B75 [M63.87-] ☑
    forearm B75 [M63.83-] ☑
    hand B75 [M63.84-] ☑
    lower leg B75 [M63.86-] ☑
    multiple sites B75 [M63.89]
    pelvic region B75 [M63.85-] ☑
    shoulder region B75 [M63.81-] ☑
    specified site NEC B75 [M63.88]
    thigh B75 [M63.85-] ☑
    upper arm B75 [M63.82-] ☑
Trichobezoar T18.9 ☑
  intestine T18.3 ☑
  stomach T18.2 ☑
Trichocephaliasis, trichocephalosis B79
Trichocephalus infestation B79
Trichoclasis L67.8
Trichoepithelioma (*see also* Neoplasm, skin, benign)
  malignant — *see* Neoplasm, skin, malignant
Trichofolliculoma — *see* Neoplasm, skin, benign
Tricholemmoma — *see* Neoplasm, skin, benign
Trichomoniasis A59.9
  bladder A59.03
  cervix A59.09
  intestinal A07.8
  prostate A59.02
  seminal vesicles A59.09
  specified site NEC A59.8
  urethra A59.03
  urogenitalis A59.00
  vagina A59.01
  vulva A59.01
Trichomycosis
  axillaris A48.8
  nodosa, nodularis B36.8
Trichonodosis L67.8
Trichophytid, trichophyton infection — *see* Dermatophytosis
Trichophytobezoar T18.9 ☑
  intestine T18.3 ☑
  stomach T18.2 ☑
Trichophytosis — *see* Dermatophytosis
Trichoptilosis L67.8
Trichorrhexis (nodosa) (invaginata) L67.0
Trichosis axillaris A48.8
Trichosporosis nodosa B36.2
Trichostasis spinulosa (congenital) Q84.1
Trichostrongyliasis, trichostrongylosis (small intestine) B81.2
Trichostrongylus infection B81.2
Trichotillomania F63.3
Trichromat, trichromatopsia, anomalous (congenital) H53.55
Trichuriasis B79
Trichuris trichiura (infection) (infestation) (any site) B79
Tricuspid (valve) — *see* condition
Trifid (*see also* Accessory)
  kidney (pelvis) Q63.8
  tongue Q38.3
Trigeminal neuralgia — *see* Neuralgia, trigeminal
Trigeminy R00.8
Trigger finger (acquired) M65.30
  congenital Q74.0
  index finger M65.32- ☑

Trigger finger — *continued*
little finger M65.35- ☑
middle finger M65.33- ☑
ring finger M65.34- ☑
thumb M65.31- ☑
Trigonitis (bladder) (chronic) (pseudomembranous) N30.30
with hematuria N30.31
Trigonocephaly Q75.0
Trilocular heart — *see* Cor triloculare
Trimethylaminuria E72.52
Tripartite placenta O43.19- ☑
Triphalangeal thumb Q74.0
Triple (*see also* Accessory)
kidneys Q63.0
uteri Q51.818
X, female Q97.0
Triplegia G83.89
congenital G80.8
Triplet (newborn) (*see also* Newborn, triplet)
complicating pregnancy — *see* Pregnancy, triplet
Triplication — *see* Accessory
Triploidy Q92.7
Trismus R25.2
neonatorum A33
newborn A33
Trisomy (syndrome) Q92.9
13 (partial) Q91.7
meiotic nondisjunction Q91.4
mitotic nondisjunction Q91.5
mosaicism Q91.5
translocation Q91.6
18 (partial) Q91.3
meiotic nondisjunction Q91.0
mitotic nondisjunction Q91.1
mosaicism Q91.1
translocation Q91.2
20 Q92.8
21 (partial) Q90.9
meiotic nondisjunction Q90.0
mitotic nondisjunction Q90.1
mosaicism Q90.1
translocation Q90.2
22 Q92.8
autosomes Q92.9
chromosome specified NEC Q92.8
partial Q92.2
due to unbalanced translocation Q92.5
specified NEC Q92.8
whole (nonsex chromosome)
meiotic nondisjunction Q92.0
mitotic nondisjunction Q92.1
mosaicism Q92.1
due to
dicentrics — *see* Extra, marker chromosomes
extra rings — *see* Extra, marker chromosomes
isochromosomes — *see* Extra, marker chromosomes
specified NEC Q92.8
whole chromosome Q92.9
meiotic nondisjunction Q92.0
mitotic nondisjunction Q92.1
mosaicism Q92.1
partial Q92.9
specified NEC Q92.8
Tritanomaly, tritanopia H53.55
Trombiculosis, trombiculiasis, trombidiosis B88.0
Trophedema (congenital) (hereditary) Q82.0
Trophoblastic disease (*see also* Mole, hydatidiform) O01.9
Tropholymphedema Q82.0
Trophoneurosis NEC G96.8
disseminated M34.9
Tropical — *see* condition
Trouble (*see also* Disease)
heart — *see* Disease, heart
kidney — *see* Disease, renal
nervous R45.0
sinus — *see* Sinusitis
Trousseau's syndrome (thrombophlebitis migrans) I82.1
Truancy, childhood
from school Z72.810
Truncus
arteriosus (persistent) Q20.0
communis Q20.0
Trunk — *see* condition

Trypanosomiasis
African B56.9
by Trypanosoma brucei
gambiense B56.0
rhodiense B56.1
American — *see* Chagas' disease
Brazilian — *see* Chagas' disease
by Trypanosoma
brucei gambiense B56.0
brucei rhodesiense B56.1
cruzi — *see* Chagas' disease
gambiensis, Gambian B56.0
rhodesiensis, Rhodesian B56.1
South American — *see* Chagas' disease
where
African trypanosomiasis is prevalent B56.9
Chagas' disease is prevalent B57.2
T-shaped incisors K00.2
Tsutsugamushi (disease) (fever) A75.3
Tube, tubal, tubular — *see* condition
Tubercle (*see also* Tuberculosis)
brain, solitary A17.81
Darwin's Q17.8
Ghon, primary infection A15.7
Tuberculid, tuberculide (indurating, subcutaneous) (lichenoid) (miliary) (papulonecrotic) (primary) (skin) A18.4
Tuberculoma (*see also* Tuberculosis)
brain A17.81
meninges (cerebral) (spinal) A17.1
spinal cord A17.81
Tuberculosis, tubercular, tuberculous (calcification) (calcified) (caseous) (chromogenic acid-fast bacilli) (degeneration) (fibrocaseous) (fistula) (interstitial) (isolated circumscribed lesions) (necrosis) (parenchymatous) (ulcerative) A15.9
with pneumoconiosis (any condition in J60-J64) J65
abdomen (lymph gland) A18.39
abscess (respiratory) A15.9
bone A18.03
hip A18.02
knee A18.02
sacrum A18.01
specified site NEC A18.03
spinal A18.01
vertebra A18.01
brain A17.81
breast A18.89
Cowper's gland A18.15
dura (mater) (cerebral) (spinal) A17.81
epidural (cerebral) (spinal) A17.81
female pelvis A18.17
frontal sinus A15.8
genital organs NEC A18.10
genitourinary A18.10
gland (lymphatic) — *see* Tuberculosis, lymph gland
hip A18.02
intestine A18.32
ischiorectal A18.32
joint NEC A18.02
hip A18.02
knee A18.02
specified NEC A18.02
vertebral A18.01
kidney A18.11
knee A18.02
latent R76.11
lumbar (spine) A18.01
lung — *see* Tuberculosis, pulmonary
meninges (cerebral) (spinal) A17.0
muscle A18.09
perianal (fistula) A18.32
perinephritic A18.11
perirectal A18.32
rectum A18.32
retropharyngeal A15.8
sacrum A18.01
scrofulous A18.2
scrotum A18.15
skin (primary) A18.4
spinal cord A17.81
spine or vertebra (column) A18.01
subdiaphragmatic A18.31
testis A18.15
urinary A18.13
uterus A18.17
accessory sinus — *see* Tuberculosis, sinus
Addison's disease A18.7

Tuberculosis, tubercular, tuberculous — *continued*
adenitis — *see* Tuberculosis, lymph gland
adenoids A15.8
adenopathy — *see* Tuberculosis, lymph gland
adherent pericardium A18.84
adnexa (uteri) A18.17
adrenal (capsule) (gland) A18.7
alimentary canal A18.32
anemia A18.89
ankle (joint) (bone) A18.02
anus A18.32
apex, apical — *see* Tuberculosis, pulmonary
appendicitis, appendix A18.32
arachnoid A17.0
artery, arteritis A18.89
cerebral A18.89
arthritis (chronic) (synovial) A18.02
spine or vertebra (column) A18.01
articular — *see* Tuberculosis, joint
ascites A18.31
asthma — *see* Tuberculosis, pulmonary
axilla, axillary (gland) A18.2
bladder A18.12
bone A18.03
hip A18.02
knee A18.02
limb NEC A18.03
sacrum A18.01
spine or vertebral column A18.01
bowel (miliary) A18.32
brain A17.81
breast A18.89
broad ligament A18.17
bronchi, bronchial, bronchus A15.5
ectasia, ectasis (bronchiectasis) — *see* Tuberculosis, pulmonary
fistula A15.5
primary (progressive) A15.7
gland or node A15.4
primary (progressive) A15.7
lymph gland or node A15.4
primary (progressive) A15.7
bronchiectasis — *see* Tuberculosis, pulmonary
bronchitis A15.5
bronchopleural A15.6
bronchopneumonia, bronchopneumonic — *see* Tuberculosis, pulmonary
bronchorrhagia A15.5
bronchotracheal A15.5
bronze disease A18.7
buccal cavity A18.83
bulbourethral gland A18.15
bursa A18.09
cachexia A15.9
cardiomyopathy A18.84
caries — *see* Tuberculosis, bone
cartilage A18.02
intervertebral A18.01
catarrhal — *see* Tuberculosis, respiratory
cecum A18.32
cellulitis (primary) A18.4
cerebellum A17.81
cerebral, cerebrum A17.81
cerebrospinal A17.81
meninges A17.0
cervical (lymph gland or node) A18.2
cervicitis, cervix (uteri) A18.16
chest — *see* Tuberculosis, respiratory
chorioretinitis A18.53
choroid, choroiditis A18.53
ciliary body A18.54
colitis A18.32
collier's J65
colliquativa (primary) A18.4
colon A18.32
complex, primary A15.7
congenital P37.0
conjunctiva A18.59
connective tissue (systemic) A18.89
contact Z20.1
cornea (ulcer) A18.52
Cowper's gland A18.15
coxae A18.02
coxalgia A18.02
cul-de-sac of Douglas A18.17
curvature, spine A18.01
cutis (colliquativa) (primary) A18.4
cyst, ovary A18.18

☑ **Additional Character Required** — Refer to the Tabular List for Character Selection   ▽ **Subterms under main terms may continue to next column or page**

Tuberculosis, tubercular, tuberculous — *continued*
- cystitis A18.12
- dactylitis A18.03
- diarrhea A18.32
- diffuse — *see* Tuberculosis, miliary
- digestive tract A18.32
- disseminated — *see* Tuberculosis, miliary
- duodenum A18.32
- dura (mater) (cerebral) (spinal) A17.0
  - abscess (cerebral) (spinal) A17.81
- dysentery A18.32
- ear (inner) (middle) A18.6
  - bone A18.03
  - external (primary) A18.4
  - skin (primary) A18.4
- elbow A18.02
- emphysema — *see* Tuberculosis, pulmonary
- empyema A15.6
- encephalitis A17.82
- endarteritis A18.89
- endocarditis A18.84
  - aortic A18.84
  - mitral A18.84
  - pulmonary A18.84
  - tricuspid A18.84
- endocrine glands NEC A18.82
- endometrium A18.17
- enteric, enterica, enteritis A18.32
- enterocolitis A18.32
- epididymis, epididymitis A18.15
- epidural abscess (cerebral) (spinal) A17.81
- epiglottis A15.5
- episcleritis A18.51
- erythema (induratum) (nodosum) (primary) A18.4
- esophagus A18.83
- eustachian tube A18.6
- exposure (to) Z20.1
- exudative — *see* Tuberculosis, pulmonary
- eye A18.50
- eyelid (primary) (lupus) A18.4
- fallopian tube (acute) (chronic) A18.17
- fascia A18.09
- fauces A15.8
- female pelvic inflammatory disease A18.17
- finger A18.03
- first infection A15.7
- gallbladder A18.83
- ganglion A18.09
- gastritis A18.83
- gastrocolic fistula A18.32
- gastroenteritis A18.32
- gastrointestinal tract A18.32
- general, generalized — *see* Tuberculosis, miliary
- genital organs A18.10
- genitourinary A18.10
- genu A18.02
- glandula suprarenalis A18.7
- glandular, general A18.2
- glottis A15.5
- grinder's J65
- gum A18.83
- hand A18.03
- heart A18.84
- hematogenous — *see* Tuberculosis, miliary
- hemoptysis — *see* Tuberculosis, pulmonary
- hemorrhage NEC — *see* Tuberculosis, pulmonary
- hemothorax A15.6
- hepatitis A18.83
- hilar lymph nodes A15.4
  - primary (progressive) A15.7
- hip (joint) (disease) (bone) A18.02
- hydropneumothorax A15.6
- hydrothorax A15.6
- hypoadrenalism A18.7
- hypopharynx A15.8
- ileocecal (hyperplastic) A18.32
- ileocolitis A18.32
- ileum A18.32
- iliac spine (superior) A18.03
- immunological findings only A15.7
- indurativa (primary) A18.4
- infantile A15.7
- infection A15.9
  - without clinical manifestations A15.7
- infraclavicular gland A18.2
- inguinal gland A18.2
- inguinalis A18.2
- intestine (any part) A18.32

Tuberculosis, tubercular, tuberculous — *continued*
- iridocyclitis A18.54
- iris, iritis A18.54
- ischiorectal A18.32
- jaw A18.03
- jejunum A18.32
- joint A18.02
  - vertebral A18.01
- keratitis (interstitial) A18.52
- keratoconjunctivitis A18.52
- kidney A18.11
- knee (joint) A18.02
- kyphosis, kyphoscoliosis A18.01
- laryngitis A15.5
- larynx A15.5
- latent R76.11
- leptomeninges, leptomeningitis (cerebral) (spinal) A17.0
- lichenoides (primary) A18.4
- linguae A18.83
- lip A18.83
- liver A18.83
- lordosis A18.01
- lung — *see* Tuberculosis, pulmonary
- lupus vulgaris A18.4
- lymph gland or node (peripheral) A18.2
  - abdomen A18.39
  - bronchial A15.4
    - primary (progressive) A15.7
  - cervical A18.2
  - hilar A15.4
    - primary (progressive) A15.7
  - intrathoracic A15.4
    - primary (progressive) A15.7
  - mediastinal A15.4
    - primary (progressive) A15.7
  - mesenteric A18.39
  - retroperitoneal A18.39
  - tracheobronchial A15.4
    - primary (progressive) A15.7
- lymphadenitis — *see* Tuberculosis, lymph gland
- lymphangitis — *see* Tuberculosis, lymph gland
- lymphatic (gland) (vessel) — *see* Tuberculosis, lymph gland
- mammary gland A18.89
- marasmus A15.9
- mastoiditis A18.03
- mediastinal lymph gland or node A15.4
  - primary (progressive) A15.7
- mediastinitis A15.8
  - primary (progressive) A15.7
- mediastinum A15.8
  - primary (progressive) A15.7
- medulla A17.81
- melanosis, Addisonian A18.7
- menges, meningitis (basilar) (cerebral) (cerebrospinal) (spinal) A17.0
- meningoencephalitis A17.82
- mesentery, mesenteric (gland or node) A18.39
- miliary A19.9
  - acute A19.2
    - multiple sites A19.1
    - single specified site A19.0
  - chronic A19.8
  - specified NEC A19.8
- millstone makers' J65
- miner's J65
- molder's J65
- mouth A18.83
- multiple A19.9
  - acute A19.1
  - chronic A19.8
- muscle A18.09
- myelitis A17.82
- myocardium, myocarditis A18.84
- nasal (passage) (sinus) A15.8
- nasopharynx A15.8
- neck gland A18.2
- nephritis A18.11
- nerve (mononeuropathy) A17.83
- nervous system A17.9
- nose (septum) A15.8
- ocular A18.50
- omentum A18.31
- oophoritis (acute) (chronic) A18.17
- optic (nerve trunk) (papilla) A18.59
- orbit A18.59
- orchitis A18.15
- organ, specified NEC A18.89

Tuberculosis, tubercular, tuberculous — *continued*
- osseous — *see* Tuberculosis, bone
- osteitis — *see* Tuberculosis, bone
- osteomyelitis — *see* Tuberculosis, bone
- otitis media A18.6
- ovary, ovaritis (acute) (chronic) A18.17
- oviduct (acute) (chronic) A18.17
- pachymeningitis A17.0
- palate (soft) A18.83
- pancreas A18.83
- papulonecrotic (a) (primary) A18.4
- parathyroid glands A18.82
- paronychia (primary) A18.4
- parotid gland or region A18.83
- pelvis (bony) A18.03
- penis A18.15
- peribronchitis A15.5
- pericardium, pericarditis A18.84
- perichondritis, larynx A15.5
- periostitis — *see* Tuberculosis, bone
- perirectal fistula A18.32
- peritoneum NEC A18.31
- peritonitis A18.31
- pharynx, pharyngitis A15.8
- phlyctenulosis (keratoconjunctivitis) A18.52
- phthisis NEC — *see* Tuberculosis, pulmonary
- pituitary gland A18.82
- pleura, pleural, pleurisy, pleuritis (fibrinous) (obliterative) (purulent) (simple plastic) (with effusion) A15.6
  - primary (progressive) A15.7
- pneumonia, pneumonic — *see* Tuberculosis, pulmonary
- pneumothorax (spontaneous) (tense valvular) — *see* Tuberculosis, pulmonary
- polyneuropathy A17.89
- polyserositis A19.9
  - acute A19.1
  - chronic A19.8
- potter's J65
- prepuce A18.15
- primary (complex) A15.7
- proctitis A18.32
- prostate, prostatitis A18.14
- pulmonalis — *see* Tuberculosis, pulmonary
- pulmonary (cavitated) (fibrotic) (infiltrative) (nodular) A15.0
  - childhood type or first infection A15.7
  - primary (complex) A15.7
- pyelitis A18.11
- pyelonephritis A18.11
- pyemia — *see* Tuberculosis, miliary
- pyonephrosis A18.11
- pyopneumothorax A15.6
- pyothorax A15.6
- rectum (fistula) (with abscess) A18.32
- reinfection stage — *see* Tuberculosis, pulmonary
- renal A18.11
- renis A18.11
- respiratory A15.9
  - primary A15.7
  - specified site NEC A15.8
- retina, retinitis A18.53
- retroperitoneal (lymph gland or node) A18.39
- rheumatism NEC A18.09
- rhinitis A15.8
- sacroiliac (joint) A18.01
- sacrum A18.01
- salivary gland A18.83
- salpingitis (acute) (chronic) A18.17
- sandblaster's J65
- sclera A18.51
- scoliosis A18.01
- scrofulous A18.2
- scrotum A18.15
- seminal tract or vesicle A18.15
- senile A15.9
- septic — *see* Tuberculosis, miliary
- shoulder (joint) A18.02
  - blade A18.03
- sigmoid A18.32
- sinus (any nasal) A15.8
  - bone A18.03
  - epididymis A18.15
- skeletal NEC A18.03
- skin (any site) (primary) A18.4
- small intestine A18.32
- soft palate A18.83

Tuberculosis, tubercular, tuberculous — *continued*
  spermatic cord A18.15
  spine, spinal (column) A18.Ø1
    cord A17.81
    medulla A17.81
    membrane A17.Ø
    meninges A17.Ø
  spleen, splenitis A18.85
  spondylitis A18.Ø1
  sternoclavicular joint A18.Ø2
  stomach A18.83
  stonemason's J65
  subcutaneous tissue (cellular) (primary) A18.4
  subcutis (primary) A18.4
  subdeltoid bursa A18.83
  submaxillary (region) A18.83
  supraclavicular gland A18.2
  suprarenal (capsule) (gland) A18.7
  swelling, joint (*see also* category MØ1) (*see also* Tuberculosis, joint) A18.Ø2
  symphysis pubis A18.Ø2
  synovitis A18.Ø9
    articular A18.Ø2
    spine or vertebra A18.Ø1
  systemic — *see* Tuberculosis, miliary
  tarsitis A18.4
  tendon (sheath) — *see* Tuberculosis, tenosynovitis
  tenosynovitis A18.Ø9
    spine or vertebra A18.Ø1
  testis A18.15
  throat A15.8
  thymus gland A18.82
  thyroid gland A18.81
  tongue A18.83
  tonsil, tonsillitis A15.8
  trachea, tracheal A15.5
    lymph gland or node A15.4
      primary (progressive) A15.7
  tracheobronchial A15.5
    lymph gland or node A15.4
      primary (progressive) A15.7
  tubal (acute) (chronic) A18.17
  tunica vaginalis A18.15
  ulcer (skin) (primary) A18.4
    bowel or intestine A18.32
    specified NEC — *see* Tuberculosis, by site
  unspecified site A15.9
  ureter A18.11
  urethra, urethral (gland) A18.13
  urinary organ or tract A18.13
  uterus A18.17
  uveal tract A18.54
  uvula A18.83
  vagina A18.18
  vas deferens A18.15
  verruca, verrucosa (cutis) (primary) A18.4
  vertebra (column) A18.Ø1
  vesiculitis A18.15
  vulva A18.18
  wrist (joint) A18.Ø2
Tuberculum
  Carabelli — *see* Excludes Note at KØØ.2
  occlusal — *see* Excludes Note at KØØ.2
  paramolare KØØ.2
Tuberosity, enitre maxillary M26.Ø7
Tuberous sclerosis (brain) Q85.1
Tubo-ovarian — *see* condition
Tuboplasty, after previous sterilization Z31.Ø
  aftercare Z31.42
Tubotympanitis, catarrhal (chronic) — *see* Otitis, media, nonsuppurative, chronic, serous
Tularemia A21.9
  with
    conjunctivitis A21.1
    pneumonia A21.2
  abdominal A21.3
  bronchopneumonic A21.2
  conjunctivitis A21.1
  cryptogenic A21.3
  enteric A21.3
  gastrointestinal A21.3
  generalized A21.7
  ingestion A21.3
  intestinal A21.3
  oculoglandular A21.1
  ophthalmic A21.1
  pneumonia (any), pneumonic A21.2
  pulmonary A21.2

Tularemia — *continued*
  sepsis A21.7
  specified NEC A21.8
  typhoidal A21.7
  ulceroglandular A21.Ø
Tularensis conjunctivitis A21.1
Tumefaction (*see also* Swelling)
  liver — *see* Hypertrophy, liver
Tumor (*see also* Neoplasm, unspecified behavior, by site)
  acinar cell — *see* Neoplasm, uncertain behavior, by site
  acinic cell — *see* Neoplasm, uncertain behavior, by site
  adenocarcinoid — *see* Neoplasm, malignant, by site
  adenomatoid (*see also* Neoplasm, benign, by site)
    odontogenic — *see* Cyst, calcifying odontogenic
  adnexal (skin) — *see* Neoplasm, skin, benign, by site
  adrenal
    cortical (benign) D35.Ø- ☑
      malignant C74.Ø- ☑
    rest — *see* Neoplasm, benign, by site
  alpha-cell
    malignant
      pancreas C25.4
      specified site NEC — *see* Neoplasm, malignant, by site
      unspecified site C25.4
    pancreas D13.7
    specified site NEC — *see* Neoplasm, benign, by site
    unspecified site D13.7
  aneurysmal — *see* Aneurysm
  aortic body D44.7
    malignant C75.5
  Askin's — *see* Neoplasm, connective tissue, malignant
  basal cell (*see also* Neoplasm, skin, uncertain behavior) D48.5
  Bednar — *see* Neoplasm, skin, malignant
  benign (unclassified) — *see* Neoplasm, benign, by site
  beta-cell
    malignant
      pancreas C25.4
      specified site NEC — *see* Neoplasm, malignant, by site
      unspecified site C25.4
    pancreas D13.7
    specified site NEC — *see* Neoplasm, benign, by site
    unspecified site D13.7
  Brenner D27.9
    borderline malignancy D39.1- ☑
    malignant C56- ☑
    proliferating D39.1- ☑
  bronchial alveolar, intravascular D38.1
  Brooke's — *see* Neoplasm, skin, benign
  brown fat — *see* Lipoma
  Burkitt — *see* Lymphoma, Burkitt
  calcifying epithelial odontogenic — *see* Cyst, calcifying odontogenic
  carcinoid
    benign D3A.ØØ (*following* D36)
      appendix D3A.Ø2Ø (*following* D36)
      ascending colon D3A.Ø22 (*following* D36)
      bronchus (lung) D3A.Ø9Ø (*following* D36)
      cecum D3A.Ø21 (*following* D36)
      colon D3A.Ø29 (*following* D36)
      descending colon D3A.Ø24 (*following* D36)
      duodenum D3A.Ø1Ø (*following* D36)
      foregut NOS D3A.Ø94 (*following* D36)
      hindgut NOS D3A.Ø96 (*following* D36)
      ileum D3A.Ø12 (*following* D36)
      jejunum D3A.Ø11 (*following* D36)
      kidney D3A.Ø93 (*following* D36)
      large intestine D3A.Ø29 (*following* D36)
      lung (bronchus) D3A.Ø9Ø (*following* D36)
      midgut NOS D3A.Ø95 (*following* D36)
      rectum D3A.Ø26 (*following* D36)
      sigmoid colon D3A.Ø25 (*following* D36)
      small intestine D3A.Ø19 (*following* D36)
      specified NEC D3A.Ø98 (*following* D36)
      stomach D3A.Ø92 (*following* D36)
      thymus D3A.Ø91 (*following* D36)
      transverse colon D3A.Ø23 (*following* D36)
    malignant C7A.ØØ (*following* C75)
      appendix C7A.Ø2Ø (*following* C75)
      ascending colon C7A.Ø22 (*following* C75)
      bronchus (lung) C7A.Ø9Ø (*following* C75)
      cecum C7A.Ø21 (*following* C75)
      colon C7A.Ø29 (*following* C75)
      descending colon C7A.Ø24 (*following* C75)

Tumor — *continued*
  carcinoid — *continued*
    malignant — *continued*
      duodenum C7A.Ø1Ø (*following* C75)
      foregut NOS C7A.Ø94 (*following* C75)
      hindgut NOS C7A.Ø96 (*following* C75)
      ileum C7A.Ø12 (*following* C75)
      jejunum C7A.Ø11 (*following* C75)
      kidney C7A.Ø93 (*following* C75)
      large intestine C7A.Ø29 (*following* C75)
      lung (bronchus) C7A.Ø9Ø (*following* C75)
      midgut NOS C7A.Ø95 (*following* C75)
      rectum C7A.Ø26 (*following* C75)
      sigmoid colon C7A.Ø25 (*following* C75)
      small intestine C7A.Ø19 (*following* C75)
      specified NEC C7A.Ø98 (*following* C75)
      stomach C7A.Ø92 (*following* C75)
      thymus C7A.Ø91 (*following* C75)
      transverse colon C7A.Ø23 (*following* C75)
    mesentery metastasis C7B.Ø4 (*following* C75)
    secondary C7B.ØØ (*following* C75)
      bone C7B.Ø3 (*following* C75)
      distant lymph nodes C7B.Ø1 (*following* C75)
      liver C7B.Ø2 (*following* C75)
      peritoneum C7B.Ø4 (*following* C75)
      specified NEC C7B.Ø9 (*following* C75)
  carotid body D44.6
    malignant C75.4
  cells (*see also* Neoplasm, unspecified behavior, by site)
    benign — *see* Neoplasm, benign, by site
    malignant — *see* Neoplasm, malignant, by site
    uncertain whether benign or malignant — *see* Neoplasm, uncertain behavior, by site
  cervix, in pregnancy or childbirth — *see* Pregnancy, complicated by, tumor, cervix
  chondromatous giant cell — *see* Neoplasm, bone, benign
  chromaffin (*see also* Neoplasm, benign, by site)
    malignant — *see* Neoplasm, malignant, by site
  Cock's peculiar L72.3
  Codman's — *see* Neoplasm, bone, benign
  dentigerous, mixed — *see* Cyst, calcifying odontogenic
  dermoid — *see* Neoplasm, benign, by site
    with malignant transformation C56- ☑
  desmoid (extra-abdominal) (*see also* Neoplasm, connective tissue, uncertain behavior)
    abdominal — *see* Neoplasm, connective tissue, uncertain behavior
  embolus — *see* Neoplasm, secondary, by site
  embryonal (mixed) (*see also* Neoplasm, uncertain behavior, by site)
    liver C22.7
  endodermal sinus
    specified site — *see* Neoplasm, malignant, by site
    unspecified site
      female C56.- ☑
      male C62.9Ø
  epithelial
    benign — *see* Neoplasm, benign, by site
    malignant — *see* Neoplasm, malignant, by site
  Ewing's — *see* Neoplasm, bone, malignant, by site
  fatty — *see* Lipoma
  fibroid — *see* Leiomyoma
  G cell
    malignant
      pancreas C25.4
      specified site NEC — *see* Neoplasm, malignant, by site
      unspecified site C25.4
    specified site — *see* Neoplasm, uncertain behavior, by site
    unspecified site D37.8
  germ cell (*see also* Neoplasm, malignant, by site)
    mixed — *see* Neoplasm, malignant, by site
  ghost cell, odontogenic — *see* Cyst, calcifying odontogenic
  giant cell (*see also* Neoplasm, uncertain behavior, by site)
    bone D48.Ø
      malignant — *see* Neoplasm, bone, malignant
    chondromatous — *see* Neoplasm, bone, benign
    malignant — *see* Neoplasm, malignant, by site
    soft parts — *see* Neoplasm, connective tissue, uncertain behavior
      malignant — *see* Neoplasm, connective tissue, malignant
  glomus D18.ØØ
    intra-abdominal D18.Ø3

Tumor — *continued*
　glomus — *continued*
　　intracranial D18.02
　　jugulare D44.7
　　　malignant C75.5
　　skin D18.01
　　specified site NEC D18.09
　gonadal stromal — *see* Neoplasm, uncertain behavior, by site
　granular cell (*see also* Neoplasm, connective tissue, benign)
　　malignant — *see* Neoplasm, connective tissue, malignant
　granulosa cell D39.1- ☑
　　juvenile D39.1- ☑
　　malignant C56- ☑
　granulosa cell-theca cell D39.1- ☑
　　malignant C56- ☑
　Grawitz's C64- ☑
　hemorrhoidal — *see* Hemorrhoids
　hilar cell D27- ☑
　hilus cell D27- ☑
　Hurthle cell (benign) D34
　　malignant C73
　hydatid — *see* Echinococcus
　hypernephroid (*see also* Neoplasm, uncertain behavior, by site)
　interstitial cell (*see also* Neoplasm, uncertain behavior, by site)
　　benign — *see* Neoplasm, benign, by site
　　malignant — *see* Neoplasm, malignant, by site
　intravascular bronchial alveolar D38.1
　islet cell — *see* Neoplasm, benign, by site
　　malignant — *see* Neoplasm, malignant, by site
　　　pancreas C25.4
　　　specified site NEC — *see* Neoplasm, malignant, by site
　　　unspecified site C25.4
　　pancreas D13.7
　　specified site NEC — *see* Neoplasm, benign, by site
　　unspecified site D13.7
　juxtaglomerular D41.0- ☑
　Klatskin's C22.1
　Krukenberg's C79.6- ☑
　Leydig cell — *see* Neoplasm, uncertain behavior, by site
　　benign — *see* Neoplasm, benign, by site
　　　specified site — *see* Neoplasm, benign, by site
　　　unspecified site
　　　　female D27.9
　　　　male D29.20
　　malignant — *see* Neoplasm, malignant, by site
　　　specified site — *see* Neoplasm, malignant, by site
　　　unspecified site
　　　　female C56.9
　　　　male C62.90
　　specified site — *see* Neoplasm, uncertain behavior, by site
　　unspecified site
　　　female D39.10
　　　male D40.10
　lipid cell, ovary D27- ☑
　lipoid cell, ovary D27- ☑
　malignant (*see also* Neoplasm, malignant, by site) C80.1
　　fusiform cell (type) C80.1
　　giant cell (type) C80.1
　　localized, plasma cell — *see* Plasmacytoma, solitary
　　mixed NEC C80.1
　　small cell (type) C80.1
　　spindle cell (type) C80.1
　　unclassified C80.1
　mast cell D47.09
　melanotic, neuroectodermal — *see* Neoplasm, benign, by site
　Merkel cell — *see* Carcinoma, Merkel cell
　mesenchymal
　　malignant — *see* Neoplasm, connective tissue, malignant
　　mixed — *see* Neoplasm, connective tissue, uncertain behavior
　mesodermal, mixed (*see also* Neoplasm, malignant, by site)
　　liver C22.4

Tumor — *continued*
　mesonephric (*see also* Neoplasm, uncertain behavior, by site)
　　malignant — *see* Neoplasm, malignant, by site
　metastatic
　　from specified site — *see* Neoplasm, malignant, by site
　　of specified site — *see* Neoplasm, malignant, by site
　　to specified site — *see* Neoplasm, secondary, by site
　mixed NEC (*see also* Neoplasm, benign, by site)
　　malignant — *see* Neoplasm, malignant, by site
　mucinous of low malignant potential
　　specified site — *see* Neoplasm, malignant, by site
　　unspecified site C56.9
　mucocarcinoid
　　specified site — *see* Neoplasm, malignant, by site
　　unspecified site C18.1
　mucoepidermoid — *see* Neoplasm, uncertain behavior, by site
　Müllerian, mixed
　　specified site — *see* Neoplasm, malignant, by site
　　unspecified site C54.9
　myoepithelial — *see* Neoplasm, benign, by site
　neuroectodermal (peripheral) — *see* Neoplasm, malignant, by site
　　primitive
　　　specified site — *see* Neoplasm, malignant, by site
　　　unspecified site C71.9
　neuroendocrine D3A.8 (*following* D36)
　　malignant poorly differentiated C7A.1 (*following* C75)
　　secondary NEC C7B.8 (*following* C75)
　　specified NEC C7A.8 (*following* C75)
　neurogenic olfactory C30.0
　nonencapsulated sclerosing C73
　odontogenic (adenomatoid) (benign) (calcifying epithelial) (keratocystic) (squamous) — *see* Cyst, calcifying odontogenic
　　malignant C41.1
　　　upper jaw (bone) C41.0
　ovarian stromal D39.1- ☑
　ovary, in pregnancy — *see* Pregnancy, complicated by
　pacinian — *see* Neoplasm, skin, benign
　Pancoast's — *see* Pancoast's syndrome
　papillary (*see also* Papilloma)
　　cystic D37.9
　　mucinous of low malignant potential C56- ☑
　　　specified site — *see* Neoplasm, malignant, by site
　　　unspecified site C56.9
　　serous of low malignant potential
　　　specified site — *see* Neoplasm, malignant, by site
　　　unspecified site C56.9
　pelvic, in pregnancy or childbirth — *see* Pregnancy, complicated by
　phantom F45.8
　phyllodes D48.6- ☑
　　benign D24- ☑
　　malignant — *see* Neoplasm, breast, malignant
　Pindborg — *see* Cyst, calcifying odontogenic
　placental site trophoblastic D39.2
　plasma cell (malignant) (localized) — *see* Plasmacytoma, solitary
　polyvesicular vitelline
　　specified site — *see* Neoplasm, malignant, by site
　　unspecified site
　　　female C56.9
　　　male C62.90
　Pott's puffy — *see* Osteomyelitis, specified NEC
　Rathke's pouch D44.3
　retinal anlage — *see* Neoplasm, benign, by site
　salivary gland type, mixed — *see* Neoplasm, salivary gland, benign
　　malignant — *see* Neoplasm, salivary gland, malignant
　Sampson's N80.1
　Schmincke's — *see* Neoplasm, nasopharynx, malignant
　sclerosing stromal D27- ☑
　sebaceous — *see* Cyst, sebaceous
　secondary — *see* Neoplasm, secondary, by site
　　carcinoid C7B.00 (*following* C75)
　　　bone C7B.03 (*following* C75)
　　　distant lymph nodes C7B.01 (*following* C75)

Tumor — *continued*
　secondary — *see* Neoplasm, secondary, by site — *continued*
　　carcinoid — *continued*
　　　liver C7B.02 (*following* C75)
　　　peritoneum C7B.04 (*following* C75)
　　　specified NEC C7B.09 (*following* C75)
　　neuroendocrine NEC C7B.8 (*following* C75)
　serous of low malignant potential
　　specified site — *see* Neoplasm, malignant, by site
　　unspecified site C56.9
　Sertoli cell (*see also* Neoplasm, benign, by site
　　with lipid storage
　　　specified site — *see* Neoplasm, benign, by site
　　　unspecified site
　　　　female D27.9
　　　　male D29.20
　　specified site — *see* Neoplasm, benign, by site
　　unspecified site
　　　female D27.9
　　　male D29.20
　Sertoli-Leydig cell — *see* Neoplasm, benign, by site
　　specified site — *see* Neoplasm, benign, by site
　　unspecified site
　　　female D27.9
　　　male D29.20
　sex cord (-stromal) — *see* Neoplasm, uncertain behavior, by site
　　with annular tubules D39.1- ☑
　skin appendage — *see* Neoplasm, skin, benign
　smooth muscle — *see* Neoplasm, connective tissue, uncertain behavior
　soft tissue
　　benign — *see* Neoplasm, connective tissue, benign
　　malignant — *see* Neoplasm, connective tissue, malignant
　sternomastoid (congenital) Q68.0
　stromal
　　endometrial D39.0
　　gastric D48.1
　　　benign D21.4
　　　malignant C16.9
　　　uncertain behavior D48.1
　　gastrointestinal C49.A- ☑
　　　benign D21.4
　　　esophagus C49.A1
　　　malignant C49.A0
　　　　colon C49.A4
　　　　duodenum C49.A3
　　　　esophagus C49.A1
　　　　ileum C49.A3
　　　　jejunum C49.A3
　　　　large intestine C49.A4
　　　　Meckel diverticulum C49.A3
　　　　omentum C49.A9
　　　　peritoneum C49.A9
　　　　rectum C49.A5
　　　　small intestine C49.A3
　　　　specified site NEC C49.A9
　　　　stomach C49.A2
　　　rectum C49.A5
　　　small intestine C49.A3
　　　specified site NEC C49.A9
　　　stomach C49.A2
　　　uncertain behavior D48.1
　　intestine
　　　benign D21.4
　　　malignant
　　　　large C49.A4
　　　　small C49.A3
　　　uncertain behavior D48.1
　　ovarian D39.1- ☑
　　stomach C49.A2
　　　benign D21.4
　　　malignant C49.A2
　　　uncertain behavior D48.1
　sweat gland (*see also* Neoplasm, skin, uncertain behavior)
　　benign — *see* Neoplasm, skin, benign
　　malignant — *see* Neoplasm, skin, malignant
　syphilitic, brain A52.17
　testicular D40.10
　testicular stromal D40.1- ☑
　theca cell D27.- ☑
　theca cell-granulosa cell D39.1- ☑
　Triton, malignant — *see* Neoplasm, nerve, malignant
　trophoblastic, placental site D39.2
　turban D23.4

Tumor — *continued*
uterus (body), in pregnancy or childbirth — *see* Pregnancy, complicated by, tumor, uterus
vagina, in pregnancy or childbirth — *see* Pregnancy, complicated by
varicose — *see* Varix
von Recklinghausen's — *see* Neurofibromatosis
vulva or perineum, in pregnancy or childbirth — *see* Pregnancy, complicated by
causing obstructed labor O65.5
Warthin's — *see* Neoplasm, salivary gland, benign
Wilms' C64- ☑
yolk sac — *see* Neoplasm, malignant, by site
specified site — *see* Neoplasm, malignant, by site
unspecified site
female C56.9
male C62.90
Tumor lysis syndrome (following antineoplastic chemotherapy) (spontaneous) NEC E88.3
Tumorlet — *see* Neoplasm, uncertain behavior, by site
Tungiasis B88.1
Tunica vasculosa lentis Q12.2
Turban tumor D23.4
Türck's trachoma J37.0
Turner-Kieser syndrome Q87.2
Turner-like syndrome Q87.1
Turner's
hypoplasia (tooth) K00.4
syndrome Q96.9
specified NEC Q96.8
tooth K00.4
Turner-Ullrich syndrome Q96.9
Tussis convulsiva — *see* Whooping cough
Twiddler's syndrome (due to)
automatic implantable defibrillatorT82.198
cardiac pacemaker T82.198 ☑
Twilight state
epileptic F05
psychogenic F44.89
Twin (newborn) (*see also* Newborn, twin)
conjoined Q89.4
pregnancy — *see* Pregnancy, twin
Twinning, teeth K00.2
Twist, twisted
bowel, colon or intestine K56.2
hair (congenital) Q84.1
mesentery K56.2
omentum K56.2
organ or site, congenital NEC — *see* Anomaly, by site
ovarian pedicle — *see* Torsion, ovary
Twitching R25.3
Tylosis (acquired) L84
buccalis K13.29
linguae K13.29
palmaris et plantaris (congenital) (inherited) Q82.8
acquired L85.1
Tympanism R14.0
Tympanites (abdominal) (intestinal) R14.0
Tympanitis — *see* Myringitis
Tympanosclerosis H74.0 ☑
Tympanum — *see* condition
Tympany
abdomen R14.0
chest R09.89
Type A behavior pattern Z73.1
Typhlitis — *see* Appendicitis
Typhoenteritis — *see* Typhoid
Typhoid (abortive) (ambulant) (any site) (clinical) (fever) (hemorrhagic) (infection) (intermittent) (malignant) (rheumatic) (Widal negative) A01.00
with pneumonia A01.03
abdominal A01.09
arthritis A01.04
carrier (suspected) of Z22.0
cholecystitis (current) A01.09
endocarditis A01.02
heart involvement A01.02
inoculation reaction — *see* Complications, vaccination
meningitis A01.01
mesenteric lymph nodes A01.09
myocarditis A01.02
osteomyelitis A01.05
perichondritis, larynx A01.09
pneumonia A01.03
specified NEC A01.09
spine A01.05
ulcer (perforating) A01.09

Typhomalaria (fever) — *see* Malaria
Typhomania A01.00
Typhoperitonitis A01.09
Typhus (fever) A75.9
abdominal, abdominalis — *see* Typhoid
African tick A77.1
amarillic A95.9
brain A75.9 [G94]
cerebral A75.9 [G94]
classical A75.0
due to Rickettsia
prowazekii A75.0
recrudescent A75.1
tsutsugamushi A75.3
typhi A75.2
endemic (flea-borne) A75.2
epidemic (louse-borne) A75.0
exanthematicus SAI A75.0
brillii SAI A75.1
mexicanus SAI A75.2
typhus murinus A75.2
exanthematic NEC A75.0
flea-borne A75.2
India tick A77.1
Kenya (tick) A77.1
louse-borne A75.0
Mexican A75.2
mite-borne A75.3
murine A75.2
North Asian tick-borne A77.2
petechial A75.9
Queensland tick A77.3
rat A75.2
recrudescent A75.1
recurrens — *see* Fever, relapsing
Sao Paulo A77.0
scrub (China) (India) (Malaysia) (New Guinea) A75.3
shop (of Malaysia) A75.2
Siberian tick A77.2
tick-borne A77.9
tropical (mite-borne) A75.3
Tyrosinemia E70.21
newborn, transitory P74.5
Tyrosinosis E70.21
Tyrosinuria E70.29

U

Uhl's anomaly or disease Q24.8
Ulcer, ulcerated, ulcerating, ulceration, ulcerative
alveolar process M27.3
amebic (intestine) A06.1
skin A06.7
anastomotic — *see* Ulcer, gastrojejunal
anorectal K62.6
antral — *see* Ulcer, stomach
anus (sphincter) (solitary) K62.6
aorta — *see* Aneurysm
aphthous (oral) (recurrent) K12.0
genital organ(s)
female N76.6
male N50.89
artery I77.2
atrophic — *see* Ulcer, skin
decubitus — *see* Ulcer, pressure, by site
back L98.429
with
bone involvement without evidence of necrosis L98.426
bone necrosis L98.424
exposed fat layer L98.422
muscle involvement without evidence of necrosis L98.425
muscle necrosis L98.423
skin breakdown only L98.421
specified severity NEC L98.428
Barrett's (esophagus) K22.10
with bleeding K22.11
bile duct (common) (hepatic) K83.8
bladder (solitary) (sphincter) NEC N32.89
bilharzial B65.9 [N33]
in schistosomiasis (bilharzial) B65.9 [N33]
submucosal — *see* Cystitis, interstitial
tuberculous A18.12
bleeding K27.4
bone — *see* Osteomyelitis, specified type NEC
bowel — *see* Ulcer, intestine
breast N61.1

Ulcer, ulcerated, ulcerating, ulceration, ulcerative — *continued*
bronchus J98.09
buccal (cavity) (traumatic) K12.1
Buruli A31.1
buttock L98.419
with
bone involvement without evidence of necrosis L98.416
bone necrosis L98.414
exposed fat layer L98.412
muscle involvement without evidence of necrosis L98.415
muscle necrosis L98.413
skin breakdown only L98.411
specified severity NEC L98.418
cancerous — *see* Neoplasm, malignant, by site
cardia K22.10
with bleeding K22.11
cardioesophageal (peptic) K22.10
with bleeding K22.11
cecum — *see* Ulcer, intestine
cervix (uteri) (decubitus) (trophic) N86
with cervicitis N72
chancroidal A57
chiclero B55.1
chronic (cause unknown) — *see* Ulcer, skin
Cochin-China B55.1
colon — *see* Ulcer, intestine
conjunctiva H10.89
cornea H16.00- ☑
with hypopyon H16.03- ☑
central H16.01- ☑
dendritic (herpes simplex) B00.52
marginal H16.04- ☑
Mooren's H16.05- ☑
mycotic H16.06- ☑
perforated H16.07- ☑
ring H16.02- ☑
tuberculous (phlyctenular) A18.52
corpus cavernosum (chronic) N48.5
crural — *see* Ulcer, lower limb
Curling's — *see* Ulcer, peptic, acute
Cushing's — *see* Ulcer, peptic, acute
cystic duct K82.8
cystitis (interstitial) — *see* Cystitis, interstitial
decubitus — *see* Ulcer, pressure, by site
dendritic, cornea (herpes simplex) B00.52
diabetes, diabetic — *see* Diabetes, ulcer
Dieulafoy's K25.0
due to
infection NEC — *see* Ulcer, skin
radiation NEC L59.8
trophic disturbance (any region) — *see* Ulcer, skin
X-ray L58.1
duodenum, duodenal (eroded) (peptic) K26.9
with
hemorrhage K26.4
and perforation K26.6
perforation K26.5
acute K26.3
with
hemorrhage K26.0
and perforation K26.2
perforation K26.1
chronic K26.7
with
hemorrhage K26.4
and perforation K26.6
perforation K26.5
dysenteric A09
elusive — *see* Cystitis, interstitial
endocarditis (acute) (chronic) (subacute) I28.8
epiglottis J38.7
esophagus (peptic) K22.10
with bleeding K22.11
due to
aspirin K22.10
with bleeding K22.11
gastrointestinal reflux disease K21.0
ingestion of chemical or medicament K22.10
with bleeding K22.11
fungal K22.10
with bleeding K22.11
infective K22.10
with bleeding K22.11
varicose — *see* Varix, esophagus
eyelid (region) H01.8

Ulcer, ulcerated, ulcerating, ulceration, ulcerative
— *continued*
   fauces J39.2
   Fenwick (-Hunner) (solitary) — *see* Cystitis, interstitial
   fistulous — *see* Ulcer, skin
   foot (indolent) (trophic) — *see* Ulcer, lower limb
   frambesial, initial A66.0
   frenum (tongue) K14.0
   gallbladder or duct K82.8
   gangrenous — *see* Gangrene
   gastric — *see* Ulcer, stomach
   gastrocolic — *see* Ulcer, gastrojejunal
   gastroduodenal — *see* Ulcer, peptic
   gastroesophageal — *see* Ulcer, stomach
   gastrointestinal — *see* Ulcer, gastrojejunal
   gastrojejunal (peptic) K28.9
      with
         hemorrhage K28.4
            and perforation K28.6
         perforation K28.5
      acute K28.3
         with
            hemorrhage K28.0
               and perforation K28.2
            perforation K28.1
      chronic K28.7
         with
            hemorrhage K28.4
               and perforation K28.6
            perforation K28.5
   gastrojejunocolic — *see* Ulcer, gastrojejunal
   gingiva K06.8
   gingivitis K05.10
      nonplaque induced K05.11
      plaque induced K05.10
   glottis J38.7
   granuloma of pudenda A58
   gum K06.8
   gumma, due to yaws A66.4
   heel — *see* Ulcer, lower limb
   hemorrhoid (*see also* Hemorrhoids, by degree) K64.8
   Hunner's — *see* Cystitis, interstitial
   hypopharynx J39.2
   hypopyon (chronic) (subacute) — *see* Ulcer, cornea,
      with hypopyon
   hypostaticum — *see* Ulcer, varicose
   ileum — *see* Ulcer, intestine
   intestine, intestinal K63.3
      with perforation K63.1
      amebic A06.1
      duodenal — *see* Ulcer, duodenum
      granulocytopenic (with hemorrhage) — *see* Neu-
         tropenia
      marginal — *see* Ulcer, gastrojejunal
      perforating K63.1
         newborn P78.0
      primary, small intestine K63.3
      rectum K62.6
      stercoraceous, stercoral K63.3
      tuberculous A18.32
      typhoid (fever) — *see* Typhoid
      varicose I86.8
   jejunum, jejunal — *see* Ulcer, gastrojejunal
   keratitis — *see* Ulcer, cornea
   knee — *see* Ulcer, lower limb
   labium (majus) (minus) N76.6
   laryngitis — *see* Laryngitis
   larynx (aphthous) (contact) J38.7
      diphtheritic A36.2
   leg — *see* Ulcer, lower limb
   lip K13.0
   Lipschütz's N76.6
   lower limb (atrophic) (chronic) (neurogenic) (perforat-
      ing) (pyogenic) (trophic) (tropical) L97.909
      with
         bone involvement without evidence of necrosis
            L97.906
         bone necrosis L97.904
         exposed fat layer L97.902
         muscle involvement without evidence of
            necrosis L97.905
         muscle necrosis L97.903
         skin breakdown only L97.901
         specified severity NEC L97.908
      ankle L97.309
         with
            bone involvement without evidence of
               necrosis L97.306

Ulcer, ulcerated, ulcerating, ulceration, ulcerative
— *continued*
   lower limb — *continued*
      ankle — *continued*
         with — *continued*
            bone necrosis L97.304
            exposed fat layer L97.302
            muscle involvement without evidence of
               necrosis L97.305
            muscle necrosis L97.303
            skin breakdown only L97.301
            specified severity NEC L97.308
         left L97.329
            with
               bone involvement without evidence of
                  necrosis L97.326
               bone necrosis L97.324
               exposed fat layer L97.322
               muscle involvement without evidence
                  of necrosis L97.325
               muscle necrosis L97.323
               skin breakdown only L97.321
               specified severity NEC L97.328
         right L97.319
            with
               bone involvement without evidence of
                  necrosis L97.316
               bone necrosis L97.314
               exposed fat layer L97.312
               muscle involvement without evidence
                  of necrosis L97.315
               muscle necrosis L97.313
               skin breakdown only L97.311
               specified severity NEC L97.318
      calf L97.209
         with
            bone involvement without evidence of
               necrosis L97.206
            bone necrosis L97.204
            exposed fat layer L97.202
            muscle involvement without evidence of
               necrosis L97.205
            muscle necrosis L97.203
            skin breakdown only L97.201
            specified severity NEC L97.208
         left L97.229
            with
               bone involvement without evidence of
                  necrosis L97.226
               bone necrosis L97.224
               exposed fat layer L97.222
               muscle involvement without evidence
                  of necrosis L97.225
               muscle necrosis L97.223
               skin breakdown only L97.221
               specified severity NEC L97.228
         right L97.219
            with
               bone involvement without evidence of
                  necrosis L97.216
               bone necrosis L97.214
               exposed fat layer L97.212
               muscle involvement without evidence
                  of necrosis L97.215
               muscle necrosis L97.213
               skin breakdown only L97.211
               specified severity NEC L97.218
      decubitus — *see* Ulcer, pressure, by site
      foot specified NEC L97.509
         with
            bone involvement without evidence of
               necrosis L97.506
            bone necrosis L97.504
            exposed fat layer L97.502
            muscle involvement without evidence of
               necrosis L97.505
            muscle necrosis L97.503
            skin breakdown only L97.501
            specified severity NEC L97.508
         left L97.529
            with
               bone involvement without evidence of
                  necrosis L97.526
               bone necrosis L97.524
               exposed fat layer L97.522
               muscle involvement without evidence
                  of necrosis L97.525
               muscle necrosis L97.523
               skin breakdown only L97.521

Ulcer, ulcerated, ulcerating, ulceration, ulcerative
— *continued*
   lower limb — *continued*
      foot specified — *continued*
         left — *continued*
            with — *continued*
               specified severity NEC L97.528
            right L97.519
               with
                  bone involvement without evidence of
                     necrosis L97.516
                  bone necrosis L97.514
                  exposed fat layer L97.512
                  muscle involvement without evidence
                     of necrosis L97.515
                  muscle necrosis L97.513
                  skin breakdown only L97.511
                  specified severity NEC L97.518
      heel L97.409
         with
            bone involvement without evidence of
               necrosis L97.406
            bone necrosis L97.404
            exposed fat layer L97.402
            muscle involvement without evidence of
               necrosis L97.405
            muscle necrosis L97.403
            skin breakdown only L97.401
            specified severity NEC L97.408
         left L97.429
            with
               bone involvement without evidence of
                  necrosis L97.426
               bone necrosis L97.424
               exposed fat layer L97.422
               muscle involvement without evidence
                  of necrosis L97.425
               muscle necrosis L97.423
               skin breakdown only L97.421
               specified severity NEC L97.428
         right L97.419
            with
               bone involvement without evidence of
                  necrosis L97.416
               bone necrosis L97.414
               exposed fat layer L97.412
               muscle involvement without evidence
                  of necrosis L97.415
               muscle necrosis L97.413
               skin breakdown only L97.411
               specified severity NEC L97.418
      left L97.929
         with
            bone involvement without evidence of
               necrosis L97.926
            bone necrosis L97.924
            exposed fat layer L97.922
            muscle involvement without evidence of
               necrosis L97.925
            muscle necrosis L97.923
            skin breakdown only L97.921
            specified severity NEC L97.928
      leprous A30.1
      lower leg NOS L97.909
         with
            bone involvement without evidence of
               necrosis L97.906
            bone necrosis L97.904
            exposed fat layer L97.902
            muscle involvement without evidence of
               necrosis L97.905
            muscle necrosis L97.903
            skin breakdown only L97.901
            specified severity NEC L97.908
         left L97.929
            with
               bone involvement without evidence of
                  necrosis L97.926
               bone necrosis L97.924
               exposed fat layer L97.922
               muscle involvement without evidence
                  of necrosis L97.925
               muscle necrosis L97.923
               skin breakdown only L97.921
               specified severity NEC L97.928
         right L97.919
            with
               bone involvement without evidence of
                  necrosis L97.916

Ulcer, ulcerated, ulcerating, ulceration, ulcerative
— *continued*
  lower limb — *continued*
    lower leg — *continued*
      right — *continued*
        with — *continued*
          bone necrosis L97.914
          exposed fat layer L97.912
          muscle involvement without evidence of necrosis L97.915
          muscle necrosis L97.913
          skin breakdown only L97.911
          specified severity NEC L97.918
      specified site NEC L97.809
        with
          bone involvement without evidence of necrosis L97.806
          bone necrosis L97.804
          exposed fat layer L97.802
          muscle involvement without evidence of necrosis L97.805
          muscle necrosis L97.803
          skin breakdown only L97.801
          specified severity NEC L97.808
      left L97.829
        with
          bone involvement without evidence of necrosis L97.826
          bone necrosis L97.824
          exposed fat layer L97.822
          muscle involvement without evidence of necrosis L97.825
          muscle necrosis L97.823
          skin breakdown only L97.821
          specified severity NEC L97.828
      right L97.819
        with
          bone involvement without evidence of necrosis L97.816
          bone necrosis L97.814
          exposed fat layer L97.812
          muscle involvement without evidence of necrosis L97.815
          muscle necrosis L97.813
          skin breakdown only L97.811
          specified severity NEC L97.818
    midfoot L97.409
      with
        bone involvement without evidence of necrosis L97.406
        bone necrosis L97.404
        exposed fat layer L97.402
        muscle involvement without evidence of necrosis L97.405
        muscle necrosis L97.403
        skin breakdown only L97.401
        specified severity NEC L97.408
      left L97.429
        with
          bone involvement without evidence of necrosis L97.426
          bone necrosis L97.424
          exposed fat layer L97.422
          muscle involvement without evidence of necrosis L97.425
          muscle necrosis L97.423
          skin breakdown only L97.421
          specified severity NEC L97.428
      right L97.419
        with
          bone involvement without evidence of necrosis L97.416
          bone necrosis L97.414
          exposed fat layer L97.412
          muscle involvement without evidence of necrosis L97.415
          muscle necrosis L97.413
          skin breakdown only L97.411
          specified severity NEC L97.418
    right L97.919
      with
        bone involvement without evidence of necrosis L97.916
        bone necrosis L97.914
        exposed fat layer L97.912
        muscle involvement without evidence of necrosis L97.915
        muscle necrosis L97.913
        skin breakdown only L97.911

Ulcer, ulcerated, ulcerating, ulceration, ulcerative
— *continued*
  lower limb — *continued*
    right — *continued*
      with — *continued*
        specified severity NEC L97.918
      syphilitic A52.19
    thigh L97.109
      with
        bone involvement without evidence of necrosis L97.106
        bone necrosis L97.104
        exposed fat layer L97.102
        muscle involvement without evidence of necrosis L97.105
        muscle necrosis L97.103
        skin breakdown only L97.101
        specified severity NEC L97.108
      left L97.129
        with
          bone involvement without evidence of necrosis L97.126
          bone necrosis L97.124
          exposed fat layer L97.122
          muscle involvement without evidence of necrosis L97.125
          muscle necrosis L97.123
          skin breakdown only L97.121
          specified severity NEC L97.128
      right L97.119
        with
          bone involvement without evidence of necrosis L97.116
          bone necrosis L97.114
          exposed fat layer L97.112
          muscle involvement without evidence of necrosis L97.115
          muscle necrosis L97.113
          skin breakdown only L97.111
          specified severity NEC L97.118
    toe L97.509
      with
        bone involvement without evidence of necrosis L97.506
        bone necrosis L97.504
        exposed fat layer L97.502
        muscle involvement without evidence of necrosis L97.505
        muscle necrosis L97.503
        skin breakdown only L97.501
        specified severity NEC L97.508
      left L97.529
        with
          bone involvement without evidence of necrosis L97.526
          bone necrosis L97.524
          exposed fat layer L97.522
          muscle involvement without evidence of necrosis L97.525
          muscle necrosis L97.523
          skin breakdown only L97.521
          specified severity NEC L97.528
      right L97.519
        with
          bone involvement without evidence of necrosis L97.516
          bone necrosis L97.514
          exposed fat layer L97.512
          muscle involvement without evidence of necrosis L97.515
          muscle necrosis L97.513
          skin breakdown only L97.511
          specified severity NEC L97.518
    varicose — *see* Varix, leg, with, ulcer
  luetic — *see* Ulcer, syphilitic
  lung J98.4
    tuberculous — *see* Tuberculosis, pulmonary
  malignant — *see* Neoplasm, malignant, by site
  marginal NEC — *see* Ulcer, gastrojejunal
  meatus (urinarius) N34.2
  Meckel's diverticulum Q43.0
    malignant — *see* Table of Neoplasms, small intestine, malignant
  Meleney's (chronic undermining) — *see* Ulcer, skin
  Mooren's (cornea) — *see* Ulcer, cornea, Mooren's
  mycobacterial (skin) A31.1
  nasopharynx J39.2
  neck, uterus N86

Ulcer, ulcerated, ulcerating, ulceration, ulcerative
— *continued*
  neurogenic NEC — *see* Ulcer, skin
  nose, nasal (passage) (infective) (septum) J34.0
    skin — *see* Ulcer, skin
    spirochetal A69.8
    varicose (bleeding) I86.8
  oral mucosa (traumatic) K12.1
  palate (soft) K12.1
  penis (chronic) N48.5
  peptic (site unspecified) K27.9
    with
      hemorrhage K27.4
        and perforation K27.6
      perforation K27.5
    acute K27.3
      with
        hemorrhage K27.0
          and perforation K27.2
        perforation K27.1
    chronic K27.7
      with
        hemorrhage K27.4
          and perforation K27.6
        perforation K27.5
    esophagus K22.10
      with bleeding K22.11
    newborn P78.82
  perforating K27.5
    skin — *see* Ulcer, skin
  peritonsillar J35.8
  phagedenic (tropical) — *see* Ulcer, skin
  pharynx J39.2
  phlebitis — *see* Phlebitis
  plaster — *see* Ulcer, pressure, by site
  popliteal space — *see* Ulcer, lower limb
  postpyloric — *see* Ulcer, duodenum
  prepuce N47.7
  prepyloric — *see* Ulcer, stomach
  pressure (pressure area) L89.9- ☑
    ankle L89.5- ☑
    back L89.1- ☑
    buttock L89.3- ☑
    coccyx L89.15- ☑
    contiguous site of back, buttock, hip L89.4- ☑
    elbow L89.0- ☑
    face L89.81- ☑
    head L89.81- ☑
    heel L89.6- ☑
    hip L89.2- ☑
    sacral region (tailbone) L89.15- ☑
    specified site NEC L89.89- ☑
    stage 1 (healing) (pre-ulcer skin changes limited to persistent focal edema)
      ankle L89.5- ☑
      back L89.1- ☑
      buttock L89.3- ☑
      coccyx L89.15- ☑
      contiguous site of back, buttock, hip L89.4- ☑
      elbow L89.0- ☑
      face L89.81- ☑
      head L89.81- ☑
      heel L89.6- ☑
      hip L89.2- ☑
      sacral region (tailbone) L89.15- ☑
      specified site NEC L89.89- ☑
    stage 2 (healing) (abrasion, blister, partial thickness skin loss involving epidermis and/or dermis)
      ankle L89.5- ☑
      back L89.1- ☑
      buttock L89.3- ☑
      coccyx L89.15- ☑
      contiguous site of back, buttock, hip L89.4- ☑
      elbow L89.0- ☑
      face L89.81- ☑
      head L89.81- ☑
      heel L89.6- ☑
      hip L89.2- ☑
      sacral region (tailbone) L89.15- ☑
      specified site NEC L89.89- ☑
    stage 3 (healing) (full thickness skin loss involving damage or necrosis of subcutaneous tissue)
      ankle L89.5- ☑
      back L89.1- ☑
      buttock L89.3- ☑
      coccyx L89.15- ☑
      contiguous site of back, buttock, hip L89.4- ☑

Ulcer, ulcerated, ulcerating, ulceration, ulcerative
  — continued
  pressure — continued
    stage 3 — continued
      elbow L89.0- ☑
      face L89.81- ☑
      head L89.81- ☑
      heel L89.6- ☑
      hip L89.2- ☑
      sacral region (tailbone) L89.15- ☑
      specified site NEC L89.89- ☑
    stage 4 (healing) (necrosis of soft tissues through
      to underlying muscle, tendon, or bone)
      ankle L89.5- ☑
      back L89.1- ☑
      buttock L89.3- ☑
      coccyx L89.15- ☑
      contiguous site of back, buttock, hip L89.4- ☑
      elbow L89.0- ☑
      face L89.81- ☑
      head L89.81- ☑
      heel L89.6- ☑
      hip L89.2- ☑
      sacral region (tailbone) L89.15- ☑
      specified site NEC L89.89- ☑
    unspecified stage
      ankle L89.5- ☑
      back L89.1- ☑
      buttock L89.3- ☑
      coccyx L89.15- ☑
      contiguous site of back, buttock, hip L89.4- ☑
      elbow L89.0- ☑
      face L89.81- ☑
      head L89.81- ☑
      heel L89.6- ☑
      hip L89.2- ☑
      sacral region (tailbone) L89.15- ☑
      specified site NEC L89.89- ☑
    unstageable
      ankle L89.5- ☑
      back L89.1- ☑
      buttock L89.3- ☑
      coccyx L89.15- ☑
      contiguous site of back, buttock, hip L89.4- ☑
      elbow L89.0- ☑
      face L89.81- ☑
      head L89.81- ☑
      heel L89.6- ☑
      hip L89.2- ☑
      sacral region (tailbone) L89.15- ☑
      specified site NEC L89.89- ☑
  primary of intestine K63.3
    with perforation K63.1
  prostate N41.9
  pyloric — see Ulcer, stomach
  rectosigmoid K63.3
    with perforation K63.1
  rectum (sphincter) (solitary) K62.6
    stercoraceous, stercoral K62.6
  retina — see Inflammation, chorioretinal
  rodent (see also Neoplasm, skin, malignant)
  sclera — see Scleritis
  scrofulous (tuberculous) A18.2
  scrotum N50.89
    tuberculous A18.15
    varicose I86.1
  seminal vesicle N50.89
  sigmoid — see Ulcer, intestine
  skin (atrophic) (chronic) (neurogenic) (non-healing)
    (perforating) (pyogenic) (trophic) (tropical)
    L98.499
    with gangrene — see Gangrene
    amebic A06.7
    back — see Ulcer, back
    buttock — see Ulcer, buttock
    decubitus — see Ulcer, pressure
    lower limb — see Ulcer, lower limb
    mycobacterial A31.1
    specified site NEC L98.499
      with
        bone involvement without evidence of
          necrosis L98.496
        bone necrosis L98.494
        exposed fat layer L98.492
        muscle involvement without evidence of
          necrosis L98.495
        muscle necrosis L98.493

Ulcer, ulcerated, ulcerating, ulceration, ulcerative
  — continued
  skin — continued
    specified site — continued
      with — continued
        skin breakdown only L98.491
        specified severity NEC L98.498
      tuberculous (primary) A18.4
      varicose — see Ulcer, varicose
  sloughing — see Ulcer, skin
  solitary, anus or rectum (sphincter) K62.6
  sore throat J02.9
    streptococcal J02.0
  spermatic cord N50.89
  spine (tuberculous) A18.01
  stasis (venous) — see Varix, leg, with, ulcer
    without varicose veins I87.2
  stercoraceous, stercoral K63.3
    with perforation K63.1
    anus or rectum K62.6
  stoma, stomal — see Ulcer, gastrojejunal
  stomach (eroded) (peptic) (round) K25.9
    with
      hemorrhage K25.4
        and perforation K25.6
      perforation K25.5
    acute K25.3
      with
        hemorrhage K25.0
          and perforation K25.2
        perforation K25.1
    chronic K25.7
      with
        hemorrhage K25.4
          and perforation K25.6
        perforation K25.5
  stomal — see Ulcer, gastrojejunal
  stomatitis K12.1
  stress — see Ulcer, peptic
  strumous (tuberculous) A18.2
  submucosal, bladder — see Cystitis, interstitial
  syphilitic (any site) (early) (secondary) A51.39
    late A52.79
    perforating A52.79
      foot A52.11
  testis N50.89
  thigh — see Ulcer, lower limb
  throat J39.2
    diphtheritic A36.0
  toe — see Ulcer, lower limb
  tongue (traumatic) K14.0
  tonsil J35.8
    diphtheritic A36.0
  trachea J39.8
  trophic — see Ulcer, skin
  tropical — see Ulcer, skin
  tuberculous — see Tuberculosis, ulcer
  tunica vaginalis N50.89
  turbinate J34.89
  typhoid (perforating) — see Typhoid
  unspecified site — see Ulcer, skin
  urethra (meatus) — see Urethritis
  uterus N85.8
    cervix N86
      with cervicitis N72
    neck N86
      with cervicitis N72
  vagina N76.5
    in Behçet's disease M35.2 [N77.0]
    pessary N89.8
  valve, heart I33.0
  varicose (lower limb, any part) (see also Varix, leg, with,
    ulcer)
    broad ligament I86.2
    esophagus — see Varix, esophagus
    inflamed or infected — see Varix, leg, with ulcer,
      with inflammation
    nasal septum I86.8
    perineum I86.3
    scrotum I86.1
    specified site NEC I86.8
    sublingual I86.0
    vulva I86.3
  vas deferens N50.89
  vulva (acute) (infectional) N76.6
    in (due to)
      Behçet's disease M35.2 [N77.0]
      herpesviral (herpes simplex) infection A60.04

Ulcer, ulcerated, ulcerating, ulceration, ulcerative
  — continued
  vulva — continued
    in — continued
      tuberculosis A18.18
    vulvobuccal, recurring N76.6
    X-ray L58.1
    yaws A66.4
Ulcerosa scarlatina A38.8
Ulcus (see also Ulcer)
  cutis tuberculosum A18.4
  duodeni — see Ulcer, duodenum
  durum (syphilitic) A51.0
    extragenital A51.2
  gastrojejunale — see Ulcer, gastrojejunal
  hypostaticum — see Ulcer, varicose
  molle (cutis) (skin) A57
  serpens corneae — see Ulcer, cornea, central
  ventriculi — see Ulcer, stomach
Ulegyria Q04.8
Ulerythema
  ophryogenes, congenital Q84.2
  sycosiforme L73.8
Ullrich (-Bonnevie)(-Turner) **syndrome** (see also Turner's
  syndrome) Q87.1
Ullrich-Feichtiger syndrome Q87.0
Ulnar — see condition
Ulorrhagia, ulorrhea K06.8
Umbilicus, umbilical — see condition
Unacceptable
  contours of tooth K08.54
  morphology of tooth K08.54
Unavailability (of)
  bed at medical facility Z75.1
  health service-related agencies Z75.4
  medical facilities (at) Z75.3
    due to
      investigation by social service agency Z75.2
      lack of services at home Z75.0
      remoteness from facility Z75.3
      waiting list Z75.1
    home Z75.0
    outpatient clinic Z75.3
  schooling Z55.1
  social service agencies Z75.4
Uncinaria americana infestation B76.1
Uncinariasis B76.9
Uncongenial work Z56.5
Unconscious (ness) — see Coma
Under observation — see Observation
Underachievement in school Z55.3
Underdevelopment (see also Undeveloped)
  nose Q30.1
  sexual E30.0
Underdosing (see also Table of Drugs and Chemicals,
  categories T36-T50, with final character 6) Z91.14
  intentional NEC Z91.128
    due to financial hardship of patient Z91.120
  unintentional NEC Z91.138
    due to patient's age related debility Z91.130
Underfeeding, newborn P92.3
Underfill, endodontic M27.53
Underimmunization status Z28.3
Undernourishment — see Malnutrition
Undernutrition — see Malnutrition
Underweight R63.6
  for gestational age — see Light for dates
Underwood's disease P83.0
Undescended (see also Malposition, congenital)
  cecum Q43.3
  colon Q43.3
  testicle — see Cryptorchid
Undeveloped, undevelopment (see also Hypoplasia)
  brain (congenital) Q02
  cerebral (congenital) Q02
  heart Q24.8
  lung Q33.6
  testis E29.1
  uterus E30.0
Undiagnosed (disease) R69
Undulant fever — see Brucellosis
Unemployment, anxiety concerning Z56.0
  threatened Z56.2
Unequal length (acquired) (limb) (see also Deformity,
  limb, unequal length)
  leg (see also Deformity, limb, unequal length)
    congenital Q72.9- ☑

Unextracted dental root KØ8.3
Unguis incarnatus L6Ø.Ø
Unhappiness R45.2
Unicornate uterus Q51.4
  in pregnancy or childbirth O34.ØØ
Unilateral (*see also* condition)
  development, breast N64.89
  organ or site, congenital NEC — *see* Agenesis, by site
Unilocular heart Q2Ø.8
Union, abnormal (*see also* Fusion)
  larynx and trachea Q34.8
Universal mesentery Q43.3
Unrepairable overhanging of dental restorative materials KØ8.52
Unsatisfactory
  restoration of tooth KØ8.5Ø
    specified NEC KØ8.59
  sample of cytologic smear
    anus R85.615
    cervix R87.615
    vagina R87.625
  surroundings Z59.1
  work Z56.5
Unsoundness of mind — *see* Psychosis
Unstable
  back NEC — *see* Instability, joint, spine
  hip (congenital) Q65.6
    acquired — *see* Derangement, joint, specified type NEC, hip
  joint — *see* Instability, joint
    secondary to removal of joint prosthesis M96.89
  lie (mother) O32.Ø ☑
  lumbosacral joint (congenital)
    acquired — *see* subcategory M53.2 ☑
  sacroiliac — *see* subcategory M53.2 ☑
  spine NEC — *see* Instability, joint, spine
Unsteadiness on feet R26.81
Untruthfulness, child problem F91.8
Unverricht (-Lundborg) **disease or epilepsy** — *see* Epilepsy, generalized, idiopathic
Unwanted pregnancy Z64.Ø
Upbringing, institutional Z62.22
  away from parents NEC Z62.29
  in care of non-parental family member Z62.21
  in foster care Z62.21
  in orphanage or group home Z62.22
  in welfare custody Z62.21
Upper respiratory — *see* condition
Upset
  gastric K3Ø
  gastrointestinal K3Ø
    psychogenic F45.8
  intestinal (large) (small) K59.9
    psychogenic F45.8
  menstruation N93.9
  mental F48.9
  stomach K3Ø
    psychogenic F45.8
Urachus (*see also* condition)
  patent or persistent Q64.4
Urbach-Oppenheim disease (necrobiosis lipoidica diabeticorum) — *see* EØ8-E13 with .62Ø
Urbach's lipoid proteinosis E78.89
Urbach-Wiethe disease E78.89
Urban yellow fever A95.1
Urea
  blood, high — *see* Uremia
  cycle metabolism disorder — *see* Disorder, urea cycle metabolism
Uremia, uremic N19
  with
    ectopic or molar pregnancy OØ8.4
    polyneuropathy N18.9 [G63]
  chronic NOS (*see also* Disease, kidney, chronic) N18.9
    due to hypertension — *see* Hypertensive, kidney
  complicating
    ectopic or molar pregnancy OØ8.4
  congenital P96.Ø
  extrarenal R39.2
  following ectopic or molar pregnancy OØ8.4
  newborn P96.Ø
  prerenal R39.2
Ureter, ureteral — *see* condition
Ureteralgia N23
Ureterectasis — *see* Hydroureter
Ureteritis N28.89
  cystica N28.86

Ureteritis — *continued*
  due to calculus N2Ø.1
    with calculus, kidney N2Ø.2
      with hydronephrosis N13.2
  gonococcal (acute) (chronic) A54.21
  nonspecific N28.89
Ureterocele N28.89
  congenital (orthotopic) Q62.31
  ectopic Q62.32
Ureterolith, ureterolithiasis — *see* Calculus, ureter
Ureterostomy
  attention to Z43.6
  status Z93.6
Urethra, urethral — *see* condition
Urethralgia R39.89
Urethritis (anterior) (posterior) N34.2
  calculous N21.1
  candidal B37.41
  chlamydial A56.Ø1
  diplococcal (gonococcal) A54.Ø1
    with abscess (accessory gland) (periurethral) A54.1
  gonococcal A54.Ø1
    with abscess (accessory gland) (periurethral) A54.1
  nongonococcal N34.1
    Reiter's — *see* Reiter's disease
  nonspecific N34.1
  nonvenereal N34.1
  postmenopausal N34.2
  puerperal O86.22
  Reiter's — *see* Reiter's disease
  specified NEC N34.2
  trichomonal or due to Trichomonas (vaginalis) A59.Ø3
Urethrocele N81.Ø
  with
    cystocele — *see* Cystocele
    prolapse of uterus — *see* Prolapse, uterus
Urethrolithiasis (with colic or infection) N21.1
Urethrorectal — *see* condition
Urethrorrhagia N36.8
Urethrorrhea R36.9
Urethrostomy
  attention to Z43.6
  status Z93.6
Urethrotrigonitis — *see* Trigonitis
Urethrovaginal — *see* condition
Urgency
  fecal R15.2
  hypertensive — *see* Hypertension
  urinary R39.15
Urhidrosis, uridrosis L74.8
Uric acid in blood (increased) E79.Ø
Uricacidemia (asymptomatic) E79.Ø
Uricemia (asymptomatic) E79.Ø
Uricosuria R82.99
Urinary — *see* condition
Urination
  frequent R35.Ø
  painful R3Ø.9
Urine
  blood in — *see* Hematuria
  discharge, excessive R35.8
  enuresis, nonorganic origin F98.Ø
  extravasation R39.Ø
  frequency R35.Ø
  incontinence R32
    nonorganic origin F98.Ø
  intermittent stream R39.198
  pus in N39.Ø
  retention or stasis R33.9
    organic R33.8
      drug-induced R33.Ø
    psychogenic F45.8
  secretion
    deficient R34
    excessive R35.8
    frequency R35.Ø
  stream
    intermittent R39.198
    slowing R39.198
    splitting R39.13
    weak R39.12
Urinemia — *see* Uremia
Urinoma, urethra N36.8
Uroarthritis, infectious (Reiter's) — *see* Reiter's disease
Urodialysis R34
Urolithiasis — *see* Calculus, urinary
Uronephrosis — *see* Hydronephrosis
Uropathy N39.9

Uropathy — *continued*
  obstructive N13.9
    specified NEC N13.8
  reflux N13.9
    specified NEC N13.8
  vesicoureteral reflux-associated — *see* Reflux, vesicoureteral
Urosepsis — *code to* condition
Urticaria L5Ø.9
  with angioneurotic edema T78.3 ☑
    hereditary D84.1
  allergic L5Ø.Ø
  cholinergic L5Ø.5
  chronic L5Ø.8
  cold, familial L5Ø.2
  contact L5Ø.6
  dermatographic L5Ø.3
  due to
    cold or heat L5Ø.2
    drugs L5Ø.Ø
    food L5Ø.Ø
    inhalants L5Ø.Ø
    plants L5Ø.6
    serum (*see also* Reaction, serum) T8Ø.69 ☑
  factitial L5Ø.3
  familial cold MØ4.2
  giant T78.3 ☑
    hereditary D84.1
  gigantea T78.3 ☑
  idiopathic L5Ø.1
  larynx T78.3 ☑
    hereditary D84.1
  neonatorum P83.88
  nonallergic L5Ø.1
  papulosa (Hebra) L28.2
  pigmentosa D47.Ø1
    congenital Q82.2
    of neonatal onset Q82.2
    of newborn onset Q82.2
  recurrent periodic L5Ø.8
  serum (*see also* Reaction, serum) T8Ø.69 ☑
  solar L56.3
  specified type NEC L5Ø.8
  thermal (cold) (heat) L5Ø.2
  vibratory L5Ø.4
  xanthelasmoidea — *see* Urticaria pigmentosa
Use (of)
  alcohol Z72.89
    with
      intoxication F1Ø.929
      sleep disorder F1Ø.982
    harmful — *see* Abuse, alcohol
  amphetamines — *see* Use, stimulant NEC
  caffeine — *see* Use, stimulant NEC
  cannabis F12.9Ø
    with
      anxiety disorder F12.98Ø
      intoxication F12.929
        with
          delirium F12.921
          perceptual disturbance F12.922
        uncomplicated F12.92Ø
      other specified disorder F12.988
      psychosis F12.959
        delusions F12.95Ø
        hallucinations F12.951
      unspecified disorder F12.99
  cocaine F14.9Ø
    with
      anxiety disorder F14.98Ø
      intoxication F14.929
        with
          delirium F14.921
          perceptual disturbance F14.922
        uncomplicated F14.92Ø
      other specified disorder F14.988
      psychosis F14.959
        delusions F14.95Ø
        hallucinations F14.951
      sexual dysfunction F14.981
      sleep disorder F14.982
      unspecified disorder F14.99
    harmful — *see* Abuse, drug, cocaine
  drug(s) NEC F19.9Ø
    with sleep disorder F19.982
    harmful — *see* Abuse, drug, by type
  hallucinogen NEC F16.9Ø

Use — *continued*
  hallucinogen — *continued*
    with
      anxiety disorder F16.980
      intoxication F16.929
        with
          delirium F16.921
        uncomplicated F16.920
      mood disorder F16.94
      other specified disorder F16.988
      perception disorder (flashbacks) F16.983
      psychosis F16.959
        delusions F16.950
        hallucinations F16.951
      unspecified disorder F16.99
    harmful — *see* Abuse, drug, hallucinogen NEC
  inhalants F18.90
    with
      anxiety disorder F18.980
      intoxication F18.929
        with delirium F18.921
        uncomplicated F18.920
      mood disorder F18.94
      other specified disorder F18.988
      persisting dementia F18.97
      psychosis F18.959
        delusions F18.950
        hallucinations F18.951
      unspecified disorder F18.99
    harmful — *see* Abuse, drug, inhalant
  methadone — *see* Use, opioid
  nonprescribed drugs F19.90
    harmful — *see* Abuse, non-psychoactive substance
  opioid F11.90
    with
      disorder F11.99
        mood F11.94
        sleep F11.982
        specified type NEC F11.988
      intoxication F11.929
        with
          delirium F11.921
          perceptual disturbance F11.922
        uncomplicated F11.920
      withdrawal F11.93
    harmful — *see* Abuse, drug, opioid
  patent medicines F19.90
    harmful — *see* Abuse, non-psychoactive substance
  psychoactive drug NEC F19.90
    with
      anxiety disorder F19.980
      intoxication F19.929
        with
          delirium F19.921
          perceptual disturbance F19.922
        uncomplicated F19.920
      mood disorder F19.94
      other specified disorder F19.988
      persisting
        amnestic disorder F19.96
        dementia F19.97
      psychosis F19.959
        delusions F19.950
        hallucinations F19.951
      sexual dysfunction F19.981
      sleep disorder F19.982
      unspecified disorder F19.99
      withdrawal F19.939
        with
          delirium F19.931
          perceptual disturbance F19.932
        uncomplicated F19.930
    harmful — *see* Abuse, drug NEC, psychoactive NEC
  sedative, hypnotic, or anxiolytic F13.90
    with
      anxiety disorder F13.980
      intoxication F13.929
        with
          delirium F13.921
        uncomplicated F13.920
      other specified disorder F13.988
      persisting
        amnestic disorder F13.96
        dementia F13.97
      psychosis F13.959
        delusions F13.950
        hallucinations F13.951
      sexual dysfunction F13.981

Use — *continued*
  sedative, hypnotic, or anxiolytic — *continued*
    with — *continued*
      sleep disorder F13.982
      unspecified disorder F13.99
    harmful — *see* Abuse, drug, sedative, hypnotic, or anxiolytic
  stimulant NEC F15.90
    with
      anxiety disorder F15.980
      intoxication F15.929
        with
          delirium F15.921
          perceptual disturbance F15.922
        uncomplicated F15.920
      mood disorder F15.94
      other specified disorder F15.988
      psychosis F15.959
        delusions F15.950
        hallucinations F15.951
      sexual dysfunction F15.981
      sleep disorder F15.982
      unspecified disorder F15.99
      withdrawal F15.93
    harmful — *see* Abuse, drug, stimulant NEC
  tobacco Z72.0
    with dependence — *see* Dependence, drug, nicotine
  volatile solvents (*see also* Use, inhalant) F18.90
    harmful — *see* Abuse, drug, inhalant
Usher-Senear disease or syndrome L10.4
Uta B55.1
Uteromegaly N85.2
Uterovaginal — *see* condition
Uterovesical — *see* condition
Uveal — *see* condition
Uveitis (anterior) (*see also* Iridocyclitis)
  acute — *see* Iridocyclitis, acute
  chronic — *see* Iridocyclitis, chronic
  due to toxoplasmosis (acquired) B58.09
    congenital P37.1
  granulomatous — *see* Iridocyclitis, chronic
  heterochromic — *see* Cyclitis, Fuchs' heterochromic
  lens-induced — *see* Iridocyclitis, lens-induced
  posterior — *see* Chorioretinitis
  sympathetic H44.13- ☑
  syphilitic (secondary) A51.43
    congenital (early) A50.01
    late A52.71
  tuberculous A18.54
Uveoencephalitis — *see* Inflammation, chorioretinal
Uveokeratitis — *see* Iridocyclitis
Uveoparotitis D86.89
Uvula — *see* condition
Uvulitis (acute) (catarrhal) (chronic) (membranous) (suppurative) (ulcerative) K12.2

V

Vaccination (prophylactic)
  complication or reaction — *see* Complications, vaccination
  delayed Z28.9
  encounter for Z23
  not done — *see* Immunization, not done, because (of)
Vaccinia (generalized) (localized) T88.1 ☑
  without vaccination B08.011
  congenital P35.8
Vacuum, in sinus (accessory) (nasal) J34.89
Vagabond, vagabondage Z59.0
Vagabond's disease B85.1
Vagina, vaginal — *see* condition
Vaginalitis (tunica) (testis) N49.1
Vaginismus (reflex) N94.2
  functional F52.5
  nonorganic F52.5
  psychogenic F52.5
  secondary N94.2
Vaginitis (acute) (circumscribed) (diffuse) (emphysematous) (nonvenereal) (ulcerative) N76.0
  with ectopic or molar pregnancy O08.0
  amebic A06.82
  atrophic, postmenopausal N95.2
  bacterial N76.0
  blennorrhagic (gonococcal) A54.02
  candidal B37.3
  chlamydial A56.02

Vaginitis — *continued*
  chronic N76.1
  due to Trichomonas (vaginalis) A59.01
  following ectopic or molar pregnancy O08.0
  gonococcal A54.02
    with abscess (accessory gland) (periurethral) A54.1
  granuloma A58
  in (due to)
    candidiasis B37.3
    herpesviral (herpes simplex) infection A60.04
    pinworm infection B80 [N77.1]
  monilial B37.3
  mycotic (candidal) B37.3
  postmenopausal atrophic N95.2
  puerperal (postpartum) O86.13
  senile (atrophic) N95.2
  subacute or chronic N76.1
  syphilitic (early) A51.0
    late A52.76
  trichomonal A59.01
  tuberculous A18.18
Vaginosis — *see* Vaginitis
Vagotonia G52.2
Vagrancy Z59.0
VAIN — *see* Neoplasia, intraepithelial, vagina
Vallecula — *see* condition
Valley fever B38.0
Valsuani's disease — *see* Anemia, obstetric
Valve, valvular (formation) (*see also* condition)
  cerebral ventricle (communicating) in situ Z98.2
  cervix, internal os Q51.828
  congenital NEC — *see* Atresia, by site
  ureter (pelvic junction) (vesical orifice) Q62.39
  urethra (congenital) (posterior) Q64.2
Valvulitis (chronic) — *see* Endocarditis
Valvulopathy — *see* Endocarditis
Van Bogaert's leukoencephalopathy (sclerosing) (subacute) A81.1
Van Bogaert-Scherer-Epstein disease or syndrome E75.5
Van Buchem's syndrome M85.2
Van Creveld-von Gierke disease E74.01
Van der Hoeve (-de Kleyn) **syndrome** Q78.0
Van der Woude's syndrome Q38.0
Van Neck's disease or osteochondrosis M91.0
Vanishing lung J44.9
Vapor asphyxia or suffocation T59.9 ☑
  specified agent — *see* Table of Drugs and Chemicals
Variance, lethal ball, prosthetic heart valve T82.09 ☑
Variants, thalassemic D56.8
Variations in hair color L67.1
Varicella B01.9
  with
    complications NEC B01.89
    encephalitis B01.11
    encephalomyelitis B01.11
    meningitis B01.0
    myelitis B01.12
    pneumonia B01.2
  congenital P35.8
Varices — *see* Varix
Varicocele (scrotum) (thrombosed) I86.1
  ovary I86.2
  perineum I86.3
  spermatic cord (ulcerated) I86.1
Varicose
  aneurysm (ruptured) I77.0
  dermatitis — *see* Varix, leg, with, inflammation
  eczema — *see* Varix, leg, with, inflammation
  phlebitis — *see* Varix, with, inflammation
  tumor — *see* Varix
  ulcer (lower limb, any part) (*see also* Varix, leg, with, ulcer)
    anus (*see also* Hemorrhoids) K64.8
    esophagus — *see* Varix, esophagus
    inflamed or infected — *see* Varix, leg, with ulcer, with inflammation
    nasal septum I86.8
    perineum I86.3
    scrotum I86.1
    specified site NEC I86.8
  vein — *see* Varix
  vessel — *see* Varix, leg
Varicosis, varicosities, varicosity — *see* Varix
Variola (major) (minor) B03
Varioloid B03
Varix (lower limb) (ruptured) I83.90

Varix — *continued*
  with
    edema I83.899
    inflammation I83.10
      with ulcer (venous) I83.209
    pain I83.819
    specified complication NEC I83.899
    stasis dermatitis I83.10
      with ulcer (venous) I83.209
    swelling I83.899
    ulcer I83.009
      with inflammation I83.209
  aneurysmal I77.0
  asymptomatic I83.9- ☑
  bladder I86.2
  broad ligament I86.2
  complicating
    childbirth (lower extremity) O87.4
      anus or rectum O87.2
      genital (vagina, vulva or perineum) O87.8
    pregnancy (lower extremity) O22.0- ☑
      anus or rectum O22.4- ☑
      genital (vagina, vulva or perineum) O22.1- ☑
    puerperium (lower extremity) O87.4
      anus or rectum O87.2
      genital (vagina, vulva, perineum) O87.8
  congenital (any site) Q27.8
  esophagus (idiopathic) (primary) (ulcerated) I85.00
    bleeding I85.01
    congenital Q27.8
    in (due to)
      alcoholic liver disease I85.10
        bleeding I85.11
      cirrhosis of liver I85.10
        bleeding I85.11
      portal hypertension I85.10
        bleeding I85.11
      schistosomiasis I85.10
        bleeding I85.11
      toxic liver disease I85.10
        bleeding I85.11
    secondary I85.10
      bleeding I85.11
  gastric I86.4
  inflamed or infected I83.10
    ulcerated I83.209
  labia (majora) I86.3
  leg (asymptomatic) I83.90
    with
      edema I83.899
      inflammation I83.10
        with ulcer — *see* Varix, leg, with, ulcer, with inflammation by site
      pain I83.819
      specified complication NEC I83.899
      swelling I83.899
      ulcer I83.009
        with inflammation I83.209
        ankle I83.003
          with inflammation I83.203
        calf I83.002
          with inflammation I83.202
        foot NEC I83.005
          with inflammation I83.205
        heel I83.004
          with inflammation I83.204
        lower leg NEC I83.008
          with inflammation I83.208
        midfoot I83.004
          with inflammation I83.204
        thigh I83.001
          with inflammation I83.201
    bilateral (asymptomatic) I83.93
      with
        edema I83.893
        pain I83.813
        specified complication NEC I83.893
        swelling I83.893
        ulcer I83.0- ☑
          with inflammation I83.209
    left (asymptomatic) I83.92
      with
        edema I83.892
        inflammation I83.12
          with ulcer — *see* Varix, leg, with, ulcer, with inflammation by site
        pain I83.812
        specified complication NEC I83.892

Varix — *continued*
  leg — *continued*
    left — *continued*
      with — *continued*
        swelling I83.892
        ulcer I83.029
          with inflammation I83.229
          ankle I83.023
            with inflammation I83.223
          calf I83.022
            with inflammation I83.222
          foot NEC I83.025
            with inflammation I83.225
          heel I83.024
            with inflammation I83.224
          lower leg NEC I83.028
            with inflammation I83.228
          midfoot I83.024
            with inflammation I83.224
          thigh I83.021
            with inflammation I83.221
    right (asymptomatic) I83.91
      with
        edema I83.891
        inflammation I83.11
          with ulcer — *see* Varix, leg, with, ulcer, with inflammation by site
        pain I83.811
        specified complication NEC I83.891
        swelling I83.891
        ulcer I83.019
          with inflammation I83.219
          ankle I83.013
            with inflammation I83.213
          calf I83.012
            with inflammation I83.212
          foot NEC I83.015
            with inflammation I83.215
          heel I83.014
            with inflammation I83.214
          lower leg NEC I83.018
            with inflammation I83.218
          midfoot I83.014
            with inflammation I83.214
          thigh I83.011
            with inflammation I83.211
  nasal septum I86.8
  orbit I86.8
    congenital Q27.8
  ovary I86.2
  papillary I78.1
  pelvis I86.2
  perineum I86.3
  pharynx I86.8
  placenta O43.89- ☑
  renal papilla I86.8
  retina H35.09
  scrotum (ulcerated) I86.1
  sigmoid colon I86.8
  specified site NEC I86.8
  spinal (cord) (vessels) I86.8
  spleen, splenic (vein) (with phlebolith) I86.8
  stomach I86.4
  sublingual I86.0
  ulcerated I83.009
    inflamed or infected I83.209
  uterine ligament I86.2
  vagina I86.8
  vocal cord I86.8
  vulva I86.3
Vas deferens — *see* condition
Vas deferentitis N49.1
Vasa previa O69.4 ☑
  hemorrhage from, affecting newborn P50.0
Vascular (*see also* condition)
  loop on optic papilla Q14.2
  spasm I73.9
  spider I78.1
Vascularization, cornea — *see* Neovascularization, cornea
Vasculitis I77.6
  allergic D69.0
  cryoglobulinemic D89.1
  disseminated I77.6
  hypocomplementemic M31.8
  kidney I77.89
  livedoid L95.0
  nodular L95.8

Vasculitis — *continued*
  retina H35.06- ☑
  rheumatic — *see* Fever, rheumatic
  rheumatoid — *see* Rheumatoid, vasculitis
  skin (limited to) L95.9
    specified NEC L95.8
  systemic M31.8
Vasculopathy, necrotizing M31.9
  cardiac allograft T86.290
  specified NEC M31.8
Vasitis (nodosa) N49.1
  tuberculous A18.15
Vasodilation I73.9
Vasomotor — *see* condition
Vasoplasty, after previous sterilization Z31.0
  aftercare Z31.42
Vasospasm (vasoconstriction) I73.9
  cerebral (cerebrovascular) (artery) I67.848
    reversible I67.841
  coronary I20.1
  nerve
    arm — *see* Mononeuropathy, upper limb
    brachial plexus G54.0
    cervical plexus G54.2
    leg — *see* Mononeuropathy, lower limb
  peripheral NOS I73.9
  retina (artery) — *see* Occlusion, artery, retina
Vasospastic — *see* condition
Vasovagal attack (paroxysmal) R55
  psychogenic F45.8
VATER syndrome Q87.2
Vater's ampulla — *see* condition
Vegetation, vegetative
  adenoid (nasal fossa) J35.8
  endocarditis (acute) (any valve) (subacute) I33.0
  heart (mycotic) (valve) I33.0
Veil
  Jackson's Q43.3
Vein, venous — *see* condition
Veldt sore — *see* Ulcer, skin
Velpeau's hernia — *see* Hernia, femoral
Venereal
  bubo A55
  disease A64
  granuloma inguinale A58
  lymphogranuloma (Durand-Nicolas-Favre) A55
Venofibrosis I87.8
Venom, venomous — *see* Table of Drugs and Chemicals, by animal or substance, poisoning
Venous — *see* condition
Ventilator lung, newborn P27.8
Ventral — *see* condition
Ventricle, ventricular (*see also* condition)
  escape I49.3
  inversion Q20.5
Ventriculitis (cerebral) (*see also* Encephalitis) G04.90
Ventriculostomy status Z98.2
Vernet's syndrome G52.7
Verneuil's disease (syphilitic bursitis) A52.78
Verruca (due to HPV) (filiformis) (simplex) (viral) (vulgaris) B07.9
  acuminata A63.0
  necrogenica (primary) (tuberculosa) A18.4
  plana B07.8
  plantaris B07.0
  seborrheica L82.1
    inflamed L82.0
  senile (seborrheic) L82.1
    inflamed L82.0
  tuberculosa (primary) A18.4
  venereal A63.0
Verrucosities — *see* Verruca
Verruga peruana, peruviana A44.1
Version
  with extraction
  cervix — *see* Malposition, uterus
  uterus (postinfectional) (postpartal, old) — *see* Malposition, uterus
Vertebra, vertebral — *see* condition
Vertical talus (congenital) Q66.80
  left foot Q66.82
  right foot Q66.81
Vertigo R42
  auditory — *see* Vertigo, aural
  aural H81.31- ☑
  benign paroxysmal (positional) H81.1- ☑
  central (origin) H81.4- ☑

Vertigo — *continued*
  cerebral H81.4- ☑
  Dix and Hallpike (epidemic) — *see* Neuronitis, vestibular
  due to infrasound T75.23 ☑
  epidemic A88.1
    Dix and Hallpike — *see* Neuronitis, vestibular
    Pedersen's — *see* Neuronitis, vestibular
    vestibular neuronitis — *see* Neuronitis, vestibular
  hysterical F44.89
  infrasound T75.23 ☑
  labyrinthine — *see* subcategory H81.0 ☑
  laryngeal R05
  malignant positional H81.4- ☑
  Ménière's — *see* subcategory H81.0 ☑
  menopausal N95.1
  otogenic — *see* Vertigo, aural
  paroxysmal positional, benign — *see* Vertigo, benign paroxysmal
  Pedersen's (epidemic) — *see* Neuronitis, vestibular
  peripheral NEC H81.39- ☑
  positional
    benign paroxysmal — *see* Vertigo, benign paroxysmal
    malignant H81.4- ☑
Very-low-density-lipoprotein-type (VLDL) **hyperlipoproteinemia** E78.1
Vesania — *see* Psychosis
Vesical — *see* condition
Vesicle
  cutaneous R23.8
  seminal — *see* condition
  skin R23.8
Vesicocolic — *see* condition
Vesicoperineal — *see* condition
Vesicorectal — *see* condition
Vesicourethrorectal — *see* condition
Vesicovaginal — *see* condition
Vesicular — *see* condition
Vesiculitis (seminal) N49.0
  amebic A06.82
  gonorrheal (acute) (chronic) A54.23
  trichomonal A59.09
  tuberculous A18.15
Vestibulitis (ear) (*see also* subcategory) H83.0 ☑
  nose (external) J34.89
  vulvar N94.810
Vestibulopathy , acute peripheral (recurrent) — *see* Neuronitis, vestibular
Vestige, vestigial (*see also* Persistence)
  branchial Q18.0
  structures in vitreous Q14.0
Vibration
  adverse effects T75.20 ☑
    pneumatic hammer syndrome T75.21 ☑
    specified effect NEC T75.29 ☑
    vasospastic syndrome T75.22 ☑
    vertigo from infrasound T75.23 ☑
  exposure (occupational) Z57.7
  vertigo T75.23 ☑
Vibriosis A28.9
Victim (of)
  crime Z65.4
  disaster Z65.5
  terrorism Z65.4
  torture Z65.4
  war Z65.5
Vidal's disease L28.0
Villaret's syndrome G52.7
Villous — *see* condition
VIN — *see* Neoplasia, intraepithelial, vulva
Vincent's infection (angina) (gingivitis) A69.1
  stomatitis NEC A69.1
Vinson-Plummer syndrome D50.1
Violence, physical R45.6
Viosterol deficiency — *see* Deficiency, calciferol
Vipoma — *see* Neoplasm, malignant, by site
Viremia B34.9
Virilism (adrenal) E25.9
  congenital E25.0
Virilization (female) (suprarenal) E25.9
  congenital E25.0
  isosexual E28.2
Virulent bubo A57
Virus, viral (*see also* condition)
  as cause of disease classified elsewhere B97.89
  cytomegalovirus B25.9

Virus, viral — *continued*
  human immunodeficiency (HIV) — *see* Human, immunodeficiency virus (HIV) disease
  infection — *see* Infection, virus
  specified NEC B34.8
  swine influenza (viruses that normally cause infections in pigs) (*see also* Influenza, due to, identified novel influenza A virus) J09.X2
  West Nile (fever) A92.30
    with
      complications NEC A92.39
      cranial nerve disorders A92.32
      encephalitis A92.31
      encephalomyelitis A92.31
      neurologic manifestation NEC A92.32
      optic neuritis A92.32
      polyradiculitis A92.32
Viscera, visceral — *see* condition
Visceroptosis K63.4
Visible peristalsis R19.2
Vision, visual
  binocular, suppression H53.34
  blurred, blurring H53.8
    hysterical F44.6
  defect, defective NEC H54.7
  disorientation (syndrome) H53.8
  disturbance H53.9
    hysterical F44.6
  double H53.2
  examination Z01.00
    with abnormal findings Z01.01
  field, limitation (defect) — *see* Defect, visual field
  hallucinations R44.1
  halos H53.19
  loss — *see* Loss, vision
    sudden — *see* Disturbance, vision, subjective, loss, sudden
  low (both eyes) — *see* Low, vision
  perception, simultaneous without fusion H53.33
Vitality, lack or want of R53.83
  newborn P96.89
Vitamin deficiency — *see* Deficiency, vitamin
Vitelline duct, persistent Q43.0
Vitiligo L80
  eyelid H02.739
    left H02.736
      lower H02.735
      upper H02.734
    right H02.733
      lower H02.732
      upper H02.731
  pinta A67.2
  vulva N90.89
Vitreal corneal syndrome H59.01- ☑
Vitreoretinopathy, proliferative (*see also* Retinopathy, proliferative)
  with retinal detachment — *see* Detachment, retina, traction
Vitreous (*see also* condition)
  touch syndrome — *see* Complication, postprocedural, following cataract surgery
Vocal cord — *see* condition
Vogt-Koyanagi syndrome H20.82- ☑
Vogt's disease or syndrome G80.3
Vogt-Spielmeyer amaurotic idiocy or disease E75.4
Voice
  change R49.9
    specified NEC R49.8
  loss — *see* Aphonia
Volhynian fever A79.0
Volkmann's ischemic contracture or paralysis (complicating trauma) T79.6 ☑
Volvulus (bowel) (colon) (intestine) K56.2
  with perforation K56.2
  congenital Q43.8
  duodenum K31.5
  fallopian tube — *see* Torsion, fallopian tube
  oviduct — *see* Torsion, fallopian tube
  stomach (due to absence of gastrocolic ligament) K31.89
Vomiting R11.10
  with nausea R11.2
  without nausea R11.11
  asphyxia — *see* Foreign body, by site, causing asphyxia, gastric contents
  bilious (cause unknown) R11.14
    following gastro-intestinal surgery K91.0
    in newborn P92.01

Vomiting — *continued*
  blood — *see* Hematemesis
  causing asphyxia, choking, or suffocation — *see* Foreign body, by site
  cyclical G43.A0 (*following* G43.7)
    with refractory migraine G43.A1 (*following* G43.7)
    without refractory migraine G43.A0 (*following* G43.7)
    intractable G43.A1 (*following* G43.7)
    not intractable G43.A0 (*following* G43.7)
    psychogenic F50.89
  fecal mater R11.13
  following gastrointestinal surgery K91.0
    psychogenic F50.89
  functional K31.89
  hysterical F50.89
  nervous F50.89
  neurotic F50.89
  newborn NEC P92.09
    bilious P92.01
  periodic R11.10
    psychogenic F50.89
  projectile R11.12
  psychogenic F50.89
  uremic — *see* Uremia
Vomito negro — *see* Fever, yellow
Von Bezold's abscess — *see* Mastoiditis, acute
Von Economo-Cruchet disease A85.8
Von Eulenburg's disease G71.19
Von Gierke's disease E74.01
Von Hippel (-Lindau) **disease or syndrome** Q85.8
Von Jaksch's anemia or disease D64.89
Von Recklinghausen
  disease (neurofibromatosis) Q85.01
    bones E21.0
Von Schroetter's syndrome I82.890
Von Willebrand (-Jurgens)(-Minot) **disease or syndrome** D68.0
Von Zumbusch's disease L40.1
Voyeurism F65.3
Vrolik's disease Q78.0
Vulva — *see* condition
Vulvismus N94.2
Vulvitis (acute) (allergic) (atrophic) (hypertrophic) (intertriginous) (senile) N76.2
  with ectopic or molar pregnancy O08.0
  adhesive, congenital Q52.79
  blennorrhagic (gonococcal) A54.02
  candidal B37.3
  chlamydial A56.02
  due to Haemophilus ducreyi A57
  following ectopic or molar pregnancy O08.0
  gonococcal A54.02
    with abscess (accessory gland) (periurethral) A54.1
  herpesviral A60.04
  leukoplakic N90.4
  monilial B37.3
  puerperal (postpartum) O86.19
  subacute or chronic N76.3
  syphilitic (early) A51.0
    late A52.76
  trichomonal A59.01
  tuberculous A18.18
Vulvodynia N94.819
  specified NEC N94.818
Vulvorectal — *see* condition
Vulvovaginitis (acute) — *see* Vaginitis

W

Waiting list, person on Z75.1
  for organ transplant Z76.82
  undergoing social agency investigation Z75.2
Waldenström
  hypergammaglobulinemia D89.0
  syndrome or macroglobulinemia C88.0
Waldenström-Kjellberg syndrome D50.1
Walking
  difficulty R26.2
    psychogenic F44.4
  sleep F51.3
    hysterical F44.89
Wall, abdominal — *see* condition
Wallenberg's disease or syndrome G46.3
Wallgren's disease I87.8
Wandering
  gallbladder, congenital Q44.1
  in diseases classified elsewhere Z91.83

Wandering — *continued*
kidney, congenital Q63.8
organ or site, congenital NEC — *see* Malposition, congenital, by site
pacemaker (heart) I49.8
spleen D73.89
War neurosis F48.8
Wart (due to HPV) (filiform) (infectious) (viral) B07.9
anogenital region (venereal) A63.0
common B07.8
external genital organs (venereal) A63.0
flat B07.8
Hassal-Henle's (of cornea) H18.49
Peruvian A44.1
plantar B07.0
prosector (tuberculous) A18.4
seborrheic L82.1
inflamed L82.0
senile (seborrheic) L82.1
inflamed L82.0
tuberculous A18.4
venereal A63.0
Warthin's tumor — *see* Neoplasm, salivary gland, benign
Wassilieff's disease A27.0
Wasting
disease R64
due to malnutrition E41
extreme (due to malnutrition) E41
muscle NEC — *see* Atrophy, muscle
Water
clefts (senile cataract) — *see* Cataract, senile, incipient
deprivation of T73.1 ☑
intoxication E87.79
itch B76.9
lack of T73.1 ☑
loading E87.70
on
brain — *see* Hydrocephalus
chest J94.8
poisoning E87.79
Waterbrash R12
Waterhouse (-Friderichsen) **syndrome or disease** (meningococcal) A39.1
Water-losing nephritis N25.89
Watermelon stomach K31.819
with hemorrhage K31.811
without hemorrhage K31.819
Watsoniasis B66.8
Wax in ear — *see* Impaction, cerumen
Weak, weakening, weakness (generalized) R53.1
arches (acquired) (*see also* Deformity, limb, flat foot)
bladder (sphincter) R32
facial R29.810
following
cerebrovascular disease I69.992
cerebral infarction I69.392
intracerebral hemorrhage I69.192
nontraumatic intracranial hemorrhage NEC I69.292
specified disease NEC I69.892
stroke I69.392
subarachnoid hemorrhage I69.092
foot (double) — *see* Weak, arches
heart, cardiac — *see* Failure, heart
mind F70
muscle M62.81
myocardium — *see* Failure, heart
newborn P96.89
pelvic fundus N81.89
pubocervical tissue N81.82
rectovaginal tissue N81.83
senile R54
urinary stream R39.12
valvular — *see* Endocarditis
Wear, worn (with normal or routine use)
articular bearing surface of internal joint prosthesis — *see* Complications, joint prosthesis, mechanical, wear of articular bearing surfaces, by site
device, implant or graft — *see* Complications, by site, mechanical complication
tooth, teeth (approximal) (hard tissues) (interproximal) (occlusal) K03.0
Weather, weathered
effects of
cold T69.9 ☑
specified effect NEC T69.8 ☑
hot — *see* Heat
skin L57.8

Weaver's syndrome Q87.3
Web, webbed (congenital)
duodenal Q43.8
esophagus Q39.4
fingers Q70.1- ☑
larynx (glottic) (subglottic) Q31.0
neck (pterygium colli) Q18.3
Paterson-Kelly D50.1
popliteal syndrome Q87.89
toes Q70.3- ☑
Weber-Christian disease M35.6
Weber-Cockayne syndrome (epidermolysis bullosa) Q81.8
Weber-Gubler syndrome G46.3
Weber-Leyden syndrome G46.3
Weber-Osler syndrome I78.0
Weber's paralysis or syndrome G46.3
Wedge-shaped or wedging vertebra — *see* Collapse, vertebra NEC
Wegener's granulomatosis or syndrome M31.30
with
kidney involvement M31.31
lung involvement M31.30
with kidney involvement M31.31
Wegner's disease A50.02
Weight
1000-2499 grams at birth (low) — *see* Low, birth-weight
999 grams or less at birth (extremely low) — *see* Low, birthweight, extreme
and length below 10th percentile for gestational age P05.1- ☑
below but length above 10th percentile for gestational age P05.0- ☑
gain (abnormal) (excessive) R63.5
in pregnancy — *see* Pregnancy, complicated by, excessive weight gain
low — *see* Pregnancy, complicated by, insufficient, weight gain
loss (abnormal) (cause unknown) R63.4
Weightlessness (effect of) T75.82 ☑
Weil (I)-**Marchesani syndrome** Q87.1
Weil's disease A27.0
Weingarten's syndrome J82
Weir Mitchell's disease I73.81
Weiss-Baker syndrome G90.09
Wells' disease L98.3
Wen — *see* Cyst, sebaceous
Wenckebach's block or phenomenon I44.1
Werdnig-Hoffmann syndrome (muscular atrophy) G12.0
Werlhof's disease D69.3
Wermer's disease or syndrome E31.21
Werner-His disease A79.0
Werner's disease or syndrome E34.8
Wernicke-Korsakoff's syndrome or psychosis (alcoholic) F10.96
with dependence F10.26
drug-induced
due to drug abuse — *see* Abuse, drug, by type, with amnestic disorder
due to drug dependence — *see* Dependence, drug, by type, with amnestic disorder
nonalcoholic F04
Wernicke-Posadas disease B38.9
Wernicke's
developmental aphasia F80.2
disease or syndrome E51.2
encephalopathy E51.2
polioencephalitis, superior E51.2
West African fever B50.8
Westphal-Strümpell syndrome E83.01
West's syndrome — *see* Epilepsy, spasms
Wet
feet, tropical (maceration) (syndrome) — *see* Immersion, foot
lung (syndrome), newborn P22.1
Wharton's duct — *see* condition
Wheal — *see* Urticaria
Wheezing R06.2
Whiplash injury S13.4 ☑
Whipple's disease (*see also* subcategory M14.8-) K90.81
Whipworm (disease) (infection) (infestation) B79
Whistling face Q87.0
White (*see also* condition)
kidney, small N03.9
leg, puerperal, postpartum, childbirth O87.1

White — *continued*
mouth B37.0
patches of mouth K13.29
spot lesions, teeth
chewing surface K02.51
pit and fissure surface K02.51
smooth surface K02.61
Whitehead L70.0
Whitlow (*see also* Cellulitis, digit)
with lymphangitis — *see* Lymphangitis, acute, digit
herpesviral B00.89
Whitmore's disease or fever — *see* Melioidosis
Whooping cough A37.90
with pneumonia A37.91
due to Bordetella
bronchiseptica A37.81
parapertussis A37.11
pertussis A37.01
specified organism NEC A37.81
due to
Bordetella
bronchiseptica A37.80
with pneumonia A37.81
parapertussis A37.10
with pneumonia A37.11
pertussis A37.00
with pneumonia A37.01
specified NEC A37.80
with pneumonia A37.81
Wichman's asthma J38.5
Wide cranial sutures, newborn P96.3
Widening aorta — *see* Ectasia, aorta
with aneurysm — *see* Aneurysm, aorta
Wilkie's disease or syndrome K55.1
Wilkinson-Sneddon disease or syndrome L13.1
Willebrand (-Jürgens) **thrombopathy** D68.0
Willige-Hunt disease or syndrome G23.1
Wilms' tumor C64- ☑
Wilson-Mikity syndrome P27.0
Wilson's
disease or syndrome E83.01
hepatolenticular degeneration E83.01
lichen ruber L43.9
Window (*see also* Imperfect, closure)
aorticopulmonary Q21.4
Winter — *see* condition
Wiskott-Aldrich syndrome D82.0
Withdrawal state (*see also* Dependence, drug by type, with withdrawal)
alcohol
with perceptual disturbances F10.232
without perceptual disturbances F10.239
caffeine F15.93
cannabis F12.288
newborn
correct therapeutic substance properly administered P96.2
infant of dependent mother P96.1
therapeutic substance, neonatal P96.2
Witts' anemia D50.8
Witzelsucht F07.0
Woakes' ethmoiditis or syndrome J33.1
Wolff-Hirschorn syndrome Q93.3
Wolff-Parkinson-White syndrome I45.6
Wolhynian fever A79.0
Wolman's disease E75.5
Wood lung or pneumonitis J67.8
Woolly, wooly hair (congenital) (nevus) Q84.1
Woolsorter's disease A22.1
Word
blindness (congenital) (developmental) F81.0
deafness (congenital) (developmental) H93.25
Worm(s) (infection) (infestation) (*see also* Infestation, helminth)
guinea B72
in intestine NEC B82.0
Worm-eaten soles A66.3
Worn out — *see* Exhaustion
cardiac
defibrillator (with synchronous cardiace pacemaker) Z45.02
pacemaker
battery Z45.010
lead Z45.018
device, implant or graft — *see* Complications, by site, mechanical
Worried well Z71.1
Worries R45.82

☑ **Additional Character Required** — Refer to the Tabular List for Character Selection ▼ Subterms under main terms may continue to next column or page

Wound, open — *continued*
  head — *continued*
    eyelid — *see* Wound, open, eyelid
    laceration — *see* Laceration, head
    lip — *see* Wound, open, lip
    nose S01.20 ☑
    oral cavity — *see* Wound, open, oral cavity
    puncture — *see* Puncture, head
    scalp — *see* Wound, open, scalp
    specified site NEC S01.80 ☑
    temporomandibular area — *see* Wound, open, cheek
  heel — *see* Wound, open, foot
  hip S71.00- ☑
    with amputation — *see* Amputation, traumatic, hip
    bite — *see* Bite, hip
    laceration — *see* Laceration, hip
    puncture — *see* Puncture, hip
  hymen S31.40 ☑
    bite — *see* Bite, vulva
    laceration — *see* Laceration, vagina
    puncture — *see* Puncture, vagina
  hypochondrium S31.109 ☑
    bite — *see* Bite, hypochondrium
    laceration — *see* Laceration, hypochondrium
    puncture — *see* Puncture, hypochondrium
  hypogastric region S31.109 ☑
    bite — *see* Bite, hypogastric region
    laceration — *see* Laceration, hypogastric region
    puncture — *see* Puncture, hypogastric region
  iliac (region) — *see* Wound, open, inguinal region
  inguinal region S31.109 ☑
    bite — *see* Bite, abdomen, wall, lower quadrant
    laceration — *see* Laceration, inguinal region
    puncture — *see* Puncture, inguinal region
  instep — *see* Wound, open, foot
  interscapular region — *see* Wound, open, thorax, back
  intraocular — *see* Wound, open, ocular
  iris — *see* Wound, open, ocular
  jaw — *see* Wound, open, head, specified site NEC
  knee S81.00- ☑
    bite — *see* Bite, knee
    laceration — *see* Laceration, knee
    puncture — *see* Puncture, knee
  labium (majus) (minus) — *see* Wound, open, vulva
  laceration — *see* Laceration, by site
  lacrimal duct — *see* Wound, open, eyelid
  larynx S11.019 ☑
    bite — *see* Bite, larynx
    laceration — *see* Laceration, larynx
    puncture — *see* Puncture, larynx
  left
    lower quadrant S31.104 ☑
      with penetration into peritoneal cavity S31.604 ☑
      bite — *see* Bite, abdomen, wall, left, lower quadrant
      laceration — *see* Laceration, abdomen, wall, left, lower quadrant
      puncture — *see* Puncture, abdomen, wall, left, lower quadrant
    upper quadrant S31.101 ☑
      with penetration into peritoneal cavity S31.601 ☑
      bite — *see* Bite, abdomen, wall, left, upper quadrant
      laceration — *see* Laceration, abdomen, wall, left, upper quadrant
      puncture — *see* Puncture, abdomen, wall, left, upper quadrant
  leg (lower) S81.80- ☑
    with amputation — *see* Amputation, traumatic, leg
    ankle — *see* Wound, open, ankle
    bite — *see* Bite, leg
    foot — *see* Wound, open, foot
    knee — *see* Wound, open, knee
    laceration — *see* Laceration, leg
    puncture — *see* Puncture, leg
    toe — *see* Wound, open, toe
    upper — *see* Wound, open, thigh
  lip S01.501 ☑
    bite — *see* Bite, lip
    laceration — *see* Laceration, lip
    puncture — *see* Puncture, lip

Wound, open — *continued*
  loin S31.109 ☑
    bite — *see* Bite, abdomen, wall
    laceration — *see* Laceration, loin
    puncture — *see* Puncture, loin
  lower back — *see* Wound, open, back, lower
  lumbar region — *see* Wound, open, back, lower
  malar region — *see* Wound, open, head, specified site NEC
  mammary — *see* Wound, open, breast
  mastoid region — *see* Wound, open, head, specified site NEC
  mouth — *see* Wound, open, oral cavity
  nail
    finger — *see* Wound, open, finger, with damage to nail
    toe — *see* Wound, open, toe, with damage to nail
  nape (neck) — *see* Wound, open, neck
  nasal (septum) (sinus) — *see* Wound, open, nose
  nasopharynx — *see* Wound, open, head, specified site NEC
  neck S11.90 ☑
    bite — *see* Bite, neck
    involving
      cervical esophagus S11.20 ☑
      larynx — *see* Wound, open, larynx
      pharynx S11.20 ☑
      thyroid S11.10 ☑
      trachea (cervical) S11.029 ☑
        bite — *see* Bite, trachea
        laceration S11.021 ☑
          with foreign body S11.022 ☑
        puncture S11.023 ☑
          with foreign body S11.024 ☑
    laceration — *see* Laceration, neck
    puncture — *see* Puncture, neck
    specified site NEC S11.80 ☑
      specified type NEC S11.89 ☑
  nose (septum) (sinus) S01.20 ☑
    with amputation — *see* Amputation, traumatic, nose
    bite — *see* Bite, nose
    laceration — *see* Laceration, nose
    puncture — *see* Puncture, nose
  ocular S05.90 ☑
    avulsion (traumatic enucleation) S05.7- ☑
    eyeball S05.6- ☑
      with foreign body S05.5- ☑
    eyelid — *see* Wound, open, eyelid
    laceration and rupture S05.3- ☑
      with prolapse or loss of intraocular tissue S05.2- ☑
    orbit (penetrating) (with or without foreign body) S05.4- ☑
    periocular area — *see* Wound, open, eyelid
    specified NEC S05.8X- ☑
  oral cavity S01.502 ☑
    bite S01.552 ☑
    laceration — *see* Laceration, oral cavity
    puncture — *see* Puncture, oral cavity
  orbit — *see* Wound, open, ocular, orbit
  palate — *see* Wound, open, oral cavity
  palm — *see* Wound, open, hand
  pelvis, pelvic (*see also* Wound, open, back, lower)
    girdle — *see* Wound, open, hip
  penetrating — *see* Puncture, by site
  penis S31.20 ☑
    with amputation — *see* Amputation, traumatic, penis
    bite S31.25 ☑
    laceration — *see* Laceration, penis
    puncture — *see* Puncture, penis
  perineum
    bite — *see* Bite, perineum
    female S31.502 ☑
    laceration — *see* Laceration, perineum
    male S31.501 ☑
    puncture — *see* Puncture, perineum
  periocular area (with or without lacrimal passages) — *see* Wound, open, eyelid
  periumbilic region S31.105 ☑
    with penetration into peritoneal cavity S31.605 ☑
    bite — *see* Bite, abdomen, wall, periumbilic region
    laceration — *see* Laceration, abdomen, wall, periumbilic region

Wound, open — *continued*
  periumbilic region — *continued*
    puncture — *see* Puncture, abdomen, wall, periumbilic region
  phalanges
    finger — *see* Wound, open, finger
    toe — *see* Wound, open, toe
  pharynx S11.20 ☑
  pinna — *see* Wound, open, ear
  popliteal space — *see* Wound, open, knee
  prepuce — *see* Wound, open, penis
  pubic region — *see* Wound, open, back, lower
  pudendum — *see* Wound, open, genital organs, external
  puncture wound — *see* Puncture
  rectovaginal septum — *see* Wound, open, vagina
  right
    lower quadrant S31.103 ☑
      with penetration into peritoneal cavity S31.603 ☑
      bite — *see* Bite, abdomen, wall, right, lower quadrant
      laceration — *see* Laceration, abdomen, wall, right, lower quadrant
      puncture — *see* Puncture, abdomen, wall, right, lower quadrant
    upper quadrant S31.100 ☑
      with penetration into peritoneal cavity S31.600 ☑
      bite — *see* Bite, abdomen, wall, right, upper quadrant
      laceration — *see* Laceration, abdomen, wall, right, upper quadrant
      puncture — *see* Puncture, abdomen, wall, right, upper quadrant
  sacral region — *see* Wound, open, back, lower
  sacroiliac region — *see* Wound, open, back, lower
  salivary gland — *see* Wound, open, oral cavity
  scalp S01.00 ☑
    bite S01.05 ☑
    laceration — *see* Laceration, scalp
    puncture — *see* Puncture, scalp
  scalpel, newborn (birth injury) P15.8
  scapular region — *see* Wound, open, shoulder
  sclera — *see* Wound, open, ocular
  scrotum S31.30 ☑
    with amputation — *see* Amputation, traumatic, scrotum
    bite S31.35 ☑
    laceration — *see* Laceration, scrotum
    puncture — *see* Puncture, scrotum
  shin — *see* Wound, open, leg
  shoulder S41.00- ☑
    with amputation — *see* Amputation, traumatic, arm
    bite — *see* Bite, shoulder
    laceration — *see* Laceration, shoulder
    puncture — *see* Puncture, shoulder
  skin NOS T14.8 ☑
  spermatic cord — *see* Wound, open, testis
  sternal region — *see* Wound, open, thorax, front wall
  submaxillary region — *see* Wound, open, head, specified site NEC
  submental region — *see* Wound, open, head, specified site NEC
  subungual
    finger(s) — *see* Wound, open, finger
    toe(s) — *see* Wound, open, toe
  supraclavicular region — *see* Wound, open, neck, specified site NEC
  temple, temporal region — *see* Wound, open, head, specified site NEC
  temporomandibular area — *see* Wound, open, cheek
  testis S31.30 ☑
    with amputation — *see* Amputation, traumatic, testes
    bite S31.35 ☑
    laceration — *see* Laceration, testis
    puncture — *see* Puncture, testis
  thigh S71.10- ☑
    with amputation — *see* Amputation, traumatic, hip
    bite — *see* Bite, thigh
    laceration — *see* Laceration, thigh
    puncture — *see* Puncture, thigh
  thorax, thoracic (wall) S21.90 ☑
    back S21.20- ☑

Wound, open — *continued*
  thorax, thoracic — *continued*
    back — *continued*
      with penetration S21.40 ☑
    bite — *see* Bite, thorax
    breast — *see* Wound, open, breast
    front S21.10- ☑
      with penetration S21.30 ☑
    laceration — *see* Laceration, thorax
    puncture — *see* Puncture, thorax
  throat — *see* Wound, open, neck
  thumb S61.009 ☑
    with
      amputation — *see* Amputation, traumatic, thumb
      damage to nail S61.109 ☑
    bite — *see* Bite, thumb
    laceration — *see* Laceration, thumb
    left S61.002 ☑
      with
        damage to nail S61.102 ☑
      puncture — *see* Puncture, thumb
    right S61.001 ☑
      with
        damage to nail S61.101 ☑
  thyroid (gland) — *see* Wound, open, neck, thyroid
  toe(s) S91.109 ☑
    with
      amputation — *see* Amputation, traumatic, toe
      damage to nail S91.209 ☑
    bite — *see* Bite, toe
    great S91.103 ☑
      with
        damage to nail S91.203 ☑
      left S91.102 ☑
        with
          damage to nail S91.202 ☑
      right S91.101 ☑
        with
          damage to nail S91.201 ☑
    laceration — *see* Laceration, toe
    lesser S91.106 ☑
      with
        damage to nail S91.206 ☑
      left S91.105 ☑
        with
          damage to nail S91.205 ☑
      right S91.104 ☑
        with
          damage to nail S91.204 ☑
    puncture — *see* Puncture, toe
  tongue — *see* Wound, open, oral cavity
  trachea (cervical region) — *see* Wound, open, neck, trachea
  tunica vaginalis — *see* Wound, open, testis
  tympanum, tympanic membrane S09.2- ☑
    laceration — *see* Laceration, ear, drum
    puncture — *see* Puncture, tympanum
  umbilical region — *see* Wound, open, abdomen, wall, periumbilic region
  uvula — *see* Wound, open, oral cavity
  vagina S31.40 ☑
    bite S31.45 ☑
    laceration — *see* Laceration, vagina
    puncture — *see* Puncture, vagina
  vitreous (humor) — *see* Wound, open, ocular
  vocal cord S11.039 ☑
    bite — *see* Bite, vocal cord
    laceration S11.031 ☑
      with foreign body S11.032 ☑
    puncture S11.033 ☑
      with foreign body S11.034 ☑
  vulva S31.40 ☑
    with amputation — *see* Amputation, traumatic, vulva
    bite S31.45 ☑
    laceration — *see* Laceration, vulva
    puncture — *see* Puncture, vulva
  wrist S61.50- ☑
    bite — *see* Bite, wrist
    laceration — *see* Laceration, wrist
    puncture — *see* Puncture, wrist
Wound, superficial — *see* Injury (*see also* specified injury type)

Wright's syndrome G54.0
Wrist — *see* condition
Wrong drug (by accident) (given in error) — *see* Table of Drugs and Chemicals, by drug, poisoning
Wry neck — *see* Torticollis
Wuchereria (bancrofti) **infestation** B74.0
Wuchereriasis B74.0
Wuchernde Struma Langhans C73

X

Xanthelasma (eyelid) (palpebrarum) H02.60
  left H02.66
    lower H02.65
    upper H02.64
  right H02.63
    lower H02.62
    upper H02.61
Xanthelasmatosis (essential) E78.2
Xanthinuria, hereditary E79.8
Xanthoastrocytoma
  specified site — *see* Neoplasm, malignant, by site
  unspecified site C71.9
Xanthofibroma — *see* Neoplasm, connective tissue, benign
Xanthogranuloma D76.3
Xanthoma(s), xanthomatosis (primary) (familial) (hereditary) E75.5
  with
    hyperlipoproteinemia
      Type I E78.3
      Type III E78.2
      Type IV E78.1
      Type V E78.3
  bone (generalisata) C96.5
  cerebrotendinous E75.5
  cutaneotendinous E75.5
  disseminatum (skin) E78.2
  eruptive E78.2
  hypercholesterinemic E78.00
  hypercholesterolemic E78.00
  hyperlipidemic E78.5
  joint E75.5
  multiple (skin) E78.2
  tendon (sheath) E75.5
  tuberosum E78.2
  tuberous E78.2
  tubo-eruptive E78.2
  verrucous, oral mucosa K13.4
Xanthosis R23.8
Xenophobia F40.10
Xeroderma (*see also* Ichthyosis)
  acquired L85.0
  eyelid H01.149
    left H01.146
      lower H01.145
      upper H01.144
    right H01.143
      lower H01.142
      upper H01.141
  pigmentosum Q82.1
  vitamin A deficiency E50.8
Xerophthalmia (vitamin A deficiency) E50.7
  unrelated to vitamin A deficiency — *see* Keratoconjunctivitis
Xerosis
  conjunctiva H11.14- ☑
    with Bitot's spots (*see also* Pigmentation, conjunctiva)
      vitamin A deficiency E50.1
    vitamin A deficiency E50.0
  cornea H18.89- ☑
    with ulceration — *see* Ulcer, cornea
      vitamin A deficiency E50.3
    vitamin A deficiency E50.2
  cutis L85.3
  skin L85.3
Xerostomia K11.7
Xiphopagus Q89.4
XO syndrome Q96.9
X-ray (of)
  abnormal findings — *see* Abnormal, diagnostic imaging
  breast (mammogram) (routine) Z12.31

X-ray — *continued*
  chest
    routine (as part of a general medical examination) Z00.00
      with abnormal findings Z00.01
  routine (as part of a general medical examination) Z00.00
    with abnormal findings Z00.01
XXXXY syndrome Q98.1
XXY syndrome Q98.0

Y

Yaba pox (virus disease) B08.72
Yatapoxvirus B08.70
  specified NEC B08.79
Yawning R06.89
  psychogenic F45.8
Yaws A66.9
  cutaneous, less than five years after infection A66.2
  bone lesions A66.6
  butter A66.1
  chancre A66.0
  early (cutaneous) (macular) (maculopapular) (micropapular) (papular) A66.2
    frambeside A66.2
    skin lesions NEC A66.2
  eyelid A66.2
  ganglion A66.6
  gangosis, gangosa A66.5
  gumma, gummata A66.4
    bone A66.6
  gummatous
    frambeside A66.4
    osteitis A66.6
    periostitis A66.6
  hydrarthrosis (*see also* subcategory M14.8-) A66.6
  hyperkeratosis (early) (late) A66.3
  initial lesions A66.0
  joint lesions (*see also* subcategory M14.8-) A66.6
  juxta-articular nodules A66.7
  late nodular (ulcerated) A66.4
  latent (without clinical manifestations) (with positive serology) A66.8
  mother A66.0
  mucosal A66.7
  multiple papillomata A66.1
  nodular, late (ulcerated) A66.4
  osteitis A66.6
  papilloma, plantar or palmar A66.1
  periostitis (hypertrophic) A66.6
  specified NEC A66.7
  ulcers A66.4
  wet crab A66.1
Yeast infection (*see also* Candidiasis) B37.9
Yellow
  atrophy (liver) — *see* Failure, hepatic
  fever — *see* Fever, yellow
  jack — *see* Fever, yellow
  jaundice — *see* Jaundice
  nail syndrome L60.5
Yersiniosis (*see also* Infection, Yersinia)
  extraintestinal A28.2
  intestinal A04.6

Z

Zahorsky's syndrome (herpangina) B08.5
Zellweger's syndrome Q87.89
Zenker's diverticulum (esophagus) K22.5
Ziehen-Oppenheim disease G24.1
Zieve's syndrome K70.0
Zika NOS A92.5
Zinc
  deficiency, dietary E60
  metabolism disorder E83.2
Zollinger-Ellison syndrome E16.4
Zona — *see* Herpes, zoster
Zoophobia F40.218
Zoster (herpes) — *see* Herpes, zoster
Zygomycosis B46.9
  specified NEC B46.8
Zymotic — *see* condition

	Malignant Primary	Malignant Secondary	Ca in situ	Benign	Uncertain	Unspecified Behavior

Note: The list below gives the code number for neoplasms by anatomical site. For each site there are six possible code numbers according to whether the neoplasm in question is malignant, benign, in situ, of uncertain behavior, or of unspecified nature. The description of the neoplasm will often indicate which of the six columns is appropriate; e.g., malignant melanoma of skin, benign fibroadenoma of breast, carcinoma in situ of cervix uteri. Where such descriptors are not present, the remainder of the Index should be consulted where guidance is given to the appropriate column for each morphological (histological) variety listed; e.g., Mesonephroma – see Neoplasm, malignant; Embryoma (see also Neoplasm, uncertain behavior); Disease, Bowen's – see Neoplasm, skin, in situ. However, the guidance in the Index can be overridden if one of the descriptors mentioned above is present; e.g., malignant adenoma of colon is coded to C18.9 and not to D12.6 as the adjective "malignant" overrides the Index entry "Adenoma (see also Neoplasm, benign, by site)." Codes listed with a dash -, following the code have a required additional character for laterality. The tabular list must be reviewed for the complete code.

	Malignant Primary	Malignant Secondary	Ca in situ	Benign	Uncertain	Unspecified Behavior
Neoplasm, neoplastic	C80.1	C79.9	D09.9	D36.9	D48.9	D49.9
abdomen,						
abdominal	C76.2	C79.8-✓	D09.8	D36.7	D48.7	D49.89
cavity	C76.2	C79.8-✓	D09.8	D36.7	D48.7	D49.89
organ	C76.2	C79.8-✓	D09.8	D36.7	D48.7	D49.89
viscera	C76.2	C79.8-✓	D09.8	D36.7	D48.7	D49.89
wall — see also Neoplasm, abdomen, wall, skin	C44.509	C79.2	D04.5	D23.5	D48.5	D49.2
connective tissue	C49.4	C79.8-✓	—	D21.4	D48.1	D49.2
skin	C44.509	—	—	—	—	—
basal cell carcinoma	C44.519	—	—	—	—	—
specified type NEC	C44.599	—	—	—	—	—
squamous cell carcinoma	C44.529	—	—	—	—	—
abdominopelvic	C76.8	C79.8-✓	—	D36.7	D48.7	D49.89
accessory sinus — see Neoplasm, sinus						
acoustic nerve	C72.4-✓	C79.49	—	D33.3	D43.3	D49.7
adenoid (pharynx) (tissue)	C11.1	C79.89	D00.08	D10.6	D37.05	D49.0
adipose tissue — see also Neoplasm, connective tissue	C49.4	C79.89	—	D21.9	D48.1	D49.2
adnexa (uterine)	C57.4	C79.89	D07.39	D28.7	D39.8	D49.59
adrenal	C74.9-✓	C79.7-✓	D09.3	D35.0-✓	D44.1-✓	D49.7
capsule	C74.9-✓	C79.7-✓	D09.3	D35.0-✓	D44.1-✓	D49.7
cortex	C74.0-✓	C79.7-✓	D09.3	D35.0-✓	D44.1-✓	D49.7
gland	C74.9-✓	C79.7-✓	D09.3	D35.0-✓	D44.1-✓	D49.7
medulla	C74.1-✓	C79.7-✓	D09.3	D35.0-✓	D44.1-✓	D49.7
ala nasi (external) — see also Neoplasm, skin, nose	C44.301	C79.2	D04.39	D23.39	D48.5	D49.2
alimentary canal or tract NEC	C26.9	C78.80	D01.9	D13.9	D37.9	D49.0
alveolar	C03.9	C79.89	D00.03	D10.39	D37.09	D49.0
mucosa	C03.9	C79.89	D00.03	D10.39	D37.09	D49.0
lower	C03.1	C79.89	D00.03	D10.39	D37.09	D49.0
upper	C03.0	C79.89	D00.03	D10.39	D37.09	D49.0
ridge or process	C41.1	C79.51	—	D16.5	D48.0	D49.2
carcinoma	C03.9	C79.8-✓	—	—	—	—
lower	C03.1	C79.8-✓	—	—	—	—
upper	C03.0	C79.8-✓	—	—	—	—
lower	C41.1	C79.51	—	D16.5	D48.0	D49.2
mucosa	C03.9	C79.89	D00.03	D10.39	D37.09	D49.0
lower	C03.1	C79.89	D00.03	D10.39	D37.09	D49.0
upper	C03.0	C79.89	D00.03	D10.39	D37.09	D49.0
upper	C41.0	C79.51	—	D16.4	D48.0	D49.2
sulcus	C06.1	C79.89	D00.02	D10.39	D37.09	D49.0
alveolus	C03.9	C79.89	D00.03	D10.39	D37.09	D49.0
lower	C03.1	C79.89	D00.03	D10.39	D37.09	D49.0
upper	C03.0	C79.89	D00.03	D10.39	D37.09	D49.0
ampulla of Vater	C24.1	C78.89	D01.5	D13.5	D37.6	D49.0
ankle NEC	C76.5-✓	C79.89	D04.7-✓	D36.7	D48.7	D49.89
anorectum, anorectal (junction)	C21.8	C78.5	D01.3	D12.9	D37.8	D49.0
antecubital fossa or space	C76.4-✓	C79.89	D04.6-✓	D36.7	D48.7	D49.89

	Malignant Primary	Malignant Secondary	Ca in situ	Benign	Uncertain	Unspecified Behavior
Neoplasm, neoplastic — continued						
antrum (Highmore) (maxillary)	C31.0	C78.39	D02.3	D14.0	D38.5	D49.1
pyloric	C16.3	C78.89	D00.2	D13.1	D37.1	D49.0
tympanicum	C30.1	C78.39	D02.3	D14.0	D38.5	D49.1
anus, anal	C21.0	C78.5	D01.3	D12.9	D37.8	D49.0
canal	C21.1	C78.5	D01.3	D12.9	D37.8	D49.0
cloacogenic zone	C21.2	C78.5	D01.3	D12.9	D37.8	D49.0
margin — see also Neoplasm, anus, skin	C44.500	C79.2	D04.5	D23.5	D48.5	D49.2
overlapping lesion with rectosigmoid junction or rectum	C21.8	—	—	—	—	—
skin	C44.500	C79.2	D04.5	D23.5	D48.5	D49.2
basal cell carcinoma	C44.510	—	—	—	—	—
specified type NEC	C44.590	—	—	—	—	—
squamous cell carcinoma	C44.520	—	—	—	—	—
sphincter	C21.1	C78.5	D01.3	D12.9	D37.8	D49.0
aorta (thoracic)	C49.3	C79.89	—	D21.3	D48.1	D49.2
abdominal	C49.4	C79.89	—	D21.4	D48.1	D49.2
aortic body	C75.5	C79.89	—	D35.6	D44.7	D49.7
aponeurosis	C49.9	C79.89	—	D21.9	D48.1	D49.2
palmar	C49.1-✓	C79.89	—	D21.1-✓	D48.1	D49.2
plantar	C49.2-✓	C79.89	—	D21.2-✓	D48.1	D49.2
appendix	C18.1	C78.5	D01.0	D12.1	D37.3	D49.0
arachnoid	C70.9	C79.49	—	D32.9	D42.9	D49.7
cerebral	C70.0	C79.32	—	D32.0	D42.0	D49.7
spinal	C70.1	C79.49	—	D32.1	D42.1	D49.7
areola	C50.0-✓	C79.81	D05-✓	D24-✓	D48.6-✓	D49.3
arm NEC	C76.4-✓	C79.89	D04.6-✓	D36.7	D48.7	D49.89
artery — see Neoplasm, connective tissue						
aryepiglottic fold	C13.1	C79.89	D00.08	D10.7	D37.05	D49.0
hypopharyngeal aspect	C13.1	C79.89	D00.08	D10.7	D37.05	D49.0
laryngeal aspect	C32.1	C78.39	D02.0	D14.1	D38.0	D49.1
marginal zone	C13.1	C79.89	D00.08	D10.7	D37.05	D49.0
arytenoid (cartilage)	C32.3	C78.39	D02.0	D14.1	D38.0	D49.1
fold — see Neoplasm, aryepiglottic						
associated with transplanted organ	C80.2	—	—	—	—	—
atlas	C41.2	C79.51	—	D16.6	D48.0	D49.2
atrium, cardiac	C38.0	C79.89	—	D15.1	D48.7	D49.89
auditory						
canal (external) (skin)	C44.20-✓	C79.2	D04.2-✓	D23.2-✓	D48.5	D49.2
internal	C30.1	C78.39	D02.3	D14.0	D38.5	D49.1
nerve	C72.4-✓	C79.49	—	D33.3	D43.3	D49.7
tube	C30.1	C78.39	D02.3	D14.0	D38.5	D49.1
opening	C11.2	C79.89	D00.08	D10.6	D37.05	D49.0
auricle, ear — see also Neoplasm, skin, ear	C44.20-✓	C79.2	D04.2-✓	D23.2-✓	D48.5	D49.2
auricular canal (external) — see also Neoplasm, skin, ear	C44.20-✓	C79.2	D04.2-✓	D23.2-✓	D48.5	D49.2
internal	C30.1	C78.39	D02.3	D14.0	D38.5	D49.2
autonomic nerve or nervous system NEC (see Neoplasm, nerve, peripheral)						
axilla, axillary	C76.1	C79.89	D09.8	D36.7	D48.7	D49.89
fold — see also Neoplasm, skin, trunk	C44.509	C79.2	D04.5	D23.5	D48.5	D49.2
back NEC	C76.8	C79.89	D04.5	D36.7	D48.7	D49.89
Bartholin's gland	C51.0	C79.82	D07.1	D28.0	D39.8	D49.59
basal ganglia	C71.0	C79.31	—	D33.0	D43.0	D49.6
basis pedunculi	C71.7	C79.31	—	D33.1	D43.1	D49.6
bile or biliary (tract)	C24.9	C78.89	D01.5	D13.5	D37.6	D49.0
canaliculi (biliferi) (intrahepatic)	C22.1	C78.7	D01.5	D13.4	D37.6	D49.0
canals, interlobular	C22.1	C78.89	D01.5	D13.4	D37.6	D49.0

	Malignant Primary	Malignant Secondary	Ca in situ	Benign	Uncertain	Unspecified Behavior
Neoplasm, neoplastic —						
continued						
bile or biliary —						
continued						
duct or passage						
(common) (cystic)						
(extrahepatic)	C24.0	C78.89	D01.5	D13.5	D37.6	D49.0
interlobular	C22.1	C78.89	D01.5	D13.4	D37.6	D49.0
intrahepatic	C22.1	C78.7	D01.5	D13.4	D37.6	D49.0
and						
extrahepatic	C24.8	C78.89	D01.5	D13.5	D37.6	D49.0
bladder (urinary)	C67.9	C79.11	D09.0	D30.3	D41.4	D49.4
dome	C67.1	C79.11	D09.0	D30.3	D41.4	D49.4
neck	C67.5	C79.11	D09.0	D30.3	D41.4	D49.4
orifice	C67.9	C79.11	D09.0	D30.3	D41.4	D49.4
ureteric	C67.6	C79.11	D09.0	D30.3	D41.4	D49.4
urethral	C67.5	C79.11	D09.0	D30.3	D41.4	D49.4
overlapping lesion	C67.8	—	—	—	—	—
sphincter	C67.8	C79.11	D09.0	D30.3	D41.4	D49.4
trigone	C67.0	C79.11	D09.0	D30.3	D41.4	D49.4
urachus	C67.7	C79.11	D09.0	D30.3	D41.4	D49.4
wall	C67.9	C79.11	D09.0	D30.3	D41.4	D49.4
anterior	C67.3	C79.11	D09.0	D30.3	D41.4	D49.4
lateral	C67.2	C79.11	D09.0	D30.3	D41.4	D49.4
posterior	C67.4	C79.11	D09.0	D30.3	D41.4	D49.4
blood vessel — *see*						
Neoplasm, connective						
tissue						
bone (periosteum)	C41.9	C79.51	—	D16.9	D48.0	D49.2
acetabulum	C41.4	C79.51	—	D16.8	D48.0	D49.2
ankle	C40.3-☑	C79.51	—	D16.3-☑	—	—
arm NEC	C40.0-☑	C79.51	—	D16.0-☑	—	—
astragalus	C40.3-☑	C79.51	—	D16.3-☑	—	—
atlas	C41.2	C79.51	—	D16.6	D48.0	D49.2
axis	C41.2	C79.51	—	D16.6	D48.0	D49.2
back NEC	C41.2	C79.51	—	D16.6	D48.0	D49.2
calcaneus	C40.3-☑	C79.51	—	D16.3-☑	—	—
calvarium	C41.0	C79.51	—	D16.4	D48.0	D49.2
carpus (any)	C40.1-☑	C79.51	—	D16.1-☑	—	—
cartilage NEC	C41.9	C79.51	—	D16.9	D48.0	D49.2
clavicle	C41.3	C79.51	—	D16.7	D48.0	D49.2
clivus	C41.0	C79.51	—	D16.4	D48.0	D49.2
coccygeal vertebra	C41.4	C79.51	—	D16.8	D48.0	D49.2
coccyx	C41.4	C79.51	—	D16.8	D48.0	D49.2
costal cartilage	C41.3	C79.51	—	D16.7	D48.0	D49.2
costovertebral						
joint	C41.3	C79.51	—	D16.7	D48.0	D49.2
cranial	C41.0	C79.51	—	D16.4	D48.0	D49.2
cuboid	C40.3-☑	C79.51	—	D16.3-☑	—	—
cuneiform	C41.9	C79.51	—	D16.9	D48.0	D49.2
elbow	C40.0-☑	C79.51	—	D16.0-☑	—	—
ethmoid						
(labyrinth)	C41.0	C79.51	—	D16.4	D48.0	D49.2
face	C41.0	C79.51	—	D16.4	D48.0	D49.2
femur (any part)	C40.2-☑	C79.51	—	D16.2-☑	—	—
fibula (any part)	C40.2-☑	C79.51	—	D16.2-☑	—	—
finger (any)	C40.1-☑	C79.51	—	D16.1-☑	—	—
foot	C40.3-☑	C79.51	—	D16.3-☑	—	—
forearm	C40.0-☑	C79.51	—	D16.0-☑	—	—
frontal	C41.0	C79.51	—	D16.4	D48.0	D49.2
hand	C40.1-☑	C79.51	—	D16.1-☑	—	—
heel	C40.3-☑	C79.51	—	D16.3-☑	—	—
hip	C41.4	C79.51	—	D16.8	D48.0	D49.2
humerus (any part)	C40.0-☑	C79.51	—	D16.0-☑	—	—
hyoid	C41.0	C79.51	—	D16.4	D48.0	D49.2
ilium	C41.4	C79.51	—	D16.8	D48.0	D49.2
innominate	C41.4	C79.51	—	D16.8	D48.0	D49.2
intervertebral cartilage or disc	C41.2	C79.51	—	D16.6	D48.0	D49.2
ischium	C41.4	C79.51	—	D16.8	D48.0	D49.2
jaw (lower)	C41.1	C79.51	—	D16.5	D48.0	D49.2
knee	C40.2-☑	C79.51	—	D16.2-☑	—	—
leg NEC	C40.2-☑	C79.51	—	D16.2-☑	—	—
limb NEC	C40.9-☑	C79.51	—	D16.9	—	—
lower (long bones)	C40.2-☑	C79.51	—	D16.2-☑	—	—
short bones	C40.3-☑	C79.51	—	D16.3-☑	—	—
upper (long bones)	C40.0-☑	C79.51	—	D16.0-☑	—	—
short bones	C40.1-☑	C79.51	—	D16.1-☑	—	—
malar	C41.0	C79.51	—	D16.4	D48.0	D49.2

	Malignant Primary	Malignant Secondary	Ca in situ	Benign	Uncertain	Unspecified Behavior
Neoplasm, neoplastic —						
continued						
bone — *continued*						
mandible	C41.1	C79.51	—	D16.5	D48.0	D49.2
marrow NEC (any bone)	C96.9	C79.52	—	—	D47.9	D49.89
mastoid	C41.0	C79.51	—	D16.4	D48.0	D49.2
maxilla, maxillary (superior)	C41.0	C79.51	—	D16.4	D48.0	D49.2
inferior	C41.1	C79.51	—	D16.5	D48.0	D49.2
metacarpus (any)	C40.1-☑	C79.51	—	D16.1-☑	—	—
metatarsus (any)	C40.3-☑	C79.51	—	D16.3-☑	—	—
navicular						
ankle	C40.3-☑	C79.51	—	—	—	—
hand	C40.1-☑	C79.51	—	—	—	—
nose, nasal	C41.0	C79.51	—	D16.4	D48.0	D49.2
occipital	C41.0	C79.51	—	D16.4	D48.0	D49.2
orbit	C41.0	C79.51	—	D16.4	D48.0	D49.2
overlapping sites	C40.8-☑	—	—	—	—	—
parietal	C41.0	C79.51	—	D16.4	D48.0	D49.2
patella	C40.2-☑	C79.51	—	—	—	—
pelvic	C41.4	C79.51	—	D16.8	D48.0	D49.2
phalanges						
foot	C40.3-☑	C79.51	—	—	—	—
hand	C40.1-☑	C79.51	—	—	—	—
pubic	C41.4	C79.51	—	D16.8	D48.0	D49.2
radius (any part)	C40.0-☑	C79.51	—	D16.0-☑	—	—
rib	C41.3	C79.51	—	D16.7	D48.0	D49.2
sacral vertebra	C41.4	C79.51	—	D16.8	D48.0	D49.2
sacrum	C41.4	C79.51	—	D16.8	D48.0	D49.2
scaphoid						
of ankle	C40.3-☑	C79.51	—	—	—	—
of hand	C40.1-☑	C79.51	—	—	—	—
scapula (any part)	C40.0-☑	C79.51	—	D16.0-☑	—	—
sella turcica	C41.0	C79.51	—	D16.4	D48.0	D49.2
shoulder	C40.0-☑	C79.51	—	D16.0-☑	—	—
skull	C41.0	C79.51	—	D16.4	D48.0	D49.2
sphenoid	C41.0	C79.51	—	D16.4	D48.0	D49.2
spine, spinal (column)	C41.2	C79.51	—	D16.6	D48.0	D49.2
coccyx	C41.4	C79.51	—	D16.8	D48.0	D49.2
sacrum	C41.4	C79.51	—	D16.8	D48.0	D49.2
sternum	C41.3	C79.51	—	D16.7	D48.0	D49.2
tarsus (any)	C40.3-☑	C79.51	—	—	—	—
temporal	C41.0	C79.51	—	D16.4	D48.0	D49.2
thumb	C40.1-☑	C79.51	—	—	—	—
tibia (any part)	C40.2-☑	C79.51	—	—	—	—
toe (any)	C40.3-☑	C79.51	—	—	—	—
trapezium	C40.1-☑	C79.51	—	—	—	—
trapezoid	C40.1-☑	C79.51	—	—	—	—
turbinate	C41.0	C79.51	—	D16.4	D48.0	D49.2
ulna (any part)	C40.0-☑	C79.51	—	D16.0-☑	—	—
unciform	C40.1-☑	C79.51	—	—	—	—
vertebra (column)	C41.2	C79.51	—	D16.6	D48.0	D49.2
coccyx	C41.4	C79.51	—	D16.8	D48.0	D49.2
sacrum	C41.4	C79.51	—	D16.8	D48.0	D49.2
vomer	C41.0	C79.51	—	D16.4	D48.0	D49.2
wrist	C40.1-☑	C79.51	—	—	—	—
xiphoid process	C41.3	C79.51	—	D16.7	D48.0	D49.2
zygomatic	C41.0	C79.51	—	D16.4	D48.0	D49.2
book-leaf (mouth) — *ventral surface of tongue and floor of mouth*	C06.89	C79.89	D00.00	D10.39	D37.09	D49.0
bowel — *see* Neoplasm, intestine						
brachial plexus	C47.1-☑	C79.89	—	D36.12	D48.2	D49.2
brain NEC	C71.9	C79.31	—	D33.2	D43.2	D49.6
basal ganglia	C71.0	C79.31	—	D33.0	D43.0	D49.6
cerebellopontine angle	C71.6	C79.31	—	D33.1	D43.1	D49.6
cerebellum NOS	C71.6	C79.31	—	D33.1	D43.1	D49.6
cerebrum	C71.0	C79.31	—	D33.0	D43.0	D49.6
choroid plexus	C71.7	C79.31	—	D33.1	D43.1	D49.6
corpus callosum	C71.8	C79.31	—	D33.2	D43.2	D49.6
corpus striatum	C71.0	C79.31	—	D33.0	D43.0	D49.6
cortex (cerebral)	C71.0	C79.31	—	D33.0	D43.0	D49.6
frontal lobe	C71.1	C79.31	—	D33.0	D43.0	D49.6
globus pallidus	C71.0	C79.31	—	D33.0	D43.0	D49.6
hippocampus	C71.2	C79.31	—	D33.0	D43.0	D49.6
hypothalamus	C71.0	C79.31	—	D33.0	D43.0	D49.6
internal capsule	C71.0	C79.31	—	D33.0	D43.0	D49.6

☑ **Additional Character Required** — Refer to the Tabular List for Character Selection   ⩔ **Subterms under main terms may continue to next column or page**

Neoplasm, neoplastic — continued

	Malignant Primary	Malignant Secondary	Ca in situ	Benign	Uncertain	Unspecified Behavior
brain — *continued*						
medulla						
oblongata	C71.7	C79.31	—	D33.1	D43.1	D49.6
meninges	C70.0	C79.32	—	D32.0	D42.0	D49.7
midbrain	C71.7	C79.31	—	D33.1	D43.1	D49.6
occipital lobe	C71.4	C79.31	—	D33.0	D43.0	D49.6
overlapping lesion	C71.8	C79.31	—	—	—	—
parietal lobe	C71.3	C79.31	—	D33.0	D43.0	D49.6
peduncle	C71.7	C79.31	—	D33.1	D43.1	D49.6
pons	C71.7	C79.31	—	D33.1	D43.1	D49.6
stem	C71.7	C79.31	—	D33.1	D43.1	D49.6
tapetum	C71.8	C79.31	—	D33.2	D43.2	D49.6
temporal lobe	C71.2	C79.31	—	D33.0	D43.0	D49.6
thalamus	C71.0	C79.31	—	D33.0	D43.0	D49.6
uncus	C71.2	C79.31	—	D33.0	D43.0	D49.6
ventricle (floor)	C71.5	C79.31	—	D33.0	D43.0	D49.6
fourth	C71.7	C79.31	—	D33.1	D43.1	D49.6
branchial (cleft) (cyst) (vestiges)	C10.4	C79.89	D00.08	D10.5	D37.05	D49.0
breast (connective tissue) (glandular tissue) (soft parts)	C50.9-☑	C79.81	D05.-☑	D24.-☑	D48.6-☑	D49.3
areola	C50.0-☑	C79.81	D05.-☑	D24.-☑	D48.6-☑	D49.3
axillary tail	C50.6-☑	C79.81	D05.-☑	D24.-☑	D48.6-☑	D49.3
central portion	C50.1-☑	C79.81	D05.-☑	D24.-☑	D48.6-☑	D49.3
inner	C50.8-☑	C79.81	D05.-☑	D24.-☑	D48.6-☑	D49.3
lower	C50.8-☑	C79.81	D05.-☑	D24.-☑	D48.6-☑	D49.3
lower-inner quadrant	C50.3-☑	C79.81	D05.-☑	D24.-☑	D48.6-☑	D49.3
lower-outer quadrant	C50.5-☑	C79.81	D05.-☑	D24.-☑	D48.6-☑	D49.3
mastectomy site (skin) — *see also* Neoplasm, breast, skin	C44.501	C79.2	—	—	—	—
specified as breast tissue	C50.8-☑	C79.81	—	—	—	—
midline	C50.8-☑	C79.81	D05.-☑	D24.-☑	D48.6-☑	D49.3
nipple	C50.0-☑	C79.81	D05.-☑	D24.-☑	D48.6-☑	D49.3
outer	C50.8-☑	C79.81	D05.-☑	D24.-☑	D48.6-☑	D49.3
overlapping lesion	C50.8-☑					
skin	C44.501	C79.2	D04.5	D23.5	D48.5	D49.2
basal cell carcinoma	C44.511	—	—	—	—	—
specified type NEC	C44.591	—	—	—	—	—
squamous cell carcinoma	C44.521	—	—	—	—	—
tail (axillary)	C50.6-☑	C79.81	D05.-☑	D24.-☑	D48.6-☑	D49.3
upper	C50.8-☑	C79.81	D05.-☑	D24.-☑	D48.6-☑	D49.3
upper-inner quadrant	C50.2-☑	C79.81	D05.-☑	D24.-☑	D48.6-☑	D49.3
upper-outer quadrant	C50.4-☑	C79.81	D05.-☑	D24.-☑	D48.6-☑	D49.3
broad ligament	C57.1-☑	C79.82	D07.39	D28.2	D39.8	D49.59
bronchiogenic, bronchogenic (lung)	C34.9-☑	C78.0-☑	D02.2-☑	D14.3-☑	D38.1	D49.1
bronchiole	C34.9-☑	C78.0-☑	D02.2-☑	D14.3-☑	D38.1	D49.1
bronchus	C34.9-☑	C78.0-☑	D02.2-☑	D14.3-☑	D38.1	D49.1
carina	C34.0-☑	C78.0-☑	D02.2-☑	D14.3-☑	D38.1	D49.1
lower lobe of lung	C34.3-☑	C78.0-☑	D02.2-☑	D14.3-☑	D38.1	D49.1
main	C34.0-☑	C78.0-☑	D02.2-☑	D14.3-☑	D38.1	D49.1
middle lobe of lung	C34.2	C78.0-☑	D02.21	D14.31	D38.1	D49.1
overlapping lesion	C34.8-☑	—	—	—	—	—
upper lobe of lung	C34.1-☑	C78.0-☑	D02.2-☑	D14.3-☑	D38.1	D49.1
brow	C44.309	C79.2	D04.39	D23.39	D48.5	D49.2
basal cell carcinoma	C44.319	—	—	—	—	—
specified type NEC	C44.399	—	—	—	—	—
squamous cell carcinoma	C44.329	—	—	—	—	—
buccal (cavity)	C06.9	C79.89	D00.00	D10.39	D37.09	D49.0
commissure	C06.0	C79.89	D00.02	D10.39	D37.09	D49.0
groove (lower) (upper)	C06.1	C79.89	D00.02	D10.39	D37.09	D49.0
mucosa	C06.0	C79.89	D00.02	D10.39	D37.09	D49.0
sulcus (lower) (upper)	C06.1	C79.89	D00.02	D10.39	D37.09	D49.0

Neoplasm, neoplastic — continued

	Malignant Primary	Malignant Secondary	Ca in situ	Benign	Uncertain	Unspecified Behavior
bulbourethral gland	C68.0	C79.19	D09.19	D30.4	D41.3	D49.59
bursa — *see* Neoplasm, connective tissue						
buttock NEC	C76.3	C79.89	D04.5	D36.7	D48.7	D49.89
calf	C76.5-☑	C79.89	D04.7-☑	D36.7	D48.7	D49.89
calvarium	C41.0	C79.51	—	D16.4	D48.0	D49.2
calyx, renal	C65.-☑	C79.0-☑	D09.19	D30.1-☑	D41.1-☑	D49.51-☑
canal						
anal	C21.1	C78.5	D01.3	D12.9	D37.8	D49.0
auditory (external) — *see also* Neoplasm, skin, ear	C44.20-☑	C79.2	D04.2-☑	D23.2-☑	D48.5	D49.2
auricular (external) — *see also* Neoplasm, skin, ear	C44.20-☑	C79.2	D04.2-☑	D23.2-☑	D48.5	D49.2
canaliculi, biliary (biliferi) (intrahepatic)	C22.1	C78.7	D01.5	D13.4	D37.6	D49.0
canthus (eye) (inner) (outer)	C44.10-☑	C79.2	D04.1-☑	D23.1-☑	D48.5	D49.2
basal cell carcinoma	C44.11-☑	—	—	—	—	—
specified type NEC	C44.19-☑	—	—	—	—	—
squamous cell carcinoma	C44.12-☑	—	—	—	—	—
capillary — *see* Neoplasm, connective tissue						
caput coli	C18.0	C78.5	D01.0	D12.0	D37.4	D49.0
carcinoid — *see* Tumor, carcinoid						
cardia (gastric)	C16.0	C78.89	D00.2	D13.1	D37.1	D49.0
cardiac orifice (stomach)	C16.0	C78.89	D00.2	D13.1	D37.1	D49.0
cardio-esophageal junction	C16.0	C78.89	D00.2	D13.1	D37.1	D49.0
cardio-esophagus	C16.0	C78.89	D00.2	D13.1	D37.1	D49.0
carina (bronchus)	C34.0-☑	C78.0-☑	D02.2-☑	D14.3-☑	D38.1	D49.1
carotid (artery)	C49.0	C79.89	—	D21.0	D48.1	D49.2
body	C75.4	C79.89	—	D35.5	D44.6	D49.7
carpus (any bone)	C40.1-☑	C79.51	—	D16.1-☑	—	—
cartilage (articular) (joint) NEC — *see also* Neoplasm, bone	C41.9	C79.51		D16.9	D48.0	D49.2
arytenoid	C32.3	C78.39	D02.0	D14.1	D38.0	D49.1
auricular	C49.0	C79.89	—	D21.0	D48.1	D49.2
bronchi	C34.0-☑	C78.39	—	D14.3-☑	D38.1	D49.1
costal	C41.3	C79.51	—	D16.7	D48.0	D49.2
cricoid	C32.3	C78.39	D02.0	D14.1	D38.0	D49.1
cuneiform	C32.3	C78.39	D02.0	D14.1	D38.0	D49.1
ear (external)	C49.0	C79.89	—	D21.0	D48.1	D49.2
ensiform	C41.3	C79.51	—	D16.7	D48.0	D49.2
epiglottis	C32.1	C78.39	D02.0	D14.1	D38.0	D49.1
anterior surface	C10.1	C78.39	D00.08	D10.5	D37.05	D49.0
eyelid	C49.0	C79.89	—	D21.0	D48.1	D49.2
intervertebral	C41.2	C79.51	—	D16.6	D48.0	D49.2
larynx, laryngeal	C32.3	C78.39	D02.0	D14.1	D38.0	D49.1
nose, nasal	C30.0	C78.39	D02.3	D14.0	D38.5	D49.1
pinna	C49.0	C79.89	—	D21.0	D48.1	D49.2
rib	C41.3	C79.51	—	D16.7	D48.0	D49.2
semilunar (knee)	C40.2-☑	C79.51	—	D16.2-☑	D48.0	D49.2
thyroid	C32.3	C78.39	D02.0	D14.1	D38.0	D49.1
trachea	C33	C78.39	D02.1	D14.2	D38.1	D49.1
cauda equina	C72.1	C79.49	—	D33.4	D43.4	D49.7
cavity						
buccal	C06.9	C79.89	D00.00	D10.30	D37.09	D49.0
nasal	C30.0	C78.39	D02.3	D14.0	D38.5	D49.1
oral	C06.9	C79.89	D00.00	D10.30	D37.09	D49.0
peritoneal	C48.2	C78.6	—	D20.1	D48.4	D49.0
tympanic	C30.1	C78.39	D02.3	D14.0	D38.5	D49.1
cecum	C18.0	C78.5	D01.0	D12.0	D37.4	D49.0
central nervous system	C72.9	C79.40	—	—	—	—
cerebellopontine (angle)	C71.6	C79.31	—	D33.1	D43.1	D49.6
cerebellum, cerebellar	C71.6	C79.31	—	D33.1	D43.1	D49.6
cerebrum, cerebral (cortex) (hemisphere) (white matter)	C71.0	C79.31	—	D33.0	D43.0	D49.6
meninges	C70.0	C79.32	—	D32.0	D42.0	D49.7
peduncle	C71.7	C79.31	—	D33.1	D43.1	D49.6

Left column table

	Malignant Primary	Malignant Secondary	Ca in situ	Benign	Uncertain	Unspecified Behavior
Neoplasm, neoplastic — *continued*						
cerebrum, cerebral — *continued*						
ventricle	C71.5	C79.31	—	D33.0	D43.0	D49.6
fourth	C71.7	C79.31	—	D33.1	D43.1	D49.6
cervical region	C76.0	C79.89	D09.8	D36.7	D48.7	D49.89
cervix (cervical) (uteri) (uterus)	C53.9	C79.82	D06.9	D26.0	D39.0	D49.59
canal	C53.0	C79.82	D06.0	D26.0	D39.0	D49.59
endocervix (canal) (gland)	C53.0	C79.82	D06.0	D26.0	D39.0	D49.59
exocervix	C53.1	C79.82	D06.1	D26.0	D39.0	D49.59
external os	C53.1	C79.82	D06.1	D26.0	D39.0	D49.59
internal os	C53.0	C79.82	D06.0	D26.0	D39.0	D49.59
nabothian gland	C53.0	C79.82	D06.0	D26.0	D39.0	D49.59
overlapping lesion	C53.8	—	—	—	—	—
squamocolumnar junction	C53.8	C79.82	D06.7	D26.0	D39.0	D49.59
stump	C53.8	C79.82	D06.7	D26.0	D39.0	D49.59
cheek	C76.0	C79.89	D09.8	D36.7	D48.7	D49.89
external	C44.309	C79.2	D04.39	D23.39	D48.5	D49.2
basal cell carcinoma	C44.319	—	—	—	—	—
specified type NEC	C44.399	—	—	—	—	—
squamous cell carcinoma	C44.329	—	—	—	—	—
inner aspect	C06.0	C79.89	D00.02	D10.39	D37.09	D49.0
internal	C06.0	C79.89	D00.02	D10.39	D37.09	D49.0
mucosa	C06.0	C79.89	D00.02	D10.39	D37.09	D49.0
chest (wall) NEC	C76.1	C79.89	D09.8	D36.7	D48.7	D49.89
chiasma opticum	C72.3-☑	C79.49	—	D33.3	D43.3	D49.7
chin	C44.309	C79.2	D04.39	D23.39	D48.5	D49.2
basal cell carcinoma	C44.319	—	—	—	—	—
specified type NEC	C44.399	—	—	—	—	—
squamous cell carcinoma	C44.329	—	—	—	—	—
choana	C11.3	C79.89	D00.08	D10.6	D37.05	D49.0
cholangiole	C22.1	C78.89	D01.5	D13.4	D37.6	D49.0
choledochal duct	C24.0	C78.89	D01.5	D13.5	D37.6	D49.0
choroid	C69.3-☑	C79.49	D09.2-☑	D31.3-☑	D48.7	D49.81
plexus	C71.5	C79.31	—	D33.0	D43.0	D49.6
ciliary body	C69.4-☑	C79.49	D09.2-☑	D31.4-☑	D48.7	D49.89
clavicle	C41.3	C79.51	—	D16.7	D48.0	D49.2
clitoris	C51.2	C79.82	D07.1	D28.0	D39.8	D49.59
clivus	C41.0	C79.51	—	D16.4	D48.0	D49.2
cloacogenic zone	C21.2	C78.5	D01.3	D12.9	D37.8	D49.0
coccygeal						
body or glomus	C49.5	C79.89	—	D21.5	D48.1	D49.2
vertebra	C41.4	C79.51	—	D16.8	D48.0	D49.2
coccyx	C41.4	C79.51	—	D16.8	D48.0	D49.2
colon — *see also* Neoplasm, intestine, large	C18.9	C78.5	—	—	—	—
with rectum	C19	C78.5	D01.1	D12.7	D37.5	D49.0
columnella — *see also* Neoplasm, skin, face	C44.390	C79.2	D04.39	D23.39	D48.5	D49.2
column, spinal — *see* Neoplasm, spine						
commissure						
labial, lip	C00.6	C79.89	D00.01	D10.39	D37.01	D49.0
laryngeal	C32.0	C78.39	D02.0	D14.1	D38.0	D49.1
common (bile) duct	C24.0	C78.89	D01.5	D13.5	D37.6	D49.0
concha — *see also* Neoplasm, skin, ear	C44.20-☑	C79.2	D04.2-☑	D23.2-☑	D48.5	D49.2
nose	C30.0	C78.39	D02.3	D14.0	D38.5	D49.1
conjunctiva	C69.0-☑	C79.49	D09.2-☑	D31.0-☑	D48.7	D49.89

Right column table

	Malignant Primary	Malignant Secondary	Ca in situ	Benign	Uncertain	Unspecified Behavior
Neoplasm, neoplastic — *continued*						
connective tissue NEC	C49.9	C79.89	—	D21.9	D48.1	D49.2

Note: For neoplasms of connective tissue (blood vessel, bursa, fascia, ligament, muscle, peripheral nerves, sympathetic and parasympathetic nerves and ganglia, synovia, tendon, etc.) or of morphological types that indicate connective tissue, code according to the list under "Neoplasm, connective tissue". For sites that do not appear in this list, code to neoplasm of that site; e.g., fibrosarcoma, pancreas (C25.9)

Note: Morphological types that indicate connective tissue appear in their proper place in the alphabetic index with the instruction "see Neoplasm, connective tissue ...."

	Malignant Primary	Malignant Secondary	Ca in situ	Benign	Uncertain	Unspecified Behavior
abdomen	C49.4	C79.89	—	D21.4	D48.1	D49.2
abdominal wall	C49.4	C79.89	—	D21.4	D48.1	D49.2
ankle	C49.2-☑	C79.89	—	D21.2-☑	D48.1	D49.2
antecubital fossa or space	C49.1-☑	C79.89	—	D21.1-☑	D48.1	D49.2
arm	C49.1-☑	C79.89	—	D21.1-☑	D48.1	D49.2
auricle (ear)	C49.0	C79.89	—	D21.0	D48.1	D49.2
axilla	C49.3	C79.89	—	D21.3	D48.1	D49.2
back	C49.6	C79.89	—	D21.6	D48.1	D49.2
breast — *see* Neoplasm, breast						
buttock	C49.5	C79.89	—	D21.5	D48.1	D49.2
calf	C49.2-☑	C79.89	—	D21.2-☑	D48.1	D49.2
cervical region	C49.0	C79.89	—	D21.0	D48.1	D49.2
cheek	C49.0	C79.89	—	D21.0	D48.1	D49.2
chest (wall)	C49.3	C79.89	—	D21.3	D48.1	D49.2
chin	C49.0	C79.89	—	D21.0	D48.1	D49.2
diaphragm	C49.3	C79.89	—	D21.3	D48.1	D49.2
ear (external)	C49.0	C79.89	—	D21.0	D48.1	D49.2
elbow	C49.1-☑	C79.89	—	D21.1-☑	D48.1	D49.2
extrarectal	C49.5	C79.89	—	D21.5	D48.1	D49.2
extremity	C49.9	C79.89	—	D21.9	D48.1	D49.2
lower	C49.2-☑	C79.89	—	D21.2-☑	D48.1	D49.2
upper	C49.1-☑	C79.89	—	D21.1-☑	D48.1	D49.2
eyelid	C49.0	C79.89	—	D21.0	D48.1	D49.2
face	C49.0	C79.89	—	D21.0	D48.1	D49.2
finger	C49.1-☑	C79.89	—	D21.1-☑	D48.1	D49.2
flank	C49.6	C79.89	—	D21.6	D48.1	D49.2
foot	C49.2-☑	C79.89	—	D21.2-☑	D48.1	D49.2
forearm	C49.1-☑	C79.89	—	D21.1-☑	D48.1	D49.2
forehead	C49.0	C79.89	—	D21.0	D48.1	D49.2
gastric	C49.4	C79.89	—	D21.4	D48.1	D49.2
gastrointestinal	C49.4	C79.89	—	D21.4	D48.1	D49.2
gluteal region	C49.5	C79.89	—	D21.5	D48.1	D49.2
great vessels NEC	C49.3	C79.89	—	D21.3	D48.1	D49.2
groin	C49.5	C79.89	—	D21.5	D48.1	D49.2
hand	C49.1-☑	C79.89	—	D21.1-☑	D48.1	D49.2
head	C49.0	C79.89	—	D21.0	D48.1	D49.2
heel	C49.2-☑	C79.89	—	D21.2-☑	D48.1	D49.2
hip	C49.2-☑	C79.89	—	D21.2-☑	D48.1	D49.2
hypochondrium	C49.4	C79.89	—	D21.4	D48.1	D49.2
iliopsoas muscle	C49.5	C79.89	—	D21.5	D48.1	D49.2
infraclavicular region	C49.3	C79.89	—	D21.3	D48.1	D49.2
inguinal (canal) (region)	C49.5	C79.89	—	D21.5	D48.1	D49.2
intestinal	C49.4	C79.89	—	D21.4	D48.1	D49.2
intrathoracic	C49.3	C79.89	—	D21.3	D48.1	D49.2
ischiorectal fossa	C49.5	C79.89	—	D21.5	D48.1	D49.2
jaw	C03.9	C79.89	D00.03	D10.39	D48.1	D49.0
knee	C49.2-☑	C79.89	—	D21.2-☑	D48.1	D49.2
leg	C49.2-☑	C79.89	—	D21.2-☑	D48.1	D49.2
limb NEC	C49.9	C79.89	—	D21.9	D48.1	D49.2
lower	C49.2-☑	C79.89	—	D21.2-☑	D48.1	D49.2
upper	C49.1-☑	C79.89	—	D21.1-☑	D48.1	D49.2
nates	C49.5	C79.89	—	D21.5	D48.1	D49.2
neck	C49.0	C79.89	—	D21.0	D48.1	D49.2
orbit	C69.6-☑	C79.49	D09.2-☑	D31.6-☑	D48.1	D49.89
overlapping lesion	C49.8	—	—	—	—	—
pararectal	C49.5	C79.89	—	D21.5	D48.1	D49.2
para-urethral	C49.5	C79.89	—	D21.5	D48.1	D49.2
paravaginal	C49.5	C79.89	—	D21.5	D48.1	D49.2
pelvis (floor)	C49.5	C79.89	—	D21.5	D48.1	D49.2
pelvo-abdominal	C49.8	C79.89	—	D21.6	D48.1	D49.2
perineum	C49.5	C79.89	—	D21.5	D48.1	D49.2
perirectal (tissue)	C49.5	C79.89	—	D21.5	D48.1	D49.2

☑ **Additional Character Required — Refer to the Tabular List for Character Selection**   ▽ Subterms under main terms may continue to next column or page

	Malignant Primary	Malignant Secondary	Ca in situ	Benign	Uncertain	Unspecified Behavior
Neoplasm, neoplastic —						
continued						
connective tissue —						
continued						
periurethral						
(tissue)	C49.5	C79.89	—	D21.5	D48.1	D49.2
popliteal fossa or						
space	C49.2-☑	C79.89	—	D21.2-☑	D48.1	D49.2
presacral	C49.5	C79.89	—	D21.5	D48.1	D49.2
psoas muscle	C49.4	C79.89	—	D21.4	D48.1	D49.2
pterygoid fossa	C49.0	C79.89	—	D21.0	D48.1	D49.2
rectovaginal septum or						
wall	C49.5	C79.89	—	D21.5	D48.1	D49.2
rectovesical	C49.5	C79.89	—	D21.5	D48.1	D49.2
retroperitoneum	C48.0	C78.6	—	D20.0	D48.3	D49.0
sacrococcygeal						
region	C49.5	C79.89	—	D21.5	D48.1	D49.2
scalp	C49.0	C79.89	—	D21.0	D48.1	D49.2
scapular region	C49.3	C79.89	—	D21.3	D48.1	D49.2
shoulder	C49.1-☑	C79.89	—	D21.1-☑	D48.1	D49.2
skin (dermis) NEC — *see*						
also Neoplasm, skin,						
by site	C44.90	C79.2	D04.9	D23.9	D48.5	D49.2
stomach	C49.4	C79.89	—	D21.4	D48.1	D49.2
submental	C49.0	C79.89	—	D21.0	D48.1	D49.2
supraclavicular						
region	C49.0	C79.89	—	D21.0	D48.1	D49.2
temple	C49.0	C79.89	—	D21.0	D48.1	D49.2
temporal region	C49.0	C79.89	—	D21.0	D48.1	D49.2
thigh	C49.2-☑	C79.89	—	D21.2-☑	D48.1	D49.2
thoracic (duct)						
(wall)	C49.3	C79.89	—	D21.3	D48.1	D49.2
thorax	C49.3	C79.89	—	D21.3	D48.1	D49.2
thumb	C49.1-☑	C79.89	—	D21.1-☑	D48.1	D49.2
toe	C49.2-☑	C79.89	—	D21.2-☑	D48.1	D49.2
trunk	C49.6	C79.89	—	D21.6	D48.1	D49.2
umbilicus	C49.4	C79.89	—	D21.4	D48.1	D49.2
vesicorectal	C49.5	C79.89	—	D21.5	D48.1	D49.2
wrist	C49.1-☑	C79.89	—	D21.1-☑	D48.1	D49.2
conus medullaris	C72.0	C79.49	—	D33.4	D43.4	D49.7
cord (true) (vocal)	C32.0	C78.39	D02.0	D14.1	D38.0	D49.1
false	C32.1	C78.39	D02.0	D14.1	D38.0	D49.1
spermatic	C63.1-☑	C79.82	D07.69	D29.8	D40.8	D49.59
spinal (cervical)						
(lumbar)						
(thoracic)	C72.0	C79.49	—	D33.4	D43.4	D49.7
cornea (limbus)	C69.1-☑	C79.49	D09.2-☑	D31.1-☑	D48.7	D49.89
corpus						
albicans	C56.-☑	C79.6-☑	D07.39	D27.-☑	D39.1-☑	D49.59
callosum, brain	C71.0	C79.31	—	D33.2	D43.2	D49.6
cavernosum	C60.2	C79.82	D07.4	D29.0	D40.8	D49.59
gastric	C16.2	C78.89	D00.2	D13.1	D37.1	D49.0
overlapping sites	C54.8	—	—	—	—	—
penis	C60.2	C79.82	D07.4	D29.0	D40.8	D49.59
striatum,						
cerebrum	C71.0	C79.31	—	D33.0	D43.0	D49.6
uteri	C54.9	C79.82	D07.0	D26.1	D39.0	D49.59
isthmus	C54.0	C79.82	D07.0	D26.1	D39.0	D49.59
cortex						
adrenal	C74.0-☑	C79.7-☑	D09.3	D35.0-☑	D44.1-☑	D49.7
cerebral	C71.0	C79.31	—	D33.0	D43.0	D49.6
costal cartilage	C41.3	C79.51	—	D16.7	D48.0	D49.2
costovertebral joint	C41.3	C79.51	—	D16.7	D48.0	D49.2
Cowper's gland	C68.0	C79.19	D09.19	D30.4	D41.3	D49.59
cranial (fossa, any)	C71.9	C79.31	—	D33.2	D43.2	D49.6
meninges	C70.0	C79.32	—	D32.0	D42.0	D49.7
nerve	C72.50	C79.49	—	D33.3	D43.3	D49.7
specified NEC	C72.59	C79.49	—	D33.3	D43.3	D49.7
craniobuccal pouch	C75.2	C79.89	D09.3	D35.2	D44.3	D49.7
craniopharyngeal (duct)						
(pouch)	C75.2	C79.89	D09.3	D35.3	D44.4	D49.7
cricoid	C13.0	C79.89	D00.08	D10.7	D37.05	D49.0
cartilage	C32.3	C78.39	D02.0	D14.1	D38.0	D49.1
cricopharynx	C13.0	C79.89	D00.08	D10.7	D37.05	D49.0
crypt of Morgagni	C21.8	C78.5	D01.3	D12.9	D37.8	D49.0
crystalline lens	C69.4-☑	C79.49	D09.2-☑	D31.4-☑	D48.7	D49.89
cul-de-sac						
(Douglas')	C48.1	C78.6	—	D20.1	D48.4	D49.0
cuneiform cartilage	C32.3	C78.39	D02.0	D14.1	D38.0	D49.1
cutaneous — *see*						
Neoplasm, skin						
cutis — *see* Neoplasm,						
skin						
Neoplasm, neoplastic —						
continued						
cystic (bile) duct						
(common)	C24.0	C78.89	D01.5	D13.5	D37.6	D49.0
dermis — *see* Neoplasm,						
skin						
diaphragm	C49.3	C79.89	—	D21.3	D48.1	D49.2
digestive organs, system,						
tube, or tract						
NEC	C26.9	C78.89	D01.9	D13.9	D37.9	D49.0
disc, intervertebral	C41.2	C79.51	—	D16.6	D48.0	D49.2
disease, generalized	C80.0	—	—	—	—	—
disseminated	C80.0	—	—	—	—	—
Douglas' cul-de-sac or						
pouch	C48.1	C78.6		D20.1	D48.4	D49.0
duodenojejunal						
junction	C17.8	C78.4	D01.49	D13.39	D37.2	D49.0
duodenum	C17.0	C78.4	D01.49	D13.2	D37.2	D49.0
dura (cranial)						
(mater)	C70.9	C79.49	—	D32.9	D42.9	D49.7
cerebral	C70.0	C79.32	—	D32.0	D42.0	D49.7
spinal	C70.1	C79.49	—	D32.1	D42.1	D49.7
ear (external) — *see also*						
Neoplasm, skin,						
ear	C44.20-☑	C79.2	D04.2-☑	D23.2-☑	D48.5	D49.2
auricle or auris — *see*						
also Neoplasm, skin,						
ear	C44.20-☑	C79.2	D04.2-☑	D23.2-☑	D48.5	D49.2
canal, external — *see*						
also Neoplasm, skin,						
ear	C44.20-☑	C79.2	D04.2-☑	D23.2-☑	D48.5	D49.2
cartilage	C49.0	C79.89	—	D21.0	D48.1	D49.2
external meatus — *see*						
also Neoplasm, skin,						
ear	C44.20-☑	C79.2	D04.2-☑	D23.2-☑	D48.5	D49.2
inner	C30.1	C78.39	D02.3	D14.0	D38.5	D49.1
lobule — *see also*						
Neoplasm, skin,						
ear	C44.20-☑	C79.2	D04.2-☑	D23.2-☑	D48.5	D49.2
middle	C30.1	C78.39	D02.3	D14.0	D38.5	D49.1
overlapping lesion with						
accessory						
sinuses	C31.8	—	—	—	—	—
skin	C44.20-☑	C79.2	D04.2-☑	D23.2-☑	D48.5	D49.2
basal cell						
carcinoma	C44.21-☑	—				
specified type						
NEC	C44.29-☑					
squamous cell						
carcinoma	C44.22-☑					
earlobe	C44.20-☑	C79.2	D04.2-☑	D23.2-☑	D48.5	D49.2
basal cell						
carcinoma	C44.21-☑	—				
specified type NEC	C44.29-☑					
squamous cell						
carcinoma	C44.22-☑					
ejaculatory duct	C63.7	C79.82	D07.69	D29.8	D40.8	D49.59
elbow NEC	C76.4-☑	C79.89	D04.6-☑	D36.7	D48.7	D49.89
endocardium	C38.0	C79.89		D15.1	D48.7	D49.89
endocervix (canal)						
(gland)	C53.0	C79.82	D06.0	D26.0	D39.0	D49.59
endocrine gland						
NEC	C75.9	C79.89	D09.3	D35.9	D44.9	D49.7
pluriglandular	C75.8	C79.89	D09.3	D35.7	D44.9	D49.7
endometrium (gland)						
(stroma)	C54.1	C79.82	D07.0	D26.1	D39.0	D49.59
ensiform cartilage	C41.3	C79.51	—	D16.7	D48.0	D49.2
enteric — *see* Neoplasm,						
intestine						
ependyma (brain)	C71.5	C79.31	—	D33.0	D43.0	D49.6
fourth ventricle	C71.7	C79.31	—	D33.1	D43.1	D49.6
epicardium	C38.0	C79.89		D15.1	D48.7	D49.89
epididymis	C63.0-☑	C79.82	D07.69	D29.3-☑	D40.8	D49.59
epidural	C72.9	C79.49	—	D33.9	D43.9	D49.7
epiglottis	C32.1	C78.39	D02.0	D14.1	D38.0	D49.1
anterior aspect or						
surface	C10.1	C79.89	D00.08	D10.5	D37.05	D49.0
cartilage	C32.3	C78.39	D02.0	D14.1	D38.0	D49.1
free border						
(margin)	C10.1	C79.89	D00.08	D10.5	D37.05	D49.0
junctional region	C10.8	C79.89	D00.08	D10.5	D37.05	D49.0
posterior (laryngeal)						
surface	C32.1	C78.39	D02.0	D14.1	D38.0	D49.1

Neoplasm, neoplastic — continued	Malignant Primary	Malignant Secondary	Ca in situ	Benign	Uncertain	Unspecified Behavior
epiglottis — continued						
suprahyoid portion	C32.1	C78.39	D02.0	D14.1	D38.0	D49.1
esophagogastric junction	C16.0	C78.89	D00.2	D13.1	D37.1	D49.0
esophagus	C15.9	C78.89	D00.1	D13.0	D37.8	D49.0
abdominal	C15.5	C78.89	D00.1	D13.0	D37.8	D49.0
cervical	C15.3	C78.89	D00.1	D13.0	D37.8	D49.0
distal (third)	C15.5	C78.89	D00.1	D13.0	D37.8	D49.0
lower (third)	C15.5	C78.89	D00.1	D13.0	D37.8	D49.0
middle (third)	C15.4	C78.89	D00.1	D13.0	D37.8	D49.0
overlapping lesion	C15.8	—	—	—	—	—
proximal (third)	C15.3	C78.89	D00.1	D13.0	D37.8	D49.0
thoracic	C15.4	C78.89	D00.1	D13.0	D37.8	D49.0
upper (third)	C15.3	C78.89	D00.1	D13.0	D37.8	D49.0
ethmoid (sinus)	C31.1	C78.39	D02.3	D14.0	D38.5	D49.1
bone or labyrinth	C41.0	C79.51	—	D16.4	D48.0	D49.2
eustachian tube	C30.1	C78.39	D02.3	D14.0	D38.5	D49.1
exocervix	C53.1	C79.82	D06.1	D26.0	D39.0	D49.59
external						
meatus (ear) — see also Neoplasm, skin,						
ear	C44.20-☑	C79.2	D04.2-☑	D23.2-☑	D48.5	D49.2
os, cervix uteri	C53.1	C79.82	D06.1	D26.0	D39.0	D49.59
extradural	C72.9	C79.49	—	D33.9	D43.9	D49.7
extrahepatic (bile) duct	C24.0	C78.89	D01.5	D13.5	D37.6	D49.0
overlapping lesion with gallbladder	C24.8	—	—	—	—	—
extraocular muscle	C69.6-☑	C79.49	D09.2-☑	D31.6-☑	D48.7	D49.89
extrarectal	C76.3	C79.89	D09.8	D36.7	D48.7	D49.89
extremity	C76.8	C79.89	D04.8	D36.7	D48.7	D49.89
lower	C76.5-☑	C79.89	D04.7-☑	D36.7	D48.7	D49.89
upper	C76.4-☑	C79.89	D04.6-☑	D36.7	D48.7	D49.89
eyeball	C69.9-☑	C79.49	D09.2-☑	D31.9-☑	D48.7	D49.89
eyebrow	C44.309	C79.2	D04.39	D23.39	D48.5	D49.2
basal cell carcinoma	C44.319	—	—	—	—	—
specified type NEC	C44.399	—	—	—	—	—
squamous cell carcinoma	C44.329	—	—	—	—	—
eyelid (lower) (skin) (upper)	C44.10-☑	—	—	—	—	—
basal cell carcinoma	C44.11-☑	—	—	—	—	—
cartilage	C49.0	C79.89	—	D21.0	D48.1	D49.2
specified type NEC	C44.19-☑	—	—	—	—	—
squamous cell carcinoma	C44.12-☑	—	—	—	—	—
eye NEC	C69.9-☑	C79.49	D09.2-☑	D31.9-☑	D48.7	D49.89
overlapping sites	C69.8-☑	—	—	—	—	—
face NEC	C76.0	C79.89	D04.39	D36.7	D48.7	D49.89
fallopian tube (accessory)	C57.0-☑	C79.82	D07.39	D28.2	D39.8	D49.59
falx (cerebella) (cerebri)	C70.0	C79.32	—	D32.0	D42.0	D49.7
fascia — see also Neoplasm, connective tissue						
palmar	C49.1-☑	C79.89	—	D21.1-☑	D48.1	D49.2
plantar	C49.2-☑	C79.89	—	D21.2-☑	D48.1	D49.2
fatty tissue — see Neoplasm, connective tissue						
fauces, faucial NEC	C10.9	C79.89	D00.08	D10.5	D37.05	D49.0
pillars	C09.1	C79.89	D00.08	D10.5	D37.05	D49.0
tonsil	C09.9	C79.89	D00.08	D10.4	D37.05	D49.0
femur (any part)	C40.2-☑	—	—	D16.2-☑	—	—
fetal membrane	C58	C79.82	D07.0	D26.7	D39.2	D49.59
fibrous tissue — see Neoplasm, connective tissue						
fibula (any part)	C40.2-☑	C79.51	—	D16.2-☑	—	—
filum terminale	C72.0	C79.49	—	D33.4	D43.4	D49.7
finger NEC	C76.4-☑	C79.89	D04.6-☑	D36.7	D48.7	D49.89
flank NEC	C76.8	C79.89	D04.5	D36.7	D48.7	D49.89
follicle, nabothian	C53.0	C79.82	D06.0	D26.0	D39.0	D49.59
foot NEC	C76.5-☑	C79.89	D04.7-☑	D36.7	D48.7	D49.89
forearm NEC	C76.4-☑	C79.89	D04.6-☑	D36.7	D48.7	D49.89
forehead (skin)	C44.309	C79.2	D04.39	D23.39	D48.5	D49.2

Neoplasm, neoplastic — continued	Malignant Primary	Malignant Secondary	Ca in situ	Benign	Uncertain	Unspecified Behavior
forehead — continued						
basal cell carcinoma	C44.319	—	—	—	—	—
specified type NEC	C44.399	—	—	—	—	—
squamous cell carcinoma	C44.329	—	—	—	—	—
foreskin	C60.0	C79.82	D07.4	D29.0	D40.8	D49.59
fornix						
pharyngeal	C11.3	C79.89	D00.08	D10.6	D37.05	D49.0
vagina	C52	C79.82	D07.2	D28.1	D39.8	D49.59
fossa (of)						
anterior (cranial)	C71.9	C79.31	—	D33.2	D43.2	D49.6
cranial	C71.9	C79.31	—	D33.2	D43.2	D49.6
ischiorectal	C76.3	C79.89	D09.8	D36.7	D48.7	D49.89
middle (cranial)	C71.9	C79.31	—	D33.2	D43.2	D49.6
piriform	C12	C79.89	D00.08	D10.7	D37.05	D49.0
pituitary	C75.1	C79.89	D09.3	D35.2	D44.3	D49.7
posterior (cranial)	C71.9	C79.31	—	D33.2	D43.2	D49.6
pterygoid	C49.0	C79.89	—	D21.0	D48.1	D49.2
pyriform	C12	C79.89	D00.08	D10.7	D37.05	D49.0
Rosenmuller	C11.2	C79.89	D00.08	D10.6	D37.05	D49.0
tonsillar	C09.0	C79.89	D00.08	D10.5	D37.05	D49.0
fourchette	C51.9	C79.82	D07.1	D28.0	D39.8	D49.59
frenulum						
labii — see Neoplasm, lip, internal						
linguae	C02.2	C79.89	D00.07	D10.1	D37.02	D49.0
frontal						
bone	C41.0	C79.51	—	D16.4	D48.0	D49.2
lobe, brain	C71.1	C79.31	—	D33.0	D43.0	D49.6
pole	C71.1	C79.31	—	D33.0	D43.0	D49.6
sinus	C31.2	C78.39	D02.3	D14.0	D38.5	D49.1
fundus						
stomach	C16.1	C78.89	D00.2	D13.1	D37.1	D49.0
uterus	C54.3	C79.82	D07.0	D26.1	D39.0	D49.59
gallbladder	C23	C78.89	D01.5	D13.5	D37.6	D49.0
overlapping lesion with extrahepatic bile ducts	C24.8	—	—	—	—	—
gall duct (extrahepatic)	C24.0	C78.89	D01.5	D13.5	D37.6	D49.0
intrahepatic	C22.1	C78.7	D01.5	D13.4	D37.6	D49.0
ganglia — see also Neoplasm, nerve, peripheral	C47.9	C79.89	—	D36.10	D48.2	D49.2
basal	C71.0	C79.31	—	D33.0	D43.0	D49.6
cranial nerve	C72.50	C79.49	—	D33.3	D43.3	D49.7
Gartner's duct	C52	C79.82	D07.2	D28.1	D39.8	D49.59
gastric — see Neoplasm, stomach						
gastrocolic	C26.9	C78.89	D01.9	D13.9	D37.9	D49.0
gastroesophageal junction	C16.0	C78.89	D00.2	D13.1	D37.1	D49.0
gastrointestinal (tract) NEC	C26.9	C78.89	D01.9	D13.9	D37.9	D49.0
generalized	C80.0	—				
genital organ or tract						
female NEC	C57.9	C79.82	D07.30	D28.9	D39.9	D49.59
overlapping lesion	C57.8	—	—	—	—	—
specified site NEC	C57.7	C79.82	D07.39	D28.7	D39.8	D49.59
male NEC	C63.9	C79.82	D07.60	D29.9	D40.9	D49.59
overlapping lesion	C63.8	—	—	—	—	—
specified site NEC	C63.7	C79.82	D07.69	D29.8	D40.8	D49.59
genitourinary tract						
female	C57.9	C79.82	D07.30	D28.9	D39.9	D49.59
male	C63.9	C79.82	D07.60	D29.9	D40.9	D49.59
gingiva (alveolar) (marginal)	C03.9	C79.89	D00.03	D10.39	D37.09	D49.0
lower	C03.1	C79.89	D00.03	D10.39	D37.09	D49.0
mandibular	C03.1	C79.89	D00.03	D10.39	D37.09	D49.0
maxillary	C03.0	C79.89	D00.03	D10.39	D37.09	D49.0
upper	C03.0	C79.89	D00.03	D10.39	D37.09	D49.0
gland, glandular (lymphatic) (system) — see also Neoplasm, lymph gland						
endocrine NEC	C75.9	C79.89	D09.3	D35.9	D44.9	D49.7

☑ Additional Character Required — Refer to the Tabular List for Character Selection   Ⓦ Subterms under main terms may continue to next column or page

Neoplasm, neoplastic — *continued*	Malignant Primary	Malignant Secondary	Ca in situ	Benign	Uncertain	Unspecified Behavior
gland, glandular — *see also* Neoplasm, lymph gland — *continued*						
salivary — *see* Neoplasm, salivary gland						
glans penis	C60.1	C79.82	D07.4	D29.0	D40.8	D49.59
globus pallidus	C71.0	C79.31	—	D33.0	D43.0	D49.6
glomus						
coccygeal	C49.5	C79.89	—	D21.5	D48.1	D49.2
jugularis	C75.5	C79.89	—	D35.6	D44.7	D49.7
glosso-epiglottic fold(s)	C10.1	C79.89	D00.08	D10.5	D37.05	D49.0
glossopalatine fold	C09.1	C79.89	D00.08	D10.5	D37.05	D49.0
glossopharyngeal sulcus	C09.0	C79.89	D00.08	D10.5	D37.05	D49.0
glottis	C32.0	C78.39	D02.0	D14.1	D38.0	D49.1
gluteal region	C76.3	C79.89	D04.5	D36.7	D48.7	D49.89
great vessels NEC	C49.3	C79.89	—	D21.3	D48.1	D49.2
groin NEC	C76.3	C79.89	D04.5	D36.7	D48.7	D49.89
gum	C03.9	C79.89	D00.03	D10.39	D37.09	D49.0
lower	C03.1	C79.89	D00.03	D10.39	D37.09	D49.0
upper	C03.0	C79.89	D00.03	D10.39	D37.09	D49.0
hand NEC	C76.4-☑	C79.89	D04.6-☑	D36.7	D48.7	D49.89
head NEC	C76.0	C79.89	D04.4	D36.7	D48.7	D49.89
heart	C38.0	C79.89	—	D15.1	D48.7	D49.89
heel NEC	C76.5-☑	C79.89	D04.7-☑	D36.7	D48.7	D49.89
helix — *see also* Neoplasm, skin, ear	C44.20-☑	C79.2	D04.2-☑	D23.2-☑	D48.5	D49.2
hematopoietic, hemopoietic tissue NEC	C96.9	—	—	—	—	—
specified NEC	C96.Z	—	—	—	—	—
hemisphere, cerebral	C71.0	C79.31	—	D33.0	D43.0	D49.6
hemorrhoidal zone	C21.1	C78.5	D01.3	D12.9	D37.8	D49.0
hepatic — *see also* Index to disease, by histology	C22.9	C78.7	D01.5	D13.4	D37.6	D49.0
duct (bile)	C24.0	C78.89	D01.5	D13.5	D37.6	D49.0
flexure (colon)	C18.3	C78.5	D01.0	D12.3	D37.4	D49.0
primary	C22.8	C78.7	D01.5	D13.4	D37.6	D49.0
hepatobiliary	C24.9	C78.89	D01.5	D13.5	D37.6	D49.0
hepatoblastoma	C22.2	C78.7	D01.5	D13.4	D37.6	D49.0
hepatoma	C22.0	C78.7	D01.5	D13.4	D37.6	D49.0
hilus of lung	C34.0-☑	C78.0-☑	D02.2-☑	D14.3-☑	D38.1	D49.1
hippocampus, brain	C71.2	C79.31	—	D33.0	D43.0	D49.6
hip NEC	C76.5-☑	C79.89	D04.7-☑	D36.7	D48.7	D49.89
humerus (any part)	C40.0-☑	C79.51	—	D16.0-☑	—	—
hymen	C52	C79.82	D07.2	D28.1	D39.8	D49.59
hypopharynx, hypopharyngeal NEC	C13.9	C79.89	D00.08	D10.7	D37.05	D49.0
overlapping lesion	C13.8	—	—	—	—	—
postcricoid region	C13.0	C79.89	D00.08	D10.7	D37.05	D49.0
posterior wall	C13.2	C79.89	D00.08	D10.7	D37.05	D49.0
pyriform fossa (sinus)	C12	C79.89	D00.08	D10.7	D37.05	D49.0
hypophysis	C75.1	C79.89	D09.3	D35.2	D44.3	D49.7
hypothalamus	C71.0	C79.31	—	D33.0	D43.0	D49.6
ileocecum, ileocecal (coil) (junction) (valve)	C18.0	C78.5	D01.0	D12.0	D37.4	D49.0
ileum	C17.2	C78.4	D01.49	D13.39	D37.2	D49.0
ilium	C41.4	C79.51	—	D16.8	D48.0	D49.2
immunoproliferative NEC	C88.9	—	—	—	—	—
infraclavicular (region)	C76.1	C79.89	D04.5	D36.7	D48.7	D49.89
inguinal (region)	C76.3	C79.89	D04.5	D36.7	D48.7	D49.89
insula	C71.0	C79.31	—	D33.0	D43.0	D49.6
insular tissue (pancreas)	C25.4	C78.89	D01.7	D13.7	D37.8	D49.0
brain	C71.0	C79.31	—	D33.0	D43.0	D49.6
interarytenoid fold	C13.1	C78.39	D00.08	D10.7	D37.05	D49.0
hypopharyngeal aspect	C13.1	C79.89	D00.08	D10.7	D37.05	D49.0
laryngeal aspect	C32.1	C78.39	D02.0	D14.1	D38.0	D49.1
marginal zone	C13.1	C79.89	D00.08	D10.7	D37.05	D49.0
interdental papillae	C03.9	C79.89	D00.03	D10.39	D37.09	D49.0

Neoplasm, neoplastic — *continued*	Malignant Primary	Malignant Secondary	Ca in situ	Benign	Uncertain	Unspecified Behavior
interdental papillae — *continued*						
lower	C03.1	C79.89	D00.03	D10.39	D37.09	D49.0
upper	C03.0	C79.89	D00.03	D10.39	D37.09	D49.0
internal						
capsule	C71.0	C79.31	—	D33.0	D43.0	D49.6
os (cervix)	C53.0	C79.82	D06.0	D26.0	D39.0	D49.59
intervertebral cartilage or disc	C41.2	C79.51	—	D16.6	D48.0	D49.2
intestine, intestinal	C26.0	C78.80	D01.40	D13.9	D37.8	D49.0
large	C18.9	C78.5	D01.0	D12.6	D37.4	D49.0
appendix	C18.1	C78.5	D01.0	D12.1	D37.3	D49.0
caput coli	C18.0	C78.5	D01.0	D12.0	D37.4	D49.0
cecum	C18.0	C78.5	D01.0	D12.0	D37.4	D49.0
colon	C18.9	C78.5	D01.0	D12.6	D37.4	D49.0
and rectum	C19	C78.5	D01.1	D12.7	D37.5	D49.0
ascending	C18.2	C78.5	D01.0	D12.2	D37.4	D49.0
caput	C18.0	C78.5	D01.0	D12.0	D37.4	D49.0
descending	C18.6	C78.5	D01.0	D12.4	D37.4	D49.0
distal	C18.6	C78.5	D01.0	D12.4	D37.4	D49.0
left	C18.6	C78.5	D01.0	D12.4	D37.4	D49.0
overlapping lesion	C18.8	—	—	—	—	—
pelvic	C18.7	C78.5	D01.0	D12.5	D37.4	D49.0
right	C18.2	C78.5	D01.0	D12.2	D37.4	D49.0
sigmoid (flexure)	C18.7	C78.5	D01.0	D12.5	D37.4	D49.0
transverse	C18.4	C78.5	D01.0	D12.3	D37.4	D49.0
hepatic flexure	C18.3	C78.5	D01.0	D12.3	D37.4	D49.0
ileocecum, ileocecal (coil) (valve)	C18.0	C78.5	D01.0	D12.0	D37.4	D49.0
overlapping lesion	C18.8	—	—	—	—	—
sigmoid flexure (lower) (upper)	C18.7	C78.5	D01.0	D12.5	D37.4	D49.0
splenic flexure	C18.5	C78.5	D01.0	D12.3	D37.4	D49.0
small	C17.9	C78.4	D01.40	D13.30	D37.2	D49.0
duodenum	C17.0	C78.4	D01.49	D13.2	D37.2	D49.0
ileum	C17.2	C78.4	D01.49	D13.39	D37.2	D49.0
jejunum	C17.1	C78.4	D01.49	D13.39	D37.2	D49.0
overlapping lesion	C17.8	—	—	—	—	—
tract NEC	C26.0	C78.89	D01.40	D13.9	D37.8	D49.0
intra-abdominal	C76.2	C79.89	D09.8	D36.7	D48.7	D49.89
intracranial NEC	C71.9	C79.31	—	D33.2	D43.2	D49.6
intrahepatic (bile) duct	C22.1	C78.7	D01.5	D13.4	D37.6	D49.0
intraocular	C69.9-☑	C79.49	D09.2-☑	D31.9-☑	D48.7	D49.89
intraorbital	C69.6-☑	C79.49	D09.2-☑	D31.6-☑	D48.7	D49.89
intrasellar	C75.1	C79.89	D09.3	D35.2	D44.3	D49.7
intrathoracic (cavity) (organs)	C76.1	C79.89	D09.8	D15.9	D48.7	D49.89
specified NEC	C76.1	C79.89	D09.8	D15.7	—	—
iris	C69.4-☑	C79.49	D09.2-☑	D31.4-☑	D48.7	D49.89
ischiorectal (fossa)	C76.3	C79.89	D09.8	D36.7	D48.7	D49.89
ischium	C41.4	C79.51	—	D16.8	D48.0	D49.2
island of Reil	C71.0	C79.31	—	D33.0	D43.0	D49.6
islands or islets of Langerhans	C25.4	C78.89	D01.7	D13.7	D37.8	D49.0
isthmus uteri	C54.0	C79.82	D07.0	D26.1	D39.0	D49.59
jaw	C76.0	C79.89	D09.8	D36.7	D48.7	D49.89
bone	C41.1	C79.51	—	D16.5	D48.0	D49.2
lower	C41.1	C79.51	—	D16.5	—	—
upper	C41.0	C79.51	—	D16.4	—	—
carcinoma (any type) (lower) (upper)	C76.0	C79.89	—	—	—	—
skin — *see also* Neoplasm, skin, face	C44.309	C79.2	D04.39	D23.39	D48.5	D49.2
soft tissues	C03.9	C79.89	D00.03	D10.39	D37.09	D49.0
lower	C03.1	C79.89	D00.03	D10.39	D37.09	D49.0
upper	C03.0	C79.89	D00.03	D10.39	D37.09	D49.0
jejunum	C17.1	C78.4	D01.49	D13.39	D37.2	D49.0
joint NEC — *see also* Neoplasm, bone	C41.9	C79.51	—	D16.9	D48.0	D49.2
acromioclavicular	C40.0-☑	C79.51	—	D16.0-☑	—	—

	Malignant Primary	Malignant Secondary	Ca in situ	Benign	Uncertain	Unspecified Behavior
Neoplasm, neoplastic — *continued*						
joint — *see also* Neoplasm, bone — *continued*						
bursa or synovial membrane — *see* Neoplasm, connective tissue						
costovertebral	C41.3	C79.51	—	D16.7	D48.0	D49.2
sternocostal	C41.3	C79.51	—	D16.7	D48.0	D49.2
temporomandibular	C41.1	C79.51	—	D16.5	D48.0	D49.2
junction						
anorectal	C21.8	C78.5	D01.3	D12.9	D37.8	D49.0
cardioesophageal	C16.0	C78.89	D00.2	D13.1	D37.1	D49.0
esophagogastric	C16.0	C78.89	D00.2	D13.1	D37.1	D49.0
gastroesophageal	C16.0	C78.89	D00.2	D13.1	D37.1	D49.0
hard and soft palate	C05.9	C79.89	D00.00	D10.39	D37.09	D49.0
ileocecal	C18.0	C78.5	D01.0	D12.0	D37.4	D49.0
pelvirectal	C19	C78.5	D01.1	D12.7	D37.5	D49.0
pelviureteric	C65.-☑	C79.0-☑	D09.19	D30.1-☑	D41.1-☑	D49.59
rectosigmoid	C19	C78.5	D01.1	D12.7	D37.5	D49.0
squamocolumnar, of cervix	C53.8	C79.82	D06.7	D26.0	D39.0	D49.59
Kaposi's sarcoma — *see* Kaposi's, sarcoma						
kidney (parenchymal)	C64.-☑	C79.0-☑	D09.19	D30.0-☑	D41.0-☑	D49.51-☑
calyx	C65.-☑	C79.0-☑	D09.19	D30.1-☑	D41.1-☑	D49.51-☑
hilus	C65.-☑	C79.0-☑	D09.19	D30.1-☑	D41.1-☑	D49.51-☑
pelvis	C65.-☑	C79.0-☑	D09.19	D30.1-☑	D41.1-☑	D49.51-☑
knee NEC	C76.5-☑	C79.89	D04.7-☑	D36.7	D48.7	D49.89
labia (skin)	C51.9	C79.82	D07.1	D28.0	D39.8	D49.59
majora	C51.0	C79.82	D07.1	D28.0	D39.8	D49.59
minora	C51.1	C79.82	D07.1	D28.0	D39.8	D49.59
labial — *see also* Neoplasm, lip	C00.9	C79.89	D00.01	D10.0	D37.01	D49.0
sulcus (lower) (upper)	C06.1	C79.89	D00.02	D10.39	D37.09	D49.0
labium (skin)	C51.9	C79.82	D07.1	D28.0	D39.8	D49.59
majus	C51.0	C79.82	D07.1	D28.0	D39.8	D49.59
minus	C51.1	C79.82	D07.1	D28.0	D39.8	D49.59
lacrimal						
canaliculi	C69.5-☑	C79.49	D09.2-☑	D31.5-☑	D48.7	D49.89
duct (nasal)	C69.5-☑	C79.49	D09.2-☑	D31.5-☑	D48.7	D49.89
gland	C69.5-☑	C79.49	D09.2-☑	D31.5-☑	D48.7	D49.89
punctum	C69.5-☑	C79.49	D09.2-☑	D31.5-☑	D48.7	D49.89
sac	C69.5-☑	C79.49	D09.2-☑	D31.5-☑	D48.7	D49.89
Langerhans, islands or islets	C25.4	C78.89	D01.7	D13.7	D37.8	D49.0
laryngopharynx	C13.9	C79.89	D00.08	D10.7	D37.05	D49.0
larynx, laryngeal NEC	C32.9	C78.39	D02.0	D14.1	D38.0	D49.1
aryepiglottic fold	C32.1	C78.39	D02.0	D14.1	D38.0	D49.1
cartilage (arytenoid) (cricoid) (cuneiform) (thyroid)	C32.3	C78.39	D02.0	D14.1	D38.0	D49.1
commissure (anterior) (posterior)	C32.0	C78.39	D02.0	D14.1	D38.0	D49.1
extrinsic NEC	C32.1	C78.39	D02.0	D14.1	D38.0	D49.1
meaning hypopharynx	C13.9	C79.89	D00.08	D10.7	D37.05	D49.0
interarytenoid fold	C32.1	C78.39	D02.0	D14.1	D38.0	D49.1
intrinsic	C32.0	C78.39	D02.0	D14.1	D38.0	D49.1
overlapping lesion	C32.8	—	—	—	—	—
ventricular band	C32.1	C78.39	D02.0	D14.1	D38.0	D49.1
leg NEC	C76.5-☑	C79.89	D04.7-☑	D36.7	D48.7	D49.89
lens, crystalline	C69.4-☑	C79.49	D09.2-☑	D31.4-☑	D48.7	D49.89
lid (lower) (upper)	C44.10-☑	C79.2	D04.1-☑	D23.1-☑	D48.5	D49.2
basal cell carcinoma	C44.11-☑	—	—	—	—	—
specified type NEC	C44.19-☑	—	—	—	—	—
squamous cell carcinoma	C44.12-☑	—	—	—	—	—

	Malignant Primary	Malignant Secondary	Ca in situ	Benign	Uncertain	Unspecified Behavior
Neoplasm, neoplastic — *continued*						
ligament — *see also* Neoplasm, connective tissue						
broad	C57.1-☑	C79.82	D07.39	D28.2	D39.8	D49.59
Mackenrodt's	C57.7	C79.82	D07.39	D28.7	D39.8	D49.59
non-uterine — *see* Neoplasm, connective tissue						
round	C57.2-☑	C79.82	—	D28.2	D39.8	D49.59
sacro-uterine	C57.3	C79.82	—	D28.2	D39.8	D49.59
uterine	C57.3	C79.82	—	D28.2	D39.8	D49.59
utero-ovarian	C57.7	C79.82	D07.39	D28.2	D39.8	D49.59
uterosacral	C57.3	C79.82	—	D28.2	D39.8	D49.59
limb	C76.8	C79.89	D04.8	D36.7	D48.7	D49.89
lower	C76.5-☑	C79.89	D04.7-☑	D36.7	D48.7	D49.89
upper	C76.4-☑	C79.89	D04.6-☑	D36.7	D48.7	D49.89
limbus of cornea	C69.1-☑	C79.49	D09.2-☑	D31.1-☑	D48.7	D49.89
lingual NEC — *see also* Neoplasm, tongue	C02.9	C79.89	D00.07	D10.1	D37.02	D49.0
lingula, lung	C34.1-☑	C78.0-☑	D02.2-☑	D14.3-☑	D38.1	D49.1
lip	C00.9	C79.89	D00.01	D10.0	D37.01	D49.0
buccal aspect — *see* Neoplasm, lip, internal						
commissure	C00.6	C79.89	D00.01	D10.0	D37.01	D49.0
external	C00.2	C79.89	D00.01	D10.0	D37.01	D49.0
lower	C00.1	C79.89	D00.01	D10.0	D37.01	D49.0
upper	C00.0	C79.89	D00.01	D10.0	D37.01	D49.0
frenulum — *see* Neoplasm, lip, internal						
inner aspect — *see* Neoplasm, lip, internal						
internal	C00.5	C79.89	D00.01	D10.0	D37.01	D49.0
lower	C00.4	C79.89	D00.01	D10.0	D37.01	D49.0
upper	C00.3	C79.89	D00.01	D10.0	D37.01	D49.0
lipstick area	C00.2	C79.89	D00.01	D10.0	D37.01	D49.0
lower	C00.1	C79.89	D00.01	D10.0	D37.01	D49.0
upper	C00.0	C79.89	D00.01	D10.0	D37.01	D49.0
lower	C00.1	C79.89	D00.01	D10.0	D37.01	D49.0
internal	C00.4	C79.89	D00.01	D10.0	D37.01	D49.0
mucosa — *see* Neoplasm, lip, internal						
oral aspect — *see* Neoplasm, lip, internal						
overlapping lesion with oral cavity or pharynx	C00.8	—	—	—	—	—
	C14.8	—	—	—	—	—
skin (commissure) (lower) (upper)	C44.00	C79.2	D04.0	D23.0	D48.5	D49.2
basal cell carcinoma	C44.01	—	—	—	—	—
specified type NEC	C44.09	—	—	—	—	—
squamous cell carcinoma	C44.02	—	—	—	—	—
upper	C00.0	C79.89	D00.01	D10.0	D37.01	D49.0
internal	C00.3	C79.89	D00.01	D10.0	D37.01	D49.0
vermilion border	C00.2	C79.89	D00.01	D10.0	D37.01	D49.0
lower	C00.1	C79.89	D00.01	D10.0	D37.01	D49.0
upper	C00.0	C79.89	D00.01	D10.0	D37.01	D49.0
lipomatous — *see* Lipoma, by site						
liver — *see also* Index to disease, by histology	C22.9	C78.7	D01.5	D13.4	D37.6	D49.0
primary	C22.8	C78.7	D01.5	D13.4	D37.6	D49.0
lumbosacral plexus	C47.5	C79.89	—	D36.16	D48.2	D49.2
lung	C34.9-☑	C78.0-☑	D02.2-☑	D14.3-☑	D38.1	D49.1
azygos lobe	C34.1-☑	C78.0-☑	D02.2-☑	D14.3-☑	D38.1	D49.1
carina	C34.0-☑	C78.0-☑	D02.2-☑	D14.3-☑	D38.1	D49.1
hilus	C34.0-☑	C78.0-☑	D02.2-☑	D14.3-☑	D38.1	D49.1
lingula	C34.1-☑	C78.0-☑	D02.2-☑	D14.3-☑	D38.1	D49.1
lobe NEC	C34.9-☑	C78.0-☑	D02.2-☑	D14.3-☑	D38.1	D49.1
lower lobe	C34.3-☑	C78.0-☑	D02.2-☑	D14.3-☑	D38.1	D49.1

☑ Additional Character Required — Refer to the Tabular List for Character Selection   Subterms under main terms may continue to next column or page

Neoplasm, neoplastic — continued	Malignant Primary	Malignant Secondary	Ca in situ	Benign	Uncertain	Unspecified Behavior
lung — continued						
main bronchus	C34.0-☑	C78.0-☑	D02.2-☑	D14.3-☑	D38.1	D49.1
mesothelioma — see Mesothelioma						
middle lobe	C34.2	C78.0-☑	D02.21	D14.31	D38.1	D49.1
overlapping lesion	C34.8-☑					
upper lobe	C34.1-☑	C78.0-☑	D02.2-☑	D14.3-☑	D38.1	D49.1
lymph, lymphatic channel						
NEC	C49.9	C79.89	—	D21.9	D48.1	D49.2
gland (secondary)	—	C77.9	—	D36.0	D48.7	D49.89
abdominal	—	C77.2	—	D36.0	D48.7	D49.89
aortic	—	C77.2	—	D36.0	D48.7	D49.89
arm	—	C77.3	—	D36.0	D48.7	D49.89
auricular (anterior) (posterior)	—	C77.0	—	D36.0	D48.7	D49.89
axilla, axillary	—	C77.3	—	D36.0	D48.7	D49.89
brachial	—	C77.3	—	D36.0	D48.7	D49.89
bronchial	—	C77.1	—	D36.0	D48.7	D49.89
bronchopulmonary	—	C77.1	—	D36.0	D48.7	D49.89
celiac	—	C77.2	—	D36.0	D48.7	D49.89
cervical	—	C77.0	—	D36.0	D48.7	D49.89
cervicofacial	—	C77.0	—	D36.0	D48.7	D49.89
Cloquet	—	C77.4	—	D36.0	D48.7	D49.89
colic	—	C77.2	—	D36.0	D48.7	D49.89
common duct	—	C77.2	—	D36.0	D48.7	D49.89
cubital	—	C77.3	—	D36.0	D48.7	D49.89
diaphragmatic	—	C77.1	—	D36.0	D48.7	D49.89
epigastric, inferior	—	C77.1	—	D36.0	D48.7	D49.89
epitrochlear	—	C77.3	—	D36.0	D48.7	D49.89
esophageal	—	C77.1	—	D36.0	D48.7	D49.89
face	—	C77.0	—	D36.0	D48.7	D49.89
femoral	—	C77.4	—	D36.0	D48.7	D49.89
gastric	—	C77.2	—	D36.0	D48.7	D49.89
groin	—	C77.4	—	D36.0	D48.7	D49.89
head	—	C77.0	—	D36.0	D48.7	D49.89
hepatic	—	C77.2	—	D36.0	D48.7	D49.89
hilar (pulmonary)	—	C77.1	—	D36.0	D48.7	D49.89
splenic	—	C77.2	—	D36.0	D48.7	D49.89
hypogastric	—	C77.5	—	D36.0	D48.7	D49.89
ileocolic	—	C77.2	—	D36.0	D48.7	D49.89
iliac	—	C77.5	—	D36.0	D48.7	D49.89
infraclavicular	—	C77.3	—	D36.0	D48.7	D49.89
inguina, inguinal	—	C77.4	—	D36.0	D48.7	D49.89
innominate	—	C77.1	—	D36.0	D48.7	D49.89
intercostal	—	C77.1	—	D36.0	D48.7	D49.89
intestinal	—	C77.2	—	D36.0	D48.7	D49.89
intrabdominal	—	C77.2	—	D36.0	D48.7	D49.89
intrapelvic	—	C77.5	—	D36.0	D48.7	D49.89
intrathoracic	—	C77.1	—	D36.0	D48.7	D49.89
jugular	—	C77.0	—	D36.0	D48.7	D49.89
leg	—	C77.4	—	D36.0	D48.7	D49.89
limb lower	—	C77.4	—	D36.0	D48.7	D49.89
upper	—	C77.3	—	D36.0	D48.7	D49.89
lower limb	—	C77.4	—	D36.0	D48.7	D49.89
lumbar	—	C77.2	—	D36.0	D48.7	D49.89
mandibular	—	C77.0	—	D36.0	D48.7	D49.89
mediastinal	—	C77.1	—	D36.0	D48.7	D49.89
mesenteric (inferior) (superior)	—	C77.2	—	D36.0	D48.7	D49.89
midcolic	—	C77.2	—	D36.0	D48.7	D49.89
multiple sites in categories C77.0-C77.5	—	C77.8	—	D36.0	D48.7	D49.89
neck	—	C77.0	—	D36.0	D48.7	D49.89
obturator	—	C77.5	—	D36.0	D48.7	D49.89
occipital	—	C77.0	—	D36.0	D48.7	D49.89
pancreatic	—	C77.2	—	D36.0	D48.7	D49.89
para-aortic	—	C77.2	—	D36.0	D48.7	D49.89
paracervical	—	C77.5	—	D36.0	D48.7	D49.89
parametrial	—	C77.5	—	D36.0	D48.7	D49.89
parasternal	—	C77.1	—	D36.0	D48.7	D49.89
parotid	—	C77.0	—	D36.0	D48.7	D49.89
pectoral	—	C77.3	—	D36.0	D48.7	D49.89
pelvic	—	C77.5	—	D36.0	D48.7	D49.89
peri-aortic	—	C77.2	—	D36.0	D48.7	D49.89
peripancreatic	—	C77.2	—	D36.0	D48.7	D49.89
popliteal	—	C77.4	—	D36.0	D48.7	D49.89
porta hepatis	—	C77.2	—	D36.0	D48.7	D49.89

Neoplasm, neoplastic — continued	Malignant Primary	Malignant Secondary	Ca in situ	Benign	Uncertain	Unspecified Behavior
lymph, lymphatic channel — continued						
gland — continued						
portal	—	C77.2	—	D36.0	D48.7	D49.89
preauricular	—	C77.0	—	D36.0	D48.7	D49.89
prelaryngeal	—	C77.0	—	D36.0	D48.7	D49.89
presymphysial	—	C77.5	—	D36.0	D48.7	D49.89
pretracheal	—	C77.0	—	D36.0	D48.7	D49.89
primary (any site) NEC	C96.9	—	—	—	—	—
pulmonary (hiler)	—	C77.1	—	D36.0	D48.7	D49.89
pyloric	—	C77.2	—	D36.0	D48.7	D49.89
retroperitoneal	—	C77.2	—	D36.0	D48.7	D49.89
retropharyngeal	—	C77.0	—	D36.0	D48.7	D49.89
Rosenmuller's	—	C77.4	—	D36.0	D48.7	D49.89
sacral	—	C77.5	—	D36.0	D48.7	D49.89
scalene	—	C77.0	—	D36.0	D48.7	D49.89
site NEC	—	C77.9	—	D36.0	D48.7	D49.89
splenic (hilar)	—	C77.2	—	D36.0	D48.7	D49.89
subclavicular	—	C77.3	—	D36.0	D48.7	D49.89
subinguinal	—	C77.4	—	D36.0	D48.7	D49.89
sublingual	—	C77.0	—	D36.0	D48.7	D49.89
submandibular	—	C77.0	—	D36.0	D48.7	D49.89
submaxillary	—	C77.0	—	D36.0	D48.7	D49.89
submental	—	C77.0	—	D36.0	D48.7	D49.89
subscapular	—	C77.3	—	D36.0	D48.7	D49.89
supraclavicular	—	C77.0	—	D36.0	D48.7	D49.89
thoracic	—	C77.1	—	D36.0	D48.7	D49.89
tibial	—	C77.4	—	D36.0	D48.7	D49.89
tracheal	—	C77.1	—	D36.0	D48.7	D49.89
tracheobronchial	—	C77.1	—	D36.0	D48.7	D49.89
upper limb	—	C77.3	—	D36.0	D48.7	D49.89
Virchow's	—	C77.0	—	D36.0	D48.7	D49.89
node — see also Neoplasm, lymph gland						
primary NEC	C96.9	—	—	—	—	—
vessel — see also Neoplasm, connective tissue	C49.9	C79.89	—	D21.9	D48.1	D49.2
Mackenrodt's ligament	C57.7	C79.82	D07.39	D28.7	D39.8	D49.59
malar	C41.0	C79.51	—	D16.4	D48.0	D49.2
region — see Neoplasm, cheek						
mammary gland — see Neoplasm, breast						
mandible	C41.1	C79.51	—	D16.5	D48.0	D49.2
alveolar mucosa (carcinoma)	C03.1	C79.89	D00.03	D10.39	D37.09	D49.0
ridge or process	C41.1	C79.51	—	D16.5	D48.0	D49.2
marrow (bone) NEC	C96.9	C79.52	—	—	D47.9	D49.89
mastectomy site (skin) — see also Neoplasm, breast, skin	C44.501	C79.2	—	—	—	—
specified as breast tissue	C50.8-☑	C79.81				
mastoid (air cells) (antrum) (cavity)	C30.1	C78.39	D02.3	D14.0	D38.5	D49.1
bone or process	C41.0	C79.51	—	D16.4	D48.0	D49.2
maxilla, maxillary (superior)	C41.0	C79.51	—	D16.4	D48.0	D49.2
alveolar mucosa	C03.0	C79.89	D00.03	D10.39	D37.09	D49.0
ridge or process (carcinoma)	C41.0	C79.51	—	D16.4	D48.0	D49.2
antrum	C31.0	C78.39	D02.3	D14.0	D38.5	D49.1
carcinoma	C03.0	C79.51	—	—	—	—
inferior — see Neoplasm, mandible						
sinus	C31.0	C78.39	D02.3	D14.0	D38.5	D49.1
meatus external (ear) — see also Neoplasm, skin, ear	C44.20-☑	C79.2	D04.2-☑	D23.2-☑	D48.5	D49.2
Meckel diverticulum, malignant	C17.3	C78.4	D01.49	D13.39	D37.2	D49.0
mediastinum, mediastinal	C38.3	C78.1	—	D15.2	D38.3	D49.89

Neoplasm, neoplastic — continued	Malignant Primary	Malignant Secondary	Ca in situ	Benign	Uncertain	Unspecified Behavior
mediastinum, mediastinal — continued						
anterior	C38.1	C78.1	—	D15.2	D38.3	D49.89
posterior	C38.2	C78.1	—	D15.2	D38.3	D49.89
medulla						
adrenal	C74.1-✓	C79.7-✓	D09.3	D35.0-✓	D44.1-✓	D49.7
oblongata	C71.7	C79.31	—	D33.1	D43.1	D49.6
meibomian gland	C44.10-✓	C79.2	D04.1-✓	D23.1-✓	D48.5	D49.2
basal cell carcinoma	C44.11-✓	—	—	—	—	—
specified type NEC	C44.19-✓	—	—	—	—	—
squamous cell carcinoma	C44.12-✓	—	—	—	—	—
melanoma — see Melanoma						
meninges	C70.9	C79.49	—	D32.9	D42.9	D49.7
brain	C70.0	C79.32	—	D32.0	D42.0	D49.7
cerebral	C70.0	C79.32	—	D32.0	D42.0	D49.7
cranial	C70.0	C79.32	—	D32.0	D42.0	D49.7
intracranial	C70.0	C79.32	—	D32.0	D42.0	D49.7
spinal (cord)	C70.1	C79.49	—	D32.1	D42.1	D49.7
meniscus, knee joint (lateral) (medial)	C40.2-✓	C79.51	—	D16.2-✓	D48.0	D49.2
Merkel cell — see Carcinoma, Merkel cell						
mesentery, mesenteric	C48.1	C78.6	—	D20.1	D48.4	D49.0
mesoappendix	C48.1	C78.6	—	D20.1	D48.4	D49.0
mesocolon	C48.1	C78.6	—	D20.1	D48.4	D49.0
mesopharynx — see Neoplasm, oropharynx						
mesosalpinx	C57.1-✓	C79.82	D07.39	D28.2	D39.8	D49.59
mesothelial tissue — see Mesothelioma						
mesothelioma — see Mesothelioma						
mesovarium	C57.1-✓	C79.82	D07.39	D28.2	D39.8	D49.59
metacarpus (any bone)	C40.1-✓	C79.51	—	D16.1-✓	—	—
metastatic NEC — see also Neoplasm, by site, secondary	—	C79.9	—	—	—	—
metatarsus (any bone)	C40.3-✓	C79.51	—	D16.3-✓	—	—
midbrain	C71.7	C79.31	—	D33.1	D43.1	D49.6
milk duct — see Neoplasm, breast						
mons						
pubis	C51.9	C79.82	D07.1	D28.0	D39.8	D49.59
veneris	C51.9	C79.82	D07.1	D28.0	D39.8	D49.59
motor tract	C72.9	C79.49	—	D33.9	D43.9	D49.7
brain	C71.9	C79.31	—	D33.2	D43.2	D49.6
cauda equina	C72.1	C79.49	—	D33.4	D43.4	D49.7
spinal	C72.0	C79.49	—	D33.4	D43.4	D49.7
mouth	C06.9	C79.89	D00.00	D10.30	D37.09	D49.0
book-leaf	C06.89	C79.89	—	—	—	—
floor	C04.9	C79.89	D00.06	D10.2	D37.09	D49.0
anterior portion	C04.0	C79.89	D00.06	D10.2	D37.09	D49.0
lateral portion	C04.1	C79.89	D00.06	D10.2	D37.09	D49.0
overlapping lesion	C04.8	—	—	—	—	—
overlapping NEC	C06.80	—	—	—	—	—
roof	C05.9	C79.89	D00.00	D10.39	D37.09	D49.0
specified part NEC	C06.89	C79.89	D00.00	D10.39	D37.09	D49.0
vestibule	C06.1	C79.89	D00.00	D10.39	D37.09	D49.0
mucosa						
alveolar (ridge or process)	C03.9	C79.89	D00.03	D10.39	D37.09	D49.0
lower	C03.1	C79.89	D00.03	D10.39	D37.09	D49.0
upper	C03.0	C79.89	D00.03	D10.39	D37.09	D49.0
buccal	C06.0	C79.89	D00.02	D10.39	D37.09	D49.0
cheek	C06.0	C79.89	D00.02	D10.39	D37.09	D49.0
lip — see Neoplasm, lip, internal						
nasal	C30.0	C78.39	D02.3	D14.0	D38.5	D49.1
oral	C06.0	C79.89	D00.02	D10.39	D37.09	D49.0
Mullerian duct						
female	C57.7	C79.82	D07.39	D28.7	D39.8	D49.59
male	C63.7	C79.82	D07.69	D29.8	D40.8	D49.59

Neoplasm, neoplastic — continued	Malignant Primary	Malignant Secondary	Ca in situ	Benign	Uncertain	Unspecified Behavior
muscle — see also Neoplasm, connective tissue						
extraocular	C69.6-✓	C79.49	D09.2-✓	D31.6-✓	D48.7	D49.89
myocardium	C38.0	C79.89	—	D15.1	D48.7	D49.89
myometrium	C54.2	C79.82	D07.0	D26.1	D39.0	D49.59
myopericardium	C38.0	C79.89	—	D15.1	D48.7	D49.89
nabothian gland (follicle)	C53.0	C79.82	D06.0	D26.0	D39.0	D49.59
nail — see also Neoplasm, skin, limb	C44.90	C79.2	D04.9	D23.9	D48.5	D49.2
finger — see also Neoplasm, skin, limb, upper	C44.60-✓	C79.2	D04.6-✓	D23.6-✓	D48.5	D49.2
toe — see also Neoplasm, skin, limb, lower	C44.70-✓	C79.2	D04.7-✓	D23.7-✓	D48.5	D49.2
nares, naris (anterior) (posterior)	C30.0	C78.39	D02.3	D14.0	D38.5	D49.1
nasal — see Neoplasm, nose						
nasolabial groove — see also Neoplasm, skin, face	C44.309	C79.2	D04.39	D23.39	D48.5	D49.2
nasolacrimal duct	C69.5-✓	C79.49	D09.2-✓	D31.5-✓	D48.7	D49.89
nasopharynx, nasopharyngeal	C11.9	C79.89	D00.08	D10.6	D37.05	D49.0
floor	C11.3	C79.89	D00.08	D10.6	D37.05	D49.0
overlapping lesion	C11.8	—	—	—	—	—
roof	C11.0	C79.89	D00.08	D10.6	D37.05	D49.0
wall	C11.9	C79.89	D00.08	D10.6	D37.05	D49.0
anterior	C11.3	C79.89	D00.08	D10.6	D37.05	D49.0
lateral	C11.2	C79.89	D00.08	D10.6	D37.05	D49.0
posterior	C11.1	C79.89	D00.08	D10.6	D37.05	D49.0
superior	C11.0	C79.89	D00.08	D10.6	D37.05	D49.0
nates — see also Neoplasm, skin, trunk	C44.509	C79.2	D04.5	D23.5	D48.5	D49.2
neck NEC	C76.0	C79.89	D09.8	D36.7	D48.7	D49.89
skin	C44.40	—	—	—	—	—
basal cell carcinoma	C44.41	—	—	—	—	—
specified type NEC	C44.49	—	—	—	—	—
squamous cell carcinoma	C44.42	—	—	—	—	—
nerve (ganglion)	C47.9	C79.89	—	D36.10	D48.2	D49.2
abducens	C72.59	C79.49	—	D33.3	D43.3	D49.7
accessory (spinal)	C72.59	C79.49	—	D33.3	D43.3	D49.7
acoustic	C72.4-✓	C79.49	—	D33.3	D43.3	D49.7
auditory	C72.4-✓	C79.49	—	D33.3	D43.3	D49.7
autonomic NEC — see also Neoplasm, nerve, peripheral	C47.9	C79.89	—	D36.10	D48.2	D49.2
brachial	C47.1-✓	C79.89	—	D36.12	D48.2	D49.2
cranial	C72.50	C79.49	—	D33.3	D43.3	D49.7
specified NEC	C72.59	C79.49	—	D33.3	D43.3	D49.7
facial	C72.59	C79.49	—	D33.3	D43.3	D49.7
femoral	C47.2-✓	C79.89	—	D36.13	D48.2	D49.2
ganglion NEC — see also Neoplasm, nerve, peripheral	C47.9	C79.89	—	D36.10	D48.2	D49.2
glossopharyngeal	C72.59	C79.49	—	D33.3	D43.3	D49.7
hypoglossal	C72.59	C79.49	—	D33.3	D43.3	D49.7
intercostal	C47.3	C79.89	—	D36.14	D48.2	D49.2
lumbar	C47.6	C79.89	—	D36.17	D48.2	D49.2
median	C47.1-✓	C79.89	—	D36.12	D48.2	D49.2
obturator	C47.2-✓	C79.89	—	D36.13	D48.2	D49.2
oculomotor	C72.59	C79.49	—	D33.3	D43.3	D49.7
olfactory	C47.2-✓	C79.49	—	D33.3	D43.3	D49.7
optic	C72.3-✓	C79.49	—	D33.3	D43.3	D49.7
parasympathetic NEC	C47.9	C79.89	—	D36.10	D48.2	D49.2
peripheral NEC	C47.9	C79.89	—	D36.10	D48.2	D49.2
abdomen	C47.4	C79.89	—	D36.15	D48.2	D49.2
abdominal wall	C47.4	C79.89	—	D36.15	D48.2	D49.2
ankle	C47.2-✓	C79.89	—	D36.13	D48.2	D49.2
antecubital fossa or space	C47.1-✓	C79.89	—	D36.12	D48.2	D49.2

✓ Additional Character Required — Refer to the Tabular List for Character Selection

▽ Subterms under main terms may continue to next column or page

	Malignant Primary	Malignant Secondary	Ca in situ	Benign	Uncertain	Unspecified Behavior
Neoplasm, neoplastic —						
continued						
nerve — *continued*						
peripheral — *continued*						
arm	C47.1-☑	C79.89	—	D36.12	D48.2	D49.2
auricle (ear)	C47.0	C79.89	—	D36.11	D48.2	D49.2
axilla	C47.3	C79.89	—	D36.12	D48.2	D49.2
back	C47.6	C79.89	—	D36.17	D48.2	D49.2
buttock	C47.5	C79.89	—	D36.16	D48.2	D49.2
calf	C47.2-☑	C79.89	—	D36.13	D48.2	D49.2
cervical region	C47.0	C79.89	—	D36.11	D48.2	D49.2
cheek	C47.0	C79.89	—	D36.11	D48.2	D49.2
chest (wall)	C47.3	C79.89	—	D36.14	D48.2	D49.2
chin	C47.0	C79.89	—	D36.11	D48.2	D49.2
ear (external)	C47.0	C79.89	—	D36.11	D48.2	D49.2
elbow	C47.1-☑	C79.89	—	D36.12	D48.2	D49.2
extrarectal	C47.5	C79.89	—	D36.16	D48.2	D49.2
extremity	C47.9	C79.89	—	D36.10	D48.2	D49.2
lower	C47.2-☑	C79.89	—	D36.13	D48.2	D49.2
upper	C47.1-☑	C79.89	—	D36.12	D48.2	D49.2
eyelid	C47.0	C79.89	—	D36.11	D48.2	D49.2
face	C47.0	C79.89	—	D36.11	D48.2	D49.2
finger	C47.1-☑	C79.89	—	D36.12	D48.2	D49.2
flank	C47.6	C79.89	—	D36.17	D48.2	D49.2
foot	C47.2-☑	C79.89	—	D36.13	D48.2	D49.2
forearm	C47.1-☑	C79.89	—	D36.12	D48.2	D49.2
forehead	C47.0	C79.89	—	D36.11	D48.2	D49.2
gluteal region	C47.5	C79.89	—	D36.16	D48.2	D49.2
groin	C47.5	C79.89	—	D36.16	D48.2	D49.2
hand	C47.1-☑	C79.89	—	D36.12	D48.2	D49.2
head	C47.0	C79.89	—	D36.11	D48.2	D49.2
heel	C47.2-☑	C79.89	—	D36.13	D48.2	D49.2
hip	C47.2-☑	C79.89	—	D36.13	D48.2	D49.2
infraclavicular region	C47.3	C79.89	—	D36.14	D48.2	D49.2
inguinal (canal) (region)	C47.5	C79.89	—	D36.16	D48.2	D49.2
intrathoracic	C47.3	C79.89	—	D36.14	D48.2	D49.2
ischiorectal fossa	C47.5	C79.89	—	D36.16	D48.2	D49.2
knee	C47.2-☑	C79.89	—	D36.13	D48.2	D49.2
leg	C47.2-☑	C79.89	—	D36.13	D48.2	D49.2
limb NEC	C47.9	C79.89	—	D36.10	D48.2	D49.2
lower	C47.2-☑	C79.89	—	D36.13	D48.2	D49.2
upper	C47.1-☑	C79.89	—	D36.12	D48.2	D49.2
nates	C47.5	C79.89	—	D36.16	D48.2	D49.2
neck	C47.0	C79.89	—	D36.11	D48.2	D49.2
orbit	C69.6-☑	C79.49	—	D31.6-☑	D48.7	D49.2
pararectal	C47.5	C79.89	—	D36.16	D48.2	D49.2
paraurethral	C47.5	C79.89	—	D36.16	D48.2	D49.2
paravaginal	C47.5	C79.89	—	D36.16	D48.2	D49.2
pelvis (floor)	C47.5	C79.89	—	D36.16	D48.2	D49.2
pelvoabdominal	C47.8	C79.89	—	D36.17	D48.2	D49.2
perineum	C47.5	C79.89	—	D36.16	D48.2	D49.2
perirectal (tissue)	C47.5	C79.89	—	D36.16	D48.2	D49.2
periurethral (tissue)	C47.5	C79.89	—	D36.16	D48.2	D49.2
popliteal fossa or space	C47.2-☑	C79.89	—	D36.13	D48.2	D49.2
presacral	C47.5	C79.89	—	D36.16	D48.2	D49.2
pterygoid fossa	C47.0	C79.89	—	D36.11	D48.2	D49.2
rectovaginal septum or wall	C47.5	C79.89	—	D36.16	D48.2	D49.2
rectovesical	C47.5	C79.89	—	D36.16	D48.2	D49.2
sacrococcygeal region	C47.5	C79.89	—	D36.16	D48.2	D49.2
scalp	C47.0	C79.89	—	D36.11	D48.2	D49.2
scapular region	C47.3	C79.89	—	D36.14	D48.2	D49.2
shoulder	C47.1-☑	C79.89	—	D36.12	D48.2	D49.2
submental	C47.0	C79.89	—	D36.11	D48.2	D49.2
supraclavicular region	C47.0	C79.89	—	D36.11	D48.2	D49.2
temple	C47.0	C79.89	—	D36.11	D48.2	D49.2
temporal region	C47.0	C79.89	—	D36.11	D48.2	D49.2
thigh	C47.2-☑	C79.89	—	D36.13	D48.2	D49.2
thoracic (duct) (wall)	C47.3	C79.89	—	D36.14	D48.2	D49.2
thorax	C47.3	C79.89	—	D36.14	D48.2	D49.2
thumb	C47.1-☑	C79.89	—	D36.12	D48.2	D49.2
toe	C47.2-☑	C79.89	—	D36.13	D48.2	D49.2
trunk	C47.6	C79.89	—	D36.17	D48.2	D49.2

	Malignant Primary	Malignant Secondary	Ca in situ	Benign	Uncertain	Unspecified Behavior
Neoplasm, neoplastic —						
continued						
nerve — *continued*						
peripheral — *continued*						
umbilicus	C47.4	C79.89	—	D36.15	D48.2	D49.2
vesicorectal	C47.5	C79.89	—	D36.16	D48.2	D49.2
wrist	C47.1-☑	C79.89	—	D36.12	D48.2	D49.2
radial	C47.1-☑	C79.89	—	D36.12	D48.2	D49.2
sacral	C47.5	C79.89	—	D36.16	D48.2	D49.2
sciatic	C47.2-☑	C79.89	—	D36.13	D48.2	D49.2
spinal NEC	C47.9	C79.89	—	D36.10	D48.2	D49.2
accessory	C72.59	C79.49		D33.3	D43.3	D49.7
sympathetic NEC — *see also* Neoplasm, nerve, peripheral	C47.9	C79.89	—	D36.10	D48.2	D49.2
trigeminal	C72.59	C79.49		D33.3	D43.3	D49.7
trochlear	C72.59	C79.49		D33.3	D43.3	D49.7
ulnar	C47.1-☑	C79.89	—	D36.12	D48.2	D49.2
vagus	C72.59	C79.49		D33.3	D43.3	D49.7
nervous system (central)	C72.9	C79.40		D33.9	D43.9	D49.7
autonomic — *see* Neoplasm, nerve, peripheral						
parasympathetic — *see* Neoplasm, nerve, peripheral						
specified site NEC	—	C79.49		D33.7	D43.8	
sympathetic — *see* Neoplasm, nerve, peripheral						
nevus — *see* Nevus						
nipple	C50.0-☑	C79.81	D05.-☑	D24.-☑	—	—
nose, nasal	C76.0	C79.89	D09.8	D36.7	D48.7	D49.89
ala (external) (nasi) — *see also* Neoplasm, nose, skin	C44.301	C79.2	D04.39	D23.39	D48.5	D49.2
bone	C41.0	C79.51	—	D16.4	D48.0	D49.2
cartilage	C30.0	C78.39	D02.3	D14.0	D38.5	D49.1
cavity	C30.0	C78.39	D02.3	D14.0	D38.5	D49.1
choana	C11.3	C79.89	D00.08	D10.6	D37.05	D49.0
external (skin) — *see also* Neoplasm, nose, skin	C44.301	C79.2	D04.39	D23.39	D48.5	D49.2
fossa	C30.0	C78.39	D02.3	D14.0	D38.5	D49.1
internal	C30.0	C78.39	D02.3	D14.0	D38.5	D49.1
mucosa	C30.0	C78.39	D02.3	D14.0	D38.5	D49.1
septum	C30.0	C78.39	D02.3	D14.0	D38.5	D49.1
posterior margin	C11.3	C79.89	D00.08	D10.6	D37.05	D49.0
sinus — *see* Neoplasm, sinus						
skin	C44.301	C79.2	D04.39	D23.39	D48.5	D49.2
basal cell carcinoma	C44.311	—	—	—	—	—
specified type NEC	C44.391	—	—	—	—	—
squamous cell carcinoma	C44.321	—	—	—	—	—
turbinate (mucosa)	C30.0	C78.39	D02.3	D14.0	D38.5	D49.1
bone	C41.0	C79.51	—	D16.4	D48.0	D49.2
vestibule	C30.0	C78.39	D02.3	D14.0	D38.5	D49.1
nostril	C30.0	C78.39	D02.3	D14.0	D38.5	D49.1
nucleus pulposus	C41.2	C79.51	—	D16.6	D48.0	D49.2
occipital						
bone	C41.0	C79.51	—	D16.4	D48.0	D49.2
lobe or pole, brain	C71.4	C79.31	—	D33.0	D43.0	D49.6
odontogenic — *see* Neoplasm, jaw bone						
olfactory nerve or bulb	C72.2-☑	C79.49	—	D33.3	D43.3	D49.7
olive (brain)	C71.7	C79.31	—	D33.1	D43.1	D49.6
omentum	C48.1	C78.6	—	D20.1	D48.4	D49.0
operculum (brain)	C71.0	C79.31	—	D33.0	D43.0	D49.6
optic nerve, chiasm, or tract	C72.3-☑	C79.49	—	D33.3	D43.3	D49.7
oral (cavity)	C06.9	C79.89	D00.00	D10.30	D37.09	D49.0
ill-defined	C14.8	C79.89	D00.00	D10.30	D37.09	D49.0
mucosa	C06.0	C79.89	D00.02	D10.39	D37.09	D49.0
orbit	C69.6-☑	C79.49	D09.2-☑	D31.6-☑	D48.7	D49.89
autonomic nerve	C69.6-☑	C79.49		D31.6-☑	D48.7	D49.2
bone	C41.0	C79.51	—	D16.4	D48.0	D49.2

Neoplasm, neoplastic — continued

orbit — continued

	Malignant Primary	Malignant Secondary	Ca in situ	Benign	Uncertain	Unspecified Behavior
eye	C69.6-✓	C79.49	D09.2-✓	D31.6-✓	D48.7	D49.89
peripheral nerves	C69.6-✓	C79.49	—	D31.6-✓	D48.7	D49.2
soft parts	C69.6-✓	C79.49	D09.2-✓	D31.6-✓	D48.7	D49.89
organ of Zuckerkandl	C75.5	C79.89	—	D35.6	D44.7	D49.7
oropharynx	C10.9	C79.89	D00.08	D10.5	D37.05	D49.0
branchial cleft (vestige)	C10.4	C79.89	D00.08	D10.5	D37.05	D49.0
junctional region	C10.8	C79.89	D00.08	D10.5	D37.05	D49.0
lateral wall	C10.2	C79.89	D00.08	D10.5	D37.05	D49.0
overlapping lesion	C10.8	—	—	—	—	—
pillars or fauces	C09.1	C79.89	D00.08	D10.5	D37.05	D49.0
posterior wall	C10.3	C79.89	D00.08	D10.5	D37.05	D49.0
vallecula	C10.0	C79.89	D00.08	D10.5	D37.05	D49.0
os						
external	C53.1	C79.82	D06.1	D26.0	D39.0	D49.59
internal	C53.0	C79.82	D06.0	D26.0	D39.0	D49.59
ovary	C56.-✓	C79.6-✓	D07.39	D27.-✓	D39.1-✓	D49.59
oviduct	C57.0-✓	C79.82	D07.39	D28.2	D39.8	D49.59
palate	C05.9	C79.89	D00.00	D10.39	D37.09	D49.0
hard	C05.0	C79.89	D00.05	D10.39	D37.09	D49.0
junction of hard and soft palate	C05.9	C79.89	D00.00	D10.39	D37.09	D49.0
overlapping lesions	C05.8	—	—	—	—	—
soft	C05.1	C79.89	D00.04	D10.39	D37.09	D49.0
nasopharyngeal surface	C11.3	C79.89	D00.08	D10.6	D37.05	D49.0
posterior surface	C11.3	C79.89	D00.08	D10.6	D37.05	D49.0
superior surface	C11.3	C79.89	D00.08	D10.6	D37.05	D49.0
palatoglossal arch	C09.1	C79.89	D00.00	D10.5	D37.09	D49.0
palatopharyngeal arch	C09.1	C79.89	D00.00	D10.5	D37.09	D49.0
pallium	C71.0	C79.31	—	D33.0	D43.0	D49.6
palpebra	C44.10-✓	C79.2	D04.1-✓	D23.1-✓	D48.5	D49.2
basal cell carcinoma	C44.11-✓	—	—	—	—	—
specified type NEC	C44.19-✓	—	—	—	—	—
squamous cell carcinoma	C44.12-✓	—	—	—	—	—
pancreas	C25.9	C78.89	D01.7	D13.6	D37.8	D49.0
body	C25.1	C78.89	D01.7	D13.6	D37.8	D49.0
duct (of Santorini) (of Wirsung)	C25.3	C78.89	D01.7	D13.6	D37.8	D49.0
ectopic tissue	C25.7	C78.89	—	D13.6	D37.8	D49.0
head	C25.0	C78.89	D01.7	D13.6	D37.8	D49.0
islet cells	C25.4	C78.89	D01.7	D13.7	D37.8	D49.0
neck	C25.7	C78.89	D01.7	D13.6	D37.8	D49.0
overlapping lesion	C25.8	—	—	—	—	—
tail	C25.2	C78.89	D01.7	D13.6	D37.8	D49.0
para-aortic body	C75.5	C79.89	—	D35.6	D44.7	D49.7
paraganglion NEC	C75.5	C79.89	—	D35.6	D44.7	D49.7
parametrium	C57.3	C79.82	—	D28.2	D39.8	D49.59
paranephric	C48.0	C78.6	—	D20.0	D48.3	D49.0
pararectal	C76.3	C79.89	—	D36.7	D48.7	D49.89
parasagittal (region)	C76.0	C79.89	D09.8	D36.7	D48.7	D49.89
parasellar	C72.9	C79.49	—	D33.9	D43.8	D49.7
parathyroid (gland)	C75.0	C79.89	D09.3	D35.1	D44.2	D49.7
paraurethral	C76.3	C79.89	—	D36.7	D48.7	D49.89
gland	C68.1	C79.19	D09.19	D30.8	D41.8	D49.59
paravaginal	C76.3	C79.89	—	D36.7	D48.7	D49.89
parenchyma, kidney	C64.-✓	C79.0-✓	D09.19	D30.0-✓	D41.0-✓	D49.51-✓
parietal						
bone	C41.0	C79.51	—	D16.4	D48.0	D49.2
lobe, brain	C71.3	C79.31	—	D33.0	D43.0	D49.6
paroophoron	C57.1-✓	C79.82	D07.39	D28.2	D39.8	D49.59
parotid (duct) (gland)	C07	C79.89	D00.00	D11.0	D37.030	D49.0
parovarium	C57.1-✓	C79.82	D07.39	D28.2	D39.8	D49.59
patella	C40.20	C79.51	—			
peduncle, cerebral	C71.7	C79.31	—	D33.1	D43.1	D49.6
pelvirectal junction	C19	C78.5	D01.1	D12.7	D37.5	D49.0
pelvis, pelvic	C76.3	C79.89	D09.8	D36.7	D48.7	D49.89
bone	C41.4	C79.51	—	D16.8	D48.0	D49.2
floor	C76.3	C79.89	D09.8	D36.7	D48.7	D49.89
renal	C65.-✓	C79.0-✓	D09.19	D30.1-✓	D41.1-✓	D49.51-✓
viscera	C76.3	C79.89	D09.8	D36.7	D48.7	D49.89
wall	C76.3	C79.89	D09.8	D36.7	D48.7	D49.89
pelvo-abdominal	C76.8	C79.89	D09.8	D36.7	D48.7	D49.89
penis	C60.9	C79.82	D07.4	D29.0	D40.8	D49.59

Neoplasm, neoplastic — continued

penis — continued

	Malignant Primary	Malignant Secondary	Ca in situ	Benign	Uncertain	Unspecified Behavior
body	C60.2	C79.82	D07.4	D29.0	D40.8	D49.59
corpus (cavernosum)	C60.2	C79.82	D07.4	D29.0	D40.8	D49.59
glans	C60.1	C79.82	D07.4	D29.0	D40.8	D49.59
overlapping sites	C60.8	—	—	—	—	—
skin NEC	C60.9	C79.82	D07.4	D29.0	D40.8	D49.59
periadrenal (tissue)	C48.0	C78.6	—	D20.0	D48.3	D49.0
perianal (skin) — see also Neoplasm, anus, skin						
skin	C44.500	C79.2	D04.5	D23.5	D48.5	D49.2
pericardium	C38.0	C79.89	—	D15.1	D48.7	D49.89
perinephric	C48.0	C78.6	—	D20.0	D48.3	D49.0
perineum	C76.3	C79.89	D09.8	D36.7	D48.7	D49.89
periodontal tissue NEC	C03.9	C79.89	D00.03	D10.39	D37.09	D49.0
periosteum — see Neoplasm, bone						
peripancreatic	C48.0	C78.6	—	D20.0	D48.3	D49.0
peripheral nerve NEC	C47.9	C79.89	—	D36.10	D48.2	D49.2
perirectal (tissue)	C76.3	C79.89	—	D36.7	D48.7	D49.89
perirenal (tissue)	C48.0	C78.6	—	D20.0	D48.3	D49.0
peritoneum, peritoneal (cavity)	C48.2	C78.6	—	D20.1	D48.4	D49.0
benign mesothelial tissue — see Mesothelioma, benign						
overlapping lesion with digestive organs	C48.8	—	—	—	—	—
	C26.9	—	—	—	—	—
parietal	C48.1	C78.6	—	D20.1	D48.4	D49.0
pelvic	C48.1	C78.6	—	D20.1	D48.4	D49.0
specified part NEC	C48.1	C78.6	—	D20.1	D48.4	D49.0
peritonsillar (tissue)	C76.0	C79.89	D09.8	D36.7	D48.7	D49.89
periurethral tissue	C76.3	C79.89	—	D36.7	D48.7	D49.89
phalanges						
foot	C40.3-✓	C79.51	—	D16.3-✓	—	—
hand	C40.1-✓	C79.51	—	D16.1-✓	—	—
pharynx, pharyngeal	C14.0	C79.89	D00.08	D10.9	D37.05	D49.0
bursa	C11.1	C79.89	D00.08	D10.6	D37.05	D49.0
fornix	C11.3	C79.89	D00.08	D10.6	D37.05	D49.0
recess	C11.2	C79.89	D00.08	D10.6	D37.05	D49.0
region	C14.0	C79.89	D00.08	D10.9	D37.05	D49.0
tonsil	C11.1	C79.89	D00.08	D10.6	D37.05	D49.0
wall (lateral) (posterior)	C14.0	C79.89	D00.08	D10.9	D37.05	D49.0
pia mater	C70.9	C79.40	—	D32.9	D42.9	D49.7
cerebral	C70.0	C79.32	—	D32.0	D42.0	D49.7
cranial	C70.0	C79.32	—	D32.0	D42.0	D49.7
spinal	C70.1	C79.49	—	D32.1	D42.1	D49.7
pillars of fauces	C09.1	C79.89	D00.08	D10.5	D37.05	D49.0
pineal (body) (gland)	C75.3	C79.89	D09.3	D35.4	D44.5	D49.7
pinna (ear) NEC — see also Neoplasm, skin, ear						
ear	C44.20-✓	C79.2	D04.2-✓	D23.2-✓	D48.5	D49.2
piriform fossa or sinus	C12	C79.89	D00.08	D10.7	D37.05	D49.0
pituitary (body) (fossa) (gland) (lobe)	C75.1	C79.89	D09.3	D35.2	D44.3	D49.7
placenta	C58	C79.82	D07.0	D26.7	D39.2	D49.59
pleura, pleural (cavity)	C38.4	C78.2	—	D19.0	D38.2	D49.1
overlapping lesion with heart or mediastinum	C38.8	—	—	—	—	—
parietal	C38.4	C78.2	—	D19.0	D38.2	D49.1
visceral	C38.4	C78.2	—	D19.0	D38.2	D49.1
plexus						
brachial	C47.1-✓	C79.89	—	D36.12	D48.2	D49.2
cervical	C47.0	C79.89	—	D36.11	D48.2	D49.2
choroid	C71.5	C79.31	—	D33.0	D43.0	D49.6
lumbosacral	C47.5	C79.89	—	D36.16	D48.2	D49.2
sacral	C47.5	C79.89	—	D36.16	D48.2	D49.2
pluriendocrine	C75.8	C79.89	D09.3	D35.7	D44.9	D49.7
pole						
frontal	C71.1	C79.31	—	D33.0	D43.0	D49.6
occipital	C71.4	C79.31	—	D33.0	D43.0	D49.6
pons (varolii)	C71.7	C79.31	—	D33.1	D43.1	D49.6

Neoplasm, neoplastic — *continued*

	Malignant Primary	Malignant Secondary	Ca in situ	Benign	Uncertain	Unspecified Behavior
popliteal fossa or space	C76.5-✓	C79.89	D04.7-✓	D36.7	D48.7	D49.89
postcricoid (region)	C13.0	C79.89	D00.08	D10.7	D37.05	D49.0
posterior fossa (cranial)	C71.9	C79.31	—	D33.2	D43.2	D49.6
postnasal space	C11.9	C79.89	D00.08	D10.6	D37.05	D49.0
prepuce	C60.0	C79.82	D07.4	D29.0	D40.8	D49.59
prepylorus	C16.4	C78.89	D00.2	D13.1	D37.1	D49.0
presacral (region)	C76.3	C79.89	—	D48.7	D48.7	D49.89
prostate (gland)	C61	C79.82	D07.5	D29.1	D40.0	D49.59
utricle	C68.0	C79.19	D09.19	D30.4	D41.3	D49.59
pterygoid fossa	C49.0	C79.89		D21.0	D48.1	D49.2
pubic bone	C41.4	C79.51		D16.8	D48.0	D49.2
pudenda, pudendum (female)	C51.9	C79.82	D07.1	D28.0	D39.8	D49.59
pulmonary — see also Neoplasm, lung	C34.9-✓	C78.0-✓	D02.2-✓	D14.3-✓	D38.1	D49.1
putamen	C71.0	C79.31		D33.0	D43.0	D49.6
pyloric						
antrum	C16.3	C78.89	D00.2	D13.1	D37.1	D49.0
canal	C16.4	C78.89	D00.2	D13.1	D37.1	D49.0
pylorus	C16.4	C78.89	D00.2	D13.1	D37.1	D49.0
pyramid (brain)	C71.7	C79.31		D33.1	D43.1	D49.6
pyriform fossa or sinus	C12	C79.89	D00.08	D10.7	D37.05	D49.0
radius (any part)	C40.0-✓	C79.51		D16.0-✓	—	—
Rathke's pouch	C75.1	C79.89	D09.3	D35.2	D44.3	D49.7
rectosigmoid (junction)	C19	C78.5	D01.1	D12.7	D37.5	D49.0
overlapping lesion with anus or rectum	C21.8	—	—	—	—	—
rectouterine pouch	C48.1	C78.6	—	D20.1	D48.4	D49.0
rectovaginal septum or wall	C76.3	C79.89	D09.8	D36.7	D48.7	D49.89
rectovesical septum	C76.3	C79.89	D09.8	D36.7	D48.7	D49.89
rectum (ampulla)	C20	C78.5	D01.2	D12.8	D37.5	D49.0
and colon	C19	C78.5	D01.1	D12.7	D37.5	D49.0
overlapping lesion with anus or rectosigmoid junction	C21.8	—	—	—	—	—
renal	C64.-✓	C79.0-✓	D09.19	D30.0-✓	D41.0-✓	D49.51-✓
calyx	C65.-✓	C79.0-✓	D09.19	D30.1-✓	D41.1-✓	D49.51-✓
hilus	C65.-✓	C79.0-✓	D09.19	D30.1-✓	D41.1-✓	D49.51-✓
parenchyma	C64.-✓	C79.0-✓	D09.19	D30.0-✓	D41.0-✓	D49.51-✓
pelvis	C65.-✓	C79.0-✓	D09.19	D30.1-✓	D41.1-✓	D49.51-✓
respiratory						
organs or system NEC	C39.9	C78.30	D02.4	D14.4	D38.6	D49.1
tract NEC	C39.9	C78.30	D02.4	D14.4	D38.5	D49.1
upper	C39.0	C78.30	D02.4	D14.4	D38.5	D49.1
retina	C69.2-✓	C79.49	D09.2-✓	D31.2-✓	D48.7	D49.81
retrobulbar	C69.6-✓	C79.49	—	D31.6-✓	D48.7	D49.89
retrocecal	C48.0	C78.6		D20.0	D48.3	D49.0
retromolar (area) (triangle) (trigone)	C06.2	C79.89	D00.00	D10.39	D37.09	D49.0
retro-orbital	C76.0	C79.89	D09.8	D36.7	D48.7	D49.89
retroperitoneal (space) (tissue)	C48.0	C78.6	—	D20.0	D48.3	D49.0
retroperitoneum	C48.0	C78.6	—	D20.0	D48.3	D49.0
retropharyngeal	C14.0	C79.89	D00.08	D10.9	D37.05	D49.0
retrovesical (septum)	C76.3	C79.89	D09.8	D36.7	D48.7	D49.89
rhinencephalon	C71.0	C79.31	—	D33.0	D43.0	D49.6
rib	C41.3	C79.51	—	D16.7	D48.0	D49.2
Rosenmuller's fossa	C11.2	C79.89	D00.08	D10.6	D37.05	D49.0
round ligament	C57.2-✓	C79.82	—	D28.2	D39.8	D49.59
sacrococcyx, sacrococcygeal	C41.4	C79.51	—	D16.8	D48.0	D49.2
region	C76.3	C79.89	D09.8	D36.7	D48.7	D49.89
sacrouterine ligament	C57.3	C79.82	—	D28.2	D39.8	D49.59
sacrum, sacral (vertebra)	C41.4	C79.51	—	D16.8	D48.0	D49.2
salivary gland or duct (major)	C08.9	C79.89	D00.00	D11.9	D37.039	D49.0
minor NEC	C06.9	C79.89	D00.00	D10.39	D37.04	D49.0
overlapping lesion	C08.9	—	—	—	—	—
parotid	C07	C79.89	D00.00	D11.0	D37.030	D49.0

Neoplasm, neoplastic — *continued*
salivary gland or duct — *continued*

	Malignant Primary	Malignant Secondary	Ca in situ	Benign	Uncertain	Unspecified Behavior
pluriglandular	C08.9	C79.89	D00.00	D11.9	D37.039	D49.0
sublingual	C08.1	C79.89	D00.00	D11.7	D37.031	D49.0
submandibular	C08.0	C79.89	D00.00	D11.7	D37.032	D49.0
submaxillary	C08.0	C79.89	D00.00	D11.7	D37.032	D49.0
salpinx (uterine)	C57.0-✓	C79.82	D07.39	D28.2	D39.8	D49.59
Santorini's duct	C25.3	C78.89	D01.7	D13.6	D37.8	D49.0
scalp	C44.40	C79.2	D04.4	D23.4	D48.5	D49.2
basal cell carcinoma	C44.41	—	—	—	—	—
specified type NEC	C44.49	—	—	—	—	—
squamous cell carcinoma	C44.42	—	—	—	—	—
scapula (any part)	C40.0-✓	C79.51	—	D16.0-✓	—	—
scapular region	C76.1	C79.89	D09.8	D36.7	D48.7	D49.89
scar NEC — see also Neoplasm, skin, by site	C44.90	C79.2	D04.9	D23.9	D48.5	D49.2
sciatic nerve	C47.2-✓	C79.89		D36.13	D48.2	D49.2
sclera	C69.4-✓	C79.49	D09.2-✓	D31.4-✓	D48.7	D49.89
scrotum (skin)	C63.2	C79.82	D07.61	D29.4	D40.8	D49.59
sebaceous gland — see Neoplasm, skin						
sella turcica	C75.1	C79.89	D09.3	D35.2	D44.3	D49.7
bone	C41.0	C79.51	—	D16.4	D48.0	D49.2
semilunar cartilage (knee)	C40.2-✓	C79.51	—	D16.2-✓	D48.0	D49.2
seminal vesicle	C63.7	C79.82	D07.69	D29.8	D40.8	D49.59
septum						
nasal	C30.0	C78.39	D02.3	D14.0	D38.5	D49.1
posterior margin	C11.3	C79.89	D00.08	D10.6	D37.05	D49.0
rectovaginal	C76.3	C79.89	D09.8	D36.7	D48.7	D49.89
rectovesical	C76.3	C79.89	D09.8	D36.7	D48.7	D49.89
urethrovaginal	C57.9	C79.82	D07.30	D28.9	D39.9	D49.59
vesicovaginal	C57.9	C79.82	D07.30	D28.9	D39.9	D49.59
shoulder NEC	C76.4-✓	C79.89	D04.6-✓	D36.7	D48.7	D49.89
sigmoid flexure (lower) (upper)	C18.7	C78.5	D01.0	D12.5	D37.4	D49.0
sinus (accessory)	C31.9	C78.39	D02.3	D14.0	D38.5	D49.1
bone (any)	C41.0	C79.51		D16.4	D48.0	D49.2
ethmoidal	C31.1	C78.39	D02.3	D14.0	D38.5	D49.1
frontal	C31.2	C78.39	D02.3	D14.0	D38.5	D49.1
maxillary	C31.0	C78.39	D02.3	D14.0	D38.5	D49.1
nasal, paranasal NEC	C31.9	C78.39	D02.3	D14.0	D38.5	D49.1
overlapping lesion	C31.8	—	—	—	—	—
pyriform	C12	C79.89	D00.08	D10.7	D37.05	D49.0
sphenoid	C31.3	C78.39	D02.3	D14.0	D38.5	D49.1
skeleton, skeletal NEC	C41.9	C79.51	—	D16.9	D48.0	D49.2
Skene's gland	C68.1	C79.19	D09.19	D30.8	D41.8	D49.59
skin NOS	C44.90	C79.2	D04.9	D23.9	D48.5	D49.2
abdominal wall	C44.509	C79.2	D04.5	D23.5	D48.5	D49.2
basal cell carcinoma	C44.519	—	—	—	—	—
specified type NEC	C44.599	—	—	—	—	—
squamous cell carcinoma	C44.529	—	—	—	—	—
ala nasi — see also Neoplasm, nose, skin	C44.301	C79.2	D04.39	D23.39	D48.5	D49.2
ankle — see also Neoplasm, skin, limb, lower	C44.70-✓	C79.2	D04.7-✓	D23.7-✓	D48.5	D49.2
antecubital space — see also Neoplasm, skin, limb, upper	C44.60-✓	C79.2	D04.6-✓	D23.6-✓	D48.5	D49.2
anus	C44.500	C79.2	D04.5	D23.5	D48.5	D49.2
basal cell carcinoma	C44.510	—	—	—	—	—
specified type NEC	C44.590	—	—	—	—	—
squamous cell carcinoma	C44.520	—	—	—	—	—
arm — see also Neoplasm, skin, limb, upper	C44.60-✓	C79.2	D04.6-✓	D23.6-✓	D48.5	D49.2

Neoplasm, neoplastic — continued skin — continued	Malignant Primary	Malignant Secondary	Ca in situ	Benign	Uncertain	Unspecified Behavior
auditory canal (external) — see also Neoplasm, skin, ear	C44.20-☑	C79.2	D04.2-☑	D23.2-☑	D48.5	D49.2
auricle (ear) — see also Neoplasm, skin, ear	C44.20-☑	C79.2	D04.2-☑	D23.2-☑	D48.5	D49.2
auricular canal (external) — see also Neoplasm, skin, ear	C44.20-☑	C79.2	D04.2-☑	D23.2-☑	D48.5	D49.2
axilla, axillary fold — see also Neoplasm, skin, trunk	C44.509	C79.2	D04.5	D23.5	D48.5	D49.2
back — see also Neoplasm, skin, trunk	C44.509	C79.2	D04.5	D23.5	D48.5	D49.2
basal cell carcinoma	C44.91	—	—	—	—	—
breast	C44.501	C79.2	D04.5	D23.5	D48.5	D49.2
basal cell carcinoma	C44.511	—	—	—	—	—
specified type NEC	C44.591	—	—	—	—	—
squamous cell carcinoma	C44.521	—	—	—	—	—
brow — see also Neoplasm, skin, face	C44.309	C79.2	D04.39	D23.39	D48.5	D49.2
buttock — see also Neoplasm, skin, trunk	C44.509	C79.2	D04.5	D23.5	D48.5	D49.2
calf — see also Neoplasm, skin, limb, lower	C44.70-☑	C79.2	D04.7-☑	D23.7-☑	D48.5	D49.2
canthus (eye) (inner) (outer)	C44.10-☑	C79.2	D04.1-☑	D23.1-☑	D48.5	D49.2
basal cell carcinoma	C44.11-☑	—	—	—	—	—
specified type NEC	C44.19-☑	—	—	—	—	—
squamous cell carcinoma	C44.12-☑	—	—	—	—	—
cervical region — see also Neoplasm, skin, neck	C44.40	C79.2	D04.4	D23.4	D48.5	D49.2
cheek (external) — see also Neoplasm, skin, face	C44.309	C79.2	D04.39	D23.39	D48.5	D49.2
chest (wall) — see also Neoplasm, skin, trunk	C44.509	C79.2	D04.5	D23.5	D48.5	D49.2
chin — see also Neoplasm, skin, face	C44.309	C79.2	D04.39	D23.39	D48.5	D49.2
clavicular area — see also Neoplasm, skin, trunk	C44.509	C79.2	D04.5	D23.5	D48.5	D49.2
clitoris	C51.2	C79.82	D07.1	D28.0	D39.8	D49.59
columnella — see also Neoplasm, skin, face	C44.309	C79.2	D04.39	D23.39	D48.5	D49.2
concha — see also Neoplasm, skin, ear	C44.20-☑	C79.2	D04.2-☑	D23.2-☑	D48.5	D49.2
ear (external)	C44.20-☑	C79.2	D04.2-☑	D23.2-☑	D48.5	D49.2
basal cell carcinoma	C44.21-☑	—	—	—	—	—
specified type NEC	C44.29-☑	—	—	—	—	—
squamous cell carcinoma	C44.22-☑	—	—	—	—	—
elbow — see also Neoplasm, skin, limb, upper	C44.60-☑	C79.2	D04.6-☑	D23.6-☑	D48.5	D49.2
eyebrow — see also Neoplasm, skin, face	C44.309	C79.2	D04.39	D23.39	D48.5	D49.2
eyelid	C44.10-☑	C79.2	D04.1-☑	D23.1-☑	D48.5	D49.2

Neoplasm, neoplastic — continued skin — continued	Malignant Primary	Malignant Secondary	Ca in situ	Benign	Uncertain	Unspecified Behavior
eyelid — continued						
basal cell carcinoma	C44.11-☑	—	—	—	—	—
specified type NEC	C44.19-☑	—	—	—	—	—
squamous cell carcinoma	C44.12-☑	—	—	—	—	—
face NOS	C44.300	C79.2	D04.30	D23.30	D48.5	D49.2
basal cell carcinoma	C44.310	—	—	—	—	—
specified type NEC	C44.390	—	—	—	—	—
squamous cell carcinoma	C44.320	—	—	—	—	—
female genital organs (external)	C51.9	C79.82	D07.1	D28.0	D39.8	D49.59
clitoris	C51.2	C79.82	D07.1	D28.0	D39.8	D49.59
labium NEC	C51.9	C79.82	D07.1	D28.0	D39.8	D49.59
majus	C51.0	C79.82	D07.1	D28.0	D39.8	D49.59
minus	C51.1	C79.82	D07.1	D28.0	D39.8	D49.59
pudendum	C51.9	C79.82	D07.1	D28.0	D39.8	D49.59
vulva	C51.9	C79.82	D07.1	D28.0	D39.8	D49.59
finger — see also Neoplasm, skin, limb, upper	C44.60-☑	C79.2	D04.6-☑	D23.6-☑	D48.5	D49.2
flank — see also Neoplasm, skin, trunk	C44.509	C79.2	D04.5	D23.5	D48.5	D49.2
foot — see also Neoplasm, skin, limb, lower	C44.70-☑	C79.2	D04.7-☑	D23.7-☑	D48.5	D49.2
forearm — see also Neoplasm, skin, limb, upper	C44.60-☑	C79.2	D04.6-☑	D23.6-☑	D48.5	D49.2
forehead — see also Neoplasm, skin, face	C44.309	C79.2	D04.39	D23.39	D48.5	D49.2
glabella — see also Neoplasm, skin, face	C44.309	C79.2	D04.39	D23.39	D48.5	D49.2
gluteal region — see also Neoplasm, skin, trunk	C44.509	C79.2	D04.5	D23.5	D48.5	D49.2
groin — see also Neoplasm, skin, trunk	C44.509	C79.2	D04.5	D23.5	D48.5	D49.2
hand — see also Neoplasm, skin, limb, upper	C44.60-☑	C79.2	D04.6-☑	D23.6-☑	D48.5	D49.2
head NEC — see also Neoplasm, skin, scalp	C44.40	C79.2	D04.4	D23.4	D48.5	D49.2
heel — see also Neoplasm, skin, limb, lower	C44.70-☑	C79.2	D04.7-☑	D23.7-☑	D48.5	D49.2
helix — see also Neoplasm, skin, ear	C44.20-☑	C79.2	D04.2-☑	D23.2-☑	D48.5	D49.2
hip — see also Neoplasm, skin, limb, lower	C44.70-☑	C79.2	D04.7-☑	D23.7-☑	D48.5	D49.2
infraclavicular region — see also Neoplasm, skin, trunk	C44.509	C79.2	D04.5	D23.5	D48.5	D49.2
inguinal region — see also Neoplasm, skin, trunk	C44.509	C79.2	D04.5	D23.5	D48.5	D49.2
jaw — see also Neoplasm, skin, face	C44.309	C79.2	D04.39	D23.39	D48.5	D49.2
Kaposi's sarcoma — see Kaposi's, sarcoma, skin						
knee — see also Neoplasm, skin, limb, lower	C44.70-☑	C79.2	D04.7-☑	D23.7-☑	D48.5	D49.2
labia						
majora	C51.0	C79.82	D07.1	D28.0	D39.8	D49.59
minora	C51.1	C79.82	D07.1	D28.0	D39.8	D49.59

Neoplasm, neoplastic — continued / skin — continued

	Malignant Primary	Malignant Secondary	Ca in situ	Benign	Uncertain	Unspecified Behavior
leg — see also Neoplasm, skin, limb, lower	C44.70-✓	C79.2	D04.7-✓	D23.7-✓	D48.5	D49.2
lid (lower) (upper)	C44.10-✓	C79.2	D04.1-✓	D23.1-✓	D48.5	D49.2
basal cell carcinoma	C44.11-✓	—	—	—	—	—
specified type NEC	C44.19-✓	—	—	—	—	—
squamous cell carcinoma	C44.12-✓	—	—	—	—	—
limb NEC	C44.90	C79.2	D04.9	D23.9	D48.5	D49.2
basal cell carcinoma	C44.91	—	—	—	—	—
lower	C44.70-✓	C79.2	D04.7-✓	D23.7-✓	D48.5	D49.2
basal cell carcinoma	C44.71-✓	—	—	—	—	—
specified type NEC	C44.79-✓	—	—	—	—	—
squamous cell carcinoma	C44.72-✓	—	—	—	—	—
upper	C44.60-✓	C79.2	D04.6-✓	D23.6-✓	D48.5	D49.2
basal cell carcinoma	C44.61-✓	—	—	—	—	—
specified type NEC	C44.69-✓	—	—	—	—	—
squamous cell carcinoma	C44.62-✓	—	—	—	—	—
lip (lower) (upper)	C44.00	C79.2	D04.0	D23.0	D48.5	D49.2
basal cell carcinoma	C44.01	—	—	—	—	—
specified type NEC	C44.09	—	—	—	—	—
squamous cell carcinoma	C44.02	—	—	—	—	—
male genital organs	C63.9	C79.82	D07.60	D29.9	D40.8	D49.59
penis	C60.9	C79.82	D07.4	D29.0	D40.8	D49.59
prepuce	C60.0	C79.82	D07.4	D29.0	D40.8	D49.59
scrotum	C63.2	C79.82	D07.61	D29.4	D40.8	D49.59
mastectomy site (skin) — see also Neoplasm, skin, breast	C44.501	C79.2	—	—	—	—
specified as breast tissue	C50.8-✓	C79.81	—	—	—	—
meatus, acoustic (external) — see also Neoplasm, skin, ear	C44.20-✓	C79.2	D04.2-✓	D23.2-✓	D48.5	D49.2
melanotic — see Melanoma						
Merkel cell — see Carcinoma, Merkel cell						
nates — see also Neoplasm, skin, trunk	C44.509	C79.2	D04.5	D23.5	D48.5	D49.2
neck	C44.40	C79.2	D04.4	D23.4	D48.5	D49.2
basal cell carcinoma	C44.41	—	—	—	—	—
specified type NEC	C44.49	—	—	—	—	—
squamous cell carcinoma	C44.42	—	—	—	—	—
nevus — see Nevus, skin						
nose (external) — see also Neoplasm, nose, skin	C44.301	C79.2	D04.39	D23.39	D48.5	D49.2
overlapping lesion	C44.80	—	—	—	—	—
basal cell carcinoma	C44.81	—	—	—	—	—
specified type NEC	C44.89	—	—	—	—	—
squamous cell carcinoma	C44.82	—	—	—	—	—
palm — see also Neoplasm, skin, limb, upper	C44.60-✓	C79.2	D04.6-✓	D23.6-✓	D48.5	D49.2
palpebra	C44.10-✓	C79.2	D04.1-✓	D23.1-✓	D48.5	D49.2

Neoplasm, neoplastic — continued / skin — continued / palpebra — continued

	Malignant Primary	Malignant Secondary	Ca in situ	Benign	Uncertain	Unspecified Behavior
basal cell carcinoma	C44.11-✓	—	—	—	—	—
specified type NEC	C44.19-✓	—	—	—	—	—
squamous cell carcinoma	C44.12-✓	—	—	—	—	—
penis NEC	C60.9	C79.82	D07.4	D29.0	D40.8	D49.59
perianal — see also Neoplasm, skin, anus	C44.500	C79.2	D04.5	D23.5	D48.5	D49.2
perineum — see also Neoplasm, skin, anus	C44.500	C79.2	D04.5	D23.5	D48.5	D49.2
pinna — see also Neoplasm, skin, ear	C44.20-✓	C79.2	D04.2-✓	D23.2-✓	D48.5	D49.2
plantar — see also Neoplasm, skin, limb, lower	C44.70-✓	C79.2	D04.7-✓	D23.7-✓	D48.5	D49.2
popliteal fossa or space — see also Neoplasm, skin, limb, lower	C44.70-✓	C79.2	D04.7-✓	D23.7-✓	D48.5	D49.2
prepuce	C60.0	C79.82	D07.4	D29.0	D40.8	D49.59
pubes — see also Neoplasm, skin, trunk	C44.509	C79.2	D04.5	D23.5	D48.5	D49.2
sacrococcygeal region — see also Neoplasm, skin, trunk	C44.509	C79.2	D04.5	D23.5	D48.5	D49.2
scalp	C44.40	C79.2	D04.4	D23.4	D48.5	D49.2
basal cell carcinoma	C44.41	—	—	—	—	—
specified type NEC	C44.49	—	—	—	—	—
squamous cell carcinoma	C44.42	—	—	—	—	—
scapular region — see also Neoplasm, skin, trunk	C44.509	C79.2	D04.5	D23.5	D48.5	D49.2
scrotum	C63.2	C79.82	D07.61	D29.4	D40.8	D49.59
shoulder — see also Neoplasm, skin, limb, upper	C44.60-✓	C79.2	D04.6-✓	D23.6-✓	D48.5	D49.2
sole (foot) — see also Neoplasm, skin, limb, lower	C44.70-✓	C79.2	D04.7-✓	D23.7-✓	D48.5	D49.2
specified sites NEC	C44.80	C79.2	D04.8	D23.9	D48.5	D49.2
basal cell carcinoma	C44.81	—	—	—	—	—
specified type NEC	C44.89	—	—	—	—	—
squamous cell carcinoma	C44.82	—	—	—	—	—
specified type NEC	C44.99	—	—	—	—	—
squamous cell carcinoma	C44.92	—	—	—	—	—
submammary fold — see also Neoplasm, skin, trunk	C44.509	C79.2	D04.5	D23.5	D48.5	D49.2
supraclavicular region — see also Neoplasm, skin, neck	C44.40	C79.2	D04.4	D23.4	D48.5	D49.2
temple — see also Neoplasm, skin, face	C44.309	C79.2	D04.39	D23.39	D48.5	D49.2
thigh — see also Neoplasm, skin, limb, lower	C44.70-✓	C79.2	D04.7-✓	D23.7-✓	D48.5	D49.2
thoracic wall — see also Neoplasm, skin, trunk	C44.509	C79.2	D04.5	D23.5	D48.5	D49.2
thumb — see also Neoplasm, skin, limb, upper	C44.60-✓	C79.2	D04.6-✓	D23.6-✓	D48.5	D49.2
toe — see also Neoplasm, skin, limb, lower	C44.70-✓	C79.2	D04.7-✓	D23.7-✓	D48.5	D49.2

Neoplasm, neoplastic — continued	Malignant Primary	Malignant Secondary	Ca in situ	Benign	Uncertain	Unspecified Behavior
skin — continued						
tragus — see also Neoplasm, skin, ear	C44.20-☑	C79.2	D04.2-☑	D23.2-☑	D48.5	D49.2
trunk	C44.509	C79.2	D04.5	D23.5	D48.5	D49.2
basal cell carcinoma	C44.519	—	—	—	—	—
specified type NEC	C44.599	—	—	—	—	—
squamous cell carcinoma	C44.529	—	—	—	—	—
umbilicus — see also Neoplasm, skin, trunk	C44.509	C79.2	D04.5	D23.5	D48.5	D49.2
vulva	C51.9	C79.82	D07.1	D28.0	D39.8	D49.59
overlapping lesion	C51.8	—	—	—	—	—
wrist — see also Neoplasm, skin, limb, upper	C44.60-☑	C79.2	D04.6-☑	D23.6-☑	D48.5	D49.2
skull	C41.0	C79.51	—	D16.4	D48.0	D49.2
soft parts or tissues — see Neoplasm, connective tissue						
specified site NEC	C76.8	C79.89	D09.8	D36.7	D48.7	D49.89
spermatic cord	C63.1-☑	C79.82	D07.69	D29.8	D40.8	D49.59
sphenoid	C31.3	C78.39	D02.3	D14.0	D38.5	D49.1
bone	C41.0	C79.51	—	D16.4	D48.0	D49.2
sinus	C31.3	C78.39	D02.3	D14.0	D38.5	D49.1
sphincter						
anal	C21.1	C78.5	D01.3	D12.9	D37.8	D49.0
of Oddi	C24.0	C78.89	D01.5	D13.5	D37.6	D49.0
spine, spinal (column)	C41.2	C79.51	—	D16.6	D48.0	D49.2
bulb	C71.7	C79.31	—	D33.1	D43.1	D49.6
coccyx	C41.4	C79.51	—	D16.8	D48.0	D49.2
cord (cervical) (lumbar) (sacral) (thoracic)	C72.0	C79.49	—	D33.4	D43.4	D49.7
dura mater	C70.1	C79.49	—	D32.1	D42.1	D49.7
lumbosacral	C41.2	C79.51	—	D16.6	D48.0	D49.2
marrow NEC	C96.9	C79.52	—	—	D47.9	D49.89
membrane	C70.1	C79.49	—	D32.1	D42.1	D49.7
meninges	C70.1	C79.49	—	D32.1	D42.1	D49.7
nerve (root)	C47.9	C79.89	—	D36.10	D48.2	D49.2
pia mater	C70.1	C79.49	—	D32.1	D42.1	D49.7
root	C47.9	C79.89	—	D36.10	D48.2	D49.2
sacrum	C41.4	C79.51	—	D16.8	D48.0	D49.2
spleen, splenic NEC	C26.1	C78.89	D01.7	D13.9	D37.8	D49.0
flexure (colon)	C18.5	C78.5	D01.0	D12.3	D37.4	D49.0
stem, brain	C71.7	C79.31	—	D33.1	D43.1	D49.6
Stensen's duct	C07	C79.89	D00.00	D11.0	D37.030	D49.0
sternum	C41.3	C79.51	—	D16.7	D48.0	D49.2
stomach	C16.9	C78.89	D00.2	D13.1	D37.1	D49.0
antrum (pyloric)	C16.3	C78.89	D00.2	D13.1	D37.1	D49.0
body	C16.2	C78.89	D00.2	D13.1	D37.1	D49.0
cardia	C16.0	C78.89	D00.2	D13.1	D37.1	D49.0
cardiac orifice	C16.0	C78.89	D00.2	D13.1	D37.1	D49.0
corpus	C16.2	C78.89	D00.2	D13.1	D37.1	D49.0
fundus	C16.1	C78.89	D00.2	D13.1	D37.1	D49.0
greater curvature NEC	C16.6	C78.89	D00.2	D13.1	D37.1	D49.0
lesser curvature NEC	C16.5	C78.89	D00.2	D13.1	D37.1	D49.0
overlapping lesion	C16.8	—	—	—	—	—
prepylorus	C16.4	C78.89	D00.2	D13.1	D37.1	D49.0
pylorus	C16.4	C78.89	D00.2	D13.1	D37.1	D49.0
wall NEC	C16.9	C78.89	D00.2	D13.1	D37.1	D49.0
anterior NEC	C16.8	C78.89	D00.2	D13.1	D37.1	D49.0
posterior NEC	C16.8	C78.89	D00.2	D13.1	D37.1	D49.0
stroma, endometrial	C54.1	C79.82	D07.0	D26.1	D39.0	D49.59
stump, cervical	C53.8	C79.82	D06.7	D26.0	D39.0	D49.59
subcutaneous (nodule) (tissue) NEC — see Neoplasm, connective tissue						
subdural	C70.9	C79.32	—	D32.9	D42.9	D49.7
subglottis, subglottic	C32.2	C78.39	D02.0	D14.1	D38.0	D49.1
sublingual	C04.9	C79.89	D00.06	D10.2	D37.09	D49.0
gland or duct	C08.1	C79.89	D00.00	D11.7	D37.031	D49.0

Neoplasm, neoplastic — continued	Malignant Primary	Malignant Secondary	Ca in situ	Benign	Uncertain	Unspecified Behavior
submandibular gland	C08.0	C79.89	D00.00	D11.7	D37.032	D49.0
submaxillary gland or duct	C08.0	C79.89	D00.00	D11.7	D37.032	D49.0
submental	C76.0	C79.89	D09.8	D36.7	D48.7	D49.89
subpleural	C34.9-☑	C78.0-☑	D02.2-☑	D14.3-☑	D38.1	D49.1
substernal	C38.1	C78.1	—	D15.2	D38.3	D49.89
sudoriferous, sudoriparous gland, site unspecified	C44.90	C79.2	D04.9	D23.9	D48.5	D49.2
specified site — see Neoplasm, skin						
supraclavicular region	C76.0	C79.89	D09.8	D36.7	D48.7	D49.89
supraglottis	C32.1	C78.39	D02.0	D14.1	D38.0	D49.1
suprarenal	C74.9-☑	C79.7-☑	D09.3	D35.0-☑	D44.1-☑	D49.7
capsule	C74.9-☑	C79.7-☑	D09.3	D35.0-☑	D44.1-☑	D49.7
cortex	C74.0-☑	C79.7-☑	D09.3	D35.0-☑	D44.1-☑	D49.7
gland	C74.9-☑	C79.7-☑	D09.3	D35.0-☑	D44.1-☑	D49.7
medulla	C74.1-☑	C79.7-☑	D09.3	D35.0-☑	D44.1-☑	D49.7
suprasellar (region)	C71.9	C79.31	—	D33.2	D43.2	D49.6
supratentorial (brain) NEC	C71.0	C79.31	—	D33.0	D43.0	D49.6
sweat gland (apocrine) (eccrine), site unspecified	C44.90	C79.2	D04.9	D23.9	D48.5	D49.2
specified site — see Neoplasm, skin						
sympathetic nerve or nervous system NEC	C47.9	C79.89	—	D36.10	D48.2	D49.2
symphysis pubis	C41.4	C79.51	—	D16.8	D48.0	D49.2
synovial membrane — see Neoplasm, connective tissue						
tapetum, brain	C71.8	C79.31	—	D33.2	D43.2	D49.6
tarsus (any bone)	C40.3-☑	C79.51	—	D16.3-☑	—	—
temple (skin) — see also Neoplasm, skin, face	C44.309	C79.2	D04.39	D23.39	D48.5	D49.2
temporal						
bone	C41.0	C79.51	—	D16.4	D48.0	D49.2
lobe or pole	C71.2	C79.31	—	D33.0	D43.0	D49.6
region	C76.0	C79.89	D09.8	D36.7	D48.7	D49.89
skin — see also Neoplasm, skin, face	C44.309	C79.2	D04.39	D23.39	D48.5	D49.2
tendon (sheath) — see Neoplasm, connective tissue						
tentorium (cerebelli)	C70.0	C79.32	—	D32.0	D42.0	D49.7
testis, testes	C62.9-☑	C79.82	D07.69	D29.2-☑	D40.1-☑	D49.59
descended	C62.1-☑	C79.82	D07.69	D29.2-☑	D40.1-☑	D49.59
ectopic	C62.0-☑	C79.82	D07.69	D29.2-☑	D40.1-☑	D49.59
retained	C62.0-☑	C79.82	D07.69	D29.2-☑	D40.1-☑	D49.59
scrotal	C62.1-☑	C79.82	D07.69	D29.2-☑	D40.1-☑	D49.59
undescended	C62.0-☑	C79.82	D07.69	D29.2-☑	D40.1-☑	D49.59
unspecified whether descended or undescended	C62.9-☑	C79.82	D07.69	D29.2-☑	D40.1-☑	D49.59
thalamus	C71.0	C79.31	—	D33.0	D43.0	D49.6
thigh NEC	C76.5-☑	C79.89	D04.7-☑	D36.7	D48.7	D49.89
thorax, thoracic (cavity) (organs NEC)	C76.1	C79.89	D09.8	D36.7	D48.7	D49.89
duct	C49.3	C79.89	—	D21.3	D48.1	D49.2
wall NEC	C76.1	C79.89	D09.8	D36.7	D48.7	D49.89
throat	C14.0	C79.89	D00.08	D10.9	D37.05	D49.0
thumb NEC	C76.4-☑	C79.89	D04.6-☑	D36.7	D48.7	D49.89
thymus (gland)	C37	C79.89	D09.3	D15.0	D38.4	D49.89
thyroglossal duct	C73	C79.89	D09.3	D34	D44.0	D49.7
thyroid (gland)	C73	C79.89	D09.3	D34	D44.0	D49.7
cartilage	C32.3	C78.39	D02.0	D14.1	D38.0	D49.1
tibia (any part)	C40.2-☑	C79.51	—	D16.2-☑	—	—
toe NEC	C76.5-☑	C79.89	D04.7-☑	D36.7	D48.7	D49.89
tongue	C02.9	C79.89	D00.07	D10.1	D37.02	D49.0
anterior (two-thirds) NEC	C02.3	C79.89	D00.07	D10.1	D37.02	D49.0
dorsal surface	C02.0	C79.89	D00.07	D10.1	D37.02	D49.0
ventral surface	C02.2	C79.89	D00.07	D10.1	D37.02	D49.0

☑ Additional Character Required — Refer to the Tabular List for Character Selection   Subterms under main terms may continue to next column or page

Neoplasm, neoplastic — continued

	Malignant Primary	Malignant Secondary	Ca in situ	Benign	Uncertain	Unspecified Behavior
tongue — continued						
base (dorsal surface)	C01	C79.89	D00.07	D10.1	D37.02	D49.0
border (lateral)	C02.1	C79.89	D00.07	D10.1	D37.02	D49.0
dorsal surface NEC	C02.0	C79.89	D00.07	D10.1	D37.02	D49.0
fixed part NEC	C01	C79.89	D00.07	D10.1	D37.02	D49.0
foreamen cecum	C02.0	C79.89	D00.07	D10.1	D37.02	D49.0
frenulum linguae	C02.2	C79.89	D00.07	D10.1	D37.02	D49.0
junctional zone	C02.8	C79.89	D00.07	D10.1	D37.02	D49.0
margin (lateral)	C02.1	C79.89	D00.07	D10.1	D37.02	D49.0
midline NEC	C02.0	C79.89	D00.07	D10.1	D37.02	D49.0
mobile part NEC	C02.3	C79.89	D00.07	D10.1	D37.02	D49.0
overlapping lesion	C02.8	—	—	—	—	—
posterior (third)	C01	C79.89	D00.07	D10.1	D37.02	D49.0
root	C01	C79.89	D00.07	D10.1	D37.02	D49.0
surface (dorsal)	C02.0	C79.89	D00.07	D10.1	D37.02	D49.0
base	C01	C79.89	D00.07	D10.1	D37.02	D49.0
ventral	C02.2	C79.89	D00.07	D10.1	D37.02	D49.0
tip	C02.1	C79.89	D00.07	D10.1	D37.02	D49.0
tonsil	C02.4	C79.89	D00.07	D10.1	D37.02	D49.0
tonsil	C09.9	C79.89	D00.08	D10.4	D37.05	D49.0
fauces, faucial	C09.9	C79.89	D00.08	D10.4	D37.05	D49.0
lingual	C02.4	C79.89	D00.07	D10.1	D37.02	D49.0
overlapping sites	C09.8	—	—	—	—	—
palatine	C09.9	C79.89	D00.08	D10.4	D37.05	D49.0
pharyngeal	C11.1	C79.89	D00.08	D10.6	D37.05	D49.0
pillar (anterior) (posterior)	C09.1	C79.89	D00.08	D10.5	D37.05	D49.0
tonsillar fossa	C09.0	C79.89	D00.08	D10.5	D37.05	D49.0
tooth socket NEC	C03.9	C79.89	D00.03	D10.39	D37.09	D49.0
trachea (cartilage) (mucosa)	C33	C78.39	D02.1	D14.2	D38.1	D49.1
overlapping lesion with bronchus or lung	C34.8-☑	—	—	—	—	—
tracheobronchial	C34.8-☑	C78.39	D02.1	D14.2	D38.1	D49.1
overlapping lesion with lung	C34.8-☑	—	—	—	—	—
tragus — see also Neoplasm, skin, ear	C44.20-☑	C79.2	D04.2-☑	D23.2-☑	D48.5	D49.2
trunk NEC	C76.8	C79.89	D04.5	D36.7	D48.7	D49.89
tubo-ovarian	C57.8	C79.82	D07.39	D28.7	D39.8	D49.59
tunica vaginalis	C63.7	C79.82	D07.69	D29.8	D40.8	D49.59
turbinate (bone)	C41.0	C79.51		D16.4	D48.0	D49.2
nasal	C30.0	C78.39	D02.3	D14.0	D38.5	D49.1
tympanic cavity	C30.1	C78.39	D02.3	D14.0	D38.5	D49.1
ulna (any part)	C40.0-☑	C79.51	—	D16.0-☑		
umbilicus, umbilical — see also Neoplasm, skin, trunk	C44.509	C79.2	D04.5	D23.5	D48.5	D49.2
uncus, brain	C71.2	C79.31	—	D33.0	D43.0	D49.6
unknown site or unspecified	C80.1	C79.9	D09.9	D36.9	D48.9	D49.9
urachus	C67.7	C79.11	D09.0	D30.3	D41.4	D49.4
ureter-bladder (junction)	C67.6	C79.11	D09.0	D30.3	D41.4	D49.4
ureter, ureteral	C66.-☑	C79.19	D09.19	D30.2-☑	D41.2-☑	D49.59
orifice (bladder)	C67.6	C79.11	D09.0	D30.3	D41.4	D49.4
urethra, urethral (gland)	C68.0	C79.19	D09.19	D30.4	D41.3	D49.59
orifice, internal	C67.5	C79.11	D09.0	D30.3	D41.4	D49.4
urethrovaginal (septum)	C57.9	C79.82	D07.30	D28.9	D39.8	D49.59
urinary organ or system	C68.9	C79.10	D09.10	D30.9	D41.9	D49.59
bladder — see Neoplasm, bladder						
overlapping lesion	C68.8	—	—	—	—	—
specified sites NEC	C68.8	C79.19	D09.19	D30.8	D41.8	D49.59
utero-ovarian	C57.8	C79.82	D07.39	D28.7	D39.8	D49.59
ligament	C57.1-☑	C79.82	D07.39	D28.2	D39.8	D49.59
uterosacral ligament	C57.3	C79.82	—	D28.2	D39.8	D49.59
uterus, uteri, uterine	C55	C79.82	D07.0	D26.9	D39.0	D49.59
adnexa NEC	C57.4	C79.82	D07.39	D28.7	D39.8	D49.59
body	C54.9	C79.82	D07.0	D26.1	D39.0	D49.59
cervix	C53.9	C79.82	D06.9	D26.0	D39.0	D49.59
cornu	C54.9	C79.82	D07.0	D26.1	D39.0	D49.59
corpus	C54.9	C79.82	D07.0	D26.1	D39.0	D49.59
endocervix (canal) (gland)	C53.0	C79.82	D06.0	D26.0	D39.0	D49.59

Neoplasm, neoplastic — continued

	Malignant Primary	Malignant Secondary	Ca in situ	Benign	Uncertain	Unspecified Behavior
uterus, uteri, uterine — continued						
endometrium	C54.1	C79.82	D07.0	D26.1	D39.0	D49.59
exocervix	C53.1	C79.82	D06.1	D26.0	D39.0	D49.59
external os	C53.1	C79.82	D06.1	D26.0	D39.0	D49.59
fundus	C54.3	C79.82	D07.0	D26.1	D39.0	D49.59
internal os	C53.0	C79.82	D06.0	D26.0	D39.0	D49.59
isthmus	C54.0	C79.82	D07.0	D26.1	D39.0	D49.59
ligament	C57.3	C79.82	—	D28.2	D39.8	D49.59
broad	C57.1-☑	C79.82	D07.39	D28.2	D39.8	D49.59
round	C57.2-☑	C79.82	—	D28.2	D39.8	D49.59
lower segment	C54.0	C79.82	D07.0	D26.1	D39.0	D49.59
myometrium	C54.2	C79.82	D07.0	D26.1	D39.0	D49.59
overlapping sites	C54.8	—	—	—	—	—
squamocolumnar junction	C53.8	C79.82	D06.7	D26.0	D39.0	D49.59
tube	C57.0-☑	C79.82	D07.39	D28.2	D39.8	D49.59
utricle, prostatic	C68.0	C79.19	D09.19	D30.4	D41.3	D49.59
uveal tract	C69.4-☑	C79.49	D09.2-☑	D31.4-☑	D48.7	D49.89
uvula	C05.2	C79.89	D00.04	D10.39	D37.09	D49.0
vagina, vaginal (fornix) (vault) (wall)	C52	C79.82	D07.2	D28.1	D39.8	D49.59
vaginovesical	C57.9	C79.82	D07.30	D28.9	D39.9	D49.59
septum	C57.9	C79.82	D07.30	D28.9	D39.9	D49.59
vallecula (epigiottis)	C10.0	C79.89	D00.08	D10.5	D37.05	D49.0
vascular — see Neoplasm, connective tissue						
vas deferens	C63.1-☑	C79.82	D07.69	D29.8	D40.8	D49.59
Vater's ampulla	C24.1	C78.89	D01.5	D13.5	D37.6	D49.0
vein, venous — see Neoplasm, connective tissue						
vena cava (abdominal) (inferior)	C49.4	C79.89	—	D21.4	D48.1	D49.2
superior	C49.3	C79.89	—	D21.3	D48.1	D49.2
ventricle (cerebral) (floor) (lateral) (third)	C71.5	C79.31		D33.0	D43.0	D49.6
cardiac (left) (right)	C38.0	C79.89		D15.1	D48.7	D49.89
fourth	C71.7	C79.31		D33.1	D43.1	D49.6
ventricular band of larynx	C32.1	C78.39	D02.0	D14.1	D38.0	D49.1
ventriculus — see Neoplasm, stomach						
vermillion border — see Neoplasm, lip						
vermis, cerebellum	C71.6	C79.31	—	D33.1	D43.1	D49.6
vertebra (column)	C41.2	C79.51	—	D16.6	D48.0	D49.2
coccyx	C41.4	C79.51	—	D16.8	D48.0	D49.2
marrow NEC	C96.9	C79.52	—	—	D47.9	D49.89
sacrum	C41.4	C79.51	—	D16.8	D48.0	D49.2
vesical — see Neoplasm, bladder						
vesicle, seminal	C63.7	C79.82	D07.69	D29.8	D40.8	D49.59
vesicocervical tissue	C57.9	C79.82	D07.30	D28.9	D39.9	D49.59
vesicorectal	C76.3	C79.82	D09.8	D36.7	D48.7	D49.89
vesicovaginal	C57.9	C79.82	D07.30	D28.9	D39.9	D49.59
septum	C57.9	C79.82	D07.30	D28.9	D39.8	D49.59
vessel (blood) — see Neoplasm, connective tissue						
vestibular gland, greater	C51.0	C79.82	D07.1	D28.0	D39.8	D49.59
vestibule						
mouth	C06.1	C79.89	D00.00	D10.39	D37.09	D49.0
nose	C30.0	C78.39	D02.3	D14.0	D38.5	D49.1
Virchow's gland	C77.0	C77.0	—	D36.0	D48.7	D49.89
viscera NEC	C76.8	C79.89	D09.8	D36.7	D48.7	D49.89
vocal cords (true)	C32.0	C78.39	D02.0	D14.1	D38.0	D49.1
false	C32.1	C78.39	D02.0	D14.1	D38.0	D49.1
vomer	C41.0	C79.51	—	D16.4	D48.0	D49.2
vulva	C51.9	C79.82	D07.1	D28.0	D39.8	D49.59
vulvovaginal gland	C51.0	C79.82	D07.1	D28.0	D39.8	D49.59
Waldeyer's ring	C14.2	C79.89	D00.08	D10.9	D37.05	D49.0
Wharton's duct	C08.0	C79.89	D00.00	D11.7	D37.032	D49.0
white matter (central) (cerebral)	C71.0	C79.31	—	D33.0	D43.0	D49.6
windpipe	C33	C78.39	D02.1	D14.2	D38.1	D49.1
Wirsung's duct	C25.3	C78.89	D01.7	D13.6	D37.8	D49.0
wolffian (body) (duct) female	C57.7	C79.82	D07.39	D28.7	D39.8	D49.59

	Malignant Primary	Malignant Secondary	Ca in situ	Benign	Uncertain	Unspecified Behavior
Neoplasm, neoplastic — *continued*						
wolffian — *continued*						
male	C63.7	C79.82	D07.69	D29.8	D40.8	D49.59
womb — *see* Neoplasm, uterus						
wrist NEC	C76.4-☑	C79.89	D04.6-☑	D36.7	D48.7	D49.89
xiphoid process	C41.3	C79.51	—	D16.7	D48.0	D49.2
Zuckerkandl organ	C75.5	C79.89	—	D35.6	D44.7	D49.7

Substance	Poisoning, Accidental (unintentional)	Poisoning, Intentional Self-harm	Poisoning, Assault	Poisoning, Undetermined	Adverse Effect	Under-dosing
14-Hydroxydihydromorphinone	T40.2X1	T40.2X2	T40.2X3	T40.2X4	T40.2X5	T40.2X6
1-Propanol	T51.3X1	T51.3X2	T51.3X3	T51.3X4	—	—
2,3,7,8-Tetrachlorodibenzo-p-dioxin	T53.7X1	T53.7X2	T53.7X3	T53.7X4	—	—
2,4,5-T (trichlorophenoxyacetic acid)	T60.1X1	T60.1X2	T60.1X3	T60.1X4	—	—
2,4,5-Trichlorophenoxyacetic acid	T60.3X1	T60.3X2	T60.3X3	T60.3X4	—	—
2,4-D (dichlorophenoxyacetic acid)	T60.3X1	T60.3X2	T60.3X3	T60.3X4	—	—
2,4-Toluene diisocyanate	T65.0X1	T65.0X2	T65.0X3	T65.0X4	—	—
2-Deoxy-5-fluorouridine	T45.1X1	T45.1X2	T45.1X3	T45.1X4	T45.1X5	T45.1X6
2-Ethoxyethanol	T52.3X1	T52.3X2	T52.3X3	T52.3X4	—	—
2-Methoxyethanol	T52.3X1	T52.3X2	T52.3X3	T52.3X4	—	—
2-Propanol	T51.2X1	T51.2X2	T51.2X3	T51.2X4	—	—
4-Aminobutyric acid	T43.8X1	T43.8X2	T43.8X3	T43.8X4	T43.8X5	T43.8X6
4-Aminophenol derivatives	T39.1X1	T39.1X2	T39.1X3	T39.1X4	T39.1X5	T39.1X6
5-Deoxy-5-fluorouridine	T45.1X1	T45.1X2	T45.1X3	T45.1X4	T45.1X5	T45.1X6
5-Methoxypsoralen (5-MOP)	T50.991	T50.992	T50.993	T50.994	T50.995	T50.996
8-Aminoquinoline drugs	T37.2X1	T37.2X2	T37.2X3	T37.2X4	T37.2X5	T37.2X6
8-Methoxypsoralen (8-MOP)	T50.991	T50.992	T50.993	T50.994	T50.995	T50.996
ABOB	T37.5X1	T37.5X2	T37.5X3	T37.5X4	T37.5X5	T37.5X6
Abrine	T62.2X1	T62.2X2	T62.2X3	T62.2X4	—	—
Abrus (seed)	T62.2X1	T62.2X2	T62.2X3	T62.2X4	—	—
Absinthe	T51.0X1	T51.0X2	T51.0X3	T51.0X4	—	—
beverage	T51.0X1	T51.0X2	T51.0X3	T51.0X4	—	—
Acaricide	T60.8X1	T60.8X2	T60.8X3	T60.8X4	—	—
Acebutolol	T44.7X1	T44.7X2	T44.7X3	T44.7X4	T44.7X5	T44.7X6
Acecarbromal	T42.6X1	T42.6X2	T42.6X3	T42.6X4	T42.6X5	T42.6X6
Aceclidine	T44.1X1	T44.1X2	T44.1X3	T44.1X4	T44.1X5	T44.1X6
Acedapsone	T37.0X1	T37.0X2	T37.0X3	T37.0X4	T37.0X5	T37.0X6
Acefylline piperazine	T48.6X1	T48.6X2	T48.6X3	T48.6X4	T48.6X5	T48.6X6
Acemorphan	T40.2X1	T40.2X2	T40.2X3	T40.2X4	—	—
Acenocoumarin	T45.511	T45.512	T45.513	T45.514	T45.515	T45.516
Acenocoumarol	T45.511	T45.512	T45.513	T45.514	T45.515	T45.516
Acepifylline	T48.6X1	T48.6X2	T48.6X3	T48.6X4	T48.6X5	T48.6X6
Acepromazine	T43.3X1	T43.3X2	T43.3X3	T43.3X4	T43.3X5	T43.3X6
Acesulfamethoxypyridazine	T37.0X1	T37.0X2	T37.0X3	T37.0X4	T37.0X5	T37.0X6
Acetal	T52.8X1	T52.8X2	T52.8X3	T52.8X4	—	—
Acetaldehyde (vapor)	T52.8X1	T52.8X2	T52.8X3	T52.8X4	—	—
liquid	T65.891	T65.892	T65.893	T65.894	—	—
Acetaminophen	T39.1X1	T39.1X2	T39.1X3	T39.1X4	T39.1X5	T39.1X6
Acetaminosalol	T39.1X1	T39.1X2	T39.1X3	T39.1X4	T39.1X5	T39.1X6
Acetanilide	T39.1X1	T39.1X2	T39.1X3	T39.1X4	T39.1X5	T39.1X6
Acetarsol	T37.3X1	T37.3X2	T37.3X3	T37.3X4	T37.3X5	T37.3X6
Acetazolamide	T50.2X1	T50.2X2	T50.2X3	T50.2X4	T50.2X5	T50.2X6
Acetiamine	T45.2X1	T45.2X2	T45.2X3	T45.2X4	T45.2X5	T45.2X6
Acetic						
acid	T54.2X1	T54.2X2	T54.2X3	T54.2X4	—	—
with sodium acetate (ointment)	T49.3X1	T49.3X2	T49.3X3	T49.3X4	T49.3X5	T49.3X6
ester (solvent)(vapor)	T52.8X1	T52.8X2	T52.8X3	T52.8X4	—	—
irrigating solution	T50.3X1	T50.3X2	T50.3X3	T50.3X4	T50.3X5	T50.3X6
medicinal (lotion)	T49.2X1	T49.2X2	T49.2X3	T49.2X4	T49.2X5	T49.2X6
anhydride	T65.891	T65.892	T65.893	T65.894	—	—
ether (vapor)	T52.8X1	T52.8X2	T52.8X3	T52.8X4	—	—
Acetohexamide	T38.3X1	T38.3X2	T38.3X3	T38.3X4	T38.3X5	T38.3X6
Acetohydroxamic acid	T50.991	T50.992	T50.993	T50.994	T50.995	T50.996
Acetomenaphthone	T45.7X1	T45.7X2	T45.7X3	T45.7X4	T45.7X5	T45.7X6
Acetomorphine	T40.1X1	T40.1X2	T40.1X3	T40.1X4	—	—
Acetone (oils)	T52.4X1	T52.4X2	T52.4X3	T52.4X4	—	—
chlorinated	T52.4X1	T52.4X2	T52.4X3	T52.4X4	—	—
vapor	T52.4X1	T52.4X2	T52.4X3	T52.4X4	—	—
Acetonitrile	T52.8X1	T52.8X2	T52.8X3	T52.8X4	—	—
Acetophenazine	T43.3X1	T43.3X2	T43.3X3	T43.3X4	T43.3X5	T43.3X6
Acetophenetedin	T39.1X1	T39.1X2	T39.1X3	T39.1X4	T39.1X5	T39.1X6
Acetophenone	T52.4X1	T52.4X2	T52.4X3	T52.4X4	—	—
Acetorphine	T40.2X1	T40.2X2	T40.2X3	T40.2X4	—	—
Acetosulfone (sodium)	T37.1X1	T37.1X2	T37.1X3	T37.1X4	T37.1X5	T37.1X6
Acetrizoate (sodium)	T50.8X1	T50.8X2	T50.8X3	T50.8X4	T50.8X5	T50.8X6
Acetrizoic acid	T50.8X1	T50.8X2	T50.8X3	T50.8X4	T50.8X5	T50.8X6
Acetyl						
bromide	T53.6X1	T53.6X2	T53.6X3	T53.6X4	—	—
chloride	T53.6X1	T53.6X2	T53.6X3	T53.6X4	—	—
Acetylcarbromal	T42.6X1	T42.6X2	T42.6X3	T42.6X4	T42.6X5	T42.6X6
Acetylcholine						
chloride	T44.1X1	T44.1X2	T44.1X3	T44.1X4	T44.1X5	T44.1X6
derivative	T44.1X1	T44.1X2	T44.1X3	T44.1X4	T44.1X5	T44.1X6
Acetylcysteine	T48.4X1	T48.4X2	T48.4X3	T48.4X4	T48.4X5	T48.4X6
Acetyldigitoxin	T46.0X1	T46.0X2	T46.0X3	T46.0X4	T46.0X5	T46.0X6
Acetyldigoxin	T46.0X1	T46.0X2	T46.0X3	T46.0X4	T46.0X5	T46.0X6

Substance	Poisoning, Accidental (unintentional)	Poisoning, Intentional Self-harm	Poisoning, Assault	Poisoning, Undetermined	Adverse Effect	Under-dosing
Acetyldihydrocodeine	T40.2X1	T40.2X2	T40.2X3	T40.2X4	—	—
Acetyldihydrocodeinone	T40.2X1	T40.2X2	T40.2X3	T40.2X4	—	—
Acetylene (gas)	T59.891	T59.892	T59.893	T59.894	—	—
dichloride	T53.6X1	T53.6X2	T53.6X3	T53.6X4	—	—
incomplete combustion of	T58.11	T58.12	T58.13	T58.14	—	—
industrial	T59.891	T59.892	T59.893	T59.894	—	—
tetrachloride	T53.6X1	T53.6X2	T53.6X3	T53.6X4	—	—
vapor	T53.6X1	T53.6X2	T53.6X3	T53.6X4	—	—
Acetylpheneturide	T42.6X1	T42.6X2	T42.6X3	T42.6X4	T42.6X5	T42.6X6
Acetylphenylhydrazine	T39.8X1	T39.8X2	T39.8X3	T39.8X4	T39.8X5	T39.8X6
Acetylsalicylic acid (salts)	T39.011	T39.012	T39.013	T39.014	T39.015	T39.016
enteric coated	T39.011	T39.012	T39.013	T39.014	T39.015	T39.016
Acetylsulfamethoxypyridazine	T37.0X1	T37.0X2	T37.0X3	T37.0X4	T37.0X5	T37.0X6
Achromycin	T36.4X1	T36.4X2	T36.4X3	T36.4X4	T36.4X5	T36.4X6
ophthalmic preparation	T49.5X1	T49.5X2	T49.5X3	T49.5X4	T49.5X5	T49.5X6
topical NEC	T49.0X1	T49.0X2	T49.0X3	T49.0X4	T49.0X5	T49.0X6
Aciclovir	T37.5X1	T37.5X2	T37.5X3	T37.5X4	T37.5X5	T37.5X6
Acidifying agent NEC	T50.901	T50.902	T50.903	T50.904	T50.905	T50.906
Acid (corrosive) NEC	T54.2X1	T54.2X2	T54.2X3	T54.2X4	—	—
Acipimox	T46.6X1	T46.6X2	T46.6X3	T46.6X4	T46.6X5	T46.6X6
Acitretin	T50.991	T50.992	T50.993	T50.994	T50.995	T50.996
Aclarubicin	T45.1X1	T45.1X2	T45.1X3	T45.1X4	T45.1X5	T45.1X6
Aclatonium napadisilate	T48.1X1	T48.1X2	T48.1X3	T48.1X4	T48.1X5	T48.1X6
Aconite (wild)	T46.991	T46.992	T46.993	T46.994	T46.995	T46.996
Aconitine	T46.991	T46.992	T46.993	T46.994	T46.995	T46.996
Aconitum ferox	T46.991	T46.992	T46.993	T46.994	T46.995	T46.996
Acridine	T65.6X1	T65.6X2	T65.6X3	T65.6X4	—	—
vapor	T59.891	T59.892	T59.893	T59.894	—	—
Acriflavine	T37.91	T37.92	T37.93	T37.94	T37.95	T37.96
Acriflavinium chloride	T49.0X1	T49.0X2	T49.0X3	T49.0X4	T49.0X5	T49.0X6
Acrinol	T49.0X1	T49.0X2	T49.0X3	T49.0X4	T49.0X5	T49.0X6
Acrisorcin	T49.0X1	T49.0X2	T49.0X3	T49.0X4	T49.0X5	T49.0X6
Acrivastine	T45.0X1	T45.0X2	T45.0X3	T45.0X4	T45.0X5	T45.0X6
Acrolein (gas)	T59.891	T59.892	T59.893	T59.894	—	—
liquid	T54.1X1	T54.1X2	T54.1X3	T54.1X4	—	—
Acrylamide	T65.891	T65.892	T65.893	T65.894	—	—
Acrylic resin	T49.3X1	T49.3X2	T49.3X3	T49.3X4	T49.3X5	T49.3X6
Acrylonitrile	T65.891	T65.892	T65.893	T65.894	—	—
Actaea spicata	T62.2X1	T62.2X2	T62.2X3	T62.2X4	—	—
berry	T62.1X1	T62.1X2	T62.1X3	T62.1X4	—	—
Acterol	T37.3X1	T37.3X2	T37.3X3	T37.3X4	T37.3X5	T37.3X6
ACTH	T38.811	T38.812	T38.813	T38.814	T38.815	T38.816
Actinomycin C	T45.1X1	T45.1X2	T45.1X3	T45.1X4	T45.1X5	T45.1X6
Actinomycin D	T45.1X1	T45.1X2	T45.1X3	T45.1X4	T45.1X5	T45.1X6
Activated charcoal — see also Charcoal, medicinal	T47.6X1	T47.6X2	T47.6X3	T47.6X4	T47.6X5	T47.6X6
Acyclovir	T37.5X1	T37.5X2	T37.5X3	T37.5X4	T37.5X5	T37.5X6
Adenine	T45.2X1	T45.2X2	T45.2X3	T45.2X4	T45.2X5	T45.2X6
arabinoside	T37.5X1	T37.5X2	T37.5X3	T37.5X4	T37.5X5	T37.5X6
Adenosine (phosphate)	T46.2X1	T46.2X2	T46.2X3	T46.2X4	T46.2X5	T46.2X6
ADH	T38.891	T38.892	T38.893	T38.894	T38.895	T38.896
Adhesive NEC	T65.891	T65.892	T65.893	T65.894	—	—
Adicillin	T36.0X1	T36.0X2	T36.0X3	T36.0X4	T36.0X5	T36.0X6
Adiphenine	T44.3X1	T44.3X2	T44.3X3	T44.3X4	T44.3X5	T44.3X6
Adipiodone	T50.8X1	T50.8X2	T50.8X3	T50.8X4	T50.8X5	T50.8X6
Adjunct, pharmaceutical	T50.901	T50.902	T50.903	T50.904	T50.905	T50.906
Adrenal (extract, cortex or medulla) (glucocorticoids) (hormones) (mineralocorticoids)	T38.0X1	T38.0X2	T38.0X3	T38.0X4	T38.0X5	T38.0X6
ENT agent	T49.6X1	T49.6X2	T49.6X3	T49.6X4	T49.6X5	T49.6X6
ophthalmic preparation	T49.5X1	T49.5X2	T49.5X3	T49.5X4	T49.5X5	T49.5X6
topical NEC	T49.0X1	T49.0X2	T49.0X3	T49.0X4	T49.0X5	T49.0X6
Adrenalin — see Adrenaline						
Adrenaline	T44.5X1	T44.5X2	T44.5X3	T44.5X4	T44.5X5	T44.5X6
Adrenergic NEC	T44.901	T44.902	T44.903	T44.904	T44.905	T44.906
blocking agent NEC	T44.8X1	T44.8X2	T44.8X3	T44.8X4	T44.8X5	T44.8X6
beta, heart	T44.7X1	T44.7X2	T44.7X3	T44.7X4	T44.7X5	T44.7X6
specified NEC	T44.991	T44.992	T44.993	T44.994	T44.995	T44.996
Adrenochrome						
derivative	T46.991	T46.992	T46.993	T46.994	T46.995	T46.996
(mono) semicarbazone	T46.991	T46.992	T46.993	T46.994	T46.995	T46.996
Adrenocorticotrophic hormone	T38.811	T38.812	T38.813	T38.814	T38.815	T38.816
Adrenocorticotrophin	T38.811	T38.812	T38.813	T38.814	T38.815	T38.816
Adriamycin	T45.1X1	T45.1X2	T45.1X3	T45.1X4	T45.1X5	T45.1X6
Aerosol spray NEC	T65.91	T65.92	T65.93	T65.94	—	—
Aerosporin	T36.8X1	T36.8X2	T36.8X3	T36.8X4	T36.8X5	T36.8X6
ENT agent	T49.6X1	T49.6X2	T49.6X3	T49.6X4	T49.6X5	T49.6X6
ophthalmic preparation	T49.5X1	T49.5X2	T49.5X3	T49.5X4	T49.5X5	T49.5X6
topical NEC	T49.0X1	T49.0X2	T49.0X3	T49.0X4	T49.0X5	T49.0X6
Aethusa cynapium	T62.2X1	T62.2X2	T62.2X3	T62.2X4	—	—
Afghanistan black	T40.7X1	T40.7X2	T40.7X3	T40.7X4	T40.7X5	T40.7X6

Table of Drugs and Chemicals

Aflatoxin — Amanita phalloides

Substance	Poisoning, Accidental (unintentional)	Poisoning, Intentional Self-harm	Poisoning, Assault	Poisoning, Undetermined	Adverse Effect	Under-dosing
Aflatoxin	T64.01	T64.02	T64.03	T64.04	—	—
Afloqualone	T42.8X1	T42.8X2	T42.8X3	T42.8X4	T42.8X5	T42.8X6
African boxwood	T62.2X1	T62.2X2	T62.2X3	T62.2X4	—	—
Agar	T47.4X1	T47.4X2	T47.4X3	T47.4X4	T47.4X5	T47.4X6
Agonist						
predominantly						
alpha-adrenoreceptor	T44.4X1	T44.4X2	T44.4X3	T44.4X4	T44.4X5	T44.4X6
beta-adrenoreceptor	T44.5X1	T44.5X2	T44.5X3	T44.5X4	T44.5X5	T44.5X6
Agricultural agent NEC	T65.91	T65.92	T65.93	T65.94	—	—
Agrypnal	T42.3X1	T42.3X2	T42.3X3	T42.3X4	T42.3X5	T42.3X6
AHLG	T50.Z11	T50.Z12	T50.Z13	T50.Z14	T50.Z15	T50.Z16
Air contaminant(s), source/type NOS	T65.91	T65.92	T65.93	T65.94	—	—
Ajmaline	T46.2X1	T46.2X2	T46.2X3	T46.2X4	T46.2X5	T46.2X6
Akee	T62.1X1	T62.1X2	T62.1X3	T62.1X4	—	—
Akrinol	T49.0X1	T49.0X2	T49.0X3	T49.0X4	T49.0X5	T49.0X6
Akritoin	T37.8X1	T37.8X2	T37.8X3	T37.8X4	T37.8X5	T37.8X6
Alacepril	T46.4X1	T46.4X2	T46.4X3	T46.4X4	T46.4X5	T46.4X6
Alantolactone	T37.4X1	T37.4X2	T37.4X3	T37.4X4	T37.4X5	T37.4X6
Albamycin	T36.8X1	T36.8X2	T36.8X3	T36.8X4	T36.8X5	T36.8X6
Albendazole	T37.4X1	T37.4X2	T37.4X3	T37.4X4	T37.4X5	T37.4X6
Albumin						
bovine	T45.8X1	T45.8X2	T45.8X3	T45.8X4	T45.8X5	T45.8X6
human serum	T45.8X1	T45.8X2	T45.8X3	T45.8X4	T45.8X5	T45.8X6
salt-poor	T45.8X1	T45.8X2	T45.8X3	T45.8X4	T45.8X5	T45.8X6
normal human serum	T45.8X1	T45.8X2	T45.8X3	T45.8X4	T45.8X5	T45.8X6
Albuterol	T48.6X1	T48.6X2	T48.6X3	T48.6X4	T48.6X5	T48.6X6
Albutoin	T42.0X1	T42.0X2	T42.0X3	T42.0X4	T42.0X5	T42.0X6
Alclometasone	T49.0X1	T49.0X2	T49.0X3	T49.0X4	T49.0X5	T49.0X6
Alcohol	T51.91	T51.92	T51.93	T51.94	—	—
absolute	T51.0X1	T51.0X2	T51.0X3	T51.0X4	—	—
beverage	T51.0X1	T51.0X2	T51.0X3	T51.0X4	—	—
allyl	T51.8X1	T51.8X2	T51.8X3	T51.8X4	—	—
amyl	T51.3X1	T51.3X2	T51.3X3	T51.3X4	—	—
antifreeze	T51.1X1	T51.1X2	T51.1X3	T51.1X4	—	—
beverage	T51.0X1	T51.0X2	T51.0X3	T51.0X4	—	—
butyl	T51.3X1	T51.3X2	T51.3X3	T51.3X4	—	—
dehydrated	T51.0X1	T51.0X2	T51.0X3	T51.0X4	—	—
beverage	T51.0X1	T51.0X2	T51.0X3	T51.0X4	—	—
denatured	T51.0X1	T51.0X2	T51.0X3	T51.0X4	—	—
deterrent NEC	T50.6X1	T50.6X2	T50.6X3	T50.6X4	T50.6X5	T50.6X6
diagnostic (gastric function)	T50.8X1	T50.8X2	T50.8X3	T50.8X4	T50.8X5	T50.8X6
ethyl	T51.0X1	T51.0X2	T51.0X3	T51.0X4	—	—
beverage	T51.0X1	T51.0X2	T51.0X3	T51.0X4	—	—
grain	T51.0X1	T51.0X2	T51.0X3	T51.0X4	—	—
beverage	T51.0X1	T51.0X2	T51.0X3	T51.0X4	—	—
industrial	T51.0X1	T51.0X2	T51.0X3	T51.0X4	—	—
isopropyl	T51.2X1	T51.2X2	T51.2X3	T51.2X4	—	—
methyl	T51.1X1	T51.1X2	T51.1X3	T51.1X4	—	—
preparation for consumption	T51.0X1	T51.0X2	T51.0X3	T51.0X4	—	—
propyl	T51.3X1	T51.3X2	T51.3X3	T51.3X4	—	—
secondary	T51.2X1	T51.2X2	T51.2X3	T51.2X4	—	—
radiator	T51.1X1	T51.1X2	T51.1X3	T51.1X4	—	—
rubbing	T51.2X1	T51.2X2	T51.2X3	T51.2X4	—	—
specified type NEC	T51.8X1	T51.8X2	T51.8X3	T51.8X4	—	—
surgical	T51.0X1	T51.0X2	T51.0X3	T51.0X4	—	—
vapor (from any type of Alcohol)	T59.891	T59.892	T59.893	T59.894	—	—
wood	T51.1X1	T51.1X2	T51.1X3	T51.1X4	—	—
Alcuronium (chloride)	T48.1X1	T48.1X2	T48.1X3	T48.1X4	T48.1X5	T48.1X6
Aldactone	T50.0X1	T50.0X2	T50.0X3	T50.0X4	T50.0X5	T50.0X6
Aldesulfone sodium	T37.1X1	T37.1X2	T37.1X3	T37.1X4	T37.1X5	T37.1X6
Aldicarb	T60.0X1	T60.0X2	T60.0X3	T60.0X4	—	—
Aldomet	T46.5X1	T46.5X2	T46.5X3	T46.5X4	T46.5X5	T46.5X6
Aldosterone	T50.0X1	T50.0X2	T50.0X3	T50.0X4	T50.0X5	T50.0X6
Aldrin (dust)	T60.1X1	T60.1X2	T60.1X3	T60.1X4	—	—
Aleve — see Naproxen						
Alexitol sodium	T47.1X1	T47.1X2	T47.1X3	T47.1X4	T47.1X5	T47.1X6
Alfacalcidol	T45.2X1	T45.2X2	T45.2X3	T45.2X4	T45.2X5	T45.2X6
Alfadolone	T41.1X1	T41.1X2	T41.1X3	T41.1X4	T41.1X5	T41.1X6
Alfaxalone	T41.1X1	T41.1X2	T41.1X3	T41.1X4	T41.1X5	T41.1X6
Alfentanil	T40.4X1	T40.4X2	T40.4X3	T40.4X4	T40.4X5	T40.4X6
Alfuzosin (hydrochloride)	T44.8X1	T44.8X2	T44.8X3	T44.8X4	T44.8X5	T44.8X6
Algae (harmful) (toxin)	T65.821	T65.822	T65.823	T65.824	—	—
Algeldrate	T47.1X1	T47.1X2	T47.1X3	T47.1X4	T47.1X5	T47.1X6
Algin	T47.8X1	T47.8X2	T47.8X3	T47.8X4	T47.8X5	T47.8X6
Alglucerase	T45.3X1	T45.3X2	T45.3X3	T45.3X4	T45.3X5	T45.3X6
Alidase	T45.3X1	T45.3X2	T45.3X3	T45.3X4	T45.3X5	T45.3X6
Alimemazine	T43.3X1	T43.3X2	T43.3X3	T43.3X4	T43.3X5	T43.3X6
Aliphatic thiocyanates	T65.0X1	T65.0X2	T65.0X3	T65.0X4	—	—
Alizapride	T45.0X1	T45.0X2	T45.0X3	T45.0X4	T45.0X5	T45.0X6

Substance	Poisoning, Accidental (unintentional)	Poisoning, Intentional Self-harm	Poisoning, Assault	Poisoning, Undetermined	Adverse Effect	Under-dosing
Alkali (caustic)	T54.3X1	T54.3X2	T54.3X3	T54.3X4	—	—
Alkaline antiseptic solution (aromatic)	T49.6X1	T49.6X2	T49.6X3	T49.6X4	T49.6X5	T49.6X6
Alkalinizing agents (medicinal)	T50.901	T50.902	T50.903	T50.904	T50.905	T50.906
Alkalizing agent NEC	T50.901	T50.902	T50.903	T50.904	T50.905	T50.906
Alka-seltzer	T39.011	T39.012	T39.013	T39.014	T39.015	T39.016
Alkavervir	T46.5X1	T46.5X2	T46.5X3	T46.5X4	T46.5X5	T46.5X6
Alkonium (bromide)	T49.0X1	T49.0X2	T49.0X3	T49.0X4	T49.0X5	T49.0X6
Alkylating drug NEC	T45.1X1	T45.1X2	T45.1X3	T45.1X4	T45.1X5	T45.1X6
antimyeloproliferative	T45.1X1	T45.1X2	T45.1X3	T45.1X4	T45.1X5	T45.1X6
lymphatic	T45.1X1	T45.1X2	T45.1X3	T45.1X4	T45.1X5	T45.1X6
Alkylisocyanate	T65.0X1	T65.0X2	T65.0X3	T65.0X4	—	—
Allantoin	T49.4X1	T49.4X2	T49.4X3	T49.4X4	T49.4X5	T49.4X6
Allegron	T43.011	T43.012	T43.013	T43.014	T43.015	T43.016
Allethrin	T49.0X1	T49.0X2	T49.0X3	T49.0X4	T49.0X5	T49.0X6
Allobarbital	T42.3X1	T42.3X2	T42.3X3	T42.3X4	T42.3X5	T42.3X6
Allopurinol	T50.4X1	T50.4X2	T50.4X3	T50.4X4	T50.4X5	T50.4X6
Allyl						
alcohol	T51.8X1	T51.8X2	T51.8X3	T51.8X4	—	—
disulfide	T46.6X1	T46.6X2	T46.6X3	T46.6X4	T46.6X5	T46.6X6
Allylestrenol	T38.5X1	T38.5X2	T38.5X3	T38.5X4	T38.5X5	T38.5X6
Allylisopropylacetylurea	T42.6X1	T42.6X2	T42.6X3	T42.6X4	T42.6X5	T42.6X6
Allylisopropylmalonylurea	T42.3X1	T42.3X2	T42.3X3	T42.3X4	T42.3X5	T42.3X6
Allylthiourea	T49.3X1	T49.3X2	T49.3X3	T49.3X4	T49.3X5	T49.3X6
Allyltribromide	T42.6X1	T42.6X2	T42.6X3	T42.6X4	T42.6X5	T42.6X6
Allypropymal	T42.3X1	T42.3X2	T42.3X3	T42.3X4	T42.3X5	T42.3X6
Almagate	T47.1X1	T47.1X2	T47.1X3	T47.1X4	T47.1X5	T47.1X6
Almasilate	T47.1X1	T47.1X2	T47.1X3	T47.1X4	T47.1X5	T47.1X6
Almitrine	T50.7X1	T50.7X2	T50.7X3	T50.7X4	T50.7X5	T50.7X6
Aloes	T47.2X1	T47.2X2	T47.2X3	T47.2X4	T47.2X5	T47.2X6
Aloglutamol	T47.1X1	T47.1X2	T47.1X3	T47.1X4	T47.1X5	T47.1X6
Aloin	T47.2X1	T47.2X2	T47.2X3	T47.2X4	T47.2X5	T47.2X6
Aloxidone	T42.2X1	T42.2X2	T42.2X3	T42.2X4	T42.2X5	T42.2X6
Alpha						
acetyldigoxin	T46.0X1	T46.0X2	T46.0X3	T46.0X4	T46.0X5	T46.0X6
adrenergic blocking drug	T44.6X1	T44.6X2	T44.6X3	T44.6X4	T44.6X5	T44.6X6
amylase	T45.3X1	T45.3X2	T45.3X3	T45.3X4	T45.3X5	T45.3X6
tocoferol (acetate)	T45.2X1	T45.2X2	T45.2X3	T45.2X4	T45.2X5	T45.2X6
tocopherol	T45.2X1	T45.2X2	T45.2X3	T45.2X4	T45.2X5	T45.2X6
Alphadolone	T41.1X1	T41.1X2	T41.1X3	T41.1X4	T41.1X5	T41.1X6
Alphaprodine	T40.4X1	T40.4X2	T40.4X3	T40.4X4	T40.4X5	T40.4X6
Alphaxalone	T41.1X1	T41.1X2	T41.1X3	T41.1X4	T41.1X5	T41.1X6
Alprazolam	T42.4X1	T42.4X2	T42.4X3	T42.4X4	T42.4X5	T42.4X6
Alprenolol	T44.7X1	T44.7X2	T44.7X3	T44.7X4	T44.7X5	T44.7X6
Alprostadil	T46.7X1	T46.7X2	T46.7X3	T46.7X4	T46.7X5	T46.7X6
Alsactide	T38.811	T38.812	T38.813	T38.814	T38.815	T38.816
Alseroxylon	T46.5X1	T46.5X2	T46.5X3	T46.5X4	T46.5X5	T46.5X6
Alteplase	T45.611	T45.612	T45.613	T45.614	T45.615	T45.616
Altizide	T50.2X1	T50.2X2	T50.2X3	T50.2X4	T50.2X5	T50.2X6
Altretamine	T45.1X1	T45.1X2	T45.1X3	T45.1X4	T45.1X5	T45.1X6
Alum (medicinal)	T49.4X1	T49.4X2	T49.4X3	T49.4X4	T49.4X5	T49.4X6
nonmedicinal (ammonium) (potassium)	T56.891	T56.892	T56.893	T56.894	—	—
Aluminium, aluminum						
acetate	T49.2X1	T49.2X2	T49.2X3	T49.2X4	T49.2X5	T49.2X6
solution	T49.0X1	T49.0X2	T49.0X3	T49.0X4	T49.0X5	T49.0X6
aspirin	T39.011	T39.012	T39.013	T39.014	T39.015	T39.016
bis (acetylsalicylate)	T39.011	T39.012	T39.013	T39.014	T39.015	T39.016
carbonate (gel, basic)	T47.1X1	T47.1X2	T47.1X3	T47.1X4	T47.1X5	T47.1X6
chlorhydroxide-complex	T47.1X1	T47.1X2	T47.1X3	T47.1X4	T47.1X5	T47.1X6
chloride	T49.2X1	T49.2X2	T49.2X3	T49.2X4	T49.2X5	T49.2X6
clofibrate	T46.6X1	T46.6X2	T46.6X3	T46.6X4	T46.6X5	T46.6X6
diacetate	T49.2X1	T49.2X2	T49.2X3	T49.2X4	T49.2X5	T49.2X6
glycinate	T47.1X1	T47.1X2	T47.1X3	T47.1X4	T47.1X5	T47.1X6
hydroxide (gel)	T47.1X1	T47.1X2	T47.1X3	T47.1X4	T47.1X5	T47.1X6
hydroxide-magnesium carb. gel	T47.1X1	T47.1X2	T47.1X3	T47.1X4	T47.1X5	T47.1X6
magnesium silicate	T47.1X1	T47.1X2	T47.1X3	T47.1X4	T47.1X5	T47.1X6
nicotinate	T46.7X1	T46.7X2	T46.7X3	T46.7X4	T46.7X5	T46.7X6
ointment (surgical) (topical)	T49.3X1	T49.3X2	T49.3X3	T49.3X4	T49.3X5	T49.3X6
phosphate	T47.1X1	T47.1X2	T47.1X3	T47.1X4	T47.1X5	T47.1X6
salicylate	T39.091	T39.092	T39.093	T39.094	T39.095	T39.096
silicate	T47.1X1	T47.1X2	T47.1X3	T47.1X4	T47.1X5	T47.1X6
sodium silicate	T47.1X1	T47.1X2	T47.1X3	T47.1X4	T47.1X5	T47.1X6
subacetate	T49.2X1	T49.2X2	T49.2X3	T49.2X4	T49.2X5	T49.2X6
sulfate	T49.0X1	T49.0X2	T49.0X3	T49.0X4	T49.0X5	T49.0X6
tannate	T47.6X1	T47.6X2	T47.6X3	T47.6X4	T47.6X5	T47.6X6
topical NEC	T49.3X1	T49.3X2	T49.3X3	T49.3X4	T49.3X5	T49.3X6
Alurate	T42.3X1	T42.3X2	T42.3X3	T42.3X4	T42.3X5	T42.3X6
Alverine	T44.3X1	T44.3X2	T44.3X3	T44.3X4	T44.3X5	T44.3X6
Alvodine	T40.2X1	T40.2X2	T40.2X3	T40.2X4	T40.2X5	T40.2X6
Amanita phalloides	T62.0X1	T62.0X2	T62.0X3	T62.0X4	—	—

Additional Character May Be Required — Refer to the Tabular List for Character Selection   ▽ Subterms under main terms may continue to next column or page

Substance	Poisoning, Accidental (unintentional)	Poisoning, Intentional Self-harm	Poisoning, Assault	Poisoning, Undetermined	Adverse Effect	Under-dosing
Amanitine	T62.0X1	T62.0X2	T62.0X3	T62.0X4	—	—
Amantadine	T42.8X1	T42.8X2	T42.8X3	T42.8X4	T42.8X5	T42.8X6
Ambazone	T49.6X1	T49.6X2	T49.6X3	T49.6X4	T49.6X5	T49.6X6
Ambenonium (chloride)	T44.0X1	T44.0X2	T44.0X3	T44.0X4	T44.0X5	T44.0X6
Ambroxol	T48.4X1	T48.4X2	T48.4X3	T48.4X4	T48.4X5	T48.4X6
Ambuphylline	T48.6X1	T48.6X2	T48.6X3	T48.6X4	T48.6X5	T48.6X6
Ambutonium bromide	T44.3X1	T44.3X2	T44.3X3	T44.3X4	T44.3X5	T44.3X6
Amcinonide	T49.0X1	T49.0X2	T49.0X3	T49.0X4	T49.0X5	T49.0X6
Amdinocilline	T36.0X1	T36.0X2	T36.0X3	T36.0X4	T36.0X5	T36.0X6
Ametazole	T50.8X1	T50.8X2	T50.8X3	T50.8X4	T50.8X5	T50.8X6
Amethocaine	T41.3X1	T41.3X2	T41.3X3	T41.3X4	T41.3X5	T41.3X6
regional	T41.3X1	T41.3X2	T41.3X3	T41.3X4	T41.3X5	T41.3X6
spinal	T41.3X1	T41.3X2	T41.3X3	T41.3X4	T41.3X5	T41.3X6
Amethopterin	T45.1X1	T45.1X2	T45.1X3	T45.1X4	T45.1X5	T45.1X6
Amezinium metilsulfate	T44.991	T44.992	T44.993	T44.994	T44.995	T44.996
Amfebutamone	T43.291	T43.292	T43.293	T43.294	T43.295	T43.296
Amfepramone	T50.5X1	T50.5X2	T50.5X3	T50.5X4	T50.5X5	T50.5X6
Amfetamine	T43.621	T43.622	T43.623	T43.624	T43.625	T43.626
Amfetaminil	T43.621	T43.622	T43.623	T43.624	T43.625	T43.626
Amfomycin	T36.8X1	T36.8X2	T36.8X3	T36.8X4	T36.8X5	T36.8X6
Amidefrine mesilate	T48.5X1	T48.5X2	T48.5X3	T48.5X4	T48.5X5	T48.5X6
Amidone	T40.3X1	T40.3X2	T40.3X3	T40.3X4	T40.3X5	T40.3X6
Amidopyrine	T39.2X1	T39.2X2	T39.2X3	T39.2X4	T39.2X5	T39.2X6
Amidotrizoate	T50.8X1	T50.8X2	T50.8X3	T50.8X4	T50.8X5	T50.8X6
Amiflamine	T43.1X1	T43.1X2	T43.1X3	T43.1X4	T43.1X5	T43.1X6
Amikacin	T36.5X1	T36.5X2	T36.5X3	T36.5X4	T36.5X5	T36.5X6
Amikhelline	T46.3X1	T46.3X2	T46.3X3	T46.3X4	T46.3X5	T46.3X6
Amiloride	T50.2X1	T50.2X2	T50.2X3	T50.2X4	T50.2X5	T50.2X6
Aminacrine	T49.0X1	T49.0X2	T49.0X3	T49.0X4	T49.0X5	T49.0X6
Amineptine	T43.011	T43.012	T43.013	T43.014	T43.015	T43.016
Aminitrozole	T37.3X1	T37.3X2	T37.3X3	T37.3X4	T37.3X5	T37.3X6
Aminoacetic acid (derivatives)	T50.3X1	T50.3X2	T50.3X3	T50.3X4	T50.3X5	T50.3X6
Amino acids	T50.3X1	T50.3X2	T50.3X3	T50.3X4	T50.3X5	T50.3X6
Aminoacridine	T49.0X1	T49.0X2	T49.0X3	T49.0X4	T49.0X5	T49.0X6
Aminobenzoic acid (-p)	T49.3X1	T49.3X2	T49.3X3	T49.3X4	T49.3X5	T49.3X6
Aminocaproic acid	T45.621	T45.622	T45.623	T45.624	T45.625	T45.626
Aminoethylisothiourium	T45.8X1	T45.8X2	T45.8X3	T45.8X4	T45.8X5	T45.8X6
Aminofenazone	T39.2X1	T39.2X2	T39.2X3	T39.2X4	T39.2X5	T39.2X6
Aminoglutethimide	T45.1X1	T45.1X2	T45.1X3	T45.1X4	T45.1X5	T45.1X6
Aminohippuric acid	T50.8X1	T50.8X2	T50.8X3	T50.8X4	T50.8X5	T50.8X6
Aminomethylbenzoic acid	T45.691	T45.692	T45.693	T45.694	T45.695	T45.696
Aminometradine	T50.2X1	T50.2X2	T50.2X3	T50.2X4	T50.2X5	T50.2X6
Aminopentamide	T44.3X1	T44.3X2	T44.3X3	T44.3X4	T44.3X5	T44.3X6
Aminophenazone	T39.2X1	T39.2X2	T39.2X3	T39.2X4	T39.2X5	T39.2X6
Aminophenol	T54.0X1	T54.0X2	T54.0X3	T54.0X4	—	—
Aminophenylpyridone	T43.591	T43.592	T43.593	T43.594	T43.595	T43.596
Aminophylline	T48.6X1	T48.6X2	T48.6X3	T48.6X4	T48.6X5	T48.6X6
Aminopterin sodium	T45.1X1	T45.1X2	T45.1X3	T45.1X4	T45.1X5	T45.1X6
Aminopyrine	T39.2X1	T39.2X2	T39.2X3	T39.2X4	T39.2X5	T39.2X6
Aminorex	T50.5X1	T50.5X2	T50.5X3	T50.5X4	T50.5X5	T50.5X6
Aminosalicylic acid	T37.1X1	T37.1X2	T37.1X3	T37.1X4	T37.1X5	T37.1X6
Aminosalylum	T37.1X1	T37.1X2	T37.1X3	T37.1X4	T37.1X5	T37.1X6
Amiodarone	T46.2X1	T46.2X2	T46.2X3	T46.2X4	T46.2X5	T46.2X6
Amiphenazole	T50.7X1	T50.7X2	T50.7X3	T50.7X4	T50.7X5	T50.7X6
Amiquinsin	T46.5X1	T46.5X2	T46.5X3	T46.5X4	T46.5X5	T46.5X6
Amisometradine	T50.2X1	T50.2X2	T50.2X3	T50.2X4	T50.2X5	T50.2X6
Amisulpride	T43.591	T43.592	T43.593	T43.594	T43.595	T43.596
Amitriptyline	T43.011	T43.012	T43.013	T43.014	T43.015	T43.016
Amitriptylinoxide	T43.011	T43.012	T43.013	T43.014	T43.015	T43.016
Amlexanox	T48.6X1	T48.6X2	T48.6X3	T48.6X4	T48.6X5	T48.6X6
Ammonia (fumes) (gas) (vapor)	T59.891	T59.892	T59.893	T59.894	—	—
aromatic spirit	T48.991	T48.992	T48.993	T48.994	T48.995	T48.996
liquid (household)	T54.3X1	T54.3X2	T54.3X3	T54.3X4	—	—
Ammoniated mercury	T49.0X1	T49.0X2	T49.0X3	T49.0X4	T49.0X5	T49.0X6
Ammonium						
acid tartrate	T49.5X1	T49.5X2	T49.5X3	T49.5X4	T49.5X5	T49.5X6
bromide	T42.6X1	T42.6X2	T42.6X3	T42.6X4	T42.6X5	T42.6X6
carbonate	T54.3X1	T54.3X2	T54.3X3	T54.3X4	—	—
chloride	T50.991	T50.992	T50.993	T50.994	T50.995	T50.996
expectorant	T48.4X1	T48.4X2	T48.4X3	T48.4X4	T48.4X5	T48.4X6
compounds (household) NEC	T54.3X1	T54.3X2	T54.3X3	T54.3X4	—	—
fumes (any usage)	T59.891	T59.892	T59.893	T59.894	—	—
industrial	T54.3X1	T54.3X2	T54.3X3	T54.3X4	—	—
ichthyosulronate	T49.4X1	T49.4X2	T49.4X3	T49.4X4	T49.4X5	T49.4X6
mandelate	T37.91	T37.92	T37.93	T37.94	T37.95	T37.96
sulfamate	T60.3X1	T60.3X2	T60.3X3	T60.3X4	—	—
sulfonate resin	T47.8X1	T47.8X2	T47.8X3	T47.8X4	T47.8X5	T47.8X6
Amobarbital (sodium)	T42.3X1	T42.3X2	T42.3X3	T42.3X4	T42.3X5	T42.3X6
Amodiaquine	T37.2X1	T37.2X2	T37.2X3	T37.2X4	T37.2X5	T37.2X6
Amopyroquin (e)	T37.2X1	T37.2X2	T37.2X3	T37.2X4	T37.2X5	T37.2X6

Substance	Poisoning, Accidental (unintentional)	Poisoning, Intentional Self-harm	Poisoning, Assault	Poisoning, Undetermined	Adverse Effect	Under-dosing
Amoxapine	T43.011	T43.012	T43.013	T43.014	T43.015	T43.016
Amoxicillin	T36.0X1	T36.0X2	T36.0X3	T36.0X4	T36.0X5	T36.0X6
Amperozide	T43.591	T43.592	T43.593	T43.594	T43.595	T43.596
Amphenidone	T43.591	T43.592	T43.593	T43.594	T43.595	T43.596
Amphetamine NEC	T43.621	T43.622	T43.623	T43.624	T43.625	T43.626
Amphomycin	T36.8X1	T36.8X2	T36.8X3	T36.8X4	T36.8X5	T36.8X6
Amphotalide	T37.4X1	T37.4X2	T37.4X3	T37.4X4	T37.4X5	T37.4X6
Amphotericin B	T36.7X1	T36.7X2	T36.7X3	T36.7X4	T36.7X5	T36.7X6
topical	T49.0X1	T49.0X2	T49.0X3	T49.0X4	T49.0X5	T49.0X6
Ampicillin	T36.0X1	T36.0X2	T36.0X3	T36.0X4	T36.0X5	T36.0X6
Amprotropine	T44.3X1	T44.3X2	T44.3X3	T44.3X4	T44.3X5	T44.3X6
Amsacrine	T45.1X1	T45.1X2	T45.1X3	T45.1X4	T45.1X5	T45.1X6
Amygdaline	T62.2X1	T62.2X2	T62.2X3	T62.2X4	—	—
Amyl						
acetate	T52.8X1	T52.8X2	T52.8X3	T52.8X4	—	—
vapor	T59.891	T59.892	T59.893	T59.894	—	—
alcohol	T51.3X1	T51.3X2	T51.3X3	T51.3X4	—	—
chloride	T53.6X1	T53.6X2	T53.6X3	T53.6X4	—	—
formate	T52.8X1	T52.8X2	T52.8X3	T52.8X4	—	—
nitrite	T46.3X1	T46.3X2	T46.3X3	T46.3X4	T46.3X5	T46.3X6
propionate	T65.891	T65.892	T65.893	T65.894	—	—
Amylase	T47.5X1	T47.5X2	T47.5X3	T47.5X4	T47.5X5	T47.5X6
Amyleine, regional	T41.3X1	T41.3X2	T41.3X3	T41.3X4	T41.3X5	T41.3X6
Amylene						
dichloride	T53.6X1	T53.6X2	T53.6X3	T53.6X4	—	—
hydrate	T51.3X1	T51.3X2	T51.3X3	T51.3X4	—	—
Amylmetacresol	T49.6X1	T49.6X2	T49.6X3	T49.6X4	T49.6X5	T49.6X6
Amylobarbitone	T42.3X1	T42.3X2	T42.3X3	T42.3X4	T42.3X5	T42.3X6
Amylocaine, regional	T41.3X1	T41.3X2	T41.3X3	T41.3X4	T41.3X5	T41.3X6
infiltration (subcutaneous)	T41.3X1	T41.3X2	T41.3X3	T41.3X4	T41.3X5	T41.3X6
nerve block (peripheral) (plexus)	T41.3X1	T41.3X2	T41.3X3	T41.3X4	T41.3X5	T41.3X6
spinal	T41.3X1	T41.3X2	T41.3X3	T41.3X4	T41.3X5	T41.3X6
topical (surface)	T41.3X1	T41.3X2	T41.3X3	T41.3X4	T41.3X5	T41.3X6
Amylopectin	T47.6X1	T47.6X2	T47.6X3	T47.6X4	T47.6X5	T47.6X6
Amytal (sodium)	T42.3X1	T42.3X2	T42.3X3	T42.3X4	T42.3X5	T42.3X6
Anabolic steroid	T38.7X1	T38.7X2	T38.7X3	T38.7X4	T38.7X5	T38.7X6
Analeptic NEC	T50.7X1	T50.7X2	T50.7X3	T50.7X4	T50.7X5	T50.7X6
Analgesic	T39.91	T39.92	T39.93	T39.94	T39.95	T39.96
anti-inflammatory NEC	T39.91	T39.92	T39.93	T39.94	T39.95	T39.96
propionic acid derivative	T39.311	T39.312	T39.313	T39.314	T39.315	T39.316
antirheumatic NEC	T39.4X1	T39.4X2	T39.4X3	T39.4X4	T39.4X5	T39.4X6
aromatic NEC	T39.1X1	T39.1X2	T39.1X3	T39.1X4	T39.1X5	T39.1X6
narcotic NEC	T40.601	T40.602	T40.603	T40.604	T40.605	T40.606
combination	T40.601	T40.602	T40.603	T40.604	T40.605	T40.606
obstetric	T40.601	T40.602	T40.603	T40.604	T40.605	T40.606
non-narcotic NEC	T39.91	T39.92	T39.93	T39.94	T39.95	T39.96
combination	T39.91	T39.92	T39.93	T39.94	T39.95	T39.96
pyrazole	T39.2X1	T39.2X2	T39.2X3	T39.2X4	T39.2X5	T39.2X6
specified NEC	T39.8X1	T39.8X2	T39.8X3	T39.8X4	T39.8X5	T39.8X6
Analgin	T39.2X1	T39.2X2	T39.2X3	T39.2X4	T39.2X5	T39.2X6
Anamirta cocculus	T62.1X1	T62.1X2	T62.1X3	T62.1X4	—	—
Ancillin	T36.0X1	T36.0X2	T36.0X3	T36.0X4	T36.0X5	T36.0X6
Ancrod	T45.691	T45.692	T45.693	T45.694	T45.695	T45.696
Androgen	T38.7X1	T38.7X2	T38.7X3	T38.7X4	T38.7X5	T38.7X6
Androgen-estrogen mixture	T38.7X1	T38.7X2	T38.7X3	T38.7X4	T38.7X5	T38.7X6
Androstalone	T38.7X1	T38.7X2	T38.7X3	T38.7X4	T38.7X5	T38.7X6
Androstanolone	T38.7X1	T38.7X2	T38.7X3	T38.7X4	T38.7X5	T38.7X6
Androsterone	T38.7X1	T38.7X2	T38.7X3	T38.7X4	T38.7X5	T38.7X6
Anemone pulsatilla	T62.2X1	T62.2X2	T62.2X3	T62.2X4	—	—
Anesthesia						
caudal	T41.3X1	T41.3X2	T41.3X3	T41.3X4	T41.3X5	T41.3X6
endotracheal	T41.0X1	T41.0X2	T41.0X3	T41.0X4	T41.0X5	T41.0X6
epidural	T41.3X1	T41.3X2	T41.3X3	T41.3X4	T41.3X5	T41.3X6
inhalation	T41.0X1	T41.0X2	T41.0X3	T41.0X4	T41.0X5	T41.0X6
local	T41.3X1	T41.3X2	T41.3X3	T41.3X4	T41.3X5	T41.3X6
mucosal	T41.3X1	T41.3X2	T41.3X3	T41.3X4	T41.3X5	T41.3X6
muscle relaxation	T48.1X1	T48.1X2	T48.1X3	T48.1X4	T48.1X5	T48.1X6
nerve blocking	T41.3X1	T41.3X2	T41.3X3	T41.3X4	T41.3X5	T41.3X6
plexus blocking	T41.3X1	T41.3X2	T41.3X3	T41.3X4	T41.3X5	T41.3X6
potentiated	T41.201	T41.202	T41.203	T41.204	T41.205	T41.206
rectal	T41.201	T41.202	T41.203	T41.204	T41.205	T41.206
general	T41.201	T41.202	T41.203	T41.204	T41.205	T41.206
local	T41.3X1	T41.3X2	T41.3X3	T41.3X4	T41.3X5	T41.3X6
regional	T41.3X1	T41.3X2	T41.3X3	T41.3X4	T41.3X5	T41.3X6
surface	T41.3X1	T41.3X2	T41.3X3	T41.3X4	T41.3X5	T41.3X6
Anesthetic NEC — see also Anesthesia	T41.41	T41.42	T41.43	T41.44	T41.45	T41.46
with muscle relaxant	T41.201	T41.202	T41.203	T41.204	T41.205	T41.206
general	T41.201	T41.202	T41.203	T41.204	T41.205	T41.206
local	T41.3X1	T41.3X2	T41.3X3	T41.3X4	T41.3X5	T41.3X6
gaseous NEC	T41.0X1	T41.0X2	T41.0X3	T41.0X4	T41.0X5	T41.0X6

Table of Drugs and Chemicals

Substance	Poisoning, Accidental (unintentional)	Poisoning, Intentional Self-harm	Poisoning, Assault	Poisoning, Undetermined	Adverse Effect	Under-dosing
Anesthetic — *see also* Anesthesia — continued						
general NEC	T41.201	T41.202	T41.203	T41.204	T41.205	T41.206
halogenated hydrocarbon derivatives NEC	T41.0X1	T41.0X2	T41.0X3	T41.0X4	T41.0X5	T41.0X6
infiltration NEC	T41.3X1	T41.3X2	T41.3X3	T41.3X4	T41.3X5	T41.3X6
intravenous NEC	T41.1X1	T41.1X2	T41.1X3	T41.1X4	T41.1X5	T41.1X6
local NEC	T41.3X1	T41.3X2	T41.3X3	T41.3X4	T41.3X5	T41.3X6
rectal	T41.201	T41.202	T41.203	T41.204	T41.205	T41.206
general	T41.201	T41.202	T41.203	T41.204	T41.205	T41.206
local	T41.3X1	T41.3X2	T41.3X3	T41.3X4	T41.3X5	T41.3X6
regional NEC	T41.3X1	T41.3X2	T41.3X3	T41.3X4	T41.3X5	T41.3X6
spinal NEC	T41.3X1	T41.3X2	T41.3X3	T41.3X4	T41.3X5	T41.3X6
thiobarbiturate	T41.1X1	T41.1X2	T41.1X3	T41.1X4	T41.1X5	T41.1X6
topical	T41.3X1	T41.3X2	T41.3X3	T41.3X4	T41.3X5	T41.3X6
Aneurine	T45.2X1	T45.2X2	T45.2X3	T45.2X4	T45.2X5	T45.2X6
Angio-Conray	T50.8X1	T50.8X2	T50.8X3	T50.8X4	T50.8X5	T50.8X6
Angiotensin	T44.5X1	T44.5X2	T44.5X3	T44.5X4	T44.5X5	T44.5X6
Angiotensinamide	T44.991	T44.992	T44.993	T44.994	T44.995	T44.996
Anhydrohydroxy-progesterone	T38.5X1	T38.5X2	T38.5X3	T38.5X4	T38.5X5	T38.5X6
Anhydron	T50.2X1	T50.2X2	T50.2X3	T50.2X4	T50.2X5	T50.2X6
Anileridine	T40.4X1	T40.4X2	T40.4X3	T40.4X4	T40.4X5	T40.4X6
Aniline (dye) (liquid)	T65.3X1	T65.3X2	T65.3X3	T65.3X4	—	—
analgesic	T39.1X1	T39.1X2	T39.1X3	T39.1X4	T39.1X5	T39.1X6
derivatives, therapeutic NEC	T39.1X1	T39.1X2	T39.1X3	T39.1X4	T39.1X5	T39.1X6
vapor	T65.3X1	T65.3X2	T65.3X3	T65.3X4	—	—
Aniscoropine	T44.3X1	T44.3X2	T44.3X3	T44.3X4	T44.3X5	T44.3X6
Anise oil	T47.5X1	T47.5X2	T47.5X3	T47.5X4	T47.5X5	T47.5X6
Anisidine	T65.3X1	T65.3X2	T65.3X3	T65.3X4	—	—
Anisindione	T45.511	T45.512	T45.513	T45.514	T45.515	T45.516
Anisotropine methyl-bromide	T44.3X1	T44.3X2	T44.3X3	T44.3X4	T44.3X5	T44.3X6
Anistreplase	T45.611	T45.612	T45.613	T45.614	T45.615	T45.616
Anorexiant (central)	T50.5X1	T50.5X2	T50.5X3	T50.5X4	T50.5X5	T50.5X6
Anorexic agents	T50.5X1	T50.5X2	T50.5X3	T50.5X4	T50.5X5	T50.5X6
Ansamycin	T36.6X1	T36.6X2	T36.6X3	T36.6X4	T36.6X5	T36.6X6
Ant (bite) (sting)	T63.421	T63.422	T63.423	T63.424	—	—
Antabuse	T50.6X1	T50.6X2	T50.6X3	T50.6X4	T50.6X5	T50.6X6
Antacid NEC	T47.1X1	T47.1X2	T47.1X3	T47.1X4	T47.1X5	T47.1X6
Antagonist						
Aldosterone	T50.0X1	T50.0X2	T50.0X3	T50.0X4	T50.0X5	T50.0X6
alpha-adrenoreceptor	T44.6X1	T44.6X2	T44.6X3	T44.6X4	T44.6X5	T44.6X6
anticoagulant	T45.7X1	T45.7X2	T45.7X3	T45.7X4	T45.7X5	T45.7X6
beta-adrenoreceptor	T44.7X1	T44.7X2	T44.7X3	T44.7X4	T44.7X5	T44.7X6
extrapyramidal NEC	T44.3X1	T44.3X2	T44.3X3	T44.3X4	T44.3X5	T44.3X6
folic acid	T45.1X1	T45.1X2	T45.1X3	T45.1X4	T45.1X5	T45.1X6
H2 receptor	T47.0X1	T47.0X2	T47.0X3	T47.0X4	T47.0X5	T47.0X6
heavy metal	T45.8X1	T45.8X2	T45.8X3	T45.8X4	T45.8X5	T45.8X6
narcotic analgesic	T50.7X1	T50.7X2	T50.7X3	T50.7X4	T50.7X5	T50.7X6
opiate	T50.7X1	T50.7X2	T50.7X3	T50.7X4	T50.7X5	T50.7X6
pyrimidine	T45.1X1	T45.1X2	T45.1X3	T45.1X4	T45.1X5	T45.1X6
serotonin	T46.5X1	T46.5X2	T46.5X3	T46.5X4	T46.5X5	T46.5X6
Antazolin(e)	T45.0X1	T45.0X2	T45.0X3	T45.0X4	T45.0X5	T45.0X6
Anterior pituitary hormone NEC	T38.811	T38.812	T38.813	T38.814	T38.815	T38.816
Anthelmintic NEC	T37.4X1	T37.4X2	T37.4X3	T37.4X4	T37.4X5	T37.4X6
Anthiolimine	T37.4X1	T37.4X2	T37.4X3	T37.4X4	T37.4X5	T37.4X6
Anthralin	T49.4X1	T49.4X2	T49.4X3	T49.4X4	T49.4X5	T49.4X6
Anthramycin	T45.1X1	T45.1X2	T45.1X3	T45.1X4	T45.1X5	T45.1X6
Antiadrenergic NEC	T44.8X1	T44.8X2	T44.8X3	T44.8X4	T44.8X5	T44.8X6
Antiallergic NEC	T45.0X1	T45.0X2	T45.0X3	T45.0X4	T45.0X5	T45.0X6
Antiandrogen NEC	T38.6X1	T38.6X2	T38.6X3	T38.6X4	T38.6X5	T38.6X6
Anti-anemic (drug) (preparation)	T45.8X1	T45.8X2	T45.8X3	T45.8X4	T45.8X5	T45.8X6
Antianxiety drug NEC	T43.501	T43.502	T43.503	T43.504	T43.505	T43.506
Antiaris toxicaria	T65.891	T65.892	T65.893	T65.894	—	—
Antiarteriosclerotic drug	T46.6X1	T46.6X2	T46.6X3	T46.6X4	T46.6X5	T46.6X6
Antiasthmatic drug NEC	T48.6X1	T48.6X2	T48.6X3	T48.6X4	T48.6X5	T48.6X6
Antibiotic NEC	T36.91	T36.92	T36.93	T36.94	T36.95	T36.96
aminoglycoside	T36.5X1	T36.5X2	T36.5X3	T36.5X4	T36.5X5	T36.5X6
anticancer	T45.1X1	T45.1X2	T45.1X3	T45.1X4	T45.1X5	T45.1X6
antifungal	T36.7X1	T36.7X2	T36.7X3	T36.7X4	T36.7X5	T36.7X6
antimycobacterial	T36.5X1	T36.5X2	T36.5X3	T36.5X4	T36.5X5	T36.5X6
antineoplastic	T45.1X1	T45.1X2	T45.1X3	T45.1X4	T45.1X5	T45.1X6
b-lactam NEC	T36.1X1	T36.1X2	T36.1X3	T36.1X4	T36.1X5	T36.1X6
cephalosporin (group)	T36.1X1	T36.1X2	T36.1X3	T36.1X4	T36.1X5	T36.1X6
chloramphenicol (group)	T36.2X1	T36.2X2	T36.2X3	T36.2X4	T36.2X5	T36.2X6
ENT	T49.6X1	T49.6X2	T49.6X3	T49.6X4	T49.6X5	T49.6X6
eye	T49.5X1	T49.5X2	T49.5X3	T49.5X4	T49.5X5	T49.5X6
fungicidal (local)	T49.0X1	T49.0X2	T49.0X3	T49.0X4	T49.0X5	T49.0X6
intestinal	T36.8X1	T36.8X2	T36.8X3	T36.8X4	T36.8X5	T36.8X6
local	T49.0X1	T49.0X2	T49.0X3	T49.0X4	T49.0X5	T49.0X6
Antibiotic — continued						
macrolides	T36.3X1	T36.3X2	T36.3X3	T36.3X4	T36.3X5	T36.3X6
polypeptide	T36.8X1	T36.8X2	T36.8X3	T36.8X4	T36.8X5	T36.8X6
specified NEC	T36.8X1	T36.8X2	T36.8X3	T36.8X4	T36.8X5	T36.8X6
tetracycline (group)	T36.4X1	T36.4X2	T36.4X3	T36.4X4	T36.4X5	T36.4X6
throat	T49.6X1	T49.6X2	T49.6X3	T49.6X4	T49.6X5	T49.6X6
Anticancer agents NEC	T45.1X1	T45.1X2	T45.1X3	T45.1X4	T45.1X5	T45.1X6
Anticholesterolemic drug NEC	T46.6X1	T46.6X2	T46.6X3	T46.6X4	T46.6X5	T46.6X6
Anticholinergic NEC	T44.3X1	T44.3X2	T44.3X3	T44.3X4	T44.3X5	T44.3X6
Anticholinesterase						
organophosphorus	T44.0X1	T44.0X2	T44.0X3	T44.0X4	T44.0X5	T44.0X6
insecticide	T60.0X1	T60.0X2	T60.0X3	T60.0X4	—	—
nerve gas	T59.891	T59.892	T59.893	T59.894	—	—
reversible	T44.0X1	T44.0X2	T44.0X3	T44.0X4	T44.0X5	T44.0X6
ophthalmological	T49.5X1	T49.5X2	T49.5X3	T49.5X4	T49.5X5	T49.5X6
Anticoagulant NEC	T45.511	T45.512	T45.513	T45.514	T45.515	T45.516
Antagonist	T45.7X1	T45.7X2	T45.7X3	T45.7X4	T45.7X5	T45.7X6
Anti-common-cold drug NEC	T48.5X1	T48.5X2	T48.5X3	T48.5X4	T48.5X5	T48.5X6
Anticonvulsant	T42.71	T42.72	T42.73	T42.74	T42.75	T42.76
barbiturate	T42.3X1	T42.3X2	T42.3X3	T42.3X4	T42.3X5	T42.3X6
combination (with barbiturate)	T42.3X1	T42.3X2	T42.3X3	T42.3X4	T42.3X5	T42.3X6
hydantoin	T42.0X1	T42.0X2	T42.0X3	T42.0X4	T42.0X5	T42.0X6
hypnotic NEC	T42.6X1	T42.6X2	T42.6X3	T42.6X4	T42.6X5	T42.6X6
oxazolidinedione	T42.2X1	T42.2X2	T42.2X3	T42.2X4	T42.2X5	T42.2X6
pyrimidinedione	T42.6X1	T42.6X2	T42.6X3	T42.6X4	T42.6X5	T42.6X6
specified NEC	T42.6X1	T42.6X2	T42.6X3	T42.6X4	T42.6X5	T42.6X6
succinimide	T42.2X1	T42.2X2	T42.2X3	T42.2X4	T42.2X5	T42.2X6
Antidepressant	T43.201	T43.202	T43.203	T43.204	T43.205	T43.206
monoamine oxidase inhibitor	T43.1X1	T43.1X2	T43.1X3	T43.1X4	T43.1X5	T43.1X6
selective serotonin norepinephrine reuptake inhibitor	T43.211	T43.212	T43.213	T43.214	T43.215	T43.216
selective serotonin reuptake inhibitor	T43.221	T43.222	T43.223	T43.224	T43.225	T43.226
specified NEC	T43.291	T43.292	T43.293	T43.294	T43.295	T43.296
tetracyclic	T43.021	T43.022	T43.023	T43.024	T43.025	T43.026
triazolopyridine	T43.211	T43.212	T43.213	T43.214	T43.215	T43.216
tricyclic	T43.011	T43.012	T43.013	T43.014	T43.015	T43.016
Antidiabetic NEC	T38.3X1	T38.3X2	T38.3X3	T38.3X4	T38.3X5	T38.3X6
biguanide	T38.3X1	T38.3X2	T38.3X3	T38.3X4	T38.3X5	T38.3X6
and sulfonyl combined	T38.3X1	T38.3X2	T38.3X3	T38.3X4	T38.3X5	T38.3X6
combined	T38.3X1	T38.3X2	T38.3X3	T38.3X4	T38.3X5	T38.3X6
sulfonylurea	T38.3X1	T38.3X2	T38.3X3	T38.3X4	T38.3X5	T38.3X6
Antidiarrheal drug NEC	T47.6X1	T47.6X2	T47.6X3	T47.6X4	T47.6X5	T47.6X6
absorbent	T47.6X1	T47.6X2	T47.6X3	T47.6X4	T47.6X5	T47.6X6
Anti-D immunoglobulin (human)	T50.Z11	T50.Z12	T50.Z13	T50.Z14	T50.Z15	T50.Z16
Antidiphtheria serum	T50.Z11	T50.Z12	T50.Z13	T50.Z14	T50.Z15	T50.Z16
Antidiuretic hormone	T38.891	T38.892	T38.893	T38.894	T38.895	T38.896
Antidote NEC	T50.6X1	T50.6X2	T50.6X3	T50.6X4	T50.6X5	T50.6X6
heavy metal	T45.8X1	T45.8X2	T45.8X3	T45.8X4	T45.8X5	T45.8X6
Antidysrhythmic NEC	T46.2X1	T46.2X2	T46.2X3	T46.2X4	T46.2X5	T46.2X6
Antiemetic drug	T45.0X1	T45.0X2	T45.0X3	T45.0X4	T45.0X5	T45.0X6
Antiepilepsy agent	T42.71	T42.72	T42.73	T42.74	T42.75	T42.76
combination	T42.5X1	T42.5X2	T42.5X3	T42.5X4	T42.5X5	T42.5X6
mixed	T42.5X1	T42.5X2	T42.5X3	T42.5X4	T42.5X5	T42.5X6
specified, NEC	T42.6X1	T42.6X2	T42.6X3	T42.6X4	T42.6X5	T42.6X6
Antiestrogen NEC	T38.6X1	T38.6X2	T38.6X3	T38.6X4	T38.6X5	T38.6X6
Antifertility pill	T38.4X1	T38.4X2	T38.4X3	T38.4X4	T38.4X5	T38.4X6
Antifibrinolytic drug	T45.621	T45.622	T45.623	T45.624	T45.625	T45.626
Antifilarial drug	T37.4X1	T37.4X2	T37.4X3	T37.4X4	T37.4X5	T37.4X6
Antiflatulent	T47.5X1	T47.5X2	T47.5X3	T47.5X4	T47.5X5	T47.5X6
Antifreeze	T65.91	T65.92	T65.93	T65.94	—	—
alcohol	T51.1X1	T51.1X2	T51.1X3	T51.1X4	—	—
ethylene glycol	T51.8X1	T51.8X2	T51.8X3	T51.8X4	—	—
Antifungal						
antibiotic (systemic)	T36.7X1	T36.7X2	T36.7X3	T36.7X4	T36.7X5	T36.7X6
anti-infective NEC	T37.91	T37.92	T37.93	T37.94	T37.95	T37.96
disinfectant, local	T49.0X1	T49.0X2	T49.0X3	T49.0X4	T49.0X5	T49.0X6
nonmedicinal (spray)	T60.3X1	T60.3X2	T60.3X3	T60.3X4	—	—
topical	T49.0X1	T49.0X2	T49.0X3	T49.0X4	T49.0X5	T49.0X6
Anti-gastric-secretion drug NEC	T47.1X1	T47.1X2	T47.1X3	T47.1X4	T47.1X5	T47.1X6
Antigonadotrophin NEC	T38.6X1	T38.6X2	T38.6X3	T38.6X4	T38.6X5	T38.6X6
Antihallucinogen	T43.501	T43.502	T43.503	T43.504	T43.505	T43.506
Antihelmintics	T37.4X1	T37.4X2	T37.4X3	T37.4X4	T37.4X5	T37.4X6
Antihemophilic						
factor	T45.8X1	T45.8X2	T45.8X3	T45.8X4	T45.8X5	T45.8X6
fraction	T45.8X1	T45.8X2	T45.8X3	T45.8X4	T45.8X5	T45.8X6

Additional Character May Be Required — Refer to the Tabular List for Character Selection

▽ Subterms under main terms may continue to next column or page

Substance	Poisoning, Accidental (unintentional)	Poisoning, Intentional Self-harm	Poisoning, Assault	Poisoning, Undetermined	Adverse Effect	Under-dosing
Antihemophilic — continued						
globulin concentrate	T45.7X1	T45.7X2	T45.7X3	T45.7X4	T45.7X5	T45.7X6
human plasma	T45.8X1	T45.8X2	T45.8X3	T45.8X4	T45.8X5	T45.8X6
plasma, dried	T45.7X1	T45.7X2	T45.7X3	T45.7X4	T45.7X5	T45.7X6
Antihemorrhoidal preparation	T49.2X1	T49.2X2	T49.2X3	T49.2X4	T49.2X5	T49.2X6
Antiheparin drug	T45.7X1	T45.7X2	T45.7X3	T45.7X4	T45.7X5	T45.7X6
Antihistamine	T45.0X1	T45.0X2	T45.0X3	T45.0X4	T45.0X5	T45.0X6
Antihookworm drug	T37.4X1	T37.4X2	T37.4X3	T37.4X4	T37.4X5	T37.4X6
Anti-human lymphocytic globulin	T50.Z11	T50.Z12	T50.Z13	T50.Z14	T50.Z15	T50.Z16
Antihyperlipidemic drug	T46.6X1	T46.6X2	T46.6X3	T46.6X4	T46.6X5	T46.6X6
Antihypertensive drug NEC	T46.5X1	T46.5X2	T46.5X3	T46.5X4	T46.5X5	T46.5X6
Anti-infective NEC	T37.91	T37.92	T37.93	T37.94	T37.95	T37.96
anthelmintic	T37.4X1	T37.4X2	T37.4X3	T37.4X4	T37.4X5	T37.4X6
antibiotics	T36.91	T36.92	T36.93	T36.94	T36.95	T36.96
specified NEC	T36.8X1	T36.8X2	T36.8X3	T36.8X4	T36.8X5	T36.8X6
antimalarial	T37.2X1	T37.2X2	T37.2X3	T37.2X4	T37.2X5	T37.2X6
antimycobacterial NEC	T37.1X1	T37.1X2	T37.1X3	T37.1X4	T37.1X5	T37.1X6
antibiotics	T36.5X1	T36.5X2	T36.5X3	T36.5X4	T36.5X5	T36.5X6
antiprotozoal NEC	T37.3X1	T37.3X2	T37.3X3	T37.3X4	T37.3X5	T37.3X6
blood	T37.2X1	T37.2X2	T37.2X3	T37.2X4	T37.2X5	T37.2X6
antiviral	T37.5X1	T37.5X2	T37.5X3	T37.5X4	T37.5X5	T37.5X6
arsenical	T37.8X1	T37.8X2	T37.8X3	T37.8X4	T37.8X5	T37.8X6
bismuth, local	T49.0X1	T49.0X2	T49.0X3	T49.0X4	T49.0X5	T49.0X6
ENT	T49.6X1	T49.6X2	T49.6X3	T49.6X4	T49.6X5	T49.6X6
eye NEC	T49.5X1	T49.5X2	T49.5X3	T49.5X4	T49.5X5	T49.5X6
heavy metals NEC	T37.8X1	T37.8X2	T37.8X3	T37.8X4	T37.8X5	T37.8X6
local NEC	T49.0X1	T49.0X2	T49.0X3	T49.0X4	T49.0X5	T49.0X6
specified NEC	T49.0X1	T49.0X2	T49.0X3	T49.0X4	T49.0X5	T49.0X6
mixed	T37.91	T37.92	T37.93	T37.94	T37.95	T37.96
ophthalmic preparation	T49.5X1	T49.5X2	T49.5X3	T49.5X4	T49.5X5	T49.5X6
topical NEC	T49.0X1	T49.0X2	T49.0X3	T49.0X4	T49.0X5	T49.0X6
Anti-inflammatory drug NEC	T39.391	T39.392	T39.393	T39.394	T39.395	T39.396
local	T49.0X1	T49.0X2	T49.0X3	T49.0X4	T49.0X5	T49.0X6
nonsteroidal NEC	T39.391	T39.392	T39.393	T39.394	T39.395	T39.396
propionic acid derivative	T39.311	T39.312	T39.313	T39.314	T39.315	T39.316
specified NEC	T39.391	T39.392	T39.393	T39.394	T39.395	T39.396
Antikaluretic	T50.3X1	T50.3X2	T50.3X3	T50.3X4	T50.3X5	T50.3X6
Antiknock (tetraethyl lead)	T56.0X1	T56.0X2	T56.0X3	T56.0X4	—	—
Antilipemic drug NEC	T46.6X1	T46.6X2	T46.6X3	T46.6X4	T46.6X5	T46.6X6
Antimalarial	T37.2X1	T37.2X2	T37.2X3	T37.2X4	T37.2X5	T37.2X6
prophylactic NEC	T37.2X1	T37.2X2	T37.2X3	T37.2X4	T37.2X5	T37.2X6
pyrimidine derivative	T37.2X1	T37.2X2	T37.2X3	T37.2X4	T37.2X5	T37.2X6
Antimetabolite	T45.1X1	T45.1X2	T45.1X3	T45.1X4	T45.1X5	T45.1X6
Antimitotic agent	T45.1X1	T45.1X2	T45.1X3	T45.1X4	T45.1X5	T45.1X6
Antimony (compounds) (vapor) **NEC**	T56.891	T56.892	T56.893	T56.894	—	—
anti-infectives	T37.8X1	T37.8X2	T37.8X3	T37.8X4	T37.8X5	T37.8X6
dimercaptosuccinate	T37.3X1	T37.3X2	T37.3X3	T37.3X4	T37.3X5	T37.3X6
hydride	T56.891	T56.892	T56.893	T56.894	—	—
pesticide (vapor)	T60.8X1	T60.8X2	T60.8X3	T60.8X4	—	—
potassium (sodium) tartrate	T37.8X1	T37.8X2	T37.8X3	T37.8X4	T37.8X5	T37.8X6
sodium dimercaptosuccinate	T37.3X1	T37.3X2	T37.3X3	T37.3X4	T37.3X5	T37.3X6
tartrated	T37.8X1	T37.8X2	T37.8X3	T37.8X4	T37.8X5	T37.8X6
Antimuscarinic NEC	T44.3X1	T44.3X2	T44.3X3	T44.3X4	T44.3X5	T44.3X6
Antimycobacterial drug NEC	T37.1X1	T37.1X2	T37.1X3	T37.1X4	T37.1X5	T37.1X6
antibiotics	T36.5X1	T36.5X2	T36.5X3	T36.5X4	T36.5X5	T36.5X6
combination	T37.1X1	T37.1X2	T37.1X3	T37.1X4	T37.1X5	T37.1X6
Antinausea drug	T45.0X1	T45.0X2	T45.0X3	T45.0X4	T45.0X5	T45.0X6
Antinematode drug	T37.4X1	T37.4X2	T37.4X3	T37.4X4	T37.4X5	T37.4X6
Antineoplastic NEC	T45.1X1	T45.1X2	T45.1X3	T45.1X4	T45.1X5	T45.1X6
alkaloidal	T45.1X1	T45.1X2	T45.1X3	T45.1X4	T45.1X5	T45.1X6
antibiotics	T45.1X1	T45.1X2	T45.1X3	T45.1X4	T45.1X5	T45.1X6
combination	T45.1X1	T45.1X2	T45.1X3	T45.1X4	T45.1X5	T45.1X6
estrogen	T38.5X1	T38.5X2	T38.5X3	T38.5X4	T38.5X5	T38.5X6
steroid	T38.7X1	T38.7X2	T38.7X3	T38.7X4	T38.7X5	T38.7X6
Antiparasitic drug (systemic)	T37.91	T37.92	T37.93	T37.94	T37.95	T37.96
local	T49.0X1	T49.0X2	T49.0X3	T49.0X4	T49.0X5	T49.0X6
specified NEC	T37.8X1	T37.8X2	T37.8X3	T37.8X4	T37.8X5	T37.8X6
Antiparkinsonism drug NEC	T42.8X1	T42.8X2	T42.8X3	T42.8X4	T42.8X5	T42.8X6
Antiperspirant NEC	T49.2X1	T49.2X2	T49.2X3	T49.2X4	T49.2X5	T49.2X6
Antiphlogistic NEC	T39.4X1	T39.4X2	T39.4X3	T39.4X4	T39.4X5	T39.4X6
Antiplatyhelmintic drug	T37.4X1	T37.4X2	T37.4X3	T37.4X4	T37.4X5	T37.4X6
Antiprotozoal drug NEC	T37.3X1	T37.3X2	T37.3X3	T37.3X4	T37.3X5	T37.3X6
blood	T37.2X1	T37.2X2	T37.2X3	T37.2X4	T37.2X5	T37.2X6
local	T49.0X1	T49.0X2	T49.0X3	T49.0X4	T49.0X5	T49.0X6

Substance	Poisoning, Accidental (unintentional)	Poisoning, Intentional Self-harm	Poisoning, Assault	Poisoning, Undetermined	Adverse Effect	Under-dosing
Antipruritic drug NEC	T49.1X1	T49.1X2	T49.1X3	T49.1X4	T49.1X5	T49.1X6
Antipsychotic drug	T43.501	T43.502	T43.503	T43.504	T43.505	T43.506
specified NEC	T43.591	T43.592	T43.593	T43.594	T43.595	T43.596
Antipyretic	T39.91	T39.92	T39.93	T39.94	T39.95	T39.96
specified NEC	T39.8X1	T39.8X2	T39.8X3	T39.8X4	T39.8X5	T39.8X6
Antipyrine	T39.2X1	T39.2X2	T39.2X3	T39.2X4	T39.2X5	T39.2X6
Antirabies hyperimmune serum	T50.Z11	T50.Z12	T50.Z13	T50.Z14	T50.Z15	T50.Z16
Antirheumatic NEC	T39.4X1	T39.4X2	T39.4X3	T39.4X4	T39.4X5	T39.4X6
Antirigidity drug NEC	T42.8X1	T42.8X2	T42.8X3	T42.8X4	T42.8X5	T42.8X6
Antischistosomal drug	T37.4X1	T37.4X2	T37.4X3	T37.4X4	T37.4X5	T37.4X6
Antiscorpion sera	T50.Z11	T50.Z12	T50.Z13	T50.Z14	T50.Z15	T50.Z16
Antiseborrheics	T49.4X1	T49.4X2	T49.4X3	T49.4X4	T49.4X5	T49.4X6
Antiseptics (external) (medicinal)	T49.0X1	T49.0X2	T49.0X3	T49.0X4	T49.0X5	T49.0X6
Antistine	T45.0X1	T45.0X2	T45.0X3	T45.0X4	T45.0X5	T45.0X6
Antitapeworm drug	T37.4X1	T37.4X2	T37.4X3	T37.4X4	T37.4X5	T37.4X6
Antitetanus immunoglobulin	T50.Z11	T50.Z12	T50.Z13	T50.Z14	T50.Z15	T50.Z16
Antithrombotic	T45.521	T45.522	T45.523	T45.524	T45.525	T45.526
Antithyroid drug NEC	T38.2X1	T38.2X2	T38.2X3	T38.2X4	T38.2X5	T38.2X6
Antitoxin	T50.Z11	T50.Z12	T50.Z13	T50.Z14	T50.Z15	T50.Z16
diphtheria	T50.Z11	T50.Z12	T50.Z13	T50.Z14	T50.Z15	T50.Z16
gas gangrene	T50.Z11	T50.Z12	T50.Z13	T50.Z14	T50.Z15	T50.Z16
tetanus	T50.Z11	T50.Z12	T50.Z13	T50.Z14	T50.Z15	T50.Z16
Antitrichomonal drug	T37.3X1	T37.3X2	T37.3X3	T37.3X4	T37.3X5	T37.3X6
Antituberculars	T37.1X1	T37.1X2	T37.1X3	T37.1X4	T37.1X5	T37.1X6
antibiotics	T36.5X1	T36.5X2	T36.5X3	T36.5X4	T36.5X5	T36.5X6
Antitussive NEC	T48.3X1	T48.3X2	T48.3X3	T48.3X4	T48.3X5	T48.3X6
codeine mixture	T40.2X1	T40.2X2	T40.2X3	T40.2X4	T40.2X5	T40.2X6
opiate	T40.2X1	T40.2X2	T40.2X3	T40.2X4	T40.2X5	T40.2X6
Antivaricose drug	T46.8X1	T46.8X2	T46.8X3	T46.8X4	T46.8X5	T46.8X6
Antivenin, antivenom (sera)	T50.Z11	T50.Z12	T50.Z13	T50.Z14	T50.Z15	T50.Z16
crotaline	T50.Z11	T50.Z12	T50.Z13	T50.Z14	T50.Z15	T50.Z16
spider bite	T50.Z11	T50.Z12	T50.Z13	T50.Z14	T50.Z15	T50.Z16
Antivertigo drug	T45.0X1	T45.0X2	T45.0X3	T45.0X4	T45.0X5	T45.0X6
Antiviral drug NEC	T37.5X1	T37.5X2	T37.5X3	T37.5X4	T37.5X5	T37.5X6
eye	T49.5X1	T49.5X2	T49.5X3	T49.5X4	T49.5X5	T49.5X6
Antiwhipworm drug	T37.4X1	T37.4X2	T37.4X3	T37.4X4	T37.4X5	T37.4X6
Ant poison — see Insecticide						
Antrol — see also by specific chemical substance	T60.91	T60.92	T60.93	T60.94	—	—
fungicide	T60.91	T60.92	T60.93	T60.94	—	—
ANTU (alpha naphthylthiourea)	T60.4X1	T60.4X2	T60.4X3	T60.4X4	—	—
Apalcillin	T36.0X1	T36.0X2	T36.0X3	T36.0X4	T36.0X5	T36.0X6
APC	T48.5X1	T48.5X2	T48.5X3	T48.5X4	T48.5X5	T48.5X6
Aplonidine	T44.4X1	T44.4X2	T44.4X3	T44.4X4	T44.4X5	T44.4X6
Apomorphine	T47.7X1	T47.7X2	T47.7X3	T47.7X4	T47.7X5	T47.7X6
Appetite depressants, central	T50.5X1	T50.5X2	T50.5X3	T50.5X4	T50.5X5	T50.5X6
Apraclonidine (hydrochloride)	T44.4X1	T44.4X2	T44.4X3	T44.4X4	T44.4X5	T44.4X6
Apresoline	T46.5X1	T46.5X2	T46.5X3	T46.5X4	T46.5X5	T46.5X6
Aprindine	T46.2X1	T46.2X2	T46.2X3	T46.2X4	T46.2X5	T46.2X6
Aprobarbital	T42.3X1	T42.3X2	T42.3X3	T42.3X4	T42.3X5	T42.3X6
Apronalide	T42.6X1	T42.6X2	T42.6X3	T42.6X4	T42.6X5	T42.6X6
Aprotinin	T45.621	T45.622	T45.623	T45.624	T45.625	T45.626
Aptocaine	T41.3X1	T41.3X2	T41.3X3	T41.3X4	T41.3X5	T41.3X6
Aqua fortis	T54.2X1	T54.2X2	T54.2X3	T54.2X4	—	—
Ara-A	T37.5X1	T37.5X2	T37.5X3	T37.5X4	—	T37.5X6
Ara-C	T45.1X1	T45.1X2	T45.1X3	T45.1X4	T45.1X5	T45.1X6
Arachis oil	T49.3X1	T49.3X2	T49.3X3	T49.3X4	T49.3X5	T49.3X6
cathartic	T47.4X1	T47.4X2	T47.4X3	T47.4X4	T47.4X5	T47.4X6
Aralen	T37.2X1	T37.2X2	T37.2X3	T37.2X4	T37.2X5	T37.2X6
Arecoline	T44.1X1	T44.1X2	T44.1X3	T44.1X4	T44.1X5	T44.1X6
Arginine	T50.991	T50.992	T50.993	T50.994	T50.995	T50.996
glutamate	T50.991	T50.992	T50.993	T50.994	T50.995	T50.996
Argyrol	T49.0X1	T49.0X2	T49.0X3	T49.0X4	T49.0X5	T49.0X6
ENT agent	T49.6X1	T49.6X2	T49.6X3	T49.6X4	T49.6X5	T49.6X6
ophthalmic preparation	T49.5X1	T49.5X2	T49.5X3	T49.5X4	T49.5X5	T49.5X6
Aristocort	T38.0X1	T38.0X2	T38.0X3	T38.0X4	T38.0X5	T38.0X6
ENT agent	T49.6X1	T49.6X2	T49.6X3	T49.6X4	T49.6X5	T49.6X6
ophthalmic preparation	T49.5X1	T49.5X2	T49.5X3	T49.5X4	T49.5X5	T49.5X6
topical NEC	T49.0X1	T49.0X2	T49.0X3	T49.0X4	T49.0X5	T49.0X6
Aromatics, corrosive	T54.1X1	T54.1X2	T54.1X3	T54.1X4	—	—
disinfectants	T54.1X1	T54.1X2	T54.1X3	T54.1X4	—	—
Arsenate of lead	T57.0X1	T57.0X2	T57.0X3	T57.0X4	—	—
herbicide	T57.0X1	T57.0X2	T57.0X3	T57.0X4	—	—
Arsenic, arsenicals (compounds) (dust) (vapor) **NEC**	T57.0X1	T57.0X2	T57.0X3	T57.0X4	—	—
anti-infectives	T37.8X1	T37.8X2	T37.8X3	T37.8X4	T37.8X5	T37.8X6
pesticide (dust) (fumes)	T57.0X1	T57.0X2	T57.0X3	T57.0X4	—	—

Table of Drugs and Chemicals

Antihemophilic — Arsenic, arsenicals

Substance	Poisoning, Accidental (unintentional)	Poisoning, Intentional Self-harm	Poisoning, Assault	Poisoning, Undetermined	Adverse Effect	Under-dosing
Arsine (gas)	T57.0X1	T57.0X2	T57.0X3	T57.0X4		
Arsphenamine (silver)	T37.8X1	T37.8X2	T37.8X3	T37.8X4	T37.8X5	T37.8X6
Arsthinol	T37.3X1	T37.3X2	T37.3X3	T37.3X4	T37.3X5	T37.3X6
Artane	T44.3X1	T44.3X2	T44.3X3	T44.3X4	T44.3X5	T44.3X6
Arthropod (venomous) NEC	T63.481	T63.482	T63.483	T63.484		
Articaine	T41.3X1	T41.3X2	T41.3X3	T41.3X4	T41.3X5	T41.3X6
Asbestos	T57.8X1	T57.8X2	T57.8X3	T57.8X4		
Ascaridole	T37.4X1	T37.4X2	T37.4X3	T37.4X4	T37.4X5	T37.4X6
Ascorbic acid	T45.2X1	T45.2X2	T45.2X3	T45.2X4	T45.2X5	T45.2X6
Asiaticoside	T49.0X1	T49.0X2	T49.0X3	T49.0X4	T49.0X5	T49.0X6
Asparaginase	T45.1X1	T45.1X2	T45.1X3	T45.1X4	T45.1X5	T45.1X6
Aspidium (oleoresin)	T37.4X1	T37.4X2	T37.4X3	T37.4X4	T37.4X5	T37.4X6
Aspirin (aluminum) (soluble)	T39.011	T39.012	T39.013	T39.014	T39.015	T39.016
Aspoxicillin	T36.0X1	T36.0X2	T36.0X3	T36.0X4	T36.0X5	T36.0X6
Astemizole	T45.0X1	T45.0X2	T45.0X3	T45.0X4	T45.0X5	T45.0X6
Astringent (local)	T49.2X1	T49.2X2	T49.2X3	T49.2X4	T49.2X5	T49.2X6
specified NEC	T49.2X1	T49.2X2	T49.2X3	T49.2X4	T49.2X5	T49.2X6
Astromicin	T36.5X1	T36.5X2	T36.5X3	T36.5X4	T36.5X5	T36.5X6
Ataractic drug NEC	T43.501	T43.502	T43.503	T43.504	T43.505	T43.506
Atenolol	T44.7X1	T44.7X2	T44.7X3	T44.7X4	T44.7X5	T44.7X6
Atonia drug, intestinal	T47.4X1	T47.4X2	T47.4X3	T47.4X4	T47.4X5	T47.4X6
Atophan	T50.4X1	T50.4X2	T50.4X3	T50.4X4	T50.4X5	T50.4X6
Atracurium besilate	T48.1X1	T48.1X2	T48.1X3	T48.1X4	T48.1X5	T48.1X6
Atropine	T44.3X1	T44.3X2	T44.3X3	T44.3X4	T44.3X5	T44.3X6
derivative	T44.3X1	T44.3X2	T44.3X3	T44.3X4	T44.3X5	T44.3X6
methonitrate	T44.3X1	T44.3X2	T44.3X3	T44.3X4	T44.3X5	T44.3X6
Attapulgite	T47.6X1	T47.6X2	T47.6X3	T47.6X4	T47.6X5	T47.6X6
Auramine	T65.891	T65.892	T65.893	T65.894	—	—
dye	T65.6X1	T65.6X2	T65.6X3	T65.6X4	—	—
fungicide	T60.3X1	T60.3X2	T60.3X3	T60.3X4	—	—
Auranofin	T39.4X1	T39.4X2	T39.4X3	T39.4X4	T39.4X5	T39.4X6
Aurantiin	T46.991	T46.992	T46.993	T46.994	T46.995	T46.996
Aureomycin	T36.4X1	T36.4X2	T36.4X3	T36.4X4	T36.4X5	T36.4X6
ophthalmic preparation	T49.5X1	T49.5X2	T49.5X3	T49.5X4	T49.5X5	T49.5X6
topical NEC	T49.0X1	T49.0X2	T49.0X3	T49.0X4	T49.0X5	T49.0X6
Aurothioglucose	T39.4X1	T39.4X2	T39.4X3	T39.4X4	T39.4X5	T39.4X6
Aurothioglycanide	T39.4X1	T39.4X2	T39.4X3	T39.4X4	T39.4X5	T39.4X6
Aurothiomalate sodium	T39.4X1	T39.4X2	T39.4X3	T39.4X4	T39.4X5	T39.4X6
Aurotioprol	T39.4X1	T39.4X2	T39.4X3	T39.4X4	T39.4X5	T39.4X6
Automobile fuel	T52.0X1	T52.0X2	T52.0X3	T52.0X4	—	—
Autonomic nervous system agent NEC	T44.901	T44.902	T44.903	T44.904	T44.905	T44.906
Avlosulfon	T37.1X1	T37.1X2	T37.1X3	T37.1X4	T37.1X5	T37.1X6
Avomine	T42.6X1	T42.6X2	T42.6X3	T42.6X4	T42.6X5	T42.6X6
Axerophthol	T45.2X1	T45.2X2	T45.2X3	T45.2X4	T45.2X5	T45.2X6
Azacitidine	T45.1X1	T45.1X2	T45.1X3	T45.1X4	T45.1X5	T45.1X6
Azacyclonol	T43.591	T43.592	T43.593	T43.594	T43.595	T43.596
Azadirachta	T60.2X1	T60.2X2	T60.2X3	T60.2X4	—	—
Azanidazole	T37.3X1	T37.3X2	T37.3X3	T37.3X4	T37.3X5	T37.3X6
Azapetine	T46.7X1	T46.7X2	T46.7X3	T46.7X4	T46.7X5	T46.7X6
Azapropazone	T39.2X1	T39.2X2	T39.2X3	T39.2X4	T39.2X5	T39.2X6
Azaribine	T45.1X1	T45.1X2	T45.1X3	T45.1X4	T45.1X5	T45.1X6
Azaserine	T45.1X1	T45.1X2	T45.1X3	T45.1X4	T45.1X5	T45.1X6
Azatadine	T45.0X1	T45.0X2	T45.0X3	T45.0X4	T45.0X5	T45.0X6
Azatepa	T45.1X1	T45.1X2	T45.1X3	T45.1X4	T45.1X5	T45.1X6
Azathioprine	T45.1X1	T45.1X2	T45.1X3	T45.1X4	T45.1X5	T45.1X6
Azelaic acid	T49.0X1	T49.0X2	T49.0X3	T49.0X4	T49.0X5	T49.0X6
Azelastine	T45.0X1	T45.0X2	T45.0X3	T45.0X4	T45.0X5	T45.0X6
Azidocillin	T36.0X1	T36.0X2	T36.0X3	T36.0X4	T36.0X5	T36.0X6
Azidothymidine	T37.5X1	T37.5X2	T37.5X3	T37.5X4	T37.5X5	T37.5X6
Azinphos (ethyl) (methyl)	T60.0X1	T60.0X2	T60.0X3	T60.0X4		
Aziridine (chelating)	T54.1X1	T54.1X2	T54.1X3	T54.1X4	—	—
Azithromycin	T36.3X1	T36.3X2	T36.3X3	T36.3X4	T36.3X5	T36.3X6
Azlocillin	T36.0X1	T36.0X2	T36.0X3	T36.0X4	T36.0X5	T36.0X6
Azobenzene smoke	T65.3X1	T65.3X2	T65.3X3	T65.3X4	—	—
acaricide	T60.8X1	T60.8X2	T60.8X3	T60.8X4	—	—
Azosulfamide	T37.0X1	T37.0X2	T37.0X3	T37.0X4	T37.0X5	T37.0X6
AZT	T37.5X1	T37.5X2	T37.5X3	T37.5X4	T37.5X5	T37.5X6
Aztreonam	T36.1X1	T36.1X2	T36.1X3	T36.1X4	T36.1X5	T36.1X6
Azulfidine	T37.0X1	T37.0X2	T37.0X3	T37.0X4	T37.0X5	T37.0X6
Azuresin	T50.8X1	T50.8X2	T50.8X3	T50.8X4	T50.8X5	T50.8X6
b-acetyldigoxin	T46.0X1	T46.0X2	T46.0X3	T46.0X4	T46.0X5	T46.0X6
P-Acetamidophenol	T39.1X1	T39.1X2	T39.1X3	T39.1X4	T39.1X5	T39.1X6
Bacampicillin	T36.0X1	T36.0X2	T36.0X3	T36.0X4	T36.0X5	T36.0X6
Bacillus						
lactobacillus	T47.8X1	T47.8X2	T47.8X3	T47.8X4	T47.8X5	T47.8X6
subtilis	T47.6X1	T47.6X2	T47.6X3	T47.6X4	T47.6X5	T47.6X6
Bacimycin	T49.0X1	T49.0X2	T49.0X3	T49.0X4	T49.0X5	T49.0X6
ophthalmic preparation	T49.5X1	T49.5X2	T49.5X3	T49.5X4	T49.5X5	T49.5X6
Bacitracin zinc	T49.0X1	T49.0X2	T49.0X3	T49.0X4	T49.0X5	T49.0X6
with neomycin	T49.0X1	T49.0X2	T49.0X3	T49.0X4	T49.0X5	T49.0X6
ENT agent	T49.6X1	T49.6X2	T49.6X3	T49.6X4	T49.6X5	T49.6X6
ophthalmic preparation	T49.5X1	T49.5X2	T49.5X3	T49.5X4	T49.5X5	T49.5X6

Substance	Poisoning, Accidental (unintentional)	Poisoning, Intentional Self-harm	Poisoning, Assault	Poisoning, Undetermined	Adverse Effect	Under-dosing
Bacitracin zinc — continued						
topical NEC	T49.0X1	T49.0X2	T49.0X3	T49.0X4	T49.0X5	T49.0X6
Baclofen	T42.8X1	T42.8X2	T42.8X3	T42.8X4	T42.8X5	T42.8X6
Baking soda	T50.991	T50.992	T50.993	T50.994	T50.995	T50.996
BAL	T45.8X1	T45.8X2	T45.8X3	T45.8X4	T45.8X5	T45.8X6
Bambuterol	T48.6X1	T48.6X2	T48.6X3	T48.6X4	T48.6X5	T48.6X6
Bamethan (sulfate)	T46.7X1	T46.7X2	T46.7X3	T46.7X4	T46.7X5	T46.7X6
Bamifylline	T48.6X1	T48.6X2	T48.6X3	T48.6X4	T48.6X5	T48.6X6
Bamipine	T45.0X1	T45.0X2	T45.0X3	T45.0X4	T45.0X5	T45.0X6
Baneberry — see Actaea spicata						
Banewort — see Belladonna						
Barbenyl	T42.3X1	T42.3X2	T42.3X3	T42.3X4	T42.3X5	T42.3X6
Barbexaclone	T42.6X1	T42.6X2	T42.6X3	T42.6X4	T42.6X5	T42.6X6
Barbital	T42.3X1	T42.3X2	T42.3X3	T42.3X4	T42.3X5	T42.3X6
sodium	T42.3X1	T42.3X2	T42.3X3	T42.3X4	T42.3X5	T42.3X6
Barbitone	T42.3X1	T42.3X2	T42.3X3	T42.3X4	T42.3X5	T42.3X6
Barbiturate NEC	T42.3X1	T42.3X2	T42.3X3	T42.3X4	T42.3X5	T42.3X6
with tranquilizer	T42.3X1	T42.3X2	T42.3X3	T42.3X4	T42.3X5	T42.3X6
anesthetic (intravenous)	T41.1X1	T41.1X2	T41.1X3	T41.1X4	T41.1X5	T41.1X6
Barium (carbonate) (chloride) (sulfite)	T57.8X1	T57.8X2	T57.8X3	T57.8X4		
diagnostic agent	T50.8X1	T50.8X2	T50.8X3	T50.8X4	T50.8X5	T50.8X6
pesticide	T60.4X1	T60.4X2	T60.4X3	T60.4X4	—	—
rodenticide	T60.4X1	T60.4X2	T60.4X3	T60.4X4	—	—
sulfate (medicinal)	T50.8X1	T50.8X2	T50.8X3	T50.8X4	T50.8X5	T50.8X6
Barrier cream	T49.3X1	T49.3X2	T49.3X3	T49.3X4	T49.3X5	T49.3X6
Basic fuchsin	T49.0X1	T49.0X2	T49.0X3	T49.0X4	T49.0X5	T49.0X6
Battery acid or fluid	T54.2X1	T54.2X2	T54.2X3	T54.2X4	—	—
Bay rum	T51.8X1	T51.8X2	T51.8X3	T51.8X4	—	—
b-benzalbutyramide	T46.6X1	T46.6X2	T46.6X3	T46.6X4	T46.6X5	T46.6X6
BCG (vaccine)	T50.A91	T50.A92	T50.A93	T50.A94	T50.A95	T50.A96
BCNU	T45.1X1	T45.1X2	T45.1X3	T45.1X4	T45.1X5	T45.1X6
Bearsfoot	T62.2X1	T62.2X2	T62.2X3	T62.2X4	—	—
Beclamide	T42.6X1	T42.6X2	T42.6X3	T42.6X4	T42.6X5	T42.6X6
Beclomethasone	T44.5X1	T44.5X2	T44.5X3	T44.5X4	T44.5X5	T44.5X6
Bee (sting) (venom)	T63.441	T63.442	T63.443	T63.444	—	—
Befunolol	T49.5X1	T49.5X2	T49.5X3	T49.5X4	T49.5X5	T49.5X6
Bekanamycin	T36.5X1	T36.5X2	T36.5X3	T36.5X4	T36.5X5	T36.5X6
Belladonna — see also Nightshade						
alkaloids	T44.3X1	T44.3X2	T44.3X3	T44.3X4	T44.3X5	T44.3X6
extract	T44.3X1	T44.3X2	T44.3X3	T44.3X4	T44.3X5	T44.3X6
herb	T44.3X1	T44.3X2	T44.3X3	T44.3X4	T44.3X5	T44.3X6
Bemegride	T50.7X1	T50.7X2	T50.7X3	T50.7X4	T50.7X5	T50.7X6
Benactyzine	T44.3X1	T44.3X2	T44.3X3	T44.3X4	T44.3X5	T44.3X6
Benadryl	T45.0X1	T45.0X2	T45.0X3	T45.0X4	T45.0X5	T45.0X6
Benaprizine	T44.3X1	T44.3X2	T44.3X3	T44.3X4	T44.3X5	T44.3X6
Benazepril	T46.4X1	T46.4X2	T46.4X3	T46.4X4	T46.4X5	T46.4X6
Bencyclane	T46.7X1	T46.7X2	T46.7X3	T46.7X4	T46.7X5	T46.7X6
Bendazol	T46.3X1	T46.3X2	T46.3X3	T46.3X4	T46.3X5	T46.3X6
Bendrofluazide	T50.2X1	T50.2X2	T50.2X3	T50.2X4	T50.2X5	T50.2X6
Bendroflumethiazide	T50.2X1	T50.2X2	T50.2X3	T50.2X4	T50.2X5	T50.2X6
Benemid	T50.4X1	T50.4X2	T50.4X3	T50.4X4	T50.4X5	T50.4X6
Benethamine penicillin	T36.0X1	T36.0X2	T36.0X3	T36.0X4	T36.0X5	T36.0X6
Benexate	T47.1X1	T47.1X2	T47.1X3	T47.1X4	T47.1X5	T47.1X6
Benfluorex	T46.6X1	T46.6X2	T46.6X3	T46.6X4	T46.6X5	T46.6X6
Benfotiamine	T45.2X1	T45.2X2	T45.2X3	T45.2X4	T45.2X5	T45.2X6
Benisone	T49.0X1	T49.0X2	T49.0X3	T49.0X4	T49.0X5	T49.0X6
Benomyl	T60.0X1	T60.0X2	T60.0X3	T60.0X4	—	—
Benoquin	T49.8X1	T49.8X2	T49.8X3	T49.8X4	T49.8X5	T49.8X6
Benoxinate	T41.3X1	T41.3X2	T41.3X3	T41.3X4	T41.3X5	T41.3X6
Benperidol	T43.4X1	T43.4X2	T43.4X3	T43.4X4	T43.4X5	T43.4X6
Benproperine	T48.3X1	T48.3X2	T48.3X3	T48.3X4	T48.3X5	T48.3X6
Benserazide	T42.8X1	T42.8X2	T42.8X3	T42.8X4	T42.8X5	T42.8X6
Bentazepam	T42.4X1	T42.4X2	T42.4X3	T42.4X4	T42.4X5	T42.4X6
Bentiromide	T50.8X1	T50.8X2	T50.8X3	T50.8X4	T50.8X5	T50.8X6
Bentonite	T49.3X1	T49.3X2	T49.3X3	T49.3X4	T49.3X5	T49.3X6
Benzalbutyramide	T46.6X1	T46.6X2	T46.6X3	T46.6X4	T46.6X5	T46.6X6
Benzalkonium (chloride)	T49.0X1	T49.0X2	T49.0X3	T49.0X4	T49.0X5	T49.0X6
ophthalmic preparation	T49.5X1	T49.5X2	T49.5X3	T49.5X4	T49.5X5	T49.5X6
Benzamidosalicylate (calcium)	T37.1X1	T37.1X2	T37.1X3	T37.1X4	T37.1X5	T37.1X6
Benzamine	T41.3X1	T41.3X2	T41.3X3	T41.3X4	T41.3X5	T41.3X6
lactate	T49.1X1	T49.1X2	T49.1X3	T49.1X4	T49.1X5	T49.1X6
Benzamphetamine	T50.5X1	T50.5X2	T50.5X3	T50.5X4	T50.5X5	T50.5X6
Benzapril hydrochloride	T46.5X1	T46.5X2	T46.5X3	T46.5X4	T46.5X5	T46.5X6
Benzathine benzylpenicillin	T36.0X1	T36.0X2	T36.0X3	T36.0X4	T36.0X5	T36.0X6
Benzathine penicillin	T36.0X1	T36.0X2	T36.0X3	T36.0X4	T36.0X5	T36.0X6
Benzatropine	T42.8X1	T42.8X2	T42.8X3	T42.8X4	T42.8X5	T42.8X6
Benzbromarone	T50.4X1	T50.4X2	T50.4X3	T50.4X4	T50.4X5	T50.4X6
Benzcarbimine	T45.1X1	T45.1X2	T45.1X3	T45.1X4	T45.1X5	T45.1X6
Benzedrex	T44.991	T44.992	T44.993	T44.994	T44.995	T44.996

Additional Character May Be Required — Refer to the Tabular List for Character Selection   ▽ Subterms under main terms may continue to next column or page

Substance	Poisoning, Accidental (unintentional)	Poisoning, Intentional Self-harm	Poisoning, Assault	Poisoning, Undetermined	Adverse Effect	Under-dosing
Benzedrine (amphetamine)	T43.621	T43.622	T43.623	T43.624	T43.625	T43.626
Benzenamine	T65.3X1	T65.3X2	T65.3X3	T65.3X4	—	—
Benzene	T52.1X1	T52.1X2	T52.1X3	T52.1X4	—	—
homologues (acetyl) (dimethyl) (methyl) (solvent)	T52.2X1	T52.2X2	T52.2X3	T52.2X4	—	—
Benzethonium (chloride)	T49.0X1	T49.0X2	T49.0X3	T49.0X4	T49.0X5	T49.0X6
Benzfetamine	T50.5X1	T50.5X2	T50.5X3	T50.5X4	T50.5X5	T50.5X6
Benzhexol	T44.3X1	T44.3X2	T44.3X3	T44.3X4	T44.3X5	T44.3X6
Benzhydramine (chloride)	T45.0X1	T45.0X2	T45.0X3	T45.0X4	T45.0X5	T45.0X6
Benzidine	T65.891	T65.892	T65.893	T65.894	—	—
Benzilonium bromide	T44.3X1	T44.3X2	T44.3X3	T44.3X4	T44.3X5	T44.3X6
Benzimidazole	T60.3X1	T60.3X2	T60.3X3	T60.3X4	—	—
Benzin (e) — see Ligroin						
Benziodarone	T46.3X1	T46.3X2	T46.3X3	T46.3X4	T46.3X5	T46.3X6
Benznidazole	T37.3X1	T37.3X2	T37.3X3	T37.3X4	T37.3X5	T37.3X6
Benzocaine	T41.3X1	T41.3X2	T41.3X3	T41.3X4	T41.3X5	T41.3X6
Benzodiapin	T42.4X1	T42.4X2	T42.4X3	T42.4X4	T42.4X5	T42.4X6
Benzodiazepine NEC	T42.4X1	T42.4X2	T42.4X3	T42.4X4	T42.4X5	T42.4X6
Benzoic acid	T49.0X1	T49.0X2	T49.0X3	T49.0X4	T49.0X5	T49.0X6
with salicylic acid	T49.0X1	T49.0X2	T49.0X3	T49.0X4	T49.0X5	T49.0X6
Benzoin (tincture)	T48.5X1	T48.5X2	T48.5X3	T48.5X4	T48.5X5	T48.5X6
Benzol (benzene)	T52.1X1	T52.1X2	T52.1X3	T52.1X4	—	—
vapor	T52.0X1	T52.0X2	T52.0X3	T52.0X4	—	—
Benzomorphan	T40.2X1	T40.2X2	T40.2X3	T40.2X4	T40.2X5	T40.2X6
Benzonatate	T48.3X1	T48.3X2	T48.3X3	T48.3X4	T48.3X5	T48.3X6
Benzophenones	T49.3X1	T49.3X2	T49.3X3	T49.3X4	T49.3X5	T49.3X6
Benzopyrone	T46.991	T46.992	T46.993	T46.994	T46.995	T46.996
Benzothiadiazides	T50.2X1	T50.2X2	T50.2X3	T50.2X4	T50.2X5	T50.2X6
Benzoxonium chloride	T49.0X1	T49.0X2	T49.0X3	T49.0X4	T49.0X5	T49.0X6
Benzoylpas calcium	T37.1X1	T37.1X2	T37.1X3	T37.1X4	T37.1X5	T37.1X6
Benzoyl peroxide	T49.0X1	T49.0X2	T49.0X3	T49.0X4	T49.0X5	T49.0X6
Benzperidin	T43.591	T43.592	T43.593	T43.594	T43.595	T43.596
Benzperidol	T43.591	T43.592	T43.593	T43.594	T43.595	T43.596
Benzphetamine	T50.5X1	T50.5X2	T50.5X3	T50.5X4	T50.5X5	T50.5X6
Benzpyrinium bromide	T44.1X1	T44.1X2	T44.1X3	T44.1X4	T44.1X5	T44.1X6
Benzquinamide	T45.0X1	T45.0X2	T45.0X3	T45.0X4	T45.0X5	T45.0X6
Benzthiazide	T50.2X1	T50.2X2	T50.2X3	T50.2X4	T50.2X5	T50.2X6
Benztropine						
anticholinergic	T44.3X1	T44.3X2	T44.3X3	T44.3X4	T44.3X5	T44.3X6
antiparkinson	T42.8X1	T42.8X2	T42.8X3	T42.8X4	T42.8X5	T42.8X6
Benzydamine	T49.0X1	T49.0X2	T49.0X3	T49.0X4	T49.0X5	T49.0X6
Benzyl						
acetate	T52.8X1	T52.8X2	T52.8X3	T52.8X4	—	—
alcohol	T49.0X1	T49.0X2	T49.0X3	T49.0X4	T49.0X5	T49.0X6
benzoate	T49.0X1	T49.0X2	T49.0X3	T49.0X4	T49.0X5	T49.0X6
Benzoic acid	T49.0X1	T49.0X2	T49.0X3	T49.0X4	T49.0X5	T49.0X6
morphine	T40.2X1	T40.2X2	T40.2X3	T40.2X4	—	—
nicotinate	T46.6X1	T46.6X2	T46.6X3	T46.6X4	T46.6X5	T46.6X6
penicillin	T36.0X1	T36.0X2	T36.0X3	T36.0X4	T36.0X5	T36.0X6
Benzylhydrochlorthiazide	T50.2X1	T50.2X2	T50.2X3	T50.2X4	T50.2X5	T50.2X6
Benzylpenicillin	T36.0X1	T36.0X2	T36.0X3	T36.0X4	T36.0X5	T36.0X6
Benzylthiouracil	T38.2X1	T38.2X2	T38.2X3	T38.2X4	T38.2X5	T38.2X6
Bephenium	T37.4X1	T37.4X2	T37.4X3	T37.4X4	T37.4X5	T37.4X6
hydroxynaphthoate						
Bepridil	T46.1X1	T46.1X2	T46.1X3	T46.1X4	T46.1X5	T46.1X6
Bergamot oil	T65.891	T65.892	T65.893	T65.894	—	—
Bergapten	T50.991	T50.992	T50.993	T50.994	T50.995	T50.996
Berries, poisonous	T62.1X1	T62.1X2	T62.1X3	T62.1X4	—	—
Beryllium (compounds)	T56.7X1	T56.7X2	T56.7X3	T56.7X4	—	—
beta adrenergic blocking agent, heart	T44.7X1	T44.7X2	T44.7X3	T44.7X4	T44.7X5	T44.7X6
Betacarotene	T45.2X1	T45.2X2	T45.2X3	T45.2X4	T45.2X5	T45.2X6
Beta-Chlor	T42.6X1	T42.6X2	T42.6X3	T42.6X4	T42.6X5	T42.6X6
Betahistine	T46.7X1	T46.7X2	T46.7X3	T46.7X4	T46.7X5	T46.7X6
Betaine	T47.5X1	T47.5X2	T47.5X3	T47.5X4	T47.5X5	T47.5X6
Betamethasone	T49.0X1	T49.0X2	T49.0X3	T49.0X4	T49.0X5	T49.0X6
topical	T49.0X1	T49.0X2	T49.0X3	T49.0X4	T49.0X5	T49.0X6
Betamicin	T36.8X1	T36.8X2	T36.8X3	T36.8X4	T36.8X5	T36.8X6
Betanidine	T46.5X1	T46.5X2	T46.5X3	T46.5X4	T46.5X5	T46.5X6
Betaxolol	T44.7X1	T44.7X2	T44.7X3	T44.7X4	T44.7X5	T44.7X6
Betazole	T50.8X1	T50.8X2	T50.8X3	T50.8X4	T50.8X5	T50.8X6
Bethanechol	T44.1X1	T44.1X2	T44.1X3	T44.1X4	T44.1X5	T44.1X6
chloride	T44.1X1	T44.1X2	T44.1X3	T44.1X4	T44.1X5	T44.1X6
Bethanidine	T46.5X1	T46.5X2	T46.5X3	T46.5X4	T46.5X5	T46.5X6
Betoxycaine	T41.3X1	T41.3X2	T41.3X3	T41.3X4	T41.3X5	T41.3X6
Betula oil	T49.3X1	T49.3X2	T49.3X3	T49.3X4	T49.3X5	T49.3X6
Bevantolol	T44.7X1	T44.7X2	T44.7X3	T44.7X4	T44.7X5	T44.7X6
Bevonium metilsulfate	T44.3X1	T44.3X2	T44.3X3	T44.3X4	T44.3X5	T44.3X6
Bezafibrate	T46.6X1	T46.6X2	T46.6X3	T46.6X4	T46.6X5	T46.6X6
Bezitramide	T40.4X1	T40.4X2	T40.4X3	T40.4X4	T40.4X5	T40.4X6
BHA	T50.991	T50.992	T50.993	T50.994	T50.995	T50.996
Bhang	T40.7X1	T40.7X2	T40.7X3	T40.7X4	T40.7X5	T40.7X6
BHC (medicinal)	T49.0X1	T49.0X2	T49.0X3	T49.0X4	T49.0X5	T49.0X6
BHC — continued						
nonmedicinal (vapor)	T53.6X1	T53.6X2	T53.6X3	T53.6X4	—	—
Bialamicol	T37.3X1	T37.3X2	T37.3X3	T37.3X4	T37.3X5	T37.3X6
Bibenzonium bromide	T48.3X1	T48.3X2	T48.3X3	T48.3X4	T48.3X5	T48.3X6
Bibrocathol	T49.5X1	T49.5X2	T49.5X3	T49.5X4	T49.5X5	T49.5X6
Bichloride of mercury — see Mercury, chloride						
Bichromates (calcium) (potassium)(sodium) (crystals)	T57.8X1	T57.8X2	T57.8X3	T57.8X4	—	—
fumes	T56.2X1	T56.2X2	T56.2X3	T56.2X4	—	—
Biclotymol	T49.6X1	T49.6X2	T49.6X3	T49.6X4	T49.6X5	T49.6X6
Bicucculine	T50.7X1	T50.7X2	T50.7X3	T50.7X4	T50.7X5	T50.7X6
Bifemelane	T43.291	T43.292	T43.294	T43.294	T43.295	T43.296
Biguanide derivatives, oral	T38.3X1	T38.3X2	T38.3X3	T38.3X4	T38.3X5	T38.3X6
Bile salts	T47.5X1	T47.5X2	T47.5X3	T47.5X4	T47.5X5	T47.5X6
Biligrafin	T50.8X1	T50.8X2	T50.8X3	T50.8X4	T50.8X5	T50.8X6
Bilopaque	T50.8X1	T50.8X2	T50.8X3	T50.8X4	T50.8X5	T50.8X6
Binifibrate	T46.6X1	T46.6X2	T46.6X3	T46.6X4	T46.6X5	T46.6X6
Binitrobenzol	T65.3X1	T65.3X2	T65.3X3	T65.3X4	—	—
Bioflavonoid(s)	T46.991	T46.992	T46.993	T46.994	T46.995	T46.996
Biological substance NEC	T50.901	T50.902	T50.903	T50.904	T50.905	T50.906
Biotin	T45.2X1	T45.2X2	T45.2X3	T45.2X4	T45.2X5	T45.2X6
Biperiden	T44.3X1	T44.3X2	T44.3X3	T44.3X4	T44.3X5	T44.3X6
Bisacodyl	T47.2X1	T47.2X2	T47.2X3	T47.2X4	T47.2X5	T47.2X6
Bisbentiamine	T45.2X1	T45.2X2	T45.2X3	T45.2X4	T45.2X5	T45.2X6
Bisbutiamine	T45.2X1	T45.2X2	T45.2X3	T45.2X4	T45.2X5	T45.2X6
Bisdequalinium (salts) (diacetate)	T49.6X1	T49.6X2	T49.6X3	T49.6X4	T49.6X5	T49.6X6
Bishydroxycoumarin	T45.511	T45.512	T45.513	T45.514	T45.515	T45.516
Bismarsen	T37.8X1	T37.8X2	T37.8X3	T37.8X4	T37.8X5	T37.8X6
Bismuth salts	T47.6X1	T47.6X2	T47.6X3	T47.6X4	T47.6X5	T47.6X6
aluminate	T47.1X1	T47.1X2	T47.1X3	T47.1X4	T47.1X5	T47.1X6
anti-infectives	T37.8X1	T37.8X2	T37.8X3	T37.8X4	T37.8X5	T37.8X6
formic iodide	T49.0X1	T49.0X2	T49.0X3	T49.0X4	T49.0X5	T49.0X6
glycolylarsenate	T49.0X1	T49.0X2	T49.0X3	T49.0X4	T49.0X5	T49.0X6
nonmedicinal (compounds) NEC	T65.91	T65.92	T65.93	T65.94	—	—
subcarbonate	T47.6X1	T47.6X2	T47.6X3	T47.6X4	T47.6X5	T47.6X6
subsalicylate	T37.8X1	T37.8X2	T37.8X3	T37.8X4	T37.8X5	T37.8X6
sulfarsphenamine	T37.8X1	T37.8X2	T37.8X3	T37.8X4	T37.8X5	T37.8X6
Bisoprolol	T44.7X1	T44.7X2	T44.7X3	T44.7X4	T44.7X5	T44.7X6
Bisoxatin	T47.2X1	T47.2X2	T47.2X3	T47.2X4	T47.2X5	T47.2X6
Bisulepin (hydrochloride)	T45.0X1	T45.0X2	T45.0X3	T45.0X4	T45.0X5	T45.0X6
Bithionol	T37.8X1	T37.8X2	T37.8X3	T37.8X4	T37.8X5	T37.8X6
anthelminthic	T37.4X1	T37.4X2	T37.4X3	T37.4X4	T37.4X5	T37.4X6
Bitolterol	T48.6X1	T48.6X2	T48.6X3	T48.6X4	T48.6X5	T48.6X6
Bitoscanate	T37.4X1	T37.4X2	T37.4X3	T37.4X4	T37.4X5	T37.4X6
Bitter almond oil	T62.8X1	T62.8X2	T62.8X3	T62.8X4	—	—
Bittersweet	T62.2X1	T62.2X2	T62.2X3	T62.2X4	—	—
Black						
flag	T60.91	T60.92	T60.93	T60.94	—	—
henbane	T62.2X1	T62.2X2	T62.2X3	T62.2X4	—	—
leaf (40)	T60.91	T60.92	T60.93	T60.94	—	—
widow spider (bite)	T63.311	T63.312	T63.313	T63.314	—	—
antivenin	T50.Z11	T50.Z12	T50.Z13	T50.Z14	T50.Z15	T50.Z16
Blast furnace gas (carbon monoxide from)	T58.8X1	T58.8X2	T58.8X3	T58.8X4	—	—
Bleach	T54.91	T54.92	T54.93	T54.94	—	—
Bleaching agent (medicinal)	T49.4X1	T49.4X2	T49.4X3	T49.4X4	T49.4X5	T49.4X6
Bleomycin	T45.1X1	T45.1X2	T45.1X3	T45.1X4	T45.1X5	T45.1X6
Blockain	T41.3X1	T41.3X2	T41.3X3	T41.3X4	T41.3X5	T41.3X6
infiltration (subcutaneous)	T41.3X1	T41.3X2	T41.3X3	T41.3X4	T41.3X5	T41.3X6
nerve block (peripheral) (plexus)	T41.3X1	T41.3X2	T41.3X3	T41.3X4	T41.3X5	T41.3X6
topical (surface)	T41.3X1	T41.3X2	T41.3X3	T41.3X4	T41.3X5	T41.3X6
Blockers, calcium channel	T46.1X1	T46.1X2	T46.1X3	T46.1X4	T46.1X5	T46.1X6
Blood (derivatives) (natural) (plasma) (whole)	T45.8X1	T45.8X2	T45.8X3	T45.8X4	T45.8X5	T45.8X6
dried	T45.8X1	T45.8X2	T45.8X3	T45.8X4	T45.8X5	T45.8X6
drug affecting NEC	T45.91	T45.92	T45.93	T45.94	T45.95	T45.96
expander NEC	T45.8X1	T45.8X2	T45.8X3	T45.8X4	T45.8X5	T45.8X6
fraction NEC	T45.8X1	T45.8X2	T45.8X3	T45.8X4	T45.8X5	T45.8X6
substitute (macromolecular)	T45.8X1	T45.8X2	T45.8X3	T45.8X4	T45.8X5	T45.8X6
Blue velvet	T40.2X1	T40.2X2	T40.2X3	T40.2X4	—	—
Bone meal	T62.8X1	T62.8X2	T62.8X3	T62.8X4	—	—
Bonine	T45.0X1	T45.0X2	T45.0X3	T45.0X4	T45.0X5	T45.0X6
Bopindolol	T44.7X1	T44.7X2	T44.7X3	T44.7X4	T44.7X5	T44.7X6
Boracic acid	T49.0X1	T49.0X2	T49.0X3	T49.0X4	T49.0X5	T49.0X6
ENT agent	T49.6X1	T49.6X2	T49.6X3	T49.6X4	T49.6X5	T49.6X6
ophthalmic preparation	T49.5X1	T49.5X2	T49.5X3	T49.5X4	T49.5X5	T49.5X6
Borane complex	T57.8X1	T57.8X2	T57.8X3	T57.8X4	—	—

▽ Subterms under main terms may continue to next column or page   Additional Character May Be Required — Refer to the Tabular List for Character Selection   355

Benzedrine — Borane complex

Table of Drugs and Chemicals

Substance	Poisoning, Accidental (unintentional)	Poisoning, Intentional Self-harm	Poisoning, Assault	Poisoning, Undetermined	Adverse Effect	Under-dosing
Borate(s)	T57.8X1	T57.8X2	T57.8X3	T57.8X4	—	—
buffer	T50.991	T50.992	T50.993	T50.994	T50.995	T50.996
cleanser	T54.91	T54.92	T54.93	T54.94	—	—
sodium	T57.8X1	T57.8X2	T57.8X3	T57.8X4	—	—
Borax (cleanser)	T54.91	T54.92	T54.93	T54.94	—	—
Bordeaux mixture	T60.3X1	T60.3X2	T60.3X3	T60.3X4	—	—
Boric acid	T49.0X1	T49.0X2	T49.0X3	T49.0X4	T49.0X5	T49.0X6
ENT agent	T49.6X1	T49.6X2	T49.6X3	T49.6X4	T49.6X5	T49.6X6
ophthalmic preparation	T49.5X1	T49.5X2	T49.5X3	T49.5X4	T49.5X5	T49.5X6
Bornaprine	T44.3X1	T44.3X2	T44.3X3	T44.3X4	T44.3X5	T44.3X6
Boron	T57.8X1	T57.8X2	T57.8X3	T57.8X4	—	—
hydride NEC	T57.8X1	T57.8X2	T57.8X3	T57.8X4	—	—
fumes or gas	T57.8X1	T57.8X2	T57.8X3	T57.8X4	—	—
trifluoride	T59.891	T59.892	T59.893	T59.894	—	—
Botox	T48.291	T48.292	T48.293	T48.294	T48.295	T48.296
Botulinus anti-toxin (type A, B)	T50.Z11	T50.Z12	T50.Z13	T50.Z14	T50.Z15	T50.Z16
Brake fluid vapor	T59.891	T59.892	T59.893	T59.894	—	—
Brallobarbital	T42.3X1	T42.3X2	T42.3X3	T42.3X4	T42.3X5	T42.3X6
Bran (wheat)	T47.4X1	T47.4X2	T47.4X3	T47.4X4	T47.4X5	T47.4X6
Brass (fumes)	T56.891	T56.892	T56.893	T56.894	—	—
Brasso	T52.0X1	T52.0X2	T52.0X3	T52.0X4	—	—
Bretylium tosilate	T46.2X1	T46.2X2	T46.2X3	T46.2X4	T46.2X5	T46.2X6
Brevital (sodium)	T41.1X1	T41.1X2	T41.1X3	T41.1X4	T41.1X5	T41.1X6
Brinase	T45.3X1	T45.3X2	T45.3X3	T45.3X4	T45.3X5	T45.3X6
British antilewisite	T45.8X1	T45.8X2	T45.8X3	T45.8X4	T45.8X5	T45.8X6
Brodifacoum	T60.4X1	T60.4X2	T60.4X3	T60.4X4	—	—
Bromal (hydrate)	T42.6X1	T42.6X2	T42.6X3	T42.6X4	T42.6X5	T42.6X6
Bromazepam	T42.4X1	T42.4X2	T42.4X3	T42.4X4	T42.4X5	T42.4X6
Bromazine	T45.0X1	T45.0X2	T45.0X3	T45.0X4	T45.0X5	T45.0X6
Brombenzylcyanide	T59.3X1	T59.3X2	T59.3X3	T59.3X4	—	—
Bromelains	T45.3X1	T45.3X2	T45.3X3	T45.3X4	T45.3X5	T45.3X6
Bromethalin	T60.4X1	T60.4X2	T60.4X3	T60.4X4	—	—
Bromhexine	T48.4X1	T48.4X2	T48.4X3	T48.4X4	T48.4X5	T48.4X6
Bromide salts	T42.6X1	T42.6X2	T42.6X3	T42.6X4	T42.6X5	T42.6X6
Bromindione	T45.511	T45.512	T45.513	T45.514	T45.515	T45.516
Bromine						
compounds (medicinal)	T42.6X1	T42.6X2	T42.6X3	T42.6X4	T42.6X5	T42.6X6
sedative	T42.6X1	T42.6X2	T42.6X3	T42.6X4	T42.6X5	T42.6X6
vapor	T59.891	T59.892	T59.893	T59.894	—	—
Bromisoval	T42.6X1	T42.6X2	T42.6X3	T42.6X4	T42.6X5	T42.6X6
Bromisovalum	T42.6X1	T42.6X2	T42.6X3	T42.6X4	T42.6X5	T42.6X6
Bromobenzylcyanide	T59.3X1	T59.3X2	T59.3X3	T59.3X4	—	—
Bromochlorosalicylani-lide	T49.0X1	T49.0X2	T49.0X3	T49.0X4	T49.0X5	T49.0X6
Bromocriptine	T42.8X1	T42.8X2	T42.8X3	T42.8X4	T42.8X5	T42.8X6
Bromodiphenhydramine	T45.0X1	T45.0X2	T45.0X3	T45.0X4	T45.0X5	T45.0X6
Bromoform	T42.6X1	T42.6X2	T42.6X3	T42.6X4	T42.6X5	T42.6X6
Bromophenol blue reagent	T50.991	T50.992	T50.993	T50.994	T50.995	T50.996
Bromopride	T47.8X1	T47.8X2	T47.8X3	T47.8X4	T47.8X5	T47.8X6
Bromosalicylchloranitide	T49.0X1	T49.0X2	T49.0X3	T49.0X4	T49.0X5	T49.0X6
Bromosalicylhydroxamic acid	T37.1X1	T37.1X2	T37.1X3	T37.1X4	T37.1X5	T37.1X6
Bromo-seltzer	T39.1X1	T39.1X2	T39.1X3	T39.1X4	T39.1X5	T39.1X6
Bromoxynil	T60.3X1	T60.3X2	T60.3X3	T60.3X4	—	—
Bromperidol	T43.4X1	T43.4X2	T43.4X3	T43.4X4	T43.4X5	T43.4X6
Brompheniramine	T45.0X1	T45.0X2	T45.0X3	T45.0X4	T45.0X5	T45.0X6
Bromsulfophthalein	T50.8X1	T50.8X2	T50.8X3	T50.8X4	T50.8X5	T50.8X6
Bromural	T42.6X1	T42.6X2	T42.6X3	T42.6X4	T42.6X5	T42.6X6
Bromvaletone	T42.6X1	T42.6X2	T42.6X3	T42.6X4	T42.6X5	T42.6X6
Bronchodilator NEC	T48.6X1	T48.6X2	T48.6X3	T48.6X4	T48.6X5	T48.6X6
Brotizolam	T42.4X1	T42.4X2	T42.4X3	T42.4X4	T42.4X5	T42.4X6
Brovincamine	T46.7X1	T46.7X2	T46.7X3	T46.7X4	T46.7X5	T46.7X6
Brown recluse spider (bite) (venom)	T63.331	T63.332	T63.333	T63.334	—	—
Brown spider (bite) (venom)	T63.391	T63.392	T63.393	T63.394	—	—
Broxaterol	T48.6X1	T48.6X2	T48.6X3	T48.6X4	T48.6X5	T48.6X6
Broxuridine	T45.1X1	T45.1X2	T45.1X3	T45.1X4	T45.1X5	T45.1X6
Broxyquinoline	T37.8X1	T37.8X2	T37.8X3	T37.8X4	T37.8X5	T37.8X6
Bruceine	T48.291	T48.292	T48.293	T48.294	T48.295	T48.296
Brucia	T62.2X1	T62.2X2	T62.2X3	T62.2X4	—	—
Brucine	T65.1X1	T65.1X2	T65.1X3	T65.1X4	—	—
Brunswick green — see Copper						
Bruten — see Ibuprofen						
Bryonia	T47.2X1	T47.2X2	T47.2X3	T47.2X4	T47.2X5	T47.2X6
Buclizine	T45.0X1	T45.0X2	T45.0X3	T45.0X4	T45.0X5	T45.0X6
Buclosamide	T49.0X1	T49.0X2	T49.0X3	T49.0X4	T49.0X5	T49.0X6
Budesonide	T44.5X1	T44.5X2	T44.5X3	T44.5X4	T44.5X5	T44.5X6
Budralazine	T46.5X1	T46.5X2	T46.5X3	T46.5X4	T46.5X5	T46.5X6
Bufferin	T39.011	T39.012	T39.013	T39.014	T39.015	T39.016
Buflomedil	T46.7X1	T46.7X2	T46.7X3	T46.7X4	T46.7X5	T46.7X6
Buformin	T38.3X1	T38.3X2	T38.3X3	T38.3X4	T38.3X5	T38.3X6
Bufotenine	T40.991	T40.992	T40.993	T40.994	—	—
Bufrolin	T48.6X1	T48.6X2	T48.6X3	T48.6X4	T48.6X5	T48.6X6

Substance	Poisoning, Accidental (unintentional)	Poisoning, Intentional Self-harm	Poisoning, Assault	Poisoning, Undetermined	Adverse Effect	Under-dosing
Bufylline	T48.6X1	T48.6X2	T48.6X3	T48.6X4	T48.6X5	T48.6X6
Bulk filler	T50.5X1	T50.5X2	T50.5X3	T50.5X4	T50.5X5	T50.5X6
cathartic	T47.4X1	T47.4X2	T47.4X3	T47.4X4	T47.4X5	T47.4X6
Bumetanide	T50.1X1	T50.1X2	T50.1X3	T50.1X4	T50.1X5	T50.1X6
Bunaftine	T46.2X1	T46.2X2	T46.2X3	T46.2X4	T46.2X5	T46.2X6
Bunamiodyl	T50.8X1	T50.8X2	T50.8X3	T50.8X4	T50.8X5	T50.8X6
Bunazosin	T44.6X1	T44.6X2	T44.6X3	T44.6X4	T44.6X5	T44.6X6
Bunitrolol	T44.7X1	T44.7X2	T44.7X3	T44.7X4	T44.7X5	T44.7X6
Buphenine	T46.7X1	T46.7X2	T46.7X3	T46.7X4	T46.7X5	T46.7X6
Bupivacaine	T41.3X1	T41.3X2	T41.3X3	T41.3X4	T41.3X5	T41.3X6
infiltration (subcutaneous)	T41.3X1	T41.3X2	T41.3X3	T41.3X4	T41.3X5	T41.3X6
nerve block (peripheral) (plexus)	T41.3X1	T41.3X2	T41.3X3	T41.3X4	T41.3X5	T41.3X6
spinal	T41.3X1	T41.3X2	T41.3X3	T41.3X4	T41.3X5	T41.3X6
Bupranolol	T44.7X1	T44.7X2	T44.7X3	T44.7X4	T44.7X5	T44.7X6
Buprenorphine	T40.4X1	T40.4X2	T40.4X3	T40.4X4	T40.4X5	T40.4X6
Bupropion	T43.291	T43.292	T43.293	T43.294	T43.295	T43.296
Burimamide	T47.1X1	T47.1X2	T47.1X3	T47.1X4	T47.1X5	T47.1X6
Buserelin	T38.891	T38.892	T38.893	T38.894	T38.895	T38.896
Buspirone	T43.591	T43.592	T43.593	T43.594	T43.595	T43.596
Busulfan, busulphan	T45.1X1	T45.1X2	T45.1X3	T45.1X4	T45.1X5	T45.1X6
Butabarbital (sodium)	T42.3X1	T42.3X2	T42.3X3	T42.3X4	T42.3X5	T42.3X6
Butabarbitone	T42.3X1	T42.3X2	T42.3X3	T42.3X4	T42.3X5	T42.3X6
Butabarpal	T42.3X1	T42.3X2	T42.3X3	T42.3X4	T42.3X5	T42.3X6
Butacaine	T41.3X1	T41.3X2	T41.3X3	T41.3X4	T41.3X5	T41.3X6
Butalamine	T46.7X1	T46.7X2	T46.7X3	T46.7X4	T46.7X5	T46.7X6
Butalbital	T42.3X1	T42.3X2	T42.3X3	T42.3X4	T42.3X5	T42.3X6
Butallylonal	T42.3X1	T42.3X2	T42.3X3	T42.3X4	T42.3X5	T42.3X6
Butamben	T41.3X1	T41.3X2	T41.3X3	T41.3X4	T41.3X5	T41.3X6
Butamirate	T48.3X1	T48.3X2	T48.3X3	T48.3X4	T48.3X5	T48.3X6
Butane (distributed in mobile container)	T59.891	T59.892	T59.893	T59.894	—	—
distributed through pipes	T59.891	T59.892	T59.893	T59.894	—	—
incomplete combustion	T58.11	T58.12	T58.13	T58.14	—	—
Butanilicaine	T41.3X1	T41.3X2	T41.3X3	T41.3X4	T41.3X5	T41.3X6
Butanol	T51.3X1	T51.3X2	T51.3X3	T51.3X4	—	—
Butanone, 2-butanone	T52.4X1	T52.4X2	T52.4X3	T52.4X4	—	—
Butantrone	T49.4X1	T49.4X2	T49.4X3	T49.4X4	T49.4X5	T49.4X6
Butaperazine	T43.3X1	T43.3X2	T43.3X3	T43.3X4	T43.3X5	T43.3X6
Butazolidin	T39.2X1	T39.2X2	T39.2X3	T39.2X4	T39.2X5	T39.2X6
Butetamate	T48.6X1	T48.6X2	T48.6X3	T48.6X4	T48.6X5	T48.6X6
Butethal	T42.3X1	T42.3X2	T42.3X3	T42.3X4	T42.3X5	T42.3X6
Butethamate	T44.3X1	T44.3X2	T44.3X3	T44.3X4	T44.3X5	T44.3X6
Buthalitone (sodium)	T41.1X1	T41.1X2	T41.1X3	T41.1X4	T41.1X5	T41.1X6
Butisol (sodium)	T42.3X1	T42.3X2	T42.3X3	T42.3X4	T42.3X5	T42.3X6
Butizide	T50.2X1	T50.2X2	T50.2X3	T50.2X4	T50.2X5	T50.2X6
Butobarbital	T42.3X1	T42.3X2	T42.3X3	T42.3X4	T42.3X5	T42.3X6
sodium	T42.3X1	T42.3X2	T42.3X3	T42.3X4	T42.3X5	T42.3X6
Butobarbitone	T42.3X1	T42.3X2	T42.3X3	T42.3X4	T42.3X5	T42.3X6
Butoconazole (nitrate)	T49.0X1	T49.0X2	T49.0X3	T49.0X4	T49.0X5	T49.0X6
Butorphanol	T40.4X1	T40.4X2	T40.4X3	T40.4X4	T40.4X5	T40.4X6
Butriptyline	T43.011	T43.012	T43.013	T43.014	T43.015	T43.016
Butropium bromide	T44.3X1	T44.3X2	T44.3X3	T44.3X4	T44.3X5	T44.3X6
Buttercups	T62.2X1	T62.2X2	T62.2X3	T62.2X4	—	—
Butter of antimony — see Antimony						
Butyl						
acetate (secondary)	T52.8X1	T52.8X2	T52.8X3	T52.8X4	—	—
alcohol	T51.3X1	T51.3X2	T51.3X3	T51.3X4	—	—
aminobenzoate	T41.3X1	T41.3X2	T41.3X3	T41.3X4	T41.3X5	T41.3X6
butyrate	T52.8X1	T52.8X2	T52.8X3	T52.8X4	—	—
carbinol	T51.3X1	T51.3X2	T51.3X3	T51.3X4	—	—
carbitol	T52.3X1	T52.3X2	T52.3X3	T52.3X4	—	—
cellosolve	T52.3X1	T52.3X2	T52.3X3	T52.3X4	—	—
chloral (hydrate)	T42.6X1	T42.6X2	T42.6X3	T42.6X4	T42.6X5	T42.6X6
formate	T52.8X1	T52.8X2	T52.8X3	T52.8X4	—	—
lactate	T52.8X1	T52.8X2	T52.8X3	T52.8X4	—	—
propionate	T52.8X1	T52.8X2	T52.8X3	T52.8X4	—	—
scopolamine bromide	T44.3X1	T44.3X2	T44.3X3	T44.3X4	T44.3X5	T44.3X6
thiobarbital sodium	T41.1X1	T41.1X2	T41.1X3	T41.1X4	T41.1X5	T41.1X6
Butylated hydroxyanisole	T50.991	T50.992	T50.993	T50.994	T50.995	T50.996
Butylchloral hydrate	T42.6X1	T42.6X2	T42.6X3	T42.6X4	T42.6X5	T42.6X6
Butyltoluene	T52.2X1	T52.2X2	T52.2X3	T52.2X4	—	—
Butyn	T41.3X1	T41.3X2	T41.3X3	T41.3X4	T41.3X5	T41.3X6
Butyrophenone (-based tranquilizers)	T43.4X1	T43.4X2	T43.4X3	T43.4X4	T43.4X5	T43.4X6
Cabergoline	T42.8X1	T42.8X2	T42.8X3	T42.8X4	T42.8X5	T42.8X6
Cacodyl, cacodylic acid	T57.0X1	T57.0X2	T57.0X3	T57.0X4	—	—
Cactinomycin	T45.1X1	T45.1X2	T45.1X3	T45.1X4	T45.1X5	T45.1X6
Cade oil	T49.4X1	T49.4X2	T49.4X3	T49.4X4	T49.4X5	T49.4X6
Cadexomer iodine	T49.0X1	T49.0X2	T49.0X3	T49.0X4	T49.0X5	T49.0X6
Cadmium (chloride) (fumes) (oxide)	T56.3X1	T56.3X2	T56.3X3	T56.3X4	—	—

Additional Character May Be Required — Refer to the Tabular List for Character Selection   ▽ Subterms under main terms may continue to next column or page

Substance	Poisoning, Accidental (unintentional)	Poisoning, Intentional Self-harm	Poisoning, Assault	Poisoning, Undetermined	Adverse Effect	Under-dosing
Cadmium — *continued*						
sulfide (medicinal) NEC	T49.4X1	T49.4X2	T49.4X3	T49.4X4	T49.4X5	T49.4X6
Cadralazine	T46.5X1	T46.5X2	T46.5X3	T46.5X4	T46.5X5	T46.5X6
Caffeine	T43.611	T43.612	T43.613	T43.614	T43.615	T43.616
Calabar bean	T62.2X1	T62.2X2	T62.2X3	T62.2X4	—	—
Caladium seguinum	T62.2X1	T62.2X2	T62.2X3	T62.2X4	—	—
Calamine (lotion)	T49.3X1	T49.3X2	T49.3X3	T49.3X4	T49.3X5	T49.3X6
Calcifediol	T45.2X1	T45.2X2	T45.2X3	T45.2X4	T45.2X5	T45.2X6
Calciferol	T45.2X1	T45.2X2	T45.2X3	T45.2X4	T45.2X5	T45.2X6
Calcitonin	T50.991	T50.992	T50.993	T50.994	T50.995	T50.996
Calcitriol	T45.2X1	T45.2X2	T45.2X3	T45.2X4	T45.2X5	T45.2X6
Calcium	T50.3X1	T50.3X2	T50.3X3	T50.3X4	T50.3X5	T50.3X6
actylsalicylate	T39.011	T39.012	T39.013	T39.014	T39.015	T39.016
benzamidosalicylate	T37.1X1	T37.1X2	T37.1X3	T37.1X4	T37.1X5	T37.1X6
bromide	T42.6X1	T42.6X2	T42.6X3	T42.6X4	T42.6X5	T42.6X6
bromolactobionate	T42.6X1	T42.6X2	T42.6X3	T42.6X4	T42.6X5	T42.6X6
carbaspirin	T39.011	T39.012	T39.013	T39.014	T39.015	T39.016
carbimide	T50.6X1	T50.6X2	T50.6X3	T50.6X4	T50.6X5	T50.6X6
carbonate	T47.1X1	T47.1X2	T47.1X3	T47.1X4	T47.1X5	T47.1X6
chloride	T50.991	T50.992	T50.993	T50.994	T50.995	T50.996
anhydrous	T50.991	T50.992	T50.993	T50.994	T50.995	T50.996
cyanide	T57.8X1	T57.8X2	T57.8X3	T57.8X4	—	—
dioctyl sulfosuccinate	T47.4X1	T47.4X2	T47.4X3	T47.4X4	T47.4X5	T47.4X6
disodium edathamil	T45.8X1	T45.8X2	T45.8X3	T45.8X4	T45.8X5	T45.8X6
disodium edetate	T45.8X1	T45.8X2	T45.8X3	T45.8X4	T45.8X5	T45.8X6
dobesilate	T46.991	T46.992	T46.993	T46.994	T46.995	T46.996
EDTA	T45.8X1	T45.8X2	T45.8X3	T45.8X4	T45.8X5	T45.8X6
ferrous citrate	T45.4X1	T45.4X2	T45.4X3	T45.4X4	T45.4X5	T45.4X6
folinate	T45.8X1	T45.8X2	T45.8X3	T45.8X4	T45.8X5	T45.8X6
glubionate	T50.3X1	T50.3X2	T50.3X3	T50.3X4	T50.3X5	T50.3X6
gluconate	T50.3X1	T50.3X2	T50.3X3	T50.3X4	T50.3X5	T50.3X6
gluconogalactogluconate	T50.3X1	T50.3X2	T50.3X3	T50.3X4	T50.3X5	T50.3X6
hydrate, hydroxide	T54.3X1	T54.3X2	T54.3X3	T54.3X4	—	—
hypochlorite	T54.3X1	T54.3X2	T54.3X3	T54.3X4	—	—
iodide	T48.4X1	T48.4X2	T48.4X3	T48.4X4	T48.4X5	T48.4X6
ipodate	T50.8X1	T50.8X2	T50.8X3	T50.8X4	T50.8X5	T50.8X6
lactate	T50.3X1	T50.3X2	T50.3X3	T50.3X4	T50.3X5	T50.3X6
leucovorin	T45.8X1	T45.8X2	T45.8X3	T45.8X4	T45.8X5	T45.8X6
mandelate	T37.91	T37.92	T37.93	T37.94	T37.95	T37.96
oxide	T54.3X1	T54.3X2	T54.3X3	T54.3X4	—	—
pantothenate	T45.2X1	T45.2X2	T45.2X3	T45.2X4	T45.2X5	T45.2X6
phosphate	T50.3X1	T50.3X2	T50.3X3	T50.3X4	T50.3X5	T50.3X6
salicylate	T39.091	T39.092	T39.093	T39.094	T39.095	T39.096
salts	T50.3X1	T50.3X2	T50.3X3	T50.3X4	T50.3X5	T50.3X6
Calculus-dissolving drug	T50.991	T50.992	T50.993	T50.994	T50.995	T50.996
Calomel	T49.0X1	T49.0X2	T49.0X3	T49.0X4	T49.0X5	T49.0X6
Caloric agent	T50.3X1	T50.3X2	T50.3X3	T50.3X4	T50.3X5	T50.3X6
Calusterone	T38.7X1	T38.7X2	T38.7X3	T38.7X4	T38.7X5	T38.7X6
Camazepam	T42.4X1	T42.4X2	T42.4X3	T42.4X4	T42.4X5	T42.4X6
Camomile	T49.0X1	T49.0X2	T49.0X3	T49.0X4	T49.0X5	T49.0X6
Camoquin	T37.2X1	T37.2X2	T37.2X3	T37.2X4	T37.2X5	T37.2X6
Camphor						
insecticide	T60.2X1	T60.2X2	T60.2X3	T60.2X4	—	—
medicinal	T49.8X1	T49.8X2	T49.8X3	T49.8X4	T49.8X5	T49.8X6
Camylofin	T44.3X1	T44.3X2	T44.3X3	T44.3X4	T44.3X5	T44.3X6
Cancer chemotherapy drug regimen	T45.1X1	T45.1X2	T45.1X3	T45.1X4	T45.1X5	T45.1X6
Candeptin	T49.0X1	T49.0X2	T49.0X3	T49.0X4	T49.0X5	T49.0X6
Candicidin	T49.0X1	T49.0X2	T49.0X3	T49.0X4	T49.0X5	T49.0X6
Cannabinol	T40.7X1	T40.7X2	T40.7X3	T40.7X4	T40.7X5	T40.7X6
Cannabis (derivatives)	T40.7X1	T40.7X2	T40.7X3	T40.7X4	T40.7X5	T40.7X6
Canned heat	T51.1X1	T51.1X2	T51.1X3	T51.1X4	—	—
Canrenoic acid	T50.0X1	T50.0X2	T50.0X3	T50.0X4	T50.0X5	T50.0X6
Canrenone	T50.0X1	T50.0X2	T50.0X3	T50.0X4	T50.0X5	T50.0X6
Cantharides, cantharidin, cantharis	T49.8X1	T49.8X2	T49.8X3	T49.8X4	T49.8X5	T49.8X6
Canthaxanthin	T50.991	T50.992	T50.993	T50.994	T50.995	T50.996
Capillary-active drug NEC	T46.901	T46.902	T46.903	T46.904	T46.905	T46.906
Capreomycin	T36.8X1	T36.8X2	T36.8X3	T36.8X4	T36.8X5	T36.8X6
Capsicum	T49.4X1	T49.4X2	T49.4X3	T49.4X4	T49.4X5	T49.4X6
Captafol	T60.3X1	T60.3X2	T60.3X3	T60.3X4	—	—
Captan	T60.3X1	T60.3X2	T60.3X3	T60.3X4	—	—
Captodiame, captodiamine	T43.591	T43.592	T43.593	T43.594	T43.595	T43.596
Captopril	T46.4X1	T46.4X2	T46.4X3	T46.4X4	T46.4X5	T46.4X6
Caramiphen	T44.3X1	T44.3X2	T44.3X3	T44.3X4	T44.3X5	T44.3X6
Carazolol	T44.7X1	T44.7X2	T44.7X3	T44.7X4	T44.7X5	T44.7X6
Carbachol	T44.1X1	T44.1X2	T44.1X3	T44.1X4	T44.1X5	T44.1X6
Carbacrylamine (resin)	T50.3X1	T50.3X2	T50.3X3	T50.3X4	T50.3X5	T50.3X6
Carbamate (insecticide)	T60.0X1	T60.0X2	T60.0X3	T60.0X4	—	—
Carbamate (sedative)	T42.6X1	T42.6X2	T42.6X3	T42.6X4	T42.6X5	T42.6X6
herbicide	T60.0X1	T60.0X2	T60.0X3	T60.0X4	—	—
insecticide	T60.0X1	T60.0X2	T60.0X3	T60.0X4	—	—
Carbamazepine	T42.1X1	T42.1X2	T42.1X3	T42.1X4	T42.1X5	T42.1X6

Substance	Poisoning, Accidental (unintentional)	Poisoning, Intentional Self-harm	Poisoning, Assault	Poisoning, Undetermined	Adverse Effect	Under-dosing
Carbamide	T47.3X1	T47.3X2	T47.3X3	T47.3X4	T47.3X5	T47.3X6
peroxide	T49.0X1	T49.0X2	T49.0X3	T49.0X4	T49.0X5	T49.0X6
topical	T49.8X1	T49.8X2	T49.8X3	T49.8X4	T49.8X5	T49.8X6
Carbamylcholine chloride	T44.1X1	T44.1X2	T44.1X3	T44.1X4	T44.1X5	T44.1X6
Carbaril	T60.0X1	T60.0X2	T60.0X3	T60.0X4	—	—
Carbarsone	T37.3X1	T37.3X2	T37.3X3	T37.3X4	T37.3X5	T37.3X6
Carbaryl	T60.0X1	T60.0X2	T60.0X3	T60.0X4	—	—
Carbaspirin	T39.011	T39.012	T39.013	T39.014	T39.015	T39.016
Carbazochrome (salicylate) (sodium sulfonate)	T49.4X1	T49.4X2	T49.4X3	T49.4X4	T49.4X5	T49.4X6
Carbenicillin	T36.0X1	T36.0X2	T36.0X3	T36.0X4	T36.0X5	T36.0X6
Carbenoxolone	T47.1X1	T47.1X2	T47.1X3	T47.1X4	T47.1X5	T47.1X6
Carbetapentane	T48.3X1	T48.3X2	T48.3X3	T48.3X4	T48.3X5	T48.3X6
Carbethyl salicylate	T39.091	T39.092	T39.093	T39.094	T39.095	T39.096
Carbidopa (with levodopa)	T42.8X1	T42.8X2	T42.8X3	T42.8X4	T42.8X5	T42.8X6
Carbimazole	T38.2X1	T38.2X2	T38.2X3	T38.2X4	T38.2X5	T38.2X6
Carbinol	T51.1X1	T51.1X2	T51.1X3	T51.1X4	—	—
Carbinoxamine	T45.0X1	T45.0X2	T45.0X3	T45.0X4	T45.0X5	T45.0X6
Carbiphene	T39.8X1	T39.8X2	T39.8X3	T39.8X4	T39.8X5	T39.8X6
Carbitol	T52.3X1	T52.3X2	T52.3X3	T52.3X4	—	—
Carbocaine	T41.3X1	T41.3X2	T41.3X3	T41.3X4	T41.3X5	T41.3X6
infiltration (subcutaneous)	T41.3X1	T41.3X2	T41.3X3	T41.3X4	T41.3X5	T41.3X6
nerve block (peripheral) (plexus)	T41.3X1	T41.3X2	T41.3X3	T41.3X4	T41.3X5	T41.3X6
topical (surface)	T41.3X1	T41.3X2	T41.3X3	T41.3X4	T41.3X5	T41.3X6
Carbocisteine	T48.4X1	T48.4X2	T48.4X3	T48.4X4	T48.4X5	T48.4X6
Carbocromen	T46.3X1	T46.3X2	T46.3X3	T46.3X4	T46.3X5	T46.3X6
Carbol fuchsin	T49.0X1	T49.0X2	T49.0X3	T49.0X4	T49.0X5	T49.0X6
Carbolic acid — *see also* Phenol	T54.0X1	T54.0X2	T54.0X3	T54.0X4	—	—
Carbolonium (bromide)	T48.1X1	T48.1X2	T48.1X3	T48.1X4	T48.1X5	T48.1X6
Carbo medicinalis	T47.6X1	T47.6X2	T47.6X3	T47.6X4	T47.6X5	T47.6X6
Carbomycin	T36.8X1	T36.8X2	T36.8X3	T36.8X4	T36.8X5	T36.8X6
Carbon						
bisulfide (liquid)	T65.4X1	T65.4X2	T65.4X3	T65.4X4	—	—
vapor	T65.4X1	T65.4X2	T65.4X3	T65.4X4	—	—
dioxide (gas)	T59.7X1	T59.7X2	T59.7X3	T59.7X4	—	—
medicinal	T41.5X1	T41.5X2	T41.5X3	T41.5X4	T41.5X5	T41.5X6
nonmedicinal	T59.7X1	T59.7X2	T59.7X3	T59.7X4	—	—
snow	T49.4X1	T49.4X2	T49.4X3	T49.4X4	T49.4X5	T49.4X6
disulfide (liquid)	T65.4X1	T65.4X2	T65.4X3	T65.4X4	—	—
vapor	T65.4X1	T65.4X2	T65.4X3	T65.4X4	—	—
monoxide (from incomplete combustion)	T58.91	T58.92	T58.93	T58.94	—	—
blast furnace gas	T58.8X1	T58.8X2	T58.8X3	T58.8X4	—	—
butane (distributed in mobile container)	T58.11	T58.12	T58.13	T58.14	—	—
distributed through pipes	T58.11	T58.12	T58.13	T58.14	—	—
charcoal fumes	T58.2X1	T58.2X2	T58.2X3	T58.2X4	—	—
coal	T58.2X1	T58.2X2	T58.2X3	T58.2X4	—	—
coke (in domestic stoves, fireplaces)	T58.2X1	T58.2X2	T58.2X3	T58.2X4	—	—
exhaust gas (motor) not in transit	T58.01	T58.02	T58.03	T58.04	—	—
combustion engine, any not in watercraft	T58.01	T58.02	T58.03	T58.04	—	—
farm tractor, not in transit	T58.01	T58.02	T58.03	T58.04	—	—
gas engine	T58.01	T58.02	T58.03	T58.04	—	—
motor pump	T58.01	T58.02	T58.03	T58.04	—	—
motor vehicle, not in transit	T58.01	T58.02	T58.03	T58.04	—	—
fuel (in domestic use)	T58.2X1	T58.2X2	T58.2X3	T58.2X4	—	—
gas (piped)	T58.11	T58.12	T58.13	T58.14	—	—
in mobile container	T58.11	T58.12	T58.13	T58.14	—	—
piped (natural)	T58.11	T58.12	T58.13	T58.14	—	—
utility	T58.11	T58.12	T58.13	T58.14	—	—
in mobile container	T58.11	T58.12	T58.13	T58.14	—	—
gas (piped)	T58.11	T58.12	T58.13	T58.14	—	—
illuminating gas	T58.11	T58.12	T58.13	T58.14	—	—
industrial fuels or gases, any	T58.8X1	T58.8X2	T58.8X3	T58.8X4	—	—
kerosene (in domestic stoves, fireplaces)	T58.2X1	T58.2X2	T58.2X3	T58.2X4	—	—
kiln gas or vapor	T58.8X1	T58.8X2	T58.8X3	T58.8X4	—	—
motor exhaust gas, not in transit	T58.01	T58.02	T58.03	T58.04	—	—
piped gas (manufactured) (natural)	T58.11	T58.12	T58.13	T58.14	—	—
producer gas	T58.8X1	T58.8X2	T58.8X3	T58.8X4	—	—
propane (distributed in mobile container)	T58.11	T58.12	T58.13	T58.14	—	—

Subterms under main terms may continue to next column or page   Additional Character May Be Required — Refer to the Tabular List for Character Selection   357

Cadmium — Carbon

Substance	Poisoning, Accidental (unintentional)	Poisoning, Intentional Self-harm	Poisoning, Assault	Poisoning, Undetermined	Adverse Effect	Under-dosing
Carbon — *continued*						
monoxide — *continued*						
propane — *continued*						
distributed through pipes	T58.11	T58.12	T58.13	T58.14	—	—
solid (in domestic stoves, fireplaces)	T58.2X1	T58.2X2	T58.2X3	T58.2X4	—	—
specified source NEC	T58.8X1	T58.8X2	T58.8X3	T58.8X4	—	—
stove gas	T58.11	T58.12	T58.13	T58.14	—	—
piped	T58.11	T58.12	T58.13	T58.14	—	—
utility gas	T58.11	T58.12	T58.13	T58.14	—	—
piped	T58.11	T58.12	T58.13	T58.14	—	—
water gas	T58.11	T58.12	T58.13	T58.14	—	—
wood (in domestic stoves, fireplaces)	T58.2X1	T58.2X2	T58.2X3	T58.2X4	—	—
tetrachloride (vapor) NEC	T53.0X1	T53.0X2	T53.0X3	T53.0X4	—	—
liquid (cleansing agent) NEC	T53.0X1	T53.0X2	T53.0X3	T53.0X4	—	—
solvent	T53.0X1	T53.0X2	T53.0X3	T53.0X4	—	—
Carbonic acid gas	T59.7X1	T59.7X2	T59.7X3	T59.7X4	—	—
anhydrase inhibitor NEC	T50.2X1	T50.2X2	T50.2X3	T50.2X4	T50.2X5	T50.2X6
Carbophenothion	T60.0X1	T60.0X2	T60.0X3	T60.0X4	—	—
Carboplatin	T45.1X1	T45.1X2	T45.1X3	T45.1X4	T45.1X5	T45.1X6
Carboprost	T48.0X1	T48.0X2	T48.0X3	T48.0X4	T48.0X5	T48.0X6
Carboquone	T45.1X1	T45.1X2	T45.1X3	T45.1X4	T45.1X5	T45.1X6
Carbowax	T49.3X1	T49.3X2	T49.3X3	T49.3X4	T49.3X5	T49.3X6
Carboxymethylcellulose	T47.4X1	T47.4X2	T47.4X3	T47.4X4	T47.4X5	T47.4X6
Carbrital	T42.3X1	T42.3X2	T42.3X3	T42.3X4	T42.3X5	T42.3X6
Carbromal	T42.6X1	T42.6X2	T42.6X3	T42.6X4	T42.6X5	T42.6X6
Carbutamide	T38.3X1	T38.3X2	T38.3X3	T38.3X4	T38.3X5	T38.3X6
Carbuterol	T48.6X1	T48.6X2	T48.6X3	T48.6X4	T48.6X5	T48.6X6
Cardiac						
depressants	T46.2X1	T46.2X2	T46.2X3	T46.2X4	T46.2X5	T46.2X6
rhythm regulator	T46.2X1	T46.2X2	T46.2X3	T46.2X4	T46.2X5	T46.2X6
specified NEC	T46.2X1	T46.2X2	T46.2X3	T46.2X4	T46.2X5	T46.2X6
Cardiografin	T50.8X1	T50.8X2	T50.8X3	T50.8X4	T50.8X5	T50.8X6
Cardiogreen	T50.8X1	T50.8X2	T50.8X3	T50.8X4	T50.8X5	T50.8X6
Cardiotonic (glycoside) **NEC**	T46.0X1	T46.0X2	T46.0X3	T46.0X4	T46.0X5	T46.0X6
Cardiovascular drug NEC	T46.901	T46.902	T46.903	T46.904	T46.905	T46.906
Cardrase	T50.2X1	T50.2X2	T50.2X3	T50.2X4	T50.2X5	T50.2X6
Carfecillin	T36.0X1	T36.0X2	T36.0X3	T36.0X4	T36.0X5	T36.0X6
Carfenazine	T43.3X1	T43.3X2	T43.3X3	T43.3X4	T43.3X5	T43.3X6
Carfusin	T49.0X1	T49.0X2	T49.0X3	T49.0X4	T49.0X5	T49.0X6
Carindacillin	T36.0X1	T36.0X2	T36.0X3	T36.0X4	T36.0X5	T36.0X6
Carisoprodol	T42.8X1	T42.8X2	T42.8X3	T42.8X4	T42.8X5	T42.8X6
Carmellose	T47.4X1	T47.4X2	T47.4X3	T47.4X4	T47.4X5	T47.4X6
Carminative	T47.5X1	T47.5X2	T47.5X3	T47.5X4	T47.5X5	T47.5X6
Carmofur	T45.1X1	T45.1X2	T45.1X3	T45.1X4	T45.1X5	T45.1X6
Carmustine	T45.1X1	T45.1X2	T45.1X3	T45.1X4	T45.1X5	T45.1X6
Carotene	T45.2X1	T45.2X2	T45.2X3	T45.2X4	T45.2X5	T45.2X6
Carphenazine	T43.3X1	T43.3X2	T43.3X3	T43.3X4	T43.3X5	T43.3X6
Carpipramine	T42.4X1	T42.4X2	T42.4X3	T42.4X4	T42.4X5	T42.4X6
Carprofen	T39.311	T39.312	T39.313	T39.314	T39.315	T39.316
Carpronium chloride	T44.3X1	T44.3X2	T44.3X3	T44.3X4	T44.3X5	T44.3X6
Carrageenan	T47.8X1	T47.8X2	T47.8X3	T47.8X4	T47.8X5	T47.8X6
Carteolol	T44.7X1	T44.7X2	T44.7X3	T44.7X4	T44.7X5	T44.7X6
Carter's Little Pills	T47.2X1	T47.2X2	T47.2X3	T47.2X4	T47.2X5	T47.2X6
Cascara (sagrada)	T47.2X1	T47.2X2	T47.2X3	T47.2X4	T47.2X5	T47.2X6
Cassava	T62.2X1	T62.2X2	T62.2X3	T62.2X4	—	—
Castellani's paint	T49.0X1	T49.0X2	T49.0X3	T49.0X4	T49.0X5	T49.0X6
Castor						
bean	T62.2X1	T62.2X2	T62.2X3	T62.2X4	—	—
oil	T47.2X1	T47.2X2	T47.2X3	T47.2X4	T47.2X5	T47.2X6
Catalase	T45.3X1	T45.3X2	T45.3X3	T45.3X4	T45.3X5	T45.3X6
Caterpillar (sting)	T63.431	T63.432	T63.433	T63.434	—	—
Catha (edulis) (tea)	T43.691	T43.692	T43.693	T43.694	—	—
Cathartic NEC	T47.4X1	T47.4X2	T47.4X3	T47.4X4	T47.4X5	T47.4X6
anthracene derivative	T47.2X1	T47.2X2	T47.2X3	T47.2X4	T47.2X5	T47.2X6
bulk	T47.4X1	T47.4X2	T47.4X3	T47.4X4	T47.4X5	T47.4X6
contact	T47.2X1	T47.2X2	T47.2X3	T47.2X4	T47.2X5	T47.2X6
emollient NEC	T47.4X1	T47.4X2	T47.4X3	T47.4X4	T47.4X5	T47.4X6
irritant NEC	T47.2X1	T47.2X2	T47.2X3	T47.2X4	T47.2X5	T47.2X6
mucilage	T47.4X1	T47.4X2	T47.4X3	T47.4X4	T47.4X5	T47.4X6
saline	T47.3X1	T47.3X2	T47.3X3	T47.3X4	T47.3X5	T47.3X6
vegetable	T47.2X1	T47.2X2	T47.2X3	T47.2X4	T47.2X5	T47.2X6
Cathine	T50.5X1	T50.5X2	T50.5X3	T50.5X4	T50.5X5	T50.5X6
Cathomycin	T36.8X1	T36.8X2	T36.8X3	T36.8X4	T36.8X5	T36.8X6
Cation exchange resin	T50.3X1	T50.3X2	T50.3X3	T50.3X4	T50.3X5	T50.3X6
Caustic(s) NEC	T54.91	T54.92	T54.93	T54.94	—	—
alkali	T54.3X1	T54.3X2	T54.3X3	T54.3X4	—	—
hydroxide	T54.3X1	T54.3X2	T54.3X3	T54.3X4	—	—
potash	T54.3X1	T54.3X2	T54.3X3	T54.3X4	—	—
soda	T54.3X1	T54.3X2	T54.3X3	T54.3X4	—	—

Substance	Poisoning, Accidental (unintentional)	Poisoning, Intentional Self-harm	Poisoning, Assault	Poisoning, Undetermined	Adverse Effect	Under-dosing
Caustic(s) NEC — *continued*						
specified NEC	T54.91	T54.92	T54.93	T54.94	—	—
Ceepryn	T49.0X1	T49.0X2	T49.0X3	T49.0X4	T49.0X5	T49.0X6
ENT agent	T49.6X1	T49.6X2	T49.6X3	T49.6X4	T49.6X5	T49.6X6
lozenges	T49.6X1	T49.6X2	T49.6X3	T49.6X4	T49.6X5	T49.6X6
Cefacetrile	T36.1X1	T36.1X2	T36.1X3	T36.1X4	T36.1X5	T36.1X6
Cefaclor	T36.1X1	T36.1X2	T36.1X3	T36.1X4	T36.1X5	T36.1X6
Cefadroxil	T36.1X1	T36.1X2	T36.1X3	T36.1X4	T36.1X5	T36.1X6
Cefalexin	T36.1X1	T36.1X2	T36.1X3	T36.1X4	T36.1X5	T36.1X6
Cefaloglycin	T36.1X1	T36.1X2	T36.1X3	T36.1X4	T36.1X5	T36.1X6
Cefaloridine	T36.1X1	T36.1X2	T36.1X3	T36.1X4	T36.1X5	T36.1X6
Cefalosporins	T36.1X1	T36.1X2	T36.1X3	T36.1X4	T36.1X5	T36.1X6
Cefalotin	T36.1X1	T36.1X2	T36.1X3	T36.1X4	T36.1X5	T36.1X6
Cefamandole	T36.1X1	T36.1X2	T36.1X3	T36.1X4	T36.1X5	T36.1X6
Cefamycin antibiotic	T36.1X1	T36.1X2	T36.1X3	T36.1X4	T36.1X5	T36.1X6
Cefapirin	T36.1X1	T36.1X2	T36.1X3	T36.1X4	T36.1X5	T36.1X6
Cefatrizine	T36.1X1	T36.1X2	T36.1X3	T36.1X4	T36.1X5	T36.1X6
Cefazedone	T36.1X1	T36.1X2	T36.1X3	T36.1X4	T36.1X5	T36.1X6
Cefazolin	T36.1X1	T36.1X2	T36.1X3	T36.1X4	T36.1X5	T36.1X6
Cefbuperazone	T36.1X1	T36.1X2	T36.1X3	T36.1X4	T36.1X5	T36.1X6
Cefetamet	T36.1X1	T36.1X2	T36.1X3	T36.1X4	T36.1X5	T36.1X6
Cefixime	T36.1X1	T36.1X2	T36.1X3	T36.1X4	T36.1X5	T36.1X6
Cefmenoxime	T36.1X1	T36.1X2	T36.1X3	T36.1X4	T36.1X5	T36.1X6
Cefmetazole	T36.1X1	T36.1X2	T36.1X3	T36.1X4	T36.1X5	T36.1X6
Cefminox	T36.1X1	T36.1X2	T36.1X3	T36.1X4	T36.1X5	T36.1X6
Cefonicid	T36.1X1	T36.1X2	T36.1X3	T36.1X4	T36.1X5	T36.1X6
Cefoperazone	T36.1X1	T36.1X2	T36.1X3	T36.1X4	T36.1X5	T36.1X6
Ceforanide	T36.1X1	T36.1X2	T36.1X3	T36.1X4	T36.1X5	T36.1X6
Cefotaxime	T36.1X1	T36.1X2	T36.1X3	T36.1X4	T36.1X5	T36.1X6
Cefotetan	T36.1X1	T36.1X2	T36.1X3	T36.1X4	T36.1X5	T36.1X6
Cefotiam	T36.1X1	T36.1X2	T36.1X3	T36.1X4	T36.1X5	T36.1X6
Cefoxitin	T36.1X1	T36.1X2	T36.1X3	T36.1X4	T36.1X5	T36.1X6
Cefpimizole	T36.1X1	T36.1X2	T36.1X3	T36.1X4	T36.1X5	T36.1X6
Cefpiramide	T36.1X1	T36.1X2	T36.1X3	T36.1X4	T36.1X5	T36.1X6
Cefradine	T36.1X1	T36.1X2	T36.1X3	T36.1X4	T36.1X5	T36.1X6
Cefroxadine	T36.1X1	T36.1X2	T36.1X3	T36.1X4	T36.1X5	T36.1X6
Cefsulodin	T36.1X1	T36.1X2	T36.1X3	T36.1X4	T36.1X5	T36.1X6
Ceftazidime	T36.1X1	T36.1X2	T36.1X3	T36.1X4	T36.1X5	T36.1X6
Cefteram	T36.1X1	T36.1X2	T36.1X3	T36.1X4	T36.1X5	T36.1X6
Ceftezole	T36.1X1	T36.1X2	T36.1X3	T36.1X4	T36.1X5	T36.1X6
Ceftizoxime	T36.1X1	T36.1X2	T36.1X3	T36.1X4	T36.1X5	T36.1X6
Ceftriaxone	T36.1X1	T36.1X2	T36.1X3	T36.1X4	T36.1X5	T36.1X6
Cefuroxime	T36.1X1	T36.1X2	T36.1X3	T36.1X4	T36.1X5	T36.1X6
Cefuzonam	T36.1X1	T36.1X2	T36.1X3	T36.1X4	T36.1X5	T36.1X6
Celestone	T38.0X1	T38.0X2	T38.0X3	T38.0X4	T38.0X5	T38.0X6
topical	T49.0X1	T49.0X2	T49.0X3	T49.0X4	T49.0X5	T49.0X6
Celiprolol	T44.7X1	T44.7X2	T44.7X3	T44.7X4	T44.7X5	T44.7X6
Cellosolve	T52.91	T52.92	T52.93	T52.94	—	—
Cell stimulants and proliferants	T49.8X1	T49.8X2	T49.8X3	T49.8X4	T49.8X5	T49.8X6
Cellulose						
cathartic	T47.4X1	T47.4X2	T47.4X3	T47.4X4	T47.4X5	T47.4X6
hydroxyethyl	T47.4X1	T47.4X2	T47.4X3	T47.4X4	T47.4X5	T47.4X6
nitrates (topical)	T49.3X1	T49.3X2	T49.3X3	T49.3X4	T49.3X5	T49.3X6
oxidized	T49.4X1	T49.4X2	T49.4X3	T49.4X4	T49.4X5	T49.4X6
Centipede (bite)	T63.411	T63.412	T63.413	T63.414	—	—
Central nervous system						
depressants	T42.71	T42.72	T42.73	T42.74	T42.75	T42.76
anesthetic (general) NEC	T41.201	T41.202	T41.203	T41.204	T41.205	T41.206
gases NEC	T41.0X1	T41.0X2	T41.0X3	T41.0X4	T41.0X5	T41.0X6
intravenous	T41.1X1	T41.1X2	T41.1X3	T41.1X4	T41.1X5	T41.1X6
barbiturates	T42.3X1	T42.3X2	T42.3X3	T42.3X4	T42.3X5	T42.3X6
benzodiazepines	T42.4X1	T42.4X2	T42.4X3	T42.4X4	T42.4X5	T42.4X6
bromides	T42.6X1	T42.6X2	T42.6X3	T42.6X4	T42.6X5	T42.6X6
cannabis sativa	T40.7X1	T40.7X2	T40.7X3	T40.7X4	T40.7X5	T40.7X6
chloral hydrate	T42.6X1	T42.6X2	T42.6X3	T42.6X4	T42.6X5	T42.6X6
ethanol	T51.0X1	T51.0X2	T51.0X3	T51.0X4	—	—
hallucinogenics	T40.901	T40.902	T40.903	T40.904	T40.905	T40.906
hypnotics	T42.71	T42.72	T42.73	T42.74	T42.75	T42.76
specified NEC	T42.6X1	T42.6X2	T42.6X3	T42.6X4	T42.6X5	T42.6X6
muscle relaxants	T42.8X1	T42.8X2	T42.8X3	T42.8X4	T42.8X5	T42.8X6
paraldehyde	T42.6X1	T42.6X2	T42.6X3	T42.6X4	T42.6X5	T42.6X6
sedatives	T42.71	T42.72	T42.73	T42.74	T42.75	T42.76
sedative-hypnotics						
mixed NEC	T42.6X1	T42.6X2	T42.6X3	T42.6X4	T42.6X5	T42.6X6
specified NEC	T42.6X1	T42.6X2	T42.6X3	T42.6X4	T42.6X5	T42.6X6
muscle-tone depressants	T42.8X1	T42.8X2	T42.8X3	T42.8X4	T42.8X5	T42.8X6
stimulants	T43.601	T43.602	T43.603	T43.604	T43.605	T43.606
amphetamines	T43.621	T43.622	T43.623	T43.624	T43.625	T43.626
analeptics	T50.7X1	T50.7X2	T50.7X3	T50.7X4	T50.7X5	T50.7X6
antidepressants	T43.201	T43.202	T43.203	T43.204	T43.205	T43.206
opiate antagonists	T50.7X1	T50.7X2	T50.7X3	T50.7X4	T50.7X5	T50.7X6
specified NEC	T43.691	T43.692	T43.693	T43.694	T43.695	T43.696

Substance	Poisoning, Accidental (unintentional)	Poisoning, Intentional Self-harm	Poisoning, Assault	Poisoning, Undetermined	Adverse Effect	Under-dosing
Cephalexin	T36.1X1	T36.1X2	T36.1X3	T36.1X4	T36.1X5	T36.1X6
Cephaloglycin	T36.1X1	T36.1X2	T36.1X3	T36.1X4	T36.1X5	T36.1X6
Cephaloridine	T36.1X1	T36.1X2	T36.1X3	T36.1X4	T36.1X5	T36.1X6
Cephalosporins	T36.1X1	T36.1X2	T36.1X3	T36.1X4	T36.1X5	T36.1X6
N (adicillin)	T36.0X1	T36.0X2	T36.0X3	T36.0X4	T36.0X5	T36.0X6
Cephalothin	T36.1X1	T36.1X2	T36.1X3	T36.1X4	T36.1X5	T36.1X6
Cephalotin	T36.1X1	T36.1X2	T36.1X3	T36.1X4	T36.1X5	T36.1X6
Cephradine	T36.1X1	T36.1X2	T36.1X3	T36.1X4	T36.1X5	T36.1X6
Cerbera (odallam)	T62.2X1	T62.2X2	T62.2X3	T62.2X4	—	—
Cerberin	T46.0X1	T46.0X2	T46.0X3	T46.0X4	T46.0X5	T46.0X6
Cerebral stimulants	T43.601	T43.602	T43.603	T43.604	T43.605	T43.606
psychotherapeutic	T43.601	T43.602	T43.603	T43.604	T43.605	T43.606
specified NEC	T43.691	T43.692	T43.693	T43.694	T43.695	T43.696
Cerium oxalate	T45.0X1	T45.0X2	T45.0X3	T45.0X4	T45.0X5	T45.0X6
Cerous oxalate	T45.0X1	T45.0X2	T45.0X3	T45.0X4	T45.0X5	T45.0X6
Ceruletide	T50.8X1	T50.8X2	T50.8X3	T50.8X4	T50.8X5	T50.8X6
Cetalkonium (chloride)	T49.0X1	T49.0X2	T49.0X3	T49.0X4	T49.0X5	T49.0X6
Cethexonium chloride	T49.0X1	T49.0X2	T49.0X3	T49.0X4	T49.0X5	T49.0X6
Cetiedil	T46.7X1	T46.7X2	T46.7X3	T46.7X4	T46.7X5	T46.7X6
Cetirizine	T45.0X1	T45.0X2	T45.0X3	T45.0X4	T45.0X5	T45.0X6
Cetomacrogol	T50.991	T50.992	T50.993	T50.994	T50.995	T50.996
Cetotiamine	T45.2X1	T45.2X2	T45.2X3	T45.2X4	T45.2X5	T45.2X6
Cetoxime	T45.0X1	T45.0X2	T45.0X3	T45.0X4	T45.0X5	T45.0X6
Cetraxate	T47.1X1	T47.1X2	T47.1X3	T47.1X4	T47.1X5	T47.1X6
Cetrimide	T49.0X1	T49.0X2	T49.0X3	T49.0X4	T49.0X5	T49.0X6
Cetrimonium (bromide)	T49.0X1	T49.0X2	T49.0X3	T49.0X4	T49.0X5	T49.0X6
Cetylpyridinium chloride	T49.0X1	T49.0X2	T49.0X3	T49.0X4	T49.0X5	T49.0X6
ENT agent	T49.6X1	T49.6X2	T49.6X3	T49.6X4	T49.6X5	T49.6X6
lozenges	T49.6X1	T49.6X2	T49.6X3	T49.6X4	T49.6X5	T49.6X6
Cevadilla — see Sabadilla						
Cevitamic acid	T45.2X1	T45.2X2	T45.2X3	T45.2X4	T45.2X5	T45.2X6
Chalk, precipitated	T47.1X1	T47.1X2	T47.1X3	T47.1X4	T47.1X5	T47.1X6
Chamomile	T49.0X1	T49.0X2	T49.0X3	T49.0X4	T49.0X5	T49.0X6
Ch'an su	T46.0X1	T46.0X2	T46.0X3	T46.0X4	T46.0X5	T46.0X6
Charcoal	T47.6X1	T47.6X2	T47.6X3	T47.6X4	T47.6X5	T47.6X6
activated — see also Charcoal, medicinal	T47.6X1	T47.6X2	T47.6X3	T47.6X4	T47.6X5	T47.6X6
fumes (Carbon monoxide)	T58.2X1	T58.2X2	T58.2X3	T58.2X4	—	—
industrial	T58.8X1	T58.8X2	T58.8X3	T58.8X4	—	—
medicinal (activated)	T47.6X1	T47.6X2	T47.6X3	T47.6X4	T47.6X5	T47.6X6
antidiarrheal	T47.6X1	T47.6X2	T47.6X3	T47.6X4	T47.6X5	T47.6X6
poison control	T47.8X1	T47.8X2	T47.8X3	T47.8X4	T47.8X5	T47.8X6
specified use other than for diarrhea	T47.8X1	T47.8X2	T47.8X3	T47.8X4	T47.8X5	T47.8X6
topical	T49.8X1	T49.8X2	T49.8X3	T49.8X4	T49.8X5	T49.8X6
Chaulmosulfone	T37.1X1	T37.1X2	T37.1X3	T37.1X4	T37.1X5	T37.1X6
Chelating agent NEC	T50.6X1	T50.6X2	T50.6X3	T50.6X4	T50.6X5	T50.6X6
Chelidonium majus	T62.2X1	T62.2X2	T62.2X3	T62.2X4	—	—
Chemical substance NEC	T65.91	T65.92	T65.93	T65.94	—	—
Chenodeoxycholic acid	T47.5X1	T47.5X2	T47.5X3	T47.5X4	T47.5X5	T47.5X6
Chenodiol	T47.5X1	T47.5X2	T47.5X3	T47.5X4	T47.5X5	T47.5X6
Chenopodium	T37.4X1	T37.4X2	T37.4X3	T37.4X4	T37.4X5	T37.4X6
Cherry laurel	T62.2X1	T62.2X2	T62.2X3	T62.2X4	—	—
Chinidin (e)	T46.2X1	T46.2X2	T46.2X3	T46.2X4	T46.2X5	T46.2X6
Chiniofon	T37.8X1	T37.8X2	T37.8X3	T37.8X4	T37.8X5	T37.8X6
Chlophedianol	T48.3X1	T48.3X2	T48.3X3	T48.3X4	T48.3X5	T48.3X6
Chloral	T42.6X1	T42.6X2	T42.6X3	T42.6X4	T42.6X5	T42.6X6
derivative	T42.6X1	T42.6X2	T42.6X3	T42.6X4	T42.6X5	T42.6X6
hydrate	T42.6X1	T42.6X2	T42.6X3	T42.6X4	T42.6X5	T42.6X6
Chloralamide	T42.6X1	T42.6X2	T42.6X3	T42.6X4	T42.6X5	T42.6X6
Chloralodol	T42.6X1	T42.6X2	T42.6X3	T42.6X4	T42.6X5	T42.6X6
Chloralose	T60.4X1	T60.4X2	T60.4X3	T60.4X4	—	—
Chlorambucil	T45.1X1	T45.1X2	T45.1X3	T45.1X4	T45.1X5	T45.1X6
Chloramine	T57.8X1	T57.8X2	T57.8X3	T57.8X4	—	—
T	T49.0X1	T49.0X2	T49.0X3	T49.0X4	T49.0X5	T49.0X6
topical	T49.0X1	T49.0X2	T49.0X3	T49.0X4	T49.0X5	T49.0X6
Chloramphenicol	T36.2X1	T36.2X2	T36.2X3	T36.2X4	T36.2X5	T36.2X6
ENT agent	T49.6X1	T49.6X2	T49.6X3	T49.6X4	T49.6X5	T49.6X6
ophthalmic preparation	T49.5X1	T49.5X2	T49.5X3	T49.5X4	T49.5X5	T49.5X6
topical NEC	T49.0X1	T49.0X2	T49.0X3	T49.0X4	T49.0X5	T49.0X6
Chlorate (potassium) (sodium) NEC	T60.3X1	T60.3X2	T60.3X3	T60.3X4	—	—
herbicide	T60.3X1	T60.3X2	T60.3X3	T60.3X4	—	—
Chlorazanil	T50.2X1	T50.2X2	T50.2X3	T50.2X4	T50.2X5	T50.2X6
Chlorbenzene, chlorbenzol	T53.7X1	T53.7X2	T53.7X3	T53.7X4	—	—
Chlorbenzoxamine	T44.3X1	T44.3X2	T44.3X3	T44.3X4	T44.3X5	T44.3X6
Chlorbutol	T42.6X1	T42.6X2	T42.6X3	T42.6X4	T42.6X5	T42.6X6
Chlorcyclizine	T45.0X1	T45.0X2	T45.0X3	T45.0X4	T45.0X5	T45.0X6
Chlordan (e) (dust)	T60.1X1	T60.1X2	T60.1X3	T60.1X4	—	—
Chlordantoin	T49.0X1	T49.0X2	T49.0X3	T49.0X4	T49.0X5	T49.0X6
Chlordiazepoxide	T42.4X1	T42.4X2	T42.4X3	T42.4X4	T42.4X5	T42.4X6
Chlordiethyl benzamide	T49.3X1	T49.3X2	T49.3X3	T49.3X4	T49.3X5	T49.3X6
Chloresium	T49.8X1	T49.8X2	T49.8X3	T49.8X4	T49.8X5	T49.8X6

Substance	Poisoning, Accidental (unintentional)	Poisoning, Intentional Self-harm	Poisoning, Assault	Poisoning, Undetermined	Adverse Effect	Under-dosing
Chlorethiazol	T42.6X1	T42.6X2	T42.6X3	T42.6X4	T42.6X5	T42.6X6
Chlorethyl — see Ethyl chloride						
Chloretone	T42.6X1	T42.6X2	T42.6X3	T42.6X4	T42.6X5	T42.6X6
Chlorex	T53.6X1	T53.6X2	T53.6X3	T53.6X4	—	—
insecticide	T60.1X1	T60.1X2	T60.1X3	T60.1X4	—	—
Chlorfenvinphos	T60.0X1	T60.0X2	T60.0X3	T60.0X4	—	—
Chlorhexadol	T42.6X1	T42.6X2	T42.6X3	T42.6X4	T42.6X5	T42.6X6
Chlorhexamide	T45.1X1	T45.1X2	T45.1X3	T45.1X4	T45.1X5	T45.1X6
Chlorhexidine	T49.0X1	T49.0X2	T49.0X3	T49.0X4	T49.0X5	T49.0X6
Chlorhydroxyquinolin	T49.0X1	T49.0X2	T49.0X3	T49.0X4	T49.0X5	T49.0X6
Chloride of lime (bleach)	T54.3X1	T54.3X2	T54.3X3	T54.3X4	—	—
Chlorimipramine	T43.011	T43.012	T43.013	T43.014	T43.015	T43.016
Chlorinated						
camphene	T53.6X1	T53.6X2	T53.6X3	T53.6X4	—	—
diphenyl	T53.7X1	T53.7X2	T53.7X3	T53.7X4	—	—
hydrocarbons NEC	T53.91	T53.92	T53.93	T53.94	—	—
solvents	T53.91	T53.92	T53.93	T53.94	—	—
lime (bleach)	T54.3X1	T54.3X2	T54.3X3	T54.3X4	—	—
and boric acid solution	T49.0X1	T49.0X2	T49.0X3	T49.0X4	T49.0X5	T49.0X6
naphthalene (insecticide)	T60.1X1	T60.1X2	T60.1X3	T60.1X4	—	—
industrial (non-pesticide)	T53.7X1	T53.7X2	T53.7X3	T53.7X4	—	—
pesticide NEC	T60.8X1	T60.8X2	T60.8X3	T60.8X4	—	—
soda — see also sodium hypochlorite						
solution	T49.0X1	T49.0X2	T49.0X3	T49.0X4	T49.0X5	T49.0X6
Chlorine (fumes) (gas)	T59.4X1	T59.4X2	T59.4X3	T59.4X4	—	—
bleach	T54.3X1	T54.3X2	T54.3X3	T54.3X4	—	—
compound gas NEC	T59.4X1	T59.4X2	T59.4X3	T59.4X4	—	—
disinfectant	T59.4X1	T59.4X2	T59.4X3	T59.4X4	—	—
releasing agents NEC	T59.4X1	T59.4X2	T59.4X3	T59.4X4	—	—
Chlorisondamine chloride	T46.991	T46.992	T46.993	T46.994	T46.995	T46.996
Chlormadinone	T38.5X1	T38.5X2	T38.5X3	T38.5X4	T38.5X5	T38.5X6
Chlormephos	T60.0X1	T60.0X2	T60.0X3	T60.0X4	—	—
Chlormerodrin	T50.2X1	T50.2X2	T50.2X3	T50.2X4	T50.2X5	T50.2X6
Chlormethiazole	T42.6X1	T42.6X2	T42.6X3	T42.6X4	T42.6X5	T42.6X6
Chlormethine	T45.1X1	T45.1X2	T45.1X3	T45.1X4	T45.1X5	T45.1X6
Chlormethylenecycline	T36.4X1	T36.4X2	T36.4X3	T36.4X4	T36.4X5	T36.4X6
Chlormezanone	T42.6X1	T42.6X2	T42.6X3	T42.6X4	T42.6X5	T42.6X6
Chloroacetic acid	T60.3X1	T60.3X2	T60.3X3	T60.3X4	—	—
Chloroacetone	T59.3X1	T59.3X2	T59.3X3	T59.3X4	—	—
Chloroacetophenone	T59.3X1	T59.3X2	T59.3X3	T59.3X4	—	—
Chloroaniline	T53.7X1	T53.7X2	T53.7X3	T53.7X4	—	—
Chlorobenzene, chlorobenzol	T53.7X1	T53.7X2	T53.7X3	T53.7X4	—	—
Chlorobromomethane (fire extinguisher)	T53.6X1	T53.6X2	T53.6X3	T53.6X4	—	—
Chlorobutanol	T49.0X1	T49.0X2	T49.0X3	T49.0X4	T49.0X5	T49.0X6
Chlorocresol	T49.0X1	T49.0X2	T49.0X3	T49.0X4	T49.0X5	T49.0X6
Chlorodehydromethyltestosterone	T38.7X1	T38.7X2	T38.7X3	T38.7X4	T38.7X5	T38.7X6
Chlorodinitrobenzene	T53.7X1	T53.7X2	T53.7X3	T53.7X4	—	—
dust or vapor	T53.7X1	T53.7X2	T53.7X3	T53.7X4	—	—
Chlorodiphenyl	T53.7X1	T53.7X2	T53.7X3	T53.7X4	—	—
Chloroethane — see Ethyl chloride						
Chloroethylene	T53.6X1	T53.6X2	T53.6X3	T53.6X4	—	—
Chlorofluorocarbons	T53.5X1	T53.5X2	T53.5X3	T53.5X4	—	—
Chloroform (fumes) (vapor)	T53.1X1	T53.1X2	T53.1X3	T53.1X4	—	—
anesthetic	T41.0X1	T41.0X2	T41.0X3	T41.0X4	T41.0X5	T41.0X6
solvent	T53.1X1	T53.1X2	T53.1X3	T53.1X4	—	—
water, concentrated	T41.0X1	T41.0X2	T41.0X3	T41.0X4	T41.0X5	T41.0X6
Chloroguanide	T37.2X1	T37.2X2	T37.2X3	T37.2X4	T37.2X5	T37.2X6
Chloromycetin	T36.2X1	T36.2X2	T36.2X3	T36.2X4	T36.2X5	T36.2X6
ENT agent	T49.6X1	T49.6X2	T49.6X3	T49.6X4	T49.6X5	T49.6X6
ophthalmic preparation	T49.5X1	T49.5X2	T49.5X3	T49.5X4	T49.5X5	T49.5X6
otic solution	T49.6X1	T49.6X2	T49.6X3	T49.6X4	T49.6X5	T49.6X6
topical NEC	T49.0X1	T49.0X2	T49.0X3	T49.0X4	T49.0X5	T49.0X6
Chloronitrobenzene	T53.7X1	T53.7X2	T53.7X3	T53.7X4	—	—
dust or vapor	T53.7X1	T53.7X2	T53.7X3	T53.7X4	—	—
Chlorophacinone	T60.4X1	T60.4X2	T60.4X3	T60.4X4	—	—
Chlorophenol	T53.7X1	T53.7X2	T53.7X3	T53.7X4	—	—
Chlorophenothane	T60.1X1	T60.1X2	T60.1X3	T60.1X4	—	—
Chlorophyll	T50.991	T50.992	T50.993	T50.994	T50.995	T50.996
Chloropicrin (fumes)	T53.6X1	T53.6X2	T53.6X3	T53.6X4	—	—
fumigant	T60.8X1	T60.8X2	T60.8X3	T60.8X4	—	—
fungicide	T60.3X1	T60.3X2	T60.3X3	T60.3X4	—	—
pesticide	T60.8X1	T60.8X2	T60.8X3	T60.8X4	—	—
Chloroprocaine	T41.3X1	T41.3X2	T41.3X3	T41.3X4	T41.3X5	T41.3X6
infiltration (subcutaneous)	T41.3X1	T41.3X2	T41.3X3	T41.3X4	T41.3X5	T41.3X6
nerve block (peripheral) (plexus)	T41.3X1	T41.3X2	T41.3X3	T41.3X4	T41.3X5	T41.3X6
spinal	T41.3X1	T41.3X2	T41.3X3	T41.3X4	T41.3X5	T41.3X6
Chloroptic	T49.5X1	T49.5X2	T49.5X3	T49.5X4	T49.5X5	T49.5X6
Chloropurine	T45.1X1	T45.1X2	T45.1X3	T45.1X4	T45.1X5	T45.1X6

Table of Drugs and Chemicals

Substance	Poisoning, Accidental (unintentional)	Poisoning, Intentional Self-harm	Poisoning, Assault	Poisoning, Undetermined	Adverse Effect	Under-dosing
Chloropyramine	T45.0X1	T45.0X2	T45.0X3	T45.0X4	T45.0X5	T45.0X6
Chloropyrifos	T60.0X1	T60.0X2	T60.0X3	T60.0X4	—	—
Chloropyrilene	T45.0X1	T45.0X2	T45.0X3	T45.0X4	T45.0X5	T45.0X6
Chloroquine	T37.2X1	T37.2X2	T37.2X3	T37.2X4	T37.2X5	T37.2X6
Chlorothalonil	T60.3X1	T60.3X2	T60.3X3	T60.3X4	—	—
Chlorothen	T45.0X1	T45.0X2	T45.0X3	T45.0X4	T45.0X5	T45.0X6
Chlorothiazide	T50.2X1	T50.2X2	T50.2X3	T50.2X4	T50.2X5	T50.2X6
Chlorothymol	T49.4X1	T49.4X2	T49.4X3	T49.4X4	T49.4X5	T49.4X6
Chlorotrianisene	T38.5X1	T38.5X2	T38.5X3	T38.5X4	T38.5X5	T38.5X6
Chlorovinyldichloroarsine, not in war	T57.0X1	T57.0X2	T57.0X3	T57.0X4	—	—
Chloroxine	T49.4X1	T49.4X2	T49.4X3	T49.4X4	T49.4X5	T49.4X6
Chloroxylenol	T49.0X1	T49.0X2	T49.0X3	T49.0X4	T49.0X5	T49.0X6
Chlorphenamine	T45.0X1	T45.0X2	T45.0X3	T45.0X4	T45.0X5	T45.0X6
Chlorphenesin	T42.8X1	T42.8X2	T42.8X3	T42.8X4	T42.8X5	T42.8X6
topical (antifungal)	T49.0X1	T49.0X2	T49.0X3	T49.0X4	T49.0X5	T49.0X6
Chlorpheniramine	T45.0X1	T45.0X2	T45.0X3	T45.0X4	T45.0X5	T45.0X6
Chlorphenoxamine	T45.0X1	T45.0X2	T45.0X3	T45.0X4	T45.0X5	T45.0X6
Chlorphentermine	T50.5X1	T50.5X2	T50.5X3	T50.5X4	T50.5X5	T50.5X6
Chlorprocaine — see Chloroprocaine						
Chlorproguanil	T37.2X1	T37.2X2	T37.2X3	T37.2X4	T37.2X5	T37.2X6
Chlorpromazine	T43.3X1	T43.3X2	T43.3X3	T43.3X4	T43.3X5	T43.3X6
Chlorpropamide	T38.3X1	T38.3X2	T38.3X3	T38.3X4	T38.3X5	T38.3X6
Chlorprothixene	T43.4X1	T43.4X2	T43.4X3	T43.4X4	T43.4X5	T43.4X6
Chlorquinaldol	T49.0X1	T49.0X2	T49.0X3	T49.0X4	T49.0X5	T49.0X6
Chlorquinol	T49.0X1	T49.0X2	T49.0X3	T49.0X4	T49.0X5	T49.0X6
Chlortalidone	T50.2X1	T50.2X2	T50.2X3	T50.2X4	T50.2X5	T50.2X6
Chlortetracycline	T36.4X1	T36.4X2	T36.4X3	T36.4X4	T36.4X5	T36.4X6
Chlorthalidone	T50.2X1	T50.2X2	T50.2X3	T50.2X4	T50.2X5	T50.2X6
Chlorthion	T60.0X1	T60.0X2	T60.0X3	T60.0X4	—	—
Chlorthiophos	T60.0X1	T60.0X2	T60.0X3	T60.0X4	—	—
Chlortrianisene	T38.5X1	T38.5X2	T38.5X3	T38.5X4	T38.5X5	T38.5X6
Chlor-Trimeton	T45.0X1	T45.0X2	T45.0X3	T45.0X4	T45.0X5	T45.0X6
Chlorzoxazone	T42.8X1	T42.8X2	T42.8X3	T42.8X4	T42.8X5	T42.8X6
Choke damp	T59.7X1	T59.7X2	T59.7X3	T59.7X4	—	—
Cholagogues	T47.5X1	T47.5X2	T47.5X3	T47.5X4	T47.5X5	T47.5X6
Cholebrine	T50.8X1	T50.8X2	T50.8X3	T50.8X4	T50.8X5	T50.8X6
Cholecalciferol	T45.2X1	T45.2X2	T45.2X3	T45.2X4	T45.2X5	T45.2X6
Cholecystokinin	T50.8X1	T50.8X2	T50.8X3	T50.8X4	T50.8X5	T50.8X6
Cholera vaccine	T50.A91	T50.A92	T50.A93	T50.A94	T50.A95	T50.A96
Choleretic	T47.5X1	T47.5X2	T47.5X3	T47.5X4	T47.5X5	T47.5X6
Cholesterol-lowering agents	T46.6X1	T46.6X2	T46.6X3	T46.6X4	T46.6X5	T46.6X6
Cholestyramine (resin)	T46.6X1	T46.6X2	T46.6X3	T46.6X4	T46.6X5	T46.6X6
Cholic acid	T47.5X1	T47.5X2	T47.5X3	T47.5X4	T47.5X5	T47.5X6
Choline	T48.6X1	T48.6X2	T48.6X3	T48.6X4	T48.6X5	T48.6X6
chloride	T50.991	T50.992	T50.993	T50.994	T50.995	T50.996
dihydrogen citrate	T50.991	T50.992	T50.993	T50.994	T50.995	T50.996
salicylate	T39.091	T39.092	T39.093	T39.094	T39.095	T39.096
theophyllinate	T48.6X1	T48.6X2	T48.6X3	T48.6X4	T48.6X5	T48.6X6
Cholinergic (drug) NEC	T44.1X1	T44.1X2	T44.1X3	T44.1X4	T44.1X5	T44.1X6
muscle tone enhancer	T44.1X1	T44.1X2	T44.1X3	T44.1X4	T44.1X5	T44.1X6
organophosphorus	T44.0X1	T44.0X2	T44.0X3	T44.0X4	T44.0X5	T44.0X6
insecticide	T60.0X1	T60.0X2	T60.0X3	T60.0X4	—	—
nerve gas	T59.891	T59.892	T59.893	T59.894	—	—
trimethyl ammonium propanediol	T44.1X1	T44.1X2	T44.1X3	T44.1X4	T44.1X5	T44.1X6
Cholinesterase reactivator	T50.6X1	T50.6X2	T50.6X3	T50.6X4	T50.6X5	T50.6X6
Cholografin	T50.8X1	T50.8X2	T50.8X3	T50.8X4	T50.8X5	T50.8X6
Chorionic gonadotropin	T38.891	T38.892	T38.893	T38.894	T38.895	T38.896
Chromate	T56.2X1	T56.2X2	T56.2X3	T56.2X4	—	—
dust or mist	T56.2X1	T56.2X2	T56.2X3	T56.2X4	—	—
lead — see also lead	T56.0X1	T56.0X2	T56.0X3	T56.0X4	—	—
paint	T56.0X1	T56.0X2	T56.0X3	T56.0X4	—	—
Chromic						
acid	T56.2X1	T56.2X2	T56.2X3	T56.2X4	—	—
dust or mist	T56.2X1	T56.2X2	T56.2X3	T56.2X4	—	—
phosphate 32P	T45.1X1	T45.1X2	T45.1X3	T45.1X4	T45.1X5	T45.1X6
Chromium	T56.2X1	T56.2X2	T56.2X3	T56.2X4	—	—
compounds — see Chromate						
sesquioxide	T50.8X1	T50.8X2	T50.8X3	T50.8X4	T50.8X5	T50.8X6
Chromomycin A3	T45.1X1	T45.1X2	T45.1X3	T45.1X4	T45.1X5	T45.1X6
Chromonar	T46.3X1	T46.3X2	T46.3X3	T46.3X4	T46.3X5	T46.3X6
Chromyl chloride	T56.2X1	T56.2X2	T56.2X3	T56.2X4	—	—
Chrysarobin	T49.4X1	T49.4X2	T49.4X3	T49.4X4	T49.4X5	T49.4X6
Chrysazin	T47.2X1	T47.2X2	T47.2X3	T47.2X4	T47.2X5	T47.2X6
Chymar	T45.3X1	T45.3X2	T45.3X3	T45.3X4	T45.3X5	T45.3X6
ophthalmic preparation	T49.5X1	T49.5X2	T49.5X3	T49.5X4	T49.5X5	T49.5X6
Chymopapain	T45.3X1	T45.3X2	T45.3X3	T45.3X4	T45.3X5	T45.3X6
Chymotrypsin	T45.3X1	T45.3X2	T45.3X3	T45.3X4	T45.3X5	T45.3X6
ophthalmic preparation	T49.5X1	T49.5X2	T49.5X3	T49.5X4	T49.5X5	T49.5X6
Cianidanol	T50.991	T50.992	T50.993	T50.994	T50.995	T50.996

Substance	Poisoning, Accidental (unintentional)	Poisoning, Intentional Self-harm	Poisoning, Assault	Poisoning, Undetermined	Adverse Effect	Under-dosing
Cianopramine	T43.011	T43.012	T43.013	T43.014	T43.015	T43.016
Cibenzoline	T46.2X1	T46.2X2	T46.2X3	T46.2X4	T46.2X5	T46.2X6
Ciclacillin	T36.0X1	T36.0X2	T36.0X3	T36.0X4	T36.0X5	T36.0X6
Ciclobarbital — see Hexobarbital						
Ciclonicate	T46.7X1	T46.7X2	T46.7X3	T46.7X4	T46.7X5	T46.7X6
Ciclopirox (olamine)	T49.0X1	T49.0X2	T49.0X3	T49.0X4	T49.0X5	T49.0X6
Ciclosporin	T45.1X1	T45.1X2	T45.1X3	T45.1X4	T45.1X5	T45.1X6
Cicuta maculata or virosa	T62.2X1	T62.2X2	T62.2X3	T62.2X4	—	—
Cicutoxin	T62.2X1	T62.2X2	T62.2X3	T62.2X4	—	—
Cigarette lighter fluid	T52.0X1	T52.0X2	T52.0X3	T52.0X4	—	—
Cigarettes (tobacco)	T65.221	T65.222	T65.223	T65.224	—	—
Ciguatoxin	T61.01	T61.02	T61.03	T61.04	—	—
Cilazapril	T46.4X1	T46.4X2	T46.4X3	T46.4X4	T46.4X5	T46.4X6
Cimetidine	T47.0X1	T47.0X2	T47.0X3	T47.0X4	T47.0X5	T47.0X6
Cimetropium bromide	T44.3X1	T44.3X2	T44.3X3	T44.3X4	T44.3X5	T44.3X6
Cinchocaine	T41.3X1	T41.3X2	T41.3X3	T41.3X4	T41.3X5	T41.3X6
topical (surface)	T41.3X1	T41.3X2	T41.3X3	T41.3X4	T41.3X5	T41.3X6
Cinchona	T37.2X1	T37.2X2	T37.2X3	T37.2X4	T37.2X5	T37.2X6
Cinchonine alkaloids	T37.2X1	T37.2X2	T37.2X3	T37.2X4	T37.2X5	T37.2X6
Cinchophen	T50.4X1	T50.4X2	T50.4X3	T50.4X4	T50.4X5	T50.4X6
Cinepazide	T46.7X1	T46.7X2	T46.7X3	T46.7X4	T46.7X5	T46.7X6
Cinnamedrine	T48.5X1	T48.5X2	T48.5X3	T48.5X4	T48.5X5	T48.5X6
Cinnarizine	T45.0X1	T45.0X2	T45.0X3	T45.0X4	T45.0X5	T45.0X6
Cinoxacin	T37.8X1	T37.8X2	T37.8X3	T37.8X4	T37.8X5	T37.8X6
Ciprofibrate	T46.6X1	T46.6X2	T46.6X3	T46.6X4	T46.6X5	T46.6X6
Ciprofloxacin	T36.8X1	T36.8X2	T36.8X3	T36.8X4	T36.8X5	T36.8X6
Cisapride	T47.8X1	T47.8X2	T47.8X3	T47.8X4	T47.8X5	T47.8X6
Cisplatin	T45.1X1	T45.1X2	T45.1X3	T45.1X4	T45.1X5	T45.1X6
Citalopram	T43.221	T43.222	T43.223	T43.224	T43.225	T43.226
Citanest	T41.3X1	T41.3X2	T41.3X3	T41.3X4	T41.3X5	T41.3X6
infiltration (subcutaneous)	T41.3X1	T41.3X2	T41.3X3	T41.3X4	T41.3X5	T41.3X6
nerve block (peripheral) (plexus)	T41.3X1	T41.3X2	T41.3X3	T41.3X4	T41.3X5	T41.3X6
Citric acid	T47.5X1	T47.5X2	T47.5X3	T47.5X4	T47.5X5	T47.5X6
Citrovorum (factor)	T45.8X1	T45.8X2	T45.8X3	T45.8X4	T45.8X5	T45.8X6
Claviceps purpurea	T62.2X1	T62.2X2	T62.2X3	T62.2X4	—	—
Clavulanic acid	T36.1X1	T36.1X2	T36.1X3	T36.1X4	T36.1X5	T36.1X6
Cleaner, cleansing agent, type not specified	T65.891	T65.892	T65.893	T65.894	—	—
of paint or varnish	T52.91	T52.92	T52.93	T52.94	—	—
specified type NEC	T65.891	T65.892	T65.893	T65.894	—	—
Clebopride	T47.8X1	T47.8X2	T47.8X3	T47.8X4	T47.8X5	T47.8X6
Clefamide	T37.3X1	T37.3X2	T37.3X3	T37.3X4	T37.3X5	T37.3X6
Clemastine	T45.0X1	T45.0X2	T45.0X3	T45.0X4	T45.0X5	T45.0X6
Clematis vitalba	T62.2X1	T62.2X2	T62.2X3	T62.2X4	—	—
Clemizole	T45.0X1	T45.0X2	T45.0X3	T45.0X4	T45.0X5	T45.0X6
penicillin	T36.0X1	T36.0X2	T36.0X3	T36.0X4	T36.0X5	T36.0X6
Clenbuterol	T48.6X1	T48.6X2	T48.6X3	T48.6X4	T48.6X5	T48.6X6
Clidinium bromide	T44.3X1	T44.3X2	T44.3X3	T44.3X4	T44.3X5	T44.3X6
Clindamycin	T36.8X1	T36.8X2	T36.8X3	T36.8X4	T36.8X5	T36.8X6
Clinofibrate	T46.6X1	T46.6X2	T46.6X3	T46.6X4	T46.6X5	T46.6X6
Clioquinol	T37.8X1	T37.8X2	T37.8X3	T37.8X4	T37.8X5	T37.8X6
Cliradon	T40.2X1	T40.2X2	T40.2X3	T40.2X4	—	—
Clobazam	T42.4X1	T42.4X2	T42.4X3	T42.4X4	T42.4X5	T42.4X6
Clobenzorex	T50.5X1	T50.5X2	T50.5X3	T50.5X4	T50.5X5	T50.5X6
Clobetasol	T49.0X1	T49.0X2	T49.0X3	T49.0X4	T49.0X5	T49.0X6
Clobetasone	T49.0X1	T49.0X2	T49.0X3	T49.0X4	T49.0X5	T49.0X6
Clobutinol	T48.3X1	T48.3X2	T48.3X3	T48.3X4	T48.3X5	T48.3X6
Clocortolone	T38.0X1	T38.0X2	T38.0X3	T38.0X4	T38.0X5	T38.0X6
Clodantoin	T49.0X1	T49.0X2	T49.0X3	T49.0X4	T49.0X5	T49.0X6
Clodronic acid	T50.991	T50.992	T50.993	T50.994	T50.995	T50.996
Clofazimine	T37.1X1	T37.1X2	T37.1X3	T37.1X4	T37.1X5	T37.1X6
Clofedanol	T48.3X1	T48.3X2	T48.3X3	T48.3X4	T48.3X5	T48.3X6
Clofenamide	T50.2X1	T50.2X2	T50.2X3	T50.2X4	T50.2X5	T50.2X6
Clofenotane	T49.0X1	T49.0X2	T49.0X3	T49.0X4	T49.0X5	T49.0X6
Clofezone	T39.2X1	T39.2X2	T39.2X3	T39.2X4	T39.2X5	T39.2X6
Clofibrate	T46.6X1	T46.6X2	T46.6X3	T46.6X4	T46.6X5	T46.6X6
Clofibride	T46.6X1	T46.6X2	T46.6X3	T46.6X4	T46.6X5	T46.6X6
Cloforex	T50.5X1	T50.5X2	T50.5X3	T50.5X4	T50.5X5	T50.5X6
Clomethiazole	T42.6X1	T42.6X2	T42.6X3	T42.6X4	T42.6X5	T42.6X6
Clometocillin	T36.0X1	T36.0X2	T36.0X3	T36.0X4	T36.0X5	T36.0X6
Clomifene	T38.5X1	T38.5X2	T38.5X3	T38.5X4	T38.5X5	T38.5X6
Clomiphene	T38.5X1	T38.5X2	T38.5X3	T38.5X4	T38.5X5	T38.5X6
Clomipramine	T43.011	T43.012	T43.013	T43.014	T43.015	T43.016
Clomocycline	T36.4X1	T36.4X2	T36.4X3	T36.4X4	T36.4X5	T36.4X6
Clonazepam	T42.4X1	T42.4X2	T42.4X3	T42.4X4	T42.4X5	T42.4X6
Clonidine	T46.5X1	T46.5X2	T46.5X3	T46.5X4	T46.5X5	T46.5X6
Clonixin	T39.8X1	T39.8X2	T39.8X3	T39.8X4	T39.8X5	T39.8X6
Clopamide	T50.2X1	T50.2X2	T50.2X3	T50.2X4	T50.2X5	T50.2X6
Clopenthixol	T43.4X1	T43.4X2	T43.4X3	T43.4X4	T43.4X5	T43.4X6
Cloperastine	T48.3X1	T48.3X2	T48.3X3	T48.3X4	T48.3X5	T48.3X6
Clophedianol	T48.3X1	T48.3X2	T48.3X3	T48.3X4	T48.3X5	T48.3X6
Cloponone	T36.2X1	T36.2X2	T36.2X3	T36.2X4	T36.2X5	T36.2X6

Chloropyramine — Cloponone

Substance	Poisoning, Accidental (unintentional)	Poisoning, Intentional Self-harm	Poisoning, Assault	Poisoning, Undetermined	Adverse Effect	Under-dosing
Cloprednol	T38.0X1	T38.0X2	T38.0X3	T38.0X4	T38.0X5	T38.0X6
Cloral betaine	T42.6X1	T42.6X2	T42.6X3	T42.6X4	T42.6X5	T42.6X6
Cloramfenicol	T36.2X1	T36.2X2	T36.2X3	T36.2X4	T36.2X5	T36.2X6
Clorazepate (dipotassium)	T42.4X1	T42.4X2	T42.4X3	T42.4X4	T42.4X5	T42.4X6
Clorexolone	T50.2X1	T50.2X2	T50.2X3	T50.2X4	T50.2X5	T50.2X6
Clorfenamine	T45.0X1	T45.0X2	T45.0X3	T45.0X4	T45.0X5	T45.0X6
Clorgiline	T43.1X1	T43.1X2	T43.1X3	T43.1X4	T43.1X5	T43.1X6
Clorotepine	T44.3X1	T44.3X2	T44.3X3	T44.3X4	T44.3X5	T44.3X6
Clorox (bleach)	T54.91	T54.92	T54.93	T54.94	—	—
Clorprenaline	T48.6X1	T48.6X2	T48.6X3	T48.6X4	T48.6X5	T48.6X6
Clortermine	T50.5X1	T50.5X2	T50.5X3	T50.5X4	T50.5X5	T50.5X6
Clotiapine	T43.591	T43.592	T43.593	T43.594	T43.595	T43.596
Clotiazepam	T42.4X1	T42.4X2	T42.4X3	T42.4X4	T42.4X5	T42.4X6
Clotibric acid	T46.6X1	T46.6X2	T46.6X3	T46.6X4	T46.6X5	T46.6X6
Clotrimazole	T49.0X1	T49.0X2	T49.0X3	T49.0X4	T49.0X5	T49.0X6
Cloxacillin	T36.0X1	T36.0X2	T36.0X3	T36.0X4	T36.0X5	T36.0X6
Cloxazolam	T42.4X1	T42.4X2	T42.4X3	T42.4X4	T42.4X5	T42.4X6
Cloxiquine	T49.0X1	T49.0X2	T49.0X3	T49.0X4	T49.0X5	T49.0X6
Clozapine	T42.4X1	T42.4X2	T42.4X3	T42.4X4	T42.4X5	T42.4X6
Coagulant NEC	T45.7X1	T45.7X2	T45.7X3	T45.7X4	T45.7X5	T45.7X6
Coal (carbon monoxide from) — see also Carbon, monoxide, coal	T58.2X1	T58.2X2	T58.2X3	T58.2X4		
oil — see Kerosene						
tar	T49.1X1	T49.1X2	T49.1X3	T49.1X4	T49.1X5	T49.1X6
fumes	T59.891	T59.892	T59.893	T59.894		
medicinal (ointment)	T49.4X1	T49.4X2	T49.4X3	T49.4X4	T49.4X5	T49.4X6
analgesics NEC	T39.2X1	T39.2X2	T39.2X3	T39.2X4	T39.2X5	T39.2X6
naphtha (solvent)	T52.0X1	T52.0X2	T52.0X3	T52.0X4		
Cobalamine	T45.2X1	T45.2X2	T45.2X3	T45.2X4	T45.2X5	T45.2X6
Cobalt (nonmedicinal) (fumes) (industrial)	T56.891	T56.892	T56.893	T56.894		
medicinal (trace) (chloride)	T45.8X1	T45.8X2	T45.8X3	T45.8X4	T45.8X5	T45.8X6
Cobra (venom)	T63.041	T63.042	T63.043	T63.044		
Coca (leaf)	T40.5X1	T40.5X2	T40.5X3	T40.5X4	T40.5X5	T40.5X6
Cocaine	T40.5X1	T40.5X2	T40.5X3	T40.5X4	T40.5X5	T40.5X6
topical anesthetic	T41.3X1	T41.3X2	T41.3X3	T41.3X4	T41.3X5	T41.3X6
Cocarboxylase	T45.3X1	T45.3X2	T45.3X3	T45.3X4	T45.3X5	T45.3X6
Coccidioidin	T50.8X1	T50.8X2	T50.8X3	T50.8X4	T50.8X5	T50.8X6
Cocculus indicus	T62.1X1	T62.1X2	T62.1X3	T62.1X4	—	—
Cochineal	T65.6X1	T65.6X2	T65.6X3	T65.6X4	—	—
medicinal products	T50.991	T50.992	T50.993	T50.994	T50.995	T50.996
Codeine	T40.2X1	T40.2X2	T40.2X3	T40.2X4	T40.2X5	T40.2X6
Cod-liver oil	T45.2X1	T45.2X2	T45.2X3	T45.2X4	T45.2X5	T45.2X6
Coenzyme A	T50.991	T50.992	T50.993	T50.994	T50.995	T50.996
Coffee	T62.8X1	T62.8X2	T62.8X3	T62.8X4	—	—
Cogalactoisomerase	T50.991	T50.992	T50.993	T50.994	T50.995	T50.996
Cogentin	T44.3X1	T44.3X2	T44.3X3	T44.3X4	T44.3X5	T44.3X6
Coke fumes or gas (carbon monoxide)	T58.2X1	T58.2X2	T58.2X3	T58.2X4		
industrial use	T58.8X1	T58.8X2	T58.8X3	T58.8X4	—	—
Colace	T47.4X1	T47.4X2	T47.4X3	T47.4X4	T47.4X5	T47.4X6
Colaspase	T45.1X1	T45.1X2	T45.1X3	T45.1X4	T45.1X5	T45.1X6
Colchicine	T50.4X1	T50.4X2	T50.4X3	T50.4X4	T50.4X5	T50.4X6
Colchicum	T62.2X1	T62.2X2	T62.2X3	T62.2X4	—	—
Cold cream	T49.3X1	T49.3X2	T49.3X3	T49.3X4	T49.3X5	T49.3X6
Colecalciferol	T45.2X1	T45.2X2	T45.2X3	T45.2X4	T45.2X5	T45.2X6
Colestipol	T46.6X1	T46.6X2	T46.6X3	T46.6X4	T46.6X5	T46.6X6
Colestyramine	T46.6X1	T46.6X2	T46.6X3	T46.6X4	T46.6X5	T46.6X6
Colimycin	T36.8X1	T36.8X2	T36.8X3	T36.8X4	T36.8X5	T36.8X6
Colistimethate	T36.8X1	T36.8X2	T36.8X3	T36.8X4	T36.8X5	T36.8X6
Colistin	T36.8X1	T36.8X2	T36.8X3	T36.8X4	T36.8X5	T36.8X6
sulfate (eye preparation)	T49.5X1	T49.5X2	T49.5X3	T49.5X4	T49.5X5	T49.5X6
Collagen	T50.991	T50.992	T50.993	T50.994	T50.995	T50.996
Collagenase	T49.4X1	T49.4X2	T49.4X3	T49.4X4	T49.4X5	T49.4X6
Collodion	T49.3X1	T49.3X2	T49.3X3	T49.3X4	T49.3X5	T49.3X6
Colocynth	T47.2X1	T47.2X2	T47.2X3	T47.2X4	T47.2X5	T47.2X6
Colophony adhesive	T49.3X1	T49.3X2	T49.3X3	T49.3X4	T49.3X5	T49.3X6
Colorant — see also Dye						
Coloring matter — see Dye(s)						
Combustion gas (after combustion) — see Carbon, monoxide						
prior to combustion	T59.891	T59.892	T59.893	T59.894	—	—
Compazine	T43.3X1	T43.3X2	T43.3X3	T43.3X4	T43.3X5	T43.3X6
Compound						
42 (warfarin)	T60.4X1	T60.4X2	T60.4X3	T60.4X4	—	—
269 (endrin)	T60.1X1	T60.1X2	T60.1X3	T60.1X4	—	—
497 (dieldrin)	T60.1X1	T60.1X2	T60.1X3	T60.1X4	—	—
1080 (sodium fluoroacetate)	T60.4X1	T60.4X2	T60.4X3	T60.4X4	—	—
3422 (parathion)	T60.0X1	T60.0X2	T60.0X3	T60.0X4	—	—
3911 (phorate)	T60.0X1	T60.0X2	T60.0X3	T60.0X4	—	—

Substance	Poisoning, Accidental (unintentional)	Poisoning, Intentional Self-harm	Poisoning, Assault	Poisoning, Undetermined	Adverse Effect	Under-dosing
Compound — continued						
3956 (toxaphene)	T60.1X1	T60.1X2	T60.1X3	T60.1X4	—	—
4049 (malathion)	T60.0X1	T60.0X2	T60.0X3	T60.0X4	—	—
4069 (malathion)	T60.0X1	T60.0X2	T60.0X3	T60.0X4	—	—
4124 (dicapthon)	T60.0X1	T60.0X2	T60.0X3	T60.0X4	—	—
E (cortisone)	T38.0X1	T38.0X2	T38.0X3	T38.0X4	T38.0X5	T38.0X6
F (hydrocortisone)	T38.0X1	T38.0X2	T38.0X3	T38.0X4	T38.0X5	T38.0X6
Congener, anabolic	T38.7X1	T38.7X2	T38.7X3	T38.7X4	T38.7X5	T38.7X6
Congo red	T50.8X1	T50.8X2	T50.8X3	T50.8X4	T50.8X5	T50.8X6
Coniine, conine	T62.2X1	T62.2X2	T62.2X3	T62.2X4	—	—
Conium (maculatum)	T62.2X1	T62.2X2	T62.2X3	T62.2X4	—	—
Conjugated estrogenic substances	T38.5X1	T38.5X2	T38.5X3	T38.5X4	T38.5X5	T38.5X6
Contac	T48.5X1	T48.5X2	T48.5X3	T48.5X4	T48.5X5	T48.5X6
Contact lens solution	T49.5X1	T49.5X2	T49.5X3	T49.5X4	T49.5X5	T49.5X6
Contraceptive (oral)	T38.4X1	T38.4X2	T38.4X3	T38.4X4	T38.4X5	T38.4X6
vaginal	T49.8X1	T49.8X2	T49.8X3	T49.8X4	T49.8X5	T49.8X6
Contrast medium, radiography	T50.8X1	T50.8X2	T50.8X3	T50.8X4	T50.8X5	T50.8X6
Convallaria glycosides	T46.0X1	T46.0X2	T46.0X3	T46.0X4	T46.0X5	T46.0X6
Convallaria majalis	T62.2X1	T62.2X2	T62.2X3	T62.2X4	—	—
berry	T62.1X1	T62.1X2	T62.1X3	T62.1X4	—	—
Copperhead snake (bite) (venom)	T63.061	T63.062	T63.063	T63.064	—	—
Copper (dust) (fumes) (nonmedicinal) NEC	T56.4X1	T56.4X2	T56.4X3	T56.4X4		
arsenate, arsenite	T57.0X1	T57.0X2	T57.0X3	T57.0X4	—	—
insecticide	T60.2X1	T60.2X2	T60.2X3	T60.2X4	—	—
emetic	T47.7X1	T47.7X2	T47.7X3	T47.7X4	T47.7X5	T47.7X6
fungicide	T60.3X1	T60.3X2	T60.3X3	T60.3X4	—	—
gluconate	T49.0X1	T49.0X2	T49.0X3	T49.0X4	T49.0X5	T49.0X6
insecticide	T60.2X1	T60.2X2	T60.2X3	T60.2X4	—	—
medicinal (trace)	T45.8X1	T45.8X2	T45.8X3	T45.8X4	T45.8X5	T45.8X6
oleate	T49.0X1	T49.0X2	T49.0X3	T49.0X4	T49.0X5	T49.0X6
sulfate	T56.4X1	T56.4X2	T56.4X3	T56.4X4	—	—
cupric	T56.4X1	T56.4X2	T56.4X3	T56.4X4	—	—
fungicide	T60.3X1	T60.3X2	T60.3X3	T60.3X4		
medicinal						
ear	T49.6X1	T49.6X2	T49.6X3	T49.6X4	T49.6X5	T49.6X6
emetic	T47.7X1	T47.7X2	T47.7X3	T47.7X4	T47.7X5	T47.7X6
eye	T49.5X1	T49.5X2	T49.5X3	T49.5X4	T49.5X5	T49.5X6
cuprous	T56.4X1	T56.4X2	T56.4X3	T56.4X4	—	—
fungicide	T60.3X1	T60.3X2	T60.3X3	T60.3X4	—	—
medicinal						
ear	T49.6X1	T49.6X2	T49.6X3	T49.6X4	T49.6X5	T49.6X6
emetic	T47.7X1	T47.7X2	T47.7X3	T47.7X4	T47.7X5	T47.7X6
eye	T49.5X1	T49.5X2	T49.5X3	T49.5X4	T49.5X5	T49.5X6
Coral (sting)	T63.691	T63.692	T63.693	T63.694	—	—
snake (bite) (venom)	T63.021	T63.022	T63.023	T63.024	—	—
Corbadrine	T49.6X1	T49.6X2	T49.6X3	T49.6X4	T49.6X5	T49.6X6
Cordite	T65.891	T65.892	T65.893	T65.894	—	—
vapor	T59.891	T59.892	T59.893	T59.894	—	—
Cordran	T49.0X1	T49.0X2	T49.0X3	T49.0X4	T49.0X5	T49.0X6
Corn cures	T49.4X1	T49.4X2	T49.4X3	T49.4X4	T49.4X5	T49.4X6
Cornhusker's lotion	T49.3X1	T49.3X2	T49.3X3	T49.3X4	T49.3X5	T49.3X6
Corn starch	T49.3X1	T49.3X2	T49.3X3	T49.3X4	T49.3X5	T49.3X6
Coronary vasodilator NEC	T46.3X1	T46.3X2	T46.3X3	T46.3X4	T46.3X5	T46.3X6
Corrosive NEC	T54.91	T54.92	T54.93	T54.94	—	—
acid NEC	T54.2X1	T54.2X2	T54.2X3	T54.2X4	—	—
aromatics	T54.1X1	T54.1X2	T54.1X3	T54.1X4	—	—
disinfectant	T54.1X1	T54.1X2	T54.1X3	T54.1X4	—	—
fumes NEC	T54.91	T54.92	T54.93	T54.94	—	—
specified NEC	T54.91	T54.92	T54.93	T54.94	—	—
sublimate	T56.1X1	T56.1X2	T56.1X3	T56.1X4	—	—
Cortate	T38.0X1	T38.0X2	T38.0X3	T38.0X4	T38.0X5	T38.0X6
Cort-Dome	T38.0X1	T38.0X2	T38.0X3	T38.0X4	T38.0X5	T38.0X6
ENT agent	T49.6X1	T49.6X2	T49.6X3	T49.6X4	T49.6X5	T49.6X6
ophthalmic preparation	T49.5X1	T49.5X2	T49.5X3	T49.5X4	T49.5X5	T49.5X6
topical NEC	T49.0X1	T49.0X2	T49.0X3	T49.0X4	T49.0X5	T49.0X6
Cortef	T38.0X1	T38.0X2	T38.0X3	T38.0X4	T38.0X5	T38.0X6
ENT agent	T49.6X1	T49.6X2	T49.6X3	T49.6X4	T49.6X5	T49.6X6
ophthalmic preparation	T49.5X1	T49.5X2	T49.5X3	T49.5X4	T49.5X5	T49.5X6
topical NEC	T49.0X1	T49.0X2	T49.0X3	T49.0X4	T49.0X5	T49.0X6
Corticosteroid	T38.0X1	T38.0X2	T38.0X3	T38.0X4	T38.0X5	T38.0X6
ENT agent	T49.6X1	T49.6X2	T49.6X3	T49.6X4	T49.6X5	T49.6X6
mineral	T50.0X1	T50.0X2	T50.0X3	T50.0X4	T50.0X5	T50.0X6
ophthalmic	T49.5X1	T49.5X2	T49.5X3	T49.5X4	T49.5X5	T49.5X6
topical NEC	T49.0X1	T49.0X2	T49.0X3	T49.0X4	T49.0X5	T49.0X6
Corticotropin	T38.811	T38.812	T38.813	T38.814	T38.815	T38.816
Cortisol	T49.0X1	T49.0X2	T49.0X3	T49.0X4	T49.0X5	T49.0X6
ENT agent	T49.6X1	T49.6X2	T49.6X3	T49.6X4	T49.6X5	T49.6X6
ophthalmic preparation	T49.5X1	T49.5X2	T49.5X3	T49.5X4	T49.5X5	T49.5X6
topical NEC	T49.0X1	T49.0X2	T49.0X3	T49.0X4	T49.0X5	T49.0X6

Substance	Poisoning, Accidental (unintentional)	Poisoning, Intentional Self-harm	Poisoning, Assault	Poisoning, Undetermined	Adverse Effect	Under-dosing
Cortisone (acetate)	T38.0X1	T38.0X2	T38.0X3	T38.0X4	T38.0X5	T38.0X6
ENT agent	T49.6X1	T49.6X2	T49.6X3	T49.6X4	T49.6X5	T49.6X6
ophthalmic preparation	T49.5X1	T49.5X2	T49.5X3	T49.5X4	T49.5X5	T49.5X6
topical NEC	T49.0X1	T49.0X2	T49.0X3	T49.0X4	T49.0X5	T49.0X6
Cortivazol	T38.0X1	T38.0X2	T38.0X3	T38.0X4	T38.0X5	T38.0X6
Cortogen	T38.0X1	T38.0X2	T38.0X3	T38.0X4	T38.0X5	T38.0X6
ENT agent	T49.6X1	T49.6X2	T49.6X3	T49.6X4	T49.6X5	T49.6X6
ophthalmic preparation	T49.5X1	T49.5X2	T49.5X3	T49.5X4	T49.5X5	T49.5X6
Cortone	T38.0X1	T38.0X2	T38.0X3	T38.0X4	T38.0X5	T38.0X6
ENT agent	T49.6X1	T49.6X2	T49.6X3	T49.6X4	T49.6X5	T49.6X6
ophthalmic preparation	T49.5X1	T49.5X2	T49.5X3	T49.5X4	T49.5X5	T49.5X6
Cortril	T38.0X1	T38.0X2	T38.0X3	T38.0X4	T38.0X5	T38.0X6
ENT agent	T49.6X1	T49.6X2	T49.6X3	T49.6X4	T49.6X5	T49.6X6
ophthalmic preparation	T49.5X1	T49.5X2	T49.5X3	T49.5X4	T49.5X5	T49.5X6
topical NEC	T49.0X1	T49.0X2	T49.0X3	T49.0X4	T49.0X5	T49.0X6
Corynebacterium parvum	T45.1X1	T45.1X2	T45.1X3	T45.1X4	T45.1X5	T45.1X6
Cosmetic preparation	T49.8X1	T49.8X2	T49.8X3	T49.8X4	T49.8X5	T49.8X6
Cosmetics	T49.8X1	T49.8X2	T49.8X3	T49.8X4	T49.8X5	T49.8X6
Cosyntropin	T38.811	T38.812	T38.813	T38.814	T38.815	T38.816
Cotarnine	T45.7X1	T45.7X2	T45.7X3	T45.7X4	T45.7X5	T45.7X6
Co-trimoxazole	T36.8X1	T36.8X2	T36.8X3	T36.8X4	T36.8X5	T36.8X6
Cottonseed oil	T49.3X1	T49.3X2	T49.3X3	T49.3X4	T49.3X5	T49.3X6
Cough mixture (syrup)	T48.4X1	T48.4X2	T48.4X3	T48.4X4	T48.4X5	T48.4X6
containing opiates	T40.2X1	T40.2X2	T40.2X3	T40.2X4	T40.2X5	T40.2X6
expectorants	T48.4X1	T48.4X2	T48.4X3	T48.4X4	T48.4X5	T48.4X6
Coumadin	T45.511	T45.512	T45.513	T45.514	T45.515	T45.516
rodenticide	T60.4X1	T60.4X2	T60.4X3	T60.4X4	—	—
Coumaphos	T60.0X1	T60.0X2	T60.0X3	T60.0X4	—	—
Coumarin	T45.511	T45.512	T45.513	T45.514	T45.515	T45.516
Coumetarol	T45.511	T45.512	T45.513	T45.514	T45.515	T45.516
Cowbane	T62.2X1	T62.2X2	T62.2X3	T62.2X4	—	—
Cozyme	T45.2X1	T45.2X2	T45.2X3	T45.2X4	T45.2X5	T45.2X6
Crack	T40.5X1	T40.5X2	T40.5X3	T40.5X4	—	—
Crataegus extract	T46.0X1	T46.0X2	T46.0X3	T46.0X4	T46.0X5	T46.0X6
Creolin	T54.1X1	T54.1X2	T54.1X3	T54.1X4	—	—
disinfectant	T54.1X1	T54.1X2	T54.1X3	T54.1X4	—	—
Creosol (compound)	T49.0X1	T49.0X2	T49.0X3	T49.0X4	T49.0X5	T49.0X6
Creosote (coal tar)	T49.0X1	T49.0X2	T49.0X3	T49.0X4	T49.0X5	T49.0X6
(beechwood)						
medicinal (expectorant)	T48.4X1	T48.4X2	T48.4X3	T48.4X4	T48.4X5	T48.4X6
syrup	T48.4X1	T48.4X2	T48.4X3	T48.4X4	T48.4X5	T48.4X6
Cresol(s)	T49.0X1	T49.0X2	T49.0X3	T49.0X4	T49.0X5	T49.0X6
and soap solution	T49.0X1	T49.0X2	T49.0X3	T49.0X4	T49.0X5	T49.0X6
Cresyl acetate	T49.0X1	T49.0X2	T49.0X3	T49.0X4	T49.0X5	T49.0X6
Cresylic acid	T49.0X1	T49.0X2	T49.0X3	T49.0X4	T49.0X5	T49.0X6
Crimidine	T60.4X1	T60.4X2	T60.4X3	T60.4X4	—	—
Croconazole	T37.8X1	T37.8X2	T37.8X3	T37.8X4	T37.8X5	T37.8X6
Cromoglicic acid	T48.6X1	T48.6X2	T48.6X3	T48.6X4	T48.6X5	T48.6X6
Cromolyn	T48.6X1	T48.6X2	T48.6X3	T48.6X4	T48.6X5	T48.6X6
Cromonar	T46.3X1	T46.3X2	T46.3X3	T46.3X4	T46.3X5	T46.3X6
Cropropamide	T39.8X1	T39.8X2	T39.8X3	T39.8X4	T39.8X5	T39.8X6
with crotethamide	T50.7X1	T50.7X2	T50.7X3	T50.7X4	T50.7X5	T50.7X6
Crotamiton	T49.0X1	T49.0X2	T49.0X3	T49.0X4	T49.0X5	T49.0X6
Crotethamide	T39.8X1	T39.8X2	T39.8X3	T39.8X4	T39.8X5	T39.8X6
with cropropamide	T50.7X1	T50.7X2	T50.7X3	T50.7X4	T50.7X5	T50.7X6
Croton (oil)	T47.2X1	T47.2X2	T47.2X3	T47.2X4	T47.2X5	T47.2X6
chloral	T42.6X1	T42.6X2	T42.6X3	T42.6X4	T42.6X5	T42.6X6
Crude oil	T52.0X1	T52.0X2	T52.0X3	T52.0X4	—	—
Cryogenine	T39.8X1	T39.8X2	T39.8X3	T39.8X4	T39.8X5	T39.8X6
Cryolite (vapor)	T60.1X1	T60.1X2	T60.1X3	T60.1X4	—	—
insecticide	T60.1X1	T60.1X2	T60.1X3	T60.1X4	—	—
Cryptenamine (tannates)	T46.5X1	T46.5X2	T46.5X3	T46.5X4	T46.5X5	T46.5X6
Crystal violet	T49.0X1	T49.0X2	T49.0X3	T49.0X4	T49.0X5	T49.0X6
Cuckoopint	T62.2X1	T62.2X2	T62.2X3	T62.2X4	—	—
Cumetharol	T45.511	T45.512	T45.513	T45.514	T45.515	T45.516
Cupric						
acetate	T60.3X1	T60.3X2	T60.3X3	T60.3X4	—	—
acetoarsenite	T57.0X1	T57.0X2	T57.0X3	T57.0X4	—	—
arsenate	T57.0X1	T57.0X2	T57.0X3	T57.0X4	—	—
gluconate	T49.0X1	T49.0X2	T49.0X3	T49.0X4	T49.0X5	T49.0X6
oleate	T49.0X1	T49.0X2	T49.0X3	T49.0X4	T49.0X5	T49.0X6
sulfate	T56.4X1	T56.4X2	T56.4X3	T56.4X4	—	—
Cuprous sulfate — see also Copper sulfate	T56.4X1	T56.4X2	T56.4X3	T56.4X4	—	—
Curare, curarine	T48.1X1	T48.1X2	T48.1X3	T48.1X4	T48.1X5	T48.1X6
Cyamemazine	T43.3X1	T43.3X2	T43.3X3	T43.3X4	T43.3X5	T43.3X6
Cyamopsis tetragonoloba	T46.6X1	T46.6X2	T46.6X3	T46.6X4	T46.6X5	T46.6X6
Cyanacetyl hydrazide	T37.1X1	T37.1X2	T37.1X3	T37.1X4	T37.1X5	T37.1X6
Cyanic acid (gas)	T59.891	T59.892	T59.893	T59.894		
Cyanide(s) (compounds) (potassium) (sodium)	T65.0X1	T65.0X2	T65.0X3	T65.0X4	—	—
NEC						
dust or gas (inhalation) NEC	T57.3X1	T57.3X2	T57.3X3	T57.3X4		
Cyanide(s) (compounds) (potassium) (sodium) **NEC** — *continued*						
fumigant	T65.0X1	T65.0X2	T65.0X3	T65.0X4	—	—
hydrogen	T57.3X1	T57.3X2	T57.3X3	T57.3X4	—	—
mercuric — see Mercury						
pesticide (dust) (fumes)	T65.0X1	T65.0X2	T65.0X3	T65.0X4	—	—
Cyanoacrylate adhesive	T49.3X1	T49.3X2	T49.3X3	T49.3X4	T49.3X5	T49.3X6
Cyanocobalamin	T45.8X1	T45.8X2	T45.8X3	T45.8X4	T45.8X5	T45.8X6
Cyanogen (chloride) (gas) NEC	T59.891	T59.892	T59.893	T59.894	—	—
Cyclacillin	T36.0X1	T36.0X2	T36.0X3	T36.0X4	T36.0X5	T36.0X6
Cyclaine	T41.3X1	T41.3X2	T41.3X3	T41.3X4	T41.3X5	T41.3X6
Cyclamate	T50.991	T50.992	T50.993	T50.994	T50.995	T50.996
Cyclamen europaeum	T62.2X1	T62.2X2	T62.2X3	T62.2X4	—	—
Cyclandelate	T46.7X1	T46.7X2	T46.7X3	T46.7X4	T46.7X5	T46.7X6
Cyclazocine	T50.7X1	T50.7X2	T50.7X3	T50.7X4	T50.7X5	T50.7X6
Cyclizine	T45.0X1	T45.0X2	T45.0X3	T45.0X4	T45.0X5	T45.0X6
Cyclobarbital	T42.3X1	T42.3X2	T42.3X3	T42.3X4	T42.3X5	T42.3X6
Cyclobarbitone	T42.3X1	T42.3X2	T42.3X3	T42.3X4	T42.3X5	T42.3X6
Cyclobenzaprine	T48.1X1	T48.1X2	T48.1X3	T48.1X4	T48.1X5	T48.1X6
Cyclodrine	T44.3X1	T44.3X2	T44.3X3	T44.3X4	T44.3X5	T44.3X6
Cycloguanil embonate	T37.2X1	T37.2X2	T37.2X3	T37.2X4	T37.2X5	T37.2X6
Cyclohexane	T52.8X1	T52.8X2	T52.8X3	T52.8X4	—	—
Cyclohexanol	T51.8X1	T51.8X2	T51.8X3	T51.8X4	—	—
Cyclohexanone	T52.4X1	T52.4X2	T52.4X3	T52.4X4	—	—
Cycloheximide	T60.3X1	T60.3X2	T60.3X3	T60.3X4	—	—
Cyclohexyl acetate	T52.8X1	T52.8X2	T52.8X3	T52.8X4	—	—
Cycloleucin	T45.1X1	T45.1X2	T45.1X3	T45.1X4	T45.1X5	T45.1X6
Cyclomethycaine	T41.3X1	T41.3X2	T41.3X3	T41.3X4	T41.3X5	T41.3X6
Cyclopentamine	T44.4X1	T44.4X2	T44.4X3	T44.4X4	T44.4X5	T44.4X6
Cyclopenthiazide	T50.2X1	T50.2X2	T50.2X3	T50.2X4	T50.2X5	T50.2X6
Cyclopentolate	T44.3X1	T44.3X2	T44.3X3	T44.3X4	T44.3X5	T44.3X6
Cyclophosphamide	T45.1X1	T45.1X2	T45.1X3	T45.1X4	T45.1X5	T45.1X6
Cycloplegic drug	T49.5X1	T49.5X2	T49.5X3	T49.5X4	T49.5X5	T49.5X6
Cyclopropane	T41.291	T41.292	T41.293	T41.294	T41.295	T41.296
Cyclopyrabital	T39.8X1	T39.8X2	T39.8X3	T39.8X4	T39.8X5	T39.8X6
Cycloserine	T37.1X1	T37.1X2	T37.1X3	T37.1X4	T37.1X5	T37.1X6
Cyclosporin	T45.1X1	T45.1X2	T45.1X3	T45.1X4	T45.1X5	T45.1X6
Cyclothiazide	T50.2X1	T50.2X2	T50.2X3	T50.2X4	T50.2X5	T50.2X6
Cycrimine	T44.3X1	T44.3X2	T44.3X3	T44.3X4	T44.3X5	T44.3X6
Cyhalothrin	T60.1X1	T60.1X2	T60.1X3	T60.1X4	—	—
Cymarin	T46.0X1	T46.0X2	T46.0X3	T46.0X4	T46.0X5	T46.0X6
Cypermethrin	T60.1X1	T60.1X2	T60.1X3	T60.1X4	—	—
Cyphenothrin	T60.2X1	T60.2X2	T60.2X3	T60.2X4	—	—
Cyproheptadine	T45.0X1	T45.0X2	T45.0X3	T45.0X4	T45.0X5	T45.0X6
Cyproterone	T38.6X1	T38.6X2	T38.6X3	T38.6X4	T38.6X5	T38.6X6
Cysteamine	T50.6X1	T50.6X2	T50.6X3	T50.6X4	T50.6X5	T50.6X6
Cytarabine	T45.1X1	T45.1X2	T45.1X3	T45.1X4	T45.1X5	T45.1X6
Cytisus						
laburnum	T62.2X1	T62.2X2	T62.2X3	T62.2X4	—	—
scoparius	T62.2X1	T62.2X2	T62.2X3	T62.2X4	—	—
Cytochrome C	T47.5X1	T47.5X2	T47.5X3	T47.5X4	T47.5X5	T47.5X6
Cytomel	T38.1X1	T38.1X2	T38.1X3	T38.1X4	T38.1X5	T38.1X6
Cytosine arabinoside	T45.1X1	T45.1X2	T45.1X3	T45.1X4	T45.1X5	T45.1X6
Cytoxan	T45.1X1	T45.1X2	T45.1X3	T45.1X4	T45.1X5	T45.1X6
Cytozyme	T45.7X1	T45.7X2	T45.7X3	T45.7X4	T45.7X5	T45.7X6
S-Carboxymethylcysteine	T48.4X1	T48.4X2	T48.4X3	T48.4X4	T48.4X5	T48.4X6
Dacarbazine	T45.1X1	T45.1X2	T45.1X3	T45.1X4	T45.1X5	T45.1X6
Dactinomycin	T45.1X1	T45.1X2	T45.1X3	T45.1X4	T45.1X5	T45.1X6
DADPS	T37.1X1	T37.1X2	T37.1X3	T37.1X4	T37.1X5	T37.1X6
Dakin's solution	T49.0X1	T49.0X2	T49.0X3	T49.0X4	T49.0X5	T49.0X6
Dalapon (sodium)	T60.3X1	T60.3X2	T60.3X3	T60.3X4	—	—
Dalmane	T42.4X1	T42.4X2	T42.4X3	T42.4X4	T42.4X5	T42.4X6
Danazol	T38.6X1	T38.6X2	T38.6X3	T38.6X4	T38.6X5	T38.6X6
Danilone	T45.511	T45.512	T45.513	T45.514	T45.515	T45.516
Danthron	T47.2X1	T47.2X2	T47.2X3	T47.2X4	T47.2X5	T47.2X6
Dantrolene	T42.8X1	T42.8X2	T42.8X3	T42.8X4	T42.8X5	T42.8X6
Dantron	T47.2X1	T47.2X2	T47.2X3	T47.2X4	T47.2X5	T47.2X6
Daphne (gnidium) (mezereum)	T62.2X1	T62.2X2	T62.2X3	T62.2X4	—	—
berry	T62.1X1	T62.1X2	T62.1X3	T62.1X4	—	—
Dapsone	T37.1X1	T37.1X2	T37.1X3	T37.1X4	T37.1X5	T37.1X6
Daraprim	T37.2X1	T37.2X2	T37.2X3	T37.2X4	T37.2X5	T37.2X6
Darnel	T62.2X1	T62.2X2	T62.2X3	T62.2X4	—	—
Darvon	T39.8X1	T39.8X2	T39.8X3	T39.8X4	T39.8X5	T39.8X6
Daunomycin	T45.1X1	T45.1X2	T45.1X3	T45.1X4	T45.1X5	T45.1X6
Daunorubicin	T45.1X1	T45.1X2	T45.1X3	T45.1X4	T45.1X5	T45.1X6
DBI	T38.3X1	T38.3X2	T38.3X3	T38.3X4	T38.3X5	T38.3X6
D-Con	T60.91	T60.92	T60.93	T60.94	—	—
insecticide	T60.2X1	T60.2X2	T60.2X3	T60.2X4	—	—
rodenticide	T60.4X1	T60.4X2	T60.4X3	T60.4X4	—	—
DDAVP	T38.891	T38.892	T38.893	T38.894	T38.895	T38.896

Substance	Poisoning, Accidental (unintentional)	Poisoning, Intentional Self-harm	Poisoning, Assault	Poisoning, Undetermined	Adverse Effect	Under-dosing
DDE (bis(chlorophenyl)-dichloroethylene)	T60.2X1	T60.2X2	T60.2X3	T60.2X4	—	—
DDS	T37.1X1	T37.1X2	T37.1X3	T37.1X4	T37.1X5	T37.1X6
DDT (dust)	T60.1X1	T60.1X2	T60.1X3	T60.1X4	—	—
Deadly nightshade — see also Belladonna	T62.2X1	T62.2X2	T62.2X3	T62.2X4	—	—
berry	T62.1X1	T62.1X2	T62.1X3	T62.1X4	—	—
Deamino-D-arginine vasopressin	T38.891	T38.892	T38.893	T38.894	T38.895	T38.896
Deanol (aceglumate)	T50.991	T50.992	T50.993	T50.994	T50.995	T50.996
Debrisoquine	T46.5X1	T46.5X2	T46.5X3	T46.5X4	T46.5X5	T46.5X6
Decaborane	T57.8X1	T57.8X2	T57.8X3	T57.8X4	—	—
fumes	T59.891	T59.892	T59.893	T59.894	—	—
Decadron	T38.0X1	T38.0X2	T38.0X3	T38.0X4	T38.0X5	T38.0X6
ENT agent	T49.6X1	T49.6X2	T49.6X3	T49.6X4	T49.6X5	T49.6X6
ophthalmic preparation	T49.5X1	T49.5X2	T49.5X3	T49.5X4	T49.5X5	T49.5X6
topical NEC	T49.0X1	T49.0X2	T49.0X3	T49.0X4	T49.0X5	T49.0X6
Decahydronaphthalene	T52.8X1	T52.8X2	T52.8X3	T52.8X4	—	—
Decalin	T52.8X1	T52.8X2	T52.8X3	T52.8X4	—	—
Decamethonium (bromide)	T48.1X1	T48.1X2	T48.1X3	T48.1X4	T48.1X5	T48.1X6
Decholin	T47.5X1	T47.5X2	T47.5X3	T47.5X4	T47.5X5	T47.5X6
Declomycin	T36.4X1	T36.4X2	T36.4X3	T36.4X4	T36.4X5	T36.4X6
Decongestant, nasal (mucosa)	T48.5X1	T48.5X2	T48.5X3	T48.5X4	T48.5X5	T48.5X6
combination	T48.5X1	T48.5X2	T48.5X3	T48.5X4	T48.5X5	T48.5X6
Deet	T60.8X1	T60.8X2	T60.8X3	T60.8X4	—	—
Deferoxamine	T45.8X1	T45.8X2	T45.8X3	T45.8X4	T45.8X5	T45.8X6
Deflazacort	T38.0X1	T38.0X2	T38.0X3	T38.0X4	T38.0X5	T38.0X6
Deglycyrrhizinized extract of licorice	T48.4X1	T48.4X2	T48.4X3	T48.4X4	T48.4X5	T48.4X6
Dehydrocholic acid	T47.5X1	T47.5X2	T47.5X3	T47.5X4	T47.5X5	T47.5X6
Dehydroemetine	T37.3X1	T37.3X2	T37.3X3	T37.3X4	T37.3X5	T37.3X6
Dekalin	T52.8X1	T52.8X2	T52.8X3	T52.8X4	—	—
Delalutin	T38.5X1	T38.5X2	T38.5X3	T38.5X4	T38.5X5	T38.5X6
Delorazepam	T42.4X1	T42.4X2	T42.4X3	T42.4X4	T42.4X5	T42.4X6
Delphinium	T62.2X1	T62.2X2	T62.2X3	T62.2X4	—	—
Deltamethrin	T60.1X1	T60.1X2	T60.1X3	T60.1X4	—	—
Deltasone	T38.0X1	T38.0X2	T38.0X3	T38.0X4	T38.0X5	T38.0X6
Deltra	T38.0X1	T38.0X2	T38.0X3	T38.0X4	T38.0X5	T38.0X6
Delvinal	T42.3X1	T42.3X2	T42.3X3	T42.3X4	T42.3X5	T42.3X6
Demecarium (bromide)	T49.5X1	T49.5X2	T49.5X3	T49.5X4	T49.5X5	T49.5X6
Demeclocycline	T36.4X1	T36.4X2	T36.4X3	T36.4X4	T36.4X5	T36.4X6
Demecolcine	T45.1X1	T45.1X2	T45.1X3	T45.1X4	T45.1X5	T45.1X6
Demegestone	T38.5X1	T38.5X2	T38.5X3	T38.5X4	T38.5X5	T38.5X6
Demelanizing agents	T49.8X1	T49.8X2	T49.8X3	T49.8X4	T49.8X5	T49.8X6
Demephion -O and -S	T60.0X1	T60.0X2	T60.0X3	T60.0X4	—	—
Demerol	T40.2X1	T40.2X2	T40.2X3	T40.2X4	T40.2X5	T40.2X6
Demethylchlortetracycline	T36.4X1	T36.4X2	T36.4X3	T36.4X4	T36.4X5	T36.4X6
Demethyltetracycline	T36.4X1	T36.4X2	T36.4X3	T36.4X4	T36.4X5	T36.4X6
Demeton -O and -S	T60.0X1	T60.0X2	T60.0X3	T60.0X4	—	—
Demulcent (external)	T49.3X1	T49.3X2	T49.3X3	T49.3X4	T49.3X5	T49.3X6
specified NEC	T49.3X1	T49.3X2	T49.3X3	T49.3X4	T49.3X5	T49.3X6
Demulen	T38.4X1	T38.4X2	T38.4X3	T38.4X4	T38.4X5	T38.4X6
Denatured alcohol	T51.0X1	T51.0X2	T51.0X3	T51.0X4	—	—
Dendrid	T49.5X1	T49.5X2	T49.5X3	T49.5X4	T49.5X5	T49.5X6
Dental drug, topical application NEC	T49.7X1	T49.7X2	T49.7X3	T49.7X4	T49.7X5	T49.7X6
Dentifrice	T49.7X1	T49.7X2	T49.7X3	T49.7X4	T49.7X5	T49.7X6
Deodorant spray (feminine hygiene)	T49.8X1	T49.8X2	T49.8X3	T49.8X4	T49.8X5	T49.8X6
Deoxycortone	T50.0X1	T50.0X2	T50.0X3	T50.0X4	T50.0X5	T50.0X6
Deoxyribonuclease (pancreatic)	T45.3X1	T45.3X2	T45.3X3	T45.3X4	T45.3X5	T45.3X6
Depilatory	T49.4X1	T49.4X2	T49.4X3	T49.4X4	T49.4X5	T49.4X6
Deprenalin	T42.8X1	T42.8X2	T42.8X3	T42.8X4	T42.8X5	T42.8X6
Deprenyl	T42.8X1	T42.8X2	T42.8X3	T42.8X4	T42.8X5	T42.8X6
Depressant						
appetite (central)	T50.5X1	T50.5X2	T50.5X3	T50.5X4	T50.5X5	T50.5X6
cardiac	T46.2X1	T46.2X2	T46.2X3	T46.2X4	T46.2X5	T46.2X6
central nervous system (anesthetic) — see also Central nervous system, depressants	T42.71	T42.72	T42.73	T42.74	T42.75	T42.76
general anesthetic	T41.201	T41.202	T41.203	T41.204	T41.205	T41.206
muscle tone	T42.8X1	T42.8X2	T42.8X3	T42.8X4	T42.8X5	T42.8X6
muscle tone, central	T42.8X1	T42.8X2	T42.8X3	T42.8X4	T42.8X5	T42.8X6
psychotherapeutic	T43.501	T43.502	T43.503	T43.504	T43.505	T43.506
Depressant, appetite	T50.5X1	T50.5X2	T50.5X3	T50.5X4	T50.5X5	T50.5X6
Deptropine	T45.0X1	T45.0X2	T45.0X3	T45.0X4	T45.0X5	T45.0X6
Dequalinium (chloride)	T49.0X1	T49.0X2	T49.0X3	T49.0X4	T49.0X5	T49.0X6
Derris root	T60.2X1	T60.2X2	T60.2X3	T60.2X4	—	—
Deserpidine	T46.5X1	T46.5X2	T46.5X3	T46.5X4	T46.5X5	T46.5X6
Desferrioxamine	T45.8X1	T45.8X2	T45.8X3	T45.8X4	T45.8X5	T45.8X6
Desipramine	T43.011	T43.012	T43.013	T43.014	T43.015	T43.016
Deslanoside	T46.0X1	T46.0X2	T46.0X3	T46.0X4	T46.0X5	T46.0X6
Desloughing agent	T49.4X1	T49.4X2	T49.4X3	T49.4X4	T49.4X5	T49.4X6
Desmethylimipramine	T43.011	T43.012	T43.013	T43.014	T43.015	T43.016
Desmopressin	T38.891	T38.892	T38.893	T38.894	T38.895	T38.896
Desocodeine	T40.2X1	T40.2X2	T40.2X3	T40.2X4	T40.2X5	T40.2X6
Desogestrel	T38.5X1	T38.5X2	T38.5X3	T38.5X4	T38.5X5	T38.5X6
Desomorphine	T40.2X1	T40.2X2	T40.2X3	T40.2X4	—	—
Desonide	T49.0X1	T49.0X2	T49.0X3	T49.0X4	T49.0X5	T49.0X6
Desoximetasone	T49.0X1	T49.0X2	T49.0X3	T49.0X4	T49.0X5	T49.0X6
Desoxycorticosteroid	T50.0X1	T50.0X2	T50.0X3	T50.0X4	T50.0X5	T50.0X6
Desoxycortone	T50.0X1	T50.0X2	T50.0X3	T50.0X4	T50.0X5	T50.0X6
Desoxyephedrine	T43.621	T43.622	T43.623	T43.624	T43.625	T43.626
Detajmium	T46.6X1	T46.6X2	T46.6X3	T46.6X4	T46.6X5	T46.6X6
Detergent	T49.2X1	T49.2X2	T49.2X3	T49.2X4	T49.2X5	T49.2X6
external medication	T49.2X1	T49.2X2	T49.2X3	T49.2X4	T49.2X5	T49.2X6
local	T49.2X1	T49.2X2	T49.2X3	T49.2X4	T49.2X5	T49.2X6
medicinal	T49.2X1	T49.2X2	T49.2X3	T49.2X4	T49.2X5	T49.2X6
nonmedicinal	T55.1X1	T55.1X2	T55.1X3	T55.1X4	—	—
specified NEC	T55.1X1	T55.1X2	T55.1X3	T55.1X4	—	—
Deterrent, alcohol	T50.6X1	T50.6X2	T50.6X3	T50.6X4	T50.6X5	T50.6X6
Detoxifying agent	T50.6X1	T50.6X2	T50.6X3	T50.6X4	T50.6X5	T50.6X6
Detrothyronine	T38.1X1	T38.1X2	T38.1X3	T38.1X4	T38.1X5	T38.1X6
Dettol (external medication)	T49.0X1	T49.0X2	T49.0X3	T49.0X4	T49.0X5	T49.0X6
Dexamethasone	T38.0X1	T38.0X2	T38.0X3	T38.0X4	T38.0X5	T38.0X6
ENT agent	T49.6X1	T49.6X2	T49.6X3	T49.6X4	T49.6X5	T49.6X6
ophthalmic preparation	T49.5X1	T49.5X2	T49.5X3	T49.5X4	T49.5X5	T49.5X6
topical NEC	T49.0X1	T49.0X2	T49.0X3	T49.0X4	T49.0X5	T49.0X6
Dexamfetamine	T43.621	T43.622	T43.623	T43.624	T43.625	T43.626
Dexamphetamine	T43.621	T43.622	T43.623	T43.624	T43.625	T43.626
Dexbrompheniramine	T45.0X1	T45.0X2	T45.0X3	T45.0X4	T45.0X5	T45.0X6
Dexchlorpheniramine	T45.0X1	T45.0X2	T45.0X3	T45.0X4	T45.0X5	T45.0X6
Dexedrine	T43.621	T43.622	T43.623	T43.624	T43.625	T43.626
Dexetimide	T44.3X1	T44.3X2	T44.3X3	T44.3X4	T44.3X5	T44.3X6
Dexfenfluramine	T50.5X1	T50.5X2	T50.5X3	T50.5X4	T50.5X5	T50.5X6
Dexpanthenol	T45.2X1	T45.2X2	T45.2X3	T45.2X4	T45.2X5	T45.2X6
Dextran (40) (70) (150)	T45.8X1	T45.8X2	T45.8X3	T45.8X4	T45.8X5	T45.8X6
Dextriferron	T45.4X1	T45.4X2	T45.4X3	T45.4X4	T45.4X5	T45.4X6
Dextroamphetamine	T43.621	T43.622	T43.623	T43.624	T43.625	T43.626
Dextro calcium pantothenate	T45.2X1	T45.2X2	T45.2X3	T45.2X4	T45.2X5	T45.2X6
Dextromethorphan	T48.3X1	T48.3X2	T48.3X3	T48.3X4	T48.3X5	T48.3X6
Dextromoramide	T40.4X1	T40.4X2	T40.4X3	T40.4X4	—	—
topical	T49.8X1	T49.8X2	T49.8X3	T49.8X4	T49.8X5	T49.8X6
Dextro pantothenyl alcohol	T45.2X1	T45.2X2	T45.2X3	T45.2X4	T45.2X5	T45.2X6
Dextropropoxyphene	T40.4X1	T40.4X2	T40.4X3	T40.4X4	T40.4X5	T40.4X6
Dextrorphan	T40.2X1	T40.2X2	T40.2X3	T40.2X4	T40.2X5	T40.2X6
Dextrose	T50.3X1	T50.3X2	T50.3X3	T50.3X4	T50.3X5	T50.3X6
concentrated solution, intravenous	T46.8X1	T46.8X2	T46.8X3	T46.8X4	T46.8X5	T46.8X6
Dextrothyroxin	T38.1X1	T38.1X2	T38.1X3	T38.1X4	T38.1X5	T38.1X6
Dextrothyroxine sodium	T38.1X1	T38.1X2	T38.1X3	T38.1X4	T38.1X5	T38.1X6
DFP	T44.0X1	T44.0X2	T44.0X3	T44.0X4	T44.0X5	T44.0X6
DHE	T37.3X1	T37.3X2	T37.3X3	T37.3X4	T37.3X5	T37.3X6
45	T46.5X1	T46.5X2	T46.5X3	T46.5X4	T46.5X5	T46.5X6
Diabinese	T38.3X1	T38.3X2	T38.3X3	T38.3X4	T38.3X5	T38.3X6
Diacetone alcohol	T52.4X1	T52.4X2	T52.4X3	T52.4X4	—	—
Diacetyl monoxime	T50.991	T50.992	T50.993	T50.994	—	—
Diacetylmorphine	T40.1X1	T40.1X2	T40.1X3	T40.1X4	—	—
Diachylon plaster	T49.4X1	T49.4X2	T49.4X3	T49.4X4	T49.4X5	T49.4X6
Diaethylstilboestrolum	T38.5X1	T38.5X2	T38.5X3	T38.5X4	T38.5X5	T38.5X6
Diagnostic agent NEC	T50.8X1	T50.8X2	T50.8X3	T50.8X4	T50.8X5	T50.8X6
Dial (soap)	T49.2X1	T49.2X2	T49.2X3	T49.2X4	T49.2X5	T49.2X6
sedative	T42.3X1	T42.3X2	T42.3X3	T42.3X4	T42.3X5	T42.3X6
Dialkyl carbonate	T52.91	T52.92	T52.93	T52.94	—	—
Diallylbarbituric acid	T42.3X1	T42.3X2	T42.3X3	T42.3X4	T42.3X5	T42.3X6
Diallymal	T42.3X1	T42.3X2	T42.3X3	T42.3X4	T42.3X5	T42.3X6
Dialysis solution (intraperitoneal)	T50.3X1	T50.3X2	T50.3X3	T50.3X4	T50.3X5	T50.3X6
Diaminodiphenylsulfone	T37.1X1	T37.1X2	T37.1X3	T37.1X4	T37.1X5	T37.1X6
Diamorphine	T40.1X1	T40.1X2	T40.1X3	T40.1X4	—	—
Diamox	T50.2X1	T50.2X2	T50.2X3	T50.2X4	T50.2X5	T50.2X6
Diamthazole	T49.0X1	T49.0X2	T49.0X3	T49.0X4	T49.0X5	T49.0X6
Dianthone	T47.2X1	T47.2X2	T47.2X3	T47.2X4	T47.2X5	T47.2X6
Diaphenylsulfone	T37.0X1	T37.0X2	T37.0X3	T37.0X4	T37.0X5	T37.0X6
Diasone (sodium)	T37.1X1	T37.1X2	T37.1X3	T37.1X4	T37.1X5	T37.1X6
Diastase	T47.5X1	T47.5X2	T47.5X3	T47.5X4	T47.5X5	T47.5X6
Diatrizoate	T50.8X1	T50.8X2	T50.8X3	T50.8X4	T50.8X5	T50.8X6
Diazepam	T42.4X1	T42.4X2	T42.4X3	T42.4X4	T42.4X5	T42.4X6
Diazinon	T60.0X1	T60.0X2	T60.0X3	T60.0X4	—	—
Diazomethane (gas)	T59.891	T59.892	T59.893	T59.894	—	—
Diazoxide	T46.5X1	T46.5X2	T46.5X3	T46.5X4	T46.5X5	T46.5X6
Dibekacin	T36.5X1	T36.5X2	T36.5X3	T36.5X4	T36.5X5	T36.5X6

⬇ Subterms under main terms may continue to next column or page　　Additional Character May Be Required — Refer to the Tabular List for Character Selection　　363

DDE — Dibekacin

Substance	Poisoning, Accidental (unintentional)	Poisoning, Intentional Self-harm	Poisoning, Assault	Poisoning, Undetermined	Adverse Effect	Under-dosing
Dibenamine	T44.6X1	T44.6X2	T44.6X3	T44.6X4	T44.6X5	T44.6X6
Dibenzepin	T43.011	T43.012	T43.013	T43.014	T43.015	T43.016
Dibenzheptropine	T45.0X1	T45.0X2	T45.0X3	T45.0X4	T45.0X5	T45.0X6
Dibenzyline	T44.6X1	T44.6X2	T44.6X3	T44.6X4	T44.6X5	T44.6X6
Diborane (gas)	T59.891	T59.892	T59.893	T59.894	—	—
Dibromochloropropane	T60.8X1	T60.8X2	T60.8X3	T60.8X4	—	—
Dibromodulcitol	T45.1X1	T45.1X2	T45.1X3	T45.1X4	T45.1X5	T45.1X6
Dibromoethane	T53.6X1	T53.6X2	T53.6X3	T53.6X4	—	—
Dibromomannitol	T45.1X1	T45.1X2	T45.1X3	T45.1X4	T45.1X5	T45.1X6
Dibromopropamidine isethionate	T49.0X1	T49.0X2	T49.0X3	T49.0X4	T49.0X5	T49.0X6
Dibrompropamidine	T49.0X1	T49.0X2	T49.0X3	T49.0X4	T49.0X5	T49.0X6
Dibucaine	T41.3X1	T41.3X2	T41.3X3	T41.3X4	T41.3X5	T41.3X6
topical (surface)	T41.3X1	T41.3X2	T41.3X3	T41.3X4	T41.3X5	T41.3X6
Dibunate sodium	T48.3X1	T48.3X2	T48.3X3	T48.3X4	T48.3X5	T48.3X6
Dibutoline sulfate	T44.3X1	T44.3X2	T44.3X3	T44.3X4	T44.3X5	T44.3X6
Dicamba	T60.3X1	T60.3X2	T60.3X3	T60.3X4	—	—
Dicapthon	T60.0X1	T60.0X2	T60.0X3	T60.0X4	—	—
Dichlobenil	T60.3X1	T60.3X2	T60.3X3	T60.3X4	—	—
Dichlone	T60.3X1	T60.3X2	T60.3X3	T60.3X4	—	—
Dichloralphenozone	T42.6X1	T42.6X2	T42.6X3	T42.6X4	T42.6X5	T42.6X6
Dichlorbenzidine	T65.3X1	T65.3X2	T65.3X3	T65.3X4	—	—
Dichlorhydrin	T52.8X1	T52.8X2	T52.8X3	T52.8X4	—	—
Dichlorhydroxyquinoline	T37.8X1	T37.8X2	T37.8X3	T37.8X4	T37.8X5	T37.8X6
Dichlorobenzene	T53.7X1	T53.7X2	T53.7X3	T53.7X4	—	—
Dichlorobenzyl alcohol	T49.6X1	T49.6X2	T49.6X3	T49.6X4	T49.6X5	T49.6X6
Dichlorodifluoromethane	T53.5X1	T53.5X2	T53.5X3	T53.5X4	—	—
Dichloroethane	T52.8X1	T52.8X2	T52.8X3	T52.8X4	—	—
Dichloroethylene	T53.6X1	T53.6X2	T53.6X3	T53.6X4	—	—
Dichloroethyl sulfide, not in war	T59.891	T59.892	T59.893	T59.894	—	—
Dichloroformoxine, not in war	T59.891	T59.892	T59.893	T59.894	—	—
Dichlorohydrin, alpha-dichlorohydrin	T52.8X1	T52.8X2	T52.8X3	T52.8X4	—	—
Dichloromethane (solvent)	T53.4X1	T53.4X2	T53.4X3	T53.4X4	—	—
vapor	T53.4X1	T53.4X2	T53.4X3	T53.4X4	—	—
Dichloronaphthoquinone	T60.3X1	T60.3X2	T60.3X3	T60.3X4	—	—
Dichlorophen	T37.4X1	T37.4X2	T37.4X3	T37.4X4	T37.4X5	T37.4X6
Dichloropropene	T60.3X1	T60.3X2	T60.3X3	T60.3X4	—	—
Dichloropropionic acid	T60.3X1	T60.3X2	T60.3X3	T60.3X4	—	—
Dichlorphenamide	T50.2X1	T50.2X2	T50.2X3	T50.2X4	T50.2X5	T50.2X6
Dichlorvos	T60.0X1	T60.0X2	T60.0X3	T60.0X4	—	—
Diclofenac	T39.391	T39.392	T39.393	T39.394	T39.395	T39.396
Diclofenamide	T50.2X1	T50.2X2	T50.2X3	T50.2X4	T50.2X5	T50.2X6
Diclofensine	T43.291	T43.292	T43.293	T43.294	T43.295	T43.296
Diclonixine	T39.8X1	T39.8X2	T39.8X3	T39.8X4	T39.8X5	T39.8X6
Dicloxacillin	T36.0X1	T36.0X2	T36.0X3	T36.0X4	T36.0X5	T36.0X6
Dicophane	T49.0X1	T49.0X2	T49.0X3	T49.0X4	T49.0X5	T49.0X6
Dicoumarol, dicoumarin, dicumarol	T45.511	T45.512	T45.513	T45.514	T45.515	T45.516
Dicrotophos	T60.0X1	T60.0X2	T60.0X3	T60.0X4	—	—
Dicyanogen (gas)	T65.0X1	T65.0X2	T65.0X3	T65.0X4	—	—
Dicyclomine	T44.3X1	T44.3X2	T44.3X3	T44.3X4	T44.3X5	T44.3X6
Dicycloverine	T44.3X1	T44.3X2	T44.3X3	T44.3X4	T44.3X5	T44.3X6
Dideoxycytidine	T37.5X1	T37.5X2	T37.5X3	T37.5X4	T37.5X5	T37.5X6
Dideoxyinosine	T37.5X1	T37.5X2	T37.5X3	T37.5X4	T37.5X5	T37.5X6
Dieldrin (vapor)	T60.1X1	T60.1X2	T60.1X3	T60.1X4	—	—
Diemal	T42.3X1	T42.3X2	T42.3X3	T42.3X4	T42.3X5	T42.3X6
Dienestrol	T38.5X1	T38.5X2	T38.5X3	T38.5X4	T38.5X5	T38.5X6
Dienoestrol	T38.5X1	T38.5X2	T38.5X3	T38.5X4	T38.5X5	T38.5X6
Dietetic drug NEC	T50.901	T50.902	T50.903	T50.904	T50.905	T50.906
Diethazine	T42.8X1	T42.8X2	T42.8X3	T42.8X4	T42.8X5	T42.8X6
Diethyl						
barbituric acid	T42.3X1	T42.3X2	T42.3X3	T42.3X4	T42.3X5	T42.3X6
carbamazine	T37.4X1	T37.4X2	T37.4X3	T37.4X4	T37.4X5	T37.4X6
carbinol	T51.3X1	T51.3X2	T51.3X3	T51.3X4	—	—
carbonate	T52.8X1	T52.8X2	T52.8X3	T52.8X4	—	—
ether (vapor) — see also ether	T41.0X1	T41.0X2	T41.0X3	T41.0X4	T41.0X5	T41.0X6
oxide	T52.8X1	T52.8X2	T52.8X3	T52.8X4	—	—
propion	T50.5X1	T50.5X2	T50.5X3	T50.5X4	T50.5X5	T50.5X6
stilbestrol	T38.5X1	T38.5X2	T38.5X3	T38.5X4	T38.5X5	T38.5X6
toluamide (nonmedicinal)	T60.8X1	T60.8X2	T60.8X3	T60.8X4	—	—
medicinal	T49.3X1	T49.3X2	T49.3X3	T49.3X4	T49.3X5	T49.3X6
Diethylcarbamazine	T37.4X1	T37.4X2	T37.4X3	T37.4X4	T37.4X5	T37.4X6
Diethylene						
dioxide	T52.8X1	T52.8X2	T52.8X3	T52.8X4	—	—
glycol (monoacetate) (monobutyl ether) (monoethyl ether)	T52.3X1	T52.3X2	T52.3X3	T52.3X4	—	—
Diethylhexylphthalate	T65.891	T65.892	T65.893	T65.894	—	—
Diethylpropion	T50.5X1	T50.5X2	T50.5X3	T50.5X4	T50.5X5	T50.5X6

Substance	Poisoning, Accidental (unintentional)	Poisoning, Intentional Self-harm	Poisoning, Assault	Poisoning, Undetermined	Adverse Effect	Under-dosing
Diethylstilbestrol	T38.5X1	T38.5X2	T38.5X3	T38.5X4	T38.5X5	T38.5X6
Diethylstilboestrol	T38.5X1	T38.5X2	T38.5X3	T38.5X4	T38.5X5	T38.5X6
Diethylsulfone-diethylmethane	T42.6X1	T42.6X2	T42.6X3	T42.6X4	T42.6X5	T42.6X6
Diethyltoluamide	T49.0X1	T49.0X2	T49.0X3	T49.0X4	T49.0X5	T49.0X6
Diethyltryptamine (DET)	T40.991	T40.992	T40.993	T40.994	—	—
Difebarbamate	T42.3X1	T42.3X2	T42.3X3	T42.3X4	T42.3X5	T42.3X6
Difencloxazine	T40.2X1	T40.2X2	T40.2X3	T40.2X4	T40.2X5	T40.2X6
Difenidol	T45.0X1	T45.0X2	T45.0X3	T45.0X4	T45.0X5	T45.0X6
Difenoxin	T47.6X1	T47.6X2	T47.6X3	T47.6X4	T47.6X5	T47.6X6
Difetarsone	T37.3X1	T37.3X2	T37.3X3	T37.3X4	T37.3X5	T37.3X6
Diffusin	T45.3X1	T45.3X2	T45.3X3	T45.3X4	T45.3X5	T45.3X6
Diflorasone	T49.0X1	T49.0X2	T49.0X3	T49.0X4	T49.0X5	T49.0X6
Diflos	T44.0X1	T44.0X2	T44.0X3	T44.0X4	T44.0X5	T44.0X6
Diflubenzuron	T60.1X1	T60.1X2	T60.1X3	T60.1X4	—	—
Diflucortolone	T49.0X1	T49.0X2	T49.0X3	T49.0X4	T49.0X5	T49.0X6
Diflunisal	T39.091	T39.092	T39.093	T39.094	T39.095	T39.096
Difluoromethyldopa	T42.8X1	T42.8X2	T42.8X3	T42.8X4	T42.8X5	T42.8X6
Difluorophate	T44.0X1	T44.0X2	T44.0X3	T44.0X4	T44.0X5	T44.0X6
Digestant NEC	T47.5X1	T47.5X2	T47.5X3	T47.5X4	T47.5X5	T47.5X6
Digitalin (e)	T46.0X1	T46.0X2	T46.0X3	T46.0X4	T46.0X5	T46.0X6
Digitalis (leaf)(glycoside)	T46.0X1	T46.0X2	T46.0X3	T46.0X4	T46.0X5	T46.0X6
lanata	T46.0X1	T46.0X2	T46.0X3	T46.0X4	T46.0X5	T46.0X6
purpurea	T46.0X1	T46.0X2	T46.0X3	T46.0X4	T46.0X5	T46.0X6
Digitoxin	T46.0X1	T46.0X2	T46.0X3	T46.0X4	T46.0X5	T46.0X6
Digitoxose	T46.0X1	T46.0X2	T46.0X3	T46.0X4	T46.0X5	T46.0X6
Digoxin	T46.0X1	T46.0X2	T46.0X3	T46.0X4	T46.0X5	T46.0X6
Digoxine	T46.0X1	T46.0X2	T46.0X3	T46.0X4	T46.0X5	T46.0X6
Dihydralazine	T46.5X1	T46.5X2	T46.5X3	T46.5X4	T46.5X5	T46.5X6
Dihydrazine	T46.5X1	T46.5X2	T46.5X3	T46.5X4	T46.5X5	T46.5X6
Dihydrocodeine	T40.2X1	T40.2X2	T40.2X3	T40.2X4	T40.2X5	T40.2X6
Dihydrocodeinone	T40.2X1	T40.2X2	T40.2X3	T40.2X4	T40.2X5	T40.2X6
Dihydroergocornine	T46.7X1	T46.7X2	T46.7X3	T46.7X4	T46.7X5	T46.7X6
Dihydroergocristine (mesilate)	T46.7X1	T46.7X2	T46.7X3	T46.7X4	T46.7X5	T46.7X6
Dihydroergokryptine	T46.7X1	T46.7X2	T46.7X3	T46.7X4	T46.7X5	T46.7X6
Dihydroergotamine	T46.5X1	T46.5X2	T46.5X3	T46.5X4	T46.5X5	T46.5X6
Dihydroergotoxine	T46.7X1	T46.7X2	T46.7X3	T46.7X4	T46.7X5	T46.7X6
mesilate	T46.7X1	T46.7X2	T46.7X3	T46.7X4	T46.7X5	T46.7X6
Dihydrohydroxycodeinone	T40.2X1	T40.2X2	T40.2X3	T40.2X4	T40.2X5	T40.2X6
Dihydrohydroxymorphinone	T40.2X1	T40.2X2	T40.2X3	T40.2X4	T40.2X5	T40.2X6
Dihydroisocodeine	T40.2X1	T40.2X2	T40.2X3	T40.2X4	T40.2X5	T40.2X6
Dihydromorphine	T40.2X1	T40.2X2	T40.2X3	T40.2X4	—	—
Dihydromorphinone	T40.2X1	T40.2X2	T40.2X3	T40.2X4	T40.2X5	T40.2X6
Dihydrostreptomycin	T36.5X1	T36.5X2	T36.5X3	T36.5X4	T36.5X5	T36.5X6
Dihydrotachysterol	T45.2X1	T45.2X2	T45.2X3	T45.2X4	T45.2X5	T45.2X6
Dihydroxyaluminum aminoacetate	T47.1X1	T47.1X2	T47.1X3	T47.1X4	T47.1X5	T47.1X6
Dihydroxyaluminum sodium carbonate	T47.1X1	T47.1X2	T47.1X3	T47.1X4	T47.1X5	T47.1X6
Dihydroxyanthraquinone	T47.2X1	T47.2X2	T47.2X3	T47.2X4	T47.2X5	T47.2X6
Dihydroxycodeinone	T40.2X1	T40.2X2	T40.2X3	T40.2X4	T40.2X5	T40.2X6
Dihydroxypropyl theophylline	T50.2X1	T50.2X2	T50.2X3	T50.2X4	T50.2X5	T50.2X6
Diiodohydroxyquin	T37.8X1	T37.8X2	T37.8X3	T37.8X4	T37.8X5	T37.8X6
topical	T49.0X1	T49.0X2	T49.0X3	T49.0X4	T49.0X5	T49.0X6
Diiodohydroxyquinoline	T37.8X1	T37.8X2	T37.8X3	T37.8X4	T37.8X5	T37.8X6
Diiodotyrosine	T38.2X1	T38.2X2	T38.2X3	T38.2X4	T38.2X5	T38.2X6
Diisopromine	T44.3X1	T44.3X2	T44.3X3	T44.3X4	T44.3X5	T44.3X6
Diisopropylamine	T46.3X1	T46.3X2	T46.3X3	T46.3X4	T46.3X5	T46.3X6
Diisopropylfluorophosphonate	T44.0X1	T44.0X2	T44.0X3	T44.0X4	T44.0X5	T44.0X6
Dilantin	T42.0X1	T42.0X2	T42.0X3	T42.0X4	T42.0X5	T42.0X6
Dilaudid	T40.2X1	T40.2X2	T40.2X3	T40.2X4	T40.2X5	T40.2X6
Dilazep	T46.3X1	T46.3X2	T46.3X3	T46.3X4	T46.3X5	T46.3X6
Dill	T47.5X1	T47.5X2	T47.5X3	T47.5X4	T47.5X5	T47.5X6
Diloxanide	T37.3X1	T37.3X2	T37.3X3	T37.3X4	T37.3X5	T37.3X6
Diltiazem	T46.1X1	T46.1X2	T46.1X3	T46.1X4	T46.1X5	T46.1X6
Dimazole	T49.0X1	T49.0X2	T49.0X3	T49.0X4	T49.0X5	T49.0X6
Dimefline	T50.7X1	T50.7X2	T50.7X3	T50.7X4	T50.7X5	T50.7X6
Dimefox	T60.0X1	T60.0X2	T60.0X3	T60.0X4	—	—
Dimemorfan	T48.3X1	T48.3X2	T48.3X3	T48.3X4	T48.3X5	T48.3X6
Dimenhydrinate	T45.0X1	T45.0X2	T45.0X3	T45.0X4	T45.0X5	T45.0X6
Dimercaprol (British anti-lewisite)	T45.8X1	T45.8X2	T45.8X3	T45.8X4	T45.8X5	T45.8X6
Dimercaptopropanol	T45.8X1	T45.8X2	T45.8X3	T45.8X4	T45.8X5	T45.8X6
Dimestrol	T38.5X1	T38.5X2	T38.5X3	T38.5X4	T38.5X5	T38.5X6
Dimetane	T45.0X1	T45.0X2	T45.0X3	T45.0X4	T45.0X5	T45.0X6
Dimethicone	T47.1X1	T47.1X2	T47.1X3	T47.1X4	T47.1X5	T47.1X6
Dimethindene	T45.0X1	T45.0X2	T45.0X3	T45.0X4	T45.0X5	T45.0X6
Dimethisoquin	T49.1X1	T49.1X2	T49.1X3	T49.1X4	T49.1X5	T49.1X6
Dimethisterone	T38.5X1	T38.5X2	T38.5X3	T38.5X4	T38.5X5	T38.5X6
Dimethoate	T60.0X1	T60.0X2	T60.0X3	T60.0X4	—	—
Dimethocaine	T41.3X1	T41.3X2	T41.3X3	T41.3X4	T41.3X5	T41.3X6
Dimethoxanate	T48.3X1	T48.3X2	T48.3X3	T48.3X4	T48.3X5	T48.3X6

Substance	Poisoning, Accidental (unintentional)	Poisoning, Intentional Self-harm	Poisoning, Assault	Poisoning, Undetermined	Adverse Effect	Under-dosing
Dimethyl						
arsine, arsinic acid	T57.0X1	T57.0X2	T57.0X3	T57.0X4	—	—
carbinol	T51.2X1	T51.2X2	T51.2X3	T51.2X4	—	—
carbonate	T52.8X1	T52.8X2	T52.8X3	T52.8X4	—	—
diguanide	T38.3X1	T38.3X2	T38.3X3	T38.3X4	T38.3X5	T38.3X6
ketone	T52.4X1	T52.4X2	T52.4X3	T52.4X4	—	—
vapor	T52.4X1	T52.4X2	T52.4X3	T52.4X4	—	—
meperidine	T40.2X1	T40.2X2	T40.2X3	T40.2X4	T40.2X5	T40.2X6
parathion	T60.0X1	T60.0X2	T60.0X3	T60.0X4	—	—
phthlate	T49.3X1	T49.3X2	T49.3X3	T49.3X4	T49.3X5	T49.3X6
polysiloxane	T47.8X1	T47.8X2	T47.8X3	T47.8X4	T47.8X5	T47.8X6
sulfate (fumes)	T59.891	T59.892	T59.893	T59.894	—	—
liquid	T65.891	T65.892	T65.893	T65.894	—	—
sulfoxide (nonmedicinal)	T52.8X1	T52.8X2	T52.8X3	T52.8X4	—	—
medicinal	T49.4X1	T49.4X2	T49.4X3	T49.4X4	T49.4X5	T49.4X6
tryptamine	T40.991	T40.992	T40.993	T40.994	—	—
tubocurarine	T48.1X1	T48.1X2	T48.1X3	T48.1X4	T48.1X5	T48.1X6
Dimethylamine sulfate	T49.4X1	T49.4X2	T49.4X3	T49.4X4	T49.4X5	T49.4X6
Dimethylformamide	T52.8X1	T52.8X2	T52.8X3	T52.8X4	—	—
Dimethyltubocurarinium chloride	T48.1X1	T48.1X2	T48.1X3	T48.1X4	T48.1X5	T48.1X6
Dimeticone	T47.1X1	T47.1X2	T47.1X3	T47.1X4	T47.1X5	T47.1X6
Dimetilan	T60.0X1	T60.0X2	T60.0X3	T60.0X4	—	—
Dimetindene	T45.0X1	T45.0X2	T45.0X3	T45.0X4	T45.0X5	T45.0X6
Dimetotiazine	T43.3X1	T43.3X2	T43.3X3	T43.3X4	T43.3X5	T43.3X6
Dimorpholamine	T50.7X1	T50.7X2	T50.7X3	T50.7X4	T50.7X5	T50.7X6
Dimoxyline	T46.3X1	T46.3X2	T46.3X3	T46.3X4	T46.3X5	T46.3X6
Dinitrobenzene	T65.3X1	T65.3X2	T65.3X3	T65.3X4	—	—
vapor	T59.891	T59.892	T59.893	T59.894	—	—
Dinitrobenzol	T65.3X1	T65.3X2	T65.3X3	T65.3X4	—	—
vapor	T59.891	T59.892	T59.893	T59.894	—	—
Dinitrobutylphenol	T65.3X1	T65.3X2	T65.3X3	T65.3X4	—	—
Dinitro (-ortho-)cresol (pesticide) (spray)	T65.3X1	T65.3X2	T65.3X3	T65.3X4	—	—
Dinitrocyclohexylphenol	T65.3X1	T65.3X2	T65.3X3	T65.3X4	—	—
Dinitrophenol	T65.3X1	T65.3X2	T65.3X3	T65.3X4	—	—
Dinoprost	T48.0X1	T48.0X2	T48.0X3	T48.0X4	T48.0X5	T48.0X6
Dinoprostone	T48.0X1	T48.0X2	T48.0X3	T48.0X4	T48.0X5	T48.0X6
Dinoseb	T60.3X1	T60.3X2	T60.3X3	T60.3X4	—	—
Dioctyl sulfosuccinate (calcium) (sodium)	T47.4X1	T47.4X2	T47.4X3	T47.4X4	T47.4X5	T47.4X6
Diodone	T50.8X1	T50.8X2	T50.8X3	T50.8X4	T50.8X5	T50.8X6
Diodoquin	T37.8X1	T37.8X2	T37.8X3	T37.8X4	T37.8X5	T37.8X6
Dionin	T40.2X1	T40.2X2	T40.2X3	T40.2X4	T40.2X5	T40.2X6
Diosmin	T46.991	T46.992	T46.993	T46.994	T46.995	T46.996
Dioxane	T52.8X1	T52.8X2	T52.8X3	T52.8X4	—	—
Dioxathion	T60.0X1	T60.0X2	T60.0X3	T60.0X4	—	—
Dioxin	T53.7X1	T53.7X2	T53.7X3	T53.7X4	—	—
Dioxopromethazine	T43.3X1	T43.3X2	T43.3X3	T43.3X4	T43.3X5	T43.3X6
Dioxyline	T46.3X1	T46.3X2	T46.3X3	T46.3X4	T46.3X5	T46.3X6
Dipentene	T52.8X1	T52.8X2	T52.8X3	T52.8X4	—	—
Diperodon	T41.3X1	T41.3X2	T41.3X3	T41.3X4	T41.3X5	T41.3X6
Diphacinone	T60.4X1	T60.4X2	T60.4X3	T60.4X4	—	—
Diphemanil	T44.3X1	T44.3X2	T44.3X3	T44.3X4	T44.3X5	T44.3X6
metilsulfate	T44.3X1	T44.3X2	T44.3X3	T44.3X4	T44.3X5	T44.3X6
Diphenadione	T45.511	T45.512	T45.513	T45.514	T45.515	T45.516
rodenticide	T60.4X1	T60.4X2	T60.4X3	T60.4X4	—	—
Diphenhydramine	T45.0X1	T45.0X2	T45.0X3	T45.0X4	T45.0X5	T45.0X6
Diphenidol	T45.0X1	T45.0X2	T45.0X3	T45.0X4	T45.0X5	T45.0X6
Diphenoxylate	T47.6X1	T47.6X2	T47.6X3	T47.6X4	T47.6X5	T47.6X6
Diphenylamine	T65.3X1	T65.3X2	T65.3X3	T65.3X4	—	—
Diphenylbutazone	T39.2X1	T39.2X2	T39.2X3	T39.2X4	T39.2X5	T39.2X6
Diphenylchloroarsine, not in war	T57.0X1	T57.0X2	T57.0X3	T57.0X4	—	—
Diphenylhydantoin	T42.0X1	T42.0X2	T42.0X3	T42.0X4	T42.0X5	T42.0X6
Diphenylmethane dye	T52.1X1	T52.1X2	T52.1X3	T52.1X4	—	—
Diphenylpyraline	T45.0X1	T45.0X2	T45.0X3	T45.0X4	T45.0X5	T45.0X6
Diphtheria						
antitoxin	T50.Z11	T50.Z12	T50.Z13	T50.Z14	T50.Z15	T50.Z16
toxoid	T50.A91	T50.A92	T50.A93	T50.A94	T50.A95	T50.A96
with tetanus toxoid	T50.A21	T50.A22	T50.A23	T50.A24	T50.A25	T50.A26
with pertussis component	T50.A11	T50.A12	T50.A13	T50.A14	T50.A15	T50.A16
vaccine	T50.A91	T50.A92	T50.A93	T50.A94	T50.A95	T50.A96
combination						
without pertussis	T50.A21	T50.A22	T50.A23	T50.A24	T50.A25	T50.A26
including pertussis	T50.A11	T50.A12	T50.A13	T50.A14	T50.A15	T50.A16
Diphylline	T50.2X1	T50.2X2	T50.2X3	T50.2X4	T50.2X5	T50.2X6
Dipipanone	T40.4X1	T40.4X2	T40.4X3	T40.4X4	—	—
Dipivefrine	T49.5X1	T49.5X2	T49.5X3	T49.5X4	T49.5X5	T49.5X6
Diplovax	T50.B91	T50.B92	T50.B93	T50.B94	T50.B95	T50.B96
Diprophylline	T50.2X1	T50.2X2	T50.2X3	T50.2X4	T50.2X5	T50.2X6
Dipropyline	T48.291	T48.292	T48.293	T48.294	T48.295	T48.296

Substance	Poisoning, Accidental (unintentional)	Poisoning, Intentional Self-harm	Poisoning, Assault	Poisoning, Undetermined	Adverse Effect	Under-dosing
Dipyridamole	T46.3X1	T46.3X2	T46.3X3	T46.3X4	T46.3X5	T46.3X6
Dipyrone	T39.2X1	T39.2X2	T39.2X3	T39.2X4	T39.2X5	T39.2X6
Diquat (dibromide)	T60.3X1	T60.3X2	T60.3X3	T60.3X4	—	—
Disinfectant	T65.891	T65.892	T65.893	T65.894	—	—
alkaline	T54.3X1	T54.3X2	T54.3X3	T54.3X4	—	—
aromatic	T54.1X1	T54.1X2	T54.1X3	T54.1X4	—	—
intestinal	T37.8X1	T37.8X2	T37.8X3	T37.8X4	T37.8X5	T37.8X6
Disipal	T42.8X1	T42.8X2	T42.8X3	T42.8X4	T42.8X5	T42.8X6
Disodium edetate	T50.6X1	T50.6X2	T50.6X3	T50.6X4	T50.6X5	T50.6X6
Disoprofol	T41.291	T41.292	T41.293	T41.294	T41.295	T41.296
Disopyramide	T46.2X1	T46.2X2	T46.2X3	T46.2X4	T46.2X5	T46.2X6
Distigmine (bromide)	T44.0X1	T44.0X2	T44.0X3	T44.0X4	T44.0X5	T44.0X6
Disulfamide	T50.2X1	T50.2X2	T50.2X3	T50.2X4	T50.2X5	T50.2X6
Disulfanilamide	T37.0X1	T37.0X2	T37.0X3	T37.0X4	T37.0X5	T37.0X6
Disulfiram	T50.6X1	T50.6X2	T50.6X3	T50.6X4	T50.6X5	T50.6X6
Disulfoton	T60.0X1	T60.0X2	T60.0X3	T60.0X4	—	—
Dithiazanine iodide	T37.4X1	T37.4X2	T37.4X3	T37.4X4	T37.4X5	T37.4X6
Dithiocarbamate	T60.0X1	T60.0X2	T60.0X3	T60.0X4	—	—
Dithranol	T49.4X1	T49.4X2	T49.4X3	T49.4X4	T49.4X5	T49.4X6
Diucardin	T50.2X1	T50.2X2	T50.2X3	T50.2X4	T50.2X5	T50.2X6
Diupres	T50.2X1	T50.2X2	T50.2X3	T50.2X4	T50.2X5	T50.2X6
Diuretic NEC	T50.2X1	T50.2X2	T50.2X3	T50.2X4	T50.2X5	T50.2X6
benzothiadiazine	T50.2X1	T50.2X2	T50.2X3	T50.2X4	T50.2X5	T50.2X6
carbonic acid anhydrase inhibitors	T50.2X1	T50.2X2	T50.2X3	T50.2X4	T50.2X5	T50.2X6
furfuryl NEC	T50.2X1	T50.2X2	T50.2X3	T50.2X4	T50.2X5	T50.2X6
loop (high-ceiling)	T50.1X1	T50.1X2	T50.1X3	T50.1X4	T50.1X5	T50.1X6
mercurial NEC	T50.2X1	T50.2X2	T50.2X3	T50.2X4	T50.2X5	T50.2X6
osmotic	T50.2X1	T50.2X2	T50.2X3	T50.2X4	T50.2X5	T50.2X6
purine NEC	T50.2X1	T50.2X2	T50.2X3	T50.2X4	T50.2X5	T50.2X6
saluretic NEC	T50.2X1	T50.2X2	T50.2X3	T50.2X4	T50.2X5	T50.2X6
sulfonamide	T50.2X1	T50.2X2	T50.2X3	T50.2X4	T50.2X5	T50.2X6
thiazide NEC	T50.2X1	T50.2X2	T50.2X3	T50.2X4	T50.2X5	T50.2X6
xanthine	T50.2X1	T50.2X2	T50.2X3	T50.2X4	T50.2X5	T50.2X6
Diurgin	T50.2X1	T50.2X2	T50.2X3	T50.2X4	T50.2X5	T50.2X6
Diuril	T50.2X1	T50.2X2	T50.2X3	T50.2X4	T50.2X5	T50.2X6
Diuron	T60.3X1	T60.3X2	T60.3X3	T60.3X4	—	—
Divalproex	T42.6X1	T42.6X2	T42.6X3	T42.6X4	T42.6X5	T42.6X6
Divinyl ether	T41.0X1	T41.0X2	T41.0X3	T41.0X4	T41.0X5	T41.0X6
Dixanthogen	T49.0X1	T49.0X2	T49.0X3	T49.0X4	T49.0X5	T49.0X6
Dixyrazine	T43.3X1	T43.3X2	T43.3X3	T43.3X4	T43.3X5	T43.3X6
D-lysergic acid diethylamide	T40.8X1	T40.8X2	T40.8X3	T40.8X4	—	—
DMCT	T36.4X1	T36.4X2	T36.4X3	T36.4X4	T36.4X5	T36.4X6
DMSO — see Dimethyl sulfoxide						
DNBP	T60.3X1	T60.3X2	T60.3X3	T60.3X4	—	—
DNOC	T65.3X1	T65.3X2	T65.3X3	T65.3X4	—	—
Dobutamine	T44.5X1	T44.5X2	T44.5X3	T44.5X4	T44.5X5	T44.5X6
DOCA	T38.0X1	T38.0X2	T38.0X3	T38.0X4	T38.0X5	T38.0X6
Docusate sodium	T47.4X1	T47.4X2	T47.4X3	T47.4X4	T47.4X5	T47.4X6
Dodicin	T49.0X1	T49.0X2	T49.0X3	T49.0X4	T49.0X5	T49.0X6
Dofamium chloride	T49.0X1	T49.0X2	T49.0X3	T49.0X4	T49.0X5	T49.0X6
Dolophine	T40.3X1	T40.3X2	T40.3X3	T40.3X4	T40.3X5	T40.3X6
Doloxene	T39.8X1	T39.8X2	T39.8X3	T39.8X4	T39.8X5	T39.8X6
Domestic gas (after combustion) — see Gas, utility						
prior to combustion	T59.891	T59.892	T59.893	T59.894	—	—
Domiodol	T48.4X1	T48.4X2	T48.4X3	T48.4X4	T48.4X5	T48.4X6
Domiphen (bromide)	T49.0X1	T49.0X2	T49.0X3	T49.0X4	T49.0X5	T49.0X6
Domperidone	T45.0X1	T45.0X2	T45.0X3	T45.0X4	T45.0X5	T45.0X6
Dopa	T42.8X1	T42.8X2	T42.8X3	T42.8X4	T42.8X5	T42.8X6
Dopamine	T44.991	T44.992	T44.993	T44.994	T44.995	T44.996
Doriden	T42.6X1	T42.6X2	T42.6X3	T42.6X4	T42.6X5	T42.6X6
Dormiral	T42.3X1	T42.3X2	T42.3X3	T42.3X4	T42.3X5	T42.3X6
Dormison	T42.6X1	T42.6X2	T42.6X3	T42.6X4	T42.6X5	T42.6X6
Dornase	T48.4X1	T48.4X2	T48.4X3	T48.4X4	T48.4X5	T48.4X6
Dorsacaine	T41.3X1	T41.3X2	T41.3X3	T41.3X4	T41.3X5	T41.3X6
Dosulepin	T43.011	T43.012	T43.013	T43.014	T43.015	T43.016
Dothiepin	T43.011	T43.012	T43.013	T43.014	T43.015	T43.016
Doxantrazole	T48.6X1	T48.6X2	T48.6X3	T48.6X4	T48.6X5	T48.6X6
Doxapram	T50.7X1	T50.7X2	T50.7X3	T50.7X4	T50.7X5	T50.7X6
Doxazosin	T44.6X1	T44.6X2	T44.6X3	T44.6X4	T44.6X5	T44.6X6
Doxepin	T43.011	T43.012	T43.013	T43.014	T43.015	T43.016
Doxifluridine	T45.1X1	T45.1X2	T45.1X3	T45.1X4	T45.1X5	T45.1X6
Doxorubicin	T45.1X1	T45.1X2	T45.1X3	T45.1X4	T45.1X5	T45.1X6
Doxycycline	T36.4X1	T36.4X2	T36.4X3	T36.4X4	T36.4X5	T36.4X6
Doxylamine	T45.0X1	T45.0X2	T45.0X3	T45.0X4	T45.0X5	T45.0X6
Dramamine	T45.0X1	T45.0X2	T45.0X3	T45.0X4	T45.0X5	T45.0X6
Drano (drain cleaner)	T54.3X1	T54.3X2	T54.3X3	T54.3X4	—	—
Dressing, live pulp	T49.7X1	T49.7X2	T49.7X3	T49.7X4	T49.7X5	T49.7X6
Drocode	T40.2X1	T40.2X2	T40.2X3	T40.2X4	T40.2X5	T40.2X6
Dromoran	T40.2X1	T40.2X2	T40.2X3	T40.2X4	T40.2X5	T40.2X6
Dromostanolone	T38.7X1	T38.7X2	T38.7X3	T38.7X4	T38.7X5	T38.7X6

▽ Subterms under main terms may continue to next column or page   Additional Character May Be Required — Refer to the Tabular List for Character Selection

Table of Drugs and Chemicals

Dronabinol — Etambutol

Substance	Poisoning, Accidental (unintentional)	Poisoning, Intentional Self-harm	Poisoning, Assault	Poisoning, Undetermined	Adverse Effect	Under-dosing
Dronabinol	T40.7X1	T40.7X2	T40.7X3	T40.7X4	T40.7X5	T40.7X6
Droperidol	T43.591	T43.592	T43.593	T43.594	T43.595	T43.596
Dropropizine	T48.3X1	T48.3X2	T48.3X3	T48.3X4	T48.3X5	T48.3X6
Drostanolone	T38.7X1	T38.7X2	T38.7X3	T38.7X4	T38.7X5	T38.7X6
Drotaverine	T44.3X1	T44.3X2	T44.3X3	T44.3X4	T44.3X5	T44.3X6
Drotrecogin alfa	T45.511	T45.512	T45.513	T45.514	T45.515	T45.516
Drug NEC	T50.901	T50.902	T50.903	T50.904	T50.905	T50.906
specified NEC	T50.991	T50.992	T50.993	T50.994	T50.995	T50.996
DTIC	T45.1X1	T45.1X2	T45.1X3	T45.1X4	T45.1X5	T45.1X6
Duboisine	T44.3X1	T44.3X2	T44.3X3	T44.3X4	T44.3X5	T44.3X6
Dulcolax	T47.2X1	T47.2X2	T47.2X3	T47.2X4	T47.2X5	T47.2X6
Duponol (C) (EP)	T49.2X1	T49.2X2	T49.2X3	T49.2X4	T49.2X5	T49.2X6
Durabolin	T38.7X1	T38.7X2	T38.7X3	T38.7X4	T38.7X5	T38.7X6
Dyclone	T41.3X1	T41.3X2	T41.3X3	T41.3X4	T41.3X5	T41.3X6
Dyclonine	T41.3X1	T41.3X2	T41.3X3	T41.3X4	T41.3X5	T41.3X6
Dydrogesterone	T38.5X1	T38.5X2	T38.5X3	T38.5X4	T38.5X5	T38.5X6
Dye NEC	T65.6X1	T65.6X2	T65.6X3	T65.6X4	—	—
antiseptic	T49.0X1	T49.0X2	T49.0X3	T49.0X4	T49.0X5	T49.0X6
diagnostic agents	T50.8X1	T50.8X2	T50.8X3	T50.8X4	T50.8X5	T50.8X6
pharmaceutical NEC	T50.901	T50.902	T50.903	T50.904	T50.905	T50.906
Dyflos	T44.0X1	T44.0X2	T44.0X3	T44.0X4	T44.0X5	T44.0X6
Dymelor	T38.3X1	T38.3X2	T38.3X3	T38.3X4	T38.3X5	T38.3X6
Dynamite	T65.3X1	T65.3X2	T65.3X3	T65.3X4	—	—
fumes	T59.891	T59.892	T59.893	T59.894	—	—
Dyphylline	T44.3X1	T44.3X2	T44.3X3	T44.3X4	T44.3X5	T44.3X6
b-eucaine	T49.1X1	T49.1X2	T49.1X3	T49.1X4	T49.1X5	T49.1X6
Ear drug NEC	T49.6X1	T49.6X2	T49.6X3	T49.6X4	T49.6X5	T49.6X6
Ear preparations	T49.6X1	T49.6X2	T49.6X3	T49.6X4	T49.6X5	T49.6X6
Echothiophate, echothiopate, ecothiopate	T49.5X1	T49.5X2	T49.5X3	T49.5X4	T49.5X5	T49.5X6
Econazole	T49.0X1	T49.0X2	T49.0X3	T49.0X4	T49.0X5	T49.0X6
Ecothiopate iodide	T49.5X1	T49.5X2	T49.5X3	T49.5X4	T49.5X5	T49.5X6
Ecstasy	T43.621	T43.622	T43.623	T43.624	T43.625	T43.626
Ectylurea	T42.6X1	T42.6X2	T42.6X3	T42.6X4	T42.6X5	T42.6X6
Edathamil disodium	T45.8X1	T45.8X2	T45.8X3	T45.8X4	T45.8X5	T45.8X6
Edecrin	T50.1X1	T50.1X2	T50.1X3	T50.1X4	T50.1X5	T50.1X6
Edetate, disodium (calcium)	T45.8X1	T45.8X2	T45.8X3	T45.8X4	T45.8X5	T45.8X6
Edoxudine	T49.5X1	T49.5X2	T49.5X3	T49.5X4	T49.5X5	T49.5X6
Edrophonium	T44.0X1	T44.0X2	T44.0X3	T44.0X4	T44.0X5	T44.0X6
chloride	T44.0X1	T44.0X2	T44.0X3	T44.0X4	T44.0X5	T44.0X6
EDTA	T50.6X1	T50.6X2	T50.6X3	T50.6X4	T50.6X5	T50.6X6
Eflornithine	T37.2X1	T37.2X2	T37.2X3	T37.2X4	T37.2X5	T37.2X6
Efloxate	T46.3X1	T46.3X2	T46.3X3	T46.3X4	T46.3X5	T46.3X6
Elase	T49.8X1	T49.8X2	T49.8X3	T49.8X4	T49.8X5	T49.8X6
Elastase	T47.5X1	T47.5X2	T47.5X3	T47.5X4	T47.5X5	T47.5X6
Elaterium	T47.2X1	T47.2X2	T47.2X3	T47.2X4	T47.2X5	T47.2X6
Elcatonin	T50.991	T50.992	T50.993	T50.994	T50.995	T50.996
Elder	T62.2X1	T62.2X2	T62.2X3	T62.2X4	—	—
berry, (unripe)	T62.1X1	T62.1X2	T62.1X3	T62.1X4	—	—
Electrolyte balance drug	T50.3X1	T50.3X2	T50.3X3	T50.3X4	T50.3X5	T50.3X6
Electrolytes NEC	T50.3X1	T50.3X2	T50.3X3	T50.3X4	T50.3X5	T50.3X6
Electrolytic agent NEC	T50.3X1	T50.3X2	T50.3X3	T50.3X4	T50.3X5	T50.3X6
Elemental diet	T50.901	T50.902	T50.903	T50.904	T50.905	T50.906
Elliptinium acetate	T45.1X1	T45.1X2	T45.1X3	T45.1X4	T45.1X5	T45.1X6
Embramine	T45.0X1	T45.0X2	T45.0X3	T45.0X4	T45.0X5	T45.0X6
Emepronium (salts)	T44.3X1	T44.3X2	T44.3X3	T44.3X4	T44.3X5	T44.3X6
bromide	T44.3X1	T44.3X2	T44.3X3	T44.3X4	T44.3X5	T44.3X6
Emetic NEC	T47.7X1	T47.7X2	T47.7X3	T47.7X4	T47.7X5	T47.7X6
Emetine	T37.3X1	T37.3X2	T37.3X3	T37.3X4	T37.3X5	T37.3X6
Emollient NEC	T49.3X1	T49.3X2	T49.3X3	T49.3X4	T49.3X5	T49.3X6
Emorfazone	T39.8X1	T39.8X2	T39.8X3	T39.8X4	T39.8X5	T39.8X6
Emylcamate	T43.591	T43.592	T43.593	T43.594	T43.595	T43.596
Enalapril	T46.4X1	T46.4X2	T46.4X3	T46.4X4	T46.4X5	T46.4X6
Enalaprilat	T46.4X1	T46.4X2	T46.4X3	T46.4X4	T46.4X5	T46.4X6
Encainide	T46.2X1	T46.2X2	T46.2X3	T46.2X4	T46.2X5	T46.2X6
Endocaine	T41.3X1	T41.3X2	T41.3X3	T41.3X4	T41.3X5	T41.3X6
Endosulfan	T60.2X1	T60.2X2	T60.2X3	T60.2X4	—	—
Endothall	T60.3X1	T60.3X2	T60.3X3	T60.3X4	—	—
Endralazine	T46.5X1	T46.5X2	T46.5X3	T46.5X4	T46.5X5	T46.5X6
Endrin	T60.1X1	T60.1X2	T60.1X3	T60.1X4	—	—
Enflurane	T41.0X1	T41.0X2	T41.0X3	T41.0X4	T41.0X5	T41.0X6
Enhexymal	T42.3X1	T42.3X2	T42.3X3	T42.3X4	T42.3X5	T42.3X6
Enocitabine	T45.1X1	T45.1X2	T45.1X3	T45.1X4	T45.1X5	T45.1X6
Enovid	T38.4X1	T38.4X2	T38.4X3	T38.4X4	T38.4X5	T38.4X6
Enoxacin	T36.8X1	T36.8X2	T36.8X3	T36.8X4	T36.8X5	T36.8X6
Enoxaparin (sodium)	T45.511	T45.512	T45.513	T45.514	T45.515	T45.516
Enpiprazole	T43.591	T43.592	T43.593	T43.594	T43.595	T43.596
Enprofylline	T48.6X1	T48.6X2	T48.6X3	T48.6X4	T48.6X5	T48.6X6
Enprostil	T47.1X1	T47.1X2	T47.1X3	T47.1X4	T47.1X5	T47.1X6
Enterogastrone	T38.891	T38.892	T38.893	T38.894	T38.895	T38.896
ENT preparations (anti-infectives)	T49.6X1	T49.6X2	T49.6X3	T49.6X4	T49.6X5	T49.6X6
Enviomycin	T36.8X1	T36.8X2	T36.8X3	T36.8X4	T36.8X5	T36.8X6

Substance	Poisoning, Accidental (unintentional)	Poisoning, Intentional Self-harm	Poisoning, Assault	Poisoning, Undetermined	Adverse Effect	Under-dosing
Enzodase	T45.3X1	T45.3X2	T45.3X3	T45.3X4	T45.3X5	T45.3X6
Enzyme NEC	T45.3X1	T45.3X2	T45.3X3	T45.3X4	T45.3X5	T45.3X6
depolymerizing	T49.8X1	T49.8X2	T49.8X3	T49.8X4	T49.8X5	T49.8X6
fibrolytic	T45.3X1	T45.3X2	T45.3X3	T45.3X4	T45.3X5	T45.3X6
gastric	T47.5X1	T47.5X2	T47.5X3	T47.5X4	T47.5X5	T47.5X6
intestinal	T47.5X1	T47.5X2	T47.5X3	T47.5X4	T47.5X5	T47.5X6
local action	T49.4X1	T49.4X2	T49.4X3	T49.4X4	T49.4X5	T49.4X6
proteolytic	T49.4X1	T49.4X2	T49.4X3	T49.4X4	T49.4X5	T49.4X6
thrombolytic	T45.3X1	T45.3X2	T45.3X3	T45.3X4	T45.3X5	T45.3X6
EPAB	T41.3X1	T41.3X2	T41.3X3	T41.3X4	T41.3X5	T41.3X6
Epanutin	T42.0X1	T42.0X2	T42.0X3	T42.0X4	T42.0X5	T42.0X6
Ephedra	T44.991	T44.992	T44.993	T44.994	T44.995	T44.996
Ephedrine	T44.991	T44.992	T44.993	T44.994	T44.995	T44.996
Epichlorhydrin, epichlorohydrin	T52.8X1	T52.8X2	T52.8X3	T52.8X4	—	—
Epicillin	T36.0X1	T36.0X2	T36.0X3	T36.0X4	T36.0X5	T36.0X6
Epiestriol	T38.5X1	T38.5X2	T38.5X3	T38.5X4	T38.5X5	T38.5X6
Epilim — see Sodium valproate						
Epimestrol	T38.5X1	T38.5X2	T38.5X3	T38.5X4	T38.5X5	T38.5X6
Epinephrine	T44.5X1	T44.5X2	T44.5X3	T44.5X4	T44.5X5	T44.5X6
Epirubicin	T45.1X1	T45.1X2	T45.1X3	T45.1X4	T45.1X5	T45.1X6
Epitiostanol	T38.7X1	T38.7X2	T38.7X3	T38.7X4	T38.7X5	T38.7X6
Epitizide	T50.2X1	T50.2X2	T50.2X3	T50.2X4	T50.2X5	T50.2X6
EPN	T60.0X1	T60.0X2	T60.0X3	T60.0X4	—	—
EPO	T45.8X1	T45.8X2	T45.8X3	T45.8X4	T45.8X5	T45.8X6
Epoetin alpha	T45.8X1	T45.8X2	T45.8X3	T45.8X4	T45.8X5	T45.8X6
Epomediol	T50.991	T50.992	T50.993	T50.994	T50.995	T50.996
Epoprostenol	T45.521	T45.522	T45.523	T45.524	T45.525	T45.526
Epoxy resin	T65.891	T65.892	T65.893	T65.894	—	—
Eprazinone	T48.4X1	T48.4X2	T48.4X3	T48.4X4	T48.4X5	T48.4X6
Epsilon aminocaproic acid	T45.621	T45.622	T45.623	T45.624	T45.625	T45.626
Epsom salt	T47.3X1	T47.3X2	T47.3X3	T47.3X4	T47.3X5	T47.3X6
Eptazocine	T40.4X1	T40.4X2	T40.4X3	T40.4X4	T40.4X5	T40.4X6
Equanil	T43.591	T43.592	T43.593	T43.594	T43.595	T43.596
Equisetum	T62.2X1	T62.2X2	T62.2X3	T62.2X4	—	—
diuretic	T50.2X1	T50.2X2	T50.2X3	T50.2X4	T50.2X5	T50.2X6
Ergobasine	T48.0X1	T48.0X2	T48.0X3	T48.0X4	T48.0X5	T48.0X6
Ergocalciferol	T45.2X1	T45.2X2	T45.2X3	T45.2X4	T45.2X5	T45.2X6
Ergoloid mesylates	T46.7X1	T46.7X2	T46.7X3	T46.7X4	T46.7X5	T46.7X6
Ergometrine	T48.0X1	T48.0X2	T48.0X3	T48.0X4	T48.0X5	T48.0X6
Ergonovine	T48.0X1	T48.0X2	T48.0X3	T48.0X4	T48.0X5	T48.0X6
Ergotamine	T46.5X1	T46.5X2	T46.5X3	T46.5X4	T46.5X5	T46.5X6
Ergotocine	T48.0X1	T48.0X2	T48.0X3	T48.0X4	T48.0X5	T48.0X6
Ergotrate	T48.0X1	T48.0X2	T48.0X3	T48.0X4	T48.0X5	T48.0X6
Ergot NEC	T64.81	T64.82	T64.83	T64.84	—	—
derivative	T48.0X1	T48.0X2	T48.0X3	T48.0X4	T48.0X5	T48.0X6
medicinal (alkaloids)	T48.0X1	T48.0X2	T48.0X3	T48.0X4	T48.0X5	T48.0X6
prepared	T48.0X1	T48.0X2	T48.0X3	T48.0X4	T48.0X5	T48.0X6
Eritrityl tetranitrate	T46.3X1	T46.3X2	T46.3X3	T46.3X4	T46.3X5	T46.3X6
Erythrityl tetranitrate	T46.3X1	T46.3X2	T46.3X3	T46.3X4	T46.3X5	T46.3X6
Erythrol tetranitrate	T46.3X1	T46.3X2	T46.3X3	T46.3X4	T46.3X5	T46.3X6
Erythromycin (salts)	T36.3X1	T36.3X2	T36.3X3	T36.3X4	T36.3X5	T36.3X6
ophthalmic preparation	T49.5X1	T49.5X2	T49.5X3	T49.5X4	T49.5X5	T49.5X6
topical NEC	T49.0X1	T49.0X2	T49.0X3	T49.0X4	T49.0X5	T49.0X6
Erythropoietin	T45.8X1	T45.8X2	T45.8X3	T45.8X4	T45.8X5	T45.8X6
human	T45.8X1	T45.8X2	T45.8X3	T45.8X4	T45.8X5	T45.8X6
Escin	T46.991	T46.992	T46.993	T46.994	T46.995	T46.996
Esculin	T45.2X1	T45.2X2	T45.2X3	T45.2X4	T45.2X5	T45.2X6
Esculoside	T45.2X1	T45.2X2	T45.2X3	T45.2X4	T45.2X5	T45.2X6
ESDT (ether-soluble tar distillate)	T49.1X1	T49.1X2	T49.1X3	T49.1X4	T49.1X5	T49.1X6
Eserine	T49.5X1	T49.5X2	T49.5X3	T49.5X4	T49.5X5	T49.5X6
Esflurbiprofen	T39.311	T39.312	T39.313	T39.314	T39.315	T39.316
Eskabarb	T42.3X1	T42.3X2	T42.3X3	T42.3X4	T42.3X5	T42.3X6
Eskalith	T43.8X1	T43.8X2	T43.8X3	T43.8X4	T43.8X5	T43.8X6
Esmolol	T44.7X1	T44.7X2	T44.7X3	T44.7X4	T44.7X5	T44.7X6
Estanozolol	T38.7X1	T38.7X2	T38.7X3	T38.7X4	T38.7X5	T38.7X6
Estazolam	T42.4X1	T42.4X2	T42.4X3	T42.4X4	T42.4X5	T42.4X6
Estradiol	T38.5X1	T38.5X2	T38.5X3	T38.5X4	T38.5X5	T38.5X6
with testosterone	T38.7X1	T38.7X2	T38.7X3	T38.7X4	T38.7X5	T38.7X6
benzoate	T38.5X1	T38.5X2	T38.5X3	T38.5X4	T38.5X5	T38.5X6
Estramustine	T45.1X1	T45.1X2	T45.1X3	T45.1X4	T45.1X5	T45.1X6
Estriol	T38.5X1	T38.5X2	T38.5X3	T38.5X4	T38.5X5	T38.5X6
Estrogen	T38.5X1	T38.5X2	T38.5X3	T38.5X4	T38.5X5	T38.5X6
with progesterone	T38.5X1	T38.5X2	T38.5X3	T38.5X4	T38.5X5	T38.5X6
conjugated	T38.5X1	T38.5X2	T38.5X3	T38.5X4	T38.5X5	T38.5X6
Estrone	T38.5X1	T38.5X2	T38.5X3	T38.5X4	T38.5X5	T38.5X6
Estropipate	T38.5X1	T38.5X2	T38.5X3	T38.5X4	T38.5X5	T38.5X6
Etacrynate sodium	T50.1X1	T50.1X2	T50.1X3	T50.1X4	T50.1X5	T50.1X6
Etacrynic acid	T50.1X1	T50.1X2	T50.1X3	T50.1X4	T50.1X5	T50.1X6
Etafedrine	T48.6X1	T48.6X2	T48.6X3	T48.6X4	T48.6X5	T48.6X6
Etafenone	T46.3X1	T46.3X2	T46.3X3	T46.3X4	T46.3X5	T46.3X6
Etambutol	T37.1X1	T37.1X2	T37.1X3	T37.1X4	T37.1X5	T37.1X6

Substance	Poisoning, Accidental (unintentional)	Poisoning, Intentional Self-harm	Poisoning, Assault	Poisoning, Undetermined	Adverse Effect	Under-dosing
Etamiphyllin	T48.6X1	T48.6X2	T48.6X3	T48.6X4	T48.6X5	T48.6X6
Etamivan	T50.7X1	T50.7X2	T50.7X3	T50.7X4	T50.7X5	T50.7X6
Etamsylate	T45.7X1	T45.7X2	T45.7X3	T45.7X4	T45.7X5	T45.7X6
Etebenecid	T50.4X1	T50.4X2	T50.4X3	T50.4X4	T50.4X5	T50.4X6
Ethacridine	T49.0X1	T49.0X2	T49.0X3	T49.0X4	T49.0X5	T49.0X6
Ethacrynic acid	T50.1X1	T50.1X2	T50.1X3	T50.1X4	T50.1X5	T50.1X6
Ethadione	T42.2X1	T42.2X2	T42.2X3	T42.2X4	T42.2X5	T42.2X6
Ethambutol	T37.1X1	T37.1X2	T37.1X3	T37.1X4	T37.1X5	T37.1X6
Ethamide	T50.2X1	T50.2X2	T50.2X3	T50.2X4	T50.2X5	T50.2X6
Ethamivan	T50.7X1	T50.7X2	T50.7X3	T50.7X4	T50.7X5	T50.7X6
Ethamsylate	T45.7X1	T45.7X2	T45.7X3	T45.7X4	T45.7X5	T45.7X6
Ethanol	T51.0X1	T51.0X2	T51.0X3	T51.0X4	—	—
beverage	T51.0X1	T51.0X2	T51.0X3	T51.0X4	—	—
Ethanolamine oleate	T46.8X1	T46.8X2	T46.8X3	T46.8X4	T46.8X5	T46.8X6
Ethaverine	T44.3X1	T44.3X2	T44.3X3	T44.3X4	T44.3X5	T44.3X6
Ethchlorvynol	T42.6X1	T42.6X2	T42.6X3	T42.6X4	T42.6X5	T42.6X6
Ethebenecid	T50.4X1	T50.4X2	T50.4X3	T50.4X4	T50.4X5	T50.4X6
Ether (vapor)	T41.0X1	T41.0X2	T41.0X3	T41.0X4	T41.0X5	T41.0X6
anesthetic	T41.0X1	T41.0X2	T41.0X3	T41.0X4	T41.0X5	T41.0X6
divinyl	T41.0X1	T41.0X2	T41.0X3	T41.0X4	T41.0X5	T41.0X6
ethyl (medicinal)	T41.0X1	T41.0X2	T41.0X3	T41.0X4	T41.0X5	T41.0X6
nonmedicinal	T52.8X1	T52.8X2	T52.8X3	T52.8X4	—	—
petroleum — see Ligroin						
solvent	T52.8X1	T52.8X2	T52.8X3	T52.8X4	—	—
Ethiazide	T50.2X1	T50.2X2	T50.2X3	T50.2X4	T50.2X5	T50.2X6
Ethidium chloride (vapor)	T59.891	T59.892	T59.893	T59.894		
Ethinamate	T42.6X1	T42.6X2	T42.6X3	T42.6X4	T42.6X5	T42.6X6
Ethinylestradiol, ethinyloestradiol	T38.5X1	T38.5X2	T38.5X3	T38.5X4	T38.5X5	T38.5X6
with						
levonorgestrel	T38.4X1	T38.4X2	T38.4X3	T38.4X4	T38.4X5	T38.4X6
norethisterone	T38.4X1	T38.4X2	T38.4X3	T38.4X4	T38.4X5	T38.4X6
Ethiodized oil (131 I)	T50.8X1	T50.8X2	T50.8X3	T50.8X4	T50.8X5	T50.8X6
Ethion	T60.0X1	T60.0X2	T60.0X3	T60.0X4	—	—
Ethionamide	T37.1X1	T37.1X2	T37.1X3	T37.1X4	T37.1X5	T37.1X6
Ethioniamide	T37.1X1	T37.1X2	T37.1X3	T37.1X4	T37.1X5	T37.1X6
Ethisterone	T38.5X1	T38.5X2	T38.5X3	T38.5X4	T38.5X5	T38.5X6
Ethobral	T42.3X1	T42.3X2	T42.3X3	T42.3X4	T42.3X5	T42.3X6
Ethocaine (infiltration) (topical)	T41.3X1	T41.3X2	T41.3X3	T41.3X4	T41.3X5	T41.3X6
nerve block (peripheral) (plexus)	T41.3X1	T41.3X2	T41.3X3	T41.3X4	T41.3X5	T41.3X6
spinal	T41.3X1	T41.3X2	T41.3X3	T41.3X4	T41.3X5	T41.3X6
Ethoheptazine	T40.4X1	T40.4X2	T40.4X3	T40.4X4	T40.4X5	T40.4X6
Ethopropazine	T44.3X1	T44.3X2	T44.3X3	T44.3X4	T44.3X5	T44.3X6
Ethosuximide	T42.2X1	T42.2X2	T42.2X3	T42.2X4	T42.2X5	T42.2X6
Ethotoin	T42.0X1	T42.0X2	T42.0X3	T42.0X4	T42.0X5	T42.0X6
Ethoxazene	T37.91	T37.92	T37.93	T37.94	T37.95	T37.96
Ethoxazorutoside	T46.991	T46.992	T46.993	T46.994	T46.995	T46.996
Ethoxzolamide	T50.2X1	T50.2X2	T50.2X3	T50.2X4	T50.2X5	T50.2X6
Ethyl						
acetate	T52.8X1	T52.8X2	T52.8X3	T52.8X4	—	—
alcohol	T51.0X1	T51.0X2	T51.0X3	T51.0X4	—	—
beverage	T51.0X1	T51.0X2	T51.0X3	T51.0X4	—	—
aldehyde (vapor)	T59.891	T59.892	T59.893	T59.894	—	—
liquid	T52.8X1	T52.8X2	T52.8X3	T52.8X4	—	—
aminobenzoate	T41.3X1	T41.3X2	T41.3X3	T41.3X4	T41.3X5	T41.3X6
aminophenothiazine	T43.3X1	T43.3X2	T43.3X3	T43.3X4	T43.3X5	T43.3X6
benzoate	T52.8X1	T52.8X2	T52.8X3	T52.8X4	—	—
biscoumacetate	T45.511	T45.512	T45.513	T45.514	T45.515	T45.516
bromide (anesthetic)	T41.0X1	T41.0X2	T41.0X3	T41.0X4	T41.0X5	T41.0X6
carbamate	T45.1X1	T45.1X2	T45.1X3	T45.1X4	T45.1X5	T45.1X6
carbinol	T51.3X1	T51.3X2	T51.3X3	T51.3X4	—	—
carbonate	T52.8X1	T52.8X2	T52.8X3	T52.8X4	—	—
chaulmoograte	T37.1X1	T37.1X2	T37.1X3	T37.1X4	T37.1X5	T37.1X6
chloride (anesthetic)	T41.0X1	T41.0X2	T41.0X3	T41.0X4	T41.0X5	T41.0X6
anesthetic (local)	T41.3X1	T41.3X2	T41.3X3	T41.3X4	T41.3X5	T41.3X6
inhaled	T41.0X1	T41.0X2	T41.0X3	T41.0X4	T41.0X5	T41.0X6
local	T49.4X1	T49.4X2	T49.4X3	T49.4X4	T49.4X5	T49.4X6
solvent	T53.6X1	T53.6X2	T53.6X3	T53.6X4	—	—
dibunate	T48.3X1	T48.3X2	T48.3X3	T48.3X4	T48.3X5	T48.3X6
dichloroarsine (vapor)	T57.0X1	T57.0X2	T57.0X3	T57.0X4	—	—
estranol	T38.7X1	T38.7X2	T38.7X3	T38.7X4	T38.7X5	T38.7X6
ether — see also ether	T52.8X1	T52.8X2	T52.8X3	T52.8X4	—	—
formate NEC (solvent)	T52.0X1	T52.0X2	T52.0X3	T52.0X4	—	—
fumarate	T49.4X1	T49.4X2	T49.4X3	T49.4X4	T49.4X5	T49.4X6
hydroxyisobutyrate NEC (solvent)	T52.8X1	T52.8X2	T52.8X3	T52.8X4	—	—
iodoacetate	T59.3X1	T59.3X2	T59.3X3	T59.3X4	—	—
lactate NEC (solvent)	T52.8X1	T52.8X2	T52.8X3	T52.8X4	—	—
loflazepate	T42.4X1	T42.4X2	T42.4X3	T42.4X4	T42.4X5	T42.4X6
mercuric chloride	T56.1X1	T56.1X2	T56.1X3	T56.1X4	—	—
methylcarbinol	T51.8X1	T51.8X2	T51.8X3	T51.8X4	—	—

Substance	Poisoning, Accidental (unintentional)	Poisoning, Intentional Self-harm	Poisoning, Assault	Poisoning, Undetermined	Adverse Effect	Under-dosing
Ethyl — continued						
morphine	T40.2X1	T40.2X2	T40.2X3	T40.2X4	T40.2X5	T40.2X6
noradrenaline	T48.6X1	T48.6X2	T48.6X3	T48.6X4	T48.6X5	T48.6X6
oxybutyrate NEC (solvent)	T52.8X1	T52.8X2	T52.8X3	T52.8X4	—	—
Ethylene (gas)	T59.891	T59.892	T59.893	T59.894		
anesthetic (general)	T41.0X1	T41.0X2	T41.0X3	T41.0X4	T41.0X5	T41.0X6
chlorohydrin	T52.8X1	T52.8X2	T52.8X3	T52.8X4	—	—
vapor	T53.6X1	T53.6X2	T53.6X3	T53.6X4	—	—
dichloride	T52.8X1	T52.8X2	T52.8X3	T52.8X4	—	—
vapor	T53.6X1	T53.6X2	T53.6X3	T53.6X4	—	—
dinitrate	T52.3X1	T52.3X2	T52.3X3	T52.3X4	—	—
glycol(s)	T52.8X1	T52.8X2	T52.8X3	T52.8X4	—	—
dinitrate	T52.3X1	T52.3X2	T52.3X3	T52.3X4	—	—
monobutyl ether	T52.3X1	T52.3X2	T52.3X3	T52.3X4	—	—
imine	T54.1X1	T54.1X2	T54.1X3	T54.1X4	—	—
oxide (fumigant) (nonmedicinal)	T59.891	T59.892	T59.893	T59.894	—	—
medicinal	T49.0X1	T49.0X2	T49.0X3	T49.0X4	T49.0X5	T49.0X6
Ethylenediaminetetra-acetic acid	T50.6X1	T50.6X2	T50.6X3	T50.6X4	T50.6X5	T50.6X6
Ethylenediamine theophylline	T48.6X1	T48.6X2	T48.6X3	T48.6X4	T48.6X5	T48.6X6
Ethylenedinitrilotetra-acetate	T50.6X1	T50.6X2	T50.6X3	T50.6X4	T50.6X5	T50.6X6
Ethylestrenol	T38.7X1	T38.7X2	T38.7X3	T38.7X4	T38.7X5	T38.7X6
Ethylhydroxycellulose	T47.4X1	T47.4X2	T47.4X3	T47.4X4	T47.4X5	T47.4X6
Ethylidene						
chloride NEC	T53.6X1	T53.6X2	T53.6X3	T53.6X4	—	—
diacetate	T60.3X1	T60.3X2	T60.3X3	T60.3X4	—	—
dicoumarin	T45.511	T45.512	T45.513	T45.514	T45.515	T45.516
dicoumarol	T45.511	T45.512	T45.513	T45.514	T45.515	T45.516
diethyl ether	T52.0X1	T52.0X2	T52.0X3	T52.0X4	—	—
Ethylmorphine	T40.2X1	T40.2X2	T40.2X3	T40.2X4	T40.2X5	T40.2X6
Ethylnorepinephrine	T48.6X1	T48.6X2	T48.6X3	T48.6X4	T48.6X5	T48.6X6
Ethylparachlorophen-oxyisobutyrate	T46.6X1	T46.6X2	T46.6X3	T46.6X4	T46.6X5	T46.6X6
Ethynodiol	T38.4X1	T38.4X2	T38.4X3	T38.4X4	T38.4X5	T38.4X6
with mestranol diacetate	T38.4X1	T38.4X2	T38.4X3	T38.4X4	T38.4X5	T38.4X6
Etidocaine	T41.3X1	T41.3X2	T41.3X3	T41.3X4	T41.3X5	T41.3X6
infiltration (subcutaneous)	T41.3X1	T41.3X2	T41.3X3	T41.3X4	T41.3X5	T41.3X6
nerve (peripheral) (plexus)	T41.3X1	T41.3X2	T41.3X3	T41.3X4	T41.3X5	T41.3X6
Etidronate	T50.991	T50.992	T50.993	T50.994	T50.995	T50.996
Etidronic acid (disodium salt)	T50.991	T50.992	T50.993	T50.994	T50.995	T50.996
Etifoxine	T42.6X1	T42.6X2	T42.6X3	T42.6X4	T42.6X5	T42.6X6
Etilefrine	T44.4X1	T44.4X2	T44.4X3	T44.4X4	T44.4X5	T44.4X6
Etilfen	T42.3X1	T42.3X2	T42.3X3	T42.3X4	T42.3X5	T42.3X6
Etinodiol	T38.4X1	T38.4X2	T38.4X3	T38.4X4	T38.4X5	T38.4X6
Etiroxate	T46.6X1	T46.6X2	T46.6X3	T46.6X4	T46.6X5	T46.6X6
Etizolam	T42.4X1	T42.4X2	T42.4X3	T42.4X4	T42.4X5	T42.4X6
Etodolac	T39.391	T39.392	T39.393	T39.394	T39.395	T39.396
Etofamide	T37.3X1	T37.3X2	T37.3X3	T37.3X4	T37.3X5	T37.3X6
Etofibrate	T46.6X1	T46.6X2	T46.6X3	T46.6X4	T46.6X5	T46.6X6
Etofylline	T46.7X1	T46.7X2	T46.7X3	T46.7X4	T46.7X5	T46.7X6
clofibrate	T46.6X1	T46.6X2	T46.6X3	T46.6X4	T46.6X5	T46.6X6
Etoglucid	T45.1X1	T45.1X2	T45.1X3	T45.1X4	T45.1X5	T45.1X6
Etomidate	T41.1X1	T41.1X2	T41.1X3	T41.1X4	T41.1X5	T41.1X6
Etomide	T39.8X1	T39.8X2	T39.8X3	T39.8X4	T39.8X5	T39.8X6
Etomidoline	T44.3X1	T44.3X2	T44.3X3	T44.3X4	T44.3X5	T44.3X6
Etoposide	T45.1X1	T45.1X2	T45.1X3	T45.1X4	T45.1X5	T45.1X6
Etorphine	T40.2X1	T40.2X2	T40.2X3	T40.2X4	T40.2X5	T40.2X6
Etoval	T42.3X1	T42.3X2	T42.3X3	T42.3X4	T42.3X5	T42.3X6
Etozolin	T50.1X1	T50.1X2	T50.1X3	T50.1X4	T50.1X5	T50.1X6
Etretinate	T50.991	T50.992	T50.993	T50.994	T50.995	T50.996
Etryptamine	T43.691	T43.692	T43.693	T43.694	T43.695	T43.696
Etybenzatropine	T44.3X1	T44.3X2	T44.3X3	T44.3X4	T44.3X5	T44.3X6
Etynodiol	T38.4X1	T38.4X2	T38.4X3	T38.4X4	T38.4X5	T38.4X6
Eucaine	T41.3X1	T41.3X2	T41.3X3	T41.3X4	T41.3X5	T41.3X6
Eucalyptus oil	T49.7X1	T49.7X2	T49.7X3	T49.7X4	T49.7X5	T49.7X6
Eucatropine	T49.5X1	T49.5X2	T49.5X3	T49.5X4	T49.5X5	T49.5X6
Eucodal	T40.2X1	T40.2X2	T40.2X3	T40.2X4	T40.2X5	T40.2X6
Euneryl	T42.3X1	T42.3X2	T42.3X3	T42.3X4	T42.3X5	T42.3X6
Euphthalmine	T44.3X1	T44.3X2	T44.3X3	T44.3X4	T44.3X5	T44.3X6
Eurax	T49.0X1	T49.0X2	T49.0X3	T49.0X4	T49.0X5	T49.0X6
Euresol	T49.4X1	T49.4X2	T49.4X3	T49.4X4	T49.4X5	T49.4X6
Euthroid	T38.1X1	T38.1X2	T38.1X3	T38.1X4	T38.1X5	T38.1X6
Evans blue	T50.8X1	T50.8X2	T50.8X3	T50.8X4	T50.8X5	T50.8X6
Evipal	T42.3X1	T42.3X2	T42.3X3	T42.3X4	T42.3X5	T42.3X6
sodium	T41.1X1	T41.1X2	T41.1X3	T41.1X4	T41.1X5	T41.1X6
Evipan	T42.3X1	T42.3X2	T42.3X3	T42.3X4	T42.3X5	T42.3X6
sodium	T41.1X1	T41.1X2	T41.1X3	T41.1X4	T41.1X5	T41.1X6
Exalamide	T49.0X1	T49.0X2	T49.0X3	T49.0X4	T49.0X5	T49.0X6
Exalgin	T39.1X1	T39.1X2	T39.1X3	T39.1X4	T39.1X5	T39.1X6
Excipients, pharmaceutical	T50.901	T50.902	T50.903	T50.904	T50.905	T50.906

▽ Subterms under main terms may continue to next column or page   Additional Character May Be Required — Refer to the Tabular List for Character Selection   367

Etamiphyllin — Excipients, pharmaceutical

Table of Drugs and Chemicals

Exhaust gas — Fluorinated corticosteroids

Substance	Poisoning, Accidental (unintentional)	Poisoning, Intentional Self-harm	Poisoning, Assault	Poisoning, Undetermined	Adverse Effect	Under-dosing
Exhaust gas (engine) (motor vehicle)	T58.01	T58.02	T58.03	T58.04	—	—
Ex-Lax (phenolphthalein)	T47.2X1	T47.2X2	T47.2X3	T47.2X4	T47.2X5	T47.2X6
Expectorant NEC	T48.4X1	T48.4X2	T48.4X3	T48.4X4	T48.4X5	T48.4X6
Extended insulin zinc suspension	T38.3X1	T38.3X2	T38.3X3	T38.3X4	T38.3X5	T38.3X6
External medications (skin) (mucous membrane)	T49.91	T49.92	T49.93	T49.94	T49.95	T49.96
dental agent	T49.7X1	T49.7X2	T49.7X3	T49.7X4	T49.7X5	T49.7X6
ENT agent	T49.6X1	T49.6X2	T49.6X3	T49.6X4	T49.6X5	T49.6X6
ophthalmic preparation	T49.5X1	T49.5X2	T49.5X3	T49.5X4	T49.5X5	T49.5X6
specified NEC	T49.8X1	T49.8X2	T49.8X3	T49.8X4	T49.8X5	T49.8X6
Extrapyramidal antagonist NEC	T44.3X1	T44.3X2	T44.3X3	T44.3X4	T44.3X5	T44.3X6
Eye agents (anti-infective)	T49.5X1	T49.5X2	T49.5X3	T49.5X4	T49.5X5	T49.5X6
Eye drug NEC	T49.5X1	T49.5X2	T49.5X3	T49.5X4	T49.5X5	T49.5X6
FAC (fluorouracil + doxorubicin + cyclophosphamide)	T45.1X1	T45.1X2	T45.1X3	T45.1X4	T45.1X5	T45.1X6
Factor						
I (fibrinogen)	T45.8X1	T45.8X2	T45.8X3	T45.8X4	T45.8X5	T45.8X6
III (thromboplastin)	T45.8X1	T45.8X2	T45.8X3	T45.8X4	T45.8X5	T45.8X6
VIII (antihemophilic Factor) (concentrate)	T45.8X1	T45.8X2	T45.8X3	T45.8X4	T45.8X5	T45.8X6
IX complex	T45.7X1	T45.7X2	T45.7X3	T45.7X4	T45.7X5	T45.7X6
human	T45.8X1	T45.8X2	T45.8X3	T45.8X4	T45.8X5	T45.8X6
Famotidine	T47.0X1	T47.0X2	T47.0X3	T47.0X4	T47.0X5	T47.0X6
Fat suspension, intravenous	T50.991	T50.992	T50.993	T50.994	T50.995	T50.996
Fazadinium bromide	T48.1X1	T48.1X2	T48.1X3	T48.1X4	T48.1X5	T48.1X6
Febarbamate	T42.3X1	T42.3X2	T42.3X3	T42.3X4	T42.3X5	T42.3X6
Fecal softener	T47.4X1	T47.4X2	T47.4X3	T47.4X4	T47.4X5	T47.4X6
Fedrilate	T48.3X1	T48.3X2	T48.3X3	T48.3X4	T48.3X5	T48.3X6
Felodipine	T46.1X1	T46.1X2	T46.1X3	T46.1X4	T46.1X5	T46.1X6
Felypressin	T38.891	T38.892	T38.893	T38.894	T38.895	T38.896
Femoxetine	T43.221	T43.222	T43.223	T43.224	T43.225	T43.226
Fenalcomine	T46.3X1	T46.3X2	T46.3X3	T46.3X4	T46.3X5	T46.3X6
Fenamisal	T37.1X1	T37.1X2	T37.1X3	T37.1X4	T37.1X5	T37.1X6
Fenazone	T39.2X1	T39.2X2	T39.2X3	T39.2X4	T39.2X5	T39.2X6
Fenbendazole	T37.4X1	T37.4X2	T37.4X3	T37.4X4	T37.4X5	T37.4X6
Fenbutrazate	T50.5X1	T50.5X2	T50.5X3	T50.5X4	T50.5X5	T50.5X6
Fencamfamine	T43.691	T43.692	T43.693	T43.694	T43.695	T43.696
Fendiline	T46.1X1	T46.1X2	T46.1X3	T46.1X4	T46.1X5	T46.1X6
Fenetylline	T43.691	T43.692	T43.693	T43.694	T43.695	T43.696
Fenflumizole	T39.391	T39.392	T39.393	T39.394	T39.395	T39.396
Fenfluramine	T50.5X1	T50.5X2	T50.5X3	T50.5X4	T50.5X5	T50.5X6
Fenobarbital	T42.3X1	T42.3X2	T42.3X3	T42.3X4	T42.3X5	T42.3X6
Fenofibrate	T46.6X1	T46.6X2	T46.6X3	T46.6X4	T46.6X5	T46.6X6
Fenoprofen	T39.311	T39.312	T39.313	T39.314	T39.315	T39.316
Fenoterol	T48.6X1	T48.6X2	T48.6X3	T48.6X4	T48.6X5	T48.6X6
Fenoverine	T44.3X1	T44.3X2	T44.3X3	T44.3X4	T44.3X5	T44.3X6
Fenoxazoline	T48.5X1	T48.5X2	T48.5X3	T48.5X4	T48.5X5	T48.5X6
Fenproporex	T50.5X1	T50.5X2	T50.5X3	T50.5X4	T50.5X5	T50.5X6
Fenquizone	T50.2X1	T50.2X2	T50.2X3	T50.2X4	T50.2X5	T50.2X6
Fentanyl	T40.4X1	T40.4X2	T40.4X3	T40.4X4	T40.4X5	T40.4X6
Fentazin	T43.3X1	T43.3X2	T43.3X3	T43.3X4	T43.3X5	T43.3X6
Fenthion	T60.0X1	T60.0X2	T60.0X3	T60.0X4	—	—
Fenticlor	T49.0X1	T49.0X2	T49.0X3	T49.0X4	T49.0X5	T49.0X6
Fenylbutazone	T39.2X1	T39.2X2	T39.2X3	T39.2X4	T39.2X5	T39.2X6
Feprazone	T39.2X1	T39.2X2	T39.2X3	T39.2X4	T39.2X5	T39.2X6
Fer de lance (bite) (venom)	T63.061	T63.062	T63.063	T63.064	—	—
Ferric — see also Iron						
chloride	T45.4X1	T45.4X2	T45.4X3	T45.4X4	T45.4X5	T45.4X6
citrate	T45.4X1	T45.4X2	T45.4X3	T45.4X4	T45.4X5	T45.4X6
hydroxide						
colloidal	T45.4X1	T45.4X2	T45.4X3	T45.4X4	T45.4X5	T45.4X6
polymaltose	T45.4X1	T45.4X2	T45.4X3	T45.4X4	T45.4X5	T45.4X6
pyrophosphate	T45.4X1	T45.4X2	T45.4X3	T45.4X4	T45.4X5	T45.4X6
Ferritin	T45.4X1	T45.4X2	T45.4X3	T45.4X4	T45.4X5	T45.4X6
Ferrocholinate	T45.4X1	T45.4X2	T45.4X3	T45.4X4	T45.4X5	T45.4X6
Ferrodextrane	T45.4X1	T45.4X2	T45.4X3	T45.4X4	T45.4X5	T45.4X6
Ferropolimaler	T45.4X1	T45.4X2	T45.4X3	T45.4X4	T45.4X5	T45.4X6
Ferrous — see also Iron						
phosphate	T45.4X1	T45.4X2	T45.4X3	T45.4X4	T45.4X5	T45.4X6
salt	T45.4X1	T45.4X2	T45.4X3	T45.4X4	T45.4X5	T45.4X6
with folic acid	T45.4X1	T45.4X2	T45.4X3	T45.4X4	T45.4X5	T45.4X6
Ferrous fumerate, gluconate, lactate, salt NEC, sulfate (medicinal)	T45.4X1	T45.4X2	T45.4X3	T45.4X4	T45.4X5	T45.4X6
Ferrovanadium (fumes)	T59.891	T59.892	T59.893	T59.894	—	—
Ferrum — see Iron						
Fertilizers NEC	T65.891	T65.892	T65.893	T65.894	—	—
with herbicide mixture	T60.3X1	T60.3X2	T60.3X3	T60.3X4	—	—
Fetoxilate	T47.6X1	T47.6X2	T47.6X3	T47.6X4	T47.6X5	T47.6X6
Fiber, dietary	T47.4X1	T47.4X2	T47.4X3	T47.4X4	T47.4X5	T47.4X6
Fiberglass	T65.831	T65.832	T65.833	T65.834	—	—
Fibrinogen (human)	T45.8X1	T45.8X2	T45.8X3	T45.8X4	T45.8X5	T45.8X6
Fibrinolysin (human)	T45.691	T45.692	T45.693	T45.694	T45.695	T45.696
Fibrinolysis						
affecting drug	T45.601	T45.602	T45.603	T45.604	T45.605	T45.606
inhibitor NEC	T45.621	T45.622	T45.623	T45.624	T45.625	T45.626
Fibrinolytic drug	T45.611	T45.612	T45.613	T45.614	T45.615	T45.616
Filix mas	T37.4X1	T37.4X2	T37.4X3	T37.4X4	T37.4X5	T37.4X6
Filtering cream	T49.3X1	T49.3X2	T49.3X3	T49.3X4	T49.3X5	T49.3X6
Fiorinal	T39.011	T39.012	T39.013	T39.014	T39.015	T39.016
Firedamp	T59.891	T59.892	T59.893	T59.894	—	—
Fish, noxious, nonbacterial	T61.91	T61.92	T61.93	T61.94	—	—
ciguatera	T61.01	T61.02	T61.03	T61.04	—	—
scombroid	T61.11	T61.12	T61.13	T61.14	—	—
shell	T61.781	T61.782	T61.783	T61.784	—	—
specified NEC	T61.771	T61.772	T61.773	T61.774	—	—
Flagyl	T37.3X1	T37.3X2	T37.3X3	T37.3X4	T37.3X5	T37.3X6
Flavine adenine dinucleotide	T45.2X1	T45.2X2	T45.2X3	T45.2X4	T45.2X5	T45.2X6
Flavodic acid	T46.991	T46.992	T46.993	T46.994	T46.995	T46.996
Flavoxate	T44.3X1	T44.3X2	T44.3X3	T44.3X4	T44.3X5	T44.3X6
Flaxedil	T48.1X1	T48.1X2	T48.1X3	T48.1X4	T48.1X5	T48.1X6
Flaxseed (medicinal)	T49.3X1	T49.3X2	T49.3X3	T49.3X4	T49.3X5	T49.3X6
Flecainide	T46.2X1	T46.2X2	T46.2X3	T46.2X4	T46.2X5	T46.2X6
Fleroxacin	T36.8X1	T36.8X2	T36.8X3	T36.8X4	T36.8X5	T36.8X6
Floctafenine	T39.8X1	T39.8X2	T39.8X3	T39.8X4	T39.8X5	T39.8X6
Flomax	T44.6X1	T44.6X2	T44.6X3	T44.6X4	T44.6X5	T44.6X6
Flomoxef	T36.1X1	T36.1X2	T36.1X3	T36.1X4	T36.1X5	T36.1X6
Flopropione	T44.3X1	T44.3X2	T44.3X3	T44.3X4	T44.3X5	T44.3X6
Florantyrone	T47.5X1	T47.5X2	T47.5X3	T47.5X4	T47.5X5	T47.5X6
Floraquin	T37.8X1	T37.8X2	T37.8X3	T37.8X4	T37.8X5	T37.8X6
Florinef	T38.0X1	T38.0X2	T38.0X3	T38.0X4	T38.0X5	T38.0X6
ENT agent	T49.6X1	T49.6X2	T49.6X3	T49.6X4	T49.6X5	T49.6X6
ophthalmic preparation	T49.5X1	T49.5X2	T49.5X3	T49.5X4	T49.5X5	T49.5X6
topical NEC	T49.0X1	T49.0X2	T49.0X3	T49.0X4	T49.0X5	T49.0X6
Flowers of sulfur	T49.4X1	T49.4X2	T49.4X3	T49.4X4	T49.4X5	T49.4X6
Floxuridine	T45.1X1	T45.1X2	T45.1X3	T45.1X4	T45.1X5	T45.1X6
Fluanisone	T43.4X1	T43.4X2	T43.4X3	T43.4X4	T43.4X5	T43.4X6
Flubendazole	T37.4X1	T37.4X2	T37.4X3	T37.4X4	T37.4X5	T37.4X6
Fluclorolone acetonide	T49.0X1	T49.0X2	T49.0X3	T49.0X4	T49.0X5	T49.0X6
Flucloxacillin	T36.0X1	T36.0X2	T36.0X3	T36.0X4	T36.0X5	T36.0X6
Fluconazole	T37.8X1	T37.8X2	T37.8X3	T37.8X4	T37.8X5	T37.8X6
Flucytosine	T37.8X1	T37.8X2	T37.8X3	T37.8X4	T37.8X5	T37.8X6
Fludeoxyglucose (18F)	T50.8X1	T50.8X2	T50.8X3	T50.8X4	T50.8X5	T50.8X6
Fludiazepam	T42.4X1	T42.4X2	T42.4X3	T42.4X4	T42.4X5	T42.4X6
Fludrocortisone	T50.0X1	T50.0X2	T50.0X3	T50.0X4	T50.0X5	T50.0X6
ENT agent	T49.6X1	T49.6X2	T49.6X3	T49.6X4	T49.6X5	T49.6X6
ophthalmic preparation	T49.5X1	T49.5X2	T49.5X3	T49.5X4	T49.5X5	T49.5X6
topical NEC	T49.0X1	T49.0X2	T49.0X3	T49.0X4	T49.0X5	T49.0X6
Fludroxycortide	T49.0X1	T49.0X2	T49.0X3	T49.0X4	T49.0X5	T49.0X6
Flufenamic acid	T39.391	T39.392	T39.393	T39.394	T39.395	T39.396
Fluindione	T45.511	T45.512	T45.513	T45.514	T45.515	T45.516
Flumequine	T37.8X1	T37.8X2	T37.8X3	T37.8X4	T37.8X5	T37.8X6
Flumethasone	T49.0X1	T49.0X2	T49.0X3	T49.0X4	T49.0X5	T49.0X6
Flumethiazide	T50.2X1	T50.2X2	T50.2X3	T50.2X4	T50.2X5	T50.2X6
Flumidin	T37.5X1	T37.5X2	T37.5X3	T37.5X4	T37.5X5	T37.5X6
Flunarizine	T46.7X1	T46.7X2	T46.7X3	T46.7X4	T46.7X5	T46.7X6
Flunidazole	T37.8X1	T37.8X2	T37.8X3	T37.8X4	T37.8X5	T37.8X6
Flunisolide	T48.6X1	T48.6X2	T48.6X3	T48.6X4	T48.6X5	T48.6X6
Flunitrazepam	T42.4X1	T42.4X2	T42.4X3	T42.4X4	T42.4X5	T42.4X6
Fluocinolone (acetonide)	T49.0X1	T49.0X2	T49.0X3	T49.0X4	T49.0X5	T49.0X6
Fluocinonide	T49.0X1	T49.0X2	T49.0X3	T49.0X4	T49.0X5	T49.0X6
Fluocortin (butyl)	T49.0X1	T49.0X2	T49.0X3	T49.0X4	T49.0X5	T49.0X6
Fluocortolone	T49.0X1	T49.0X2	T49.0X3	T49.0X4	T49.0X5	T49.0X6
Fluohydrocortisone	T38.0X1	T38.0X2	T38.0X3	T38.0X4	T38.0X5	T38.0X6
ENT agent	T49.6X1	T49.6X2	T49.6X3	T49.6X4	T49.6X5	T49.6X6
ophthalmic preparation	T49.5X1	T49.5X2	T49.5X3	T49.5X4	T49.5X5	T49.5X6
topical NEC	T49.0X1	T49.0X2	T49.0X3	T49.0X4	T49.0X5	T49.0X6
Fluonid	T49.0X1	T49.0X2	T49.0X3	T49.0X4	T49.0X5	T49.0X6
Fluopromazine	T43.3X1	T43.3X2	T43.3X3	T43.3X4	T43.3X5	T43.3X6
Fluoracetate	T60.8X1	T60.8X2	T60.8X3	T60.8X4	—	—
Fluorescein	T50.8X1	T50.8X2	T50.8X3	T50.8X4	T50.8X5	T50.8X6
Fluorhydrocortisone	T50.0X1	T50.0X2	T50.0X3	T50.0X4	T50.0X5	T50.0X6
Fluoride (nonmedicinal) (pesticide) (sodium) NEC	T60.8X1	T60.8X2	T60.8X3	T60.8X4	—	—
hydrogen — see Hydrofluoric acid						
medicinal NEC	T50.991	T50.992	T50.993	T50.994	T50.995	T50.996
dental use	T49.7X1	T49.7X2	T49.7X3	T49.7X4	ICD49.7X5	T49.7X6
not pesticide NEC	T54.91	T54.92	T54.93	T54.94	—	—
stannous	T49.7X1	T49.7X2	T49.7X3	T49.7X4	T49.7X5	T49.7X6
Fluorinated corticosteroids	T38.0X1	T38.0X2	T38.0X3	T38.0X4	T38.0X5	T38.0X6

Substance	Poisoning, Accidental (unintentional)	Poisoning, Intentional Self-harm	Poisoning, Assault	Poisoning, Undetermined	Adverse Effect	Under-dosing
Fluorine (gas)	T59.5X1	T59.5X2	T59.5X3	T59.5X4	—	—
salt — see Fluoride(s)						
Fluoristan	T49.7X1	T49.7X2	T49.7X3	T49.7X4	T49.7X5	T49.7X6
Fluormetholone	T49.0X1	T49.0X2	T49.0X3	T49.0X4	T49.0X5	T49.0X6
Fluoroacetate	T60.8X1	T60.8X2	T60.8X3	T60.8X4	—	—
Fluorocarbon monomer	T53.6X1	T53.6X2	T53.6X3	T53.6X4	—	—
Fluorocytosine	T37.8X1	T37.8X2	T37.8X3	T37.8X4	T37.8X5	T37.8X6
Fluorodeoxyuridine	T45.1X1	T45.1X2	T45.1X3	T45.1X4	T45.1X5	T45.1X6
Fluorometholone	T49.0X1	T49.0X2	T49.0X3	T49.0X4	T49.0X5	T49.0X6
ophthalmic preparation	T49.5X1	T49.5X2	T49.5X3	T49.5X4	T49.5X5	T49.5X6
Fluorophosphate insecticide	T60.0X1	T60.0X2	T60.0X3	T60.0X4	—	—
Fluorosol	T46.3X1	T46.3X2	T46.3X3	T46.3X4	T46.3X5	T46.3X6
Fluorouracil	T45.1X1	T45.1X2	T45.1X3	T45.1X4	T45.1X5	T45.1X6
Fluorphenylalanine	T49.5X1	T49.5X2	T49.5X3	T49.5X4	T49.5X5	T49.5X6
Fluothane	T41.0X1	T41.0X2	T41.0X3	T41.0X4	T41.0X5	T41.0X6
Fluoxetine	T43.221	T43.222	T43.223	T43.224	T43.225	T43.226
Fluoxymesterone	T38.7X1	T38.7X2	T38.7X3	T38.7X4	T38.7X5	T38.7X6
Flupenthixol	T43.4X1	T43.4X2	T43.4X3	T43.4X4	T43.4X5	T43.4X6
Flupentixol	T43.4X1	T43.4X2	T43.4X3	T43.4X4	T43.4X5	T43.4X6
Fluphenazine	T43.3X1	T43.3X2	T43.3X3	T43.3X4	T43.3X5	T43.3X6
Fluprednidene	T49.0X1	T49.0X2	T49.0X3	T49.0X4	T49.0X5	T49.0X6
Fluprednisolone	T38.0X1	T38.0X2	T38.0X3	T38.0X4	T38.0X5	T38.0X6
Fluradoline	T39.8X1	T39.8X2	T39.8X3	T39.8X4	T39.8X5	T39.8X6
Flurandrenolide	T49.0X1	T49.0X2	T49.0X3	T49.0X4	T49.0X5	T49.0X6
Flurandrenolone	T49.0X1	T49.0X2	T49.0X3	T49.0X4	T49.0X5	T49.0X6
Flurazepam	T42.4X1	T42.4X2	T42.4X3	T42.4X4	T42.4X5	T42.4X6
Flurbiprofen	T39.311	T39.312	T39.313	T39.314	T39.315	T39.316
Flurobate	T49.0X1	T49.0X2	T49.0X3	T49.0X4	T49.0X5	T49.0X6
Fluroxene	T41.0X1	T41.0X2	T41.0X3	T41.0X4	T41.0X5	T41.0X6
Fluspirilene	T43.591	T43.592	T43.593	T43.594	T43.595	T43.596
Flutamide	T38.6X1	T38.6X2	T38.6X3	T38.6X4	T38.6X5	T38.6X6
Flutazolam	T38.0X1	T38.0X2	T38.0X3	T38.0X4	T38.0X5	T38.0X6
Fluticasone propionate	T38.0X1	T38.0X2	T38.0X3	T38.0X4	T38.0X5	T38.0X6
Flutoprazepam	T42.4X1	T42.4X2	T42.4X3	T42.4X4	T42.4X5	T42.4X6
Flutropium bromide	T48.6X1	T48.6X2	T48.6X3	T48.6X4	T48.6X5	T48.6X6
Fluvoxamine	T43.221	T43.222	T43.223	T43.224	T43.225	T43.226
Folacin	T45.8X1	T45.8X2	T45.8X3	T45.8X4	T45.8X5	T45.8X6
Folic acid	T45.8X1	T45.8X2	T45.8X3	T45.8X4	T45.8X5	T45.8X6
with ferrous salt	T45.2X1	T45.2X2	T45.2X3	T45.2X4	T45.2X5	T45.2X6
antagonist	T45.1X1	T45.1X2	T45.1X3	T45.1X4	T45.1X5	T45.1X6
Folinic acid	T45.8X1	T45.8X2	T45.8X3	T45.8X4	T45.8X5	T45.8X6
Folium stramoniae	T48.6X1	T48.6X2	T48.6X3	T48.6X4	T48.6X5	T48.6X6
Follicle-stimulating hormone, human	T38.811	T38.812	T38.813	T38.814	T38.815	T38.816
Folpet	T60.3X1	T60.3X2	T60.3X3	T60.3X4	—	—
Fominoben	T48.3X1	T48.3X2	T48.3X3	T48.3X4	T48.3X5	T48.3X6
Food, foodstuffs, noxious, nonbacterial, NEC	T62.91	T62.92	T62.93	T62.94	—	—
berries	T62.1X1	T62.1X2	T62.1X3	T62.1X4	—	—
fish — see also Fish	T61.91	T61.92	T61.93	T61.94	—	—
mushrooms	T62.0X1	T62.0X2	T62.0X3	T62.0X4	—	—
plants	T62.2X1	T62.2X2	T62.2X3	T62.2X4	—	—
seafood	T61.91	T61.92	T61.93	T61.94	—	—
specified NEC	T61.8X1	T61.8X2	T61.8X3	T61.8X4	—	—
seeds	T62.2X1	T62.2X2	T62.2X3	T62.2X4	—	—
shellfish	T61.781	T61.782	T61.783	T61.784	—	—
specified NEC	T62.8X1	T62.8X2	T62.8X3	T62.8X4	—	—
Fool's parsley	T62.2X1	T62.2X2	T62.2X3	T62.2X4	—	—
Formaldehyde (solution), gas or vapor	T59.2X1	T59.2X2	T59.2X3	T59.2X4	—	—
fungicide	T60.3X1	T60.3X2	T60.3X3	T60.3X4	—	—
Formalin	T59.2X1	T59.2X2	T59.2X3	T59.2X4	—	—
fungicide	T60.3X1	T60.3X2	T60.3X3	T60.3X4	—	—
vapor	T59.2X1	T59.2X2	T59.2X3	T59.2X4	—	—
Formic acid	T54.2X1	T54.2X2	T54.2X3	T54.2X4	—	—
vapor	T59.891	T59.892	T59.893	T59.894	—	—
Foscarnet sodium	T37.5X1	T37.5X2	T37.5X3	T37.5X4	T37.5X5	T37.5X6
Fosfestrol	T38.5X1	T38.5X2	T38.5X3	T38.5X4	T38.5X5	T38.5X6
Fosfomycin	T36.8X1	T36.8X2	T36.8X3	T36.8X4	T36.8X5	T36.8X6
Fosfonet sodium	T37.5X1	T37.5X2	T37.5X3	T37.5X4	T37.5X5	T37.5X6
Fosinopril	T46.4X1	T46.4X2	T46.4X3	T46.4X4	T46.4X5	T46.4X6
sodium	T46.4X1	T46.4X2	T46.4X3	T46.4X4	T46.4X5	T46.4X6
Fowler's solution	T57.0X1	T57.0X2	T57.0X3	T57.0X4	—	—
Foxglove	T62.2X1	T62.2X2	T62.2X3	T62.2X4	—	—
Framycetin	T36.5X1	T36.5X2	T36.5X3	T36.5X4	T36.5X5	T36.5X6
Frangula	T47.2X1	T47.2X2	T47.2X3	T47.2X4	T47.2X5	T47.2X6
extract	T47.2X1	T47.2X2	T47.2X3	T47.2X4	T47.2X5	T47.2X6
Frei antigen	T50.8X1	T50.8X2	T50.8X3	T50.8X4	T50.8X5	T50.8X6
Freon	T53.5X1	T53.5X2	T53.5X3	T53.5X4	—	—
Fructose	T50.3X1	T50.3X2	T50.3X3	T50.3X4	T50.3X5	T50.3X6
Frusemide	T50.1X1	T50.1X2	T50.1X3	T50.1X4	T50.1X5	T50.1X6
FSH	T38.811	T38.812	T38.813	T38.814	T38.815	T38.816
Ftorafur	T45.1X1	T45.1X2	T45.1X3	T45.1X4	T45.1X5	T45.1X6
Fuel						
automobile	T52.0X1	T52.0X2	T52.0X3	T52.0X4	—	—
exhaust gas, not in transit	T58.01	T58.02	T58.03	T58.04	—	—
vapor NEC	T52.0X1	T52.0X2	T52.0X3	T52.0X4	—	—
gas (domestic use) — see also Carbon, monoxide, fuel, utility	T59.891	T59.892	T59.893	T59.894	—	—
utility	T59.891	T59.892	T59.893	T59.894	—	—
incomplete combustion of — see Carbon, monoxide, fuel, utility						
in mobile container	T59.891	T59.892	T59.893	T59.894	—	—
piped (natural)	T59.891	T59.892	T59.893	T59.894	—	—
industrial, incomplete combustion	T58.8X1	T58.8X2	T58.8X3	T58.8X4	—	—
Fugillin	T36.8X1	T36.8X2	T36.8X3	T36.8X4	T36.8X5	T36.8X6
Fulminate of mercury	T56.1X1	T56.1X2	T56.1X3	T56.1X4	—	—
Fulvicin	T36.7X1	T36.7X2	T36.7X3	T36.7X4	T36.7X5	T36.7X6
Fumadil	T36.8X1	T36.8X2	T36.8X3	T36.8X4	T36.8X5	T36.8X6
Fumagillin	T36.8X1	T36.8X2	T36.8X3	T36.8X4	T36.8X5	T36.8X6
Fumaric acid	T49.4X1	T49.4X2	T49.4X3	T49.4X4	T49.4X5	T49.4X6
Fumes (from)	T59.91	T59.92	T59.93	T59.94	—	—
carbon monoxide — see Carbon, monoxide						
charcoal (domestic use) — see Charcoal, fumes						
chloroform — see Chloroform						
coke (in domestic stoves, fireplaces) — see Coke fumes						
corrosive NEC	T54.91	T54.92	T54.93	T54.94	—	—
ether — see ether						
freons	T53.5X1	T53.5X2	T53.5X3	T53.5X4	—	—
hydrocarbons	T59.891	T59.892	T59.893	T59.894	—	—
petroleum (liquefied)	T59.891	T59.892	T59.893	T59.894	—	—
distributed through pipes (pure or mixed with air)	T59.891	T59.892	T59.893	T59.894	—	—
lead — see lead						
metal — see Metals, or the specified metal						
nitrogen dioxide	T59.0X1	T59.0X2	T59.0X3	—	—	—
pesticides — see Pesticides						
petroleum (liquefied)	T59.891	T59.892	T59.893	T59.894	—	—
distributed through pipes (pure or mixed with air)	T59.891	T59.892	T59.893	T59.894	—	—
polyester	T59.891	T59.892	T59.893	T59.894	—	—
specified source NEC — see also substance specified	T59.891	T59.892	T59.893	T59.894	—	—
sulfur dioxide	T59.1X1	T59.1X2	T59.1X3	T59.1X4	—	—
Fumigant NEC	T60.91	T60.92	T60.93	T60.94	—	—
Fungicide NEC (nonmedicinal)	T60.3X1	T60.3X2	T60.3X3	T60.3X4	—	—
Fungi, noxious, used as food	T62.0X1	T62.0X2	T62.0X3	T62.0X4	—	—
Fungizone	T36.7X1	T36.7X2	T36.7X3	T36.7X4	T36.7X5	T36.7X6
topical	T49.0X1	T49.0X2	T49.0X3	T49.0X4	T49.0X5	T49.0X6
Furacin	T49.0X1	T49.0X2	T49.0X3	T49.0X4	T49.0X5	T49.0X6
Furadantin	T37.91	T37.92	T37.93	T37.94	T37.95	T37.96
Furazolidone	T37.8X1	T37.8X2	T37.8X3	T37.8X4	T37.8X5	T37.8X6
Furazolium chloride	T49.0X1	T49.0X2	T49.0X3	T49.0X4	T49.0X5	T49.0X6
Furfural	T52.8X1	T52.8X2	T52.8X3	T52.8X4	—	—
Furnace (coal burning) (domestic), gas from	T58.2X1	T58.2X2	T58.2X3	T58.2X4	—	—
industrial	T58.8X1	T58.8X2	T58.8X3	T58.8X4	—	—
Furniture polish	T65.891	T65.892	T65.893	T65.894	—	—
Furosemide	T50.1X1	T50.1X2	T50.1X3	T50.1X4	T50.1X5	T50.1X6
Furoxone	T37.91	T37.92	T37.93	T37.94	T37.95	T37.96
Fursultiamine	T45.2X1	T45.2X2	T45.2X3	T45.2X4	T45.2X5	T45.2X6
Fusafungine	T36.8X1	T36.8X2	T36.8X3	T36.8X4	T36.8X5	T36.8X6
Fusel oil (any) (amyl) (butyl) (propyl), vapor	T51.3X1	T51.3X2	T51.3X3	T51.3X4	—	—
Fusidate (ethanolamine) (sodium)	T36.8X1	T36.8X2	T36.8X3	T36.8X4	T36.8X5	T36.8X6
Fusidic acid	T36.8X1	T36.8X2	T36.8X3	T36.8X4	T36.8X5	T36.8X6
Fytic acid, nonasodium	T50.6X1	T50.6X2	T50.6X3	T50.6X4	T50.6X5	T50.6X6
b-Galactosidase	T47.5X1	T47.5X2	T47.5X3	T47.5X4	T47.5X5	T47.5X6
GABA	T43.8X1	T43.8X2	T43.8X3	T43.8X4	T43.8X5	T43.8X6
Gadopentetic acid	T50.8X1	T50.8X2	T50.8X3	T50.8X4	T50.8X5	T50.8X6
Galactose	T50.3X1	T50.3X2	T50.3X3	T50.3X4	T50.3X5	T50.3X6
Galantamine	T44.0X1	T44.0X2	T44.0X3	T44.0X4	T44.0X5	T44.0X6

Subterms under main terms may continue to next column or page   Additional Character May Be Required — Refer to the Tabular List for Character Selection   369

Fluorine — Galantamine

Substance	Poisoning, Accidental (unintentional)	Poisoning, Intentional Self-harm	Poisoning, Assault	Poisoning, Undetermined	Adverse Effect	Under-dosing
Gallamine (triethiodide)	T48.1X1	T48.1X2	T48.1X3	T48.1X4	T48.1X5	T48.1X6
Gallium citrate	T50.991	T50.992	T50.993	T50.994	T50.995	T50.996
Gallopamil	T46.1X1	T46.1X2	T46.1X3	T46.1X4	T46.1X5	T46.1X6
Gamboge	T47.2X1	T47.2X2	T47.2X3	T47.2X4	T47.2X5	T47.2X6
Gamimune	T50.Z11	T50.Z12	T50.Z13	T50.Z14	T50.Z15	T50.Z16
Gamma-aminobutyric acid	T43.8X1	T43.8X2	T43.8X3	T43.8X4	T43.8X5	T43.8X6
Gamma-benzene hexachloride (medicinal)	T49.0X1	T49.0X2	T49.0X3	T49.0X4	T49.0X5	T49.0X6
nonmedicinal, vapor	T53.6X1	T53.6X2	T53.6X3	T53.6X4	—	—
Gamma-BHC (medicinal) — see also Gamma-benzene hexachloride	T49.0X1	T49.0X2	T49.0X3	T49.0X4	T49.0X5	T49.0X6
Gamma globulin	T50.Z11	T50.Z12	T50.Z13	T50.Z14	T50.Z15	T50.Z16
Gamulin	T50.Z11	T50.Z12	T50.Z13	T50.Z14	T50.Z15	T50.Z16
Ganciclovir (sodium)	T37.5X1	T37.5X2	T37.5X3	T37.5X4	T37.5X5	T37.5X6
Ganglionic blocking drug NEC	T44.2X1	T44.2X2	T44.2X3	T44.2X4	T44.2X5	T44.2X6
specified NEC	T44.2X1	T44.2X2	T44.2X3	T44.2X4	T44.2X5	T44.2X6
Ganja	T40.7X1	T40.7X2	T40.7X3	T40.7X4	T40.7X5	T40.7X6
Garamycin	T36.5X1	T36.5X2	T36.5X3	T36.5X4	T36.5X5	T36.5X6
ophthalmic preparation	T49.5X1	T49.5X2	T49.5X3	T49.5X4	T49.5X5	T49.5X6
topical NEC	T49.0X1	T49.0X2	T49.0X3	T49.0X4	T49.0X5	T49.0X6
Gardenal	T42.3X1	T42.3X2	T42.3X3	T42.3X4	T42.3X5	T42.3X6
Gardepanyl	T42.3X1	T42.3X2	T42.3X3	T42.3X4	T42.3X5	T42.3X6
Gaseous substance — see Gas						
Gasoline	T52.0X1	T52.0X2	T52.0X3	T52.0X4	—	—
vapor	T52.0X1	T52.0X2	T52.0X3	T52.0X4	—	—
Gastric enzymes	T47.5X1	T47.5X2	T47.5X3	T47.5X4	T47.5X5	T47.5X6
Gastrografin	T50.8X1	T50.8X2	T50.8X3	T50.8X4	T50.8X5	T50.8X6
Gastrointestinal drug	T47.91	T47.92	T47.93	T47.94	T47.95	T47.96
biological	T47.8X1	T47.8X2	T47.8X3	T47.8X4	T47.8X5	T47.8X6
specified NEC	T47.8X1	T47.8X2	T47.8X3	T47.8X4	T47.8X5	T47.8X6
Gas NEC	T59.91	T59.92	T59.93	T59.94	—	—
acetylene	T59.891	T59.892	T59.893	T59.894	—	—
incomplete combustion of	T58.11	T58.12	T58.13	T58.14	—	—
air contaminants, source or type not specified	T59.91	T59.92	T59.93	T59.94	—	—
anesthetic	T41.0X1	T41.0X2	T41.0X3	T41.0X4	T41.0X5	T41.0X6
blast furnace	T58.8X1	T58.8X2	T58.8X3	T58.8X4	—	—
butane — see butane						
carbon monoxide — see Carbon, monoxide						
chlorine	T59.4X1	T59.4X2	T59.4X3	T59.4X4	—	—
coal	T58.2X1	T58.2X2	T58.2X3	T58.2X4	—	—
cyanide	T57.3X1	T57.3X2	T57.3X3	T57.3X4	—	—
dicyanogen	T65.0X1	T65.0X2	T65.0X3	T65.0X4	—	—
domestic — see Domestic gas						
exhaust	T58.01	T58.02	T58.03	T58.04	—	—
from utility (for cooking, heating, or lighting) (after combustion) — see Carbon, monoxide, fuel, utility						
prior to combustion	T59.891	T59.892	T59.893	T59.894	—	—
from wood- or coal-burning stove or fireplace	T58.2X1	T58.2X2	T58.2X3	T58.2X4	—	—
fuel (domestic use) (after combustion) — see also Carbon, monoxide, fuel						
industrial use	T58.8X1	T58.8X2	T58.8X3	T58.8X4	—	—
prior to combustion	T59.891	T59.892	T59.893	T59.894	—	—
utility	T59.891	T59.892	T59.893	T59.894	—	—
incomplete combustion of — see Carbon, monoxide, fuel, utility						
in mobile container	T59.891	T59.892	T59.893	T59.894	—	—
piped (natural)	T59.891	T59.892	T59.893	T59.894	—	—
garage	T58.01	T58.02	T58.03	T58.04	—	—
hydrocarbon NEC	T59.891	T59.892	T59.893	T59.894	—	—
incomplete combustion of — see Carbon, monoxide, fuel, utility						
liquefied — see butane						
piped	T59.891	T59.892	T59.893	T59.894	—	—
hydrocyanic acid	T65.0X1	T65.0X2	T65.0X3	T65.0X4	—	—
illuminating (after combustion)	T58.11	T58.12	T58.13	T58.14	—	—
prior to combustion	T59.891	T59.892	T59.893	T59.894	—	—
incomplete combustion, any — see Carbon, monoxide						
kiln	T58.8X1	T58.8X2	T58.8X3	T58.8X4	—	—
lacrimogenic	T59.3X1	T59.3X2	T59.3X3	T59.3X4	—	—

Substance	Poisoning, Accidental (unintentional)	Poisoning, Intentional Self-harm	Poisoning, Assault	Poisoning, Undetermined	Adverse Effect	Under-dosing
Gas — continued						
liquefied petroleum — see butane						
marsh	T59.891	T59.892	T59.893	T59.894	—	—
motor exhaust, not in transit	T58.01	T58.02	T58.03	T58.04	—	—
mustard, not in war	T59.891	T59.892	T59.893	T59.894	—	—
natural	T59.891	T59.892	T59.893	T59.894	—	—
nerve, not in war	T59.91	T59.92	T59.93	T59.94	—	—
oil	T52.0X1	T52.0X2	T52.0X3	T52.0X4	—	—
petroleum (liquefied) (distributed in mobile containers)	T59.891	T59.892	T59.893	T59.894	—	—
piped (pure or mixed with air)	T59.891	T59.892	T59.893	T59.894	—	—
piped (manufactured) (natural) NEC	T59.891	T59.892	T59.893	T59.894	—	—
producer	T58.8X1	T58.8X2	T58.8X3	T58.8X4	—	—
propane — see propane						
refrigerant (chlorofluoro-carbon)	T53.5X1	T53.5X2	T53.5X3	T53.5X4	—	—
not chlorofluoro-carbon	T59.891	T59.892	T59.893	T59.894	—	—
sewer	T59.91	T59.92	T59.93	T59.94	—	—
specified source NEC	T59.91	T59.92	T59.93	T59.94	—	—
stove (after combustion)	T58.11	T58.12	T58.13	T58.14	—	—
prior to combustion	T59.891	T59.892	T59.893	T59.894	—	—
tear	T59.3X1	T59.3X2	T59.3X3	T59.3X4	—	—
therapeutic	T41.5X1	T41.5X2	T41.5X3	T41.5X4	T41.5X5	T41.5X6
utility (for cooking, heating, or lighting) (piped) NEC	T59.891	T59.892	T59.893	T59.894	—	—
incomplete combustion of — see Carbon, monoxide, fuel, utilty						
in mobile container	T59.891	T59.892	T59.893	T59.894	—	—
piped (natural)	T59.891	T59.892	T59.893	T59.894	—	—
water	T58.11	T58.12	T58.13	T58.14	—	—
incomplete combustion of — see Carbon, monoxide, fuel, utility						
Gaultheria procumbens	T62.2X1	T62.2X2	T62.2X3	T62.2X4	—	—
Gefarnate	T44.3X1	T44.3X2	T44.3X3	T44.3X4	T44.3X5	T44.3X6
Gelatin (intravenous)	T45.8X1	T45.8X2	T45.8X3	T45.8X4	T45.8X5	T45.8X6
absorbable (sponge)	T45.7X1	T45.7X2	T45.7X3	T45.7X4	T45.7X5	T45.7X6
Gelfilm	T49.8X1	T49.8X2	T49.8X3	T49.8X4	T49.8X5	T49.8X6
Gelfoam	T45.7X1	T45.7X2	T45.7X3	T45.7X4	T45.7X5	T45.7X6
Gelsemine	T50.991	T50.992	T50.993	T50.994	T50.995	T50.996
Gelsemium (sempervirens)	T62.2X1	T62.2X2	T62.2X3	T62.2X4	—	—
Gemeprost	T48.0X1	T48.0X2	T48.0X3	T48.0X4	T48.0X5	T48.0X6
Gemfibrozil	T46.6X1	T46.6X2	T46.6X3	T46.6X4	T46.6X5	T46.6X6
Gemonil	T42.3X1	T42.3X2	T42.3X3	T42.3X4	T42.3X5	T42.3X6
Gentamicin	T36.5X1	T36.5X2	T36.5X3	T36.5X4	T36.5X5	T36.5X6
ophthalmic preparation	T49.5X1	T49.5X2	T49.5X3	T49.5X4	T49.5X5	T49.5X6
topical NEC	T49.0X1	T49.0X2	T49.0X3	T49.0X4	T49.0X5	T49.0X6
Gentian	T47.5X1	T47.5X2	T47.5X3	T47.5X4	T47.5X5	T47.5X6
violet	T49.0X1	T49.0X2	T49.0X3	T49.0X4	T49.0X5	T49.0X6
Gepefrine	T44.4X1	T44.4X2	T44.4X3	T44.4X4	T44.4X5	T44.4X6
Gestonorone caproate	T38.5X1	T38.5X2	T38.5X3	T38.5X4	T38.5X5	T38.5X6
Gexane	T49.0X1	T49.0X2	T49.0X3	T49.0X4	T49.0X5	T49.0X6
Gila monster (venom)	T63.111	T63.112	T63.113	T63.114	—	—
Ginger	T47.5X1	T47.5X2	T47.5X3	T47.5X4	T47.5X5	T47.5X6
Jamaica — see Jamaica, ginger						
Gitalin	T46.0X1	T46.0X2	T46.0X3	T46.0X4	T46.0X5	T46.0X6
amorphous	T46.0X1	T46.0X2	T46.0X3	T46.0X4	T46.0X5	T46.0X6
Gitaloxin	T46.0X1	T46.0X2	T46.0X3	T46.0X4	T46.0X5	T46.0X6
Gitoxin	T46.0X1	T46.0X2	T46.0X3	T46.0X4	T46.0X5	T46.0X6
Glafenine	T39.8X1	T39.8X2	T39.8X3	T39.8X4	T39.8X5	T39.8X6
Glandular extract (medicinal) NEC	T50.Z91	T50.Z92	T50.Z93	T50.Z94	T50.Z95	T50.Z96
Glaucarubin	T37.3X1	T37.3X2	T37.3X3	T37.3X4	T37.3X5	T37.3X6
Glibenclamide	T38.3X1	T38.3X2	T38.3X3	T38.3X4	T38.3X5	T38.3X6
Glibornuride	T38.3X1	T38.3X2	T38.3X3	T38.3X4	T38.3X5	T38.3X6
Gliclazide	T38.3X1	T38.3X2	T38.3X3	T38.3X4	T38.3X5	T38.3X6
Glimidine	T38.3X1	T38.3X2	T38.3X3	T38.3X4	T38.3X5	T38.3X6
Glipizide	T38.3X1	T38.3X2	T38.3X3	T38.3X4	T38.3X5	T38.3X6
Gliquidone	T38.3X1	T38.3X2	T38.3X3	T38.3X4	T38.3X5	T38.3X6
Glisolamide	T38.3X1	T38.3X2	T38.3X3	T38.3X4	T38.3X5	T38.3X6
Glisoxepide	T38.3X1	T38.3X2	T38.3X3	T38.3X4	T38.3X5	T38.3X6
Globin zinc insulin	T38.3X1	T38.3X2	T38.3X3	T38.3X4		
Globulin						
antilymphocytic	T50.Z11	T50.Z12	T50.Z13	T50.Z14	T50.Z15	T50.Z16
antirhesus	T50.Z11	T50.Z12	T50.Z13	T50.Z14	T50.Z15	T50.Z16
antivenin	T50.Z11	T50.Z12	T50.Z13	T50.Z14	T50.Z15	T50.Z16
antiviral	T50.Z11	T50.Z12	T50.Z13	T50.Z14	T50.Z15	T50.Z16

Substance	Poisoning, Accidental (unintentional)	Poisoning, Intentional Self-harm	Poisoning, Assault	Poisoning, Undetermined	Adverse Effect	Under-dosing
Glucagon	T38.3X1	T38.3X2	T38.3X3	T38.3X4	T38.3X5	T38.3X6
Glucocorticoids	T38.0X1	T38.0X2	T38.0X3	T38.0X4	T38.0X5	T38.0X6
Glucocorticosteroid	T38.0X1	T38.0X2	T38.0X3	T38.0X4	T38.0X5	T38.0X6
Gluconic acid	T50.991	T50.992	T50.993	T50.994	T50.995	T50.996
Glucosamine sulfate	T39.4X1	T39.4X2	T39.4X3	T39.4X4	T39.4X5	T39.4X6
Glucose	T50.3X1	T50.3X2	T50.3X3	T50.3X4	T50.3X5	T50.3X6
with sodium chloride	T50.3X1	T50.3X2	T50.3X3	T50.3X4	T50.3X5	T50.3X6
Glucosulfone sodium	T37.1X1	T37.1X2	T37.1X3	T37.1X4	T37.1X5	T37.1X6
Glucurolactone	T47.8X1	T47.8X2	T47.8X3	T47.8X4	T47.8X5	T47.8X6
Glue NEC	T52.8X1	T52.8X2	T52.8X3	T52.8X4	—	—
Glutamic acid	T47.5X1	T47.5X2	T47.5X3	T47.5X4	T47.5X5	T47.5X6
Glutaral (medicinal)	T49.0X1	T49.0X2	T49.0X3	T49.0X4	T49.0X5	T49.0X6
nonmedicinal	T65.891	T65.892	T65.893	T65.894	—	—
Glutaraldehyde (nonmedicinal)	T65.891	T65.892	T65.893	T65.894	—	—
medicinal	T49.0X1	T49.0X2	T49.0X3	T49.0X4	T49.0X5	T49.0X6
Glutathione	T50.6X1	T50.6X2	T50.6X3	T50.6X4	T50.6X5	T50.6X6
Glutethimide	T42.6X1	T42.6X2	T42.6X3	T42.6X4	T42.6X5	T42.6X6
Glyburide	T38.3X1	T38.3X2	T38.3X3	T38.3X4	T38.3X5	T38.3X6
Glycerin	T47.4X1	T47.4X2	T47.4X3	T47.4X4	T47.4X5	T47.4X6
Glycerol	T47.4X1	T47.4X2	T47.4X3	T47.4X4	T47.4X5	T47.4X6
borax	T49.6X1	T49.6X2	T49.6X3	T49.6X4	T49.6X5	T49.6X6
intravenous	T50.3X1	T50.3X2	T50.3X3	T50.3X4	T50.3X5	T50.3X6
iodinated	T48.4X1	T48.4X2	T48.4X3	T48.4X4	T48.4X5	T48.4X6
Glycerophosphate	T50.991	T50.992	T50.993	T50.994	T50.995	T50.996
Glyceryl						
gualacolate	T48.4X1	T48.4X2	T48.4X3	T48.4X4	T48.4X5	T48.4X6
nitrate	T46.3X1	T46.3X2	T46.3X3	T46.3X4	T46.3X5	T46.3X6
triacetate (topical)	T49.0X1	T49.0X2	T49.0X3	T49.0X4	T49.0X5	T49.0X6
trinitrate	T46.3X1	T46.3X2	T46.3X3	T46.3X4	T46.3X5	T46.3X6
Glycine	T50.3X1	T50.3X2	T50.3X3	T50.3X4	T50.3X5	T50.3X6
Glyclopyramide	T38.3X1	T38.3X2	T38.3X3	T38.3X4	T38.3X5	T38.3X6
Glycobiarsol	T37.3X1	T37.3X2	T37.3X3	T37.3X4	T37.3X5	T37.3X6
Glycols (ether)	T52.3X1	T52.3X2	T52.3X3	T52.3X4	—	—
Glyconiazide	T37.1X1	T37.1X2	T37.1X3	T37.1X4	T37.1X5	T37.1X6
Glycopyrrolate	T44.3X1	T44.3X2	T44.3X3	T44.3X4	T44.3X5	T44.3X6
Glycopyrronium	T44.3X1	T44.3X2	T44.3X3	T44.3X4	T44.3X5	T44.3X6
bromide	T44.3X1	T44.3X2	T44.3X3	T44.3X4	T44.3X5	T44.3X6
Glycoside, cardiac	T46.0X1	T46.0X2	T46.0X3	T46.0X4	T46.0X5	T46.0X6
(stimulant)						
Glycyclamide	T38.3X1	T38.3X2	T38.3X3	T38.3X4	T38.3X5	T38.3X6
Glycyrrhiza extract	T48.4X1	T48.4X2	T48.4X3	T48.4X4	T48.4X5	T48.4X6
Glycyrrhizic acid	T48.4X1	T48.4X2	T48.4X3	T48.4X4	T48.4X5	T48.4X6
Glycyrrhizinate potassium	T48.4X1	T48.4X2	T48.4X3	T48.4X4	T48.4X5	T48.4X6
Glymidine sodium	T38.3X1	T38.3X2	T38.3X3	T38.3X4	T38.3X5	T38.3X6
Glyphosate	T60.3X1	T60.3X2	T60.3X3	T60.3X4	—	—
Glyphylline	T48.6X1	T48.6X2	T48.6X3	T48.6X4	T48.6X5	T48.6X6
Gold						
colloidal (I98Au)	T45.1X1	T45.1X2	T45.1X3	T45.1X4	T45.1X5	T45.1X6
salts	T39.4X1	T39.4X2	T39.4X3	T39.4X4	T39.4X5	T39.4X6
Golden sulfide of antimony	T56.891	T56.892	T56.893	T56.894	—	—
Goldylocks	T62.2X1	T62.2X2	T62.2X3	T62.2X4	—	—
Gonadal tissue extract	T38.901	T38.902	T38.903	T38.904	T38.905	T38.906
female	T38.5X1	T38.5X2	T38.5X3	T38.5X4	T38.5X5	T38.5X6
male	T38.7X1	T38.7X2	T38.7X3	T38.7X4	T38.7X5	T38.7X6
Gonadorelin	T38.891	T38.892	T38.893	T38.894	T38.895	T38.896
Gonadotropin	T38.891	T38.892	T38.893	T38.894	T38.895	T38.896
chorionic	T38.891	T38.892	T38.893	T38.894	T38.895	T38.896
pituitary	T38.811	T38.812	T38.813	T38.814	T38.815	T38.816
Goserelin	T45.1X1	T45.1X2	T45.1X3	T45.1X4	T45.1X5	T45.1X6
Grain alcohol	T51.0X1	T51.0X2	T51.0X3	T51.0X4	—	—
Gramicidin	T49.0X1	T49.0X2	T49.0X3	T49.0X4	T49.0X5	T49.0X6
Granisetron	T45.0X1	T45.0X2	T45.0X3	T45.0X4	T45.0X5	T45.0X6
Gratiola officinalis	T62.2X1	T62.2X2	T62.2X3	T62.2X4	—	—
Grease	T65.891	T65.892	T65.893	T65.894	—	—
Green hellebore	T62.2X1	T62.2X2	T62.2X3	T62.2X4	—	—
Green soap	T49.2X1	T49.2X2	T49.2X3	T49.2X4	T49.2X5	T49.2X6
Grifulvin	T36.7X1	T36.7X2	T36.7X3	T36.7X4	T36.7X5	T36.7X6
Griseofulvin	T36.7X1	T36.7X2	T36.7X3	T36.7X4	T36.7X5	T36.7X6
Growth hormone	T38.811	T38.812	T38.813	T38.814	T38.815	T38.816
Guaiacol derivatives	T48.4X1	T48.4X2	T48.4X3	T48.4X4	T48.4X5	T48.4X6
Guaiac reagent	T50.991	T50.992	T50.993	T50.994	T50.995	T50.996
Guaifenesin	T48.4X1	T48.4X2	T48.4X3	T48.4X4	T48.4X5	T48.4X6
Guaimesal	T48.4X1	T48.4X2	T48.4X3	T48.4X4	T48.4X5	T48.4X6
Guaiphenesin	T48.4X1	T48.4X2	T48.4X3	T48.4X4	T48.4X5	T48.4X6
Guamecycline	T36.4X1	T36.4X2	T36.4X3	T36.4X4	T36.4X5	T36.4X6
Guanabenz	T46.5X1	T46.5X2	T46.5X3	T46.5X4	T46.5X5	T46.5X6
Guanacline	T46.5X1	T46.5X2	T46.5X3	T46.5X4	T46.5X5	T46.5X6
Guanadrel	T46.5X1	T46.5X2	T46.5X3	T46.5X4	T46.5X5	T46.5X6
Guanatol	T37.2X1	T37.2X2	T37.2X3	T37.2X4	T37.2X5	T37.2X6
Guanethidine	T46.5X1	T46.5X2	T46.5X3	T46.5X4	T46.5X5	T46.5X6
Guanfacine	T46.5X1	T46.5X2	T46.5X3	T46.5X4	T46.5X5	T46.5X6
Guano	T65.891	T65.892	T65.893	T65.894	—	—
Guanochlor	T46.5X1	T46.5X2	T46.5X3	T46.5X4	T46.5X5	T46.5X6
Guanoclor	T46.5X1	T46.5X2	T46.5X3	T46.5X4	T46.5X5	T46.5X6
Guanoctine	T46.5X1	T46.5X2	T46.5X3	T46.5X4	T46.5X5	T46.5X6
Guanoxabenz	T46.5X1	T46.5X2	T46.5X3	T46.5X4	T46.5X5	T46.5X6
Guanoxan	T46.5X1	T46.5X2	T46.5X3	T46.5X4	T46.5X5	T46.5X6
Guar gum (medicinal)	T46.6X1	T46.6X2	T46.6X3	T46.6X4	T46.6X5	T46.6X6
Hachimycin	T36.7X1	T36.7X2	T36.7X3	T36.7X4	T36.7X5	T36.7X6
Hair						
dye	T49.4X1	T49.4X2	T49.4X3	T49.4X4	T49.4X5	T49.4X6
preparation NEC	T49.4X1	T49.4X2	T49.4X3	T49.4X4	T49.4X5	T49.4X6
Halazepam	T42.4X1	T42.4X2	T42.4X3	T42.4X4	T42.4X5	T42.4X6
Halcinolone	T49.0X1	T49.0X2	T49.0X3	T49.0X4	T49.0X5	T49.0X6
Halcinonide	T49.0X1	T49.0X2	T49.0X3	T49.0X4	T49.0X5	T49.0X6
Halethazole	T49.0X1	T49.0X2	T49.0X3	T49.0X4	T49.0X5	T49.0X6
Hallucinogen NEC	T40.901	T40.902	T40.903	T40.904	T40.905	T40.906
Halofantrine	T37.2X1	T37.2X2	T37.2X3	T37.2X4	T37.2X5	T37.2X6
Halofenate	T46.6X1	T46.6X2	T46.6X3	T46.6X4	T46.6X5	T46.6X6
Halometasone	T49.0X1	T49.0X2	T49.0X3	T49.0X4	T49.0X5	T49.0X6
Haloperidol	T43.4X1	T43.4X2	T43.4X3	T43.4X4	T43.4X5	T43.4X6
Haloprogin	T49.0X1	T49.0X2	T49.0X3	T49.0X4	T49.0X5	T49.0X6
Halotex	T49.0X1	T49.0X2	T49.0X3	T49.0X4	T49.0X5	T49.0X6
Halothane	T41.0X1	T41.0X2	T41.0X3	T41.0X4	T41.0X5	T41.0X6
Haloxazolam	T42.4X1	T42.4X2	T42.4X3	T42.4X4	T42.4X5	T42.4X6
Halquinols	T49.0X1	T49.0X2	T49.0X3	T49.0X4	T49.0X5	T49.0X6
Hamamelis	T49.2X1	T49.2X2	T49.2X3	T49.2X4	T49.2X5	T49.2X6
Haptendextran	T45.8X1	T45.8X2	T45.8X3	T45.8X4	T45.8X5	T45.8X6
Harmonyl	T46.5X1	T46.5X2	T46.5X3	T46.5X4	T46.5X5	T46.5X6
Hartmann's solution	T50.3X1	T50.3X2	T50.3X3	T50.3X4	T50.3X5	T50.3X6
Hashish	T40.7X1	T40.7X2	T40.7X3	T40.7X4	T40.7X5	T40.7X6
Hawaiian Woodrose seeds	T40.991	T40.992	T40.993	T40.994	—	—
HCB	T60.3X1	T60.3X2	T60.3X3	T60.3X4	—	—
HCH	T53.6X1	T53.6X2	T53.6X3	T53.6X4	—	—
medicinal	T49.0X1	T49.0X2	T49.0X3	T49.0X4	T49.0X5	T49.0X6
HCN	T57.3X1	T57.3X2	T57.3X3	T57.3X4	—	—
Headache cures, drugs, powders NEC	T50.901	T50.902	T50.903	T50.904	T50.905	T50.906
Heavenly Blue (morning glory)	T40.991	T40.992	T40.993	T40.994	—	—
Heavy metal antidote	T45.8X1	T45.8X2	T45.8X3	T45.8X4	T45.8X5	T45.8X6
Hedaquinium	T49.0X1	T49.0X2	T49.0X3	T49.0X4	T49.0X5	T49.0X6
Hedge hyssop	T62.2X1	T62.2X2	T62.2X3	T62.2X4	—	—
Heet	T49.8X1	T49.8X2	T49.8X3	T49.8X4	T49.8X5	T49.8X6
Helenin	T37.4X1	T37.4X2	T37.4X3	T37.4X4	T37.4X5	T37.4X6
Helium (nonmedicinal) NEC	T59.891	T59.892	T59.893	T59.894	—	—
medicinal	T48.991	T48.992	T48.993	T48.994	T48.995	T48.996
Hellebore (black) (green) (white)	T62.2X1	T62.2X2	T62.2X3	T62.2X4	—	—
Hematin	T45.8X1	T45.8X2	T45.8X3	T45.8X4	T45.8X5	T45.8X6
Hematinic preparation	T45.8X1	T45.8X2	T45.8X3	T45.8X4	T45.8X5	T45.8X6
Hematological agent	T45.91	T45.92	T45.93	T45.94	T45.95	T45.96
specified NEC	T45.8X1	T45.8X2	T45.8X3	T45.8X4	T45.8X5	T45.8X6
Hemlock	T62.2X1	T62.2X2	T62.2X3	T62.2X4	—	—
Hemostatic	T45.621	T45.622	T45.623	T45.624	T45.625	T45.626
drug, systemic	T45.621	T45.622	T45.623	T45.624	T45.625	T45.626
Hemostyptic	T49.4X1	T49.4X2	T49.4X3	T49.4X4	T49.4X5	T49.4X6
Henbane	T62.2X1	T62.2X2	T62.2X3	T62.2X4	—	—
Heparin (sodium)	T45.511	T45.512	T45.513	T45.514	T45.515	T45.516
action reverser	T45.7X1	T45.7X2	T45.7X3	T45.7X4	T45.7X5	T45.7X6
Heparin-fraction	T45.511	T45.512	T45.513	T45.514	T45.515	T45.516
Heparinoid (systemic)	T45.511	T45.512	T45.513	T45.514	T45.515	T45.516
Hepatic secretion stimulant	T47.8X1	T47.8X2	T47.8X3	T47.8X4	T47.8X5	T47.8X6
Hepatitis B						
immune globulin	T50.Z11	T50.Z12	T50.Z13	T50.Z14	T50.Z15	T50.Z16
vaccine	T50.B91	T50.B92	T50.B93	T50.B94	T50.B95	T50.B96
Hepronicate	T46.7X1	T46.7X2	T46.7X3	T46.7X4	T46.7X5	T46.7X6
Heptabarb	T42.3X1	T42.3X2	T42.3X3	T42.3X4	T42.3X5	T42.3X6
Heptabarbital	T42.3X1	T42.3X2	T42.3X3	T42.3X4	T42.3X5	T42.3X6
Heptabarbitone	T42.3X1	T42.3X2	T42.3X3	T42.3X4	T42.3X5	T42.3X6
Heptachlor	T60.1X1	T60.1X2	T60.1X3	T60.1X4	—	—
Heptalgin	T40.2X1	T40.2X2	T40.2X3	T40.2X4	T40.2X5	T40.2X6
Heptaminol	T46.3X1	T46.3X2	T46.3X3	T46.3X4	T46.3X5	T46.3X6
Herbicide NEC	T60.3X1	T60.3X2	T60.3X3	T60.3X4	—	—
Heroin	T40.1X1	T40.1X2	T40.1X3	T40.1X4	—	—
Herplex	T49.5X1	T49.5X2	T49.5X3	T49.5X4	T49.5X5	T49.5X6
HES	T45.8X1	T45.8X2	T45.8X3	T45.8X4	T45.8X5	T45.8X6
Hesperidin	T46.991	T46.992	T46.993	T46.994	T46.995	T46.996
Hetacillin	T36.0X1	T36.0X2	T36.0X3	T36.0X4	T36.0X5	T36.0X6
Hetastarch	T45.8X1	T45.8X2	T45.8X3	T45.8X4	T45.8X5	T45.8X6
HETP	T60.0X1	T60.0X2	T60.0X3	T60.0X4	—	—
Hexachlorobenzene (vapor)	T60.3X1	T60.3X2	T60.3X3	T60.3X4	—	—
Hexachlorocyclohexane	T53.6X1	T53.6X2	T53.6X3	T53.6X4	—	—
Hexachlorophene	T49.0X1	T49.0X2	T49.0X3	T49.0X4	T49.0X5	T49.0X6

Table of Drugs and Chemicals

Hexadiline — Hydroxyprogesterone

Substance	Poisoning, Accidental (unintentional)	Poisoning, Intentional Self-harm	Poisoning, Assault	Poisoning, Undetermined	Adverse Effect	Under-dosing
Hexadiline	T46.3X1	T46.3X2	T46.3X3	T46.3X4	T46.3X5	T46.3X6
Hexadimethrine (bromide)	T45.7X1	T45.7X2	T45.7X3	T45.7X4	T45.7X5	T45.7X6
Hexadylamine	T46.3X1	T46.3X2	T46.3X3	T46.3X4	T46.3X5	T46.3X6
Hexaethyl tetraphosphate	T60.0X1	T60.0X2	T60.0X3	T60.0X4	—	—
Hexafluorenium bromide	T48.1X1	T48.1X2	T48.1X3	T48.1X4	T48.1X5	T48.1X6
Hexafluronium (bromide)	T48.1X1	T48.1X2	T48.1X3	T48.1X4	T48.1X5	T48.1X6
Hexa-germ	T49.2X1	T49.2X2	T49.2X3	T49.2X4	T49.2X5	T49.2X6
Hexahydrobenzol	T52.8X1	T52.8X2	T52.8X3	T52.8X4	—	—
Hexahydrocresol(s)	T51.8X1	T51.8X2	T51.8X3	T51.8X4	—	—
arsenide	T57.0X1	T57.0X2	T57.0X3	T57.0X4	—	—
arseniurated	T57.0X1	T57.0X2	T57.0X3	T57.0X4	—	—
cyanide	T57.3X1	T57.3X2	T57.3X3	T57.3X4	—	—
gas	T59.891	T59.892	T59.893	T59.894	—	—
Fluoride (liquid)	T57.8X1	T57.8X2	T57.8X3	T57.8X4	—	—
vapor	T59.891	T59.892	T59.893	T59.894	—	—
phophorated	T60.0X1	T60.0X2	T60.0X3	T60.0X4	—	—
sulfate	T57.8X1	T57.8X2	T57.8X3	T57.8X4	—	—
sulfide (gas)	T59.6X1	T59.6X2	T59.6X3	T59.6X4	—	—
arseniurated	T57.0X1	T57.0X2	T57.0X3	T57.0X4	—	—
sulfurated	T57.8X1	T57.8X2	T57.8X3	T57.8X4	—	—
Hexahydrophenol	T51.8X1	T51.8X2	T51.8X3	T51.8X4	—	—
Hexalen	T51.8X1	T51.8X2	T51.8X3	T51.8X4	—	—
Hexamethonium bromide	T44.2X1	T44.2X2	T44.2X3	T44.2X4	T44.2X5	T44.2X6
Hexamethylene	T52.8X1	T52.8X2	T52.8X3	T52.8X4	—	—
Hexamethylmelamine	T45.1X1	T45.1X2	T45.1X3	T45.1X4	T45.1X5	T45.1X6
Hexamidine	T49.0X1	T49.0X2	T49.0X3	T49.0X4	T49.0X5	T49.0X6
Hexamine (mandelate)	T37.8X1	T37.8X2	T37.8X3	T37.8X4	T37.8X5	T37.8X6
Hexanone, 2-hexanone	T52.4X1	T52.4X2	T52.4X3	T52.4X4	—	—
Hexanuorenium	T48.1X1	T48.1X2	T48.1X3	T48.1X4	T48.1X5	T48.1X6
Hexapropymate	T42.6X1	T42.6X2	T42.6X3	T42.6X4	T42.6X5	T42.6X6
Hexasonium iodide	T44.3X1	T44.3X2	T44.3X3	T44.3X4	T44.3X5	T44.3X6
Hexcarbacholine bromide	T48.1X1	T48.1X2	T48.1X3	T48.1X4	T48.1X5	T48.1X6
Hexemal	T42.3X1	T42.3X2	T42.3X3	T42.3X4	T42.3X5	T42.3X6
Hexestrol	T38.5X1	T38.5X2	T38.5X3	T38.5X4	T38.5X5	T38.5X6
Hexethal (sodium)	T42.3X1	T42.3X2	T42.3X3	T42.3X4	T42.3X5	T42.3X6
Hexetidine	T37.8X1	T37.8X2	T37.8X3	T37.8X4	T37.8X5	T37.8X6
Hexobarbital	T42.3X1	T42.3X2	T42.3X3	T42.3X4	T42.3X5	T42.3X6
rectal	T41.291	T41.292	T41.293	T41.294	T41.295	T41.296
sodium	T41.1X1	T41.1X2	T41.1X3	T41.1X4	T41.1X5	T41.1X6
Hexobendine	T46.3X1	T46.3X2	T46.3X3	T46.3X4	T46.3X5	T46.3X6
Hexocyclium	T44.3X1	T44.3X2	T44.3X3	T44.3X4	T44.3X5	T44.3X6
metilsulfate	T44.3X1	T44.3X2	T44.3X3	T44.3X4	T44.3X5	T44.3X6
Hexoestrol	T38.5X1	T38.5X2	T38.5X3	T38.5X4	T38.5X5	T38.5X6
Hexone	T52.4X1	T52.4X2	T52.4X3	T52.4X4	—	—
Hexoprenaline	T48.6X1	T48.6X2	T48.6X3	T48.6X4	T48.6X5	T48.6X6
Hexylcaine	T41.3X1	T41.3X2	T41.3X3	T41.3X4	T41.3X5	T41.3X6
Hexylresorcinol	T52.2X1	T52.2X2	T52.2X3	T52.2X4	—	—
HGH (human growth hormone)	T38.811	T38.812	T38.813	T38.814	T38.815	T38.816
Hinkle's pills	T47.2X1	T47.2X2	T47.2X3	T47.2X4	T47.2X5	T47.2X6
Histalog	T50.8X1	T50.8X2	T50.8X3	T50.8X4	T50.8X5	T50.8X6
Histamine (phosphate)	T50.8X1	T50.8X2	T50.8X3	T50.8X4	T50.8X5	T50.8X6
Histoplasmin	T50.8X1	T50.8X2	T50.8X3	T50.8X4	T50.8X5	T50.8X6
Holly berries	T62.2X1	T62.2X2	T62.2X3	T62.2X4	—	—
Homatropine	T44.3X1	T44.3X2	T44.3X3	T44.3X4	T44.3X5	T44.3X6
methylbromide	T44.3X1	T44.3X2	T44.3X3	T44.3X4	T44.3X5	T44.3X6
Homochlorcyclizine	T45.0X1	T45.0X2	T45.0X3	T45.0X4	T45.0X5	T45.0X6
Homosalate	T49.3X1	T49.3X2	T49.3X3	T49.3X4	T49.3X5	T49.3X6
Homo-tet	T50.Z11	T50.Z12	T50.Z13	T50.Z14	T50.Z15	T50.Z16
Hormone	T38.801	T38.802	T38.803	T38.804	T38.805	T38.806
adrenal cortical steroids	T38.0X1	T38.0X2	T38.0X3	T38.0X4	T38.0X5	T38.0X6
androgenic	T38.7X1	T38.7X2	T38.7X3	T38.7X4	T38.7X5	T38.7X6
anterior pituitary NEC	T38.811	T38.812	T38.813	T38.814	T38.815	T38.816
antidiabetic agents	T38.3X1	T38.3X2	T38.3X3	T38.3X4	T38.3X5	T38.3X6
antidiuretic	T38.891	T38.892	T38.893	T38.894	T38.895	T38.896
cancer therapy	T45.1X1	T45.1X2	T45.1X3	T45.1X4	T45.1X5	T45.1X6
follicle stimulating	T38.811	T38.812	T38.813	T38.814	T38.815	T38.816
gonadotropic	T38.891	T38.892	T38.893	T38.894	T38.895	T38.896
pituitary	T38.811	T38.812	T38.813	T38.814	T38.815	T38.816
growth	T38.811	T38.812	T38.813	T38.814	T38.815	T38.816
luteinizing	T38.811	T38.812	T38.813	T38.814	T38.815	T38.816
ovarian	T38.5X1	T38.5X2	T38.5X3	T38.5X4	T38.5X5	T38.5X6
oxytocic	T48.0X1	T48.0X2	T48.0X3	T48.0X4	T48.0X5	T48.0X6
parathyroid (derivatives)	T50.991	T50.992	T50.993	T50.994	T50.995	T50.996
pituitary (posterior) NEC	T38.891	T38.892	T38.893	T38.894	T38.895	T38.896
anterior	T38.811	T38.812	T38.813	T38.814	T38.815	T38.816
specified, NEC	T38.891	T38.892	T38.893	T38.894	T38.895	T38.896
thyroid	T38.1X1	T38.1X2	T38.1X3	T38.1X4	T38.1X5	T38.1X6
Hornet (sting)	T63.451	T63.452	T63.453	T63.454	—	—
Horse anti-human lymphocytic serum	T50.Z11	T50.Z12	T50.Z13	T50.Z14	T50.Z15	T50.Z16
Horticulture agent NEC	T65.91	T65.92	T65.93	T65.94	—	—
with pesticide	T60.91	T60.92	T60.93	T60.94	—	—

Substance	Poisoning, Accidental (unintentional)	Poisoning, Intentional Self-harm	Poisoning, Assault	Poisoning, Undetermined	Adverse Effect	Under-dosing
Human						
albumin	T45.8X1	T45.8X2	T45.8X3	T45.8X4	T45.8X5	T45.8X6
growth hormone (HGH)	T38.811	T38.812	T38.813	T38.814	T38.815	T38.816
immune serum	T50.Z11	T50.Z12	T50.Z13	T50.Z14	T50.Z15	T50.Z16
Hyaluronidase	T45.3X1	T45.3X2	T45.3X3	T45.3X4	T45.3X5	T45.3X6
Hyazyme	T45.3X1	T45.3X2	T45.3X3	T45.3X4	T45.3X5	T45.3X6
Hycodan	T40.2X1	T40.2X2	T40.2X3	T40.2X4	T40.2X5	T40.2X6
Hydantoin derivative NEC	T42.0X1	T42.0X2	T42.0X3	T42.0X4	T42.0X5	T42.0X6
Hydeltra	T38.0X1	T38.0X2	T38.0X3	T38.0X4	T38.0X5	T38.0X6
Hydergine	T44.6X1	T44.6X2	T44.6X3	T44.6X4	T44.6X5	T44.6X6
Hydrabamine penicillin	T36.0X1	T36.0X2	T36.0X3	T36.0X4	T36.0X5	T36.0X6
Hydralazine	T46.5X1	T46.5X2	T46.5X3	T46.5X4	T46.5X5	T46.5X6
Hydrargaphen	T49.0X1	T49.0X2	T49.0X3	T49.0X4	T49.0X5	T49.0X6
Hydrargyri aminochloridum	T49.0X1	T49.0X2	T49.0X3	T49.0X4	T49.0X5	T49.0X6
Hydrastine	T48.291	T48.292	T48.293	T48.294	T48.295	T48.296
Hydrazine	T54.1X1	T54.1X2	T54.1X3	T54.1X4	—	—
monoamine oxidase inhibitors	T43.1X1	T43.1X2	T43.1X3	T43.1X4	T43.1X5	T43.1X6
Hydrazoic acid, azides	T54.2X1	T54.2X2	T54.2X3	T54.2X4	—	—
Hydriodic acid	T48.4X1	T48.4X2	T48.4X3	T48.4X4	T48.4X5	T48.4X6
Hydrocarbon gas	T59.891	T59.892	T59.893	T59.894	—	—
incomplete combustion of — *see* Carbon, monoxide, fuel, utility						
liquefied (mobile container)	T59.891	T59.892	T59.893	T59.894	—	—
piped (natural)	T59.891	T59.892	T59.893	T59.894	—	—
Hydrochloric acid (liquid)	T54.2X1	T54.2X2	T54.2X3	T54.2X4	—	—
medicinal (digestant)	T47.5X1	T47.5X2	T47.5X3	T47.5X4	T47.5X5	T47.5X6
vapor	T59.891	T59.892	T59.893	T59.894	—	—
Hydrochlorothiazide	T50.2X1	T50.2X2	T50.2X3	T50.2X4	T50.2X5	T50.2X6
Hydrocodone	T40.2X1	T40.2X2	T40.2X3	T40.2X4	T40.2X5	T40.2X6
Hydrocortisone (derivatives)	T38.0X1	T38.0X2	T38.0X3	T38.0X4	T38.0X5	T38.0X6
aceponate	T49.0X1	T49.0X2	T49.0X3	T49.0X4	T49.0X5	T49.0X6
ENT agent	T49.6X1	T49.6X2	T49.6X3	T49.6X4	T49.6X5	T49.6X6
ophthalmic preparation	T49.5X1	T49.5X2	T49.5X3	T49.5X4	T49.5X5	T49.5X6
topical NEC	T49.0X1	T49.0X2	T49.0X3	T49.0X4	T49.0X5	T49.0X6
Hydrocortone	T38.0X1	T38.0X2	T38.0X3	T38.0X4	T38.0X5	T38.0X6
ENT agent	T49.6X1	T49.6X2	T49.6X3	T49.6X4	T49.6X5	T49.6X6
ophthalmic preparation	T49.5X1	T49.5X2	T49.5X3	T49.5X4	T49.5X5	T49.5X6
topical NEC	T49.0X1	T49.0X2	T49.0X3	T49.0X4	T49.0X5	T49.0X6
Hydrocyanic acid (liquid)	T57.3X1	T57.3X2	T57.3X3	T57.3X4	—	—
gas	T65.0X1	T65.0X2	T65.0X3	T65.0X4	—	—
Hydroflumethiazide	T50.2X1	T50.2X2	T50.2X3	T50.2X4	T50.2X5	T50.2X6
Hydrofluoric acid (liquid)	T54.2X1	T54.2X2	T54.2X3	T54.2X4	—	—
vapor	T59.891	T59.892	T59.893	T59.894	—	—
Hydrogen	T59.891	T59.892	T59.893	T59.894	—	—
arsenide	T57.0X1	T57.0X2	T57.0X3	T57.0X4	—	—
arseniureted	T57.0X1	T57.0X2	T57.0X3	T57.0X4	—	—
chloride	T57.8X1	T57.8X2	T57.8X3	T57.8X4	—	—
cyanide (salts)	T57.3X1	T57.3X2	T57.3X3	T57.3X4	—	—
gas	T57.3X1	T57.3X2	T57.3X3	T57.3X4	—	—
Fluoride	T59.5X1	T59.5X2	T59.5X3	T59.5X4	—	—
vapor	T59.5X1	T59.5X2	T59.5X3	T59.5X4	—	—
peroxide	T49.0X1	T49.0X2	T49.0X3	T49.0X4	T49.0X5	T49.0X6
phosphureted	T57.1X1	T57.1X2	T57.1X3	T57.1X4	—	—
sulfide	T59.6X1	T59.6X2	T59.6X3	T59.6X4	—	—
arseniureted	T57.0X1	T57.0X2	T57.0X3	T57.0X4	—	—
sulfureted	T59.6X1	T59.6X2	T59.6X3	T59.6X4	—	—
Hydromethylpyridine	T46.7X1	T46.7X2	T46.7X3	T46.7X4	T46.7X5	T46.7X6
Hydromorphinol	T40.2X1	T40.2X2	T40.2X3	T40.2X4	—	—
Hydromorphinone	T40.2X1	T40.2X2	T40.2X3	T40.2X4	T40.2X5	T40.2X6
Hydromorphone	T40.2X1	T40.2X2	T40.2X3	T40.2X4	T40.2X5	T40.2X6
Hydromox	T50.2X1	T50.2X2	T50.2X3	T50.2X4	T50.2X5	T50.2X6
Hydrophilic lotion	T49.3X1	T49.3X2	T49.3X3	T49.3X4	T49.3X5	T49.3X6
Hydroquinidine	T46.2X1	T46.2X2	T46.2X3	T46.2X4	T46.2X5	T46.2X6
Hydroquinone	T52.2X1	T52.2X2	T52.2X3	T52.2X4	—	—
vapor	T59.891	T59.892	T59.893	T59.894	—	—
Hydrosulfuric acid (gas)	T59.6X1	T59.6X2	T59.6X3	T59.6X4	—	—
Hydrotalcite	T47.1X1	T47.1X2	T47.1X3	T47.1X4	T47.1X5	T47.1X6
Hydrous wool fat	T49.3X1	T49.3X2	T49.3X3	T49.3X4	T49.3X5	T49.3X6
Hydroxide, caustic	T54.3X1	T54.3X2	T54.3X3	T54.3X4	—	—
Hydroxocobalamin	T45.8X1	T45.8X2	T45.8X3	T45.8X4	T45.8X5	T45.8X6
Hydroxyamphetamine	T49.5X1	T49.5X2	T49.5X3	T49.5X4	T49.5X5	T49.5X6
Hydroxycarbamide	T45.1X1	T45.1X2	T45.1X3	T45.1X4	T45.1X5	T45.1X6
Hydroxychloroquine	T37.8X1	T37.8X2	T37.8X3	T37.8X4	T37.8X5	T37.8X6
Hydroxydihydrocodeinone	T40.2X1	T40.2X2	T40.2X3	T40.2X4	T40.2X5	T40.2X6
Hydroxyestrone	T38.5X1	T38.5X2	T38.5X3	T38.5X4	T38.5X5	T38.5X6
Hydroxyethyl starch	T45.8X1	T45.8X2	T45.8X3	T45.8X4	T45.8X5	T45.8X6
Hydroxymethylpentanone	T52.4X1	T52.4X2	T52.4X3	T52.4X4	—	—
Hydroxyphenamate	T43.591	T43.592	T43.593	T43.594	T43.595	T43.596
Hydroxyphenylbutazone	T39.2X1	T39.2X2	T39.2X3	T39.2X4	T39.2X5	T39.2X6
Hydroxyprogesterone	T38.5X1	T38.5X2	T38.5X3	T38.5X4	T38.5X5	T38.5X6

Substance	Poisoning, Accidental (unintentional)	Poisoning, Intentional Self-harm	Poisoning, Assault	Poisoning, Undetermined	Adverse Effect	Under-dosing
Hydroxyprogesterone — *continued*						
caproate	T38.5X1	T38.5X2	T38.5X3	T38.5X4	T38.5X5	T38.5X6
Hydroxyquinoline (derivatives) **NEC**	T37.8X1	T37.8X2	T37.8X3	T37.8X4	T37.8X5	T37.8X6
Hydroxystilbamidine	T37.3X1	T37.3X2	T37.3X3	T37.3X4	T37.3X5	T37.3X6
Hydroxytoluene (nonmedicinal)	T54.0X1	T54.0X2	T54.0X3	T54.0X4	—	—
medicinal	T49.0X1	T49.0X2	T49.0X3	T49.0X4	T49.0X5	T49.0X6
Hydroxyurea	T45.1X1	T45.1X2	T45.1X3	T45.1X4	T45.1X5	T45.1X6
Hydroxyzine	T43.591	T43.592	T43.593	T43.594	T43.595	T43.596
Hyoscine	T44.3X1	T44.3X2	T44.3X3	T44.3X4	T44.3X5	T44.3X6
Hyoscyamine	T44.3X1	T44.3X2	T44.3X3	T44.3X4	T44.3X5	T44.3X6
Hyoscyamus	T44.3X1	T44.3X2	T44.3X3	T44.3X4	T44.3X5	T44.3X6
dry extract	T44.3X1	T44.3X2	T44.3X3	T44.3X4	T44.3X5	T44.3X6
Hypaque	T50.8X1	T50.8X2	T50.8X3	T50.8X4	T50.8X5	T50.8X6
Hypertussis	T50.Z11	T50.Z12	T50.Z13	T50.Z14	T50.Z15	T50.Z16
Hypnotic	T42.71	T42.72	T42.73	T42.74	T42.75	T42.76
anticonvulsant	T42.71	T42.72	T42.73	T42.74	T42.75	T42.76
specified NEC	T42.6X1	T42.6X2	T42.6X3	T42.6X4	T42.6X5	T42.6X6
Hypochlorite	T49.0X1	T49.0X2	T49.0X3	T49.0X4	T49.0X5	T49.0X6
Hypophysis, posterior	T38.891	T38.892	T38.893	T38.894	T38.895	T38.896
Hypotensive NEC	T46.5X1	T46.5X2	T46.5X3	T46.5X4	T46.5X5	T46.5X6
Hypromellose	T49.5X1	T49.5X2	T49.5X3	T49.5X4	T49.5X5	T49.5X6
Ibacitabine	T37.5X1	T37.5X2	T37.5X3	T37.5X4	T37.5X5	T37.5X6
Ibopamine	T44.991	T44.992	T44.993	T44.994	T44.995	T44.996
Ibufenac	T39.311	T39.312	T39.313	T39.314	T39.315	T39.316
Ibuprofen	T39.311	T39.312	T39.313	T39.314	T39.315	T39.316
Ibuproxam	T39.311	T39.312	T39.313	T39.314	T39.315	T39.316
Ibuterol	T48.6X1	T48.6X2	T48.6X3	T48.6X4	T48.6X5	T48.6X6
Ichthammol	T49.0X1	T49.0X2	T49.0X3	T49.0X4	T49.0X5	T49.0X6
Ichthyol	T49.4X1	T49.4X2	T49.4X3	T49.4X4	T49.4X5	T49.4X6
Idarubicin	T45.1X1	T45.1X2	T45.1X3	T45.1X4	T45.1X5	T45.1X6
Idrocilamide	T42.8X1	T42.8X2	T42.8X3	T42.8X4	T42.8X5	T42.8X6
Ifenprodil	T46.7X1	T46.7X2	T46.7X3	T46.7X4	T46.7X5	T46.7X6
Ifosfamide	T45.1X1	T45.1X2	T45.1X3	T45.1X4	T45.1X5	T45.1X6
Iletin	T38.3X1	T38.3X2	T38.3X3	T38.3X4	T38.3X5	T38.3X6
Ilex	T62.2X1	T62.2X2	T62.2X3	T62.2X4	—	—
Illuminating gas (after combustion)	T58.11	T58.12	T58.13	T58.14	—	—
prior to combustion	T59.891	T59.892	T59.893	T59.894	—	—
Ilopan	T45.2X1	T45.2X2	T45.2X3	T45.2X4	T45.2X5	T45.2X6
Iloprost	T46.7X1	T46.7X2	T46.7X3	T46.7X4	T46.7X5	T46.7X6
Ilotycin	T36.3X1	T36.3X2	T36.3X3	T36.3X4	T36.3X5	T36.3X6
ophthalmic preparation	T49.5X1	T49.5X2	T49.5X3	T49.5X4	T49.5X5	T49.5X6
topical NEC	T49.0X1	T49.0X2	T49.0X3	T49.0X4	T49.0X5	T49.0X6
Imidazole-4-carboxamide	T45.1X1	T45.1X2	T45.1X3	T45.1X4	T45.1X5	T45.1X6
Iminostilbene	T42.1X1	T42.1X2	T42.1X3	T42.1X4	T42.1X5	T42.1X6
Imipenem	T36.0X1	T36.0X2	T36.0X3	T36.0X4	T36.0X5	T36.0X6
Imipramine	T43.011	T43.012	T43.013	T43.014	T43.015	T43.016
Immu-G	T50.Z11	T50.Z12	T50.Z13	T50.Z14	T50.Z15	T50.Z16
Immuglobin	T50.Z11	T50.Z12	T50.Z13	T50.Z14	T50.Z15	T50.Z16
Immune						
globulin	T50.Z11	T50.Z12	T50.Z13	T50.Z14	T50.Z15	T50.Z16
serum globulin	T50.Z11	T50.Z12	T50.Z13	T50.Z14	T50.Z15	T50.Z16
Immunoglobulin human (intravenous) (normal)	T50.Z11	T50.Z12	T50.Z13	T50.Z14	T50.Z15	T50.Z16
unmodified	T50.Z11	T50.Z12	T50.Z13	T50.Z14	T50.Z15	T50.Z16
Immunosuppressive drug	T45.1X1	T45.1X2	T45.1X3	T45.1X4	T45.1X5	T45.1X6
Immu-tetanus	T50.Z11	T50.Z12	T50.Z13	T50.Z14	T50.Z15	T50.Z16
Indalpine	T43.221	T43.222	T43.223	T43.224	T43.225	T43.226
Indanazoline	T48.5X1	T48.5X2	T48.5X3	T48.5X4	T48.5X5	T48.5X6
Indandione (derivatives)	T45.511	T45.512	T45.513	T45.514	T45.515	T45.516
Indapamide	T46.5X1	T46.5X2	T46.5X3	T46.5X4	T46.5X5	T46.5X6
Indendione (derivatives)	T45.511	T45.512	T45.513	T45.514	T45.515	T45.516
Indenolol	T44.7X1	T44.7X2	T44.7X3	T44.7X4	T44.7X5	T44.7X6
Inderal	T44.7X1	T44.7X2	T44.7X3	T44.7X4	T44.7X5	T44.7X6
Indian						
hemp	T40.7X1	T40.7X2	T40.7X3	T40.7X4	T40.7X5	T40.7X6
tobacco	T62.2X1	T62.2X2	T62.2X3	T62.2X4	—	—
Indigo carmine	T50.8X1	T50.8X2	T50.8X3	T50.8X4	T50.8X5	T50.8X6
Indobufen	T45.521	T45.522	T45.523	T45.524	T45.525	T45.526
Indocin	T39.2X1	T39.2X2	T39.2X3	T39.2X4	T39.2X5	T39.2X6
Indocyanine green	T50.8X1	T50.8X2	T50.8X3	T50.8X4	T50.8X5	T50.8X6
Indometacin	T39.391	T39.392	T39.393	T39.394	T39.395	T39.396
Indomethacin	T39.391	T39.392	T39.393	T39.394	T39.395	T39.396
farnesil	T39.4X1	T39.4X2	T39.4X3	T39.4X4	T39.4X5	T39.4X6
Indoramin	T44.6X1	T44.6X2	T44.6X3	T44.6X4	T44.6X5	T44.6X6
Industrial						
alcohol	T51.0X1	T51.0X2	T51.0X3	T51.0X4	—	—
fumes	T59.891	T59.892	T59.893	T59.894	—	—
solvents (fumes) (vapors)	T52.91	T52.92	T52.93	T52.94	—	—
Influenza vaccine	T50.B91	T50.B92	T50.B93	T50.B94	T50.B95	T50.B96

Substance	Poisoning, Accidental (unintentional)	Poisoning, Intentional Self-harm	Poisoning, Assault	Poisoning, Undetermined	Adverse Effect	Under-dosing
Ingested substance NEC	T65.91	T65.92	T65.93	T65.94	—	—
INH	T37.1X1	T37.1X2	T37.1X3	T37.1X4	T37.1X5	T37.1X6
Inhalation, gas (noxious) — *see* Gas						
Inhibitor						
angiotensin-converting enzyme	T46.4X1	T46.4X2	T46.4X3	T46.4X4	T46.4X5	T46.4X6
carbonic anhydrase	T50.2X1	T50.2X2	T50.2X3	T50.2X4	T50.2X5	T50.2X6
fibrinolysis	T45.621	T45.622	T45.623	T45.624	T45.625	T45.626
monoamine oxidase NEC	T43.1X1	T43.1X2	T43.1X3	T43.1X4	T43.1X5	T43.1X6
hydrazine	T43.1X1	T43.1X2	T43.1X3	T43.1X4	T43.1X5	T43.1X6
postsynaptic	T43.8X1	T43.8X2	T43.8X3	T43.8X4	T43.8X5	T43.8X6
prothrombin synthesis	T45.511	T45.512	T45.513	T45.514	T45.515	T45.516
Ink	T65.891	T65.892	T65.893	T65.894	—	—
Inorganic substance NEC	T57.91	T57.92	T57.93	T57.94	—	—
Inosine pranobex	T37.5X1	T37.5X2	T37.5X3	T37.5X4	T37.5X5	T37.5X6
Inositol	T50.991	T50.992	T50.993	T50.994	T50.995	T50.996
nicotinate	T46.7X1	T46.7X2	T46.7X3	T46.7X4	T46.7X5	T46.7X6
Inproquone	T45.1X1	T45.1X2	T45.1X3	T45.1X4	T45.1X5	T45.1X6
Insecticide NEC	T60.91	T60.92	T60.93	T60.94	—	—
carbamate	T60.0X1	T60.0X2	T60.0X3	T60.0X4	—	—
chlorinated	T60.1X1	T60.1X2	T60.1X3	T60.1X4	—	—
mixed	T60.91	T60.92	T60.93	T60.94	—	—
organochlorine	T60.1X1	T60.1X2	T60.1X3	T60.1X4	—	—
organophosphorus	T60.0X1	T60.0X2	T60.0X3	T60.0X4	—	—
Insect (sting), venomous	T63.481	T63.482	T63.483	T63.484	—	—
ant	T63.421	T63.422	T63.423	T63.424	—	—
bee	T63.441	T63.442	T63.443	T63.444	—	—
caterpillar	T63.431	T63.432	T63.433	T63.434	—	—
hornet	T63.451	T63.452	T63.453	T63.454	—	—
wasp	T63.461	T63.462	T63.463	T63.464	—	—
Insular tissue extract	T38.3X1	T38.3X2	T38.3X3	T38.3X4	T38.3X5	T38.3X6
Insulin (amorphous) (globin) (isophane) (Lente) (NPH) (Semilente) (Ultralente)	T38.3X1	T38.3X2	T38.3X3	T38.3X4	T38.3X5	T38.3X6
defalan	T38.3X1	T38.3X2	T38.3X3	T38.3X4	T38.3X5	T38.3X6
human	T38.3X1	T38.3X2	T38.3X3	T38.3X4	T38.3X5	T38.3X6
injection, soluble	T38.3X1	T38.3X2	T38.3X3	T38.3X4	T38.3X5	T38.3X6
biphasic	T38.3X1	T38.3X2	T38.3X3	T38.3X4	T38.3X5	T38.3X6
intermediate acting	T38.3X1	T38.3X2	T38.3X3	T38.3X4	T38.3X5	T38.3X6
protamine zinc	T38.3X1	T38.3X2	T38.3X3	T38.3X4	T38.3X5	T38.3X6
slow acting	T38.3X1	T38.3X2	T38.3X3	T38.3X4	T38.3X5	T38.3X6
zinc						
protamine injection	T38.3X1	T38.3X2	T38.3X3	T38.3X4	T38.3X5	T38.3X6
suspension (amorphous) (crystalline)	T38.3X1	T38.3X2	T38.3X3	T38.3X4	T38.3X5	T38.3X6
Interferon (alpha) (beta) (gamma)	T37.5X1	T37.5X2	T37.5X3	T37.5X4	T37.5X5	T37.5X6
Intestinal motility control drug	T47.6X1	T47.6X2	T47.6X3	T47.6X4	T47.6X5	T47.6X6
biological	T47.8X1	T47.8X2	T47.8X3	T47.8X4	T47.8X5	T47.8X6
Intranarcon	T41.1X1	T41.1X2	T41.1X3	T41.1X4	T41.1X5	T41.1X6
Intravenous						
amino acids	T50.991	T50.992	T50.993	T50.994	T50.995	T50.996
fat suspension	T50.991	T50.992	T50.993	T50.994	T50.995	T50.996
Inulin	T50.8X1	T50.8X2	T50.8X3	T50.8X4	T50.8X5	T50.8X6
Invert sugar	T50.3X1	T50.3X2	T50.3X3	T50.3X4	T50.3X5	T50.3X6
Inza — *see* Naproxen						
Iobenzamic acid	T50.8X1	T50.8X2	T50.8X3	T50.8X4	T50.8X5	T50.8X6
Iocarmic acid	T50.8X1	T50.8X2	T50.8X3	T50.8X4	T50.8X5	T50.8X6
Iocetamic acid	T50.8X1	T50.8X2	T50.8X3	T50.8X4	T50.8X5	T50.8X6
Iodamide	T50.8X1	T50.8X2	T50.8X3	T50.8X4	T50.8X5	T50.8X6
Iodide NEC — *see also* Iodine	T49.0X1	T49.0X2	T49.0X3	T49.0X4	T49.0X5	T49.0X6
mercury (ointment)	T49.0X1	T49.0X2	T49.0X3	T49.0X4	T49.0X5	T49.0X6
methylate	T49.0X1	T49.0X2	T49.0X3	T49.0X4	T49.0X5	T49.0X6
potassium (expectorant) NEC	T48.4X1	T48.4X2	T48.4X3	T48.4X4	T48.4X5	T48.4X6
Iodinated						
contrast medium	T50.8X1	T50.8X2	T50.8X3	T50.8X4	T50.8X5	T50.8X6
glycerol	T48.4X1	T48.4X2	T48.4X3	T48.4X4	T48.4X5	T48.4X6
human serum albumin (131I)	T50.8X1	T50.8X2	T50.8X3	T50.8X4	T50.8X5	T50.8X6
Iodine (antiseptic, external) (tincture) **NEC**	T49.0X1	T49.0X2	T49.0X3	T49.0X4	T49.0X5	T49.0X6
125 — *see also* Radiation sickness, and Exposure to radioactive isotopes	T50.8X1	T50.8X2	T50.8X3	T50.8X4	T50.8X5	T50.8X6
therapeutic	T50.991	T50.992	T50.993	T50.994	T50.995	T50.996
131 — *see also* Radiation sickness, and Exposure to radioactive isotopes	T50.8X1	T50.8X2	T50.8X3	T50.8X4	T50.8X5	T50.8X6
therapeutic	T38.2X1	T38.2X2	T38.2X3	T38.2X4	T38.2X5	T38.2X6
diagnostic	T50.8X1	T50.8X2	T50.8X3	T50.8X4	T50.8X5	T50.8X6

Substance	Poisoning, Accidental (unintentional)	Poisoning, Intentional Self-harm	Poisoning, Assault	Poisoning, Undetermined	Adverse Effect	Under-dosing
Iodine (antiseptic, external) (tincture) **NEC** — *continued*						
for thyroid conditions (antithyroid)	T38.2X1	T38.2X2	T38.2X3	T38.2X4	T38.2X5	T38.2X6
solution	T49.0X1	T49.0X2	T49.0X3	T49.0X4	T49.0X5	T49.0X6
vapor	T59.891	T59.892	T59.893	T59.894		
Iodipamide	T50.8X1	T50.8X2	T50.8X3	T50.8X4	T50.8X5	T50.8X6
Iodized (poppy seed) oil	T50.8X1	T50.8X2	T50.8X3	T50.8X4	T50.8X5	T50.8X6
Iodobismitol	T37.8X1	T37.8X2	T37.8X3	T37.8X4	T37.8X5	T37.8X6
Iodochlorhydroxyquin	T37.8X1	T37.8X2	T37.8X3	T37.8X4	T37.8X5	T37.8X6
topical	T49.0X1	T49.0X2	T49.0X3	T49.0X4	T49.0X5	T49.0X6
Iodochlorhydroxyquinoline	T37.8X1	T37.8X2	T37.8X3	T37.8X4	T37.8X5	T37.8X6
Iodocholesterol (131I)	T50.8X1	T50.8X2	T50.8X3	T50.8X4	T50.8X5	T50.8X6
Iodoform	T49.0X1	T49.0X2	T49.0X3	T49.0X4	T49.0X5	T49.0X6
Iodohippuric acid	T50.8X1	T50.8X2	T50.8X3	T50.8X4	T50.8X5	T50.8X6
Iodopanoic acid	T50.8X1	T50.8X2	T50.8X3	T50.8X4	T50.8X5	T50.8X6
Iodophthalein (sodium)	T50.8X1	T50.8X2	T50.8X3	T50.8X4	T50.8X5	T50.8X6
Iodopyracet	T50.8X1	T50.8X2	T50.8X3	T50.8X4	T50.8X5	T50.8X6
Iodoquinol	T37.8X1	T37.8X2	T37.8X3	T37.8X4	T37.8X5	T37.8X6
Iodoxamic acid	T50.8X1	T50.8X2	T50.8X3	T50.8X4	T50.8X5	T50.8X6
Iofendylate	T50.8X1	T50.8X2	T50.8X3	T50.8X4	T50.8X5	T50.8X6
Ioglycamic acid	T50.8X1	T50.8X2	T50.8X3	T50.8X4	T50.8X5	T50.8X6
Iohexol	T50.8X1	T50.8X2	T50.8X3	T50.8X4	T50.8X5	T50.8X6
Ion exchange resin						
anion	T47.8X1	T47.8X2	T47.8X3	T47.8X4	T47.8X5	T47.8X6
cation	T50.3X1	T50.3X2	T50.3X3	T50.3X4	T50.3X5	T50.3X6
cholestyramine	T46.6X1	T46.6X2	T46.6X3	T46.6X4	T46.6X5	T46.6X6
intestinal	T47.8X1	T47.8X2	T47.8X3	T47.8X4	T47.8X5	T47.8X6
Iopamidol	T50.8X1	T50.8X2	T50.8X3	T50.8X4	T50.8X5	T50.8X6
Iopanoic acid	T50.8X1	T50.8X2	T50.8X3	T50.8X4	T50.8X5	T50.8X6
Iophenoic acid	T50.8X1	T50.8X2	T50.8X3	T50.8X4	T50.8X5	T50.8X6
Iopodate, sodium	T50.8X1	T50.8X2	T50.8X3	T50.8X4	T50.8X5	T50.8X6
Iopodic acid	T50.8X1	T50.8X2	T50.8X3	T50.8X4	T50.8X5	T50.8X6
Iopromide	T50.8X1	T50.8X2	T50.8X3	T50.8X4	T50.8X5	T50.8X6
Iopydol	T50.8X1	T50.8X2	T50.8X3	T50.8X4	T50.8X5	T50.8X6
Iotalamic acid	T50.8X1	T50.8X2	T50.8X3	T50.8X4	T50.8X5	T50.8X6
Iothalamate	T50.8X1	T50.8X2	T50.8X3	T50.8X4	T50.8X5	T50.8X6
Iothiouracil	T38.2X1	T38.2X2	T38.2X3	T38.2X4	T38.2X5	T38.2X6
Iotrol	T50.8X1	T50.8X2	T50.8X3	T50.8X4	T50.8X5	T50.8X6
Iotrolan	T50.8X1	T50.8X2	T50.8X3	T50.8X4	T50.8X5	T50.8X6
Iotroxate	T50.8X1	T50.8X2	T50.8X3	T50.8X4	T50.8X5	T50.8X6
Iotroxic acid	T50.8X1	T50.8X2	T50.8X3	T50.8X4	T50.8X5	T50.8X6
Ioversol	T50.8X1	T50.8X2	T50.8X3	T50.8X4	T50.8X5	T50.8X6
Ioxaglate	T50.8X1	T50.8X2	T50.8X3	T50.8X4	T50.8X5	T50.8X6
Ioxaglic acid	T50.8X1	T50.8X2	T50.8X3	T50.8X4	T50.8X5	T50.8X6
Ioxitalamic acid	T50.8X1	T50.8X2	T50.8X3	T50.8X4	T50.8X5	T50.8X6
Ipecac	T47.7X1	T47.7X2	T47.7X3	T47.7X4	T47.7X5	T47.7X6
Ipecacuanha	T48.4X1	T48.4X2	T48.4X3	T48.4X4	T48.4X5	T48.4X6
Ipodate, calcium	T50.8X1	T50.8X2	T50.8X3	T50.8X4	T50.8X5	T50.8X6
Ipral	T42.3X1	T42.3X2	T42.3X3	T42.3X4	T42.3X5	T42.3X6
Ipratropium (bromide)	T48.6X1	T48.6X2	T48.6X3	T48.6X4	T48.6X5	T48.6X6
Ipriflavone	T46.3X1	T46.3X2	T46.3X3	T46.3X4	T46.3X5	T46.3X6
Iprindole	T43.011	T43.012	T43.013	T43.014	T43.015	T43.016
Iproclozide	T43.1X1	T43.1X2	T43.1X3	T43.1X4	T43.1X5	T43.1X6
Iprofenin	T50.8X1	T50.8X2	T50.8X3	T50.8X4	T50.8X5	T50.8X6
Iproheptine	T49.2X1	T49.2X2	T49.2X3	T49.2X4	T49.2X5	T49.2X6
Iproniazid	T43.1X1	T43.1X2	T43.1X3	T43.1X4	T43.1X5	T43.1X6
Iproplatin	T45.1X1	T45.1X2	T45.1X3	T45.1X4	T45.1X5	T45.1X6
Iproveratril	T46.1X1	T46.1X2	T46.1X3	T46.1X4	T46.1X5	T46.1X6
Iron (compounds) (medicinal) **NEC**	T45.4X1	T45.4X2	T45.4X3	T45.4X4	T45.4X5	T45.4X6
ammonium	T45.4X1	T45.4X2	T45.4X3	T45.4X4	T45.4X5	T45.4X6
dextran injection	T45.4X1	T45.4X2	T45.4X3	T45.4X4	T45.4X5	T45.4X6
nonmedicinal	T56.891	T56.892	T56.893	T56.894		
salts	T45.4X1	T45.4X2	T45.4X3	T45.4X4	T45.4X5	T45.4X6
sorbitex	T45.4X1	T45.4X2	T45.4X3	T45.4X4	T45.4X5	T45.4X6
sorbitol citric acid complex	T45.4X1	T45.4X2	T45.4X3	T45.4X4	T45.4X5	T45.4X6
Irrigating fluid (vaginal)	T49.8X1	T49.8X2	T49.8X3	T49.8X4	T49.8X5	T49.8X6
eye	T49.5X1	T49.5X2	T49.5X3	T49.5X4	T49.5X5	T49.5X6
Isepamicin	T36.5X1	T36.5X2	T36.5X3	T36.5X4	T36.5X5	T36.5X6
Isoaminile (citrate)	T48.3X1	T48.3X2	T48.3X3	T48.3X4	T48.3X5	T48.3X6
Isoamyl nitrite	T46.3X1	T46.3X2	T46.3X3	T46.3X4	T46.3X5	T46.3X6
Isobenzan	T60.1X1	T60.1X2	T60.1X3	T60.1X4		
Isobutyl acetate	T52.8X1	T52.8X2	T52.8X3	T52.8X4		
Isocarboxazid	T43.1X1	T43.1X2	T43.1X3	T43.1X4	T43.1X5	T43.1X6
Isoconazole	T49.0X1	T49.0X2	T49.0X3	T49.0X4	T49.0X5	T49.0X6
Isocyanate	T65.0X1	T65.0X2	T65.0X3	T65.0X4		
Isoephedrine	T44.991	T44.992	T44.993	T44.994	T44.995	T44.996
Isoetarine	T48.6X1	T48.6X2	T48.6X3	T48.6X4	T48.6X5	T48.6X6
Isoethadione	T42.2X1	T42.2X2	T42.2X3	T42.2X4	T42.2X5	T42.2X6
Isoetharine	T44.5X1	T44.5X2	T44.5X3	T44.5X4	T44.5X5	T44.5X6
Isoflurane	T41.0X1	T41.0X2	T41.0X3	T41.0X4	T41.0X5	T41.0X6
Isoflurophate	T44.0X1	T44.0X2	T44.0X3	T44.0X4	T44.0X5	T44.0X6
Isomaltose, ferric complex	T45.4X1	T45.4X2	T45.4X3	T45.4X4	T45.4X5	T45.4X6
Isometheptene	T44.3X1	T44.3X2	T44.3X3	T44.3X4	T44.3X5	T44.3X6
Isoniazid	T37.1X1	T37.1X2	T37.1X3	T37.1X4	T37.1X5	T37.1X6
with						
rifampicin	T36.6X1	T36.6X2	T36.6X3	T36.6X4	T36.6X5	T36.6X6
thioacetazone	T37.1X1	T37.1X2	T37.1X3	T37.1X4	T37.1X5	T37.1X6
Isonicotinic acid hydrazide	T37.1X1	T37.1X2	T37.1X3	T37.1X4	T37.1X5	T37.1X6
Isonipecaine	T40.4X1	T40.4X2	T40.4X3	T40.4X4	T40.4X5	T40.4X6
Isopentaquine	T37.2X1	T37.2X2	T37.2X3	T37.2X4	T37.2X5	T37.2X6
Isophane insulin	T38.3X1	T38.3X2	T38.3X3	T38.3X4	T38.3X5	T38.3X6
Isophorone	T65.891	T65.892	T65.893	T65.894		
Isophosphamide	T45.1X1	T45.1X2	T45.1X3	T45.1X4	T45.1X5	T45.1X6
Isopregnenone	T38.5X1	T38.5X2	T38.5X3	T38.5X4	T38.5X5	T38.5X6
Isoprenaline	T48.6X1	T48.6X2	T48.6X3	T48.6X4	T48.6X5	T48.6X6
Isopromethazine	T43.3X1	T43.3X2	T43.3X3	T43.3X4	T43.3X5	T43.3X6
Isopropamide	T44.3X1	T44.3X2	T44.3X3	T44.3X4	T44.3X5	T44.3X6
iodide	T44.3X1	T44.3X2	T44.3X3	T44.3X4	T44.3X5	T44.3X6
Isopropanol	T51.2X1	T51.2X2	T51.2X3	T51.2X4		
Isopropyl						
acetate	T52.8X1	T52.8X2	T52.8X3	T52.8X4		
alcohol	T51.2X1	T51.2X2	T51.2X3	T51.2X4		
medicinal	T49.4X1	T49.4X2	T49.4X3	T49.4X4	T49.4X5	T49.4X6
ether	T52.8X1	T52.8X2	T52.8X3	T52.8X4		
Isopropylaminophenazone	T39.2X1	T39.2X2	T39.2X3	T39.2X4	T39.2X5	T39.2X6
Isoproterenol	T48.6X1	T48.6X2	T48.6X3	T48.6X4	T48.6X5	T48.6X6
Isosorbide dinitrate	T46.3X1	T46.3X2	T46.3X3	T46.3X4	T46.3X5	T46.3X6
Isothipendyl	T45.0X1	T45.0X2	T45.0X3	T45.0X4	T45.0X5	T45.0X6
Isotretinoin	T50.991	T50.992	T50.993	T50.994	T50.995	T50.996
Isoxazolyl penicillin	T36.0X1	T36.0X2	T36.0X3	T36.0X4	T36.0X5	T36.0X6
Isoxicam	T39.391	T39.392	T39.393	T39.394	T39.395	T39.396
Isoxsuprine	T46.7X1	T46.7X2	T46.7X3	T46.7X4	T46.7X5	T46.7X6
Ispagula	T47.4X1	T47.4X2	T47.4X3	T47.4X4	T47.4X5	T47.4X6
husk	T47.4X1	T47.4X2	T47.4X3	T47.4X4	T47.4X5	T47.4X6
Isradipine	T46.1X1	T46.1X2	T46.1X3	T46.1X4	T46.1X5	T46.1X6
I-thyroxine sodium	T38.1X1	T38.1X2	T38.1X3	T38.1X4	T38.1X5	T38.1X6
Itraconazole	T37.8X1	T37.8X2	T37.8X3	T37.8X4	T37.8X5	T37.8X6
Itramin tosilate	T46.3X1	T46.3X2	T46.3X3	T46.3X4	T46.3X5	T46.3X6
Ivermectin	T37.4X1	T37.4X2	T37.4X3	T37.4X4	T37.4X5	T37.4X6
Izoniazid	T37.1X1	T37.1X2	T37.1X3	T37.1X4	T37.1X5	T37.1X6
with thioacetazone	T37.1X1	T37.1X2	T37.1X3	T37.1X4	T37.1X5	T37.1X6
Jalap	T47.2X1	T47.2X2	T47.2X3	T47.2X4	T47.2X5	T47.2X6
Jamaica						
dogwood (bark)	T39.8X1	T39.8X2	T39.8X3	T39.8X4	T39.8X5	T39.8X6
ginger	T65.891	T65.892	T65.893	T65.894		
root	T62.2X1	T62.2X2	T62.2X3	T62.2X4		
Jatropha	T62.2X1	T62.2X2	T62.2X3	T62.2X4		
curcas	T62.2X1	T62.2X2	T62.2X3	T62.2X4		
Jectofer	T45.4X1	T45.4X2	T45.4X3	T45.4X4	T45.4X5	T45.4X6
Jellyfish (sting)	T63.621	T63.622	T63.623	T63.624		
Jequirity (bean)	T62.2X1	T62.2X2	T62.2X3	T62.2X4		
Jimson weed (stramonium)	T62.2X1	T62.2X2	T62.2X3	T62.2X4		
seeds	T62.2X1	T62.2X2	T62.2X3	T62.2X4		
Josamycin	T36.3X1	T36.3X2	T36.3X3	T36.3X4	T36.3X5	T36.3X6
Juniper tar	T49.1X1	T49.1X2	T49.1X3	T49.1X4	T49.1X5	T49.1X6
Kallidinogenase	T46.7X1	T46.7X2	T46.7X3	T46.7X4	T46.7X5	T46.7X6
Kallikrein	T46.7X1	T46.7X2	T46.7X3	T46.7X4	T46.7X5	T46.7X6
Kanamycin	T36.5X1	T36.5X2	T36.5X3	T36.5X4	T36.5X5	T36.5X6
Kantrex	T36.5X1	T36.5X2	T36.5X3	T36.5X4	T36.5X5	T36.5X6
Kaolin	T47.6X1	T47.6X2	T47.6X3	T47.6X4	T47.6X5	T47.6X6
light	T47.6X1	T47.6X2	T47.6X3	T47.6X4	T47.6X5	T47.6X6
Karaya (gum)	T47.4X1	T47.4X2	T47.4X3	T47.4X4	T47.4X5	T47.4X6
Kebuzone	T39.2X1	T39.2X2	T39.2X3	T39.2X4	T39.2X5	T39.2X6
Kelevan	T60.1X1	T60.1X2	T60.1X3	T60.1X4		
Kemithal	T41.1X1	T41.1X2	T41.1X3	T41.1X4	T41.1X5	T41.1X6
Kenacort	T38.0X1	T38.0X2	T38.0X3	T38.0X4	T38.0X5	T38.0X6
Keratolytic drug NEC	T49.4X1	T49.4X2	T49.4X3	T49.4X4	T49.4X5	T49.4X6
anthracene	T49.4X1	T49.4X2	T49.4X3	T49.4X4	T49.4X5	T49.4X6
Keratoplastic NEC	T49.4X1	T49.4X2	T49.4X3	T49.4X4	T49.4X5	T49.4X6
Kerosene, kerosine (fuel) (solvent) **NEC**	T52.0X1	T52.0X2	T52.0X3	T52.0X4		
insecticide	T52.0X1	T52.0X2	T52.0X3	T52.0X4		
vapor	T52.0X1	T52.0X2	T52.0X3	T52.0X4		
Ketamine	T41.291	T41.292	T41.293	T41.294	T41.295	T41.296
Ketazolam	T42.4X1	T42.4X2	T42.4X3	T42.4X4	T42.4X5	T42.4X6
Ketazon	T39.2X1	T39.2X2	T39.2X3	T39.2X4	T39.2X5	T39.2X6
Ketobemidone	T40.4X1	T40.4X2	T40.4X3	T40.4X4		
Ketoconazole	T49.0X1	T49.0X2	T49.0X3	T49.0X4	T49.0X5	T49.0X6
Ketols	T52.4X1	T52.4X2	T52.4X3	T52.4X4		
Ketone oils	T52.4X1	T52.4X2	T52.4X3	T52.4X4		
Ketoprofen	T39.311	T39.312	T39.313	T39.314	T39.315	T39.316
Ketorolac	T39.8X1	T39.8X2	T39.8X3	T39.8X4	T39.8X5	T39.8X6
Ketotifen	T45.0X1	T45.0X2	T45.0X3	T45.0X4	T45.0X5	T45.0X6
Khat	T43.691	T43.692	T43.693	T43.694		

374

Additional Character May Be Required — Refer to the Tabular List for Character Selection · Subterms under main terms may continue to next column or page

Substance	Poisoning, Accidental (unintentional)	Poisoning, Intentional Self-harm	Poisoning, Assault	Poisoning, Undetermined	Adverse Effect	Under-dosing
Khellin	T46.3X1	T46.3X2	T46.3X3	T46.3X4	T46.3X5	T46.3X6
Khelloside	T46.3X1	T46.3X2	T46.3X3	T46.3X4	T46.3X5	T46.3X6
Kiln gas or vapor (carbon monoxide)	T58.8X1	T58.8X2	T58.8X3	T58.8X4	—	—
Kitasamycin	T36.3X1	T36.3X2	T36.3X3	T36.3X4	T36.3X5	T36.3X6
Konsyl	T47.4X1	T47.4X2	T47.4X3	T47.4X4	T47.4X5	T47.4X6
Kosam seed	T62.2X1	T62.2X2	T62.2X3	T62.2X4	—	—
Krait (venom)	T63.091	T63.092	T63.093	T63.094	—	—
Kwell (insecticide)	T60.1X1	T60.1X2	T60.1X3	T60.1X4	—	—
anti-infective (topical)	T49.0X1	T49.0X2	T49.0X3	T49.0X4	T49.0X5	T49.0X6
Labetalol	T44.8X1	T44.8X2	T44.8X3	T44.8X4	T44.8X5	T44.8X6
Laburnum (seeds)	T62.2X1	T62.2X2	T62.2X3	T62.2X4	—	—
leaves	T62.2X1	T62.2X2	T62.2X3	T62.2X4	—	—
Lachesine	T49.5X1	T49.5X2	T49.5X3	T49.5X4	T49.5X5	T49.5X6
Lacidipine	T46.5X1	T46.5X2	T46.5X3	T46.5X4	T46.5X5	T46.5X6
Lacquer	T65.6X1	T65.6X2	T65.6X3	T65.6X4	—	—
Lacrimogenic gas	T59.3X1	T59.3X2	T59.3X3	T59.3X4	—	—
Lactated potassic saline	T50.3X1	T50.3X2	T50.3X3	T50.3X4	T50.3X5	T50.3X6
Lactic acid	T49.8X1	T49.8X2	T49.8X3	T49.8X4	T49.8X5	T49.8X6
Lactobacillus						
acidophilus	T47.6X1	T47.6X2	T47.6X3	T47.6X4	T47.6X5	T47.6X6
compound	T47.6X1	T47.6X2	T47.6X3	T47.6X4	T47.6X5	T47.6X6
bifidus, lyophilized	T47.6X1	T47.6X2	T47.6X3	T47.6X4	T47.6X5	T47.6X6
bulgaricus	T47.6X1	T47.6X2	T47.6X3	T47.6X4	T47.6X5	T47.6X6
sporogenes	T47.6X1	T47.6X2	T47.6X3	T47.6X4	T47.6X5	T47.6X6
Lactoflavin	T45.2X1	T45.2X2	T45.2X3	T45.2X4	T45.2X5	T45.2X6
Lactose (as excipient)	T50.901	T50.902	T50.903	T50.904	T50.905	T50.906
Lactuca (virosa) (extract)	T42.6X1	T42.6X2	T42.6X3	T42.6X4	T42.6X5	T42.6X6
Lactucarium	T42.6X1	T42.6X2	T42.6X3	T42.6X4	T42.6X5	T42.6X6
Lactulose	T47.3X1	T47.3X2	T47.3X3	T47.3X4	T47.3X5	T47.3X6
Laevo — see Levo-						
Lanatosides	T46.0X1	T46.0X2	T46.0X3	T46.0X4	T46.0X5	T46.0X6
Lanolin	T49.3X1	T49.3X2	T49.3X3	T49.3X4	T49.3X5	T49.3X6
Largactil	T43.3X1	T43.3X2	T43.3X3	T43.3X4	T43.3X5	T43.3X6
Larkspur	T62.2X1	T62.2X2	T62.2X3	T62.2X4	—	—
Laroxyl	T43.011	T43.012	T43.013	T43.014	T43.015	T43.016
Lasix	T50.1X1	T50.1X2	T50.1X3	T50.1X4	T50.1X5	T50.1X6
Lassar's paste	T49.4X1	T49.4X2	T49.4X3	T49.4X4	T49.4X5	T49.4X6
Latamoxef	T36.1X1	T36.1X2	T36.1X3	T36.1X4	T36.1X5	T36.1X6
Latex	T65.811	T65.812	T65.813	T65.814	—	—
Lathyrus (seed)	T62.2X1	T62.2X2	T62.2X3	T62.2X4	—	—
Laudanum	T40.0X1	T40.0X2	T40.0X3	T40.0X4	T40.0X5	T40.0X6
Laudexium	T48.1X1	T48.1X2	T48.1X3	T48.1X4	T48.1X5	T48.1X6
Laughing gas	T41.0X1	T41.0X2	T41.0X3	T41.0X4	T41.0X5	T41.0X6
Laurel, black or cherry	T62.2X1	T62.2X2	T62.2X3	T62.2X4	—	—
Laurolinium	T49.0X1	T49.0X2	T49.0X3	T49.0X4	T49.0X5	T49.0X6
Lauryl sulfoacetate	T49.2X1	T49.2X2	T49.2X3	T49.2X4	T49.2X5	T49.2X6
Laxative NEC	T47.4X1	T47.4X2	T47.4X3	T47.4X4	T47.4X5	T47.4X6
osmotic	T47.3X1	T47.3X2	T47.3X3	T47.3X4	T47.3X5	T47.3X6
saline	T47.3X1	T47.3X2	T47.3X3	T47.3X4	T47.3X5	T47.3X6
stimulant	T47.2X1	T47.2X2	T47.2X3	T47.2X4	T47.2X5	T47.2X6
L-dopa	T42.8X1	T42.8X2	T42.8X3	T42.8X4	T42.8X5	T42.8X6
Lead (dust) (fumes) (vapor)	T56.0X1	T56.0X2	T56.0X3	T56.0X4	—	—
NEC						
acetate	T49.2X1	T49.2X2	T49.2X3	T49.2X4	T49.2X5	T49.2X6
alkyl (fuel additive)	T56.0X1	T56.0X2	T56.0X3	T56.0X4	—	—
anti-infectives	T37.8X1	T37.8X2	T37.8X3	T37.8X4	T37.8X5	T37.8X6
antiknock compound (tetraethyl)	T56.0X1	T56.0X2	T56.0X3	T56.0X4	—	—
arsenate, arsenite (dust)(herbicide) (insecticide) (vapor)	T57.0X1	T57.0X2	T57.0X3	T57.0X4	—	—
carbonate	T56.0X1	T56.0X2	T56.0X3	T56.0X4	—	—
paint	T56.0X1	T56.0X2	T56.0X3	T56.0X4	—	—
chromate	T56.0X1	T56.0X2	T56.0X3	T56.0X4	—	—
paint	T56.0X1	T56.0X2	T56.0X3	T56.0X4	—	—
dioxide	T56.0X1	T56.0X2	T56.0X3	T56.0X4	—	—
inorganic	T56.0X1	T56.0X2	T56.0X3	T56.0X4	—	—
iodide	T56.0X1	T56.0X2	T56.0X3	T56.0X4	—	—
pigment (paint)	T56.0X1	T56.0X2	T56.0X3	T56.0X4	—	—
monoxide (dust)	T56.0X1	T56.0X2	T56.0X3	T56.0X4	—	—
paint	T56.0X1	T56.0X2	T56.0X3	T56.0X4	—	—
organic	T56.0X1	T56.0X2	T56.0X3	T56.0X4	—	—
oxide	T56.0X1	T56.0X2	T56.0X3	T56.0X4	—	—
paint	T56.0X1	T56.0X2	T56.0X3	T56.0X4	—	—
paint	T56.0X1	T56.0X2	T56.0X3	T56.0X4	—	—
salts	T56.0X1	T56.0X2	T56.0X3	T56.0X4	—	—
specified compound NEC	T56.0X1	T56.0X2	T56.0X3	T56.0X4	—	—
tetra-ethyl	T56.0X1	T56.0X2	T56.0X3	T56.0X4	—	—
Lebanese red	T40.7X1	T40.7X2	T40.7X3	T40.7X4	T40.7X5	T40.7X6
Lefetamine	T39.8X1	T39.8X2	T39.8X3	T39.8X4	T39.8X5	T39.8X6
Lenperone	T43.4X1	T43.4X2	T43.4X3	T43.4X4	T43.4X5	T43.4X6
Lente lietin (insulin)	T38.3X1	T38.3X2	T38.3X3	T38.3X4	T38.3X5	T38.3X6
Leptazol	T50.7X1	T50.7X2	T50.7X3	T50.7X4	T50.7X5	T50.7X6
Leptophos	T60.0X1	T60.0X2	T60.0X3	T60.0X4	—	—
Leritine	T40.2X1	T40.2X2	T40.2X3	T40.2X4	T40.2X5	T40.2X6
Letosteine	T48.4X1	T48.4X2	T48.4X3	T48.4X4	T48.4X5	T48.4X6
Letter	T38.1X1	T38.1X2	T38.1X3	T38.1X4	T38.1X5	T38.1X6
Lettuce opium	T42.6X1	T42.6X2	T42.6X3	T42.6X4	T42.6X5	T42.6X6
Leucinocaine	T41.3X1	T41.3X2	T41.3X3	T41.3X4	T41.3X5	T41.3X6
Leucocianidol	T46.991	T46.992	T46.993	T46.994	T46.995	T46.996
Leucovorin (factor)	T45.8X1	T45.8X2	T45.8X3	T45.8X4	T45.8X5	T45.8X6
Leukeran	T45.1X1	T45.1X2	T45.1X3	T45.1X4	T45.1X5	T45.1X6
Leuprolide	T38.891	T38.892	T38.893	T38.894	T38.895	T38.896
Levalbuterol	T48.6X1	T48.6X2	T48.6X3	T48.6X4	T48.6X5	T48.6X6
Levallorphan	T50.7X1	T50.7X2	T50.7X3	T50.7X4	T50.7X5	T50.7X6
Levamisole	T37.4X1	T37.4X2	T37.4X3	T37.4X4	T37.4X5	T37.4X6
Levanil	T42.6X1	T42.6X2	T42.6X3	T42.6X4	T42.6X5	T42.6X6
Levarterenol	T44.4X1	T44.4X2	T44.4X3	T44.4X4	T44.4X5	T44.4X6
Levdropropizine	T48.3X1	T48.3X2	T48.3X3	T48.3X4	T48.3X5	T48.3X6
Levobunolol	T49.5X1	T49.5X2	T49.5X3	T49.5X4	T49.5X5	T49.5X6
Levocabastine (hydrochloride)	T45.0X1	T45.0X2	T45.0X3	T45.0X4	T45.0X5	T45.0X6
Levocarnitine	T50.991	T50.992	T50.993	T50.994	T50.995	T50.996
Levodopa	T42.8X1	T42.8X2	T42.8X3	T42.8X4	T42.8X5	T42.8X6
with carbidopa	T42.8X1	T42.8X2	T42.8X3	T42.8X4	T42.8X5	T42.8X6
Levo-dromoran	T40.2X1	T40.2X2	T40.2X3	T40.2X4	T40.2X5	T40.2X6
Levoglutamide	T50.991	T50.992	T50.993	T50.994	T50.995	T50.996
Levoid	T38.1X1	T38.1X2	T38.1X3	T38.1X4	T38.1X5	T38.1X6
Levo-isomethadone	T40.3X1	T40.3X2	T40.3X3	T40.3X4	T40.3X5	T40.3X6
Levomepromazine	T43.3X1	T43.3X2	T43.3X3	T43.3X4	T43.3X5	T43.3X6
Levonordefrin	T49.6X1	T49.6X2	T49.6X3	T49.6X4	T49.6X5	T49.6X6
Levonorgestrel	T38.4X1	T38.4X2	T38.4X3	T38.4X4	T38.4X5	T38.4X6
with ethinylestradiol	T38.5X1	T38.5X2	T38.5X3	T38.5X4	T38.5X5	T38.5X6
Levopromazine	T43.3X1	T43.3X2	T43.3X3	T43.3X4	T43.3X5	T43.3X6
Levoprome	T42.6X1	T42.6X2	T42.6X3	T42.6X4	T42.6X5	T42.6X6
Levopropoxyphene	T40.4X1	T40.4X2	T40.4X3	T40.4X4	T40.4X5	T40.4X6
Levopropylhexedrine	T50.5X1	T50.5X2	T50.5X3	T50.5X4	T50.5X5	T50.5X6
Levoproxyphylline	T48.6X1	T48.6X2	T48.6X3	T48.6X4	T48.6X5	T48.6X6
Levorphanol	T40.4X1	T40.4X2	T40.4X3	T40.4X4	T40.4X5	T40.4X6
Levothyroxine	T38.1X1	T38.1X2	T38.1X3	T38.1X4	T38.1X5	T38.1X6
sodium	T38.1X1	T38.1X2	T38.1X3	T38.1X4	T38.1X5	T38.1X6
Levsin	T44.3X1	T44.3X2	T44.3X3	T44.3X4	T44.3X5	T44.3X6
Levulose	T50.3X1	T50.3X2	T50.3X3	T50.3X4	T50.3X5	T50.3X6
Lewisite (gas), not in war	T57.0X1	T57.0X2	T57.0X3	T57.0X4	—	—
Librium	T42.4X1	T42.4X2	T42.4X3	T42.4X4	T42.4X5	T42.4X6
Lidex	T49.0X1	T49.0X2	T49.0X3	T49.0X4	T49.0X5	T49.0X6
Lidocaine	T41.3X1	T41.3X2	T41.3X3	T41.3X4	T41.3X5	T41.3X6
regional	T41.3X1	T41.3X2	T41.3X3	T41.3X4	T41.3X5	T41.3X6
spinal	T41.3X1	T41.3X2	T41.3X3	T41.3X4	T41.3X5	T41.3X6
Lidofenin	T50.8X1	T50.8X2	T50.8X3	T50.8X4	T50.8X5	T50.8X6
Lidoflazine	T46.1X1	T46.1X2	T46.1X3	T46.1X4	T46.1X5	T46.1X6
Lighter fluid	T52.0X1	T52.0X2	T52.0X3	T52.0X4	—	—
Lignin hemicellulose	T47.6X1	T47.6X2	T47.6X3	T47.6X4	T47.6X5	T47.6X6
Lignocaine	T41.3X1	T41.3X2	T41.3X3	T41.3X4	T41.3X5	T41.3X6
regional	T41.3X1	T41.3X2	T41.3X3	T41.3X4	T41.3X5	T41.3X6
spinal	T41.3X1	T41.3X2	T41.3X3	T41.3X4	T41.3X5	T41.3X6
Ligroin (e) (solvent)	T52.0X1	T52.0X2	T52.0X3	T52.0X4	—	—
vapor	T59.891	T59.892	T59.893	T59.894	—	—
Ligustrum vulgare	T62.2X1	T62.2X2	T62.2X3	T62.2X4	—	—
Lily of the valley	T62.2X1	T62.2X2	T62.2X3	T62.2X4	—	—
Lime (chloride)	T54.3X1	T54.3X2	T54.3X3	T54.3X4	—	—
Limonene	T52.8X1	T52.8X2	T52.8X3	T52.8X4	—	—
Lincomycin	T36.8X1	T36.8X2	T36.8X3	T36.8X4	T36.8X5	T36.8X6
Lindane (insecticide) (nonmedicinal) (vapor)	T53.6X1	T53.6X2	T53.6X3	T53.6X4	—	—
medicinal	T49.0X1	T49.0X2	T49.0X3	T49.0X4	T49.0X5	T49.0X6
Liniments NEC	T49.91	T49.92	T49.93	T49.94	T49.95	T49.96
Linoleic acid	T46.6X1	T46.6X2	T46.6X3	T46.6X4	T46.6X5	T46.6X6
Linolenic acid	T46.6X1	T46.6X2	T46.6X3	T46.6X4	T46.6X5	T46.6X6
Linseed	T47.4X1	T47.4X2	T47.4X3	T47.4X4	T47.4X5	T47.4X6
Liothyronine	T38.1X1	T38.1X2	T38.1X3	T38.1X4	T38.1X5	T38.1X6
Liotrix	T38.1X1	T38.1X2	T38.1X3	T38.1X4	T38.1X5	T38.1X6
Lipancreatin	T47.5X1	T47.5X2	T47.5X3	T47.5X4	T47.5X5	T47.5X6
Lipo-alprostadil	T46.7X1	T46.7X2	T46.7X3	T46.7X4	T46.7X5	T46.7X6
Lipo-Lutin	T38.5X1	T38.5X2	T38.5X3	T38.5X4	T38.5X5	T38.5X6
Lipotropic drug NEC	T50.901	T50.902	T50.903	T50.904	T50.905	T50.906
Liquefied petroleum gases	T59.891	T59.892	T59.893	T59.894	—	—
piped (pure or mixed with air)	T59.891	T59.892	T59.893	T59.894	—	—
Liquid						
paraffin	T47.4X1	T47.4X2	T47.4X3	T47.4X4	T47.4X5	T47.4X6
petrolatum	T47.4X1	T47.4X2	T47.4X3	T47.4X4	T47.4X5	T47.4X6
topical	T49.3X1	T49.3X2	T49.3X3	T49.3X4	T49.3X5	T49.3X6
specified NEC	T65.891	T65.892	T65.893	T65.894	—	—
substance	T65.91	T65.92	T65.93	T65.94	—	—

🔎 Subterms under main terms may continue to next column or page

Additional Character May Be Required — Refer to the Tabular List for Character Selection

Substance	Poisoning, Accidental (unintentional)	Poisoning, Intentional Self-harm	Poisoning, Assault	Poisoning, Undetermined	Adverse Effect	Under-dosing
Liquor creosolis compositus	T65.891	T65.892	T65.893	T65.894	—	—
Liquorice	T48.4X1	T48.4X2	T48.4X3	T48.4X4	T48.4X5	T48.4X6
extract	T47.8X1	T47.8X2	T47.8X3	T47.8X4	T47.8X5	T47.8X6
Lisinopril	T46.4X1	T46.4X2	T46.4X3	T46.4X4	T46.4X5	T46.4X6
Lisuride	T42.8X1	T42.8X2	T42.8X3	T42.8X4	T42.8X5	T42.8X6
Lithane	T43.8X1	T43.8X2	T43.8X3	T43.8X4	T43.8X5	T43.8X6
Lithium	T56.891	T56.892	T56.893	T56.894	—	—
gluconate	T43.591	T43.592	T43.593	T43.594	T43.595	T43.596
salts (carbonate)	T43.591	T43.592	T43.593	T43.594	T43.595	T43.596
Lithonate	T43.8X1	T43.8X2	T43.8X3	T43.8X4	T43.8X5	T43.8X6
Liver						
extract	T45.8X1	T45.8X2	T45.8X3	T45.8X4	T45.8X5	T45.8X6
for parenteral use	T45.8X1	T45.8X2	T45.8X3	T45.8X4	T45.8X5	T45.8X6
fraction 1	T45.8X1	T45.8X2	T45.8X3	T45.8X4	T45.8X5	T45.8X6
hydrolysate	T45.8X1	T45.8X2	T45.8X3	T45.8X4	T45.8X5	T45.8X6
Lizard (bite) (venom)	T63.121	T63.122	T63.123	T63.124	—	—
LMD	T45.8X1	T45.8X2	T45.8X3	T45.8X4	T45.8X5	T45.8X6
Lobelia	T62.2X1	T62.2X2	T62.2X3	T62.2X4		
Lobeline	T50.7X1	T50.7X2	T50.7X3	T50.7X4	T50.7X5	T50.7X6
Local action drug NEC	T49.8X1	T49.8X2	T49.8X3	T49.8X4	T49.8X5	T49.8X6
Locorten	T49.0X1	T49.0X2	T49.0X3	T49.0X4	T49.0X5	T49.0X6
Lofepramine	T43.011	T43.012	T43.013	T43.014	T43.015	T43.016
Lolium temulentum	T62.2X1	T62.2X2	T62.2X3	T62.2X4	—	—
Lomotil	T47.6X1	T47.6X2	T47.6X3	T47.6X4	T47.6X5	T47.6X6
Lomustine	T45.1X1	T45.1X2	T45.1X3	T45.1X4	T45.1X5	T45.1X6
Lonidamine	T45.1X1	T45.1X2	T45.1X3	T45.1X4	T45.1X5	T45.1X6
Loperamide	T47.6X1	T47.6X2	T47.6X3	T47.6X4	T47.6X5	T47.6X6
Loprazolam	T42.4X1	T42.4X2	T42.4X3	T42.4X4	T42.4X5	T42.4X6
Lorajmine	T46.2X1	T46.2X2	T46.2X3	T46.2X4	T46.2X5	T46.2X6
Loratadine	T45.0X1	T45.0X2	T45.0X3	T45.0X4	T45.0X5	T45.0X6
Lorazepam	T42.4X1	T42.4X2	T42.4X3	T42.4X4	T42.4X5	T42.4X6
Lorcainide	T46.2X1	T46.2X2	T46.2X3	T46.2X4	T46.2X5	T46.2X6
Lormetazepam	T42.4X1	T42.4X2	T42.4X3	T42.4X4	T42.4X5	T42.4X6
Lotions NEC	T49.91	T49.92	T49.93	T49.94	T49.95	T49.96
Lotusate	T42.3X1	T42.3X2	T42.3X3	T42.3X4	T42.3X5	T42.3X6
Lovastatin	T46.6X1	T46.6X2	T46.6X3	T46.6X4	T46.6X5	T46.6X6
Lowila	T49.2X1	T49.2X2	T49.2X3	T49.2X4	T49.2X5	T49.2X6
Loxapine	T43.591	T43.592	T43.593	T43.594	T43.595	T43.596
Lozenges (throat)	T49.6X1	T49.6X2	T49.6X3	T49.6X4	T49.6X5	T49.6X6
LSD	T40.8X1	T40.8X2	T40.8X3	T40.8X4	—	—
L-Tryptophan — see amino acid						
Lubricant, eye	T49.5X1	T49.5X2	T49.5X3	T49.5X4	T49.5X5	T49.5X6
Lubricating oil NEC	T52.0X1	T52.0X2	T52.0X3	T52.0X4		
Lucanthone	T37.4X1	T37.4X2	T37.4X3	T37.4X4	T37.4X5	T37.4X6
Luminal	T42.3X1	T42.3X2	T42.3X3	T42.3X4	T42.3X5	T42.3X6
Lung irritant (gas) NEC	T59.91	T59.92	T59.93	T59.94	—	—
Luteinizing hormone	T38.811	T38.812	T38.813	T38.814	T38.815	T38.816
Lutocylol	T38.5X1	T38.5X2	T38.5X3	T38.5X4	T38.5X5	T38.5X6
Lutromone	T38.5X1	T38.5X2	T38.5X3	T38.5X4	T38.5X5	T38.5X6
Lututrin	T48.291	T48.292	T48.293	T48.294	T48.295	T48.296
Lye (concentrated)	T54.3X1	T54.3X2	T54.3X3	T54.3X4	—	—
Lygranum (skin test)	T50.8X1	T50.8X2	T50.8X3	T50.8X4	T50.8X5	T50.8X6
Lymecycline	T36.4X1	T36.4X2	T36.4X3	T36.4X4	T36.4X5	T36.4X6
Lymphogranuloma venereum antigen	T50.8X1	T50.8X2	T50.8X3	T50.8X4	T50.8X5	T50.8X6
Lynestrenol	T38.4X1	T38.4X2	T38.4X3	T38.4X4	T38.4X5	T38.4X6
Lyovac Sodium Edecrin	T50.1X1	T50.1X2	T50.1X3	T50.1X4	T50.1X5	T50.1X6
Lypressin	T38.891	T38.892	T38.893	T38.894	T38.895	T38.896
Lysergic acid diethylamide	T40.8X1	T40.8X2	T40.8X3	T40.8X4		
Lysergide	T40.8X1	T40.8X2	T40.8X3	T40.8X4		
Lysine vasopressin	T38.891	T38.892	T38.893	T38.894	T38.895	T38.896
Lysol	T54.1X1	T54.1X2	T54.1X3	T54.1X4	—	—
Lysozyme	T49.0X1	T49.0X2	T49.0X3	T49.0X4	T49.0X5	T49.0X6
Lytta (vitatta)	T49.8X1	T49.8X2	T49.8X3	T49.8X4	T49.8X5	T49.8X6
Mace	T59.3X1	T59.3X2	T59.3X3	T59.3X4		
Macrogol	T50.991	T50.992	T50.993	T50.994	T50.995	T50.996
Macrolide						
anabolic drug	T38.7X1	T38.7X2	T38.7X3	T38.7X4	T38.7X5	T38.7X6
antibiotic	T36.3X1	T36.3X2	T36.3X3	T36.3X4	T36.3X5	T36.3X6
Mafenide	T49.0X1	T49.0X2	T49.0X3	T49.0X4	T49.0X5	T49.0X6
Magaldrate	T47.1X1	T47.1X2	T47.1X3	T47.1X4	T47.1X5	T47.1X6
Magic mushroom	T40.991	T40.992	T40.993	T40.994	—	—
Magnamycin	T36.8X1	T36.8X2	T36.8X3	T36.8X4	T36.8X5	T36.8X6
Magnesia magma	T47.1X1	T47.1X2	T47.1X3	T47.1X4	T47.1X5	T47.1X6
Magnesium NEC	T56.891	T56.892	T56.893	T56.894	—	—
carbonate	T47.1X1	T47.1X2	T47.1X3	T47.1X4	T47.1X5	T47.1X6
citrate	T47.4X1	T47.4X2	T47.4X3	T47.4X4	T47.4X5	T47.4X6
hydroxide	T47.1X1	T47.1X2	T47.1X3	T47.1X4	T47.1X5	T47.1X6
oxide	T47.1X1	T47.1X2	T47.1X3	T47.1X4	T47.1X5	T47.1X6
peroxide	T49.0X1	T49.0X2	T49.0X3	T49.0X4	T49.0X5	T49.0X6
salicylate	T39.091	T39.092	T39.093	T39.094	T39.095	T39.096
silicofluoride	T50.3X1	T50.3X2	T50.3X3	T50.3X4	T50.3X5	T50.3X6

Substance	Poisoning, Accidental (unintentional)	Poisoning, Intentional Self-harm	Poisoning, Assault	Poisoning, Undetermined	Adverse Effect	Under-dosing
Magnesium — continued						
sulfate	T47.4X1	T47.4X2	T47.4X3	T47.4X4	T47.4X5	T47.4X6
thiosulfate	T45.0X1	T45.0X2	T45.0X3	T45.0X4	T45.0X5	T45.0X6
trisilicate	T47.1X1	T47.1X2	T47.1X3	T47.1X4	T47.1X5	T47.1X6
Malathion (medicinal)	T49.0X1	T49.0X2	T49.0X3	T49.0X4	T49.0X5	T49.0X6
insecticide	T60.0X1	T60.0X2	T60.0X3	T60.0X4	—	—
Male fern extract	T37.4X1	T37.4X2	T37.4X3	T37.4X4	T37.4X5	T37.4X6
M-AMSA	T45.1X1	T45.1X2	T45.1X3	T45.1X4	T45.1X5	T45.1X6
Mandelic acid	T37.8X1	T37.8X2	T37.8X3	T37.8X4	T37.8X5	T37.8X6
Manganese (dioxide) (salts)	T57.2X1	T57.2X2	T57.2X3	T57.2X4		
medicinal	T50.991	T50.992	T50.993	T50.994	T50.995	T50.996
Mannitol	T47.3X1	T47.3X2	T47.3X3	T47.3X4	T47.3X5	T47.3X6
hexanitrate	T46.3X1	T46.3X2	T46.3X3	T46.3X4	T46.3X5	T46.3X6
Mannomustine	T45.1X1	T45.1X2	T45.1X3	T45.1X4	T45.1X5	T45.1X6
MAO inhibitors	T43.1X1	T43.1X2	T43.1X3	T43.1X4	T43.1X5	T43.1X6
Mapharsen	T37.8X1	T37.8X2	T37.8X3	T37.8X4	T37.8X5	T37.8X6
Maphenide	T49.0X1	T49.0X2	T49.0X3	T49.0X4	T49.0X5	T49.0X6
Maprotiline	T43.021	T43.022	T43.023	T43.024	T43.025	T43.026
Marcaine	T41.3X1	T41.3X2	T41.3X3	T41.3X4	T41.3X5	T41.3X6
infiltration (subcutaneous)	T41.3X1	T41.3X2	T41.3X3	T41.3X4	T41.3X5	T41.3X6
nerve block (peripheral) (plexus)	T41.3X1	T41.3X2	T41.3X3	T41.3X4	T41.3X5	T41.3X6
Marezine	T45.0X1	T45.0X2	T45.0X3	T45.0X4	T45.0X5	T45.0X6
Marihuana	T40.7X1	T40.7X2	T40.7X3	T40.7X4	T40.7X5	T40.7X6
Marijuana	T40.7X1	T40.7X2	T40.7X3	T40.7X4	T40.7X5	T40.7X6
Marine (sting)	T63.691	T63.692	T63.693	T63.694	—	—
animals (sting)	T63.691	T63.692	T63.693	T63.694	—	—
plants (sting)	T63.711	T63.712	T63.713	T63.714	—	—
Marplan	T43.1X1	T43.1X2	T43.1X3	T43.1X4	T43.1X5	T43.1X6
Marsh gas	T59.891	T59.892	T59.893	T59.894		
Marsilid	T43.1X1	T43.1X2	T43.1X3	T43.1X4	T43.1X5	T43.1X6
Matulane	T45.1X1	T45.1X2	T45.1X3	T45.1X4	T45.1X5	T45.1X6
Mazindol	T50.5X1	T50.5X2	T50.5X3	T50.5X4	T50.5X5	T50.5X6
MCPA	T60.3X1	T60.3X2	T60.3X3	T60.3X4		
MDMA	T43.621	T43.622	T43.623	T43.624	T43.625	T43.626
Meadow saffron	T62.2X1	T62.2X2	T62.2X3	T62.2X4		
Measles virus vaccine (attenuated)	T50.B91	T50.B92	T50.B93	T50.B94	T50.B95	T50.B96
Meat, noxious	T62.8X1	T62.8X2	T62.8X3	T62.8X4		
Meballymal	T42.3X1	T42.3X2	T42.3X3	T42.3X4	T42.3X5	T42.3X6
Mebanazine	T43.1X1	T43.1X2	T43.1X3	T43.1X4	T43.1X5	T43.1X6
Mebaral	T42.3X1	T42.3X2	T42.3X3	T42.3X4	T42.3X5	T42.3X6
Mebendazole	T37.4X1	T37.4X2	T37.4X3	T37.4X4	T37.4X5	T37.4X6
Mebeverine	T44.3X1	T44.3X2	T44.3X3	T44.3X4	T44.3X5	T44.3X6
Mebhydrolin	T45.0X1	T45.0X2	T45.0X3	T45.0X4	T45.0X5	T45.0X6
Mebumal	T42.3X1	T42.3X2	T42.3X3	T42.3X4	T42.3X5	T42.3X6
Mebutamate	T43.591	T43.592	T43.593	T43.594	T43.595	T43.596
Mecamylamine	T44.2X1	T44.2X2	T44.2X3	T44.2X4	T44.2X5	T44.2X6
Mechlorethamine	T45.1X1	T45.1X2	T45.1X3	T45.1X4	T45.1X5	T45.1X6
Mecillinam	T36.0X1	T36.0X2	T36.0X3	T36.0X4	T36.0X5	T36.0X6
Meclizine (hydrochloride)	T45.0X1	T45.0X2	T45.0X3	T45.0X4	T45.0X5	T45.0X6
Meclocycline	T36.4X1	T36.4X2	T36.4X3	T36.4X4	T36.4X5	T36.4X6
Meclofenamate	T39.391	T39.392	T39.393	T39.394	T39.395	T39.396
Meclofenamic acid	T39.391	T39.392	T39.393	T39.394	T39.395	T39.396
Meclofenoxate	T43.691	T43.692	T43.693	T43.694	T43.695	T43.696
Meclozine	T45.0X1	T45.0X2	T45.0X3	T45.0X4	T45.0X5	T45.0X6
Mecobalamin	T45.8X1	T45.8X2	T45.8X3	T45.8X4	T45.8X5	T45.8X6
Mecoprop	T60.3X1	T60.3X2	T60.3X3	T60.3X4	—	—
Mecrilate	T49.3X1	T49.3X2	T49.3X3	T49.3X4	T49.3X5	T49.3X6
Mecysteine	T48.4X1	T48.4X2	T48.4X3	T48.4X4	T48.4X5	T48.4X6
Medazepam	T42.4X1	T42.4X2	T42.4X3	T42.4X4	T42.4X5	T42.4X6
Medicament NEC	T50.901	T50.902	T50.903	T50.904	T50.905	T50.906
Medinal	T42.3X1	T42.3X2	T42.3X3	T42.3X4	T42.3X5	T42.3X6
Medomin	T42.3X1	T42.3X2	T42.3X3	T42.3X4	T42.3X5	T42.3X6
Medrogestone	T38.5X1	T38.5X2	T38.5X3	T38.5X4	T38.5X5	T38.5X6
Medroxalol	T44.8X1	T44.8X2	T44.8X3	T44.8X4	T44.8X5	T44.8X6
Medroxyprogesterone acetate (depot)	T38.5X1	T38.5X2	T38.5X3	T38.5X4	T38.5X5	T38.5X6
Medrysone	T49.0X1	T49.0X2	T49.0X3	T49.0X4	T49.0X5	T49.0X6
Mefenamic acid	T39.391	T39.392	T39.393	T39.394	T39.395	T39.396
Mefenorex	T50.5X1	T50.5X2	T50.5X3	T50.5X4	T50.5X5	T50.5X6
Mefloquine	T37.2X1	T37.2X2	T37.2X3	T37.2X4	T37.2X5	T37.2X6
Mefruside	T50.2X1	T50.2X2	T50.2X3	T50.2X4	T50.2X5	T50.2X6
Megahallucinogen	T40.901	T40.902	T40.903	T40.904	T40.905	T40.906
Megestrol	T38.5X1	T38.5X2	T38.5X3	T38.5X4	T38.5X5	T38.5X6
Meglumine						
antimoniate	T37.8X1	T37.8X2	T37.8X3	T37.8X4	T37.8X5	T37.8X6
diatrizoate	T50.8X1	T50.8X2	T50.8X3	T50.8X4	T50.8X5	T50.8X6
iodipamide	T50.8X1	T50.8X2	T50.8X3	T50.8X4	T50.8X5	T50.8X6
iotroxate	T50.8X1	T50.8X2	T50.8X3	T50.8X4	T50.8X5	T50.8X6
MEK (methyl ethyl ketone)	T52.4X1	T52.4X2	T52.4X3	T52.4X4	—	—
Meladinin	T49.3X1	T49.3X2	T49.3X3	T49.3X4	T49.3X5	T49.3X6
Meladrazine	T44.3X1	T44.3X2	T44.3X3	T44.3X4	T44.3X5	T44.3X6

Substance	Poisoning, Accidental (unintentional)	Poisoning, Intentional Self-harm	Poisoning, Assault	Poisoning, Undetermined	Adverse Effect	Under-dosing
Melaleuca alternifolia oil	T49.0X1	T49.0X2	T49.0X3	T49.0X4	T49.0X5	T49.0X6
Melanizing agents	T49.3X1	T49.3X2	T49.3X3	T49.3X4	T49.3X5	T49.3X6
Melanocyte-stimulating hormone	T38.891	T38.892	T38.893	T38.894	T38.895	T38.896
Melarsonyl potassium	T37.3X1	T37.3X2	T37.3X3	T37.3X4	T37.3X5	T37.3X6
Melarsoprol	T37.3X1	T37.3X2	T37.3X3	T37.3X4	T37.3X5	T37.3X6
Melia azedarach	T62.2X1	T62.2X2	T62.2X3	T62.2X4	—	—
Melitracen	T43.011	T43.012	T43.013	T43.014	T43.015	T43.016
Mellaril	T43.3X1	T43.3X2	T43.3X3	T43.3X4	T43.3X5	T43.3X6
Meloxine	T49.3X1	T49.3X2	T49.3X3	T49.3X4	T49.3X5	T49.3X6
Melperone	T43.4X1	T43.4X2	T43.4X3	T43.4X4	T43.4X5	T43.4X6
Melphalan	T45.1X1	T45.1X2	T45.1X3	T45.1X4	T45.1X5	T45.1X6
Memantine	T43.8X1	T43.8X2	T43.8X3	T43.8X4	T43.8X5	T43.8X6
Menadiol	T45.7X1	T45.7X2	T45.7X3	T45.7X4	T45.7X5	T45.7X6
sodium sulfate	T45.7X1	T45.7X2	T45.7X3	T45.7X4	T45.7X5	T45.7X6
Menadione	T45.7X1	T45.7X2	T45.7X3	T45.7X4	T45.7X5	T45.7X6
sodium bisulfite	T45.7X1	T45.7X2	T45.7X3	T45.7X4	T45.7X5	T45.7X6
Menaphthone	T45.7X1	T45.7X2	T45.7X3	T45.7X4	T45.7X5	T45.7X6
Menaquinone	T45.7X1	T45.7X2	T45.7X3	T45.7X4	T45.7X5	T45.7X6
Menatetrenone	T45.7X1	T45.7X2	T45.7X3	T45.7X4	T45.7X5	T45.7X6
Meningococcal vaccine	T50.A91	T50.A92	T50.A93	T50.A94	T50.A95	T50.A96
Meningovax (-AC) (-C)	T50.A91	T50.A92	T50.A93	T50.A94	T50.A95	T50.A96
Menotropins	T38.811	T38.812	T38.813	T38.814	T38.815	T38.816
Menthol	T48.5X1	T48.5X2	T48.5X3	T48.5X4	T48.5X5	T48.5X6
Mepacrine	T37.2X1	T37.2X2	T37.2X3	T37.2X4	T37.2X5	T37.2X6
Meparfynol	T42.6X1	T42.6X2	T42.6X3	T42.6X4	T42.6X5	T42.6X6
Mepartricin	T36.7X1	T36.7X2	T36.7X3	T36.7X4	T36.7X5	T36.7X6
Mepazine	T43.3X1	T43.3X2	T43.3X3	T43.3X4	T43.3X5	T43.3X6
Mepenzolate	T44.3X1	T44.3X2	T44.3X3	T44.3X4	T44.3X5	T44.3X6
bromide	T44.3X1	T44.3X2	T44.3X3	T44.3X4	T44.3X5	T44.3X6
Meperidine	T40.4X1	T40.4X2	T40.4X3	T40.4X4	T40.4X5	T40.4X6
Mephebarbital	T42.3X1	T42.3X2	T42.3X3	T42.3X4	T42.3X5	T42.3X6
Mephenamin (e)	T42.8X1	T42.8X2	T42.8X3	T42.8X4	T42.8X5	T42.8X6
Mephenesin	T42.8X1	T42.8X2	T42.8X3	T42.8X4	T42.8X5	T42.8X6
Mephenhydramine	T45.0X1	T45.0X2	T45.0X3	T45.0X4	T45.0X5	T45.0X6
Mephenoxalone	T42.8X1	T42.8X2	T42.8X3	T42.8X4	T42.8X5	T42.8X6
Mephentermine	T44.991	T44.992	T44.993	T44.994	T44.995	T44.996
Mephenytoin	T42.0X1	T42.0X2	T42.0X3	T42.0X4	T42.0X5	T42.0X6
with phenobarbital	T42.3X1	T42.3X2	T42.3X3	T42.3X4	T42.3X5	T42.3X6
Mephobarbital	T42.3X1	T42.3X2	T42.3X3	T42.3X4	T42.3X5	T42.3X6
Mephosfolan	T60.0X1	T60.0X2	T60.0X3	T60.0X4	—	—
Mepindolol	T44.7X1	T44.7X2	T44.7X3	T44.7X4	T44.7X5	T44.7X6
Mepiperphenidol	T44.3X1	T44.3X2	T44.3X3	T44.3X4	T44.3X5	T44.3X6
Mepitiostane	T38.7X1	T38.7X2	T38.7X3	T38.7X4	T38.7X5	T38.7X6
Mepivacaine	T41.3X1	T41.3X2	T41.3X3	T41.3X4	T41.3X5	T41.3X6
epidural	T41.3X1	T41.3X2	T41.3X3	T41.3X4	T41.3X5	T41.3X6
Meprednisone	T38.0X1	T38.0X2	T38.0X3	T38.0X4	T38.0X5	T38.0X6
Meprobam	T43.591	T43.592	T43.593	T43.594	T43.595	T43.596
Meprobamate	T43.591	T43.592	T43.593	T43.594	T43.595	T43.596
Meproscillarin	T46.0X1	T46.0X2	T46.0X3	T46.0X4	T46.0X5	T46.0X6
Meprylcaine	T41.3X1	T41.3X2	T41.3X3	T41.3X4	T41.3X5	T41.3X6
Meptazinol	T39.8X1	T39.8X2	T39.8X3	T39.8X4	T39.8X5	T39.8X6
Mepyramine	T45.0X1	T45.0X2	T45.0X3	T45.0X4	T45.0X5	T45.0X6
Mequitazine	T43.3X1	T43.3X2	T43.3X3	T43.3X4	T43.3X5	T43.3X6
Meralluride	T50.2X1	T50.2X2	T50.2X3	T50.2X4	T50.2X5	T50.2X6
Merbaphen	T50.2X1	T50.2X2	T50.2X3	T50.2X4	T50.2X5	T50.2X6
Merbromin	T49.0X1	T49.0X2	T49.0X3	T49.0X4	T49.0X5	T49.0X6
Mercaptobenzothiazole salts	T49.0X1	T49.0X2	T49.0X3	T49.0X4	T49.0X5	T49.0X6
Mercaptomerin	T50.2X1	T50.2X2	T50.2X3	T50.2X4	T50.2X5	T50.2X6
Mercaptopurine	T45.1X1	T45.1X2	T45.1X3	T45.1X4	T45.1X5	T45.1X6
Mercumatilin	T50.2X1	T50.2X2	T50.2X3	T50.2X4	T50.2X5	T50.2X6
Mercuramide	T50.2X1	T50.2X2	T50.2X3	T50.2X4	T50.2X5	T50.2X6
Mercurochrome	T49.0X1	T49.0X2	T49.0X3	T49.0X4	T49.0X5	T49.0X6
Mercurophylline	T50.2X1	T50.2X2	T50.2X3	T50.2X4	T50.2X5	T50.2X6
Mercury, mercurial, mercuric, mercurous (compounds) (cyanide) (fumes) (nonmedicinal) (vapor) NEC	T56.1X1	T56.1X2	T56.1X3	T56.1X4	—	—
ammoniated	T49.0X1	T49.0X2	T49.0X3	T49.0X4	T49.0X5	T49.0X6
anti-infective						
local	T49.0X1	T49.0X2	T49.0X3	T49.0X4	T49.0X5	T49.0X6
systemic	T37.8X1	T37.8X2	T37.8X3	T37.8X4	T37.8X5	T37.8X6
topical	T49.0X1	T49.0X2	T49.0X3	T49.0X4	T49.0X5	T49.0X6
chloride (ammoniated)	T49.0X1	T49.0X2	T49.0X3	T49.0X4	T49.0X5	T49.0X6
fungicide	T56.1X1	T56.1X2	T56.1X3	T56.1X4	—	—
diuretic NEC	T50.2X1	T50.2X2	T50.2X3	T50.2X4	T50.2X5	T50.2X6
fungicide	T56.1X1	T56.1X2	T56.1X3	T56.1X4	—	—
organic (fungicide)	T56.1X1	T56.1X2	T56.1X3	T56.1X4	—	—
oxide, yellow	T49.0X1	T49.0X2	T49.0X3	T49.0X4	T49.0X5	T49.0X6
Mersalyl	T50.2X1	T50.2X2	T50.2X3	T50.2X4	T50.2X5	T50.2X6
Merthiolate	T49.0X1	T49.0X2	T49.0X3	T49.0X4	T49.0X5	T49.0X6
Merthiolate — continued						
ophthalmic preparation	T49.5X1	T49.5X2	T49.5X3	T49.5X4	T49.5X5	T49.5X6
Meruvax	T50.B91	T50.B92	T50.B93	T50.B94	T50.B95	T50.B96
Mesalazine	T47.8X1	T47.8X2	T47.8X3	T47.8X4	T47.8X5	T47.8X6
Mescal buttons	T40.991	T40.992	T40.993	T40.994	—	—
Mescaline	T40.991	T40.992	T40.993	T40.994	—	—
Mesna	T48.4X1	T48.4X2	T48.4X3	T48.4X4	T48.4X5	T48.4X6
Mesoglycan	T46.6X1	T46.6X2	T46.6X3	T46.6X4	T46.6X5	T46.6X6
Mesoridazine	T43.3X1	T43.3X2	T43.3X3	T43.3X4	T43.3X5	T43.3X6
Mestanolone	T38.7X1	T38.7X2	T38.7X3	T38.7X4	T38.7X5	T38.7X6
Mesterolone	T38.7X1	T38.7X2	T38.7X3	T38.7X4	T38.7X5	T38.7X6
Mestranol	T38.5X1	T38.5X2	T38.5X3	T38.5X4	T38.5X5	T38.5X6
Mesulergine	T42.8X1	T42.8X2	T42.8X3	T42.8X4	T42.8X5	T42.8X6
Mesulfen	T49.0X1	T49.0X2	T49.0X3	T49.0X4	T49.0X5	T49.0X6
Mesuximide	T42.2X1	T42.2X2	T42.2X3	T42.2X4	T42.2X5	T42.2X6
Metabutethamine	T41.3X1	T41.3X2	T41.3X3	T41.3X4	T41.3X5	T41.3X6
Metactesylacetate	T49.0X1	T49.0X2	T49.0X3	T49.0X4	T49.0X5	T49.0X6
Metacycline	T36.4X1	T36.4X2	T36.4X3	T36.4X4	T36.4X5	T36.4X6
Metaldehyde (snail killer) NEC	T60.8X1	T60.8X2	T60.8X3	T60.8X4		
Metals (heavy) (nonmedicinal)	T56.91	T56.92	T56.93	T56.94	—	—
dust, fumes, or vapor NEC	T56.91	T56.92	T56.93	T56.94	—	—
light NEC	T56.91	T56.92	T56.93	T56.94	—	—
dust, fumes, or vapor NEC	T56.91	T56.92	T56.93	T56.94	—	—
specified NEC	T56.891	T56.892	T56.893	T56.894	—	—
thallium	T56.811	T56.812	T56.813	T56.814	—	—
Metamfetamine	T43.621	T43.622	T43.623	T43.624	T43.625	T43.626
Metamizole sodium	T39.2X1	T39.2X2	T39.2X3	T39.2X4	T39.2X5	T39.2X6
Metampicillin	T36.0X1	T36.0X2	T36.0X3	T36.0X4	T36.0X5	T36.0X6
Metamucil	T47.4X1	T47.4X2	T47.4X3	T47.4X4	T47.4X5	T47.4X6
Metandienone	T38.7X1	T38.7X2	T38.7X3	T38.7X4	T38.7X5	T38.7X6
Metandrostenolone	T38.7X1	T38.7X2	T38.7X3	T38.7X4	T38.7X5	T38.7X6
Metaphen	T49.0X1	T49.0X2	T49.0X3	T49.0X4	T49.0X5	T49.0X6
Metaphos	T60.0X1	T60.0X2	T60.0X3	T60.0X4		
Metapramine	T43.011	T43.012	T43.013	T43.014	T43.015	T43.016
Metaproterenol	T48.291	T48.292	T48.293	T48.294	T48.295	T48.296
Metaraminol	T44.4X1	T44.4X2	T44.4X3	T44.4X4	T44.4X5	T44.4X6
Metaxalone	T42.8X1	T42.8X2	T42.8X3	T42.8X4	T42.8X5	T42.8X6
Metenolone	T38.7X1	T38.7X2	T38.7X3	T38.7X4	T38.7X5	T38.7X6
Metergoline	T42.8X1	T42.8X2	T42.8X3	T42.8X4	T42.8X5	T42.8X6
Metescufylline	T46.991	T46.992	T46.993	T46.994	T46.995	T46.996
Metetoin	T42.0X1	T42.0X2	T42.0X3	T42.0X4	T42.0X5	T42.0X6
Metformin	T38.3X1	T38.3X2	T38.3X3	T38.3X4	T38.3X5	T38.3X6
Methacholine	T44.1X1	T44.1X2	T44.1X3	T44.1X4	T44.1X5	T44.1X6
Methacycline	T36.4X1	T36.4X2	T36.4X3	T36.4X4	T36.4X5	T36.4X6
Methadone	T40.3X1	T40.3X2	T40.3X3	T40.3X4	T40.3X5	T40.3X6
Methallenestril	T38.5X1	T38.5X2	T38.5X3	T38.5X4	T38.5X5	T38.5X6
Methallenoestril	T38.5X1	T38.5X2	T38.5X3	T38.5X4	T38.5X5	T38.5X6
Methamphetamine	T43.621	T43.622	T43.623	T43.624	T43.625	T43.626
Methampyrone	T39.2X1	T39.2X2	T39.2X3	T39.2X4	T39.2X5	T39.2X6
Methandienone	T38.7X1	T38.7X2	T38.7X3	T38.7X4	T38.7X5	T38.7X6
Methandriol	T38.7X1	T38.7X2	T38.7X3	T38.7X4	T38.7X5	T38.7X6
Methandrostenolone	T38.7X1	T38.7X2	T38.7X3	T38.7X4	T38.7X5	T38.7X6
Methane	T59.891	T59.892	T59.893	T59.894	—	—
Methanethiol	T59.891	T59.892	T59.893	T59.894	—	—
Methaniazide	T37.1X1	T37.1X2	T37.1X3	T37.1X4	T37.1X5	T37.1X6
Methanol (vapor)	T51.1X1	T51.1X2	T51.1X3	T51.1X4	—	—
Methantheline	T44.3X1	T44.3X2	T44.3X3	T44.3X4	T44.3X5	T44.3X6
Methanthelinium bromide	T44.3X1	T44.3X2	T44.3X3	T44.3X4	T44.3X5	T44.3X6
Methaphenilene	T45.0X1	T45.0X2	T45.0X3	T45.0X4	T45.0X5	T45.0X6
Methapyrilene	T45.0X1	T45.0X2	T45.0X3	T45.0X4	T45.0X5	T45.0X6
Methaqualone (compound)	T42.6X1	T42.6X2	T42.6X3	T42.6X4	T42.6X5	T42.6X6
Metharbital	T42.3X1	T42.3X2	T42.3X3	T42.3X4	T42.3X5	T42.3X6
Methazolamide	T50.2X1	T50.2X2	T50.2X3	T50.2X4	T50.2X5	T50.2X6
Methdilazine	T43.3X1	T43.3X2	T43.3X3	T43.3X4	T43.3X5	T43.3X6
Methedrine	T43.621	T43.622	T43.623	T43.624	T43.625	T43.626
Methenamine (mandelate)	T37.8X1	T37.8X2	T37.8X3	T37.8X4	T37.8X5	T37.8X6
Methenolone	T38.7X1	T38.7X2	T38.7X3	T38.7X4	T38.7X5	T38.7X6
Methergine	T48.0X1	T48.0X2	T48.0X3	T48.0X4	T48.0X5	T48.0X6
Methetoin	T42.0X1	T42.0X2	T42.0X3	T42.0X4	T42.0X5	T42.0X6
Methiacil	T38.2X1	T38.2X2	T38.2X3	T38.2X4	T38.2X5	T38.2X6
Methicillin	T36.0X1	T36.0X2	T36.0X3	T36.0X4	T36.0X5	T36.0X6
Methimazole	T38.2X1	T38.2X2	T38.2X3	T38.2X4	T38.2X5	T38.2X6
Methiodal sodium	T50.8X1	T50.8X2	T50.8X3	T50.8X4	T50.8X5	T50.8X6
Methionine	T50.991	T50.992	T50.993	T50.994	T50.995	T50.996
Methisazone	T37.5X1	T37.5X2	T37.5X3	T37.5X4	T37.5X5	T37.5X6
Methisoprinol	T37.5X1	T37.5X2	T37.5X3	T37.5X4	T37.5X5	T37.5X6
Methitural	T42.3X1	T42.3X2	T42.3X3	T42.3X4	T42.3X5	T42.3X6
Methixene	T44.3X1	T44.3X2	T44.3X3	T44.3X4	T44.3X5	T44.3X6
Methobarbital, methobarbitone	T42.3X1	T42.3X2	T42.3X3	T42.3X4	T42.3X5	T42.3X6
Methocarbamol	T42.8X1	T42.8X2	T42.8X3	T42.8X4	T42.8X5	T42.8X6

Substance	Poisoning, Accidental (unintentional)	Poisoning, Intentional Self-harm	Poisoning, Assault	Poisoning, Undetermined	Adverse Effect	Under-dosing
Methocarbamol — *continued*						
skeletal muscle relaxant	T48.1X1	T48.1X2	T48.1X3	T48.1X4	T48.1X5	T48.1X6
Methohexital	T41.1X1	T41.1X2	T41.1X3	T41.1X4	T41.1X5	T41.1X6
Methohexitone	T41.1X1	T41.1X2	T41.1X3	T41.1X4	T41.1X5	T41.1X6
Methoin	T42.0X1	T42.0X2	T42.0X3	T42.0X4	T42.0X5	T42.0X6
Methopholine	T39.8X1	T39.8X2	T39.8X3	T39.8X4	T39.8X5	T39.8X6
Methopromazine	T43.3X1	T43.3X2	T43.3X3	T43.3X4	T43.3X5	T43.3X6
Methorate	T48.3X1	T48.3X2	T48.3X3	T48.3X4	T48.3X5	T48.3X6
Methoserpidine	T46.5X1	T46.5X2	T46.5X3	T46.5X4	T46.5X5	T46.5X6
Methotrexate	T45.1X1	T45.1X2	T45.1X3	T45.1X4	T45.1X5	T45.1X6
Methotrimeprazine	T43.3X1	T43.3X2	T43.3X3	T43.3X4	T43.3X5	T43.3X6
Methoxa-Dome	T49.3X1	T49.3X2	T49.3X3	T49.3X4	T49.3X5	T49.3X6
Methoxamine	T44.4X1	T44.4X2	T44.4X3	T44.4X4	T44.4X5	T44.4X6
Methoxsalen	T50.991	T50.992	T50.993	T50.994	T50.995	T50.996
Methoxyaniline	T65.3X1	T65.3X2	T65.3X3	T65.3X4	—	—
Methoxybenzyl penicillin	T36.0X1	T36.0X2	T36.0X3	T36.0X4	T36.0X5	T36.0X6
Methoxychlor	T53.7X1	T53.7X2	T53.7X3	T53.7X4	—	—
Methoxy-DDT	T53.7X1	T53.7X2	T53.7X3	T53.7X4	—	—
Methoxyflurane	T41.0X1	T41.0X2	T41.0X3	T41.0X4	T41.0X5	T41.0X6
Methoxyphenamine	T48.6X1	T48.6X2	T48.6X3	T48.6X4	T48.6X5	T48.6X6
Methoxypromazine	T43.3X1	T43.3X2	T43.3X3	T43.3X4	T43.3X5	T43.3X6
Methscopolamine bromide	T44.3X1	T44.3X2	T44.3X3	T44.3X4	T44.3X5	T44.3X6
Methsuximide	T42.2X1	T42.2X2	T42.2X3	T42.2X4	T42.2X5	T42.2X6
Methyclothiazide	T50.2X1	T50.2X2	T50.2X3	T50.2X4	T50.2X5	T50.2X6
Methyl						
acetate	T52.4X1	T52.4X2	T52.4X3	T52.4X4	—	—
acetone	T52.4X1	T52.4X2	T52.4X3	T52.4X4	—	—
acrylate	T65.891	T65.892	T65.893	T65.894	—	—
alcohol	T51.1X1	T51.1X2	T51.1X3	T51.1X4	—	—
aminophenol	T65.3X1	T65.3X2	T65.3X3	T65.3X4	—	—
amphetamine	T43.621	T43.622	T43.623	T43.624	T43.625	T43.626
androstanolone	T38.7X1	T38.7X2	T38.7X3	T38.7X4	T38.7X5	T38.7X6
atropine	T44.3X1	T44.3X2	T44.3X3	T44.3X4	T44.3X5	T44.3X6
benzene	T52.2X1	T52.2X2	T52.2X3	T52.2X4	—	—
benzoate	T52.8X1	T52.8X2	T52.8X3	T52.8X4	—	—
benzol	T52.2X1	T52.2X2	T52.2X3	T52.2X4	—	—
bromide (gas)	T59.891	T59.892	T59.893	T59.894	—	—
fumigant	T60.8X1	T60.8X2	T60.8X3	T60.8X4	—	—
butanol	T51.3X1	T51.3X2	T51.3X3	T51.3X4	—	—
carbinol	T51.1X1	T51.1X2	T51.1X3	T51.1X4	—	—
carbonate	T52.8X1	T52.8X2	T52.8X3	T52.8X4	—	—
CCNU	T45.1X1	T45.1X2	T45.1X3	T45.1X4	T45.1X5	T45.1X6
cellosolve	T52.91	T52.92	T52.93	T52.94	—	—
cellulose	T47.4X1	T47.4X2	T47.4X3	T47.4X4	T47.4X5	T47.4X6
chloride (gas)	T59.891	T59.892	T59.893	T59.894	—	—
chloroformate	T59.3X1	T59.3X2	T59.3X3	T59.3X4	—	—
cyclohexane	T52.8X1	T52.8X2	T52.8X3	T52.8X4	—	—
cyclohexanol	T51.8X1	T51.8X2	T51.8X3	T51.8X4	—	—
cyclohexanone	T52.8X1	T52.8X2	T52.8X3	T52.8X4	—	—
cyclohexyl acetate	T52.8X1	T52.8X2	T52.8X3	T52.8X4	—	—
demeton	T60.0X1	T60.0X2	T60.0X3	T60.0X4	—	—
dihydromorphinone	T40.2X1	T40.2X2	T40.2X3	T40.2X4	T40.2X5	T40.2X6
ergometrine	T48.0X1	T48.0X2	T48.0X3	T48.0X4	T48.0X5	T48.0X6
ergonovine	T48.0X1	T48.0X2	T48.0X3	T48.0X4	T48.0X5	T48.0X6
ethyl ketone	T52.4X1	T52.4X2	T52.4X3	T52.4X4	—	—
glucamine antimonate	T37.8X1	T37.8X2	T37.8X3	T37.8X4	T37.8X5	T37.8X6
hydrazine	T65.891	T65.892	T65.893	T65.894	—	—
iodide	T65.891	T65.892	T65.893	T65.894	—	—
isobutyl ketone	T52.4X1	T52.4X2	T52.4X3	T52.4X4	—	—
isothiocyanate	T60.3X1	T60.3X2	T60.3X3	T60.3X4	—	—
mercaptan	T59.891	T59.892	T59.893	T59.894	—	—
morphine NEC	T40.2X1	T40.2X2	T40.2X3	T40.2X4	T40.2X5	T40.2X6
nicotinate	T49.4X1	T49.4X2	T49.4X3	T49.4X4	T49.4X5	T49.4X6
paraben	T49.0X1	T49.0X2	T49.0X3	T49.0X4	T49.0X5	T49.0X6
parafynol	T42.6X1	T42.6X2	T42.6X3	T42.6X4	T42.6X5	T42.6X6
parathion	T60.0X1	T60.0X2	T60.0X3	T60.0X4	—	—
peridol	T43.4X1	T43.4X2	T43.4X3	T43.4X4	T43.4X5	T43.4X6
phenidate	T43.631	T43.632	T43.633	T43.634	T43.635	T43.636
prednisolone	T38.0X1	T38.0X2	T38.0X3	T38.0X4	T38.0X5	T38.0X6
ENT agent	T49.6X1	T49.6X2	T49.6X3	T49.6X4	T49.6X5	T49.6X6
ophthalmic preparation	T49.5X1	T49.5X2	T49.5X3	T49.5X4	T49.5X5	T49.5X6
topical NEC	T49.0X1	T49.0X2	T49.0X3	T49.0X4	T49.0X5	T49.0X6
propylcarbinol	T51.3X1	T51.3X2	T51.3X3	T51.3X4	—	—
rosaniline NEC	T49.0X1	T49.0X2	T49.0X3	T49.0X4	T49.0X5	T49.0X6
salicylate	T49.2X1	T49.2X2	T49.2X3	T49.2X4	T49.2X5	T49.2X6
sulfate (fumes)	T59.891	T59.892	T59.893	T59.894	—	—
liquid	T52.8X1	T52.8X2	T52.8X3	T52.8X4	—	—
sulfonal	T42.6X1	T42.6X2	T42.6X3	T42.6X4	T42.6X5	T42.6X6
testosterone	T38.7X1	T38.7X2	T38.7X3	T38.7X4	T38.7X5	T38.7X6
thiouracil	T38.2X1	T38.2X2	T38.2X3	T38.2X4	T38.2X5	T38.2X6
Methylamphetamine	T43.621	T43.622	T43.623	T43.624	T43.625	T43.626
Methylated spirit	T51.1X1	T51.1X2	T51.1X3	T51.1X4	—	—
Methylatropine nitrate	T44.3X1	T44.3X2	T44.3X3	T44.3X4	T44.3X5	T44.3X6

Substance	Poisoning, Accidental (unintentional)	Poisoning, Intentional Self-harm	Poisoning, Assault	Poisoning, Undetermined	Adverse Effect	Under-dosing
Methylbenactyzium bromide	T44.3X1	T44.3X2	T44.3X3	T44.3X4	T44.3X5	T44.3X6
Methylbenzethonium chloride	T49.0X1	T49.0X2	T49.0X3	T49.0X4	T49.0X5	T49.0X6
Methylcellulose	T47.4X1	T47.4X2	T47.4X3	T47.4X4	T47.4X5	T47.4X6
laxative	T47.4X1	T47.4X2	T47.4X3	T47.4X4	T47.4X5	T47.4X6
Methylchlorophenoxyacetic acid	T60.3X1	T60.3X2	T60.3X3	T60.3X4	—	—
Methyldopa	T46.5X1	T46.5X2	T46.5X3	T46.5X4	T46.5X5	T46.5X6
Methyldopate	T46.5X1	T46.5X2	T46.5X3	T46.5X4	T46.5X5	T46.5X6
Methylene						
blue	T50.6X1	T50.6X2	T50.6X3	T50.6X4	T50.6X5	T50.6X6
chloride or dichloride (solvent) NEC	T53.4X1	T53.4X2	T53.4X3	T53.4X4	—	—
Methylenedioxyamphetamine	T43.621	T43.622	T43.623	T43.624	T43.625	T43.626
Methylenedioxymethamphetamine	T43.621	T43.622	T43.623	T43.624	T43.625	T43.626
Methylergometrine	T48.0X1	T48.0X2	T48.0X3	T48.0X4	T48.0X5	T48.0X6
Methylergonovine	T48.0X1	T48.0X2	T48.0X3	T48.0X4	T48.0X5	T48.0X6
Methylestrenolone	T38.5X1	T38.5X2	T38.5X3	T38.5X4	T38.5X5	T38.5X6
Methylethyl cellulose	T50.991	T50.992	T50.993	T50.994	T50.995	T50.996
Methylhexabital	T42.3X1	T42.3X2	T42.3X3	T42.3X4	T42.3X5	T42.3X6
Methylmorphine	T40.2X1	T40.2X2	T40.2X3	T40.2X4	T40.2X5	T40.2X6
Methylparaben (ophthalmic)	T49.5X1	T49.5X2	T49.5X3	T49.5X4	T49.5X5	T49.5X6
Methylparafynol	T42.6X1	T42.6X2	T42.6X3	T42.6X4	T42.6X5	T42.6X6
Methylpentynol, methylpenthynol	T42.6X1	T42.6X2	T42.6X3	T42.6X4	T42.6X5	T42.6X6
Methylphenidate	T43.631	T43.632	T43.633	T43.634	T43.635	T43.636
Methylphenobarbital	T42.3X1	T42.3X2	T42.3X3	T42.3X4	T42.3X5	T42.3X6
Methylpolysiloxane	T47.1X1	T47.1X2	T47.1X3	T47.1X4	T47.1X5	T47.1X6
Methylprednisolone — *see* Methyl, prednisolone						
Methylrosaniline	T49.0X1	T49.0X2	T49.0X3	T49.0X4	T49.0X5	T49.0X6
Methylrosanilinium chloride	T49.0X1	T49.0X2	T49.0X3	T49.0X4	T49.0X5	T49.0X6
Methyltestosterone	T38.7X1	T38.7X2	T38.7X3	T38.7X4	T38.7X5	T38.7X6
Methylthionine chloride	T50.6X1	T50.6X2	T50.6X3	T50.6X4	T50.6X5	T50.6X6
Methylthioninium chloride	T50.6X1	T50.6X2	T50.6X3	T50.6X4	T50.6X5	T50.6X6
Methylthiouracil	T38.2X1	T38.2X2	T38.2X3	T38.2X4	T38.2X5	T38.2X6
Methyprylon	T42.6X1	T42.6X2	T42.6X3	T42.6X4	T42.6X5	T42.6X6
Methysergide	T46.5X1	T46.5X2	T46.5X3	T46.5X4	T46.5X5	T46.5X6
Metiamide	T47.1X1	T47.1X2	T47.1X3	T47.1X4	T47.1X5	T47.1X6
Meticillin	T36.0X1	T36.0X2	T36.0X3	T36.0X4	T36.0X5	T36.0X6
Meticrane	T50.2X1	T50.2X2	T50.2X3	T50.2X4	T50.2X5	T50.2X6
Metildigoxin	T46.0X1	T46.0X2	T46.0X3	T46.0X4	T46.0X5	T46.0X6
Metipranolol	T49.5X1	T49.5X2	T49.5X3	T49.5X4	T49.5X5	T49.5X6
Metirosine	T46.5X1	T46.5X2	T46.5X3	T46.5X4	T46.5X5	T46.5X6
Metisazone	T37.5X1	T37.5X2	T37.5X3	T37.5X4	T37.5X5	T37.5X6
Metixene	T44.3X1	T44.3X2	T44.3X3	T44.3X4	T44.3X5	T44.3X6
Metizoline	T48.5X1	T48.5X2	T48.5X3	T48.5X4	T48.5X5	T48.5X6
Metoclopramide	T45.0X1	T45.0X2	T45.0X3	T45.0X4	T45.0X5	T45.0X6
Metofenazate	T43.3X1	T43.3X2	T43.3X3	T43.3X4	T43.3X5	T43.3X6
Metofoline	T39.8X1	T39.8X2	T39.8X3	T39.8X4	T39.8X5	T39.8X6
Metolazone	T50.2X1	T50.2X2	T50.2X3	T50.2X4	T50.2X5	T50.2X6
Metopon	T40.2X1	T40.2X2	T40.2X3	T40.2X4	T40.2X5	T40.2X6
Metoprine	T45.1X1	T45.1X2	T45.1X3	T45.1X4	T45.1X5	T45.1X6
Metoprolol	T44.7X1	T44.7X2	T44.7X3	T44.7X4	T44.7X5	T44.7X6
Metrifonate	T60.0X1	T60.0X2	T60.0X3	T60.0X4	—	—
Metrizamide	T50.8X1	T50.8X2	T50.8X3	T50.8X4	T50.8X5	T50.8X6
Metrizoic acid	T50.8X1	T50.8X2	T50.8X3	T50.8X4	T50.8X5	T50.8X6
Metronidazole	T37.8X1	T37.8X2	T37.8X3	T37.8X4	T37.8X5	T37.8X6
Metycaine	T41.3X1	T41.3X2	T41.3X3	T41.3X4	T41.3X5	T41.3X6
infiltration (subcutaneous)	T41.3X1	T41.3X2	T41.3X3	T41.3X4	T41.3X5	T41.3X6
nerve block (peripheral) (plexus)	T41.3X1	T41.3X2	T41.3X3	T41.3X4	T41.3X5	T41.3X6
topical (surface)	T41.3X1	T41.3X2	T41.3X3	T41.3X4	T41.3X5	T41.3X6
Metyrapone	T50.8X1	T50.8X2	T50.8X3	T50.8X4	T50.8X5	T50.8X6
Mevinphos	T60.0X1	T60.0X2	T60.0X3	T60.0X4	—	—
Mexazolam	T42.4X1	T42.4X2	T42.4X3	T42.4X4	T42.4X5	T42.4X6
Mexenone	T49.3X1	T49.3X2	T49.3X3	T49.3X4	T49.3X5	T49.3X6
Mexiletine	T46.2X1	T46.2X2	T46.2X3	T46.2X4	T46.2X5	T46.2X6
Mezereon	T62.2X1	T62.2X2	T62.2X3	T62.2X4	—	—
berries	T62.1X1	T62.1X2	T62.1X3	T62.1X4	—	—
Mezlocillin	T36.0X1	T36.0X2	T36.0X3	T36.0X4	T36.0X5	T36.0X6
Mianserin	T43.021	T43.022	T43.023	T43.024	T43.025	T43.026
Micatin	T49.0X1	T49.0X2	T49.0X3	T49.0X4	T49.0X5	T49.0X6
Miconazole	T49.0X1	T49.0X2	T49.0X3	T49.0X4	T49.0X5	T49.0X6
Micronomicin	T36.5X1	T36.5X2	T36.5X3	T36.5X4	T36.5X5	T36.5X6
Midazolam	T42.4X1	T42.4X2	T42.4X3	T42.4X4	T42.4X5	T42.4X6
Midecamycin	T36.3X1	T36.3X2	T36.3X3	T36.3X4	T36.3X5	T36.3X6
Mifepristone	T38.6X1	T38.6X2	T38.6X3	T38.6X4	T38.6X5	T38.6X6
Milk of magnesia	T47.1X1	T47.1X2	T47.1X3	T47.1X4	T47.1X5	T47.1X6

Substance	Poisoning, Accidental (unintentional)	Poisoning, Intentional Self-harm	Poisoning, Assault	Poisoning, Undetermined	Adverse Effect	Under-dosing
Millipede (tropical)	T63.411	T63.412	T63.413	T63.414	—	—
(venomous)						
Miltown	T43.591	T43.592	T43.593	T43.594	T43.595	T43.596
Milverine	T44.3X1	T44.3X2	T44.3X3	T44.3X4	T44.3X5	T44.3X6
Minaprine	T43.291	T43.292	T43.293	T43.294	T43.295	T43.296
Minaxolone	T41.291	T41.292	T41.293	T41.294	T41.295	T41.296
Mineral						
acids	T54.2X1	T54.2X2	T54.2X3	T54.2X4	—	—
oil (laxative)(medicinal)	T47.4X1	T47.4X2	T47.4X3	T47.4X4	T47.4X5	T47.4X6
emulsion	T47.2X1	T47.2X2	T47.2X3	T47.2X4	T47.2X5	T47.2X6
nonmedicinal	T52.0X1	T52.0X2	T52.0X3	T52.0X4	—	—
topical	T49.3X1	T49.3X2	T49.3X3	T49.3X4	T49.3X5	T49.3X6
salt NEC	T50.3X1	T50.3X2	T50.3X3	T50.3X4	T50.3X5	T50.3X6
spirits	T52.0X1	T52.0X2	T52.0X3	T52.0X4	—	—
Mineralocorticosteroid	T50.0X1	T50.0X2	T50.0X3	T50.0X4	T50.0X5	T50.0X6
Minocycline	T36.4X1	T36.4X2	T36.4X3	T36.4X4	T36.4X5	T36.4X6
Minoxidil	T46.7X1	T46.7X2	T46.7X3	T46.7X4	T46.7X5	T46.7X6
Miokamycin	T36.3X1	T36.3X2	T36.3X3	T36.3X4	T36.3X5	T36.3X6
Miotic drug	T49.5X1	T49.5X2	T49.5X3	T49.5X4	T49.5X5	T49.5X6
Mipafox	T60.0X1	T60.0X2	T60.0X3	T60.0X4	—	—
Mirex	T60.1X1	T60.1X2	T60.1X3	T60.1X4	—	—
Mirtazapine	T43.021	T43.022	T43.023	T43.024	T43.025	T43.026
Misonidazole	T37.3X1	T37.3X2	T37.3X3	T37.3X4	T37.3X5	T37.3X6
Misoprostol	T47.1X1	T47.1X2	T47.1X3	T47.1X4	T47.1X5	T47.1X6
Mithramycin	T45.1X1	T45.1X2	T45.1X3	T45.1X4	T45.1X5	T45.1X6
Mitobronitol	T45.1X1	T45.1X2	T45.1X3	T45.1X4	T45.1X5	T45.1X6
Mitoguazone	T45.1X1	T45.1X2	T45.1X3	T45.1X4	T45.1X5	T45.1X6
Mitolactol	T45.1X1	T45.1X2	T45.1X3	T45.1X4	T45.1X5	T45.1X6
Mitomycin	T45.1X1	T45.1X2	T45.1X3	T45.1X4	T45.1X5	T45.1X6
Mitopodozide	T45.1X1	T45.1X2	T45.1X3	T45.1X4	T45.1X5	T45.1X6
Mitotane	T45.1X1	T45.1X2	T45.1X3	T45.1X4	T45.1X5	T45.1X6
Mitoxantrone	T45.1X1	T45.1X2	T45.1X3	T45.1X4	T45.1X5	T45.1X6
Mivacurium chloride	T48.1X1	T48.1X2	T48.1X3	T48.1X4	T48.1X5	T48.1X6
Miyari bacteria	T47.6X1	T47.6X2	T47.6X3	T47.6X4	T47.6X5	T47.6X6
Moclobemide	T43.1X1	T43.1X2	T43.1X3	T43.1X4	T43.1X5	T43.1X6
Moderil	T46.5X1	T46.5X2	T46.5X3	T46.5X4	T46.5X5	T46.5X6
Mofebutazone	T39.2X1	T39.2X2	T39.2X3	T39.2X4	T39.2X5	T39.2X6
Mogadon — see Nitrazepam						
Molindone	T43.591	T43.592	T43.593	T43.594	T43.595	T43.596
Molsidomine	T46.3X1	T46.3X2	T46.3X3	T46.3X4	T46.3X5	T46.3X6
Mometasone	T49.0X1	T49.0X2	T49.0X3	T49.0X4	T49.0X5	T49.0X6
Monistat	T49.0X1	T49.0X2	T49.0X3	T49.0X4	T49.0X5	T49.0X6
Monkshood	T62.2X1	T62.2X2	T62.2X3	T62.2X4	—	—
Monoamine oxidase inhibitor NEC	T43.1X1	T43.1X2	T43.1X3	T43.1X4	T43.1X5	T43.1X6
hydrazine	T43.1X1	T43.1X2	T43.1X3	T43.1X4	T43.1X5	T43.1X6
Monobenzone	T49.4X1	T49.4X2	T49.4X3	T49.4X4	T49.4X5	T49.4X6
Monochloroacetic acid	T60.3X1	T60.3X2	T60.3X3	T60.3X4	—	—
Monochlorobenzene	T53.7X1	T53.7X2	T53.7X3	T53.7X4	—	—
Monoethanolamine	T46.8X1	T46.8X2	T46.8X3	T46.8X4	T46.8X5	T46.8X6
oleate	T46.8X1	T46.8X2	T46.8X3	T46.8X4	T46.8X5	T46.8X6
Monooctanoin	T50.991	T50.992	T50.993	T50.994	T50.995	T50.996
Monophenylbutazone	T39.2X1	T39.2X2	T39.2X3	T39.2X4	T39.2X5	T39.2X6
Monosodium glutamate	T65.891	T65.892	T65.893	T65.894	—	—
Monosulfiram	T49.0X1	T49.0X2	T49.0X3	T49.0X4	T49.0X5	T49.0X6
Monoxide, carbon — see Carbon, monoxide						
Monoxidine hydrochloride	T46.1X1	T46.1X2	T46.1X3	T46.1X4	T46.1X5	T46.1X6
Monuron	T60.3X1	T60.3X2	T60.3X3	T60.3X4	—	—
Moperone	T43.4X1	T43.4X2	T43.4X3	T43.4X4	T43.4X5	T43.4X6
Mopidamol	T45.1X1	T45.1X2	T45.1X3	T45.1X4	T45.1X5	T45.1X6
MOPP (mechloreth-amine + vincristine + prednisone + procarba-zine)	T45.1X1	T45.1X2	T45.1X3	T45.1X4	T45.1X5	T45.1X6
Morfin	T40.2X1	T40.2X2	T40.2X3	T40.2X4	T40.2X5	T40.2X6
Morinamide	T37.1X1	T37.1X2	T37.1X3	T37.1X4	T37.1X5	T37.1X6
Morning glory seeds	T40.991	T40.992	T40.993	T40.994	—	—
Moroxydine	T37.5X1	T37.5X2	T37.5X3	T37.5X4	T37.5X5	T37.5X6
Morphazinamide	T37.1X1	T37.1X2	T37.1X3	T37.1X4	T37.1X5	T37.1X6
Morphine	T40.2X1	T40.2X2	T40.2X3	T40.2X4	T40.2X5	T40.2X6
antagonist	T50.7X1	T50.7X2	T50.7X3	T50.7X4		T50.7X6
Morpholinylethylmorphine	T40.2X1	T40.2X2	T40.2X3	T40.2X4	—	—
Morsuximide	T42.2X1	T42.2X2	T42.2X3	T42.2X4	T42.2X5	T42.2X6
Mosapramine	T43.591	T43.592	T43.593	T43.594	T43.595	T43.596
Moth balls — see also Pesticides						
naphthalene	T60.2X1	T60.2X2	T60.2X3	T60.2X4	—	—
paradichlorobenzene	T60.1X1	T60.1X2	T60.1X3	T60.1X4	—	—
Motor exhaust gas	T58.01	T58.02	T58.03	T58.04	—	—
Mouthwash (antiseptic) (zinc chloride)	T49.6X1	T49.6X2	T49.6X3	T49.6X4	T49.6X5	T49.6X6
Moxastine	T45.0X1	T45.0X2	T45.0X3	T45.0X4	T45.0X5	T45.0X6
Moxaverine	T44.3X1	T44.3X2	T44.3X3	T44.3X4	T44.3X5	T44.3X6
Moxisylyte	T46.7X1	T46.7X2	T46.7X3	T46.7X4	T46.7X5	T46.7X6
Mucilage, plant	T47.4X1	T47.4X2	T47.4X3	T47.4X4	T47.4X5	T47.4X6
Mucolytic drug	T48.4X1	T48.4X2	T48.4X3	T48.4X4	T48.4X5	T48.4X6
Mucomyst	T48.4X1	T48.4X2	T48.4X3	T48.4X4	T48.4X5	T48.4X6
Mucous membrane agents (external)	T49.91	T49.92	T49.93	T49.94	T49.95	T49.96
specified NEC	T49.8X1	T49.8X2	T49.8X3	T49.8X4	T49.8X5	T49.8X6
Mumps						
immune globulin (human)	T50.Z11	T50.Z12	T50.Z13	T50.Z14	T50.Z15	T50.Z16
skin test antigen	T50.8X1	T50.8X2	T50.8X3	T50.8X4	T50.8X5	T50.8X6
vaccine	T50.B91	T50.B92	T50.B93	T50.B94	T50.B95	T50.B96
Mumpsvax	T50.B91	T50.B92	T50.B93	T50.B94	T50.B95	T50.B96
Mupirocin	T49.0X1	T49.0X2	T49.0X3	T49.0X4	T49.0X5	T49.0X6
Muriatic acid — see Hydrochloric acid						
Muromonab-CD3	T45.1X1	T45.1X2	T45.1X3	T45.1X4	T45.1X5	T45.1X6
Muscle-action drug NEC	T48.201	T48.202	T48.203	T48.204	T48.205	T48.206
Muscle affecting agents NEC	T48.201	T48.202	T48.203	T48.204	T48.205	T48.206
oxytocic	T48.0X1	T48.0X2	T48.0X3	T48.0X4	T48.0X5	T48.0X6
relaxants	T48.201	T48.202	T48.203	T48.204	T48.205	T48.206
central nervous system	T42.8X1	T42.8X2	T42.8X3	T42.8X4	T42.8X5	T42.8X6
skeletal	T48.1X1	T48.1X2	T48.1X3	T48.1X4	T48.1X5	T48.1X6
smooth	T44.3X1	T44.3X2	T44.3X3	T44.3X4	T44.3X5	T44.3X6
Muscle relaxant — see Relaxant, muscle						
Muscle-tone depressant, central NEC	T42.8X1	T42.8X2	T42.8X3	T42.8X4	T42.8X5	T42.8X6
specified NEC	T42.8X1	T42.8X2	T42.8X3	T42.8X4	T42.8X5	T42.8X6
Mushroom, noxious	T62.0X1	T62.0X2	T62.0X3	T62.0X4	—	—
Mussel, noxious	T61.781	T61.782	T61.783	T61.784	—	—
Mustard (emetic)	T47.7X1	T47.7X2	T47.7X3	T47.7X4	T47.7X5	T47.7X6
black	T47.7X1	T47.7X2	T47.7X3	T47.7X4	T47.7X5	T47.7X6
gas, not in war	T59.91	T59.92	T59.93	T59.94	—	—
nitrogen	T45.1X1	T45.1X2	T45.1X3	T45.1X4	T45.1X5	T45.1X6
Mustine	T45.1X1	T45.1X2	T45.1X3	T45.1X4	T45.1X5	T45.1X6
M-vac	T45.1X1	T45.1X2	T45.1X3	T45.1X4	T45.1X5	T45.1X6
Mycifradin	T36.5X1	T36.5X2	T36.5X3	T36.5X4	T36.5X5	T36.5X6
topical	T49.0X1	T49.0X2	T49.0X3	T49.0X4	T49.0X5	T49.0X6
Mycitracin	T36.8X1	T36.8X2	T36.8X3	T36.8X4	T36.8X5	T36.8X6
ophthalmic preparation	T49.5X1	T49.5X2	T49.5X3	T49.5X4	T49.5X5	T49.5X6
Mycostatin	T36.7X1	T36.7X2	T36.7X3	T36.7X4	T36.7X5	T36.7X6
topical	T49.0X1	T49.0X2	T49.0X3	T49.0X4	T49.0X5	T49.0X6
Mycotoxins	T64.81	T64.82	T64.83	T64.84	—	—
aflatoxin	T64.01	T64.02	T64.03	T64.04	—	—
specified NEC	T64.81	T64.82	T64.83	T64.84	—	—
Mydriacyl	T44.3X1	T44.3X2	T44.3X3	T44.3X4	T44.3X5	T44.3X6
Mydriatic drug	T49.5X1	T49.5X2	T49.5X3	T49.5X4	T49.5X5	T49.5X6
Myelobromal	T45.1X1	T45.1X2	T45.1X3	T45.1X4	T45.1X5	T45.1X6
Myleran	T45.1X1	T45.1X2	T45.1X3	T45.1X4	T45.1X5	T45.1X6
Myochrysin (e)	T39.2X1	T39.2X2	T39.2X3	T39.2X4	T39.2X5	T39.2X6
Myoneural blocking agents	T48.1X1	T48.1X2	T48.1X3	T48.1X4	T48.1X5	T48.1X6
Myralact	T49.0X1	T49.0X2	T49.0X3	T49.0X4	T49.0X5	T49.0X6
Myristica fragrans	T62.2X1	T62.2X2	T62.2X3	T62.2X4	—	—
Myristicin	T65.891	T65.892	T65.893	T65.894	—	—
Mysoline	T42.3X1	T42.3X2	T42.3X3	T42.3X4	T42.3X5	T42.3X6
Nabilone	T40.7X1	T40.7X2	T40.7X3	T40.7X4	T40.7X5	T40.7X6
Nabumetone	T39.391	T39.392	T39.393	T39.394	T39.395	T39.396
Nadolol	T44.7X1	T44.7X2	T44.7X3	T44.7X4	T44.7X5	T44.7X6
Nafcillin	T36.0X1	T36.0X2	T36.0X3	T36.0X4	T36.0X5	T36.0X6
Nafoxidine	T38.6X1	T38.6X2	T38.6X3	T38.6X4	T38.6X5	T38.6X6
Naftazone	T46.991	T46.992	T46.993	T46.994	T46.995	T46.996
Naftidrofuryl (oxalate)	T46.7X1	T46.7X2	T46.7X3	T46.7X4	T46.7X5	T46.7X6
Naftifine	T49.0X1	T49.0X2	T49.0X3	T49.0X4	T49.0X5	T49.0X6
Nail polish remover	T52.91	T52.92	T52.93	T52.94	—	—
Nalbuphine	T40.4X1	T40.4X2	T40.4X3	T40.4X4	T40.4X5	T40.4X6
Naled	T60.0X1	T60.0X2	T60.0X3	T60.0X4	—	—
Nalidixic acid	T37.8X1	T37.8X2	T37.8X3	T37.8X4	T37.8X5	T37.8X6
Nalorphine	T50.7X1	T50.7X2	T50.7X3	T50.7X4	T50.7X5	T50.7X6
Naloxone	T50.7X1	T50.7X2	T50.7X3	T50.7X4	T50.7X5	T50.7X6
Naltrexone	T50.7X1	T50.7X2	T50.7X3	T50.7X4	T50.7X5	T50.7X6
Namenda	T43.8X1	T43.8X2	T43.8X3	T43.8X4	T43.8X5	T43.8X6
Nandrolone	T38.7X1	T38.7X2	T38.7X3	T38.7X4	T38.7X5	T38.7X6
Naphazoline	T48.5X1	T48.5X2	T48.5X3	T48.5X4	T48.5X5	T48.5X6
Naphtha (painters') (petroleum)	T52.0X1	T52.0X2	T52.0X3	T52.0X4	—	—
solvent	T52.0X1	T52.0X2	T52.0X3	T52.0X4	—	—
vapor	T52.0X1	T52.0X2	T52.0X3	T52.0X4	—	—
Naphthalene (non-chlorinated)	T60.2X1	T60.2X2	T60.2X3	T60.2X4	—	—
chlorinated	T60.1X1	T60.1X2	T60.1X3	T60.1X4	—	—
vapor	T60.1X1	T60.1X2	T60.1X3	T60.1X4	—	—

▼ Subterms under main terms may continue to next column or page   Additional Character May Be Required — Refer to the Tabular List for Character Selection   379

Millipede — Naphthalene

Table of Drugs and Chemicals

Naphthalene — Nonoxinol

Substance	Poisoning, Accidental (unintentional)	Poisoning, Intentional Self-harm	Poisoning, Assault	Poisoning, Undetermined	Adverse Effect	Under-dosing
Naphthalene — continued						
insecticide or moth repellent	T60.2X1	T60.2X2	T60.2X3	T60.2X4	—	—
chlorinated	T60.1X1	T60.1X2	T60.1X3	T60.1X4	—	—
vapor	T60.2X1	T60.2X2	T60.2X3	T60.2X4	—	—
chlorinated	T60.1X1	T60.1X2	T60.1X3	T60.1X4	—	—
Naphthol	T65.891	T65.892	T65.893	T65.894	—	—
Naphthylamine	T65.891	T65.892	T65.893	T65.894	—	—
Naphthylthiourea (ANTU)	T60.4X1	T60.4X2	T60.4X3	T60.4X4	—	—
Naprosyn — see Naproxen						
Naproxen	T39.311	T39.312	T39.313	T39.314	T39.315	T39.316
Narcotic (drug)	T40.601	T40.602	T40.603	T40.604	T40.605	T40.606
analgesic NEC	T40.601	T40.602	T40.603	T40.604	T40.605	T40.606
antagonist	T50.7X1	T50.7X2	T50.7X3	T50.7X4	T50.7X5	T50.7X6
specified NEC	T40.691	T40.692	T40.693	T40.694	T40.695	T40.696
synthetic	T40.4X1	T40.4X2	T40.4X3	T40.4X4	T40.4X5	T40.4X6
Narcotine	T48.3X1	T48.3X2	T48.3X3	T48.3X4	T48.3X5	T48.3X6
Nardil	T43.1X1	T43.1X2	T43.1X3	T43.1X4	T43.1X5	T43.1X6
Nasal drug NEC	T49.6X1	T49.6X2	T49.6X3	T49.6X4	T49.6X5	T49.6X6
Natamycin	T49.0X1	T49.0X2	T49.0X3	T49.0X4	T49.0X5	T49.0X6
Natrium cyanide — see Cyanide(s)						
Natural						
blood (product)	T45.8X1	T45.8X2	T45.8X3	T45.8X4	T45.8X5	T45.8X6
gas (piped)	T59.891	T59.892	T59.893	T59.894	—	—
incomplete combustion	T58.11	T58.12	T58.13	T58.14	—	—
Nealbarbital	T42.3X1	T42.3X2	T42.3X3	T42.3X4	T42.3X5	T42.3X6
Nectadon	T48.3X1	T48.3X2	T48.3X3	T48.3X4	T48.3X5	T48.3X6
Nedocromil	T48.6X1	T48.6X2	T48.6X3	T48.6X4	T48.6X5	T48.6X6
Nefopam	T39.8X1	T39.8X2	T39.8X3	T39.8X4	T39.8X5	T39.8X6
Nematocyst (sting)	T63.691	T63.692	T63.693	T63.694	—	—
Nembutal	T42.3X1	T42.3X2	T42.3X3	T42.3X4	T42.3X5	T42.3X6
Nemonapride	T43.591	T43.592	T43.593	T43.594	T43.595	T43.596
Neoarsphenamine	T37.8X1	T37.8X2	T37.8X3	T37.8X4	T37.8X5	T37.8X6
Neocinchophen	T50.4X1	T50.4X2	T50.4X3	T50.4X4	T50.4X5	T50.4X6
Neomycin (derivatives)	T36.5X1	T36.5X2	T36.5X3	T36.5X4	T36.5X5	T36.5X6
with						
bacitracin	T49.0X1	T49.0X2	T49.0X3	T49.0X4	T49.0X5	T49.0X6
neostigmine	T44.0X1	T44.0X2	T44.0X3	T44.0X4	T44.0X5	T44.0X6
ENT agent	T49.6X1	T49.6X2	T49.6X3	T49.6X4	T49.6X5	T49.6X6
ophthalmic preparation	T49.5X1	T49.5X2	T49.5X3	T49.5X4	T49.5X5	T49.5X6
topical NEC	T49.0X1	T49.0X2	T49.0X3	T49.0X4	T49.0X5	T49.0X6
Neonal	T42.3X1	T42.3X2	T42.3X3	T42.3X4	T42.3X5	T42.3X6
Neoprontosil	T37.0X1	T37.0X2	T37.0X3	T37.0X4	T37.0X5	T37.0X6
Neosalvarsan	T37.8X1	T37.8X2	T37.8X3	T37.8X4	T37.8X5	T37.8X6
Neosilversalvarsan	T37.8X1	T37.8X2	T37.8X3	T37.8X4	T37.8X5	T37.8X6
Neosporin	T36.8X1	T36.8X2	T36.8X3	T36.8X4	T36.8X5	T36.8X6
ENT agent	T49.6X1	T49.6X2	T49.6X3	T49.6X4	T49.6X5	T49.6X6
opthalmic preparation	T49.5X1	T49.5X2	T49.5X3	T49.5X4	T49.5X5	T49.5X6
topical NEC	T49.0X1	T49.0X2	T49.0X3	T49.0X4	T49.0X5	T49.0X6
Neostigmine bromide	T44.0X1	T44.0X2	T44.0X3	T44.0X4	T44.0X5	T44.0X6
Neraval	T42.3X1	T42.3X2	T42.3X3	T42.3X4	T42.3X5	T42.3X6
Neravan	T42.3X1	T42.3X2	T42.3X3	T42.3X4	T42.3X5	T42.3X6
Nerium oleander	T62.2X1	T62.2X2	T62.2X3	T62.2X4	—	—
Nerve gas, not in war	T59.91	T59.92	T59.93	T59.94	—	—
Nesacaine	T41.3X1	T41.3X2	T41.3X3	T41.3X4	T41.3X5	T41.3X6
infiltration (subcutaneous)	T41.3X1	T41.3X2	T41.3X3	T41.3X4	T41.3X5	T41.3X6
nerve block (peripheral) (plexus)	T41.3X1	T41.3X2	T41.3X3	T41.3X4	T41.3X5	T41.3X6
Netilmicin	T36.5X1	T36.5X2	T36.5X3	T36.5X4	T36.5X5	T36.5X6
Neurobarb	T42.3X1	T42.3X2	T42.3X3	T42.3X4	T42.3X5	T42.3X6
Neuroleptic drug NEC	T43.501	T43.502	T43.503	T43.504	T43.505	T43.506
Neuromuscular blocking drug	T48.1X1	T48.1X2	T48.1X3	T48.1X4	T48.1X5	T48.1X6
Neutral insulin injection	T38.3X1	T38.3X2	T38.3X3	T38.3X4	T38.3X5	T38.3X6
Neutral spirits	T51.0X1	T51.0X2	T51.0X3	T51.0X4	—	—
beverage	T51.0X1	T51.0X2	T51.0X3	T51.0X4	—	—
Niacin	T46.7X1	T46.7X2	T46.7X3	T46.7X4	T46.7X5	T46.7X6
Niacinamide	T45.2X1	T45.2X2	T45.2X3	T45.2X4	T45.2X5	T45.2X6
Nialamide	T43.1X1	T43.1X2	T43.1X3	T43.1X4	T43.1X5	T43.1X6
Niaprazine	T42.6X1	T42.6X2	T42.6X3	T42.6X4	T42.6X5	T42.6X6
Nicametate	T46.7X1	T46.7X2	T46.7X3	T46.7X4	T46.7X5	T46.7X6
Nicardipine	T46.1X1	T46.1X2	T46.1X3	T46.1X4	T46.1X5	T46.1X6
Nicergoline	T46.7X1	T46.7X2	T46.7X3	T46.7X4	T46.7X5	T46.7X6
Nickel (carbonyl) (tetra-carbonyl) (fumes) (vapor)	T56.891	T56.892	T56.893	T56.894	—	—
Nickelocene	T56.891	T56.892	T56.893	T56.894	—	—
Niclosamide	T37.4X1	T37.4X2	T37.4X3	T37.4X4	T37.4X5	T37.4X6
Nicofuranose	T46.7X1	T46.7X2	T46.7X3	T46.7X4	T46.7X5	T46.7X6
Nicomorphine	T40.2X1	T40.2X2	T40.2X3	T40.2X4	—	—
Nicorandil	T46.3X1	T46.3X2	T46.3X3	T46.3X4	T46.3X5	T46.3X6
Nicotiana (plant)	T62.2X1	T62.2X2	T62.2X3	T62.2X4	—	—
Nicotinamide	T45.2X1	T45.2X2	T45.2X3	T45.2X4	T45.2X5	T45.2X6

Substance	Poisoning, Accidental (unintentional)	Poisoning, Intentional Self-harm	Poisoning, Assault	Poisoning, Undetermined	Adverse Effect	Under-dosing
Nicotine (insecticide) (spray) (sulfate) **NEC**	T60.2X1	T60.2X2	T60.2X3	T60.2X4	—	—
from tobacco	T65.291	T65.292	T65.293	T65.294	—	—
cigarettes	T65.221	T65.222	T65.223	T65.224	—	—
not insecticide	T65.291	T65.292	T65.293	T65.294	—	—
Nicotinic acid	T46.7X1	T46.7X2	T46.7X3	T46.7X4	T46.7X5	T46.7X6
Nicotinyl alcohol	T46.7X1	T46.7X2	T46.7X3	T46.7X4	T46.7X5	T46.7X6
Nicoumalone	T45.511	T45.512	T45.513	T45.514	T45.515	T45.516
Nifedipine	T46.1X1	T46.1X2	T46.1X3	T46.1X4	T46.1X5	T46.1X6
Nifenazone	T39.2X1	T39.2X2	T39.2X3	T39.2X4	T39.2X5	T39.2X6
Nifuraldezone	T37.91	T37.92	T37.93	T37.94	T37.95	T37.96
Nifuratel	T37.8X1	T37.8X2	T37.8X3	T37.8X4	T37.8X5	T37.8X6
Nifurtimox	T37.3X1	T37.3X2	T37.3X3	T37.3X4	T37.3X5	T37.3X6
Nifurtoinol	T37.8X1	T37.8X2	T37.8X3	T37.8X4	T37.8X5	T37.8X6
Nightshade, deadly (solanum) — see also Belladonna	T62.2X1	T62.2X2	T62.2X3	T62.2X4	—	—
berry	T62.1X1	T62.1X2	T62.1X3	T62.1X4	—	—
Nikethamide	T50.7X1	T50.7X2	T50.7X3	T50.7X4	T50.7X5	T50.7X6
Nilstat	T36.7X1	T36.7X2	T36.7X3	T36.7X4	T36.7X5	T36.7X6
topical	T49.0X1	T49.0X2	T49.0X3	T49.0X4	T49.0X5	T49.0X6
Nilutamide	T38.6X1	T38.6X2	T38.6X3	T38.6X4	T38.6X5	T38.6X6
Nimesulide	T39.391	T39.392	T39.393	T39.394	T39.395	T39.396
Nimetazepam	T42.4X1	T42.4X2	T42.4X3	T42.4X4	T42.4X5	T42.4X6
Nimodipine	T46.1X1	T46.1X2	T46.1X3	T46.1X4	T46.1X5	T46.1X6
Nimorazole	T37.3X1	T37.3X2	T37.3X3	T37.3X4	T37.3X5	T37.3X6
Nimustine	T45.1X1	T45.1X2	T45.1X3	T45.1X4	T45.1X5	T45.1X6
Niridazole	T37.4X1	T37.4X2	T37.4X3	T37.4X4	T37.4X5	T37.4X6
Nisentil	T40.2X1	T40.2X2	T40.2X3	T40.2X4	T40.2X5	T40.2X6
Nisoldipine	T46.1X1	T46.1X2	T46.1X3	T46.1X4	T46.1X5	T46.1X6
Nitramine	T65.3X1	T65.3X2	T65.3X3	T65.3X4	—	—
Nitrate, organic	T46.3X1	T46.3X2	T46.3X3	T46.3X4	T46.3X5	T46.3X6
Nitrazepam	T42.4X1	T42.4X2	T42.4X3	T42.4X4	T42.4X5	T42.4X6
Nitrefazole	T50.6X1	T50.6X2	T50.6X3	T50.6X4	T50.6X5	T50.6X6
Nitrendipine	T46.1X1	T46.1X2	T46.1X3	T46.1X4	T46.1X5	T46.1X6
Nitric						
acid (liquid)	T54.2X1	T54.2X2	T54.2X3	T54.2X4	—	—
vapor	T59.891	T59.892	T59.893	T59.894	—	—
oxide (gas)	T59.0X1	T59.0X2	T59.0X3	T59.0X4	—	—
Nitrimidazine	T37.3X1	T37.3X2	T37.3X3	T37.3X4	T37.3X5	T37.3X6
Nitrite, amyl (medicinal) (vapor)	T46.3X1	T46.3X2	T46.3X3	T46.3X4	T46.3X5	T46.3X6
Nitroaniline	T65.3X1	T65.3X2	T65.3X3	T65.3X4	—	—
vapor	T59.891	T59.892	T59.893	T59.894	—	—
Nitrobenzene, nitrobenzol	T65.3X1	T65.3X2	T65.3X3	T65.3X4	—	—
vapor	T65.3X1	T65.3X2	T65.3X3	T65.3X4	—	—
Nitrocellulose	T65.891	T65.892	T65.893	T65.894	—	—
lacquer	T65.891	T65.892	T65.893	T65.894	—	—
Nitrodiphenyl	T65.3X1	T65.3X2	T65.3X3	T65.3X4	—	—
Nitrofural	T49.0X1	T49.0X2	T49.0X3	T49.0X4	T49.0X5	T49.0X6
Nitrofurantoin	T37.8X1	T37.8X2	T37.8X3	T37.8X4	T37.8X5	T37.8X6
Nitrofurazone	T49.0X1	T49.0X2	T49.0X3	T49.0X4	T49.0X5	T49.0X6
Nitrogen	T59.0X1	T59.0X2	T59.0X3	T59.0X4	—	—
mustard	T45.1X1	T45.1X2	T45.1X3	T45.1X4	T45.1X5	T45.1X6
Nitroglycerin, nitroglycerol (medicinal)	T46.3X1	T46.3X2	T46.3X3	T46.3X4	T46.3X5	T46.3X6
nonmedicinal	T65.5X1	T65.5X2	T65.5X3	T65.5X4	—	—
fumes	T65.5X1	T65.5X2	T65.5X3	T65.5X4	—	—
Nitroglycol	T52.3X1	T52.3X2	T52.3X3	T52.3X4	—	—
Nitrohydrochloric acid	T54.2X1	T54.2X2	T54.2X3	T54.2X4	—	—
Nitromersol	T49.0X1	T49.0X2	T49.0X3	T49.0X4	T49.0X5	T49.0X6
Nitronaphthalene	T65.891	T65.892	T65.893	T65.894	—	—
Nitrophenol	T54.0X1	T54.0X2	T54.0X3	T54.0X4	—	—
Nitropropane	T52.8X1	T52.8X2	T52.8X3	T52.8X4	—	—
Nitroprusside	T46.5X1	T46.5X2	T46.5X3	T46.5X4	T46.5X5	T46.5X6
Nitrosodimethylamine	T65.3X1	T65.3X2	T65.3X3	T65.3X4	—	—
Nitrothiazol	T37.4X1	T37.4X2	T37.4X3	T37.4X4	T37.4X5	T37.4X6
Nitrotoluene, nitrotoluol	T65.3X1	T65.3X2	T65.3X3	T65.3X4	—	—
vapor	T65.3X1	T65.3X2	T65.3X3	T65.3X4	—	—
Nitrous						
acid (liquid)	T54.2X1	T54.2X2	T54.2X3	T54.2X4	—	—
fumes	T59.891	T59.892	T59.893	T59.894	—	—
ether spirit	T46.3X1	T46.3X2	T46.3X3	T46.3X4	T46.3X5	T46.3X6
oxide	T41.0X1	T41.0X2	T41.0X3	T41.0X4	T41.0X5	T41.0X6
Nitroxoline	T37.8X1	T37.8X2	T37.8X3	T37.8X4	T37.8X5	T37.8X6
Nitrozone	T49.0X1	T49.0X2	T49.0X3	T49.0X4	T49.0X5	T49.0X6
Nizatidine	T47.0X1	T47.0X2	T47.0X3	T47.0X4	T47.0X5	T47.0X6
Nizofenone	T43.8X1	T43.8X2	T43.8X3	T43.8X4	T43.8X5	T43.8X6
Noctec	T42.6X1	T42.6X2	T42.6X3	T42.6X4	T42.6X5	T42.6X6
Noludar	T42.6X1	T42.6X2	T42.6X3	T42.6X4	T42.6X5	T42.6X6
Nomegestrol	T38.5X1	T38.5X2	T38.5X3	T38.5X4	T38.5X5	T38.5X6
Nomifensine	T43.291	T43.292	T43.293	T43.294	T43.295	T43.296
Nonoxinol	T49.8X1	T49.8X2	T49.8X3	T49.8X4	T49.8X5	T49.8X6

Additional Character May Be Required — Refer to the Tabular List for Character Selection ⚐ Subterms under main terms may continue to next column or page

Substance	Poisoning, Accidental (unintentional)	Poisoning, Intentional Self-harm	Poisoning, Assault	Poisoning, Undetermined	Adverse Effect	Under-dosing
Nonylphenoxy	T49.8X1	T49.8X2	T49.8X3	T49.8X4	T49.8X5	T49.8X6
(polyethoxyethanol)						
Noptil	T42.3X1	T42.3X2	T42.3X3	T42.3X4	T42.3X5	T42.3X6
Noradrenaline	T44.4X1	T44.4X2	T44.4X3	T44.4X4	T44.4X5	T44.4X6
Noramidopyrine	T39.2X1	T39.2X2	T39.2X3	T39.2X4	T39.2X5	T39.2X6
methanesulfonate sodium	T39.2X1	T39.2X2	T39.2X3	T39.2X4	T39.2X5	T39.2X6
Norbormide	T60.4X1	T60.4X2	T60.4X3	T60.4X4	—	—
Nordazepam	T42.4X1	T42.4X2	T42.4X3	T42.4X4	T42.4X5	T42.4X6
Norepinephrine	T44.4X1	T44.4X2	T44.4X3	T44.4X4	T44.4X5	T44.4X6
Norethandrolone	T38.7X1	T38.7X2	T38.7X3	T38.7X4	T38.7X5	T38.7X6
Norethindrone	T38.4X1	T38.4X2	T38.4X3	T38.4X4	T38.4X5	T38.4X6
Norethisterone (acetate)	T38.4X1	T38.4X2	T38.4X3	T38.4X4	T38.4X5	T38.4X6
(enantate)						
with ethinylestradiol	T38.5X1	T38.5X2	T38.5X3	T38.5X4	T38.5X5	T38.5X6
Noretynodrel	T38.5X1	T38.5X2	T38.5X3	T38.5X4	T38.5X5	T38.5X6
Norfenefrine	T44.4X1	T44.4X2	T44.4X3	T44.4X4	T44.4X5	T44.4X6
Norfloxacin	T36.8X1	T36.8X2	T36.8X3	T36.8X4	T36.8X5	T36.8X6
Norgestrel	T38.4X1	T38.4X2	T38.4X3	T38.4X4	T38.4X5	T38.4X6
Norgestrienone	T38.4X1	T38.4X2	T38.4X3	T38.4X4	T38.4X5	T38.4X6
Norlestrin	T38.4X1	T38.4X2	T38.4X3	T38.4X4	T38.4X5	T38.4X6
Norlutin	T38.4X1	T38.4X2	T38.4X3	T38.4X4	T38.4X5	T38.4X6
Normal serum albumin (human),	T45.8X1	T45.8X2	T45.8X3	T45.8X4	T45.8X5	T45.8X6
salt-poor						
Normethandrone	T38.5X1	T38.5X2	T38.5X3	T38.5X4	T38.5X5	T38.5X6
Normison — see						
Benzodiazepines						
Normorphine	T40.2X1	T40.2X2	T40.2X3	T40.2X4	—	—
Norpseudoephedrine	T50.5X1	T50.5X2	T50.5X3	T50.5X4	T50.5X5	T50.5X6
Nortestosterone	T38.7X1	T38.7X2	T38.7X3	T38.7X4	T38.7X5	T38.7X6
(furanpropionate)						
Nortriptyline	T43.011	T43.012	T43.013	T43.014	T43.015	T43.016
Noscapine	T48.3X1	T48.3X2	T48.3X3	T48.3X4	T48.3X5	T48.3X6
Nose preparations	T49.6X1	T49.6X2	T49.6X3	T49.6X4	T49.6X5	T49.6X6
Novobiocin	T36.5X1	T36.5X2	T36.5X3	T36.5X4	T36.5X5	T36.5X6
Novocain (infiltration)	T41.3X1	T41.3X2	T41.3X3	T41.3X4	T41.3X5	T41.3X6
(topical)						
nerve block (peripheral)	T41.3X1	T41.3X2	T41.3X3	T41.3X4	T41.3X5	T41.3X6
(plexus)						
spinal	T41.3X1	T41.3X2	T41.3X3	T41.3X4	T41.3X5	T41.3X6
Noxious foodstuff	T62.91	T62.92	T62.93	T62.94	—	—
specified NEC	T62.8X1	T62.8X2	T62.8X3	T62.8X4	—	—
Noxiptiline	T43.011	T43.012	T43.013	T43.014	T43.015	T43.016
Noxytiolin	T49.0X1	T49.0X2	T49.0X3	T49.0X4	T49.0X5	T49.0X6
NPH lletin (insulin)	T38.3X1	T38.3X2	T38.3X3	T38.3X4	T38.3X5	T38.3X6
Numorphan	T40.2X1	T40.2X2	T40.2X3	T40.2X4	T40.2X5	T40.2X6
Nunol	T42.3X1	T42.3X2	T42.3X3	T42.3X4	T42.3X5	T42.3X6
Nupercaine (spinal	T41.3X1	T41.3X2	T41.3X3	T41.3X4	T41.3X5	T41.3X6
anesthetic)						
topical (surface)	T41.3X1	T41.3X2	T41.3X3	T41.3X4	T41.3X5	T41.3X6
Nutmeg oil (liniment)	T49.3X1	T49.3X2	T49.3X3	T49.3X4	T49.3X5	T49.3X6
Nutritional supplement	T50.901	T50.902	T50.903	T50.904	T50.905	T50.906
Nux vomica	T65.1X1	T65.1X2	T65.1X3	T65.1X4	—	—
Nydrazid	T37.1X1	T37.1X2	T37.1X3	T37.1X4	T37.1X5	T37.1X6
Nylidrin	T46.7X1	T46.7X2	T46.7X3	T46.7X4	T46.7X5	T46.7X6
Nystatin	T36.7X1	T36.7X2	T36.7X3	T36.7X4	T36.7X5	T36.7X6
topical	T49.0X1	T49.0X2	T49.0X3	T49.0X4	T49.0X5	T49.0X6
Nytol	T45.0X1	T45.0X2	T45.0X3	T45.0X4	T45.0X5	T45.0X6
Obidoxime chloride	T50.6X1	T50.6X2	T50.6X3	T50.6X4	T50.6X5	T50.6X6
Octafonium (chloride)	T49.3X1	T49.3X2	T49.3X3	T49.3X4	T49.3X5	T49.3X6
Octamethyl	T60.0X1	T60.0X2	T60.0X3	T60.0X4	—	—
pyrophosphoramide						
Octanoin	T50.991	T50.992	T50.993	T50.994	T50.995	T50.996
Octatropine	T44.3X1	T44.3X2	T44.3X3	T44.3X4	T44.3X5	T44.3X6
methylbromide						
Octotiamine	T45.2X1	T45.2X2	T45.2X3	T45.2X4	T45.2X5	T45.2X6
Octoxinol (9)	T49.8X1	T49.8X2	T49.8X3	T49.8X4	T49.8X5	T49.8X6
Octreotide	T38.991	T38.992	T38.993	T38.994	T38.995	T38.996
Octyl nitrite	T46.3X1	T46.3X2	T46.3X3	T46.3X4	T46.3X5	T46.3X6
Oestradiol	T38.5X1	T38.5X2	T38.5X3	T38.5X4	T38.5X5	T38.5X6
Oestriol	T38.5X1	T38.5X2	T38.5X3	T38.5X4	T38.5X5	T38.5X6
Oestrogen	T38.5X1	T38.5X2	T38.5X3	T38.5X4	T38.5X5	T38.5X6
Oestrone	T38.5X1	T38.5X2	T38.5X3	T38.5X4	T38.5X5	T38.5X6
Ofloxacin	T36.8X1	T36.8X2	T36.8X3	T36.8X4	T36.8X5	T36.8X6
Oil (of)	T65.891	T65.892	T65.893	T65.894	—	—
bitter almond	T62.8X1	T62.8X2	T62.8X3	T62.8X4	—	—
cloves	T49.7X1	T49.7X2	T49.7X3	T49.7X4	T49.7X5	T49.7X6
colors	T65.6X1	T65.6X2	T65.6X3	T65.6X4	—	—
fumes	T59.891	T59.892	T59.893	T59.894	—	—
lubricating	T52.0X1	T52.0X2	T52.0X3	T52.0X4	—	—
Niobe	T52.8X1	T52.8X2	T52.8X3	T52.8X4	—	—
vitriol (liquid)	T54.2X1	T54.2X2	T54.2X3	T54.2X4	—	—
fumes	T54.2X1	T54.2X2	T54.2X3	T54.2X4	—	—
wintergreen (bitter) NEC	T49.3X1	T49.3X2	T49.3X3	T49.3X4	T49.3X5	T49.3X6

Substance	Poisoning, Accidental (unintentional)	Poisoning, Intentional Self-harm	Poisoning, Assault	Poisoning, Undetermined	Adverse Effect	Under-dosing
Oily preparation (for skin)	T49.3X1	T49.3X2	T49.3X3	T49.3X4	T49.3X5	T49.3X6
Ointment NEC	T49.3X1	T49.3X2	T49.3X3	T49.3X4	T49.3X5	T49.3X6
Olanzapine	T43.591	T43.592	T43.593	T43.594	T43.595	T43.596
Oleander	T62.2X1	T62.2X2	T62.2X3	T62.2X4	—	—
Oleandomycin	T36.3X1	T36.3X2	T36.3X3	T36.3X4	T36.3X5	T36.3X6
Oleandrin	T46.0X1	T46.0X2	T46.0X3	T46.0X4	T46.0X5	T46.0X6
Oleic acid	T46.6X1	T46.6X2	T46.6X3	T46.6X4	T46.6X5	T46.6X6
Oleovitamin A	T45.2X1	T45.2X2	T45.2X3	T45.2X4	T45.2X5	T45.2X6
Oleum ricini	T47.2X1	T47.2X2	T47.2X3	T47.2X4	T47.2X5	T47.2X6
Olive oil (medicinal) NEC	T47.4X1	T47.4X2	T47.4X3	T47.4X4	T47.4X5	T47.4X6
Olivomycin	T45.1X1	T45.1X2	T45.1X3	T45.1X4	T45.1X5	T45.1X6
Olsalazine	T47.8X1	T47.8X2	T47.8X3	T47.8X4	T47.8X5	T47.8X6
Omeprazole	T47.1X1	T47.1X2	T47.1X3	T47.1X4	T47.1X5	T47.1X6
OMPA	T60.0X1	T60.0X2	T60.0X3	T60.0X4	—	—
Oncovin	T45.1X1	T45.1X2	T45.1X3	T45.1X4	T45.1X5	T45.1X6
Ondansetron	T45.0X1	T45.0X2	T45.0X3	T45.0X4	T45.0X5	T45.0X6
Ophthaine	T41.3X1	T41.3X2	T41.3X3	T41.3X4	T41.3X5	T41.3X6
Ophthetic	T41.3X1	T41.3X2	T41.3X3	T41.3X4	T41.3X5	T41.3X6
Opiate NEC	T40.601	T40.602	T40.603	T40.604	T40.605	T40.606
antagonists	T50.7X1	T50.7X2	T50.7X3	T50.7X4	T50.7X5	T50.7X6
Opioid NEC	T40.2X1	T40.2X2	T40.2X3	T40.2X4	T40.2X5	T40.2X6
Opipramol	T43.011	T43.012	T43.013	T43.014	T43.015	T43.016
Opium alkaloids (total)	T40.0X1	T40.0X2	T40.0X3	T40.0X4	T40.0X5	T40.0X6
standardized powdered	T40.0X1	T40.0X2	T40.0X3	T40.0X4	T40.0X5	T40.0X6
tincture (camphorated)	T40.0X1	T40.0X2	T40.0X3	T40.0X4	T40.0X5	T40.0X6
Oracon	T38.4X1	T38.4X2	T38.4X3	T38.4X4	T38.4X5	T38.4X6
Oragrafin	T50.8X1	T50.8X2	T50.8X3	T50.8X4	T50.8X5	T50.8X6
Oral contraceptives	T38.4X1	T38.4X2	T38.4X3	T38.4X4	T38.4X5	T38.4X6
Oral rehydration salts	T50.3X1	T50.3X2	T50.3X3	T50.3X4	T50.3X5	T50.3X6
Orazamide	T50.991	T50.992	T50.993	T50.994	T50.995	T50.996
Orciprenaline	T48.291	T48.292	T48.293	T48.294	T48.295	T48.296
Organidin	T48.4X1	T48.4X2	T48.4X3	T48.4X4	T48.4X5	T48.4X6
Organonitrate NEC	T46.3X1	T46.3X2	T46.3X3	T46.3X4	T46.3X5	T46.3X6
Organophosphates	T60.0X1	T60.0X2	T60.0X3	T60.0X4	—	—
Orimune	T50.B91	T50.B92	T50.B93	T50.B94	T50.B95	T50.B96
Orinase	T38.3X1	T38.3X2	T38.3X3	T38.3X4	T38.3X5	T38.3X6
Ormeloxifene	T38.6X1	T38.6X2	T38.6X3	T38.6X4	T38.6X5	T38.6X6
Ornidazole	T37.3X1	T37.3X2	T37.3X3	T37.3X4	T37.3X5	T37.3X6
Ornithine aspartate	T50.991	T50.992	T50.993	T50.994	T50.995	T50.996
Ornoprostil	T47.1X1	T47.1X2	T47.1X3	T47.1X4	T47.1X5	T47.1X6
Orphenadrine	T42.8X1	T42.8X2	T42.8X3	T42.8X4	T42.8X5	T42.8X6
(hydrochloride)						
Ortal (sodium)	T42.3X1	T42.3X2	T42.3X3	T42.3X4	T42.3X5	T42.3X6
Orthoboric acid	T49.0X1	T49.0X2	T49.0X3	T49.0X4	T49.0X5	T49.0X6
ENT agent	T49.6X1	T49.6X2	T49.6X3	T49.6X4	T49.6X5	T49.6X6
ophthalmic preparation	T49.5X1	T49.5X2	T49.5X3	T49.5X4	T49.5X5	T49.5X6
Orthocaine	T41.3X1	T41.3X2	T41.3X3	T41.3X4	T41.3X5	T41.3X6
Orthodichlorobenzene	T53.7X1	T53.7X2	T53.7X3	T53.7X4	—	—
Ortho-Novum	T38.4X1	T38.4X2	T38.4X3	T38.4X4	T38.4X5	T38.4X6
Orthotolidine (reagent)	T54.2X1	T54.2X2	T54.2X3	T54.2X4	—	—
Osmic acid (liquid)	T54.2X1	T54.2X2	T54.2X3	T54.2X4	—	—
fumes	T54.2X1	T54.2X2	T54.2X3	T54.2X4	—	—
Osmotic diuretics	T50.2X1	T50.2X2	T50.2X3	T50.2X4	T50.2X5	T50.2X6
Otilonium bromide	T44.3X1	T44.3X2	T44.3X3	T44.3X4	T44.3X5	T44.3X6
Otorhinolaryngological drug NEC	T49.6X1	T49.6X2	T49.6X3	T49.6X4	T49.6X5	T49.6X6
Ouabain (e)	T46.0X1	T46.0X2	T46.0X3	T46.0X4	T46.0X5	T46.0X6
Ovarian						
hormone	T38.5X1	T38.5X2	T38.5X3	T38.5X4	T38.5X5	T38.5X6
stimulant	T38.5X1	T38.5X2	T38.5X3	T38.5X4	T38.5X5	T38.5X6
Ovral	T38.4X1	T38.4X2	T38.4X3	T38.4X4	T38.4X5	T38.4X6
Ovulen	T38.4X1	T38.4X2	T38.4X3	T38.4X4	T38.4X5	T38.4X6
Oxacillin	T36.0X1	T36.0X2	T36.0X3	T36.0X4	T36.0X5	T36.0X6
Oxalic acid	T54.2X1	T54.2X2	T54.2X3	T54.2X4	—	—
ammonium salt	T50.991	T50.992	T50.993	T50.994	T50.995	T50.996
Oxamniquine	T37.4X1	T37.4X2	T37.4X3	T37.4X4	T37.4X5	T37.4X6
Oxanamide	T43.591	T43.592	T43.593	T43.594	T43.595	T43.596
Oxandrolone	T38.7X1	T38.7X2	T38.7X3	T38.7X4	T38.7X5	T38.7X6
Oxantel	T37.4X1	T37.4X2	T37.4X3	T37.4X4	T37.4X5	T37.4X6
Oxapium iodide	T44.3X1	T44.3X2	T44.3X3	T44.3X4	T44.3X5	T44.3X6
Oxaprotiline	T43.021	T43.022	T43.023	T43.024	T43.025	T43.026
Oxaprozin	T39.311	T39.312	T39.313	T39.314	T39.315	T39.316
Oxatomide	T45.0X1	T45.0X2	T45.0X3	T45.0X4	T45.0X5	T45.0X6
Oxazepam	T42.4X1	T42.4X2	T42.4X3	T42.4X4	T42.4X5	T42.4X6
Oxazimedrine	T50.5X1	T50.5X2	T50.5X3	T50.5X4	T50.5X5	T50.5X6
Oxazolam	T42.4X1	T42.4X2	T42.4X3	T42.4X4	T42.4X5	T42.4X6
Oxazolidine derivatives	T42.2X1	T42.2X2	T42.2X3	T42.2X4	T42.2X5	T42.2X6
Oxazolidinedione	T42.2X1	T42.2X2	T42.2X3	T42.2X4	T42.2X5	T42.2X6
(derivative)						
Ox bile extract	T47.5X1	T47.5X2	T47.5X3	T47.5X4	T47.5X5	T47.5X6
Oxcarbazepine	T42.1X1	T42.1X2	T42.1X3	T42.1X4	T42.1X5	T42.1X6
Oxedrine	T44.4X1	T44.4X2	T44.4X3	T44.4X4	T44.4X5	T44.4X6
Oxeladin (citrate)	T48.3X1	T48.3X2	T48.3X3	T48.3X4	T48.3X5	T48.3X6

Substance	Poisoning, Accidental (unintentional)	Poisoning, Intentional Self-harm	Poisoning, Assault	Poisoning, Undetermined	Adverse Effect	Under-dosing
Oxendolone	T38.5X1	T38.5X2	T38.5X3	T38.5X4	T38.5X5	T38.5X6
Oxetacaine	T41.3X1	T41.3X2	T41.3X3	T41.3X4	T41.3X5	T41.3X6
Oxethazine	T41.3X1	T41.3X2	T41.3X3	T41.3X4	T41.3X5	T41.3X6
Oxetorone	T39.8X1	T39.8X2	T39.8X3	T39.8X4	T39.8X5	T39.8X6
Oxiconazole	T49.0X1	T49.0X2	T49.0X3	T49.0X4	T49.0X5	T49.0X6
Oxidizing agent NEC	T54.91	T54.92	T54.93	T54.94	—	—
Oxipurinol	T50.4X1	T50.4X2	T50.4X3	T50.4X4	T50.4X5	T50.4X6
Oxitriptan	T43.291	T43.292	T43.293	T43.294	T43.295	T43.296
Oxitropium bromide	T48.6X1	T48.6X2	T48.6X3	T48.6X4	T48.6X5	T48.6X6
Oxodipine	T46.1X1	T46.1X2	T46.1X3	T46.1X4	T46.1X5	T46.1X6
Oxolamine	T48.3X1	T48.3X2	T48.3X3	T48.3X4	T48.3X5	T48.3X6
Oxolinic acid	T37.8X1	T37.8X2	T37.8X3	T37.8X4	T37.8X5	T37.8X6
Oxomemazine	T43.3X1	T43.3X2	T43.3X3	T43.3X4	T43.3X5	T43.3X6
Oxophenarsine	T37.3X1	T37.3X2	T37.3X3	T37.3X4	T37.3X5	T37.3X6
Oxprenolol	T44.7X1	T44.7X2	T44.7X3	T44.7X4	T44.7X5	T44.7X6
Oxsoralen	T49.3X1	T49.3X2	T49.3X3	T49.3X4	T49.3X5	T49.3X6
Oxtriphylline	T48.6X1	T48.6X2	T48.6X3	T48.6X4	T48.6X5	T48.6X6
Oxybate sodium	T41.291	T41.292	T41.293	T41.294	T41.295	T41.296
Oxybuprocaine	T41.3X1	T41.3X2	T41.3X3	T41.3X4	T41.3X5	T41.3X6
Oxybutynin	T44.3X1	T44.3X2	T44.3X3	T44.3X4	T44.3X5	T44.3X6
Oxychlorosene	T49.0X1	T49.0X2	T49.0X3	T49.0X4	T49.0X5	T49.0X6
Oxycodone	T40.2X1	T40.2X2	T40.2X3	T40.2X4	T40.2X5	T40.2X6
Oxyfedrine	T46.3X1	T46.3X2	T46.3X3	T46.3X4	T46.3X5	T46.3X6
Oxygen	T41.5X1	T41.5X2	T41.5X3	T41.5X4	T41.5X5	T41.5X6
Oxylone	T49.0X1	T49.0X2	T49.0X3	T49.0X4	T49.0X5	T49.0X6
ophthalmic preparation	T49.5X1	T49.5X2	T49.5X3	T49.5X4	T49.5X5	T49.5X6
Oxymesterone	T38.7X1	T38.7X2	T38.7X3	T38.7X4	T38.7X5	T38.7X6
Oxymetazoline	T48.5X1	T48.5X2	T48.5X3	T48.5X4	T48.5X5	T48.5X6
Oxymetholone	T38.7X1	T38.7X2	T38.7X3	T38.7X4	T38.7X5	T38.7X6
Oxymorphone	T40.2X1	T40.2X2	T40.2X3	T40.2X4	T40.2X5	T40.2X6
Oxypertine	T43.591	T43.592	T43.593	T43.594	T43.595	T43.596
Oxyphenbutazone	T39.2X1	T39.2X2	T39.2X3	T39.2X4	T39.2X5	T39.2X6
Oxyphencyclimine	T44.3X1	T44.3X2	T44.3X3	T44.3X4	T44.3X5	T44.3X6
Oxyphenisatine	T47.2X1	T47.2X2	T47.2X3	T47.2X4	T47.2X5	T47.2X6
Oxyphenonium bromide	T44.3X1	T44.3X2	T44.3X3	T44.3X4	T44.3X5	T44.3X6
Oxypolygelatin	T45.8X1	T45.8X2	T45.8X3	T45.8X4	T45.8X5	T45.8X6
Oxyquinoline (derivatives)	T37.8X1	T37.8X2	T37.8X3	T37.8X4	T37.8X5	T37.8X6
Oxytetracycline	T36.4X1	T36.4X2	T36.4X3	T36.4X4	T36.4X5	T36.4X6
Oxytocic drug NEC	T48.0X1	T48.0X2	T48.0X3	T48.0X4	T48.0X5	T48.0X6
Oxytocin (synthetic)	T48.0X1	T48.0X2	T48.0X3	T48.0X4	T48.0X5	T48.0X6
Ozone	T59.891	T59.892	T59.893	T59.894	—	—
PABA	T49.3X1	T49.3X2	T49.3X3	T49.3X4	T49.3X5	T49.3X6
Packed red cells	T45.8X1	T45.8X2	T45.8X3	T45.8X4	T45.8X5	T45.8X6
Padimate	T49.3X1	T49.3X2	T49.3X3	T49.3X4	T49.3X5	T49.3X6
Paint NEC	T65.6X1	T65.6X2	T65.6X3	T65.6X4	—	—
cleaner	T52.91	T52.92	T52.93	T52.94	—	—
fumes NEC	T59.891	T59.892	T59.893	T59.894	—	—
lead (fumes)	T56.0X1	T56.0X2	T56.0X3	T56.0X4	—	—
solvent NEC	T52.8X1	T52.8X2	T52.8X3	T52.8X4	—	—
stripper	T52.8X1	T52.8X2	T52.8X3	T52.8X4	—	—
Palfium	T40.2X1	T40.2X2	T40.2X3	T40.2X4	—	—
Palm kernel oil	T50.991	T50.992	T50.993	T50.994	T50.995	T50.996
Paludrine	T37.2X1	T37.2X2	T37.2X3	T37.2X4	T37.2X5	T37.2X6
PAM (pralidoxime)	T50.6X1	T50.6X2	T50.6X3	T50.6X4	T50.6X5	T50.6X6
Pamaquine (naphthoute)	T37.2X1	T37.2X2	T37.2X3	T37.2X4	T37.2X5	T37.2X6
Panadol	T39.1X1	T39.1X2	T39.1X3	T39.1X4	T39.1X5	T39.1X6
Pancreatic						
digestive secretion stimulant	T47.8X1	T47.8X2	T47.8X3	T47.8X4	T47.8X5	T47.8X6
dornase	T45.3X1	T45.3X2	T45.3X3	T45.3X4	T45.3X5	T45.3X6
Pancreatin	T47.5X1	T47.5X2	T47.5X3	T47.5X4	T47.5X5	T47.5X6
Pancrelipase	T47.5X1	T47.5X2	T47.5X3	T47.5X4	T47.5X5	T47.5X6
Pancuronium (bromide)	T48.1X1	T48.1X2	T48.1X3	T48.1X4	T48.1X5	T48.1X6
Pangamic acid	T45.2X1	T45.2X2	T45.2X3	T45.2X4	T45.2X5	T45.2X6
Panthenol	T45.2X1	T45.2X2	T45.2X3	T45.2X4	T45.2X5	T45.2X6
topical	T49.8X1	T49.8X2	T49.8X3	T49.8X4	T49.8X5	T49.8X6
Pantopon	T40.0X1	T40.0X2	T40.0X3	T40.0X4	T40.0X5	T40.0X6
Pantothenic acid	T45.2X1	T45.2X2	T45.2X3	T45.2X4	T45.2X5	T45.2X6
Panwarfin	T45.511	T45.512	T45.513	T45.514	T45.515	T45.516
Papain	T47.5X1	T47.5X2	T47.5X3	T47.5X4	T47.5X5	T47.5X6
digestant	T47.5X1	T47.5X2	T47.5X3	T47.5X4	T47.5X5	T47.5X6
Papaveretum	T40.0X1	T40.0X2	T40.0X3	T40.0X4	T40.0X5	T40.0X6
Papaverine	T44.3X1	T44.3X2	T44.3X3	T44.3X4	T44.3X5	T44.3X6
Para-acetamidophenol	T39.1X1	T39.1X2	T39.1X3	T39.1X4	T39.1X5	T39.1X6
Para-aminobenzoic acid	T49.3X1	T49.3X2	T49.3X3	T49.3X4	T49.3X5	T49.3X6
Para-aminophenol derivatives	T39.1X1	T39.1X2	T39.1X3	T39.1X4	T39.1X5	T39.1X6
Para-aminosalicylic acid	T37.1X1	T37.1X2	T37.1X3	T37.1X4	T37.1X5	T37.1X6
Paracetaldehyde	T42.6X1	T42.6X2	T42.6X3	T42.6X4	T42.6X5	T42.6X6
Paracetamol	T39.1X1	T39.1X2	T39.1X3	T39.1X4	T39.1X5	T39.1X6
Parachlorophenol (camphorated)	T49.0X1	T49.0X2	T49.0X3	T49.0X4	T49.0X5	T49.0X6
Paracodin	T40.2X1	T40.2X2	T40.2X3	T40.2X4	T40.2X5	T40.2X6

Substance	Poisoning, Accidental (unintentional)	Poisoning, Intentional Self-harm	Poisoning, Assault	Poisoning, Undetermined	Adverse Effect	Under-dosing
Paradione	T42.2X1	T42.2X2	T42.2X3	T42.2X4	T42.2X5	T42.2X6
Paraffin(s) (wax)	T52.0X1	T52.0X2	T52.0X3	T52.0X4	—	—
liquid (medicinal)	T47.4X1	T47.4X2	T47.4X3	T47.4X4	T47.4X5	T47.4X6
nonmedicinal	T52.0X1	T52.0X2	T52.0X3	T52.0X4	—	—
Paraformaldehyde	T60.3X1	T60.3X2	T60.3X3	T60.3X4	—	—
Paraldehyde	T42.6X1	T42.6X2	T42.6X3	T42.6X4	T42.6X5	T42.6X6
Paramethadione	T42.2X1	T42.2X2	T42.2X3	T42.2X4	T42.2X5	T42.2X6
Paramethasone	T38.0X1	T38.0X2	T38.0X3	T38.0X4	T38.0X5	T38.0X6
acetate	T49.0X1	T49.0X2	T49.0X3	T49.0X4	T49.0X5	T49.0X6
Paraoxon	T60.0X1	T60.0X2	T60.0X3	T60.0X4	—	—
Paraquat	T60.3X1	T60.3X2	T60.3X3	T60.3X4	—	—
Parasympatholytic NEC	T44.3X1	T44.3X2	T44.3X3	T44.3X4	T44.3X5	T44.3X6
Parasympathomimetic drug NEC	T44.1X1	T44.1X2	T44.1X3	T44.1X4	T44.1X5	T44.1X6
Parathion	T60.0X1	T60.0X2	T60.0X3	T60.0X4	—	—
Parathormone	T50.991	T50.992	T50.993	T50.994	T50.995	T50.996
Parathyroid extract	T50.991	T50.992	T50.993	T50.994	T50.995	T50.996
Paratyphoid vaccine	T50.A91	T50.A92	T50.A93	T50.A94	T50.A95	T50.A96
Paredrine	T44.4X1	T44.4X2	T44.4X3	T44.4X4	T44.4X5	T44.4X6
Paregoric	T40.0X1	T40.0X2	T40.0X3	T40.0X4	T40.0X5	T40.0X6
Pargyline	T46.5X1	T46.5X2	T46.5X3	T46.5X4	T46.5X5	T46.5X6
Paris green	T57.0X1	T57.0X2	T57.0X3	T57.0X4	—	—
insecticide	T57.0X1	T57.0X2	T57.0X3	T57.0X4	—	—
Parnate	T43.1X1	T43.1X2	T43.1X3	T43.1X4	T43.1X5	T43.1X6
Paromomycin	T36.5X1	T36.5X2	T36.5X3	T36.5X4	T36.5X5	T36.5X6
Paroxypropione	T45.1X1	T45.1X2	T45.1X3	T45.1X4	T45.1X5	T45.1X6
Parzone	T40.2X1	T40.2X2	T40.2X3	T40.2X4	T40.2X5	T40.2X6
PAS	T37.1X1	T37.1X2	T37.1X3	T37.1X4	T37.1X5	T37.1X6
Pasiniazid	T37.1X1	T37.1X2	T37.1X3	T37.1X4	T37.1X5	T37.1X6
PBB (polybrominated biphenyls)	T65.891	T65.892	T65.893	T65.894	—	—
PCB	T65.891	T65.892	T65.893	T65.894	—	—
PCP						
meaning pentachlorophenol	T60.1X1	T60.1X2	T60.1X3	T60.1X4		
fungicide	T60.3X1	T60.3X2	T60.3X3	T60.3X4		
herbicide	T60.3X1	T60.3X2	T60.3X3	T60.3X4		
insecticide	T60.1X1	T60.1X2	T60.1X3	T60.1X4		
meaning phencyclidine	T40.991	T40.992	T40.993	T40.994		
Peach kernel oil (emulsion)	T47.4X1	T47.4X2	T47.4X3	T47.4X4	T47.4X5	T47.4X6
Peanut oil (emulsion) NEC	T47.4X1	T47.4X2	T47.4X3	T47.4X4	T47.4X5	T47.4X6
topical	T49.3X1	T49.3X2	T49.3X3	T49.3X4	T49.3X5	T49.3X6
Pearly Gates (morning glory seeds)	T40.991	T40.992	T40.993	T40.994	—	—
Pecazine	T43.3X1	T43.3X2	T43.3X3	T43.3X4	T43.3X5	T43.3X6
Pectin	T47.6X1	T47.6X2	T47.6X3	T47.6X4	T47.6X5	T47.6X6
Pefloxacin	T37.8X1	T37.8X2	T37.8X3	T37.8X4	T37.8X5	T37.8X6
Pegademase, bovine	T50.Z91	T50.Z92	T50.Z93	T50.Z94	T50.Z95	T50.Z96
Pelletierine tannate	T37.4X1	T37.4X2	T37.4X3	T37.4X4	T37.4X5	T37.4X6
Pemirolast (potassium)	T48.6X1	T48.6X2	T48.6X3	T48.6X4	T48.6X5	T48.6X6
Pemoline	T50.7X1	T50.7X2	T50.7X3	T50.7X4	T50.7X5	T50.7X6
Pempidine	T44.2X1	T44.2X2	T44.2X3	T44.2X4	T44.2X5	T44.2X6
Penamecillin	T36.0X1	T36.0X2	T36.0X3	T36.0X4	T36.0X5	T36.0X6
Penbutolol	T44.7X1	T44.7X2	T44.7X3	T44.7X4	T44.7X5	T44.7X6
Penethamate	T36.0X1	T36.0X2	T36.0X3	T36.0X4	T36.0X5	T36.0X6
Penfluridol	T43.591	T43.592	T43.593	T43.594	T43.595	T43.596
Penflutizide	T50.2X1	T50.2X2	T50.2X3	T50.2X4	T50.2X5	T50.2X6
Pengitoxin	T46.0X1	T46.0X2	T46.0X3	T46.0X4	T46.0X5	T46.0X6
Penicillamine	T50.6X1	T50.6X2	T50.6X3	T50.6X4	T50.6X5	T50.6X6
Penicillin (any)	T36.0X1	T36.0X2	T36.0X3	T36.0X4	T36.0X5	T36.0X6
Penicillinase	T45.3X1	T45.3X2	T45.3X3	T45.3X4	T45.3X5	T45.3X6
Penicilloyl polylysine	T50.8X1	T50.8X2	T50.8X3	T50.8X4	T50.8X5	T50.8X6
Penimepicycline	T36.4X1	T36.4X2	T36.4X3	T36.4X4	T36.4X5	T36.4X6
Pentachloroethane	T53.6X1	T53.6X2	T53.6X3	T53.6X4	—	—
Pentachloronaphthalene	T53.7X1	T53.7X2	T53.7X3	T53.7X4	—	—
Pentachlorophenol (pesticide)	T60.1X1	T60.1X2	T60.1X3	T60.1X4	—	—
fungicide	T60.3X1	T60.3X2	T60.3X3	T60.3X4	—	—
herbicide	T60.3X1	T60.3X2	T60.3X3	T60.3X4	—	—
insecticide	T60.1X1	T60.1X2	T60.1X3	T60.1X4	—	—
Pentaerythritol	T46.3X1	T46.3X2	T46.3X3	T46.3X4	T46.3X5	T46.3X6
chloral	T42.6X1	T42.6X2	T42.6X3	T42.6X4	T42.6X5	T42.6X6
tetranitrate NEC	T46.3X1	T46.3X2	T46.3X3	T46.3X4	T46.3X5	T46.3X6
Pentaerythrityl tetranitrate	T46.3X1	T46.3X2	T46.3X3	T46.3X4	T46.3X5	T46.3X6
Pentagastrin	T50.8X1	T50.8X2	T50.8X3	T50.8X4	T50.8X5	T50.8X6
Pentalin	T53.6X1	T53.6X2	T53.6X3	T53.6X4	—	—
Pentamethonium bromide	T44.2X1	T44.2X2	T44.2X3	T44.2X4	T44.2X5	T44.2X6
Pentamidine	T37.3X1	T37.3X2	T37.3X3	T37.3X4	T37.3X5	T37.3X6
Pentanol	T51.3X1	T51.3X2	T51.3X3	T51.3X4	—	—
Pentapyrrolinium (bitartrate)	T44.2X1	T44.2X2	T44.2X3	T44.2X4	T44.2X5	T44.2X6
Pentaquine	T37.2X1	T37.2X2	T37.2X3	T37.2X4	T37.2X5	T37.2X6

Additional Character May Be Required — Refer to the Tabular List for Character Selection ▽ Subterms under main terms may continue to next column or page

Substance	Poisoning, Accidental (unintentional)	Poisoning, Intentional Self-harm	Poisoning, Assault	Poisoning, Undetermined	Adverse Effect	Under-dosing
Pentazocine	T40.4X1	T40.4X2	T40.4X3	T40.4X4	T40.4X5	T40.4X6
Pentetrazole	T50.7X1	T50.7X2	T50.7X3	T50.7X4	T50.7X5	T50.7X6
Penthienate bromide	T44.3X1	T44.3X2	T44.3X3	T44.3X4	T44.3X5	T44.3X6
Pentifylline	T46.7X1	T46.7X2	T46.7X3	T46.7X4	T46.7X5	T46.7X6
Pentobarbital	T42.3X1	T42.3X2	T42.3X3	T42.3X4	T42.3X5	T42.3X6
sodium	T42.3X1	T42.3X2	T42.3X3	T42.3X4	T42.3X5	T42.3X6
Pentobarbitone	T42.3X1	T42.3X2	T42.3X3	T42.3X4	T42.3X5	T42.3X6
Pentolonium tartrate	T44.2X1	T44.2X2	T44.2X3	T44.2X4	T44.2X5	T44.2X6
Pentosan polysulfate (sodium)	T39.8X1	T39.8X2	T39.8X3	T39.8X4	T39.8X5	T39.8X6
Pentostatin	T45.1X1	T45.1X2	T45.1X3	T45.1X4	T45.1X5	T45.1X6
Pentothal	T41.1X1	T41.1X2	T41.1X3	T41.1X4	T41.1X5	T41.1X6
Pentoxifylline	T46.7X1	T46.7X2	T46.7X3	T46.7X4	T46.7X5	T46.7X6
Pentoxyverine	T48.3X1	T48.3X2	T48.3X3	T48.3X4	T48.3X5	T48.3X6
Pentrinat	T46.3X1	T46.3X2	T46.3X3	T46.3X4	T46.3X5	T46.3X6
Pentylenetetrazole	T50.7X1	T50.7X2	T50.7X3	T50.7X4	T50.7X5	T50.7X6
Pentylsalicylamide	T37.1X1	T37.1X2	T37.1X3	T37.1X4	T37.1X5	T37.1X6
Pentymal	T42.3X1	T42.3X2	T42.3X3	T42.3X4	T42.3X5	T42.3X6
Peplomycin	T45.1X1	T45.1X2	T45.1X3	T45.1X4	T45.1X5	T45.1X6
Peppermint (oil)	T47.5X1	T47.5X2	T47.5X3	T47.5X4	T47.5X5	T47.5X6
Pepsin	T47.5X1	T47.5X2	T47.5X3	T47.5X4	T47.5X5	T47.5X6
digestant	T47.5X1	T47.5X2	T47.5X3	T47.5X4	T47.5X5	T47.5X6
Pepstatin	T47.1X1	T47.1X2	T47.1X3	T47.1X4	T47.1X5	T47.1X6
Peptavlon	T50.8X1	T50.8X2	T50.8X3	T50.8X4	T50.8X5	T50.8X6
Perazine	T43.3X1	T43.3X2	T43.3X3	T43.3X4	T43.3X5	T43.3X6
Percaine (spinal)	T41.3X1	T41.3X2	T41.3X3	T41.3X4	T41.3X5	T41.3X6
topical (surface)	T41.3X1	T41.3X2	T41.3X3	T41.3X4	T41.3X5	T41.3X6
Perchloroethylene	T53.3X1	T53.3X2	T53.3X3	T53.3X4	—	—
medicinal	T37.4X1	T37.4X2	T37.4X3	T37.4X4	T37.4X5	T37.4X6
vapor	T53.3X1	T53.3X2	T53.3X3	T53.3X4	—	—
Percodan	T40.2X1	T40.2X2	T40.2X3	T40.2X4	T40.2X5	T40.2X6
Percogesic — see also acetaminophen	T45.0X1	T45.0X2	T45.0X3	T45.0X4	T45.0X5	T45.0X6
Percorten	T38.0X1	T38.0X2	T38.0X3	T38.0X4	T38.0X5	T38.0X6
Pergolide	T42.8X1	T42.8X2	T42.8X3	T42.8X4	T42.8X5	T42.8X6
Pergonal	T38.811	T38.812	T38.813	T38.814	T38.815	T38.816
Perhexilene	T46.3X1	T46.3X2	T46.3X3	T46.3X4	T46.3X5	T46.3X6
Perhexiline (maleate)	T46.3X1	T46.3X2	T46.3X3	T46.3X4	T46.3X5	T46.3X6
Periactin	T45.0X1	T45.0X2	T45.0X3	T45.0X4	T45.0X5	T45.0X6
Periciazine	T43.3X1	T43.3X2	T43.3X3	T43.3X4	T43.3X5	T43.3X6
Periclor	T42.6X1	T42.6X2	T42.6X3	T42.6X4	T42.6X5	T42.6X6
Perindopril	T46.4X1	T46.4X2	T46.4X3	T46.4X4	T46.4X5	T46.4X6
Perisoxal	T39.8X1	T39.8X2	T39.8X3	T39.8X4	T39.8X5	T39.8X6
Peritoneal dialysis solution	T50.3X1	T50.3X2	T50.3X3	T50.3X4	T50.3X5	T50.3X6
Peritrate	T46.3X1	T46.3X2	T46.3X3	T46.3X4	T46.3X5	T46.3X6
Perlapine	T42.4X1	T42.4X2	T42.4X3	T42.4X4	T42.4X5	T42.4X6
Permanganate	T65.891	T65.892	T65.893	T65.894	—	—
Permethrin	T60.1X1	T60.1X2	T60.1X3	T60.1X4	—	—
Pernocton	T42.3X1	T42.3X2	T42.3X3	T42.3X4	T42.3X5	T42.3X6
Pernoston	T42.3X1	T42.3X2	T42.3X3	T42.3X4	T42.3X5	T42.3X6
Peronine	T40.2X1	T40.2X2	T40.2X3	T40.2X4	—	—
Perphenazine	T43.3X1	T43.3X2	T43.3X3	T43.3X4	T43.3X5	T43.3X6
Pertofrane	T43.011	T43.012	T43.013	T43.014	T43.015	T43.016
Pertussis						
immune serum (human)	T50.Z11	T50.Z12	T50.Z13	T50.Z14	T50.Z15	T50.Z16
vaccine (with diphtheria toxoid) (with tetanus toxoid)	T50.A11	T50.A12	T50.A13	T50.A14	T50.A15	T50.A16
Peruvian balsam	T49.0X1	T49.0X2	T49.0X3	T49.0X4	T49.0X5	T49.0X6
Peruvoside	T46.0X1	T46.0X2	T46.0X3	T46.0X4	T46.0X5	T46.0X6
Pesticide (dust) (fumes) (vapor) NEC	T60.91	T60.92	T60.93	T60.94	—	—
arsenic	T57.0X1	T57.0X2	T57.0X3	T57.0X4	—	—
chlorinated	T60.1X1	T60.1X2	T60.1X3	T60.1X4	—	—
cyanide	T65.0X1	T65.0X2	T65.0X3	T65.0X4	—	—
kerosene	T52.0X1	T52.0X2	T52.0X3	T52.0X4	—	—
mixture (of compounds)	T60.91	T60.92	T60.93	T60.94	—	—
naphthalene	T60.2X1	T60.2X2	T60.2X3	T60.2X4	—	—
organochlorine (compounds)	T60.1X1	T60.1X2	T60.1X3	T60.1X4	—	—
petroleum (distillate) (products) NEC	T60.8X1	T60.8X2	T60.8X3	T60.8X4	—	—
specified ingredient NEC	T60.8X1	T60.8X2	T60.8X3	T60.8X4	—	—
strychnine	T65.1X1	T65.1X2	T65.1X3	T65.1X4	—	—
thallium	T60.4X1	T60.4X2	T60.4X3	T60.4X4	—	—
Pethidine	T40.4X1	T40.4X2	T40.4X3	T40.4X4	T40.4X5	T40.4X6
Petrichloral	T42.6X1	T42.6X2	T42.6X3	T42.6X4	T42.6X5	T42.6X6
Petrol	T52.0X1	T52.0X2	T52.0X3	T52.0X4	—	—
vapor	T52.0X1	T52.0X2	T52.0X3	T52.0X4	—	—
Petrolatum	T49.3X1	T49.3X2	T49.3X3	T49.3X4	T49.3X5	T49.3X6
hydrophilic	T49.3X1	T49.3X2	T49.3X3	T49.3X4	T49.3X5	T49.3X6
liquid	T47.4X1	T47.4X2	T47.4X3	T47.4X4	T47.4X5	T47.4X6
topical	T49.3X1	T49.3X2	T49.3X3	T49.3X4	T49.3X5	T49.3X6
nonmedicinal	T52.0X1	T52.0X2	T52.0X3	T52.0X4	—	—

Substance	Poisoning, Accidental (unintentional)	Poisoning, Intentional Self-harm	Poisoning, Assault	Poisoning, Undetermined	Adverse Effect	Under-dosing
Petrolatum — continued						
red veterinary	T49.3X1	T49.3X2	T49.3X3	T49.3X4	T49.3X5	T49.3X6
white	T49.3X1	T49.3X2	T49.3X3	T49.3X4	T49.3X5	T49.3X6
Petroleum (products) NEC	T52.0X1	T52.0X2	T52.0X3	T52.0X4	—	—
benzine(s) — see Ligroin						
ether — see Ligroin						
jelly — see Petrolatum						
naphtha — see Ligroin						
pesticide	T60.8X1	T60.8X2	T60.8X3	T60.8X4	—	—
solids	T52.0X1	T52.0X2	T52.0X3	T52.0X4	—	—
solvents	T52.0X1	T52.0X2	T52.0X3	T52.0X4	—	—
vapor	T52.0X1	T52.0X2	T52.0X3	T52.0X4	—	—
Peyote	T40.991	T40.992	T40.993	T40.994	—	—
Phanodorm, phanodorn	T42.3X1	T42.3X2	T42.3X3	T42.3X4	T42.3X5	T42.3X6
Phanquinone	T37.3X1	T37.3X2	T37.3X3	T37.3X4	T37.3X5	T37.3X6
Phanquone	T37.3X1	T37.3X2	T37.3X3	T37.3X4	T37.3X5	T37.3X6
Pharmaceutical						
adjunct NEC	T50.901	T50.902	T50.903	T50.904	T50.905	T50.906
excipient NEC	T50.901	T50.902	T50.903	T50.904	T50.905	T50.906
sweetener	T50.901	T50.902	T50.903	T50.904	T50.905	T50.906
viscous agent	T50.901	T50.902	T50.903	T50.904	T50.905	T50.906
Phemitone	T42.3X1	T42.3X2	T42.3X3	T42.3X4	T42.3X5	T42.3X6
Phenacaine	T41.3X1	T41.3X2	T41.3X3	T41.3X4	T41.3X5	T41.3X6
Phenacemide	T42.6X1	T42.6X2	T42.6X3	T42.6X4	T42.6X5	T42.6X6
Phenacetin	T39.1X1	T39.1X2	T39.1X3	T39.1X4	T39.1X5	T39.1X6
Phenadoxone	T40.2X1	T40.2X2	T40.2X3	T40.2X4	—	—
Phenaglycodol	T43.591	T43.592	T43.593	T43.594	T43.595	T43.596
Phenantoin	T42.0X1	T42.0X2	T42.0X3	T42.0X4	T42.0X5	T42.0X6
Phenaphthazine reagent	T50.991	T50.992	T50.993	T50.994	T50.995	T50.996
Phenazocine	T40.4X1	T40.4X2	T40.4X3	T40.4X4	T40.4X5	T40.4X6
Phenazone	T39.2X1	T39.2X2	T39.2X3	T39.2X4	T39.2X5	T39.2X6
Phenazopyridine	T39.8X1	T39.8X2	T39.8X3	T39.8X4	T39.8X5	T39.8X6
Phenbenicillin	T36.0X1	T36.0X2	T36.0X3	T36.0X4	T36.0X5	T36.0X6
Phenbutrazate	T50.5X1	T50.5X2	T50.5X3	T50.5X4	T50.5X5	T50.5X6
Phencyclidine	T40.991	T40.992	T40.993	T40.994	T40.995	T40.996
Phendimetrazine	T50.5X1	T50.5X2	T50.5X3	T50.5X4	T50.5X5	T50.5X6
Phenelzine	T43.1X1	T43.1X2	T43.1X3	T43.1X4	T43.1X5	T43.1X6
Phenemal	T42.3X1	T42.3X2	T42.3X3	T42.3X4	T42.3X5	T42.3X6
Phenergan	T42.6X1	T42.6X2	T42.6X3	T42.6X4	T42.6X5	T42.6X6
Phenethicillin	T36.0X1	T36.0X2	T36.0X3	T36.0X4	T36.0X5	T36.0X6
Pheneticillin	T36.0X1	T36.0X2	T36.0X3	T36.0X4	T36.0X5	T36.0X6
Pheneturide	T42.6X1	T42.6X2	T42.6X3	T42.6X4	T42.6X5	T42.6X6
Phenformin	T38.3X1	T38.3X2	T38.3X3	T38.3X4	T38.3X5	T38.3X6
Phenglutarimide	T44.3X1	T44.3X2	T44.3X3	T44.3X4	T44.3X5	T44.3X6
Phenicarbazide	T39.8X1	T39.8X2	T39.8X3	T39.8X4	T39.8X5	T39.8X6
Phenindamine	T45.0X1	T45.0X2	T45.0X3	T45.0X4	T45.0X5	T45.0X6
Phenindione	T45.511	T45.512	T45.513	T45.514	T45.515	T45.516
Pheniprazine	T43.1X1	T43.1X2	T43.1X3	T43.1X4	T43.1X5	T43.1X6
Pheniramine	T45.0X1	T45.0X2	T45.0X3	T45.0X4	T45.0X5	T45.0X6
Phenisatin	T47.2X1	T47.2X2	T47.2X3	T47.2X4	T47.2X5	T47.2X6
Phenmetrazine	T50.5X1	T50.5X2	T50.5X3	T50.5X4	T50.5X5	T50.5X6
Phenobal	T42.3X1	T42.3X2	T42.3X3	T42.3X4	T42.3X5	T42.3X6
Phenobarbital	T42.3X1	T42.3X2	T42.3X3	T42.3X4	T42.3X5	T42.3X6
with						
mephenytoin	T42.3X1	T42.3X2	T42.3X3	T42.3X4	T42.3X5	T42.3X6
phenytoin	T42.3X1	T42.3X2	T42.3X3	T42.3X4	T42.3X5	T42.3X6
sodium	T42.3X1	T42.3X2	T42.3X3	T42.3X4	T42.3X5	T42.3X6
Phenobarbitone	T42.3X1	T42.3X2	T42.3X3	T42.3X4	T42.3X5	T42.3X6
Phenobutiodil	T50.8X1	T50.8X2	T50.8X3	T50.8X4	T50.8X5	T50.8X6
Phenoctide	T49.0X1	T49.0X2	T49.0X3	T49.0X4	T49.0X5	T49.0X6
Phenol	T49.0X1	T49.0X2	T49.0X3	T49.0X4	T49.0X5	T49.0X6
disinfectant	T54.0X1	T54.0X2	T54.0X3	T54.0X4	—	—
in oil injection	T46.8X1	T46.8X2	T46.8X3	T46.8X4	T46.8X5	T46.8X6
medicinal	T49.1X1	T49.1X2	T49.1X3	T49.1X4	T49.1X5	T49.1X6
nonmedicinal NEC	T54.0X1	T54.0X2	T54.0X3	T54.0X4	—	—
pesticide	T60.8X1	T60.8X2	T60.8X3	T60.8X4	—	—
red	T50.8X1	T50.8X2	T50.8X3	T50.8X4	T50.8X5	T50.8X6
Phenolic preparation	T49.1X1	T49.1X2	T49.1X3	T49.1X4	T49.1X5	T49.1X6
Phenolphthalein	T47.2X1	T47.2X2	T47.2X3	T47.2X4	T47.2X5	T47.2X6
Phenolsulfonphthalein	T50.8X1	T50.8X2	T50.8X3	T50.8X4	T50.8X5	T50.8X6
Phenomorphan	T40.2X1	T40.2X2	T40.2X3	T40.2X4	—	—
Phenonyl	T42.3X1	T42.3X2	T42.3X3	T42.3X4	T42.3X5	T42.3X6
Phenoperidine	T40.4X1	T40.4X2	T40.4X3	T40.4X4	—	—
Phenopyrazone	T46.991	T46.992	T46.993	T46.994	T46.995	T46.996
Phenoquin	T50.4X1	T50.4X2	T50.4X3	T50.4X4	T50.4X5	T50.4X6
Phenothiazine (psychotropic) NEC	T43.3X1	T43.3X2	T43.3X3	T43.3X4	T43.3X5	T43.3X6
insecticide	T60.2X1	T60.2X2	T60.2X3	T60.2X4	—	—
Phenothrin	T49.0X1	T49.0X2	T49.0X3	T49.0X4	T49.0X5	T49.0X6
Phenoxybenzamine	T46.7X1	T46.7X2	T46.7X3	T46.7X4	T46.7X5	T46.7X6
Phenoxyethanol	T49.0X1	T49.0X2	T49.0X3	T49.0X4	T49.0X5	T49.0X6
Phenoxymethyl penicillin	T36.0X1	T36.0X2	T36.0X3	T36.0X4	T36.0X5	T36.0X6
Phenprobamate	T42.8X1	T42.8X2	T42.8X3	T42.8X4	T42.8X5	T42.8X6
Phenprocoumon	T45.511	T45.512	T45.513	T45.514	T45.515	T45.516

Substance	Poisoning, Accidental (unintentional)	Poisoning, Intentional Self-harm	Poisoning, Assault	Poisoning, Undetermined	Adverse Effect	Under-dosing
Phensuximide	T42.2X1	T42.2X2	T42.2X3	T42.2X4	T42.2X5	T42.2X6
Phentermine	T50.5X1	T50.5X2	T50.5X3	T50.5X4	T50.5X5	T50.5X6
Phenthicillin	T36.0X1	T36.0X2	T36.0X3	T36.0X4	T36.0X5	T36.0X6
Phentolamine	T46.7X1	T46.7X2	T46.7X3	T46.7X4	T46.7X5	T46.7X6
Phenyl						
butazone	T39.2X1	T39.2X2	T39.2X3	T39.2X4	T39.2X5	T39.2X6
enediamine	T65.3X1	T65.3X2	T65.3X3	T65.3X4	—	—
hydrazine	T65.3X1	T65.3X2	T65.3X3	T65.3X4	—	—
antineoplastic	T45.1X1	T45.1X2	T45.1X3	T45.1X4	T45.1X5	T45.1X6
mercuric compounds — see Mercury						
salicylate	T49.3X1	T49.3X2	T49.3X3	T49.3X4	T49.3X5	T49.3X6
Phenylalanine mustard	T45.1X1	T45.1X2	T45.1X3	T45.1X4	T45.1X5	T45.1X6
Phenylbutazone	T39.2X1	T39.2X2	T39.2X3	T39.2X4	T39.2X5	T39.2X6
Phenylenediamine	T65.3X1	T65.3X2	T65.3X3	T65.3X4	—	—
Phenylephrine	T44.4X1	T44.4X2	T44.4X3	T44.4X4	T44.4X5	T44.4X6
Phenylethylbiguanide	T38.3X1	T38.3X2	T38.3X3	T38.3X4	T38.3X5	T38.3X6
Phenylmercuric						
acetate	T49.0X1	T49.0X2	T49.0X3	T49.0X4	T49.0X5	T49.0X6
borate	T49.0X1	T49.0X2	T49.0X3	T49.0X4	T49.0X5	T49.0X6
nitrate	T49.0X1	T49.0X2	T49.0X3	T49.0X4	T49.0X5	T49.0X6
Phenylmethylbarbitone	T42.3X1	T42.3X2	T42.3X3	T42.3X4	T42.3X5	T42.3X6
Phenylpropanol	T47.5X1	T47.5X2	T47.5X3	T47.5X4	T47.5X5	T47.5X6
Phenylpropanolamine	T44.991	T44.992	T44.993	T44.994	T44.995	T44.996
Phenylsulfthion	T60.0X1	T60.0X2	T60.0X3	T60.0X4	—	—
Phenyltoloxamine	T45.0X1	T45.0X2	T45.0X3	T45.0X4	T45.0X5	T45.0X6
Phenyramidol, phenyramidon	T39.8X1	T39.8X2	T39.8X3	T39.8X4	T39.8X5	T39.8X6
Phenytoin	T42.0X1	T42.0X2	T42.0X3	T42.0X4	T42.0X5	T42.0X6
with Phenobarbital	T42.3X1	T42.3X2	T42.3X3	T42.3X4	T42.3X5	T42.3X6
pHisoHex	T49.2X1	T49.2X2	T49.2X3	T49.2X4	T49.2X5	T49.2X6
Pholcodine	T48.3X1	T48.3X2	T48.3X3	T48.3X4	T48.3X5	T48.3X6
Pholedrine	T46.991	T46.992	T46.993	T46.994	T46.995	T46.996
Phorate	T60.0X1	T60.0X2	T60.0X3	T60.0X4	—	—
Phosdrin	T60.0X1	T60.0X2	T60.0X3	T60.0X4	—	—
Phosfolan	T60.0X1	T60.0X2	T60.0X3	T60.0X4	—	—
Phosgene (gas)	T59.891	T59.892	T59.893	T59.894	—	—
Phosphamidon	T60.0X1	T60.0X2	T60.0X3	T60.0X4	—	—
Phosphate	T65.891	T65.892	T65.893	T65.894	—	—
laxative	T47.4X1	T47.4X2	T47.4X3	T47.4X4	T47.4X5	T47.4X6
organic	T60.0X1	T60.0X2	T60.0X3	T60.0X4	—	—
solvent	T52.91	T52.92	T52.93	T52.94	—	—
tricresyl	T65.891	T65.892	T65.893	T65.894	—	—
Phosphine	T57.1X1	T57.1X2	T57.1X3	T57.1X4	—	—
fumigant	T57.1X1	T57.1X2	T57.1X3	T57.1X4	—	—
Phospholine	T49.5X1	T49.5X2	T49.5X3	T49.5X4	T49.5X5	T49.5X6
Phosphoric acid	T54.2X1	T54.2X2	T54.2X3	T54.2X4	—	—
Phosphorus (compound) NEC	T57.1X1	T57.1X2	T57.1X3	T57.1X4	—	—
pesticide	T60.0X1	T60.0X2	T60.0X3	T60.0X4	—	—
Phthalates	T65.891	T65.892	T65.893	T65.894	—	—
Phthalic anhydride	T65.891	T65.892	T65.893	T65.894	—	—
Phthalimidoglutarimide	T42.6X1	T42.6X2	T42.6X3	T42.6X4	T42.6X5	T42.6X6
Phthalylsulfathiazole	T37.0X1	T37.0X2	T37.0X3	T37.0X4	T37.0X5	T37.0X6
Phylloquinone	T45.7X1	T45.7X2	T45.7X3	T45.7X4	T45.7X5	T45.7X6
Physeptone	T40.3X1	T40.3X2	T40.3X3	T40.3X4	T40.3X5	T40.3X6
Physostigma venenosum	T62.2X1	T62.2X2	T62.2X3	T62.2X4	—	—
Physostigmine	T49.5X1	T49.5X2	T49.5X3	T49.5X4	T49.5X5	T49.5X6
Phytolacca decandra	T62.2X1	T62.2X2	T62.2X3	T62.2X4	—	—
berries	T62.1X1	T62.1X2	T62.1X3	T62.1X4	—	—
Phytomenadione	T45.7X1	T45.7X2	T45.7X3	T45.7X4	T45.7X5	T45.7X6
Phytonadione	T45.7X1	T45.7X2	T45.7X3	T45.7X4	T45.7X5	T45.7X6
Picoperine	T48.3X1	T48.3X2	T48.3X3	T48.3X4	T48.3X5	T48.3X6
Picosulfate (sodium)	T47.2X1	T47.2X2	T47.2X3	T47.2X4	T47.2X5	T47.2X6
Picric (acid)	T54.2X1	T54.2X2	T54.2X3	T54.2X4	—	—
Picrotoxin	T50.7X1	T50.7X2	T50.7X3	T50.7X4	T50.7X5	T50.7X6
Piketoprofen	T49.0X1	T49.0X2	T49.0X3	T49.0X4	T49.0X5	T49.0X6
Pilocarpine	T44.1X1	T44.1X2	T44.1X3	T44.1X4	T44.1X5	T44.1X6
Pilocarpus (jaborandi)	T44.1X1	T44.1X2	T44.1X3	T44.1X4	T44.1X5	T44.1X6
extract						
Pilsicainide (hydrochloride)	T46.2X1	T46.2X2	T46.2X3	T46.2X4	T46.2X5	T46.2X6
Pimaricin	T36.7X1	T36.7X2	T36.7X3	T36.7X4	T36.7X5	T36.7X6
Pimeclone	T50.7X1	T50.7X2	T50.7X3	T50.7X4	T50.7X5	T50.7X6
Pimelic ketone	T52.8X1	T52.8X2	T52.8X3	T52.8X4	—	—
Pimethixene	T45.0X1	T45.0X2	T45.0X3	T45.0X4	T45.0X5	T45.0X6
Piminodine	T40.2X1	T40.2X2	T40.2X3	T40.2X4	T40.2X5	T40.2X6
Pimozide	T43.591	T43.592	T43.593	T43.594	T43.595	T43.596
Pinacidil	T46.5X1	T46.5X2	T46.5X3	T46.5X4	T46.5X5	T46.5X6
Pinaverium bromide	T44.3X1	T44.3X2	T44.3X3	T44.3X4	T44.3X5	T44.3X6
Pinazepam	T42.4X1	T42.4X2	T42.4X3	T42.4X4	T42.4X5	T42.4X6
Pindolol	T44.7X1	T44.7X2	T44.7X3	T44.7X4	T44.7X5	T44.7X6
Pindone	T60.4X1	T60.4X2	T60.4X3	T60.4X4	—	—
Pine oil (disinfectant)	T65.891	T65.892	T65.893	T65.894	—	—
Pinkroot	T37.4X1	T37.4X2	T37.4X3	T37.4X4	T37.4X5	T37.4X6
Pipadone	T40.2X1	T40.2X2	T40.2X3	T40.2X4	—	—
Pipamazine	T45.0X1	T45.0X2	T45.0X3	T45.0X4	T45.0X5	T45.0X6
Pipamperone	T43.4X1	T43.4X2	T43.4X3	T43.4X4	T43.4X5	T43.4X6
Pipazetate	T48.3X1	T48.3X2	T48.3X3	T48.3X4	T48.3X5	T48.3X6
Pipemidic acid	T37.8X1	T37.8X2	T37.8X3	T37.8X4	T37.8X5	T37.8X6
Pipenzolate bromide	T44.3X1	T44.3X2	T44.3X3	T44.3X4	T44.3X5	T44.3X6
Piperacetazine	T43.3X1	T43.3X2	T43.3X3	T43.3X4	T43.3X5	T43.3X6
Piperacillin	T36.0X1	T36.0X2	T36.0X3	T36.0X4	T36.0X5	T36.0X6
Piperazine	T37.4X1	T37.4X2	T37.4X3	T37.4X4	T37.4X5	T37.4X6
estrone sulfate	T38.5X1	T38.5X2	T38.5X3	T38.5X4	T38.5X5	T38.5X6
Piper cubeba	T62.2X1	T62.2X2	T62.2X3	T62.2X4	—	—
Piperidione	T48.3X1	T48.3X2	T48.3X3	T48.3X4	T48.3X5	T48.3X6
Piperidolate	T44.3X1	T44.3X2	T44.3X3	T44.3X4	T44.3X5	T44.3X6
Piperocaine	T41.3X1	T41.3X2	T41.3X3	T41.3X4	T41.3X5	T41.3X6
infiltration (subcutaneous)	T41.3X1	T41.3X2	T41.3X3	T41.3X4	T41.3X5	T41.3X6
nerve block (peripheral) (plexus)	T41.3X1	T41.3X2	T41.3X3	T41.3X4	T41.3X5	T41.3X6
topical (surface)	T41.3X1	T41.3X2	T41.3X3	T41.3X4	T41.3X5	T41.3X6
Piperonyl butoxide	T60.8X1	T60.8X2	T60.8X3	T60.8X4	—	—
Pipethanate	T44.3X1	T44.3X2	T44.3X3	T44.3X4	T44.3X5	T44.3X6
Pipobroman	T45.1X1	T45.1X2	T45.1X3	T45.1X4	T45.1X5	T45.1X6
Pipotiazine	T43.3X1	T43.3X2	T43.3X3	T43.3X4	T43.3X5	T43.3X6
Pipoxizine	T45.0X1	T45.0X2	T45.0X3	T45.0X4	T45.0X5	T45.0X6
Pipradrol	T43.691	T43.692	T43.693	T43.694	T43.695	T43.696
Piprinhydrinate	T45.0X1	T45.0X2	T45.0X3	T45.0X4	T45.0X5	T45.0X6
Pirarubicin	T45.1X1	T45.1X2	T45.1X3	T45.1X4	T45.1X5	T45.1X6
Pirazinamide	T37.1X1	T37.1X2	T37.1X3	T37.1X4	T37.1X5	T37.1X6
Pirbuterol	T48.6X1	T48.6X2	T48.6X3	T48.6X4	T48.6X5	T48.6X6
Pirenzepine	T47.1X1	T47.1X2	T47.1X3	T47.1X4	T47.1X5	T47.1X6
Piretanide	T50.1X1	T50.1X2	T50.1X3	T50.1X4	T50.1X5	T50.1X6
Piribedil	T42.8X1	T42.8X2	T42.8X3	T42.8X4	T42.8X5	T42.8X6
Piridoxilate	T46.3X1	T46.3X2	T46.3X3	T46.3X4	T46.3X5	T46.3X6
Piritramide	T40.4X1	T40.4X2	T40.4X3	T40.4X4	—	—
Piromidic acid	T37.8X1	T37.8X2	T37.8X3	T37.8X4	T37.8X5	T37.8X6
Piroxicam	T39.391	T39.392	T39.393	T39.394	T39.395	T39.396
beta-cyclodextrin complex	T39.8X1	T39.8X2	T39.8X3	T39.8X4	T39.8X5	T39.8X6
Pirozadil	T46.6X1	T46.6X2	T46.6X3	T46.6X4	T46.6X5	T46.6X6
Piscidia (bark) (erythrina)	T39.8X1	T39.8X2	T39.8X3	T39.8X4	T39.8X5	T39.8X6
Pitch	T65.891	T65.892	T65.893	T65.894	—	—
Pitkin's solution	T41.3X1	T41.3X2	T41.3X3	T41.3X4	T41.3X5	T41.3X6
Pitocin	T48.0X1	T48.0X2	T48.0X3	T48.0X4	T48.0X5	T48.0X6
Pitressin (tannate)	T38.891	T38.892	T38.893	T38.894	T38.895	T38.896
Pituitary extracts (posterior)	T38.891	T38.892	T38.893	T38.894	T38.895	T38.896
anterior	T38.811	T38.812	T38.813	T38.814	T38.815	T38.816
Pituitrin	T38.891	T38.892	T38.893	T38.894	T38.895	T38.896
Pivampicillin	T36.0X1	T36.0X2	T36.0X3	T36.0X4	T36.0X5	T36.0X6
Pivmecillinam	T36.0X1	T36.0X2	T36.0X3	T36.0X4	T36.0X5	T36.0X6
Placental hormone	T38.891	T38.892	T38.893	T38.894	T38.895	T38.896
Placidyl	T42.6X1	T42.6X2	T42.6X3	T42.6X4	T42.6X5	T42.6X6
Plague vaccine	T50.A91	T50.A92	T50.A93	T50.A94	T50.A95	T50.A96
Plant						
food or fertilizer NEC	T65.891	T65.892	T65.893	T65.894	—	—
containing herbicide	T60.3X1	T60.3X2	T60.3X3	T60.3X4	—	—
noxious, used as food	T62.2X1	T62.2X2	T62.2X3	T62.2X4	—	—
berries	T62.1X1	T62.1X2	T62.1X3	T62.1X4	—	—
seeds	T62.2X1	T62.2X2	T62.2X3	T62.2X4	—	—
specified type NEC	T62.2X1	T62.2X2	T62.2X3	T62.2X4	—	—
Plasma	T45.8X1	T45.8X2	T45.8X3	T45.8X4	T45.8X5	T45.8X6
expander NEC	T45.8X1	T45.8X2	T45.8X3	T45.8X4	T45.8X5	T45.8X6
protein fraction (human)	T45.8X1	T45.8X2	T45.8X3	T45.8X4	T45.8X5	T45.8X6
Plasmanate	T45.8X1	T45.8X2	T45.8X3	T45.8X4	T45.8X5	T45.8X6
Plasminogen (tissue) activator	T45.611	T45.612	T45.613	T45.614	T45.615	T45.616
Plaster dressing	T49.3X1	T49.3X2	T49.3X3	T49.3X4	T49.3X5	T49.3X6
Plastic dressing	T49.3X1	T49.3X2	T49.3X3	T49.3X4	T49.3X5	T49.3X6
Plegicil	T43.3X1	T43.3X2	T43.3X3	T43.3X4	T43.3X5	T43.3X6
Plicamycin	T45.1X1	T45.1X2	T45.1X3	T45.1X4	T45.1X5	T45.1X6
Podophyllotoxin	T49.8X1	T49.8X2	T49.8X3	T49.8X4	T49.8X5	T49.8X6
Podophyllum (resin)	T49.4X1	T49.4X2	T49.4X3	T49.4X4	T49.4X5	T49.4X6
Poisonous berries	T62.1X1	T62.1X2	T62.1X3	T62.1X4	—	—
Poison NEC	T65.91	T65.92	T65.93	T65.94	—	—
Pokeweed (any part)	T62.2X1	T62.2X2	T62.2X3	T62.2X4	—	—
Poldine metilsulfate	T44.3X1	T44.3X2	T44.3X3	T44.3X4	T44.3X5	T44.3X6
Polidexide (sulfate)	T46.6X1	T46.6X2	T46.6X3	T46.6X4	T46.6X5	T46.6X6
Polidocanol	T46.8X1	T46.8X2	T46.8X3	T46.8X4	T46.8X5	T46.8X6
Poliomyelitis vaccine	T50.B91	T50.B92	T50.B93	T50.B94	T50.B95	T50.B96
Polish (car) (floor) (furniture) (metal) (porcelain) (silver)	T65.891	T65.892	T65.893	T65.894	—	—
abrasive	T65.891	T65.892	T65.893	T65.894	—	—
porcelain	T65.891	T65.892	T65.893	T65.894	—	—
Poloxalkol	T47.4X1	T47.4X2	T47.4X3	T47.4X4	T47.4X5	T47.4X6
Poloxamer	T47.4X1	T47.4X2	T47.4X3	T47.4X4	T47.4X5	T47.4X6

Substance	Poisoning, Accidental (unintentional)	Poisoning, Intentional Self-harm	Poisoning, Assault	Poisoning, Undetermined	Adverse Effect	Under-dosing
Polyaminostyrene resins	T50.3X1	T50.3X2	T50.3X3	T50.3X4	T50.3X5	T50.3X6
Polycarbophil	T47.4X1	T47.4X2	T47.4X3	T47.4X4	T47.4X5	T47.4X6
Polychlorinated biphenyl	T65.891	T65.892	T65.893	T65.894	—	—
Polycycline	T36.4X1	T36.4X2	T36.4X3	T36.4X4	T36.4X5	T36.4X6
Polyester fumes	T59.891	T59.892	T59.893	T59.894	—	—
Polyester resin hardener	T52.91	T52.92	T52.93	T52.94	—	—
fumes	T59.891	T59.892	T59.893	T59.894	—	—
Polyestradiol phosphate	T38.5X1	T38.5X2	T38.5X3	T38.5X4	T38.5X5	T38.5X6
Polyethanolamine alkyl sulfate	T49.2X1	T49.2X2	T49.2X3	T49.2X4	T49.2X5	T49.2X6
Polyethylene adhesive	T49.3X1	T49.3X2	T49.3X3	T49.3X4	T49.3X5	T49.3X6
Polyferose	T45.4X1	T45.4X2	T45.4X3	T45.4X4	T45.4X5	T45.4X6
Polygeline	T45.8X1	T45.8X2	T45.8X3	T45.8X4	T45.8X5	T45.8X6
Polymyxin	T36.8X1	T36.8X2	T36.8X3	T36.8X4	T36.8X5	T36.8X6
B	T36.8X1	T36.8X2	T36.8X3	T36.8X4	T36.8X5	T36.8X6
ENT agent	T49.6X1	T49.6X2	T49.6X3	T49.6X4	T49.6X5	T49.6X6
ophthalmic preparation	T49.5X1	T49.5X2	T49.5X3	T49.5X4	T49.5X5	T49.5X6
topical NEC	T49.0X1	T49.0X2	T49.0X3	T49.0X4	T49.0X5	T49.0X6
E sulfate (eye preparation)	T49.5X1	T49.5X2	T49.5X3	T49.5X4	T49.5X5	T49.5X6
Polynoxylin	T49.0X1	T49.0X2	T49.0X3	T49.0X4	T49.0X5	T49.0X6
Polyoestradiol phosphate	T38.5X1	T38.5X2	T38.5X3	T38.5X4	T38.5X5	T38.5X6
Polyoxymethyleneurea	T49.0X1	T49.0X2	T49.0X3	T49.0X4	T49.0X5	T49.0X6
Polysilane	T47.8X1	T47.8X2	T47.8X3	T47.8X4	T47.8X5	T47.8X6
Polytetrafluoroethylene (inhaled)	T59.891	T59.892	T59.893	T59.894	—	—
Polythiazide	T50.2X1	T50.2X2	T50.2X3	T50.2X4	T50.2X5	T50.2X6
Polyvidone	T45.8X1	T45.8X2	T45.8X3	T45.8X4	T45.8X5	T45.8X6
Polyvinylpyrrolidone	T45.8X1	T45.8X2	T45.8X3	T45.8X4	T45.8X5	T45.8X6
Pontocaine (hydrochloride) (infiltration) (topical)	T41.3X1	T41.3X2	T41.3X3	T41.3X4	T41.3X5	T41.3X6
nerve block (peripheral) (plexus)	T41.3X1	T41.3X2	T41.3X3	T41.3X4	T41.3X5	T41.3X6
spinal	T41.3X1	T41.3X2	T41.3X3	T41.3X4	T41.3X5	T41.3X6
Porfiromycin	T45.1X1	T45.1X2	T45.1X3	T45.1X4	T45.1X5	T45.1X6
Posterior pituitary hormone NEC	T38.891	T38.892	T38.893	T38.894	T38.895	T38.896
Pot	T40.7X1	T40.7X2	T40.7X3	T40.7X4	T40.7X5	T40.7X6
Potash (caustic)	T54.3X1	T54.3X2	T54.3X3	T54.3X4	—	—
Potassic saline injection (lactated)	T50.3X1	T50.3X2	T50.3X3	T50.3X4	T50.3X5	T50.3X6
Potassium-removing resin	T50.3X1	T50.3X2	T50.3X3	T50.3X4	T50.3X5	T50.3X6
Potassium-retaining drug	T50.3X1	T50.3X2	T50.3X3	T50.3X4	T50.3X5	T50.3X6
Potassium (salts) NEC	T50.3X1	T50.3X2	T50.3X3	T50.3X4	T50.3X5	T50.3X6
aminobenzoate	T45.8X1	T45.8X2	T45.8X3	T45.8X4	T45.8X5	T45.8X6
aminosalicylate	T37.1X1	T37.1X2	T37.1X3	T37.1X4	T37.1X5	T37.1X6
antimony ' tartrate'	T37.8X1	T37.8X2	T37.8X3	T37.8X4	T37.8X5	T37.8X6
arsenite (solution)	T57.0X1	T57.0X2	T57.0X3	T57.0X4	—	—
bichromate	T56.2X1	T56.2X2	T56.2X3	T56.2X4	—	—
bisulfate	T47.3X1	T47.3X2	T47.3X3	T47.3X4	T47.3X5	T47.3X6
bromide	T42.6X1	T42.6X2	T42.6X3	T42.6X4	T42.6X5	T42.6X6
canrenoate	T50.0X1	T50.0X2	T50.0X3	T50.0X4	T50.0X5	T50.0X6
carbonate	T54.3X1	T54.3X2	T54.3X3	T54.3X4	—	—
chlorate NEC	T65.891	T65.892	T65.893	T65.894	—	—
chloride	T50.3X1	T50.3X2	T50.3X3	T50.3X4	T50.3X5	T50.3X6
citrate	T50.991	T50.992	T50.993	T50.994	T50.995	T50.996
cyanide	T65.0X1	T65.0X2	T65.0X3	T65.0X4	—	—
ferric hexacyanoferrate (medicinal)	T50.6X1	T50.6X2	T50.6X3	T50.6X4	T50.6X5	T50.6X6
nonmedicinal	T65.891	T65.892	T65.893	T65.894	—	—
Fluoride	T57.8X1	T57.8X2	T57.8X3	T57.8X4	—	—
glucaldrate	T47.1X1	T47.1X2	T47.1X3	T47.1X4	T47.1X5	T47.1X6
hydroxide	T54.3X1	T54.3X2	T54.3X3	T54.3X4	—	—
iodate	T49.0X1	T49.0X2	T49.0X3	T49.0X4	T49.0X5	T49.0X6
iodide	T48.4X1	T48.4X2	T48.4X3	T48.4X4	T48.4X5	T48.4X6
nitrate	T57.8X1	T57.8X2	T57.8X3	T57.8X4	—	—
oxalate	T65.891	T65.892	T65.893	T65.894	—	—
perchlorate (nonmedicinal) NEC	T65.891	T65.892	T65.893	T65.894	—	—
antithyroid	T38.2X1	T38.2X2	T38.2X3	T38.2X4	T38.2X5	T38.2X6
medicinal	T38.2X1	T38.2X2	T38.2X3	T38.2X4	T38.2X5	T38.2X6
Permanganate (nonmedicinal)	T65.891	T65.892	T65.893	T65.894	—	—
medicinal	T49.0X1	T49.0X2	T49.0X3	T49.0X4	T49.0X5	T49.0X6
sulfate	T47.2X1	T47.2X2	T47.2X3	T47.2X4	T47.2X5	T47.2X6
Povidone	T45.8X1	T45.8X2	T45.8X3	T45.8X4	T45.8X5	T45.8X6
iodine	T49.0X1	T49.0X2	T49.0X3	T49.0X4	T49.0X5	T49.0X6
Practolol	T44.7X1	T44.7X2	T44.7X3	T44.7X4	T44.7X5	T44.7X6
Prajmalium bitartrate	T46.2X1	T46.2X2	T46.2X3	T46.2X4	T46.2X5	T46.2X6
Pralidoxime (iodide)	T50.6X1	T50.6X2	T50.6X3	T50.6X4	T50.6X5	T50.6X6
chloride	T50.6X1	T50.6X2	T50.6X3	T50.6X4	T50.6X5	T50.6X6
Pramiverine	T44.3X1	T44.3X2	T44.3X3	T44.3X4		T44.3X6
Pramocaine	T49.1X1	T49.1X2	T49.1X3	T49.1X4	T49.1X5	T49.1X6
Pramoxine	T49.1X1	T49.1X2	T49.1X3	T49.1X4	T49.1X5	T49.1X6
Prasterone	T38.7X1	T38.7X2	T38.7X3	T38.7X4	T38.7X5	T38.7X6
Pravastatin	T46.6X1	T46.6X2	T46.6X3	T46.6X4	T46.6X5	T46.6X6
Prazepam	T42.4X1	T42.4X2	T42.4X3	T42.4X4	T42.4X5	T42.4X6
Praziquantel	T37.4X1	T37.4X2	T37.4X3	T37.4X4	T37.4X5	T37.4X6
Prazitone	T43.291	T43.292	T43.293	T43.294	T43.295	T43.296
Prazosin	T44.6X1	T44.6X2	T44.6X3	T44.6X4	T44.6X5	T44.6X6
Prednicarbate	T49.0X1	T49.0X2	T49.0X3	T49.0X4	T49.0X5	T49.0X6
Prednimustine	T45.1X1	T45.1X2	T45.1X3	T45.1X4	T45.1X5	T45.1X6
Prednisolone	T38.0X1	T38.0X2	T38.0X3	T38.0X4	T38.0X5	T38.0X6
ENT agent	T49.6X1	T49.6X2	T49.6X3	T49.6X4	T49.6X5	T49.6X6
ophthalmic preparation	T49.5X1	T49.5X2	T49.5X3	T49.5X4	T49.5X5	T49.5X6
steaglate	T49.0X1	T49.0X2	T49.0X3	T49.0X4	T49.0X5	T49.0X6
topical NEC	T49.0X1	T49.0X2	T49.0X3	T49.0X4	T49.0X5	T49.0X6
Prednisone	T38.0X1	T38.0X2	T38.0X3	T38.0X4	T38.0X5	T38.0X6
Prednylidene	T38.0X1	T38.0X2	T38.0X3	T38.0X4	T38.0X5	T38.0X6
Pregnandiol	T38.5X1	T38.5X2	T38.5X3	T38.5X4	T38.5X5	T38.5X6
Pregneninolone	T38.5X1	T38.5X2	T38.5X3	T38.5X4	T38.5X5	T38.5X6
Preludin	T43.691	T43.692	T43.693	T43.694	T43.695	T43.696
Premarin	T38.5X1	T38.5X2	T38.5X3	T38.5X4	T38.5X5	T38.5X6
Premedication anesthetic	T41.201	T41.202	T41.203	T41.204	T41.205	T41.206
Prenalterol	T44.5X1	T44.5X2	T44.5X3	T44.5X4	T44.5X5	T44.5X6
Prenoxdiazine	T48.3X1	T48.3X2	T48.3X3	T48.3X4	T48.3X5	T48.3X6
Prenylamine	T46.3X1	T46.3X2	T46.3X3	T46.3X4	T46.3X5	T46.3X6
Preparation H	T49.8X1	T49.8X2	T49.8X3	T49.8X4	T49.8X5	T49.8X6
Preparation, local	T49.4X1	T49.4X2	T49.4X3	T49.4X4	T49.4X5	T49.4X6
Preservative (nonmedicinal)	T65.891	T65.892	T65.893	T65.894	—	—
medicinal	T50.901	T50.902	T50.903	T50.904	T50.905	T50.906
wood	T60.91	T60.92	T60.93	T60.94	—	—
Prethcamide	T50.7X1	T50.7X2	T50.7X3	T50.7X4	T50.7X5	T50.7X6
Pride of China	T62.2X1	T62.2X2	T62.2X3	T62.2X4	—	—
Pridinol	T44.3X1	T44.3X2	T44.3X3	T44.3X4	T44.3X5	T44.3X6
Prifinium bromide	T44.3X1	T44.3X2	T44.3X3	T44.3X4	T44.3X5	T44.3X6
Prilocaine	T41.3X1	T41.3X2	T41.3X3	T41.3X4	T41.3X5	T41.3X6
infiltration (subcutaneous)	T41.3X1	T41.3X2	T41.3X3	T41.3X4	T41.3X5	T41.3X6
nerve block (peripheral) (plexus)	T41.3X1	T41.3X2	T41.3X3	T41.3X4	T41.3X5	T41.3X6
regional	T41.3X1	T41.3X2	T41.3X3	T41.3X4	T41.3X5	T41.3X6
Primaquine	T37.2X1	T37.2X2	T37.2X3	T37.2X4	T37.2X5	T37.2X6
Primidone	T42.6X1	T42.6X2	T42.6X3	T42.6X4	T42.6X5	T42.6X6
Primula (veris)	T62.2X1	T62.2X2	T62.2X3	T62.2X4	—	—
Prinadol	T40.2X1	T40.2X2	T40.2X3	T40.2X4	T40.2X5	T40.2X6
Priscol, Priscoline	T44.6X1	T44.6X2	T44.6X3	T44.6X4	T44.6X5	T44.6X6
Pristinamycin	T36.3X1	T36.3X2	T36.3X3	T36.3X4	T36.3X5	T36.3X6
Privet	T62.2X1	T62.2X2	T62.2X3	T62.2X4	—	—
berries	T62.1X1	T62.1X2	T62.1X3	T62.1X4	—	—
Privine	T44.4X1	T44.4X2	T44.4X3	T44.4X4	T44.4X5	T44.4X6
Pro-Banthine	T44.3X1	T44.3X2	T44.3X3	T44.3X4	T44.3X5	T44.3X6
Probarbital	T42.3X1	T42.3X2	T42.3X3	T42.3X4	T42.3X5	T42.3X6
Probenecid	T50.4X1	T50.4X2	T50.4X3	T50.4X4	T50.4X5	T50.4X6
Probucol	T46.6X1	T46.6X2	T46.6X3	T46.6X4	T46.6X5	T46.6X6
Procainamide	T46.2X1	T46.2X2	T46.2X3	T46.2X4	T46.2X5	T46.2X6
Procaine	T41.3X1	T41.3X2	T41.3X3	T41.3X4	T41.3X5	T41.3X6
benzylpenicillin	T36.0X1	T36.0X2	T36.0X3	T36.0X4	T36.0X5	T36.0X6
nerve block (periphreal) (plexus)	T41.3X1	T41.3X2	T41.3X3	T41.3X4	T41.3X5	T41.3X6
penicillin G	T36.0X1	T36.0X2	T36.0X3	T36.0X4	T36.0X5	T36.0X6
regional	T41.3X1	T41.3X2	T41.3X3	T41.3X4	T41.3X5	T41.3X6
spinal	T41.3X1	T41.3X2	T41.3X3	T41.3X4	T41.3X5	T41.3X6
Procalmidol	T43.591	T43.592	T43.593	T43.594	T43.595	T43.596
Procarbazine	T45.1X1	T45.1X2	T45.1X3	T45.1X4	T45.1X5	T45.1X6
Procaterol	T44.5X1	T44.5X2	T44.5X3	T44.5X4	T44.5X5	T44.5X6
Prochlorperazine	T43.3X1	T43.3X2	T43.3X3	T43.3X4	T43.3X5	T43.3X6
Procyclidine	T44.3X1	T44.3X2	T44.3X3	T44.3X4	T44.3X5	T44.3X6
Producer gas	T58.8X1	T58.8X2	T58.8X3	T58.8X4	—	—
Profadol	T40.4X1	T40.4X2	T40.4X3	T40.4X4	T40.4X5	T40.4X6
Profenamine	T44.3X1	T44.3X2	T44.3X3	T44.3X4	T44.3X5	T44.3X6
Profenil	T44.3X1	T44.3X2	T44.3X3	T44.3X4	T44.3X5	T44.3X6
Proflavine	T49.0X1	T49.0X2	T49.0X3	T49.0X4	T49.0X5	T49.0X6
Progabide	T42.6X1	T42.6X2	T42.6X3	T42.6X4	T42.6X5	T42.6X6
Progesterone	T38.5X1	T38.5X2	T38.5X3	T38.5X4	T38.5X5	T38.5X6
Progestin	T38.5X1	T38.5X2	T38.5X3	T38.5X4	T38.5X5	T38.5X6
oral contraceptive	T38.4X1	T38.4X2	T38.4X3	T38.4X4	T38.4X5	T38.4X6
Progestogen NEC	T38.5X1	T38.5X2	T38.5X3	T38.5X4	T38.5X5	T38.5X6
Progestone	T38.5X1	T38.5X2	T38.5X3	T38.5X4	T38.5X5	T38.5X6
Proglumide	T47.1X1	T47.1X2	T47.1X3	T47.1X4	T47.1X5	T47.1X6
Proguanil	T37.2X1	T37.2X2	T37.2X3	T37.2X4	T37.2X5	T37.2X6
Prolactin	T38.811	T38.812	T38.813	T38.814	T38.815	T38.816
Prolintane	T43.691	T43.692	T43.693	T43.694	T43.695	T43.696
Proloid	T38.1X1	T38.1X2	T38.1X3	T38.1X4	T38.1X5	T38.1X6
Proluton	T38.5X1	T38.5X2	T38.5X3	T38.5X4	T38.5X5	T38.5X6
Promacetin	T37.1X1	T37.1X2	T37.1X3	T37.1X4	T37.1X5	T37.1X6
Promazine	T43.3X1	T43.3X2	T43.3X3	T43.3X4	T43.3X5	T43.3X6
Promedol	T40.2X1	T40.2X2	T40.2X3	T40.2X4	—	—

⌄ Subterms under main terms may continue to next column or page — Additional Character May Be Required — Refer to the Tabular List for Character Selection

Substance	Poisoning, Accidental (unintentional)	Poisoning, Intentional Self-harm	Poisoning, Assault	Poisoning, Undetermined	Adverse Effect	Under-dosing
Promegestone	T38.5X1	T38.5X2	T38.5X3	T38.5X4	T38.5X5	T38.5X6
Promethazine (teoclate)	T43.3X1	T43.3X2	T43.3X3	T43.3X4	T43.3X5	T43.3X6
Promin	T37.1X1	T37.1X2	T37.1X3	T37.1X4	T37.1X5	T37.1X6
Pronase	T45.3X1	T45.3X2	T45.3X3	T45.3X4	T45.3X5	T45.3X6
Pronestyl (hydrochloride)	T46.2X1	T46.2X2	T46.2X3	T46.2X4	T46.2X5	T46.2X6
Pronetalol	T44.7X1	T44.7X2	T44.7X3	T44.7X4	T44.7X5	T44.7X6
Prontosil	T37.0X1	T37.0X2	T37.0X3	T37.0X4	T37.0X5	T37.0X6
Propachlor	T60.3X1	T60.3X2	T60.3X3	T60.3X4	—	—
Propafenone	T46.2X1	T46.2X2	T46.2X3	T46.2X4	T46.2X5	T46.2X6
Propallylonal	T42.3X1	T42.3X2	T42.3X3	T42.3X4	T42.3X5	T42.3X6
Propamidine	T49.0X1	T49.0X2	T49.0X3	T49.0X4	T49.0X5	T49.0X6
Propane (distributed in mobile container)	T59.891	T59.892	T59.893	T59.894	—	—
distributed through pipes	T59.891	T59.892	T59.893	T59.894	—	—
incomplete combustion	T58.11	T58.12	T58.13	T58.14	—	—
Propanidid	T41.291	T41.292	T41.293	T41.294	T41.295	T41.296
Propanil	T60.3X1	T60.3X2	T60.3X3	T60.3X4	—	—
Propantheline	T44.3X1	T44.3X2	T44.3X3	T44.3X4	T44.3X5	T44.3X6
bromide	T44.3X1	T44.3X2	T44.3X3	T44.3X4	T44.3X5	T44.3X6
Proparacaine	T41.3X1	T41.3X2	T41.3X3	T41.3X4	T41.3X5	T41.3X6
Propatylnitrate	T46.3X1	T46.3X2	T46.3X3	T46.3X4	T46.3X5	T46.3X6
Propicillin	T36.0X1	T36.0X2	T36.0X3	T36.0X4	T36.0X5	T36.0X6
Propiolactone	T49.0X1	T49.0X2	T49.0X3	T49.0X4	T49.0X5	T49.0X6
Propiomazine	T45.0X1	T45.0X2	T45.0X3	T45.0X4	T45.0X5	T45.0X6
Propionaldehyde (medicinal)	T42.6X1	T42.6X2	T42.6X3	T42.6X4	T42.6X5	T42.6X6
Propionate (calcium) (sodium)	T49.0X1	T49.0X2	T49.0X3	T49.0X4	T49.0X5	T49.0X6
Propion gel	T49.0X1	T49.0X2	T49.0X3	T49.0X4	T49.0X5	T49.0X6
Propitocaine	T41.3X1	T41.3X2	T41.3X3	T41.3X4	T41.3X5	T41.3X6
infiltration (subcutaneous)	T41.3X1	T41.3X2	T41.3X3	T41.3X4	T41.3X5	T41.3X6
nerve block (peripheral) (plexus)	T41.3X1	T41.3X2	T41.3X3	T41.3X4	T41.3X5	T41.3X6
Propofol	T41.291	T41.292	T41.293	T41.294	T41.295	T41.296
Propoxur	T60.0X1	T60.0X2	T60.0X3	T60.0X4	—	—
Propoxycaine	T41.3X1	T41.3X2	T41.3X3	T41.3X4	T41.3X5	T41.3X6
infiltration (subcutaneous)	T41.3X1	T41.3X2	T41.3X3	T41.3X4	T41.3X5	T41.3X6
nerve block (peripheral) (plexus)	T41.3X1	T41.3X2	T41.3X3	T41.3X4	T41.3X5	T41.3X6
topical (surface)	T41.3X1	T41.3X2	T41.3X3	T41.3X4	T41.3X5	T41.3X6
Propoxyphene	T40.4X1	T40.4X2	T40.4X3	T40.4X4	T40.4X5	T40.4X6
Propranolol	T44.7X1	T44.7X2	T44.7X3	T44.7X4	T44.7X5	T44.7X6
Propyl						
alcohol	T51.3X1	T51.3X2	T51.3X3	T51.3X4	—	—
carbinol	T51.3X1	T51.3X2	T51.3X3	T51.3X4	—	—
hexadrine	T44.4X1	T44.4X2	T44.4X3	T44.4X4	T44.4X5	T44.4X6
iodone	T50.8X1	T50.8X2	T50.8X3	T50.8X4	T50.8X5	T50.8X6
thiouracil	T38.2X1	T38.2X2	T38.2X3	T38.2X4	T38.2X5	T38.2X6
Propylaminophenothiazine	T43.3X1	T43.3X2	T43.3X3	T43.3X4	T43.3X5	T43.3X6
Propylene	T59.891	T59.892	T59.893	T59.894	—	—
Propylhexedrine	T48.5X1	T48.5X2	T48.5X3	T48.5X4	T48.5X5	T48.5X6
Propyliodone	T50.8X1	T50.8X2	T50.8X3	T50.8X4	T50.8X5	T50.8X6
Propylparaben (ophthalmic)	T49.5X1	T49.5X2	T49.5X3	T49.5X4	T49.5X5	T49.5X6
Propylthiouracil	T38.2X1	T38.2X2	T38.2X3	T38.2X4	T38.2X5	T38.2X6
Propyphenazone	T39.2X1	T39.2X2	T39.2X3	T39.2X4	T39.2X5	T39.2X6
Proquazone	T39.391	T39.392	T39.393	T39.394	T39.395	T39.396
Proscillaridin	T46.0X1	T46.0X2	T46.0X3	T46.0X4	T46.0X5	T46.0X6
Prostacyclin	T45.521	T45.522	T45.523	T45.524	T45.525	T45.526
Prostaglandin (I2)	T45.521	T45.522	T45.523	T45.524	T45.525	T45.526
E1	T46.7X1	T46.7X2	T46.7X3	T46.7X4	T46.7X5	T46.7X6
E2	T48.0X1	T48.0X2	T48.0X3	T48.0X4	T48.0X5	T48.0X6
F2 alpha	T48.0X1	T48.0X2	T48.0X3	T48.0X4	T48.0X5	T48.0X6
Prostigmin	T44.0X1	T44.0X2	T44.0X3	T44.0X4	T44.0X5	T44.0X6
Prosultiamine	T45.2X1	T45.2X2	T45.2X3	T45.2X4	T45.2X5	T45.2X6
Protamine sulfate	T45.7X1	T45.7X2	T45.7X3	T45.7X4	T45.7X5	T45.7X6
zinc insulin	T38.3X1	T38.3X2	T38.3X3	T38.3X4	T38.3X5	T38.3X6
Protease	T47.5X1	T47.5X2	T47.5X3	T47.5X4	T47.5X5	T47.5X6
Protectant, skin NEC	T49.3X1	T49.3X2	T49.3X3	T49.3X4	T49.3X5	T49.3X6
Protein hydrolysate	T50.991	T50.992	T50.993	T50.994	T50.995	T50.996
Prothiaden — see Dothiepin hydrochloride						
Prothionamide	T37.1X1	T37.1X2	T37.1X3	T37.1X4	T37.1X5	T37.1X6
Prothipendyl	T43.591	T43.592	T43.593	T43.594	T43.595	T43.596
Prothoate	T60.0X1	T60.0X2	T60.0X3	T60.0X4	—	—
Prothrombin						
activator	T45.7X1	T45.7X2	T45.7X3	T45.7X4	T45.7X5	T45.7X6
synthesis inhibitor	T45.511	T45.512	T45.513	T45.514	T45.515	T45.516
Protionamide	T37.1X1	T37.1X2	T37.1X3	T37.1X4	T37.1X5	T37.1X6
Protirelin	T38.891	T38.892	T38.893	T38.894	T38.895	T38.896
Protokylol	T48.6X1	T48.6X2	T48.6X3	T48.6X4	T48.6X5	T48.6X6
Protopam	T50.6X1	T50.6X2	T50.6X3	T50.6X4	T50.6X5	T50.6X6
Protoveratrine(s) (A) (B)	T46.5X1	T46.5X2	T46.5X3	T46.5X4	T46.5X5	T46.5X6
Protriptyline	T43.011	T43.012	T43.013	T43.014	T43.015	T43.016

Substance	Poisoning, Accidental (unintentional)	Poisoning, Intentional Self-harm	Poisoning, Assault	Poisoning, Undetermined	Adverse Effect	Under-dosing
Provera	T38.5X1	T38.5X2	T38.5X3	T38.5X4	T38.5X5	T38.5X6
Provitamin A	T45.2X1	T45.2X2	T45.2X3	T45.2X4	T45.2X5	T45.2X6
Proxibarbal	T42.3X1	T42.3X2	T42.3X3	T42.3X4	T42.3X5	T42.3X6
Proxymetacaine	T41.3X1	T41.3X2	T41.3X3	T41.3X4	T41.3X5	T41.3X6
Proxyphylline	T48.6X1	T48.6X2	T48.6X3	T48.6X4	T48.6X5	T48.6X6
Prozac — see Fluoxetine hydrochloride						
Prunus						
laurocerasus	T62.2X1	T62.2X2	T62.2X3	T62.2X4	—	—
virginiana	T62.2X1	T62.2X2	T62.2X3	T62.2X4	—	—
Prussian blue						
commercial	T65.891	T65.892	T65.893	T65.894	—	—
therapeutic	T50.6X1	T50.6X2	T50.6X3	T50.6X4	T50.6X5	T50.6X6
Prussic acid	T65.0X1	T65.0X2	T65.0X3	T65.0X4	—	—
vapor	T57.3X1	T57.3X2	T57.3X3	T57.3X4	—	—
Pseudoephedrine	T44.991	T44.992	T44.993	T44.994	T44.995	T44.996
Psilocin	T40.991	T40.992	T40.993	T40.994	—	—
Psilocybin	T40.991	T40.992	T40.993	T40.994	—	—
Psilocybine	T40.991	T40.992	T40.993	T40.994	—	—
Psoralene (nonmedicinal)	T65.891	T65.892	T65.893	T65.894	—	—
Psoralens (medicinal)	T50.991	T50.992	T50.993	T50.994	T50.995	T50.996
PSP (phenolsulfonphthalein)	T50.8X1	T50.8X2	T50.8X3	T50.8X4	T50.8X5	T50.8X6
Psychodysleptic drug NEC	T40.901	T40.902	T40.903	T40.904	T40.905	T40.906
Psychostimulant	T43.601	T43.602	T43.603	T43.604	T43.605	T43.606
amphetamine	T43.621	T43.622	T43.623	T43.624	T43.625	T43.626
caffeine	T43.611	T43.612	T43.613	T43.614	T43.615	T43.616
methylphenidate	T43.631	T43.632	T43.633	T43.634	T43.635	T43.636
specified NEC	T43.691	T43.692	T43.693	T43.694	T43.695	T43.696
Psychotherapeutic drug NEC	T43.91	T43.92	T43.93	T43.94	T43.95	T43.96
antidepressants — see also Antidepressant	T43.201	T43.202	T43.203	T43.204	T43.205	T43.206
specified NEC	T43.8X1	T43.8X2	T43.8X3	T43.8X4	T43.8X5	T43.8X6
tranquilizers NEC	T43.501	T43.502	T43.503	T43.504	T43.505	T43.506
Psychotomimetic agents	T40.901	T40.902	T40.903	T40.904	T40.905	T40.906
Psychotropic drug NEC	T43.91	T43.92	T43.93	T43.94	T43.95	T43.96
specified NEC	T43.8X1	T43.8X2	T43.8X3	T43.8X4	T43.8X5	T43.8X6
Psyllium hydrophilic mucilloid	T47.4X1	T47.4X2	T47.4X3	T47.4X4	T47.4X5	T47.4X6
Pteroylglutamic acid	T45.8X1	T45.8X2	T45.8X3	T45.8X4	T45.8X5	T45.8X6
Pteroyltriglutamate	T45.1X1	T45.1X2	T45.1X3	T45.1X4	T45.1X5	T45.1X6
PTFE — see Polytetrafluoroethylene						
Pulp						
devitalizing paste	T49.7X1	T49.7X2	T49.7X3	T49.7X4	T49.7X5	T49.7X6
dressing	T49.7X1	T49.7X2	T49.7X3	T49.7X4	T49.7X5	T49.7X6
Pulsatilla	T62.2X1	T62.2X2	T62.2X3	T62.2X4	—	—
Pumpkin seed extract	T37.4X1	T37.4X2	T37.4X3	T37.4X4	T37.4X5	T37.4X6
Purex (bleach)	T54.91	T54.92	T54.93	T54.94	—	—
Purgative NEC — see also Cathartic	T47.4X1	T47.4X2	T47.4X3	T47.4X4	T47.4X5	T47.4X6
Purine analogue (antineoplastic)	T45.1X1	T45.1X2	T45.1X3	T45.1X4	T45.1X5	T45.1X6
Purine diuretics	T50.2X1	T50.2X2	T50.2X3	T50.2X4	T50.2X5	T50.2X6
Purinethol	T45.1X1	T45.1X2	T45.1X3	T45.1X4	T45.1X5	T45.1X6
PVP	T45.8X1	T45.8X2	T45.8X3	T45.8X4	T45.8X5	T45.8X6
Pyrabital	T39.8X1	T39.8X2	T39.8X3	T39.8X4	T39.8X5	T39.8X6
Pyramidon	T39.2X1	T39.2X2	T39.2X3	T39.2X4	T39.2X5	T39.2X6
Pyrantel	T37.4X1	T37.4X2	T37.4X3	T37.4X4	T37.4X5	T37.4X6
Pyrathiazine	T45.0X1	T45.0X2	T45.0X3	T45.0X4	T45.0X5	T45.0X6
Pyrazinamide	T37.1X1	T37.1X2	T37.1X3	T37.1X4	T37.1X5	T37.1X6
Pyrazinoic acid (amide)	T37.1X1	T37.1X2	T37.1X3	T37.1X4	T37.1X5	T37.1X6
Pyrazole (derivatives)	T39.2X1	T39.2X2	T39.2X3	T39.2X4	T39.2X5	T39.2X6
Pyrazolone analgesic NEC	T39.2X1	T39.2X2	T39.2X3	T39.2X4	T39.2X5	T39.2X6
Pyrethrin, pyrethrum (nonmedicinal)	T60.2X1	T60.2X2	T60.2X3	T60.2X4	—	—
Pyrethrum extract	T49.0X1	T49.0X2	T49.0X3	T49.0X4	T49.0X5	T49.0X6
Pyribenzamine	T45.0X1	T45.0X2	T45.0X3	T45.0X4	T45.0X5	T45.0X6
Pyridine	T52.8X1	T52.8X2	T52.8X3	T52.8X4	—	—
aldoxime methiodide	T50.6X1	T50.6X2	T50.6X3	T50.6X4	T50.6X5	T50.6X6
aldoxime methyl chloride	T50.6X1	T50.6X2	T50.6X3	T50.6X4	T50.6X5	T50.6X6
vapor	T59.891	T59.892	T59.893	T59.894	—	—
Pyridium	T39.8X1	T39.8X2	T39.8X3	T39.8X4	T39.8X5	T39.8X6
Pyridostigmine bromide	T44.0X1	T44.0X2	T44.0X3	T44.0X4	T44.0X5	T44.0X6
Pyridoxal phosphate	T45.2X1	T45.2X2	T45.2X3	T45.2X4	T45.2X5	T45.2X6
Pyridoxine	T45.2X1	T45.2X2	T45.2X3	T45.2X4	T45.2X5	T45.2X6
Pyrilamine	T45.0X1	T45.0X2	T45.0X3	T45.0X4	T45.0X5	T45.0X6
Pyrimethamine	T37.2X1	T37.2X2	T37.2X3	T37.2X4	T37.2X5	T37.2X6
with sulfadoxine	T37.2X1	T37.2X2	T37.2X3	T37.2X4	T37.2X5	T37.2X6
Pyrimidine antagonist	T45.1X1	T45.1X2	T45.1X3	T45.1X4	IC45.1X5	T45.1X6
Pyriminil	T60.4X1	T60.4X2	T60.4X3	T60.4X4	—	—
Pyrithione zinc	T49.4X1	T49.4X2	T49.4X3	T49.4X4	T49.4X5	T49.4X6
Pyrithyldione	T42.6X1	T42.6X2	T42.6X3	T42.6X4	T42.6X5	T42.6X6

386

Additional Character May Be Required — Refer to the Tabular List for Character Selection   ▽ Subterms under main terms may continue to next column or page

Substance	Poisoning, Accidental (unintentional)	Poisoning, Intentional Self-harm	Poisoning, Assault	Poisoning, Undetermined	Adverse Effect	Under-dosing
Pyrogallic acid	T49.0X1	T49.0X2	T49.0X3	T49.0X4	T49.0X5	T49.0X6
Pyrogallol	T49.0X1	T49.0X2	T49.0X3	T49.0X4	T49.0X5	T49.0X6
Pyroxylin	T49.3X1	T49.3X2	T49.3X3	T49.3X4	T49.3X5	T49.3X6
Pyrrobutamine	T45.0X1	T45.0X2	T45.0X3	T45.0X4	T45.0X5	T45.0X6
Pyrrolizidine alkaloids	T62.8X1	T62.8X2	T62.8X3	T62.8X4	—	—
Pyrvinium chloride	T37.4X1	T37.4X2	T37.4X3	T37.4X4	T37.4X5	T37.4X6
PZI	T38.3X1	T38.3X2	T38.3X3	T38.3X4	T38.3X5	T38.3X6
Quaalude	T42.6X1	T42.6X2	T42.6X3	T42.6X4	T42.6X5	T42.6X6
Quarternary ammonium						
anti-infective	T49.0X1	T49.0X2	T49.0X3	T49.0X4	T49.0X5	T49.0X6
ganglion blocking	T44.2X1	T44.2X2	T44.2X3	T44.2X4	T44.2X5	T44.2X6
parasympatholytic	T44.3X1	T44.3X2	T44.3X3	T44.3X4	T44.3X5	T44.3X6
Quazepam	T42.4X1	T42.4X2	T42.4X3	T42.4X4	T42.4X5	T42.4X6
Quicklime	T54.3X1	T54.3X2	T54.3X3	T54.3X4	—	—
Quillaja extract	T48.4X1	T48.4X2	T48.4X3	T48.4X4	T48.4X5	T48.4X6
Quinacrine	T37.2X1	T37.2X2	T37.2X3	T37.2X4	T37.2X5	T37.2X6
Quinaglute	T46.2X1	T46.2X2	T46.2X3	T46.2X4	T46.2X5	T46.2X6
Quinalbarbital	T42.3X1	T42.3X2	T42.3X3	T42.3X4	T42.3X5	T42.3X6
Quinalbarbitone sodium	T42.3X1	T42.3X2	T42.3X3	T42.3X4	T42.3X5	T42.3X6
Quinalphos	T60.0X1	T60.0X2	T60.0X3	T60.0X4	—	—
Quinapril	T46.4X1	T46.4X2	T46.4X3	T46.4X4	T46.4X5	T46.4X6
Quinestradiol	T38.5X1	T38.5X2	T38.5X3	T38.5X4	T38.5X5	T38.5X6
Quinestradol	T38.5X1	T38.5X2	T38.5X3	T38.5X4	T38.5X5	T38.5X6
Quinestrol	T38.5X1	T38.5X2	T38.5X3	T38.5X4	T38.5X5	T38.5X6
Quinethazone	T50.2X1	T50.2X2	T50.2X3	T50.2X4	T50.2X5	T50.2X6
Quingestanol	T38.4X1	T38.4X2	T38.4X3	T38.4X4	T38.4X5	T38.4X6
Quinidine	T46.2X1	T46.2X2	T46.2X3	T46.2X4	T46.2X5	T46.2X6
Quinine	T37.2X1	T37.2X2	T37.2X3	T37.2X4	T37.2X5	T37.2X6
Quiniobine	T37.8X1	T37.8X2	T37.8X3	T37.8X4	T37.8X5	T37.8X6
Quinisocaine	T49.1X1	T49.1X2	T49.1X3	T49.1X4	T49.1X5	T49.1X6
Quinocide	T37.2X1	T37.2X2	T37.2X3	T37.2X4	T37.2X5	T37.2X6
Quinoline (derivatives) NEC	T37.8X1	T37.8X2	T37.8X3	T37.8X4	T37.8X5	T37.8X6
Quinupramine	T43.011	T43.012	T43.013	T43.014	T43.015	T43.016
Quotane	T41.3X1	T41.3X2	T41.3X3	T41.3X4	T41.3X5	T41.3X6
Rabies						
immune globulin (human)	T50.Z11	T50.Z12	T50.Z13	T50.Z14	T50.Z15	T50.Z16
vaccine	T50.B91	T50.B92	T50.B93	T50.B94	T50.B95	T50.B96
Racemoramide	T40.2X1	T40.2X2	T40.2X3	T40.2X4	—	—
Racemorphan	T40.2X1	T40.2X2	T40.2X3	T40.2X4	T40.2X5	T40.2X6
Racepinefrin	T44.5X1	T44.5X2	T44.5X3	T44.5X4	T44.5X5	T44.5X6
Raclopride	T43.591	T43.592	T43.593	T43.594	T43.595	T43.596
Radiator alcohol	T51.1X1	T51.1X2	T51.1X3	T51.1X4		
Radioactive drug NEC	T50.8X1	T50.8X2	T50.8X3	T50.8X4	T50.8X5	T50.8X6
Radio-opaque (drugs) (materials)	T50.8X1	T50.8X2	T50.8X3	T50.8X4	T50.8X5	T50.8X6
Ramifenazone	T39.2X1	T39.2X2	T39.2X3	T39.2X4	T39.2X5	T39.2X6
Ramipril	T46.4X1	T46.4X2	T46.4X3	T46.4X4	T46.4X5	T46.4X6
Ranitidine	T47.0X1	T47.0X2	T47.0X3	T47.0X4	T47.0X5	T47.0X6
Ranunculus	T62.2X1	T62.2X2	T62.2X3	T62.2X4	—	—
Rat poison NEC	T60.4X1	T60.4X2	T60.4X3	T60.4X4	—	—
Rattlesnake (venom)	T63.011	T63.012	T63.013	T63.014	—	—
Raubasine	T46.7X1	T46.7X2	T46.7X3	T46.7X4	T46.7X5	T46.7X6
Raudixin	T46.5X1	T46.5X2	T46.5X3	T46.5X4	T46.5X5	T46.5X6
Rautensin	T46.5X1	T46.5X2	T46.5X3	T46.5X4	T46.5X5	T46.5X6
Rautina	T46.5X1	T46.5X2	T46.5X3	T46.5X4	T46.5X5	T46.5X6
Rautotal	T46.5X1	T46.5X2	T46.5X3	T46.5X4	T46.5X5	T46.5X6
Rauwiloid	T46.5X1	T46.5X2	T46.5X3	T46.5X4	T46.5X5	T46.5X6
Rauwoldin	T46.5X1	T46.5X2	T46.5X3	T46.5X4	T46.5X5	T46.5X6
Rauwolfia (alkaloids)	T46.5X1	T46.5X2	T46.5X3	T46.5X4	T46.5X5	T46.5X6
Razoxane	T45.1X1	T45.1X2	T45.1X3	T45.1X4	T45.1X5	T45.1X6
Realgar	T57.0X1	T57.0X2	T57.0X3	T57.0X4	—	—
Recombinant (R) — see specific protein						
Red blood cells, packed	T45.8X1	T45.8X2	T45.8X3	T45.8X4	T45.8X5	T45.8X6
Red squill (scilliroside)	T60.4X1	T60.4X2	T60.4X3	T60.4X4	—	—
Reducing agent, industrial NEC	T65.891	T65.892	T65.893	T65.894		
Refrigerant gas (chlorofluorocarbon)	T53.5X1	T53.5X2	T53.5X3	T53.5X4	—	—
not chlorofluorocarbon	T59.891	T59.892	T59.893	T59.894	—	—
Regroton	T50.2X1	T50.2X2	T50.2X3	T50.2X4	T50.2X5	T50.2X6
Rehydration salts (oral)	T50.3X1	T50.3X2	T50.3X3	T50.3X4	T50.3X5	T50.3X6
Rela	T42.8X1	T42.8X2	T42.8X3	T42.8X4	T42.8X5	T42.8X6
Relaxant, muscle						
anesthetic	T48.1X1	T48.1X2	T48.1X3	T48.1X4	T48.1X5	T48.1X6
central nervous system	T42.8X1	T42.8X2	T42.8X3	T42.8X4	T42.8X5	T42.8X6
skeletal NEC	T48.1X1	T48.1X2	T48.1X3	T48.1X4	T48.1X5	T48.1X6
smooth NEC	T44.3X1	T44.3X2	T44.3X3	T44.3X4	T44.3X5	T44.3X6
Remoxipride	T43.591	T43.592	T43.593	T43.594	T43.595	T43.596
Renese	T50.2X1	T50.2X2	T50.2X3	T50.2X4	T50.2X5	T50.2X6
Renografin	T50.8X1	T50.8X2	T50.8X3	T50.8X4	T50.8X5	T50.8X6
Replacement solution	T50.3X1	T50.3X2	T50.3X3	T50.3X4	T50.3X5	T50.3X6
Reproterol	T48.6X1	T48.6X2	T48.6X3	T48.6X4	T48.6X5	T48.6X6
Rescinnamine	T46.5X1	T46.5X2	T46.5X3	T46.5X4	T46.5X5	T46.5X6
Reserpin (e)	T46.5X1	T46.5X2	T46.5X3	T46.5X4	T46.5X5	T46.5X6
Resorcin, resorcinol (nonmedicinal)	T65.891	T65.892	T65.893	T65.894	—	—
medicinal	T49.4X1	T49.4X2	T49.4X3	T49.4X4	T49.4X5	T49.4X6
Respaire	T48.4X1	T48.4X2	T48.4X3	T48.4X4	T48.4X5	T48.4X6
Respiratory drug NEC	T48.901	T48.902	T48.903	T48.904	T48.905	T48.906
antiasthmatic NEC	T48.6X1	T48.6X2	T48.6X3	T48.6X4	T48.6X5	T48.6X6
anti-common-cold NEC	T48.5X1	T48.5X2	T48.5X3	T48.5X4	T48.5X5	T48.5X6
expectorant NEC	T48.4X1	T48.4X2	T48.4X3	T48.4X4	T48.4X5	T48.4X6
stimulant	T48.901	T48.902	T48.903	T48.904	T48.905	T48.906
Retinoic acid	T49.0X1	T49.0X2	T49.0X3	T49.0X4	T49.0X5	T49.0X6
Retinol	T45.2X1	T45.2X2	T45.2X3	T45.2X4	T45.2X5	T45.2X6
Rh (D) immune globulin (human)	T50.Z11	T50.Z12	T50.Z13	T50.Z14	T50.Z15	T50.Z16
Rhodine	T39.011	T39.012	T39.013	T39.014	T39.015	T39.016
RhoGAM	T50.Z11	T50.Z12	T50.Z13	T50.Z14	T50.Z15	T50.Z16
Rhubarb						
dry extract	T47.2X1	T47.2X2	T47.2X3	T47.2X4	T47.2X5	T47.2X6
tincture, compound	T47.2X1	T47.2X2	T47.2X3	T47.2X4	T47.2X5	T47.2X6
Ribavirin	T37.5X1	T37.5X2	T37.5X3	T37.5X4	T37.5X5	T37.5X6
Riboflavin	T45.2X1	T45.2X2	T45.2X3	T45.2X4	T45.2X5	T45.2X6
Ribostamycin	T36.5X1	T36.5X2	T36.5X3	T36.5X4	T36.5X5	T36.5X6
Ricin	T62.2X1	T62.2X2	T62.2X3	T62.2X4	—	—
Ricinus communis	T62.2X1	T62.2X2	T62.2X3	T62.2X4	—	—
Rickettsial vaccine NEC	T50.A91	T50.A92	T50.A93	T50.A94	T50.A95	T50.A96
Rifabutin	T36.6X1	T36.6X2	T36.6X3	T36.6X4	T36.6X5	T36.6X6
Rifamide	T36.6X1	T36.6X2	T36.6X3	T36.6X4	T36.6X5	T36.6X6
Rifampicin	T36.6X1	T36.6X2	T36.6X3	T36.6X4	T36.6X5	T36.6X6
with isoniazid	T37.1X1	T37.1X2	T37.1X3	T37.1X4	T37.1X5	T37.1X6
Rifampin	T36.6X1	T36.6X2	T36.6X3	T36.6X4	T36.6X5	T36.6X6
Rifamycin	T36.6X1	T36.6X2	T36.6X3	T36.6X4	T36.6X5	T36.6X6
Rifaximin	T36.6X1	T36.6X2	T36.6X3	T36.6X4	T36.6X5	T36.6X6
Rimantadine	T37.5X1	T37.5X2	T37.5X3	T37.5X4	T37.5X5	T37.5X6
Rimazolium metilsulfate	T39.8X1	T39.8X2	T39.8X3	T39.8X4	T39.8X5	T39.8X6
Rimifon	T37.1X1	T37.1X2	T37.1X3	T37.1X4	T37.1X5	T37.1X6
Rimiterol	T48.6X1	T48.6X2	T48.6X3	T48.6X4	T48.6X5	T48.6X6
Ringer (lactate) solution	T50.3X1	T50.3X2	T50.3X3	T50.3X4	T50.3X5	T50.3X6
Ristocetin	T36.8X1	T36.8X2	T36.8X3	T36.8X4	T36.8X5	T36.8X6
Ritalin	T43.631	T43.632	T43.633	T43.634	T43.635	T43.636
Ritodrine	T44.5X1	T44.5X2	T44.5X3	T44.5X4	T44.5X5	T44.5X6
Roach killer — see Insecticide						
Rociverine	T44.3X1	T44.3X2	T44.3X3	T44.3X4	T44.3X5	T44.3X6
Rocky Mountain spotted fever vaccine	T50.A91	T50.A92	T50.A93	T50.A94	T50.A95	T50.A96
Rodenticide NEC	T60.4X1	T60.4X2	T60.4X3	T60.4X4	—	—
Rohypnol	T42.4X1	T42.4X2	T42.4X3	T42.4X4	T42.4X5	T42.4X6
Rokitamycin	T36.3X1	T36.3X2	T36.3X3	T36.3X4	T36.3X5	T36.3X6
Rolaids	T47.1X1	T47.1X2	T47.1X3	T47.1X4	T47.1X5	T47.1X6
Rolitetracycline	T36.4X1	T36.4X2	T36.4X3	T36.4X4	T36.4X5	T36.4X6
Romilar	T48.3X1	T48.3X2	T48.3X3	T48.3X4	T48.3X5	T48.3X6
Ronifibrate	T46.6X1	T46.6X2	T46.6X3	T46.6X4	T46.6X5	T46.6X6
Rosaprostol	T47.1X1	T47.1X2	T47.1X3	T47.1X4	T47.1X5	T47.1X6
Rose bengal sodium (131I)	T50.8X1	T50.8X2	T50.8X3	T50.8X4	T50.8X5	T50.8X6
Rose water ointment	T49.3X1	T49.3X2	T49.3X3	T49.3X4	T49.3X5	T49.3X6
Rosoxacin	T37.8X1	T37.8X2	T37.8X3	T37.8X4	T37.8X5	T37.8X6
Rotenone	T60.2X1	T60.2X2	T60.2X3	T60.2X4	—	—
Rotoxamine	T45.0X1	T45.0X2	T45.0X3	T45.0X4	T45.0X5	T45.0X6
Rough-on-rats	T60.4X1	T60.4X2	T60.4X3	T60.4X4	—	—
Roxatidine	T47.0X1	T47.0X2	T47.0X3	T47.0X4	T47.0X5	T47.0X6
Roxithromycin	T36.3X1	T36.3X2	T36.3X3	T36.3X4	T36.3X5	T36.3X6
Rt-PA	T45.611	T45.612	T45.613	T45.614	T45.615	T45.616
Rubbing alcohol	T51.2X1	T51.2X2	T51.2X3	T51.2X4		
Rubefacient	T49.4X1	T49.4X2	T49.4X3	T49.4X4	T49.4X5	T49.4X6
Rubella vaccine	T50.B91	T50.B92	T50.B93	T50.B94	T50.B95	T50.B96
Rubeola vaccine	T50.B91	T50.B92	T50.B93	T50.B94	T50.B95	T50.B96
Rubidium chloride Rb82	T50.8X1	T50.8X2	T50.8X3	T50.8X4	T50.8X5	T50.8X6
Rubidomycin	T45.1X1	T45.1X2	T45.1X3	T45.1X4	T45.1X5	T45.1X6
Rue	T62.2X1	T62.2X2	T62.2X3	T62.2X4	—	—
Rufocromomycin	T45.1X1	T45.1X2	T45.1X3	T45.1X4	T45.1X5	T45.1X6
Russel's viper venin	T45.7X1	T45.7X2	T45.7X3	T45.7X4	T45.7X5	T45.7X6
Ruta (graveolens)	T62.2X1	T62.2X2	T62.2X3	T62.2X4	—	—
Rutinum	T46.991	T46.992	T46.993	T46.994	T46.995	T46.996
Rutoside	T46.991	T46.992	T46.993	T46.994	T46.995	T46.996
b-sitosterol(s)	T46.6X1	T46.6X2	T46.6X3	T46.6X4	T46.6X5	T46.6X6
Sabadilla (plant)	T62.2X1	T62.2X2	T62.2X3	T62.2X4	—	—
pesticide	T60.2X1	T60.2X2	T60.2X3	T60.2X4	—	—
Saccharated iron oxide	T45.8X1	T45.8X2	T45.8X3	T45.8X4	T45.8X5	T45.8X6
Saccharin	T50.901	T50.902	T50.903	T50.904	T50.905	T50.906
Saccharomyces boulardii	T47.6X1	T47.6X2	T47.6X3	T47.6X4	T47.6X5	T47.6X6
Safflower oil	T46.6X1	T46.6X2	T46.6X3	T46.6X4	T46.6X5	T46.6X6
Safrazine	T43.1X1	T43.1X2	T43.1X3	T43.1X4	T43.1X5	T43.1X6
Salazosulfapyridine	T37.0X1	T37.0X2	T37.0X3	T37.0X4	T37.0X5	T37.0X6

Subterms under main terms may continue to next column or page   Additional Character May Be Required — Refer to the Tabular List for Character Selection   387

Pyrogallic acid — Salazosulfapyridine

Substance	Poisoning, Accidental (unintentional)	Poisoning, Intentional Self-harm	Poisoning, Assault	Poisoning, Undetermined	Adverse Effect	Under-dosing
Salbutamol	T48.6X1	T48.6X2	T48.6X3	T48.6X4	T48.6X5	T48.6X6
Salicylamide	T39.091	T39.092	T39.093	T39.094	T39.095	T39.096
Salicylate NEC	T39.091	T39.092	T39.093	T39.094	T39.095	T39.096
methyl	T49.3X1	T49.3X2	T49.3X3	T49.3X4	T49.3X5	T49.3X6
theobromine calcium	T50.2X1	T50.2X2	T50.2X3	T50.2X4	T50.2X5	T50.2X6
Salicylazosulfapyridine	T37.0X1	T37.0X2	T37.0X3	T37.0X4	T37.0X5	T37.0X6
Salicylhydroxamic acid	T49.0X1	T49.0X2	T49.0X3	T49.0X4	T49.0X5	T49.0X6
Salicylic acid	T49.4X1	T49.4X2	T49.4X3	T49.4X4	T49.4X5	T49.4X6
with benzoic acid	T49.4X1	T49.4X2	T49.4X3	T49.4X4	T49.4X5	T49.4X6
congeners	T39.091	T39.092	T39.093	T39.094	T39.095	T39.096
derivative	T39.091	T39.092	T39.093	T39.094	T39.095	T39.096
salts	T39.091	T39.092	T39.093	T39.094	T39.095	T39.096
Salinazid	T37.1X1	T37.1X2	T37.1X3	T37.1X4	T37.1X5	T37.1X6
Salmeterol	T48.6X1	T48.6X2	T48.6X3	T48.6X4	T48.6X5	T48.6X6
Salol	T49.3X1	T49.3X2	T49.3X3	T49.3X4	T49.3X5	T49.3X6
Salsalate	T39.091	T39.092	T39.093	T39.094	T39.095	T39.096
Salt-replacing drug	T50.901	T50.902	T50.903	T50.904	T50.905	T50.906
Salt-retaining mineralocorticoid	T50.0X1	T50.0X2	T50.0X3	T50.0X4	T50.0X5	T50.0X6
Salt substitute	T50.901	T50.902	T50.903	T50.904	T50.905	T50.906
Saluretic NEC	T50.2X1	T50.2X2	T50.2X3	T50.2X4	T50.2X5	T50.2X6
Saluron	T50.2X1	T50.2X2	T50.2X3	T50.2X4	T50.2X5	T50.2X6
Salvarsan 606 (neosilver) (silver)	T37.8X1	T37.8X2	T37.8X3	T37.8X4	T37.8X5	T37.8X6
Sambucus canadensis	T62.2X1	T62.2X2	T62.2X3	T62.2X4	—	—
berry	T62.1X1	T62.1X2	T62.1X3	T62.1X4	—	—
Sandril	T46.5X1	T46.5X2	T46.5X3	T46.5X4	T46.5X5	T46.5X6
Sanguinaria canadensis	T62.2X1	T62.2X2	T62.2X3	T62.2X4	—	—
Saniflush (cleaner)	T54.2X1	T54.2X2	T54.2X3	T54.2X4	—	—
Santonin	T37.4X1	T37.4X2	T37.4X3	T37.4X4	T37.4X5	T37.4X6
Santyl	T49.8X1	T49.8X2	T49.8X3	T49.8X4	T49.8X5	T49.8X6
Saralasin	T46.5X1	T46.5X2	T46.5X3	T46.5X4	T46.5X5	T46.5X6
Sarcolysin	T45.1X1	T45.1X2	T45.1X3	T45.1X4	T45.1X5	T45.1X6
Sarkomycin	T45.1X1	T45.1X2	T45.1X3	T45.1X4	T45.1X5	T45.1X6
Saroten	T43.011	T43.012	T43.013	T43.014	T43.015	T43.016
Saturnine — *see* Lead						
Savin (oil)	T49.4X1	T49.4X2	T49.4X3	T49.4X4	T49.4X5	T49.4X6
Scammony	T47.2X1	T47.2X2	T47.2X3	T47.2X4	T47.2X5	T47.2X6
Scarlet red	T49.8X1	T49.8X2	T49.8X3	T49.8X4	T49.8X5	T49.8X6
Scheele's green	T57.0X1	T57.0X2	T57.0X3	T57.0X4	—	—
insecticide	T57.0X1	T57.0X2	T57.0X3	T57.0X4		
Schizontozide (blood)	T37.2X1	T37.2X2	T37.2X3	T37.2X4	T37.2X5	T37.2X6
(tissue)						
Schradan	T60.0X1	T60.0X2	T60.0X3	T60.0X4	—	—
Schweinfurth green	T57.0X1	T57.0X2	T57.0X3	T57.0X4	—	—
insecticide	T57.0X1	T57.0X2	T57.0X3	T57.0X4		
Scilla, rat poison	T60.4X1	T60.4X2	T60.4X3	T60.4X4	—	—
Scillaren	T60.4X1	T60.4X2	T60.4X3	T60.4X4	—	—
Sclerosing agent	T46.8X1	T46.8X2	T46.8X3	T46.8X4	T46.8X5	T46.8X6
Scombrotoxin	T61.11	T61.12	T61.13	T61.14		
Scopolamine	T44.3X1	T44.3X2	T44.3X3	T44.3X4	T44.3X5	T44.3X6
Scopolia extract	T44.3X1	T44.3X2	T44.3X3	T44.3X4	T44.3X5	T44.3X6
Scouring powder	T65.891	T65.892	T65.893	T65.894	—	—
Sea						
anemone (sting)	T63.631	T63.632	T63.633	T63.634	—	—
cucumber (sting)	T63.691	T63.692	T63.693	T63.694	—	—
snake (bite) (venom)	T63.091	T63.092	T63.093	T63.094	—	—
urchin spine (puncture)	T63.691	T63.692	T63.693	T63.694	—	—
Seafood	T61.91	T61.92	T61.93	T61.94	—	—
specified NEC	T61.8X1	T61.8X2	T61.8X3	T61.8X4	—	—
Secbutabarbital	T42.3X1	T42.3X2	T42.3X3	T42.3X4	T42.3X5	T42.3X6
Secbutabarbitone	T42.3X1	T42.3X2	T42.3X3	T42.3X4	T42.3X5	T42.3X6
Secnidazole	T37.3X1	T37.3X2	T37.3X3	T37.3X4	T37.3X5	T37.3X6
Secobarbital	T42.3X1	T42.3X2	T42.3X3	T42.3X4	T42.3X5	T42.3X6
Seconal	T42.3X1	T42.3X2	T42.3X3	T42.3X4	T42.3X5	T42.3X6
Secretin	T50.8X1	T50.8X2	T50.8X3	T50.8X4	T50.8X5	T50.8X6
Sedative NEC	T42.71	T42.72	T42.73	T42.74	T42.75	T42.76
mixed NEC	T42.6X1	T42.6X2	T42.6X3	T42.6X4	T42.6X5	T42.6X6
Sedormid	T42.6X1	T42.6X2	T42.6X3	T42.6X4	T42.6X5	T42.6X6
Seed disinfectant or dressing	T60.8X1	T60.8X2	T60.8X3	T60.8X4	—	—
Seeds (poisonous)	T62.2X1	T62.2X2	T62.2X3	T62.2X4	—	—
Selegiline	T42.8X1	T42.8X2	T42.8X3	T42.8X4	T42.8X5	T42.8X6
Selenium NEC	T56.891	T56.892	T56.893	T56.894	—	—
disulfide or sulfide	T49.4X1	T49.4X2	T49.4X3	T49.4X4	T49.4X5	T49.4X6
fumes	T59.891	T59.892	T59.893	T59.894	—	—
sulfide	T49.4X1	T49.4X2	T49.4X3	T49.4X4	T49.4X5	T49.4X6
Selenomethionine (75Se)	T50.8X1	T50.8X2	T50.8X3	T50.8X4	T50.8X5	T50.8X6
Selsun	T49.4X1	T49.4X2	T49.4X3	T49.4X4	T49.4X5	T49.4X6
Semustine	T45.1X1	T45.1X2	T45.1X3	T45.1X4	T45.1X5	T45.1X6
Senega syrup	T48.4X1	T48.4X2	T48.4X3	T48.4X4	T48.4X5	T48.4X6
Senna	T47.2X1	T47.2X2	T47.2X3	T47.2X4	T47.2X5	T47.2X6
Sennoside A+B	T47.2X1	T47.2X2	T47.2X3	T47.2X4	T47.2X5	T47.2X6

Substance	Poisoning, Accidental (unintentional)	Poisoning, Intentional Self-harm	Poisoning, Assault	Poisoning, Undetermined	Adverse Effect	Under-dosing
Septisol	T49.2X1	T49.2X2	T49.2X3	T49.2X4	T49.2X5	T49.2X6
Seractide	T38.811	T38.812	T38.813	T38.814	T38.815	T38.816
Serax	T42.4X1	T42.4X2	T42.4X3	T42.4X4	T42.4X5	T42.4X6
Serenesil	T42.6X1	T42.6X2	T42.6X3	T42.6X4	T42.6X5	T42.6X6
Serenium (hydrochloride)	T37.91	T37.92	T37.93	T37.94	T37.95	T37.96
Serepax — *see* Oxazepam						
Sermorelin	T38.891	T38.892	T38.893	T38.894	T38.895	T38.896
Sernyl	T41.1X1	T41.1X2	T41.1X3	T41.1X4	T41.1X5	T41.1X6
Serotonin	T50.991	T50.992	T50.993	T50.994	T50.995	T50.996
Serpasil	T46.5X1	T46.5X2	T46.5X3	T46.5X4	T46.5X5	T46.5X6
Serrapeptase	T45.3X1	T45.3X2	T45.3X3	T45.3X4	T45.3X5	T45.3X6
Serum						
antibotulinus	T50.Z11	T50.Z12	T50.Z13	T50.Z14	T50.Z15	T50.Z16
anticytotoxic	T50.Z11	T50.Z12	T50.Z13	T50.Z14	T50.Z15	T50.Z16
antidiphtheria	T50.Z11	T50.Z12	T50.Z13	T50.Z14	T50.Z15	T50.Z16
antimeningococcus	T50.Z11	T50.Z12	T50.Z13	T50.Z14	T50.Z15	T50.Z16
anti-Rh	T50.Z11	T50.Z12	T50.Z13	T50.Z14	T50.Z15	T50.Z16
anti-snake-bite	T50.Z11	T50.Z12	T50.Z13	T50.Z14	T50.Z15	T50.Z16
antitetanic	T50.Z11	T50.Z12	T50.Z13	T50.Z14	T50.Z15	T50.Z16
antitoxic	T50.Z11	T50.Z12	T50.Z13	T50.Z14	T50.Z15	T50.Z16
complement (inhibitor)	T45.8X1	T45.8X2	T45.8X3	T45.8X4	T45.8X5	T45.8X6
convalescent	T50.Z11	T50.Z12	T50.Z13	T50.Z14	T50.Z15	T50.Z16
hemolytic complement	T45.8X1	T45.8X2	T45.8X3	T45.8X4	T45.8X5	T45.8X6
immune (human)	T50.Z11	T50.Z12	T50.Z13	T50.Z14	T50.Z15	T50.Z16
protective NEC	T50.Z11	T50.Z12	T50.Z13	T50.Z14	T50.Z15	T50.Z16
Setastine	T45.0X1	T45.0X2	T45.0X3	T45.0X4	T45.0X5	T45.0X6
Setoperone	T43.591	T43.592	T43.593	T43.594	T43.595	T43.596
Sewer gas	T59.91	T59.92	T59.93	T59.94	—	—
Shampoo	T55.0X1	T55.0X2	T55.0X3	T55.0X4	—	—
Shellfish, noxious, nonbacterial	T61.781	T61.782	T61.783	T61.784	—	—
Sildenafil	T46.7X1	T46.7X2	T46.7X3	T46.7X4	T46.7X5	T46.7X6
Silibinin	T50.991	T50.992	T50.993	T50.994	T50.995	T50.996
Silicone NEC	T65.891	T65.892	T65.893	T65.894		
medicinal	T49.3X1	T49.3X2	T49.3X3	T49.3X4	T49.3X5	T49.3X6
Silvadene	T49.0X1	T49.0X2	T49.0X3	T49.0X4	T49.0X5	T49.0X6
Silver	T49.0X1	T49.0X2	T49.0X3	T49.0X4	T49.0X5	T49.0X6
anti-infectives	T49.0X1	T49.0X2	T49.0X3	T49.0X4	T49.0X5	T49.0X6
arsphenamine	T37.8X1	T37.8X2	T37.8X3	T37.8X4	T37.8X5	T37.8X6
colloidal	T49.0X1	T49.0X2	T49.0X3	T49.0X4	T49.0X5	T49.0X6
nitrate	T49.0X1	T49.0X2	T49.0X3	T49.0X4	T49.0X5	T49.0X6
ophthalmic preparation	T49.5X1	T49.5X2	T49.5X3	T49.5X4	T49.5X5	T49.5X6
toughened (keratolytic)	T49.4X1	T49.4X2	T49.4X3	T49.4X4	T49.4X5	T49.4X6
nonmedicinal (dust)	T56.891	T56.892	T56.893	T56.894	—	—
protein	T49.5X1	T49.5X2	T49.5X3	T49.5X4	T49.5X5	T49.5X6
salvarsan	T37.8X1	T37.8X2	T37.8X3	T37.8X4	T37.8X5	T37.8X6
sulfadiazine	T49.4X1	T49.4X2	T49.4X3	T49.4X4	T49.4X5	T49.4X6
Silymarin	T50.991	T50.992	T50.993	T50.994	T50.995	T50.996
Simaldrate	T47.1X1	T47.1X2	T47.1X3	T47.1X4	T47.1X5	T47.1X6
Simazine	T60.3X1	T60.3X2	T60.3X3	T60.3X4	—	—
Simethicone	T47.1X1	T47.1X2	T47.1X3	T47.1X4	T47.1X5	T47.1X6
Simfibrate	T46.6X1	T46.6X2	T46.6X3	T46.6X4	T46.6X5	T46.6X6
Simvastatin	T46.6X1	T46.6X2	T46.6X3	T46.6X4	T46.6X5	T46.6X6
Sincalide	T50.8X1	T50.8X2	T50.8X3	T50.8X4	T50.8X5	T50.8X6
Sinequan	T43.011	T43.012	T43.013	T43.014	T43.015	T43.016
Singoserp	T46.5X1	T46.5X2	T46.5X3	T46.5X4	T46.5X5	T46.5X6
Sintrom	T45.511	T45.512	T45.513	T45.514	T45.515	T45.516
Sisomicin	T36.5X1	T36.5X2	T36.5X3	T36.5X4	T36.5X5	T36.5X6
Sitosterols	T46.6X1	T46.6X2	T46.6X3	T46.6X4	T46.6X5	T46.6X6
Skeletal muscle relaxants	T48.1X1	T48.1X2	T48.1X3	T48.1X4	T48.1X5	T48.1X6
Skin						
agents (external)	T49.91	T49.92	T49.93	T49.94	T49.95	T49.96
specified NEC	T49.8X1	T49.8X2	T49.8X3	T49.8X4	T49.8X5	T49.8X6
test antigen	T50.8X1	T50.8X2	T50.8X3	T50.8X4	T50.8X5	T50.8X6
Sleep-eze	T45.0X1	T45.0X2	T45.0X3	T45.0X4	T45.0X5	T45.0X6
Sleeping draught, pill	T42.71	T42.72	T42.73	T42.74	T42.75	T42.76
Smallpox vaccine	T50.B11	T50.B12	T50.B13	T50.B14	T50.B15	T50.B16
Smelter fumes NEC	T56.91	T56.92	T56.93	T56.94	—	—
Smog	T59.1X1	T59.1X2	T59.1X3	T59.1X4	—	—
Smoke NEC	T59.811	T59.812	T59.813	T59.814	—	—
Smooth muscle relaxant	T44.3X1	T44.3X2	T44.3X3	T44.3X4	T44.3X5	T44.3X6
Snail killer NEC	T60.8X1	T60.8X2	T60.8X3	T60.8X4	—	—
Snake venom or bite	T63.001	T63.002	T63.003	T63.004	—	—
hemocoagulase	T45.7X1	T45.7X2	T45.7X3	T45.7X4	T45.7X5	T45.7X6
Snuff	T65.211	T65.212	T65.213	T65.214	—	—
Soap (powder) (product)	T55.0X1	T55.0X2	T55.0X3	T55.0X4	—	—
enema	T47.4X1	T47.4X2	T47.4X3	T47.4X4	T47.4X5	T47.4X6
medicinal, soft	T49.2X1	T49.2X2	T49.2X3	T49.2X4	T49.2X5	T49.2X6
superfatted	T49.2X1	T49.2X2	T49.2X3	T49.2X4	T49.2X5	T49.2X6
Sobrerol	T48.4X1	T48.4X2	T48.4X3	T48.4X4	T48.4X5	T48.4X6
Soda (caustic)	T54.3X1	T54.3X2	T54.3X3	T54.3X4	—	—
bicarb	T47.1X1	T47.1X2	T47.1X3	T47.1X4	T47.1X5	T47.1X6

Substance	Poisoning, Accidental (unintentional)	Poisoning, Intentional Self-harm	Poisoning, Assault	Poisoning, Undetermined	Adverse Effect	Under-dosing
Soda — continued						
chlorinated — see Sodium, hypochlorite						
Sodium						
acetosulfone	T37.1X1	T37.1X2	T37.1X3	T37.1X4	T37.1X5	T37.1X6
acetrizoate	T50.8X1	T50.8X2	T50.8X3	T50.8X4	T50.8X5	T50.8X6
acid phosphate	T50.3X1	T50.3X2	T50.3X3	T50.3X4	T50.3X5	T50.3X6
alginate	T47.8X1	T47.8X2	T47.8X3	T47.8X4	T47.8X5	T47.8X6
amidotrizoate	T50.8X1	T50.8X2	T50.8X3	T50.8X4	T50.8X5	T50.8X6
aminopterin	T45.1X1	T45.1X2	T45.1X3	T45.1X4	T45.1X5	T45.1X6
amylosulfate	T47.8X1	T47.8X2	T47.8X3	T47.8X4	T47.8X5	T47.8X6
amytal	T42.3X1	T42.3X2	T42.3X3	T42.3X4	T42.3X5	T42.3X6
antimony gluconate	T37.3X1	T37.3X2	T37.3X3	T37.3X4	T37.3X5	T37.3X6
arsenate	T57.0X1	T57.0X2	T57.0X3	T57.0X4	—	—
aurothiomalate	T39.4X1	T39.4X2	T39.4X3	T39.4X4	T39.4X5	T39.4X6
aurothiosulfate	T39.4X1	T39.4X2	T39.4X3	T39.4X4	T39.4X5	T39.4X6
barbiturate	T42.3X1	T42.3X2	T42.3X3	T42.3X4	T42.3X5	T42.3X6
basic phosphate	T47.4X1	T47.4X2	T47.4X3	T47.4X4	T47.4X5	T47.4X6
bicarbonate	T47.1X1	T47.1X2	T47.1X3	T47.1X4	T47.1X5	T47.1X6
bichromate	T57.8X1	T57.8X2	T57.8X3	T57.8X4	—	—
biphosphate	T50.3X1	T50.3X2	T50.3X3	T50.3X4	T50.3X5	T50.3X6
bisulfate	T65.891	T65.892	T65.893	T65.894	—	—
borate						
cleanser	T57.8X1	T57.8X2	T57.8X3	T57.8X4	—	—
eye	T49.5X1	T49.5X2	T49.5X3	T49.5X4	T49.5X5	T49.5X6
therapeutic	T49.8X1	T49.8X2	T49.8X3	T49.8X4	T49.8X5	T49.8X6
bromide	T42.6X1	T42.6X2	T42.6X3	T42.6X4	T42.6X5	T42.6X6
cacodylate (nonmedicinal) NEC	T50.8X1	T50.8X2	T50.8X3	T50.8X4	T50.8X5	T50.8X6
anti-infective	T37.8X1	T37.8X2	T37.8X3	T37.8X4	T37.8X5	T37.8X6
herbicide	T60.3X1	T60.3X2	T60.3X3	T60.3X4	—	—
calcium edetate	T45.8X1	T45.8X2	T45.8X3	T45.8X4	T45.8X5	T45.8X6
carbonate NEC	T54.3X1	T54.3X2	T54.3X3	T54.3X4	—	—
chlorate NEC	T65.891	T65.892	T65.893	T65.894	—	—
herbicide	T54.91	T54.92	T54.93	T54.94	—	—
chloride	T50.3X1	T50.3X2	T50.3X3	T50.3X4	T50.3X5	T50.3X6
with glucose	T50.3X1	T50.3X2	T50.3X3	T50.3X4	T50.3X5	T50.3X6
chromate	T65.891	T65.892	T65.893	T65.894	—	—
citrate	T50.991	T50.992	T50.993	T50.994	T50.995	T50.996
cromoglicate	T48.6X1	T48.6X2	T48.6X3	T48.6X4	T48.6X5	T48.6X6
cyanide	T65.0X1	T65.0X2	T65.0X3	T65.0X4	—	—
cyclamate	T50.3X1	T50.3X2	T50.3X3	T50.3X4	T50.3X5	T50.3X6
dehydrocholate	T45.8X1	T45.8X2	T45.8X3	T45.8X4	T45.8X5	T45.8X6
diatrizoate	T50.8X1	T50.8X2	T50.8X3	T50.8X4	T50.8X5	T50.8X6
dibunate	T48.4X1	T48.4X2	T48.4X3	T48.4X4	T48.4X5	T48.4X6
dioctyl sulfosuccinate	T47.4X1	T47.4X2	T47.4X3	T47.4X4	T47.4X5	T47.4X6
dipantoyl ferrate	T45.8X1	T45.8X2	T45.8X3	T45.8X4	T45.8X5	T45.8X6
edetate	T45.8X1	T45.8X2	T45.8X3	T45.8X4	T45.8X5	T45.8X6
ethacrynate	T50.1X1	T50.1X2	T50.1X3	T50.1X4	T50.1X5	T50.1X6
feredetate	T45.8X1	T45.8X2	T45.8X3	T45.8X4	T45.8X5	T45.8X6
Fluoride — see Fluoride						
fluoroacetate (dust) (pesticide)	T60.4X1	T60.4X2	T60.4X3	T60.4X4	—	—
free salt	T50.3X1	T50.3X2	T50.3X3	T50.3X4	T50.3X5	T50.3X6
fusidate	T36.8X1	T36.8X2	T36.8X3	T36.8X4	T36.8X5	T36.8X6
glucaldrate	T47.1X1	T47.1X2	T47.1X3	T47.1X4	T47.1X5	T47.1X6
glucosulfone	T37.1X1	T37.1X2	T37.1X3	T37.1X4	T37.1X5	T37.1X6
glutamate	T45.8X1	T45.8X2	T45.8X3	T45.8X4	T45.8X5	T45.8X6
hydrogen carbonate	T50.3X1	T50.3X2	T50.3X3	T50.3X4	T50.3X5	T50.3X6
hydroxide	T54.3X1	T54.3X2	T54.3X3	T54.3X4	—	—
hypochlorite (bleach) NEC	T54.3X1	T54.3X2	T54.3X3	T54.3X4	—	—
disinfectant	T54.3X1	T54.3X2	T54.3X3	T54.3X4	—	—
medicinal (anti-infective) (external)	T49.0X1	T49.0X2	T49.0X3	T49.0X4	T49.0X5	T49.0X6
vapor	T54.3X1	T54.3X2	T54.3X3	T54.3X4	—	—
hyposulfite	T49.0X1	T49.0X2	T49.0X3	T49.0X4	T49.0X5	T49.0X6
indigotin disulfonate	T50.8X1	T50.8X2	T50.8X3	T50.8X4	T50.8X5	T50.8X6
iodide	T50.991	T50.992	T50.993	T50.994	T50.995	T50.996
I-131	T50.8X1	T50.8X2	T50.8X3	T50.8X4	T50.8X5	T50.8X6
therapeutic	T38.2X1	T38.2X2	T38.2X3	T38.2X4	T38.2X5	T38.2X6
iodohippurate (131I)	T50.8X1	T50.8X2	T50.8X3	T50.8X4	T50.8X5	T50.8X6
iopodate	T50.8X1	T50.8X2	T50.8X3	T50.8X4	T50.8X5	T50.8X6
iothalamate	T50.8X1	T50.8X2	T50.8X3	T50.8X4	T50.8X5	T50.8X6
iron edetate	T45.4X1	T45.4X2	T45.4X3	T45.4X4	T45.4X5	T45.4X6
lactate (compound solution)	T45.8X1	T45.8X2	T45.8X3	T45.8X4	T45.8X5	T45.8X6
lauryl (sulfate)	T49.2X1	T49.2X2	T49.2X3	T49.2X4	T49.2X5	T49.2X6
L-triiodothyronine	T38.1X1	T38.1X2	T38.1X3	T38.1X4	T38.1X5	T38.1X6
magnesium citrate	T50.991	T50.992	T50.993	T50.994	T50.995	T50.996
mersalate	T50.2X1	T50.2X2	T50.2X3	T50.2X4	T50.2X5	T50.2X6
metasilicate	T65.891	T65.892	T65.893	T65.894	—	—
metrizoate	T50.8X1	T50.8X2	T50.8X3	T50.8X4	T50.8X5	T50.8X6
Sodium — continued						
monofluoroacetate (pesticide)	T60.1X1	T60.1X2	T60.1X3	T60.1X4	—	—
morrhuate	T46.8X1	T46.8X2	T46.8X3	T46.8X4	T46.8X5	T46.8X6
nafcillin	T36.0X1	T36.0X2	T36.0X3	T36.0X4	T36.0X5	T36.0X6
nitrate (oxidizing agent)	T65.891	T65.892	T65.893	T65.894	—	—
nitrite	T50.6X1	T50.6X2	T50.6X3	T50.6X4	T50.6X5	T50.6X6
nitroferricyanide	T46.5X1	T46.5X2	T46.5X3	T46.5X4	T46.5X5	T46.5X6
nitroprusside	T46.5X1	T46.5X2	T46.5X3	T46.5X4	T46.5X5	T46.5X6
oxalate	T65.891	T65.892	T65.893	T65.894	—	—
oxide/peroxide	T65.891	T65.892	T65.893	T65.894	—	—
oxybate	T41.291	T41.292	T41.293	T41.294	T41.295	T41.296
para-aminohippurate	T50.8X1	T50.8X2	T50.8X3	T50.8X4	T50.8X5	T50.8X6
perborate (nonmedicinal) NEC	T65.891	T65.892	T65.893	T65.894	—	—
medicinal	T49.0X1	T49.0X2	T49.0X3	T49.0X4	T49.0X5	T49.0X6
soap	T55.0X1	T55.0X2	T55.0X3	T55.0X4	—	—
percarbonate — see Sodium, perborate						
pertechnetate Tc99m	T50.8X1	T50.8X2	T50.8X3	T50.8X4	T50.8X5	T50.8X6
phosphate						
cellulose	T45.8X1	T45.8X2	T45.8X3	T45.8X4	T45.8X5	T45.8X6
dibasic	T47.2X1	T47.2X2	T47.2X3	T47.2X4	T47.2X5	T47.2X6
monobasic	T47.2X1	T47.2X2	T47.2X3	T47.2X4	T47.2X5	T47.2X6
phytate	T50.6X1	T50.6X2	T50.6X3	T50.6X4	T50.6X5	T50.6X6
picosulfate	T47.2X1	T47.2X2	T47.2X3	T47.2X4	T47.2X5	T47.2X6
polyhydroxyaluminium monocarbonate	T47.1X1	T47.1X2	T47.1X3	T47.1X4	T47.1X5	T47.1X6
polystyrene sulfonate	T50.3X1	T50.3X2	T50.3X3	T50.3X4	T50.3X5	T50.3X6
propionate	T49.0X1	T49.0X2	T49.0X3	T49.0X4	T49.0X5	T49.0X6
propyl hydroxybenzoate	T50.991	T50.992	T50.993	T50.994	T50.995	T50.996
psylliate	T46.8X1	T46.8X2	T46.8X3	T46.8X4	T46.8X5	T46.8X6
removing resins	T50.3X1	T50.3X2	T50.3X3	T50.3X4	T50.3X5	T50.3X6
salicylate	T39.091	T39.092	T39.093	T39.094	T39.095	T39.096
salt NEC	T50.3X1	T50.3X2	T50.3X3	T50.3X4	T50.3X5	T50.3X6
selenate	T60.2X1	T60.2X2	T60.2X3	T60.2X4	—	—
stibogluconate	T37.3X1	T37.3X2	T37.3X3	T37.3X4	T37.3X5	T37.3X6
sulfate	T47.4X1	T47.4X2	T47.4X3	T47.4X4	T47.4X5	T47.4X6
sulfoxone	T37.1X1	T37.1X2	T37.1X3	T37.1X4	T37.1X5	T37.1X6
tetradecyl sulfate	T46.8X1	T46.8X2	T46.8X3	T46.8X4	T46.8X5	T46.8X6
thiopental	T41.1X1	T41.1X2	T41.1X3	T41.1X4	T41.1X5	T41.1X6
thiosalicylate	T39.091	T39.092	T39.093	T39.094	T39.095	T39.096
thiosulfate	T50.6X1	T50.6X2	T50.6X3	T50.6X4	T50.6X5	T50.6X6
tolbutamide	T38.3X1	T38.3X2	T38.3X3	T38.3X4	T38.3X5	T38.3X6
(L)-triiodothyronine	T38.1X1	T38.1X2	T38.1X3	T38.1X4	T38.1X5	T38.1X6
tyropanoate	T50.8X1	T50.8X2	T50.8X3	T50.8X4	T50.8X5	T50.8X6
valproate	T42.6X1	T42.6X2	T42.6X3	T42.6X4	T42.6X5	T42.6X6
versenate	T50.6X1	T50.6X2	T50.6X3	T50.6X4	T50.6X5	T50.6X6
Sodium-free salt	T50.901	T50.902	T50.903	T50.904	T50.905	T50.906
Sodium-removing resin	T50.3X1	T50.3X2	T50.3X3	T50.3X4	T50.3X5	T50.3X6
Soft soap	T55.0X1	T55.0X2	T55.0X3	T55.0X4	—	—
Solanine	T62.2X1	T62.2X2	T62.2X3	T62.2X4	—	—
berries	T62.1X1	T62.1X2	T62.1X3	T62.1X4	—	—
Solanum dulcamara	T62.2X1	T62.2X2	T62.2X3	T62.2X4	—	—
berries	T62.1X1	T62.1X2	T62.1X3	T62.1X4	—	—
Solapsone	T37.1X1	T37.1X2	T37.1X3	T37.1X4	T37.1X5	T37.1X6
Solar lotion	T49.3X1	T49.3X2	T49.3X3	T49.3X4	T49.3X5	T49.3X6
Solasulfone	T37.1X1	T37.1X2	T37.1X3	T37.1X4	T37.1X5	T37.1X6
Soldering fluid	T65.891	T65.892	T65.893	T65.894	—	—
Solid substance	T65.91	T65.92	T65.93	T65.94	—	—
specified NEC	T65.891	T65.892	T65.893	T65.894	—	—
Solvent, industrial NEC	T52.91	T52.92	T52.93	T52.94	—	—
naphtha	T52.0X1	T52.0X2	T52.0X3	T52.0X4	—	—
petroleum	T52.0X1	T52.0X2	T52.0X3	T52.0X4	—	—
specified NEC	T52.8X1	T52.8X2	T52.8X3	T52.8X4	—	—
Soma	T42.8X1	T42.8X2	T42.8X3	T42.8X4	T42.8X5	T42.8X6
Somatorelin	T38.891	T38.892	T38.893	T38.894	T38.895	T38.896
Somatostatin	T38.991	T38.992	T38.993	T38.994	T38.995	T38.996
Somatotropin	T38.811	T38.812	T38.813	T38.814	T38.815	T38.816
Somatrem	T38.811	T38.812	T38.813	T38.814	T38.815	T38.816
Somatropin	T38.811	T38.812	T38.813	T38.814	T38.815	T38.816
Sominex	T45.0X1	T45.0X2	T45.0X3	T45.0X4	T45.0X5	T45.0X6
Somnos	T42.6X1	T42.6X2	T42.6X3	T42.6X4	T42.6X5	T42.6X6
Somonal	T42.3X1	T42.3X2	T42.3X3	T42.3X4	T42.3X5	T42.3X6
Soneryl	T42.3X1	T42.3X2	T42.3X3	T42.3X4	T42.3X5	T42.3X6
Soothing syrup	T50.901	T50.902	T50.903	T50.904	T50.905	T50.906
Sopor	T42.6X1	T42.6X2	T42.6X3	T42.6X4	T42.6X5	T42.6X6
Soporific	T42.71	T42.72	T42.73	T42.74	T42.75	T42.76
Soporific drug	T42.71	T42.72	T42.73	T42.74	T42.75	T42.76
specified type NEC	T42.6X1	T42.6X2	T42.6X3	T42.6X4	T42.6X5	T42.6X6
Sorbide nitrate	T46.3X1	T46.3X2	T46.3X3	T46.3X4	T46.3X5	T46.3X6
Sorbitol	T47.4X1	T47.4X2	T47.4X3	T47.4X4	T47.4X5	T47.4X6
Sotalol	T44.7X1	T44.7X2	T44.7X3	T44.7X4	T44.7X5	T44.7X6

Substance	Poisoning, Accidental (unintentional)	Poisoning, Intentional Self-harm	Poisoning, Assault	Poisoning, Undetermined	Adverse Effect	Under-dosing
Sotradecol	T46.8X1	T46.8X2	T46.8X3	T46.8X4	T46.8X5	T46.8X6
Soysterol	T46.6X1	T46.6X2	T46.6X3	T46.6X4	T46.6X5	T46.6X6
Spacoline	T44.3X1	T44.3X2	T44.3X3	T44.3X4	T44.3X5	T44.3X6
Spanish fly	T49.8X1	T49.8X2	T49.8X3	T49.8X4	T49.8X5	T49.8X6
Sparine	T43.3X1	T43.3X2	T43.3X3	T43.3X4	T43.3X5	T43.3X6
Sparteine	T48.0X1	T48.0X2	T48.0X3	T48.0X4	T48.0X5	T48.0X6
Spasmolytic						
anticholinergics	T44.3X1	T44.3X2	T44.3X3	T44.3X4	T44.3X5	T44.3X6
autonomic	T44.3X1	T44.3X2	T44.3X3	T44.3X4	T44.3X5	T44.3X6
bronchial NEC	T48.6X1	T48.6X2	T48.6X3	T48.6X4	T48.6X5	T48.6X6
quaternary ammonium	T44.3X1	T44.3X2	T44.3X3	T44.3X4	T44.3X5	T44.3X6
skeletal muscle NEC	T48.1X1	T48.1X2	T48.1X3	T48.1X4	T48.1X5	T48.1X6
Spectinomycin	T36.5X1	T36.5X2	T36.5X3	T36.5X4	T36.5X5	T36.5X6
Speed	T43.621	T43.622	T43.623	T43.624	T43.625	T43.626
Spermicide	T49.8X1	T49.8X2	T49.8X3	T49.8X4	T49.8X5	T49.8X6
Spider (bite) (venom)	T63.391	T63.392	T63.393	T63.394		
antivenin	T50.Z11	T50.Z12	T50.Z13	T50.Z14	T50.Z15	T50.Z16
Spigelia (root)	T37.4X1	T37.4X2	T37.4X3	T37.4X4	T37.4X5	T37.4X6
Spindle inactivator	T50.4X1	T50.4X2	T50.4X3	T50.4X4	T50.4X5	T50.4X6
Spiperone	T43.4X1	T43.4X2	T43.4X3	T43.4X4	T43.4X5	T43.4X6
Spiramycin	T36.3X1	T36.3X2	T36.3X3	T36.3X4	T36.3X5	T36.3X6
Spirapril	T46.4X1	T46.4X2	T46.4X3	T46.4X4	T46.4X5	T46.4X6
Spirilene	T43.591	T43.592	T43.593	T43.594	T43.595	T43.596
Spirit(s) (neutral) **NEC**	T51.0X1	T51.0X2	T51.0X3	T51.0X4	—	—
beverage	T51.0X1	T51.0X2	T51.0X3	T51.0X4	—	—
industrial	T51.0X1	T51.0X2	T51.0X3	T51.0X4	—	—
mineral	T52.0X1	T52.0X2	T52.0X3	T52.0X4	—	—
of salt — *see* Hydrochloric acid						
surgical	T51.0X1	T51.0X2	T51.0X3	T51.0X4	—	—
Spironolactone	T50.0X1	T50.0X2	T50.0X3	T50.0X4	T50.0X5	T50.0X6
Spiroperidol	T43.4X1	T43.4X2	T43.4X3	T43.4X4	T43.4X5	T43.4X6
Sponge, absorbable (gelatin)	T45.7X1	T45.7X2	T45.7X3	T45.7X4	T45.7X5	T45.7X6
Sporostacin	T49.0X1	T49.0X2	T49.0X3	T49.0X4	T49.0X5	T49.0X6
Spray (aerosol)	T65.91	T65.92	T65.93	T65.94	—	—
cosmetic	T65.891	T65.892	T65.893	T65.894	—	—
medicinal NEC	T50.901	T50.902	T50.903	T50.904	T50.905	T50.906
pesticides — *see* Pesticides						
specified content — *see* specific substance						
Spurge flax	T62.2X1	T62.2X2	T62.2X3	T62.2X4	—	—
Spurges	T62.2X1	T62.2X2	T62.2X3	T62.2X4	—	—
Sputum viscosity-lowering drug	T48.4X1	T48.4X2	T48.4X3	T48.4X4	T48.4X5	T48.4X6
Squill	T46.0X1	T46.0X2	T46.0X3	T46.0X4	T46.0X5	T46.0X6
rat poison	T60.4X1	T60.4X2	T60.4X3	T60.4X4		
Squirting cucumber (cathartic)	T47.2X1	T47.2X2	T47.2X3	T47.2X4	T47.2X5	T47.2X6
Stains	T65.6X1	T65.6X2	T65.6X3	T65.6X4		
Stannous fluoride	T49.7X1	T49.7X2	T49.7X3	T49.7X4	T49.7X5	T49.7X6
Stanolone	T38.7X1	T38.7X2	T38.7X3	T38.7X4	T38.7X5	T38.7X6
Stanozolol	T38.7X1	T38.7X2	T38.7X3	T38.7X4	T38.7X5	T38.7X6
Staphisagria or stavesacre (pediculicide)	T49.0X1	T49.0X2	T49.0X3	T49.0X4	T49.0X5	T49.0X6
Starch	T50.901	T50.902	T50.903	T50.904	T50.905	T50.906
Stelazine	T43.3X1	T43.3X2	T43.3X3	T43.3X4	T43.3X5	T43.3X6
Stemetil	T43.3X1	T43.3X2	T43.3X3	T43.3X4	T43.3X5	T43.3X6
Stepronin	T48.4X1	T48.4X2	T48.4X3	T48.4X4	T48.4X5	T48.4X6
Sterculia	T47.4X1	T47.4X2	T47.4X3	T47.4X4	T47.4X5	T47.4X6
Sternutator gas	T59.891	T59.892	T59.893	T59.894	—	—
Steroid	T38.0X1	T38.0X2	T38.0X3	T38.0X4	T38.0X5	T38.0X6
anabolic	T38.7X1	T38.7X2	T38.7X3	T38.7X4	T38.7X5	T38.7X6
androgenic	T38.7X1	T38.7X2	T38.7X3	T38.7X4	T38.7X5	T38.7X6
antineoplastic, hormone	T38.7X1	T38.7X2	T38.7X3	T38.7X4	T38.7X5	T38.7X6
estrogen	T38.5X1	T38.5X2	T38.5X3	T38.5X4	T38.5X5	T38.5X6
ENT agent	T49.6X1	T49.6X2	T49.6X3	T49.6X4	T49.6X5	T49.6X6
ophthalmic preparation	T49.5X1	T49.5X2	T49.5X3	T49.5X4	T49.5X5	T49.5X6
topical NEC	T49.0X1	T49.0X2	T49.0X3	T49.0X4	T49.0X5	T49.0X6
Stibine	T56.891	T56.892	T56.893	T56.894	—	—
Stibogluconate	T37.3X1	T37.3X2	T37.3X3	T37.3X4	T37.3X5	T37.3X6
Stibophen	T37.4X1	T37.4X2	T37.4X3	T37.4X4	T37.4X5	T37.4X6
Stilbamidine (isetionate)	T37.3X1	T37.3X2	T37.3X3	T37.3X4	T37.3X5	T37.3X6
Stilbestrol	T38.5X1	T38.5X2	T38.5X3	T38.5X4	T38.5X5	T38.5X6
Stilboestrol	T38.5X1	T38.5X2	T38.5X3	T38.5X4	T38.5X5	T38.5X6
Stimulant						
central nervous system — *see also* Psychostimulant	T43.601	T43.602	T43.603	T43.604	T43.605	T43.606
analeptics	T50.7X1	T50.7X2	T50.7X3	T50.7X4	T50.7X5	T50.7X6
opiate antagonist	T50.7X1	T50.7X2	T50.7X3	T50.7X4	T50.7X5	T50.7X6
psychotherapeutic NEC — *see also* Psychotherapeutic drug	T43.601	T43.602	T43.603	T43.604	T43.605	T43.606
specified NEC	T43.691	T43.692	T43.693	T43.694	T43.695	T43.696

Substance	Poisoning, Accidental (unintentional)	Poisoning, Intentional Self-harm	Poisoning, Assault	Poisoning, Undetermined	Adverse Effect	Under-dosing
Stimulant — *continued*						
respiratory	T48.901	T48.902	T48.903	T48.904	T48.905	T48.906
Stone-dissolving drug	T50.901	T50.902	T50.903	T50.904	T50.905	T50.906
Storage battery (cells) (acid)	T54.2X1	T54.2X2	T54.2X3	T54.2X4		
Stovaine	T41.3X1	T41.3X2	T41.3X3	T41.3X4	T41.3X5	T41.3X6
infiltration (subcutaneous)	T41.3X1	T41.3X2	T41.3X3	T41.3X4	T41.3X5	T41.3X6
nerve block (peripheral) (plexus)	T41.3X1	T41.3X2	T41.3X3	T41.3X4	T41.3X5	T41.3X6
spinal	T41.3X1	T41.3X2	T41.3X3	T41.3X4	T41.3X5	T41.3X6
topical (surface)	T41.3X1	T41.3X2	T41.3X3	T41.3X4	T41.3X5	T41.3X6
Stovarsal	T37.8X1	T37.8X2	T37.8X3	T37.8X4	T37.8X5	T37.8X6
Stove gas — *see* Gas, stove						
Stoxil	T49.5X1	T49.5X2	T49.5X3	T49.5X4	T49.5X5	T49.5X6
Stramonium	T48.6X1	T48.6X2	T48.6X3	T48.6X4	T48.6X5	T48.6X6
natural state	T62.2X1	T62.2X2	T62.2X3	T62.2X4	—	—
Streptodornase	T45.3X1	T45.3X2	T45.3X3	T45.3X4	T45.3X5	T45.3X6
Streptoduocin	T36.5X1	T36.5X2	T36.5X3	T36.5X4	T36.5X5	T36.5X6
Streptokinase	T45.611	T45.612	T45.613	T45.614	T45.615	T45.616
Streptomycin (derivative)	T36.5X1	T36.5X2	T36.5X3	T36.5X4	T36.5X5	T36.5X6
Streptonivicin	T36.5X1	T36.5X2	T36.5X3	T36.5X4	T36.5X5	T36.5X6
Streptovarycin	T36.5X1	T36.5X2	T36.5X3	T36.5X4	T36.5X5	T36.5X6
Streptozocin	T45.1X1	T45.1X2	T45.1X3	T45.1X4	T45.1X5	T45.1X6
Streptozotocin	T45.1X1	T45.1X2	T45.1X3	T45.1X4	T45.1X5	T45.1X6
Stripper (paint) (solvent)	T52.8X1	T52.8X2	T52.8X3	T52.8X4	—	—
Strobane	T60.1X1	T60.1X2	T60.1X3	T60.1X4	—	—
Strofantina	T46.0X1	T46.0X2	T46.0X3	T46.0X4	T46.0X5	T46.0X6
Strophanthin (g) (k)	T46.0X1	T46.0X2	T46.0X3	T46.0X4	T46.0X5	T46.0X6
Strophanthus	T46.0X1	T46.0X2	T46.0X3	T46.0X4	T46.0X5	T46.0X6
Strophantin	T46.0X1	T46.0X2	T46.0X3	T46.0X4	T46.0X5	T46.0X6
Strophantin-g	T46.0X1	T46.0X2	T46.0X3	T46.0X4	T46.0X5	T46.0X6
Strychnine (nonmedicinal) (pesticide) (salts)	T65.1X1	T65.1X2	T65.1X3	T65.1X4	—	—
medicinal	T48.291	T48.292	T48.293	T48.294	T48.295	T48.296
Strychnos (ignatii) — *see* Strychnine						
Styramate	T42.8X1	T42.8X2	T42.8X3	T42.8X4	T42.8X5	T42.8X6
Styrene	T65.891	T65.892	T65.893	T65.894	—	—
Succinimide, antiepileptic or anticonvulsant	T42.2X1	T42.2X2	T42.2X3	T42.2X4	T42.2X5	T42.2X6
mercuric — *see* Mercury						
Succinylcholine	T48.1X1	T48.1X2	T48.1X3	T48.1X4	T48.1X5	T48.1X6
Succinylsulfathiazole	T37.0X1	T37.0X2	T37.0X3	T37.0X4	T37.0X5	T37.0X6
Sucralfate	T47.1X1	T47.1X2	T47.1X3	T47.1X4	T47.1X5	T47.1X6
Sucrose	T50.3X1	T50.3X2	T50.3X3	T50.3X4	T50.3X5	T50.3X6
Sufentanil	T40.4X1	T40.4X2	T40.4X3	T40.4X4	T40.4X5	T40.4X6
Sulbactam	T36.0X1	T36.0X2	T36.0X3	T36.0X4	T36.0X5	T36.0X6
Sulbenicillin	T36.0X1	T36.0X2	T36.0X3	T36.0X4	T36.0X5	T36.0X6
Sulbentine	T49.0X1	T49.0X2	T49.0X3	T49.0X4	T49.0X5	T49.0X6
Sulfacetamide	T49.0X1	T49.0X2	T49.0X3	T49.0X4	T49.0X5	T49.0X6
ophthalmic preparation	T49.5X1	T49.5X2	T49.5X3	T49.5X4	T49.5X5	T49.5X6
Sulfachlorpyridazine	T37.0X1	T37.0X2	T37.0X3	T37.0X4	T37.0X5	T37.0X6
Sulfacitine	T37.0X1	T37.0X2	T37.0X3	T37.0X4	T37.0X5	T37.0X6
Sulfadiasulfone sodium	T37.0X1	T37.0X2	T37.0X3	T37.0X4	T37.0X5	T37.0X6
Sulfadiazine	T37.0X1	T37.0X2	T37.0X3	T37.0X4	T37.0X5	T37.0X6
silver (topical)	T49.0X1	T49.0X2	T49.0X3	T49.0X4	T49.0X5	T49.0X6
Sulfadimethoxine	T37.0X1	T37.0X2	T37.0X3	T37.0X4	T37.0X5	T37.0X6
Sulfadimidine	T37.0X1	T37.0X2	T37.0X3	T37.0X4	T37.0X5	T37.0X6
Sulfadoxine	T37.0X1	T37.0X2	T37.0X3	T37.0X4	T37.0X5	T37.0X6
with pyrimethamine	T37.2X1	T37.2X2	T37.2X3	T37.2X4	T37.2X5	T37.2X6
Sulfaethidole	T37.0X1	T37.0X2	T37.0X3	T37.0X4	T37.0X5	T37.0X6
Sulfafurazole	T37.0X1	T37.0X2	T37.0X3	T37.0X4	T37.0X5	T37.0X6
Sulfaguanidine	T37.0X1	T37.0X2	T37.0X3	T37.0X4	T37.0X5	T37.0X6
Sulfalene	T37.0X1	T37.0X2	T37.0X3	T37.0X4	T37.0X5	T37.0X6
Sulfaloxate	T37.0X1	T37.0X2	T37.0X3	T37.0X4	T37.0X5	T37.0X6
Sulfaloxic acid	T37.0X1	T37.0X2	T37.0X3	T37.0X4	T37.0X5	T37.0X6
Sulfamazone	T39.2X1	T39.2X2	T39.2X3	T39.2X4	T39.2X5	T39.2X6
Sulfamerazine	T37.0X1	T37.0X2	T37.0X3	T37.0X4	T37.0X5	T37.0X6
Sulfameter	T37.0X1	T37.0X2	T37.0X3	T37.0X4	T37.0X5	T37.0X6
Sulfamethazine	T37.0X1	T37.0X2	T37.0X3	T37.0X4	T37.0X5	T37.0X6
Sulfamethizole	T37.0X1	T37.0X2	T37.0X3	T37.0X4	T37.0X5	T37.0X6
Sulfamethoxazole	T37.0X1	T37.0X2	T37.0X3	T37.0X4	T37.0X5	T37.0X6
with trimethoprim	T36.8X1	T36.8X2	T36.8X3	T36.8X4	T36.8X5	T36.8X6
Sulfamethoxydiazine	T37.0X1	T37.0X2	T37.0X3	T37.0X4	T37.0X5	T37.0X6
Sulfamethoxypyridazine	T37.0X1	T37.0X2	T37.0X3	T37.0X4	T37.0X5	T37.0X6
Sulfamethylthiazole	T37.0X1	T37.0X2	T37.0X3	T37.0X4	T37.0X5	T37.0X6
Sulfametoxydiazine	T37.0X1	T37.0X2	T37.0X3	T37.0X4	T37.0X5	T37.0X6
Sulfamidopyrine	T39.2X1	T39.2X2	T39.2X3	T39.2X4	T39.2X5	T39.2X6
Sulfamonomethoxine	T37.0X1	T37.0X2	T37.0X3	T37.0X4	T37.0X5	T37.0X6
Sulfamoxole	T37.0X1	T37.0X2	T37.0X3	T37.0X4	T37.0X5	T37.0X6
Sulfamylon	T49.0X1	T49.0X2	T49.0X3	T49.0X4	T49.0X5	T49.0X6
Sulfan blue (diagnostic dye)	T50.8X1	T50.8X2	T50.8X3	T50.8X4	T50.8X5	T50.8X6
Sulfanilamide	T37.0X1	T37.0X2	T37.0X3	T37.0X4	T37.0X5	T37.0X6
Sulfanilylguanidine	T37.0X1	T37.0X2	T37.0X3	T37.0X4	T37.0X5	T37.0X6

Additional Character May Be Required — Refer to the Tabular List for Character Selection   ▽ **Subterms under main terms may continue to next column or page**

Substance	Poisoning, Accidental (unintentional)	Poisoning, Intentional Self-harm	Poisoning, Assault	Poisoning, Undetermined	Adverse Effect	Under-dosing
Sulfaperin	T37.0X1	T37.0X2	T37.0X3	T37.0X4	T37.0X5	T37.0X6
Sulfaphenazole	T37.0X1	T37.0X2	T37.0X3	T37.0X4	T37.0X5	T37.0X6
Sulfaphenylthiazole	T37.0X1	T37.0X2	T37.0X3	T37.0X4	T37.0X5	T37.0X6
Sulfaproxyline	T37.0X1	T37.0X2	T37.0X3	T37.0X4	T37.0X5	T37.0X6
Sulfapyridine	T37.0X1	T37.0X2	T37.0X3	T37.0X4	T37.0X5	T37.0X6
Sulfapyrimidine	T37.0X1	T37.0X2	T37.0X3	T37.0X4	T37.0X5	T37.0X6
Sulfarsphenamine	T37.8X1	T37.8X2	T37.8X3	T37.8X4	T37.8X5	T37.8X6
Sulfasalazine	T37.0X1	T37.0X2	T37.0X3	T37.0X4	T37.0X5	T37.0X6
Sulfasuxidine	T37.0X1	T37.0X2	T37.0X3	T37.0X4	T37.0X5	T37.0X6
Sulfasymazine	T37.0X1	T37.0X2	T37.0X3	T37.0X4	T37.0X5	T37.0X6
Sulfated amylopectin	T47.8X1	T47.8X2	T47.8X3	T47.8X4	T47.8X5	T47.8X6
Sulfathiazole	T37.0X1	T37.0X2	T37.0X3	T37.0X4	T37.0X5	T37.0X6
Sulfatostearate	T49.2X1	T49.2X2	T49.2X3	T49.2X4	T49.2X5	T49.2X6
Sulfinpyrazone	T50.4X1	T50.4X2	T50.4X3	T50.4X4	T50.4X5	T50.4X6
Sulfiram	T49.0X1	T49.0X2	T49.0X3	T49.0X4	T49.0X5	T49.0X6
Sulfisomidine	T37.0X1	T37.0X2	T37.0X3	T37.0X4	T37.0X5	T37.0X6
Sulfisoxazole	T37.0X1	T37.0X2	T37.0X3	T37.0X4	T37.0X5	T37.0X6
ophthalmic preparation	T49.5X1	T49.5X2	T49.5X3	T49.5X4	T49.5X5	T49.5X6
Sulfobromophthalein	T50.8X1	T50.8X2	T50.8X3	T50.8X4	T50.8X5	T50.8X6
(sodium)						
Sulfobromphthalein	T50.8X1	T50.8X2	T50.8X3	T50.8X4	T50.8X5	T50.8X6
Sulfogaiacol	T48.4X1	T48.4X2	T48.4X3	T48.4X4	T48.4X5	T48.4X6
Sulfomyxin	T36.8X1	T36.8X2	T36.8X3	T36.8X4	T36.8X5	T36.8X6
Sulfonal	T42.6X1	T42.6X2	T42.6X3	T42.6X4	T42.6X5	T42.6X6
Sulfonamide NEC	T37.0X1	T37.0X2	T37.0X3	T37.0X4	T37.0X5	T37.0X6
eye	T49.5X1	T49.5X2	T49.5X3	T49.5X4	T49.5X5	T49.5X6
Sulfonazide	T37.1X1	T37.1X2	T37.1X3	T37.1X4	T37.1X5	T37.1X6
Sulfones	T37.1X1	T37.1X2	T37.1X3	T37.1X4	T37.1X5	T37.1X6
Sulfonethylmethane	T42.6X1	T42.6X2	T42.6X3	T42.6X4	T42.6X5	T42.6X6
Sulfonmethane	T42.6X1	T42.6X2	T42.6X3	T42.6X4	T42.6X5	T42.6X6
Sulfonphthal, sulfonphthol	T50.8X1	T50.8X2	T50.8X3	T50.8X4	T50.8X5	T50.8X6
Sulfonylurea derivatives, oral	T38.3X1	T38.3X2	T38.3X3	T38.3X4	T38.3X5	T38.3X6
Sulforidazine	T43.3X1	T43.3X2	T43.3X3	T43.3X4	T43.3X5	T43.3X6
Sulfoxone	T37.1X1	T37.1X2	T37.1X3	T37.1X4	T37.1X5	T37.1X6
Sulfuric acid	T54.2X1	T54.2X2	T54.2X3	T54.2X4	—	—
Sulfur, sulfurated, sulfuric, sulfurous, sulfuryl	T49.4X1	T49.4X2	T49.4X3	T49.4X4	T49.4X5	T49.4X6
(compounds NEC) (medicinal)						
acid	T54.2X1	T54.2X2	T54.2X3	T54.2X4	—	—
dioxide (gas)	T59.1X1	T59.1X2	T59.1X3	T59.1X4	—	—
ether — see Ether(s)						
hydrogen	T59.6X1	T59.6X2	T59.6X3	T59.6X4	—	—
medicinal (keratolytic) (ointment) NEC	T49.4X1	T49.4X2	T49.4X3	T49.4X4	T49.4X5	T49.4X6
ointment	T49.0X1	T49.0X2	T49.0X3	T49.0X4	T49.0X5	T49.0X6
pesticide (vapor)	T60.91	T60.92	T60.93	T60.94	—	—
vapor NEC	T59.891	T59.892	T59.893	T59.894	—	—
Sulglicotide	T47.1X1	T47.1X2	T47.1X3	T47.1X4	T47.1X5	T47.1X6
Sulindac	T39.391	T39.392	T39.393	T39.394	T39.395	T39.396
Sulisatin	T47.2X1	T47.2X2	T47.2X3	T47.2X4	T47.2X5	T47.2X6
Sulisobenzone	T49.3X1	T49.3X2	T49.3X3	T49.3X4	T49.3X5	T49.3X6
Sulkowitch's reagent	T50.8X1	T50.8X2	T50.8X3	T50.8X4	T50.8X5	T50.8X6
Sulmetozine	T44.3X1	T44.3X2	T44.3X3	T44.3X4	T44.3X5	T44.3X6
Suloctidil	T46.7X1	T46.7X2	T46.7X3	T46.7X4	T46.7X5	T46.7X6
Sulph- — see also Sulf-						
Sulphadiazine	T37.0X1	T37.0X2	T37.0X3	T37.0X4	T37.0X5	T37.0X6
Sulphadimethoxine	T37.0X1	T37.0X2	T37.0X3	T37.0X4	T37.0X5	T37.0X6
Sulphadimidine	T37.0X1	T37.0X2	T37.0X3	T37.0X4	T37.0X5	T37.0X6
Sulphadione	T37.1X1	T37.1X2	T37.1X3	T37.1X4	T37.1X5	T37.1X6
Sulphafurazole	T37.0X1	T37.0X2	T37.0X3	T37.0X4	T37.0X5	T37.0X6
Sulphamethizole	T37.0X1	T37.0X2	T37.0X3	T37.0X4	T37.0X5	T37.0X6
Sulphamethoxazole	T37.0X1	T37.0X2	T37.0X3	T37.0X4	T37.0X5	T37.0X6
Sulphan blue	T50.8X1	T50.8X2	T50.8X3	T50.8X4	T50.8X5	T50.8X6
Sulphaphenazole	T37.0X1	T37.0X2	T37.0X3	T37.0X4	T37.0X5	T37.0X6
Sulphapyridine	T37.0X1	T37.0X2	T37.0X3	T37.0X4	T37.0X5	T37.0X6
Sulphasalazine	T37.0X1	T37.0X2	T37.0X3	T37.0X4	T37.0X5	T37.0X6
Sulphinpyrazone	T50.4X1	T50.4X2	T50.4X3	T50.4X4	T50.4X5	T50.4X6
Sulpiride	T43.591	T43.592	T43.593	T43.594	T43.595	T43.596
Sulprostone	T48.0X1	T48.0X2	T48.0X3	T48.0X4	T48.0X5	T48.0X6
Sulpyrine	T39.2X1	T39.2X2	T39.2X3	T39.2X4	T39.2X5	T39.2X6
Sultamicillin	T36.0X1	T36.0X2	T36.0X3	T36.0X4	T36.0X5	T36.0X6
Sulthiame	T42.6X1	T42.6X2	T42.6X3	T42.6X4	T42.6X5	T42.6X6
Sultiame	T42.6X1	T42.6X2	T42.6X3	T42.6X4	T42.6X5	T42.6X6
Sultopride	T43.591	T43.592	T43.593	T43.594	T43.595	T43.596
Sumatriptan	T39.8X1	T39.8X2	T39.8X3	T39.8X4	T39.8X5	T39.8X6
Sunflower seed oil	T46.6X1	T46.6X2	T46.6X3	T46.6X4	T46.6X5	T46.6X6
Superinone	T48.4X1	T48.4X2	T48.4X3	T48.4X4	T48.4X5	T48.4X6
Suprofen	T39.311	T39.312	T39.313	T39.314	T39.315	T39.316
Suramin (sodium)	T37.4X1	T37.4X2	T37.4X3	T37.4X4	T37.4X5	T37.4X6
Surfacaine	T41.3X1	T41.3X2	T41.3X3	T41.3X4	T41.3X5	T41.3X6
Surital	T41.1X1	T41.1X2	T41.1X3	T41.1X4	T41.1X5	T41.1X6
Sutilains	T45.3X1	T45.3X2	T45.3X3	T45.3X4	T45.3X5	T45.3X6
Suxamethonium (chloride)	T48.1X1	T48.1X2	T48.1X3	T48.1X4	T48.1X5	T48.1X6
Suxethonium (chloride)	T48.1X1	T48.1X2	T48.1X3	T48.1X4	T48.1X5	T48.1X6
Suxibuzone	T39.2X1	T39.2X2	T39.2X3	T39.2X4	T39.2X5	T39.2X6
Sweetener	T50.901	T50.902	T50.903	T50.904	T50.905	T50.906
Sweet niter spirit	T46.3X1	T46.3X2	T46.3X3	T46.3X4	T46.3X5	T46.3X6
Sweet oil (birch)	T49.3X1	T49.3X2	T49.3X3	T49.3X4	T49.3X5	T49.3X6
Sym-dichloroethyl ether	T53.6X1	T53.6X2	T53.6X3	T53.6X4	—	—
Sympatholytic NEC	T44.8X1	T44.8X2	T44.8X3	T44.8X4	T44.8X5	T44.8X6
haloalkylamine	T44.8X1	T44.8X2	T44.8X3	T44.8X4	T44.8X5	T44.8X6
Sympathomimetic NEC	T44.901	T44.902	T44.903	T44.904	T44.905	T44.906
anti-common-cold	T48.5X1	T48.5X2	T48.5X3	T48.5X4	T48.5X5	T48.5X6
bronchodilator	T48.6X1	T48.6X2	T48.6X3	T48.6X4	T48.6X5	T48.6X6
specified NEC	T44.991	T44.992	T44.993	T44.994	T44.995	T44.996
Synagis	T50.B91	T50.B92	T50.B93	T50.B94	T50.B95	T50.B96
Synalar	T49.0X1	T49.0X2	T49.0X3	T49.0X4	T49.0X5	T49.0X6
Synthroid	T38.1X1	T38.1X2	T38.1X3	T38.1X4	T38.1X5	T38.1X6
Syntocinon	T48.0X1	T48.0X2	T48.0X3	T48.0X4	T48.0X5	T48.0X6
Syrosingopine	T46.5X1	T46.5X2	T46.5X3	T46.5X4	T46.5X5	T46.5X6
Systemic drug	T45.91	T45.92	T45.93	T45.94	T45.95	T45.96
specified NEC	T45.8X1	T45.8X2	T45.8X3	T45.8X4	T45.8X5	T45.8X6
Tablets — see also specified substance	T50.901	T50.902	T50.903	T50.904	T50.905	T50.906
Tace	T38.5X1	T38.5X2	T38.5X3	T38.5X4	T38.5X5	T38.5X6
Tacrine	T44.0X1	T44.0X2	T44.0X3	T44.0X4	T44.0X5	T44.0X6
Tadalafil	T46.7X1	T46.7X2	T46.7X3	T46.7X4	T46.7X5	T46.7X6
Talampicillin	T36.0X1	T36.0X2	T36.0X3	T36.0X4	T36.0X5	T36.0X6
Talbutal	T42.3X1	T42.3X2	T42.3X3	T42.3X4	T42.3X5	T42.3X6
Talc powder	T49.3X1	T49.3X2	T49.3X3	T49.3X4	T49.3X5	T49.3X6
Talcum	T49.3X1	T49.3X2	T49.3X3	T49.3X4	T49.3X5	T49.3X6
Taleranol	T38.6X1	T38.6X2	T38.6X3	T38.6X4	T38.6X5	T38.6X6
Tamoxifen	T38.6X1	T38.6X2	T38.6X3	T38.6X4	T38.6X5	T38.6X6
Tamsulosin	T44.6X1	T44.6X2	T44.6X3	T44.6X4	T44.6X5	T44.6X6
Tandearil, tanderil	T39.2X1	T39.2X2	T39.2X3	T39.2X4	T39.2X5	T39.2X6
Tannic acid	T49.2X1	T49.2X2	T49.2X3	T49.2X4	T49.2X5	T49.2X6
medicinal (astringent)	T49.2X1	T49.2X2	T49.2X3	T49.2X4	T49.2X5	T49.2X6
Tannin — see Tannic acid						
Tansy	T62.2X1	T62.2X2	T62.2X3	T62.2X4	—	—
TAO	T36.3X1	T36.3X2	T36.3X3	T36.3X4	T36.3X5	T36.3X6
Tapazole	T38.2X1	T38.2X2	T38.2X3	T38.2X4	T38.2X5	T38.2X6
Taractan	T43.591	T43.592	T43.593	T43.594	T43.595	T43.596
Tarantula (venomous)	T63.321	T63.322	T63.323	T63.324		
Tartar emetic	T37.8X1	T37.8X2	T37.8X3	T37.8X4	T37.8X5	T37.8X6
Tartaric acid	T65.891	T65.892	T65.893	T65.894	—	—
Tartrated antimony (anti-infective)	T37.8X1	T37.8X2	T37.8X3	T37.8X4	T37.8X5	T37.8X6
Tartrate, laxative	T47.4X1	T47.4X2	T47.4X3	T47.4X4	T47.4X5	T47.4X6
Tar NEC	T52.0X1	T52.0X2	T52.0X3	T52.0X4	—	—
camphor	T60.1X1	T60.1X2	T60.1X3	T60.1X4		
distillate	T49.1X1	T49.1X2	T49.1X3	T49.1X4	T49.1X5	T49.1X6
fumes	T59.891	T59.892	T59.893	T59.894		
medicinal	T49.1X1	T49.1X2	T49.1X3	T49.1X4	T49.1X5	T49.1X6
ointment	T49.1X1	T49.1X2	T49.1X3	T49.1X4	T49.1X5	T49.1X6
Tauromustine	T45.1X1	T45.1X2	T45.1X3	T45.1X4	T45.1X5	T45.1X6
TCA — see Trichloroacetic acid						
TCDD	T53.7X1	T53.7X2	T53.7X3	T53.7X4	—	—
TDI (vapor)	T65.0X1	T65.0X2	T65.0X3	T65.0X4	—	—
Tear						
gas	T59.3X1	T59.3X2	T59.3X3	T59.3X4	—	—
solution	T49.5X1	T49.5X2	T49.5X3	T49.5X4	T49.5X5	T49.5X6
Teclothiazide	T50.2X1	T50.2X2	T50.2X3	T50.2X4	T50.2X5	T50.2X6
Teclozan	T37.3X1	T37.3X2	T37.3X3	T37.3X4	T37.3X5	T37.3X6
Tegafur	T45.1X1	T45.1X2	T45.1X3	T45.1X4	T45.1X5	T45.1X6
Tegretol	T42.1X1	T42.1X2	T42.1X3	T42.1X4	T42.1X5	T42.1X6
Teicoplanin	T36.8X1	T36.8X2	T36.8X3	T36.8X4	T36.8X5	T36.8X6
Telepaque	T50.8X1	T50.8X2	T50.8X3	T50.8X4	T50.8X5	T50.8X6
Tellurium	T56.891	T56.892	T56.893	T56.894	—	—
fumes	T56.891	T56.892	T56.893	T56.894	—	—
TEM	T45.1X1	T45.1X2	T45.1X3	T45.1X4	T45.1X5	T45.1X6
Temazepam	T42.4X1	T42.4X2	T42.4X3	T42.4X4	T42.4X5	T42.4X6
Temocillin	T36.0X1	T36.0X2	T36.0X3	T36.0X4	T36.0X5	T36.0X6
Tenamfetamine	T43.621	T43.622	T43.623	T43.624	T43.625	T43.626
Teniposide	T45.1X1	T45.1X2	T45.1X3	T45.1X4	T45.1X5	T45.1X6
Tenitramine	T46.3X1	T46.3X2	T46.3X3	T46.3X4	T46.3X5	T46.3X6
Tenoglicin	T48.4X1	T48.4X2	T48.4X3	T48.4X4	T48.4X5	T48.4X6
Tenonitrozole	T37.3X1	T37.3X2	T37.3X3	T37.3X4	T37.3X5	T37.3X6
Tenoxicam	T39.391	T39.392	T39.393	T39.394	T39.395	T39.396
TEPA	T45.1X1	T45.1X2	T45.1X3	T45.1X4	T45.1X5	T45.1X6
TEPP	T60.0X1	T60.0X2	T60.0X3	T60.0X4	—	—
Teprotide	T46.5X1	T46.5X2	T46.5X3	T46.5X4	T46.5X5	T46.5X6
Terazosin	T44.6X1	T44.6X2	T44.6X3	T44.6X4	T44.6X5	T44.6X6
Terbufos	T60.0X1	T60.0X2	T60.0X3	T60.0X4	—	—
Terbutaline	T48.6X1	T48.6X2	T48.6X3	T48.6X4	T48.6X5	T48.6X6

Substance	Poisoning, Accidental (unintentional)	Poisoning, Intentional Self-harm	Poisoning, Assault	Poisoning, Undetermined	Adverse Effect	Under-dosing
Terconazole	T49.0X1	T49.0X2	T49.0X3	T49.0X4	T49.0X5	T49.0X6
Terfenadine	T45.0X1	T45.0X2	T45.0X3	T45.0X4	T45.0X5	T45.0X6
Teriparatide (acetate)	T50.991	T50.992	T50.993	T50.994	T50.995	T50.996
Terizidone	T37.1X1	T37.1X2	T37.1X3	T37.1X4	T37.1X5	T37.1X6
Terlipressin	T38.891	T38.892	T38.893	T38.894	T38.895	T38.896
Terodiline	T46.3X1	T46.3X2	T46.3X3	T46.3X4	T46.3X5	T46.3X6
Teroxalene	T37.4X1	T37.4X2	T37.4X3	T37.4X4	T37.4X5	T37.4X6
Terpin (cis) hydrate	T48.4X1	T48.4X2	T48.4X3	T48.4X4	T48.4X5	T48.4X6
Terramycin	T36.4X1	T36.4X2	T36.4X3	T36.4X4	T36.4X5	T36.4X6
Tertatolol	T44.7X1	T44.7X2	T44.7X3	T44.7X4	T44.7X5	T44.7X6
Tessalon	T48.3X1	T48.3X2	T48.3X3	T48.3X4	T48.3X5	T48.3X6
Testolactone	T38.7X1	T38.7X2	T38.7X3	T38.7X4	T38.7X5	T38.7X6
Testosterone	T38.7X1	T38.7X2	T38.7X3	T38.7X4	T38.7X5	T38.7X6
Tetanus toxoid or vaccine	T50.A91	T50.A92	T50.A93	T50.A94	T50.A95	T50.A96
antitoxin	T50.Z11	T50.Z12	T50.Z13	T50.Z14	T50.Z15	T50.Z16
immune globulin (human)	T50.Z11	T50.Z12	T50.Z13	T50.Z14	T50.Z15	T50.Z16
toxoid	T50.A91	T50.A92	T50.A93	T50.A94	T50.A95	T50.A96
with diphtheria toxoid	T50.A21	T50.A22	T50.A23	T50.A24	T50.A25	T50.A26
with pertussis	T50.A11	T50.A12	T50.A13	T50.A14	T50.A15	T50.A16
Tetrabenazine	T43.591	T43.592	T43.593	T43.594	T43.595	T43.596
Tetracaine	T41.3X1	T41.3X2	T41.3X3	T41.3X4	T41.3X5	T41.3X6
nerve block (peripheral) (plexus)	T41.3X1	T41.3X2	T41.3X3	T41.3X4	T41.3X5	T41.3X6
regional	T41.3X1	T41.3X2	T41.3X3	T41.3X4	T41.3X5	T41.3X6
spinal	T41.3X1	T41.3X2	T41.3X3	T41.3X4	T41.3X5	T41.3X6
Tetrachlorethylene — see Tetrachloroethylene						
Tetrachlormethiazide	T50.2X1	T50.2X2	T50.2X3	T50.2X4	T50.2X5	T50.2X6
Tetrachloroethane	T53.6X1	T53.6X2	T53.6X3	T53.6X4	—	—
vapor	T53.6X1	T53.6X2	T53.6X3	T53.6X4	—	—
paint or varnish	T53.6X1	T53.6X2	T53.6X3	T53.6X4	—	—
Tetrachloroethylene (liquid)	T53.3X1	T53.3X2	T53.3X3	T53.3X4	—	—
medicinal	T37.4X1	T37.4X2	T37.4X3	T37.4X4	T37.4X5	T37.4X6
vapor	T53.3X1	T53.3X2	T53.3X3	T53.3X4	—	—
Tetrachloromethane — see Carbon tetrachloride						
Tetracosactide	T38.811	T38.812	T38.813	T38.814	T38.815	T38.816
Tetracosactrin	T38.811	T38.812	T38.813	T38.814	T38.815	T38.816
Tetracycline	T36.4X1	T36.4X2	T36.4X3	T36.4X4	T36.4X5	T36.4X6
ophthalmic preparation	T49.5X1	T49.5X2	T49.5X3	T49.5X4	T49.5X5	T49.5X6
topical NEC	T49.0X1	T49.0X2	T49.0X3	T49.0X4	T49.0X5	T49.0X6
Tetradifon	T60.8X1	T60.8X2	T60.8X3	T60.8X4	—	—
Tetradotoxin	T61.771	T61.772	T61.773	T61.774	—	—
Tetraethyl						
lead	T56.0X1	T56.0X2	T56.0X3	T56.0X4	—	—
pyrophosphate	T60.0X1	T60.0X2	T60.0X3	T60.0X4	—	—
Tetraethylammonium chloride	T44.2X1	T44.2X2	T44.2X3	T44.2X4	T44.2X5	T44.2X6
Tetraethylthiuram disulfide	T50.6X1	T50.6X2	T50.6X3	T50.6X4	T50.6X5	T50.6X6
Tetrahydroaminoacridine	T44.0X1	T44.0X2	T44.0X3	T44.0X4	T44.0X5	T44.0X6
Tetrahydrocannabinol	T40.7X1	T40.7X2	T40.7X3	T40.7X4	T40.7X5	T40.7X6
Tetrahydrofuran	T52.8X1	T52.8X2	T52.8X3	T52.8X4	—	—
Tetrahydronaphthalene	T52.8X1	T52.8X2	T52.8X3	T52.8X4	—	—
Tetrahydrozoline	T49.5X1	T49.5X2	T49.5X3	T49.5X4	T49.5X5	T49.5X6
Tetralin	T52.8X1	T52.8X2	T52.8X3	T52.8X4	—	—
Tetramethrin	T60.2X1	T60.2X2	T60.2X3	T60.2X4	—	—
Tetramethylthiuram (disulfide) NEC	T60.3X1	T60.3X2	T60.3X3	T60.3X4	—	—
medicinal	T49.0X1	T49.0X2	T49.0X3	T49.0X4	T49.0X5	T49.0X6
Tetramisole	T37.4X1	T37.4X2	T37.4X3	T37.4X4	T37.4X5	T37.4X6
Tetranicotinoyl fructose	T46.7X1	T46.7X2	T46.7X3	T46.7X4	T46.7X5	T46.7X6
Tetrazepam	T42.4X1	T42.4X2	T42.4X3	T42.4X4	T42.4X5	T42.4X6
Tetronal	T42.6X1	T42.6X2	T42.6X3	T42.6X4	T42.6X5	T42.6X6
Tetryl	T65.3X1	T65.3X2	T65.3X3	T65.3X4	—	—
Tetrylammonium chloride	T44.2X1	T44.2X2	T44.2X3	T44.2X4	T44.2X5	T44.2X6
Tetryzoline	T49.5X1	T49.5X2	T49.5X3	T49.5X4	T49.5X5	T49.5X6
Thalidomide	T45.1X1	T45.1X2	T45.1X3	T45.1X4	T45.1X5	T45.1X6
Thallium (compounds) (dust) NEC	T56.811	T56.812	T56.813	T56.814	—	—
pesticide	T60.4X1	T60.4X2	T60.4X3	T60.4X4	—	—
THC	T40.7X1	T40.7X2	T40.7X3	T40.7X4	T40.7X5	T40.7X6
Thebacon	T48.3X1	T48.3X2	T48.3X3	T48.3X4	T48.3X5	T48.3X6
Thebaine	T40.2X1	T40.2X2	T40.2X3	T40.2X4	T40.2X5	T40.2X6
Thenoic acid	T49.6X1	T49.6X2	T49.6X3	T49.6X4	T49.6X5	T49.6X6
Thenyldiamine	T45.0X1	T45.0X2	T45.0X3	T45.0X4	T45.0X5	T45.0X6
Theobromine (calcium salicylate)	T48.6X1	T48.6X2	T48.6X3	T48.6X4	T48.6X5	T48.6X6
sodium salicylate	T48.6X1	T48.6X2	T48.6X3	T48.6X4	T48.6X5	T48.6X6
Theophyllamine	T48.6X1	T48.6X2	T48.6X3	T48.6X4	T48.6X5	T48.6X6
Theophylline	T48.6X1	T48.6X2	T48.6X3	T48.6X4	T48.6X5	T48.6X6
aminobenzoic acid	T48.6X1	T48.6X2	T48.6X3	T48.6X4	T48.6X5	T48.6X6
Theophylline — continued						
ethylenediamine	T48.6X1	T48.6X2	T48.6X3	T48.6X4	T48.6X5	T48.6X6
piperazine	T48.6X1	T48.6X2	T48.6X3	T48.6X4	T48.6X5	T48.6X6
p-amino-benzoate						
Thiabendazole	T37.4X1	T37.4X2	T37.4X3	T37.4X4	T37.4X5	T37.4X6
Thialbarbital	T41.1X1	T41.1X2	T41.1X3	T41.1X4	T41.1X5	T41.1X6
Thiamazole	T38.2X1	T38.2X2	T38.2X3	T38.2X4	T38.2X5	T38.2X6
Thiambutosine	T37.1X1	T37.1X2	T37.1X3	T37.1X4	T37.1X5	T37.1X6
Thiamine	T45.2X1	T45.2X2	T45.2X3	T45.2X4	T45.2X5	T45.2X6
Thiamphenicol	T36.2X1	T36.2X2	T36.2X3	T36.2X4	T36.2X5	T36.2X6
Thiamylal	T41.1X1	T41.1X2	T41.1X3	T41.1X4	T41.1X5	T41.1X6
sodium	T41.1X1	T41.1X2	T41.1X3	T41.1X4	T41.1X5	T41.1X6
Thiazesim	T43.291	T43.292	T43.293	T43.294	T43.295	T43.296
Thiazides (diuretics)	T50.2X1	T50.2X2	T50.2X3	T50.2X4	T50.2X5	T50.2X6
Thiazinamium metilsulfate	T43.3X1	T43.3X2	T43.3X3	T43.3X4	T43.3X5	T43.3X6
Thiethylperazine	T43.3X1	T43.3X2	T43.3X3	T43.3X4	T43.3X5	T43.3X6
Thimerosal	T49.0X1	T49.0X2	T49.0X3	T49.0X4	T49.0X5	T49.0X6
ophthalmic preparation	T49.5X1	T49.5X2	T49.5X3	T49.5X4	T49.5X5	T49.5X6
Thioacetazone	T37.1X1	T37.1X2	T37.1X3	T37.1X4	T37.1X5	T37.1X6
with isoniazid	T37.1X1	T37.1X2	T37.1X3	T37.1X4	T37.1X5	T37.1X6
Thiobarbital sodium	T41.1X1	T41.1X2	T41.1X3	T41.1X4	T41.1X5	T41.1X6
Thiobarbiturate anesthetic	T41.1X1	T41.1X2	T41.1X3	T41.1X4	T41.1X5	T41.1X6
Thiobismol	T37.8X1	T37.8X2	T37.8X3	T37.8X4	T37.8X5	T37.8X6
Thiobutabarbital sodium	T41.1X1	T41.1X2	T41.1X3	T41.1X4	T41.1X5	T41.1X6
Thiocarbamate (insecticide)	T60.0X1	T60.0X2	T60.0X3	T60.0X4	—	—
Thiocarbamide	T38.2X1	T38.2X2	T38.2X3	T38.2X4	T38.2X5	T38.2X6
Thiocarbarsone	T37.8X1	T37.8X2	T37.8X3	T37.8X4	T37.8X5	T37.8X6
Thiocarlide	T37.1X1	T37.1X2	T37.1X3	T37.1X4	T37.1X5	T37.1X6
Thioctamide	T50.991	T50.992	T50.993	T50.994	T50.995	T50.996
Thioctic acid	T50.991	T50.992	T50.993	T50.994	T50.995	T50.996
Thiofos	T60.0X1	T60.0X2	T60.0X3	T60.0X4	—	—
Thioglycolate	T49.4X1	T49.4X2	T49.4X3	T49.4X4	T49.4X5	T49.4X6
Thioglycolic acid	T65.891	T65.892	T65.893	T65.894	—	—
Thioguanine	T45.1X1	T45.1X2	T45.1X3	T45.1X4	T45.1X5	T45.1X6
Thiomercaptomerin	T50.2X1	T50.2X2	T50.2X3	T50.2X4	T50.2X5	T50.2X6
Thiomerin	T50.2X1	T50.2X2	T50.2X3	T50.2X4	T50.2X5	T50.2X6
Thiomersal	T49.0X1	T49.0X2	T49.0X3	T49.0X4	T49.0X5	T49.0X6
Thionazin	T60.0X1	T60.0X2	T60.0X3	T60.0X4	—	—
Thiopental (sodium)	T41.1X1	T41.1X2	T41.1X3	T41.1X4	T41.1X5	T41.1X6
Thiopentone (sodium)	T41.1X1	T41.1X2	T41.1X3	T41.1X4	T41.1X5	T41.1X6
Thiopropazate	T43.3X1	T43.3X2	T43.3X3	T43.3X4	T43.3X5	T43.3X6
Thioproperazine	T43.3X1	T43.3X2	T43.3X3	T43.3X4	T43.3X5	T43.3X6
Thioridazine	T43.3X1	T43.3X2	T43.3X3	T43.3X4	T43.3X5	T43.3X6
Thiosinamine	T49.3X1	T49.3X2	T49.3X3	T49.3X4	T49.3X5	T49.3X6
Thiotepa	T45.1X1	T45.1X2	T45.1X3	T45.1X4	T45.1X5	T45.1X6
Thiothixene	T43.4X1	T43.4X2	T43.4X3	T43.4X4	T43.4X5	T43.4X6
Thiouracil (benzyl) (methyl) (propyl)	T38.2X1	T38.2X2	T38.2X3	T38.2X4	T38.2X5	T38.2X6
Thiourea	T38.2X1	T38.2X2	T38.2X3	T38.2X4	T38.2X5	T38.2X6
Thiphenamil	T44.3X1	T44.3X2	T44.3X3	T44.3X4	T44.3X5	T44.3X6
Thiram	T60.3X1	T60.3X2	T60.3X3	T60.3X4	—	—
medicinal	T49.2X1	T49.2X2	T49.2X3	T49.2X4	T49.2X5	T49.2X6
Thonzylamine (systemic)	T45.0X1	T45.0X2	T45.0X3	T45.0X4	T45.0X5	T45.0X6
mucosal decongestant	T48.5X1	T48.5X2	T48.5X3	T48.5X4	T48.5X5	T48.5X6
Thorazine	T43.3X1	T43.3X2	T43.3X3	T43.3X4	T43.3X5	T43.3X6
Thorium dioxide suspension	T50.8X1	T50.8X2	T50.8X3	T50.8X4	T50.8X5	T50.8X6
Thornapple	T62.2X1	T62.2X2	T62.2X3	T62.2X4	—	—
Throat drug NEC	T49.6X1	T49.6X2	T49.6X3	T49.6X4	T49.6X5	T49.6X6
Thrombin	T45.7X1	T45.7X2	T45.7X3	T45.7X4	T45.7X5	T45.7X6
Thrombolysin	T45.611	T45.612	T45.613	T45.614	T45.615	T45.616
Thromboplastin	T45.7X1	T45.7X2	T45.7X3	T45.7X4	T45.7X5	T45.7X6
Thurfyl nicotinate	T46.7X1	T46.7X2	T46.7X3	T46.7X4	T46.7X5	T46.7X6
Thymol	T49.0X1	T49.0X2	T49.0X3	T49.0X4	T49.0X5	T49.0X6
Thymopentin	T37.5X1	T37.5X2	T37.5X3	T37.5X4	T37.5X5	T37.5X6
Thymoxamine	T46.7X1	T46.7X2	T46.7X3	T46.7X4	T46.7X5	T46.7X6
Thymus extract	T38.891	T38.892	T38.893	T38.894	T38.895	T38.896
Thyreotrophic hormone	T38.811	T38.812	T38.813	T38.814	T38.815	T38.816
Thyroglobulin	T38.1X1	T38.1X2	T38.1X3	T38.1X4	T38.1X5	T38.1X6
Thyroid (hormone)	T38.1X1	T38.1X2	T38.1X3	T38.1X4	T38.1X5	T38.1X6
Thyrolar	T38.1X1	T38.1X2	T38.1X3	T38.1X4	T38.1X5	T38.1X6
Thyrotrophin	T38.811	T38.812	T38.813	T38.814	T38.815	T38.816
Thyrotropic hormone	T38.811	T38.812	T38.813	T38.814	T38.815	T38.816
Thyroxine	T38.1X1	T38.1X2	T38.1X3	T38.1X4	T38.1X5	T38.1X6
Tiabendazole	T37.4X1	T37.4X2	T37.4X3	T37.4X4	T37.4X5	T37.4X6
Tiamizide	T50.2X1	T50.2X2	T50.2X3	T50.2X4	T50.2X5	T50.2X6
Tianeptine	T43.291	T43.292	T43.293	T43.294	T43.295	T43.296
Tiapamil	T46.1X1	T46.1X2	T46.1X3	T46.1X4	T46.1X5	T46.1X6
Tiapride	T43.591	T43.592	T43.593	T43.594	T43.595	T43.596
Tiaprofenic acid	T39.311	T39.312	T39.313	T39.314	T39.315	T39.316
Tiaramide	T39.8X1	T39.8X2	T39.8X3	T39.8X4	T39.8X5	T39.8X6
Ticarcillin	T36.0X1	T36.0X2	T36.0X3	T36.0X4	T36.0X5	T36.0X6
Ticlatone	T49.0X1	T49.0X2	T49.0X3	T49.0X4	T49.0X5	T49.0X6

Additional Character May Be Required — Refer to the Tabular List for Character Selection

▽ Subterms under main terms may continue to next column or page

Substance	Poisoning, Accidental (unintentional)	Poisoning, Intentional Self-harm	Poisoning, Assault	Poisoning, Undetermined	Adverse Effect	Under-dosing
Ticlopidine	T45.521	T45.522	T45.523	T45.524	T45.525	T45.526
Ticrynafen	T50.1X1	T50.1X2	T50.1X3	T50.1X4	T50.1X5	T50.1X6
Tidiacic	T50.991	T50.992	T50.993	T50.994	T50.995	T50.996
Tiemonium	T44.3X1	T44.3X2	T44.3X3	T44.3X4	T44.3X5	T44.3X6
iodide	T44.3X1	T44.3X2	T44.3X3	T44.3X4	T44.3X5	T44.3X6
Tienilic acid	T50.1X1	T50.1X2	T50.1X3	T50.1X4	T50.1X5	T50.1X6
Tifenamil	T44.3X1	T44.3X2	T44.3X3	T44.3X4	T44.3X5	T44.3X6
Tigan	T45.0X1	T45.0X2	T45.0X3	T45.0X4	T45.0X5	T45.0X6
Tigloidine	T44.3X1	T44.3X2	T44.3X3	T44.3X4	T44.3X5	T44.3X6
Tilactase	T47.5X1	T47.5X2	T47.5X3	T47.5X4	T47.5X5	T47.5X6
Tiletamine	T41.291	T41.292	T41.293	T41.294	T41.295	T41.296
Tilidine	T40.4X1	T40.4X2	T40.4X3	T40.4X4	—	—
Timepidium bromide	T44.3X1	T44.3X2	T44.3X3	T44.3X4	T44.3X5	T44.3X6
Timiperone	T43.4X1	T43.4X2	T43.4X3	T43.4X4	T43.4X5	T43.4X6
Timolol	T44.7X1	T44.7X2	T44.7X3	T44.7X4	T44.7X5	T44.7X6
Tincture, iodine — see Iodine						
Tindal	T43.3X1	T43.3X2	T43.3X3	T43.3X4	T43.3X5	T43.3X6
Tinidazole	T37.3X1	T37.3X2	T37.3X3	T37.3X4	T37.3X5	T37.3X6
Tinoridine	T39.8X1	T39.8X2	T39.8X3	T39.8X4	T39.8X5	T39.8X6
Tin (chloride) (dust) (oxide) NEC	T56.6X1	T56.6X2	T56.6X3	T56.6X4	—	—
anti-infectives	T37.8X1	T37.8X2	T37.8X3	T37.8X4	T37.8X5	T37.8X6
Tiocarlide	T37.1X1	T37.1X2	T37.1X3	T37.1X4	T37.1X5	T37.1X6
Tioclomarol	T45.511	T45.512	T45.513	T45.514	T45.515	T45.516
Tioconazole	T49.0X1	T49.0X2	T49.0X3	T49.0X4	T49.0X5	T49.0X6
Tioguanine	T45.1X1	T45.1X2	T45.1X3	T45.1X4	T45.1X5	T45.1X6
Tiopronin	T50.991	T50.992	T50.993	T50.994	T50.995	T50.996
Tiotixene	T43.4X1	T43.4X2	T43.4X3	T43.4X4	T43.4X5	T43.4X6
Tioxolone	T49.4X1	T49.4X2	T49.4X3	T49.4X4	T49.4X5	T49.4X6
Tipepidine	T48.3X1	T48.3X2	T48.3X3	T48.3X4	T48.3X5	T48.3X6
Tiquizium bromide	T44.3X1	T44.3X2	T44.3X3	T44.3X4	T44.3X5	T44.3X6
Tiratricol	T38.1X1	T38.1X2	T38.1X3	T38.1X4	T38.1X5	T38.1X6
Tisopurine	T50.4X1	T50.4X2	T50.4X3	T50.4X4	T50.4X5	T50.4X6
Titanium (compounds) (vapor)	T56.891	T56.892	T56.893	T56.894	—	—
dioxide	T49.3X1	T49.3X2	T49.3X3	T49.3X4	T49.3X5	T49.3X6
ointment	T49.3X1	T49.3X2	T49.3X3	T49.3X4	T49.3X5	T49.3X6
oxide	T49.3X1	T49.3X2	T49.3X3	T49.3X4	T49.3X5	T49.3X6
tetrachloride	T56.891	T56.892	T56.893	T56.894	—	—
Titanocene	T56.891	T56.892	T56.893	T56.894	—	—
Titroid	T38.1X1	T38.1X2	T38.1X3	T38.1X4	T38.1X5	T38.1X6
Tizanidine	T42.8X1	T42.8X2	T42.8X3	T42.8X4	T42.8X5	T42.8X6
TMTD	T60.3X1	T60.3X2	T60.3X3	T60.3X4	—	—
TNT (fumes)	T65.3X1	T65.3X2	T65.3X3	T65.3X4	—	—
Toadstool	T62.0X1	T62.0X2	T62.0X3	T62.0X4	—	—
Tobacco NEC	T65.291	T65.292	T65.293	T65.294	—	—
cigarettes	T65.221	T65.222	T65.223	T65.224	—	—
Indian	T62.2X1	T62.2X2	T62.2X3	T62.2X4	—	—
smoke, second-hand	T65.221	T65.222	T65.223	T65.224	—	—
Tobramycin	T36.5X1	T36.5X2	T36.5X3	T36.5X4	T36.5X5	T36.5X6
Tocainide	T46.2X1	T46.2X2	T46.2X3	T46.2X4	T46.2X5	T46.2X6
Tocoferol	T45.2X1	T45.2X2	T45.2X3	T45.2X4	T45.2X5	T45.2X6
Tocopherol	T45.2X1	T45.2X2	T45.2X3	T45.2X4	T45.2X5	T45.2X6
acetate	T45.2X1	T45.2X2	T45.2X3	T45.2X4	T45.2X5	T45.2X6
Tocosamine	T48.0X1	T48.0X2	T48.0X3	T48.0X4	T48.0X5	T48.0X6
Todralazine	T46.5X1	T46.5X2	T46.5X3	T46.5X4	T46.5X5	T46.5X6
Tofisopam	T42.4X1	T42.4X2	T42.4X3	T42.4X4	T42.4X5	T42.4X6
Tofranil	T43.011	T43.012	T43.013	T43.014	T43.015	T43.016
Toilet deodorizer	T65.891	T65.892	T65.893	T65.894	—	—
Tolamolol	T44.7X1	T44.7X2	T44.7X3	T44.7X4	T44.7X5	T44.7X6
Tolazamide	T38.3X1	T38.3X2	T38.3X3	T38.3X4	T38.3X5	T38.3X6
Tolazoline	T46.7X1	T46.7X2	T46.7X3	T46.7X4	T46.7X5	T46.7X6
Tolbutamide (sodium)	T38.3X1	T38.3X2	T38.3X3	T38.3X4	T38.3X5	T38.3X6
Tolciclate	T49.0X1	T49.0X2	T49.0X3	T49.0X4	T49.0X5	T49.0X6
Tolmetin	T39.391	T39.392	T39.393	T39.394	T39.395	T39.396
Tolnaftate	T49.0X1	T49.0X2	T49.0X3	T49.0X4	T49.0X5	T49.0X6
Tolonidine	T46.5X1	T46.5X2	T46.5X3	T46.5X4	T46.5X5	T46.5X6
Toloxatone	T42.6X1	T42.6X2	T42.6X3	T42.6X4	T42.6X5	T42.6X6
Tolperisone	T44.3X1	T44.3X2	T44.3X3	T44.3X4	T44.3X5	T44.3X6
Tolserol	T42.8X1	T42.8X2	T42.8X3	T42.8X4	T42.8X5	T42.8X6
Toluene (liquid)	T52.2X1	T52.2X2	T52.2X3	T52.2X4	—	—
diisocyanate	T65.0X1	T65.0X2	T65.0X3	T65.0X4	—	—
Toluidine	T65.891	T65.892	T65.893	T65.894	—	—
vapor	T59.891	T59.892	T59.893	T59.894	—	—
Toluol (liquid)	T52.2X1	T52.2X2	T52.2X3	T52.2X4	—	—
vapor	T52.2X1	T52.2X2	T52.2X3	T52.2X4	—	—
Toluylenediamine	T65.3X1	T65.3X2	T65.3X3	T65.3X4	—	—
Tolylene-2,4-diisocyanate	T65.0X1	T65.0X2	T65.0X3	T65.0X4	—	—
Tonic NEC	T50.901	T50.902	T50.903	T50.904	T50.905	T50.906
Topical action drug NEC	T49.91	T49.92	T49.93	T49.94	T49.95	T49.96
ear, nose or throat	T49.6X1	T49.6X2	T49.6X3	T49.6X4	T49.6X5	T49.6X6
eye	T49.5X1	T49.5X2	T49.5X3	T49.5X4	T49.5X5	T49.5X6
skin	T49.91	T49.92	T49.93	T49.94	T49.95	T49.96
Topical action drug — continued						
specified NEC	T49.8X1	T49.8X2	T49.8X3	T49.8X4	T49.8X5	T49.8X6
Toquizine	T44.3X1	T44.3X2	T44.3X3	T44.3X4	T44.3X5	T44.3X6
Toremifene	T38.6X1	T38.6X2	T38.6X3	T38.6X4	T38.6X5	T38.6X6
Tosylchloramide sodium	T49.8X1	T49.8X2	T49.8X3	T49.8X4	T49.8X5	T49.8X6
Toxaphene (dust) (spray)	T60.1X1	T60.1X2	T60.1X3	T60.1X4	—	—
Toxin, diphtheria (Schick Test)	T50.8X1	T50.8X2	T50.8X3	T50.8X4	T50.8X5	T50.8X6
Toxoid						
combined	T50.A21	T50.A22	T50.A23	T50.A24	T50.A25	T50.A26
diphtheria	T50.A91	T50.A92	T50.A93	T50.A94	T50.A95	T50.A96
tetanus	T50.A91	T50.A92	T50.A93	T50.A94	T50.A95	T50.A96
Trace element NEC	T45.8X1	T45.8X2	T45.8X3	T45.8X4	T45.8X5	T45.8X6
Tractor fuel NEC	T52.0X1	T52.0X2	T52.0X3	T52.0X4	—	—
Tragacanth	T50.991	T50.992	T50.993	T50.994	T50.995	T50.996
Tramadol	T40.4X1	T40.4X2	T40.4X3	T40.4X4	T40.4X5	T40.4X6
Tramazoline	T48.5X1	T48.5X2	T48.5X3	T48.5X4	T48.5X5	T48.5X6
Tranexamic acid	T45.621	T45.622	T45.623	T45.624	T45.625	T45.626
Tranexamic acid	T45.0X1	T45.0X2	T45.0X3	T45.0X4	T45.0X5	T45.0X6
Tranilast	T45.0X1	T45.0X2	T45.0X3	T45.0X4	T45.0X5	T45.0X6
Tranquilizer NEC	T43.501	T43.502	T43.503	T43.504	T43.505	T43.506
with hypnotic or sedative	T42.6X1	T42.6X2	T42.6X3	T42.6X4	T42.6X5	T42.6X6
benzodiazepine NEC	T42.4X1	T42.4X2	T42.4X3	T42.4X4	T42.4X5	T42.4X6
butyrophenone NEC	T43.4X1	T43.4X2	T43.4X3	T43.4X4	T43.4X5	T43.4X6
carbamate	T43.591	T43.592	T43.593	T43.594	T43.595	T43.596
dimethylamine	T43.3X1	T43.3X2	T43.3X3	T43.3X4	T43.3X5	T43.3X6
ethylamine	T43.3X1	T43.3X2	T43.3X3	T43.3X4	T43.3X5	T43.3X6
hydroxyzine	T43.591	T43.592	T43.593	T43.594	T43.595	T43.596
major NEC	T43.501	T43.502	T43.503	T43.504	T43.505	T43.506
penothiazine NEC	T43.3X1	T43.3X2	T43.3X3	T43.3X4	T43.3X5	T43.3X6
phenothiazine-based	T43.3X1	T43.3X2	T43.3X3	T43.3X4	T43.3X5	T43.3X6
piperazine NEC	T43.3X1	T43.3X2	T43.3X3	T43.3X4	T43.3X5	T43.3X6
piperidine	T43.3X1	T43.3X2	T43.3X3	T43.3X4	T43.3X5	T43.3X6
propylamine	T43.3X1	T43.3X2	T43.3X3	T43.3X4	T43.3X5	T43.3X6
specified NEC	T43.591	T43.592	T43.593	T43.594	T43.595	T43.596
thioxanthene NEC	T43.591	T43.592	T43.593	T43.594	T43.595	T43.596
Tranxene	T42.4X1	T42.4X2	T42.4X3	T42.4X4	T42.4X5	T42.4X6
Tranylcypromine	T43.1X1	T43.1X2	T43.1X3	T43.1X4	T43.1X5	T43.1X6
Trapidil	T46.3X1	T46.3X2	T46.3X3	T46.3X4	T46.3X5	T46.3X6
Trasentine	T44.3X1	T44.3X2	T44.3X3	T44.3X4	T44.3X5	T44.3X6
Travert	T50.3X1	T50.3X2	T50.3X3	T50.3X4	T50.3X5	T50.3X6
Trazodone	T43.211	T43.212	T43.213	T43.214	T43.215	T43.216
Trecator	T37.1X1	T37.1X2	T37.1X3	T37.1X4	T37.1X5	T37.1X6
Treosulfan	T45.1X1	T45.1X2	T45.1X3	T45.1X4	T45.1X5	T45.1X6
Tretamine	T45.1X1	T45.1X2	T45.1X3	T45.1X4	T45.1X5	T45.1X6
Tretinoin	T49.0X1	T49.0X2	T49.0X3	T49.0X4	T49.0X5	T49.0X6
Tretoquinol	T48.6X1	T48.6X2	T48.6X3	T48.6X4	T48.6X5	T48.6X6
Triacetin	T49.0X1	T49.0X2	T49.0X3	T49.0X4	T49.0X5	T49.0X6
Triacetoxyanthracene	T49.4X1	T49.4X2	T49.4X3	T49.4X4	T49.4X5	T49.4X6
Triacetyloleandomycin	T36.3X1	T36.3X2	T36.3X3	T36.3X4	T36.3X5	T36.3X6
Triamcinolone	T38.0X1	T38.0X2	T38.0X3	T38.0X4	T38.0X5	T38.0X6
ENT agent	T49.6X1	T49.6X2	T49.6X3	T49.6X4	T49.6X5	T49.6X6
hexacetonide	T49.0X1	T49.0X2	T49.0X3	T49.0X4	T49.0X5	T49.0X6
ophthalmic preparation	T49.5X1	T49.5X2	T49.5X3	T49.5X4	T49.5X5	T49.5X6
topical NEC	T49.0X1	T49.0X2	T49.0X3	T49.0X4	T49.0X5	T49.0X6
Triampyzine	T44.3X1	T44.3X2	T44.3X3	T44.3X4	T44.3X5	T44.3X6
Triamterene	T50.2X1	T50.2X2	T50.2X3	T50.2X4	T50.2X5	T50.2X6
Triazine (herbicide)	T60.3X1	T60.3X2	T60.3X3	T60.3X4	—	—
Triaziquone	T45.1X1	T45.1X2	T45.1X3	T45.1X4	T45.1X5	T45.1X6
Triazolam	T42.4X1	T42.4X2	T42.4X3	T42.4X4	T42.4X5	T42.4X6
Triazole (herbicide)	T60.3X1	T60.3X2	T60.3X3	T60.3X4	—	—
Tribenoside	T46.991	T46.992	T46.993	T46.994	T46.995	T46.996
Tribromacetaldehyde	T42.6X1	T42.6X2	T42.6X3	T42.6X4	T42.6X5	T42.6X6
Tribromoethanol, rectal	T41.291	T41.292	T41.293	T41.294	T41.295	T41.296
Tribromomethane	T42.6X1	T42.6X2	T42.6X3	T42.6X4	T42.6X5	T42.6X6
Trichlorethane	T53.2X1	T53.2X2	T53.2X3	T53.2X4		
Trichlorethylene	T53.2X1	T53.2X2	T53.2X3	T53.2X4		
Trichlorfon	T60.0X1	T60.0X2	T60.0X3	T60.0X4		
Trichlormethiazide	T50.2X1	T50.2X2	T50.2X3	T50.2X4	T50.2X5	T50.2X6
Trichlormethine	T45.1X1	T45.1X2	T45.1X3	T45.1X4	T45.1X5	T45.1X6
Trichloroacetic acid, Trichloracetic acid	T54.2X1	T54.2X2	T54.2X3	T54.2X4		
medicinal	T49.4X1	T49.4X2	T49.4X3	T49.4X4	T49.4X5	T49.4X6
Trichloroethane	T53.2X1	T53.2X2	T53.2X3	T53.2X4		
Trichloroethanol	T42.6X1	T42.6X2	T42.6X3	T42.6X4	T42.6X5	T42.6X6
Trichloroethylene (liquid) (vapor)	T53.2X1	T53.2X2	T53.2X3	T53.2X4		
anesthetic (gas)	T41.0X1	T41.0X2	T41.0X3	T41.0X4	T41.0X5	T41.0X6
vapor NEC	T53.2X1	T53.2X2	T53.2X3	T53.2X4		
Trichloroethyl phosphate	T42.6X1	T42.6X2	T42.6X3	T42.6X4	T42.6X5	T42.6X6
Trichlorofluoromethane NEC	T53.5X1	T53.5X2	T53.5X3	T53.5X4		
Trichloronate	T60.0X1	T60.0X2	T60.0X3	T60.0X4	—	—
Trichloropropane	T53.6X1	T53.6X2	T53.6X3	T53.6X4		

Table of Drugs and Chemicals

Substance	Poisoning, Accidental (unintentional)	Poisoning, Intentional Self-harm	Poisoning, Assault	Poisoning, Undetermined	Adverse Effect	Under-dosing
Trichlorotriethylamine	T45.1X1	T45.1X2	T45.1X3	T45.1X4	T45.1X5	T45.1X6
Trichomonacides NEC	T37.3X1	T37.3X2	T37.3X3	T37.3X4	T37.3X5	T37.3X6
Trichomycin	T36.7X1	T36.7X2	T36.7X3	T36.7X4	T36.7X5	T36.7X6
Triclobisonium chloride	T49.0X1	T49.0X2	T49.0X3	T49.0X4	T49.0X5	T49.0X6
Triclocarban	T49.0X1	T49.0X2	T49.0X3	T49.0X4	T49.0X5	T49.0X6
Triclofos	T42.6X1	T42.6X2	T42.6X3	T42.6X4	T42.6X5	T42.6X6
Triclosan	T49.0X1	T49.0X2	T49.0X3	T49.0X4	T49.0X5	T49.0X6
Tricresyl phosphate	T65.891	T65.892	T65.893	T65.894	—	—
solvent	T52.91	T52.92	T52.93	T52.94		
Tricyclamol chloride	T44.3X1	T44.3X2	T44.3X3	T44.3X4	T44.3X5	T44.3X6
Tridesilon	T49.0X1	T49.0X2	T49.0X3	T49.0X4	T49.0X5	T49.0X6
Tridihexethyl iodide	T44.3X1	T44.3X2	T44.3X3	T44.3X4	T44.3X5	T44.3X6
Tridione	T42.2X1	T42.2X2	T42.2X3	T42.2X4	T42.2X5	T42.2X6
Trientine	T45.8X1	T45.8X2	T45.8X3	T45.8X4	T45.8X5	T45.8X6
Triethanolamine NEC	T54.3X1	T54.3X2	T54.3X3	T54.3X4	—	—
detergent	T54.3X1	T54.3X2	T54.3X3	T54.3X4	—	—
trinitrate (biphosphate)	T46.3X1	T46.3X2	T46.3X3	T46.3X4	T46.3X5	T46.3X6
Triethanomelamine	T45.1X1	T45.1X2	T45.1X3	T45.1X4	T45.1X5	T45.1X6
Triethylenemelamine	T45.1X1	T45.1X2	T45.1X3	T45.1X4	T45.1X5	T45.1X6
Triethylenephosphoramide	T45.1X1	T45.1X2	T45.1X3	T45.1X4	T45.1X5	T45.1X6
Triethylenethiophosphoramide	T45.1X1	T45.1X2	T45.1X3	T45.1X4	T45.1X5	T45.1X6
Trifluoperazine	T43.3X1	T43.3X2	T43.3X3	T43.3X4	T43.3X5	T43.3X6
Trifluoroethyl vinyl ether	T41.0X1	T41.0X2	T41.0X3	T41.0X4	T41.0X5	T41.0X6
Trifluperidol	T43.4X1	T43.4X2	T43.4X3	T43.4X4	T43.4X5	T43.4X6
Triflupromazine	T43.3X1	T43.3X2	T43.3X3	T43.3X4	T43.3X5	T43.3X6
Trifluridine	T37.5X1	T37.5X2	T37.5X3	T37.5X4	T37.5X5	T37.5X6
Triflusal	T45.521	T45.522	T45.523	T45.524	T45.525	T45.526
Trihexyphenidyl	T44.3X1	T44.3X2	T44.3X3	T44.3X4	T44.3X5	T44.3X6
Triiodothyronine	T38.1X1	T38.1X2	T38.1X3	T38.1X4	T38.1X5	T38.1X6
Trilene	T41.0X1	T41.0X2	T41.0X3	T41.0X4	T41.0X5	T41.0X6
Trilostane	T38.991	T38.992	T38.993	T38.994	T38.995	T38.996
Trimebutine	T44.3X1	T44.3X2	T44.3X3	T44.3X4	T44.3X5	T44.3X6
Trimecaine	T41.3X1	T41.3X2	T41.3X3	T41.3X4	T41.3X5	T41.3X6
Trimeprazine (tartrate)	T44.3X1	T44.3X2	T44.3X3	T44.3X4	T44.3X5	T44.3X6
Trimetaphan camsilate	T44.2X1	T44.2X2	T44.2X3	T44.2X4	T44.2X5	T44.2X6
Trimetazidine	T46.7X1	T46.7X2	T46.7X3	T46.7X4	T46.7X5	T46.7X6
Trimethadione	T42.2X1	T42.2X2	T42.2X3	T42.2X4	T42.2X5	T42.2X6
Trimethaphan	T44.2X1	T44.2X2	T44.2X3	T44.2X4	T44.2X5	T44.2X6
Trimethidinium	T44.2X1	T44.2X2	T44.2X3	T44.2X4	T44.2X5	T44.2X6
Trimethobenzamide	T45.0X1	T45.0X2	T45.0X3	T45.0X4	T45.0X5	T45.0X6
Trimethoprim	T37.8X1	T37.8X2	T37.8X3	T37.8X4	T37.8X5	T37.8X6
with sulfamethoxazole	T36.8X1	T36.8X2	T36.8X3	T36.8X4	T36.8X5	T36.8X6
Trimethylcarbinol	T51.3X1	T51.3X2	T51.3X3	T51.3X4		
Trimethylpsoralen	T49.3X1	T49.3X2	T49.3X3	T49.3X4	T49.3X5	T49.3X6
Trimeton	T45.0X1	T45.0X2	T45.0X3	T45.0X4	T45.0X5	T45.0X6
Trimetrexate	T45.1X1	T45.1X2	T45.1X3	T45.1X4	T45.1X5	T45.1X6
Trimipramine	T43.011	T43.012	T43.013	T43.014	T43.015	T43.016
Trimustine	T45.1X1	T45.1X2	T45.1X3	T45.1X4	T45.1X5	T45.1X6
Trinitrine	T46.3X1	T46.3X2	T46.3X3	T46.3X4	T46.3X5	T46.3X6
Trinitrobenzol	T65.3X1	T65.3X2	T65.3X3	T65.3X4	—	—
Trinitrophenol	T65.3X1	T65.3X2	T65.3X3	T65.3X4	—	—
Trinitrotoluene (fumes)	T65.3X1	T65.3X2	T65.3X3	T65.3X4	—	—
Trional	T42.6X1	T42.6X2	T42.6X3	T42.6X4	T42.6X5	T42.6X6
Triorthocresyl phosphate	T65.891	T65.892	T65.893	T65.894	—	—
Trioxide of arsenic	T57.0X1	T57.0X2	T57.0X3	T57.0X4	—	—
Trioxysalen	T49.4X1	T49.4X2	T49.4X3	T49.4X4	T49.4X5	T49.4X6
Tripamide	T50.2X1	T50.2X2	T50.2X3	T50.2X4	T50.2X5	T50.2X6
Triparanol	T46.6X1	T46.6X2	T46.6X3	T46.6X4	T46.6X5	T46.6X6
Tripelennamine	T45.0X1	T45.0X2	T45.0X3	T45.0X4	T45.0X5	T45.0X6
Triperiden	T44.3X1	T44.3X2	T44.3X3	T44.3X4	T44.3X5	T44.3X6
Triperidol	T43.4X1	T43.4X2	T43.4X3	T43.4X4	T43.4X5	T43.4X6
Triphenylphosphate	T65.891	T65.892	T65.893	T65.894	—	—
Triple						
bromides	T42.6X1	T42.6X2	T42.6X3	T42.6X4	T42.6X5	T42.6X6
carbonate	T47.1X1	T47.1X2	T47.1X3	T47.1X4	T47.1X5	T47.1X6
vaccine						
DPT	T50.A11	T50.A12	T50.A13	T50.A14	T50.A15	T50.A16
including pertussis	T50.A11	T50.A12	T50.A13	T50.A14	T50.A15	T50.A16
MMR	T50.B91	T50.B92	T50.B93	T50.B94	T50.B95	T50.B96
Triprolidine	T45.0X1	T45.0X2	T45.0X3	T45.0X4	T45.0X5	T45.0X6
Trisodium hydrogen edetate	T50.6X1	T50.6X2	T50.6X3	T50.6X4	T50.6X5	T50.6X6
Trisoralen	T49.3X1	T49.3X2	T49.3X3	T49.3X4	T49.3X5	T49.3X6
Trisulfapyrimidines	T37.0X1	T37.0X2	T37.0X3	T37.0X4	T37.0X5	T37.0X6
Trithiozine	T44.3X1	T44.3X2	T44.3X3	T44.3X4	T44.3X5	T44.3X6
Tritiozine	T44.3X1	T44.3X2	T44.3X3	T44.3X4	T44.3X5	T44.3X6
Tritoqualine	T45.0X1	T45.0X2	T45.0X3	T45.0X4	T45.0X5	T45.0X6
Trofosfamide	T45.1X1	T45.1X2	T45.1X3	T45.1X4	T45.1X5	T45.1X6
Troleandomycin	T36.3X1	T36.3X2	T36.3X3	T36.3X4	T36.3X5	T36.3X6
Trolnitrate (phosphate)	T46.3X1	T46.3X2	T46.3X3	T46.3X4	T46.3X5	T46.3X6
Tromantadine	T37.5X1	T37.5X2	T37.5X3	T37.5X4	T37.5X5	T37.5X6
Trometamol	T50.2X1	T50.2X2	T50.2X3	T50.2X4	T50.2X5	T50.2X6
Tromethamine	T50.2X1	T50.2X2	T50.2X3	T50.2X4	T50.2X5	T50.2X6

Substance	Poisoning, Accidental (unintentional)	Poisoning, Intentional Self-harm	Poisoning, Assault	Poisoning, Undetermined	Adverse Effect	Under-dosing
Tronothane	T41.3X1	T41.3X2	T41.3X3	T41.3X4	T41.3X5	T41.3X6
Tropacine	T44.3X1	T44.3X2	T44.3X3	T44.3X4	T44.3X5	T44.3X6
Tropatepine	T44.3X1	T44.3X2	T44.3X3	T44.3X4	T44.3X5	T44.3X6
Tropicamide	T44.3X1	T44.3X2	T44.3X3	T44.3X4	T44.3X5	T44.3X6
Trospium chloride	T44.3X1	T44.3X2	T44.3X3	T44.3X4	T44.3X5	T44.3X6
Troxerutin	T46.991	T46.992	T46.993	T46.994	T46.995	T46.996
Troxidone	T42.2X1	T42.2X2	T42.2X3	T42.2X4	T42.2X5	T42.2X6
Tryparsamide	T37.3X1	T37.3X2	T37.3X3	T37.3X4	T37.3X5	T37.3X6
Trypsin	T45.3X1	T45.3X2	T45.3X3	T45.3X4	T45.3X5	T45.3X6
Tryptizol	T43.011	T43.012	T43.013	T43.014	T43.015	T43.016
TSH	T38.811	T38.812	T38.813	T38.814	T38.815	T38.816
Tuaminoheptane	T48.5X1	T48.5X2	T48.5X3	T48.5X4	T48.5X5	T48.5X6
Tuberculin, purified protein derivative (PPD)	T50.8X1	T50.8X2	T50.8X3	T50.8X4	T50.8X5	T50.8X6
Tubocurare	T48.1X1	T48.1X2	T48.1X3	T48.1X4	T48.1X5	T48.1X6
Tubocurarine (chloride)	T48.1X1	T48.1X2	T48.1X3	T48.1X4	T48.1X5	T48.1X6
Tulobuterol	T48.6X1	T48.6X2	T48.6X3	T48.6X4	T48.6X5	T48.6X6
Turpentine (spirits of)	T52.8X1	T52.8X2	T52.8X3	T52.8X4		
vapor	T52.8X1	T52.8X2	T52.8X3	T52.8X4	—	—
Tybamate	T43.591	T43.592	T43.593	T43.594	T43.595	T43.596
Tyloxapol	T48.4X1	T48.4X2	T48.4X3	T48.4X4	T48.4X5	T48.4X6
Tymazoline	T48.5X1	T48.5X2	T48.5X3	T48.5X4	T48.5X5	T48.5X6
Typhoid-paratyphoid vaccine	T50.A91	T50.A92	T50.A93	T50.A94	T50.A95	T50.A96
Typhus vaccine	T50.A91	T50.A92	T50.A93	T50.A94	T50.A95	T50.A96
Tyropanoate	T50.8X1	T50.8X2	T50.8X3	T50.8X4	T50.8X5	T50.8X6
Tyrothricin	T49.6X1	T49.6X2	T49.6X3	T49.6X4	T49.6X5	T49.6X6
ENT agent	T49.6X1	T49.6X2	T49.6X3	T49.6X4	T49.6X5	T49.6X6
ophthalmic preparation	T49.5X1	T49.5X2	T49.5X3	T49.5X4	T49.5X5	T49.5X6
Ufenamate	T39.391	T39.392	T39.393	T39.394	T39.395	T39.396
Ultraviolet light protectant	T49.3X1	T49.3X2	T49.3X3	T49.3X4	T49.3X5	T49.3X6
Undecenoic acid	T49.0X1	T49.0X2	T49.0X3	T49.0X4	T49.0X5	T49.0X6
Undecoylium	T49.0X1	T49.0X2	T49.0X3	T49.0X4	T49.0X5	T49.0X6
Undecylenic acid (derivatives)	T49.0X1	T49.0X2	T49.0X3	T49.0X4	T49.0X5	T49.0X6
Unna's boot	T49.3X1	T49.3X2	T49.3X3	T49.3X4	T49.3X5	T49.3X6
Unsaturated fatty acid	T46.6X1	T46.6X2	T46.6X3	T46.6X4	T46.6X5	T46.6X6
Uracil mustard	T45.1X1	T45.1X2	T45.1X3	T45.1X4	T45.1X5	T45.1X6
Uramustine	T45.1X1	T45.1X2	T45.1X3	T45.1X4	T45.1X5	T45.1X6
Urapidil	T46.5X1	T46.5X2	T46.5X3	T46.5X4	T46.5X5	T46.5X6
Urari	T48.1X1	T48.1X2	T48.1X3	T48.1X4	T48.1X5	T48.1X6
Urate oxidase	T50.4X1	T50.4X2	T50.4X3	T50.4X4	T50.4X5	T50.4X6
Urea	T47.3X1	T47.3X2	T47.3X3	T47.3X4	T47.3X5	T47.3X6
peroxide	T49.0X1	T49.0X2	T49.0X3	T49.0X4	T49.0X5	T49.0X6
stibamine	T37.4X1	T37.4X2	T37.4X3	T37.4X4	T37.4X5	T37.4X6
topical	T49.8X1	T49.8X2	T49.8X3	T49.8X4	T49.8X5	T49.8X6
Urethane	T45.1X1	T45.1X2	T45.1X3	T45.1X4	T45.1X5	T45.1X6
Urginea (maritima) (scilla) — see Squill						
Uric acid metabolism drug NEC	T50.4X1	T50.4X2	T50.4X3	T50.4X4	T50.4X5	T50.4X6
Uricosuric agent	T50.4X1	T50.4X2	T50.4X3	T50.4X4	T50.4X5	T50.4X6
Urinary anti-infective	T37.8X1	T37.8X2	T37.8X3	T37.8X4	T37.8X5	T37.8X6
Urofollitropin	T38.811	T38.812	T38.813	T38.814	T38.815	T38.816
Urokinase	T45.611	T45.612	T45.613	T45.614	T45.615	T45.616
Urokon	T50.8X1	T50.8X2	T50.8X3	T50.8X4	T50.8X5	T50.8X6
Ursodeoxycholic acid	T50.991	T50.992	T50.993	T50.994	T50.995	T50.996
Ursodiol	T50.991	T50.992	T50.993	T50.994	T50.995	T50.996
Urtica	T62.2X1	T62.2X2	T62.2X3	T62.2X4	—	—
Utility gas — see Gas, utility						
Vaccine NEC	T50.Z91	T50.Z92	T50.Z93	T50.Z94	T50.Z95	T50.Z96
antineoplastic	T50.Z91	T50.Z92	T50.Z93	T50.Z94	T50.Z95	T50.Z96
bacterial NEC	T50.A91	T50.A92	T50.A93	T50.A94	T50.A95	T50.A96
with						
other bacterial component	T50.A21	T50.A22	T50.A23	T50.A24	T50.A25	T50.A26
pertussis component	T50.A11	T50.A12	T50.A13	T50.A14	T50.A15	T50.A16
viral-rickettsial component	T50.A21	T50.A22	T50.A23	T50.A24	T50.A25	T50.A26
mixed NEC	T50.A21	T50.A22	T50.A23	T50.A24	T50.A25	T50.A26
BCG	T50.A91	T50.A92	T50.A93	T50.A94	T50.A95	T50.A96
cholera	T50.A91	T50.A92	T50.A93	T50.A94	T50.A95	T50.A96
diphtheria	T50.A91	T50.A92	T50.A93	T50.A94	T50.A95	T50.A96
with tetanus	T50.A21	T50.A22	T50.A23	T50.A24	T50.A25	T50.A26
and pertussis	T50.A11	T50.A12	T50.A13	T50.A14	T50.A15	T50.A16
influenza	T50.B91	T50.B92	T50.B93	T50.B94	T50.B95	T50.B96
measles	T50.B91	T50.B92	T50.B93	T50.B94	T50.B95	T50.B96
with mumps and rubella	T50.B91	T50.B92	T50.B93	T50.B94	T50.B95	T50.B96
meningococcal	T50.A91	T50.A92	T50.A93	T50.A94	T50.A95	T50.A96
mumps	T50.B91	T50.B92	T50.B93	T50.B94	T50.B95	T50.B96
paratyphoid	T50.A91	T50.A92	T50.A93	T50.A94	T50.A95	T50.A96
pertussis	T50.A11	T50.A12	T50.A13	T50.A14	T50.A15	T50.A16
with diphtheria	T50.A11	T50.A12	T50.A13	T50.A14	T50.A15	T50.A16

Additional Character May Be Required — Refer to the Tabular List for Character Selection

▽ Subterms under main terms may continue to next column or page

Trichlorotriethylamine — Vaccine NEC

Substance	Poisoning, Accidental (unintentional)	Poisoning, Intentional Self-harm	Poisoning, Assault	Poisoning, Undetermined	Adverse Effect	Under-dosing
Vaccine — *continued*						
pertussis — *continued*						
with diphtheria — *continued*						
and tetanus	T50.A11	T50.A12	T50.A13	T50.A14	T50.A15	T50.A16
with other component	T50.A11	T50.A12	T50.A13	T50.A14	T50.A15	T50.A16
plague	T50.A91	T50.A92	T50.A93	T50.A94	T50.A95	T50.A96
poliomyelitis	T50.B91	T50.B92	T50.B93	T50.B94	T50.B95	T50.B96
poliovirus	T50.B91	T50.B92	T50.B93	T50.B94	T50.B95	T50.B96
rabies	T50.B91	T50.B92	T50.B93	T50.B94	T50.B95	T50.B96
respiratory syncytial virus	T50.B91	T50.B92	T50.B93	T50.B94	T50.B95	T50.B96
rickettsial NEC	T50.A91	T50.A92	T50.A93	T50.A94	T50.A95	T50.A96
with						
bacterial component	T50.A21	T50.A22	T50.A23	T50.A24	T50.A25	T50.A26
Rocky Mountain spotted fever	T50.A91	T50.A92	T50.A93	T50.A94	T50.A95	T50.A96
rubella	T50.B91	T50.B92	T50.B93	T50.B94	T50.B95	T50.B96
sabin oral	T50.B91	T50.B92	T50.B93	T50.B94	T50.B95	T50.B96
smallpox	T50.B11	T50.B12	T50.B13	T50.B14	T50.B15	T50.B16
TAB	T50.A91	T50.A92	T50.A93	T50.A94	T50.A95	T50.A96
tetanus	T50.A91	T50.A92	T50.A93	T50.A94	T50.A95	T50.A96
typhoid	T50.A91	T50.A92	T50.A93	T50.A94	T50.A95	T50.A96
typhus	T50.A91	T50.A92	T50.A93	T50.A94	T50.A95	T50.A96
viral NEC	T50.B91	T50.B92	T50.B93	T50.B94	T50.B95	T50.B96
yellow fever	T50.B91	T50.B92	T50.B93	T50.B94	T50.B95	T50.B96
Vaccinia immune globulin	T50.Z11	T50.Z12	T50.Z13	T50.Z14	T50.Z15	T50.Z16
Vaginal contraceptives	T49.8X1	T49.8X2	T49.8X3	T49.8X4	T49.8X5	T49.8X6
Valerian						
root	T42.6X1	T42.6X2	T42.6X3	T42.6X4	T42.6X5	T42.6X6
tincture	T42.6X1	T42.6X2	T42.6X3	T42.6X4	T42.6X5	T42.6X6
Valethamate bromide	T44.3X1	T44.3X2	T44.3X3	T44.3X4	T44.3X5	T44.3X6
Valisone	T49.0X1	T49.0X2	T49.0X3	T49.0X4	T49.0X5	T49.0X6
Valium	T42.4X1	T42.4X2	T42.4X3	T42.4X4	T42.4X5	T42.4X6
Valmid	T42.6X1	T42.6X2	T42.6X3	T42.6X4	T42.6X5	T42.6X6
Valnoctamide	T42.6X1	T42.6X2	T42.6X3	T42.6X4	T42.6X5	T42.6X6
Valproate (sodium)	T42.6X1	T42.6X2	T42.6X3	T42.6X4	T42.6X5	T42.6X6
Valproic acid	T42.6X1	T42.6X2	T42.6X3	T42.6X4	T42.6X5	T42.6X6
Valpromide	T42.6X1	T42.6X2	T42.6X3	T42.6X4	T42.6X5	T42.6X6
Vanadium	T56.891	T56.892	T56.893	T56.894	—	—
Vancomycin	T36.8X1	T36.8X2	T36.8X3	T36.8X4	T36.8X5	T36.8X6
Vapor — *see also* Gas	T59.91	T59.92	T59.93	T59.94	—	—
kiln (carbon monoxide)	T58.8X1	T58.8X2	T58.8X3	T58.8X4	—	—
lead — *see* lead						
specified source NEC	T59.891	T59.892	T59.893	T59.894	—	—
Vardenafil	T46.7X1	T46.7X2	T46.7X3	T46.7X4	T46.7X5	T46.7X6
Varicose reduction drug	T46.8X1	T46.8X2	T46.8X3	T46.8X4	T46.8X5	T46.8X6
Varnish	T65.4X1	T65.4X2	T65.4X3	T65.4X4	—	—
cleaner	T52.91	T52.92	T52.93	T52.94	—	—
Vaseline	T49.3X1	T49.3X2	T49.3X3	T49.3X4	T49.3X5	T49.3X6
Vasodilan	T46.7X1	T46.7X2	T46.7X3	T46.7X4	T46.7X5	T46.7X6
Vasodilator						
coronary NEC	T46.3X1	T46.3X2	T46.3X3	T46.3X4	T46.3X5	T46.3X6
peripheral NEC	T46.7X1	T46.7X2	T46.7X3	T46.7X4	T46.7X5	T46.7X6
Vasopressin	T38.891	T38.892	T38.893	T38.894	T38.895	T38.896
Vasopressor drugs	T38.891	T38.892	T38.893	T38.894	T38.895	T38.896
Vecuronium bromide	T48.1X1	T48.1X2	T48.1X3	T48.1X4	T48.1X5	T48.1X6
Vegetable extract, astringent	T49.2X1	T49.2X2	T49.2X3	T49.2X4	T49.2X5	T49.2X6
Venlafaxine	T43.211	T43.212	T43.213	T43.214	T43.215	T43.216
Venom, venomous (bite) (sting)	T63.91	T63.92	T63.93	T63.94	—	—
amphibian NEC	T63.831	T63.832	T63.833	T63.834	—	—
animal NEC	T63.891	T63.892	T63.893	T63.894	—	—
ant	T63.421	T63.422	T63.423	T63.424	—	—
arthropod NEC	T63.481	T63.482	T63.483	T63.484	—	—
bee	T63.441	T63.442	T63.443	T63.444	—	—
centipede	T63.411	T63.412	T63.413	T63.414	—	—
fish	T63.591	T63.592	T63.593	T63.594	—	—
frog	T63.811	T63.812	T63.813	T63.814	—	—
hornet	T63.451	T63.452	T63.453	T63.454	—	—
insect NEC	T63.481	T63.482	T63.483	T63.484	—	—
lizard	T63.121	T63.122	T63.123	T63.124	—	—
marine						
animals	T63.691	T63.692	T63.693	T63.694	—	—
bluebottle	T63.611	T63.612	T63.613	T63.614	—	—
jellyfish NEC	T63.621	T63.622	T63.623	T63.624	—	—
Portugese Man-o-war	T63.611	T63.612	T63.613	T63.614	—	—
sea anemone	T63.631	T63.632	T63.633	T63.634	—	—
specified NEC	T63.691	T63.692	T63.693	T63.694	—	—
fish	T63.591	T63.592	T63.593	T63.594	—	—
plants	T63.711	T63.712	T63.713	T63.714	—	—
sting ray	T63.511	T63.512	T63.513	T63.514	—	—
millipede (tropical)	T63.411	T63.412	T63.413	T63.414	—	—
plant NEC	T63.791	T63.792	T63.793	T63.794	—	—

Substance	Poisoning, Accidental (unintentional)	Poisoning, Intentional Self-harm	Poisoning, Assault	Poisoning, Undetermined	Adverse Effect	Under-dosing
Venom, venomous — *continued*						
plant — *continued*						
marine	T63.711	T63.712	T63.713	T63.714	—	—
reptile	T63.191	T63.192	T63.193	T63.194	—	—
gila monster	T63.111	T63.112	T63.113	T63.114	—	—
lizard NEC	T63.121	T63.122	T63.123	T63.124	—	—
scorpion	T63.2X1	T63.2X2	T63.2X3	T63.2X4	—	—
snake	T63.001	T63.002	T63.003	T63.004	—	—
African NEC	T63.081	T63.082	T63.083	T63.084	—	—
American (North) (South) NEC	T63.061	T63.062	T63.063	T63.064	—	—
Asian	T63.081	T63.082	T63.083	T63.084	—	—
Australian	T63.071	T63.072	T63.073	T63.074	—	—
cobra	T63.041	T63.042	T63.043	T63.044	—	—
coral snake	T63.021	T63.022	T63.023	T63.024	—	—
rattlesnake	T63.011	T63.012	T63.013	T63.014	—	—
specified NEC	T63.091	T63.092	T63.093	T63.094	—	—
taipan	T63.031	T63.032	T63.033	T63.034	—	—
specified NEC	T63.891	T63.892	T63.893	T63.894	—	—
spider	T63.301	T63.302	T63.303	T63.304	—	—
black widow	T63.311	T63.312	T63.313	T63.314	—	—
brown recluse	T63.331	T63.332	T63.333	T63.334	—	—
specified NEC	T63.391	T63.392	T63.393	T63.394	—	—
tarantula	T63.321	T63.322	T63.323	T63.324	—	—
sting ray	T63.511	T63.512	T63.513	T63.514	—	—
toad	T63.821	T63.822	T63.823	T63.824	—	—
wasp	T63.461	T63.462	T63.463	T63.464	—	—
Venous sclerosing drug NEC	T46.8X1	T46.8X2	T46.8X3	T46.8X4	T46.8X5	T46.8X6
Ventolin — *see* Albuterol						
Veramon	T42.3X1	T42.3X2	T42.3X3	T42.3X4	T42.3X5	T42.3X6
Verapamil	T46.1X1	T46.1X2	T46.1X3	T46.1X4	T46.1X5	T46.1X6
Veratrine	T46.5X1	T46.5X2	T46.5X3	T46.5X4	T46.5X5	T46.5X6
Veratrum						
album	T62.2X1	T62.2X2	T62.2X3	T62.2X4	—	—
alkaloids	T46.5X1	T46.5X2	T46.5X3	T46.5X4	T46.5X5	T46.5X6
viride	T62.2X1	T62.2X2	T62.2X3	T62.2X4	—	—
Verdigris	T60.3X1	T60.3X2	T60.3X3	T60.3X4	—	—
Veronal	T42.3X1	T42.3X2	T42.3X3	T42.3X4	T42.3X5	T42.3X6
Veroxil	T37.4X1	T37.4X2	T37.4X3	T37.4X4	T37.4X5	T37.4X6
Versenate	T50.6X1	T50.6X2	T50.6X3	T50.6X4	T50.6X5	T50.6X6
Versidyne	T39.8X1	T39.8X2	T39.8X3	T39.8X4	T39.8X5	T39.8X6
Vetrabutine	T48.0X1	T48.0X2	T48.0X3	T48.0X4	T48.0X5	T48.0X6
Vidarabine	T37.5X1	T37.5X2	T37.5X3	T37.5X4	T37.5X5	T37.5X6
Vienna						
green	T57.0X1	T57.0X2	T57.0X3	T57.0X4	—	—
insecticide	T60.2X1	T60.2X2	T60.2X3	T60.2X4	—	—
red	T57.0X1	T57.0X2	T57.0X3	T57.0X4	—	—
pharmaceutical dye	T50.991	T50.992	T50.993	T50.994	T50.995	T50.996
Vigabatrin	T42.6X1	T42.6X2	T42.6X3	T42.6X4	T42.6X5	T42.6X6
Viloxazine	T43.291	T43.292	T43.293	T43.294	T43.295	T43.296
Viminol	T39.8X1	T39.8X2	T39.8X3	T39.8X4	T39.8X5	T39.8X6
Vinbarbital, vinbarbitone	T42.3X1	T42.3X2	T42.3X3	T42.3X4	T42.3X5	T42.3X6
Vinblastine	T45.1X1	T45.1X2	T45.1X3	T45.1X4	T45.1X5	T45.1X6
Vinburnine	T46.7X1	T46.7X2	T46.7X3	T46.7X4	T46.7X5	T46.7X6
Vincamine	T45.1X1	T45.1X2	T45.1X3	T45.1X4	T45.1X5	T45.1X6
Vincristine	T45.1X1	T45.1X2	T45.1X3	T45.1X4	T45.1X5	T45.1X6
Vindesine	T45.1X1	T45.1X2	T45.1X3	T45.1X4	T45.1X5	T45.1X6
Vinesthene, vinethene	T41.0X1	T41.0X2	T41.0X3	T41.0X4	T41.0X5	T41.0X6
Vinorelbine tartrate	T45.1X1	T45.1X2	T45.1X3	T45.1X4	T45.1X5	T45.1X6
Vinpocetine	T46.7X1	T46.7X2	T46.7X3	T46.7X4	T46.7X5	T46.7X6
Vinyl						
acetate	T65.891	T65.892	T65.893	T65.894	—	—
bital	T42.3X1	T42.3X2	T42.3X3	T42.3X4	T42.3X5	T42.3X6
bromide	T65.891	T65.892	T65.893	T65.894	—	—
chloride	T59.891	T59.892	T59.893	T59.894	—	—
ether	T41.0X1	T41.0X2	T41.0X3	T41.0X4	T41.0X5	T41.0X6
Vinylbital	T42.3X1	T42.3X2	T42.3X3	T42.3X4	T42.3X5	T42.3X6
Vinylidene chloride	T65.891	T65.892	T65.893	T65.894	—	—
Vioform	T37.8X1	T37.8X2	T37.8X3	T37.8X4	T37.8X5	T37.8X6
topical	T49.0X1	T49.0X2	T49.0X3	T49.0X4	T49.0X5	T49.0X6
Viomycin	T36.8X1	T36.8X2	T36.8X3	T36.8X4	T36.8X5	T36.8X6
Viosterol	T45.2X1	T45.2X2	T45.2X3	T45.2X4	T45.2X5	T45.2X6
Viper (venom)	T63.091	T63.092	T63.093	T63.094	—	—
Viprynium	T37.4X1	T37.4X2	T37.4X3	T37.4X4	T37.4X5	T37.4X6
Viquidil	T46.7X1	T46.7X2	T46.7X3	T46.7X4	T46.7X5	T46.7X6
Viral vaccine NEC	T50.B91	T50.B92	T50.B93	T50.B94	T50.B95	T50.B96
Virginiamycin	T36.8X1	T36.8X2	T36.8X3	T36.8X4	T36.8X5	T36.8X6
Virugon	T37.5X1	T37.5X2	T37.5X3	T37.5X4	T37.5X5	T37.5X6
Viscous agent	T50.901	T50.902	T50.903	T50.904	T50.905	T50.906
Visine	T49.5X1	T49.5X2	T49.5X3	T49.5X4	T49.5X5	T49.5X6
Visnadine	T46.3X1	T46.3X2	T46.3X3	T46.3X4	T46.3X5	T46.3X6
Vitamin NEC	T45.2X1	T45.2X2	T45.2X3	T45.2X4	T45.2X5	T45.2X6

Substance	Poisoning, Accidental (unintentional)	Poisoning, Intentional Self-harm	Poisoning, Assault	Poisoning, Undetermined	Adverse Effect	Under-dosing
Vitamin — *continued*						
A	T45.2X1	T45.2X2	T45.2X3	T45.2X4	T45.2X5	T45.2X6
B1	T45.2X1	T45.2X2	T45.2X3	T45.2X4	T45.2X5	T45.2X6
B2	T45.2X1	T45.2X2	T45.2X3	T45.2X4	T45.2X5	T45.2X6
B6	T45.2X1	T45.2X2	T45.2X3	T45.2X4	T45.2X5	T45.2X6
B12	T45.2X1	T45.2X2	T45.2X3	T45.2X4	T45.2X5	T45.2X6
B15	T45.2X1	T45.2X2	T45.2X3	T45.2X4	T45.2X5	T45.2X6
B NEC	T45.2X1	T45.2X2	T45.2X3	T45.2X4	T45.2X5	T45.2X6
nicotinic acid	T46.7X1	T46.7X2	T46.7X3	T46.7X4	T46.7X5	T46.7X6
C	T45.2X1	T45.2X2	T45.2X3	T45.2X4	T45.2X5	T45.2X6
D	T45.2X1	T45.2X2	T45.2X3	T45.2X4	T45.2X5	T45.2X6
D2	T45.2X1	T45.2X2	T45.2X3	T45.2X4	T45.2X5	T45.2X6
D3	T45.2X1	T45.2X2	T45.2X3	T45.2X4	T45.2X5	T45.2X6
E	T45.2X1	T45.2X2	T45.2X3	T45.2X4	T45.2X5	T45.2X6
E acetate	T45.2X1	T45.2X2	T45.2X3	T45.2X4	T45.2X5	T45.2X6
hematopoietic	T45.8X1	T45.8X2	T45.8X3	T45.8X4	T45.8X5	T45.8X6
K1	T45.7X1	T45.7X2	T45.7X3	T45.7X4	T45.7X5	T45.7X6
K2	T45.7X1	T45.7X2	T45.7X3	T45.7X4	T45.7X5	T45.7X6
K NEC	T45.7X1	T45.7X2	T45.7X3	T45.7X4	T45.7X5	T45.7X6
PP	T45.2X1	T45.2X2	T45.2X3	T45.2X4	T45.2X5	T45.2X6
ulceroprotectant	T47.1X1	T47.1X2	T47.1X3	T47.1X4	T47.1X5	T47.1X6
Vleminckx's solution	T49.4X1	T49.4X2	T49.4X3	T49.4X4	T49.4X5	T49.4X6
Voltaren — *see* Diclofenac sodium						
Warfarin	T45.511	T45.512	T45.513	T45.514	T45.515	T45.516
rodenticide	T45.511	T45.512	T45.513	T45.514	T45.515	T45.516
sodium	T45.511	T45.512	T45.513	T45.514	T45.515	T45.516
Wasp (sting)	T63.461	T63.462	T63.463	T63.464	—	—
Water						
balance drug	T50.3X1	T50.3X2	T50.3X3	T50.3X4	T50.3X5	T50.3X6
distilled	T50.3X1	T50.3X2	T50.3X3	T50.3X4	T50.3X5	T50.3X6
gas — *see* Gas, water						
incomplete combustion of — *see* Carbon, monoxide, fuel, utility						
hemlock	T62.2X1	T62.2X2	T62.2X3	T62.2X4	—	—
moccasin (venom)	T63.061	T63.062	T63.063	T63.064	—	—
purified	T50.3X1	T50.3X2	T50.3X3	T50.3X4	T50.3X5	T50.3X6
Wax (paraffin) (petroleum)	T52.0X1	T52.0X2	T52.0X3	T52.0X4	—	—
automobile	T65.891	T65.892	T65.893	T65.894	—	—
floor	T52.0X1	T52.0X2	T52.0X3	T52.0X4	—	—
Weed killers NEC	T60.3X1	T60.3X2	T60.3X3	T60.3X4	—	—
Welldorm	T42.6X1	T42.6X2	T42.6X3	T42.6X4	T42.6X5	T42.6X6
White						
arsenic	T57.0X1	T57.0X2	T57.0X3	T57.0X4	—	—
hellebore	T62.2X1	T62.2X2	T62.2X3	T62.2X4	—	—
lotion (keratolytic)	T49.4X1	T49.4X2	T49.4X3	T49.4X4	T49.4X5	T49.4X6
spirit	T52.0X1	T52.0X2	T52.0X3	T52.0X4	—	—
Whitewash	T65.891	T65.892	T65.893	T65.894	—	—
Whole blood (human)	T45.8X1	T45.8X2	T45.8X3	T45.8X4	T45.8X5	T45.8X6
Wild						
black cherry	T62.2X1	T62.2X2	T62.2X3	T62.2X4	—	—
poisonous plants NEC	T62.2X1	T62.2X2	T62.2X3	T62.2X4	—	—
Window cleaning fluid	T65.891	T65.892	T65.893	T65.894	—	—
Wintergreen (oil)	T49.3X1	T49.3X2	T49.3X3	T49.3X4	T49.3X5	T49.3X6
Wisterine	T62.2X1	T62.2X2	T62.2X3	T62.2X4	—	—
Witch hazel	T49.2X1	T49.2X2	T49.2X3	T49.2X4	T49.2X5	T49.2X6
Wood alcohol or spirit	T51.1X1	T51.1X2	T51.1X3	T51.1X4	—	—
Wool fat (hydrous)	T49.3X1	T49.3X2	T49.3X3	T49.3X4	T49.3X5	T49.3X6
Woorali	T48.1X1	T48.1X2	T48.1X3	T48.1X4	T48.1X5	T48.1X6
Wormseed, American	T37.4X1	T37.4X2	T37.4X3	T37.4X4	T37.4X5	T37.4X6
Xamoterol	T44.5X1	T44.5X2	T44.5X3	T44.5X4	T44.5X5	T44.5X6
Xanthine diuretics	T50.2X1	T50.2X2	T50.2X3	T50.2X4	T50.2X5	T50.2X6
Xanthinol nicotinate	T46.7X1	T46.7X2	T46.7X3	T46.7X4	T46.7X5	T46.7X6
Xanthotoxin	T49.3X1	T49.3X2	T49.3X3	T49.3X4	T49.3X5	T49.3X6
Xantinol nicotinate	T46.7X1	T46.7X2	T46.7X3	T46.7X4	T46.7X5	T46.7X6
Xantocillin	T36.0X1	T36.0X2	T36.0X3	T36.0X4	T36.0X5	T36.0X6
Xenon (127Xe) (133Xe)	T50.8X1	T50.8X2	T50.8X3	T50.8X4	T50.8X5	T50.8X6
Xenysalate	T49.4X1	T49.4X2	T49.4X3	T49.4X4	T49.4X5	T49.4X6
Xibornol	T37.8X1	T37.8X2	T37.8X3	T37.8X4	T37.8X5	T37.8X6
Xigris	T45.511	T45.512	T45.513	T45.514	T45.515	T45.516
Xipamide	T50.2X1	T50.2X2	T50.2X3	T50.2X4	T50.2X5	T50.2X6
Xylene (vapor)	T52.2X1	T52.2X2	T52.2X3	T52.2X4	—	—
Xylocaine (infiltration) (topical)	T41.3X1	T41.3X2	T41.3X3	T41.3X4	T41.3X5	T41.3X6
nerve block (peripheral) (plexus)	T41.3X1	T41.3X2	T41.3X3	T41.3X4	T41.3X5	T41.3X6
spinal	T41.3X1	T41.3X2	T41.3X3	T41.3X4	T41.3X5	T41.3X6
Xylol (vapor)	T52.2X1	T52.2X2	T52.2X3	T52.2X4	—	—
Xylometazoline	T48.5X1	T48.5X2	T48.5X3	T48.5X4	T48.5X5	T48.5X6
Yeast	T45.2X1	T45.2X2	T45.2X3	T45.2X4	T45.2X5	T45.2X6
dried	T45.2X1	T45.2X2	T45.2X3	T45.2X4	T45.2X5	T45.2X6

Substance	Poisoning, Accidental (unintentional)	Poisoning, Intentional Self-harm	Poisoning, Assault	Poisoning, Undetermined	Adverse Effect	Under-dosing
Yellow						
fever vaccine	T50.B91	T50.B92	T50.B93	T50.B94	T50.B95	T50.B96
jasmine	T62.2X1	T62.2X2	T62.2X3	T62.2X4	—	—
phenolphthalein	T47.2X1	T47.2X2	T47.2X3	T47.2X4	T47.2X5	T47.2X6
Yew	T62.2X1	T62.2X2	T62.2X3	T62.2X4	—	—
Yohimbic acid	T40.991	T40.992	T40.993	T40.994	T40.995	T40.996
Zactane	T39.8X1	T39.8X2	T39.8X3	T39.8X4	T39.8X5	T39.8X6
Zalcitabine	T37.5X1	T37.5X2	T37.5X3	T37.5X4	T37.5X5	T37.5X6
Zaroxolyn	T50.2X1	T50.2X2	T50.2X3	T50.2X4	T50.2X5	T50.2X6
Zephiran (topical)	T49.0X1	T49.0X2	T49.0X3	T49.0X4	T49.0X5	T49.0X6
ophthalmic preparation	T49.5X1	T49.5X2	T49.5X3	T49.5X4	T49.5X5	T49.5X6
Zeranol	T38.7X1	T38.7X2	T38.7X3	T38.7X4	T38.7X5	T38.7X6
Zerone	T51.1X1	T51.1X2	T51.1X3	T51.1X4	—	—
Zidovudine	T37.5X1	T37.5X2	T37.5X3	T37.5X4	T37.5X5	T37.5X6
Zimeldine	T43.221	T43.222	T43.223	T43.224	T43.225	T43.226
Zinc (compounds) (fumes) (vapor)	T56.5X1	T56.5X2	T56.5X3	T56.5X4	—	—
NEC						
anti-infectives	T49.0X1	T49.0X2	T49.0X3	T49.0X4	T49.0X5	T49.0X6
antivaricose	T46.8X1	T46.8X2	T46.8X3	T46.8X4	T46.8X5	T46.8X6
bacitracin	T49.0X1	T49.0X2	T49.0X3	T49.0X4	T49.0X5	T49.0X6
chloride (mouthwash)	T49.6X1	T49.6X2	T49.6X3	T49.6X4	T49.6X5	T49.6X6
chromate	T56.5X1	T56.5X2	T56.5X3	T56.5X4	—	—
gelatin	T49.3X1	T49.3X2	T49.3X3	T49.3X4	T49.3X5	T49.3X6
oxide	T49.3X1	T49.3X2	T49.3X3	T49.3X4	T49.3X5	T49.3X6
plaster	T49.3X1	T49.3X2	T49.3X3	T49.3X4	T49.3X5	T49.3X6
peroxide	T49.0X1	T49.0X2	T49.0X3	T49.0X4	T49.0X5	T49.0X6
pesticides	T56.5X1	T56.5X2	T56.5X3	T56.5X4	—	—
phosphide	T60.4X1	T60.4X2	T60.4X3	T60.4X4	—	—
pyrithionate	T49.4X1	T49.4X2	T49.4X3	T49.4X4	T49.4X5	T49.4X6
stearate	T49.3X1	T49.3X2	T49.3X3	T49.3X4	T49.3X5	T49.3X6
sulfate	T49.5X1	T49.5X2	T49.5X3	T49.5X4	T49.5X5	T49.5X6
ENT agent	T49.6X1	T49.6X2	T49.6X3	T49.6X4	T49.6X5	T49.6X6
ophthalmic solution	T49.5X1	T49.5X2	T49.5X3	T49.5X4	T49.5X5	T49.5X6
topical NEC	T49.0X1	T49.0X2	T49.0X3	T49.0X4	T49.0X5	T49.0X6
undecylenate	T49.0X1	T49.0X2	T49.0X3	T49.0X4	T49.0X5	T49.0X6
Zineb	T60.0X1	T60.0X2	T60.0X3	T60.0X4	—	—
Zinostatin	T45.1X1	T45.1X2	T45.1X3	T45.1X4	T45.1X5	T45.1X6
Zipeprol	T48.3X1	T48.3X2	T48.3X3	T48.3X4	T48.3X5	T48.3X6
Zofenopril	T46.4X1	T46.4X2	T46.4X3	T46.4X4	T46.4X5	T46.4X6
Zolpidem	T42.6X1	T42.6X2	T42.6X3	T42.6X4	T42.6X5	T42.6X6
Zomepirac	T39.391	T39.392	T39.393	T39.394	T39.395	T39.396
Zopiclone	T42.6X1	T42.6X2	T42.6X3	T42.6X4	T42.6X5	T42.6X6
Zorubicin	T45.1X1	T45.1X2	T45.1X3	T45.1X4	T45.1X5	T45.1X6
Zotepine	T43.591	T43.592	T43.593	T43.594	T43.595	T43.596
Zovant	T45.511	T45.512	T45.513	T45.514	T45.515	T45.516
Zoxazolamine	T42.8X1	T42.8X2	T42.8X3	T42.8X4	T42.8X5	T42.8X6
Zuclopenthixol	T43.4X1	T43.4X2	T43.4X3	T43.4X4	T43.4X5	T43.4X6
Zygadenus (venenosus)	T62.2X1	T62.2X2	T62.2X3	T62.2X4	—	—
Zyprexa	T43.591	T43.592	T43.593	T43.594	T43.595	T43.596

Additional Character May Be Required — Refer to the Tabular List for Character Selection ▽ Subterms under main terms may continue to next column or page

A

Abandonment (causing exposure to weather conditions) (with intent to injure or kill) NEC X58 ☑
Abuse (adult) (child) (mental) (physical) (sexual) X58 ☑
Accident (to) X58 ☑
  aircraft (in transit) (powered) (*see also* Accident, transport, aircraft)
    due to, caused by cataclysm — *see* Forces of nature, by type
  animal-drawn vehicle — *see* Accident, transport, animal-drawn vehicle occupant
  animal-rider — *see* Accident, transport, animal-rider
  automobile — *see* Accident, transport, car occupant
  bare foot water skier V94.4 ☑
  boat, boating (*see also* Accident, watercraft)
    striking swimmer
      powered V94.11 ☑
      unpowered V94.12 ☑
  bus — *see* Accident, transport, bus occupant
  cable car, not on rails V98.0 ☑
    on rails — *see* Accident, transport, streetcar occupant
  car — *see* Accident, transport, car occupant
  caused by, due to
    animal NEC W64 ☑
    chain hoist W24.0 ☑
    cold (excessive) — *see* Exposure, cold
    corrosive liquid, substance — *see* Table of Drugs and Chemicals
    cutting or piercing instrument — *see* Contact, with, by type of instrument
    drive belt W24.0 ☑
    electric
      current — *see* Exposure, electric current
      motor (*see also* Contact, with, by type of machine) W31.3 ☑
      current (of) W86.8 ☑
    environmental factor NEC X58 ☑
    explosive material — *see* Explosion
    fire, flames — *see* Exposure, fire
    firearm missile — *see* Discharge, firearm by type
    heat (excessive) — *see* Heat
    hot — *see* Contact, with, hot
    ignition — *see* Ignition
    lifting device W24.0 ☑
    lightning — *see* subcategory T75.0 ☑
      causing fire — *see* Exposure, fire
    machine, machinery — *see* Contact, with, by type of machine
    natural factor NEC X58 ☑
    pulley (block) W24.0 ☑
    radiation — *see* Radiation
    steam X13.1
      inhalation X13.0 ☑
      pipe X16 ☑
    thunderbolt — *see* subcategory T75.0 ☑
      causing fire — *see* Exposure, fire
    transmission device W24.1 ☑
  coach — *see* Accident, transport, bus occupant
  coal car — *see* Accident, transport, industrial vehicle occupant
  diving (*see also* Fall, into, water)
    with
      drowning or submersion — *see* Drowning
  forklift — *see* Accident, transport, industrial vehicle occupant
  heavy transport vehicle NOS — *see* Accident, transport, truck occupant
  ice yacht V98.2 ☑
  in
    medical, surgical procedure
      as, or due to misadventure — *see* Misadventure
      causing an abnormal reaction or later complication without mention of misadventure (*see also* Complication of or following, by type of procedure) Y84.9
  land yacht V98.1 ☑
  late effect of — *see* W00-X58 with 7th character S
  logging car — *see* Accident, transport, industrial vehicle occupant
  machine, machinery (*see also* Contact, with, by type of machine)
    on board watercraft V93.69 ☑
      explosion — *see* Explosion, in, watercraft

Accident — *continued*
  machine, machinery (*see also* Contact, with, by type of machine) — *continued*
    on board watercraft — *continued*
      fire — *see* Burn, on board watercraft
      powered craft V93.63 ☑
        ferry boat V93.61 ☑
        fishing boat V93.62 ☑
        jetskis V93.63 ☑
        liner V93.61 ☑
        merchant ship V93.60 ☑
        passenger ship V93.61 ☑
        sailboat V93.64 ☑
  mine tram — *see* Accident, transport, industrial vehicle occupant
  mobility scooter (motorized) — *see* Accident, transport, pedestrian, conveyance, specified type NEC
  motor scooter — *see* Accident, transport, motorcyclist
  motor vehicle NOS (traffic) (*see also* Accident, transport) V89.2 ☑
    nontraffic V89.0 ☑
    three-wheeled NOS — *see* Accident, transport, three-wheeled motor vehicle occupant
  motorcycle NOS — *see* Accident, transport, motorcyclist
  nonmotor vehicle NOS (nontraffic) (*see also* Accident, transport) V89.1 ☑
    traffic NOS V89.3 ☑
  nontraffic (victim's mode of transport NOS) V88.9 ☑
    collision (between) V88.7 ☑
      bus and truck V88.5 ☑
      car and:
        bus V88.3 ☑
        pickup V88.2 ☑
        three-wheeled motor vehicle V88.0 ☑
        train V88.6 ☑
        truck V88.4 ☑
        two-wheeled motor vehicle V88.0 ☑
        van V88.2 ☑
      specified vehicle NEC and:
        three-wheeled motor vehicle V88.1 ☑
        two-wheeled motor vehicle V88.1 ☑
    known mode of transport — *see* Accident, transport, by type of vehicle
    noncollision V88.8 ☑
  on board watercraft V93.89 ☑
    powered craft V93.83 ☑
      ferry boat V93.81 ☑
      fishing boat V93.82 ☑
      jetskis V93.83 ☑
      liner V93.81 ☑
      merchant ship V93.80 ☑
      passenger ship V93.81 ☑
    unpowered craft V93.88 ☑
      canoe V93.85 ☑
      inflatable V93.86 ☑
        in tow
          recreational V94.31 ☑
          specified NEC V94.32 ☑
      kayak V93.85 ☑
      sailboat V93.84 ☑
      surf-board V93.88 ☑
      water skis V93.87 ☑
      windsurfer V93.88 ☑
  parachutist V97.29 ☑
    entangled in object V97.21 ☑
    injured on landing V97.22 ☑
  pedal cycle — *see* Accident, transport, pedal cyclist
  pedestrian (on foot)
    with
      another pedestrian W51 ☑
        with fall W03 ☑
          due to ice or snow W00.0 ☑
      on pedestrian conveyance NEC V00.09 ☑
      roller skater (in-line) V00.01 ☑
      skate boarder V00.02 ☑
      transport vehicle — *see* Accident, transport
    on pedestrian conveyance — *see* Accident, transport, pedestrian, conveyance
  pick-up truck or van — *see* Accident, transport, pickup truck occupant
  quarry truck — *see* Accident, transport, industrial vehicle occupant
  railway vehicle (any) (in motion) — *see* Accident, transport, railway vehicle occupant
    due to cataclysm — *see* Forces of nature, by type

Accident — *continued*
  scooter (non-motorized) — *see* Accident, transport, pedestrian, conveyance, scooter
  sequelae of — *see* categories W00-X58 with 7th character S
  skateboard — *see* Accident, transport, pedestrian, conveyance, skateboard
  ski(ing) — *see* Accident, transport, pedestrian, conveyance
    lift V98.3 ☑
  specified cause NEC X58 ☑
  streetcar — *see* Accident, transport, streetcar occupant
  traffic (victim's mode of transport NOS) V87.9 ☑
    collision (between) V87.7 ☑
      bus and truck V87.5 ☑
      car and:
        bus V87.3 ☑
        pickup V87.2 ☑
        three-wheeled motor vehicle V87.0 ☑
        train V87.6 ☑
        truck V87.4 ☑
        two-wheeled motor vehicle V87.0 ☑
        van V87.2 ☑
      specified vehicle NEC and:
        three-wheeled motor vehicle V87.1 ☑
        two-wheeled motor vehicle V87.1 ☑
    known mode of transport — *see* Accident, transport, by type of vehicle
    noncollision V87.8 ☑
  transport (involving injury to) V99 ☑
    18 wheeler — *see* Accident, transport, truck occupant
    agricultural vehicle occupant (nontraffic) V84.9 ☑
      driver V84.5 ☑
      hanger-on V84.7 ☑
      passenger V84.6 ☑
      traffic V84.3 ☑
        driver V84.0 ☑
        hanger-on V84.2 ☑
        passenger V84.1 ☑
      while boarding or alighting V84.4 ☑
    aircraft NEC V97.89 ☑
      military NEC V97.818 ☑
        with civlian aircraft V97.810 ☑
        civilian injured by V97.811 ☑
      occupant injured (in)
        nonpowered craft accident V96.9 ☑
          balloon V96.00 ☑
            collision V96.03 ☑
            crash V96.01 ☑
            explosion V96.05 ☑
            fire V96.04 ☑
            forced landing V96.02 ☑
            specified type NEC V96.09 ☑
          glider V96.20 ☑
            collision V96.23 ☑
            crash V96.21 ☑
            explosion V96.25 ☑
            fire V96.24 ☑
            forced landing V96.22 ☑
            specified type NEC V96.29 ☑
          hang glider V96.10 ☑
            collision V96.13 ☑
            crash V96.11 ☑
            explosion V96.15 ☑
            fire V96.14 ☑
            forced landing V96.12 ☑
            specified type NEC V96.19 ☑
          specified craft NEC V96.8 ☑
        powered craft accident V95.9 ☑
          fixed wing NEC
            commercial V95.30 ☑
              collision V95.33 ☑
              crash V95.31 ☑
              explosion V95.35 ☑
              fire V95.34 ☑
              forced landing V95.32 ☑
              specified type NEC V95.39 ☑
            private V95.20 ☑
              collision V95.23 ☑
              crash V95.21 ☑
              explosion V95.25 ☑
              fire V95.24 ☑
              forced landing V95.22 ☑
              specified type NEC V95.29 ☑
          glider V95.10 ☑

Accident — *continued*
  transport — *continued*
    aircraft — *continued*
      occupant injured — *continued*
        powered craft accident — *continued*
          glider — *continued*
            collision V95.13 ☑
            crash V95.11 ☑
            explosion V95.15 ☑
            fire V95.14 ☑
            forced landing V95.12 ☑
            specified type NEC V95.19 ☑
          helicopter V95.00 ☑
            collision V95.03 ☑
            crash V95.01 ☑
            explosion V95.05 ☑
            fire V95.04 ☑
            forced landing V95.02 ☑
            specified type NEC V95.09 ☑
          spacecraft V95.40 ☑
            collision V95.43 ☑
            crash V95.41 ☑
            explosion V95.45 ☑
            fire V95.44 ☑
            forced landing V95.42 ☑
            specified type NEC V95.49 ☑
          specified craft NEC V95.8 ☑
          ultralight V95.10 ☑
            collision V95.13 ☑
            crash V95.11 ☑
            explosion V95.15 ☑
            fire V95.14 ☑
            forced landing V95.12 ☑
            specified type NEC V95.19 ☑
      specified accident NEC V97.0 ☑
      while boarding or alighting V97.1 ☑
    person (injured by)
      falling from, in or on aircraft V97.0 ☑
      machinery on aircraft V97.89 ☑
      on ground with aircraft involvement V97.39 ☑
      rotating propeller V97.32 ☑
      struck by object falling from aircraft V97.31 ☑
      sucked into aircraft jet V97.33 ☑
      while boarding or alighting aircraft V97.1 ☑
    airport (battery-powered) passenger vehicle — *see* Accident, transport, industrial vehicle occupant
    all-terrain vehicle occupant (nontraffic) V86.95 ☑
      driver V86.55 ☑
      dune buggy — *see* Accident, transport, dune buggy occupant
      hanger-on V86.75 ☑
      passenger V86.65 ☑
      snowmobile — *see* Accident, transport, snowmobile occupant
      specified type NEC V86.99 ☑
      traffic V86.35 ☑
        driver V86.05 ☑
        hanger-on V86.25 ☑
        passenger V86.15 ☑
      while boarding or alighting V86.45 ☑
    ambulance occupant (traffic) V86.31 ☑
      driver V86.01 ☑
      hanger-on V86.21 ☑
      nontraffic V86.91 ☑
        driver V86.51 ☑
        hanger-on V86.71 ☑
        passenger V86.61 ☑
      passenger V86.11 ☑
      while boarding or alighting V86.41 ☑
    animal-drawn vehicle occupant (in) V80.929 ☑
      collision (with)
        animal V80.12 ☑
          being ridden V80.711 ☑
        animal-drawn vehicle V80.721 ☑
        bus V80.42 ☑
        car V80.42 ☑
        fixed or stationary object V80.82 ☑
        military vehicle V80.920 ☑
        nonmotor vehicle V80.791 ☑
        pedal cycle V80.22 ☑
        pedestrian V80.12 ☑
        pickup V80.42 ☑
        railway train or vehicle V80.62 ☑

Accident — *continued*
  transport — *continued*
    animal-drawn vehicle occupant — *continued*
      collision — *continued*
        specified motor vehicle NEC V80.52 ☑
        streetcar V80.731 ☑
        truck V80.42 ☑
        two- or three-wheeled motor vehicle V80.32 ☑
        van V80.42 ☑
      noncollision V80.02 ☑
      specified circumstance NEC V80.928 ☑
    animal-rider V80.919 ☑
      collision (with)
        animal V80.11 ☑
          being ridden V80.710 ☑
        animal-drawn vehicle V80.720 ☑
        bus V80.41 ☑
        car V80.41 ☑
        fixed or stationary object V80.81 ☑
        military vehicle V80.910 ☑
        nonmotor vehicle V80.790 ☑
        pedal cycle V80.21 ☑
        pedestrian V80.11 ☑
        pickup V80.41 ☑
        railway train or vehicle V80.61 ☑
        specified motor vehicle NEC V80.51 ☑
        streetcar V80.730 ☑
        truck V80.41 ☑
        two- or three-wheeled motor vehicle V80.31 ☑
        van V80.41 ☑
      noncollision V80.018 ☑
        specified as horse rider V80.010 ☑
      specified circumstance NEC V80.918 ☑
    armored car — *see* Accident, transport, truck occupant
    battery-powered truck (baggage) (mail) — *see* Accident, transport, industrial vehicle occupant
    bus occupant V79.9 ☑
      collision (with)
        animal (traffic) V70.9 ☑
          being ridden (traffic) V76.9 ☑
            nontraffic V76.3 ☑
            while boarding or alighting V76.4 ☑
          nontraffic V70.3 ☑
          while boarding or alighting V70.4 ☑
        animal-drawn vehicle (traffic) V76.9 ☑
          nontraffic V76.3 ☑
          while boarding or alighting V76.4 ☑
        bus (traffic) V74.9 ☑
          nontraffic V74.3 ☑
          while boarding or alighting V74.4 ☑
        car (traffic) V73.9 ☑
          nontraffic V73.3 ☑
          while boarding or alighting V73.4 ☑
        motor vehicle NOS (traffic) V79.60 ☑
          nontraffic V79.20 ☑
          specified type NEC (traffic) V79.69 ☑
            nontraffic V79.29 ☑
        pedal cycle (traffic) V71.9 ☑
          nontraffic V71.3 ☑
          while boarding or alighting V71.4 ☑
        pickup truck (traffic) V73.9 ☑
          nontraffic V73.3 ☑
          while boarding or alighting V73.4 ☑
        railway vehicle (traffic) V75.9 ☑
          nontraffic V75.3 ☑
          while boarding or alighting V75.4 ☑
        specified vehicle NEC (traffic) V76.9 ☑
          nontraffic V76.3 ☑
          while boarding or alighting V76.4 ☑
        stationary object (traffic) V77.9 ☑
          nontraffic V77.3 ☑
          while boarding or alighting V77.4 ☑
        streetcar (traffic) V76.9 ☑
          nontraffic V76.3 ☑
          while boarding or alighting V76.4 ☑
        three wheeled motor vehicle (traffic) V72.9 ☑
          nontraffic V72.3 ☑
          while boarding or alighting V72.4 ☑
        truck (traffic) V74.9 ☑
          nontraffic V74.3 ☑
          while boarding or alighting V74.4 ☑

Accident — *continued*
  transport — *continued*
    bus occupant — *continued*
      collision — *continued*
        two wheeled motor vehicle (traffic) V72.9 ☑
          nontraffic V72.3 ☑
          while boarding or alighting V72.4 ☑
        van (traffic) V73.9 ☑
          nontraffic V73.3 ☑
          while boarding or alighting V73.4 ☑
      driver
        collision (with)
          animal (traffic) V70.5 ☑
            being ridden (traffic) V76.5 ☑
              nontraffic V76.0 ☑
            nontraffic V70.0 ☑
          animal-drawn vehicle (traffic) V76.5 ☑
            nontraffic V76.0 ☑
          bus (traffic) V74.5 ☑
            nontraffic V74.0 ☑
          car (traffic) V73.5 ☑
            nontraffic V73.0 ☑
          motor vehicle NOS (traffic) V79.40 ☑
            nontraffic V79.00 ☑
            specified type NEC (traffic) V79.49 ☑
              nontraffic V79.09 ☑
          pedal cycle (traffic) V71.5 ☑
            nontraffic V71.0 ☑
          pickup truck (traffic) V73.5 ☑
            nontraffic V73.0 ☑
          railway vehicle (traffic) V75.5 ☑
            nontraffic V75.0 ☑
          specified vehicle NEC (traffic) V76.5 ☑
            nontraffic V76.0 ☑
          stationary object (traffic) V77.5 ☑
            nontraffic V77.0 ☑
          streetcar (traffic) V76.5 ☑
            nontraffic V76.0 ☑
          three wheeled motor vehicle (traffic) V72.5 ☑
            nontraffic V72.0 ☑
          truck (traffic) V74.5 ☑
            nontraffic V74.0 ☑
          two wheeled motor vehicle (traffic) V72.5 ☑
            nontraffic V72.0 ☑
          van (traffic) V73.5 ☑
            nontraffic V73.0 ☑
        noncollision accident (traffic) V78.5 ☑
          nontraffic V78.0 ☑
      hanger-on
        collision (with)
          animal (traffic) V70.7 ☑
            being ridden (traffic) V76.7 ☑
              nontraffic V76.2 ☑
            nontraffic V70.2 ☑
          animal-drawn vehicle (traffic) V76.7 ☑
            nontraffic V76.2 ☑
          bus (traffic) V74.7 ☑
            nontraffic V74.2 ☑
          car (traffic) V73.7 ☑
            nontraffic V73.2 ☑
          pedal cycle (traffic) V71.7 ☑
            nontraffic V71.2 ☑
          pickup truck (traffic) V73.7 ☑
            nontraffic V73.2 ☑
          railway vehicle (traffic) V75.7 ☑
            nontraffic V75.2 ☑
          specified vehicle NEC (traffic) V76.7 ☑
            nontraffic V76.2 ☑
          stationary object (traffic) V77.7 ☑
            nontraffic V77.2 ☑
          streetcar (traffic) V76.7 ☑
            nontraffic V76.2 ☑
          three wheeled motor vehicle (traffic) V72.7 ☑
            nontraffic V72.2 ☑
          truck (traffic) V74.7 ☑
            nontraffic V74.2 ☑
          two wheeled motor vehicle (traffic) V72.7 ☑
            nontraffic V72.2 ☑
          van (traffic) V73.7 ☑
            nontraffic V73.2 ☑
        noncollision accident (traffic) V78.7 ☑
          nontraffic V78.2 ☑

Accident — *continued*
  transport — *continued*
    bus occupant — *continued*
      noncollision accident (traffic) V78.9 ☑
        nontraffic V78.3 ☑
        while boarding or alighting V78.4 ☑
      nontraffic V79.3 ☑
      passenger
        collision (with)
          animal (traffic) V70.6 ☑
            being ridden (traffic) V76.6 ☑
              nontraffic V76.1 ☑
            nontraffic V70.1 ☑
          animal-drawn vehicle (traffic) V76.6 ☑
            nontraffic V76.1 ☑
          bus (traffic) V74.6 ☑
            nontraffic V74.1 ☑
          car (traffic) V73.6 ☑
            nontraffic V73.1 ☑
          motor vehicle NOS (traffic) V79.50 ☑
            nontraffic V79.10 ☑
            specified type NEC (traffic) V79.59 ☑
              nontraffic V79.19 ☑
          pedal cycle (traffic) V71.6 ☑
            nontraffic V71.1 ☑
          pickup truck (traffic) V73.6 ☑
            nontraffic V73.1 ☑
          railway vehicle (traffic) V75.6 ☑
            nontraffic V75.1 ☑
          specified vehicle NEC (traffic) V76.6 ☑
            nontraffic V76.1 ☑
          stationary object (traffic) V77.6 ☑
            nontraffic V77.1 ☑
          streetcar (traffic) V76.6 ☑
            nontraffic V76.1 ☑
          three wheeled motor vehicle (traffic)
            V72.6 ☑
            nontraffic V72.1 ☑
          truck (traffic) V74.6 ☑
            nontraffic V74.1 ☑
          two wheeled motor vehicle (traffic)
            V72.6 ☑
            nontraffic V72.1 ☑
          van (traffic) V73.6 ☑
            nontraffic V73.1 ☑
      noncollision accident (traffic) V78.6 ☑
        nontraffic V78.1 ☑
    specified type NEC V79.88 ☑
    military vehicle V79.81 ☑
  cable car, not on rails V98.0 ☑
    on rails — *see* Accident, transport, streetcar
      occupant
  car occupant V49.9 ☑
    ambulance occupant — *see* Accident, transport,
      ambulance occupant
    collision (with)
      animal (traffic) V40.9 ☑
        being ridden (traffic) V46.9 ☑
          nontraffic V46.3 ☑
          while boarding or alighting V46.4 ☑
        nontraffic V40.3 ☑
        while boarding or alighting V40.4 ☑
      animal-drawn vehicle (traffic) V46.9 ☑
        nontraffic V46.3 ☑
        while boarding or alighting V46.4 ☑
      bus (traffic) V44.9 ☑
        nontraffic V44.3 ☑
        while boarding or alighting V44.4 ☑
      car (traffic) V43.92 ☑
        nontraffic V43.32 ☑
        while boarding or alighting V43.42 ☑
      motor vehicle NOS (traffic) V49.60 ☑
        nontraffic V49.20 ☑
        specified type NEC (traffic) V49.69 ☑
          nontraffic V49.29 ☑
      pedal cycle (traffic) V41.9 ☑
        nontraffic V41.3 ☑
        while boarding or alighting V41.4 ☑
      pickup truck (traffic) V43.93 ☑
        nontraffic V43.33 ☑
        while boarding or alighting V43.43 ☑
      railway vehicle (traffic) V45.9 ☑
        nontraffic V45.3 ☑
        while boarding or alighting V45.4 ☑
      specified vehicle NEC (traffic) V46.9 ☑
        nontraffic V46.3 ☑

Accident — *continued*
  transport — *continued*
    car occupant — *continued*
      collision — *continued*
        specified vehicle — *continued*
          while boarding or alighting V46.4 ☑
        sport utility vehicle (traffic) V43.91 ☑
          nontraffic V43.31 ☑
          while boarding or alighting V43.41 ☑
        stationary object (traffic) V47.9 ☑
          nontraffic V47.3 ☑
          while boarding or alighting V47.4 ☑
        streetcar (traffic) V46.9 ☑
          nontraffic V46.3 ☑
          while boarding or alighting V46.4 ☑
        three wheeled motor vehicle (traffic)
          V42.9 ☑
          nontraffic V42.3 ☑
          while boarding or alighting V42.4 ☑
        truck (traffic) V44.9 ☑
          nontraffic V44.3 ☑
          while boarding or alighting V44.4 ☑
        two wheeled motor vehicle (traffic) V42.9 ☑
          nontraffic V42.3 ☑
          while boarding or alighting V42.4 ☑
        van (traffic) V43.94 ☑
          nontraffic V43.34 ☑
          while boarding or alighting V43.44 ☑
      driver
        collision (with)
          animal (traffic) V40.5 ☑
            being ridden (traffic) V46.5 ☑
              nontraffic V46.0 ☑
            nontraffic V40.0 ☑
          animal-drawn vehicle (traffic) V46.5 ☑
            nontraffic V46.0 ☑
          bus (traffic) V44.5 ☑
            nontraffic V44.0 ☑
          car (traffic) V43.52 ☑
            nontraffic V43.02 ☑
          motor vehicle NOS (traffic) V49.40 ☑
            nontraffic V49.00 ☑
            specified type NEC (traffic) V49.49 ☑
              nontraffic V49.09 ☑
          pedal cycle (traffic) V41.5 ☑
            nontraffic V41.0 ☑
          pickup truck (traffic) V43.53 ☑
            nontraffic V43.03 ☑
          railway vehicle (traffic) V45.5 ☑
            nontraffic V45.0 ☑
          specified vehicle NEC (traffic) V46.5 ☑
            nontraffic V46.0 ☑
          sport utility vehicle (traffic) V43.51 ☑
            nontraffic V43.01 ☑
          stationary object (traffic) V47.5 ☑
            nontraffic V47.0 ☑
          streetcar (traffic) V46.5 ☑
            nontraffic V46.0 ☑
          three wheeled motor vehicle (traffic)
            V42.5 ☑
            nontraffic V42.0 ☑
          truck (traffic) V44.5 ☑
            nontraffic V44.0 ☑
          two wheeled motor vehicle (traffic)
            V42.5 ☑
            nontraffic V42.0 ☑
          van (traffic) V43.54 ☑
            nontraffic V43.04 ☑
        noncollision accident (traffic) V48.5 ☑
          nontraffic V48.0 ☑
      hanger-on
        collision (with)
          animal (traffic) V40.7 ☑
            being ridden (traffic) V46.7 ☑
              nontraffic V46.2 ☑
            nontraffic V40.2 ☑
          animal-drawn vehicle (traffic) V46.7 ☑
            nontraffic V46.2 ☑
          bus (traffic) V44.7 ☑
            nontraffic V44.2 ☑
          car (traffic) V43.72 ☑
            nontraffic V43.22 ☑
          pedal cycle (traffic) V41.7 ☑
            nontraffic V41.2 ☑
          pickup truck (traffic) V43.73 ☑
            nontraffic V43.23 ☑

Accident — *continued*
  transport — *continued*
    car occupant — *continued*
      hanger-on — *continued*
        collision — *continued*
          railway vehicle (traffic) V45.7 ☑
            nontraffic V45.2 ☑
          specified vehicle NEC (traffic) V46.7 ☑
            nontraffic V46.2 ☑
          sport utility vehicle (traffic) V43.71 ☑
            nontraffic V43.21 ☑
          stationary object (traffic) V47.7 ☑
            nontraffic V47.2 ☑
          streetcar (traffic) V46.7 ☑
            nontraffic V46.2 ☑
          three wheeled motor vehicle (traffic)
            V42.7 ☑
            nontraffic V42.2 ☑
          truck (traffic) V44.7 ☑
            nontraffic V44.2 ☑
          two wheeled motor vehicle (traffic)
            V42.7 ☑
            nontraffic V42.2 ☑
          van (traffic) V43.74 ☑
            nontraffic V43.24 ☑
        noncollision accident (traffic) V48.7 ☑
          nontraffic V48.2 ☑
      noncollision accident (traffic) V48.9 ☑
        nontraffic V48.3 ☑
        while boarding or alighting V48.4 ☑
      nontraffic V49.3 ☑
      passenger
        collision (with)
          animal (traffic) V40.6 ☑
            being ridden (traffic) V46.6 ☑
              nontraffic V46.1 ☑
            nontraffic V40.1 ☑
          animal-drawn vehicle (traffic) V46.6 ☑
            nontraffic V46.1 ☑
          bus (traffic) V44.6 ☑
            nontraffic V44.1 ☑
          car (traffic) V43.62 ☑
            nontraffic V43.12 ☑
          motor vehicle NOS (traffic) V49.50 ☑
            nontraffic V49.10 ☑
            specified type NEC (traffic) V49.59 ☑
              nontraffic V49.19 ☑
          pedal cycle (traffic) V41.6 ☑
            nontraffic V41.1 ☑
          pickup truck (traffic) V43.63 ☑
            nontraffic V43.13 ☑
          railway vehicle (traffic) V45.6 ☑
            nontraffic V45.1 ☑
          specified vehicle NEC (traffic) V46.6 ☑
            nontraffic V46.1 ☑
          sport utility vehicle (traffic) V43.61 ☑
            nontraffic V43.11 ☑
          stationary object (traffic) V47.6 ☑
            nontraffic V47.1 ☑
          streetcar (traffic) V46.6 ☑
            nontraffic V46.1 ☑
          three wheeled motor vehicle (traffic)
            V42.6 ☑
            nontraffic V42.1 ☑
          truck (traffic) V44.6 ☑
            nontraffic V44.1 ☑
          two wheeled motor vehicle (traffic)
            V42.6 ☑
            nontraffic V42.1 ☑
          van (traffic) V43.64 ☑
            nontraffic V43.14 ☑
        noncollision accident (traffic) V48.6 ☑
          nontraffic V48.1 ☑
      specified type NEC V49.88 ☑
      military vehicle V49.81 ☑
    coal car — *see* Accident, transport, industrial vehi-
      cle occupant
    construction vehicle occupant (nontraffic) V85.9 ☑
      driver V85.5 ☑
      hanger-on V85.7 ☑
      passenger V85.6 ☑
      traffic V85.3 ☑
        driver V85.0 ☑
        hanger-on V85.2 ☑
        passenger V85.1 ☑
      while boarding or alighting V85.4 ☑

Accident — *continued*
  transport — *continued*
    dirt bike rider (nontraffic) V86.96 ☑
      driver V86.56 ☑
      hanger-on V86.76 ☑
      passenger V86.66 ☑
      traffic V86.36 ☑
        driver V86.06 ☑
        hanger-on V86.26 ☑
        passenger V86.16 ☑
      while boarding or alighting V86.46 ☑
    due to cataclysm — *see* Forces of nature, by type
    dune buggy occupant (nontraffic) V86.93 ☑
      driver V86.53 ☑
      hanger-on V86.73 ☑
      passenger V86.63 ☑
      traffic V86.33 ☑
        driver V86.03 ☑
        hanger-on V86.23 ☑
        passenger V86.13 ☑
      while boarding or alighting V86.43 ☑
    forklift — *see* Accident, transport, industrial vehicle occupant
    go cart — *see* Accident, transport, all-terrain vehicle occupant
    golf cart — *see* Accident, transport, all-terrain vehicle occupant
    heavy transport vehicle occupant — *see* Accident, transport, truck occupant
    ice yacht V98.2 ☑
    industrial vehicle occupant (nontraffic) V83.9 ☑
      driver V83.5 ☑
      hanger-on V83.7 ☑
      passenger V83.6 ☑
      traffic V83.3 ☑
        driver V83.0 ☑
        hanger-on V83.2 ☑
        passenger V83.1 ☑
      while boarding or alighting V83.4 ☑
    interurban electric car — *see* Accident, transport, streetcar
    land yacht V98.1 ☑
    logging car — *see* Accident, transport, industrial vehicle occupant
    military vehicle occupant (traffic) V86.34 ☑
      driver V86.04 ☑
      hanger-on V86.24 ☑
      nontraffic V86.94 ☑
        driver V86.54 ☑
        hanger-on V86.74 ☑
        passenger V86.64 ☑
      passenger V86.14 ☑
      while boarding or alighting V86.44 ☑
    mine tram — *see* Accident, transport, industrial vehicle occupant
    motor vehicle NEC occupant (traffic) V89.2 ☑
    motorcoach — *see* Accident, transport, bus occupant
    motor/cross bike rider (*see also* Accident, transport, dirt bike rider) V86.96 ☑
    motorcyclist V29.9 ☑
      collision (with)
        animal (traffic) V20.9 ☑
          being ridden (traffic) V26.9 ☑
            nontraffic V26.2 ☑
            while boarding or alighting V26.3 ☑
          nontraffic V20.2 ☑
          while boarding or alighting V20.3 ☑
        animal-drawn vehicle (traffic) V26.9 ☑
          nontraffic V26.2 ☑
          while boarding or alighting V26.3 ☑
        bus (traffic) V24.9 ☑
          nontraffic V24.2 ☑
          while boarding or alighting V24.3 ☑
        car (traffic) V23.9 ☑
          nontraffic V23.2 ☑
          while boarding or alighting V23.3 ☑
        motor vehicle NOS (traffic) V29.60 ☑
          nontraffic V29.20 ☑
          specified type NEC (traffic) V29.69 ☑
            nontraffic V29.29 ☑
        pedal cycle (traffic) V21.9 ☑
          nontraffic V21.2 ☑
          while boarding or alighting V21.3 ☑
        pickup truck (traffic) V23.9 ☑
          nontraffic V23.2 ☑

Accident — *continued*
  transport — *continued*
    motorcyclist — *continued*
      collision — *continued*
        pickup truck — *continued*
          while boarding or alighting V23.3 ☑
        railway vehicle (traffic) V25.9 ☑
          nontraffic V25.2 ☑
          while boarding or alighting V25.3 ☑
        specified vehicle NEC (traffic) V26.9 ☑
          nontraffic V26.2 ☑
          while boarding or alighting V26.3 ☑
        stationary object (traffic) V27.9 ☑
          nontraffic V27.2 ☑
          while boarding or alighting V27.3 ☑
        streetcar (traffic) V26.9 ☑
          nontraffic V26.2 ☑
          while boarding or alighting V26.3 ☑
        three wheeled motor vehicle (traffic) V22.9 ☑
          nontraffic V22.2 ☑
          while boarding or alighting V22.3 ☑
        truck (traffic) V24.9 ☑
          nontraffic V24.2 ☑
          while boarding or alighting V24.3 ☑
        two wheeled motor vehicle (traffic) V22.9 ☑
          nontraffic V22.2 ☑
          while boarding or alighting V22.3 ☑
        van (traffic) V23.9 ☑
          nontraffic V23.2 ☑
          while boarding or alighting V23.3 ☑
      driver
        collision (with)
          animal (traffic) V20.4 ☑
            being ridden (traffic) V26.4 ☑
              nontraffic V26.0 ☑
            nontraffic V20.0 ☑
          animal-drawn vehicle (traffic) V26.4 ☑
            nontraffic V26.0 ☑
          bus (traffic) V24.4 ☑
            nontraffic V24.0 ☑
          car (traffic) V23.4 ☑
            nontraffic V23.0 ☑
          motor vehicle NOS (traffic) V29.40 ☑
            nontraffic V29.00 ☑
            specified type NEC (traffic) V29.49 ☑
              nontraffic V29.09 ☑
          pedal cycle (traffic) V21.4 ☑
            nontraffic V21.0 ☑
          pickup truck (traffic) V23.4 ☑
            nontraffic V23.0 ☑
          railway vehicle (traffic) V25.4 ☑
            nontraffic V25.0 ☑
          specified vehicle NEC (traffic) V26.4 ☑
            nontraffic V26.0 ☑
          stationary object (traffic) V27.4 ☑
            nontraffic V27.0 ☑
          streetcar (traffic) V26.4 ☑
            nontraffic V26.0 ☑
          three wheeled motor vehicle (traffic) V22.4 ☑
            nontraffic V22.0 ☑
          truck (traffic) V24.4 ☑
            nontraffic V24.0 ☑
          two wheeled motor vehicle (traffic) V22.4 ☑
            nontraffic V22.0 ☑
          van (traffic) V23.4 ☑
            nontraffic V23.0 ☑
        noncollision accident (traffic) V28.4 ☑
          nontraffic V28.0 ☑
      noncollision accident (traffic) V28.9 ☑
        nontraffic V28.2 ☑
        while boarding or alighting V28.3 ☑
      nontraffic V29.3 ☑
      passenger
        collision (with)
          animal (traffic) V20.5 ☑
            being ridden (traffic) V26.5 ☑
              nontraffic V26.1 ☑
            nontraffic V20.1 ☑
          animal-drawn vehicle (traffic) V26.5 ☑
            nontraffic V26.1 ☑
          bus (traffic) V24.5 ☑
            nontraffic V24.1 ☑
          car (traffic) V23.5 ☑

Accident — *continued*
  transport — *continued*
    motorcyclist — *continued*
      passenger — *continued*
        collision — *continued*
          car — *continued*
            nontraffic V23.1 ☑
          motor vehicle NOS (traffic) V29.50 ☑
            nontraffic V29.10 ☑
            specified type NEC (traffic) V29.59 ☑
              nontraffic V29.19 ☑
          pedal cycle (traffic) V21.5 ☑
            nontraffic V21.1 ☑
          pickup truck (traffic) V23.5 ☑
            nontraffic V23.1 ☑
          railway vehicle (traffic) V25.5 ☑
            nontraffic V25.1 ☑
          specified vehicle NEC (traffic) V26.5 ☑
            nontraffic V26.1 ☑
          stationary object (traffic) V27.5 ☑
            nontraffic V27.1 ☑
          streetcar (traffic) V26.5 ☑
            nontraffic V26.1 ☑
          three wheeled motor vehicle (traffic) V22.5 ☑
            nontraffic V22.1 ☑
          truck (traffic) V24.5 ☑
            nontraffic V24.1 ☑
          two wheeled motor vehicle (traffic) V22.5 ☑
            nontraffic V22.1 ☑
          van (traffic) V23.5 ☑
            nontraffic V23.1 ☑
        noncollision accident (traffic) V28.5 ☑
          nontraffic V28.1 ☑
    specified type NEC V29.88 ☑
      military vehicle V29.81 ☑
    occupant (of)
      aircraft (powered) V95.9 ☑
        fixed wing
          commercial — *see* Accident, transport, aircraft, occupant, powered, fixed wing, commercial
          private — *see* Accident, transport, aircraft, occupant, powered, fixed wing, private
        nonpowered V96.9 ☑
        specified NEC V95.8 ☑
      airport battery-powered vehicle — *see* Accident, transport, industrial vehicle occupant
      all-terrain vehicle (ATV) — *see* Accident, transport, all-terrain vehicle occupant
      animal-drawn vehicle — *see* Accident, transport, animal-drawn vehicle occupant
      automobile — *see* Accident, transport, car occupant
      balloon V96.00 ☑
      battery-powered vehicle — *see* Accident, transport, industrial vehicle occupant
      bicycle — *see* Accident, transport, pedal cyclist
        motorized — *see* Accident, transport, motorcycle rider
      boat NEC — *see* Accident, watercraft
      bulldozer — *see* Accident, transport, construction vehicle occupant
      bus — *see* Accident, transport, bus occupant
      cable car (on rails) (*see also* Accident, transport, streetcar occupant)
        not on rails V98.0 ☑
      car (*see also* Accident, transport, car occupant)
        cable (on rails) (*see also* Accident, transport, streetcar occupant)
        not on rails V98.0 ☑
      coach — *see* Accident, transport, bus occupant
      coal-car — *see* Accident, transport, industrial vehicle occupant
      digger — *see* Accident, transport, construction vehicle occupant
      dump truck — *see* Accident, transport, construction vehicle occupant
      earth-leveler — *see* Accident, transport, construction vehicle occupant
      farm machinery (self-propelled) — *see* Accident, transport, agricultural vehicle occupant

Accident — *continued*
  transport — *continued*
    occupant — *continued*
      forklift — *see* Accident, transport, industrial vehicle occupant
      glider (unpowered) V96.20 ☑
        hang V96.10 ☑
        powered (microlight) (ultralight) — *see* Accident, transport, aircraft, occupant, powered, glider
      glider (unpowered) NEC V96.20 ☑
      hang-glider V96.10 ☑
      harvester — *see* Accident, transport, agricultural vehicle occupant
      heavy (transport) vehicle — *see* Accident, transport, truck occupant
      helicopter — *see* Accident, transport, aircraft, occupant, helicopter
      ice-yacht V98.2 ☑
      kite (carrying person) V96.8 ☑
      land-yacht V98.1 ☑
      logging car — *see* Accident, transport, industrial vehicle occupant
      mechanical shovel — *see* Accident, transport, construction vehicle occupant
      microlight — *see* Accident, transport, aircraft, occupant, powered, glider
      minibus — *see* Accident, transport, pickup truck occupant
      minivan — *see* Accident, transport, pickup truck occupant
      moped — *see* Accident, transport, motorcycle
      motor scooter — *see* Accident, transport, motorcycle
      motorcycle (with sidecar) — *see* Accident, transport, motorcycle
      off-road motor-vehicle (*see also* Accident, transport, all-terrain vehicle occupant) V86.99 ☑
      pedal cycle (*see also* Accident, transport, pedal cyclist)
      pick-up (truck) — *see* Accident, transport, pickup truck occupant
      railway (train) (vehicle) (subterranean) (elevated) — *see* Accident, transport, railway vehicle occupant
      rickshaw — *see* Accident, transport, pedal cycle
        motorized — *see* Accident, transport, three-wheeled motor vehicle
        pedal driven — *see* Accident, transport, pedal cyclist
      road-roller — *see* Accident, transport, construction vehicle occupant
      ship NOS V94.9 ☑
      ski-lift (chair) (gondola) V98.3 ☑
      snowmobile — *see* Accident, transport, snowmobile occupant
      spacecraft, spaceship — *see* Accident, transport, aircraft, occupant, spacecraft
      sport utility vehicle — *see* Accident, transport, pickup truck occupant
      streetcar (interurban) (operating on public street or highway) — *see* Accident, transport, streetcar occupant
      SUV — *see* Accident, transport, pickup truck occupant
      téléférique V98.0 ☑
      three-wheeled vehicle (motorized) (*see also* Accident, transport, three-wheeled motor vehicle occupant)
        nonmotorized — *see* Accident, transport, pedal cycle
      tractor (farm) (and trailer) — *see* Accident, transport, agricultural vehicle occupant
      train — *see* Accident, transport, railway vehicle occupant
      tram — *see* Accident, transport, streetcar occupant
        in mine or quarry — *see* Accident, transport, industrial vehicle occupant
      tricycle — *see* Accident, transport, pedal cycle
        motorized — *see* Accident, transport, three-wheeled motor vehicle
      trolley — *see* Accident, transport, streetcar occupant
        in mine or quarry — *see* Accident, transport, industrial vehicle occupant

Accident — *continued*
  transport — *continued*
    occupant — *continued*
      tub, in mine or quarry — *see* Accident, transport, industrial vehicle occupant
      ultralight — *see* Accident, transport, aircraft, occupant, powered, glider
      van — *see* Accident, transport, van occupant
      vehicle NEC V89.9 ☑
        heavy transport — *see* Accident, transport, truck occupant
        motor (traffic) NEC V89.2 ☑
        nontraffic NEC V89.0 ☑
      watercraft NOS V94.9 ☑
        causing drowning — *see* Drowning, resulting from accident to boat
    off-road motor-vehicle (*see also* Accident, transport, all-terrain vehicle occupant) V86.99 ☑
    parachutist V97.29 ☑
      after accident to aircraft — *see* Accident, transport, aircraft
      entangled in object V97.21 ☑
      injured on landing V97.22 ☑
    pedal cyclist V19.9 ☑
      collision (with)
        animal (traffic) V10.9 ☑
          being ridden (traffic) V16.9 ☑
            nontraffic V16.2 ☑
            while boarding or alighting V16.3 ☑
          nontraffic V10.2 ☑
          while boarding or alighting V10.3 ☑
        animal-drawn vehicle (traffic) V16.9 ☑
          nontraffic V16.2 ☑
          while boarding or alighting V16.3 ☑
        bus (traffic) V14.9 ☑
          nontraffic V14.2 ☑
          while boarding or alighting V14.3 ☑
        car (traffic) V13.9 ☑
          nontraffic V13.2 ☑
          while boarding or alighting V13.3 ☑
        motor vehicle NOS (traffic) V19.60 ☑
          nontraffic V19.20 ☑
          specified type NEC (traffic) V19.69 ☑
            nontraffic V19.29 ☑
        pedal cycle (traffic) V11.9 ☑
          nontraffic V11.2 ☑
          while boarding or alighting V11.3 ☑
        pickup truck (traffic) V13.9 ☑
          nontraffic V13.2 ☑
          while boarding or alighting V13.3 ☑
        railway vehicle (traffic) V15.9 ☑
          nontraffic V15.2 ☑
          while boarding or alighting V15.3 ☑
        specified vehicle NEC (traffic) V16.9 ☑
          nontraffic V16.2 ☑
          while boarding or alighting V16.3 ☑
        stationary object (traffic) V17.9 ☑
          nontraffic V17.2 ☑
          while boarding or alighting V17.3 ☑
        streetcar (traffic) V16.9 ☑
          nontraffic V16.2 ☑
          while boarding or alighting V16.3 ☑
        three wheeled motor vehicle (traffic) V12.9 ☑
          nontraffic V12.2 ☑
          while boarding or alighting V12.3 ☑
        truck (traffic) V14.9 ☑
          nontraffic V14.2 ☑
          while boarding or alighting V14.3 ☑
        two wheeled motor vehicle (traffic) V12.9 ☑
          nontraffic V12.2 ☑
          while boarding or alighting V12.3 ☑
        van (traffic) V13.9 ☑
          nontraffic V13.2 ☑
          while boarding or alighting V13.3 ☑
      driver
        collision (with)
          animal (traffic) V10.4 ☑
            being ridden (traffic) V16.4 ☑
              nontraffic V16.0 ☑
            nontraffic V10.0 ☑
          animal-drawn vehicle (traffic) V16.4 ☑
            nontraffic V16.0 ☑
          bus (traffic) V14.4 ☑
            nontraffic V14.0 ☑
          car (traffic) V13.4 ☑

Accident — *continued*
  transport — *continued*
    pedal cyclist — *continued*
      driver — *continued*
        collision — *continued*
          car — *continued*
            nontraffic V13.0 ☑
          motor vehicle NOS (traffic) V19.40 ☑
            nontraffic V19.00 ☑
            specified type NEC (traffic) V19.49 ☑
              nontraffic V19.09 ☑
          pedal cycle (traffic) V11.4 ☑
            nontraffic V11.0 ☑
          pickup truck (traffic) V13.4 ☑
            nontraffic V13.0 ☑
          railway vehicle (traffic) V15.4 ☑
            nontraffic V15.0 ☑
          specified vehicle NEC (traffic) V16.4 ☑
            nontraffic V16.0 ☑
          stationary object (traffic) V17.4 ☑
            nontraffic V17.0 ☑
          streetcar (traffic) V16.4 ☑
            nontraffic V16.0 ☑
          three wheeled motor vehicle (traffic) V12.4 ☑
            nontraffic V12.0 ☑
          truck (traffic) V14.4 ☑
            nontraffic V14.0 ☑
          two wheeled motor vehicle (traffic) V12.4 ☑
            nontraffic V12.0 ☑
          van (traffic) V13.4 ☑
            nontraffic V13.0 ☑
        noncollision accident (traffic) V18.4 ☑
          nontraffic V18.0 ☑
      noncollision accident (traffic) V18.9 ☑
        nontraffic V18.2 ☑
        while boarding or alighting V18.3 ☑
      nontraffic V19.3 ☑
      passenger
        collision (with)
          animal (traffic) V10.5 ☑
            being ridden (traffic) V16.5 ☑
              nontraffic V16.1 ☑
            nontraffic V10.1 ☑
          animal-drawn vehicle (traffic) V16.5 ☑
            nontraffic V16.1 ☑
          bus (traffic) V14.5 ☑
            nontraffic V14.1 ☑
          car (traffic) V13.5 ☑
            nontraffic V13.1 ☑
          motor vehicle NOS (traffic) V19.50 ☑
            nontraffic V19.10 ☑
            specified type NEC (traffic) V19.59 ☑
              nontraffic V19.19 ☑
          pedal cycle (traffic) V11.5 ☑
            nontraffic V11.1 ☑
          pickup truck (traffic) V13.5 ☑
            nontraffic V13.1 ☑
          railway vehicle (traffic) V15.5 ☑
            nontraffic V15.1 ☑
          specified vehicle NEC (traffic) V16.5 ☑
            nontraffic V16.1 ☑
          stationary object (traffic) V17.5 ☑
            nontraffic V17.1 ☑
          streetcar (traffic) V16.5 ☑
            nontraffic V16.1 ☑
          three wheeled motor vehicle (traffic) V12.5 ☑
            nontraffic V12.1 ☑
          truck (traffic) V14.5 ☑
            nontraffic V14.1 ☑
          two wheeled motor vehicle (traffic) V12.5 ☑
            nontraffic V12.1 ☑
          van (traffic) V13.5 ☑
            nontraffic V13.1 ☑
        noncollision accident (traffic) V18.5 ☑
          nontraffic V18.1 ☑
      specified type NEC V19.88 ☑
      military vehicle V19.81 ☑
    pedestrian
      conveyance (occupant) V09.9 ☑
        babystroller V00.828 ☑
          collision (with) V09.9 ☑

Accident — *continued*
  transport — *continued*
    pedestrian — *continued*
      conveyance — *continued*
        babystroller — *continued*
          collision — *continued*
            animal being ridden or animal drawn
              vehicle V06.99 ☑
              nontraffic V06.09 ☑
              traffic V06.19 ☑
            bus or heavy transport V04.99 ☑
              nontraffic V04.09 ☑
              traffic V04.19 ☑
            car V03.99 ☑
              nontraffic V03.09 ☑
              traffic V03.19 ☑
            pedal cycle V01.99 ☑
              nontraffic V01.09 ☑
              traffic V01.19 ☑
            pick-up truck or van V03.99 ☑
              nontraffic V03.09 ☑
              traffic V03.19 ☑
            railway (train) (vehicle) V05.99 ☑
              nontraffic V05.09 ☑
              traffic V05.19 ☑
            stationary object V00.822 ☑
            streetcar V06.99 ☑
              nontraffic V06.09 ☑
              traffic V06.19 ☑
            two- or three-wheeled motor vehicle
              V02.99 ☑
              nontraffic V02.09 ☑
              traffic V02.19 ☑
            vehicle V09.9 ☑
              animal-drawn V06.99 ☑
                nontraffic V06.09 ☑
                traffic V06.19 ☑
              motor
                nontraffic V09.00 ☑
                traffic V09.20 ☑
          fall V00.821 ☑
          nontraffic V09.1 ☑
            involving motor vehicle NEC
              V09.00 ☑
          traffic V09.3 ☑
            involving motor vehicle NEC
              V09.20 ☑
        flat-bottomed NEC V00.388 ☑
          collision (with) V09.9 ☑
            animal being ridden or animal drawn
              vehicle V06.99 ☑
              nontraffic V06.09 ☑
              traffic V06.19 ☑
            bus or heavy transport V04.99 ☑
              nontraffic V04.09 ☑
              traffic V04.19 ☑
            car V03.99 ☑
              nontraffic V03.09 ☑
              traffic V03.19 ☑
            pedal cycle V01.99 ☑
              nontraffic V01.09 ☑
              traffic V01.19 ☑
            pick-up truck or van V03.99 ☑
              nontraffic V03.09 ☑
              traffic V03.19 ☑
            railway (train) (vehicle) V05.99 ☑
              nontraffic V05.09 ☑
              traffic V05.19 ☑
            stationary object V00.382 ☑
            streetcar V06.99 ☑
              nontraffic V06.09 ☑
              traffic V06.19 ☑
            two- or three-wheeled motor vehicle
              V02.99 ☑
              nontraffic V02.09 ☑
              traffic V02.19 ☑
            vehicle V09.9 ☑
              animal-drawn V06.99 ☑
                nontraffic V06.09 ☑
                traffic V06.19 ☑
              motor
                nontraffic V09.00 ☑
                traffic V09.20 ☑
          fall V00.381 ☑
          nontraffic V09.1 ☑

Accident — *continued*
  transport — *continued*
    pedestrian — *continued*
      conveyance — *continued*
        flat-bottomed — *continued*
          nontraffic — *continued*
            involving motor vehicle NEC
              V09.00 ☑
          snow
            board — *see* Accident, transport,
              pedestrian, conveyance, snow
              board
            ski — *see* Accident, transport,
              pedestrian, conveyance, skis
              (snow)
          traffic V09.3 ☑
            involving motor vehicle NEC
              V09.20 ☑
        gliding type NEC V00.288 ☑
          collision (with) V09.9 ☑
            animal being ridden or animal drawn
              vehicle V06.99 ☑
              nontraffic V06.09 ☑
              traffic V06.19 ☑
            bus or heavy transport V04.99 ☑
              nontraffic V04.09 ☑
              traffic V04.19 ☑
            car V03.99 ☑
              nontraffic V03.09 ☑
              traffic V03.19 ☑
            pedal cycle V01.99 ☑
              nontraffic V01.09 ☑
              traffic V01.19 ☑
            pick-up truck or van V03.99 ☑
              nontraffic V03.09 ☑
              traffic V03.19 ☑
            railway (train) (vehicle) V05.99 ☑
              nontraffic V05.09 ☑
              traffic V05.19 ☑
            stationary object V00.282 ☑
            streetcar V06.99 ☑
              nontraffic V06.09 ☑
              traffic V02.19 ☑
            two- or three-wheeled motor vehicle
              V02.99 ☑
              nontraffic V02.09 ☑
              traffic V02.19 ☑
            vehicle V09.9 ☑
              animal-drawn V06.99 ☑
                nontraffic V06.09 ☑
                traffic V06.19 ☑
              motor
                nontraffic V09.00 ☑
                traffic V09.20 ☑
          fall V00.281 ☑
          heelies — *see* Accident, transport,
            pedestrian, conveyance, heelies
          ice skate — *see* Accident, transport,
            pedestrian, conveyance, ice skate
          nontraffic V09.1 ☑
            involving motor vehicle NEC
              V09.00 ☑
          sled — *see* Accident, transport, pedestri-
            an, conveyance, sled
          traffic V09.3 ☑
            involving motor vehicle NEC
              V09.20 ☑
          wheelies — *see* Accident, transport,
            pedestrian, conveyance, heel-
            ies
        heelies V00.158 ☑
          colliding with stationary object
            V00.152 ☑
          fall V00.151 ☑
        ice skates V00.218 ☑
          collision (with) V09.9 ☑
            animal being ridden or animal drawn
              vehicle V06.99 ☑
              nontraffic V06.09 ☑
              traffic V06.19 ☑
            bus or heavy transport V04.99 ☑
              nontraffic V04.09 ☑
              traffic V04.19 ☑
            car V03.99 ☑
              nontraffic V03.09 ☑
              traffic V03.19 ☑

Accident — *continued*
  transport — *continued*
    pedestrian — *continued*
      conveyance — *continued*
        ice skates — *continued*
          collision — *continued*
            pedal cycle V01.99 ☑
              nontraffic V01.09 ☑
              traffic V01.19 ☑
            pick-up truck or van V03.99 ☑
              nontraffic V03.09 ☑
              traffic V03.19 ☑
            railway (train) (vehicle) V05.99 ☑
              nontraffic V05.09 ☑
              traffic V05.19 ☑
            stationary object V00.212 ☑
            streetcar V06.99 ☑
              nontraffic V06.09 ☑
              traffic V06.19 ☑
            two- or three-wheeled motor vehicle
              V02.99 ☑
              nontraffic V02.09 ☑
              traffic V02.19 ☑
            vehicle V09.9 ☑
              animal-drawn V06.99 ☑
                nontraffic V06.09 ☑
                traffic V06.19 ☑
              motor
                nontraffic V09.00 ☑
                traffic V09.20 ☑
          fall V00.211 ☑
          nontraffic V09.1 ☑
            involving motor vehicle NEC
              V09.00 ☑
          traffic V09.3 ☑
            involving motor vehicle NEC
              V09.20 ☑
        motorized mobility scooter V00.838 ☑
          collision with stationary object
            V00.832 ☑
          fall from V00.831 ☑
        nontraffic V09.1 ☑
          involving motor vehicle V09.00 ☑
            military V09.01 ☑
            specified type NEC V09.09 ☑
        roller skates (non in-line) V00.128 ☑
          collision (with) V09.9 ☑
            animal being ridden or animal drawn
              vehicle V06.91 ☑
              nontraffic V06.01 ☑
              traffic V06.11 ☑
            bus or heavy transport V04.91 ☑
              nontraffic V04.01 ☑
              traffic V04.11 ☑
            car V03.91 ☑
              nontraffic V03.01 ☑
              traffic V03.11 ☑
            pedal cycle V01.91 ☑
              nontraffic V01.01 ☑
              traffic V01.11 ☑
            pick-up truck or van V03.91 ☑
              nontraffic V03.01 ☑
              traffic V03.11 ☑
            railway (train) (vehicle) V05.91 ☑
              nontraffic V05.01 ☑
              traffic V05.11 ☑
            stationary object V00.122 ☑
            streetcar V06.91 ☑
              nontraffic V06.01 ☑
              traffic V06.11 ☑
            two- or three-wheeled motor vehicle
              V02.91 ☑
              nontraffic V02.01 ☑
              traffic V02.11 ☑
            vehicle V09.9 ☑
              animal-drawn V06.91 ☑
                nontraffic V06.01 ☑
                traffic V06.11 ☑
              motor
                nontraffic V09.00 ☑
                traffic V09.20 ☑
          fall V00.121 ☑
          in-line V00.118 ☑

Accident — *continued*
  transport — *continued*
    pedestrian — *continued*
      conveyance — *continued*
        roller skates — *continued*
          in-line — *continued*
            collision — *see also* Accident, transport, pedestrian, conveyance occupant, roller skates, collision
              with stationary object V00.112 ☑
            fall V00.111 ☑
            nontraffic V09.1 ☑
              involving motor vehicle NEC V09.00 ☑
            traffic V09.3 ☑
              involving motor vehicle NEC V09.20 ☑
        rolling shoes V00.158 ☑
          colliding with stationary object V00.152 ☑
          fall V00.151 ☑
        rolling type NEC V00.188 ☑
          collision (with) V09.9 ☑
            animal being ridden or animal drawn vehicle V06.99 ☑
              nontraffic V06.09 ☑
              traffic V06.19 ☑
            bus or heavy transport V04.99 ☑
              nontraffic V04.09 ☑
              traffic V04.19 ☑
            car V03.99 ☑
              nontraffic V03.09 ☑
              traffic V03.19 ☑
            pedal cycle V01.99 ☑
              nontraffic V01.09 ☑
              traffic V01.19 ☑
            pick-up truck or van V03.99 ☑
              nontraffic V03.09 ☑
              traffic V03.19 ☑
            railway (train) (vehicle) V05.99 ☑
              nontraffic V05.09 ☑
              traffic V05.19 ☑
            stationary object V00.182 ☑
            streetcar V06.99 ☑
              nontraffic V06.09 ☑
              traffic V06.19 ☑
            two- or three-wheeled motor vehicle V02.99 ☑
              nontraffic V02.09 ☑
              traffic V02.19 ☑
            vehicle V09.9 ☑
              animal-drawn V06.99 ☑
                nontraffic V06.09 ☑
                traffic V06.19 ☑
              motor
                nontraffic V09.00 ☑
                traffic V09.20 ☑
           fall V00.181 ☑
          in-line roller skate — *see* Accident, transport, pedestrian, conveyance, roller skate, in-line
          nontraffic V09.1 ☑
            involving motor vehicle NEC V09.00 ☑
          roller skate — *see* Accident, transport, pedestrian, conveyance, roller skate
          scooter (non-motorized) — *see* Accident, transport, pedestrian, conveyance, scooter
          skateboard — *see* Accident, transport, pedestrian, conveyance, skateboard
          traffic V09.3 ☑
            involving motor vehicle NEC V09.20 ☑
        scooter (non-motorized) V00.148 ☑
          collision (with) V09.9 ☑
            animal being ridden or animal drawn vehicle V06.99 ☑
              nontraffic V06.09 ☑
              traffic V06.19 ☑
            bus or heavy transport V04.99 ☑
              nontraffic V04.09 ☑
              traffic V04.19 ☑

Accident — *continued*
  transport — *continued*
    pedestrian — *continued*
      conveyance — *continued*
        scooter — *continued*
          collision — *continued*
           car V03.99 ☑
              nontraffic V03.09 ☑
              traffic V03.19 ☑
            pedal cycle V01.99 ☑
              nontraffic V01.09 ☑
              traffic V01.19 ☑
            pick-up truck or van V03.99 ☑
              nontraffic V03.09 ☑
              traffic V03.19 ☑
            railway (train) (vehicle) V05.99 ☑
              nontraffic V05.09 ☑
              traffic V05.19 ☑
            stationary object V00.142 ☑
            streetcar V06.99 ☑
              nontraffic V06.09 ☑
              traffic V06.19 ☑
            two- or three-wheeled motor vehicle V02.99 ☑
              nontraffic V02.09 ☑
              traffic V02.19 ☑
            vehicle V09.9 ☑
              animal-drawn V06.99 ☑
                nontraffic V06.09 ☑
                traffic V06.19 ☑
              motor
                nontraffic V09.00 ☑
                traffic V09.20 ☑
          fall V00.141 ☑
          nontraffic V09.1 ☑
            involving motor vehicle NEC V09.00 ☑
          traffic V09.3 ☑
            involving motor vehicle NEC V09.20 ☑
        skate board V00.138 ☑
          collision (with) V09.9 ☑
            animal being ridden or animal drawn vehicle V06.92 ☑
              nontraffic V06.02 ☑
              traffic V06.12 ☑
            bus or heavy transport V04.92 ☑
              nontraffic V04.02 ☑
              traffic V04.12 ☑
            car V03.92 ☑
              nontraffic V03.02 ☑
              traffic V03.12 ☑
            pedal cycle V01.92 ☑
              nontraffic V01.02 ☑
              traffic V01.12 ☑
            pick-up truck or van V03.92 ☑
              nontraffic V03.02 ☑
              traffic V03.12 ☑
            railway (train) (vehicle) V05.92 ☑
              nontraffic V05.02 ☑
              traffic V05.12 ☑
            stationary object V00.132 ☑
            streetcar V06.92 ☑
              nontraffic V06.02 ☑
              traffic V06.12 ☑
            two- or three-wheeled motor vehicle V02.92 ☑
              nontraffic V02.02 ☑
              traffic V02.12 ☑
            vehicle V09.9 ☑
              animal-drawn V06.92 ☑
                nontraffic V06.02 ☑
                traffic V06.12 ☑
              motor
                nontraffic V09.00 ☑
                traffic V09.20 ☑
          fall V00.131 ☑
          nontraffic V09.1 ☑
            involving motor vehicle NEC V09.00 ☑
          traffic V09.3 ☑
            involving motor vehicle NEC V09.20 ☑
        skis (snow) V00.328 ☑
          collision (with) V09.9 ☑

Accident — *continued*
  transport — *continued*
    pedestrian — *continued*
      conveyance — *continued*
        skis — *continued*
          collision — *continued*
            animal being ridden or animal drawn vehicle V06.99 ☑
              nontraffic V06.09 ☑
              traffic V06.19 ☑
            bus or heavy transport V04.99 ☑
              nontraffic V04.09 ☑
              traffic V04.19 ☑
            car V03.99 ☑
              nontraffic V03.09 ☑
              traffic V03.19 ☑
            pedal cycle V01.99 ☑
              nontraffic V01.09 ☑
              traffic V01.19 ☑
            pick-up truck or van V03.99 ☑
              nontraffic V03.09 ☑
              traffic V03.19 ☑
            railway (train) (vehicle) V05.99 ☑
              nontraffic V05.09 ☑
              traffic V05.19 ☑
            stationary object V00.322 ☑
            streetcar V06.99 ☑
              nontraffic V06.09 ☑
              traffic V06.19 ☑
            two- or three-wheeled motor vehicle V02.99 ☑
              nontraffic V02.09 ☑
              traffic V02.19 ☑
            vehicle V09.9 ☑
              animal-drawn V06.99 ☑
                nontraffic V06.09 ☑
                traffic V06.19 ☑
              motor
                nontraffic V09.00 ☑
                traffic V09.20 ☑
          fall V00.321 ☑
          nontraffic V09.1 ☑
            involving motor vehicle NEC V09.00 ☑
          traffic V09.3 ☑
            involving motor vehicle NEC V09.20 ☑
        sled V00.228 ☑
          collision (with) V09.9 ☑
            animal being ridden or animal drawn vehicle V06.99 ☑
              nontraffic V06.09 ☑
              traffic V06.19 ☑
            bus or heavy transport V04.99 ☑
              nontraffic V04.09 ☑
              traffic V04.19 ☑
            car V03.99 ☑
              nontraffic V03.09 ☑
              traffic V03.19 ☑
            pedal cycle V01.99 ☑
              nontraffic V01.09 ☑
              traffic V01.19 ☑
            pick-up truck or van V03.99 ☑
              nontraffic V03.09 ☑
              traffic V03.19 ☑
            railway (train) (vehicle) V05.99 ☑
              nontraffic V05.09 ☑
              traffic V05.19 ☑
            stationary object V00.222 ☑
            streetcar V06.99 ☑
              nontraffic V06.09 ☑
              traffic V06.19 ☑
            two- or three-wheeled motor vehicle V02.99 ☑
              nontraffic V02.09 ☑
              traffic V02.19 ☑
            vehicle V09.9 ☑
              animal-drawn V06.99 ☑
                nontraffic V06.09 ☑
                traffic V06.19 ☑
              motor
                nontraffic V09.00 ☑
                traffic V09.20 ☑
          fall V00.221 ☑
          nontraffic V09.1 ☑

Accident — *continued*
  transport — *continued*
    pedestrian — *continued*
      conveyance — *continued*
        sled — *continued*
          nontraffic — *continued*
            involving motor vehicle NEC
              V09.00 ☑
          traffic V09.3 ☑
            involving motor vehicle NEC
              V09.20 ☑
        snow board V00.318 ☑
          collision (with) V09.9 ☑
            animal being ridden or animal drawn
              vehicle V06.99 ☑
              nontraffic V06.09 ☑
              traffic V06.19 ☑
            bus or heavy transport V04.99 ☑
              nontraffic V04.09 ☑
              traffic V04.19 ☑
            car V03.99 ☑
              nontraffic V03.09 ☑
              traffic V03.19 ☑
            pedal cycle V01.99 ☑
              nontraffic V01.09 ☑
              traffic V01.19 ☑
            pick-up truck or van V03.99 ☑
              nontraffic V03.09 ☑
              traffic V03.19 ☑
            railway (train) (vehicle) V05.99 ☑
              nontraffic V05.09 ☑
              traffic V05.19 ☑
            stationary object V00.312 ☑
            streetcar V06.99 ☑
              nontraffic V06.09 ☑
              traffic V06.19 ☑
            two- or three-wheeled motor vehicle
              V02.99 ☑
              nontraffic V02.09 ☑
              traffic V02.19 ☑
            vehicle V09.9 ☑
              animal-drawn V06.99 ☑
                nontraffic V06.09 ☑
                traffic V06.19 ☑
              motor
                nontraffic V09.00 ☑
                traffic V09.20 ☑
          fall V00.311 ☑
          nontraffic V09.1 ☑
            involving motor vehicle NEC
              V09.00 ☑
          traffic V09.3 ☑
            involving motor vehicle NEC
              V09.20 ☑
        specified type NEC V00.898 ☑
          collision (with) V09.9 ☑
            animal being ridden or animal drawn
              vehicle V06.99 ☑
              nontraffic V06.09 ☑
              traffic V06.19 ☑
            bus or heavy transport V04.99 ☑
              nontraffic V04.09 ☑
              traffic V04.19 ☑
            car V03.99 ☑
              nontraffic V03.09 ☑
              traffic V03.19 ☑
            pedal cycle V01.99 ☑
              nontraffic V01.09 ☑
              traffic V01.19 ☑
            pick-up truck or van V03.99 ☑
              nontraffic V03.09 ☑
              traffic V03.19 ☑
            railway (train) (vehicle) V05.99 ☑
              nontraffic V05.09 ☑
              traffic V05.19 ☑
            stationary object V00.892 ☑
            streetcar V06.99 ☑
              nontraffic V06.09 ☑
              traffic V06.19 ☑
            two- or three-wheeled motor vehicle
              V02.99 ☑
              nontraffic V02.09 ☑
              traffic V02.19 ☑
            vehicle V09.9 ☑
              animal-drawn V06.99 ☑
                nontraffic V06.09 ☑

Accident — *continued*
  transport — *continued*
    pedestrian — *continued*
      conveyance — *continued*
        specified type — *continued*
          collision — *continued*
            vehicle — *continued*
              animal-drawn — *continued*
                traffic V06.19 ☑
              motor
                nontraffic V09.00 ☑
                traffic V09.20 ☑
         fall V00.891 ☑
        nontraffic V09.1 ☑
          involving motor vehicle NEC
            V09.00 ☑
        traffic V09.3 ☑
          involving motor vehicle NEC
            V09.20 ☑
      traffic V09.3 ☑
        involving motor vehicle V09.20 ☑
          military V09.21 ☑
          specified type NEC V09.29 ☑
      wheelchair (powered) V00.818 ☑
        collision (with) V09.9 ☑
          animal being ridden or animal drawn
            vehicle V06.99 ☑
            nontraffic V06.09 ☑
            traffic V06.19 ☑
          bus or heavy transport V04.99 ☑
            nontraffic V04.09 ☑
            traffic V04.19 ☑
          car V03.99 ☑
            nontraffic V03.09 ☑
            traffic V03.19 ☑
          pedal cycle V01.99 ☑
            nontraffic V01.09 ☑
            traffic V01.19 ☑
          pick-up truck or van V03.99 ☑
            nontraffic V03.09 ☑
            traffic V03.19 ☑
          railway (train) (vehicle) V05.99 ☑
            nontraffic V05.09 ☑
            traffic V05.19 ☑
          stationary object V00.812 ☑
          streetcar V06.99 ☑
            nontraffic V06.09 ☑
            traffic V06.19 ☑
          two- or three-wheeled motor vehicle
            V02.99 ☑
            nontraffic V02.09 ☑
            traffic V02.19 ☑
          vehicle V09.9 ☑
            animal-drawn V06.99 ☑
              nontraffic V06.09 ☑
              traffic V06.19 ☑
            motor
              nontraffic V09.00 ☑
              traffic V09.20 ☑
        fall V00.811 ☑
        nontraffic V09.1 ☑
          involving motor vehicle NEC
            V09.00 ☑
        traffic V09.3 ☑
          involving motor vehicle NEC
            V09.20 ☑
      wheeled shoe V00.158 ☑
        colliding with stationary object
          V00.152 ☑
        fall V00.151 ☑
     on foot (*see also* Accident, pedestrian)
        collision (with)
          animal being ridden or animal drawn
            vehicle V06.90 ☑
            nontraffic V06.00 ☑
            traffic V06.10 ☑
          bus or heavy transport V04.90 ☑
            nontraffic V04.00 ☑
            traffic V04.10 ☑
          car V03.90 ☑
            nontraffic V03.00 ☑
            traffic V03.10 ☑
          pedal cycle V01.90 ☑
            nontraffic V01.00 ☑
            traffic V01.10 ☑
          pick-up truck or van V03.90 ☑

Accident — *continued*
  transport — *continued*
    pedestrian — *continued*
      on foot (*see also* Accident, pedestrian) — *continued*
        collision — *continued*
          pick-up truck or van — *continued*
            nontraffic V03.00 ☑
            traffic V03.10 ☑
          railway (train) (vehicle) V05.90 ☑
            nontraffic V05.00 ☑
            traffic V05.10 ☑
          streetcar V06.90 ☑
            nontraffic V06.00 ☑
            traffic V06.10 ☑
          two- or three-wheeled motor vehicle
            V02.90 ☑
            nontraffic V02.00 ☑
            traffic V02.10 ☑
          vehicle V09.9 ☑
            animal-drawn V06.90 ☑
              nontraffic V06.00 ☑
              traffic V06.10 ☑
            motor
        nontraffic V09.1 ☑
          involving motor vehicle V09.00 ☑
            military V09.01 ☑
            specified type NEC V09.09 ☑
        traffic V09.3 ☑
          involving motor vehicle V09.20 ☑
            military V09.21 ☑
            specified type NEC V09.29 ☑
    person NEC (unknown way or transportation)
      V99 ☑
    collision (between)
      bus (with)
        heavy transport vehicle (traffic) V87.5 ☑
          nontraffic V88.5 ☑
      car (with)
        bus (traffic) V87.3 ☑
          nontraffic V88.3 ☑
        heavy transport vehicle (traffic) V87.4 ☑
          nontraffic V88.4 ☑
        nontraffic V88.5 ☑
        pick-up truck or van (traffic) V87.2 ☑
          nontraffic V88.2 ☑
        train or railway vehicle (traffic) V87.6 ☑
          nontraffic V88.6 ☑
        two-or three-wheeled motor vehicle
          (traffic) V87.0 ☑
          nontraffic V88.0 ☑
      motor vehicle (traffic) NEC V87.7 ☑
        nontraffic V88.7 ☑
      two-or three-wheeled vehicle (with) (traffic)
        motor vehicle NEC V87.1 ☑
          nontraffic V88.1 ☑
      nonmotor vehicle (collision) (noncollision)
        (traffic) V87.9 ☑
        nontraffic V88.9 ☑
    pickup truck occupant V59.9 ☑
      collision (with)
        animal (traffic) V50.9 ☑
          being ridden (traffic) V56.9 ☑
            nontraffic V56.3 ☑
            while boarding or alighting V56.4 ☑
          nontraffic V50.3 ☑
          while boarding or alighting V50.4 ☑
        animal-drawn vehicle (traffic) V56.9 ☑
          nontraffic V56.3 ☑
          while boarding or alighting V56.4 ☑
        bus (traffic) V54.9 ☑
          nontraffic V54.3 ☑
          while boarding or alighting V54.4 ☑
        car (traffic) V53.9 ☑
          nontraffic V53.3 ☑
          while boarding or alighting V53.4 ☑
        motor vehicle NOS (traffic) V59.60 ☑
          nontraffic V59.20 ☑
          specified type NEC (traffic) V59.69 ☑
            nontraffic V59.29 ☑
        pedal cycle (traffic) V51.9 ☑
          nontraffic V51.3 ☑
          while boarding or alighting V51.4 ☑
        pickup truck (traffic) V53.9 ☑
          nontraffic V53.3 ☑
          while boarding or alighting V53.4 ☑

☑ **Additional Character Required — Refer to the Tabular List for Character Selection**
🔻 **Subterms under main terms may continue to next column or page**

Accident — *continued*
  transport — *continued*
    pickup truck occupant — *continued*
      collision — *continued*
        railway vehicle (traffic) V55.9 ☑
          nontraffic V55.3 ☑
          while boarding or alighting V55.4 ☑
        specified vehicle NEC (traffic) V56.9 ☑
          nontraffic V56.3 ☑
          while boarding or alighting V56.4 ☑
        stationary object (traffic) V57.9 ☑
          nontraffic V57.3 ☑
          while boarding or alighting V57.4 ☑
        streetcar (traffic) V56.9 ☑
          nontraffic V56.3 ☑
          while boarding or alighting V56.4 ☑
        three wheeled motor vehicle (traffic) V52.9 ☑
          nontraffic V52.3 ☑
          while boarding or alighting V52.4 ☑
        truck (traffic) V54.9 ☑
          nontraffic V54.3 ☑
          while boarding or alighting V54.4 ☑
        two wheeled motor vehicle (traffic) V52.9 ☑
          nontraffic V52.3 ☑
          while boarding or alighting V52.4 ☑
        van (traffic) V53.9 ☑
          nontraffic V53.3 ☑
          while boarding or alighting V53.4 ☑
      driver
        collision (with)
          animal (traffic) V50.5 ☑
            being ridden (traffic) V56.5 ☑
              nontraffic V56.0 ☑
            nontraffic V50.0 ☑
          animal-drawn vehicle (traffic) V56.5 ☑
            nontraffic V56.0 ☑
          bus (traffic) V54.5 ☑
            nontraffic V54.0 ☑
          car (traffic) V53.5 ☑
            nontraffic V53.0 ☑
          motor vehicle NOS (traffic) V59.40 ☑
            nontraffic V59.00 ☑
            specified type NEC (traffic) V59.49 ☑
              nontraffic V59.09 ☑
          pedal cycle (traffic) V51.5 ☑
            nontraffic V51.0 ☑
          pickup truck (traffic) V53.5 ☑
            nontraffic V53.0 ☑
          railway vehicle (traffic) V55.5 ☑
            nontraffic V55.0 ☑
          specified vehicle NEC (traffic) V56.5 ☑
            nontraffic V56.0 ☑
          stationary object (traffic) V57.5 ☑
            nontraffic V57.0 ☑
          streetcar (traffic) V56.5 ☑
            nontraffic V56.0 ☑
          three wheeled motor vehicle (traffic) V52.5 ☑
            nontraffic V52.0 ☑
          truck (traffic) V54.5 ☑
            nontraffic V54.0 ☑
          two wheeled motor vehicle (traffic) V52.5 ☑
            nontraffic V52.0 ☑
          van (traffic) V53.5 ☑
            nontraffic V53.0 ☑
        noncollision accident (traffic) V58.5 ☑
          nontraffic V58.0 ☑
      hanger-on
        collision (with)
          animal (traffic) V50.7 ☑
            being ridden (traffic) V56.7 ☑
              nontraffic V56.2 ☑
            nontraffic V50.2 ☑
          animal-drawn vehicle (traffic) V56.7 ☑
            nontraffic V56.2 ☑
          bus (traffic) V54.7 ☑
            nontraffic V54.2 ☑
          car (traffic) V53.7 ☑
            nontraffic V53.2 ☑
          pedal cycle (traffic) V51.7 ☑
            nontraffic V51.2 ☑
          pickup truck (traffic) V53.7 ☑
            nontraffic V53.2 ☑
          railway vehicle (traffic) V55.7 ☑

Accident — *continued*
  transport — *continued*
    pickup truck occupant — *continued*
      hanger-on — *continued*
        collision — *continued*
          railway vehicle — *continued*
            nontraffic V55.2 ☑
          specified vehicle NEC (traffic) V56.7 ☑
            nontraffic V56.2 ☑
          stationary object (traffic) V57.7 ☑
            nontraffic V57.2 ☑
          streetcar (traffic) V56.7 ☑
            nontraffic V56.2 ☑
          three wheeled motor vehicle (traffic) V52.7 ☑
            nontraffic V52.2 ☑
          truck (traffic) V54.7 ☑
            nontraffic V54.2 ☑
          two wheeled motor vehicle (traffic) V52.7 ☑
            nontraffic V52.2 ☑
          van (traffic) V53.7 ☑
            nontraffic V53.2 ☑
        noncollision accident (traffic) V58.7 ☑
          nontraffic V58.2 ☑
      noncollision accident (traffic) V58.9 ☑
        nontraffic V58.3 ☑
        while boarding or alighting V58.4 ☑
      nontraffic V59.3 ☑
      passenger
        collision (with)
          animal (traffic) V50.6 ☑
            being ridden (traffic) V56.6 ☑
              nontraffic V56.1 ☑
            nontraffic V50.1 ☑
          animal-drawn vehicle (traffic) V56.6 ☑
            nontraffic V56.1 ☑
          bus (traffic) V54.6 ☑
            nontraffic V54.1 ☑
          car (traffic) V53.6 ☑
            nontraffic V53.1 ☑
          motor vehicle NOS (traffic) V59.50 ☑
            nontraffic V59.10 ☑
            specified type NEC (traffic) V59.59 ☑
              nontraffic V59.19 ☑
          pedal cycle (traffic) V51.6 ☑
            nontraffic V51.1 ☑
          pickup truck (traffic) V53.6 ☑
            nontraffic V53.1 ☑
          railway vehicle (traffic) V55.6 ☑
            nontraffic V55.1 ☑
          specified vehicle NEC (traffic) V56.6 ☑
            nontraffic V56.1 ☑
          stationary object (traffic) V57.6 ☑
            nontraffic V57.1 ☑
          streetcar (traffic) V56.6 ☑
            nontraffic V56.1 ☑
          three wheeled motor vehicle (traffic) V52.6 ☑
            nontraffic V52.1 ☑
          truck (traffic) V54.6 ☑
            nontraffic V54.1 ☑
          two wheeled motor vehicle (traffic) V52.6 ☑
            nontraffic V52.1 ☑
          van (traffic) V53.6 ☑
            nontraffic V53.1 ☑
        noncollision accident (traffic) V58.6 ☑
          nontraffic V58.1 ☑
      specified type NEC V59.88 ☑
        military vehicle V59.81 ☑
      quarry truck — *see* Accident, transport, industrial vehicle occupant
      race car — *see* Accident, transport, motor vehicle NEC occupant
    railway vehicle occupant V81.9 ☑
      collision (with) V81.3 ☑
        motor vehicle (non-military) (traffic) V81.1 ☑
          military V81.83 ☑
          nontraffic V81.0 ☑
        rolling stock V81.2 ☑
        specified object NEC V81.3 ☑
      during derailment V81.7 ☑

Accident — *continued*
  transport — *continued*
    railway vehicle occupant — *continued*
      during derailment — *continued*
        with antecedent collision — *see* Accident, transport, railway vehicle occupant, collision
      explosion V81.81 ☑
      fall (in railway vehicle) V81.5 ☑
        during derailment V81.7 ☑
          with antecedent collision — *see* Accident, transport, railway vehicle occupant, collision
        from railway vehicle V81.6 ☑
          during derailment V81.7 ☑
            with antecedent collision — *see* Accident, transport, railway vehicle occupant, collision
        while boarding or alighting V81.4 ☑
      fire V81.81 ☑
      object falling onto train V81.82 ☑
      specified type NEC V81.89 ☑
      while boarding or alighting V81.4 ☑
    ski lift V98.3 ☑
    snowmobile occupant (nontraffic) V86.92 ☑
      driver V86.52 ☑
      hanger-on V86.72 ☑
      passenger V86.62 ☑
      traffic V86.32 ☑
        driver V86.02 ☑
        hanger-on V86.22 ☑
        passenger V86.12 ☑
      while boarding or alighting V86.42 ☑
    specified NEC V98.8 ☑
    sport utility vehicle occupant (*see also* Accident, transport, pickup truck occupant)
    streetcar occupant V82.9 ☑
      collision (with) V82.3 ☑
        motor vehicle (traffic) V82.1 ☑
          nontraffic V82.0 ☑
        rolling stock V82.2 ☑
      during derailment V82.7 ☑
        with antecedent collision — *see* Accident, transport, streetcar occupant, collision
      fall (in streetcar) V82.5 ☑
        during derailment V82.7 ☑
          with antecedent collision — *see* Accident, transport, streetcar occupant, collision
        from streetcar V82.6 ☑
          during derailment V82.7 ☑
            with antecedent collision — *see* Accident, transport, streetcar occupant, collision
        while boarding or alighting V82.4 ☑
      while boarding or alighting V82.4 ☑
      specified type NEC V82.8 ☑
      while boarding or alighting V82.4 ☑
    three-wheeled motor vehicle occupant V39.9 ☑
      collision (with)
        animal (traffic) V30.9 ☑
          being ridden (traffic) V36.9 ☑
            nontraffic V36.3 ☑
            while boarding or alighting V36.4 ☑
          nontraffic V30.3 ☑
          while boarding or alighting V30.4 ☑
        animal-drawn vehicle (traffic) V36.9 ☑
          nontraffic V36.3 ☑
          while boarding or alighting V36.4 ☑
        bus (traffic) V34.9 ☑
          nontraffic V34.3 ☑
          while boarding or alighting V34.4 ☑
        car (traffic) V33.9 ☑
          nontraffic V33.3 ☑
          while boarding or alighting V33.4 ☑
        motor vehicle NOS (traffic) V39.60 ☑
          nontraffic V39.20 ☑
          specified type NEC (traffic) V39.69 ☑
            nontraffic V39.29 ☑
        pedal cycle (traffic) V31.9 ☑
          nontraffic V31.3 ☑
          while boarding or alighting V31.4 ☑
        pickup truck (traffic) V33.9 ☑
          nontraffic V33.3 ☑
          while boarding or alighting V33.4 ☑
        railway vehicle (traffic) V35.9 ☑

Accident — *continued*
  transport — *continued*
    three-wheeled motor vehicle occupant — *continued*
      collision — *continued*
        railway vehicle — *continued*
          nontraffic V35.3 ☑
          while boarding or alighting V35.4 ☑
        specified vehicle NEC (traffic) V36.9 ☑
          nontraffic V36.3 ☑
          while boarding or alighting V36.4 ☑
        stationary object (traffic) V37.9 ☑
          nontraffic V37.3 ☑
          while boarding or alighting V37.4 ☑
        streetcar (traffic) V36.9 ☑
          nontraffic V36.3 ☑
          while boarding or alighting V36.4 ☑
        three wheeled motor vehicle (traffic) V32.9 ☑
          nontraffic V32.3 ☑
          while boarding or alighting V32.4 ☑
        truck (traffic) V34.9 ☑
          nontraffic V34.3 ☑
          while boarding or alighting V34.4 ☑
        two wheeled motor vehicle (traffic) V32.9 ☑
          nontraffic V32.3 ☑
          while boarding or alighting V32.4 ☑
        van (traffic) V33.9 ☑
          nontraffic V33.3 ☑
          while boarding or alighting V33.4 ☑
      driver
        collision (with)
          animal (traffic) V30.5 ☑
            being ridden (traffic) V36.5 ☑
              nontraffic V36.0 ☑
            nontraffic V30.1 ☑
          animal-drawn vehicle (traffic) V36.5 ☑
            nontraffic V36.0 ☑
          bus (traffic) V34.5 ☑
            nontraffic V34.0 ☑
          car (traffic) V33.5 ☑
            nontraffic V33.0 ☑
          motor vehicle NOS (traffic) V39.40 ☑
            nontraffic V39.00 ☑
            specified type NEC (traffic) V39.49 ☑
              nontraffic V39.09 ☑
          pedal cycle (traffic) V31.5 ☑
            nontraffic V31.0 ☑
          pickup truck (traffic) V33.5 ☑
            nontraffic V33.0 ☑
          railway vehicle (traffic) V35.5 ☑
            nontraffic V35.0 ☑
          specified vehicle NEC (traffic) V36.5 ☑
            nontraffic V36.0 ☑
          stationary object (traffic) V37.5 ☑
            nontraffic V37.0 ☑
          streetcar (traffic) V36.5 ☑
            nontraffic V36.0 ☑
          three wheeled motor vehicle (traffic) V32.5 ☑
            nontraffic V32.0 ☑
          truck (traffic) V34.5 ☑
            nontraffic V34.0 ☑
          two wheeled motor vehicle (traffic) V32.5 ☑
            nontraffic V32.0 ☑
          van (traffic) V33.5 ☑
            nontraffic V33.0 ☑
        noncollision accident (traffic) V38.5 ☑
          nontraffic V38.0 ☑
      hanger-on
        collision (with)
          animal (traffic) V30.7 ☑
            being ridden (traffic) V36.7 ☑
              nontraffic V36.2 ☑
            nontraffic V30.2 ☑
          animal-drawn vehicle (traffic) V36.7 ☑
            nontraffic V36.2 ☑
          bus (traffic) V34.7 ☑
            nontraffic V34.2 ☑
          car (traffic) V33.7 ☑
            nontraffic V33.2 ☑
          pedal cycle (traffic) V31.7 ☑
            nontraffic V31.2 ☑
          pickup truck (traffic) V33.7 ☑
            nontraffic V33.2 ☑

Accident — *continued*
  transport — *continued*
    three-wheeled motor vehicle occupant — *continued*
      hanger-on — *continued*
        collision — *continued*
          railway vehicle (traffic) V35.7 ☑
            nontraffic V35.2 ☑
          specified vehicle NEC (traffic) V36.7 ☑
            nontraffic V36.2 ☑
          stationary object (traffic) V37.7 ☑
            nontraffic V37.2 ☑
          streetcar (traffic) V36.7 ☑
            nontraffic V36.2 ☑
          three wheeled motor vehicle (traffic) V32.7 ☑
            nontraffic V32.2 ☑
          truck (traffic) V34.7 ☑
            nontraffic V34.2 ☑
          two wheeled motor vehicle (traffic) V32.7 ☑
            nontraffic V32.2 ☑
          van (traffic) V33.7 ☑
            nontraffic V33.2 ☑
        noncollision accident (traffic) V38.7 ☑
          nontraffic V38.2 ☑
      noncollision accident (traffic) V38.9 ☑
        nontraffic V38.3 ☑
        while boarding or alighting V38.4 ☑
      nontraffic V39.3 ☑
      passenger
        collision (with)
          animal (traffic) V30.6 ☑
            being ridden (traffic) V36.6 ☑
              nontraffic V36.1 ☑
            nontraffic V30.1 ☑
          animal-drawn vehicle (traffic) V36.6 ☑
            nontraffic V36.1 ☑
          bus (traffic) V34.6 ☑
            nontraffic V34.1 ☑
          car (traffic) V33.6 ☑
            nontraffic V33.1 ☑
          motor vehicle NOS (traffic) V39.50 ☑
            nontraffic V39.10 ☑
            specified type NEC (traffic) V39.59 ☑
              nontraffic V39.19 ☑
          pedal cycle (traffic) V31.6 ☑
            nontraffic V31.1 ☑
          pickup truck (traffic) V33.6 ☑
            nontraffic V33.1 ☑
          railway vehicle (traffic) V35.6 ☑
            nontraffic V35.1 ☑
          specified vehicle NEC (traffic) V36.6 ☑
            nontraffic V36.1 ☑
          stationary object (traffic) V37.6 ☑
            nontraffic V37.1 ☑
          streetcar (traffic) V36.6 ☑
            nontraffic V36.1 ☑
          three wheeled motor vehicle (traffic) V32.6 ☑
            nontraffic V32.1 ☑
          truck (traffic) V34.6 ☑
            nontraffic V34.1 ☑
          two wheeled motor vehicle (traffic) V32.6 ☑
            nontraffic V32.1 ☑
          van (traffic) V33.6 ☑
            nontraffic V33.1 ☑
        noncollision accident (traffic) V38.6 ☑
          nontraffic V38.1 ☑
      specified type NEC V39.89 ☑
      military vehicle V39.81 ☑
    tractor (farm) (and trailer) — *see* Accident, transport, agricultural vehicle occupant
    tram — *see* Accident, transport, streetcar
      in mine or quarry — *see* Accident, transport, industrial vehicle occupant
    trolley — *see* Accident, transport, streetcar
      in mine or quarry — *see* Accident, transport, industrial vehicle occupant
    truck (heavy) occupant V69.9 ☑
      collision (with)
        animal (traffic) V60.9 ☑
          being ridden (traffic) V66.9 ☑
            nontraffic V66.3 ☑
            while boarding or alighting V66.4 ☑

Accident — *continued*
  transport — *continued*
    truck occupant — *continued*
      collision — *continued*
        animal — *continued*
          nontraffic V60.3 ☑
          while boarding or alighting V60.4 ☑
        animal-drawn vehicle (traffic) V66.9 ☑
          nontraffic V66.3 ☑
          while boarding or alighting V66.4 ☑
        bus (traffic) V64.9 ☑
          nontraffic V64.3 ☑
          while boarding or alighting V64.4 ☑
        car (traffic) V63.9 ☑
          nontraffic V63.3 ☑
          while boarding or alighting V63.4 ☑
        motor vehicle NOS (traffic) V69.60 ☑
          nontraffic V69.20 ☑
          specified type NEC (traffic) V69.69 ☑
            nontraffic V69.29 ☑
        pedal cycle (traffic) V61.9 ☑
          nontraffic V61.3 ☑
          while boarding or alighting V61.4 ☑
        pickup truck (traffic) V63.9 ☑
          nontraffic V63.3 ☑
          while boarding or alighting V63.4 ☑
        railway vehicle (traffic) V65.9 ☑
          nontraffic V65.3 ☑
          while boarding or alighting V65.4 ☑
        specified vehicle NEC (traffic) V66.9 ☑
          nontraffic V66.3 ☑
          while boarding or alighting V66.4 ☑
        stationary object (traffic) V67.9 ☑
          nontraffic V67.3 ☑
          while boarding or alighting V67.4 ☑
        streetcar (traffic) V66.9 ☑
          nontraffic V66.3 ☑
          while boarding or alighting V66.4 ☑
        three wheeled motor vehicle (traffic) V62.9 ☑
          nontraffic V62.3 ☑
          while boarding or alighting V62.4 ☑
        truck (traffic) V64.9 ☑
          nontraffic V64.3 ☑
          while boarding or alighting V64.4 ☑
        two wheeled motor vehicle (traffic) V62.9 ☑
          nontraffic V62.3 ☑
          while boarding or alighting V62.4 ☑
        van (traffic) V63.9 ☑
          nontraffic V63.3 ☑
          while boarding or alighting V63.4 ☑
      driver
        collision (with)
          animal (traffic) V60.5 ☑
            being ridden (traffic) V66.5 ☑
              nontraffic V66.0 ☑
            nontraffic V60.0 ☑
          animal-drawn vehicle (traffic) V66.5 ☑
            nontraffic V66.0 ☑
          bus (traffic) V64.5 ☑
            nontraffic V64.0 ☑
          car (traffic) V63.5 ☑
            nontraffic V63.0 ☑
          motor vehicle NOS (traffic) V69.40 ☑
            nontraffic V69.00 ☑
            specified type NEC (traffic) V69.49 ☑
              nontraffic V69.09 ☑
          pedal cycle (traffic) V61.5 ☑
            nontraffic V61.0 ☑
          pickup truck (traffic) V63.5 ☑
            nontraffic V63.0 ☑
          railway vehicle (traffic) V65.5 ☑
            nontraffic V65.0 ☑
          specified vehicle NEC (traffic) V66.5 ☑
            nontraffic V66.0 ☑
          stationary object (traffic) V67.5 ☑
            nontraffic V67.0 ☑
          streetcar (traffic) V66.5 ☑
            nontraffic V66.0 ☑
          three wheeled motor vehicle (traffic) V62.5 ☑
            nontraffic V62.0 ☑
          truck (traffic) V64.5 ☑
            nontraffic V64.0 ☑
          two wheeled motor vehicle (traffic) V62.5 ☑

External Causes Index

Accident — *continued*
　transport — *continued*
　　truck occupant — *continued*
　　　driver — *continued*
　　　　collision — *continued*
　　　　　two wheeled motor vehicle — *continued*
　　　　　　nontraffic V62.0 ☑
　　　　　van (traffic) V63.5 ☑
　　　　　　nontraffic V63.0 ☑
　　　　noncollision accident (traffic) V68.5 ☑
　　　　　nontraffic V68.0 ☑
　　　dump — *see* Accident, transport, construction vehicle occupant
　　　hanger-on
　　　　collision (with)
　　　　　animal (traffic) V60.7 ☑
　　　　　　being ridden (traffic) V66.7 ☑
　　　　　　　nontraffic V66.2 ☑
　　　　　　nontraffic V60.2 ☑
　　　　　animal-drawn vehicle (traffic) V66.7 ☑
　　　　　　nontraffic V66.2 ☑
　　　　　bus (traffic) V64.7 ☑
　　　　　　nontraffic V64.2 ☑
　　　　　car (traffic) V63.7 ☑
　　　　　　nontraffic V63.2 ☑
　　　　　pedal cycle (traffic) V61.7 ☑
　　　　　　nontraffic V61.2 ☑
　　　　　pickup truck (traffic) V63.7 ☑
　　　　　　nontraffic V63.2 ☑
　　　　　railway vehicle (traffic) V65.7 ☑
　　　　　　nontraffic V65.2 ☑
　　　　　specified vehicle NEC (traffic) V66.7 ☑
　　　　　　nontraffic V66.2 ☑
　　　　　stationary object (traffic) V67.7 ☑
　　　　　　nontraffic V67.2 ☑
　　　　　streetcar (traffic) V66.7 ☑
　　　　　　nontraffic V66.2 ☑
　　　　　three wheeled motor vehicle (traffic) V62.7 ☑
　　　　　　nontraffic V62.2 ☑
　　　　　truck (traffic) V64.7 ☑
　　　　　　nontraffic V64.2 ☑
　　　　　two wheeled motor vehicle (traffic) V62.7 ☑
　　　　　　nontraffic V62.2 ☑
　　　　　van (traffic) V63.7 ☑
　　　　　　nontraffic V63.2 ☑
　　　　noncollision accident (traffic) V68.7 ☑
　　　　　nontraffic V68.2 ☑
　　　noncollision accident (traffic) V68.9 ☑
　　　　nontraffic V68.3 ☑
　　　　while boarding or alighting V68.4 ☑
　　　nontraffic V69.3 ☑
　　　passenger
　　　　collision (with)
　　　　　animal (traffic) V60.6 ☑
　　　　　　being ridden (traffic) V66.6 ☑
　　　　　　　nontraffic V66.1- ☑
　　　　　　nontraffic V60.1 ☑
　　　　　animal-drawn vehicle (traffic) V66.6 ☑
　　　　　　nontraffic V66.1 ☑
　　　　　bus (traffic) V64.6 ☑
　　　　　　nontraffic V64.1 ☑
　　　　　car (traffic) V63.6 ☑
　　　　　　nontraffic V63.1 ☑
　　　　　motor vehicle NOS (traffic) V69.50 ☑
　　　　　　nontraffic V69.10 ☑
　　　　　　specified type NEC (traffic) V69.59 ☑
　　　　　　　nontraffic V69.19 ☑
　　　　　pedal cycle (traffic) V61.6 ☑
　　　　　　nontraffic V61.1 ☑
　　　　　pickup truck (traffic) V63.6 ☑
　　　　　　nontraffic V63.1 ☑
　　　　　railway vehicle (traffic) V65.6 ☑
　　　　　　nontraffic V65.1 ☑
　　　　　specified vehicle NEC (traffic) V66.6 ☑
　　　　　　nontraffic V66.1 ☑
　　　　　stationary object (traffic) V67.6 ☑
　　　　　　nontraffic V67.1 ☑
　　　　　streetcar (traffic) V66.6 ☑
　　　　　　nontraffic V66.1 ☑
　　　　　three wheeled motor vehicle (traffic) V62.6 ☑
　　　　　　nontraffic V62.1 ☑
　　　　　truck (traffic) V64.6 ☑

Accident — *continued*
　transport — *continued*
　　truck occupant — *continued*
　　　passenger — *continued*
　　　　collision — *continued*
　　　　　truck — *continued*
　　　　　　nontraffic V64.1 ☑
　　　　　two wheeled motor vehicle (traffic) V62.6 ☑
　　　　　　nontraffic V62.1 ☑
　　　　　van (traffic) V63.6 ☑
　　　　　　nontraffic V63.1 ☑
　　　　noncollision accident (traffic) V68.6 ☑
　　　　　nontraffic V68.1 ☑
　　　pickup — *see* Accident, transport, pickup truck occupant
　　　specified type NEC V69.88 ☑
　　　military vehicle V69.81 ☑
　　van occupant V59.9 ☑
　　　collision (with)
　　　　animal (traffic) V50.9 ☑
　　　　　being ridden (traffic) V56.9 ☑
　　　　　　nontraffic V56.3 ☑
　　　　　　while boarding or alighting V56.4 ☑
　　　　　nontraffic V50.3 ☑
　　　　　while boarding or alighting V50.4 ☑
　　　　animal-drawn vehicle (traffic) V56.9 ☑
　　　　　nontraffic V56.3 ☑
　　　　　while boarding or alighting V56.4 ☑
　　　　bus (traffic) V54.9 ☑
　　　　　nontraffic V54.3 ☑
　　　　　while boarding or alighting V54.4 ☑
　　　　car (traffic) V53.9 ☑
　　　　　nontraffic V53.3 ☑
　　　　　while boarding or alighting V53.4 ☑
　　　　motor vehicle NOS (traffic) V59.60 ☑
　　　　　nontraffic V59.20 ☑
　　　　　specified type NEC (traffic) V59.69 ☑
　　　　　　nontraffic V59.29 ☑
　　　　pedal cycle (traffic) V51.9 ☑
　　　　　nontraffic V51.3 ☑
　　　　　while boarding or alighting V51.4 ☑
　　　　pickup truck (traffic) V53.9 ☑
　　　　　nontraffic V53.3 ☑
　　　　　while boarding or alighting V53.4 ☑
　　　　railway vehicle (traffic) V55.9 ☑
　　　　　nontraffic V55.3 ☑
　　　　　while boarding or alighting V55.4 ☑
　　　　specified vehicle NEC (traffic) V56.9 ☑
　　　　　nontraffic V56.3 ☑
　　　　　while boarding or alighting V56.4 ☑
　　　　stationary object (traffic) V57.9 ☑
　　　　　nontraffic V57.3 ☑
　　　　　while boarding or alighting V57.4 ☑
　　　　streetcar (traffic) V56.9 ☑
　　　　　nontraffic V56.3 ☑
　　　　　while boarding or alighting V56.4 ☑
　　　　three wheeled motor vehicle (traffic) V52.9 ☑
　　　　　nontraffic V52.3 ☑
　　　　　while boarding or alighting V52.4 ☑
　　　　truck (traffic) V54.9 ☑
　　　　　nontraffic V54.3 ☑
　　　　　while boarding or alighting V54.4 ☑
　　　　two wheeled motor vehicle (traffic) V52.9 ☑
　　　　　nontraffic V52.3 ☑
　　　　　while boarding or alighting V52.4 ☑
　　　　van (traffic) V53.9 ☑
　　　　　nontraffic V53.3 ☑
　　　　　while boarding or alighting V53.4 ☑
　　　driver
　　　　collision (with)
　　　　　animal (traffic) V50.5 ☑
　　　　　　being ridden (traffic) V56.5 ☑
　　　　　　　nontraffic V56.0 ☑
　　　　　　nontraffic V50.0 ☑
　　　　　animal-drawn vehicle (traffic) V56.5 ☑
　　　　　　nontraffic V56.0 ☑
　　　　　bus (traffic) V54.5 ☑
　　　　　　nontraffic V54.0 ☑
　　　　　car (traffic) V53.5 ☑
　　　　　　nontraffic V53.0 ☑
　　　　　motor vehicle NOS (traffic) V59.40 ☑
　　　　　　nontraffic V59.00 ☑
　　　　　　specified type NEC (traffic) V59.49 ☑
　　　　　　　nontraffic V59.09 ☑

Accident — *continued*
　transport — *continued*
　　van occupant — *continued*
　　　driver — *continued*
　　　　collision — *continued*
　　　　　pedal cycle (traffic) V51.5 ☑
　　　　　　nontraffic V51.0 ☑
　　　　　pickup truck (traffic) V53.5 ☑
　　　　　　nontraffic V53.0 ☑
　　　　　railway vehicle (traffic) V55.5 ☑
　　　　　　nontraffic V55.0 ☑
　　　　　specified vehicle NEC (traffic) V56.5 ☑
　　　　　　nontraffic V56.0 ☑
　　　　　stationary object (traffic) V57.5 ☑
　　　　　　nontraffic V57.0 ☑
　　　　　streetcar (traffic) V56.5 ☑
　　　　　　nontraffic V56.0 ☑
　　　　　three wheeled motor vehicle (traffic) V52.5 ☑
　　　　　　nontraffic V52.0 ☑
　　　　　truck (traffic) V54.5 ☑
　　　　　　nontraffic V54.0 ☑
　　　　　two wheeled motor vehicle (traffic) V52.5 ☑
　　　　　　nontraffic V52.0 ☑
　　　　　van (traffic) V53.5 ☑
　　　　　　nontraffic V53.0 ☑
　　　　noncollision accident (traffic) V58.5 ☑
　　　　　nontraffic V58.0 ☑
　　　hanger-on
　　　　collision (with)
　　　　　animal (traffic) V50.7 ☑
　　　　　　being ridden (traffic) V56.7 ☑
　　　　　　　nontraffic V56.2 ☑
　　　　　　nontraffic V50.2 ☑
　　　　　animal-drawn vehicle (traffic) V56.7 ☑
　　　　　　nontraffic V56.2 ☑
　　　　　bus (traffic) V54.7 ☑
　　　　　　nontraffic V54.2 ☑
　　　　　car (traffic) V53.7 ☑
　　　　　　nontraffic V53.2 ☑
　　　　　pedal cycle (traffic) V51.7 ☑
　　　　　　nontraffic V51.2 ☑
　　　　　pickup truck (traffic) V53.7 ☑
　　　　　　nontraffic V53.2 ☑
　　　　　railway vehicle (traffic) V55.7 ☑
　　　　　　nontraffic V55.2 ☑
　　　　　specified vehicle NEC (traffic) V56.7 ☑
　　　　　　nontraffic V56.2 ☑
　　　　　stationary object (traffic) V57.7 ☑
　　　　　　nontraffic V57.2 ☑
　　　　　streetcar (traffic) V56.7 ☑
　　　　　　nontraffic V56.2 ☑
　　　　　three wheeled motor vehicle (traffic) V52.7 ☑
　　　　　　nontraffic V52.2 ☑
　　　　　truck (traffic) V54.7 ☑
　　　　　　nontraffic V54.2 ☑
　　　　　two wheeled motor vehicle (traffic) V52.7 ☑
　　　　　　nontraffic V52.2 ☑
　　　　　van (traffic) V53.7 ☑
　　　　　　nontraffic V53.2 ☑
　　　　noncollision accident (traffic) V58.7 ☑
　　　　　nontraffic V58.2 ☑
　　　noncollision accident (traffic) V58.9 ☑
　　　　nontraffic V58.3 ☑
　　　　while boarding or alighting V58.4 ☑
　　　nontraffic V59.3 ☑
　　　passenger
　　　　collision (with)
　　　　　animal (traffic) V50.6 ☑
　　　　　　being ridden (traffic) V56.6 ☑
　　　　　　　nontraffic V56.1 ☑
　　　　　　nontraffic V50.1 ☑
　　　　　animal-drawn vehicle (traffic) V56.6 ☑
　　　　　　nontraffic V56.1 ☑
　　　　　bus (traffic) V54.6 ☑
　　　　　　nontraffic V54.1 ☑
　　　　　car (traffic) V53.6 ☑
　　　　　　nontraffic V53.1 ☑
　　　　　motor vehicle NOS (traffic) V59.50 ☑
　　　　　　nontraffic V59.10 ☑
　　　　　　specified type NEC (traffic) V59.59 ☑
　　　　　　　nontraffic V59.19 ☑
　　　　　pedal cycle (traffic) V51.6 ☑

Accident — Accident

Accident — *continued*
  transport — *continued*
    van occupant — *continued*
      passenger — *continued*
        collision — *continued*
          pedal cycle — *continued*
            nontraffic V51.1 ☑
          pickup truck (traffic) V53.6 ☑
            nontraffic V53.1 ☑
          railway vehicle (traffic) V55.6 ☑
            nontraffic V55.1 ☑
          specified vehicle NEC (traffic) V56.6 ☑
            nontraffic V56.1 ☑
          stationary object (traffic) V57.6 ☑
            nontraffic V57.1 ☑
          streetcar (traffic) V56.6 ☑
            nontraffic V56.1 ☑
          three wheeled motor vehicle (traffic) V52.6 ☑
            nontraffic V52.1 ☑
          truck (traffic) V54.6 ☑
            nontraffic V54.1 ☑
          two wheeled motor vehicle (traffic) V52.6 ☑
            nontraffic V52.1 ☑
          van (traffic) V53.6 ☑
            nontraffic V53.1 ☑
        noncollision accident (traffic) V58.6 ☑
          nontraffic V58.1 ☑
      specified type NEC V59.88 ☑
      military vehicle V59.81 ☑
  watercraft occupant — *see* Accident, watercraft
  vehicle NEC V89.9 ☑
    animal-drawn NEC — *see* Accident, transport, animal-drawn vehicle occupant
    special
      agricultural — *see* Accident, transport, agricultural vehicle occupant
      construction — *see* Accident, transport, construction vehicle occupant
      industrial — *see* Accident, transport, industrial vehicle occupant
      three-wheeled NEC (motorized) — *see* Accident, transport, three-wheeled motor vehicle occupant
  watercraft V94.9 ☑
    causing
      drowning — *see* Drowning, due to, accident to, watercraft
      injury NEC V91.89 ☑
        crushed between craft and object V91.19 ☑
          powered craft V91.13 ☑
            ferry boat V91.11 ☑
            fishing boat V91.12 ☑
            jetskis V91.13 ☑
            liner V91.11 ☑
            merchant ship V91.10 ☑
            passenger ship V91.11 ☑
          unpowered craft V91.18 ☑
            canoe V91.15 ☑
            inflatable V91.16 ☑
            kayak V91.15 ☑
            sailboat V91.14 ☑
            surf-board V91.18 ☑
            windsurfer V91.18 ☑
        fall on board V91.29 ☑
          powered craft V91.23 ☑
            ferry boat V91.21 ☑
            fishing boat V91.22 ☑
            jetskis V91.23 ☑
            liner V91.21 ☑
            merchant ship V91.20 ☑
            passenger ship V91.21 ☑
          unpowered craft
            canoe V91.25 ☑
            inflatable V91.26 ☑
            kayak V91.25 ☑
            sailboat V91.24 ☑
        fire on board causing burn V91.09 ☑
          powered craft V91.03 ☑
            ferry boat V91.01 ☑
            fishing boat V91.02 ☑
            jetskis V91.03 ☑
            liner V91.01 ☑
            merchant ship V91.00 ☑
            passenger ship V91.01 ☑

Accident — *continued*
  watercraft — *continued*
    causing — *continued*
      injury — *continued*
        fire on board causing burn — *continued*
          unpowered craft V91.08 ☑
            canoe V91.05 ☑
            inflatable V91.06 ☑
            kayak V91.05 ☑
            sailboat V91.04 ☑
            surf-board V91.08 ☑
            water skis V91.07 ☑
            windsurfer V91.08 ☑
        hit by falling object V91.39 ☑
          powered craft V91.33 ☑
            ferry boat V91.31 ☑
            fishing boat V91.32 ☑
            jetskis V91.33 ☑
            liner V91.31 ☑
            merchant ship V91.30 ☑
            passenger ship V91.31 ☑
          unpowered craft V91.38 ☑
            canoe V91.35 ☑
            inflatable V91.36 ☑
            kayak V91.35 ☑
            sailboat V91.34 ☑
            surf-board V91.38 ☑
            water skis V91.37 ☑
            windsurfer V91.38 ☑
        specified type NEC V91.89 ☑
          powered craft V91.83 ☑
            ferry boat V91.81 ☑
            fishing boat V91.82 ☑
            jetskis V91.83 ☑
            liner V91.81 ☑
            merchant ship V91.80 ☑
            passenger ship V91.81 ☑
          unpowered craft V91.88 ☑
            canoe V91.85 ☑
            inflatable V91.86 ☑
            kayak V91.85 ☑
            sailboat V91.84 ☑
            surf-board V91.88 ☑
            water skis V91.87 ☑
            windsurfer V91.88 ☑
    due to, caused by cataclysm — *see* Forces of nature, by type
    military NEC V94.818 ☑
      with civilian watercraft V94.810 ☑
      civilian in water injured by V94.811 ☑
    nonpowered, struck by
      nonpowered vessel V94.22 ☑
      powered vessel V94.21 ☑
    specified type NEC V94.89 ☑
    striking swimmer
      powered V94.11 ☑
      unpowered V94.12 ☑
Acid throwing (assault) Y08.89 ☑
Activity (involving) (of victim at time of event) Y93.9
  aerobic and step exercise (class) Y93.A3 (*following* Y93.7)
  alpine skiing Y93.23
  animal care NEC Y93.K9 (*following* Y93.7)
  arts and handcrafts NEC Y93.D9 (*following* Y93.7)
  athletics played as a team or group NEC Y93.69
  athletics played individually NEC Y93.59
  athletics NEC Y93.79
  baking Y93.G3 (*following* Y93.7)
  ballet Y93.41
  barbells Y93.B3 (*following* Y93.7)
  BASE (Building, Antenna, Span, Earth) jumping Y93.33
  baseball Y93.64
  basketball Y93.67
  bathing (personal) Y93.E1 (*following* Y93.7)
  beach volleyball Y93.68
  bike riding Y93.55
  blackout game Y93.85
  boogie boarding Y93.18
  bowling Y93.54
  boxing Y93.71
  brass instrument playing Y93.J4 (*following* Y93.7)
  building construction Y93.H3 (*following* Y93.7)
  bungee jumping Y93.34
  calisthenics Y93.A2 (*following* Y93.7)
  canoeing (in calm and turbulent water) Y93.16
  capture the flag Y93.6A
  cardiorespiratory exercise NEC Y93.A9 (*following* Y93.7)

Activity — *continued*
  caregiving (providing) NEC Y93.F9 (*following* Y93.7)
    bathing Y93.F1 (*following* Y93.7)
    lifting Y93.F2 (*following* Y93.7)
  cellular
    communication device Y93.C2 (*following* Y93.7)
    telephone Y93.C2 (*following* Y93.7)
  challenge course Y93.A5 (*following* Y93.7)
  cheerleading Y93.45
  choking game Y93.85
  circuit training Y93.A4 (*following* Y93.7)
  cleaning
    floor Y93.E5 (*following* Y93.7)
  climbing NEC Y93.39
    mountain Y93.31
    rock Y93.31
    wall Y93.31
  clothing care and maintenance NEC Y93.E9 (*following* Y93.7)
  combatives Y93.75
  computer
    keyboarding Y93.C1 (*following* Y93.7)
    technology NEC Y93.C9 (*following* Y93.7)
  confidence course Y93.A5 (*following* Y93.7)
  construction (building) Y93.H3 (*following* Y93.7)
  cooking and baking Y93.G3 (*following* Y93.7)
  cool down exercises Y93.A2 (*following* Y93.7)
  cricket Y93.69
  crocheting Y93.D1 (*following* Y93.7)
  cross country skiing Y93.24
  dancing (all types) Y93.41
  digging
    dirt Y93.H1 (*following* Y93.7)
  dirt digging Y93.H1 (*following* Y93.7)
  dishwashing Y93.G1 (*following* Y93.7)
  diving (platform) (springboard) Y93.12
    underwater Y93.15
  dodge ball Y93.6A
  downhill skiing Y93.23
  drum playing Y93.J2 (*following* Y93.7)
  dumbbells Y93.B3 (*following* Y93.7)
  electronic
    devices NEC Y93.C9 (*following* Y93.7)
      hand held interactive Y93.C2 (*following* Y93.7)
    game playing (using) (with)
      interactive device Y93.C2 (*following* Y93.7)
      keyboard or other stationary device Y93.C1 (*following* Y93.7)
  elliptical machine Y93.A1 (*following* Y93.7)
  exercise(s)
    machines ((primarily) for)
      cardiorespiratory conditioning Y93.A1 (*following* Y93.7)
      muscle strengthening Y93.B1 (*following* Y93.7)
    muscle strengthening (non-machine) NEC Y93.B9 (*following* Y93.7)
  external motion NEC Y93.I9 (*following* Y93.7)
    rollercoaster Y93.I1 (*following* Y93.7)
  fainting game Y93.85
  field hockey Y93.65
  figure skating (pairs) (singles) Y93.21
  flag football Y93.62
  floor mopping and cleaning Y93.E5 (*following* Y93.7)
  food preparation and clean up Y93.G1 (*following* Y93.7)
  football (American) NOS Y93.61
    flag Y93.62
    tackle Y93.61
    touch Y93.62
  four square Y93.6A
  free weights Y93.B3 (*following* Y93.7)
  frisbee (ultimate) Y93.74
  furniture
    building Y93.D3 (*following* Y93.7)
    finishing Y93.D3 (*following* Y93.7)
    repair Y93.D3 (*following* Y93.7)
  game playing (electronic)
    using interactive device Y93.C2 (*following* Y93.7)
    using keyboard or other stationary device Y93.C1 (*following* Y93.7)
  gardening Y93.H2 (*following* Y93.7)
  golf Y93.53
  grass drills Y93.A6 (*following* Y93.7)
  grilling and smoking food Y93.G2 (*following* Y93.7)
  grooming and shearing an animal Y93.K3 (*following* Y93.7)
  guerilla drills Y93.A6 (*following* Y93.7)
  gymnastics (rhythmic) Y93.43
  hand held interactive electronic device Y93.C2 (*following* Y93.7)

Activity — *continued*
  handball Y93.73
  handcrafts NEC Y93.D9 (*following* Y93.7)
  hang gliding Y93.35
  hiking (on level or elevated terrain) Y93.Ø1
  hockey (ice) Y93.22
    field Y93.65
  horseback riding Y93.52
  household (interior) maintenance NEC Y93.E9 (*following* Y93.7)
  ice NEC Y93.29
    dancing Y93.21
    hockey Y93.22
    skating Y93.21
  inline roller skating Y93.51
  ironing Y93.E4 (*following* Y93.7)
  judo Y93.75
  jumping jacks Y93.A2 (*following* Y93.7)
  jumping rope Y93.56
  jumping (off) NEC Y93.39
    BASE (Building, Antenna, Span, Earth) Y93.33
    bungee Y93.34
    jacks Y93.A2 (*following* Y93.7)
    rope Y93.56
  karate Y93.75
  kayaking (in calm and turbulent water) Y93.16
  keyboarding (computer) Y93.C1 (*following* Y93.7)
  kickball Y93.6A
  knitting Y93.D1 (*following* Y93.7)
  lacrosse Y93.65
  land maintenance NEC Y93.H9 (*following* Y93.7)
  landscaping Y93.H2 (*following* Y93.7)
  laundry Y93.E2 (*following* Y93.7)
  machines (exercise)
    primarily for cardiorespiratory conditioning Y93.A1 (*following* Y93.7)
    primarily for muscle strengthening Y93.B1 (*following* Y93.7)
  maintenance
    exterior building NEC Y93.H9 (*following* Y93.7)
    household (interior) NEC Y93.E9 (*following* Y93.7)
    land Y93.H9 (*following* Y93.7)
    property Y93.H9 (*following* Y93.7)
  marching (on level or elevated terrain) Y93.Ø1
  martial arts Y93.75
  microwave oven Y93.G3 (*following* Y93.7)
  milking an animal Y93.K2 (*following* Y93.7)
  mopping (floor) Y93.E5 (*following* Y93.7)
  mountain climbing Y93.31
  muscle strengthening
    exercises (non-machine) NEC Y93.B9 (*following* Y93.7)
    machines Y93.B1 (*following* Y93.7)
  musical keyboard (electronic) playing Y93.J1 (*following* Y93.7)
  nordic skiing Y93.24
  obstacle course Y93.A5 (*following* Y93.7)
  oven (microwave) Y93.G3 (*following* Y93.7)
  packing up and unpacking in moving to a new residence Y93.E6 (*following* Y93.7)
  parasailing Y93.19
  pass out game Y93.85
  percussion instrument playing NEC Y93.J2 (*following* Y93.7)
  personal
    bathing and showering Y93.E1 (*following* Y93.7)
    hygiene NEC Y93.E8 (*following* Y93.7)
    showering Y93.E1 (*following* Y93.7)
  physical games generally associated with school recess, summer camp and children Y93.6A
  physical training NEC Y93.A9 (*following* Y93.7)
  piano playing Y93.J1 (*following* Y93.7)
  pilates Y93.B4 (*following* Y93.7)
  platform diving Y93.12
  playing musical instrument
    brass instrument Y93.J4 (*following* Y93.7)
    drum Y93.J2 (*following* Y93.7)
    musical keyboard (electronic) Y93.J1 (*following* Y93.7)
    percussion instrument NEC Y93.J2 (*following* Y93.7)
    piano Y93.J1 (*following* Y93.7)
    string instrument Y93.J3 (*following* Y93.7)
    winds instrument Y93.J4 (*following* Y93.7)
  property maintenance
    exterior NEC Y93.H9 (*following* Y93.7)
    interior NEC Y93.E9 (*following* Y93.7)
  pruning (garden and lawn) Y93.H2 (*following* Y93.7)
  pull-ups Y93.B2 (*following* Y93.7)
  push-ups Y93.B2 (*following* Y93.7)

Activity — *continued*
  racquetball Y93.73
  rafting (in calm and turbulent water) Y93.16
  raking (leaves) Y93.H1 (*following* Y93.7)
  rappelling Y93.32
  refereeing a sports activity Y93.81
  residential relocation Y93.E6 (*following* Y93.7)
  rhythmic gymnastics Y93.43
  rhythmic movement NEC Y93.49
  riding
    horseback Y93.52
    rollercoaster Y93.I1 (*following* Y93.7)
  rock climbing Y93.31
  roller skating (inline) Y93.51
  rollercoaster riding Y93.I1 (*following* Y93.7)
  rough housing and horseplay Y93.83
  rowing (in calm and turbulent water) Y93.16
  rugby Y93.63
  running Y93.Ø2
  SCUBA diving Y93.15
  sewing Y93.D2 (*following* Y93.7)
  shoveling Y93.H1 (*following* Y93.7)
    dirt Y93.H1 (*following* Y93.7)
    snow Y93.H1 (*following* Y93.7)
  showering (personal) Y93.E1 (*following* Y93.7)
  sit-ups Y93.B2 (*following* Y93.7)
  skateboarding Y93.51
  skating (ice) Y93.21
    roller Y93.51
  skiing (alpine) (downhill) Y93.23
    cross country Y93.24
    nordic Y93.24
    water Y93.17
  sledding (snow) Y93.23
  sleeping (sleep) Y93.84
  smoking and grilling food Y93.G2 (*following* Y93.7)
  snorkeling Y93.15
  snow NEC Y93.29
    boarding Y93.23
    shoveling Y93.H1 (*following* Y93.7)
    sledding Y93.23
    tubing Y93.23
  soccer Y93.66
  softball Y93.64
  specified NEC Y93.89
  spectator at an event Y93.82
  sports NEC Y93.79
    sports played as a team or group NEC Y93.69
    sports played individually NEC Y93.59
  springboard diving Y93.12
  squash Y93.73
  stationary bike Y93.A1 (*following* Y93.7)
  step (stepping) exercise (class) Y93.A3 (*following* Y93.7)
  stepper machine Y93.A1 (*following* Y93.7)
  stove Y93.G3 (*following* Y93.7)
  string instrument playing Y93.J3 (*following* Y93.7)
  surfing Y93.18
    wind Y93.18
  swimming Y93.11
  tackle football Y93.61
  tap dancing Y93.41
  tennis Y93.73
  tobogganing Y93.23
  touch football Y93.62
  track and field events (non-running) Y93.57
    running Y93.Ø2
  trampoline Y93.44
  treadmill Y93.A1 (*following* Y93.7)
  trimming shrubs Y93.H2 (*following* Y93.7)
  tubing (in calm and turbulent water) Y93.16
    snow Y93.23
  ultimate frisbee Y93.74
  underwater diving Y93.15
  unpacking in moving to a new residence Y93.E6 (*following* Y93.7)
  use of stove, oven and microwave oven Y93.G3 (*following* Y93.7)
  vacuuming Y93.E3 (*following* Y93.7)
  volleyball (beach) (court) Y93.68
  wake boarding Y93.17
  walking (on level or elevated terrain) Y93.Ø1
    an animal Y93.K1 (*following* Y93.7)
  walking an animal Y93.K1 (*following* Y93.7)
  wall climbing Y93.31
  warm up and cool down exercises Y93.A2 (*following* Y93.7)
  water NEC Y93.19
    aerobics Y93.14
    craft NEC Y93.19

Activity — *continued*
  water — *continued*
    exercise Y93.14
    polo Y93.13
    skiing Y93.17
    sliding Y93.18
    survival training and testing Y93.19
  weeding (garden and lawn) Y93.H2 (*following* Y93.7)
  wind instrument playing Y93.J4 (*following* Y93.7)
  windsurfing Y93.18
  wrestling Y93.72
  yoga Y93.42
Adverse effect of drugs — *see* Table of Drugs and Chemicals
Aerosinusitis — *see* Air, pressure
After-effect, late — *see* Sequelae
Air
  blast in war operations — *see* War operations, air blast
  pressure
    change, rapid
      during
        ascent W94.29 ☑
          while (in) (surfacing from)
            aircraft W94.23 ☑
            deep water diving W94.21 ☑
            underground W94.22 ☑
        descent W94.39 ☑
          in
            aircraft W94.31 ☑
            water W94.32 ☑
    high, prolonged W94.Ø ☑
    low, prolonged W94.12 ☑
      due to residence or long visit at high altitude W94.11 ☑
Alpine sickness W94.11 ☑
Altitude sickness W94.11 ☑
Anaphylactic shock, anaphylaxis — *see* Table of Drugs and Chemicals
Andes disease W94.11 ☑
Arachnidism, arachnoidism X58 ☑
Arson (with intent to injure or kill) X97 ☑
Asphyxia, asphyxiation
  by
    food (bone) (seed) — *see* categories T17 and T18 ☑
    gas (*see also* Table of Drugs and Chemicals)
      legal
        execution — *see* Legal, intervention, gas
        intervention — *see* Legal, intervention, gas
  from
    fire (*see also* Exposure, fire)
      in war operations — *see* War operations, fire
    ignition — *see* Ignition
    vomitus T17.81 ☑
  in war operations — *see* War operations, restriction of airway
Aspiration
  food (any type) (into respiratory tract) (with asphyxia, obstruction respiratory tract, suffocation) — *see* categories T17 and T18 ☑
  foreign body — *see* Foreign body, aspiration
  vomitus (with asphyxia, obstruction respiratory tract, suffocation) T17.81 ☑
Assassination (attempt) — *see* Assault
Assault (homicidal) (by) (in) YØ9
  arson X97 ☑
  bite (of human being) YØ4.1 ☑
  bodily force YØ4.8 ☑
    bite YØ4.1 ☑
    bumping into YØ4.2 ☑
    sexual — *see* subcategories T74.Ø, T76.Ø ☑
    unarmed fight YØ4.Ø ☑
  bomb X96.9 ☑
    antipersonnel X96.Ø ☑
    fertilizer X96.3 ☑
    gasoline X96.1 ☑
    letter X96.2 ☑
    petrol X96.1 ☑
    pipe X96.3 ☑
    specified NEC X96.8 ☑
  brawl (hand) (fists) (foot) (unarmed) YØ4.Ø ☑
  burning, burns (by fire) NEC X97 ☑
    acid YØ8.89 ☑
    caustic, corrosive substance YØ8.89 ☑
    chemical from swallowing caustic, corrosive substance — *see* Table of Drugs and Chemicals

Assault — *continued*
  burning, burns — *continued*
    cigarette(s) X97 ☑
    hot object X98.9 ☑
      fluid NEC X98.2 ☑
      household appliance X98.3 ☑
      specified NEC X98.8 ☑
      steam X98.0 ☑
      tap water X98.1 ☑
      vapors X98.0 ☑
    scalding — *see* Assault, burning
    steam X98.0 ☑
    vitriol Y08.89 ☑
  caustic, corrosive substance (gas) Y08.89 ☑
  crashing of
    aircraft Y08.81 ☑
    motor vehicle Y03.8 ☑
      pushed in front of Y02.0 ☑
      run over Y03.0 ☑
      specified NEC Y03.8 ☑
  cutting or piercing instrument X99.9 ☑
    dagger X99.2 ☑
    glass X99.0 ☑
    knife X99.1 ☑
    specified NEC X99.8 ☑
    sword X99.2 ☑
  dagger X99.2 ☑
  drowning (in) X92.9 ☑
    bathtub X92.0 ☑
    natural water X92.3 ☑
    specified NEC X92.8 ☑
    swimming pool X92.1 ☑
      following fall X92.2 ☑
  dynamite X96.8 ☑
  explosive(s) (material) X96.9 ☑
  fight (hand) (fists) (foot) (unarmed) Y04.0 ☑
    with weapon — *see* Assault, by type of weapon
  fire X97 ☑
  firearm X95.9 ☑
    airgun X95.01 ☑
    handgun X93 ☑
    hunting rifle X94.1 ☑
    larger X94.9 ☑
      specified NEC X94.8 ☑
    machine gun X94.2 ☑
    shotgun X94.0 ☑
    specified NEC X95.8 ☑
  from high place Y01 ☑
  gunshot (wound) NEC — *see* Assault, firearm, by type
  incendiary device X97 ☑
  injury Y09
    to child due to criminal abortion attempt NEC
      Y08.89 ☑
  knife X99.1 ☑
  late effect of — *see* categories X92-Y08 with 7th
    character S
  placing before moving object NEC Y02.8 ☑
    motor vehicle Y02.0 ☑
  poisoning — *see* categories T36-T65 with 7th character
    S
  puncture, any part of body — *see* Assault, cutting or
    piercing instrument
  pushing
    before moving object NEC Y02.8 ☑
      motor vehicle Y02.0 ☑
      subway train Y02.1 ☑
      train Y02.1 ☑
    from high place Y01 ☑
  rape T74.2-
  scalding — *see* Assault, burning
  sequelae of — *see* categories X92-Y08 with 7th char-
    acter S
  sexual (by bodily force) T74.2- ☑
  shooting — *see* Assault, firearm
  specified means NEC Y08.89 ☑
  stab, any part of body — *see* Assault, cutting or pierc-
    ing instrument
  steam X98.0 ☑
  striking against
    other person Y04.2 ☑
    sports equipment Y08.09 ☑
      baseball bat Y08.02 ☑
      hockey stick Y08.01 ☑
  struck by
    sports equipment Y08.09 ☑
      baseball bat Y08.02 ☑

Assault — *continued*
  struck by — *continued*
    sports equipment — *continued*
      hockey stick Y08.01 ☑
  submersion — *see* Assault, drowning
  violence Y09
  weapon Y09
    blunt Y00 ☑
    cutting or piercing — *see* Assault, cutting or
      piercing instrument
    firearm — *see* Assault, firearm
  wound Y09
    cutting — *see* Assault, cutting or piercing instru-
      ment
    gunshot — *see* Assault, firearm
    knife X99.1 ☑
    piercing — *see* Assault, cutting or piercing instru-
      ment
    puncture — *see* Assault, cutting or piercing instru-
      ment
    stab — *see* Assault, cutting or piercing instrument
Attack by mammals NEC W55.89 ☑
Avalanche — *see* Landslide
Aviator's disease — *see* Air, pressure

B

Barotitis, barodontalgia, barosinusitis, barotrauma
  (otitic) (sinus) — *see* Air, pressure
Battered (baby) (child) (person) (syndrome) X58 ☑
Bayonet wound W26.1 ☑
  in
    legal intervention — *see* Legal, intervention, sharp
      object, bayonet
    war operations — *see* War operations, combat
  stated as undetermined whether accidental or inten-
    tional Y28.8 ☑
  suicide (attempt) X78.2 ☑
Bean in nose — *see* categories T17 and T18 ☑
Bed set on fire NEC — *see* Exposure, fire, uncontrolled,
  building, bed
Beheading (by guillotine)
  homicide X99.9 ☑
  legal execution — *see* Legal, intervention
Bending, injury in (prolonged) (static) X50.1 ☑
Bends — *see* Air, pressure, change
Bite, bitten by
  alligator W58.01 ☑
  arthropod (nonvenomous) NEC W57 ☑
  bull W55.21 ☑
  cat W55.01 ☑
  cow W55.21 ☑
  crocodile W58.11 ☑
  dog W54.0 ☑
  goat W55.31 ☑
  hoof stock NEC W55.31 ☑
  horse W55.11 ☑
  human being (accidentally) W50.3 ☑
    with intent to injure or kill Y04.1 ☑
    as, or caused by, a crowd or human stampede (with
      fall) W52 ☑
    assault Y04.1 ☑
    homicide (attempt) Y04.1 ☑
    in
      fight Y04.1 ☑
  insect (nonvenomous) W57 ☑
  lizard (nonvenomous) W59.01 ☑
  mammal NEC W55.81 ☑
    marine W56.31 ☑
  marine animal (nonvenomous) W56.81 ☑
  millipede W57 ☑
  moray eel W56.51 ☑
  mouse W53.01 ☑
  person(s) (accidentally) W50.3 ☑
    with intent to injure or kill Y04.1 ☑
    as, or caused by, a crowd or human stampede (with
      fall) W52 ☑
    assault Y04.1 ☑
    homicide (attempt) Y04.1 ☑
    in
      fight Y04.1 ☑
  pig W55.41 ☑
  raccoon W55.51 ☑
  rat W53.11 ☑
  reptile W59.81 ☑
    lizard W59.01 ☑

Bite, bitten by — *continued*
  reptile — *continued*
    snake W59.11 ☑
    turtle W59.21 ☑
      terrestrial W59.81 ☑
  rodent W53.81 ☑
    mouse W53.01 ☑
    rat W53.11 ☑
    specified NEC W53.81 ☑
    squirrel W53.21 ☑
  shark W56.41 ☑
  sheep W55.31 ☑
  snake (nonvenomous) W59.11 ☑
  spider (nonvenomous) W57 ☑
  squirrel W53.21 ☑
Blast (air) in war operations — *see* War operations, blast
Blizzard X37.2 ☑
Blood alcohol level Y90.9
  less than 20mg/100ml Y90.0
  20-39mg/100ml Y90.1
  40-59mg/100ml Y90.2
  60-79mg/100ml Y90.3
  80-99mg/100ml Y90.4
  100-119mg/100ml Y90.5
  120-199mg/100ml Y90.6
  200-239mg/100ml Y90.7
  presence in blood, level not specified Y90.9
Blow X58 ☑
  by law-enforcing agent, police (on duty) — *see* Legal,
    intervention, manhandling
    blunt object — *see* Legal, intervention, blunt object
Blowing up — *see* Explosion
Brawl (hand) (fists) (foot) Y04.0 ☑
Breakage (accidental) (part of)
  ladder (causing fall) W11 ☑
  scaffolding (causing fall) W12 ☑
Broken
  glass, contact with — *see* Contact, with, glass
  power line (causing electric shock) W85 ☑
Bumping against, into (accidentally)
  object NEC W22.8 ☑
    with fall — *see* Fall, due to, bumping against, ob-
      ject
    caused by crowd or human stampede (with fall)
      W52 ☑
    sports equipment W21.9 ☑
  person(s) W51 ☑
    with fall W03 ☑
      due to ice or snow W00.0 ☑
    assault Y04.2 ☑
    caused by, a crowd or human stampede (with fall)
      W52 ☑
    homicide (attempt) Y04.2 ☑
  sports equipment W21.9 ☑
Burn, burned, burning (accidental) (by) (from) (on)
  acid NEC — *see* Table of Drugs and Chemicals
  bed linen — *see* Exposure, fire, uncontrolled, in
    building, bed
  blowtorch X08.8 ☑
    with ignition of clothing NEC X06.2 ☑
      nightwear X05 ☑
  bonfire, campfire (controlled) (*see also* Exposure, fire,
    controlled, not in building)
    uncontrolled — *see* Exposure, fire, uncontrolled,
      not in building
  candle X08.8 ☑
    with ignition of clothing NEC X06.2 ☑
      nightwear X05 ☑
  caustic liquid, substance (external) (internal) NEC —
    see Table of Drugs and Chemicals
  chemical (external) (internal) (*see also* Table of Drugs
    and Chemicals)
    in war operations — *see* War operations. fire
  cigar(s) or cigarette(s) X08.8 ☑
    with ignition of clothing NEC X06.2 ☑
      nightwear X05 ☑
  clothes, clothing NEC (from controlled fire) X06.2 ☑
    with conflagration — *see* Exposure, fire, uncon-
      trolled, building
    not in building or structure — *see* Exposure,
      fire, uncontrolled, not in building
  cooker (hot) X15.8 ☑
    stated as undetermined whether accidental or in-
      tentional Y27.3 ☑
    suicide (attempt) X77.3 ☑
  electric blanket X16 ☑

Burn, burned, burning — *continued*
- engine (hot) X17 ☑
- fire, flames — *see* Exposure, fire
- flare, Very pistol — *see* Discharge, firearm NEC
- heat
  - from appliance (electrical) (household) X15.8 ☑
    - cooker X15.8 ☑
    - hotplate X15.2 ☑
    - kettle X15.8 ☑
    - light bulb X15.8 ☑
    - saucepan X15.3 ☑
    - skillet X15.3 ☑
    - stated as undetermined whether accidental or intentional Y27.3 ☑
    - stove X15.0 ☑
    - suicide (attempt) X77.3 ☑
    - toaster X15.1 ☑
  - in local application or packing during medical or surgical procedure Y63.5
- heating
  - appliance, radiator or pipe X16 ☑
- homicide (attempt) — *see* Assault, burning
- hot
  - air X14.1 ☑
  - cooker X15.8 ☑
  - drink X10.0 ☑
  - engine X17 ☑
  - fat X10.2 ☑
  - fluid NEC X12 ☑
  - food X10.1 ☑
  - gases X14.1 ☑
  - heating appliance X16 ☑
  - household appliance NEC X15.8 ☑
  - kettle X15.8 ☑
  - liquid NEC X12 ☑
  - machinery X17 ☑
  - metal (molten) (liquid) NEC X18 ☑
  - object (not producing fire or flames) NEC X19 ☑
  - oil (cooking) X10.2 ☑
  - pipe(s) X16 ☑
  - radiator X16 ☑
  - saucepan (glass) (metal) X15.3 ☑
  - stove (kitchen) X15.0 ☑
  - substance NEC X19 ☑
    - caustic or corrosive NEC — *see* Table of Drugs and Chemicals
  - toaster X15.1 ☑
  - tool X17 ☑
  - vapor X13.1 ☑
  - water (tap) — *see* Contact, with, hot, tap water
- hotplate X15.2 ☑
  - suicide (attempt) X77.3 ☑
- ignition — *see* Ignition
- in war operations — *see* War operations, fire
- inflicted by other person X97 ☑
  - by hot objects, hot vapor, and steam — *see* Assault, burning, hot object
- internal, from swallowed caustic, corrosive liquid, substance — *see* Table of Drugs and Chemicals
- iron (hot) X15.8 ☑
  - stated as undetermined whether accidental or intentional Y27.3 ☑
  - suicide (attempt) X77.3 ☑
- kettle (hot) X15.8 ☑
  - stated as undetermined whether accidental or intentional Y27.3 ☑
  - suicide (attempt) X77.3 ☑
- lamp (flame) X08.8 ☑
  - with ignition of clothing NEC X06.2 ☑
    - nightwear X05 ☑
- lighter (cigar) (cigarette) X08.8 ☑
  - with ignition of clothing NEC X06.2 ☑
    - nightwear X05 ☑
- lightning — *see* subcategory T75.0 ☑
  - causing fire — *see* Exposure, fire
- liquid (boiling) (hot) NEC X12 ☑
  - stated as undetermined whether accidental or intentional Y27.2 ☑
  - suicide (attempt) X77.2 ☑
- local application of externally applied substance in medical or surgical care Y63.5
- machinery (hot) X17 ☑
- matches X08.8 ☑
  - with ignition of clothing NEC X06.2 ☑
    - nightwear X05 ☑

Burn, burned, burning — *continued*
- mattress — *see* Exposure, fire, uncontrolled, building, bed
- medicament, externally applied Y63.5
- metal (hot) (liquid) (molten) NEC X18 ☑
- nightwear (nightclothes, nightdress, gown, pajamas, robe) X05 ☑
- object (hot) NEC X19 ☑
- on board watercraft
  - due to
    - accident to watercraft V91.09 ☑
      - powered craft V91.03 ☑
        - ferry boat V91.01 ☑
        - fishing boat V91.02 ☑
        - jetskis V91.03 ☑
        - liner V91.01 ☑
        - merchant ship V91.00 ☑
        - passenger ship V91.01 ☑
      - unpowered craft V91.08 ☑
        - canoe V91.05 ☑
        - inflatable V91.06 ☑
        - kayak V91.05 ☑
        - sailboat V91.04 ☑
        - surf-board V91.08 ☑
        - water skis V91.07 ☑
        - windsurfer V91.08 ☑
    - fire on board V93.09 ☑
      - ferry boat V93.01 ☑
      - fishing boat V93.02 ☑
      - jetskis V93.03 ☑
      - liner V93.01 ☑
      - merchant ship V93.00 ☑
      - passenger ship V93.01 ☑
      - powered craft NEC V93.03 ☑
      - sailboat V93.04 ☑
    - specified heat source NEC on board V93.19 ☑
      - ferry boat V93.11 ☑
      - fishing boat V93.12 ☑
      - jetskis V93.13 ☑
      - liner V93.11 ☑
      - merchant ship V93.10 ☑
      - passenger ship V93.11 ☑
      - powered craft NEC V93.13 ☑
      - sailboat V93.14 ☑
- pipe (hot) X16 ☑
  - smoking X08.8 ☑
    - with ignition of clothing NEC X06.2 ☑
      - nightwear X05 ☑
- powder — *see* Powder burn
- radiator (hot) X16 ☑
- saucepan (hot) (glass) (metal) X15.3 ☑
  - stated as undetermined whether accidental or intentional Y27.3 ☑
  - suicide (attempt) X77.3 ☑
- self-inflicted X76 ☑
  - stated as undetermined whether accidental or intentional Y26 ☑
- stated as undetermined whether accidental or intentional Y27.0 ☑
- steam X13.1 ☑
  - pipe X16 ☑
    - stated as undetermined whether accidental or intentional Y27.8 ☑
  - stated as undetermined whether accidental or intentional Y27.0 ☑
  - suicide (attempt) X77.0 ☑
- stove (hot) (kitchen) X15.0 ☑
  - stated as undetermined whether accidental or intentional Y27.3 ☑
  - suicide (attempt) X77.3 ☑
- substance (hot) NEC X19 ☑
  - boiling X12 ☑
    - stated as undetermined whether accidental or intentional Y27.2 ☑
    - suicide (attempt) X77.2 ☑
  - molten (metal) X18 ☑
- suicide (attempt) NEC X76 ☑
  - hot
    - household appliance X77.3 ☑
    - object X77.9 ☑
- therapeutic misadventure
  - heat in local application or packing during medical or surgical procedure Y63.5
  - overdose of radiation Y63.2
- toaster (hot) X15.1 ☑

Burn, burned, burning — *continued*
- toaster — *continued*
  - stated as undetermined whether accidental or intentional Y27.3 ☑
  - suicide (attempt) X77.3 ☑
- tool (hot) X17 ☑
- torch, welding X08.8 ☑
  - with ignition of clothing NEC X06.2 ☑
    - nightwear X05 ☑
- trash fire (controlled) — *see* Exposure, fire, controlled, not in building
  - uncontrolled — *see* Exposure, fire, uncontrolled, not in building
- vapor (hot) X13.1 ☑
  - stated as undetermined whether accidental or intentional Y27.0 ☑
  - suicide (attempt) X77.0 ☑
- Very pistol — *see* Discharge, firearm NEC

Butted by animal W55.82 ☑
- bull W55.22 ☑
- cow W55.22 ☑
- goat W55.32 ☑
- horse W55.12 ☑
- pig W55.42 ☑
- sheep W55.32 ☑

C

Caisson disease — *see* Air, pressure, change
Campfire (exposure to) (controlled) (*see also* Exposure, fire, controlled, not in building)
- uncontrolled — *see* Exposure, fire, uncontrolled, not in building

Capital punishment (any means) — *see* Legal, intervention
Car sickness T75.3 ☑
Casualty (not due to war) NEC X58 ☑
- war — *see* War operations
Cat
- bite W55.01 ☑
- scratch W55.03 ☑
Cataclysm, cataclysmic (any injury) NEC — *see* Forces of nature
Catching fire — *see* Exposure, fire
Caught
- between
  - folding object W23.0 ☑
  - objects (moving) (stationary and moving) W23.0 ☑
    - and machinery — *see* Contact, with, by type of machine
  - stationary W23.1 ☑
  - sliding door and door frame W23.0 ☑
- by, in
  - machinery (moving parts of) — *see* Contact, with, by type of machine
  - washing-machine wringer W23.0 ☑
- under packing crate (due to losing grip) W23.1 ☑
Cave-in caused by cataclysmic earth surface movement or eruption — *see* Landslide
Change(s) in air pressure — *see* Air, pressure, change
Choked, choking (on) (any object except food or vomitus)
- food (bone) (seed) — *see* categories T17 and T18 ☑
- vomitus T17.81- ☑
Civil insurrection — *see* War operations
Cloudburst (any injury) X37.8 ☑
Cold, exposure to (accidental) (excessive) (extreme) (natural) (place) NEC — *see* Exposure, cold
Collapse
- building W20.1 ☑
  - burning (uncontrolled fire) X00.2 ☑
- dam or man-made structure (causing earth movement) X36.0 ☑
- machinery — *see* Contact, with, by type of machine
- structure W20.1 ☑
  - burning (uncontrolled fire) X00.2 ☑
Collision (accidental) NEC (*see also* Accident, transport) V89.9 ☑
- pedestrian W51 ☑
  - with fall W03 ☑
    - due to ice or snow W00.0 ☑
    - involving pedestrian conveyance — *see* Accident, transport, pedestrian, conveyance
  - and
    - crowd or human stampede (with fall) W52 ☑
    - object W22.8 ☑

Collision — *continued*
  pedestrian — *continued*
    and — *continued*
      object — *continued*
        with fall — *see* Fall, due to, bumping
          against, object
  person(s) — *see* Collision, pedestrian
  transport vehicle NEC V89.9 ☑
    and
      avalanche, fallen or not moving — *see* Accident, transport
        falling or moving — *see* Landslide
      landslide, fallen or not moving — *see* Accident, transport
        falling or moving — *see* Landslide
    due to cataclysm — *see* Forces of nature, by type
    intentional, purposeful suicide (attempt) — *see* Suicide, collision
Combustion, spontaneous — *see* Ignition
Complication (delayed) **of or following** (medical or surgical procedure) Y84.9
  with misadventure — *see* Misadventure
  amputation of limb(s) Y83.5
  anastomosis (arteriovenous) (blood vessel) (gastrojejunal) (tendon) (natural or artificial material) Y83.2
  aspiration (of fluid) Y84.4
    tissue Y84.8
  biopsy Y84.8
  blood
    sampling Y84.7
    transfusion
      procedure Y84.8
  bypass Y83.2
  catheterization (urinary) Y84.6
    cardiac Y84.0
  colostomy Y83.3
  cystostomy Y83.3
  dialysis (kidney) Y84.1
  drug — *see* Table of Drugs and Chemicals
  due to misadventure — *see* Misadventure
  duodenostomy Y83.3
  electroshock therapy Y84.3
  external stoma, creation of Y83.3
  formation of external stoma Y83.3
  gastrostomy Y83.3
  graft Y83.2
  hypothermia (medically-induced) Y84.8
  implant, implantation (of)
    artificial
      internal device (cardiac pacemaker) (electrodes in brain) (heart valve prosthesis) (orthopedic) Y83.1
      material or tissue (for anastomosis or bypass) Y83.2
        with creation of external stoma Y83.3
      natural tissues (for anastomosis or bypass) Y83.2
        with creation of external stoma Y83.3
  infusion
    procedure Y84.8
  injection — *see* Table of Drugs and Chemicals
    procedure Y84.8
  insertion of gastric or duodenal sound Y84.5
  insulin-shock therapy Y84.3
  paracentesis (abdominal) (thoracic) (aspirative) Y84.4
  procedures other than surgical operation — *see* Complication of or following, by type of procedure
  radiological procedure or therapy Y84.2
  removal of organ (partial) (total) NEC Y83.6
  sampling
    blood Y84.7
    fluid NEC Y84.4
    tissue Y84.8
  shock therapy Y84.3
  surgical operation NEC (*see also* Complication of or following, by type of operation) Y83.9
    reconstructive NEC Y83.4
      with
        anastomosis, bypass or graft Y83.2
        formation of external stoma Y83.3
    specified NEC Y83.8
  transfusion (*see also* Table of Drugs and Chemicals)
    procedure Y84.8
  transplant, transplantation (heart) (kidney) (liver) (whole organ, any) Y83.0
    partial organ Y83.4
  ureterostomy Y83.3

Complication (delayed) **of or following** — *continued*
  vaccination (*see also* Table of Drugs and Chemicals)
    procedure Y84.8
Compression
  divers' squeeze — *see* Air, pressure, change
  trachea by
    food (lodged in esophagus) — *see* categories T17 and T18 ☑
    vomitus (lodged in esophagus) T17.81- ☑
Conflagration — *see* Exposure, fire, uncontrolled
Constriction (external)
  hair W49.01 ☑
  jewelry W49.04 ☑
  ring W49.04 ☑
  rubber band W49.03 ☑
  specified item NEC W49.09 ☑
  string W49.02 ☑
  thread W49.02 ☑
Contact (accidental)
  with
    abrasive wheel (metalworking) W31.1 ☑
    alligator W58.09 ☑
      bite W58.01 ☑
      crushing W58.03 ☑
      strike W58.02 ☑
    amphibian W62.9 ☑
      frog W62.0 ☑
      toad W62.1 ☑
    animal (nonvenomous) NEC W64 ☑
      marine W56.89 ☑
        bite W56.81 ☑
        dolphin — *see* Contact, with, dolphin
        fish NEC — *see* Contact, with, fish
        mammal — *see* Contact, with, mammal, marine
        orca — *see* Contact, with, orca
        sea lion — *see* Contact, with, sea lion
        shark — *see* Contact, with, shark
        strike W56.82 ☑
    animate mechanical force NEC W64 ☑
    arrow W21.89 ☑
      not thrown, projected or falling W45.8 ☑
    arthropods (nonvenomous) W57 ☑
    axe W27.0 ☑
    band-saw (industrial) W31.2 ☑
    bayonet — *see* Bayonet wound
    bee(s) X58 ☑
    bench-saw (industrial) W31.2 ☑
    bird W61.99 ☑
      bite W61.91 ☑
      chicken — *see* Contact, with, chicken
      duck — *see* Contact, with, duck
      goose — *see* Contact, with, goose
      macaw — *see* Contact, with, macaw
      parrot — *see* Contact, with, parrot
      psittacine — *see* Contact, with, psittacine
      strike W61.92 ☑
      turkey — *see* Contact, with, turkey
    blender W29.0 ☑
    boiling water X12 ☑
      stated as undetermined whether accidental or intentional Y27.2 ☑
      suicide (attempt) X77.2 ☑
    bore, earth-drilling or mining (land) (seabed) W31.0 ☑
    buffalo — *see* Contact, with, hoof stock NEC
    bull W55.29 ☑
      bite W55.21 ☑
      gored W55.22 ☑
      strike W55.22 ☑
    bumper cars W31.81 ☑
    camel — *see* Contact, with, hoof stock NEC
    can
      lid W26.8 ☑
      opener W27.4 ☑
        powered W29.0 ☑
    cat W55.09 ☑
      bite W55.01 ☑
      scratch W55.03 ☑
    caterpillar (venomous) X58 ☑
    centipede (venomous) X58 ☑
    chain
      hoist W24.0 ☑
        agricultural operations W30.89 ☑
      saw W29.3 ☑

Contact — *continued*
  with — *continued*
    chicken W61.39 ☑
      peck W61.33 ☑
      strike W61.32 ☑
    chisel W27.0 ☑
    circular saw W31.2 ☑
    cobra X58 ☑
    combine (harvester) W30.0 ☑
    conveyer belt W24.1 ☑
    cooker (hot) X15.8 ☑
      stated as undetermined whether accidental or intentional Y27.3 ☑
      suicide (attempt) X77.3 ☑
    coral X58 ☑
    cotton gin W31.82 ☑
    cow W55.29 ☑
      bite W55.21 ☑
      strike W55.22 ☑
    crane W24.0 ☑
      agricultural operations W30.89 ☑
    crocodile W58.19 ☑
      bite W58.11 ☑
      crushing W58.13 ☑
      strike W58.12 ☑
    dagger W26.1 ☑
      stated as undetermined whether accidental or intentional Y28.2 ☑
      suicide (attempt) X78.2 ☑
    dairy equipment W31.82 ☑
    dart W21.89 ☑
      not thrown, projected or falling W45.8 ☑
    deer — *see* Contact, with, hoof stock NEC
    derrick W24.0 ☑
      agricultural operations W30.89 ☑
        hay W30.2 ☑
    dog W54.8 ☑
      bite W54.0 ☑
      strike W54.1 ☑
    dolphin W56.09 ☑
      bite W56.01 ☑
      strike W56.02 ☑
    donkey — *see* Contact, with, hoof stock NEC
    drill (powered) W29.8 ☑
      earth (land) (seabed) W31.0 ☑
      nonpowered W27.8 ☑
    drive belt W24.0 ☑
      agricultural operations W30.89 ☑
    dry ice — *see* Exposure, cold, man-made
    dryer (clothes) (powered) (spin) W29.2 ☑
    duck W61.69 ☑
      bite W61.61 ☑
      strike W61.62 ☑
    earth (-)
      drilling machine (industrial) W31.0 ☑
      scraping machine in stationary use W31.83 ☑
    edge of stiff paper W26.2 ☑
    electric
      beater W29.0 ☑
      blanket X16 ☑
      fan W29.2 ☑
        commercial W31.82 ☑
      knife W29.1 ☑
      mixer W29.0 ☑
    elevator (building) W24.0 ☑
      agricultural operations W30.89 ☑
        grain W30.3 ☑
    engine(s), hot NEC X17 ☑
    excavating machine W31.0 ☑
    farm machine W30.9 ☑
    feces — *see* Contact, with, by type of animal
    fer de lance X58 ☑
    fish W56.59 ☑
      bite W56.51 ☑
      shark — *see* Contact, with, shark
      strike W56.52 ☑
    flying horses W31.81 ☑
    forging (metalworking) machine W31.1 ☑
    fork W27.4 ☑
    forklift (truck) W24.0 ☑
      agricultural operations W30.89 ☑
    frog W62.0 ☑
    garden
      cultivator (powered) W29.3 ☑
        riding W30.89 ☑
      fork W27.1 ☑

Contact — *continued*
  with — *continued*
    gas turbine W31.3 ☑
    Gila monster X58 ☑
    giraffe — *see* Contact, with, hoof stock NEC
    glass (sharp) (broken) W25 ☑
      with subsequent fall W18.02 ☑
      assault X99.0 ☑
      due to fall — *see* Fall, by type
      stated as undetermined whether accidental or
        intentional Y28.0 ☑
      suicide (attempt) X78.0 ☑
    goat W55.39 ☑
      bite W55.31 ☑
      strike W55.32 ☑
    goose W61.59 ☑
      bite W61.51 ☑
      strike W61.52 ☑
    hand
      saw W27.0 ☑
      tool (not powered) NEC W27.8 ☑
        powered W29.8 ☑
    harvester W30.0 ☑
    hay-derrick W30.2 ☑
    heating
      appliance (hot) X16 ☑
      pad (electric) X16 ☑
    heat NEC X19 ☑
      from appliance (electrical) (household) — *see*
        Contact, with, hot, household appliance
        heating appliance X16 ☑
    hedge-trimmer (powered) W29.3 ☑
    hoe W27.1 ☑
    hoist (chain) (shaft) NEC W24.0 ☑
      agricultural W30.89 ☑
    hoof stock NEC W55.39 ☑
      bite W55.31 ☑
      strike W55.32 ☑
    hornet(s) X58 ☑
    horse W55.19 ☑
      bite W55.11 ☑
      strike W55.12 ☑
    hot
      air X14.1 ☑
        inhalation X14.0 ☑
      cooker X15.8 ☑
      drinks X10.0 ☑
      engine X17 ☑
      fats X10.2 ☑
      fluids NEC X12 ☑
        assault X98.2 ☑
        suicide (attempt) X77.2 ☑
        undetermined whether accidental or inten-
          tional Y27.2 ☑
      food X10.1 ☑
      gases X14.1 ☑
        inhalation X14.0 ☑
      heating appliance X16 ☑
      household appliance X15.8 ☑
        assault X98.3 ☑
        cooker X15.8 ☑
        hotplate X15.2 ☑
        kettle X15.8 ☑
        light bulb X15.8 ☑
        object NEC X19 ☑
          assault X98.8 ☑
          stated as undetermined whether acciden-
            tal or intentional Y27.9 ☑
          suicide (attempt) X77.8 ☑
        saucepan X15.3 ☑
        skillet X15.3 ☑
        stated as undetermined whether accidental
          or intentional Y27.3 ☑
        stove X15.0 ☑
        suicide (attempt) X77.3 ☑
        toaster X15.1 ☑
      kettle X15.8 ☑
      light bulb X15.8 ☑
      liquid NEC (*see also* Burn) X12 ☑
        drinks X10.0 ☑
        stated as undetermined whether accidental
          or intentional Y27.2 ☑
        suicide (attempt) X77.2 ☑
        tap water X11.8 ☑
          stated as undetermined whether acciden-
            tal or intentional Y27.1 ☑

Contact — *continued*
  with — *continued*
    hot — *continued*
      liquid (*see also* Burn) — *continued*
        tap water — *continued*
          suicide (attempt) X77.1 ☑
      machinery X17 ☑
      metal (molten) (liquid) NEC X18 ☑
      object (not producing fire or flames) NEC X19 ☑
      oil (cooking) X10.2 ☑
      pipe X16 ☑
      plate X15.2 ☑
      radiator X16 ☑
      saucepan (glass) (metal) X15.3 ☑
      skillet X15.3 ☑
      stove (kitchen) X15.0 ☑
      substance NEC X19 ☑
      tap-water X11.8 ☑
        assault X98.1 ☑
        heated on stove X12 ☑
          stated as undetermined whether acciden-
            tal or intentional Y27.2 ☑
          suicide (attempt) X77.2 ☑
        in bathtub X11.0 ☑
        running X11.1 ☑
        stated as undetermined whether accidental
          or intentional Y27.1 ☑
        suicide (attempt) X77.1 ☑
      toaster X15.1 ☑
      tool X17 ☑
      vapors X13.1 ☑
        inhalation X13.0 ☑
      water (tap) X11.8 ☑
        boiling X12 ☑
          stated as undetermined whether acciden-
            tal or intentional Y27.2 ☑
          suicide (attempt) X77.2 ☑
        heated on stove X12 ☑
          stated as undetermined whether acciden-
            tal or intentional Y27.2 ☑
          suicide (attempt) X77.2 ☑
        in bathtub X11.0 ☑
        running X11.1 ☑
        stated as undetermined whether accidental
          or intentional Y27.1 ☑
        suicide (attempt) X77.1 ☑
    hotplate X15.2 ☑
    ice-pick W27.4 ☑
    insect (nonvenomous) NEC W57 ☑
    kettle (hot) X15.8 ☑
    knife W26.0 ☑
      assault X99.1 ☑
      electric W29.1 ☑
      stated as undetermined whether accidental or
        intentional Y28.1 ☑
      suicide (attempt) X78.1 ☑
    lathe (metalworking) W31.1 ☑
      turnings W45.8 ☑
      woodworking W31.2 ☑
    lawnmower (powered) (ridden) W28 ☑
      causing electrocution W86.8 ☑
        suicide (attempt) X83.1 ☑
      unpowered W27.1 ☑
    lift, lifting (devices) W24.0 ☑
      agricultural operations W30.89 ☑
      shaft W24.0 ☑
    liquefied gas — *see* Exposure, cold, man-made
    liquid air, hydrogen, nitrogen — *see* Exposure, cold,
      man-made
    lizard (nonvenomous) W59.09 ☑
      bite W59.01 ☑
      strike W59.02 ☑
    llama — *see* Contact, with, hoof stock NEC
    macaw W61.19 ☑
      bite W61.11 ☑
      strike W61.12 ☑
    machine, machinery W31.9 ☑
      abrasive wheel W31.1 ☑
      agricultural including animal-powered
        W30.9 ☑
        combine harvester W30.0 ☑
        grain storage elevator W30.3 ☑
        hay derrick W30.2 ☑
        power take-off device W30.1 ☑
        reaper W30.0 ☑
        specified NEC W30.89 ☑

Contact — *continued*
  with — *continued*
    machine, machinery — *continued*
      agricultural including animal-powered — *con-*
        tinued
        thresher W30.0 ☑
        transport vehicle, stationary W30.81 ☑
      band saw W31.2 ☑
      bench saw W31.2 ☑
      circular saw W31.2 ☑
      commercial NEC W31.82 ☑
      drilling, metal (industrial) W31.1 ☑
      earth-drilling W31.0 ☑
      earthmoving or scraping W31.89 ☑
      excavating W31.89 ☑
      forging machine W31.1 ☑
      gas turbine W31.3 ☑
      hot X17 ☑
      internal combustion engine W31.3 ☑
      land drill W31.0 ☑
      lathe W31.1 ☑
      lifting (devices) W24.0 ☑
      metal drill W31.1 ☑
      metalworking (industrial) W31.1 ☑
      milling, metal W31.1 ☑
      mining W31.0 ☑
      molding W31.2 ☑
      overhead plane W31.2 ☑
      power press, metal W31.1 ☑
      prime mover W31.3 ☑
      printing W31.89 ☑
      radial saw W31.2 ☑
      recreational W31.81 ☑
      roller-coaster W31.81 ☑
      rolling mill, metal W31.1 ☑
      sander W31.2 ☑
      seabed drill W31.0 ☑
      shaft
        hoist W31.0 ☑
        lift W31.0 ☑
      specified NEC W31.89 ☑
      spinning W31.89 ☑
      steam engine W31.3 ☑
      transmission W24.1 ☑
      undercutter W31.0 ☑
      water driven turbine W31.3 ☑
      weaving W31.89 ☑
      woodworking or forming (industrial) W31.2 ☑
    mammal (feces) (urine) W55.89 ☑
      bull — *see* Contact, with, bull
      cat — *see* Contact, with, cat
      cow — *see* Contact, with, cow
      goat — *see* Contact, with, goat
      hoof stock — *see* Contact, with, hoof stock
      horse — *see* Contact, with, horse
      marine W56.39 ☑
        dolphin — *see* Contact, with, dolphin
        orca — *see* Contact, with, orca
        sea lion — *see* Contact, with, sea lion
        specified NEC W56.39 ☑
          bite W56.31 ☑
          strike W56.32 ☑
      pig — *see* Contact, with, pig
      raccoon — *see* Contact, with, raccoon
      rodent — *see* Contact, with, rodent
      sheep — *see* Contact, with, sheep
      specified NEC W55.89 ☑
        bite W55.81 ☑
        strike W55.82 ☑
    marine
      animal W56.89 ☑
        bite W56.81 ☑
        dolphin — *see* Contact, with, dolphin
        fish NEC — *see* Contact, with, fish
        mammal — *see* Contact, with, mammal,
          marine
        orca — *see* Contact, with, orca
        sea lion — *see* Contact, with, sea lion
        shark — *see* Contact, with, shark
        strike W56.82 ☑
    meat
      grinder (domestic) W29.0 ☑
        industrial W31.82 ☑
        nonpowered W27.4 ☑
      slicer (domestic) W29.0 ☑
        industrial W31.82 ☑

Contact — continued
　with — continued
　　merry go round W31.81 ☑
　　metal, hot (liquid) (molten) NEC X18 ☑
　　millipede W57 ☑
　　nail W45.0 ☑
　　　gun W29.4 ☑
　　needle (sewing) W27.3 ☑
　　　hypodermic W46.0 ☑
　　　　contaminated W46.1 ☑
　　object (blunt) NEC
　　　hot NEC X19 ☑
　　　legal intervention — see Legal, intervention, blunt object
　　　sharp NEC W45.8 ☑
　　　　inflicted by other person NEC W45.8 ☑
　　　　stated as
　　　　　intentional homicide (attempt) — see Assault, cutting or piercing instrument
　　　　legal intervention — see Legal, intervention, sharp object
　　　　self-inflicted X78.9 ☑
　　orca W56.29 ☑
　　　bite W56.21 ☑
　　　strike W56.22 ☑
　　overhead plane W31.2 ☑
　　paper (as sharp object) W26.2 ☑
　　paper-cutter W27.5 ☑
　　parrot W61.09 ☑
　　　bite W61.01 ☑
　　　strike W61.02 ☑
　　pig W55.49 ☑
　　　bite W55.41 ☑
　　　strike W55.42 ☑
　　pipe, hot X16 ☑
　　pitchfork W27.1 ☑
　　plane (metal) (wood) W27.0 ☑
　　　overhead W31.2 ☑
　　plant thorns, spines, sharp leaves or other mechanisms W60 ☑
　　powered
　　　garden cultivator W29.3 ☑
　　　household appliance, implement, or machine W29.8 ☑
　　　saw (industrial) W31.2 ☑
　　　　hand W29.8 ☑
　　printing machine W31.89 ☑
　　psittacine bird W61.29 ☑
　　　bite W61.21 ☑
　　　macaw — see Contact, with, macaw
　　　parrot — see Contact, with, parrot
　　　strike W61.22 ☑
　　pulley (block) (transmission) W24.0 ☑
　　　agricultural operations W30.89 ☑
　　raccoon W55.59 ☑
　　　bite W55.51 ☑
　　　strike W55.52 ☑
　　radial-saw (industrial) W31.2 ☑
　　radiator (hot) X16 ☑
　　rake W27.1 ☑
　　rattlesnake X58 ☑
　　reaper W30.0 ☑
　　reptile W59.89 ☑
　　　lizard — see Contact, with, lizard
　　　snake — see Contact, with, snake
　　　specified NEC W59.89 ☑
　　　　bite W59.81 ☑
　　　　crushing W59.83 ☑
　　　　strike W59.82 ☑
　　　turtle — see Contact, with, turtle
　　rivet gun (powered) W29.4 ☑
　　road scraper — see Accident, transport, construction vehicle
　　rodent (feces) (urine) W53.89 ☑
　　　bite W53.81 ☑
　　　mouse W53.09 ☑
　　　　bite W53.01 ☑
　　　rat W53.19 ☑
　　　　bite W53.11 ☑
　　　specified NEC W53.89 ☑
　　　　bite W53.81 ☑
　　　squirrel W53.29 ☑
　　　　bite W53.21 ☑
　　roller coaster W31.81 ☑
　　rope NEC W24.0 ☑

Contact — continued
　with — continued
　　rope — continued
　　　agricultural operations W30.89 ☑
　　saliva — see Contact, with, by type of animal
　　sander W29.8 ☑
　　　industrial W31.2 ☑
　　saucepan (hot) (glass) (metal) X15.3 ☑
　　saw W27.0 ☑
　　　band (industrial) W31.2 ☑
　　　bench (industrial) W31.2 ☑
　　　chain W29.3 ☑
　　　hand W27.0 ☑
　　sawing machine, metal W31.1 ☑
　　scissors W27.2 ☑
　　scorpion X58 ☑
　　screwdriver W27.0 ☑
　　　powered W29.8 ☑
　　sea
　　　anemone, cucumber or urchin (spine) X58 ☑
　　　lion W56.19 ☑
　　　　bite W56.11 ☑
　　　　strike W56.12 ☑
　　serpent — see Contact, with, snake, by type
　　sewing-machine (electric) (powered) W29.2 ☑
　　　not powered W27.8 ☑
　　shaft (hoist) (lift) (transmission) NEC W24.0 ☑
　　　agricultural W30.89 ☑
　　shark W56.49 ☑
　　　bite W56.41 ☑
　　　strike W56.42 ☑
　　sharp object(s) W26.9 ☑
　　　specified NEC W26.8 ☑
　　shears (hand) W27.2 ☑
　　　powered (industrial) W31.1 ☑
　　　　domestic W29.2 ☑
　　sheep W55.39 ☑
　　　bite W55.31 ☑
　　　strike W55.32 ☑
　　shovel W27.8 ☑
　　　steam — see Accident, transport, construction vehicle
　　snake (nonvenomous) W59.19 ☑
　　　bite W59.11 ☑
　　　crushing W59.13 ☑
　　　strike W59.12 ☑
　　spade W27.1 ☑
　　spider (venomous) X58 ☑
　　spin-drier W29.2 ☑
　　spinning machine W31.89 ☑
　　splinter W45.8 ☑
　　sports equipment W21.9 ☑
　　staple gun (powered) W29.8 ☑
　　steam X13.1 ☑
　　　engine W31.3 ☑
　　　inhalation X13.0 ☑
　　　pipe X16 ☑
　　　shovel W31.89 ☑
　　stove (hot) (kitchen) X15.0 ☑
　　substance, hot NEC X19 ☑
　　　molten (metal) X18 ☑
　　sword W26.1 ☑
　　　assault X99.2 ☑
　　　stated as undetermined whether accidental or intentional Y28.2 ☑
　　　suicide (attempt) X78.2 ☑
　　tarantula X58 ☑
　　thresher W30.0 ☑
　　tin can lid W26.8 ☑
　　toad W62.1 ☑
　　toaster (hot) X15.1 ☑
　　tool W27.8 ☑
　　　hand (not powered) W27.8 ☑
　　　　auger W27.0 ☑
　　　　axe W27.0 ☑
　　　　can opener W27.4 ☑
　　　　chisel W27.0 ☑
　　　　fork W27.4 ☑
　　　　garden W27.1 ☑
　　　　handsaw W27.0 ☑
　　　　hoe W27.1 ☑
　　　　ice-pick W27.4 ☑
　　　　kitchen utensil W27.4 ☑
　　　　manual
　　　　　lawn mower W27.1 ☑
　　　　　sewing machine W27.8 ☑

Contact — continued
　with — continued
　　tool — continued
　　　hand — continued
　　　　meat grinder W27.4 ☑
　　　　needle (sewing) W27.3 ☑
　　　　　hypodermic W46.0 ☑
　　　　　　contaminated W46.1 ☑
　　　　paper cutter W27.5 ☑
　　　　pitchfork W27.1 ☑
　　　　rake W27.1 ☑
　　　　scissors W27.2 ☑
　　　　screwdriver W27.0 ☑
　　　　specified NEC W27.8 ☑
　　　　workbench W27.0 ☑
　　　hot X17 ☑
　　　powered W29.8 ☑
　　　　blender W29.0 ☑
　　　　　commercial W31.82 ☑
　　　　can opener W29.0 ☑
　　　　　commercial W31.82 ☑
　　　　chainsaw W29.3 ☑
　　　　clothes dryer W29.2 ☑
　　　　　commercial W31.82 ☑
　　　　dishwasher W29.2 ☑
　　　　　commercial W31.82 ☑
　　　　edger W29.3 ☑
　　　　electric fan W29.2 ☑
　　　　　commercial W31.82 ☑
　　　　electric knife W29.1 ☑
　　　　food processor W29.0 ☑
　　　　　commercial W31.82 ☑
　　　　garbage disposal W29.0 ☑
　　　　　commercial W31.82 ☑
　　　　garden tool W29.3 ☑
　　　　hedge trimmer W29.3 ☑
　　　　ice maker W29.0 ☑
　　　　　commercial W31.82 ☑
　　　　kitchen appliance W29.0 ☑
　　　　　commercial W31.82 ☑
　　　　lawn mower W28 ☑
　　　　meat grinder W29.0 ☑
　　　　　commercial W31.82 ☑
　　　　mixer W29.0 ☑
　　　　　commercial W31.82 ☑
　　　　rototiller W29.3 ☑
　　　　sewing machine W29.2 ☑
　　　　　commercial W31.82 ☑
　　　　washing machine W29.2 ☑
　　　　　commercial W31.82 ☑
　　transmission device (belt, cable, chain, gear, pinion, shaft) W24.1 ☑
　　　agricultural operations W30.89 ☑
　　turbine (gas) (water-driven) W31.3 ☑
　　turkey W61.49 ☑
　　　peck W61.43 ☑
　　　strike W61.42 ☑
　　turtle (nonvenomous) W59.29 ☑
　　　bite W59.21 ☑
　　　strike W59.22 ☑
　　　terrestrial W59.89 ☑
　　　　bite W59.81 ☑
　　　　crushing W59.83 ☑
　　　　strike W59.82 ☑
　　under-cutter W31.0 ☑
　　urine — see Contact, with, by type of animal
　vehicle
　　agricultural use (transport) — see Accident, transport, agricultural vehicle
　　　not on public highway W30.81 ☑
　　industrial use (transport) — see Accident, transport, industrial vehicle
　　　not on public highway W31.83 ☑
　　off-road use (transport) — see Accident, transport, all-terrain or off-road vehicle
　　　not on public highway W31.83 ☑
　　special construction use (transport) — see Accident, transport, construction vehicle
　　　not on public highway W31.83 ☑
　venomous
　　animal X58 ☑
　　arthropods X58 ☑
　　lizard X58 ☑
　　marine animal NEC X58 ☑
　　marine plant NEC X58 ☑
　　millipedes (tropical) X58 ☑

Contact — *continued*
  with — *continued*
    venomous — *continued*
      plant(s) X58 ☑
      snake X58 ☑
      spider X58 ☑
      viper X58 ☑
      washing-machine (powered) W29.2 ☑
      wasp X58 ☑
      weaving-machine W31.89 ☑
      winch W24.0 ☑
        agricultural operations W30.89 ☑
      wire NEC W24.0 ☑
        agricultural operations W30.89 ☑
      wood slivers W45.8 ☑
      yellow jacket X58 ☑
      zebra — *see* Contact, with, hoof stock NEC
    pressure X50.9 ☑
    stress X50.9 ☑
Coup de soleil X32 ☑
Crash
  aircraft (in transit) (powered) V95.9 ☑
    balloon V96.01 ☑
    fixed wing NEC (private) V95.21 ☑
      commercial V95.31 ☑
    glider V96.21 ☑
      hang V96.11 ☑
      powered V95.11 ☑
    helicopter V95.01 ☑
    in war operations — *see* War operations, destruction of aircraft
    microlight V95.11 ☑
    nonpowered V96.9 ☑
      specified NEC V96.8 ☑
    powered NEC V95.8 ☑
    stated as
      homicide (attempt) Y08.81 ☑
      suicide (attempt) X83.0 ☑
    ultralight V95.11 ☑
  spacecraft V95.41 ☑
  transport vehicle NEC (*see also* Accident, transport) V89.9 ☑
    homicide (attempt) Y03.8 ☑
    motor NEC (traffic) V89.2 ☑
      homicide (attempt) Y03.8 ☑
    suicide (attempt) — *see* Suicide, collision
Cruelty (mental) (physical) (sexual) X58 ☑
Crushed (accidentally) X58 ☑
  between objects (moving) (stationary and moving) W23.0 ☑
    stationary W23.1 ☑
  by
    alligator W58.03 ☑
    avalanche NEC — *see* Landslide
    cave-in W20.0 ☑
      caused by cataclysmic earth surface movement — *see* Landslide
    crocodile W58.13 ☑
    crowd or human stampede W52 ☑
    falling
      aircraft V97.39 ☑
        in war operations — *see* War operations, destruction of aircraft
      earth, material W20.0 ☑
        caused by cataclysmic earth surface movement — *see* Landslide
      object NEC W20.8 ☑
    landslide NEC — *see* Landslide
    lizard (nonvenomous) W59.09 ☑
    machinery — *see* Contact, with, by type of machine
    reptile NEC W59.89 ☑
    snake (nonvenomous) W59.13 ☑
  in
    machinery — *see* Contact, with, by type of machine
Cut, cutting (any part of body) (accidental) (*see also* Contact, with, by object or machine)
  during medical or surgical treatment as misadventure — *see* Index to Diseases and Injuries, Complications
  homicide (attempt) — *see* Assault, cutting or piercing instrument
  inflicted by other person — *see* Assault, cutting or piercing instrument
  legal
    execution — *see* Legal, intervention

Cut, cutting — *continued*
  legal — *continued*
    intervention — *see* Legal, intervention, sharp object
  machine NEC (*see also* Contact, with, by type of machine) W31.9 ☑
  self-inflicted — *see* Suicide, cutting or piercing instrument
  suicide (attempt) — *see* Suicide, cutting or piercing instrument
Cyclone (any injury) X37.1 ☑

D

Decapitation (accidental circumstances) NEC X58 ☑
  homicide X99.9 ☑
  legal execution — *see* Legal, intervention
Dehydration from lack of water X58 ☑
Deprivation X58 ☑
Derailment (accidental)
  railway (rolling stock) (train) (vehicle) (without antecedent collision) V81.7 ☑
    with antecedent collision — *see* Accident, transport, railway vehicle occupant
  streetcar (without antecedent collision) V82.7 ☑
    with antecedent collision — *see* Accident, transport, streetcar occupant
Descent
  parachute (voluntary) (without accident to aircraft) V97.29 ☑
    due to accident to aircraft — *see* Accident, transport, aircraft
Desertion X58 ☑
Destitution X58 ☑
Disability, late effect or sequela of injury — *see* Sequelae
Discharge (accidental)
  airgun W34.010 ☑
    assault X95.01 ☑
    homicide (attempt) X95.01 ☑
    stated as undetermined whether accidental or intentional Y24.0 ☑
    suicide (attempt) X74.01 ☑
  BB gun — *see* Discharge, airgun
  firearm (accidental) W34.00 ☑
    assault X95.9 ☑
    handgun (pistol) (revolver) W32.0 ☑
      assault X93 ☑
      homicide (attempt) X93 ☑
      legal intervention — *see* Legal, intervention, firearm, handgun
      stated as undetermined whether accidental or intentional Y22 ☑
      suicide (attempt) X72 ☑
    homicide (attempt) X95.9 ☑
    hunting rifle W33.02 ☑
      assault X94.1 ☑
      homicide (attempt) X94.1 ☑
      legal intervention
        injuring
          bystander Y35.032 ☑
          law enforcement personnel Y35.031 ☑
          suspect Y35.033 ☑
      stated as undetermined whether accidental or intentional Y23.1 ☑
      suicide (attempt) X73.1 ☑
    larger W33.00 ☑
      assault X94.9 ☑
      homicide (attempt) X94.9 ☑
      hunting rifle — *see* Discharge, firearm, hunting rifle
      legal intervention — *see* Legal, intervention, firearm by type of firearm
      machine gun — *see* Discharge, firearm, machine gun
      shotgun — *see* Discharge, firearm, shotgun
      specified NEC W33.09 ☑
        assault X94.8 ☑
        homicide (attempt) X94.8 ☑
        legal intervention
          injuring
            bystander Y35.092 ☑
            law enforcement personnel Y35.091 ☑
            suspect Y35.093 ☑

Discharge — *continued*
  firearm — *continued*
    larger — *continued*
      specified — *continued*
        stated as undetermined whether accidental or intentional Y23.8 ☑
        suicide (attempt) X73.8 ☑
      stated as undetermined whether accidental or intentional Y23.9 ☑
      suicide (attempt) X73.9 ☑
    legal intervention
      injuring
        bystander Y35.002 ☑
        law enforcement personnel Y35.001 ☑
        suspect Y35.03 ☑
      using rubber bullet
        injuring
          bystander Y35.042 ☑
          law enforcement personnel Y35.041 ☑
          suspect Y35.043 ☑
    machine gun W33.03 ☑
      assault X94.2 ☑
      homicide (attempt) X94.2 ☑
      legal intervention — *see* Legal, intervention, firearm, machine gun
      stated as undetermined whether accidental or intentional Y23.3 ☑
      suicide (attempt) X73.2 ☑
    pellet gun — *see* Discharge, airgun
    shotgun W33.01 ☑
      assault X94.0 ☑
      homicide (attempt) X94.0 ☑
      legal intervention — *see* Legal, intervention, firearm, specified NEC
      stated as undetermined whether accidental or intentional Y23.0 ☑
      suicide (attempt) X73.0 ☑
    specified NEC W34.09 ☑
      assault X95.8 ☑
      homicide (attempt) X95.8 ☑
      legal intervention — *see* Legal, intervention, firearm, specified NEC
      stated as undetermined whether accidental or intentional Y24.8 ☑
      suicide (attempt) X74.8 ☑
    stated as undetermined whether accidental or intentional Y24.9 ☑
    suicide (attempt) X74.9 ☑
    Very pistol W34.09 ☑
      assault X95.8 ☑
      homicide (attempt) X95.8 ☑
      stated as undetermined whether accidental or intentional Y24.8 ☑
      suicide (attempt) X74.8 ☑
  firework(s) W39 ☑
    stated as undetermined whether accidental or intentional Y25 ☑
  gas-operated gun NEC W34.018 ☑
    airgun — *see* Discharge, airgun
    assault X95.09 ☑
    homicide (attempt) X95.09 ☑
    paintball gun — *see* Discharge, paintball gun
    stated as undetermined whether accidental or intentional Y24.8 ☑
    suicide (attempt) X74.09 ☑
  gun NEC (*see also* Discharge, firearm NEC)
    air — *see* Discharge, airgun
    BB — *see* Discharge, airgun
    for single hand use — *see* Discharge, firearm, handgun
    hand — *see* Discharge, firearm, handgun
    machine — *see* Discharge, firearm, machine gun
    other specified — *see* Discharge, firearm NEC
    paintball — *see* Discharge, paintball gun
    pellet — *see* Discharge, airgun
  handgun — *see* Discharge, firearm, handgun
  machine gun — *see* Discharge, firearm, machine gun
  paintball gun W34.011 ☑
    assault X95.02 ☑
    homicide (attempt) X95.02 ☑
    stated as undetermined whether accidental or intentional Y24.8 ☑
    suicide (attempt) X74.02 ☑
  pistol — *see* Discharge, firearm, handgun
    flare — *see* Discharge, firearm, Very pistol
    pellet — *see* Discharge, airgun

Discharge — continued
  pistol — see Discharge, firearm, handgun — continued
    Very — see Discharge, firearm, Very pistol
  revolver — see Discharge, firearm, handgun
  rifle (hunting) — see Discharge, firearm, hunting rifle
  shotgun — see Discharge, firearm, shotgun
  spring-operated gun NEC W34.018 ☑
    assault X95.09 ☑
    homicide (attempt) X95.09 ☑
    stated as undetermined whether accidental or intentional Y24.8 ☑
    suicide (attempt) X74.09 ☑

Disease
  Andes W94.11 ☑
  aviator's — see Air, pressure
  range W94.11 ☑

Diver's disease, palsy, paralysis, squeeze — see Air, pressure

Diving (into water) — see Accident, diving

Dog bite W54.0 ☑

Dragged by transport vehicle NEC (see also Accident, transport) V09.9 ☑

Drinking poison (accidental) — see Table of Drugs and Chemicals

Dropped (accidentally) **while being carried or supported by other person** W04 ☑

Drowning (accidental) W74 ☑
  assault X92.9 ☑
  due to
    accident (to)
      machinery — see Contact, with, by type of machine
      watercraft V90.89 ☑
        burning V90.29 ☑
          powered V90.23 ☑
            fishing boat V90.22 ☑
            jetskis V90.23 ☑
            merchant ship V90.20 ☑
            passenger ship V90.21 ☑
          unpowered V90.28 ☑
            canoe V90.25 ☑
            inflatable V90.26 ☑
            kayak V90.25 ☑
            sailboat V90.24 ☑
            water skis V90.27 ☑
        crushed V90.39 ☑
          powered V90.33 ☑
            fishing boat V90.32 ☑
            jetskis V90.33 ☑
            merchant ship V90.30 ☑
            passenger ship V90.31 ☑
          unpowered V90.38 ☑
            canoe V90.35 ☑
            inflatable V90.36 ☑
            kayak V90.35 ☑
            sailboat V90.34 ☑
            water skis V90.37 ☑
        overturning V90.09 ☑
          powered V90.03 ☑
            fishing boat V90.02 ☑
            jetskis V90.03 ☑
            merchant ship V90.00 ☑
            passenger ship V90.01 ☑
          unpowered V90.08 ☑
            canoe V90.05 ☑
            inflatable V90.06 ☑
            kayak V90.05 ☑
            sailboat V90.04 ☑
        sinking V90.19 ☑
          powered V90.13 ☑
            fishing boat V90.12 ☑
            jetskis V90.13 ☑
            merchant ship V90.10 ☑
            passenger ship V90.11 ☑
          unpowered V90.18 ☑
            canoe V90.15 ☑
            inflatable V90.16 ☑
            kayak V90.15 ☑
            sailboat V90.14 ☑
        specified type NEC V90.89 ☑
          powered V90.83 ☑
            fishing boat V90.82 ☑
            jetskis V90.83 ☑
            merchant ship V90.80 ☑
            passenger ship V90.81 ☑

Drowning — continued
  due to — continued
    accident — continued
      watercraft — continued
        specified type — continued
          unpowered V90.88 ☑
            canoe V90.85 ☑
            inflatable V90.86 ☑
            kayak V90.85 ☑
            sailboat V90.84 ☑
            water skis V90.87 ☑
    avalanche — see Landslide
    cataclysmic
      earth surface movement NEC — see Forces of nature, earth movement
      storm — see Forces of nature, cataclysmic storm
    cloudburst X37.8 ☑
    cyclone X37.1 ☑
    fall overboard (from) V92.09 ☑
      powered craft V92.03 ☑
        ferry boat V92.01 ☑
        fishing boat V92.02 ☑
        jetskis V92.03 ☑
        liner V92.01 ☑
        merchant ship V92.00 ☑
        passenger ship V92.01 ☑
      resulting from
        accident to watercraft — see Drowning, due to, accident to, watercraft
        being washed overboard (from) V92.29 ☑
          powered craft V92.23 ☑
            ferry boat V92.21 ☑
            fishing boat V92.22 ☑
            jetskis V92.23 ☑
            liner V92.21 ☑
            merchant ship V92.20 ☑
            passenger ship V92.21 ☑
          unpowered craft V92.28 ☑
            canoe V92.25 ☑
            inflatable V92.26 ☑
            kayak V92.25 ☑
            sailboat V92.24 ☑
            surf-board V92.28 ☑
            water skis V92.27 ☑
            windsurfer V92.28 ☑
        motion of watercraft V92.19 ☑
          powered craft V92.13 ☑
            ferry boat V92.11 ☑
            fishing boat V92.12 ☑
            jetskis V92.13 ☑
            liner V92.11 ☑
            merchant ship V92.10 ☑
            passenger ship V92.11 ☑
          unpowered craft V92.08 ☑
            canoe V92.15 ☑
            inflatable V92.16 ☑
            kayak V92.15 ☑
            sailboat V92.14 ☑
      unpowered craft V92.08 ☑
        canoe V92.05 ☑
        inflatable V92.06 ☑
        kayak V92.05 ☑
        sailboat V92.04 ☑
        surf-board V92.08 ☑
        water skis V92.07 ☑
        windsurfer V92.08 ☑
    hurricane X37.0 ☑
    jumping into water from watercraft (involved in accident) (see also Drowning, due to, accident to, watercraft)
      without accident to or on watercraft W16.711 ☑
    tidal wave NEC — see Forces of nature, tidal wave
    torrential rain X37.8 ☑
  following
    fall
      into
        bathtub W16.211 ☑
        bucket W16.221 ☑
        fountain — see Drowning, following, fall, into, water, specified NEC
        quarry — see Drowning, following, fall, into, water, specified NEC
        reservoir — see Drowning, following, fall, into, water, specified NEC

Drowning — continued
  following — continued
    fall — continued
      into — continued
        swimming-pool W16.011 ☑
          stated as undetermined whether accidental or intentional Y21.3 ☑
          striking
            bottom W16.021 ☑
            wall W16.031 ☑
          suicide (attempt) X71.2 ☑
        water NOS W16.41 ☑
          natural (lake) (open sea) (river) (stream) (pond) W16.111 ☑
            striking
              bottom W16.121 ☑
              side W16.131 ☑
          specified NEC W16.311 ☑
            striking
              bottom W16.321 ☑
              wall W16.331 ☑
      overboard NEC — see Drowning, due to, fall overboard
    jump or dive
      from boat W16.711 ☑
        striking bottom W16.721 ☑
      into
        fountain — see Drowning, following, jump or dive, into, water, specified NEC
        quarry — see Drowning, following, jump or dive, into, water, specified NEC
        reservoir — see Drowning, following, jump or dive, into, water, specified NEC
        swimming-pool W16.511 ☑
          striking
            bottom W16.521 ☑
            wall W16.531 ☑
          suicide (attempt) X71.2 ☑
        water NOS W16.91 ☑
          natural (lake) (open sea) (river) (stream) (pond) W16.611 ☑
          specified NEC W16.811 ☑
            bottom W16.821 ☑
            striking
              bottom W16.821 ☑
              wall W16.831 ☑
          striking
            bottom W16.821 ☑
            wall W16.831 ☑
          striking bottom W16.621 ☑
  homicide (attempt) X92.9 ☑
  in
    bathtub (accidental) W65 ☑
      assault X92.0 ☑
      following fall W16.211 ☑
        stated as undetermined whether accidental or intentional Y21.1 ☑
      stated as undetermined whether accidental or intentional Y21.0 ☑
      suicide (attempt) X71.0 ☑
    lake — see Drowning, in, natural water
    natural water (lake) (open sea) (river) (stream) (pond) W69 ☑
      assault X92.3 ☑
      following
        dive or jump W16.611 ☑
          striking bottom W16.621 ☑
        fall W16.111 ☑
          striking
            bottom W16.121 ☑
            side W16.131 ☑
      stated as undetermined whether accidental or intentional Y21.4 ☑
      suicide (attempt) X71.3 ☑
    quarry — see Drowning, in, specified place NEC
    quenching tank — see Drowning, in, specified place NEC
    reservoir — see Drowning, in, specified place NEC
    river — see Drowning, in, natural water
    sea — see Drowning, in, natural water
    specified place NEC W73 ☑
      assault X92.8 ☑
      following
        dive or jump W16.811 ☑
          striking
            bottom W16.821 ☑
            wall W16.831 ☑

☑ Additional Character Required — Refer to the Tabular List for Character Selection   ⬗ Subterms under main terms may continue to next column or page

Drowning — *continued*
in — *continued*
    specified place — *continued*
      following — *continued*
        fall W16.311 ✓
          striking
            bottom W16.321 ✓
            wall W16.331 ✓
        stated as undetermined whether accidental or
          intentional Y21.8 ✓
        suicide (attempt) X71.8 ✓
    stream — *see* Drowning, in, natural water
    swimming-pool W67 ✓
      assault X92.1 ✓
        following fall X92.2 ✓
      following
        dive or jump W16.511 ✓
          striking
            bottom W16.521 ✓
            wall W16.531 ✓
        fall W16.011 ✓
          striking
            bottom W16.021 ✓
            wall W16.031 ✓
      stated as undetermined whether accidental or
        intentional Y21.2 ✓
        following fall Y21.3 ✓
      suicide (attempt) X71.1 ✓
        following fall X71.2 ✓
    war operations — *see* War operations, restriction
      of airway
  resulting from accident to watercraft — *see* Drowning,
    due to, accident, watercraft
  self-inflicted X71.9 ✓
  stated as undetermined whether accidental or inten-
    tional Y21.9 ✓
  suicide (attempt) X71.9 ✓

E

Earth falling (on) W20.0 ✓
  caused by cataclysmic earth surface movement or
    eruption — *see* Landslide
Earth (surface) **movement NEC** — *see* Forces of nature,
  earth movement
Earthquake (any injury) X34 ✓
Effect(s) (adverse) **of**
  air pressure (any) — *see* Air, pressure
  cold, excessive (exposure to) — *see* Exposure, cold
  heat (excessive) — *see* Heat
  hot place (weather) — *see* Heat
  insolation X30 ✓
  late — *see* Sequelae
  motion — *see* Motion
  nuclear explosion or weapon in war operations — *see*
    War operations, nuclear weapon
  radiation — *see* Radiation
  travel — *see* Travel
Electric shock (accidental) (by) (in) — *see* Exposure,
  electric current
Electrocution (accidental) — *see* Exposure, electric current
Endotracheal tube wrongly placed during anesthetic
  procedure
Entanglement
  in
    bed linen, causing suffocation T71 ✓
    wheel of pedal cycle V19.88 ✓
Entry of foreign body or material — *see* Foreign body
Environmental pollution related condition — *see*
  category Z57 ✓
Execution, legal (any method) — *see* Legal, intervention
Exhaustion
  cold — *see* Exposure, cold
  due to excessive exertion (*see also* Overexertion)
    X50.9 ✓
  heat — *see* Heat
Explosion (accidental) (of) (with secondary fire) W40.9 ✓
  acetylene W40.1 ✓
  aerosol can W36.1 ✓
  air tank (compressed) (in machinery) W36.2 ✓
  aircraft (in transit) (powered) NEC V95.9 ✓
    balloon V96.05 ✓
    fixed wing NEC (private) V95.25 ✓
      commercial V95.35 ✓
    glider V96.25 ✓

Explosion — *continued*
  aircraft — *continued*
    glider — *continued*
      hang V96.15 ✓
      powered V95.15 ✓
    helicopter V95.05 ✓
    in war operations — *see* War operations, destruc-
      tion of aircraft
    microlight V95.15 ✓
    nonpowered V96.9 ✓
      specified NEC V96.8 ✓
    powered NEC V95.8 ✓
    stated as
      homicide (attempt) Y03.8 ✓
      suicide (attempt) X83.0 ✓
    ultralight V95.15 ✓
  anesthetic gas in operating room W40.1 ✓
  antipersonnel bomb W40.8 ✓
    assault X96.0 ✓
    homicide (attempt) X96.0 ✓
    suicide (attempt) X75 ✓
  assault X96.9 ✓
  bicycle tire W37.0 ✓
  blasting (cap) (materials) W40.0 ✓
  boiler (machinery), not on transport vehicle W35 ✓
    on watercraft — *see* Explosion, in, watercraft
  butane W40.1 ✓
  caused by other person X96.9 ✓
  coal gas W40.1 ✓
  detonator W40.0 ✓
  dump (munitions) W40.8 ✓
  dynamite W40.0 ✓
    in
      assault X96.8 ✓
      homicide (attempt) X96.8 ✓
      legal intervention
        injuring
          bystander Y35.112 ✓
          law enforcement personnel Y35.111 ✓
          suspect Y35.113 ✓
      suicide (attempt) X75 ✓
  explosive (material) W40.9 ✓
    gas W40.1 ✓
    in blasting operation W40.0 ✓
    specified NEC W40.8 ✓
      in
        assault X96.8 ✓
        homicide (attempt) X96.8 ✓
        legal intervention
          injuring
            bystander Y35.192 ✓
            law enforcement personnel
              Y35.191 ✓
            suspect Y35.193 ✓
        suicide (attempt) X75 ✓
  factory (munitions) W40.8 ✓
  fertilizer bomb W40.8 ✓
    assault X96.3 ✓
    homicide (attempt) X96.3 ✓
    suicide (attempt) X75 ✓
  firearm (parts) NEC W34.19 ✓
    airgun W34.110 ✓
    BB gun W34.110 ✓
    gas, air or spring-operated gun NEC W34.118 ✓
    hangun W32.1 ✓
    hunting rifle W33.12 ✓
    larger firearm W33.10 ✓
      specified NEC W33.19 ✓
    machine gun W33.13 ✓
    paintball gun W34.111 ✓
    pellet gun W34.110 ✓
    shotgun W33.11 ✓
    Very pistol [flare] W34.19 ✓
  fire-damp W40.1 ✓
  fireworks W39 ✓
  gas (coal) (explosive) W40.1 ✓
    cylinder W36.9 ✓
      aerosol can W36.1 ✓
      air tank W36.2 ✓
      pressurized W36.3 ✓
      specified NEC W36.8 ✓
  gasoline (fumes) (tank) not in moving motor vehicle
    W40.1 ✓
    bomb W40.8 ✓
      assault X96.1 ✓
      homicide (attempt) X96.1 ✓

Explosion — *continued*
  gasoline not in moving motor vehicle — *continued*
    bomb — *continued*
      suicide (attempt) X75 ✓
    in motor vehicle — *see* Accident, transport, by type
      of vehicle
  grain store W40.8 ✓
  grenade W40.8 ✓
    in
      assault X96.8 ✓
      homicide (attempt) X96.8 ✓
      legal intervention
        injuring
          bystander Y35.192 ✓
          law enforcement personnel Y35.191 ✓
          suspect Y35.193 ✓
      suicide (attempt) X75 ✓
  handgun (parts) — *see* Explosion, firearm, hangun
    (parts)
  homicide (attempt) X96.9 ✓
    antipersonnel bomb — *see* Explosion, antiperson-
      nel bomb
    fertilizer bomb — *see* Explosion, fertilizer bomb
    gasoline bomb — *see* Explosion, gasoline bomb
    letter bomb — *see* Explosion, letter bomb
    pipe bomb — *see* Explosion, pipe bomb
    specified NEC X96.8 ✓
  hose, pressurized W37.8 ✓
  hot water heater, tank (in machinery) W35 ✓
    on watercraft — *see* Explosion, in, watercraft
  in, on
    dump W40.8 ✓
    factory W40.8 ✓
    mine (of explosive gases) NEC W40.1 ✓
    watercraft V93.59 ✓
      powered craft V93.53 ✓
        ferry boat V93.51 ✓
        fishing boat V93.52 ✓
        jetskis V93.53 ✓
        liner V93.51 ✓
        merchant ship V93.50 ✓
        passenger ship V93.51 ✓
        sailboat V93.54 ✓
  letter bomb W40.8 ✓
    assault X96.2 ✓
    homicide (attempt) X96.2 ✓
    suicide (attempt) X75 ✓
  machinery (*see also* Contact, with, by type of machine)
    on board watercraft — *see* Explosion, in, watercraft
    pressure vessel — *see* Explosion, by type of vessel
  methane W40.1 ✓
  mine W40.1 ✓
  missile NEC W40.8 ✓
  mortar bomb W40.8 ✓
    in
      assault X96.8 ✓
      homicide (attempt) X96.8 ✓
      legal intervention
        injuring
          bystander Y35.192 ✓
          law enforcement personnel Y35.191 ✓
          suspect Y35.193 ✓
      suicide (attempt) X75 ✓
  munitions (dump) (factory) W40.8 ✓
  pipe, pressurized W37.8 ✓
    bomb W40.8 ✓
      assault X96.4 ✓
      homicide (attempt) X96.4 ✓
      suicide (attempt) X75 ✓
  pressure, pressurized
    cooker W38 ✓
    gas tank (in machinery) W36.3 ✓
    hose W37.8 ✓
    pipe W37.8 ✓
    specified device NEC W38 ✓
    tire W37.8 ✓
      bicycle W37.0 ✓
    vessel (in machinery) W38 ✓
  propane W40.1 ✓
  self-inflicted X75 ✓
  shell (artillery) NEC W40.8 ✓
    during war operations — *see* War operations, ex-
      plosion

Explosion — *continued*
- shell — *continued*
  - in
    - legal intervention
      - injuring
        - bystander Y35.122 ☑
        - law enforcement personnel Y35.121 ☑
        - suspect Y35.123 ☑
    - war — *see* War operations, explosion
- spacecraft V95.45 ☑
- stated as undetermined whether accidental or intentional Y25 ☑
- steam or water lines (in machinery) W37.8 ☑
- stove W40.9 ☑
- suicide (attempt) X75 ☑
- tire, pressurized W37.8 ☑
  - bicycle W37.0 ☑
- undetermined whether accidental or intentional Y25 ☑
- vehicle tire NEC W37.8 ☑
  - bicycle W37.0 ☑
- war operations — *see* War operations, explosion

Exposure (to) X58 ☑
- air pressure change — *see* Air, pressure
- cold (accidental) (excessive) (extreme) (natural) (place) X31 ☑
  - assault Y08.89 ☑
  - due to
    - man-made conditions W93.8 ☑
      - dry ice (contact) W93.01 ☑
        - inhalation W93.02 ☑
      - liquid air (contact) (hydrogen) (nitrogen) W93.11 ☑
        - inhalation W93.12 ☑
      - refrigeration unit (deep freeze) W93.2 ☑
    - suicide (attempt) X83.2 ☑
    - weather (conditions) X31 ☑
  - homicide (attempt) Y08.89 ☑
  - self-inflicted X83.2 ☑
- due to abandonment or neglect X58 ☑
- electric current W86.8 ☑
  - appliance (faulty) W86.8 ☑
    - domestic W86.0 ☑
  - caused by other person Y08.89 ☑
  - conductor (faulty) W86.1 ☑
  - control apparatus (faulty) W86.1 ☑
  - electric power generating plant, distribution station W86.1 ☑
  - electroshock gun — *see* Exposure, electric current, taser
  - high-voltage cable W85 ☑
  - homicide (attempt) Y08.89 ☑
  - legal execution — *see* Legal, intervention, specified means NEC
  - lightning — *see* subcategory T75.0 ☑
  - live rail W86.8 ☑
  - misadventure in medical or surgical procedure in electroshock therapy Y63.4
  - motor (electric) (faulty) W86.8 ☑
    - domestic W86.0 ☑
  - self-inflicted X83.1 ☑
  - specified NEC W86.8 ☑
    - domestic W86.0 ☑
  - stun gun — *see* Exposure, electric current, taser
  - suicide (attempt) X83.1 ☑
  - taser W86.8 ☑
    - assault Y08.89 ☑
    - legal intervention — *see* category Y35
    - self-harm (intentional) X83.8 ☑
    - undetermined intent Y33 ☑
  - third rail W86.8 ☑
  - transformer (faulty) W86.1 ☑
  - transmission lines W85 ☑
- environmental tobacco smoke X58 ☑
- excessive
  - cold — *see* Exposure, cold
  - heat (natural) NEC X30 ☑
    - man-made W92 ☑
- factor(s) NOS X58 ☑
  - environmental NEC X58 ☑
  - man-made NEC W99 ☑
  - natural NEC — *see* Forces of nature
  - specified NEC X58 ☑
- fire, flames (accidental) X08.8 ☑
  - assault X97 ☑

Exposure — *continued*
- fire, flames — *continued*
  - campfire — *see* Exposure, fire, controlled, not in building
  - controlled (in)
    - with ignition (of) clothing (*see also* Ignition, clothes) X06.2 ☑
      - nightwear X05 ☑
    - bonfire — *see* Exposure, fire, controlled, not in building
    - brazier (in building or structure) (*see also* Exposure, fire, controlled, building)
      - not in building or structure — *see* Exposure, fire, controlled, not in building
    - building or structure X02.0 ☑
      - with
        - fall from building X02.3 ☑
        - from building X02.5 ☑
        - injury due to building collapse X02.2 ☑
        - smoke inhalation X02.1 ☑
      - hit by object from building X02.4 ☑
      - specified mode of injury NEC X02.8 ☑
    - fireplace, furnace or stove — *see* Exposure, fire, controlled, building
    - not in building or structure X03.0 ☑
      - with
        - fall X03.3 ☑
        - smoke inhalation X03.1 ☑
      - hit by object X03.4 ☑
      - specified mode of injury NEC X03.8 ☑
    - trash — *see* Exposure, fire, controlled, not in building
  - fireplace — *see* Exposure, fire, controlled, building
  - fittings or furniture (in building or structure) (uncontrolled) — *see* Exposure, fire, uncontrolled, building
  - forest (uncontrolled) — *see* Exposure, fire, uncontrolled, not in building
  - grass (uncontrolled) — *see* Exposure, fire, uncontrolled, not in building
  - hay (uncontrolled) — *see* Exposure, fire, uncontrolled, not in building
  - homicide (attempt) X97 ☑
  - ignition of highly flammable material X04 ☑
  - in, of, on, starting in
    - machinery — *see* Contact, with, by type of machine
    - motor vehicle (in motion) (*see also* Accident, transport, occupant by type of vehicle) V87.8 ☑
      - with collision — *see* Collision
    - railway rolling stock, train, vehicle V81.81 ☑
      - with collision — *see* Accident, transport, railway vehicle occupant
    - street car (in motion) V82.8 ☑
      - with collision — *see* Accident, transport, streetcar occupant
    - transport vehicle NEC (*see also* Accident, transport)
      - with collision — *see* Collision
    - war operations (*see also* War operations, fire)
      - from nuclear explosion — *see* War operations, nuclear weapons
    - watercraft (in transit) (not in transit) V91.09 ☑
      - localized — *see* Burn, on board watercraft, due to, fire on board
      - powered craft V91.03 ☑
        - ferry boat V91.01 ☑
        - fishing boat V91.02 ☑
        - jet skis V91.03 ☑
        - liner V91.01 ☑
        - merchant ship V91.00 ☑
        - passenger ship V91.01 ☑
      - unpowered craft V91.08 ☑
        - canoe V91.05 ☑
        - inflatable V91.06 ☑
        - kayak V91.05 ☑
        - sailboat V91.04 ☑
        - surf-board V91.08 ☑
        - waterskis V91.07 ☑
        - windsurfer V91.08 ☑
  - lumber (uncontrolled) — *see* Exposure, fire, uncontrolled, not in building
  - mine (uncontrolled) — *see* Exposure, fire, uncontrolled, not in building
  - prairie (uncontrolled) — *see* Exposure, fire, uncontrolled, not in building

Exposure — *continued*
- fire, flames — *continued*
  - resulting from
    - explosion — *see* Explosion
    - lightning X08.8 ☑
  - self-inflicted X76 ☑
  - specified NEC X08.8 ☑
  - started by other person X97 ☑
  - stated as undetermined whether accidental or intentional Y26 ☑
  - stove — *see* Exposure, fire, controlled, building
  - suicide (attempt) X76 ☑
  - tunnel (uncontrolled) — *see* Exposure, fire, uncontrolled, not in building
  - uncontrolled
    - in building or structure X00.0 ☑
      - with
        - fall from building X00.3 ☑
        - injury due to building collapse X00.2 ☑
        - jump from building X00.5 ☑
        - smoke inhalation X00.1 ☑
      - bed X08.00 ☑
        - due to
          - cigarette X08.01 ☑
          - specified material NEC X08.09 ☑
      - furniture NEC X08.20 ☑
        - due to
          - cigarette X08.21 ☑
          - specified material NEC X08.29 ☑
      - hit by object from building X00.4 ☑
      - sofa X08.10 ☑
        - due to
          - cigarette X08.11 ☑
          - specified material NEC X08.19 ☑
      - specified mode of injury NEC X00.8 ☑
    - not in building or structure (any) X01.0 ☑
      - with
        - fall X01.3 ☑
        - smoke inhalation X01.1 ☑
      - hit by object X01.4 ☑
      - specified mode of injury NEC X01.8 ☑
  - undetermined whether accidental or intentional Y26 ☑
- forces of nature NEC — *see* Forces of nature
- G-forces (abnormal) W49.9 ☑
- gravitational forces (abnormal) W49.9 ☑
- heat (natural) NEC — *see* Heat
- high-pressure jet (hydraulic) (pneumatic) W49.9 ☑
- hydraulic jet W49.9 ☑
- inanimate mechanical force W49.9 ☑
- jet, high-pressure (hydraulic) (pneumatic) W49.9 ☑
- lightning — *see* subcategory T75.0 ☑
  - causing fire — *see* Exposure, fire
- mechanical forces NEC W49.9 ☑
  - animate NEC W64 ☑
  - inanimate NEC W49.9 ☑
- noise W42.9 ☑
  - supersonic W42.0 ☑
- noxious substance — *see* Table of Drugs and Chemicals
- pneumatic jet W49.9 ☑
- prolonged in deep-freeze unit or refrigerator W93.2 ☑
- radiation — *see* Radiation
- smoke (*see also* Exposure, fire)
  - tobacco, second hand Z77.22
- specified factors NEC X58 ☑
- sunlight X32 ☑
  - man-made (sun lamp) W89.8 ☑
    - tanning bed W89.1 ☑
- supersonic waves W42.0 ☑
- transmission line(s), electric W85 ☑
- vibration W49.9 ☑
- waves
  - infrasound W49.9 ☑
  - sound W42.9 ☑
  - supersonic W42.0 ☑
- weather NEC — *see* Forces of nature

External cause status Y99.9
- child assisting in compensated work for family Y99.8
- civilian activity done for financial or other compensation Y99.0
- civilian activity done for income or pay Y99.0
- family member assisting in compensated work for other family member Y99.8
- hobby not done for income Y99.8
- leisure activity Y99.8

External cause status — *continued*
military activity Y99.1
off-duty activity of military personnel Y99.8
recreation or sport not for income or while a student Y99.8
specified NEC Y99.8
student activity Y99.8
volunteer activity Y99.2

F

Factors, supplemental
alcohol
  blood level
    less than 20mg/100ml Y90.0
    20-39mg/100ml Y90.1
    40-59mg/100ml Y90.2
    60-79mg/100ml Y90.3
    80-99mg/100ml Y90.4
    100-119mg/100ml Y90.5
    120-199mg/100ml Y90.6
    200-239mg/100ml Y90.7
    240mg/100ml or more Y90.8
    presence in blood, level not specified Y90.9
  presence in blood, but level not specified Y90.9
environmental-pollution-related condition- see Z57 ☑
nosocomial condition Y95
work-related condition Y99.0

Failure
in suture or ligature during surgical procedure Y65.2
mechanical, of instrument or apparatus (any) (during any medical or surgical procedure) Y65.8
sterile precautions (during medical and surgical care) — *see* Misadventure, failure, sterile precautions, by type of procedure
to
  introduce tube or instrument Y65.4
    endotracheal tube during anesthesia Y65.3
  make curve (transport vehicle) NEC — *see* Accident, transport
  remove tube or instrument Y65.4

Fall, falling (accidental) W19 ☑
building W20.1 ☑
  burning (uncontrolled fire) X00.3 ☑
down
  embankment W17.81 ☑
  escalator W10.0 ☑
  hill W17.81 ☑
  ladder W11 ☑
  ramp W10.2 ☑
  stairs, steps W10.9 ☑
due to
  bumping against
    object W18.00 ☑
      sharp glass W18.02 ☑
      specified NEC W18.09 ☑
      sports equipment W18.01 ☑
    person W03 ☑
      due to ice or snow W00.0 ☑
      on pedestrian conveyance — *see* Accident, transport, pedestrian, conveyance
  collision with another person W03 ☑
    due to ice or snow W00.0 ☑
    involving pedestrian conveyance — *see* Accident, transport, pedestrian, conveyance
  grocery cart tipping over W17.82 ☑
  ice or snow W00.9 ☑
    from one level to another W00.2 ☑
    on stairs or steps W00.1 ☑
  involving pedestrian conveyance — *see* Accident, transport, pedestrian, conveyance
  on same level W00.0 ☑
  slipping (on moving sidewalk) W01.0 ☑
    with subsequent striking against object W01.10 ☑
      furniture W01.190 ☑
      sharp object W01.119 ☑
        glass W01.110 ☑
        power tool or machine W01.111 ☑
        specified NEC W01.118 ☑
      specified NEC W01.198 ☑
  striking against
    object W18.00 ☑
      sharp glass W18.02 ☑
      specified NEC W18.09 ☑
      sports equipment W18.01 ☑
    person W03 ☑

Fall, falling — *continued*
due to — *continued*
  striking against — *continued*
    person — *continued*
      due to ice or snow W00.0 ☑
      on pedestrian conveyance — *see* Accident, transport, pedestrian, conveyance
earth (with asphyxia or suffocation (by pressure)) — *see* Earth, falling
from, off, out of
  aircraft NEC (with accident to aircraft NEC) V97.0 ☑
    while boarding or alighting V97.1 ☑
  balcony W13.0 ☑
  bed W06 ☑
  boat, ship, watercraft NEC (with drowning or submersion) — *see* Drowning, due to, fall overboard
    with hitting bottom or object V94.0 ☑
  bridge W13.1 ☑
  building W13.9 ☑
    burning (uncontrolled fire) X00.3 ☑
  cavity W17.2 ☑
  chair W07 ☑
  cherry picker W17.89 ☑
  cliff W15 ☑
  dock W17.4 ☑
  embankment W17.81 ☑
  escalator W10.0 ☑
  flagpole W13.8 ☑
  furniture NEC W08 ☑
  grocery cart W17.82 ☑
  haystack W17.89 ☑
  high place NEC W17.89 ☑
    stated as undetermined whether accidental or intentional Y30 ☑
  hole W17.2 ☑
  incline W10.2 ☑
  ladder W11 ☑
  lifting device W17.89 ☑
  machine, machinery (*see also* Contact, with, by type of machine)
    not in operation W17.89 ☑
  manhole W17.1 ☑
  mobile elevated work platform [MEWP] W17.89 ☑
  motorized mobility scooter W05.2 ☑
  one level to another NEC W17.89 ☑
    intentional, purposeful, suicide (attempt) X80 ☑
    stated as undetermined whether accidental or intentional Y30 ☑
  pit W17.2 ☑
  playground equipment W09.8 ☑
    jungle gym W09.2 ☑
    slide W09.0 ☑
    swing W09.1 ☑
  quarry W17.89 ☑
  railing W13.9 ☑
  ramp W10.2 ☑
  roof W13.2 ☑
  scaffolding W12 ☑
  scooter (nonmotorized) W05.1 ☑
    motorized mobility W05.2 ☑
  sky lift W17.89 ☑
  stairs, steps W10.9 ☑
    curb W10.1 ☑
    due to ice or snow W00.1 ☑
    escalator W10.0 ☑
    incline W10.2 ☑
    ramp W10.2 ☑
    sidewalk curb W10.1 ☑
    specified NEC W10.8 ☑
  stepladder W11 ☑
  storm drain W17.1 ☑
  streetcar NEC V82.6 ☑
    with antecedent collision — *see* Accident, transport, streetcar occupant
    while boarding or alighting V82.4 ☑
  structure NEC W13.8 ☑
    burning (uncontrolled fire) X00.3 ☑
  table W08 ☑
  toilet W18.11 ☑
    with subsequent striking against object W18.12 ☑
  train NEC V81.6 ☑
    during derailment (without antecedent collision) V81.7 ☑

Fall, falling — *continued*
from, off, out of — *continued*
  train — *continued*
    during derailment — *continued*
      with antecedent collision — *see* Accident, transport, railway vehicle occupant
    while boarding or alighting V81.4 ☑
    transport vehicle after collision — *see* Accident, transport, by type of vehicle, collision
  tree W14 ☑
  vehicle (in motion) NEC (*see also* Accident, transport) V89.9 ☑
    motor NEC (*see also* Accident, transport, occupant, by type of vehicle) V87.8 ☑
    stationary W17.89 ☑
      while boarding or alighting — *see* Accident, transport, by type of vehicle, while boarding or alighting
  viaduct W13.8 ☑
  wall W13.8 ☑
  watercraft (*see also* Drowning, due to, fall overboard)
    with hitting bottom or object V94.0 ☑
  well W17.0 ☑
  wheelchair, non-moving W05.0 ☑
    powered — *see* Accident, transport, pedestrian, conveyance occupant, specified type NEC
  window W13.4 ☑
in, on
  aircraft NEC V97.0 ☑
    with accident to aircraft V97.0 ☑
    while boarding or alighting V97.1 ☑
  bathtub (empty) W18.2 ☑
    filled W16.212 ☑
      causing drowning W16.211 ☑
  escalator W10.0 ☑
  incline W10.2 ☑
  ladder W11 ☑
  machine, machinery — *see* Contact, with, by type of machine
  object, edged, pointed or sharp (with cut) — *see* Fall, by type
  playground equipment W09.8 ☑
    jungle gym W09.2 ☑
    slide W09.0 ☑
    swing W09.1 ☑
  ramp W10.2 ☑
  scaffolding W12 ☑
  shower W18.2 ☑
    causing drowning W16.211 ☑
  staircase, stairs, steps W10.9 ☑
    curb W10.1 ☑
    due to ice or snow W00.1 ☑
    escalator W10.0 ☑
    incline W10.2 ☑
    specified NEC W10.8 ☑
  streetcar (without antecedent collision) V82.5 ☑
    with antecedent collision — *see* Accident, transport, streetcar occupant
    while boarding or alighting V82.4 ☑
  train (without antecedent collision) V81.5 ☑
    with antecedent collision — *see* Accident, transport, railway vehicle occupant
    during derailment (without antecedent collision) V81.7 ☑
      with antecedent collision — *see* Accident, transport, railway vehicle occupant
    while boarding or alighting V81.4 ☑
  transport vehicle after collision — *see* Accident, transport, by type of vehicle, collision
  watercraft V93.39 ☑
    due to
      accident to craft V91.29 ☑
        powered craft V91.23 ☑
          ferry boat V91.21 ☑
          fishing boat V91.22 ☑
          jetskis V91.23 ☑
          liner V91.21 ☑
          merchant ship V91.20 ☑
          passenger ship V91.21 ☑
        unpowered craft
          canoe V91.25 ☑
          inflatable V91.26 ☑
          kayak V91.25 ☑
          sailboat V91.24 ☑
      powered craft V93.33 ☑

Fall, falling — *continued*
- in, on — *continued*
  - watercraft — *continued*
    - powered craft — *continued*
      - ferry boat V93.31 ☑
      - fishing boat V93.32 ☑
      - jetskis V93.33 ☑
      - liner V93.31 ☑
      - merchant ship V93.30 ☑
      - passenger ship V93.31 ☑
    - unpowered craft V93.38 ☑
      - canoe V93.35 ☑
      - inflatable V93.36 ☑
      - kayak V93.35 ☑
      - sailboat V93.34 ☑
      - surf-board V93.38 ☑
      - windsurfer V93.38 ☑
- into
  - cavity W17.2 ☑
  - dock W17.4 ☑
  - fire — *see* Exposure, fire, by type
  - haystack W17.89 ☑
  - hole W17.2 ☑
  - lake — *see* Fall, into, water
  - manhole W17.1 ☑
  - moving part of machinery — *see* Contact, with, by type of machine
  - ocean — *see* Fall, into, water
  - opening in surface NEC W17.89 ☑
  - pit W17.2 ☑
  - pond — *see* Fall, into, water
  - quarry W17.89 ☑
  - river — *see* Fall, into, water
  - shaft W17.89 ☑
  - storm drain W17.1 ☑
  - stream — *see* Fall, into, water
  - swimming pool (*see also* Fall, into, water, in, swimming pool)
    - empty W17.3 ☑
  - tank W17.89 ☑
  - water W16.42 ☑
    - causing drowning W16.41 ☑
    - from watercraft — *see* Drowning, due to, fall overboard
    - hitting diving board W21.4 ☑
    - in
      - bathtub W16.212 ☑
        - causing drowning W16.211 ☑
      - bucket W16.222 ☑
        - causing drowning W16.221 ☑
      - natural body of water W16.112 ☑
        - causing drowning W16.111 ☑
        - striking
          - bottom W16.122 ☑
            - causing drowning W16.121 ☑
          - side W16.132 ☑
            - causing drowning W16.131 ☑
      - specified water NEC W16.312 ☑
        - causing drowning W16.311 ☑
        - striking
          - bottom W16.322 ☑
            - causing drowning W16.321 ☑
          - wall W16.332 ☑
            - causing drowning W16.331 ☑
      - swimming pool W16.012 ☑
        - causing drowning W16.011 ☑
        - striking
          - bottom W16.022 ☑
            - causing drowning W16.031 ☑
          - wall W16.032 ☑
            - causing drowning W16.021 ☑
      - utility bucket W16.222 ☑
        - causing drowning W16.221 ☑
  - well W17.0 ☑
- involving
  - bed W06 ☑
  - chair W07 ☑
  - furniture NEC W08 ☑
  - glass — *see* Fall, by type
  - playground equipment W09.8 ☑
    - jungle gym W09.2 ☑
    - slide W09.0 ☑
    - swing W09.1 ☑
  - roller blades — *see* Accident, transport, pedestrian, conveyance

Fall, falling — *continued*
- involving — *continued*
  - skateboard(s) — *see* Accident, transport, pedestrian, conveyance
  - skates (ice) (in line) (roller) — *see* Accident, transport, pedestrian, conveyance
  - skis — *see* Accident, transport, pedestrian, conveyance
  - table W08 ☑
  - wheelchair, non-moving W05.0 ☑
    - powered — *see* Accident, transport, pedestrian, conveyance, specified type NEC
- object — *see* Struck by, object, falling
- off
  - toilet W18.11 ☑
    - with subsequent striking against object W18.12 ☑
- on same level W18.30 ☑
  - due to
    - specified NEC W18.39 ☑
    - stepping on an object W18.31 ☑
- out of
  - bed W06 ☑
  - building NEC W13.8 ☑
  - chair W07 ☑
  - furniture NEC W08 ☑
  - wheelchair, non-moving W05.0 ☑
    - powered — *see* Accident, transport, pedestrian, conveyance, specified type NEC
  - window W13.4 ☑
- over
  - animal W01.0 ☑
  - cliff W15 ☑
  - embankment W17.81 ☑
  - small object W01.0 ☑
- rock W20.8 ☑
- same level W18.30 ☑
  - from
    - being crushed, pushed, or stepped on by a crowd or human stampede W52 ☑
    - collision, pushing, shoving, by or with other person W03 ☑
    - slipping, stumbling, tripping W01.0 ☑
  - involving ice or snow W00.0 ☑
    - involving skates (ice) (roller), skateboard, skis — *see* Accident, transport, pedestrian, conveyance
- snowslide (avalanche) — *see* Landslide
- stone W20.8 ☑
- structure W20.1 ☑
  - burning (uncontrolled fire) X00.3 ☑
- through
  - bridge W13.1 ☑
  - floor W13.3 ☑
  - roof W13.2 ☑
  - wall W13.8 ☑
  - window W13.4 ☑
- timber W20.8 ☑
- tree (caused by lightning) W20.8 ☑
- while being carried or supported by other person(s) W04 ☑

Fallen on by
- animal (not being ridden) NEC W55.89 ☑

Felo-de-se — *see* Suicide

Fight (hand) (fists) (foot) — *see* Assault, fight

Fire (accidental) — *see* Exposure, fire

Firearm discharge — *see* Discharge, firearm

Fireball effects from nuclear explosion in war operations — *see* War operations, nuclear weapons

Fireworks (explosion) W39 ☑

Flash burns from explosion — *see* Explosion

Flood (any injury) (caused by) X38 ☑
- collapse of man-made structure causing earth movement X36.0 ☑
- tidal wave — *see* Forces of nature, tidal wave

Food (any type) **in**
- air passages (with asphyxia, obstruction, or suffocation) — *see* categories T17 and T18 ☑
- alimentary tract causing asphyxia (due to compression of trachea) — *see* categories T17 and T18 ☑

Forces of nature X39.8 ☑
- avalanche X36.1 ☑
  - causing transport accident — *see* Accident, transport, by type of vehicle
- blizzard X37.2 ☑
- cataclysmic storm X37.9 ☑

Forces of nature — *continued*
- cataclysmic storm — *continued*
  - with flood X38 ☑
  - blizzard X37.2 ☑
  - cloudburst X37.8 ☑
  - cyclone X37.1 ☑
  - dust storm X37.3 ☑
  - hurricane X37.0 ☑
  - specified storm NEC X37.8 ☑
  - storm surge X37.0 ☑
  - tornado X37.1 ☑
  - twister X37.1 ☑
  - typhoon X37.0 ☑
- cloudburst X37.8 ☑
- cold (natural) X31 ☑
- cyclone X37.1 ☑
- dam collapse causing earth movement X36.0 ☑
- dust storm X37.3 ☑
- earth movement X36.1 ☑
  - caused by dam or structure collapse X36.0 ☑
  - earthquake X34 ☑
- earthquake X34 ☑
- flood (caused by) X38 ☑
  - dam collapse X36.0 ☑
  - tidal wave — *see* Forces of nature, tidal wave
- heat (natural) X30 ☑
- hurricane X37.0 ☑
- landslide X36.1 ☑
  - causing transport accident — *see* Accident, transport, by type of vehicle
- lightning — *see* subcategory T75.0 ☑
  - causing fire — *see* Exposure, fire
- mudslide X36.1 ☑
  - causing transport accident — *see* Accident, transport, by type of vehicle
- radiation (natural) X39.08 ☑
  - radon X39.01 ☑
- radon X39.01 ☑
- specified force NEC X39.8 ☑
- storm surge X37.0 ☑
- structure collapse causing earth movement X36.0 ☑
- sunlight X32 ☑
- tidal wave X37.41 ☑
  - due to
    - earthquake X37.41 ☑
    - landslide X37.43 ☑
    - storm X37.42 ☑
    - volcanic eruption X37.41 ☑
- tornado X37.1 ☑
- tsunami X37.41 ☑
- twister X37.1 ☑
- typhoon X37.0 ☑
- volcanic eruption X35 ☑

Foreign body
- aspiration — *see* Index to Diseases and Injuries, Foreign body, respiratory tract
- embedded in skin W45 ☑
- entering through skin W45.8 ☑
  - can lid W26.8 ☑
  - nail W45.0 ☑
  - paper W26.2 ☑
  - specified NEC W45.8 ☑
  - splinter W45.8 ☑

Forest fire (exposure to) — *see* Exposure, fire, uncontrolled, not in building

Found injured X58 ☑
- from exposure (to) — *see* Exposure
- on
  - highway, road(way), street V89.9 ☑
  - railway right of way V81.9 ☑

Fracture (circumstances unknown or unspecified) X58 ☑
- due to specified cause NEC X58 ☑

Freezing — *see* Exposure, cold

Frostbite X31 ☑
- due to man-made conditions — *see* Exposure, cold, man-made

Frozen — *see* Exposure, cold

G

Gored by bull W55.22 ☑
Gunshot wound W34.00 ☑

H

Hailstones, injured by X39.8 ☑

Hanged herself or himself — *see* Hanging, self-inflicted
Hanging (accidental) (*see also* category) T71 ☑
   legal execution — *see* Legal, intervention, specified
      means NEC
Heat (effects of) (excessive) X30 ☑
   due to
      man-made conditions W92 ☑
         on board watercraft V93.29 ☑
            fishing boat V93.22 ☑
            merchant ship V93.20 ☑
            passenger ship V93.21 ☑
            sailboat V93.24 ☑
            specified powered craft NEC V93.23 ☑
      weather (conditions) X30 ☑
   from
      electric heating apparatus causing burning X16 ☑
      nuclear explosion in war operations — *see* War
         operations, nuclear weapons
   inappropriate in local application or packing in medical
      or surgical procedure Y63.5
Hemorrhage
   delayed following medical or surgical treatment
      without mention of misadventure — *see* Index
      to Diseases and Injuries, Complication(s)
   during medical or surgical treatment as misadventure
      — *see* Index to Diseases and Injuries, Complica-
      tion(s)
High
   altitude (effects) — *see* Air, pressure, low
   level of radioactivity, effects — *see* Radiation
   pressure (effects) — *see* Air, pressure, high
   temperature, effects — *see* Heat
Hit, hitting (accidental) by — *see* Struck by
Hitting against — *see* Striking against
Homicide (attempt) (justifiable) — *see* Assault
Hot
   place, effects (*see also* Heat)
   weather, effects X30 ☑
House fire (uncontrolled) — *see* Exposure, fire, uncon-
   trolled, building
Humidity, causing problem X39.8 ☑
Hunger X58 ☑
Hurricane (any injury) X37.0 ☑
Hypobarism, hypobaropathy — *see* Air, pressure, low

Ictus
   caloris (*see also* Heat)
   solaris X30 ☑
Ignition (accidental) (*see also* Exposure, fire) X08.8 ☑
   anesthetic gas in operating room W40.1 ☑
   apparel X06.2 ☑
      from highly flammable material X04 ☑
      nightwear X05 ☑
   bed linen (sheets) (spreads) (pillows) (mattress) — *see*
      Exposure, fire, uncontrolled, building, bed
   benzine X04 ☑
   clothes, clothing NEC (from controlled fire) X06.2 ☑
      from
         highly flammable material X04 ☑
   ether X04 ☑
      in operating room W40.1 ☑
   explosive material — *see* Explosion
   gasoline X04 ☑
   jewelry (plastic) (any) X06.0 ☑
   kerosene X04 ☑
   material
      explosive — *see* Explosion
      highly flammable with secondary explosion X04 ☑
   nightwear X05 ☑
   paraffin X04 ☑
   petrol X04 ☑
Immersion (accidental) (*see also* Drowning)
   hand or foot due to cold (excessive) X31 ☑
Implantation of quills of porcupine W55.89 ☑
Inanition (from) (hunger) X58 ☑
   thirst X58 ☑
Inappropriate operation performed
   correct operation on wrong side or body part (wrong
      side) (wrong site) Y65.53
   operation intended for another patient done on wrong
      patient Y65.52
   wrong operation performed on correct patient Y65.51
Inattention after, at birth (homicidal intent) (infantici-
   dal intent) X58 ☑

Incident, adverse
   device
      anesthesiology Y70.8
         accessory Y70.2
         diagnostic Y70.0
         miscellaneous Y70.8
         monitoring Y70.0
         prosthetic Y70.2
         rehabilitative Y70.1
         surgical Y70.3
         therapeutic Y70.1
      cardiovascular Y71.8
         accessory Y71.2
         diagnostic Y71.0
         miscellaneous Y71.8
         monitoring Y71.0
         prosthetic Y71.2
         rehabilitative Y71.1
         surgical Y71.3
         therapeutic Y71.1
      gastroenterology Y73.8
         accessory Y73.2
         diagnostic Y73.0
         miscellaneous Y73.8
         monitoring Y73.0
         prosthetic Y73.2
         rehabilitative Y73.1
         surgical Y73.3
         therapeutic Y73.1
      general
         hospital Y74.8
            accessory Y74.2
            diagnostic Y74.0
            miscellaneous Y74.8
            monitoring Y74.0
            prosthetic Y74.2
            rehabilitative Y74.1
            surgical Y74.3
            therapeutic Y74.1
         surgical Y81.8
            accessory Y81.2
            diagnostic Y81.0
            miscellaneous Y81.8
            monitoring Y81.0
            prosthetic Y81.2
            rehabilitative Y81.1
            surgical Y81.3
            therapeutic Y81.1
      gynecological Y76.8
         accessory Y76.2
         diagnostic Y76.0
         miscellaneous Y76.8
         monitoring Y76.0
         prosthetic Y76.2
         rehabilitative Y76.1
         surgical Y76.3
         therapeutic Y76.1
      medical Y82.9
         specified type NEC Y82.8
      neurological Y75.8
         accessory Y75.2
         diagnostic Y75.0
         miscellaneous Y75.8
         monitoring Y75.0
         prosthetic Y75.2
         rehabilitative Y75.1
         surgical Y75.3
         therapeutic Y75.1
      obstetrical Y76.8
         accessory Y76.2
         diagnostic Y76.0
         miscellaneous Y76.8
         monitoring Y76.0
         prosthetic Y76.2
         rehabilitative Y76.1
         surgical Y76.3
         therapeutic Y76.1
      ophthalmic Y77.8
         accessory Y77.2
         diagnostic Y77.0
         miscellaneous Y77.8
         monitoring Y77.0
         prosthetic Y77.2
         rehabilitative Y77.1
         surgical Y77.3
         therapeutic Y77.1
      orthopedic Y79.8
         accessory Y79.2
         diagnostic Y79.0

Incident, adverse — *continued*
   device — *continued*
      orthopedic — *continued*
         miscellaneous Y79.8
         monitoring Y79.0
         prosthetic Y79.2
         rehabilitative Y79.1
         surgical Y79.3
         therapeutic Y79.1
      otorhinolaryngological Y72.8
         accessory Y72.2
         diagnostic Y72.0
         miscellaneous Y72.8
         monitoring Y72.0
         prosthetic Y72.2
         rehabilitative Y72.1
         surgical Y72.3
         therapeutic Y72.1
      personal use Y74.8
         accessory Y74.2
         diagnostic Y74.0
         miscellaneous Y74.8
         monitoring Y74.0
         prosthetic Y74.2
         rehabilitative Y74.1
         surgical Y74.3
         therapeutic Y74.1
      physical medicine Y80.8
         accessory Y80.2
         diagnostic Y80.0
         miscellaneous Y80.8
         monitoring Y80.0
         prosthetic Y80.2
         rehabilitative Y80.1
         surgical Y80.3
         therapeutic Y80.1
      plastic surgical Y81.8
         accessory Y81.2
         diagnostic Y81.0
         miscellaneous Y81.8
         monitoring Y81.0
         prosthetic Y81.2
         rehabilitative Y81.1
         surgical Y81.3
         therapeutic Y81.1
      radiological Y78.8
         accessory Y78.2
         diagnostic Y78.0
         miscellaneous Y78.8
         monitoring Y78.0
         prosthetic Y78.2
         rehabilitative Y78.1
         surgical Y78.3
         therapeutic Y78.1
      urology Y73.8
         accessory Y73.2
         diagnostic Y73.0
         miscellaneous Y73.8
         monitoring Y73.0
         prosthetic Y73.2
         rehabilitative Y73.1
         surgical Y73.3
         therapeutic Y73.1
Incineration (accidental) — *see* Exposure, fire
Infanticide — *see* Assault
Infrasound waves (causing injury) W49.9 ☑
Ingestion
   foreign body (causing injury) (with obstruction) — *see*
      Foreign body, alimentary canal
   poisonous
      plant(s) X58 ☑
      substance NEC — *see* Table of Drugs and Chemicals
Inhalation
   excessively cold substance, man-made — *see* Expo-
      sure, cold, man-made
   food (any type) (into respiratory tract) (with asphyxia,
      obstruction respiratory tract, suffocation) — *see*
      categories T17 and T18 ☑
   foreign body — *see* Foreign body, aspiration
   gastric contents (with asphyxia, obstruction respiratory
      passage, suffocation) T17.81- ☑
   hot air or gases X14.0 ☑
   liquid air, hydrogen, nitrogen W93.12 ☑
      suicide (attempt) X83.2 ☑
   steam X13.0 ☑
      assault X98.0 ☑
      stated as undetermined whether accidental or in-
         tentional Y27.0 ☑

Inhalation — *continued*
- steam — *continued*
  - suicide (attempt) X77.0 ☑
- toxic gas — *see* Table of Drugs and Chemicals
- vomitus (with asphyxia, obstruction respiratory passage, suffocation) T17.81- ☑

Injury, injured (accidental(ly)) NOS X58 ☑
- by, caused by, from
  - assault — *see* Assault
  - law-enforcing agent, police, in course of legal intervention — *see* Legal intervention
  - suicide (attempt) X83.8 ☑
- due to, in
  - civil insurrection — *see* War operations
  - fight (*see also* Assault, fight) Y04.0 ☑
  - war operations — *see* War operations
- homicide (*see also* Assault) Y09
- inflicted (by)
  - in course of arrest (attempted), suppression of disturbance, maintenance of order, by law-enforcing agents — *see* Legal intervention
  - other person
    - stated as
      - accidental X58 ☑
      - intentional, homicide (attempt) — *see* Assault
      - undetermined whether accidental or intentional Y33 ☑
  - purposely (inflicted) by other person(s) — *see* Assault
- self-inflicted X83.8 ☑
  - stated as accidental X58 ☑
- specified cause NEC X58 ☑
- undetermined whether accidental or intentional Y33 ☑

Insolation, effects X30 ☑
Insufficient nourishment X58 ☑
Interruption of respiration (by)
- food (lodged in esophagus) — *see* categories T17 and T18 ☑
- vomitus (lodged in esophagus) T17.81- ☑

Intervention, legal — *see* Legal intervention
Intoxication
- drug — *see* Table of Drugs and Chemicals
- poison — *see* Table of Drugs and Chemicals

J

Jammed (accidentally)
- between objects (moving) (stationary and moving) W23.0 ☑
  - stationary W23.1 ☑
Jumped, jumping
- before moving object NEC X81.8 ☑
  - motor vehicle X81.0 ☑
  - subway train X81.1 ☑
  - train X81.1 ☑
  - undetermined whether accidental or intentional Y31 ☑
- from
  - boat (into water) voluntarily, without accident (to or on boat) W16.712 ☑
    - with
      - accident to or on boat — *see* Accident, watercraft
      - drowning or submersion W16.711 ☑
        - suicide (attempt) X71.3 ☑
      - striking bottom W16.722 ☑
        - causing drowning W16.721 ☑
  - building (*see also* Jumped, from, high place) W13.9 ☑
    - burning (uncontrolled fire) X00.5 ☑
  - high place NEC W17.89 ☑
    - suicide (attempt) X80 ☑
    - undetermined whether accidental or intentional Y30 ☑
  - structure (*see also* Jumped, from, high place) W13.9 ☑
    - burning (uncontrolled fire) X00.5 ☑
- into water W16.92 ☑
  - causing drowning W16.91 ☑
  - from, off watercraft — *see* Jumped, from, boat
  - in
    - natural body W16.612 ☑
      - causing drowning W16.611 ☑
      - striking bottom W16.622 ☑
        - causing drowning W16.621 ☑

Jumped, jumping — *continued*
- into water — *continued*
  - in — *continued*
    - specified place NEC W16.812 ☑
      - causing drowning W16.811 ☑
      - striking
        - bottom W16.822 ☑
          - causing drowning W16.821 ☑
        - wall W16.832 ☑
          - causing drowning W16.831 ☑
    - swimming pool W16.512 ☑
      - causing drowning W16.511 ☑
      - striking
        - bottom W16.522 ☑
          - causing drowning W16.521 ☑
        - wall W16.532 ☑
          - causing drowning W16.531 ☑
  - suicide (attempt) X71.3 ☑

K

Kicked by
- animal NEC W55.82 ☑
- person(s) (accidentally) W50.1 ☑
  - with intent to injure or kill Y04.0 ☑
  - as, or caused by, a crowd or human stampede (with fall) W52 ☑
  - assault Y04.0 ☑
  - homicide (attempt) Y04.0 ☑
  - in
    - fight Y04.0 ☑
    - legal intervention
      - injuring
        - bystander Y35.812 ☑
        - law enforcement personnel Y35.811 ☑
        - suspect Y35.813 ☑

Kicking
- against
  - object W22.8 ☑
    - sports equipment W21.9 ☑
  - stationary W22.09 ☑
    - sports equipment W21.89 ☑
  - person — *see* Striking against, person
  - sports equipment W21.9 ☑
- carpet stretcher with knee X50.3 ☑
Killed, killing (accidentally) NOS (*see also* Injury) X58 ☑
- in
  - action — *see* War operations
  - brawl, fight (hand) (fists) (foot) Y04.0 ☑
    - by weapon (*see also* Assault)
      - cutting, piercing — *see* Assault, cutting or piercing instrument
      - firearm — *see* Discharge, firearm, by type, homicide
- self
  - stated as
    - accident NOS X58 ☑
    - suicide — *see* Suicide
    - undetermined whether accidental or intentional Y33 ☑
Kneeling (prolonged (static)) X50.1 ☑
Knocked down (accidentally) (by) NOS X58 ☑
- animal (not being ridden) NEC (*see also* Struck by, by type of animal)
- crowd or human stampede W52 ☑
- person W51 ☑
  - in brawl, fight Y04.0 ☑
- transport vehicle NEC (*see also* Accident, transport) V09.9 ☑

L

Laceration NEC — *see* Injury
Lack of
- care (helpless person) (infant) (newborn) X58 ☑
- food except as result of abandonment or neglect X58 ☑
  - due to abandonment or neglect X58 ☑
- water except as result of transport accident X58 ☑
  - due to transport accident — *see* Accident, transport, by type
  - helpless person, infant, newborn X58 ☑
Landslide (falling on transport vehicle) X36.1 ☑
- caused by collapse of man-made structure X36.0 ☑
Late effect — *see* Sequelae

Legal
- execution (any method) — *see* Legal, intervention
- intervention (by)
  - baton — *see* Legal, intervention, blunt object, baton
  - bayonet — *see* Legal, intervention, sharp object, bayonet
  - blow — *see* Legal, intervention, manhandling
  - blunt object
    - baton
      - injuring
        - bystander Y35.312 ☑
        - law enforcement personnel Y35.311 ☑
        - suspect Y35.313 ☑
    - injuring
      - bystander Y35.302 ☑
      - law enforcement personnel Y35.301 ☑
      - suspect Y35.303 ☑
    - specified NEC
      - injuring
        - bystander Y35.392 ☑
        - law enforcement personnel Y35.391 ☑
        - suspect Y35.393 ☑
    - stave
      - injuring
        - bystander Y35.392 ☑
        - law enforcement personnel Y35.391 ☑
        - suspect Y35.393 ☑
  - bomb — *see* Legal, intervention, explosive
  - cutting or piercing instrument — *see* Legal, intervention, sharp object
  - dynamite — *see* Legal, intervention, explosive, dynamite
  - explosive(s)
    - dynamite
      - injuring
        - bystander Y35.112 ☑
        - law enforcement personnel Y35.111 ☑
        - suspect Y35.113 ☑
    - grenade
      - injuring
        - bystander Y35.192 ☑
        - law enforcement personnel Y35.191 ☑
        - suspect Y35.193 ☑
    - injuring
      - bystander Y35.102 ☑
      - law enforcement personnel Y35.101 ☑
      - suspect Y35.103 ☑
    - mortar bomb
      - injuring
        - bystander Y35.192 ☑
        - law enforcement personnel Y35.191 ☑
        - suspect Y35.193 ☑
    - shell
      - injuring
        - bystander Y35.122 ☑
        - law enforcement personnel Y35.121 ☑
        - suspect Y35.123 ☑
    - specified NEC
      - injuring
        - bystander Y35.192 ☑
        - law enforcement personnel Y35.191 ☑
        - suspect Y35.193 ☑
  - firearm(s) (discharge)
    - handgun
      - injuring
        - bystander Y35.022 ☑
        - law enforcement personnel Y35.021 ☑
        - suspect Y35.023 ☑
    - injuring
      - bystander Y35.002 ☑
      - law enforcement personnel Y35.001 ☑
      - suspect Y35.003 ☑
    - machine gun
      - injuring
        - bystander Y35.012 ☑
        - law enforcement personnel Y35.011 ☑
        - suspect Y35.013 ☑
    - rifle pellet
      - injuring
        - bystander Y35.032 ☑
        - law enforcement personnel Y35.031 ☑
        - suspect Y35.033 ☑
    - rubber bullet
      - injuring
        - bystander Y35.042 ☑
        - law enforcement personnel Y35.041 ☑

Legal — *continued*
  intervention — *continued*
    firearm(s) — *continued*
      rubber bullet — *continued*
        injuring — *continued*
          suspect Y35.043 ☑
      shotgun — *see* Legal, intervention, firearm, specified NEC
      specified NEC
        injuring
          bystander Y35.092 ☑
          law enforcement personnel Y35.091 ☑
          suspect Y35.093 ☑
    gas (asphyxiation) (poisoning)
      injuring
        bystander Y35.202 ☑
        law enforcement personnel Y35.201 ☑
        suspect Y35.203 ☑
      specified NEC
        injuring
          bystander Y35.292 ☑
          law enforcement personnel Y35.291 ☑
          suspect Y35.293 ☑
      tear gas
        injuring
          bystander Y35.212 ☑
          law enforcement personnel Y35.211 ☑
          suspect Y35.213 ☑
    grenade — *see* Legal, intervention, explosive, grenade
    injuring
      bystander Y35.92 ☑
      law enforcement personnel Y35.91 ☑
      suspect Y35.93 ☑
    late effect (of) — *see* with 7th character S Y35 ☑
    manhandling
      injuring
        bystander Y35.812 ☑
        law enforcement personnel Y35.811 ☑
        suspect Y35.813 ☑
    sequelae (of) — *see* with 7th character S Y35 ☑
    sharp objects
      bayonet
        injuring
          bystander Y35.412 ☑
          law enforcement personnel Y35.411 ☑
          suspect Y35.413 ☑
      injuring
        bystander Y35.402 ☑
        law enforcement personnel Y35.401 ☑
        suspect Y35.403 ☑
      specified NEC
        injuring
          bystander Y35.492 ☑
          law enforcement personnel Y35.491 ☑
          suspect Y35.493 ☑
    specified means NEC
      injuring
        bystander Y35.892 ☑
        law enforcement personnel Y35.891 ☑
        suspect Y35.893 ☑
    stabbing — *see* Legal, intervention, sharp object
    stave — *see* Legal, intervention, blunt object, stave
    tear gas — *see* Legal, intervention, gas, tear gas
    truncheon — *see* Legal, intervention, blunt object, stave
Lifting — *see also* Overexertion
  heavy objects X50.0 ☑
  weights X50.0 ☑
Lightning (shock) (stroke) (struck by) — *see* subcategory T75.0 ☑
  causing fire — *see* Exposure, fire
Loss of control (transport vehicle) NEC — *see* Accident, transport
Lost at sea NOS — *see* Drowning, due to, fall overboard
Low
  pressure (effects) — *see* Air, pressure, low
  temperature (effects) — *see* Exposure, cold
Lying before train, vehicle or other moving object X81.8 ☑
  subway train X81.1 ☑
  train X81.1 ☑
  undetermined whether accidental or intentional Y31 ☑
Lynching — *see* Assault

M

Malfunction (mechanism or component) (of)
  firearm W34.10 ☑
    airgun W34.110 ☑
    BB gun W34.110 ☑
    gas, air or spring-operated gun NEC W34.118 ☑
    handgun W32.1 ☑
    hunting rifle W33.12 ☑
    larger firearm W33.10 ☑
      specified NEC W33.19 ☑
    machine gun W33.13 ☑
    paintball gun W34.111 ☑
    pellet gun W34.110 ☑
    shotgun W33.11 ☑
    specified NEC W34.19 ☑
    Very pistol [flare] W34.19 ☑
  handgun — *see* Malfunction, firearm, handgun
Maltreatment — *see* Perpetrator
Mangled (accidentally) NOS X58 ☑
Manhandling (in brawl, fight) Y04.0 ☑
  legal intervention — *see* Legal, intervention, manhandling
Manslaughter (nonaccidental) — *see* Assault
Mauled by animal NEC W55.89 ☑
Medical procedure, complication of (delayed or as an abnormal reaction without mention of misadventure) — *see* Complication of or following, by specified type of procedure
  due to or as a result of misadventure — *see* Misadventure
Melting (due to fire) (*see also* Exposure, fire)
  apparel NEC X06.3 ☑
  clothes, clothing NEC X06.3 ☑
    nightwear X05 ☑
  fittings or furniture (burning building) (uncontrolled fire) X00.8 ☑
  nightwear X05 ☑
  plastic jewelry X06.1 ☑
Mental cruelty X58 ☑
Military operations (injuries to military and civilians occuring during peacetime on military property and during routine military exercises and operations) (by) (from) (involving) Y37.90- ☑
  air blast Y37.20- ☑
  aircraft
    destruction — *see* Military operations, destruction of aircraft
    airway restriction — *see* Military operations, restriction of airways
    asphyxiation — *see* Military operations, restriction of airways
  biological weapons Y37.6X- ☑
  blast Y37.20- ☑
  blast fragments Y37.20- ☑
  blast wave Y37.20- ☑
  blast wind Y37.20- ☑
  bomb Y37.20- ☑
    dirty Y37.50- ☑
    gasoline Y37.31- ☑
    incendiary Y37.31- ☑
    petrol Y37.31- ☑
  bullet Y37.43- ☑
    incendiary Y37.32- ☑
    rubber Y37.41- ☑
  chemical weapons Y37.7X- ☑
  combat
    hand to hand (unarmed) combat Y37.44- ☑
    using blunt or piercing object Y37.45- ☑
  conflagration — *see* Military operations, fire
  conventional warfare NEC Y37.49- ☑
  depth-charge Y37.01- ☑
  destruction of aircraft Y37.10- ☑
    due to
      air to air missile Y37.11- ☑
      collision with other aircraft Y37.12- ☑
      detonation (accidental) of onboard munitions and explosives Y37.14- ☑
      enemy fire or explosives Y37.11- ☑
      explosive placed on aircraft Y37.11- ☑
      onboard fire Y37.13- ☑
      rocket propelled grenade [RPG] Y37.11- ☑
      small arms fire Y37.11- ☑
      surface to air missile Y37.11- ☑
    specified NEC Y37.19- ☑

Military operations — *continued*
  detonation (accidental) of
    onboard marine weapons Y37.05- ☑
    own munitions or munitions launch device Y37.24- ☑
  dirty bomb Y37.50- ☑
  explosion (of) Y37.20- ☑
    aerial bomb Y37.21- ☑
    bomb NOS (*see also* Military operations, bomb(s)) Y37.20- ☑
    fragments Y37.20- ☑
    grenade Y37.29- ☑
    guided missile Y37.22- ☑
    improvised explosive device [IED] (person-borne) (roadside) (vehicle-borne) Y37.23- ☑
    land mine Y37.29- ☑
    marine mine (at sea) (in harbor) Y37.02- ☑
    marine weapon Y37.00- ☑
      specified NEC Y37.09- ☑
    own munitions or munitions launch device (accidental) Y37.24- ☑
    sea-based artillery shell Y37.03- ☑
    specified NEC Y37.29- ☑
    torpedo Y37.04- ☑
  fire Y37.30- ☑
    specified NEC Y37.39- ☑
  firearms
    discharge Y37.43- ☑
    pellets Y37.42- ☑
  flamethrower Y37.33- ☑
  fragments (from) (of)
    improvised explosive device [IED] (person-borne) (roadside) (vehicle-borne) Y37.26- ☑
    munitions Y37.25- ☑
    specified NEC Y37.29- ☑
    weapons Y37.27- ☑
  friendly fire Y37.92- ☑
  hand to hand (unarmed) combat Y37.44- ☑
  hot substances — *see* Military operations, fire
  incendiary bullet Y37.32- ☑
  nuclear weapon (effects of) Y37.50- ☑
    acute radiation exposure Y37.54- ☑
    blast pressure Y37.51- ☑
    direct blast Y37.51- ☑
    direct heat Y37.53- ☑
    fallout exposure Y37.54- ☑
    fireball Y37.53- ☑
    indirect blast (struck or crushed by blast debris) (being thrown by blast) Y37.52- ☑
    ionizing radiation (immediate exposure) Y37.54- ☑
    nuclear radiation Y37.54- ☑
    radiation
      ionizing (immediate exposure) Y37.54- ☑
      nuclear Y37.54- ☑
      thermal Y37.53- ☑
    secondary effects Y37.54- ☑
    specified NEC Y37.59- ☑
    thermal radiation Y37.53- ☑
  restriction of air (airway)
    intentional Y37.46- ☑
    unintentional Y37.47- ☑
  rubber bullets Y37.41- ☑
  shrapnel NOS Y37.29- ☑
  suffocation — *see* Military operations, restriction of airways
  unconventional warfare NEC Y37.7X- ☑
  underwater blast NOS Y37.00- ☑
  warfare
    conventional NEC Y37.49- ☑
    unconventional NEC Y37.7X- ☑
  weapon of mass destruction [WMD] Y37.91- ☑
  weapons
    biological weapons Y37.6X- ☑
    chemical Y37.7X- ☑
    nuclear (effects of) Y37.50- ☑
      acute radiation exposure Y37.54- ☑
      blast pressure Y37.51- ☑
      direct blast Y37.51- ☑
      direct heat Y37.53- ☑
      fallout exposure Y37.54- ☑
      fireball Y37.53- ☑
      radiation
        ionizing (immediate exposure) Y37.54- ☑
        nuclear Y37.54- ☑
        thermal Y37.53- ☑
      secondary effects Y37.54- ☑

Military operations — continued
weapons — continued
nuclear — continued
specified NEC Y37.59- ☑
of mass destruction [WMD] Y37.91- ☑
Misadventure(s) **to patient**(s) **during surgical or medical care** Y69
contaminated medical or biological substance (blood, drug, fluid) Y64.9
administered (by) NEC Y64.9
immunization Y64.1
infusion Y64.0
injection Y64.1
specified means NEC Y64.8
transfusion Y64.0
vaccination Y64.1
excessive amount of blood or other fluid during transfusion or infusion Y63.0
failure
in dosage Y63.9
electroshock therapy Y63.4
inappropriate temperature (too hot or too cold) in local application and packing Y63.5
infusion
excessive amount of fluid Y63.0
incorrect dilution of fluid Y63.1
insulin-shock therapy Y63.4
nonadministration of necessary drug or biological substance Y63.6
overdose — see Table of Drugs and Chemicals radiation, in therapy Y63.2
radiation
overdose Y63.2
specified procedure NEC Y63.8
transfusion
excessive amount of blood Y63.0
mechanical, of instrument or apparatus (any) (during any procedure) Y65.8
sterile precautions (during procedure) Y62.9
aspiration of fluid or tissue (by puncture or catheterization, except heart) Y62.6
biopsy (except needle aspiration) Y62.8
needle (aspirating) Y62.6
blood sampling Y62.6
catheterization Y62.6
heart Y62.5
dialysis (kidney) Y62.2
endoscopic examination Y62.4
enema Y62.8
immunization Y62.3
infusion Y62.1
injection Y62.3
needle biopsy Y62.6
paracentesis (abdominal) (thoracic) Y62.6
perfusion Y62.2
puncture (lumbar) Y62.6
removal of catheter or packing Y62.8
specified procedure NEC Y62.8
surgical operation Y62.0
transfusion Y62.1
vaccination Y62.3
suture or ligature during surgical procedure Y65.2
to introduce or to remove tube or instrument — see Failure, to
hemorrhage — see Index to Diseases and Injuries, Complication(s)
inadvertent exposure of patient to radiation Y63.3
inappropriate
operation performed — see Inappropriate operation performed
temperature (too hot or too cold) in local application or packing Y63.5
infusion (see also Misadventure, by type, infusion) Y69
excessive amount of fluid Y63.0
incorrect dilution of fluid Y63.1
wrong fluid Y65.1
mismatched blood in transfusion Y65.0
nonadministration of necessary drug or biological substance Y63.6
overdose — see Table of Drugs and Chemicals radiation (in therapy) Y63.2
perforation — see Index to Diseases and Injuries, Complication(s)
performance of inappropriate operation — see Inappropriate operation performed
puncture — see Index to Diseases and Injuries, Complication(s)
specified type NEC Y65.8

Misadventure(s) **to patient**(s) **during surgical or medical care** — continued
specified type — continued
failure
suture or ligature during surgical operation Y65.2
to introduce or to remove tube or instrument — see Failure, to
infusion of wrong fluid Y65.1
performance of inappropriate operation — see Inappropriate operation performed
transfusion of mismatched blood Y65.0
wrong
fluid in infusion Y65.1
placement of endotracheal tube during anesthetic procedure Y65.3
transfusion — see Misadventure, by type, transfusion
excessive amount of blood Y63.0
mismatched blood Y65.0
wrong
drug given in error — see Table of Drugs and Chemicals
fluid in infusion Y65.1
placement of endotracheal tube during anesthetic procedure Y65.3
Mismatched blood in transfusion Y65.0
Motion sickness T75.3 ☑
Mountain sickness W94.11 ☑
Mudslide (of cataclysmic nature) — see Landslide
Murder (attempt) — see Assault

N

Nail
contact with W45.0 ☑
gun W29.4 ☑
embedded in skin W45.0 ☑
Neglect (criminal) (homicidal intent) X58 ☑
Noise (causing injury) (pollution) W42.9 ☑
supersonic W42.0 ☑
Nonadministration (of)
drug or biological substance (necessary) Y63.6
surgical and medical care Y66
Nosocomial condition Y95

O

Object
falling
from, in, on, hitting
machinery — see Contact, with, by type of machine
set in motion by
accidental explosion or rupture of pressure vessel W38 ☑
firearm — see Discharge, firearm, by type
machine(ry) — see Contact, with, by type of machine
Overdose (drug) — see Table of Drugs and Chemicals radiation Y63.2
Overexertion X50.9 ☑
from
prolonged static or awkward postures X50.1 ☑
repetitive movements X50.3 ☑
specified strenuous movements or postures NEC X50.9 ☑
strenuous movement or load X50.0 ☑
Overexposure (accidental) (to)
cold (see also Exposure, cold) X31 ☑
due to man-made conditions — see Exposure, cold, man-made
heat (see also Heat) X30 ☑
radiation — see Radiation
radioactivity W88.0 ☑
sun (sunburn) X32 ☑
weather NEC — see Forces of nature
wind NEC — see Forces of nature
Overheated — see Heat
Overturning (accidental)
machinery — see Contact, with, by type of machine
transport vehicle NEC (see also Accident, transport) V89.9 ☑
watercraft (causing drowning, submersion) (see also Drowning, due to, accident to, watercraft, overturning)
causing injury except drowning or submersion — see Accident, watercraft, causing, injury NEC

P

Parachute descent (voluntary) (without accident to aircraft) V97.29 ☑
due to accident to aircraft — see Accident, transport, aircraft
Pecked by bird W61.99 ☑
Perforation during medical or surgical treatment as misadventure — see Index to Diseases and Injuries, Complication(s)
Perpetrator, perpetration, of assault, maltreatment and neglect (by) Y07.9
boyfriend Y07.03
brother Y07.410
stepbrother Y07.435
coach Y07.53
cousin
female Y07.491
male Y07.490
daycare provider Y07.519
at-home
adult care Y07.512
childcare Y07.510
care center
adult care Y07.513
childcare Y07.511
family member NEC Y07.499
father Y07.11
adoptive Y07.13
foster Y07.420
stepfather Y07.430
foster father Y07.420
foster mother Y07.421
girl friend Y07.04
healthcare provider Y07.529
mental health Y07.521
specified NEC Y07.528
husband Y07.01
instructor Y07.53
mother Y07.12
adoptive Y07.14
foster Y07.421
stepmother Y07.433
nonfamily member Y07.50
specified NEC Y07.59
nurse Y07.528
occupational therapist Y07.528
partner of parent
female Y07.434
male Y07.432
physical therapist Y07.528
sister Y07.411
speech therapist Y07.528
stepbrother Y07.435
stepfather Y07.430
stepmother Y07.433
stepsister Y07.436
teacher Y07.53
wife Y07.02
Piercing — see Contact, with, by type of object or machine
Pinched
between objects (moving) (stationary and moving) W23.0 ☑
stationary W23.1 ☑
Pinned under machine(ry) — see Contact, with, by type of machine
Place of occurrence Y92.9
abandoned house Y92.89
airplane Y92.813
airport Y92.520
ambulatory health services establishment NEC Y92.538
ambulatory surgery center Y92.530
amusement park Y92.831
apartment (co-op) — see Place of occurrence, residence, apartment
assembly hall Y92.29
bank Y92.510
barn Y92.71
baseball field Y92.320
basketball court Y92.310
beach Y92.832
boarding house — see Place of occurrence, residence, boarding house
boat Y92.814
bowling alley Y92.39
bridge Y92.89

Place of occurrence — *continued*
- building under construction Y92.61
- bus Y92.811
  - station Y92.521
- cafe Y92.511
- campsite Y92.833
- campus — *see* Place of occurrence, school
- canal Y92.89
- car Y92.810
- casino Y92.59
- children's home — *see* Place of occurrence, residence, institutional, orphanage
- church Y92.22
- cinema Y92.26
- clubhouse Y92.29
- coal pit Y92.64
- college (community) Y92.214
- condominium — *see* Place of occurrence, residence, apartment
- construction area — *see* Place of occurrence, industrial and construction area
- convalescent home — *see* Place of occurrence, residence, institutional, nursing home
- court-house Y92.240
- cricket ground Y92.328
- cultural building Y92.258
  - art gallery Y92.250
  - museum Y92.251
  - music hall Y92.252
  - opera house Y92.253
  - specified NEC Y92.258
  - theater Y92.254
- dancehall Y92.252
- day nursery Y92.210
- dentist office Y92.531
- derelict house Y92.89
- desert Y92.820
- dockyard Y92.62
- dock NOS Y92.89
- doctor's office Y92.531
- dormitory — *see* Place of occurrence, residence, institutional, school dormitory
- dry dock Y92.62
- factory (building) (premises) Y92.63
- farm (land under cultivation) (outbuildings) Y92.79
  - barn Y92.71
  - chicken coop Y92.72
  - field Y92.73
  - hen house Y92.72
  - house — *see* Place of occurrence, residence, house
  - orchard Y92.74
  - specified NEC Y92.79
- football field Y92.321
- forest Y92.821
- freeway Y92.411
- gallery Y92.250
- garage (commercial) Y92.59
  - boarding house Y92.044
  - military base Y92.135
  - mobile home Y92.025
  - nursing home Y92.124
  - orphanage Y92.114
  - private house Y92.015
  - reform school Y92.155
- gas station Y92.524
- gasworks Y92.69
- golf course Y92.39
- gravel pit Y92.64
- grocery Y92.512
- gymnasium Y92.39
- handball court Y92.318
- harbor Y92.89
- harness racing course Y92.39
- healthcare provider office Y92.531
- highway (interstate) Y92.411
- hill Y92.828
- hockey rink Y92.330
- home — *see* Place of occurrence, residence
- hospice — *see* Place of occurrence, residence, institutional, nursing home
- hospital Y92.239
  - cafeteria Y92.233
  - corridor Y92.232
  - operating room Y92.234
  - patient
    - bathroom Y92.231
    - room Y92.230
  - specified NEC Y92.238

Place of occurrence — *continued*
- hotel Y92.59
- house (*see also* Place of occurrence, residence)
  - abandoned Y92.89
  - under construction Y92.61
- industrial and construction area (yard) Y92.69
  - building under construction Y92.61
  - dock Y92.62
  - dry dock Y92.62
  - factory Y92.63
  - gasworks Y92.69
  - mine Y92.64
  - oil rig Y92.65
  - pit Y92.64
  - power station Y92.69
  - shipyard Y92.62
  - specified NEC Y92.69
  - tunnel under construction Y92.69
  - workshop Y92.69
- kindergarten Y92.211
- lacrosse field Y92.328
- lake Y92.828
- library Y92.241
- mall Y92.59
- market Y92.512
- marsh Y92.828
- military
  - base — *see* Place of occurrence, residence, institutional, military base
  - training ground Y92.84
- mine Y92.64
- mosque Y92.22
- motel Y92.59
- motorway (interstate) Y92.411
- mountain Y92.828
- movie-house Y92.26
- museum Y92.251
- music-hall Y92.252
- not applicable Y92.9
- nuclear power station Y92.69
- nursing home — *see* Place of occurrence, residence, institutional, nursing home
- office building Y92.59
- offshore installation Y92.65
- oil rig Y92.65
- old people's home — *see* Place of occurrence, residence, institutional, specified NEC
- opera-house Y92.253
- orphanage — *see* Place of occurrence, residence, institutional, orphanage
- outpatient surgery center Y92.530
- park (public) Y92.830
  - amusement Y92.831
- parking garage Y92.89
  - lot Y92.481
- pavement Y92.480
- physician office Y92.531
- polo field Y92.328
- pond Y92.828
- post office Y92.242
- power station Y92.69
- prairie Y92.828
- prison — *see* Place of occurrence, residence, institutional, prison
- public
  - administration building Y92.248
    - city hall Y92.243
    - courthouse Y92.240
    - library Y92.241
    - post office Y92.242
    - specified NEC Y92.248
  - building NEC Y92.29
  - hall Y92.29
  - place NOS Y92.89
- race course Y92.39
- radio station Y92.59
- railway line (bridge) Y92.85
- ranch (outbuildings) — *see* Place of occurrence, farm
- recreation area Y92.838
  - amusement park Y92.831
  - beach Y92.832
  - campsite Y92.833
  - park (public) Y92.830
  - seashore Y92.832
  - specified NEC Y92.838
- reform school - — *see* Place of occurrence, residence, institutional, reform school
- religious institution Y92.22

Place of occurrence — *continued*
- residence (non-institutional) (private) Y92.009
  - apartment Y92.039
    - bathroom Y92.031
    - bedroom Y92.032
    - kitchen Y92.030
    - specified NEC Y92.038
  - bathroom Y92.002
  - bedroom Y92.003
  - boarding house Y92.049
    - bathroom Y92.041
    - bedroom Y92.042
    - driveway Y92.043
    - garage Y92.044
    - garden Y92.046
    - kitchen Y92.040
    - specified NEC Y92.048
    - swimming pool Y92.045
    - yard Y92.046
  - dining room Y92.001
  - garden Y92.007
  - home Y92.009
  - house, single family Y92.019
    - bathroom Y92.012
    - bedroom Y92.013
    - dining room Y92.011
    - driveway Y92.014
    - garage Y92.015
    - garden Y92.017
    - kitchen Y92.010
    - specified NEC Y92.018
    - swimming pool Y92.016
    - yard Y92.017
  - institutional Y92.10
    - children's home — *see* Place of occurrence, residence, institutional, orphanage
    - hospice — *see* Place of occurrence, residence, institutional, nursing home
    - military base Y92.139
      - barracks Y92.133
      - garage Y92.135
      - garden Y92.137
      - kitchen Y92.130
      - mess hall Y92.131
      - specified NEC Y92.138
      - swimming pool Y92.136
      - yard Y92.137
    - nursing home Y92.129
      - bathroom Y92.121
      - bedroom Y92.122
      - driveway Y92.123
      - garage Y92.124
      - garden Y92.126
      - kitchen Y92.120
      - specified NEC Y92.128
      - swimming pool Y92.125
      - yard Y92.126
    - orphanage Y92.119
      - bathroom Y92.111
      - bedroom Y92.112
      - driveway Y92.113
      - garage Y92.114
      - garden Y92.116
      - kitchen Y92.110
      - specified NEC Y92.118
      - swimming pool Y92.115
      - yard Y92.116
    - prison Y92.149
      - bathroom Y92.142
      - cell Y92.143
      - courtyard Y92.147
      - dining room Y92.141
      - kitchen Y92.140
      - specified NEC Y92.148
      - swimming pool Y92.146
    - reform school Y92.159
      - bathroom Y92.152
      - bedroom Y92.153
      - dining room Y92.151
      - driveway Y92.154
      - garage Y92.155
      - garden Y92.157
      - kitchen Y92.150
      - specified NEC Y92.158
      - swimming pool Y92.156
      - yard Y92.157
    - school dormitory Y92.169
      - bathroom Y92.162
      - bedroom Y92.163

Place of occurrence — *continued*
 residence — *continued*
  institutional — *continued*
   school dormitory — *continued*
    dining room Y92.161
    kitchen Y92.160
    specified NEC Y92.168
   specified NEC Y92.199
    bathroom Y92.192
    bedroom Y92.193
    dining room Y92.191
    driveway Y92.194
    garage Y92.195
    garden Y92.197
    kitchen Y92.190
    specified NEC Y92.198
    swimming pool Y92.196
    yard Y92.197
  kitchen Y92.000
  mobile home Y92.029
   bathroom Y92.022
   bedroom Y92.023
   dining room Y92.021
   driveway Y92.024
   garage Y92.025
   garden Y92.027
   kitchen Y92.020
   specified NEC Y92.028
   swimming pool Y92.026
   yard Y92.027
  specified place in residence NEC Y92.008
  specified residence type NEC Y92.099
   bathroom Y92.091
   bedroom Y92.092
   driveway Y92.093
   garage Y92.094
   garden Y92.096
   kitchen Y92.090
   specified NEC Y92.098
   swimming pool Y92.095
   yard Y92.096
 restaurant Y92.511
 riding school Y92.39
 river Y92.828
 road Y92.488
 rodeo ring Y92.39
 rugby field Y92.328
 same day surgery center Y92.530
 sand pit Y92.64
 school (private) (public) (state) Y92.219
  college Y92.214
  daycare center Y92.210
  elementary school Y92.211
  high school Y92.213
  kindergarten Y92.211
  middle school Y92.212
  specified NEC Y92.218
  trace school Y92.215
  university Y92.214
  vocational school Y92.215
 sea (shore) Y92.832
 senior citizen center Y92.29
 service area
  airport Y92.520
  bus station Y92.521
  gas station Y92.524
  highway rest stop Y92.523
  railway station Y92.522
 shipyard Y92.62
 shop (commercial) Y92.513
 sidewalk Y92.480
 silo Y92.79
 skating rink (roller) Y92.331
  ice Y92.330
 slaughter house Y92.86
 soccer field Y92.322
 specified place NEC Y92.89
 sports area Y92.39
  athletic
   court Y92.318
    basketball Y92.310
    specified NEC Y92.318
    squash Y92.311
    tennis Y92.312
   field Y92.328
    baseball Y92.320
    cricket ground Y92.328
    football Y92.321
    hockey Y92.328

Place of occurrence — *continued*
 sports area — *continued*
  athletic — *continued*
   field — *continued*
    soccer Y92.322
    specified NEC Y92.328
  golf course Y92.39
  gymnasium Y92.39
  riding school Y92.39
  skating rink (roller) Y92.331
   ice Y92.330
  stadium Y92.39
  swimming pool Y92.34
 squash court Y92.311
 stadium Y92.39
 steeplechasing course Y92.39
 store Y92.512
 stream Y92.828
 street and highway Y92.410
  bike path Y92.482
  freeway Y92.411
  highway ramp Y92.415
  interstate highway Y92.411
  local residential or business street Y92.414
  motorway Y92.411
  parking lot Y92.481
  parkway Y92.412
  sidewalk Y92.480
  specified NEC Y92.488
  state road Y92.413
 subway car Y92.816
 supermarket Y92.512
 swamp Y92.828
 swimming pool (public) Y92.34
  private (at) Y92.095
   boarding house Y92.045
   military base Y92.136
   mobile home Y92.026
   nursing home Y92.125
   orphanage Y92.115
   prison Y92.146
   reform school Y92.156
   single family residence Y92.016
 synagogue Y92.22
 television station Y92.59
 tennis court Y92.312
 theater Y92.254
 trade area Y92.59
  bank Y92.510
  cafe Y92.511
  casino Y92.59
  garage Y92.59
  hotel Y92.59
  market Y92.512
  office building Y92.59
  radio station Y92.59
  restaurant Y92.511
  shop Y92.513
  shopping mall Y92.59
  store Y92.512
  supermarket Y92.512
  television station Y92.59
  warehouse Y92.59
 trailer park, residential — *see* Place of occurrence, residence, mobile home
 trailer site NOS Y92.89
 train Y92.815
  station Y92.522
 truck Y92.812
 tunnel under construction Y92.69
 university Y92.214
 urgent (health) care center Y92.532
 vehicle (transport) Y92.818
  airplane Y92.813
  boat Y92.814
  bus Y92.811
  car Y92.810
  specified NEC Y92.818
  subway car Y92.816
  train Y92.815
  truck Y92.812
 warehouse Y92.59
 water reservoir Y92.89
 wilderness area Y92.828
  desert Y92.820
  forest Y92.821
  marsh Y92.828
  mountain Y92.828
  prairie Y92.828

Place of occurrence — *continued*
 wilderness area — *continued*
  specified NEC Y92.828
  swamp Y92.828
 workshop Y92.69
 yard, private Y92.096
  boarding house Y92.046
  mobile home Y92.027
  single family house Y92.017
 youth center Y92.29
 zoo (zoological garden) Y92.834
Plumbism — *see* Table of Drugs and Chemicals, lead
Poisoning (accidental) (by) (*see also* Table of Drugs and Chemicals)
 by plant, thorns, spines, sharp leaves or other mechanisms NEC X58 ☑
 carbon monoxide
  generated by
   motor vehicle — *see* Accident, transport
   watercraft (in transit) (not in transit) V93.89 ☑
    ferry boat V93.81 ☑
    fishing boat V93.82 ☑
    jet skis V93.83 ☑
    liner V93.81 ☑
    merchant ship V93.80 ☑
    passenger ship V93.81 ☑
    powered craft NEC V93.83 ☑
 caused by injection of poisons into skin by plant thorns, spines, sharp leaves X58 ☑
  marine or sea plants (venomous) X58 ☑
 execution — *see* Legal, intervention, gas
  intervention
   by gas — *see* Legal, intervention, gas
   other specified means — *see* Legal, intervention, specified means NEC
 exhaust gas
  generated by
   motor vehicle — *see* Accident, transport
   watercraft (in transit) (not in transit) V93.89 ☑
    ferry boat V93.81 ☑
    fishing boat V93.82 ☑
    jet skis V93.83 ☑
    liner V93.81 ☑
    merchant ship V93.80 ☑
    passenger ship V93.81 ☑
    powered craft NEC V93.83 ☑
 fumes or smoke due to
  explosion (*see also* Explosion) W40.9 ☑
  fire — *see* Exposure, fire
  ignition — *see* Ignition
 gas
  in legal intervention — *see* Legal, intervention, gas
  legal execution — *see* Legal, intervention, gas
 in war operations — *see* War operations
 legal
Powder burn (by) (from)
 airgun W34.110 ☑
 BB gun W34.110 ☑
 firearm NEC W34.19 ☑
 gas, air or spring-operated gun NEC W34.118 ☑
 handgun W32.1 ☑
 hunting rifle W33.12 ☑
 larger firearm W33.10 ☑
  specified NEC W33.19 ☑
 machine gun W33.13 ☑
 paintball gun W34.111 ☑
 pellet gun W34.110 ☑
 shotgun W33.11 ☑
 Very pistol [flare] W34.19 ☑
Premature cessation (of) **surgical and medical care** Y66
Privation (food) (water) X58 ☑
Procedure (operation)
 correct, on wrong side or body part (wrong side) (wrong site) Y65.53
 intended for another patient done on wrong patient Y65.52
 performed on patient not scheduled for surgery Y65.52
 performed on wrong patient Y65.52
 wrong, performed on correct patient Y65.51
Prolonged
 sitting in transport vehicle — *see* Travel, by type of vehicle
 stay in
  high altitude as cause of anoxia, barodontalgia, barotitis or hypoxia W94.11 ☑
  weightless environment X52 ☑

Pulling, excessive (*see also* Overexertion) X50.9- ☑
Puncture, puncturing (*see also* Contact, with, by type
    of object or machine)
   by
      plant thorns, spines, sharp leaves or other mecha-
         nisms NEC W60 ☑
   during medical or surgical treatment as misadventure
     — *see* Index to Diseases and Injuries, Complica-
     tion(s)
Pushed, pushing (accidental) (injury in)
   by other person(s) (accidental) W51 ☑
     with fall W03 ☑
       due to ice or snow W00.0 ☑
     as, or caused by, a crowd or human stampede (with
       fall) W52 ☑
      before moving object NEC Y02.8 ☑
        motor vehicle Y02.0 ☑
        subway train Y02.1 ☑
        train Y02.1 ☑
     from
       high place NEC
         in accidental circumstances W17.89 ☑
         stated as
           intentional, homicide (attempt) Y01 ☑
           undetermined whether accidental or
             intentional Y30 ☑
       transport vehicle NEC (*see also* Accident, trans-
         port) V89.9 ☑
        stated as
          intentional, homicide (attempt)
           Y08.89 ☑
   overexertion X50.9 ☑

R

Radiation (exposure to)
   arc lamps W89.0 ☑
   atomic power plant (malfunction) NEC W88.1 ☑
   complication of or abnormal reaction to medical radio-
     therapy Y84.2
   electromagnetic, ionizing W88.0 ☑
   gamma rays W88.1 ☑
   in
     war operations (from or following nuclear explo-
       sion) — *see* War operations
   inadvertent exposure of patient (receiving test or
     therapy) Y63.3
   infrared (heaters and lamps) W90.1 ☑
     excessive heat from W92 ☑
   ionized, ionizing (particles, artificially accelerated)
     radioisotopes W88.1 ☑
     specified NEC W88.8 ☑
     x-rays W88.0 ☑
   isotopes, radioactive — *see* Radiation, radioactive
     isotopes
   laser(s) W90.2 ☑
     in war operations — *see* War operations
     misadventure in medical care Y63.2
   light sources (man-made visible and ultraviolet)
     W89.9 ☑
     natural X32 ☑
     specified NEC W89.8 ☑
     tanning bed W89.1 ☑
     welding light W89.0 ☑
   man-made visible light W89.9 ☑
     specified NEC W89.8 ☑
     tanning bed W89.1 ☑
     welding light W89.0 ☑
   microwave W90.8 ☑
   misadventure in medical or surgical procedure Y63.2
   natural NEC X39.08 ☑
     radon X39.01 ☑
   overdose (in medical or surgical procedure) Y63.2
   radar W90.0 ☑
   radioactive isotopes (any) W88.1 ☑
     atomic power plant malfunction W88.1 ☑
     misadventure in medical or surgical treatment
       Y63.2
   radiofrequency W90.0 ☑
   radium NEC W88.1 ☑
   sun X32 ☑
   ultraviolet (light) (man-made) W89.9 ☑
     natural X32 ☑
     specified NEC W89.8 ☑
     tanning bed W89.1 ☑
     welding light W89.0 ☑

Radiation — *continued*
   welding arc, torch, or light W89.0 ☑
     excessive heat from W92 ☑
   x-rays (hard) (soft) W88.0 ☑
Range disease W94.11 ☑
Rape (attempted) T74.2- ☑
Rat bite W53.11 ☑
Reaching (prolonged) (static) X50.1 ☑
Reaction, abnormal to medical procedure (*see also*
     Complication of or following, by type of procedure)
     Y84.9
   with misadventure — *see* Misadventure
   biologicals — *see* Table of Drugs and Chemicals
   drugs — *see* Table of Drugs and Chemicals
   vaccine — *see* Table of Drugs and Chemicals
Recoil
   airgun W34.110 ☑
   BB gun W34.110 ☑
   firearm NEC W34.19 ☑
   gas, air or spring-operated gun NEC W34.118 ☑
   handgun W32.1 ☑
   hunting rifle W33.12 ☑
   larger firearm W33.10 ☑
     specified NEC W33.19 ☑
   machine gun W33.13 ☑
   paintball gun W34.111 ☑
   pellet W34.110 ☑
   shotgun W33.11 ☑
   Very pistol [flare] W34.19 ☑
Reduction in
   atmospheric pressure — *see* Air, pressure, change
Rock falling on or hitting (accidentally) (person)
     W20.8 ☑
   in cave-in W20.0 ☑
Run over (accidentally) (by)
   animal (not being ridden) NEC W55.89 ☑
   machinery — *see* Contact, with, by specified type of
     machine
   transport vehicle NEC (*see also* Accident, transport)
     V09.9 ☑
     intentional homicide (attempt) Y03.0 ☑
     motor NEC V09.20 ☑
       intentional homicide (attempt) Y03.0 ☑
Running
   before moving object X81.8 ☑
     motor vehicle X81.0 ☑
Running off, away
   animal (being ridden) (*see also* Accident, transport)
     V80.918 ☑
     not being ridden W55.89 ☑
   animal-drawn vehicle NEC (*see also* Accident, trans-
     port) V80.928 ☑
   highway, road(way), street
     transport vehicle NEC (*see also* Accident, transport)
       V89.9 ☑
Rupture pressurized devices — *see* Explosion, by type
     of device

S

Saturnism — *see* Table of Drugs and Chemicals, lead
Scald, scalding (accidental) (by) (from) (in) X19 ☑
   air (hot) X14.1 ☑
   gases (hot) X14.1 ☑
   homicide (attempt) — *see* Assault, burning, hot object
   inflicted by other person
     stated as intentional, homicide (attempt) — *see*
       Assault, burning, hot object
   liquid (boiling) (hot) NEC X12 ☑
     stated as undetermined whether accidental or in-
       tentional Y27.2 ☑
     suicide (attempt) X77.2 ☑
   local application of externally applied substance in
     medical or surgical care Y63.5
   metal (molten) (liquid) (hot) NEC X18 ☑
   self-inflicted X77.9 ☑
   stated as undetermined whether accidental or inten-
     tional Y27.8 ☑
   steam X13.1 ☑
     assault X98.0 ☑
     stated as undetermined whether accidental or in-
       tentional Y27.0 ☑
     suicide (attempt) X77.0 ☑
   suicide (attempt) X77.9 ☑
   vapor (hot) X13.1 ☑
     assault X98.0 ☑

Scald, scalding — *continued*
   vapor — *continued*
     stated as undetermined whether accidental or in-
       tentional Y27.0 ☑
     suicide (attempt) X77.0 ☑
Scratched by
   cat W55.03 ☑
   person(s) (accidentally) W50.4 ☑
     with intent to injure or kill Y04.0 ☑
     as, or caused by, a crowd or human stampede (with
       fall) W52 ☑
     assault Y04.0 ☑
     homicide (attempt) Y04.0 ☑
     in
       fight Y04.0 ☑
       legal intervention
         injuring
           bystander Y35.892 ☑
           law enforcement personnel Y35.891 ☑
           suspect Y35.893 ☑
Seasickness T75.3 ☑
Self-harm NEC (*see also* External cause by type, undeter-
     mined whether accidental or intentional)
   intentional — *see* Suicide
   poisoning NEC — *see* Table of Drugs and Chemicals,
     poisoning, accidental
Self-inflicted (injury) **NEC** (*see also* External cause by
     type, undetermined whether accidental or inten-
     tional)
   intentional — *see* Suicide
   poisoning NEC — *see* Table of Drugs and Chemicals,
     poisoning, accidental
Sequelae (of)
   accident NEC — *see* W00-X58 with 7th character S
   assault (homicidal) (any means) — *see* X92-Y08 with
     7th character S
   homicide, attempt (any means) — *see* X92-Y08 with
     7th character S
   injury undetermined whether accidentally or purposely
     inflicted — *see* Y21-Y33 with 7th character S
   intentional self-harm (classifiable to X71-X83) — *see*
     X71-X83 with 7th character S
   legal intervention — *see* with 7th character S Y35 ☑
   motor vehicle accident — *see* V00-V99 with 7th char-
     acter S
   suicide, attempt (any means) — *see* X71-X83 with 7th
     character S
   transport accident — *see* V00-V99 with 7th character
     S
   war operations — *see* War operations
Shock
   electric — *see* Exposure, electric current
   from electric appliance (any) (faulty) W86.8 ☑
     domestic W86.0 ☑
     suicide (attempt) X83.1 ☑
Shooting, shot (accidental(ly)) (*see also* Discharge,
     firearm, by type)
   herself or himself — *see* Discharge, firearm by type,
     self-inflicted
   homicide (attempt) — *see* Discharge, firearm by type,
     homicide
   in war operations — *see* War operations
   inflicted by other person — *see* Discharge, firearm by
     type, homicide
     accidental — *see* Discharge, firearm, by type of
       firearm
   legal
     execution — *see* Legal, intervention, firearm
     intervention — *see* Legal, intervention, firearm
   self-inflicted — *see* Discharge, firearm by type, suicide
     accidental — *see* Discharge, firearm, by type of
       firearm
   suicide (attempt) — *see* Discharge, firearm by type,
     suicide
Shoving (accidentally) **by other person** — *see* Pushed,
     by other person
Sickness
   alpine W94.11 ☑
   motion — *see* Motion
   mountain W94.11 ☑
Sinking (accidental)
   watercraft (causing drowning, submersion) (*see also*
     Drowning, due to, accident to, watercraft, sink-
     ing)
     causing injury except drowning or submersion —
       see Accident, watercraft, causing, injury NEC
Siriasis X32 ☑

Sitting (prolonged) (static) X50.1 ☑
Slashed wrists — *see* Cut, self-inflicted
Slipping (accidental) (on same level) (with fall) W01.0 ☑
- without fall W18.40 ☑
  - due to
    - specified NEC W18.49 ☑
    - stepping from one level to another W18.43 ☑
    - stepping into hole or opening W18.42 ☑
    - stepping on object W18.41 ☑
- on
  - ice W00.0 ☑
    - with skates — *see* Accident, transport, pedestrian, conveyance
  - mud W01.0 ☑
  - oil W01.0 ☑
  - snow W00.0 ☑
    - with skis — *see* Accident, transport, pedestrian, conveyance
  - surface (slippery) (wet) NEC W01.0 ☑
Sliver, wood, contact with W45.8 ☑
Smoldering (due to fire) — *see* Exposure, fire
Sodomy (attempted) **by force** T74.2 ☑
Sound waves (causing injury) W42.9 ☑
- supersonic W42.0 ☑
Splinter, contact with W45.8 ☑
Stab, stabbing — *see* Cut
Standing (prolonged) (static) X50.1 ☑
Starvation X58 ☑
Status of external cause Y99.9
- child assisting in compensated work for family Y99.8
- civilian activity done for financial or other compensation Y99.8
- civilian activity done for income or pay Y99.0
- family member assisting in compensated work for other family member Y99.8
- hobby not done for income Y99.8
- leisure activity Y99.8
- military activity Y99.1
- off-duty activity of military personnel Y99.8
- recreation or sport not for income or while a student Y99.8
- specified NEC Y99.8
- student activity Y99.8
- volunteer activity Y99.2
Stepped on
- by
  - animal (not being ridden) NEC W55.89 ☑
  - crowd or human stampede W52 ☑
  - person W50.0 ☑
Stepping on
- object W22.8 ☑
  - with fall W18.31 ☑
  - sports equipment W21.9 ☑
  - stationary W22.09 ☑
    - sports equipment W21.89 ☑
- person W51 ☑
  - by crowd or human stampede W52 ☑
- sports equipment W21.9 ☑
Sting
- arthropod, nonvenomous W57 ☑
- insect, nonvenomous W57 ☑
Storm (cataclysmic) — *see* Forces of nature, cataclysmic storm
Straining, excessive (*see also* Overexertion) X50.9 ☑
Strangling — *see* Strangulation
Strangulation (accidental) T71 ☑
Strenuous movements (*see also* Overexertion) X50.9 ☑
Striking against
- airbag (automobile) W22.10 ☑
  - driver side W22.11 ☑
  - front passenger side W22.12 ☑
  - specified NEC W22.19 ☑
- bottom when
  - diving or jumping into water (in) W16.822 ☑
    - causing drowning W16.821 ☑
    - from boat W16.722 ☑
      - causing drowning W16.721 ☑
    - natural body W16.622 ☑
      - causing drowning W16.821 ☑
    - swimming pool W16.522 ☑
      - causing drowning W16.521 ☑
  - falling into water (in) W16.322 ☑
    - causing drowning W16.321 ☑
    - fountain — *see* Striking against, bottom when, falling into water, specified NEC
    - natural body W16.122 ☑

Striking against — *continued*
- bottom when — *continued*
  - falling into water — *continued*
    - natural body — *continued*
      - causing drowning W16.121 ☑
    - reservoir — *see* Striking against, bottom when, falling into water, specified NEC
    - specified NEC W16.322 ☑
      - causing drowning W16.321 ☑
    - swimming pool W16.022 ☑
      - causing drowning W16.021 ☑
- diving board (swimming-pool) W21.4 ☑
- object W22.8 ☑
  - with
    - drowning or submersion — *see* Drowning
    - fall — *see* Fall, due to, bumping against, object
    - caused by crowd or human stampede (with fall) W52 ☑
  - furniture W22.03 ☑
  - lamppost W22.02 ☑
  - sports equipment W21.9 ☑
  - stationary W22.09 ☑
    - sports equipment W21.89 ☑
  - wall W22.01 ☑
- person(s) W51 ☑
  - with fall W03 ☑
    - due to ice or snow W00.0 ☑
  - as, or caused by, a crowd or human stampede (with fall) W52 ☑
  - assault Y04.2 ☑
  - homicide (attempt) Y04.2 ☑
- sports equipment W21.9 ☑
- wall (when) W22.01 ☑
  - diving or jumping into water (in) W16.832 ☑
    - causing drowning W16.831 ☑
    - swimming pool W16.532 ☑
      - causing drowning W16.531 ☑
  - falling into water (in) W16.332 ☑
    - causing drowning W16.331 ☑
    - fountain — *see* Striking against, wall when, falling into water, specified NEC
    - natural body W16.132 ☑
      - causing drowning W16.131 ☑
    - reservoir — *see* Striking against, wall when, falling into water, specified NEC
    - specified NEC W16.332 ☑
      - causing drowning W16.331 ☑
    - swimming pool W16.032 ☑
      - causing drowning W16.031 ☑
  - swimming pool (when) W22.042 ☑
    - causing drowning W22.041 ☑
    - diving or jumping into water W16.532 ☑
      - causing drowning W16.531 ☑
    - falling into water W16.032 ☑
      - causing drowning W16.031 ☑
Struck (accidentally) **by**
- airbag (automobile) W22.10 ☑
  - driver side W22.11 ☑
  - front passenger side W22.12 ☑
  - specified NEC W22.19 ☑
- alligator W58.02 ☑
- animal (not being ridden) NEC W55.89 ☑
- avalanche — *see* Landslide
- ball (hit) (thrown) W21.00 ☑
  - assault Y08.09 ☑
  - baseball W21.03 ☑
  - basketball W21.05 ☑
  - football W21.01 ☑
  - golf ball W21.04 ☑
  - soccer W21.02 ☑
  - softball W21.07 ☑
  - specified NEC W21.09 ☑
  - volleyball W21.06 ☑
- bat or racquet
  - baseball bat W21.11 ☑
    - assault Y08.02 ☑
  - golf club W21.13 ☑
    - assault Y08.09 ☑
  - specified NEC W21.19 ☑
    - assault Y08.09 ☑
  - tennis racquet W21.12 ☑
    - assault Y08.09 ☑
- bullet (*see also* Discharge, firearm by type)
  - in war operations — *see* War operations
- crocodile W58.12 ☑
- dog W54.1 ☑

Struck (accidentally) **by** — *continued*
- flare, Very pistol — *see* Discharge, firearm NEC
- hailstones X39.8 ☑
- hockey (ice)
  - field
    - puck W21.221 ☑
    - stick W21.211 ☑
  - puck W21.220 ☑
  - stick W21.210 ☑
  - assault Y08.01 ☑
- landslide — *see* Landslide
- law-enforcement agent (on duty) — *see* Legal, intervention, manhandling
  - with blunt object — *see* Legal, intervention, blunt object
- lightning T75.0 ☑
  - causing fire — *see* Exposure, fire
- machine — *see* Contact, with, by type of machine
- mammal NEC W55.89 ☑
  - marine W56.32 ☑
- marine animal W56.82 ☑
- missile
  - firearm — *see* Discharge, firearm by type
  - in war operations — *see* War operations, missile
- object W22.8 ☑
  - blunt W22.8 ☑
    - assault Y00 ☑
    - suicide (attempt) X79 ☑
    - undetermined whether accidental or intentional Y29 ☑
  - falling W20.8 ☑
    - from, in, on
      - building W20.1 ☑
        - burning (uncontrolled fire) X00.4 ☑
      - cataclysmic
        - earth surface movement NEC — *see* Landslide
        - storm — *see* Forces of nature, cataclysmic storm
      - cave-in W20.0 ☑
      - earthquake X34 ☑
      - machine (in operation) — *see* Contact, with, by type of machine
      - structure W20.1 ☑
        - burning X00.4 ☑
      - transport vehicle (in motion) — *see* Accident, transport, by type of vehicle
      - watercraft V93.49 ☑
        - due to
          - accident to craft V91.39 ☑
            - powered craft V91.33 ☑
              - ferry boat V91.31 ☑
              - fishing boat V91.32 ☑
              - jetskis V91.33 ☑
              - liner V91.31 ☑
              - merchant ship V91.30 ☑
              - passenger ship V91.31 ☑
            - unpowered craft V91.38 ☑
              - canoe V91.35 ☑
              - inflatable V91.36 ☑
              - kayak V91.35 ☑
              - sailboat V91.34 ☑
              - surf-board V91.38 ☑
              - windsurfer V91.38 ☑
          - powered craft V93.43 ☑
            - ferry boat V93.41 ☑
            - fishing boat V93.42 ☑
            - jetskis V93.43 ☑
            - liner V93.41 ☑
            - merchant ship V93.40 ☑
            - passenger ship V93.41 ☑
          - unpowered craft V93.48 ☑
            - sailboat V93.44 ☑
            - surf-board V93.48 ☑
            - windsurfer V93.48 ☑
  - moving NEC W20.8 ☑
  - projected W20.8 ☑
    - assault Y00 ☑
    - in sports W21.9 ☑
      - assault Y08.09 ☑
      - ball W21.00 ☑
        - baseball W21.03 ☑
        - basketball W21.05 ☑
        - football W21.01 ☑
        - golf ball W21.04 ☑
        - soccer W21.02 ☑

Struck (accidentally) **by** — *continued*
  object — *continued*
    projected — *continued*
      in sports — *continued*
        ball — *continued*
          softball W21.07 ☑
          specified NEC W21.09 ☑
          volleyball W21.06 ☑
        bat or racquet
          baseball bat W21.11 ☑
            assault Y08.02 ☑
          golf club W21.13 ☑
            assault Y08.09 ☑
          specified NEC W21.19 ☑
            assault Y08.09 ☑
          tennis racquet W21.12 ☑
            assault Y08.09 ☑
        hockey (ice)
          field
            puck W21.221 ☑
            stick W21.211 ☑
          puck W21.220 ☑
          stick W21.210 ☑
            assault Y08.01 ☑
        specified NEC W21.89 ☑
    set in motion by explosion — *see* Explosion
    thrown W20.8 ☑
      assault Y00 ☑
      in sports W21.9 ☑
        assault Y08.09 ☑
        ball W21.00 ☑
          baseball W21.03 ☑
          basketball W21.05 ☑
          football W21.01 ☑
          golf ball W21.04 ☑
          soccer W21.02 ☑
          soft ball W21.07 ☑
          specified NEC W21.09 ☑
          volleyball W21.06 ☑
        bat or racquet
          baseball bat W21.11 ☑
            assault Y08.02 ☑
          golf club W21.13 ☑
            assault Y08.09 ☑
          specified NEC W21.19 ☑
            assault Y08.09 ☑
          tennis racquet W21.12 ☑
            assault Y08.09 ☑
        hockey (ice)
          field
            puck W21.221 ☑
            stick W21.211 ☑
          puck W21.220 ☑
          stick W21.210 ☑
            assault Y08.01 ☑
    other person(s) W50.0 ☑
      with
        blunt object W22.8 ☑
          intentional, homicide (attempt) Y00 ☑
          sports equipment W21.9 ☑
          undetermined whether accidental or intentional Y29 ☑
        fall W03 ☑
          due to ice or snow W00.0 ☑
      as, or caused by, a crowd or human stampede (with fall) W52 ☑
      assault Y04.2 ☑
      homicide (attempt) Y04.2 ☑
      in legal intervention
        injuring
          bystander Y35.812 ☑
          law enforcement personnel Y35.811 ☑
          suspect Y35.813 ☑
      sports equipment W21.9 ☑
    police (on duty) — *see* Legal, intervention, manhandling
      with blunt object — *see* Legal, intervention, blunt object
    sports equipment W21.9 ☑
      assault Y08.09 ☑
      ball W21.00 ☑
        baseball W21.03 ☑
        basketball W21.05 ☑
        football W21.01 ☑
        golf ball W21.04 ☑

Struck (accidentally) **by** — *continued*
  sports equipment — *continued*
    ball — *continued*
      soccer W21.02 ☑
      soft ball W21.07 ☑
      specified NEC W21.09 ☑
      volleyball W21.06 ☑
    bat or racquet
      baseball bat W21.11 ☑
        assault Y08.02 ☑
      golf club W21.13 ☑
        assault Y08.09 ☑
      specified NEC W21.19 ☑
      tennis racquet W21.12 ☑
        assault Y08.09 ☑
    cleats (shoe) W21.31 ☑
    foot wear NEC W21.39 ☑
    football helmet W21.81 ☑
    hockey (ice)
      field
        puck W21.221 ☑
        stick W21.211 ☑
      puck W21.220 ☑
      stick W21.210 ☑
        assault Y08.01 ☑
    skate blades W21.32 ☑
    specified NEC W21.89 ☑
      assault Y08.09 ☑
  thunderbolt — *see* subcategory T75.0 ☑
    causing fire — *see* Exposure, fire
  transport vehicle NEC (*see also* Accident, transport) V09.9 ☑
    intentional, homicide (attempt) Y03.0 ☑
    motor NEC (*see also* Accident, transport) V09.20 ☑
      homicide Y03.0 ☑
  vehicle (transport) NEC — *see* Accident, transport, by type of vehicle
    stationary (falling from jack, hydraulic lift, ramp) W20.8 ☑

Stumbling
  without fall W18.40 ☑
    due to
      specified NEC W18.49 ☑
      stepping from one level to another W18.43 ☑
      stepping into hole or opening W18.42 ☑
      stepping on object W18.41 ☑
    over
      animal NEC W01.0 ☑
        with fall W18.09 ☑
      carpet, rug or (small) object W22.8 ☑
        with fall W18.09 ☑
      person W51 ☑
        with fall W03 ☑
          due to ice or snow W00.0 ☑
Submersion (accidental) — *see* Drowning
Suffocation (accidental) (by external means) (by pressure) (mechanical) (*see also* category) T71
  due to, by
    avalanche — *see* Landslide
    explosion — *see* Explosion
    fire — *see* Exposure, fire
    food, any type (aspiration) (ingestion) (inhalation) — *see* categories T17 and T18 ☑
    ignition — *see* Ignition
    landslide — *see* Landslide
    machine(ry) — *see* Contact, with, by type of machine
    vomitus (aspiration) (inhalation) T17.81- ☑
  in
    burning building X00.8 ☑
Suicide, suicidal (attempted) (by) X83.8 ☑
  blunt object X79 ☑
  burning, burns X76 ☑
    hot object X77.9 ☑
      fluid NEC X77.2 ☑
      household appliance X77.3 ☑
      specified NEC X77.8 ☑
      steam X77.0 ☑
      tap water X77.1 ☑
      vapors X77.0 ☑
  caustic substance — *see* Table of Drugs and Chemicals
  cold, extreme X83.2 ☑
  collision of motor vehicle with
    motor vehicle X82.0 ☑
    specified NEC X82.8 ☑
    train X82.1 ☑

Suicide, suicidal — *continued*
  collision of motor vehicle with — *continued*
    tree X82.2 ☑
  crashing of aircraft X83.0 ☑
  cut (any part of body) X78.9 ☑
  cutting or piercing instrument X78.9 ☑
    dagger X78.2 ☑
    glass X78.0 ☑
    knife X78.1 ☑
    specified NEC X78.8 ☑
    sword X78.2 ☑
  drowning (in) X71.9 ☑
    bathtub X71.0 ☑
    natural water X71.3 ☑
    specified NEC X71.8 ☑
    swimming pool X71.1 ☑
      following fall X71.2 ☑
  electrocution X83.1 ☑
  explosive(s) (material) X75 ☑
  fire, flames X76 ☑
  firearm X74.9 ☑
    airgun X74.01 ☑
    handgun X72 ☑
    hunting rifle X73.1 ☑
    larger X73.9 ☑
      specified NEC X73.8 ☑
    machine gun X73.2 ☑
    shotgun X73.0 ☑
    specified NEC X74.8 ☑
  hanging X83.8 ☑
  hot object — *see* Suicide, burning, hot object
  jumping
    before moving object X81.8 ☑
      motor vehicle X81.0 ☑
      subway train X81.1 ☑
      train X81.1 ☑
    from high place X80 ☑
  late effect of attempt — *see* X71-X83 with 7th character S
  lying before moving object, train, vehicle X81.8 ☑
  poisoning — *see* Table of Drugs and Chemicals
  puncture (any part of body) — *see* Suicide, cutting or piercing instrument
  scald — *see* Suicide, burning, hot object
  sequelae of attempt — *see* X71-X83 with 7th character S
  sharp object (any) — *see* Suicide, cutting or piercing instrument
  shooting — *see* Suicide, firearm
  specified means NEC X83.8 ☑
  stab (any part of body) — *see* Suicide, cutting or piercing instrument
  steam, hot vapors X77.0 ☑
  strangulation X83.8 ☑
  submersion — *see* Suicide, drowning
  suffocation X83.8 ☑
  wound NEC X83.8 ☑
Sunstroke X32
Supersonic waves (causing injury) W42.0 ☑
Surgical procedure, complication of (delayed or as an abnormal reaction without mention of misadventure) (*see also* Complication of or following, by type of procedure)
  due to or as a result of misadventure — *see* Misadventure
Swallowed, swallowing
  foreign body — *see* Foreign body, alimentary canal
  poison — *see* Table of Drugs and Chemicals
  substance
    caustic or corrosive — *see* Table of Drugs and Chemicals
    poisonous — *see* Table of Drugs and Chemicals

T

Tackle in sport W03 ☑
Terrorism (involving) Y38.80 ☑
  biological weapons Y38.6X- ☑
  chemical weapons Y38.7X- ☑
  conflagration Y38.3X- ☑
  drowning and submersion Y38.89- ☑
  explosion Y38.2X- ☑
    destruction of aircraft Y38.1X- ☑
    marine weapons Y38.0X- ☑
  fire Y38.3X- ☑
  firearms Y38.4X- ☑

Terrorism — *continued*
    hot substances Y38.3X- ☑
    lasers Y38.89- ☑
    nuclear weapons Y38.5X- ☑
    piercing or stabbing instruments Y38.89- ☑
    secondary effects Y38.9X- ☑
    specified method NEC Y38.89- ☑
    suicide bomber Y38.81- ☑
Thirst X58 ☑
Threat to breathing
    aspiration — *see* Aspiration
    due to cave-in, falling earth or substance NEC T71 ☑
Thrown (accidentally)
    against part (any) of or object in transport vehicle (in motion) NEC (*see also* Accident, transport)
    from
        high place, homicide (attempt) Y01 ☑
        machinery — *see* Contact, with, by type of machine
        transport vehicle NEC (*see also* Accident, transport) V89.9 ☑
    off — *see* Thrown, from
Thunderbolt — *see* subcategory T75.0 ☑
    causing fire — *see* Exposure, fire
Tidal wave (any injury) **NEC** — *see* Forces of nature, tidal wave
Took
    overdose (drug) — *see* Table of Drugs and Chemicals
    poison — *see* Table of Drugs and Chemicals
Tornado (any injury) X37.1 ☑
Torrential rain (any injury) X37.8 ☑
Torture X58 ☑
Trampled by animal NEC W55.89 ☑
Trapped (accidentally)
    between objects (moving) (stationary and moving) — *see* Caught
    by part (any) of
        motorcycle V29.88 ☑
        pedal cycle V19.88 ☑
        transport vehicle NEC (*see also* Accident, transport) V89.9 ☑
Travel (effects) (sickness) T75.3 ☑
Tree falling on or hitting (accidentally) (person) W20.8 ☑
Tripping
    without fall W18.40 ☑
        due to
            specified NEC W18.49 ☑
            stepping from one level to another W18.43 ☑
            stepping into hole or opening W18.42 ☑
            stepping on object W18.41 ☑
        over
            animal W01.0 ☑
                with fall W01.0 ☑
            carpet, rug or (small) object W22.8 ☑
                with fall W18.09 ☑
            person W51 ☑
                with fall W03 ☑
                    due to ice or snow W00.0 ☑
Twisted by person(s) (accidentally) W50.2 ☑
    with intent to injure or kill Y04.0 ☑
    as, or caused by, a crowd or human stampede (with fall) W52 ☑
    assault Y04.0 ☑
    homicide (attempt) Y04.0 ☑
    in
        fight Y04.0 ☑
        legal intervention — *see* Legal, intervention, manhandling
Twisting (prolonged) (static) X50.1- ☑

U

Underdosing of necessary drugs, medicaments or biological substances Y63.6
Undetermined intent (contact) (exposure)
    automobile collision Y32 ☑
    blunt object Y29 ☑
    drowning (submersion) (in) Y21.9 ☑
        bathtub Y21.0 ☑
            after fall Y21.1 ☑
        natural water (lake) (ocean) (pond) (river) (stream) Y21.4 ☑
        specified place NEC Y21.8 ☑
        swimming pool Y21.2 ☑
            after fall Y21.3 ☑
    explosive material Y25 ☑

Undetermined intent — *continued*
    fall, jump or push from high place Y30 ☑
    falling, lying or running before moving object Y31 ☑
    fire Y26 ☑
    firearm discharge Y24.9 ☑
        airgun (BB) (pellet) Y24.0 ☑
        handgun (pistol) (revolver) Y22 ☑
        hunting rifle Y23.1 ☑
        larger Y23.9 ☑
            hunting rifle Y23.1 ☑
            machine gun Y23.3 ☑
            military Y23.2 ☑
            shotgun Y23.0 ☑
            specified type NEC Y23.8 ☑
        machine gun Y23.3 ☑
        military Y23.2 ☑
        shotgun Y23.0 ☑
        specified type NEC Y24.8 ☑
        Very pistol Y24.8 ☑
    hot object Y27.9 ☑
        fluid NEC Y27.2 ☑
        household appliance Y27.3 ☑
        specified object NEC Y27.8 ☑
        steam Y27.0 ☑
        tap water Y27.1 ☑
        vapor Y27.0 ☑
    jump, fall or push from high place Y30 ☑
    lying, falling or running before moving object Y31 ☑
    motor vehicle crash Y32 ☑
    push, fall or jump from high place Y30 ☑
    running, falling or lying before moving object Y31 ☑
    sharp object Y28.9 ☑
        dagger Y28.2 ☑
        glass Y28.0 ☑
        knife Y28.1 ☑
        specified object NEC Y28.8 ☑
        sword Y28.2 ☑
    smoke Y26 ☑
    specified event NEC Y33 ☑
Use of hand as hammer X50.3 ☑

V

Vibration (causing injury) W49.9 ☑
Victim (of)
    avalanche — *see* Landslide
    earth movements NEC — *see* Forces of nature, earth movement
    earthquake X34 ☑
    flood — *see* Flood
    landslide — *see* Landslide
    lightning — *see* subcategory T75.0 ☑
        causing fire — *see* Exposure, fire
    storm (cataclysmic) NEC — *see* Forces of nature, cataclysmic storm
    volcanic eruption X35 ☑
Volcanic eruption (any injury) X35 ☑
Vomitus, gastric contents in air passages (with asphyxia, obstruction or suffocation) T17.81- ☑

W

Walked into stationary object (any) W22.09 ☑
    furniture W22.03 ☑
    lamppost W22.02 ☑
    wall W22.01 ☑
War operations (injuries to military personnel and civilians during war, civil insurrection and peacekeeping missions) (by) (from) (involving) Y36.90 ☑
    after cessation of hostilities Y36.89- ☑
        explosion (of)
            bomb placed during war operations Y36.82- ☑
            mine placed during war operations Y36.81- ☑
            specified NEC Y36.88- ☑
    air blast Y36.20- ☑
    aircraft
        destruction — *see* War operations, destruction of aircraft
        airway restriction — *see* War operations, restriction of airways
    asphyxiation — *see* War operations, restriction of airways
    biological weapons Y36.6X- ☑
    blast Y36.20- ☑
    blast fragments Y36.20- ☑
    blast wave Y36.20- ☑

War operations — *continued*
    blast wind Y36.20- ☑
    bomb Y36.20- ☑
        dirty Y36.50- ☑
        gasoline Y36.31- ☑
        incendiary Y36.31- ☑
        petrol Y36.31- ☑
    bullet Y36.43- ☑
        incendiary Y36.32- ☑
        rubber Y36.41- ☑
    chemical weapons Y36.7X- ☑
    combat
        hand to hand (unarmed) combat Y36.44- ☑
        using blunt or piercing object Y36.45- ☑
    conflagration — *see* War operations, fire
    conventional warfare NEC Y36.49- ☑
    depth-charge Y36.01- ☑
    destruction of aircraft Y36.10- ☑
        due to
            air to air missile Y36.11- ☑
            collision with other aircraft Y36.12- ☑
            detonation (accidental) of onboard munitions and explosives Y36.14- ☑
            enemy fire or explosives Y36.11- ☑
            explosive placed on aircraft Y36.11- ☑
            onboard fire Y36.13- ☑
            rocket propelled grenade [RPG] Y36.11- ☑
            small arms fire Y36.11- ☑
            surface to air missile Y36.11- ☑
        specified NEC Y36.19- ☑
    detonation (accidental) of
        onboard marine weapons Y36.05- ☑
        own munitions or munitions launch device Y36.24- ☑
    dirty bomb Y36.50- ☑
    explosion (of) Y36.20- ☑
        aerial bomb Y36.21- ☑
        after cessation of hostilities
            bomb placed during war operations Y36.82- ☑
            mine placed during war operations Y36.81- ☑
        bomb NOS (*see also* War operations, bomb(s)) Y36.20- ☑
        fragments Y36.20- ☑
        grenade Y36.29- ☑
        guided missile Y36.22- ☑
        improvised explosive device [IED] (person-borne) (roadside) (vehicle-borne) Y36.23- ☑
        land mine Y36.29- ☑
        marine mine (at sea) (in harbor) Y36.02- ☑
        marine weapon Y36.00- ☑
            specified NEC Y36.09- ☑
        own munitions or munitions launch device (accidental) Y36.24- ☑
        sea-based artillery shell Y36.03- ☑
        specified NEC Y36.29- ☑
        torpedo Y36.04- ☑
    fire Y36.30- ☑
        specified NEC Y36.39- ☑
    firearms
        discharge Y36.43- ☑
        pellets Y36.42- ☑
    flamethrower Y36.33- ☑
    fragments (from) (of)
        improvised explosive device [IED] (person-borne) (roadside) (vehicle-borne) Y36.26- ☑
        munitions Y36.25- ☑
        specified NEC Y36.29- ☑
        weapons Y36.27- ☑
    friendly fire Y36.92 ☑
    hand to hand (unarmed) combat Y36.44- ☑
    hot substances — *see* War operations, fire
    incendiary bullet Y36.32- ☑
    nuclear weapon (effects of) Y36.50- ☑
        acute radiation exposure Y36.54- ☑
        blast pressure Y36.51- ☑
        direct blast Y36.51- ☑
        direct heat Y36.53- ☑
        fallout exposure Y36.54- ☑
        fireball Y36.53- ☑
        indirect blast (struck or crushed by blast debris) (being thrown by blast) Y36.52- ☑
        ionizing radiation (immediate exposure) Y36.54- ☑
        nuclear radiation Y36.54- ☑
        radiation
            ionizing (immediate exposure) Y36.54- ☑
            nuclear Y36.54- ☑

War operations — *continued*
   nuclear weapon — *continued*
      radiation — *continued*
         thermal Y36.53- ☑
      secondary effects Y36.54- ☑
      specified NEC Y36.59- ☑
      thermal radiation Y36.53- ☑
   restriction of air (airway)
      intentional Y36.46- ☑
      unintentional Y36.47- ☑
   rubber bullets Y36.41- ☑
   shrapnel NOS Y36.29- ☑
   suffocation — *see* War operations, restriction of airways
   unconventional warfare NEC Y36.7X- ☑
   underwater blast NOS Y36.00- ☑
   warfare
      conventional NEC Y36.49- ☑
      unconventional NEC Y36.7X- ☑

War operations — *continued*
   weapon of mass destruction [WMD] Y36.91 ☑
   weapons
      biological weapons Y36.6X- ☑
      chemical Y36.7X- ☑
      nuclear (effects of) Y36.50- ☑
         acute radiation exposure Y36.54- ☑
         blast pressure Y36.51- ☑
         direct blast Y36.51- ☑
         direct heat Y36.53- ☑
         fallout exposure Y36.54- ☑
         fireball Y36.53- ☑
         radiation
            ionizing (immediate exposure) Y36.54- ☑
            nuclear Y36.54- ☑
            thermal Y36.53- ☑
         secondary effects Y36.54- ☑
         specified NEC Y36.59- ☑
   of mass destruction [WMD] Y36.91 ☑

Washed
   away by flood — *see* Flood
   off road by storm (transport vehicle) — *see* Forces of nature, cataclysmic storm
Weather exposure NEC — *see* Forces of nature
Weightlessness (causing injury) (effects of) (in spacecraft, real or simulated) X52 ☑
Work related condition Y99.0
Wound (accidental) NEC (*see also* Injury) X58 ☑
   battle (*see also* War operations) Y36.90 ☑
   gunshot — *see* Discharge, firearm by type
Wreck transport vehicle NEC (*see also* Accident, transport) V89.9 ☑
Wrong
   device implanted into correct surgical site Y65.51
   fluid in infusion Y65.1
   patient, procedure performed on Y65.52
   procedure (operation) on correct patient Y65.51

ICD-10-CM Tabular List of Diseases and Injuries

Chapter 1. Certain Infectious and Parasitic Diseases (AØØ–B99)

Chapter Specific Guidelines with Coding Examples

The chapter specific guidelines from the ICD-10-CM Official Guidelines for Coding and Reporting have been provided below. Along with these guidelines are coding examples, contained in the shaded boxes, that have been developed to help illustrate the coding and/or sequencing guidance found in these guidelines.

a. Human immunodeficiency virus (HIV) infections

1) Code only confirmed cases

Code only confirmed cases of HIV infection/illness. This is an exception to the hospital inpatient guideline Section II, H.

In this context, "confirmation" does not require documentation of positive serology or culture for HIV; the provider's diagnostic statement that the patient is HIV positive, or has an HIV-related illness is sufficient.

> Patient being seen for hypothyroidism with possible HIV infection
>
> **EØ3.9**   **Hypothyroidism, unspecified**
>
> *Explanation:* Only the hypothyroidism is coded in this scenario because it has not been confirmed that an HIV infection is present.

2) Selection and sequencing of HIV codes

(a) Patient admitted for HIV-related condition

If a patient is admitted for an HIV-related condition, the principal diagnosis should be B2Ø, Human immunodeficiency virus [HIV] disease followed by additional diagnosis codes for all reported HIV-related conditions.

> HIV with CMV
>
> **B2Ø**   **Human immunodeficiency virus [HIV] disease**
>
> **B25.9**   **Cytomegaloviral disease, unspecified**
>
> *Explanation:* Cytomegaloviral infection is an HIV related condition, so the HIV diagnosis code is reported first, followed by the code for the CMV.

(b) Patient with HIV disease admitted for unrelated condition

If a patient with HIV disease is admitted for an unrelated condition (such as a traumatic injury), the code for the unrelated condition (e.g., the nature of injury code) should be the principal diagnosis. Other diagnoses would be B2Ø followed by additional diagnosis codes for all reported HIV-related conditions.

> Sprain of the internal collateral ligament, right ankle; HIV
>
> **S93.491A**   **Sprain of other ligament of right ankle, initial encounter**
>
> **B2Ø**   **Human immunodeficiency virus [HIV] disease**
>
> *Explanation:* The ankle sprain is not related to HIV, so it is the first-listed diagnosis code, and HIV is reported secondarily.

(c) Whether the patient is newly diagnosed

Whether the patient is newly diagnosed or has had previous admissions/encounters for HIV conditions is irrelevant to the sequencing decision.

> Newly diagnosed multiple cutaneous Kaposi's sarcoma lesions in previously diagnosed HIV disease
>
> **B2Ø**   **Human immunodeficiency virus [HIV] disease**
>
> **C46.Ø**   **Kaposi's sarcoma of skin**
>
> *Explanation:* Even though the HIV was diagnosed on a previous encounter, it is still sequenced first when coded with an HIV related condition. Kaposi's sarcoma is an HIV-related condition.

(d) Asymptomatic human immunodeficiency virus

Z21, Asymptomatic human immunodeficiency virus [HIV] infection status, is to be applied when the patient without any documentation of symptoms is listed as being "HIV positive," "known HIV," "HIV test positive," or similar terminology. Do not use this code if the term "AIDS" is used or if the patient is treated for any HIV-related illness or is described as having any condition(s) resulting from his/her HIV positive status; use B2Ø in these cases.

> Patient is being seen for iron deficiency anemia. Status positive HIV test on Atripla, with no prior symptoms
>
> **D5Ø.9**   **Iron deficiency anemia, unspecified**
>
> **Z21**   **Asymptomatic human immunodeficiency virus [HIV] infection status**
>
> *Explanation:* Code Z21 is sequenced second since documentation indicates that the patient has had a positive HIV test but has been asymptomatic. Being on medication for HIV is not an indication that code B2Ø is used instead of Z21. Unless there has been documentation that the patient has had current or prior symptoms or HIV-related complications, code B2Ø is not used. The anemia is not an AIDS-related complication and is sequenced first.

(e) Patients with inconclusive HIV serology

Patients with inconclusive HIV serology, but no definitive diagnosis or manifestations of the illness, may be assigned code R75, Inconclusive laboratory evidence of human immunodeficiency virus [HIV].

(f) Previously diagnosed HIV-related illness

Patients with any known prior diagnosis of an HIV-related illness should be coded to B2Ø. Once a patient has developed an HIV-related illness, the patient should always be assigned code B2Ø on every subsequent admission/encounter. Patients previously diagnosed with any HIV illness (B2Ø) should never be assigned to R75 or Z21, Asymptomatic human immunodeficiency virus [HIV] infection status.

(g) HIV infection in pregnancy, childbirth and the puerperium

During pregnancy, childbirth or the puerperium, a patient admitted (or presenting for a health care encounter) because of an HIV-related illness should receive a principal diagnosis code of O98.7-, Human immunodeficiency [HIV] disease complicating pregnancy, childbirth and the puerperium, followed by B2Ø and the code(s) for the HIV-related illness(es). Codes from Chapter 15 always take sequencing priority.

Patients with asymptomatic HIV infection status admitted (or presenting for a health care encounter) during pregnancy, childbirth, or the puerperium should receive codes of O98.7- and Z21.

(h) Encounters for testing for HIV

If a patient is being seen to determine his/her HIV status, use code Z11.4, Encounter for screening for human immunodeficiency virus [HIV]. Use additional codes for any associated high risk behavior.

If a patient with signs or symptoms is being seen for HIV testing, code the signs and symptoms. An additional counseling code Z71.7, Human immunodeficiency virus [HIV] counseling, may be used if counseling is provided during the encounter for the test.

When a patient returns to be informed of his/her HIV test results and the test result is negative, use code Z71.7, Human immunodeficiency virus [HIV] counseling.

If the results are positive, see previous guidelines and assign codes as appropriate.

b. Infectious agents as the cause of diseases classified to other chapters

Certain infections are classified in chapters other than Chapter 1 and no organism is identified as part of the infection code. In these instances, it is necessary to use an additional code from Chapter 1 to identify the organism. A code from category B95, Streptococcus, Staphylococcus, and Enterococcus as the cause of diseases classified to other chapters, B96, Other bacterial agents as the cause of diseases classified to other chapters, or B97, Viral agents as the cause of diseases classified to other chapters, is to be used as an additional code to identify the organism. An instructional note will be found at the infection code advising that an additional organism code is required.

Chapter 1. Certain Infectious and Parasitic Diseases

Acute *E. coli* cystitis

N30.00	**Acute cystitis without hematuria**
B96.20	**Unspecified Escherichia coli [E.coli] as the cause of diseases classified elsewhere**

Explanation: An instructional note under the category for the cystitis indicates to code also the specific organism.

c. Infections resistant to antibiotics

Many bacterial infections are resistant to current antibiotics. It is necessary to identify all infections documented as antibiotic resistant. Assign a code from category Z16, Resistance to antimicrobial drugs, following the infection code only if the infection code does not identify drug resistance.

Penicillin-resistant *Streptococcus pneumoniae* pneumonia

J13	**Pneumonia due to Streptococcus pneumoniae**
Z16.11	**Resistance to penicillins**

Explanation: Code Z16.11 is assigned as a secondary code to represent the penicillin resistance. This code includes resistance to amoxicillin and ampicillin.

d. Sepsis, severe sepsis, and septic shock

1) Coding of Sepsis and Severe Sepsis

(a) Sepsis

For a diagnosis of sepsis, assign the appropriate code for the underlying systemic infection. If the type of infection or causal organism is not further specified, assign code A41.9, Sepsis, unspecified organism.

A code from subcategory R65.2, Severe sepsis, should not be assigned unless severe sepsis or an associated acute organ dysfunction is documented.

Gram-negative sepsis

A41.50	**Gram-negative sepsis, unspecified**

Staphylococcal sepsis

A41.2	**Sepsis due to unspecified staphylococcus**

Explanation: In both examples above the organism causing the sepsis is identified, therefore A41.9 Sepsis, unspecified organism, would not be appropriate as this code would not capture the highest degree of specificity found in the documentation. Do not use an additional code for severe sepsis unless an acute organ dysfunction was also documented as "associated with" or "due to" the sepsis or the sepsis was documented as "severe."

(i) Negative or inconclusive blood cultures and sepsis

Negative or inconclusive blood cultures do not preclude a diagnosis of sepsis in patients with clinical evidence of the condition; however, the provider should be queried.

(ii) Urosepsis

The term urosepsis is a nonspecific term. It is not to be considered synonymous with sepsis. It has no default code in the Alphabetic Index. Should a provider use this term, he/she must be queried for clarification.

(iii) Sepsis with organ dysfunction

If a patient has sepsis and associated acute organ dysfunction or multiple organ dysfunction (MOD), follow the instructions for coding severe sepsis.

(iv) Acute organ dysfunction that is not clearly associated with the sepsis

If a patient has sepsis and an acute organ dysfunction, but the medical record documentation indicates that the acute organ dysfunction is related to a medical condition other than the sepsis, do not assign a code from subcategory R65.2, Severe sepsis. An acute organ dysfunction must be associated with the sepsis in order to assign the severe sepsis code. If the documentation is not clear as to whether an acute organ dysfunction is related to the sepsis or another medical condition, query the provider.

Sepsis and acute respiratory failure due to COPD exacerbation

A41.9	**Sepsis, unspecified organism**
J44.1	**Chronic obstructive pulmonary disease with (acute) exacerbation**
J96.00	**Acute respiratory failure, unspecified whether with hypoxia or hypercapnia**

Explanation: Although acute organ dysfunction is present in the form of acute respiratory failure, severe sepsis (R65.2) is not coded in this example, as the acute respiratory failure is attributed to the COPD exacerbation rather than the sepsis. Sequencing of these codes would be determined by the reason for the encounter.

(b) Severe sepsis

The coding of severe sepsis requires a minimum of 2 codes: first a code for the underlying systemic infection, followed by a code from subcategory R65.2, Severe sepsis. If the causal organism is not documented, assign code A41.9, Sepsis, unspecified organism, for the infection. Additional code(s) for the associated acute organ dysfunction are also required.

Due to the complex nature of severe sepsis, some cases may require querying the provider prior to assignment of the codes.

2) Septic shock

(a) Septic shock generally refers to circulatory failure associated with severe sepsis, and therefore, it represents a type of acute organ dysfunction.

For cases of septic shock, the code for the systemic infection should be sequenced first, followed by code R65.21, Severe sepsis with septic shock or code T81.12, Postprocedural septic shock. Any additional codes for the other acute organ dysfunctions should also be assigned. As noted in the sequencing instructions in the Tabular List, the code for septic shock cannot be assigned as a principal diagnosis.

Sepsis with septic shock

A41.9	**Sepsis, unspecified organism**
R65.21	**Severe sepsis with septic shock**

Explanation: Documentation of septic shock automatically implies severe sepsis as it is a form of acute organ dysfunction. Septic shock is not coded as the first-listed diagnosis; it is always preceded by the code for the systemic infection.

3) Sequencing of severe sepsis

If severe sepsis is present on admission, and meets the definition of principal diagnosis, the underlying systemic infection should be assigned as principal diagnosis followed by the appropriate code from subcategory R65.2 as required by the sequencing rules in the Tabular List. A code from subcategory R65.2 can never be assigned as a principal diagnosis.

When severe sepsis develops during an encounter (it was not present on admission), the underlying systemic infection and the appropriate code from subcategory R65.2 should be assigned as secondary diagnoses.

Severe sepsis may be present on admission, but the diagnosis may not be confirmed until sometime after admission. If the documentation is not clear whether severe sepsis was present on admission, the provider should be queried.

4) Sepsis and severe sepsis with a localized infection

If the reason for admission is both sepsis or severe sepsis and a localized infection, such as pneumonia or cellulitis, a code(s) for the underlying systemic infection should be assigned first and the code for the localized infection should be assigned as a secondary diagnosis. If the patient has severe sepsis, a code from subcategory R65.2 should also be assigned as a secondary diagnosis. If the patient is admitted with a localized infection, such as pneumonia, and sepsis/severe sepsis doesn't develop until after admission, the localized infection should be assigned first, followed by the appropriate sepsis/severe sepsis codes.

Patient presents with acute renal failure due to severe sepsis from *Pseudomonas pneumonia*

A41.52	Sepsis, due to Pseudomonas
J15.1	Pneumonia due to Pseudomonas
R65.20	Severe sepsis without septic shock
N17.9	Acute kidney failure, unspecified

Explanation: If all conditions are present, the systemic infection (sepsis) is sequenced first followed by the codes for the localized infection (pneumonia), severe sepsis and any organ dysfunction.

5) Sepsis due to a postprocedural infection

(a) Documentation of causal relationship

As with all postprocedural complications, code assignment is based on the provider's documentation of the relationship between the infection and the procedure.

(b) Sepsis due to a postprocedural infection

For such cases, the postprocedural infection code, such as T80.2, Infections following infusion, transfusion, and therapeutic injection, T81.4, Infection following a procedure, T88.0, Infection following immunization, or O86.0, Infection of obstetric surgical wound, should be coded first, followed by the code for the specific infection. If the patient has severe sepsis, the appropriate code from subcategory R65.2 should also be assigned with the additional code(s) for any acute organ dysfunction.

(c) Postprocedural infection and postprocedural septic shock

In cases where a postprocedural infection has occurred and has resulted in severe sepsis the code for the precipitating complication such as code T81.4, Infection following a procedure, or O86.0, Infection of obstetrical surgical wound should be coded first followed by code R65.20, Severe sepsis without septic shock. A code for the systemic infection should also be assigned.

If a postprocedural infection has resulted in postprocedural septic shock, the code for the precipitating complication such as code T81.4, Infection following a procedure, or O86.0, Infection of obstetrical surgical wound should be coded first followed by code T81.12-, Postprocedural septic shock. A code for the systemic infection should also be assigned.

6) Sepsis and severe sepsis associated with a noninfectious process (condition)

In some cases a noninfectious process (condition), such as trauma, may lead to an infection which can result in sepsis or severe sepsis. If sepsis or severe sepsis is documented as associated with a noninfectious condition, such as a burn or serious injury, and this condition meets the definition for principal diagnosis, the code for the noninfectious condition should be sequenced first, followed by the code for the resulting infection. If severe sepsis is present, a code from subcategory R65.2 should also be assigned with any associated organ dysfunction(s) codes. It is not necessary to assign a code from subcategory R65.1, Systemic inflammatory response syndrome (SIRS) of non-infectious origin, for these cases.

If the infection meets the definition of principal diagnosis, it should be sequenced before the non-infectious condition. When both the associated non-infectious condition and the infection meet the definition of principal diagnosis, either may be assigned as principal diagnosis.

Only one code from category R65, Symptoms and signs specifically associated with systemic inflammation and infection, should be assigned. Therefore, when a non-infectious condition leads to an infection resulting in severe sepsis, assign the appropriate code from subcategory R65.2, Severe sepsis. Do not additionally assign a code from subcategory R65.1, Systemic inflammatory response syndrome (SIRS) of non-infectious origin.

See Section I.C.18. SIRS due to non-infectious process

7) Sepsis and septic shock complicating abortion, pregnancy, childbirth, and the puerperium

See Section I.C.15. Sepsis and septic shock complicating abortion, pregnancy, childbirth and the puerperium

8) Newborn sepsis

See Section I.C.16. f. Bacterial sepsis of Newborn

e. Methicillin resistant *Staphylococcus aureus* (MRSA) conditions

1) Selection and sequencing of MRSA codes

(a) Combination codes for MRSA infection

When a patient is diagnosed with an infection that is due to methicillin resistant *Staphylococcus aureus* (MRSA), and that infection has a combination code that includes the causal organism (e.g., sepsis, pneumonia) assign the appropriate combination code for the condition (e.g., code A41.02, Sepsis due to Methicillin resistant Staphylococcus aureus or code J15.212, Pneumonia due to Methicillin resistant Staphylococcus aureus). Do not assign code B95.62, Methicillin resistant Staphylococcus aureus infection as the cause of diseases classified elsewhere, as an additional code, because the combination code includes the type of infection and the MRSA organism. Do not assign a code from subcategory Z16.11, Resistance to penicillins, as an additional diagnosis.

See Section C.1. for instructions on coding and sequencing of sepsis and severe sepsis.

(b) Other codes for MRSA infection

When there is documentation of a current infection (e.g., wound infection, stitch abscess, urinary tract infection) due to MRSA, and that infection does not have a combination code that includes the causal organism, assign the appropriate code to identify the condition along with code B95.62, Methicillin resistant Staphylococcus aureus infection as the cause of diseases classified elsewhere for the MRSA infection. Do not assign a code from subcategory Z16.11, Resistance to penicillins.

(c) Methicillin susceptible Staphylococcus aureus (MSSA) and MRSA colonization

The condition or state of being colonized or carrying MSSA or MRSA is called colonization or carriage, while an individual person is described as being colonized or being a carrier. Colonization means that MSSA or MSRA is present on or in the body without necessarily causing illness. A positive MRSA colonization test might be documented by the provider as "MRSA screen positive" or "MRSA nasal swab positive".

Assign code Z22.322, Carrier or suspected carrier of Methicillin resistant Staphylococcus aureus, for patients documented as having MRSA colonization. Assign code Z22.321, Carrier or suspected carrier of Methicillin susceptible Staphylococcus aureus, for patient documented as having MSSA colonization. Colonization is not necessarily indicative of a disease process or as the cause of a specific condition the patient may have unless documented as such by the provider.

(d) MRSA colonization and infection

If a patient is documented as having both MRSA colonization and infection during a hospital admission, code Z22.322, Carrier or suspected carrier of Methicillin resistant Staphylococcus aureus, and a code for the MRSA infection may both be assigned.

f. Zika virus infections

1) Code only confirmed cases

Code only a confirmed diagnosis of Zika virus (A92.5, Zika virus disease) as documented by the provider. This is an exception to the hospital inpatient guideline Section II, H.

In this context, "confirmation" does not require documentation of the type of test performed; the physician's diagnostic statement that the condition is confirmed is sufficient. This code should be assigned regardless of the stated mode of transmission.

If the provider documents "suspected", "possible" or "probable" Zika, do not assign code A92.5. Assign a code(s) explaining the reason for encounter (such as fever, rash, or joint pain) or Z20.828, Contact with and (suspected) exposure to other viral communicable diseases.

Chapter 1. Certain Infectious and Parasitic Diseases (A00–B99)

INCLUDES   diseases generally recognized as communicable or transmissible

Use additional code to identify resistance to antimicrobial drugs (Z16.-)

EXCLUDES 1   certain localized infections—see body system-related chapters

EXCLUDES 2   carrier or suspected carrier of infectious disease (Z22.-)
infectious and parasitic diseases specific to the perinatal period (P35-P39)
infectious and parasitic diseases complicating pregnancy, childbirth and the puerperium (O98.-)
influenza and other acute respiratory infections (J00-J22)

This chapter contains the following blocks:

A00-A09   Intestinal infectious diseases
A15-A19   Tuberculosis
A20-A28   Certain zoonotic bacterial diseases
A30-A49   Other bacterial diseases
A50-A64   Infections with a predominantly sexual mode of transmission
A65-A69   Other spirochetal diseases
A70-A74   Other diseases caused by chlamydiae
A75-A79   Rickettsioses
A80-A89   Viral infections of the central nervous system
A90-A99   Arthropod-borne viral fevers and viral hemorrhagic fevers
B00-B09   Viral infections characterized by skin and mucous membrane lesions
B10   Other human herpesviruses
B15-B19   Viral hepatitis
B20   Human immunodeficiency virus [HIV] disease
B25-B34   Other viral diseases
B35-B49   Mycoses
B50-B64   Protozoal diseases
B65-B83   Helminthiases
B85-B89   Pediculosis, acariasis and other infestations
B90-B94   Sequelae of infectious and parasitic diseases
B95-B97   Bacterial and viral infectious agents
B99   Other infectious diseases

Intestinal Infectious Diseases (A00-A09)

✓4ᵗʰ **A00 Cholera**

A00.0 Cholera due to Vibrio cholerae 01, biovar cholerae
Classical cholera

A00.1 Cholera due to Vibrio cholerae 01, biovar eltor
Cholera eltor

A00.9 Cholera, unspecified ▽

✓4ᵗʰ **A01 Typhoid and paratyphoid fevers**
DEF: Typhoid fever: An acute generalized illness caused by *Salmonella typhi*; clinical features are fever, headache, abdominal pain, cough, toxemia, leukopenia, abnormal pulse, rose spots on the skin, bacteremia, hyperplasia of intestinal lymph nodes, mesenteric lymphadenopathy, and Peyer's patches in the intestines.
DEF: Paratyphoid fever: A prolonged febrile illness, caused by *Salmonella* serotypes other than *S. typhi*, especially *S. enterica* serotypes paratyphi A, B, and C.

✓5ᵗʰ **A01.0 Typhoid fever**
Infection due to Salmonella typhi

A01.00 Typhoid fever, unspecified ▽

A01.01 Typhoid meningitis

A01.02 Typhoid fever with heart involvement
Typhoid endocarditis
Typhoid myocarditis

A01.03 Typhoid pneumonia HCC

A01.04 Typhoid arthritis HCC

A01.05 Typhoid osteomyelitis HCC

A01.09 Typhoid fever with other complications

A01.1 Paratyphoid fever A

A01.2 Paratyphoid fever B

A01.3 Paratyphoid fever C

A01.4 Paratyphoid fever, unspecified ▽
Infection due to Salmonella paratyphi NOS

✓4ᵗʰ **A02 Other salmonella infections**
INCLUDES   infection or foodborne intoxication due to any Salmonella species other than S. typhi and S. paratyphi

A02.0 Salmonella enteritis
Salmonellosis

A02.1 Salmonella sepsis HCC

✓5ᵗʰ **A02.2 Localized salmonella infections**

A02.20 Localized salmonella infection, unspecified ▽

A02.21 Salmonella meningitis

A02.22 Salmonella pneumonia HCC

A02.23 Salmonella arthritis HCC

A02.24 Salmonella osteomyelitis HCC

A02.25 Salmonella pyelonephritis
Salmonella tubulo-interstitial nephropathy

A02.29 Salmonella with other localized infection

A02.8 Other specified salmonella infections

A02.9 Salmonella infection, unspecified ▽

✓4ᵗʰ **A03 Shigellosis**
DEF: Infection caused by the genus *Shigella*, of the family *Enterobacteriaceae*; known to cause an acute dysenteric infection of the bowel with fever, drowsiness, anorexia, nausea, vomiting, bloody diarrhea, abdominal cramps, and distention.

A03.0 Shigellosis due to Shigella dysenteriae
Group A shigellosis [Shiga-Kruse dysentery]

A03.1 Shigellosis due to Shigella flexneri
Group B shigellosis

A03.2 Shigellosis due to Shigella boydii
Group C shigellosis

A03.3 Shigellosis due to Shigella sonnei
Group D shigellosis

A03.8 Other shigellosis

A03.9 Shigellosis, unspecified ▽
Bacillary dysentery NOS

✓4ᵗʰ **A04 Other bacterial intestinal infections**
EXCLUDES 1   bacterial foodborne intoxications, NEC (A05.-)
tuberculous enteritis (A18.32)

A04.0 Enteropathogenic Escherichia coli infection

A04.1 Enterotoxigenic Escherichia coli infection

A04.2 Enteroinvasive Escherichia coli infection

A04.3 Enterohemorrhagic Escherichia coli infection
DEF: *E. coli* infection penetrating the intestinal mucosa, producing microscopic ulceration and bleeding.

A04.4 Other intestinal Escherichia coli infections
Escherichia coli enteritis NOS

A04.5 Campylobacter enteritis

A04.6 Enteritis due to Yersinia enterocolitica
EXCLUDES 1   extraintestinal yersiniosis (A28.2)

✓5ᵗʰ **A04.7 Enterocolitis due to Clostridium difficile**
Foodborne intoxication by Clostridium difficile
Pseudomembraneous colitis

●   **A04.71 Enterocolitis due to Clostridium difficile, recurrent**

●   **A04.72 Enterocolitis due to Clostridium difficile, not specified as recurrent**

A04.8 Other specified bacterial intestinal infections

A04.9 Bacterial intestinal infection, unspecified ▽
Bacterial enteritis NOS

✓4ᵗʰ **A05 Other bacterial foodborne intoxications, not elsewhere classified**
EXCLUDES 1   Clostridium difficile foodborne intoxication and infection ▶(A04.7-)◀
Escherichia coli infection (A04.0-A04.4)
listeriosis (A32.-)
salmonella foodborne intoxication and infection (A02.-)
toxic effect of noxious foodstuffs (T61-T62)

A05.0 Foodborne staphylococcal intoxication

A05.1 Botulism food poisoning
Botulism NOS
Classical foodborne intoxication due to Clostridium botulinum
EXCLUDES 1   infant botulism (A48.51)
wound botulism (A48.52)

A05.2 Foodborne Clostridium perfringens [Clostridium welchii] intoxication
Enteritis necroticans
Pig-bel

A05.3 Foodborne Vibrio parahaemolyticus intoxication

A05.4 Foodborne Bacillus cereus intoxication

A05.5 Foodborne Vibrio vulnificus intoxication

A05.8 Other specified bacterial foodborne intoxications

A05.9 Bacterial foodborne intoxication, unspecified ▽

EXCLUDES 1   Not coded here   EXCLUDES 2   Not included here   N Newborn Age: 0   P Pediatric Age: 0-17   M Maternity Age: 12-55   A Adult Age: 15-124

✓4th A06 Amebiasis

INCLUDES   infection due to Entamoeba histolytica
EXCLUDES 1   *other protozoal intestinal diseases (A07.-)*
EXCLUDES 2   *acanthamebiasis (B60.1-)*
              Naegleriasis (B60.2)

A06.0 Acute amebic dysentery
     Acute amebiasis
     Intestinal amebiasis NOS

A06.1 Chronic intestinal amebiasis

A06.2 Amebic nondysenteric colitis

A06.3 Ameboma of intestine
     Ameboma NOS

A06.4 Amebic liver abscess
     Hepatic amebiasis

A06.5 Amebic lung abscess   HCC
     Amebic abscess of lung (and liver)

A06.6 Amebic brain abscess
     Amebic abscess of brain (and liver) (and lung)

A06.7 Cutaneous amebiasis

✓5th **A06.8 Amebic infection of other sites**

     A06.81 Amebic cystitis

     A06.82 Other amebic genitourinary infections
         Amebic balanitis
         Amebic vesiculitis
         Amebic vulvovaginitis

     A06.89 Other amebic infections
         Amebic appendicitis
         Amebic splenic abscess

A06.9 Amebiasis, unspecified   ▽

✓4th A07 Other protozoal intestinal diseases

A07.0 Balantidiasis
     Balantidial dysentery

A07.1 Giardiasis [lambliasis]

A07.2 Cryptosporidiosis   HCC

A07.3 Isosporiasis
     Infection due to Isospora belli and Isospora hominis
     Intestinal coccidiosis
     Isosporosis

A07.4 Cyclosporiasis

A07.8 Other specified protozoal intestinal diseases
     Intestinal microsporidiosis
     Intestinal trichomoniasis
     Sarcocystosis
     Sarcosporidiosis

A07.9 Protozoal intestinal disease, unspecified   ▽
     Flagellate diarrhea
     Protozoal colitis
     Protozoal diarrhea
     Protozoal dysentery

✓4th A08 Viral and other specified intestinal infections

EXCLUDES 1   *influenza with involvement of gastrointestinal tract (J09.X3, J10.2, J11.2)*

A08.0 Rotaviral enteritis

✓5th **A08.1 Acute gastroenteropathy due to Norwalk agent and other small round viruses**

     A08.11 Acute gastroenteropathy due to Norwalk agent
         Acute gastroenteropathy due to Norovirus
         Acute gastroenteropathy due to Norwalk-like agent

     A08.19 Acute gastroenteropathy due to other small round viruses
         Acute gastroenteropathy due to small round virus [SRV] NOS

A08.2 Adenoviral enteritis

✓5th **A08.3 Other viral enteritis**

     A08.31 Calicivirus enteritis

     A08.32 Astrovirus enteritis

     A08.39 Other viral enteritis
         Coxsackie virus enteritis
         Echovirus enteritis
         Enterovirus enteritis NEC
         Torovirus enteritis

A08.4 Viral intestinal infection, unspecified   ▽
     Viral enteritis NOS
     Viral gastroenteritis NOS
     Viral gastroenteropathy NOS
     AHA: 2016, 3Q, 12

A08.8 Other specified intestinal infections

A09 Infectious gastroenteritis and colitis, unspecified   ▽

     Infectious colitis NOS
     Infectious enteritis NOS
     Infectious gastroenteritis NOS
     EXCLUDES 1   *colitis NOS (K52.9)*
               diarrhea NOS (R19.7)
               enteritis NOS (K52.9)
               gastroenteritis NOS (K52.9)
               noninfective gastroenteritis and colitis, unspecified (K52.9)
     DEF: Colitis: An inflammation of mucous membranes of the colon.
     DEF: Enteritis: An inflammation of mucous membranes of the small intestine.
     DEF: Gastroenteritis: An inflammation of mucous membranes of stomach and intestines.

Tuberculosis (A15-A19)

INCLUDES   infections due to Mycobacterium tuberculosis and Mycobacterium bovis
EXCLUDES 1   *congenital tuberculosis (P37.0)*
            nonspecific reaction to test for tuberculosis without active tuberculosis (R76.1-)
            pneumoconiosis associated with tuberculosis, any type in A15 (J65)
            positive PPD (R76.11)
            positive tuberculin skin test without active tuberculosis (R76.11)
            sequelae of tuberculosis (B90.-)
            silicotuberculosis (J65)

✓4th A15 Respiratory tuberculosis

A15.0 Tuberculosis of lung
     Tuberculous bronchiectasis
     Tuberculous fibrosis of lung
     Tuberculous pneumonia
     Tuberculous pneumothorax

A15.4 Tuberculosis of intrathoracic lymph nodes
     Tuberculosis of hilar lymph nodes
     Tuberculosis of mediastinal lymph nodes
     Tuberculosis of tracheobronchial lymph nodes
     EXCLUDES 1   *tuberculosis specified as primary (A15.7)*

A15.5 Tuberculosis of larynx, trachea and bronchus
     Tuberculosis of bronchus   Tuberculosis of larynx
     Tuberculosis of glottis   Tuberculosis of trachea

A15.6 Tuberculous pleurisy
     Tuberculosis of pleura   Tuberculous empyema
     EXCLUDES 1   *primary respiratory tuberculosis (A15.7)*

A15.7 Primary respiratory tuberculosis

A15.8 Other respiratory tuberculosis
     Mediastinal tuberculosis
     Nasopharyngeal tuberculosis
     Tuberculosis of nose
     Tuberculosis of sinus [any nasal]

A15.9 Respiratory tuberculosis unspecified   ▽

✓4th A17 Tuberculosis of nervous system

A17.0 Tuberculous meningitis
     Tuberculosis of meninges (cerebral) (spinal)
     Tuberculous leptomeningitis
     EXCLUDES 1   *tuberculous meningoencephalitis (A17.82)*

A17.1 Meningeal tuberculoma
     Tuberculoma of meninges (cerebral) (spinal)
     EXCLUDES 2   *tuberculoma of brain and spinal cord (A17.81)*

Tuberculosis of Lung

Granulomas from Mycobacterium tuberculosis

☑ Additional Character Req   ✓x7th Placeholder Alert   Manifestation   HCC CMS-HCC Condition   ▽ Unspecified Code   ▶◀ Revised Text   ● New Code   ▲ Revised Code Title

ICD-10-CM 2018   437

✓5ᵗʰ **A17.8 Other tuberculosis of nervous system**

A17.81 Tuberculoma of brain and spinal cord
Tuberculous abscess of brain and spinal cord

A17.82 Tuberculous meningoencephalitis
Tuberculous myelitis

A17.83 Tuberculous neuritis
Tuberculous mononeuropathy

A17.89 Other tuberculosis of nervous system
Tuberculous polyneuropathy

A17.9 Tuberculosis of nervous system, unspecified ▽

✓4ᵗʰ **A18 Tuberculosis of other organs**

✓5ᵗʰ **A18.0 Tuberculosis of bones and joints**

A18.01 Tuberculosis of spine
Pott's disease or curvature of spine
Tuberculous arthritis
Tuberculous osteomyelitis of spine
Tuberculous spondylitis

A18.02 Tuberculous arthritis of other joints
Tuberculosis of hip (joint)
Tuberculosis of knee (joint)

A18.03 Tuberculosis of other bones
Tuberculous mastoiditis
Tuberculous osteomyelitis

A18.09 Other musculoskeletal tuberculosis
Tuberculous myositis
Tuberculous synovitis
Tuberculous tenosynovitis

✓5ᵗʰ **A18.1 Tuberculosis of genitourinary system**

A18.10 Tuberculosis of genitourinary system, unspecified ▽

A18.11 Tuberculosis of kidney and ureter

A18.12 Tuberculosis of bladder

A18.13 Tuberculosis of other urinary organs
Tuberculous urethritis

A18.14 Tuberculosis of prostate Ⓐ♂

A18.15 Tuberculosis of other male genital organs ♂

A18.16 Tuberculosis of cervix ♀

A18.17 Tuberculous female pelvic inflammatory disease ♀
Tuberculous endometritis
Tuberculous oophoritis and salpingitis

A18.18 Tuberculosis of other female genital organs ♀
Tuberculous ulceration of vulva

A18.2 Tuberculous peripheral lymphadenopathy
Tuberculous adenitis
EXCLUDES 2 *tuberculosis of bronchial and mediastinal lymph nodes (A15.4)*
tuberculosis of mesenteric and retroperitoneal lymph nodes (A18.39)
tuberculous tracheobronchial adenopathy (A15.4)

✓5ᵗʰ **A18.3 Tuberculosis of intestines, peritoneum and mesenteric glands**

A18.31 Tuberculous peritonitis
Tuberculous ascites
DEF: Tuberculous inflammation of the membrane lining the abdomen.

A18.32 Tuberculous enteritis
Tuberculosis of anus and rectum
Tuberculosis of intestine (large) (small)

A18.39 Retroperitoneal tuberculosis
Tuberculosis of mesenteric glands
Tuberculosis of retroperitoneal (lymph glands)

A18.4 Tuberculosis of skin and subcutaneous tissue
Erythema induratum, tuberculous
Lupus excedens
Lupus vulgaris NOS
Lupus vulgaris of eyelid
Scrofuloderma
Tuberculosis of external ear
EXCLUDES 2 *lupus erythematosus (L93.-)*
lupus NOS (M32.9)
systemic (M32.-)

✓5ᵗʰ **A18.5 Tuberculosis of eye**
EXCLUDES 2 *lupus vulgaris of eyelid (A18.4)*

A18.50 Tuberculosis of eye, unspecified ▽

A18.51 Tuberculous episcleritis

A18.52 Tuberculous keratitis
Tuberculous interstitial keratitis
Tuberculous keratoconjunctivitis (interstitial) (phlyctenular)

A18.53 Tuberculous chorioretinitis

A18.54 Tuberculous iridocyclitis

A18.59 Other tuberculosis of eye
Tuberculous conjunctivitis

A18.6 Tuberculosis of (inner) (middle) ear
Tuberculous otitis media
EXCLUDES 2 *tuberculosis of external ear (A18.4)*
tuberculous mastoiditis (A18.03)

A18.7 Tuberculosis of adrenal glands
Tuberculous Addison's disease

✓5ᵗʰ **A18.8 Tuberculosis of other specified organs**

A18.81 Tuberculosis of thyroid gland

A18.82 Tuberculosis of other endocrine glands
Tuberculosis of pituitary gland
Tuberculosis of thymus gland

A18.83 Tuberculosis of digestive tract organs, not elsewhere classified
EXCLUDES 1 *tuberculosis of intestine (A18.32)*

A18.84 Tuberculosis of heart
Tuberculous cardiomyopathy
Tuberculous endocarditis
Tuberculous myocarditis
Tuberculous pericarditis

A18.85 Tuberculosis of spleen

A18.89 Tuberculosis of other sites
Tuberculosis of muscle
Tuberculous cerebral arteritis

✓4ᵗʰ **A19 Miliary tuberculosis**
INCLUDES disseminated tuberculosis
generalized tuberculosis
tuberculous polyserositis

A19.0 Acute miliary tuberculosis of a single specified site

A19.1 Acute miliary tuberculosis of multiple sites

A19.2 Acute miliary tuberculosis, unspecified ▽

A19.8 Other miliary tuberculosis

A19.9 Miliary tuberculosis, unspecified ▽

Certain zoonotic bacterial diseases (A20-A28)

✓4ᵗʰ **A20 Plague**
INCLUDES infection due to Yersinia pestis

A20.0 Bubonic plague

A20.1 Cellulocutaneous plague

A20.2 Pneumonic plague HCC

A20.3 Plague meningitis

A20.7 Septicemic plague HCC

A20.8 Other forms of plague
Abortive plague
Asymptomatic plague
Pestis minor

A20.9 Plague, unspecified ▽

✓4ᵗʰ **A21 Tularemia**
INCLUDES deer-fly fever
infection due to Francisella tularensis
rabbit fever
DEF: A febrile disease transmitted to humans by the bites of deer flies, fleas, and ticks; by inhaling aerosolized *F. tularensis*; or by ingesting contaminated food or water. Patients quickly develop fever, chills, weakness, headache, backache, and malaise.

A21.0 Ulceroglandular tularemia

A21.1 Oculoglandular tularemia
Ophthalmic tularemia

A21.2 Pulmonary tularemia HCC

A21.3 Gastrointestinal tularemia
Abdominal tularemia

A21.7 Generalized tularemia

A21.8 Other forms of tularemia

A21.9 Tularemia, unspecified ▽

✓4ᵗʰ **A22 Anthrax**
INCLUDES infection due to Bacillus anthracis

A22.0 Cutaneous anthrax
Malignant carbuncle
Malignant pustule

A22.1 Pulmonary anthrax HCC
Inhalation anthrax
Ragpicker's disease
Woolsorter's disease

EXCLUDES 1 Not coded here   EXCLUDES 2 Not included here   Ⓝ Newborn Age: 0   Ⓟ Pediatric Age: 0-17   Ⓜ Maternity Age: 12-55   Ⓐ Adult Age: 15-124

438   ICD-10-CM 2018

A22.2   **Gastrointestinal anthrax**

A22.7   **Anthrax sepsis**   HCC

A22.8   **Other forms of anthrax**
Anthrax meningitis

A22.9   **Anthrax, unspecified**   ▽

✓4th **A23   Brucellosis**
INCLUDES   Malta fever
Mediterranean fever
undulant fever

A23.0   **Brucellosis due to Brucella melitensis**

A23.1   **Brucellosis due to Brucella abortus**

A23.2   **Brucellosis due to Brucella suis**

A23.3   **Brucellosis due to Brucella canis**

A23.8   **Other brucellosis**

A23.9   **Brucellosis, unspecified**   ▽

✓4th **A24   Glanders and melioidosis**

A24.0   **Glanders**
Infection due to Pseudomonas mallei
Malleus

A24.1   **Acute and fulminating melioidosis**
Melioidosis pneumonia
Melioidosis sepsis

A24.2   **Subacute and chronic melioidosis**

A24.3   **Other melioidosis**

A24.9   **Melioidosis, unspecified**   ▽
Infection due to Pseudomonas pseudomallei NOS
Whitmore's disease

✓4th **A25   Rat-bite fevers**

A25.0   **Spirillosis**
Sodoku

A25.1   **Streptobacillosis**
Epidemic arthritic erythema
Haverhill fever
Streptobacillary rat-bite fever

A25.9   **Rat-bite fever, unspecified**   ▽

✓4th **A26   Erysipeloid**

A26.0   **Cutaneous erysipeloid**
Erythema migrans

A26.7   **Erysipelothrix sepsis**   HCC

A26.8   **Other forms of erysipeloid**

A26.9   **Erysipeloid, unspecified**   ▽

✓4th **A27   Leptospirosis**

A27.0   **Leptospirosis icterohemorrhagica**
Leptospiral or spirochetal jaundice (hemorrhagic)
Weil's disease

✓5th A27.8   **Other forms of leptospirosis**

A27.81   **Aseptic meningitis in leptospirosis**

A27.89   **Other forms of leptospirosis**

A27.9   **Leptospirosis, unspecified**   ▽

✓4th **A28   Other zoonotic bacterial diseases, not elsewhere classified**

A28.0   **Pasteurellosis**

A28.1   **Cat-scratch disease**
Cat-scratch fever

A28.2   **Extraintestinal yersiniosis**
EXCLUDES 1   enteritis due to Yersinia enterocolitica (A04.6)
plague (A20.-)

A28.8   **Other specified zoonotic bacterial diseases, not elsewhere classified**

A28.9   **Zoonotic bacterial disease, unspecified**   ▽

Other bacterial diseases (A30-A49)
AHA: 2016, 3Q, 8-14

✓4th **A30   Leprosy [Hansen's disease]**
INCLUDES   infection due to Mycobacterium leprae
EXCLUDES 1   sequelae of leprosy (B92)

A30.0   **Indeterminate leprosy**
I leprosy

A30.1   **Tuberculoid leprosy**
TT leprosy

A30.2   **Borderline tuberculoid leprosy**
BT leprosy

A30.3   **Borderline leprosy**
BB leprosy

A30.4   **Borderline lepromatous leprosy**
BL leprosy

A30.5   **Lepromatous leprosy**
LL leprosy

A30.8   **Other forms of leprosy**

A30.9   **Leprosy, unspecified**   ▽

✓4th **A31   Infection due to other mycobacteria**
EXCLUDES 2   leprosy (A30.-)
tuberculosis (A15-A19)

A31.0   **Pulmonary mycobacterial infection**   HCC
Infection due to Mycobacterium avium
Infection due to Mycobacterium intracellulare [Battey bacillus]
Infection due to Mycobacterium kansasii

A31.1   **Cutaneous mycobacterial infection**
Buruli ulcer
Infection due to Mycobacterium marinum
Infection due to Mycobacterium ulcerans

A31.2   **Disseminated mycobacterium avium-intracellulare complex (DMAC)**   HCC
MAC sepsis

A31.8   **Other mycobacterial infections**

A31.9   **Mycobacterial infection, unspecified**   ▽
Atypical mycobacterial infection NOS
Mycobacteriosis NOS

✓4th **A32   Listeriosis**
INCLUDES   listerial foodborne infection
EXCLUDES 1   neonatal (disseminated) listeriosis (P37.2)

A32.0   **Cutaneous listeriosis**

✓5th A32.1   **Listerial meningitis and meningoencephalitis**

A32.11   **Listerial meningitis**

A32.12   **Listerial meningoencephalitis**

A32.7   **Listerial sepsis**   HCC

✓5th A32.8   **Other forms of listeriosis**

A32.81   **Oculoglandular listeriosis**

A32.82   **Listerial endocarditis**

A32.89   **Other forms of listeriosis**
Listerial cerebral arteritis

A32.9   **Listeriosis, unspecified**   ▽

A33   **Tetanus neonatorum**   N

A34   **Obstetrical tetanus**   M ♀

A35   **Other tetanus**
Tetanus NOS
EXCLUDES 1   obstetrical tetanus (A34)
tetanus neonatorum (A33)

✓4th **A36   Diphtheria**

A36.0   **Pharyngeal diphtheria**
Diphtheritic membranous angina
Tonsillar diphtheria

A36.1   **Nasopharyngeal diphtheria**

A36.2   **Laryngeal diphtheria**
Diphtheritic laryngotracheitis

A36.3   **Cutaneous diphtheria**
EXCLUDES 2   erythrasma (L08.1)

✓5th A36.8   **Other diphtheria**

A36.81   **Diphtheritic cardiomyopathy**   HCC
Diphtheritic myocarditis

A36.82   **Diphtheritic radiculomyelitis**

A36.83   **Diphtheritic polyneuritis**

A36.84   **Diphtheritic tubulo-interstitial nephropathy**

A36.85   **Diphtheritic cystitis**

A36.86   **Diphtheritic conjunctivitis**

A36.89   **Other diphtheritic complications**
Diphtheritic peritonitis

A36.9   **Diphtheria, unspecified**   ▽

✓4th **A37   Whooping cough**

✓5th A37.0   **Whooping cough due to Bordetella pertussis**

A37.00   **Whooping cough due to Bordetella pertussis without pneumonia**

A37.01   **Whooping cough due to Bordetella pertussis with pneumonia**

✓5th A37.1   **Whooping cough due to Bordetella parapertussis**

A37.10   **Whooping cough due to Bordetella parapertussis without pneumonia**

A37.11   **Whooping cough due to Bordetella parapertussis with pneumonia**

✓5ᵗʰ **A37.8**   **Whooping cough due to other Bordetella species**

     A37.80   **Whooping cough due to other Bordetella species without pneumonia**

     A37.81   **Whooping cough due to other Bordetella species with pneumonia**

✓5ᵗʰ **A37.9**   **Whooping cough, unspecified species**

     A37.90   **Whooping cough, unspecified species without pneumonia** ▽

     A37.91   **Whooping cough, unspecified species with pneumonia** ▽

✓4ᵗʰ **A38**   **Scarlet fever**

     INCLUDES   scarlatina

     EXCLUDES 2   *streptococcal sore throat (J02.0)*

A38.0   **Scarlet fever with otitis media**

A38.1   **Scarlet fever with myocarditis**

A38.8   **Scarlet fever with other complications**

A38.9   **Scarlet fever, uncomplicated** ▽
     Scarlet fever, NOS

✓4ᵗʰ **A39**   **Meningococcal infection**

A39.0   **Meningococcal meningitis**

A39.1   **Waterhouse-Friderichsen syndrome** HCC
     Meningococcal hemorrhagic adrenalitis
     Meningococcic adrenal syndrome

A39.2   **Acute meningococcemia** HCC

A39.3   **Chronic meningococcemia** HCC

A39.4   **Meningococcemia, unspecified** HCC ▽

✓5ᵗʰ **A39.5**   **Meningococcal heart disease**

     A39.50   **Meningococcal carditis, unspecified** ▽

     A39.51   **Meningococcal endocarditis**

     A39.52   **Meningococcal myocarditis**

     A39.53   **Meningococcal pericarditis**

✓5ᵗʰ **A39.8**   **Other meningococcal infections**

     A39.81   **Meningococcal encephalitis**

     A39.82   **Meningococcal retrobulbar neuritis**

     A39.83   **Meningococcal arthritis** HCC

     A39.84   **Postmeningococcal arthritis** HCC

     A39.89   **Other meningococcal infections**
         Meningococcal conjunctivitis

A39.9   **Meningococcal infection, unspecified** ▽
     Meningococcal disease NOS

✓4ᵗʰ **A40**   **Streptococcal sepsis**

     Code first: postprocedural streptococcal sepsis (T81.4-)
         streptococcal sepsis during labor (O75.3)
         streptococcal sepsis following abortion or ectopic or molar pregnancy (O03-O07, O08.0)
         streptococcal sepsis following immunization (T88.0)
         streptococcal sepsis following infusion, transfusion or therapeutic injection (T80.2-)

     EXCLUDES 1   *neonatal (P36.0-P36.1)*
         puerperal sepsis (O85)
         sepsis due to Streptococcus, group D (A41.81)

     AHA: 2016, 1Q, 32

A40.0   **Sepsis due to streptococcus, group A** HCC

A40.1   **Sepsis due to streptococcus, group B** HCC

A40.3   **Sepsis due to Streptococcus pneumoniae** HCC
     Pneumococcal sepsis

A40.8   **Other streptococcal sepsis** HCC

A40.9   **Streptococcal sepsis, unspecified** HCC ▽

✓4ᵗʰ **A41**   **Other sepsis**

     Code first: postprocedural sepsis (T81.4-)
         sepsis during labor (O75.3)
         sepsis following abortion, ectopic or molar pregnancy (O03-O07, O08.0)
         sepsis following immunization (T88.0)
         sepsis following infusion, transfusion or therapeutic injection (T80.2-)

     EXCLUDES 1   *bacteremia NOS (R78.81)*
         neonatal (P36.-)
         puerperal sepsis (O85)
         streptococcal sepsis (A40.-)

     EXCLUDES 2   *sepsis (due to) (in) actinomycotic (A42.7)*
         sepsis (due to) (in) anthrax (A22.7)
         sepsis (due to) (in) candidal (B37.7)
         sepsis (due to) (in) Erysipelothrix (A26.7)
         sepsis (due to) (in) extraintestinal yersiniosis (A28.2)
         sepsis (due to) (in) gonococcal (A54.86)
         sepsis (due to) (in) herpesviral (B00.7)
         sepsis (due to) (in) listerial (A32.7)
         sepsis (due to) (in) melioidosis (A24.1)
         sepsis (due to) (in) meningococcal (A39.2-A39.4)
         sepsis (due to) (in) plague (A20.7)
         sepsis (due to) (in) tularemia (A21.7)
         toxic shock syndrome (A48.3)

     AHA: 2016, 1Q, 32; 2014, 2Q, 13

✓5ᵗʰ **A41.0**   **Sepsis due to Staphylococcus aureus**

     A41.01   **Sepsis due to Methicillin susceptible Staphylococcus aureus** HCC
         MSSA sepsis
         Staphylococcus aureus sepsis NOS

     A41.02   **Sepsis due to Methicillin resistant Staphylococcus aureus** HCC

A41.1   **Sepsis due to other specified staphylococcus** HCC
     Coagulase negative staphylococcus sepsis

A41.2   **Sepsis due to unspecified staphylococcus** HCC ▽

A41.3   **Sepsis due to Hemophilus influenzae** HCC

A41.4   **Sepsis due to anaerobes** HCC
     EXCLUDES 1   *gas gangrene (A48.0)*

✓5ᵗʰ **A41.5**   **Sepsis due to other Gram-negative organisms**

     A41.50   **Gram-negative sepsis, unspecified** HCC ▽
         Gram-negative sepsis NOS

     A41.51   **Sepsis due to Escherichia coli [E. coli]** HCC

     A41.52   **Sepsis due to Pseudomonas** HCC
         Pseudomonas aeroginosa

     A41.53   **Sepsis due to Serratia** HCC

     A41.59   **Other Gram-negative sepsis** HCC

✓5ᵗʰ **A41.8**   **Other specified sepsis**

     A41.81   **Sepsis due to Enterococcus** HCC

     A41.89   **Other specified sepsis** HCC
         AHA: 2017, 1Q, 51; 2016, 3Q, 8-14

A41.9   **Sepsis, unspecified organism** HCC ▽
     Septicemia NOS

✓4ᵗʰ **A42**   **Actinomycosis**

     EXCLUDES 1   *actinomycetoma (B47.1)*

A42.0   **Pulmonary actinomycosis** HCC

A42.1   **Abdominal actinomycosis**

A42.2   **Cervicofacial actinomycosis**

A42.7   **Actinomycotic sepsis** HCC

✓5ᵗʰ **A42.8**   **Other forms of actinomycosis**

     A42.81   **Actinomycotic meningitis**

     A42.82   **Actinomycotic encephalitis**

     A42.89   **Other forms of actinomycosis**

A42.9   **Actinomycosis, unspecified** ▽

✓4ᵗʰ **A43**   **Nocardiosis**

A43.0   **Pulmonary nocardiosis** HCC

A43.1   **Cutaneous nocardiosis**

A43.8   **Other forms of nocardiosis**

A43.9   **Nocardiosis, unspecified** ▽

✓4ᵗʰ **A44**   **Bartonellosis**

A44.0   **Systemic bartonellosis**
     Oroya fever

A44.1   **Cutaneous and mucocutaneous bartonellosis**
     Verruga peruana

A44.8   **Other forms of bartonellosis**

EXCLUDES 1 Not coded here   **EXCLUDES 2** Not included here   N Newborn Age: 0   P Pediatric Age: 0-17   M Maternity Age: 12-55   A Adult Age: 15-124

440   ICD-10-CM 2018

A44.9   **Bartonellosis, unspecified** ▽

A46 Erysipelas
 EXCLUDES 1   *postpartum or puerperal erysipelas (O86.89)*
 DEF: A skin infection affecting the upper dermis and superficial dermal lymphatics; lesion edges are well-demarcated with distinct raised borders; it is often caused by group A *Streptococci*.

√4ᵗʰ **A48 Other bacterial diseases, not elsewhere classified**
 EXCLUDES 1   *actinomycetoma (B47.1)*

 A48.0 Gas gangrene   HCC
  Clostridial cellulitis
  Clostridial myonecrosis

 A48.1 Legionnaires' disease   HCC
  DEF: Severe and often fatal infection by *Legionella pneumophila*; symptoms include high fever, gastrointestinal pain, headache, myalgia, dry cough, and pneumonia; usually transmitted through airborne water droplets via air conditioning systems or hot tubs.

 A48.2 Nonpneumonic Legionnaires' disease [Pontiac fever]

 A48.3 Toxic shock syndrome   HCC
  Use additional code to identify the organism (B95, B96)
  EXCLUDES 1   *endotoxic shock NOS (R57.8)*
   sepsis NOS (A41.9)

 A48.4 Brazilian purpuric fever
  Systemic Hemophilus aegyptius infection

√5ᵗʰ **A48.5 Other specified botulism**
  Non-foodborne intoxication due to toxins of Clostridium botulinum [C. botulinum]
  EXCLUDES 1   *food poisoning due to toxins of Clostridium botulinum (A05.1)*

  A48.51 Infant botulism   P

  A48.52 Wound botulism
   Non-foodborne botulism NOS
   Use additional code for associated wound

 A48.8 Other specified bacterial diseases

√4ᵗʰ **A49 Bacterial infection of unspecified site**
 EXCLUDES 1   *bacterial agents as the cause of diseases classified elsewhere (B95-B96)*
  chlamydial infection NOS (A74.9)
  meningococcal infection NOS (A39.9)
  rickettsial infection NOS (A79.9)
  spirochetal infection NOS (A69.9)

 √5ᵗʰ **A49.0 Staphylococcal infection, unspecified site**
  A49.01 Methicillin susceptible Staphylococcus aureus infection, unspecified site
   Methicillin susceptible Staphylococcus aureus (MSSA) infection
   Staphylococcus aureus infection NOS

  A49.02 Methicillin resistant Staphylococcus aureus infection, unspecified site
   Methicillin resistant Staphylococcus aureus (MRSA) infection

 A49.1 Streptococcal infection, unspecified site
 A49.2 Hemophilus influenzae infection, unspecified site
 A49.3 Mycoplasma infection, unspecified site
 A49.8 Other bacterial infections of unspecified site
 A49.9 Bacterial infection, unspecified ▽
  EXCLUDES 1   *bacteremia NOS (R78.81)*

Infections with a predominantly sexual mode of transmission (A50-A64)

 EXCLUDES 1   *human immunodeficiency virus [HIV] disease (B20)*
  nonspecific and nongonococcal urethritis (N34.1)
  Reiter's disease (M02.3-)

√4ᵗʰ **A50 Congenital syphilis**
 √5ᵗʰ **A50.0 Early congenital syphilis, symptomatic**
  Any congenital syphilitic condition specified as early or manifest less than two years after birth.

  A50.01 Early congenital syphilitic oculopathy
  A50.02 Early congenital syphilitic osteochondropathy
  A50.03 Early congenital syphilitic pharyngitis
   Early congenital syphilitic laryngitis
  A50.04 Early congenital syphilitic pneumonia
  A50.05 Early congenital syphilitic rhinitis
  A50.06 Early cutaneous congenital syphilis
  A50.07 Early mucocutaneous congenital syphilis
  A50.08 Early visceral congenital syphilis
  A50.09 Other early congenital syphilis, symptomatic

 A50.1 Early congenital syphilis, latent
  Congenital syphilis without clinical manifestations, with positive serological reaction and negative spinal fluid test, less than two years after birth.

 A50.2 Early congenital syphilis, unspecified ▽
  Congenital syphilis NOS less than two years after birth.

 √5ᵗʰ **A50.3 Late congenital syphilitic oculopathy**
  EXCLUDES 1   *Hutchinson's triad (A50.53)*
  A50.30 Late congenital syphilitic oculopathy, unspecified ▽
  A50.31 Late congenital syphilitic interstitial keratitis
  A50.32 Late congenital syphilitic chorioretinitis
  A50.39 Other late congenital syphilitic oculopathy

 √5ᵗʰ **A50.4 Late congenital neurosyphilis [juvenile neurosyphilis]**
  Use additional code to identify any associated mental disorder
  EXCLUDES 1   *Hutchinson's triad (A50.53)*
  A50.40 Late congenital neurosyphilis, unspecified ▽
   Juvenile neurosyphilis NOS
  A50.41 Late congenital syphilitic meningitis
  A50.42 Late congenital syphilitic encephalitis
  A50.43 Late congenital syphilitic polyneuropathy
  A50.44 Late congenital syphilitic optic nerve atrophy
  A50.45 Juvenile general paresis
   Dementia paralytica juvenilis
   Juvenile tabetoparetic neurosyphilis
  A50.49 Other late congenital neurosyphilis
   Juvenile tabes dorsalis

 √5ᵗʰ **A50.5 Other late congenital syphilis, symptomatic**
  Any congenital syphilitic condition specified as late or manifest two years or more after birth.
  A50.51 Clutton's joints
  A50.52 Hutchinson's teeth
  A50.53 Hutchinson's triad
  A50.54 Late congenital cardiovascular syphilis
  A50.55 Late congenital syphilitic arthropathy   HCC
  A50.56 Late congenital syphilitic osteochondropathy
  A50.57 Syphilitic saddle nose
  A50.59 Other late congenital syphilis, symptomatic

 A50.6 Late congenital syphilis, latent
  Congenital syphilis without clinical manifestations, with positive serological reaction and negative spinal fluid test, two years or more after birth.

 A50.7 Late congenital syphilis, unspecified ▽
  Congenital syphilis NOS two years or more after birth.

 A50.9 Congenital syphilis, unspecified ▽

√4ᵗʰ **A51 Early syphilis**
 A51.0 Primary genital syphilis
  Syphilitic chancre NOS
 A51.1 Primary anal syphilis
 A51.2 Primary syphilis of other sites

 √5ᵗʰ **A51.3 Secondary syphilis of skin and mucous membranes**
  DEF: Transitory or chronic cutaneous eruptions that present within two to 10 weeks following initial syphilis infection that may include nontender lymphadenopathy along with alopecia and condylomata lata.
  A51.31 Condyloma latum
  A51.32 Syphilitic alopecia
  A51.39 Other secondary syphilis of skin
   Syphilitic leukoderma
   Syphilitic mucous patch
   EXCLUDES 1   *late syphilitic leukoderma (A52.79)*

 √5ᵗʰ **A51.4 Other secondary syphilis**
  A51.41 Secondary syphilitic meningitis
  A51.42 Secondary syphilitic female pelvic disease   ♀
  A51.43 Secondary syphilitic oculopathy
   Secondary syphilitic chorioretinitis
   Secondary syphilitic iridocyclitis, iritis
   Secondary syphilitic uveitis
  A51.44 Secondary syphilitic nephritis
  A51.45 Secondary syphilitic hepatitis
  A51.46 Secondary syphilitic osteopathy
  A51.49 Other secondary syphilitic conditions
   Secondary syphilitic lymphadenopathy
   Secondary syphilitic myositis

A51.5 Early syphilis, latent
Syphilis (acquired) without clinical manifestations, with positive serological reaction and negative spinal fluid test, less than two years after infection.

A51.9 Early syphilis, unspecified ▽

✓4ᵗʰ **A52 Late syphilis**

✓5ᵗʰ **A52.0 Cardiovascular and cerebrovascular syphilis**

A52.00 Cardiovascular syphilis, unspecified ▽

A52.01 Syphilitic aneurysm of aorta

A52.02 Syphilitic aortitis

A52.03 Syphilitic endocarditis
Syphilitic aortic valve incompetence or stenosis
Syphilitic mitral valve stenosis
Syphilitic pulmonary valve regurgitation

A52.04 Syphilitic cerebral arteritis

A52.05 Other cerebrovascular syphilis
Syphilitic cerebral aneurysm (ruptured) (non-ruptured)
Syphilitic cerebral thrombosis

A52.06 Other syphilitic heart involvement
Syphilitic coronary artery disease
Syphilitic myocarditis
Syphilitic pericarditis

A52.09 Other cardiovascular syphilis

✓5ᵗʰ **A52.1 Symptomatic neurosyphilis**

A52.10 Symptomatic neurosyphilis, unspecified ▽

A52.11 Tabes dorsalis
Locomotor ataxia (progressive)
Tabetic neurosyphilis

A52.12 Other cerebrospinal syphilis

A52.13 Late syphilitic meningitis

A52.14 Late syphilitic encephalitis

A52.15 Late syphilitic neuropathy
Late syphilitic acoustic neuritis
Late syphilitic optic (nerve) atrophy
Late syphilitic polyneuropathy
Late syphilitic retrobulbar neuritis

A52.16 Charcôt's arthropathy (tabetic)

A52.17 General paresis
Dementia paralytica

A52.19 Other symptomatic neurosyphilis
Syphilitic parkinsonism

A52.2 Asymptomatic neurosyphilis

A52.3 Neurosyphilis, unspecified ▽
Gumma (syphilitic)
Syphilis (late)
Syphiloma

✓5ᵗʰ **A52.7 Other symptomatic late syphilis**

A52.71 Late syphilitic oculopathy
Late syphilitic chorioretinitis
Late syphilitic episcleritis

A52.72 Syphilis of lung and bronchus

A52.73 Symptomatic late syphilis of other respiratory organs

A52.74 Syphilis of liver and other viscera
Late syphilitic peritonitis

A52.75 Syphilis of kidney and ureter
Syphilitic glomerular disease

A52.76 Other genitourinary symptomatic late syphilis
Late syphilitic female pelvic inflammatory disease

A52.77 Syphilis of bone and joint

A52.78 Syphilis of other musculoskeletal tissue
Late syphilitic bursitis
Syphilis [stage unspecified] of bursa
Syphilis [stage unspecified] of muscle
Syphilis [stage unspecified] of synovium
Syphilis [stage unspecified] of tendon

A52.79 Other symptomatic late syphilis
Late syphilitic leukoderma
Syphilis of adrenal gland
Syphilis of pituitary gland
Syphilis of thyroid gland
Syphilitic splenomegaly
EXCLUDES 1 syphilitic leukoderma (secondary) (A51.39)

A52.8 Late syphilis, latent
Syphilis (acquired) without clinical manifestations, with positive serological reaction and negative spinal fluid test, two years or more after infection.

A52.9 Late syphilis, unspecified ▽

✓4ᵗʰ **A53 Other and unspecified syphilis**

A53.0 Latent syphilis, unspecified as early or late
Latent syphilis NOS
Positive serological reaction for syphilis

A53.9 Syphilis, unspecified ▽
Infection due to Treponema pallidum NOS
Syphilis (acquired) NOS
EXCLUDES 1 syphilis NOS under two years of age (A50.2)

✓4ᵗʰ **A54 Gonococcal infection**

✓5ᵗʰ **A54.0 Gonococcal infection of lower genitourinary tract without periurethral or accessory gland abscess**
EXCLUDES 1 gonococcal infection with genitourinary gland abscess (A54.1)
gonococcal infection with periurethral abscess (A54.1)

A54.00 Gonococcal infection of lower genitourinary tract, unspecified ▽

A54.01 Gonococcal cystitis and urethritis, unspecified ▽

A54.02 Gonococcal vulvovaginitis, unspecified ♀▽

A54.03 Gonococcal cervicitis, unspecified ♀▽

A54.09 Other gonococcal infection of lower genitourinary tract

A54.1 Gonococcal infection of lower genitourinary tract with periurethral and accessory gland abscess
Gonococcal Bartholin's gland abscess

✓5ᵗʰ **A54.2 Gonococcal pelviperitonitis and other gonococcal genitourinary infection**

A54.21 Gonococcal infection of kidney and ureter

A54.22 Gonococcal prostatitis ♂

A54.23 Gonococcal infection of other male genital organs ♂
Gonococcal epididymitis
Gonococcal orchitis

A54.24 Gonococcal female pelvic inflammatory disease ♀
Gonococcal pelviperitonitis
EXCLUDES 1 gonococcal peritonitis (A54.85)

A54.29 Other gonococcal genitourinary infections

✓5ᵗʰ **A54.3 Gonococcal infection of eye**

A54.30 Gonococcal infection of eye, unspecified ▽

A54.31 Gonococcal conjunctivitis
Ophthalmia neonatorum due to gonococcus

A54.32 Gonococcal iridocyclitis

A54.33 Gonococcal keratitis

A54.39 Other gonococcal eye infection
Gonococcal endophthalmia

✓5ᵗʰ **A54.4 Gonococcal infection of musculoskeletal system**

A54.40 Gonococcal infection of musculoskeletal system, unspecified HCC ▽

A54.41 Gonococcal spondylopathy HCC

A54.42 Gonococcal arthritis HCC
EXCLUDES 2 gonococcal infection of spine (A54.41)

A54.43 Gonococcal osteomyelitis HCC
EXCLUDES 2 gonococcal infection of spine (A54.41)

A54.49 Gonococcal infection of other musculoskeletal tissue HCC
Gonococcal bursitis
Gonococcal myositis
Gonococcal synovitis
Gonococcal tenosynovitis

A54.5 Gonococcal pharyngitis

A54.6 Gonococcal infection of anus and rectum

✓5ᵗʰ **A54.8 Other gonococcal infections**

A54.81 Gonococcal meningitis

A54.82 Gonococcal brain abscess

A54.83 Gonococcal heart infection
Gonococcal endocarditis
Gonococcal myocarditis
Gonococcal pericarditis

A54.84 Gonococcal pneumonia HCC

A54.85 Gonococcal peritonitis HCC
EXCLUDES 1 gonococcal pelviperitonitis (A54.24)

A54.86 Gonococcal sepsis HCC

A54.89 Other gonococcal infections
Gonococcal keratoderma
Gonococcal lymphadenitis

A54.9 Gonococcal infection, unspecified ▽

A55 Chlamydial lymphogranuloma (venereum)
Climatic or tropical bubo
Durand-Nicolas-Favre disease
Esthiomene
Lymphogranuloma inguinale

☑️4th **A56 Other sexually transmitted chlamydial diseases**
INCLUDES sexually transmitted diseases due to Chlamydia trachomatis
EXCLUDES 1 neonatal chlamydial conjunctivitis (P39.1)
neonatal chlamydial pneumonia (P23.1)
EXCLUDES 2 chlamydial lymphogranuloma (A55)
conditions classified to A74-

☑️5th **A56.0 Chlamydial infection of lower genitourinary tract**

A56.00 Chlamydial infection of lower genitourinary tract, unspecified ▽

A56.01 Chlamydial cystitis and urethritis

A56.02 Chlamydial vulvovaginitis ♀

A56.09 Other chlamydial infection of lower genitourinary tract
Chlamydial cervicitis

☑️5th **A56.1 Chlamydial infection of pelviperitoneum and other genitourinary organs**

A56.11 Chlamydial female pelvic inflammatory disease ♀

A56.19 Other chlamydial genitourinary infection
Chlamydial epididymitis
Chlamydial orchitis

A56.2 Chlamydial infection of genitourinary tract, unspecified ▽

A56.3 Chlamydial infection of anus and rectum

A56.4 Chlamydial infection of pharynx

A56.8 Sexually transmitted chlamydial infection of other sites

A57 Chancroid
Ulcus molle

A58 Granuloma inguinale
Donovanosis

☑️4th **A59 Trichomoniasis**
EXCLUDES 2 intestinal trichomoniasis (A07.8)

☑️5th **A59.0 Urogenital trichomoniasis**

A59.00 Urogenital trichomoniasis, unspecified ▽
Fluor (vaginalis) due to Trichomonas
Leukorrhea (vaginalis) due to Trichomonas

A59.01 Trichomonal vulvovaginitis ♀

A59.02 Trichomonal prostatitis ♂

A59.03 Trichomonal cystitis and urethritis

A59.09 Other urogenital trichomoniasis
Trichomonas cervicitis

A59.8 Trichomoniasis of other sites

A59.9 Trichomoniasis, unspecified ▽

☑️4th **A60 Anogenital herpesviral [herpes simplex] infections**

☑️5th **A60.0 Herpesviral infection of genitalia and urogenital tract**

A60.00 Herpesviral infection of urogenital system, unspecified ▽

A60.01 Herpesviral infection of penis ♂

A60.02 Herpesviral infection of other male genital organs ♂

A60.03 Herpesviral cervicitis ♀

A60.04 Herpesviral vulvovaginitis ♀
Herpesviral [herpes simplex] ulceration
Herpesviral [herpes simplex] vaginitis
Herpesviral [herpes simplex] vulvitis

A60.09 Herpesviral infection of other urogenital tract

A60.1 Herpesviral infection of perianal skin and rectum

A60.9 Anogenital herpesviral infection, unspecified ▽

☑️4th **A63 Other predominantly sexually transmitted diseases, not elsewhere classified**
EXCLUDES 2 molluscum contagiosum (B08.1)
papilloma of cervix (D26.0)

A63.0 Anogenital (venereal) warts
Anogenital warts due to (human) papillomavirus [HPV]
Condyloma acuminatum

A63.8 Other specified predominantly sexually transmitted diseases

A64 Unspecified sexually transmitted disease ▽

Other spirochetal diseases (A65-A69)

EXCLUDES 2 leptospirosis (A27.-)
syphilis (A50-A53)

A65 Nonvenereal syphilis
Bejel   Njovera
Endemic syphilis

☑️4th **A66 Yaws**
INCLUDES bouba
frambesia (tropica)
pian

A66.0 Initial lesions of yaws
Chancre of yaws
Frambesia, initial or primary
Initial frambesial ulcer
Mother yaw

A66.1 Multiple papillomata and wet crab yaws
Frambesioma
Pianoma
Plantar or palmar papilloma of yaws

A66.2 Other early skin lesions of yaws
Cutaneous yaws, less than five years after infection
Early yaws (cutaneous) (macular) (maculopapular) (micropapular) (papular)
Frambeside of early yaws

A66.3 Hyperkeratosis of yaws
Ghoul hand
Hyperkeratosis, palmar or plantar (early) (late) due to yaws
Worm-eaten soles

A66.4 Gummata and ulcers of yaws
Gummatous frambeside
Nodular late yaws (ulcerated)

A66.5 Gangosa
Rhinopharyngitis mutilans

A66.6 Bone and joint lesions of yaws HCC
Yaws ganglion   Yaws hydrarthrosis
Yaws goundou   Yaws osteitis
Yaws gumma, bone   Yaws periostitis (hypertrophic)
Yaws gummatous osteitis
or periostitis

A66.7 Other manifestations of yaws
Juxta-articular nodules of yaws
Mucosal yaws

A66.8 Latent yaws
Yaws without clinical manifestations, with positive serology

A66.9 Yaws, unspecified ▽

☑️4th **A67 Pinta [carate]**

A67.0 Primary lesions of pinta
Chancre (primary) of pinta
Papule (primary) of pinta

A67.1 Intermediate lesions of pinta
Erythematous plaques of pinta
Hyperchromic lesions of pinta
Hyperkeratosis of pinta
Pintids

A67.2 Late lesions of pinta
Achromic skin lesions of pinta
Cicatricial skin lesions of pinta
Dyschromic skin lesions of pinta

A67.3 Mixed lesions of pinta
Achromic with hyperchromic skin lesions of pinta [carate]

A67.9 Pinta, unspecified ▽

☑️4th **A68 Relapsing fevers**
INCLUDES recurrent fever
EXCLUDES 2 Lyme disease (A69.2-)

A68.0 Louse-borne relapsing fever
Relapsing fever due to Borrelia recurrentis

A68.1 Tick-borne relapsing fever
Relapsing fever due to any Borrelia species other than Borrelia recurrentis

A68.9 Relapsing fever, unspecified ▽

☑️4th **A69 Other spirochetal infections**

A69.0 Necrotizing ulcerative stomatitis
Cancrum oris
Fusospirochetal gangrene
Noma
Stomatitis gangrenosa

☑️ Additional Character Req   ✗7th Placeholder Alert   Manifestation   HCC CMS-HCC Condition   ▽ Unspecified Code   ▶◀ Revised Text   ● New Code   ▲ Revised Code Title

ICD-10-CM 2018   443

Chapter 1. Certain Infectious and Parasitic Diseases

A55–A69.0

A69.1 Other Vincent's infections
Fusospirochetal pharyngitis
Necrotizing ulcerative (acute) gingivitis
Necrotizing ulcerative (acute) gingivostomatitis
Spirochetal stomatitis
Trench mouth
Vincent's angina
Vincent's gingivitis

✓5ᵗʰ A69.2 Lyme disease
Erythema chronicum migrans due to Borrelia burgdorferi
DEF: A recurrent multisystem disorder through tick bites; begins with lesions of erythema chronicum migrans; followed by arthritis of the large joints, myalgia, malaise, and neurological and cardiac manifestations.

     A69.20 Lyme disease, unspecified ▽
     A69.21 Meningitis due to Lyme disease
     A69.22 Other neurologic disorders in Lyme disease
        Cranial neuritis
        Meningoencephalitis
        Polyneuropathy
     A69.23 Arthritis due to Lyme disease HCC
     A69.29 Other conditions associated with Lyme disease
        Myopericarditis due to Lyme disease
        AHA: 2016, 3Q, 12

A69.8 Other specified spirochetal infections
A69.9 Spirochetal infection, unspecified ▽

Other diseases caused by chlamydiae (A70-A74)

EXCLUDES 1   *sexually transmitted chlamydial diseases (A55-A56)*

A70 Chlamydia psittaci infections
Ornithosis
Parrot fever
Psittacosis

✓4ᵗʰ A71 Trachoma
EXCLUDES 1   *sequelae of trachoma (B94.0)*

A71.0 Initial stage of trachoma
Trachoma dubium

A71.1 Active stage of trachoma
Granular conjunctivitis (trachomatous)
Trachomatous follicular conjunctivitis
Trachomatous pannus

A71.9 Trachoma, unspecified ▽

✓4ᵗʰ A74 Other diseases caused by chlamydiae
EXCLUDES 1   *neonatal chlamydial conjunctivitis (P39.1)*
        neonatal chlamydial pneumonia (P23.1)
        Reiter's disease (M02.3-)
        sexually transmitted chlamydial diseases (A55-A56)
EXCLUDES 2   *chlamydial pneumonia (J16.0)*

A74.0 Chlamydial conjunctivitis
Paratrachoma

✓5ᵗʰ A74.8 Other chlamydial diseases
     A74.81 Chlamydial peritonitis
     A74.89 Other chlamydial diseases

A74.9 Chlamydial infection, unspecified ▽
Chlamydiosis NOS

Rickettsioses (A75-A79)

✓4ᵗʰ A75 Typhus fever
EXCLUDES 1   *rickettsiosis due to Ehrlichia sennetsu (A79.81)*

A75.0 Epidemic louse-borne typhus fever due to Rickettsia prowazekii
Classical typhus (fever)
Epidemic (louse-borne) typhus

A75.1 Recrudescent typhus [Brill's disease]
Brill-Zinsser disease

A75.2 Typhus fever due to Rickettsia typhi
Murine (flea-borne) typhus

A75.3 Typhus fever due to Rickettsia tsutsugamushi
Scrub (mite-borne) typhus
Tsutsugamushi fever

A75.9 Typhus fever, unspecified ▽
Typhus (fever) NOS

✓4ᵗʰ A77 Spotted fever [tick-borne rickettsioses]

A77.0 Spotted fever due to Rickettsia rickettsii
Rocky Mountain spotted fever
Sao Paulo fever

A77.1 Spotted fever due to Rickettsia conorii
African tick typhus
Boutonneuse fever
India tick typhus
Kenya tick typhus
Marseilles fever
Mediterranean tick fever

A77.2 Spotted fever due to Rickettsia siberica
North Asian tick fever
Siberian tick typhus

A77.3 Spotted fever due to Rickettsia australis
Queensland tick typhus

✓5ᵗʰ A77.4 Ehrlichiosis
EXCLUDES 1   *Rickettsiosis due to Ehrlichia sennetsu (A79.81)*

     A77.40 Ehrlichiosis, unspecified ▽
     A77.41 Ehrlichiosis chafeensis [E. chafeensis]
     A77.49 Other ehrlichiosis

A77.8 Other spotted fevers
A77.9 Spotted fever, unspecified ▽
Tick-borne typhus NOS

A78 Q fever
Infection due to Coxiella burnetii
Nine Mile fever
Quadrilateral fever

✓4ᵗʰ A79 Other rickettsioses
A79.0 Trench fever
Quintan fever
Wolhynian fever

A79.1 Rickettsialpox due to Rickettsia akari
Kew Garden fever
Vesicular rickettsiosis

✓5ᵗʰ A79.8 Other specified rickettsioses
     A79.81 Rickettsiosis due to Ehrlichia sennetsu
     A79.89 Other specified rickettsioses

A79.9 Rickettsiosis, unspecified ▽
Rickettsial infection NOS

Viral and prion infections of the central nervous system (A80-A89)

EXCLUDES 1   *postpolio syndrome (G14)*
        sequelae of poliomyelitis (B91)
        sequelae of viral encephalitis (B94.1)

✓4ᵗʰ A80 Acute poliomyelitis
A80.0 Acute paralytic poliomyelitis, vaccine-associated
A80.1 Acute paralytic poliomyelitis, wild virus, imported
A80.2 Acute paralytic poliomyelitis, wild virus, indigenous
✓5ᵗʰ A80.3 Acute paralytic poliomyelitis, other and unspecified ▽
     A80.30 Acute paralytic poliomyelitis, unspecified
     A80.39 Other acute paralytic poliomyelitis
A80.4 Acute nonparalytic poliomyelitis
A80.9 Acute poliomyelitis, unspecified ▽

✓4ᵗʰ A81 Atypical virus infections of central nervous system
INCLUDES   diseases of the central nervous system caused by prions
Use additional code to identify:
dementia with behavioral disturbance (F02.81)
dementia without behavioral disturbance (F02.80)

✓5ᵗʰ A81.0 Creutzfeldt-Jakob disease
     A81.00 Creutzfeldt-Jakob disease, unspecified ▽
        Jakob-Creutzfeldt disease, unspecified
     A81.01 Variant Creutzfeldt-Jakob disease
        vCJD
     A81.09 Other Creutzfeldt-Jakob disease
        CJD
        Familial Creutzfeldt-Jakob disease
        Iatrogenic Creutzfeldt-Jakob disease
        Sporadic Creutzfeldt-Jakob disease
        Subacute spongiform encephalopathy (with dementia)

A81.1 Subacute sclerosing panencephalitis
Dawson's inclusion body encephalitis
Van Bogaert's sclerosing leukoencephalopathy

A81.2 Progressive multifocal leukoencephalopathy
Multifocal leukoencephalopathy NOS

EXCLUDES 1 Not coded here   EXCLUDES 2 Not included here   N Newborn Age: 0   P Pediatric Age: 0-17   M Maternity Age: 12-55   A Adult Age: 15-124

ICD-10-CM 2018

444

✓5ᵗʰ **A81.8 Other atypical virus infections of central nervous system**

    A81.81 Kuru

    A81.82 Gerstmann-Sträussler-Scheinker syndrome
        GSS syndrome

    A81.83 Fatal familial insomnia
        FFI

    A81.89 Other atypical virus infections of central nervous system

A81.9 Atypical virus infection of central nervous system, unspecified ▽
    Prion diseases of the central nervous system NOS

✓4ᵗʰ **A82 Rabies**

    A82.0 Sylvatic rabies

    A82.1 Urban rabies

    A82.9 Rabies, unspecified ▽

✓4ᵗʰ **A83 Mosquito-borne viral encephalitis**
    INCLUDES mosquito-borne viral meningoencephalitis
    EXCLUDES 2 *Venezuelan equine encephalitis (A92.2)*
        West Nile fever (A92.3-)
        West Nile virus (A92.3-)

    A83.0 Japanese encephalitis

    A83.1 Western equine encephalitis

    A83.2 Eastern equine encephalitis

    A83.3 St Louis encephalitis

    A83.4 Australian encephalitis
        Kunjin virus disease

    A83.5 California encephalitis
        California meningoencephalitis
        La Crosse encephalitis

    A83.6 Rocio virus disease

    A83.8 Other mosquito-borne viral encephalitis

    A83.9 Mosquito-borne viral encephalitis, unspecified ▽

✓4ᵗʰ **A84 Tick-borne viral encephalitis**
    INCLUDES tick-borne viral meningoencephalitis

    A84.0 Far Eastern tick-borne encephalitis [Russian spring-summer encephalitis]

    A84.1 Central European tick-borne encephalitis

    A84.8 Other tick-borne viral encephalitis
        Louping ill
        Powassan virus disease

    A84.9 Tick-borne viral encephalitis, unspecified ▽

✓4ᵗʰ **A85 Other viral encephalitis, not elsewhere classified**
    INCLUDES specified viral encephalomyelitis NEC
        specified viral meningoencephalitis NEC
    EXCLUDES 1 *benign myalgic encephalomyelitis (G93.3)*
        encephalitis due to cytomegalovirus (B25.8)
        encephalitis due to herpesvirus NEC (B10.0-)
        encephalitis due to herpesvirus [herpes simplex] (B00.4)
        encephalitis due to measles virus (B05.0)
        encephalitis due to mumps virus (B26.2)
        encephalitis due to poliomyelitis virus (A80.-)
        encephalitis due to zoster (B02.0)
        lymphocytic choriomeningitis (A87.2)

    A85.0 Enteroviral encephalitis
        Enteroviral encephalomyelitis

    A85.1 Adenoviral encephalitis
        Adenoviral meningoencephalitis

    A85.2 Arthropod-borne viral encephalitis, unspecified ▽
        EXCLUDES 1 *West nile virus with encephalitis (A92.31)*

    A85.8 Other specified viral encephalitis
        Encephalitis lethargica
        Von Economo-Cruchet disease

A86 Unspecified viral encephalitis ▽
    Viral encephalomyelitis NOS
    Viral meningoencephalitis NOS

✓4ᵗʰ **A87 Viral meningitis**
    EXCLUDES 1 *meningitis due to herpesvirus [herpes simplex] (B00.3)*
        meningitis due to measles virus (B05.1)
        meningitis due to mumps virus (B26.1)
        meningitis due to poliomyelitis virus (A80.-)
        meningitis due to zoster (B02.1)

    A87.0 Enteroviral meningitis
        Coxsackievirus meningitis
        Echovirus meningitis

    A87.1 Adenoviral meningitis

    A87.2 Lymphocytic choriomeningitis
        Lymphocytic meningoencephalitis

    A87.8 Other viral meningitis

    A87.9 Viral meningitis, unspecified ▽

✓4ᵗʰ **A88 Other viral infections of central nervous system, not elsewhere classified**
    EXCLUDES 1 *viral encephalitis NOS (A86)*
        viral meningitis NOS (A87.9)

    A88.0 Enteroviral exanthematous fever [Boston exanthem]

    A88.1 Epidemic vertigo

    A88.8 Other specified viral infections of central nervous system

A89 Unspecified viral infection of central nervous system ▽

Arthropod-borne viral fevers and viral hemorrhagic fevers (A90-A99)

A90 Dengue fever [classical dengue]
    EXCLUDES 1 *dengue hemorrhagic fever (A91)*
    AHA: 2016, 3Q, 13

A91 Dengue hemorrhagic fever

✓4ᵗʰ **A92 Other mosquito-borne viral fevers**
    EXCLUDES 1 *Ross River disease (B33.1)*

    A92.0 Chikungunya virus disease
        Chikungunya (hemorrhagic) fever

    A92.1 O'nyong-nyong fever

    A92.2 Venezuelan equine fever
        Venezuelan equine encephalitis
        Venezuelan equine encephalomyelitis virus disease

    ✓5ᵗʰ **A92.3 West Nile virus infection**
        West Nile fever
        AHA: 2016, 3Q, 12

        A92.30 West Nile virus infection, unspecified ▽
            West Nile fever NOS
            West Nile fever without complications
            West Nile virus NOS

        A92.31 West Nile virus infection with encephalitis
            West Nile encephalitis
            West Nile encephalomyelitis

        A92.32 West Nile virus infection with other neurologic manifestation
            Use additional code to specify the neurologic manifestation

        A92.39 West Nile virus infection with other complications
            Use additional code to specify the other conditions

    A92.4 Rift Valley fever

    A92.5 Zika virus disease
        Zika virus fever
        Zika virus infection
        Zika NOS

    A92.8 Other specified mosquito-borne viral fevers

    A92.9 Mosquito-borne viral fever, unspecified ▽

✓4ᵗʰ **A93 Other arthropod-borne viral fevers, not elsewhere classified**

    A93.0 Oropouche virus disease
        Oropouche fever

    A93.1 Sandfly fever
        Pappataci fever
        Phlebotomus fever

    A93.2 Colorado tick fever

    A93.8 Other specified arthropod-borne viral fevers
        Piry virus disease
        Vesicular stomatitis virus disease [Indiana fever]

A94 Unspecified arthropod-borne viral fever ▽
    Arboviral fever NOS
    Arbovirus infection NOS

✓4ᵗʰ **A95 Yellow fever**

    A95.0 Sylvatic yellow fever
        Jungle yellow fever

    A95.1 Urban yellow fever

    A95.9 Yellow fever, unspecified ▽

✓4ᵗʰ **A96 Arenaviral hemorrhagic fever**

    A96.0 Junin hemorrhagic fever
        Argentinian hemorrhagic fever

    A96.1 Machupo hemorrhagic fever
        Bolivian hemorrhagic fever

    A96.2 Lassa fever

☑ Additional Character Req   v17 Placeholder Alert   Manifestation   HCC CMS-HCC Condition   ▽ Unspecified Code   ►◄ Revised Text   ● New Code   ▲ Revised Code Title

ICD-10-CM 2018   **445**

Chapter 1. Certain Infectious and Parasitic Diseases

A81.8-A96.2

A96.8   **Other arenaviral hemorrhagic fevers**

A96.9   **Arenaviral hemorrhagic fever, unspecified** ▽

✓4ᵗʰ **A98**   **Other viral hemorrhagic fevers, not elsewhere classified**
> EXCLUDES 1   *chikungunya hemorrhagic fever (A92.0)*
> *dengue hemorrhagic fever (A91)*

A98.0   **Crimean-Congo hemorrhagic fever**
Central Asian hemorrhagic fever

A98.1   **Omsk hemorrhagic fever**

A98.2   **Kyasanur Forest disease**

A98.3   **Marburg virus disease**

A98.4   **Ebola virus disease**

A98.5   **Hemorrhagic fever with renal syndrome**
Epidemic hemorrhagic fever
Korean hemorrhagic fever
Russian hemorrhagic fever
Hantaan virus disease
Hantavirus disease with renal manifestations
Nephropathia epidemica
Songo fever
> EXCLUDES 1   *hantavirus (cardio)-pulmonary syndrome (B33.4)*

A98.8   **Other specified viral hemorrhagic fevers**

A99   **Unspecified viral hemorrhagic fever** ▽

Viral infections characterized by skin and mucous membrane lesions (B00-B09)

✓4ᵗʰ **B00**   **Herpesviral [herpes simplex] infections**
> EXCLUDES 1   *congenital herpesviral infections (P35.2)*
> EXCLUDES 2   *anogenital herpesviral infection (A60.-)*
> *gammaherpesviral mononucleosis (B27.0-)*
> *herpangina (B08.5)*

B00.0   **Eczema herpeticum**
Kaposi's varicelliform eruption

B00.1   **Herpesviral vesicular dermatitis**
Herpes simplex facialis
Herpes simplex labialis
Herpes simplex otitis externa
Vesicular dermatitis of ear
Vesicular dermatitis of lip

B00.2   **Herpesviral gingivostomatitis and pharyngotonsillitis**
Herpesviral pharyngitis

B00.3   **Herpesviral meningitis**

B00.4   **Herpesviral encephalitis**
Herpesviral meningoencephalitis
Simian B disease
> EXCLUDES 1   *herpesviral encephalitis due to herpesvirus 6 and 7 (B10.01, B10.09)*
> *non-simplex herpesviral encephalitis (B10.0-)*

✓5ᵗʰ   B00.5   **Herpesviral ocular disease**

B00.50   **Herpesviral ocular disease, unspecified** ▽

B00.51   **Herpesviral iridocyclitis**
Herpesviral iritis
Herpesviral uveitis, anterior

B00.52   **Herpesviral keratitis**
Herpesviral keratoconjunctivitis

B00.53   **Herpesviral conjunctivitis**

B00.59   **Other herpesviral disease of eye**
Herpesviral dermatitis of eyelid

B00.7   **Disseminated herpesviral disease**   HCC
Herpesviral sepsis

✓5ᵗʰ   B00.8   **Other forms of herpesviral infections**

B00.81   **Herpesviral hepatitis**

B00.82   **Herpes simplex myelitis**   HCC

B00.89   **Other herpesviral infection**
Herpesviral whitlow

B00.9   **Herpesviral infection, unspecified** ▽
Herpes simplex infection NOS

✓4ᵗʰ **B01**   **Varicella [chickenpox]**

B01.0   **Varicella meningitis**

✓5ᵗʰ   B01.1   **Varicella encephalitis, myelitis and encephalomyelitis**
Postchickenpox encephalitis, myelitis and encephalomyelitis

B01.11   **Varicella encephalitis and encephalomyelitis**
Postchickenpox encephalitis and encephalomyelitis

B01.12   **Varicella myelitis**   HCC
Postchickenpox myelitis

B01.2   **Varicella pneumonia**

✓5ᵗʰ   B01.8   **Varicella with other complications**

B01.81   **Varicella keratitis**

B01.89   **Other varicella complications**

B01.9   **Varicella without complication** ▽
Varicella NOS

✓4ᵗʰ **B02**   **Zoster [herpes zoster]**
> INCLUDES   shingles
> zona

B02.0   **Zoster encephalitis**
Zoster meningoencephalitis

B02.1   **Zoster meningitis**

✓5ᵗʰ   B02.2   **Zoster with other nervous system involvement**

B02.21   **Postherpetic geniculate ganglionitis**

B02.22   **Postherpetic trigeminal neuralgia**

B02.23   **Postherpetic polyneuropathy**

B02.24   **Postherpetic myelitis**   HCC
Herpes zoster myelitis

B02.29   **Other postherpetic nervous system involvement**
Postherpetic radiculopathy

✓5ᵗʰ   B02.3   **Zoster ocular disease**

B02.30   **Zoster ocular disease, unspecified** ▽

B02.31   **Zoster conjunctivitis**

B02.32   **Zoster iridocyclitis**

B02.33   **Zoster keratitis**
Herpes zoster keratoconjunctivitis

B02.34   **Zoster scleritis**

B02.39   **Other herpes zoster eye disease**
Zoster blepharitis

B02.7   **Disseminated zoster**

B02.8   **Zoster with other complications**
Herpes zoster otitis externa

B02.9   **Zoster without complications** ▽
Zoster NOS

B03   **Smallpox**
> NOTE   In 1980 the 33rd World Health Assembly declared that smallpox had been eradicated. The classification is maintained for surveillance purposes.

B04   **Monkeypox**

✓4ᵗʰ **B05**   **Measles**
> INCLUDES   morbilli
> EXCLUDES 1   *subacute sclerosing panencephalitis (A81.1)*

B05.0   **Measles complicated by encephalitis**
Postmeasles encephalitis

B05.1   **Measles complicated by meningitis**
Postmeasles meningitis

B05.2   **Measles complicated by pneumonia**
Postmeasles pneumonia

B05.3   **Measles complicated by otitis media**
Postmeasles otitis media

B05.4   **Measles with intestinal complications**

✓5ᵗʰ   B05.8   **Measles with other complications**

B05.81   **Measles keratitis and keratoconjunctivitis**

B05.89   **Other measles complications**

B05.9   **Measles without complication** ▽
Measles NOS

✓4ᵗʰ **B06**   **Rubella [German measles]**
> EXCLUDES 1   *congenital rubella (P35.0)*

✓5ᵗʰ   B06.0   **Rubella with neurological complications**

B06.00   **Rubella with neurological complication, unspecified** ▽

B06.01   **Rubella encephalitis**
Rubella meningoencephalitis

B06.02   **Rubella meningitis**

B06.09   **Other neurological complications of rubella**

✓5ᵗʰ   B06.8   **Rubella with other complications**

B06.81   **Rubella pneumonia**

B06.82   **Rubella arthritis**   HCC

B06.89   **Other rubella complications**

B06.9   **Rubella without complication** ▽
Rubella NOS

EXCLUDES 1 Not coded here   EXCLUDES 2 Not included here   N Newborn Age: 0   P Pediatric Age: 0-17   M Maternity Age: 12-55   A Adult Age: 15-124

446   ICD-10-CM 2018

✓4ᵗʰ **B07** **Viral warts**
    INCLUDES   verruca simplex
               verruca vulgaris
               viral warts due to human papillomavirus
    EXCLUDES 2   *anogenital (venereal) warts (A63.0)*
               papilloma of bladder (D41.4)
               papilloma of cervix (D26.0)
               papilloma larynx (D14.1)

    B07.0 **Plantar wart**
        Verruca plantaris

    B07.8 **Other viral warts**
        Common wart
        Flat wart
        Verruca plana

    B07.9 **Viral wart, unspecified** ▽

✓4ᵗʰ **B08** **Other viral infections characterized by skin and mucous membrane lesions, not elsewhere classified**
    EXCLUDES 1   *vesicular stomatitis virus disease (A93.8)*

  ✓5ᵗʰ **B08.0** **Other orthopoxvirus infections**
      EXCLUDES 2   *monkeypox (B04)*

    ✓6ᵗʰ **B08.01** **Cowpox and vaccinia not from vaccine**
        B08.010 **Cowpox**
            DEF: A disease contracted by milking infected cows; vesicles usually appear on the fingers, hands, and adjacent areas and usually disappear without scarring; other symptoms: local edema, lymphangitis, and regional lymphadenitis with or without fever.

        B08.011 **Vaccinia not from vaccine**
            EXCLUDES 1   *vaccinia (from vaccination) (generalized) (T88.1)*

    B08.02 **Orf virus disease**
        Contagious pustular dermatitis
        Ecthyma contagiosum

    B08.03 **Pseudocowpox [milker's node]**

    B08.04 **Paravaccinia, unspecified** ▽

    B08.09 **Other orthopoxvirus infections**
        Orthopoxvirus infection NOS

  B08.1 **Molluscum contagiosum**
      DEF: Benign poxvirus infection causing small bumps on the skin or conjunctiva; transmitted by close contact.

  ✓5ᵗʰ **B08.2** **Exanthema subitum [sixth disease]**
      Roseola infantum

    B08.20 **Exanthema subitum [sixth disease], unspecified** P ▽
        Roseola infantum, unspecified

    B08.21 **Exanthema subitum [sixth disease] due to human herpesvirus 6** P
        Roseola infantum due to human herpesvirus 6

    B08.22 **Exanthema subitum [sixth disease] due to human herpesvirus 7** P
        Roseola infantum due to human herpesvirus 7

  B08.3 **Erythema infectiosum [fifth disease]**

  B08.4 **Enteroviral vesicular stomatitis with exanthem**
      Hand, foot and mouth disease

  B08.5 **Enteroviral vesicular pharyngitis**
      Herpangina
      DEF: Acute infectious Coxsackie virus infection causing throat lesions, fever, and vomiting; generally affects children in summer.

  ✓5ᵗʰ **B08.6** **Parapoxvirus infections**
    B08.60 **Parapoxvirus infection, unspecified** ▽
    B08.61 **Bovine stomatitis**
    B08.62 **Sealpox**
    B08.69 **Other parapoxvirus infections**

  ✓5ᵗʰ **B08.7** **Yatapoxvirus infections**
    B08.70 **Yatapoxvirus infection, unspecified** ▽
    B08.71 **Tanapox virus disease**
    B08.72 **Yaba pox virus disease**
        Yaba monkey tumor disease
    B08.79 **Other yatapoxvirus infections**

  B08.8 **Other specified viral infections characterized by skin and mucous membrane lesions**
      Enteroviral lymphonodular pharyngitis
      Foot-and-mouth disease
      Poxvirus NEC

B09 **Unspecified viral infection characterized by skin and mucous membrane lesions** ▽
    Viral enanthema NOS
    Viral exanthema NOS

Other human herpesviruses (B10)

✓4ᵗʰ **B10** **Other human herpesviruses**
    EXCLUDES 2   *cytomegalovirus (B25.9)*
               Epstein-Barr virus (B27.0-)
               herpes NOS (B00.9)
               herpes simplex (B00.-)
               herpes zoster (B02.-)
               human herpesvirus NOS (B00.-)
               human herpesvirus 1 and 2 (B00.-)
               human herpesvirus 3 (B01.-, B02.-)
               human herpesvirus 4 (B27.0-)
               human herpesvirus (B25.-)
               varicella (B01.-)
               zoster (B02.-)

  ✓5ᵗʰ **B10.0** **Other human herpesvirus encephalitis**
      EXCLUDES 2   *herpes encephalitis NOS (B00.4)*
               herpes simplex encephalitis (B00.4)
               human herpesvirus encephalitis (B00.4)
               simian B herpes virus encephalitis (B00.4)

    B10.01 **Human herpesvirus 6 encephalitis**

    B10.09 **Other human herpesvirus encephalitis**
        Human herpesvirus 7 encephalitis

  ✓5ᵗʰ **B10.8** **Other human herpesvirus infection**
    B10.81 **Human herpesvirus 6 infection**
    B10.82 **Human herpesvirus 7 infection**
    B10.89 **Other human herpesvirus infection**
        Human herpesvirus 8 infection
        Kaposi's sarcoma-associated herpesvirus infection

Viral hepatitis (B15-B19)

    EXCLUDES 1   *sequelae of viral hepatitis (B94.2)*
    EXCLUDES 2   *cytomegaloviral hepatitis (B25.1)*
               herpesviral [herpes simplex] hepatitis (B00.81)
    DEF: Hepatitis A: HAV infection is self-limiting with flulike symptoms; transmission, fecal-oral.
    DEF: Hepatitis B: HBV infection can be chronic and systemic; transmission, bodily fluids.
    DEF: Hepatitis C: HCV infection can be chronic and systemic; transmission, blood transfusion and unidentified agents.
    DEF: Hepatitis D (delta): HDV occurs only in the presence of hepatitis B virus; transmission, contaminated blood in contact with mucous membranes.
    DEF: Hepatitis E: HEV is epidemic form; transmission, fecal-oral, most often from contaminated water.

✓4ᵗʰ **B15** **Acute hepatitis A**
    B15.0 **Hepatitis A with hepatic coma**
    B15.9 **Hepatitis A without hepatic coma**
        Hepatitis A (acute)(viral) NOS

✓4ᵗʰ **B16** **Acute hepatitis B**
    AHA: 2016, 3Q, 13
    B16.0 **Acute hepatitis B with delta-agent with hepatic coma**
    B16.1 **Acute hepatitis B with delta-agent without hepatic coma**
    B16.2 **Acute hepatitis B without delta-agent with hepatic coma**
    B16.9 **Acute hepatitis B without delta-agent and without hepatic coma**
        Hepatitis B (acute) (viral) NOS

✓4ᵗʰ **B17** **Other acute viral hepatitis**
    B17.0 **Acute delta-(super) infection of hepatitis B carrier**
  ✓5ᵗʰ **B17.1** **Acute hepatitis C**
    B17.10 **Acute hepatitis C without hepatic coma**
        Acute hepatitis C NOS
    B17.11 **Acute hepatitis C with hepatic coma**
    B17.2 **Acute hepatitis E**
    B17.8 **Other specified acute viral hepatitis**
        Hepatitis non-A non-B (acute) (viral) NEC
    B17.9 **Acute viral hepatitis, unspecified** ▽
        Acute hepatitis NOS
        Acute infectious hepatitis NOS

✓4ᵗʰ **B18** **Chronic viral hepatitis**
    INCLUDES   carrier of viral hepatitis
    AHA: 2017, 1Q, 41
    B18.0 **Chronic viral hepatitis B with delta-agent** HCC

✓ Additional Character Req   ✓7ᵗʰ Placeholder Alert   Manifestation   HCC CMS-HCC Condition   ▽ Unspecified Code   ►◄ Revised Text   ● New Code   ▲ Revised Code Title

B18.1 Chronic viral hepatitis B without delta-agent [HCC]
Carrier of viral hepatitis B
Chronic (viral) hepatitis B

B18.2 Chronic viral hepatitis C [HCC]
Carrier of viral hepatitis C

B18.8 Other chronic viral hepatitis [HCC]
Carrier of other viral hepatitis

B18.9 Chronic viral hepatitis, unspecified [HCC] ▽
Carrier of unspecified viral hepatitis

✓4ᵗʰ **B19 Unspecified viral hepatitis**

B19.0 Unspecified viral hepatitis with hepatic coma ▽

✓5ᵗʰ **B19.1 Unspecified viral hepatitis B**

B19.10 Unspecified viral hepatitis B without hepatic coma ▽
Unspecified viral hepatitis B NOS

B19.11 Unspecified viral hepatitis B with hepatic coma ▽

✓5ᵗʰ **B19.2 Unspecified viral hepatitis C**

B19.20 Unspecified viral hepatitis C without hepatic coma ▽
Viral hepatitis C NOS

B19.21 Unspecified viral hepatitis C with hepatic coma ▽

B19.9 Unspecified viral hepatitis without hepatic coma ▽
Viral hepatitis NOS

Human immunodeficiency virus [HIV] disease (B20)

B20 Human immunodeficiency virus [HIV] disease [HCC]
INCLUDES acquired immune deficiency syndrome [AIDS]
AIDS-related complex [ARC]
HIV infection, symptomatic
Code first human immunodeficiency virus [HIV] disease complicating
pregnancy, childbirth and the puerperium, if applicable (O98.7-)
Use additional code(s) to identify all manifestations of HIV infection
EXCLUDES 1 asymptomatic human immunodeficiency virus [HIV] infection
status (Z21)
exposure to HIV virus (Z20.6)
inconclusive serologic evidence of HIV (R75)

Other viral diseases (B25-B34)

✓4ᵗʰ **B25 Cytomegaloviral disease**
EXCLUDES 1 congenital cytomegalovirus infection (P35.1)
cytomegaloviral mononucleosis (B27.1-)

B25.0 Cytomegaloviral pneumonitis [HCC]

B25.1 Cytomegaloviral hepatitis [HCC]

B25.2 Cytomegaloviral pancreatitis [HCC]

B25.8 Other cytomegaloviral diseases [HCC]
Cytomegaloviral encephalitis

B25.9 Cytomegaloviral disease, unspecified [HCC] ▽

✓4ᵗʰ **B26 Mumps**
INCLUDES epidemic parotitis
infectious parotitis

B26.0 Mumps orchitis ♂

B26.1 Mumps meningitis

B26.2 Mumps encephalitis

B26.3 Mumps pancreatitis

✓5ᵗʰ **B26.8 Mumps with other complications**

B26.81 Mumps hepatitis

B26.82 Mumps myocarditis

B26.83 Mumps nephritis

B26.84 Mumps polyneuropathy

B26.85 Mumps arthritis [HCC]

B26.89 Other mumps complications

B26.9 Mumps without complication ▽
Mumps NOS
Mumps parotitis NOS

✓4ᵗʰ **B27 Infectious mononucleosis**
INCLUDES glandular fever
monocytic angina
Pfeiffer's disease

✓5ᵗʰ **B27.0 Gammaherpesviral mononucleosis**
Mononucleosis due to Epstein-Barr virus

B27.00 Gammaherpesviral mononucleosis without complication

B27.01 Gammaherpesviral mononucleosis with polyneuropathy

B27.02 Gammaherpesviral mononucleosis with meningitis

B27.09 Gammaherpesviral mononucleosis with other complications
Hepatomegaly in gammaherpesviral mononucleosis

✓5ᵗʰ **B27.1 Cytomegaloviral mononucleosis**

B27.10 Cytomegaloviral mononucleosis without complications

B27.11 Cytomegaloviral mononucleosis with polyneuropathy

B27.12 Cytomegaloviral mononucleosis with meningitis

B27.19 Cytomegaloviral mononucleosis with other complication
Hepatomegaly in cytomegaloviral mononucleosis

✓5ᵗʰ **B27.8 Other infectious mononucleosis**

B27.80 Other infectious mononucleosis without complication

B27.81 Other infectious mononucleosis with polyneuropathy

B27.82 Other infectious mononucleosis with meningitis

B27.89 Other infectious mononucleosis with other complication
Hepatomegaly in other infectious mononucleosis

✓5ᵗʰ **B27.9 Infectious mononucleosis, unspecified**

B27.90 Infectious mononucleosis, unspecified without complication ▽

B27.91 Infectious mononucleosis, unspecified with polyneuropathy ▽

B27.92 Infectious mononucleosis, unspecified with meningitis ▽

B27.99 Infectious mononucleosis, unspecified with other complication ▽
Hepatomegaly in unspecified infectious mononucleosis

✓4ᵗʰ **B30 Viral conjunctivitis**
EXCLUDES 1 herpesviral [herpes simplex] ocular disease (B00.5)
ocular zoster (B02.3)

B30.0 Keratoconjunctivitis due to adenovirus
Epidemic keratoconjunctivitis
Shipyard eye

B30.1 Conjunctivitis due to adenovirus
Acute adenoviral follicular conjunctivitis
Swimming-pool conjunctivitis

B30.2 Viral pharyngoconjunctivitis

B30.3 Acute epidemic hemorrhagic conjunctivitis (enteroviral)
Conjunctivitis due to coxsackievirus 24
Conjunctivitis due to enterovirus 70
Hemorrhagic conjunctivitis (acute)(epidemic)

B30.8 Other viral conjunctivitis
Newcastle conjunctivitis

B30.9 Viral conjunctivitis, unspecified ▽

✓4ᵗʰ **B33 Other viral diseases, not elsewhere classified**

B33.0 Epidemic myalgia
Bornholm disease

B33.1 Ross River disease
Epidemic polyarthritis and exanthema
Ross River fever

Viral Conjunctivitis

Normal conjunctiva

Inflamed conjunctiva

EXCLUDES 1 Not coded here   EXCLUDES 2 Not included here   N Newborn Age: 0   P Pediatric Age: 0-17   M Maternity Age: 12-55   A Adult Age: 15-124

448   ICD-10-CM 2018

✓5ᵗʰ **B33.2 Viral carditis**
     Coxsackie (virus) carditis

     B33.20 Viral carditis, unspecified ▽

     B33.21 Viral endocarditis

     B33.22 Viral myocarditis

     B33.23 Viral pericarditis

     B33.24 Viral cardiomyopathy HCC

B33.3 Retrovirus infections, not elsewhere classified
     Retrovirus infection NOS

B33.4 Hantavirus (cardio)-pulmonary syndrome [HPS] [HCPS]
     Hantavirus disease with pulmonary manifestations
     Sin nombre virus disease
     Use additional code to identify any associated acute kidney failure (N17.9)
     EXCLUDES 1   *hantavirus disease with renal manifestations (A98.5)*
                 hemorrhagic fever with renal manifestations (A98.5)

B33.8 Other specified viral diseases
     EXCLUDES 1   *anogenital human papillomavirus infection (A63.0)*
                 viral warts due to human papillomavirus infection (B07)

✓4ᵗʰ **B34 Viral infection of unspecified site**
     EXCLUDES 1   *anogenital human papillomavirus infection (A63.0)*
                 cytomegaloviral disease NOS (B25.9)
                 herpesvirus [herpes simplex] infection NOS (B00.9)
                 retrovirus infection NOS (B33.3)
                 viral agents as the cause of diseases classified elsewhere (B97.-)
                 viral warts due to human papillomavirus infection (B07)

     B34.0 Adenovirus infection, unspecified ▽

     B34.1 Enterovirus infection, unspecified ▽
         Coxsackievirus infection NOS
         Echovirus infection NOS

     B34.2 Coronavirus infection, unspecified ▽
         EXCLUDES 1   *pneumonia due to SARS-associated coronavirus (J12.81)*

     B34.3 Parvovirus infection, unspecified ▽

     B34.4 Papovavirus infection, unspecified ▽

     B34.8 Other viral infections of unspecified site ▽

     B34.9 Viral infection, unspecified ▽
         Viremia NOS
         AHA: 2016, 3Q, 10

Mycoses (B35-B49)

EXCLUDES 2   *hypersensitivity pneumonitis due to organic dust (J67.-)*
              mycosis fungoides (C84.0-)

✓4ᵗʰ **B35 Dermatophytosis**
     INCLUDES   favus
              infections due to species of Epidermophyton, Micro-sporum and Trichophyton
              tinea, any type except those in B36-
     DEF: Contagious superficial fungal infection of the skin that invades and grows in dead keratin.

     B35.0 Tinea barbae and tinea capitis
         Beard ringworm
         Kerion
         Scalp ringworm
         Sycosis, mycotic

     B35.1 Tinea unguium
         Dermatophytic onychia
         Dermatophytosis of nail
         Onychomycosis
         Ringworm of nails

     B35.2 Tinea manuum
         Dermatophytosis of hand
         Hand ringworm

     B35.3 Tinea pedis
         Athlete's foot
         Dermatophytosis of foot
         Foot ringworm

     B35.4 Tinea corporis
         Ringworm of the body

     B35.5 Tinea imbricata
         Tokelau

     B35.6 Tinea cruris
         Dhobi itch
         Groin ringworm
         Jock itch

     B35.8 Other dermatophytoses
         Disseminated dermatophytosis
         Granulomatous dermatophytosis

     B35.9 Dermatophytosis, unspecified ▽
         Ringworm NOS

✓4ᵗʰ **B36 Other superficial mycoses**
     B36.0 Pityriasis versicolor
         Tinea flava
         Tinea versicolor

     B36.1 Tinea nigra
         Keratomycosis nigricans palmaris
         Microsporosis nigra
         Pityriasis nigra

     B36.2 White piedra
         Tinea blanca

     B36.3 Black piedra

     B36.8 Other specified superficial mycoses

     B36.9 Superficial mycosis, unspecified ▽

✓4ᵗʰ **B37 Candidiasis**
     INCLUDES   candidosis
              moniliasis
     EXCLUDES 1   *neonatal candidiasis (P37.5)*

     B37.0 Candidal stomatitis
         Oral thrush

     B37.1 Pulmonary candidiasis HCC
         Candidal bronchitis
         Candidal pneumonia

     B37.2 Candidiasis of skin and nail
         Candidal onychia
         Candidal paronychia
         EXCLUDES 2   *diaper dermatitis (L22)*

     B37.3 Candidiasis of vulva and vagina ♀
         Candidal vulvovaginitis
         Monilial vulvovaginitis
         Vaginal thrush

✓5ᵗʰ **B37.4 Candidiasis of other urogenital sites**
         B37.41 Candidal cystitis and urethritis
         B37.42 Candidal balanitis
         B37.49 Other urogenital candidiasis
               Candidal pyelonephritis

     B37.5 Candidal meningitis

     B37.6 Candidal endocarditis

     B37.7 Candidal sepsis HCC
         Disseminated candidiasis
         Systemic candidiasis
         AHA: 2014, 4Q, 46

✓5ᵗʰ **B37.8 Candidiasis of other sites**
         B37.81 Candidal esophagitis HCC
         B37.82 Candidal enteritis
               Candidal proctitis
         B37.83 Candidal cheilitis
         B37.84 Candidal otitis externa
         B37.89 Other sites of candidiasis
               Candidal osteomyelitis

     B37.9 Candidiasis, unspecified ▽
         Thrush NOS

✓4ᵗʰ **B38 Coccidioidomycosis**
     B38.0 Acute pulmonary coccidioidomycosis HCC

     B38.1 Chronic pulmonary coccidioidomycosis HCC

     B38.2 Pulmonary coccidioidomycosis, unspecified HCC ▽

     B38.3 Cutaneous coccidioidomycosis

     B38.4 Coccidioidomycosis meningitis
         DEF: *Coccidioides immitis* infection of the lining of the brain and/or spinal cord.

     B38.7 Disseminated coccidioidomycosis
         Generalized coccidioidomycosis

✓5ᵗʰ **B38.8 Other forms of coccidioidomycosis**
         B38.81 Prostatic coccidioidomycosis ♂
         B38.89 Other forms of coccidioidomycosis

     B38.9 Coccidioidomycosis, unspecified ▽

✓ Additional Character Req   ✓x7ᵗʰ Placeholder Alert   Manifestation   HCC CMS-HCC Condition   ▽ Unspecified Code   ►◄ Revised Text   ● New Code   ▲ Revised Code Title

ICD-10-CM 2018   449

B33.2-B38.9

Histoplasmosis

Histoplasma capsulatum spores

Spores

✓4ᵗʰ B39 Histoplasmosis
Code first associated AIDS (B20)
Use additional code for any associated manifestations, such as:
   endocarditis (I39)
   meningitis (G02)
   pericarditis (I32)
   retinitits (H32)

DEF: Type of lung infection caused by breathing in fungal spores often found in the droppings of bats and birds or soil contaminated by their droppings.

- **B39.0 Acute pulmonary histoplasmosis capsulati**   HCC
- **B39.1 Chronic pulmonary histoplasmosis capsulati**   HCC
- **B39.2 Pulmonary histoplasmosis capsulati, unspecified**   HCC ▽
- **B39.3 Disseminated histoplasmosis capsulati**
   Generalized histoplasmosis capsulati
- **B39.4 Histoplasmosis capsulati, unspecified**   ▽
   American histoplasmosis
- **B39.5 Histoplasmosis duboisii**
   African histoplasmosis
- **B39.9 Histoplasmosis, unspecified**   ▽

✓4ᵗʰ B40 Blastomycosis
   EXCLUDES 1 *Brazilian blastomycosis (B41.-)*
   keloidal blastomycosis (B48.0)

- **B40.0 Acute pulmonary blastomycosis**   HCC
- **B40.1 Chronic pulmonary blastomycosis**   HCC
- **B40.2 Pulmonary blastomycosis, unspecified**   HCC ▽
- **B40.3 Cutaneous blastomycosis**
- **B40.7 Disseminated blastomycosis**
   Generalized blastomycosis
- ✓5ᵗʰ **B40.8 Other forms of blastomycosis**
   - **B40.81 Blastomycotic meningoencephalitis**
      Meningomyelitis due to blastomycosis
   - **B40.89 Other forms of blastomycosis**
- **B40.9 Blastomycosis, unspecified**   ▽

✓4ᵗʰ B41 Paracoccidioidomycosis
   INCLUDES Brazilian blastomycosis
      Lutz' disease

- **B41.0 Pulmonary paracoccidioidomycosis**   HCC
- **B41.7 Disseminated paracoccidioidomycosis**
   Generalized paracoccidioidomycosis
- **B41.8 Other forms of paracoccidioidomycosis**
- **B41.9 Paracoccidioidomycosis, unspecified**   ▽

✓4ᵗʰ B42 Sporotrichosis
- **B42.0 Pulmonary sporotrichosis**
- **B42.1 Lymphocutaneous sporotrichosis**
- **B42.7 Disseminated sporotrichosis**
   Generalized sporotrichosis

- ✓5ᵗʰ **B42.8 Other forms of sporotrichosis**
   - **B42.81 Cerebral sporotrichosis**
      Meningitis due to sporotrichosis
   - **B42.82 Sporotrichosis arthritis**   HCC
   - **B42.89 Other forms of sporotrichosis**
- **B42.9 Sporotrichosis, unspecified**   ▽

✓4ᵗʰ B43 Chromomycosis and pheomycotic abscess
- **B43.0 Cutaneous chromomycosis**
   Dermatitis verrucosa
- **B43.1 Pheomycotic brain abscess**
   Cerebral chromomycosis
- **B43.2 Subcutaneous pheomycotic abscess and cyst**
- **B43.8 Other forms of chromomycosis**
- **B43.9 Chromomycosis, unspecified**   ▽

✓4ᵗʰ B44 Aspergillosis
   INCLUDES aspergilloma
- **B44.0 Invasive pulmonary aspergillosis**   HCC
- **B44.1 Other pulmonary aspergillosis**   HCC
- **B44.2 Tonsillar aspergillosis**   HCC
- **B44.7 Disseminated aspergillosis**   HCC
   Generalized aspergillosis
- ✓5ᵗʰ **B44.8 Other forms of aspergillosis**
   - **B44.81 Allergic bronchopulmonary aspergillosis**   HCC
   - **B44.89 Other forms of aspergillosis**   HCC
- **B44.9 Aspergillosis, unspecified**   HCC ▽

✓4ᵗʰ B45 Cryptococcosis
- **B45.0 Pulmonary cryptococcosis**   HCC
- **B45.1 Cerebral cryptococcosis**   HCC
   Cryptococcal meningitis
   Cryptococcosis meningocerebralis
- **B45.2 Cutaneous cryptococcosis**   HCC
- **B45.3 Osseous cryptococcosis**   HCC
- **B45.7 Disseminated cryptococcosis**   HCC
   Generalized cryptococcosis
- **B45.8 Other forms of cryptococcosis**   HCC
- **B45.9 Cryptococcosis, unspecified**   HCC ▽

✓4ᵗʰ B46 Zygomycosis
- **B46.0 Pulmonary mucormycosis**   HCC
- **B46.1 Rhinocerebral mucormycosis**   HCC
- **B46.2 Gastrointestinal mucormycosis**   HCC
- **B46.3 Cutaneous mucormycosis**   HCC
   Subcutaneous mucormycosis
- **B46.4 Disseminated mucormycosis**   HCC
   Generalized mucormycosis
- **B46.5 Mucormycosis, unspecified**   HCC ▽
- **B46.8 Other zygomycoses**   HCC
   Entomophthoromycosis
- **B46.9 Zygomycosis, unspecified**   HCC ▽
   Phycomycosis NOS

✓4ᵗʰ B47 Mycetoma
- **B47.0 Eumycetoma**
   Madura foot, mycotic
   Maduromycosis
- **B47.1 Actinomycetoma**
- **B47.9 Mycetoma, unspecified**   ▽
   Madura foot NOS

✓4ᵗʰ B48 Other mycoses, not elsewhere classified
- **B48.0 Lobomycosis**
   Keloidal blastomycosis
   Lobo's disease
- **B48.1 Rhinosporidiosis**
- **B48.2 Allescheriasis**
   Infection due to Pseudallescheria boydii
   EXCLUDES 1 *eumycetoma (B47.0)*
- **B48.3 Geotrichosis**
   Geotrichum stomatitis
- **B48.4 Penicillosis**   HCC

B48.8 Other specified mycoses `HCC`
Adiaspiromycosis
Infection of tissue and organs by Alternaria
Infection of tissue and organs by Drechslera
Infection of tissue and organs by Fusarium
Infection of tissue and organs by saprophytic fungi NEC
AHA: 2014, 4Q, 46; 2014, 2Q, 13

B49 Unspecified mycosis ▽
Fungemia NOS

Protozoal diseases (B50-B64)

EXCLUDES 1   amebiasis (A06.-)
other protozoal intestinal diseases (A07.-)

✓4ᵗʰ **B50 Plasmodium falciparum malaria**
INCLUDES   mixed infections of Plasmodium falciparum with any other Plasmodium species

B50.0 Plasmodium falciparum malaria with cerebral complications
Cerebral malaria NOS

B50.8 Other severe and complicated Plasmodium falciparum malaria
Severe or complicated Plasmodium falciparum malaria NOS

B50.9 Plasmodium falciparum malaria, unspecified ▽

✓4ᵗʰ **B51 Plasmodium vivax malaria**
INCLUDES   mixed infections of Plasmodium vivax with other Plasmodium species, except Plasmodium falciparum
EXCLUDES 1   plasmodium vivax with Plasmodium falciparum (B50.-)

B51.0 Plasmodium vivax malaria with rupture of spleen

B51.8 Plasmodium vivax malaria with other complications

B51.9 Plasmodium vivax malaria without complication ▽
Plasmodium vivax malaria NOS

✓4ᵗʰ **B52 Plasmodium malariae malaria**
INCLUDES   mixed infections of Plasmodium malariae with other Plasmodium species, except Plasmodium falciparum and Plasmodium vivax
EXCLUDES 1   Plasmodium falciparum (B50.-)
Plasmodium vivax (B51.-)

B52.0 Plasmodium malariae malaria with nephropathy

B52.8 Plasmodium malariae malaria with other complications

B52.9 Plasmodium malariae malaria without complication ▽
Plasmodium malariae malaria NOS

✓4ᵗʰ **B53 Other specified malaria**
B53.0 Plasmodium ovale malaria
EXCLUDES 1   Plasmodium ovale with Plasmodium falciparum (B50.-)
Plasmodium ovale with Plasmodium malariae (B52.-)
Plasmodium ovale with Plasmodium vivax (B51.-)

B53.1 Malaria due to simian plasmodia
EXCLUDES 1   Malaria due to simian plasmodia with Plasmodium falciparum (B50.-)
Malaria due to simian plasmodia with Plasmodium malariae (B52.-)
Malaria due to simian plasmodia with Plasmodium ovale (B53.0)
Malaria due to simian plasmodia with Plasmodium vivax (B51.-)

B53.8 Other malaria, not elsewhere classified

B54 Unspecified malaria ▽

✓4ᵗʰ **B55 Leishmaniasis**
B55.0 Visceral leishmaniasis
Kala-azar
Post-kala-azar dermal leishmaniasis

B55.1 Cutaneous leishmaniasis

B55.2 Mucocutaneous leishmaniasis

B55.9 Leishmaniasis, unspecified ▽

✓4ᵗʰ **B56 African trypanosomiasis**
B56.0 Gambiense trypanosomiasis
Infection due to Trypanosoma brucei gambiense
West African sleeping sickness

B56.1 Rhodesiense trypanosomiasis
East African sleeping sickness
Infection due to Trypanosoma brucei rhodesiense

B56.9 African trypanosomiasis, unspecified ▽
Sleeping sickness NOS

✓4ᵗʰ **B57 Chagas' disease**
INCLUDES   American trypanosomiasis
infection due to Trypanosoma cruzi

B57.0 Acute Chagas' disease with heart involvement
Acute Chagas' disease with myocarditis

B57.1 Acute Chagas' disease without heart involvement
Acute Chagas' disease NOS

B57.2 Chagas' disease (chronic) with heart involvement
American trypanosomiasis NOS
Chagas' disease (chronic) NOS
Chagas' disease (chronic) with myocarditis
Trypanosomiasis NOS

✓5ᵗʰ **B57.3 Chagas' disease (chronic) with digestive system involvement**
B57.30 Chagas' disease with digestive system involvement, unspecified ▽
B57.31 Megaesophagus in Chagas' disease
B57.32 Megacolon in Chagas' disease
B57.39 Other digestive system involvement in Chagas' disease

✓5ᵗʰ **B57.4 Chagas' disease (chronic) with nervous system involvement**
B57.40 Chagas' disease with nervous system involvement, unspecified ▽
B57.41 Meningitis in Chagas' disease
B57.42 Meningoencephalitis in Chagas' disease
B57.49 Other nervous system involvement in Chagas' disease

B57.5 Chagas' disease (chronic) with other organ involvement

✓4ᵗʰ **B58 Toxoplasmosis**
INCLUDES   infection due to Toxoplasma gondii
EXCLUDES 1   congenital toxoplasmosis (P37.1)

✓5ᵗʰ **B58.0 Toxoplasma oculopathy**
B58.00 Toxoplasma oculopathy, unspecified ▽
B58.01 Toxoplasma chorioretinitis
B58.09 Other toxoplasma oculopathy
Toxoplasma uveitis

B58.1 Toxoplasma hepatitis

B58.2 Toxoplasma meningoencephalitis `HCC`

B58.3 Pulmonary toxoplasmosis `HCC`

✓5ᵗʰ **B58.8 Toxoplasmosis with other organ involvement**
B58.81 Toxoplasma myocarditis
B58.82 Toxoplasma myositis
B58.83 Toxoplasma tubulo-interstitial nephropathy
Toxoplasma pyelonephritis
B58.89 Toxoplasmosis with other organ involvement

B58.9 Toxoplasmosis, unspecified ▽

B59 Pneumocystosis `HCC`
Pneumonia due to Pneumocystis carinii
Pneumonia due to Pneumocystis jiroveci

✓4ᵗʰ **B60 Other protozoal diseases, not elsewhere classified**
EXCLUDES 1   cryptosporidiosis (A07.2)
intestinal microsporidiosis (A07.8)
isosporiasis (A07.3)

B60.0 Babesiosis
Piroplasmosis

✓5ᵗʰ **B60.1 Acanthamebiasis**
B60.10 Acanthamebiasis, unspecified ▽
B60.11 Meningoencephalitis due to Acanthamoeba (culbertsoni)
B60.12 Conjunctivitis due to Acanthamoeba
B60.13 Keratoconjunctivitis due to Acanthamoeba
B60.19 Other acanthamebic disease

B60.2 Naegleriasis
Primary amebic meningoencephalitis

B60.8 Other specified protozoal diseases
Microsporidiosis

B64 Unspecified protozoal disease ▽

☑ Additional Character Req   ✓x7ᵗʰ Placeholder Alert   Manifestation   `HCC` CMS-HCC Condition   ▽ Unspecified Code   ▶◀ Revised Text   ● New Code   ▲ Revised Code Title

Helminthiases (B65-B83)

✓4ᵗʰ B65　Schistosomiasis [bilharziasis]
　　INCLUDES　snail fever

B65.0　Schistosomiasis due to Schistosoma haematobium [urinary schistosomiasis]

B65.1　Schistosomiasis due to Schistosoma mansoni [intestinal schistosomiasis]

B65.2　Schistosomiasis due to Schistosoma japonicum
　　Asiatic schistosomiasis

B65.3　Cercarial dermatitis
　　Swimmer's itch

B65.8　Other schistosomiasis
　　Infection due to Schistosoma intercalatum
　　Infection due to Schistosoma mattheei
　　Infection due to Schistosoma mekongi

B65.9　Schistosomiasis, unspecified ▽

✓4ᵗʰ B66　Other fluke infections

B66.0　Opisthorchiasis
　　Infection due to cat liver fluke
　　Infection due to Opisthorchis (felineus)(viverrini)

B66.1　Clonorchiasis
　　Chinese liver fluke disease
　　Infection due to Clonorchis sinensis
　　Oriental liver fluke disease

B66.2　Dicroceliasis
　　Infection due to Dicrocoelium dendriticum
　　Lancet fluke infection

B66.3　Fascioliasis
　　Infection due to Fasciola gigantica
　　Infection due to Fasciola hepatica
　　Infection due to Fasciola indica
　　Sheep liver fluke disease

B66.4　Paragonimiasis HCC
　　Infection due to Paragonimus species
　　Lung fluke disease
　　Pulmonary distomiasis

B66.5　Fasciolopsiasis
　　Infection due to Fasciolopsis buski
　　Intestinal distomiasis

B66.8　Other specified fluke infections
　　Echinostomiasis
　　Heterophyiasis
　　Metagonimiasis
　　Nanophyetiasis
　　Watsoniasis

B66.9　Fluke infection, unspecified ▽

✓4ᵗʰ B67　Echinococcosis
　　INCLUDES　hydatidosis

B67.0　Echinococcus granulosus infection of liver

B67.1　Echinococcus granulosus infection of lung HCC

B67.2　Echinococcus granulosus infection of bone

✓5ᵗʰ B67.3　Echinococcus granulosus infection, other and multiple sites

　　B67.31　Echinococcus granulosus infection, thyroid gland

　　B67.32　Echinococcus granulosus infection, multiple sites

　　B67.39　Echinococcus granulosus infection, other sites

B67.4　Echinococcus granulosus infection, unspecified ▽
　　Dog tapeworm (infection)

B67.5　Echinococcus multilocularis infection of liver

✓5ᵗʰ B67.6　Echinococcus multilocularis infection, other and multiple sites

　　B67.61　Echinococcus multilocularis infection, multiple sites

　　B67.69　Echinococcus multilocularis infection, other sites

B67.7　Echinococcus multilocularis infection, unspecified ▽

B67.8　Echinococcosis, unspecified, of liver ▽

✓5ᵗʰ B67.9　Echinococcosis, other and unspecified

　　B67.90　Echinococcosis, unspecified ▽
　　　　Echinococcosis NOS

　　B67.99　Other echinococcosis

✓4ᵗʰ B68　Taeniasis
　　EXCLUDES 1　cysticercosis (B69.-)

B68.0　Taenia solium taeniasis
　　Pork tapeworm (infection)

B68.1　Taenia saginata taeniasis
　　Beef tapeworm (infection)
　　Infection due to adult tapeworm Taenia saginata

B68.9　Taeniasis, unspecified ▽

✓4ᵗʰ B69　Cysticercosis
　　INCLUDES　cysticerciasis infection due to larval form of Taenia solium

B69.0　Cysticercosis of central nervous system

B69.1　Cysticercosis of eye

✓5ᵗʰ B69.8　Cysticercosis of other sites

　　B69.81　Myositis in cysticercosis

　　B69.89　Cysticercosis of other sites

B69.9　Cysticercosis, unspecified ▽

✓4ᵗʰ B70　Diphyllobothriasis and sparganosis

B70.0　Diphyllobothriasis
　　Diphyllobothrium (adult) (latum) (pacificum) infection
　　Fish tapeworm (infection)
　　EXCLUDES 2　larval diphyllobothriasis (B70.1)

B70.1　Sparganosis
　　Infection due to Sparganum (mansoni) (proliferum)
　　Infection due to Spirometra larva
　　Larval diphyllobothriasis
　　Spirometrosis

✓4ᵗʰ B71　Other cestode infections

B71.0　Hymenolepiasis
　　Dwarf tapeworm infection
　　Rat tapeworm (infection)

B71.1　Dipylidiasis

B71.8　Other specified cestode infections
　　Coenurosis

B71.9　Cestode infection, unspecified ▽
　　Tapeworm (infection) NOS

B72　Dracunculiasis
　　INCLUDES　guinea worm infection
　　　　infection due to Dracunculus medinensis

✓4ᵗʰ B73　Onchocerciasis
　　INCLUDES　onchocerca volvulus infection
　　　　onchocercosis
　　　　river blindness

✓5ᵗʰ B73.0　Onchocerciasis with eye disease

　　B73.00　Onchocerciasis with eye involvement, unspecified ▽

　　B73.01　Onchocerciasis with endophthalmitis

　　B73.02　Onchocerciasis with glaucoma

　　B73.09　Onchocerciasis with other eye involvement
　　　　Infestation of eyelid due to onchocerciasis

B73.1　Onchocerciasis without eye disease

✓4ᵗʰ B74　Filariasis
　　EXCLUDES 2　onchocerciasis (B73)
　　　　tropical (pulmonary) eosinophilia NOS (J82)

B74.0　Filariasis due to Wuchereria bancrofti
　　Bancroftian elephantiasis
　　Bancroftian filariasis

B74.1　Filariasis due to Brugia malayi

B74.2　Filariasis due to Brugia timori

B74.3　Loiasis
　　Calabar swelling
　　Eyeworm disease of Africa
　　Loa loa infection

B74.4　Mansonelliasis
　　Infection due to Mansonella ozzardi
　　Infection due to Mansonella perstans
　　Infection due to Mansonella streptocerca

B74.8　Other filariases
　　Dirofilariasis

B74.9　Filariasis, unspecified ▽

B75　Trichinellosis
　　INCLUDES　infection due to Trichinella species
　　　　trichiniasis

✓4ᵗʰ B76　Hookworm diseases
　　INCLUDES　uncinariasis

B76.0　Ancylostomiasis
　　Infection due to Ancylostoma species

B76.1　Necatoriasis
　　Infection due to Necator americanus

B76.8　Other hookworm diseases

B76.9　Hookworm disease, unspecified ▽
　　Cutaneous larva migrans NOS

EXCLUDES 1　Not coded here　　　EXCLUDES 2　Not included here　　　N Newborn Age: 0　　　P Pediatric Age: 0-17　　　M Maternity Age: 12-55　　　A Adult Age: 15-124

452　　　　　　　　　　　　　　　　　　　　　　　　　　　　　　　　　　ICD-10-CM 2018

☑4ᵗʰ **B77 Ascariasis**
   INCLUDES   ascaridiasis
             roundworm infection

   B77.0 Ascariasis with intestinal complications

☑5ᵗʰ   **B77.8 Ascariasis with other complications**
       B77.81 Ascariasis pneumonia
       B77.89 Ascariasis with other complications

   B77.9 Ascariasis, unspecified ▽

☑4ᵗʰ **B78 Strongyloidiasis**
   EXCLUDES 1   trichostrongyliasis (B81.2)

   B78.0 Intestinal strongyloidiasis

   B78.1 Cutaneous strongyloidiasis

   B78.7 Disseminated strongyloidiasis

   B78.9 Strongyloidiasis, unspecified ▽

B79 Trichuriasis
   INCLUDES   trichocephaliasis
             whipworm (disease)(infection)

B80 Enterobiasis
   INCLUDES   oxyuriasis
             pinworm infection
             threadworm infection

☑4ᵗʰ **B81 Other intestinal helminthiases, not elsewhere classified**
   EXCLUDES 1 ►angiostrongyliasis due to:
         angiostrongylus cantonensis (B83.2)
         parastrongylus cantonensis (B83.2) ◄

   B81.0 Anisakiasis
        Infection due to Anisakis larva

   B81.1 Intestinal capillariasis
        Capillariasis NOS
        Infection due to Capillaria philippinensis
       EXCLUDES 2   hepatic capillariasis (B83.8)

   B81.2 Trichostrongyliasis

   B81.3 Intestinal angiostrongyliasis
        ►Angiostrongyliasis due to:
         angiostrongylus costaricensis
         parastrongylus costaricensis◄

   B81.4 Mixed intestinal helminthiases
        Infection due to intestinal helminths classified to more than one
         of the categories B65.0-B81.3 and B81.8
        Mixed helminthiasis NOS

   B81.8 Other specified intestinal helminthiases
        Infection due to Oesophagostomum species
         [esophagostomiasis]
        Infection due to Ternidens diminutus [ternidensiasis]

☑4ᵗʰ **B82 Unspecified intestinal parasitism**
   B82.0 Intestinal helminthiasis, unspecified ▽
   B82.9 Intestinal parasitism, unspecified ▽

☑4ᵗʰ **B83 Other helminthiases**
   EXCLUDES 1   capillariasis NOS (B81.1)
   EXCLUDES 2   intestinal capillariasis (B81.1)

   B83.0 Visceral larva migrans
        Toxocariasis

   B83.1 Gnathostomiasis
        Wandering swelling

   B83.2 Angiostrongyliasis due to Parastrongylus cantonensis
        Eosinophilic meningoencephalitis due to Parastrongylus
         cantonensis
       EXCLUDES 2   intestinal angiostrongyliasis (B81.3)

   B83.3 Syngamiasis
        Syngamosis

   B83.4 Internal hirudiniasis
       EXCLUDES 2   external hirudiniasis (B88.3)

   B83.8 Other specified helminthiases
        Acanthocephaliasis
        Gongylonemiasis
        Hepatic capillariasis
        Metastrongyliasis
        Thelaziasis

   B83.9 Helminthiasis, unspecified ▽
        Worms NOS
       EXCLUDES 1   intestinal helminthiasis NOS (B82.0)

Pediculosis, acariasis and other infestations (B85-B89)

☑4ᵗʰ **B85 Pediculosis and phthiriasis**

   B85.0 Pediculosis due to Pediculus humanus capitis
        Head-louse infestation

   B85.1 Pediculosis due to Pediculus humanus corporis
        Body-louse infestation

   B85.2 Pediculosis, unspecified ▽

   B85.3 Phthiriasis
        Infestation by crab-louse
        Infestation by Phthirus pubis

   B85.4 Mixed pediculosis and phthiriasis
        Infestation classifiable to more than one of the categories
         B85.0- B85.3

B86 Scabies
      Sarcoptic itch

☑4ᵗʰ **B87 Myiasis**
   INCLUDES   infestation by larva of flies

   B87.0 Cutaneous myiasis
        Creeping myiasis

   B87.1 Wound myiasis
        Traumatic myiasis

   B87.2 Ocular myiasis

   B87.3 Nasopharyngeal myiasis
        Laryngeal myiasis

   B87.4 Aural myiasis

☑5ᵗʰ   **B87.8 Myiasis of other sites**
       B87.81 Genitourinary myiasis
       B87.82 Intestinal myiasis
       B87.89 Myiasis of other sites

   B87.9 Myiasis, unspecified ▽

☑4ᵗʰ **B88 Other infestations**

   B88.0 Other acariasis
        Acarine dermatitis
        Dermatitis due to Demodex species
        Dermatitis due to Dermanyssus gallinae
        Dermatitis due to Liponyssoides sanguineus
        Trombiculosis
       EXCLUDES 2   scabies (B86)

   B88.1 Tungiasis [sandflea infestation]

   B88.2 Other arthropod infestations
        Scarabiasis

   B88.3 External hirudiniasis
        Leech infestation NOS
       EXCLUDES 2   internal hirudiniasis (B83.4)

   B88.8 Other specified infestations
        Ichthyoparasitism due to Vandellia cirrhosa
        Linguatulosis
        Porocephaliasis

   B88.9 Infestation, unspecified ▽
        Infestation (skin) NOS
        Infestation by mites NOS
        Skin parasites NOS

B89 Unspecified parasitic disease ▽

Sequelae of infectious and parasitic diseases (B90-B94)

   NOTE   Categories B90-B94 are to be used to indicate conditions in
        categories A00-B89 as the cause of sequelae, which are themselves
        classified elsewhere. The "sequelae" include conditions specified as
        such; they also include residuals of diseases classifiable to the above
        categories if there is no evidence that the disease itself is no longer
        present. Codes from these categories are not to be used for chronic
        infections. Code chronic current infections to active infectious
        disease as appropriate.

Code first condition resulting from (sequela) the infectious or parasitic disease

☑4ᵗʰ **B90 Sequelae of tuberculosis**

   B90.0 Sequelae of central nervous system tuberculosis

   B90.1 Sequelae of genitourinary tuberculosis

   B90.2 Sequelae of tuberculosis of bones and joints

   B90.8 Sequelae of tuberculosis of other organs
       EXCLUDES 2   sequelae of respiratory tuberculosis (B90.9)

   B90.9 Sequelae of respiratory and unspecified tuberculosis ▽
        Sequelae of tuberculosis NOS

B91 Sequelae of poliomyelitis
  EXCLUDES 1　postpolio syndrome (G14)

B92 Sequelae of leprosy

✓4th **B94 Sequelae of other and unspecified infectious and parasitic diseases**

　B94.0 **Sequelae of trachoma**

　B94.1 **Sequelae of viral encephalitis**

　B94.2 **Sequelae of viral hepatitis**

　B94.8 **Sequelae of other specified infectious and parasitic diseases**

　B94.9 **Sequelae of unspecified infectious and parasitic disease** ▽

Bacterial and viral infectious agents (B95-B97)

NOTE　These categories are provided for use as supplementary or additional codes to identify the infectious agent(s) in diseases classified elsewhere.

✓4th **B95 Streptococcus, Staphylococcus, and Enterococcus as the cause of diseases classified elsewhere**

　B95.0 **Streptococcus, group A, as the cause of diseases classified elsewhere**

　B95.1 **Streptococcus, group B, as the cause of diseases classified elsewhere**

　B95.2 **Enterococcus as the cause of diseases classified elsewhere**

　B95.3 **Streptococcus pneumoniae as the cause of diseases classified elsewhere**

　B95.4 **Other streptococcus as the cause of diseases classified elsewhere**

　B95.5 **Unspecified streptococcus as the cause of diseases classified elsewhere** ▽

　✓5th B95.6 **Staphylococcus aureus as the cause of diseases classified elsewhere**

　　B95.61 **Methicillin susceptible Staphylococcus aureus infection as the cause of diseases classified elsewhere**
　　　Methicillin susceptible Staphylococcus aureus (MSSA) infection as the cause of diseases classified elsewhere
　　　Staphylococcus aureus infection NOS as the cause of diseases classified elsewhere

　　B95.62 **Methicillin resistant Staphylococcus aureus infection as the cause of diseases classified elsewhere**
　　　Methicillin resistant Staphylococcus aureus (MRSA) infection as the cause of diseases classified elsewhere
　　　AHA: 2016, 1Q, 12

　B95.7 **Other staphylococcus as the cause of diseases classified elsewhere**

　B95.8 **Unspecified staphylococcus as the cause of diseases classified elsewhere** ▽

✓4th **B96 Other bacterial agents as the cause of diseases classified elsewhere**

　B96.0 **Mycoplasma pneumoniae [M. pneumoniae] as the cause of diseases classified elsewhere**
　　Pleuro-pneumonia-like-organism [PPLO]

　B96.1 **Klebsiella pneumoniae [K. pneumoniae] as the cause of diseases classified elsewhere**

　✓5th B96.2 **Escherichia coli [E. coli] as the cause of diseases classified elsewhere**

　　B96.20 **Unspecified Escherichia coli [E. coli] as the cause of diseases classified elsewhere** ▽
　　　Escherichia coli [E. coli] NOS

　　B96.21 **Shiga toxin-producing Escherichia coli [E. coli] (STEC) O157 as the cause of diseases classified elsewhere**
　　　E. coli O157:H- (nonmotile) with confirmation of Shiga toxin
　　　E. coli O157 with confirmation of Shiga toxin when H antigen is unknown, or is not H7
　　　O157:H7 Escherichia coli [E.coli] with or without confirmation of Shiga toxin-production
　　　Shiga toxin-producing Escherichia coli [E.coli] O157:H7 with or without confirmation of Shiga toxin-production
　　　STEC O157:H7 with or without confirmation of Shiga toxin-production

　　B96.22 **Other specified Shiga toxin-producing Escherichia coli [E. coli] (STEC) as the cause of diseases classified elsewhere**
　　　Non-O157 Shiga toxin-producing Escherichia coli [E.coli]
　　　Non-O157 Shiga toxin-producing Escherichia coli [E.coli] with known O group

　　B96.23 **Unspecified Shiga toxin-producing Escherichia coli [E. coli] (STEC) as the cause of diseases classified elsewhere** ▽
　　　Shiga toxin-producing Escherichia coli [E. coli] with unspecified O group
　　　STEC NOS

　　B96.29 **Other Escherichia coli [E. coli] as the cause of diseases classified elsewhere**
　　　Non-Shiga toxin-producing E. coli

　B96.3 **Hemophilus influenzae [H. influenzae] as the cause of diseases classified elsewhere**

　B96.4 **Proteus (mirabilis) (morganii) as the cause of diseases classified elsewhere**

　B96.5 **Pseudomonas (aeruginosa) (mallei) (pseudomallei) as the cause of diseases classified elsewhere**
　　AHA: 2015, 1Q, 18

　B96.6 **Bacteroides fragilis [B. fragilis] as the cause of diseases classified elsewhere**

　B96.7 **Clostridium perfringens [C. perfringens] as the cause of diseases classified elsewhere**

　✓5th B96.8 **Other specified bacterial agents as the cause of diseases classified elsewhere**

　　B96.81 **Helicobacter pylori [H. pylori] as the cause of diseases classified elsewhere**

　　B96.82 **Vibrio vulnificus as the cause of diseases classified elsewhere**

　　B96.89 **Other specified bacterial agents as the cause of diseases classified elsewhere**

✓4th **B97 Viral agents as the cause of diseases classified elsewhere**
　AHA: 2016, 3Q, 8-10, 14

　B97.0 **Adenovirus as the cause of diseases classified elsewhere**

　✓5th B97.1 **Enterovirus as the cause of diseases classified elsewhere**

　　B97.10 **Unspecified enterovirus as the cause of diseases classified elsewhere** ▽

　　B97.11 **Coxsackievirus as the cause of diseases classified elsewhere**

　　B97.12 **Echovirus as the cause of diseases classified elsewhere**

　　B97.19 **Other enterovirus as the cause of diseases classified elsewhere**

　✓5th B97.2 **Coronavirus as the cause of diseases classified elsewhere**

　　B97.21 **SARS-associated coronavirus as the cause of diseases classified elsewhere**
　　　EXCLUDES 1　pneumonia due to SARS-associated coronavirus (J12.81)

　　B97.29 **Other coronavirus as the cause of diseases classified elsewhere**

　✓5th B97.3 **Retrovirus as the cause of diseases classified elsewhere**
　　EXCLUDES 1　human immunodeficiency virus [HIV} disease (B20)

　　B97.30 **Unspecified retrovirus as the cause of diseases classified elsewhere** ▽

　　B97.31 **Lentivirus as the cause of diseases classified elsewhere**

　　B97.32 **Oncovirus as the cause of diseases classified elsewhere**

　　B97.33 **Human T-cell lymphotrophic virus, type I [HTLV-I] as the cause of diseases classified elsewhere**

　　B97.34 **Human T-cell lymphotrophic virus, type II [HTLV-II] as the cause of diseases classified elsewhere**

　　B97.35 **Human immunodeficiency virus, type 2 [HIV 2] as the cause of diseases classified elsewhere** HCC

　　B97.39 **Other retrovirus as the cause of diseases classified elsewhere**

　B97.4 **Respiratory syncytial virus as the cause of diseases classified elsewhere**

　B97.5 **Reovirus as the cause of diseases classified elsewhere**

　B97.6 **Parvovirus as the cause of diseases classified elsewhere**

　B97.7 **Papillomavirus as the cause of diseases classified elsewhere**

EXCLUDES 1 Not coded here　　　EXCLUDES 2 Not included here　　　N Newborn Age: 0　　　P Pediatric Age: 0-17　　　M Maternity Age: 12-55　　　A Adult Age: 15-124

454　　　　　　　　　　　　　　　　　　　　　　　　　　　　　　　　　　　ICD-10-CM 2018

☑5ᵗʰ **B97.8** **Other viral agents as the cause of diseases classified elsewhere**

    B97.81 Human metapneumovirus as the cause of diseases classified elsewhere

    B97.89 Other viral agents as the cause of diseases classified elsewhere

Other infectious diseases (B99)

☑4ᵗʰ **B99** **Other and unspecified infectious diseases**

    B99.8 Other infectious disease

    B99.9 Unspecified infectious disease   ▽

☑ Additional Character Req   ✓x7ᵗʰ Placeholder Alert   Manifestation   HCC CMS-HCC Condition   ▽ Unspecified Code   ►◄ Revised Text   ● New Code   ▲ Revised Code Title

ICD-10-CM 2018   **455**

Chapter 2. Neoplasms (C00–D49)

Chapter Specific Guidelines with Coding Examples

The chapter specific guidelines from the ICD-10-CM Official Guidelines for Coding and Reporting have been provided below. Along with these guidelines are coding examples, contained in the shaded boxes, that have been developed to help illustrate the coding and/or sequencing guidance found in these guidelines.

General guidelines

Chapter 2 of the ICD-10-CM contains the codes for most benign and all malignant neoplasms. Certain benign neoplasms, such as prostatic adenomas, may be found in the specific body system chapters. To properly code a neoplasm it is necessary to determine from the record if the neoplasm is benign, in-situ, malignant, or of uncertain histologic behavior. If malignant, any secondary (metastatic) sites should also be determined.

Primary malignant neoplasms overlapping site boundaries

A primary malignant neoplasm that overlaps two or more contiguous (next to each other) sites should be classified to the subcategory/code .8 ('overlapping lesion'), unless the combination is specifically indexed elsewhere. For multiple neoplasms of the same site that are not contiguous such as tumors in different quadrants of the same breast, codes for each site should be assigned.

> A 62-year-old female with a malignant lesion of the upper lip that extends from the lipstick area to the labial frenulum
>
> **C00.8**   **Malignant neoplasm of overlapping sites of lip**
>
> *Explanation*: Because this is a single lesion that overlaps two contiguous sites, a single code for overlapping sites is assigned.

> A 74-year-old male is treated for two distinct malignant lesions, one in the mucosa of the upper lip and a second in the mucosa of the lower lip.
>
> **C00.3**   **Malignant neoplasm of upper lip, inner aspect**
>
> **C00.4**   **Malignant neoplasm of lower lip, inner aspect**
>
> *Explanation*: This patient has two distinct malignant lesions of the upper and lower lips. Because the lesions are not contiguous, two codes are reported.

Malignant neoplasm of ectopic tissue

Malignant neoplasms of ectopic tissue are to be coded to the site of origin mentioned, e.g., ectopic pancreatic malignant neoplasms involving the stomach are coded to **malignant neoplasm of** pancreas, unspecified (C25.9).

The neoplasm table in the Alphabetic Index should be referenced first. However, if the histological term is documented, that term should be referenced first, rather than going immediately to the Neoplasm Table, in order to determine which column in the Neoplasm Table is appropriate. For example, if the documentation indicates "adenoma," refer to the term in the Alphabetic Index to review the entries under this term and the instructional note to "see also neoplasm, by site, benign." The table provides the proper code based on the type of neoplasm and the site. It is important to select the proper column in the table that corresponds to the type of neoplasm. The Tabular List should then be referenced to verify that the correct code has been selected from the table and that a more specific site code does not exist.

See Section I.C.21. Factors influencing health status and contact with health services, Status, for information regarding Z15.0, codes for genetic susceptibility to cancer.

a. Treatment directed at the malignancy

If the treatment is directed at the malignancy, designate the malignancy as the principal diagnosis.

The only exception to this guideline is if a patient admission/encounter is solely for the administration of chemotherapy, immunotherapy or **external beam** radiation therapy, assign the appropriate Z51.-- code as the first-listed or principal diagnosis, and the diagnosis or problem for which the service is being performed as a secondary diagnosis.

b. Treatment of secondary site

When a patient is admitted because of a primary neoplasm with metastasis and treatment is directed toward the secondary site only, the secondary neoplasm is designated as the principal diagnosis even though the primary malignancy is still present.

> Patient with primary prostate cancer with metastasis to lungs presents for wedge resection of mass in right lung
>
> **C78.01**   **Secondary malignant neoplasm of right lung**
>
> **C61**   **Malignant neoplasm of prostate**
>
> *Explanation*: Since the encounter is for treatment of the lung metastasis, the secondary lung metastasis is sequenced before the primary prostate cancer.

c. Coding and sequencing of complications

Coding and sequencing of complications associated with the malignancies or with the therapy thereof are subject to the following guidelines:

1) Anemia associated with malignancy

When admission/encounter is for management of an anemia associated with the malignancy, and the treatment is only for anemia, the appropriate code for the malignancy is sequenced as the principal or first-listed diagnosis followed by the appropriate code for the anemia (such as code D63.0, Anemia in neoplastic disease).

> Patient is seen for treatment of anemia in advanced primary liver cancer
>
> **C22.8**   **Malignant neoplasm of liver, primary, unspecified as to type**
>
> **D63.0**   **Anemia in neoplastic disease**
>
> *Explanation*: Even though the admission was solely to treat the anemia, this guideline indicates that the code for the malignancy is sequenced first.

2) Anemia associated with chemotherapy, immunotherapy and radiation therapy

When the admission/encounter is for management of an anemia associated with an adverse effect of the administration of chemotherapy or immunotherapy and the only treatment is for the anemia, the anemia code is sequenced first followed by the appropriate codes for the neoplasm and the adverse effect (T45.1X5, Adverse effect of antineoplastic and immunosuppressive drugs).

> A 56-year-old Hispanic male with grade II follicular lymphoma involving multiple lymph node sites referred for blood transfusion to treat anemia due to chemotherapy
>
> **D64.81**   **Anemia due to antineoplastic chemotherapy**
>
> **C82.18**   **Follicular lymphoma grade II, lymph nodes of multiple sites**
>
> **T45.1X5A**   **Adverse effect of antineoplastic and immunosuppressive drugs, initial encounter**
>
> *Explanation*: The code for the anemia is sequenced first followed by the code for the malignant neoplasm and lastly the code for the adverse effect.

When the admission/encounter is for management of an anemia associated with an adverse effect of radiotherapy, the anemia code should be sequenced first, followed by the appropriate neoplasm code and code Y84.2, Radiological procedure and radiotherapy as the cause of abnormal reaction of the patient, or of later complication, without mention of misadventure at the time of the procedure.

A 55-year-old male with a large malignant rectal tumor has been receiving external radiation therapy to shrink the tumor prior to planned surgery. He is referred today for a blood transfusion to treat anemia related to radiation therapy.

D64.89	Other specified anemias
C20	Malignant neoplasm of rectum
Y84.2	Radiological procedure and radiotherapy as the cause of abnormal reaction of the patient, or of later complication, without mention of misadventure at the time of the procedure

Explanation: The code for the anemia is sequenced first, followed by the code for the malignancy, and lastly the code for the abnormal reaction due to radiotherapy.

3) Management of dehydration due to the malignancy

When the admission/encounter is for management of dehydration due to the malignancy and only the dehydration is being treated (intravenous rehydration), the dehydration is sequenced first, followed by the code(s) for the malignancy.

4) Treatment of a complication resulting from a surgical procedure

When the admission/encounter is for treatment of a complication resulting from a surgical procedure, designate the complication as the principal or first-listed diagnosis if treatment is directed at resolving the complication.

d. Primary malignancy previously excised

When a primary malignancy has been previously excised or eradicated from its site and there is no further treatment directed to that site and there is no evidence of any existing primary malignancy, a code from category Z85, Personal history of malignant neoplasm, should be used to indicate the former site of the malignancy. Any mention of extension, invasion, or metastasis to another site is coded as a secondary malignant neoplasm to that site. The secondary site may be the principal or first-listed with the Z85 code used as a secondary code.

History of lung cancer, left upper lobectomy 18 months ago with no current treatment; MRI of the brain shows metastatic disease in the brain

C79.31	Secondary malignant neoplasm of brain
Z85.118	Personal history of other other malignant neoplasm of bronchifus and bronchfuls and lung

Explanation: The patient has undergone a diagnostic procedure that revealed metastatic lung cancer in the brain. The code for the secondary (metastatic) site is sequenced first, followed by a personal history code to identify the former site of the primary malignancy.

e. Admissions/encounters involving chemotherapy, immunotherapy and radiation therapy

1) Episode of care involves surgical removal of neoplasm

When an episode of care involves the surgical removal of a neoplasm, primary or secondary site, followed by adjunct chemotherapy or radiation treatment during the same episode of care, the code for the neoplasm should be assigned as principal or first-listed diagnosis.

2) Patient admission/encounter solely for administration of chemotherapy, immunotherapy and radiation therapy

If a patient admission/encounter is solely for the administration of chemotherapy, immunotherapy or **external beam** radiation therapy assign code Z51.0, Encounter for antineoplastic radiation therapy, or Z51.11, Encounter for antineoplastic chemotherapy, or Z51.12, Encounter for antineoplastic immunotherapy as the first-listed or principal diagnosis. If a patient receives more than one of these therapies during the same admission more than one of these codes may be assigned, in any sequence.

The malignancy for which the therapy is being administered should be assigned as a secondary diagnosis.

If a patient admission/encounter is for the insertion or implantation of radioactive elements (e.g., brachytherapy) the appropriate code for the malignancy is sequenced as the principal or first-listed diagnosis. Code Z51.0 should not be assigned.

Patient presents for second round of rituximab and fludarabine for his chronic B cell lymphocytic leukemia

Z51.11	Encounter for antineoplastic chemotherapy
Z51.12	Encounter for antineoplastic immunotherapy
C91.10	Chronic lymphocytic leukemia of B-cell type not having achieved remission

Explanation: Rituximab is an antineoplastic immunotherapy while fludarabine is an antineoplastic chemotherapy. The two treatments are often used together. The encounter was solely for the purpose of administering this treatment and either can be sequenced first, before the neoplastic condition.

3) Patient admitted for radiation therapy, chemotherapy or immunotherapy and develops complications

When a patient is admitted for the purpose of **external beam** radiotherapy, immunotherapy or chemotherapy and develops complications such as uncontrolled nausea and vomiting or dehydration, the principal or first-listed diagnosis is Z51.0, Encounter for antineoplastic radiation therapy, or Z51.11, Encounter for antineoplastic chemotherapy, or Z51.12, Encounter for antineoplastic immunotherapy followed by any codes for the complications.

When a patient is admitted for the purpose of insertion or implantation of radioactive elements (e.g., brachytherapy)and develops complications such as uncontrolled nausea and vomiting or dehydration, the principal or first-listed diagnosis is the appropriate code for the malignancy followed by any codes for the complications.

f. Admission/encounter to determine extent of malignancy

When the reason for admission/encounter is to determine the extent of the malignancy, or for a procedure such as paracentesis or thoracentesis, the primary malignancy or appropriate metastatic site is designated as the principal or first-listed diagnosis, even though chemotherapy or radiotherapy is administered.

Patient with left lung cancer with malignant pleural effusion being seen for paracentesis and initiation/administration of chemotherapy

C34.92	Malignant neoplasm of unspecified part of left bronchus or lung
J91.0	Malignant pleural effusion
Z51.11	Encounter for antineoplastic chemotherapy

Explanation: The lung cancer is sequenced before the chemotherapy in this instance because the paracentesis for the malignant effusion is also being performed. An instructional note under the malignant effusion instructs that the lung cancer be sequenced first.

g. Symptoms, signs, and abnormal findings listed in Chapter 18 associated with neoplasms

Symptoms, signs, and ill-defined conditions listed in Chapter 18 characteristic of, or associated with, an existing primary or secondary site malignancy cannot be used to replace the malignancy as principal or first-listed diagnosis, regardless of the number of admissions or encounters for treatment and care of the neoplasm.

See Section I.C.21. Factors influencing health status and contact with health services, Encounter for prophylactic organ removal.

h. Admission/encounter for pain control/management

See Section I.C.6. for information on coding admission/encounter for pain control/management.

i. Malignancy in two or more noncontiguous sites

A patient may have more than one malignant tumor in the same organ. These tumors may represent different primaries or metastatic disease, depending on the site. Should the documentation be unclear, the provider should be queried as to the status of each tumor so that the correct codes can be assigned.

Chapter 2. Neoplasms

j. Disseminated malignant neoplasm, unspecified

Code C80.0, Disseminated malignant neoplasm, unspecified, is for use only in those cases where the patient has advanced metastatic disease and no known primary or secondary sites are specified. It should not be used in place of assigning codes for the primary site and all known secondary sites.

> Patient who has had no medical care for many years is seen today and diagnosed with carcinomatosis
>
> **C80.0**   **Disseminated malignant neoplasm, unspecified**
>
> *Explanation*: Carcinomatosis NOS is an "includes" note under this code. Should seldom be used but is available for use in cases such as this.

k. Malignant neoplasm without specification of site

Code C80.1, Malignant (primary) neoplasm, unspecified, equates to Cancer, unspecified. This code should only be used when no determination can be made as to the primary site of a malignancy. This code should rarely be used in the inpatient setting.

> Evaluation of painful hip leads to diagnosis of a metastatic bone lesion from an unknown primary neoplasm source
>
> **C79.51**   **Secondary malignant neoplasm of bone**
>
> **C80.1**   **Malignant (primary) neoplasm, unspecified**
>
> *Explanation*: If only the secondary site is known, use code C80.1 for the unknown primary site.

l. Sequencing of neoplasm codes

1) Encounter for treatment of primary malignancy

If the reason for the encounter is for treatment of a primary malignancy, assign the malignancy as the principal/first-listed diagnosis. The primary site is to be sequenced first, followed by any metastatic sites.

2) Encounter for treatment of secondary malignancy

When an encounter is for a primary malignancy with metastasis and treatment is directed toward the metastatic (secondary) site(s) only, the metastatic site(s) is designated as the principal/first-listed diagnosis. The primary malignancy is coded as an additional code.

> Patient has primary colon cancer with metastasis to rib and is evaluated for possible excision of portion of rib bone
>
> **C79.51**   **Secondary malignant neoplasm of bone**
>
> **C18.9**   **Malignant neoplasm of colon, unspecified**
>
> *Explanation*: The treatment for this encounter is focused on the metastasis to the rib bone rather than the primary colon cancer, thus indicating that the bone metastasis is sequenced as the first-listed code.

3) Malignant neoplasm in a pregnant patient

When a pregnant woman has a malignant neoplasm, a code from subcategory O9A.1-, Malignant neoplasm complicating pregnancy, childbirth, and the puerperium, should be sequenced first, followed by the appropriate code from Chapter 2 to indicate the type of neoplasm.

> A 30-year-old pregnant female in first trimester evaluated for pituitary gland malignancy
>
> **O9A.111**   **Malignant neoplasm complicating pregnancy, first trimester**
>
> **C75.1**   **Malignant neoplasm of pituitary gland**
>
> *Explanation*: Codes from chapter 15 describing complications of pregnancy are sequenced as first-listed codes, further specified by codes from other chapters such as neoplastic, unless the pregnancy is documented as incidental to the condition. See also guideline 1.C.15.a.1.

4) Encounter for complication associated with a neoplasm

When an encounter is for management of a complication associated with a neoplasm, such as dehydration, and the treatment is only for the complication, the complication is coded first, followed by the appropriate code(s) for the neoplasm.

The exception to this guideline is anemia. When the admission/encounter is for management of an anemia associated with the malignancy, and the treatment is only for anemia, the appropriate code for the malignancy is sequenced as the principal or first-listed diagnosis followed by code D63.0, Anemia in neoplastic disease.

> Patient with pancreatic cancer is seen for initiation of TPN for cancer-related moderate protein-calorie malnutrition
>
> **E44.0**   **Moderate protein-calorie malnutrition**
>
> **C25.9**   **Malignant neoplasm of pancreas, unspecified**
>
> *Explanation*: The encounter is to initiate treatment for malnutrition, a common complication of many types of neoplasms, and is sequenced first.

5) Complication from surgical procedure for treatment of a neoplasm

When an encounter is for treatment of a complication resulting from a surgical procedure performed for the treatment of the neoplasm, designate the complication as the principal/first-listed diagnosis. See guideline regarding the coding of a current malignancy versus personal history to determine if the code for the neoplasm should also be assigned.

6) Pathologic fracture due to a neoplasm

When an encounter is for a pathological fracture due to a neoplasm, and the focus of treatment is the fracture, a code from subcategory M84.5, Pathological fracture in neoplastic disease, should be sequenced first, followed by the code for the neoplasm.

If the focus of treatment is the neoplasm with an associated pathological fracture, the neoplasm code should be sequenced first, followed by a code from M84.5 for the pathological fracture.

m. Current malignancy versus personal history of malignancy

When a primary malignancy has been excised but further treatment, such as an additional surgery for the malignancy, radiation therapy or chemotherapy is directed to that site, the primary malignancy code should be used until treatment is completed.

When a primary malignancy has been previously excised or eradicated from its site, there is no further treatment (of the malignancy) directed to that site, and there is no evidence of any existing primary malignancy, a code from category Z85, Personal history of malignant neoplasm, should be used to indicate the former site of the malignancy.

See Section I.C.21. Factors influencing health status and contact with health services, History (of)

> Female patient with ongoing chemotherapy after right mastectomy for breast cancer
>
> **C50.911**   **Malignant neoplasm of unspecified site of right female breast**
>
> **Z90.11**   **Acquired absence of right breast and nipple**
>
> *Explanation*: Even though the breast has been removed, the breast cancer is still being treated with chemotherapy and therefore is still coded as a current condition rather than personal history.

n. Leukemia, multiple myeloma, and malignant plasma cell neoplasms in remission versus personal history

The categories for leukemia, and category C90, Multiple myeloma and malignant plasma cell neoplasms, have codes indicating whether or not the leukemia has achieved remission. There are also codes Z85.6, Personal history of leukemia, and Z85.79, Personal history of other malignant neoplasms of lymphoid, hematopoietic and related tissues. If the documentation is unclear as to whether the leukemia has achieved remission, the provider should be queried.

See Section I.C.21. Factors influencing health status and contact with health services, History (of)

o. Aftercare following surgery for neoplasm

See Section I.C.21. Factors influencing health status and contact with health services, Aftercare

p. Follow-up care for completed treatment of a malignancy

See Section I.C.21. Factors influencing health status and contact with health services, Follow-up

q. Prophylactic organ removal for prevention of malignancy

See Section I.C. 21, Factors influencing health status and contact with health services, Prophylactic organ removal

r. Malignant neoplasm associated with transplanted organ

A malignant neoplasm of a transplanted organ should be coded as a transplant complication. Assign first the appropriate code from category T86.-, Complications of transplanted organs and tissue, followed by code C80.2, Malignant neoplasm associated with transplanted organ. Use an additional code for the specific malignancy.

Chapter 2. Neoplasms (C00-D49)

NOTE

Functional activity

All neoplasms are classified in this chapter, whether they are functionally active or not. An additional code from Chapter 4 may be used, to identify functional activity associated with any neoplasm.

Morphology [Histology]

Chapter 2 classifies neoplasms primarily by site (topography), with broad groupings for behavior, malignant, in situ, benign, etc. The Table of Neoplasms should be used to identify the correct topography code. In a few cases, such as for malignant melanoma and certain neuroendocrine tumors, the morphology (histologic type) is included in the category and codes.

Primary malignant neoplasms overlapping site boundaries

A primary malignant neoplasm that overlaps two or more contiguous (next to each other) sites should be classified to the subcategory/code .8 ("overlapping lesion"), unless the combination is specifically indexed elsewhere. For multiple neoplasms of the same site that are not contiguous, such as tumors in different quadrants of the same breast, codes for each site should be assigned.

Malignant neoplasm of ectopic tissue

Malignant neoplasms of ectopic tissue are to be coded to the site mentioned, e.g., ectopic pancreatic malignant neoplasms are coded to pancreas, unspecified (C25.9).

AHA: 2017, 1Q, 4, 5-6, 8

This chapter contains the following blocks:

C00-C14	Malignant neoplasms of lip, oral cavity and pharynx
C15-C26	Malignant neoplasms of digestive organs
C30-C39	Malignant neoplasms of respiratory and intrathoracic organs
C40-C41	Malignant neoplasms of bone and articular cartilage
C43-C44	Melanoma and other malignant neoplasms of skin
C45-C49	Malignant neoplasms of mesothelial and soft tissue
C50	Malignant neoplasms of breast
C51-C58	Malignant neoplasms of female genital organs
C60-C63	Malignant neoplasms of male genital organs
C64-C68	Malignant neoplasms of urinary tract
C69-C72	Malignant neoplasms of eye, brain and other parts of central nervous system
C73-C75	Malignant neoplasms of thyroid and other endocrine glands
C7A	Malignant neuroendocrine tumors
C7B	Secondary neuroendocrine tumors
C76-C80	Malignant neoplasms of ill-defined, other secondary and unspecified sites
C81-C96	Malignant neoplasms of lymphoid, hematopoietic and related tissue
D00-D09	In situ neoplasms
D10-D36	Benign neoplasms, except benign neuroendocrine tumors
D3A	Benign neuroendocrine tumors
D37-D48	Neoplasms of uncertain behavior, polycythemia vera and myelodysplastic syndromes
D49	Neoplasms of unspecified behavior

MALIGNANT NEOPLASMS (C00-C96)

Malignant neoplasms, stated or presumed to be primary (of specified sites), and certain specified histologies, except neuroendocrine, and of lymphoid, hematopoietic and related tissue (C00-C75)

Malignant neoplasms of lip, oral cavity and pharynx (C00-C14)

✓4ᵗʰ C00   Malignant neoplasm of lip

Use additional code to identify:
alcohol abuse and dependence (F10.-)
history of tobacco dependence (Z87.891)
tobacco dependence (F17.-)
tobacco use (Z72.0)

EXCLUDES 1   malignant melanoma of lip (C43.0)
Merkel cell carcinoma of lip (C4A.0)
other and unspecified malignant neoplasm of skin of lip (C44.0-)

C00.0   Malignant neoplasm of external upper lip
Malignant neoplasm of lipstick area of upper lip
Malignant neoplasm of upper lip NOS
Malignant neoplasm of vermilion border of upper lip

C00.1   Malignant neoplasm of external lower lip
Malignant neoplasm of lower lip NOS
Malignant neoplasm of lipstick area of lower lip
Malignant neoplasm of vermilion border of lower lip

C00.2   Malignant neoplasm of external lip, unspecified ▽
Malignant neoplasm of vermilion border of lip NOS

Malignant Neoplasm of Tongue

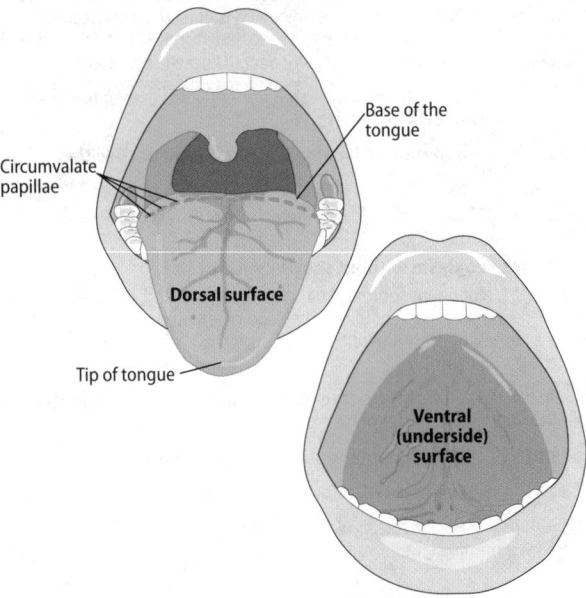

Circumvalate papillae
Base of the tongue
Dorsal surface
Tip of tongue
Ventral (underside) surface

C00.3   Malignant neoplasm of upper lip, inner aspect
Malignant neoplasm of buccal aspect of upper lip
Malignant neoplasm of frenulum of upper lip
Malignant neoplasm of mucosa of upper lip
Malignant neoplasm of oral aspect of upper lip

C00.4   Malignant neoplasm of lower lip, inner aspect
Malignant neoplasm of buccal aspect of lower lip
Malignant neoplasm of frenulum of lower lip
Malignant neoplasm of mucosa of lower lip
Malignant neoplasm of oral aspect of lower lip

C00.5   Malignant neoplasm of lip, unspecified, inner aspect ▽
Malignant neoplasm of buccal aspect of lip, unspecified
Malignant neoplasm of frenulum of lip, unspecified
Malignant neoplasm of mucosa of lip, unspecified
Malignant neoplasm of oral aspect of lip, unspecified

C00.6   Malignant neoplasm of commissure of lip, unspecified ▽

C00.8   Malignant neoplasm of overlapping sites of lip

C00.9   Malignant neoplasm of lip, unspecified ▽

C01   Malignant neoplasm of base of tongue   HCC
Malignant neoplasm of dorsal surface of base of tongue
Malignant neoplasm of fixed part of tongue NOS
Malignant neoplasm of posterior third of tongue

Use additional code to identify:
alcohol abuse and dependence (F10.-)
history of tobacco dependence (Z87.891)
tobacco dependence (F17.-)
tobacco use (Z72.0)

✓4ᵗʰ C02   Malignant neoplasm of other and unspecified parts of tongue

Use additional code to identify:
alcohol abuse and dependence (F10.-)
history of tobacco dependence (Z87.891)
tobacco dependence (F17.-)
tobacco use (Z72.0)

C02.0   Malignant neoplasm of dorsal surface of tongue   HCC
Malignant neoplasm of anterior two-thirds of tongue, dorsal surface

EXCLUDES 2   malignant neoplasm of dorsal surface of base of tongue (C01)

C02.1   Malignant neoplasm of border of tongue   HCC
Malignant neoplasm of tip of tongue

C02.2   Malignant neoplasm of ventral surface of tongue   HCC
Malignant neoplasm of anterior two-thirds of tongue, ventral surface
Malignant neoplasm of frenulum linguae

C02.3   Malignant neoplasm of anterior two-thirds of tongue, part unspecified   HCC
Malignant neoplasm of middle third of tongue NOS
Malignant neoplasm of mobile part of tongue NOS

C02.4   Malignant neoplasm of lingual tonsil   HCC
EXCLUDES 2   malignant neoplasm of tonsil NOS (C09.9)

C02.8   Malignant neoplasm of overlapping sites of tongue   HCC
Malignant neoplasm of two or more contiguous sites of tongue

EXCLUDES 1 Not coded here   **EXCLUDES 2** Not included here   N Newborn Age: 0   P Pediatric Age: 0-17   M Maternity Age: 12-55   A Adult Age: 15-124

460   ICD-10-CM 2018

C02.9   Malignant neoplasm of tongue, unspecified   HCC ▽

✓4ᵗʰ **C03**   **Malignant neoplasm of gum**
    INCLUDES   malignant neoplasm of alveolar (ridge) mucosa
                 malignant neoplasm of gingiva
    Use additional code to identify:
      alcohol abuse and dependence (F10.-)
      history of tobacco dependence (Z87.891)
      tobacco dependence (F17.-)
      tobacco use (Z72.0)
    EXCLUDES 2   malignant odontogenic neoplasms (C41.0-C41.1)

    C03.0   Malignant neoplasm of upper gum   HCC
    C03.1   Malignant neoplasm of lower gum   HCC
    C03.9   Malignant neoplasm of gum, unspecified   HCC ▽

✓4ᵗʰ **C04**   **Malignant neoplasm of floor of mouth**
    Use additional code to identify:
      alcohol abuse and dependence (F10.-)
      history of tobacco dependence (Z87.891)
      tobacco dependence (F17.-)
      tobacco use (Z72.0)

    C04.0   Malignant neoplasm of anterior floor of mouth   HCC
       Malignant neoplasm of anterior to the premolar-canine junction
    C04.1   Malignant neoplasm of lateral floor of mouth   HCC
    C04.8   Malignant neoplasm of overlapping sites of floor of mouth   HCC
    C04.9   Malignant neoplasm of floor of mouth, unspecified   HCC ▽

✓4ᵗʰ **C05**   **Malignant neoplasm of palate**
    Use additional code to identify:
      alcohol abuse and dependence (F10.-)
      history of tobacco dependence (Z87.891)
      tobacco dependence (F17.-)
      tobacco use (Z72.0)
    EXCLUDES 1   Kaposi's sarcoma of palate (C46.2)

    C05.0   Malignant neoplasm of hard palate   HCC
    C05.1   Malignant neoplasm of soft palate   HCC
       EXCLUDES 2   malignant neoplasm of nasopharyngeal surface of soft palate (C11.3)
    C05.2   Malignant neoplasm of uvula   HCC
    C05.8   Malignant neoplasm of overlapping sites of palate   HCC
    C05.9   Malignant neoplasm of palate, unspecified   HCC ▽
       Malignant neoplasm of roof of mouth

✓4ᵗʰ **C06**   **Malignant neoplasm of other and unspecified parts of mouth**
    Use additional code to identify:
      alcohol abuse and dependence (F10.-)
      history of tobacco dependence (Z87.891)
      tobacco dependence (F17.-)
      tobacco use (Z72.0)

    C06.0   Malignant neoplasm of cheek mucosa   HCC
       Malignant neoplasm of buccal mucosa NOS
       Malignant neoplasm of internal cheek
    C06.1   Malignant neoplasm of vestibule of mouth   HCC
       Malignant neoplasm of buccal sulcus (upper) (lower)
       Malignant neoplasm of labial sulcus (upper) (lower)
    C06.2   Malignant neoplasm of retromolar area   HCC
    ✓5ᵗʰ **C06.8**   Malignant neoplasm of overlapping sites of other and unspecified parts of mouth
      C06.80   Malignant neoplasm of overlapping sites of unspecified parts of mouth   HCC ▽
      C06.89   Malignant neoplasm of overlapping sites of other parts of mouth   HCC
         "book leaf" neoplasm [ventral surface of tongue and floor of mouth]
    C06.9   Malignant neoplasm of mouth, unspecified   HCC ▽
       Malignant neoplasm of minor salivary gland, unspecified site
       Malignant neoplasm of oral cavity NOS

C07   **Malignant neoplasm of parotid gland**   HCC
    Use additional code to identify:
      alcohol abuse and dependence (F10.-)
      exposure to environmental tobacco smoke (Z77.22)
      exposure to tobacco smoke in the perinatal period (P96.81)
      history of tobacco dependence (Z87.891)
      occupational exposure to environmental tobacco smoke (Z57.31)
      tobacco dependence (F17.-)
      tobacco use (Z72.0)

✓4ᵗʰ **C08**   **Malignant neoplasm of other and unspecified major salivary glands**
    INCLUDES   malignant neoplasm of salivary ducts
    Use additional code to identify:
      alcohol abuse and dependence (F10.-)
      exposure to environmental tobacco smoke (Z77.22)
      exposure to tobacco smoke in the perinatal period (P96.81)
      history of tobacco dependence (Z87.891)
      occupational exposure to environmental tobacco smoke (Z57.31)
      tobacco dependence (F17.-)
      tobacco use (Z72.0)
    EXCLUDES 1   malignant neoplasms of specified minor salivary glands which are classified according to their anatomical location
    EXCLUDES 2   malignant neoplasms of minor salivary glands NOS (C06.9)
               malignant neoplasm of parotid gland (C07)

    C08.0   Malignant neoplasm of submandibular gland   HCC
       Malignant neoplasm of submaxillary gland
    C08.1   Malignant neoplasm of sublingual gland   HCC
    C08.9   Malignant neoplasm of major salivary gland, unspecified   HCC ▽
       Malignant neoplasm of salivary gland (major) NOS

✓4ᵗʰ **C09**   **Malignant neoplasm of tonsil**
    Use additional code to identify:
      alcohol abuse and dependence (F10.-)
      exposure to environmental tobacco smoke (Z77.22)
      exposure to tobacco smoke in the perinatal period (P96.81)
      history of tobacco dependence (Z87.891)
      occupational exposure to environmental tobacco smoke (Z57.31)
      tobacco dependence (F17.-)
      tobacco use (Z72.0)
    EXCLUDES 2   malignant neoplasm of lingual tonsil (C02.4)
               malignant neoplasm of pharyngeal tonsil (C11.1)

    C09.0   Malignant neoplasm of tonsillar fossa   HCC
    C09.1   Malignant neoplasm of tonsillar pillar (anterior) (posterior)   HCC
    C09.8   Malignant neoplasm of overlapping sites of tonsil   HCC
    C09.9   Malignant neoplasm of tonsil, unspecified   HCC ▽
       Malignant neoplasm of tonsil NOS
       Malignant neoplasm of faucial tonsils
       Malignant neoplasm of palatine tonsils

✓4ᵗʰ **C10**   **Malignant neoplasm of oropharynx**
    Use additional code to identify:
      alcohol abuse and dependence (F10.-)
      exposure to environmental tobacco smoke (Z77.22)
      exposure to tobacco smoke in the perinatal period (P96.81)
      history of tobacco dependence (Z87.891)
      occupational exposure to environmental tobacco smoke (Z57.31)
      tobacco dependence (F17.-)
      tobacco use (Z72.0)
    EXCLUDES 2   malignant neoplasm of tonsil (C09.-)

    C10.0   Malignant neoplasm of vallecula   HCC
    C10.1   Malignant neoplasm of anterior surface of epiglottis   HCC
       Malignant neoplasm of epiglottis, free border [margin]
       Malignant neoplasm of glossoepiglottic fold(s)
       EXCLUDES 2   malignant neoplasm of epiglottis (suprahyoid portion) NOS (C32.1)
    C10.2   Malignant neoplasm of lateral wall of oropharynx   HCC
    C10.3   Malignant neoplasm of posterior wall of oropharynx   HCC
    C10.4   Malignant neoplasm of branchial cleft   HCC
       Malignant neoplasm of branchial cyst [site of neoplasm]
    C10.8   Malignant neoplasm of overlapping sites of oropharynx   HCC
       Malignant neoplasm of junctional region of oropharynx
    C10.9   Malignant neoplasm of oropharynx, unspecified   HCC ▽

✓4ᵗʰ **C11**   **Malignant neoplasm of nasopharynx**
    Use additional code to identify:
      exposure to environmental tobacco smoke (Z77.22)
      exposure to tobacco smoke in the perinatal period (P96.81)
      history of tobacco dependence (Z87.891)
      occupational exposure to environmental tobacco smoke (Z57.31)
      tobacco dependence (F17.-)
      tobacco use (Z72.0)

    C11.0   Malignant neoplasm of superior wall of nasopharynx   HCC
       Malignant neoplasm of roof of nasopharynx
    C11.1   Malignant neoplasm of posterior wall of nasopharynx   HCC
       Malignant neoplasm of adenoid
       Malignant neoplasm of pharyngeal tonsil

✓ Additional Character Req   ✓x7ᵗʰ Placeholder Alert   Manifestation   HCC CMS-HCC Condition   ▽ Unspecified Code   ►◄ Revised Text   ● New Code   ▲ Revised Code Title

ICD-10-CM 2018   **461**

C11.2 Malignant neoplasm of lateral wall of nasopharynx HCC
 Malignant neoplasm of fossa of Rosenmüller
 Malignant neoplasm of opening of auditory tube
 Malignant neoplasm of pharyngeal recess

C11.3 Malignant neoplasm of anterior wall of nasopharynx HCC
 Malignant neoplasm of floor of nasopharynx
 Malignant neoplasm of nasopharyngeal (anterior) (posterior) surface of soft palate
 Malignant neoplasm of posterior margin of nasal choana
 Malignant neoplasm of posterior margin of nasal septum

C11.8 Malignant neoplasm of overlapping sites of nasopharynx HCC

C11.9 Malignant neoplasm of nasopharynx, unspecified HCC ▽
 Malignant neoplasm of nasopharyngeal wall NOS

C12 Malignant neoplasm of pyriform sinus HCC
 Malignant neoplasm of pyriform fossa
 Use additional code to identify:
  exposure to environmental tobacco smoke (Z77.22)
  exposure to tobacco smoke in the perinatal period (P96.81)
  history of tobacco dependence (Z87.891)
  occupational exposure to environmental tobacco smoke (Z57.31)
  tobacco dependence (F17.-)
  tobacco use (Z72.0)

✓4ᵗʰ C13 Malignant neoplasm of hypopharynx
 Use additional code to identify:
  exposure to environmental tobacco smoke (Z77.22)
  exposure to tobacco smoke in the perinatal period (P96.81)
  history of tobacco dependence (Z87.891)
  occupational exposure to environmental tobacco smoke (Z57.31)
  tobacco dependence (F17.-)
  tobacco use (Z72.0)
 EXCLUDES 2 *malignant neoplasm of pyriform sinus (C12)*

C13.0 Malignant neoplasm of postcricoid region HCC

C13.1 Malignant neoplasm of aryepiglottic fold, hypopharyngeal aspect HCC
 Malignant neoplasm of aryepiglottic fold, marginal zone
 Malignant neoplasm of aryepiglottic fold NOS
 Malignant neoplasm of interarytenoid fold, marginal zone
 Malignant neoplasm of interarytenoid fold NOS
 EXCLUDES 2 *malignant neoplasm of aryepiglottic fold or interarytenoid fold, laryngeal aspect (C32.1)*

C13.2 Malignant neoplasm of posterior wall of hypopharynx HCC

C13.8 Malignant neoplasm of overlapping sites of hypopharynx HCC

C13.9 Malignant neoplasm of hypopharynx, unspecified HCC ▽
 Malignant neoplasm of hypopharyngeal wall NOS

✓4ᵗʰ C14 Malignant neoplasm of other and ill-defined sites in the lip, oral cavity and pharynx
 Use additional code to identify:
  alcohol abuse and dependence (F10.-)
  exposure to environmental tobacco smoke (Z77.22)
  exposure to tobacco smoke in the perinatal period (P96.81)
  history of tobacco dependence (Z87.891)
  occupational exposure to environmental tobacco smoke (Z57.31)
  tobacco dependence (F17.-)
  tobacco use (Z72.0)
 EXCLUDES 1 *malignant neoplasm of oral cavity NOS (C06.9)*

C14.0 Malignant neoplasm of pharynx, unspecified HCC ▽

C14.2 Malignant neoplasm of Waldeyer's ring HCC

C14.8 Malignant neoplasm of overlapping sites of lip, oral cavity and pharynx HCC
 Primary malignant neoplasm of two or more contiguous sites of lip, oral cavity and pharynx
 EXCLUDES 1 *"book leaf" neoplasm [ventral surface of tongue and floor of mouth] (C06.89)*

Malignant neoplasms of digestive organs (C15-C26)

EXCLUDES 1 *Kaposi's sarcoma of gastrointestinal sites (C46.4)*
EXCLUDES 2 *gastrointestinal stromal tumors (C49.A-)*

✓4ᵗʰ C15 Malignant neoplasm of esophagus
 Use additional code to identify:
  alcohol abuse and dependence (F10.-)

C15.3 Malignant neoplasm of upper third of esophagus HCC

C15.4 Malignant neoplasm of middle third of esophagus HCC

C15.5 Malignant neoplasm of lower third of esophagus HCC
 EXCLUDES 1 *malignant neoplasm of cardio-esophageal junction (C16.0)*

C15.8 Malignant neoplasm of overlapping sites of esophagus HCC

C15.9 Malignant neoplasm of esophagus, unspecified HCC ▽

✓4ᵗʰ C16 Malignant neoplasm of stomach
 Use additional code to identify:
  alcohol abuse and dependence (F10.-)
 EXCLUDES 2 *malignant carcinoid tumor of the stomach (C7A.092)*

C16.0 Malignant neoplasm of cardia HCC
 Malignant neoplasm of cardiac orifice
 Malignant neoplasm of cardio-esophageal junction
 Malignant neoplasm of esophagus and stomach
 Malignant neoplasm of gastro-esophageal junction

C16.1 Malignant neoplasm of fundus of stomach HCC

C16.2 Malignant neoplasm of body of stomach HCC

C16.3 Malignant neoplasm of pyloric antrum HCC
 Malignant neoplasm of gastric antrum

C16.4 Malignant neoplasm of pylorus HCC
 Malignant neoplasm of prepylorus
 Malignant neoplasm of pyloric canal

C16.5 Malignant neoplasm of lesser curvature of stomach, unspecified HCC ▽
 Malignant neoplasm of lesser curvature of stomach, not classifiable to C16.1-C16.4

C16.6 Malignant neoplasm of greater curvature of stomach, unspecified HCC ▽
 Malignant neoplasm of greater curvature of stomach, not classifiable to C16.0-C16.4

C16.8 Malignant neoplasm of overlapping sites of stomach HCC

C16.9 Malignant neoplasm of stomach, unspecified HCC ▽
 Gastric cancer NOS

✓4ᵗʰ C17 Malignant neoplasm of small intestine
 EXCLUDES 1 *malignant carcinoid tumors of the small intestine (C7A.01)*
 AHA: 2016, 1Q, 19

C17.0 Malignant neoplasm of duodenum HCC

C17.1 Malignant neoplasm of jejunum HCC

C17.2 Malignant neoplasm of ileum HCC
 EXCLUDES 1 *malignant neoplasm of ileocecal valve (C18.0)*

C17.3 Meckel's diverticulum, malignant HCC
 EXCLUDES 1 *Meckel's diverticulum, congenital (Q43.0)*

C17.8 Malignant neoplasm of overlapping sites of small intestine HCC

C17.9 Malignant neoplasm of small intestine, unspecified HCC ▽

✓4ᵗʰ C18 Malignant neoplasm of colon
 EXCLUDES 1 *malignant carcinoid tumors of the colon (C7A.02-)*

C18.0 Malignant neoplasm of cecum HCC
 Malignant neoplasm of ileocecal valve

C18.1 Malignant neoplasm of appendix HCC

C18.2 Malignant neoplasm of ascending colon HCC

C18.3 Malignant neoplasm of hepatic flexure HCC

C18.4 Malignant neoplasm of transverse colon HCC

C18.5 Malignant neoplasm of splenic flexure HCC

C18.6 Malignant neoplasm of descending colon HCC

C18.7 Malignant neoplasm of sigmoid colon HCC
 Malignant neoplasm of sigmoid (flexure)
 EXCLUDES 1 *malignant neoplasm of rectosigmoid junction (C19)*

C18.8 Malignant neoplasm of overlapping sites of colon HCC

C18.9 Malignant neoplasm of colon, unspecified HCC ▽
 Malignant neoplasm of large intestine NOS

C19 Malignant neoplasm of rectosigmoid junction HCC
 Malignant neoplasm of colon with rectum
 Malignant neoplasm of rectosigmoid (colon)
 EXCLUDES 1 *malignant carcinoid tumors of the colon (C7A.02-)*

C20 Malignant neoplasm of rectum HCC
 Malignant neoplasm of rectal ampulla
 EXCLUDES 1 *malignant carcinoid tumor of the rectum (C7A.026)*

✓4ᵗʰ C21 Malignant neoplasm of anus and anal canal
 EXCLUDES 2 *malignant carcinoid tumors of the colon (C7A.02-)*
  malignant melanoma of anal margin (C43.51)
  malignant melanoma of anal skin (C43.51)
  malignant melanoma of perianal skin (C43.51)
  other and unspecified malignant neoplasm of anal margin (C44.500, C44.510, C44.520, C44.590)
  other and unspecified malignant neoplasm of anal skin (C44.500, C44.510, C44.520, C44.590)
  other and unspecified malignant neoplasm of perianal skin (C44.500, C44.510, C44.520, C44.590)

C21.0 Malignant neoplasm of anus, unspecified HCC ▽

EXCLUDES 1 Not coded here   *EXCLUDES 2* Not included here   N Newborn Age: 0   P Pediatric Age: 0-17   M Maternity Age: 12-55   A Adult Age: 15-124

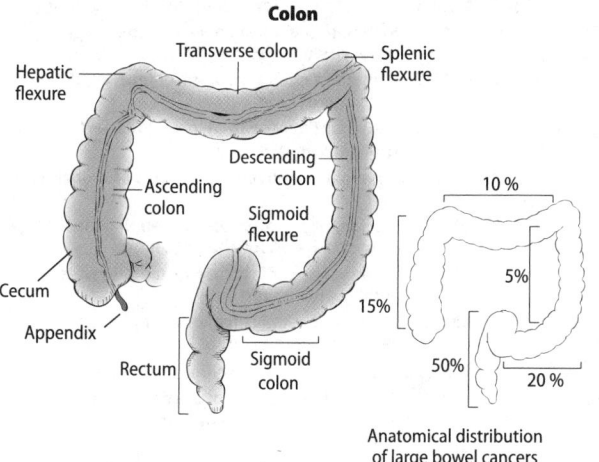

Colon

Transverse colon

Hepatic flexure

Splenic flexure

Descending colon

Ascending colon

Sigmoid flexure

Cecum

Appendix

Rectum

Sigmoid colon

10 %
5%
15%
50%
20 %

Anatomical distribution of large bowel cancers

Pancreas

Head   Neck   Body   Tail   Spleen

Common bile duct

Accesory pancreatic duct

Pancreatic duct (of Wirsung)

Uncinate process

Duodenum

Superior mesenteric artery and vein

C21.1   **Malignant neoplasm of** anal canal   HCC
      Malignant neoplasm of anal sphincter

C21.2   **Malignant neoplasm of** cloacogenic zone   HCC

C21.8   **Malignant neoplasm of** overlapping sites **of rectum,**   HCC
      anus and anal canal
      Malignant neoplasm of anorectal junction
      Malignant neoplasm of anorectum
      Primary malignant neoplasm of two or more contiguous sites of rectum, anus and anal canal

✓4ᵗʰ **C22**   **Malignant neoplasm of** liver and intrahepatic bile ducts
      Use additional code to identify:
      alcohol abuse and dependence (F10.-)
      hepatitis B (B16.-, B18.0-B18.1)
      hepatitis C (B17.1-, B18.2)
      EXCLUDES 1   *malignant neoplasm of biliary tract NOS (C24.9)*
            secondary malignant neoplasm of liver and intrahepatic bile duct (C78.7)

   C22.0   **Liver cell carcinoma**   HCC
      Hepatocellular carcinoma   Hepatoma
      AHA: 2016, 1Q, 18

   C22.1   **Intrahepatic bile duct carcinoma**   HCC
      Cholangiocarcinoma
      EXCLUDES 1   *malignant neoplasm of hepatic duct (C24.0)*

   C22.2   **Hepatoblastoma**   HCC

   C22.3   **Angiosarcoma of liver**   HCC
      Kupffer cell sarcoma

   C22.4   **Other** sarcomas **of liver**   HCC

   C22.7   **Other specified carcinomas of liver**   HCC

   C22.8   **Malignant neoplasm of liver, primary, unspecified**   HCC ▽
      as to type

   C22.9   **Malignant neoplasm of liver, not specified as primary**   HCC ▽
      or secondary

C23   **Malignant neoplasm of** gallbladder   HCC

✓4ᵗʰ **C24**   **Malignant neoplasm of** other and unspecified parts of biliary **tract**
      EXCLUDES 1   *malignant neoplasm of intrahepatic bile duct (C22.1)*

   C24.0   **Malignant neoplasm of** extrahepatic bile duct   HCC
      Malignant neoplasm of biliary duct or passage NOS
      Malignant neoplasm of common bile duct
      Malignant neoplasm of cystic duct
      Malignant neoplasm of hepatic duct

   C24.1   **Malignant neoplasm of** ampulla of Vater   HCC
      DEF: Malignant neoplasm in the area of dilation at the juncture of the common bile and pancreatic ducts near the opening into the lumen of the duodenum.

   C24.8   **Malignant neoplasm of** overlapping sites **of biliary tract**   HCC
      Malignant neoplasm involving both intrahepatic and extrahepatic bile ducts
      Primary malignant neoplasm of two or more contiguous sites of biliary tract

   C24.9   **Malignant neoplasm of biliary tract, unspecified**   HCC ▽

✓4ᵗʰ **C25**   **Malignant neoplasm of** pancreas
      Code also exocrine pancreatic insufficiency (K86.81)
      Use additional code to identify:
      alcohol abuse and dependence (F10.-)

   C25.0   **Malignant neoplasm of** head **of pancreas**   HCC

   C25.1   **Malignant neoplasm of** body **of pancreas**   HCC

   C25.2   **Malignant neoplasm of** tail **of pancreas**   HCC

   C25.3   **Malignant neoplasm of** pancreatic duct   HCC

   C25.4   **Malignant neoplasm of** endocrine **pancreas**   HCC
      Malignant neoplasm of islets of Langerhans
      Use additional code to identify any functional activity

   C25.7   **Malignant neoplasm of other parts of pancreas**   HCC
      Malignant neoplasm of neck of pancreas

   C25.8   **Malignant neoplasm of** overlapping sites **of pancreas**   HCC

   C25.9   **Malignant neoplasm of pancreas, unspecified**   HCC ▽

✓4ᵗʰ **C26**   **Malignant neoplasm of other and ill-defined digestive organs**
      EXCLUDES 1   *malignant neoplasm of peritoneum and retroperitoneum (C48.-)*

   C26.0   **Malignant neoplasm of** intestinal tract,   HCC ▽
      part unspecified
      Malignant neoplasm of intestine NOS

   C26.1   **Malignant neoplasm of** spleen   HCC
      EXCLUDES 1   *Hodgkin lymphoma (C81.-)*
            non-Hodgkin lymphoma (C82-C85)

   C26.9   **Malignant neoplasm of** ill-defined sites **within the**   HCC ▽
      digestive system
      Malignant neoplasm of alimentary canal or tract NOS
      Malignant neoplasm of gastrointestinal tract NOS
      EXCLUDES 1   *malignant neoplasm of abdominal NOS (C76.2)*
            malignant neoplasm of intra-abdominal NOS (C76.2)

Malignant neoplasms of respiratory and intrathoracic organs (C30-C39)

      INCLUDES   malignant neoplasm of middle ear
      EXCLUDES 1   *mesothelioma (C45.-)*

✓4ᵗʰ **C30**   **Malignant neoplasm of** nasal cavity and middle ear

   C30.0   **Malignant neoplasm of** nasal cavity   HCC
      Malignant neoplasm of cartilage of nose
      Malignant neoplasm of nasal concha
      Malignant neoplasm of internal nose
      Malignant neoplasm of septum of nose
      Malignant neoplasm of vestibule of nose
      EXCLUDES 1   *malignant melanoma of skin of nose (C43.31)*
            malignant neoplasm of nasal bone (C41.0)
            malignant neoplasm of nose NOS (C76.0)
            malignant neoplasm of olfactory bulb (C72.2-)
            malignant neoplasm of posterior margin of nasal septum and choana (C11.3)
            malignant neoplasm of turbinates (C41.0)
            other and unspecified malignant neoplasm of skin of nose (C44.301, C44.311, C44.321, C44.391)

   C30.1   **Malignant neoplasm of** middle ear   HCC
      Malignant neoplasm of antrum tympanicum
      Malignant neoplasm of auditory tube
      Malignant neoplasm of eustachian tube
      Malignant neoplasm of inner ear
      Malignant neoplasm of mastoid air cells
      Malignant neoplasm of tympanic cavity
      EXCLUDES 1   *malignant melanoma of skin of (external) ear (C43.2-)*
            malignant neoplasm of auricular canal (external) (C43.2-,C44.2-)
            malignant neoplasm of bone of ear (meatus) (C41.0)
            malignant neoplasm of cartilage of ear (C49.0)
            other and unspecified malignant neoplasm of skin of (external) ear (C44.2-)

✓ Additional Character Req   Placeholder Alert   Manifestation   HCC CMS-HCC Condition   ▽ Unspecified Code   ►◄ Revised Text   ● New Code   ▲ Revised Code Title

ICD-10-CM 2018   **463**

C21.1–C30.1

Chapter 2. Neoplasms

✓4ᵗʰ **C31 Malignant neoplasm of accessory sinuses**

C31.0 Malignant neoplasm of maxillary sinus `HCC`
Malignant neoplasm of antrum (Highmore) (maxillary)

C31.1 Malignant neoplasm of ethmoidal sinus `HCC`

C31.2 Malignant neoplasm of frontal sinus `HCC`

C31.3 Malignant neoplasm of sphenoid sinus `HCC`

C31.8 Malignant neoplasm of overlapping sites of accessory sinuses `HCC`

C31.9 Malignant neoplasm of accessory sinus, unspecified `HCC` ▽

✓4ᵗʰ **C32 Malignant neoplasm of larynx**
Use additional code to identify:
alcohol abuse and dependence (F10.-)
exposure to environmental tobacco smoke (Z77.22)
exposure to tobacco smoke in the perinatal period (P96.81)
history of tobacco dependence (Z87.891)
occupational exposure to environmental tobacco smoke (Z57.31)
tobacco dependence (F17.-)
tobacco use (Z72.0)

C32.0 Malignant neoplasm of glottis `HCC`
Malignant neoplasm of intrinsic larynx
Malignant neoplasm of laryngeal commissure (anterior)(posterior)
Malignant neoplasm of vocal cord (true) NOS

C32.1 Malignant neoplasm of supraglottis `HCC`
Malignant neoplasm of aryepiglottic fold or interarytenoid fold, laryngeal aspect
Malignant neoplasm of epiglottis (suprahyoid portion) NOS
Malignant neoplasm of extrinsic larynx
Malignant neoplasm of false vocal cord
Malignant neoplasm of posterior (laryngeal) surface of epiglottis
Malignant neoplasm of ventricular bands
EXCLUDES 2 *malignant neoplasm of anterior surface of epiglottis (C10.1)*
malignant neoplasm of aryepiglottic fold or interarytenoid fold, hypopharyngeal aspect (C13.1)
malignant neoplasm of aryepiglottic fold or interarytenoid fold, marginal zone (C13.1)
malignant neoplasm of aryepiglottic fold or interarytenoid fold NOS (C13.1)

C32.2 Malignant neoplasm of subglottis `HCC`

C32.3 Malignant neoplasm of laryngeal cartilage `HCC`

C32.8 Malignant neoplasm of overlapping sites of larynx `HCC`

C32.9 Malignant neoplasm of larynx, unspecified `HCC` ▽

C33 Malignant neoplasm of trachea `HCC`
Use additional code to identify:
exposure to environmental tobacco smoke (Z77.22)
exposure to tobacco smoke in the perinatal period (P96.81)
history of tobacco dependence (Z87.891)
occupational exposure to environmental tobacco smoke (Z57.31)
tobacco dependence (F17.-)
tobacco use (Z72.0)

✓4ᵗʰ **C34 Malignant neoplasm of bronchus and lung**
Use additional code to identify:
exposure to environmental tobacco smoke (Z77.22)
exposure to tobacco smoke in the perinatal period (P96.81)
history of tobacco dependence (Z87.891)
occupational exposure to environmental tobacco smoke (Z57.31)
tobacco dependence (F17.-)
tobacco use (Z72.0)
EXCLUDES 1 *Kaposi's sarcoma of lung (C46.5-)*
malignant carcinoid tumor of the bronchus and lung (C7A.090)

✓5ᵗʰ **C34.0 Malignant neoplasm of main bronchus**
Malignant neoplasm of carina
Malignant neoplasm of hilus (of lung)

C34.00 Malignant neoplasm of unspecified main bronchus `HCC` ▽

C34.01 Malignant neoplasm of right main bronchus `HCC`

C34.02 Malignant neoplasm of left main bronchus `HCC`

✓5ᵗʰ **C34.1 Malignant neoplasm of upper lobe, bronchus or lung**

C34.10 Malignant neoplasm of upper lobe, unspecified bronchus or lung `HCC` ▽

C34.11 Malignant neoplasm of upper lobe, right bronchus or lung `HCC`

C34.12 Malignant neoplasm of upper lobe, left bronchus or lung `HCC`

C34.2 Malignant neoplasm of middle lobe, bronchus or lung `HCC`

✓5ᵗʰ **C34.3 Malignant neoplasm of lower lobe, bronchus or lung**

C34.30 Malignant neoplasm of lower lobe, unspecified bronchus or lung `HCC` ▽

C34.31 Malignant neoplasm of lower lobe, right bronchus or lung `HCC`

C34.32 Malignant neoplasm of lower lobe, left bronchus or lung `HCC`

✓5ᵗʰ **C34.8 Malignant neoplasm of overlapping sites of bronchus and lung**

C34.80 Malignant neoplasm of overlapping sites of unspecified bronchus and lung `HCC` ▽

C34.81 Malignant neoplasm of overlapping sites of right bronchus and lung `HCC`

C34.82 Malignant neoplasm of overlapping sites of left bronchus and lung `HCC`

✓5ᵗʰ **C34.9 Malignant neoplasm of unspecified part of bronchus or lung**

C34.90 Malignant neoplasm of unspecified part of unspecified bronchus or lung `HCC` ▽
Lung cancer NOS

C34.91 Malignant neoplasm of unspecified part of right bronchus or lung `HCC` ▽

C34.92 Malignant neoplasm of unspecified part of left bronchus or lung `HCC` ▽

C37 Malignant neoplasm of thymus `HCC`
EXCLUDES 1 *malignant carcinoid tumor of the thymus (C7A.091)*

✓4ᵗʰ **C38 Malignant neoplasm of heart, mediastinum and pleura**
EXCLUDES 1 *mesothelioma (C45.-)*

C38.0 Malignant neoplasm of heart `HCC`
Malignant neoplasm of pericardium
EXCLUDES 1 *malignant neoplasm of great vessels (C49.3)*

C38.1 Malignant neoplasm of anterior mediastinum `HCC`

C38.2 Malignant neoplasm of posterior mediastinum `HCC`

C38.3 Malignant neoplasm of mediastinum, part unspecified `HCC` ▽

C38.4 Malignant neoplasm of pleura `HCC`

C38.8 Malignant neoplasm of overlapping sites of heart, mediastinum and pleura `HCC`

✓4ᵗʰ **C39 Malignant neoplasm of other and ill-defined sites in the respiratory system and intrathoracic organs**
Use additional code to identify:
exposure to environmental tobacco smoke (Z77.22)
exposure to tobacco smoke in the perinatal period (P96.81)
history of tobacco dependence (Z87.891)
occupational exposure to environmental tobacco smoke (Z57.31)
tobacco dependence (F17.-)
tobacco use (Z72.0)
EXCLUDES 1 *intrathoracic malignant neoplasm NOS (C76.1)*
thoracic malignant neoplasm NOS (C76.1)

C39.0 Malignant neoplasm of upper respiratory tract, part unspecified `HCC` ▽

C39.9 Malignant neoplasm of lower respiratory tract, part unspecified `HCC` ▽
Malignant neoplasm of respiratory tract NOS

Malignant neoplasms of bone and articular cartilage (C40-C41)

INCLUDES malignant neoplasm of cartilage (articular) (joint)
malignant neoplasm of periosteum
EXCLUDES 1 *malignant neoplasm of bone marrow NOS (C96.9)*
malignant neoplasm of synovia (C49.-)

✓4ᵗʰ **C40 Malignant neoplasm of bone and articular cartilage of limbs**
Use additional code to identify major osseous defect, if applicable (M89.7-)

✓5ᵗʰ **C40.0 Malignant neoplasm of scapula and long bones of upper limb**

C40.00 Malignant neoplasm of scapula and long bones of unspecified upper limb `HCC` ▽

C40.01 Malignant neoplasm of scapula and long bones of right upper limb `HCC`

C40.02 Malignant neoplasm of scapula and long bones of left upper limb `HCC`

✓5ᵗʰ **C40.1 Malignant neoplasm of short bones of upper limb**

C40.10 Malignant neoplasm of short bones of unspecified upper limb `HCC` ▽

C40.11 Malignant neoplasm of short bones of right upper limb `HCC`

C40.12 Malignant neoplasm of short bones of left upper limb `HCC`

EXCLUDES 1 Not coded here   *EXCLUDES 2* Not included here   N Newborn Age: 0   P Pediatric Age: 0-17   M Maternity Age: 12-55   A Adult Age: 15-124

464   ICD-10-CM 2018

C40.2 Malignant neoplasm of long bones of lower limb ✓5ᵗʰ

    C40.20 Malignant neoplasm of long bones of unspecified lower limb   HCC ▽

    C40.21 Malignant neoplasm of long bones of right lower limb   HCC

    C40.22 Malignant neoplasm of long bones of left lower limb   HCC

C40.3 Malignant neoplasm of short bones of lower limb ✓5ᵗʰ

    C40.30 Malignant neoplasm of short bones of unspecified lower limb   HCC ▽

    C40.31 Malignant neoplasm of short bones of right lower limb   HCC

    C40.32 Malignant neoplasm of short bones of left lower limb   HCC

C40.8 Malignant neoplasm of overlapping sites of bone and articular cartilage of limb ✓5ᵗʰ

    C40.80 Malignant neoplasm of overlapping sites of bone and articular cartilage of unspecified limb   HCC ▽

    C40.81 Malignant neoplasm of overlapping sites of bone and articular cartilage of right limb   HCC

    C40.82 Malignant neoplasm of overlapping sites of bone and articular cartilage of left limb   HCC

C40.9 Malignant neoplasm of unspecified bones and articular cartilage of limb ✓5ᵗʰ

    C40.90 Malignant neoplasm of unspecified bones and articular cartilage of unspecified limb   HCC ▽

    C40.91 Malignant neoplasm of unspecified bones and articular cartilage of right limb   HCC ▽

    C40.92 Malignant neoplasm of unspecified bones and articular cartilage of left limb   HCC ▽

C41 Malignant neoplasm of bone and articular cartilage of other and unspecified sites ✓4ᵗʰ

    EXCLUDES 1   malignant neoplasm of bones of limbs (C40.-)
                 malignant neoplasm of cartilage of ear (C49.0)
                 malignant neoplasm of cartilage of eyelid (C49.0)
                 malignant neoplasm of cartilage of larynx (C32.3)
                 malignant neoplasm of cartilage of limbs (C40.-)
                 malignant neoplasm of cartilage of nose (C30.0)

    C41.0 Malignant neoplasm of bones of skull and face   HCC
         Malignant neoplasm of maxilla (superior)
         Malignant neoplasm of orbital bone
         EXCLUDES 2   carcinoma, any type except intraosseous or odontogenic of:
                 maxillary sinus (C31.0)
                 upper jaw (C03.0)
                 malignant neoplasm of jaw bone (lower) (C41.1)

    C41.1 Malignant neoplasm of mandible   HCC
         Malignant neoplasm of inferior maxilla
         Malignant neoplasm of lower jaw bone
         EXCLUDES 2   carcinoma, any type except intraosseous or odontogenic of:
                 jaw NOS (C03.9)
                 lower (C03.1)
                 malignant neoplasm of upper jaw bone (C41.0)

    C41.2 Malignant neoplasm of vertebral column   HCC
         EXCLUDES 1   malignant neoplasm of sacrum and coccyx (C41.4)

    C41.3 Malignant neoplasm of ribs, sternum and clavicle   HCC

    C41.4 Malignant neoplasm of pelvic bones, sacrum and coccyx   HCC

    C41.9 Malignant neoplasm of bone and articular cartilage, unspecified   HCC ▽

Melanoma and other malignant neoplasms of skin (C43-C44)

C43 Malignant melanoma of skin ✓4ᵗʰ

    EXCLUDES 1   melanoma in situ (D03.-)
    EXCLUDES 2   malignant melanoma of skin of genital organs (C51-C52, C60.-, C63.-)
                 Merkel cell carcinoma (C4A.-)
                 sites other than skin—code to malignant neoplasm of the site

    C43.0 Malignant melanoma of lip   HCC
         EXCLUDES 1   malignant neoplasm of vermilion border of lip (C00.0-C00.2)

    C43.1 Malignant melanoma of eyelid, including canthus ✓5ᵗʰ

        C43.10 Malignant melanoma of unspecified eyelid, including canthus   HCC ▽

        C43.11 Malignant melanoma of right eyelid, including canthus   HCC

        C43.12 Malignant melanoma of left eyelid, including canthus   HCC

C43.2 Malignant melanoma of ear and external auricular canal ✓5ᵗʰ

    C43.20 Malignant melanoma of unspecified ear and external auricular canal   HCC ▽

    C43.21 Malignant melanoma of right ear and external auricular canal   HCC

    C43.22 Malignant melanoma of left ear and external auricular canal   HCC

C43.3 Malignant melanoma of other and unspecified parts of face ✓5ᵗʰ

    C43.30 Malignant melanoma of unspecified part of face   HCC ▽

    C43.31 Malignant melanoma of nose   HCC

    C43.39 Malignant melanoma of other parts of face   HCC

C43.4 Malignant melanoma of scalp and neck   HCC

C43.5 Malignant melanoma of trunk ✓5ᵗʰ

    EXCLUDES 2   malignant neoplasm of anus NOS (C21.0)
                 malignant neoplasm of scrotum (C63.2)

    C43.51 Malignant melanoma of anal skin   HCC
         Malignant melanoma of anal margin
         Malignant melanoma of perianal skin

    C43.52 Malignant melanoma of skin of breast   HCC

    C43.59 Malignant melanoma of other part of trunk   HCC

C43.6 Malignant melanoma of upper limb, including shoulder ✓5ᵗʰ

    C43.60 Malignant melanoma of unspecified upper limb, including shoulder   HCC ▽

    C43.61 Malignant melanoma of right upper limb, including shoulder   HCC

    C43.62 Malignant melanoma of left upper limb, including shoulder   HCC

C43.7 Malignant melanoma of lower limb, including hip ✓5ᵗʰ

    C43.70 Malignant melanoma of unspecified lower limb, including hip   HCC ▽

    C43.71 Malignant melanoma of right lower limb, including hip   HCC

    C43.72 Malignant melanoma of left lower limb, including hip   HCC

C43.8 Malignant melanoma of overlapping sites of skin   HCC

C43.9 Malignant melanoma of skin, unspecified   HCC ▽
     Malignant melanoma of unspecified site of skin
     Melanoma (malignant) NOS

C4A Merkel cell carcinoma ✓4ᵗʰ

    DEF: Malignant cutaneous cancer predominantly found in elderly patients with sun exposure that usually presents as a flesh-colored or bluish-red lump typically seen on the neck, head and face.

    C4A.0 Merkel cell carcinoma of lip   HCC
         EXCLUDES 1   malignant neoplasm of vermilion border of lip (C00.0-C00.2)

    C4A.1 Merkel cell carcinoma of eyelid, including canthus ✓5ᵗʰ

        C4A.10 Merkel cell carcinoma of unspecified eyelid, including canthus   HCC ▽

        C4A.11 Merkel cell carcinoma of right eyelid, including canthus   HCC

        C4A.12 Merkel cell carcinoma of left eyelid, including canthus   HCC

    C4A.2 Merkel cell carcinoma of ear and external auricular canal ✓5ᵗʰ

        C4A.20 Merkel cell carcinoma of unspecified ear and external auricular canal   HCC ▽

        C4A.21 Merkel cell carcinoma of right ear and external auricular canal   HCC

        C4A.22 Merkel cell carcinoma of left ear and external auricular canal   HCC

    C4A.3 Merkel cell carcinoma of other and unspecified parts of face ✓5ᵗʰ

        C4A.30 Merkel cell carcinoma of unspecified part of face   HCC ▽

        C4A.31 Merkel cell carcinoma of nose   HCC

        C4A.39 Merkel cell carcinoma of other parts of face   HCC

    C4A.4 Merkel cell carcinoma of scalp and neck   HCC

    C4A.5 Merkel cell carcinoma of trunk ✓5ᵗʰ

         EXCLUDES 2   malignant neoplasm of anus NOS (C21.0)
                 malignant neoplasm of scrotum (C63.2)

        C4A.51 Merkel cell carcinoma of anal skin   HCC
                Merkel cell carcinoma of anal margin
                Merkel cell carcinoma of perianal skin

✓ Additional Character Req   ✓x7ᵗʰ Placeholder Alert   Manifestation   HCC CMS-HCC Condition   ▽ Unspecified Code   ►◄ Revised Text   ● New Code   ▲ Revised Code Title

Chapter 2. Neoplasms

    C4A.52   Merkel cell carcinoma of skin of breast   HCC

    C4A.59   Merkel cell carcinoma of other part of trunk   HCC

✓5ᵗʰ **C4A.6**   Merkel cell carcinoma of upper limb, including shoulder

    C4A.60   Merkel cell carcinoma of unspecified upper limb, including shoulder   HCC ▽

    C4A.61   Merkel cell carcinoma of right upper limb, including shoulder   HCC

    C4A.62   Merkel cell carcinoma of left upper limb, including shoulder   HCC

✓5ᵗʰ **C4A.7**   Merkel cell carcinoma of lower limb, including hip

    C4A.70   Merkel cell carcinoma of unspecified lower limb, including hip   HCC ▽

    C4A.71   Merkel cell carcinoma of right lower limb, including hip   HCC

    C4A.72   Merkel cell carcinoma of left lower limb, including hip   HCC

C4A.8   Merkel cell carcinoma of overlapping sites   HCC

C4A.9   Merkel cell carcinoma, unspecified   HCC ▽
     Merkel cell carcinoma of unspecified site

✓4ᵗʰ **C44**   **Other and unspecified malignant neoplasm** of skin

     INCLUDES   malignant neoplasm of sebaceous glands
               malignant neoplasm of sweat glands

     EXCLUDES 1   Kaposi's sarcoma of skin (C46.0)
               malignant melanoma of skin (C43.-)
               malignant neoplasm of skin of genital organs (C51-C52, C60-, C63.2)
               Merkel cell carcinoma (C4A.-)

     DEF: Basal cell carcinoma: An abnormal growth of skin cells that arises from the deepest layer of the epidermis and may present as an open sore, red patches, pink growth, or scar. One of the most common forms of skin cancer, typically caused by sun exposure.
     DEF: Squamous cell carcinoma: An uncontrolled growth of abnormal skin cells that arises from the skin's outer layers (epidermis) and may present as an open sore; firm, red nodule; elevated growth with a central depression; or flat sore with a scaly crust.

✓5ᵗʰ **C44.0**   Other and unspecified malignant neoplasm of skin of lip

     EXCLUDES 1   malignant neoplasm of lip (C00.-)

    C44.00   Unspecified malignant neoplasm of skin of lip   ▽

    C44.01   Basal cell carcinoma of skin of lip

    C44.02   Squamous cell carcinoma of skin of lip

    C44.09   Other specified malignant neoplasm of skin of lip

✓5ᵗʰ **C44.1**   Other and unspecified malignant neoplasm of skin of eyelid, including canthus

     EXCLUDES 1   connective tissue of eyelid (C49.0)

     ✓6ᵗʰ **C44.10**   Unspecified malignant neoplasm of skin of eyelid, including canthus

        C44.101   Unspecified malignant neoplasm of skin of unspecified eyelid, including canthus   ▽

        C44.102   Unspecified malignant neoplasm of skin of right eyelid, including canthus   ▽

        C44.109   Unspecified malignant neoplasm of skin of left eyelid, including canthus   ▽

     ✓6ᵗʰ **C44.11**   Basal cell carcinoma of skin of eyelid, including canthus

        C44.111   Basal cell carcinoma of skin of unspecified eyelid, including canthus   ▽

        C44.112   Basal cell carcinoma of skin of right eyelid, including canthus

        C44.119   Basal cell carcinoma of skin of left eyelid, including canthus

     ✓6ᵗʰ **C44.12**   Squamous cell carcinoma of skin of eyelid, including canthus

        C44.121   Squamous cell carcinoma of skin of unspecified eyelid, including canthus   ▽

        C44.122   Squamous cell carcinoma of skin of right eyelid, including canthus

        C44.129   Squamous cell carcinoma of skin of left eyelid, including canthus

     ✓6ᵗʰ **C44.19**   Other specified malignant neoplasm of skin of eyelid, including canthus

        C44.191   Other specified malignant neoplasm of skin of unspecified eyelid, including canthus   ▽

        C44.192   Other specified malignant neoplasm of skin of right eyelid, including canthus

        C44.199   Other specified malignant neoplasm of skin of left eyelid, including canthus

✓5ᵗʰ **C44.2**   Other and unspecified malignant neoplasm of skin of ear and external auricular canal

     EXCLUDES 1   connective tissue of ear (C49.0)

     ✓6ᵗʰ **C44.20**   Unspecified malignant neoplasm of skin of ear and external auricular canal

        C44.201   Unspecified malignant neoplasm of skin of unspecified ear and external auricular canal   ▽

        C44.202   Unspecified malignant neoplasm of skin of right ear and external auricular canal   ▽

        C44.209   Unspecified malignant neoplasm of skin of left ear and external auricular canal   ▽

     ✓6ᵗʰ **C44.21**   Basal cell carcinoma of skin of ear and external auricular canal

        C44.211   Basal cell carcinoma of skin of unspecified ear and external auricular canal   ▽

        C44.212   Basal cell carcinoma of skin of right ear and external auricular canal

        C44.219   Basal cell carcinoma of skin of left ear and external auricular canal

     ✓6ᵗʰ **C44.22**   Squamous cell carcinoma of skin of ear and external auricular canal

        C44.221   Squamous cell carcinoma of skin of unspecified ear and external auricular canal   ▽

        C44.222   Squamous cell carcinoma of skin of right ear and external auricular canal

        C44.229   Squamous cell carcinoma of skin of left ear and external auricular canal

     ✓6ᵗʰ **C44.29**   Other specified malignant neoplasm of skin of ear and external auricular canal

        C44.291   Other specified malignant neoplasm of skin of unspecified ear and external auricular canal   ▽

        C44.292   Other specified malignant neoplasm of skin of right ear and external auricular canal

        C44.299   Other specified malignant neoplasm of skin of left ear and external auricular canal

✓5ᵗʰ **C44.3**   Other and unspecified malignant neoplasm of skin of other and unspecified parts of face

     ✓6ᵗʰ **C44.30**   Unspecified malignant neoplasm of skin of other and unspecified parts of face

        C44.300   Unspecified malignant neoplasm of skin of unspecified part of face   ▽

        C44.301   Unspecified malignant neoplasm of skin of nose   ▽

        C44.309   Unspecified malignant neoplasm of skin of other parts of face   ▽

     ✓6ᵗʰ **C44.31**   Basal cell carcinoma of skin of other and unspecified parts of face

        C44.310   Basal cell carcinoma of skin of unspecified parts of face   ▽

        C44.311   Basal cell carcinoma of skin of nose

        C44.319   Basal cell carcinoma of skin of other parts of face

     ✓6ᵗʰ **C44.32**   Squamous cell carcinoma of skin of other and unspecified parts of face

        C44.320   Squamous cell carcinoma of skin of unspecified parts of face

        C44.321   Squamous cell carcinoma of skin of nose

        C44.329   Squamous cell carcinoma of skin of other parts of face

     ✓6ᵗʰ **C44.39**   Other specified malignant neoplasm of skin of other and unspecified parts of face

        C44.390   Other specified malignant neoplasm of skin of unspecified parts of face   ▽

        C44.391   Other specified malignant neoplasm of skin of nose

        C44.399   Other specified malignant neoplasm of skin of other parts of face

✓5ᵗʰ **C44.4**   Other and unspecified malignant neoplasm of skin of scalp and neck

    C44.40   Unspecified malignant neoplasm of skin of scalp and neck   ▽

EXCLUDES 1 Not coded here   **EXCLUDES 2** Not included here   N Newborn Age: 0   P Pediatric Age: 0-17   M Maternity Age: 12-55   A Adult Age: 15-124

466   ICD-10-CM 2018

C4A.52–C44.40

    C44.41   Basal cell carcinoma of skin of scalp and neck

    C44.42   Squamous cell carcinoma of skin of scalp and neck

    C44.49   Other specified malignant neoplasm of skin of scalp and neck

✓5th **C44.5**   **Other and unspecified malignant neoplasm of** skin of trunk
> EXCLUDES 1   anus NOS (C21.0)
>   scrotum (C63.2)

  ✓6th **C44.50**   Unspecified malignant neoplasm of skin of trunk

    C44.500   Unspecified malignant neoplasm of anal skin ▽
> Unspecified malignant neoplasm of anal margin
> Unspecified malignant neoplasm of perianal skin

    C44.501   Unspecified malignant neoplasm of skin of breast ▽

    C44.509   Unspecified malignant neoplasm of skin of other part of trunk ▽

  ✓6th **C44.51**   Basal cell carcinoma of skin of trunk

    C44.510   Basal cell carcinoma of anal skin
> Basal cell carcinoma of anal margin
> Basal cell carcinoma of perianal skin

    C44.511   Basal cell carcinoma of skin of breast

    C44.519   Basal cell carcinoma of skin of other part of trunk

  ✓6th **C44.52**   Squamous cell carcinoma of skin of trunk

    C44.520   Squamous cell carcinoma of anal skin
> Squamous cell carcinoma of anal margin
> Squamous cell carcinoma of perianal skin

    C44.521   Squamous cell carcinoma of skin of breast

    C44.529   Squamous cell carcinoma of skin of other part of trunk

  ✓6th **C44.59**   Other specified malignant neoplasm of skin of trunk

    C44.590   Other specified malignant neoplasm of anal skin
> Other specified malignant neoplasm of anal margin
> Other specified malignant neoplasm of perianal skin

    C44.591   Other specified malignant neoplasm of skin of breast

    C44.599   Other specified malignant neoplasm of skin of other part of trunk

✓5th **C44.6**   **Other and unspecified malignant neoplasm of skin of** upper limb, including shoulder

  ✓6th **C44.60**   Unspecified malignant neoplasm of skin of upper limb, including shoulder

    C44.601   Unspecified malignant neoplasm of skin of unspecified upper limb, including shoulder ▽

    C44.602   Unspecified malignant neoplasm of skin of right upper limb, including shoulder ▽

    C44.609   Unspecified malignant neoplasm of skin of left upper limb, including shoulder ▽

  ✓6th **C44.61**   Basal cell carcinoma of skin of upper limb, including shoulder

    C44.611   Basal cell carcinoma of skin of unspecified upper limb, including shoulder ▽

    C44.612   Basal cell carcinoma of skin of right upper limb, including shoulder

    C44.619   Basal cell carcinoma of skin of left upper limb, including shoulder

  ✓6th **C44.62**   Squamous cell carcinoma of skin of upper limb, including shoulder

    C44.621   Squamous cell carcinoma of skin of unspecified upper limb, including shoulder ▽

    C44.622   Squamous cell carcinoma of skin of right upper limb, including shoulder

    C44.629   Squamous cell carcinoma of skin of left upper limb, including shoulder

  ✓6th **C44.69**   Other specified malignant neoplasm of skin of upper limb, including shoulder

    C44.691   Other specified malignant neoplasm of skin of unspecified upper limb, including shoulder ▽

    C44.692   Other specified malignant neoplasm of skin of right upper limb, including shoulder

    C44.699   Other specified malignant neoplasm of skin of left upper limb, including shoulder

✓5th **C44.7**   **Other and unspecified malignant neoplasm of skin of** lower limb, including hip

  ✓6th **C44.70**   Unspecified malignant neoplasm of skin of lower limb, including hip

    C44.701   Unspecified malignant neoplasm of skin of unspecified lower limb, including hip ▽

    C44.702   Unspecified malignant neoplasm of skin of right lower limb, including hip ▽

    C44.709   Unspecified malignant neoplasm of skin of left lower limb, including hip ▽

  ✓6th **C44.71**   Basal cell carcinoma of skin of lower limb, including hip

    C44.711   Basal cell carcinoma of skin of unspecified lower limb, including hip ▽

    C44.712   Basal cell carcinoma of skin of right lower limb, including hip

    C44.719   Basal cell carcinoma of skin of left lower limb, including hip

  ✓6th **C44.72**   Squamous cell carcinoma of skin of lower limb, including hip

    C44.721   Squamous cell carcinoma of skin of unspecified lower limb, including hip ▽

    C44.722   Squamous cell carcinoma of skin of right lower limb, including hip

    C44.729   Squamous cell carcinoma of skin of left lower limb, including hip

  ✓6th **C44.79**   Other specified malignant neoplasm of skin of lower limb, including hip

    C44.791   Other specified malignant neoplasm of skin of unspecified lower limb, including hip ▽

    C44.792   Other specified malignant neoplasm of skin of right lower limb, including hip

    C44.799   Other specified malignant neoplasm of skin of left lower limb, including hip

✓5th **C44.8**   **Other and unspecified malignant neoplasm of** overlapping sites of skin

    C44.80   Unspecified malignant neoplasm of overlapping sites of skin ▽

    C44.81   Basal cell carcinoma of overlapping sites of skin

    C44.82   Squamous cell carcinoma of overlapping sites of skin

    C44.89   Other specified malignant neoplasm of overlapping sites of skin

✓5th **C44.9**   **Other and unspecified malignant neoplasm of skin, unspecified**

    C44.90   Unspecified malignant neoplasm of skin, unspecified ▽
> Malignant neoplasm of unspecified site of skin

    C44.91   Basal cell carcinoma of skin, unspecified ▽

    C44.92   Squamous cell carcinoma of skin, unspecified ▽

    C44.99   Other specified malignant neoplasm of skin, unspecified ▽

Malignant neoplasms of mesothelial and soft tissue (C45-C49)

✓4th **C45**   **Mesothelioma**
> **DEF:** Rare type of cancer that forms in the thin layer of protective tissue that covers the majority of internal organs (mesothelium).

  C45.0   **Mesothelioma of pleura**   HCC
> EXCLUDES 1   other malignant neoplasm of pleura (C38.4)
> **AHA:** 2017, 2Q, 11

  C45.1   **Mesothelioma of peritoneum**   HCC
> Mesothelioma of cul-de-sac   Mesothelioma of omentum
> Mesothelioma of mesentery   Mesothelioma of peritoneum
> Mesothelioma of mesocolon   (parietal) (pelvic)
> EXCLUDES 1   other malignant neoplasm of soft tissue of peritoneum (C48.-)

  C45.2   **Mesothelioma of pericardium**   HCC
> EXCLUDES 1   other malignant neoplasm of pericardium (C38.0)

  C45.7   **Mesothelioma of other sites**   HCC

  C45.9   **Mesothelioma, unspecified**   HCC ▽

☑ Additional Character Req   ✓x7th Placeholder Alert   Manifestation   HCC CMS-HCC Condition   ▽ Unspecified Code   ►◄ Revised Text   ● New Code   ▲ Revised Code Title

ICD-10-CM 2018   467

C44.41–C45.9

Chapter 2. Neoplasms

✓4ᵗʰ C46 Kaposi's sarcoma

Code first any human immunodeficiency virus [HIV] disease (B20)

DEF: Malignant neoplasm that causes patches of abnormal tissue to grow under the skin, in the lining of the mouth, nose, and throat, in lymph nodes, or in other visceral organs. Kaposi's sarcoma is caused by human herpesvirus8 (HHV8).

C46.0 Kaposi's sarcoma of skin `HCC`

C46.1 Kaposi's sarcoma of soft tissue `HCC`
Kaposi's sarcoma of blood vessel
Kaposi's sarcoma of connective tissue
Kaposi's sarcoma of fascia
Kaposi's sarcoma of ligament
Kaposi's sarcoma of lymphatic(s) NEC
Kaposi's sarcoma of muscle
EXCLUDES 2   *Kaposi's sarcoma of lymph glands and nodes (C46.3)*

C46.2 Kaposi's sarcoma of palate `HCC`

C46.3 Kaposi's sarcoma of lymph nodes `HCC`

C46.4 Kaposi's sarcoma of gastrointestinal sites `HCC`

✓5ᵗʰ C46.5 Kaposi's sarcoma of lung

    C46.50 Kaposi's sarcoma of unspecified lung `HCC` ▽

    C46.51 Kaposi's sarcoma of right lung `HCC`

    C46.52 Kaposi's sarcoma of left lung `HCC`

C46.7 Kaposi's sarcoma of other sites `HCC`

C46.9 Kaposi's sarcoma, unspecified `HCC` ▽
Kaposi's sarcoma of unspecified site

✓4ᵗʰ C47 Malignant neoplasm of peripheral nerves and autonomic nervous system
INCLUDES   malignant neoplasm of sympathetic and parasympathetic nerves and ganglia
EXCLUDES 1   *Kaposi's sarcoma of soft tissue (C46.1)*

C47.0 Malignant neoplasm of peripheral nerves of head, face and neck `HCC`
EXCLUDES 1   *malignant neoplasm of peripheral nerves of orbit (C69.6-)*

✓5ᵗʰ C47.1 Malignant neoplasm of peripheral nerves of upper limb, including shoulder

    C47.10 Malignant neoplasm of peripheral nerves of unspecified upper limb, including shoulder `HCC` ▽

    C47.11 Malignant neoplasm of peripheral nerves of right upper limb, including shoulder `HCC`

    C47.12 Malignant neoplasm of peripheral nerves of left upper limb, including shoulder `HCC`

✓5ᵗʰ C47.2 Malignant neoplasm of peripheral nerves of lower limb, including hip

    C47.20 Malignant neoplasm of peripheral nerves of unspecified lower limb, including hip `HCC` ▽

    C47.21 Malignant neoplasm of peripheral nerves of right lower limb, including hip `HCC`

    C47.22 Malignant neoplasm of peripheral nerves of left lower limb, including hip `HCC`

C47.3 Malignant neoplasm of peripheral nerves of thorax `HCC`

C47.4 Malignant neoplasm of peripheral nerves of abdomen `HCC`

C47.5 Malignant neoplasm of peripheral nerves of pelvis `HCC`

C47.6 Malignant neoplasm of peripheral nerves of trunk, unspecified `HCC` ▽
Malignant neoplasm of peripheral nerves of unspecified part of trunk

C47.8 Malignant neoplasm of overlapping sites of peripheral nerves and autonomic nervous system `HCC`

C47.9 Malignant neoplasm of peripheral nerves and autonomic nervous system, unspecified `HCC` ▽
Malignant neoplasm of unspecified site of peripheral nerves and autonomic nervous system

✓4ᵗʰ C48 Malignant neoplasm of retroperitoneum and peritoneum
EXCLUDES 1   *Kaposi's sarcoma of connective tissue (C46.1)*
mesothelioma (C45.-)

C48.0 Malignant neoplasm of retroperitoneum `HCC`

C48.1 Malignant neoplasm of specified parts of peritoneum `HCC`
Malignant neoplasm of cul-de-sac
Malignant neoplasm of mesentery
Malignant neoplasm of mesocolon
Malignant neoplasm of omentum
Malignant neoplasm of parietal peritoneum
Malignant neoplasm of pelvic peritoneum

C48.2 Malignant neoplasm of peritoneum, unspecified `HCC` ▽

C48.8 Malignant neoplasm of overlapping sites of retroperitoneum and peritoneum `HCC`

✓4ᵗʰ C49 Malignant neoplasm of other connective and soft tissue
INCLUDES   malignant neoplasm of blood vessel
malignant neoplasm of bursa
malignant neoplasm of cartilage
malignant neoplasm of fascia
malignant neoplasm of fat
malignant neoplasm of ligament, except uterine
malignant neoplasm of lymphatic vessel
malignant neoplasm of muscle
malignant neoplasm of synovia
malignant neoplasm of tendon (sheath)
EXCLUDES 1   *malignant neoplasm of cartilage (of):*
articular (C40-C41)
larynx (C32.3)
nose (C30.0)
malignant neoplasm of connective tissue of breast (C50.-)
EXCLUDES 2   *Kaposi's sarcoma of soft tissue (C46.1)*
malignant neoplasm of heart (C38.0)
malignant neoplasm of peripheral nerves and autonomic nervous system (C47.-)
malignant neoplasm of peritoneum (C48.2)
malignant neoplasm of retroperitoneum (C48.0)
malignant neoplasm of uterine ligament (C57.3)
mesothelioma (C45.-)

C49.0 Malignant neoplasm of connective and soft tissue of head, face and neck `HCC`
Malignant neoplasm of connective tissue of ear
Malignant neoplasm of connective tissue of eyelid
EXCLUDES 1   *connective tissue of orbit (C69.6-)*

✓5ᵗʰ C49.1 Malignant neoplasm of connective and soft tissue of upper limb, including shoulder

    C49.10 Malignant neoplasm of connective and soft tissue of unspecified upper limb, including shoulder `HCC` ▽

    C49.11 Malignant neoplasm of connective and soft tissue of right upper limb, including shoulder `HCC`

    C49.12 Malignant neoplasm of connective and soft tissue of left upper limb, including shoulder `HCC`

✓5ᵗʰ C49.2 Malignant neoplasm of connective and soft tissue of lower limb, including hip

    C49.20 Malignant neoplasm of connective and soft tissue of unspecified lower limb, including hip `HCC` ▽

    C49.21 Malignant neoplasm of connective and soft tissue of right lower limb, including hip `HCC`

    C49.22 Malignant neoplasm of connective and soft tissue of left lower limb, including hip `HCC`

C49.3 Malignant neoplasm of connective and soft tissue of thorax `HCC`
Malignant neoplasm of axilla
Malignant neoplasm of diaphragm
Malignant neoplasm of great vessels
EXCLUDES 1   *malignant neoplasm of breast (C50.-)*
malignant neoplasm of heart (C38.0)
malignant neoplasm of mediastinum (C38.1-C38.3)
malignant neoplasm of thymus (C37)
AHA: 2015, 3Q, 19

C49.4 Malignant neoplasm of connective and soft tissue of abdomen `HCC`
Malignant neoplasm of abdominal wall
Malignant neoplasm of hypochondrium

C49.5 Malignant neoplasm of connective and soft tissue of pelvis `HCC`
Malignant neoplasm of buttock
Malignant neoplasm of groin
Malignant neoplasm of perineum

C49.6 Malignant neoplasm of connective and soft tissue of trunk, unspecified `HCC` ▽
Malignant neoplasm of back NOS

C49.8 Malignant neoplasm of overlapping sites of connective and soft tissue `HCC`
Primary malignant neoplasm of two or more contiguous sites of connective and soft tissue

C49.9 Malignant neoplasm of connective and soft tissue, unspecified `HCC` ▽

✓5ᵗʰ C49.A Gastrointestinal stromal tumor

    C49.A0 Gastrointestinal stromal tumor, unspecified site `HCC` ▽

    C49.A1 Gastrointestinal stromal tumor of esophagus `HCC`

    C49.A2 Gastrointestinal stromal tumor of stomach `HCC`

    C49.A3 Gastrointestinal stromal tumor of small intestine `HCC`

EXCLUDES 1 Not coded here   *EXCLUDES 2* Not included here   N Newborn Age: 0   P Pediatric Age: 0-17   M Maternity Age: 12-55   A Adult Age: 15-124

C49.A4   **Gastrointestinal stromal tumor of** large intestine ᴴᶜᶜ

C49.A5   **Gastrointestinal stromal tumor of** rectum   ᴴᶜᶜ

C49.A9   **Gastrointestinal stromal tumor of other sites**   ᴴᶜᶜ

Malignant neoplasms of breast (C50)

✓4ᵗʰ **C50 Malignant neoplasm of** breast
> **INCLUDES** connective tissue of breast
> Paget's disease of breast
> Paget's disease of nipple
>
> Use additional code to identify estrogen receptor status (Z17.0, Z17.1)
> **EXCLUDES 1** *skin of breast (C44.501, C44.511, C44.521, C44.591)*

✓5ᵗʰ **C50.0 Malignant neoplasm of** nipple and areola

✓6ᵗʰ **C50.01   Malignant neoplasm of nipple and areola,** female

C50.011   **Malignant neoplasm of nipple and** ᴴᶜᶜ ♀
areola, **right female breast**

C50.012   **Malignant neoplasm of nipple and** ᴴᶜᶜ ♀
areola, **left female breast**

C50.019   **Malignant neoplasm of nipple** ᴴᶜᶜ ♀▽
and areola, **unspecified female breast**

✓6ᵗʰ **C50.02   Malignant neoplasm of nipple and areola,** male

C50.021   **Malignant neoplasm of nipple and** ᴴᶜᶜ ♂
areola, **right male breast**

C50.022   **Malignant neoplasm of nipple and** ᴴᶜᶜ ♂
areola, **left male breast**

C50.029   **Malignant neoplasm of nipple** ᴴᶜᶜ ♂▽
and areola, **unspecified male breast**

✓5ᵗʰ **C50.1 Malignant neoplasm of** central portion of breast

✓6ᵗʰ **C50.11   Malignant neoplasm of central portion of breast,** female

C50.111   **Malignant neoplasm of central** ᴴᶜᶜ ♀
portion of **right female breast**

C50.112   **Malignant neoplasm of central** ᴴᶜᶜ ♀
portion of **left female breast**

C50.119   **Malignant neoplasm of central** ᴴᶜᶜ ♀▽
portion of **unspecified female breast**

✓6ᵗʰ **C50.12   Malignant neoplasm of central portion of breast,** male

C50.121   **Malignant neoplasm of central** ᴴᶜᶜ ♂
portion of **right male breast**

C50.122   **Malignant neoplasm of central** ᴴᶜᶜ ♂
portion of **left male breast**

C50.129   **Malignant neoplasm of central** ᴴᶜᶜ ♂▽
portion of **unspecified male breast**

✓5ᵗʰ **C50.2 Malignant neoplasm of** upper-inner quadrant of breast

✓6ᵗʰ **C50.21   Malignant neoplasm of upper-inner quadrant of breast,** female

C50.211   **Malignant neoplasm of upper-inner** ᴴᶜᶜ ♀
quadrant of **right female breast**

C50.212   **Malignant neoplasm of upper-inner** ᴴᶜᶜ ♀
quadrant of **left female breast**

C50.219   **Malignant neoplasm of** ᴴᶜᶜ ♀▽
**upper-inner quadrant of unspecified
female breast**

✓6ᵗʰ **C50.22   Malignant neoplasm of upper-inner quadrant of breast,** male

C50.221   **Malignant neoplasm of upper-inner** ᴴᶜᶜ ♂
quadrant of **right male breast**

C50.222   **Malignant neoplasm of upper-inner** ᴴᶜᶜ ♂
quadrant of **left male breast**

C50.229   **Malignant neoplasm of** ᴴᶜᶜ ♂▽
**upper-inner quadrant of
unspecified male breast**

✓5ᵗʰ **C50.3 Malignant neoplasm of** lower-inner quadrant of breast

✓6ᵗʰ **C50.31   Malignant neoplasm of lower-inner quadrant of breast,** female

C50.311   **Malignant neoplasm of lower-inner** ᴴᶜᶜ ♀
quadrant of **right female breast**

C50.312   **Malignant neoplasm of lower-inner** ᴴᶜᶜ ♀
quadrant of **left female breast**

C50.319   **Malignant neoplasm of** ᴴᶜᶜ ♀▽
**lower-inner quadrant of unspecified
female breast**

✓6ᵗʰ **C50.32   Malignant neoplasm of lower-inner quadrant of breast,** male

C50.321   **Malignant neoplasm of lower-inner** ᴴᶜᶜ ♂
quadrant of **right male breast**

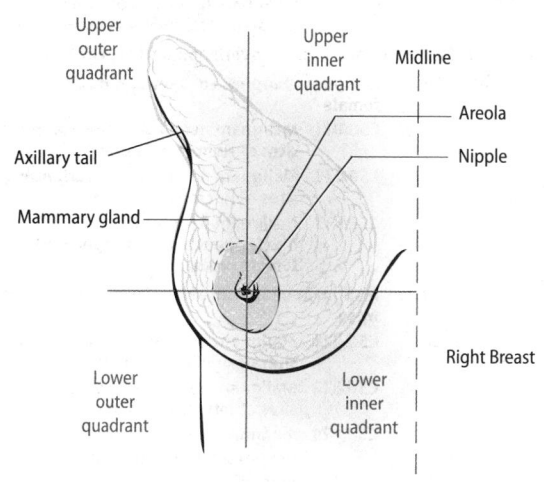

Female Breast

Upper outer quadrant
Upper inner quadrant
Midline
Areola
Axillary tail
Nipple
Mammary gland
Right Breast
Lower outer quadrant
Lower inner quadrant

C50.322   **Malignant neoplasm of lower-inner** ᴴᶜᶜ ♂
quadrant of **left male breast**

C50.329   **Malignant neoplasm of lower-** ᴴᶜᶜ ♂▽
inner quadrant of **unspecified male breast**

✓5ᵗʰ **C50.4 Malignant neoplasm of** upper-outer quadrant of breast

✓6ᵗʰ **C50.41   Malignant neoplasm of upper-outer quadrant of breast,** female

C50.411   **Malignant neoplasm of upper-outer** ᴴᶜᶜ ♀
quadrant of **right female breast**

C50.412   **Malignant neoplasm of upper-outer** ᴴᶜᶜ ♀
quadrant of **left female breast**

C50.419   **Malignant neoplasm of** ᴴᶜᶜ ♀▽
**upper-outer quadrant of unspecified
female breast**

✓6ᵗʰ **C50.42   Malignant neoplasm of upper-outer quadrant of breast,** male

C50.421   **Malignant neoplasm of upper-outer** ᴴᶜᶜ ♂
quadrant of **right male breast**

C50.422   **Malignant neoplasm of upper-outer** ᴴᶜᶜ ♂
quadrant of **left male breast**

C50.429   **Malignant neoplasm of** ᴴᶜᶜ ♂▽
**upper-outer quadrant of unspecified
male breast**

✓5ᵗʰ **C50.5 Malignant neoplasm of** lower-outer quadrant of breast

✓6ᵗʰ **C50.51   Malignant neoplasm of lower-outer quadrant of breast,** female

C50.511   **Malignant neoplasm of lower-outer** ᴴᶜᶜ ♀
quadrant of **right female breast**

C50.512   **Malignant neoplasm of lower-outer** ᴴᶜᶜ ♀
quadrant of **left female breast**

C50.519   **Malignant neoplasm of** ᴴᶜᶜ ♀▽
**lower-outer quadrant of unspecified
female breast**

✓6ᵗʰ **C50.52   Malignant neoplasm of lower-outer quadrant of breast,** male

C50.521   **Malignant neoplasm of lower-outer** ᴴᶜᶜ ♂
quadrant of **right male breast**

C50.522   **Malignant neoplasm of lower-outer** ᴴᶜᶜ ♂
quadrant of **left male breast**

C50.529   **Malignant neoplasm of** ᴴᶜᶜ ♂▽
**lower-outer quadrant of unspecified
male breast**

✓5ᵗʰ **C50.6 Malignant neoplasm of** axillary tail of breast

✓6ᵗʰ **C50.61   Malignant neoplasm of axillary tail of breast,** female

C50.611   **Malignant neoplasm of axillary tail** ᴴᶜᶜ ♀
of **right female breast**

C50.612   **Malignant neoplasm of axillary tail** ᴴᶜᶜ ♀
of **left female breast**

C50.619   **Malignant neoplasm of axillary** ᴴᶜᶜ ♀▽
tail of **unspecified female breast**

✓6ᵗʰ **C50.62   Malignant neoplasm of axillary tail of breast,** male

C50.621   **Malignant neoplasm of axillary tail** ᴴᶜᶜ ♂
of **right male breast**

☑ Additional Character Req   ✓ₓ7ᵗʰ Placeholder Alert   Manifestation   ᴴᶜᶜ CMS-HCC Condition   ▽ Unspecified Code   ►◄ Revised Text   ● New Code   ▲ Revised Code Title

C50.622 Malignant neoplasm of axillary tail of **left** male breast   HCC ♂

C50.629 Malignant neoplasm of axillary tail of unspecified male breast   HCC ♂ ▽

✓5th **C50.8** Malignant neoplasm of **overlapping sites** of breast

   ✓6th **C50.81** Malignant neoplasm of overlapping sites of breast, **female**

C50.811 Malignant neoplasm of overlapping sites of **right** female breast   HCC ♀

C50.812 Malignant neoplasm of overlapping sites of **left** female breast   HCC ♀

C50.819 Malignant neoplasm of overlapping sites of unspecified female breast   HCC ♀ ▽

   ✓6th **C50.82** Malignant neoplasm of overlapping sites of breast, **male**

C50.821 Malignant neoplasm of overlapping sites of **right** male breast   HCC ♂

C50.822 Malignant neoplasm of overlapping sites of **left** male breast   HCC ♂

C50.829 Malignant neoplasm of overlapping sites of unspecified male breast   HCC ♂ ▽

✓5th **C50.9** Malignant neoplasm of breast of unspecified site

   ✓6th **C50.91** Malignant neoplasm of breast of unspecified site, **female**

C50.911 Malignant neoplasm of unspecified site of **right** female breast   HCC ♀

C50.912 Malignant neoplasm of unspecified site of **left** female breast   HCC ♀

C50.919 Malignant neoplasm of unspecified site of unspecified female breast   HCC ♀ ▽

   ✓6th **C50.92** Malignant neoplasm of breast of unspecified site, **male**

C50.921 Malignant neoplasm of unspecified site of **right** male breast   HCC ♂

C50.922 Malignant neoplasm of unspecified site of **left** male breast   HCC ♂

C50.929 Malignant neoplasm of unspecified site of unspecified male breast   HCC ♂ ▽

Malignant neoplasms of female genital organs (C51-C58)

INCLUDES malignant neoplasm of skin of female genital organs

✓4th **C51** **Malignant neoplasm of vulva**

   EXCLUDES 1 carcinoma in situ of vulva (D07.1)

C51.0 Malignant neoplasm of **labium majus**   HCC ♀
   Malignant neoplasm of Bartholin's [greater vestibular] gland

C51.1 Malignant neoplasm of **labium minus**   HCC ♀

C51.2 Malignant neoplasm of **clitoris**   HCC ♀

C51.8 Malignant neoplasm of **overlapping sites** of vulva   HCC ♀

C51.9 Malignant neoplasm of **vulva, unspecified**   HCC ♀ ▽
   Malignant neoplasm of external female genitalia NOS
   Malignant neoplasm of pudendum

C52 **Malignant neoplasm of vagina**   HCC ♀

   EXCLUDES 1 carcinoma in situ of vagina (D07.2)

✓4th **C53** **Malignant neoplasm of cervix uteri**

   EXCLUDES 1 carcinoma in situ of cervix uteri (D06.-)

C53.0 Malignant neoplasm of **endocervix**   HCC ♀

C53.1 Malignant neoplasm of **exocervix**   HCC ♀

C53.8 Malignant neoplasm of **overlapping sites** of cervix uteri   HCC ♀

C53.9 Malignant neoplasm of cervix uteri, unspecified   HCC ♀ ▽

✓4th **C54** **Malignant neoplasm of corpus uteri**

C54.0 Malignant neoplasm of **isthmus uteri**   HCC ♀
   Malignant neoplasm of lower uterine segment

C54.1 Malignant neoplasm of **endometrium**   HCC ♀

C54.2 Malignant neoplasm of **myometrium**   HCC ♀

C54.3 Malignant neoplasm of **fundus uteri**   HCC ♀

C54.8 Malignant neoplasm of **overlapping sites** of corpus uteri   HCC ♀

C54.9 Malignant neoplasm of corpus uteri, unspecified   HCC ♀ ▽

C55 **Malignant neoplasm of uterus, part unspecified**   HCC ♀ ▽

✓4th **C56** **Malignant neoplasm of ovary**
   Use additional code to identify any functional activity

C56.1 Malignant neoplasm of **right** ovary   HCC

C56.2 Malignant neoplasm of **left** ovary   HCC

C56.9 Malignant neoplasm of unspecified ovary   HCC ♀ ▽

✓4th **C57** **Malignant neoplasm of other and unspecified female genital organs**

   ✓5th **C57.0** Malignant neoplasm of **fallopian tube**
     Malignant neoplasm of oviduct
     Malignant neoplasm of uterine tube

C57.00 Malignant neoplasm of unspecified fallopiantube   HCC ♀ ▽

C57.01 Malignant neoplasm of **right** fallopian tube   HCC ♀

C57.02 Malignant neoplasm of **left** fallopian tube   HCC ♀

   ✓5th **C57.1** Malignant neoplasm of **broad ligament**

C57.10 Malignant neoplasm of unspecified broad ligament   HCC ♀ ▽

C57.11 Malignant neoplasm of **right** broad ligament   HCC ♀

C57.12 Malignant neoplasm of **left** broad ligament   HCC ♀

   ✓5th **C57.2** Malignant neoplasm of **round ligament**

C57.20 Malignant neoplasm of unspecified round ligament   HCC ♀ ▽

C57.21 Malignant neoplasm of **right** round ligament   HCC ♀

C57.22 Malignant neoplasm of **left** round ligament   HCC ♀

C57.3 Malignant neoplasm of **parametrium**   HCC ♀
   Malignant neoplasm of uterine ligament NOS

C57.4 Malignant neoplasm of **uterine adnexa, unspecified**   HCC ♀ ▽

C57.7 Malignant neoplasm of **other specified** female genital organs   HCC ♀
   Malignant neoplasm of wolffian body or duct

C57.8 Malignant neoplasm of **overlapping sites** of female genital organs   HCC ♀
   Primary malignant neoplasm of two or more contiguous sites of the female genital organs whose point of origin cannot be determined
   Primary tubo-ovarian malignant neoplasm whose point of origin cannot be determined
   Primary utero-ovarian malignant neoplasm whose point of origin cannot be determined

C57.9 Malignant neoplasm of female genital organ, unspecified   HCC ♀ ▽
   Malignant neoplasm of female genitourinary tract NOS

C58 **Malignant neoplasm of placenta**   HCC M ♀
   INCLUDES choriocarcinoma NOS
     chorionepithelioma NOS
   EXCLUDES 1 chorioadenoma (destruens) (D39.2)
     hydatidiform mole NOS (O01.9)
     invasive hydatidiform mole (D39.2)
     male choriocarcinoma NOS (C62.9-)
     malignant hydatidiform mole (D39.2)

Malignant neoplasms of male genital organs (C60-C63)

INCLUDES malignant neoplasm of skin of male genital organs

✓4th **C60** **Malignant neoplasm of penis**

C60.0 Malignant neoplasm of **prepuce**   HCC ♂
   Malignant neoplasm of foreskin

C60.1 Malignant neoplasm of **glans** penis   HCC ♂

C60.2 Malignant neoplasm of **body of penis**   HCC ♂
   Malignant neoplasm of corpus cavernosum

C60.8 Malignant neoplasm of **overlapping sites** of penis   HCC ♂

C60.9 Malignant neoplasm of **penis, unspecified**   HCC ♂ ▽
   Malignant neoplasm of skin of penis NOS

C61 **Malignant neoplasm of prostate**   HCC ♂
   Use additional code to identify:
     hormone sensitivity status (Z19.1-Z19.2)
     rising PSA following treatment for malignant neoplasm of prostate (R97.21)
   EXCLUDES 1 malignant neoplasm of seminal vesicle (C63.7)
   AHA: 2017, 1Q, 17

EXCLUDES 1 Not coded here   EXCLUDES 2 Not included here   N Newborn Age: 0   P Pediatric Age: 0-17   M Maternity Age: 12-55   A Adult Age: 15-124

470   ICD-10-CM 2018

C50.622–C61

Chapter 2. Neoplasms

☑4ᵗʰ **C62** **Malignant neoplasm of testis**
Use additional code to identify any functional activity

☑5ᵗʰ **C62.0** **Malignant neoplasm of undescended testis**
Malignant neoplasm of ectopic testis
Malignant neoplasm of retained testis

C62.00 **Malignant neoplasm of unspecified undescended testis**   HCC ♂ ▽

C62.01 **Malignant neoplasm of undescended right testis**   HCC ♂

C62.02 **Malignant neoplasm of undescended left testis**   HCC ♂

☑5ᵗʰ **C62.1** **Malignant neoplasm of descended testis**
Malignant neoplasm of scrotal testis

C62.10 **Malignant neoplasm of unspecified descended testis**   HCC ♂ ▽

C62.11 **Malignant neoplasm of descended right testis**   HCC ♂

C62.12 **Malignant neoplasm of descended left testis**   HCC ♂

☑5ᵗʰ **C62.9** **Malignant neoplasm of testis, unspecified whether descended or undescended**

C62.90 **Malignant neoplasm of unspecified testis, unspecified whether descended or undescended**   HCC ♂ ▽
Malignant neoplasm of testis NOS

C62.91 **Malignant neoplasm of right testis, unspecified whether descended or undescended**   HCC ♂ ▽

C62.92 **Malignant neoplasm of left testis, unspecified whether descended or undescended**   HCC ♂ ▽

☑4ᵗʰ **C63** **Malignant neoplasm of other and unspecified male genital organs**

☑5ᵗʰ **C63.0** **Malignant neoplasm of epididymis**

C63.00 **Malignant neoplasm of unspecified epididymis**   HCC ♂ ▽

C63.01 **Malignant neoplasm of right epididymis**   HCC ♂

C63.02 **Malignant neoplasm of left epididymis**   HCC ♂

☑5ᵗʰ **C63.1** **Malignant neoplasm of spermatic cord**

C63.10 **Malignant neoplasm of unspecified spermatic cord**   HCC ♂ ▽

C63.11 **Malignant neoplasm of right spermatic cord**   HCC ♂

C63.12 **Malignant neoplasm of left spermatic cord**   HCC ♂

C63.2 **Malignant neoplasm of scrotum**   HCC ♂
Malignant neoplasm of skin of scrotum

C63.7 **Malignant neoplasm of other specified male genital organs**   HCC ♂
Malignant neoplasm of seminal vesicle
Malignant neoplasm of tunica vaginalis

C63.8 **Malignant neoplasm of overlapping sites of male genital organs**   HCC ♂
Primary malignant neoplasm of two or more contiguous sites of male genital organs whose point of origin cannot be determined

C63.9 **Malignant neoplasm of male genital organ, unspecified**   HCC ♂ ▽
Malignant neoplasm of male genitourinary tract NOS

Malignant neoplasms of urinary tract (C64-C68)

☑4ᵗʰ **C64** **Malignant neoplasm of kidney, except renal pelvis**
EXCLUDES 1   malignant carcinoid tumor of the kidney (C7A.093)
malignant neoplasm of renal calyces (C65.-)
malignant neoplasm of renal pelvis (C65.-)

C64.1 **Malignant neoplasm of right kidney, except renal pelvis**   HCC

C64.2 **Malignant neoplasm of left kidney, except renal pelvis**   HCC

C64.9 **Malignant neoplasm of unspecified kidney, except renal pelvis**   HCC ▽

☑4ᵗʰ **C65** **Malignant neoplasm of renal pelvis**
INCLUDES   malignant neoplasm of pelviureteric junction
malignant neoplasm of renal calyces

C65.1 **Malignant neoplasm of right renal pelvis**   HCC

C65.2 **Malignant neoplasm of left renal pelvis**   HCC

C65.9 **Malignant neoplasm of unspecified renal pelvis**   HCC ▽

☑4ᵗʰ **C66** **Malignant neoplasm of ureter**
EXCLUDES 1   malignant neoplasm of ureteric orifice of bladder (C67.6)

C66.1 **Malignant neoplasm of right ureter**   HCC

C66.2 **Malignant neoplasm of left ureter**   HCC

C66.9 **Malignant neoplasm of unspecified ureter**   HCC ▽

☑4ᵗʰ **C67** **Malignant neoplasm of bladder**

C67.0 **Malignant neoplasm of trigone of bladder**   HCC

C67.1 **Malignant neoplasm of dome of bladder**   HCC

C67.2 **Malignant neoplasm of lateral wall of bladder**   HCC

C67.3 **Malignant neoplasm of anterior wall of bladder**   HCC

C67.4 **Malignant neoplasm of posterior wall of bladder**   HCC

C67.5 **Malignant neoplasm of bladder neck**   HCC
Malignant neoplasm of internal urethral orifice

C67.6 **Malignant neoplasm of ureteric orifice**   HCC

C67.7 **Malignant neoplasm of urachus**   HCC

C67.8 **Malignant neoplasm of overlapping sites of bladder**   HCC

C67.9 **Malignant neoplasm of bladder, unspecified**   HCC ▽
AHA: 2016, 1Q, 19

☑4ᵗʰ **C68** **Malignant neoplasm of other and unspecified urinary organs**
EXCLUDES 1   malignant neoplasm of female genitourinary tract NOS (C57.9)
malignant neoplasm of male genitourinary tract NOS (C63.9)

C68.0 **Malignant neoplasm of urethra**   HCC
EXCLUDES 1   malignant neoplasm of urethral orifice of bladder (C67.5)

C68.1 **Malignant neoplasm of paraurethral glands**   HCC

C68.8 **Malignant neoplasm of overlapping sites of urinary organs**   HCC
Primary malignant neoplasm of two or more contiguous sites of urinary organs whose point of origin cannot be determined

C68.9 **Malignant neoplasm of urinary organ, unspecified**   HCC ▽
Malignant neoplasm of urinary system NOS

Malignant neoplasms of eye, brain and other parts of central nervous system (C69-C72)

☑4ᵗʰ **C69** **Malignant neoplasm of eye and adnexa**
EXCLUDES 1   malignant neoplasm of connective tissue of eyelid (C49.0)
malignant neoplasm of eyelid (skin) (C43.1-, C44.1-)
malignant neoplasm of optic nerve (C72.3-)

☑5ᵗʰ **C69.0** **Malignant neoplasm of conjunctiva**

C69.00 **Malignant neoplasm of unspecified conjunctiva**   HCC ▽

C69.01 **Malignant neoplasm of right conjunctiva**   HCC

C69.02 **Malignant neoplasm of left conjunctiva**   HCC

☑5ᵗʰ **C69.1** **Malignant neoplasm of cornea**

C69.10 **Malignant neoplasm of unspecified cornea**   HCC ▽

C69.11 **Malignant neoplasm of right cornea**   HCC

C69.12 **Malignant neoplasm of left cornea**   HCC

☑5ᵗʰ **C69.2** **Malignant neoplasm of retina**
EXCLUDES 1   dark area on retina (D49.81)
neoplasm of unspecified behavior of retina and choroid (D49.81)
retinal freckle (D49.81)

C69.20 **Malignant neoplasm of unspecified retina**   HCC ▽

C69.21 **Malignant neoplasm of right retina**   HCC

C69.22 **Malignant neoplasm of left retina**   HCC

☑5ᵗʰ **C69.3** **Malignant neoplasm of choroid**

C69.30 **Malignant neoplasm of unspecified choroid**   HCC ▽

C69.31 **Malignant neoplasm of right choroid**   HCC

C69.32 **Malignant neoplasm of left choroid**   HCC

☑5ᵗʰ **C69.4** **Malignant neoplasm of ciliary body**

C69.40 **Malignant neoplasm of unspecified ciliary body**   HCC ▽

C69.41 **Malignant neoplasm of right ciliary body**   HCC

C69.42 **Malignant neoplasm of left ciliary body**   HCC

☑5ᵗʰ **C69.5** **Malignant neoplasm of lacrimal gland and duct**
Malignant neoplasm of lacrimal sac
Malignant neoplasm of nasolacrimal duct

C69.50 **Malignant neoplasm of unspecified lacrimal gland and duct**   HCC ▽

C69.51 **Malignant neoplasm of right lacrimal gland and duct**   HCC

C69.52 **Malignant neoplasm of left lacrimal gland and duct**   HCC

Chapter 2. Neoplasms

C62–C69.52

☑ Additional Character Req   ☑x7ᵗʰ Placeholder Alert   Manifestation   HCC CMS-HCC Condition   ▽ Unspecified Code   ►◄ Revised Text   ● New Code   ▲ Revised Code Title

✓5ᵗʰ **C69.6 Malignant neoplasm of orbit**
Malignant neoplasm of connective tissue of orbit
Malignant neoplasm of extraocular muscle
Malignant neoplasm of peripheral nerves of orbit
Malignant neoplasm of retrobulbar tissue
Malignant neoplasm of retro-ocular tissue
    EXCLUDES 1   malignant neoplasm of orbital bone (C41.0)

   C69.60 Malignant neoplasm of unspecified orbit   HCC ▽
   C69.61 Malignant neoplasm of right orbit   HCC
   C69.62 Malignant neoplasm of left orbit   HCC

✓5ᵗʰ **C69.8 Malignant neoplasm of overlapping sites of eye and adnexa**
   C69.80 Malignant neoplasm of overlapping sites of unspecified eye and adnexa   HCC ▽
   C69.81 Malignant neoplasm of overlapping sites of right eye and adnexa   HCC
   C69.82 Malignant neoplasm of overlapping sites of left eye and adnexa   HCC

✓5ᵗʰ **C69.9 Malignant neoplasm of unspecified site of eye**
Malignant neoplasm of eyeball
   C69.90 Malignant neoplasm of unspecified site of unspecified eye   HCC ▽
   C69.91 Malignant neoplasm of unspecified site of right eye   HCC ▽
   C69.92 Malignant neoplasm of unspecified site of left eye   HCC ▽

✓4ᵗʰ **C70 Malignant neoplasm of meninges**
   C70.0 Malignant neoplasm of cerebral meninges   HCC
   C70.1 Malignant neoplasm of spinal meninges   HCC
   C70.9 Malignant neoplasm of meninges, unspecified   HCC ▽

✓4ᵗʰ **C71 Malignant neoplasm of brain**
    EXCLUDES 1   malignant neoplasm of cranial nerves (C72.2-C72.5)
         retrobulbar malignant neoplasm (C69.6-)

   C71.0 Malignant neoplasm of cerebrum, except lobes and ventricles   HCC
Malignant neoplasm of supratentorial NOS
   C71.1 Malignant neoplasm of frontal lobe   HCC
   C71.2 Malignant neoplasm of temporal lobe   HCC
   C71.3 Malignant neoplasm of parietal lobe   HCC
   C71.4 Malignant neoplasm of occipital lobe   HCC
   C71.5 Malignant neoplasm of cerebral ventricle   HCC
    EXCLUDES 1   malignant neoplasm of fourth cerebral ventricle (C71.7)
   C71.6 Malignant neoplasm of cerebellum   HCC
   C71.7 Malignant neoplasm of brain stem   HCC
Malignant neoplasm of fourth cerebral ventricle
Infratentorial malignant neoplasm NOS
   C71.8 Malignant neoplasm of overlapping sites of brain   HCC
   C71.9 Malignant neoplasm of brain, unspecified   HCC ▽
     AHA: 2014, 3Q, 3

✓4ᵗʰ **C72 Malignant neoplasm of spinal cord, cranial nerves and other parts of central nervous system**
    EXCLUDES 1   malignant neoplasm of meninges (C70.-)
         malignant neoplasm of peripheral nerves and autonomic nervous system (C47.-)

   C72.0 Malignant neoplasm of spinal cord   HCC
   C72.1 Malignant neoplasm of cauda equina   HCC
✓5ᵗʰ **C72.2 Malignant neoplasm of olfactory nerve**
Malignant neoplasm of olfactory bulb
   C72.20 Malignant neoplasm of unspecified olfactory nerve   HCC ▽
   C72.21 Malignant neoplasm of right olfactory nerve   HCC
   C72.22 Malignant neoplasm of left olfactory nerve   HCC
✓5ᵗʰ **C72.3 Malignant neoplasm of optic nerve**
   C72.30 Malignant neoplasm of unspecified optic nerve   HCC ▽
   C72.31 Malignant neoplasm of right optic nerve   HCC
   C72.32 Malignant neoplasm of left optic nerve   HCC
✓5ᵗʰ **C72.4 Malignant neoplasm of acoustic nerve**
   C72.40 Malignant neoplasm of unspecified acoustic nerve   HCC ▽
   C72.41 Malignant neoplasm of right acoustic nerve   HCC
   C72.42 Malignant neoplasm of left acoustic nerve   HCC

Lobes of the Brain

Frontal lobe
Parietal lobe
Occipital lobe
Temporal lobe
Brain stem
Cerebellum

✓5ᵗʰ **C72.5 Malignant neoplasm of other and unspecified cranial nerves**
   C72.50 Malignant neoplasm of unspecified cranial nerve   HCC ▽
Malignant neoplasm of cranial nerve NOS
   C72.59 Malignant neoplasm of other cranial nerves   HCC
   C72.9 Malignant neoplasm of central nervous system, unspecified   HCC ▽
Malignant neoplasm of unspecified site of central nervous system
Malignant neoplasm of nervous system NOS

Malignant neoplasms of thyroid and other endocrine glands (C73-C75)

C73 Malignant neoplasm of thyroid gland   HCC
Use additional code to identify any functional activity

✓4ᵗʰ **C74 Malignant neoplasm of adrenal gland**
✓5ᵗʰ **C74.0 Malignant neoplasm of cortex of adrenal gland**
   C74.00 Malignant neoplasm of cortex of unspecified adrenal gland   HCC ▽
   C74.01 Malignant neoplasm of cortex of right adrenal gland   HCC
   C74.02 Malignant neoplasm of cortex of left adrenal gland   HCC
✓5ᵗʰ **C74.1 Malignant neoplasm of medulla of adrenal gland**
   C74.10 Malignant neoplasm of medulla of unspecified adrenal gland   HCC ▽
   C74.11 Malignant neoplasm of medulla of right adrenal gland   HCC
   C74.12 Malignant neoplasm of medulla of left adrenal gland   HCC
✓5ᵗʰ **C74.9 Malignant neoplasm of unspecified part of adrenal gland**
   C74.90 Malignant neoplasm of unspecified part of unspecified adrenal gland   HCC ▽
   C74.91 Malignant neoplasm of unspecified part of right adrenal gland   HCC ▽
   C74.92 Malignant neoplasm of unspecified part of left adrenal gland   HCC ▽

✓4ᵗʰ **C75 Malignant neoplasm of other endocrine glands and related structures**
    EXCLUDES 1   malignant carcinoid tumors (C7A.0-)
         malignant neoplasm of adrenal gland (C74.-)
         malignant neoplasm of endocrine pancreas (C25.4)
         malignant neoplasm of islets of Langerhans (C25.4)
         malignant neoplasm of ovary (C56.-)
         malignant neoplasm of testis (C62.-)
         malignant neoplasm of thymus (C37)
         malignant neoplasm of thyroid gland (C73)
         malignant neuroendocrine tumors (C7A.-)

   C75.0 Malignant neoplasm of parathyroid gland   HCC
   C75.1 Malignant neoplasm of pituitary gland   HCC
   C75.2 Malignant neoplasm of craniopharyngeal duct   HCC
   C75.3 Malignant neoplasm of pineal gland   HCC
   C75.4 Malignant neoplasm of carotid body   HCC

EXCLUDES 1 Not coded here   **EXCLUDES 2** Not included here   N Newborn Age: 0   P Pediatric Age: 0-17   M Maternity Age: 12-55   A Adult Age: 15-124

472   ICD-10-CM 2018

C75.5   **Malignant neoplasm of aortic body and other**   `HCC`
       paraganglia

C75.8   **Malignant neoplasm with pluriglandular involvement,**   `HCC` ▽
       unspecified

C75.9   **Malignant neoplasm of endocrine gland, unspecified**   `HCC` ▽

Malignant neuroendocrine tumors (C7A)

✓⁴ᵗʰ **C7A**   **Malignant neuroendocrine tumors**
       Code also any associated multiple endocrine neoplasia [MEN]
         syndromes (E31.2-)
       Use additional code to identify any associated endocrine syndrome,
         such as:
         carcinoid syndrome (E34.0)
       EXCLUDES 2   malignant pancreatic islet cell tumors (C25.4)
               Merkel cell carcinoma (C4A.-)

✓⁵ᵗʰ **C7A.0**   **Malignant carcinoid tumors**

     C7A.00   **Malignant carcinoid tumor of unspecified site**   `HCC` ▽

   ✓⁶ᵗʰ **C7A.01**   **Malignant carcinoid tumors of the small intestine**

         C7A.010   **Malignant carcinoid tumor of the**   `HCC`
                 duodenum

         C7A.011   **Malignant carcinoid tumor of the**   `HCC`
                 jejunum

         C7A.012   **Malignant carcinoid tumor of the**   `HCC`
                 ileum

         C7A.019   **Malignant carcinoid tumor of the**   `HCC` ▽
                 small intestine, unspecified portion

   ✓⁶ᵗʰ **C7A.02**   **Malignant carcinoid tumors of the appendix, large**
        intestine, and rectum

         C7A.020   **Malignant carcinoid tumor of the**   `HCC`
                 appendix

         C7A.021   **Malignant carcinoid tumor of the**   `HCC`
                 cecum

         C7A.022   **Malignant carcinoid tumor of the**   `HCC`
                 ascending colon

         C7A.023   **Malignant carcinoid tumor of the**   `HCC`
                 transverse colon

         C7A.024   **Malignant carcinoid tumor of the**   `HCC`
                 descending colon

         C7A.025   **Malignant carcinoid tumor of the**   `HCC`
                 sigmoid colon

         C7A.026   **Malignant carcinoid tumor of the**   `HCC`
                 rectum

         C7A.029   **Malignant carcinoid tumor of the**   `HCC` ▽
                 large intestine, unspecified portion
                   Malignant carcinoid tumor of the colon
                     NOS

   ✓⁶ᵗʰ **C7A.09**   **Malignant carcinoid tumors of other sites**

         C7A.090   **Malignant carcinoid tumor of the**   `HCC`
                 bronchus and lung

         C7A.091   **Malignant carcinoid tumor of the**   `HCC`
                 thymus

         C7A.092   **Malignant carcinoid tumor of the**   `HCC`
                 stomach

         C7A.093   **Malignant carcinoid tumor of the**   `HCC`
                 kidney

         C7A.094   **Malignant carcinoid tumor of the**   `HCC` ▽
                 foregut unspecified

         C7A.095   **Malignant carcinoid tumor of the**   `HCC` ▽
                 midgut unspecified

         C7A.096   **Malignant carcinoid tumor of the**   `HCC` ▽
                 hindgut unspecified

         C7A.098   **Malignant carcinoid tumors of**   `HCC`
                 other sites

C7A.1   **Malignant poorly differentiated neuroendocrine tumors**   `HCC`
       High grade neuroendocrine carcinoma, any site
       Malignant poorly differentiated neuroendocrine tumor NOS
       Malignant poorly differentiated neuroendocrine carcinoma,
         any site

C7A.8   **Other malignant neuroendocrine tumors**   `HCC`

Secondary neuroendocrine tumors (C7B)

✓⁴ᵗʰ **C7B**   **Secondary neuroendocrine tumors**
       Use additional code to identify any functional activity

✓⁵ᵗʰ **C7B.0**   **Secondary carcinoid tumors**

     C7B.00   **Secondary carcinoid tumors, unspecified site**   `HCC` ▽

     C7B.01   **Secondary carcinoid tumors of distant lymph**   `HCC`
         nodes

     C7B.02   **Secondary carcinoid tumors of liver**   `HCC`

     C7B.03   **Secondary carcinoid tumors of bone**   `HCC`

     C7B.04   **Secondary carcinoid tumors of peritoneum**   `HCC`
         Mesentery metastasis of carcinoid tumor

     C7B.09   **Secondary carcinoid tumors of other sites**   `HCC`

C7B.1   **Secondary Merkel cell carcinoma**   `HCC`
       Merkel cell carcinoma nodal presentation
       Merkel cell carcinoma visceral metastatic presentation

C7B.8   **Other secondary neuroendocrine tumors**   `HCC`

Malignant neoplasms of ill-defined, other secondary and unspecified sites (C76-C80)

✓⁴ᵗʰ **C76**   **Malignant neoplasm of other and ill-defined sites**
       EXCLUDES 1   malignant neoplasm of female genitourinary tract NOS (C57.9)
               malignant neoplasm of male genitourinary tract NOS (C63.9)
               malignant neoplasm of lymphoid, hematopoietic and related
                  tissue (C81-C96)
               malignant neoplasm of skin (C44.-)
               malignant neoplasm of unspecified site NOS (C80.1)

C76.0   **Malignant neoplasm of head, face and neck**   `HCC`
       Malignant neoplasm of cheek NOS
       Malignant neoplasm of nose NOS

C76.1   **Malignant neoplasm of thorax**   `HCC`
       Intrathoracic malignant neoplasm NOS
       Malignant neoplasm of axilla NOS
       Thoracic malignant neoplasm NOS

C76.2   **Malignant neoplasm of abdomen**   `HCC`

C76.3   **Malignant neoplasm of pelvis**   `HCC`
       Malignant neoplasm of groin NOS
       Malignant neoplasm of sites overlapping systems within the
         pelvis
       Rectovaginal (septum) malignant neoplasm
       Rectovesical (septum) malignant neoplasm

✓⁵ᵗʰ **C76.4**   **Malignant neoplasm of upper limb**

     C76.40   **Malignant neoplasm of unspecified upper**   `HCC` ▽
         limb

     C76.41   **Malignant neoplasm of right upper limb**   `HCC`

     C76.42   **Malignant neoplasm of left upper limb**   `HCC`

✓⁵ᵗʰ **C76.5**   **Malignant neoplasm of lower limb**

     C76.50   **Malignant neoplasm of unspecified lower**   `HCC` ▽
         limb

     C76.51   **Malignant neoplasm of right lower limb**   `HCC`

     C76.52   **Malignant neoplasm of left lower limb**   `HCC`

C76.8   **Malignant neoplasm of other specified ill-defined sites**   `HCC`
       Malignant neoplasm of overlapping ill-defined sites

✓⁴ᵗʰ **C77**   **Secondary and unspecified malignant neoplasm of lymph nodes**
       EXCLUDES 1   malignant neoplasm of lymph nodes, specified as primary
               (C81-C86, C88, C96.-)
               mesentery metastasis of carcinoid tumor (C7B.04)
               secondary carcinoid tumors of distant lymph nodes (C7B.01)

C77.0   **Secondary and unspecified malignant neoplasm of**   `HCC`
       lymph nodes of head, face and neck
       Secondary and unspecified malignant neoplasm of
         supraclavicular lymph nodes

C77.1   **Secondary and unspecified malignant neoplasm of**   `HCC`
       intrathoracic lymph nodes

C77.2   **Secondary and unspecified malignant neoplasm of**   `HCC`
       intra-abdominal lymph nodes

C77.3   **Secondary and unspecified malignant neoplasm of**   `HCC`
       axilla and upper limb lymph nodes
       Secondary and unspecified malignant neoplasm of pectoral
         lymph nodes

C77.4   **Secondary and unspecified malignant neoplasm of**   `HCC`
       inguinal and lower limb lymph nodes

C77.5   **Secondary and unspecified malignant neoplasm of**   `HCC`
       intrapelvic lymph nodes

C77.8   **Secondary and unspecified malignant neoplasm of**   `HCC`
       lymph nodes of multiple regions

C77.9   **Secondary and unspecified malignant neoplasm of**   `HCC` ▽
       lymph node, unspecified

☑ Additional Character Req   ✓⁷ᵗʰ Placeholder Alert   Manifestation   `HCC` CMS-HCC Condition   ▽ Unspecified Code   ►◄ Revised Text   ● New Code   ▲ Revised Code Title

ICD-10-CM 2018   **473**

✓4ᵗʰ **C78** **Secondary malignant neoplasm of respiratory and digestive organs**
> EXCLUDES 1   *secondary carcinoid tumors of liver (C7B.Ø2)*
> *secondary carcinoid tumors of peritoneum (C7B.Ø4)*
> EXCLUDES 2   *lymph node metastases (C77.Ø)*

✓5ᵗʰ **C78.Ø** **Secondary malignant neoplasm of lung**
- **C78.ØØ** **Secondary malignant neoplasm of unspecified lung** HCC ▽
- **C78.Ø1** **Secondary malignant neoplasm of right lung** HCC
- **C78.Ø2** **Secondary malignant neoplasm of left lung** HCC

C78.1 **Secondary malignant neoplasm of mediastinum** HCC

C78.2 **Secondary malignant neoplasm of pleura** HCC

✓5ᵗʰ **C78.3** **Secondary malignant neoplasm of other and unspecified respiratory organs**
- **C78.3Ø** **Secondary malignant neoplasm of unspecified respiratory organ** HCC ▽
- **C78.39** **Secondary malignant neoplasm of other respiratory organs** HCC

C78.4 **Secondary malignant neoplasm of small intestine** HCC

C78.5 **Secondary malignant neoplasm of large intestine and rectum** HCC

C78.6 **Secondary malignant neoplasm of retroperitoneum and peritoneum** HCC
> AHA: 2017, 2Q, 12

C78.7 **Secondary malignant neoplasm of liver and intrahepatic bile duct** HCC

✓5ᵗʰ **C78.8** **Secondary malignant neoplasm of other and unspecified digestive organs**
- **C78.8Ø** **Secondary malignant neoplasm of unspecified digestive organ** HCC ▽
- **C78.89** **Secondary malignant neoplasm of other digestive organs** HCC
  > Code also exocrine pancreatic insufficiency (K86.81)

✓4ᵗʰ **C79** **Secondary malignant neoplasm of other and unspecified sites**
> EXCLUDES 1   *secondary carcinoid tumors (C7B.-)*
> *secondary neuroendocrine tumors (C7B.-)*
> EXCLUDES 2   *lymph node metastases (C77.Ø)*

✓5ᵗʰ **C79.Ø** **Secondary malignant neoplasm of kidney and renal pelvis**
- **C79.ØØ** **Secondary malignant neoplasm of unspecified kidney and renal pelvis** HCC ▽
- **C79.Ø1** **Secondary malignant neoplasm of right kidney and renal pelvis** HCC
- **C79.Ø2** **Secondary malignant neoplasm of left kidney and renal pelvis** HCC

✓5ᵗʰ **C79.1** **Secondary malignant neoplasm of bladder and other and unspecified urinary organs**
- **C79.1Ø** **Secondary malignant neoplasm of unspecified urinary organs** HCC ▽
- **C79.11** **Secondary malignant neoplasm of bladder** HCC
  > EXCLUDES 2 ▶*lymph node metastases (C77.Ø)*◀
- **C79.19** **Secondary malignant neoplasm of other urinary organs** HCC

C79.2 **Secondary malignant neoplasm of skin** HCC
> EXCLUDES 1   *secondary Merkel cell carcinoma (C7B.1)*

✓5ᵗʰ **C79.3** **Secondary malignant neoplasm of brain and cerebral meninges**
- **C79.31** **Secondary malignant neoplasm of brain** HCC
- **C79.32** **Secondary malignant neoplasm of cerebral meninges** HCC

✓5ᵗʰ **C79.4** **Secondary malignant neoplasm of other and unspecified parts of nervous system**
- **C79.4Ø** **Secondary malignant neoplasm of unspecified part of nervous system** HCC ▽
- **C79.49** **Secondary malignant neoplasm of other parts of nervous system** HCC

✓5ᵗʰ **C79.5** **Secondary malignant neoplasm of bone and bone marrow**
> EXCLUDES 1   *secondary carcinoid tumors of bone (C7B.Ø3)*
- **C79.51** **Secondary malignant neoplasm of bone** HCC
- **C79.52** **Secondary malignant neoplasm of bone marrow** HCC

✓5ᵗʰ **C79.6** **Secondary malignant neoplasm of ovary**
- **C79.6Ø** **Secondary malignant neoplasm of unspecified ovary** HCC ♀▽
- **C79.61** **Secondary malignant neoplasm of right ovary** HCC ♀
- **C79.62** **Secondary malignant neoplasm of left ovary** HCC ♀

✓5ᵗʰ **C79.7** **Secondary malignant neoplasm of adrenal gland**
- **C79.7Ø** **Secondary malignant neoplasm of unspecified adrenal gland** HCC ▽
- **C79.71** **Secondary malignant neoplasm of right adrenal gland** HCC
- **C79.72** **Secondary malignant neoplasm of left adrenal gland** HCC

✓5ᵗʰ **C79.8** **Secondary malignant neoplasm of other specified sites**
- **C79.81** **Secondary malignant neoplasm of breast** HCC
- **C79.82** **Secondary malignant neoplasm of genital organs** HCC
- **C79.89** **Secondary malignant neoplasm of other specified sites** HCC
  > AHA: 2017, 2Q, 11

C79.9 **Secondary malignant neoplasm of unspecified site** HCC ▽
> Metastatic cancer NOS
> Metastatic disease NOS
> EXCLUDES 1   *carcinomatosis NOS (C80.Ø)*
> *generalized cancer NOS (C80.Ø)*
> *malignant (primary) neoplasm of unspecified site (C80.1)*

✓4ᵗʰ **C80** **Malignant neoplasm without specification of site**
> EXCLUDES 1   *malignant carcinoid tumor of unspecified site (C7A.ØØ)*
> *malignant neoplasm of specified multiple sites—code to each site*

C80.Ø **Disseminated malignant neoplasm, unspecified** HCC ▽
> Carcinomatosis NOS
> Generalized cancer, unspecified site (primary) (secondary)
> Generalized malignancy, unspecified site (primary) (secondary)

C80.1 **Malignant (primary) neoplasm, unspecified** HCC ▽
> Cancer NOS
> Cancer unspecified site (primary)
> Carcinoma unspecified site (primary)
> Malignancy unspecified site (primary)
> EXCLUDES 1   *secondary malignant neoplasm of unspecified site (C79.9)*

C80.2 **Malignant neoplasm associated with transplanted organ** HCC
> Code first complication of transplanted organ (T86.-)
> Use additional code to identify the specific malignancy

Malignant neoplasms of lymphoid, hematopoietic and related tissue (C81-C96)

> EXCLUDES 2   *Kaposi's sarcoma of lymph nodes (C46.3)*
> *secondary and unspecified neoplasm of lymph nodes (C77.-)*
> *secondary neoplasm of bone marrow (C79.52)*
> *secondary neoplasm of spleen (C78.89)*

✓4ᵗʰ **C81** **Hodgkin lymphoma**
> EXCLUDES 1   *personal history of Hodgkin lymphoma (Z85.71)*

✓5ᵗʰ **C81.Ø** **Nodular lymphocyte predominant Hodgkin lymphoma**
- **C81.ØØ** **Nodular lymphocyte predominant Hodgkin lymphoma, unspecified site** HCC ▽
- **C81.Ø1** **Nodular lymphocyte predominant Hodgkin lymphoma, lymph nodes of head, face, and neck** HCC
- **C81.Ø2** **Nodular lymphocyte predominant Hodgkin lymphoma, intrathoracic lymph nodes** HCC
- **C81.Ø3** **Nodular lymphocyte predominant Hodgkin lymphoma, intra-abdominal lymph nodes** HCC
- **C81.Ø4** **Nodular lymphocyte predominant Hodgkin lymphoma, lymph nodes of axilla and upper limb** HCC
- **C81.Ø5** **Nodular lymphocyte predominant Hodgkin lymphoma, lymph nodes of inguinal region and lower limb** HCC
- **C81.Ø6** **Nodular lymphocyte predominant Hodgkin lymphoma, intrapelvic lymph nodes** HCC
- **C81.Ø7** **Nodular lymphocyte predominant Hodgkin lymphoma, spleen** HCC
- **C81.Ø8** **Nodular lymphocyte predominant Hodgkin lymphoma, lymph nodes of multiple sites** HCC
- **C81.Ø9** **Nodular lymphocyte predominant Hodgkin lymphoma, extranodal and solid organ sites** HCC

✓5ᵗʰ **C81.1** **Nodular sclerosis Hodgkin lymphoma**
> Nodular sclerosis classical Hodgkin lymphoma
- **C81.1Ø** **Nodular sclerosis Hodgkin lymphoma, unspecified site** HCC ▽
- **C81.11** **Nodular sclerosis Hodgkin lymphoma, lymph nodes of head, face, and neck** HCC

EXCLUDES 1 Not coded here   EXCLUDES 2 Not included here   N Newborn Age: 0   P Pediatric Age: 0-17   M Maternity Age: 12-55   A Adult Age: 15-124

474   ICD-10-CM 2018

C81.12 **Nodular sclerosis Hodgkin lymphoma, intrathoracic lymph nodes** `HCC`

C81.13 **Nodular sclerosis Hodgkin lymphoma, intra-abdominal lymph nodes** `HCC`

C81.14 **Nodular sclerosis Hodgkin lymphoma, lymph nodes of axilla and upper limb** `HCC`

C81.15 **Nodular sclerosis Hodgkin lymphoma, lymph nodes of inguinal region and lower limb** `HCC`

C81.16 **Nodular sclerosis Hodgkin lymphoma, intrapelvic lymph nodes** `HCC`

C81.17 **Nodular sclerosis Hodgkin lymphoma, spleen** `HCC`

C81.18 **Nodular sclerosis Hodgkin lymphoma, lymph nodes of multiple sites** `HCC`

C81.19 **Nodular sclerosis Hodgkin lymphoma, extranodal and solid organ sites** `HCC`

√5ᵗʰ **C81.2 Mixed cellularity Hodgkin lymphoma**
Mixed cellularity classical Hodgkin lymphoma

C81.20 **Mixed cellularity Hodgkin lymphoma, unspecified site** `HCC` ▽

C81.21 **Mixed cellularity Hodgkin lymphoma, lymph nodes of head, face, and neck** `HCC`

C81.22 **Mixed cellularity Hodgkin lymphoma, intrathoracic lymph nodes** `HCC`

C81.23 **Mixed cellularity Hodgkin lymphoma, intra-abdominal lymph nodes** `HCC`

C81.24 **Mixed cellularity Hodgkin lymphoma, lymph nodes of axilla and upper limb** `HCC`

C81.25 **Mixed cellularity Hodgkin lymphoma, lymph nodes of inguinal region and lower limb** `HCC`

C81.26 **Mixed cellularity Hodgkin lymphoma, intrapelvic lymph nodes** `HCC`

C81.27 **Mixed cellularity Hodgkin lymphoma, spleen** `HCC`

C81.28 **Mixed cellularity Hodgkin lymphoma, lymph nodes of multiple sites** `HCC`

C81.29 **Mixed cellularity Hodgkin lymphoma, extranodal and solid organ sites** `HCC`

√5ᵗʰ **C81.3 Lymphocyte depleted Hodgkin lymphoma**
Lymphocyte depleted classical Hodgkin lymphoma

C81.30 **Lymphocyte depleted Hodgkin lymphoma, unspecified site** `HCC` ▽

C81.31 **Lymphocyte depleted Hodgkin lymphoma, lymph nodes of head, face, and neck** `HCC`

C81.32 **Lymphocyte depleted Hodgkin lymphoma, intrathoracic lymph nodes** `HCC`

C81.33 **Lymphocyte depleted Hodgkin lymphoma, intra-abdominal lymph nodes** `HCC`

C81.34 **Lymphocyte depleted Hodgkin lymphoma, lymph nodes of axilla and upper limb** `HCC`

C81.35 **Lymphocyte depleted Hodgkin lymphoma, lymph nodes of inguinal region and lower limb** `HCC`

C81.36 **Lymphocyte depleted Hodgkin lymphoma, intrapelvic lymph nodes** `HCC`

C81.37 **Lymphocyte depleted Hodgkin lymphoma, spleen** `HCC`

C81.38 **Lymphocyte depleted Hodgkin lymphoma, lymph nodes of multiple sites** `HCC`

C81.39 **Lymphocyte depleted Hodgkin lymphoma, extranodal and solid organ sites** `HCC`

√5ᵗʰ **C81.4 Lymphocyte-rich Hodgkin lymphoma**
Lymphocyte-rich classical Hodgkin lymphoma
EXCLUDES 1 *nodular lymphocyte predominant Hodgkin lymphoma (C81.0-)*

C81.40 **Lymphocyte-rich Hodgkin lymphoma, unspecified site** `HCC` ▽

C81.41 **Lymphocyte-rich Hodgkin lymphoma, lymph nodes of head, face, and neck** `HCC`

C81.42 **Lymphocyte-rich Hodgkin lymphoma, intrathoracic lymph nodes** `HCC`

C81.43 **Lymphocyte-rich Hodgkin lymphoma, intra-abdominal lymph nodes** `HCC`

C81.44 **Lymphocyte-rich Hodgkin lymphoma, lymph nodes of axilla and upper limb** `HCC`

C81.45 **Lymphocyte-rich Hodgkin lymphoma, lymph nodes of inguinal region and lower limb** `HCC`

C81.46 **Lymphocyte-rich Hodgkin lymphoma, intrapelvic lymph nodes** `HCC`

C81.47 **Lymphocyte-rich Hodgkin lymphoma, spleen** `HCC`

C81.48 **Lymphocyte-rich Hodgkin lymphoma, lymph nodes of multiple sites** `HCC`

C81.49 **Lymphocyte-rich Hodgkin lymphoma, extranodal and solid organ sites** `HCC`

√5ᵗʰ **C81.7 Other Hodgkin lymphoma**
Classical Hodgkin lymphoma NOS
Other classical Hodgkin lymphoma

C81.70 **Other Hodgkin lymphoma, unspecified site** `HCC` ▽

C81.71 **Other Hodgkin lymphoma, lymph nodes of head, face, and neck** `HCC`

C81.72 **Other Hodgkin lymphoma, intrathoracic lymph nodes** `HCC`

C81.73 **Other Hodgkin lymphoma, intra-abdominal lymph nodes** `HCC`

C81.74 **Other Hodgkin lymphoma, lymph nodes of axilla and upper limb** `HCC`

C81.75 **Other Hodgkin lymphoma, lymph nodes of inguinal region and lower limb** `HCC`

C81.76 **Other Hodgkin lymphoma, intrapelvic lymph nodes** `HCC`

C81.77 **Other Hodgkin lymphoma, spleen** `HCC`

C81.78 **Other Hodgkin lymphoma, lymph nodes of multiple sites** `HCC`

C81.79 **Other Hodgkin lymphoma, extranodal and solid organ sites** `HCC`

√5ᵗʰ **C81.9 Hodgkin lymphoma, unspecified**

C81.90 **Hodgkin lymphoma, unspecified, unspecified site** `HCC` ▽

C81.91 **Hodgkin lymphoma, unspecified, lymph nodes of head, face, and neck** `HCC` ▽

C81.92 **Hodgkin lymphoma, unspecified, intrathoracic lymph nodes** `HCC` ▽

C81.93 **Hodgkin lymphoma, unspecified, intra-abdominal lymph nodes** `HCC` ▽

C81.94 **Hodgkin lymphoma, unspecified, lymph nodes of axilla and upper limb** `HCC` ▽

C81.95 **Hodgkin lymphoma, unspecified, lymph nodes of inguinal region and lower limb** `HCC` ▽

C81.96 **Hodgkin lymphoma, unspecified, intrapelvic lymph nodes** `HCC` ▽

C81.97 **Hodgkin lymphoma, unspecified, spleen** `HCC` ▽

C81.98 **Hodgkin lymphoma, unspecified, lymph nodes of multiple sites** `HCC` ▽

C81.99 **Hodgkin lymphoma, unspecified, extranodal and solid organ sites** `HCC` ▽

√4ᵗʰ **C82 Follicular lymphoma**
INCLUDES follicular lymphoma with or without diffuse areas
EXCLUDES 1 *mature T/NK-cell lymphomas (C84.-)*
personal history of non-Hodgkin lymphoma (Z85.72)

√5ᵗʰ **C82.0 Follicular lymphoma grade I**

C82.00 **Follicular lymphoma grade I, unspecified site** `HCC` ▽

C82.01 **Follicular lymphoma grade I, lymph nodes of head, face, and neck** `HCC`

C82.02 **Follicular lymphoma grade I, intrathoracic lymph nodes** `HCC`

C82.03 **Follicular lymphoma grade I, intra-abdominal lymph nodes** `HCC`

C82.04 **Follicular lymphoma grade I, lymph nodes of axilla and upper limb** `HCC`

C82.05 **Follicular lymphoma grade I, lymph nodes of inguinal region and lower limb** `HCC`

C82.06 **Follicular lymphoma grade I, intrapelvic lymph nodes** `HCC`

C82.07 **Follicular lymphoma grade I, spleen** `HCC`

C82.08 **Follicular lymphoma grade I, lymph nodes of multiple sites** `HCC`

C82.09 **Follicular lymphoma grade I, extranodal and solid organ sites** `HCC`

√5ᵗʰ **C82.1 Follicular lymphoma grade II**

C82.10 **Follicular lymphoma grade II, unspecified site** `HCC` ▽

C82.11 **Follicular lymphoma grade II, lymph nodes of head, face, and neck** `HCC`

C82.12 **Follicular lymphoma grade II, intrathoracic lymph nodes** `HCC`

C82.13 **Follicular lymphoma grade II, intra-abdominal lymph nodes** `HCC`

C82.14 Follicular lymphoma grade II, lymph nodes of axilla and upper limb `HCC`

C82.15 Follicular lymphoma grade II, lymph nodes of inguinal region and lower limb `HCC`

C82.16 Follicular lymphoma grade II, intrapelvic lymph nodes `HCC`

C82.17 Follicular lymphoma grade II, spleen `HCC`

C82.18 Follicular lymphoma grade II, lymph nodes of multiple sites `HCC`

C82.19 Follicular lymphoma grade II, extranodal and solid organ sites `HCC`

✓5ᵗʰ **C82.2** Follicular lymphoma grade III, unspecified

C82.20 Follicular lymphoma grade III, unspecified, unspecified site `HCC` ▽

C82.21 Follicular lymphoma grade III, unspecified, lymph nodes of head, face, and neck `HCC` ▽

C82.22 Follicular lymphoma grade III, unspecified, intrathoracic lymph nodes `HCC` ▽

C82.23 Follicular lymphoma grade III, unspecified, intra-abdominal lymph nodes `HCC` ▽

C82.24 Follicular lymphoma grade III, unspecified, lymph nodes of axilla and upper limb `HCC` ▽

C82.25 Follicular lymphoma grade III, unspecified, lymph nodes of inguinal region and lower limb `HCC` ▽

C82.26 Follicular lymphoma grade III, unspecified, intrapelvic lymph nodes `HCC` ▽

C82.27 Follicular lymphoma grade III, unspecified, spleen `HCC` ▽

C82.28 Follicular lymphoma grade III, unspecified, lymph nodes of multiple sites `HCC` ▽

C82.29 Follicular lymphoma grade III, unspecified, extranodal and solid organ sites `HCC` ▽

✓5ᵗʰ **C82.3** Follicular lymphoma grade IIIa

C82.30 Follicular lymphoma grade IIIa, unspecified site `HCC` ▽

C82.31 Follicular lymphoma grade IIIa, lymph nodes of head, face, and neck `HCC`

C82.32 Follicular lymphoma grade IIIa, intrathoracic lymph nodes `HCC`

C82.33 Follicular lymphoma grade IIIa, intra-abdominal lymph nodes `HCC`

C82.34 Follicular lymphoma grade IIIa, lymph nodes of axilla and upper limb `HCC`

C82.35 Follicular lymphoma grade IIIa, lymph nodes of inguinal region and lower limb `HCC`

C82.36 Follicular lymphoma grade IIIa, intrapelvic lymph nodes `HCC`

C82.37 Follicular lymphoma grade IIIa, spleen `HCC`

C82.38 Follicular lymphoma grade IIIa, lymph nodes of multiple sites `HCC`

C82.39 Follicular lymphoma grade IIIa, extranodal and solid organ sites `HCC`

✓5ᵗʰ **C82.4** Follicular lymphoma grade IIIb

C82.40 Follicular lymphoma grade IIIb, unspecified site `HCC` ▽

C82.41 Follicular lymphoma grade IIIb, lymph nodes of head, face, and neck `HCC`

C82.42 Follicular lymphoma grade IIIb, intrathoracic lymph nodes `HCC`

C82.43 Follicular lymphoma grade IIIb, intra-abdominal lymph nodes `HCC`

C82.44 Follicular lymphoma grade IIIb, lymph nodes of axilla and upper limb `HCC`

C82.45 Follicular lymphoma grade IIIb, lymph nodes of inguinal region and lower limb `HCC`

C82.46 Follicular lymphoma grade IIIb, intrapelvic lymph nodes `HCC`

C82.47 Follicular lymphoma grade IIIb, spleen `HCC`

C82.48 Follicular lymphoma grade IIIb, lymph nodes of multiple sites `HCC`

C82.49 Follicular lymphoma grade IIIb, extranodal and solid organ sites `HCC`

✓5ᵗʰ **C82.5** Diffuse follicle center lymphoma

C82.50 Diffuse follicle center lymphoma, unspecified site `HCC` ▽

C82.51 Diffuse follicle center lymphoma, lymph nodes of head, face, and neck `HCC`

C82.52 Diffuse follicle center lymphoma, intrathoracic lymph nodes `HCC`

C82.53 Diffuse follicle center lymphoma, intra-abdominal lymph nodes `HCC`

C82.54 Diffuse follicle center lymphoma, lymph nodes of axilla and upper limb `HCC`

C82.55 Diffuse follicle center lymphoma, lymph nodes of inguinal region and lower limb `HCC`

C82.56 Diffuse follicle center lymphoma, intrapelvic lymph nodes `HCC`

C82.57 Diffuse follicle center lymphoma, spleen `HCC`

C82.58 Diffuse follicle center lymphoma, lymph nodes of multiple sites `HCC`

C82.59 Diffuse follicle center lymphoma, extranodal and solid organ sites `HCC`

✓5ᵗʰ **C82.6** Cutaneous follicle center lymphoma

C82.60 Cutaneous follicle center lymphoma, unspecified site `HCC` ▽

C82.61 Cutaneous follicle center lymphoma, lymph nodes of head, face, and neck `HCC`

C82.62 Cutaneous follicle center lymphoma, intrathoracic lymph nodes `HCC`

C82.63 Cutaneous follicle center lymphoma, intra-abdominal lymph nodes `HCC`

C82.64 Cutaneous follicle center lymphoma, lymph nodes of axilla and upper limb `HCC`

C82.65 Cutaneous follicle center lymphoma, lymph nodes of inguinal region and lower limb `HCC`

C82.66 Cutaneous follicle center lymphoma, intrapelvic lymph nodes `HCC`

C82.67 Cutaneous follicle center lymphoma, spleen `HCC`

C82.68 Cutaneous follicle center lymphoma, lymph nodes of multiple sites `HCC`

C82.69 Cutaneous follicle center lymphoma, extranodal and solid organ sites `HCC`

✓5ᵗʰ **C82.8** Other types of follicular lymphoma

C82.80 Other types of follicular lymphoma, unspecified site `HCC` ▽

C82.81 Other types of follicular lymphoma, lymph nodes of head, face, and neck `HCC`

C82.82 Other types of follicular lymphoma, intrathoracic lymph nodes `HCC`

C82.83 Other types of follicular lymphoma, intra-abdominal lymph nodes `HCC`

C82.84 Other types of follicular lymphoma, lymph nodes of axilla and upper limb `HCC`

C82.85 Other types of follicular lymphoma, lymph nodes of inguinal region and lower limb `HCC`

C82.86 Other types of follicular lymphoma, intrapelvic lymph nodes `HCC`

C82.87 Other types of follicular lymphoma, spleen `HCC`

C82.88 Other types of follicular lymphoma, lymph nodes of multiple sites `HCC`

C82.89 Other types of follicular lymphoma, extranodal and solid organ sites `HCC`

✓5ᵗʰ **C82.9** Follicular lymphoma, unspecified

C82.90 Follicular lymphoma, unspecified, unspecified site `HCC` ▽

C82.91 Follicular lymphoma, unspecified, lymph nodes of head, face, and neck `HCC` ▽

C82.92 Follicular lymphoma, unspecified, intrathoracic lymph nodes `HCC` ▽

C82.93 Follicular lymphoma, unspecified, intra-abdominal lymph nodes `HCC` ▽

C82.94 Follicular lymphoma, unspecified, lymph nodes of axilla and upper limb `HCC` ▽

C82.95 Follicular lymphoma, unspecified, lymph nodes of inguinal region and lower limb `HCC` ▽

C82.96 Follicular lymphoma, unspecified, intrapelvic lymph nodes `HCC` ▽

C82.97 Follicular lymphoma, unspecified, spleen `HCC` ▽

EXCLUDES 1 Not coded here   **EXCLUDES 2** Not included here   **N** Newborn Age: 0   **P** Pediatric Age: 0-17   **M** Maternity Age: 12-55   **A** Adult Age: 15-124

476   ICD-10-CM 2018

C82.98   **Follicular lymphoma, unspecified, lymph nodes of multiple sites**   HCC ▽

C82.99   **Follicular lymphoma, unspecified, extranodal and solid organ sites**   HCC ▽

✓4ᵗʰ **C83**   **Non-follicular lymphoma**
> EXCLUDES 1   *personal history of non-Hodgkin lymphoma (Z85.72)*

✓5ᵗʰ **C83.0**   **Small cell B-cell lymphoma**
Lymphoplasmacytic lymphoma
Nodal marginal zone lymphoma
Non-leukemic variant of B-CLL
Splenic marginal zone lymphoma
> EXCLUDES 1   *chronic lymphocytic leukemia (C91.1)*
> *mature T/NK-cell lymphomas (C84.-)*
> *Waldenström macroglobulinemia (C88.0)*

C83.00   **Small cell B-cell lymphoma, unspecified site**   HCC ▽

C83.01   **Small cell B-cell lymphoma, lymph nodes of head, face, and neck**   HCC

C83.02   **Small cell B-cell lymphoma, intrathoracic lymph nodes**   HCC

C83.03   **Small cell B-cell lymphoma, intra-abdominal lymph nodes**   HCC

C83.04   **Small cell B-cell lymphoma, lymph nodes of axilla and upper limb**   HCC

C83.05   **Small cell B-cell lymphoma, lymph nodes of inguinal region and lower limb**   HCC

C83.06   **Small cell B-cell lymphoma, intrapelvic lymph nodes**   HCC

C83.07   **Small cell B-cell lymphoma, spleen**   HCC

C83.08   **Small cell B-cell lymphoma, lymph nodes of multiple sites**   HCC

C83.09   **Small cell B-cell lymphoma, extranodal and solid organ sites**   HCC

✓5ᵗʰ **C83.1**   **Mantle cell lymphoma**
Centrocytic lymphoma
Malignant lymphomatous polyposis
DEF: Rare form of B-cell non-Hodgkin lymphoma named for the location of tumor cell production, the mantle zone of the lymph nodes.

C83.10   **Mantle cell lymphoma, unspecified site**   HCC ▽

C83.11   **Mantle cell lymphoma, lymph nodes of head, face, and neck**   HCC

C83.12   **Mantle cell lymphoma, intrathoracic lymph nodes**   HCC

C83.13   **Mantle cell lymphoma, intra-abdominal lymph nodes**   HCC

C83.14   **Mantle cell lymphoma, lymph nodes of axilla and upper limb**   HCC

C83.15   **Mantle cell lymphoma, lymph nodes of inguinal region and lower limb**   HCC

C83.16   **Mantle cell lymphoma, intrapelvic lymph nodes**   HCC

C83.17   **Mantle cell lymphoma, spleen**   HCC

C83.18   **Mantle cell lymphoma, lymph nodes of multiple sites**   HCC

C83.19   **Mantle cell lymphoma, extranodal and solid organ sites**   HCC

✓5ᵗʰ **C83.3**   **Diffuse large B-cell lymphoma**
Anaplastic diffuse large B-cell lymphoma
CD30-positive diffuse large B-cell lymphoma
Centroblastic diffuse large B-cell lymphoma
Diffuse large B-cell lymphoma, subtype not specified
Immunoblastic diffuse large B-cell lymphoma
Plasmablastic diffuse large B-cell lymphoma
T-cell rich diffuse large B-cell lymphoma
> EXCLUDES 1   *mature T/NK-cell lymphomas (C84.-)*
> *mediastinal (thymic) large B-cell lymphoma (C85.2-)*

C83.30   **Diffuse large B-cell lymphoma, unspecified site**   HCC ▽

C83.31   **Diffuse large B-cell lymphoma, lymph nodes of head, face, and neck**   HCC

C83.32   **Diffuse large B-cell lymphoma, intrathoracic lymph nodes**   HCC

C83.33   **Diffuse large B-cell lymphoma, intra-abdominal lymph nodes**   HCC

C83.34   **Diffuse large B-cell lymphoma, lymph nodes of axilla and upper limb**   HCC

C83.35   **Diffuse large B-cell lymphoma, lymph nodes of inguinal region and lower limb**   HCC

C83.36   **Diffuse large B-cell lymphoma, intrapelvic lymph nodes**   HCC

C83.37   **Diffuse large B-cell lymphoma, spleen**   HCC

C83.38   **Diffuse large B-cell lymphoma, lymph nodes of multiple sites**   HCC

C83.39   **Diffuse large B-cell lymphoma, extranodal and solid organ sites**   HCC

✓5ᵗʰ **C83.5**   **Lymphoblastic (diffuse) lymphoma**
B-precursor lymphoma
Lymphoblastic B-cell lymphoma
Lymphoblastic lymphoma NOS
Lymphoblastic T-cell lymphoma
T-precursor lymphoma

C83.50   **Lymphoblastic (diffuse) lymphoma, unspecified site**   HCC ▽

C83.51   **Lymphoblastic (diffuse) lymphoma, lymph nodes of head, face, and neck**   HCC

C83.52   **Lymphoblastic (diffuse) lymphoma, intrathoracic lymph nodes**   HCC

C83.53   **Lymphoblastic (diffuse) lymphoma, intra-abdominal lymph nodes**   HCC

C83.54   **Lymphoblastic (diffuse) lymphoma, lymph nodes of axilla and upper limb**   HCC

C83.55   **Lymphoblastic (diffuse) lymphoma, lymph nodes of inguinal region and lower limb**   HCC

C83.56   **Lymphoblastic (diffuse) lymphoma, intrapelvic lymph nodes**   HCC

C83.57   **Lymphoblastic (diffuse) lymphoma, spleen**   HCC

C83.58   **Lymphoblastic (diffuse) lymphoma, lymph nodes of multiple sites**   HCC

C83.59   **Lymphoblastic (diffuse) lymphoma, extranodal and solid organ sites**   HCC

✓5ᵗʰ **C83.7**   **Burkitt lymphoma**
Atypical Burkitt lymphoma
Burkitt-like lymphoma
> EXCLUDES 1   *mature B-cell leukemia Burkitt type (C91.A-)*
DEF: Malignancy of the lymphatic system, most often seen as a large bone-deteriorating lesion within the jaw or as an abdominal mass. It is a form of non-Hodgkin's lymphoma and is recognized as the fastest growing human tumor.

C83.70   **Burkitt lymphoma, unspecified site**   HCC ▽

C83.71   **Burkitt lymphoma, lymph nodes of head, face, and neck**   HCC

C83.72   **Burkitt lymphoma, intrathoracic lymph nodes**   HCC

C83.73   **Burkitt lymphoma, intra-abdominal lymph nodes**   HCC

C83.74   **Burkitt lymphoma, lymph nodes of axilla and upper limb**   HCC

C83.75   **Burkitt lymphoma, lymph nodes of inguinal region and lower limb**   HCC

C83.76   **Burkitt lymphoma, intrapelvic lymph nodes**   HCC

C83.77   **Burkitt lymphoma, spleen**   HCC

C83.78   **Burkitt lymphoma, lymph nodes of multiple sites**   HCC

C83.79   **Burkitt lymphoma, extranodal and solid organ sites**   HCC

✓5ᵗʰ **C83.8**   **Other non-follicular lymphoma**
Intravascular large B-cell lymphoma
Lymphoid granulomatosis
Primary effusion B-cell lymphoma
> EXCLUDES 1   *mediastinal (thymic) large B-cell lymphoma (C85.2-)*
> *T-cell rich B-cell lymphoma (C83.3-)*

C83.80   **Other non-follicular lymphoma, unspecified site**   HCC ▽

C83.81   **Other non-follicular lymphoma, lymph nodes of head, face, and neck**   HCC

C83.82   **Other non-follicular lymphoma, intrathoracic lymph nodes**   HCC

C83.83   **Other non-follicular lymphoma, intra-abdominal lymph nodes**   HCC

C83.84   **Other non-follicular lymphoma, lymph nodes of axilla and upper limb**   HCC

C83.85   **Other non-follicular lymphoma, lymph nodes of inguinal region and lower limb**   HCC

✓ Additional Character Req   ✓x7ᵗʰ Placeholder Alert   Manifestation   HCC CMS-HCC Condition   ▽ Unspecified Code   ▶◀ Revised Text   ● New Code   ▲ Revised Code Title

C83.86   **Other non-follicular lymphoma, intrapelvic lymph nodes** `HCC`

C83.87   **Other non-follicular lymphoma, spleen** `HCC`

C83.88   **Other non-follicular lymphoma, lymph nodes of multiple sites** `HCC`

C83.89   **Other non-follicular lymphoma, extranodal and solid organ sites** `HCC`

√5ᵗʰ **C83.9   Non-follicular (diffuse) lymphoma, unspecified**

C83.90   **Non-follicular (diffuse) lymphoma, unspecified, unspecified site** `HCC` ▽

C83.91   **Non-follicular (diffuse) lymphoma, unspecified, lymph nodes of head, face, and neck** `HCC` ▽

C83.92   **Non-follicular (diffuse) lymphoma, unspecified, intrathoracic lymph nodes** `HCC` ▽

C83.93   **Non-follicular (diffuse) lymphoma, unspecified, intra-abdominal lymph nodes** `HCC` ▽

C83.94   **Non-follicular (diffuse) lymphoma, unspecified, lymph nodes of axilla and upper limb** `HCC` ▽

C83.95   **Non-follicular (diffuse) lymphoma, unspecified, lymph nodes of inguinal region and lower limb** `HCC` ▽

C83.96   **Non-follicular (diffuse) lymphoma, unspecified, intrapelvic lymph nodes** `HCC` ▽

C83.97   **Non-follicular (diffuse) lymphoma, unspecified, spleen** `HCC` ▽

C83.98   **Non-follicular (diffuse) lymphoma, unspecified, lymph nodes of multiple sites** `HCC` ▽

C83.99   **Non-follicular (diffuse) lymphoma, unspecified, extranodal and solid organ sites** `HCC` ▽

√4ᵗʰ **C84   Mature T/NK-cell lymphomas**

> *EXCLUDES 1*   personal history of non-Hodgkin lymphoma (Z85.72)

√5ᵗʰ **C84.0   Mycosis fungoides**

> *EXCLUDES 1*   peripheral T-cell lymphoma, not classified (C84.4-)
> **DEF:** Most common form of cutaneous T-cell lymphoma, also known as Alibert-Bazin syndrome. A type of non-Hodgkin lymphoma in which white blood cells become cancerous and affect the skin and sometimes internal organs.

C84.00   **Mycosis fungoides, unspecified site** `HCC` ▽

C84.01   **Mycosis fungoides, lymph nodes of head, face, and neck** `HCC`

C84.02   **Mycosis fungoides, intrathoracic lymph nodes** `HCC`

C84.03   **Mycosis fungoides, intra-abdominal lymph nodes** `HCC`

C84.04   **Mycosis fungoides, lymph nodes of axilla and upper limb** `HCC`

C84.05   **Mycosis fungoides, lymph nodes of inguinal region and lower limb** `HCC`

C84.06   **Mycosis fungoides, intrapelvic lymph nodes** `HCC`

C84.07   **Mycosis fungoides, spleen** `HCC`

C84.08   **Mycosis fungoides, lymph nodes of multiple sites** `HCC`

C84.09   **Mycosis fungoides, extranodal and solid organ sites** `HCC`

√5ᵗʰ **C84.1   Sézary disease**

C84.10   **Sézary disease, unspecified site** `HCC` ▽

C84.11   **Sézary disease, lymph nodes of head, face, and neck** `HCC`

C84.12   **Sézary disease, intrathoracic lymph nodes** `HCC`

C84.13   **Sézary disease, intra-abdominal lymph nodes** `HCC`

C84.14   **Sézary disease, lymph nodes of axilla and upper limb** `HCC`

C84.15   **Sézary disease, lymph nodes of inguinal region and lower limb** `HCC`

C84.16   **Sézary disease, intrapelvic lymph nodes** `HCC`

C84.17   **Sézary disease, spleen** `HCC`

C84.18   **Sézary disease, lymph nodes of multiple sites** `HCC`

C84.19   **Sézary disease, extranodal and solid organ sites** `HCC`

√5ᵗʰ **C84.4   Peripheral T-cell lymphoma, not classified**

> Lennert's lymphoma
> Lymphoepithelioid lymphoma
> Mature T-cell lymphoma, not elsewhere classified

C84.40   **Peripheral T-cell lymphoma, not classified, unspecified site** `HCC` ▽

C84.41   **Peripheral T-cell lymphoma, not classified, lymph nodes of head, face, and neck** `HCC`

C84.42   **Peripheral T-cell lymphoma, not classified, intrathoracic lymph nodes** `HCC`

C84.43   **Peripheral T-cell lymphoma, not classified, intra-abdominal lymph nodes** `HCC`

C84.44   **Peripheral T-cell lymphoma, not classified, lymph nodes of axilla and upper limb** `HCC`

C84.45   **Peripheral T-cell lymphoma, not classified, lymph nodes of inguinal region and lower limb** `HCC`

C84.46   **Peripheral T-cell lymphoma, not classified, intrapelvic lymph nodes** `HCC`

C84.47   **Peripheral T-cell lymphoma, not classified, spleen** `HCC`

C84.48   **Peripheral T-cell lymphoma, not classified, lymph nodes of multiple sites** `HCC`

C84.49   **Peripheral T-cell lymphoma, not classified, extranodal and solid organ sites** `HCC`

√5ᵗʰ **C84.6   Anaplastic large cell lymphoma, ALK-positive**

> Anaplastic large cell lymphoma, CD30-positive

C84.60   **Anaplastic large cell lymphoma, ALK-positive, unspecified site** `HCC` ▽

C84.61   **Anaplastic large cell lymphoma, ALK-positive, lymph nodes of head, face, and neck** `HCC`

C84.62   **Anaplastic large cell lymphoma, ALK-positive, intrathoracic lymph nodes** `HCC`

C84.63   **Anaplastic large cell lymphoma, ALK-positive, intra-abdominal lymph nodes** `HCC`

C84.64   **Anaplastic large cell lymphoma, ALK-positive, lymph nodes of axilla and upper limb** `HCC`

C84.65   **Anaplastic large cell lymphoma, ALK-positive, lymph nodes of inguinal region and lower limb** `HCC`

C84.66   **Anaplastic large cell lymphoma, ALK-positive, intrapelvic lymph nodes** `HCC`

C84.67   **Anaplastic large cell lymphoma, ALK-positive, spleen** `HCC`

C84.68   **Anaplastic large cell lymphoma, ALK-positive, lymph nodes of multiple sites** `HCC`

C84.69   **Anaplastic large cell lymphoma, ALK-positive, extranodal and solid organ sites** `HCC`

√5ᵗʰ **C84.7   Anaplastic large cell lymphoma, ALK-negative**

> *EXCLUDES 1*   primary cutaneous CD30-positive T-cell proliferations (C86.6-)

C84.70   **Anaplastic large cell lymphoma, ALK-negative, unspecified site** `HCC` ▽

C84.71   **Anaplastic large cell lymphoma, ALK-negative, lymph nodes of head, face, and neck** `HCC`

C84.72   **Anaplastic large cell lymphoma, ALK-negative, intrathoracic lymph nodes** `HCC`

C84.73   **Anaplastic large cell lymphoma, ALK-negative, intra-abdominal lymph nodes** `HCC`

C84.74   **Anaplastic large cell lymphoma, ALK-negative, lymph nodes of axilla and upper limb** `HCC`

C84.75   **Anaplastic large cell lymphoma, ALK-negative, lymph nodes of inguinal region and lower limb** `HCC`

C84.76   **Anaplastic large cell lymphoma, ALK-negative, intrapelvic lymph nodes** `HCC`

C84.77   **Anaplastic large cell lymphoma, ALK-negative, spleen** `HCC`

C84.78   **Anaplastic large cell lymphoma, ALK-negative, lymph nodes of multiple sites** `HCC`

C84.79   **Anaplastic large cell lymphoma, ALK-negative, extranodal and solid organ sites** `HCC`

√5ᵗʰ **C84.A   Cutaneous T-cell lymphoma, unspecified**

C84.A0   **Cutaneous T-cell lymphoma, unspecified, unspecified site** `HCC` ▽

C84.A1   **Cutaneous T-cell lymphoma, unspecified, lymph nodes of head, face, and neck** `HCC` ▽

C84.A2   **Cutaneous T-cell lymphoma, unspecified, intrathoracic lymph nodes** `HCC` ▽

C84.A3   **Cutaneous T-cell lymphoma, unspecified, intra-abdominal lymph nodes** `HCC` ▽

C84.A4   **Cutaneous T-cell lymphoma, unspecified, lymph nodes of axilla and upper limb** `HCC` ▽

C84.A5   **Cutaneous T-cell lymphoma, unspecified, lymph nodes of inguinal region and lower limb** `HCC` ▽

C84.A6   **Cutaneous T-cell lymphoma, unspecified, intrapelvic lymph nodes** `HCC` ▽

EXCLUDES 1 Not coded here   *EXCLUDES 2* Not included here   N Newborn Age: 0   P Pediatric Age: 0-17   M Maternity Age: 12-55   A Adult Age: 15-124

478   ICD-10-CM 2018

C84.A7   Cutaneous T-cell lymphoma, unspecified, spleen   HCC ▽

C84.A8   Cutaneous T-cell lymphoma, unspecified, lymph nodes of multiple sites   HCC ▽

C84.A9   Cutaneous T-cell lymphoma, unspecified, extranodal and solid organ sites   HCC ▽

✓5th **C84.Z**   **Other mature T/NK-cell lymphomas**

> NOTE   If T-cell lineage or involvement is mentioned in conjunction with a specific lymphoma, code to the more specific description.

> EXCLUDES 1   angioimmunoblastic T-cell lymphoma (C86.5)
> blastic NK-cell lymphoma (C86.4)
> enteropathy-type T-cell lymphoma (C86.2)
> extranodal NK-cell lymphoma, nasal type (C86.0)
> hepatosplenic T-cell lymphoma (C86.1)
> primary cutaneous CD30-positive T-cell proliferations (C86.6)
> subcutaneous panniculitis-like T-cell lymphoma (C86.3)
> T-cell leukemia (C91.1-)

C84.Z0   Other mature T/NK-cell lymphomas, unspecified site   HCC ▽

C84.Z1   Other mature T/NK-cell lymphomas, lymph nodes of head, face, and neck   HCC

C84.Z2   Other mature T/NK-cell lymphomas, intrathoracic lymph nodes   HCC

C84.Z3   Other mature T/NK-cell lymphomas, intra-abdominal lymph nodes   HCC

C84.Z4   Other mature T/NK-cell lymphomas, lymph nodes of axilla and upper limb   HCC

C84.Z5   Other mature T/NK-cell lymphomas, lymph nodes of inguinal region and lower limb   HCC

C84.Z6   Other mature T/NK-cell lymphomas, intrapelvic lymph nodes   HCC

C84.Z7   Other mature T/NK-cell lymphomas, spleen   HCC

C84.Z8   Other mature T/NK-cell lymphomas, lymph nodes of multiple sites   HCC

C84.Z9   Other mature T/NK-cell lymphomas, extranodal and solid organ sites   HCC

✓5th **C84.9**   **Mature T/NK-cell lymphomas, unspecified**
NK/T cell lymphoma NOS

> EXCLUDES 1   mature T-cell lymphoma, not elsewhere classified (C84.4-)

C84.90   Mature T/NK-cell lymphomas, unspecified, unspecified site   HCC ▽

C84.91   Mature T/NK-cell lymphomas, unspecified, lymph nodes of head, face, and neck   HCC ▽

C84.92   Mature T/NK-cell lymphomas, unspecified, intrathoracic lymph nodes   HCC ▽

C84.93   Mature T/NK-cell lymphomas, unspecified, intra-abdominal lymph nodes   HCC ▽

C84.94   Mature T/NK-cell lymphomas, unspecified, lymph nodes of axilla and upper limb   HCC ▽

C84.95   Mature T/NK-cell lymphomas, unspecified, lymph nodes of inguinal region and lower limb   HCC ▽

C84.96   Mature T/NK-cell lymphomas, unspecified, intrapelvic lymph nodes   HCC ▽

C84.97   Mature T/NK-cell lymphomas, unspecified, spleen   HCC ▽

C84.98   Mature T/NK-cell lymphomas, unspecified, lymph nodes of multiple sites   HCC ▽

C84.99   Mature T/NK-cell lymphomas, unspecified, extranodal and solid organ sites   HCC ▽

✓4th **C85**   **Other specified and unspecified types of non-Hodgkin lymphoma**

> EXCLUDES 1   other specified types of T/NK-cell lymphoma (C86.-)
> personal history of non-Hodgkin lymphoma (Z85.72)

✓5th **C85.1**   **Unspecified B-cell lymphoma**

> NOTE   If B-cell lineage or involvement is mentioned in conjunction with a specific lymphoma, code to the more specific description.

C85.10   Unspecified B-cell lymphoma, unspecified site   HCC ▽

C85.11   Unspecified B-cell lymphoma, lymph nodes of head, face, and neck   HCC ▽

C85.12   Unspecified B-cell lymphoma, intrathoracic lymph nodes   HCC ▽

C85.13   Unspecified B-cell lymphoma, intra-abdominal lymph nodes   HCC ▽

C85.14   Unspecified B-cell lymphoma, lymph nodes of axilla and upper limb   HCC ▽

C85.15   Unspecified B-cell lymphoma, lymph nodes of inguinal region and lower limb   HCC ▽

C85.16   Unspecified B-cell lymphoma, intrapelvic lymph nodes   HCC ▽

C85.17   Unspecified B-cell lymphoma, spleen   HCC ▽

C85.18   Unspecified B-cell lymphoma, lymph nodes of multiple sites   HCC ▽

C85.19   Unspecified B-cell lymphoma, extranodal and solid organ sites   HCC ▽

✓5th **C85.2**   **Mediastinal (thymic) large B-cell lymphoma**

C85.20   Mediastinal (thymic) large B-cell lymphoma, unspecified site   HCC ▽

C85.21   Mediastinal (thymic) large B-cell lymphoma, lymph nodes of head, face, and neck   HCC

C85.22   Mediastinal (thymic) large B-cell lymphoma, intrathoracic lymph nodes   HCC

C85.23   Mediastinal (thymic) large B-cell lymphoma, intra-abdominal lymph nodes   HCC

C85.24   Mediastinal (thymic) large B-cell lymphoma, lymph nodes of axilla and upper limb   HCC

C85.25   Mediastinal (thymic) large B-cell lymphoma, lymph nodes of inguinal region and lower limb   HCC

C85.26   Mediastinal (thymic) large B-cell lymphoma, intrapelvic lymph nodes   HCC

C85.27   Mediastinal (thymic) large B-cell lymphoma, spleen   HCC

C85.28   Mediastinal (thymic) large B-cell lymphoma, lymph nodes of multiple sites   HCC

C85.29   Mediastinal (thymic) large B-cell lymphoma, extranodal and solid organ sites   HCC

✓5th **C85.8**   **Other specified types of non-Hodgkin lymphoma**

C85.80   Other specified types of non-Hodgkin lymphoma, unspecified site   HCC ▽

C85.81   Other specified types of non-Hodgkin lymphoma, lymph nodes of head, face, and neck   HCC

C85.82   Other specified types of non-Hodgkin lymphoma, intrathoracic lymph nodes   HCC

C85.83   Other specified types of non-Hodgkin lymphoma, intra-abdominal lymph nodes   HCC

C85.84   Other specified types of non-Hodgkin lymphoma, lymph nodes of axilla and upper limb   HCC

C85.85   Other specified types of non-Hodgkin lymphoma, lymph nodes of inguinal region and lower limb   HCC

C85.86   Other specified types of non-Hodgkin lymphoma, intrapelvic lymph nodes   HCC

C85.87   Other specified types of non-Hodgkin lymphoma, spleen   HCC

C85.88   Other specified types of non-Hodgkin lymphoma, lymph nodes of multiple sites   HCC

C85.89   Other specified types of non-Hodgkin lymphoma, extranodal and solid organ sites   HCC

✓5th **C85.9**   **Non-Hodgkin lymphoma, unspecified**
Lymphoma NOS
Malignant lymphoma NOS
Non-Hodgkin lymphoma NOS

C85.90   Non-Hodgkin lymphoma, unspecified, unspecified site   HCC ▽

C85.91   Non-Hodgkin lymphoma, unspecified, lymph nodes of head, face, and neck   HCC ▽

C85.92   Non-Hodgkin lymphoma, unspecified, intrathoracic lymph nodes   HCC ▽

C85.93   Non-Hodgkin lymphoma, unspecified, intra-abdominal lymph nodes   HCC ▽

C85.94   Non-Hodgkin lymphoma, unspecified, lymph nodes of axilla and upper limb   HCC ▽

C85.95   Non-Hodgkin lymphoma, unspecified, lymph nodes of inguinal region and lower limb   HCC ▽

C85.96   Non-Hodgkin lymphoma, unspecified, intrapelvic lymph nodes   HCC ▽

C85.97   Non-Hodgkin lymphoma, unspecified, spleen   HCC ▽

C85.98   Non-Hodgkin lymphoma, unspecified, lymph nodes of multiple sites   HCC ▽

C85.99   Non-Hodgkin lymphoma, unspecified, extranodal and solid organ sites   HCC ▽

☑ Additional Character Req   ✓x7th Placeholder Alert   Manifestation   HCC CMS-HCC Condition   ▽ Unspecified Code   ►◄ Revised Text   ● New Code   ▲ Revised Code Title

Chapter 2. Neoplasms

✓4th C86 Other specified types of T/NK-cell lymphoma

> **EXCLUDES 1**   anaplastic large cell lymphoma, ALK negative (C84.7-)
> anaplastic large cell lymphoma, ALK positive (C84.6-)
> mature T/NK-cell lymphomas (C84.-)
> other specified types of non-Hodgkin lymphoma (C85.8-)

C86.0 Extranodal NK/T-cell lymphoma, nasal type   HCC

C86.1 Hepatosplenic T-cell lymphoma   HCC
    Alpha-beta and gamma delta types

C86.2 Enteropathy-type (intestinal) T-cell lymphoma   HCC
    Enteropathy associated T-cell lymphoma

C86.3 Subcutaneous panniculitis-like T-cell lymphoma   HCC

C86.4 Blastic NK-cell lymphoma   HCC
    ▶Blastic plasmacytoid dendritic cell neoplasm (BPDCN)◀

C86.5 Angioimmunoblastic T-cell lymphoma   HCC
    Angioimmunoblastic lymphadenopathy with dysproteinemia [AILD]

C86.6 Primary cutaneous CD30-positive T-cell proliferations   HCC
    Lymphomatoid papulosis
    Primary cutaneous anaplastic large cell lymphoma
    Primary cutaneous CD30-positive large T-cell lymphoma

✓4th C88 Malignant immunoproliferative diseases and certain other B-cell lymphomas

> **EXCLUDES 1**   B-cell lymphoma, unspecified (C85.1-)
> personal history of other malignant neoplasms of lymphoid, hematopoietic and related tissues (Z85.79)

C88.0 Waldenström macroglobulinemia   HCC
    Lymphoplasmacytic lymphoma with IgM-production
    Macroglobulinemia (idiopathic) (primary)
> **EXCLUDES 1**   small cell B-cell lymphoma (C83.0)

C88.2 Heavy chain disease   HCC
    Franklin disease
    Gamma heavy chain disease
    Mu heavy chain disease

C88.3 Immunoproliferative small intestinal disease   HCC
    Alpha heavy chain disease
    Mediterranean lymphoma

C88.4 Extranodal marginal zone B-cell lymphoma of mucosa-associated lymphoid tissue [MALT-lymphoma]   HCC
    Lymphoma of skin-associated lymphoid tissue [SALT-lymphoma]
    Lymphoma of bronchial-associated lymphoid tissue [BALT-lymphoma]
> **EXCLUDES 1**   high malignant (diffuse large B-cell) lymphoma (C83.3-)

C88.8 Other malignant immunoproliferative diseases   HCC

C88.9 Malignant immunoproliferative disease, unspecified   HCC ▽
    Immunoproliferative disease NOS

✓4th C90 Multiple myeloma and malignant plasma cell neoplasms

> **EXCLUDES 1**   personal history of other malignant neoplasms of lymphoid, hematopoietic and related tissues (Z85.79)

✓5th C90.0 Multiple myeloma
    Kahler's disease   Myelomatosis
    Medullary plasmacytoma   Plasma cell myeloma
> **EXCLUDES 1**   solitary myeloma (C90.3-)
> solitary plasmacytoma (C90.3-)

    C90.00 Multiple myeloma not having achieved remission   HCC
       Multiple myeloma with failed remission
       Multiple myeloma NOS

    C90.01 Multiple myeloma in remission   HCC

    C90.02 Multiple myeloma in relapse   HCC

✓5th C90.1 Plasma cell leukemia
    Plasmacytic leukemia

    C90.10 Plasma cell leukemia not having achieved remission   HCC
       Plasma cell leukemia with failed remission
       Plasma cell leukemia NOS

    C90.11 Plasma cell leukemia in remission   HCC

    C90.12 Plasma cell leukemia in relapse   HCC

✓5th C90.2 Extramedullary plasmacytoma

    C90.20 Extramedullary plasmacytoma not having achieved remission   HCC
       Extramedullary plasmacytoma with failed remission
       Extramedullary plasmacytoma NOS

    C90.21 Extramedullary plasmacytoma in remission   HCC

    C90.22 Extramedullary plasmacytoma in relapse   HCC

✓5th C90.3 Solitary plasmacytoma
    Localized malignant plasma cell tumor NOS
    Plasmacytoma NOS
    Solitary myeloma

    C90.30 Solitary plasmacytoma not having achieved remission   HCC
       Solitary plasmacytoma with failed remission
       Solitary plasmacytoma NOS

    C90.31 Solitary plasmacytoma in remission   HCC

    C90.32 Solitary plasmacytoma in relapse   HCC

✓4th C91 Lymphoid leukemia

> **EXCLUDES 1**   personal history of leukemia (Z85.6)

✓5th C91.0 Acute lymphoblastic leukemia [ALL]
> **NOTE**   Code C91.0 should only be used for T-cell and B-cell precursor leukemia.

    C91.00 Acute lymphoblastic leukemia not having achieved remission   HCC
       Acute lymphoblastic leukemia with failed remission
       Acute lymphoblastic leukemia NOS

    C91.01 Acute lymphoblastic leukemia, in remission   HCC

    C91.02 Acute lymphoblastic leukemia, in relapse   HCC

✓5th C91.1 Chronic lymphocytic leukemia of B-cell type
    Lymphoplasmacytic leukemia
    Richter syndrome
> **EXCLUDES 1**   lymphoplasmacytic lymphoma (C83.0-)

    C91.10 Chronic lymphocytic leukemia of B-cell type not having achieved remission   HCC
       Chronic lymphocytic leukemia of B-cell type with failed remission
       Chronic lymphocytic leukemia of B-cell type NOS

    C91.11 Chronic lymphocytic leukemia of B-cell type in remission   HCC

    C91.12 Chronic lymphocytic leukemia of B-cell type in relapse   HCC

✓5th C91.3 Prolymphocytic leukemia of B-cell type

    C91.30 Prolymphocytic leukemia of B-cell type not having achieved remission   HCC
       Prolymphocytic leukemia of B-cell type with failed remission
       Prolymphocytic leukemia of B-cell type NOS

    C91.31 Prolymphocytic leukemia of B-cell type, in remission   HCC

    C91.32 Prolymphocytic leukemia of B-cell type, in relapse   HCC

✓5th C91.4 Hairy cell leukemia
    Leukemic reticuloendotheliosis

    C91.40 Hairy cell leukemia not having achieved remission   HCC
       Hairy cell leukemia with failed remission
       Hairy cell leukemia NOS

    C91.41 Hairy cell leukemia, in remission   HCC

    C91.42 Hairy cell leukemia, in relapse   HCC

✓5th C91.5 Adult T-cell lymphoma/leukemia (HTLV-1-associated)
    Acute variant of adult T-cell lymphoma/leukemia (HTLV-1-associated)
    Chronic variant of adult T-cell lymphoma/leukemia (HTLV-1-associated)
    Lymphomatoid variant of adult T-cell lymphoma/leukemia (HTLV-1-associated)
    Smouldering variant of adult T-cell lymphoma/leukemia (HTLV-1-associated)

    C91.50 Adult T-cell lymphoma/leukemia (HTLV-1-associated) not having achieved remission   HCC A
       Adult T-cell lymphoma/leukemia (HTLV-1-associated) with failed remission
       Adult T-cell lymphoma/leukemia (HTLV-1-associated) NOS

    C91.51 Adult T-cell lymphoma/leukemia (HTLV-1-associated), in remission   HCC A

    C91.52 Adult T-cell lymphoma/leukemia (HTLV-1-associated), in relapse   HCC A

✓5th C91.6 Prolymphocytic leukemia of T-cell type

    C91.60 Prolymphocytic leukemia of T-cell type not having achieved remission   HCC
       Prolymphocytic leukemia of T-cell type with failed remission
       Prolymphocytic leukemia of T-cell type NOS

EXCLUDES 1 Not coded here   **EXCLUDES 2** Not included here   N Newborn Age: 0   P Pediatric Age: 0-17   M Maternity Age: 12-55   A Adult Age: 15-124

480   ICD-10-CM 2018

C91.61 **Prolymphocytic leukemia of T-cell type, in remission** `HCC`

C91.62 **Prolymphocytic leukemia of T-cell type, in relapse** `HCC`

☑5th **C91.A** **Mature B-cell leukemia Burkitt-type**
> EXCLUDES 1 *Burkitt lymphoma (C83.7-)*

C91.A0 **Mature B-cell leukemia Burkitt-type not having achieved remission** `HCC`
> Mature B-cell leukemia Burkitt-type with failed remission
> Mature B-cell leukemia Burkitt-type NOS

C91.A1 **Mature B-cell leukemia Burkitt-type, in remission** `HCC`

C91.A2 **Mature B-cell leukemia Burkitt-type, in relapse** `HCC`

☑5th **C91.Z** **Other lymphoid leukemia**
> T-cell large granular lymphocytic leukemia (associated with rheumatoid arthritis)

C91.Z0 **Other lymphoid leukemia not having achieved remission** `HCC`
> Other lymphoid leukemia with failed remission
> Other lymphoid leukemia NOS

C91.Z1 **Other lymphoid leukemia, in remission** `HCC`

C91.Z2 **Other lymphoid leukemia, in relapse** `HCC`

☑5th **C91.9** **Lymphoid leukemia, unspecified**

C91.90 **Lymphoid leukemia, unspecified not having achieved remission** `HCC` ▽
> Lymphoid leukemia with failed remission
> Lymphoid leukemia NOS

C91.91 **Lymphoid leukemia, unspecified, in remission** `HCC` ▽

C91.92 **Lymphoid leukemia, unspecified, in relapse** `HCC` ▽

☑4th **C92** **Myeloid leukemia**
> INCLUDES   granulocytic leukemia
>   myelogenous leukemia
> EXCLUDES 1 *personal history of leukemia (Z85.6)*

☑5th **C92.0** **Acute myeloblastic leukemia**
> Acute myeloblastic leukemia, minimal differentiation
> Acute myeloblastic leukemia (with maturation)
> Acute myeloblastic leukemia 1/ETO
> Acute myeloblastic leukemia M0
> Acute myeloblastic leukemia M1
> Acute myeloblastic leukemia M2
> Acute myeloblastic leukemia with t(8;21)
> Acute myeloblastic leukemia (without a FAB classification) NOS
> Refractory anemia with excess blasts in transformation [RAEB T]
> EXCLUDES 1 *acute exacerbation of chronic myeloid leukemia (C92.10)*
> *refractory anemia with excess of blasts not in transformation (D46.2-)*

C92.00 **Acute myeloblastic leukemia, not having achieved remission** `HCC`
> Acute myeloblastic leukemia with failed remission
> Acute myeloblastic leukemia NOS

C92.01 **Acute myeloblastic leukemia, in remission** `HCC`

C92.02 **Acute myeloblastic leukemia, in relapse** `HCC`

☑5th **C92.1** **Chronic myeloid leukemia, BCR/ABL-positive**
> Chronic myelogenous leukemia, Philadelphia chromosome (Ph1) positive
> Chronic myelogenous leukemia, t(9;22) (q34;q11)
> Chronic myelogenous leukemia with crisis of blast cells
> EXCLUDES 1 *atypical chronic myeloid leukemia BCR/ABL-negative (C92.2-)*
> *chronic myelomonocytic leukemia (C93.1-)*
> *chronic myeloproliferative disease (D47.1)*

C92.10 **Chronic myeloid leukemia, BCR/ABL-positive, not having achieved remission** `HCC`
> Chronic myeloid leukemia, BCR/ABL-positive with failed remission
> Chronic myeloid leukemia, BCR/ABL-positive NOS

C92.11 **Chronic myeloid leukemia, BCR/ABL-positive, in remission** `HCC`

C92.12 **Chronic myeloid leukemia, BCR/ABL-positive, in relapse** `HCC`

☑5th **C92.2** **Atypical chronic myeloid leukemia, BCR/ABL-negative**

C92.20 **Atypical chronic myeloid leukemia, BCR/ABL-negative, not having achieved remission** `HCC`
> Atypical chronic myeloid leukemia, BCR/ABL-negative with failed remission
> Atypical chronic myeloid leukemia, BCR/ABL-negative NOS

C92.21 **Atypical chronic myeloid leukemia, BCR/ABL-negative, in remission** `HCC`

C92.22 **Atypical chronic myeloid leukemia, BCR/ABL-negative, in relapse** `HCC`

☑5th **C92.3** **Myeloid sarcoma**
> A malignant tumor of immature myeloid cells
> Chloroma
> Granulocytic sarcoma

C92.30 **Myeloid sarcoma, not having achieved remission** `HCC`
> Myeloid sarcoma with failed remission
> Myeloid sarcoma NOS

C92.31 **Myeloid sarcoma, in remission** `HCC`

C92.32 **Myeloid sarcoma, in relapse** `HCC`

☑5th **C92.4** **Acute promyelocytic leukemia**
> AML M3
> AML Me with t(15;17) and variants

C92.40 **Acute promyelocytic leukemia, not having achieved remission** `HCC`
> Acute promyelocytic leukemia with failed remission
> Acute promyelocytic leukemia NOS

C92.41 **Acute promyelocytic leukemia, in remission** `HCC`

C92.42 **Acute promyelocytic leukemia, in relapse** `HCC`

☑5th **C92.5** **Acute myelomonocytic leukemia**
> AML M4
> AML M4 Eo with inv(16) or t(16;16)

C92.50 **Acute myelomonocytic leukemia, not having achieved remission** `HCC`
> Acute myelomonocytic leukemia with failed remission
> Acute myelomonocytic leukemia NOS

C92.51 **Acute myelomonocytic leukemia, in remission** `HCC`

C92.52 **Acute myelomonocytic leukemia, in relapse** `HCC`

☑5th **C92.6** **Acute myeloid leukemia with 11q23-abnormality**
> Acute myeloid leukemia with variation of MLL-gene

C92.60 **Acute myeloid leukemia with 11q23-abnormality not having achieved remission** `HCC`
> Acute myeloid leukemia with 11q23-abnormality with failed remission
> Acute myeloid leukemia with 11q23-abnormality NOS

C92.61 **Acute myeloid leukemia with 11q23-abnormality in remission** `HCC`

C92.62 **Acute myeloid leukemia with 11q23-abnormality in relapse** `HCC`

☑5th **C92.A** **Acute myeloid leukemia with multilineage dysplasia**
> Acute myeloid leukemia with dysplasia of remaining hematopoesis and/or myelodysplastic disease in its history

C92.A0 **Acute myeloid leukemia with multilineage dysplasia, not having achieved remission** `HCC`
> Acute myeloid leukemia with multilineage dysplasia with failed remission
> Acute myeloid leukemia with multilineage dysplasia NOS

C92.A1 **Acute myeloid leukemia with multilineage dysplasia, in remission** `HCC`

C92.A2 **Acute myeloid leukemia with multilineage dysplasia, in relapse** `HCC`

☑5th **C92.Z** **Other myeloid leukemia**

C92.Z0 **Other myeloid leukemia not having achieved remission** `HCC`
> Myeloid leukemia NEC with failed remission
> Myeloid leukemia NEC

C92.Z1 **Other myeloid leukemia, in remission** `HCC`

C92.Z2 **Other myeloid leukemia, in relapse** `HCC`

☑5th **C92.9** **Myeloid leukemia, unspecified**

C92.90 **Myeloid leukemia, unspecified, not having achieved remission** `HCC` ▽
> Myeloid leukemia, unspecified with failed remission
> Myeloid leukemia, unspecified NOS

C92.91 **Myeloid leukemia, unspecified in remission** `HCC` ▽

C92.92 **Myeloid leukemia, unspecified in relapse** `HCC` ▽

☑ Additional Character Req   ✔x7th Placeholder Alert   Manifestation   `HCC` CMS-HCC Condition   ▽ Unspecified Code   ▶◀ Revised Text   ● New Code   ▲ Revised Code Title

✓4ᵗʰ **C93 Monocytic leukemia**
    INCLUDES monocytoid leukemia
    EXCLUDES1 personal history of leukemia (Z85.6)

  ✓5ᵗʰ **C93.0 Acute monoblastic/monocytic leukemia**
    AML M5   AML M5b
    AML M5a

    C93.00 Acute monoblastic/monocytic leukemia, HCC
      not having achieved remission
      Acute monoblastic/monocytic leukemia with failed remission
      Acute monoblastic/monocytic leukemia NOS

    C93.01 Acute monoblastic/monocytic leukemia, HCC
      in remission

    C93.02 Acute monoblastic/monocytic leukemia, HCC
      in relapse

  ✓5ᵗʰ **C93.1 Chronic myelomonocytic leukemia**
    Chronic monocytic leukemia
    CMML-1
    CMML-2
    CMML with eosinophilia

    C93.10 Chronic myelomonocytic leukemia not having HCC
      achieved remission
      Chronic myelomonocytic leukemia with failed remission
      Chronic myelomonocytic leukemia NOS

    C93.11 Chronic myelomonocytic leukemia, in remission HCC
    C93.12 Chronic myelomonocytic leukemia, in relapse HCC

  ✓5ᵗʰ **C93.3 Juvenile myelomonocytic leukemia**

    C93.30 Juvenile myelomonocytic leukemia, HCC P
      not having achieved remission
      Juvenile myelomonocytic leukemia with failed remission
      Juvenile myelomonocytic leukemia NOS

    C93.31 Juvenile myelomonocytic leukemia, HCC P
      in remission

    C93.32 Juvenile myelomonocytic leukemia, HCC P
      in relapse

  ✓5ᵗʰ **C93.Z Other monocytic leukemia**

    C93.Z0 Other monocytic leukemia, not having HCC
      achieved remission
      Other monocytic leukemia NOS

    C93.Z1 Other monocytic leukemia, in remission HCC
    C93.Z2 Other monocytic leukemia, in relapse HCC

  ✓5ᵗʰ **C93.9 Monocytic leukemia, unspecified**

    C93.90 Monocytic leukemia, unspecified, not having HCC ▽
      achieved remission
      Monocytic leukemia, unspecified with failed remission
      Monocytic leukemia, unspecified NOS

    C93.91 Monocytic leukemia, unspecified in remission HCC ▽
    C93.92 Monocytic leukemia, unspecified in relapse HCC ▽

✓4ᵗʰ **C94 Other leukemias of specified cell type**
    EXCLUDES1 leukemic reticuloendotheliosis (C91.4-)
      myelodysplastic syndromes (D46.-)
      personal history of leukemia (Z85.6)
      plasma cell leukemia (C90.1-)

  ✓5ᵗʰ **C94.0 Acute erythroid leukemia**
    Acute myeloid leukemia M6(a)(b)
    Erythroleukemia
    DEF: Erythroleukemia: A malignant blood dyscrasia (a myeloproliferative disorder).

    C94.00 Acute erythroid leukemia, not having achieved HCC
      remission
      Acute erythroid leukemia with failed remission
      Acute erythroid leukemia NOS

    C94.01 Acute erythroid leukemia, in remission HCC
    C94.02 Acute erythroid leukemia, in relapse HCC

  ✓5ᵗʰ **C94.2 Acute megakaryoblastic leukemia**
    Acute myeloid leukemia M7
    Acute megakaryocytic leukemia

    C94.20 Acute megakaryoblastic leukemia not having HCC
      achieved remission
      Acute megakaryoblastic leukemia with failed remission
      Acute megakaryoblastic leukemia NOS

    C94.21 Acute megakaryoblastic leukemia, in remission HCC
    C94.22 Acute megakaryoblastic leukemia, in relapse HCC

  ✓5ᵗʰ **C94.3 Mast cell leukemia**

    C94.30 Mast cell leukemia not having achieved HCC
      remission
      Mast cell leukemia with failed remission
      Mast cell leukemia NOS

    C94.31 Mast cell leukemia, in remission HCC
    C94.32 Mast cell leukemia, in relapse HCC

  ✓5ᵗʰ **C94.4 Acute panmyelosis with myelofibrosis**
    Acute myelofibrosis
    EXCLUDES1 myelofibrosis NOS (D75.81)
      secondary myelofibrosis NOS (D75.81)

    C94.40 Acute panmyelosis with myelofibrosis not HCC
      having achieved remission
      Acute myelofibrosis NOS
      Acute panmyelosis with myelofibrosis with failed remission
      Acute panmyelosis NOS

    C94.41 Acute panmyelosis with myelofibrosis, HCC
      in remission

    C94.42 Acute panmyelosis with myelofibrosis, HCC
      in relapse

  C94.6 Myelodysplastic disease, not classified HCC
    Myeloproliferative disease, not classified

  ✓5ᵗʰ **C94.8 Other specified leukemias**
    Aggressive NK-cell leukemia
    Acute basophilic leukemia

    C94.80 Other specified leukemias not having HCC
      achieved remission
      Other specified leukemia with failed remission
      Other specified leukemias NOS

    C94.81 Other specified leukemias, in remission HCC
    C94.82 Other specified leukemias, in relapse HCC

✓4ᵗʰ **C95 Leukemia of unspecified cell type**
    EXCLUDES1 personal history of leukemia (Z85.6)

  ✓5ᵗʰ **C95.0 Acute leukemia of unspecified cell type**
    Acute bilineal leukemia
    Acute mixed lineage leukemia
    Biphenotypic acute leukemia
    Stem cell leukemia of unclear lineage
    EXCLUDES1 acute exacerbation of unspecified chronic leukemia (C95.10)

    C95.00 Acute leukemia of unspecified cell type HCC
      not having achieved remission
      Acute leukemia of unspecified cell type with failed remission
      Acute leukemia NOS

    C95.01 Acute leukemia of unspecified cell type, HCC
      in remission

    C95.02 Acute leukemia of unspecified cell type, HCC
      in relapse

  ✓5ᵗʰ **C95.1 Chronic leukemia of unspecified cell type**

    C95.10 Chronic leukemia of unspecified cell type HCC
      not having achieved remission
      Chronic leukemia of unspecified cell type with failed remission
      Chronic leukemia NOS

    C95.11 Chronic leukemia of unspecified cell type, HCC
      in remission

    C95.12 Chronic leukemia of unspecified cell type, HCC
      in relapse

  ✓5ᵗʰ **C95.9 Leukemia, unspecified**

    C95.90 Leukemia, unspecified not having achieved HCC ▽
      remission
      Leukemia, unspecified with failed remission
      Leukemia NOS

    C95.91 Leukemia, unspecified, in remission HCC ▽
    C95.92 Leukemia, unspecified, in relapse HCC ▽

EXCLUDES1 Not coded here   **EXCLUDES2** Not included here   **N** Newborn Age: 0   **P** Pediatric Age: 0-17   **M** Maternity Age: 12-55   **A** Adult Age: 15-124

482   ICD-10-CM 2018

☑4th **C96 Other and unspecified malignant neoplasms of lymphoid, hematopoietic and related tissue**
> EXCLUDES 1   *personal history of other malignant neoplasms of lymphoid, hematopoietic and related tissues (Z85.79)*

C96.0 Multifocal and multisystemic (disseminated) Langerhans-cell histiocytosis HCC
Histiocytosis X, multisystemic
Letterer-Siwe disease
> EXCLUDES 1   *adult pulmonary Langerhans cell histiocytosis (J84.82)*
> *multifocal and unisystemic Langerhans-cell histiocytosis (C96.5)*
> *unifocal Langerhans-cell histiocytosis (C96.6)*

▲ ☑5th **C96.2 Malignant mast cell neoplasm**
~~Aggressive systemic mastocytosis~~
Mast cell sarcoma
> EXCLUDES 1   *indolent mastocytosis ▶(D47.02)◀*
> *mast cell leukemia (C94.30)*
> *mastocytosis (congenital) (cutaneous) (Q82.2)*

●   **C96.20 Malignant mast cell neoplasm, unspecified** ▽
●   **C96.21 Aggressive systemic mastocytosis**
●   **C96.22 Mast cell sarcoma**
●   **C96.29 Other malignant mast cell neoplasm**

C96.4 Sarcoma of dendritic cells (accessory cells) HCC
Follicular dendritic cell sarcoma
Interdigitating dendritic cell sarcoma
Langerhans cell sarcoma

C96.5 Multifocal and unisystemic Langerhans-cell histiocytosis HCC
Hand-Schüller-Christian disease
Histiocytosis X, multifocal
> EXCLUDES 1   *multifocal and multisystemic (disseminated) Langerhans-cell histiocytosis (C96.0)*
> *unifocal Langerhans-cell histiocytosis (C96.6)*

C96.6 Unifocal Langerhans-cell histiocytosis HCC
Eosinophilic granuloma
Histiocytosis X, unifocal
Histiocytosis X NOS
Langerhans-cell histiocytosis NOS
> EXCLUDES 1   *multifocal and multisysemic (disseminated) Langerhans-cell histiocytosis (C96.0)*
> *multifocal and unisystemic Langerhans-cell histiocytosis (C96.5)*

C96.A Histiocytic sarcoma HCC
Malignant histiocytosis

C96.Z Other specified malignant neoplasms of lymphoid, hematopoietic and related tissue HCC

C96.9 Malignant neoplasm of lymphoid, hematopoietic and related tissue, unspecified HCC ▽

In situ neoplasms (D00-D09)

INCLUDES   Bowen's disease
erythroplasia
grade III intraepithelial neoplasia
Queyrat's erythroplasia

☑4th **D00 Carcinoma in situ of oral cavity, esophagus and stomach**
> EXCLUDES 1   *melanoma in situ (D03.-)*

☑5th **D00.0 Carcinoma in situ of lip, oral cavity and pharynx**
Use additional code to identify:
exposure to environmental tobacco smoke (Z77.22)
exposure to tobacco smoke in the perinatal period (P96.81)
history of tobacco dependence (Z87.891)
occupational exposure to environmental tobacco smoke (Z57.31)
tobacco dependence (F17.-)
tobacco use (Z72.0)
> EXCLUDES 1   *carcinoma in situ of aryepiglottic fold or interarytenoid fold, laryngeal aspect (D02.0)*
> *carcinoma in situ of epiglottis NOS (D02.0)*
> *carcinoma in situ of epiglottis suprahyoid portion (D02.0)*
> *carcinoma in situ of skin of lip (D03.0, D04.0)*

   D00.00 Carcinoma in situ of oral cavity, unspecified site ▽
   D00.01 Carcinoma in situ of labial mucosa and vermilion border
   D00.02 Carcinoma in situ of buccal mucosa
   D00.03 Carcinoma in situ of gingiva and edentulous alveolar ridge
   D00.04 Carcinoma in situ of soft palate
   D00.05 Carcinoma in situ of hard palate
   D00.06 Carcinoma in situ of floor of mouth

   D00.07 Carcinoma in situ of tongue
   D00.08 Carcinoma in situ of pharynx
Carcinoma in situ of aryepiglottic fold NOS
Carcinoma in situ of hypopharyngeal aspect of aryepiglottic fold
Carcinoma in situ of marginal zone of aryepiglottic fold

D00.1 Carcinoma in situ of esophagus
D00.2 Carcinoma in situ of stomach

☑4th **D01 Carcinoma in situ of other and unspecified digestive organs**
> EXCLUDES 1   *melanoma in situ (D03.-)*

D01.0 Carcinoma in situ of colon
> EXCLUDES 1   *carcinoma in situ of rectosigmoid junction (D01.1)*

D01.1 Carcinoma in situ of rectosigmoid junction
D01.2 Carcinoma in situ of rectum
D01.3 Carcinoma in situ of anus and anal canal
Anal intraepithelial neoplasia III [AIN III]
Severe dysplasia of anus
> EXCLUDES 1   *anal intraepithelial neoplasia I and II [AIN I and AIN II] (K62.82)*
> *carcinoma in situ of anal margin (D04.5)*
> *carcinoma in situ of anal skin (D04.5)*
> *carcinoma in situ of perianal skin (D04.5)*

☑5th **D01.4 Carcinoma in situ of other and unspecified parts of intestine**
> EXCLUDES 1   *carcinoma in situ of ampulla of Vater (D01.5)*

   D01.40 Carcinoma in situ of unspecified part of intestine ▽
   D01.49 Carcinoma in situ of other parts of intestine

D01.5 Carcinoma in situ of liver, gallbladder and bile ducts
Carcinoma in situ of ampulla of Vater

D01.7 Carcinoma in situ of other specified digestive organs
Carcinoma in situ of pancreas

D01.9 Carcinoma in situ of digestive organ, unspecified ▽

☑4th **D02 Carcinoma in situ of middle ear and respiratory system**
Use additional code to identify:
exposure to environmental tobacco smoke (Z77.22)
exposure to tobacco smoke in the perinatal period (P96.81)
history of tobacco dependence(Z87.891)
occupational exposure to environmental tobacco smoke (Z57.31)
tobacco dependence (F17.-)
tobacco use (Z72.0)
> EXCLUDES 1   *melanoma in situ (D03.-)*

D02.0 Carcinoma in situ of larynx
Carcinoma in situ of aryepiglottic fold or interarytenoid fold, laryngeal aspect
Carcinoma in situ of epiglottis (suprahyoid portion)
> EXCLUDES 1   *carcinoma in situ of aryepiglottic fold or interarytenoid fold NOS (D00.08)*
> *carcinoma in situ of hypopharyngeal aspect (D00.08)*
> *carcinoma in situ of marginal zone (D00.08)*

D02.1 Carcinoma in situ of trachea

☑5th **D02.2 Carcinoma in situ of bronchus and lung**
   D02.20 Carcinoma in situ of unspecified bronchus and lung ▽
   D02.21 Carcinoma in situ of right bronchus and lung
   D02.22 Carcinoma in situ of left bronchus and lung

D02.3 Carcinoma in situ of other parts of respiratory system
Carcinoma in situ of accessory sinuses
Carcinoma in situ of middle ear
Carcinoma in situ of nasal cavities
> EXCLUDES 1   *carcinoma in situ of ear (external) (skin) (D04.2-)*
> *carcinoma in situ of nose NOS (D09.8)*
> *carcinoma in situ of skin of nose (D04.3)*

D02.4 Carcinoma in situ of respiratory system, unspecified ▽

☑4th **D03 Melanoma in situ**
D03.0 Melanoma in situ of lip HCC

☑5th **D03.1 Melanoma in situ of eyelid, including canthus**
   D03.10 Melanoma in situ of unspecified eyelid, including canthus HCC ▽
   D03.11 Melanoma in situ of right eyelid, including canthus HCC
   D03.12 Melanoma in situ of left eyelid, including canthus HCC

☑5th **D03.2 Melanoma in situ of ear and external auricular canal**
   D03.20 Melanoma in situ of unspecified ear and external auricular canal HCC ▽

☑ Additional Character Req   ✔7th Placeholder Alert   Manifestation   HCC CMS-HCC Condition   ▽ Unspecified Code   ▶◀ Revised Text   ● New Code   ▲ Revised Code Title

Chapter 2. Neoplasms

D03.21 Melanoma in situ of right ear and external auricular canal   `HCC`

D03.22 Melanoma in situ of left ear and external auricular canal   `HCC`

✓5ᵗʰ **D03.3** Melanoma in situ of other and unspecified parts of face

D03.30 Melanoma in situ of unspecified part of face   `HCC` ▽

D03.39 Melanoma in situ of other parts of face   `HCC`

D03.4 Melanoma in situ of scalp and neck

✓5ᵗʰ **D03.5** Melanoma in situ of trunk

D03.51 Melanoma in situ of anal skin   `HCC`
Melanoma in situ of anal margin
Melanoma in situ of perianal skin

D03.52 Melanoma in situ of breast (skin) (soft tissue)   `HCC`

D03.59 Melanoma in situ of other part of trunk   `HCC`

✓5ᵗʰ **D03.6** Melanoma in situ of upper limb, including shoulder

D03.60 Melanoma in situ of unspecified upper limb, including shoulder   `HCC` ▽

D03.61 Melanoma in situ of right upper limb, including shoulder   `HCC`

D03.62 Melanoma in situ of left upper limb, including shoulder   `HCC`

✓5ᵗʰ **D03.7** Melanoma in situ of lower limb, including hip

D03.70 Melanoma in situ of unspecified lower limb, including hip   `HCC` ▽

D03.71 Melanoma in situ of right lower limb, including hip   `HCC`

D03.72 Melanoma in situ of left lower limb, including hip   `HCC`

D03.8 Melanoma in situ of other sites   `HCC`
Melanoma in situ of scrotum
EXCLUDES 1   carcinoma in situ of scrotum (D07.61)

D03.9 Melanoma in situ, unspecified   `HCC` ▽

✓4ᵗʰ **D04** Carcinoma in situ of skin
EXCLUDES 1   erythroplasia of Queyrat (penis) NOS (D07.4)
melanoma in situ (D03.-)

D04.0 Carcinoma in situ of skin of lip
EXCLUDES 1   carcinoma in situ of vermilion border of lip (D00.01)

✓5ᵗʰ **D04.1** Carcinoma in situ of skin of eyelid, including canthus

D04.10 Carcinoma in situ of skin of unspecified eyelid, including canthus   ▽

D04.11 Carcinoma in situ of skin of right eyelid, including canthus

D04.12 Carcinoma in situ of skin of left eyelid, including canthus

✓5ᵗʰ **D04.2** Carcinoma in situ of skin of ear and external auricular canal

D04.20 Carcinoma in situ of skin of unspecified ear and external auricular canal   ▽

D04.21 Carcinoma in situ of skin of right ear and external auricular canal

D04.22 Carcinoma in situ of skin of left ear and external auricular canal

✓5ᵗʰ **D04.3** Carcinoma in situ of skin of other and unspecified parts of face

D04.30 Carcinoma in situ of skin of unspecified part of face   ▽

D04.39 Carcinoma in situ of skin of other parts of face

D04.4 Carcinoma in situ of skin of scalp and neck

D04.5 Carcinoma in situ of skin of trunk
Carcinoma in situ of anal margin
Carcinoma in situ of anal skin
Carcinoma in situ of perianal skin
Carcinoma in situ of skin of breast
EXCLUDES 1   carcinoma in situ of anus NOS (D01.3)
carcinoma in situ of scrotum (D07.61)
carcinoma in situ of skin of genital organs (D07.-)

✓5ᵗʰ **D04.6** Carcinoma in situ of skin of upper limb, including shoulder

D04.60 Carcinoma in situ of skin of unspecified upper limb, including shoulder   ▽

D04.61 Carcinoma in situ of skin of right upper limb, including shoulder

D04.62 Carcinoma in situ of skin of left upper limb, including shoulder

✓5ᵗʰ **D04.7** Carcinoma in situ of skin of lower limb, including hip

D04.70 Carcinoma in situ of skin of unspecified lower limb, including hip   ▽

D04.71 Carcinoma in situ of skin of right lower limb, including hip

D04.72 Carcinoma in situ of skin of left lower limb, including hip

D04.8 Carcinoma in situ of skin of other sites

D04.9 Carcinoma in situ of skin, unspecified   ▽

✓4ᵗʰ **D05** Carcinoma in situ of breast
EXCLUDES 1   carcinoma in situ of skin of breast (D04.5)
melanoma in situ of breast (skin) (D03.5)
Paget's disease of breast or nipple (C50.-)

✓5ᵗʰ **D05.0** Lobular carcinoma in situ of breast

D05.00 Lobular carcinoma in situ of unspecified breast   ▽

D05.01 Lobular carcinoma in situ of right breast

D05.02 Lobular carcinoma in situ of left breast

✓5ᵗʰ **D05.1** Intraductal carcinoma in situ of breast

D05.10 Intraductal carcinoma in situ of unspecified breast   ▽

D05.11 Intraductal carcinoma in situ of right breast

D05.12 Intraductal carcinoma in situ of left breast

✓5ᵗʰ **D05.8** Other specified type of carcinoma in situ of breast

D05.80 Other specified type of carcinoma in situ of unspecified breast   ▽

D05.81 Other specified type of carcinoma in situ of right breast

D05.82 Other specified type of carcinoma in situ of left breast

✓5ᵗʰ **D05.9** Unspecified type of carcinoma in situ of breast

D05.90 Unspecified type of carcinoma in situ of unspecified breast   ▽

D05.91 Unspecified type of carcinoma in situ of right breast   ▽

D05.92 Unspecified type of carcinoma in situ of left breast   ▽

✓4ᵗʰ **D06** Carcinoma in situ of cervix uteri
INCLUDES   cervical adenocarcinoma in situ
cervical intraepithelial glandular neoplasia
cervical intraepithelial neoplasia III [CIN III]
severe dysplasia of cervix uteri
EXCLUDES 1   cervical intraepithelial neoplasia II [CIN II] (N87.1)
cytologic evidence of malignancy of cervix without histologic confirmation (R87.614)
high grade squamous intraepithelial lesion (HGSIL) of cervix (R87.613)
melanoma in situ of cervix (D03.5)
moderate cervical dysplasia (N87.1)

D06.0 Carcinoma in situ of endocervix   ♀

D06.1 Carcinoma in situ of exocervix   ♀

D06.7 Carcinoma in situ of other parts of cervix   ♀

D06.9 Carcinoma in situ of cervix, unspecified   ♀▽

✓4ᵗʰ **D07** Carcinoma in situ of other and unspecified genital organs
EXCLUDES 1   melanoma in situ of trunk (D03.5)

D07.0 Carcinoma in situ of endometrium   ♀

D07.1 Carcinoma in situ of vulva   ♀
Severe dysplasia of vulva
Vulvar intraepithelial neoplasia III [VIN III]
EXCLUDES 1   moderate dysplasia of vulva (N90.1)
vulvar intraepithelial neoplasia II [VIN II] (N90.1)

D07.2 Carcinoma in situ of vagina   ♀
Severe dysplasia of vagina
Vaginal intraepithelial neoplasia III [VAIN III]
EXCLUDES 1   moderate dysplasia of vagina (N89.1)
vaginal intraepithelial neoplasia II [VIN II] (N89.1)

✓5ᵗʰ **D07.3** Carcinoma in situ of other and unspecified female genital organs

D07.30 Carcinoma in situ of unspecified female genital organs   ♀▽

D07.39 Carcinoma in situ of other female genital organs   ♀

D07.4 Carcinoma in situ of penis   ♂
Erythroplasia of Queyrat NOS

D07.5 Carcinoma in situ of prostate   ♂
Prostatic intraepithelial neoplasia III (PIN III)
Severe dysplasia of prostate
EXCLUDES 1   dysplasia (mild) (moderate) of prostate (N42.3-)
prostatic intraepithelial neoplasia II [PIN II] (N42.3-)

✓5ᵗʰ **D07.6** **Carcinoma in situ of other and unspecified** male genital **organs**

     D07.60 **Carcinoma in situ of unspecified male genital** ♂▽ **organs**

     D07.61 **Carcinoma in situ of** scrotum   ♂

     D07.69 **Carcinoma in situ of other male genital organs**   ♂

✓4ᵗʰ **D09** **Carcinoma in situ of other and unspecified** sites

     EXCLUDES 1   melanoma in situ (D03.-)

     D09.0 **Carcinoma in situ of** bladder

✓5ᵗʰ **D09.1** **Carcinoma in situ of other and unspecified** urinary organs ▽

     D09.10 **Carcinoma in situ of unspecified urinary organ** ▽

     D09.19 **Carcinoma in situ of other urinary organs**

✓5ᵗʰ **D09.2** **Carcinoma in situ of** eye

     EXCLUDES 1   carcinoma in situ of skin of eyelid (D04.1-)

     D09.20 **Carcinoma in situ of unspecified eye** ▽

     D09.21 **Carcinoma in situ of** right **eye**

     D09.22 **Carcinoma in situ of** left **eye**

     D09.3 **Carcinoma in situ of** thyroid **and other** endocrine glands

     EXCLUDES 1   carcinoma in situ of endocrine pancreas (D01.7)

               carcinoma in situ of ovary (D07.39)

               carcinoma in situ of testis (D07.69)

     D09.8 **Carcinoma in situ of other specified sites**

     D09.9 **Carcinoma in situ, unspecified** ▽

Benign neoplasms, except benign neuroendocrine tumors (D10-D36)

✓4ᵗʰ **D10** **Benign neoplasm of** mouth and pharynx

     D10.0 **Benign neoplasm of** lip

     Benign neoplasm of lip (frenulum) (inner aspect) (mucosa) (vermilion border)

     EXCLUDES 1   benign neoplasm of skin of lip (D22.0, D23.0)

     D10.1 **Benign neoplasm of** tongue

     Benign neoplasm of lingual tonsil

     D10.2 **Benign neoplasm of** floor **of mouth**

✓5ᵗʰ **D10.3** **Benign neoplasm** of other and unspecified parts of mouth

     D10.30 **Benign neoplasm of unspecified part of mouth** ▽

     D10.39 **Benign neoplasm of other parts of mouth**

         Benign neoplasm of minor salivary gland NOS

         EXCLUDES 1   benign odontogenic neoplasms (D16.4-D16.5)

               benign neoplasm of mucosa of lip (D10.0)

               benign neoplasm of nasopharyngeal surface of soft palate (D10.6)

     D10.4 **Benign neoplasm of** tonsil

     Benign neoplasm of tonsil (faucial) (palatine)

     EXCLUDES 1   benign neoplasm of lingual tonsil (D10.1)

               benign neoplasm of pharyngeal tonsil (D10.6)

               benign neoplasm of tonsillar fossa (D10.5)

               benign neoplasm of tonsillar pillars (D10.5)

     D10.5 **Benign neoplasm of other parts of** oropharynx

     Benign neoplasm of epiglottis, anterior aspect

     Benign neoplasm of tonsillar fossa

     Benign neoplasm of tonsillar pillars

     Benign neoplasm of vallecula

     EXCLUDES 1   benign neoplasm of epiglottis NOS (D14.1)

               benign neoplasm of epiglottis, suprahyoid portion (D14.1)

     D10.6 **Benign neoplasm of** nasopharynx

     Benign neoplasm of pharyngeal tonsil

     Benign neoplasm of posterior margin of septum and choanae

     D10.7 **Benign neoplasm of** hypopharynx

     D10.9 **Benign neoplasm of pharynx, unspecified** ▽

✓4ᵗʰ **D11** **Benign neoplasm of** major salivary glands

     EXCLUDES 1   benign neoplasms of minor salivary glands NOS (D10.39)

               benign neoplasms of specified minor salivary glands which are classified according to their anatomical location

     D11.0 **Benign neoplasm of** parotid gland

     D11.7 **Benign neoplasm of other major salivary glands**

     Benign neoplasm of sublingual salivary gland

     Benign neoplasm of submandibular salivary gland

     D11.9 **Benign neoplasm of major salivary gland, unspecified** ▽

✓4ᵗʰ **D12** **Benign neoplasm of** colon, rectum, anus and anal canal

     EXCLUDES 1   benign carcinoid tumors of the large intestine, and rectum (D3A.02-)

     AHA: 2017, 1Q, 15; 2015, 2Q, 14

     D12.0 **Benign neoplasm of** cecum

     Benign neoplasm of ileocecal valve

     D12.1 **Benign neoplasm of** appendix

     EXCLUDES 1   benign carcinoid tumor of the appendix (D3A.020)

     D12.2 **Benign neoplasm of** ascending colon

     D12.3 **Benign neoplasm of** transverse colon

     Benign neoplasm of hepatic flexure

     Benign neoplasm of splenic flexure

     AHA: 2017, 1Q, 16

     D12.4 **Benign neoplasm of** descending colon

     D12.5 **Benign neoplasm of** sigmoid colon

     D12.6 **Benign neoplasm of** colon, unspecified ▽

     Adenomatosis of colon

     Benign neoplasm of large intestine NOS

     Polyposis (hereditary) of colon

     EXCLUDES 1   inflammatory polyp of colon (K51.4-)

               polyp of colon NOS (K63.5)

     D12.7 **Benign neoplasm of** rectosigmoid junction

     D12.8 **Benign neoplasm of** rectum

     EXCLUDES 1   benign carcinoid tumor of the rectum (D3A.026)

     D12.9 **Benign neoplasm of** anus and anal canal

     Benign neoplasm of anus NOS

     EXCLUDES 1   benign neoplasm of anal margin (D22.5, D23.5)

               benign neoplasm of anal skin (D22.5, D23.5)

               benign neoplasm of perianal skin (D22.5, D23.5)

✓4ᵗʰ **D13** **Benign neoplasm of other and ill-defined parts of** digestive system

     EXCLUDES 1   benign stromal tumors of digestive system (D21.4)

     D13.0 **Benign neoplasm of** esophagus

     D13.1 **Benign neoplasm of** stomach

     EXCLUDES 1   benign carcinoid tumor of the stomach (D3A.092)

     D13.2 **Benign neoplasm of** duodenum

     EXCLUDES 1   benign carcinoid tumor of the duodenum (D3A.010)

✓5ᵗʰ **D13.3** **Benign neoplasm of other and unspecified parts of** small intestine

     EXCLUDES 1   benign carcinoid tumors of the small intestine (D3A.01-)

               benign neoplasm of ileocecal valve (D12.0)

     D13.30 **Benign neoplasm of unspecified part of small** ▽ **intestine**

     D13.39 **Benign neoplasm of other parts of small intestine**

     D13.4 **Benign neoplasm of** liver

     Benign neoplasm of intrahepatic bile ducts

     D13.5 **Benign neoplasm of** extrahepatic bile ducts

     D13.6 **Benign neoplasm of** pancreas

     EXCLUDES 1   benign neoplasm of endocrine pancreas (D13.7)

     D13.7 **Benign neoplasm of** endocrine pancreas

     Islet cell tumor

     Benign neoplasm of islets of Langerhans

     Use additional code to identify any functional activity

     D13.9 **Benign neoplasm of** ill-defined sites **within the digestive system**

     Benign neoplasm of digestive system NOS

     Benign neoplasm of intestine NOS

     Benign neoplasm of spleen

✓4ᵗʰ **D14** **Benign neoplasm of** middle ear and respiratory system

     D14.0 **Benign neoplasm of** middle ear, nasal cavity and accessory sinuses

     Benign neoplasm of cartilage of nose

     EXCLUDES 1   benign neoplasm of auricular canal (external) (D22.2-, D23.2-)

               benign neoplasm of bone of ear (D16.4)

               benign neoplasm of bone of nose (D16.4)

               benign neoplasm of cartilage of ear (D21.0)

               benign neoplasm of ear (external)(skin) (D22.2-, D23.2-)

               benign neoplasm of nose NOS (D36.7)

               benign neoplasm of skin of nose (D22.39, D23.39)

               benign neoplasm of olfactory bulb (D33.3)

               benign neoplasm of posterior margin of septum and choanae (D10.6)

               polyp of accessory sinus (J33.8)

               polyp of ear (middle) (H74.4)

               polyp of nasal (cavity) (J33.-)

✓ Additional Character Req   ✓ˣ⁷ᵗʰ Placeholder Alert   Manifestation   ᴴᶜᶜ CMS-HCC Condition   ▽ Unspecified Code   ▶◀ Revised Text   ● New Code   ▲ Revised Code Title

ICD-10-CM 2018   485

D07.6–D14.0

D14.1   Benign neoplasm of larynx
Adenomatous polyp of larynx
Benign neoplasm of epiglottis (suprahyoid portion)
EXCLUDES 1   benign neoplasm of epiglottis, anterior aspect (D10.5)
polyp (nonadenomatous) of vocal cord or larynx
(J38.1)

D14.2   Benign neoplasm of trachea

✓5ᵗʰ **D14.3   Benign neoplasm of** bronchus and lung
EXCLUDES 1   benign carcinoid tumor of the bronchus and lung
(D3A.090)

    **D14.30   Benign neoplasm of unspecified bronchus   ▽
and lung**

    D14.31   Benign neoplasm of right **bronchus and lung**

    D14.32   Benign neoplasm of left **bronchus and lung**

D14.4   Benign neoplasm of respiratory system, unspecified   ▽

✓4ᵗʰ **D15   Benign neoplasm of other and unspecified** intrathoracic organs
EXCLUDES 1   benign neoplasm of mesothelial tissue (D19.-)

D15.0   Benign neoplasm of thymus
EXCLUDES 1   benign carcinoid tumor of the thymus (D3A.091)

D15.1   Benign neoplasm of heart
EXCLUDES 1   benign neoplasm of great vessels (D21.3)

D15.2   Benign neoplasm of mediastinum

D15.7   Benign neoplasm of other specified intrathoracic organs

D15.9   Benign neoplasm of intrathoracic organ, unspecified   ▽

✓4ᵗʰ **D16   Benign neoplasm of** bone and articular cartilage
EXCLUDES 1   benign neoplasm of connective tissue of ear (D21.0)
benign neoplasm of connective tissue of eyelid (D21.0)
benign neoplasm of connective tissue of larynx (D14.1)
benign neoplasm of connective tissue of nose (D14.0)
benign neoplasm of synovia (D21.-)

✓5ᵗʰ **D16.0   Benign neoplasm of** scapula and long bones of upper limb
    **D16.00   Benign neoplasm of scapula and long bones of   ▽
unspecified upper limb**
    D16.01   Benign neoplasm of scapula and long bones of right
upper limb
    D16.02   Benign neoplasm of scapula and long bones of left
upper limb

✓5ᵗʰ **D16.1   Benign neoplasm of** short bones of upper limb
    **D16.10   Benign neoplasm of short bones of unspecified   ▽
upper limb**
    D16.11   Benign neoplasm of short bones of right **upper limb**
    D16.12   Benign neoplasm of short bones of left **upper limb**

✓5ᵗʰ **D16.2   Benign neoplasm of** long bones of lower limb
    **D16.20   Benign neoplasm of long bones of unspecified   ▽
lower limb**
    D16.21   Benign neoplasm of long bones of right **lower limb**
    D16.22   Benign neoplasm of long bones of left **lower limb**

✓5ᵗʰ **D16.3   Benign neoplasm of** short bones of lower limb
    **D16.30   Benign neoplasm of short bones of unspecified   ▽
lower limb**
    D16.31   Benign neoplasm of short bones of right **lower limb**
    D16.32   Benign neoplasm of short bones of left **lower limb**

D16.4   Benign neoplasm of bones of skull and face
Benign neoplasm of maxilla (superior)
Benign neoplasm of orbital bone
Keratocyst of maxilla
Keratocystic odontogenic tumor of maxilla
EXCLUDES 2   benign neoplasm of lower jaw bone (D16.5)

D16.5   Benign neoplasm of lower jaw bone
Keratocyst of mandible
Keratocystic odontogenic tumor of mandible

D16.6   Benign neoplasm of vertebral column
EXCLUDES 1   benign neoplasm of sacrum and coccyx (D16.8)

D16.7   Benign neoplasm of ribs, sternum and clavicle

D16.8   Benign neoplasm of pelvic bones, sacrum and coccyx

**D16.9   Benign neoplasm of bone and articular cartilage,   ▽
unspecified**

✓4ᵗʰ **D17   Benign** lipomatous **neoplasm**

D17.0   Benign lipomatous neoplasm of skin and subcutaneous tissue
of head, face and neck

D17.1   Benign lipomatous neoplasm of skin and subcutaneous tissue
of trunk

✓5ᵗʰ **D17.2   Benign lipomatous neoplasm of** skin and subcutaneous tissue
of limb
    **D17.20   Benign lipomatous neoplasm of skin and   ▽
subcutaneous tissue of unspecified limb**
    **D17.21   Benign lipomatous neoplasm of skin and
subcutaneous tissue of** right **arm**
    **D17.22   Benign lipomatous neoplasm of skin and
subcutaneous tissue of** left **arm**
    **D17.23   Benign lipomatous neoplasm of skin and
subcutaneous tissue of** right **leg**
    **D17.24   Benign lipomatous neoplasm of skin and
subcutaneous tissue of** left **leg**

✓5ᵗʰ **D17.3   Benign lipomatous neoplasm of** skin and subcutaneous tissue
of other and unspecified sites
    **D17.30   Benign lipomatous neoplasm of skin and   ▽
subcutaneous tissue of unspecified sites**
    **D17.39   Benign lipomatous neoplasm of skin and
subcutaneous tissue of other sites**

D17.4   Benign lipomatous neoplasm of intrathoracic organs

D17.5   Benign lipomatous neoplasm of intra-abdominal organs
EXCLUDES 1   benign lipomatous neoplasm of peritoneum and
retroperitoneum (D17.79)

D17.6   Benign lipomatous neoplasm of spermatic cord   ♂

✓5ᵗʰ **D17.7   Benign lipomatous neoplasm of other sites**
    D17.71   Benign lipomatous neoplasm of kidney
    D17.72   Benign lipomatous neoplasm of other genitourinary
organ
    D17.79   Benign lipomatous neoplasm of other sites
Benign lipomatous neoplasm of peritoneum
Benign lipomatous neoplasm of retroperitoneum

D17.9   Benign lipomatous neoplasm, unspecified   ▽
Lipoma NOS

✓4ᵗʰ **D18   Hemangioma and lymphangioma, any site**
EXCLUDES 1   benign neoplasm of glomus jugulare (D35.6)
blue or pigmented nevus (D22.-)
nevus NOS (D22.-)
vascular nevus (Q82.5)

✓5ᵗʰ **D18.0   Hemangioma**
Angioma NOS
Cavernous nevus
DEF: A common benign tumor usually occurring in infancy;
composed of newly formed blood vessels due to malformation of
angioblastic tissue.
    D18.00   Hemangioma unspecified site   ▽
    D18.01   Hemangioma of skin and subcutaneous tissue
    D18.02   Hemangioma of intracranial structures   HCC
    D18.03   Hemangioma of intra-abdominal structures
    D18.09   Hemangioma of other sites

D18.1   Lymphangioma, any site

✓4ᵗʰ **D19   Benign neoplasm of** mesothelial tissue

D19.0   Benign neoplasm of mesothelial tissue of pleura

D19.1   Benign neoplasm of mesothelial tissue of peritoneum

D19.7   Benign neoplasm of mesothelial tissue of other sites

D19.9   Benign neoplasm of mesothelial tissue, unspecified   ▽
Benign mesothelioma NOS

✓4ᵗʰ **D20   Benign neoplasm of soft tissue of** retroperitoneum and
peritoneum
EXCLUDES 1   benign lipomatous neoplasm of peritoneum and
retroperitoneum (D17.79)
benign neoplasm of mesothelial tissue (D19.-)

D20.0   Benign neoplasm of soft tissue of retroperitoneum

D20.1   Benign neoplasm of soft tissue of peritoneum

✓4ᵗʰ **D21 Other benign neoplasms of connective and other soft tissue**

    INCLUDES benign neoplasm of blood vessel
                  benign neoplasm of bursa
                  benign neoplasm of cartilage
                  benign neoplasm of fascia
                  benign neoplasm of fat
                  benign neoplasm of ligament, except uterine
                  benign neoplasm of lymphatic channel
                  benign neoplasm of muscle
                  benign neoplasm of synovia
                  benign neoplasm of tendon (sheath)
                  benign stromal tumors

    EXCLUDES1 *benign neoplasm of articular cartilage (D16.-)*
                  benign neoplasm of cartilage of larynx (D14.1)
                  benign neoplasm of cartilage of nose (D14.0)
                  benign neoplasm of connective tissue of breast (D24.-)
                  benign neoplasm of peripheral nerves and autonomic nervous
                    system (D36.1-)
                  benign neoplasm of peritoneum (D20.1)
                  benign neoplasm of retroperitoneum (D20.0)
                  benign neoplasm of uterine ligament, any (D28.2)
                  benign neoplasm of vascular tissue (D18.-)
                  hemangioma (D18.0-)
                  lipomatous neoplasm (D17.-)
                  lymphangioma (D18.1)
                  uterine leiomyoma (D25.-)

D21.0 Benign neoplasm of connective and other soft tissue of head, face and neck
    Benign neoplasm of connective tissue of ear
    Benign neoplasm of connective tissue of eyelid
    EXCLUDES1 *benign neoplasm of connective tissue of orbit (D31.6-)*

✓5ᵗʰ **D21.1 Benign neoplasm of connective and other soft tissue of upper limb, including shoulder**

    **D21.10 Benign neoplasm of connective and other soft ▽
tissue of unspecified upper limb, including shoulder**

    D21.11 Benign neoplasm of connective and other soft tissue of right upper limb, including shoulder

    D21.12 Benign neoplasm of connective and other soft tissue of left upper limb, including shoulder

✓5ᵗʰ **D21.2 Benign neoplasm of connective and other soft tissue of lower limb, including hip**

    **D21.20 Benign neoplasm of connective and other soft ▽
tissue of unspecified lower limb, including hip**

    D21.21 Benign neoplasm of connective and other soft tissue of right lower limb, including hip

    D21.22 Benign neoplasm of connective and other soft tissue of left lower limb, including hip

D21.3 Benign neoplasm of connective and other soft tissue of thorax
    Benign neoplasm of axilla
    Benign neoplasm of diaphragm
    Benign neoplasm of great vessels
    EXCLUDES1 *benign neoplasm of heart (D15.1)*
                  benign neoplasm of mediastinum (D15.2)
                  benign neoplasm of thymus (D15.0)

D21.4 Benign neoplasm of connective and other soft tissue of abdomen
    Benign stromal tumors of abdomen

D21.5 Benign neoplasm of connective and other soft tissue of pelvis
    EXCLUDES1 *benign neoplasm of any uterine ligament (D28.2)*
                  uterine leiomyoma (D25.-)

**D21.6 Benign neoplasm of connective and other soft tissue of ▽
trunk, unspecified**
    Benign neoplasm of back NOS

**D21.9 Benign neoplasm of connective and other soft tissue, ▽
unspecified**

✓4ᵗʰ **D22 Melanocytic nevi**
    INCLUDES atypical nevus
                  blue hairy pigmented nevus
                  nevus NOS

D22.0 Melanocytic nevi of lip

✓5ᵗʰ **D22.1 Melanocytic nevi of eyelid, including canthus**

    **D22.10 Melanocytic nevi of unspecified eyelid, including ▽
canthus**

    D22.11 Melanocytic nevi of right eyelid, including canthus

    D22.12 Melanocytic nevi of left eyelid, including canthus

✓5ᵗʰ **D22.2 Melanocytic nevi of ear and external auricular canal**

    **D22.20 Melanocytic nevi of unspecified ear and external ▽
auricular canal**

    D22.21 Melanocytic nevi of right ear and external auricular canal

    D22.22 Melanocytic nevi of left ear and external auricular canal

✓5ᵗʰ **D22.3 Melanocytic nevi of other and unspecified parts of face**

    D22.30 Melanocytic nevi of unspecified part of face ▽

    D22.39 Melanocytic nevi of other parts of face

D22.4 Melanocytic nevi of scalp and neck

D22.5 Melanocytic nevi of trunk
    Melanocytic nevi of anal margin
    Melanocytic nevi of anal skin
    Melanocytic nevi of perianal skin
    Melanocytic nevi of skin of breast

✓5ᵗʰ **D22.6 Melanocytic nevi of upper limb, including shoulder**

    **D22.60 Melanocytic nevi of unspecified upper limb, ▽
including shoulder**

    D22.61 Melanocytic nevi of right upper limb, including shoulder

    D22.62 Melanocytic nevi of left upper limb, including shoulder

✓5ᵗʰ **D22.7 Melanocytic nevi of lower limb, including hip**

    **D22.70 Melanocytic nevi of unspecified lower limb, ▽
including hip**

    D22.71 Melanocytic nevi of right lower limb, including hip

    D22.72 Melanocytic nevi of left lower limb, including hip

D22.9 Melanocytic nevi, unspecified ▽

✓4ᵗʰ **D23 Other benign neoplasms of skin**
    INCLUDES benign neoplasm of hair follicles
                  benign neoplasm of sebaceous glands
                  benign neoplasm of sweat glands
    EXCLUDES1 *benign lipomatous neoplasms of skin (D17.0-D17.3)*
                  melanocytic nevi (D22.-)

D23.0 Other benign neoplasm of skin of lip
    EXCLUDES1 *benign neoplasm of vermilion border of lip (D10.0)*

✓5ᵗʰ **D23.1 Other benign neoplasm of skin of eyelid, including canthus**

    **D23.10 Other benign neoplasm of skin of unspecified ▽
eyelid, including canthus**

    D23.11 Other benign neoplasm of skin of right eyelid, including canthus

    D23.12 Other benign neoplasm of skin of left eyelid, including canthus

✓5ᵗʰ **D23.2 Other benign neoplasm of skin of ear and external auricular canal**

    **D23.20 Other benign neoplasm of skin of unspecified ▽
ear and external auricular canal**

    D23.21 Other benign neoplasm of skin of right ear and external auricular canal

    D23.22 Other benign neoplasm of skin of left ear and external auricular canal

✓5ᵗʰ **D23.3 Other benign neoplasm of skin of other and unspecified parts of face**

    **D23.30 Other benign neoplasm of skin of unspecified ▽
part of face**

    D23.39 Other benign neoplasm of skin of other parts of face

D23.4 Other benign neoplasm of skin of scalp and neck

D23.5 Other benign neoplasm of skin of trunk
    Other benign neoplasm of anal margin
    Other benign neoplasm of anal skin
    Other benign neoplasm of perianal skin
    Other benign neoplasm of skin of breast
    EXCLUDES1 *benign neoplasm of anus NOS (D12.9)*

✓5ᵗʰ **D23.6 Other benign neoplasm of skin of upper limb, including shoulder**

    **D23.60 Other benign neoplasm of skin of unspecified ▽
upper limb, including shoulder**

    D23.61 Other benign neoplasm of skin of right upper limb, including shoulder

    D23.62 Other benign neoplasm of skin of left upper limb, including shoulder

✓5ᵗʰ **D23.7 Other benign neoplasm of skin of lower limb, including hip**

    **D23.70 Other benign neoplasm of skin of unspecified ▽
lower limb, including hip**

    D23.71 Other benign neoplasm of skin of right lower limb, including hip

    D23.72 Other benign neoplasm of skin of left lower limb, including hip

---

✓ Additional Character Req   ✓x7ᵗʰ Placeholder Alert   Manifestation   HCC CMS-HCC Condition   ▽ Unspecified Code   ►◄ Revised Text   ● New Code   ▲ Revised Code Title

D23.9   Other benign neoplasm of skin, unspecified   ▽

✓4th D24   Benign neoplasm of breast
INCLUDES   benign neoplasm of connective tissue of breast
benign neoplasm of soft parts of breast
fibroadenoma of breast

EXCLUDES 2   adenofibrosis of breast (N60.2)
benign cyst of breast (N60.-)
benign mammary dysplasia (N60.-)
benign neoplasm of skin of breast (D22.5, D23.5)
fibrocystic disease of breast (N60.-)

D24.1   Benign neoplasm of right breast
D24.2   Benign neoplasm of left breast
D24.9   Benign neoplasm of unspecified breast   ▽

✓4th D25   Leiomyoma of uterus
INCLUDES   uterine fibroid
uterine fibromyoma
uterine myoma

D25.0   Submucous leiomyoma of uterus   ♀
D25.1   Intramural leiomyoma of uterus   ♀
       Interstitial leiomyoma of uterus
D25.2   Subserosal leiomyoma of uterus   ♀
       Subperitoneal leiomyoma of uterus
D25.9   Leiomyoma of uterus, unspecified   ♀▽

✓4th D26   Other benign neoplasms of uterus
D26.0   Other benign neoplasm of cervix uteri   ♀
D26.1   Other benign neoplasm of corpus uteri   ♀
D26.7   Other benign neoplasm of other parts of uterus   ♀
D26.9   Other benign neoplasm of uterus, unspecified   ♀▽

✓4th D27   Benign neoplasm of ovary
Use additional code to identify any functional activity
EXCLUDES 2   corpus albicans cyst (N83.2-)
corpus luteum cyst (N83.1-)
endometrial cyst (N80.1)
follicular (atretic) cyst (N83.0-)
graafian follicle cyst (N83.0-)
ovarian cyst NEC (N83.2-)
ovarian retention cyst (N83.2-)

D27.0   Benign neoplasm of right ovary   ♀
D27.1   Benign neoplasm of left ovary   ♀
D27.9   Benign neoplasm of unspecified ovary   ♀▽

✓4th D28   Benign neoplasm of other and unspecified female genital organs
INCLUDES   adenomatous polyp
benign neoplasm of skin of female genital organs
benign teratoma

EXCLUDES 1   epoophoron cyst (Q50.5)
fimbrial cyst (Q50.4)
Gartner's duct cyst (Q52.4)
parovarian cyst (Q50.5)

D28.0   Benign neoplasm of vulva   ♀
D28.1   Benign neoplasm of vagina   ♀
D28.2   Benign neoplasm of uterine tubes and ligaments   ♀
       Benign neoplasm of fallopian tube
       Benign neoplasm of uterine ligament (broad) (round)
D28.7   Benign neoplasm of other specified female genital organs   ♀
D28.9   Benign neoplasm of female genital organ, unspecified   ♀▽

Uterine Leiomyomas (Fibroids)

✓4th D29   Benign neoplasm of male genital organs
INCLUDES   benign neoplasm of skin of male genital organs

D29.0   Benign neoplasm of penis   ♂
D29.1   Benign neoplasm of prostate   ♂
       EXCLUDES 1   enlarged prostate (N40.-)

✓5th D29.2   Benign neoplasm of testis
       Use additional code to identify any functional activity
       D29.20   Benign neoplasm of unspecified testis   ♂▽
       D29.21   Benign neoplasm of right testis   ♂
       D29.22   Benign neoplasm of left testis   ♂

✓5th D29.3   Benign neoplasm of epididymis
       D29.30   Benign neoplasm of unspecified epididymis   ♂▽
       D29.31   Benign neoplasm of right epididymis   ♂
       D29.32   Benign neoplasm of left epididymis   ♂

D29.4   Benign neoplasm of scrotum   ♂
       Benign neoplasm of skin of scrotum
D29.8   Benign neoplasm of other specified male genital organs   ♂
       Benign neoplasm of seminal vesicle
       Benign neoplasm of spermatic cord
       Benign neoplasm of tunica vaginalis
D29.9   Benign neoplasm of male genital organ, unspecified   ♂▽

✓4th D30   Benign neoplasm of urinary organs
✓5th D30.0   Benign neoplasm of kidney
       EXCLUDES 1   benign carcinoid tumor of the kidney (D3A.093)
             benign neoplasm of renal calyces (D30.1-)
             benign neoplasm of renal pelvis (D30.1-)
       D30.00   Benign neoplasm of unspecified kidney   ▽
       D30.01   Benign neoplasm of right kidney
       D30.02   Benign neoplasm of left kidney

✓5th D30.1   Benign neoplasm of renal pelvis
       D30.10   Benign neoplasm of unspecified renal pelvis   ▽
       D30.11   Benign neoplasm of right renal pelvis
       D30.12   Benign neoplasm of left renal pelvis

✓5th D30.2   Benign neoplasm of ureter
       EXCLUDES 1   benign neoplasm of ureteric orifice of bladder (D30.3)
       D30.20   Benign neoplasm of unspecified ureter   ▽
       D30.21   Benign neoplasm of right ureter
       D30.22   Benign neoplasm of left ureter

D30.3   Benign neoplasm of bladder
       Benign neoplasm of ureteric orifice of bladder
       Benign neoplasm of urethral orifice of bladder
D30.4   Benign neoplasm of urethra
       EXCLUDES 1   benign neoplasm of urethral orifice of bladder (D30.3)
D30.8   Benign neoplasm of other specified urinary organs
       Benign neoplasm of paraurethral glands
D30.9   Benign neoplasm of urinary organ, unspecified   ▽
       Benign neoplasm of urinary system NOS

✓4th D31   Benign neoplasm of eye and adnexa
EXCLUDES 1   benign neoplasm of connective tissue of eyelid (D21.0)
           benign neoplasm of optic nerve (D33.3)
           benign neoplasm of skin of eyelid (D22.1-, D23.1-)

✓5th D31.0   Benign neoplasm of conjunctiva
       D31.00   Benign neoplasm of unspecified conjunctiva   ▽
       D31.01   Benign neoplasm of right conjunctiva
       D31.02   Benign neoplasm of left conjunctiva

✓5th D31.1   Benign neoplasm of cornea
       D31.10   Benign neoplasm of unspecified cornea   ▽
       D31.11   Benign neoplasm of right cornea
       D31.12   Benign neoplasm of left cornea

✓5th D31.2   Benign neoplasm of retina
       EXCLUDES 1   dark area on retina (D49.81)
           hemangioma of retina (D49.81)
           neoplasm of unspecified behavior of retina and
               choroid (D49.81)
           retinal freckle (D49.81)
       D31.20   Benign neoplasm of unspecified retina   ▽
       D31.21   Benign neoplasm of right retina
       D31.22   Benign neoplasm of left retina

✓5th D31.3   Benign neoplasm of choroid
       D31.30   Benign neoplasm of unspecified choroid   ▽
       D31.31   Benign neoplasm of right choroid
       D31.32   Benign neoplasm of left choroid

EXCLUDES 1 Not coded here   EXCLUDES 2 Not included here   N Newborn Age: 0   P Pediatric Age: 0-17   M Maternity Age: 12-55   A Adult Age: 15-124

488   ICD-10-CM 2018

Caption labels in figure: Cornual, Pedunculated, Uterine cavity, Intramural, Subserosal, Submucosal, Cervical

✓5ᵗʰ **D31.4 Benign neoplasm of ciliary body**

    D31.40 Benign neoplasm of unspecified ciliary body ▽

    D31.41 Benign neoplasm of right ciliary body

    D31.42 Benign neoplasm of left ciliary body

✓5ᵗʰ **D31.5 Benign neoplasm of lacrimal gland and duct**
    Benign neoplasm of lacrimal sac
    Benign neoplasm of nasolacrimal duct

    D31.50 Benign neoplasm of unspecified lacrimal gland and duct ▽

    D31.51 Benign neoplasm of right lacrimal gland and duct

    D31.52 Benign neoplasm of left lacrimal gland and duct

✓5ᵗʰ **D31.6 Benign neoplasm of unspecified site of orbit**
    Benign neoplasm of connective tissue of orbit
    Benign neoplasm of extraocular muscle
    Benign neoplasm of peripheral nerves of orbit
    Benign neoplasm of retrobulbar tissue
    Benign neoplasm of retro-ocular tissue
    EXCLUDES 1 benign neoplasm of orbital bone (D16.4)

    D31.60 Benign neoplasm of unspecified site of unspecified orbit ▽

    D31.61 Benign neoplasm of unspecified site of right orbit

    D31.62 Benign neoplasm of unspecified site of left orbit

✓5ᵗʰ **D31.9 Benign neoplasm of unspecified part of eye**
    Benign neoplasm of eyeball

    D31.90 Benign neoplasm of unspecified part of unspecified eye ▽

    D31.91 Benign neoplasm of unspecified part of right eye

    D31.92 Benign neoplasm of unspecified part of left eye

✓4ᵗʰ **D32 Benign neoplasm of meninges**

    D32.0 Benign neoplasm of cerebral meninges   HCC

    D32.1 Benign neoplasm of spinal meninges   HCC

    D32.9 Benign neoplasm of meninges, unspecified   HCC ▽
    Meningioma NOS

✓4ᵗʰ **D33 Benign neoplasm of brain and other parts of central nervous system**
    EXCLUDES 1 angioma (D18.0-)
        benign neoplasm of meninges (D32.-)
        benign neoplasm of peripheral nerves and autonomic nervous system (D36.1-)
        hemangioma (D18.0-)
        neurofibromatosis (Q85.0-)
        retro-ocular benign neoplasm (D31.6-)

    D33.0 Benign neoplasm of brain, supratentorial   HCC
    Benign neoplasm of cerebral ventricle
    Benign neoplasm of cerebrum
    Benign neoplasm of frontal lobe
    Benign neoplasm of occipital lobe
    Benign neoplasm of parietal lobe
    Benign neoplasm of temporal lobe
    EXCLUDES 1 benign neoplasm of fourth ventricle (D33.1)

    D33.1 Benign neoplasm of brain, infratentorial   HCC
    Benign neoplasm of brain stem
    Benign neoplasm of cerebellum
    Benign neoplasm of fourth ventricle

    D33.2 Benign neoplasm of brain, unspecified   HCC ▽

    D33.3 Benign neoplasm of cranial nerves   HCC
    Benign neoplasm of olfactory bulb

    D33.4 Benign neoplasm of spinal cord   HCC

    D33.7 Benign neoplasm of other specified parts of central nervous system   HCC

    D33.9 Benign neoplasm of central nervous system, unspecified   HCC ▽
    Benign neoplasm of nervous system (central) NOS

D34 Benign neoplasm of thyroid gland
    Use additional code to identify any functional activity

✓4ᵗʰ **D35 Benign neoplasm of other and unspecified endocrine glands**
    Use additional code to identify any functional activity
    EXCLUDES 1 benign neoplasm of endocrine pancreas (D13.7)
        benign neoplasm of ovary (D27.-)
        benign neoplasm of testis (D29.2-)
        benign neoplasm of thymus (D15.0)

✓5ᵗʰ **D35.0 Benign neoplasm of adrenal gland**

    D35.00 Benign neoplasm of unspecified adrenal gland ▽

    D35.01 Benign neoplasm of right adrenal gland

    D35.02 Benign neoplasm of left adrenal gland

    D35.1 Benign neoplasm of parathyroid gland

    D35.2 Benign neoplasm of pituitary gland   HCC
    AHA: 2014, 3Q, 22

    D35.3 Benign neoplasm of craniopharyngeal duct   HCC

    D35.4 Benign neoplasm of pineal gland   HCC

    D35.5 Benign neoplasm of carotid body

    D35.6 Benign neoplasm of aortic body and other paraganglia
    Benign tumor of glomus jugulare

    D35.7 Benign neoplasm of other specified endocrine glands

    D35.9 Benign neoplasm of endocrine gland, unspecified ▽
    Benign neoplasm of unspecified endocrine gland

✓4ᵗʰ **D36 Benign neoplasm of other and unspecified sites**

    D36.0 Benign neoplasm of lymph nodes
    EXCLUDES 1 lymphangioma (D18.1)

✓5ᵗʰ   **D36.1** Benign neoplasm of peripheral nerves and autonomic nervous system
    EXCLUDES 1 benign neoplasm of peripheral nerves of orbit (D31.6-)
        neurofibromatosis (Q85.0-)

    D36.10 Benign neoplasm of peripheral nerves and autonomic nervous system, unspecified ▽

    D36.11 Benign neoplasm of peripheral nerves and autonomic nervous system of face, head, and neck

    D36.12 Benign neoplasm of peripheral nerves and autonomic nervous system, upper limb, including shoulder

    D36.13 Benign neoplasm of peripheral nerves and autonomic nervous system of lower limb, including hip

    D36.14 Benign neoplasm of peripheral nerves and autonomic nervous system of thorax

    D36.15 Benign neoplasm of peripheral nerves and autonomic nervous system of abdomen

    D36.16 Benign neoplasm of peripheral nerves and autonomic nervous system of pelvis

    D36.17 Benign neoplasm of peripheral nerves and autonomic nervous system of trunk, unspecified ▽

    D36.7 Benign neoplasm of other specified sites
    Benign neoplasm of nose NOS

    D36.9 Benign neoplasm, unspecified site ▽

Benign neuroendocrine tumors (D3A)

✓4ᵗʰ **D3A Benign neuroendocrine tumors**
    Code also any associated multiple endocrine neoplasia [MEN] syndromes (E31.2-)
    Use additional code to identify any associated endocrine syndrome, such as:
    carcinoid syndrome (E34.0)
    EXCLUDES 2 benign pancreatic islet cell tumors (D13.7)

✓5ᵗʰ   **D3A.0 Benign carcinoid tumors**

    D3A.00 Benign carcinoid tumor of unspecified site ▽
    Carcinoid tumor NOS

✓6ᵗʰ   **D3A.01** Benign carcinoid tumors of the small intestine
    D3A.010 Benign carcinoid tumor of the duodenum
    D3A.011 Benign carcinoid tumor of the jejunum
    D3A.012 Benign carcinoid tumor of the ileum
    D3A.019 Benign carcinoid tumor of the small intestine, unspecified portion ▽

✓6ᵗʰ   **D3A.02** Benign carcinoid tumors of the appendix, large intestine, and rectum
    D3A.020 Benign carcinoid tumor of the appendix
    D3A.021 Benign carcinoid tumor of the cecum
    D3A.022 Benign carcinoid tumor of the ascending colon
    D3A.023 Benign carcinoid tumor of the transverse colon
    D3A.024 Benign carcinoid tumor of the descending colon
    D3A.025 Benign carcinoid tumor of the sigmoid colon
    D3A.026 Benign carcinoid tumor of the rectum
    D3A.029 Benign carcinoid tumor of the large intestine, unspecified portion ▽
    Benign carcinoid tumor of the colon NOS

✓6ᵗʰ   **D3A.09** Benign carcinoid tumors of other sites
    D3A.090 Benign carcinoid tumor of the bronchus and lung
    D3A.091 Benign carcinoid tumor of the thymus

✓ Additional Character Req   ✓x7ᵗʰ Placeholder Alert   Manifestation   HCC CMS-HCC Condition   ▽ Unspecified Code   ►◄ Revised Text   ● New Code   ▲ Revised Code Title

ICD-10-CM 2018   489

D31.4–D3A.091

D3A.Ø92 Benign carcinoid tumor of the **stomach**

D3A.Ø93 Benign carcinoid tumor of the **kidney**

D3A.Ø94 Benign carcinoid tumor of the **foregut,** ▽ **unspecified**

D3A.Ø95 Benign carcinoid tumor of the **midgut,** ▽ **unspecified**

D3A.Ø96 Benign carcinoid tumor of the **hindgut,** ▽ **unspecified**

D3A.Ø98 Benign carcinoid tumors of other sites

D3A.8 Other benign neuroendocrine tumors
Neuroendocrine tumor NOS

Neoplasms of uncertain behavior, polycythemia vera and myelodysplastic syndromes (D37-D48)

NOTE Categories D37-D44, and D48 classify by site neoplasms of uncertain behavior, i.e., histologic confirmation whether the neoplasm is malignant or benign cannot be made.

EXCLUDES 1 neoplasms of unspecified behavior (D49.-)

✓4ᵗʰ **D37 Neoplasm of uncertain behavior of oral cavity and digestive organs**

EXCLUDES 1 stromal tumors of uncertain behavior of digestive system (D48.1)

✓5ᵗʰ **D37.Ø Neoplasm of uncertain behavior of lip, oral cavity and pharynx**

EXCLUDES 1 neoplasm of uncertain behavior of aryepiglottic fold or interarytenoid fold, laryngeal aspect (D38.Ø)
neoplasm of uncertain behavior of epiglottis NOS (D38.Ø)
neoplasm of uncertain behavior of skin of lip (D48.5)
neoplasm of uncertain behavior of suprahyoid portion of epiglottis (D38.Ø)

D37.Ø1 Neoplasm of uncertain behavior of lip
Neoplasm of uncertain behavior of vermilion border of lip

D37.Ø2 Neoplasm of uncertain behavior of tongue

✓6ᵗʰ **D37.Ø3 Neoplasm of uncertain behavior of the major salivary glands**

D37.Ø3Ø Neoplasm of uncertain behavior of the parotid salivary glands

D37.Ø31 Neoplasm of uncertain behavior of the sublingual salivary glands

D37.Ø32 Neoplasm of uncertain behavior of the submandibular salivary glands

D37.Ø39 Neoplasm of uncertain behavior of ▽ **the major salivary glands, unspecified**

D37.Ø4 Neoplasm of uncertain behavior of the minor salivary glands
Neoplasm of uncertain behavior of submucosal salivary glands of lip
Neoplasm of uncertain behavior of submucosal salivary glands of cheek
Neoplasm of uncertain behavior of submucosal salivary glands of hard palate
Neoplasm of uncertain behavior of submucosal salivary glands of soft palate

D37.Ø5 Neoplasm of uncertain behavior of pharynx
Neoplasm of uncertain behavior of aryepiglottic fold of pharynx NOS
Neoplasm of uncertain behavior of hypopharyngeal aspect of aryepiglottic fold of pharynx
Neoplasm of uncertain behavior of marginal zone of aryepiglottic fold of pharynx

D37.Ø9 Neoplasm of uncertain behavior of other specified sites of the oral cavity

D37.1 Neoplasm of uncertain behavior of stomach

D37.2 Neoplasm of uncertain behavior of small intestine

D37.3 Neoplasm of uncertain behavior of appendix

D37.4 Neoplasm of uncertain behavior of colon

D37.5 Neoplasm of uncertain behavior of rectum
Neoplasm of uncertain behavior of rectosigmoid junction

D37.6 Neoplasm of uncertain behavior of liver, gallbladder and bile ducts
Neoplasm of uncertain behavior of ampulla of Vater

D37.8 Neoplasm of uncertain behavior of other specified digestive organs
Neoplasm of uncertain behavior of anal canal
Neoplasm of uncertain behavior of anal sphincter
Neoplasm of uncertain behavior of anus NOS
Neoplasm of uncertain behavior of esophagus
Neoplasm of uncertain behavior of intestine NOS
Neoplasm of uncertain behavior of pancreas

EXCLUDES 1 neoplasm of uncertain behavior of anal margin (D48.5)
neoplasm of uncertain behavior of anal skin (D48.5)
neoplasm of uncertain behavior of perianal skin (D48.5)

D37.9 Neoplasm of uncertain behavior of digestive organ, ▽ **unspecified**

✓4ᵗʰ **D38 Neoplasm of uncertain behavior of middle ear and respiratory and intrathoracic organs**

EXCLUDES 1 neoplasm of uncertain behavior of heart (D48.7)

D38.Ø Neoplasm of uncertain behavior of larynx
Neoplasm of uncertain behavior of aryepiglottic fold or interarytenoid fold, laryngeal aspect
Neoplasm of uncertain behavior of epiglottis (suprahyoid portion)

EXCLUDES 1 neoplasm of uncertain behavior of aryepiglottic fold or interarytenoid fold NOS (D37.Ø5)
neoplasm of uncertain behavior of hypopharyngeal aspect of aryepiglottic fold (D37.Ø5)
neoplasm of uncertain behavior of marginal zone of aryepiglottic fold (D37.Ø5)

D38.1 Neoplasm of uncertain behavior of trachea, bronchus and lung

D38.2 Neoplasm of uncertain behavior of pleura

D38.3 Neoplasm of uncertain behavior of mediastinum

D38.4 Neoplasm of uncertain behavior of thymus

D38.5 Neoplasm of uncertain behavior of other respiratory organs
Neoplasm of uncertain behavior of accessory sinuses
Neoplasm of uncertain behavior of cartilage of nose
Neoplasm of uncertain behavior of middle ear
Neoplasm of uncertain behavior of nasal cavities

EXCLUDES 1 neoplasm of uncertain behavior of ear (external) (skin) (D48.5)
neoplasm of uncertain behavior of nose NOS (D48.7)
neoplasm of uncertain behavior of skin of nose (D48.5)

D38.6 Neoplasm of uncertain behavior of respiratory organ, ▽ **unspecified**

✓4ᵗʰ **D39 Neoplasm of uncertain behavior of female genital organs**

D39.Ø Neoplasm of uncertain behavior of uterus ♀

✓5ᵗʰ **D39.1 Neoplasm of uncertain behavior of ovary**
Use additional code to identify any functional activity

D39.1Ø Neoplasm of uncertain behavior of unspecified ♀▽ **ovary**

D39.11 Neoplasm of uncertain behavior of right ovary ♀

D39.12 Neoplasm of uncertain behavior of left ovary ♀

D39.2 Neoplasm of uncertain behavior of placenta Ⓜ♀
Chorioadenoma destruens
Invasive hydatidiform mole
Malignant hydatidiform mole

EXCLUDES 1 hydatidiform mole NOS (OØ1.9)

D39.8 Neoplasm of uncertain behavior of other specified ♀ **female genital organs**
Neoplasm of uncertain behavior of skin of female genital organs

D39.9 Neoplasm of uncertain behavior of female genital organ, ♀▽ **unspecified**

✓4ᵗʰ **D4Ø Neoplasm of uncertain behavior of male genital organs**

D4Ø.Ø Neoplasm of uncertain behavior of prostate ♂

✓5ᵗʰ **D4Ø.1 Neoplasm of uncertain behavior of testis**

D4Ø.1Ø Neoplasm of uncertain behavior of unspecified ♂▽ **testis**

D4Ø.11 Neoplasm of uncertain behavior of right testis ♂

D4Ø.12 Neoplasm of uncertain behavior of left testis ♂

D4Ø.8 Neoplasm of uncertain behavior of other specified male ♂ **genital organs**
Neoplasm of uncertain behavior of skin of male genital organs

D4Ø.9 Neoplasm of uncertain behavior of male genital organ, ♂▽ **unspecified**

✓4ᵗʰ **D41 Neoplasm of uncertain behavior of urinary organs**

   ✓5ᵗʰ **D41.0 Neoplasm of uncertain behavior of kidney**

       EXCLUDES 1   *neoplasm of uncertain behavior of renal pelvis (D41.1-)*

       D41.00 Neoplasm of uncertain behavior of unspecified kidney ▽

       D41.01 Neoplasm of uncertain behavior of right kidney

       D41.02 Neoplasm of uncertain behavior of left kidney

   ✓5ᵗʰ **D41.1 Neoplasm of uncertain behavior of renal pelvis**

       D41.10 Neoplasm of uncertain behavior of unspecified renal pelvis ▽

       D41.11 Neoplasm of uncertain behavior of right renal pelvis

       D41.12 Neoplasm of uncertain behavior of left renal pelvis

   ✓5ᵗʰ **D41.2 Neoplasm of uncertain behavior of ureter**

       D41.20 Neoplasm of uncertain behavior of unspecified ureter ▽

       D41.21 Neoplasm of uncertain behavior of right ureter

       D41.22 Neoplasm of uncertain behavior of left ureter

   D41.3 Neoplasm of uncertain behavior of urethra

   D41.4 Neoplasm of uncertain behavior of bladder

   D41.8 Neoplasm of uncertain behavior of other specified urinary organs

   D41.9 Neoplasm of uncertain behavior of unspecified urinary organ ▽

✓4ᵗʰ **D42 Neoplasm of uncertain behavior of meninges**

   D42.0 Neoplasm of uncertain behavior of cerebral meninges HCC

   D42.1 Neoplasm of uncertain behavior of spinal meninges HCC

   D42.9 Neoplasm of uncertain behavior of meninges, unspecified HCC ▽

✓4ᵗʰ **D43 Neoplasm of uncertain behavior of brain and central nervous system**

       EXCLUDES 1   *neoplasm of uncertain behavior of peripheral nerves and autonomic nervous system (D48.2)*

   D43.0 Neoplasm of uncertain behavior of brain, supratentorial HCC

       Neoplasm of uncertain behavior of cerebral ventricle

       Neoplasm of uncertain behavior of cerebrum

       Neoplasm of uncertain behavior of frontal lobe

       Neoplasm of uncertain behavior of occipital lobe

       Neoplasm of uncertain behavior of parietal lobe

       Neoplasm of uncertain behavior of temporal lobe

       EXCLUDES 1   *neoplasm of uncertain behavior of fourth ventricle (D43.1)*

   D43.1 Neoplasm of uncertain behavior of brain, infratentorial HCC

       Neoplasm of uncertain behavior of brain stem

       Neoplasm of uncertain behavior of cerebellum

       Neoplasm of uncertain behavior of fourth ventricle

   D43.2 Neoplasm of uncertain behavior of brain, unspecified HCC ▽

   D43.3 Neoplasm of uncertain behavior of cranial nerves HCC

   D43.4 Neoplasm of uncertain behavior of spinal cord HCC

   D43.8 Neoplasm of uncertain behavior of other specified parts of central nervous system HCC

   D43.9 Neoplasm of uncertain behavior of central nervous system, unspecified HCC ▽

       Neoplasm of uncertain behavior of nervous system (central) NOS

✓4ᵗʰ **D44 Neoplasm of uncertain behavior of endocrine glands**

       EXCLUDES 1   *multiple endocrine adenomatosis (E31.2-)*

              multiple endocrine neoplasia (E31.2-)

              neoplasm of uncertain behavior of endocrine pancreas (D37.8)

              neoplasm of uncertain behavior of ovary (D39.1-)

              neoplasm of uncertain behavior of testis (D40.1-)

              neoplasm of uncertain behavior of thymus (D38.4)

   D44.0 Neoplasm of uncertain behavior of thyroid gland

   ✓5ᵗʰ **D44.1 Neoplasm of uncertain behavior of adrenal gland**

       Use additional code to identify any functional activity

       D44.10 Neoplasm of uncertain behavior of unspecified adrenal gland ▽

       D44.11 Neoplasm of uncertain behavior of right adrenal gland

       D44.12 Neoplasm of uncertain behavior of left adrenal gland

   D44.2 Neoplasm of uncertain behavior of parathyroid gland

   D44.3 Neoplasm of uncertain behavior of pituitary gland HCC

       Use additional code to identify any functional activity

   D44.4 Neoplasm of uncertain behavior of craniopharyngeal duct HCC

   D44.5 Neoplasm of uncertain behavior of pineal gland HCC

   D44.6 Neoplasm of uncertain behavior of carotid body HCC

   D44.7 Neoplasm of uncertain behavior of aortic body and other paraganglia HCC

   D44.9 Neoplasm of uncertain behavior of unspecified endocrine gland ▽

D45 Polycythemia vera HCC

       EXCLUDES 1   *familial polycythemia (D75.0)*

              secondary polycythemia (D75.1)

   DEF: Abnormal proliferation of all bone marrow elements, increased red cell mass, and total blood volume; unknown etiology, frequently associated with splenomegaly, leukocytosis, and thrombocythemia.

✓4ᵗʰ **D46 Myelodysplastic syndromes**

    Use additional code for adverse effect, if applicable, to identify drug (T36-T50 with fifth or sixth character 5)

       EXCLUDES 2   *drug-induced aplastic anemia (D61.1)*

   D46.0 Refractory anemia without ring sideroblasts, so stated HCC

       Refractory anemia without sideroblasts, without excess of blasts

   D46.1 Refractory anemia with ring sideroblasts HCC

       RARS

   ✓5ᵗʰ **D46.2 Refractory anemia with excess of blasts [RAEB]**

       D46.20 Refractory anemia with excess of blasts, unspecified HCC ▽

          RAEB NOS

       D46.21 Refractory anemia with excess of blasts 1 HCC

          RAEB 1

       D46.22 Refractory anemia with excess of blasts 2 HCC

          RAEB 2

   D46.A Refractory cytopenia with multilineage dysplasia HCC

   D46.B Refractory cytopenia with multilineage dysplasia and ring sideroblasts HCC

       RCMD RS

   D46.C Myelodysplastic syndrome with isolated del(5q) chromosomal abnormality HCC

       Myelodysplastic syndrome with 5q deletion

       5q minus syndrome NOS

   D46.4 Refractory anemia, unspecified HCC ▽

   D46.Z Other myelodysplastic syndromes HCC

       EXCLUDES 1   *chronic myelomonocytic leukemia (C93.1-)*

   D46.9 Myelodysplastic syndrome, unspecified HCC ▽

       Myelodysplasia NOS

✓4ᵗʰ **D47 Other neoplasms of uncertain behavior of lymphoid, hematopoietic and related tissue**

▲ ✓5ᵗʰ **D47.0 Mast cell neoplasms of uncertain behavior**

       ~~Indolent systemic mastocytosis~~

       ~~Mast cell tumor NOS~~

       ~~Mastocytoma NOS~~

       EXCLUDES 1 ▶*congenital cutaneous mastocytosis (Q82.2-)*

              histiocytic neoplasms of uncertain behavior (D47.Z9)

              malignant mast cell neoplasm (C96.2-)◀

              ~~*mastocytosis (congenital) (cutaneous) (Q82.2)*~~

●   **D47.01 Cutaneous mastocytosis**

       Diffuse cutaneous mastocytosis

       Maculopapular cutaneous mastocytosis

       Solitary mastocytoma

       Telangiectasia macularis eruptiva perstans

       Urticaria pigmentosa

       EXCLUDES 1   *congenital (diffuse) (maculopapular) cutaneous mastocytosis (Q82.2)*

              congenital urticaria pigmentosa (Q82.2)

              extracutaneous mastocytoma (D47.09)

✓ Additional Character Req   ✓7ᵗʰ Placeholder Alert   Manifestation   HCC CMS-HCC Condition   ▽ Unspecified Code   ▶◀ Revised Text   ● New Code   ▲ Revised Code Title

Chapter 2. Neoplasms

D47.Ø2 Systemic mastocytosis
Indolent systemic mastocytosis
Isolated bone marrow mastocytosis
Smoldering systemic mastocytosis
Systemic mastocytosis, with an associated
hematological non-mast cell lineage disease
(SM-AHNMD)
Code also, if applicable, any associated hematological
non-mast cell lineage disease, such as:
acute myeloid leukemia (C92.6-, C92.A-)
chronic myelomonocytic leukemia (C93.1-)
essential thrombocytosis (D47.3)
hypereosinophilic syndrome (D72.1)
myelodysplastic syndrome (D46.9)
myeloproliferative syndrome (D47.1)
non-Hodgkin lymphoma (C82-C85)
plasma cell myeloma (C90.Ø-)
polycythemia vera (D45)
EXCLUDES 1   *aggressive systemic mastocytosis (C96.21)*
mast cell leukemia (C94.3-)

D47.Ø9 Other mast cell neoplasms of uncertain behavior
Extracutaneous mastocytoma
Mast cell tumor NOS
Mastocytoma NOS
Mastocytosis NOS

D47.1 Chronic myeloproliferative disease   `HCC`
Chronic neutrophilic leukemia
Myeloproliferative disease, unspecified
EXCLUDES 1   *atypical chronic myeloid leukemia BCR/ABL-negative*
(C92.2-)
chronic myeloid leukemia BCR/ABL-positive (C92.1-)
myelofibrosis NOS (D75.81)
myelophthisic anemia (D61.82)
myelophthisis (D61.82)
secondary myelofibrosis NOS (D75.81)

D47.2 Monoclonal gammopathy
Monoclonal gammopathy of undetermined significance [MGUS]

D47.3 Essential (hemorrhagic) thrombocythemia   `HCC`
Essential thrombocytosis
Idiopathic hemorrhagic thrombocythemia

D47.4 Osteomyelofibrosis   `HCC`
Chronic idiopathic myelofibrosis
Myelofibrosis (idiopathic) (with myeloid metaplasia)
Myelosclerosis (megakaryocytic) with myeloid metaplasia
Secondary myelofibrosis in myeloproliferative disease
EXCLUDES 1   *acute myelofibrosis (C94.4-)*

√5ᵗʰ D47.Z Other specified neoplasms of uncertain behavior of lymphoid, hematopoietic and related tissue

D47.Z1 Post-transplant lymphoproliferative disorder (PTLD)   `HCC`
Code first complications of transplanted organs and tissue (T86.-)
DEF: Excessive proliferation of B-cell lymphocytes following Epstein-Barr virus infection in organ transplant patients; may progress to non-Hodgkin lymphoma.

D47.Z2 Castleman disease   `HCC`
Code also if applicable human herpesvirus 8 infection (B1Ø.89)
EXCLUDES 2   *Kaposi's sarcoma (C46-)*

D47.Z9 Other specified neoplasms of uncertain behavior of lymphoid, hematopoietic and related tissue   `HCC`
Histiocytic tumors of uncertain behavior

D47.9 Neoplasm of uncertain behavior of lymphoid, hematopoietic and related tissue, unspecified   `HCC` ▽
Lymphoproliferative disease NOS

√4ᵗʰ D48 Neoplasm of uncertain behavior of other and unspecified sites
EXCLUDES 1   *neurofibromatosis (nonmalignant) (Q85.Ø-)*

D48.Ø Neoplasm of uncertain behavior of bone and articular cartilage
EXCLUDES 1   *neoplasm of uncertain behavior of cartilage of ear*
(D48.1)
neoplasm of uncertain behavior of cartilage of larynx
(D38.Ø)
neoplasm of uncertain behavior of cartilage of nose
(D38.5)
neoplasm of uncertain behavior of connective tissue of
eyelid (D48.1)
neoplasm of uncertain behavior of synovia (D48.1)

D48.1 Neoplasm of uncertain behavior of connective and other soft tissue
Neoplasm of uncertain behavior of connective tissue of ear
Neoplasm of uncertain behavior of connective tissue of eyelid
Stromal tumors of uncertain behavior of digestive system
EXCLUDES 1   *neoplasm of uncertain behavior of articular cartilage*
(D48.Ø)
neoplasm of uncertain behavior of cartilage of larynx
(D38.Ø)
neoplasm of uncertain behavior of cartilage of nose
(D38.5)
neoplasm of uncertain behavior of connective tissue of
breast (D48.6-)

D48.2 Neoplasm of uncertain behavior of peripheral nerves and autonomic nervous system
EXCLUDES 1   *neoplasm of uncertain behavior of peripheral nerves of*
orbit (D48.7)

D48.3 Neoplasm of uncertain behavior of retroperitoneum

D48.4 Neoplasm of uncertain behavior of peritoneum

D48.5 Neoplasm of uncertain behavior of skin
Neoplasm of uncertain behavior of anal margin
Neoplasm of uncertain behavior of anal skin
Neoplasm of uncertain behavior of perianal skin
Neoplasm of uncertain behavior of skin of breast
EXCLUDES 1   *neoplasm of uncertain behavior of anus NOS (D37.8)*
neoplasm of uncertain behavior of skin of genital
organs (D39.8, D4Ø.8)
neoplasm of uncertain behavior of vermilion border of
lip (D37.Ø)

√5ᵗʰ D48.6 Neoplasm of uncertain behavior of breast
Neoplasm of uncertain behavior of connective tissue of breast
Cystosarcoma phyllodes
EXCLUDES 1   *neoplasm of uncertain behavior of skin of breast*
(D48.5)

D48.6Ø Neoplasm of uncertain behavior of unspecified breast ▽

D48.61 Neoplasm of uncertain behavior of right breast

D48.62 Neoplasm of uncertain behavior of left breast

D48.7 Neoplasm of uncertain behavior of other specified sites
Neoplasm of uncertain behavior of eye
Neoplasm of uncertain behavior of heart
Neoplasm of uncertain behavior of peripheral nerves of orbit
EXCLUDES 1   *neoplasm of uncertain behavior of connective tissue*
(D48.1)
neoplasm of uncertain behavior of skin of eyelid
(D48.5)

D48.9 Neoplasm of uncertain behavior, unspecified ▽

Neoplasms of unspecified behavior (D49)

√4ᵗʰ D49 Neoplasms of unspecified behavior
`NOTE`   Category D49 classifies by site neoplasms of unspecified morphology and behavior. The term "mass", unless otherwise stated, is not to be regarded as a neoplastic growth.
`INCLUDES`   "growth" NOS
neoplasm NOS
new growth NOS
tumor NOS
EXCLUDES 1   *neoplasms of uncertain behavior (D37-D44, D48)*

D49.Ø Neoplasm of unspecified behavior of digestive system
EXCLUDES 1   *neoplasm of unspecified behavior of margin of anus*
(D49.2)
neoplasm of unspecified behavior of perianal skin
(D49.2)
neoplasm of unspecified behavior of skin of anus
(D49.2)

D49.1 Neoplasm of unspecified behavior of respiratory system

EXCLUDES 1 Not coded here   *EXCLUDES 2* Not included here   N Newborn Age: 0   P Pediatric Age: 0-17   M Maternity Age: 12-55   A Adult Age: 15-124

492   ICD-10-CM 2018

D47.Ø2–D49.1

D49.2 Neoplasm of unspecified behavior of bone, soft tissue, and skin
> EXCLUDES 1   *neoplasm of unspecified behavior of anal canal (D49.0)*
> *neoplasm of unspecified behavior of anus NOS (D49.0)*
> *neoplasm of unspecified behavior of bone marrow (D49.89)*
> *neoplasm of unspecified behavior of cartilage of larynx (D49.1)*
> *neoplasm of unspecified behavior of cartilage of nose (D49.1)*
> *neoplasm of unspecified behavior of connective tissue of breast (D49.3)*
> *neoplasm of unspecified behavior of skin of genital organs (D49.59)*
> *neoplasm of unspecified behavior of vermilion border of lip (D49.0)*

D49.3 Neoplasm of unspecified behavior of breast
> EXCLUDES 1   *neoplasm of unspecified behavior of skin of breast (D49.2)*

D49.4 Neoplasm of unspecified behavior of bladder

D49.5 Neoplasm of unspecified behavior of other genitourinary organs
> **D49.51 Neoplasm of unspecified behavior of** kidney
> > **D49.511 Neoplasm of unspecified behavior of** right kidney
> > **D49.512 Neoplasm of unspecified behavior of** left kidney
> > **D49.519 Neoplasm of unspecified behavior of** unspecified kidney ▽
> **D49.59 Neoplasm of unspecified behavior of other** genitourinary organ

D49.6 Neoplasm of unspecified behavior of brain HCC
> EXCLUDES 1   *neoplasm of unspecified behavior of cerebral meninges (D49.7)*
> *neoplasm of unspecified behavior of cranial nerves (D49.7)*

D49.7 Neoplasm of unspecified behavior of endocrine glands and other parts of nervous system
> EXCLUDES 1   *neoplasm of unspecified behavior of peripheral, sympathetic, and parasympathetic nerves and ganglia (D49.2)*

D49.8 Neoplasm of unspecified behavior of other specified sites
> EXCLUDES 1   *neoplasm of unspecified behavior of eyelid (skin) (D49.2)*
> *neoplasm of unspecified behavior of eyelid cartilage (D49.2)*
> *neoplasm of unspecified behavior of great vessels (D49.2)*
> *neoplasm of unspecified behavior of optic nerve (D49.7)*
> **D49.81 Neoplasm of unspecified behavior of** retina and choroid
> > Dark area on retina
> > Retinal freckle
> **D49.89 Neoplasm of unspecified behavior of other specified sites**

D49.9 Neoplasm of unspecified behavior of unspecified site ▽

Chapter 3. Disease of the Blood and Blood-Forming Organs and Certain Disorders Involving the Immune Mechanism (D5Ø–D89)

Chapter Specific Coding Guidelines and Examples
Reserved for future guideline expansion.

Chapter 3. Diseases of the Blood and Blood-forming Organs and Certain Disorders Involving the Immune Mechanism (D50-D89)

EXCLUDES 2   autoimmune disease (systemic) NOS (M35.9)
certain conditions originating in the perinatal period (P00-P96)
complications of pregnancy, childbirth and the puerperium (O00-O9A)
congenital malformations, deformations and chromosomal abnormalities (Q00-Q99)
endocrine, nutritional and metabolic diseases (E00-E88)
human immunodeficiency virus [HIV] disease (B20)
injury, poisoning and certain other consequences of external causes (S00-T88)
neoplasms (C00-D49)
symptoms, signs and abnormal clinical and laboratory findings, not elsewhere classified (R00-R94)

This chapter contains the following blocks:

D50-D53   Nutritional anemias
D55-D59   Hemolytic anemias
D60-D64   Aplastic and other anemias and other bone marrow failure syndromes
D65-D69   Coagulation defects, purpura and other hemorrhagic conditions
D70-D77   Other disorders of blood and blood-forming organs
D78   Intraoperative and postprocedural complications of the spleen
D80-D89   Certain disorders involving the immune mechanism

Nutritional anemias (D50-D53)

✓4ᵗʰ D50   Iron deficiency anemia
   INCLUDES   asiderotic anemia
               hypochromic anemia

  D50.0   Iron deficiency anemia secondary to blood loss (chronic)
     Posthemorrhagic anemia (chronic)
     EXCLUDES 1   acute posthemorrhagic anemia (D62)
             congenital anemia from fetal blood loss (P61.3)

  D50.1   Sideropenic dysphagia
     Kelly-Paterson syndrome
     Plummer-Vinson syndrome

  D50.8   Other iron deficiency anemias
     Iron deficiency anemia due to inadequate dietary iron intake

  D50.9   Iron deficiency anemia, unspecified   ▽

✓4ᵗʰ D51   Vitamin B12 deficiency anemia
   EXCLUDES 1   vitamin B12 deficiency (E53.8)

  D51.0   Vitamin B12 deficiency anemia due to intrinsic factor deficiency
     Addison anemia
     Biermer anemia
     Pernicious (congenital) anemia
     Congenital intrinsic factor deficiency
     DEF: Chronic progressive anemia due to vitamin B12 malabsorption; caused by lack of secretion of intrinsic factor, which is produced by the gastric mucosa of the stomach.

  D51.1   Vitamin B12 deficiency anemia due to selective vitamin B12 malabsorption with proteinuria
     Imerslund (Gräsbeck) syndrome
     Megaloblastic hereditary anemia

  D51.2   Transcobalamin II deficiency

  D51.3   Other dietary vitamin B12 deficiency anemia
     Vegan anemia

  D51.8   Other vitamin B12 deficiency anemias

  D51.9   Vitamin B12 deficiency anemia, unspecified   ▽

✓4ᵗʰ D52   Folate deficiency anemia
   EXCLUDES 1   folate deficiency without anemia (E53.8)

  D52.0   Dietary folate deficiency anemia
     Nutritional megaloblastic anemia
     DEF: The result of a poor diet with inadequate intake of folate, which is needed to produce healthy red blood cells.

  D52.1   Drug-induced folate deficiency anemia
     Use additional code for adverse effect, if applicable, to identify drug (T36-T50 with fifth or sixth character 5)

  D52.8   Other folate deficiency anemias

  D52.9   Folate deficiency anemia, unspecified   ▽
     Folic acid deficiency anemia NOS

✓4ᵗʰ D53   Other nutritional anemias
   INCLUDES   megaloblastic anemia unresponsive to vitamin B12 or folate therapy

  D53.0   Protein deficiency anemia
     Amino-acid deficiency anemia
     Orotaciduric anemia
     EXCLUDES 1   Lesch-Nyhan syndrome (E79.1)

  D53.1   Other megaloblastic anemias, not elsewhere classified
     Megaloblastic anemia NOS
     EXCLUDES 1   Di Guglielmo's disease (C94.0)

  D53.2   Scorbutic anemia
     EXCLUDES 1   scurvy (E54)

  D53.8   Other specified nutritional anemias
     Anemia associated with deficiency of copper
     Anemia associated with deficiency of molybdenum
     Anemia associated with deficiency of zinc
     EXCLUDES 1   nutritional deficiencies without anemia, such as:
           copper deficiency NOS (E61.0)
           molybdenum deficiency NOS (E61.5)
           zinc deficiency NOS (E60)

  D53.9   Nutritional anemia, unspecified   ▽
     Simple chronic anemia
     EXCLUDES 1   anemia NOS (D64.9)

Hemolytic anemias (D55-D59)

✓4ᵗʰ D55   Anemia due to enzyme disorders
   EXCLUDES 1   drug-induced enzyme deficiency anemia (D59.2)

  D55.0   Anemia due to glucose-6-phosphate dehydrogenase [G6PD] deficiency   **HCC**
     Favism
     G6PD deficiency anemia

  D55.1   Anemia due to other disorders of glutathione metabolism   **HCC**
     Anemia (due to) enzyme deficiencies, except G6PD, related to the hexose monophosphate [HMP] shunt pathway
     Anemia (due to) hemolytic nonspherocytic (hereditary), type I

  D55.2   Anemia due to disorders of glycolytic enzymes   **HCC**
     Hemolytic nonspherocytic (hereditary) anemia, type II
     Hexokinase deficiency anemia
     Pyruvate kinase [PK] deficiency anemia
     Triose-phosphate isomerase deficiency anemia
     EXCLUDES 1   disorders of glycolysis not associated with anemia (E74.8)

  D55.3   Anemia due to disorders of nucleotide metabolism   **HCC**

  D55.8   Other anemias due to enzyme disorders   **HCC**

  D55.9   Anemia due to enzyme disorder, unspecified   **HCC** ▽

✓4ᵗʰ D56   Thalassemia
   EXCLUDES 1   sickle-cell thalassemia (D57.4-)

  D56.0   Alpha thalassemia   **HCC**
     Alpha thalassemia major
     Hemoglobin H Constant Spring
     Hemoglobin H disease
     Hydrops fetalis due to alpha thalassemia
     Severe alpha thalassemia
     Triple gene defect alpha thalassemia
     Use additional code, if applicable, for hydrops fetalis due to alpha thalassemia (P56.99)
     EXCLUDES 1   alpha thalassemia trait or minor (D56.3)
           asymptomatic alpha thalassemia (D56.3)
           hydrops fetalis due to isoimmunization (P56.0)
           hydrops fetalis not due to immune hemolysis (P83.2)
     DEF: HBA1 and HBA2 genetic variant of chromosome 16 prevalent among those of African and Southeast Asian descent; associated with a wide spectrum of anemic presentation; includes hemoglobin H disease subtypes.

  D56.1   Beta thalassemia   **HCC**
     Beta thalassemia major
     Cooley's anemia
     Homozygous beta thalassemia
     Severe beta thalassemia
     Thalassemia intermedia
     Thalassemia major
     EXCLUDES 1   beta thalassemia minor (D56.3)
           beta thalassemia trait (D56.3)
           delta-beta thalassemia (D56.2)
           hemoglobin E-beta thalassemia (D56.5)
           sickle-cell beta thalassemia (D57.4-)

EXCLUDES 1 Not coded here   **EXCLUDES 2** Not included here   **N** Newborn Age: 0   **P** Pediatric Age: 0-17   **M** Maternity Age: 12-55   **A** Adult Age: 15-124

496   ICD-10-CM 2018

D50-D56.1

Thalassemia

Misshapen RBC

Misshapen RBC

Healthy RBC

Sickle cell

Sickle cells

Normal RBCs

D56.2 **Delta-beta** thalassemia   HCC
Homozygous delta-beta thalassemia
EXCLUDES 1   *delta-beta thalassemia minor (D56.3)*
delta-beta thalassemia trait (D56.3)

D56.3 **Thalassemia** minor
Alpha thalassemia minor
Alpha thalassemia silent carrier
Alpha thalassemia trait
Beta thalassemia minor
Beta thalassemia trait
Delta-beta thalassemia minor
Delta-beta thalassemia trait
Thalassemia trait NOS
EXCLUDES 1   *alpha thalassemia (D56.0)*
beta thalassemia (D56.1)
delta-beta thalassemia (D56.2)
hemoglobin E-beta thalassemia (D56.5)
sickle-cell trait (D57.3)
DEF: Solitary abnormal gene that identifies a carrier of the disease, yet with an absence of symptoms or a clinically mild anemic presentation.

D56.4 **Hereditary persistence of fetal hemoglobin [HPFH]**   HCC

D56.5 **Hemoglobin E-beta** thalassemia   HCC
EXCLUDES 1   *beta thalassemia (D56.1)*
beta thalassemia minor (D56.3)
beta thalassemia trait (D56.3)
delta-beta thalassemia (D56.2)
delta-beta thalassemia trait (D56.3)
hemoglobin E disease (D58.2)
other hemoglobinopathies (D58.2)
sickle-cell beta thalassemia (D57.4-)

D56.8 **Other thalassemias**   HCC
Dominant thalassemia
Hemoglobin C thalassemia
Mixed thalassemia
Thalassemia with other hemoglobinopathy
EXCLUDES 1   *hemoglobin C disease (D58.2)*
hemoglobin E disease (D58.2)
other hemoglobinopathies (D58.2)
sickle-cell anemia (D57.-)
sickle-cell thalassemia (D57.4)

D56.9 **Thalassemia, unspecified**   ▽
Mediterranean anemia (with other hemoglobinopathy)

✓4th **D57** **Sickle-cell disorders**
Use additional code for any associated fever (R50.81)
EXCLUDES 1   *other hemoglobinopathies (D58.-)*

✓5th **D57.0** **Hb-SS disease** with crisis
Sickle-cell disease NOS with crisis
Hb-SS disease with vasoocclusive pain
     D57.00 **Hb-SS disease with** crisis, unspecified   HCC ▽
     D57.01 **Hb-SS disease with** acute chest syndrome   HCC
     D57.02 **Hb-SS disease with** splenic sequestration   HCC

D57.1 **Sickle-cell disease** without crisis   HCC ▽
Hb-SS disease without crisis
Sickle-cell anemia NOS
Sickle-cell disease NOS
Sickle-cell disorder NOS

✓5th **D57.2** **Sickle-cell/Hb-C disease**
Hb-SC disease
Hb-S/Hb-C disease
     D57.20 **Sickle-cell/Hb-C disease** without crisis   HCC ▽
✓6th   **D57.21** **Sickle-cell/Hb-C disease** with crisis
         D57.211 **Sickle-cell/Hb-C disease with** acute chest syndrome   HCC
         D57.212 **Sickle-cell/Hb-C disease with** splenic sequestration   HCC
         D57.219 **Sickle-cell/Hb-C disease with crisis,** unspecified   HCC ▽
Sickle-cell/Hb-C disease with crisis NOS

D57.3 **Sickle-cell** trait   HCC
Hb-S trait
Heterozygous hemoglobin S
DEF: Heterozygous genetic makeup characterized by one gene for normal hemoglobin and one for sickle-cell hemoglobin; clinical disease rarely present.

✓5th **D57.4** **Sickle-cell** thalassemia
Sickle-cell beta thalassemia
Thalassemia Hb-S disease
     D57.40 **Sickle-cell thalassemia** without crisis   HCC ▽
Microdrepanocytosis
Sickle-cell thalassemia NOS
✓6th   **D57.41** **Sickle-cell thalassemia** with crisis
Sickle-cell thalassemia with vasoocclusive pain
         D57.411 **Sickle-cell thalassemia with** acute chest syndrome   HCC
         D57.412 **Sickle-cell thalassemia with** splenic sequestration   HCC
         D57.419 **Sickle-cell thalassemia with crisis,** unspecified   HCC ▽
Sickle-cell thalassemia with crisis NOS

✓5th **D57.8** **Other sickle-cell disorders**
Hb-SD disease
Hb-SE disease
     D57.80 **Other sickle-cell disorders** without crisis   HCC ▽
✓6th   **D57.81** **Other sickle-cell disorders** with crisis
         D57.811 **Other sickle-cell disorders with** acute chest syndrome   HCC
         D57.812 **Other sickle-cell disorders with** splenic sequestration   HCC
         D57.819 **Other sickle-cell disorders with crisis,** unspecified   HCC ▽
Other sickle-cell disorders with crisis NOS

✓4th **D58** **Other** hereditary hemolytic anemias
EXCLUDES 1   *hemolytic anemia of the newborn (P55.-)*

D58.0 **Hereditary** spherocytosis   HCC
Acholuric (familial) jaundice
Congenital (spherocytic) hemolytic icterus
Minkowski-Chauffard syndrome

D58.1 **Hereditary** elliptocytosis   HCC
Elliptocytosis (congenital)
Ovalocytosis (congenital) (hereditary)

☑ Additional Character Req   ✓x7th Placeholder Alert   Manifestation   HCC CMS-HCC Condition   ▽ Unspecified Code   ►◄ Revised Text   ● New Code   ▲ Revised Code Title

ICD-10-CM 2018   497

D58.2 Other hemoglobinopathies `HCC`
    Abnormal hemoglobin NOS
    Congenital Heinz body anemia
    Hb-C disease
    Hb-D disease
    Hb-E disease
    Hemoglobinopathy NOS
    Unstable hemoglobin hemolytic disease
    EXCLUDES 1 *familial polycythemia (D75.0)*
        Hb-M disease (D74.0)
        hemoglobin E-beta thalassemia (D56.5)
        hereditary persistence of fetal hemoglobin [HPFH]
          (D56.4)
        high-altitude polycythemia (D75.1)
        methemoglobinemia (D74.-)
        other hemoglobinopathies with thalassemia (D56.8)

D58.8 Other specified hereditary hemolytic anemias `HCC`
    Stomatocytosis

D58.9 Hereditary hemolytic anemia, unspecified `HCC` ▽

✓4ᵗʰ **D59 Acquired hemolytic anemia**
    DEF: Non-hereditary anemia characterized by premature destruction of red blood cells; caused by infectious organisms, poisons, and physical agents.

D59.0 Drug-induced autoimmune hemolytic anemia `HCC`
    Use additional code for adverse effect, if applicable, to identify drug (T36-T50 with fifth or sixth character 5)

D59.1 Other autoimmune hemolytic anemias `HCC`
    Autoimmune hemolytic disease (cold type) (warm type)
    Chronic cold hemagglutinin disease
    Cold agglutinin disease
    Cold agglutinin hemoglobinuria
    Cold type (secondary) (symptomatic) hemolytic anemia
    Warm type (secondary) (symptomatic) hemolytic anemia
    EXCLUDES 1 *Evans syndrome (D69.41)*
        hemolytic disease of newborn (P55.-)
        paroxysmal cold hemoglobinuria (D59.6)

D59.2 Drug-induced nonautoimmune hemolytic anemia `HCC`
    Drug-induced enzyme deficiency anemia
    Use additional code for adverse effect, if applicable, to identify drug (T36-T50 with fifth or sixth character 5)

D59.3 Hemolytic-uremic syndrome `HCC`
    Use additional code to identify associated:
      E. coli infection (B96.2-)
      Pneumococcal pneumonia (J13)
      Shigella dysenteriae (A03.9)

D59.4 Other nonautoimmune hemolytic anemias `HCC`
    Mechanical hemolytic anemia
    Microangiopathic hemolytic anemia
    Toxic hemolytic anemia

D59.5 Paroxysmal nocturnal hemoglobinuria [Marchiafava-Micheli] `HCC`
    EXCLUDES 1 *hemoglobinuria NOS (R82.3)*

D59.6 Hemoglobinuria due to hemolysis from other external causes `HCC`
    Hemoglobinuria from exertion
    March hemoglobinuria
    Paroxysmal cold hemoglobinuria
    Use additional code (Chapter 20) to identify external cause
    EXCLUDES 1 *hemoglobinuria NOS (R82.3)*

D59.8 Other acquired hemolytic anemias `HCC`

D59.9 Acquired hemolytic anemia, unspecified `HCC` ▽
    Idiopathic hemolytic anemia, chronic

Aplastic and other anemias and other bone marrow failure syndromes (D60-D64)

✓4ᵗʰ **D60 Acquired pure red cell aplasia [erythroblastopenia]**
    INCLUDES red cell aplasia (acquired) (adult) (with thymoma)
    EXCLUDES 1 *congenital red cell aplasia (D61.01)*

D60.0 Chronic acquired pure red cell aplasia `HCC`

D60.1 Transient acquired pure red cell aplasia `HCC`

D60.8 Other acquired pure red cell aplasias `HCC`

D60.9 Acquired pure red cell aplasia, unspecified `HCC` ▽

✓4ᵗʰ **D61 Other aplastic anemias and other bone marrow failure syndromes**
    EXCLUDES 1 *neutropenia (D70.-)*
    AHA: 2014, 4Q, 22

✓5ᵗʰ **D61.0 Constitutional aplastic anemia**

D61.01 Constitutional (pure) red blood cell aplasia `HCC`
    Blackfan-Diamond syndrome
    Congenital (pure) red cell aplasia
    Familial hypoplastic anemia
    Primary (pure) red cell aplasia
    Red cell (pure) aplasia of infants
    EXCLUDES 1 *acquired red cell aplasia (D60.9)*

D61.09 Other constitutional aplastic anemia `HCC`
    Fanconi's anemia
    Pancytopenia with malformations

D61.1 Drug-induced aplastic anemia `HCC`
    Use additional code for adverse effect, if applicable, to identify drug (T36-T50 with fifth or sixth character 5)

D61.2 Aplastic anemia due to other external agents `HCC`
    Code first, if applicable, toxic effects of substances chiefly nonmedicinal as to source (T51-T65)

D61.3 Idiopathic aplastic anemia `HCC`

✓5ᵗʰ **D61.8 Other specified aplastic anemias and other bone marrow failure syndromes**

✓6ᵗʰ **D61.81 Pancytopenia**
    EXCLUDES 1 *pancytopenia (due to) (with) aplastic anemia (D61.9)*
        pancytopenia (due to) (with) bone marrow infiltration (D61.82)
        pancytopenia (due to) (with) congenital (pure) red cell aplasia (D61.01)
        pancytopenia (due to) (with) hairy cell leukemia (C91.4-)
        pancytopenia (due to) (with) human immunodeficiency virus disease (B20)
        pancytopenia (due to) (with) leukoerythroblastic anemia (D61.82)
        pancytopenia (due to) (with) myeloproliferative disease (D47.1)
    EXCLUDES 2 *pancytopenia (due to) (with) myelodysplastic syndromes (D46.-)*
    DEF: Occurs when a person has a shortage of all three blood cells: white, red, and platelets.

D61.810 Antineoplastic chemotherapy induced pancytopenia `HCC`
    EXCLUDES 2 *aplastic anemia due to antineoplastic chemotherapy (D61.1)*

D61.811 Other drug-induced pancytopenia `HCC`
    EXCLUDES 2 *aplastic anemia due to drugs (D61.1)*

D61.818 Other pancytopenia `HCC`

D61.82 Myelophthisis `HCC`
    Leukoerythroblastic anemia
    Myelophthisic anemia
    Panmyelophthisis
    Code also the underlying disorder, such as:
      malignant neoplasm of breast (C50.-)
      tuberculosis (A15.-)
    EXCLUDES 1 *idiopathic myelofibrosis (D47.1)*
        myelofibrosis NOS (D75.81)
        myelofibrosis with myeloid metaplasia (D47.4)
        primary myelofibrosis (D47.1)
        secondary myelofibrosis (D75.81)

D61.89 Other specified aplastic anemias and other bone marrow failure syndromes `HCC`

D61.9 Aplastic anemia, unspecified `HCC` ▽
    Hypoplastic anemia NOS
    Medullary hypoplasia

D62 Acute posthemorrhagic anemia
    EXCLUDES 1 *anemia due to chronic blood loss (D50.0)*
        blood loss anemia NOS (D50.0)
        congenital anemia from fetal blood loss (P61.3)

EXCLUDES 1 Not coded here   **EXCLUDES 2** Not included here   N Newborn Age: 0   P Pediatric Age: 0-17   M Maternity Age: 12-55   A Adult Age: 15-124

498   ICD-10-CM 2018

✓4ᵗʰ **D63** **Anemia in chronic diseases classified elsewhere**

D63.0 *Anemia in neoplastic disease*
   Code first neoplasm (C00-D49)
   EXCLUDES 1 *anemia due to antineoplastic chemotherapy (D64.81)*
      aplastic anemia due to antineoplastic chemotherapy (D61.1)
   EXCLUDES 2 ►*anemia due to antineoplastic chemotherapy (D64.81)*◄

D63.1 **Anemia in chronic kidney disease**
   Erythropoietin resistant anemia (EPO resistant anemia)
   Code first underlying chronic kidney disease (CKD) (N18.-)

D63.8 *Anemia in other chronic diseases classified elsewhere*
   Code first underlying disease, such as:
      diphyllobothriasis (B70.0)
      hookworm disease (B76.0-B76.9)
      hypothyroidism (E00.0-E03.9)
      malaria (B50.0-B54)
      symptomatic late syphilis (A52.79)
      tuberculosis (A18.89)

✓4ᵗʰ **D64** **Other anemias**
   EXCLUDES 1 *refractory anemia (D46.-)*
      refractory anemia with excess blasts in transformation [RAEB T] (C92.0-)

D64.0 **Hereditary sideroblastic anemia**   HCC
   Sex-linked hypochromic sideroblastic anemia

D64.1 *Secondary sideroblastic anemia due to disease*   HCC
   Code first underlying disease

D64.2 **Secondary sideroblastic anemia due to drugs and toxins**   HCC
   Code first poisoning due to drug or toxin, if applicable (T36-T65 with fifth or sixth character 1-4 or 6)
   Use additional code for adverse effect, if applicable, to identify drug (T36-T50 with fifth or sixth character 5)

D64.3 **Other sideroblastic anemias**   HCC
   Sideroblastic anemia NOS
   Pyridoxine-responsive sideroblastic anemia NEC

D64.4 **Congenital dyserythropoietic anemia**
   Dyshematopoietic anemia (congenital)
   EXCLUDES 1 *Blackfan-Diamond syndrome (D61.01)*
      Di Guglielmo's disease (C94.0)

✓5ᵗʰ **D64.8** **Other specified anemias**

D64.81 **Anemia due to antineoplastic chemotherapy**
   Antineoplastic chemotherapy induced anemia
   EXCLUDES 1 *aplastic anemia due to antineoplastic chemotherapy (D61.1)*
   EXCLUDES 2 *anemia in neoplastic disease (D63.0)*
   AHA: 2014, 4Q, 22
   DEF: Reversible adverse effect of chemotherapy, causing inhibition of bone marrow production; decrease in red blood cell production prevents adequate oxygenation of the tissues and organs causing fatigue, SOB, and exacerbation of other medical conditions.

D64.89 **Other specified anemias**
   Infantile pseudoleukemia

D64.9 **Anemia, unspecified**   ▽
   AHA: 2017, 1Q, 7

Coagulation defects, purpura and other hemorrhagic conditions (D65-D69)

D65 **Disseminated intravascular coagulation [defibrination syndrome]**   HCC
   Afibrinogenemia, acquired
   Consumption coagulopathy
   Diffuse or disseminated intravascular coagulation [DIC]
   Fibrinolytic hemorrhage, acquired
   Fibrinolytic purpura
   Purpura fulminans
   EXCLUDES 1 *disseminated intravascular coagulation (complicating):*
      abortion or ectopic or molar pregnancy (O00-O07, O08.1)
      in newborn (P60)
      pregnancy, childbirth and the puerperium (O45.0, O46.0, O67.0, O72.3)

Coagulation

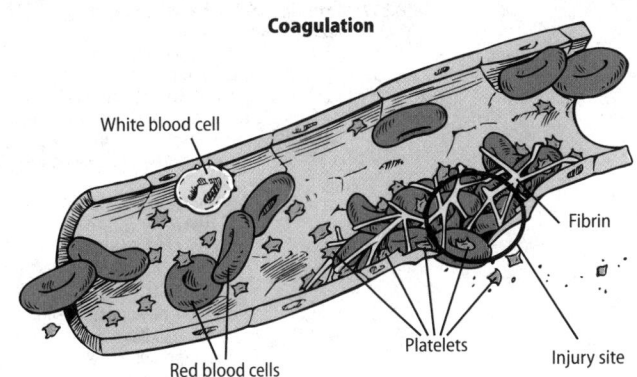

White blood cell
Fibrin
Red blood cells
Platelets
Injury site

D66 **Hereditary factor VIII deficiency**   HCC
   Classical hemophilia
   Deficiency factor VIII (with functional defect)
   Hemophilia A
   Hemophilia NOS
   EXCLUDES 1 *factor VIII deficiency with vascular defect (D68.0)*
   DEF: Hereditary, sex-linked lack of antihemophilic globulin (AHG) (factor VIII); causes abnormal coagulation characterized by increased bleeding, large bruises of skin, bleeding in mouth, nose, gastrointestinal tract; hemorrhages into joints, resulting in swelling and impaired function.

D67 **Hereditary factor IX deficiency**   HCC
   Christmas disease
   Factor IX deficiency (with functional defect)
   Hemophilia B
   Plasma thromboplastin component [PTC] deficiency

✓4ᵗʰ **D68** **Other coagulation defects**
   EXCLUDES 1 *abnormal coagulation profile (R79.1)*
      coagulation defects complicating abortion or ectopic or molar pregnancy (O00-O07, O08.1)
      coagulation defects complicating pregnancy, childbirth and the puerperium (O45.0, O46.0, O67.0, O72.3)
   AHA: 2016, 1Q, 14

D68.0 **Von Willebrand's disease**   HCC
   Angiohemophilia
   Factor VIII deficiency with vascular defect
   Vascular hemophilia
   EXCLUDES 1 *capillary fragility (hereditary) (D69.8)*
      factor VIII deficiency NOS (D66)
      factor VIII deficiency with functional defect (D66)
   DEF: Abnormal blood coagulation caused by deficient blood factor VII; congenital; symptoms include excess or prolonged bleeding.

D68.1 **Hereditary factor XI deficiency**   HCC
   Hemophilia C
   Plasma thromboplastin antecedent [PTA] deficiency
   Rosenthal's disease

D68.2 **Hereditary deficiency of other clotting factors**   HCC
   AC globulin deficiency
   Congenital afibrinogenemia
   Deficiency of factor I [fibrinogen]
   Deficiency of factor II [prothrombin]
   Deficiency of factor V [labile]
   Deficiency of factor VII [stable]
   Deficiency of factor X [Stuart-Prower]
   Deficiency of factor XII [Hageman]
   Deficiency of factor XIII [fibrin stabilizing]
   Dysfibrinogenemia (congenital)
   Hypoproconvertinemia
   Owren's disease
   Proaccelerin deficiency

✓5ᵗʰ **D68.3** **Hemorrhagic disorder due to circulating anticoagulants**

✓6ᵗʰ **D68.31** **Hemorrhagic disorder due to intrinsic circulating anticoagulants, antibodies, or inhibitors**

D68.311 **Acquired hemophilia**   HCC
   Autoimmune hemophilia
   Autoimmune inhibitors to clotting factors
   Secondary hemophilia

✓ Additional Character Req   ✓7ᵗʰ Placeholder Alert   Manifestation   HCC CMS-HCC Condition   ▽ Unspecified Code   ►◄ Revised Text   ● New Code   ▲ Revised Code Title

ICD-10-CM 2018   **499**

D68.312 Antiphospholipid antibody with hemorrhagic disorder HCC
Lupus anticoagulant (LAC) with hemorrhagic disorder
Systemic lupus erythematosus [SLE] inhibitor with hemorrhagic disorder
EXCLUDES 1 antiphospholipid antibody, finding without diagnosis (R76.0)
antiphospholipid antibody syndrome (D68.61)
antiphospholipid antibody with hypercoagulable state (D68.61)
lupus anticoagulant (LAC) finding without diagnosis (R76.0)
lupus anticoagulant (LAC) with hypercoagulable state (D68.62)
systemic lupus erythematosus [SLE] inhibitor finding without diagnosis (R76.0)
systemic lupus erythematosus [SLE] inhibitor with hypercoagulable state (D68.62)

D68.318 Other hemorrhagic disorder due to intrinsic circulating anticoagulants, antibodies, or inhibitors HCC
Antithromboplastinemia
Antithromboplastinogenemia
Hemorrhagic disorder due to intrinsic increase in antithrombin
Hemorrhagic disorder due to intrinsic increase in anti-VIIIa
Hemorrhagic disorder due to intrinsic increase in anti-IXa
Hemorrhagic disorder due to intrinsic increase in anti-XIa

D68.32 Hemorrhagic disorder due to extrinsic circulating anticoagulants HCC
Drug-induced hemorrhagic disorder
Hemorrhagic disorder due to increase in anti-IIa
Hemorrhagic disorder due to increase in anti-Xa
Hyperheparinemia
Use additional code for adverse effect, if applicable, to identify drug (T45.515, T45.525)
AHA: 2016, 1Q, 14-15

D68.4 Acquired coagulation factor deficiency HCC
Deficiency of coagulation factor due to liver disease
Deficiency of coagulation factor due to vitamin K deficiency
EXCLUDES 1 vitamin K deficiency of newborn (P53)

D68.5 Primary thrombophilia
Primary hypercoagulable states
EXCLUDES 1 antiphospholipid syndrome (D68.61)
lupus anticoagulant (D68.62)
secondary activated protein C resistance (D68.69)
secondary antiphospholipid antibody syndrome (D68.69)
secondary lupus anticoagulant with hypercoagulable state (D68.69)
secondary systemic lupus erythematosus [SLE] inhibitor with hypercoagulable state (D68.69)
systemic lupus erythematosus [SLE] inhibitor finding without diagnosis (R76.0)
systemic lupus erythematosus [SLE] inhibitor with hemorrhagic disorder (D68.312)
thrombotic thrombocytopenic purpura (M31.1)

D68.51 Activated protein C resistance HCC
Factor V Leiden mutation

D68.52 Prothrombin gene mutation HCC

D68.59 Other primary thrombophilia HCC
Antithrombin III deficiency
Hypercoagulable state NOS
Primary hypercoagulable state NEC
Primary thrombophilia NEC
Protein C deficiency
Protein S deficiency
Thrombophilia NOS

D68.6 Other thrombophilia
Other hypercoagulable states
EXCLUDES 1 diffuse or disseminated intravascular coagulation [DIC] (D65)
heparin induced thrombocytopenia (HIT) (D75.82)
hyperhomocysteinemia (E72.11)

D68.61 Antiphospholipid syndrome HCC
Anticardiolipin syndrome
Antiphospholipid antibody syndrome
EXCLUDES 1 antiphospholipid antibody, finding without diagnosis (R76.0)
antiphospholipid antibody with hemorrhagic disorder (D68.312)
lupus anticoagulant syndrome (D68.62)

D68.62 Lupus anticoagulant syndrome HCC
Lupus anticoagulant
Presence of systemic lupus erythematosus [SLE] inhibitor
EXCLUDES 1 anticardiolipin syndrome (D68.61)
antiphospholipid syndrome (D68.61)
lupus anticoagulant (LAC) finding without diagnosis (R76.0)
lupus anticoagulant (LAC) with hemorrhagic disorder (D68.312)

D68.69 Other thrombophilia HCC
Hypercoagulable states NEC
Secondary hypercoagulable state NOS

D68.8 Other specified coagulation defects HCC
EXCLUDES 1 hemorrhagic disease of newborn (P53)

D68.9 Coagulation defect, unspecified HCC ▽

D69 Purpura and other hemorrhagic conditions
EXCLUDES 1 benign hypergammaglobulinemic purpura (D89.0)
cryoglobulinemic purpura (D89.1)
essential (hemorrhagic) thrombocythemia (D47.3)
hemorrhagic thrombocythemia (D47.3)
purpura fulminans (D65)
thrombotic thrombocytopenic purpura (M31.1)
Waldenström hypergammaglobulinemic purpura (D89.0)

D69.0 Allergic purpura HCC
Allergic vasculitis
Nonthrombocytopenic hemorrhagic purpura
Nonthrombocytopenic idiopathic purpura
Purpura anaphylactoid
Purpura Henoch(-Schönlein)
Purpura rheumatica
Vascular purpura
EXCLUDES 1 thrombocytopenic hemorrhagic purpura (D69.3)
DEF: Any hemorrhagic condition, thrombocytic or nonthrombocytopenic in origin, caused by a presumed allergic reaction.

D69.1 Qualitative platelet defects HCC
Bernard-Soulier [giant platelet] syndrome
Glanzmann's disease
Grey platelet syndrome
Thromboasthenia (hemorrhagic) (hereditary)
Thrombocytopathy
EXCLUDES 1 von Willebrand's disease (D68.0)

D69.2 Other nonthrombocytopenic purpura HCC
Purpura NOS
Purpura simplex
Senile purpura

D69.3 Immune thrombocytopenic purpura HCC
Hemorrhagic (thrombocytopenic) purpura
Idiopathic thrombocytopenic purpura
Tidal platelet dysgenesis
DEF: Tidal platelet dysgenesis: Platelet counts fluctuate from normal to very low within periods of 20 to 40 days and may involve autoimmune platelet destruction.

D69.4 Other primary thrombocytopenia
EXCLUDES 1 transient neonatal thrombocytopenia (P61.0)
Wiskott-Aldrich syndrome (D82.0)

D69.41 Evans syndrome HCC

D69.42 Congenital and hereditary thrombocytopenia purpura HCC
Congenital thrombocytopenia
Hereditary thrombocytopenia
Code first congenital or hereditary disorder, such as:
thrombocytopenia with absent radius (TAR syndrome) (Q87.2)

D69.49 Other primary thrombocytopenia HCC
Megakaryocytic hypoplasia
Primary thrombocytopenia NOS

✓5th **D69.5 Secondary thrombocytopenia**
   EXCLUDES 1 *heparin induced thrombocytopenia (HIT) (D75.82)*
     transient thrombocytopenia of newborn (P61.0)

   D69.51 Posttransfusion purpura
     Posttransfusion purpura from whole blood (fresh) or blood products
     PTP

   D69.59 Other secondary thrombocytopenia
     AHA: 2014, 4Q, 22

D69.6 Thrombocytopenia, unspecified   HCC ▽

D69.8 Other specified hemorrhagic conditions   HCC
   Capillary fragility (hereditary)
   Vascular pseudohemophilia

D69.9 Hemorrhagic condition, unspecified   HCC ▽

Other disorders of blood and blood-forming organs (D70-D77)

✓4th **D70 Neutropenia**
   INCLUDES agranulocytosis
     decreased absolute neurophile count (ANC)
   Use additional code for any associated:
     fever (R50.81)
     mucositis (J34.81, K12.3-, K92.81, N76.81)
   EXCLUDES 1 *neutropenic splenomegaly (D73.81)*
     transient neonatal neutropenia (P61.5)

   D70.0 Congenital agranulocytosis   HCC
     Congenital neutropenia   Kostmann's disease
     Infantile genetic agranulocytosis

   D70.1 Agranulocytosis secondary to cancer chemotherapy   HCC
     Code also underlying neoplasm
     Use additional code for adverse effect, if applicable, to identify drug (T45.1X5)
     AHA: 2014, 4Q, 22

   D70.2 Other drug-induced agranulocytosis   HCC
     Use additional code for adverse effect, if applicable, to identify drug (T36-T50 with fifth or sixth character 5)

   D70.3 Neutropenia due to infection   HCC

   D70.4 Cyclic neutropenia   HCC
     Cyclic hematopoiesis
     Periodic neutropenia

   D70.8 Other neutropenia   HCC

   D70.9 Neutropenia, unspecified   HCC ▽

D71 Functional disorders of polymorphonuclear neutrophils   HCC
   Cell membrane receptor complex [CR3] defect
   Chronic (childhood) granulomatous disease
   Congenital dysphagocytosis
   Progressive septic granulomatosis

✓4th **D72 Other disorders of white blood cells**
   EXCLUDES 1 *basophilia (D72.824)*
     immunity disorders (D80-D89)
     neutropenia (D70)
     preleukemia (syndrome) (D46.9)

   D72.0 Genetic anomalies of leukocytes   HCC
     Alder (granulation) (granulocyte) anomaly
     Alder syndrome
     Hereditary leukocytic hypersegmentation
     Hereditary leukocytic hyposegmentation
     Hereditary leukomelanopathy
     May-Hegglin (granulation) (granulocyte) anomaly
     May-Hegglin syndrome
     Pelger-Huët (granulation) (granulocyte) anomaly
     Pelger-Huët syndrome
     EXCLUDES 1 *Chédiak (-Steinbrinck)-Higashi syndrome (E70.330)*

   D72.1 Eosinophilia
     Allergic eosinophilia   Hereditary eosinophilia
     EXCLUDES 1 *Löffler's syndrome (J82)*
      pulmonary eosinophilia (J82)

✓5th   **D72.8 Other specified disorders of white blood cells**
     EXCLUDES 1 *leukemia (C91-C95)*

✓6th   **D72.81 Decreased white blood cell count**
      EXCLUDES 1 *neutropenia (D70.-)*

     D72.810 Lymphocytopenia
      Decreased lymphocytes

     D72.818 Other decreased white blood cell count
      Basophilic leukopenia
      Eosinophilic leukopenia
      Monocytopenia
      Other decreased leukocytes
      Plasmacytopenia

     D72.819 Decreased white blood cell count, unspecified ▽
      Decreased leukocytes, unspecified
      Leukocytopenia, unspecified
      Leukopenia
      EXCLUDES 1 *malignant leukopenia (D70.9)*

✓6th   **D72.82 Elevated white blood cell count**
      EXCLUDES 1 *eosinophilia (D72.1)*

     D72.820 Lymphocytosis (symptomatic)
      Elevated lymphocytes

     D72.821 Monocytosis (symptomatic)
      EXCLUDES 1 *infectious mononucleosis (B27.-)*

     D72.822 Plasmacytosis

     D72.823 Leukemoid reaction
      Basophilic leukemoid reaction
      Leukemoid reaction NOS
      Lymphocytic leukemoid reaction
      Monocytic leukemoid reaction
      Myelocytic leukemoid reaction
      Neutrophilic leukemoid reaction

     D72.824 Basophilia

     D72.825 Bandemia
      Bandemia without diagnosis of specific infection
      EXCLUDES 1 *confirmed infection—code to infection*
      leukemia (C91.-, C92.-, C93.-, C94.-, C95.-)
      DEF: Increase in early neutrophil cells, called band cells; may indicate infection.

     D72.828 Other elevated white blood cell count

     D72.829 Elevated white blood cell count, unspecified ▽
      Elevated leukocytes, unspecified
      Leukocytosis, unspecified

   D72.89 Other specified disorders of white blood cells
     Abnormality of white blood cells NEC

   D72.9 Disorder of white blood cells, unspecified ▽
     Abnormal leukocyte differential NOS

✓4th **D73 Diseases of spleen**
   D73.0 Hyposplenism
     Atrophy of spleen
     EXCLUDES 1 *asplenia (congenital) (Q89.01)*
      postsurgical absence of spleen (Z90.81)

   D73.1 Hypersplenism
     EXCLUDES 1 *neutropenic splenomegaly (D73.81)*
      primary splenic neutropenia (D73.81)
      splenitis, splenomegaly in late syphilis (A52.79)
      splenitis, splenomegaly in tuberculosis (A18.85)
      splenomegaly NOS (R16.1)
      splenomegaly congenital (Q89.0)

   D73.2 Chronic congestive splenomegaly

   D73.3 Abscess of spleen

   D73.4 Cyst of spleen

   D73.5 Infarction of spleen
     Splenic rupture, nontraumatic
     Torsion of spleen
     EXCLUDES 1 *rupture of spleen due to Plasmodium vivax malaria (B51.0)*
      traumatic rupture of spleen (S36.03-)

✓5th   **D73.8 Other diseases of spleen**
     D73.81 Neutropenic splenomegaly
      Werner-Schultz disease

     D73.89 Other diseases of spleen
      Fibrosis of spleen NOS
      Perisplenitis
      Splenitis NOS

   D73.9 Disease of spleen, unspecified ▽

✓4th **D74 Methemoglobinemia**
   D74.0 Congenital methemoglobinemia
     Congenital NADH-methemoglobin reductase deficiency
     Hemoglobin-M [Hb-M] disease
     Methemoglobinemia, hereditary

   D74.8 Other methemoglobinemias
     Acquired methemoglobinemia (with sulfhemoglobinemia)
     Toxic methemoglobinemia

   D74.9 Methemoglobinemia, unspecified ▽

✓ Additional Character Req   ✓x7th Placeholder Alert   Manifestation   HCC CMS-HCC Condition   ▽ Unspecified Code   ▶◀ Revised Text   ● New Code   ▲ Revised Code Title

Chapter 3. Disease of the Blood and Blood-Forming Organs

D75–D80.5

✓4ᵗʰ **D75** **Other and unspecified diseases of blood and blood-forming organs**

> *EXCLUDES 2*   *acute lymphadenitis (L04.-)*
> *chronic lymphadenitis (I88.1)*
> *enlarged lymph nodes (R59.-)*
> *hypergammaglobulinemia NOS (D89.2)*
> *lymphadenitis NOS (I88.9)*
> *mesenteric lymphadenitis (acute) (chronic) (I88.0)*

D75.0 **Familial erythrocytosis**
> Benign polycythemia
> Familial polycythemia
> > *EXCLUDES 1*   *hereditary ovalocytosis (D58.1)*

D75.1 **Secondary polycythemia**
> Acquired polycythemia
> Emotional polycythemia
> Erythrocytosis NOS
> Hypoxemic polycythemia
> Nephrogenous polycythemia
> Polycythemia due to erythropoietin
> Polycythemia due to fall in plasma volume
> Polycythemia due to high altitude
> Polycythemia due to stress
> Polycythemia NOS
> Relative polycythemia
> > *EXCLUDES 1*   *polycythemia neonatorum (P61.1)*
> > *polycythemia vera (D45)*
>
> **DEF:** Elevated number of red blood cells in circulating blood as a result of reduced oxygen supply to the tissues.

✓5ᵗʰ **D75.8** **Other specified diseases of blood and blood-forming organs**

> **D75.81** **Myelofibrosis**   HCC
> > Myelofibrosis NOS
> > Secondary myelofibrosis NOS
> > Code first the underlying disorder, such as:
> >   malignant neoplasm of breast (C50.-)
> > Use additional code, if applicable, for associated therapy-related myelodysplastic syndrome (D46.-)
> > Use additional code for adverse effect, if applicable, to identify drug (T45.1X5)
> > > *EXCLUDES 1*   *acute myelofibrosis (C94.4-)*
> > > *idiopathic myelofibrosis (D47.1)*
> > > *leukoerythroblastic anemia (D61.82)*
> > > *myelofibrosis with myeloid metaplasia (D47.4)*
> > > *myelophthisic anemia (D61.82)*
> > > *myelophthisis (D61.82)*
> > > *primary myelofibrosis (D47.1)*
>
> **D75.82** **Heparin induced thrombocytopenia (HIT)**   HCC
> > **DEF:** Immune-mediated reaction to heparin therapy causing an abrupt fall in platelet count and serious complications such as pulmonary embolism, stroke, AMI, or DVT.
>
> **D75.89** **Other specified diseases of blood and blood-forming organs**

D75.9 **Disease of blood and blood-forming organs, unspecified**   ▽

✓4ᵗʰ **D76** **Other specified diseases with participation of lymphoreticular and reticulohistiocytic tissue**

> *EXCLUDES 1*   *(Abt-) Letterer-Siwe disease (C96.0)*
> *eosinophilic granuloma (C96.6)*
> *Hand-Schüller-Christian disease (C96.5)*
> *histiocytic medullary reticulosis (C96.9)*
> *histiocytic sarcoma (C96.A)*
> *histiocytosis X, multifocal (C96.5)*
> *histiocytosis X, unifocal (C96.6)*
> *Langerhans-cell histiocytosis, multifocal (C96.5)*
> *Langerhans-cell histiocytosis NOS (C96.6)*
> *Langerhans-cell histiocytosis, unifocal (C96.6)*
> *leukemic reticuloendotheliosis (C91.4-)*
> *lipomelanotic reticulosis (I89.8)*
> *malignant histiocytosis (C96.A)*
> *malignant reticulosis (C86.0)*
> *nonlipid reticuloendotheliosis (C96.0)*

D76.1 **Hemophagocytic lymphohistiocytosis**   HCC
> Familial hemophagocytic reticulosis
> Histiocytoses of mononuclear phagocytes

D76.2 **Hemophagocytic syndrome, infection-associated**   HCC
> Use additional code to identify infectious agent or disease

D76.3 **Other histiocytosis syndromes**   HCC
> Reticulohistiocytoma (giant-cell)
> Sinus histiocytosis with massive lymphadenopathy
> Xanthogranuloma

D77 **Other disorders of blood and blood-forming organs in diseases classified elsewhere**

> Code first underlying disease, such as:
>   amyloidosis (E85.-)
>   congenital early syphilis (A50.0)
>   echinococcosis (B67.0-B67.9)
>   malaria (B50.0-B54)
>   schistosomiasis [bilharziasis] (B65.0-B65.9)
>   vitamin C deficiency (E54)
> > *EXCLUDES 1*   *rupture of spleen due to Plasmodium vivax malaria (B51.0)*
> > *splenitis, splenomegaly in late syphilis (A52.79)*
> > *splenitis, splenomegaly in tuberculosis (A18.85)*

Intraoperative and postprocedural complications of the spleen (D78)

✓4ᵗʰ **D78** **Intraoperative and postprocedural complications of the spleen**

✓5ᵗʰ **D78.0** **Intraoperative hemorrhage and hematoma of the spleen complicating a procedure**
> > *EXCLUDES 1*   *intraoperative hemorrhage and hematoma of the spleen due to accidental puncture or laceration during a procedure (D78.1-)*
>
> **D78.01** **Intraoperative hemorrhage and hematoma of the spleen complicating a procedure on the spleen**
>
> **D78.02** **Intraoperative hemorrhage and hematoma of the spleen complicating other procedure**

✓5ᵗʰ **D78.1** **Accidental puncture and laceration of the spleen during a procedure**
> **D78.11** **Accidental puncture and laceration of the spleen during a procedure on the spleen**
>
> **D78.12** **Accidental puncture and laceration of the spleen during other procedure**

✓5ᵗʰ **D78.2** **Postprocedural hemorrhage of the spleen following a procedure**
> **D78.21** **Postprocedural hemorrhage of the spleen following a procedure on the spleen**
>
> **D78.22** **Postprocedural hemorrhage of the spleen following other procedure**

✓5ᵗʰ **D78.3** **Postprocedural hematoma and seroma of the spleen following a procedure**
> **D78.31** **Postprocedural hematoma of the spleen following a procedure on the spleen**
>
> **D78.32** **Postprocedural hematoma of the spleen following other procedure**
>
> **D78.33** **Postprocedural seroma of the spleen following a procedure on the spleen**
>
> **D78.34** **Postprocedural seroma of the spleen following other procedure**

✓5ᵗʰ **D78.8** **Other intraoperative and postprocedural complications of the spleen**
> Use additional code, if applicable, to further specify disorder
>
> **D78.81** **Other intraoperative complications of the spleen**
>
> **D78.89** **Other postprocedural complications of the spleen**

Certain disorders involving the immune mechanism (D80-D89)

> INCLUDES   defects in the complement system
> immunodeficiency disorders, except human immunodeficiency virus [HIV] disease
> sarcoidosis
>
> *EXCLUDES 1*   *autoimmune disease (systemic) NOS (M35.9)*
> *functional disorders of polymorphonuclear neutrophils (D71)*
> *human immunodeficiency virus [HIV] disease (B20)*

✓4ᵗʰ **D80** **Immunodeficiency with predominantly antibody defects**

D80.0 **Hereditary hypogammaglobulinemia**   HCC
> Autosomal recessive agammaglobulinemia (Swiss type)
> X-linked agammaglobulinemia [Bruton] (with growth hormone deficiency)

D80.1 **Nonfamilial hypogammaglobulinemia**   HCC
> Agammaglobulinemia with immunoglobulin-bearing B-lymphocytes
> Common variable agammaglobulinemia [CVAgamma]
> Hypogammaglobulinemia NOS

D80.2 **Selective deficiency of immunoglobulin A [IgA]**   HCC

D80.3 **Selective deficiency of immunoglobulin G [IgG] subclasses**   HCC

D80.4 **Selective deficiency of immunoglobulin M [IgM]**   HCC

D80.5 **Immunodeficiency with increased immunoglobulin M [IgM]**   HCC

EXCLUDES 1 Not coded here   *EXCLUDES 2* Not included here   N Newborn Age: 0   P Pediatric Age: 0-17   M Maternity Age: 12-55   A Adult Age: 15-124

502   ICD-10-CM 2018

D80.6   **Antibody deficiency with** near-normal immunoglobulins or with hyperimmunoglobulinemia   HCC

D80.7   **Transient hypogammaglobulinemia of infancy**   HCC

D80.8   **Other immunodeficiencies with predominantly antibody defects**   HCC
Kappa light chain deficiency

D80.9   **Immunodeficiency with predominantly antibody defects, unspecified**   HCC ▽

✓4th **D81**   **Combined immunodeficiencies**
EXCLUDES 1   autosomal recessive agammaglobulinemia (Swiss type) (D80.0)

D81.0   **Severe combined immunodeficiency [SCID] with reticular dysgenesis**   HCC

D81.1   **Severe combined immunodeficiency [SCID] with low T- and B-cell numbers**   HCC

D81.2   **Severe combined immunodeficiency [SCID] with low or normal B-cell numbers**   HCC

D81.3   **Adenosine deaminase [ADA] deficiency**   HCC

D81.4   **Nezelof's syndrome**   HCC

D81.5   **Purine nucleoside phosphorylase [PNP] deficiency**   HCC

D81.6   **Major histocompatibility complex class I deficiency**   HCC
Bare lymphocyte syndrome

D81.7   **Major histocompatibility complex class II deficiency**   HCC

✓5th **D81.8**   **Other combined immunodeficiencies**

   ✓6th **D81.81**   **Biotin-dependent carboxylase deficiency**
Multiple carboxylase deficiency
EXCLUDES 1   biotin-dependent carboxylase deficiency due to dietary deficiency of biotin (E53.8)

     D81.810   **Biotinidase deficiency**

     D81.818   **Other biotin-dependent carboxylase deficiency**
Holocarboxylase synthetase deficiency
Other multiple carboxylase deficiency

     D81.819   **Biotin-dependent carboxylase deficiency, unspecified**   ▽
Multiple carboxylase deficiency, unspecified

   D81.89   **Other combined immunodeficiencies**   HCC

D81.9   **Combined immunodeficiency, unspecified**   HCC ▽
Severe combined immunodeficiency disorder [SCID] NOS

✓4th **D82**   **Immunodeficiency associated with other major defects**
EXCLUDES 1   ataxia telangiectasia [Louis-Bar] (G11.3)

D82.0   **Wiskott-Aldrich syndrome**   HCC
Immunodeficiency with thrombocytopenia and eczema

D82.1   **Di George's syndrome**   HCC
Pharyngeal pouch syndrome
Thymic alymphoplasia
Thymic aplasia or hypoplasia with immunodeficiency

D82.2   **Immunodeficiency with short-limbed stature**   HCC

D82.3   **Immunodeficiency following hereditary defective response to Epstein-Barr virus**   HCC
X-linked lymphoproliferative disease

D82.4   **Hyperimmunoglobulin E [IgE] syndrome**   HCC

D82.8   **Immunodeficiency associated with other specified major defects**   HCC

D82.9   **Immunodeficiency associated with major defect, unspecified**   HCC ▽

✓4th **D83**   **Common variable immunodeficiency**

D83.0   **Common variable immunodeficiency with predominant abnormalities of B-cell numbers and function**   HCC

D83.1   **Common variable immunodeficiency with predominant immunoregulatory T-cell disorders**   HCC

D83.2   **Common variable immunodeficiency with autoantibodies to B- or T-cells**   HCC

D83.8   **Other common variable immunodeficiencies**   HCC

D83.9   **Common variable immunodeficiency, unspecified**   HCC ▽

✓4th **D84**   **Other immunodeficiencies**

D84.0   **Lymphocyte function antigen-1 [LFA-1] defect**   HCC

D84.1   **Defects in the complement system**   HCC
C1 esterase inhibitor [C1-INH] deficiency

D84.8   **Other specified immunodeficiencies**   HCC

D84.9   **Immunodeficiency, unspecified**   HCC ▽

✓4th **D86**   **Sarcoidosis**

D86.0   **Sarcoidosis of lung**   HCC

D86.1   **Sarcoidosis of lymph nodes**

D86.2   **Sarcoidosis of lung with sarcoidosis of lymph nodes**   HCC

D86.3   **Sarcoidosis of skin**

✓5th **D86.8**   **Sarcoidosis of other sites**

   D86.81   **Sarcoid meningitis**

   D86.82   **Multiple cranial nerve palsies in sarcoidosis**   HCC

   D86.83   **Sarcoid iridocyclitis**

   D86.84   **Sarcoid pyelonephritis**
Tubulo-interstitial nephropathy in sarcoidosis

   D86.85   **Sarcoid myocarditis**

   D86.86   **Sarcoid arthropathy**
Polyarthritis in sarcoidosis

   D86.87   **Sarcoid myositis**

   D86.89   **Sarcoidosis of other sites**
Hepatic granuloma
Uveoparotid fever [Heerfordt]

D86.9   **Sarcoidosis, unspecified**   ▽

✓4th **D89**   **Other disorders involving the immune mechanism, not elsewhere classified**
EXCLUDES 1   hyperglobulinemia NOS (R77.1)
monoclonal gammopathy (of undetermined significance) (D47.2)
EXCLUDES 2   transplant failure and rejection (T86.-)

D89.0   **Polyclonal hypergammaglobulinemia**
Benign hypergammaglobulinemic purpura
Polyclonal gammopathy NOS

D89.1   **Cryoglobulinemia**   HCC
Cryoglobulinemic purpura   Mixed cryoglobulinemia
Cryoglobulinemic vasculitis   Primary cryoglobulinemia
Essential cryoglobulinemia   Secondary cryoglobulinemia
Idiopathic cryoglobulinemia

D89.2   **Hypergammaglobulinemia, unspecified**   ▽

D89.3   **Immune reconstitution syndrome**   HCC
Immune reconstitution inflammatory syndrome [IRIS]
Use additional code for adverse effect, if applicable, to identify drug (T36-T50 with fifth or sixth character 5)

✓5th **D89.4**   **Mast cell activation syndrome and related disorders**
EXCLUDES 1   aggressive systemic mastocytosis ▶(C96.21)◀
▶congenital cutaneous mastocytosis◀ (Q82.2)
▶(non-congenital) cutaneous mastocytosis (D47.01)◀
(indolent) systemic mastocytosis (D47.02)
malignant mast cell neoplasm (C96.2-)◀
malignant mastocytoma ▶(C96.29)◀
mast cell leukemia (C94.3-)
▶mast cell sarcoma (C96.22)
mastocytoma NOS (D47.09)
other mast cell neoplasms of uncertain behavior (D47.09)◀
systemic mastocytosis associated with a clonal hematologic non-mast cell lineage disease (SM-AHNMD)▶(D47.02)◀

   D89.40   **Mast cell activation, unspecified**   HCC ▽
Mast cell activation disorder, unspecified
Mast cell activation syndrome, NOS

   D89.41   **Monoclonal mast cell activation syndrome**   HCC

   D89.42   **Idiopathic mast cell activation syndrome**   HCC

   D89.43   **Secondary mast cell activation**   HCC
Secondary mast cell activation syndrome
Code also underlying etiology, if known

   D89.49   **Other mast cell activation disorder**   HCC
Other mast cell activation syndrome

✓5th **D89.8**   **Other specified disorders involving the immune mechanism, not elsewhere classified**

   ✓6th **D89.81**   **Graft-versus-host disease**
Code first underlying cause, such as:
complications of transplanted organs and tissue (T86.-)
complications of blood transfusion (T80.89)
Use additional code to identify associated manifestations, such as:
desquamative dermatitis (L30.8)
diarrhea (R19.7)
elevated bilirubin (R17)
hair loss (L65.9)

     D89.810   **Acute graft-versus-host disease**   HCC

     D89.811   **Chronic graft-versus-host disease**   HCC

     D89.812   **Acute on chronic graft-versus-host disease**   HCC

     D89.813   **Graft-versus-host disease, unspecified**   HCC ▽

✓ Additional Character Req   ✓x7th Placeholder Alert   Manifestation   HCC CMS-HCC Condition   ▽ Unspecified Code   ▶◀ Revised Text   ● New Code   ▲ Revised Code Title

D89.82 Autoimmune lymphoproliferative syndrome [ALPS] HCC

DEF: Rare genetic alteration of the Fas protein; impairs normal cellular apoptosis (normal cell death), causing abnormal accumulation of lymphocytes in the lymph glands, liver, and spleen; symptoms include neutropenia, anemia, and thrombocytopenia.

D89.89 Other specified disorders involving the immune mechanism, not elsewhere classified HCC

EXCLUDES 1   human immunodeficiency virus disease (B20)

D89.9 Disorder involving the immune mechanism, unspecified HCC ▽

Immune disease NOS

AHA: 2015, 3Q, 22

EXCLUDES 1 Not coded here   EXCLUDES 2 Not included here   N Newborn Age: 0   P Pediatric Age: 0-17   M Maternity Age: 12-55   A Adult Age: 15-124

504   ICD-10-CM 2018

Chapter 3. Disease of the Blood and Blood-Forming Organs

D89.82–D89.9

Chapter 4. Endocrine, Nutritional, and Metabolic Diseases (E00–E89)

Chapter Specific Guidelines with Coding Examples

The chapter specific guidelines from the ICD-10-CM Official Guidelines for Coding and Reporting have been provided below. Along with these guidelines are coding examples, contained in the shaded boxes, that have been developed to help illustrate the coding and/or sequencing guidance found in these guidelines.

a. Diabetes mellitus

The diabetes mellitus codes are combination codes that include the type of diabetes mellitus, the body system affected, and the complications affecting that body system. As many codes within a particular category as are necessary to describe all of the complications of the disease may be used. They should be sequenced based on the reason for a particular encounter. Assign as many codes from categories E08–E13 as needed to identify all of the associated conditions that the patient has.

Patient is seen for uncontrolled diabetes, type 2, with diabetic nephropathy and diabetic gastroparesis.

E11.65   **Type 2 diabetes mellitus with hyperglycemia**

E11.21   **Type 2 diabetes mellitus with diabetic nephropathy**

E11.43   **Type 2 diabetes mellitus with diabetic automomic (poly)neuropathy**

Explanation: Use as many codes to describe the diabetic complications as needed. Many are combination codes that describe more than one condition. Code first the reason for the encounter. "Uncontrolled" is described as "with hyperglycemia."

---

1) Type of diabetes

The age of a patient is not the sole determining factor, though most type 1 diabetics develop the condition before reaching puberty. For this reason type 1 diabetes mellitus is also referred to as juvenile diabetes.

A 45-year-old patient is diagnosed with type 1 diabetes

E10.9   **Type 1 diabetes mellitus without complications**

Explanation: Although most type 1 diabetics are diagnosed in childhood or adolescence, it can also begin in adults.

---

2) Type of diabetes mellitus not documented

If the type of diabetes mellitus is not documented in the medical record the default is E11.-, Type 2 diabetes mellitus.

Office visit lists diabetic retinopathy with macular edema and hypertension on patient problem list

E11.311   **Type 2 diabetes mellitus with unspecified diabetic retinopathy with macular edema**

I10   **Essential (primary) hypertension**

Explanation: Since the type of diabetes was not documented, default to category E11.

---

3) Diabetes mellitus and the use of insulin and oral hypoglycemics

If the documentation in a medical record does not indicate the type of diabetes but does indicate that the patient uses insulin, code E11-, Type 2 diabetes mellitus, should be assigned. **An additional code should be assigned from category Z79 to identify the long-term (current) use of insulin or oral hypoglycemic drugs. If the patient is treated with both oral medications and insulin, only the code for long-term (current) use of insulin should be assigned. Code Z79.4 should not be assigned if insulin is given temporarily to bring a type 2 patient's blood sugar under control during an encounter.**

Office visit lists chronic diabetes with daily insulin use on patient problem list

E11.9   **Type 2 diabetes mellitus without complications**

Z79.4   **Long term (current) use of insulin**

Explanation: Do not assume that a patient on insulin must have type 1 diabetes. The default for diabetes without further specification defaults to type 2. Add the code for long term use of insulin.

---

4) Diabetes mellitus in pregnancy and gestational diabetes

See Section I.C.15. Diabetes mellitus in pregnancy.

See Section I.C.15. Gestational (pregnancy induced) diabetes

5) Complications due to insulin pump malfunction

(a) Underdose of insulin due to insulin pump failure

An underdose of insulin due to an insulin pump failure should be assigned to a code from subcategory T85.6, Mechanical complication of other specified internal and external prosthetic devices, implants and grafts, that specifies the type of pump malfunction, as the principal or first-listed code, followed by code T38.3X6-, Underdosing of insulin and oral hypoglycemic [antidiabetic] drugs. Additional codes for the type of diabetes mellitus and any associated complications due to the underdosing should also be assigned.

A 24-year-old type 1 diabetic male treated in for hyperglycemia; insulin pump found to be malfunctioning and underdosing

T85.614A   **Breakdown (mechanical) of insulin pump, initial encounter**

T38.3X6A   **Underdosing of insulin and oral hypoglycemic [antidiabetic] drugs, initial encounter**

E10.65   **Type 1 diabetes mellitus with hyperglycemia**

Explanation: The complication code for the mechanical breakdown of the pump is sequenced first, followed by the underdosing code and type of diabetes with complication. Code all other diabetic complication codes necessary to describe the patient's condition.

(b) Overdose of insulin due to insulin pump failure

The principal or first-listed code for an encounter due to an insulin pump malfunction resulting in an overdose of insulin, should also be T85.6-, Mechanical complication of other specified internal and external prosthetic devices, implants and grafts, followed by code T38.3X1-, Poisoning by insulin and oral hypoglycemic [antidiabetic] drugs, accidental (unintentional).

A 24-year-old type 1 diabetic male found down with diabetic coma, brought into ED and treated for hypoglycemia; insulin pump found to be malfunctioning and overdosing

T85.614A   **Breakdown (mechanical) of insulin pump, initial encounter**

T38.3X1A   **Poisoning by insulin and oral hypoglycemic [antidiabetic] drugs, accidental (unintentional), initial encounter**

E10.641   **Type 1 diabetes mellitus with hypoglycemia with coma**

Explanation: The complication code for the mechanical breakdown of the pump is sequenced first, followed by the poisoning code and type of diabetes with complication. All the characters in the combination code must be used to form a valid code and to fully describe the type of diabetes, the hypoglycemia, and the coma.

---

6) Secondary diabetes mellitus

Codes under categories E08, Diabetes mellitus due to underlying condition, E09, Drug or chemical induced diabetes mellitus, and E13, Other specified diabetes mellitus, identify complications/manifestations associated with secondary diabetes mellitus. Secondary diabetes is always caused by another condition or event (e.g., cystic fibrosis, malignant neoplasm of pancreas, pancreatectomy, adverse effect of drug, or poisoning).

(a) Secondary diabetes mellitus and the use of insulin or *oral* hypoglycemic drugs

For patients with secondary diabetes mellitus who routinely use insulin or oral hypoglycemic drugs, an additional code from category Z79 should be assigned to identify the long-term (current) use of insulin or oral hypoglycemic drugs. If the patient is treated with both oral medications and insulin, only the code for long-term (current) use of insulin should be assigned. Code Z79.4 should not be assigned if insulin is given temporarily to bring a type 2 patient's blood sugar under control during an encounter.

Type 2 diabetic with no complications, normally only on oral metformin, is given insulin for three days to maintain glucose control while in the hospital recovering from surgery

E11.9   **Type 2 diabetes mellitus without complications**

Z79.84   **Long term (current) use of oral hypoglycemic drugs**

Explanation: Although the patient was given insulin for a short time during his hospital stay, the intent was only to maintain the patient's glucose levels while off his regular oral hypoglycemic medication, not for long term use. No code is needed for long term use of insulin, but a Z code for long term use of an oral hypoglycemic should be added to identify the chronic use of this drug.

Type 2 diabetic with diabetic polyneuropathy on insulin

E11.42   **Type 2 diabetes mellitus with diabetic polyneuropathy**

Z79.4   **Long term (current) use of insulin**

Explanation: Add the Z code for the long term use of insulin because the insulin is taken chronically.

(b) Assigning and sequencing secondary diabetes codes and its causes

The sequencing of the secondary diabetes codes in relationship to codes for the cause of the diabetes is based on the Tabular List instructions for categories E08, E09 and E13.

(i) Secondary diabetes mellitus due to pancreatectomy

For postpancreatectomy diabetes mellitus (lack of insulin due to the surgical removal of all or part of the pancreas), assign code E89.1, Postprocedural hypoinsulinemia. Assign a code from category E13 and a code from subcategory Z90.41-, Acquired absence of pancreas, as additional codes.

Patient with newly diagnosed diabetes after surgical removal of part of pancreas

E89.1   **Postprocedural hypoinsulinemia**

E13.9   **Other specified diabetes mellitus without complications**

Z90.411   **Acquired partial absence of pancreas**

Explanation: Sequence the postprocedural complication of the hypoinsulinemia due to the partial removal of the pancreas as the first-listed code, followed by the other specified diabetes (NEC) with or without complications and the partial or total acquired absence of the pancreas.

(ii) Secondary diabetes due to drugs

Secondary diabetes may be caused by an adverse effect of correctly administered medications, poisoning or sequela of poisoning.

See section I.C.19.e for coding of adverse effects and poisoning, and section I.C.20 for external cause code reporting.

Initial encounter for corticosteroid-induced diabetes mellitus

E09.9   **Drug or chemical induced diabetes mellitus without complications**

T38.0X5A   **Adverse effect of glucocorticoids and synthetic analogues, initial encounter**

Explanation: If the diabetes is caused by an adverse effect of a drug, the diabetic condition is coded first. If it occurs from a poisoning or overdose, the poisoning code causing the diabetes is sequenced first.

Chapter 4. Endocrine, Nutritional and Metabolic Diseases (E00-E89)

> **NOTE** All neoplasms, whether functionally active or not, are classified in Chapter 2. Appropriate codes in this chapter (i.e. E05.8, E07.0, E16-E31, E34-) may be used as additional codes to indicate either functional activity by neoplasms and ectopic endocrine tissue or hyperfunction and hypofunction of endocrine glands associated with neoplasms and other conditions classified elsewhere.

> **EXCLUDES 1** *transitory endocrine and metabolic disorders specific to newborn (P70-P74)*

This chapter contains the following blocks:

E00-E07   Disorders of thyroid gland
E08-E13   Diabetes mellitus
E15-E16   Other disorders of glucose regulation and pancreatic internal secretion
E20-E35   Disorders of other endocrine glands
E36   Intraoperative complications of endocrine system
E40-E46   Malnutrition
E50-E64   Other nutritional deficiencies
E65-E68   Overweight, obesity and other hyperalimentation
E70-E88   Metabolic disorders
E89   Postprocedural endocrine and metabolic complications and disorders, not elsewhere classified

Disorders of thyroid gland (E00-E07)

✓4ᵗʰ E00   Congenital iodine-deficiency syndrome
   Use additional code (F70-F79) to identify associated intellectual disabilities
   > **EXCLUDES 1** *subclinical iodine-deficiency hypothyroidism (E02)*

   E00.0   Congenital iodine-deficiency syndrome, neurological type
      Endemic cretinism, neurological type

   E00.1   Congenital iodine-deficiency syndrome, myxedematous type
      Endemic hypothyroid cretinism
      Endemic cretinism, myxedematous type

   E00.2   Congenital iodine-deficiency syndrome, mixed type
      Endemic cretinism, mixed type

   E00.9   Congenital iodine-deficiency syndrome, unspecified   ▽
      Congenital iodine-deficiency hypothyroidism NOS
      Endemic cretinism NOS

✓4ᵗʰ E01   Iodine-deficiency related thyroid disorders and allied conditions
   > **EXCLUDES 1** *congenital iodine-deficiency syndrome (E00.-)*
   > *subclinical iodine-deficiency hypothyroidism (E02)*

   E01.0   Iodine-deficiency related diffuse (endemic) goiter

   E01.1   Iodine-deficiency related multinodular (endemic) goiter
      Iodine-deficiency related nodular goiter

   E01.2   Iodine-deficiency related (endemic) goiter, unspecified   ▽
      Endemic goiter NOS

   E01.8   Other iodine-deficiency related thyroid disorders and allied conditions
      Acquired iodine-deficiency hypothyroidism NOS

E02   Subclinical iodine-deficiency hypothyroidism

✓4ᵗʰ E03   Other hypothyroidism
   > **EXCLUDES 1** *iodine-deficiency related hypothyroidism (E00-E02)*
   > *postprocedural hypothyroidism (E89.0)*

   E03.0   Congenital hypothyroidism with diffuse goiter
      Congenital parenchymatous goiter (nontoxic)
      Congenital goiter (nontoxic) NOS
      > **EXCLUDES 1** *transitory congenital goiter with normal function (P72.0)*

   E03.1   Congenital hypothyroidism without goiter
      Aplasia of thyroid (with myxedema)
      Congenital atrophy of thyroid
      Congenital hypothyroidism NOS

   E03.2   Hypothyroidism due to medicaments and other exogenous substances
      Code first poisoning due to drug or toxin, if applicable (T36-T65 with fifth or sixth character 1-4 or 6)
      Use additional code for adverse effect, if applicable, to identify drug (T36-T50 with fifth or sixth character 5)

   E03.3   Postinfectious hypothyroidism

   E03.4   Atrophy of thyroid (acquired)
      > **EXCLUDES 1** *congenital atrophy of thyroid (E03.1)*

   E03.5   Myxedema coma   HCC

   E03.8   Other specified hypothyroidism

   E03.9   Hypothyroidism, unspecified   ▽
      Myxedema NOS

Goiter

Pyramidal lobe
Thyroid cartilage
Healthy thyroid
Goiter (hyperfunctioning thyroid)

✓4ᵗʰ E04   Other nontoxic goiter
   > **EXCLUDES 1** *congenital goiter (NOS) (diffuse) (parenchymatous) (E03.0)*
   > *iodine-deficiency related goiter (E00-E02)*

   E04.0   Nontoxic diffuse goiter
      Diffuse (colloid) nontoxic goiter
      Simple nontoxic goiter

   E04.1   Nontoxic single thyroid nodule
      Colloid nodule (cystic) (thyroid)
      Nontoxic uninodular goiter
      Thyroid (cystic) nodule NOS
      DEF: Enlarged thyroid, commonly due to decreased thyroid production, with single nodule; no clinical hypothyroidism.

   E04.2   Nontoxic multinodular goiter
      Cystic goiter NOS
      Multinodular (cystic) goiter NOS
      DEF: Enlarged thyroid, commonly due to decreased thyroid production with multiple nodules; no clinical hypothyroidism.

   E04.8   Other specified nontoxic goiter

   E04.9   Nontoxic goiter, unspecified   ▽
      Goiter NOS
      Nodular goiter (nontoxic) NOS

✓4ᵗʰ E05   Thyrotoxicosis [hyperthyroidism]
   > **EXCLUDES 1** *chronic thyroiditis with transient thyrotoxicosis (E06.2)*
   > *neonatal thyrotoxicosis (P72.1)c*

   ✓5ᵗʰ E05.0   Thyrotoxicosis with diffuse goiter
      Exophthalmic or toxic goiter NOS   Graves' disease
                                               Toxic diffuse goiter
      DEF: Diffuse thyroid enlargement accompanied by hyperthyroidism, bulging eyes, and dermopathy.

      E05.00   Thyrotoxicosis with diffuse goiter without thyrotoxic crisis or storm

      E05.01   Thyrotoxicosis with diffuse goiter with thyrotoxic crisis or storm

   ✓5ᵗʰ E05.1   Thyrotoxicosis with toxic single thyroid nodule
      Thyrotoxicosis with toxic uninodular goiter
      DEF: Symptomatic hyperthyroidism with a single nodule on the enlarged thyroid gland. Abrupt onset of symptoms include extreme nervousness, insomnia, weight loss, tremors, and psychosis or coma.

      E05.10   Thyrotoxicosis with toxic single thyroid nodule without thyrotoxic crisis or storm

      E05.11   Thyrotoxicosis with toxic single thyroid nodule with thyrotoxic crisis or storm

   ✓5ᵗʰ E05.2   Thyrotoxicosis with toxic multinodular goiter
      Toxic nodular goiter NOS

      E05.20   Thyrotoxicosis with toxic multinodular goiter without thyrotoxic crisis or storm

      E05.21   Thyrotoxicosis with toxic multinodular goiter with thyrotoxic crisis or storm

   ✓5ᵗʰ E05.3   Thyrotoxicosis from ectopic thyroid tissue

      E05.30   Thyrotoxicosis from ectopic thyroid tissue without thyrotoxic crisis or storm

      E05.31   Thyrotoxicosis from ectopic thyroid tissue with thyrotoxic crisis or storm

   ✓5ᵗʰ E05.4   Thyrotoxicosis factitia

      E05.40   Thyrotoxicosis factitia without thyrotoxic crisis or storm

      E05.41   Thyrotoxicosis factitia with thyrotoxic crisis or storm

---

☑ Additional Character Req   ✓x7ᵗʰ Placeholder Alert   ░Manifestation   HCC CMS-HCC Condition   ▽ Unspecified Code   ►◄ Revised Text   ● New Code   ▲ Revised Code Title

✓5ᵗʰ E05.8   **Other thyrotoxicosis**
Overproduction of thyroid-stimulating hormone

     E05.80   **Other thyrotoxicosis without thyrotoxic crisis or storm**

     E05.81   **Other thyrotoxicosis with thyrotoxic crisis or storm**

✓5ᵗʰ E05.9   **Thyrotoxicosis, unspecified**
Hyperthyroidism NOS

     E05.90   **Thyrotoxicosis, unspecified without thyrotoxic crisis or storm** ▽

     E05.91   **Thyrotoxicosis, unspecified with thyrotoxic crisis or storm** ▽

✓4ᵗʰ E06   **Thyroiditis**
     EXCLUDES 1   *postpartum thyroiditis (O90.5)*

   E06.0   **Acute thyroiditis**
Abscess of thyroid
Pyogenic thyroiditis
Suppurative thyroiditis
Use additional code (B95-B97) to identify infectious agent

   E06.1   **Subacute thyroiditis**
de Quervain thyroiditis
Giant-cell thyroiditis
Granulomatous thyroiditis
Nonsuppurative thyroiditis
Viral thyroiditis
     EXCLUDES 1   *autoimmune thyroiditis (E06.3)*

   E06.2   **Chronic thyroiditis with transient thyrotoxicosis**
     EXCLUDES 1   *autoimmune thyroiditis (E06.3)*

   E06.3   **Autoimmune thyroiditis**
Hashimoto's thyroiditis
Hashitoxicosis (transient)
Lymphadenoid goiter
Lymphocytic thyroiditis
Struma lymphomatosa

   E06.4   **Drug-induced thyroiditis**
Use additional code for adverse effect, if applicable, to identify drug (T36-T50 with fifth or sixth character 5)

   E06.5   **Other chronic thyroiditis**
Chronic fibrous thyroiditis
Chronic thyroiditis NOS
Ligneous thyroiditis
Riedel thyroiditis

   E06.9   **Thyroiditis, unspecified** ▽

✓4ᵗʰ E07   **Other disorders of thyroid**
   E07.0   **Hypersecretion of calcitonin**
C-cell hyperplasia of thyroid
Hypersecretion of thyrocalcitonin

   E07.1   **Dyshormogenetic goiter**
Familial dyshormogenetic goiter
Pendred's syndrome
     EXCLUDES 1   *transitory congenital goiter with normal function (P72.0)*

✓5ᵗʰ E07.8   **Other specified disorders of thyroid**
     E07.81   **Sick-euthyroid syndrome**
Euthyroid sick-syndrome

     E07.89   **Other specified disorders of thyroid**
Abnormality of thyroid-binding globulin
Hemorrhage of thyroid
Infarction of thyroid

   E07.9   **Disorder of thyroid, unspecified** ▽

Diabetes mellitus (E08-E13)
AHA: 2017, 1Q, 42; 2016, 2Q, 36; 2016, 1Q, 11-13

✓4ᵗʰ E08   **Diabetes mellitus due to underlying condition**
Code first the underlying condition, such as:
   congenital rubella (P35.0)
   Cushing's syndrome (E24.-)
   cystic fibrosis (E84.-)
   malignant neoplasm (C00-C96)
   malnutrition (E40-E46)
   pancreatitis and other diseases of the pancreas (K85.-, K86.-)
Use additional code to identify control using:
   insulin (Z79.4)
   oral antidiabetic drugs (Z79.84)
   oral hypoglycemic drugs (Z79.84)
     EXCLUDES 1   *drug or chemical induced diabetes mellitus (E09.-)*
         gestational diabetes (O24.4-)
         neonatal diabetes mellitus (P70.2)
         postpancreatectomy diabetes mellitus (E13.-)
         postprocedural diabetes mellitus (E13.-)
         secondary diabetes mellitus NEC (E13.-)
         type 1 diabetes mellitus (E10.-)
         type 2 diabetes mellitus (E11.-)
AHA: 2013, 4Q, 114; 2013, 3Q, 20

✓5ᵗʰ E08.0   **Diabetes mellitus due to underlying condition with hyperosmolarity**
     E08.00   ***Diabetes mellitus due to underlying condition with hyperosmolarity without nonketotic hyperglycemic-hyperosmolar coma (NKHHC)*** `HCC`

     E08.01   ***Diabetes mellitus due to underlying condition with hyperosmolarity with coma*** `HCC`

✓5ᵗʰ E08.1   **Diabetes mellitus due to underlying condition with ketoacidosis**
     E08.10   ***Diabetes mellitus due to underlying condition with ketoacidosis without coma*** `HCC`

     E08.11   ***Diabetes mellitus due to underlying condition with ketoacidosis with coma*** `HCC`

✓5ᵗʰ E08.2   **Diabetes mellitus due to underlying condition with kidney complications**
     E08.21   ***Diabetes mellitus due to underlying condition with diabetic nephropathy*** `HCC`
Diabetes mellitus due to underlying condition with intercapillary glomerulosclerosis
Diabetes mellitus due to underlying condition with intracapillary glomerulonephrosis
Diabetes mellitus due to underlying condition with Kimmelstiel-Wilson disease

     E08.22   ***Diabetes mellitus due to underlying condition with diabetic chronic kidney disease*** `HCC`
Use additional code to identify stage of chronic kidney disease (N18.1-N18.6)

     E08.29   ***Diabetes mellitus due to underlying condition with other diabetic kidney complication*** `HCC`
Renal tubular degeneration in diabetes mellitus due to underlying condition

✓5ᵗʰ E08.3   **Diabetes mellitus due to underlying condition with ophthalmic complications**

One of the following 7th characters is to be assigned to codes in subcategories E08.32, E08.33, E08.34, E08.35, and E08.37 to designate laterality of the disease:
1   right eye
2   left eye
3   bilateral
9   unspecified eye

     ✓6ᵗʰ E08.31   **Diabetes mellitus due to underlying condition with unspecified diabetic retinopathy**
       E08.311   ***Diabetes mellitus due to underlying condition with unspecified diabetic retinopathy with macular edema*** `HCC` ▽

       E08.319   ***Diabetes mellitus due to underlying condition with unspecified diabetic retinopathy without macular edema*** `HCC` ▽

     ✓6ᵗʰ E08.32   **Diabetes mellitus due to underlying condition with mild nonproliferative diabetic retinopathy**
Diabetes mellitus due to underlying condition with nonproliferative diabetic retinopathy NOS

       ✓7ᵗʰ E08.321   ***Diabetes mellitus due to underlying condition with mild nonproliferative diabetic retinopathy with macular edema*** `HCC`

EXCLUDES 1 Not coded here   *EXCLUDES 2* Not included here   **N** Newborn Age: 0   **P** Pediatric Age: 0-17   **M** Maternity Age: 12-55   **A** Adult Age: 15-124

508   ICD-10-CM 2018

√6th E08.33 Diabetes mellitus due to underlying condition with moderate nonproliferative diabetic retinopathy

√7th **E08.329** *Diabetes mellitus due to underlying condition with mild nonproliferative diabetic retinopathy without macular edema* HCC

√7th **E08.331** *Diabetes mellitus due to underlying condition with moderate nonproliferative diabetic retinopathy with macular edema* HCC

√7th **E08.339** *Diabetes mellitus due to underlying condition with moderate nonproliferative diabetic retinopathy without macular edema* HCC

√6th E08.34 Diabetes mellitus due to underlying condition with severe nonproliferative diabetic retinopathy

√7th **E08.341** *Diabetes mellitus due to underlying condition with severe nonproliferative diabetic retinopathy with macular edema* HCC

√7th **E08.349** *Diabetes mellitus due to underlying condition with severe nonproliferative diabetic retinopathy without macular edema* HCC

√6th E08.35 Diabetes mellitus due to underlying condition with proliferative diabetic retinopathy

√7th **E08.351** *Diabetes mellitus due to underlying condition with proliferative diabetic retinopathy with macular edema* HCC

√7th **E08.352** *Diabetes mellitus due to underlying condition with proliferative diabetic retinopathy with traction retinal detachment involving the macula* HCC

√7th **E08.353** *Diabetes mellitus due to underlying condition with proliferative diabetic retinopathy with traction retinal detachment not involving the macula* HCC

√7th **E08.354** *Diabetes mellitus due to underlying condition with proliferative diabetic retinopathy with combined traction retinal detachment and rhegmatogenous retinal detachment* HCC

√7th **E08.355** *Diabetes mellitus due to underlying condition with stable proliferative diabetic retinopathy* HCC

√7th **E08.359** *Diabetes mellitus due to underlying condition with proliferative diabetic retinopathy without macular edema* HCC

E08.36 *Diabetes mellitus due to underlying condition with diabetic cataract* HCC
AHA: 2016, 4Q, 142

√x7th **E08.37** *Diabetes mellitus due to underlying condition with diabetic macular edema, resolved following treatment* HCC

E08.39 *Diabetes mellitus due to underlying condition with other diabetic ophthalmic complication* HCC
Use additional code to identify manifestation, such as: diabetic glaucoma (H40-H42)

√5th E08.4 Diabetes mellitus due to underlying condition with neurological complications

E08.40 *Diabetes mellitus due to underlying condition with diabetic neuropathy, unspecified* HCC ▽

E08.41 *Diabetes mellitus due to underlying condition with diabetic mononeuropathy* HCC

E08.42 *Diabetes mellitus due to underlying condition with diabetic polyneuropathy* HCC
Diabetes mellitus due to underlying condition with diabetic neuralgia

E08.43 *Diabetes mellitus due to underlying condition with diabetic autonomic (poly)neuropathy* HCC
Diabetes mellitus due to underlying condition with diabetic gastroparesis
AHA: 2013, 4Q, 114

E08.44 *Diabetes mellitus due to underlying condition with diabetic amyotrophy* HCC

E08.49 *Diabetes mellitus due to underlying condition with other diabetic neurological complication* HCC

√5th E08.5 Diabetes mellitus due to underlying condition with circulatory complications

E08.51 *Diabetes mellitus due to underlying condition with diabetic peripheral angiopathy without gangrene* HCC

E08.52 *Diabetes mellitus due to underlying condition with diabetic peripheral angiopathy with gangrene* HCC
Diabetes mellitus due to underlying condition with diabetic gangrene

E08.59 *Diabetes mellitus due to underlying condition with other circulatory complications* HCC

√5th E08.6 Diabetes mellitus due to underlying condition with other specified complications

√6th E08.61 Diabetes mellitus due to underlying condition with diabetic arthropathy

E08.610 *Diabetes mellitus due to underlying condition with diabetic neuropathic arthropathy* HCC
Diabetes mellitus due to underlying condition with Charcôt's joints

E08.618 *Diabetes mellitus due to underlying condition with other diabetic arthropathy* HCC

√6th E08.62 Diabetes mellitus due to underlying condition with skin complications

E08.620 *Diabetes mellitus due to underlying condition with diabetic dermatitis* HCC
Diabetes mellitus due to underlying condition with diabetic necrobiosis lipoidica

E08.621 *Diabetes mellitus due to underlying condition with foot ulcer* HCC
Use additional code to identify site of ulcer (L97.4-, L97.5-)

E08.622 *Diabetes mellitus due to underlying condition with other skin ulcer* HCC
Use additional code to identify site of ulcer (L97.1-L97.9, L98.41-L98.49)

E08.628 *Diabetes mellitus due to underlying condition with other skin complications* HCC

√6th E08.63 Diabetes mellitus due to underlying condition with oral complications

E08.630 *Diabetes mellitus due to underlying condition with periodontal disease* HCC

E08.638 *Diabetes mellitus due to underlying condition with other oral complications* HCC

√6th E08.64 Diabetes mellitus due to underlying condition with hypoglycemia

E08.641 *Diabetes mellitus due to underlying condition with hypoglycemia with coma* HCC

E08.649 *Diabetes mellitus due to underlying condition with hypoglycemia without coma* HCC
AHA: 2016, 3Q, 42; 2015, 3Q, 21

E08.65 *Diabetes mellitus due to underlying condition with hyperglycemia* HCC

E08.69 *Diabetes mellitus due to underlying condition with other specified complication* HCC
Use additional code to identify complication
AHA: 2016, 4Q, 141; 2016, 1Q, 13

E08.8 *Diabetes mellitus due to underlying condition with unspecified complications* HCC ▽

E08.9 *Diabetes mellitus due to underlying condition without complications* HCC

√4th E09 Drug or chemical induced diabetes mellitus
Code first poisoning due to drug or toxin, if applicable (T36-T65 with fifth or sixth character 1-4 or 6)
Use additional code for adverse effect, if applicable, to identify drug (T36-T50 with fifth or sixth character 5)
Use additional code to identify control using:
insulin (Z79.4)
oral antidiabetic drugs (Z79.84)
oral hypoglycemic drugs (Z79.84)
EXCLUDES 1   diabetes mellitus due to underlying condition (E08.-)
gestational diabetes (O24.4-)
neonatal diabetes mellitus (P70.2)
postpancreatectomy diabetes mellitus (E13.-)
postprocedural diabetes mellitus (E13.-)
secondary diabetes mellitus NEC (E13.-)
type 1 diabetes mellitus (E10.-)
type 2 diabetes mellitus (E11.-)
AHA: 2013, 4Q, 114; 2013, 3Q, 20

√5th E09.0 Drug or chemical induced diabetes mellitus with hyperosmolarity

E09.00 Drug or chemical induced diabetes mellitus with hyperosmolarity without nonketotic hyperglycemic-hyperosmolar coma (NKHHC) HCC

E09.01 Drug or chemical induced diabetes mellitus with hyperosmolarity with coma `HCC`

✓5ᵗʰ **E09.1** Drug or chemical induced diabetes mellitus with ketoacidosis

E09.10 Drug or chemical induced diabetes mellitus with ketoacidosis without coma `HCC`

E09.11 Drug or chemical induced diabetes mellitus with ketoacidosis with coma `HCC`

✓5ᵗʰ **E09.2** Drug or chemical induced diabetes mellitus with kidney complications

E09.21 Drug or chemical induced diabetes mellitus with diabetic nephropathy `HCC`
  Drug or chemical induced diabetes mellitus with intercapillary glomerulosclerosis
  Drug or chemical induced diabetes mellitus with intracapillary glomerulonephrosis
  Drug or chemical induced diabetes mellitus with Kimmelstiel-Wilson disease

E09.22 Drug or chemical induced diabetes mellitus with diabetic chronic kidney disease `HCC`
  Use additional code to identify stage of chronic kidney disease (N18.1-N18.6)

E09.29 Drug or chemical induced diabetes mellitus with other diabetic kidney complication `HCC`
  Drug or chemical induced diabetes mellitus with renal tubular degeneration

✓5ᵗʰ **E09.3** Drug or chemical induced diabetes mellitus with ophthalmic complications

One of the following 7th characters is to be assigned to codes in subcategories E09.32, E09.33, E09.34, E09.35, and E09.37 to designate laterality of the disease:
1   right eye
2   left eye
3   bilateral
9   unspecified eye

✓6ᵗʰ **E09.31** Drug or chemical induced diabetes mellitus with unspecified diabetic retinopathy

E09.311 Drug or chemical induced diabetes mellitus with unspecified diabetic retinopathy with macular edema `HCC` ▽

E09.319 Drug or chemical induced diabetes mellitus with unspecified diabetic retinopathy without macular edema `HCC` ▽

✓6ᵗʰ **E09.32** Drug or chemical induced diabetes mellitus with mild nonproliferative diabetic retinopathy
  Drug or chemical induced diabetes mellitus with nonproliferative diabetic retinopathy NOS

✓7ᵗʰ **E09.321** Drug or chemical induced diabetes mellitus with mild nonproliferative diabetic retinopathy with macular edema `HCC`

✓7ᵗʰ **E09.329** Drug or chemical induced diabetes mellitus with mild nonproliferative diabetic retinopathy without macular edema `HCC`

✓6ᵗʰ **E09.33** Drug or chemical induced diabetes mellitus with moderate nonproliferative diabetic retinopathy

✓7ᵗʰ **E09.331** Drug or chemical induced diabetes mellitus with moderate nonproliferative diabetic retinopathy with macular edema `HCC`

✓7ᵗʰ **E09.339** Drug or chemical induced diabetes mellitus with moderate nonproliferative diabetic retinopathy without macular edema `HCC`

✓6ᵗʰ **E09.34** Drug or chemical induced diabetes mellitus with severe nonproliferative diabetic retinopathy

✓7ᵗʰ **E09.341** Drug or chemical induced diabetes mellitus with severe nonproliferative diabetic retinopathy with macular edema `HCC`

✓7ᵗʰ **E09.349** Drug or chemical induced diabetes mellitus with severe nonproliferative diabetic retinopathy without macular edema `HCC`

✓6ᵗʰ **E09.35** Drug or chemical induced diabetes mellitus with proliferative diabetic retinopathy

✓7ᵗʰ **E09.351** Drug or chemical induced diabetes mellitus with proliferative diabetic retinopathy with macular edema `HCC`

✓7ᵗʰ **E09.352** Drug or chemical induced diabetes mellitus with proliferative diabetic retinopathy with traction retinal detachment involving the macula `HCC`

✓7ᵗʰ **E09.353** Drug or chemical induced diabetes mellitus with proliferative diabetic retinopathy with traction retinal detachment not involving the macula `HCC`

✓7ᵗʰ **E09.354** Drug or chemical induced diabetes mellitus with proliferative diabetic retinopathy with combined traction retinal detachment and rhegmatogenous retinal detachment `HCC`

✓7ᵗʰ **E09.355** Drug or chemical induced diabetes mellitus with stable proliferative diabetic retinopathy `HCC`

✓7ᵗʰ **E09.359** Drug or chemical induced diabetes mellitus with proliferative diabetic retinopathy without macular edema `HCC`

E09.36 Drug or chemical induced diabetes mellitus with diabetic cataract `HCC`
  AHA: 2016, 4Q, 142

✓x7ᵗʰ **E09.37** Drug or chemical induced diabetes mellitus with diabetic macular edema, resolved following treatment `HCC`

E09.39 Drug or chemical induced diabetes mellitus with other diabetic ophthalmic complication `HCC`
  Use additional code to identify manifestation, such as: diabetic glaucoma (H40-H42)

✓5ᵗʰ **E09.4** Drug or chemical induced diabetes mellitus with neurological complications

E09.40 Drug or chemical induced diabetes mellitus with neurological complications with diabetic neuropathy, unspecified `HCC` ▽

E09.41 Drug or chemical induced diabetes mellitus with neurological complications with diabetic mononeuropathy `HCC`

E09.42 Drug or chemical induced diabetes mellitus with neurological complications with diabetic polyneuropathy `HCC`
  Drug or chemical induced diabetes mellitus with diabetic neuralgia

E09.43 Drug or chemical induced diabetes mellitus with neurological complications with diabetic autonomic (poly)neuropathy `HCC`
  Drug or chemical induced diabetes mellitus with diabetic gastroparesis
  AHA: 2013, 4Q, 114

E09.44 Drug or chemical induced diabetes mellitus with neurological complications with diabetic amyotrophy `HCC`

E09.49 Drug or chemical induced diabetes mellitus with neurological complications with other diabetic neurological complication `HCC`

✓5ᵗʰ **E09.5** Drug or chemical induced diabetes mellitus with circulatory complications

E09.51 Drug or chemical induced diabetes mellitus with diabetic peripheral angiopathy without gangrene `HCC`

E09.52 Drug or chemical induced diabetes mellitus with diabetic peripheral angiopathy with gangrene `HCC`
  Drug or chemical induced diabetes mellitus with diabetic gangrene

E09.59 Drug or chemical induced diabetes mellitus with other circulatory complications `HCC`

✓5ᵗʰ **E09.6** Drug or chemical induced diabetes mellitus with other specified complications

✓6ᵗʰ **E09.61** Drug or chemical induced diabetes mellitus with diabetic arthropathy

E09.610 Drug or chemical induced diabetes mellitus with diabetic neuropathic arthropathy `HCC`
  Drug or chemical induced diabetes mellitus with Charcôt's joints

E09.618 Drug or chemical induced diabetes mellitus with other diabetic arthropathy `HCC`

☑6ᵗʰ **E09.62** **Drug or chemical induced diabetes mellitus with skin complications**

> **E09.620** **Drug or chemical induced diabetes** ᴴᶜᶜ
> **mellitus with** diabetic dermatitis
> > Drug or chemical induced diabetes mellitus with diabetic necrobiosis lipoidica

> **E09.621** **Drug or chemical induced diabetes** ᴴᶜᶜ
> **mellitus with** foot ulcer
> > Use additional code to identify site of ulcer (L97.4-, L97.5-)

> **E09.622** **Drug or chemical induced diabetes** ᴴᶜᶜ
> **mellitus with** other skin ulcer
> > Use additional code to identify site of ulcer (L97.1-L97.9, L98.41-L98.49)

> **E09.628** **Drug or chemical induced diabetes** ᴴᶜᶜ
> **mellitus with other skin complications**

☑6ᵗʰ **E09.63** **Drug or chemical induced diabetes mellitus with** oral complications

> **E09.630** **Drug or chemical induced diabetes** ᴴᶜᶜ
> **mellitus with** periodontal disease

> **E09.638** **Drug or chemical induced diabetes** ᴴᶜᶜ
> **mellitus with other oral complications**

☑6ᵗʰ **E09.64** **Drug or chemical induced diabetes mellitus with** hypoglycemia

> **E09.641** **Drug or chemical induced diabetes** ᴴᶜᶜ
> **mellitus with hypoglycemia** with coma

> **E09.649** **Drug or chemical induced diabetes** ᴴᶜᶜ
> **mellitus with hypoglycemia** without coma
> > **AHA:** 2016, 3Q, 42; 2015, 3Q, 21

> **E09.65** **Drug or chemical induced diabetes mellitus** ᴴᶜᶜ
> **with** hyperglycemia

> **E09.69** **Drug or chemical induced diabetes mellitus** ᴴᶜᶜ
> **with other specified complication**
> > Use additional code to identify complication
> > **AHA:** 2016, 4Q, 141; 2016, 1Q, 13

E09.8 **Drug or chemical induced diabetes mellitus with** ᴴᶜᶜ ▽
unspecified complications

E09.9 **Drug or chemical induced diabetes mellitus** without ᴴᶜᶜ
complications

☑4ᵗʰ **E10** **Type 1 diabetes mellitus**

> INCLUDES   brittle diabetes (mellitus)
> diabetes (mellitus) due to autoimmune process
> diabetes (mellitus) due to immune mediated pancreatic islet beta-cell destruction
> idiopathic diabetes (mellitus)
> juvenile onset diabetes (mellitus)
> ketosis-prone diabetes (mellitus)

> EXCLUDES 1   *diabetes mellitus due to underlying condition (E08.-)*
> *drug or chemical induced diabetes mellitus (E09.-)*
> *gestational diabetes (O24.4-)*
> *hyperglycemia NOS (R73.9)*
> *neonatal diabetes mellitus (P70.2)*
> *postpancreatectomy diabetes mellitus (E13.-)*
> *postprocedural diabetes mellitus (E13.-)*
> *secondary diabetes mellitus NEC (E13.-)*
> *type 2 diabetes mellitus (E11.-)*

> **AHA:** 2013, 4Q, 114; 2013, 3Q, 20

☑5ᵗʰ **E10.1** **Type 1 diabetes mellitus with** ketoacidosis
> **AHA:** 2013, 3Q, 20

> **E10.10** **Type 1 diabetes mellitus with ketoacidosis** ᴴᶜᶜ
> **without coma**

> **E10.11** **Type 1 diabetes mellitus with ketoacidosis** ᴴᶜᶜ
> **with coma**

☑5ᵗʰ **E10.2** **Type 1 diabetes mellitus with** kidney complications

> **E10.21** **Type 1 diabetes mellitus with diabetic** ᴴᶜᶜ
> **nephropathy**
> > Type 1 diabetes mellitus with intercapillary glomerulosclerosis
> > Type 1 diabetes mellitus with intracapillary glomerulonephrosis
> > Type 1 diabetes mellitus with Kimmelstiel-Wilson disease

> **E10.22** **Type 1 diabetes mellitus with diabetic** chronic ᴴᶜᶜ
> **kidney disease**
> > Use additional code to identify stage of chronic kidney disease (N18.1-N18.6)

> **E10.29** **Type 1 diabetes mellitus with other diabetic** ᴴᶜᶜ
> **kidney complication**
> > Type 1 diabetes mellitus with renal tubular degeneration
> > **AHA:** 2016, 1Q, 13

☑5ᵗʰ **E10.3** **Type 1 diabetes mellitus with** ophthalmic complications

> One of the following 7th characters is to be assigned to codes in subcategories E10.32, E10.33, E10.34, E10.35, and E10.37 to designate laterality of the disease:
> 1   right eye
> 2   left eye
> 3   bilateral
> 9   unspecified eye

☑6ᵗʰ **E10.31** **Type 1 diabetes mellitus with unspecified diabetic retinopathy**

> **E10.311** **Type 1 diabetes mellitus with** ᴴᶜᶜ ▽
> **unspecified diabetic retinopathy with macular edema**

> **E10.319** **Type 1 diabetes mellitus with** ᴴᶜᶜ ▽
> **unspecified diabetic retinopathy without macular edema**

☑6ᵗʰ **E10.32** **Type 1 diabetes mellitus with** mild nonproliferative
diabetic retinopathy
> Type 1 diabetes mellitus with nonproliferative diabetic retinopathy NOS

> ☑7ᵗʰ **E10.321** **Type 1 diabetes mellitus with mild** ᴴᶜᶜ
> **nonproliferative diabetic retinopathy with macular edema**

> ☑7ᵗʰ **E10.329** **Type 1 diabetes mellitus with mild** ᴴᶜᶜ
> **nonproliferative diabetic retinopathy without macular edema**

☑6ᵗʰ **E10.33** **Type 1 diabetes mellitus with** moderate
nonproliferative **diabetic** retinopathy

> ☑7ᵗʰ **E10.331** **Type 1 diabetes mellitus with** ᴴᶜᶜ
> **moderate nonproliferative diabetic retinopathy with macular edema**

> ☑7ᵗʰ **E10.339** **Type 1 diabetes mellitus with** ᴴᶜᶜ
> **moderate nonproliferative diabetic retinopathy without macular edema**

☑6ᵗʰ **E10.34** **Type 1 diabetes mellitus with** severe
nonproliferative **diabetic** retinopathy

> ☑7ᵗʰ **E10.341** **Type 1 diabetes mellitus with severe** ᴴᶜᶜ
> **nonproliferative diabetic retinopathy with macular edema**

> ☑7ᵗʰ **E10.349** **Type 1 diabetes mellitus with severe** ᴴᶜᶜ
> **nonproliferative diabetic retinopathy without macular edema**

☑6ᵗʰ **E10.35** **Type 1 diabetes mellitus with** proliferative **diabetic** retinopathy

> ☑7ᵗʰ **E10.351** **Type 1 diabetes mellitus with** ᴴᶜᶜ
> **proliferative diabetic retinopathy with macular edema**

> ☑7ᵗʰ **E10.352** **Type 1 diabetes mellitus with** ᴴᶜᶜ
> **proliferative diabetic retinopathy with traction retinal detachment involving the macula**

> ☑7ᵗʰ **E10.353** **Type 1 diabetes mellitus with** ᴴᶜᶜ
> **proliferative diabetic retinopathy with traction retinal detachment not involving the macula**

> ☑7ᵗʰ **E10.354** **Type 1 diabetes mellitus with** ᴴᶜᶜ
> **proliferative diabetic retinopathy with combined traction retinal detachment and rhegmatogenous retinal detachment**

> ☑7ᵗʰ **E10.355** **Type 1 diabetes mellitus with stable** ᴴᶜᶜ
> **proliferative diabetic retinopathy**

> ☑7ᵗʰ **E10.359** **Type 1 diabetes mellitus with** ᴴᶜᶜ
> **proliferative diabetic retinopathy without macular edema**

> **E10.36** **Type 1 diabetes mellitus with diabetic** cataract ᴴᶜᶜ
> > **AHA:** 2016, 4Q, 142

☑x7ᵗʰ **E10.37** **Type 1 diabetes mellitus with diabetic** macular ᴴᶜᶜ
edema, resolved following treatment

> **E10.39** **Type 1 diabetes mellitus with** other diabetic ᴴᶜᶜ
> **ophthalmic complication**
> > Use additional code to identify manifestation, such as: diabetic glaucoma (H40-H42)

☑5ᵗʰ **E10.4** **Type 1 diabetes mellitus with** neurological complications

> **E10.40** **Type 1 diabetes mellitus with diabetic** ᴴᶜᶜ ▽
> **neuropathy, unspecified**

> **E10.41** **Type 1 diabetes mellitus with diabetic** ᴴᶜᶜ
> **mononeuropathy**

☑ Additional Character Req   ✓ˣ7ᵗʰ Placeholder Alert   Manifestation   ᴴᶜᶜ CMS-HCC Condition   ▽ Unspecified Code   ▶◀ Revised Text   ● New Code   ▲ Revised Code Title

E10.42   **Type 1 diabetes mellitus with diabetic polyneuropathy**   `HCC`
Type 1 diabetes mellitus with diabetic neuralgia

E10.43   **Type 1 diabetes mellitus with diabetic autonomic (poly)neuropathy**   `HCC`
Type 1 diabetes mellitus with diabetic gastroparesis
AHA: 2013, 4Q, 114

E10.44   **Type 1 diabetes mellitus with diabetic amyotrophy**   `HCC`

E10.49   **Type 1 diabetes mellitus with other diabetic neurological complication**   `HCC`

√5th **E10.5**   **Type 1 diabetes mellitus with circulatory complications**

E10.51   **Type 1 diabetes mellitus with diabetic peripheral angiopathy without gangrene**   `HCC`

E10.52   **Type 1 diabetes mellitus with diabetic peripheral angiopathy with gangrene**   `HCC`
Type 1 diabetes mellitus with diabetic gangrene

E10.59   **Type 1 diabetes mellitus with other circulatory complications**   `HCC`

√5th **E10.6**   **Type 1 diabetes mellitus with other specified complications**

√6th **E10.61**   **Type 1 diabetes mellitus with diabetic arthropathy**

E10.610   **Type 1 diabetes mellitus with diabetic neuropathic arthropathy**   `HCC`
Type 1 diabetes mellitus with Charcôt's joints

E10.618   **Type 1 diabetes mellitus with other diabetic arthropathy**   `HCC`

√6th **E10.62**   **Type 1 diabetes mellitus with skin complications**

E10.620   **Type 1 diabetes mellitus with diabetic dermatitis**   `HCC`
Type 1 diabetes mellitus with diabetic necrobiosis lipoidica

E10.621   **Type 1 diabetes mellitus with foot ulcer**   `HCC`
Use additional code to identify site of ulcer (L97.4-, L97.5-)

E10.622   **Type 1 diabetes mellitus with other skin ulcer**   `HCC`
Use additional code to identify site of ulcer (L97.1-L97.9, L98.41-L98.49)

E10.628   **Type 1 diabetes mellitus with other skin complications**   `HCC`

√6th **E10.63**   **Type 1 diabetes mellitus with oral complications**

E10.630   **Type 1 diabetes mellitus with periodontal disease**   `HCC`

E10.638   **Type 1 diabetes mellitus with other oral complications**   `HCC`

√6th **E10.64**   **Type 1 diabetes mellitus with hypoglycemia**

E10.641   **Type 1 diabetes mellitus with hypoglycemia with coma**   `HCC`

E10.649   **Type 1 diabetes mellitus with hypoglycemia without coma**   `HCC`
AHA: 2016, 3Q, 42; 2016, 1Q, 13; 2015, 3Q, 21

E10.65   **Type 1 diabetes mellitus with hyperglycemia**   `HCC`
AHA: 2013, 3Q, 20

E10.69   **Type 1 diabetes mellitus with other specified complication**   `HCC`
Use additional code to identify complication
AHA: 2016, 4Q, 141; 2016, 1Q, 13

E10.8   **Type 1 diabetes mellitus with unspecified complications**   `HCC` ▽

E10.9   **Type 1 diabetes mellitus without complications**   `HCC`

√4th **E11**   **Type 2 diabetes mellitus**
`INCLUDES`   diabetes (mellitus) due to insulin secretory defect
diabetes NOS
insulin resistant diabetes (mellitus)
Use additional code to identify control using:
insulin (Z79.4)
oral antidiabetic drugs (Z79.84)
oral hypoglycemic drugs (Z79.84)
`EXCLUDES 1`   *diabetes mellitus due to underlying condition (E08.-)*
drug or chemical induced diabetes mellitus (E09.-)
gestational diabetes (O24.4-)
neonatal diabetes mellitus (P70.2)
postpancreatectomy diabetes mellitus (E13.-)
postprocedural diabetes mellitus (E13.-)
secondary diabetes mellitus NEC (E13.-)
type 1 diabetes mellitus (E10.-)
AHA: 2016, 2Q, 10; 2013, 4Q, 114; 2013, 3Q, 20; 2013, 1Q, 26

√5th **E11.0**   **Type 2 diabetes mellitus with hyperosmolarity**

E11.00   **Type 2 diabetes mellitus with hyperosmolarity without nonketotic hyperglycemic-hyperosmolar coma (NKHHC)**   `HCC`

E11.01   **Type 2 diabetes mellitus with hyperosmolarity with coma**   `HCC`

● √5th **E11.1**   **Type 2 diabetes mellitus with ketoacidosis**

●   **E11.10**   **Type 2 diabetes mellitus with ketoacidosis without coma**

●   **E11.11**   **Type 2 diabetes mellitus with ketoacidosis with coma**

√5th **E11.2**   **Type 2 diabetes mellitus with kidney complications**

E11.21   **Type 2 diabetes mellitus with diabetic nephropathy**   `HCC`
Type 2 diabetes mellitus with intercapillary glomerulosclerosis
Type 2 diabetes mellitus with intracapillary glomerulonephrosis
Type 2 diabetes mellitus with Kimmelstiel-Wilson disease

E11.22   **Type 2 diabetes mellitus with diabetic chronic kidney disease**   `HCC`
Use additional code to identify stage of chronic kidney disease (N18.1-N18.6)
AHA: 2016, 1Q, 12

E11.29   **Type 2 diabetes mellitus with other diabetic kidney complication**   `HCC`
Type 2 diabetes mellitus with renal tubular degeneration

√5th **E11.3**   **Type 2 diabetes mellitus with ophthalmic complications**

One of the following 7th characters is to be assigned to codes in subcategories E11.32, E11.33, E11.34, E11.35, and E11.37 to designate laterality of the disease:
1   right eye
2   left eye
3   bilateral
9   unspecified eye

√6th **E11.31**   **Type 2 diabetes mellitus with unspecified diabetic retinopathy**

E11.311   **Type 2 diabetes mellitus with unspecified diabetic retinopathy with macular edema**   `HCC` ▽

E11.319   **Type 2 diabetes mellitus with unspecified diabetic retinopathy without macular edema**   `HCC` ▽

√6th **E11.32**   **Type 2 diabetes mellitus with mild nonproliferative diabetic retinopathy**
Type 2 diabetes mellitus with nonproliferative diabetic retinopathy NOS

√7th **E11.321**   **Type 2 diabetes mellitus with mild nonproliferative diabetic retinopathy with macular edema**   `HCC`

√7th **E11.329**   **Type 2 diabetes mellitus with mild nonproliferative diabetic retinopathy without macular edema**   `HCC`

√6th **E11.33**   **Type 2 diabetes mellitus with moderate nonproliferative diabetic retinopathy**

√7th **E11.331**   **Type 2 diabetes mellitus with moderate nonproliferative diabetic retinopathy with macular edema**   `HCC`

√7th **E11.339**   **Type 2 diabetes mellitus with moderate nonproliferative diabetic retinopathy without macular edema**   `HCC`

`EXCLUDES 1` Not coded here   `EXCLUDES 2` Not included here   N Newborn Age: 0   P Pediatric Age: 0-17   M Maternity Age: 12-55   A Adult Age: 15-124

512   ICD-10-CM 2018

☑6ᵗʰ **E11.34**   **Type 2 diabetes mellitus with** severe nonproliferative **diabetic** retinopathy

     ☑7ᵗʰ **E11.341**   **Type 2 diabetes mellitus with severe nonproliferative diabetic retinopathy with macular edema**   HCC

     ☑7ᵗʰ **E11.349**   **Type 2 diabetes mellitus with severe nonproliferative diabetic retinopathy without macular edema**   HCC

☑6ᵗʰ **E11.35**   **Type 2 diabetes mellitus with** proliferative diabetic retinopathy

     ☑7ᵗʰ **E11.351**   **Type 2 diabetes mellitus with proliferative diabetic retinopathy with macular edema**   HCC

     ☑7ᵗʰ **E11.352**   **Type 2 diabetes mellitus with proliferative diabetic retinopathy with traction retinal detachment involving the macula**   HCC

     ☑7ᵗʰ **E11.353**   **Type 2 diabetes mellitus with proliferative diabetic retinopathy with traction retinal detachment not involving the macula**   HCC

     ☑7ᵗʰ **E11.354**   **Type 2 diabetes mellitus with proliferative diabetic retinopathy** with **combined traction retinal detachment and rhegmatogenous retinal detachment**   HCC

     ☑7ᵗʰ **E11.355**   **Type 2 diabetes mellitus with** stable **proliferative diabetic retinopathy**   HCC

     ☑7ᵗʰ **E11.359**   **Type 2 diabetes mellitus with proliferative diabetic retinopathy without macular edema**   HCC

E11.36   **Type 2 diabetes mellitus with diabetic** cataract   HCC
     AHA: 2016, 4Q, 142

☑x7ᵗʰ **E11.37**   **Type 2 diabetes mellitus with diabetic** macular **edema, resolved following treatment**   HCC

E11.39   **Type 2 diabetes mellitus with other diabetic ophthalmic complication**   HCC
     Use additional code to identify manifestation, such as: diabetic glaucoma (H40-H42)

☑5ᵗʰ **E11.4**   **Type 2 diabetes mellitus with** neurological complications

     E11.40   **Type 2 diabetes mellitus with diabetic neuropathy, unspecified**   HCC ▽
         AHA: 2013, 4Q, 129

     E11.41   **Type 2 diabetes mellitus with diabetic mononeuropathy**   HCC

     E11.42   **Type 2 diabetes mellitus with diabetic polyneuropathy**   HCC
         Type 2 diabetes mellitus with diabetic neuralgia
         AHA: 2016, 1Q, 12

     E11.43   **Type 2 diabetes mellitus with diabetic autonomic (poly)neuropathy**   HCC
         Type 2 diabetes mellitus with diabetic gastroparesis
         AHA: 2013, 4Q, 114

     E11.44   **Type 2 diabetes mellitus with diabetic amyotrophy**   HCC

     E11.49   **Type 2 diabetes mellitus with other diabetic neurological complication**   HCC

☑5ᵗʰ **E11.5**   **Type 2 diabetes mellitus with** circulatory complications

     E11.51   **Type 2 diabetes mellitus with diabetic peripheral angiopathy without gangrene**   HCC

     E11.52   **Type 2 diabetes mellitus with diabetic peripheral angiopathy with gangrene**   HCC
         Type 2 diabetes mellitus with diabetic gangrene

     E11.59   **Type 2 diabetes mellitus with other circulatory complications**   HCC

☑5ᵗʰ **E11.6**   **Type 2 diabetes mellitus with other specified complications**

     ☑6ᵗʰ **E11.61**   **Type 2 diabetes mellitus with diabetic** arthropathy

         E11.610   **Type 2 diabetes mellitus with diabetic neuropathic arthropathy**   HCC
             Type 2 diabetes mellitus with Charcôt's joints

         E11.618   **Type 2 diabetes mellitus with other diabetic arthropathy**   HCC

     ☑6ᵗʰ **E11.62**   **Type 2 diabetes mellitus with** skin complications

         E11.620   **Type 2 diabetes mellitus with diabetic dermatitis**   HCC
             Type 2 diabetes mellitus with diabetic necrobiosis lipoidica

         E11.621   **Type 2 diabetes mellitus with foot ulcer**   HCC
             Use additional code to identify site of ulcer (L97.4-, L97.5-)
             AHA: 2016, 1Q, 12

         E11.622   **Type 2 diabetes mellitus with other skin ulcer**   HCC
             Use additional code to identify site of ulcer (L97.1-L97.9, L98.41-L98.49)

         E11.628   **Type 2 diabetes mellitus with other skin complications**   HCC

     ☑6ᵗʰ **E11.63**   **Type 2 diabetes mellitus with** oral complications

         E11.630   **Type 2 diabetes mellitus with periodontal disease**   HCC

         E11.638   **Type 2 diabetes mellitus with other oral complications**   HCC

     ☑6ᵗʰ **E11.64**   **Type 2 diabetes mellitus with** hypoglycemia

         E11.641   **Type 2 diabetes mellitus with hypoglycemia with coma**   HCC

         E11.649   **Type 2 diabetes mellitus with hypoglycemia without coma**   HCC
             AHA: 2016, 3Q, 42; 2015, 3Q, 21

     E11.65   **Type 2 diabetes mellitus with** hyperglycemia   HCC
         AHA: 2013, 3Q, 20

     E11.69   **Type 2 diabetes mellitus with other specified complication**   HCC
         Use additional code to identify complication
         AHA: 2016, 4Q, 141; 2016, 1Q, 13

E11.8   **Type 2 diabetes mellitus with unspecified complications**   HCC ▽

E11.9   **Type 2 diabetes mellitus** without complications   HCC

☑4ᵗʰ **E13**   **Other specified diabetes mellitus**

     INCLUDES   diabetes mellitus due to genetic defects of beta-cell function
            diabetes mellitus due to genetic defects in insulin action
            postpancreatectomy diabetes mellitus
            postprocedural diabetes mellitus
            secondary diabetes mellitus NEC

     Use additional code to identify control using:
         insulin (Z79.4)
         oral antidiabetic drugs (Z79.84)
         oral hypoglycemic drugs (Z79.84)

     EXCLUDES 1   *diabetes (mellitus) due to autoimmune process (E10.-)*
            diabetes (mellitus) due to immune mediated pancreatic islet beta-cell destruction (E10.-)
            diabetes mellitus due to underlying condition (E08.-)
            drug or chemical induced diabetes mellitus (E09.-)
            gestational diabetes (O24.4-)
            neonatal diabetes mellitus (P70.2)
            type 1 diabetes mellitus (E10.-)
            ~~*type 2 diabetes mellitus (E11.-)*~~
     AHA: 2013, 4Q, 114; 2013, 3Q, 20

☑5ᵗʰ **E13.0**   **Other specified diabetes mellitus with** hyperosmolarity

     E13.00   **Other specified diabetes mellitus with hyperosmolarity without nonketotic hyperglycemic-hyperosmolar coma (NKHHC)**   HCC
         EXCLUDES 2   ►*type 2 diabetes mellitus (E11.-)*◄

     E13.01   **Other specified diabetes mellitus with hyperosmolarity with coma**   HCC

☑5ᵗʰ **E13.1**   **Other specified diabetes mellitus with** ketoacidosis
     AHA: 2016, 2Q, 10; 2013, 1Q, 26

     E13.10   **Other specified diabetes mellitus with ketoacidosis without coma**   HCC

     E13.11   **Other specified diabetes mellitus with ketoacidosis with coma**   HCC

☑5ᵗʰ **E13.2**   **Other specified diabetes mellitus with** kidney complications

     E13.21   **Other specified diabetes mellitus with diabetic nephropathy**   HCC
         Other specified diabetes mellitus with intercapillary glomerulosclerosis
         Other specified diabetes mellitus with intracapillary glomerulonephrosis
         Other specified diabetes mellitus with Kimmelstiel-Wilson disease

     E13.22   **Other specified diabetes mellitus with diabetic chronic kidney disease**   HCC
         Use additional code to identify stage of chronic kidney disease (N18.1-N18.6)

☑ Additional Character Req   ☑x7ᵗʰ Placeholder Alert   Manifestation   HCC CMS-HCC Condition   ▽ Unspecified Code   ►◄ Revised Text   ● New Code   ▲ Revised Code Title

E13.29   **Other specified diabetes mellitus with other diabetic kidney complication**   HCC
Other specified diabetes mellitus with renal tubular degeneration

✓5ᵗʰ **E13.3**   **Other specified diabetes mellitus with ophthalmic complications**

One of the following 7th characters is to be assigned to codes in subcategories E13.32, E13.33, E13.34, E13.35, and E13.37 to designate laterality of the disease:
1   right eye
2   left eye
3   bilateral
9   unspecified eye

✓6ᵗʰ **E13.31**   **Other specified diabetes mellitus with unspecified diabetic retinopathy**

    E13.311   **Other specified diabetes mellitus with unspecified diabetic retinopathy with macular edema**   HCC ▽

    E13.319   **Other specified diabetes mellitus with unspecified diabetic retinopathy without macular edema**   HCC ▽

✓6ᵗʰ **E13.32**   **Other specified diabetes mellitus with mild nonproliferative diabetic retinopathy**
Other specified diabetes mellitus with nonproliferative diabetic retinopathy NOS

    ✓7ᵗʰ **E13.321**   **Other specified diabetes mellitus with mild nonproliferative diabetic retinopathy with macular edema**   HCC

    ✓7ᵗʰ **E13.329**   **Other specified diabetes mellitus with mild nonproliferative diabetic retinopathy without macular edema**   HCC

✓6ᵗʰ **E13.33**   **Other specified diabetes mellitus with moderate nonproliferative diabetic retinopathy**

    ✓7ᵗʰ **E13.331**   **Other specified diabetes mellitus with moderate nonproliferative diabetic retinopathy with macular edema**   HCC

    ✓7ᵗʰ **E13.339**   **Other specified diabetes mellitus with moderate nonproliferative diabetic retinopathy without macular edema**   HCC

✓6ᵗʰ **E13.34**   **Other specified diabetes mellitus with severe nonproliferative diabetic retinopathy**

    ✓7ᵗʰ **E13.341**   **Other specified diabetes mellitus with severe nonproliferative diabetic retinopathy with macular edema**   HCC

    ✓7ᵗʰ **E13.349**   **Other specified diabetes mellitus with severe nonproliferative diabetic retinopathy without macular edema**   HCC

✓6ᵗʰ **E13.35**   **Other specified diabetes mellitus with proliferative diabetic retinopathy**

    ✓7ᵗʰ **E13.351**   **Other specified diabetes mellitus with proliferative diabetic retinopathy with macular edema**   HCC

    ✓7ᵗʰ **E13.352**   **Other specified diabetes mellitus with proliferative diabetic retinopathy with traction retinal detachment involving the macula**   HCC

    ✓7ᵗʰ **E13.353**   **Other specified diabetes mellitus with proliferative diabetic retinopathy with traction retinal detachment not involving the macula**   HCC

    ✓7ᵗʰ **E13.354**   **Other specified diabetes mellitus with proliferative diabetic retinopathy with combined traction retinal detachment and rhegmatogenous retinal detachment**   HCC

    ✓7ᵗʰ **E13.355**   **Other specified diabetes mellitus with stable proliferative diabetic retinopathy**   HCC

    ✓7ᵗʰ **E13.359**   **Other specified diabetes mellitus with proliferative diabetic retinopathy without macular edema**   HCC

E13.36   **Other specified diabetes mellitus with diabetic cataract**   HCC
AHA: 2016, 4Q, 142

✓x7ᵗʰ **E13.37**   **Other specified diabetes mellitus with diabetic macular edema, resolved following treatment**   HCC

E13.39   **Other specified diabetes mellitus with other diabetic ophthalmic complication**   HCC
Use additional code to identify manifestation, such as: diabetic glaucoma (H40-H42)

✓5ᵗʰ **E13.4**   **Other specified diabetes mellitus with neurological complications**

    E13.40   **Other specified diabetes mellitus with diabetic neuropathy, unspecified**   HCC ▽

    E13.41   **Other specified diabetes mellitus with diabetic mononeuropathy**

    E13.42   **Other specified diabetes mellitus with diabetic polyneuropathy**   HCC
Other specified diabetes mellitus with diabetic neuralgia

    E13.43   **Other specified diabetes mellitus with diabetic autonomic (poly)neuropathy**   HCC
Other specified diabetes mellitus with diabetic gastroparesis
AHA: 2013, 4Q, 114

    E13.44   **Other specified diabetes mellitus with diabetic amyotrophy**   HCC

    E13.49   **Other specified diabetes mellitus with other diabetic neurological complication**   HCC

✓5ᵗʰ **E13.5**   **Other specified diabetes mellitus with circulatory complications**

    E13.51   **Other specified diabetes mellitus with diabetic peripheral angiopathy without gangrene**   HCC

    E13.52   **Other specified diabetes mellitus with diabetic peripheral angiopathy with gangrene**   HCC
Other specified diabetes mellitus with diabetic gangrene

    E13.59   **Other specified diabetes mellitus with other circulatory complications**   HCC

✓5ᵗʰ **E13.6**   **Other specified diabetes mellitus with other specified complications**

    ✓6ᵗʰ **E13.61**   **Other specified diabetes mellitus with diabetic arthropathy**

      E13.610   **Other specified diabetes mellitus with diabetic neuropathic arthropathy**   HCC
Other specified diabetes mellitus with Charcôt's joints

      E13.618   **Other specified diabetes mellitus with other diabetic arthropathy**   HCC

    ✓6ᵗʰ **E13.62**   **Other specified diabetes mellitus with skin complications**

      E13.620   **Other specified diabetes mellitus with diabetic dermatitis**   HCC
Other specified diabetes mellitus with diabetic necrobiosis lipoidica

      E13.621   **Other specified diabetes mellitus with foot ulcer**   HCC
Use additional code to identify site of ulcer (L97.4-, L97.5-)

      E13.622   **Other specified diabetes mellitus with other skin ulcer**   HCC
Use additional code to identify site of ulcer (L97.1-L97.9, L98.41-L98.49)

      E13.628   **Other specified diabetes mellitus with other skin complications**   HCC

    ✓6ᵗʰ **E13.63**   **Other specified diabetes mellitus with oral complications**

      E13.630   **Other specified diabetes mellitus with periodontal disease**   HCC

      E13.638   **Other specified diabetes mellitus with other oral complications**   HCC

    ✓6ᵗʰ **E13.64**   **Other specified diabetes mellitus with hypoglycemia**

      E13.641   **Other specified diabetes mellitus with hypoglycemia with coma**   HCC

      E13.649   **Other specified diabetes mellitus with hypoglycemia without coma**   HCC
AHA: 2016, 3Q, 42; 2015, 3Q, 21

    E13.65   **Other specified diabetes mellitus with hyperglycemia**   HCC

    E13.69   **Other specified diabetes mellitus with other specified complication**   HCC
Use additional code to identify complication
AHA: 2016, 4Q, 141; 2016, 1Q, 13

E13.8   **Other specified diabetes mellitus with unspecified complications**   HCC ▽

E13.9   **Other specified diabetes mellitus without complications**   HCC

EXCLUDES 1 Not coded here   **EXCLUDES 2** Not included here   **N** Newborn Age: 0   **P** Pediatric Age: 0-17   **M** Maternity Age: 12-55   **A** Adult Age: 15-124

514   ICD-10-CM 2018

Other disorders of glucose regulation and pancreatic internal secretion (E15-E16)

E15 Nondiabetic hypoglycemic coma `HCC`
> INCLUDES drug-induced insulin coma in nondiabetic
> hyperinsulinism with hypoglycemic coma
> hypoglycemic coma NOS

✓4th E16 Other disorders of pancreatic internal secretion

E16.0 Drug-induced hypoglycemia without coma
> Use additional code for adverse effect, if applicable, to identify drug (T36-T50 with fifth or sixth character 5)
> EXCLUDES 1 diabetes with hypoglycemia without coma ▶(E09.649)◄

E16.1 Other hypoglycemia
> Functional hyperinsulinism
> Functional nonhyperinsulinemic hypoglycemia
> Hyperinsulinism NOS
> Hyperplasia of pancreatic islet beta cells NOS
> EXCLUDES 1 diabetes with hypoglycemia (E08.649, E10.649, E11.649, E13.649)
> hypoglycemia in infant of diabetic mother (P70.1)
> neonatal hypoglycemia (P70.4)

E16.2 Hypoglycemia, unspecified ▽
> EXCLUDES 1 diabetes with hypoglycemia (E08.649, E10.649, E11.649, E13.649)
> AHA: 2016, 3Q, 42

E16.3 Increased secretion of glucagon
> Hyperplasia of pancreatic endocrine cells with glucagon excess

E16.4 Increased secretion of gastrin
> Hypergastrinemia
> Hyperplasia of pancreatic endocrine cells with gastrin excess
> Zollinger-Ellison syndrome

E16.8 Other specified disorders of pancreatic internal secretion
> Increased secretion from endocrine pancreas of growth hormone-releasing hormone
> Increased secretion from endocrine pancreas of pancreatic polypeptide
> Increased secretion from endocrine pancreas of somatostatin
> Increased secretion from endocrine pancreas of vasoactive-intestinal polypeptide

E16.9 Disorder of pancreatic internal secretion, unspecified ▽
> Islet-cell hyperplasia NOS
> Pancreatic endocrine cell hyperplasia NOS

Disorders of other endocrine glands (E20-E35)

> EXCLUDES 1 galactorrhea (N64.3)
> gynecomastia (N62)

✓4th E20 Hypoparathyroidism
> EXCLUDES 1 Di George's syndrome (D82.1)
> postprocedural hypoparathyroidism (E89.2)
> tetany NOS (R29.0)
> transitory neonatal hypoparathyroidism (P71.4)

E20.0 Idiopathic hypoparathyroidism `HCC`
> DEF: Abnormally low secretion of parathyroid hormones, with unknown cause, which causes decreased calcium and increased phosphorus in the blood, resulting in muscle cramps, tetany, tingling, or burning in lips, fingers, and toes, and cataracts.

E20.1 Pseudohypoparathyroidism

E20.8 Other hypoparathyroidism `HCC`

E20.9 Hypoparathyroidism, unspecified `HCC` ▽
> Parathyroid tetany

✓4th E21 Hyperparathyroidism and other disorders of parathyroid gland
> EXCLUDES 1 adult osteomalacia (M83.-)
> ectopic hyperparathyroidism (E34.2)
> familial hypocalciuric hypercalcemia (E83.52)
> hungry bone syndrome (E83.81)
> infantile and juvenile osteomalacia (E55.0)

E21.0 Primary hyperparathyroidism `HCC`
> Hyperplasia of parathyroid
> Osteitis fibrosa cystica generalisata [von Recklinghausen's disease of bone]
> DEF: Parathyroid dysfunction commonly caused by hyperplasia of two or more glands; characteristic hypercalcemia and increased parathyroid hormone levels.

E21.1 Secondary hyperparathyroidism, not elsewhere classified `HCC`
> EXCLUDES 1 secondary hyperparathyroidism of renal origin (N25.81)

E21.2 Other hyperparathyroidism `HCC`
> Tertiary hyperparathyroidism
> EXCLUDES 1 familial hypocalciuric hypercalcemia (E83.52)

E21.3 Hyperparathyroidism, unspecified `HCC` ▽

E21.4 Other specified disorders of parathyroid gland `HCC`

E21.5 Disorder of parathyroid gland, unspecified `HCC` ▽

✓4th E22 Hyperfunction of pituitary gland
> EXCLUDES 1 Cushing's syndrome (E24.-)
> Nelson's syndrome (E24.1)
> overproduction of ACTH not associated with Cushing's disease (E27.0)
> overproduction of pituitary ACTH (E24.0)
> overproduction of thyroid-stimulating hormone (E05.8-)

E22.0 Acromegaly and pituitary gigantism `HCC`
> Overproduction of growth hormone
> EXCLUDES 1 constitutional gigantism (E34.4)
> constitutional tall stature (E34.4)
> increased secretion from endocrine pancreas of growth hormone-releasing hormone (E16.8)

E22.1 Hyperprolactinemia `HCC`
> Use additional code for adverse effect, if applicable, to identify drug (T36-T50 with fifth or sixth character 5)

E22.2 Syndrome of inappropriate secretion of antidiuretic hormone `HCC`

E22.8 Other hyperfunction of pituitary gland `HCC`
> Central precocious puberty

E22.9 Hyperfunction of pituitary gland, unspecified `HCC` ▽

✓4th E23 Hypofunction and other disorders of the pituitary gland
> INCLUDES the listed conditions whether the disorder is in the pituitary or the hypothalamus
> EXCLUDES 1 postprocedural hypopituitarism (E89.3)

E23.0 Hypopituitarism `HCC`
> Fertile eunuch syndrome
> Hypogonadotropic hypogonadism
> Idiopathic growth hormone deficiency
> Isolated deficiency of gonadotropin
> Isolated deficiency of growth hormone
> Isolated deficiency of pituitary hormone
> Kallmann's syndrome
> Lorain-Levi short stature
> Necrosis of pituitary gland (postpartum)
> Panhypopituitarism
> Pituitary cachexia
> Pituitary insufficiency NOS
> Pituitary short stature
> Sheehan's syndrome
> Simmonds' disease

E23.1 Drug-induced hypopituitarism `HCC`
> Use additional code for adverse effect, if applicable, to identify drug (T36-T50 with fifth or sixth character 5)

E23.2 Diabetes insipidus `HCC`
> EXCLUDES 1 nephrogenic diabetes insipidus (N25.1)

E23.3 Hypothalamic dysfunction, not elsewhere classified `HCC`
> EXCLUDES 1 Prader-Willi syndrome (Q87.1)
> Russell-Silver syndrome (Q87.1)

E23.6 Other disorders of pituitary gland `HCC`
> Abscess of pituitary   Adiposogenital dystrophy

E23.7 Disorder of pituitary gland, unspecified `HCC` ▽

✓4th E24 Cushing's syndrome
> EXCLUDES 1 congenital adrenal hyperplasia (E25.0)

E24.0 Pituitary-dependent Cushing's disease `HCC`
> Overproduction of pituitary ACTH
> Pituitary-dependent hypercorticalism

E24.1 Nelson's syndrome `HCC`

E24.2 Drug-induced Cushing's syndrome `HCC`
> Use additional code for adverse effect, if applicable, to identify drug (T36-T50 with fifth or sixth character 5)

E24.3 Ectopic ACTH syndrome `HCC`

E24.4 Alcohol-induced pseudo-Cushing's syndrome `HCC`

E24.8 Other Cushing's syndrome `HCC`

E24.9 Cushing's syndrome, unspecified `HCC` ▽

☑ Additional Character Req   ✓7th Placeholder Alert   Manifestation   `HCC` CMS-HCC Condition   ▽ Unspecified Code   ▶◄ Revised Text   ● New Code   ▲ Revised Code Title

Chapter 4. Endocrine, Nutritional, and Metabolic Diseases

E25–E31.1

✓4ᵗʰ E25 Adrenogenital disorders

INCLUDES adrenogenital syndromes, virilizing or feminizing, whether acquired or due to adrenal hyperplasia
consequent on inborn enzyme defects in hormone synthesis
female adrenal pseudohermaphroditism
female heterosexual precocious pseudopuberty
male isosexual precocious pseudopuberty
male macrogenitosomia praecox
male sexual precocity with adrenal hyperplasia
male virilization (female)

EXCLUDES 1 indeterminate sex and pseudohermaphroditism (Q56)
chromosomal abnormalities (Q90-Q99)

E25.0 Congenital adrenogenital disorders associated with enzyme deficiency HCC
Congenital adrenal hyperplasia
21-Hydroxylase deficiency
Salt-losing congenital adrenal hyperplasia

E25.8 Other adrenogenital disorders HCC
Idiopathic adrenogenital disorder
Use additional code for adverse effect, if applicable, to identify drug (T36-T50 with fifth or sixth character 5)

E25.9 Adrenogenital disorder, unspecified HCC ▽
Adrenogenital syndrome NOS

✓4ᵗʰ E26 Hyperaldosteronism

✓5ᵗʰ E26.0 Primary hyperaldosteronism

E26.01 Conn's syndrome HCC
Code also adrenal adenoma (D35.0-)

E26.02 Glucocorticoid-remediable aldosteronism HCC
Familial aldosteronism type I
DEF: Rare autosomal dominant familial form of primary aldosteronism in which the secretion of aldosterone is under the influence of adrenocorticotrophic hormone (ACTH) rather than the renin-angiotensin mechanism; moderate hypersecretion of aldosterone and suppressed plasma renin activity that are rapidly reversed by administration of glucosteroids; symptoms include hypertension and mild hypokalemia.

E26.09 Other primary hyperaldosteronism HCC
Primary aldosteronism due to adrenal hyperplasia (bilateral)

E26.1 Secondary hyperaldosteronism HCC

✓5ᵗʰ E26.8 Other hyperaldosteronism

E26.81 Bartter's syndrome HCC

E26.89 Other hyperaldosteronism HCC

E26.9 Hyperaldosteronism, unspecified HCC ▽
Aldosteronism NOS
Hyperaldosteronism NOS

✓4ᵗʰ E27 Other disorders of adrenal gland

E27.0 Other adrenocortical overactivity HCC
Overproduction of ACTH, not associated with Cushing's disease
Premature adrenarche
EXCLUDES 1 Cushing's syndrome (E24.-)

E27.1 Primary adrenocortical insufficiency HCC
Addison's disease
Autoimmune adrenalitis
EXCLUDES 1 Addison only phenotype adrenoleukodystrophy (E71.528)
amyloidosis (E85.-)
tuberculous Addison's disease (A18.7)
Waterhouse-Friderichsen syndrome (A39.1)

E27.2 Addisonian crisis HCC
Adrenal crisis
Adrenocortical crisis

E27.3 Drug-induced adrenocortical insufficiency HCC
Use additional code for adverse effect, if applicable, to identify drug (T36-T50 with fifth or sixth character 5)

✓5ᵗʰ E27.4 Other and unspecified adrenocortical insufficiency
EXCLUDES 1 adrenoleukodystrophy [Addison-Schilder] (E71.528)
Waterhouse-Friderichsen syndrome (A39.1)

E27.40 Unspecified adrenocortical insufficiency HCC ▽
Adrenocortical insufficiency NOS
Hypoaldosteronism

E27.49 Other adrenocortical insufficiency HCC
Adrenal hemorrhage
Adrenal infarction

E27.5 Adrenomedullary hyperfunction HCC
Adrenomedullary hyperplasia
Catecholamine hypersecretion

E27.8 Other specified disorders of adrenal gland HCC
Abnormality of cortisol-binding globulin

E27.9 Disorder of adrenal gland, unspecified HCC ▽

✓4ᵗʰ E28 Ovarian dysfunction

EXCLUDES 1 isolated gonadotropin deficiency (E23.0)
postprocedural ovarian failure (E89.4-)

E28.0 Estrogen excess ♀
Use additional code for adverse effect, if applicable, to identify drug (T36-T50 with fifth or sixth character 5)

E28.1 Androgen excess ♀
Hypersecretion of ovarian androgens
Use additional code for adverse effect, if applicable, to identify drug (T36-T50 with fifth or sixth character 5)

E28.2 Polycystic ovarian syndrome ♀
Sclerocystic ovary syndrome
Stein-Leventhal syndrome

✓5ᵗʰ E28.3 Primary ovarian failure
EXCLUDES 1 pure gonadal dysgenesis (Q99.1)
Turner's syndrome (Q96.-)

✓6ᵗʰ E28.31 Premature menopause

E28.310 Symptomatic premature menopause Ⓐ♀
Symptoms such as flushing, sleeplessness, headache, lack of concentration, associated with premature menopause

E28.319 Asymptomatic premature menopause Ⓐ♀
Premature menopause NOS

E28.39 Other primary ovarian failure ♀
Decreased estrogen
Resistant ovary syndrome

E28.8 Other ovarian dysfunction ♀
Ovarian hyperfunction NOS
EXCLUDES 1 postprocedural ovarian failure (E89.4-)

E28.9 Ovarian dysfunction, unspecified ♀▽

✓4ᵗʰ E29 Testicular dysfunction

EXCLUDES 1 androgen insensitivity syndrome (E34.5-)
azoospermia or oligospermia NOS (N46.0-N46.1)
isolated gonadotropin deficiency (E23.0)
Klinefelter's syndrome (Q98.0-Q98.1, Q98.4)

E29.0 Testicular hyperfunction ♂
Hypersecretion of testicular hormones

E29.1 Testicular hypofunction ♂
Defective biosynthesis of testicular androgen NOS
5-delta-Reductase deficiency (with male pseudohermaphroditism)
Testicular hypogonadism NOS
Use additional code for adverse effect, if applicable, to identify drug (T36-T50 with fifth or sixth character 5)
EXCLUDES 1 postprocedural testicular hypofunction (E89.5)

E29.8 Other testicular dysfunction ♂

E29.9 Testicular dysfunction, unspecified ♂▽

✓4ᵗʰ E30 Disorders of puberty, not elsewhere classified

E30.0 Delayed puberty
Constitutional delay of puberty
Delayed sexual development

E30.1 Precocious puberty Ⓟ
Precocious menstruation
EXCLUDES 1 Albright (-McCune) (-Sternberg) syndrome (Q78.1)
central precocious puberty (E22.8)
congenital adrenal hyperplasia (E25.0)
female heterosexual precocious pseudopuberty (E25.-)
male isosexual precocious pseudopuberty (E25.-)

E30.8 Other disorders of puberty Ⓟ
Premature thelarche

E30.9 Disorder of puberty, unspecified ▽

✓4ᵗʰ E31 Polyglandular dysfunction

EXCLUDES 1 ataxia telangiectasia [Louis-Bar] (G11.3)
dystrophia myotonica [Steinert] (G71.11)
pseudohypoparathyroidism (E20.1)

E31.0 Autoimmune polyglandular failure HCC
Schmidt's syndrome

E31.1 Polyglandular hyperfunction HCC
EXCLUDES 1 multiple endocrine adenomatosis (E31.2-)
multiple endocrine neoplasia (E31.2-)

EXCLUDES 1 Not coded here   **EXCLUDES 2** Not included here   Ⓝ Newborn Age: 0   Ⓟ Pediatric Age: 0-17   Ⓜ Maternity Age: 12-55   Ⓐ Adult Age: 15-124

516   ICD-10-CM 2018

✓5ᵗʰ E31.2 Multiple endocrine neoplasia [MEN] syndromes
Multiple endocrine adenomatosis
Code also any associated malignancies and other conditions associated with the syndromes

    E31.20 Multiple endocrine neoplasia [MEN] syndrome, unspecified   HCC ▽
        Multiple endocrine adenomatosis NOS
        Multiple endocrine neoplasia [MEN] syndrome NOS

    E31.21 Multiple endocrine neoplasia [MEN] type I   HCC
        Wermer's syndrome

    E31.22 Multiple endocrine neoplasia [MEN] type IIA   HCC
        Sipple's syndrome

    E31.23 Multiple endocrine neoplasia [MEN] type IIB   HCC

E31.8 Other polyglandular dysfunction   HCC
E31.9 Polyglandular dysfunction, unspecified   HCC ▽

✓4ᵗʰ E32 Diseases of thymus
EXCLUDES 1   aplasia or hypoplasia of thymus with immunodeficiency (D82.1)
        myasthenia gravis (G70.0)

E32.0 Persistent hyperplasia of thymus   HCC
    Hypertrophy of thymus

E32.1 Abscess of thymus   HCC
E32.8 Other diseases of thymus   HCC
EXCLUDES 1   aplasia or hypoplasia with immunodeficiency (D82.1)
        thymoma (D15.0)

E32.9 Disease of thymus, unspecified   HCC ▽

✓4ᵗʰ E34 Other endocrine disorders
EXCLUDES 1   pseudohypoparathyroidism (E20.1)

E34.0 Carcinoid syndrome   HCC
    NOTE   May be used as an additional code to identify functional activity associated with a carcinoid tumor.

E34.1 Other hypersecretion of intestinal hormones
E34.2 Ectopic hormone secretion, not elsewhere classified
EXCLUDES 1   ectopic ACTH syndrome (E24.3)

E34.3 Short stature due to endocrine disorder
Constitutional short stature
Laron-type short stature
EXCLUDES 1   achondroplastic short stature (Q77.4)
        hypochondroplastic short stature (Q77.4)
        nutritional short stature (E45)
        pituitary short stature (E23.0)
        progeria (E34.8)
        renal short stature (N25.0)
        Russell-Silver syndrome (Q87.1)
        short-limbed stature with immunodeficiency (D82.2)
        short stature in specific dysmorphic syndromes— code to syndrome—see Alphabetical Index
        short stature NOS (R62.52)

E34.4 Constitutional tall stature   HCC
    Constitutional gigantism

✓5ᵗʰ E34.5 Androgen insensitivity syndrome
    E34.50 Androgen insensitivity syndrome, unspecified   ▽
        Androgen insensitivity NOS

    E34.51 Complete androgen insensitivity syndrome
        Complete androgen insensitivity
        de Quervain syndrome
        Goldberg-Maxwell syndrome

    E34.52 Partial androgen insensitivity syndrome
        Partial androgen insensitivity
        Reifenstein syndrome

E34.8 Other specified endocrine disorders
Pineal gland dysfunction
Progeria
EXCLUDES 2   pseudohypoparathyroidism (E20.1)

E34.9 Endocrine disorder, unspecified   ▽
Endocrine disturbance NOS
Hormone disturbance NOS

E35 Disorders of endocrine glands in diseases classified elsewhere
Code first underlying disease, such as:
    late congenital syphilis of thymus gland [Dubois disease] (A50.5)
Use additional code, if applicable, to identify:
    sequelae of tuberculosis of other organs (B90.8)
EXCLUDES 1   Echinococcus granulosus infection of thyroid gland (B67.3)
        meningococcal hemorrhagic adrenalitis (A39.1)
        syphilis of endocrine gland (A52.79)
        tuberculosis of adrenal gland, except calcification (A18.7)
        tuberculosis of endocrine gland NEC (A18.82)
        tuberculosis of thyroid gland (A18.81)
        Waterhouse-Friderichsen syndrome (A39.1)

Intraoperative complications of endocrine system (E36)

✓4ᵗʰ E36 Intraoperative complications of endocrine system
EXCLUDES 2   postprocedural endocrine and metabolic complications and disorders, not elsewhere classified (E89.-)

✓5ᵗʰ E36.0 Intraoperative hemorrhage and hematoma of an endocrine system organ or structure complicating a procedure
EXCLUDES 1   intraoperative hemorrhage and hematoma of an endocrine system organ or structure due to accidental puncture or laceration during a procedure (E36.1-)

    E36.01 Intraoperative hemorrhage and hematoma of an endocrine system organ or structure complicating an endocrine system procedure

    E36.02 Intraoperative hemorrhage and hematoma of an endocrine system organ or structure complicating other procedure

✓5ᵗʰ E36.1 Accidental puncture and laceration of an endocrine system organ or structure during a procedure
    E36.11 Accidental puncture and laceration of an endocrine system organ or structure during an endocrine system procedure

    E36.12 Accidental puncture and laceration of an endocrine system organ or structure during other procedure

E36.8 Other intraoperative complications of endocrine system
Use additional code, if applicable, to further specify disorder

Malnutrition (E40-E46)

EXCLUDES 1   intestinal malabsorption (K90.-)
        sequelae of protein-calorie malnutrition (E64.0)
EXCLUDES 2   nutritional anemias (D50-D53)
        starvation (T73.0)

E40 Kwashiorkor   HCC
Severe malnutrition with nutritional edema with dyspigmentation of skin and hair
EXCLUDES 1   marasmic kwashiorkor (E42)

E41 Nutritional marasmus   HCC
Severe malnutrition with marasmus
EXCLUDES 1   marasmic kwashiorkor (E42)
DEF: Protein-calorie malabsorption or malnutrition in children; characterized by tissue wasting, dehydration, and subcutaneous fat depletion; may occur with infectious disease; also called infantile atrophy.

E42 Marasmic kwashiorkor   HCC
Intermediate form severe protein-calorie malnutrition
Severe protein-calorie malnutrition with signs of both kwashiorkor and marasmus

E43 Unspecified severe protein-calorie malnutrition   HCC ▽
Starvation edema

✓4ᵗʰ E44 Protein-calorie malnutrition of moderate and mild degree
    E44.0 Moderate protein-calorie malnutrition   HCC
    E44.1 Mild protein-calorie malnutrition   HCC

E45 Retarded development following protein-calorie malnutrition   HCC
Nutritional short stature
Nutritional stunting
Physical retardation due to malnutrition

E46 Unspecified protein-calorie malnutrition   HCC ▽
Malnutrition NOS
Protein-calorie imbalance NOS
EXCLUDES 1   nutritional deficiency NOS (E63.9)

Other nutritional deficiencies (E50-E64)

EXCLUDES 2   nutritional anemias (D50-D53)

✓4ᵗʰ E50 Vitamin A deficiency
EXCLUDES 1   sequelae of vitamin A deficiency (E64.1)

    E50.0 Vitamin A deficiency with conjunctival xerosis
    E50.1 Vitamin A deficiency with Bitot's spot and conjunctival xerosis
        Bitot's spot in the young child
        DEF: Vitamin A deficiency with conjunctival dryness, superficial spots of keratinized epithelium.

    E50.2 Vitamin A deficiency with corneal xerosis
    E50.3 Vitamin A deficiency with corneal ulceration and xerosis
    E50.4 Vitamin A deficiency with keratomalacia
        DEF: Vitamin A deficiency creating corneal dryness; progresses to corneal insensitivity, softness, and necrosis; usually bilateral.

Chapter 4. Endocrine, Nutritional, and Metabolic Diseases

E5Ø.5–E66.1

E5Ø.5   **Vitamin A deficiency with night blindness**

E5Ø.6   **Vitamin A deficiency with xerophthalmic scars of cornea**

E5Ø.7   **Other ocular manifestations of vitamin A deficiency**
Xerophthalmia NOS

E5Ø.8   **Other manifestations of vitamin A deficiency**
Follicular keratosis
Xeroderma

E5Ø.9   **Vitamin A deficiency, unspecified** ▽
Hypovitaminosis A NOS

✓4ᵗʰ **E51**   **Thiamine deficiency**
EXCLUDES 1   *sequelae of thiamine deficiency (E64.8)*

    ✓5ᵗʰ **E51.1**   **Beriberi**

E51.11   **Dry beriberi**
Beriberi NOS
Beriberi with polyneuropathy

E51.12   **Wet beriberi**
Beriberi with cardiovascular manifestations
Cardiovascular beriberi
Shoshin disease

E51.2   **Wernicke's encephalopathy**

E51.8   **Other manifestations of thiamine deficiency**

E51.9   **Thiamine deficiency, unspecified** ▽

E52   **Niacin deficiency [pellagra]**
Niacin (-tryptophan) deficiency
Nicotinamide deficiency
Pellagra (alcoholic)
EXCLUDES 1   *sequelae of niacin deficiency (E64.8)*

✓4ᵗʰ **E53**   **Deficiency of other B group vitamins**
EXCLUDES 1   *sequelae of vitamin B deficiency (E64.8)*

E53.Ø   **Riboflavin deficiency**
Ariboflavinosis
Vitamin B2 deficiency

E53.1   **Pyridoxine deficiency**
Vitamin B6 deficiency
EXCLUDES 1   *pyridoxine-responsive sideroblastic anemia (D64.3)*

E53.8   **Deficiency of other specified B group vitamins**
Biotin deficiency
Cyanocobalamin deficiency
Folate deficiency
Folic acid deficiency
Pantothenic acid deficiency
Vitamin B12 deficiency
EXCLUDES 1   *folate deficiency anemia (D52.-)*
                vitamin B12 deficiency anemia (D51.-)

E53.9   **Vitamin B deficiency, unspecified** ▽

E54   **Ascorbic acid deficiency**
Deficiency of vitamin C
Scurvy
EXCLUDES 1   *scorbutic anemia (D53.2)*
                sequelae of vitamin C deficiency (E64.2)
DEF: Vitamin C deficiency causing swollen gums, myalgia, weight loss, and weakness.

✓4ᵗʰ **E55**   **Vitamin D deficiency**
EXCLUDES 1   *adult osteomalacia (M83.-)*
                osteoporosis (M8Ø.-)
                sequelae of rickets (E64.3)

E55.Ø   **Rickets, active**
Infantile osteomalacia
Juvenile osteomalacia
EXCLUDES 1   *celiac rickets (K9Ø.Ø)*
                Crohn's rickets (K5Ø.-)
                hereditary vitamin D-dependent rickets (E83.32)
                inactive rickets (E64.3)
                renal rickets (N25.Ø)
                sequelae of rickets (E64.3)
                vitamin D-resistant rickets (E83.31)

E55.9   **Vitamin D deficiency, unspecified** ▽
Avitaminosis D

✓4ᵗʰ **E56**   **Other vitamin deficiencies**
EXCLUDES 1   *sequelae of other vitamin deficiencies (E64.8)*

E56.Ø   **Deficiency of vitamin E**

E56.1   **Deficiency of vitamin K**
EXCLUDES 1   *deficiency of coagulation factor due to vitamin K deficiency (D68.4)*
                vitamin K deficiency of newborn (P53)

E56.8   **Deficiency of other vitamins**

E56.9   **Vitamin deficiency, unspecified** ▽

E58   **Dietary calcium deficiency**
EXCLUDES 1   *disorders of calcium metabolism (E83.5-)*
                sequelae of calcium deficiency (E64.8)

E59   **Dietary selenium deficiency**
Keshan disease
EXCLUDES 1   *sequelae of selenium deficiency (E64.8)*

E6Ø   **Dietary zinc deficiency**

✓4ᵗʰ **E61**   **Deficiency of other nutrient elements**
Use additional code for adverse effect, if applicable, to identify drug (T36-T5Ø with fifth or sixth character 5)
EXCLUDES 1   *disorders of mineral metabolism (E83.-)*
                iodine deficiency related thyroid disorders (EØØ-EØ2)
                sequelae of malnutrition and other nutritional deficiencies (E64.-)

E61.Ø   **Copper deficiency**

E61.1   **Iron deficiency**
EXCLUDES 1   *iron deficiency anemia (D5Ø.-)*

E61.2   **Magnesium deficiency**

E61.3   **Manganese deficiency**

E61.4   **Chromium deficiency**

E61.5   **Molybdenum deficiency**

E61.6   **Vanadium deficiency**

E61.7   **Deficiency of multiple nutrient elements**

E61.8   **Deficiency of other specified nutrient elements**

E61.9   **Deficiency of nutrient element, unspecified** ▽

✓4ᵗʰ **E63**   **Other nutritional deficiencies**
EXCLUDES 1   *dehydration (E86.Ø)*
                failure to thrive, adult (R62.7)
                failure to thrive, child (R62.51)
                feeding problems in newborn (P92.-)
                sequelae of malnutrition and other nutritional deficiencies (E64.-)

E63.Ø   **Essential fatty acid [EFA] deficiency**

E63.1   **Imbalance of constituents of food intake**

E63.8   **Other specified nutritional deficiencies**

E63.9   **Nutritional deficiency, unspecified** ▽

✓4ᵗʰ **E64**   **Sequelae of malnutrition and other nutritional deficiencies**
NOTE   This category is to be used to indicate conditions in categories E43, E44, E46, E5Ø-E63 as the cause of sequelae, which are themselves classified elsewhere. The 'sequelae' include conditions specified as such; they also include the late effects of diseases classifiable to the above categories if the disease itself is no longer present.
Code first condition resulting from (sequela) of malnutrition and other nutritional deficiencies

E64.Ø   **Sequelae of protein-calorie malnutrition**   HCC
EXCLUDES 2   *retarded development following protein-calorie malnutrition (E45)*

E64.1   **Sequelae of vitamin A deficiency**

E64.2   **Sequelae of vitamin C deficiency**

E64.3   **Sequelae of rickets**

E64.8   **Sequelae of other nutritional deficiencies**

E64.9   **Sequelae of unspecified nutritional deficiency** ▽

Overweight, obesity and other hyperalimentation (E65-E68)

E65   **Localized adiposity**
Fat pad

✓4ᵗʰ **E66**   **Overweight and obesity**
Code first obesity complicating pregnancy, childbirth and the puerperium, if applicable (O99.21-)
Use additional code to identify body mass index (BMI), if known (Z68.-)
EXCLUDES 1   *adiposogenital dystrophy (E23.6)*
                lipomatosis NOS (E88.2)
                lipomatosis dolorosa [Dercum] (E88.2)
                Prader-Willi syndrome (Q87.1)

    ✓5ᵗʰ **E66.Ø**   **Obesity due to excess calories**

E66.Ø1   **Morbid (severe) obesity due to excess calories**   HCC
EXCLUDES 1   *morbid (severe) obesity with alveolar hypoventilation (E66.2)*

E66.Ø9   **Other obesity due to excess calories**

E66.1   **Drug-induced obesity**
Use additional code for adverse effect, if applicable, to identify drug (T36-T5Ø with fifth or sixth character 5)

EXCLUDES 1 Not coded here   *EXCLUDES 2* Not included here   N Newborn Age: 0   P Pediatric Age: 0-17   M Maternity Age: 12-55   A Adult Age: 15-124

518   ICD-10-CM 2018

E66.2 Morbid (severe) obesity with alveolar hypoventilation   HCC
     Obesity hypoventilation syndrome (OHS)
     Pickwickian syndrome

E66.3 Overweight

E66.8 Other obesity

E66.9 Obesity, unspecified   ▽
     Obesity NOS

✓4ᵗʰ **E67** Other hyperalimentation
     EXCLUDES 1   hyperalimentation NOS (R63.2)
              sequelae of hyperalimentation (E68)

E67.0 Hypervitaminosis A

E67.1 Hypercarotinemia

E67.2 Megavitamin-B6 syndrome

E67.3 Hypervitaminosis D

E67.8 Other specified hyperalimentation

E68 Sequelae of hyperalimentation
     Code first condition resulting from (sequela) of hyperalimentation

Metabolic disorders (E70-E88)

EXCLUDES 1   androgen insensitivity syndrome (E34.5-)
          congenital adrenal hyperplasia (E25.0)
          Ehlers-Danlos syndrome (Q79.6)
          hemolytic anemias attributable to enzyme disorders (D55.-)
          Marfan's syndrome (Q87.4)
          5-alpha-reductase deficiency (E29.1)

✓4ᵗʰ **E70** Disorders of aromatic amino-acid metabolism

E70.0 Classical phenylketonuria   HCC

E70.1 Other hyperphenylalaninemias   HCC

✓5ᵗʰ **E70.2** Disorders of tyrosine metabolism
     EXCLUDES 1   transitory tyrosinemia of newborn (P74.5)

     E70.20 Disorder of tyrosine metabolism, unspecified   HCC ▽

     E70.21 Tyrosinemia   HCC
         Hypertyrosinemia

     E70.29 Other disorders of tyrosine metabolism   HCC
         Alkaptonuria
         Ochronosis

✓5ᵗʰ **E70.3** Albinism

     E70.30 Albinism, unspecified   HCC ▽

     ✓6ᵗʰ **E70.31** Ocular albinism

         E70.310 X-linked ocular albinism   HCC

         E70.311 Autosomal recessive ocular albinism   HCC

         E70.318 Other ocular albinism   HCC

         E70.319 Ocular albinism, unspecified   HCC ▽

     ✓6ᵗʰ **E70.32** Oculocutaneous albinism
         EXCLUDES 1   Chediak-Higashi syndrome (E70.330)
               Hermansky-Pudlak syndrome (E70.331)

         E70.320 Tyrosinase negative oculocutaneous albinism   HCC
             Albinism I
             Oculocutaneous albinism ty-neg

         E70.321 Tyrosinase positive oculocutaneous albinism   HCC
             Albinism II
             Oculocutaneous albinism ty-pos

         E70.328 Other oculocutaneous albinism   HCC
             Cross syndrome

         E70.329 Oculocutaneous albinism, unspecified   HCC ▽

     ✓6ᵗʰ **E70.33** Albinism with hematologic abnormality

         E70.330 Chediak-Higashi syndrome   HCC

         E70.331 Hermansky-Pudlak syndrome   HCC

         E70.338 Other albinism with hematologic abnormality   HCC

         E70.339 Albinism with hematologic abnormality, unspecified   HCC ▽

     E70.39 Other specified albinism   HCC
         Piebaldism

✓5ᵗʰ **E70.4** Disorders of histidine metabolism

     E70.40 Disorders of histidine metabolism, unspecified   HCC ▽

     E70.41 Histidinemia   HCC

     E70.49 Other disorders of histidine metabolism   HCC

E70.5 Disorders of tryptophan metabolism   HCC

E70.8 Other disorders of aromatic amino-acid metabolism   HCC

E70.9 Disorder of aromatic amino-acid metabolism, unspecified   HCC ▽

✓4ᵗʰ **E71** Disorders of branched-chain amino-acid metabolism and fatty-acid metabolism

E71.0 Maple-syrup-urine disease   HCC

✓5ᵗʰ **E71.1** Other disorders of branched-chain amino-acid metabolism

     ✓6ᵗʰ **E71.11** Branched-chain organic acidurias

         E71.110 Isovaleric acidemia   HCC

         E71.111 3-methylglutaconic aciduria   HCC

         E71.118 Other branched-chain organic acidurias   HCC

     ✓6ᵗʰ **E71.12** Disorders of propionate metabolism

         E71.120 Methylmalonic acidemia   HCC

         E71.121 Propionic acidemia   HCC

         E71.128 Other disorders of propionate metabolism   HCC

     E71.19 Other disorders of branched-chain amino-acid metabolism   HCC
         Hyperleucine-isoleucinemia
         Hypervalinemia

E71.2 Disorder of branched-chain amino-acid metabolism, unspecified   HCC ▽

✓5ᵗʰ **E71.3** Disorders of fatty-acid metabolism
     EXCLUDES 1   peroxisomal disorders (E71.5)
               Refsum's disease (G60.1)
               Schilder's disease (G37.0)
     EXCLUDES 2   carnitine deficiency due to inborn error of metabolism (E71.42)

     E71.30 Disorder of fatty-acid metabolism, unspecified   ▽

     ✓6ᵗʰ **E71.31** Disorders of fatty-acid oxidation

         E71.310 Long chain/very long chain acyl CoA dehydrogenase deficiency   HCC
             LCAD   VLCAD

         E71.311 Medium chain acyl CoA dehydrogenase deficiency   HCC
             MCAD

         E71.312 Short chain acyl CoA dehydrogenase deficiency   HCC
             SCAD

         E71.313 Glutaric aciduria type II   HCC
             Glutaric aciduria type II A
             Glutaric aciduria type II B
             Glutaric aciduria type II C
             EXCLUDES 1   glutaric aciduria (type 1) NOS (E72.3)

         E71.314 Muscle carnitine palmitoyltransferase deficiency   HCC

         E71.318 Other disorders of fatty-acid oxidation   HCC

     E71.32 Disorders of ketone metabolism   HCC

     E71.39 Other disorders of fatty-acid metabolism   HCC

✓5ᵗʰ **E71.4** Disorders of carnitine metabolism
     EXCLUDES 1   muscle carnitine palmitoyltransferase deficiency (E71.314)

     E71.40 Disorder of carnitine metabolism, unspecified   HCC ▽

     E71.41 Primary carnitine deficiency   HCC

     E71.42 Carnitine deficiency due to inborn errors of metabolism   HCC
         Code also associated inborn error or metabolism

     E71.43 Iatrogenic carnitine deficiency   HCC
         Carnitine deficiency due to hemodialysis
         Carnitine deficiency due to Valproic acid therapy

     ✓6ᵗʰ **E71.44** Other secondary carnitine deficiency

         E71.440 Ruvalcaba-Myhre-Smith syndrome   HCC

         E71.448 Other secondary carnitine deficiency   HCC

✓5ᵗʰ **E71.5** Peroxisomal disorders
     EXCLUDES 1   Schilder's disease (G37.0)

     E71.50 Peroxisomal disorder, unspecified   HCC ▽

     ✓6ᵗʰ **E71.51** Disorders of peroxisome biogenesis
         Group 1 peroxisomal disorders
         EXCLUDES 1   Refsum's disease (G60.1)

         E71.510 Zellweger syndrome   HCC

         E71.511 Neonatal adrenoleukodystrophy   HCC
             EXCLUDES 1   X-linked adrenoleuko- dystrophy (E71.52-)

         E71.518 Other disorders of peroxisome biogenesis   HCC

☑ Additional Character Req   ✓x7ᵗʰ Placeholder Alert   Manifestation   HCC CMS-HCC Condition   ▽ Unspecified Code   ◄► Revised Text   ● New Code   ▲ Revised Code Title

✓6ᵗʰ **E71.52** **X-linked adrenoleukodystrophy**

     E71.520 **Childhood cerebral X-linked** HCC
         adrenoleukodystrophy

     E71.521 **Adolescent X-linked** HCC
         adrenoleukodystrophy

     E71.522 **Adrenomyeloneuropathy** HCC

     E71.528 **Other X-linked adrenoleukodystrophy** HCC
         Addison only phenotype
           adrenoleukodystrophy
         Addison-Schilder adrenoleukodystrophy

     E71.529 **X-linked adrenoleukodystrophy,** HCC ▽
         unspecified type

E71.53 **Other group 2 peroxisomal disorders** HCC

✓6ᵗʰ **E71.54** **Other peroxisomal disorders**

     E71.540 **Rhizomelic chondrodysplasia** HCC
         punctata
         EXCLUDES 1   *chondrodysplasia punctata NOS*
             (Q77.3)

     E71.541 **Zellweger-like syndrome** HCC

     E71.542 **Other group 3 peroxisomal disorders** HCC

     E71.548 **Other peroxisomal disorders** HCC

✓4ᵗʰ **E72** **Other disorders of amino-acid metabolism**

     EXCLUDES 1   *disorders of:*
         aromatic amino-acid metabolism (E70.-)
         branched-chain amino-acid metabolism (E71.0-E71.2)
         fatty-acid metabolism (E71.3)
         purine and pyrimidine metabolism (E79.-)
         gout (M1A.-, M10.-)

✓5ᵗʰ **E72.0** **Disorders of amino-acid transport**

     EXCLUDES 1   *disorders of tryptophan metabolism (E70.5)*

     E72.00 **Disorders of amino-acid transport,** HCC ▽
         unspecified

     E72.01 **Cystinuria** HCC

     E72.02 **Hartnup's disease** HCC

     E72.03 **Lowe's syndrome**
         Use additional code for associated glaucoma (H42)

     E72.04 **Cystinosis**
         Fanconi (-de Toni) (-Debré) syndrome with cystinosis
         EXCLUDES 1   *Fanconi (-de Toni) (-Debré) syndrome*
             without cystinosis (E72.09)

     E72.09 **Other disorders of amino-acid transport** HCC
         Fanconi (-de Toni) (-Debré) syndrome, unspecified

✓5ᵗʰ **E72.1** **Disorders of sulfur-bearing amino-acid metabolism**

     EXCLUDES 1   *cystinosis (E72.04)*
         cystinuria (E72.01)
         transcobalamin II deficiency (D51.2)

     E72.10 **Disorders of sulfur-bearing amino-acid** HCC ▽
         metabolism, unspecified

     E72.11 **Homocystinuria** HCC
         Cystathionine synthase deficiency

     E72.12 **Methylenetetrahydrofolate reductase deficiency** HCC

     E72.19 **Other disorders of sulfur-bearing amino-acid** HCC
         metabolism
         Cystathioninuria
         Methioninemia
         Sulfite oxidase deficiency

✓5ᵗʰ **E72.2** **Disorders of urea cycle metabolism**

     EXCLUDES 1   *disorders of ornithine metabolism (E72.4)*

     E72.20 **Disorder of urea cycle metabolism,** HCC ▽
         unspecified
         Hyperammonemia
         EXCLUDES 1   *hyperammonemia- hyperornithinemia-*
             homocitrullinemia syndrome (E72.4)
             transient hyperammonemia of newborn
               (P74.6)

     E72.21 **Argininemia** HCC

     E72.22 **Arginosuccinic aciduria** HCC

     E72.23 **Citrullinemia** HCC

     E72.29 **Other disorders of urea cycle metabolism** HCC

E72.3 **Disorders of lysine and hydroxylysine metabolism** HCC
     Glutaric aciduria NOS   Hydroxylysinemia
     Glutaric aciduria (type I)   Hyperlysinemia
     EXCLUDES 1   *glutaric aciduria type II (E71.313)*
         Refsum's disease (G60.1)
         Zellweger syndrome (E71.510)

E72.4 **Disorders of ornithine metabolism** HCC
     Hyperammonemia-hyperornithinemia-homocitrullinemia
       syndrome
     Ornithinemia (types I, II)
     Ornithine transcarbamylase deficiency
     EXCLUDES 1   *hereditary choroidal dystrophy (H31.2-)*

✓5ᵗʰ **E72.5** **Disorders of glycine metabolism**

     E72.50 **Disorder of glycine metabolism, unspecified** HCC ▽

     E72.51 **Non-ketotic hyperglycinemia** HCC

     E72.52 **Trimethylaminuria** HCC

     E72.53 **Hyperoxaluria** HCC
         Oxalosis
         Oxaluria

     E72.59 **Other disorders of glycine metabolism** HCC
         D-glycericacidemia
         Hyperhydroxyprolinemia
         Hyperprolinemia (types I, II)
         Sarcosinemia

E72.8 **Other specified disorders of amino-acid metabolism** HCC
     Disorders of beta-amino-acid metabolism
     Disorders of gamma-glutamyl cycle

E72.9 **Disorder of amino-acid metabolism, unspecified** HCC ▽

✓4ᵗʰ **E73** **Lactose intolerance**

E73.0 **Congenital lactase deficiency**

E73.1 **Secondary lactase deficiency**

E73.8 **Other lactose intolerance**

E73.9 **Lactose intolerance, unspecified** ▽

✓4ᵗʰ **E74** **Other disorders of carbohydrate metabolism**

     EXCLUDES 1   *diabetes mellitus (E08-E13)*
         hypoglycemia NOS (E16.2)
         increased secretion of glucagon (E16.3)
         mucopolysaccharidosis (E76.0-E76.3)

✓5ᵗʰ **E74.0** **Glycogen storage disease**

     E74.00 **Glycogen storage disease, unspecified** HCC ▽

     E74.01 **von Gierke disease** HCC
         Type I glycogen storage disease

     E74.02 **Pompe disease** HCC
         Cardiac glycogenosis
         Type II glycogen storage disease

     E74.03 **Cori disease** HCC
         Forbes disease
         Type III glycogen storage disease

     E74.04 **McArdle disease** HCC
         Type V glycogen storage disease

     E74.09 **Other glycogen storage disease** HCC
         Andersen disease
         Hers disease
         Tauri disease
         Glycogen storage disease, types 0, IV, VI-XI
         Liver phosphorylase deficiency
         Muscle phosphofructokinase deficiency

✓5ᵗʰ **E74.1** **Disorders of fructose metabolism**

     EXCLUDES 1   *muscle phosphofructokinase deficiency (E74.09)*

     E74.10 **Disorder of fructose metabolism, unspecified** ▽

     E74.11 **Essential fructosuria**
         Fructokinase deficiency

     E74.12 **Hereditary fructose intolerance**
         Fructosemia

     E74.19 **Other disorders of fructose metabolism**
         Fructose-1, 6-diphosphatase deficiency

✓5ᵗʰ **E74.2** **Disorders of galactose metabolism**

     E74.20 **Disorders of galactose metabolism,** HCC ▽
         unspecified

     E74.21 **Galactosemia** HCC
         DEF: Any of three genetic disorders due to defective
         galactose metabolism; symptoms include failure to
         thrive in infancy, jaundice, liver and spleen damage,
         cataracts, and mental retardation.

     E74.29 **Other disorders of galactose metabolism** HCC
         Galactokinase deficiency

✓5ᵗʰ **E74.3** **Other disorders of intestinal carbohydrate absorption**

     EXCLUDES 2   *lactose intolerance (E73.-)*

     E74.31 **Sucrase-isomaltase deficiency**

Tay-Sachs Disease

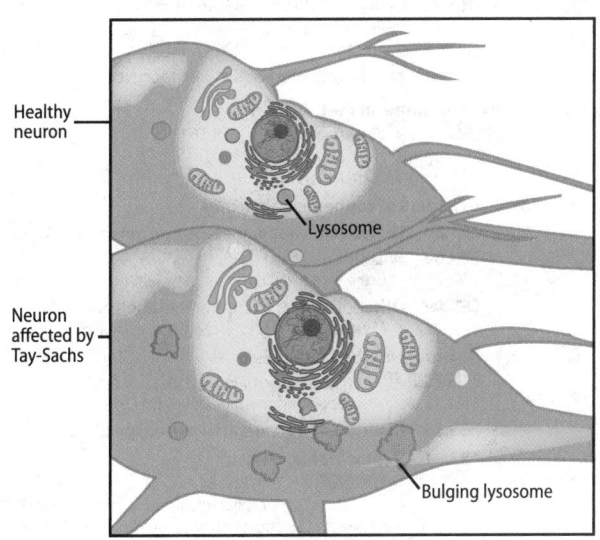

Healthy neuron

Lysosome

Neuron affected by Tay-Sachs

Bulging lysosome

E74.39 Other disorders of intestinal carbohydrate absorption
Disorder of intestinal carbohydrate absorption NOS
Glucose-galactose malabsorption
Sucrase deficiency

E74.4 Disorders of pyruvate metabolism and gluconeogenesis ᴴᶜᶜ
Deficiency of phosphoenolpyruvate carboxykinase
Deficiency of pyruvate carboxylase
Deficiency of pyruvate dehydrogenase
EXCLUDES 1 *disorders of pyruvate metabolism and gluconeogenesis with anemia (D55.-)*
Leigh's syndrome (G31.82)

E74.8 Other specified disorders of carbohydrate metabolism ᴴᶜᶜ
Essential pentosuria
Renal glycosuria

E74.9 Disorder of carbohydrate metabolism, unspecified ᴴᶜᶜ ▽

✓4ᵗʰ **E75 Disorders of sphingolipid metabolism and other lipid storage disorders**
EXCLUDES 1 *mucolipidosis, types I-III (E77.0-E77.1)*
Refsum's disease (G60.1)

✓5ᵗʰ **E75.0 GM2 gangliosidosis**

E75.00 GM2 gangliosidosis, unspecified ▽

E75.01 Sandhoff disease

E75.02 Tay-Sachs disease
DEF: Genetic mutation of the HEXA gene that inhibits the breakdown of a toxic substance called ganglioside. The accumulation of ganglioside results in destruction of the neurons in the brain and spinal cord.

E75.09 Other GM2 gangliosidosis
Adult GM2 gangliosidosis
Juvenile GM2 gangliosidosis

✓5ᵗʰ **E75.1 Other and unspecified gangliosidosis**

E75.10 Unspecified gangliosidosis ▽
Gangliosidosis NOS

E75.11 Mucolipidosis IV

E75.19 Other gangliosidosis
GM1 gangliosidosis
GM3 gangliosidosis

✓5ᵗʰ **E75.2 Other sphingolipidosis**
EXCLUDES 1 *adrenoleukodystrophy [Addison-Schilder] (E71.528)*

E75.21 Fabry (-Anderson) disease ᴴᶜᶜ

E75.22 Gaucher disease ᴴᶜᶜ

E75.23 Krabbe disease

✓6ᵗʰ **E75.24 Niemann-Pick disease**

E75.240 Niemann-Pick disease type A ᴴᶜᶜ

E75.241 Niemann-Pick disease type B ᴴᶜᶜ

E75.242 Niemann-Pick disease type C ᴴᶜᶜ

E75.243 Niemann-Pick disease type D ᴴᶜᶜ

E75.248 Other Niemann-Pick disease ᴴᶜᶜ

E75.249 Niemann-Pick disease, unspecified ᴴᶜᶜ ▽

E75.25 Metachromatic leukodystrophy

E75.29 Other sphingolipidosis
Farber's syndrome
Sulfatase deficiency
Sulfatide lipidosis

E75.3 Sphingolipidosis, unspecified ᴴᶜᶜ ▽

E75.4 Neuronal ceroid lipofuscinosis
Batten disease   Kufs disease
Bielschowsky-Jansky disease   Spielmeyer-Vogt disease

E75.5 Other lipid storage disorders
Cerebrotendinous cholesterosis [van Bogaert-Scherer-Epstein]
Wolman's disease

E75.6 Lipid storage disorder, unspecified ▽

✓4ᵗʰ **E76 Disorders of glycosaminoglycan metabolism**

✓5ᵗʰ **E76.0 Mucopolysaccharidosis, type I**

E76.01 Hurler's syndrome ᴴᶜᶜ

E76.02 Hurler-Scheie syndrome ᴴᶜᶜ

E76.03 Scheie's syndrome ᴴᶜᶜ

E76.1 Mucopolysaccharidosis, type II ᴴᶜᶜ
Hunter's syndrome

✓5ᵗʰ **E76.2 Other mucopolysaccharidoses**

✓6ᵗʰ **E76.21 Morquio mucopolysaccharidoses**

E76.210 Morquio A mucopolysaccharidoses ᴴᶜᶜ
Classic Morquio syndrome
Morquio syndrome A
Mucopolysaccharidosis, type IVA

E76.211 Morquio B mucopolysaccharidoses ᴴᶜᶜ
Morquio-like mucopolysaccharidoses
Morquio-like syndrome
Morquio syndrome B
Mucopolysaccharidosis, type IVB

E76.219 Morquio mucopolysaccharidoses, unspecified ᴴᶜᶜ ▽
Morquio syndrome
Mucopolysaccharidosis, type IV

E76.22 Sanfilippo mucopolysaccharidoses ᴴᶜᶜ
Mucopolysaccharidosis, type III (A) (B) (C) (D)
Sanfilippo A syndrome
Sanfilippo B syndrome
Sanfilippo C syndrome
Sanfilippo D syndrome

E76.29 Other mucopolysaccharidoses ᴴᶜᶜ
beta-Glucuronidase deficiency
Maroteaux-Lamy (mild) (severe) syndrome
Mucopolysaccharidosis, types VI, VII

E76.3 Mucopolysaccharidosis, unspecified ᴴᶜᶜ ▽

E76.8 Other disorders of glycosaminoglycan metabolism ᴴᶜᶜ

E76.9 Glucosaminoglycan metabolism disorder, unspecified ᴴᶜᶜ ▽

✓4ᵗʰ **E77 Disorders of glycoprotein metabolism**

E77.0 Defects in post-translational modification of lysosomal enzymes ᴴᶜᶜ
Mucolipidosis II [I-cell disease]
Mucolipidosis III [pseudo-Hurler polydystrophy]

E77.1 Defects in glycoprotein degradation ᴴᶜᶜ
Aspartylglucosaminuria
Fucosidosis
Mannosidosis
Sialidosis [mucolipidosis I]

E77.8 Other disorders of glycoprotein metabolism ᴴᶜᶜ

E77.9 Disorder of glycoprotein metabolism, unspecified ᴴᶜᶜ ▽

✓4ᵗʰ **E78 Disorders of lipoprotein metabolism and other lipidemias**
EXCLUDES 1 *sphingolipidosis (E75.0-E75.3)*

✓5ᵗʰ **E78.0 Pure hypercholesterolemia**

E78.00 Pure hypercholesterolemia, unspecified ▽
Fredrickson's hyperlipoproteinemia, type IIa
Hyperbetalipoproteinemia
Low-density-lipoprotein-type [LDL] hyperlipoproteinemia
▶(Pure) hypercholesterolemia NOS◀

E78.01 Familial hypercholesterolemia

E78.1 Pure hyperglyceridemia
Elevated fasting triglycerides
Endogenous hyperglyceridemia
Fredrickson's hyperlipoproteinemia, type IV
Hyperlipidemia, group B
Hyperprebetalipoproteinemia
Very-low-density-lipoprotein-type [VLDL] hyperlipoproteinemia

---

✓ Additional Character Req   ✓7ᵗʰ Placeholder Alert   Manifestation   ᴴᶜᶜ CMS-HCC Condition   ▽ Unspecified Code   ▶◀ Revised Text   ● New Code   ▲ Revised Code Title

E78.2 **Mixed hyperlipidemia**
Broad- or floating-betalipoproteinemia
Combined hyperlipidemia NOS
Elevated cholesterol with elevated triglycerides NEC
Fredrickson's hyperlipoproteinemia, type IIb or III
Hyperbetalipoproteinemia with prebetalipoproteinemia
Hypercholesteremia with endogenous hyperglyceridemia
Hyperlipidemia, group C
Tubo-eruptive xanthoma
Xanthoma tuberosum
> EXCLUDES 1   *cerebrotendinous cholesterosis [van Bogaert-Scherer-Epstein] (E75.5)*
> *familial combined hyperlipidemia (E78.4)*

E78.3 **Hyperchylomicronemia**
Chylomicron retention disease
Fredrickson's hyperlipoproteinemia, type I or V
Hyperlipidemia, group D
Mixed hyperglyceridemia

E78.4 **Other hyperlipidemia**
Familial combined hyperlipidemia

E78.5 **Hyperlipidemia, unspecified**   ▽

E78.6 **Lipoprotein deficiency**
Abetalipoproteinemia
Depressed HDL cholesterol
High-density lipoprotein deficiency
Hypoalphalipoproteinemia
Hypobetalipoproteinemia (familial)
Lecithin cholesterol acyltransferase deficiency
Tangier disease

✓5ᵗʰ **E78.7** **Disorders of bile acid and cholesterol metabolism**
> EXCLUDES 1   *Niemann-Pick disease type C (E75.242)*

    E78.70 **Disorder of bile acid and cholesterol metabolism,** ▽
            unspecified

    E78.71 **Barth syndrome**

    E78.72 **Smith-Lemli-Opitz syndrome**

    E78.79 **Other disorders of bile acid and cholesterol**
            metabolism

✓5ᵗʰ **E78.8** **Other disorders of lipoprotein metabolism**
    E78.81 **Lipoid dermatoarthritis**
    E78.89 **Other lipoprotein metabolism disorders**

E78.9 **Disorder of lipoprotein metabolism, unspecified**   ▽

✓4ᵗʰ **E79** **Disorders of purine and pyrimidine metabolism**
> EXCLUDES 1   *Ataxia-telangiectasia (Q87.1)*
> *Bloom's syndrome (Q82.8)*
> *Cockayne's syndrome (Q87.1)*
> *calculus of kidney (N20.0)*
> *combined immunodeficiency disorders (D81.-)*
> *Fanconi's anemia (D61.09)*
> *gout (M1A.-, M10.-)*
> *orotaciduric anemia (D53.0)*
> *progeria (E34.8)*
> *Werner's syndrome (E34.8)*
> *xeroderma pigmentosum (Q82.1)*

E79.0 **Hyperuricemia without signs of inflammatory arthritis and**
tophaceous disease
Asymptomatic hyperuricemia

E79.1 **Lesch-Nyhan syndrome**   HCC
HGPRT deficiency

E79.2 **Myoadenylate deaminase deficiency**   HCC

E79.8 **Other disorders of purine and pyrimidine metabolism**   HCC
Hereditary xanthinuria

E79.9 **Disorder of purine and pyrimidine metabolism,**   HCC ▽
unspecified

✓4ᵗʰ **E80** **Disorders of porphyrin and bilirubin metabolism**
> INCLUDES   defects of catalase and peroxidase

E80.0 **Hereditary erythropoietic porphyria**   HCC
Congenital erythropoietic porphyria
Erythropoietic protoporphyria

E80.1 **Porphyria cutanea tarda**   HCC

✓5ᵗʰ **E80.2** **Other and unspecified porphyria**
    E80.20 **Unspecified porphyria**   HCC ▽
            Porphyria NOS

    E80.21 **Acute intermittent (hepatic) porphyria**   HCC

    E80.29 **Other porphyria**   HCC
            Hereditary coproporphyria

E80.3 **Defects of catalase and peroxidase**   HCC
Acatalasia [Takahara]

E80.4 **Gilbert syndrome**

E80.5 **Crigler-Najjar syndrome**

E80.6 **Other disorders of bilirubin metabolism**
Dubin-Johnson syndrome
Rotor's syndrome

E80.7 **Disorder of bilirubin metabolism, unspecified**   ▽

✓4ᵗʰ **E83** **Disorders of mineral metabolism**
> EXCLUDES 1   *dietary mineral deficiency (E58-E61)*
> *parathyroid disorders (E20-E21)*
> *vitamin D deficiency (E55.-)*

✓5ᵗʰ **E83.0** **Disorders of copper metabolism**
    E83.00 **Disorder of copper metabolism, unspecified**   ▽

    E83.01 **Wilson's disease**
            Code also associated Kayser Fleischer ring (H18.04-)

    E83.09 **Other disorders of copper metabolism**
            Menkes' (kinky hair) (steely hair) disease

✓5ᵗʰ **E83.1** **Disorders of iron metabolism**
> EXCLUDES 1   *iron deficiency anemia (D50.-)*
> *sideroblastic anemia (D64.0-D64.3)*

    E83.10 **Disorder of iron metabolism, unspecified**   ▽

✓6ᵗʰ   **E83.11** **Hemochromatosis**
> EXCLUDES 1   ▶*GALD (P78.84)*
> *gestational alloimmune liver disease (P78.84)*
> *neonatal hemochromatosis (P78.84)*◀

        E83.110 **Hereditary hemochromatosis**   HCC
                Bronzed diabetes
                Pigmentary cirrhosis (of liver)
                Primary (hereditary) hemochromatosis

        E83.111 **Hemochromatosis due to repeated red**
             blood cell transfusions
                Iron overload due to repeated red blood
                    cell transfusions
                Transfusion (red blood cell) associated
                    hemochromatosis

        E83.118 **Other hemochromatosis**
        E83.119 **Hemochromatosis, unspecified**   ▽

    E83.19 **Other disorders of iron metabolism**
            Use additional code, if applicable, for idiopathic
                pulmonary hemosiderosis (J84.03)

E83.2 **Disorders of zinc metabolism**
Acrodermatitis enteropathica

✓5ᵗʰ **E83.3** **Disorders of phosphorus metabolism and phosphatases**
> EXCLUDES 1   *adult osteomalacia (M83.-)*
> *osteoporosis (M80.-)*

    E83.30 **Disorder of phosphorus metabolism, unspecified** ▽

    E83.31 **Familial hypophosphatemia**
            Vitamin D-resistant osteomalacia
            Vitamin D-resistant rickets
>   EXCLUDES 1   *vitamin D-deficiency rickets (E55.0)*

    E83.32 **Hereditary vitamin D-dependent rickets (type 1)**
            (type 2)
            25-hydroxyvitamin D 1-alpha-hydroxylase deficiency
            Pseudovitamin D deficiency
            Vitamin D receptor defect

    E83.39 **Other disorders of phosphorus metabolism**
            Acid phosphatase deficiency
            Hypophosphatasia

✓5ᵗʰ **E83.4** **Disorders of magnesium metabolism**
    E83.40 **Disorders of magnesium metabolism, unspecified** ▽
    E83.41 **Hypermagnesemia**
    E83.42 **Hypomagnesemia**
    E83.49 **Other disorders of magnesium metabolism**

✓5ᵗʰ **E83.5** **Disorders of calcium metabolism**
> EXCLUDES 1   *chondrocalcinosis (M11.1-M11.2)*
> *hungry bone syndrome (E83.81)*
> *hyperparathyroidism (E20.0-E21.3)*

    E83.50 **Unspecified disorder of calcium metabolism**   ▽
    E83.51 **Hypocalcemia**
    E83.52 **Hypercalcemia**
            Familial hypocalciuric hypercalcemia
    E83.59 **Other disorders of calcium metabolism**
            Idiopathic hypercalciuria

✓5ᵗʰ **E83.8** **Other disorders of mineral metabolism**
    E83.81 **Hungry bone syndrome**
    E83.89 **Other disorders of mineral metabolism**

E83.9 **Disorder of mineral metabolism, unspecified**   ▽

EXCLUDES 1 Not coded here   EXCLUDES 2 Not included here   N Newborn Age: 0   P Pediatric Age: 0-17   M Maternity Age: 12-55   A Adult Age: 15-124

522   ICD-10-CM 2018

✓4th **E84 Cystic fibrosis**
    INCLUDES mucoviscidosis
    Code also exocrine pancreatic insufficiency (K86.81)

    E84.0 Cystic fibrosis with pulmonary manifestations HCC
          Use additional code to identify any infectious organism present, such as:
            Pseudomonas (B96.5)

    ✓5th **E84.1 Cystic fibrosis with intestinal manifestations**

        E84.11 Meconium ileus in cystic fibrosis HCC N
            EXCLUDES 1 *meconium ileus not due to cystic fibrosis (P76.0)*

        E84.19 Cystic fibrosis with other intestinal manifestations HCC
            Distal intestinal obstruction syndrome

    E84.8 Cystic fibrosis with other manifestations HCC

    E84.9 Cystic fibrosis, unspecified HCC ▽

✓4th **E85 Amyloidosis**
    EXCLUDES 1 Alzheimer's disease (G30.0-)
    EXCLUDES 2 ▶*Alzheimer's disease (G30.0-)*◀
    DEF: Conditions of diverse etiologies characterized by the accumulation of insoluble fibrillar proteins (amyloid) in various organs and tissues of the body, compromising vital functions.

    E85.0 Non-neuropathic heredofamilial amyloidosis HCC
          Hereditary amyloid nephropathy
          ▶Code also associated disorders, such as:
            autoinflammatory syndromes (M04.-)◀
          EXCLUDES 2 ▶*transthyretin-related (ATTR) familial amyloid cardiomyopathy (E85.4)*◀

    E85.1 Neuropathic heredofamilial amyloidosis HCC
          Amyloid polyneuropathy (Portuguese)
          ▶Transthyretin-related (ATTR) familial amyloid polyneuropathy◀
          AHA: 2012, 4Q, 99

    E85.2 Heredofamilial amyloidosis, unspecified HCC ▽

    E85.3 Secondary systemic amyloidosis HCC
          Hemodialysis-associated amyloidosis

    E85.4 Organ-limited amyloidosis HCC
          Localized amyloidosis
          ▶Transthyretin-related (ATTR) familial amyloid cardiomyopathy◀

    ✓5th **E85.8 Other amyloidosis**

  ●   **E85.81 Light chain (AL) amyloidosis**

  ●   **E85.82 Wild-type transthyretin-related (ATTR) amyloidosis**
            Senile systemic amyloidosis (SSA)

  ●   **E85.89 Other amyloidosis**

    E85.9 Amyloidosis, unspecified HCC

✓4th **E86 Volume depletion**
    Use additional code(s) for any associated disorders of electrolyte and acid-base balance (E87.-)
    EXCLUDES 1 *dehydration of newborn (P74.1)*
            hypovolemic shock NOS (R57.1)
            postprocedural hypovolemic shock (T81.19)
            traumatic hypovolemic shock (T79.4)

    E86.0 Dehydration
          AHA: 2014, 1Q, 7

    E86.1 Hypovolemia
          Depletion of volume of plasma

    E86.9 Volume depletion, unspecified ▽
          DEF: Depletion of total body water (dehydration) and/or contraction of total intravascular plasma (hypovolemia).

✓4th **E87 Other disorders of fluid, electrolyte and acid-base balance**
    EXCLUDES 1 ▶*diabetes insipidus (E23.2)*
            electrolyte imbalance associated with hyperemesis gravidarum (O21.1)
            electrolyte imbalance following ectopic or molar pregnancy (O08.5)
            familial periodic paralysis (G72.3)

    E87.0 Hyperosmolality and hypernatremia
          Sodium [Na] excess
          Sodium [Na] overload
          AHA: 2014, 1Q, 7

    E87.1 Hypo-osmolality and hyponatremia
          Sodium [Na] deficiency
          EXCLUDES 1 *syndrome of inappropriate secretion of antidiuretic hormone (E22.2)*
          AHA: 2014, 1Q, 7

    E87.2 Acidosis
          Acidosis NOS   Metabolic acidosis
          Lactic acidosis   Respiratory acidosis
          EXCLUDES 1 *diabetic acidosis—see categories E08-E10, E13 with ketoacidosis*

    E87.3 Alkalosis
          Alkalosis NOS   Respiratory alkalosis
          Metabolic alkalosis

    E87.4 Mixed disorder of acid-base balance

    E87.5 Hyperkalemia
          Potassium [K] excess   Potassium [K] overload

    E87.6 Hypokalemia
          Potassium [K] deficiency

    ✓5th **E87.7 Fluid overload**
          EXCLUDES 1 *edema NOS (R60.9)*
             fluid retention (R60.9)

        E87.70 Fluid overload, unspecified ▽

        E87.71 Transfusion associated circulatory overload
            Fluid overload due to transfusion (blood) (blood components)
            TACO

        E87.79 Other fluid overload

    E87.8 Other disorders of electrolyte and fluid balance, not elsewhere classified
          Electrolyte imbalance NOS
          Hyperchloremia
          Hypochloremia

✓4th **E88 Other and unspecified metabolic disorders**
    Use additional codes for associated conditions
    EXCLUDES 1 *histiocytosis X (chronic) (C96.6)*

    ✓5th **E88.0 Disorders of plasma-protein metabolism, not elsewhere classified**
          EXCLUDES 1 *disorder of lipoprotein metabolism (E78.-)*
             monoclonal gammopathy (of undetermined significance) (D47.2)
             polyclonal hypergammaglobulinemia (D89.0)
             Waldenström's macroglobulinemia (C88.0)

        E88.01 Alpha-1-antitrypsin deficiency HCC
            AAT deficiency

        E88.09 Other disorders of plasma-protein metabolism, not elsewhere classified
            Bisalbuminemia

    E88.1 Lipodystrophy, not elsewhere classified
          Lipodystrophy NOS
          EXCLUDES 1 *Whipple's disease (K90.81)*

    E88.2 Lipomatosis, not elsewhere classified
          Lipomatosis NOS
          Lipomatosis (Check) dolorosa [Dercum]

    E88.3 Tumor lysis syndrome
          Tumor lysis syndrome (spontaneous)
          Tumor lysis syndrome following antineoplastic drug chemotherapy
          Use additional code for adverse effect, if applicable, to identify drug (T45.1X5)
          DEF: A potentially fatal metabolic complication of tumor necrosis caused by either spontaneous or treatment-related accumulation of byproducts from dying cancer cells; symptoms include hyperkalemia, hyperphosphatemia, hypocalcemia, hyperuricemia, and hyperuricosuria.

    ✓5th **E88.4 Mitochondrial metabolism disorders**
          EXCLUDES 1 *disorders of pyruvate metabolism (E74.4)*
             Kearns-Sayre syndrome (H49.81)
             Leber's disease (H47.22)
             Leigh's encephalopathy (G31.82)
             Mitochondrial myopathy, NEC (G71.3)
             Reye's syndrome (G93.7)

        E88.40 Mitochondrial metabolism disorder, unspecified HCC ▽

        E88.41 MELAS syndrome HCC
            Mitochondrial myopathy, encephalopathy, lactic acidosis and stroke-like episodes

        E88.42 MERRF syndrome HCC
            Myoclonic epilepsy associated with ragged-red fibers
            Code also progressive myoclonic epilepsy (G40.3-)

        E88.49 Other mitochondrial metabolism disorders HCC

✔ Additional Character Req   ✔7th Placeholder Alert   Manifestation   HCC CMS-HCC Condition   ▽ Unspecified Code   ▶◀ Revised Text   ● New Code   ▲ Revised Code Title

✓5ᵗʰ **E88.8 Other specified metabolic disorders**

    E88.81 Metabolic syndrome
        Dysmetabolic syndrome X
        Use additional codes for associated manifestations,
            such as:
            obesity (E66.-)

    E88.89 Other specified metabolic disorders   `HCC`
        Launois-Bensaude adenolipomatosis
        EXCLUDES 1 adult pulmonary Langerhans cell
               histiocytosis (J84.82)

E88.9 Metabolic disorder, unspecified   ▽

Postprocedural endocrine and metabolic complications and disorders, not elsewhere classified (E89)

✓4ᵗʰ **E89 Postprocedural endocrine and metabolic complications and disorders, not elsewhere classified**
    EXCLUDES 2 intraoperative complications of endocrine system organ or
          structure (E36.0-, E36.1-, E36.8)

E89.0 Postprocedural hypothyroidism
    Postirradiation hypothyroidism
    Postsurgical hypothyroidism

E89.1 Postprocedural hypoinsulinemia
    Postpancreatectomy hyperglycemia
    Postsurgical hypoinsulinemia
    Use additional code, if applicable, to identify:
        acquired absence of pancreas (Z90.41-)
        diabetes mellitus (postpancreatectomy) (postprocedural)
           (E13.-)
        insulin use (Z79.4)
    EXCLUDES 1 transient postprocedural hyperglycemia (R73.9)
              transient postprocedural hypoglycemia (E16.2)

E89.2 Postprocedural hypoparathyroidism   `HCC`
    Parathyroprival tetany

E89.3 Postprocedural hypopituitarism   `HCC`
    Postirradiation hypopituitarism

✓5ᵗʰ **E89.4 Postprocedural ovarian failure**

    E89.40 Asymptomatic postprocedural ovarian failure   ♀
        Postprocedural ovarian failure NOS

    E89.41 Symptomatic postprocedural ovarian failure   ♀
        Symptoms such as flushing, sleeplessness, headache,
            lack of concentration, associated with
            postprocedural menopause

E89.5 Postprocedural testicular hypofunction   ♂

E89.6 Postprocedural adrenocortical (-medullary) hypofunction `HCC`

✓5ᵗʰ **E89.8 Other postprocedural endocrine and metabolic complications and disorders**

    ✓6ᵗʰ **E89.81 Postprocedural hemorrhage of an endocrine system organ or structure following a procedure**
        E89.810 Postprocedural hemorrhage of an endocrine system organ or structure following an endocrine system procedure
        E89.811 Postprocedural hemorrhage of an endocrine system organ or structure following other procedure

    ✓6ᵗʰ **E89.82 Postprocedural hematoma and seroma of an endocrine system organ or structure following a procedure**
        E89.820 Postprocedural hematoma of an endocrine system organ or structure following an endocrine system procedure
        E89.821 Postprocedural hematoma of an endocrine system organ or structure following other procedure
        E89.822 Postprocedural seroma of an endocrine system organ or structure following an endocrine system procedure
        E89.823 Postprocedural seroma of an endocrine system organ or structure following other procedure

    E89.89 Other postprocedural endocrine and metabolic complications and disorders
        Use additional code, if applicable, to further specify
           disorder

EXCLUDES 1 Not coded here   *EXCLUDES 2* Not included here   N Newborn Age: 0   P Pediatric Age: 0-17   M Maternity Age: 12-55   A Adult Age: 15-124

524   ICD-10-CM 2018

Chapter 5. Mental, Behavioral and Neurodevelopmental Disorders (F01–F99)

Chapter Specific Guidelines with Coding Examples

The chapter specific guidelines from the ICD-10-CM Official Guidelines for Coding and Reporting have been provided below. Along with these guidelines are coding examples, contained in the shaded boxes, that have been developed to help illustrate the coding and/or sequencing guidance found in these guidelines.

a. Pain disorders related to psychological factors

Assign code F45.41, for pain that is exclusively related to psychological disorders. As indicated by the Excludes 1 note under category G89, a code from category G89 should not be assigned with code F45.41.

Chest pain determined to be persistent somatoform pain disorder

F45.41   Pain disorder exclusively related to psychological factors

Explanation: This pain was diagnosed as being exclusively psychological; therefore, no code from category G89 is added.

Code F45.42, Pain disorders with related psychological factors, should be used with a code from category G89, Pain, not elsewhere classified, if there is documentation of a psychological component for a patient with acute or chronic pain.

See Section I.C.6. Pain

b. Mental and behavioral disorders due to psychoactive substance use

1) In remission

Selection of codes for "in remission" for categories F10-F19, Mental and behavioral disorders due to psychoactive substance use (categories F10-F19 with -.11, -.21) requires the provider's clinical judgment. The appropriate codes for "in remission" are assigned only on the basis of provider documentation (as defined in the Official Guidelines for Coding and Reporting), **unless otherwise instructed by the classification.**

Mild substance use disorders in early or sustained remission are classified to the appropriate codes for substance abuse in remission, and moderate or severe substance use disorders in early or sustained remission are classified to the appropriate codes for substance dependence in remission.

2) Psychoactive substance use, abuse and dependence

When the provider documentation refers to use, abuse and dependence of the same substance (e.g. alcohol, opioid, cannabis, etc.), only one code should be assigned to identify the pattern of use based on the following hierarchy:

- If both use and abuse are documented, assign only the code for abuse
  If both abuse and dependence are documented, assign only the code for dependence
- If use, abuse and dependence are all documented, assign only the code for dependence
- If both use and dependence are documented, assign only the code for dependence.

History and physical notes cannabis dependence and ongoing cannabis abuse

F12.20   Cannabis dependence, uncomplicated

Explanation: In the hierarchy, the dependence code is used if both abuse and dependence are documented.

Current problem list indicates daily opioid use with opioid abuse.

F11.10   Opioid abuse, uncomplicated

Explanation: In the hierarchy, the abuse code is used if both abuse and use are documented.

3) Psychoactive substance use *disorders*

As with all other diagnoses, the codes for psychoactive substance use **disorders** (F10.9-, F11.9-, F12.9-, F13.9-, F14.9-, F15.9-, F16.9-) should only be assigned based on provider documentation and when they meet the definition of a reportable diagnosis (see Section III, Reporting Additional Diagnoses). The codes are to be used only when the psychoactive substance use is associated with a **physical,** mental or behavioral disorder, and such a relationship is documented by the provider.

ED reports that a 27-year-old female tripped and twisted and broke her right ankle. Her friends reported that they were drinking and dancing at a nightclub.

S82.891A   Other fracture of right lower leg, initial encounter for closed fracture

W18.40XA   Slipping, tripping and stumbling without falling, unspecified, initial encounter

Y92.252   Music hall as the place of occurrence of the external cause

Y93.41   Activity, dancing

Explanation: Note that no code was added for alcohol use or abuse. Unless it is specifically associated with a diagnosis by provider documentation and meets the definition of a reportable diagnosis, it is not assigned. However, if the documentation from the provider stated: "The patient tripped, and twisted and fractured her right ankle while dancing due to her elevated blood alcohol, consistent with her ongoing alcohol abuse," the following code would be added:

F10.10   Alcohol abuse, uncomplicated

Chapter 5. Mental, Behavioral, and Neurodevelopmental Disorders (F01-F99)

INCLUDES   disorders of psychological development
EXCLUDES 2   *symptoms, signs and abnormal clinical laboratory findings, not elsewhere classified (R00-R99)*

This chapter contains the following blocks:

F01-F09	Mental disorders due to known physiological conditions
F10-F19	Mental and behavioral disorders due to psychoactive substance use
F20-F29	Schizophrenia, schizotypal, delusional, and other non-mood psychotic disorders
F30-F39	Mood [affective] disorders
F40-F48	Anxiety, dissociative, stress-related, somatoform and other nonpsychotic mental disorders
F50-F59	Behavioral syndromes associated with physiological disturbances and physical factors
F60-F69	Disorders of adult personality and behavior
F70-F79	Intellectual disabilities
F80-F89	Pervasive and specific developmental disorders
F90-F98	Behavioral and emotional disorders with onset usually occurring in childhood and adolescence
F99	Unspecified mental disorder

Mental disorders due to known physiological conditions (F01-F09)

NOTE   This block comprises a range of mental disorders grouped together on the basis of their having in common a demonstrable etiology in cerebral disease, brain injury, or other insult leading to cerebral dysfunction. The dysfunction may be primary, as in diseases, injuries, and insults that affect the brain directly and selectively; or secondary, as in systemic diseases and disorders that attack the brain only as one of the multiple organs or systems of the body that are involved.

✓4ᵗʰ **F01   Vascular dementia**

Vascular dementia as a result of infarction of the brain due to vascular disease, including hypertensive cerebrovascular disease.
INCLUDES   arteriosclerotic dementia
Code first the underlying physiological condition or sequelae of cerebrovascular disease.

✓5ᵗʰ **F01.5   Vascular dementia**

     F01.50   Vascular dementia without behavioral disturbance   A
         Major neurocognitive disorder without behavioral disturbance

     F01.51   Vascular dementia with behavioral disturbance   A
         Major neurocognitive disorder due to vascular disease, with behavioral disturbance
         Major neurocognitive disorder with aggressive behavior
         Major neurocognitive disorder with combative behavior
         Major neurocognitive disorder with violent behavior
         Vascular dementia with aggressive behavior
         Vascular dementia with combative behavior
         Vascular dementia with violent behavior
         Use additional code, if applicable, to identify wandering in vascular dementia (Z91.83)

✓4ᵗʰ **F02   Dementia in other diseases classified elsewhere**

INCLUDES   major neurocognitive disorder in other diseases classified elsewhere
Code first the underlying physiological condition, such as:
     Alzheimer's (G30.-)
     cerebral lipidosis (E75.4)
     Creutzfeldt-Jakob disease (A81.0-)
     dementia with Lewy bodies (G31.83)
     dementia with Parkinsonism (G31.83)
     epilepsy and recurrent seizures (G40.-)
     frontotemporal dementia (G31.09)
     hepatolenticular degeneration (E83.0)
     human immunodeficiency virus [HIV] disease (B20)
     Huntington's disease (G10)
     hypercalcemia (E83.52)
     hypothyroidism, acquired (E00-E03.-)
     intoxications (T36-T65)
     Jakob-Creutzfeldt disease (A81.0-)
     multiple sclerosis (G35)
     neurosyphilis (A52.17)
     niacin deficiency [pellagra] (E52)
     Parkinson's disease (G20)
     Pick's disease (G31.01)
     polyarteritis nodosa (M30.0)
     prion disease (A81.9)
     systemic lupus erythematosus (M32.-)
     traumatic brain injury (S06.-)
     trypanosomiasis (B56.-, B57.-)
     vitamin B deficiency (E53.8)
EXCLUDES 2   *dementia in alcohol and psychoactive substance disorders (F10-F19, with .17, .27, .97)*
         vascular dementia (F01.5-)

✓5ᵗʰ **F02.8   Dementia in other diseases classified elsewhere**
AHA: 2017, 2Q, 7; 2016, 4Q, 141; 2016, 2Q, 6

     F02.80   *Dementia in other diseases classified elsewhere without behavioral disturbance*
         Dementia in other diseases classified elsewhere NOS
         Major neurocognitive disorder in other diseases classified elsewhere

     F02.81   *Dementia in other diseases classified elsewhere with behavioral disturbance*
         Dementia in other diseases classified elsewhere with aggressive behavior
         Dementia in other diseases classified elsewhere with combative behavior
         Dementia in other diseases classified elsewhere with violent behavior
         Major neurocognitive disorder in other diseases classified elsewhere with aggressive behavior
         Major neurocognitive disorder in other diseases classified elsewhere with combative behavior
         Major neurocognitive disorder in other diseases classified elsewhere with violent behavior
         Use additional code, if applicable, to identify wandering in dementia in conditions classified elsewhere (Z91.83)

✓4ᵗʰ **F03   Unspecified dementia**

     Presenile dementia NOS
     Presenile psychosis NOS
     Primary degenerative dementia NOS
     Senile dementia NOS
     Senile dementia depressed or paranoid type
     Senile psychosis NOS
EXCLUDES 1   *senility NOS (R41.81)*
EXCLUDES 2   *mild memory disturbance due to known physiological condition (F06.8)*
         senile dementia with delirium or acute confusional state (F05)

✓5ᵗʰ **F03.9   Unspecified dementia**

     F03.90   Unspecified dementia without behavioral disturbance   A ▽
         Dementia NOS
         AHA: 2012, 4Q, 92

     F03.91   Unspecified dementia with behavioral disturbance   A ▽
         Unspecified dementia with aggressive behavior
         Unspecified dementia with combative behavior
         Unspecified dementia with violent behavior
         Use additional code, if applicable, to identify wandering in unspecified dementia (Z91.83)

EXCLUDES 1 Not coded here   **EXCLUDES 2** Not included here   N Newborn Age: 0   P Pediatric Age: 0-17   M Maternity Age: 12-55   A Adult Age: 15-124

526   ICD-10-CM 2018

F04　Amnestic disorder due to known physiological condition
Korsakov's psychosis or syndrome, nonalcoholic
Code first the underlying physiological condition
EXCLUDES 1　amnesia NOS (R41.3)
　　　　　　anterograde amnesia (R41.1)
　　　　　　dissociative amnesia (F44.0)
　　　　　　retrograde amnesia (R41.2)
EXCLUDES 2　alcohol-induced or unspecified Korsakov's syndrome (F10.26,
　　　　　　F10.96)
　　　　　　Korsakov's syndrome induced by other psychoactive substances
　　　　　　(F13.26, F13.96, F19.16, F19.26, F19.96)

F05　Delirium due to known physiological condition
Acute or subacute brain syndrome
Acute or subacute confusional state (nonalcoholic)
Acute or subacute infective psychosis
Acute or subacute organic reaction
Acute or subacute psycho-organic syndrome
Delirium of mixed etiology
Delirium superimposed on dementia
Sundowning
Code first the underlying physiological condition
EXCLUDES 1　delirium NOS (R41.0)
EXCLUDES 2　delirium tremens alcohol-induced or unspecified (F10.231,
　　　　　　F10.921)

✓4th **F06　Other mental disorders due to known physiological condition**
[INCLUDES]　mental disorders due to endocrine disorder
　　　　　mental disorders due to exogenous hormone
　　　　　mental disorders due to exogenous toxic substance
　　　　　mental disorders due to primary cerebral disease
　　　　　mental disorders due to somatic illness
　　　　　mental disorders due to systemic disease affecting the brain
Code first the underlying physiological condition
EXCLUDES 1　unspecified dementia (F03)
EXCLUDES 2　delirium due to known physiological condition (F05)
　　　　　　dementia as classified in F01-F02
　　　　　　other mental disorders associated with alcohol and other
　　　　　　psychoactive substances (F10-F19)

**F06.0　Psychotic disorder with hallucinations due to known
physiological condition**
Organic hallucinatory state (nonalcoholic)
EXCLUDES 2　hallucinations and perceptual disturbance induced by
　　　　　　alcohol and other psychoactive substances
　　　　　　(F10-F19 with .151, .251, .951)
　　　　　　schizophrenia (F20.-)

F06.1　Catatonic disorder due to known physiological condition
Catatonia associated with another mental disorder
Catatonia NOS
EXCLUDES 1　catatonic stupor (R40.1)
　　　　　　stupor NOS (R40.1)
EXCLUDES 2　catatonic schizophrenia (F20.2)
　　　　　　dissociative stupor (F44.2)

**F06.2　Psychotic disorder with delusions due to known physiological
condition**
Paranoid and paranoid-hallucinatory organic states
Schizophrenia-like psychosis in epilepsy
EXCLUDES 2　alcohol and drug-induced psychotic disorder (F10-F19
　　　　　　with .150, .250, .950)
　　　　　　brief psychotic disorder (F23)
　　　　　　delusional disorder (F22)
　　　　　　schizophrenia (F20.-)

✓5th **F06.3　Mood disorder due to known physiological condition**
EXCLUDES 2　mood disorders due to alcohol and other psychoactive
　　　　　　substances (F10-F19 with .14, .24, .94)
　　　　　　mood disorders, not due to known physiological
　　　　　　condition or unspecified (F30-F39)

　　**F06.30　Mood disorder due to known physiological　　▽
　　　　　condition, unspecified**

　　**F06.31　Mood disorder due to known physiological
　　　　　condition with depressive features**
　　　　　▶Depressive disorder due to known physiological
　　　　　condition, with depressive features◀

　　**F06.32　Mood disorder due to known physiological
　　　　　condition with major depressive-like episode**
　　　　　▶Depressive disorder due to known physiological
　　　　　condition, with major depressive–like episode◀

　　**F06.33　Mood disorder due to known physiological
　　　　　condition with manic features**
　　　　　▶Bipolar and related disorder due to a known
　　　　　physiological condition, with manic features
　　　　　Bipolar and related disorder due to known
　　　　　physiological condition, with manic- or
　　　　　hypomanic-like episodes◀

　　**F06.34　Mood disorder due to known physiological
　　　　　condition with mixed features**
　　　　　▶Bipolar and related disorder due to known
　　　　　physiological condition, with mixed features
　　　　　Depressive disorder due to known physiological
　　　　　condition, with mixed features◀

F06.4　Anxiety disorder due to known physiological condition
EXCLUDES 2　anxiety disorders due to alcohol and other psychoactive
　　　　　　substances (F10-F19 with .180, .280, .980)
　　　　　　anxiety disorders, not due to known physiological
　　　　　　condition or unspecified (F40.-, F41.-)

**F06.8　Other specified mental disorders due to known physiological
condition**
Epileptic psychosis NOS
▶Obsessive-compulsive and related disorder due to a known
physiological condition◀
Organic dissociative disorder
Organic emotionally labile [asthenic] disorder

✓4th **F07　Personality and behavioral disorders due to known
physiological condition**
Code first the underlying physiological condition

F07.0　Personality change due to known physiological condition
Frontal lobe syndrome
Limbic epilepsy personality syndrome
Lobotomy syndrome
Organic personality disorder
Organic pseudopsychopathic personality
Organic pseudoretarded personality
Postleucotomy syndrome
Code first underlying physiological condition
EXCLUDES 1　mild cognitive impairment (G31.84)
　　　　　　postconcussional syndrome (F07.81)
　　　　　　postencephalitic syndrome (F07.89)
　　　　　　signs and symptoms involving emotional state (R45.-)
EXCLUDES 2　specific personality disorder (F60.-)

✓5th **F07.8　Other personality and behavioral disorders due to known
physiological condition**

　　F07.81　Postconcussional syndrome
　　　　　Postcontusional syndrome (encephalopathy)
　　　　　Post-traumatic brain syndrome, nonpsychotic
　　　　　Use additional code to identify associated
　　　　　post-traumatic headache, if applicable (G44.3-)
　　　　　EXCLUDES 1　current concussion (brain) (S06.0-)
　　　　　　　　　　postencephalitic syndrome (F07.89)

　　**F07.89　Other personality and behavioral disorders due to
　　　　　known physiological condition**
　　　　　Postencephalitic syndrome
　　　　　Right hemispheric organic affective disorder

**F07.9　Unspecified personality and behavioral disorder due to　　▽
known physiological condition**
Organic psychosyndrome

**F09　Unspecified mental disorder due to known physiological　　▽
condition**
Mental disorder NOS due to known physiological condition
Organic brain syndrome NOS
Organic mental disorder NOS
Organic psychosis NOS
Symptomatic psychosis NOS
Code first the underlying physiological condition
EXCLUDES 1　psychosis NOS (F29)

**Mental and behavioral disorders due to
psychoactive substance use (F10-F19)**
AHA: 2017, 2Q, 27

✓4th **F10　Alcohol related disorders**
Use additional code for blood alcohol level, if applicable (Y90.-)

✓5th **F10.1　Alcohol abuse**
EXCLUDES 1　alcohol dependence (F10.2-)
　　　　　　alcohol use, unspecified (F10.9-)
AHA: 2015, 2Q, 15

　　F10.10　Alcohol abuse, uncomplicated
　　　　　Alcohol use disorder, mild

✓ Additional Character Req　　✓x7th Placeholder Alert　　Manifestation　　HCC CMS-HCC Condition　　▽ Unspecified Code　　▶◀ Revised Text　　● New Code　　▲ Revised Code Title

Chapter 5. Mental, Behavioral and Neurodevelopmental Disorders

- **F10.11**   **Alcohol abuse, in remission**
  Alcohol use disorder, mild, in early remission
  Alcohol use disorder, mild, in sustained remission

✓6ᵗʰ **F10.12**   **Alcohol abuse with intoxication**

     F10.120   **Alcohol abuse with intoxication, uncomplicated**   HCC

     F10.121   **Alcohol abuse with intoxication delirium**   HCC

     F10.129   **Alcohol abuse with intoxication, unspecified**   HCC ▽

     F10.14   **Alcohol abuse with alcohol-induced mood disorder**   HCC
Alcohol use disorder, mild, with alcohol-induced bipolar or related disorder
Alcohol use disorder, mild, with alcohol-induced depressive disorder

✓6ᵗʰ **F10.15**   **Alcohol abuse with alcohol-induced psychotic disorder**

     F10.150   **Alcohol abuse with alcohol-induced psychotic disorder with delusions**   HCC

     F10.151   **Alcohol abuse with alcohol-induced psychotic disorder with hallucinations**   HCC
       DEF: Psychosis lasting less than six months with slight or no clouding of consciousness in which auditory hallucinations predominate.

     F10.159   **Alcohol abuse with alcohol-induced psychotic disorder, unspecified**   HCC ▽

✓6ᵗʰ **F10.18**   **Alcohol abuse with other alcohol-induced disorders**

     F10.180   **Alcohol abuse with alcohol-induced anxiety disorder**   HCC

     F10.181   **Alcohol abuse with alcohol-induced sexual dysfunction**   HCC

     F10.182   **Alcohol abuse with alcohol-induced sleep disorder**   HCC

     F10.188   **Alcohol abuse with other alcohol-induced disorder**   HCC

     F10.19   **Alcohol abuse with unspecified alcohol-induced disorder**   HCC ▽

✓5ᵗʰ **F10.2**   **Alcohol dependence**
     EXCLUDES 1   alcohol abuse (F10.1-)
              alcohol use, unspecified (F10.9-)
     EXCLUDES 2   toxic effect of alcohol (T51.0-)

     F10.20   **Alcohol dependence, uncomplicated**   HCC
Alcohol use disorder, moderate
Alcohol use disorder, severe

     F10.21   **Alcohol dependence, in remission**   HCC
▶Alcohol use disorder, moderate, in early remission
Alcohol use disorder, moderate, in sustained remission
Alcohol use disorder, severe, in early remission
Alcohol use disorder, severe, in sustained remission◀

✓6ᵗʰ **F10.22**   **Alcohol dependence with intoxication**
Acute drunkenness (in alcoholism)
     EXCLUDES 2   alcohol dependence with withdrawal (F10.23-)

     F10.220   **Alcohol dependence with intoxication, uncomplicated**   HCC

     F10.221   **Alcohol dependence with intoxication delirium**   HCC

     F10.229   **Alcohol dependence with intoxication, unspecified**   HCC ▽

✓6ᵗʰ **F10.23**   **Alcohol dependence with withdrawal**
     EXCLUDES 2   alcohol dependence with withdrawal (F10.22-)
     AHA: 2015, 2Q, 15

     F10.230   **Alcohol dependence with withdrawal, uncomplicated**   HCC

     F10.231   **Alcohol dependence with withdrawal delirium**   HCC

     F10.232   **Alcohol dependence with withdrawal with perceptual disturbance**   HCC

     F10.239   **Alcohol dependence with withdrawal, unspecified**   HCC ▽

     F10.24   **Alcohol dependence with alcohol-induced mood disorder**   HCC
Alcohol use disorder, moderate, with alcohol-induced bipolar or related disorder
Alcohol use disorder, moderate, with alcohol-induced depressive disorder
Alcohol use disorder, severe, with alcohol-induced bipolar or related disorder
Alcohol use disorder, severe, with alcohol-induced depressive disorder

✓6ᵗʰ **F10.25**   **Alcohol dependence with alcohol-induced psychotic disorder**

     F10.250   **Alcohol dependence with alcohol-induced psychotic disorder with delusions**   HCC

     F10.251   **Alcohol dependence with alcohol-induced psychotic disorder with hallucinations**   HCC

     F10.259   **Alcohol dependence with alcohol-induced psychotic disorder, unspecified**   HCC ▽

     F10.26   **Alcohol dependence with alcohol-induced persisting amnestic disorder**   HCC
Alcohol use disorder, moderate, with alcohol-induced major neurocognitive disorder, amnestic-confabulatory type
Alcohol use disorder, severe, with alcohol-induced major neurocognitive disorder, amnestic-confabulatory type
       DEF: Prominent and lasting reduced memory span, disordered time appreciation and confabulation, occurs in alcoholics as sequel to acute alcoholic psychosis.

     F10.27   **Alcohol dependence with alcohol-induced persisting dementia**   HCC
Alcohol use disorder, moderate, with alcohol-induced major neurocognitive disorder, nonamnestic-confabulatory type
Alcohol use disorder, severe, with alcohol-induced major neurocognitive disorder, nonamnestic-confabulatory type

✓6ᵗʰ **F10.28**   **Alcohol dependence with other alcohol-induced disorders**

     F10.280   **Alcohol dependence with alcohol-induced anxiety disorder**   HCC

     F10.281   **Alcohol dependence with alcohol-induced sexual dysfunction**   HCC

     F10.282   **Alcohol dependence with alcohol-induced sleep disorder**   HCC

     F10.288   **Alcohol dependence with other alcohol-induced disorder**   HCC
Alcohol use disorder, moderate, with alcohol-induced mild neurocognitive disorder
Alcohol use disorder, severe, with alcohol-induced mild neurocognitive disorder

     F10.29   **Alcohol dependence with unspecified alcohol-induced disorder**   HCC ▽

✓5ᵗʰ **F10.9**   **Alcohol use, unspecified**
     EXCLUDES 1   alcohol abuse (F10.1-)
              alcohol dependence (F10.2-)

✓6ᵗʰ **F10.92**   **Alcohol use, unspecified with intoxication**

     F10.920   **Alcohol use, unspecified with intoxication, uncomplicated**   HCC

     F10.921   **Alcohol use, unspecified with intoxication delirium**   HCC

     F10.929   **Alcohol use, unspecified with intoxication, unspecified**   HCC ▽

     F10.94   **Alcohol use, unspecified with alcohol-induced mood disorder**   HCC
Alcohol induced bipolar or related disorder, without use disorder
Alcohol induced depressive disorder, without use disorder

✓6ᵗʰ **F10.95**   **Alcohol use, unspecified with alcohol-induced psychotic disorder**

     F10.950   **Alcohol use, unspecified with alcohol-induced psychotic disorder with delusions**   HCC

     F10.951   **Alcohol use, unspecified with alcohol-induced psychotic disorder with hallucinations**   HCC

EXCLUDES 1 Not coded here   **EXCLUDES 2** Not included here   N Newborn Age: 0   P Pediatric Age: 0-17   M Maternity Age: 12-55   A Adult Age: 15-124

528   ICD-10-CM 2018

F10.959   **Alcohol use, unspecified with alcohol-induced psychotic disorder, unspecified**   HCC ▽
Alcohol-induced psychotic disorder without use disorder

F10.96   **Alcohol use, unspecified with alcohol-induced persisting amnestic disorder**   HCC
Alcohol-induced major neurocognitive disorder, amnestic-confabulatory type, without use disorder

F10.97   **Alcohol use, unspecified with alcohol-induced persisting dementia**   HCC
Alcohol-induced major neurocognitive disorder, amnestic-confabulatory type, without use disorder

√6th   F10.98   **Alcohol use, unspecified with other alcohol-induced disorders**

F10.980   **Alcohol use, unspecified with alcohol-induced anxiety disorder**   HCC
Alcohol induced anxiety disorder, without use disorder

F10.981   **Alcohol use, unspecified with alcohol-induced sexual dysfunction**   HCC
Alcohol induced sexual dysfunction, without use disorder

F10.982   **Alcohol use, unspecified with alcohol-induced sleep disorder**   HCC
Alcohol induced sleep disorder, without use disorder

F10.988   **Alcohol use, unspecified with other alcohol-induced disorder**   HCC
Alcohol induced mild neurocognitive disorder, without use disorder

F10.99   **Alcohol use, unspecified with unspecified alcohol-induced disorder**   HCC ▽

√4th   **F11   Opioid related disorders**

√5th   F11.1   **Opioid abuse**
EXCLUDES 1   opioid dependence (F11.2-)
opioid use, unspecified (F11.9-)

F11.10   **Opioid abuse, uncomplicated**
Opioid use disorder, mild

●   F11.11   **Opioid abuse, in remission**
Opioid use disorder, mild, in early remission
Opioid use disorder, mild, in sustained remission

√6th   F11.12   **Opioid abuse with intoxication**

F11.120   **Opioid abuse with intoxication, uncomplicated**   HCC

F11.121   **Opioid abuse with intoxication delirium**   HCC

F11.122   **Opioid abuse with intoxication with perceptual disturbance**   HCC

F11.129   **Opioid abuse with intoxication, unspecified**   HCC ▽

F11.14   **Opioid abuse with opioid-induced mood disorder**   HCC
Opioid use disorder, mild, with opioid-induced depressive disorder

√6th   F11.15   **Opioid abuse with opioid-induced psychotic disorder**

F11.150   **Opioid abuse with opioid-induced psychotic disorder with delusions**   HCC

F11.151   **Opioid abuse with opioid-induced psychotic disorder with hallucinations**   HCC

F11.159   **Opioid abuse with opioid-induced psychotic disorder, unspecified**   HCC ▽

√6th   F11.18   **Opioid abuse with other opioid-induced disorder**

F11.181   **Opioid abuse with opioid-induced sexual dysfunction**   HCC

F11.182   **Opioid abuse with opioid-induced sleep disorder**   HCC

F11.188   **Opioid abuse with other opioid-induced disorder**   HCC

F11.19   **Opioid abuse with unspecified opioid-induced disorder**   HCC ▽

√5th   F11.2   **Opioid dependence**
EXCLUDES 1   opioid abuse (F11.1-)
opioid use, unspecified (F11.9-)
EXCLUDES 2   opioid poisoning (T40.0-T40.2-)

F11.20   **Opioid dependence, uncomplicated**   HCC
Opioid use disorder, moderate
Opioid use disorder, severe

F11.21   **Opioid dependence, in remission**   HCC
▶Opioid use disorder, moderate, in early remission
Opioid use disorder, moderate, in sustained remission
Opioid use disorder, severe, in early remission
Opioid use disorder, severe, in sustained remission◀

√6th   F11.22   **Opioid dependence with intoxication**
EXCLUDES 1   opioid dependence with withdrawal (F11.23)

F11.220   **Opioid dependence with intoxication, uncomplicated**   HCC

F11.221   **Opioid dependence with intoxication delirium**   HCC

F11.222   **Opioid dependence with intoxication with perceptual disturbance**   HCC

F11.229   **Opioid dependence with intoxication, unspecified**   HCC ▽

F11.23   **Opioid dependence with withdrawal**   HCC
EXCLUDES 1   opioid dependence with intoxication (F11.22-)

F11.24   **Opioid dependence with opioid-induced mood disorder**   HCC
Opioid use disorder, moderate, with opioid induced depressive disorder

√6th   F11.25   **Opioid dependence with opioid-induced psychotic disorder**

F11.250   **Opioid dependence with opioid-induced psychotic disorder with delusions**   HCC

F11.251   **Opioid dependence with opioid-induced psychotic disorder with hallucinations**   HCC

F11.259   **Opioid dependence with opioid-induced psychotic disorder, unspecified**   HCC ▽

√6th   F11.28   **Opioid dependence with other opioid-induced disorder**

F11.281   **Opioid dependence with opioid-induced sexual dysfunction**   HCC

F11.282   **Opioid dependence with opioid-induced sleep disorder**   HCC

F11.288   **Opioid dependence with other opioid-induced disorder**   HCC

F11.29   **Opioid dependence with unspecified opioid-induced disorder**   HCC ▽

√5th   F11.9   **Opioid use, unspecified**
EXCLUDES 1   opioid abuse (F11.1-)
opioid dependence (F11.2-)

F11.90   **Opioid use, unspecified, uncomplicated**

√6th   F11.92   **Opioid use, unspecified with intoxication**
EXCLUDES 1   opioid use, unspecified with withdrawal (F11.93)

F11.920   **Opioid use, unspecified with intoxication, uncomplicated**   HCC

F11.921   **Opioid use, unspecified with intoxication delirium**   HCC
Opioid-induced delirium

F11.922   **Opioid use, unspecified with intoxication with perceptual disturbance**   HCC

F11.929   **Opioid use, unspecified with intoxication, unspecified**   HCC ▽

F11.93   **Opioid use, unspecified with withdrawal**   HCC
EXCLUDES 1   opioid use, unspecified with intoxication (F11.92-)

F11.94   **Opioid use, unspecified with opioid-induced mood disorder**   HCC
Opioid induced depressive disorder, without use disorder

√6th   F11.95   **Opioid use, unspecified with opioid-induced psychotic disorder**

F11.950   **Opioid use, unspecified with opioid-induced psychotic disorder with delusions**   HCC

☑ Additional Character Req   √×7th Placeholder Alert   Manifestation   HCC CMS-HCC Condition   ▽ Unspecified Code   ▶◀ Revised Text   ● New Code   ▲ Revised Code Title

ICD-10-CM 2018   529

F11.951   **Opioid use, unspecified with** HCC
opioid-induced psychotic disorder with
hallucinations

F11.959   **Opioid use, unspecified with** HCC ▽
opioid-induced psychotic disorder,
unspecified

✓6ᵗʰ F11.98   **Opioid use, unspecified with other specified**
opioid-induced disorder

F11.981   **Opioid use, unspecified with** HCC
opioid-induced sexual dysfunction
Opioid induced sexual dysfunction, without
use disorder

F11.982   **Opioid use, unspecified with** HCC
opioid-induced sleep disorder
Opioid induced sleep disorder, without use
disorder

F11.988   **Opioid use, unspecified with other** HCC
opioid-induced disorder
Opioid induced anxiety disorder, without
use disorder

F11.99   **Opioid use, unspecified with unspecified** HCC ▽
opioid-induced disorder

✓4ᵗʰ **F12   Cannabis related disorders**
INCLUDES   marijuana

✓5ᵗʰ **F12.1   Cannabis abuse**
EXCLUDES 1   *cannabis dependence (F12.2-)*
cannabis use, unspecified (F12.9-)

F12.10   **Cannabis abuse, uncomplicated**
Cannabis use disorder, mild

●   F12.11   **Cannabis abuse, in remission**
Cannabis use disorder, mild, in early remission
Cannabis use disorder, mild, in sustained remission

✓6ᵗʰ F12.12   **Cannabis abuse with intoxication**

F12.120   **Cannabis abuse with intoxication,** HCC
uncomplicated

F12.121   **Cannabis abuse with intoxication** HCC
delirium

F12.122   **Cannabis abuse with intoxication** HCC
with perceptual disturbance

F12.129   **Cannabis abuse with intoxication,** HCC ▽
unspecified

✓6ᵗʰ F12.15   **Cannabis abuse with psychotic disorder**

F12.150   **Cannabis abuse with psychotic** HCC
disorder with delusions

F12.151   **Cannabis abuse with psychotic** HCC
disorder with hallucinations

F12.159   **Cannabis abuse with psychotic** HCC ▽
disorder, unspecified

✓6ᵗʰ F12.18   **Cannabis abuse with other cannabis-induced**
disorder

F12.180   **Cannabis abuse with cannabis-** HCC
induced anxiety disorder

F12.188   **Cannabis abuse with other** HCC
cannabis-induced disorder
Cannabis use disorder, mild, with
cannabis-induced sleep disorder

F12.19   **Cannabis abuse with unspecified cannabis-** HCC ▽
induced disorder

✓5ᵗʰ **F12.2   Cannabis dependence**
EXCLUDES 1   *cannabis abuse (F12.1-)*
cannabis use, unspecified (F12.9-)
EXCLUDES 2   *cannabis poisoning (T40.7-)*

F12.20   **Cannabis dependence, uncomplicated** HCC
Cannabis use disorder, moderate
Cannabis use disorder, severe

F12.21   **Cannabis dependence, in remission** HCC
▶Cannabis use disorder, moderate, in early remission
Cannabis use disorder, moderate, in sustained
remission
Cannabis use disorder, severe, in early remission
Cannabis use disorder, severe, in sustained remission◀

✓6ᵗʰ F12.22   **Cannabis dependence with intoxication**

F12.220   **Cannabis dependence with** HCC
intoxication, uncomplicated

F12.221   **Cannabis dependence with** HCC
intoxication delirium

F12.222   **Cannabis dependence with** HCC
intoxication with perceptual disturbance

F12.229   **Cannabis dependence with** HCC ▽
intoxication, unspecified

✓6ᵗʰ F12.25   **Cannabis dependence with psychotic disorder**

F12.250   **Cannabis dependence with psychotic** HCC
disorder with delusions

F12.251   **Cannabis dependence with psychotic** HCC
disorder with hallucinations

F12.259   **Cannabis dependence with** HCC
psychotic disorder, unspecified

✓6ᵗʰ F12.28   **Cannabis dependence with other cannabis-induced**
disorder

F12.280   **Cannabis dependence with** HCC
cannabis-induced anxiety disorder

F12.288   **Cannabis dependence with other** HCC
cannabis-induced disorder
Cannabis use disorder, moderate, with
cannabis-induced sleep disorder
Cannabis use disorder, severe, with
cannabis-induced sleep disorder
Cannabis withdrawal

F12.29   **Cannabis dependence with unspecified** HCC ▽
cannabis-induced disorder

✓5ᵗʰ **F12.9   Cannabis use, unspecified**
EXCLUDES 1   *cannabis abuse (F12.1-)*
cannabis dependence (F12.2-)

F12.90   **Cannabis use, unspecified, uncomplicated**

✓6ᵗʰ F12.92   **Cannabis use, unspecified with intoxication**

F12.920   **Cannabis use, unspecified with** HCC
intoxication, uncomplicated

F12.921   **Cannabis use, unspecified with** HCC
intoxication delirium

F12.922   **Cannabis use, unspecified with** HCC
intoxication with perceptual disturbance

F12.929   **Cannabis use, unspecified with** HCC ▽
intoxication, unspecified

✓6ᵗʰ F12.95   **Cannabis use, unspecified with psychotic disorder**

F12.950   **Cannabis use, unspecified with** HCC
psychotic disorder with delusions

F12.951   **Cannabis use, unspecified with** HCC
psychotic disorder with hallucinations

F12.959   **Cannabis use, unspecified with** HCC ▽
psychotic disorder, unspecified
Cannabis induced psychotic disorder,
without use disorder

✓6ᵗʰ F12.98   **Cannabis use, unspecified with other**
cannabis-induced disorder

F12.980   **Cannabis use, unspecified with** HCC
anxiety disorder
Cannabis induced anxiety disorder, without
use disorder

F12.988   **Cannabis use, unspecified with** HCC
other cannabis-induced disorder
Cannabis induced sleep disorder, without
use disorder

F12.99   **Cannabis use, unspecified with unspecified** HCC ▽
cannabis-induced disorder

✓4ᵗʰ **F13   Sedative, hypnotic, or anxiolytic related disorders**

✓5ᵗʰ **F13.1   Sedative, hypnotic or anxiolytic-related abuse**
EXCLUDES 1   *sedative, hypnotic or anxiolytic-related dependence*
(F13.2-)
sedative, hypnotic, or anxiolytic use, unspecified
(F13.9-)

F13.10   **Sedative, hypnotic or anxiolytic abuse,**
uncomplicated
Sedative, hypnotic, or anxiolytic use disorder, mild

●   F13.11   **Sedative, hypnotic or anxiolytic abuse, in remission**
Sedative, hypnotic or anxiolytic use disorder, mild, in
early remission
Sedative, hypnotic or anxiolytic use disorder, mild, in
sustained remission

✓6ᵗʰ F13.12   **Sedative, hypnotic or anxiolytic abuse with**
intoxication

F13.120   **Sedative, hypnotic or anxiolytic** HCC
abuse with intoxication, uncomplicated

F13.121   **Sedative, hypnotic or anxiolytic** HCC
abuse with intoxication delirium

F13.129   **Sedative, hypnotic or anxiolytic** HCC ▽
abuse with intoxication, unspecified

EXCLUDES 1 Not coded here   EXCLUDES 2 Not included here   N Newborn Age: 0   P Pediatric Age: 0-17   M Maternity Age: 12-55   A Adult Age: 15-124

530   ICD-10-CM 2018

F13.14   **Sedative, hypnotic or anxiolytic abuse with sedative, hypnotic or anxiolytic-induced mood disorder**   `HCC`
> ►Sedative, hypnotic, or anxiolytic use disorder, mild, with sedative, hypnotic, or anxiolytic-induced bipolar or related disorder
> Sedative, hypnotic, or anxiolytic use disorder, mild, with sedative, hypnotic, or anxiolytic-induced depressive disorder◄

✓6ᵗʰ **F13.15**   **Sedative, hypnotic or anxiolytic abuse with sedative, hypnotic or anxiolytic-induced psychotic disorder**

     F13.150   **Sedative, hypnotic or anxiolytic abuse with sedative, hypnotic or anxiolytic-induced psychotic disorder with delusions**   `HCC`

     F13.151   **Sedative, hypnotic or anxiolytic abuse with sedative, hypnotic or anxiolytic-induced psychotic disorder with hallucinations**   `HCC`

     F13.159   **Sedative, hypnotic or anxiolytic abuse with sedative, hypnotic or anxiolytic-induced psychotic disorder, unspecified**   `HCC` ▽

✓6ᵗʰ **F13.18**   **Sedative, hypnotic or anxiolytic abuse with other sedative, hypnotic or anxiolytic-induced disorders**

     F13.180   **Sedative, hypnotic or anxiolytic abuse with sedative, hypnotic or anxiolytic-induced anxiety disorder**   `HCC`

     F13.181   **Sedative, hypnotic or anxiolytic abuse with sedative, hypnotic or anxiolytic-induced sexual dysfunction**   `HCC`

     F13.182   **Sedative, hypnotic or anxiolytic abuse with sedative, hypnotic or anxiolytic-induced sleep disorder**   `HCC`

     F13.188   **Sedative, hypnotic or anxiolytic abuse with other sedative, hypnotic or anxiolytic-induced disorder**   `HCC`

F13.19   **Sedative, hypnotic or anxiolytic abuse with unspecified sedative, hypnotic or anxiolytic-induced disorder**   `HCC` ▽

✓5ᵗʰ **F13.2**   **Sedative, hypnotic or anxiolytic-related dependence**
> EXCLUDES 1   *sedative, hypnotic or anxiolytic-related abuse (F13.1-)*
> *sedative, hypnotic, or anxiolytic use, unspecified (F13.9-)*
> EXCLUDES 2   *sedative, hypnotic, or anxiolytic poisoning (T42.-)*

F13.20   **Sedative, hypnotic or anxiolytic dependence, uncomplicated**   `HCC`

F13.21   **Sedative, hypnotic or anxiolytic dependence, in remission**   `HCC`
> ►Sedative, hypnotic or anxiolytic use disorder, moderate, in early remission
> Sedative, hypnotic or anxiolytic use disorder, moderate, in sustained remission
> Sedative, hypnotic or anxiolytic use disorder, severe, in early remission
> Sedative, hypnotic or anxiolytic use disorder, severe, in sustained remission◄

✓6ᵗʰ **F13.22**   **Sedative, hypnotic or anxiolytic dependence with intoxication**
> EXCLUDES 1   *sedative, hypnotic or anxiolytic dependence with withdrawal (F13.23-)*

     F13.220   **Sedative, hypnotic or anxiolytic dependence with intoxication, uncomplicated**   `HCC`

     F13.221   **Sedative, hypnotic or anxiolytic dependence with intoxication delirium**   `HCC`

     F13.229   **Sedative, hypnotic or anxiolytic dependence with intoxication, unspecified**   `HCC` ▽

✓6ᵗʰ **F13.23**   **Sedative, hypnotic or anxiolytic dependence with withdrawal**
> Sedative, hypnotic, or anxiolytic use disorder, moderate
> Sedative, hypnotic, or anxiolytic use disorder, severe
> EXCLUDES 1   *sedative, hypnotic or anxiolytic dependence with intoxication (F13.22-)*

     F13.230   **Sedative, hypnotic or anxiolytic dependence with withdrawal, uncomplicated**   `HCC`

     F13.231   **Sedative, hypnotic or anxiolytic dependence with withdrawal delirium**   `HCC`

     F13.232   **Sedative, hypnotic or anxiolytic dependence with withdrawal with perceptual disturbance**   `HCC`
> Sedative, hypnotic, or anxiolytic withdrawal with perceptual disturbances

     F13.239   **Sedative, hypnotic or anxiolytic dependence with withdrawal, unspecified**   `HCC` ▽
> Sedative, hypnotic, or anxiolytic withdrawal without perceptual disturbances

F13.24   **Sedative, hypnotic or anxiolytic dependence with sedative, hypnotic or anxiolytic-induced mood disorder**   `HCC`
> ►Sedative, hypnotic, or anxiolytic use disorder, moderate, with sedative, hypnotic, or anxiolytic-induced bipolar or related disorder
> Sedative, hypnotic, or anxiolytic use disorder, moderate, with sedative, hypnotic, or anxiolytic-induced depressive disorder◄
> Sedative, hypnotic, or anxiolytic use disorder, severe, with sedative, hypnotic, or anxiolytic-induced bipolar or related disorder
> ►Sedative, hypnotic, or anxiolytic use disorder, severe, with sedative, hypnotic, or anxiolytic-induced depressive disorder◄

✓6ᵗʰ **F13.25**   **Sedative, hypnotic or anxiolytic dependence with sedative, hypnotic or anxiolytic-induced psychotic disorder**

     F13.250   **Sedative, hypnotic or anxiolytic dependence with sedative, hypnotic or anxiolytic-induced psychotic disorder with delusions**   `HCC`

     F13.251   **Sedative, hypnotic or anxiolytic dependence with sedative, hypnotic or anxiolytic-induced psychotic disorder with hallucinations**   `HCC`

     F13.259   **Sedative, hypnotic or anxiolytic dependence with sedative, hypnotic or anxiolytic-induced psychotic disorder, unspecified**   `HCC` ▽

F13.26   **Sedative, hypnotic or anxiolytic dependence with sedative, hypnotic or anxiolytic-induced persisting amnestic disorder**   `HCC`

F13.27   **Sedative, hypnotic or anxiolytic dependence with sedative, hypnotic or anxiolytic-induced persisting dementia**   `HCC`
> ►Sedative, hypnotic, or anxiolytic use disorder, moderate, with sedative, hypnotic, or anxiolytic-induced major neurocognitive disorder◄
> Sedative, hypnotic, or anxiolytic use disorder, severe, with sedative, hypnotic, or anxiolytic-induced major neurocognitive disorder

✓6ᵗʰ **F13.28**   **Sedative, hypnotic or anxiolytic dependence with other sedative, hypnotic or anxiolytic-induced disorders**

     F13.280   **Sedative, hypnotic or anxiolytic dependence with sedative, hypnotic or anxiolytic-induced anxiety disorder**   `HCC`

     F13.281   **Sedative, hypnotic or anxiolytic dependence with sedative, hypnotic or anxiolytic-induced sexual dysfunction**   `HCC`

     F13.282   **Sedative, hypnotic or anxiolytic dependence with sedative, hypnotic or anxiolytic-induced sleep disorder**   `HCC`

     F13.288   **Sedative, hypnotic or anxiolytic dependence with other sedative, hypnotic or anxiolytic-induced disorder**   `HCC`
> ►Sedative, hypnotic, or anxiolytic use disorder, moderate, with sedative, hypnotic, or anxiolytic-induced mild neurocognitive disorder
> Sedative, hypnotic, or anxiolytic use disorder, severe, with sedative, hypnotic, or anxiolytic-induced mild neurocognitive disorder◄

F13.29   **Sedative, hypnotic or anxiolytic dependence with unspecified sedative, hypnotic or anxiolytic-induced disorder**   `HCC` ▽

✓ Additional Character Req   ✓x7ᵗʰ Placeholder Alert   Manifestation   `HCC` CMS-HCC Condition   ▽ Unspecified Code   ►◄ Revised Text   ● New Code   ▲ Revised Code Title

✓5ᵗʰ **F13.9** **Sedative, hypnotic or anxiolytic-related use, unspecified**
> EXCLUDES 1   *sedative, hypnotic or anxiolytic-related abuse (F13.1-)*
> *sedative, hypnotic or anxiolytic-related dependence (F13.2-)*

F13.90 **Sedative, hypnotic, or anxiolytic use, unspecified, uncomplicated**

✓6ᵗʰ **F13.92** **Sedative, hypnotic or anxiolytic use, unspecified with intoxication**
> EXCLUDES 1   *sedative, hypnotic or anxiolytic use, unspecified with withdrawal (F13.93-)*

F13.920 **Sedative, hypnotic or anxiolytic use, unspecified with intoxication, uncomplicated** HCC

F13.921 **Sedative, hypnotic or anxiolytic use, unspecified with intoxication delirium** HCC
Sedative, hypnotic, or anxiolytic-induced delirium

F13.929 **Sedative, hypnotic or anxiolytic use, unspecified with intoxication, unspecified** HCC ▽

✓6ᵗʰ **F13.93** **Sedative, hypnotic or anxiolytic use, unspecified with withdrawal**
> EXCLUDES 1   *sedative, hypnotic or anxiolytic use, unspecified with intoxication (F13.92-)*

F13.930 **Sedative, hypnotic or anxiolytic use, unspecified with withdrawal, uncomplicated** HCC

F13.931 **Sedative, hypnotic or anxiolytic use, unspecified with withdrawal delirium** HCC

F13.932 **Sedative, hypnotic or anxiolytic use, unspecified with withdrawal with perceptual disturbances** HCC

F13.939 **Sedative, hypnotic or anxiolytic use, unspecified with withdrawal, unspecified** HCC ▽

F13.94 **Sedative, hypnotic or anxiolytic use, unspecified with sedative, hypnotic or anxiolytic-induced mood disorder** HCC ▽
Sedative, hypnotic, or anxiolytic-induced bipolar or related disorder, without use disorder
Sedative, hypnotic, or anxiolytic-induced depressive disorder, without use disorder

✓6ᵗʰ **F13.95** **Sedative, hypnotic or anxiolytic use, unspecified with sedative, hypnotic or anxiolytic-induced psychotic disorder**

F13.950 **Sedative, hypnotic or anxiolytic use, unspecified with sedative, hypnotic or anxiolytic-induced psychotic disorder with delusions** HCC

F13.951 **Sedative, hypnotic or anxiolytic use, unspecified with sedative, hypnotic or anxiolytic-induced psychotic disorder with hallucinations** HCC

F13.959 **Sedative, hypnotic or anxiolytic use, unspecified with sedative, hypnotic or anxiolytic-induced psychotic disorder, unspecified** HCC ▽
▶Sedative, hypnotic, or anxiolytic-induced psychotic disorder, without use disorder◀

F13.96 **Sedative, hypnotic or anxiolytic use, unspecified with sedative, hypnotic or anxiolytic-induced persisting amnestic disorder** HCC

F13.97 **Sedative, hypnotic or anxiolytic use, unspecified with sedative, hypnotic or anxiolytic-induced persisting dementia** HCC
▶Sedative, hypnotic, or anxiolytic-induced major neurocognitive disorder, without use disorder◀

✓6ᵗʰ **F13.98** **Sedative, hypnotic or anxiolytic use, unspecified with other sedative, hypnotic or anxiolytic-induced disorders**

F13.980 **Sedative, hypnotic or anxiolytic use, unspecified with sedative, hypnotic or anxiolytic-induced anxiety disorder** HCC
▶Sedative, hypnotic, or anxiolytic-induced anxiety disorder, without use disorder◀

F13.981 **Sedative, hypnotic or anxiolytic use, unspecified with sedative, hypnotic or anxiolytic-induced sexual dysfunction** HCC
▶Sedative, hypnotic, or anxiolytic-induced sexual dysfunction disorder, without use disorder◀

F13.982 **Sedative, hypnotic or anxiolytic use, unspecified with sedative, hypnotic or anxiolytic-induced sleep disorder** HCC
▶Sedative, hypnotic, or anxiolytic-induced sleep disorder, without use disorder◀

F13.988 **Sedative, hypnotic or anxiolytic use, unspecified with other sedative, hypnotic or anxiolytic-induced disorder** HCC
▶Sedative, hypnotic, or anxiolytic-induced mild neurocognitive disorder◀

F13.99 **Sedative, hypnotic or anxiolytic use, unspecified with unspecified sedative, hypnotic or anxiolytic-induced disorder** HCC ▽

✓4ᵗʰ **F14** **Cocaine related disorders**
> EXCLUDES 2   *other stimulant-related disorders (F15.-)*

✓5ᵗʰ **F14.1** **Cocaine abuse**
> EXCLUDES 1   *cocaine dependence (F14.2-)*
> *cocaine use, unspecified (F14.9-)*

F14.10 **Cocaine abuse, uncomplicated**
Cocaine use disorder, mild

● **F14.11** **Cocaine abuse, in remission**
Cocaine use disorder, mild, in early remission
Cocaine use disorder, mild, in sustained remission

✓6ᵗʰ **F14.12** **Cocaine abuse with intoxication**

F14.120 **Cocaine abuse with intoxication, uncomplicated** HCC

F14.121 **Cocaine abuse with intoxication with delirium** HCC

F14.122 **Cocaine abuse with intoxication with perceptual disturbance** HCC

F14.129 **Cocaine abuse with intoxication, unspecified** HCC ▽

F14.14 **Cocaine abuse with cocaine-induced mood disorder** HCC
Cocaine use disorder, mild, with cocaine-induced bipolar or related disorder
Cocaine use disorder, mild, with cocaine-induced depressive disorder

✓6ᵗʰ **F14.15** **Cocaine abuse with cocaine-induced psychotic disorder**

F14.150 **Cocaine abuse with cocaine-induced psychotic disorder with delusions** HCC

F14.151 **Cocaine abuse with cocaine-induced psychotic disorder with hallucinations** HCC

F14.159 **Cocaine abuse with cocaine-induced psychotic disorder, unspecified** HCC ▽

✓6ᵗʰ **F14.18** **Cocaine abuse with other cocaine-induced disorder**

F14.180 **Cocaine abuse with cocaine-induced anxiety disorder** HCC

F14.181 **Cocaine abuse with cocaine-induced sexual dysfunction** HCC

F14.182 **Cocaine abuse with cocaine-induced sleep disorder** HCC

F14.188 **Cocaine abuse with other cocaine-induced disorder** HCC
Cocaine use disorder, mild, with cocaine-induced obsessive compulsive or related disorder

F14.19 **Cocaine abuse with unspecified cocaine-induced disorder** HCC ▽

✓5ᵗʰ **F14.2** **Cocaine dependence**
> EXCLUDES 1   *cocaine abuse (F14.1-)*
> *cocaine use, unspecified (F14.9-)*
> EXCLUDES 2   *cocaine poisoning (T40.5-)*

F14.20 **Cocaine dependence, uncomplicated** HCC
Cocaine use disorder, moderate
Cocaine use disorder, severe

F14.21 **Cocaine dependence, in remission** HCC
▶Cocaine use disorder, moderate, in early remission
Cocaine use disorder, moderate, in sustained remission
Cocaine use disorder, severe, in early remission
Cocaine use disorder, severe, in sustained remission◀

✓6ᵗʰ **F14.22** **Cocaine dependence with intoxication**
> EXCLUDES 1   *cocaine dependence with withdrawal (F14.23)*

F14.220 **Cocaine dependence with intoxication, uncomplicated** HCC

EXCLUDES 1 Not coded here   EXCLUDES 2 Not included here   N Newborn Age: 0   P Pediatric Age: 0-17   M Maternity Age: 12-55   A Adult Age: 15-124

532   ICD-10-CM 2018

F13.9–F14.220

F14.221   **Cocaine dependence with intoxication delirium** `HCC`

F14.222   **Cocaine dependence with intoxication with perceptual disturbance** `HCC`

F14.229   **Cocaine dependence with intoxication, unspecified** `HCC` ▽

F14.23   **Cocaine dependence with withdrawal** `HCC`
> *EXCLUDES 1*   *cocaine dependence with intoxication (F14.22-)*

F14.24   **Cocaine dependence with cocaine-induced mood disorder** `HCC`
> Cocaine use disorder, moderate, with cocaine-induced bipolar or related disorder
> Cocaine use disorder, moderate, with cocaine-induced depressive disorder
> Cocaine use disorder, severe, with cocaine-induced bipolar or related disorder
> Cocaine use disorder, severe, with cocaine-induced depressive disorder

√6th F14.25   **Cocaine dependence with cocaine-induced psychotic disorder**

F14.250   **Cocaine dependence with cocaine-induced psychotic disorder with delusions** `HCC`

F14.251   **Cocaine dependence with cocaine-induced psychotic disorder with hallucinations** `HCC`

F14.259   **Cocaine dependence with cocaine-induced psychotic disorder, unspecified** `HCC` ▽

√6th F14.28   **Cocaine dependence with other cocaine-induced disorder**

F14.280   **Cocaine dependence with cocaine-induced anxiety disorder** `HCC`

F14.281   **Cocaine dependence with cocaine-induced sexual dysfunction** `HCC`

F14.282   **Cocaine dependence with cocaine-induced sleep disorder** `HCC`

F14.288   **Cocaine dependence with other cocaine-induced disorder** `HCC`
> Cocaine use disorder, moderate, with cocaine-induced obsessive compulsive or related disorder
> Cocaine use disorder, severe, with cocaine-induced obsessive compulsive or related disorder

F14.29   **Cocaine dependence with unspecified cocaine-induced disorder** `HCC` ▽

√5th F14.9   **Cocaine use, unspecified**
> *EXCLUDES 1*   *cocaine abuse (F14.1-)*
> *cocaine dependence (F14.2-)*

F14.90   **Cocaine use, unspecified, uncomplicated**

√6th F14.92   **Cocaine use, unspecified with intoxication**

F14.920   **Cocaine use, unspecified with intoxication, uncomplicated** `HCC`

F14.921   **Cocaine use, unspecified with intoxication delirium** `HCC`

F14.922   **Cocaine use, unspecified with intoxication with perceptual disturbance** `HCC`

F14.929   **Cocaine use, unspecified with intoxication, unspecified** `HCC` ▽

F14.94   **Cocaine use, unspecified with cocaine-induced mood disorder** `HCC`
> Cocaine induced bipolar or related disorder, without use disorder
> Cocaine induced depressive disorder, without use disorder

√6th F14.95   **Cocaine use, unspecified with cocaine-induced psychotic disorder**

F14.950   **Cocaine use, unspecified with cocaine-induced psychotic disorder with delusions** `HCC`

F14.951   **Cocaine use, unspecified with cocaine-induced psychotic disorder with hallucinations** `HCC`

F14.959   **Cocaine use, unspecified with cocaine-induced psychotic disorder, unspecified** `HCC` ▽
> Cocaine induced psychotic disorder, without use disorder

F14.98   **Cocaine use, unspecified with other specified cocaine-induced disorder**

F14.980   **Cocaine use, unspecified with cocaine-induced anxiety disorder** `HCC`
> Cocaine induced anxiety disorder, without use disorder

F14.981   **Cocaine use, unspecified with cocaine-induced sexual dysfunction** `HCC`
> Cocaine induced sexual dysfunction, without use disorder

F14.982   **Cocaine use, unspecified with cocaine-induced sleep disorder** `HCC`
> Cocaine induced sleep disorder, without use disorder

F14.988   **Cocaine use, unspecified with other cocaine-induced disorder** `HCC`
> Cocaine induced obsessive compulsive or related disorder

F14.99   **Cocaine use, unspecified with unspecified cocaine-induced disorder** `HCC` ▽

√4th **F15**   **Other stimulant related disorders**
> *INCLUDES*   amphetamine-related disorders
> caffeine
> *EXCLUDES 2*   *cocaine-related disorders (F14.-)*

√5th F15.1   **Other stimulant abuse**
> *EXCLUDES 1*   *other stimulant dependence (F15.2-)*
> *other stimulant use, unspecified (F15.9-)*

F15.10   **Other stimulant abuse, uncomplicated**
> Amphetamine type substance use disorder, mild
> Other or unspecified stimulant use disorder, mild

● F15.11   **Other stimulant abuse, in remission**
> Amphetamine type substance use disorder, mild, in early remission
> Amphetamine type substance use disorder, mild, in sustained remission
> Other or unspecified stimulant use disorder, mild, in early remission
> Other or unspecified stimulant use disorder, mild, in sustained remission

√6th F15.12   **Other stimulant abuse with intoxication**

F15.120   **Other stimulant abuse with intoxication, uncomplicated** `HCC`

F15.121   **Other stimulant abuse with intoxication delirium** `HCC`

F15.122   **Other stimulant abuse with intoxication with perceptual disturbance** `HCC`
> Amphetamine or other stimulant use disorder, mild, with amphetamine or other stimulant intoxication, with perceptual disturbances

F15.129   **Other stimulant abuse with intoxication, unspecified** `HCC` ▽
> Amphetamine or other stimulant use disorder, mild, with amphetamine or other stimulant intoxication, without perceptual disturbances

F15.14   **Other stimulant abuse with stimulant-induced mood disorder** `HCC`
> Amphetamine or other stimulant use disorder, mild, with amphetamine or other stimulant induced bipolar or related disorder
> Amphetamine or other stimulant use disorder, mild, with amphetamine or other stimulant induced depressive disorder

√6th F15.15   **Other stimulant abuse with stimulant-induced psychotic disorder**

F15.150   **Other stimulant abuse with stimulant-induced psychotic disorder with delusions** `HCC`

F15.151   **Other stimulant abuse with stimulant-induced psychotic disorder with hallucinations** `HCC`

F15.159   **Other stimulant abuse with stimulant-induced psychotic disorder, unspecified** `HCC` ▽

√6th F15.18   **Other stimulant abuse with other stimulant-induced disorder**

F15.180   **Other stimulant abuse with stimulant-induced anxiety disorder** `HCC`

F15.181   **Other stimulant abuse with stimulant-induced sexual dysfunction** `HCC`

☑ Additional Character Req   √7th Placeholder Alert   Manifestation   `HCC` CMS-HCC Condition   ▽ Unspecified Code   ▶◀ Revised Text   ● New Code   ▲ Revised Code Title

ICD-10-CM 2018   533

F15.182   **Other stimulant abuse with** `HCC` **stimulant-induced sleep disorder**

F15.188   **Other stimulant abuse with other** `HCC` **stimulant-induced disorder**
Amphetamine or other stimulant use disorder, mild, with amphetamine or other stimulant induced obsessive-compulsive or related disorder

F15.19   **Other stimulant abuse with unspecified** `HCC` ▽ **stimulant-induced disorder**

✓5ᵗʰ **F15.2**   **Other stimulant dependence**
EXCLUDES 1   *other stimulant abuse (F15.1-)*
other stimulant use, unspecified (F15.9-)

F15.20   **Other stimulant dependence, uncomplicated** `HCC`
Amphetamine type substance use disorder, moderate
Amphetamine type substance use disorder, severe
Other or unspecified stimulant use disorder, moderate
Other or unspecified stimulant use disorder, severe

F15.21   **Other stimulant dependence, in remission** `HCC`
▶Amphetamine type substance use disorder, moderate, in early remission
Amphetamine type substance use disorder, moderate, in sustained remission
Amphetamine type substance use disorder, severe, in early remission
Amphetamine type substance use disorder, severe, in sustained remission
Other or unspecified stimulant use disorder, moderate, in early remission
Other or unspecified stimulant use disorder, moderate, in sustained remission
Other or unspecified stimulant use disorder, severe, in early remission
Other or unspecified stimulant use disorder, severe, in sustained remission◀

✓6ᵗʰ **F15.22**   **Other stimulant dependence with intoxication**
EXCLUDES 1   *other stimulant dependence with withdrawal (F15.23)*

F15.220   **Other stimulant dependence with** `HCC` **intoxication, uncomplicated**

F15.221   **Other stimulant dependence with** `HCC` **intoxication delirium**

F15.222   **Other stimulant dependence with** `HCC` **intoxication with perceptual disturbance**
Amphetamine or other stimulant use disorder, moderate, with amphetamine or other stimulant intoxication, with perceptual disturbances
Amphetamine or other stimulant use disorder, severe, with amphetamine or other stimulant intoxication, with perceptual disturbances

F15.229   **Other stimulant dependence with** `HCC` ▽ **intoxication, unspecified**
Amphetamine or other stimulant use disorder, moderate, with amphetamine or other stimulant intoxication, without perceptual disturbances
Amphetamine or other stimulant use disorder, severe, with amphetamine or other stimulant intoxication, without perceptual disturbances

F15.23   **Other stimulant dependence with withdrawal** `HCC`
Amphetamine or other stimulant withdrawal
EXCLUDES 1   *other stimulant dependence with intoxication (F15.22-)*

F15.24   **Other stimulant dependence with** `HCC` **stimulant-induced mood disorder**
Amphetamine or other stimulant use disorder, moderate, with amphetamine or other stimulant-induced bipolar or related disorder
Amphetamine or other stimulant use disorder, moderate, with amphetamine or other stimulant induced depressive disorder
Amphetamine or other stimulant use disorder, severe, with amphetamine or other stimulant-induced bipolar or related disorder
Amphetamine or other stimulant use disorder, severe, with amphetamine or other stimulant-induced depressive disorder

✓6ᵗʰ **F15.25**   **Other stimulant dependence with stimulant-induced psychotic disorder**

F15.250   **Other stimulant dependence with** `HCC` **stimulant-induced psychotic disorder with delusions**

F15.251   **Other stimulant dependence with** `HCC` **stimulant-induced psychotic disorder with hallucinations**

F15.259   **Other stimulant dependence with** `HCC` ▽ **stimulant-induced psychotic disorder, unspecified**

✓6ᵗʰ **F15.28**   **Other stimulant dependence with other stimulant-induced disorder**

F15.280   **Other stimulant dependence with** `HCC` **stimulant-induced anxiety disorder**

F15.281   **Other stimulant dependence with** `HCC` **stimulant-induced sexual dysfunction**

F15.282   **Other stimulant dependence with** `HCC` **stimulant-induced sleep disorder**

F15.288   **Other stimulant dependence with** `HCC` **other stimulant-induced disorder**
▶Amphetamine or other stimulant use disorder, moderate, with amphetamine or other stimulant induced obsessive compulsive or related disorder
Amphetamine or other stimulant use disorder, severe, with amphetamine or other stimulant induced obsessive compulsive or related disorder◀

F15.29   **Other stimulant dependence with unspecified** `HCC` ▽ **stimulant-induced disorder**

✓5ᵗʰ **F15.9**   **Other stimulant use, unspecified**
EXCLUDES 1   *other stimulant abuse (F15.1-)*
other stimulant dependence (F15.2-)

F15.90   **Other stimulant use, unspecified, uncomplicated**

✓6ᵗʰ **F15.92**   **Other stimulant use, unspecified with intoxication**
EXCLUDES 1   *other stimulant use, unspecified with withdrawal (F15.93)*

F15.920   **Other stimulant use, unspecified with** `HCC` **intoxication, uncomplicated**

F15.921   **Other stimulant use, unspecified with** `HCC` **intoxication delirium**
Amphetamine or other stimulant-induced delirium

F15.922   **Other stimulant use, unspecified with** `HCC` **intoxication with perceptual disturbance**

F15.929   **Other stimulant use, unspecified** `HCC` ▽ **with intoxication, unspecified**
Caffeine intoxication

F15.93   **Other stimulant use, unspecified with** `HCC` **withdrawal**
Caffeine withdrawal
EXCLUDES 1   *other stimulant use, unspecified with intoxication (F15.92-)*

F15.94   **Other stimulant use, unspecified with** `HCC` **stimulant-induced mood disorder**
Amphetamine or other stimulant-induced bipolar or related disorder, without use disorder
Amphetamine or other stimulant-induced depressive disorder, without use disorder

✓6ᵗʰ **F15.95**   **Other stimulant use, unspecified with stimulant-induced psychotic disorder**

F15.950   **Other stimulant use, unspecified with** `HCC` **stimulant-induced p sychotic disorder with delusions**

F15.951   **Other stimulant use, unspecified with** `HCC` **stimulant-induced p sychotic disorder with hallucinations**

F15.959   **Other stimulant use, unspecified** `HCC` ▽ **with stimulant-induced psychotic disorder, unspecified**
▶Amphetamine or other stimulant-induced psychotic disorder, without use disorder◀

EXCLUDES 1 Not coded here   *EXCLUDES 2* Not included here   N Newborn Age: 0   P Pediatric Age: 0-17   M Maternity Age: 12-55   A Adult Age: 15-124

534   ICD-10-CM 2018

✓6ᵗʰ **F15.98 Other stimulant use, unspecified with other stimulant-induced disorder**

F15.980 Other stimulant use, unspecified with ᴴᶜᶜ **stimulant-induced anxiety disorder**
Amphetamine or other stimulant-induced anxiety disorder, without use disorder
Caffeine induced anxiety disorder, without use disorder

F15.981 Other stimulant use, unspecified with ᴴᶜᶜ **stimulant-induced sexual dysfunction**
Amphetamine or other stimulant-induced sexual dysfunction, without use disorder

F15.982 Other stimulant use, unspecified with ᴴᶜᶜ **stimulant-induced sleep disorder**
Amphetamine or other stimulant-induced sleep disorder, without use disorder
Caffeine induced sleep disorder, without use disorder

F15.988 Other stimulant use, unspecified with ᴴᶜᶜ **other stimulant-induced disorder**
Amphetamine or other stimulant-induced obsessive compulsive or related disorder, without use disorder

F15.99 Other stimulant use, unspecified with ᴴᶜᶜ ▽ **unspecified stimulant-induced disorder**

✓4ᵗʰ **F16 Hallucinogen related disorders**
INCLUDES ecstasy
PCP
phencyclidine

✓5ᵗʰ **F16.1 Hallucinogen abuse**
EXCLUDES 1 hallucinogen dependence (F16.2-)
hallucinogen use, unspecified (F16.9-)

F16.10 Hallucinogen abuse, uncomplicated
Other hallucinogen use disorder, mild
Phencyclidine use disorder, mild

● **F16.11 Hallucinogen abuse, in remission**
Other hallucinogen use disorder, mild, in early remission
Other hallucinogen use disorder, mild, in sustained remission
Phencyclidine use disorder, mild, in early remission
Phencyclidine use disorder, mild, in sustained remission

✓6ᵗʰ **F16.12 Hallucinogen abuse with intoxication**

F16.120 Hallucinogen abuse with intoxication, ᴴᶜᶜ **uncomplicated**

F16.121 Hallucinogen abuse with intoxication ᴴᶜᶜ **with delirium**

F16.122 Hallucinogen abuse with intoxication ᴴᶜᶜ **with perceptual disturbance**

F16.129 Hallucinogen abuse with ᴴᶜᶜ ▽ **intoxication, unspecified**

F16.14 Hallucinogen abuse with hallucinogen-induced mood disorder
Other hallucinogen use disorder, mild, with other hallucinogen induced bipolar or related disorder
Other hallucinogen use disorder, mild, with other hallucinogen induced depressive disorder
Phencyclidine use disorder, mild, with phencyclidine induced bipolar or related disorder
Phencyclidine use disorder, mild, with phencyclidine induced depressive disorder

✓6ᵗʰ **F16.15 Hallucinogen abuse with hallucinogen-induced psychotic disorder**

F16.150 Hallucinogen abuse with ᴴᶜᶜ **hallucinogen-induced psychotic disorder with delusions**

F16.151 Hallucinogen abuse with ᴴᶜᶜ **hallucinogen-induced psychotic disorder with hallucinations**

F16.159 Hallucinogen abuse with ᴴᶜᶜ ▽ **hallucinogen-induced psychotic disorder, unspecified**

✓6ᵗʰ **F16.18 Hallucinogen abuse with other hallucinogen-induced disorder**

F16.180 Hallucinogen abuse with ᴴᶜᶜ **hallucinogen-induced anxiety disorder**

F16.183 Hallucinogen abuse with ᴴᶜᶜ **hallucinogen persisting perception disorder (flashbacks)**

F16.188 Hallucinogen abuse with other ᴴᶜᶜ **hallucinogen-induced disorder**

F16.19 Hallucinogen abuse with unspecified ᴴᶜᶜ ▽ **hallucinogen-induced disorder**

✓5ᵗʰ **F16.2 Hallucinogen dependence**
EXCLUDES 1 hallucinogen abuse (F16.1-)
hallucinogen use, unspecified (F16.9-)

F16.20 Hallucinogen dependence, uncomplicated ᴴᶜᶜ
Other hallucinogen use disorder, moderate
Other hallucinogen use disorder, severe
Phencyclidine use disorder, moderate
Phencyclidine use disorder, severe

F16.21 Hallucinogen dependence, in remission ᴴᶜᶜ
▶Other hallucinogen use disorder, moderate, in early remission
Other hallucinogen use disorder, moderate, in sustained remission
Other hallucinogen use disorder, severe, in early remission
Other hallucinogen use disorder, severe, in sustained remission
Phencyclidine use disorder, moderate, in early remission
Phencyclidine use disorder, moderate, in sustained remission
Phencyclidine use disorder, severe, in early remission
Phencyclidine use disorder, severe, in sustained remission◀

✓6ᵗʰ **F16.22 Hallucinogen dependence with intoxication**

F16.220 Hallucinogen dependence with ᴴᶜᶜ **intoxication, uncomplicated**

F16.221 Hallucinogen dependence with ᴴᶜᶜ **intoxication with delirium**

F16.229 Hallucinogen dependence with ᴴᶜᶜ ▽ **intoxication, unspecified**

F16.24 Hallucinogen dependence with ᴴᶜᶜ **hallucinogen-induced mood disorder**
Other hallucinogen use disorder, moderate, with other hallucinogen induced bipolar or related disorder
Other hallucinogen use disorder, moderate, with other hallucinogen induced depressive disorder
Other hallucinogen use disorder, severe, with other hallucinogen-induced bipolar or related disorder
Other hallucinogen use disorder, severe, with other hallucinogen-induced depressive disorder
Phencyclidine use disorder, moderate, with phencyclidine induced bipolar or related disorder
Phencyclidine use disorder, moderate, with phencyclidine induced depressive disorder
Phencyclidine use disorder, severe, with phencyclidine induced bipolar or related disorder
Phencyclidine use disorder, severe, with phencyclidine-induced depressive disorder

✓6ᵗʰ **F16.25 Hallucinogen dependence with hallucinogen-induced psychotic disorder**

F16.250 Hallucinogen dependence with ᴴᶜᶜ **hallucinogen-induced psychotic disorder with delusions**

F16.251 Hallucinogen dependence with ᴴᶜᶜ **hallucinogen-induced psychotic disorder with hallucinations**

F16.259 Hallucinogen dependence with ᴴᶜᶜ ▽ **hallucinogen-induced psychotic disorder, unspecified**

✓6ᵗʰ **F16.28 Hallucinogen dependence with other hallucinogen-induced disorder**

F16.280 Hallucinogen dependence with ᴴᶜᶜ **hallucinogen-induced anxiety disorder**

F16.283 Hallucinogen dependence with ᴴᶜᶜ **hallucinogen persisting perception disorder (flashbacks)**

F16.288 Hallucinogen dependence with other ᴴᶜᶜ **hallucinogen-induced disorder**

F16.29 Hallucinogen dependence with unspecified ᴴᶜᶜ ▽ **hallucinogen-induced disorder**

✓5ᵗʰ **F16.9 Hallucinogen use, unspecified**
EXCLUDES 1 hallucinogen abuse (F16.1-)
hallucinogen dependence (F16.2-)

F16.90 Hallucinogen use, unspecified, uncomplicated

☑ Additional Character Req   ✓ˣ⁷ᵗʰ Placeholder Alert   Manifestation   ᴴᶜᶜ CMS-HCC Condition   ▽ Unspecified Code   ▶◀ Revised Text   ● New Code   ▲ Revised Code Title

ICD-10-CM 2018   535

Chapter 5. Mental, Behavioral and Neurodevelopmental Disorders

✓6ᵗʰ **F16.92 Hallucinogen use, unspecified with intoxication**

F16.920 Hallucinogen use, unspecified with ᴴᶜᶜ
intoxication, uncomplicated

F16.921 Hallucinogen use, unspecified with ᴴᶜᶜ
intoxication with delirium
Other hallucinogen intoxication delirium

F16.929 Hallucinogen use, unspecified with ᴴᶜᶜ ▽
intoxication, unspecified

F16.94 Hallucinogen use, unspecified with ᴴᶜᶜ
hallucinogen-induced mood disorder
Other hallucinogen induced bipolar or related
disorder, without use disorder
Other hallucinogen induced depressive disorder,
without use disorder
Phencyclidine induced bipolar or related disorder,
without use disorder
Phencyclidine induced depressive disorder, without
use disorder

✓6ᵗʰ **F16.95 Hallucinogen use, unspecified with**
hallucinogen-induced psychotic disorder

F16.950 Hallucinogen use, unspecified with ᴴᶜᶜ
hallucinogen-induced psychotic disorder
with delusions

F16.951 Hallucinogen use, unspecified with ᴴᶜᶜ
hallucinogen-induced psychotic disorder
with hallucinations

F16.959 Hallucinogen use, unspecified with ᴴᶜᶜ ▽
hallucinogen-induced psychotic disorder,
unspecified
Other hallucinogen induced psychotic
disorder, without use disorder
Phencyclidine induced psychotic disorder,
without use disorder

✓6ᵗʰ **F16.98 Hallucinogen use, unspecified with other specified**
hallucinogen-induced disorder

F16.980 Hallucinogen use, unspecified with ᴴᶜᶜ
hallucinogen-induced anxiety disorder
Other hallucinogen-induced anxiety
disorder, without use disorder
Phencyclidine induced anxiety disorder,
without use disorder

F16.983 Hallucinogen use, unspecified with ᴴᶜᶜ
hallucinogen persisting perception
disorder (flashbacks)

F16.988 Hallucinogen use, unspecified with ᴴᶜᶜ
other hallucinogen-induced disorder

F16.99 Hallucinogen use, unspecified with ᴴᶜᶜ ▽
unspecified hallucinogen-induced disorder

✓4ᵗʰ **F17 Nicotine dependence**
EXCLUDES 1 history of tobacco dependence (Z87.891)
tobacco use NOS (Z72.0)
EXCLUDES 2 tobacco use (smoking) during pregnancy, childbirth and the
puerperium (O99.33-)
toxic effect of nicotine (T65.2-)
AHA: 2013, 4Q, 108-109

✓5ᵗʰ **F17.2 Nicotine dependence**

✓6ᵗʰ **F17.20 Nicotine dependence, unspecified**

F17.200 Nicotine dependence, unspecified, ▽
uncomplicated
Tobacco use disorder, mild
Tobacco use disorder, moderate
Tobacco use disorder, severe
AHA: 2016, 1Q, 36

F17.201 Nicotine dependence, unspecified, in ▽
remission
▶Tobacco use disorder, mild, in early
remission
Tobacco use disorder, mild, in sustained
remission
Tobacco use disorder, moderate, in early
remission
Tobacco use disorder, moderate, in
sustained remission
Tobacco use disorder, severe, in early
remission
Tobacco use disorder, severe, in sustained
remission◀

F17.203 Nicotine dependence unspecified, ▽
with withdrawal
Tobacco withdrawal

F17.208 Nicotine dependence, unspecified, ▽
with other nicotine-induced disorders

F17.209 Nicotine dependence, unspecified, ▽
with unspecified nicotine-induced
disorders

✓6ᵗʰ **F17.21 Nicotine dependence, cigarettes**

F17.210 Nicotine dependence, cigarettes,
uncomplicated
AHA: 2017, 2Q, 28-29

F17.211 Nicotine dependence, cigarettes, in
remission
▶Tobacco use disorder, cigarettes, mild, in
early remission
Tobacco use disorder, cigarettes, mild, in
sustained remission
Tobacco use disorder, cigarettes, moderate,
in early remission
Tobacco use disorder, cigarettes, moderate,
in sustained remission
Tobacco use disorder, cigarettes, severe, in
early remission
Tobacco use disorder, cigarettes, severe, in
sustained remission◀

F17.213 Nicotine dependence, cigarettes, with
withdrawal

F17.218 Nicotine dependence, cigarettes, with
other nicotine-induced disorders

F17.219 Nicotine dependence, cigarettes, with ▽
unspecified nicotine-induced disorders

✓6ᵗʰ **F17.22 Nicotine dependence, chewing tobacco**

F17.220 Nicotine dependence, chewing tobacco,
uncomplicated

F17.221 Nicotine dependence, chewing tobacco, in
remission
▶Tobacco use disorder, chewing tobacco,
mild, in early remission
Tobacco use disorder, chewing tobacco,
mild, in sustained remission
Tobacco use disorder, chewing tobacco,
moderate, in early remission
Tobacco use disorder, chewing tobacco,
moderate, in sustained remission
Tobacco use disorder, chewing tobacco,
severe, in early remission
Tobacco use disorder, chewing tobacco,
severe, in sustained remission◀

F17.223 Nicotine dependence, chewing tobacco,
with withdrawal

F17.228 Nicotine dependence, chewing tobacco,
with other nicotine-induced disorders

F17.229 Nicotine dependence, chewing ▽
tobacco, with unspecified
nicotine-induced disorders

✓6ᵗʰ **F17.29 Nicotine dependence, other tobacco product**

F17.290 Nicotine dependence, other tobacco
product, uncomplicated
AHA: 2017, 2Q, 28-29

F17.291 Nicotine dependence, other tobacco
product, in remission
▶Tobacco use disorder, other tobacco
product, mild, in early remission
Tobacco use disorder, other tobacco
product, mild, in sustained remission
Tobacco use disorder, other tobacco
product, moderate, in early remission
Tobacco use disorder, other tobacco
product, moderate, in sustained
remission
Tobacco use disorder, other tobacco
product, severe, in early remission
Tobacco use disorder, other tobacco
product, severe, in sustained
remission◀

F17.293 Nicotine dependence, other tobacco
product, with withdrawal

F17.298 Nicotine dependence, other tobacco
product, with other nicotine-induced
disorders

F17.299 Nicotine dependence, other tobacco ▽
product, with unspecified
nicotine-induced disorders

EXCLUDES 1 Not coded here   EXCLUDES 2 Not included here   N Newborn Age: 0   P Pediatric Age: 0-17   M Maternity Age: 12-55   A Adult Age: 15-124

536   ICD-10-CM 2018

Chapter 5. Mental, Behavioral and Neurodevelopmental Disorders

✓4th **F18** **Inhalant related disorders**
     INCLUDES volatile solvents

✓5th **F18.1** **Inhalant abuse**
     EXCLUDES 1 *inhalant dependence (F18.2-)*
         inhalant use, unspecified (F18.9-)

    F18.10 **Inhalant abuse, uncomplicated**
        Inhalant use disorder, mild

●   **F18.11** **Inhalant abuse, in remission**
        Inhalant use disorder, mild, in early remission
        Inhalant use disorder, mild, in sustained remission

✓6th **F18.12** **Inhalant abuse with intoxication**
       F18.120 **Inhalant abuse with intoxication,**   HCC
          uncomplicated
       F18.121 **Inhalant abuse with intoxication**   HCC
          delirium
       F18.129 **Inhalant abuse with intoxication,**   HCC ▽
          unspecified

    F18.14 **Inhalant abuse with inhalant-induced mood**   HCC
        disorder
        Inhalant use disorder, mild, with inhalant induced
          depressive disorder

✓6th **F18.15** **Inhalant abuse with inhalant-induced psychotic**
        disorder
       F18.150 **Inhalant abuse with inhalant-induced**   HCC
          psychotic disorder with delusions
       F18.151 **Inhalant abuse with inhalant-induced**   HCC
          psychotic disorder with hallucinations
       F18.159 **Inhalant abuse with inhalant-**   HCC ▽
          induced psychotic disorder, unspecified

    F18.17 **Inhalant abuse with inhalant-induced dementia**   HCC
        Inhalant use disorder, mild, with inhalant induced
          major neurocognitive disorder

✓6th **F18.18** **Inhalant abuse with other inhalant-induced**
        disorders
       F18.180 **Inhalant abuse with inhalant-induced**   HCC
          anxiety disorder
       F18.188 **Inhalant abuse with other**   HCC
          inhalant-induced disorder
          Inhalant use disorder, mild, with inhalant
            induced mild neurocognitive disorder

    F18.19 **Inhalant abuse with unspecified inhalant-**   HCC ▽
        induced disorder

✓5th **F18.2** **Inhalant dependence**
     EXCLUDES 1 *inhalant abuse (F18.1-)*
         inhalant use, unspecified (F18.9-)

    F18.20 **Inhalant dependence, uncomplicated**   HCC
        Inhalant use disorder, moderate
        Inhalant use disorder, severe

    F18.21 **Inhalant dependence, in remission**   HCC
        ▶Inhalant use disorder, moderate, in early remission
        Inhalant use disorder, moderate, in sustained
          remission
        Inhalant use disorder, severe, in early remission
        Inhalant use disorder, severe, in sustained remission◀

✓6th **F18.22** **Inhalant dependence with intoxication**
       F18.220 **Inhalant dependence with in**   HCC
          toxication, uncomplicated
       F18.221 **Inhalant dependence with**   HCC
          intoxication delirium
       F18.229 **Inhalant dependence with**   HCC ▽
          intoxication, unspecified

    F18.24 **Inhalant dependence with inhalant-induced**   HCC
        mood disorder
        Inhalant use disorder, moderate, with inhalant
          induced depressive disorder
        Inhalant use disorder, severe, with inhalant induced
          depressive disorder

✓6th **F18.25** **Inhalant dependence with inhalant-induced**
        psychotic disorder
       F18.250 **Inhalant dependence with**   HCC
          inhalant-induced psychotic disorder
          with delusions
       F18.251 **Inhalant dependence with**   HCC
          inhalant-induced psychotic disorder
          with hallucinations
       F18.259 **Inhalant dependence with**   HCC ▽
          inhalant-induced psychotic disorder,
          unspecified

    F18.27 **Inhalant dependence with inhalant-induced**   HCC
        dementia
        Inhalant use disorder, moderate, with inhalant
          induced major neurocognitive disorder
        Inhalant use disorder, severe, with inhalant induced
          major neurocognitive disorder

✓6th **F18.28** **Inhalant dependence with other inhalant-induced**
        disorders
       F18.280 **Inhalant dependence with**   HCC
          inhalant-induced anxiety disorder
       F18.288 **Inhalant dependence with other**   HCC
          inhalant-induced disorder
          Inhalant use disorder, moderate, with
            inhalant-induced mild neurocognitive
            disorder
          Inhalant use disorder, severe, with
            inhalant-induced mild neurocognitive
            disorder

    F18.29 **Inhalant dependence with unspecified**   HCC ▽
        inhalant-induced disorder

✓5th **F18.9** **Inhalant use, unspecified**
     EXCLUDES 1 *inhalant abuse (F18.1-)*
         inhalant dependence (F18.2-)

    F18.90 **Inhalant use, unspecified, uncomplicated**

✓6th **F18.92** **Inhalant use, unspecified with intoxication**
       F18.920 **Inhalant use, unspecified with**   HCC
          intoxication, uncomplicated
       F18.921 **Inhalant use, unspecified with**   HCC
          intoxication with delirium
       F18.929 **Inhalant use, unspecified with**   HCC ▽
          intoxication, unspecified

    F18.94 **Inhalant use, unspecified with inhalant-induced**   HCC
        mood disorder
        Inhalant induced depressive disorder

✓6th **F18.95** **Inhalant use, unspecified with inhalant-induced**
        psychotic disorder
       F18.950 **Inhalant use, unspecified with**   HCC
          inhalant-induced psychotic disorder
          with delusions
       F18.951 **Inhalant use, unspecified with**   HCC
          inhalant-induced psychotic disorder
          with hallucinations
       F18.959 **Inhalant use, unspecified with**   HCC ▽
          inhalant-induced psychotic disorder,
          unspecified

    F18.97 **Inhalant use, unspecified with inhalant-**   HCC
        induced persisting dementia
        Inhalant-induced major neurocognitive disorder

✓6th **F18.98** **Inhalant use, unspecified with other**
        inhalant-induced disorders
       F18.980 **Inhalant use, unspecified with**   HCC
          inhalant-induced anxiety disorder
       F18.988 **Inhalant use, unspecified with other**   HCC
          inhalant-induced disorder
          Inhalant-induced mild neurocognitive
            disorder

    F18.99 **Inhalant use, unspecified with unspecified**   HCC ▽
        inhalant-induced disorder

✓4th **F19** **Other psychoactive substance related disorders**
     INCLUDES polysubstance drug use (indiscriminate drug use)

✓5th **F19.1** **Other psychoactive substance abuse**
     EXCLUDES 1 *other psychoactive substance dependence (F19.2-)*
         other psychoactive substance use, unspecified (F19.9-)

    F19.10 **Other psychoactive substance abuse, uncomplicated**
        Other (or unknown) substance use disorder, mild

●   **F19.11** **Other psychoactive substance abuse, in remission**
        Other (or unknown) substance use disorder, mild, in
          early remission
        Other (or unknown) substance use disorder, mild, in
          sustained remission

✓6th **F19.12** **Other psychoactive substance abuse with**
        intoxication
       F19.120 **Other psychoactive substance abuse**
          with intoxication, uncomplicated
       F19.121 **Other psychoactive substance abuse**   HCC
          with intoxication delirium

✓ Additional Character Req   ✓x7th Placeholder Alert   Manifestation   HCC CMS-HCC Condition   ▽ Unspecified Code   ▶◀ Revised Text   ● New Code   ▲ Revised Code Title

ICD-10-CM 2018   537

Chapter 5. Mental, Behavioral and Neurodevelopmental Disorders

F18–F19.121

Chapter 5. Mental, Behavioral and Neurodevelopmental Disorders

F19.122 Other psychoactive substance abuse with intoxication with perceptual disturbances `HCC`

F19.129 Other psychoactive substance abuse with intoxication, unspecified `HCC` ▽

F19.14 Other psychoactive substance abuse with psychoactive substance-induced mood disorder `HCC`
Other (or unknown) substance use disorder, mild, with other (or unknown) substance-induced bipolar or related disorder
Other (or unknown) substance use disorder, mild, with other (or unknown) substance-induced depressive disorder

✓6ᵗʰ **F19.15** Other psychoactive substance abuse with psychoactive substance-induced psychotic disorder

F19.150 Other psychoactive substance abuse with psychoactive substance-induced psychotic disorder with delusions `HCC`

F19.151 Other psychoactive substance abuse with psychoactive substance-induced psychotic disorder with hallucinations `HCC`

F19.159 Other psychoactive substance abuse with psychoactive substance-induced psychotic disorder, unspecified `HCC` ▽

F19.16 Other psychoactive substance abuse with psychoactive substance-induced persisting amnestic disorder `HCC`

F19.17 Other psychoactive substance abuse with psychoactive substance-induced persisting dementia `HCC`
Other (or unknown) substance use disorder, mild, with other (or unknown) substance-induced major neurocognitive disorder

✓6ᵗʰ **F19.18** Other psychoactive substance abuse with other psychoactive substance-induced disorders

F19.180 Other psychoactive substance abuse with psychoactive substance-induced anxiety disorder `HCC`

F19.181 Other psychoactive substance abuse with psychoactive substance-induced sexual dysfunction `HCC`

F19.182 Other psychoactive substance abuse with psychoactive substance-induced sleep disorder `HCC`

F19.188 Other psychoactive substance abuse with other psychoactive substance-induced disorder `HCC`
Other (or unknown) substance use disorder, mild, with other (or unknown) substance induced mild neurocognitive disorder
Other (or unknown) substance use disorder, mild, with other (or unknown) substance induced obsessive-compulsive or related disorder

F19.19 Other psychoactive substance abuse with unspecified psychoactive substance-induced disorder `HCC` ▽

✓5ᵗʰ **F19.2** Other psychoactive substance dependence
EXCLUDES1 other psychoactive substance abuse (F19.1-)
other psychoactive substance use, unspecified (F19.9-)

F19.20 Other psychoactive substance dependence, uncomplicated `HCC`
Other (or unknown) substance use disorder, moderate
Other (or unknown) substance use disorder, severe

F19.21 Other psychoactive substance dependence, in remission `HCC`
▶Other (or unknown) substance use disorder, moderate, in early remission
Other (or unknown) substance use disorder, moderate, in sustained remission
Other (or unknown) substance use disorder, severe, in early remission
Other (or unknown) substance use, severe, in sustained remission◀

✓6ᵗʰ **F19.22** Other psychoactive substance dependence with intoxication
EXCLUDES1 other psychoactive substance dependence with withdrawal (F19.23-)

F19.220 Other psychoactive substance dependence with intoxication, uncomplicated `HCC`

F19.221 Other psychoactive substance dependence with intoxication delirium `HCC`

F19.222 Other psychoactive substance dependence with intoxication with perceptual disturbance `HCC`

F19.229 Other psychoactive substance dependence with intoxication, unspecified `HCC` ▽

✓6ᵗʰ **F19.23** Other psychoactive substance dependence with withdrawal
EXCLUDES1 other psychoactive substance dependence with intoxication (F19.22-)

F19.230 Other psychoactive substance dependence with withdrawal, uncomplicated `HCC`

F19.231 Other psychoactive substance dependence with withdrawal delirium `HCC`

F19.232 Other psychoactive substance dependence with withdrawal with perceptual disturbance `HCC`

F19.239 Other psychoactive substance dependence with withdrawal, unspecified `HCC` ▽

F19.24 Other psychoactive substance dependence with psychoactive substance-induced mood disorder `HCC`
Other (or unknown) substance use disorder, moderate, with other (or unknown) substance induced bipolar or related disorder
Other (or unknown) substance use disorder, moderate, with other (or unknown) substance induced depressive disorder
Other (or unknown) use disorder, severe, with other (or unknown) substance induced bipolar or related disorder
Other (or unknown) substance use disorder, severe, with other (or unknown) substance induced depressive disorder

✓6ᵗʰ **F19.25** Other psychoactive substance dependence with psychoactive substance-induced psychotic disorder

F19.250 Other psychoactive substance dependence with psychoactive substance-induced psychotic disorder with delusions `HCC`

F19.251 Other psychoactive substance dependence with psychoactive substance-induced psychotic disorder with hallucinations `HCC`

F19.259 Other psychoactive substance dependence with psychoactive substance-induce d psychotic disorder, unspecified `HCC` ▽

F19.26 Other psychoactive substance dependence with psychoactive substance-induced persisting amnestic disorder `HCC`

F19.27 Other psychoactive substance dependence with psychoactive substance-induced persisting dementia `HCC`
Other (or unknown) substance use disorder, moderate, with other (or unknown) substance induced major neurocognitive disorder
Other (or unknown) substance use disorder, severe, with other (or unknown) substance induced major neurocognitive disorder

✓6ᵗʰ **F19.28** Other psychoactive substance dependence with other psychoactive substance-induced disorders

F19.280 Other psychoactive substance dependence with psychoactive substance-induced anxiety disorder `HCC`

F19.281 Other psychoactive substance dependence with psychoactive substance-induced sexual dysfunction `HCC`

F19.282 Other psychoactive substance dependence with psychoactive substance-induced sleep disorder `HCC`

F19.288 Other psychoactive substance dependence with other psychoactive substance-induced disorder   HCC
Other (or unknown) substance use disorder, moderate, with other (or unknown) substance induced mild neurocognitive disorder
Other (or unknown) substance use disorder, severe, with other (or unknown) substance induced mild neurocognitive disorder
Other (or unknown) substance use disorder, moderate, with other (or unknown) substance induced obsessive compulsive or related disorder
Other (or unknown) substance use disorder, severe, with other (or unknown) substance induced obsessive-compulsive or related disorder

F19.29 Other psychoactive substance dependence with unspecified psychoactive substance-induced disorder   HCC ▽

✓5th **F19.9 Other psychoactive substance use, unspecified**
EXCLUDES 1   *other psychoactive substance abuse (F19.1-)*
other psychoactive substance dependence (F19.2-)

F19.90 Other psychoactive substance use, unspecified, uncomplicated

✓6th **F19.92 Other psychoactive substance use, unspecified with intoxication**
EXCLUDES 1   *other psychoactive substance use, unspecified with withdrawal (F19.93)*

F19.920 Other psychoactive substance use, unspecified with intoxication, uncomplicated   HCC

F19.921 Other psychoactive substance use, unspecified with intoxication with delirium   HCC
Other (or unknown) substance-induced delirium

F19.922 Other psychoactive substance use, unspecified with intoxication with perceptual disturbance   HCC

F19.929 Other psychoactive substance use, unspecified with intoxication, unspecified   HCC ▽

✓6th **F19.93 Other psychoactive substance use, unspecified with withdrawal**
EXCLUDES 1   *other psychoactive substance use, unspecified with intoxication (F19.92-)*

F19.930 Other psychoactive substance use, unspecified with withdrawal, uncomplicated   HCC

F19.931 Other psychoactive substance use, unspecified with withdrawal delirium   HCC

F19.932 Other psychoactive substance use, unspecified with withdrawal with perceptual disturbance   HCC

F19.939 Other psychoactive substance use, unspecified with withdrawal, unspecified   HCC ▽

F19.94 Other psychoactive substance use, unspecified with psychoactive substance-induced mood disorder   HCC
Other (or unknown) substance-induced bipolar or related disorder, without use disorder
Other (or unknown) substance-induced depressive disorder, without use disorder

✓6th **F19.95 Other psychoactive substance use, unspecified with psychoactive substance-induced psychotic disorder**

F19.950 Other psychoactive substance use, unspecified with psychoactive substance-induced psychotic disorder with delusions   HCC

F19.951 Other psychoactive substance use, unspecified with psychoactive substance-induced psychotic disorder with hallucinations   HCC

F19.959 Other psychoactive substance use, unspecified with psychoactive substance-induced psychotic disorder, unspecified   HCC ▽
Other or unknown substance-induced psychotic disorder, without use disorder

F19.96 Other psychoactive substance use, unspecified with psychoactive substance-induced persisting amnestic disorder   HCC

F19.97 Other psychoactive substance use, unspecified with psychoactive substance-induced persisting dementia   HCC
Other (or unknown) substance-induced major neurocognitive disorder, without use disorder

✓6th **F19.98 Other psychoactive substance use, unspecified with other psychoactive substance-induced disorders**

F19.980 Other psychoactive substance use, unspecified with psychoactive substance-induced anxiety disorder   HCC
Other (or unknown) substance-induced anxiety disorder, without use disorder

F19.981 Other psychoactive substance use, unspecified with psychoactive substance-induced sexual dysfunction   HCC
Other (or unknown) substance-induced sexual dysfunction, without use disorder

F19.982 Other psychoactive substance use, unspecified with psychoactive substance-induced sleep disorder   HCC
Other (or unknown) substance-induced sleep disorder, without use disorder

F19.988 Other psychoactive substance use, unspecified with other psychoactive substance-induced disorder   HCC
Other (or unknown) substance-induced mild neurocognitive disorder, without use disorder
Other (or unknown) substance-induced obsessive-compulsive or related disorder, without use disorder

F19.99 Other psychoactive substance use, unspecified with unspecified psychoactive substance-induced disorder   HCC ▽

Schizophrenia, schizotypal, delusional, and other non-mood psychotic disorders (F20-F29)

✓4th **F20 Schizophrenia**
EXCLUDES 1   *brief psychotic disorder (F23)*
cyclic schizophrenia (F25.0)
mood [affective] disorders with psychotic symptoms (F30.2, F31.2, F31.5, F31.64, F32.3, F33.3)
schizoaffective disorder (F25.-)
schizophrenic reaction NOS (F23)
EXCLUDES 2   *schizophrenic reaction in:*
alcoholism (F10.15-, F10.25-, F10.95-)
brain disease (F06.2)
epilepsy (F06.2)
psychoactive drug use (F11-F19 with .15..25, .95)
schizotypal disorder (F21)
DEF: Group of disorders with disturbances in thought (delusions, hallucinations), mood (blunted, flattened, inappropriate affect), sense of self; also bizarre, purposeless behavior, repetitive activity, or inactivity.

F20.0 Paranoid schizophrenia   HCC
Paraphrenic schizophrenia
EXCLUDES 1   *involutional paranoid state (F22)*
paranoia (F22)
DEF: Preoccupied with delusional suspicions and auditory hallucinations related to single theme; usually hostile, grandiose, threatening, persecutory, occasionally hypochondriacal.

F20.1 Disorganized schizophrenia   HCC
Hebephrenic schizophrenia
Hebephrenia

F20.2 Catatonic schizophrenia   HCC
Schizophrenic catalepsy
Schizophrenic catatonia
Schizophrenic flexibilitas cerea
EXCLUDES 1   *catatonic stupor (R40.1)*
DEF: Extreme changes in motor activity; one extreme is decreased response or reaction to the environment and the other is spontaneous activity.

☑ Additional Character Req   ✓x7th Placeholder Alert   Manifestation   HCC CMS-HCC Condition   ▽ Unspecified Code   ►◄ Revised Text   ● New Code   ▲ Revised Code Title

ICD-10-CM 2018   539

F20.3 Undifferentiated schizophrenia `HCC`
Atypical schizophrenia
EXCLUDES 1 *acute schizophrenia-like psychotic disorder (F23)*
EXCLUDES 2 *post-schizophrenic depression (F32.89)*

F20.5 Residual schizophrenia `HCC`
Restzustand (schizophrenic)
Schizophrenic residual state

√5ᵗʰ **F20.8 Other schizophrenia**

F20.81 Schizophreniform disorder `HCC`
Schizophreniform psychosis NOS

F20.89 Other schizophrenia `HCC`
Cenesthopathic schizophrenia
Simple schizophrenia

F20.9 Schizophrenia, unspecified `HCC` ▽

F21 Schizotypal disorder
Borderline schizophrenia   Prodromal schizophrenia
Latent schizophrenia   Pseudoneurotic schizophrenia
Latent schizophrenic reaction   Pseudopsychopathic schizophrenia
Prepsychotic schizophrenia   Schizotypal personality disorder
EXCLUDES 2 *Asperger's syndrome (F84.5)*
schizoid personality disorder (F60.1)

F22 Delusional disorders `HCC`
Delusional dysmorphophobia   Paranoid psychosis
Involutional paranoid state   Paranoid state
Paranoia   Paraphrenia (late)
Paranoia querulans   Sensitiver Beziehungswahn
EXCLUDES 1 *mood [affective] disorders with psychotic symptoms (F30.2, F31.2, F31.5, F31.64, F32.3, F33.3)*
paranoid schizophrenia (F20.0)
EXCLUDES 2 *paranoid personality disorder (F60.0)*
paranoid psychosis, psychogenic (F23)
paranoid reaction (F23)

F23 Brief psychotic disorder
Paranoid reaction
Psychogenic paranoid psychosis
EXCLUDES 2 *mood [affective] disorders with psychotic symptoms (F30.2, F31.2, F31.5, F31.64, F32.3, F33.3)*

F24 Shared psychotic disorder `HCC`
Folie à deux
Induced paranoid disorder
Induced psychotic disorder

√4ᵗʰ **F25 Schizoaffective disorders**
EXCLUDES 1 *mood [affective] disorders with psychotic symptoms (F30.2, F31.2, F31.5, F31.64, F32.3, F33.3)*
schizophrenia (F20.-)

F25.0 Schizoaffective disorder, bipolar type `HCC`
Cyclic schizophrenia
Schizoaffective disorder, manic type
Schizoaffective disorder, mixed type
Schizoaffective psychosis, bipolar type
~~Schizophreniform psychosis, manic type~~

F25.1 Schizoaffective disorder, depressive type `HCC`
Schizoaffective psychosis, depressive type
~~Schizophreniform psychosis, depressive type~~

F25.8 Other schizoaffective disorders `HCC`

F25.9 Schizoaffective disorder, unspecified `HCC` ▽
Schizoaffective psychosis NOS

F28 Other psychotic disorder not due to a substance or known physiological condition
Chronic hallucinatory psychosis
▶Other specified schizophrenia spectrum and other psychotic disorder◀

F29 Unspecified psychosis not due to a substance or known physiological condition ▽
Psychosis NOS
▶Unspecified schizophrenia spectrum and other psychotic disorder◀
EXCLUDES 1 *mental disorder NOS (F99)*
unspecified mental disorder due to known physiological condition (F09)

Mood [affective] disorders (F30-F39)

√4ᵗʰ **F30 Manic episode**
INCLUDES bipolar disorder, single manic episode
mixed affective episode
EXCLUDES 1 *bipolar disorder (F31.-)*
major depressive disorder, recurrent (F33.-)
major depressive disorder, single episode (F32.-)

√5ᵗʰ **F30.1 Manic episode without psychotic symptoms**

F30.10 Manic episode without psychotic symptoms, unspecified `HCC` ▽

F30.11 Manic episode without psychotic symptoms, mild `HCC`

F30.12 Manic episode without psychotic symptoms, moderate `HCC`

F30.13 Manic episode, severe, without psychotic symptoms `HCC`

F30.2 Manic episode, severe with psychotic symptoms `HCC`
Manic stupor
Mania with mood-congruent psychotic symptoms
Mania with mood-incongruent psychotic symptoms

F30.3 Manic episode in partial remission `HCC`

F30.4 Manic episode in full remission `HCC`

F30.8 Other manic episodes `HCC`
Hypomania

F30.9 Manic episode, unspecified `HCC` ▽
Mania NOS

√4ᵗʰ **F31 Bipolar disorder**
INCLUDES ▶bipolar I disorder
bipolar type I disorder◀
manic-depressive illness
manic-depressive psychosis
manic-depressive reaction
EXCLUDES 1 *bipolar disorder, single manic episode (F30.-)*
major depressive disorder, single episode (F32.-)
major depressive disorder, recurrent (F33.-)
EXCLUDES 2 *cyclothymia (F34.0)*

F31.0 Bipolar disorder, current episode hypomanic `HCC`

√5ᵗʰ **F31.1 Bipolar disorder, current episode manic without psychotic features**

F31.10 Bipolar disorder, current episode manic without psychotic features, unspecified `HCC` ▽

F31.11 Bipolar disorder, current episode manic without psychotic features, mild `HCC`

F31.12 Bipolar disorder, current episode manic without psychotic features, moderate `HCC`

F31.13 Bipolar disorder, current episode manic without psychotic features, severe `HCC`

F31.2 Bipolar disorder, current episode manic severe with psychotic features `HCC`
Bipolar disorder, current episode manic with mood-congruent psychotic symptoms
Bipolar disorder, current episode manic with mood-incongruent psychotic symptoms
▶Bipolar I disorder, current or most recent episode manic with psychotic features◀

√5ᵗʰ **F31.3 Bipolar disorder, current episode depressed, mild or moderate severity**

F31.30 Bipolar disorder, current episode depressed, mild or moderate severity, unspecified `HCC` ▽

F31.31 Bipolar disorder, current episode depressed, mild `HCC`

F31.32 Bipolar disorder, current episode depressed, moderate `HCC`

F31.4 Bipolar disorder, current episode depressed, severe, without psychotic features `HCC`

F31.5 Bipolar disorder, current episode depressed, severe, with psychotic features `HCC`
Bipolar disorder, current episode depressed with mood-incongruent psychotic symptoms
Bipolar disorder, current episode depressed with mood-congruent psychotic symptoms
▶Bipolar I disorder, current or most recent episode depressed, with psychotic features◀

√5ᵗʰ **F31.6 Bipolar disorder, current episode mixed**

F31.60 Bipolar disorder, current episode mixed, unspecified `HCC` ▽

F31.61 Bipolar disorder, current episode mixed, mild `HCC`

EXCLUDES 1 Not coded here   *EXCLUDES 2* Not included here   N Newborn Age: 0   P Pediatric Age: 0-17   M Maternity Age: 12-55   A Adult Age: 15-124

540   ICD-10-CM 2018

F31.62   **Bipolar disorder, current episode mixed, moderate**   HCC

F31.63   **Bipolar disorder, current episode mixed, severe, without psychotic features**   HCC

F31.64   **Bipolar disorder, current episode mixed, severe, with psychotic features**   HCC
Bipolar disorder, current episode mixed with mood-congruent psychotic symptoms
Bipolar disorder, current episode mixed with mood-incongruent psychotic symptoms

√5ᵗʰ **F31.7**   **Bipolar disorder, currently in remission**

F31.70   **Bipolar disorder, currently in remission, most recent episode unspecified**   HCC ▽

F31.71   **Bipolar disorder, in partial remission, most recent episode hypomanic**   HCC

F31.72   **Bipolar disorder, in full remission, most recent episode hypomanic**   HCC

F31.73   **Bipolar disorder, in partial remission, most recent episode manic**   HCC

F31.74   **Bipolar disorder, in full remission, most recent episode manic**   HCC

F31.75   **Bipolar disorder, in partial remission, most recent episode depressed**   HCC

F31.76   **Bipolar disorder, in full remission, most recent episode depressed**   HCC

F31.77   **Bipolar disorder, in partial remission, most recent episode mixed**   HCC

F31.78   **Bipolar disorder, in full remission, most recent episode mixed**   HCC

√5ᵗʰ **F31.8**   **Other bipolar disorders**

F31.81   **Bipolar II disorder**   HCC
▶Bipolar disorder, type 2◀

F31.89   **Other bipolar disorder**   HCC
Recurrent manic episodes NOS

F31.9   **Bipolar disorder, unspecified**   HCC ▽
▶Manic depression◀

√4ᵗʰ **F32**   **Major depressive disorder, single episode**
INCLUDES   single episode of agitated depression
single episode of depressive reaction
single episode of major depression
single episode of psychogenic depression
single episode of reactive depression
single episode of vital depression
EXCLUDES 1   bipolar disorder (F31.-)
manic episode (F30.-)
recurrent depressive disorder (F33.-)
EXCLUDES 2   adjustment disorder (F43.2)
DEF: Mood disorder that produces depression; may exhibit as sadness, low self-esteem, or guilt feelings; other manifestations may be withdrawal from friends and family and interrupted sleep.

F32.0   **Major depressive disorder, single episode, mild**   HCC

F32.1   **Major depressive disorder, single episode, moderate**   HCC

F32.2   **Major depressive disorder, single episode, severe without psychotic features**   HCC

F32.3   **Major depressive disorder, single episode, severe with psychotic features**   HCC
Single episode of major depression with mood-congruent psychotic symptoms
Single episode of major depression with mood-incongruent psychotic symptoms
Single episode of major depression with psychotic symptoms
Single episode of psychogenic depressive psychosis
Single episode of psychotic depression
Single episode of reactive depressive psychosis

F32.4   **Major depressive disorder, single episode, in partial remission**   HCC

F32.5   **Major depressive disorder, single episode, in full remission**   HCC

√5ᵗʰ **F32.8**   **Other depressive episodes**

F32.81   **Premenstrual dysphoric disorder**   ♀
EXCLUDES 1   premenstrual tension syndrome (N94.3)

F32.89   **Other specified depressive episodes**
Atypical depression
Post-schizophrenic depression
Single episode of 'masked' depression NOS

F32.9   **Major depressive disorder, single episode, unspecified**   ▽
Depression NOS
Depressive disorder NOS
Major depression NOS
AHA: 2013, 4Q, 107

√4ᵗʰ **F33**   **Major depressive disorder, recurrent**
Recurrent episodes of depressive reaction
Recurrent episodes of endogenous depression
Recurrent episodes of major depression
Recurrent episodes of psychogenic depression
Recurrent episodes of reactive depression
Recurrent episodes of seasonal depressive disorder
Recurrent episodes of vital depression
EXCLUDES 1   bipolar disorder (F31.-)
manic episode (F30.-)

F33.0   **Major depressive disorder, recurrent, mild**   HCC

F33.1   **Major depressive disorder, recurrent, moderate**   HCC

F33.2   **Major depressive disorder, recurrent, severe without psychotic features**   HCC

F33.3   **Major depressive disorder, recurrent, severe with psychotic symptoms**   HCC
Endogenous depression with psychotic symptoms
▶Major depressive disorder, recurrent, with psychotic features◀
Recurrent severe episodes of major depression with mood-congruent psychotic symptoms
Recurrent severe episodes of major depression with mood-incongruent psychotic symptoms
Recurrent severe episodes of major depression with psychotic symptoms
Recurrent severe episodes of psychogenic depressive psychosis
Recurrent severe episodes of psychotic depression
Recurrent severe episodes of reactive depressive psychosis

√5ᵗʰ **F33.4**   **Major depressive disorder, recurrent, in remission**

F33.40   **Major depressive disorder, recurrent, in remission, unspecified**   HCC ▽

F33.41   **Major depressive disorder, recurrent, in partial remission**   HCC

F33.42   **Major depressive disorder, recurrent, in full remission**   HCC

F33.8   **Other recurrent depressive disorders**   HCC
Recurrent brief depressive episodes

F33.9   **Major depressive disorder, recurrent, unspecified**   HCC ▽
Monopolar depression NOS

√4ᵗʰ **F34**   **Persistent mood [affective] disorders**

F34.0   **Cyclothymic disorder**
Affective personality disorder
Cycloid personality
Cyclothymia
Cyclothymic personality

F34.1   **Dysthymic disorder**
Depressive neurosis
Depressive personality disorder
Dysthymia
Neurotic depression
Persistent anxiety depression
Persistent depressive disorder
EXCLUDES 2   anxiety depression (mild or not persistent) (F41.8)
DEF: Depression without psychosis; less severe but persistent depression; is considered a mild to moderate chronic form of depression.

√5ᵗʰ **F34.8**   **Other persistent mood [affective] disorders**

F34.81   **Disruptive mood dysregulation disorder**   HCC

F34.89   **Other specified persistent mood disorders**   HCC

F34.9   **Persistent mood [affective] disorder, unspecified**   HCC ▽

F39   **Unspecified mood [affective] disorder**   HCC ▽
Affective psychosis NOS

Anxiety, dissociative, stress-related, somatoform and other nonpsychotic mental disorders (F40-F48)

√4ᵗʰ **F40**   **Phobic anxiety disorders**

√5ᵗʰ **F40.0**   **Agoraphobia**
DEF: Profound anxiety or fear of leaving familiar settings like home, or being in unfamiliar locations or with strangers or crowds; may or may not be preceded by recurrent panic attacks.

F40.00   **Agoraphobia, unspecified**   ▽

F40.01   **Agoraphobia with panic disorder**
Panic disorder with agoraphobia
EXCLUDES 1   panic disorder without agoraphobia (F41.0)

☑ Additional Character Req   √xᵗʰ Placeholder Alert   Manifestation   HCC CMS-HCC Condition   ▽ Unspecified Code   ▶◀ Revised Text   ● New Code   ▲ Revised Code Title

F40.02   Agoraphobia without panic disorder

✓5th   F40.1   Social phobias
Anthropophobia
▶Social anxiety disorder◀
Social anxiety disorder of childhood
Social neurosis

F40.10   Social phobia, unspecified   ▽

F40.11   Social phobia, generalized

✓5th   F40.2   Specific (isolated) phobias
EXCLUDES 2   dysmorphophobia (nondelusional) (F45.22)
nosophobia (F45.22)

✓6th   F40.21   Animal type phobia
F40.210   Arachnophobia
Fear of spiders
F40.218   Other animal type phobia

✓6th   F40.22   Natural environment type phobia
F40.220   Fear of thunderstorms
F40.228   Other natural environment type phobia

✓6th   F40.23   Blood, injection, injury type phobia
F40.230   Fear of blood
F40.231   Fear of injections and transfusions
F40.232   Fear of other medical care
F40.233   Fear of injury

✓6th   F40.24   Situational type phobia
F40.240   Claustrophobia
F40.241   Acrophobia
F40.242   Fear of bridges
F40.243   Fear of flying
F40.248   Other situational type phobia

✓6th   F40.29   Other specified phobia
F40.290   Androphobia
Fear of men
F40.291   Gynephobia
Fear of women
F40.298   Other specified phobia

F40.8   Other phobic anxiety disorders
Phobic anxiety disorder of childhood

F40.9   Phobic anxiety disorder, unspecified   ▽
Phobia NOS
Phobic state NOS

✓4th   F41   Other anxiety disorders
EXCLUDES 2   anxiety in:
acute stress reaction (F43.0)
transient adjustment reaction (F43.2)
neurasthenia (F48.8)
psychophysiologic disorders (F45.-)
separation anxiety (F93.0)

▲   **F41.0   Panic disorder [episodic paroxysmal anxiety]**
Panic attack
Panic state
EXCLUDES 1   panic disorder with agoraphobia (F40.01)
DEF: Neurotic disorder characterized by recurrent panic or anxiety, apprehension, fear, or terror; symptoms include shortness of breath, palpitations, dizziness, shakiness; fear of dying may persist.

F41.1   Generalized anxiety disorder
Anxiety neurosis   Anxiety state
Anxiety reaction   Overanxious disorder
EXCLUDES 2   neurasthenia (F48.8)

F41.3   Other mixed anxiety disorders

F41.8   Other specified anxiety disorders
Anxiety depression (mild or not persistent)
Anxiety hysteria
Mixed anxiety and depressive disorder

F41.9   Anxiety disorder, unspecified   ▽
Anxiety NOS

✓4th   F42   Obsessive-compulsive disorder
EXCLUDES 2   obsessive-compulsive personality (disorder) (F60.5)
obsessive-compulsive symptoms occurring in depression (F32-F33)
obsessive-compulsive symptoms occurring in schizophrenia (F20.-)

F42.2   Mixed obsessional thoughts and acts

F42.3   Hoarding disorder

F42.4   Excoriation (skin-picking) disorder
EXCLUDES 1   factitial dermatitis (L98.1)
other specified behavioral and emotional disorders with onset usually occurring in early childhood and adolescence (F98.8)

F42.8   Other obsessive-compulsive disorder
Anancastic neurosis
Obsessive-compulsive neurosis

F42.9   Obsessive-compulsive disorder, unspecified   ▽

✓4th   F43   Reaction to severe stress, and adjustment disorders
F43.0   Acute stress reaction
Acute crisis reaction
Acute reaction to stress
Combat and operational stress reaction
Combat fatigue
Crisis state
Psychic shock

✓5th   F43.1   Post-traumatic stress disorder (PTSD)
Traumatic neurosis
DEF: Preoccupation with traumatic events beyond normal experience; i.e., rape, personal assault, etc.; also recurring flashbacks of trauma; symptoms include difficulty remembering, sleeping, or concentrating, and guilt feelings for surviving.

F43.10   Post-traumatic stress disorder, unspecified   ▽

F43.11   Post-traumatic stress disorder, acute

F43.12   Post-traumatic stress disorder, chronic

✓5th   F43.2   Adjustment disorders
Culture shock
Grief reaction
Hospitalism in children
EXCLUDES 2   separation anxiety disorder of childhood (F93.0)

F43.20   Adjustment disorder, unspecified   ▽

F43.21   Adjustment disorder with depressed mood
AHA: 2014, 1Q, 25

F43.22   Adjustment disorder with anxiety

F43.23   Adjustment disorder with mixed anxiety and depressed mood

F43.24   Adjustment disorder with disturbance of conduct

F43.25   Adjustment disorder with mixed disturbance of emotions and conduct

F43.29   Adjustment disorder with other symptoms

F43.8   Other reactions to severe stress
Other specified trauma and stressor-related disorder

F43.9   Reaction to severe stress, unspecified   ▽
Trauma and stressor-related disorder, NOS

✓4th   F44   Dissociative and conversion disorders
INCLUDES   conversion hysteria
conversion reaction
hysteria
hysterical psychosis
EXCLUDES 2   malingering [conscious simulation] (Z76.5)

F44.0   Dissociative amnesia
EXCLUDES 1   amnesia NOS (R41.3)
anterograde amnesia (R41.1)
dissociative amnesia with dissociative fugue (F44.1)
retrograde amnesia (R41.2)
EXCLUDES 2   alcohol-or other psychoactive substance-induced amnestic disorder (F10, F13, F19 with .26, .96)
amnestic disorder due to known physiological condition (F04)
postictal amnesia in epilepsy (G40.-)

F44.1   Dissociative fugue
Dissociative amnesia with dissociative fugue
EXCLUDES 2   postictal fugue in epilepsy (G40.-)
DEF: Dissociative hysteria; identified by loss of memory, flight from familiar surroundings to a completely separate environment, episodes may last hours or days; conscious activity is not associated with perception of surroundings and there is no later memory of episode.

F44.2   Dissociative stupor
EXCLUDES 1   catatonic stupor (R40.1)
stupor NOS (R40.1)
EXCLUDES 2   catatonic disorder due to known physiological condition (F06.1)
depressive stupor (F32, F33)
manic stupor (F30, F31)

F44.4 Conversion disorder with motor symptom or deficit
▶Conversion disorder with abnormal movement
Conversion disorder with speech symptoms
Conversion disorder with swallowing symptoms
Conversion disorder with weakness/paralysis◀
Dissociative motor disorders
Psychogenic aphonia
Psychogenic dysphonia

F44.5 Conversion disorder with seizures or convulsions
▶Conversion disorder with attacks or seizures◀
Dissociative convulsions

F44.6 Conversion disorder with sensory symptom or deficit
▶Conversion disorder with anesthesia or sensory loss
Conversion disorder with special sensory symptoms◀
Dissociative anesthesia and sensory loss
Psychogenic deafness

F44.7 Conversion disorder with mixed symptom presentation

✓5ᵗʰ **F44.8 Other dissociative and conversion disorders**

  F44.81 Dissociative identity disorder
    Multiple personality disorder

  F44.89 Other dissociative and conversion disorders
    Ganser's syndrome
    Psychogenic confusion
    Psychogenic twilight state
    Trance and possession disorders

F44.9 Dissociative and conversion disorder, unspecified ▽
Dissociative disorder NOS

✓4ᵗʰ **F45 Somatoform disorders**

  EXCLUDES 2   *dissociative and conversion disorders (F44.-)*
    factitious disorders (F68.1-)
    hair-plucking (F63.3)
    lalling (F80.0)
    lisping (F80.0)
    malingering [conscious simulation] (Z76.5)
    nail-biting (F98.8)
    psychological or behavioral factors associated with disorders or
      diseases classified elsewhere (F54)
    sexual dysfunction, not due to a substance or known
      physiological condition (F52.-)
    thumb-sucking (F98.8)
    tic disorders (in childhood and adolescence) (F95.-)
    Tourette's syndrome (F95.2)
    trichotillomania (F63.3)

F45.0 Somatization disorder
Briquet's disorder
Multiple psychosomatic disorder

F45.1 Undifferentiated somatoform disorder
Somatic symptom disorder
Undifferentiated psychosomatic disorder

✓5ᵗʰ **F45.2 Hypochondriacal disorders**
  EXCLUDES 2   *delusional dysmorphophobia (F22)*
    fixed delusions about bodily functions or shape (F22)

  F45.20 Hypochondriacal disorder, unspecified ▽

  F45.21 Hypochondriasis
    Hypochondriacal neurosis
    Illness anxiety disorder

  F45.22 Body dysmorphic disorder
    Dysmorphophobia (nondelusional)
    Nosophobia

  F45.29 Other hypochondriacal disorders

✓5ᵗʰ **F45.4 Pain disorders related to psychological factors**
  EXCLUDES 1   *pain NOS (R52)*

  F45.41 Pain disorder exclusively related to psychological factors
    Somatoform pain disorder (persistent)

  F45.42 Pain disorder with related psychological factors
    Code also associated acute or chronic pain (G89.-)

F45.8 Other somatoform disorders
Psychogenic dysmenorrhea
Psychogenic dysphagia, including "globus hystericus"
Psychogenic pruritus
Psychogenic torticollis
Somatoform autonomic dysfunction
Teeth grinding
  EXCLUDES 1   *sleep related teeth grinding (G47.63)*

F45.9 Somatoform disorder, unspecified ▽
Psychosomatic disorder NOS

✓4ᵗʰ **F48 Other nonpsychotic mental disorders**

F48.1 Depersonalization-derealization syndrome

F48.2 Pseudobulbar affect
Involuntary emotional expression disorder
Code first underlying cause, if known, such as:
  amyotrophic lateral sclerosis (G12.21)
  multiple sclerosis (G35)
  sequelae of cerebrovascular disease (I69.-)
  sequelae of traumatic intracranial injury (S06.-)

F48.8 Other specified nonpsychotic mental disorders
Dhat syndrome
Neurasthenia
Occupational neurosis, including writer's cramp
Psychasthenia
Psychasthenic neurosis
Psychogenic syncope

F48.9 Nonpsychotic mental disorder, unspecified ▽
Neurosis NOS

Behavioral syndromes associated with physiological disturbances and physical factors (F50-F59)

✓4ᵗʰ **F50 Eating disorders**
  EXCLUDES 1   *anorexia NOS (R63.0)*
    feeding difficulties (R63.3)
    ▶*feeding problems of newborn (P92.-)*◀
    polyphagia (R63.2)
  EXCLUDES 2   *feeding disorder in infancy or childhood (F98.2-)*

✓5ᵗʰ **F50.0 Anorexia nervosa**
  EXCLUDES 1   *loss of appetite (R63.0)*
    psychogenic loss of appetite (F50.89)

  F50.00 Anorexia nervosa, unspecified ▽

  F50.01 Anorexia nervosa, restricting type

  F50.02 Anorexia nervosa, binge eating/purging type
    EXCLUDES 1   *bulimia nervosa (F50.2)*

F50.2 Bulimia nervosa
Bulimia NOS
Hyperorexia nervosa
  EXCLUDES 1   *anorexia nervosa, binge eating/purging type (F50.02)*

✓5ᵗʰ **F50.8 Other eating disorders**
  EXCLUDES 2   *pica of infancy and childhood (F98.3)*

  F50.81 Binge eating disorder

  ● **F50.82 Avoidant/restrictive food intake disorder**

  F50.89 Other specified eating disorder
    Pica in adults
    Psychogenic loss of appetite

F50.9 Eating disorder, unspecified ▽
Atypical anorexia nervosa
Atypical bulimia nervosa
▶Feeding or eating disorder, unspecified
Other specified feeding disorder ◀

✓4ᵗʰ **F51 Sleep disorders not due to a substance or known physiological condition**
  EXCLUDES 2   *organic sleep disorders (G47.-)*

✓5ᵗʰ **F51.0 Insomnia not due to a substance or known physiological condition**
  EXCLUDES 2   *alcohol related insomnia (F10.182, F10.282, F10.982)*
    drug-related insomnia (F11.182, F11.282, F11.982,
      F13.182, F13.282, F13.982, F14.182, F14.282,
      F14.982, F15.182, F15.282, F15.982, F19.182,
      F19.282, F19.982)
    insomnia NOS (G47.0-)
    insomnia due to known physiological condition
      (G47.0-)
    organic insomnia (G47.0-)
    sleep deprivation (Z72.820)

  F51.01 Primary insomnia
    Idiopathic insomnia

  F51.02 Adjustment insomnia

  F51.03 Paradoxical insomnia

  F51.04 Psychophysiologic insomnia

  F51.05 Insomnia due to other mental disorder
    Code also associated mental disorder

  F51.09 Other insomnia not due to a substance or known physiological condition

---

✓ Additional Character Req   ✓xᵗʰ Placeholder Alert   Manifestation   HCC CMS-HCC Condition   ▽ Unspecified Code   ▶◀ Revised Text   ● New Code   ▲ Revised Code Title

✓6th F51.1 Hypersomnia not due to a substance or known physiological condition
    EXCLUDES 2   alcohol related hypersomnia (F10.182, F10.282, F10.982)
      drug-related hypersomnia (F11.182, F11.282, F11.982, F13.182, F13.282, F13.982, F14.182, F14.282, F14.982, F15.182, F15.282, F15.982, F19.182, F19.282, F19.982)
      hypersomnia NOS (G47.10)
      hypersomnia due to known physiological condition (G47.10)
      idiopathic hypersomnia (G47.11, G47.12)
      narcolepsy (G47.4-)

F51.11 Primary hypersomnia

F51.12 Insufficient sleep syndrome
    EXCLUDES 1   sleep deprivation (Z72.820)

F51.13 Hypersomnia due to other mental disorder
    Code also associated mental disorder

F51.19 Other hypersomnia not due to a substance or known physiological condition

F51.3 Sleepwalking [somnambulism]
    ▶Non–rapid eye movement sleep arousal disorders, sleepwalking type◀

F51.4 Sleep terrors [night terrors]
    ▶Non–rapid eye movement sleep arousal disorders, sleep terror type◀

F51.5 Nightmare disorder
    Dream anxiety disorder

F51.8 Other sleep disorders not due to a substance or known physiological condition

F51.9 Sleep disorder not due to a substance or known physiological condition, unspecified   ▽
    Emotional sleep disorder NOS

✓4th F52 Sexual dysfunction not due to a substance or known physiological condition
    EXCLUDES 2   Dhat syndrome (F48.8)

F52.0 Hypoactive sexual desire disorder
    Lack or loss of sexual desire
    ▶Male hypoactive sexual desire disorder◀
    Sexual anhedonia
    EXCLUDES 1   decreased libido (R68.82)

F52.1 Sexual aversion disorder
    Sexual aversion and lack of sexual enjoyment

✓5th F52.2 Sexual arousal disorders
    Failure of genital response

F52.21 Male erectile disorder   ♂
    ▶Erectile disorder◀
    Psychogenic impotence
    EXCLUDES 1   impotence of organic origin (N52.-)
      impotence NOS (N52.-)

F52.22 Female sexual arousal disorder   ♀
    ▶Female sexual interest/arousal disorder◀

✓5th F52.3 Orgasmic disorder
    Inhibited orgasm
    Psychogenic anorgasmy

F52.31 Female orgasmic disorder   ♀

F52.32 Male orgasmic disorder   ♂
    Delayed ejaculation

F52.4 Premature ejaculation   ♂

F52.5 Vaginismus not due to a substance or known physiological condition   ♀
    Psychogenic vaginismus
    EXCLUDES 2   vaginismus (due to a known physiological condition) (N94.2)
    DEF: Psychogenic response resulting in painful contractions of vaginal canal muscles; can be severe enough to prevent sexual intercourse.

F52.6 Dyspareunia not due to a substance or known physiological condition   ♀
    Genito-pelvic pain or penetration disorder
    Psychogenic dyspareunia
    EXCLUDES 2   dyspareunia (due to a known physiological condition) (N94.1-)

F52.8 Other sexual dysfunction not due to a substance or known physiological condition
    Excessive sexual drive
    Nymphomania
    Satyriasis

F52.9 Unspecified sexual dysfunction not due to a substance or known physiological condition   ▽
    Sexual dysfunction NOS

F53 Puerperal psychosis   M♀
    Postpartum depression
    EXCLUDES 1   mood disorders with psychotic features (F30.2, F31.2, F31.5, F31.64, F32.3, F33.3)
      postpartum dysphoria (O90.6)
      psychosis in schizophrenia, schizotypal, delusional, and other psychotic disorders (F20-F29)

F54 *Psychological and behavioral factors associated with disorders or diseases classified elsewhere*
    Psychological factors affecting physical conditions
    Code first the associated physical disorder, such as:
      asthma (J45.-)
      dermatitis (L23-L25)
      gastric ulcer (K25.-)
      mucous colitis (K58.-)
      ulcerative colitis (K51.-)
      urticaria (L50.-)
    EXCLUDES 2   tension-type headache (G44.2)

✓4th F55 Abuse of non-psychoactive substances
    EXCLUDES 2   abuse of psychoactive substances (F10-F19)

F55.0 Abuse of antacids

F55.1 Abuse of herbal or folk remedies

F55.2 Abuse of laxatives

F55.3 Abuse of steroids or hormones

F55.4 Abuse of vitamins

F55.8 Abuse of other non-psychoactive substances

F59 Unspecified behavioral syndromes associated with physiological disturbances and physical factors   ▽
    Psychogenic physiological dysfunction NOS

Disorders of adult personality and behavior (F60-F69)

✓4th F60 Specific personality disorders

F60.0 Paranoid personality disorder
    Expansive paranoid personality (disorder)
    Fanatic personality (disorder)
    Paranoid personality (disorder)
    Querulant personality (disorder)
    Sensitive paranoid personality (disorder)
    EXCLUDES 2   paranoia (F22)
      paranoia querulans (F22)
      paranoid psychosis (F22)
      paranoid schizophrenia (F20.0)
      paranoid state (F22)

F60.1 Schizoid personality disorder
    EXCLUDES 2   Asperger's syndrome (F84.5)
      delusional disorder (F22)
      schizoid disorder of childhood (F84.5)
      schizophrenia (F20.-)
      schizotypal disorder (F21)

F60.2 Antisocial personality disorder
    Amoral personality (disorder)
    Asocial personality (disorder)
    Dissocial personality disorder
    Psychopathic personality (disorder)
    Sociopathic personality (disorder)
    EXCLUDES 1   conduct disorders (F91.-)
    EXCLUDES 2   borderline personality disorder (F60.3)

F60.3 Borderline personality disorder
    Aggressive personality (disorder)
    Emotionally unstable personality disorder
    Explosive personality (disorder)
    EXCLUDES 2   antisocial personality disorder (F60.2)

F60.4 Histrionic personality disorder
    Hysterical personality (disorder)
    Psychoinfantile personality (disorder)

F60.5 Obsessive-compulsive personality disorder
    Anankastic personality (disorder)
    Compulsive personality (disorder)
    Obsessional personality (disorder)
    EXCLUDES 2   obsessive-compulsive disorder (F42-)

F60.6 Avoidant personality disorder
    Anxious personality disorder

F60.7 Dependent personality disorder
    Asthenic personality (disorder)
    Inadequate personality (disorder)
    Passive personality (disorder)

EXCLUDES 1 Not coded here   *EXCLUDES 2* Not included here   N Newborn Age: 0   P Pediatric Age: 0-17   M Maternity Age: 12-55   A Adult Age: 15-124

544   ICD-10-CM 2018

✓5ᵗʰ **F60.8 Other specific personality disorders**

     F60.81 Narcissistic personality disorder

     F60.89 Other specific personality disorders
         Eccentric personality disorder
         "Haltlose" type personality disorder
         Immature personality disorder
         Passive-aggressive personality disorder
         Psychoneurotic personality disorder
         Self-defeating personality disorder

F60.9 Personality disorder, unspecified ▽
     Character disorder NOS
     Character neurosis NOS
     Pathological personality NOS

✓4ᵗʰ **F63 Impulse disorders**

     EXCLUDES 2   *habitual excessive use of alcohol or psychoactive substances (F10–F19)*
                impulse disorders involving sexual behavior (F65.-)

F63.0 Pathological gambling
     Compulsive gambling
     ▶Gambling disorder◀
     EXCLUDES 1   *gambling and betting NOS (Z72.6)*
     EXCLUDES 2   *excessive gambling by manic patients (F30, F31)*
                gambling in antisocial personality disorder (F60.2)

F63.1 Pyromania
     Pathological fire-setting
     EXCLUDES 2   *fire-setting (by) (in):*
                adult with antisocial personality disorder (F60.2)
                alcohol or psychoactive substance intoxication (F10–F19)
                conduct disorders (F91.-)
                mental disorders due to known physiological condition (F01-F09)
                schizophrenia (F20.-)

F63.2 Kleptomania
     Pathological stealing
     EXCLUDES 1   *shoplifting as the reason for observation for suspected mental disorder (Z03.8)*
     EXCLUDES 2   *depressive disorder with stealing (F31-F33)*
                stealing due to underlying mental condition—code to mental condition
                stealing in mental disorders due to known physiological condition (F01-F09)

F63.3 Trichotillomania
     Hair plucking
     EXCLUDES 2   *other stereotyped movement disorder (F98.4)*

✓5ᵗʰ **F63.8 Other impulse disorders**

     F63.81 Intermittent explosive disorder

     F63.89 Other impulse disorders

F63.9 Impulse disorder, unspecified ▽
     Impulse control disorder NOS

✓4ᵗʰ **F64 Gender identity disorders**

F64.0 Transsexualism
     Gender identity disorder in adolescence and adulthood
     Gender dysphoria in adolescents and adults

F64.1 Dual role transvestism
     Use additional code to identify sex reassignment status (Z87.890)
     EXCLUDES 1   *gender identity disorder in childhood (F64.2)*
     EXCLUDES 2   *fetishistic transvestism (F65.1)*

F64.2 Gender identity disorder of childhood Ⓟ
     Gender dysphoria in children
     EXCLUDES 1   *gender identity disorder in adolescence and adulthood (F64.0)*
     EXCLUDES 2   *sexual maturation disorder (F66)*

F64.8 Other gender identity disorders
     ▶Other specified gender dysphoria◀

F64.9 Gender identity disorder, unspecified ▽
     ▶Gender dysphoria, unspecified◀
     Gender-role disorder NOS

✓4ᵗʰ **F65 Paraphilias**

F65.0 Fetishism
     ▶Fetishistic disorder◀

F65.1 Transvestic fetishism
     Fetishistic transvestism
     ▶Transvestic disorder◀

F65.2 Exhibitionism
     ▶Exhibitionistic disorder◀

F65.3 Voyeurism
     ▶Voyeuristic disorder◀

F65.4 Pedophilia
     ▶Pedophilic disorder◀

✓5ᵗʰ **F65.5 Sadomasochism** ▽

     F65.50 Sadomasochism, unspecified

     F65.51 Sexual masochism
         ▶Sexual masochism disorder◀

     F65.52 Sexual sadism
         ▶Sexual sadism disorder◀

✓5ᵗʰ **F65.8 Other paraphilias**

     F65.81 Frotteurism
         ▶Frotteuristic disorder◀

     F65.89 Other paraphilias
         Necrophilia
         ▶Other specified paraphilic disorder◀

F65.9 Paraphilia, unspecified ▽
     ▶Paraphilic disorder, unspecified◀
     Sexual deviation NOS

F66 Other sexual disorders
     Sexual maturation disorder
     Sexual relationship disorder

✓4ᵗʰ **F68 Other disorders of adult personality and behavior**

✓5ᵗʰ **F68.1 Factitious disorder**
     Compensation neurosis
     Elaboration of physical symptoms for psychological reasons
     Hospital hopper syndrome
     Münchhausen's syndrome
     Peregrinating patient
     EXCLUDES 2   *factitial dermatitis (L98.1)*
                person feigning illness (with obvious motivation) (Z76.5)

     F68.10 Factitious disorder, unspecified ▽

     F68.11 Factitious disorder with predominantly psychological signs and symptoms

     F68.12 Factitious disorder with predominantly physical signs and symptoms

     F68.13 Factitious disorder with combined psychological and physical signs and symptoms

F68.8 Other specified disorders of adult personality and behavior

F69 Unspecified disorder of adult personality and behavior ▲▽

Intellectual Disabilities (F70-F79)

Code first any associated physical or developmental disorders
EXCLUDES 1   *borderline intellectual functioning, IQ above 70 to 84 (R41.83)*

F70 Mild intellectual disabilities
     IQ level 50-55 to approximately 70
     Mild mental subnormality

F71 Moderate intellectual disabilities
     IQ level 35-40 to 50-55
     Moderate mental subnormality

F72 Severe intellectual disabilities
     IQ 20-25 to 35-40
     Severe mental subnormality

F73 Profound intellectual disabilities
     IQ level below 20-25
     Profound mental subnormality

F78 Other intellectual disabilities

F79 Unspecified intellectual disabilities ▽
     Mental deficiency NOS
     Mental subnormality NOS

✓ Additional Character Req   ✓7ᵗʰ Placeholder Alert   Manifestation   HCC CMS-HCC Condition   ▽ Unspecified Code   ▶◀ Revised Text   ● New Code   ▲ Revised Code Title

ICD-10-CM 2018   **545**

Chapter 5. Mental, Behavioral and Neurodevelopmental Disorders *(sidebar)*

Pervasive and specific developmental disorders (F80-F89)

✓4th F80 Specific developmental disorders of speech and language

F80.0 Phonological disorder
Dyslalia
Functional speech articulation disorder
Lalling
Lisping
Phonological developmental disorder
Speech articulation developmental disorder
Speech-sound disorder
EXCLUDES1 speech articulation impairment due to aphasia NOS (R47.01)
speech articulation impairment due to apraxia (R48.2)
EXCLUDES2 speech articulation impairment due to hearing loss (F80.4)
speech articulation impairment due to intellectual disabilities (F70-F79)
speech articulation impairment with expressive language developmental disorder (F80.1)
speech articulation impairment with mixed receptive expressive language developmental disorder (F80.2)

F80.1 Expressive language disorder
Developmental dysphasia or aphasia, expressive type
EXCLUDES1 dysphasia and aphasia NOS (R47.-)
mixed receptive-expressive language disorder (F80.2)
EXCLUDES2 acquired aphasia with epilepsy [Landau-Kleffner] (G40.80-)
intellectual disabilities (F70-F79)
pervasive developmental disorders (F84.-)
selective mutism (F94.0)

F80.2 Mixed receptive-expressive language disorder
Developmental dysphasia or aphasia, receptive type
Developmental Wernicke's aphasia
EXCLUDES1 central auditory processing disorder (H93.25)
dysphasia or aphasia NOS (R47.-)
expressive language disorder (F80.1)
expressive type dysphasia or aphasia (F80.1)
word deafness (H93.25)
EXCLUDES2 acquired aphasia with epilepsy [Landau-Kleffner] (G40.80-)
intellectual disabilities (F70-F79)
pervasive developmental disorders (F84.-)
selective mutism (F94.0)

F80.4 Speech and language development delay due to hearing loss
Code also type of hearing loss (H90.-, H91.-)

✓5th F80.8 Other developmental disorders of speech and language
AHA: 2017, 1Q, 27

F80.81 Childhood onset fluency disorder
Cluttering NOS
Stuttering NOS
EXCLUDES1 adult onset fluency disorder (F98.5)
fluency disorder in conditions classified elsewhere (R47.82)
fluency disorder (stuttering) following cerebrovascular disease (I69. with final characters-23)

F80.82 Social pragmatic communication disorder
EXCLUDES1 Asperger's syndrome (F84.5)
autistic disorder (F84.0)

F80.89 Other developmental disorders of speech and language

F80.9 Developmental disorder of speech and language, unspecified ▽
Communication disorder NOS
Language disorder NOS

✓4th F81 Specific developmental disorders of scholastic skills

F81.0 Specific reading disorder
"Backward reading"
Developmental dyslexia
▶Specific learning disorder, with impairment in reading◀
Specific reading retardation
EXCLUDES1 alexia NOS (R48.0)
dyslexia NOS (R48.0)
DEF: Serious impairment of reading skills unexplained in relation to general intelligence and teaching processes.

F81.2 Mathematics disorder
Developmental acalculia
Developmental arithmetical disorder
Developmental Gerstmann's syndrome
▶Specific learning disorder, with impairment in mathmatics◀
EXCLUDES1 acalculia NOS (R48.8)
EXCLUDES2 arithmetical difficulties associated with a reading disorder (F81.0)
arithmetical difficulties associated with a spelling disorder (F81.81)
arithmetical difficulties due to inadequate teaching (Z55.8)

✓5th F81.8 Other developmental disorders of scholastic skills

F81.81 Disorder of written expression
▶Specific learning disorder, with impairment in written expression◀
Specific spelling disorder

F81.89 Other developmental disorders of scholastic skills

F81.9 Developmental disorder of scholastic skills, unspecified ▽
Knowledge acquisition disability NOS
Learning disability NOS
Learning disorder NOS

F82 Specific developmental disorder of motor function
Clumsy child syndrome
Developmental coordination disorder
Developmental dyspraxia
EXCLUDES1 abnormalities of gait and mobility (R26.-)
lack of coordination (R27.-)
EXCLUDES2 lack of coordination secondary to intellectual disabilities (F70-F79)

✓4th F84 Pervasive developmental disorders
Use additional code to identify any associated medical condition and intellectual disabilities

F84.0 Autistic disorder
Autism spectrum disorder
Infantile autism
Infantile psychosis
Kanner's syndrome
EXCLUDES1 Asperger's syndrome (F84.5)
AHA: 2017, 1Q, 27

F84.2 Rett's syndrome
EXCLUDES1 Asperger's syndrome (F84.5)
Autistic disorder (F84.0)
Other childhood disintegrative disorder (F84.3)

F84.3 Other childhood disintegrative disorder P
Dementia infantilis
Disintegrative psychosis
Heller's syndrome
Symbiotic psychosis
Use additional code to identify any associated neurological condition
EXCLUDES1 Asperger's syndrome (F84.5)
Autistic disorder (F84.0)
Rett's syndrome (F84.2)

F84.5 Asperger's syndrome
Asperger's disorder
Autistic psychopathy
Schizoid disorder of childhood

F84.8 Other pervasive developmental disorders
Overactive disorder associated with intellectual disabilities and stereotyped movements

F84.9 Pervasive developmental disorder, unspecified ▽
Atypical autism

F88 Other disorders of psychological development
Developmental agnosia
Global development delay
Other specified neurodevelopmental disorder

F89 Unspecified disorder of psychological development ▽
Developmental disorder NOS
Neurodevelopmental disorder NOS

Behavioral and emotional disorders with onset usually occurring in childhood and adolescence (F90-F98)

> **NOTE**   Codes within categories F90-F98 may be used regardless of the age of a patient. These disorders generally have onset within the childhood or adolescent years, but may continue throughout life or not be diagnosed until adulthood.

✓4ᵗʰ F90   Attention-deficit hyperactivity disorders

> **INCLUDES**   attention deficit disorder with hyperactivity
> attention deficit syndrome with hyperactivity
> **EXCLUDES 2**   *anxiety disorders (F40.-, F41.-)*
> *mood [affective] disorders (F30-F39)*
> *pervasive developmental disorders (F84.-)*
> *schizophrenia (F20.-)*

F90.0   **Attention-deficit hyperactivity disorder, predominantly inattentive type**
▶Attention-deficit/hyperactivity disorder, predominantly inattentive presentation◀

F90.1   **Attention-deficit hyperactivity disorder, predominantly hyperactive type**
▶Attention-deficit/hyperactivity disorder, predominantly hyperactive impulsive presentation◀

F90.2   **Attention-deficit hyperactivity disorder, combined type**
▶Attention-deficit/hyperactivity disorder, combined presentation◀

F90.8   **Attention-deficit hyperactivity disorder, other type**

F90.9   **Attention-deficit hyperactivity disorder, unspecified type** ▽
Attention-deficit hyperactivity disorder of childhood or adolescence NOS
Attention-deficit hyperactivity disorder NOS

✓4ᵗʰ F91   Conduct disorders

> **EXCLUDES 1**   *antisocial behavior (Z72.81-)*
> *antisocial personality disorder (F60.2)*
> **EXCLUDES 2**   *conduct problems associated with attention-deficit hyperactivity disorder (F90.-)*
> *mood [affective] disorders (F30-F39)*
> *pervasive developmental disorders (F84.-)*
> *schizophrenia (F20.-)*

F91.0   **Conduct disorder confined to family context**

F91.1   **Conduct disorder, childhood-onset type**
Unsocialized conduct disorder
Conduct disorder, solitary aggressive type
Unsocialized aggressive disorder

F91.2   **Conduct disorder, adolescent-onset type**
Socialized conduct disorder
Conduct disorder, group type

F91.3   **Oppositional defiant disorder**

F91.8   **Other conduct disorders**
Other specified conduct disorder
Other specified disruptive disorder

F91.9   **Conduct disorder, unspecified** ▽
Behavioral disorder NOS
Conduct disorder NOS
Disruptive behavior disorder NOS
Disruptive disorder NOS

✓4ᵗʰ F93   Emotional disorders with onset specific to childhood

F93.0   **Separation anxiety disorder of childhood**
> **EXCLUDES 2**   *mood [affective] disorders (F30-F39)*
> *nonpsychotic mental disorders (F40-F48)*
> *phobic anxiety disorder of childhood (F40.8)*
> *social phobia (F40.1)*

F93.8   **Other childhood emotional disorders**
Identity disorder
> **EXCLUDES 2**   *gender identity disorder of childhood (F64.2)*

F93.9   **Childhood emotional disorder, unspecified** ▽

✓4ᵗʰ F94   Disorders of social functioning with onset specific to childhood and adolescence

F94.0   **Selective mutism**
Elective mutism
> **EXCLUDES 2**   *pervasive developmental disorders (F84.-)*
> *schizophrenia (F20.-)*
> *specific developmental disorders of speech and language (F80.-)*
> *transient mutism as part of separation anxiety in young children (F93.0)*

F94.1   **Reactive attachment disorder of childhood**
Use additional code to identify any associated failure to thrive or growth retardation
> **EXCLUDES 1**   *disinhibited attachment disorder of childhood (F94.1)*
> *normal variation in pattern of selective attachment*
> **EXCLUDES 2**   *Asperger's syndrome (F84.5)*
> *maltreatment syndromes (T74.-)*
> *sexual or physical abuse in childhood, resulting in psychosocial problems (Z62.81-)*

F94.2   **Disinhibited attachment disorder of childhood**
Affectionless psychopathy
Institutional syndrome
> **EXCLUDES 1**   *reactive attachment disorder of childhood (F94.1)*
> **EXCLUDES 2**   *Asperger's syndrome (F84.5)*
> *attention-deficit hyperactivity disorders (F90.-)*
> *hospitalism in children (F43.2-)*

F94.8   **Other childhood disorders of social functioning**

F94.9   **Childhood disorder of social functioning, unspecified** ▽

✓4ᵗʰ F95   Tic disorder

F95.0   **Transient tic disorder**
Provisional tic disorder

F95.1   **Chronic motor or vocal tic disorder**

F95.2   **Tourette's disorder**
Combined vocal and multiple motor tic disorder [de la Tourette]
Tourette's syndrome

F95.8   **Other tic disorders**

F95.9   **Tic disorder, unspecified** ▽
Tic NOS

✓4ᵗʰ F98   Other behavioral and emotional disorders with onset usually occurring in childhood and adolescence

> **EXCLUDES 2**   *breath-holding spells (R06.89)*
> *gender identity disorder of childhood (F64.2)*
> *Kleine-Levin syndrome (G47.13)*
> *obsessive-compulsive disorder (F42-)*
> *sleep disorders not due to a substance or known physiological condition (F51.-)*

F98.0   **Enuresis not due to a substance or known physiological condition**
Enuresis (primary) (secondary) of nonorganic origin
Functional enuresis
Psychogenic enuresis
Urinary incontinence of nonorganic origin
> **EXCLUDES 1**   *enuresis NOS (R32)*

F98.1   **Encopresis not due to a substance or known physiological condition**
Functional encopresis
Incontinence of feces of nonorganic origin
Psychogenic encopresis
Use additional code to identify the cause of any coexisting constipation
> **EXCLUDES 1**   *encopresis NOS (R15.-)*

✓5ᵗʰ F98.2   Other feeding disorders of infancy and childhood
> **EXCLUDES 1**   *feeding difficulties (R63.3)*
> **EXCLUDES 2**   *anorexia nervosa and other eating disorders (F50.-)*
> *feeding problems of newborn (P92.-)*
> *pica of infancy or childhood (F98.3)*

F98.21   **Rumination disorder of infancy**

F98.29   **Other feeding disorders of infancy and early childhood**

F98.3   **Pica of infancy and childhood**

F98.4   **Stereotyped movement disorders**
Stereotype/habit disorder
> **EXCLUDES 1**   *abnormal involuntary movements (R25.-)*
> **EXCLUDES 2**   *compulsions in obsessive-compulsive disorder (F42-)*
> *hair plucking (F63.3)*
> *movement disorders of organic origin (G20-G25)*
> *nail-biting (F98.8)*
> *nose-picking (F98.8)*
> *stereotypies that are part of a broader psychiatric condition (F01-F95)*
> *thumb-sucking (F98.8)*
> *tic disorders (F95.-)*
> *trichotillomania (F63.3)*

☑ Additional Character Req   ✓x7ᵗʰ Placeholder Alert   **Manifestation**   **HCC** CMS-HCC Condition   ▽ Unspecified Code   ▶◀ Revised Text   ● New Code   ▲ Revised Code Title

ICD-10-CM 2018   547

F98.5 Adult onset fluency disorder

> EXCLUDES 1   *childhood onset fluency disorder (F80.81)*
> *dysphasia (R47.02)*
> *fluency disorder in conditions classified elsewhere (R47.82)*
> *fluency disorder (stuttering) following cerebrovascular disease (I69. with final characters -23)*
> *tic disorders (F95.-)*

F98.8 Other specified behavioral and emotional disorders with onset usually occurring in childhood and adolescence

Excessive masturbation

Nail-biting

Nose-picking

Thumb-sucking

F98.9 Unspecified behavioral and emotional disorders with onset usually occurring in childhood and adolescence   ▽

Unspecified mental disorder (F99)

F99 Mental disorder, not otherwise specified

Mental illness NOS

> EXCLUDES 1   *unspecified mental disorder due to known physiological condition (F09)*

EXCLUDES 1 Not coded here   EXCLUDES 2 Not included here   N Newborn Age: 0   P Pediatric Age: 0-17   M Maternity Age: 12-55   A Adult Age: 15-124

Chapter 6. Diseases of the Nervous System (G00-G99)

Chapter Specific Guidelines with Coding Examples

The chapter specific guidelines from the ICD-10-CM Official Guidelines for Coding and Reporting have been provided below. Along with these guidelines are coding examples, contained in the shaded boxes, that have been developed to help illustrate the coding and/or sequencing guidance found in these guidelines.

a. Dominant/nondominant side

Codes from category G81, Hemiplegia and hemiparesis, and subcategories G83.1, Monoplegia of lower limb, G83.2, Monoplegia of upper limb, and G83.3, Monoplegia, unspecified, identify whether the dominant or nondominant side is affected. Should the affected side be documented, but not specified as dominant or nondominant, and the classification system does not indicate a default, code selection is as follows:

- For ambidextrous patients, the default should be dominant.
- If the left side is affected, the default is non-dominant.
- If the right side is affected, the default is dominant.

Hemiplegia affecting left side of ambidextrous patient

G81.92   Hemiplegia, unspecified affecting left dominant side

Explanation: Documentation states that the left side is affected and dominant is used for ambidextrous persons.

Right spastic hemiplegia, unknown whether patient is right- or left-handed

G81.11   Spastic hemiplegia affecting right dominant side

Explanation: Since it is unknown whether the patient is right- or left-handed, if the right side is affected, the default is dominant.

---

b. Pain—Category G89

1) General coding information

Codes in category G89, Pain, not elsewhere classified, may be used in conjunction with codes from other categories and chapters to provide more detail about acute or chronic pain and neoplasm-related pain, unless otherwise indicated below.

If the pain is not specified as acute or chronic, post-thoracotomy, postprocedural, or neoplasm-related, do not assign codes from category G89.

A code from category G89 should not be assigned if the underlying (definitive) diagnosis is known, unless the reason for the encounter is pain control/ management and not management of the underlying condition.

When an admission or encounter is for a procedure aimed at treating the underlying condition (e.g., spinal fusion, kyphoplasty), a code for the underlying condition (e.g., vertebral fracture, spinal stenosis) should be assigned as the principal diagnosis. No code from category G89 should be assigned.

Elderly patient with back pain is admitted for outpatient kyphoplasty for age-related osteopathic compression fracture at vertebra T3

M80.08XA   Age-related osteoporosis with current pathological fracture, vertebra(e), initial encounter for fracture

Explanation: No code is assigned for the pain as it is inherent in the underlying condition being treated.

(a) Category G89 codes as principal or first-listed diagnosis

Category G89 codes are acceptable as principal diagnosis or the first-listed code:

- When pain control or pain management is the reason for the admission/encounter (e.g., a patient with displaced intervertebral disc, nerve impingement and severe back pain presents for injection of steroid into the spinal canal). The underlying cause of the pain should be reported as an additional diagnosis, if known.

Patient presents for steroid injection in the right elbow due to chronic pain associated with primary degenerative joint disease.

G89.29   Other chronic pain

M19.021   Primary osteoarthritis, right elbow

Explanation: Since the encounter is for control of pain, not treating the underlying condition, the pain code is sequenced first followed by the underlying condition. The M25 pain code is not necessary as the underlying condition code represents the specific site.

- When a patient is admitted for the insertion of a neurostimulator for pain control, assign the appropriate pain code as the principal or first-listed diagnosis. When an admission or encounter is for a procedure aimed at treating the underlying condition and a neurostimulator is inserted for pain control during the same admission/encounter, a code for the underlying condition should be assigned as the principal diagnosis and the appropriate pain code should be assigned as a secondary diagnosis.

(b) Use of category G89 codes in conjunction with site specific pain codes

(i) Assigning category G89 and site-specific pain codes

Codes from category G89 may be used in conjunction with codes that identify the site of pain (including codes from chapter 18) if the category G89 code provides additional information. For example, if the code describes the site of the pain, but does not fully describe whether the pain is acute or chronic, then both codes should be assigned.

Patient is seen to evaluate chronic right knee pain

M25.561   Pain in right knee

G89.29   Other chronic pain

Explanation: No underlying condition has been determined yet so the pain would be the reason for the visit. The M25 pain code in this instance does not fully describe the condition as it does not represent that the pain is chronic. The G89 chronic pain code is assigned to provide specificity.

(ii) Sequencing of category G89 codes with site-specific pain codes

The sequencing of category G89 codes with site-specific pain codes (including chapter 18 codes), is dependent on the circumstances of the encounter/admission as follows:

- If the encounter is for pain control or pain management, assign the code from category G89 followed by the code identifying the specific site of pain (e.g., encounter for pain management for acute neck pain from trauma is assigned code G89.11, Acute pain due to trauma, followed by code M54.2, Cervicalgia, to identify the site of pain).

Management of acute, traumatic left shoulder pain

G89.11   Acute pain due to trauma

M25.512   Pain in left shoulder

Explanation: The reason for the encounter is to manage or control the pain, not to treat or evaluate an underlying condition. The G89 pain code is assigned as the first-listed diagnosis but in this instance does not fully describe the condition as it does not include the site and laterality. The M25 pain code is added to provide this information.

- If the encounter is for any other reason except pain control or pain management, and a related definitive diagnosis has not been established (confirmed) by the provider, assign the code for the specific site of pain first, followed by the appropriate code from category G89.

> Tests are performed to investigate the source of the patient's chronic epigastric abdominal pain
>
> **R10.13**   **Epigastric pain**
>
> **G89.29**   **Other chronic pain**
>
> *Explanation*: In this instance the patient's epigastric pain is not being treated; rather the source of the pain is being investigated. A code from chapter 18 for epigastric pain is sequenced before the additional specificity of the G89 code for the chronic pain.

2) Pain due to devices, implants and grafts

See Section I.C.19. Pain due to medical devices

3) Postoperative Pain

The provider's documentation should be used to guide the coding of postoperative pain, as well as *Section III. Reporting Additional Diagnoses* and *Section IV. Diagnostic Coding and Reporting in the Outpatient Setting*.

The default for post-thoracotomy and other postoperative pain not specified as acute or chronic is the code for the acute form.

Routine or expected postoperative pain immediately after surgery should not be coded.

> Pain pump dose is increased for the patient's unexpected, extreme post-thoracotomy
>
> **G89.12**   **Acute post-thoracotomy pain**
>
> *Explanation*: When acute or chronic is not documented, default to acute. The use of "unexpected, extreme" and the increase of medication dosage indicate that the pain was more than routine or expected.

(a) Postoperative pain not associated with specific postoperative complication

Postoperative pain not associated with a specific postoperative complication is assigned to the appropriate postoperative pain code in category G89.

(b) Postoperative pain associated with specific postoperative complication

Postoperative pain associated with a specific postoperative complication (such as painful wire sutures) is assigned to the appropriate code(s) found in Chapter 19, Injury, poisoning, and certain other consequences of external causes. If appropriate, use additional code(s) from category G89 to identify acute or chronic pain (G89.18 or G89.28).

4) Chronic pain

Chronic pain is classified to subcategory G89.2. There is no time frame defining when pain becomes chronic pain. The provider's documentation should be used to guide use of these codes.

5) Neoplasm related pain

Code G89.3 is assigned to pain documented as being related, associated or due to cancer, primary or secondary malignancy, or tumor. This code is assigned regardless of whether the pain is acute or chronic.

This code may be assigned as the principal or first-listed code when the stated reason for the admission/encounter is documented as pain control/pain management. The underlying neoplasm should be reported as an additional diagnosis.

> Patient referred today for pain management due to acute pain related to malignancy of the right breast.
>
> **G89.3**   **Neoplasm related pain (acute)(chronic)**
>
> **C50.911**   **Malignant neoplasm of unspecified site of right female breast**
>
> *Explanation*: Since the encounter was for pain medication management, the pain, rather than the neoplasm, was the reason for the encounter and is sequenced first. This "neoplasm-related pain" code includes both acute and chronic pain.

When the reason for the admission/encounter is management of the neoplasm and the pain associated with the neoplasm is also documented, code G89.3 may be assigned as an additional diagnosis. It is not necessary to assign an additional code for the site of the pain.

See Section I.C.2 for instructions on the sequencing of neoplasms for all other stated reasons for the admission/encounter (except for pain control/pain management).

> Patient with lung cancer presents with acute hip pain and is evaluated and found to have iliac bone metastasis
>
> **C79.51**   **Secondary malignant neoplasm of bone**
>
> **C34.90**   **Malignant neoplasm of unspecified part of unspecified bronchus or lung**
>
> **G89.3**   **Neoplasm related pain (acute)(chronic)**
>
> *Explanation*: The reason for the encounter was the evaluation and diagnosis of the bone metastasis, whose code would be assigned as first-listed, followed by codes for the primary neoplasm and the pain due to the iliac bone metastasis.

6) Chronic pain syndrome

Central pain syndrome (G89.0) and chronic pain syndrome (G89.4) are different than the term "chronic pain," and therefore codes should only be used when the provider has specifically documented this condition.

See Section I.C.5. Pain disorders related to psychological factors

Chapter 6. Diseases of the Nervous System (G00-G99)

EXCLUDES 2   *certain conditions originating in the perinatal period (P04-P96)*
certain infectious and parasitic diseases (A00-B99)
complications of pregnancy, childbirth and the puerperium (O00-O9A)
congenital malformations, deformations, and chromosomal abnormalities (Q00-Q99)
endocrine, nutritional and metabolic diseases (E00-E88)
injury, poisoning and certain other consequences of external causes (S00-T88)
neoplasms (C00-D49)
symptoms, signs and abnormal clinical and laboratory findings, not elsewhere classified (R00-R94)

This chapter contains the following blocks:

G00-G09   Inflammatory diseases of the central nervous system
G10-G14   Systemic atrophies primarily affecting the central nervous system
G20-G26   Extrapyramidal and movement disorders
G30-G32   Other degenerative diseases of the nervous system
G35-G37   Demyelinating diseases of the central nervous system
G40-G47   Episodic and paroxysmal disorders
G50-G59   Nerve, nerve root and plexus disorders
G60-G65   Polyneuropathies and other disorders of the peripheral nervous system
G70-G73   Diseases of myoneural junction and muscle
G80-G83   Cerebral palsy and other paralytic syndromes
G89-G99   Other disorders of the nervous system

Inflammatory diseases of the central nervous system (G00-G09)

✓4ᵗʰ G00   Bacterial meningitis, not elsewhere classified
INCLUDES   bacterial arachnoiditis
bacterial leptomeningitis
bacterial meningitis
bacterial pachymeningitis
EXCLUDES 1   ▶*bacterial meningoencephalitis◀ (G04.2)*
▶*bacterial meningomyelitis◀ (G04.2)*

G00.0   Hemophilus meningitis
Meningitis due to Hemophilus influenzae

G00.1   Pneumococcal meningitis
Meningtitis due to Streptococcal pneumoniae

G00.2   Streptococcal meningitis
Use additional code to further identify organism (B95.0-B95.5)

G00.3   Staphylococcal meningitis
Use additional code to further identify organism (B95.61-B95.8)

G00.8   Other bacterial meningitis
Meningitis due to Escherichia coli
Meningitis due to Friedländer's bacillus
Meningitis due to Klebsiella
Use additional code to further identify organism (B96.-)

G00.9   Bacterial meningitis, unspecified   ▽
Meningitis due to gram-negative bacteria, unspecified
Purulent meningitis NOS
Pyogenic meningitis NOS
Suppurative meningitis NOS

G01   Meningitis in bacterial diseases classified elsewhere
Code first underlying disease
EXCLUDES 1   *meningitis (in):*
gonococcal (A54.81)
leptospirosis (A27.81)
listeriosis (A32.11)
Lyme disease (A69.21)
meningococcal (A39.0)
neurosyphilis (A52.13)
tuberculosis (A17.0)
meningoencephalitis and meningomyelitis in bacterial diseases classified elsewhere (G05)

G02   Meningitis in other infectious and parasitic diseases classified elsewhere
Code first underlying disease, such as:
African trypanosomiasis (B56.-)
poliovirus infection (A80.-)
EXCLUDES 1   *candidal meningitis (B37.5)*
coccidioidomycosis meningitis (B38.4)
cryptococcal meningitis (B45.1)
herpesviral [herpes simplex] meningitis (B00.3)
infectious mononucleosis complicated by meningitis (B27.- with fourth character 2)
measles complicated by meningitis (B05.1)
meningoencephalitis and meningomyelitis in other infectious and parasitic diseases classified elsewhere (G05)
mumps meningitis (B26.1)
rubella meningitis (B06.02)
varicella [chickenpox] meningitis (B01.0)
zoster meningitis (B02.1)

✓4ᵗʰ G03   Meningitis due to other and unspecified causes
INCLUDES   arachnoiditis NOS
leptomeningitis NOS
meningitis NOS
pachymeningitis NOS
EXCLUDES 1   *meningoencephalitis (G04.-)*
meningomyelitis (G04.-)

G03.0   Nonpyogenic meningitis
Aseptic meningitis
Nonbacterial meningitis

G03.1   Chronic meningitis

G03.2   Benign recurrent meningitis [Mollaret]

G03.8   Meningitis due to other specified causes

G03.9   Meningitis, unspecified   ▽
Arachnoiditis (spinal) NOS

✓4ᵗʰ G04   Encephalitis, myelitis and encephalomyelitis
INCLUDES   acute ascending myelitis
meningoencephalitis
meningomyelitis
EXCLUDES 1   *encephalopathy NOS (G93.40)*
EXCLUDES 2   *acute transverse myelitis (G37.3-)*
alcoholic encephalopathy (G31.2)
benign myalgic encephalomyelitis (G93.3)
multiple sclerosis (G35)
subacute necrotizing myelitis (G37.4)
toxic encephalitis (G92)
toxic encephalopathy (G92)

✓5ᵗʰ G04.0   Acute disseminated encephalitis and encephalomyelitis (ADEM)
EXCLUDES 1   *acute necrotizing hemorrhagic encephalopathy (G04.3-)*
other noninfectious acute disseminated encephalomyelitis (noninfectious ADEM) (G04.81)

G04.00   Acute disseminated encephalitis and encephalomyelitis, unspecified   ▽

G04.01   Postinfectious acute disseminated encephalitis and encephalomyelitis (postinfectious ADEM)
EXCLUDES 1   *post chickenpox encephalitis (B01.1)*
post measles encephalitis (B05.0)
post measles myelitis (B05.1)

G04.02   Postimmunization acute disseminated encephalitis, myelitis and encephalomyelitis
Encephalitis, postimmunization
Encephalomyelitis, postimmunization
Use additional code to identify the vaccine (T50.A-, T50.B-, T50.Z-)

G04.1   Tropical spastic paraplegia   HCC

G04.2   Bacterial meningoencephalitis and meningomyelitis, not elsewhere classified

✓5ᵗʰ G04.3   Acute necrotizing hemorrhagic encephalopathy
EXCLUDES 1   *acute disseminated encephalitis and encephalomyelitis (G04.0-)*

G04.30   Acute necrotizing hemorrhagic encephalopathy, unspecified   ▽

G04.31   Postinfectious acute necrotizing hemorrhagic encephalopathy

G04.32   Postimmunization acute necrotizing hemorrhagic encephalopathy
Use additional code to identify the vaccine (T50.A-, T50.B-, T50.Z-)

☑ Additional Character Req   ✓x7ᵗʰ Placeholder Alert   Manifestation   HCC CMS-HCC Condition   ▽ Unspecified Code   ▶◀ Revised Text   ● New Code   ▲ Revised Code Title

ICD-10-CM 2018   551

G04.39 Other acute necrotizing hemorrhagic encephalopathy
Code also underlying etiology, if applicable

✓5th **G04.8 Other encephalitis, myelitis and encephalomyelitis**
Code also any associated seizure (G40.-, R56.9)

G04.81 Other encephalitis and encephalomyelitis
Noninfectious acute disseminated encephalomyelitis (noninfectious ADEM)

G04.89 Other myelitis HCC

✓5th **G04.9 Encephalitis, myelitis and encephalomyelitis, unspecified**

G04.90 Encephalitis and encephalomyelitis, unspecified ▽
Ventriculitis (cerebral) NOS

G04.91 Myelitis, unspecified HCC ▽

✓4th **G05 Encephalitis, myelitis and encephalomyelitis in diseases classified elsewhere**
Code first underlying disease, such as:
human immunodeficiency virus [HIV] disease (B20)
poliovirus (A80.-)
suppurative otitis media (H66.01-H66.4)
trichinellosis (B75)
EXCLUDES 1 *adenoviral encephalitis, myelitis and encephalomyelitis (A85.1)*
congenital toxoplasmosis encephalitis, myelitis and encephalomyelitis (P37.1)
cytomegaloviral encephalitis, myelitis and encephalomyelitis (B25.8)
encephalitis, myelitis and encephalomyelitis (in) measles (B05.0)
encephalitis, myelitis and encephalomyelitis (in) systemic lupus erythematosus (M32.19)
enteroviral encephalitis, myelitis and encephalomyelitis (A85.0)
eosinophilic meningoencephalitis (B83.2)
herpesviral [herpes simplex] encephalitis, myelitis and encephalomyelitis (B00.4)
listerial encephalitis, myelitis and encephalomyelitis (A32.12)
meningococcal encephalitis, myelitis and encephalomyelitis (A39.81)
mumps encephalitis, myelitis and encephalomyelitis (B26.2)
postchickenpox encephalitis, myelitis and encephalomyelitis (B01.1-)
rubella encephalitis, myelitis and encephalomyelitis (B06.01)
toxoplasmosis encephalitis, myelitis and encephalomyelitis (B58.2)
zoster encephalitis, myelitis and encephalomyelitis (B02.0)

G05.3 Encephalitis and encephalomyelitis in diseases classified elsewhere
Meningoencephalitis in diseases classified elsewhere

G05.4 Myelitis in diseases classified elsewhere HCC
Meningomyelitis in diseases classified elsewhere

✓4th **G06 Intracranial and intraspinal abscess and granuloma**
Use additional code (B95-B97) to identify infectious agent

G06.0 Intracranial abscess and granuloma
Brain [any part] abscess (embolic)
Cerebellar abscess (embolic)
Cerebral abscess (embolic)
Intracranial epidural abscess or granuloma
Intracranial extradural abscess or granuloma
Intracranial subdural abscess or granuloma
Otogenic abscess (embolic)
EXCLUDES 1 *tuberculous intracranial abscess and granuloma (A17.81)*

G06.1 Intraspinal abscess and granuloma
Abscess (embolic) of spinal cord [any part]
Intraspinal epidural abscess or granuloma
Intraspinal extradural abscess or granuloma
Intraspinal subdural abscess or granuloma
EXCLUDES 1 *tuberculous intraspinal abscess and granuloma (A17.81)*

G06.2 Extradural and subdural abscess, unspecified ▽

G07 Intracranial and intraspinal abscess and granuloma in diseases classified elsewhere
Code first underlying disease, such as:
schistosomiasis granuloma of brain (B65.-)
EXCLUDES 1 *abscess of brain:*
amebic (A06.6)
chromomycotic (B43.1)
gonococcal (A54.82)
tuberculous (A17.81)
tuberculoma of meninges (A17.1)

G08 Intracranial and intraspinal phlebitis and thrombophlebitis
Septic embolism of intracranial or intraspinal venous sinuses and veins
Septic endophlebitis of intracranial or intraspinal venous sinuses and veins
Septic phlebitis of intracranial or intraspinal venous sinuses and veins
Septic thrombophlebitis of intracranial or intraspinal venous sinuses and veins
Septic thrombosis of intracranial or intraspinal venous sinuses and veins
EXCLUDES 1 *intracranial phlebitis and thrombophlebitis complicating:*
abortion, ectopic or molar pregnancy (O00-O07, O08.7)
pregnancy, childbirth and the puerperium (O22.5, O87.3)
nonpyogenic intracranial phlebitis and thrombophlebitis (I67.6)
EXCLUDES 2 *intracranial phlebitis and thrombophlebitis complicating nonpyogenic intraspinal phlebitis and thrombophlebitis (G95.1)*
DEF: Inflammation and formation of blood clot in a vein within the brain or spine, or their linings.

G09 Sequelae of inflammatory diseases of central nervous system
NOTE   Category G09 is to be used to indicate conditions whose primary classification is to G00-G08 as the cause of sequelae, themselves classifiable elsewhere. The "sequelae" include conditions specified as residuals.
Code first condition resulting from (sequela) of inflammatory diseases of central nervous system

Systemic atrophies primarily affecting the central nervous system (G10-G14)

G10 Huntington's disease HCC
Huntington's chorea
Huntington's dementia
▶Code also dementia in other diseases classified elsewhere without behavioral disturbance (F02.80)◀
DEF: Genetic disease caused by degeneration of nerve cells in the brain, characterized by chronic progressive mental deterioration; dementia and death within 15 to 20 years of onset.

✓4th **G11 Hereditary ataxia**
EXCLUDES 2 *cerebral palsy (G80.-)*
hereditary and idiopathic neuropathy (G60.-)
metabolic disorders (E70-E88)

G11.0 Congenital nonprogressive ataxia HCC

G11.1 Early-onset cerebellar ataxia HCC
Early-onset cerebellar ataxia with essential tremor
Early-onset cerebellar ataxia with myoclonus [Hunt's ataxia]
Early-onset cerebellar ataxia with retained tendon reflexes
Friedreich's ataxia (autosomal recessive)
X-linked recessive spinocerebellar ataxia

G11.2 Late-onset cerebellar ataxia HCC A

G11.3 Cerebellar ataxia with defective DNA repair HCC
Ataxia telangiectasia [Louis-Bar]
EXCLUDES 2 *Cockayne's syndrome (Q87.1)*
other disorders of purine and pyrimidine metabolism (E79.-)
xeroderma pigmentosum (Q82.1)

G11.4 Hereditary spastic paraplegia HCC

G11.8 Other hereditary ataxias HCC

G11.9 Hereditary ataxia, unspecified HCC ▽
Hereditary cerebellar ataxia NOS
Hereditary cerebellar degeneration
Hereditary cerebellar disease
Hereditary cerebellar syndrome

✓4th **G12 Spinal muscular atrophy and related syndromes**

G12.0 Infantile spinal muscular atrophy, type I [Werdnig-Hoffman] HCC

G12.1 Other inherited spinal muscular atrophy HCC
Adult form spinal muscular atrophy
Childhood form, type II spinal muscular atrophy
Distal spinal muscular atrophy
Juvenile form, type III spinal muscular atrophy [Kugelberg-Welander]
Progressive bulbar palsy of childhood [Fazio-Londe]
Scapuloperoneal form spinal muscular atrophy

✓5th **G12.2 Motor neuron disease**

G12.20 Motor neuron disease, unspecified HCC ▽

G12.21 Amyotrophic lateral sclerosis HCC A
~~Progressive spinal muscle atrophy~~

G12.22 Progressive bulbar palsy HCC

● **G12.23 Primary lateral sclerosis**

● **G12.24 Familial motor neuron disease**

● **G12.25 Progressive spinal muscle atrophy**

EXCLUDES 1 Not coded here   EXCLUDES 2 Not included here   N Newborn Age: 0   P Pediatric Age: 0-17   M Maternity Age: 12-55   A Adult Age: 15-124

552   ICD-10-CM 2018

G12.29   **Other motor neuron disease**   HCC
~~Familial motor neuron disease~~
Primary lateral sclerosis

G12.8   **Other spinal muscular atrophies and related syndromes**   HCC

G12.9   **Spinal muscular atrophy, unspecified**   HCC ▽

✓4th **G13   Systemic atrophies primarily affecting central nervous system in diseases classified elsewhere**

     G13.0   Paraneoplastic neuromyopathy and neuropathy   HCC
         Carcinomatous neuromyopathy
         Sensorial paraneoplastic neuropathy [Denny Brown]
         Code first underlying neoplasm (C00-D49)

     G13.1   Other systemic atrophy primarily affecting central nervous system in neoplastic disease   HCC
         Paraneoplastic limbic encephalopathy
         Code first underlying neoplasm (C00-D49)

     G13.2   Systemic atrophy primarily affecting the central nervous system in myxedema
         Code first underlying disease, such as:
           hypothyroidism (E03.-)
           myxedematous congenital iodine deficiency (E00.1)

     G13.8   Systemic atrophy primarily affecting central nervous system in other diseases classified elsewhere
         Code first underlying disease

G14   Postpolio syndrome
     Postpolio myelitic syndrome
     EXCLUDES 1   *sequelae of poliomyelitis (B91)*

Extrapyramidal and movement disorders (G20-G26)

G20   Parkinson's disease   HCC
     Hemiparkinsonism
     Idiopathic Parkinsonism or Parkinson's disease
     Paralysis agitans
     Parkinsonism or Parkinson's disease NOS
     Primary Parkinsonism or Parkinson's disease
     EXCLUDES 1   *dementia with Parkinsonism (G31.83)*
     AHA: 2017, 2Q, 7; 2016, 2Q, 6

✓4th **G21   Secondary parkinsonism**
     EXCLUDES 1   *dementia with Parkinsonism (G31.83)*
               Huntington's disease (G10)
               Shy-Drager syndrome (G90.3)
               syphilitic Parkinsonism (A52.19)

     G21.0   Malignant neuroleptic syndrome
         Use additional code for adverse effect, if applicable, to identify drug (T43.3X5, T43.4X5, T43.505, T43.595)
         EXCLUDES 1   *neuroleptic induced parkinsonism (G21.11)*

     ✓5th **G21.1   Other drug-induced secondary parkinsonism**

         G21.11   Neuroleptic induced parkinsonism   HCC
             Use additional code for adverse effect, if applicable, to identify drug (T43.3X5, T43.4X5, T43.505, T43.595)
             EXCLUDES 1   *malignant neuroleptic syndrome (G21.0)*

         G21.19   Other drug induced secondary parkinsonism   HCC
             ▶Other medication-induced parkinsonism◀
             Use additional code for adverse effect, if applicable, to identify drug (T36-T50 with fifth or sixth character 5)

     G21.2   Secondary parkinsonism due to other external agents   HCC
         Code first (T51-T65) to identify external agent

     G21.3   Postencephalitic parkinsonism   HCC

     G21.4   Vascular parkinsonism   HCC

     G21.8   Other secondary parkinsonism   HCC

     G21.9   Secondary parkinsonism, unspecified   HCC ▽

✓4th **G23   Other degenerative diseases of basal ganglia**
     EXCLUDES 2   *multi-system degeneration of the autonomic nervous system (G90.3)*

     G23.0   Hallervorden-Spatz disease   HCC
         Pigmentary pallidal degeneration

     G23.1   Progressive supranuclear ophthalmoplegia [Steele-Richardson-Olszewski]   HCC
         Progressive supranuclear palsy

     G23.2   Striatonigral degeneration   HCC

     G23.8   Other specified degenerative diseases of basal ganglia   HCC
         Calcification of basal ganglia

     G23.9   Degenerative disease of basal ganglia, unspecified   HCC ▽

✓4th **G24   Dystonia**
     INCLUDES   dyskinesia
     EXCLUDES 2   *athetoid cerebral palsy (G80.3)*

     ✓5th **G24.0   Drug induced dystonia**
         Use additional code for adverse effect, if applicable, to identify drug (T36-T50 with fifth or sixth character5)

         G24.01   Drug induced subacute dyskinesia
             Drug induced blepharospasm
             Drug induced orofacial dyskinesia
             Neuroleptic induced tardive dyskinesia
             Tardive dyskinesia

         G24.02   Drug induced acute dystonia
             Acute dystonic reaction to drugs
             Neuroleptic induced acute dystonia

         G24.09   Other drug induced dystonia

     G24.1   Genetic torsion dystonia
         Dystonia deformans progressiva
         Dystonia musculorum deformans
         Familial torsion dystonia
         Idiopathic familial dystonia
         Idiopathic (torsion) dystonia NOS
         (Schwalbe-) Ziehen-Oppenheim disease

     G24.2   Idiopathic nonfamilial dystonia

     G24.3   Spasmodic torticollis
         EXCLUDES 1   *congenital torticollis (Q68.0)*
               hysterical torticollis (F44.4)
               ocular torticollis (R29.891)
               psychogenic torticollis (F45.8)
               torticollis NOS (M43.6)
               traumatic recurrent torticollis (S13.4)

     G24.4   Idiopathic orofacial dystonia
         Orofacial dyskinesia
         EXCLUDES 1   *drug induced orofacial dyskinesia (G24.01)*

     G24.5   Blepharospasm
         EXCLUDES 1   *drug induced blepharospasm (G24.01)*

     G24.8   Other dystonia
         Acquired torsion dystonia NOS

     G24.9   Dystonia, unspecified   ▽
         Dyskinesia NOS

✓4th **G25   Other extrapyramidal and movement disorders**
     EXCLUDES 2   *sleep related movement disorders (G47.6-)*

     G25.0   Essential tremor
         Familial tremor
         EXCLUDES 1   *tremor NOS (R25.1)*

     G25.1   Drug-induced tremor
         Use additional code for adverse effect, if applicable, to identify drug (T36-T50 with fifth or sixth character 5)

     G25.2   Other specified forms of tremor
         Intention tremor

     G25.3   Myoclonus
         Drug-induced myoclonus
         Palatal myoclonus
         Use additional code for adverse effect, if applicable, to identify drug (T36-T50 with fifth or sixth character 5)
         EXCLUDES 1   *facial myokymia (G51.4)*
               myoclonic epilepsy (G40.-)

     G25.4   Drug-induced chorea
         Use additional code for adverse effect, if applicable, to identify drug (T36-T50 with fifth or sixth character 5)

     G25.5   Other chorea
         Chorea NOS
         EXCLUDES 1   *chorea NOS with heart involvement (I02.0)*
               Huntington's chorea (G10)
               rheumatic chorea (I02.-)
               Sydenham's chorea (I02.-)

     ✓5th **G25.6   Drug induced tics and other tics of organic origin**

         G25.61   Drug induced tics
             Use additional code for adverse effect, if applicable, to identify drug (T36-T50 with fifth or sixth character 5)

         G25.69   Other tics of organic origin
             EXCLUDES 1   *habit spasm (F95.9)*
                 tic NOS (F95.9)
                 Tourette's syndrome (F95.2)

     ✓5th **G25.7   Other and unspecified drug induced movement disorders**
         Use additional code for adverse effect, if applicable, to identify drug (T36-T50 with fifth or sixth character 5)

         G25.70   Drug induced movement disorder, unspecified   ▽

☑ Additional Character Req   ✓x7th Placeholder Alert   Manifestation   HCC CMS-HCC Condition   ▽ Unspecified Code   ▶◀ Revised Text   ● New Code   ▲ Revised Code Title

ICD-10-CM 2018   553

Chapter 6. Diseases of the Nervous System

G25.71–G35

G25.71 Drug induced akathisia
Drug induced acathisia
Neuroleptic induced acute akathisia
▶Tardive akathisia◀

G25.79 Other drug induced movement disorders

✓5ᵗʰ **G25.8 Other specified extrapyramidal and movement disorders**

G25.81 Restless legs syndrome
DEF: Neurological disorder of unknown etiology creating an irresistible urge to move the legs, which may temporarily relieve the symptoms; is accompanied by motor restlessness and sensations of pain, burning, prickling, or tingling.

G25.82 Stiff-man syndrome

G25.83 Benign shuddering attacks

G25.89 Other specified extrapyramidal and movement disorders

G25.9 Extrapyramidal and movement disorder, unspecified ▽

G26 Extrapyramidal and movement disorders in diseases classified elsewhere
Code first underlying disease

Other degenerative diseases of the nervous system (G30-G32)

✓4ᵗʰ **G30 Alzheimer's disease**
INCLUDES Alzheimer's dementia senile and presenile forms
Use additional code to identify:
delirium, if applicable (F05)
dementia with behavioral disturbance (F02.81)
dementia without behavioral disturbance (F02.80)
EXCLUDES 1 senile degeneration of brain NEC (G31.1)
senile dementia NOS (F03)
senility NOS (R41.81)
AHA: 2017, 1Q, 43

G30.0 Alzheimer's disease with early onset

G30.1 Alzheimer's disease with late onset Ⓐ

G30.8 Other Alzheimer's disease

G30.9 Alzheimer's disease, unspecified ▽
AHA: 2016, 2Q, 6; 2012, 4Q, 95

✓4ᵗʰ **G31 Other degenerative diseases of nervous system, not elsewhere classified**
Use additional code to identify:
dementia with behavioral disturbance (F02.81)
dementia without behavioral disturbance (F02.80)
EXCLUDES 2 Reye's syndrome (G93.7)

✓5ᵗʰ **G31.0 Frontotemporal dementia**

G31.01 Pick's disease
Primary progressive aphasia
Progressive isolated aphasia
DEF: A progressive frontotemporal dementia with asymmetrical atrophy of the frontal and temporal regions of the cerebral cortex, abnormal rounded brain cells called Pick cells with the presence of abnormal staining of protein (called tau); symptoms include prominent apathy, behavioral changes such as disinhibition and restlessness, echolalia, impairment of language, memory, and intellect, increased carelessness, poor personal hygiene, and decreased attention span.

G31.09 Other frontotemporal dementia
Frontal dementia

G31.1 Senile degeneration of brain, not elsewhere classified
EXCLUDES 1 Alzheimer's disease (G30.-)
senility NOS (R41.81)

G31.2 Degeneration of nervous system due to alcohol
Alcoholic cerebellar ataxia
Alcoholic cerebellar degeneration
Alcoholic cerebral degeneration
Alcoholic encephalopathy
Dysfunction of the autonomic nervous system due to alcohol
Code also associated alcoholism (F10.-)

✓5ᵗʰ **G31.8 Other specified degenerative diseases of nervous system**

G31.81 Alpers disease
Grey-matter degeneration

G31.82 Leigh's disease
Subacute necrotizing encephalopathy

G31.83 Dementia with Lewy bodies
Dementia with Parkinsonism
Lewy body dementia
Lewy body disease
AHA: 2017, 2Q, 7; 2016, 4Q, 141
DEF: A cerebral dementia with neurophysiologic changes, increased hippocampal volume, hypoperfusion in the occipital lobes, beta amyloid deposits with neurofibrillary tangles, and atrophy of cortex and brainstem. Hallmark neuropsychological characteristics include fluctuating cognition with pronounced variation in attention and alertness; recurrent hallucinations; and Parkinsonism.

G31.84 Mild cognitive impairment, so stated
▶Mild neurocognitive disorder◀
EXCLUDES 1 age related cognitive decline (R41.81)
altered mental status (R41.82)
cerebral degeneration (G31.9)
change in mental status (R41.82)
cognitive deficits following (sequelae of) cerebral hemorrhage or infarction (I69.01-, I69.11-, I69.21-, I69.31-, I69.81-, I69.91-)
cognitive impairment due to intracranial or head injury (S06.-)
dementia (F01.-, F02.-, F03)
mild memory disturbance (F06.8)
neurologic neglect syndrome (R41.4)
personality change, nonpsychotic (F68.8)

G31.85 Corticobasal degeneration

G31.89 Other specified degenerative diseases of nervous system

G31.9 Degenerative disease of nervous system, unspecified ▽

✓4ᵗʰ **G32 Other degenerative disorders of nervous system in diseases classified elsewhere**

G32.0 Subacute combined degeneration of spinal cord in diseases HCC **classified elsewhere**
Dana-Putnam syndrome
Sclerosis of spinal cord (combined) (dorsolateral) (posterolateral)
Code first underlying disease, such as:
vitamin B12 deficiency (E53.8)
vitamin B12 deficiency:
anemia (D51.9)
dietary (D51.3)
pernicious (D51.0)
EXCLUDES 1 syphilitic combined degeneration of spinal cord (A52.11)

✓5ᵗʰ **G32.8 Other specified degenerative disorders of nervous system in diseases classified elsewhere**
Code first underlying disease, such as:
amyloidosis cerebral degeneration (E85.-)
cerebral degeneration (due to) hypothyroidism (E00.0-E03.9)
cerebral degeneration (due to) neoplasm (C00-D49)
cerebral degeneration (due to) vitamin B deficiency, except thiamine (E52-E53.-)
EXCLUDES 1 superior hemorrhagic polioencephalitis [Wernicke's encephalopathy] (E51.2)

G32.81 Cerebellar ataxia in diseases classified elsewhere HCC
Code first underlying disease, such as:
celiac disease (with gluten ataxia) (K90.0)
cerebellar ataxia (in) neoplastic disease (paraneoplastic cerebellar degeneration) (C00-D49)
non-celiac gluten ataxia (M35.9)
EXCLUDES 1 systemic atrophy primarily affecting the central nervous system in alcoholic cerebellar ataxia (G31.2)
systemic atrophy primarily affecting the central nervous system in myxedema (G13.2)

G32.89 Other specified degenerative disorders of nervous system in diseases classified elsewhere
Degenerative encephalopathy in diseases classified elsewhere

Demyelinating diseases of the central nervous system (G35-G37)

G35 Multiple sclerosis HCC
Disseminated multiple sclerosis
Generalized multiple sclerosis
Multiple sclerosis NOS
Multiple sclerosis of brain stem
Multiple sclerosis of cord

✓4ᵗʰ **G36 Other acute disseminated demyelination**
     EXCLUDES 1   postinfectious encephalitis and encephalomyelitis NOS (G04.01)

     G36.0 Neuromyelitis optica [Devic]   HCC
         Demyelination in optic neuritis
         EXCLUDES 1   optic neuritis NOS (H46)

     G36.1 Acute and subacute hemorrhagic leukoencephalitis [Hurst]   HCC

     G36.8 Other specified acute disseminated demyelination   HCC

     G36.9 Acute disseminated demyelination, unspecified   HCC ▽

✓4ᵗʰ **G37 Other demyelinating diseases of central nervous system**

     G37.0 Diffuse sclerosis of central nervous system   HCC
         Periaxial encephalitis
         Schilder's disease
         EXCLUDES 1   X linked adrenoleukodystrophy (E71.52-)

     G37.1 Central demyelination of corpus callosum   HCC

     G37.2 Central pontine myelinolysis   HCC

     G37.3 Acute transverse myelitis in demyelinating disease of central nervous system   HCC
         Acute transverse myelitis NOS
         Acute transverse myelopathy
         EXCLUDES 1   multiple sclerosis (G35)
                     neuromyelitis optica [Devic] (G36.0)

     G37.4 Subacute necrotizing myelitis of central nervous system   HCC

     G37.5 Concentric sclerosis [Balo] of central nervous system   HCC

     G37.8 Other specified demyelinating diseases of central nervous system   HCC

     G37.9 Demyelinating disease of central nervous system, unspecified   HCC ▽

Episodic and paroxysmal disorders (G40-G47)

✓4ᵗʰ **G40 Epilepsy and recurrent seizures**
     NOTE   The following terms are to be considered equivalent to intractable: pharmacoresistant (pharmacologically resistant), treatment resistant, refractory (medically) and poorly controlled

     EXCLUDES 1   conversion disorder with seizures (F44.5)
                     convulsions NOS (R56.9)
                     post traumatic seizures (R56.1)
                     seizure (convulsive) NOS (R56.9)
                     seizure of newborn (P90)

     EXCLUDES 2   hippocampal sclerosis (G93.81)
                     mesial temporal sclerosis (G93.81)
                     temporal sclerosis (G93.81)
                     Todd's paralysis (G83.84)

     ✓5ᵗʰ **G40.0 Localization-related (focal) (partial) idiopathic epilepsy and epileptic syndromes with seizures of localized onset**
         Benign childhood epilepsy with centrotemporal EEG spikes
         Childhood epilepsy with occipital EEG paroxysms
         EXCLUDES 1   adult onset localization-related epilepsy (G40.1-, G40.2-)

         ✓6ᵗʰ **G40.00 Localization-related (focal) (partial) idiopathic epilepsy and epileptic syndromes with seizures of localized onset, not intractable**
             Localization-related (focal) (partial) idiopathic epilepsy and epileptic syndromes with seizures of localized onset without intractability

             G40.001 Localization-related (focal) (partial) idiopathic epilepsy and epileptic syndromes with seizures of localized onset, not intractable, with status epilepticus   HCC

             G40.009 Localization-related (focal) (partial) idiopathic epilepsy and epileptic syndromes with seizures of localized onset, not intractable, without status epilepticus   HCC
                 Localization-related (focal) (partial) idiopathic epilepsy and epileptic syndromes with seizures of localized onset NOS

         ✓6ᵗʰ **G40.01 Localization-related (focal) (partial) idiopathic epilepsy and epileptic syndromes with seizures of localized onset, intractable**

             G40.011 Localization-related (focal) (partial) idiopathic epilepsy and epileptic syndromes with seizures of localized onset, intractable, with status epilepticus   HCC

             G40.019 Localization-related (focal) (partial) idiopathic epilepsy and epileptic syndromes with seizures of localized onset, intractable, without status epilepticus   HCC

     ✓5ᵗʰ **G40.1 Localization-related (focal) (partial) symptomatic epilepsy and epileptic syndromes with simple partial seizures**
         Attacks without alteration of consciousness
         Epilepsia partialis continua [Kozhevnikof]
         Simple partial seizures developing into secondarily generalized seizures

         ✓6ᵗʰ **G40.10 Localization-related (focal) (partial) symptomatic epilepsy and epileptic syndromes with simple partial seizures, not intractable**
             Localization-related (focal) (partial) symptomatic epilepsy and epileptic syndromes with simple partial seizures without intractability

             G40.101 Localization-related (focal) (partial) symptomatic epilepsy and epileptic syndromes with simple partial seizures, not intractable, with status epilepticus   HCC

             G40.109 Localization-related (focal) (partial) symptomatic epilepsy and epileptic syndromes with simple partial seizures, not intractable, without status epilepticus   HCC
                 Localization-related (focal) (partial) symptomatic epilepsy and epileptic syndromes with simple partial seizures NOS

         ✓6ᵗʰ **G40.11 Localization-related (focal) (partial) symptomatic epilepsy and epileptic syndromes with simple partial seizures, intractable**

             G40.111 Localization-related (focal) (partial) symptomatic epilepsy and epileptic syndromes with simple partial seizures, intractable, with status epilepticus   HCC

             G40.119 Localization-related (focal) (partial) symptomatic epilepsy and epileptic syndromes with simple partial seizures, intractable, without status epilepticus   HCC

     ✓5ᵗʰ **G40.2 Localization-related (focal) (partial) symptomatic epilepsy and epileptic syndromes with complex partial seizures**
         Attacks with alteration of consciousness, often with automatisms
         Complex partial seizures developing into secondarily generalized seizures

         ✓6ᵗʰ **G40.20 Localization-related (focal) (partial) symptomatic epilepsy and epileptic syndromes with complex partial seizures, not intractable**
             Localization-related (focal) (partial) symptomatic epilepsy and epileptic syndromes with complex partial seizures without intractability

             G40.201 Localization-related (focal) (partial) symptomatic epilepsy and epileptic syndromes with complex partial seizures, not intractable, with status epilepticus   HCC

             G40.209 Localization-related (focal) (partial) symptomatic epilepsy and epileptic syndromes with complex partial seizures, not intractable, without status epilepticus   HCC
                 Localization-related (focal) (partial) symptomatic epilepsy and epileptic syndromes with complex partial seizures NOS

         ✓6ᵗʰ **G40.21 Localization-related (focal) (partial) symptomatic epilepsy and epileptic syndromes with complex partial seizures, intractable**

             G40.211 Localization-related (focal) (partial) symptomatic epilepsy and epileptic syndromes with complex partial seizures, intractable, with status epilepticus   HCC

             G40.219 Localization-related (focal) (partial) symptomatic epilepsy and epileptic syndromes with complex partial seizures, intractable, without status epilepticus   HCC

     ✓5ᵗʰ **G40.3 Generalized idiopathic epilepsy and epileptic syndromes**
         Code also MERRF syndrome, if applicable (E88.42)

         ✓6ᵗʰ **G40.30 Generalized idiopathic epilepsy and epileptic syndromes, not intractable**
             Generalized idiopathic epilepsy and epileptic syndromes without intractability

---

✓ Additional Character Req   ✓x7ᵗʰ Placeholder Alert   Manifestation   HCC CMS-HCC Condition   ▽ Unspecified Code   ►◄ Revised Text   ● New Code   ▲ Revised Code Title

ICD-10-CM 2018   555

G40.301   Generalized idiopathic epilepsy and epileptic syndromes, not intractable, with status epilepticus `HCC`

G40.309   Generalized idiopathic epilepsy and epileptic syndromes, not intractable, without status epilepticus `HCC`
Generalized idiopathic epilepsy and epileptic syndromes NOS

✓6ᵗʰ **G40.31**   Generalized idiopathic epilepsy and epileptic syndromes, intractable

G40.311   Generalized idiopathic epilepsy and epileptic syndromes, intractable, with status epilepticus `HCC`

G40.319   Generalized idiopathic epilepsy and epileptic syndromes, intractable, without status epilepticus `HCC`

✓5ᵗʰ **G40.A**   Absence epileptic syndrome
Childhood absence epilepsy [pyknolepsy]
Juvenile absence epilepsy
Absence epileptic syndrome, NOS

✓6ᵗʰ **G40.A0**   Absence epileptic syndrome, not intractable

G40.A01   Absence epileptic syndrome, not intractable, with status epilepticus `HCC`

G40.A09   Absence epileptic syndrome, not intractable, without status epilepticus `HCC`

✓6ᵗʰ **G40.A1**   Absence epileptic syndrome, intractable

G40.A11   Absence epileptic syndrome, intractable, with status epilepticus `HCC`

G40.A19   Absence epileptic syndrome, intractable, without status epilepticus `HCC`

✓5ᵗʰ **G40.B**   Juvenile myoclonic epilepsy [impulsive petit mal]

✓6ᵗʰ **G40.B0**   Juvenile myoclonic epilepsy, not intractable

G40.B01   Juvenile myoclonic epilepsy, not intractable, with status epilepticus `HCC`

G40.B09   Juvenile myoclonic epilepsy, not intractable, without status epilepticus `HCC`

✓6ᵗʰ **G40.B1**   Juvenile myoclonic epilepsy, intractable

G40.B11   Juvenile myoclonic epilepsy, intractable, with status epilepticus `HCC`

G40.B19   Juvenile myoclonic epilepsy, intractable, without status epilepticus `HCC`

✓5ᵗʰ **G40.4**   Other generalized epilepsy and epileptic syndromes
Epilepsy with grand mal seizures on awakening
Epilepsy with myoclonic absences
Epilepsy with myoclonic-astatic seizures
Grand mal seizure NOS
Nonspecific atonic epileptic seizures
Nonspecific clonic epileptic seizures
Nonspecific myoclonic epileptic seizures
Nonspecific tonic epileptic seizures
Nonspecific tonic-clonic epileptic seizures
Symptomatic early myoclonic encephalopathy

✓6ᵗʰ **G40.40**   Other generalized epilepsy and epileptic syndromes, not intractable
Other generalized epilepsy and epileptic syndromes without intractability
Other generalized epilepsy and epileptic syndromes NOS

G40.401   Other generalized epilepsy and epileptic syndromes, not intractable, with status epilepticus `HCC`

G40.409   Other generalized epilepsy and epileptic syndromes, not intractable, without status epilepticus `HCC`

✓6ᵗʰ **G40.41**   Other generalized epilepsy and epileptic syndromes, intractable

G40.411   Other generalized epilepsy and epileptic syndromes, intractable, with status epilepticus `HCC`

G40.419   Other generalized epilepsy and epileptic syndromes, intractable, without status epilepticus `HCC`

✓5ᵗʰ **G40.5**   Epileptic seizures related to external causes
Epileptic seizures related to alcohol
Epileptic seizures related to drugs
Epileptic seizures related to hormonal changes
Epileptic seizures related to sleep deprivation
Epileptic seizures related to stress
Code also, if applicable, associated epilepsy and recurrent seizures (G40.-)
Use additional code for adverse effect, if applicable, to identify drug (T36-T50 with fifth or sixth character 5)

✓6ᵗʰ **G40.50**   Epileptic seizures related to external causes, not intractable

G40.501   Epileptic seizures related to external causes, not intractable, with status epilepticus `HCC`

G40.509   Epileptic seizures related to external causes, not intractable, without status epilepticus `HCC`
Epileptic seizures related to external causes, NOS

✓5ᵗʰ **G40.8**   Other epilepsy and recurrent seizures
Epilepsies and epileptic syndromes undetermined as to whether they are focal or generalized
Landau-Kleffner syndrome

✓6ᵗʰ **G40.80**   Other epilepsy

G40.801   Other epilepsy, not intractable, with status epilepticus `HCC`
Other epilepsy without intractability with status epilepticus

G40.802   Other epilepsy, not intractable, without status epilepticus `HCC`
Other epilepsy NOS
Other epilepsy without intractability without status epilepticus

G40.803   Other epilepsy, intractable, with status epilepticus `HCC`

G40.804   Other epilepsy, intractable, without status epilepticus `HCC`

✓6ᵗʰ **G40.81**   Lennox-Gastaut syndrome

G40.811   Lennox-Gastaut syndrome, not intractable, with status epilepticus `HCC`

G40.812   Lennox-Gastaut syndrome, not intractable, without status epilepticus `HCC`

G40.813   Lennox-Gastaut syndrome, intractable, with status epilepticus `HCC`

G40.814   Lennox-Gastaut syndrome, intractable, without status epilepticus `HCC`

✓6ᵗʰ **G40.82**   Epileptic spasms
Infantile spasms
Salaam attacks
West's syndrome

G40.821   Epileptic spasms, not intractable, with status epilepticus `HCC`

G40.822   Epileptic spasms, not intractable, without status epilepticus `HCC`

G40.823   Epileptic spasms, intractable, with status epilepticus `HCC`

G40.824   Epileptic spasms, intractable, without status epilepticus `HCC`

G40.89   Other seizures `HCC`
EXCLUDES 1   post traumatic seizures (R56.1)
recurrent seizures NOS (G40.909)
seizure NOS (R56.9)

✓5ᵗʰ **G40.9**   Epilepsy, unspecified

✓6ᵗʰ **G40.90**   Epilepsy, unspecified, not intractable
Epilepsy, unspecified, without intractability

G40.901   Epilepsy, unspecified, not intractable, with status epilepticus `HCC` ▽

G40.909   Epilepsy, unspecified, not intractable, without status epilepticus `HCC` ▽
Epilepsy NOS
Epileptic convulsions NOS
Epileptic fits NOS
Epileptic seizures NOS
Recurrent seizures NOS
Seizure disorder NOS

EXCLUDES 1 Not coded here   **EXCLUDES 2** Not included here   N Newborn Age: 0   P Pediatric Age: 0-17   M Maternity Age: 12-55   A Adult Age: 15-124

✓6ᵗʰ **G40.91** **Epilepsy, unspecified, intractable**
     Intractable seizure disorder NOS

     G40.911 **Epilepsy, unspecified, intractable,** HCC ▽
         with status epilepticus

     G40.919 **Epilepsy, unspecified, intractable,** HCC ▽
         without status epilepticus

✓4ᵗʰ **G43** **Migraine**
    NOTE   The following terms are to be considered equivalent to
       intractable: pharmacoresistant (pharmacologically resistant),
       treatment resistant, refractory (medically) and poorly
       controlled.
     Use additional code for adverse effect, if applicable, to identify drug
       (T36-T50 with fifth or sixth character 5)
    EXCLUDES 1   headache NOS (R51)
        lower half migraine (G44.00)
    EXCLUDES 2   headache syndromes (G44.-)

✓5ᵗʰ **G43.0** **Migraine** without aura
     Common migraine
    EXCLUDES 1   chronic migraine without aura (G43.7-)

   ✓6ᵗʰ **G43.00** **Migraine without aura, not intractable**
     Migraine without aura without mention of refractory
     migraine

     G43.001 **Migraine without aura, not intractable,**
       with status migrainosus

     G43.009 **Migraine without aura, not intractable,**
       without status migrainosus
       Migraine without aura NOS

   ✓6ᵗʰ **G43.01** **Migraine without aura, intractable**
     Migraine without aura with refractory migraine

     G43.011 **Migraine without aura, intractable, with**
       status migrainosus

     G43.019 **Migraine without aura, intractable,**
       without status migrainosus

✓5ᵗʰ **G43.1** **Migraine** with aura
     Basilar migraine
     Classical migraine
     Migraine equivalents
     Migraine preceded or accompanied by transient focal
       neurological phenomena
     Migraine triggered seizures
     Migraine with acute-onset aura
     Migraine with aura without headache (migraine equivalents)
     Migraine with prolonged aura
     Migraine with typical aura
     Retinal migraine
     Code also any associated seizure (G40.-, R56.9)
    EXCLUDES 1   persistent migraine aura (G43.5-, G43.6-)

   ✓6ᵗʰ **G43.10** **Migraine with aura, not intractable**
     Migraine with aura without mention of refractory
     migraine

     G43.101 **Migraine with aura, not intractable, with**
       status migrainosus

     G43.109 **Migraine with aura, not intractable,**
       without status migrainosus
       Migraine with aura NOS

   ✓6ᵗʰ **G43.11** **Migraine with aura, intractable**
     Migraine with aura with refractory migraine

     G43.111 **Migraine with aura, intractable, with**
       status migrainosus

     G43.119 **Migraine with aura, intractable, without**
       status migrainosus

✓5ᵗʰ **G43.4** Hemiplegic **migraine**
     Familial migraine
     Sporadic migraine

   ✓6ᵗʰ **G43.40** **Hemiplegic migraine,** not intractable
     Hemiplegic migraine without refractory migraine

     G43.401 **Hemiplegic migraine, not intractable,** with
       status migrainosus

     G43.409 **Hemiplegic migraine, not intractable,**
       without status migrainosus
       Hemiplegic migraine NOS

   ✓6ᵗʰ **G43.41** **Hemiplegic migraine,** intractable
     Hemiplegic migraine with refractory migraine

     G43.411 **Hemiplegic migraine, intractable,** with
       status migrainosus

     G43.419 **Hemiplegic migraine, intractable, without**
       status migrainosus

✓5ᵗʰ **G43.5** Persistent **migraine** aura without cerebral infarction

   ✓6ᵗʰ **G43.50** **Persistent migraine aura without cerebral infarction,**
     not intractable
     Persistent migraine aura without cerebral infarction,
     without refractory migraine

     G43.501 **Persistent migraine aura without cerebral**
       infarction, not intractable, with status
       migrainosus

     G43.509 **Persistent migraine aura without cerebral**
       infarction, not intractable, without status
       migrainosus
       Persistent migraine aura NOS

   ✓6ᵗʰ **G43.51** **Persistent migraine aura without cerebral infarction,**
     intractable
     Persistent migraine aura without cerebral infarction,
     with refractory migraine

     G43.511 **Persistent migraine aura without cerebral**
       infarction, intractable, with status
       migrainosus

     G43.519 **Persistent migraine aura without cerebral**
       infarction, intractable, without status
       migrainosus

✓5ᵗʰ **G43.6** Persistent **migraine** aura with cerebral infarction
     Code also the type of cerebral infarction (I63.-)

   ✓6ᵗʰ **G43.60** **Persistent migraine aura with cerebral infarction,**
     not intractable
     Persistent migraine aura with cerebral infarction,
     without refractory migraine

     G43.601 **Persistent migraine aura with cerebral**
       infarction, not intractable, with status
       migrainosus

     G43.609 **Persistent migraine aura with cerebral**
       infarction, not intractable, without status
       migrainosus

   ✓6ᵗʰ **G43.61** **Persistent migraine aura with cerebral infarction,**
     intractable
     Persistent migraine aura with cerebral infarction, with
     refractory migraine

     G43.611 **Persistent migraine aura with cerebral**
       infarction, intractable, with status
       migrainosus

     G43.619 **Persistent migraine aura with cerebral**
       infarction, intractable, without status
       migrainosus

✓5ᵗʰ **G43.7** Chronic **migraine** without aura
     Transformed migraine
    EXCLUDES 1   migraine without aura (G43.0-)

   ✓6ᵗʰ **G43.70** **Chronic migraine without aura,** not intractable
     Chronic migraine without aura, without refractory
     migraine

     G43.701 **Chronic migraine without aura, not**
       intractable, with status migrainosus

     G43.709 **Chronic migraine without aura, not**
       intractable, without status migrainosus
       Chronic migraine without aura NOS

   ✓6ᵗʰ **G43.71** **Chronic migraine without aura,** intractable
     Chronic migraine without aura, with refractory
     migraine

     G43.711 **Chronic migraine without aura,**
       intractable, with status migrainosus

     G43.719 **Chronic migraine without aura,**
       intractable, without status migrainosus

✓5ᵗʰ **G43.A** Cyclical vomiting

     G43.A0 **Cyclical vomiting,** not intractable
       Cyclical vomiting, without refractory migraine

     G43.A1 **Cyclical vomiting,** intractable
       Cyclical vomiting, with refractory migraine

✓5ᵗʰ **G43.B** Ophthalmoplegic **migraine**

     G43.B0 **Ophthalmoplegic migraine,** not intractable
       Ophthalmoplegic migraine, without refractory
       migraine

     G43.B1 **Ophthalmoplegic migraine,** intractable
       Ophthalmoplegic migraine, with refractory migraine

✓5ᵗʰ **G43.C** Periodic headache **syndromes in child or adult**

     G43.C0 **Periodic headache syndromes in child or adult,** not
     intractable
       Periodic headache syndromes in child or adult,
       without refractory migraine

☑ Additional Character Req   ✓x7ᵗʰ Placeholder Alert   Manifestation   HCC CMS-HCC Condition   ▽ Unspecified Code   ►◄ Revised Text   ● New Code   ▲ Revised Code Title

G43.C1 Periodic headache syndromes in child or adult, intractable
Periodic headache syndromes in child or adult, with refractory migraine

✓5th **G43.D Abdominal migraine**

G43.D0 Abdominal migraine, not intractable
Abdominal migraine, without refractory migraine

G43.D1 Abdominal migraine, intractable
Abdominal migraine, with refractory migraine

✓5th **G43.8 Other migraine**

✓6th **G43.80 Other migraine, not intractable**
Other migraine, without refractory migraine

G43.801 Other migraine, not intractable, with status migrainosus

G43.809 Other migraine, not intractable, without status migrainosus

✓6th **G43.81 Other migraine, intractable**
Other migraine, with refractory migraine

G43.811 Other migraine, intractable, with status migrainosus

G43.819 Other migraine, intractable, without status migrainosus

✓6th **G43.82 Menstrual migraine, not intractable**
Menstrual headache, not intractable
Menstrual migraine, without refractory migraine
Menstrually related migraine, not intractable
Pre-menstrual headache, not intractable
Pre-menstrual migraine, not intractable
Pure menstrual migraine, not intractable
Code also associated premenstrual tension syndrome (N94.3)

G43.821 Menstrual migraine, not intractable, with status migrainosus ♀

G43.829 Menstrual migraine, not intractable, without status migrainosus ♀
Menstrual migraine NOS

✓6th **G43.83 Menstrual migraine, intractable**
Menstrual headache, intractable
Menstrual migraine, with refractory migraine
Menstrually related migraine, intractable
Pre-menstrual headache, intractable
Pre-menstrual migraine, intractable
Pure menstrual migraine, intractable
Code also associated premenstrual tension syndrome (N94.3)

G43.831 Menstrual migraine, intractable, with status migrainosus ♀

G43.839 Menstrual migraine, intractable, without status migrainosus ♀

✓5th **G43.9 Migraine, unspecified**

✓6th **G43.90 Migraine, unspecified, not intractable**
Migraine, unspecified, without refractory migraine

G43.901 Migraine, unspecified, not intractable, with status migrainosus ▽
Status migrainosus NOS

G43.909 Migraine, unspecified, not intractable, without status migrainosus ▽
Migraine NOS

✓6th **G43.91 Migraine, unspecified, intractable**
Migraine, unspecified, with refractory migraine

G43.911 Migraine, unspecified, intractable, with status migrainosus ▽

G43.919 Migraine, unspecified, intractable, without status migrainosus ▽

✓4th **G44 Other headache syndromes**
EXCLUDES 1 headache NOS (R51)
EXCLUDES 2 atypical facial pain (G50.1)
headache due to lumbar puncture (G97.1)
migraines (G43.-)
trigeminal neuralgia (G50.0)

✓5th **G44.0 Cluster headaches and other trigeminal autonomic cephalgias (TAC)**

✓6th **G44.00 Cluster headache syndrome, unspecified**
Ciliary neuralgia
Cluster headache NOS
Histamine cephalgia
Lower half migraine
Migrainous neuralgia

G44.001 Cluster headache syndrome, unspecified, intractable ▽

G44.009 Cluster headache syndrome, unspecified, not intractable ▽
Cluster headache syndrome NOS

✓6th **G44.01 Episodic cluster headache**

G44.011 Episodic cluster headache, intractable

G44.019 Episodic cluster headache, not intractable
Episodic cluster headache NOS

✓6th **G44.02 Chronic cluster headache**

G44.021 Chronic cluster headache, intractable

G44.029 Chronic cluster headache, not intractable
Chronic cluster headache NOS

✓6th **G44.03 Episodic paroxysmal hemicrania**
Paroxysmal hemicrania NOS

G44.031 Episodic paroxysmal hemicrania, intractable

G44.039 Episodic paroxysmal hemicrania, not intractable
Episodic paroxysmal hemicrania NOS

✓6th **G44.04 Chronic paroxysmal hemicrania**

G44.041 Chronic paroxysmal hemicrania, intractable

G44.049 Chronic paroxysmal hemicrania, not intractable
Chronic paroxysmal hemicrania NOS

✓6th **G44.05 Short lasting unilateral neuralgiform headache with conjunctival injection and tearing (SUNCT)**

G44.051 Short lasting unilateral neuralgiform headache with conjunctival injection and tearing (SUNCT), intractable

G44.059 Short lasting unilateral neuralgiform headache with conjunctival injection and tearing (SUNCT), not intractable
Short lasting unilateral neuralgiform headache with conjunctival injection and tearing (SUNCT) NOS

✓6th **G44.09 Other trigeminal autonomic cephalgias (TAC)**

G44.091 Other trigeminal autonomic cephalgias (TAC), intractable

G44.099 Other trigeminal autonomic cephalgias syndrome (TAC), not intractable

G44.1 Vascular headache, not elsewhere classified
EXCLUDES 2 cluster headache (G44.0)
complicated headache syndromes (G44.5-)
drug-induced headache (G44.4-)
migraine (G43.-)
other specified headache syndromes (G44.8-)
post-traumatic headache (G44.3-)
tension-type headache (G44.2-)

✓5th **G44.2 Tension-type headache**

✓6th **G44.20 Tension-type headache, unspecified**

G44.201 Tension-type headache, unspecified, intractable ▽

G44.209 Tension-type headache, unspecified, not intractable ▽
Tension headache NOS

✓6th **G44.21 Episodic tension-type headache**

G44.211 Episodic tension-type headache, intractable

G44.219 Episodic tension-type headache, not intractable
Episodic tension-type headache NOS

✓6th **G44.22**   Chronic tension-type headache

     G44.221   Chronic tension-type headache, intractable

     G44.229   Chronic tension-type headache, not intractable
         Chronic tension-type headache NOS

✓5th **G44.3**   Post-traumatic headache

     ✓6th **G44.30**   Post-traumatic headache, unspecified

         G44.301   Post-traumatic headache, unspecified, ▽ intractable

         G44.309   Post-traumatic headache, unspecified, ▽ not intractable
             Post-traumatic headache NOS

     ✓6th **G44.31**   Acute post-traumatic headache

         G44.311   Acute post-traumatic headache, intractable

         G44.319   Acute post-traumatic headache, not intractable
             Acute post-traumatic headache NOS

     ✓6th **G44.32**   Chronic post-traumatic headache

         G44.321   Chronic post-traumatic headache, intractable

         G44.329   Chronic post-traumatic headache, not intractable
             Chronic post-traumatic headache NOS

✓5th **G44.4**   Drug-induced headache, not elsewhere classified
     Medication overuse headache
     Use additional code for adverse effect, if applicable, to identify drug (T36-T50 with fifth or sixth character 5)

     G44.40   Drug-induced headache, not elsewhere classified, not intractable

     G44.41   Drug-induced headache, not elsewhere classified, intractable

✓5th **G44.5**   Complicated headache syndromes

     G44.51   Hemicrania continua

     G44.52   New daily persistent headache (NDPH)

     G44.53   Primary thunderclap headache

     G44.59   Other complicated headache syndrome

✓5th **G44.8**   Other specified headache syndromes

     G44.81   Hypnic headache

     G44.82   Headache associated with sexual activity
         Orgasmic headache
         Preorgasmic headache

     G44.83   Primary cough headache

     G44.84   Primary exertional headache

     G44.85   Primary stabbing headache

     G44.89   Other headache syndrome

✓4th **G45**   **Transient cerebral ischemic attacks and related syndromes**
     EXCLUDES 1   neonatal cerebral ischemia (P91.0)
             transient retinal artery occlusion (H34.0-)

     G45.0   Vertebro-basilar artery syndrome

     G45.1   Carotid artery syndrome (hemispheric)

     G45.2   Multiple and bilateral precerebral artery syndromes

     G45.3   Amaurosis fugax

     G45.4   Transient global amnesia
         EXCLUDES 1   amnesia NOS (R41.3)

     G45.8   Other transient cerebral ischemic attacks and related syndromes

     G45.9   Transient cerebral ischemic attack, unspecified   ▽
         Spasm of cerebral artery
         TIA
         Transient cerebral ischemia NOS

✓4th **G46**   **Vascular syndromes of brain in cerebrovascular diseases**
     Code first underlying cerebrovascular disease (I60-I69)

     G46.0   Middle cerebral artery syndrome

     G46.1   Anterior cerebral artery syndrome

     G46.2   Posterior cerebral artery syndrome

     G46.3   Brain stem stroke syndrome
         Benedikt syndrome
         Claude syndrome
         Foville syndrome
         Millard-Gubler syndrome
         Wallenberg syndrome
         Weber syndrome

     G46.4   Cerebellar stroke syndrome

     G46.5   Pure motor lacunar syndrome

     G46.6   Pure sensory lacunar syndrome

     G46.7   Other lacunar syndromes

     G46.8   Other vascular syndromes of brain in cerebrovascular diseases

✓4th **G47**   **Sleep disorders**
     EXCLUDES 2   nightmares (F51.5)
             nonorganic sleep disorders (F51.-)
             sleep terrors (F51.4)
             sleepwalking (F51.3)

     ✓5th **G47.0**   Insomnia
         EXCLUDES 2   alcohol related insomnia (F10.182, F10.282, F10.982)
             drug-related insomnia (F11.182, F11.282, F11.982, F13.182, F13.282, F13.982, F14.182, F14.282,F14.982, F15.182, F15.282, F15.982, F19.182, F19.282, F19.982)
             idiopathic insomnia (F51.01)
             insomnia due to a mental disorder (F51.05)
             insomnia not due to a substance or known physiological condition (F51.0-)
             nonorganic insomnia (F51.0-)
             primary insomnia (F51.01)
             sleep apnea (G47.3-)

         G47.00   Insomnia, unspecified   ▽
             Insomnia NOS

         G47.01   Insomnia due to medical condition
             Code also associated medical condition

         G47.09   Other insomnia

     ✓5th **G47.1**   Hypersomnia
         EXCLUDES 2   alcohol-related hypersomnia (F10.182, F10.282, F10.982)
             drug-related hypersomnia (F11.182, F11.282, F11.982, F13.182, F13.282, F13.982, F14.182,F14.282, F14.982, F15.182, F15.282, F15.982, F19.182, F19.282, F19.982)
             hypersomnia due to a mental disorder (F51.13)
             hypersomnia not due to a substance or known physiological condition (F51.1-)
             primary hypersomnia (F51.11)
             sleep apnea (G47.3-)

         G47.10   Hypersomnia, unspecified   ▽
             Hypersomnia NOS

         G47.11   Idiopathic hypersomnia with long sleep time
             Idiopathic hypersomnia NOS

         G47.12   Idiopathic hypersomnia without long sleep time

         G47.13   Recurrent hypersomnia
             Kleine-Levin syndrome
             Menstrual related hypersomnia

         G47.14   Hypersomnia due to medical condition
             Code also associated medical condition

         G47.19   Other hypersomnia

     ✓5th **G47.2**   Circadian rhythm sleep disorders
         Disorders of the sleep wake schedule
         Inversion of nyctohemeral rhythm
         Inversion of sleep rhythm

         G47.20   Circadian rhythm sleep disorder, unspecified type ▽
             Sleep wake schedule disorder NOS

         G47.21   Circadian rhythm sleep disorder, delayed sleep phase type
             Delayed sleep phase syndrome

         G47.22   Circadian rhythm sleep disorder, advanced sleep phase type

         G47.23   Circadian rhythm sleep disorder, irregular sleep wake type
             Irregular sleep-wake pattern

         G47.24   Circadian rhythm sleep disorder, free running type
             ▶Circadian rhythm sleep disorder, non-24-hour sleep-wake type◀

         G47.25   Circadian rhythm sleep disorder, jet lag type

         G47.26   Circadian rhythm sleep disorder, shift work type

         G47.27   *Circadian rhythm sleep disorder in conditions classified elsewhere*
             Code first underlying condition

         G47.29   Other circadian rhythm sleep disorder

✓   Additional Character Req   ✓x7th   Placeholder Alert   Manifestation   HCC   CMS-HCC Condition   ▽ Unspecified Code   ▶◀ Revised Text   ● New Code   ▲ Revised Code Title

✓5ᵗʰ **G47.3** **Sleep apnea**
Code also any associated underlying condition
     EXCLUDES 1   *apnea NOS (R06.81)*
         Cheyne-Stokes breathing (R06.3)
         pickwickian syndrome (E66.2)
         sleep apnea of newborn (P28.3)

     G47.30   **Sleep apnea, unspecified** ▽
               Sleep apnea NOS

     G47.31   **Primary central sleep apnea**
               ▶Idiopathic central sleep apnea◀

     G47.32   **High altitude periodic breathing**

     G47.33   **Obstructive sleep apnea (adult) (pediatric)**
               ▶Obstructive sleep apnea hypopnea◀
               EXCLUDES 1   *obstructive sleep apnea of newborn (P28.3)*

     G47.34   **Idiopathic sleep related nonobstructive alveolar hypoventilation**
               Sleep related hypoxia

     G47.35   **Congenital central alveolar hypoventilation syndrome**

     G47.36   *Sleep related hypoventilation in conditions classified elsewhere*
               Sleep related hypoxemia in conditions classified elsewhere
               Code first underlying condition

     G47.37   *Central sleep apnea in conditions classified elsewhere*
               Code first underlying condition

     G47.39   **Other sleep apnea**

✓5ᵗʰ **G47.4** **Narcolepsy and cataplexy**

     ✓6ᵗʰ **G47.41**   **Narcolepsy**
               G47.411   **Narcolepsy with cataplexy**
               G47.419   **Narcolepsy without cataplexy**
                       Narcolepsy NOS

     ✓6ᵗʰ **G47.42**   **Narcolepsy in conditions classified elsewhere**
               Code first underlying condition
               G47.421   *Narcolepsy in conditions classified elsewhere with cataplexy*
               G47.429   *Narcolepsy in conditions classified elsewhere without cataplexy*

✓5ᵗʰ **G47.5** **Parasomnia**
     EXCLUDES 1   *alcohol induced parasomnia (F10.182, F10.282, F10.982)*
         drug induced parasomnia (F11.182, F11.282, F11.982, F13.182, F13.282, F13.982, F14.182, F14.282, F14.982, F15.182, F15.282, F15.982, F19.182, F19.282, F19.982)
         parasomnia not due to a substance or known physiological condition (F51.8)

     G47.50   **Parasomnia, unspecified** ▽
               Parasomnia NOS

     G47.51   **Confusional arousals**

     G47.52   **REM sleep behavior disorder**

     G47.53   **Recurrent isolated sleep paralysis**

     G47.54   *Parasomnia in conditions classified elsewhere*
               Code first underlying condition

     G47.59   **Other parasomnia**

✓5ᵗʰ **G47.6** **Sleep related movement disorders**
     EXCLUDES 2   *restless legs syndrome (G25.81)*

     G47.61   **Periodic limb movement disorder**
               ~~Periodic limb movement disorder~~

     G47.62   **Sleep related leg cramps**

     G47.63   **Sleep related bruxism**
               EXCLUDES 1   *psychogenic bruxism (F45.8)*

     G47.69   **Other sleep related movement disorders**

   G47.8 **Other sleep disorders**
         ▶Other specified sleep-wake disorder◀

   G47.9 **Sleep disorder, unspecified** ▽
         Sleep disorder NOS
         ▶Unspecified sleep-wake disorder◀

Trigeminal and Facial Nerve Branches

Supratrochlear nerve
Supraorbital nerve
V1 branch
V2 branch
Trigeminal nerve (CN V) branches in infratemporal fossa
Infraorbital nerve
V3 branch
Mental nerve
Mental foramen

Nerve, nerve root and plexus disorders (G50-G59)

   EXCLUDES 1   *current traumatic nerve, nerve root and plexus disorders—see Injury, nerve by body region*
         neuralgia NOS (M79.2)
         neuritis NOS (M79.2)
         peripheral neuritis in pregnancy (O26.82-)
         radiculitis NOS (M54.1-)

✓4ᵗʰ **G50** **Disorders of trigeminal nerve**
     INCLUDES   disorders of 5th cranial nerve

     G50.0   **Trigeminal neuralgia**
             Syndrome of paroxysmal facial pain
             Tic douloureux

     G50.1   **Atypical facial pain**

     G50.8   **Other disorders of trigeminal nerve**

     G50.9   **Disorder of trigeminal nerve, unspecified** ▽

✓4ᵗʰ **G51** **Facial nerve disorders**
     INCLUDES   disorders of 7th cranial nerve

     G51.0   **Bell's palsy**
             Facial palsy

     G51.1   **Geniculate ganglionitis**
             EXCLUDES 1   *postherpetic geniculate ganglionitis (B02.21)*

     G51.2   **Melkersson's syndrome**
             Melkersson-Rosenthal syndrome

     G51.3   **Clonic hemifacial spasm**

     G51.4   **Facial myokymia**

     G51.8   **Other disorders of facial nerve**

     G51.9   **Disorder of facial nerve, unspecified** ▽

✓4ᵗʰ **G52** **Disorders of other cranial nerves**
     EXCLUDES 2   *disorders of acoustic [8th] nerve (H93.3)*
         disorders of optic [2nd] nerve (H46, H47.0)
         paralytic strabismus due to nerve palsy (H49.0-H49.2)

     G52.0   **Disorders of olfactory nerve**
             Disorders of 1st cranial nerve

     G52.1   **Disorders of glossopharyngeal nerve**
             Disorder of 9th cranial nerve
             Glossopharyngeal neuralgia

     G52.2   **Disorders of vagus nerve**
             Disorders of pneumogastric [10th] nerve

     G52.3   **Disorders of hypoglossal nerve**
             Disorders of 12th cranial nerve

     G52.7   **Disorders of multiple cranial nerves**
             Polyneuritis cranialis

     G52.8   **Disorders of other specified cranial nerves**

     G52.9   **Cranial nerve disorder, unspecified** ▽

   G53   *Cranial nerve disorders in diseases classified elsewhere*
         Code first underlying disease, such as:
         neoplasm (C00-D49)
         EXCLUDES 1   *multiple cranial nerve palsy in sarcoidosis (D86.82)*
            multiple cranial nerve palsy in syphilis (A52.15)
            postherpetic geniculate ganglionitis (B02.21)
            postherpetic trigeminal neuralgia (B02.22)

EXCLUDES 1 Not coded here   EXCLUDES 2 Not included here   N Newborn Age: 0   P Pediatric Age: 0-17   M Maternity Age: 12-55   A Adult Age: 15-124

560   ICD-10-CM 2018

☑️4ᵗʰ **G54 Nerve root and plexus disorders**

> *EXCLUDES 1*   current traumatic nerve root and plexus disorders—see nerve
> injury by body region
> intervertebral disc disorders (M50-M51)
> neuralgia or neuritis NOS (M79.2)
> neuritis or radiculitis brachial NOS (M54.13)
> neuritis or radiculitis lumbar NOS (M54.16)
> neuritis or radiculitis lumbosacral NOS (M54.17)
> neuritis or radiculitis thoracic NOS (M54.14)
> radiculitis NOS (M54.10)
> radiculopathy NOS (M54.10)
> spondylosis (M47.-)

G54.0 Brachial plexus disorders
Thoracic outlet syndrome
DEF: Acquired disorder affecting the spinal nerves that send
signals to the shoulder, arm, and hand; causes corresponding
motor and sensory dysfunction; characterized by regional
paresthesia, pain, and muscle weakness, and in severe cases
paralysis.

G54.1 Lumbosacral plexus disorders

G54.2 Cervical root disorders, not elsewhere classified

G54.3 Thoracic root disorders, not elsewhere classified

G54.4 Lumbosacral root disorders, not elsewhere classified

G54.5 Neuralgic amyotrophy
Parsonage-Aldren-Turner syndrome
Shoulder-girdle neuritis
> *EXCLUDES 1*   neuralgic amyotrophy in diabetes mellitus (E08-E13
> with .44)

G54.6 Phantom limb syndrome with pain   HCC

G54.7 Phantom limb syndrome without pain   HCC
Phantom limb syndrome NOS

G54.8 Other nerve root and plexus disorders

G54.9 Nerve root and plexus disorder, unspecified   ▽

*G55 Nerve root and plexus compressions in diseases classified
elsewhere*

> Code first underlying disease, such as:
> neoplasm (C00-D49)
> *EXCLUDES 1*   nerve root compression (due to) (in) ankylosing spondylitis
> (M45.-)
> nerve root compression (due to) (in) dorsopathies (M53.-, M54.-)
> nerve root compression (due to) (in) intervertebral disc
> disorders (M50.1-, M51.1-)
> nerve root compression (due to) (in) spondylopathies
> (M46.-, M48.-)

☑️4ᵗʰ **G56 Mononeuropathies of upper limb**

> *EXCLUDES 1*   current traumatic nerve disorder—see nerve injury by body
> region

☑️5ᵗʰ **G56.0 Carpal tunnel syndrome**

G56.00 Carpal tunnel syndrome, unspecified upper limb   ▽

G56.01 Carpal tunnel syndrome, right upper limb

G56.02 Carpal tunnel syndrome, left upper limb

G56.03 Carpal tunnel syndrome, bilateral upper limbs

☑️5ᵗʰ **G56.1 Other lesions of median nerve**

G56.10 Other lesions of median nerve, unspecified   ▽
upper limb

G56.11 Other lesions of median nerve, right upper limb

G56.12 Other lesions of median nerve, left upper limb

G56.13 Other lesions of median nerve, bilateral upper limbs

☑️5ᵗʰ **G56.2 Lesion of ulnar nerve**
Tardy ulnar nerve palsy

G56.20 Lesion of ulnar nerve, unspecified upper limb   ▽

G56.21 Lesion of ulnar nerve, right upper limb

G56.22 Lesion of ulnar nerve, left upper limb

G56.23 Lesion of ulnar nerve, bilateral upper limbs

☑️5ᵗʰ **G56.3 Lesion of radial nerve**

G56.30 Lesion of radial nerve, unspecified upper limb   ▽

G56.31 Lesion of radial nerve, right upper limb

G56.32 Lesion of radial nerve, left upper limb

G56.33 Lesion of radial nerve, bilateral upper limbs

Nerves of Upper Limb

Radial

Deep branch of radial

Ulnar

Superficial branch of radial

Median

☑️5ᵗʰ **G56.4 Causalgia of upper limb**
Complex regional pain syndrome II of upper limb
> *EXCLUDES 1*   complex regional pain syndrome I of lower limb (G90.52-)
> complex regional pain syndrome I of upper limb (G90.51-)
> complex regional pain syndrome II of lower limb (G57.7-)
> reflex sympathetic dystrophy of lower limb (G90.52-)
> reflex sympathetic dystrophy of upper limb (G90.51-)

G56.40 Causalgia of unspecified upper limb   ▽

G56.41 Causalgia of right upper limb

G56.42 Causalgia of left upper limb

G56.43 Causalgia of bilateral upper limbs

☑️5ᵗʰ **G56.8 Other specified mononeuropathies of upper limb**
Interdigital neuroma of upper limb

G56.80 Other specified mononeuropathies of   ▽
unspecified upper limb

**G56.81 Other specified mononeuropathies of right upper
limb**

**G56.82 Other specified mononeuropathies of left upper
limb**

**G56.83 Other specified mononeuropathies of bilateral
upper limbs**

☑️5ᵗʰ **G56.9 Unspecified mononeuropathy of upper limb**

G56.90 Unspecified mononeuropathy of unspecified   ▽
upper limb

G56.91 Unspecified mononeuropathy of right upper   ▽
limb

G56.92 Unspecified mononeuropathy of left upper   ▽
limb

G56.93 Unspecified mononeuropathy of bilateral   ▽
upper limbs

☑️4ᵗʰ **G57 Mononeuropathies of lower limb**

> *EXCLUDES 1*   current traumatic nerve disorder—see nerve injury by body
> region

☑️5ᵗʰ **G57.0 Lesion of sciatic nerve**
> *EXCLUDES 1*   sciatica NOS (M54.3-)
> *EXCLUDES 2*   sciatica attributed to intervertebral disc disorder
> (M51.1-)

G57.00 Lesion of sciatic nerve, unspecified lower limb   ▽

G57.01 Lesion of sciatic nerve, right lower limb

G57.02 Lesion of sciatic nerve, left lower limb

G57.03 Lesion of sciatic nerve, bilateral lower limbs

☑️5ᵗʰ **G57.1 Meralgia paresthetica**
Lateral cutaneous nerve of thigh syndrome

G57.10 Meralgia paresthetica, unspecified lower limb   ▽

G57.11 Meralgia paresthetica, right lower limb

G57.12 Meralgia paresthetica, left lower limb

G57.13 Meralgia paresthetica, bilateral lower limbs

☑️ Additional Character Req   ⁻ˣ⁷⁻ Placeholder Alert   Manifestation   HCC CMS-HCC Condition   ▽ Unspecified Code   ►◄ Revised Text   ● New Code   ▲ Revised Code Title

Nerves of Lower Limb

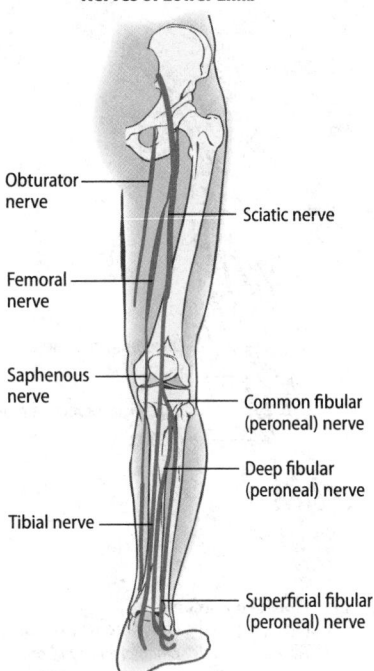

Obturator nerve

Sciatic nerve

Femoral nerve

Saphenous nerve

Common fibular (peroneal) nerve

Deep fibular (peroneal) nerve

Tibial nerve

Superficial fibular (peroneal) nerve

✓5ᵗʰ **G57.2 Lesion of** femoral nerve
- **G57.20 Lesion of femoral nerve, unspecified lower limb** ▽
- **G57.21 Lesion of femoral nerve, right lower limb**
- **G57.22 Lesion of femoral nerve, left lower limb**
- **G57.23 Lesion of femoral nerve, bilateral lower limbs**

✓5ᵗʰ **G57.3 Lesion of** lateral popliteal nerve
Peroneal nerve palsy
- **G57.30 Lesion of lateral popliteal nerve, unspecified lower limb** ▽
- **G57.31 Lesion of lateral popliteal nerve, right lower limb**
- **G57.32 Lesion of lateral popliteal nerve, left lower limb**
- **G57.33 Lesion of lateral popliteal nerve, bilateral lower limbs**

✓5ᵗʰ **G57.4 Lesion of** medial popliteal nerve
- **G57.40 Lesion of medial popliteal nerve, unspecified lower limb** ▽
- **G57.41 Lesion of medial popliteal nerve, right lower limb**
- **G57.42 Lesion of medial popliteal nerve, left lower limb**
- **G57.43 Lesion of medial popliteal nerve, bilateral lower limbs**

✓5ᵗʰ **G57.5 Tarsal tunnel syndrome**
- **G57.50 Tarsal tunnel syndrome, unspecified lower limb** ▽
- **G57.51 Tarsal tunnel syndrome, right lower limb**
- **G57.52 Tarsal tunnel syndrome, left lower limb**
- **G57.53 Tarsal tunnel syndrome, bilateral lower limbs**

✓5ᵗʰ **G57.6 Lesion of** plantar nerve
Morton's metatarsalgia
- **G57.60 Lesion of plantar nerve, unspecified lower limb** ▽
- **G57.61 Lesion of plantar nerve, right lower limb**
- **G57.62 Lesion of plantar nerve, left lower limb**
- **G57.63 Lesion of plantar nerve, bilateral lower limbs**

✓5ᵗʰ **G57.7 Causalgia of** lower limb
Complex regional pain syndrome II of lower limb
EXCLUDES 1   complex regional pain syndrome I of lower limb (G90.52-)
complex regional pain syndrome I of upper limb (G90.51-)
complex regional pain syndrome II of upper limb (G56.4-)
reflex sympathetic dystrophy of lower limb (G90.52-)
reflex sympathetic dystrophy of upper limb (G90.51-)
- **G57.70 Causalgia of unspecified lower limb** ▽
- **G57.71 Causalgia of right lower limb**
- **G57.72 Causalgia of left lower limb**
- **G57.73 Causalgia of bilateral lower limbs**

✓5ᵗʰ **G57.8 Other specified mononeuropathies of lower limb**
Interdigital neuroma of lower limb
- **G57.80 Other specified mononeuropathies of unspecified lower limb** ▽
- **G57.81 Other specified mononeuropathies of right lower limb**
- **G57.82 Other specified mononeuropathies of left lower limb**
- **G57.83 Other specified mononeuropathies of bilateral lower limbs**

✓5ᵗʰ **G57.9 Unspecified mononeuropathy of lower limb**
- **G57.90 Unspecified mononeuropathy of unspecified lower limb** ▽
- **G57.91 Unspecified mononeuropathy of right lower limb** ▽
- **G57.92 Unspecified mononeuropathy of left lower limb** ▽
- **G57.93 Unspecified mononeuropathy of bilateral lower limbs** ▽

✓4ᵗʰ **G58 Other mononeuropathies**
- **G58.0 Intercostal neuropathy**
- **G58.7 Mononeuritis multiplex**
- **G58.8 Other specified mononeuropathies**
- **G58.9 Mononeuropathy, unspecified** ▽

G59 *Mononeuropathy in diseases classified elsewhere*
Code first underlying disease
EXCLUDES 1   diabetic mononeuropathy (E08-E13 with .41)
syphilitic nerve paralysis (A52.19)
syphilitic neuritis (A52.15)
tuberculous mononeuropathy (A17.83)

Polyneuropathies and other disorders of the peripheral nervous system (G60-G65)

EXCLUDES 1   neuralgia NOS (M79.2)
neuritis NOS (M79.2)
peripheral neuritis in pregnancy (O26.82-)
radiculitis NOS (M54.10)

✓4ᵗʰ **G60 Hereditary and idiopathic neuropathy**
- **G60.0 Hereditary motor and sensory neuropathy**
  Charcôt-Marie-Tooth disease
  Déjérine-Sottas disease
  Hereditary motor and sensory neuropathy, types I-IV
  Hypertrophic neuropathy of infancy
  Peroneal muscular atrophy (axonal type) (hypertrophic type)
  Roussy-Levy syndrome
- **G60.1 Refsum's disease**
  Infantile Refsum disease
  DEF: Genetic disorder of lipid metabolism; characterized by retinitis pigmentosa, degenerative nerve disease, ataxia, and dry, rough, scaly skin.
- **G60.2 Neuropathy in association with hereditary ataxia**
- **G60.3 Idiopathic progressive neuropathy**
- **G60.8 Other hereditary and idiopathic neuropathies**
  Dominantly inherited sensory neuropathy
  Morvan's disease
  Nelaton's syndrome
  Recessively inherited sensory neuropathy
- **G60.9 Hereditary and idiopathic neuropathy, unspecified** ▽

✓4ᵗʰ **G61 Inflammatory polyneuropathy**
- **G61.0 Guillain-Barre syndrome**   HCC
  Acute (post-)infective polyneuritis
  Miller Fisher syndrome
  AHA: 2014, 2Q, 4
- **G61.1 Serum neuropathy**   HCC
  Use additional code for adverse effect, if applicable, to identify serum (T50.-)
- ✓5ᵗʰ **G61.8 Other inflammatory polyneuropathies**
  - **G61.81 Chronic inflammatory demyelinating polyneuritis**   HCC
  - **G61.82 Multifocal motor neuropathy**   HCC
    MMN
  - **G61.89 Other inflammatory polyneuropathies**   HCC
- **G61.9 Inflammatory polyneuropathy, unspecified**   HCC ▽

EXCLUDES 1 Not coded here   EXCLUDES 2 Not included here   N Newborn Age: 0   P Pediatric Age: 0-17   M Maternity Age: 12-55   A Adult Age: 15-124

562   ICD-10-CM 2018

☑4ᵗʰ **G62 Other and unspecified polyneuropathies**

G62.0 Drug-induced polyneuropathy `HCC`
> Use additional code for adverse effect, if applicable, to identify drug (T36-T50 with fifth or sixth character 5)

G62.1 Alcoholic polyneuropathy `HCC`

G62.2 Polyneuropathy due to other toxic agents `HCC`
> Code first (T51-T65) to identify toxic agent

☑5ᵗʰ **G62.8 Other specified polyneuropathies**

G62.81 Critical illness polyneuropathy `HCC`
> Acute motor neuropathy

G62.82 Radiation-induced polyneuropathy `HCC`
> Use additional external cause code (W88-W90, X39.0-) to identify cause

G62.89 Other specified polyneuropathies
> AHA: 2016, 2Q, 11

G62.9 Polyneuropathy, unspecified ▽
> Neuropathy NOS

G63 *Polyneuropathy in diseases classified elsewhere* `HCC`
> Code first underlying disease, such as:
> amyloidosis (E85.-)
> endocrine disease, except diabetes (E00-E07, E15-E16, E20-E34)
> metabolic diseases (E70-E88)
> neoplasm (C00-D49)
> nutritional deficiency (E40-E64)
>
> `EXCLUDES 1`   *polyneuropathy (in):*
>   *diabetes mellitus (E08-E13 with .42)*
>   *diphtheria (A36.83)*
>   *infectious mononucleosis (B27.0-B27.9 with 1)*
>   *Lyme disease (A69.22)*
>   *mumps (B26.84)*
>   *postherpetic (B02.23)*
>   *rheumatoid arthritis (M05.33)*
>   *scleroderma (M34.83)*
>   *systemic lupus erythematosus (M32.19)*
> AHA: 2012, 4Q, 99

G64 Other disorders of peripheral nervous system
> Disorder of peripheral nervous system NOS

☑4ᵗʰ **G65 Sequelae of inflammatory and toxic polyneuropathies**
> Code first condition resulting from (sequela) of inflammatory and toxic polyneuropathies

G65.0 Sequelae of Guillain-Barré syndrome `HCC`

G65.1 Sequelae of other inflammatory polyneuropathy `HCC`

G65.2 Sequelae of toxic polyneuropathy `HCC`

Diseases of myoneural junction and muscle (G70-G73)

☑4ᵗʰ **G70 Myasthenia gravis and other myoneural disorders**
> `EXCLUDES 1`   *botulism (A05.1, A48.51-A48.52)*
>   *transient neonatal myasthenia gravis (P94.0)*

☑5ᵗʰ **G70.0 Myasthenia gravis**

G70.00 Myasthenia gravis without (acute) exacerbation `HCC`
> Myasthenia gravis NOS

G70.01 Myasthenia gravis with (acute) exacerbation `HCC`
> Myasthenia gravis in crisis

G70.1 Toxic myoneural disorders `HCC`
> Code first (T51-T65) to identify toxic agent

G70.2 Congenital and developmental myasthenia `HCC`

☑5ᵗʰ **G70.8 Other specified myoneural disorders**

G70.80 Lambert-Eaton syndrome, unspecified `HCC` ▽
> Lambert-Eaton syndrome NOS

G70.81 *Lambert-Eaton syndrome in disease classified elsewhere* `HCC`
> Code first underlying disease
> `EXCLUDES 1`   *Lambert-Eaton syndrome in neoplastic disease (G73.1)*

G70.89 Other specified myoneural disorders `HCC`

G70.9 Myoneural disorder, unspecified `HCC` ▽

☑4ᵗʰ **G71 Primary disorders of muscles**
> `EXCLUDES 2`   *arthrogryposis multiplex congenita (Q74.3)*
>   *metabolic disorders (E70-E88)*
>   *myositis (M60.-)*

G71.0 Muscular dystrophy `HCC`
> Autosomal recessive, childhood type, muscular dystrophy resembling Duchenne or Becker muscular dystrophy
> Benign [Becker] muscular dystrophy
> Benign scapuloperoneal muscular dystrophy with early contractures [Emery-Dreifuss]
> Congenital muscular dystrophy NOS
> Congenital muscular dystrophy with specific morphological abnormalities of the muscle fiber
> Distal muscular dystrophy
> Facioscapulohumeral muscular dystrophy
> Limb-girdle muscular dystrophy
> Ocular muscular dystrophy
> Oculopharyngeal muscular dystrophy
> Scapuloperoneal muscular dystrophy
> Severe [Duchenne] muscular dystrophy

☑5ᵗʰ **G71.1 Myotonic disorders**

G71.11 Myotonic muscular dystrophy `HCC`
> Dystrophia myotonica [Steinert]
> Myotonia atrophica
> Myotonic dystrophy
> Proximal myotonic myopathy (PROMM)
> Steinert disease

G71.12 Myotonia congenita
> Acetazolamide responsive myotonia congenita
> Dominant myotonia congenita [Thomsen disease]
> Myotonia levior
> Recessive myotonia congenita [Becker disease]

G71.13 Myotonic chondrodystrophy
> Chondrodystrophic myotonia
> Congenital myotonic chondrodystrophy
> Schwartz-Jampel disease

G71.14 Drug induced myotonia
> Use additional code for adverse effect, if applicable, to identify drug (T36-T50 with fifth or sixth character 5)

G71.19 Other specified myotonic disorders
> Myotonia fluctuans
> Myotonia permanens
> Neuromyotonia [Isaacs]
> Paramyotonia congenita (of von Eulenburg)
> Pseudomyotonia
> Symptomatic myotonia

G71.2 Congenital myopathies `HCC`
> Central core disease
> Fiber-type disproportion
> Minicore disease
> Multicore disease
> Myotubular (centronuclear) myopathy
> Nemaline myopathy
> `EXCLUDES 1`   *arthrogryposis multiplex congenita (Q74.3)*

G71.3 Mitochondrial myopathy, not elsewhere classified
> `EXCLUDES 1`   *Kearns-Sayre syndrome (H49.81)*
>   *Leber's disease (H47.21)*
>   *Leigh's encephalopathy (G31.82)*
>   *mitochondrial metabolism disorders (E88.4-)*
>   *Reye's syndrome (G93.7)*

G71.8 Other primary disorders of muscles

G71.9 Primary disorder of muscle, unspecified ▽
> Hereditary myopathy NOS

☑4ᵗʰ **G72 Other and unspecified myopathies**
> `EXCLUDES 1`   *arthrogryposis multiplex congenita (Q74.3)*
>   *dermatopolymyositis (M33.-)*
>   *ischemic infarction of muscle (M62.2-)*
>   *myositis (M60.-)*
>   *polymyositis (M33.2-)*

G72.0 Drug-induced myopathy
> Use additional code for adverse effect, if applicable, to identify drug (T36-T50 with fifth or sixth character 5)

G72.1 Alcoholic myopathy
> Use additional code to identify alcoholism (F10.-)

G72.2 Myopathy due to other toxic agents
> Code first (T51-T65) to identify toxic agent

☑ Additional Character Req   `xT` Placeholder Alert   Manifestation   `HCC` CMS-HCC Condition   ▽ Unspecified Code   ►◄ Revised Text   ● New Code   ▲ Revised Code Title

ICD-10-CM 2018   563

G62–G72.2

G72.3 Periodic paralysis
Familial periodic paralysis
Hyperkalemic periodic paralysis (familial)
Hypokalemic periodic paralysis (familial)
Myotonic periodic paralysis (familial)
Normokalemic paralysis (familial)
Potassium sensitive periodic paralysis
EXCLUDES 1 paramyotonia congenita (of von Eulenburg) (G71.19)

✓5th G72.4 Inflammatory and immune myopathies, not elsewhere classified
G72.41 Inclusion body myositis [IBM]
G72.49 Other inflammatory and immune myopathies, not elsewhere classified
Inflammatory myopathy NOS

✓5th G72.8 Other specified myopathies
G72.81 Critical illness myopathy
Acute necrotizing myopathy
Acute quadriplegic myopathy
Intensive care (ICU) myopathy
Myopathy of critical illness
G72.89 Other specified myopathies

G72.9 Myopathy, unspecified ▽

✓4th G73 Disorders of myoneural junction and muscle in diseases classified elsewhere
G73.1 Lambert-Eaton syndrome in neoplastic disease HCC
Code first underlying neoplasm (C00-D49)
EXCLUDES 1 Lambert-Eaton syndrome not associated with neoplasm (G70.80-G70.81)
G73.3 Myasthenic syndromes in other diseases classified elsewhere HCC
Code first underlying disease, such as:
neoplasm (C00-D49)
thyrotoxicosis (E05.-)
G73.7 Myopathy in diseases classified elsewhere
Code first underlying disease, such as:
hyperparathyroidism (E21.0, E21.3)
hypoparathyroidism (E20.-)
glycogen storage disease (E74.0)
lipid storage disorders (E75.-)
EXCLUDES 1 myopathy in:
rheumatoid arthritis (M05.4-)
sarcoidosis (D86.87)
scleroderma (M34.82)
sicca syndrome [Sjögren] (M35.03)
systemic lupus erythematosus (M32.19)

Cerebral palsy and other paralytic syndromes (G80-G83)

✓4th G80 Cerebral palsy
EXCLUDES 1 hereditary spastic paraplegia (G11.4)
G80.0 Spastic quadriplegic cerebral palsy HCC
Congenital spastic paralysis (cerebral)
G80.1 Spastic diplegic cerebral palsy HCC
Spastic cerebral palsy NOS
G80.2 Spastic hemiplegic cerebral palsy HCC
G80.3 Athetoid cerebral palsy HCC
Double athetosis (syndrome)
Dyskinetic cerebral palsy
Dystonic cerebral palsy
Vogt disease
G80.4 Ataxic cerebral palsy HCC
G80.8 Other cerebral palsy HCC
Mixed cerebral palsy syndromes
G80.9 Cerebral palsy, unspecified HCC ▽
Cerebral palsy NOS

✓4th G81 Hemiplegia and hemiparesis
NOTE This category is to be used only when hemiplegia (complete)(incomplete) is reported without further specification, or is stated to be old or longstanding but of unspecified cause. The category is also for use in multiple coding to identify these types of hemiplegia resulting from any cause.
EXCLUDES 1 congenital cerebral palsy (G80.-)
hemiplegia and hemiparesis due to sequela of cerebrovascular disease (I69.05-, I69.15-, I69.25-, I69.35-, I69.85-, I69.95-)
AHA: 2015, 1Q, 25

✓5th G81.0 Flaccid hemiplegia
G81.00 Flaccid hemiplegia affecting unspecified side HCC ▽
G81.01 Flaccid hemiplegia affecting right dominant side HCC
G81.02 Flaccid hemiplegia affecting left dominant side HCC
G81.03 Flaccid hemiplegia affecting right nondominant side HCC
G81.04 Flaccid hemiplegia affecting left nondominant side HCC

✓5th G81.1 Spastic hemiplegia
G81.10 Spastic hemiplegia affecting unspecified side HCC ▽
G81.11 Spastic hemiplegia affecting right dominant side HCC
G81.12 Spastic hemiplegia affecting left dominant side HCC
G81.13 Spastic hemiplegia affecting right nondominant side HCC
G81.14 Spastic hemiplegia affecting left nondominant side HCC

✓5th G81.9 Hemiplegia, unspecified
AHA: 2014, 1Q, 23
G81.90 Hemiplegia, unspecified affecting unspecified side HCC ▽
G81.91 Hemiplegia, unspecified affecting right dominant side HCC ▽
G81.92 Hemiplegia, unspecified affecting left dominant side HCC ▽
G81.93 Hemiplegia, unspecified affecting right nondominant side HCC ▽
G81.94 Hemiplegia, unspecified affecting left nondominant side HCC ▽

✓4th G82 Paraplegia (paraparesis) and quadriplegia (quadriparesis)
NOTE This category is to be used only when the listed conditions are reported without further specification, or are stated to be old or longstanding but of unspecified cause. The category is also for use in multiple coding to identify these conditions resulting from any cause
EXCLUDES 1 congenital cerebral palsy (G80.-)
functional quadriplegia (R53.2)
hysterical paralysis (F44.4)

✓5th G82.2 Paraplegia
Paralysis of both lower limbs NOS
Paraparesis (lower) NOS
Paraplegia (lower) NOS
G82.20 Paraplegia, unspecified HCC ▽
G82.21 Paraplegia, complete HCC
G82.22 Paraplegia, incomplete HCC

✓5th G82.5 Quadriplegia
G82.50 Quadriplegia, unspecified HCC ▽
G82.51 Quadriplegia, C1-C4 complete HCC
G82.52 Quadriplegia, C1-C4 incomplete HCC
G82.53 Quadriplegia, C5-C7 complete HCC
G82.54 Quadriplegia, C5-C7 incomplete HCC

✓4th G83 Other paralytic syndromes
NOTE This category is to be used only when the listed conditions are reported without further specification, or are stated to be old or longstanding but of unspecified cause. The category is also for use in multiple coding to identify these conditions resulting from any cause.
INCLUDES paralysis (complete) (incomplete), except as in G80-G82
G83.0 Diplegia of upper limbs HCC
Diplegia (upper)
Paralysis of both upper limbs
✓5th G83.1 Monoplegia of lower limb
Paralysis of lower limb
EXCLUDES 1 monoplegia of lower limbs due to sequela of cerebrovascular disease (I69.04-, I69.14-, I69.24-, I69.34-, I69.84-, I69.94-)
G83.10 Monoplegia of lower limb affecting unspecified side HCC ▽
G83.11 Monoplegia of lower limb affecting right dominant side HCC
G83.12 Monoplegia of lower limb affecting left dominant side HCC
G83.13 Monoplegia of lower limb affecting right nondominant side HCC
G83.14 Monoplegia of lower limb affecting left nondominant side HCC

√5th **G83.2 Monoplegia of** upper limb
     Paralysis of upper limb
     EXCLUDES 1   *monoplegia of upper limbs due to sequela of*
           cerebrovascular disease (I69.03-, I69.13-, I69.23-,
           I69.33-, I69.83-, I69.93-)

     G83.20 Monoplegia of upper limb affecting   HCC ▽
         unspecified side

     G83.21 Monoplegia of upper limb affecting right   HCC
         dominant side

     G83.22 Monoplegia of upper limb affecting left   HCC
         dominant side

     G83.23 Monoplegia of upper limb affecting right   HCC
         nondominant side

     G83.24 Monoplegia of upper limb affecting left   HCC
         nondominant side

√5th **G83.3 Monoplegia, unspecified**

     G83.30 Monoplegia, unspecified affecting   HCC ▽
         unspecified side

     G83.31 Monoplegia, unspecified affecting right   HCC ▽
         dominant side

     G83.32 Monoplegia, unspecified affecting left   HCC ▽
         dominant side

     G83.33 Monoplegia, unspecified affecting right   HCC ▽
         nondominant side

     G83.34 Monoplegia, unspecified affecting left   HCC ▽
         nondominant side

G83.4 Cauda equina syndrome   HCC
     Neurogenic bladder due to cauda equina syndrome
     EXCLUDES 1   *cord bladder NOS (G95.89)*
           neurogenic bladder NOS (N31.9)

G83.5 Locked-in state   HCC

√5th **G83.8 Other specified paralytic syndromes**
     EXCLUDES 1   *paralytic syndromes due to current spinal cord*
           injury—code to spinal cord injury (S14, S24, S34)

     G83.81 Brown-Séquard syndrome   HCC
     G83.82 Anterior cord syndrome   HCC
     G83.83 Posterior cord syndrome   HCC
     G83.84 Todd's paralysis (postepileptic)   HCC
     G83.89 Other specified paralytic syndromes   HCC

G83.9 Paralytic syndrome, unspecified   HCC ▽

Other disorders of the nervous system (G89-G99)

√4th **G89 Pain, not elsewhere classified**
     Code also related psychological factors associated with pain (F45.42)
     EXCLUDES 1   *generalized pain NOS (R52)*
           pain disorders exclusively related to psychological factors
             (F45.41)
           pain NOS (R52)
     EXCLUDES 2   *atypical face pain (G50.1)*
           headache syndromes (G44.-)
           localized pain, unspecified type—code to pain by site, such as:
             abdomen pain (R10.-)
             back pain (M54.9)
             breast pain (N64.4)
             chest pain (R07.1-R07.9)
             ear pain (H92.0-)
             eye pain (H57.1)
             headache (R51)
             joint pain (M25.5-)
             limb pain (M79.6-)
             lumbar region pain (M54.5)
             painful urination (R30.9)
             pelvic and perineal pain (R10.2)
             renal colic (N23)
             shoulder pain (M25.51-)
             spine pain (M54.-)
             throat pain (R07.0)
             tongue pain (K14.6)
             tooth pain (K08.8)
            migraines (G43.-)
            myalgia (M79.1)
            pain from prosthetic devices, implants, and grafts (T82.84,
             T83.84, T84.84, T85.84-)
           phantom limb syndrome with pain (G54.6)
           vulvar vestibulitis (N94.810)
           vulvodynia (N94.81-)

G89.0 Central pain syndrome
     Déjérine-Roussy syndrome
     Myelopathic pain syndrome
     Thalamic pain syndrome (hyperesthetic)

√5th **G89.1 Acute pain, not elsewhere classified**
     G89.11 Acute pain due to trauma
     G89.12 Acute post-thoracotomy pain
         Post-thoracotomy pain NOS
     G89.18 Other acute postprocedural pain
         Postoperative pain NOS
         Postprocedural pain NOS

√5th **G89.2 Chronic pain, not elsewhere classified**
     EXCLUDES 1   *causalgia, lower limb (G57.7-)*
           causalgia, upper limb (G56.4-)
           central pain syndrome (G89.0)
           chronic pain syndrome (G89.4)
           complex regional pain syndrome II, lower limb (G57.7-)
           complex regional pain syndrome II, upper limb (G56.4-)
           neoplasm related chronic pain (G89.3)
           reflex sympathetic dystrophy (G90.5-)

     G89.21 Chronic pain due to trauma
     G89.22 Chronic post-thoracotomy pain
     G89.28 Other chronic postprocedural pain
         Other chronic postoperative pain
     G89.29 Other chronic pain

G89.3 Neoplasm related pain (acute) (chronic)
     Cancer associated pain
     Pain due to malignancy (primary) (secondary)
     Tumor associated pain

G89.4 Chronic pain syndrome
     Chronic pain associated with significant psychosocial
     dysfunction

√4th **G90 Disorders of autonomic nervous system**
     EXCLUDES 1   *dysfunction of the autonomic nervous system due to alcohol*
           (G31.2)

√5th **G90.0 Idiopathic peripheral autonomic neuropathy**
     G90.01 Carotid sinus syncope
         Carotid sinus syndrome
         DEF: Vagal activation caused by pressure on the carotid
         sinus baroreceptors; sympathetic nerve impulses may
         cause sinus arrest or AV block.

     G90.09 Other idiopathic peripheral autonomic neuropathy
         Idiopathic peripheral autonomic neuropathy NOS

G90.1 Familial dysautonomia [Riley-Day]   HCC

G90.2 Horner's syndrome
     Bernard(-Horner) syndrome
     Cervical sympathetic dystrophy or paralysis

G90.3 Multi-system degeneration of the autonomic nervous   HCC
system
     Neurogenic orthostatic hypotension [Shy-Drager]
     EXCLUDES 1   *orthostatic hypotension NOS (I95.1)*

G90.4 Autonomic dysreflexia
     Use additional code to identify the cause, such as:
         fecal impaction (K56.41)
         pressure ulcer (pressure area) (L89.-)
         urinary tract infection (N39.0)

√5th **G90.5 Complex regional pain syndrome I (CRPS I)**
     Reflex sympathetic dystrophy
     EXCLUDES 1   *causalgia of lower limb (G57.7-)*
           causalgia of upper limb (G56.4-)
           complex regional pain syndrome II of lower limb
             (G57.7-)
           complex regional pain syndrome II of upper limb
             (G56.4-)

     G90.50 Complex regional pain syndrome I, unspecified   ▽

√6th   **G90.51 Complex regional pain syndrome I of upper limb**
         G90.511 Complex regional pain syndrome I of
             right upper limb
         G90.512 Complex regional pain syndrome I of
             left upper limb
         G90.513 Complex regional pain syndrome I of
             upper limb, bilateral
         G90.519 Complex regional pain syndrome I of   ▽
             unspecified upper limb

√6th   **G90.52 Complex regional pain syndrome I of lower limb**
         G90.521 Complex regional pain syndrome I of
             right lower limb

Chapter 6. Diseases of the Nervous System

Hydrocephalus (Acquired)

Normal ventricles   Hydrocephalic ventricles

G90.522   **Complex regional pain syndrome I of left lower limb**

G90.523   **Complex regional pain syndrome I of lower limb, bilateral**

G90.529   **Complex regional pain syndrome I of unspecified lower limb** ▽

G90.59   **Complex regional pain syndrome I of other specified site**

G90.8   **Other disorders of autonomic nervous system**

G90.9   **Disorder of the autonomic nervous system, unspecified** ▽

✓4ᵗʰ **G91 Hydrocephalus**
- INCLUDES   acquired hydrocephalus
- EXCLUDES 1   *Arnold-Chiari syndrome with hydrocephalus (Q07.-)*
  congenital hydrocephalus (Q03.-)
  spina bifida with hydrocephalus (Q05.-)

G91.0   **Communicating hydrocephalus**
Secondary normal pressure hydrocephalus

G91.1   **Obstructive hydrocephalus**
DEF: Obstruction of cerebrospinal fluid passage from brain into spinal canal; characterized by headaches, drowsiness, poor coordination, urinary incontinence, nausea, vomiting, and papilledema.

G91.2   **(Idiopathic) normal pressure hydrocephalus**
Normal pressure hydrocephalus NOS

G91.3   **Post-traumatic hydrocephalus, unspecified**

G91.4   *Hydrocephalus in diseases classified elsewhere*
Code first underlying condition, such as:
   congenital syphilis (A50.4-)
   neoplasm (C00-D49)
- EXCLUDES 1   *hydrocephalus due to congenital toxoplasmosis (P37.1)*

AHA: 2014, 3Q, 3

G91.8   **Other hydrocephalus**

G91.9   **Hydrocephalus, unspecified** ▽

G92 Toxic encephalopathy
Toxic encephalitis
Toxic metabolic encephalopathy
►Code first, if applicable, drug induced (T36-T50)◄
Code first (T51-T65) to identify toxic agent
AHA: 2017, 1Q, 39-40
DEF: Brain tissue degeneration due to toxic substance.

✓4ᵗʰ **G93 Other disorders of brain**

G93.0   **Cerebral cysts**
Arachnoid cyst
Porencephalic cyst, acquired
- EXCLUDES 1   *acquired periventricular cysts of newborn (P91.1)*
  congenital cerebral cysts (Q04.6)

G93.1   **Anoxic brain damage, not elsewhere classified** HCC
- EXCLUDES 1   *cerebral anoxia due to anesthesia during labor and delivery (O74.3)*
  cerebral anoxia due to anesthesia during the puerperium (O89.2)
  neonatal anoxia (P84)

DEF: Brain injury not resulting from birth trauma that is due to lack of oxygen. Brain cells, when deprived of oxygen, begin to expire after 4 minutes.

G93.2   **Benign intracranial hypertension**
- EXCLUDES 1   *hypertensive encephalopathy (I67.4)*

G93.3   **Postviral fatigue syndrome**
Benign myalgic encephalomyelitis
- EXCLUDES 1   *chronic fatigue syndrome NOS (R53.82)*

✓5ᵗʰ **G93.4**   **Other and unspecified encephalopathy**
- EXCLUDES 1   *alcoholic encephalopathy (G31.2)*
  encephalopathy in diseases classified elsewhere (G94)
  hypertensive encephalopathy (I67.4)
  toxic (metabolic) encephalopathy (G92)

G93.40   **Encephalopathy, unspecified** ▽
AHA: 2017, 2Q, 8

G93.41   **Metabolic encephalopathy**
Septic encephalopathy
AHA: 2017, 2Q, 8; 2016, 3Q, 42; 2015, 3Q, 21

G93.49   **Other encephalopathy**
Encephalopathy NEC
AHA: 2017, 2Q, 9

G93.5   **Compression of brain** HCC
Arnold-Chiari type 1 compression of brain
Compression of brain (stem)
Herniation of brain (stem)
- EXCLUDES 1   *diffuse traumatic compression of brain (S06.2-)*
  focal traumatic compression of brain (S06.3-)

G93.6   **Cerebral edema** HCC
- EXCLUDES 1   *cerebral edema due to birth injury (P11.0)*
  traumatic cerebral edema (S06.1-)

G93.7   **Reye's syndrome** P
Code first (T39.0-), if salicylates-induced
►Code first poisoning due to salicylates, if applicable (T39.0-, with sixth character 1-4)◄
►Use additional code for adverse effect due to salicylates, if applicable (T39.0-, with sixth character 5)◄
DEF: Rare childhood illness often developed after a viral upper respiratory infection; characterized by vomiting, elevated serum transaminase, brain swelling, disturbances of consciousness, seizures, and changes in liver and other viscera; can be fatal.

✓5ᵗʰ **G93.8**   **Other specified disorders of brain**

G93.81   **Temporal sclerosis**
Hippocampal sclerosis
Mesial temporal sclerosis

G93.82   **Brain death**

G93.89   **Other specified disorders of brain**
Postradiation encephalopathy

G93.9   **Disorder of brain, unspecified** ▽

G94 *Other disorders of brain in diseases classified elsewhere*
Code first underlying disease
- EXCLUDES 1   *encephalopathy in congenital syphilis (A50.49)*
  encephalopathy in influenza (J09.X9, J10.81, J11.81)
  encephalopathy in syphilis (A52.19)
  hydrocephalus in diseases classified elsewhere (G91.4)

✓4ᵗʰ **G95 Other and unspecified diseases of spinal cord**
- EXCLUDES 2   *myelitis (G04.-)*

G95.0   **Syringomyelia and syringobulbia** HCC

✓5ᵗʰ **G95.1**   **Vascular myelopathies**
- EXCLUDES 2   *intraspinal phlebitis and thrombophlebitis, except non-pyogenic (G08)*

G95.11   **Acute infarction of spinal cord (embolic) (nonembolic)** HCC
Anoxia of spinal cord
Arterial thrombosis of spinal cord

G95.19   **Other vascular myelopathies** HCC
Edema of spinal cord
Hematomyelia
Nonpyogenic intraspinal phlebitis and thrombophlebitis
Subacute necrotic myelopathy

✓5ᵗʰ **G95.2**   **Other and unspecified cord compression**

G95.20   **Unspecified cord compression** HCC ▽

G95.29   **Other cord compression** HCC

✓5ᵗʰ **G95.8**   **Other specified diseases of spinal cord**
- EXCLUDES 1   *neurogenic bladder NOS (N31.9)*
  neurogenic bladder due to cauda equina syndrome (G83.4)
  neuromuscular dysfunction of bladder without spinal cord lesion (N31.-)

G95.81   **Conus medullaris syndrome** HCC

EXCLUDES 1 Not coded here   EXCLUDES 2 Not included here   N Newborn Age: 0   P Pediatric Age: 0-17   M Maternity Age: 12-55   A Adult Age: 15-124

566   ICD-10-CM 2018

G90.522–G95.81

G95.89 Other specified diseases of spinal cord `HCC`
Cord bladder NOS
Drug-induced myelopathy
Radiation-induced myelopathy
EXCLUDES 1   *myelopathy NOS (G95.9)*

G95.9 Disease of spinal cord, unspecified `HCC` ▽
Myelopathy NOS

✓4ᵗʰ **G96 Other disorders of central nervous system**

G96.0 Cerebrospinal fluid leak
EXCLUDES 1   *cerebrospinal fluid leak from spinal puncture (G97.0)*
DEF: Cerebrospinal fluid discharging from the nose or the ear; caused by fracture of frontal bone with tearing of dura mater and arachnoid; characterized by watery drainage usually from only one side of the nose or one ear, headache, vision changes, and hearing loss.

✓5ᵗʰ **G96.1 Disorders of meninges, not elsewhere classified**

G96.11 Dural tear
EXCLUDES 1   *accidental puncture or laceration of dura during a procedure (G97.41)*
AHA: 2014, 4Q, 24

G96.12 Meningeal adhesions (cerebral) (spinal)

G96.19 Other disorders of meninges, not elsewhere classified

G96.8 Other specified disorders of central nervous system

G96.9 Disorder of central nervous system, unspecified ▽

✓4ᵗʰ **G97 Intraoperative and postprocedural complications and disorders of nervous system, not elsewhere classified**
EXCLUDES 2   *intraoperative and postprocedural cerebrovascular infarction (I97.81-, I97.82-)*

G97.0 Cerebrospinal fluid leak from spinal puncture

G97.1 Other reaction to spinal and lumbar puncture
Headache due to lumbar puncture

G97.2 Intracranial hypotension following ventricular shunting

✓5ᵗʰ **G97.3 Intraoperative hemorrhage and hematoma of a nervous system organ or structure complicating a procedure**
EXCLUDES 1   *intraoperative hemorrhage and hematoma of a nervous system organ or structure due to accidental puncture and laceration during a procedure (G97.4-)*

G97.31 Intraoperative hemorrhage and hematoma of a nervous system organ or structure complicating a nervous system procedure

G97.32 Intraoperative hemorrhage and hematoma of a nervous system organ or structure complicating other procedure

✓5ᵗʰ **G97.4 Accidental puncture and laceration of a nervous system organ or structure during a procedure**

G97.41 Accidental puncture or laceration of dura during a procedure
Incidental (inadvertent) durotomy
AHA: 2014, 4Q, 24

G97.48 Accidental puncture and laceration of other nervous system organ or structure during a nervous system procedure

G97.49 Accidental puncture and laceration of other nervous system organ or structure during other procedure

Spinal Puncture

- Spinal cord
- Epidural space
- Subarachnoid space
- Vertebra
- Spinal needle

- Lumbar area

✓5ᵗʰ **G97.5 Postprocedural hemorrhage of a nervous system organ or structure following a procedure**

G97.51 Postprocedural hemorrhage of a nervous system organ or structure following a nervous system procedure

G97.52 Postprocedural hemorrhage of a nervous system organ or structure following other procedure

✓5ᵗʰ **G97.6 Postprocedural hematoma and seroma of a nervous system organ or structure following a procedure**

G97.61 Postprocedural hematoma of a nervous system organ or structure following a nervous system procedure

G97.62 Postprocedural hematoma of a nervous system organ or structure following other procedure

G97.63 Postprocedural seroma of a nervous system organ or structure following a nervous system procedure

G97.64 Postprocedural seroma of a nervous system organ or structure following other procedure

✓5ᵗʰ **G97.8 Other intraoperative and postprocedural complications and disorders of nervous system**
Use additional code to further specify disorder

G97.81 Other intraoperative complications of nervous system

G97.82 Other postprocedural complications and disorders of nervous system

✓4ᵗʰ **G98 Other disorders of nervous system not elsewhere classified**
`INCLUDES`   nervous system disorder NOS

G98.0 Neurogenic arthritis, not elsewhere classified
Nonsyphilitic neurogenic arthropathy NEC
Nonsyphilitic neurogenic spondylopathy NEC
EXCLUDES 1   *spondylopathy (in):*
    syringomyelia and syringobulbia (G95.0)
    tabes dorsalis (A52.11)

G98.8 Other disorders of nervous system
Nervous system disorder NOS

✓4ᵗʰ **G99 Other disorders of nervous system in diseases classified elsewhere**

G99.0 Autonomic neuropathy in diseases classified elsewhere
Code first underlying disease, such as:
    amyloidosis (E85.-)
    gout (M1A.-, M10.-)
    hyperthyroidism (E05.-)
EXCLUDES 1   *diabetic autonomic neuropathy (E08-E13 with .43)*

G99.2 Myelopathy in diseases classified elsewhere `HCC`
Code first underlying disease, such as:
    neoplasm (C00-D49)
EXCLUDES 1   *myelopathy in:*
    intervertebral disease (M50.0-, M51.0-)
    spondylosis (M47.0-, M47.1-)

G99.8 Other specified disorders of nervous system in diseases classified elsewhere
Code first underlying disorder, such as:
    amyloidosis (E85.-)
    avitaminosis (E56.9)
EXCLUDES 1   *nervous system involvement in:*
    cysticercosis (B69.0)
    rubella (B06.0-)
    syphilis (A52.1-)

☑ Additional Character Req   ✓x7ᵗʰ Placeholder Alert   Manifestation   `HCC` CMS-HCC Condition   ▽ Unspecified Code   ▶◀ Revised Text   ● New Code   ▲ Revised Code Title

Chapter 7. Diseases of the Eye and Adnexa (H00–H59)

Chapter Specific Guidelines with Coding Examples

The chapter specific guidelines from the ICD-10-CM Official Guidelines for Coding and Reporting have been provided below. Along with these guidelines are coding examples, contained in the shaded boxes, that have been developed to help illustrate the coding and/or sequencing guidance found in these guidelines.

a. Glaucoma

1) Assigning glaucoma codes

Assign as many codes from category H40, Glaucoma, as needed to identify the type of glaucoma, the affected eye, and the glaucoma stage.

2) Bilateral glaucoma with same type and stage

When a patient has bilateral glaucoma and both eyes are documented as being the same type and stage, and there is a code for bilateral glaucoma, report only the code for the type of glaucoma, bilateral, with the seventh character for the stage.

> Bilateral mild stage primary open-angle glaucoma
>
> **H40.1131   Primary open-angle glaucoma, bilateral, mild stage**
>
> *Explanation*: In this scenario, the patient has the same type and stage of glaucoma in both eyes. As this type of glaucoma has a code for bilateral, assign only the code for the bilateral glaucoma with the seventh character for the stage.

When a patient has bilateral glaucoma and both eyes are documented as being the same type and stage, and the classification does not provide a code for bilateral glaucoma (i.e. subcategories H40.10, H40.11 and H40.20) report only one code for the type of glaucoma with the appropriate seventh character for the stage.

> Bilateral open-angle glaucoma, severe stage; not specified as to type
>
> **H40.10X3   Unspecified open-angle glaucoma, severe stage**
>
> *Explanation*: In this scenario, the patient has glaucoma of the same type and stage of both eyes, but there is no code specifically for bilateral glaucoma. Only one code is assigned with the appropriate seventh character for the stage.

3) Bilateral glaucoma stage with different types or stages

When a patient has bilateral glaucoma and each eye is documented as having a different type or stage, and the classification distinguishes laterality, assign the appropriate code for each eye rather than the code for bilateral glaucoma.

> Bilateral chronic angle-closure glaucoma; right eye is documented as mild stage and left eye as moderate stage
>
> **H40.2211   Chronic angle-closure glaucoma, right eye, mild stage**
>
> **H40.2222   Chronic angle-closure glaucoma, left eye, moderate stage**
>
> *Explanation*: In this scenario the patient has the same type of glaucoma in both eyes, but each eye is at a different stage. Because the subcategory for this condition identifies laterality, one code is assigned for the right eye and one code is assigned for the left eye, each with the appropriate seventh character for the stage appended.

When a patient has bilateral glaucoma and each eye is documented as having a different type, and the classification does not distinguish laterality (i.e. subcategories H40.10, H40.11 and H40.20), assign one code for each type of glaucoma with the appropriate seventh character for the stage.

> Documentation relates mild, unspecified primary angle-closure glaucoma of the left eye with mild unspecified open-angle glaucoma of the right eye
>
> **H40.20X1   Unspecified primary angle-closure glaucoma, mild stage**
>
> **H40.10X1   Unspecified open-angle glaucoma, mild stage**
>
> *Explanation*: In this scenario the patient has a different type of glaucoma in each eye and the classification does not distinguish laterality. A code for each type of glaucoma is assigned, each with the appropriate seventh character for the stage.

When a patient has bilateral glaucoma and each eye is documented as having the same type, but different stage, and the classification does not distinguish laterality (i.e. subcategories H40.10, H40.11 and H40.20), assign a code for the type of glaucoma for each eye with the seventh character for the specific glaucoma stage documented for each eye.

> Bilateral open-angle glaucoma, not specified as to type; the right eye is documented to be in mild stage and the left eye as being in moderate stage
>
> **H40.10X1   Unspecified open-angle glaucoma, mild stage**
>
> **H40.10X2   Unspecified open-angle glaucoma, moderate stage**
>
> *Explanation*: In this scenario the patient has the same type of glaucoma in each eye but each eye is at a different stage, and the classification does not distinguish laterality at this subcategory level. Two codes are assigned; both codes represent the same type of glaucoma but each has a different seventh character identifying the appropriate stage for each eye.

4) Patient admitted with glaucoma and stage evolves during the admission

If a patient is admitted with glaucoma and the stage progresses during the admission, assign the code for highest stage documented.

5) Indeterminate stage glaucoma

Assignment of the seventh character "4" for "indeterminate stage" should be based on the clinical documentation. The seventh character "4" is used for glaucomas whose stage cannot be clinically determined. This seventh character should not be confused with the seventh character "0", unspecified, which should be assigned when there is no documentation regarding the stage of the glaucoma.

b. Blindness

If "blindness" or "low vision" of both eyes is documented but the visual impairment category is not documented, assign code H54.3, Unqualified visual loss, both eyes. If "blindness" or "low vision" in one eye is documented but the visual impairment category is not documented, assign a code from H54.6-, Unqualified visual loss, one eye. If "blindness" or "visual loss" is documented without any information about whether one or both eyes are affected, assign code H54.7, Unspecified visual loss.

Chapter 7. Diseases of the Eye and Adnexa (H00–H59)

NOTE   Use an external cause code following the code for the eye condition, if applicable, to identify the cause of the eye condition.

EXCLUDES 2 *certain conditions originating in the perinatal period (P04-P96)*
certain infectious and parasitic diseases (A00-B99)
complications of pregnancy, childbirth and the puerperium (O00-O9A)
congenital malformations, deformations, and chromosomal abnormalities (Q00-Q99)
diabetes mellitus related eye conditions (E09.3-, E10.3-, E11.3-, E13.3-)
endocrine, nutritional and metabolic diseases (E00-E88)
injury (trauma) of eye and orbit (S05.-)
injury, poisoning and certain other consequences of external causes (S00-T88)
neoplasms (C00-D49)
symptoms, signs and abnormal clinical and laboratory findings, not elsewhere classified (R00-R94)
syphilis related eye disorders (A50.01, A50.3-, A51.43, A52.71)

This chapter contains the following blocks:

H00-H05	Disorders of eyelid, lacrimal system and orbit
H10-H11	Disorders of conjunctiva
H15-H22	Disorders of sclera, cornea, iris and ciliary body
H25-H28	Disorders of lens
H30-H36	Disorders of choroid and retina
H40-H42	Glaucoma
H43-H44	Disorders of vitreous body and globe
H46-H47	Disorders of optic nerve and visual pathways
H49-H52	Disorders of ocular muscles, binocular movement, accommodation and refraction
H53-H54	Visual disturbances and blindness
H55-H57	Other disorders of eye and adnexa
H59	Intraoperative and postprocedural complications and disorders of eye and adnexa, not elsewhere classified

Disorders of eyelid, lacrimal system and orbit (H00-H05)

EXCLUDES 2 *open wound of eyelid (S01.1-)*
superficial injury of eyelid (S00.1-, S00.2-)

✓4ᵗʰ **H00 Hordeolum and chalazion**

  ✓5ᵗʰ **H00.0** Hordeolum (externum) (internum) of eyelid

    ✓6ᵗʰ **H00.01 Hordeolum externum**
      Hordeolum NOS
      Stye

      H00.011   Hordeolum externum right upper eyelid
      H00.012   Hordeolum externum right lower eyelid
      H00.013   Hordeolum externum right eye, unspecified eyelid ▽
      H00.014   Hordeolum externum left upper eyelid
      H00.015   Hordeolum externum left lower eyelid
      H00.016   Hordeolum externum left eye, unspecified eyelid ▽
      H00.019   Hordeolum externum unspecified eye, unspecified eyelid ▽

    ✓6ᵗʰ **H00.02 Hordeolum internum**
      Infection of meibomian gland

      H00.021   Hordeolum internum right upper eyelid
      H00.022   Hordeolum internum right lower eyelid
      H00.023   Hordeolum internum right eye, unspecified eyelid ▽
      H00.024   Hordeolum internum left upper eyelid
      H00.025   Hordeolum internum left lower eyelid
      H00.026   Hordeolum internum left eye, unspecified eyelid ▽
      H00.029   Hordeolum internum unspecified eye, unspecified eyelid ▽

    ✓6ᵗʰ **H00.03 Abscess of eyelid**
      Furuncle of eyelid

      H00.031   Abscess of right upper eyelid
      H00.032   Abscess of right lower eyelid
      H00.033   Abscess of eyelid right eye, unspecified eyelid ▽
      H00.034   Abscess of left upper eyelid
      H00.035   Abscess of left lower eyelid
      H00.036   Abscess of eyelid left eye, unspecified eyelid ▽
      H00.039   Abscess of eyelid unspecified eye, unspecified eyelid ▽

✓5ᵗʰ **H00.1 Chalazion**
  Meibomian (gland) cyst
  EXCLUDES 2 *infected meibomian gland (H00.02-)*

  H00.11   **Chalazion right upper eyelid**
  H00.12   **Chalazion right lower eyelid**
  H00.13   **Chalazion right eye, unspecified eyelid** ▽
  H00.14   **Chalazion left upper eyelid**
  H00.15   **Chalazion left lower eyelid**
  H00.16   **Chalazion left eye, unspecified eyelid** ▽
  H00.19   **Chalazion unspecified eye, unspecified eyelid** ▽

✓4ᵗʰ **H01 Other inflammation of eyelid**

  ✓5ᵗʰ **H01.0 Blepharitis**
    EXCLUDES 1 *blepharoconjunctivitis (H10.5-)*

    ✓6ᵗʰ **H01.00 Unspecified blepharitis**
      H01.001   Unspecified blepharitis right upper eyelid ▽
      H01.002   Unspecified blepharitis right lower eyelid ▽
      H01.003   Unspecified blepharitis right eye, unspecified eyelid ▽
      H01.004   Unspecified blepharitis left upper eyelid ▽
      H01.005   Unspecified blepharitis left lower eyelid ▽
      H01.006   Unspecified blepharitis left eye, unspecified eyelid ▽
      H01.009   Unspecified blepharitis unspecified eye, unspecified eyelid ▽

    ✓6ᵗʰ **H01.01 Ulcerative blepharitis**
      H01.011   Ulcerative blepharitis right upper eyelid
      H01.012   Ulcerative blepharitis right lower eyelid
      H01.013   Ulcerative blepharitis right eye, unspecified eyelid ▽
      H01.014   Ulcerative blepharitis left upper eyelid
      H01.015   Ulcerative blepharitis left lower eyelid
      H01.016   Ulcerative blepharitis left eye, unspecified eyelid ▽
      H01.019   Ulcerative blepharitis unspecified eye, unspecified eyelid ▽

    ✓6ᵗʰ **H01.02 Squamous blepharitis**
      H01.021   Squamous blepharitis right upper eyelid
      H01.022   Squamous blepharitis right lower eyelid
      H01.023   Squamous blepharitis right eye, unspecified eyelid ▽
      H01.024   Squamous blepharitis left upper eyelid
      H01.025   Squamous blepharitis left lower eyelid
      H01.026   Squamous blepharitis left eye, unspecified eyelid ▽
      H01.029   Squamous blepharitis unspecified eye, unspecified eyelid ▽

  ✓5ᵗʰ **H01.1 Noninfectious dermatoses of eyelid**

    ✓6ᵗʰ **H01.11 Allergic dermatitis of eyelid**
      Contact dermatitis of eyelid

      H01.111   Allergic dermatitis of right upper eyelid
      H01.112   Allergic dermatitis of right lower eyelid
      H01.113   Allergic dermatitis of right eye, unspecified eyelid ▽
      H01.114   Allergic dermatitis of left upper eyelid
      H01.115   Allergic dermatitis of left lower eyelid
      H01.116   Allergic dermatitis of left eye, unspecified eyelid ▽
      H01.119   Allergic dermatitis of unspecified eye, unspecified eyelid ▽

    ✓6ᵗʰ **H01.12 Discoid lupus erythematosus of eyelid**
      H01.121   Discoid lupus erythematosus of right upper eyelid
      H01.122   Discoid lupus erythematosus of right lower eyelid
      H01.123   Discoid lupus erythematosus of right eye, unspecified eyelid ▽
      H01.124   Discoid lupus erythematosus of left upper eyelid
      H01.125   Discoid lupus erythematosus of left lower eyelid

EXCLUDES 1 Not coded here   **EXCLUDES 2** Not included here   **N** Newborn Age: 0   **P** Pediatric Age: 0-17   **M** Maternity Age: 12-55   **A** Adult Age: 15-124

570   ICD-10-CM 2018

H01.126   Discoid lupus erythematosus of left eye, unspecified eyelid ▽

H01.129   Discoid lupus erythematosus of unspecified eye, unspecified eyelid ▽

✓6ᵗʰ H01.13   Eczematous dermatitis of eyelid

H01.131   Eczematous dermatitis of right upper eyelid

H01.132   Eczematous dermatitis of right lower eyelid

H01.133   Eczematous dermatitis of right eye, unspecified eyelid

H01.134   Eczematous dermatitis of left upper eyelid

H01.135   Eczematous dermatitis of left lower eyelid

H01.136   Eczematous dermatitis of left eye, unspecified eyelid ▽

H01.139   Eczematous dermatitis of unspecified eye, unspecified eyelid ▽

✓6ᵗʰ H01.14   Xeroderma of eyelid

H01.141   Xeroderma of right upper eyelid

H01.142   Xeroderma of right lower eyelid

H01.143   Xeroderma of right eye, unspecified eyelid ▽

H01.144   Xeroderma of left upper eyelid

H01.145   Xeroderma of left lower eyelid

H01.146   Xeroderma of left eye, unspecified eyelid ▽

H01.149   Xeroderma of unspecified eye, unspecified eyelid ▽

H01.8   Other specified inflammations of eyelid

H01.9   Unspecified inflammation of eyelid ▽
     Inflammation of eyelid NOS

✓4ᵗʰ **H02**   **Other disorders of eyelid**
     EXCLUDES 1   congenital malformations of eyelid (Q10.0-Q10.3)

✓5ᵗʰ H02.0   Entropion and trichiasis of eyelid

✓6ᵗʰ H02.00   Unspecified entropion of eyelid

H02.001   Unspecified entropion of right upper eyelid ▽

H02.002   Unspecified entropion of right lower eyelid ▽

H02.003   Unspecified entropion of right eye, unspecified eyelid ▽

H02.004   Unspecified entropion of left upper eyelid ▽

H02.005   Unspecified entropion of left lower eyelid ▽

H02.006   Unspecified entropion of left eye, unspecified eyelid ▽

H02.009   Unspecified entropion of unspecified eye, unspecified eyelid ▽

✓6ᵗʰ H02.01   Cicatricial entropion of eyelid

H02.011   Cicatricial entropion of right upper eyelid

H02.012   Cicatricial entropion of right lower eyelid

H02.013   Cicatricial entropion of right eye, unspecified eyelid ▽

H02.014   Cicatricial entropion of left upper eyelid

H02.015   Cicatricial entropion of left lower eyelid

H02.016   Cicatricial entropion of left eye, unspecified eyelid ▽

H02.019   Cicatricial entropion of unspecified eye, unspecified eyelid ▽

✓6ᵗʰ H02.02   Mechanical entropion of eyelid

H02.021   Mechanical entropion of right upper eyelid

H02.022   Mechanical entropion of right lower eyelid

H02.023   Mechanical entropion of right eye, unspecified eyelid ▽

H02.024   Mechanical entropion of left upper eyelid

H02.025   Mechanical entropion of left lower eyelid

H02.026   Mechanical entropion of left eye, unspecified eyelid ▽

H02.029   Mechanical entropion of unspecified eye, unspecified eyelid ▽

✓6ᵗʰ H02.03   Senile entropion of eyelid

H02.031   Senile entropion of right upper eyelid Ⓐ

H02.032   Senile entropion of right lower eyelid Ⓐ

H02.033   Senile entropion of right eye, unspecified eyelid Ⓐ▽

H02.034   Senile entropion of left upper eyelid Ⓐ

H02.035   Senile entropion of left lower eyelid Ⓐ

H02.036   Senile entropion of left eye, unspecified eyelid Ⓐ▽

H02.039   Senile entropion of unspecified eye, unspecified eyelid Ⓐ▽

✓6ᵗʰ H02.04   Spastic entropion of eyelid

H02.041   Spastic entropion of right upper eyelid

H02.042   Spastic entropion of right lower eyelid

H02.043   Spastic entropion of right eye, unspecified eyelid ▽

H02.044   Spastic entropion of left upper eyelid

H02.045   Spastic entropion of left lower eyelid

H02.046   Spastic entropion of left eye, unspecified eyelid ▽

H02.049   Spastic entropion of unspecified eye, unspecified eyelid ▽

▲ ✓6ᵗʰ H02.05   Trichiasis without entropion

▲   H02.051   Trichiasis without entropion right upper eyelid

▲   H02.052   Trichiasis without entropion right lower eyelid

▲   H02.053   Trichiasis without entropion right eye, unspecified eyelid ▽

▲   H02.054   Trichiasis without entropion left upper eyelid

▲   H02.055   Trichiasis without entropion left lower eyelid

▲   H02.056   Trichiasis without entropion left eye, unspecified eyelid ▽

▲   H02.059   Trichiasis without entropion unspecified eye, unspecified eyelid ▽

✓5ᵗʰ H02.1   Ectropion of eyelid

✓6ᵗʰ H02.10   Unspecified ectropion of eyelid

H02.101   Unspecified ectropion of right upper eyelid ▽

H02.102   Unspecified ectropion of right lower eyelid ▽

H02.103   Unspecified ectropion of right eye, unspecified eyelid ▽

H02.104   Unspecified ectropion of left upper eyelid ▽

H02.105   Unspecified ectropion of left lower eyelid ▽

H02.106   Unspecified ectropion of left eye, unspecified eyelid ▽

H02.109   Unspecified ectropion of unspecified eye, unspecified eyelid ▽

✓6ᵗʰ H02.11   Cicatricial ectropion of eyelid

H02.111   Cicatricial ectropion of right upper eyelid

H02.112   Cicatricial ectropion of right lower eyelid

H02.113   Cicatricial ectropion of right eye, unspecified eyelid ▽

H02.114   Cicatricial ectropion of left upper eyelid

H02.115   Cicatricial ectropion of left lower eyelid

H02.116   Cicatricial ectropion of left eye, unspecified eyelid ▽

H02.119   Cicatricial ectropion of unspecified eye, unspecified eyelid ▽

Entropion and Ectropion

Normal eyelid   Entropion   Ectropion

✓ Additional Character Req   ✓x7ᵗʰ Placeholder Alert   Manifestation   HCC CMS-HCC Condition   ▽ Unspecified Code   ▶◀ Revised Text   ● New Code   ▲ Revised Code Title

ICD-10-CM 2018   571

✓6ᵗʰ **H02.12 Mechanical ectropion of eyelid**
 H02.121 Mechanical ectropion of right upper eyelid
 H02.122 Mechanical ectropion of right lower eyelid
 H02.123 Mechanical ectropion of right eye, unspecified eyelid ▽
 H02.124 Mechanical ectropion of left upper eyelid
 H02.125 Mechanical ectropion of left lower eyelid
 H02.126 Mechanical ectropion of left eye, unspecified eyelid ▽
 H02.129 Mechanical ectropion of unspecified eye, unspecified eyelid ▽

✓6ᵗʰ **H02.13 Senile ectropion of eyelid**
 H02.131 Senile ectropion of right upper eyelid Ⓐ
 H02.132 Senile ectropion of right lower eyelid Ⓐ
 H02.133 Senile ectropion of right eye, unspecified eyelid Ⓐ▽
 H02.134 Senile ectropion of left upper eyelid Ⓐ
 H02.135 Senile ectropion of left lower eyelid Ⓐ
 H02.136 Senile ectropion of left eye, unspecified eyelid Ⓐ▽
 H02.139 Senile ectropion of unspecified eye, unspecified eyelid Ⓐ▽

✓6ᵗʰ **H02.14 Spastic ectropion of eyelid**
 H02.141 Spastic ectropion of right upper eyelid
 H02.142 Spastic ectropion of right lower eyelid
 H02.143 Spastic ectropion of right eye, unspecified eyelid ▽
 H02.144 Spastic ectropion of left upper eyelid
 H02.145 Spastic ectropion of left lower eyelid
 H02.146 Spastic ectropion of left eye, unspecified eyelid ▽
 H02.149 Spastic ectropion of unspecified eye, unspecified eyelid ▽

✓5ᵗʰ **H02.2 Lagophthalmos**
✓6ᵗʰ **H02.20 Unspecified lagophthalmos**
 H02.201 Unspecified lagophthalmos right upper eyelid ▽
 H02.202 Unspecified lagophthalmos right lower eyelid ▽
 H02.203 Unspecified lagophthalmos right eye, unspecified eyelid ▽
 H02.204 Unspecified lagophthalmos left upper eyelid ▽
 H02.205 Unspecified lagophthalmos left lower eyelid ▽
 H02.206 Unspecified lagophthalmos left eye, unspecified eyelid ▽
 H02.209 Unspecified lagophthalmos unspecified eye, unspecified eyelid ▽

✓6ᵗʰ **H02.21 Cicatricial lagophthalmos**
 H02.211 Cicatricial lagophthalmos right upper eyelid
 H02.212 Cicatricial lagophthalmos right lower eyelid
 H02.213 Cicatricial lagophthalmos right eye, unspecified eyelid ▽
 H02.214 Cicatricial lagophthalmos left upper eyelid
 H02.215 Cicatricial lagophthalmos left lower eyelid
 H02.216 Cicatricial lagophthalmos left eye, unspecified eyelid ▽
 H02.219 Cicatricial lagophthalmos unspecified eye, unspecified eyelid ▽

✓6ᵗʰ **H02.22 Mechanical lagophthalmos**
 H02.221 Mechanical lagophthalmos right upper eyelid
 H02.222 Mechanical lagophthalmos right lower eyelid
 H02.223 Mechanical lagophthalmos right eye, unspecified eyelid ▽
 H02.224 Mechanical lagophthalmos left upper eyelid
 H02.225 Mechanical lagophthalmos left lower eyelid
 H02.226 Mechanical lagophthalmos left eye, unspecified eyelid ▽
 H02.229 Mechanical lagophthalmos unspecified eye, unspecified eyelid ▽

✓6ᵗʰ **H02.23 Paralytic lagophthalmos**
 H02.231 Paralytic lagophthalmos right upper eyelid
 H02.232 Paralytic lagophthalmos right lower eyelid
 H02.233 Paralytic lagophthalmos right eye, unspecified eyelid ▽
 H02.234 Paralytic lagophthalmos left upper eyelid
 H02.235 Paralytic lagophthalmos left lower eyelid
 H02.236 Paralytic lagophthalmos left eye, unspecified eyelid ▽
 H02.239 Paralytic lagophthalmos unspecified eye, unspecified eyelid ▽

✓5ᵗʰ **H02.3 Blepharochalasis**
 Pseudoptosis
 H02.30 Blepharochalasis unspecified eye, unspecified eyelid ▽
 H02.31 Blepharochalasis right upper eyelid
 H02.32 Blepharochalasis right lower eyelid
 H02.33 Blepharochalasis right eye, unspecified eyelid ▽
 H02.34 Blepharochalasis left upper eyelid
 H02.35 Blepharochalasis left lower eyelid
 H02.36 Blepharochalasis left eye, unspecified eyelid ▽

✓5ᵗʰ **H02.4 Ptosis of eyelid**
✓6ᵗʰ **H02.40 Unspecified ptosis of eyelid**
 H02.401 Unspecified ptosis of right eyelid ▽
 H02.402 Unspecified ptosis of left eyelid ▽
 H02.403 Unspecified ptosis of bilateral eyelids ▽
 H02.409 Unspecified ptosis of unspecified eyelid ▽

✓6ᵗʰ **H02.41 Mechanical ptosis of eyelid**
 H02.411 Mechanical ptosis of right eyelid
 H02.412 Mechanical ptosis of left eyelid
 H02.413 Mechanical ptosis of bilateral eyelids
 H02.419 Mechanical ptosis of unspecified eyelid ▽

✓6ᵗʰ **H02.42 Myogenic ptosis of eyelid**
 H02.421 Myogenic ptosis of right eyelid
 H02.422 Myogenic ptosis of left eyelid
 H02.423 Myogenic ptosis of bilateral eyelids
 H02.429 Myogenic ptosis of unspecified eyelid ▽

✓6ᵗʰ **H02.43 Paralytic ptosis of eyelid**
 Neurogenic ptosis of eyelid
 H02.431 Paralytic ptosis of right eyelid
 H02.432 Paralytic ptosis of left eyelid
 H02.433 Paralytic ptosis of bilateral eyelids
 H02.439 Paralytic ptosis unspecified eyelid ▽

✓5ᵗʰ **H02.5 Other disorders affecting eyelid function**
 EXCLUDES 2 blepharospasm (G24.5)
    organic tic (G25.69)
    psychogenic tic (F95.-)

✓6ᵗʰ **H02.51 Abnormal innervation syndrome**
 H02.511 Abnormal innervation syndrome right upper eyelid
 H02.512 Abnormal innervation syndrome right lower eyelid
 H02.513 Abnormal innervation syndrome right eye, unspecified eyelid ▽
 H02.514 Abnormal innervation syndrome left upper eyelid
 H02.515 Abnormal innervation syndrome left lower eyelid
 H02.516 Abnormal innervation syndrome left eye, unspecified eyelid ▽
 H02.519 Abnormal innervation syndrome unspecified eye, unspecified eyelid ▽

✓6ᵗʰ **H02.52 Blepharophimosis**
 Ankyloblepharon
 H02.521 Blepharophimosis right upper eyelid
 H02.522 Blepharophimosis right lower eyelid
 H02.523 Blepharophimosis right eye, unspecified eyelid ▽
 H02.524 Blepharophimosis left upper eyelid
 H02.525 Blepharophimosis left lower eyelid
 H02.526 Blepharophimosis left eye, unspecified eyelid ▽

EXCLUDES 1 Not coded here *EXCLUDES 2* Not included here Ⓝ Newborn Age: 0 Ⓟ Pediatric Age: 0-17 Ⓜ Maternity Age: 12-55 Ⓐ Adult Age: 15-124

572   ICD-10-CM 2018

H02.529   **Blepharophimosis unspecified eye, unspecified lid** ▽

✓6ᵗʰ **H02.53   Eyelid retraction**
Eyelid lag

H02.531   **Eyelid retraction** right upper **eyelid**

H02.532   **Eyelid retraction** right lower **eyelid**

H02.533   **Eyelid retraction** right eye, unspecified **eyelid** ▽

H02.534   **Eyelid retraction** left upper **eyelid**

H02.535   **Eyelid retraction** left lower **eyelid**

H02.536   **Eyelid retraction** left eye, unspecified **eyelid** ▽

H02.539   **Eyelid retraction unspecified eye, unspecified lid** ▽

H02.59   **Other disorders affecting eyelid function**
Deficient blink reflex
Sensory disorders

✓5ᵗʰ **H02.6   Xanthelasma of eyelid**

H02.60   **Xanthelasma of unspecified eye, unspecified eyelid** ▽

H02.61   **Xanthelasma of** right upper **eyelid**

H02.62   **Xanthelasma of** right lower **eyelid**

H02.63   **Xanthelasma of** right eye, unspecified **eyelid** ▽

H02.64   **Xanthelasma of** left upper **eyelid**

H02.65   **Xanthelasma of** left lower **eyelid**

H02.66   **Xanthelasma of** left eye, unspecified **eyelid** ▽

✓5ᵗʰ **H02.7   Other and unspecified degenerative disorders of eyelid and periocular area**

H02.70   **Unspecified degenerative disorders of eyelid and periocular area** ▽

✓6ᵗʰ **H02.71   Chloasma of eyelid and periocular area**
Dyspigmentation of eyelid
Hyperpigmentation of eyelid

H02.711   **Chloasma of** right upper **eyelid and periocular area**

H02.712   **Chloasma of** right lower **eyelid and periocular area**

H02.713   **Chloasma of** right eye, unspecified **eyelid and periocular area** ▽

H02.714   **Chloasma of** left upper **eyelid and periocular area**

H02.715   **Chloasma of** left lower **eyelid and periocular area**

H02.716   **Chloasma of** left eye, unspecified **eyelid and periocular area** ▽

H02.719   **Chloasma of unspecified eye, unspecified eyelid and periocular area** ▽

✓6ᵗʰ **H02.72   Madarosis of eyelid and periocular area**
Hypotrichosis of eyelid

H02.721   **Madarosis of** right upper **eyelid and periocular area**

H02.722   **Madarosis of** right lower **eyelid and periocular area**

H02.723   **Madarosis of** right eye, unspecified **eyelid and periocular area** ▽

H02.724   **Madarosis of** left upper **eyelid and periocular area**

H02.725   **Madarosis of** left lower **eyelid and periocular area**

H02.726   **Madarosis of** left eye, unspecified **eyelid and periocular area** ▽

H02.729   **Madarosis of unspecified eye, unspecified eyelid and periocular area** ▽

✓6ᵗʰ **H02.73   Vitiligo of eyelid and periocular area**
Hypopigmentation of eyelid

H02.731   **Vitiligo of** right upper **eyelid and periocular area**

H02.732   **Vitiligo of** right lower **eyelid and periocular area**

H02.733   **Vitiligo of** right eye, unspecified **eyelid and periocular area** ▽

H02.734   **Vitiligo of** left upper **eyelid and periocular area**

H02.735   **Vitiligo of** left lower **eyelid and periocular area**

H02.736   **Vitiligo of** left eye, unspecified **eyelid and periocular area** ▽

H02.739   **Vitiligo of unspecified eye, unspecified eyelid and periocular area** ▽

H02.79   **Other degenerative disorders of eyelid and periocular area**

✓5ᵗʰ **H02.8   Other specified disorders of eyelid**

✓6ᵗʰ **H02.81   Retained foreign body in eyelid**
Use additional code to identify the type of retained foreign body (Z18.-)

EXCLUDES 1   laceration of eyelid with foreign body (S01.12-)
retained intraocular foreign body (H44.6-, H44.7-)
superficial foreign body of eyelid and periocular area (S00.25-)

H02.811   **Retained foreign body in** right upper **eyelid**

H02.812   **Retained foreign body in** right lower **eyelid**

H02.813   **Retained foreign body in** right eye, unspecified **eyelid** ▽

H02.814   **Retained foreign body in** left upper **eyelid**

H02.815   **Retained foreign body in** left lower **eyelid**

H02.816   **Retained foreign body in** left eye, unspecified **eyelid** ▽

H02.819   **Retained foreign body in unspecified eye, unspecified eyelid** ▽

✓6ᵗʰ **H02.82   Cysts of eyelid**
Sebaceous cyst of eyelid

H02.821   **Cysts of** right upper **eyelid**

H02.822   **Cysts of** right lower **eyelid**

H02.823   **Cysts of** right eye, unspecified **eyelid** ▽

H02.824   **Cysts of** left upper **eyelid**

H02.825   **Cysts of** left lower **eyelid**

H02.826   **Cysts of** left eye, unspecified **eyelid** ▽

H02.829   **Cysts of unspecified eye, unspecified eyelid** ▽

✓6ᵗʰ **H02.83   Dermatochalasis of eyelid**
DEF: Acquired form of connective tissue disorder associated with decreased elastic tissue and abnormal elastin formation, resulting in loss of elasticity of the skin of the eyelid; generally associated with aging.

H02.831   **Dermatochalasis of** right upper **eyelid**

H02.832   **Dermatochalasis of** right lower **eyelid**

H02.833   **Dermatochalasis of** right eye, unspecified **eyelid** ▽

H02.834   **Dermatochalasis of** left upper **eyelid**

H02.835   **Dermatochalasis of** left lower **eyelid**

H02.836   **Dermatochalasis of** left eye, unspecified **eyelid** ▽

H02.839   **Dermatochalasis of unspecified eye, unspecified eyelid** ▽

✓6ᵗʰ **H02.84   Edema of eyelid**
Hyperemia of eyelid

H02.841   **Edema of** right upper **eyelid**

H02.842   **Edema of** right lower **eyelid**

H02.843   **Edema of** right eye, unspecified **eyelid** ▽

H02.844   **Edema of** left upper **eyelid**

H02.845   **Edema of** left lower **eyelid**

H02.846   **Edema of** left eye, unspecified **eyelid** ▽

H02.849   **Edema of unspecified eye, unspecified eyelid** ▽

✓6ᵗʰ **H02.85   Elephantiasis of eyelid**

H02.851   **Elephantiasis of** right upper **eyelid**

H02.852   **Elephantiasis of** right lower **eyelid**

H02.853   **Elephantiasis of** right eye, unspecified **eyelid** ▽

H02.854   **Elephantiasis of** left upper **eyelid**

H02.855   **Elephantiasis of** left lower **eyelid**

H02.856   **Elephantiasis of** left eye, unspecified **eyelid** ▽

H02.859   **Elephantiasis of unspecified eye, unspecified eyelid** ▽

✓6ᵗʰ **H02.86   Hypertrichosis of eyelid**

H02.861   **Hypertrichosis of** right upper **eyelid**

H02.862   **Hypertrichosis of** right lower **eyelid**

H02.863   **Hypertrichosis of** right eye, unspecified **eyelid** ▽

☑ Additional Character Req   ✓x7ᵗʰ Placeholder Alert   Manifestation   HCC CMS-HCC Condition   ▽ Unspecified Code   ►◄ Revised Text   ● New Code   ▲ Revised Code Title

ICD-10-CM 2018   573

H02.864   **Hypertrichosis of** left upper **eyelid**

H02.865   **Hypertrichosis of** left lower **eyelid**

H02.866   **Hypertrichosis of** left **eye,** ▽
unspecified **eyelid**

H02.869   **Hypertrichosis of unspecified eye,** ▽
unspecified eyelid

✓6ᵗʰ **H02.87**   Vascular anomalies **of eyelid**

H02.871   **Vascular anomalies of** right upper **eyelid**

H02.872   **Vascular anomalies of** right lower **eyelid**

H02.873   **Vascular anomalies of** right eye, ▽
unspecified eyelid

H02.874   **Vascular anomalies of** left upper **eyelid**

H02.875   **Vascular anomalies of** left lower **eyelid**

H02.876   **Vascular anomalies of** left eye, ▽
unspecified eyelid

H02.879   **Vascular anomalies of unspecified** ▽
eye, unspecified eyelid

H02.89   **Other specified disorders of eyelid**
Hemorrhage of eyelid

H02.9   **Unspecified disorder of eyelid** ▽
Disorder of eyelid NOS

✓4ᵗʰ **H04**   **Disorders of lacrimal system**
EXCLUDES 1   *congenital malformations of lacrimal system (Q10.4-Q10.6)*

✓5ᵗʰ **H04.0**   **Dacryoadenitis**

✓6ᵗʰ **H04.00**   **Unspecified dacryoadenitis**

H04.001   **Unspecified dacryoadenitis,** right ▽
lacrimal gland

H04.002   **Unspecified dacryoadenitis,** left ▽
lacrimal gland

H04.003   **Unspecified dacryoadenitis,** ▽
bilateral **lacrimal glands**

H04.009   **Unspecified dacryoadenitis,** ▽
unspecified lacrimal gland

✓6ᵗʰ **H04.01**   Acute **dacryoadenitis**

H04.011   **Acute dacryoadenitis,** right **lacrimal gland**

H04.012   **Acute dacryoadenitis,** left **lacrimal gland**

H04.013   **Acute dacryoadenitis,** bilateral **lacrimal glands**

H04.019   **Acute dacryoadenitis, unspecified** ▽
lacrimal gland

✓6ᵗʰ **H04.02**   Chronic **dacryoadenitis**

H04.021   **Chronic dacryoadenitis,** right **lacrimal gland**

H04.022   **Chronic dacryoadenitis,** left **lacrimal gland**

H04.023   **Chronic dacryoadenitis,** bilateral **lacrimal glands**

H04.029   **Chronic dacryoadenitis, unspecified** ▽
lacrimal gland

✓6ᵗʰ **H04.03**   **Chronic enlargement of lacrimal gland**

H04.031   **Chronic enlargement of** right **lacrimal gland**

H04.032   **Chronic enlargement of** left **lacrimal gland**

H04.033   **Chronic enlargement of** bilateral **lacrimal glands**

H04.039   **Chronic enlargement of unspecified** ▽
lacrimal gland

✓5ᵗʰ **H04.1**   **Other disorders of lacrimal gland**

✓6ᵗʰ **H04.11**   **Dacryops**

H04.111   **Dacryops of** right **lacrimal gland**

H04.112   **Dacryops of** left **lacrimal gland**

H04.113   **Dacryops of** bilateral **lacrimal glands**

H04.119   **Dacryops of unspecified lacrimal gland** ▽

✓6ᵗʰ **H04.12**   **Dry eye syndrome**
Tear film insufficiency, NOS

H04.121   **Dry eye syndrome of** right **lacrimal gland**

H04.122   **Dry eye syndrome of** left **lacrimal gland**

H04.123   **Dry eye syndrome of** bilateral **lacrimal glands**

H04.129   **Dry eye syndrome of unspecified** ▽
lacrimal gland

✓6ᵗʰ **H04.13**   Lacrimal cyst
Lacrimal cystic degeneration

H04.131   **Lacrimal cyst,** right **lacrimal gland**

H04.132   **Lacrimal cyst,** left **lacrimal gland**

H04.133   **Lacrimal cyst,** bilateral **lacrimal glands**

H04.139   **Lacrimal cyst, unspecified lacrimal** ▽
gland

✓6ᵗʰ **H04.14**   Primary **lacrimal gland atrophy**

H04.141   **Primary lacrimal gland atrophy,** right
lacrimal gland

H04.142   **Primary lacrimal gland atrophy,** left
lacrimal gland

H04.143   **Primary lacrimal gland atrophy,** bilateral
lacrimal glands

H04.149   **Primary lacrimal gland atrophy,** ▽
unspecified lacrimal gland

✓6ᵗʰ **H04.15**   Secondary **lacrimal gland atrophy**

H04.151   **Secondary lacrimal gland atrophy,** right
lacrimal gland

H04.152   **Secondary lacrimal gland atrophy,** left
lacrimal gland

H04.153   **Secondary lacrimal gland atrophy,**
bilateral **lacrimal glands**

H04.159   **Secondary lacrimal gland atrophy,** ▽
unspecified lacrimal gland

✓6ᵗʰ **H04.16**   **Lacrimal gland dislocation**

H04.161   **Lacrimal gland dislocation,** right **lacrimal**
gland

H04.162   **Lacrimal gland dislocation,** left **lacrimal**
gland

H04.163   **Lacrimal gland dislocation,** bilateral
lacrimal glands

H04.169   **Lacrimal gland dislocation,** ▽
unspecified lacrimal gland

H04.19   **Other specified disorders of lacrimal gland**

✓5ᵗʰ **H04.2**   **Epiphora**

✓6ᵗʰ **H04.20**   **Unspecified epiphora**

H04.201   **Unspecified epiphora,** right **lacrimal** ▽
gland

H04.202   **Unspecified epiphora,** left **lacrimal** ▽
gland

H04.203   **Unspecified epiphora,** bilateral ▽
lacrimal glands

H04.209   **Unspecified epiphora, unspecified** ▽
lacrimal gland

✓6ᵗʰ **H04.21**   **Epiphora** due to excess lacrimation

H04.211   **Epiphora due to excess lacrimation,** right
lacrimal gland

H04.212   **Epiphora due to excess lacrimation,** left
lacrimal gland

H04.213   **Epiphora due to excess lacrimation,**
bilateral **lacrimal glands**

H04.219   **Epiphora due to excess lacrimation,** ▽
unspecified lacrimal gland

✓6ᵗʰ **H04.22**   **Epiphora** due to insufficient drainage

H04.221   **Epiphora due to insufficient drainage,**
right **lacrimal gland**

H04.222   **Epiphora due to insufficient drainage,** left
lacrimal gland

H04.223   **Epiphora due to insufficient drainage,**
bilateral **lacrimal glands**

H04.229   **Epiphora due to insufficient drainage,** ▽
unspecified lacrimal gland

✓5ᵗʰ **H04.3**   **Acute and unspecified inflammation of lacrimal passages**
EXCLUDES 1   *neonatal dacryocystitis (P39.1)*

✓6ᵗʰ **H04.30**   **Unspecified dacryocystitis**

H04.301   **Unspecified dacryocystitis of** right ▽
lacrimal passage

H04.302   **Unspecified dacryocystitis of** left ▽
lacrimal passage

H04.303   **Unspecified dacryocystitis of** bilateral ▽
lacrimal passages

H04.309   **Unspecified dacryocystitis of** ▽
unspecified lacrimal passage

✓6ᵗʰ **H04.31**   Phlegmonous **dacryocystitis**

H04.311   **Phlegmonous dacryocystitis of** right
lacrimal passage

H04.312   **Phlegmonous dacryocystitis of** left
lacrimal passage

H04.313   **Phlegmonous dacryocystitis of** bilateral
lacrimal passages

EXCLUDES 1 Not coded here   *EXCLUDES 2* Not included here   N Newborn Age: 0   P Pediatric Age: 0-17   M Maternity Age: 12-55   A Adult Age: 15-124

574   ICD-10-CM 2018

　　　　H04.319 **Phlegmonous dacryocystitis of** ▽
　　　　　　　　　unspecified lacrimal passage

✓6ᵗʰ **H04.32** Acute **dacryocystitis**
　　　　　Acute dacryopericystitis
　　　　H04.321 **Acute dacryocystitis of right lacrimal**
　　　　　　　　　passage
　　　　H04.322 **Acute dacryocystitis of left lacrimal**
　　　　　　　　　passage
　　　　H04.323 **Acute dacryocystitis of bilateral lacrimal**
　　　　　　　　　passages
　　　　H04.329 **Acute dacryocystitis of unspecified** ▽
　　　　　　　　　lacrimal passage

✓6ᵗʰ **H04.33** Acute **lacrimal** canaliculitis
　　　　H04.331 **Acute lacrimal canaliculitis of right**
　　　　　　　　　lacrimal passage
　　　　H04.332 **Acute lacrimal canaliculitis of left lacrimal**
　　　　　　　　　passage
　　　　H04.333 **Acute lacrimal canaliculitis of bilateral**
　　　　　　　　　lacrimal passages
　　　　H04.339 **Acute lacrimal canaliculitis of** ▽
　　　　　　　　　unspecified lacrimal passage

✓5ᵗʰ **H04.4** **Chronic inflammation of lacrimal passages**
　✓6ᵗʰ **H04.41** Chronic **dacryocystitis**
　　　　H04.411 **Chronic dacryocystitis of right lacrimal**
　　　　　　　　　passage
　　　　H04.412 **Chronic dacryocystitis of left lacrimal**
　　　　　　　　　passage
　　　　H04.413 **Chronic dacryocystitis of bilateral lacrimal**
　　　　　　　　　passages
　　　　H04.419 **Chronic dacryocystitis of unspecified** ▽
　　　　　　　　　lacrimal passage

　✓6ᵗʰ **H04.42** Chronic **lacrimal** canaliculitis
　　　　H04.421 **Chronic lacrimal canaliculitis of right**
　　　　　　　　　lacrimal passage
　　　　H04.422 **Chronic lacrimal canaliculitis of left**
　　　　　　　　　lacrimal passage
　　　　H04.423 **Chronic lacrimal canaliculitis of bilateral**
　　　　　　　　　lacrimal passages
　　　　H04.429 **Chronic lacrimal canaliculitis of** ▽
　　　　　　　　　unspecified lacrimal passage

　✓6ᵗʰ **H04.43** Chronic **lacrimal** mucocele
　　　　H04.431 **Chronic lacrimal mucocele of right**
　　　　　　　　　lacrimal passage
　　　　H04.432 **Chronic lacrimal mucocele of left lacrimal**
　　　　　　　　　passage
　　　　H04.433 **Chronic lacrimal mucocele of bilateral**
　　　　　　　　　lacrimal passages
　　　　H04.439 **Chronic lacrimal mucocele of** ▽
　　　　　　　　　unspecified lacrimal passage

✓5ᵗʰ **H04.5** **Stenosis and insufficiency of lacrimal passages**
　✓6ᵗʰ **H04.51** Dacryolith
　　　　H04.511 **Dacryolith of right lacrimal passage**
　　　　H04.512 **Dacryolith of left lacrimal passage**
　　　　H04.513 **Dacryolith of bilateral lacrimal passages**
　　　　H04.519 **Dacryolith of unspecified lacrimal** ▽
　　　　　　　　　passage

　✓6ᵗʰ **H04.52** Eversion **of lacrimal** punctum
　　　　H04.521 **Eversion of right lacrimal punctum**
　　　　H04.522 **Eversion of left lacrimal punctum**
　　　　H04.523 **Eversion of bilateral lacrimal punctum**
　　　　H04.529 **Eversion of unspecified lacrimal** ▽
　　　　　　　　　punctum

　✓6ᵗʰ **H04.53** Neonatal **obstruction of nasolacrimal duct**
　　　　　EXCLUDES 1 congenital stenosis and stricture of lacrimal
　　　　　　　　　duct (Q10.5)
　　　　H04.531 **Neonatal obstruction of right** N
　　　　　　　　　nasolacrimal duct
　　　　H04.532 **Neonatal obstruction of left** N
　　　　　　　　　nasolacrimal duct
　　　　H04.533 **Neonatal obstruction of bilateral** N
　　　　　　　　　nasolacrimal duct
　　　　H04.539 **Neonatal obstruction of unspecified** N▽
　　　　　　　　　nasolacrimal duct

　✓6ᵗʰ **H04.54** **Stenosis of lacrimal** canaliculi
　　　　H04.541 **Stenosis of right lacrimal canaliculi**
　　　　H04.542 **Stenosis of left lacrimal canaliculi**

　　　　H04.543 **Stenosis of bilateral lacrimal canaliculi**
　　　　H04.549 **Stenosis of unspecified lacrimal** ▽
　　　　　　　　　canaliculi

　✓6ᵗʰ **H04.55** **Acquired stenosis of nasolacrimal duct**
　　　　H04.551 **Acquired stenosis of right nasolacrimal**
　　　　　　　　　duct
　　　　H04.552 **Acquired stenosis of left nasolacrimal duct**
　　　　H04.553 **Acquired stenosis of bilateral nasolacrimal**
　　　　　　　　　duct
　　　　H04.559 **Acquired stenosis of unspecified** ▽
　　　　　　　　　nasolacrimal duct

　✓6ᵗʰ **H04.56** **Stenosis of lacrimal** punctum
　　　　H04.561 **Stenosis of right lacrimal punctum**
　　　　H04.562 **Stenosis of left lacrimal punctum**
　　　　H04.563 **Stenosis of bilateral lacrimal punctum**
　　　　H04.569 **Stenosis of unspecified lacrimal** ▽
　　　　　　　　　punctum

　✓6ᵗʰ **H04.57** **Stenosis of lacrimal** sac
　　　　H04.571 **Stenosis of right lacrimal sac**
　　　　H04.572 **Stenosis of left lacrimal sac**
　　　　H04.573 **Stenosis of bilateral lacrimal sac**
　　　　H04.579 **Stenosis of unspecified lacrimal sac** ▽

✓5ᵗʰ **H04.6** **Other changes of lacrimal passages**
　✓6ᵗʰ **H04.61** Lacrimal fistula
　　　　H04.611 **Lacrimal fistula right lacrimal passage**
　　　　H04.612 **Lacrimal fistula left lacrimal passage**
　　　　H04.613 **Lacrimal fistula bilateral lacrimal passages**
　　　　H04.619 **Lacrimal fistula unspecified lacrimal** ▽
　　　　　　　　　passage
　　　H04.69 **Other changes of lacrimal passages**

✓5ᵗʰ **H04.8** **Other disorders of lacrimal system**
　✓6ᵗʰ **H04.81** Granuloma **of lacrimal passages**
　　　　H04.811 **Granuloma of right lacrimal passage**
　　　　H04.812 **Granuloma of left lacrimal passage**
　　　　H04.813 **Granuloma of bilateral lacrimal passages**
　　　　H04.819 **Granuloma of unspecified lacrimal** ▽
　　　　　　　　　passage
　　　H04.89 **Other disorders of lacrimal system**
　H04.9 **Disorder of lacrimal system, unspecified** ▽

✓4ᵗʰ **H05** **Disorders of orbit**
　　　EXCLUDES 1 congenital malformation of orbit (Q10.7)
　✓5ᵗʰ **H05.0** Acute **inflammation** of orbit
　　　H05.00 **Unspecified acute inflammation of orbit** ▽
　　✓6ᵗʰ **H05.01** Cellulitis **of orbit**
　　　　　Abscess of orbit
　　　　H05.011 **Cellulitis of right orbit**
　　　　H05.012 **Cellulitis of left orbit**
　　　　H05.013 **Cellulitis of bilateral orbits**
　　　　H05.019 **Cellulitis of unspecified orbit** ▽
　　✓6ᵗʰ **H05.02** Osteomyelitis **of orbit**
　　　　H05.021 **Osteomyelitis of right orbit**
　　　　H05.022 **Osteomyelitis of left orbit**
　　　　H05.023 **Osteomyelitis of bilateral orbits**
　　　　H05.029 **Osteomyelitis of unspecified orbit** ▽
　　✓6ᵗʰ **H05.03** Periostitis **of orbit**
　　　　H05.031 **Periostitis of right orbit**
　　　　H05.032 **Periostitis of left orbit**
　　　　H05.033 **Periostitis of bilateral orbits**
　　　　H05.039 **Periostitis of unspecified orbit** ▽
　　✓6ᵗʰ **H05.04** Tenonitis **of orbit**
　　　　H05.041 **Tenonitis of right orbit**
　　　　H05.042 **Tenonitis of left orbit**
　　　　H05.043 **Tenonitis of bilateral orbits**
　　　　H05.049 **Tenonitis of unspecified orbit** ▽
　✓5ᵗʰ **H05.1** **Chronic inflammatory disorders of orbit**
　　　H05.10 **Unspecified chronic inflammatory disorders** ▽
　　　　　of orbit
　　✓6ᵗʰ **H05.11** Granuloma **of orbit**
　　　　　Pseudotumor (inflammatory) of orbit
　　　　H05.111 **Granuloma of right orbit**
　　　　H05.112 **Granuloma of left orbit**
　　　　H05.113 **Granuloma of bilateral orbits**

          H05.119   **Granuloma of unspecified orbit** ▽

✓6th   **H05.12**   **Orbital myositis**
          H05.121   **Orbital myositis, right orbit**
          H05.122   **Orbital myositis, left orbit**
          H05.123   **Orbital myositis, bilateral**
          H05.129   **Orbital myositis, unspecified orbit** ▽

✓5th   **H05.2**   **Exophthalmic conditions**
     H05.20   **Unspecified exophthalmos** ▽
   ✓6th   **H05.21**   **Displacement (lateral) of globe**
          H05.211   **Displacement (lateral) of globe, right eye**
          H05.212   **Displacement (lateral) of globe, left eye**
          H05.213   **Displacement (lateral) of globe, bilateral**
          H05.219   **Displacement (lateral) of globe, unspecified eye** ▽
   ✓6th   **H05.22**   **Edema of orbit**
          Orbital congestion
          H05.221   **Edema of right orbit**
          H05.222   **Edema of left orbit**
          H05.223   **Edema of bilateral orbit**
          H05.229   **Edema of unspecified orbit** ▽
   ✓6th   **H05.23**   **Hemorrhage of orbit**
          H05.231   **Hemorrhage of right orbit**
          H05.232   **Hemorrhage of left orbit**
          H05.233   **Hemorrhage of bilateral orbit**
          H05.239   **Hemorrhage of unspecified orbit** ▽
   ✓6th   **H05.24**   **Constant exophthalmos**
          H05.241   **Constant exophthalmos, right eye**
          H05.242   **Constant exophthalmos, left eye**
          H05.243   **Constant exophthalmos, bilateral**
          H05.249   **Constant exophthalmos, unspecified eye** ▽
   ✓6th   **H05.25**   **Intermittent exophthalmos**
          H05.251   **Intermittent exophthalmos, right eye**
          H05.252   **Intermittent exophthalmos, left eye**
          H05.253   **Intermittent exophthalmos, bilateral**
          H05.259   **Intermittent exophthalmos, unspecified eye** ▽
   ✓6th   **H05.26**   **Pulsating exophthalmos**
          H05.261   **Pulsating exophthalmos, right eye**
          H05.262   **Pulsating exophthalmos, left eye**
          H05.263   **Pulsating exophthalmos, bilateral**
          H05.269   **Pulsating exophthalmos, unspecified eye** ▽

✓5th   **H05.3**   **Deformity of orbit**
     EXCLUDES 1   congenital deformity of orbit (Q10.7)
                 hypertelorism (Q75.2)
     H05.30   **Unspecified deformity of orbit** ▽
   ✓6th   **H05.31**   **Atrophy of orbit**
          H05.311   **Atrophy of right orbit**
          H05.312   **Atrophy of left orbit**
          H05.313   **Atrophy of bilateral orbit**
          H05.319   **Atrophy of unspecified orbit** ▽
   ✓6th   **H05.32**   **Deformity of orbit due to bone disease**
          Code also associated bone disease
          H05.321   **Deformity of right orbit due to bone disease**
          H05.322   **Deformity of left orbit due to bone disease**
          H05.323   **Deformity of bilateral orbits due to bone disease**
          H05.329   **Deformity of unspecified orbit due to bone disease** ▽
   ✓6th   **H05.33**   **Deformity of orbit due to trauma or surgery**
          H05.331   **Deformity of right orbit due to trauma or surgery**
          H05.332   **Deformity of left orbit due to trauma or surgery**
          H05.333   **Deformity of bilateral orbits due to trauma or surgery**
          H05.339   **Deformity of unspecified orbit due to trauma or surgery** ▽
   ✓6th   **H05.34**   **Enlargement of orbit**
          H05.341   **Enlargement of right orbit**
          H05.342   **Enlargement of left orbit**
          H05.343   **Enlargement of bilateral orbits**
          H05.349   **Enlargement of unspecified orbit** ▽
   ✓6th   **H05.35**   **Exostosis of orbit**
          H05.351   **Exostosis of right orbit**
          H05.352   **Exostosis of left orbit**
          H05.353   **Exostosis of bilateral orbits**
          H05.359   **Exostosis of unspecified orbit** ▽

✓5th   **H05.4**   **Enophthalmos**
   ✓6th   **H05.40**   **Unspecified enophthalmos**
          H05.401   **Unspecified enophthalmos, right eye** ▽
          H05.402   **Unspecified enophthalmos, left eye** ▽
          H05.403   **Unspecified enophthalmos, bilateral** ▽
          H05.409   **Unspecified enophthalmos, unspecified eye** ▽
   ✓6th   **H05.41**   **Enophthalmos due to atrophy of orbital tissue**
          H05.411   **Enophthalmos due to atrophy of orbital tissue, right eye**
          H05.412   **Enophthalmos due to atrophy of orbital tissue, left eye**
          H05.413   **Enophthalmos due to atrophy of orbital tissue, bilateral**
          H05.419   **Enophthalmos due to atrophy of orbital tissue, unspecified eye** ▽
   ✓6th   **H05.42**   **Enophthalmos due to trauma or surgery**
          H05.421   **Enophthalmos due to trauma or surgery, right eye**
          H05.422   **Enophthalmos due to trauma or surgery, left eye**
          H05.423   **Enophthalmos due to trauma or surgery, bilateral**
          H05.429   **Enophthalmos due to trauma or surgery, unspecified eye** ▽

✓5th   **H05.5**   **Retained (old) foreign body following penetrating wound of orbit**
     Retrobulbar foreign body
     Use additional code to identify the type of retained foreign body (Z18.-)
     EXCLUDES 1   current penetrating wound of orbit (S05.4-)
     EXCLUDES 2   retained foreign body of eyelid (H02.81-)
                 retained intraocular foreign body (H44.6-, H44.7-)
     H05.50   **Retained (old) foreign body following penetrating wound of unspecified orbit** ▽
     H05.51   **Retained (old) foreign body following penetrating wound of right orbit**
     H05.52   **Retained (old) foreign body following penetrating wound of left orbit**
     H05.53   **Retained (old) foreign body following penetrating wound of bilateral orbits**

✓5th   **H05.8**   **Other disorders of orbit**
   ✓6th   **H05.81**   **Cyst of orbit**
          Encephalocele of orbit
          H05.811   **Cyst of right orbit**
          H05.812   **Cyst of left orbit**
          H05.813   **Cyst of bilateral orbits**
          H05.819   **Cyst of unspecified orbit** ▽
   ✓6th   **H05.82**   **Myopathy of extraocular muscles**
          H05.821   **Myopathy of extraocular muscles, right orbit**
          H05.822   **Myopathy of extraocular muscles, left orbit**
          H05.823   **Myopathy of extraocular muscles, bilateral**
          H05.829   **Myopathy of extraocular muscles, unspecified orbit** ▽
     H05.89   **Other disorders of orbit**
     H05.9   **Unspecified disorder of orbit** ▽

Disorders of conjunctiva (H10-H11)

✓4th   **H10**   **Conjunctivitis**
     EXCLUDES 1   keratoconjunctivitis (H16.2-)
   ✓5th   **H10.0**   **Mucopurulent conjunctivitis**
     ✓6th   **H10.01**   **Acute follicular conjunctivitis**
          H10.011   **Acute follicular conjunctivitis, right eye**
          H10.012   **Acute follicular conjunctivitis, left eye**
          H10.013   **Acute follicular conjunctivitis, bilateral**

H10.019   Acute follicular conjunctivitis, unspecified eye ▽

✓6ᵗʰ H10.02   Other mucopurulent conjunctivitis

H10.021   Other mucopurulent conjunctivitis, right eye

H10.022   Other mucopurulent conjunctivitis, left eye

H10.023   Other mucopurulent conjunctivitis, bilateral

H10.029   Other mucopurulent conjunctivitis, unspecified eye ▽

✓5ᵗʰ H10.1   Acute atopic conjunctivitis
Acute papillary conjunctivitis

H10.10   Acute atopic conjunctivitis, unspecified eye ▽

H10.11   Acute atopic conjunctivitis, right eye

H10.12   Acute atopic conjunctivitis, left eye

H10.13   Acute atopic conjunctivitis, bilateral

✓5ᵗʰ H10.2   Other acute conjunctivitis

✓6ᵗʰ H10.21   Acute toxic conjunctivitis
Acute chemical conjunctivitis
Code first (T51-T65) to identify chemical and intent
EXCLUDES 1   burn and corrosion of eye and adnexa (T26.-)

H10.211   Acute toxic conjunctivitis, right eye

H10.212   Acute toxic conjunctivitis, left eye

H10.213   Acute toxic conjunctivitis, bilateral

H10.219   Acute toxic conjunctivitis, unspecified eye ▽

✓6ᵗʰ H10.22   Pseudomembranous conjunctivitis

H10.221   Pseudomembranous conjunctivitis, right eye

H10.222   Pseudomembranous conjunctivitis, left eye

H10.223   Pseudomembranous conjunctivitis, bilateral

H10.229   Pseudomembranous conjunctivitis, unspecified eye ▽

✓6ᵗʰ H10.23   Serous conjunctivitis, except viral
EXCLUDES 1   viral conjunctivitis (B30.-)

H10.231   Serous conjunctivitis, except viral, right eye

H10.232   Serous conjunctivitis, except viral, left eye

H10.233   Serous conjunctivitis, except viral, bilateral

H10.239   Serous conjunctivitis, except viral, unspecified eye ▽

✓5ᵗʰ H10.3   Unspecified acute conjunctivitis
EXCLUDES 1   ophthalmia neonatorum NOS (P39.1)

H10.30   Unspecified acute conjunctivitis, unspecified eye ▽

H10.31   Unspecified acute conjunctivitis, right eye ▽

H10.32   Unspecified acute conjunctivitis, left eye ▽

H10.33   Unspecified acute conjunctivitis, bilateral ▽

✓5ᵗʰ H10.4   Chronic conjunctivitis

✓6ᵗʰ H10.40   Unspecified chronic conjunctivitis

H10.401   Unspecified chronic conjunctivitis, right eye ▽

H10.402   Unspecified chronic conjunctivitis, left eye ▽

H10.403   Unspecified chronic conjunctivitis, bilateral ▽

H10.409   Unspecified chronic conjunctivitis, unspecified eye ▽

✓6ᵗʰ H10.41   Chronic giant papillary conjunctivitis

H10.411   Chronic giant papillary conjunctivitis, right eye

H10.412   Chronic giant papillary conjunctivitis, left eye

H10.413   Chronic giant papillary conjunctivitis, bilateral

H10.419   Chronic giant papillary conjunctivitis, unspecified eye ▽

✓6ᵗʰ H10.42   Simple chronic conjunctivitis

H10.421   Simple chronic conjunctivitis, right eye

H10.422   Simple chronic conjunctivitis, left eye

H10.423   Simple chronic conjunctivitis, bilateral

H10.429   Simple chronic conjunctivitis, unspecified eye ▽

✓6ᵗʰ H10.43   Chronic follicular conjunctivitis

H10.431   Chronic follicular conjunctivitis, right eye

H10.432   Chronic follicular conjunctivitis, left eye

H10.433   Chronic follicular conjunctivitis, bilateral

H10.439   Chronic follicular conjunctivitis, unspecified eye ▽

H10.44   Vernal conjunctivitis
EXCLUDES 1   vernal keratoconjunctivitis with limbar and corneal involvement (H16.26-)

H10.45   Other chronic allergic conjunctivitis

✓5ᵗʰ H10.5   Blepharoconjunctivitis

✓6ᵗʰ H10.50   Unspecified blepharoconjunctivitis

H10.501   Unspecified blepharoconjunctivitis, right eye ▽

H10.502   Unspecified blepharoconjunctivitis, left eye ▽

H10.503   Unspecified blepharoconjunctivitis, bilateral ▽

H10.509   Unspecified blepharoconjunctivitis, unspecified eye ▽

✓6ᵗʰ H10.51   Ligneous conjunctivitis

H10.511   Ligneous conjunctivitis, right eye

H10.512   Ligneous conjunctivitis, left eye

H10.513   Ligneous conjunctivitis, bilateral

H10.519   Ligneous conjunctivitis, unspecified eye ▽

✓6ᵗʰ H10.52   Angular blepharoconjunctivitis

H10.521   Angular blepharoconjunctivitis, right eye

H10.522   Angular blepharoconjunctivitis, left eye

H10.523   Angular blepharoconjunctivitis, bilateral

H10.529   Angular blepharoconjunctivitis, unspecified eye ▽

✓6ᵗʰ H10.53   Contact blepharoconjunctivitis

H10.531   Contact blepharoconjunctivitis, right eye

H10.532   Contact blepharoconjunctivitis, left eye

H10.533   Contact blepharoconjunctivitis, bilateral

H10.539   Contact blepharoconjunctivitis, unspecified eye ▽

✓5ᵗʰ H10.8   Other conjunctivitis

✓6ᵗʰ H10.81   Pingueculitis
EXCLUDES 1   pinguecula (H11.15-)

H10.811   Pingueculitis, right eye

H10.812   Pingueculitis, left eye

H10.813   Pingueculitis, bilateral

H10.819   Pingueculitis, unspecified eye ▽

H10.89   Other conjunctivitis

H10.9   Unspecified conjunctivitis ▽

✓4ᵗʰ H11   Other disorders of conjunctiva
EXCLUDES 1   keratoconjunctivitis (H16.2-)

✓5ᵗʰ H11.0   Pterygium of eye
EXCLUDES 1   pseudopterygium (H11.81-)

✓6ᵗʰ H11.00   Unspecified pterygium of eye

H11.001   Unspecified pterygium of right eye ▽

H11.002   Unspecified pterygium of left eye ▽

H11.003   Unspecified pterygium of eye, bilateral ▽

H11.009   Unspecified pterygium of unspecified eye ▽

Pterygium

Pterygium

✓ Additional Character Req   ✓7ᵗʰ Placeholder Alert   Manifestation   HCC CMS-HCC Condition   ▽ Unspecified Code   ►◄ Revised Text   ● New Code   ▲ Revised Code Title

Chapter 7. Diseases of the Eye and Adnexa

✓6ᵗʰ **H11.01 Amyloid** pterygium
    H11.011 Amyloid pterygium of right eye
    H11.012 Amyloid pterygium of left eye
    H11.013 Amyloid pterygium of eye, bilateral
    H11.019 Amyloid pterygium of unspecified eye ▽

✓6ᵗʰ **H11.02 Central** pterygium of eye
    H11.021 Central pterygium of right eye
    H11.022 Central pterygium of left eye
    H11.023 Central pterygium of eye, bilateral
    H11.029 Central pterygium of unspecified eye ▽

✓6ᵗʰ **H11.03 Double** pterygium of eye
    H11.031 Double pterygium of right eye
    H11.032 Double pterygium of left eye
    H11.033 Double pterygium of eye, bilateral
    H11.039 Double pterygium of unspecified eye ▽

✓6ᵗʰ **H11.04 Peripheral** pterygium of eye, stationary
    H11.041 Peripheral pterygium, stationary, right eye
    H11.042 Peripheral pterygium, stationary, left eye
    H11.043 Peripheral pterygium, stationary, bilateral
    H11.049 Peripheral pterygium, stationary, unspecified eye ▽

✓6ᵗʰ **H11.05 Peripheral** pterygium of eye, progressive
    H11.051 Peripheral pterygium, progressive, right eye
    H11.052 Peripheral pterygium, progressive, left eye
    H11.053 Peripheral pterygium, progressive, bilateral
    H11.059 Peripheral pterygium, progressive, unspecified eye ▽

✓6ᵗʰ **H11.06 Recurrent** pterygium of eye
    H11.061 Recurrent pterygium of right eye
    H11.062 Recurrent pterygium of left eye
    H11.063 Recurrent pterygium of eye, bilateral
    H11.069 Recurrent pterygium of unspecified eye ▽

✓5ᵗʰ **H11.1 Conjunctival degenerations and deposits**
    EXCLUDES 2   pseudopterygium (H11.81)
    H11.10 Unspecified conjunctival degenerations ▽

✓6ᵗʰ **H11.11 Conjunctival** deposits
    H11.111 Conjunctival deposits, right eye
    H11.112 Conjunctival deposits, left eye
    H11.113 Conjunctival deposits, bilateral
    H11.119 Conjunctival deposits, unspecified eye ▽

✓6ᵗʰ **H11.12 Conjunctival** concretions
    H11.121 Conjunctival concretions, right eye
    H11.122 Conjunctival concretions, left eye
    H11.123 Conjunctival concretions, bilateral
    H11.129 Conjunctival concretions, unspecified eye ▽

✓6ᵗʰ **H11.13 Conjunctival** pigmentations
    Conjunctival argyrosis [argyria]
    H11.131 Conjunctival pigmentations, right eye
    H11.132 Conjunctival pigmentations, left eye
    H11.133 Conjunctival pigmentations, bilateral
    H11.139 Conjunctival pigmentations, unspecified eye ▽

✓6ᵗʰ **H11.14 Conjunctival xerosis, unspecified**
    EXCLUDES 1   xerosis of conjunctiva due to vitamin A deficiency (E50.0, E50.1)
    DEF: Abnormal dryness of conjunctiva due to lack of insufficient tears or conjunctival secretions.
    H11.141 Conjunctival xerosis, unspecified, right eye ▽
    H11.142 Conjunctival xerosis , unspecified, left eye ▽
    H11.143 Conjunctival xerosis, unspecified, bilateral ▽
    H11.149 Conjunctival xerosis, unspecified, unspecified eye ▽

✓6ᵗʰ **H11.15 Pinguecula**
    EXCLUDES 1   pingueculitis (H10.81-)
    H11.151 Pinguecula, right eye

Pinguecula

Pinguecula

    H11.152 Pinguecula, left eye
    H11.153 Pinguecula, bilateral
    H11.159 Pinguecula, unspecified eye ▽

✓5ᵗʰ **H11.2 Conjunctival scars**

✓6ᵗʰ **H11.21 Conjunctival** adhesions and strands (localized)
    H11.211 Conjunctival adhesions and strands (localized), right eye
    H11.212 Conjunctival adhesions and strands (localized), left eye
    H11.213 Conjunctival adhesions and strands (localized), bilateral
    H11.219 Conjunctival adhesions and strands (localized), unspecified eye ▽

✓6ᵗʰ **H11.22 Conjunctival** granuloma
    H11.221 Conjunctival granuloma, right eye
    H11.222 Conjunctival granuloma, left eye
    H11.223 Conjunctival granuloma, bilateral
    H11.229 Conjunctival granuloma, unspecified ▽

✓6ᵗʰ **H11.23 Symblepharon**
    H11.231 Symblepharon, right eye
    H11.232 Symblepharon, left eye
    H11.233 Symblepharon, bilateral
    H11.239 Symblepharon, unspecified eye ▽

✓6ᵗʰ **H11.24 Scarring** of conjunctiva
    H11.241 Scarring of conjunctiva, right eye
    H11.242 Scarring of conjunctiva, left eye
    H11.243 Scarring of conjunctiva, bilateral
    H11.249 Scarring of conjunctiva, unspecified eye ▽

✓5ᵗʰ **H11.3 Conjunctival hemorrhage**
    Subconjunctival hemorrhage
    H11.30 Conjunctival hemorrhage, unspecified eye ▽
    H11.31 Conjunctival hemorrhage, right eye
    H11.32 Conjunctival hemorrhage, left eye
    H11.33 Conjunctival hemorrhage, bilateral

✓5ᵗʰ **H11.4 Other conjunctival vascular disorders and cysts**

✓6ᵗʰ **H11.41 Vascular abnormalities** of conjunctiva
    Conjunctival aneurysm
    H11.411 Vascular abnormalities of conjunctiva, right eye
    H11.412 Vascular abnormalities of conjunctiva, left eye
    H11.413 Vascular abnormalities of conjunctiva, bilateral
    H11.419 Vascular abnormalities of conjunctiva, unspecified eye ▽

✓6ᵗʰ **H11.42 Conjunctival** edema
    H11.421 Conjunctival edema, right eye
    H11.422 Conjunctival edema, left eye
    H11.423 Conjunctival edema, bilateral
    H11.429 Conjunctival edema, unspecified eye ▽

✓6ᵗʰ **H11.43 Conjunctival** hyperemia
    H11.431 Conjunctival hyperemia, right eye
    H11.432 Conjunctival hyperemia, left eye
    H11.433 Conjunctival hyperemia, bilateral
    H11.439 Conjunctival hyperemia, unspecified eye ▽

EXCLUDES 1 Not coded here   EXCLUDES 2 Not included here   N Newborn Age: 0   P Pediatric Age: 0-17   M Maternity Age: 12-55   A Adult Age: 15-124

578   ICD-10-CM 2018

✓6ᵗʰ **H11.44 Conjunctival cysts**
     H11.441 Conjunctival cysts, right eye
     H11.442 Conjunctival cysts, left eye
     H11.443 Conjunctival cysts, bilateral
     H11.449 Conjunctival cysts, unspecified eye ▽

✓5ᵗʰ **H11.8 Other specified disorders of conjunctiva**
   ✓6ᵗʰ **H11.81 Pseudopterygium of conjunctiva**
     H11.811 Pseudopterygium of conjunctiva, right eye
     H11.812 Pseudopterygium of conjunctiva, left eye
     H11.813 Pseudopterygium of conjunctiva, bilateral
     H11.819 Pseudopterygium of conjunctiva, unspecified eye ▽
   ✓6ᵗʰ **H11.82 Conjunctivochalasis**
     H11.821 Conjunctivochalasis, right eye
     H11.822 Conjunctivochalasis, left eye
     H11.823 Conjunctivochalasis, bilateral
     H11.829 Conjunctivochalasis, unspecified eye ▽
     H11.89 Other specified disorders of conjunctiva
  H11.9 Unspecified disorder of conjunctiva ▽

Disorders of sclera, cornea, iris and ciliary body (H15-H22)

✓4ᵗʰ **H15 Disorders of sclera**
  ✓5ᵗʰ **H15.0 Scleritis**
   ✓6ᵗʰ **H15.00 Unspecified scleritis**
     H15.001 Unspecified scleritis, right eye ▽
     H15.002 Unspecified scleritis, left eye ▽
     H15.003 Unspecified scleritis, bilateral ▽
     H15.009 Unspecified scleritis, unspecified eye ▽
   ✓6ᵗʰ **H15.01 Anterior scleritis**
     H15.011 Anterior scleritis, right eye
     H15.012 Anterior scleritis, left eye
     H15.013 Anterior scleritis, bilateral
     H15.019 Anterior scleritis, unspecified eye ▽
   ✓6ᵗʰ **H15.02 Brawny scleritis**
     H15.021 Brawny scleritis, right eye
     H15.022 Brawny scleritis, left eye
     H15.023 Brawny scleritis, bilateral
     H15.029 Brawny scleritis, unspecified eye ▽
   ✓6ᵗʰ **H15.03 Posterior scleritis**
     Sclerotenonitis
     H15.031 Posterior scleritis, right eye
     H15.032 Posterior scleritis, left eye
     H15.033 Posterior scleritis, bilateral
     H15.039 Posterior scleritis, unspecified eye ▽
   ✓6ᵗʰ **H15.04 Scleritis with corneal involvement**
     H15.041 Scleritis with corneal involvement, right eye
     H15.042 Scleritis with corneal involvement, left eye
     H15.043 Scleritis with corneal involvement, bilateral
     H15.049 Scleritis with corneal involvement, unspecified eye ▽
   ✓6ᵗʰ **H15.05 Scleromalacia perforans**
     H15.051 Scleromalacia perforans, right eye
     H15.052 Scleromalacia perforans, left eye
     H15.053 Scleromalacia perforans, bilateral
     H15.059 Scleromalacia perforans, unspecified eye ▽
   ✓6ᵗʰ **H15.09 Other scleritis**
     Scleral abscess
     H15.091 Other scleritis, right eye
     H15.092 Other scleritis, left eye
     H15.093 Other scleritis, bilateral
     H15.099 Other scleritis, unspecified eye ▽
  ✓5ᵗʰ **H15.1 Episcleritis**
   ✓6ᵗʰ **H15.10 Unspecified episcleritis**
     H15.101 Unspecified episcleritis, right eye ▽
     H15.102 Unspecified episcleritis, left eye ▽
     H15.103 Unspecified episcleritis, bilateral ▽
     H15.109 Unspecified episcleritis, unspecified eye ▽

   ✓6ᵗʰ **H15.11 Episcleritis periodica fugax**
     H15.111 Episcleritis periodica fugax, right eye
     H15.112 Episcleritis periodica fugax, left eye
     H15.113 Episcleritis periodica fugax, bilateral
     H15.119 Episcleritis periodica fugax, unspecified eye ▽
   ✓6ᵗʰ **H15.12 Nodular episcleritis**
     H15.121 Nodular episcleritis, right eye
     H15.122 Nodular episcleritis, left eye
     H15.123 Nodular episcleritis, bilateral
     H15.129 Nodular episcleritis, unspecified eye ▽
  ✓5ᵗʰ **H15.8 Other disorders of sclera**
     EXCLUDES 2   blue sclera (Q13.5)
          degenerative myopia (H44.2-)
   ✓6ᵗʰ **H15.81 Equatorial staphyloma**
     H15.811 Equatorial staphyloma, right eye
     H15.812 Equatorial staphyloma, left eye
     H15.813 Equatorial staphyloma, bilateral
     H15.819 Equatorial staphyloma, unspecified eye ▽
   ✓6ᵗʰ **H15.82 Localized anterior staphyloma**
     H15.821 Localized anterior staphyloma, right eye
     H15.822 Localized anterior staphyloma, left eye
     H15.823 Localized anterior staphyloma, bilateral
     H15.829 Localized anterior staphyloma, unspecified eye ▽
   ✓6ᵗʰ **H15.83 Staphyloma posticum**
     H15.831 Staphyloma posticum, right eye
     H15.832 Staphyloma posticum, left eye
     H15.833 Staphyloma posticum, bilateral
     H15.839 Staphyloma posticum, unspecified eye ▽
   ✓6ᵗʰ **H15.84 Scleral ectasia**
     H15.841 Scleral ectasia, right eye
     H15.842 Scleral ectasia, left eye
     H15.843 Scleral ectasia, bilateral
     H15.849 Scleral ectasia, unspecified eye ▽
   ✓6ᵗʰ **H15.85 Ring staphyloma**
     H15.851 Ring staphyloma, right eye
     H15.852 Ring staphyloma, left eye
     H15.853 Ring staphyloma, bilateral
     H15.859 Ring staphyloma, unspecified eye ▽
     H15.89 Other disorders of sclera
  H15.9 Unspecified disorder of sclera ▽

✓4ᵗʰ **H16 Keratitis**
  ✓5ᵗʰ **H16.0 Corneal ulcer**
   ✓6ᵗʰ **H16.00 Unspecified corneal ulcer**
     H16.001 Unspecified corneal ulcer, right eye ▽
     H16.002 Unspecified corneal ulcer, left eye ▽
     H16.003 Unspecified corneal ulcer, bilateral ▽
     H16.009 Unspecified corneal ulcer, unspecified eye ▽
   ✓6ᵗʰ **H16.01 Central corneal ulcer**
     H16.011 Central corneal ulcer, right eye
     H16.012 Central corneal ulcer, left eye
     H16.013 Central corneal ulcer, bilateral
     H16.019 Central corneal ulcer, unspecified eye ▽
   ✓6ᵗʰ **H16.02 Ring corneal ulcer**
     H16.021 Ring corneal ulcer, right eye
     H16.022 Ring corneal ulcer, left eye
     H16.023 Ring corneal ulcer, bilateral
     H16.029 Ring corneal ulcer, unspecified eye ▽
   ✓6ᵗʰ **H16.03 Corneal ulcer with hypopyon**
     H16.031 Corneal ulcer with hypopyon, right eye
     H16.032 Corneal ulcer with hypopyon, left eye
     H16.033 Corneal ulcer with hypopyon, bilateral
     H16.039 Corneal ulcer with hypopyon, unspecified eye ▽
   ✓6ᵗʰ **H16.04 Marginal corneal ulcer**
     H16.041 Marginal corneal ulcer, right eye
     H16.042 Marginal corneal ulcer, left eye
     H16.043 Marginal corneal ulcer, bilateral
     H16.049 Marginal corneal ulcer, unspecified eye ▽

☑ Additional Character Req   ✓x7ᵗʰ Placeholder Alert   Manifestation   HCC CMS-HCC Condition   ▽ Unspecified Code   ▶◀ Revised Text   ● New Code   ▲ Revised Code Title

✓6ᵗʰ **H16.05** **Mooren's** corneal ulcer
     H16.051   Mooren's corneal ulcer, **right eye**
     H16.052   Mooren's corneal ulcer, **left eye**
     H16.053   Mooren's corneal ulcer, **bilateral**
     H16.059   Mooren's corneal ulcer, **unspecified eye** ▽

✓6ᵗʰ **H16.06** **Mycotic** corneal ulcer
     H16.061   Mycotic corneal ulcer, **right eye**
     H16.062   Mycotic corneal ulcer, **left eye**
     H16.063   Mycotic corneal ulcer, **bilateral**
     H16.069   Mycotic corneal ulcer, **unspecified eye** ▽

✓6ᵗʰ **H16.07** **Perforated** corneal ulcer
     H16.071   Perforated corneal ulcer, **right eye**
     H16.072   Perforated corneal ulcer, **left eye**
     H16.073   Perforated corneal ulcer, **bilateral**
     H16.079   Perforated corneal ulcer, **unspecified eye** ▽

✓5ᵗʰ **H16.1** **Other and unspecified superficial keratitis without conjunctivitis**

✓6ᵗʰ **H16.10** **Unspecified** superficial keratitis
     H16.101   Unspecified superficial keratitis, **right eye** ▽
     H16.102   Unspecified superficial keratitis, **left eye** ▽
     H16.103   Unspecified superficial keratitis, **bilateral** ▽
     H16.109   Unspecified superficial keratitis, **unspecified eye** ▽

✓6ᵗʰ **H16.11** **Macular** keratitis
     Areolar keratitis
     Nummular keratitis
     Stellate keratitis
     Striate keratitis
     H16.111   Macular keratitis, **right eye**
     H16.112   Macular keratitis, **left eye**
     H16.113   Macular keratitis, **bilateral**
     H16.119   Macular keratitis, **unspecified eye** ▽

✓6ᵗʰ **H16.12** **Filamentary** keratitis
     H16.121   Filamentary keratitis, **right eye**
     H16.122   Filamentary keratitis, **left eye**
     H16.123   Filamentary keratitis, **bilateral**
     H16.129   Filamentary keratitis, **unspecified eye** ▽

✓6ᵗʰ **H16.13** **Photokeratitis**
     Snow blindness
     Welders keratitis
     H16.131   Photokeratitis, **right eye**
     H16.132   Photokeratitis, **left eye**
     H16.133   Photokeratitis, **bilateral**
     H16.139   Photokeratitis, **unspecified eye** ▽

✓6ᵗʰ **H16.14** **Punctate** keratitis
     H16.141   Punctate keratitis, **right eye**
     H16.142   Punctate keratitis, **left eye**
     H16.143   Punctate keratitis, **bilateral**
     H16.149   Punctate keratitis, **unspecified eye** ▽

✓5ᵗʰ **H16.2** **Keratoconjunctivitis**

✓6ᵗʰ **H16.20** **Unspecified** keratoconjunctivitis
     Superficial keratitis with conjunctivitis NOS
     H16.201   Unspecified keratoconjunctivitis, **right eye** ▽
     H16.202   Unspecified keratoconjunctivitis, **left eye** ▽
     H16.203   Unspecified keratoconjunctivitis, **bilateral** ▽
     H16.209   Unspecified keratoconjunctivitis, **unspecified eye** ▽

✓6ᵗʰ **H16.21** **Exposure** keratoconjunctivitis
     H16.211   Exposure keratoconjunctivitis, **right eye**
     H16.212   Exposure keratoconjunctivitis, **left eye**
     H16.213   Exposure keratoconjunctivitis, **bilateral**
     H16.219   Exposure keratoconjunctivitis, **unspecified eye**

✓6ᵗʰ **H16.22** **Keratoconjunctivitis sicca, not specified as Sjögren's**
     EXCLUDES 1   *Sjögren's syndrome (M35.01)*
     H16.221   Keratoconjunctivitis sicca, not specified as Sjögren's, **right eye**

H16.222   Keratoconjunctivitis sicca, not specified as Sjögren's, **left eye**
H16.223   Keratoconjunctivitis sicca, not specified as Sjögren's, **bilateral**
H16.229   Keratoconjunctivitis sicca, not specified as Sjögren's, **unspecified eye** ▽

✓6ᵗʰ **H16.23** **Neurotrophic** keratoconjunctivitis
     H16.231   Neurotrophic keratoconjunctivitis, **right eye**
     H16.232   Neurotrophic keratoconjunctivitis, **left eye**
     H16.233   Neurotrophic keratoconjunctivitis, **bilateral**
     H16.239   Neurotrophic keratoconjunctivitis, **unspecified eye** ▽

✓6ᵗʰ **H16.24** **Ophthalmia nodosa**
     H16.241   Ophthalmia nodosa, **right eye**
     H16.242   Ophthalmia nodosa, **left eye**
     H16.243   Ophthalmia nodosa, **bilateral**
     H16.249   Ophthalmia nodosa, **unspecified eye** ▽

✓6ᵗʰ **H16.25** **Phlyctenular** keratoconjunctivitis
     H16.251   Phlyctenular keratoconjunctivitis, **right eye**
     H16.252   Phlyctenular keratoconjunctivitis, **left eye**
     H16.253   Phlyctenular keratoconjunctivitis, **bilateral**
     H16.259   Phlyctenular keratoconjunctivitis, **unspecified eye** ▽

✓6ᵗʰ **H16.26** **Vernal keratoconjunctivitis, with limbar and corneal involvement**
     EXCLUDES 1   *vernal conjunctivitis without limbar and corneal involvement (H10.44)*
     H16.261   Vernal keratoconjunctivitis, with limbar and corneal involvement, **right eye**
     H16.262   Vernal keratoconjunctivitis, with limbar and corneal involvement, **left eye**
     H16.263   Vernal keratoconjunctivitis, with limbar and corneal involvement, **bilateral**
     H16.269   Vernal keratoconjunctivitis, with limbar and corneal involvement, **unspecified eye** ▽

✓6ᵗʰ **H16.29** **Other keratoconjunctivitis**
     H16.291   Other keratoconjunctivitis, **right eye**
     H16.292   Other keratoconjunctivitis, **left eye**
     H16.293   Other keratoconjunctivitis, **bilateral**
     H16.299   Other keratoconjunctivitis, **unspecified eye** ▽

✓5ᵗʰ **H16.3** **Interstitial and deep keratitis**

✓6ᵗʰ **H16.30** **Unspecified** interstitial keratitis
     H16.301   Unspecified interstitial keratitis, **right eye** ▽
     H16.302   Unspecified interstitial keratitis, **left eye** ▽
     H16.303   Unspecified interstitial keratitis, **bilateral** ▽
     H16.309   Unspecified interstitial keratitis, **unspecified eye** ▽

✓6ᵗʰ **H16.31** **Corneal abscess**
     H16.311   Corneal abscess, **right eye**
     H16.312   Corneal abscess, **left eye**
     H16.313   Corneal abscess, **bilateral**
     H16.319   Corneal abscess, **unspecified eye** ▽

✓6ᵗʰ **H16.32** **Diffuse interstitial keratitis**
     Cogan's syndrome
     H16.321   Diffuse interstitial keratitis, **right eye**
     H16.322   Diffuse interstitial keratitis, **left eye**
     H16.323   Diffuse interstitial keratitis, **bilateral**
     H16.329   Diffuse interstitial keratitis, **unspecified eye** ▽

✓6ᵗʰ **H16.33** **Sclerosing keratitis**
     H16.331   Sclerosing keratitis, **right eye**
     H16.332   Sclerosing keratitis, **left eye**
     H16.333   Sclerosing keratitis, **bilateral**
     H16.339   Sclerosing keratitis, **unspecified eye** ▽

✓6ᵗʰ **H16.39** **Other interstitial and deep keratitis**
- **H16.391** Other interstitial and deep keratitis, **right eye**
- **H16.392** Other interstitial and deep keratitis, **left eye**
- **H16.393** Other interstitial and deep keratitis, **bilateral**
- **H16.399** Other interstitial and deep keratitis, **unspecified eye** ▽

✓5ᵗʰ **H16.4** **Corneal neovascularization**

✓6ᵗʰ **H16.40** **Unspecified corneal neovascularization**
- **H16.401** Unspecified corneal neovascularization, **right eye** ▽
- **H16.402** Unspecified corneal neovascularization, **left eye** ▽
- **H16.403** Unspecified corneal neovascularization, **bilateral** ▽
- **H16.409** Unspecified corneal neovascularization, **unspecified eye** ▽

✓6ᵗʰ **H16.41** **Ghost vessels (corneal)**
- **H16.411** Ghost vessels (corneal), **right eye**
- **H16.412** Ghost vessels (corneal), **left eye**
- **H16.413** Ghost vessels (corneal), **bilateral**
- **H16.419** Ghost vessels (corneal), **unspecified eye** ▽

✓6ᵗʰ **H16.42** **Pannus (corneal)**
- **H16.421** Pannus (corneal), **right eye**
- **H16.422** Pannus (corneal), **left eye**
- **H16.423** Pannus (corneal), **bilateral**
- **H16.429** Pannus (corneal), **unspecified eye** ▽

✓6ᵗʰ **H16.43** **Localized vascularization of cornea**
- **H16.431** Localized vascularization of cornea, **right eye**
- **H16.432** Localized vascularization of cornea, **left eye**
- **H16.433** Localized vascularization of cornea, **bilateral**
- **H16.439** Localized vascularization of cornea, **unspecified eye** ▽

✓6ᵗʰ **H16.44** **Deep vascularization of cornea**
- **H16.441** Deep vascularization of cornea, **right eye**
- **H16.442** Deep vascularization of cornea, **left eye**
- **H16.443** Deep vascularization of cornea, **bilateral**
- **H16.449** Deep vascularization of cornea, **unspecified eye** ▽

H16.8 **Other keratitis**

H16.9 **Unspecified keratitis** ▽

✓4ᵗʰ **H17** **Corneal scars and opacities**

✓5ᵗʰ **H17.0** **Adherent leukoma**
- **H17.00** Adherent leukoma, **unspecified eye** ▽
- **H17.01** Adherent leukoma, **right eye**
- **H17.02** Adherent leukoma, **left eye**
- **H17.03** Adherent leukoma, **bilateral**

✓5ᵗʰ **H17.1** **Central corneal opacity**
- **H17.10** Central corneal opacity, **unspecified eye** ▽
- **H17.11** Central corneal opacity, **right eye**
- **H17.12** Central corneal opacity, **left eye**
- **H17.13** Central corneal opacity, **bilateral**

✓5ᵗʰ **H17.8** **Other corneal scars and opacities**

✓6ᵗʰ **H17.81** **Minor opacity of cornea**
Corneal nebula
- **H17.811** Minor opacity of cornea, **right eye**
- **H17.812** Minor opacity of cornea, **left eye**
- **H17.813** Minor opacity of cornea, **bilateral**
- **H17.819** Minor opacity of cornea, **unspecified eye** ▽

✓6ᵗʰ **H17.82** **Peripheral opacity of cornea**
- **H17.821** Peripheral opacity of cornea, **right eye**
- **H17.822** Peripheral opacity of cornea, **left eye**
- **H17.823** Peripheral opacity of cornea, **bilateral**
- **H17.829** Peripheral opacity of cornea, **unspecified eye** ▽

H17.89 **Other corneal scars and opacities**

H17.9 **Unspecified corneal scar and opacity** ▽

✓4ᵗʰ **H18** **Other disorders of cornea**

✓5ᵗʰ **H18.0** **Corneal pigmentations and deposits**

✓6ᵗʰ **H18.00** **Unspecified corneal deposit**
- **H18.001** Unspecified corneal deposit, **right eye** ▽
- **H18.002** Unspecified corneal deposit, **left eye** ▽
- **H18.003** Unspecified corneal deposit, **bilateral** ▽
- **H18.009** Unspecified corneal deposit, **unspecified eye** ▽

✓6ᵗʰ **H18.01** **Anterior corneal pigmentations**
Staehli's line
- **H18.011** Anterior corneal pigmentations, **right eye**
- **H18.012** Anterior corneal pigmentations, **left eye**
- **H18.013** Anterior corneal pigmentations, **bilateral**
- **H18.019** Anterior corneal pigmentations, **unspecified eye** ▽

✓6ᵗʰ **H18.02** **Argentous corneal deposits**
- **H18.021** Argentous corneal deposits, **right eye**
- **H18.022** Argentous corneal deposits, **left eye**
- **H18.023** Argentous corneal deposits, **bilateral**
- **H18.029** Argentous corneal deposits, **unspecified eye** ▽

✓6ᵗʰ **H18.03** **Corneal deposits in metabolic disorders**
Code also associated metabolic disorder
- **H18.031** Corneal deposits in metabolic disorders, **right eye**
- **H18.032** Corneal deposits in metabolic disorders, **left eye**
- **H18.033** Corneal deposits in metabolic disorders, **bilateral**
- **H18.039** Corneal deposits in metabolic disorders, **unspecified eye** ▽

✓6ᵗʰ **H18.04** **Kayser-Fleischer ring**
Code also associated Wilson's disease (E83.01)
- **H18.041** Kayser-Fleischer ring, **right eye**
- **H18.042** Kayser-Fleischer ring, **left eye**
- **H18.043** Kayser-Fleischer ring, **bilateral**
- **H18.049** Kayser-Fleischer ring, **unspecified eye** ▽

✓6ᵗʰ **H18.05** **Posterior corneal pigmentations**
Krukenberg's spindle
- **H18.051** Posterior corneal pigmentations, **right eye**
- **H18.052** Posterior corneal pigmentations, **left eye**
- **H18.053** Posterior corneal pigmentations, **bilateral**
- **H18.059** Posterior corneal pigmentations, **unspecified eye** ▽

✓6ᵗʰ **H18.06** **Stromal corneal pigmentations**
Hematocornea
- **H18.061** Stromal corneal pigmentations, **right eye**
- **H18.062** Stromal corneal pigmentations, **left eye**
- **H18.063** Stromal corneal pigmentations, **bilateral**
- **H18.069** Stromal corneal pigmentations, **unspecified eye** ▽

✓5ᵗʰ **H18.1** **Bullous keratopathy**
DEF: Corneal swelling due to damaged corneal endothelium; characterized by recurring, rupturing epithelial "blisters"; occurs in glaucoma, iridocyclitis and Fuchs dystrophy.
- **H18.10** Bullous keratopathy, **unspecified eye** ▽
- **H18.11** Bullous keratopathy, **right eye**
- **H18.12** Bullous keratopathy, **left eye**
- **H18.13** Bullous keratopathy, **bilateral**

✓5ᵗʰ **H18.2** **Other and unspecified corneal edema**
- **H18.20** Unspecified corneal edema ▽

✓6ᵗʰ **H18.21** **Corneal edema secondary to contact lens**
EXCLUDES 2 other corneal disorders due to contact lens (H18.82-)
- **H18.211** Corneal edema secondary to contact lens, **right eye**
- **H18.212** Corneal edema secondary to contact lens, **left eye**
- **H18.213** Corneal edema secondary to contact lens, **bilateral**
- **H18.219** Corneal edema secondary to contact lens, **unspecified eye** ▽

| ✓ Additional Character Req | ✓7ᵗʰ Placeholder Alert | Manifestation | HCC CMS-HCC Condition | ▽ Unspecified Code | ▶◀ Revised Text | ● New Code | ▲ Revised Code Title |

ICD-10-CM 2018   581

√6ᵗʰ **H18.22** **Idiopathic** corneal edema
    H18.221 **Idiopathic** corneal edema, **right** eye
    H18.222 **Idiopathic** corneal edema, **left** eye
    H18.223 **Idiopathic** corneal edema, **bilateral**
    H18.229 **Idiopathic** corneal edema, **unspecified** ▽
         eye

√6ᵗʰ **H18.23** **Secondary** corneal edema
    H18.231 **Secondary** corneal edema, **right** eye
    H18.232 **Secondary** corneal edema, **left** eye
    H18.233 **Secondary** corneal edema, **bilateral**
    H18.239 **Secondary** corneal edema, **unspecified** ▽
         eye

√5ᵗʰ **H18.3** **Changes of corneal membranes**
    H18.30 **Unspecified corneal membrane change** ▽

√6ᵗʰ **H18.31** **Folds and rupture in** Bowman's membrane
    H18.311 **Folds and rupture in Bowman's membrane, right** eye
    H18.312 **Folds and rupture in Bowman's membrane, left** eye
    H18.313 **Folds and rupture in Bowman's membrane, bilateral**
    H18.319 **Folds and rupture in Bowman's** ▽
         membrane, unspecified eye

√6ᵗʰ **H18.32** **Folds in** Descemet's membrane
    H18.321 **Folds in Descemet's membrane, right** eye
    H18.322 **Folds in Descemet's membrane, left** eye
    H18.323 **Folds in Descemet's membrane, bilateral**
    H18.329 **Folds in Descemet's membrane,** ▽
         unspecified eye

√6ᵗʰ **H18.33** **Rupture** in Descemet's membrane
    H18.331 **Rupture in Descemet's membrane, right** eye
    H18.332 **Rupture in Descemet's membrane, left** eye
    H18.333 **Rupture in Descemet's membrane, bilateral**
    H18.339 **Rupture in Descemet's membrane,** ▽
         unspecified eye

√5ᵗʰ **H18.4** **Corneal degeneration**
    EXCLUDES 1   *Mooren's ulcer (H16.0-)*
              recurrent erosion of cornea (H18.83-)
    H18.40 **Unspecified corneal degeneration** ▽

√6ᵗʰ **H18.41** **Arcus senilis**
         Senile corneal changes
    H18.411 **Arcus senilis, right** eye
    H18.412 **Arcus senilis, left** eye
    H18.413 **Arcus senilis, bilateral**
    H18.419 **Arcus senilis, unspecified** eye ▽

√6ᵗʰ **H18.42** **Band** keratopathy
    H18.421 **Band keratopathy, right** eye
    H18.422 **Band keratopathy, left** eye
    H18.423 **Band keratopathy, bilateral**
    H18.429 **Band keratopathy, unspecified** eye ▽

    H18.43 **Other calcerous corneal degeneration**

√6ᵗʰ **H18.44** **Keratomalacia**
    EXCLUDES 1   *keratomalacia due to vitamin A deficiency (E50.4)*
    H18.441 **Keratomalacia, right** eye
    H18.442 **Keratomalacia, left** eye
    H18.443 **Keratomalacia, bilateral**
    H18.449 **Keratomalacia, unspecified** eye ▽

√6ᵗʰ **H18.45** **Nodular** corneal degeneration
    H18.451 **Nodular corneal degeneration, right** eye
    H18.452 **Nodular corneal degeneration, left** eye
    H18.453 **Nodular corneal degeneration, bilateral**
    H18.459 **Nodular corneal degeneration,** ▽
         unspecified eye

√6ᵗʰ **H18.46** **Peripheral** corneal degeneration
    H18.461 **Peripheral corneal degeneration, right** eye
    H18.462 **Peripheral corneal degeneration, left** eye
    H18.463 **Peripheral corneal degeneration, bilateral**
    H18.469 **Peripheral corneal degeneration,** ▽
         unspecified eye

    H18.49 **Other corneal degeneration**

√5ᵗʰ **H18.5** **Hereditary corneal dystrophies**
    H18.50 **Unspecified hereditary corneal dystrophies** ▽
    H18.51 **Endothelial corneal dystrophy**
         Fuchs' dystrophy
    H18.52 **Epithelial (juvenile) corneal dystrophy**
    H18.53 **Granular corneal dystrophy**
    H18.54 **Lattice corneal dystrophy**
    H18.55 **Macular corneal dystrophy**
    H18.59 **Other hereditary corneal dystrophies**

√5ᵗʰ **H18.6** **Keratoconus**
√6ᵗʰ **H18.60** **Keratoconus, unspecified**
    H18.601 **Keratoconus, unspecified, right** eye ▽
    H18.602 **Keratoconus, unspecified, left** eye ▽
    H18.603 **Keratoconus, unspecified, bilateral** ▽
    H18.609 **Keratoconus, unspecified,** ▽
         unspecified eye

√6ᵗʰ **H18.61** **Keratoconus, stable**
    H18.611 **Keratoconus, stable, right** eye
    H18.612 **Keratoconus, stable, left** eye
    H18.613 **Keratoconus, stable, bilateral**
    H18.619 **Keratoconus, stable, unspecified** eye ▽

√6ᵗʰ **H18.62** **Keratoconus, unstable**
         Acute hydrops
    H18.621 **Keratoconus, unstable, right** eye
    H18.622 **Keratoconus, unstable, left** eye
    H18.623 **Keratoconus, unstable, bilateral**
    H18.629 **Keratoconus, unstable, unspecified** eye ▽

√5ᵗʰ **H18.7** **Other and unspecified corneal deformities**
    EXCLUDES 1   *congenital malformations of cornea (Q13.3-Q13.4)*
    H18.70 **Unspecified corneal deformity** ▽

√6ᵗʰ **H18.71** **Corneal ectasia**
    H18.711 **Corneal ectasia, right** eye
    H18.712 **Corneal ectasia, left** eye
    H18.713 **Corneal ectasia, bilateral**
    H18.719 **Corneal ectasia, unspecified** eye ▽

√6ᵗʰ **H18.72** **Corneal staphyloma**
    H18.721 **Corneal staphyloma, right** eye
    H18.722 **Corneal staphyloma, left** eye
    H18.723 **Corneal staphyloma, bilateral**
    H18.729 **Corneal staphyloma, unspecified** eye ▽

√6ᵗʰ **H18.73** **Descemetocele**
    H18.731 **Descemetocele, right** eye
    H18.732 **Descemetocele, left** eye
    H18.733 **Descemetocele, bilateral**
    H18.739 **Descemetocele, unspecified** eye ▽

√6ᵗʰ **H18.79** **Other corneal deformities**
    H18.791 **Other corneal deformities, right** eye
    H18.792 **Other corneal deformities, left** eye
    H18.793 **Other corneal deformities, bilateral**
    H18.799 **Other corneal deformities,** ▽
         unspecified eye

√5ᵗʰ **H18.8** **Other specified disorders of cornea**
√6ᵗʰ **H18.81** **Anesthesia and hypoesthesia of cornea**
    H18.811 **Anesthesia and hypoesthesia of cornea, right** eye
    H18.812 **Anesthesia and hypoesthesia of cornea, left** eye
    H18.813 **Anesthesia and hypoesthesia of cornea, bilateral**
    H18.819 **Anesthesia and hypoesthesia of** ▽
         cornea, unspecified eye

√6ᵗʰ **H18.82** **Corneal disorder due to contact lens**
    EXCLUDES 2   *corneal edema due to contact lens (H18.21-)*
    H18.821 **Corneal disorder due to contact lens, right** eye
    H18.822 **Corneal disorder due to contact lens, left** eye
    H18.823 **Corneal disorder due to contact lens, bilateral**
    H18.829 **Corneal disorder due to contact lens,** ▽
         unspecified eye

EXCLUDES 1 Not coded here   **EXCLUDES 2** Not included here   Ⓝ Newborn Age: 0   Ⓟ Pediatric Age: 0-17   Ⓜ Maternity Age: 12-55   Ⓐ Adult Age: 15-124

582   ICD-10-CM 2018

✓6th **H18.83** **Recurrent erosion of cornea**
     H18.831   **Recurrent erosion of cornea, right eye**
     H18.832   **Recurrent erosion of cornea, left eye**
     H18.833   **Recurrent erosion of cornea, bilateral**
     H18.839   **Recurrent erosion of cornea, unspecified eye** ▽

✓6th **H18.89** **Other specified disorders of cornea**
     H18.891   **Other specified disorders of cornea, right eye**
     H18.892   **Other specified disorders of cornea, left eye**
     H18.893   **Other specified disorders of cornea, bilateral**
     H18.899   **Other specified disorders of cornea, unspecified eye** ▽

H18.9   **Unspecified disorder of cornea** ▽

✓4th **H20**   **Iridocyclitis**

✓5th **H20.0**   **Acute and subacute iridocyclitis**
     Acute anterior uveitis
     Acute cyclitis
     Acute iritis
     Subacute anterior uveitis
     Subacute cyclitis
     Subacute iritis
     EXCLUDES 1   *iridocyclitis, iritis, uveitis (due to) (in) diabetes mellitus (E08-E13 with .39)*
                 iridocyclitis, iritis, uveitis (due to) (in) diphtheria (A36.89)
                 iridocyclitis, iritis, uveitis (due to) (in) gonococcal (A54.32)
                 iridocyclitis, iritis, uveitis (due to) (in) herpes (simplex) (B00.51)
                 iridocyclitis, iritis, uveitis (due to) (in) herpes zoster (B02.32)
                 iridocyclitis, iritis, uveitis (due to) (in) late congenital syphilis (A50.39)
                 iridocyclitis, iritis, uveitis (due to) (in) late syphilis (A52.71)
                 iridocyclitis, iritis, uveitis (due to) (in) sarcoidosis (D86.83)
                 iridocyclitis, iritis, uveitis (due to) (in) syphilis (A51.43)
                 iridocyclitis, iritis, uveitis (due to) (in) toxoplasmosis (B58.09)
                 iridocyclitis, iritis, uveitis (due to) (in) tuberculosis (A18.54)

     H20.00   **Unspecified acute and subacute iridocyclitis** ▽

✓6th **H20.01**   **Primary iridocyclitis**
     H20.011   **Primary iridocyclitis, right eye**
     H20.012   **Primary iridocyclitis, left eye**
     H20.013   **Primary iridocyclitis, bilateral**
     H20.019   **Primary iridocyclitis, unspecified eye** ▽

✓6th **H20.02**   **Recurrent acute iridocyclitis**
     H20.021   **Recurrent acute iridocyclitis, right eye**
     H20.022   **Recurrent acute iridocyclitis, left eye**
     H20.023   **Recurrent acute iridocyclitis, bilateral**
     H20.029   **Recurrent acute iridocyclitis, unspecified eye** ▽

✓6th **H20.03**   **Secondary infectious iridocyclitis**
     H20.031   **Secondary infectious iridocyclitis, right eye**
     H20.032   **Secondary infectious iridocyclitis, left eye**
     H20.033   **Secondary infectious iridocyclitis, bilateral**
     H20.039   **Secondary infectious iridocyclitis, unspecified eye** ▽

✓6th **H20.04**   **Secondary noninfectious iridocyclitis**
     H20.041   **Secondary noninfectious iridocyclitis, right eye**
     H20.042   **Secondary noninfectious iridocyclitis, left eye**
     H20.043   **Secondary noninfectious iridocyclitis, bilateral**
     H20.049   **Secondary noninfectious iridocyclitis, unspecified eye** ▽

✓6th **H20.05**   **Hypopyon**
     H20.051   **Hypopyon, right eye**
     H20.052   **Hypopyon, left eye**
     H20.053   **Hypopyon, bilateral**

     H20.059   **Hypopyon, unspecified eye**

✓5th **H20.1**   **Chronic iridocyclitis**
     Use additional code for any associated cataract (H26.21-)
     EXCLUDES 2   *posterior cyclitis (H30.2-)*
     H20.10   **Chronic iridocyclitis, unspecified eye** ▽
     H20.11   **Chronic iridocyclitis, right eye**
     H20.12   **Chronic iridocyclitis, left eye**
     H20.13   **Chronic iridocyclitis, bilateral**

✓5th **H20.2**   **Lens-induced iridocyclitis**
     H20.20   **Lens-induced iridocyclitis, unspecified eye** ▽
     H20.21   **Lens-induced iridocyclitis, right eye**
     H20.22   **Lens-induced iridocyclitis, left eye**
     H20.23   **Lens-induced iridocyclitis, bilateral**

✓5th **H20.8**   **Other iridocyclitis**
     EXCLUDES 2   *glaucomatocyclitis crises (H40.4-)*
                posterior cyclitis (H30.2-)
                sympathetic uveitis (H44.13-)

✓6th **H20.81**   **Fuchs' heterochromic cyclitis**
     H20.811   **Fuchs' heterochromic cyclitis, right eye**
     H20.812   **Fuchs' heterochromic cyclitis, left eye**
     H20.813   **Fuchs' heterochromic cyclitis, bilateral**
     H20.819   **Fuchs' heterochromic cyclitis, unspecified eye** ▽

✓6th **H20.82**   **Vogt-Koyanagi syndrome**
     H20.821   **Vogt-Koyanagi syndrome, right eye**
     H20.822   **Vogt-Koyanagi syndrome, left eye**
     H20.823   **Vogt-Koyanagi syndrome, bilateral**
     H20.829   **Vogt-Koyanagi syndrome, unspecified eye** ▽

H20.9   **Unspecified iridocyclitis** ▽
     Uveitis NOS

✓4th **H21**   **Other disorders of iris and ciliary body**
     EXCLUDES 2   *sympathetic uveitis (H44.1-)*

✓5th **H21.0**   **Hyphema**
     EXCLUDES 1   *traumatic hyphema (S05.1-)*
     H21.00   **Hyphema, unspecified eye** ▽
     H21.01   **Hyphema, right eye**
     H21.02   **Hyphema, left eye**
     H21.03   **Hyphema, bilateral**

✓5th **H21.1**   **Other vascular disorders of iris and ciliary body**
     Neovascularization of iris or ciliary body
     Rubeosis iridis
     Rubeosis of iris

✓6th **H21.1X**   **Other vascular disorders of iris and ciliary body**
     H21.1X1   **Other vascular disorders of iris and ciliary body, right eye**
     H21.1X2   **Other vascular disorders of iris and ciliary body, left eye**
     H21.1X3   **Other vascular disorders of iris and ciliary body, bilateral**
     H21.1X9   **Other vascular disorders of iris and ciliary body, unspecified eye** ▽

✓5th **H21.2**   **Degeneration of iris and ciliary body**
✓6th **H21.21**   **Degeneration of chamber angle**
     H21.211   **Degeneration of chamber angle, right eye**
     H21.212   **Degeneration of chamber angle, left eye**
     H21.213   **Degeneration of chamber angle, bilateral**
     H21.219   **Degeneration of chamber angle, unspecified eye** ▽

Hyphema

Iris
Cornea
Hyphema

Chapter 7. Diseases of the Eye and Adnexa

H21.22–H21.559

✓6th **H21.22** **Degeneration of ciliary body**
- H21.221 Degeneration of ciliary body, right eye
- H21.222 Degeneration of ciliary body, left eye
- H21.223 Degeneration of ciliary body, bilateral
- H21.229 Degeneration of ciliary body, unspecified eye ▽

✓6th **H21.23** **Degeneration of iris (pigmentary)**
Translucency of iris
- H21.231 Degeneration of iris (pigmentary), right eye
- H21.232 Degeneration of iris (pigmentary), left eye
- H21.233 Degeneration of iris (pigmentary), bilateral
- H21.239 Degeneration of iris (pigmentary), unspecified eye ▽

✓6th **H21.24** **Degeneration of pupillary margin**
- H21.241 Degeneration of pupillary margin, right eye
- H21.242 Degeneration of pupillary margin, left eye
- H21.243 Degeneration of pupillary margin, bilateral
- H21.249 Degeneration of pupillary margin, unspecified eye ▽

✓6th **H21.25** **Iridoschisis**
- H21.251 Iridoschisis, right eye
- H21.252 Iridoschisis, left eye
- H21.253 Iridoschisis, bilateral
- H21.259 Iridoschisis, unspecified eye ▽

✓6th **H21.26** **Iris atrophy (essential) (progressive)**
- H21.261 Iris atrophy (essential) (progressive), right eye
- H21.262 Iris atrophy (essential) (progressive), left eye
- H21.263 Iris atrophy (essential) (progressive), bilateral
- H21.269 Iris atrophy (essential) (progressive), unspecified eye ▽

✓6th **H21.27** **Miotic pupillary cyst**
- H21.271 Miotic pupillary cyst, right eye
- H21.272 Miotic pupillary cyst, left eye
- H21.273 Miotic pupillary cyst, bilateral
- H21.279 Miotic pupillary cyst, unspecified eye ▽

H21.29 **Other iris atrophy**

✓5th **H21.3** **Cyst of iris, ciliary body and anterior chamber**
EXCLUDES 2   miotic pupillary cyst (H21.27-)

✓6th **H21.30** **Idiopathic cysts of iris, ciliary body or anterior chamber**
Cyst of iris, ciliary body or anterior chamber NOS
- H21.301 Idiopathic cysts of iris, ciliary body or anterior chamber, right eye
- H21.302 Idiopathic cysts of iris, ciliary body or anterior chamber, left eye
- H21.303 Idiopathic cysts of iris, ciliary body or anterior chamber, bilateral
- H21.309 Idiopathic cysts of iris, ciliary body or anterior chamber, unspecified eye ▽

✓6th **H21.31** **Exudative cysts of iris or anterior chamber**
- H21.311 Exudative cysts of iris or anterior chamber, right eye
- H21.312 Exudative cysts of iris or anterior chamber, left eye
- H21.313 Exudative cysts of iris or anterior chamber, bilateral
- H21.319 Exudative cysts of iris or anterior chamber, unspecified eye ▽

✓6th **H21.32** **Implantation cysts of iris, ciliary body or anterior chamber**
- H21.321 Implantation cysts of iris, ciliary body or anterior chamber, right eye
- H21.322 Implantation cysts of iris, ciliary body or anterior chamber, left eye
- H21.323 Implantation cysts of iris, ciliary body or anterior chamber, bilateral
- H21.329 Implantation cysts of iris, ciliary body or anterior chamber, unspecified eye ▽

✓6th **H21.33** **Parasitic cyst of iris, ciliary body or anterior chamber**
- H21.331 Parasitic cyst of iris, ciliary body or anterior chamber, right eye
- H21.332 Parasitic cyst of iris, ciliary body or anterior chamber, left eye
- H21.333 Parasitic cyst of iris, ciliary body or anterior chamber, bilateral
- H21.339 Parasitic cyst of iris, ciliary body or anterior chamber, unspecified eye ▽

✓6th **H21.34** **Primary cyst of pars plana**
- H21.341 Primary cyst of pars plana, right eye
- H21.342 Primary cyst of pars plana, left eye
- H21.343 Primary cyst of pars plana, bilateral
- H21.349 Primary cyst of pars plana, unspecified eye ▽

✓6th **H21.35** **Exudative cyst of pars plana**
DEF: Protein, fatty-filled bullous elevation of nonpigmented outermost ciliary epithelium of pars plana; due to fluid leak from blood vessels.
- H21.351 Exudative cyst of pars plana, right eye
- H21.352 Exudative cyst of pars plana, left eye
- H21.353 Exudative cyst of pars plana, bilateral
- H21.359 Exudative cyst of pars plana, unspecified eye ▽

✓5th **H21.4** **Pupillary membranes**
Iris bombé
Pupillary occlusion
Pupillary seclusion
EXCLUDES 1   congenital pupillary membranes (Q13.8)
- H21.40 Pupillary membranes, unspecified eye ▽
- H21.41 Pupillary membranes, right eye
- H21.42 Pupillary membranes, left eye
- H21.43 Pupillary membranes, bilateral

✓5th **H21.5** **Other and unspecified adhesions and disruptions of iris and ciliary body**
EXCLUDES 1   corectopia (Q13.2)

✓6th **H21.50** **Unspecified adhesions of iris**
Synechia (iris) NOS
- H21.501 Unspecified adhesions of iris, right eye ▽
- H21.502 Unspecified adhesions of iris, left eye ▽
- H21.503 Unspecified adhesions of iris, bilateral ▽
- H21.509 Unspecified adhesions of iris and ciliary body, unspecified eye ▽

✓6th **H21.51** **Anterior synechiae (iris)**
- H21.511 Anterior synechiae (iris), right eye
- H21.512 Anterior synechiae (iris), left eye
- H21.513 Anterior synechiae (iris), bilateral
- H21.519 Anterior synechiae (iris), unspecified eye ▽

✓6th **H21.52** **Goniosynechiae**
- H21.521 Goniosynechiae, right eye
- H21.522 Goniosynechiae, left eye
- H21.523 Goniosynechiae, bilateral
- H21.529 Goniosynechiae, unspecified eye ▽

✓6th **H21.53** **Iridodialysis**
- H21.531 Iridodialysis, right eye
- H21.532 Iridodialysis, left eye
- H21.533 Iridodialysis, bilateral
- H21.539 Iridodialysis, unspecified eye ▽

✓6th **H21.54** **Posterior synechiae (iris)**
- H21.541 Posterior synechiae (iris), right eye
- H21.542 Posterior synechiae (iris), left eye
- H21.543 Posterior synechiae (iris), bilateral
- H21.549 Posterior synechiae (iris), unspecified eye ▽

✓6th **H21.55** **Recession of chamber angle**
- H21.551 Recession of chamber angle, right eye
- H21.552 Recession of chamber angle, left eye
- H21.553 Recession of chamber angle, bilateral
- H21.559 Recession of chamber angle, unspecified eye ▽

EXCLUDES 1 Not coded here   EXCLUDES 2 Not included here   N Newborn Age: 0   P Pediatric Age: 0-17   M Maternity Age: 12-55   A Adult Age: 15-124

584   ICD-10-CM 2018

√6ᵗʰ H21.56 Pupillary abnormalities
Deformed pupil
Ectopic pupil
Rupture of sphincter, pupil
EXCLUDES 1 congenital deformity of pupil (Q13.2-)

     H21.561 Pupillary abnormality, **right eye**
     H21.562 Pupillary abnormality, **left eye**
     H21.563 Pupillary abnormality, **bilateral**
     H21.569 Pupillary abnormality, **unspecified eye** ▽

√5ᵗʰ H21.8 Other specified disorders of iris and ciliary body
     H21.81 **Floppy iris syndrome**
Intraoperative floppy iris syndrome (IFIS)
Use additional code for adverse effect, if applicable, to identify drug (T36-T50 with fifth or sixth character 5)

     H21.82 **Plateau iris syndrome (post-iridectomy) (postprocedural)**

     H21.89 **Other specified disorders of iris and ciliary body**
H21.9 **Unspecified disorder of iris and ciliary body** ▽

H22 Disorders of iris and ciliary body in diseases classified elsewhere
Code first underlying disease, such as:
gout (M1A.-, M10.-)
leprosy (A30.-)
parasitic disease (B89)

Disorders of lens (H25-H28)

√4ᵗʰ H25 Age-related cataract
Senile cataract
EXCLUDES 2 capsular glaucoma with pseudoexfoliation of lens (H40.1-)

√5ᵗʰ H25.0 Age-related incipient cataract
     √6ᵗʰ H25.01 Cortical age-related cataract
         H25.011 Cortical age-related cataract, **right eye** Ⓐ
         H25.012 Cortical age-related cataract, **left eye** Ⓐ
         H25.013 Cortical age-related cataract, **bilateral** Ⓐ
         H25.019 Cortical age-related cataract, **unspecified eye** Ⓐ▽

     √6ᵗʰ H25.03 Anterior subcapsular polar age-related cataract
         H25.031 Anterior subcapsular polar age-related cataract, **right eye** Ⓐ
         H25.032 Anterior subcapsular polar age-related cataract, **left eye** Ⓐ
         H25.033 Anterior subcapsular polar age-related cataract, **bilateral** Ⓐ
         H25.039 Anterior subcapsular polar age-related cataract, **unspecified eye** Ⓐ▽

     √6ᵗʰ H25.04 Posterior subcapsular polar age-related cataract
         H25.041 Posterior subcapsular polar age-related cataract, **right eye** Ⓐ
         H25.042 Posterior subcapsular polar age-related cataract, **left eye** Ⓐ
         H25.043 Posterior subcapsular polar age-related cataract, **bilateral** Ⓐ
         H25.049 Posterior subcapsular polar age-related cataract, **unspecified eye** Ⓐ▽

     √6ᵗʰ H25.09 Other age-related incipient cataract
Coronary age-related cataract
Punctate age-related cataract
Water clefts
         H25.091 Other age-related incipient cataract, **right eye** Ⓐ
         H25.092 Other age-related incipient cataract, **left eye** Ⓐ
         H25.093 Other age-related incipient cataract, **bilateral** Ⓐ
         H25.099 Other age-related incipient cataract, **unspecified eye** Ⓐ▽

√5ᵗʰ H25.1 Age-related nuclear cataract
Cataracta brunescens
Nuclear sclerosis cataract
AHA: 2016, 1Q, 36
     H25.10 Age-related nuclear cataract, **unspecified eye** Ⓐ▽
     H25.11 Age-related nuclear cataract, **right eye** Ⓐ
     H25.12 Age-related nuclear cataract, **left eye** Ⓐ
     H25.13 Age-related nuclear cataract, **bilateral** Ⓐ

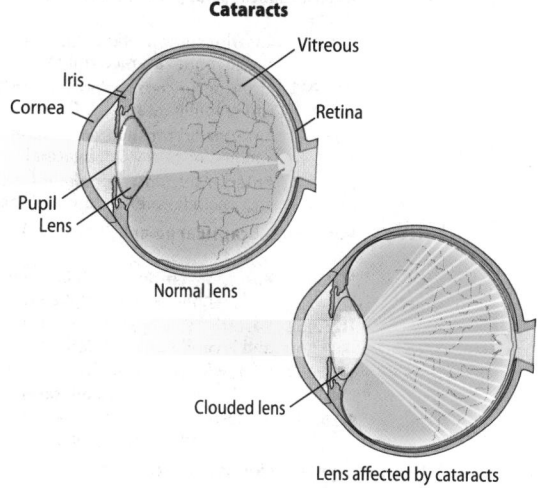

Cataracts

Vitreous
Iris
Cornea
Retina
Pupil
Lens

Normal lens

Clouded lens

Lens affected by cataracts

√5ᵗʰ H25.2 Age-related cataract, morgagnian type
Age-related hypermature cataract
     H25.20 Age-related cataract, morgagnian type, **unspecified eye** Ⓐ▽
     H25.21 Age-related cataract, morgagnian type, **right eye** Ⓐ
     H25.22 Age-related cataract, morgagnian type, **left eye** Ⓐ
     H25.23 Age-related cataract, morgagnian type, **bilateral** Ⓐ

√5ᵗʰ H25.8 Other age-related cataract
     √6ᵗʰ H25.81 Combined forms of age-related cataract
         H25.811 Combined forms of age-related cataract, **right eye** Ⓐ
         H25.812 Combined forms of age-related cataract, **left eye** Ⓐ
         H25.813 Combined forms of age-related cataract, **bilateral** Ⓐ
         H25.819 Combined forms of age-related cataract, **unspecified eye** Ⓐ▽
     H25.89 **Other age-related cataract** Ⓐ
H25.9 **Unspecified age-related cataract** Ⓐ▽

√4ᵗʰ H26 Other cataract
EXCLUDES 1 congenital cataract (Q12.0)

√5ᵗʰ H26.0 Infantile and juvenile cataract
     √6ᵗʰ H26.00 Unspecified infantile and juvenile cataract
         H26.001 Unspecified infantile and juvenile cataract, **right eye** Ⓟ▽
         H26.002 Unspecified infantile and juvenile cataract, **left eye** Ⓟ▽
         H26.003 Unspecified infantile and juvenile cataract, **bilateral** Ⓟ▽
         H26.009 Unspecified infantile and juvenile cataract, **unspecified eye** Ⓟ▽

     √6ᵗʰ H26.01 Infantile and juvenile cortical, lamellar, or zonular cataract
         H26.011 Infantile and juvenile cortical, lamellar, or zonular cataract, **right eye** Ⓟ
         H26.012 Infantile and juvenile cortical, lamellar, or zonular cataract, **left eye** Ⓟ
         H26.013 Infantile and juvenile cortical, lamellar, or zonular cataract, **bilateral** Ⓟ
         H26.019 Infantile and juvenile cortical, lamellar, or zonular cataract, **unspecified eye** Ⓟ▽

     √6ᵗʰ H26.03 Infantile and juvenile nuclear cataract
         H26.031 Infantile and juvenile nuclear cataract, **right eye** Ⓟ
         H26.032 Infantile and juvenile nuclear cataract, **left eye** Ⓟ
         H26.033 Infantile and juvenile nuclear cataract, **bilateral** Ⓟ
         H26.039 Infantile and juvenile nuclear cataract, **unspecified eye** Ⓟ▽

☑ Additional Character Req   ✓x7ᵗʰ Placeholder Alert   Manifestation   ᴴᶜᶜ CMS-HCC Condition   ▽ Unspecified Code   ▶◀ Revised Text   ● New Code   ▲ Revised Code Title

✓6ᵗʰ **H26.04** **Anterior subcapsular polar infantile and juvenile cataract**

    H26.041 **Anterior subcapsular polar infantile and juvenile cataract, right eye** P

    H26.042 **Anterior subcapsular polar infantile and juvenile cataract, left eye** P

    H26.043 **Anterior subcapsular polar infantile and juvenile cataract, bilateral** P

    H26.049 **Anterior subcapsular polar infantile and juvenile cataract, unspecified eye** P ▽

✓6ᵗʰ **H26.05** **Posterior subcapsular polar infantile and juvenile cataract**

    H26.051 **Posterior subcapsular polar infantile and juvenile cataract, right eye** P

    H26.052 **Posterior subcapsular polar infantile and juvenile cataract, left eye** P

    H26.053 **Posterior subcapsular polar infantile and juvenile cataract, bilateral** P

    H26.059 **Posterior subcapsular polar infantile and juvenile cataract, unspecified eye** P ▽

✓6ᵗʰ **H26.06** **Combined forms of infantile and juvenile cataract**

    H26.061 **Combined forms of infantile and juvenile cataract, right eye** P

    H26.062 **Combined forms of infantile and juvenile cataract, left eye** P

    H26.063 **Combined forms of infantile and juvenile cataract, bilateral** P

    H26.069 **Combined forms of infantile and juvenile cataract, unspecified eye** P ▽

    H26.09 **Other infantile and juvenile cataract** P

✓5ᵗʰ **H26.1** **Traumatic cataract**

    Use additional code (Chapter 20) to identify external cause

✓6ᵗʰ **H26.10** **Unspecified traumatic cataract**

    H26.101 **Unspecified traumatic cataract, right eye** ▽

    H26.102 **Unspecified traumatic cataract, left eye** ▽

    H26.103 **Unspecified traumatic cataract, bilateral** ▽

    H26.109 **Unspecified traumatic cataract, unspecified eye** ▽

✓6ᵗʰ **H26.11** **Localized traumatic opacities**

    H26.111 **Localized traumatic opacities, right eye**

    H26.112 **Localized traumatic opacities, left eye**

    H26.113 **Localized traumatic opacities, bilateral**

    H26.119 **Localized traumatic opacities, unspecified eye** ▽

✓6ᵗʰ **H26.12** **Partially resolved traumatic cataract**

    H26.121 **Partially resolved traumatic cataract, right eye**

    H26.122 **Partially resolved traumatic cataract, left eye**

    H26.123 **Partially resolved traumatic cataract, bilateral**

    H26.129 **Partially resolved traumatic cataract, unspecified eye** ▽

✓6ᵗʰ **H26.13** **Total traumatic cataract**

    H26.131 **Total traumatic cataract, right eye**

    H26.132 **Total traumatic cataract, left eye**

    H26.133 **Total traumatic cataract, bilateral**

    H26.139 **Total traumatic cataract, unspecified eye** ▽

✓5ᵗʰ **H26.2** **Complicated cataract**

    H26.20 **Unspecified complicated cataract** ▽
      Cataracta complicata NOS

✓6ᵗʰ **H26.21** **Cataract with neovascularization**
      Code also associated condition, such as:
      chronic iridocyclitis (H20.1-)

    H26.211 **Cataract with neovascularization, right eye**

    H26.212 **Cataract with neovascularization, left eye**

    H26.213 **Cataract with neovascularization, bilateral**

    H26.219 **Cataract with neovascularization, unspecified eye** ▽

✓6ᵗʰ **H26.22** **Cataract secondary to ocular disorders (degenerative) (inflammatory)**
      Code also associated ocular disorder

    H26.221 **Cataract secondary to ocular disorders (degenerative) (inflammatory), right eye**

    H26.222 **Cataract secondary to ocular disorders (degenerative) (inflammatory), left eye**

    H26.223 **Cataract secondary to ocular disorders (degenerative) (inflammatory), bilateral**

    H26.229 **Cataract secondary to ocular disorders (degenerative) (inflammatory), unspecified** ▽

✓6ᵗʰ **H26.23** **Glaucomatous flecks (subcapsular)**
      Code first underlying glaucoma (H40-H42)

    H26.231 **Glaucomatous flecks (subcapsular), right eye**

    H26.232 **Glaucomatous flecks (subcapsular), left eye**

    H26.233 **Glaucomatous flecks (subcapsular), bilateral**

    H26.239 **Glaucomatous flecks (subcapsular), unspecified eye** ▽

✓5ᵗʰ **H26.3** **Drug-induced cataract**
      Toxic cataract
      Use additional code for adverse effect, if applicable, to identify drug (T36-T50 with fifth or sixth character 5)

    H26.30 **Drug-induced cataract, unspecified eye** ▽

    H26.31 **Drug-induced cataract, right eye**

    H26.32 **Drug-induced cataract, left eye**

    H26.33 **Drug-induced cataract, bilateral**

✓5ᵗʰ **H26.4** **Secondary cataract**

    H26.40 **Unspecified secondary cataract** ▽

✓6ᵗʰ **H26.41** **Soemmering's ring**

    H26.411 **Soemmering's ring, right eye**

    H26.412 **Soemmering's ring, left eye**

    H26.413 **Soemmering's ring, bilateral**

    H26.419 **Soemmering's ring, unspecified eye** ▽

✓6ᵗʰ **H26.49** **Other secondary cataract**

    H26.491 **Other secondary cataract, right eye**

    H26.492 **Other secondary cataract, left eye**

    H26.493 **Other secondary cataract, bilateral**

    H26.499 **Other secondary cataract, unspecified eye** ▽

    H26.8 **Other specified cataract**

    H26.9 **Unspecified cataract** ▽

✓4ᵗʰ **H27** **Other disorders of lens**
      EXCLUDES 1 *congenital lens malformations (Q12.-)*
      mechanical complications of intraocular lens implant (T85.2)
      pseudophakia (Z96.1)

✓5ᵗʰ **H27.0** **Aphakia**
      Acquired absence of lens
      Acquired aphakia
      Aphakia due to trauma
      EXCLUDES 1 *cataract extraction status (Z98.4-)*
      congenital absence of lens (Q12.3)
      congenital aphakia (Q12.3)

    H27.00 **Aphakia, unspecified eye** ▽

    H27.01 **Aphakia, right eye**

    H27.02 **Aphakia, left eye**

    H27.03 **Aphakia, bilateral**

✓5ᵗʰ **H27.1** **Dislocation of lens**

    H27.10 **Unspecified dislocation of lens** ▽

✓6ᵗʰ **H27.11** **Subluxation of lens**

    H27.111 **Subluxation of lens, right eye**

    H27.112 **Subluxation of lens, left eye**

    H27.113 **Subluxation of lens, bilateral**

    H27.119 **Subluxation of lens, unspecified eye** ▽

✓6ᵗʰ **H27.12** **Anterior dislocation of lens**

    H27.121 **Anterior dislocation of lens, right eye**

    H27.122 **Anterior dislocation of lens, left eye**

    H27.123 **Anterior dislocation of lens, bilateral**

    H27.129 **Anterior dislocation of lens, unspecified eye** ▽

EXCLUDES 1 Not coded here   **EXCLUDES 2** Not included here   N Newborn Age: 0   P Pediatric Age: 0-17   M Maternity Age: 12-55   A Adult Age: 15-124

586   ICD-10-CM 2018

✓6th **H27.13 Posterior dislocation of lens**

    H27.131 Posterior dislocation of lens, right eye

    H27.132 Posterior dislocation of lens, left eye

    H27.133 Posterior dislocation of lens, bilateral

    H27.139 Posterior dislocation of lens, unspecified eye ▽

H27.8 Other specified disorders of lens

H27.9 Unspecified disorder of lens ▽

H28 Cataract in diseases classified elsewhere

Code first underlying disease, such as:
  hypoparathyroidism (E20.-)
  myotonia (G71.1-)
  myxedema (E03.-)
  protein-calorie malnutrition (E40-E46)

  EXCLUDES 1   *cataract in diabetes mellitus (E08.36, E09.36, E10.36, E11.36, E13.36)*

Disorders of choroid and retina (H30-H36)

✓4th **H30 Chorioretinal inflammation**

✓5th **H30.0 Focal chorioretinal inflammation**

  Focal chorioretinitis
  Focal choroiditis
  Focal retinitis
  Focal retinochoroiditis

✓6th **H30.00 Unspecified focal chorioretinal inflammation**

  Focal chorioretinitis NOS
  Focal choroiditis NOS
  Focal retinitis NOS
  Focal retinochoroiditis NOS

    H30.001 Unspecified focal chorioretinal inflammation, right eye ▽

    H30.002 Unspecified focal chorioretinal inflammation, left eye ▽

    H30.003 Unspecified focal chorioretinal inflammation, bilateral ▽

    H30.009 Unspecified focal chorioretinal inflammation, unspecified eye ▽

✓6th **H30.01 Focal chorioretinal inflammation, juxtapapillary**

    H30.011 Focal chorioretinal inflammation, juxtapapillary, right eye

    H30.012 Focal chorioretinal inflammation, juxtapapillary, left eye

    H30.013 Focal chorioretinal inflammation, juxtapapillary, bilateral

    H30.019 Focal chorioretinal inflammation, juxtapapillary, unspecified eye ▽

✓6th **H30.02 Focal chorioretinal inflammation of posterior pole**

    H30.021 Focal chorioretinal inflammation of posterior pole, right eye

    H30.022 Focal chorioretinal inflammation of posterior pole, left eye

    H30.023 Focal chorioretinal inflammation of posterior pole, bilateral

    H30.029 Focal chorioretinal inflammation of posterior pole, unspecified eye ▽

✓6th **H30.03 Focal chorioretinal inflammation, peripheral**

    H30.031 Focal chorioretinal inflammation, peripheral, right eye

    H30.032 Focal chorioretinal inflammation, peripheral, left eye

    H30.033 Focal chorioretinal inflammation, peripheral, bilateral

    H30.039 Focal chorioretinal inflammation, peripheral, unspecified eye ▽

✓6th **H30.04 Focal chorioretinal inflammation, macular or paramacular**

    H30.041 Focal chorioretinal inflammation, macular or paramacular, right eye

    H30.042 Focal chorioretinal inflammation, macular or paramacular, left eye

    H30.043 Focal chorioretinal inflammation, macular or paramacular, bilateral

    H30.049 Focal chorioretinal inflammation, macular or paramacular, unspecified eye ▽

✓5th **H30.1 Disseminated chorioretinal inflammation**

  Disseminated chorioretinitis
  Disseminated choroiditis
  Disseminated retinitis
  Disseminated retinochoroiditis

  EXCLUDES 2   *exudative retinopathy (H35.02-)*

✓6th **H30.10 Unspecified disseminated chorioretinal inflammation**

  Disseminated chorioretinitis NOS
  Disseminated choroiditis NOS
  Disseminated retinitis NOS
  Disseminated retinochoroiditis NOS

    H30.101 Unspecified disseminated chorioretinal inflammation, right eye ▽

    H30.102 Unspecified disseminated chorioretinal inflammation, left eye ▽

    H30.103 Unspecified disseminated chorioretinal inflammation, bilateral ▽

    H30.109 Unspecified disseminated chorioretinal inflammation, unspecified eye ▽

✓6th **H30.11 Disseminated chorioretinal inflammation of posterior pole**

    H30.111 Disseminated chorioretinal inflammation of posterior pole, right eye

    H30.112 Disseminated chorioretinal inflammation of posterior pole, left eye

    H30.113 Disseminated chorioretinal inflammation of posterior pole, bilateral

    H30.119 Disseminated chorioretinal inflammation of posterior pole, unspecified eye ▽

✓6th **H30.12 Disseminated chorioretinal inflammation, peripheral**

    H30.121 Disseminated chorioretinal inflammation, peripheral right eye

    H30.122 Disseminated chorioretinal inflammation, peripheral, left eye

    H30.123 Disseminated chorioretinal inflammation, peripheral, bilateral

    H30.129 Disseminated chorioretinal inflammation, peripheral, unspecified eye ▽

✓6th **H30.13 Disseminated chorioretinal inflammation, generalized**

    H30.131 Disseminated chorioretinal inflammation, generalized, right eye

    H30.132 Disseminated chorioretinal inflammation, generalized, left eye

    H30.133 Disseminated chorioretinal inflammation, generalized, bilateral

    H30.139 Disseminated chorioretinal inflammation, generalized, unspecified eye ▽

✓6th **H30.14 Acute posterior multifocal placoid pigment epitheliopathy**

    H30.141 Acute posterior multifocal placoid pigment epitheliopathy, right eye

    H30.142 Acute posterior multifocal placoid pigment epitheliopathy, left eye

    H30.143 Acute posterior multifocal placoid pigment epitheliopathy, bilateral

    H30.149 Acute posterior multifocal placoid pigment epitheliopathy, unspecified eye ▽

✓5th **H30.2 Posterior cyclitis**

  Pars planitis

    H30.20 Posterior cyclitis, unspecified eye ▽

    H30.21 Posterior cyclitis, right eye

    H30.22 Posterior cyclitis, left eye

    H30.23 Posterior cyclitis, bilateral

✓5th **H30.8 Other chorioretinal inflammations**

✓6th **H30.81 Harada's disease**

    H30.811 Harada's disease, right eye

    H30.812 Harada's disease, left eye

    H30.813 Harada's disease, bilateral

    H30.819 Harada's disease, unspecified eye ▽

✓ Additional Character Req   ✓x7th Placeholder Alert   Manifestation   HCC CMS-HCC Condition   ▽ Unspecified Code   ▶◀ Revised Text   ● New Code   ▲ Revised Code Title

✓6ᵗʰ **H30.89**   **Other chorioretinal inflammations**
    H30.891   **Other chorioretinal inflammations, right eye**
    H30.892   **Other chorioretinal inflammations, left eye**
    H30.893   **Other chorioretinal inflammations, bilateral**
    H30.899   **Other chorioretinal inflammations, unspecified eye** ▽

✓5ᵗʰ **H30.9**   **Unspecified chorioretinal inflammation**
    Chorioretinitis NOS   Retinitis NOS
    Choroiditis NOS   Retinochoroiditis NOS
    Neuroretinitis NOS
    H30.90   **Unspecified chorioretinal inflammation, unspecified eye** ▽
    H30.91   **Unspecified chorioretinal inflammation, right eye** ▽
    H30.92   **Unspecified chorioretinal inflammation, left eye** ▽
    H30.93   **Unspecified chorioretinal inflammation, bilateral** ▽

✓4ᵗʰ **H31**   **Other disorders of choroid**

✓5ᵗʰ **H31.0**   **Chorioretinal scars**
    EXCLUDES 2   *postsurgical chorioretinal scars (H59.81-)*

    ✓6ᵗʰ **H31.00**   **Unspecified chorioretinal scars**
      H31.001   **Unspecified chorioretinal scars, right eye** ▽
      H31.002   **Unspecified chorioretinal scars, left eye** ▽
      H31.003   **Unspecified chorioretinal scars, bilateral** ▽
      H31.009   **Unspecified chorioretinal scars, unspecified eye** ▽

    ✓6ᵗʰ **H31.01**   **Macula scars of posterior pole (postinflammatory) (post-traumatic)**
      EXCLUDES 1   *postprocedural chorioretinal scar (H59.81-)*
      H31.011   **Macula scars of posterior pole (postinflammatory) (post-traumatic), right eye**
      H31.012   **Macula scars of posterior pole (postinflammatory) (post-traumatic), left eye**
      H31.013   **Macula scars of posterior pole (postinflammatory) (post-traumatic), bilateral**
      H31.019   **Macula scars of posterior pole (postinflammatory) (post-traumatic), unspecified eye** ▽

    ✓6ᵗʰ **H31.02**   **Solar retinopathy**
      H31.021   **Solar retinopathy, right eye**
      H31.022   **Solar retinopathy, left eye**
      H31.023   **Solar retinopathy, bilateral**
      H31.029   **Solar retinopathy, unspecified eye** ▽

    ✓6ᵗʰ **H31.09**   **Other chorioretinal scars**
      H31.091   **Other chorioretinal scars, right eye**
      H31.092   **Other chorioretinal scars, left eye**
      H31.093   **Other chorioretinal scars, bilateral**
      H31.099   **Other chorioretinal scars, unspecified eye** ▽

✓5ᵗʰ **H31.1**   **Choroidal degeneration**
    EXCLUDES 2   *angioid streaks of macula (H35.33)*

    ✓6ᵗʰ **H31.10**   **Unspecified choroidal degeneration**
      Choroidal sclerosis NOS
      H31.101   **Choroidal degeneration, unspecified, right eye** ▽
      H31.102   **Choroidal degeneration, unspecified, left eye** ▽
      H31.103   **Choroidal degeneration, unspecified, bilateral** ▽
      H31.109   **Choroidal degeneration, unspecified, unspecified eye** ▽

    ✓6ᵗʰ **H31.11**   **Age-related choroidal atrophy**
      H31.111   **Age-related choroidal atrophy, right eye** Ⓐ
      H31.112   **Age-related choroidal atrophy, left eye** Ⓐ
      H31.113   **Age-related choroidal atrophy, bilateral** Ⓐ
      H31.119   **Age-related choroidal atrophy, unspecified eye** Ⓐ ▽

    ✓6ᵗʰ **H31.12**   **Diffuse secondary atrophy of choroid**
      H31.121   **Diffuse secondary atrophy of choroid, right eye**
      H31.122   **Diffuse secondary atrophy of choroid, left eye**
      H31.123   **Diffuse secondary atrophy of choroid, bilateral**
      H31.129   **Diffuse secondary atrophy of choroid, unspecified eye** ▽

✓5ᵗʰ **H31.2**   **Hereditary choroidal dystrophy**
    EXCLUDES 2   *hyperornithinemia (E72.4)*
               ornithinemia (E72.4)
    H31.20   **Hereditary choroidal dystrophy, unspecified** ▽
    H31.21   **Choroideremia**
    H31.22   **Choroidal dystrophy (central areolar) (generalized) (peripapillary)**
    H31.23   **Gyrate atrophy, choroid**
    H31.29   **Other hereditary choroidal dystrophy**

✓5ᵗʰ **H31.3**   **Choroidal hemorrhage and rupture**

    ✓6ᵗʰ **H31.30**   **Unspecified choroidal hemorrhage**
      H31.301   **Unspecified choroidal hemorrhage, right eye** ▽
      H31.302   **Unspecified choroidal hemorrhage, left eye** ▽
      H31.303   **Unspecified choroidal hemorrhage, bilateral** ▽
      H31.309   **Unspecified choroidal hemorrhage, unspecified eye** ▽

    ✓6ᵗʰ **H31.31**   **Expulsive choroidal hemorrhage**
      H31.311   **Expulsive choroidal hemorrhage, right eye**
      H31.312   **Expulsive choroidal hemorrhage, left eye**
      H31.313   **Expulsive choroidal hemorrhage, bilateral**
      H31.319   **Expulsive choroidal hemorrhage, unspecified eye**

    ✓6ᵗʰ **H31.32**   **Choroidal rupture**
      H31.321   **Choroidal rupture, right eye**
      H31.322   **Choroidal rupture, left eye**
      H31.323   **Choroidal rupture, bilateral**
      H31.329   **Choroidal rupture, unspecified eye** ▽

✓5ᵗʰ **H31.4**   **Choroidal detachment**

    ✓6ᵗʰ **H31.40**   **Unspecified choroidal detachment**
      H31.401   **Unspecified choroidal detachment, right eye** ▽
      H31.402   **Unspecified choroidal detachment, left eye** ▽
      H31.403   **Unspecified choroidal detachment, bilateral** ▽
      H31.409   **Unspecified choroidal detachment, unspecified eye** ▽

    ✓6ᵗʰ **H31.41**   **Hemorrhagic choroidal detachment**
      H31.411   **Hemorrhagic choroidal detachment, right eye**
      H31.412   **Hemorrhagic choroidal detachment, left eye**
      H31.413   **Hemorrhagic choroidal detachment, bilateral**
      H31.419   **Hemorrhagic choroidal detachment, unspecified eye** ▽

    ✓6ᵗʰ **H31.42**   **Serous choroidal detachment**
      H31.421   **Serous choroidal detachment, right eye**
      H31.422   **Serous choroidal detachment, left eye**
      H31.423   **Serous choroidal detachment, bilateral**
      H31.429   **Serous choroidal detachment, unspecified eye** ▽

    H31.8   **Other specified disorders of choroid**
    H31.9   **Unspecified disorder of choroid** ▽

H32   *Chorioretinal disorders in diseases classified elsewhere*
    Code first underlying disease, such as:
      congenital toxoplasmosis (P37.1)
      histoplasmosis (B39.-)
      leprosy (A30.-)
    EXCLUDES 1   *chorioretinitis (in):*
        toxoplasmosis (acquired) (B58.01)
        tuberculosis (A18.53)

EXCLUDES 1 Not coded here   *EXCLUDES 2* Not included here   Ⓝ Newborn Age: 0   Ⓟ Pediatric Age: 0-17   Ⓜ Maternity Age: 12-55   Ⓐ Adult Age: 15-124

588   ICD-10-CM 2018

Chapter 7. Diseases of the Eye and Adnexa

Retinal Detachment

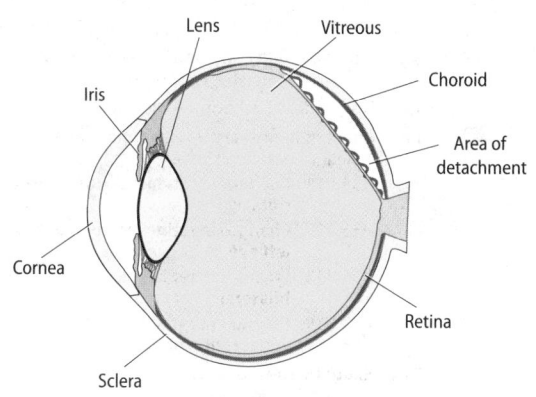

Lens
Vitreous
Iris
Choroid
Area of detachment
Cornea
Retina
Sclera

✓4th **H33** **Retinal detachments and breaks**
> EXCLUDES 1   *detachment of retinal pigment epithelium (H35.72-, H35.73-)*

✓5th **H33.0** **Retinal detachment** with retinal break
Rhegmatogenous retinal detachment
> EXCLUDES 1   *serous retinal detachment (without retinal break) (H33.2-)*

  ✓6th **H33.00** **Unspecified retinal detachment with retinal break**
     H33.001   Unspecified retinal detachment with retinal break, right eye ▽
     H33.002   Unspecified retinal detachment with retinal break, left eye ▽
     H33.003   Unspecified retinal detachment with retinal break, bilateral ▽
     H33.009   Unspecified retinal detachment with retinal break, unspecified eye ▽

  ✓6th **H33.01** **Retinal detachment with** single break
     H33.011   Retinal detachment with single break, right eye
     H33.012   Retinal detachment with single break, left eye
     H33.013   Retinal detachment with single break, bilateral
     H33.019   Retinal detachment with single break, unspecified eye ▽

  ✓6th **H33.02** **Retinal detachment with** multiple breaks
     H33.021   Retinal detachment with multiple breaks, right eye
     H33.022   Retinal detachment with multiple breaks, left eye
     H33.023   Retinal detachment with multiple breaks, bilateral
     H33.029   Retinal detachment with multiple breaks, unspecified eye ▽

  ✓6th **H33.03** **Retinal detachment with** giant retinal tear
     H33.031   Retinal detachment with giant retinal tear, right eye
     H33.032   Retinal detachment with giant retinal tear, left eye
     H33.033   Retinal detachment with giant retinal tear, bilateral
     H33.039   Retinal detachment with giant retinal tear, unspecified eye ▽

  ✓6th **H33.04** **Retinal detachment with** retinal dialysis
     H33.041   Retinal detachment with retinal dialysis, right eye
     H33.042   Retinal detachment with retinal dialysis, left eye
     H33.043   Retinal detachment with retinal dialysis, bilateral
     H33.049   Retinal detachment with retinal dialysis, unspecified eye ▽

  ✓6th **H33.05** **Total retinal detachment**
     H33.051   Total retinal detachment, right eye
     H33.052   Total retinal detachment, left eye
     H33.053   Total retinal detachment, bilateral

     H33.059   Total retinal detachment, unspecified eye ▽

✓5th **H33.1** **Retinoschisis and retinal cysts**
> EXCLUDES 1   *congenital retinoschisis (Q14.1)*
> *microcystoid degeneration of retina (H35.42-)*

  ✓6th **H33.10** **Unspecified retinoschisis**
     H33.101   Unspecified retinoschisis, right eye ▽
     H33.102   Unspecified retinoschisis, left eye ▽
     H33.103   Unspecified retinoschisis, bilateral ▽
     H33.109   Unspecified retinoschisis, unspecified eye ▽

  ✓6th **H33.11** **Cyst of ora serrata**
     H33.111   Cyst of ora serrata, right eye
     H33.112   Cyst of ora serrata, left eye
     H33.113   Cyst of ora serrata, bilateral
     H33.119   Cyst of ora serrata, unspecified eye ▽

  ✓6th **H33.12** **Parasitic cyst of retina**
     H33.121   Parasitic cyst of retina, right eye
     H33.122   Parasitic cyst of retina, left eye
     H33.123   Parasitic cyst of retina, bilateral
     H33.129   Parasitic cyst of retina, unspecified eye ▽

  ✓6th **H33.19** **Other retinoschisis and retinal cysts**
Pseudocyst of retina
     H33.191   Other retinoschisis and retinal cysts, right eye
     H33.192   Other retinoschisis and retinal cysts, left eye
     H33.193   Other retinoschisis and retinal cysts, bilateral
     H33.199   Other retinoschisis and retinal cysts, unspecified eye ▽

✓5th **H33.2** **Serous retinal detachment**
Retinal detachment NOS
Retinal detachment without retinal break
> EXCLUDES 1   *central serous chorioretinopathy (H35.71-)*

     H33.20   Serous retinal detachment, unspecified eye ▽
     H33.21   Serous retinal detachment, right eye
     H33.22   Serous retinal detachment, left eye
     H33.23   Serous retinal detachment, bilateral

✓5th **H33.3** **Retinal breaks without detachment**
> EXCLUDES 1   *chorioretinal scars after surgery for detachment (H59.81-)*
> *peripheral retinal degeneration without break (H35.4-)*

  ✓6th **H33.30** **Unspecified retinal break**
     H33.301   Unspecified retinal break, right eye ▽
     H33.302   Unspecified retinal break, left eye ▽
     H33.303   Unspecified retinal break, bilateral ▽
     H33.309   Unspecified retinal break, unspecified eye ▽

  ✓6th **H33.31** **Horseshoe tear of retina without detachment**
Operculum of retina without detachment
     H33.311   Horseshoe tear of retina without detachment, right eye
     H33.312   Horseshoe tear of retina without detachment, left eye
     H33.313   Horseshoe tear of retina without detachment, bilateral
     H33.319   Horseshoe tear of retina without detachment, unspecified eye ▽

  ✓6th **H33.32** **Round hole of retina without detachment**
     H33.321   Round hole, right eye
     H33.322   Round hole, left eye
     H33.323   Round hole, bilateral
     H33.329   Round hole, unspecified eye ▽

  ✓6th **H33.33** **Multiple defects of retina without detachment**
     H33.331   Multiple defects of retina without detachment, right eye
     H33.332   Multiple defects of retina without detachment, left eye
     H33.333   Multiple defects of retina without detachment, bilateral
     H33.339   Multiple defects of retina without detachment, unspecified eye ▽

☑ Additional Character Req   ✓x7th Placeholder Alert   Manifestation   HCC CMS-HCC Condition   ▽ Unspecified Code   ►◄ Revised Text   ● New Code   ▲ Revised Code Title

√5th **H33.4 Traction detachment of retina**
Proliferative vitreo-retinopathy with retinal detachment

     H33.40 Traction detachment of retina, unspecified eye ▽
     H33.41 Traction detachment of retina, right eye
     H33.42 Traction detachment of retina, left eye
     H33.43 Traction detachment of retina, bilateral

H33.8 Other retinal detachments

√4th **H34 Retinal vascular occlusions**
     EXCLUDES 1   amaurosis fugax (G45.3)

√5th **H34.0 Transient retinal artery occlusion**

     H34.00 Transient retinal artery occlusion, unspecified eye ▽
     H34.01 Transient retinal artery occlusion, right eye
     H34.02 Transient retinal artery occlusion, left eye
     H34.03 Transient retinal artery occlusion, bilateral

√5th **H34.1 Central retinal artery occlusion**

     H34.10 Central retinal artery occlusion, unspecified eye ▽
     H34.11 Central retinal artery occlusion, right eye
     H34.12 Central retinal artery occlusion, left eye
     H34.13 Central retinal artery occlusion, bilateral

√5th **H34.2 Other retinal artery occlusions**

     √6th **H34.21 Partial retinal artery occlusion**
       Hollenhorst's plaque
       Retinal microembolism
       H34.211 Partial retinal artery occlusion, right eye
       H34.212 Partial retinal artery occlusion, left eye
       H34.213 Partial retinal artery occlusion, bilateral
       H34.219 Partial retinal artery occlusion, unspecified eye ▽

     √6th **H34.23 Retinal artery branch occlusion**
       H34.231 Retinal artery branch occlusion, right eye
       H34.232 Retinal artery branch occlusion, left eye
       H34.233 Retinal artery branch occlusion, bilateral
       H34.239 Retinal artery branch occlusion, unspecified eye ▽

√5th **H34.8 Other retinal vascular occlusions**

     √6th **H34.81 Central retinal vein occlusion**

> One of the following 7th characters is to be assigned to codes in subcategory H34.81 to designate the severity of the occlusion:
> Ø   with macular edema
> 1   with retinal neovascularization
> 2   stable
>   old central retinal vein occlusion

       √7th **H34.811 Central retinal vein occlusion, right eye**
       √7th **H34.812 Central retinal vein occlusion, left eye**
       √7th **H34.813 Central retinal vein occlusion, bilateral**
       √7th **H34.819 Central retinal vein occlusion, unspecified eye** ▽

     √6th **H34.82 Venous engorgement**
       Incipient retinal vein occlusion
       Partial retinal vein occlusion
       H34.821 Venous engorgement, right eye
       H34.822 Venous engorgement, left eye
       H34.823 Venous engorgement, bilateral
       H34.829 Venous engorgement, unspecified eye ▽

     √6th **H34.83 Tributary (branch) retinal vein occlusion**

> One of the following 7th characters is to be assigned to codes in subcategory H34.83 to designate the severity of the occlusion:
> Ø   with macular edema
> 1   with retinal neovascularization
> 2   stable
>   old tributary (branch) retinal vein occlusion

       √7th **H34.831 Tributary (branch) retinal vein occlusion, right eye**
       √7th **H34.832 Tributary (branch) retinal vein occlusion, left eye**
       √7th **H34.833 Tributary (branch) retinal vein occlusion, bilateral**
       √7th **H34.839 Tributary (branch) retinal vein occlusion, unspecified eye** ▽

H34.9 Unspecified retinal vascular occlusion ▽

√4th **H35 Other retinal disorders**
     EXCLUDES 2   diabetic retinal disorders (E08.311- E08.359, E09.311- E09.359, E10.311- E10.359, E11.311- E11.359, E13.311- E13.359)

√5th **H35.0 Background retinopathy and retinal vascular changes**
Code also any associated hypertension (I10.-)

     H35.00 Unspecified background retinopathy ▽

     √6th **H35.01 Changes in retinal vascular appearance**
       Retinal vascular sheathing
       H35.011 Changes in retinal vascular appearance, right eye
       H35.012 Changes in retinal vascular appearance, left eye
       H35.013 Changes in retinal vascular appearance, bilateral
       H35.019 Changes in retinal vascular appearance, unspecified eye ▽

     √6th **H35.02 Exudative retinopathy**
       Coats retinopathy
       H35.021 Exudative retinopathy, right eye
       H35.022 Exudative retinopathy, left eye
       H35.023 Exudative retinopathy, bilateral
       H35.029 Exudative retinopathy, unspecified eye ▽

     √6th **H35.03 Hypertensive retinopathy**
       H35.031 Hypertensive retinopathy, right eye
       H35.032 Hypertensive retinopathy, left eye
       H35.033 Hypertensive retinopathy, bilateral
       H35.039 Hypertensive retinopathy, unspecified eye ▽

     √6th **H35.04 Retinal micro-aneurysms, unspecified**
       H35.041 Retinal micro-aneurysms, unspecified, right eye ▽
       H35.042 Retinal micro-aneurysms, unspecified, left eye ▽
       H35.043 Retinal micro-aneurysms, unspecified, bilateral ▽
       H35.049 Retinal micro-aneurysms, unspecified, unspecified eye ▽

     √6th **H35.05 Retinal neovascularization, unspecified**
       H35.051 Retinal neovascularization, unspecified, right eye ▽
       H35.052 Retinal neovascularization, unspecified, left eye ▽
       H35.053 Retinal neovascularization, unspecified, bilateral ▽
       H35.059 Retinal neovascularization, unspecified, unspecified eye ▽

     √6th **H35.06 Retinal vasculitis**
       Eales disease
       Retinal perivasculitis
       DEF: Sight-threatening intraocular inflammation of the retinal blood vessels; causes minimal, partial, or even complete blindness.
       H35.061 Retinal vasculitis, right eye
       H35.062 Retinal vasculitis, left eye
       H35.063 Retinal vasculitis, bilateral
       H35.069 Retinal vasculitis, unspecified eye ▽

     √6th **H35.07 Retinal telangiectasis**
       H35.071 Retinal telangiectasis, right eye
       H35.072 Retinal telangiectasis, left eye
       H35.073 Retinal telangiectasis, bilateral
       H35.079 Retinal telangiectasis, unspecified eye ▽

     H35.09 Other intraretinal microvascular abnormalities
       Retinal varices

√5th **H35.1 Retinopathy of prematurity**

     √6th **H35.10 Retinopathy of prematurity, unspecified**
       Retinopathy of prematurity NOS
       H35.101 Retinopathy of prematurity, unspecified, right eye ▽
       H35.102 Retinopathy of prematurity, unspecified, left eye ▽
       H35.103 Retinopathy of prematurity, unspecified, bilateral ▽
       H35.109 Retinopathy of prematurity, unspecified, unspecified eye ▽

EXCLUDES 1 Not coded here   EXCLUDES 2 Not included here   N Newborn Age: 0   P Pediatric Age: 0-17   M Maternity Age: 12-55   A Adult Age: 15-124

590   ICD-10-CM 2018

✓6ᵗʰ **H35.11** **Retinopathy of prematurity,** stage Ø

   H35.111 **Retinopathy of prematurity, stage Ø, right eye**

   H35.112 **Retinopathy of prematurity, stage Ø, left eye**

   H35.113 **Retinopathy of prematurity, stage Ø, bilateral**

   H35.119 **Retinopathy of prematurity, stage Ø, unspecified eye** ▽

✓6ᵗʰ **H35.12** **Retinopathy of prematurity,** stage 1

   H35.121 **Retinopathy of prematurity, stage 1, right eye**

   H35.122 **Retinopathy of prematurity, stage 1, left eye**

   H35.123 **Retinopathy of prematurity, stage 1, bilateral**

   H35.129 **Retinopathy of prematurity, stage 1, unspecified eye** ▽

✓6ᵗʰ **H35.13** **Retinopathy of prematurity,** stage 2

   H35.131 **Retinopathy of prematurity, stage 2, right eye**

   H35.132 **Retinopathy of prematurity, stage 2, left eye**

   H35.133 **Retinopathy of prematurity, stage 2, bilateral**

   H35.139 **Retinopathy of prematurity, stage 2, unspecified eye** ▽

✓6ᵗʰ **H35.14** **Retinopathy of prematurity,** stage 3

   H35.141 **Retinopathy of prematurity, stage 3, right eye**

   H35.142 **Retinopathy of prematurity, stage 3, left eye**

   H35.143 **Retinopathy of prematurity, stage 3, bilateral**

   H35.149 **Retinopathy of prematurity, stage 3, unspecified eye** ▽

✓6ᵗʰ **H35.15** **Retinopathy of prematurity,** stage 4

   H35.151 **Retinopathy of prematurity, stage 4, right eye**

   H35.152 **Retinopathy of prematurity, stage 4, left eye**

   H35.153 **Retinopathy of prematurity, stage 4, bilateral**

   H35.159 **Retinopathy of prematurity, stage 4, unspecified eye** ▽

✓6ᵗʰ **H35.16** **Retinopathy of prematurity,** stage 5

   H35.161 **Retinopathy of prematurity, stage 5, right eye**

   H35.162 **Retinopathy of prematurity, stage 5, left eye**

   H35.163 **Retinopathy of prematurity, stage 5, bilateral**

   H35.169 **Retinopathy of prematurity, stage 5, unspecified eye** ▽

✓6ᵗʰ **H35.17** **Retrolental fibroplasia**

   H35.171 **Retrolental fibroplasia, right eye**

   H35.172 **Retrolental fibroplasia, left eye**

   H35.173 **Retrolental fibroplasia, bilateral**

   H35.179 **Retrolental fibroplasia, unspecified eye** ▽

✓5ᵗʰ **H35.2** **Other non-diabetic proliferative retinopathy**
   Proliferative vitreo-retinopathy
   EXCLUDES 1 *proliferative vitreo-retinopathy with retinal detachment (H33.4-)*

   H35.2Ø **Other non-diabetic proliferative retinopathy, unspecified eye** ▽

   H35.21 **Other non-diabetic proliferative retinopathy, right eye**

   H35.22 **Other non-diabetic proliferative retinopathy, left eye**

   H35.23 **Other non-diabetic proliferative retinopathy, bilateral**

✓5ᵗʰ **H35.3** **Degeneration of macula and posterior pole**

   H35.3Ø **Unspecified macular degeneration** A ▽
     Age-related macular degeneration

✓6ᵗʰ **H35.31** **Nonexudative age-related macular degeneration**
   Atrophic age-related macular degeneration
   Dry age-related macular degeneration
   AHA: 2016, 4Q, 21

   One of the following 7th characters is to be assigned to codes in subcategory H35.31 to designate the stage of the disease:
   Ø   stage unspecified
   1   early dry stage
   2   intermediate dry stage
   3   advanced atrophic without subfoveal involvement
      advanced dry stage
   4   advanced atrophic with subfoveal involvement

   ✓7ᵗʰ **H35.311** **Nonexudative age-related macular degeneration, right eye** A

   ✓7ᵗʰ **H35.312** **Nonexudative age-related macular degeneration, left eye** A

   ✓7ᵗʰ **H35.313** **Nonexudative age-related macular degeneration, bilateral** A

   ✓7ᵗʰ **H35.319** **Nonexudative age-related macular degeneration, unspecified eye** A ▽

✓6ᵗʰ **H35.32** **Exudative age-related macular degeneration**
   Wet age-related macular degeneration

   One of the following 7th characters is to be assigned to codes in subcategory H35.32 to designate the stage of the disease:
   Ø   stage unspecified
   1   with active choroidal neovascularization
   2   with inactive choroidal neovascularization
      with involuted or regressed neovascularization
   3   with inactive scar

   ✓7ᵗʰ **H35.321** **Exudative age-related macular degeneration, right eye** HCC A

   ✓7ᵗʰ **H35.322** **Exudative age-related macular degeneration, left eye** HCC A

   ✓7ᵗʰ **H35.323** **Exudative age-related macular degeneration, bilateral** HCC A

   ✓7ᵗʰ **H35.329** **Exudative age-related macular degeneration, unspecified eye** HCC A ▽

   H35.33 **Angioid streaks of macula**
     DEF: Degeneration of choroid; characterized by broad, irregular, dark brown streaks radiating from optic disc; occurs with pseudoxanthoma elasticum or Paget's disease.

✓6ᵗʰ **H35.34** **Macular cyst, hole, or pseudohole**

   H35.341 **Macular cyst, hole, or pseudohole, right eye**

   H35.342 **Macular cyst, hole, or pseudohole, left eye**

   H35.343 **Macular cyst, hole, or pseudohole, bilateral**

   H35.349 **Macular cyst, hole, or pseudohole, unspecified eye** ▽

✓6ᵗʰ **H35.35** **Cystoid macular degeneration**
   EXCLUDES 1 *cystoid macular edema following cataract surgery (H59.Ø3-)*

   H35.351 **Cystoid macular degeneration, right eye**

   H35.352 **Cystoid macular degeneration, left eye**

   H35.353 **Cystoid macular degeneration, bilateral**

   H35.359 **Cystoid macular degeneration, unspecified eye** ▽

✓6ᵗʰ **H35.36** **Drusen (degenerative) of macula**
   AHA: 2017, 1Q, 51; 2016, 4Q, 21

   H35.361 **Drusen (degenerative) of macula, right eye**

   H35.362 **Drusen (degenerative) of macula, left eye**

   H35.363 **Drusen (degenerative) of macula, bilateral**

   H35.369 **Drusen (degenerative) of macula, unspecified eye** ▽

✓6ᵗʰ **H35.37** **Puckering of macula**

   H35.371 **Puckering of macula, right eye**

   H35.372 **Puckering of macula, left eye**

   H35.373 **Puckering of macula, bilateral**

   H35.379 **Puckering of macula, unspecified eye** ▽

☑ Additional Character Req   ✓x7ᵗʰ Placeholder Alert   Manifestation   HCC CMS-HCC Condition   ▽ Unspecified Code   ►◄ Revised Text   ● New Code   ▲ Revised Code Title

√6ᵗʰ H35.38 Toxic maculopathy
  Code first poisoning due to drug or toxin, if applicable
  (T36-T65 with fifth or sixth character 1-4 or 6)
  Use additional code for adverse effect, if applicable,
  to identify drug (T36-T50 with fifth or sixth
  character 5)

  H35.381 Toxic maculopathy, right eye
  H35.382 Toxic maculopathy, left eye
  H35.383 Toxic maculopathy, bilateral
  H35.389 Toxic maculopathy, unspecified eye ▽

√5ᵗʰ H35.4 Peripheral retinal degeneration
  EXCLUDES 1   hereditary retinal degeneration (dystrophy) (H35.5-)
        peripheral retinal degeneration with retinal break
        (H33.3-)

  H35.40 Unspecified peripheral retinal degeneration ▽

  √6ᵗʰ H35.41 Lattice degeneration of retina
    Palisade degeneration of retina
    DEF: Degeneration of retina; often bilateral, usually
    benign; characterized by lines intersecting at irregular
    intervals in peripheral retina; retinal thinning and retinal
    holes may occur.

    H35.411 Lattice degeneration of retina, right eye
    H35.412 Lattice degeneration of retina, left eye
    H35.413 Lattice degeneration of retina, bilateral
    H35.419 Lattice degeneration of retina, unspecified eye ▽

  √6ᵗʰ H35.42 Microcystoid degeneration of retina
    H35.421 Microcystoid degeneration of retina, right eye
    H35.422 Microcystoid degeneration of retina, left eye
    H35.423 Microcystoid degeneration of retina, bilateral
    H35.429 Microcystoid degeneration of retina, unspecified eye ▽

  √6ᵗʰ H35.43 Paving stone degeneration of retina
    H35.431 Paving stone degeneration of retina, right eye
    H35.432 Paving stone degeneration of retina, left eye
    H35.433 Paving stone degeneration of retina, bilateral
    H35.439 Paving stone degeneration of retina, unspecified eye ▽

  √6ᵗʰ H35.44 Age-related reticular degeneration of retina
    H35.441 Age-related reticular degeneration of retina, right eye Ⓐ
    H35.442 Age-related reticular degeneration of retina, left eye Ⓐ
    H35.443 Age-related reticular degeneration of retina, bilateral Ⓐ
    H35.449 Age-related reticular degeneration of retina, unspecified eye Ⓐ▽

  √6ᵗʰ H35.45 Secondary pigmentary degeneration
    H35.451 Secondary pigmentary degeneration, right eye
    H35.452 Secondary pigmentary degeneration, left eye
    H35.453 Secondary pigmentary degeneration, bilateral
    H35.459 Secondary pigmentary degeneration, unspecified eye ▽

  √6ᵗʰ H35.46 Secondary vitreoretinal degeneration
    H35.461 Secondary vitreoretinal degeneration, right eye
    H35.462 Secondary vitreoretinal degeneration, left eye
    H35.463 Secondary vitreoretinal degeneration, bilateral
    H35.469 Secondary vitreoretinal degeneration, unspecified eye ▽

√5ᵗʰ H35.5 Hereditary retinal dystrophy
  EXCLUDES 1   dystrophies primarily involving Bruch's membrane
        (H31.1-)

  H35.50 Unspecified hereditary retinal dystrophy ▽
  H35.51 Vitreoretinal dystrophy

H35.52 Pigmentary retinal dystrophy
  Albipunctate retinal dystrophy
  Retinitis pigmentosa
  Tapetoretinal dystrophy

H35.53 Other dystrophies primarily involving the sensory retina
  Stargardt's disease

H35.54 Dystrophies primarily involving the retinal pigment epithelium
  Vitelliform retinal dystrophy

√5ᵗʰ H35.6 Retinal hemorrhage
  H35.60 Retinal hemorrhage, unspecified eye ▽
  H35.61 Retinal hemorrhage, right eye
  H35.62 Retinal hemorrhage, left eye
  H35.63 Retinal hemorrhage, bilateral

√5ᵗʰ H35.7 Separation of retinal layers
  EXCLUDES 1   retinal detachment (serous) (H33.2-)
        rhegmatogenous retinal detachment (H33.0-)

  H35.70 Unspecified separation of retinal layers ▽

  √6ᵗʰ H35.71 Central serous chorioretinopathy
    H35.711 Central serous chorioretinopathy, right eye
    H35.712 Central serous chorioretinopathy, left eye
    H35.713 Central serous chorioretinopathy, bilateral
    H35.719 Central serous chorioretinopathy, unspecified eye ▽

  √6ᵗʰ H35.72 Serous detachment of retinal pigment epithelium
    H35.721 Serous detachment of retinal pigment epithelium, right eye
    H35.722 Serous detachment of retinal pigment epithelium, left eye
    H35.723 Serous detachment of retinal pigment epithelium, bilateral
    H35.729 Serous detachment of retinal pigment epithelium, unspecified eye ▽

  √6ᵗʰ H35.73 Hemorrhagic detachment of retinal pigment epithelium
    H35.731 Hemorrhagic detachment of retinal pigment epithelium, right eye
    H35.732 Hemorrhagic detachment of retinal pigment epithelium, left eye
    H35.733 Hemorrhagic detachment of retinal pigment epithelium, bilateral
    H35.739 Hemorrhagic detachment of retinal pigment epithelium, unspecified eye ▽

√5ᵗʰ H35.8 Other specified retinal disorders
  EXCLUDES 2   retinal hemorrhage (H35.6-)

  H35.81 Retinal edema
    Retinal cotton wool spots
  H35.82 Retinal ischemia
  H35.89 Other specified retinal disorders

H35.9 Unspecified retinal disorder ▽

H36 Retinal disorders in diseases classified elsewhere
  Code first underlying disease, such as:
  lipid storage disorders (E75.-)
  sickle-cell disorders (D57.-)
  EXCLUDES 1   arteriosclerotic retinopathy (H35.0-)
        diabetic retinopathy (E08.3-, E09.3-, E10.3-, E11.3-, E13.3-)

Glaucoma (H40-H42)

√4ᵗʰ H40 Glaucoma
  EXCLUDES 1   absolute glaucoma (H44.51-)
        congenital glaucoma (Q15.0)
        traumatic glaucoma due to birth injury (P15.3)

  √5ᵗʰ H40.0 Glaucoma suspect
    √6ᵗʰ H40.00 Preglaucoma, unspecified
      H40.001 Preglaucoma, unspecified, right eye ▽
      H40.002 Preglaucoma, unspecified, left eye ▽
      H40.003 Preglaucoma, unspecified, bilateral ▽
      H40.009 Preglaucoma, unspecified, unspecified eye ▽

EXCLUDES 1 Not coded here   EXCLUDES 2 Not included here   Ⓝ Newborn Age: 0   Ⓟ Pediatric Age: 0-17   Ⓜ Maternity Age: 12-55   Ⓐ Adult Age: 15-124

592   ICD-10-CM 2018

✓6ᵗʰ **H40.01**   Open angle **with borderline findings,** low risk
    Open angle, low risk

   H40.011   Open angle with borderline findings, low risk, **right eye**

   H40.012   Open angle with borderline findings, low risk, **left eye**

   H40.013   Open angle with borderline findings, low risk, **bilateral**

   H40.019   Open angle with borderline findings, low risk, unspecified eye ▽

✓6ᵗʰ **H40.02**   Open angle **with borderline findings,** high risk
    Open angle, high risk

   H40.021   Open angle with borderline findings, high risk, **right eye**

   H40.022   Open angle with borderline findings, high risk, **left eye**

   H40.023   Open angle with borderline findings, high risk, **bilateral**

   H40.029   Open angle with borderline findings, high risk, unspecified eye ▽

✓6ᵗʰ **H40.03**   Anatomical narrow **angle**
    Primary angle closure suspect

   H40.031   Anatomical narrow angle, **right eye**

   H40.032   Anatomical narrow angle, **left eye**

   H40.033   Anatomical narrow angle, **bilateral**

   H40.039   Anatomical narrow angle, unspecified eye ▽

✓6ᵗʰ **H40.04**   Steroid responder

   H40.041   Steroid responder, **right eye**

   H40.042   Steroid responder, **left eye**

   H40.043   Steroid responder, **bilateral**

   H40.049   Steroid responder, unspecified eye ▽

✓6ᵗʰ **H40.05**   Ocular hypertension

   H40.051   Ocular hypertension, **right eye**

   H40.052   Ocular hypertension, **left eye**

   H40.053   Ocular hypertension, **bilateral**

   H40.059   Ocular hypertension, unspecified eye ▽

✓6ᵗʰ **H40.06**   Primary angle **closure** without glaucoma damage

   H40.061   Primary angle closure without glaucoma damage, **right eye**

   H40.062   Primary angle closure without glaucoma damage, **left eye**

   H40.063   Primary angle closure without glaucoma damage, **bilateral**

   H40.069   Primary angle closure without glaucoma damage, unspecified eye ▽

✓5ᵗʰ **H40.1**   Open-angle glaucoma

One of the following 7th characters is to be assigned to each code in subcategories H40.10, H40.11-, H40.12-, H40.13-, and H40.14- to designate the stage of glaucoma.
0   stage unspecified
1   mild stage
2   moderate stage
3   severe stage
4   indeterminate stage

✓x7ᵗʰ **H40.10**   Unspecified open-angle glaucoma ▽

✓6ᵗʰ **H40.11**   Primary **open-angle glaucoma**
    Chronic simple glaucoma

   ✓7ᵗʰ **H40.111**   Primary open-angle glaucoma, **right eye**

   ✓7ᵗʰ **H40.112**   Primary open-angle glaucoma, **left eye**

   ✓7ᵗʰ **H40.113**   Primary open-angle glaucoma, **bilateral**

   ✓7ᵗʰ **H40.119**   Primary open-angle glaucoma, unspecified eye ▽

✓6ᵗʰ **H40.12**   Low-tension **glaucoma**

   ✓7ᵗʰ **H40.121**   Low-tension glaucoma, **right eye**

   ✓7ᵗʰ **H40.122**   Low-tension glaucoma, **left eye**

   ✓7ᵗʰ **H40.123**   Low-tension glaucoma, **bilateral**

   ✓7ᵗʰ **H40.129**   Low-tension glaucoma, unspecified eye ▽

✓6ᵗʰ **H40.13**   Pigmentary **glaucoma**

   ✓7ᵗʰ **H40.131**   Pigmentary glaucoma, **right eye**

   ✓7ᵗʰ **H40.132**   Pigmentary glaucoma, **left eye**

   ✓7ᵗʰ **H40.133**   Pigmentary glaucoma, **bilateral**

   ✓7ᵗʰ **H40.139**   Pigmentary glaucoma, unspecified eye ▽

Open Angle/Angle Closure Glaucoma

Open angle — Closed angle — Fluid flow — Lens — Lens — Iris — Cornea — Fluid flow — Drainage canal

✓6ᵗʰ **H40.14**   Capsular glaucoma with pseudoexfoliation **of lens**

   ✓7ᵗʰ **H40.141**   Capsular glaucoma with pseudoexfoliation of lens, **right eye**

   ✓7ᵗʰ **H40.142**   Capsular glaucoma with pseudoexfoliation of lens, **left eye**

   ✓7ᵗʰ **H40.143**   Capsular glaucoma with pseudoexfoliation of lens, **bilateral**

   ✓7ᵗʰ **H40.149**   Capsular glaucoma with pseudoexfoliation of lens, unspecified eye ▽

✓6ᵗʰ **H40.15**   Residual stage **of open-angle glaucoma**

   H40.151   Residual stage of open-angle glaucoma, **right eye**

   H40.152   Residual stage of open-angle glaucoma, **left eye**

   H40.153   Residual stage of open-angle glaucoma, **bilateral**

   H40.159   Residual stage of open-angle glaucoma, unspecified eye ▽

✓5ᵗʰ **H40.2**   Primary angle-closure glaucoma

   EXCLUDES 1   *aqueous misdirection (H40.83-)*
           malignant glaucoma (H40.83-)

One of the following 7th characters is to be assigned to each code in subcategories H40.20 and H40.22- to designate the stage of glaucoma.
0   stage unspecified
1   mild stage
2   moderate stage
3   severe stage
4   indeterminate stage

✓x7ᵗʰ **H40.20**   Unspecified primary angle-closure glaucoma ▽

✓6ᵗʰ **H40.21**   Acute **angle-closure glaucoma**
    Acute angle-closure glaucoma attack
    Acute angle-closure glaucoma crisis

   H40.211   Acute angle-closure glaucoma, **right eye**

   H40.212   Acute angle-closure glaucoma, **left eye**

   H40.213   Acute angle-closure glaucoma, **bilateral**

   H40.219   Acute angle-closure glaucoma, unspecified eye ▽

✓6ᵗʰ **H40.22**   Chronic **angle-closure glaucoma**
    Chronic primary angle-closure glaucoma

   ✓7ᵗʰ **H40.221**   Chronic angle-closure glaucoma, **right eye**

   ✓7ᵗʰ **H40.222**   Chronic angle-closure glaucoma, **left eye**

   ✓7ᵗʰ **H40.223**   Chronic angle-closure glaucoma, **bilateral**

   ✓7ᵗʰ **H40.229**   Chronic angle-closure glaucoma, unspecified eye ▽

✓6ᵗʰ **H40.23**   Intermittent **angle-closure glaucoma**

   H40.231   Intermittent angle-closure glaucoma, **right eye**

   H40.232   Intermittent angle-closure glaucoma, **left eye**

   H40.233   Intermittent angle-closure glaucoma, **bilateral**

   H40.239   Intermittent angle-closure glaucoma, unspecified eye ▽

✓6ᵗʰ **H40.24**   Residual stage **of angle-closure glaucoma**

   H40.241   Residual stage of angle-closure glaucoma, **right eye**

   H40.242   Residual stage of angle-closure glaucoma, **left eye**

✅ Additional Character Req   ✓x7ᵗʰ Placeholder Alert   Manifestation   HCC CMS-HCC Condition   ▽ Unspecified Code   ▶◀ Revised Text   ● New Code   ▲ Revised Code Title

ICD-10-CM 2018   593

H40.243   **Residual stage of angle-closure glaucoma, bilateral**

H40.249   **Residual stage of angle-closure glaucoma, unspecified eye** ▽

√5ᵗʰ **H40.3**   **Glaucoma secondary to eye trauma**
Code also underlying condition

> One of the following 7th characters is to be assigned to each code in subcategory H40.3- to designate the stage of glaucoma.
> 0   stage unspecified
> 1   mild stage
> 2   moderate stage
> 3   severe stage
> 4   indeterminate stage

√x7ᵗʰ **H40.30**   **Glaucoma secondary to eye trauma, unspecified eye** ▽

√x7ᵗʰ **H40.31**   **Glaucoma secondary to eye trauma, right eye**

√x7ᵗʰ **H40.32**   **Glaucoma secondary to eye trauma, left eye**

√x7ᵗʰ **H40.33**   **Glaucoma secondary to eye trauma, bilateral**

√5ᵗʰ **H40.4**   **Glaucoma secondary to eye inflammation**
Code also underlying condition

> One of the following 7th characters is to be assigned to each code in subcategory H40.4- to designate the stage of glaucoma.
> 0   stage unspecified
> 1   mild stage
> 2   moderate stage
> 3   severe stage
> 4   indeterminate stage

√x7ᵗʰ **H40.40**   **Glaucoma secondary to eye inflammation, unspecified eye** ▽

√x7ᵗʰ **H40.41**   **Glaucoma secondary to eye inflammation, right eye**

√x7ᵗʰ **H40.42**   **Glaucoma secondary to eye inflammation, left eye**

√x7ᵗʰ **H40.43**   **Glaucoma secondary to eye inflammation, bilateral**

√5ᵗʰ **H40.5**   **Glaucoma secondary to other eye disorders**
Code also underlying eye disorder

> One of the following 7th characters is to be assigned to each code in subcategory H40.5- to designate the stage of glaucoma.
> 0   stage unspecified
> 1   mild stage
> 2   moderate stage
> 3   severe stage
> 4   indeterminate stage

√x7ᵗʰ **H40.50**   **Glaucoma secondary to other eye disorders, unspecified eye** ▽

√x7ᵗʰ **H40.51**   **Glaucoma secondary to other eye disorders, right eye**

√x7ᵗʰ **H40.52**   **Glaucoma secondary to other eye disorders, left eye**

√x7ᵗʰ **H40.53**   **Glaucoma secondary to other eye disorders, bilateral**

√5ᵗʰ **H40.6**   **Glaucoma secondary to drugs**
Use additional code for adverse effect, if applicable, to identify drug (T36-T50 with fifth or sixth character 5)

> One of the following 7th characters is to be assigned to each code in subcategory H40.6- to designate the stage of glaucoma.
> 0   stage unspecified
> 1   mild stage
> 2   moderate stage
> 3   severe stage
> 4   indeterminate stage

√x7ᵗʰ **H40.60**   **Glaucoma secondary to drugs, unspecified eye** ▽

√x7ᵗʰ **H40.61**   **Glaucoma secondary to drugs, right eye**

√x7ᵗʰ **H40.62**   **Glaucoma secondary to drugs, left eye**

√x7ᵗʰ **H40.63**   **Glaucoma secondary to drugs, bilateral**

√5ᵗʰ **H40.8**   **Other glaucoma**

√6ᵗʰ **H40.81**   **Glaucoma with increased episcleral venous pressure**

H40.811   **Glaucoma with increased episcleral venous pressure, right eye**

H40.812   **Glaucoma with increased episcleral venous pressure, left eye**

H40.813   **Glaucoma with increased episcleral venous pressure, bilateral**

H40.819   **Glaucoma with increased episcleral venous pressure, unspecified eye** ▽

√6ᵗʰ **H40.82**   **Hypersecretion glaucoma**

H40.821   **Hypersecretion glaucoma, right eye**

H40.822   **Hypersecretion glaucoma, left eye**

H40.823   **Hypersecretion glaucoma, bilateral**

H40.829   **Hypersecretion glaucoma, unspecified eye** ▽

√6ᵗʰ **H40.83**   **Aqueous misdirection**
Malignant glaucoma

H40.831   **Aqueous misdirection, right eye**

H40.832   **Aqueous misdirection, left eye**

H40.833   **Aqueous misdirection, bilateral**

H40.839   **Aqueous misdirection, unspecified eye** ▽

H40.89   **Other specified glaucoma**

H40.9   **Unspecified glaucoma** ▽

H42   *Glaucoma in diseases classified elsewhere*
Code first underlying condition, such as:
    amyloidosis (E85.-)
    aniridia (Q13.1)
 ▶glaucoma (in) diabetes mellitus (E08.39, E09.39, E10.39, E11.39, E13.39)◀
    Lowe's syndrome (E72.03)
    Reiger's anomaly (Q13.81)
    specified metabolic disorder (E70-E88)

> EXCLUDES 1   *glaucoma (in) onchocerciasis (B73.02)*
> *glaucoma (in) syphilis (A52.71)*
> *glaucoma (in) tuberculous (A18.59)*
> EXCLUDES 2   ~~*glaucoma (in) diabetes mellitus (E08.39, E09.39, E10.39, E11.39, E13.39)*~~

Disorders of vitreous body and globe (H43-H44)

√4ᵗʰ **H43**   **Disorders of vitreous body**

√5ᵗʰ **H43.0**   **Vitreous prolapse**

> EXCLUDES 1   *traumatic vitreous prolapse (S05.2-)*
> *vitreous syndrome following cataract surgery (H59.0-)*

H43.00   **Vitreous prolapse, unspecified eye** ▽

H43.01   **Vitreous prolapse, right eye**

H43.02   **Vitreous prolapse, left eye**

H43.03   **Vitreous prolapse, bilateral**

√5ᵗʰ **H43.1**   **Vitreous hemorrhage**

H43.10   **Vitreous hemorrhage, unspecified eye** HCC ▽

H43.11   **Vitreous hemorrhage, right eye** HCC

H43.12   **Vitreous hemorrhage, left eye** HCC

H43.13   **Vitreous hemorrhage, bilateral** HCC

√5ᵗʰ **H43.2**   **Crystalline deposits in vitreous body**

H43.20   **Crystalline deposits in vitreous body, unspecified eye** ▽

H43.21   **Crystalline deposits in vitreous body, right eye**

H43.22   **Crystalline deposits in vitreous body, left eye**

H43.23   **Crystalline deposits in vitreous body, bilateral**

√5ᵗʰ **H43.3**   **Other vitreous opacities**

√6ᵗʰ **H43.31**   **Vitreous membranes and strands**

H43.311   **Vitreous membranes and strands, right eye**

H43.312   **Vitreous membranes and strands, left eye**

H43.313   **Vitreous membranes and strands, bilateral**

H43.319   **Vitreous membranes and strands, unspecified eye** ▽

√6ᵗʰ **H43.39**   **Other vitreous opacities**
Vitreous floaters

H43.391   **Other vitreous opacities, right eye**

H43.392   **Other vitreous opacities, left eye**

H43.393   **Other vitreous opacities, bilateral**

H43.399   **Other vitreous opacities, unspecified eye** ▽

√5ᵗʰ **H43.8**   **Other disorders of vitreous body**

> EXCLUDES 1   *proliferative vitreo-retinopathy with retinal detachment (H33.4-)*
> EXCLUDES 2   *vitreous abscess (H44.02-)*

√6ᵗʰ **H43.81**   **Vitreous degeneration**
Vitreous detachment

H43.811   **Vitreous degeneration, right eye**

        H43.812   **Vitreous degeneration,** left **eye**

        H43.813   **Vitreous degeneration,** bilateral

        H43.819   **Vitreous degeneration,** unspecified **eye** ▽

  ✓6ᵗʰ **H43.82** **Vitreomacular** adhesion
             Vitreomacular traction

        H43.821   **Vitreomacular adhesion,** right **eye** Ⓐ

        H43.822   **Vitreomacular adhesion,** left **eye** Ⓐ

        H43.823   **Vitreomacular adhesion,** bilateral Ⓐ

        H43.829   **Vitreomacular adhesion,** unspecified Ⓐ ▽
                eye

      H43.89 **Other disorders of vitreous body**

   H43.9 **Unspecified disorder of vitreous body**   ▽

✓4ᵗʰ **H44** **Disorders of globe**
     INCLUDES   disorders affecting multiple structures of eye

  ✓5ᵗʰ **H44.0** **Purulent endophthalmitis**
       Use additional code to identify organism
       EXCLUDES 1   bleb associated endophthalmitis (H59.4-)

   ✓6ᵗʰ **H44.00** **Unspecified purulent endophthalmitis**

        H44.001 **Unspecified purulent endophthalmitis,** ▽
               right **eye**

        H44.002 **Unspecified purulent endophthalmitis,** ▽
               left **eye**

        H44.003 **Unspecified purulent endophthalmitis,** ▽
               bilateral

        H44.009 **Unspecified purulent endophthalmitis,** ▽
               unspecified eye

   ✓6ᵗʰ **H44.01** **Panophthalmitis (acute)**

        H44.011 **Panophthalmitis (acute),** right **eye**

        H44.012 **Panophthalmitis (acute),** left **eye**

        H44.013 **Panophthalmitis (acute),** bilateral

        H44.019 **Panophthalmitis (acute),** unspecified ▽
               eye

   ✓6ᵗʰ **H44.02** **Vitreous abscess (chronic)**

        H44.021 **Vitreous abscess (chronic),** right **eye**

        H44.022 **Vitreous abscess (chronic),** left **eye**

        H44.023 **Vitreous abscess (chronic),** bilateral

        H44.029 **Vitreous abscess (chronic),** unspecified ▽
               eye

  ✓5ᵗʰ **H44.1** **Other endophthalmitis**
       EXCLUDES 1   bleb associated endophthalmitis (H59.4-)
       EXCLUDES 2   ophthalmia nodosa (H16.2-)

   ✓6ᵗʰ **H44.11** **Panuveitis**
         DEF: Inflammation of all layers of uvea of eye, including
         choroid, iris, and ciliary body; also typically involves lens,
         retina, optic nerve, and vitreous; causes reduced vision
         or blindness.

        H44.111 **Panuveitis,** right **eye**

        H44.112 **Panuveitis,** left **eye**

        H44.113 **Panuveitis,** bilateral

        H44.119 **Panuveitis, unspecified eye**   ▽

   ✓6ᵗʰ **H44.12** **Parasitic endophthalmitis, unspecified**

        H44.121 **Parasitic endophthalmitis, unspecified,** ▽
               right **eye**

        H44.122 **Parasitic endophthalmitis, unspecified,** ▽
               left **eye**

        H44.123 **Parasitic endophthalmitis, unspecified,** ▽
               bilateral

        H44.129 **Parasitic endophthalmitis, unspecified,** ▽
               unspecified eye

   ✓6ᵗʰ **H44.13** **Sympathetic uveitis**

        H44.131 **Sympathetic uveitis,** right **eye**

        H44.132 **Sympathetic uveitis,** left **eye**

        H44.133 **Sympathetic uveitis,** bilateral

        H44.139 **Sympathetic uveitis, unspecified eye**   ▽

      H44.19 **Other endophthalmitis**

  ✓5ᵗʰ **H44.2** **Degenerative myopia**
        Malignant myopia

      H44.20 **Degenerative myopia, unspecified eye**   ▽

      H44.21 **Degenerative myopia,** right **eye**

      H44.22 **Degenerative myopia,** left **eye**

      H44.23 **Degenerative myopia,** bilateral

   ✓6ᵗʰ **H44.2A** **Degenerative myopia** with choroidal
          neovascularization
          Use additional code for any associated choroid
          disorders (H31.-)

        H44.2A1 **Degenerative myopia with choroidal**
               neovascularization, right **eye**

        H44.2A2 **Degenerative myopia with choroidal**
               neovascularization, left **eye**

        H44.2A3 **Degenerative myopia with choroidal**
               neovascularization, bilateral **eye**

        H44.2A9 **Degenerative myopia with choroidal** ▽
               neovascularization, unspecified **eye**

   ✓6ᵗʰ **H44.2B** **Degenerative myopia** with macular hole

        H44.2B1 **Degenerative myopia with macular hole,**
               right **eye**

        H44.2B2 **Degenerative myopia with macular hole,**
               left **eye**

        H44.2B3 **Degenerative myopia with macular hole,**
               bilateral eye

        H44.2B9 **Degenerative myopia with macular** ▽
               hole, unspecified eye

   ✓6ᵗʰ **H44.2C** **Degenerative myopia** with retinal detachment
          Use additional code to identify the retinal detachment
          (H33.-)

        H44.2C1 **Degenerative myopia with retinal**
               detachment, right **eye**

        H44.2C2 **Degenerative myopia with retinal**
               detachment, left **eye**

        H44.2C3 **Degenerative myopia with retinal**
               detachment, bilateral **eye**

        H44.2C9 **Degenerative myopia with retinal** ▽
               detachment, unspecified eye

   ✓6ᵗʰ **H44.2D** **Degenerative myopia** with foveoschisis

        H44.2D1 **Degenerative myopia with foveoschisis,**
               right **eye**

        H44.2D2 **Degenerative myopia with foveoschisis,**
               left **eye**

        H44.2D3 **Degenerative myopia with foveoschisis,**
               bilateral eye

        H44.2D9 **Degenerative myopia with** ▽
               foveoschisis, unspecified eye

   ✓6ᵗʰ **H44.2E** **Degenerative myopia** with other maculopathy

        H44.2E1 **Degenerative myopia with other**
               maculopathy, right **eye**

        H44.2E2 **Degenerative myopia with other**
               maculopathy, left **eye**

        H44.2E3 **Degenerative myopia with other**
               maculopathy, bilateral **eye**

        H44.2E9 **Degenerative myopia with other** ▽
               maculopathy, unspecified eye

  ✓5ᵗʰ **H44.3** **Other and unspecified degenerative disorders of globe**

      H44.30 **Unspecified degenerative disorder of globe**   ▽

   ✓6ᵗʰ **H44.31** **Chalcosis**

        H44.311 **Chalcosis,** right **eye**

        H44.312 **Chalcosis,** left **eye**

        H44.313 **Chalcosis,** bilateral

        H44.319 **Chalcosis, unspecified eye**   ▽

   ✓6ᵗʰ **H44.32** **Siderosis of eye**
         DEF: Iron pigment deposits within tissue of eyeball;
         caused by high iron content of blood; characterized by
         cataract, rust-colored anterior subcapsular deposits, iris
         heterochromia, pupillary mydriasis, and depressed
         electroretinogram amplitudes.

        H44.321 **Siderosis of eye,** right **eye**

        H44.322 **Siderosis of eye,** left **eye**

        H44.323 **Siderosis of eye,** bilateral

        H44.329 **Siderosis of eye, unspecified eye**   ▽

   ✓6ᵗʰ **H44.39** **Other degenerative disorders of globe**

        H44.391 **Other degenerative disorders of globe,**
               right **eye**

        H44.392 **Other degenerative disorders of globe,**
               left **eye**

        H44.393 **Other degenerative disorders of globe,**
               bilateral

        H44.399 **Other degenerative disorders of globe,** ▽
               unspecified eye

| ☑ Additional Character Req | ✓ₓ7ᵗʰ Placeholder Alert | Manifestation | HCC CMS-HCC Condition | ▽ Unspecified Code | ▶◀ Revised Text | ● New Code | ▲ Revised Code Title |

ICD-10-CM 2018   **595**

H43.812-H44.399

✓5ᵗʰ **H44.4 Hypotony of eye**

     H44.40 Unspecified hypotony of eye ▽

✓6ᵗʰ **H44.41 Flat anterior chamber hypotony of eye**

     H44.411 Flat anterior chamber hypotony of right eye

     H44.412 Flat anterior chamber hypotony of left eye

     H44.413 Flat anterior chamber hypotony of eye, bilateral

     H44.419 Flat anterior chamber hypotony of unspecified eye ▽

✓6ᵗʰ **H44.42 Hypotony of eye due to ocular fistula**

     H44.421 Hypotony of right eye due to ocular fistula

     H44.422 Hypotony of left eye due to ocular fistula

     H44.423 Hypotony of eye due to ocular fistula, bilateral

     H44.429 Hypotony of unspecified eye due to ocular fistula ▽

✓6ᵗʰ **H44.43 Hypotony of eye due to other ocular disorders**

     H44.431 Hypotony of eye due to other ocular disorders, right eye

     H44.432 Hypotony of eye due to other ocular disorders, left eye

     H44.433 Hypotony of eye due to other ocular disorders, bilateral

     H44.439 Hypotony of eye due to other ocular disorders, unspecified eye ▽

✓6ᵗʰ **H44.44 Primary hypotony of eye**

     H44.441 Primary hypotony of right eye

     H44.442 Primary hypotony of left eye

     H44.443 Primary hypotony of eye, bilateral

     H44.449 Primary hypotony of unspecified eye ▽

✓5ᵗʰ **H44.5 Degenerated conditions of globe**

     H44.50 Unspecified degenerated conditions of globe ▽

✓6ᵗʰ **H44.51 Absolute glaucoma**

     H44.511 Absolute glaucoma, right eye

     H44.512 Absolute glaucoma, left eye

     H44.513 Absolute glaucoma, bilateral

     H44.519 Absolute glaucoma, unspecified eye ▽

✓6ᵗʰ **H44.52 Atrophy of globe**

     Phthisis bulbi

     H44.521 Atrophy of globe, right eye

     H44.522 Atrophy of globe, left eye

     H44.523 Atrophy of globe, bilateral

     H44.529 Atrophy of globe, unspecified eye ▽

✓6ᵗʰ **H44.53 Leucocoria**

     H44.531 Leucocoria, right eye

     H44.532 Leucocoria, left eye

     H44.533 Leucocoria, bilateral

     H44.539 Leucocoria, unspecified eye ▽

✓5ᵗʰ **H44.6 Retained (old) intraocular foreign body, magnetic**

     Use additional code to identify magnetic foreign body (Z18.11)

     EXCLUDES 1   *current intraocular foreign body (S05.-)*

     EXCLUDES 2   *retained foreign body in eyelid (H02.81-)*

         retained (old) foreign body following penetrating wound of orbit (H05.5-)

         retained (old) intraocular foreign body, nonmagnetic (H44.7-)

✓6ᵗʰ **H44.60 Unspecified retained (old) intraocular foreign body, magnetic**

     H44.601 Unspecified retained (old) intraocular foreign body, magnetic, right eye ▽

     H44.602 Unspecified retained (old) intraocular foreign body, magnetic, left eye ▽

     H44.603 Unspecified retained (old) intraocular foreign body, magnetic, bilateral ▽

     H44.609 Unspecified retained (old) intraocular foreign body, magnetic, unspecified eye ▽

✓6ᵗʰ **H44.61 Retained (old) magnetic foreign body in anterior chamber**

     H44.611 Retained (old) magnetic foreign body in anterior chamber, right eye

     H44.612 Retained (old) magnetic foreign body in anterior chamber, left eye

     H44.613 Retained (old) magnetic foreign body in anterior chamber, bilateral

     H44.619 Retained (old) magnetic foreign body in anterior chamber, unspecified eye ▽

✓6ᵗʰ **H44.62 Retained (old) magnetic foreign body in iris or ciliary body**

     H44.621 Retained (old) magnetic foreign body in iris or ciliary body, right eye

     H44.622 Retained (old) magnetic foreign body in iris or ciliary body, left eye

     H44.623 Retained (old) magnetic foreign body in iris or ciliary body, bilateral

     H44.629 Retained (old) magnetic foreign body in iris or ciliary body, unspecified eye ▽

✓6ᵗʰ **H44.63 Retained (old) magnetic foreign body in lens**

     H44.631 Retained (old) magnetic foreign body in lens, right eye

     H44.632 Retained (old) magnetic foreign body in lens, left eye

     H44.633 Retained (old) magnetic foreign body in lens, bilateral

     H44.639 Retained (old) magnetic foreign body in lens, unspecified eye ▽

✓6ᵗʰ **H44.64 Retained (old) magnetic foreign body in posterior wall of globe**

     H44.641 Retained (old) magnetic foreign body in posterior wall of globe, right eye

     H44.642 Retained (old) magnetic foreign body in posterior wall of globe, left eye

     H44.643 Retained (old) magnetic foreign body in posterior wall of globe, bilateral

     H44.649 Retained (old) magnetic foreign body in posterior wall of globe, unspecified eye ▽

✓6ᵗʰ **H44.65 Retained (old) magnetic foreign body in vitreous body**

     H44.651 Retained (old) magnetic foreign body in vitreous body, right eye

     H44.652 Retained (old) magnetic foreign body in vitreous body, left eye

     H44.653 Retained (old) magnetic foreign body in vitreous body, bilateral

     H44.659 Retained (old) magnetic foreign body in vitreous body, unspecified eye ▽

✓6ᵗʰ **H44.69 Retained (old) intraocular foreign body, magnetic, in other or multiple sites**

     H44.691 Retained (old) intraocular foreign body, magnetic, in other or multiple sites, right eye

     H44.692 Retained (old) intraocular foreign body, magnetic, in other or multiple sites, left eye

     H44.693 Retained (old) intraocular foreign body, magnetic, in other or multiple sites, bilateral

     H44.699 Retained (old) intraocular foreign body, magnetic, in other or multiple sites, unspecified eye ▽

✓5ᵗʰ **H44.7 Retained (old) intraocular foreign body, nonmagnetic**

     Use additional code to identify nonmagnetic foreign body (Z18.01-Z18.10, Z18.12, Z18.2-Z18.9)

     EXCLUDES 1   *current intraocular foreign body (S05.-)*

     EXCLUDES 2   *retained foreign body in eyelid (H02.81-)*

         retained (old) foreign body following penetrating wound of orbit (H05.5-)

         retained (old) intraocular foreign body, magnetic (H44.6-)

✓6ᵗʰ **H44.70 Unspecified retained (old) intraocular foreign body, nonmagnetic**

     H44.701 Unspecified retained (old) intraocular foreign body, nonmagnetic, right eye ▽

     H44.702 Unspecified retained (old) intraocular foreign body, nonmagnetic, left eye ▽

     H44.703 Unspecified retained (old) intraocular foreign body, nonmagnetic, bilateral ▽

     H44.709 Unspecified retained (old) intraocular foreign body, nonmagnetic, unspecified eye ▽

         Retained (old) intraocular foreign body NOS

EXCLUDES 1 Not coded here   **EXCLUDES 2** Not included here   N Newborn Age: 0   P Pediatric Age: 0-17   M Maternity Age: 12-55   A Adult Age: 15-124

596   ICD-10-CM 2018

✓6ᵗʰ **H44.71** Retained (nonmagnetic) (old) foreign body in anterior chamber

     H44.711 Retained (nonmagnetic) (old) foreign body in anterior chamber, right eye

     H44.712 Retained (nonmagnetic) (old) foreign body in anterior chamber, left eye

     H44.713 Retained (nonmagnetic) (old) foreign body in anterior chamber, bilateral

     H44.719 Retained (nonmagnetic) (old) foreign body in anterior chamber, unspecified eye ▽

✓6ᵗʰ **H44.72** Retained (nonmagnetic) (old) foreign body in iris or ciliary body

     H44.721 Retained (nonmagnetic) (old) foreign body in iris or ciliary body, right eye

     H44.722 Retained (nonmagnetic) (old) foreign body in iris or ciliary body, left eye

     H44.723 Retained (nonmagnetic) (old) foreign body in iris or ciliary body, bilateral

     H44.729 Retained (nonmagnetic) (old) foreign body in iris or ciliary body, unspecified eye ▽

✓6ᵗʰ **H44.73** Retained (nonmagnetic) (old) foreign body in lens

     H44.731 Retained (nonmagnetic) (old) foreign body in lens, right eye

     H44.732 Retained (nonmagnetic) (old) foreign body in lens, left eye

     H44.733 Retained (nonmagnetic) (old) foreign body in lens, bilateral

     H44.739 Retained (nonmagnetic) (old) foreign body in lens, unspecified eye ▽

✓6ᵗʰ **H44.74** Retained (nonmagnetic) (old) foreign body in posterior wall of globe

     H44.741 Retained (nonmagnetic) (old) foreign body in posterior wall of globe, right eye

     H44.742 Retained (nonmagnetic) (old) foreign body in posterior wall of globe, left eye

     H44.743 Retained (nonmagnetic) (old) foreign body in posterior wall of globe, bilateral

     H44.749 Retained (nonmagnetic) (old) foreign body in posterior wall of globe, unspecified eye ▽

✓6ᵗʰ **H44.75** Retained (nonmagnetic) (old) foreign body in vitreous body

     H44.751 Retained (nonmagnetic) (old) foreign body in vitreous body, right eye

     H44.752 Retained (nonmagnetic) (old) foreign body in vitreous body, left eye

     H44.753 Retained (nonmagnetic) (old) foreign body in vitreous body, bilateral

     H44.759 Retained (nonmagnetic) (old) foreign body in vitreous body, unspecified eye ▽

✓6ᵗʰ **H44.79** Retained (old) intraocular foreign body, nonmagnetic, in other or multiple sites

     H44.791 Retained (old) intraocular foreign body, nonmagnetic, in other or multiple sites, right eye

     H44.792 Retained (old) intraocular foreign body, nonmagnetic, in other or multiple sites, left eye

     H44.793 Retained (old) intraocular foreign body, nonmagnetic, in other or multiple sites, bilateral

     H44.799 Retained (old) intraocular foreign body, nonmagnetic, in other or multiple sites, unspecified eye ▽

✓5ᵗʰ **H44.8** Other disorders of globe

✓6ᵗʰ **H44.81** Hemophthalmos

     DEF: Pool of blood within eyeball, not from current injury.

     H44.811 Hemophthalmos, right eye

     H44.812 Hemophthalmos, left eye

     H44.813 Hemophthalmos, bilateral

     H44.819 Hemophthalmos, unspecified eye ▽

✓6ᵗʰ **H44.82** Luxation of globe

     H44.821 Luxation of globe, right eye

     H44.822 Luxation of globe, left eye

     H44.823 Luxation of globe, bilateral

     H44.829 Luxation of globe, unspecified eye ▽

     H44.89 Other disorders of globe

H44.9 Unspecified disorder of globe ▽

Disorders of optic nerve and visual pathways (H46-H47)

✓4ᵗʰ **H46** Optic neuritis

     EXCLUDES 2   ischemic optic neuropathy (H47.01-)
                neuromyelitis optica [Devic] (G36.0)

✓5ᵗʰ **H46.0** Optic papillitis

     H46.00 Optic papillitis, unspecified eye ▽

     H46.01 Optic papillitis, right eye

     H46.02 Optic papillitis, left eye

     H46.03 Optic papillitis, bilateral

✓5ᵗʰ **H46.1** Retrobulbar neuritis

     Retrobulbar neuritis NOS

     EXCLUDES 1   syphilitic retrobulbar neuritis (A52.15)

     H46.10 Retrobulbar neuritis, unspecified eye ▽

     H46.11 Retrobulbar neuritis, right eye

     H46.12 Retrobulbar neuritis, left eye

     H46.13 Retrobulbar neuritis, bilateral

H46.2 Nutritional optic neuropathy

H46.3 Toxic optic neuropathy

     Code first (T51-T65) to identify cause

H46.8 Other optic neuritis

H46.9 Unspecified optic neuritis ▽

✓4ᵗʰ **H47** Other disorders of optic [2nd] nerve and visual pathways

✓5ᵗʰ **H47.0** Disorders of optic nerve, not elsewhere classified

✓6ᵗʰ **H47.01** Ischemic optic neuropathy

     H47.011 Ischemic optic neuropathy, right eye

     H47.012 Ischemic optic neuropathy, left eye

     H47.013 Ischemic optic neuropathy, bilateral

     H47.019 Ischemic optic neuropathy, unspecified eye ▽

✓6ᵗʰ **H47.02** Hemorrhage in optic nerve sheath

     H47.021 Hemorrhage in optic nerve sheath, right eye

     H47.022 Hemorrhage in optic nerve sheath, left eye

     H47.023 Hemorrhage in optic nerve sheath, bilateral

     H47.029 Hemorrhage in optic nerve sheath, unspecified eye ▽

✓6ᵗʰ **H47.03** Optic nerve hypoplasia

     H47.031 Optic nerve hypoplasia, right eye

     H47.032 Optic nerve hypoplasia, left eye

     H47.033 Optic nerve hypoplasia, bilateral

     H47.039 Optic nerve hypoplasia, unspecified eye ▽

✓6ᵗʰ **H47.09** Other disorders of optic nerve, not elsewhere classified

     Compression of optic nerve

     H47.091 Other disorders of optic nerve, not elsewhere classified, right eye

     H47.092 Other disorders of optic nerve, not elsewhere classified, left eye

     H47.093 Other disorders of optic nerve, not elsewhere classified, bilateral

     H47.099 Other disorders of optic nerve, not elsewhere classified, unspecified eye ▽

✓5ᵗʰ **H47.1** Papilledema

     H47.10 Unspecified papilledema ▽

     H47.11 Papilledema associated with increased intracranial pressure

     H47.12 Papilledema associated with decreased ocular pressure

     H47.13 Papilledema associated with retinal disorder

✓6ᵗʰ **H47.14** Foster-Kennedy syndrome

     H47.141 Foster-Kennedy syndrome, right eye

     H47.142 Foster-Kennedy syndrome, left eye

     H47.143 Foster-Kennedy syndrome, bilateral

     H47.149 Foster-Kennedy syndrome, unspecified eye ▽

✓5ᵗʰ **H47.2** Optic atrophy

     H47.20 Unspecified optic atrophy ▽

✓ Additional Character Req   ✕7ᵗʰ Placeholder Alert   Manifestation   HCC CMS-HCC Condition   ▽ Unspecified Code   ►◄ Revised Text   ● New Code   ▲ Revised Code Title

Chapter 7. Diseases of the Eye and Adnexa

✓6ᵗʰ **H47.21** **Primary** optic atrophy
     H47.211 **Primary** optic atrophy, **right** eye
     H47.212 **Primary** optic atrophy, **left** eye
     H47.213 **Primary** optic atrophy, **bilateral**
     H47.219 **Primary** optic atrophy, **unspecified** eye ▽

H47.22 **Hereditary** optic atrophy
     Leber's optic atrophy

✓6ᵗʰ **H47.23** **Glaucomatous** optic atrophy
     H47.231 **Glaucomatous** optic atrophy, **right** eye
     H47.232 **Glaucomatous** optic atrophy, **left** eye
     H47.233 **Glaucomatous** optic atrophy, **bilateral**
     H47.239 **Glaucomatous** optic atrophy, **unspecified** eye ▽

✓6ᵗʰ **H47.29** **Other** optic atrophy
     Temporal pallor of optic disc
     H47.291 **Other** optic atrophy, **right** eye
     H47.292 **Other** optic atrophy, **left** eye
     H47.293 **Other** optic atrophy, **bilateral**
     H47.299 **Other** optic atrophy, **unspecified** eye ▽

✓5ᵗʰ **H47.3** **Other disorders of optic disc**
     ✓6ᵗʰ **H47.31** **Coloboma** of optic disc
         H47.311 **Coloboma** of optic disc, **right** eye
         H47.312 **Coloboma** of optic disc, **left** eye
         H47.313 **Coloboma** of optic disc, **bilateral**
         H47.319 **Coloboma** of optic disc, **unspecified** eye ▽

     ✓6ᵗʰ **H47.32** **Drusen** of optic disc
         H47.321 **Drusen** of optic disc, **right** eye
         H47.322 **Drusen** of optic disc, **left** eye
         H47.323 **Drusen** of optic disc, **bilateral**
         H47.329 **Drusen** of optic disc, **unspecified** eye ▽

     ✓6ᵗʰ **H47.33** **Pseudopapilledema** of optic disc
         H47.331 **Pseudopapilledema** of optic disc, **right** eye
         H47.332 **Pseudopapilledema** of optic disc, **left** eye
         H47.333 **Pseudopapilledema** of optic disc, **bilateral**
         H47.339 **Pseudopapilledema** of optic disc, **unspecified** eye ▽

     ✓6ᵗʰ **H47.39** **Other disorders of optic disc**
         H47.391 **Other disorders of optic disc, right** eye
         H47.392 **Other disorders of optic disc, left** eye
         H47.393 **Other disorders of optic disc, bilateral**
         H47.399 **Other disorders of optic disc, unspecified** eye ▽

✓5ᵗʰ **H47.4** **Disorders of optic chiasm**
     Code also underlying condition
     H47.41 **Disorders of optic chiasm in (due to) inflammatory disorders**
     H47.42 **Disorders of optic chiasm in (due to) neoplasm**
     H47.43 **Disorders of optic chiasm in (due to) vascular disorders**
     H47.49 **Disorders of optic chiasm in (due to) other disorders**

✓5ᵗʰ **H47.5** **Disorders of other visual pathways**
     Disorders of optic tracts, geniculate nuclei and optic radiations
     Code also underlying condition
     ✓6ᵗʰ **H47.51** **Disorders of visual pathways in (due to) inflammatory disorders**
         H47.511 **Disorders of visual pathways in (due to) inflammatory disorders, right** side
         H47.512 **Disorders of visual pathways in (due to) inflammatory disorders, left** side
         H47.519 **Disorders of visual pathways in (due to)** ▽ **inflammatory disorders, unspecified** side

     ✓6ᵗʰ **H47.52** **Disorders of visual pathways in (due to) neoplasm**
         H47.521 **Disorders of visual pathways in (due to) neoplasm, right** side
         H47.522 **Disorders of visual pathways in (due to) neoplasm, left** side
         H47.529 **Disorders of visual pathways in (due to)** ▽ **neoplasm, unspecified** side

     ✓6ᵗʰ **H47.53** **Disorders of visual pathways in (due to) vascular disorders**
         H47.531 **Disorders of visual pathways in (due to) vascular disorders, right** side
         H47.532 **Disorders of visual pathways in (due to) vascular disorders, left** side

         H47.539 **Disorders of visual pathways in (due to)** ▽ **vascular disorders, unspecified** side

✓5ᵗʰ **H47.6** **Disorders of visual cortex**
     Code also underlying condition
     EXCLUDES 1 injury to visual cortex S04.04
     ✓6ᵗʰ **H47.61** **Cortical blindness**
         H47.611 **Cortical blindness, right** side of brain
         H47.612 **Cortical blindness, left** side of brain
         H47.619 **Cortical blindness, unspecified** side of ▽ **brain**

     ✓6ᵗʰ **H47.62** **Disorders of visual cortex in (due to) inflammatory disorders**
         H47.621 **Disorders of visual cortex in (due to) inflammatory disorders, right** side of brain
         H47.622 **Disorders of visual cortex in (due to) inflammatory disorders, left** side of brain
         H47.629 **Disorders of visual cortex in (due to)** ▽ **inflammatory disorders, unspecified** side of brain

     ✓6ᵗʰ **H47.63** **Disorders of visual cortex in (due to) neoplasm**
         H47.631 **Disorders of visual cortex in (due to) neoplasm, right** side of brain
         H47.632 **Disorders of visual cortex in (due to) neoplasm, left** side of brain
         H47.639 **Disorders of visual cortex in (due to)** ▽ **neoplasm, unspecified** side of brain

     ✓6ᵗʰ **H47.64** **Disorders of visual cortex in (due to) vascular disorders**
         H47.641 **Disorders of visual cortex in (due to) vascular disorders, right** side of brain
         H47.642 **Disorders of visual cortex in (due to) vascular disorders, left** side of brain
         H47.649 **Disorders of visual cortex in (due to)** ▽ **vascular disorders, unspecified** side of brain

     H47.9 **Unspecified disorder of visual pathways** ▽

Disorders of ocular muscles, binocular movement, accommodation and refraction (H49-H52)

EXCLUDES 2 nystagmus and other irregular eye movements (H55)

✓4ᵗʰ **H49** **Paralytic strabismus**
     EXCLUDES 2 internal ophthalmoplegia (H52.51-)
         internuclear ophthalmoplegia (H51.2-)
         progressive supranuclear ophthalmoplegia (G23.1)

✓5ᵗʰ **H49.0** **Third [oculomotor] nerve palsy**
     H49.00 **Third [oculomotor] nerve palsy, unspecified** eye ▽
     H49.01 **Third [oculomotor] nerve palsy, right** eye
     H49.02 **Third [oculomotor] nerve palsy, left** eye
     H49.03 **Third [oculomotor] nerve palsy, bilateral**

✓5ᵗʰ **H49.1** **Fourth [trochlear] nerve palsy**
     H49.10 **Fourth [trochlear] nerve palsy, unspecified** eye ▽
     H49.11 **Fourth [trochlear] nerve palsy, right** eye
     H49.12 **Fourth [trochlear] nerve palsy, left** eye
     H49.13 **Fourth [trochlear] nerve palsy, bilateral**

✓5ᵗʰ **H49.2** **Sixth [abducent] nerve palsy**
     H49.20 **Sixth [abducent] nerve palsy, unspecified** eye ▽
     H49.21 **Sixth [abducent] nerve palsy, right** eye
     H49.22 **Sixth [abducent] nerve palsy, left** eye
     H49.23 **Sixth [abducent] nerve palsy, bilateral**

✓5ᵗʰ **H49.3** **Total (external) ophthalmoplegia**
     H49.30 **Total (external) ophthalmoplegia, unspecified** eye ▽
     H49.31 **Total (external) ophthalmoplegia, right** eye
     H49.32 **Total (external) ophthalmoplegia, left** eye
     H49.33 **Total (external) ophthalmoplegia, bilateral**

✓5ᵗʰ **H49.4** **Progressive external ophthalmoplegia**
     EXCLUDES 1 Kearns-Sayre syndrome (H49.81-)
     H49.40 **Progressive external ophthalmoplegia, unspecified** eye ▽
     H49.41 **Progressive external ophthalmoplegia, right** eye
     H49.42 **Progressive external ophthalmoplegia, left** eye
     H49.43 **Progressive external ophthalmoplegia, bilateral**

EXCLUDES 1 Not coded here   **EXCLUDES 2** Not included here   **N** Newborn Age: 0   **P** Pediatric Age: 0-17   **M** Maternity Age: 12-55   **A** Adult Age: 15-124

598   ICD-10-CM 2018

✓5th **H49.8 Other paralytic strabismus**

  ✓6th **H49.81 Kearns-Sayre syndrome**
    Progressive external ophthalmoplegia with pigmentary retinopathy
    Use additional code for other manifestation, such as: heart block (I45.9)

    H49.811 Kearns-Sayre syndrome, right eye `HCC`
    H49.812 Kearns-Sayre syndrome, left eye `HCC`
    H49.813 Kearns-Sayre syndrome, bilateral `HCC`
    H49.819 Kearns-Sayre syndrome, unspecified eye `HCC` ▽

  ✓6th **H49.88 Other paralytic strabismus**
    External ophthalmoplegia NOS
    H49.881 Other paralytic strabismus, right eye
    H49.882 Other paralytic strabismus, left eye
    H49.883 Other paralytic strabismus, bilateral
    H49.889 Other paralytic strabismus, unspecified eye ▽

H49.9 Unspecified paralytic strabismus ▽

✓4th **H50 Other strabismus**

  ✓5th **H50.0 Esotropia**
    Convergent concomitant strabismus
    EXCLUDES 1 intermittent esotropia (H50.31-, H50.32)

    H50.00 Unspecified esotropia ▽

  ✓6th **H50.01 Monocular esotropia**
    H50.011 Monocular esotropia, right eye
    H50.012 Monocular esotropia, left eye

  ✓6th **H50.02 Monocular esotropia with A pattern**
    H50.021 Monocular esotropia with A pattern, right eye
    H50.022 Monocular esotropia with A pattern, left eye

  ✓6th **H50.03 Monocular esotropia with V pattern**
    H50.031 Monocular esotropia with V pattern, right eye
    H50.032 Monocular esotropia with V pattern, left eye

  ✓6th **H50.04 Monocular esotropia with other noncomitancies**
    H50.041 Monocular esotropia with other noncomitancies, right eye
    H50.042 Monocular esotropia with other noncomitancies, left eye

    H50.05 Alternating esotropia
    H50.06 Alternating esotropia with A pattern
    H50.07 Alternating esotropia with V pattern
    H50.08 Alternating esotropia with other noncomitancies

  ✓5th **H50.1 Exotropia**
    Divergent concomitant strabismus
    EXCLUDES 1 intermittent exotropia (H50.33-, H50.34)

    H50.10 Unspecified exotropia ▽

Eye Muscle Diseases

R.   L.
Monocular (one eye only) esotropia (inward)

Monocular exotropia (outward)

Monocular hypertropia (upward)

  ✓6th **H50.11 Monocular exotropia**
    H50.111 Monocular exotropia, right eye
    H50.112 Monocular exotropia, left eye

  ✓6th **H50.12 Monocular exotropia with A pattern**
    H50.121 Monocular exotropia with A pattern, right eye
    H50.122 Monocular exotropia with A pattern, left eye

  ✓6th **H50.13 Monocular exotropia with V pattern**
    H50.131 Monocular exotropia with V pattern, right eye
    H50.132 Monocular exotropia with V pattern, left eye

  ✓6th **H50.14 Monocular exotropia with other noncomitancies**
    H50.141 Monocular exotropia with other noncomitancies, right eye
    H50.142 Monocular exotropia with other noncomitancies, left eye

    H50.15 Alternating exotropia
    H50.16 Alternating exotropia with A pattern
    H50.17 Alternating exotropia with V pattern
    H50.18 Alternating exotropia with other noncomitancies

  ✓5th **H50.2 Vertical strabismus**
    Hypertropia
    H50.21 Vertical strabismus, right eye
    H50.22 Vertical strabismus, left eye

  ✓5th **H50.3 Intermittent heterotropia**
    H50.30 Unspecified intermittent heterotropia ▽

  ✓6th **H50.31 Intermittent monocular esotropia**
    H50.311 Intermittent monocular esotropia, right eye
    H50.312 Intermittent monocular esotropia, left eye
    H50.32 Intermittent alternating esotropia

  ✓6th **H50.33 Intermittent monocular exotropia**
    H50.331 Intermittent monocular exotropia, right eye
    H50.332 Intermittent monocular exotropia, left eye
    H50.34 Intermittent alternating exotropia

  ✓5th **H50.4 Other and unspecified heterotropia**
    H50.40 Unspecified heterotropia ▽

  ✓6th **H50.41 Cyclotropia**
    H50.411 Cyclotropia, right eye
    H50.412 Cyclotropia, left eye
    H50.42 Monofixation syndrome
    H50.43 Accommodative component in esotropia

  ✓5th **H50.5 Heterophoria**
    H50.50 Unspecified heterophoria ▽
    H50.51 Esophoria
    H50.52 Exophoria
    H50.53 Vertical heterophoria
    H50.54 Cyclophoria
    H50.55 Alternating heterophoria

  ✓5th **H50.6 Mechanical strabismus**
    H50.60 Mechanical strabismus, unspecified ▽

  ✓6th **H50.61 Brown's sheath syndrome**
    H50.611 Brown's sheath syndrome, right eye
    H50.612 Brown's sheath syndrome, left eye
    H50.69 Other mechanical strabismus
      Strabismus due to adhesions
      Traumatic limitation of duction of eye muscle

  ✓5th **H50.8 Other specified strabismus**
  ✓6th **H50.81 Duane's syndrome**
    H50.811 Duane's syndrome, right eye
    H50.812 Duane's syndrome, left eye
    H50.89 Other specified strabismus

H50.9 Unspecified strabismus ▽

✓4th **H51 Other disorders of binocular movement**
  H51.0 Palsy (spasm) of conjugate gaze

  ✓5th **H51.1 Convergence insufficiency and excess**
    H51.11 Convergence insufficiency
    H51.12 Convergence excess

☑ Additional Character Req   ✓x7th Placeholder Alert   Manifestation   `HCC` CMS-HCC Condition   ▽ Unspecified Code   ▶◀ Revised Text   ● New Code   ▲ Revised Code Title

Chapter 7. Diseases of the Eye and Adnexa

H51.2–H53.413

✓5ᵗʰ **H51.2 Internuclear ophthalmoplegia**
    H51.20 Internuclear ophthalmoplegia, unspecified eye ▽
    H51.21 Internuclear ophthalmoplegia, right eye
    H51.22 Internuclear ophthalmoplegia, left eye
    H51.23 Internuclear ophthalmoplegia, bilateral
  H51.8 Other specified disorders of binocular movement
  H51.9 Unspecified disorder of binocular movement ▽

✓4ᵗʰ **H52 Disorders of refraction and accommodation**
  ✓5ᵗʰ **H52.0 Hypermetropia**
    H52.00 Hypermetropia, unspecified eye ▽
    H52.01 Hypermetropia, right eye
    H52.02 Hypermetropia, left eye
    H52.03 Hypermetropia, bilateral
  ✓5ᵗʰ **H52.1 Myopia**
    EXCLUDES 1   *degenerative myopia (H44.2-)*
    H52.10 Myopia, unspecified eye ▽
    H52.11 Myopia, right eye
    H52.12 Myopia, left eye
    H52.13 Myopia, bilateral
  ✓5ᵗʰ **H52.2 Astigmatism**
    ✓6ᵗʰ H52.20 Unspecified astigmatism
      H52.201 Unspecified astigmatism, right eye ▽
      H52.202 Unspecified astigmatism, left eye ▽
      H52.203 Unspecified astigmatism, bilateral ▽
      H52.209 Unspecified astigmatism, unspecified eye ▽
    ✓6ᵗʰ H52.21 Irregular astigmatism
      H52.211 Irregular astigmatism, right eye
      H52.212 Irregular astigmatism, left eye
      H52.213 Irregular astigmatism, bilateral
      H52.219 Irregular astigmatism, unspecified eye ▽
    ✓6ᵗʰ H52.22 Regular astigmatism
      H52.221 Regular astigmatism, right eye
      H52.222 Regular astigmatism, left eye
      H52.223 Regular astigmatism, bilateral
      H52.229 Regular astigmatism, unspecified eye ▽
  ✓5ᵗʰ **H52.3 Anisometropia and aniseikonia**
    H52.31 Anisometropia
    H52.32 Aniseikonia
  H52.4 Presbyopia
  ✓5ᵗʰ **H52.5 Disorders of accommodation**
    ✓6ᵗʰ H52.51 Internal ophthalmoplegia (complete) (total)
      H52.511 Internal ophthalmoplegia (complete) (total), right eye
      H52.512 Internal ophthalmoplegia (complete) (total), left eye
      H52.513 Internal ophthalmoplegia (complete) (total), bilateral
      H52.519 Internal ophthalmoplegia (complete) (total), unspecified eye ▽
    ✓6ᵗʰ H52.52 Paresis of accommodation
      H52.521 Paresis of accommodation, right eye
      H52.522 Paresis of accommodation, left eye
      H52.523 Paresis of accommodation, bilateral
      H52.529 Paresis of accommodation, unspecified eye ▽
    ✓6ᵗʰ H52.53 Spasm of accommodation
      H52.531 Spasm of accommodation, right eye
      H52.532 Spasm of accommodation, left eye
      H52.533 Spasm of accommodation, bilateral
      H52.539 Spasm of accommodation, unspecified eye ▽
  H52.6 Other disorders of refraction
  H52.7 Unspecified disorder of refraction ▽

      Visual disturbances and blindness (H53-H54)

✓4ᵗʰ **H53 Visual disturbances**
  ✓5ᵗʰ **H53.0 Amblyopia ex anopsia**
    EXCLUDES 1   *amblyopia due to vitamin A deficiency (E50.5)*
    ✓6ᵗʰ H53.00 Unspecified amblyopia
      H53.001 Unspecified amblyopia, right eye ▽

      H53.002 Unspecified amblyopia, left eye ▽
      H53.003 Unspecified amblyopia, bilateral ▽
      H53.009 Unspecified amblyopia, unspecified eye ▽
    ✓6ᵗʰ H53.01 Deprivation amblyopia
      H53.011 Deprivation amblyopia, right eye
      H53.012 Deprivation amblyopia, left eye
      H53.013 Deprivation amblyopia, bilateral
      H53.019 Deprivation amblyopia, unspecified eye ▽
    ✓6ᵗʰ H53.02 Refractive amblyopia
      H53.021 Refractive amblyopia, right eye
      H53.022 Refractive amblyopia, left eye
      H53.023 Refractive amblyopia, bilateral
      H53.029 Refractive amblyopia, unspecified eye ▽
    ✓6ᵗʰ H53.03 Strabismic amblyopia
      EXCLUDES 1   *strabismus (H50.-)*
      H53.031 Strabismic amblyopia, right eye
      H53.032 Strabismic amblyopia, left eye
      H53.033 Strabismic amblyopia, bilateral
      H53.039 Strabismic amblyopia, unspecified eye ▽
    ✓6ᵗʰ H53.04 Amblyopia suspect
      H53.041 Amblyopia suspect, right eye
      H53.042 Amblyopia suspect, left eye
      H53.043 Amblyopia suspect, bilateral
      H53.049 Amblyopia suspect, unspecified eye ▽
  ✓5ᵗʰ **H53.1 Subjective visual disturbances**
    EXCLUDES 1   *subjective visual disturbances due to vitamin A deficiency (E50.5)*
                visual hallucinations (R44.1)
    H53.10 Unspecified subjective visual disturbances ▽
    H53.11 Day blindness
      Hemeralopia
    ✓6ᵗʰ H53.12 Transient visual loss
      Scintillating scotoma
      EXCLUDES 1   *amaurosis fugax (G45.3-)*
              transient retinal artery occlusion (H34.0-)
      H53.121 Transient visual loss, right eye
      H53.122 Transient visual loss, left eye
      H53.123 Transient visual loss, bilateral
      H53.129 Transient visual loss, unspecified eye ▽
    ✓6ᵗʰ H53.13 Sudden visual loss
      H53.131 Sudden visual loss, right eye
      H53.132 Sudden visual loss, left eye
      H53.133 Sudden visual loss, bilateral
      H53.139 Sudden visual loss, unspecified eye ▽
    ✓6ᵗʰ H53.14 Visual discomfort
      Asthenopia   Photophobia
      H53.141 Visual discomfort, right eye
      H53.142 Visual discomfort, left eye
      H53.143 Visual discomfort, bilateral
      H53.149 Visual discomfort, unspecified ▽
    H53.15 Visual distortions of shape and size
      Metamorphopsia
    H53.16 Psychophysical visual disturbances
    H53.19 Other subjective visual disturbances
      Visual halos
  H53.2 Diplopia
    Double vision
  ✓5ᵗʰ **H53.3 Other and unspecified disorders of binocular vision**
    H53.30 Unspecified disorder of binocular vision ▽
    H53.31 Abnormal retinal correspondence
    H53.32 Fusion with defective stereopsis
    H53.33 Simultaneous visual perception without fusion
    H53.34 Suppression of binocular vision
  ✓5ᵗʰ **H53.4 Visual field defects**
    H53.40 Unspecified visual field defects ▽
    ✓6ᵗʰ H53.41 Scotoma involving central area
      Central scotoma
      H53.411 Scotoma involving central area, right eye
      H53.412 Scotoma involving central area, left eye
      H53.413 Scotoma involving central area, bilateral

EXCLUDES 1 Not coded here   EXCLUDES 2 Not included here   N Newborn Age: 0   P Pediatric Age: 0-17   M Maternity Age: 12-55   A Adult Age: 15-124

600   ICD-10-CM 2018

H53.419 Scotoma involving central area, unspecified eye ▽

✓6th **H53.42** Scotoma of blind spot area
Enlarged blind spot
     H53.421 Scotoma of blind spot area, right eye
     H53.422 Scotoma of blind spot area, left eye
     H53.423 Scotoma of blind spot area, bilateral
     H53.429 Scotoma of blind spot area, unspecified eye ▽

✓6th **H53.43** Sector or arcuate defects
Arcuate scotoma
Bjerrum scotoma
     H53.431 Sector or arcuate defects, right eye
     H53.432 Sector or arcuate defects, left eye
     H53.433 Sector or arcuate defects, bilateral
     H53.439 Sector or arcuate defects, unspecified eye ▽

✓6th **H53.45** Other localized visual field defect
Peripheral visual field defect
Ring scotoma NOS
Scotoma NOS
     H53.451 Other localized visual field defect, right eye
     H53.452 Other localized visual field defect, left eye
     H53.453 Other localized visual field defect, bilateral
     H53.459 Other localized visual field defect, unspecified eye ▽

✓6th **H53.46** Homonymous bilateral field defects
Homonymous hemianopia
Homonymous hemianopsia
Quadrant anopia
Quadrant anopsia
     H53.461 Homonymous bilateral field defects, right side
     H53.462 Homonymous bilateral field defects, left side
     H53.469 Homonymous bilateral field defects, unspecified side ▽
         Homonymous bilateral field defects NOS

     H53.47 Heteronymous bilateral field defects
Heteronymous hemianop(s)ia

✓6th **H53.48** Generalized contraction of visual field
     H53.481 Generalized contraction of visual field, right eye
     H53.482 Generalized contraction of visual field, left eye
     H53.483 Generalized contraction of visual field, bilateral
     H53.489 Generalized contraction of visual field, unspecified eye ▽

✓5th **H53.5** Color vision deficiencies
Color blindness
EXCLUDES 2   day blindness (H53.11)
     H53.50 Unspecified color vision deficiencies ▽
Color blindness NOS
     H53.51 Achromatopsia
         DEF: Nonprogressive genetic visual disorder; characterized by complete color blindness, decreased vision, and light sensitivity.
     H53.52 Acquired color vision deficiency
     H53.53 Deuteranomaly
         Deuteranopia
         DEF: Male-only genetic disorder; difficulty in distinguishing green and red, no shortened spectrum.
     H53.54 Protanomaly
         Protanopia
     H53.55 Tritanomaly
         Tritanopia
     H53.59 Other color vision deficiencies

✓5th **H53.6** Night blindness
EXCLUDES 1   night blindness due to vitamin A deficiency (E50.5)
     H53.60 Unspecified night blindness ▽
     H53.61 Abnormal dark adaptation curve
     H53.62 Acquired night blindness
     H53.63 Congenital night blindness
     H53.69 Other night blindness

✓5th **H53.7** Vision sensitivity deficiencies
     H53.71 Glare sensitivity
     H53.72 Impaired contrast sensitivity
H53.8 Other visual disturbances
H53.9 Unspecified visual disturbance ▽

✓4th **H54** Blindness and low vision
NOTE   For definition of visual impairment categories see table below
Code first any associated underlying cause of the blindness
EXCLUDES 1   amaurosis fugax (G45.3)

✓5th **H54.0** Blindness, both eyes
Visual impairment categories 3, 4, 5 in both eyes
   ✓6th **H54.0X** Blindness, both eyes, different category levels
     ✓7th **H54.0X3** Blindness right eye, category 3
         H54.0X33 Blindness right eye category 3, blindness left eye category 3
         H54.0X34 Blindness right eye category 3, blindness left eye category 4
         H54.0X35 Blindness right eye category 3, blindness left eye category 5
     ✓7th **H54.0X4** Blindness right eye, category 4
         H54.0X43 Blindness right eye category 4, blindness left eye category 3
         H54.0X44 Blindness right eye category 4, blindness left eye category 4
         H54.0X45 Blindness right eye category 4, blindness left eye category 5
     ✓7th **H54.0X5** Blindness right eye, category 5
         H54.0X53 Blindness right eye category 5, blindness left eye category 3
         H54.0X54 Blindness right eye category 5, blindness left eye category 4
         H54.0X55 Blindness right eye category 5, blindness left eye category 5

✓5th **H54.1** Blindness, one eye, low vision other eye
Visual impairment categories 3, 4, 5 in one eye, with categories 1 or 2 in the other eye.
     H54.10 Blindness, one eye, low vision other eye, unspecified eyes ▽
   ✓6th **H54.11** Blindness, right eye, low vision left eye
     ✓7th **H54.113** Blindness right eye category 3, low vision left eye
         H54.1131 Blindness right eye category 3, low vision left eye category 1
         H54.1132 Blindness right eye category 3, low vision left eye category 2
     ✓7th **H54.114** Blindness right eye category 4, low vision left eye
         H54.1141 Blindness right eye category 4, low vision left eye category 1
         H54.1142 Blindness right eye category 4, low vision left eye category 2
     ✓7th **H54.115** Blindness right eye category 5, low vision left eye
         H54.1151 Blindness right eye category 5, low vision left eye category 1
         H54.1152 Blindness right eye category 5, low vision left eye category 2
   ✓6th **H54.12** Blindness, left eye, low vision right eye
     ✓7th **H54.121** Low vision right eye category 1, blindness left eye
         H54.1213 Low vision right eye category 1, blindness left eye category 3
         H54.1214 Low vision right eye category 1, blindness left eye category 4
         H54.1215 Low vision right eye category 1, blindness left eye category 5

    H54.122   **Low vision right eye category 2, blindness left eye**

        H54.1223   Low vision right eye category 2, blindness left eye category 3

        H54.1224   Low vision right eye category 2, blindness left eye category 4

        H54.1225   Low vision right eye category 2, blindness left eye category 5

√5ᵗʰ H54.2   **Low vision, both eyes**
    Visual impairment categories 1 or 2 in both eyes

    √6ᵗʰ H54.2X   **Low vision, both eyes, different category levels**

        √7ᵗʰ H54.2X1   **Low vision, right eye, category 1**

            H54.2X11   Low vision right eye category 1, low vision left eye category 1

            H54.2X12   Low vision right eye category 1, low vision left eye category 2

        √7ᵗʰ H54.2X2   **Low vision, right eye, category 2**

            H54.2X21   Low vision right eye category 2, low vision left eye category 1

            H54.2X22   Low vision right eye category 2, low vision left eye category 2

H54.3   **Unqualified visual loss, both eyes**
    Visual impairment category 9 in both eyes.

√5ᵗʰ H54.4   **Blindness, one eye**
    Visual impairment categories 3, 4, 5 in one eye [normal vision in other eye]

    H54.40   **Blindness, one eye, unspecified eye**   ▽

    √6ᵗʰ H54.41   **Blindness, right eye, normal vision left eye**

        √7ᵗʰ H54.413   **Blindness, right eye, category 3**

            H54.413A   **Blindness right eye category 3, normal vision left eye**

        √7ᵗʰ H54.414   **Blindness, right eye, category 4**

            H54.414A   **Blindness right eye category 4, normal vision left eye**

        √7ᵗʰ H54.415   **Blindness, right eye, category 5**

            H54.415A   **Blindness right eye category 5, normal vision left eye**

    √6ᵗʰ H54.42   **Blindness, left eye, normal vision right eye**

        √7ᵗʰ H54.42A   **Blindness, left eye, category 3-5**

            H54.42A3   **Blindness left eye category 3, normal vision right eye**

            H54.42A4   **Blindness left eye category 4, normal vision right eye**

            H54.42A5   **Blindness left eye category 5, normal vision right eye**

√5ᵗʰ H54.5   **Low vision, one eye**
    Visual impairment categories 1 or 2 in one eye [normal vision in other eye]

    H54.50   **Low vision, one eye, unspecified eye**   ▽

    √6ᵗʰ H54.51   **Low vision, right eye, normal vision left eye**

        √7ᵗʰ H54.511   **Low vision, right eye, category 1-2**

            H54.511A   **Low vision right eye category 1, normal vision left eye**

            H54.512A   **Low vision right eye category 2, normal vision left eye**

    √6ᵗʰ H54.52   **Low vision, left eye, normal vision right eye**

        √7ᵗʰ H54.52A   **Low vision, left eye, category 1-2**

            H54.52A1   **Low vision left eye category 1, normal vision right eye**

            H54.52A2   **Low vision left eye category 2, normal vision right eye**

√5ᵗʰ H54.6   **Unqualified visual loss, one eye**
    Visual impairment category 9 in one eye [normal vision in other eye].

    H54.60   **Unqualified visual loss, one eye, unspecified**   ▽

    H54.61   **Unqualified visual loss, right eye, normal vision left eye**

    H54.62   **Unqualified visual loss, left eye, normal vision right eye**

H54.7   **Unspecified visual loss**   ▽
    Visual impairment category 9 NOS

H54.8   **Legal blindness, as defined in USA**
    Blindness NOS according to USA definition
    EXCLUDES 1   *legal blindness with specification of impairment level (H54.0-H54.7)*

NOTE   The table below gives a classification of severity of visual impairment recommended by a WHO Study Group on the Prevention of Blindness, Geneva, 6-10 November 1972.

The term "low vision" in category H54 comprises categories 1 and 2 of the table, the term "blindness" categories 3, 4 and 5, and the term "unqualified visual loss" category 9.

If the extent of the visual field is taken into account, patients with a field no greater than 10 but greater than 5 around central fixation should be placed in category 3 and patients with a field greater than 5 around central fixation should be placed in category 4, even if the central acuity is not impaired.

Category of visual impairment	Visual acuity with best possible correction	
	Maximum less than:	**Minimum equal to or better than:**
1	6/18 3/10 (0.3) 20/70	6/60 1/10 (0.1) 20/200
2	6/60 1/10 (0.1) 20/200	3/60 1/20 (0.05) 20/400
3	3/60 1/200 (0.05) 20/400	1/60 (finger counting at one meter) 1/50 (0.02) 5/300 (20/1200)
4	1/60 (finger counting at one meter) 1/50 (0.02) 5/300	Light perception
5	No light perception	
9	Undetermined or unspecified	

Other disorders of eye and adnexa (H55-H57)

√4ᵗʰ H55   **Nystagmus and other irregular eye movements**

    √5ᵗʰ H55.0   **Nystagmus**

        H55.00   **Unspecified nystagmus**   ▽

        H55.01   **Congenital nystagmus**

        H55.02   **Latent nystagmus**

        H55.03   **Visual deprivation nystagmus**

        H55.04   **Dissociated nystagmus**

        H55.09   **Other forms of nystagmus**

    √5ᵗʰ H55.8   **Other irregular eye movements**

        H55.81   **Saccadic eye movements**

        H55.89   **Other irregular eye movements**

√4ᵗʰ H57   **Other disorders of eye and adnexa**

    √5ᵗʰ H57.0   **Anomalies of pupillary function**

        H57.00   **Unspecified anomaly of pupillary function**   ▽

        H57.01   **Argyll Robertson pupil, atypical**
            EXCLUDES 1   *syphilitic Argyll Robertson pupil (A52.19)*

        H57.02   **Anisocoria**

        H57.03   **Miosis**

        H57.04   **Mydriasis**

        √6ᵗʰ H57.05   **Tonic pupil**

            H57.051   **Tonic pupil, right eye**

            H57.052   **Tonic pupil, left eye**

            H57.053   **Tonic pupil, bilateral**

            H57.059   **Tonic pupil, unspecified eye**   ▽

        H57.09   **Other anomalies of pupillary function**

    √5ᵗʰ H57.1   **Ocular pain**

        H57.10   **Ocular pain, unspecified eye**   ▽

        H57.11   **Ocular pain, right eye**

        H57.12   **Ocular pain, left eye**

        H57.13   **Ocular pain, bilateral**

EXCLUDES 1 Not coded here   **EXCLUDES 2** Not included here   N Newborn Age: 0   P Pediatric Age: 0-17   M Maternity Age: 12-55   A Adult Age: 15-124

602   ICD-10-CM 2018

H57.8   Other specified disorders of eye and adnexa

H57.9   Unspecified disorder of eye and adnexa   ▽

Intraoperative and postprocedural complications and disorders of eye and adnexa, not elsewhere classified (H59)

✓4ᵗʰ H59   **Intraoperative and postprocedural complications and disorders of eye and adnexa, not elsewhere classified**

     EXCLUDES 1   mechanical complication of intraocular lens (T85.2)
         mechanical complication of other ocular prosthetic devices, implants and grafts (T85.3)
         pseudophakia (Z96.1)
         secondary cataracts (H26.4-)

✓5ᵗʰ H59.0   **Disorders of the eye following cataract surgery**

   ✓6ᵗʰ H59.01   **Keratopathy (bullous aphakic) following cataract surgery**
       Vitreal corneal syndrome
       Vitreous (touch) syndrome

     H59.011   Keratopathy (bullous aphakic) following cataract surgery, right eye
     H59.012   Keratopathy (bullous aphakic) following cataract surgery, left eye
     H59.013   Keratopathy (bullous aphakic) following cataract surgery, bilateral
     H59.019   Keratopathy (bullous aphakic) following cataract surgery, unspecified eye   ▽

   ✓6ᵗʰ H59.02   **Cataract (lens) fragments in eye following cataract surgery**
     H59.021   Cataract (lens) fragments in eye following cataract surgery, right eye
     H59.022   Cataract (lens) fragments in eye following cataract surgery, left eye
     H59.023   Cataract (lens) fragments in eye following cataract surgery, bilateral
     H59.029   Cataract (lens) fragments in eye following cataract surgery, unspecified eye   ▽

   ✓6ᵗʰ H59.03   **Cystoid macular edema following cataract surgery**
     H59.031   Cystoid macular edema following cataract surgery, right eye
     H59.032   Cystoid macular edema following cataract surgery, left eye
     H59.033   Cystoid macular edema following cataract surgery, bilateral
     H59.039   Cystoid macular edema following cataract surgery, unspecified eye   ▽

   ✓6ᵗʰ H59.09   **Other disorders of the eye following cataract surgery**
     H59.091   Other disorders of the right eye following cataract surgery
     H59.092   Other disorders of the left eye following cataract surgery
     H59.093   Other disorders of the eye following cataract surgery, bilateral
     H59.099   Other disorders of unspecified eye following cataract surgery   ▽

✓5ᵗʰ H59.1   **Intraoperative hemorrhage and hematoma of eye and adnexa complicating a procedure**

     EXCLUDES 1   intraoperative hemorrhage and hematoma of eye and adnexa due to accidental puncture or laceration during a procedure (H59.2-)

   ✓6ᵗʰ H59.11   **Intraoperative hemorrhage and hematoma of eye and adnexa complicating an ophthalmic procedure**
     H59.111   Intraoperative hemorrhage and hematoma of right eye and adnexa complicating an ophthalmic procedure
     H59.112   Intraoperative hemorrhage and hematoma of left eye and adnexa complicating an ophthalmic procedure
     H59.113   Intraoperative hemorrhage and hematoma of eye and adnexa complicating an ophthalmic procedure, bilateral
     H59.119   Intraoperative hemorrhage and hematoma of unspecified eye and adnexa complicating an ophthalmic procedure   ▽

   ✓6ᵗʰ H59.12   **Intraoperative hemorrhage and hematoma of eye and adnexa complicating other procedure**
     H59.121   Intraoperative hemorrhage and hematoma of right eye and adnexa complicating other procedure
     H59.122   Intraoperative hemorrhage and hematoma of left eye and adnexa complicating other procedure
     H59.123   Intraoperative hemorrhage and hematoma of eye and adnexa complicating other procedure, bilateral
     H59.129   Intraoperative hemorrhage and hematoma of unspecified eye and adnexa complicating other procedure   ▽

✓5ᵗʰ H59.2   **Accidental puncture and laceration of eye and adnexa during a procedure**

   ✓6ᵗʰ H59.21   **Accidental puncture and laceration of eye and adnexa during an ophthalmic procedure**
     H59.211   Accidental puncture and laceration of right eye and adnexa during an ophthalmic procedure
     H59.212   Accidental puncture and laceration of left eye and adnexa during an ophthalmic procedure
     H59.213   Accidental puncture and laceration of eye and adnexa during an ophthalmic procedure, bilateral
     H59.219   Accidental puncture and laceration of unspecified eye and adnexa during an ophthalmic procedure   ▽

   ✓6ᵗʰ H59.22   **Accidental puncture and laceration of eye and adnexa during other procedure**
     H59.221   Accidental puncture and laceration of right eye and adnexa during other procedure
     H59.222   Accidental puncture and laceration of left eye and adnexa during other procedure
     H59.223   Accidental puncture and laceration of eye and adnexa during other procedure, bilateral
     H59.229   Accidental puncture and laceration of unspecified eye and adnexa during other procedure   ▽

✓5ᵗʰ H59.3   **Postprocedural hemorrhage, hematoma, and seroma of eye and adnexa following a procedure**

   ✓6ᵗʰ H59.31   **Postprocedural hemorrhage of eye and adnexa following an ophthalmic procedure**
     H59.311   Postprocedural hemorrhage of right eye and adnexa following an ophthalmic procedure
     H59.312   Postprocedural hemorrhage of left eye and adnexa following an ophthalmic procedure
     H59.313   Postprocedural hemorrhage of eye and adnexa following an ophthalmic procedure, bilateral
     H59.319   Postprocedural hemorrhage of unspecified eye and adnexa following an ophthalmic procedure   ▽

   ✓6ᵗʰ H59.32   **Postprocedural hemorrhage of eye and adnexa following other procedure**
     H59.321   Postprocedural hemorrhage of right eye and adnexa following other procedure
     H59.322   Postprocedural hemorrhage of left eye and adnexa following other procedure
     H59.323   Postprocedural hemorrhage of eye and adnexa following other procedure, bilateral
     H59.329   Postprocedural hemorrhage of unspecified eye and adnexa following other procedure   ▽

   ✓6ᵗʰ H59.33   **Postprocedural hematoma of eye and adnexa following an ophthalmic procedure**
     H59.331   Postprocedural hematoma of right eye and adnexa following an ophthalmic procedure
     H59.332   Postprocedural hematoma of left eye and adnexa following an ophthalmic procedure

✓ Additional Character Req   ✓x7ᵗʰ Placeholder Alert   Manifestation   HCC CMS-HCC Condition   ▽ Unspecified Code   ►◄ Revised Text   ● New Code   ▲ Revised Code Title

ICD-10-CM 2018   603

        H59.333   Postprocedural hematoma of eye and adnexa following an ophthalmic procedure, **bilateral**

        H59.339   Postprocedural hematoma of unspecified eye and adnexa following an ophthalmic procedure   ▽

✓6ᵗʰ **H59.34** Postprocedural **hematoma** of eye and adnexa following **other procedure**

        H59.341   Postprocedural hematoma of **right** eye and adnexa following other procedure

        H59.342   Postprocedural hematoma of **left** eye and adnexa following other procedure

        H59.343   Postprocedural hematoma of eye and adnexa following other procedure, **bilateral**

        H59.349   Postprocedural hematoma of unspecified eye and adnexa following other procedure   ▽

✓6ᵗʰ **H59.35** Postprocedural **seroma** of eye and adnexa following an **ophthalmic procedure**

        H59.351   Postprocedural seroma of **right** eye and adnexa following an ophthalmic procedure

        H59.352   Postprocedural seroma of **left** eye and adnexa following an ophthalmic procedure

        H59.353   Postprocedural seroma of eye and adnexa following an ophthalmic procedure, **bilateral**

        H59.359   Postprocedural seroma of unspecified eye and adnexa following an ophthalmic procedure   ▽

✓6ᵗʰ **H59.36** Postprocedural **seroma** of eye and adnexa following **other procedure**

        H59.361   Postprocedural seroma of **right** eye and adnexa following other procedure

        H59.362   Postprocedural seroma of **left** eye and adnexa following other procedure

        H59.363   Postprocedural seroma of eye and adnexa following other procedure, **bilateral**

        H59.369   Postprocedural seroma of unspecified eye and adnexa following other procedure   ▽

✓5ᵗʰ **H59.4** Inflammation (infection) of **postprocedural bleb**
Postprocedural blebitis

    EXCLUDES 1   *filtering (vitreous) bleb after glaucoma surgery status (Z98.83)*

    H59.40 Inflammation (infection) of postprocedural bleb, unspecified   ▽

    H59.41 Inflammation (infection) of postprocedural bleb, stage 1

    H59.42 Inflammation (infection) of postprocedural bleb, stage 2

    H59.43 Inflammation (infection) of postprocedural bleb, stage 3
        Bleb endophthalmitis

✓5ᵗʰ **H59.8** Other intraoperative and postprocedural complications and disorders of eye and adnexa, not elsewhere classified

    ✓6ᵗʰ **H59.81** Chorioretinal scars after surgery for detachment

        H59.811   Chorioretinal scars after surgery for detachment, **right** eye

        H59.812   Chorioretinal scars after surgery for detachment, **left** eye

        H59.813   Chorioretinal scars after surgery for detachment, **bilateral**

        H59.819   Chorioretinal scars after surgery for detachment, unspecified eye   ▽

    H59.88 Other intraoperative complications of eye and adnexa, not elsewhere classified

    H59.89 Other postprocedural complications and disorders of eye and adnexa, not elsewhere classified

EXCLUDES 1 Not coded here   **EXCLUDES 2** Not included here   N Newborn Age: 0   P Pediatric Age: 0-17   M Maternity Age: 12-55   A Adult Age: 15-124

604   ICD-10-CM 2018

H59.333–H59.89

Chapter 8. Diseases of the Ear and Mastoid Process (H60–H95)

Chapter Specific Coding Guidelines and Examples
Reserved for future guideline expansion.

Chapter 8. Diseases of the Ear and Mastoid Process (H60–H95)

Chapter 8. Diseases of the Ear and Mastoid Process (H60-H95)

NOTE Use an external cause code following the code for the ear condition, if applicable, to identify the cause of the ear condition.

EXCLUDES 2 *certain conditions originating in the perinatal period (P04-P96)*
certain infectious and parasitic diseases (A00-B99)
complications of pregnancy, childbirth and the puerperium (O00-O9A)
congenital malformations, deformations and chromosomal abnormalities (Q00-Q99)
endocrine, nutritional and metabolic diseases (E00-E88)
injury, poisoning and certain other consequences of external causes (S00-T88)
neoplasms (C00-D49)
symptoms, signs and abnormal clinical and laboratory findings, not elsewhere classified (R00-R94)

This chapter contains the following blocks:
H60-H62   Diseases of external ear
H65-H75   Diseases of middle ear and mastoid
H80-H83   Diseases of inner ear
H90-H94   Other disorders of ear
H95   Intraoperative and postprocedural complications and disorders of ear and mastoid process, not elsewhere classified

Diseases of external ear (H60-H62)

✓4ᵗʰ H60 Otitis externa

✓5ᵗʰ H60.0 Abscess of external ear
Boil of external ear
Carbuncle of auricle or external auditory canal
Furuncle of external ear
    H60.00   Abscess of external ear, unspecified ear ▽
    H60.01   Abscess of **right** external ear
    H60.02   Abscess of **left** external ear
    H60.03   Abscess of external ear, **bilateral**

✓5ᵗʰ H60.1 Cellulitis of external ear
Cellulitis of auricle
Cellulitis of external auditory canal
    H60.10   Cellulitis of external ear, unspecified ear ▽
    H60.11   Cellulitis of **right** external ear
    H60.12   Cellulitis of **left** external ear
    H60.13   Cellulitis of external ear, **bilateral**

✓5ᵗʰ H60.2 Malignant otitis externa
    H60.20   Malignant otitis externa, unspecified ear ▽
    H60.21   Malignant otitis externa, **right** ear
    H60.22   Malignant otitis externa, **left** ear
    H60.23   Malignant otitis externa, **bilateral**

✓5ᵗʰ H60.3 Other infective otitis externa
  ✓6ᵗʰ H60.31 Diffuse otitis externa
    H60.311   Diffuse otitis externa, **right** ear
    H60.312   Diffuse otitis externa, **left** ear
    H60.313   Diffuse otitis externa, **bilateral**
    H60.319   Diffuse otitis externa, unspecified ear ▽
  ✓6ᵗʰ H60.32 Hemorrhagic otitis externa
    H60.321   Hemorrhagic otitis externa, **right** ear
    H60.322   Hemorrhagic otitis externa, **left** ear
    H60.323   Hemorrhagic otitis externa, **bilateral**
    H60.329   Hemorrhagic otitis externa, unspecified ear ▽
  ✓6ᵗʰ H60.33 Swimmer's ear
    DEF: Otitis externa; commonly occurs when water gets trapped in the ear after swimming.
    H60.331   Swimmer's ear, **right** ear
    H60.332   Swimmer's ear, **left** ear
    H60.333   Swimmer's ear, **bilateral**
    H60.339   Swimmer's ear, unspecified ear ▽
  ✓6ᵗʰ H60.39 Other infective otitis externa
    H60.391   Other infective otitis externa, **right** ear
    H60.392   Other infective otitis externa, **left** ear
    H60.393   Other infective otitis externa, **bilateral**
    H60.399   Other infective otitis externa, unspecified ear ▽

✓5ᵗʰ H60.4 Cholesteatoma of external ear
Keratosis obturans of external ear (canal)
    EXCLUDES 2 *cholesteatoma of middle ear (H71.-)*
                recurrent cholesteatoma of postmastoidectomy cavity (H95.0-)
    H60.40   Cholesteatoma of external ear, unspecified ear ▽
    H60.41   Cholesteatoma of **right** external ear
    H60.42   Cholesteatoma of **left** external ear
    H60.43   Cholesteatoma of external ear, **bilateral**

✓5ᵗʰ H60.5 Acute noninfective otitis externa
  ✓6ᵗʰ H60.50 Unspecified acute noninfective otitis externa
    Acute otitis externa NOS
    H60.501   Unspecified acute noninfective otitis externa, **right** ear ▽
    H60.502   Unspecified acute noninfective otitis externa, **left** ear ▽
    H60.503   Unspecified acute noninfective otitis externa, **bilateral** ▽
    H60.509   Unspecified acute noninfective otitis externa, unspecified ear ▽
  ✓6ᵗʰ H60.51 Acute actinic otitis externa
    H60.511   Acute actinic otitis externa, **right** ear
    H60.512   Acute actinic otitis externa, **left** ear
    H60.513   Acute actinic otitis externa, **bilateral**
    H60.519   Acute actinic otitis externa, unspecified ear ▽
  ✓6ᵗʰ H60.52 Acute chemical otitis externa
    H60.521   Acute chemical otitis externa, **right** ear
    H60.522   Acute chemical otitis externa, **left** ear
    H60.523   Acute chemical otitis externa, **bilateral**
    H60.529   Acute chemical otitis externa, unspecified ear ▽
  ✓6ᵗʰ H60.53 Acute contact otitis externa
    H60.531   Acute contact otitis externa, **right** ear
    H60.532   Acute contact otitis externa, **left** ear
    H60.533   Acute contact otitis externa, **bilateral**
    H60.539   Acute contact otitis externa, unspecified ear ▽
  ✓6ᵗʰ H60.54 Acute eczematoid otitis externa
    H60.541   Acute eczematoid otitis externa, **right** ear
    H60.542   Acute eczematoid otitis externa, **left** ear
    H60.543   Acute eczematoid otitis externa, **bilateral**
    H60.549   Acute eczematoid otitis externa, unspecified ear
  ✓6ᵗʰ H60.55 Acute reactive otitis externa
    H60.551   Acute reactive otitis externa, **right** ear
    H60.552   Acute reactive otitis externa, **left** ear
    H60.553   Acute reactive otitis externa, **bilateral**
    H60.559   Acute reactive otitis externa, unspecified ear ▽
  ✓6ᵗʰ H60.59 Other noninfective acute otitis externa
    H60.591   Other noninfective acute otitis externa, **right** ear
    H60.592   Other noninfective acute otitis externa, **left** ear
    H60.593   Other noninfective acute otitis externa, **bilateral**
    H60.599   Other noninfective acute otitis externa, unspecified ear ▽

✓5ᵗʰ H60.6 Unspecified chronic otitis externa
    H60.60   Unspecified chronic otitis externa, unspecified ear ▽
    H60.61   Unspecified chronic otitis externa, **right** ear ▽
    H60.62   Unspecified chronic otitis externa, **left** ear ▽
    H60.63   Unspecified chronic otitis externa, **bilateral** ▽

✓5ᵗʰ H60.8 Other otitis externa
  ✓6ᵗʰ H60.8X Other otitis externa
    H60.8X1   Other otitis externa, **right** ear
    H60.8X2   Other otitis externa, **left** ear
    H60.8X3   Other otitis externa, **bilateral**
    H60.8X9   Other otitis externa, unspecified ear ▽

✓5ᵗʰ H60.9 Unspecified otitis externa
    H60.90   Unspecified otitis externa, unspecified ear ▽
    H60.91   Unspecified otitis externa, **right** ear ▽

EXCLUDES 1 Not coded here   **EXCLUDES 2** Not included here   N Newborn Age: 0   P Pediatric Age: 0-17   M Maternity Age: 12-55   A Adult Age: 15-124

606   ICD-10-CM 2018

H60.92　Unspecified otitis externa, **left** ear ▽
H60.93　Unspecified otitis externa, **bilateral** ▽

✓4th **H61**　**Other disorders of external ear**

✓5th **H61.0**　**Chondritis and perichondritis of external ear**
Chondrodermatitis nodularis chronica helicis
Perichondritis of auricle
Perichondritis of pinna

✓6th **H61.00**　**Unspecified perichondritis of external ear**
H61.001　Unspecified perichondritis of **right** external ear ▽
H61.002　Unspecified perichondritis of **left** external ear ▽
H61.003　Unspecified perichondritis of external ear, **bilateral** ▽
H61.009　Unspecified perichondritis of external ear, unspecified ear ▽

✓6th **H61.01**　**Acute perichondritis of external ear**
H61.011　Acute perichondritis of **right** external ear
H61.012　Acute perichondritis of **left** external ear
H61.013　Acute perichondritis of external ear, **bilateral**
H61.019　Acute perichondritis of external ear, unspecified ear ▽

✓6th **H61.02**　**Chronic perichondritis of external ear**
H61.021　Chronic perichondritis of **right** external ear
H61.022　Chronic perichondritis of **left** external ear
H61.023　Chronic perichondritis of external ear, **bilateral**
H61.029　Chronic perichondritis of external ear, unspecified ear ▽

✓6th **H61.03**　**Chondritis of external ear**
Chondritis of auricle
Chondritis of pinna
AHA: 2015, 1Q, 18
DEF: Infection that has progressed into the cartilage; presents as indurated and edematous skin over the pinna; vascular compromise occurs with tissue necrosis and deformity.
H61.031　Chondritis of **right** external ear
H61.032　Chondritis of **left** external ear
H61.033　Chondritis of external ear, **bilateral**
H61.039　Chondritis of external ear, unspecified ear ▽

✓5th **H61.1**　**Noninfective disorders of pinna**
EXCLUDES 2　cauliflower ear (M95.1-)
gouty tophi of ear (M1A.-)

✓6th **H61.10**　**Unspecified noninfective disorders of pinna**
Disorder of pinna NOS
H61.101　Unspecified noninfective disorders of pinna, **right** ear ▽
H61.102　Unspecified noninfective disorders of pinna, **left** ear ▽
H61.103　Unspecified noninfective disorders of pinna, **bilateral** ▽
H61.109　Unspecified noninfective disorders of pinna, unspecified ear ▽

✓6th **H61.11**　**Acquired deformity of pinna**
Acquired deformity of auricle
EXCLUDES 2　cauliflower ear (M95.1-)
H61.111　Acquired deformity of pinna, **right** ear
H61.112　Acquired deformity of pinna, **left** ear
H61.113　Acquired deformity of pinna, **bilateral**
H61.119　Acquired deformity of pinna, unspecified ear ▽

✓6th **H61.12**　**Hematoma of pinna**
Hematoma of auricle
H61.121　Hematoma of pinna, **right** ear
H61.122　Hematoma of pinna, **left** ear
H61.123　Hematoma of pinna, **bilateral**
H61.129　Hematoma of pinna, unspecified ear ▽

✓6th **H61.19**　**Other noninfective disorders of pinna**
H61.191　Noninfective disorders of pinna, **right** ear
H61.192　Noninfective disorders of pinna, **left** ear
H61.193　Noninfective disorders of pinna, **bilateral**
H61.199　Noninfective disorders of pinna, unspecified ear ▽

✓5th **H61.2**　**Impacted cerumen**
Wax in ear
H61.20　Impacted cerumen, unspecified ear ▽
H61.21　Impacted cerumen, **right** ear
H61.22　Impacted cerumen, **left** ear
H61.23　Impacted cerumen, **bilateral**

✓5th **H61.3**　**Acquired stenosis of external ear canal**
Collapse of external ear canal
EXCLUDES 1　postprocedural stenosis of external ear canal (H95.81-)

✓6th **H61.30**　**Acquired stenosis of external ear canal, unspecified**
H61.301　Acquired stenosis of **right** external ear canal, unspecified ▽
H61.302　Acquired stenosis of **left** external ear canal, unspecified ▽
H61.303　Acquired stenosis of external ear canal, unspecified, **bilateral** ▽
H61.309　Acquired stenosis of external ear canal, unspecified, unspecified ear ▽

✓6th **H61.31**　**Acquired stenosis of external ear canal secondary to trauma**
H61.311　Acquired stenosis of **right** external ear canal secondary to trauma
H61.312　Acquired stenosis of **left** external ear canal secondary to trauma
H61.313　Acquired stenosis of external ear canal secondary to trauma, **bilateral**
H61.319　Acquired stenosis of external ear canal secondary to trauma, unspecified ear ▽

✓6th **H61.32**　**Acquired stenosis of external ear canal secondary to inflammation and infection**
DEF: Narrowing of the external ear canal; due to chronic inflammation or infection.
H61.321　Acquired stenosis of **right** external ear canal secondary to inflammation and infection
H61.322　Acquired stenosis of **left** external ear canal secondary to inflammation and infection
H61.323　Acquired stenosis of external ear canal secondary to inflammation and infection, **bilateral**
H61.329　Acquired stenosis of external ear canal secondary to inflammation and infection, unspecified ear ▽

✓6th **H61.39**　**Other acquired stenosis of external ear canal**
H61.391　Other acquired stenosis of **right** external ear canal
H61.392　Other acquired stenosis of **left** external ear canal
H61.393　Other acquired stenosis of external ear canal, **bilateral**
H61.399　Other acquired stenosis of external ear canal, unspecified ear ▽

✓5th **H61.8**　**Other specified disorders of external ear**

✓6th **H61.81**　**Exostosis of external canal**
H61.811　Exostosis of **right** external canal
H61.812　Exostosis of **left** external canal
H61.813　Exostosis of external canal, **bilateral**
H61.819　Exostosis of external canal, unspecified ear ▽

✓6th **H61.89**　**Other specified disorders of external ear**
H61.891　Other specified disorders of **right** external ear
H61.892　Other specified disorders of **left** external ear
H61.893　Other specified disorders of external ear, **bilateral**
H61.899　Other specified disorders of external ear, unspecified ear ▽

✓5th **H61.9**　**Disorder of external ear, unspecified**
H61.90　Disorder of external ear, unspecified, unspecified ear ▽
H61.91　Disorder of **right** external ear, unspecified ▽
H61.92　Disorder of **left** external ear, unspecified ▽
H61.93　Disorder of external ear, unspecified, **bilateral** ▽

✓4ᵗʰ **H62 Disorders of external ear in diseases classified elsewhere**

✓5ᵗʰ **H62.4 Otitis externa in other diseases classified elsewhere**

Code first underlying disease, such as:
erysipelas (A46)
impetigo (L01.0)

EXCLUDES 1   otitis externa (in):
candidiasis (B37.84)
herpes viral [herpes simplex] (B00.1)
herpes zoster (B02.8)

H62.40 *Otitis externa in other diseases classified elsewhere, unspecified ear* ▽

H62.41 *Otitis externa in other diseases classified elsewhere, right ear*

H62.42 *Otitis externa in other diseases classified elsewhere, left ear*

H62.43 *Otitis externa in other diseases classified elsewhere, bilateral*

✓5ᵗʰ **H62.8 Other disorders of external ear in diseases classified elsewhere**

Code first underlying disease, such as:
gout (M1A.-, M10.-)

✓6ᵗʰ **H62.8X Other disorders of external ear in diseases classified elsewhere**

H62.8X1 *Other disorders of right external ear in diseases classified elsewhere*

H62.8X2 *Other disorders of left external ear in diseases classified elsewhere*

H62.8X3 *Other disorders of external ear in diseases classified elsewhere, bilateral*

H62.8X9 *Other disorders of external ear in diseases classified elsewhere, unspecified ear* ▽

Diseases of middle ear and mastoid (H65-H75)

✓4ᵗʰ **H65 Nonsuppurative otitis media**

INCLUDES   nonsuppurative otitis media with myringitis

Use additional code for any associated perforated tympanic membrane (H72.-)

Use additional code to identify:
exposure to environmental tobacco smoke (Z77.22)
exposure to tobacco smoke in the perinatal period (P96.81)
history of tobacco dependence (Z87.891)
occupational exposure to environmental tobacco smoke (Z57.31)
tobacco dependence (F17.-)
tobacco use (Z72.0)

✓5ᵗʰ **H65.0 Acute serous otitis media**

Acute and subacute secretory otitis

H65.00 Acute serous otitis media, unspecified ear ▽

H65.01 Acute serous otitis media, right ear

H65.02 Acute serous otitis media, left ear

H65.03 Acute serous otitis media, bilateral

H65.04 Acute serous otitis media, recurrent, right ear

H65.05 Acute serous otitis media, recurrent, left ear

H65.06 Acute serous otitis media, recurrent, bilateral

H65.07 Acute serous otitis media, recurrent, unspecified ear ▽

✓5ᵗʰ **H65.1 Other acute nonsuppurative otitis media**

EXCLUDES 1   otitic barotrauma (T70.0)
otitis media (acute) NOS (H66.9)

✓6ᵗʰ **H65.11 Acute and subacute allergic otitis media (mucoid) (sanguinous) (serous)**

H65.111 Acute and subacute allergic otitis media (mucoid) (sanguinous) (serous), right ear

H65.112 Acute and subacute allergic otitis media (mucoid) (sanguinous) (serous), left ear

H65.113 Acute and subacute allergic otitis media (mucoid) (sanguinous) (serous), bilateral

H65.114 Acute and subacute allergic otitis media (mucoid) (sanguinous) (serous), recurrent, right ear

H65.115 Acute and subacute allergic otitis media (mucoid) (sanguinous) (serous), recurrent, left ear

H65.116 Acute and subacute allergic otitis media (mucoid) (sanguinous) (serous), recurrent, bilateral

H65.117 Acute and subacute allergic otitis media (mucoid) (sanguinous) (serous), recurrent, unspecified ear ▽

H65.119 Acute and subacute allergic otitis media (mucoid) (sanguinous) (serous), unspecified ear ▽

✓6ᵗʰ **H65.19 Other acute nonsuppurative otitis media**

Acute and subacute mucoid otitis media
Acute and subacute nonsuppurative otitis media NOS
Acute and subacute sanguinous otitis media
Acute and subacute seromucinous otitis media

H65.191 Other acute nonsuppurative otitis media, right ear

H65.192 Other acute nonsuppurative otitis media, left ear

H65.193 Other acute nonsuppurative otitis media, bilateral

H65.194 Other acute nonsuppurative otitis media, recurrent, right ear

H65.195 Other acute nonsuppurative otitis media, recurrent, left ear

H65.196 Other acute nonsuppurative otitis media, recurrent, bilateral

H65.197 Other acute nonsuppurative otitis media recurrent, unspecified ear ▽

H65.199 Other acute nonsuppurative otitis media, unspecified ear ▽

✓5ᵗʰ **H65.2 Chronic serous otitis media**

Chronic tubotympanal catarrh

H65.20 Chronic serous otitis media, unspecified ear ▽

H65.21 Chronic serous otitis media, right ear

H65.22 Chronic serous otitis media, left ear

H65.23 Chronic serous otitis media, bilateral

✓5ᵗʰ **H65.3 Chronic mucoid otitis media**

Chronic mucinous otitis media
Chronic secretory otitis media
Chronic transudative otitis media
Glue ear

EXCLUDES 1   adhesive middle ear disease (H74.1)

H65.30 Chronic mucoid otitis media, unspecified ear ▽

H65.31 Chronic mucoid otitis media, right ear

H65.32 Chronic mucoid otitis media, left ear

H65.33 Chronic mucoid otitis media, bilateral

✓5ᵗʰ **H65.4 Other chronic nonsuppurative otitis media**

✓6ᵗʰ **H65.41 Chronic allergic otitis media**

H65.411 Chronic allergic otitis media, right ear

H65.412 Chronic allergic otitis media, left ear

H65.413 Chronic allergic otitis media, bilateral

H65.419 Chronic allergic otitis media, unspecified ear ▽

✓6ᵗʰ **H65.49 Other chronic nonsuppurative otitis media**

Chronic exudative otitis media
Chronic nonsuppurative otitis media NOS
Chronic otitis media with effusion (nonpurulent)
Chronic seromucinous otitis media

H65.491 Other chronic nonsuppurative otitis media, right ear

H65.492 Other chronic nonsuppurative otitis media, left ear

H65.493 Other chronic nonsuppurative otitis media, bilateral

H65.499 Other chronic nonsuppurative otitis media, unspecified ear ▽

✓5ᵗʰ **H65.9 Unspecified nonsuppurative otitis media**

Allergic otitis media NOS
Catarrhal otitis media NOS
Exudative otitis media NOS
Mucoid otitis media NOS
Otitis media with effusion (nonpurulent) NOS

Secretory otitis media NOS
Seromucinous otitis media NOS
Serous otitis media NOS
Transudative otitis media NOS

H65.90 Unspecified nonsuppurative otitis media, unspecified ear ▽

H65.91 Unspecified nonsuppurative otitis media, right ear ▽

H65.92 Unspecified nonsuppurative otitis media, left ear ▽

H65.93 Unspecified nonsuppurative otitis media, bilateral ▽

EXCLUDES 1 Not coded here   **EXCLUDES 2** Not included here   **N** Newborn Age: 0   **P** Pediatric Age: 0-17   **M** Maternity Age: 12-55   **A** Adult Age: 15-124

✓4th **H66 Suppurative and unspecified otitis media**
     INCLUDES suppurative and unspecified otitis media with myringitis
     Use additional code to identify:
       exposure to environmental tobacco smoke (Z77.22)
       exposure to tobacco smoke in the perinatal period (P96.81)
       history of tobacco dependence (Z87.891)
       occupational exposure to environmental tobacco smoke (Z57.31)
       tobacco dependence (F17.-)
       tobacco use (Z72.0)
     AHA: 2016, 1Q, 34

   ✓5th **H66.0 Acute suppurative otitis media**

     ✓6th **H66.00 Acute suppurative otitis media without spontaneous rupture of ear drum**
       H66.001 Acute suppurative otitis media without spontaneous rupture of ear drum, right ear
       H66.002 Acute suppurative otitis media without spontaneous rupture of ear drum, left ear
       H66.003 Acute suppurative otitis media without spontaneous rupture of ear drum, bilateral
       H66.004 Acute suppurative otitis media without spontaneous rupture of ear drum, recurrent, right ear
       H66.005 Acute suppurative otitis media without spontaneous rupture of ear drum, recurrent, left ear
       H66.006 Acute suppurative otitis media without spontaneous rupture of ear drum, recurrent, bilateral
       H66.007 Acute suppurative otitis media without spontaneous rupture of ear drum, recurrent, unspecified ear ▽
       H66.009 Acute suppurative otitis media without spontaneous rupture of ear drum, unspecified ear ▽

     ✓6th **H66.01 Acute suppurative otitis media with spontaneous rupture of ear drum**
       DEF: Sudden, severe inflammation of middle ear, with pressure causing the perforation of ear drum tissue.
       H66.011 Acute suppurative otitis media with spontaneous rupture of ear drum, right ear
       H66.012 Acute suppurative otitis media with spontaneous rupture of ear drum, left ear
       H66.013 Acute suppurative otitis media with spontaneous rupture of ear drum, bilateral
       H66.014 Acute suppurative otitis media with spontaneous rupture of ear drum, recurrent, right ear
       H66.015 Acute suppurative otitis media with spontaneous rupture of ear drum, recurrent, left ear
       H66.016 Acute suppurative otitis media with spontaneous rupture of ear drum, recurrent, bilateral
       H66.017 Acute suppurative otitis media with spontaneous rupture of ear drum, recurrent, unspecified ear ▽
       H66.019 Acute suppurative otitis media with spontaneous rupture of ear drum, unspecified ear ▽

   ✓5th **H66.1 Chronic tubotympanic suppurative otitis media**
     Benign chronic suppurative otitis media
     Chronic tubotympanic disease
     Use additional code for any associated perforated tympanic membrane (H72.-)
     H66.10 Chronic tubotympanic suppurative otitis media, unspecified ▽
     H66.11 Chronic tubotympanic suppurative otitis media, right ear
     H66.12 Chronic tubotympanic suppurative otitis media, left ear
     H66.13 Chronic tubotympanic suppurative otitis media, bilateral

   ✓5th **H66.2 Chronic atticoantral suppurative otitis media**
     Chronic atticoantral disease
     Use additional code for any associated perforated tympanic membrane (H72.-)
     H66.20 Chronic atticoantral suppurative otitis media, unspecified ear ▽
     H66.21 Chronic atticoantral suppurative otitis media, right ear
     H66.22 Chronic atticoantral suppurative otitis media, left ear
     H66.23 Chronic atticoantral suppurative otitis media, bilateral

   ✓5th **H66.3 Other chronic suppurative otitis media**
     Chronic suppurative otitis media NOS
     Use additional code for any associated perforated tympanic membrane (H72.-)
     EXCLUDES 1 tuberculous otitis media (A18.6)
     ✓6th **H66.3X Other chronic suppurative otitis media**
       H66.3X1 Other chronic suppurative otitis media, right ear
       H66.3X2 Other chronic suppurative otitis media, left ear
       H66.3X3 Other chronic suppurative otitis media, bilateral
       H66.3X9 Other chronic suppurative otitis media, unspecified ear ▽

   ✓5th **H66.4 Suppurative otitis media, unspecified**
     Purulent otitis media NOS
     Use additional code for any associated perforated tympanic membrane (H72.-)
     H66.40 Suppurative otitis media, unspecified, unspecified ear ▽
     H66.41 Suppurative otitis media, unspecified, right ear
     H66.42 Suppurative otitis media, unspecified, left ear
     H66.43 Suppurative otitis media, unspecified, bilateral

   ✓5th **H66.9 Otitis media, unspecified**
     Otitis media NOS
     Acute otitis media NOS
     Chronic otitis media NOS
     Use additional code for any associated perforated tympanic membrane (H72.-)
     H66.90 Otitis media, unspecified, unspecified ear ▽
     H66.91 Otitis media, unspecified, right ear ▽
     H66.92 Otitis media, unspecified, left ear ▽
     H66.93 Otitis media, unspecified, bilateral ▽

✓4th **H67 Otitis media in diseases classified elsewhere**
     Code first underlying disease, such as:
       viral disease NEC (B00-B34)
     Use additional code for any associated perforated tympanic membrane (H72.-)
     EXCLUDES 1 otitis media in:
       influenza (J09.X9, J10.83, J11.83)
       measles (B05.3)
       scarlet fever (A38.0)
       tuberculosis (A18.6)
     H67.1 Otitis media in diseases classified elsewhere, right ear
     H67.2 Otitis media in diseases classified elsewhere, left ear
     H67.3 Otitis media in diseases classified elsewhere, bilateral
     H67.9 Otitis media in diseases classified elsewhere, unspecified ear ▽

✓4th **H68 Eustachian salpingitis and obstruction**
   ✓5th **H68.0 Eustachian salpingitis**
     ✓6th **H68.00 Unspecified Eustachian salpingitis**
       H68.001 Unspecified Eustachian salpingitis, right ear ▽
       H68.002 Unspecified Eustachian salpingitis, left ear ▽
       H68.003 Unspecified Eustachian salpingitis, bilateral ▽
       H68.009 Unspecified Eustachian salpingitis, unspecified ear ▽
     ✓6th **H68.01 Acute Eustachian salpingitis**
       H68.011 Acute Eustachian salpingitis, right ear
       H68.012 Acute Eustachian salpingitis, left ear
       H68.013 Acute Eustachian salpingitis, bilateral

✓ Additional Character Req   ✓x7th Placeholder Alert   Manifestation   HCC CMS-HCC Condition   ▽ Unspecified Code   ►◄ Revised Text   ● New Code   ▲ Revised Code Title

ICD-10-CM 2018   609

H66–H68.013

H68.019   Acute Eustachian salpingitis, unspecified ear ▽

√6ᵗʰ **H68.02**   Chronic Eustachian salpingitis
- H68.021   Chronic Eustachian salpingitis, right ear
- H68.022   Chronic Eustachian salpingitis, left ear
- H68.023   Chronic Eustachian salpingitis, bilateral
- H68.029   Chronic Eustachian salpingitis, unspecified ear ▽

√5ᵗʰ **H68.1**   Obstruction of Eustachian tube
Stenosis of Eustachian tube   Stricture of Eustachian tube

√6ᵗʰ **H68.10**   Unspecified obstruction of Eustachian tube
- H68.101   Unspecified obstruction of Eustachian tube, right ear ▽
- H68.102   Unspecified obstruction of Eustachian tube, left ear ▽
- H68.103   Unspecified obstruction of Eustachian tube, bilateral ▽
- H68.109   Unspecified obstruction of Eustachian tube, unspecified ear ▽

√6ᵗʰ **H68.11**   Osseous obstruction of Eustachian tube
- H68.111   Osseous obstruction of Eustachian tube, right ear
- H68.112   Osseous obstruction of Eustachian tube, left ear
- H68.113   Osseous obstruction of Eustachian tube, bilateral
- H68.119   Osseous obstruction of Eustachian tube, unspecified ear ▽

√6ᵗʰ **H68.12**   Intrinsic cartilagenous obstruction of Eustachian tube
- H68.121   Intrinsic cartilagenous obstruction of Eustachian tube, right ear
- H68.122   Intrinsic cartilagenous obstruction of Eustachian tube, left ear
- H68.123   Intrinsic cartilagenous obstruction of Eustachian tube, bilateral
- H68.129   Intrinsic cartilagenous obstruction of Eustachian tube, unspecified ear ▽

√6ᵗʰ **H68.13**   Extrinsic cartilagenous obstruction of Eustachian tube
Compression of Eustachian tube
- H68.131   Extrinsic cartilagenous obstruction of Eustachian tube, right ear
- H68.132   Extrinsic cartilagenous obstruction of Eustachian tube, left ear
- H68.133   Extrinsic cartilagenous obstruction of Eustachian tube, bilateral
- H68.139   Extrinsic cartilagenous obstruction of Eustachian tube, unspecified ear ▽

√4ᵗʰ **H69**   Other and unspecified disorders of Eustachian tube

√5ᵗʰ **H69.0**   Patulous Eustachian tube
- H69.00   Patulous Eustachian tube, unspecified ear ▽
- H69.01   Patulous Eustachian tube, right ear
- H69.02   Patulous Eustachian tube, left ear
- H69.03   Patulous Eustachian tube, bilateral

√5ᵗʰ **H69.8**   Other specified disorders of Eustachian tube
- H69.80   Other specified disorders of Eustachian tube, unspecified ear ▽
- H69.81   Other specified disorders of Eustachian tube, right ear
- H69.82   Other specified disorders of Eustachian tube, left ear
- H69.83   Other specified disorders of Eustachian tube, bilateral

√5ᵗʰ **H69.9**   Unspecified Eustachian tube disorder
- H69.90   Unspecified Eustachian tube disorder, unspecified ear ▽
- H69.91   Unspecified Eustachian tube disorder, right ear ▽
- H69.92   Unspecified Eustachian tube disorder, left ear ▽
- H69.93   Unspecified Eustachian tube disorder, bilateral ▽

√4ᵗʰ **H70**   Mastoiditis and related conditions

√5ᵗʰ **H70.0**   Acute mastoiditis
Abscess of mastoid
Empyema of mastoid

√6ᵗʰ **H70.00**   Acute mastoiditis without complications
- H70.001   Acute mastoiditis without complications, right ear
- H70.002   Acute mastoiditis without complications, left ear
- H70.003   Acute mastoiditis without complications, bilateral
- H70.009   Acute mastoiditis without complications, unspecified ear ▽

√6ᵗʰ **H70.01**   Subperiosteal abscess of mastoid
- H70.011   Subperiosteal abscess of mastoid, right ear
- H70.012   Subperiosteal abscess of mastoid, left ear
- H70.013   Subperiosteal abscess of mastoid, bilateral
- H70.019   Subperiosteal abscess of mastoid, unspecified ear ▽

√6ᵗʰ **H70.09**   Acute mastoiditis with other complications
- H70.091   Acute mastoiditis with other complications, right ear
- H70.092   Acute mastoiditis with other complications, left ear
- H70.093   Acute mastoiditis with other complications, bilateral
- H70.099   Acute mastoiditis with other complications, unspecified ear ▽

√5ᵗʰ **H70.1**   Chronic mastoiditis
Caries of mastoid
Fistula of mastoid
EXCLUDES 1   *tuberculous mastoiditis (A18.03)*
- H70.10   Chronic mastoiditis, unspecified ear ▽
- H70.11   Chronic mastoiditis, right ear
- H70.12   Chronic mastoiditis, left ear
- H70.13   Chronic mastoiditis, bilateral

√5ᵗʰ **H70.2**   Petrositis
Inflammation of petrous bone

√6ᵗʰ **H70.20**   Unspecified petrositis
- H70.201   Unspecified petrositis, right ear ▽
- H70.202   Unspecified petrositis, left ear ▽
- H70.203   Unspecified petrositis, bilateral ▽
- H70.209   Unspecified petrositis, unspecified ear ▽

√6ᵗʰ **H70.21**   Acute petrositis
DEF: Sudden, severe inflammation of petrous temporal bone behind the ear; associated with middle ear infection.
- H70.211   Acute petrositis, right ear
- H70.212   Acute petrositis, left ear
- H70.213   Acute petrositis, bilateral
- H70.219   Acute petrositis, unspecified ear ▽

√6ᵗʰ **H70.22**   Chronic petrositis
- H70.221   Chronic petrositis, right ear
- H70.222   Chronic petrositis, left ear
- H70.223   Chronic petrositis, bilateral
- H70.229   Chronic petrositis, unspecified ear ▽

√5ᵗʰ **H70.8**   Other mastoiditis and related conditions
EXCLUDES 1   *preauricular sinus and cyst (Q18.1)*
sinus, fistula, and cyst of branchial cleft (Q18.0)

√6ᵗʰ **H70.81**   Postauricular fistula
- H70.811   Postauricular fistula, right ear
- H70.812   Postauricular fistula, left ear
- H70.813   Postauricular fistula, bilateral
- H70.819   Postauricular fistula, unspecified ear ▽

√6ᵗʰ **H70.89**   Other mastoiditis and related conditions
- H70.891   Other mastoiditis and related conditions, right ear
- H70.892   Other mastoiditis and related conditions, left ear
- H70.893   Other mastoiditis and related conditions, bilateral
- H70.899   Other mastoiditis and related conditions, unspecified ear ▽

Cholesteatoma of Middle Ear

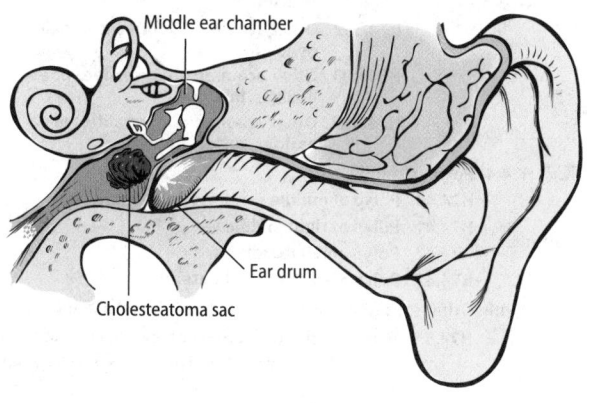

Middle ear chamber

Ear drum

Cholesteatoma sac

✓5th **H70.9 Unspecified mastoiditis**
　H70.90　Unspecified mastoiditis, unspecified ear　▽
　H70.91　Unspecified mastoiditis, **right** ear　▽
　H70.92　Unspecified mastoiditis, **left** ear　▽
　H70.93　Unspecified mastoiditis, **bilateral**　▽

✓4th **H71 Cholesteatoma of middle ear**
　EXCLUDES 2　cholesteatoma of external ear (H60.4-)
　　　　　recurrent cholesteatoma of postmastoidectomy cavity (H95.0-)

✓5th **H71.0 Cholesteatoma of attic**
　H71.00　Cholesteatoma of attic, unspecified ear　▽
　H71.01　Cholesteatoma of attic, **right** ear
　H71.02　Cholesteatoma of attic, **left** ear
　H71.03　Cholesteatoma of attic, **bilateral**

✓5th **H71.1 Cholesteatoma of tympanum**
　H71.10　Cholesteatoma of tympanum, unspecified ear　▽
　H71.11　Cholesteatoma of tympanum, **right** ear
　H71.12　Cholesteatoma of tympanum, **left** ear
　H71.13　Cholesteatoma of tympanum, **bilateral**

✓5th **H71.2 Cholesteatoma of mastoid**
　H71.20　Cholesteatoma of mastoid, unspecified ear　▽
　H71.21　Cholesteatoma of mastoid, **right** ear
　H71.22　Cholesteatoma of mastoid, **left** ear
　H71.23　Cholesteatoma of mastoid, **bilateral**

✓5th **H71.3 Diffuse cholesteatosis**
　H71.30　Diffuse cholesteatosis, unspecified ear　▽
　H71.31　Diffuse cholesteatosis, **right** ear
　H71.32　Diffuse cholesteatosis, **left** ear
　H71.33　Diffuse cholesteatosis, **bilateral**

✓5th **H71.9 Unspecified cholesteatoma**
　H71.90　Unspecified cholesteatoma, unspecified ear　▽
　H71.91　Unspecified cholesteatoma, **right** ear　▽
　H71.92　Unspecified cholesteatoma, **left** ear　▽
　H71.93　Unspecified cholesteatoma, **bilateral**　▽

✓4th **H72 Perforation of tympanic membrane**
　INCLUDES　persistent post-traumatic perforation of ear drum
　　　　　postinflammatory perforation of ear drum
　Code first any associated otitis media (H65.-, H66.1-, H66.2-, H66.3-,
　　H66.4-, H66.9-, H67.-)
　EXCLUDES 1　acute suppurative otitis media with rupture of the tympanic
　　　　　membrane (H66.01-)
　　　　　traumatic rupture of ear drum (S09.2-)

✓5th **H72.0 Central perforation of tympanic membrane**
　H72.00　Central perforation of tympanic membrane,　▽
　　　　　unspecified ear
　H72.01　Central perforation of tympanic membrane, **right**
　　　　　ear
　H72.02　Central perforation of tympanic membrane, **left** ear
　H72.03　Central perforation of tympanic membrane,
　　　　　bilateral

✓5th **H72.1 Attic perforation of tympanic membrane**
　Perforation of pars flaccida
　H72.10　Attic perforation of tympanic membrane,　▽
　　　　　unspecified ear

H72.11　Attic perforation of tympanic membrane, **right** ear
H72.12　Attic perforation of tympanic membrane, **left** ear
H72.13　Attic perforation of tympanic membrane, **bilateral**

✓5th **H72.2 Other marginal perforations of tympanic membrane**
　✓6th **H72.2X Other marginal perforations of tympanic membrane**
　　H72.2X1　Other marginal perforations of tympanic
　　　　　membrane, **right** ear
　　H72.2X2　Other marginal perforations of tympanic
　　　　　membrane, **left** ear
　　H72.2X3　Other marginal perforations of tympanic
　　　　　membrane, **bilateral**
　　H72.2X9　Other marginal perforations of　▽
　　　　　tympanic membrane, unspecified ear

✓5th **H72.8 Other perforations of tympanic membrane**
　✓6th **H72.81 Multiple perforations of tympanic membrane**
　　H72.811　Multiple perforations of tympanic
　　　　　membrane, **right** ear
　　H72.812　Multiple perforations of tympanic
　　　　　membrane, **left** ear
　　H72.813　Multiple perforations of tympanic
　　　　　membrane, **bilateral**
　　H72.819　Multiple perforations of tympanic　▽
　　　　　membrane, unspecified ear
　✓6th **H72.82 Total perforations of tympanic membrane**
　　H72.821　Total perforations of tympanic
　　　　　membrane, **right** ear
　　H72.822　Total perforations of tympanic
　　　　　membrane, **left** ear
　　H72.823　Total perforations of tympanic
　　　　　membrane, **bilateral**
　　H72.829　Total perforations of tympanic　▽
　　　　　membrane, unspecified ear

✓5th **H72.9 Unspecified perforation of tympanic membrane**
　H72.90　Unspecified perforation of tympanic membrane,　▽
　　　　　unspecified ear
　H72.91　Unspecified perforation of tympanic membrane,　▽
　　　　　right ear
　H72.92　Unspecified perforation of tympanic membrane,　▽
　　　　　left ear
　H72.93　Unspecified perforation of tympanic membrane,　▽
　　　　　bilateral

✓4th **H73 Other disorders of tympanic membrane**
　✓5th **H73.0 Acute myringitis**
　　EXCLUDES 1　acute myringitis with otitis media (H65, H66)
　　✓6th **H73.00 Unspecified acute myringitis**
　　　Acute tympanitis NOS
　　　H73.001　Acute myringitis, **right** ear
　　　H73.002　Acute myringitis, **left** ear
　　　H73.003　Acute myringitis, **bilateral**
　　　H73.009　Acute myringitis, unspecified ear　▽
　　✓6th **H73.01 Bullous myringitis**
　　　DEF: Bacterial or viral otitis media; characterized by the
　　　appearance of serous or hemorrhagic blebs on the ear
　　　drum and sudden onset of severe pain in ear.
　　　H73.011　Bullous myringitis, **right** ear
　　　H73.012　Bullous myringitis, **left** ear
　　　H73.013　Bullous myringitis, **bilateral**
　　　H73.019　Bullous myringitis, unspecified ear　▽
　　✓6th **H73.09 Other acute myringitis**
　　　H73.091　Other acute myringitis, **right** ear
　　　H73.092　Other acute myringitis, **left** ear
　　　H73.093　Other acute myringitis, **bilateral**
　　　H73.099　Other acute myringitis, unspecified ear　▽
　✓5th **H73.1 Chronic myringitis**
　　Chronic tympanitis
　　EXCLUDES 1　chronic myringitis with otitis media (H65, H66)
　　H73.10　Chronic myringitis, unspecified ear　▽
　　H73.11　Chronic myringitis, **right** ear
　　H73.12　Chronic myringitis, **left** ear
　　H73.13　Chronic myringitis, **bilateral**
　✓5th **H73.2 Unspecified myringitis**
　　H73.20　Unspecified myringitis, unspecified ear　▽
　　H73.21　Unspecified myringitis, **right** ear　▽
　　H73.22　Unspecified myringitis, **left** ear　▽

✓ Additional Character Req　✓x7th Placeholder Alert　Manifestation　HCC CMS-HCC Condition　▽ Unspecified Code　►◄ Revised Text　● New Code　▲ Revised Code Title
ICD-10-CM 2018　　611

H70.9–H73.22

Chapter 8. Diseases of the Ear and Mastoid Process

H73.23   **Unspecified myringitis**, bilateral ▽

✓5ᵗʰ **H73.8   Other specified disorders of tympanic membrane**

  ✓6ᵗʰ **H73.81   Atrophic flaccid tympanic membrane**

    H73.811   **Atrophic flaccid tympanic membrane, right ear**

    H73.812   **Atrophic flaccid tympanic membrane, left ear**

    H73.813   **Atrophic flaccid tympanic membrane, bilateral**

    H73.819   **Atrophic flaccid tympanic membrane, unspecified ear** ▽

  ✓6ᵗʰ **H73.82   Atrophic nonflaccid tympanic membrane**

    H73.821   **Atrophic nonflaccid tympanic membrane, right ear**

    H73.822   **Atrophic nonflaccid tympanic membrane, left ear**

    H73.823   **Atrophic nonflaccid tympanic membrane, bilateral**

    H73.829   **Atrophic nonflaccid tympanic membrane, unspecified ear** ▽

  ✓6ᵗʰ **H73.89   Other specified disorders of tympanic membrane**

    H73.891   **Other specified disorders of tympanic membrane, right ear**

    H73.892   **Other specified disorders of tympanic membrane, left ear**

    H73.893   **Other specified disorders of tympanic membrane, bilateral**

    H73.899   **Other specified disorders of tympanic membrane, unspecified ear** ▽

✓5ᵗʰ **H73.9   Unspecified disorder of tympanic membrane**

  H73.90   **Unspecified disorder of tympanic membrane, unspecified ear** ▽

  H73.91   **Unspecified disorder of tympanic membrane, right ear** ▽

  H73.92   **Unspecified disorder of tympanic membrane, left ear** ▽

  H73.93   **Unspecified disorder of tympanic membrane, bilateral** ▽

✓4ᵗʰ **H74   Other disorders of middle ear mastoid**

  EXCLUDES 2   mastoiditis (H70.-)

✓5ᵗʰ **H74.0   Tympanosclerosis**

  DEF: Calcification of tissue in the ear drum, middle ear bones, and middle ear canal.

  H74.01   **Tympanosclerosis, right ear**

  H74.02   **Tympanosclerosis, left ear**

  H74.03   **Tympanosclerosis, bilateral**

  H74.09   **Tympanosclerosis, unspecified ear** ▽

✓5ᵗʰ **H74.1   Adhesive middle ear disease**

  Adhesive otitis

  EXCLUDES 1   glue ear (H65.3-)

  H74.11   **Adhesive right middle ear disease**

  H74.12   **Adhesive left middle ear disease**

  H74.13   **Adhesive middle ear disease, bilateral**

  H74.19   **Adhesive middle ear disease, unspecified ear** ▽

✓5ᵗʰ **H74.2   Discontinuity and dislocation of ear ossicles**

  H74.20   **Discontinuity and dislocation of ear ossicles, unspecified ear** ▽

  H74.21   **Discontinuity and dislocation of right ear ossicles**

  H74.22   **Discontinuity and dislocation of left ear ossicles**

  H74.23   **Discontinuity and dislocation of ear ossicles, bilateral**

✓5ᵗʰ **H74.3   Other acquired abnormalities of ear ossicles**

  ✓6ᵗʰ **H74.31   Ankylosis of ear ossicles**

    H74.311   **Ankylosis of ear ossicles, right ear**

    H74.312   **Ankylosis of ear ossicles, left ear**

    H74.313   **Ankylosis of ear ossicles, bilateral**

    H74.319   **Ankylosis of ear ossicles, unspecified ear** ▽

  ✓6ᵗʰ **H74.32   Partial loss of ear ossicles**

    H74.321   **Partial loss of ear ossicles, right ear**

    H74.322   **Partial loss of ear ossicles, left ear**

    H74.323   **Partial loss of ear ossicles, bilateral**

    H74.329   **Partial loss of ear ossicles, unspecified ear** ▽

  ✓6ᵗʰ **H74.39   Other acquired abnormalities of ear ossicles**

    H74.391   **Other acquired abnormalities of right ear ossicles**

    H74.392   **Other acquired abnormalities of left ear ossicles**

    H74.393   **Other acquired abnormalities of ear ossicles, bilateral**

    H74.399   **Other acquired abnormalities of ear ossicles, unspecified ear** ▽

✓5ᵗʰ **H74.4   Polyp of middle ear**

  H74.40   **Polyp of middle ear, unspecified ear** ▽

  H74.41   **Polyp of right middle ear**

  H74.42   **Polyp of left middle ear**

  H74.43   **Polyp of middle ear, bilateral**

✓5ᵗʰ **H74.8   Other specified disorders of middle ear and mastoid**

  ✓6ᵗʰ **H74.8X   Other specified disorders of middle ear and mastoid**

    H74.8X1   **Other specified disorders of right middle ear and mastoid**

    H74.8X2   **Other specified disorders of left middle ear and mastoid**

    H74.8X3   **Other specified disorders of middle ear and mastoid, bilateral**

    H74.8X9   **Other specified disorders of middle ear and mastoid, unspecified ear** ▽

✓5ᵗʰ **H74.9   Unspecified disorder of middle ear and mastoid**

  H74.90   **Unspecified disorder of middle ear and mastoid, unspecified ear** ▽

  H74.91   **Unspecified disorder of right middle ear and mastoid** ▽

  H74.92   **Unspecified disorder of left middle ear and mastoid** ▽

  H74.93   **Unspecified disorder of middle ear and mastoid, bilateral** ▽

✓4ᵗʰ **H75   Other disorders of middle ear and mastoid in diseases classified elsewhere**

  Code first underlying disease

✓5ᵗʰ **H75.0   Mastoiditis in infectious and parasitic diseases classified elsewhere**

  EXCLUDES 1   mastoiditis (in):

    syphilis (A52.77)

    tuberculosis (A18.03)

  H75.00   *Mastoiditis in infectious and parasitic diseases classified elsewhere, unspecified ear* ▽

  H75.01   *Mastoiditis in infectious and parasitic diseases classified elsewhere, right ear*

  H75.02   *Mastoiditis in infectious and parasitic diseases classified elsewhere, left ear*

  H75.03   *Mastoiditis in infectious and parasitic diseases classified elsewhere, bilateral*

✓5ᵗʰ **H75.8   Other specified disorders of middle ear and mastoid in diseases classified elsewhere**

  H75.80   *Other specified disorders of middle ear and mastoid in diseases classified elsewhere, unspecified ear* ▽

  H75.81   *Other specified disorders of right middle ear and mastoid in diseases classified elsewhere*

  H75.82   *Other specified disorders of left middle ear and mastoid in diseases classified elsewhere*

  H75.83   *Other specified disorders of middle ear and mastoid in diseases classified elsewhere, bilateral*

Diseases of inner ear (H80-H83)

✓4ᵗʰ **H80   Otosclerosis**

  INCLUDES   otospongiosis

✓5ᵗʰ **H80.0   Otosclerosis involving oval window, nonobliterative**

  H80.00   **Otosclerosis involving oval window, nonobliterative, unspecified ear** ▽

  H80.01   **Otosclerosis involving oval window, nonobliterative, right ear**

  H80.02   **Otosclerosis involving oval window, nonobliterative, left ear**

  H80.03   **Otosclerosis involving oval window, nonobliterative, bilateral**

EXCLUDES 1 Not coded here   *EXCLUDES 2* Not included here   N Newborn Age: 0   P Pediatric Age: 0-17   M Maternity Age: 12-55   A Adult Age: 15-124

612   ICD-10-CM 2018

✓5th **H80.1 Otosclerosis involving oval window,** obliterative

     H80.10 Otosclerosis involving oval window, obliterative, unspecified ear ▽

     H80.11 Otosclerosis involving oval window, obliterative, right ear

     H80.12 Otosclerosis involving oval window, obliterative, left ear

     H80.13 Otosclerosis involving oval window, obliterative, bilateral

✓5th **H80.2 Cochlear otosclerosis**
     Otosclerosis involving otic capsule
     Otosclerosis involving round window

     H80.20 Cochlear otosclerosis, unspecified ear ▽

     H80.21 Cochlear otosclerosis, right ear

     H80.22 Cochlear otosclerosis, left ear

     H80.23 Cochlear otosclerosis, bilateral

✓5th **H80.8 Other otosclerosis**

     H80.80 Other otosclerosis, unspecified ear ▽

     H80.81 Other otosclerosis, right ear

     H80.82 Other otosclerosis, left ear

     H80.83 Other otosclerosis, bilateral

✓5th **H80.9 Unspecified otosclerosis**

     H80.90 Unspecified otosclerosis, unspecified ear ▽

     H80.91 Unspecified otosclerosis, right ear ▽

     H80.92 Unspecified otosclerosis, left ear ▽

     H80.93 Unspecified otosclerosis, bilateral ▽

✓4th **H81 Disorders of vestibular function**
     EXCLUDES 1   epidemic vertigo (A88.1)
               vertigo NOS (R42)

✓5th **H81.0 Ménière's disease**
     Labyrinthine hydrops
     Ménière's syndrome or vertigo

     H81.01 Ménière's disease, right ear

     H81.02 Ménière's disease, left ear

     H81.03 Ménière's disease, bilateral

     H81.09 Ménière's disease, unspecified ear ▽

✓5th **H81.1 Benign paroxysmal vertigo**

     H81.10 Benign paroxysmal vertigo, unspecified ear ▽

     H81.11 Benign paroxysmal vertigo, right ear

     H81.12 Benign paroxysmal vertigo, left ear

     H81.13 Benign paroxysmal vertigo, bilateral

✓5th **H81.2 Vestibular neuronitis**
     DEF: Transient benign vertigo, caused by inflammation of the vestibular nerve; characterized by response to caloric stimulation on one side, nystagmus with rhythmic movement of eyes; normal auditory function present.

     H81.20 Vestibular neuronitis, unspecified ear ▽

     H81.21 Vestibular neuronitis, right ear

     H81.22 Vestibular neuronitis, left ear

     H81.23 Vestibular neuronitis, bilateral

✓5th **H81.3 Other peripheral vertigo**

     ✓6th **H81.31 Aural vertigo**

         H81.311 Aural vertigo, right ear

         H81.312 Aural vertigo, left ear

         H81.313 Aural vertigo, bilateral

         H81.319 Aural vertigo, unspecified ear ▽

     ✓6th **H81.39 Other peripheral vertigo**
         Lermoyez' syndrome
         Otogenic vertigo
         Peripheral vertigo NOS

         H81.391 Other peripheral vertigo, right ear

         H81.392 Other peripheral vertigo, left ear

         H81.393 Other peripheral vertigo, bilateral

         H81.399 Other peripheral vertigo, unspecified ear ▽

✓5th **H81.4 Vertigo of central origin**
     Central positional nystagmus

     H81.41 Vertigo of central origin, right ear

     H81.42 Vertigo of central origin, left ear

     H81.43 Vertigo of central origin, bilateral

     H81.49 Vertigo of central origin, unspecified ear ▽

✓5th **H81.8 Other disorders of vestibular function**

     ✓6th **H81.8X Other disorders of vestibular function**

         H81.8X1 Other disorders of vestibular function, right ear

         H81.8X2 Other disorders of vestibular function, left ear

         H81.8X3 Other disorders of vestibular function, bilateral

         H81.8X9 Other disorders of vestibular function, unspecified ear ▽

✓5th **H81.9 Unspecified disorder of vestibular function**
     Vertiginous syndrome NOS

     H81.90 Unspecified disorder of vestibular function, unspecified ear ▽

     H81.91 Unspecified disorder of vestibular function, right ear ▽

     H81.92 Unspecified disorder of vestibular function, left ear ▽

     H81.93 Unspecified disorder of vestibular function, bilateral ▽

✓4th **H82 Vertiginous syndromes in diseases classified elsewhere**
     Code first underlying disease
     EXCLUDES 1   epidemic vertigo (A88.1)

     H82.1 Vertiginous syndromes in diseases classified elsewhere, right ear

     H82.2 Vertiginous syndromes in diseases classified elsewhere, left ear

     H82.3 Vertiginous syndromes in diseases classified elsewhere, bilateral

     H82.9 Vertiginous syndromes in diseases classified elsewhere, unspecified ear ▽

✓4th **H83 Other diseases of inner ear**

     ✓5th **H83.0 Labyrinthitis**
         DEF: Inflammation of the inner ear, or labyrinth; characterized by pus, vertigo, dizziness, nausea, and hearing loss.

         H83.01 Labyrinthitis, right ear

         H83.02 Labyrinthitis, left ear

         H83.03 Labyrinthitis, bilateral

         H83.09 Labyrinthitis, unspecified ear ▽

     ✓5th **H83.1 Labyrinthine fistula**

         H83.11 Labyrinthine fistula, right ear

         H83.12 Labyrinthine fistula, left ear

         H83.13 Labyrinthine fistula, bilateral

         H83.19 Labyrinthine fistula, unspecified ear ▽

     ✓5th **H83.2 Labyrinthine dysfunction**
         Labyrinthine hypersensitivity
         Labyrinthine hypofunction
         Labyrinthine loss of function
         DEF: Decreased function of the labyrinth sensors.

         ✓6th **H83.2X Labyrinthine dysfunction**

             H83.2X1 Labyrinthine dysfunction, right ear

             H83.2X2 Labyrinthine dysfunction, left ear

             H83.2X3 Labyrinthine dysfunction, bilateral

             H83.2X9 Labyrinthine dysfunction, unspecified ear ▽

     ✓5th **H83.3 Noise effects on inner ear**
         Acoustic trauma of inner ear
         Noise-induced hearing loss of inner ear

         ✓6th **H83.3X Noise effects on inner ear**

             H83.3X1 Noise effects on right inner ear

             H83.3X2 Noise effects on left inner ear

             H83.3X3 Noise effects on inner ear, bilateral

             H83.3X9 Noise effects on inner ear, unspecified ear ▽

     ✓5th **H83.8 Other specified diseases of inner ear**

         ✓6th **H83.8X Other specified diseases of inner ear**

             H83.8X1 Other specified diseases of right inner ear

             H83.8X2 Other specified diseases of left inner ear

             H83.8X3 Other specified diseases of inner ear, bilateral

             H83.8X9 Other specified diseases of inner ear, unspecified ear ▽

✓ Additional Character Req   ✓x7th Placeholder Alert   Manifestation   HCC CMS-HCC Condition   ▽ Unspecified Code   ►◄ Revised Text   ● New Code   ▲ Revised Code Title

ICD-10-CM 2018   613

✓5th **H83.9** **Unspecified disease of inner ear**
　　H83.90 Unspecified disease of inner ear, unspecified ear ▽
　　H83.91 Unspecified disease of right inner ear ▽
　　H83.92 Unspecified disease of left inner ear ▽
　　H83.93 Unspecified disease of inner ear, bilateral ▽

Other disorders of ear (H90-H94)

✓4th **H90** **Conductive and sensorineural hearing loss**
　　EXCLUDES 1 *deaf nonspeaking NEC (H91.3)*
　　　　deafness NOS (H91.9-)
　　　　hearing loss NOS (H91.9-)
　　　　noise-induced hearing loss (H83.3-)
　　　　ototoxic hearing loss (H91.0-)
　　　　sudden (idiopathic) hearing loss (H91.2-)
　　AHA: 2015, 2Q, 7

H90.0 Conductive hearing loss, bilateral

✓5th **H90.1** Conductive hearing loss, unilateral with unrestricted hearing on the contralateral side
　　H90.11 Conductive hearing loss, unilateral, right ear, with unrestricted hearing on the contralateral side
　　H90.12 Conductive hearing loss, unilateral, left ear, with unrestricted hearing on the contralateral side

H90.2 Conductive hearing loss, unspecified ▽
　　Conductive deafness NOS

H90.3 Sensorineural hearing loss, bilateral

✓5th **H90.4** Sensorineural hearing loss, unilateral with unrestricted hearing on the contralateral side
　　H90.41 Sensorineural hearing loss, unilateral, right ear, with unrestricted hearing on the contralateral side
　　H90.42 Sensorineural hearing loss, unilateral, left ear, with unrestricted hearing on the contralateral side

H90.5 Unspecified sensorineural hearing loss ▽
　　Central hearing loss NOS
　　Congenital deafness NOS
　　Neural hearing loss NOS
　　Perceptive hearing loss NOS
　　Sensorineural deafness NOS
　　Sensory hearing loss NOS
　　　EXCLUDES 1 *abnormal auditory perception (H93.2-)*
　　　　　psychogenic deafness (F44.6)

H90.6 Mixed conductive and sensorineural hearing loss, bilateral
　　AHA: 2015, 2Q, 7

✓5th **H90.7** Mixed conductive and sensorineural hearing loss, unilateral with unrestricted hearing on the contralateral side
　　H90.71 Mixed conductive and sensorineural hearing loss, unilateral, right ear, with unrestricted hearing on the contralateral side
　　H90.72 Mixed conductive and sensorineural hearing loss, unilateral, left ear, with unrestricted hearing on the contralateral side

H90.8 Mixed conductive and sensorineural hearing loss, unspecified ▽

✓5th **H90.A** Conductive and sensorineural hearing loss with restricted hearing on the contralateral side
　　✓6th **H90.A1** Conductive hearing loss, unilateral, with restricted hearing on the contralateral side
　　　　H90.A11 Conductive hearing loss, unilateral, right ear with restricted hearing on the contralateral side
　　　　H90.A12 Conductive hearing loss, unilateral, left ear with restricted hearing on the contralateral side
　　✓6th **H90.A2** Sensorineural hearing loss, unilateral, with restricted hearing on the contralateral side
　　　　H90.A21 Sensorineural hearing loss, unilateral, right ear, with restricted hearing on the contralateral side
　　　　H90.A22 Sensorineural hearing loss, unilateral, left ear, with restricted hearing on the contralateral side
　　✓6th **H90.A3** Mixed conductive and sensorineural hearing loss, unilateral with restricted hearing on the contralateral side
　　　　H90.A31 Mixed conductive and sensorineural hearing loss, unilateral, right ear with restricted hearing on the contralateral side

H90.A32 Mixed conductive and sensorineural hearing loss, unilateral, left ear with restricted hearing on the contralateral side

✓4th **H91** **Other and unspecified hearing loss**
　　EXCLUDES 1 *abnormal auditory perception (H93.2-)*
　　　　hearing loss as classified in H90-
　　　　impacted cerumen (H61.2-)
　　　　noise-induced hearing loss (H83.3-)
　　　　psychogenic deafness (F44.6)
　　　　transient ischemic deafness (H93.01-)

✓5th **H91.0** Ototoxic hearing loss
　　Code first poisoning due to drug or toxin, if applicable (T36-T65 with fifth or sixth character 1-4 or 6)
　　Use additional code for adverse effect, if applicable, to identify drug (T36-T50 with fifth or sixth character 5)
　　H91.01 Ototoxic hearing loss, right ear
　　H91.02 Ototoxic hearing loss, left ear
　　H91.03 Ototoxic hearing loss, bilateral
　　H91.09 Ototoxic hearing loss, unspecified ear ▽

✓5th **H91.1** Presbycusis
　　Presbyacusia
　　H91.10 Presbycusis, unspecified ear ▽
　　H91.11 Presbycusis, right ear
　　H91.12 Presbycusis, left ear
　　H91.13 Presbycusis, bilateral

✓5th **H91.2** Sudden idiopathic hearing loss
　　Sudden hearing loss NOS
　　H91.20 Sudden idiopathic hearing loss, unspecified ear ▽
　　H91.21 Sudden idiopathic hearing loss, right ear
　　H91.22 Sudden idiopathic hearing loss, left ear
　　H91.23 Sudden idiopathic hearing loss, bilateral

H91.3 Deaf nonspeaking, not elsewhere classified

✓5th **H91.8** Other specified hearing loss
　　✓6th **H91.8X** Other specified hearing loss
　　　　H91.8X1 Other specified hearing loss, right ear
　　　　H91.8X2 Other specified hearing loss, left ear
　　　　H91.8X3 Other specified hearing loss, bilateral
　　　　H91.8X9 Other specified hearing loss, unspecified ear ▽

✓5th **H91.9** Unspecified hearing loss
　　Deafness NOS
　　High frequency deafness
　　Low frequency deafness
　　H91.90 Unspecified hearing loss, unspecified ear ▽
　　H91.91 Unspecified hearing loss, right ear ▽
　　H91.92 Unspecified hearing loss, left ear ▽
　　H91.93 Unspecified hearing loss, bilateral ▽

✓4th **H92** **Otalgia and effusion of ear**
　　✓5th **H92.0** Otalgia
　　　　H92.01 Otalgia, right ear
　　　　H92.02 Otalgia, left ear
　　　　H92.03 Otalgia, bilateral
　　　　H92.09 Otalgia, unspecified ear ▽
　　✓5th **H92.1** Otorrhea
　　　　EXCLUDES 1 *leakage of cerebrospinal fluid through ear (G96.0)*
　　　　H92.10 Otorrhea, unspecified ear ▽
　　　　H92.11 Otorrhea, right ear
　　　　H92.12 Otorrhea, left ear
　　　　H92.13 Otorrhea, bilateral
　　✓5th **H92.2** Otorrhagia
　　　　EXCLUDES 1 *traumatic otorrhagia—code to injury*
　　　　H92.20 Otorrhagia, unspecified ear ▽
　　　　H92.21 Otorrhagia, right ear
　　　　H92.22 Otorrhagia, left ear
　　　　H92.23 Otorrhagia, bilateral

✓4th **H93** **Other disorders of ear, not elsewhere classified**
　　✓5th **H93.0** Degenerative and vascular disorders of ear
　　　　EXCLUDES 1 *presbycusis (H91.1)*
　　　　✓6th **H93.01** Transient ischemic deafness
　　　　　　H93.011 Transient ischemic deafness, right ear
　　　　　　H93.012 Transient ischemic deafness, left ear

H93.013   Transient ischemic deafness, bilateral

H93.019   Transient ischemic deafness, unspecified ear

✓6th **H93.09**   Unspecified degenerative and vascular disorders of ear

H93.091   Unspecified degenerative and vascular disorders of right ear

H93.092   Unspecified degenerative and vascular disorders of left ear

H93.093   Unspecified degenerative and vascular disorders of ear, bilateral

H93.099   Unspecified degenerative and vascular disorders of unspecified ear

✓5th **H93.1**   Tinnitus

H93.11   Tinnitus, right ear

H93.12   Tinnitus, left ear

H93.13   Tinnitus, bilateral

H93.19   Tinnitus, unspecified ear

✓5th **H93.A**   Pulsatile Tinnitus

H93.A1   Pulsatile tinnitus, right ear

H93.A2   Pulsatile tinnitus, left ear

H93.A3   Pulsatile tinnitus, bilateral

H93.A9   Pulsatile tinnitus, unspecified ear

✓5th **H93.2**   Other abnormal auditory perceptions

EXCLUDES 2   auditory hallucinations (R44.0)

✓6th **H93.21**   Auditory recruitment

H93.211   Auditory recruitment, right ear

H93.212   Auditory recruitment, left ear

H93.213   Auditory recruitment, bilateral

H93.219   Auditory recruitment, unspecified ear

✓6th **H93.22**   Diplacusis

H93.221   Diplacusis, right ear

H93.222   Diplacusis, left ear

H93.223   Diplacusis, bilateral

H93.229   Diplacusis, unspecified ear

✓6th **H93.23**   Hyperacusis

DEF: Exceptionally acute sense of hearing caused by such conditions as Bell's palsy; this term may also refer to painful sensitivity to sounds.

H93.231   Hyperacusis, right ear

H93.232   Hyperacusis, left ear

H93.233   Hyperacusis, bilateral

H93.239   Hyperacusis, unspecified ear

✓6th **H93.24**   Temporary auditory threshold shift

H93.241   Temporary auditory threshold shift, right ear

H93.242   Temporary auditory threshold shift, left ear

H93.243   Temporary auditory threshold shift, bilateral

H93.249   Temporary auditory threshold shift, unspecified ear

H93.25   Central auditory processing disorder

Congenital auditory imperception

Word deafness

EXCLUDES 1   mixed receptive-expressive language disorder (F80.2)

✓6th **H93.29**   Other abnormal auditory perceptions

H93.291   Other abnormal auditory perceptions, right ear

H93.292   Other abnormal auditory perceptions, left ear

H93.293   Other abnormal auditory perceptions, bilateral

H93.299   Other abnormal auditory perceptions, unspecified ear

✓5th **H93.3**   Disorders of acoustic nerve

Disorder of 8th cranial nerve

EXCLUDES 1   acoustic neuroma (D33.3)

syphilitic acoustic neuritis (A52.15)

✓6th **H93.3X**   Disorders of acoustic nerve

H93.3X1   Disorders of right acoustic nerve

H93.3X2   Disorders of left acoustic nerve

H93.3X3   Disorders of bilateral acoustic nerves

H93.3X9   Disorders of unspecified acoustic nerve

✓5th **H93.8**   Other specified disorders of ear

✓6th **H93.8X**   Other specified disorders of ear

H93.8X1   Other specified disorders of right ear

H93.8X2   Other specified disorders of left ear

H93.8X3   Other specified disorders of ear, bilateral

H93.8X9   Other specified disorders of ear, unspecified ear

✓5th **H93.9**   Unspecified disorder of ear

H93.90   Unspecified disorder of ear, unspecified ear

H93.91   Unspecified disorder of right ear

H93.92   Unspecified disorder of left ear

H93.93   Unspecified disorder of ear, bilateral

✓4th **H94**   Other disorders of ear in diseases classified elsewhere

✓5th **H94.0**   Acoustic neuritis in infectious and parasitic diseases classified elsewhere

Code first underlying disease, such as:

parasitic disease (B65-B89)

EXCLUDES 1   acoustic neuritis (in):

herpes zoster (B02.29)

syphilis (A52.15)

H94.00   Acoustic neuritis in infectious and parasitic diseases classified elsewhere, unspecified ear

H94.01   Acoustic neuritis in infectious and parasitic diseases classified elsewhere, right ear

H94.02   Acoustic neuritis in infectious and parasitic diseases classified elsewhere, left ear

H94.03   Acoustic neuritis in infectious and parasitic diseases classified elsewhere, bilateral

✓5th **H94.8**   Other specified disorders of ear in diseases classified elsewhere

Code first underlying disease, such as:

congenital syphilis (A50.0)

EXCLUDES 1   aural myiasis (B87.4)

syphilitic labyrinthitis (A52.79)

H94.80   Other specified disorders of ear in diseases classified elsewhere, unspecified ear

H94.81   Other specified disorders of right ear in diseases classified elsewhere

H94.82   Other specified disorders of left ear in diseases classified elsewhere

H94.83   Other specified disorders of ear in diseases classified elsewhere, bilateral

Intraoperative and postprocedural complications and disorders of ear and mastoid process, not elsewhere classified (H95)

✓4th **H95**   Intraoperative and postprocedural complications and disorders of ear and mastoid process, not elsewhere classified

✓5th **H95.0**   Recurrent cholesteatoma of postmastoidectomy cavity

H95.00   Recurrent cholesteatoma of postmastoidectomy cavity, unspecified ear

H95.01   Recurrent cholesteatoma of postmastoidectomy cavity, right ear

H95.02   Recurrent cholesteatoma of postmastoidectomy cavity, left ear

H95.03   Recurrent cholesteatoma of postmastoidectomy cavity, bilateral ears

✓5th **H95.1**   Other disorders of ear and mastoid process following mastoidectomy

✓6th **H95.11**   Chronic inflammation of postmastoidectomy cavity

H95.111   Chronic inflammation of postmastoidectomy cavity, right ear

H95.112   Chronic inflammation of postmastoidectomy cavity, left ear

H95.113   Chronic inflammation of postmastoidectomy cavity, bilateral ears

H95.119   Chronic inflammation of postmastoidectomy cavity, unspecified ear

✓6th **H95.12**   Granulation of postmastoidectomy cavity

H95.121   Granulation of postmastoidectomy cavity, right ear

H95.122   Granulation of postmastoidectomy cavity, left ear

H95.123   Granulation of postmastoidectomy cavity, bilateral ears

✓ Additional Character Req   ✓x7th Placeholder Alert   Manifestation   HCC CMS-HCC Condition   ▽ Unspecified Code   ►◄ Revised Text   ● New Code   ▲ Revised Code Title

    H95.129 **Granulation of postmastoidectomy cavity, unspecified ear** ▽

✓6ᵗʰ **H95.13** **Mucosal cyst of postmastoidectomy cavity**

    H95.131 **Mucosal cyst of postmastoidectomy cavity, right ear**

    H95.132 **Mucosal cyst of postmastoidectomy cavity, left ear**

    H95.133 **Mucosal cyst of postmastoidectomy cavity, bilateral ears**

    H95.139 **Mucosal cyst of postmastoidectomy cavity, unspecified ear** ▽

✓6ᵗʰ **H95.19** **Other disorders following mastoidectomy**

    H95.191 **Other disorders following mastoidectomy, right ear**

    H95.192 **Other disorders following mastoidectomy, left ear**

    H95.193 **Other disorders following mastoidectomy, bilateral ears**

    H95.199 **Other disorders following mastoidectomy, unspecified ear** ▽

✓5ᵗʰ **H95.2** **Intraoperative hemorrhage and hematoma of ear and mastoid process complicating a procedure**

    EXCLUDES 1 *intraoperative hemorrhage and hematoma of ear and mastoid process due to accidental puncture or laceration during a procedure (H95.3-)*

    H95.21 **Intraoperative hemorrhage and hematoma of ear and mastoid process complicating a procedure on the ear and mastoid process**

    H95.22 **Intraoperative hemorrhage and hematoma of ear and mastoid process complicating other procedure**

✓5ᵗʰ **H95.3** **Accidental puncture and laceration of ear and mastoid process during a procedure**

    H95.31 **Accidental puncture and laceration of the ear and mastoid process during a procedure on the ear and mastoid process**

    H95.32 **Accidental puncture and laceration of the ear and mastoid process during other procedure**

✓5ᵗʰ **H95.4** **Postprocedural hemorrhage of ear and mastoid process following a procedure**

    H95.41 **Postprocedural hemorrhage of ear and mastoid process following a procedure on the ear and mastoid process**

    H95.42 **Postprocedural hemorrhage of ear and mastoid process following other procedure**

✓5ᵗʰ **H95.5** **Postprocedural hematoma and seroma of ear and mastoid process following a procedure**

    H95.51 **Postprocedural hematoma of ear and mastoid process following a procedure on the ear and mastoid process**

    H95.52 **Postprocedural hematoma of ear and mastoid process following other procedure**

    H95.53 **Postprocedural seroma of ear and mastoid process following a procedure on the ear and mastoid process**

    H95.54 **Postprocedural seroma of ear and mastoid process following other procedure**

✓5ᵗʰ **H95.8** **Other intraoperative and postprocedural complications and disorders of the ear and mastoid process, not elsewhere classified**

    EXCLUDES 2 *postprocedural complications and disorders following mastoidectomy (H95.0-, H95.1-)*

✓6ᵗʰ **H95.81** **Postprocedural stenosis of external ear canal**

    H95.811 **Postprocedural stenosis of right external ear canal**

    H95.812 **Postprocedural stenosis of left external ear canal**

    H95.813 **Postprocedural stenosis of external ear canal, bilateral**

    H95.819 **Postprocedural stenosis of unspecified external ear canal** ▽

    H95.88 **Other intraoperative complications and disorders of the ear and mastoid process, not elsewhere classified**

    Use additional code, if applicable, to further specify disorder

    H95.89 **Other postprocedural complications and disorders of the ear and mastoid process, not elsewhere classified**

    Use additional code, if applicable, to further specify disorder

EXCLUDES 1 Not coded here   **EXCLUDES 2** Not included here   N Newborn Age: 0   P Pediatric Age: 0-17   M Maternity Age: 12-55   A Adult Age: 15-124

616   ICD-10-CM 2018

H95.129–H95.89

Chapter 9. Diseases of the Circulatory System (I00–I99)

Chapter Specific Guidelines with Coding Examples

The chapter specific guidelines from the ICD-10-CM Official Guidelines for Coding and Reporting have been provided below. Along with these guidelines are coding examples, contained in the shaded boxes, that have been developed to help illustrate the coding and/or sequencing guidance found in these guidelines.

a. Hypertension

The classification presumes a causal relationship between hypertension and heart involvement and between hypertension and kidney involvement, as the two conditions are linked by the term "with" in the Alphabetic Index. These conditions should be coded as related even in the absence of provider documentation explicitly linking them, unless the documentation clearly states the conditions are unrelated.

For hypertension and conditions not specifically linked by relational terms such as "with," "associated with" or "due to" in the classification, provider documentation must link the conditions in order to code them as related.

1) Hypertension with heart disease

Hypertension with heart conditions classified to I50.- or I51.4-I51.9, are assigned to a code from category I11, Hypertensive heart disease. Use additional code(s) from category I50, Heart failure, to identify the type(s) of heart failure in those patients with heart failure.

The same heart conditions (I50.-, I51.4-I51.9) with hypertension are coded separately if the provider has specifically documented a different cause. Sequence according to the circumstances of the admission/encounter.

> Patient is treated for left heart failure. Patient also has a history of hypertension managed by medication.
>
> **I11.0**   **Hypertensive heart disease with heart failure**
>
> **I50.1**   **Left ventricular failure, unspecified**
>
> *Explanation*: Without a diagnostic statement to the contrary, hypertension and heart failure have an assumed causal relationship, and a combination code should be used. An additional code to identify the type of heart failure (I50.-) should also be provided.

2) Hypertensive chronic kidney disease

Assign codes from category I12, Hypertensive chronic kidney disease, when both hypertension and a condition classifiable to category N18, Chronic kidney disease (CKD), are present. CKD should not be coded as hypertensive if the physician has specifically documented a different cause.

The appropriate code from category N18 should be used as a secondary code with a code from category I12 to identify the stage of chronic kidney disease.

See Section I.C.14. Chronic kidney disease.

If a patient has hypertensive chronic kidney disease and acute renal failure, an additional code for the acute renal failure is required.

> Patient presents with stage IV chronic kidney disease (CKD). The patient also has documented hypertension secondary to primary hyperparathyroidism.
>
> **N18.4**   **Chronic kidney disease, stage 4 (severe)**
>
> **I10**   **Essential (primary) hypertension**
>
> **E21.0**   **Primary hyperparathyroidism**
>
> *Explanation*: A combination code describing a relationship between hypertension and CKD is not used due to the physician documentation identifying the primary hyperparathyroidism as the cause for the hypertension.

3) Hypertensive heart and chronic kidney disease

Assign codes from combination category I13, Hypertensive heart and chronic kidney disease, when there is hypertension with both heart and kidney involvement. If heart failure is present, assign an additional code from category I50 to identify the type of heart failure.

The appropriate code from category N18, Chronic kidney disease, should be used as a secondary code with a code from category I13 to identify the stage of chronic kidney disease.

See Section I.C.14. Chronic kidney disease.

The codes in category I13, Hypertensive heart and chronic kidney disease, are combination codes that include hypertension, heart disease and chronic kidney disease. The Includes note at I13 specifies that the conditions included at I11 and I12 are included together in I13. If a patient has hypertension, heart disease and chronic kidney disease, then a code

from I13 should be used, not individual codes for hypertension, heart disease and chronic kidney disease, or codes from I11 or I12.

For patients with both acute renal failure and chronic kidney disease, an additional code for acute renal failure is required.

> Hypertensive heart and kidney disease with congestive heart failure and stage 2 chronic kidney disease
>
> **I13.0**   **Hypertensive heart and chronic kidney disease with heart failure and stage 1 through stage 4 chronic kidney disease, or unspecified chronic kidney disease**
>
> **I50.9**   **Heart failure, unspecified**
>
> **N18.2**   **Chronic kidney disease, stage 2 (mild)**
>
> *Explanation*: Combination codes in category I13 are used to report conditions classifiable to *both* categories I11 and I12. Do not report conditions classifiable to I11 and I12 separately. Use additional codes to report type of heart failure and stage of CKD.

4) Hypertensive cerebrovascular disease

For hypertensive cerebrovascular disease, first assign the appropriate code from categories I60-I69, followed by the appropriate hypertension code.

> Rupture of cerebral aneurysm caused by malignant hypertension
>
> **I60.7**   **Nontraumatic subarachnoid hemorrhage from unspecified introcranial artery**
>
> **I10**   **Essential (primary) hypertension**
>
> *Explanation*: Hypertensive cerebrovascular disease requires two codes: the appropriate I60–I69 code followed by the appropriate hypertension code.

5) Hypertensive retinopathy

Subcategory H35.0, Background retinopathy and retinal vascular changes, should be used with a code from category I10 – I15, Hypertensive disease to include the systemic hypertension. The sequencing is based on the reason for the encounter.

> Hypertensive retinopathy of the right eye
>
> **H35.031**   **Hypertensive retinopathy, right eye**
>
> **I10**   **Essential (primary) hypertension**
>
> *Explanation*: Hypertensive retinopathy requires two codes: the appropriate subcategory H35.0 code and a code for the hypertension.

6) Hypertension, secondary

Secondary hypertension is due to an underlying condition. Two codes are required: one to identify the underlying etiology and one from category I15 to identify the hypertension. Sequencing of codes is determined by the reason for admission/encounter.

> Renovascular hypertension due to renal artery atherosclerosis
>
> **I15.0**   **Renovascular hypertension**
>
> **I70.1**   **Atherosclerosis of renal artery**
>
> *Explanation*: Secondary hypertension requires two codes: a code to identify the etiology and the appropriate I15 code.

7) Hypertension, transient

Assign code R03.0, Elevated blood pressure reading without diagnosis of hypertension, unless patient has an established diagnosis of hypertension. Assign code O13.-, Gestational [pregnancy-induced] hypertension without significant proteinuria, or O14.-, Pre-eclampsia, for transient hypertension of pregnancy.

8) Hypertension, controlled

This diagnostic statement usually refers to an existing state of hypertension under control by therapy. Assign the appropriate code from categories I10-I15, Hypertensive diseases.

9) Hypertension, uncontrolled

Uncontrolled hypertension may refer to untreated hypertension or hypertension not responding to current therapeutic regimen. In either case, assign the appropriate code from categories I10-I15, Hypertensive diseases.

10) Hypertensive Crisis

Assign a code from category I16, Hypertensive crisis, for documented hypertensive urgency, hypertensive emergency or unspecified

Chapter 9. Diseases of the Circulatory System

hypertensive crisis. Code also any identified hypertensive disease (I10-I15). The sequencing is based on the reason for the encounter.

10) Pulmonary hypertension

Pulmonary hypertension is classified to category I27, Other pulmonary heart diseases. For secondary pulmonary hypertension (I27.1, I27.2-), code also any associated conditions or adverse effects of drugs or toxins. The sequencing is based on the reason for the encounter.

b. Atherosclerotic coronary artery disease and angina

ICD-10-CM has combination codes for atherosclerotic heart disease with angina pectoris. The subcategories for these codes are I25.11, Atherosclerotic heart disease of native coronary artery with angina pectoris and I25.7, Atherosclerosis of coronary artery bypass graft(s) and coronary artery of transplanted heart with angina pectoris.

When using one of these combination codes it is not necessary to use an additional code for angina pectoris. A causal relationship can be assumed in a patient with both atherosclerosis and angina pectoris, unless the documentation indicates the angina is due to something other than the atherosclerosis.

If a patient with coronary artery disease is admitted due to an acute myocardial infarction (AMI), the AMI should be sequenced before the coronary artery disease.

See Section I.C.9. Acute myocardial infarction (AMI)

> Patient is being seen for spastic angina pectoris. She also has a documented history of progressive coronary artery disease of the native vessels.
>
> **I25.111**   **Atherosclerotic heart disease of native coronary artery with angina pectoris with documented spasm**
>
> *Explanation*: Report the combination code for atherosclerotic heart disease (coronary artery disease) with angina pectoris. A causal relationship is assumed in a patient with both atherosclerosis and angina pectoris, unless the documentation indicates the angina is due to something other than the atherosclerosis. When using one of these combination codes, it is not necessary to use an additional code for angina pectoris.

c. Intraoperative and postprocedural cerebrovascular accident

Medical record documentation should clearly specify the cause- and- effect relationship between the medical intervention and the cerebrovascular accident in order to assign a code for intraoperative or postprocedural cerebrovascular accident.

Proper code assignment depends on whether it was an infarction or hemorrhage and whether it occurred intraoperatively or postoperatively. If it was a cerebral hemorrhage, code assignment depends on the type of procedure performed.

> Embolic cerebral infarction of the right middle cerebral artery that occurred during hip replacement surgery. The surgeon documented as due to the surgery.
>
> **I97.811**   **Intraoperative cerebrovascular infarction during other surgery**
>
> **I63.411**   **Cerebral infarction due to embolism of right middle cerebral artery**
>
> *Explanation*: Code assignment for intraoperative or postprocedural cerebrovascular accident is based on the provider's documentation of a cause-and-effect relationship between the condition and the procedure. Proper code assignment also depends on whether the cerebrovascular accident was an infarction or hemorrhage, occurred intraoperatively or postoperatively, and the type of procedure performed.

d. Sequelae of cerebrovascular disease

1) Category I69, Sequelae of cerebrovascular disease

Category I69 is used to indicate conditions classifiable to categories I60-I67 as the causes of sequela (neurologic deficits), themselves classified elsewhere. These "late effects" include neurologic deficits that persist after initial onset of conditions classifiable to categories I60-I67. The neurologic deficits caused by cerebrovascular disease may be present from the onset or may arise at any time after the onset of the condition classifiable to categories I60-I67.

Codes from category I69, Sequelae of cerebrovascular disease, that specify hemiplegia, hemiparesis and monoplegia identify whether the dominant or nondominant side is affected. Should the affected side be documented, but not specified as dominant or nondominant, and the classification system does not indicate a default, code selection is as follows:

- For ambidextrous patients, the default should be dominant.
- If the left side is affected, the default is non-dominant.

- If the right side is affected, the default is dominant.

2) Codes from category I69 with codes from I60–I67

Codes from category I69 may be assigned on a health care record with codes from I60-I67, if the patient has a current cerebrovascular disease and deficits from an old cerebrovascular disease.

3) Codes from category I69 and personal history of transient ischemic attack (TIA) and cerebral infarction (Z86.73)

Codes from category I69 should not be assigned if the patient does not have neurologic deficits.

See Section I.C.21. 4. History (of) for use of personal history codes

e. Acute myocardial infarction (AMI)

1) Type 1 ST elevation myocardial infarction (STEMI) and non-ST elevation myocardial infarction (NSTEMI)

The ICD-10-CM codes for **type 1** acute myocardial infarction (AMI) identify the site, such as anterolateral wall or true posterior wall. Subcategories I21.0-I21.2 and code I21.3 are used for **type 1** ST elevation myocardial infarction (STEMI). Code I21.4, Non-ST elevation (NSTEMI) myocardial infarction, is used for **type 1** non ST elevation myocardial infarction (NSTEMI) and nontransmural MIs.

If **a type 1** NSTEMI evolves to STEMI, assign the STEMI code. If **a type 1** STEMI converts to NSTEMI due to thrombolytic therapy, it is still coded as STEMI.

For encounters occurring while the myocardial infarction is equal to, or less than, four weeks old, including transfers to another acute setting or a postacute setting, and the myocardial infarction meets the definition for "other diagnoses" (see Section III, Reporting Additional Diagnoses), codes from category I21 may continue to be reported. For encounters after the 4 week time frame and the patient is still receiving care related to the myocardial infarction, the appropriate aftercare code should be assigned, rather than a code from category I21. For old or healed myocardial infarctions not requiring further care, code I25.2, Old myocardial infarction, may be assigned.

2) Acute myocardial infarction, unspecified

Code **I21.9, Acute myocardial infarction, unspecified,** is the default for unspecified acute myocardial infarction **or unspecified type**. If only type 1 STEMI or transmural MI without the site is documented, assign code I21.3, **ST elevation (STEMI) myocardial infarction of unspecified site**.

3) AMI documented as nontransmural or subendocardial but site provided

If an AMI is documented as nontransmural or subendocardial, but the site is provided, it is still coded as a subendocardial AMI.

See Section I.C.21.3 for information on coding status post administration of tPA in a different facility within the last 24 hours.

> Acute inferior subendocardial myocardial infarction (NSTEMI)
>
> **I21.4**   **Non-ST elevation (NSTEMI) myocardial infarction**
>
> *Explanation*: An AMI documented as subendocardial or nontransmural is coded as such (I21.4, I22.2), even if the site of infarction is specified.

4) Subsequent acute myocardial infarction

A code from category I22, Subsequent ST elevation (STEMI) and non-ST elevation (NSTEMI) myocardial infarction, is to be used when a patient who has suffered **a type 1 or unspecified** AMI has a new AMI within the 4 week time frame of the initial AMI. A code from category I22 must be used in conjunction with a code from category I21. The sequencing of the I22 and I21 codes depends on the circumstances of the encounter.

Do not assign code I22 for subsequent myocardial infarctions other than type 1 or unspecified. For subsequent type 2 AMI assign only code I21.A1. For subsequent type 4 or type 5 AMI, assign only code I21.A9.

5) Other Types of Myocardial Infarction

The ICD-10-CM provides codes for different types of myocardial infarction. Type 1 myocardial infarctions are assigned to codes I21.0-I21.4.

Type 2 myocardial infarction, and myocardial infarction due to demand ischemia or secondary to ischemic balance, is assigned to code I21.A1, Myocardial infarction type 2 with a code for the underlying cause. Do not assign code I24.8, Other forms of acute ischemic heart disease for the demand ischemia. Sequencing of type 2 AMI or the underlying cause is dependent on the circumstances of admission. When a type 2 AMI code is described as NSTEMI or STEMI, only assign code I21.A1. Codes I21.01-I21.4 should only be assigned for type 1 AMIs.

Acute myocardial infarctions type 3, 4a, 4b, 4c and 5 are assigned to code I21.A9, Other myocardial infarction type.

The "Code also" and "Code first" notes should be followed related to complications, and for coding of postprocedural myocardial infarctions during or following cardiac surgery.

Chapter 9. Diseases of the Circulatory System (I00-I99)

EXCLUDES 2   certain conditions originating in the perinatal period (P04-P96)
certain infectious and parasitic diseases (A00-B99)
complications of pregnancy, childbirth and the puerperium (O00-O9A)
congenital malformations, deformations, and chromosomal abnormalities (Q00-Q99)
endocrine, nutritional and metabolic diseases (E00-E88)
injury, poisoning and certain other consequences of external causes (S00-T88)
neoplasms (C00-D49)
symptoms, signs and abnormal clinical and laboratory findings, not elsewhere classified (R00-R94)
systemic connective tissue disorders (M30-M36)
transient cerebral ischemic attacks and related syndromes (G45.-)

This chapter contains the following blocks:

I00-I02   Acute rheumatic fever
I05-I09   Chronic rheumatic heart diseases
I10-I16   Hypertensive diseases
I20-I25   Ischemic heart diseases
I26-I28   Pulmonary heart disease and diseases of pulmonary circulation
I30-I52   Other forms of heart disease
I60-I69   Cerebrovascular diseases
I70-I79   Diseases of arteries, arterioles and capillaries
I80-I89   Diseases of veins, lymphatic vessels and lymph nodes, not elsewhere classified
I95-I99   Other and unspecified disorders of the circulatory system

Acute rheumatic fever (I00-I02)

I00   **Rheumatic fever without heart involvement**
INCLUDES   arthritis, rheumatic, acute or subacute
EXCLUDES 1   rheumatic fever with heart involvement (I01.0-I01.9)

✓4ᵗʰ **I01**   **Rheumatic fever with heart involvement**
EXCLUDES 1   chronic diseases of rheumatic origin (I05-I09) unless rheumatic fever is also present or there is evidence of reactivation or activity of the rheumatic process.

   I01.0   **Acute rheumatic pericarditis**
     Any condition in I00 with pericarditis
     Rheumatic pericarditis (acute)
     EXCLUDES 1   acute pericarditis not specified as rheumatic (I30.-)

   I01.1   **Acute rheumatic endocarditis**
     Any condition in I00 with endocarditis or valvulitis
     Acute rheumatic valvulitis

   I01.2   **Acute rheumatic myocarditis**
     Any condition in I00 with myocarditis

   I01.8   **Other acute rheumatic heart disease**
     Any condition in I00 with other or multiple types of heart involvement
     Acute rheumatic pancarditis

   I01.9   **Acute rheumatic heart disease, unspecified**   ▽
     Any condition in I00 with unspecified type of heart involvement
     Rheumatic carditis, acute
     Rheumatic heart disease, active or acute

✓4ᵗʰ **I02**   **Rheumatic chorea**
INCLUDES   Sydenham's chorea
EXCLUDES 1   chorea NOS (G25.5)
     Huntington's chorea (G10)

   I02.0   **Rheumatic chorea with heart involvement**
     Chorea NOS with heart involvement
     Rheumatic chorea with heart involvement of any type classifiable under I01-

   I02.9   **Rheumatic chorea without heart involvement**
     Rheumatic chorea NOS

Chronic rheumatic heart diseases (I05-I09)

✓4ᵗʰ **I05**   **Rheumatic mitral valve diseases**
INCLUDES   conditions classifiable to both I05.0 and I05.2-I05.9, whether specified as rheumatic or not
EXCLUDES 1   mitral valve disease specified as nonrheumatic (I34.-)
     mitral valve disease with aortic and/or tricuspid valve involvement (I08.-)

   I05.0   **Rheumatic mitral stenosis**
     Mitral (valve) obstruction (rheumatic)
     DEF: Narrowing of mitral valve between left atrium and left ventricle; due to rheumatic fever; characterized by shortness of breath during or after exercise, fatigue, palpitations, chest discomfort, and swelling of feet or legs.

   I05.1   **Rheumatic mitral insufficiency**
     Rheumatic mitral incompetence
     Rheumatic mitral regurgitation
     EXCLUDES 1   mitral insufficiency not specified as rheumatic (I34.0)

   I05.2   **Rheumatic mitral stenosis with insufficiency**
     Rheumatic mitral stenosis with incompetence or regurgitation

   I05.8   **Other rheumatic mitral valve diseases**
     Rheumatic mitral (valve) failure

   I05.9   **Rheumatic mitral valve disease, unspecified**   ▽
     Rheumatic mitral (valve) disorder (chronic) NOS

✓4ᵗʰ **I06**   **Rheumatic aortic valve diseases**
EXCLUDES 1   aortic valve disease not specified as rheumatic (I35.-)
     aortic valve disease with mitral and/or tricuspid valve involvement (I08.-)

   I06.0   **Rheumatic aortic stenosis**
     Rheumatic aortic (valve) obstruction

   I06.1   **Rheumatic aortic insufficiency**
     Rheumatic aortic incompetence
     Rheumatic aortic regurgitation

   I06.2   **Rheumatic aortic stenosis with insufficiency**
     Rheumatic aortic stenosis with incompetence or regurgitation

   I06.8   **Other rheumatic aortic valve diseases**

   I06.9   **Rheumatic aortic valve disease, unspecified**   ▽
     Rheumatic aortic (valve) disease NOS

✓4ᵗʰ **I07**   **Rheumatic tricuspid valve diseases**
INCLUDES   rheumatic tricuspid valve diseases specified as rheumatic or unspecified
EXCLUDES 1   tricuspid valve disease specified as nonrheumatic (I36.-)
     tricuspid valve disease with aortic and/or mitral valve involvement (I08.-)

   I07.0   **Rheumatic tricuspid stenosis**
     Tricuspid (valve) stenosis (rheumatic)

   I07.1   **Rheumatic tricuspid insufficiency**
     Tricuspid (valve) insufficiency (rheumatic)

   I07.2   **Rheumatic tricuspid stenosis and insufficiency**

   I07.8   **Other rheumatic tricuspid valve diseases**

   I07.9   **Rheumatic tricuspid valve disease, unspecified**   ▽
     Rheumatic tricuspid valve disorder NOS

✓4ᵗʰ **I08**   **Multiple valve diseases**
INCLUDES   multiple valve diseases specified as rheumatic or unspecified
EXCLUDES 1   endocarditis, valve unspecified (I38)
     multiple valve disease specified a nonrheumatic (I34.-, I35.-, I36.-, I37.-, I38.-, Q22.-, Q23.-, Q24.8-)
     rheumatic valve disease NOS (I09.1)

   I08.0   **Rheumatic disorders of both mitral and aortic valves**
     Involvement of both mitral and aortic valves specified as rheumatic or unspecified

   I08.1   **Rheumatic disorders of both mitral and tricuspid valves**

   I08.2   **Rheumatic disorders of both aortic and tricuspid valves**

   I08.3   **Combined rheumatic disorders of mitral, aortic and tricuspid valves**

   I08.8   **Other rheumatic multiple valve diseases**

   I08.9   **Rheumatic multiple valve disease, unspecified**   ▽

✓4ᵗʰ **I09**   **Other rheumatic heart diseases**

   I09.0   **Rheumatic myocarditis**
     EXCLUDES 1   myocarditis not specified as rheumatic (I51.4)

   I09.1   **Rheumatic diseases of endocardium, valve unspecified**   ▽
     Rheumatic endocarditis (chronic)
     Rheumatic valvulitis (chronic)
     EXCLUDES 1   endocarditis, valve unspecified (I38)

   I09.2   **Chronic rheumatic pericarditis**
     Adherent pericardium, rheumatic
     Chronic rheumatic mediastinopericarditis
     Chronic rheumatic myopericarditis
     EXCLUDES 1   chronic pericarditis not specified as rheumatic (I31.-)

✓5ᵗʰ   **I09.8**   **Other specified rheumatic heart diseases**

     I09.81   **Rheumatic heart failure**   HCC
       Use additional code to identify type of heart failure (I50.-)
       DEF: Decreased cardiac output, edema, and hypertension; due to rheumatic heart disease.

     I09.89   **Other specified rheumatic heart diseases**
       Rheumatic disease of pulmonary valve

   I09.9   **Rheumatic heart disease, unspecified**   ▽
     Rheumatic carditis
     EXCLUDES 1   rheumatoid carditis (M05.31)

✓ Additional Character Req   ✓7ᵗʰ Placeholder Alert   Manifestation   HCC CMS-HCC Condition   ▽ Unspecified Code   ▶◀ Revised Text   ● New Code   ▲ Revised Code Title

Chapter 9. Diseases of the Circulatory System

Hypertensive diseases (I10-I16)

Use additional code to identify:
  exposure to environmental tobacco smoke (Z77.22)
  history of tobacco dependence (Z87.891)
  occupational exposure to environmental tobacco smoke (Z57.31)
  tobacco dependence (F17.-)
  tobacco use (Z72.0)

EXCLUDES 1   *neonatal hypertension (P29.2)*
    primary pulmonary hypertension (I27.0)

EXCLUDES 2   *hypertensive disease complicating pregnancy, childbirth and the*
    puerperium (O10-O11, O13-O16)

I10   Essential (primary) hypertension

INCLUDES   high blood pressure
    hypertension (arterial) (benign) (essential) (malignant)
    (primary) (systemic)

EXCLUDES 1   *hypertensive disease complicating pregnancy, childbirth and*
    the puerperium (O10-O11, O13-O16)

EXCLUDES 2   *essential (primary) hypertension involving vessels of brain*
    (I60-I69)
    essential (primary) hypertension involving vessels of eye
    (H35.0-)

AHA: 2016, 4Q, 27

✓4th I11   Hypertensive heart disease

INCLUDES   ►any condition in I50.-, I51.4-I51.9 due to hypertension◄

I11.0   Hypertensive heart disease with heart failure   HCC
    Hypertensive heart failure
    Use additional code to identify type of heart failure (I50.-)
    AHA: 2017, 1Q, 47

I11.9   Hypertensive heart disease without heart failure   ▽
    Hypertensive heart disease NOS

✓4th I12   Hypertensive chronic kidney disease

INCLUDES   any condition in N18- and N26- due to hypertension
    arteriosclerosis of kidney
    arteriosclerotic nephritis (chronic) (interstitial)
    hypertensive nephropathy
    nephrosclerosis

EXCLUDES 1   *hypertension due to kidney disease (I15.0, I15.1)*
    renovascular hypertension (I15.0)
    secondary hypertension (I15.-)

EXCLUDES 2   *acute kidney failure (N17.-)*

AHA: 2016, 3Q, 22

I12.0   Hypertensive chronic kidney disease with stage 5   HCC
chronic kidney disease or end stage renal disease
    Use additional code to identify the stage of chronic kidney
    disease (N18.5, N18.6)

I12.9   Hypertensive chronic kidney disease with stage 1 through   ▽
stage 4 chronic kidney disease, or unspecified chronic kidney
disease
    Hypertensive chronic kidney disease NOS
    Hypertensive renal disease NOS
    Use additional code to identify the stage of chronic kidney
    disease (N18.1-N18.4, N18.9)

✓4th I13   Hypertensive heart and chronic kidney disease

INCLUDES   any condition in I11- with any condition in I12-
    cardiorenal disease
    cardiovascular renal disease

I13.0   Hypertensive heart and chronic kidney disease with   HCC
heart failure and stage 1 through stage 4 chronic kidney
disease, or unspecified chronic kidney disease
    Use additional code to identify type of heart failure (I50.-)
    Use additional code to identify stage of chronic kidney disease
    (N18.1-N18.4, N18.9)

✓5th I13.1   Hypertensive heart and chronic kidney disease without heart
failure

I13.10   Hypertensive heart and chronic kidney disease   ▽
without heart failure, with stage 1 through stage 4
chronic kidney disease, or unspecified chronic
kidney disease
    Hypertensive heart disease and hypertensive chronic
    kidney disease NOS
    Use additional code to identify the stage of chronic
    kidney disease (N18.1-N18.4, N18.9)

I13.11   Hypertensive heart and chronic kidney disease   HCC
without heart failure, with stage 5 chronic kidney
disease, or end stage renal disease
    Use additional code to identify the stage of chronic
    kidney disease (N18.5, N18.6)

I13.2   Hypertensive heart and chronic kidney disease with   HCC
heart failure and with stage 5 chronic kidney disease,
or end stage renal disease
    Use additional code to identify type of heart failure (I50.-)
    Use additional code to identify the stage of chronic kidney
    disease (N18.5, N18.6)

✓4th I15   Secondary hypertension

Code also underlying condition

EXCLUDES 1   *postprocedural hypertension (I97.3)*

EXCLUDES 2   *secondary hypertension involving vessels of brain (I60-I69)*
    secondary hypertension involving vessels of eye (H35.0-)

I15.0   Renovascular hypertension

I15.1   Hypertension secondary to other renal disorders
    AHA: 2016, 3Q, 22

I15.2   Hypertension secondary to endocrine disorders

I15.8   Other secondary hypertension

I15.9   Secondary hypertension, unspecified   ▽

✓4th I16   Hypertensive crisis

Code also any identified hypertensive disease (I10-I15)
AHA: 2016, 4Q, 27

I16.0   Hypertensive urgency

I16.1   Hypertensive emergency

I16.9   Hypertensive crisis, unspecified   ▽

Ischemic heart diseases (I20-I25)

Use additional code to identify presence of hypertension (I10-I16)

✓4th I20   Angina pectoris

Use additional code to identify:
  exposure to environmental tobacco smoke (Z77.22)
  history of tobacco dependence (Z87.891)
  occupational exposure to environmental tobacco smoke (Z57.31)
  tobacco dependence (F17.-)
  tobacco use (Z72.0)

EXCLUDES 1   *angina pectoris with atherosclerotic heart disease of native*
    coronary arteries (I25.1-)
    atherosclerosis of coronary artery bypass graft(s) and coronary
    artery of transplanted heart with angina pectoris (I25.7-)
    postinfarction angina (I23.7)

I20.0   Unstable angina   HCC
    Accelerated angina
    Crescendo angina
    De novo effort angina
    Intermediate coronary syndrome
    Preinfarction syndrome
    Worsening effort angina
    DEF: A condition representing an intermediate stage between
    angina of effort and acute myocardial infarction.

I20.1   Angina pectoris with documented spasm   HCC
    Angiospastic angina
    Prinzmetal angina
    Spasm-induced angina
    Variant angina

I20.8   Other forms of angina pectoris   HCC
    Angina equivalent
    Angina of effort
    Coronary slow flow syndrome
    Stable angina
    Stenocardia
    Use additional code(s) for symptoms associated with angina
    equivalent

I20.9   Angina pectoris, unspecified   HCC ▽
    Angina NOS
    Anginal syndrome
    Cardiac angina
    Ischemic chest pain

EXCLUDES 1 Not coded here   EXCLUDES 2 Not included here   N Newborn Age: 0   P Pediatric Age: 0-17   M Maternity Age: 12-55   A Adult Age: 15-124

620   ICD-10-CM 2018

▲ ✓4th I21 Acute myocardial infarction

    INCLUDES   cardiac infarction
             coronary (artery) embolism
             coronary (artery) occlusion
             coronary (artery) rupture
             coronary (artery) thrombosis
             infarction of heart, myocardium, or ventricle
             myocardial infarction specified as acute or with a stated
                duration of 4 weeks (28 days) or less from onset

Use additional code, if applicable, to identify:
   exposure to environmental tobacco smoke (Z77.22)
   history of tobacco dependence (Z87.891)
   occupational exposure to environmental tobacco smoke (Z57.31)
   status post administration of tPA (rtPA) in a different facility within
     the last 24 hours prior to admission to current facility (Z92.82)
   tobacco dependence (F17.-)
   tobacco use (Z72.0)

    EXCLUDES 2   old myocardial infarction (I25.2)
              postmyocardial infarction syndrome (I24.1)
              ▶subsequent type 1 myocardial infarction◀ (I22.-)
   AHA: 2017, 1Q, 44-45; 2016, 4Q, 140; 2015, 2Q, 16; 2013, 1Q, 25; 2012, 4Q, 96, 102-103

✓5th I21.0 ST elevation (STEMI) myocardial infarction of anterior wall
     ▶Type 1 ST elevation myocardial infarction of anterior wall◀

     I21.01 ST elevation (STEMI) myocardial infarction   HCC
           involving left main coronary artery

     I21.02 ST elevation (STEMI) myocardial infarction   HCC
           involving left anterior descending coronary artery
             ST elevation (STEMI) myocardial infarction involving
               diagonal coronary artery
             AHA: 2013, 1Q, 25

     I21.09 ST elevation (STEMI) myocardial infarction   HCC
           involving other coronary artery of anterior wall
             Acute transmural myocardial infarction of anterior wall
             Anteroapical transmural (Q wave) infarction (acute)
             Anterolateral transmural (Q wave) infarction (acute)
             Anteroseptal transmural (Q wave) infarction (acute)
             Transmural (Q wave) infarction (acute) (of) anterior
               (wall) NOS
             AHA: 2012, 4Q, 102-103

✓5th I21.1 ST elevation (STEMI) myocardial infarction of inferior wall
     ▶Type 1 ST elevation myocardial infarction of inferior wall◀

     I21.11 ST elevation (STEMI) myocardial infarction   HCC
           involving right coronary artery
             Inferoposterior transmural (Q wave) infarction (acute)

     I21.19 ST elevation (STEMI) myocardial infarction   HCC
           involving other coronary artery of inferior wall
             Acute transmural myocardial infarction of inferior wall
             Inferolateral transmural (Q wave) infarction (acute)
             Transmural (Q wave) infarction (acute) (of)
               diaphragmatic wall
             Transmural (Q wave) infarction (acute) (of) inferior
               (wall) NOS
            EXCLUDES 2   ST elevation (STEMI) myocardial infarction
                  involving left circumflex coronary artery
                  (I21.21)
             AHA: 2012, 4Q, 96

✓5th I21.2 ST elevation (STEMI) myocardial infarction of other sites
     ▶Type 1 ST elevation myocardial infarction of other sites◀

     I21.21 ST elevation (STEMI) myocardial infarction   HCC
           involving left circumflex coronary artery
             ST elevation (STEMI) myocardial infarction involving
               oblique marginal coronary artery

     I21.29 ST elevation (STEMI) myocardial infarction   HCC
           involving other sites
             Acute transmural myocardial infarction of other sites
             Apical-lateral transmural (Q wave) infarction (acute)
             Basal-lateral transmural (Q wave) infarction (acute)
             High lateral transmural (Q wave) infarction (acute)
             Lateral (wall) NOS transmural (Q wave) infarction
               (acute)
             Posterior (true) transmural (Q wave) infarction (acute)
             Posterobasal transmural (Q wave) infarction (acute)
             Posterolateral transmural (Q wave) infarction (acute)
             Posteroseptal transmural (Q wave) infarction (acute)
             Septal transmural (Q wave) infarction (acute) NOS

I21.3 ST elevation (STEMI) myocardial infarction of   HCC ▽
unspecified site
     Acute transmural myocardial infarction of unspecified site
     ~~Myocardial infarction (acute) NOS~~
     Transmural (Q wave) myocardial infarction NOS
     ▶Type 1 ST elevation myocardial infarction of unspecified site◀

I21.4 Non-ST elevation (NSTEMI) myocardial infarction   HCC
     Acute subendocardial myocardial infarction
     Non-Q wave myocardial infarction NOS
     Nontransmural myocardial infarction NOS
     ▶Type 1 non-ST elevation myocardial infarction◀
     AHA: 2017, 1Q, 44-45

● **I21.9 Acute myocardial infarction, unspecified**   ▽
     Myocardial infarction (acute) NOS

● **✓5th I21.A Other type of myocardial infarction**

●   **I21.A1 Myocardial infarction type 2**
             Myocardial infarction due to demand ischemia
             Myocardial infarction secondary to ischemic
               imbalance
             Code also the underlying cause, if known and
               applicable, such as:
             anemia (D50.0-D64.9)
             chronic obstructive pulmonary disease (J44.-)
             heart failure (I50.-)
             paroxysmal tachycardia (I47.0-I47.9)
             renal failure (N17.0-N19)
             shock (R57.0-R57.9)

●   **I21.A9 Other myocardial infarction type**
             Myocardial infarction associated with
               revascularization procedure
             Myocardial infarction type 3
             Myocardial infarction type 4a
             Myocardial infarction type 4b
             Myocardial infarction type 4c
             Myocardial infarction type 5
             Code first, if applicable, postprocedural myocardial
               infarction following cardiac surgery (I97.190), or
               postprocedural myocardial infarction during
               cardiac surgery (I97.790)
             Code also complication, if known and applicable, such
               as:
             (acute) stent occlusion (T82.897-)
             (acute) stent stenosis (T82.857-)
             (acute) stent thrombosis (T82.867-)
             cardiac arrest due to underlying cardiac condition
               (I46.2)
             complication of percutaneous coronary
               intervention (PCI) (I97.89)
             occlusion of coronary artery bypass graft (T82.218-)

✓4th I22 Subsequent ST elevation (STEMI) and non-ST elevation (NSTEMI) myocardial infarction

    INCLUDES   acute myocardial infarction occurring within four weeks (28
              days) of a previous acute myocardial infarction,
              regardless of site
             cardiac infarction
             coronary (artery) embolism
             coronary (artery) occlusion
             coronary (artery) rupture
             coronary (artery) thrombosis
             infarction of heart, myocardium, or ventricle
             recurrent myocardial infarction
             reinfarction of myocardium
             rupture of heart, myocardium, or ventricle
             ▶subsequent type 1 myocardial infarction◀

Use additional code, if applicable, to identify:
   exposure to environmental tobacco smoke (Z77.22)
   history of tobacco dependence (Z87.891)
   occupational exposure to environmental tobacco smoke (Z57.31)
   status post administration of tPA (rtPA) in a different facility within
     the last 24 hours prior to admission to current facility (Z92.82)
   tobacco dependence (F17.-)
   tobacco use (Z72.0)

    EXCLUDES 1   ▶subsequent myocardial infarction, type 2 (I21.A1)
              subsequent myocardial infarction of other type (type 3) (type 4)
              (type 5) (I21.A9)◀
   AHA: 2017, 2Q, 11; 2013, 1Q, 25; 2012, 4Q, 97, 102-103

I22.0 Subsequent ST elevation (STEMI) myocardial infarction   HCC
of anterior wall
     Subsequent acute transmural myocardial infarction of anterior
       wall
     Subsequent transmural (Q wave) infarction (acute)(of) anterior
       (wall) NOS
     Subsequent anteroapical transmural (Q wave) infarction (acute)
     Subsequent anterolateral transmural (Q wave) infarction (acute)
     Subsequent anteroseptal transmural (Q wave) infarction (acute)

✓ Additional Character Req   ✓x7th Placeholder Alert   Manifestation   HCC CMS-HCC Condition   ▽ Unspecified Code   ▶◀ Revised Text   ● New Code   ▲ Revised Code Title

I22.1   Subsequent ST elevation (STEMI) myocardial infarction HCC
of inferior wall
  Subsequent acute transmural myocardial infarction of inferior
    wall
  Subsequent transmural (Q wave) infarction (acute)(of)
    diaphragmatic wall
  Subsequent transmural (Q wave) infarction (acute)(of) inferior
    (wall) NOS
  Subsequent inferolateral transmural (Q wave) infarction (acute)
  Subsequent inferoposterior transmural (Q wave) infarction
    (acute)
  AHA: 2012, 4Q, 102

I22.2   Subsequent non-ST elevation (NSTEMI) myocardial HCC
infarction
  Subsequent acute subendocardial myocardial infarction
  Subsequent non-Q wave myocardial infarction NOS
  Subsequent nontransmural myocardial infarction NOS

I22.8   Subsequent ST elevation (STEMI) myocardial infarction HCC
of other sites
  Subsequent acute transmural myocardial infarction of other
    sites
  Subsequent apical-lateral transmural (Q wave) myocardial
    infarction (acute)
  Subsequent basal-lateral transmural (Q wave) myocardial
    infarction (acute)
  Subsequent high lateral transmural (Q wave) myocardial
    infarction (acute)
  Subsequent transmural (Q wave) myocardial infarction
    (acute)(of) lateral (wall) NOS
  Subsequent posterior (true)transmural (Q wave) myocardial
    infarction (acute)
  Subsequent posterobasal transmural (Q wave) myocardial
    infarction (acute)
  Subsequent posterolateral transmural (Q wave) myocardial
    infarction (acute)
  Subsequent posteroseptal transmural (Q wave) myocardial
    infarction (acute)
  Subsequent septal NOS transmural (Q wave) myocardial
    infarction (acute)

I22.9   Subsequent ST elevation (STEMI) myocardial infarction HCC ▽
of unspecified site
  Subsequent acute myocardial infarction of unspecified site
  Subsequent myocardial infarction (acute) NOS

✓4th **I23   Certain current complications following ST elevation (STEMI)**
and non-ST elevation (NSTEMI) myocardial infarction (within the
28 day period)
  AHA: 2017, 2Q, 11

I23.0   Hemopericardium as current complication following HCC
acute myocardial infarction
  EXCLUDES 1   hemopericardium not specified as current
    complication following acute myocardial
    infarction (I31.2)

I23.1   Atrial septal defect as current complication following HCC A
acute myocardial infarction
  EXCLUDES 1   acquired atrial septal defect not specified as current
    complication following acute myocardial
    infarction (I51.0)

I23.2   Ventricular septal defect as current complication HCC A
following acute myocardial infarction
  EXCLUDES 1   acquired ventricular septal defect not specified as
    current complication following acute myocardial
    infarction (I51.0)

I23.3   Rupture of cardiac wall without hemopericardium as HCC A
current complication following acute myocardial infarction

I23.4   Rupture of chordae tendineae as current complication HCC
following acute myocardial infarction
  EXCLUDES 1   rupture of chordae tendineae not specified as current
    complication following acute myocardial
    infarction (I51.1)

I23.5   Rupture of papillary muscle as current complication HCC
following acute myocardial infarction
  EXCLUDES 1   rupture of papillary muscle not specified as current
    complication following acute myocardial
    infarction (I51.2)

I23.6   Thrombosis of atrium, auricular appendage, and HCC A
ventricle as current complications following acute
myocardial infarction
  EXCLUDES 1   thrombosis of atrium, auricular appendage, and
    ventricle not specified as current complication
    following acute myocardial infarction (I51.3)

I23.7   Postinfarction angina HCC A
  AHA: 2015, 2Q, 16

I23.8   Other current complications following acute HCC A
myocardial infarction

✓4th **I24   Other acute ischemic heart diseases**
  EXCLUDES 1   angina pectoris (I20.-)
    transient myocardial ischemia in newborn (P29.4)

I24.0   Acute coronary thrombosis not resulting in myocardial HCC
infarction
  Acute coronary (artery) (vein) embolism not resulting in
    myocardial infarction
  Acute coronary (artery) (vein) occlusion not resulting in
    myocardial infarction
  Acute coronary (artery) (vein) thromboembolism not
    resulting in myocardial infarction
  EXCLUDES 1   atherosclerotic heart disease (I25.1-)
  AHA: 2013, 1Q, 24

I24.1   Dressler's syndrome HCC
  Postmyocardial infarction syndrome
  EXCLUDES 1   postinfarction angina (I23.7)

I24.8   Other forms of acute ischemic heart disease HCC
  EXCLUDES 1 ▶myocardial infarction due to demand ischemia
    (I21.A1)◀

I24.9   Acute ischemic heart disease, unspecified HCC ▽
  EXCLUDES 1   ischemic heart disease (chronic) NOS (I25.9)

✓4th **I25   Chronic ischemic heart disease**
  Use additional code to identify:
    chronic total occlusion of coronary artery (I25.82)
    exposure to environmental tobacco smoke (Z77.22)
    history of tobacco dependence (Z87.891)
    occupational exposure to environmental tobacco smoke (Z57.31)
    tobacco dependence (F17.-)
    tobacco use (Z72.0)

✓5th **I25.1   Atherosclerotic heart disease of native coronary artery**
  Atherosclerotic cardiovascular disease
  Coronary (artery) atheroma
  Coronary (artery) atherosclerosis
  Coronary (artery) disease
  Coronary (artery) sclerosis
  Use additional code, if applicable, to identify:
    coronary atherosclerosis due to calcified coronary lesion (I25.84)
    coronary atherosclerosis due to lipid rich plaque (I25.83)
  EXCLUDES 2   atheroembolism (I75.-)
    atherosclerosis of coronary artery bypass graft(s) and
    transplanted heart (I25.7-)

I25.10   Atherosclerotic heart disease of native coronary A
artery without angina pectoris
  Atherosclerotic heart disease NOS
  AHA: 2015, 2Q, 16; 2012, 4Q, 92

✓6th **I25.11   Atherosclerotic heart disease of native coronary**
artery with angina pectoris

I25.110   Atherosclerotic heart disease of HCC A
native coronary artery with unstable
angina pectoris
  EXCLUDES 1   unstable angina without
    atherosclerotic heart disease
    (I20.0)

I25.111   Atherosclerotic heart disease of HCC A
native coronary artery with angina
pectoris
with documented spasm
  EXCLUDES 1   angina pectoris with documented
    spasm without
    atherosclerotic heart disease
    (I20.1)

Atheromas

Atheromas (fatty tissue
  and/or plaque)

Lumen

EXCLUDES 1 Not coded here   EXCLUDES 2 Not included here   N Newborn Age: 0   P Pediatric Age: 0-17   M Maternity Age: 12-55   A Adult Age: 15-124

622   ICD-10-CM 2018

I25.118   **Atherosclerotic heart disease of** `HCC` `A`
native coronary artery with other forms of
angina pectoris
> *EXCLUDES 1*   *other forms of angina pectoris*
> *without atherosclerotic*
> *heart disease (I20.8)*

     AHA: 2015, 2Q, 16

I25.119   **Atherosclerotic heart disease of** `HCC` `A` ▽
native coronary artery with unspecified
angina pectoris
> Atherosclerotic heart disease with angina
> NOS
> Atherosclerotic heart disease with ischemic
> chest pain
> *EXCLUDES 1*   *unspecified angina pectoris*
> *without atherosclerotic*
> *heart disease (I20.9)*

I25.2   **Old myocardial infarction**
> Healed myocardial infarction
> Past myocardial infarction diagnosed by ECG or other
> investigation, but currently presenting no symptoms

I25.3   **Aneurysm of heart**
> Mural aneurysm
> Ventricular aneurysm

✓5ᵗʰ **I25.4**   **Coronary artery aneurysm and dissection**

I25.41   **Coronary artery aneurysm**
> Coronary arteriovenous fistula, acquired
> *EXCLUDES 1*   *congenital coronary (artery) aneurysm*
> *(Q24.5)*

I25.42   **Coronary artery dissection**
> **DEF:** A tear in the intimal arterial wall of a coronary
> artery resulting in the sudden intrusion of blood within
> the layers of the wall.

I25.5   **Ischemic cardiomyopathy**
> *EXCLUDES 2*   *coronary atherosclerosis (I25.1-, I25.7-)*

I25.6   **Silent myocardial ischemia**

✓5ᵗʰ **I25.7**   **Atherosclerosis of coronary artery bypass graft(s) and**
coronary artery of transplanted heart with angina pectoris
> Use additional code, if applicable, to identify:
> coronary atherosclerosis due to calcified coronary lesion
> (I25.84)
> coronary atherosclerosis due to lipid rich plaque (I25.83)
> *EXCLUDES 1*   *atherosclerosis of bypass graft(s) of transplanted heart*
> *without angina pectoris (I25.812)*
> *atherosclerosis of coronary artery bypass graft(s)*
> *without angina pectoris (I25.810)*
> *atherosclerosis of native coronary artery of*
> *transplanted heart without angina pectoris*
> *(I25.811)*
> ~~*embolism or thrombus of coronary artery bypass*~~
> ~~*graft(s) (T82.8-)*~~

✓6ᵗʰ **I25.70**   **Atherosclerosis of coronary artery bypass graft(s),**
unspecified, with angina pectoris

I25.700   **Atherosclerosis of coronary** `HCC` `A` ▽
artery bypass graft(s), unspecified, with
unstable angina pectoris
> *EXCLUDES 1*   *unstable angina pectoris without*
> *atherosclerosis of coronary*
> *artery bypass graft (I20.0)*

I25.701   **Atherosclerosis of coronary** `HCC` `A` ▽
artery bypass graft(s), unspecified, with
angina pectoris with documented spasm
> *EXCLUDES 1*   *angina pectoris with documented*
> *spasm without*
> *atherosclerosis of coronary*
> *artery bypass graft (I20.1)*

I25.708   **Atherosclerosis of coronary** `HCC` `A` ▽
artery bypass graft(s), unspecified, with
other forms of angina pectoris
> *EXCLUDES 1*   *other forms of angina pectoris*
> *without atherosclerosis of*
> *coronary artery bypass graft*
> *(I20.8)*

I25.709   **Atherosclerosis of coronary** `HCC` `A` ▽
artery bypass graft(s), unspecified, with
unspecified angina pectoris
> *EXCLUDES 1*   *unspecified angina pectoris*
> *without atherosclerosis of*
> *coronary artery bypass graft*
> *(I20.9)*

✓6ᵗʰ **I25.71**   **Atherosclerosis of autologous vein coronary artery**
bypass graft(s) with angina pectoris

I25.710   **Atherosclerosis of autologous vein** `HCC` `A`
coronary artery bypass graft(s) with
unstable angina pectoris
> *EXCLUDES 1*   *unstable angina without*
> *atherosclerosis of*
> *autologous vein coronary*
> *artery bypass graft(s) (I20.0)*
> *EXCLUDES 2* ▸*embolism or thrombus of*
> *coronary artery bypass*
> *graft(s) (T82.8-)*◂

I25.711   **Atherosclerosis of autologous vein** `HCC` `A`
coronary artery bypass graft(s) with
angina pectoris with documented spasm
> *EXCLUDES 1*   *angina pectoris with documented*
> *spasm without*
> *atherosclerosis of*
> *autologous vein coronary*
> *artery bypass graft(s) (I20.1)*

I25.718   **Atherosclerosis of autologous vein** `HCC` `A`
coronary artery bypass graft(s) with
other forms of angina pectoris
> *EXCLUDES 1*   *other forms of angina pectoris*
> *without atherosclerosis of*
> *autologous vein coronary*
> *artery bypass graft(s) (I20.8)*

I25.719   **Atherosclerosis of autologous** `HCC` `A` ▽
vein coronary artery bypass graft(s) with
unspecified angina pectoris
> *EXCLUDES 1*   *unspecified angina pectoris*
> *without atherosclerosis of*
> *autologous vein coronary*
> *artery bypass graft(s) (I20.9)*

✓6ᵗʰ **I25.72**   **Atherosclerosis of autologous artery coronary artery**
bypass graft(s) with angina pectoris
> Atherosclerosis of internal mammary artery graft with
> angina pectoris

I25.720   **Atherosclerosis of autologous artery** `HCC` `A`
coronary artery bypass graft(s) with
unstable angina pectoris
> *EXCLUDES 1*   *unstable angina without*
> *atherosclerosis of*
> *autologous artery coronary*
> *artery bypass graft(s) (I20.0)*

I25.721   **Atherosclerosis of autologous artery** `HCC` `A`
coronary artery bypass graft(s) with
angina pectoris with documented spasm
> *EXCLUDES 1*   *angina pectoris with documented*
> *spasm without*
> *atherosclerosis of*
> *autologous artery coronary*
> *artery bypass graft(s) (I20.1)*

I25.728   **Atherosclerosis of autologous artery** `HCC` `A`
coronary artery bypass graft(s) with
other forms of angina pectoris
> *EXCLUDES 1*   *other forms of angina pectoris*
> *without atherosclerosis of*
> *autologous artery coronary*
> *artery bypass graft(s) (I20.8)*

I25.729   **Atherosclerosis of autologous** `HCC` `A` ▽
artery coronary artery bypass graft(s)
with unspecified angina pectoris
> *EXCLUDES 1*   *unspecified angina pectoris*
> *without atherosclerosis of*
> *autologous artery coronary*
> *artery bypass graft(s) (I20.9)*

✓6ᵗʰ **I25.73**   **Atherosclerosis of nonautologous biological**
coronary artery bypass graft(s) with angina pectoris

I25.730   **Atherosclerosis of nonautologous** `HCC` `A`
biological coronary artery bypass graft(s)
with unstable angina pectoris
> *EXCLUDES 1*   *unstable angina without*
> *atherosclerosis of*
> *nonautologous biological*
> *coronary artery bypass*
> *graft(s) (I20.0)*

☑ Additional Character Req   ✓x7ᵗʰ Placeholder Alert   Manifestation   `HCC` CMS-HCC Condition   ▽ Unspecified Code   ▸◂ Revised Text   ● New Code   ▲ Revised Code Title

ICD-10-CM 2018   623

Chapter 9. Diseases of the Circulatory System

I25.731   Atherosclerosis of nonautologous `HCC` `A`
biological coronary artery bypass graft(s)
with angina pectoris with documented
spasm
    EXCLUDES 1   angina pectoris with documented
spasm without
atherosclerosis of
nonautologous biological
coronary artery bypass
graft(s) (I20.1)

I25.738   Atherosclerosis of nonautologous `HCC` `A`
biological coronary artery bypass graft(s)
with other forms of angina pectoris
    EXCLUDES 1   other forms of angina pectoris
without atherosclerosis of
nonautologous biological
coronary artery bypass
graft(s) (I20.8)

I25.739   Atherosclerosis of nonautologous `HCC` `A` ▽
biological coronary artery bypass graft(s)
with unspecified angina pectoris
    EXCLUDES 1   unspecified angina pectoris
without atherosclerosis of
nonautologous biological
coronary artery bypass
graft(s) (I20.9)

✓6th   I25.75   Atherosclerosis of native coronary artery of
transplanted heart with angina pectoris
    EXCLUDES 1   atherosclerosis of native coronary artery of
transplanted heart without angina
pectoris (I25.811)

I25.750   Atherosclerosis of native coronary `HCC`
artery of transplanted heart with
unstable angina

I25.751   Atherosclerosis of native coronary `HCC`
artery of transplanted heart with
angina pectoris with documented
spasm

I25.758   Atherosclerosis of native coronary `HCC`
artery of transplanted heart with
other forms of angina pectoris

I25.759   Atherosclerosis of native coronary `HCC` ▽
artery of transplanted heart with
unspecified angina pectoris

✓6th   I25.76   Atherosclerosis of bypass graft of coronary artery of
transplanted heart with angina pectoris
    EXCLUDES 1   atherosclerosis of bypass graft of coronary
artery of transplanted heart without
angina pectoris (I25.812)

I25.760   Atherosclerosis of bypass graft of `HCC` `A`
coronary artery of transplanted heart
with unstable angina

I25.761   Atherosclerosis of bypass graft of `HCC` `A`
coronary artery of transplanted heart
with angina pectoris with documented
spasm

I25.768   Atherosclerosis of bypass graft of `HCC` `A`
coronary artery of transplanted heart
with other forms of angina pectoris

I25.769   Atherosclerosis of bypass graft of `HCC` `A` ▽
coronary artery of transplanted heart
with unspecified angina pectoris

✓6th   I25.79   Atherosclerosis of other coronary artery bypass
graft(s) with angina pectoris

I25.790   Atherosclerosis of other coronary `HCC` `A`
artery bypass graft(s) with unstable
angina pectoris
    EXCLUDES 1   unstable angina without
atherosclerosis of other
coronary artery bypass
graft(s) (I20.0)

I25.791   Atherosclerosis of other coronary `HCC` `A`
artery bypass graft(s) with angina
pectoris with documented spasm
    EXCLUDES 1   angina pectoris with documented
spasm without
atherosclerosis of other
coronary artery bypass
graft(s) (I20.1)

I25.798   Atherosclerosis of other coronary `HCC` `A`
artery bypass graft(s) with other
forms of angina pectoris
    EXCLUDES 1   other forms of angina pectoris
without atherosclerosis of
other coronary artery bypass
graft(s) (I20.8)

I25.799   Atherosclerosis of other coronary `HCC` `A` ▽
artery bypass graft(s) with unspecified
angina pectoris
    EXCLUDES 1   unspecified angina pectoris
without atherosclerosis of
other coronary artery bypass
graft(s) (I20.9)

✓5th   I25.8   Other forms of chronic ischemic heart disease

✓6th   I25.81   Atherosclerosis of other coronary vessels without
angina pectoris
Use additional code, if applicable, to identify:
coronary atherosclerosis due to calcified coronary
lesion (I25.84)
coronary atherosclerosis due to lipid rich plaque
(I25.83)
    EXCLUDES 1   atherosclerotic heart disease of native
coronary artery without angina pectoris
(I25.10)

I25.810   Atherosclerosis of coronary artery `A`
bypass graft(s) without angina pectoris
Atherosclerosis of coronary artery bypass
graft NOS
    EXCLUDES 1   atherosclerosis of coronary
bypass graft(s) with angina
pectoris (I25.70--I25.73-,
I25.79-)

I25.811   Atherosclerosis of native coronary
artery of transplanted heart without
angina pectoris
Atherosclerosis of native coronary artery of
transplanted heart NOS
    EXCLUDES 1   atherosclerosis of native coronary
artery of transplanted heart
with angina pectoris
(I25.75-)

I25.812   Atherosclerosis of bypass graft of `A`
coronary artery of transplanted heart
without angina pectoris
Atherosclerosis of bypass graft of
transplanted heart NOS
    EXCLUDES 1   atherosclerosis of bypass graft of
transplanted heart with
angina pectoris (I25.76)

I25.82   Chronic total occlusion of coronary artery
Complete occlusion of coronary artery
Total occlusion of coronary artery
Code first coronary atherosclerosis (I25.1-, I25.7-,
I25.81-)
    EXCLUDES 1 ▶acute coronary occlusion with myocardial
infarction (I21.0-I21.9, I22.-)◀
▶acute coronary occlusion without
myocardial infarction◀ (I24.0)
    DEF: Complete blockage of coronary artery due to
plaque accumulation over an extended period of time;
results in substantial reduction of blood flow;
characterized by angina or chest pain.

I25.83   Coronary atherosclerosis due to lipid rich plaque `A`
Code first coronary atherosclerosis (I25.1-, I25.7-,
I25.81-)

I25.84   Coronary atherosclerosis due to calcified coronary
lesion
Coronary atherosclerosis due to severely calcified
coronary lesion
Code first coronary atherosclerosis (I25.1-, I25.7-,
I25.81-)

I25.89   Other forms of chronic ischemic heart disease

I25.9   Chronic ischemic heart disease, unspecified   ▽
Ischemic heart disease (chronic) NOS

Pulmonary heart disease and diseases of pulmonary circulation (I26-I28)

✓4ᵗʰ **I26   Pulmonary embolism**

     INCLUDES   pulmonary (acute) (artery)(vein) infarction
                 pulmonary (acute) (artery)(vein) thromboembolism
                 pulmonary (acute) (artery)(vein) thrombosis

     EXCLUDES 2   *chronic pulmonary embolism (I27.82)*
                 personal history of pulmonary embolism (Z86.711)
                 pulmonary embolism complicating abortion, ectopic or molar
                   pregnancy (O00-O07, O08.2)
                 pulmonary embolism complicating pregnancy, childbirth and
                   the puerperium (O88.-)
                 pulmonary embolism due to complications of surgical and
                   medical care (T80.0, T81.7-, T82.8-)
                 pulmonary embolism due to trauma (T79.0, T79.1)
                 septic (non-pulmonary) arterial embolism (I76)

✓5ᵗʰ **I26.0   Pulmonary embolism with acute cor pulmonale**

     I26.01   Septic pulmonary embolism with acute cor pulmonale   HCC
         Code first underlying infection

     I26.02   Saddle embolus of pulmonary artery with acute cor pulmonale   HCC

     I26.09   Other pulmonary embolism with acute cor pulmonale   HCC
         Acute cor pulmonale NOS
         AHA: 2014, 4Q, 21

✓5ᵗʰ **I26.9   Pulmonary embolism without acute cor pulmonale**

     I26.90   Septic pulmonary embolism without acute cor pulmonale   HCC
         Code first underlying infection

     I26.92   Saddle embolus of pulmonary artery without acute cor pulmonale   HCC

     I26.99   Other pulmonary embolism without acute cor pulmonale   HCC
         Acute pulmonary embolism NOS
         Pulmonary embolism NOS

✓4ᵗʰ **I27   Other pulmonary heart diseases**

     I27.0   Primary pulmonary hypertension   HCC
         ▶Heritable pulmonary arterial hypertension
         Idiopathic pulmonary arterial hypertension
         Primary group 1 pulmonary hypertension
         Primary pulmonary arterial hypertension◀
         EXCLUDES 1 ▶*persistent pulmonary hypertension of newborn*
                 (P29.30)◀
                 pulmonary hypertension NOS ▶*(I27.20)*◀
                 ▶*secondary pulmonary arterial hypertension (I27.21)*◀
                 secondary pulmonary hypertension ▶*(I27.29)*◀

     I27.1   Kyphoscoliotic heart disease   HCC

     ✓5ᵗʰ **I27.2   Other secondary pulmonary hypertension**
         ~~Pulmonary hypertension NOS~~
         Code also associated underlying condition
         EXCLUDES 1 ▶*Eisenmenger's syndrome (I27.83)*◀
         AHA: 2014, 4Q, 21

     ● **I27.20   Pulmonary hypertension, unspecified**   ▽
         Pulmonary hypertension NOS

     ● **I27.21   Secondary pulmonary arterial hypertension**
         (Associated) (drug-induced) (toxin-induced)
             pulmonary arterial hypertension NOS
         (Associated) (drug-induced) (toxin-induced)
             (secondary) group 1 pulmonary hypertension
         Code also associated conditions if applicable, or
             adverse effects of drugs or toxins, such as:
             adverse effect of appetite depressants (T50.5X5)
             congenital heart disease (Q20-Q28)
             human immunodeficiency virus [HIV] disease (B20)
             polymyositis (M33.2-)
             portal hypertension (K76.6)
             rheumatoid arthritis (M05.-)
             schistosomiasis (B65.-)
             Sjögren syndrome (M35.0-)
             systemic sclerosis (M34.-)

     ● **I27.22   Pulmonary hypertension due to left heart disease**
         Group 2 pulmonary hypertension
         Code also associated left heart disease, if known, such
             as:
             multiple valve disease (I08.-)
             rheumatic mitral valve diseases (I05.-)
             rheumatic aortic valve diseases (I06.-)

     ● **I27.23   Pulmonary hypertension due to lung diseases and hypoxia**
         Group 3 pulmonary hypertension
         Code also associated lung disease, if known, such as:
             bronchiectasis (J47.-)
             cystic fibrosis with pulmonary manifestations
                 (E84.0)
             interstitial lung disease (J84.-)
             pleural effusion (J90)
             sleep apnea (G47.3-)

     ● **I27.24   Chronic thromboembolic pulmonary hypertension**
         Group 4 pulmonary hypertension
         Code also associated pulmonary embolism, if
             applicable (I26.-, I27.82)

     ● **I27.29   Other secondary pulmonary hypertension**
         Group 5 pulmonary hypertension
         Pulmonary hypertension with unclear multifactorial
             mechanisms
         Pulmonary hypertension due to hematologic
             disorders
         Pulmonary hypertension due to metabolic disorders
         Pulmonary hypertension due to other systemic
             disorders
         Code also other associated disorders, if known, such
             as:
             chronic myeloid leukemia (C92.10- C92.22)
             essential thrombocythemia (D47.3)
             Gaucher disease (E75.22)
             hypertensive chronic kidney disease with end stage
                 renal disease (I12.0, I12.11, I13.2)
             hyperthyroidism (E05.-)
             hypothyroidism (E00-E03)
             polycythemia vera (D45)
             sarcoidosis (D86.-)
         AHA: 2016, 2Q, 8

     ✓5ᵗʰ **I27.8   Other specified pulmonary heart diseases**

     I27.81   Cor pulmonale (chronic)   HCC
         Cor pulmonale NOS
         EXCLUDES 1   *acute cor pulmonale (I26.0-)*
         AHA: 2014, 4Q, 21

     I27.82   Chronic pulmonary embolism   HCC
         Use additional code, if applicable, for associated
             long-term (current) use of anticoagulants
             (Z79.01)
         EXCLUDES 1   *personal history of pulmonary embolism*
                 (Z86.711)
         DEF: A long-standing condition commonly associated
         with pulmonary hypertension in which small blood clots
         travel to the lungs repeatedly over many weeks,
         months, or years, requiring continuation of established
         anticoagulant or thrombolytic therapy.

     I27.83   Eisenmenger's syndrome
         Eisenmenger's complex
         (Irreversible) Eisenmenger's disease
         Pulmonary hypertension with right to left shunt
             related to congenital heart disease
         Code also underlying heart defect, if known, such as:
             atrial septal defect (Q21.1)
             Eisenmenger's defect (Q21.8)
             patent ductus arteriosus (Q25.0)
             ventricular septal defect (Q21.0)

     I27.89   Other specified pulmonary heart diseases   HCC
         ~~Eisenmenger's complex~~
         ~~Eisenmenger's syndrome~~
         EXCLUDES 1   *Eisenmenger's defect (Q21.8)*

     I27.9   Pulmonary heart disease, unspecified   HCC ▽
         Chronic cardiopulmonary disease

✓4ᵗʰ **I28   Other diseases of pulmonary vessels**

     I28.0   Arteriovenous fistula of pulmonary vessels   HCC
         EXCLUDES 1   *congenital arteriovenous fistula (Q25.72)*

     I28.1   Aneurysm of pulmonary artery   HCC
         EXCLUDES 1   *congenital aneurysm (Q25.79)*
                 congenital arteriovenous aneurysm (Q25.72)

     I28.8   Other diseases of pulmonary vessels   HCC
         Pulmonary arteritis
         Pulmonary endarteritis
         Rupture of pulmonary vessels
         Stenosis of pulmonary vessels
         Stricture of pulmonary vessels

     I28.9   Disease of pulmonary vessels, unspecified   HCC ▽

✓ Additional Character Req   ✓x7ᵗʰ Placeholder Alert   Manifestation   HCC CMS-HCC Condition   ▽ Unspecified Code   ▶◀ Revised Text   ● New Code   ▲ Revised Code Title

Other forms of heart disease (I30-I52)

✓4ᵗʰ I30 Acute pericarditis

INCLUDES acute mediastinopericarditis
acute myopericarditis
acute pericardial effusion
acute pleuropericarditis
acute pneumopericarditis

EXCLUDES 1 Dressler's syndrome (I24.1)
rheumatic pericarditis (acute) (I01.0)
▶viral pericarditis due to Coxsakie virus (B33.23)◄

I30.0 Acute nonspecific idiopathic pericarditis

I30.1 Infective pericarditis
Pneumococcal pericarditis
Pneumopyopericardium
Purulent pericarditis
Pyopericarditis
Pyopericardium
Pyopneumopericardium
Staphylococcal pericarditis
Streptococcal pericarditis
Suppurative pericarditis
Viral pericarditis
Use additional code (B95-B97) to identify infectious agent

I30.8 Other forms of acute pericarditis

I30.9 Acute pericarditis, unspecified ▽

✓4ᵗʰ I31 Other diseases of pericardium

EXCLUDES 1 diseases of pericardium specified as rheumatic (I09.2)
postcardiotomy syndrome (I97.0)
traumatic injury to pericardium (S26.-)

I31.0 Chronic adhesive pericarditis
Accretio cordis
Adherent pericardium
Adhesive mediastinopericarditis

I31.1 Chronic constrictive pericarditis
Concretio cordis
Pericardial calcification

I31.2 Hemopericardium, not elsewhere classified
EXCLUDES 1 hemopericardium as current complication following acute myocardial infarction (I23.0)
DEF: Presence of blood in the pericardial sac (pericardium). It can lead to potentially fatal cardiac tamponade if enough blood enters the pericardial cavity.

I31.3 Pericardial effusion (noninflammatory)
Chylopericardium
EXCLUDES 1 acute pericardial effusion (I30.9)

I31.4 Cardiac tamponade
Code first underlying cause

I31.8 Other specified diseases of pericardium
Epicardial plaques
Focal pericardial adhesions

I31.9 Disease of pericardium, unspecified ▽
Pericarditis (chronic) NOS

Cardiac Tamponade

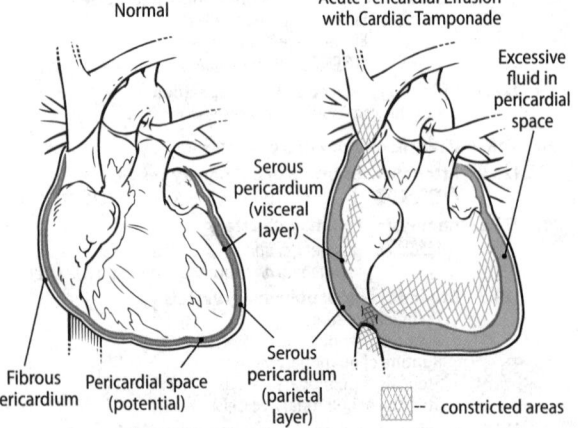

Normal

Acute Pericardial Effusion with Cardiac Tamponade

Excessive fluid in pericardial space

Serous pericardium (visceral layer)

Serous pericardium (parietal layer)

Fibrous pericardium

Pericardial space (potential)

constricted areas

I32 Pericarditis in diseases classified elsewhere
Code first underlying disease
EXCLUDES 1 pericarditis (in):
coxsackie (virus) (B33.23)
gonococcal (A54.83)
meningococcal (A39.53)
rheumatoid (arthritis) (M05.31)
syphilitic (A52.06)
systemic lupus erythematosus (M32.12)
tuberculosis (A18.84)

✓4ᵗʰ I33 Acute and subacute endocarditis
EXCLUDES 1 acute rheumatic endocarditis (I01.1)
endocarditis NOS (I38)

I33.0 Acute and subacute infective endocarditis
Bacterial endocarditis (acute) (subacute)
Infective endocarditis (acute) (subacute) NOS
Endocarditis lenta (acute) (subacute)
Malignant endocarditis (acute) (subacute)
Purulent endocarditis (acute) (subacute)
Septic endocarditis (acute) (subacute)
Ulcerative endocarditis (acute) (subacute)
Vegetative endocarditis (acute) (subacute)
Use additional code (B95-B97) to identify infectious agent

I33.9 Acute and subacute endocarditis, unspecified ▽
Acute endocarditis NOS
Acute myoendocarditis NOS
Acute periendocarditis NOS
Subacute endocarditis NOS
Subacute myoendocarditis NOS
Subacute periendocarditis NOS

✓4ᵗʰ I34 Nonrheumatic mitral valve disorders
EXCLUDES 1 mitral valve disease (I05.9)
mitral valve failure (I05.8)
mitral valve stenosis (I05.0)
mitral valve disorder of unspecified cause with diseases of aortic and/or tricuspid valve(s) (I08.-)
mitral valve disorder of unspecified cause with mitral stenosis or obstruction (I05.0)
mitral valve disorder specified as congenital ▶(Q23.2, Q23.9)◄
mitral valve disorder specified as rheumatic (I05.-)

I34.0 Nonrheumatic mitral (valve) insufficiency
Nonrheumatic mitral (valve) incompetence NOS
Nonrheumatic mitral (valve) regurgitation NOS

I34.1 Nonrheumatic mitral (valve) prolapse
Floppy nonrheumatic mitral valve syndrome
EXCLUDES 1 Marfan's syndrome (Q87.4-)

I34.2 Nonrheumatic mitral (valve) stenosis

I34.8 Other nonrheumatic mitral valve disorders

I34.9 Nonrheumatic mitral valve disorder, unspecified ▽

✓4ᵗʰ I35 Nonrheumatic aortic valve disorders
EXCLUDES 1 aortic valve disorder of unspecified cause but with diseases of mitral and/or tricuspid valve(s) (I08.-)
aortic valve disorder specified as congenital (Q23.0, Q23.1)
aortic valve disorder specified as rheumatic (I06.-)
hypertrophic subaortic stenosis (I42.1)

I35.0 Nonrheumatic aortic (valve) stenosis

I35.1 Nonrheumatic aortic (valve) insufficiency
Nonrheumatic aortic (valve) incompetence NOS
Nonrheumatic aortic (valve) regurgitation NOS

I35.2 Nonrheumatic aortic (valve) stenosis with insufficiency

I35.8 Other nonrheumatic aortic valve disorders

I35.9 Nonrheumatic aortic (valve) disorder, unspecified ▽

✓4ᵗʰ I36 Nonrheumatic tricuspid valve disorders
EXCLUDES 1 tricuspid valve disorders of unspecified cause (I07.-)
tricuspid valve disorders specified as congenital (Q22.4, Q22.8, Q22.9)
tricuspid valve disorders specified as rheumatic (I07.-)
tricuspid valve disorders with aortic and/or mitral valve involvement (I08.-)

I36.0 Nonrheumatic tricuspid (valve) stenosis

I36.1 Nonrheumatic tricuspid (valve) insufficiency
Nonrheumatic tricuspid (valve) incompetence
Nonrheumatic tricuspid (valve) regurgitation

I36.2 Nonrheumatic tricuspid (valve) stenosis with insufficiency

I36.8 Other nonrheumatic tricuspid valve disorders

I36.9 Nonrheumatic tricuspid valve disorder, unspecified ▽

EXCLUDES 1 Not coded here   EXCLUDES 2 Not included here   N Newborn Age: 0   P Pediatric Age: 0-17   M Maternity Age: 12-55   A Adult Age: 15-124

626

ICD-10-CM 2018

✓4ᵗʰ **I37**   **Nonrheumatic pulmonary valve disorders**
- **EXCLUDES 1**   *pulmonary valve disorder specified as congenital (Q22.1, Q22.2, Q22.3)*
  - *pulmonary valve disorder specified as rheumatic (I09.89)*

I37.0   **Nonrheumatic pulmonary valve stenosis**

I37.1   **Nonrheumatic pulmonary valve insufficiency**
- Nonrheumatic pulmonary valve incompetence
- Nonrheumatic pulmonary valve regurgitation

I37.2   **Nonrheumatic pulmonary valve stenosis with insufficiency**

I37.8   **Other nonrheumatic pulmonary valve disorders**

I37.9   **Nonrheumatic pulmonary valve disorder, unspecified** ▽

I38   **Endocarditis, valve unspecified** ▽
- **INCLUDES**   endocarditis (chronic) NOS
  - valvular incompetence NOS
  - valvular insufficiency NOS
  - valvular regurgitation NOS
  - valvular stenosis NOS
  - valvulitis (chronic) NOS
- **EXCLUDES 1**   *congenital insufficiency of cardiac valve NOS (Q24.8)*
  - *congenital stenosis of cardiac valve NOS (Q24.8)*
  - *endocardial fibroelastosis (I42.4)*
  - *endocarditis specified as rheumatic (I09.1)*

I39   ***Endocarditis and heart valve disorders in diseases classified elsewhere***
- Code first underlying disease, such as:
  - Q fever (A78)
- **EXCLUDES 1**   *endocardial involvement in:*
  - *candidiasis (B37.6)*
  - *gonococcal infection (A54.83)*
  - *Libman-Sacks disease (M32.11)*
  - *listerosis (A32.82)*
  - *meningococcal infection (A39.51)*
  - *rheumatoid arthritis (M05.31)*
  - *syphilis (A52.03)*
  - *tuberculosis (A18.84)*
  - *typhoid fever (A01.02)*

✓4ᵗʰ **I40**   **Acute myocarditis**
- **INCLUDES**   subacute myocarditis
- **EXCLUDES 1**   *acute rheumatic myocarditis (I01.2)*

I40.0   **Infective myocarditis**
- Septic myocarditis
- Use additional code (B95-B97) to identify infectious agent

I40.1   **Isolated myocarditis**
- Fiedler's myocarditis
- Giant cell myocarditis
- Idiopathic myocarditis

I40.8   **Other acute myocarditis**

I40.9   **Acute myocarditis, unspecified** ▽

I41   ***Myocarditis in diseases classified elsewhere***
- Code first underlying disease, such as:
  - typhus (A75.0-A75.9)
- **EXCLUDES 1**   *myocarditis (in):*
  - *Chagas' disease (chronic) (B57.2)*
    - *acute (B57.0)*
  - *coxsackie (virus) infection (B33.22)*
  - *diphtheritic (A36.81)*
  - *gonococcal (A54.83)*
  - *influenzal (J09.X9, J10.82, J11.82)*
  - *meningococcal (A39.52)*
  - *mumps (B26.82)*
  - *rheumatoid arthritis (M05.31)*
  - *sarcoid (D86.85)*
  - *syphilis (A52.06)*
  - *toxoplasmosis (B58.81)*
  - *tuberculous (A18.84)*

✓4ᵗʰ **I42**   **Cardiomyopathy**
- **INCLUDES**   myocardiopathy
- Code first pre-existing cardiomyopathy complicating pregnancy and puerperium (O99.4)
- **EXCLUDES 2**   *ischemic cardiomyopathy (I25.5)*
  - *peripartum cardiomyopathy (O90.3)*
  - *ventricular hypertrophy (I51.7)*

I42.0   **Dilated cardiomyopathy** HCC
- Congestive cardiomyopathy

I42.1   **Obstructive hypertrophic cardiomyopathy** HCC
- Hypertrophic subaortic stenosis (idiopathic)
- **DEF:** Cardiomyopathy marked by left ventricle hypertrophy, enlarged septum; results in obstructed blood flow, arrhythmias, mitral regurgitation, and sudden cardiac death.

I42.2   **Other hypertrophic cardiomyopathy** HCC
- Nonobstructive hypertrophic cardiomyopathy

I42.3   **Endomyocardial (eosinophilic) disease** HCC
- Endomyocardial (tropical) fibrosis
- Löffler's endocarditis

I42.4   **Endocardial fibroelastosis** HCC
- Congenital cardiomyopathy
- Elastomyofibrosis

I42.5   **Other restrictive cardiomyopathy** HCC
- Constrictive cardiomyopathy NOS

I42.6   **Alcoholic cardiomyopathy** HCC
- Code also presence of alcoholism (F10.-)

I42.7   **Cardiomyopathy due to drug and external agent** HCC
- Code first poisoning due to drug or toxin, if applicable (T36-T65 with fifth or sixth character 1-4 or 6)
- Use additional code for adverse effect, if applicable, to identify drug (T36-T50 with fifth or sixth character 5)

I42.8   **Other cardiomyopathies** HCC

I42.9   **Cardiomyopathy, unspecified** HCC ▽
- Cardiomyopathy (primary) (secondary) NOS

I43   ***Cardiomyopathy in diseases classified elsewhere*** HCC
- Code first underlying disease, such as:
  - amyloidosis (E85.-)
  - glycogen storage disease (E74.0)
  - gout (M10.0-)
  - thyrotoxicosis (E05.0-E05.9-)
- **EXCLUDES 1**   *cardiomyopathy (in):*
  - *coxsackie (virus) (B33.24)*
  - *diphtheria (A36.81)*
  - *sarcoidosis (D86.85)*
  - *tuberculosis (A18.84)*

✓4ᵗʰ **I44**   **Atrioventricular and left bundle-branch block**

I44.0   **Atrioventricular block, first degree**

I44.1   **Atrioventricular block, second degree**
- Atrioventricular block, type I and II
- Möbitz block, type I and II
- Second degree block, type I and II
- Wenckebach's block

I44.2   **Atrioventricular block, complete** HCC
- Complete heart block NOS
- Third degree block

✓5ᵗʰ **I44.3**   **Other and unspecified atrioventricular block**
- Atrioventricular block NOS

     I44.30   **Unspecified atrioventricular block** ▽

     I44.39   **Other atrioventricular block**

I44.4   **Left anterior fascicular block**

I44.5   **Left posterior fascicular block**

✓5ᵗʰ **I44.6**   **Other and unspecified fascicular block**

     I44.60   **Unspecified fascicular block** ▽
- Left bundle-branch hemiblock NOS

     I44.69   **Other fascicular block**

I44.7   **Left bundle-branch block, unspecified** ▽

✓4ᵗʰ **I45**   **Other conduction disorders**

I45.0   **Right fascicular block**

✓5ᵗʰ **I45.1**   **Other and unspecified right bundle-branch block**

     I45.10   **Unspecified right bundle-branch block** ▽
- Right bundle-branch block NOS

     I45.19   **Other right bundle-branch block**

I45.2   **Bifascicular block**

I45.3   **Trifascicular block**

I45.4   **Nonspecific intraventricular block**
- Bundle-branch block NOS

I45.5   **Other specified heart block**
- Sinoatrial block
- Sinoauricular block
- **EXCLUDES 1**   *heart block NOS (I45.9)*

I45.6   **Pre-excitation syndrome**
- Accelerated atrioventricular conduction
- Accessory atrioventricular conduction
- Anomalous atrioventricular excitation
- Lown-Ganong-Levine syndrome
- Pre-excitation atrioventricular conduction
- Wolff-Parkinson-White syndrome

☑ Additional Character Req   ✓ₓ7ᵗʰ Placeholder Alert   Manifestation   HCC CMS-HCC Condition   ▽ Unspecified Code   ▶◀ Revised Text   ● New Code   ▲ Revised Code Title

Conduction Disorders

Sinoatrial node (pacemaker)

Internodal tracts:
Anterior
Middle
Posterior

Bachmann's bundle

Left bundle branch block

Left bundle branch:
Anterior fascicle
Posterior fascicle

Atrioventricular node
Atrioventricular bundle (of His)
Atrioventricular block
Accessory bundle (of Kent)
Right bundle branch
Right bundle branch block
Moderator band
Purkinje fibers

Left bundle branch hemiblock

✓5th **I45.8** **Other specified conduction disorders**

I45.81 **Long QT syndrome**
DEF: Condition characterized by recurrent syncope, malignant arrhythmias, and sudden death; characteristic prolonged Q-T interval on electrocardiogram.

I45.89 **Other specified conduction disorders**
Atrioventricular [AV] dissociation
Interference dissociation
Isorhythmic dissociation
Nonparoxysmal AV nodal tachycardia
AHA: 2013, 2Q, 31

I45.9 **Conduction disorder, unspecified** ▽
Heart block NOS
Stokes-Adams syndrome

✓4th **I46** **Cardiac arrest**
EXCLUDES 1   cardiogenic shock (R57.0)

I46.2 **Cardiac arrest due to underlying cardiac condition** HCC
Code first underlying cardiac condition

I46.8 **Cardiac arrest due to other underlying condition** HCC
Code first underlying condition

I46.9 **Cardiac arrest, cause unspecified** HCC ▽

✓4th **I47** **Paroxysmal tachycardia**
Code first tachycardia complicating:
abortion or ectopic or molar pregnancy (O00-O07, O08.8)
obstetric surgery and procedures (O75.4)
EXCLUDES 1   tachycardia NOS (R00.0)
sinoauricular tachycardia NOS (R00.0)
sinus [sinusal] tachycardia NOS (R00.0)

I47.0 **Re-entry ventricular arrhythmia** HCC

I47.1 **Supraventricular tachycardia** HCC
Atrial (paroxysmal) tachycardia
Atrioventricular [AV] (paroxysmal) tachycardia
Atrioventricular re-entrant (nodal) tachycardia [AVNRT] [AVRT]
Junctional (paroxysmal) tachycardia
Nodal (paroxysmal) tachycardia

I47.2 **Ventricular tachycardia** HCC
AHA: 2013, 3Q, 23

I47.9 **Paroxysmal tachycardia, unspecified** HCC ▽
Bouveret (-Hoffman) syndrome

✓4th **I48** **Atrial fibrillation and flutter**

I48.0 **Paroxysmal atrial fibrillation** HCC

I48.1 **Persistent atrial fibrillation** HCC

I48.2 **Chronic atrial fibrillation** HCC
Permanent atrial fibrillation

I48.3 **Typical atrial flutter** HCC
Type I atrial flutter

I48.4 **Atypical atrial flutter** HCC
Type II atrial flutter

✓5th **I48.9** **Unspecified atrial fibrillation and atrial flutter**

I48.91 **Unspecified atrial fibrillation** HCC ▽

I48.92 **Unspecified atrial flutter** HCC ▽

✓4th **I49** **Other cardiac arrhythmias**
Code first cardiac arrhythmia complicating:
abortion or ectopic or molar pregnancy (O00-O07, O08.8)
obstetric surgery and procedures (O75.4)
EXCLUDES 1   bradycardia NOS (R00.1)
neonatal dysrhythmia (P29.1-)
sinoatrial bradycardia (R00.1)
sinus bradycardia (R00.1)
vagal bradycardia (R00.1)
EXCLUDES 2 ▶bradycardia NOS (R00.1)◀

✓5th **I49.0** **Ventricular fibrillation and flutter**

I49.01 **Ventricular fibrillation** HCC

I49.02 **Ventricular flutter** HCC

I49.1 **Atrial premature depolarization**
Atrial premature beats

I49.2 **Junctional premature depolarization** HCC

I49.3 **Ventricular premature depolarization**

✓5th **I49.4** **Other and unspecified premature depolarization**

I49.40 **Unspecified premature depolarization** ▽
Premature beats NOS

I49.49 **Other premature depolarization**
Ectopic beats
Extrasystoles
Extrasystolic arrhythmias
Premature contractions

I49.5 **Sick sinus syndrome** HCC
Tachycardia-bradycardia syndrome

I49.8 **Other specified cardiac arrhythmias**
▶Brugada syndrome◀
Coronary sinus rhythm disorder
Ectopic rhythm disorder
Nodal rhythm disorder

I49.9 **Cardiac arrhythmia, unspecified** ▽
Arrhythmia (cardiac) NOS

✓4th **I50** **Heart failure**
Code first:
heart failure complicating abortion or ectopic or molar pregnancy (O00-O07, O08.8)
heart failure due to hypertension (I11.0)
heart failure due to hypertension with chronic kidney disease (I13.-)
heart failure following surgery (I97.13-)
obstetric surgery and procedures (O75.4)
rheumatic heart failure (I09.81)
EXCLUDES 1   neonatal cardiac failure (P29.0)
EXCLUDES 2   cardiac arrest (I46.-)
AHA: 2017, 1Q, 47; 2014, 1Q, 25; 2013, 2Q, 33

▲ **I50.1** **Left ventricular failure, unspecified** HCC ▽
Cardiac asthma
Edema of lung with heart disease NOS
Edema of lung with heart failure
Left heart failure
Pulmonary edema with heart disease NOS
Pulmonary edema with heart failure
EXCLUDES 1   edema of lung without heart disease or heart failure (J81.-)
pulmonary edema without heart disease or failure (J81.-)

✓5th **I50.2** **Systolic (congestive) heart failure**
▶Heart failure with reduced ejection fraction [HFrEF]
Systolic left ventricular heart failure◀
▶Code also end stage heart failure, if applicable (I50.84)◀
AHA: 2017, 1Q, 46; 2016, 1Q, 10

I50.20 **Unspecified systolic (congestive) heart failure** HCC ▽

I50.21 **Acute systolic (congestive) heart failure** HCC

I50.22 **Chronic systolic (congestive) heart failure** HCC

I50.23 **Acute on chronic systolic (congestive) heart failure** HCC

✓5th **I50.3** **Diastolic (congestive) heart failure**
▶Diastolic left ventricular heart failure
Heart failure with normal ejection fraction
Heart failure with preserved ejection fraction [HFpEF]◀
▶Code also end stage heart failure, if applicable (I50.84)◀
EXCLUDES 1   combined systolic (congestive) and diastolic (congestive) heart failure (I50.4-)
AHA: 2017, 1Q, 46; 2016, 1Q, 10

EXCLUDES 1 Not coded here   *EXCLUDES 2* Not included here   N Newborn Age: 0   P Pediatric Age: 0-17   M Maternity Age: 12-55   A Adult Age: 15-124

628   ICD-10-CM 2018

I50.30   **Unspecified diastolic (congestive) heart failure**   HCC ▽

I50.31   **Acute diastolic (congestive) heart failure**   HCC

I50.32   **Chronic diastolic (congestive) heart failure**   HCC

I50.33   **Acute on chronic diastolic (congestive) heart failure**   HCC

✓5th **I50.4**   **Combined systolic (congestive) and diastolic (congestive) heart failure**
▶Combined systolic and diastolic left ventricular heart failure
Heart failure with reduced ejection fraction and diastolic dysfunction◀
▶Code also end stage heart failure, if applicable (I50.84)◀
AHA: 2017, 1Q, 46; 2016, 1Q, 10

I50.40   **Unspecified combined systolic (congestive) and diastolic (congestive) heart failure**   HCC ▽

I50.41   **Acute combined systolic (congestive) and diastolic (congestive) heart failure**   HCC

I50.42   **Chronic combined systolic (congestive) and diastolic (congestive) heart failure**   HCC

I50.43   **Acute on chronic combined systolic (congestive) and diastolic (congestive) heart failure**   HCC

● ✓5th **I50.8**   **Other heart failure**

●   ✓6th **I50.81**   **Right heart failure**
Right ventricular failure

●   **I50.810**   **Right heart failure, unspecified**   ▽
Right heart failure without mention of left heart failure
Right ventricular failure NOS

●   **I50.811**   **Acute right heart failure**
Acute isolated right heart failure
Acute (isolated) right ventricular failure

●   **I50.812**   **Chronic right heart failure**
Chronic isolated right heart failure
Chronic (isolated) right ventricular failure

●   **I50.813**   **Acute on chronic right heart failure**
Acute on chronic isolated right heart failure
Acute on chronic (isolated) right ventricular failure
Acute decompensation of chronic (isolated) right ventricular failure
Acute exacerbation of chronic (isolated) right ventricular failure

●   **I50.814**   **Right heart failure due to left heart failure**
Right ventricular failure secondary to left ventricular failure
Code also the type of left ventricular failure, if known (I50.2-I50.43)
EXCLUDES 1   right heart failure with but not due to left heart failure (I50.82)

●   **I50.82**   **Biventricular heart failure**
Code also the type of left ventricular failure as systolic, diastolic, or combined, if known (I50.2-I50.43)

●   **I50.83**   **High output heart failure**

●   **I50.84**   **End stage heart failure**
Stage D heart failure
Code also the type of heart failure as systolic, diastolic, or combined, if known (I50.2-I50.43)

●   **I50.89**   **Other heart failure**

I50.9   **Heart failure, unspecified**   HCC ▽
~~Biventricular (heart) failure NOS~~
Cardiac, heart or myocardial failure NOS
Congestive heart disease
Congestive heart failure NOS
~~Right ventricular failure (secondary to left heart failure)~~
EXCLUDES 2   fluid overload (E87.70)
AHA: 2017, 1Q, 45-46; 2014, 4Q, 21; 2012, 4Q, 92

✓4th **I51**   **Complications and ill-defined descriptions of heart disease**
EXCLUDES 1   any condition in I51.4-I51.9 due to hypertension (I11.-)
any condition in I51.4-I51.9 due to hypertension and chronic kidney disease (I13.-)
heart disease specified as rheumatic (I00-I09)

I51.0   **Cardiac septal defect, acquired**   A
Acquired septal atrial defect (old)
Acquired septal auricular defect (old)
Acquired septal ventricular defect (old)
EXCLUDES 1   cardiac septal defect as current complication following acute myocardial infarction (I23.1, I23.2)
DEF: Abnormal communication between opposite heart chambers due to defect of septum; not present at birth.

I51.1   **Rupture of chordae tendineae, not elsewhere classified**   HCC
EXCLUDES 1   rupture of chordae tendineae as current complication following acute myocardial infarction (I23.4)

I51.2   **Rupture of papillary muscle, not elsewhere classified**   HCC
EXCLUDES 1   rupture of papillary muscle as current complication following acute myocardial infarction (I23.5)

I51.3   **Intracardiac thrombosis, not elsewhere classified**
Apical thrombosis (old)   Mural thrombosis (old)
Atrial thrombosis (old)   Ventricular thrombosis (old)
Auricular thrombosis (old)
EXCLUDES 1   intracardiac thrombosis as current complication following acute myocardial infarction (I23.6)
AHA: 2013, 1Q, 24

I51.4   **Myocarditis, unspecified**   HCC ▽
Chronic (interstitial) myocarditis
Myocardial fibrosis
Myocarditis NOS
EXCLUDES 1   acute or subacute myocarditis (I40.-)

I51.5   **Myocardial degeneration**   HCC
Fatty degeneration of heart or myocardium
Myocardial disease
Senile degeneration of heart or myocardium

I51.7   **Cardiomegaly**
Cardiac dilatation
Cardiac hypertrophy
Ventricular dilatation

✓5th **I51.8**   **Other ill-defined heart diseases**

I51.81   **Takotsubo syndrome**
Reversible left ventricular dysfunction following sudden emotional stress
Stress induced cardiomyopathy
Takotsubo cardiomyopathy
Transient left ventricular apical ballooning syndrome

I51.89   **Other ill-defined heart diseases**
Carditis (acute)(chronic)
Pancarditis (acute)(chronic)

I51.9   **Heart disease, unspecified**   ▽

I52   ***Other heart disorders in diseases classified elsewhere***
Code first underlying disease, such as:
congenital syphilis (A50.5)
mucopolysaccharidosis (E76.3)
schistosomiasis (B65.0-B65.9)
EXCLUDES 1   heart disease (in):
gonococcal infection (A54.83)
meningococcal infection (A39.50)
rheumatoid arthritis (M05.31)
syphilis (A52.06)

Cerebrovascular diseases (I60-I69)

Use additional code to identify presence of:
alcohol abuse and dependence (F10.-)
exposure to environmental tobacco smoke (Z77.22)
history of tobacco dependence (Z87.891)
hypertension (I10-I15)
occupational exposure to environmental tobacco smoke (Z57.31)
tobacco dependence (F17.-)
tobacco use (Z72.0)
EXCLUDES 1   ~~transient cerebral ischemic attacks and related syndromes (G45.-)~~
traumatic intracranial hemorrhage (S06.-)
AHA: 2014, 3Q, 5; 2012, 4Q, 91-92

✓4th **I60**   **Nontraumatic subarachnoid hemorrhage**
INCLUDES   ~~ruptured cerebral aneurysm~~
EXCLUDES 1   syphilitic ruptured cerebral aneurysm (A52.05)
EXCLUDES 2   sequelae of subarachnoid hemorrhage (I69.0-)

✓5th **I60.0**   **Nontraumatic subarachnoid hemorrhage from carotid siphon and bifurcation**

I60.00   **Nontraumatic subarachnoid hemorrhage from unspecified carotid siphon and bifurcation**   HCC ▽

I60.01   **Nontraumatic subarachnoid hemorrhage from right carotid siphon and bifurcation**   HCC

I60.02   **Nontraumatic subarachnoid hemorrhage from left carotid siphon and bifurcation**   HCC

✓5ᵗʰ **I60.1** **Nontraumatic subarachnoid hemorrhage from** middle cerebral artery

     I60.10 **Nontraumatic subarachnoid hemorrhage from unspecified middle cerebral artery** HCC ▽

     I60.11 **Nontraumatic subarachnoid hemorrhage from** right **middle cerebral artery** HCC

     I60.12 **Nontraumatic subarachnoid hemorrhage from** left **middle cerebral artery** HCC

I60.2 **Nontraumatic subarachnoid hemorrhage from** anterior **communicating artery** HCC

✓5ᵗʰ **I60.3** **Nontraumatic subarachnoid hemorrhage from** posterior **communicating artery**

     I60.30 **Nontraumatic subarachnoid hemorrhage from unspecified posterior communicating artery** HCC ▽

     I60.31 **Nontraumatic subarachnoid hemorrhage from** right **posterior communicating artery** HCC

     I60.32 **Nontraumatic subarachnoid hemorrhage from** left **posterior communicating artery** HCC

I60.4 **Nontraumatic subarachnoid hemorrhage from** basilar artery HCC

✓5ᵗʰ **I60.5** **Nontraumatic subarachnoid hemorrhage from** vertebral artery

     I60.50 **Nontraumatic subarachnoid hemorrhage from unspecified vertebral artery** HCC ▽

     I60.51 **Nontraumatic subarachnoid hemorrhage from** right **vertebral artery** HCC

     I60.52 **Nontraumatic subarachnoid hemorrhage from** left **vertebral artery** HCC

I60.6 **Nontraumatic subarachnoid hemorrhage from other intracranial arteries** HCC

I60.7 **Nontraumatic subarachnoid hemorrhage from unspecified intracranial artery** HCC ▽

     Ruptured (congenital) berry aneurysm
     Ruptured (congenital) cerebral aneurysm
     Subarachnoid hemorrhage (nontraumatic) from cerebral artery NOS
     Subarachnoid hemorrhage (nontraumatic) from communicating artery NOS

     EXCLUDES 1 berry aneurysm, nonruptured (I67.1)

I60.8 **Other nontraumatic subarachnoid hemorrhage** HCC
     Meningeal hemorrhage
     Rupture of cerebral arteriovenous malformation

I60.9 **Nontraumatic subarachnoid hemorrhage, unspecified** HCC ▽

✓4ᵗʰ **I61** **Nontraumatic intracerebral hemorrhage**
     EXCLUDES 2 sequelae of intracerebral hemorrhage (I69.1-)
     AHA: 2017, 2Q, 9-10

I61.0 **Nontraumatic intracerebral hemorrhage in** hemisphere, subcortical HCC
     Deep intracerebral hemorrhage (nontraumatic)

I61.1 **Nontraumatic intracerebral hemorrhage in** hemisphere, cortical HCC
     Cerebral lobe hemorrhage (nontraumatic)
     Superficial intracerebral hemorrhage (nontraumatic)

I61.2 **Nontraumatic intracerebral hemorrhage in** hemisphere, unspecified HCC ▽

I61.3 **Nontraumatic intracerebral hemorrhage in** brain stem HCC

I61.4 **Nontraumatic intracerebral hemorrhage in** cerebellum HCC

I61.5 **Nontraumatic intracerebral hemorrhage, intraventricular** HCC

I61.6 **Nontraumatic intracerebral hemorrhage,** multiple localized HCC

I61.8 **Other nontraumatic intracerebral hemorrhage** HCC

I61.9 **Nontraumatic intracerebral hemorrhage, unspecified** HCC ▽

✓4ᵗʰ **I62** **Other and unspecified** nontraumatic intracranial **hemorrhage**
     EXCLUDES 2 sequelae of intracranial hemorrhage (I69.2)

✓5ᵗʰ **I62.0** **Nontraumatic** subdural **hemorrhage**

     I62.00 **Nontraumatic subdural hemorrhage, unspecified** HCC ▽

     I62.01 **Nontraumatic** acute **subdural hemorrhage** HCC

     I62.02 **Nontraumatic** subacute **subdural hemorrhage** HCC

     I62.03 **Nontraumatic** chronic **subdural hemorrhage** HCC

I62.1 **Nontraumatic** extradural **hemorrhage** HCC
     Nontraumatic epidural hemorrhage

I62.9 **Nontraumatic intracranial hemorrhage, unspecified** HCC ▽

✓4ᵗʰ **I63** **Cerebral infarction**
     INCLUDES occlusion and stenosis of cerebral and precerebral arteries, resulting in cerebral infarction
     Use additional code, if applicable, to identify status post administration of tPA (rtPA) in a different facility within the last 24 hours prior to admission to current facility (Z92.82)
     Use additional code, if known, to indicate National Institutes of Health Stroke Scale (NIHSS) score (R29.7-)
     EXCLUDES 2 sequelae of cerebral infarction (I69.3-)
     AHA: 2017, 2Q, 9-10; 2014, 1Q, 23

✓5ᵗʰ **I63.0** **Cerebral infarction due to** thrombosis of precerebral **arteries**

     I63.00 **Cerebral infarction due to thrombosis of unspecified precerebral artery** HCC ▽

✓6ᵗʰ   **I63.01** **Cerebral infarction due to thrombosis of** vertebral artery

         I63.011 **Cerebral infarction due to thrombosis of** right **vertebral artery** HCC

         I63.012 **Cerebral infarction due to thrombosis of** left **vertebral artery** HCC

         I63.013 **Cerebral infarction due to thrombosis of** bilateral **vertebral arteries** HCC

         I63.019 **Cerebral infarction due to thrombosis of unspecified vertebral artery** HCC ▽

     I63.02 **Cerebral infarction due to thrombosis of** basilar **artery** HCC

✓6ᵗʰ   **I63.03** **Cerebral infarction due to thrombosis of** carotid artery

         I63.031 **Cerebral infarction due to thrombosis of** right **carotid artery** HCC

         I63.032 **Cerebral infarction due to thrombosis of** left **carotid artery** HCC

         I63.033 **Cerebral infarction due to thrombosis of** bilateral **carotid arteries** HCC

         I63.039 **Cerebral infarction due to thrombosis of unspecified carotid artery** HCC ▽

     I63.09 **Cerebral infarction due to thrombosis of other** precerebral **artery** HCC

✓5ᵗʰ **I63.1** **Cerebral infarction due to** embolism of precerebral **arteries**

     I63.10 **Cerebral infarction due to embolism of unspecified precerebral artery** HCC ▽

✓6ᵗʰ   **I63.11** **Cerebral infarction due to embolism of** vertebral artery

         I63.111 **Cerebral infarction due to embolism of** right **vertebral artery** HCC

         I63.112 **Cerebral infarction due to embolism of** left **vertebral artery** HCC

         I63.113 **Cerebral infarction due to embolism of** bilateral **vertebral arteries** HCC

         I63.119 **Cerebral infarction due to embolism of unspecified vertebral artery** HCC ▽

     I63.12 **Cerebral infarction due to embolism of** basilar **artery** HCC

✓6ᵗʰ   **I63.13** **Cerebral infarction due to embolism of** carotid artery

         I63.131 **Cerebral infarction due to embolism of** right **carotid artery** HCC

         I63.132 **Cerebral infarction due to embolism of** left **carotid artery** HCC

         I63.133 **Cerebral infarction due to embolism of** bilateral **carotid arteries** HCC

         I63.139 **Cerebral infarction due to embolism of unspecified carotid artery** HCC ▽

     I63.19 **Cerebral infarction due to embolism of other** precerebral artery HCC

✓5ᵗʰ **I63.2** **Cerebral infarction due to unspecified** occlusion or stenosis of precerebral **arteries**

     I63.20 **Cerebral infarction due to unspecified occlusion or stenosis of unspecified precerebral arteries** HCC ▽

✓6ᵗʰ   **I63.21** **Cerebral infarction due to unspecified occlusion or stenosis of** vertebral **arteries**

         ▲ **I63.211** **Cerebral infarction due to unspecified occlusion or stenosis of** right **vertebral artery** HCC

         ▲ **I63.212** **Cerebral infarction due to unspecified occlusion or stenosis of** left **vertebral artery** HCC

EXCLUDES 1 Not coded here   *EXCLUDES 2* Not included here   N Newborn Age: 0   P Pediatric Age: 0-17   M Maternity Age: 12-55   A Adult Age: 15-124

I63.213 **Cerebral infarction due to unspecified occlusion or stenosis of bilateral vertebral arteries** HCC

I63.219 **Cerebral infarction due to unspecified occlusion or stenosis of unspecified vertebral arteries** HCC ▽

▲   I63.22 **Cerebral infarction due to unspecified occlusion or stenosis of basilar artery** HCC

✓6th I63.23 **Cerebral infarction due to unspecified occlusion or stenosis of carotid arteries**

I63.231 **Cerebral infarction due to unspecified occlusion or stenosis of right carotid arteries** HCC

I63.232 **Cerebral infarction due to unspecified occlusion or stenosis of left carotid arteries** HCC

I63.233 **Cerebral infarction due to unspecified occlusion or stenosis of bilateral carotid arteries** HCC

I63.239 **Cerebral infarction due to unspecified occlusion or stenosis of unspecified carotid arteries** HCC ▽

I63.29 **Cerebral infarction due to unspecified occlusion or stenosis of other precerebral arteries** HCC ▽

✓5th I63.3 **Cerebral infarction due to thrombosis of cerebral arteries**

I63.30 **Cerebral infarction due to thrombosis of unspecified cerebral artery** HCC ▽

✓6th I63.31 **Cerebral infarction due to thrombosis of middle cerebral artery**

I63.311 **Cerebral infarction due to thrombosis of right middle cerebral artery** HCC

I63.312 **Cerebral infarction due to thrombosis of left middle cerebral artery** HCC

I63.313 **Cerebral infarction due to thrombosis of bilateral middle cerebral arteries** HCC

I63.319 **Cerebral infarction due to thrombosis of unspecified middle cerebral artery** HCC ▽

✓6th I63.32 **Cerebral infarction due to thrombosis of anterior cerebral artery**

I63.321 **Cerebral infarction due to thrombosis of right anterior cerebral artery** HCC

I63.322 **Cerebral infarction due to thrombosis of left anterior cerebral artery** HCC

I63.323 **Cerebral infarction due to thrombosis of bilateral anterior cerebral arteries** HCC

I63.329 **Cerebral infarction due to thrombosis of unspecified anterior cerebral artery** HCC ▽

✓6th I63.33 **Cerebral infarction due to thrombosis of posterior cerebral artery**

I63.331 **Cerebral infarction due to thrombosis of right posterior cerebral artery** HCC

I63.332 **Cerebral infarction due to thrombosis of left posterior cerebral artery** HCC

I63.333 **Cerebral infarction to thrombosis of bilateral posterior cerebral arteries** HCC

I63.339 **Cerebral infarction due to thrombosis of unspecified posterior cerebral artery** HCC ▽

✓6th I63.34 **Cerebral infarction due to thrombosis of cerebellar artery**

I63.341 **Cerebral infarction due to thrombosis of right cerebellar artery** HCC

I63.342 **Cerebral infarction due to thrombosis of left cerebellar artery** HCC

I63.343 **Cerebral infarction to thrombosis of bilateral cerebellar arteries** HCC

I63.349 **Cerebral infarction due to thrombosis of unspecified cerebellar artery** HCC ▽

I63.39 **Cerebral infarction due to thrombosis of other cerebral artery** HCC

✓5th I63.4 **Cerebral infarction due to embolism of cerebral arteries**

I63.40 **Cerebral infarction due to embolism of unspecified cerebral artery** HCC ▽

✓6th I63.41 **Cerebral infarction due to embolism of middle cerebral artery**

I63.411 **Cerebral infarction due to embolism of right middle cerebral artery** HCC

I63.412 **Cerebral infarction due to embolism of left middle cerebral artery** HCC

I63.413 **Cerebral infarction due to embolism of bilateral middle cerebral arteries** HCC

I63.419 **Cerebral infarction due to embolism of unspecified middle cerebral artery** HCC ▽

✓6th I63.42 **Cerebral infarction due to embolism of anterior cerebral artery**

I63.421 **Cerebral infarction due to embolism of right anterior cerebral artery** HCC

I63.422 **Cerebral infarction due to embolism of left anterior cerebral artery** HCC

I63.423 **Cerebral infarction due to embolism of bilateral anterior cerebral arteries** HCC

I63.429 **Cerebral infarction due to embolism of unspecified anterior cerebral artery** HCC ▽

✓6th I63.43 **Cerebral infarction due to embolism of posterior cerebral artery**

I63.431 **Cerebral infarction due to embolism of right posterior cerebral artery** HCC

I63.432 **Cerebral infarction due to embolism of left posterior cerebral artery** HCC

I63.433 **Cerebral infarction due to embolism of bilateral posterior cerebral arteries** HCC

I63.439 **Cerebral infarction due to embolism of unspecified posterior cerebral artery** HCC ▽

✓6th I63.44 **Cerebral infarction due to embolism of cerebellar artery**

I63.441 **Cerebral infarction due to embolism of right cerebellar artery** HCC

I63.442 **Cerebral infarction due to embolism of left cerebellar artery** HCC

I63.443 **Cerebral infarction due to embolism of bilateral cerebellar arteries** HCC

I63.449 **Cerebral infarction due to embolism of unspecified cerebellar artery** HCC ▽

I63.49 **Cerebral infarction due to embolism of other cerebral artery** HCC

✓5th I63.5 **Cerebral infarction due to unspecified occlusion or stenosis of cerebral arteries**

I63.50 **Cerebral infarction due to unspecified occlusion or stenosis of unspecified cerebral artery** HCC ▽

✓6th I63.51 **Cerebral infarction due to unspecified occlusion or stenosis of middle cerebral artery**

I63.511 **Cerebral infarction due to unspecified occlusion or stenosis of right middle cerebral artery** HCC

I63.512 **Cerebral infarction due to unspecified occlusion or stenosis of left middle cerebral artery** HCC

▲   I63.513 **Cerebral infarction due to unspecified occlusion or stenosis of bilateral middle cerebral arteries** HCC

I63.519 **Cerebral infarction due to unspecified occlusion or stenosis of unspecified middle cerebral artery** HCC ▽

✓6th I63.52 **Cerebral infarction due to unspecified occlusion or stenosis of anterior cerebral artery**

I63.521 **Cerebral infarction due to unspecified occlusion or stenosis of right anterior cerebral artery** HCC

I63.522 **Cerebral infarction due to unspecified occlusion or stenosis of left anterior cerebral artery** HCC

▲   I63.523 **Cerebral infarction due to unspecified occlusion or stenosis of bilateral anterior cerebral arteries** HCC

I63.529 **Cerebral infarction due to unspecified occlusion or stenosis of unspecified anterior cerebral artery** HCC ▽

☑ Additional Character Req   v×7 Placeholder Alert   Manifestation   HCC CMS-HCC Condition   ▽ Unspecified Code   ▶◀ Revised Text   ● New Code   ▲ Revised Code Title

ICD-10-CM 2018   631

✓6ᵗʰ **I63.53** **Cerebral infarction due to unspecified occlusion or stenosis of posterior cerebral artery**

     I63.531 Cerebral infarction due to unspecified occlusion or stenosis of right posterior cerebral artery   HCC

     I63.532 Cerebral infarction due to unspecified occlusion or stenosis of left posterior cerebral artery   HCC

     I63.533 Cerebral infarction due to unspecified occlusion or stenosis of bilateral posterior cerebral arteries   HCC

     I63.539 Cerebral infarction due to unspecified occlusion or stenosis of unspecified posterior cerebral artery   HCC ▽

✓6ᵗʰ **I63.54** **Cerebral infarction due to unspecified occlusion or stenosis of cerebellar artery**

     I63.541 Cerebral infarction due to unspecified occlusion or stenosis of right cerebellar artery   HCC

     I63.542 Cerebral infarction due to unspecified occlusion or stenosis of left cerebellar artery   HCC

     I63.543 Cerebral infarction due to unspecified occlusion or stenosis of bilateral cerebellar arteries   HCC

     I63.549 Cerebral infarction due to unspecified occlusion or stenosis of unspecified cerebellar artery   HCC ▽

    I63.59 Cerebral infarction due to unspecified occlusion or stenosis of other cerebral artery   HCC ▽

    I63.6 **Cerebral infarction due to cerebral venous thrombosis, nonpyogenic**   HCC

    I63.8 **Other cerebral infarction**   HCC

    I63.9 **Cerebral infarction, unspecified**   HCC ▽
     Stroke NOS
     EXCLUDES 2 ▶transient cerebral ischemic attacks and related syndromes (G45.-)◀
     AHA: 2015, 1Q, 25

✓4ᵗʰ **I65** **Occlusion and stenosis of precerebral arteries, not resulting in cerebral infarction**
     INCLUDES embolism of precerebral artery
         narrowing of precerebral artery
         obstruction (complete) (partial) of precerebral artery
         thrombosis of precerebral artery
     EXCLUDES 1 insufficiency, NOS, of precerebral artery (G45.-)
         insufficiency of precerebral arteries causing cerebral infarction (I63.0–I63.2)

    ✓5ᵗʰ **I65.0** **Occlusion and stenosis of vertebral artery**

     I65.01 Occlusion and stenosis of right vertebral artery

     I65.02 Occlusion and stenosis of left vertebral artery

     I65.03 Occlusion and stenosis of bilateral vertebral arteries

     I65.09 Occlusion and stenosis of unspecified vertebral artery ▽

    I65.1 **Occlusion and stenosis of basilar artery**

    ✓5ᵗʰ **I65.2** **Occlusion and stenosis of carotid artery**

     I65.21 Occlusion and stenosis of right carotid artery

     I65.22 Occlusion and stenosis of left carotid artery

     I65.23 Occlusion and stenosis of bilateral carotid arteries

     I65.29 Occlusion and stenosis of unspecified carotid artery ▽

    I65.8 **Occlusion and stenosis of other precerebral arteries**

    I65.9 **Occlusion and stenosis of unspecified precerebral artery** ▽
     Occlusion and stenosis of precerebral artery NOS

✓4ᵗʰ **I66** **Occlusion and stenosis of cerebral arteries, not resulting in cerebral infarction**
     INCLUDES embolism of cerebral artery
         narrowing of cerebral artery
         obstruction (complete) (partial) of cerebral artery
         thrombosis of cerebral artery
     EXCLUDES 1 occlusion and stenosis of cerebral artery causing cerebral infarction (I63.3–I63.5)

    ✓5ᵗʰ **I66.0** **Occlusion and stenosis of middle cerebral artery**

     I66.01 Occlusion and stenosis of right middle cerebral artery

     I66.02 Occlusion and stenosis of left middle cerebral artery

     I66.03 Occlusion and stenosis of bilateral middle cerebral arteries

     I66.09 Occlusion and stenosis of unspecified middle cerebral artery ▽

    ✓5ᵗʰ **I66.1** **Occlusion and stenosis of anterior cerebral artery**

     I66.11 Occlusion and stenosis of right anterior cerebral artery

     I66.12 Occlusion and stenosis of left anterior cerebral artery

     I66.13 Occlusion and stenosis of bilateral anterior cerebral arteries

     I66.19 Occlusion and stenosis of unspecified anterior cerebral artery ▽

    ✓5ᵗʰ **I66.2** **Occlusion and stenosis of posterior cerebral artery**

     I66.21 Occlusion and stenosis of right posterior cerebral artery

     I66.22 Occlusion and stenosis of left posterior cerebral artery

     I66.23 Occlusion and stenosis of bilateral posterior cerebral arteries

     I66.29 Occlusion and stenosis of unspecified posterior cerebral artery ▽

    I66.3 **Occlusion and stenosis of cerebellar arteries**

    I66.8 **Occlusion and stenosis of other cerebral arteries**
     Occlusion and stenosis of perforating arteries

    I66.9 **Occlusion and stenosis of unspecified cerebral artery** ▽

✓4ᵗʰ **I67** **Other cerebrovascular diseases**
     EXCLUDES 2 sequelae of the listed conditions (I69.8)

    I67.0 **Dissection of cerebral arteries, nonruptured**   HCC
     EXCLUDES 1 ruptured cerebral arteries (I60.7)

    I67.1 **Cerebral aneurysm, nonruptured**
     Cerebral aneurysm NOS
     Cerebral arteriovenous fistula, acquired
     Internal carotid artery aneurysm, intracranial portion
     Internal carotid artery aneurysm, NOS
     EXCLUDES 1 congenital cerebral aneurysm, nonruptured (Q28.-)
         ruptured cerebral aneurysm (I60.7)

    I67.2 **Cerebral atherosclerosis**   A
     Atheroma of cerebral and precerebral arteries

    I67.3 **Progressive vascular leukoencephalopathy**
     Binswanger's disease

    I67.4 **Hypertensive encephalopathy**
     EXCLUDES 2 ▶insufficiency, NOS, of precerebral arteries (G45.2)◀

Berry Aneurysm

Berry aneurysms form at the site of a weakness in an arterial wall, often at a junction

Berry aneurysm

Anterior communicating artery

Anterior cerebral artery

Internal carotid

Posterior cerebral artery

Basilar artery

Posterior communicating artery

Middle cerebral artery

40%

34%

20%

4%

Common sites of berry aneurysms in the circle of Willis arteries

EXCLUDES 1 Not coded here   *EXCLUDES 2* Not included here   N Newborn Age: 0   P Pediatric Age: 0-17   M Maternity Age: 12-55   A Adult Age: 15-124

632   ICD-10-CM 2018

I67.5 **Moyamoya disease**
DEF: Cerebrovascular ischemia; vessels occlude and rupture, causing tiny hemorrhages at base of brain; affects predominantly Japanese people.

I67.6 **Nonpyogenic thrombosis of intracranial venous system**
Nonpyogenic thrombosis of cerebral vein
Nonpyogenic thrombosis of intracranial venous sinus
EXCLUDES 1 nonpyogenic thrombosis of intracranial venous system causing infarction (I63.6)

I67.7 **Cerebral arteritis, not elsewhere classified**
Granulomatous angiitis of the nervous system
EXCLUDES 1 allergic granulomatous angiitis (M30.1)

√5th I67.8 **Other specified cerebrovascular diseases**

I67.81 **Acute cerebrovascular insufficiency**
Acute cerebrovascular insufficiency unspecified as to location or reversibility

I67.82 **Cerebral ischemia**
Chronic cerebral ischemia

I67.83 **Posterior reversible encephalopathy syndrome**
PRES

√6th I67.84 **Cerebral vasospasm and vasoconstriction**

I67.841 **Reversible cerebrovascular vasoconstriction syndrome**
Call-Fleming syndrome
Code first underlying condition, if applicable, such as eclampsia (O15.00-O15.9)

I67.848 **Other cerebrovascular vasospasm and vasoconstriction**

I67.89 **Other cerebrovascular disease**

I67.9 **Cerebrovascular disease, unspecified** ▽

√4th I68 **Cerebrovascular disorders in diseases classified elsewhere**

I68.0 *Cerebral amyloid angiopathy*
Code first underlying amyloidosis (E85.-)

I68.2 *Cerebral arteritis in other diseases classified elsewhere*
Code first underlying disease
EXCLUDES 1 cerebral arteritis (in):
listerosis (A32.89)
systemic lupus erythematosus (M32.19)
syphilis (A52.04)
tuberculosis (A18.89)

I68.8 *Other cerebrovascular disorders in diseases classified elsewhere*
Code first underlying disease
EXCLUDES 1 syphilitic cerebral aneurysm (A52.05)

√4th I69 **Sequelae of cerebrovascular disease**
NOTE Category I69 is to be used to indicate conditions in I60-I67 as the cause of sequelae. The "sequelae" include conditions specified as such or as residuals which may occur at any time after the onset of the causal condition
EXCLUDES 1 personal history of cerebral infarction without residual deficit (Z86.73)
personal history of prolonged reversible ischemic neurologic deficit (PRIND) (Z86.73)
personal history of reversible ischemic neurologcial deficit (RIND) (Z86.73)
sequelae of traumatic intracranial injury (S06.-)
~~transient ischemic attack (TIA) (G45.9)~~
AHA: 2017, 1Q, 47; 2015, 1Q, 25; 2012, 4Q, 106

√5th I69.0 **Sequelae of nontraumatic subarachnoid hemorrhage**

I69.00 **Unspecified sequelae of nontraumatic subarachnoid hemorrhage** ▽

√6th I69.01 **Cognitive deficits following nontraumatic subarachnoid hemorrhage**

I69.010 **Attention and concentration deficit following nontraumatic subarachnoid hemorrhage**

I69.011 **Memory deficit following nontraumatic subarachnoid hemorrhage**

I69.012 **Visuospatial deficit and spatial neglect following nontraumatic subarachnoid hemorrhage**

I69.013 **Psychomotor deficit following nontraumatic subarachnoid hemorrhage**

I69.014 **Frontal lobe and executive function deficit following nontraumatic subarachnoid hemorrhage**

I69.015 **Cognitive social or emotional deficit following nontraumatic subarachnoid hemorrhage**

I69.018 **Other symptoms and signs involving cognitive functions following nontraumatic subarachnoid hemorrhage**

I69.019 **Unspecified symptoms and signs involving cognitive functions following nontraumatic subarachnoid hemorrhage** ▽

√6th I69.02 **Speech and language deficits following nontraumatic subarachnoid hemorrhage**

I69.020 **Aphasia following nontraumatic subarachnoid hemorrhage**

I69.021 **Dysphasia following nontraumatic subarachnoid hemorrhage**

I69.022 **Dysarthria following nontraumatic subarachnoid hemorrhage**

I69.023 **Fluency disorder following nontraumatic subarachnoid hemorrhage**
Stuttering following nontraumatic subarachnoid hemorrhage

I69.028 **Other speech and language deficits following nontraumatic subarachnoid hemorrhage**

√6th I69.03 **Monoplegia of upper limb following nontraumatic subarachnoid hemorrhage**
AHA: 2017, 1Q, 47

I69.031 **Monoplegia of upper limb following nontraumatic subarachnoid hemorrhage affecting right dominant side** HCC

I69.032 **Monoplegia of upper limb following nontraumatic subarachnoid hemorrhage affecting left dominant side** HCC

I69.033 **Monoplegia of upper limb following nontraumatic subarachnoid hemorrhage affecting right non-dominant side** HCC

I69.034 **Monoplegia of upper limb following nontraumatic subarachnoid hemorrhage affecting left non-dominant side** HCC

I69.039 **Monoplegia of upper limb following nontraumatic subarachnoid hemorrhage affecting unspecified side** HCC ▽

√6th I69.04 **Monoplegia of lower limb following nontraumatic subarachnoid hemorrhage**
AHA: 2017, 1Q, 47

I69.041 **Monoplegia of lower limb following nontraumatic subarachnoid hemorrhage affecting right dominant side** HCC

I69.042 **Monoplegia of lower limb following nontraumatic subarachnoid hemorrhage affecting left dominant side** HCC

I69.043 **Monoplegia of lower limb following nontraumatic subarachnoid hemorrhage affecting right non-dominant side** HCC

I69.044 **Monoplegia of lower limb following nontraumatic subarachnoid hemorrhage affecting left non-dominant side** HCC

I69.049 **Monoplegia of lower limb following nontraumatic subarachnoid hemorrhage affecting unspecified side** HCC ▽

√6th I69.05 **Hemiplegia and hemiparesis following nontraumatic subarachnoid hemorrhage**
AHA: 2015, 1Q, 25

I69.051 **Hemiplegia and hemiparesis following nontraumatic subarachnoid hemorrhage affecting right dominant side** HCC

I69.052 **Hemiplegia and hemiparesis following nontraumatic subarachnoid hemorrhage affecting left dominant side** HCC

I69.053 **Hemiplegia and hemiparesis following nontraumatic subarachnoid hemorrhage affecting right non-dominant side** HCC

I69.054 **Hemiplegia and hemiparesis following nontraumatic subarachnoid hemorrhage affecting left non-dominant side** HCC

I69.059 **Hemiplegia and hemiparesis following nontraumatic subarachnoid hemorrhage affecting unspecified side** HCC ▽

✓6th **I69.06** **Other paralytic syndrome following nontraumatic subarachnoid hemorrhage**
Use additional code to identify type of paralytic syndrome, such as:
locked-in state (G83.5)
quadriplegia (G82.5-)

EXCLUDES 1   hemiplegia/hemiparesis following nontraumatic subarachnoid hemorrhage (I69.05-)
monoplegia of lower limb following nontraumatic subarachnoid hemorrhage (I69.04-)
monoplegia of upper limb following nontraumatic subarachnoid hemorrhage (I69.03-)

I69.061 **Other paralytic syndrome following** HCC **nontraumatic subarachnoid hemorrhage affecting right dominant side**

I69.062 **Other paralytic syndrome following** HCC **nontraumatic subarachnoid hemorrhage affecting left dominant side**

I69.063 **Other paralytic syndrome following** HCC **nontraumatic subarachnoid hemorrhage affecting right non-dominant side**

I69.064 **Other paralytic syndrome following** HCC **nontraumatic subarachnoid hemorrhage affecting left non-dominant side**

I69.065 **Other paralytic syndrome following** HCC **nontraumatic subarachnoid hemorrhage, bilateral**

I69.069 **Other paralytic syndrome following** HCC ▽ **nontraumatic subara chnoid hemorrhage affecting unspecified side**

✓6th **I69.09** **Other sequelae of nontraumatic subarachnoid hemorrhage**

I69.090 **Apraxia following nontraumatic subarachnoid hemorrhage**

I69.091 **Dysphagia following nontraumatic subarachnoid hemorrhage**
Use additional code to identify the type of dysphagia, if known (R13.1-)

I69.092 **Facial weakness following nontraumatic subarachnoid hemorrhage**
Facial droop following nontraumatic subarachnoid hemorrhage

I69.093 **Ataxia following nontraumatic subarachnoid hemorrhage**

I69.098 **Other sequelae following nontraumatic subarachnoid hemorrhage**
Alterations of sensation following nontraumatic subarachnoid hemorrhage
Disturbance of vision following nontraumatic subarachnoid hemorrhage
Use additional code to identify the sequelae

✓5th **I69.1** **Sequelae of nontraumatic intracerebral hemorrhage**

I69.10 **Unspecified sequelae of nontraumatic intracerebral hemorrhage** ▽

✓6th **I69.11** **Cognitive deficits following nontraumatic intracerebral hemorrhage**

I69.110 **Attention and concentration deficit following nontraumatic intracerebral hemorrhage**

I69.111 **Memory deficit following nontraumatic intracerebral hemorrhage**

I69.112 **Visuospatial deficit and spatial neglect following nontraumatic intracerebral hemorrhage**

I69.113 **Psychomotor deficit following nontraumatic intracerebral hemorrhage**

I69.114 **Frontal lobe and executive function deficit following nontraumatic intracerebral hemorrhage**

I69.115 **Cognitive social or emotional deficit following nontraumatic intracerebral hemorrhage**

I69.118 **Other symptoms and signs involving cognitive functions following nontraumatic intracerebral hemorrhage**

I69.119 **Unspecified symptoms and signs** ▽ **involving cognitive functions following nontraumatic intracerebral hemorrhage**

✓6th **I69.12** **Speech and language deficits following nontraumatic intracerebral hemorrhage**

I69.120 **Aphasia following nontraumatic intracerebral hemorrhage**

I69.121 **Dysphasia following nontraumatic intracerebral hemorrhage**

I69.122 **Dysarthria following nontraumatic intracerebral hemorrhage**

I69.123 **Fluency disorder following nontraumatic intracerebral hemorrhage**
Stuttering following nontraumatic intracerebral hemorrhage

I69.128 **Other speech and language deficits following nontraumatic intracerebral hemorrhage**

✓6th **I69.13** **Monoplegia of upper limb following nontraumatic intracerebral hemorrhage**
AHA: 2017, 1Q, 47

I69.131 **Monoplegia of upper limb following** HCC **nontraumatic intracerebral hemorrhage affecting right dominant side**

I69.132 **Monoplegia of upper limb following** HCC **nontraumatic intracerebral hemorrhage affecting left dominant side**

I69.133 **Monoplegia of upper limb following** HCC **nontraumatic intracerebral hemorrhage affecting right non-dominant side**

I69.134 **Monoplegia of upper limb following** HCC **nontraumatic intracerebral hemorrhage affecting left non-dominant side**

I69.139 **Monoplegia of upper limb** HCC ▽ **following nontraumatic intracerebral hemorrhage affecting unspecified side**

✓6th **I69.14** **Monoplegia of lower limb following nontraumatic intracerebral hemorrhage**
AHA: 2017, 1Q, 47

I69.141 **Monoplegia of lower limb following** HCC **nontraumatic intracerebral hemorrhage affecting right dominant side**

I69.142 **Monoplegia of lower limb following** HCC **nontraumatic intracerebral hemorrhage affecting left dominant side**

I69.143 **Monoplegia of lower limb following** HCC **nontraumatic intracerebral hemorrhage affecting right non-dominant side**

I69.144 **Monoplegia of lower limb following** HCC **nontraumatic intracerebral hemorrhage affecting left non-dominant side**

I69.149 **Monoplegia of lower limb following** HCC ▽ **nontraumatic intracerebral hemorrhage affecting unspecified side**

✓6th **I69.15** **Hemiplegia and hemiparesis following nontraumatic intracerebral hemorrhage**
AHA: 2015, 1Q, 25

I69.151 **Hemiplegia and hemiparesis following** HCC **nontraumatic intracerebral hemorrhage affecting right dominant side**

I69.152 **Hemiplegia and hemiparesis following** HCC **nontraumatic intracerebral hemorrhage affecting left dominant side**

I69.153 **Hemiplegia and hemiparesis following** HCC **nontraumatic intracerebral hemorrhage affecting right non-dominant side**

I69.154 **Hemiplegia and hemiparesis following** HCC **nontraumatic intracerebral hemorrhage affecting left non-dominant side**

I69.159 **Hemiplegia and hemiparesis** HCC ▽ **following nontraumatic intracerebral hemorrhage affecting unspecified side**

☑6ᵗʰ I69.16   **Other paralytic syndrome following nontraumatic intracerebral hemorrhage**

Use additional code to identify type of paralytic syndrome, such as:
locked-in state (G83.5)
quadriplegia (G82.5-)

EXCLUDES 1   hemiplegia/hemiparesis following nontraumatic intracerebral hemorrhage (I69.15-)
monoplegia of lower limb following nontraumatic intracerebral hemorrhage (I69.14-)
monoplegia of upper limb following nontraumatic intracerebral hemorrhage (I69.13-)

I69.161   **Other paralytic syndrome following nontraumatic intracerebral hemorrhage affecting right dominant side**   HCC

I69.162   **Other paralytic syndrome following nontraumatic intracerebral hemorrhage affecting left dominant side**   HCC

I69.163   **Other paralytic syndrome following nontraumatic intracerebral hemorrhage affecting right non-dominant side**   HCC

I69.164   **Other paralytic syndrome following nontraumatic intracerebral hemorrhage affecting left non-dominant side**   HCC

I69.165   **Other paralytic syndrome following nontraumatic intracerebral hemorrhage, bilateral**   HCC

I69.169   **Other paralytic syndrome following nontraumatic intracerebral hemorrhage affecting unspecified side**   HCC ▽

☑6ᵗʰ I69.19   **Other sequelae of nontraumatic intracerebral hemorrhage**

I69.190   **Apraxia following nontraumatic intracerebral hemorrhage**

I69.191   **Dysphagia following nontraumatic intracerebral hemorrhage**
Use additional code to identify the type of dysphagia, if known (R13.1-)

I69.192   **Facial weakness following nontraumatic intracerebral hemorrhage**
Facial droop following nontraumatic intracerebral hemorrhage

I69.193   **Ataxia following nontraumatic intracerebral hemorrhage**

I69.198   **Other sequelae of nontraumatic intracerebral hemorrhage**
Alteration of sensations following nontraumatic intracerebral hemorrhage
Disturbance of vision following nontraumatic intracerebral hemorrhage
Use additional code to identify the sequelae

☑5ᵗʰ I69.2   **Sequelae of other nontraumatic intracranial hemorrhage**

I69.20   **Unspecified sequelae of other nontraumatic intracranial hemorrhage**   ▽

☑6ᵗʰ I69.21   **Cognitive deficits following other nontraumatic intracranial hemorrhage**

I69.210   **Attention and concentration deficit following other nontraumatic intracranial hemorrhage**

I69.211   **Memory deficit following other nontraumatic intracranial hemorrhage**

I69.212   **Visuospatial deficit and spatial neglect following other nontraumatic intracranial hemorrhage**

I69.213   **Psychomotor deficit following other nontraumatic intracranial hemorrhage**

I69.214   **Frontal lobe and executive function deficit following other nontraumatic intracranial hemorrhage**

I69.215   **Cognitive social or emotional deficit following other nontraumatic intracranial hemorrhage**

I69.218   **Other symptoms and signs involving cognitive functions following other nontraumatic intracranial hemorrhage**

I69.219   **Unspecified symptoms and signs involving cognitive functions following other nontraumatic intracranial hemorrhage**   ▽

☑6ᵗʰ I69.22   **Speech and language deficits following other nontraumatic intracranial hemorrhage**

I69.220   **Aphasia following other nontraumatic intracranial hemorrhage**

I69.221   **Dysphasia following other nontraumatic intracranial hemorrhage**

I69.222   **Dysarthria following other nontraumatic intracranial hemorrhage**

I69.223   **Fluency disorder following other nontraumatic intracranial hemorrhage**
Stuttering following nontraumatic intracerebral hemorrhage

I69.228   **Other speech and language deficits following other nontraumatic intracranial hemorrhage**

☑6ᵗʰ I69.23   **Monoplegia of upper limb following other nontraumatic intracranial hemorrhage**
AHA: 2017, 1Q, 47

I69.231   **Monoplegia of upper limb following other nontraumatic intracranial hemorrhage affecting right dominant side**   HCC

I69.232   **Monoplegia of upper limb following other nontraumatic intracranial hemorrhage affecting left dominant side**   HCC

I69.233   **Monoplegia of upper limb following other nontraumatic intracranial hemorrhage affecting right non-dominant side**   HCC

I69.234   **Monoplegia of upper limb following other nontraumatic intracranial hemorrhage affecting left non-dominant side**   HCC

I69.239   **Monoplegia of upper limb following other nontraumatic intracranial hemorrhage affecting unspecified side**   HCC ▽

☑6ᵗʰ I69.24   **Monoplegia of lower limb following other nontraumatic intracranial hemorrhage**
AHA: 2017, 1Q, 47

I69.241   **Monoplegia of lower limb following other nontraumatic intracranial hemorrhage affecting right dominant side**   HCC

I69.242   **Monoplegia of lower limb following other nontraumatic intracranial hemorrhage affecting left dominant side**   HCC

I69.243   **Monoplegia of lower limb following other nontraumatic intracranial hemorrhage affecting right non-dominant side**   HCC

I69.244   **Monoplegia of lower limb following other nontraumatic intracranial hemorrhage affecting left non-dominant side**   HCC

I69.249   **Monoplegia of lower limb following other nontraumatic intracranial hemorrhage affecting unspecified side**   HCC ▽

☑6ᵗʰ I69.25   **Hemiplegia and hemiparesis following other nontraumatic intracranial hemorrhage**
AHA: 2015, 1Q, 25

I69.251   **Hemiplegia and hemiparesis following other nontraumatic intracranial hemorrhage affecting right dominant side**   HCC

I69.252   **Hemiplegia and hemiparesis following other nontraumatic intracranial hemorrhage affecting left dominant side**   HCC

I69.253   **Hemiplegia and hemiparesis following other nontraumatic intracranial hemorrhage affecting right non-dominant side**   HCC

I69.254   **Hemiplegia and hemiparesis following other nontraumatic intracranial hemorrhage affecting left non-dominant side**   HCC

I69.259   **Hemiplegia and hemiparesis following other nontraumatic intracranial hemorrhage affecting unspecified side**   HCC ▽

☑ Additional Character Req   ☑x7ᵗʰ Placeholder Alert   Manifestation   HCC CMS-HCC Condition   ▽ Unspecified Code   ▶◀ Revised Text   ● New Code   ▲ Revised Code Title

ICD-10-CM 2018   635

Chapter 9. Diseases of the Circulatory System

I69.26–I69.36

✓6ᵗʰ **I69.26** **Other paralytic syndrome following other nontraumatic intracranial hemorrhage**
Use additional code to identify type of paralytic syndrome, such as:
locked-in state (G83.5)
quadriplegia (G82.5-)
EXCLUDES 1   *hemiplegia/hemiparesis following other nontraumatic intracranial hemorrhage (I69.25-)*
monoplegia of lower limb following other nontraumatic intracranial hemorrhage (I69.24-)
monoplegia of upper limb following other nontraumatic intracranial hemorrhage (I69.23-)

     I69.261 **Other paralytic syndrome following other nontraumatic intracranial hemorrhage affecting right dominant side** `HCC`

     I69.262 **Other paralytic syndrome following other nontraumatic intracranial hemorrhage affecting left dominant side** `HCC`

     I69.263 **Other paralytic syndrome following other nontraumatic intracranial hemorrhage affecting right non-dominant side** `HCC`

     I69.264 **Other paralytic syndrome following other nontraumatic intracranial hemorrhage affecting left non-dominant side** `HCC`

     I69.265 **Other paralytic syndrome following other nontraumatic intracranial hemorrhage, bilateral** `HCC`

     I69.269 **Other paralytic syndrome following other nontraumatic intracranial hemorrhage affecting unspecified side** `HCC` ▽

✓6ᵗʰ **I69.29** **Other sequelae of other nontraumatic intracranial hemorrhage**

     I69.290 **Apraxia following other nontraumatic intracranial hemorrhage**

     I69.291 **Dysphagia following other nontraumatic intracranial hemorrhage**
Use additional code to identify the type of dysphagia, if known (R13.1-)

     I69.292 **Facial weakness following other nontraumatic intracranial hemorrhage**
Facial droop following other nontraumatic intracranial hemorrhage

     I69.293 **Ataxia following other nontraumatic intracranial hemorrhage**

     I69.298 **Other sequelae of other nontraumatic intracranial hemorrhage**
Alteration of sensation following other nontraumatic intracranial hemorrhage
Disturbance of vision following other nontraumatic intracranial hemorrhage
Use additional code to identify the sequelae

✓5ᵗʰ **I69.3** **Sequelae of cerebral infarction**
Sequelae of stroke NOS
AHA: 2013, 4Q, 127-128; 2012, 4Q, 92, 94

     I69.30 **Unspecified sequelae of cerebral infarction** ▽

✓6ᵗʰ **I69.31** **Cognitive deficits following cerebral infarction**

     I69.310 **Attention and concentration deficit following cerebral infarction**

     I69.311 **Memory deficit following cerebral infarction**

     I69.312 **Visuospatial deficit and spatial neglect following cerebral infarction**

     I69.313 **Psychomotor deficit following cerebral infarction**

     I69.314 **Frontal lobe and executive function deficit following cerebral infarction**

     I69.315 **Cognitive social or emotional deficit following cerebral infarction**

     I69.318 **Other symptoms and signs involving cognitive functions following cerebral infarction**

     I69.319 **Unspecified symptoms and signs involving cognitive functions following cerebral infarction** ▽

✓6ᵗʰ **I69.32** **Speech and language deficits following cerebral infarction**

     I69.320 **Aphasia following cerebral infarction**

     I69.321 **Dysphasia following cerebral infarction**
AHA: 2012, 4Q, 91

     I69.322 **Dysarthria following cerebral infarction**
EXCLUDES 2   ▶*transient ischemic attack (TIA) (G45.9)*◀

     I69.323 **Fluency disorder following cerebral infarction**
Stuttering following cerebral infarction

     I69.328 **Other speech and language deficits following cerebral infarction**

✓6ᵗʰ **I69.33** **Monoplegia of upper limb following cerebral infarction**
AHA: 2017, 1Q, 47

     I69.331 **Monoplegia of upper limb following cerebral infarction affecting right dominant side** `HCC`

     I69.332 **Monoplegia of upper limb following cerebral infarction affecting left dominant side** `HCC`

     I69.333 **Monoplegia of upper limb following cerebral infarction affecting right non-dominant side** `HCC`

     I69.334 **Monoplegia of upper limb following cerebral infarction affecting left non-dominant side** `HCC`

     I69.339 **Monoplegia of upper limb following cerebral infarction affecting unspecified side** `HCC` ▽

✓6ᵗʰ **I69.34** **Monoplegia of lower limb following cerebral infarction**
AHA: 2017, 1Q, 47

     I69.341 **Monoplegia of lower limb following cerebral infarction affecting right dominant side** `HCC`

     I69.342 **Monoplegia of lower limb following cerebral infarction affecting left dominant side** `HCC`

     I69.343 **Monoplegia of lower limb following cerebral infarction affecting right non-dominant side** `HCC`

     I69.344 **Monoplegia of lower limb following cerebral infarction affecting left non-dominant side** `HCC`

     I69.349 **Monoplegia of lower limb following cerebral infarction affecting unspecified side** `HCC` ▽

✓6ᵗʰ **I69.35** **Hemiplegia and hemiparesis following cerebral infarction**
AHA: 2015, 1Q, 25

     I69.351 **Hemiplegia and hemiparesis following cerebral infarction affecting right dominant side** `HCC`
EXCLUDES 2   ▶*transient ischemic attack (TIA) (G45.9)*◀

     I69.352 **Hemiplegia and hemiparesis following cerebral infarction affecting left dominant side** `HCC`

     I69.353 **Hemiplegia and hemiparesis following cerebral infarction affecting right non-dominant side** `HCC`

     I69.354 **Hemiplegia and hemiparesis following cerebral infarction affecting left non-dominant side** `HCC`
AHA: 2012, 4Q, 91

     I69.359 **Hemiplegia and hemiparesis following cerebral infarction affecting unspecified side** `HCC` ▽

✓6ᵗʰ **I69.36** **Other paralytic syndrome following cerebral infarction**
Use additional code to identify type of paralytic syndrome, such as:
locked-in state (G83.5)
quadriplegia (G82.5-)
EXCLUDES 1   *hemiplegia/hemiparesis following cerebral infarction (I69.35-)*
monoplegia of lower limb following cerebral infarction (I69.34-)
monoplegia of upper limb following cerebral infarction (I69.33-)

EXCLUDES 1 Not coded here   *EXCLUDES 2* Not included here   N Newborn Age: 0   P Pediatric Age: 0-17   M Maternity Age: 12-55   A Adult Age: 15-124

636   ICD-10-CM 2018

I69.361   Other paralytic syndrome following cerebral infarction affecting **right dominant** side   HCC

I69.362   Other paralytic syndrome following cerebral infarction affecting **left dominant** side   HCC

I69.363   Other paralytic syndrome following cerebral infarction affecting **right non-dominant** side   HCC

I69.364   Other paralytic syndrome following cerebral infarction affecting **left non-dominant** side   HCC

I69.365   Other paralytic syndrome following cerebral infarction, **bilateral**   HCC

I69.369   Other paralytic syndrome following cerebral infarction affecting unspecified side   HCC ▽

✓6th **I69.39**   **Other sequelae of cerebral infarction**

I69.390   **Apraxia** following cerebral infarction

I69.391   **Dysphagia** following cerebral infarction
Use additional code to identify the type of dysphagia, if known (R13.1-)

I69.392   **Facial weakness** following cerebral infarction
Facial droop following cerebral infarction

I69.393   **Ataxia** following cerebral infarction

I69.398   **Other sequelae** of cerebral infarction
Alteration of sensation following cerebral infarction
Disturbance of vision following cerebral infarction
Use additional code to identify the sequelae

✓5th **I69.8**   **Sequelae of other cerebrovascular diseases**
EXCLUDES 1   *sequelae of traumatic intracranial injury (S06.-)*

I69.80   **Unspecified sequelae of other cerebrovascular disease**   ▽

✓6th **I69.81**   **Cognitive deficits following other cerebrovascular disease**

I69.810   **Attention and concentration deficit** following other cerebrovascular disease

I69.811   **Memory deficit** following other cerebrovascular disease

I69.812   **Visuospatial deficit and spatial neglect** following other cerebrovascular disease

I69.813   **Psychomotor deficit** following other cerebrovascular disease

I69.814   **Frontal lobe and executive function deficit** following other cerebrovascular disease

I69.815   **Cognitive social or emotional deficit** following other cerebrovascular disease

I69.818   **Other symptoms and signs involving cognitive functions** following other cerebrovascular disease

I69.819   **Unspecified symptoms and signs involving cognitive functions** following other cerebrovascular disease   ▽

✓6th **I69.82**   **Speech and language deficits following other cerebrovascular disease**

I69.820   **Aphasia** following other cerebrovascular disease

I69.821   **Dysphasia** following other cerebrovascular disease

I69.822   **Dysarthria** following other cerebrovascular disease

I69.823   **Fluency disorder** following other cerebrovascular disease
Stuttering following other cerebrovascular disease

I69.828   **Other speech and language deficits** following other cerebrovascular disease

✓6th **I69.83**   **Monoplegia of upper limb following other cerebrovascular disease**
AHA: 2017, 1Q, 47

I69.831   **Monoplegia of upper limb following other cerebrovascular disease affecting right dominant** side   HCC

I69.832   **Monoplegia of upper limb following other cerebrovascular disease affecting left dominant** side   HCC

I69.833   **Monoplegia of upper limb following other cerebrovascular disease affecting right non-dominant** side   HCC

I69.834   **Monoplegia of upper limb following other cerebrovascular disease affecting left non-dominant** side   HCC

I69.839   **Monoplegia of upper limb following other cerebrovascular disease affecting unspecified side**   HCC ▽

✓6th **I69.84**   **Monoplegia of lower limb following other cerebrovascular disease**
AHA: 2017, 1Q, 47

I69.841   **Monoplegia of lower limb following other cerebrovascular disease affecting right dominant** side   HCC

I69.842   **Monoplegia of lower limb following other cerebrovascular disease affecting left dominant** side   HCC

I69.843   **Monoplegia of lower limb following other cerebrovascular disease affecting right non-dominant** side   HCC

I69.844   **Monoplegia of lower limb following other cerebrovascular disease affecting left non-dominant** side   HCC

I69.849   **Monoplegia of lower limb following other cerebrovascular disease affecting unspecified side**   HCC ▽

✓6th **I69.85**   **Hemiplegia and hemiparesis following other cerebrovascular disease**
AHA: 2015, 1Q, 25

I69.851   **Hemiplegia and hemiparesis following other cerebrovascular disease affecting right dominant** side   HCC

I69.852   **Hemiplegia and hemiparesis following other cerebrovascular disease affecting left dominant** side   HCC

I69.853   **Hemiplegia and hemiparesis following other cerebrovascular disease affecting right non-dominant** side   HCC

I69.854   **Hemiplegia and hemiparesis following other cerebrovascular disease affecting left non-dominant** side   HCC

I69.859   **Hemiplegia and hemiparesis following other cerebrovascular disease affecting unspecified side**   HCC ▽

✓6th **I69.86**   **Other paralytic syndrome following other cerebrovascular disease**
Use additional code to identify type of paralytic syndrome, such as:
locked-in state (G83.5)
quadriplegia (G82.5-)
EXCLUDES 1   *hemiplegia/hemiparesis following other cerebrovascular disease (I69.85-)*
monoplegia of lower limb following other cerebrovascular disease (I69.84-)
monoplegia of upper limb following other cerebrovascular disease (I69.83-)

I69.861   **Other paralytic syndrome following other cerebrovascular disease affecting right dominant** side   HCC

I69.862   **Other paralytic syndrome following other cerebrovascular disease affecting left dominant** side   HCC

I69.863   **Other paralytic syndrome following other cerebrovascular disease affecting right non-dominant** side   HCC

I69.864   **Other paralytic syndrome following other cerebrovascular disease affecting left non-dominant** side   HCC

I69.865   **Other paralytic syndrome following other cerebrovascular disease, bilateral**   HCC

I69.869   **Other paralytic syndrome following other cerebrovascular disease affecting unspecified side**   HCC ▽

✓6th **I69.89**   **Other sequelae of other cerebrovascular disease**

I69.890   **Apraxia** following other cerebrovascular disease

I69.891   **Dysphagia** following other cerebrovascular disease
Use additional code to identify the type of dysphagia, if known (R13.1-)

✓ Additional Character Req   ✓x7th Placeholder Alert   Manifestation   HCC CMS-HCC Condition   ▽ Unspecified Code   ▶◀ Revised Text   ● New Code   ▲ Revised Code Title

Chapter 9. Diseases of the Circulatory System

I69.892   Facial weakness following other cerebrovascular disease
Facial droop following other cerebrovascular disease

I69.893   Ataxia following other cerebrovascular disease

I69.898   Other sequelae of other cerebrovascular disease
Alteration of sensation following other cerebrovascular disease
Disturbance of vision following other cerebrovascular disease
Use additional code to identify the sequelae

✓5th I69.9   Sequelae of unspecified cerebrovascular diseases
EXCLUDES 1   sequelae of stroke (I69.3)
sequelae of traumatic intracranial injury (S06.-)

I69.90   Unspecified sequelae of unspecified cerebrovascular disease ▽

✓6th I69.91   Cognitive deficits following unspecified cerebrovascular disease

I69.910   Attention and concentration deficit following unspecified cerebrovascular disease ▽

I69.911   Memory deficit following unspecified cerebrovascular disease ▽

I69.912   Visuospatial deficit and spatial neglect following unspecified cerebrovascular disease ▽

I69.913   Psychomotor deficit following unspecified cerebrovascular disease ▽

I69.914   Frontal lobe and executive function deficit following unspecified cerebrovascular disease ▽

I69.915   Cognitive social or emotional deficit following unspecified cerebrovascular disease ▽

I69.918   Other symptoms and signs involving cognitive functions following unspecified cerebrovascular disease ▽

I69.919   Unspecified symptoms and signs involving cognitive functions following unspecified cerebrovascular disease ▽

✓6th I69.92   Speech and language deficits following unspecified cerebrovascular disease

I69.920   Aphasia following unspecified cerebrovascular disease ▽

I69.921   Dysphasia following unspecified cerebrovascular disease ▽

I69.922   Dysarthria following unspecified cerebrovascular disease ▽

I69.923   Fluency disorder following unspecified cerebrovascular disease ▽
Stuttering following unspecified cerebrovascular disease

I69.928   Other speech and language deficits following unspecified cerebrovascular disease ▽

✓6th I69.93   Monoplegia of upper limb following unspecified cerebrovascular disease
AHA: 2017, 1Q, 47

I69.931   Monoplegia of upper limb following unspecified cerebrovascular disease affecting right dominant side HCC ▽

I69.932   Monoplegia of upper limb following unspecified cerebrovascular disease affecting left dominant side HCC ▽

I69.933   Monoplegia of upper limb following unspecified cerebrovascular disease affecting right non-dominant side HCC ▽

I69.934   Monoplegia of upper limb following unspecified cerebrovascular disease affecting left non-dominant side HCC ▽

I69.939   Monoplegia of upper limb following unspecified cerebrovascular disease affecting unspecified side HCC ▽

✓6th I69.94   Monoplegia of lower limb following unspecified cerebrovascular disease
AHA: 2017, 1Q, 47

I69.941   Monoplegia of lower limb following unspecified cerebrovascular disease affecting right dominant side HCC ▽

I69.942   Monoplegia of lower limb following unspecified cerebrovascular disease affecting left dominant side HCC ▽

I69.943   Monoplegia of lower limb following unspecified cerebrovascular disease affecting right non-dominant side HCC ▽

I69.944   Monoplegia of lower limb following unspecified cerebrovascular disease affecting left non-dominant side HCC ▽

I69.949   Monoplegia of lower limb following unspecified cerebrovascular disease affecting unspecified side HCC ▽

✓6th I69.95   Hemiplegia and hemiparesis following unspecified cerebrovascular disease
AHA: 2015, 1Q, 25

I69.951   Hemiplegia and hemiparesis following unspecified cerebrovascular disease affecting right dominant side HCC ▽

I69.952   Hemiplegia and hemiparesis following unspecified cerebrovascular disease affecting left dominant side HCC ▽

I69.953   Hemiplegia and hemiparesis following unspecified cerebrovascular disease affecting right non-dominant side HCC ▽

I69.954   Hemiplegia and hemiparesis following unspecified cerebrovascular disease affecting left non-dominant side HCC ▽

I69.959   Hemiplegia and hemiparesis following unspecified cerebrovascular disease affecting unspecified side HCC ▽

✓6th I69.96   Other paralytic syndrome following unspecified cerebrovascular disease
Use additional code to identify type of paralytic syndrome, such as:
locked-in state (G83.5)
quadriplegia (G82.5-)
EXCLUDES 1   hemiplegia/hemiparesis following unspecified cerebrovascular disease (I69.95-)
monoplegia of lower limb following unspecified cerebrovascular disease (I69.94-)
monoplegia of upper limb following unspecified cerebrovascular disease (I69.93-)

I69.961   Other paralytic syndrome following unspecified cerebrovascular disease affecting right dominant side HCC ▽

I69.962   Other paralytic syndrome following unspecified cerebrovascular disease affecting left dominant side HCC ▽

I69.963   Other paralytic syndrome following unspecified cerebrovascular disease affecting right non-dominant side HCC ▽

I69.964   Other paralytic syndrome following unspecified cerebrovascular disease affecting left non-dominant side HCC ▽

I69.965   Other paralytic syndrome following unspecified cerebrovascular disease, bilateral HCC ▽

I69.969   Other paralytic syndrome following unspecified cerebrovascular disease affecting unspecified side HCC ▽

✓6th I69.99   Other sequelae of unspecified cerebrovascular disease

I69.990   Apraxia following unspecified cerebrovascular disease ▽

I69.991   Dysphagia following unspecified cerebrovascular disease ▽
Use additional code to identify the type of dysphagia, if known (R13.1-)

I69.992   Facial weakness following unspecified cerebrovascular disease ▽
Facial droop following unspecified cerebrovascular disease

I69.993   Ataxia following unspecified ▽
              cerebrovascular disease

I69.998   Other sequelae following unspecified ▽
              cerebrovascular disease
              Alteration in sensation following
                  unspecified cerebrovascular disease
              Disturbance of vision following unspecified
                  cerebrovascular disease
              Use additional code to identify the
                  sequelae

Diseases of arteries, arterioles and capillaries (I70–I79)

✓4ᵗʰ **I70   Atherosclerosis**
        INCLUDES   arteriolosclerosis
                   arterial degeneration
                   arteriosclerosis
                   arteriosclerotic vascular disease
                   arteriovascular degeneration
                   atheroma
                   endarteritis deformans or obliterans
                   senile arteritis
                   senile endarteritis
                   vascular degeneration
        Use additional code to identify:
            exposure to environmental tobacco smoke (Z77.22)
            history of tobacco dependence (Z87.891)
            occupational exposure to environmental tobacco smoke (Z57.31)
            tobacco dependence (F17.-)
            tobacco use (Z72.0)
        EXCLUDES 2   arteriosclerotic cardiovascular disease (I25.1-)
                     arteriosclerotic heart disease (I25.1-)
                     atheroembolism (I75.-)
                     cerebral atherosclerosis (I67.2)
                     coronary atherosclerosis (I25.1-)
                     mesenteric atherosclerosis (K55.1)
                     precerebral atherosclerosis (I67.2)
                     primary pulmonary atherosclerosis (I27.0)

I70.0   Atherosclerosis of aorta   HCC A

I70.1   Atherosclerosis of renal artery   HCC A
            Goldblatt's kidney
            EXCLUDES 2   atherosclerosis of renal arterioles (I12.-)

✓5ᵗʰ **I70.2   Atherosclerosis of native arteries of the extremities**
            Mönckeberg's (medial) sclerosis
            Use additional code, if applicable, to identify chronic total
                occlusion of artery of extremity (I70.92)
            EXCLUDES 2   atherosclerosis of bypass graft of extremities
                         (I70.30-I70.79)

✓6ᵗʰ **I70.20   Unspecified atherosclerosis of native arteries of
                 extremities**

        I70.201   Unspecified atherosclerosis of   HCC A ▽
                    native arteries of extremities, right leg

        I70.202   Unspecified atherosclerosis of   HCC A ▽
                    native arteries of extremities, left leg

        I70.203   Unspecified atherosclerosis of   HCC A ▽
                    **native arteries of extremities, bilateral
                    legs**

        I70.208   Unspecified atherosclerosis of   HCC A ▽
                    **native arteries of extremities,
                    other extremity**

        I70.209   Unspecified atherosclerosis of   HCC A ▽
                    **nativearteries of extremities,
                    unspecified extremity**

✓6ᵗʰ **I70.21   Atherosclerosis of native arteries of extremities with
                 intermittent claudication**

        I70.211   Atherosclerosis of native arteries   HCC A
                    **of extremities with intermittent
                    claudication, right leg**

        I70.212   Atherosclerosis of native arteries   HCC A
                    **of extremities with intermittent
                    claudication, left leg**

        I70.213   Atherosclerosis of native arteries   HCC A
                    **of extremities with intermittent
                    claudication, bilateral legs**

        I70.218   Atherosclerosis of native arteries   HCC A
                    **of extremities with intermittent
                    claudication, other extremity**

        I70.219   Atherosclerosis of native arteries   HCC A ▽
                    **of extremities with intermittent
                    claudication, unspecified extremity**

✓6ᵗʰ **I70.22   Atherosclerosis of native arteries of extremities with
                 rest pain**
            INCLUDES   any condition classifiable to I70.21-

        I70.221   Atherosclerosis of native arteries of   HCC A
                    extremities with rest pain, right leg

        I70.222   Atherosclerosis of native arteries of   HCC A
                    extremities with rest pain, left leg

        I70.223   Atherosclerosis of native arteries of   HCC A
                    extremities with rest pain, bilateral legs

        I70.228   Atherosclerosis of native arteries of   HCC A
                    **extremities with rest pain, other
                    extremity**

        I70.229   Atherosclerosis of native arteries   HCC A ▽
                    **of extremities with rest pain, unspecified
                    extremity**

✓6ᵗʰ **I70.23   Atherosclerosis of native arteries of right leg with
                 ulceration**
            INCLUDES   any condition classifiable to I70.211 and
                       I70.221
            Use additional code to identify severity of ulcer (L97.-)

        I70.231   Atherosclerosis of native arteries of   HCC A
                    right leg with ulceration of thigh

        I70.232   Atherosclerosis of native arteries of   HCC A
                    right leg with ulceration of calf

        I70.233   Atherosclerosis of native arteries of   HCC A
                    right leg with ulceration of ankle

        I70.234   Atherosclerosis of native arteries of   HCC A
                    **right leg with ulceration of heel and
                    midfoot**
                    Atherosclerosis of native arteries of right
                        leg with ulceration of plantar surface
                        of midfoot

        I70.235   Atherosclerosis of native arteries of   HCC A
                    **right leg with ulceration of other part
                    of foot**
                    Atherosclerosis of native arteries of right
                        leg extremities with ulceration of toe

        I70.238   Atherosclerosis of native arteries of   HCC A
                    **right leg with ulceration of other
                    part of lower right leg**

        I70.239   Atherosclerosis of native arteries   HCC A ▽
                    **of right leg with ulceration of unspecified
                    site**

✓6ᵗʰ **I70.24   Atherosclerosis of native arteries of left leg with
                 ulceration**
            INCLUDES   any condition classifiable to I70.212 and
                       I70.222
            Use additional code to identify severity of ulcer (L97.-)

        I70.241   Atherosclerosis of native arteries   HCC A
                    of left leg with ulceration of thigh

        I70.242   Atherosclerosis of native arteries   HCC A
                    of left leg with ulceration of calf

        I70.243   Atherosclerosis of native arteries   HCC A
                    of left leg with ulceration of ankle

        I70.244   Atherosclerosis of native arteries   HCC A
                    **of left leg with ulceration of heel and
                    midfoot**
                    Atherosclerosis of native arteries of left leg
                        with ulceration of plantar surface of
                        midfoot

        I70.245   Atherosclerosis of native arteries   HCC A
                    **of left leg with ulceration of other part of
                    foot**
                    Atherosclerosis of native arteries of left leg
                        extremities with ulceration of toe

        I70.248   Atherosclerosis of native arteries   HCC A
                    **of left leg with ulceration of other
                    part of lower left leg**

        I70.249   Atherosclerosis of native arteries   HCC A ▽
                    **of left leg with ulceration of
                    unspecified site**

I70.25   Atherosclerosis of native arteries of other   HCC A
            extremities with ulceration
            INCLUDES   an y condition classifiable to I70.218 and
                       I70.228
            Use additional code to identify the severity of the ulcer
                (L98.49-)

☑ Additional Character Req   ✓x7ᵗʰ Placeholder Alert   Manifestation   HCC CMS-HCC Condition   ▽ Unspecified Code   ►◄ Revised Text   ● New Code   ▲ Revised Code Title

√6ᵗʰ I70.26 Atherosclerosis of native arteries of extremities with gangrene

INCLUDES   any condition classifiable to I70.21-, I70.22-, I70.23-, I70.24-, and I70.25-

Use additional code to identify the severity of any ulcer (L97.-, L98.49-), if applicable

- I70.261   Atherosclerosis of native arteries of HCC A extremities with gangrene, right leg
- I70.262   Atherosclerosis of native arteries of HCC A extremities with gangrene, left leg
- I70.263   Atherosclerosis of native arteries of HCC A extremities with gangrene, bilateral legs
- I70.268   Atherosclerosis of native arteries of HCC A extremities with gangrene, other extremity
- I70.269   Atherosclerosis of native arteries HCC A ▽ of extremities with gangrene, unspecified extremity

√6ᵗʰ I70.29 Other atherosclerosis of native arteries of extremities

- I70.291   Other atherosclerosis of native HCC A arteries of extremities, right leg
- I70.292   Other atherosclerosis of native HCC A arteries of extremities, left leg
- I70.293   Other atherosclerosis of native HCC A arteries of extremities, bilateral legs
- I70.298   Other atherosclerosis of native HCC A arteries of extremities, other extremity
- I70.299   Other atherosclerosis of native HCC A ▽ arteries of extremities, unspecified extremity

√5ᵗʰ I70.3 Atherosclerosis of unspecified type of bypass graft(s) of the extremities

Use additional code, if applicable, to identify chronic total occlusion of artery of extremity (I70.92)

EXCLUDES 1   embolism or thrombus of bypass graft(s) of extremities (T82.8-)

√6ᵗʰ I70.30 Unspecified atherosclerosis of unspecified type of bypass graft(s) of the extremities

- I70.301   Unspecified atherosclerosis of HCC A ▽ unspecified type of bypass graft(s) of the extremities, right leg
- I70.302   Unspecified atherosclerosis of HCC A ▽ unspecified type of bypass graft(s) of the extremities, left leg
- I70.303   Unspecified atherosclerosis of HCC A ▽ unspecified type of bypass graft(s) of the extremities, bilateral legs
- I70.308   Unspecified atherosclerosis of HCC A ▽ unspecified type of bypass graft(s) of the extremities, other extremity
- I70.309   Unspecified atherosclerosis of HCC A ▽ unspecified type of bypass graft(s) of the extremities, unspecified extremity

√6ᵗʰ I70.31 Atherosclerosis of unspecified type of bypass graft(s) of the extremities with intermittent claudication

- I70.311   Atherosclerosis of unspecified type HCC A of bypass graft(s) of the extremities with intermittent claudication, right leg
- I70.312   Atherosclerosis of unspecified type HCC A of bypass graft(s) of the extremities with intermittent claudication, left leg
- I70.313   Atherosclerosis of unspecified type HCC A of bypass graft(s) of the extremities with intermittent claudication, bilateral legs
- I70.318   Atherosclerosis of unspecified type HCC A of bypass graft(s) of the extremities with intermittent claudication, other extremity
- I70.319   Atherosclerosis of unspecified HCC A ▽ type of bypass graft(s) of the extremities with intermittent claudication, unspecified extremity

√6ᵗʰ I70.32 Atherosclerosis of unspecified type of bypass graft(s) of the extremities with rest pain

INCLUDES   any condition classifiable to I70.31-

- I70.321   Atherosclerosis of unspecified type HCC A of bypass graft(s) of the extremities with rest pain, right leg

- I70.322   Atherosclerosis of unspecified type HCC A of bypass graft(s) of the extremities with rest pain, left leg
- I70.323   Atherosclerosis of unspecified type HCC A of bypass graft(s) of the extremities with rest pain, bilateral legs
- I70.328   Atherosclerosis of unspecified type HCC A of bypass graft(s) of the extremities with rest pain, other extremity
- I70.329   Atherosclerosis of unspecified HCC A ▽ type of bypass graft(s) of the extremities with rest pain, unspecified extremity

√6ᵗʰ I70.33 Atherosclerosis of unspecified type of bypass graft(s) of the right leg with ulceration

INCLUDES   any condition classifiable to I70.311 and I70.321

Use additional code to identify severity of ulcer (L97.-)

- I70.331   Atherosclerosis of unspecified type HCC A of bypass graft(s) of the right leg with ulceration of thigh
- I70.332   Atherosclerosis of unspecified type HCC A of bypass graft(s) of the right leg with ulceration of calf
- I70.333   Atherosclerosis of unspecified type HCC A of bypass graft(s) of the right leg with ulceration of ankle
- I70.334   Atherosclerosis of unspecified type HCC A of bypass graft(s) of the right leg with ulceration of heel and midfoot

  Atherosclerosis of unspecified type of bypass graft(s) of right leg with ulceration of plantar surface of midfoot
- I70.335   Atherosclerosis of unspecified type HCC A of bypass graft(s) of the right leg with ulceration of other part of foot

  Atherosclerosis of unspecified type of bypass graft(s) of the right leg with ulceration of toe
- I70.338   Atherosclerosis of unspecified type HCC A of bypass graft(s) of the right leg with ulceration of other part of lower leg
- I70.339   Atherosclerosis of unspecified HCC A ▽ type of bypass graft(s) of the right leg with ulceration of unspecified site

√6ᵗʰ I70.34 Atherosclerosis of unspecified type of bypass graft(s) of the left leg with ulceration

INCLUDES   any condition classifiable to I70.312 and I70.322

Use additional code to identify severity of ulcer (L97.-)

- I70.341   Atherosclerosis of unspecified type HCC A of bypass graft(s) of the left leg with ulceration of thigh
- I70.342   Atherosclerosis of unspecified type HCC A of bypass graft(s) of the left leg with ulceration of calf
- I70.343   Atherosclerosis of unspecified type HCC A of bypass graft(s) of the left leg with ulceration of ankle
- I70.344   Atherosclerosis of unspecified type HCC A of bypass graft(s) of the left leg with ulceration of heel and midfoot

  Atherosclerosis of unspecified type of bypass graft(s) of left leg with ulceration of plantar surface of midfoot
- I70.345   Atherosclerosis of unspecified type HCC A of bypass graft(s) of the left leg with ulceration of other part of foot

  Atherosclerosis of unspecified type of bypass graft(s) of the left leg with ulceration of toe
- I70.348   Atherosclerosis of unspecified type HCC A of bypass graft(s) of the left leg with ulceration of other part of lower leg
- I70.349   Atherosclerosis of unspecified HCC A ▽ type of bypass graft(s) of the left leg with ulceration of unspecified site

EXCLUDES 1 Not coded here   EXCLUDES 2 Not included here   N Newborn Age: 0   P Pediatric Age: 0-17   M Maternity Age: 12-55   A Adult Age: 15-124

640   ICD-10-CM 2018

I70.26–I70.349

I70.35   **Atherosclerosis of unspecified type of bypass** HCC A **graft(s) of other extremity with** ulceration
> **INCLUDES**   any condition classifiable to I70.318 and I70.328
> Use additional code to identify severity of ulcer (L98.49-)

√6ᵗʰ   **I70.36**   **Atherosclerosis of unspecified type of bypass graft(s) of the extremities with** gangrene
> **INCLUDES**   any condition classifiable to I70.31-, I70.32-, I70.33-, I70.34-, I70.35
> Use additional code to identify the severity of any ulcer (L97.-, L98.49-), if applicable

    I70.361   **Atherosclerosis of unspecified type** HCC A **of bypass graft(s) of the extremities with gangrene,** right leg

    I70.362   **Atherosclerosis of unspecified type** HCC A **of bypass graft(s) of the extremities with gangrene,** left leg

    I70.363   **Atherosclerosis of unspecified type** HCC A **of bypass graft(s) of the extremities with gangrene,** bilateral legs

    I70.368   **Atherosclerosis of unspecified type** HCC A **of bypass graft(s) of the extremities with gangrene,** other extremity

    I70.369   **Atherosclerosis of unspecified** HCC A ▽ **type of bypass graft(s) of the extremities with gangrene, unspecified extremity**

√6ᵗʰ   **I70.39**   **Other atherosclerosis of unspecified type of bypass graft(s) of the extremities**

    I70.391   **Other atherosclerosis of** HCC A **unspecified type of bypass graft(s) of the extremities,** right leg

    I70.392   **Other atherosclerosis of** HCC A **unspecified type of bypass graft(s) of the extremities,** left leg

    I70.393   **Other atherosclerosis of** HCC A **unspecified type of bypass graft(s) of the extremities,** bilateral legs

    I70.398   **Other atherosclerosis of** HCC A **unspecified type of bypass graft(s) of the extremities,** other extremity

    I70.399   **Other atherosclerosis of** HCC A ▽ **unspecified type of bypass graft(s) of the extremities, unspecified extremity**

√5ᵗʰ   **I70.4**   **Atherosclerosis of** autologous vein bypass graft(s) **of the extremities**
> Use additional code, if applicable, to identify chronic total occlusion of artery of extremity (I70.92)

√6ᵗʰ   **I70.40**   **Unspecified atherosclerosis of autologous vein bypass graft(s) of the extremities**

    I70.401   **Unspecified atherosclerosis of** HCC A ▽ **autologous vein bypass graft(s) of the extremities,** right leg

    I70.402   **Unspecified atherosclerosis of** HCC A ▽ **autologous vein bypass graft(s) of the extremities,** left leg

    I70.403   **Unspecified atherosclerosis of** HCC A ▽ **autologous vein bypass graft(s) of the extremities,** bilateral legs

    I70.408   **Unspecified atherosclerosis of** HCC A ▽ **autologous vein bypass graft(s) of the extremities,** other extremity

    I70.409   **Unspecified atherosclerosis of** HCC A ▽ **autologous vein bypass graft(s) of the extremities, unspecified extremity**

√6ᵗʰ   **I70.41**   **Atherosclerosis of autologous vein bypass graft(s) of the extremities with** intermittent claudication

    I70.411   **Atherosclerosis of autologous vein** HCC A **bypass graft(s) of the extremities with intermittent claudication,** right leg

    I70.412   **Atherosclerosis of autologous vein** HCC A **bypass graft(s) of the extremities with intermittent claudication,** left leg

    I70.413   **Atherosclerosis of autologous vein** HCC A **bypass graft(s) of the extremities with intermittent claudication,** bilateral legs

    I70.418   **Atherosclerosis of autologous vein** HCC A **bypass graft(s) of the extremities with intermittent claudication, other extremity**

    I70.419   **Atherosclerosis of autologous** HCC A ▽ **vein bypass graft(s) of the extremities with intermittent claudication, unspecified extremity**

√6ᵗʰ   **I70.42**   **Atherosclerosis of autologous vein bypass graft(s) of the extremities with** rest pain
> **INCLUDES**   any condition classifiable to I70.41-

    I70.421   **Atherosclerosis of autologous vein** HCC A **bypass graft(s) of the extremities with rest pain,** right leg

    I70.422   **Atherosclerosis of autologous vein** HCC A **bypass graft(s) of the extremities with rest pain,** left leg

    I70.423   **Atherosclerosis of autologous vein** HCC A **bypass graft(s) of the extremities with rest pain,** bilateral legs

    I70.428   **Atherosclerosis of autologous vein** HCC A **bypass graft(s) of the extremities with rest pain, other extremity**

    I70.429   **Atherosclerosis of autologous** HCC A ▽ **vein bypass graft(s) of the extremities with rest pain, unspecified extremity**

√6ᵗʰ   **I70.43**   **Atherosclerosis of autologous vein bypass graft(s) of the** right leg with ulceration
> **INCLUDES**   any condition classifiable to I70.411 and I70.421
> Use additional code to identify severity of ulcer (L97.-)

    I70.431   **Atherosclerosis of autologous vein** HCC A **bypass graft(s) of the right leg with ulceration of** thigh

    I70.432   **Atherosclerosis of autologous vein** HCC A **bypass graft(s) of the right leg with ulceration of** calf

    I70.433   **Atherosclerosis of autologous vein** HCC A **bypass graft(s) of the right leg with ulceration of** ankle

    I70.434   **Atherosclerosis of autologous vein** HCC A **bypass graft(s) of the right leg with ulceration of** heel and midfoot
> Atherosclerosis of autologous vein bypass graft(s) of right leg with ulceration of plantar surface of midfoot

    I70.435   **Atherosclerosis of autologous vein** HCC A **bypass graft(s) of the right leg with ulceration of other** part of foot
> Atherosclerosis of autologous vein bypass graft(s) of right leg with ulceration of toe

    I70.438   **Atherosclerosis of autologous vein** HCC A **bypass graft(s) of the right leg with ulceration of other** part of lower leg

    I70.439   **Atherosclerosis of autologous** HCC A ▽ **vein bypass graft(s) of the right leg with ulceration of unspecified site**

√6ᵗʰ   **I70.44**   **Atherosclerosis of autologous vein bypass graft(s) of the** left leg with ulceration
> **INCLUDES**   any condition classifiable to I70.412 and I70.422
> Use additional code to identify severity of ulcer (L97.-)

    I70.441   **Atherosclerosis of autologous vein** HCC A **bypass graft(s) of the left leg with ulceration of** thigh

    I70.442   **Atherosclerosis of autologous vein** HCC A **bypass graft(s) of the left leg with ulceration of** calf

    I70.443   **Atherosclerosis of autologous vein** HCC A **bypass graft(s) of the left leg with ulceration of** ankle

    I70.444   **Atherosclerosis of autologous vein** HCC A **bypass graft(s) of the left leg with ulceration of** heel and midfoot
> Atherosclerosis of autologous vein bypass graft(s) of left leg with ulceration of plantar surface of midfoot

    I70.445   **Atherosclerosis of autologous vein** HCC A **bypass graft(s) of the left leg with ulceration of other** part of foot
> Atherosclerosis of autologous vein bypass graft(s) of left leg with ulceration of toe

---

☑ Additional Character Req   √ₓ7ᵗʰ Placeholder Alert   Manifestation   HCC CMS-HCC Condition   ▽ Unspecified Code   ►◄ Revised Text   ● New Code   ▲ Revised Code Title

I70.448 Atherosclerosis of autologous vein [HCC] [A]
bypass graft(s) of the left leg with
ulceration of other part of lower leg

I70.449 Atherosclerosis of autologous [HCC] [A] ▽
vein bypass graft(s) of the left leg with
ulceration of unspecified site

I70.45 Atherosclerosis of autologous vein bypass [HCC] [A]
graft(s) of other extremity with ulceration
INCLUDES any condition classifiable to I70.418,
I70.428, and I70.438
Use additional code to identify severity of ulcer
(L98.49)

√6ᵗʰ **I70.46** Atherosclerosis of autologous vein bypass graft(s) of
the extremities with gangrene
INCLUDES any condition classifiable to I70.41-, I70.42-,
and I70.43-, I70.44-, I70.45
Use additional code to identify the severity of any
ulcer (L97.-, L98.49-), if applicable

I70.461 Atherosclerosis of autologous vein [HCC] [A]
bypass graft(s) of the extremities with
gangrene, right leg

I70.462 Atherosclerosis of autologous vein [HCC] [A]
bypass graft(s) of the extremities with
gangrene, left leg

I70.463 Atherosclerosis of autologous vein [HCC] [A]
bypass graft(s) of the extremities with
gangrene, bilateral legs

I70.468 Atherosclerosis of autologous vein [HCC] [A]
bypass graft(s) of the extremities with
gangrene, other extremity

I70.469 Atherosclerosis of autologous [HCC] [A] ▽
vein bypass graft(s) of the extremities
with gangrene, unspecified extremity

√6ᵗʰ **I70.49** Other atherosclerosis of autologous vein bypass
graft(s) of the extremities

I70.491 Other atherosclerosis of autologous [HCC] [A]
vein bypass graft(s) of the extremities,
right leg

I70.492 Other atherosclerosis of autologous [HCC] [A]
vein bypass graft(s) of the extremities,
left leg

I70.493 Other atherosclerosis of autologous [HCC] [A]
vein bypass graft(s) of the extremities,
bilateral legs

I70.498 Other atherosclerosis of autologous [HCC] [A]
vein bypass graft(s) of the extremities,
other extremity

I70.499 Other atherosclerosis of [HCC] [A] ▽
autologous vein bypass graft(s) of the
extremities, unspecified extremity

√5ᵗʰ **I70.5** Atherosclerosis of nonautologous biological bypass graft(s)
of the extremities
Use additional code, if applicable, to identify chronic total
occlusion of artery of extremity (I70.92)

√6ᵗʰ **I70.50** Unspecified atherosclerosis of nonautologous
biological bypass graft(s) of the extremities

I70.501 Unspecified atherosclerosis of [HCC] [A] ▽
nonautologous biological bypass
graft(s) of the extremities, right leg

I70.502 Unspecified atherosclerosis of [HCC] [A] ▽
nonautologous biological bypass
graft(s) of the extremities, left leg

I70.503 Unspecified atherosclerosis of [HCC] [A] ▽
nonautologous biological bypass graft(s)
of the extremities, bilateral legs

I70.508 Unspecified atherosclerosis of [HCC] [A] ▽
nonautologous biological bypass graft(s)
of the extremities, other extremity

I70.509 Unspecified atherosclerosis of [HCC] [A] ▽
nonautologous biological bypass graft(s)
of the extremities, unspecified extremity

√6ᵗʰ **I70.51** Atherosclerosis of nonautologous biological bypass
graft(s) of the extremities with intermittent
claudication

I70.511 Atherosclerosis of nonautologous [HCC] [A]
biological bypass graft(s) of the
extremities with intermittent
claudication, right leg

I70.512 Atherosclerosis of nonautologous [HCC] [A]
biological bypass graft(s) of the
extremities with intermittent
claudication, left leg

I70.513 Atherosclerosis of nonautologous [HCC] [A]
biological bypass graft(s) of the
extremities with intermittent
claudication, bilateral legs

I70.518 Atherosclerosis of nonautologous [HCC] [A]
biological bypass graft(s) of the
extremities with intermittent
claudication, other extremity

I70.519 Atherosclerosis of nonautologous [HCC] [A] ▽
biological bypass graft(s) of the
extremities with intermittent
claudication, unspecified extremity

√6ᵗʰ **I70.52** Atherosclerosis of nonautologous biological bypass
graft(s) of the extremities with rest pain
INCLUDES any condition classifiable to I70.51-

I70.521 Atherosclerosis of nonautologous [HCC] [A]
biological bypass graft(s) of the
extremities with rest pain, right leg

I70.522 Atherosclerosis of nonautologous [HCC] [A]
biological bypass graft(s) of the
extremities with rest pain, left leg

I70.523 Atherosclerosis of nonautologous [HCC] [A]
biological bypass graft(s) of the
extremities with rest pain, bilateral legs

I70.528 Atherosclerosis of nonautologous [HCC] [A]
biological bypass graft(s) of the
extremities with rest pain, other extremity

I70.529 Atherosclerosis of nonautologous [HCC] [A] ▽
biological bypass graft(s) of the
extremities with rest pain, unspecified
extremity

√6ᵗʰ **I70.53** Atherosclerosis of nonautologous biological bypass
graft(s) of the right leg with ulceration
INCLUDES any condition classifiable to I70.511 and
I70.521
Use additional code to identify severity of ulcer (L97.-)

I70.531 Atherosclerosis of nonautologous [HCC] [A]
biological bypass graft(s) of the right leg
with ulceration of thigh

I70.532 Atherosclerosis of nonautologous [HCC] [A]
biological bypass graft(s) of the right leg
with ulceration of calf

I70.533 Atherosclerosis of nonautologous [HCC] [A]
biological bypass graft(s) of the right leg
with ulceration of ankle

I70.534 Atherosclerosis of nonautologous [HCC] [A]
biological bypass graft(s) of the right leg
with ulceration of heel and midfoot
Atherosclerosis of nonautologous
biological bypass graft(s) of right leg
with ulceration of plantar surface of
midfoot

I70.535 Atherosclerosis of nonautologous [HCC] [A]
biological bypass graft(s) of the right leg
with ulceration of other part of foot
Atherosclerosis of nonautologous
biological bypass graft(s) of the right
leg with ulceration of toe

I70.538 Atherosclerosis of nonautologous [HCC] [A]
biological bypass graft(s) of the right leg
with ulceration of other part of lower leg

I70.539 Atherosclerosis of nonautologous [HCC] [A] ▽
biological bypass graft(s) of the right leg
with ulceration of unspecified site

√6ᵗʰ **I70.54** Atherosclerosis of nonautologous biological bypass
graft(s) of the left leg with ulceration
INCLUDES any condition classifiable to I70.512 and
I70.522
Use additional code to identify severity of ulcer (L97.-)

I70.541 Atherosclerosis of nonautologous [HCC] [A]
biological bypass graft(s) of the left leg
with ulceration of thigh

I70.542 Atherosclerosis of nonautologous [HCC] [A]
biological bypass graft(s) of the left leg
with ulceration of calf

I70.543 Atherosclerosis of nonautologous [HCC] [A]
biological bypass graft(s) of the left leg
with ulceration of ankle

EXCLUDES 1 Not coded here   EXCLUDES 2 Not included here   [N] Newborn Age: 0   [P] Pediatric Age: 0-17   [M] Maternity Age: 12-55   [A] Adult Age: 15-124

642   ICD-10-CM 2018

I70.544   **Atherosclerosis of nonautologous** `HCC` `A`
biological bypass graft(s) of the left leg
with ulceration of heel and midfoot
Atherosclerosis of nonautologous
biological bypass graft(s) of left leg
with ulceration of plantar surface of
midfoot

I70.545   **Atherosclerosis of nonautologous** `HCC` `A`
biological bypass graft(s) of the left leg
with ulceration of other part of foot
Atherosclerosis of nonautologous
biological bypass graft(s) of the left leg
with ulceration of toe

I70.548   **Atherosclerosis of nonautologous** `HCC` `A`
biological bypass graft(s) of the left leg
with ulceration of other part of lower leg

I70.549   **Atherosclerosis of nonautologous** `HCC` `A` `▽`
biological bypass graft(s) of the left
leg with ulceration of unspecified site

I70.55   **Atherosclerosis of nonautologous biological** `HCC` `A`
bypass graft(s) of other extremity with ulceration
> INCLUDES   any condition classifiable to I70.518,
> I70.528, and I70.538
> Use additional code to identify severity of ulcer
> (L98.49)

`✓6ᵗʰ` **I70.56**   **Atherosclerosis of nonautologous biological bypass**
graft(s) of the extremities with gangrene
> INCLUDES   any condition classifiable to I70.51-, I70.52-,
> and I70.53-, I70.54-, I70.55
> Use additional code to identify the severity of any
> ulcer (L97.-, L98.49-), if applicable

I70.561   **Atherosclerosis of nonautologous** `HCC` `A`
biological bypass graft(s) of the
extremities with gangrene, right leg

I70.562   **Atherosclerosis of nonautologous** `HCC` `A`
biological bypass graft(s) of the
extremities with gangrene, left leg

I70.563   **Atherosclerosis of nonautologous** `HCC` `A`
biological bypass graft(s) of the
extremities with gangrene, bilateral legs

I70.568   **Atherosclerosis of nonautologous** `HCC` `A`
biological bypass graft(s) of the
extremities with gangrene, other
extremity

I70.569   **Atherosclerosis of nonautologous** `HCC` `A` `▽`
biological bypass graft(s) of the
extremities with gangrene, unspecified
extremity

`✓6ᵗʰ` **I70.59**   **Other atherosclerosis of nonautologous biological**
bypass graft(s) of the extremities

I70.591   **Other atherosclerosis of** `HCC` `A`
nonautologous biological bypass graft(s)
of the extremities, right leg

I70.592   **Other atherosclerosis of** `HCC` `A`
nonautologous biological bypass graft(s)
of the extremities, left leg

I70.593   **Other atherosclerosis of** `HCC` `A`
nonautologous biological bypass graft(s)
of the extremities, bilateral legs

I70.598   **Other atherosclerosis of** `HCC` `A`
nonautologous biological bypass graft(s)
of the extremities, other extremity

I70.599   **Other atherosclerosis of non-** `HCC` `A` `▽`
autologous biological bypass graft(s) of
the extremities, unspecified extremity

`✓5ᵗʰ` **I70.6**   **Atherosclerosis of nonbiological bypass graft(s) of the**
extremities
> Use additional code, if applicable, to identify chronic total
> occlusion of artery of extremity (I70.92)

`✓6ᵗʰ` **I70.60**   **Unspecified atherosclerosis of nonbiological bypass**
graft(s) of the extremities

I70.601   **Unspecified atherosclerosis of** `HCC` `A` `▽`
nonbiological bypass graft(s) of the
extremities, right leg

I70.602   **Unspecified atherosclerosis of** `HCC` `A` `▽`
nonbiological bypass graft(s) of the
extremities, left leg

I70.603   **Unspecified atherosclerosis of** `HCC` `A` `▽`
nonbiological bypass graft(s) of the
extremities, bilateral legs

I70.608   **Unspecified atherosclerosis of** `HCC` `A` `▽`
nonbiological bypass graft(s) of the
extremities, other extremity

I70.609   **Unspecified atherosclerosis of** `HCC` `A` `▽`
nonbiological bypass graft(s) of the
extremities, unspecified extremity

`✓6ᵗʰ` **I70.61**   **Atherosclerosis of nonbiological bypass graft(s) of**
the extremities with intermittent claudication

I70.611   **Atherosclerosis of nonbiological** `HCC` `A`
bypass graft(s) of the extremities with
intermittent claudication, right leg

I70.612   **Atherosclerosis of nonbiological** `HCC` `A`
bypass graft(s) of the extremities with
intermittent claudication, left leg

I70.613   **Atherosclerosis of nonbiological** `HCC` `A`
bypass graft(s) of the extremities with
intermittent claudication, bilateral legs

I70.618   **Atherosclerosis of nonbiological** `HCC` `A`
bypass graft(s) of the extremities
with intermittent claudication, other
extremity

I70.619   **Atherosclerosis of nonbiological** `HCC` `A` `▽`
bypass graft(s) of the extremities with
intermittent claudication, unspecified
extremity

`✓6ᵗʰ` **I70.62**   **Atherosclerosis of nonbiological bypass graft(s) of**
the extremities with rest pain
> INCLUDES   any condition classifiable to I70.61-

I70.621   **Atherosclerosis of nonbiological** `HCC` `A`
bypass graft(s) of the extremities
with rest pain, right leg

I70.622   **Atherosclerosis of nonbiological** `HCC` `A`
bypass graft(s) of the extremities
with rest pain, left leg

I70.623   **Atherosclerosis of nonbiological** `HCC` `A`
bypass graft(s) of the extremities
with rest pain, bilateral legs

I70.628   **Atherosclerosis of nonbiological** `HCC` `A`
bypass graft(s) of the extremities
with rest pain, other extremity

I70.629   **Atherosclerosis of nonbiological** `HCC` `A` `▽`
bypass graft(s) of the extremities
with rest pain, unspecified extremity

`✓6ᵗʰ` **I70.63**   **Atherosclerosis of nonbiological bypass graft(s) of**
the right leg with ulceration
> INCLUDES   any condition classifiable to I70.611 and
> I70.621
> Use additional code to identify severity of ulcer (L97.-)

I70.631   **Atherosclerosis of nonbiological** `HCC` `A`
bypass graft(s) of the right leg with
ulceration of thigh

I70.632   **Atherosclerosis of nonbiological** `HCC` `A`
bypass graft(s) of the right leg with
ulceration of calf

I70.633   **Atherosclerosis of nonbiological** `HCC` `A`
bypass graft(s) of the right leg with
ulceration of ankle

I70.634   **Atherosclerosis of nonbiological** `HCC` `A`
bypass graft(s) of the right leg with
ulceration of heel and midfoot
Atherosclerosis of nonbiological bypass
graft(s) of right leg with ulceration of
plantar surface of midfoot

I70.635   **Atherosclerosis of nonbiological** `HCC` `A`
bypass graft(s) of the right leg with
ulceration of other part of foot
Atherosclerosis of nonbiological bypass
graft(s) of the right leg with ulceration
of toe

I70.638   **Atherosclerosis of nonbiological** `HCC` `A`
bypass graft(s) of the right leg with
ulceration of other part of lower leg

I70.639   **Atherosclerosis of nonbiological** `HCC` `A` `▽`
bypass graft(s) of the right leg with
ulceration of unspecified site

`✓` Additional Character Req   `✓x7ᵗʰ` Placeholder Alert   Manifestation   `HCC` CMS-HCC Condition   `▽` Unspecified Code   `▶◀` Revised Text   `●` New Code   `▲` Revised Code Title

Chapter 9. Diseases of the Circulatory System

✓6ᵗʰ **I70.64** **Atherosclerosis of nonbiological bypass graft(s) of the left leg with ulceration**
INCLUDES any condition classifiable to I70.612 and I70.622
Use additional code to identify severity of ulcer (L97.-)

I70.641 **Atherosclerosis of nonbiological bypass graft(s) of the left leg with ulceration of thigh** HCC A

I70.642 **Atherosclerosis of nonbiological bypass graft(s) of the left leg with ulceration of calf** HCC A

I70.643 **Atherosclerosis of nonbiological bypass graft(s) of the left leg with ulceration of ankle** HCC A

I70.644 **Atherosclerosis of nonbiological bypass graft(s) of the left leg with ulceration of heel and midfoot** HCC A
Atherosclerosis of nonbiological bypass graft(s) of left leg with ulceration of plantar surface of midfoot

I70.645 **Atherosclerosis of nonbiological bypassgraft(s) of the left leg with ulceration of other part of foot** HCC A
Atherosclerosis of nonbiological bypass graft(s) of the left leg with ulceration of toe

I70.648 **Atherosclerosis of nonbiological bypass graft(s) of the left leg with ulceration of other part of lower leg** HCC A

I70.649 **Atherosclerosis of nonbiological bypass graft(s) of the left leg with ulceration of unspecified site** HCC A ▽

I70.65 **Atherosclerosis of nonbiological bypass graft(s) of other extremity with ulceration** HCC A
INCLUDES any condition classifiable to I70.618 and I70.628
Use additional code to identify severity of ulcer (L98.49)

✓6ᵗʰ **I70.66** **Atherosclerosis of nonbiological bypass graft(s) of the extremities with gangrene**
INCLUDES any condition classifiable to I70.61-, I70.62-, I70.63-, I70.64-, I70.65
Use additional code to identify the severity of any ulcer (L97.-, L98.49-), if applicable

I70.661 **Atherosclerosis of nonbiological bypass graft(s) of the extremities with gangrene, right leg** HCC A

I70.662 **Atherosclerosis of nonbiological bypass graft(s) of the extremities with gangrene, left leg** HCC A

I70.663 **Atherosclerosis of nonbiological bypass graft(s) of the extremities with gangrene, bilateral legs** HCC A

I70.668 **Atherosclerosis of nonbiological bypass graft(s) of the extremities with gangrene, other extremity** HCC A

I70.669 **Atherosclerosis of nonbiological bypass graft(s) of the extremities with gangrene, unspecified extremity** HCC A ▽

✓6ᵗʰ **I70.69** **Other atherosclerosis of nonbiological bypass graft(s) of the extremities**

I70.691 **Other atherosclerosis of nonbiological bypass graft(s) of the extremities, right leg** HCC A

I70.692 **Other atherosclerosis of nonbiological bypass graft(s) of the extremities, left leg** HCC A

I70.693 **Other atherosclerosis of nonbiological bypass graft(s) of the extremities, bilateral legs** HCC A

I70.698 **Other atherosclerosis of nonbiological bypass graft(s) of the extremities, other extremity** HCC A

I70.699 **Other atherosclerosis of non-biological bypass graft(s) of the extremities, unspecified extremity** HCC A ▽

✓5ᵗʰ **I70.7** **Atherosclerosis of other type of bypass graft(s) of the extremities**
Use additional code, if applicable, to identify chronic total occlusion of artery of extremity (I70.92)

✓6ᵗʰ **I70.70** **Unspecified atherosclerosis of other type of bypass graft(s) of the extremities**

I70.701 **Unspecified atherosclerosis of other type of bypass graft(s) of the extremities, right leg** HCC A ▽

I70.702 **Unspecified atherosclerosis of other type of bypass graft(s) of the extremities, left leg** HCC A ▽

I70.703 **Unspecified atherosclerosis of other type of bypass graft(s) of the extremities, bilateral legs** HCC A ▽

I70.708 **Unspecified atherosclerosis of other type of bypass graft(s) of the extremities, other extremity** HCC A ▽

I70.709 **Unspecified atherosclerosis of other type of bypass graft(s) of the extremities, unspecified extremity** HCC A ▽

✓6ᵗʰ **I70.71** **Atherosclerosis of other type of bypass graft(s) of the extremities with intermittent claudication**

I70.711 **Atherosclerosis of other type of bypass graft(s) of the extremities with intermittent claudication, right leg** HCC A

I70.712 **Atherosclerosis of other type of bypass graft(s) of the extremities with intermittent claudication, left leg** HCC A

I70.713 **Atherosclerosis of other type of bypass graft(s) of the extremities with intermittent claudication, bilateral legs** HCC A

I70.718 **Atherosclerosis of other type of bypass graft(s) of the extremities with intermittent claudication, other extremity** HCC A

I70.719 **Atherosclerosis of other type of bypass graft(s) of the extremities withintermittent claudication, unspecified extremity** HCC A ▽

✓6ᵗʰ **I70.72** **Atherosclerosis of other type of bypass graft(s) of the extremities with rest pain**
INCLUDES any condition classifiable to I70.71-

I70.721 **Atherosclerosis of other type of bypass graft(s) of the extremities with rest pain, right leg** HCC A

I70.722 **Atherosclerosis of other type of bypass graft(s) of the extremities with rest pain, left leg** HCC A

I70.723 **Atherosclerosis of other type of bypass graft(s) of the extremities with rest pain, bilateral legs** HCC A

I70.728 **Atherosclerosis of other type of bypass graft(s) of the extremities with rest pain, other extremity** HCC A

I70.729 **Atherosclerosis of other type of bypass graft(s) of the extremities with rest pain, unspecified extremity** HCC A ▽

✓6ᵗʰ **I70.73** **Atherosclerosis of other type of bypass graft(s) of the right leg with ulceration**
INCLUDES any condition classifiable to I70.711 and I70.721
Use additional code to identify severity of ulcer (L97.-)

I70.731 **Atherosclerosis of other type of bypass graft(s) of the right leg with ulceration of thigh** HCC A

I70.732 **Atherosclerosis of other type of bypass graft(s) of the right leg with ulceration of calf** HCC A

I70.733 **Atherosclerosis of other type of bypass graft(s) of the right leg with ulceration of ankle** HCC A

I70.734 **Atherosclerosis of other type of bypass graft(s) of the right leg with ulceration of heel and midfoot** HCC A
Atherosclerosis of other type of bypass graft(s) of right leg with ulceration of plantar surface of midfoot

EXCLUDES 1 Not coded here   EXCLUDES 2 Not included here   N Newborn Age: 0   P Pediatric Age: 0-17   M Maternity Age: 12-55   A Adult Age: 15-124

644   ICD-10-CM 2018

I70.735 **Atherosclerosis of other type of bypass graft(s) of the right leg with ulceration of other part of foot** `HCC` `A`
    Atherosclerosis of other type of bypass graft(s) of right leg with ulceration of toe

I70.738 **Atherosclerosis of other type of bypass graft(s) of the right leg with ulceration of other part of lower leg** `HCC` `A`

I70.739 **Atherosclerosis of other type of bypass graft(s) of the right leg with ulceration of unspecified site** `HCC` `A` ▽

✓6ᵗʰ **I70.74** **Atherosclerosis of other type of bypass graft(s) of the left leg with ulceration**
    INCLUDES any condition classifiable to I70.712 and I70.722
    Use additional code to identify severity of ulcer (L97.-)

I70.741 **Atherosclerosis of other type of bypass graft(s) of the left leg with ulceration of thigh** `HCC` `A`

I70.742 **Atherosclerosis of other type of bypass graft(s) of the left leg with ulceration of calf** `HCC` `A`

I70.743 **Atherosclerosis of other type of bypass raft(s) of the left leg with ulceration of ankle** `HCC` `A`

I70.744 **Atherosclerosis of other type of bypass graft(s) of the left leg with ulceration of heel and midfoot** `HCC` `A`
    Atherosclerosis of other type of bypass graft(s) of left leg with ulceration of plantar surface of midfoot

I70.745 **Atherosclerosis of other type of bypass graft(s) of the left leg with ulceration of other part of foot** `HCC` `A`
    Atherosclerosis of other type of bypass graft(s) of left leg with ulceration of toe

I70.748 **Atherosclerosis of other type of bypass graft(s) of the left leg with ulceration of other part of lower leg** `HCC` `A`

I70.749 **Atherosclerosis of other type of bypass graft(s) of the left leg with ulceration of unspecified site** `HCC` `A` ▽

I70.75 **Atherosclerosis of other type of bypass graft(s) of other extremity with ulceration** `HCC` `A`
    INCLUDES any condition classifiable to I70.718 and I70.728
    Use additional code to identify severity of ulcer (L98.49)

✓6ᵗʰ **I70.76** **Atherosclerosis of other type of bypass graft(s) of the extremities with gangrene**
    INCLUDES any condition classifiable to I70.71-, I70.72-, I70.73-, I70.74-, I70.75
    Use additional code to identify the severity of any ulcer (L97.-, L98.49-), if applicable

I70.761 **Atherosclerosis of other type of bypass graft(s) of the extremities with gangrene, right leg** `HCC` `A`

I70.762 **Atherosclerosis of other type of bypass graft(s) of the extremities with gangrene, left leg** `HCC` `A`

I70.763 **Atherosclerosis of other type of bypass graft(s) of the extremities with gangrene, bilateral legs** `HCC` `A`

I70.768 **Atherosclerosis of other type of bypass graft(s) of the extremities with gangrene, other extremity** `HCC` `A`

I70.769 **Atherosclerosis of other type of bypass graft(s) of the extremities with gangrene, unspecified extremity** `HCC` `A` ▽

✓6ᵗʰ **I70.79** **Other atherosclerosis of other type of bypass graft(s) of the extremities**

I70.791 **Other atherosclerosis of other type of bypass graft(s) of the extremities, right leg** `HCC` `A`

I70.792 **Other atherosclerosis of other type of bypass graft(s) of the extremities, left leg** `HCC` `A`

I70.793 **Other atherosclerosis of other type of bypass graft(s) of the extremities, bilateral legs** `HCC` `A`

I70.798 **Other atherosclerosis of other type of bypass graft(s) of the extremities, other extremity** `HCC` `A`

I70.799 **Other atherosclerosis of other typeof bypass graft(s) of the extremities, unspecified extremity** `HCC` `A` ▽

I70.8 **Atherosclerosis of other arteries** `A`
    TIP: Arteriosclerosis of the iliac arteries is coded here.

✓5ᵗʰ **I70.9** **Other and unspecified atherosclerosis**

I70.90 **Unspecified atherosclerosis** `A` ▽

I70.91 **Generalized atherosclerosis** `A`

I70.92 **Chronic total occlusion of artery of the extremities** `HCC`
    Complete occlusion of artery of the extremities
    Total occlusion of artery of the extremities
    Code first atherosclerosis of arteries of the extremities (I70.2-, I70.3-, I70.4-, I70.5-, I70.6-, I70.7-)

✓4ᵗʰ **I71** **Aortic aneurysm and dissection**
    EXCLUDES 1 aortic ectasia (I77.81-)
       syphilitic aortic aneurysm (A52.01)
       traumatic aortic aneurysm (S25.09, S35.09)

✓5ᵗʰ **I71.0** **Dissection of aorta**

I71.00 **Dissection of unspecified site of aorta** `HCC` ▽

I71.01 **Dissection of thoracic aorta** `HCC`

I71.02 **Dissection of abdominal aorta** `HCC`

I71.03 **Dissection of thoracoabdominal aorta** `HCC`

I71.1 **Thoracic aortic aneurysm, ruptured** `HCC`

I71.2 **Thoracic aortic aneurysm, without rupture** `HCC`

I71.3 **Abdominal aortic aneurysm, ruptured** `HCC`

I71.4 **Abdominal aortic aneurysm, without rupture** `HCC`

I71.5 **Thoracoabdominal aortic aneurysm, ruptured** `HCC`

I71.6 **Thoracoabdominal aortic aneurysm, without rupture** `HCC`

I71.8 **Aortic aneurysm of unspecified site, ruptured** `HCC` ▽
    Rupture of aorta NOS

I71.9 **Aortic aneurysm of unspecified site, without rupture** `HCC` ▽
    Aneurysm of aorta
    Dilatation of aorta
    Hyaline necrosis of aorta

✓4ᵗʰ **I72** **Other aneurysm**
    INCLUDES aneurysm (cirsoid) (false) (ruptured)
    EXCLUDES 2 acquired aneurysm (I77.0)
       aneurysm (of) aorta (I71.-)
       aneurysm (of) arteriovenous NOS (Q27.3-)
       carotid artery dissection (I77.71)
       cerebral (nonruptured) aneurysm (I67.1)
       coronary aneurysm (I25.4)
       coronary artery dissection (I25.42)
       dissection of artery NEC (I77.79)
       dissection of precerebral artery, congenital (nonruptured) (Q28.1)
       heart aneurysm (I25.3)
       iliac artery dissection (I77.72)
       ▶precerebral artery, congenital (nonruptured) (Q28.1)◀
       pulmonary artery aneurysm (I28.1)
       renal artery dissection (I77.73)
       retinal aneurysm (H35.0)
       ruptured cerebral aneurysm (I60.7)
       varicose aneurysm (I77.0)
       vertebral artery dissection (I77.74)

I72.0 **Aneurysm of carotid artery** `HCC`
    Aneurysm of common carotid artery
    Aneurysm of external carotid artery
    Aneurysm of internal carotid artery, extracranial portion
    EXCLUDES 1 aneurysm of internal carotid artery, intracranial portion (I67.1)
       aneurysm of internal carotid artery NOS (I67.1)

I72.1 **Aneurysm of artery of upper extremity** `HCC`

I72.2 **Aneurysm of renal artery** `HCC`

I72.3 **Aneurysm of iliac artery** `HCC`

I72.4 **Aneurysm of artery of lower extremity** `HCC`

I72.5 **Aneurysm of other precerebral arteries** `HCC`
    Aneurysm of basilar artery (trunk)
    EXCLUDES 2 aneurysm of carotid artery (I72.0)
       aneurysm of vertebral artery (I72.6)
       dissection of carotid artery (I77.71)
       dissection of other precerebral arteries (I77.75)
       dissection of vertebral artery (I77.74)

✓ Additional Character Req   ✓x7ᵗʰ Placeholder Alert   Manifestation   `HCC` CMS-HCC Condition   ▽ Unspecified Code   ▶◀ Revised Text   ● New Code   ▲ Revised Code Title

ICD-10-CM 2018   645

Aneurysm

Layers of muscular and elastic tissue
Outer layer
Inner layer
Aneurysm

I72.6   **Aneurysm of vertebral artery**   HCC
     EXCLUDES 2   dissection of vertebral artery (I77.74)

I72.8   **Aneurysm of other specified arteries**   HCC

I72.9   **Aneurysm of unspecified site**   HCC ▽

✓4ᵗʰ **I73**   **Other peripheral vascular diseases**
     EXCLUDES 2   chilblains (T69.1)
                frostbite (T33- T34)
                immersion hand or foot (T69.0-)
                spasm of cerebral artery (G45.9)

✓5ᵗʰ **I73.0**   **Raynaud's syndrome**
         Raynaud's disease
         Raynaud's phenomenon (secondary)

     I73.00   **Raynaud's syndrome without gangrene**

     I73.01   **Raynaud's syndrome with gangrene**   HCC

I73.1   **Thromboangiitis obliterans [Buerger's disease]**   HCC
     DEF: Inflammatory disease of extremity blood vessels, mainly the lower; associated with heavy tobacco use; arteries are more affected than veins; occurs primarily in young men and leads to tissue ischemia and gangrene.

✓5ᵗʰ **I73.8**   **Other specified peripheral vascular diseases**
     EXCLUDES 1   diabetic (peripheral) angiopathy (E08-E13 with .51-.52)

     I73.81   **Erythromelalgia**   HCC

     I73.89   **Other specified peripheral vascular diseases**   HCC
         Acrocyanosis
         Erythrocyanosis
         Simple acroparesthesia [Schultze's type]
         Vasomotor acroparesthesia [Nothnagel's type]

I73.9   **Peripheral vascular disease, unspecified**   HCC ▽
     Intermittent claudication
     Peripheral angiopathy NOS
     Spasm of artery
     EXCLUDES 1   atherosclerosis of the extremities (I70.2--I70.7-)

✓4ᵗʰ **I74**   **Arterial embolism and thrombosis**
     INCLUDES   embolic infarction
               embolic occlusion
               thrombotic infarction
               thrombotic occlusion
     Code first:
         embolism and thrombosis complicating abortion or ectopic or molar pregnancy (O00-O07, O08.2)
         embolism and thrombosis complicating pregnancy, childbirth and the puerperium (O88.-)
     EXCLUDES 2   atheroembolism (I75.-)
            basilar embolism and thrombosis (I63.0-I63.2, I65.1)
            carotid embolism and thrombosis (I63.0-I63.2, I65.2)
            cerebral embolism and thrombosis (I63.3-I63.5, I66.-)
            coronary embolism and thrombosis (I21-I25)
            mesenteric embolism and thrombosis (K55.0-)
            ophthalmic embolism and thrombosis (H34.-)
            precerebral embolism and thrombosis NOS (I63.0-I63.2, I65.9)
            pulmonary embolism and thrombosis (I26.-)
            renal embolism and thrombosis (N28.0)
            retinal embolism and thrombosis (H34.-)
            septic embolism and thrombosis (I76)
            vertebral embolism and thrombosis (I63.0-I63.2, I65.0)

✓5ᵗʰ **I74.0**   **Embolism and thrombosis of abdominal aorta**

     I74.01   **Saddle embolus of abdominal aorta**   HCC

     I74.09   **Other arterial embolism and thrombosis of abdominal aorta**   HCC
         Aortic bifurcation syndrome
         Aortoiliac obstruction
         Leriche's syndrome

✓5ᵗʰ **I74.1**   **Embolism and thrombosis of other and unspecified parts of aorta**

     I74.10   **Embolism and thrombosis of unspecified parts of aorta**   HCC ▽

     I74.11   **Embolism and thrombosis of thoracic aorta**   HCC

     I74.19   **Embolism and thrombosis of other parts of aorta**   HCC

I74.2   **Embolism and thrombosis of arteries of the upper extremities**   HCC

I74.3   **Embolism and thrombosis of arteries of the lower extremities**   HCC

I74.4   **Embolism and thrombosis of arteries of extremities, unspecified**   HCC ▽
     Peripheral arterial embolism NOS

I74.5   **Embolism and thrombosis of iliac artery**   HCC

I74.8   **Embolism and thrombosis of other arteries**   HCC

I74.9   **Embolism and thrombosis of unspecified artery**   HCC ▽

✓4ᵗʰ **I75**   **Atheroembolism**
     INCLUDES   atherothrombotic microembolism
               cholesterol embolism

✓5ᵗʰ **I75.0**   **Atheroembolism of extremities**

     ✓6ᵗʰ **I75.01**   **Atheroembolism of upper extremity**

         I75.011   **Atheroembolism of right upper extremity**   HCC

         I75.012   **Atheroembolism of left upper extremity**   HCC

         I75.013   **Atheroembolism of bilateral upper extremities**   HCC

         I75.019   **Atheroembolism of unspecified upper extremity**   HCC ▽

     ✓6ᵗʰ **I75.02**   **Atheroembolism of lower extremity**

         I75.021   **Atheroembolism of right lower extremity**   HCC

         I75.022   **Atheroembolism of left lower extremity**   HCC

         I75.023   **Atheroembolism of bilateral lower extremities**   HCC

         I75.029   **Atheroembolism of unspecified lower extremity**   HCC ▽

✓5ᵗʰ **I75.8**   **Atheroembolism of other sites**

     I75.81   **Atheroembolism of kidney**   HCC
         Use additional code for any associated acute kidney failure and chronic kidney disease (N17.-, N18.-)

     I75.89   **Atheroembolism of other site**   HCC

I76   **Septic arterial embolism**   HCC
     Code first underlying infection, such as:
         infective endocarditis (I33.0)
         lung abscess (J85.-)
     Use additional code to identify the site of the embolism (I74.-)
     EXCLUDES 2   septic pulmonary embolism (I26.01, I26.90)

✓4ᵗʰ **I77**   **Other disorders of arteries and arterioles**
     EXCLUDES 2   collagen (vascular) diseases (M30-M36)
            hypersensitivity angiitis (M31.0)
            pulmonary artery (I28.-)

I77.0   **Arteriovenous fistula, acquired**   HCC
     Aneurysmal varix
     Arteriovenous aneurysm, acquired
     EXCLUDES 1   arteriovenous aneurysm NOS (Q27.3-)
           presence of arteriovenous shunt (fistula) for dialysis (Z99.2)
           traumatic—see injury of blood vessel by body region
     EXCLUDES 2   cerebral (I67.1)
           coronary (I25.4)
     DEF: Communication between an artery and vein; caused by trauma or invasive procedures.

I77.1   **Stricture of artery**   HCC
     Narrowing of artery

I77.2   **Rupture of artery**   HCC
     Erosion of artery
     Fistula of artery
     Ulcer of artery
     EXCLUDES 1   traumatic rupture of artery—see injury of blood vessel by body region

I77.3   **Arterial fibromuscular dysplasia**   HCC
     Fibromuscular hyperplasia (of) carotid artery
     Fibromuscular hyperplasia (of) renal artery

I77.4   **Celiac artery compression syndrome**   HCC

EXCLUDES 1 Not coded here   EXCLUDES 2 Not included here   N Newborn Age: 0   P Pediatric Age: 0-17   M Maternity Age: 12-55   A Adult Age: 15-124

646   ICD-10-CM 2018

I77.5   **Necrosis of artery**   HCC

I77.6   **Arteritis, unspecified**   HCC ▽
     Aortitis NOS
     Endarteritis NOS
       EXCLUDES 1   *arteritis or endarteritis:*
          aortic arch (M31.4)
          cerebral NEC (I67.7)
          coronary (I25.89)
          deformans (I70.-)
          giant cell (M31.5, M31.6)
          obliterans (I70.-)
          senile (I70.-)

√5th **I77.7**   **Other arterial dissection**
       EXCLUDES 2   *dissection of aorta (I71.0-)*
          dissection of coronary artery (I25.42)

    I77.70   **Dissection of unspecified artery**   HCC ▽

    I77.71   **Dissection of carotid artery**   HCC

    I77.72   **Dissection of iliac artery**   HCC

    I77.73   **Dissection of renal artery**   HCC

    I77.74   **Dissection of vertebral artery**   HCC
       EXCLUDES 2   *aneurysm of vertebral artery (I72.6)*

    I77.75   **Dissection of other precerebral arteries**   HCC
       Dissection of basilar artery (trunk)
       EXCLUDES 2   *aneurysm of carotid artery (I72.0)*
          aneurysm of other precerebral arteries (I72.5)
          aneurysm of vertebral artery (I72.6)
          dissection of carotid artery (I77.71)
          dissection of vertebral artery (I77.74)

    I77.76   **Dissection of artery of upper extremity**   HCC

    I77.77   **Dissection of artery of lower extremity**   HCC

    I77.79   **Dissection of other specified artery**   HCC

√5th **I77.8**   **Other specified disorders of arteries and arterioles**

   √6th **I77.81**   **Aortic ectasia**
       Ectasis aorta
       EXCLUDES 1   *aortic aneurysm and dissection (I71.0-)*

      I77.810   **Thoracic aortic ectasia**   HCC

      I77.811   **Abdominal aortic ectasia**   HCC

      I77.812   **Thoracoabdominal aortic ectasia**   HCC

      I77.819   **Aortic ectasia, unspecified site**   HCC ▽

    I77.89   **Other specified disorders of arteries and arterioles**   HCC

I77.9   **Disorder of arteries and arterioles, unspecified**   HCC ▽

√4th **I78**   **Diseases of capillaries**

   I78.0   **Hereditary hemorrhagic telangiectasia**   HCC
       Rendu-Osler-Weber disease

   I78.1   **Nevus, non-neoplastic**
       Araneus nevus
       Senile nevus
       Spider nevus
       Stellar nevus
       EXCLUDES 1   *nevus NOS (D22.-)*
          vascular NOS (Q82.5)
       EXCLUDES 2   *blue nevus (D22.-)*
          flammeus nevus (Q82.5)
          hairy nevus (D22.-)
          melanocytic nevus (D22.-)
          pigmented nevus (D22.-)
          portwine nevus (Q82.5)
          sanguineous nevus (Q82.5)
          strawberry nevus (Q82.5)
          verrucous nevus (Q82.5)

   I78.8   **Other diseases of capillaries**

   I78.9   **Disease of capillaries, unspecified**   ▽

√4th **I79**   **Disorders of arteries, arterioles and capillaries in diseases classified elsewhere**

   I79.0   *Aneurysm of aorta in diseases classified elsewhere*   HCC
       Code first underlying disease
       EXCLUDES 1   *syphilitic aneurysm (A52.01)*

   I79.1   *Aortitis in diseases classified elsewhere*   HCC
       Code first underlying disease
       EXCLUDES 1   *syphilitic aortitis (A52.02)*

I79.8   *Other disorders of arteries, arterioles and capillaries in diseases classified elsewhere*   HCC
       Code first underlying disease, such as:
       amyloidosis (E85.-)
       EXCLUDES 1   *diabetic (peripheral) angiopathy (E08-E13 with*
          .51-.52)
          syphilitic endarteritis (A52.09)
          tuberculous endarteritis (A18.89)

Diseases of veins, lymphatic vessels and lymph nodes, not elsewhere classified (I80-I89)

√4th **I80**   **Phlebitis and thrombophlebitis**
       INCLUDES   endophlebitis
          inflammation, vein
          periphlebitis
          suppurative phlebitis
       Code first:
          phlebitis and thrombophlebitis complicating abortion, ectopic or molar pregnancy (O00-O07, O08.7)
          phlebitis and thrombophlebitis complicating pregnancy, childbirth and the puerperium (O22.-, O87.-)
       EXCLUDES 1   *venous embolism and thrombosis of lower extremities ((I82.4-, I82.5-, I82.81-)*

√5th **I80.0**   **Phlebitis and thrombophlebitis of superficial vessels of lower extremities**
       Phlebitis and thrombophlebitis of femoropopliteal vein

    I80.00   **Phlebitis and thrombophlebitis of superficial vessels of unspecified lower extremity**   ▽

    I80.01   **Phlebitis and thrombophlebitis of superficial vessels of right lower extremity**

    I80.02   **Phlebitis and thrombophlebitis of superficial vessels of left lower extremity**

    I80.03   **Phlebitis and thrombophlebitis of superficial vessels of lower extremities, bilateral**

√5th **I80.1**   **Phlebitis and thrombophlebitis of femoral vein**

    I80.10   **Phlebitis and thrombophlebitis of unspecified femoral vein**   HCC ▽

    I80.11   **Phlebitis and thrombophlebitis of right femoral vein**   HCC

    I80.12   **Phlebitis and thrombophlebitis of left femoral vein**   HCC

    I80.13   **Phlebitis and thrombophlebitis of femoral vein, bilateral**   HCC

√5th **I80.2**   **Phlebitis and thrombophlebitis of other and unspecified deep vessels of lower extremities**

   √6th **I80.20**   **Phlebitis and thrombophlebitis of unspecified deep vessels of lower extremities**

      I80.201   **Phlebitis and thrombophlebitis of unspecified deep vessels of right lower extremity**   HCC

      I80.202   **Phlebitis and thrombophlebitis of unspecified deep vessels of left lower extremity**   HCC

      I80.203   **Phlebitis and thrombophlebitis of unspecified deep vessels of lower extremities, bilateral**   HCC

      I80.209   **Phlebitis and thrombophlebitis of unspecified deep vessels of unspecified lower extremity**   HCC ▽

   √6th **I80.21**   **Phlebitis and thrombophlebitis of iliac vein**

      I80.211   **Phlebitis and thrombophlebitis of right iliac vein**   HCC

      I80.212   **Phlebitis and thrombophlebitis of left iliac vein**   HCC

      I80.213   **Phlebitis and thrombophlebitis of iliac vein, bilateral**   HCC

      I80.219   **Phlebitis and thrombophlebitis of unspecified iliac vein**   HCC ▽

   √6th **I80.22**   **Phlebitis and thrombophlebitis of popliteal vein**

      I80.221   **Phlebitis and thrombophlebitis of right popliteal vein**   HCC

      I80.222   **Phlebitis and thrombophlebitis of left popliteal vein**   HCC

      I80.223   **Phlebitis and thrombophlebitis of popliteal vein, bilateral**   HCC

      I80.229   **Phlebitis and thrombophlebitis of unspecified popliteal vein**   HCC ▽

☑ Additional Character Req   √×7th Placeholder Alert   Manifestation   HCC CMS-HCC Condition   ▽ Unspecified Code   ▶◀ Revised Text   ● New Code   ▲ Revised Code Title

Chapter 9. Diseases of the Circulatory System

√6th **I80.23** **Phlebitis and thrombophlebitis of tibial vein**

     I80.231 **Phlebitis and thrombophlebitis of right tibial vein** HCC

     I80.232 **Phlebitis and thrombophlebitis of left tibial vein** HCC

     I80.233 **Phlebitis and thrombophlebitis of tibial vein, bilateral** HCC

     I80.239 **Phlebitis and thrombophlebitis of unspecified tibial vein** HCC ▽

√6th **I80.29** **Phlebitis and thrombophlebitis of other deep vessels of lower extremities**

     I80.291 **Phlebitis and thrombophlebitis of other deep vessels of right lower extremity** HCC

     I80.292 **Phlebitis and thrombophlebitis of other deep vessels of left lower extremity** HCC

     I80.293 **Phlebitis and thrombophlebitis of other deep vessels of lower extremity, bilateral** HCC

     I80.299 **Phlebitis and thrombophlebitis of other deep vessels of unspecified lower extremity** HCC ▽

I80.3 **Phlebitis and thrombophlebitis of lower extremities, unspecified** ▽

I80.8 **Phlebitis and thrombophlebitis of other sites**

I80.9 **Phlebitis and thrombophlebitis of unspecified site** ▽

I81 **Portal vein thrombosis**
Portal (vein) obstruction
EXCLUDES 2   hepatic vein thrombosis (I82.0)
     phlebitis of portal vein (K75.1)

√4th **I82** **Other venous embolism and thrombosis**
Code first venous embolism and thrombosis complicating:
abortion, ectopic or molar pregnancy (O00-O07, O08.7)
pregnancy, childbirth and the puerperium (O22.-, O87.-)
EXCLUDES 2   venous embolism and thrombosis (of):
     cerebral (I63.6, I67.6)
     coronary (I21-I25)
     intracranial and intraspinal, septic or NOS (G08)
     intracranial, nonpyogenic (I67.6)
     intraspinal, nonpyogenic (G95.1)
     mesenteric (K55.0-)
     portal (I81)
     pulmonary (I26.-)

I82.0 **Budd-Chiari syndrome** HCC
Hepatic vein thrombosis
DEF: Thrombosis or other obstruction of hepatic veins; symptoms include enlarged liver, extensive collateral vessels, intractable ascites, and severe portal hypertension.

I82.1 **Thrombophlebitis migrans**

√5th **I82.2** **Embolism and thrombosis of vena cava and other thoracic veins**

√6th **I82.21** **Embolism and thrombosis of superior vena cava**

     I82.210 **Acute embolism and thrombosis of superior vena cava** HCC
Embolism and thrombosis of superior vena cava NOS

     I82.211 **Chronic embolism and thrombosis of superior vena cava** HCC

√6th **I82.22** **Embolism and thrombosis of inferior vena cava**

     I82.220 **Acute embolism and thrombosis of inferior vena cava** HCC
Embolism and thrombosis of inferior vena cava NOS

     I82.221 **Chronic embolism and thrombosis of inferior vena cava** HCC

√6th **I82.29** **Embolism and thrombosis of other thoracic veins**
Embolism and thrombosis of brachiocephalic (innominate) vein

     I82.290 **Acute embolism and thrombosis of other thoracic veins** HCC

     I82.291 **Chronic embolism and thrombosis of other thoracic veins** HCC

I82.3 **Embolism and thrombosis of renal vein** HCC

√5th **I82.4** **Acute embolism and thrombosis of deep veins of lower extremity**

√6th **I82.40** **Acute embolism and thrombosis of unspecified deep veins of lower extremity**
Deep vein thrombosis NOS
DVT NOS
EXCLUDES 1   acute embolism and thrombosis of unspecified deep veins of distal lower extremity (I82.4Z-)
     acute embolism and thrombosis of unspecified deep veins of proximal lower extremity (I82.4Y-)

     I82.401 **Acute embolism and thrombosis of unspecified deep veins of right lower extremity** HCC ▽

     I82.402 **Acute embolism and thrombosis of unspecified deep veins of left lower extremity** HCC ▽

     I82.403 **Acute embolism and thrombosis of unspecified deep veins of lower extremity, bilateral** HCC ▽

     I82.409 **Acute embolism and thrombosis of unspecified deep veins of unspecified lower extremity** HCC ▽

√6th **I82.41** **Acute embolism and thrombosis of femoral vein**

     I82.411 **Acute embolism and thrombosis of right femoral vein** HCC

     I82.412 **Acute embolism and thrombosis of left femoral vein** HCC

     I82.413 **Acute embolism and thrombosis of femoral vein, bilateral** HCC

     I82.419 **Acute embolism and thrombosis of unspecified femoral vein** HCC ▽

√6th **I82.42** **Acute embolism and thrombosis of iliac vein**

     I82.421 **Acute embolism and thrombosis of right iliac vein** HCC

     I82.422 **Acute embolism and thrombosis of left iliac vein** HCC

     I82.423 **Acute embolism and thrombosis of iliac vein, bilateral** HCC

     I82.429 **Acute embolism and thrombosis of unspecified iliac vein** HCC ▽

√6th **I82.43** **Acute embolism and thrombosis of popliteal vein**

     I82.431 **Acute embolism and thrombosis of right popliteal vein** HCC

     I82.432 **Acute embolism and thrombosis of left popliteal vein** HCC

     I82.433 **Acute embolism and thrombosis of popliteal vein, bilateral** HCC

     I82.439 **Acute embolism and thrombosis of unspecified popliteal vein** HCC ▽

√6th **I82.44** **Acute embolism and thrombosis of tibial vein**

     I82.441 **Acute embolism and thrombosis of right tibial vein** HCC

     I82.442 **Acute embolism and thrombosis of left tibial vein** HCC

     I82.443 **Acute embolism and thrombosis of tibial vein, bilateral** HCC

     I82.449 **Acute embolism and thrombosis of unspecified tibial vein** HCC ▽

√6th **I82.49** **Acute embolism and thrombosis of other specified deep vein of lower extremity**

     I82.491 **Acute embolism and thrombosis of other specified deep vein of right lower extremity** HCC

     I82.492 **Acute embolism and thrombosis of other specified deep vein of left lower extremity** HCC

     I82.493 **Acute embolism and thrombosis of other specified deep vein of lower extremity, bilateral** HCC

     I82.499 **Acute embolism and thrombosis of other specified deep vein of unspecified lower extremity** HCC

EXCLUDES 1 Not coded here   EXCLUDES 2 Not included here   N Newborn Age: 0   P Pediatric Age: 0-17   M Maternity Age: 12-55   A Adult Age: 15-124

648   ICD-10-CM 2018

✓6ᵗʰ **I82.4Y** **Acute embolism and thrombosis of unspecified deep veins of proximal lower extremity**
　Acute embolism and thrombosis of deep vein of thigh NOS
　Acute embolism and thrombosis of deep vein of upper leg NOS

　I82.4Y1 **Acute embolism and thrombosis of** HCC ▽ **unspecified deep veins of right proximal lower extremity**

　I82.4Y2 **Acute embolism and thrombosis of** HCC ▽ **unspecified deep veins of left proximal lower extremity**

　I82.4Y3 **Acute embolism and thrombosis of** HCC ▽ **unspecified deep veins of proximal lower extremity, bilateral**

　I82.4Y9 **Acute embolism and thrombosis of** HCC ▽ **unspecified deep veins of unspecified proximal lower extremity**

✓6ᵗʰ **I82.4Z** **Acute embolism and thrombosis of unspecified deep veins of distal lower extremity**
　Acute embolism and thrombosis of deep vein of calf NOS
　Acute embolism and thrombosis of deep vein of lower leg NOS

　I82.4Z1 **Acute embolism and thrombosis of** HCC ▽ **unspecified deep veins of right distal lower extremity**

　I82.4Z2 **Acute embolism and thrombosis of** HCC ▽ **unspecified deep veins of left distal lower extremity**

　I82.4Z3 **Acute embolism and thrombosis of** HCC ▽ **unspecified deep veins of distal lower extremity, bilateral**

　I82.4Z9 **Acute embolism and thrombosis of** HCC ▽ **unspecified deep veins of unspecified distal lower extremity**

✓5ᵗʰ **I82.5** **Chronic embolism and thrombosis of deep veins of lower extremity**
　Use additional code, if applicable, for associated long-term (current) use of anticoagulants (Z79.01)
　EXCLUDES 1 personal history of venous embolism and thrombosis (Z86.718)

✓6ᵗʰ **I82.50** **Chronic embolism and thrombosis of unspecified deep veins of lower extremity**
　EXCLUDES 1 chronic embolism and thrombosis of unspecified deep veins of distal lower extremity (I82.5Z-)
　chronic embolism and thrombosis of unspecified deep veins of proximal lower extremity (I82.5Y-)

　I82.501 **Chronic embolism and thrombosis** HCC ▽ **of unspecified deep veins of right lower extremity**

　I82.502 **Chronic embolism and thrombosis** HCC ▽ **of unspecified deep veins of left lower extremity**

　I82.503 **Chronic embolism and thrombosis** HCC ▽ **of unspecified deep veins of lower extremity, bilateral**

　I82.509 **Chronic embolism and thrombosis** HCC ▽ **of unspecified deep veins of unspecified lower extremity**

✓6ᵗʰ **I82.51** **Chronic embolism and thrombosis of femoral vein**

　I82.511 **Chronic embolism and thrombosis of** HCC **right femoral vein**

　I82.512 **Chronic embolism and thrombosis of** HCC **left femoral vein**

　I82.513 **Chronic embolism and thrombosis of** HCC **femoral vein, bilateral**

　I82.519 **Chronic embolism and thrombosis** HCC ▽ **of unspecified femoral vein**

✓6ᵗʰ **I82.52** **Chronic embolism and thrombosis of iliac vein**

　I82.521 **Chronic embolism and thrombosis of** HCC **right iliac vein**

　I82.522 **Chronic embolism and thrombosis of** HCC **left iliac vein**

　I82.523 **Chronic embolism and thrombosis of** HCC **iliac vein, bilateral**

　I82.529 **Chronic embolism and thrombosis** HCC ▽ **of unspecified iliac vein**

✓6ᵗʰ **I82.53** **Chronic embolism and thrombosis of popliteal vein**

　I82.531 **Chronic embolism and thrombosis of** HCC **right popliteal vein**

　I82.532 **Chronic embolism and thrombosis of** HCC **left popliteal vein**

　I82.533 **Chronic embolism and thrombosis of** HCC **popliteal vein, bilateral**

　I82.539 **Chronic embolism and thrombosis** HCC ▽ **of unspecified popliteal vein**

✓6ᵗʰ **I82.54** **Chronic embolism and thrombosis of tibial vein**

　I82.541 **Chronic embolism and thrombosis of** HCC **right tibial vein**

　I82.542 **Chronic embolism and thrombosis of** HCC **left tibial vein**

　I82.543 **Chronic embolism and thrombosis of** HCC **tibial vein, bilateral**

　I82.549 **Chronic embolism and thrombosis** HCC ▽ **of unspecified tibial vein**

✓6ᵗʰ **I82.59** **Chronic embolism and thrombosis of other specified deep vein of lower extremity**

　I82.591 **Chronic embolism and thrombosis of** HCC **other specified deep vein of right lower extremity**

　I82.592 **Chronic embolism and thrombosis of** HCC **other specified deep vein of left lower extremity**

　I82.593 **Chronic embolism and thrombosis of** HCC **other specified deep vein of lower extremity, bilateral**

　I82.599 **Chronic embolism and thrombosis** HCC ▽ **of other specified deep vein of unspecified lower extremity**

✓6ᵗʰ **I82.5Y** **Chronic embolism and thrombosis of unspecified deep veins of proximal lower extremity**
　Chronic embolism and thrombosis of deep veins of thigh NOS
　Chronic embolism and thrombosis of deep veins of upper leg NOS

　I82.5Y1 **Chronic embolism and thrombosis** HCC ▽ **of unspecified deep veins of right proximal lower extremity**

　I82.5Y2 **Chronic embolism and thrombosis** HCC ▽ **of unspecified deep veins of left proximal lower extremity**

　I82.5Y3 **Chronic embolism and thrombosis** HCC ▽ **of unspecified deep veins of proximal lower extremity, bilateral**

　I82.5Y9 **Chronic embolism and thrombosis** HCC ▽ **of unspecified deep veins of unspecified proximal lower extremity**

✓6ᵗʰ **I82.5Z** **Chronic embolism and thrombosis of unspecified deep veins of distal lower extremity**
　Chronic embolism and thrombosis of deep veins of calf NOS
　Chronic embolism and thrombosis of deep veins of lower leg NOS

　I82.5Z1 **Chronic embolism and thrombosis** HCC ▽ **of unspecified deep veins of right distal lower extremity**

　I82.5Z2 **Chronic embolism and thrombosis** HCC ▽ **of unspecified deep veins of left distal lower extremity**

　I82.5Z3 **Chronic embolism and thrombosis** HCC ▽ **of unspecified deep veins of distal lower extremity, bilateral**

　I82.5Z9 **Chronic embolism and thrombosis** HCC ▽ **of unspecified deep veins of unspecified distal lower extremity**

✓5ᵗʰ **I82.6** **Acute embolism and thrombosis of veins of upper extremity**

✓6ᵗʰ **I82.60** **Acute embolism and thrombosis of unspecified veins of upper extremity**

　I82.601 **Acute embolism and thrombosis of** ▽ **unspecified veins of right upper extremity**

　I82.602 **Acute embolism and thrombosis of** ▽ **unspecified veins of left upper extremity**

　I82.603 **Acute embolism and thrombosis of** ▽ **unspecified veins of upper extremity, bilateral**

☑ Additional Character Req　　✓x7ᵗʰ Placeholder Alert　　Manifestation　　HCC CMS-HCC Condition　　▽ Unspecified Code　　▶◀ Revised Text　　● New Code　　▲ Revised Code Title

ICD-10-CM 2018　　　　　　　　　　　　　　　　649

Chapter 9. Diseases of the Circulatory System

I82.609   Acute embolism and thrombosis of unspecified veins of unspecified upper extremity ▽

✓6th **I82.61**   Acute embolism and thrombosis of superficial veins of upper extremity
Acute embolism and thrombosis of antecubital vein
Acute embolism and thrombosis of basilic vein
Acute embolism and thrombosis of cephalic vein

I82.611   Acute embolism and thrombosis of superficial veins of right upper extremity

I82.612   Acute embolism and thrombosis of superficial veins of left upper extremity

I82.613   Acute embolism and thrombosis of superficial veins of upper extremity, bilateral

I82.619   Acute embolism and thrombosis of superficial veins of unspecified upper extremity ▽

✓6th **I82.62**   Acute embolism and thrombosis of deep veins of upper extremity
Acute embolism and thrombosis of brachial vein
Acute embolism and thrombosis of radial vein
Acute embolism and thrombosis of ulnar vein

I82.621   Acute embolism and thrombosis of deep veins of right upper extremity   HCC

I82.622   Acute embolism and thrombosis of deep veins of left upper extremity   HCC

I82.623   Acute embolism and thrombosis of deep veins of upper extremity, bilateral   HCC

I82.629   Acute embolism and thrombosis of deep veins of unspecified upper extremity   HCC ▽

✓5th **I82.7**   Chronic embolism and thrombosis of veins of upper extremity
Use additional code, if applicable, for associated long-term (current) use of anticoagulants (Z79.01)
    EXCLUDES 1   personal history of venous embolism and thrombosis (Z86.718)

✓6th **I82.70**   Chronic embolism and thrombosis of unspecified veins of upper extremity

I82.701   Chronic embolism and thrombosis of unspecified veins of right upper extremity ▽

I82.702   Chronic embolism and thrombosis of unspecified veins of left upper extremity ▽

I82.703   Chronic embolism and thrombosis of unspecified veins of upper extremity, bilateral ▽

I82.709   Chronic embolism and thrombosis of unspecified veins of unspecified upper extremity ▽

✓6th **I82.71**   Chronic embolism and thrombosis of superficial veins of upper extremity
Chronic embolism and thrombosis of antecubital vein
Chronic embolism and thrombosis of basilic vein
Chronic embolism and thrombosis of cephalic vein

I82.711   Chronic embolism and thrombosis of superficial veins of right upper extremity

I82.712   Chronic embolism and thrombosis of superficial veins of left upper extremity

I82.713   Chronic embolism and thrombosis of superficial veins of upper extremity, bilateral

I82.719   Chronic embolism and thrombosis of superficial veins of unspecified upper extremity ▽

✓6th **I82.72**   Chronic embolism and thrombosis of deep veins of upper extremity
Chronic embolism and thrombosis of brachial vein
Chronic embolism and thrombosis of radial vein
Chronic embolism and thrombosis of ulnar vein

I82.721   Chronic embolism and thrombosis of deep veins of right upper extremity   HCC

I82.722   Chronic embolism and thrombosis of deep veins of left upper extremity   HCC

I82.723   Chronic embolism and thrombosis of deep veins of upper extremity, bilateral   HCC

I82.729   Chronic embolism and thrombosis of deep veins of unspecified upper extremity   HCC ▽

✓5th **I82.A**   Embolism and thrombosis of axillary vein

✓6th **I82.A1**   Acute embolism and thrombosis of axillary vein

I82.A11   Acute embolism and thrombosis of right axillary vein   HCC

I82.A12   Acute embolism and thrombosis of left axillary vein   HCC

I82.A13   Acute embolism and thrombosis of axillary vein, bilateral   HCC

I82.A19   Acute embolism and thrombosis of unspecified axillary vein   HCC ▽

✓6th **I82.A2**   Chronic embolism and thrombosis of axillary vein

I82.A21   Chronic embolism and thrombosis of right axillary vein   HCC

I82.A22   Chronic embolism and thrombosis of left axillary vein   HCC

I82.A23   Chronic embolism and thrombosis of axillary vein, bilateral   HCC

I82.A29   Chronic embolism and thrombosis of unspecified axillary vein   HCC ▽

✓5th **I82.B**   Embolism and thrombosis of subclavian vein

✓6th **I82.B1**   Acute embolism and thrombosis of subclavian vein

I82.B11   Acute embolism and thrombosis of right subclavian vein   HCC

I82.B12   Acute embolism and thrombosis of left subclavian vein   HCC

I82.B13   Acute embolism and thrombosis of subclavian vein, bilateral

I82.B19   Acute embolism and thrombosis of unspecified subclavian vein   HCC ▽

✓6th **I82.B2**   Chronic embolism and thrombosis of subclavian vein

I82.B21   Chronic embolism and thrombosis of right subclavian vein   HCC

I82.B22   Chronic embolism and thrombosis of left subclavian vein   HCC

I82.B23   Chronic embolism and thrombosis of subclavian vein, bilateral   HCC

I82.B29   Chronic embolism and thrombosis of unspecified subclavian vein   HCC ▽

✓5th **I82.C**   Embolism and thrombosis of internal jugular vein

✓6th **I82.C1**   Acute embolism and thrombosis of internal jugular vein

I82.C11   Acute embolism and thrombosis of right internal jugular vein   HCC

I82.C12   Acute embolism and thrombosis of left internal jugular vein   HCC

I82.C13   Acute embolism and thrombosis of internal jugular vein, bilateral   HCC

I82.C19   Acute embolism and thrombosis of unspecified internal jugular vein   HCC ▽

✓6th **I82.C2**   Chronic embolism and thrombosis of internal jugular vein

I82.C21   Chronic embolism and thrombosis of right internal jugular vein   HCC

I82.C22   Chronic embolism and thrombosis of left internal jugular vein   HCC

I82.C23   Chronic embolism and thrombosis of internal jugular vein, bilateral   HCC

I82.C29   Chronic embolism and thrombosis of unspecified internal jugular vein   HCC ▽

✓5th **I82.8**   Embolism and thrombosis of other specified veins
Use additional code, if applicable, for associated long-term (current) use of anticoagulants (Z79.01)

✓6th **I82.81**   Embolism and thrombosis of superficial veins of lower extremities
Embolism and thrombosis of saphenous vein (greater) (lesser)

▲   **I82.811**   Embolism and thrombosis of superficial veins of right lower extremity

▲   **I82.812**   Embolism and thrombosis of superficial veins of left lower extremity

I82.813   Embolism and thrombosis of superficial veins of lower extremities, bilateral

▲   **I82.819**   Embolism and thrombosis of superficial veins of unspecified lower extremity ▽

EXCLUDES 1 Not coded here   EXCLUDES 2 Not included here   N Newborn Age: 0   P Pediatric Age: 0-17   M Maternity Age: 12-55   A Adult Age: 15-124

650   ICD-10-CM 2018

I82.609–I82.819

√6th **I82.89** **Embolism and thrombosis of other specified veins**

     I82.890 Acute embolism and thrombosis of other specified veins

     I82.891 Chronic embolism and thrombosis of other specified veins

√5th **I82.9** **Embolism and thrombosis of unspecified vein**

     I82.90 Acute embolism and thrombosis of unspecified vein ▽
         Embolism of vein NOS
         Thrombosis (vein) NOS

     I82.91 Chronic embolism and thrombosis of unspecified vein ▽

√4th **I83** **Varicose veins of lower extremities**
     EXCLUDES 1   varicose veins complicating pregnancy (O22.0-)
                 varicose veins complicating the puerperium (O87.4)

√5th **I83.0** **Varicose veins of lower extremities with ulcer**
     Use additional code to identify severity of ulcer (L97.-)

     √6th **I83.00** Varicose veins of unspecified lower extremity with ulcer

         I83.001 Varicose veins of unspecified lower extremity with ulcer of thigh   HCC A ▽

         I83.002 Varicose veins of unspecified lower extremity with ulcer of calf   HCC A ▽

         I83.003 Varicose veins of unspecified lower extremity with ulcer of ankle   HCC A ▽

         I83.004 Varicose veins of unspecified lower extremity with ulcer of heel and midfoot   HCC A ▽
              Varicose veins of unspecified lower extremity with ulcer of plantar surface of midfoot

         I83.005 Varicose veins of unspecified lower extremity with ulcer other part of foot   HCC A ▽
              Varicose veins of unspecified lower extremity with ulcer of toe

         I83.008 Varicose veins of unspecified lower extremity with ulcer other part of lower leg   HCC A ▽

         I83.009 Varicose veins of unspecified lower extremity with ulcer of unspecified site   HCC A ▽

     √6th **I83.01** Varicose veins of right lower extremity with ulcer

         I83.011 Varicose veins of right lower extremity with ulcer of thigh   HCC A

         I83.012 Varicose veins of right lower extremity with ulcer of calf   HCC A

         I83.013 Varicose veins of right lower extremity with ulcer of ankle   HCC A

         I83.014 Varicose veins of right lower extremity with ulcer of heel and midfoot   HCC A
              Varicose veins of right lower extremity with ulcer of plantar surface of midfoot

         I83.015 Varicose veins of right lower extremity with ulcer other part of foot   HCC A
              Varicose veins of right lower extremity with ulcer of toe

         I83.018 Varicose veins of right lower extremity with ulcer other part of lower leg   HCC A

         I83.019 Varicose veins of right lower extremity with ulcer of unspecified site   HCC A ▽

     √6th **I83.02** Varicose veins of left lower extremity with ulcer

         I83.021 Varicose veins of left lower extremity with ulcer of thigh   HCC A

         I83.022 Varicose veins of left lower extremity with ulcer of calf   HCC A

         I83.023 Varicose veins of left lower extremity with ulcer of ankle   HCC A

         I83.024 Varicose veins of left lower extremity with ulcer of heel and midfoot   HCC A
              Varicose veins of left lower extremity with ulcer of plantar surface of midfoot

         I83.025 Varicose veins of left lower extremity with ulcer other part of foot   HCC A
              Varicose veins of left lower extremity with ulcer of toe

         I83.028 Varicose veins of left lower extremity with ulcer other part of lower leg   HCC A

         I83.029 Varicose veins of left lower extremity with ulcer of unspecified site   HCC A ▽

√5th **I83.1** **Varicose veins of lower extremities with inflammation**

     I83.10 Varicose veins of unspecified lower extremity with inflammation   A ▽

     I83.11 Varicose veins of right lower extremity with inflammation   A

     I83.12 Varicose veins of left lower extremity with inflammation   A

√5th **I83.2** **Varicose veins of lower extremities with both ulcer and inflammation**
     Use additional code to identify severity of ulcer (L97.-)

     √6th **I83.20** Varicose veins of unspecified lower extremity with both ulcer and inflammation

         I83.201 Varicose veins of unspecified lower extremity with both ulcer of thigh and inflammation   HCC A ▽

         I83.202 Varicose veins of unspecified lower extremity with both ulcer of calf and inflammation   HCC A ▽

         I83.203 Varicose veins of unspecified lower extremity with both ulcer of ankle and inflammation   HCC A ▽

         I83.204 Varicose veins of unspecified lower extremity with both ulcer of heel and midfoot and inflammation   HCC A ▽
              Varicose veins of unspecified lower extremity with both ulcer of plantar surface of midfoot and inflammation

         I83.205 Varicose veins of unspecified lower extremity with both ulcer of other part of foot and inflammation   HCC A ▽
              Varicose veins of unspecified lower extremity with both ulcer of toe and inflammation

         I83.208 Varicose veins of unspecified lower extremity with both ulcer of other part of lower extremity and inflammation   HCC A ▽

         I83.209 Varicose veins of unspecified lower extremity with both ulcer of unspecified site and inflammation   HCC A ▽

     √6th **I83.21** Varicose veins of right lower extremity with both ulcer and inflammation

         I83.211 Varicose veins of right lower extremity with both ulcer of thigh and inflammation   HCC A

         I83.212 Varicose veins of right lower extremity with both ulcer of calf and inflammation   HCC A

         I83.213 Varicose veins of right lower extremity with both ulcer of ankle and inflammation   HCC A

         I83.214 Varicose veins of right lower extremity with both ulcer of heel and midfoot and inflammation   HCC A
              Varicose veins of right lower extremity with both ulcer of plantar surface of midfoot and inflammation

         I83.215 Varicose veins of right lower extremity with both ulcer other part of foot and inflammation   HCC A
              Varicose veins of right lower extremity with both ulcer of toe and inflammation

         I83.218 Varicose veins of right lower extremity with both ulcer of other part of lower extremity and inflammation   HCC A

         I83.219 Varicose veins of right lower extremity with both ulcer of unspecified site and inflammation   HCC A ▽

     √6th **I83.22** Varicose veins of left lower extremity with both ulcer and inflammation

         I83.221 Varicose veins of left lower extremity with both ulcer of thigh and inflammation   HCC A

         I83.222 Varicose veins of left lower extremity with both ulcer of calf and inflammation   HCC A

☑ Additional Character Req   √x7th Placeholder Alert   Manifestation   HCC CMS-HCC Condition   ▽ Unspecified Code   ►◄ Revised Text   ● New Code   ▲ Revised Code Title

I83.223 Varicose veins of left lower extremity with both ulcer of ankle and inflammation HCC A

I83.224 Varicose veins of left lower extremity with both ulcer of heel and midfoot and inflammation HCC A
Varicose veins of left lower extremity with both ulcer of plantar surface of midfoot and inflammation

I83.225 Varicose veins of left lower extremity with both ulcer other part of foot and inflammation HCC A
Varicose veins of left lower extremity with both ulcer of toe and inflammation

I83.228 Varicose veins of left lower extremity with both ulcer of other part of lower extremity and inflammation HCC A

I83.229 Varicose veins of left lower extremity with both ulcer of unspecified site and inflammation HCC A ▽

✓5th **I83.8** Varicose veins of lower extremities with other complications

✓6th **I83.81** Varicose veins of lower extremities with pain

▲ **I83.811** Varicose veins of right lower extremity with pain A

▲ **I83.812** Varicose veins of left lower extremity with pain A

I83.813 Varicose veins of bilateral lower extremities with pain A

▲ **I83.819** Varicose veins of unspecified lower extremity with pain A ▽

✓6th **I83.89** Varicose veins of lower extremities with other complications
Varicose veins of lower extremities with edema
Varicose veins of lower extremities with swelling

▲ **I83.891** Varicose veins of right lower extremity with other complications A

▲ **I83.892** Varicose veins of left lower extremity with other complications A

I83.893 Varicose veins of bilateral lower extremities with other complications A

▲ **I83.899** Varicose veins of unspecified lower extremity with other complications A ▽

✓5th **I83.9** Asymptomatic varicose veins of lower extremities
Phlebectasia of lower extremities
Varicose veins of lower extremities
Varix of lower extremities

I83.90 Asymptomatic varicose veins of unspecified lower extremity A ▽
Varicose veins NOS

I83.91 Asymptomatic varicose veins of right lower extremity A

I83.92 Asymptomatic varicose veins of left lower extremity A

I83.93 Asymptomatic varicose veins of bilateral lower extremities A

✓4th **I85** Esophageal varices
Use additional code to identify:
alcohol abuse and dependence (F10.-)

✓5th **I85.0** Esophageal varices
Idiopathic esophageal varices
Primary esophageal varices

I85.00 Esophageal varices without bleeding HCC
Esophageal varices NOS

I85.01 Esophageal varices with bleeding HCC

✓5th **I85.1** Secondary esophageal varices
Esophageal varices secondary to alcoholic liver disease
Esophageal varices secondary to cirrhosis of liver
Esophageal varices secondary to schistosomiasis
Esophageal varices secondary to toxic liver disease
Code first underlying disease

I85.10 Secondary esophageal varices without bleeding HCC

I85.11 Secondary esophageal varices with bleeding HCC

✓4th **I86** Varicose veins of other sites
EXCLUDES 1 varicose veins of unspecified site (I83.9-)
EXCLUDES 2 retinal varices (H35.0-)

I86.0 Sublingual varices
DEF: Distended, tortuous veins beneath tongue.

I86.1 Scrotal varices ♂
Varicocele

I86.2 Pelvic varices

I86.3 Vulval varices ♀
EXCLUDES 1 vulval varices complicating childbirth and the puerperium (O87.8)
vulval varices complicating pregnancy (O22.1-)

I86.4 Gastric varices

I86.8 Varicose veins of other specified sites A
Varicose ulcer of nasal septum

✓4th **I87** Other disorders of veins

✓5th **I87.0** Postthrombotic syndrome
Chronic venous hypertension due to deep vein thrombosis
Postphlebitic syndrome
EXCLUDES 1 chronic venous hypertension without deep vein thrombosis (I87.3-)

✓6th **I87.00** Postthrombotic syndrome without complications
Asymptomatic postthrombotic syndrome

I87.001 Postthrombotic syndrome without complications of right lower extremity

I87.002 Postthrombotic syndrome without complications of left lower extremity

I87.003 Postthrombotic syndrome without complications of bilateral lower extremity

I87.009 Postthrombotic syndrome without complications of unspecified extremity ▽
Postthrombotic syndrome NOS

✓6th **I87.01** Postthrombotic syndrome with ulcer
Use additional code to specify site and severity of ulcer (L97.-)

I87.011 Postthrombotic syndrome with ulcer of right lower extremity HCC

I87.012 Postthrombotic syndrome with ulcer of left lower extremity HCC

I87.013 Postthrombotic syndrome with ulcer of bilateral lower extremity HCC

I87.019 Postthrombotic syndrome with ulcer of unspecified lower extremity HCC ▽

✓6th **I87.02** Postthrombotic syndrome with inflammation

I87.021 Postthrombotic syndrome with inflammation of right lower extremity

I87.022 Postthrombotic syndrome with inflammation of left lower extremity

I87.023 Postthrombotic syndrome with inflammation of bilateral lower extremity

I87.029 Postthrombotic syndrome with inflammation of unspecified lower extremity ▽

✓6th **I87.03** Postthrombotic syndrome with ulcer and inflammation
Use additional code to specify site and severity of ulcer (L97.-)

I87.031 Postthrombotic syndrome with ulcer and inflammation of right lower extremity HCC

I87.032 Postthrombotic syndrome with ulcer and inflammation of left lower extremity HCC

I87.033 Postthrombotic syndrome with ulcer and inflammation of bilateral lower extremity HCC

I87.039 Postthrombotic syndrome with ulcer and inflammation of unspecified lower extremity HCC ▽

✓6th **I87.09** Postthrombotic syndrome with other complications

I87.091 Postthrombotic syndrome with other complications of right lower extremity

I87.092 Postthrombotic syndrome with other complications of left lower extremity

I87.093 Postthrombotic syndrome with other complications of bilateral lower extremity

I87.099 Postthrombotic syndrome with other complications of unspecified lower extremity ▽

I87.1 Compression of vein
Stricture of vein
Vena cava syndrome (inferior) (superior)
EXCLUDES 2 compression of pulmonary vein (I28.8)

I87.2 Venous insufficiency (chronic) (peripheral)
Stasis dermatitis
EXCLUDES 1   stasis dermatitis with varicose veins of lower extremities (I83.1-, I83.2-)
DEF: Insufficient drainage of venous blood in any part of body; results in edema or dermatosis.

✓5ᵗʰ I87.3 Chronic venous hypertension (idiopathic)
Stasis edema
EXCLUDES 1   chronic venous hypertension due to deep vein thrombosis (I87.0-)
varicose veins of lower extremities (I83.-)

✓6ᵗʰ I87.30 Chronic venous hypertension (idiopathic) without complications
Asymptomatic chronic venous hypertension (idiopathic)
I87.301 Chronic venous hypertension (idiopathic) without complications of right lower extremity
I87.302 Chronic venous hypertension (idiopathic) without complications of left lower extremity
I87.303 Chronic venous hypertension (idiopathic) without complications of bilateral lower extremity
I87.309 Chronic venous hypertension (idiopathic) without complications of unspecified lower extremity ▽
Chronic venous hypertension NOS

✓6ᵗʰ I87.31 Chronic venous hypertension (idiopathic) with ulcer
Use additional code to specify site and severity of ulcer (L97.-)
I87.311 Chronic venous hypertension (idiopathic) with ulcer of right lower extremity HCC
I87.312 Chronic venous hypertension (idiopathic) with ulcer of left lower extremity HCC
I87.313 Chronic venous hypertension (idiopathic) with ulcer of bilateral lower extremity HCC
I87.319 Chronic venous hypertension (idiopathic) with ulcer of unspecified lower extremity HCC ▽

✓6ᵗʰ I87.32 Chronic venous hypertension (idiopathic) with inflammation
I87.321 Chronic venous hypertension (idiopathic) with inflammation of right lower extremity
I87.322 Chronic venous hypertension (idiopathic) with inflammation of left lower extremity
I87.323 Chronic venous hypertension (idiopathic) with inflammation of bilateral lower extremity
I87.329 Chronic venous hypertension (idiopathic) with inflammation of unspecified lower extremity ▽

✓6ᵗʰ I87.33 Chronic venous hypertension (idiopathic) with ulcer and inflammation
Use additional code to specify site and severity of ulcer (L97.-)
I87.331 Chronic venous hypertension (idiopathic) with ulcer and inflammation of right lower extremity HCC
I87.332 Chronic venous hypertension (idiopathic) with ulcer and inflammation of left lower extremity HCC
I87.333 Chronic venous hypertension (idiopathic) with ulcer and inflammation of bilateral lower extremity HCC
I87.339 Chronic venous hypertension (idiopathic) with ulcer and inflammation of unspecified lower extremity HCC ▽

✓6ᵗʰ I87.39 Chronic venous hypertension (idiopathic) with other complications
I87.391 Chronic venous hypertension (idiopathic) with other complications of right lower extremity
I87.392 Chronic venous hypertension (idiopathic) with other complications of left lower extremity
I87.393 Chronic venous hypertension (idiopathic) with other complications of bilateral lower extremity
I87.399 Chronic venous hypertension (idiopathic) with other complications of unspecified lower extremity ▽

I87.8 Other specified disorders of veins
Phlebosclerosis
Venofibrosis
I87.9 Disorder of vein, unspecified ▽

✓4ᵗʰ I88 Nonspecific lymphadenitis
EXCLUDES 1   acute lymphadenitis, except mesenteric (L04.-)
enlarged lymph nodes NOS (R59.-)
human immunodeficiency virus [HIV] disease resulting in generalized lymphadenopathy (B20)
I88.0 Nonspecific mesenteric lymphadenitis
Mesenteric lymphadenitis (acute)(chronic)
I88.1 Chronic lymphadenitis, except mesenteric
Adenitis
Lymphadenitis
I88.8 Other nonspecific lymphadenitis
I88.9 Nonspecific lymphadenitis, unspecified ▽
Lymphadenitis NOS

✓4ᵗʰ I89 Other noninfective disorders of lymphatic vessels and lymph nodes
EXCLUDES 1   chylocele, tunica vaginalis (nonfilarial) NOS (N50.89)
enlarged lymph nodes NOS (R59.-)
filarial chylocele (B74.-)
hereditary lymphedema (Q82.0)
I89.0 Lymphedema, not elsewhere classified
Elephantiasis (nonfilarial) NOS
Lymphangiectasis
Obliteration, lymphatic vessel
Praecox lymphedema
Secondary lymphedema
EXCLUDES 1   postmastectomy lymphedema (I97.2)
I89.1 Lymphangitis
Chronic lymphangitis
Lymphangitis NOS
Subacute lymphangitis
EXCLUDES 1   acute lymphangitis (L03.-)
I89.8 Other specified noninfective disorders of lymphatic vessels and lymph nodes
Chylocele (nonfilarial)
Chylous ascites
Chylous cyst
Lipomelanotic reticulosis
Lymph node or vessel fistula
Lymph node or vessel infarction
Lymph node or vessel rupture
I89.9 Noninfective disorder of lymphatic vessels and lymph nodes, unspecified ▽
Disease of lymphatic vessels NOS

Other and unspecified disorders of the circulatory system (I95-I99)

✓4ᵗʰ I95 Hypotension
EXCLUDES 1   cardiovascular collapse (R57.9)
maternal hypotension syndrome (O26.5-)
nonspecific low blood pressure reading NOS (R03.1)
I95.0 Idiopathic hypotension
I95.1 Orthostatic hypotension
Hypotension, postural
EXCLUDES 1   neurogenic orthostatic hypotension [Shy-Drager] (G90.3)
orthostatic hypotension due to drugs (I95.2)
I95.2 Hypotension due to drugs
Orthostatic hypotension due to drugs
Use additional code for adverse effect, if applicable, to identify drug (T36-T50 with fifth or sixth character 5)
I95.3 Hypotension of hemodialysis
Intra-dialytic hypotension
✓5ᵗʰ I95.8 Other hypotension
I95.81 Postprocedural hypotension
I95.89 Other hypotension
Chronic hypotension
I95.9 Hypotension, unspecified ▽

☑ Additional Character Req   ✔x7ᵗʰ Placeholder Alert   Manifestation   HCC CMS-HCC Condition   ▽ Unspecified Code   ▶◀ Revised Text   ● New Code   ▲ Revised Code Title

I96   Gangrene, not elsewhere classified   HCC
Gangrenous cellulitis
EXCLUDES 1   gangrene in atherosclerosis of native arteries of the extremities (I70.26)
~~gangrene in diabetes mellitus (E08-E13 with .52)~~
gangrene in hernia (K40.1, K40.4, K41.1, K41.4, K42.1, K43.1-, K44.1, K45.1, K46.1)
gangrene in other peripheral vascular diseases (I73.-)
gangrene of certain specified sites—see Alphabetical Index
gas gangrene (A48.0)
pyoderma gangrenosum (L88)
EXCLUDES 2 ▶gangrene in diabetes mellitus (E08-E13 with .52)◄
AHA: 2013, 2Q, 34

✓4th I97   Intraoperative and postprocedural complications and disorders of circulatory system, not elsewhere classified
EXCLUDES 2   postprocedural shock (T81.1-)

I97.0   Postcardiotomy syndrome

✓5th I97.1   Other postprocedural cardiac functional disturbances
EXCLUDES 2   acute pulmonary insufficiency following thoracic surgery (J95.1)
intraoperative cardiac functional disturbances (I97.7-)

    ✓6th I97.11   Postprocedural cardiac insufficiency
      I97.110   Postprocedural cardiac insufficiency following cardiac surgery
      I97.111   Postprocedural cardiac insufficiency following other surgery

    ✓6th I97.12   Postprocedural cardiac arrest
      I97.120   Postprocedural cardiac arrest following cardiac surgery
      I97.121   Postprocedural cardiac arrest following other surgery

    ✓6th I97.13   Postprocedural heart failure
      Use additional code to identify the heart failure (I50.-)
      I97.130   Postprocedural heart failure following cardiac surgery
      I97.131   Postprocedural heart failure following other surgery

    ✓6th I97.19   Other postprocedural cardiac functional disturbances
      Use additional code, if applicable, to further specify disorder
      I97.190   Other postprocedural cardiac functional disturbances following cardiac surgery
       ▶Use additional code, if applicable, for type 4 or type 5 myocardial infarction, to further specify disorder◄
      I97.191   Other postprocedural cardiac functional disturbances following other surgery

I97.2   Postmastectomy lymphedema syndrome   A
Elephantiasis due to mastectomy
Obliteration of lymphatic vessels

I97.3   Postprocedural hypertension

✓5th I97.4   Intraoperative hemorrhage and hematoma of a circulatory system organ or structure complicating a procedure
EXCLUDES 1   intraoperative hemorrhage and hematoma of a circulatory system organ or structure due to accidental puncture and laceration during a procedure (I97.5-)
EXCLUDES 2   intraoperative cerebrovascular hemorrhage complicating a procedure (G97.3-)

    ✓6th I97.41   Intraoperative hemorrhage and hematoma of a circulatory system organ or structure complicating a circulatory system procedure
      I97.410   Intraoperative hemorrhage and hematoma of a circulatory system organ or structure complicating a cardiac catheterization
      I97.411   Intraoperative hemorrhage and hematoma of a circulatory system organ or structure complicating a cardiac bypass
      I97.418   Intraoperative hemorrhage and hematoma of a circulatory system organ or structure complicating other circulatory system procedure
    I97.42   Intraoperative hemorrhage and hematoma of a circulatory system organ or structure complicating other procedure

✓5th I97.5   Accidental puncture and laceration of a circulatory system organ or structure during a procedure
EXCLUDES 2   accidental puncture and laceration of brain during a procedure (G97.4-)

    I97.51   Accidental puncture and laceration of a circulatory system organ or structure during a circulatory system procedure
    I97.52   Accidental puncture and laceration of a circulatory system organ or structure during other procedure

✓5th I97.6   Postprocedural hemorrhage, hematoma and seroma of a circulatory system organ or structure following a procedure
EXCLUDES 2   postprocedural cerebrovascular hemorrhage complicating a procedure (G97.5-)

    ✓6th I97.61   Postprocedural hemorrhage of a circulatory system organ or structure following a circulatory system procedure
      I97.610   Postprocedural hemorrhage of a circulatory system organ or structure following a cardiac catheterization
      I97.611   Postprocedural hemorrhage of a circulatory system organ or structure following cardiac bypass
      I97.618   Postprocedural hemorrhage of a circulatory system organ or structure following other circulatory system procedure

    ✓6th I97.62   Postprocedural hemorrhage, hematoma and seroma of a circulatory system organ or structure following other procedure
      I97.620   Postprocedural hemorrhage of a circulatory system organ or structure following other procedure
      I97.621   Postprocedural hematoma of a circulatory system organ or structure following other procedure
      I97.622   Postprocedural seroma of a circulatory system organ or structure following procedure

    ✓6th I97.63   Postprocedural hematoma of a circulatory system organ or structure following a circulatory system procedure
      I97.630   Postprocedural hematoma of a circulatory system organ or structure following a cardiac catheterization
      I97.631   Postprocedural hematoma of a circulatory system organ or structure following cardiac bypass
      I97.638   Postprocedural hematoma of a circulatory system organ or structure following other circulatory system procedure

    ✓6th I97.64   Postprocedural seroma of a circulatory system organ or structure following a circulatory system procedure
      I97.640   Postprocedural seroma of a circulatory system organ or structure following a cardiac catheterization
      I97.641   Postprocedural seroma of a circulatory system organ or structure following cardiac bypass
      I97.648   Postprocedural seroma of a circulatory system organ or structure following other circulatory system procedure

✓5th I97.7   Intraoperative cardiac functional disturbances
EXCLUDES 2   acute pulmonary insufficiency following thoracic surgery (J95.1)
postprocedural cardiac functional disturbances (I97.1-)

    ✓6th I97.71   Intraoperative cardiac arrest
      I97.710   Intraoperative cardiac arrest during cardiac surgery
      I97.711   Intraoperative cardiac arrest during other surgery

    ✓6th I97.79   Other intraoperative cardiac functional disturbances
      Use additional code, if applicable, to further specify disorder
      I97.790   Other intraoperative cardiac functional disturbances during cardiac surgery
      I97.791   Other intraoperative cardiac functional disturbances during other surgery

EXCLUDES 1 Not coded here   EXCLUDES 2 Not included here   N Newborn Age: 0   P Pediatric Age: 0-17   M Maternity Age: 12-55   A Adult Age: 15-124

654   ICD-10-CM 2018

✓5th **I97.8**   **Other intraoperative and postprocedural complications and disorders of the circulatory system, not elsewhere classified**
      Use additional code, if applicable, to further specify disorder

    ✓6th **I97.81**   **Intraoperative cerebrovascular infarction**

        I97.810   **Intraoperative cerebrovascular infarction during cardiac surgery** HCC

        I97.811   **Intraoperative cerebrovascular infarction during other surgery** HCC

    ✓6th **I97.82**   **Postprocedural cerebrovascular infarction**

        I97.820   **Postprocedural cerebrovascular infarction following cardiac surgery** HCC

        I97.821   **Postprocedural cerebrovascular infarction following other surgery** HCC

    I97.88   **Other intraoperative complications of the circulatory system, not elsewhere classified**

    I97.89   **Other postprocedural complications and disorders of the circulatory system, not elsewhere classified**

✓4th **I99**   **Other and unspecified disorders of circulatory system**

    I99.8   **Other disorder of circulatory system**

    I99.9   **Unspecified disorder of circulatory system**   ▽

Chapter 10. Diseases of the Respiratory System (JØØ–J99)

Chapter Specific Guidelines with Coding Examples

The chapter specific guidelines from the ICD-10-CM Official Guidelines for Coding and Reporting have been provided below. Along with these guidelines are coding examples, contained in the shaded boxes, that have been developed to help illustrate the coding and/or sequencing guidance found in these guidelines.

a. Chronic obstructive pulmonary disease [COPD] and asthma

1) Acute exacerbation of chronic obstructive bronchitis and asthma

The codes in categories J44 and J45 distinguish between uncomplicated cases and those in acute exacerbation. An acute exacerbation is a worsening or a decompensation of a chronic condition. An acute exacerbation is not equivalent to an infection superimposed on a chronic condition, though an exacerbation may be triggered by an infection.

Acute streptococcal bronchitis with acute exacerbation of COPD

J20.2   **Acute bronchitis due to streptococcus**

J44.0   **Chronic obstructive pulmonary disease with acute lower respiratory infection**

J44.1   **Chronic obstructive pulmonary disease with (acute) exacerbation**

Explanation: ICD-10-CM uses combination codes to create organism-specific classifications for acute bronchitis. Category J44 codes include combination codes with severity components, which differentiate between COPD with acute lower respiratory infection (acute bronchitis), COPD with acute exacerbation, and COPD without mention of a complication (unspecified).

An acute exacerbation is a worsening or a decompensation of a chronic condition. An acute exacerbation is not equivalent to an infection superimposed on a chronic condition, though an exacerbation may be triggered by an infection, as in this example.

Exacerbation of moderate persistent asthma with status asthmaticus

J45.42   **Moderate persistent asthma with status asthmaticus**

Explanation: Category J45 Asthma includes severity-specific subcategories and fifth-character codes to distinguish between uncomplicated cases, those in acute exacerbation, and those with status asthmaticus.

---

b. Acute respiratory failure

1) Acute respiratory failure as principal diagnosis

A code from subcategory J96.0, Acute respiratory failure, or subcategory J96.2, Acute and chronic respiratory failure, may be assigned as a principal diagnosis when it is the condition established after study to be chiefly responsible for occasioning the admission to the hospital, and the selection is supported by the Alphabetic Index and Tabular List. However, chapter-specific coding guidelines (such as obstetrics, poisoning, HIV, newborn) that provide sequencing direction take precedence.

Acute hypoxic respiratory failure due to exacerbation of chronic obstructive bronchitis

J96.01   **Acute respiratory failure with hypoxia**

J44.1   **Chronic obstructive pulmonary disease with (acute) exacerbation**

Explanation: Category J96 classifies respiratory failure with combination codes that designate the severity and the presence of hypoxia and hypercapnia. Code J96.01 is sequenced as the first-listed diagnosis, as the reason for the encounter. Respiratory failure may be assigned as a principal diagnosis when it is the condition established after study to be chiefly responsible for occasioning the encounter and the selection is supported by the Alphabetic Index and Tabular List.

---

2) Acute respiratory failure as secondary diagnosis

Respiratory failure may be listed as a secondary diagnosis if it occurs after admission, or if it is present on admission, but does not meet the definition of principal diagnosis.

Acute respiratory failure due to accidental oxycodone overdose

T40.2X1A   **Poisoning by other opioids, accidental (unintentional), initial encounter**

J96.00   **Acute respiratory failure, unspecified whether with hypoxia or hypercapnia**

Explanation: Respiratory failure may be assigned as a principal diagnosis when it is the condition established after study to be chiefly responsible for occasioning the encounter, and the selection is supported by the Alphabetic Index and Tabular List. However, chapter-specific coding guidelines, such as poisoning, that provide sequencing direction take precedence. When coding a poisoning or reaction to the improper use of a medication (e.g. overdose, wrong substance given or taken in error, wrong route of administration), first assign the appropriate code from categories T36–T50. Use additional code(s) for all manifestations of the poisoning. In this instance, the respiratory failure is a manifestation of the poisoning and is sequenced as a secondary diagnosis.

---

3) Sequencing of acute respiratory failure and another acute condition

When a patient is admitted with respiratory failure and another acute condition, (e.g., myocardial infarction, cerebrovascular accident, aspiration pneumonia), the principal diagnosis will not be the same in every situation. This applies whether the other acute condition is a respiratory or nonrespiratory condition. Selection of the principal diagnosis will be dependent on the circumstances of admission. If both the respiratory failure and the other acute condition are equally responsible for occasioning the admission to the hospital, and there are no chapter-specific sequencing rules, the guideline regarding two or more diagnoses that equally meet the definition for principal diagnosis (*Section II, C.*) may be applied in these situations.

If the documentation is not clear as to whether acute respiratory failure and another condition are equally responsible for occasioning the admission, query the provider for clarification.

Patient presents with acute pneumococcal pneumonia and acute respiratory failure

J96.00   **Acute respiratory failure, unspecified whether with hypoxia or hypercapnia**

J13   **Pneumonia due to Streptococcus pneumoniae**

Explanation: When a patient is seen for respiratory failure and another acute condition, such as a bacterial pneumonia, the principal or first-listed diagnosis is not the same in every situation. This applies whether the other acute condition is a respiratory or nonrespiratory condition. The principal diagnosis depends on the problem chiefly responsible for the encounter.

---

c. Influenza due to certain identified influenza viruses

Code only confirmed cases of influenza due to certain identified influenza viruses (category J09), and due to other identified influenza virus (category J10). This is an exception to the hospital inpatient guideline Section II, H. (Uncertain Diagnosis).

In this context, "confirmation" does not require documentation of positive laboratory testing specific for avian or other novel influenza A or other identified influenza virus. However, coding should be based on the provider's diagnostic statement that the patient has avian influenza, or other novel influenza A, for category J09, or has another particular identified strain of influenza, such as H1N1 or H3N2, but not identified as novel or variant, for category J10.

If the provider records "suspected" or "possible" or "probable" avian influenza, or novel influenza, or other identified influenza, then the appropriate influenza code from category J11, Influenza due to unidentified influenza virus, should be assigned. A code from category J09, Influenza due to certain identified influenza viruses, should not be assigned nor should a code from category J10, Influenza due to other identified influenza virus.

Influenza due to avian influenza virus with pneumonia

J09.X1   Influenza due to identified novel influenza A virus with pneumonia

Explanation: Codes in category J09 Influenza due to certain identified influenza viruses should be assigned only for confirmed cases. "Confirmation" does not require positive laboratory testing of a specific influenza virus but does need to be based on the provider's diagnostic statement, which should not include terms such as "possible," "probable," or "suspected."

d. Ventilator associated pneumonia

1) Documentation of ventilator associated pneumonia

As with all procedural or postprocedural complications, code assignment is based on the provider's documentation of the relationship between the condition and the procedure.

Code J95.851, Ventilator associated pneumonia, should be assigned only when the provider has documented ventilator associated pneumonia (VAP). An additional code to identify the organism (e.g., Pseudomonas aeruginosa, code B96.5) should also be assigned. Do not assign an additional code from categories J12-J18 to identify the type of pneumonia.

Code J95.851 should not be assigned for cases where the patient has pneumonia and is on a mechanical ventilator and the provider has not specifically stated that the pneumonia is ventilator-associated pneumonia. If the documentation is unclear as to whether the patient has a pneumonia that is a complication attributable to the mechanical ventilator, query the provider.

2) Ventilator associated pneumonia develops after admission

A patient may be admitted with one type of pneumonia (e.g., code J13, Pneumonia due to Streptococcus pneumonia) and subsequently develop VAP. In this instance, the principal diagnosis would be the appropriate code from categories J12-J18 for the pneumonia diagnosed at the time of admission. Code J95.851, Ventilator associated pneumonia, would be assigned as an additional diagnosis when the provider has also documented the presence of ventilator associated pneumonia.

Chapter 10. Diseases of the Respiratory System (J00-J99)

NOTE   When a respiratory condition is described as occurring in more than one site and is not specifically indexed, it should be classified to the lower anatomic site (e.g. tracheobronchitis to bronchitis in J40).

Use additional code, where applicable, to identify:
exposure to environmental tobacco smoke (Z77.22)
exposure to tobacco smoke in the perinatal period (P96.81)
history of tobacco dependence (Z87.891)
occupational exposure to environmental tobacco smoke (Z57.31)
tobacco dependence (F17.-)
tobacco use (Z72.0)

EXCLUDES 2   *certain conditions originating in the perinatal period (P04-P96)*
certain infectious and parasitic diseases (A00-B99)
complications of pregnancy, childbirth and the puerperium (O00-O9A)
congenital malformations, deformations and chromosomal abnormalities (Q00-Q99)
endocrine, nutritional and metabolic diseases (E00-E88)
injury, poisoning and certain other consequences of external causes (S00-T88)
neoplasms (C00-D49)
smoke inhalation (T59.81-)
symptoms, signs and abnormal clinical and laboratory findings, not elsewhere classified (R00-R94)

This chapter contains the following blocks:
J00-J06   Acute upper respiratory infections
J09-J18   Influenza and pneumonia
J20-J22   Other acute lower respiratory infections
J30-J39   Other diseases of upper respiratory tract
J40-J47   Chronic lower respiratory diseases
J60-J70   Lung diseases due to external agents
J80-J84   Other respiratory diseases principally affecting the interstitium
J85-J86   Suppurative and necrotic conditions of the lower respiratory tract
J90-J94   Other diseases of the pleura
J95   Intraoperative and postprocedural complications and disorders of respiratory system, not elsewhere classified
J96-J99   Other diseases of the respiratory system

Acute upper respiratory infections (J00-J06)

EXCLUDES 1   *chronic obstructive pulmonary disease with acute lower respiratory infection (J44.0)*
influenza virus with other respiratory manifestations (J09.X2, J10.1, J11.1)

J00   **Acute nasopharyngitis (common cold)**
Acute rhinitis
Coryza (acute)
Infective nasopharyngitis NOS
Infective rhinitis
Nasal catarrh, acute
Nasopharyngitis NOS

EXCLUDES 1   *acute pharyngitis (J02.-)*
acute sore throat NOS (J02.9)
pharyngitis NOS (J02.9)
rhinitis NOS (J31.0)
sore throat NOS (J02.9)

EXCLUDES 2   *allergic rhinitis (J30.1-J30.9)*
chronic pharyngitis (J31.2)
chronic rhinitis (J31.0)
chronic sore throat (J31.2)
nasopharyngitis, chronic (J31.1)
vasomotor rhinitis (J30.0)

DEF: Acute inflammation of mucous membranes; extends from nares to pharynx; characterized by nasal obstruction, sneezing, runny nose, and sore throat.

☑4ᵗʰ J01   **Acute sinusitis**
INCLUDES   acute abscess of sinus
acute empyema of sinus
acute infection of sinus
acute inflammation of sinus
acute suppuration of sinus
Use additional code (B95-B97) to identify infectious agent
EXCLUDES 1   *sinusitis NOS (J32.9)*
EXCLUDES 2   *chronic sinusitis (J32.0-J32.8)*

☑5ᵗʰ J01.0   **Acute maxillary sinusitis**
Acute antritis
    J01.00   **Acute maxillary sinusitis, unspecified** ▽
    J01.01   **Acute recurrent maxillary sinusitis**

☑5ᵗʰ J01.1   **Acute frontal sinusitis**
    J01.10   **Acute frontal sinusitis, unspecified** ▽
    J01.11   **Acute recurrent frontal sinusitis**

☑5ᵗʰ J01.2   **Acute ethmoidal sinusitis**
    J01.20   **Acute ethmoidal sinusitis, unspecified** ▽
    J01.21   **Acute recurrent ethmoidal sinusitis**

☑5ᵗʰ J01.3   **Acute sphenoidal sinusitis**
    J01.30   **Acute sphenoidal sinusitis, unspecified** ▽
    J01.31   **Acute recurrent sphenoidal sinusitis**

☑5ᵗʰ J01.4   **Acute pansinusitis**
    J01.40   **Acute pansinusitis, unspecified** ▽
    J01.41   **Acute recurrent pansinusitis**

☑5ᵗʰ J01.8   **Other acute sinusitis**
    J01.80   **Other acute sinusitis**
       Acute sinusitis involving more than one sinus but not pansinusitis
    J01.81   **Other acute recurrent sinusitis**
       Acute recurrent sinusitis involving more than one sinus but not pansinusitis

☑5ᵗʰ J01.9   **Acute sinusitis, unspecified**
    J01.90   **Acute sinusitis, unspecified** ▽
    J01.91   **Acute recurrent sinusitis, unspecified** ▽

☑4ᵗʰ J02   **Acute pharyngitis**
INCLUDES   acute sore throat
EXCLUDES 1   *acute laryngopharyngitis (J06.0)*
peritonsillar abscess (J36)
pharyngeal abscess (J39.1)
retropharyngeal abscess (J39.0)
EXCLUDES 2   *chronic pharyngitis (J31.2)*

J02.0   **Streptococcal pharyngitis**
Septic pharyngitis
Streptococcal sore throat
EXCLUDES 2   *scarlet fever (A38.-)*

J02.8   **Acute pharyngitis due to other specified organisms**
Use additional code (B95-B97) to identify infectious agent
EXCLUDES 1   *acute pharyngitis due to coxsackie virus (B08.5)*
acute pharyngitis due to gonococcus (A54.5)
acute pharyngitis due to herpes [simplex] virus (B00.2)
acute pharyngitis due to infectious mononucleosis (B27.-)
enteroviral vesicular pharyngitis (B08.5)

J02.9   **Acute pharyngitis, unspecified** ▽
Gangrenous pharyngitis (acute)
Infective pharyngitis (acute) NOS
Pharyngitis (acute) NOS
Sore throat (acute) NOS
Suppurative pharyngitis (acute)
Ulcerative pharyngitis (acute)

☑4ᵗʰ J03   **Acute tonsillitis**
EXCLUDES 1   *acute sore throat (J02.-)*
hypertrophy of tonsils (J35.1)
peritonsillar abscess (J36)
sore throat NOS (J02.9)
streptococcal sore throat (J02.0)
EXCLUDES 2   *chronic tonsillitis (J35.0)*

☑5ᵗʰ J03.0   **Streptococcal tonsillitis**
    J03.00   **Acute streptococcal tonsillitis, unspecified** ▽
    J03.01   **Acute recurrent streptococcal tonsillitis**

☑5ᵗʰ J03.8   **Acute tonsillitis due to other specified organisms**
Use additional code (B95-B97) to identify infectious agent
EXCLUDES 1   *diphtheritic tonsillitis (A36.0)*
herpesviral pharyngotonsillitis (B00.2)
streptococcal tonsillitis (J03.0)
tuberculous tonsillitis (A15.8)
Vincent's tonsillitis (A69.1)
    J03.80   **Acute tonsillitis due to other specified organisms**
    J03.81   **Acute recurrent tonsillitis due to other specified organisms**

☑5ᵗʰ J03.9   **Acute tonsillitis, unspecified**
Follicular tonsillitis (acute)
Gangrenous tonsillitis (acute)
Infective tonsillitis (acute)
Tonsillitis (acute) NOS
Ulcerative tonsillitis (acute)
    J03.90   **Acute tonsillitis, unspecified** ▽
    J03.91   **Acute recurrent tonsillitis, unspecified** ▽

☑ Additional Character Req   ✓7ᵗʰ Placeholder Alert   Manifestation   HCC CMS-HCC Condition   ▽ Unspecified Code   ►◄ Revised Text   ● New Code   ▲ Revised Code Title

ICD-10-CM 2018   **659**

Chapter 10. Diseases of the Respiratory System

J04–J11.00

✓4ᵗʰ **J04 Acute laryngitis and tracheitis**
Use additional code (B95-B97) to identify infectious agent
EXCLUDES 1 *acute obstructive laryngitis [croup] and epiglottitis (J05.-)*
EXCLUDES 2 *laryngismus (stridulus) (J38.5)*

J04.0 Acute laryngitis
Edematous laryngitis (acute)
Laryngitis (acute) NOS
Subglottic laryngitis (acute)
Suppurative laryngitis (acute)
Ulcerative laryngitis (acute)
EXCLUDES 1 *acute obstructive laryngitis (J05.0)*
EXCLUDES 2 *chronic laryngitis (J37.0)*

✓5ᵗʰ **J04.1 Acute tracheitis**
Acute viral tracheitis
Catarrhal tracheitis (acute)
Tracheitis (acute) NOS
EXCLUDES 2 *chronic tracheitis (J42)*

    J04.10 Acute tracheitis without obstruction
    J04.11 Acute tracheitis with obstruction

J04.2 Acute laryngotracheitis
Laryngotracheitis NOS
Tracheitis (acute) with laryngitis (acute)
EXCLUDES 1 *acute obstructive laryngotracheitis (J05.0)*
EXCLUDES 2 *chronic laryngotracheitis (J37.1)*

✓5ᵗʰ **J04.3 Supraglottitis, unspecified**
    J04.30 Supraglottitis, unspecified, without obstruction ▽
    J04.31 Supraglottitis, unspecified, with obstruction ▽

✓4ᵗʰ **J05 Acute obstructive laryngitis [croup] and epiglottitis**
Use additional code (B95-B97) to identify infectious agent

J05.0 Acute obstructive laryngitis [croup]
Obstructive laryngitis (acute) NOS
Obstructive laryngotracheitis NOS
DEF: Acute laryngeal obstruction due to allergy, foreign body, or in the majority of cases a viral infection; symptoms include harsh, barking cough, hoarseness, and persistent high-pitched respiratory sound (stridor).

✓5ᵗʰ **J05.1 Acute epiglottitis**
EXCLUDES 2 *epiglottitis, chronic (J37.0)*

    J05.10 Acute epiglottitis without obstruction
      Epiglottitis NOS
    J05.11 Acute epiglottitis with obstruction

✓4ᵗʰ **J06 Acute upper respiratory infections of multiple and unspecified sites**
EXCLUDES 1 *acute respiratory infection NOS (J22)*
streptococcal pharyngitis (J02.0)3

J06.0 Acute laryngopharyngitis

J06.9 Acute upper respiratory infection, unspecified ▽
Upper respiratory disease, acute
Upper respiratory infection NOS

Influenza and pneumonia (J09-J18)

EXCLUDES 2 *allergic or eosinophilic pneumonia (J82)*
aspiration pneumonia NOS (J69.0)
congenital pneumonia (P23.9)
lipid pneumonia (J69.1)
meconium pneumonia (P24.01)
neonatal aspiration pneumonia (P24.-)
pneumonia due to solids and liquids (J69.-)
rheumatic pneumonia (I00)
ventilator associated pneumonia (J95.851)

✓4ᵗʰ **J09 Influenza due to certain identified influenza viruses**
EXCLUDES 1 ▸*influenza A/H1N1 (J10.-)*◂
influenza due to other identified influenza virus (J10.-)
influenza due to unidentified influenza virus (J11.-)
seasonal influenza due to other identified influenza virus (J10.-)
seasonal influenza due to unidentified influenza virus (J11.-)

✓5ᵗʰ **J09.X Influenza due to identified novel influenza A virus**
Avian influenza
Bird influenza
Influenza A/H5N1
Influenza of other animal origin, not bird or swine
Swine influenza virus (viruses that normally cause infections in pigs)
AHA: 2016, 3Q, 10

    J09.X1 Influenza due to identified novel influenza A virus with pneumonia
Code also, if applicable, associated:
lung abscess (J85.1)
other specified type of pneumonia

    J09.X2 Influenza due to identified novel influenza A virus with other respiratory manifestations
Influenza due to identified novel influenza A virus NOS
Influenza due to identified novel influenza A virus with laryngitis
Influenza due to identified novel influenza A virus with pharyngitis
Influenza due to identified novel influenza A virus with upper respiratory symptoms
Use additional code, if applicable, for associated:
pleural effusion (J91.8)
sinusitis (J01.-)

    J09.X3 Influenza due to identified novel influenza A virus with gastrointestinal manifestations
Influenza due to identified novel influenza A virus gastroenteritis
EXCLUDES 1 *'intestinal flu' [viral gastroenteritis] (A08.-)*

    J09.X9 Influenza due to identified novel influenza A virus with other manifestations
Influenza due to identified novel influenza A virus with encephalopathy
Influenza due to identified novel influenza A virus with myocarditis
Influenza due to identified novel influenza A virus with otitis media
Use additional code to identify manifestation

✓4ᵗʰ **J10 Influenza due to other identified influenza virus**
EXCLUDES 1 *influenza due to avian influenza virus (J09.X-)*
influenza due to swine flu (J09.X-)
influenza due to unidentifed influenza virus (J11.-)

✓5ᵗʰ **J10.0 Influenza due to other identified influenza virus with pneumonia**
Code also associated lung abscess, if applicable (J85.1)

    J10.00 Influenza due to other identified influenza virus with unspecified type of pneumonia ▽

    J10.01 Influenza due to other identified influenza virus with the same other identified influenza virus pneumonia

    J10.08 Influenza due to other identified influenza virus with other specified pneumonia
Code also other specified type of pneumonia

J10.1 Influenza due to other identified influenza virus with other respiratory manifestations
Influenza due to other identified influenza virus NOS
Influenza due to other identified influenza virus with laryngitis
Influenza due to other identified influenza virus with pharyngitis
Influenza due to other identified influenza virus with upper respiratory symptoms
Use additional code for associated pleural effusion, if applicable (J91.8)
Use additional code for associated sinusitis, if applicable (J01.-)
AHA: 2016, 3Q, 10-11

J10.2 Influenza due to other identified influenza virus with gastrointestinal manifestations
Influenza due to other identified influenza virus gastroenteritis
EXCLUDES 1 *'intestinal flu' [viral gastroenteritis] (A08.-)*

✓5ᵗʰ **J10.8 Influenza due to other identified influenza virus with other manifestations**

    J10.81 Influenza due to other identified influenza virus with encephalopathy

    J10.82 Influenza due to other identified influenza virus with myocarditis

    J10.83 Influenza due to other identified influenza virus with otitis media
Use additional code for any associated perforated tympanic membrane (H72.-)

    J10.89 Influenza due to other identified influenza virus with other manifestations
Use additional codes to identify the manifestations

✓4ᵗʰ **J11 Influenza due to unidentified influenza virus**

✓5ᵗʰ **J11.0 Influenza due to unidentified influenza virus with pneumonia**
Code also associated lung abscess, if applicable (J85.1)
AHA: 2016, 3Q, 11

    J11.00 Influenza due to unidentified influenza virus with unspecified type of pneumonia ▽
Influenza with pneumonia NOS

EXCLUDES 1 Not coded here   **EXCLUDES 2** Not included here   N Newborn Age: 0   P Pediatric Age: 0-17   M Maternity Age: 12-55   A Adult Age: 15-124

660   ICD-10-CM 2018

J11.Ø8 Influenza due to unidentified influenza virus with specified pneumonia
Code also other specified type of pneumonia

J11.1 Influenza due to unidentified influenza virus with other respiratory manifestations
Influenza NOS
Influenzal laryngitis NOS
Influenzal pharyngitis NOS
Influenza with upper respiratory symptoms NOS
Use additional code for associated pleural effusion, if applicable (J91.8)
Use additional code for associated sinusitis, if applicable (J01.-)

J11.2 Influenza due to unidentified influenza virus with gastrointestinal manifestations
Influenza gastroenteritis NOS
EXCLUDES 1   'intestinal flu' [viral gastroenteritis] (A08.-)

☑5ᵗʰ **J11.8 Influenza due to unidentified influenza virus with other manifestations**

J11.81 Influenza due to unidentified influenza virus with encephalopathy
Influenzal encephalopathy NOS

J11.82 Influenza due to unidentified influenza virus with myocarditis
Influenzal myocarditis NOS

J11.83 Influenza due to unidentified influenza virus with otitis media
Influenzal otitis media NOS
Use additional code for any associated perforated tympanic membrane (H72.-)

J11.89 Influenza due to unidentified influenza virus with other manifestations
Use additional codes to identify the manifestations

☑4ᵗʰ **J12 Viral pneumonia, not elsewhere classified**
INCLUDES   bronchopneumonia due to viruses other than influenza viruses
Code first associated influenza, if applicable (J09.X1, J10.0-, J11.0-)
Code also associated abscess, if applicable (J85.1)
EXCLUDES 1   aspiration pneumonia due to anesthesia during labor and delivery (O74.0)
aspiration pneumonia due to anesthesia during pregnancy (O29)
aspiration pneumonia due to anesthesia during puerperium (O89.0)
aspiration pneumonia due to solids and liquids (J69.-)
aspiration pneumonia NOS (J69.0)
congenital pneumonia (P23.0)
congenital rubella pneumonitis (P35.0)
interstitial pneumonia NOS (J84.9)
lipid pneumonia (J69.1)
neonatal aspiration pneumonia (P24.-)
AHA: 2016, 3Q, 15; 2013, 4Q, 118

J12.Ø Adenoviral pneumonia

J12.1 Respiratory syncytial virus pneumonia

J12.2 Parainfluenza virus pneumonia

J12.3 Human metapneumovirus pneumonia

☑5ᵗʰ **J12.8 Other viral pneumonia**

J12.81 Pneumonia due to SARS-associated coronavirus
Severe acute respiratory syndrome NOS
DEF: A severe adult respiratory syndrome caused by the coronavirus, specified as inflammation of the lungs with consolidation.

J12.89 Other viral pneumonia

J12.9 Viral pneumonia, unspecified ▽

J13 Pneumonia due to Streptococcus pneumoniae HCC
Bronchopneumonia due to S. pneumoniae
Code first associated influenza, if applicable (J09.X1, J10.0-, J11.0-)
Code also associated lung abscess, if applicable (J85.1)
EXCLUDES 1   congenital pneumonia due to S. pneumoniae (P23.6)
lobar pneumonia, unspecified organism (J18.1)
pneumonia due to other streptococci (J15.3-J15.4)
AHA: 2016, 3Q, 15; 2013, 4Q, 118

J14 Pneumonia due to Hemophilus influenzae HCC
Bronchopneumonia due to H. influenzae
Code first associated influenza, if applicable (J09.X1, J10.0-, J11.0-)
Code also associated lung abscess, if applicable (J85.1)
EXCLUDES 1   congenital pneumonia due to H. influenzae (P23.6)
AHA: 2016, 3Q, 15; 2013, 4Q, 118

☑4ᵗʰ **J15 Bacterial pneumonia, not elsewhere classified**
INCLUDES   bronchopneumonia due to bacteria other than S. pneumoniae and H. influenzae
Code first associated influenza, if applicable (J09.X1, J10.0-, J11.0-)
Code also associated lung abscess, if applicable (J85.1)
EXCLUDES 1   chlamydial pneumonia (J16.0)
congenital pneumonia (P23.-)
Legionnaires' disease (A48.1)
spirochetal pneumonia (A69.8)
AHA: 2016, 3Q, 15; 2013, 4Q, 118

J15.Ø Pneumonia due to Klebsiella pneumoniae HCC

J15.1 Pneumonia due to Pseudomonas HCC

☑5ᵗʰ **J15.2 Pneumonia due to staphylococcus**

J15.2Ø Pneumonia due to staphylococcus, unspecified HCC ▽

☑6ᵗʰ **J15.21 Pneumonia due to Staphylococcus aureus**

J15.211 Pneumonia due to Methicillin susceptible Staphylococcus aureus HCC
MSSA pneumonia
Pneumonia due to Staphylococcus aureus NOS

J15.212 Pneumonia due to Methicillin resistant Staphylococcus aureus HCC

J15.29 Pneumonia due to other staphylococcus HCC

J15.3 Pneumonia due to streptococcus, group B HCC

J15.4 Pneumonia due to other streptococci HCC
EXCLUDES 1   pneumonia due to streptococcus, group B (J15.3)
pneumonia due to Streptococcus pneumoniae (J13)

J15.5 Pneumonia due to Escherichia coli HCC

▲ **J15.6 Pneumonia due to other Gram-negative bacteria** HCC
▶Pneumonia due to other aerobic Gram-negative bacteria◀
Pneumonia due to Serratia marcescens

J15.7 Pneumonia due to Mycoplasma pneumoniae

J15.8 Pneumonia due to other specified bacteria HCC

J15.9 Unspecified bacterial pneumonia ▽
Pneumonia due to gram-positive bacteria

☑4ᵗʰ **J16 Pneumonia due to other infectious organisms, not elsewhere classified**
Code first associated influenza, if applicable (J09.X1, J10.0-, J11.0-)
Code also associated lung abscess, if applicable (J85.1)
EXCLUDES 1   congenital pneumonia (P23.-)
ornithosis (A70)
pneumocystosis (B59)
pneumonia NOS (J18.9)
AHA: 2016, 3Q, 15; 2013, 4Q, 118

J16.Ø Chlamydial pneumonia

J16.8 Pneumonia due to other specified infectious organisms

J17   **Pneumonia in diseases classified elsewhere**
Code first underlying disease, such as:
Q fever (A78)
rheumatic fever (I00)
schistosomiasis (B65.0-B65.9)
EXCLUDES 1   candidial pneumonia (B37.1)
chlamydial pneumonia (J16.0)
gonorrheal pneumonia (A54.84)
histoplasmosis pneumonia (B39.0-B39.2)
measles pneumonia (B05.2)
nocardiosis pneumonia (A43.0)
pneumocystosis (B59)
pneumonia due to Pneumocystis carinii (B59)
pneumonia due to Pneumocystis jiroveci (B59)
pneumonia in actinomycosis (A42.0)
pneumonia in anthrax (A22.1)
pneumonia in ascariasis (B77.81)
pneumonia in aspergillosis (B44.0-B44.1)
pneumonia in coccidioidomycosis (B38.0-B38.2)
pneumonia in cytomegalovirus disease (B25.0)
pneumonia in toxoplasmosis (B58.3)
rubella pneumonia (B06.81)
salmonella pneumonia (A02.22)
spirochetal infection NEC with pneumonia (A69.8)
tularemia pneumonia (A21.2)
typhoid fever with pneumonia (A01.03)
varicella pneumonia (B01.2)
whooping cough with pneumonia (A37 with fifth-character 1)
AHA: 2016, 3Q, 15; 2013, 4Q, 118

☑ Additional Character Req   ✓x7ᵗʰ Placeholder Alert   Manifestation   HCC CMS-HCC Condition   ▽ Unspecified Code   ▶◀ Revised Text   ● New Code   ▲ Revised Code Title

✓4ᵗʰ J18   Pneumonia, unspecified organism
Code first associated influenza, if applicable (J09.X1, J10.0-, J11.0-)
> EXCLUDES 1   abscess of lung with pneumonia (J85.1)
> aspiration pneumonia due to anesthesia during labor and delivery (O74.0)
> aspiration pneumonia due to anesthesia during pregnancy (O29)
> aspiration pneumonia due to anesthesia during puerperium (O89.0)
> aspiration pneumonia due to solids and liquids (J69.-)
> aspiration pneumonia NOS (J69.0)
> congenital pneumonia (P23.0)
> drug-induced interstitial lung disorder (J70.2-J70.4)
> interstitial pneumonia NOS (J84.9)
> lipid pneumonia (J69.1)
> neonatal aspiration pneumonia (P24.-)
> pneumonitis due to external agents (J67-J70)
> pneumonitis due to fumes and vapors (J68.0)
> usual interstitial pneumonia (J84.17)

    AHA: 2016, 3Q, 15; 2013, 4Q, 118

    J18.0   Bronchopneumonia, unspecified organism ▽
> EXCLUDES 1   hypostatic bronchopneumonia (J18.2)
> lipid pneumonia (J69.1)
> EXCLUDES 2   acute bronchiolitis (J21.-)
> chronic bronchiolitis (J44.9)

    J18.1   Lobar pneumonia, unspecified organism HCC ▽
    J18.2   Hypostatic pneumonia, unspecified organism ▽
> Hypostatic bronchopneumonia
> Passive pneumonia

    J18.8   Other pneumonia, unspecified organism ▽
    J18.9   Pneumonia, unspecified organism ▽
        AHA: 2014, 3Q, 4; 2013, 4Q, 119; 2012, 4Q, 94

Other acute lower respiratory infections (J20-J22)

> EXCLUDES 2   chronic obstructive pulmonary disease with acute lower respiratory infection (J44.0)

✓4ᵗʰ J20   Acute bronchitis
> INCLUDES   acute and subacute bronchitis (with) bronchospasm
> acute and subacute bronchitis (with) tracheitis
> acute and subacute bronchitis (with) tracheobronchitis, acute
> acute and subacute fibrinous bronchitis
> acute and subacute membranous bronchitis
> acute and subacute purulent bronchitis
> acute and subacute septic bronchitis
> EXCLUDES 1   bronchitis NOS (J40)
> tracheobronchitis NOS (J40)
> EXCLUDES 2   acute bronchitis with bronchiectasis (J47.0)
> acute bronchitis with chronic obstructive asthma (J44.0)
> acute bronchitis with chronic obstructive pulmonary disease (J44.0)
> allergic bronchitis NOS (J45.909)
> bronchitis due to chemicals, fumes and vapors (J68.0)
> chronic bronchitis NOS (J42)
> chronic mucopurulent bronchitis (J41.1)
> chronic obstructive bronchitis (J44.-)
> chronic obstructive tracheobronchitis (J44.-)
> chronic simple bronchitis (J41.0)
> chronic tracheobronchitis (J42)

    AHA: 2016, 3Q, 10, 16
    DEF: Acute inflammation of main branches of bronchial tree due to infectious or irritant agents; symptoms include cough with a varied production of sputum, fever, substernal soreness, and lung rales; usually last for three to 10 days.

    J20.0   Acute bronchitis due to Mycoplasma pneumoniae
    J20.1   Acute bronchitis due to Hemophilus influenzae
    J20.2   Acute bronchitis due to streptococcus
    J20.3   Acute bronchitis due to coxsackievirus
    J20.4   Acute bronchitis due to parainfluenza virus
    J20.5   Acute bronchitis due to respiratory syncytial virus
    J20.6   Acute bronchitis due to rhinovirus
    J20.7   Acute bronchitis due to echovirus
    J20.8   Acute bronchitis due to other specified organisms
    J20.9   Acute bronchitis, unspecified ▽

✓4ᵗʰ J21   Acute bronchiolitis
> Acute bronchiolitis with bronchospasm
> EXCLUDES 2   respiratory bronchiolitis interstitial lung disease (J84.115)

    J21.0   Acute bronchiolitis due to respiratory syncytial virus
    J21.1   Acute bronchiolitis due to human metapneumovirus
    J21.8   Acute bronchiolitis due to other specified organisms

    J21.9   Acute bronchiolitis, unspecified ▽
> Bronchiolitis (acute)
> EXCLUDES 1   chronic bronchiolitis (J44.-)

J22   Unspecified acute lower respiratory infection ▽
> Acute (lower) respiratory (tract) infection NOS
> EXCLUDES 1   upper respiratory infection (acute) (J06.9)

Other diseases of upper respiratory tract (J30-J39)

✓4ᵗʰ J30   Vasomotor and allergic rhinitis
> INCLUDES   spasmodic rhinorrhea
> EXCLUDES 1   allergic rhinitis with asthma (bronchial) (J45.909)
> rhinitis NOS (J31.0)

    J30.0   Vasomotor rhinitis
    J30.1   Allergic rhinitis due to pollen
> Allergy NOS due to pollen
> Hay fever
> Pollinosis

    J30.2   Other seasonal allergic rhinitis
    J30.5   Allergic rhinitis due to food
    ✓5ᵗʰ J30.8   Other allergic rhinitis
        J30.81   Allergic rhinitis due to animal (cat) (dog) hair and dander
        J30.89   Other allergic rhinitis
> Perennial allergic rhinitis

    J30.9   Allergic rhinitis, unspecified ▽

✓4ᵗʰ J31   Chronic rhinitis, nasopharyngitis and pharyngitis
Use additional code to identify:
> exposure to environmental tobacco smoke (Z77.22)
> exposure to tobacco smoke in the perinatal period (P96.81)
> history of tobacco dependence (Z87.891)
> occupational exposure to environmental tobacco smoke (Z57.31)
> tobacco dependence (F17.-)
> tobacco use (Z72.0)

    J31.0   Chronic rhinitis
> Atrophic rhinitis (chronic)
> Granulomatous rhinitis (chronic)
> Hypertrophic rhinitis (chronic)
> Obstructive rhinitis (chronic)
> Ozena
> Purulent rhinitis (chronic)
> Rhinitis (chronic) NOS
> Ulcerative rhinitis (chronic)
> EXCLUDES 1   allergic rhinitis (J30.1-J30.9)
> vasomotor rhinitis (J30.0)
> **DEF:** Persistent inflammation of mucous membranes of nose; characterized by postnasal drip.

    J31.1   Chronic nasopharyngitis
> EXCLUDES 2   acute nasopharyngitis (J00)
> **DEF:** Persistent inflammation of mucous membranes extending from nares to pharynx; characterized by constant irritation in nasopharynx and postnasal drip.

    J31.2   Chronic pharyngitis
> Atrophic pharyngitis (chronic)
> Chronic sore throat
> Granular pharyngitis (chronic)
> Hypertrophic pharyngitis (chronic)
> EXCLUDES 2   acute pharyngitis (J02.9)

✓4ᵗʰ J32   Chronic sinusitis
> INCLUDES   sinus abscess
> sinus empyema
> sinus infection
> sinus suppuration

Use additional code to identify:
> exposure to environmental tobacco smoke (Z77.22)
> exposure to tobacco smoke in the perinatal period (P96.81)
> history of tobacco dependence (Z87.891)
> infectious agent (B95-B97)
> occupational exposure to environmental tobacco smoke (Z57.31)
> tobacco dependence (F17.-)
> tobacco use (Z72.0)
> EXCLUDES 2   acute sinusitis (J01.-)

    J32.0   Chronic maxillary sinusitis
> Antritis (chronic)
> Maxillary sinusitis NOS

    J32.1   Chronic frontal sinusitis
> Frontal sinusitis NOS

    J32.2   Chronic ethmoidal sinusitis
> Ethmoidal sinusitis NOS
> EXCLUDES 1   Woakes' ethmoiditis (J33.1)

J32.3   **Chronic sphenoidal sinusitis**
Sphenoidal sinusitis NOS

J32.4   **Chronic pansinusitis**
Pansinusitis NOS

J32.8   **Other chronic sinusitis**
Sinusitis (chronic) involving more than one sinus but not pansinusitis

J32.9   **Chronic sinusitis, unspecified**   ▽
Sinusitis (chronic) NOS

✓4ᵗʰ **J33**   **Nasal polyp**
Use additional code to identify:
exposure to environmental tobacco smoke (Z77.22)
exposure to tobacco smoke in the perinatal period (P96.81)
history of tobacco dependence (Z87.891)
occupational exposure to environmental tobacco smoke (Z57.31)
tobacco dependence (F17.-)
tobacco use (Z72.0)
EXCLUDES 1   *adenomatous polyps (D14.0)*

J33.0   **Polyp of nasal cavity**
Choanal polyp
Nasopharyngeal polyp

J33.1   **Polypoid sinus degeneration**
Woakes' syndrome or ethmoiditis

J33.8   **Other polyp of sinus**
Accessory polyp of sinus
Ethmoidal polyp of sinus
Maxillary polyp of sinus
Sphenoidal polyp of sinus

J33.9   **Nasal polyp, unspecified**   ▽

✓4ᵗʰ **J34**   **Other and unspecified disorders of nose and nasal sinuses**
EXCLUDES 2   *varicose ulcer of nasal septum (I86.8)*

J34.0   **Abscess, furuncle and carbuncle of nose**
Cellulitis of nose
Necrosis of nose
Ulceration of nose

J34.1   **Cyst and mucocele of nose and nasal sinus**

J34.2   **Deviated nasal septum**
Deflection or deviation of septum (nasal) (acquired)
EXCLUDES 1   *congenital deviated nasal septum (Q67.4)*

J34.3   **Hypertrophy of nasal turbinates**

✓5ᵗʰ **J34.8**   **Other specified disorders of nose and nasal sinuses**

     J34.81   **Nasal mucositis (ulcerative)**
Code also type of associated therapy, such as:
antineoplastic and immunosuppressive drugs (T45.1X-)
radiological procedure and radiotherapy (Y84.2)
EXCLUDES 2   *gastrointestinal mucositis (ulcerative) (K92.81)*
mucositis (ulcerative) of vagina and vulva (N76.81)
oral mucositis (ulcerative) (K12.3-)

     J34.89   **Other specified disorders of nose and nasal sinuses**
Perforation of nasal septum NOS
Rhinolith

J34.9   **Unspecified disorder of nose and nasal sinuses**   ▽

✓4ᵗʰ **J35**   **Chronic diseases of tonsils and adenoids**
Use additional code to identify:
exposure to environmental tobacco smoke (Z77.22)
exposure to tobacco smoke in the perinatal period (P96.81)
history of tobacco dependence (Z87.891)
occupational exposure to environmental tobacco smoke (Z57.31)
tobacco dependence (F17.-)
tobacco use (Z72.0)

✓5ᵗʰ **J35.0**   **Chronic tonsillitis and adenoiditis**
EXCLUDES 2   *acute tonsillitis (J03.-)*

     J35.01   **Chronic tonsillitis**

     J35.02   **Chronic adenoiditis**

     J35.03   **Chronic tonsillitis and adenoiditis**

J35.1   **Hypertrophy of tonsils**
Enlargement of tonsils
EXCLUDES 1   *hypertrophy of tonsils with tonsillitis (J35.0-)*

J35.2   **Hypertrophy of adenoids**
Enlargement of adenoids
EXCLUDES 1   *hypertrophy of adenoids with adenoiditis (J35.0-)*

J35.3   **Hypertrophy of tonsils with hypertrophy of adenoids**
EXCLUDES 1   *hypertrophy of tonsils and adenoids with tonsillitis and adenoiditis (J35.03)*

J35.8   **Other chronic diseases of tonsils and adenoids**
Adenoid vegetations
Amygdalolith
Calculus, tonsil
Cicatrix of tonsil (and adenoid)
Tonsillar tag
Ulcer of tonsil

J35.9   **Chronic disease of tonsils and adenoids, unspecified**   ▽
Disease (chronic) of tonsils and adenoids NOS

J36   **Peritonsillar abscess**
INCLUDES   abscess of tonsil
peritonsillar cellulitis
quinsy
Use additional code (B95-B97) to identify infectious agent
EXCLUDES 1   *acute tonsillitis (J03.-)*
chronic tonsillitis (J35.0)
retropharyngeal abscess (J39.0)
tonsillitis NOS (J03.9-)

✓4ᵗʰ **J37**   **Chronic laryngitis and laryngotracheitis**
Use additional code to identify:
exposure to environmental tobacco smoke (Z77.22)
exposure to tobacco smoke in the perinatal period (P96.81)
history of tobacco dependence (Z87.891)
infectious agent (B95-B97)
occupational exposure to environmental tobacco smoke (Z57.31)
tobacco dependence (F17.-)
tobacco use (Z72.0)

J37.0   **Chronic laryngitis**
Catarrhal laryngitis
Hypertrophic laryngitis
Sicca laryngitis
EXCLUDES 2   *acute laryngitis (J04.0)*
obstructive (acute) laryngitis (J05.0)

J37.1   **Chronic laryngotracheitis**
Laryngitis, chronic, with tracheitis (chronic)
Tracheitis, chronic, with laryngitis
EXCLUDES 1   *chronic tracheitis (J42)*
EXCLUDES 2   *acute laryngotracheitis (J04.2)*
acute tracheitis (J04.1)

✓4ᵗʰ **J38**   **Diseases of vocal cords and larynx, not elsewhere classified**
Use additional code to identify:
exposure to environmental tobacco smoke (Z77.22)
exposure to tobacco smoke in the perinatal period (P96.81)
history of tobacco dependence (Z87.891)
occupational exposure to environmental tobacco smoke (Z57.31)
tobacco dependence (F17.-)
tobacco use (Z72.0)
EXCLUDES 1   *congenital laryngeal stridor (P28.89)*
obstructive laryngitis (acute) (J05.0)
postprocedural subglottic stenosis (J95.5)
stridor (R06.1)
ulcerative laryngitis (J04.0)

✓5ᵗʰ **J38.0**   **Paralysis of vocal cords and larynx**
Laryngoplegia
Paralysis of glottis

     J38.00   **Paralysis of vocal cords and larynx, unspecified**   ▽

     J38.01   **Paralysis of vocal cords and larynx, unilateral**

     J38.02   **Paralysis of vocal cords and larynx, bilateral**

J38.1   **Polyp of vocal cord and larynx**
EXCLUDES 1   *adenomatous polyps (D14.1)*

J38.2   **Nodules of vocal cords**
Chorditis (fibrinous)(nodosa)(tuberosa)
Singer's nodes
Teacher's nodes

J38.3   **Other diseases of vocal cords**
Abscess of vocal cords
Cellulitis of vocal cords
Granuloma of vocal cords
Leukokeratosis of vocal cords
Leukoplakia of vocal cords

J38.4   **Edema of larynx**
Edema (of) glottis
Subglottic edema
Supraglottic edema
EXCLUDES 1   *acute obstructive laryngitis [croup] (J05.0)*
edematous laryngitis (J04.0)

J38.5   **Laryngeal spasm**
Laryngismus (stridulus)

J38.6   **Stenosis of larynx**

☑ Additional Character Req   ✓x7ᵗʰ Placeholder Alert   Manifestation   HCC CMS-HCC Condition   ▽ Unspecified Code   ►◄ Revised Text   ● New Code   ▲ Revised Code Title

J38.7   **Other diseases of larynx**
Abscess of larynx
Cellulitis of larynx
Disease of larynx NOS
Necrosis of larynx
Pachyderma of larynx
Perichondritis of larynx
Ulcer of larynx

✓4ᵗʰ J39   **Other diseases of upper respiratory tract**
> EXCLUDES 1   acute respiratory infection NOS (J22)
> acute upper respiratory infection (J06.9)
> upper respiratory inflammation due to chemicals, gases, fumes
> or vapors (J68.2)

J39.0   **Retropharyngeal and parapharyngeal abscess**
Peripharyngeal abscess
> EXCLUDES 1   peritonsillar abscess (J36)

DEF: Purulent infection behind pharynx and front of precerebral fascia; characterized by neck stiffness, cervical lymphadenopathy, sore throat, fever, and stridor.

J39.1   **Other abscess of pharynx**
Cellulitis of pharynx
Nasopharyngeal abscess

J39.2   **Other diseases of pharynx**
Cyst of pharynx
Edema of pharynx
> EXCLUDES 2   chronic pharyngitis (J31.2)
> ulcerative pharyngitis (J02.9)

J39.3   **Upper respiratory tract hypersensitivity reaction, site unspecified**   ▽
> EXCLUDES 1   hypersensitivity reaction of upper respiratory tract,
> such as:
> extrinsic allergic alveolitis (J67.9)
> pneumoconiosis (J60-J67.9)

J39.8   **Other specified diseases of upper respiratory tract**

J39.9   **Disease of upper respiratory tract, unspecified**   ▽

Chronic lower respiratory diseases (J40-J47)

> EXCLUDES 1   bronchitis due to chemicals, gases, fumes and vapors (J68.0)
> EXCLUDES 2   cystic fibrosis (E84.-)

J40   **Bronchitis, not specified as acute or chronic**   ▽
Bronchitis NOS
Bronchitis with tracheitis NOS
Catarrhal bronchitis
Tracheobronchitis NOS
Use additional code to identify:
    exposure to environmental tobacco smoke (Z77.22)
    exposure to tobacco smoke in the perinatal period (P96.81)
    history of tobacco dependence (Z87.891)
    occupational exposure to environmental tobacco smoke (Z57.31)
    tobacco dependence (F17.-)
    tobacco use (Z72.0)
> EXCLUDES 1   acute bronchitis (J20.-)
> allergic bronchitis NOS (J45.909)
> asthmatic bronchitis NOS (J45.9-)
> bronchitis due to chemicals, gases, fumes and vapors (J68.0)

✓4ᵗʰ J41   **Simple and mucopurulent chronic bronchitis**
Use additional code to identify:
    exposure to environmental tobacco smoke (Z77.22)
    exposure to tobacco smoke in the perinatal period (P96.81)
    history of tobacco dependence (Z87.891)
    occupational exposure to environmental tobacco smoke (Z57.31)
    tobacco dependence (F17.-)
    tobacco use (Z72.0)
> EXCLUDES 1   chronic bronchitis NOS (J42)
> chronic obstructive bronchitis (J44.-)

J41.0   **Simple chronic bronchitis**   HCC

J41.1   **Mucopurulent chronic bronchitis**   HCC

J41.8   **Mixed simple and mucopurulent chronic bronchitis**   HCC

Emphysema

Healthy alveoli   **Alveoli w/ Emphysema**

Patent bronchiole
Collapsed bronchiole
Well-vascularized
Dilated alveoli
Alveolar membranes break down
Excess mucus
Enlarged alveoli
Broken/ fewer capillaries

J42   **Unspecified chronic bronchitis**   HCC ▽
Chronic bronchitis NOS
Chronic tracheitis
Chronic tracheobronchitis
Use additional code to identify:
    exposure to environmental tobacco smoke (Z77.22)
    exposure to tobacco smoke in the perinatal period (P96.81)
    history of tobacco dependence (Z87.891)
    occupational exposure to environmental tobacco smoke (Z57.31)
    tobacco dependence (F17.-)
    tobacco use (Z72.0)
> EXCLUDES 1   chronic asthmatic bronchitis (J44.-)
> chronic bronchitis with airways obstruction (J44.-)
> chronic emphysematous bronchitis (J44.-)
> chronic obstructive pulmonary disease NOS (J44.9)
> simple and mucopurulent chronic bronchitis (J41.-)

✓4ᵗʰ J43   **Emphysema**
Use additional code to identify:
    exposure to environmental tobacco smoke (Z77.22)
    history of tobacco dependence (Z87.891)
    occupational exposure to environmental tobacco smoke (Z57.31)
    tobacco dependence (F17.-)
    tobacco use (Z72.0)
> EXCLUDES 1   compensatory emphysema (J98.3)
> emphysema due to inhalation of chemicals, gases, fumes or
> vapors (J68.4)
> emphysema with chronic (obstructive) bronchitis (J44.-)
> emphysematous (obstructive) bronchitis (J44.-)
> interstitial emphysema (J98.2)
> mediastinal emphysema (J98.2)
> neonatal interstitial emphysema (P25.0)
> surgical (subcutaneous) emphysema (T81.82)
> traumatic subcutaneous emphysema (T79.7)

J43.0   **Unilateral pulmonary emphysema [MacLeod's syndrome]**   HCC
Swyer-James syndrome
Unilateral emphysema
Unilateral hyperlucent lung
Unilateral pulmonary artery functional hypoplasia
Unilateral transparency of lung

J43.1   **Panlobular emphysema**   HCC
Panacinar emphysema

J43.2   **Centrilobular emphysema**   HCC

J43.8   **Other emphysema**   HCC

J43.9   **Emphysema, unspecified**   HCC ▽
Bullous emphysema (lung)(pulmonary)
Emphysema (lung)(pulmonary) NOS
Emphysematous bleb
Vesicular emphysema (lung)(pulmonary)

EXCLUDES 1 Not coded here   EXCLUDES 2 Not included here   N Newborn Age: 0   P Pediatric Age: 0-17   M Maternity Age: 12-55   A Adult Age: 15-124

664   ICD-10-CM 2018

✓4ᵗʰ J44 Other chronic obstructive pulmonary disease

INCLUDES   asthma with chronic obstructive pulmonary disease
chronic asthmatic (obstructive) bronchitis
chronic bronchitis with airways obstruction
chronic bronchitis with emphysema
chronic emphysematous bronchitis
chronic obstructive asthma
chronic obstructive bronchitis
chronic obstructive tracheobronchitis

Code also type of asthma, if applicable (J45.-)
Use additional code to identify:
  exposure to environmental tobacco smoke (Z77.22)
  history of tobacco dependence (Z87.891)
  occupational exposure to environmental tobacco smoke (Z57.31)
  tobacco dependence (F17.-)
  tobacco use (Z72.0)

EXCLUDES 1   bronchiectasis (J47.-)
chronic bronchitis NOS (J42)
chronic simple and mucopurulent bronchitis (J41.-)
chronic tracheitis (J42)
chronic tracheobronchitis (J42)
emphysema without chronic bronchitis (J43.-)

EXCLUDES 2   ~~lung diseases due to external agents (J60-J70)~~

AHA: 2017, 1Q, 25-26; 2016, 3Q, 15-16; 2013, 4Q, 109

J44.0   **Chronic obstructive pulmonary disease with acute lower respiratory infection**   HCC
  ▶Code also to identify the infection◀
  ~~Use additional code to identify the infection~~
  AHA: 2017, 1Q, 24-25

J44.1   **Chronic obstructive pulmonary disease with (acute) exacerbation**   HCC
  Decompensated COPD
  Decompensated COPD with (acute) exacerbation
  EXCLUDES 2   chronic obstructive pulmonary disease [COPD] with acute bronchitis (J44.0)
      ▶lung diseases due to external agents (J60-J70)◀
  AHA: 2017, 1Q, 26; 2016, 1Q, 35

J44.9   **Chronic obstructive pulmonary disease, unspecified**   HCC ▽
  Chronic obstructive airway disease NOS
  Chronic obstructive lung disease NOS
  EXCLUDES 2   ▶lung diseases due to external agents (J60-J70)◀
  AHA: 2016, 1Q, 36; 2014, 4Q, 21; 2013, 4Q, 129

✓4ᵗʰ J45 Asthma

INCLUDES   allergic (predominantly) asthma
allergic bronchitis nos
allergic rhinitis with asthma
atopic asthma
extrinsic allergic asthma
hay fever with asthma
idiosyncratic asthma
intrinsic nonallergic asthma
nonallergic asthma

Use additional code to identify:
  exposure to environmental tobacco smoke (Z77.22)
  exposure to tobacco smoke in the perinatal period (P96.81)
  history of tobacco dependence (Z87.891)
  occupational exposure to environmental tobacco smoke (Z57.31)
  tobacco dependence (F17.-)
  tobacco use (Z72.0)

EXCLUDES 1   detergent asthma (J69.8)
eosinophilic asthma (J82)
~~lung diseases due to external agents (J60-J70)~~
miner's asthma (J60)
wheezing NOS (R06.2)
wood asthma (J67.8)

EXCLUDES 2   asthma with chronic obstructive pulmonary disease (J44.9)
chronic asthmatic (obstructive) bronchitis (J44.9)
chronic obstructive asthma (J44.9)

AHA: 2017, 1Q, 25-26; 2012, 4Q, 99
DEF: Status asthmaticus: Severe, intractable episode of asthma that is unresponsive to normal therapeutic measures.

✓5ᵗʰ J45.2 Mild intermittent asthma

J45.20   **Mild intermittent asthma, uncomplicated**
  Mild intermittent asthma NOS

J45.21   **Mild intermittent asthma with (acute) exacerbation**

J45.22   **Mild intermittent asthma with status asthmaticus**

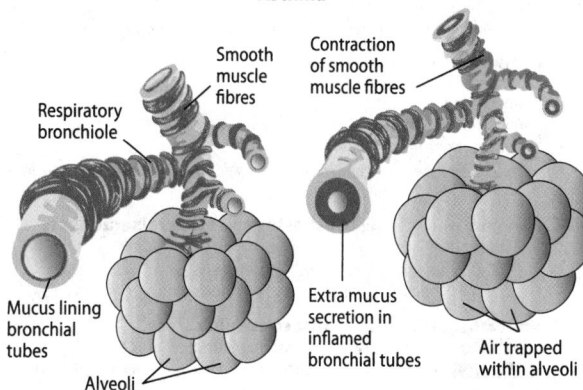

Asthma

Respiratory bronchiole
Smooth muscle fibres
Contraction of smooth muscle fibres
Mucus lining bronchial tubes
Alveoli
Extra mucus secretion in inflamed bronchial tubes
Air trapped within alveoli

Normal alveoli   Asthmatic alveoli

✓5ᵗʰ J45.3 Mild persistent asthma

J45.30   **Mild persistent asthma, uncomplicated**
  Mild persistent asthma NOS

J45.31   **Mild persistent asthma with (acute) exacerbation**
  AHA: 2016, 1Q, 35

J45.32   **Mild persistent asthma with status asthmaticus**

✓5ᵗʰ J45.4 Moderate persistent asthma

J45.40   **Moderate persistent asthma, uncomplicated**
  Moderate persistent asthma NOS

J45.41   **Moderate persistent asthma with (acute) exacerbation**
  AHA: 2017, 1Q, 26

J45.42   **Moderate persistent asthma with status asthmaticus**

✓5ᵗʰ J45.5 Severe persistent asthma

J45.50   **Severe persistent asthma, uncomplicated**
  Severe persistent asthma NOS

J45.51   **Severe persistent asthma with (acute) exacerbation**

J45.52   **Severe persistent asthma with status asthmaticus**

✓5ᵗʰ J45.9 Other and unspecified asthma

✓6ᵗʰ J45.90 Unspecified asthma
  Asthmatic bronchitis NOS
  Childhood asthma NOS
  Late onset asthma

J45.901   **Unspecified asthma with (acute) exacerbation**   ▽

J45.902   **Unspecified asthma with status asthmaticus**   ▽

J45.909   **Unspecified asthma, uncomplicated**   ▽
  Asthma NOS
  EXCLUDES 2   ▶lung diseases due to external agents (J60-J70)◀
  AHA: 2017, 1Q, 25

✓6ᵗʰ J45.99 Other asthma

J45.990   **Exercise induced bronchospasm**

J45.991   **Cough variant asthma**

J45.998   **Other asthma**

✓4ᵗʰ J47 Bronchiectasis

INCLUDES   bronchiolectasis

Use additional code to identify:
  exposure to environmental tobacco smoke (Z77.22)
  exposure to tobacco smoke in the perinatal period (P96.81)
  history of tobacco dependence (Z87.891)
  occupational exposure to environmental tobacco smoke (Z57.31)
  tobacco dependence (F17.-)
  tobacco use (Z72.0)

EXCLUDES 1   congenital bronchiectasis (Q33.4)
tuberculous bronchiectasis (current disease) (A15.0)

J47.0   **Bronchiectasis with acute lower respiratory infection**   HCC
  Bronchiectasis with acute bronchitis
  Use additional code to identify the infection

J47.1   **Bronchiectasis with (acute) exacerbation**   HCC

J47.9   **Bronchiectasis, uncomplicated**   HCC ▽
  Bronchiectasis NOS

Lung diseases due to external agents (J60-J70)

EXCLUDES 2   asthma (J45.-)
              malignant neoplasm of bronchus and lung (C34.-)

J60   Coalworker's pneumoconiosis   HCC A
Anthracosilicosis
Anthracosis
Black lung disease
Coalworker's lung
EXCLUDES 1   coalworker pneumoconiosis with tuberculosis, any type in A15
              (J65)

J61   Pneumoconiosis due to asbestos and other mineral fibers   HCC A
Asbestosis
EXCLUDES 1   pleural plaque with asbestosis (J92.0)
              pneumoconiosis with tuberculosis, any type in A15 (J65)

✓4ᵗʰ **J62   Pneumoconiosis due to dust containing silica**
INCLUDES   silicotic fibrosis (massive) of lung
EXCLUDES 1   pneumoconiosis with tuberculosis, any type in A15 (J65)

J62.0   Pneumoconiosis due to talc dust   HCC

J62.8   Pneumoconiosis due to other dust containing silica   HCC
Silicosis NOS

✓4ᵗʰ **J63   Pneumoconiosis due to other inorganic dusts**
EXCLUDES 1   pneumoconiosis with tuberculosis, any type in A15 (J65)

J63.0   Aluminosis (of lung)   HCC
J63.1   Bauxite fibrosis (of lung)   HCC
J63.2   Berylliosis   HCC
J63.3   Graphite fibrosis (of lung)   HCC
J63.4   Siderosis   HCC
J63.5   Stannosis   HCC
J63.6   Pneumoconiosis due to other specified inorganic dusts   HCC

J64   Unspecified pneumoconiosis   HCC ▽
EXCLUDES 1   pneumonoconiosis with tuberculosis, any type in A15 (J65)

J65   Pneumoconiosis associated with tuberculosis   HCC
Any condition in J60-J64 with tuberculosis, any type in A15
Silicotuberculosis

✓4ᵗʰ **J66   Airway disease due to specific organic dust**
EXCLUDES 2   allergic alveolitis (J67.-)
              asbestosis (J61)
              bagassosis (J67.1)
              farmer's lung (J67.0)
              hypersensitivity pneumonitis due to organic dust (J67.-)
              reactive airways dysfunction syndrome (J68.3)

J66.0   Byssinosis   HCC
Airway disease due to cotton dust

J66.1   Flax-dressers' disease   HCC
J66.2   Cannabinosis   HCC
J66.8   Airway disease due to other specific organic dusts   HCC

✓4ᵗʰ **J67   Hypersensitivity pneumonitis due to organic dust**
INCLUDES   allergic alveolitis and pneumonitis due to inhaled organic
            dust and particles of fungal, actinomycetic or other
            origin
EXCLUDES 1   pneumonitis due to inhalation of chemicals, gases, fumes or
              vapors (J68.0)

J67.0   Farmer's lung   HCC
Harvester's lung   Moldy hay disease
Haymaker's lung

J67.1   Bagassosis   HCC
Bagasse disease   Bagasse pneumonitis

J67.2   Bird fancier's lung   HCC
Budgerigar fancier's disease or lung
Pigeon fancier's disease or lung

J67.3   Suberosis   HCC
Corkhandler's disease or lung
Corkworker's disease or lung

J67.4   Maltworker's lung   HCC
Alveolitis due to Aspergillus clavatus

J67.5   Mushroom-worker's lung   HCC
J67.6   Maple-bark-stripper's lung   HCC
Alveolitis due to Cryptostroma corticale
Cryptostromosis

J67.7   Air conditioner and humidifier lung   HCC
Allergic alveolitis due to fungal, thermophilic actinomycetes and
other organisms growing in ventilation [air conditioning]
systems

J67.8   Hypersensitivity pneumonitis due to other organic dusts   HCC
Cheese-washer's lung   Furrier's lung
Coffee-worker's lung   Sequoiosis
Fish-meal worker's lung

J67.9   Hypersensitivity pneumonitis due to unspecified   HCC ▽
organic dust
Allergic alveolitis (extrinsic) NOS
Hypersensitivity pneumonitis NOS

✓4ᵗʰ **J68   Respiratory conditions due to inhalation of chemicals, gases,
fumes and vapors**
Code first (T51-T65) to identify cause
Use additional code to identify associated respiratory conditions, such
as:
acute respiratory failure (J96.0-)

**J68.0   Bronchitis and pneumonitis due to chemicals, gases,   HCC
fumes and vapors**
Chemical bronchitis (acute)

**J68.1   Pulmonary edema due to chemicals, gases, fumes and   HCC
vapors**
Chemical pulmonary edema (acute) (chronic)
EXCLUDES 1   pulmonary edema (acute) (chronic) NOS (J81.-)

**J68.2   Upper respiratory inflammation due to chemicals, gases,   HCC
fumes and vapors, not elsewhere classified**

**J68.3   Other acute and subacute respiratory conditions due to   HCC
chemicals, gases, fumes and vapors**
Reactive airways dysfunction syndrome

**J68.4   Chronic respiratory conditions due to chemicals, gases,   HCC
fumes and vapors**
Emphysema (diffuse) (chronic) due to inhalation of chemicals,
gases, fumes and vapors
Obliterative bronchiolitis (chronic) (subacute) due to inhalation
of chemicals, gases, fumes and vapors
Pulmonary fibrosis (chronic) due to inhalation of chemicals,
gases, fumes and vapors
EXCLUDES 1   chronic pulmonary edema due to chemicals, gases,
              fumes and vapors (J68.1)

**J68.8   Other respiratory conditions due to chemicals, gases,   HCC
fumes and vapors**

**J68.9   Unspecified respiratory condition due to chemicals,   HCC ▽
gases, fumes and vapors**

✓4ᵗʰ **J69   Pneumonitis due to solids and liquids**
EXCLUDES 1   neonatal aspiration syndromes (P24.-)
              postprocedural pneumonitis (J95.4)
AHA: 2017, 1Q, 24

J69.0   Pneumonitis due to inhalation of food and vomit   HCC
Aspiration pneumonia NOS
Aspiration pneumonia (due to) food (regurgitated)
Aspiration pneumonia (due to) gastric secretions
Aspiration pneumonia (due to) milk
Aspiration pneumonia (due to) vomit
Code also any associated foreign body in respiratory tract (T17.-)
EXCLUDES 1   chemical pneumonitis due to anesthesia (J95.4)
              obstetric aspiration pneumonitis (O74.0)

J69.1   Pneumonitis due to inhalation of oils and essences   HCC
Exogenous lipoid pneumonia
Lipid pneumonia NOS
Code first (T51-T65) to identify substance
EXCLUDES 1   endogenous lipoid pneumonia (J84.89)

J69.8   Pneumonitis due to inhalation of other solids and liquids HCC
Pneumonitis due to aspiration of blood
Pneumonitis due to aspiration of detergent
Code first (T51-T65) to identify substance

✓4ᵗʰ **J70   Respiratory conditions due to other external agents**

J70.0   Acute pulmonary manifestations due to radiation   HCC
Radiation pneumonitis
Use additional code (W88-W90, X39.0-) to identify the external
cause

**J70.1   Chronic and other pulmonary manifestations due to   HCC
radiation**
Fibrosis of lung following radiation
Use additional code (W88-W90, X39.0-) to identify the external
cause

J70.2   Acute drug-induced interstitial lung disorders   HCC
Use additional code for adverse effect, if applicable, to identify
drug (T36-T50 with fifth or sixth character 5)
EXCLUDES 1   interstitial pneumonia NOS (J84.9)
              lymphoid interstitial pneumonia (J84.2)

EXCLUDES 1 Not coded here   EXCLUDES 2 Not included here   N Newborn Age: 0   P Pediatric Age: 0-17   M Maternity Age: 12-55   A Adult Age: 15-124

J70.3 **Chronic drug-induced interstitial lung disorders** HCC
Use additional code for adverse effect, if applicable, to identify drug (T36-T50 with fifth or sixth character 5)
EXCLUDES 1 *interstitial pneumonia NOS (J84.9)*
lymphoid interstitial pneumonia (J84.2)

J70.4 **Drug-induced interstitial lung disorders, unspecified** HCC ▽
Use additional code for adverse effect, if applicable, to identify drug (T36-T50 with fifth or sixth character 5)
EXCLUDES 1 *interstitial pneumonia NOS (J84.9)*
lymphoid interstitial pneumonia (J84.2)

J70.5 **Respiratory conditions due to smoke inhalation** HCC
Smoke inhalation NOS
EXCLUDES 1 *smoke inhalation due to chemicals, gases, fumes and vapors (J68.9)*
AHA: 2013, 4Q, 121

J70.8 **Respiratory conditions due to other specified external agents** HCC
Code first (T51-T65) to identify the external agent

J70.9 **Respiratory conditions due to unspecified external agent** HCC ▽
Code first (T51-T65) to identify the external agent

Other respiratory diseases principally affecting the interstitium (J80-J84)

J80 **Acute respiratory distress syndrome** HCC
Acute respiratory distress syndrome in adult or child
Adult hyaline membrane disease
EXCLUDES 1 *respiratory distress syndrome in newborn (perinatal) (P22.0)*
AHA: 2017, 1Q, 26

✓4th **J81** **Pulmonary edema**
Use additional code to identify:
exposure to environmental tobacco smoke (Z77.22)
history of tobacco dependence (Z87.891)
occupational exposure to environmental tobacco smoke (Z57.31)
tobacco dependence (F17.-)
tobacco use (Z72.0)
EXCLUDES 1 *chemical (acute) pulmonary edema (J68.1)*
hypostatic pneumonia (J18.2)
passive pneumonia (J18.2)
pulmonary edema due to external agents (J60-J70)
pulmonary edema with heart disease NOS (I50.1)
pulmonary edema with heart failure (I50.1)

J81.0 **Acute pulmonary edema** HCC
Acute edema of lung

J81.1 **Chronic pulmonary edema**
Pulmonary congestion (chronic) (passive)
Pulmonary edema NOS

J82 **Pulmonary eosinophilia, not elsewhere classified** HCC
Allergic pneumonia   Löffler's pneumonia
Eosinophilic asthma   Tropical (pulmonary)
Eosinophilic pneumonia   eosinophilia NOS
EXCLUDES 1 *pulmonary eosinophilia due to aspergillosis (B44.-)*
pulmonary eosinophilia due to drugs (J70.2-J70.4)
pulmonary eosinophilia due to specified parasitic infection (B50-B83)
pulmonary eosinophilia due to systemic connective tissue disorders (M30-M36)
pulmonary infiltrate NOS (R91.8)

✓4th **J84** **Other interstitial pulmonary diseases**
EXCLUDES 1 *drug-induced interstitial lung disorders (J70.2-J70.4)*
interstitial emphysema (J98.2)
lung diseases due to external agents (J60-J70)
EXCLUDES 2 ▶*lung diseases due to external agents (J60-J70)*◀

✓5th **J84.0** **Alveolar and parieto-alveolar conditions**
J84.01 **Alveolar proteinosis** HCC
DEF: Reduced ventilation due to proteinaceous deposits on alveoli; symptoms include dyspnea, cough, chest pain, weakness, weight loss, and hemoptysis.

J84.02 **Pulmonary alveolar microlithiasis** HCC

J84.03 *Idiopathic pulmonary hemosiderosis* HCC
Essential brown induration of lung
Code first underlying disease, such as:
disorders of iron metabolism (E83.1-)
EXCLUDES 1 *acute idiopathic pulmonary hemorrhage in infants [AIPHI] (R04.81)*
DEF: Fibrosis of alveolar walls; marked by abnormal accumulation of iron as hemosiderin in lungs; primarily affects children; symptoms include anemia, fluid in lungs, and blood in sputum; etiology unknown.

J84.09 **Other alveolar and parieto-alveolar conditions** HCC

✓5th **J84.1** **Other interstitial pulmonary diseases with fibrosis**
EXCLUDES 1 *pulmonary fibrosis (chronic) due to inhalation of chemicals, gases, fumes or vapors (J68.4)*
pulmonary fibrosis (chronic) following radiation (J70.1)

J84.10 **Pulmonary fibrosis, unspecified** HCC ▽
Capillary fibrosis of lung
Cirrhosis of lung (chronic) NOS
Fibrosis of lung (atrophic) (chronic) (confluent) (massive) (perialveolar) (peribronchial) NOS
Induration of lung (chronic) NOS
Postinflammatory pulmonary fibrosis

✓6th **J84.11** **Idiopathic interstitial pneumonia**
EXCLUDES 1 *lymphoid interstitial pneumonia (J84.2)*
pneumocystis pneumonia (B59)

J84.111 **Idiopathic interstitial pneumonia, not otherwise specified** HCC ▽

J84.112 **Idiopathic pulmonary fibrosis** HCC
Cryptogenic fibrosing alveolitis
Idiopathic fibrosing alveolitis

J84.113 **Idiopathic non-specific interstitial pneumonitis** HCC
EXCLUDES 1 *non-specific interstitial pneumonia NOS, or due to known underlying cause (J84.89)*

J84.114 **Acute interstitial pneumonitis** HCC
Hamman-Rich syndrome
EXCLUDES 1 *pneumocystis pneumonia (B59)*

J84.115 **Respiratory bronchiolitis interstitial lung disease** HCC

J84.116 **Cryptogenic organizing pneumonia** HCC
EXCLUDES 1 *organizing pneumonia NOS, or due to known underlying cause (J84.89)*

J84.117 **Desquamative interstitial pneumonia** HCC

J84.17 *Other interstitial pulmonary diseases with fibrosis in diseases classified elsewhere* HCC
Interstitial pneumonia (nonspecific) (usual) due to collagen vascular disease
Interstitial pneumonia (nonspecific) (usual) in diseases classified elsewhere
Organizing pneumonia due to collagen vascular disease
Organizing pneumonia in diseases classified elsewhere
Code first underlying disease, such as:
progressive systemic sclerosis (M34.0)
rheumatoid arthritis (M05.00-M06.9)
systemic lupus erythematosis (M32.0-M32.9)

J84.2 **Lymphoid interstitial pneumonia** HCC
Lymphoid interstitial pneumonitis

✓5th **J84.8** **Other specified interstitial pulmonary diseases**
EXCLUDES 1 *exogenous lipoid pneumonia (J69.1)*
unspecified lipoid pneumonia (J69.1)

J84.81 **Lymphangioleiomyomatosis** HCC ♀
Lymphangiomyomatosis

J84.82 **Adult pulmonary Langerhans cell histiocytosis** HCC A
Adult PLCH

J84.83 **Surfactant mutations of the lung** HCC
DEF: Genetic disorder resulting in insufficient secretion of a complex mixture of phospholipids and proteins that reduce surface tension in the alveoli following the onset of breathing to facilitate lung expansion in the newborn; leading indication for pediatric lung transplantation.

✓6th **J84.84** **Other interstitial lung diseases of childhood**
J84.841 **Neuroendocrine cell hyperplasia of infancy** HCC

J84.842 **Pulmonary interstitial glycogenosis** HCC

J84.843 **Alveolar capillary dysplasia with vein misalignment** HCC

J84.848 **Other interstitial lung diseases of childhood** HCC

✓ Additional Character Req   ✓x7th Placeholder Alert   Manifestation   HCC CMS-HCC Condition   ▽ Unspecified Code   ▶◀ Revised Text   ● New Code   ▲ Revised Code Title

Chapter 10. Diseases of the Respiratory System

J84.89   **Other specified interstitial pulmonary diseases** `HCC`
Endogenous lipoid pneumonia
Interstitial pneumonitis
Non-specific interstitial pneumonitis NOS
Organizing pneumonia NOS
Code first, if applicable:
   poisoning due to drug or toxin (T51-T65 with fifth or
     sixth character to indicate intent), for toxic
     pneumonopathy
   underlying cause of pneumonopathy, if known
Use additional code, for adverse effect, to identify
   drug (T36-T50 with fifth or sixth character 5), if
   drug-induced
   EXCLUDES 1   *cryptogenic organizing pneumonia (J84.116)*
        idiopathic non-specific interstitial
          pneumonitis (J84.113)
        lipoid pneumonia, exogenous or unspecified
          (J69.1)
        lymphoid interstitial pneumonia (J84.2)

J84.9   **Interstitial pulmonary disease, unspecified** `HCC` ▽
Interstitial pneumonia NOS

Suppurative and necrotic conditions of the lower respiratory tract (J85-J86)

✓4ᵗʰ **J85**   **Abscess of lung and mediastinum**
Use additional code (B95-B97) to identify infectious agent.

   J85.0   **Gangrene and necrosis of lung** `HCC`

   J85.1   **Abscess of lung with pneumonia** `HCC`
       Code also the type of pneumonia

   J85.2   **Abscess of lung without pneumonia** `HCC`
       Abscess of lung NOS

   J85.3   **Abscess of mediastinum** `HCC`

✓4ᵗʰ **J86**   **Pyothorax**
Use additional code (B95-B97) to identify infectious agent
   EXCLUDES 1   *abscess of lung (J85.-)*
        pyothorax due to tuberculosis (A15.6)

   J86.0   **Pyothorax with fistula** `HCC`
       Bronchocutaneous fistula
       Bronchopleural fistula
       Hepatopleural fistula
       Mediastinal fistula
       Pleural fistula
       Thoracic fistula
       Any condition classifiable to J86.9 with fistula
       DEF: Purulent infection of respiratory cavity, with communication from cavity to another structure.

   J86.9   **Pyothorax without fistula** `HCC`
       Abscess of pleura   Pyopneumothorax
       Abscess of thorax   Septic pleurisy
       Empyema (chest) (lung) (pleura)   Seropurulent pleurisy
       Fibrinopurulent pleurisy   Suppurative pleurisy
       Purulent pleurisy

Other diseases of the pleura (J90-J94)

J90   **Pleural effusion, not elsewhere classified**
Encysted pleurisy
Pleural effusion NOS
Pleurisy with effusion (exudative) (serous)
   EXCLUDES 1   *chylous (pleural) effusion (J94.0)*
        malignant pleural effusion (J91.0))
        pleurisy NOS (R09.1)
        tuberculous pleural effusion (A15.6)

✓4ᵗʰ **J91**   **Pleural effusion in conditions classified elsewhere**
   EXCLUDES 2   *pleural effusion in heart failure (I50.-)*
        pleural effusion in systemic lupus erythematosus (M32.13)

   J91.0   *Malignant pleural effusion*
       Code first underlying neoplasm

   J91.8   *Pleural effusion in other conditions classified elsewhere*
       Code first underlying disease, such as:
         filariasis (B74.0-B74.9)
         influenza (J09.X2, J10.1, J11.1)
       AHA: 2015, 2Q, 15

Pleural Effusion

Right lung   Left lung   Pleura   Pleural space   Pleural effusion

✓4ᵗʰ **J92**   **Pleural plaque**
   `INCLUDES`   pleural thickening

   J92.0   **Pleural plaque with presence of asbestos**

   J92.9   **Pleural plaque without asbestos**
       Pleural plaque NOS

✓4ᵗʰ **J93**   **Pneumothorax and air leak**
   EXCLUDES 1   *congenital or perinatal pneumothorax (P25.1)*
        postprocedural air leak (J95.812)
        postprocedural pneumothorax (J95.811)
        traumatic pneumothorax (S27.0)
        tuberculous (current disease) pneumothorax (A15.-)
        pyopneumothorax (J86.-)

   J93.0   **Spontaneous tension pneumothorax**
       DEF: Leaking air from lung into lining, causing collapse.

✓5ᵗʰ **J93.1**   **Other spontaneous pneumothorax**

     J93.11   **Primary spontaneous pneumothorax**

     J93.12   **Secondary spontaneous pneumothorax**
         Code first underlying condition, such as:
           catamenial pneumothorax due to endometriosis
             (N80.8)
           cystic fibrosis (E84.-)
           eosinophilic pneumonia (J82)
           lymphangioleiomyomatosis (J84.81)
           malignant neoplasm of bronchus and lung (C34.-)
           Marfan's syndrome (Q87.4)
           pneumonia due to Pneumocystis carinii (B59)
           secondary malignant neoplasm of lung (C78.0-)
           spontaneous rupture of the esophagus (K22.3)

✓5ᵗʰ **J93.8**   **Other pneumothorax and air leak**

     J93.81   **Chronic pneumothorax**

     J93.82   **Other air leak**
         Persistent air leak

     J93.83   **Other pneumothorax**
         Acute pneumothorax
         Spontaneous pneumothorax NOS

   J93.9   **Pneumothorax, unspecified** ▽
       Pneumothorax NOS

✓4ᵗʰ **J94**   **Other pleural conditions**
   EXCLUDES 1   *pleurisy NOS (R09.1)*
        traumatic hemopneumothorax (S27.2)
        traumatic hemothorax (S27.1)
        tuberculous pleural conditions (current disease) (A15.-)

   J94.0   **Chylous effusion**
       Chyliform effusion

   J94.1   **Fibrothorax**

   J94.2   **Hemothorax**
       Hemopneumothorax

   J94.8   **Other specified pleural conditions**
       Hydropneumothorax
       Hydrothorax

   J94.9   **Pleural condition, unspecified** ▽

Tracheostomy

Tracheostomy
in place

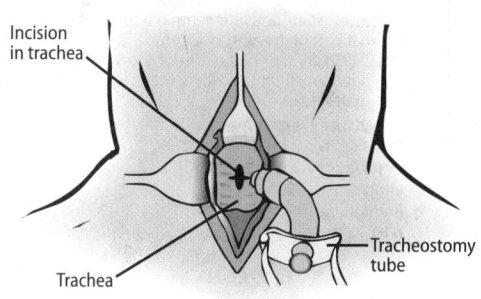

Incision
in trachea

Trachea

Tracheostomy
tube

Intraoperative and postprocedural complications and disorders of respiratory system, not elsewhere classified (J95)

☑4ᵗʰ **J95**   **Intraoperative and postprocedural complications and disorders of respiratory system, not elsewhere classified**
    EXCLUDES 2   *aspiration pneumonia (J69.-)*
       emphysema (subcutaneous) resulting from a procedure (T81.82)
       hypostatic pneumonia (J18.2)
       pulmonary manifestations due to radiation (J70.0- J70.1)

☑5ᵗʰ **J95.0**   **Tracheostomy complications**
    J95.00   **Unspecified tracheostomy complication**   HCC ▽
    J95.01   **Hemorrhage from tracheostomy stoma**   HCC
    J95.02   **Infection of tracheostomy stoma**   HCC
       Use additional code to identify type of infection, such as:
         cellulitis of neck ▶(L03.221)◀
         sepsis (A40, A41-)
    J95.03   **Malfunction of tracheostomy stoma**   HCC
       Mechanical complication of tracheostomy stoma
       Obstruction of tracheostomy airway
       Tracheal stenosis due to tracheostomy
    J95.04   **Tracheo-esophageal fistula following tracheostomy**   HCC
    J95.09   **Other tracheostomy complication**   HCC

J95.1   **Acute pulmonary insufficiency following thoracic surgery**   HCC
    EXCLUDES 2   *functional disturbances following cardiac surgery (I97.0, I97.1-)*

J95.2   **Acute pulmonary insufficiency following nonthoracic surgery**   HCC
    EXCLUDES 2   *functional disturbances following cardiac surgery (I97.0, I97.1-)*

J95.3   **Chronic pulmonary insufficiency following surgery**   HCC
    EXCLUDES 2   *functional disturbances following cardiac surgery (I97.0, I97.1-)*

J95.4   **Chemical pneumonitis due to anesthesia**
    Mendelson's syndrome
    Postprocedural aspiration pneumonia
    Use additional code for adverse effect, if applicable, to identify drug (T41.- with fifth or sixth character 5)
    EXCLUDES 1   *aspiration pneumonitis due to anesthesia complicating labor and delivery (O74.0)*
       aspiration pneumonitis due to anesthesia complicating pregnancy (O29)
       aspiration pneumonitis due to anesthesia complicating the puerperium (O89.01)

J95.5   **Postprocedural subglottic stenosis**

☑5ᵗʰ **J95.6**   **Intraoperative hemorrhage and hematoma of a respiratory system organ or structure complicating a procedure**
    EXCLUDES 1   *intraoperative hemorrhage and hematoma of a respiratory system organ or structure due to accidental puncture and laceration during procedure (J95.7-)*
    J95.61   **Intraoperative hemorrhage and hematoma of a respiratory system organ or structure complicating a respiratory system procedure**
    J95.62   **Intraoperative hemorrhage and hematoma of a respiratory system organ or structure complicating other procedure**

☑5ᵗʰ **J95.7**   **Accidental puncture and laceration of a respiratory system organ or structure during a procedure**
    EXCLUDES 2   *postprocedural pneumothorax (J95.811)*
    J95.71   **Accidental puncture and laceration of a respiratory system organ or structure during a respiratory system procedure**
    J95.72   **Accidental puncture and laceration of a respiratory system organ or structure during other procedure**

☑5ᵗʰ **J95.8**   **Other intraoperative and postprocedural complications and disorders of respiratory system, not elsewhere classified**
    ☑6ᵗʰ **J95.81**   **Postprocedural pneumothorax and air leak**
       J95.811   **Postprocedural pneumothorax**
       J95.812   **Postprocedural air leak**
    ☑6ᵗʰ **J95.82**   **Postprocedural respiratory failure**
       EXCLUDES 1   *respiratory failure in other conditions (J96.-)*
       J95.821   **Acute postprocedural respiratory failure**   HCC
         Postprocedural respiratory failure NOS
       J95.822   **Acute and chronic postprocedural respiratory failure**   HCC
    ☑6ᵗʰ **J95.83**   **Postprocedural hemorrhage of a respiratory system organ or structure following a procedure**
       J95.830   **Postprocedural hemorrhage of a respiratory system organ or structure following a respiratory system procedure**
       J95.831   **Postprocedural hemorrhage of a respiratory system organ or structure following other procedure**
    J95.84   **Transfusion-related acute lung injury (TRALI)**
       DEF: A relatively rare, but serious, pulmonary complication of blood transfusion, with acute respiratory distress, noncardiogenic pulmonary edema, cyanosis, hypoxemia, hypotension, fever, and chills.
    ☑6ᵗʰ **J95.85**   **Complication of respirator [ventilator]**
       J95.850   **Mechanical complication of respirator**   HCC
         EXCLUDES 1   *encounter for respirator [ventilator] dependence during power failure (Z99.12)*
       J95.851   **Ventilator associated pneumonia**   HCC
         Ventilator associated pneumonitis
         Use additional code to identify the organism, if known (B95.-, B96.-, B97.-)
         EXCLUDES 1   *ventilator lung in newborn (P27.8)*
         AHA: 2017, 1Q, 25
       J95.859   **Other complication of respirator [ventilator]**   HCC
    ☑6ᵗʰ **J95.86**   **Postprocedural hematoma and seroma of a respiratory system organ or structure following a procedure**
       J95.860   **Postprocedural hematoma of a respiratory system organ or structure following a respiratory system procedure**
       J95.861   **Postprocedural hematoma of a respiratory system organ or structure following other procedure**
       J95.862   **Postprocedural seroma of a respiratory system organ or structure following a respiratory system procedure**
       J95.863   **Postprocedural seroma of a respiratory system organ or structure following other procedure**
    J95.88   **Other intraoperative complications of respiratory system, not elsewhere classified**

☑ Additional Character Req   ✔x7ᵗʰ Placeholder Alert   Manifestation   HCC CMS-HCC Condition   ▽ Unspecified Code   ▶◀ Revised Text   ● New Code   ▲ Revised Code Title

J95.89   **Other postprocedural complications and disorders of respiratory system, not elsewhere classified**
Use additional code to identify disorder, such as:
aspiration pneumonia (J69.-)
bacterial or viral pneumonia (J12-J18)
EXCLUDES 2   acute pulmonary insufficiency following thoracic surgery (J95.1)
postprocedural subglottic stenosis (J95.5)

Other diseases of the respiratory system (J96-J99)

✓4ᵗʰ **J96**   **Respiratory failure, not elsewhere classified**
EXCLUDES 1   acute respiratory distress syndrome (J80)
cardiorespiratory failure (R09.2)
newborn respiratory distress syndrome (P22.0)
postprocedural respiratory failure (J95.82-)
respiratory arrest (R09.2)
respiratory arrest of newborn (P28.81)
respiratory failure of newborn (P28.5)

✓5ᵗʰ **J96.0**   **Acute respiratory failure**

J96.00   **Acute respiratory failure, unspecified whether with hypoxia or hypercapnia**   HCC ▽
AHA: 2016, 3Q, 14; 2013, 4Q, 121

J96.01   **Acute respiratory failure with hypoxia**   HCC

J96.02   **Acute respiratory failure with hypercapnia**   HCC

✓5ᵗʰ **J96.1**   **Chronic respiratory failure**

J96.10   **Chronic respiratory failure, unspecified whether with hypoxia or hypercapnia**   HCC ▽
AHA: 2016, 1Q, 38; 2015, 1Q, 21

J96.11   **Chronic respiratory failure with hypoxia**   HCC
AHA: 2013, 4Q, 129

J96.12   **Chronic respiratory failure with hypercapnia**   HCC

✓5ᵗʰ **J96.2**   **Acute and chronic respiratory failure**
Acute on chronic respiratory failure

J96.20   **Acute and chronic respiratory failure, unspecified whether with hypoxia or hypercapnia**   HCC ▽

J96.21   **Acute and chronic respiratory failure with hypoxia**   HCC

J96.22   **Acute and chronic respiratory failure with hypercapnia**   HCC

✓5ᵗʰ **J96.9**   **Respiratory failure, unspecified**

J96.90   **Respiratory failure, unspecified, unspecified whether with hypoxia or hypercapnia**   HCC ▽

J96.91   **Respiratory failure, unspecified with hypoxia**   HCC ▽

J96.92   **Respiratory failure, unspecified with hypercapnia**   HCC ▽

✓4ᵗʰ **J98**   **Other respiratory disorders**
Use additional code to identify:
exposure to environmental tobacco smoke (Z77.22)
exposure to tobacco smoke in the perinatal period (P96.81)
history of tobacco dependence (Z87.891)
occupational exposure to environmental tobacco smoke (Z57.31)
tobacco dependence (F17.-)
tobacco use (Z72.0)
EXCLUDES 1   newborn apnea (P28.4)
newborn sleep apnea (P28.3)
EXCLUDES 2   apnea NOS (R06.81)
sleep apnea (G47.3-)

✓5ᵗʰ **J98.0**   **Diseases of bronchus, not elsewhere classified**

J98.01   **Acute bronchospasm**
EXCLUDES 1   acute bronchiolitis with bronchospasm (J21.-)
acute bronchitis with bronchospasm (J20.-)
asthma (J45.-)
exercise induced bronchospasm (J45.990)

J98.09   **Other diseases of bronchus, not elsewhere classified**
Broncholithiasis
Calcification of bronchus
Stenosis of bronchus
Tracheobronchial collapse
Tracheobronchial dyskinesia
Ulcer of bronchus

✓5ᵗʰ **J98.1**   **Pulmonary collapse**
EXCLUDES 1   therapeutic collapse of lung status (Z98.3)

J98.11   **Atelectasis**
EXCLUDES 1   newborn atelectasis
tuberculous atelectasis (current disease) (A15)

J98.19   **Other pulmonary collapse**

J98.2   **Interstitial emphysema**   HCC
Mediastinal emphysema
EXCLUDES 1   emphysema NOS (J43.9)
emphysema in newborn (P25.0)
surgical emphysema (subcutaneous) (T81.82)
traumatic subcutaneous emphysema (T79.7)

J98.3   **Compensatory emphysema**   HCC
DEF: Distention of all or part of the lung caused by disease processes or surgical intervention that decreased volume in another part of the lung; overcompensation reaction to the loss of capacity in another part of the lung; occurs in association with pneumonias, pleural effusions, atelectasis, empyema, and pneumothorax.

J98.4   **Other disorders of lung**
Calcification of lung
Cystic lung disease (acquired)
Lung disease NOS
Pulmolithiasis
EXCLUDES 1   acute interstitial pneumonitis (J84.114)
pulmonary insufficiency following surgery (J95.1-J95.2)

✓5ᵗʰ **J98.5**   **Diseases of mediastinum, not elsewhere classified**
EXCLUDES 2   abscess of mediastinum (J85.3)

J98.51   **Mediastinitis**
Code first:
underlying condition, if applicable, such as postoperative mediastinitis (T81.-)

J98.59   **Other diseases of mediastinum, not elsewhere classified**
Fibrosis of mediastinum
Hernia of mediastinum
Retraction of mediastinum

J98.6   **Disorders of diaphragm**
Diaphragmatitis
Paralysis of diaphragm
Relaxation of diaphragm
EXCLUDES 1   congenital malformation of diaphragm NEC (Q79.1)
congenital diaphragmatic hernia (Q79.0)
EXCLUDES 2   diaphragmatic hernia (K44.-)

J98.8   **Other specified respiratory disorders**

J98.9   **Respiratory disorder, unspecified**   ▽
Respiratory disease (chronic) NOS

J99   **Respiratory disorders in diseases classified elsewhere**   HCC
Code first underlying disease, such as:
amyloidosis (E85.-)
ankylosing spondylitis (M45)
congenital syphilis (A50.5)
cryoglobulinemia (D89.1)
early congenital syphilis (A50.0)
schistosomiasis (B65.0-B65.9)
EXCLUDES 1   respiratory disorders in:
amebiasis (A06.5)
blastomycosis (B40.0-B40.2)
candidiasis (B37.1)
coccidioidomycosis (B38.0-B38.2)
cystic fibrosis with pulmonary manifestations (E84.0)
dermatomyositis (M33.01, M33.11)
histoplasmosis (B39.0-B39.2)
late syphilis (A52.72, A52.73)
polymyositis (M33.21)
sicca syndrome (M35.02)
systemic lupus erythematosus (M32.13)
systemic sclerosis (M34.81)
Wegener's granulomatosis (M31.30-M31.31)

EXCLUDES 1 Not coded here   EXCLUDES 2 Not included here   N Newborn Age: 0   P Pediatric Age: 0-17   M Maternity Age: 12-55   A Adult Age: 15-124

670   ICD-10-CM 2018

Chapter 11. Diseases of the Digestive System (K00–K95)

Chapter Specific Coding Guidelines and Examples
Reserved for future guideline expansion.

Chapter 11. Diseases of the Digestive System (K00-K95)

EXCLUDES 2   certain conditions originating in the perinatal period (P04-P96)
certain infectious and parasitic diseases (A00-B99)
complications of pregnancy, childbirth and the puerperium (O00-O9A)
congenital malformations, deformations and chromosomal abnormalities (Q00-Q99)
endocrine, nutritional and metabolic diseases (E00-E88)
injury, poisoning and certain other consequences of external causes (S00-T88)
neoplasms (C00-D49)
symptoms, signs and abnormal clinical and laboratory findings, not elsewhere classified (R00-R94)

This chapter contains the following blocks:

K00-K14   Diseases of oral cavity and salivary glands
K20-K31   Diseases of esophagus, stomach and duodenum
K35-K38   Diseases of appendix
K40-K46   Hernia
K50-K52   Noninfective enteritis and colitis
K55-K64   Other diseases of intestines
K65-K68   Diseases of peritoneum and retroperitoneum
K70-K77   Diseases of liver
K80-K87   Disorders of gallbladder, biliary tract and pancreas
K90-K95   Other diseases of the digestive system

Diseases of oral cavity and salivary glands (K00-K14)

✓4th **K00   Disorders of tooth development and eruption**
     EXCLUDES 2   embedded and impacted teeth (K01.-)

K00.0   Anodontia
Hypodontia
Oligodontia
EXCLUDES 1   acquired absence of teeth (K08.1-)

K00.1   Supernumerary teeth
Distomolar
Fourth molar
Mesiodens
Paramolar
Supplementary teeth
EXCLUDES 2   supernumerary roots (K00.2)

K00.2   Abnormalities of size and form of teeth
Concrescence of teeth
Dens evaginatus
Dens in dente
Dens invaginatus
Enamel pearls
Fusion of teeth
Gemination of teeth
Macrodontia
Microdontia
Peg-shaped [conical] teeth
Supernumerary roots
Taurodontism
Tuberculum paramolare
EXCLUDES 1   abnormalities of teeth due to congenital syphilis (A50.5)
tuberculum Carabelli, which is regarded as a normal variation and should not be coded

K00.3   Mottled teeth
Dental fluorosis
Mottling of enamel
Nonfluoride enamel opacities
EXCLUDES 2   deposits [accretions] on teeth (K03.6)

K00.4   Disturbances in tooth formation
Aplasia and hypoplasia of cementum
Dilaceration of tooth
Enamel hypoplasia (neonatal) (postnatal) (prenatal)
Regional odontodysplasia
Turner's tooth
EXCLUDES 1   Hutchinson's teeth and mulberry molars in congenital syphilis (A50.5)
EXCLUDES 2   mottled teeth (K00.3)

K00.5   Hereditary disturbances in tooth structure, not elsewhere classified
Amelogenesis imperfecta
Dentinogenesis imperfecta
Odontogenesis imperfecta
Dentinal dysplasia
Shell teeth

Tooth Anatomy

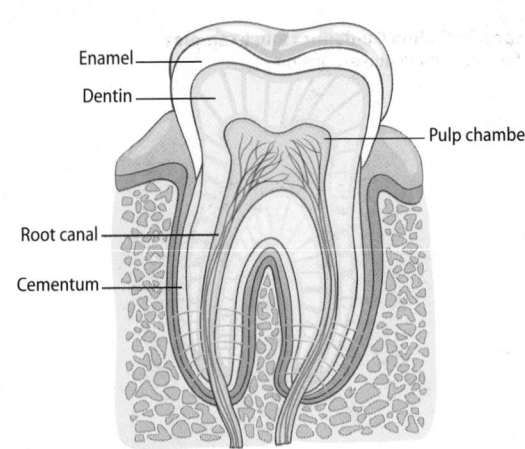

Enamel
Dentin
Pulp chamber
Root canal
Cementum

K00.6   Disturbances in tooth eruption
Dentia praecox
Natal tooth
Neonatal tooth
Premature eruption of tooth
Premature shedding of primary [deciduous] tooth
Prenatal teeth
Retained [persistent] primary tooth
EXCLUDES 2   embedded and impacted teeth (K01.-)

K00.7   Teething syndrome

K00.8   Other disorders of tooth development
Color changes during tooth formation
Intrinsic staining of teeth NOS
EXCLUDES 2   posteruptive color changes (K03.7)

K00.9   Disorder of tooth development, unspecified   ▽
Disorder of odontogenesis NOS

✓4th **K01   Embedded and impacted teeth**
     EXCLUDES 1   abnormal position of fully erupted teeth (M26.3-)

K01.0   Embedded teeth

K01.1   Impacted teeth

✓4th **K02   Dental caries**
     INCLUDES   caries of dentine
dental cavities
early childhood caries
pre-eruptive caries
recurrent caries (dentino enamel junction) (enamel) (to the pulp)
tooth decay

K02.3   Arrested dental caries
Arrested coronal and root caries

✓5th **K02.5   Dental caries on pit and fissure surface**
Dental caries on chewing surface of tooth

K02.51   Dental caries on pit and fissure surface limited to enamel
White spot lesions [initial caries] on pit and fissure surface of tooth

K02.52   Dental caries on pit and fissure surface penetrating into dentin
Primary dental caries, cervical origin)

K02.53   Dental caries on pit and fissure surface penetrating into pulp

✓5th **K02.6   Dental caries on smooth surface**

K02.61   Dental caries on smooth surface limited to enamel
White spot lesions [initial caries] on smooth surface of tooth

K02.62   Dental caries on smooth surface penetrating into dentin

K02.63   Dental caries on smooth surface penetrating into pulp

K02.7   Dental root caries

K02.9   Dental caries, unspecified   ▽

EXCLUDES 1 Not coded here   EXCLUDES 2 Not included here   N Newborn Age: 0   P Pediatric Age: 0-17   M Maternity Age: 12-55   A Adult Age: 15-124

672   ICD-10-CM 2018

✓4th K03 Other diseases of hard tissues of teeth

EXCLUDES 2   bruxism (F45.8)
       dental caries (K02.-)
       teeth-grinding NOS (F45.8)

K03.0 Excessive attrition of teeth
   Approximal wear of teeth
   Occlusal wear of teeth

K03.1 Abrasion of teeth
   Dentifrice abrasion of teeth
   Habitual abrasion of teeth
   Occupational abrasion of teeth
   Ritual abrasion of teeth
   Traditional abrasion of teeth
   Wedge defect NOS

K03.2 Erosion of teeth
   Erosion of teeth due to diet
   Erosion of teeth due to drugs and medicaments
   Erosion of teeth due to persistent vomiting
   Erosion of teeth NOS
   Idiopathic erosion of teeth
   Occupational erosion of teeth

K03.3 Pathological resorption of teeth
   Internal granuloma of pulp
   Resorption of teeth (external)

K03.4 Hypercementosis
   Cementation hyperplasia

K03.5 Ankylosis of teeth

K03.6 Deposits [accretions] on teeth
   Betel deposits [accretions] on teeth
   Black deposits [accretions] on teeth
   Extrinsic staining of teeth NOS
   Green deposits [accretions] on teeth
   Materia alba deposits [accretions] on teeth
   Orange deposits [accretions] on teeth
   Staining of teeth NOS
   Subgingival dental calculus
   Supragingival dental calculus
   Tobacco deposits [accretions] on teeth

K03.7 Posteruptive color changes of dental hard tissues
   EXCLUDES 2   deposits [accretions] on teeth (K03.6)

✓5th K03.8 Other specified diseases of hard tissues of teeth

K03.81 Cracked tooth
   EXCLUDES 1   asymptomatic craze lines in enamel—omit
          code
       broken or fractured tooth due to trauma
       (S02.5)

K03.89 Other specified diseases of hard tissues of teeth

K03.9 Disease of hard tissues of teeth, unspecified ▽

✓4th K04 Diseases of pulp and periapical tissues

✓5th K04.0 Pulpitis
   Acute pulpitis
   Chronic (hyperplastic) (ulcerative) pulpitis

K04.01 Reversible pulpitis

K04.02 Irreversible pulpitis

K04.1 Necrosis of pulp
   Pulpal gangrene

K04.2 Pulp degeneration
   Denticles
   Pulpal calcifications
   Pulpal stones

K04.3 Abnormal hard tissue formation in pulp
   Secondary or irregular dentine

K04.4 Acute apical periodontitis of pulpal origin
   Acute apical periodontitis NOS
   EXCLUDES 1   acute periodontitis (K05.2-)
   DEF: Severe inflammation of the area surrounding the tip of a
   tooth's root; often secondary to infection or trauma.

K04.5 Chronic apical periodontitis
   Apical or periapical granuloma
   Apical periodontitis NOS
   EXCLUDES 1   chronic periodontitis (K05.3-)

K04.6 Periapical abscess with sinus
   Dental abscess with sinus
   Dentoalveolar abscess with sinus

K04.7 Periapical abscess without sinus
   Dental abscess without sinus
   Dentoalveolar abscess without sinus
   ~~Periapical abscess without sinus~~

K04.8 Radicular cyst
   Apical (periodontal) cyst
   Periapical cyst
   Residual radicular cyst
   EXCLUDES 2   lateral periodontal cyst (K09.0)
   DEF: Most common odontogenic cyst in tissue around tooth apex
   due to chronic inflammation of dental pulp.

✓5th K04.9 Other and unspecified diseases of pulp and periapical tissues

K04.90 Unspecified diseases of pulp and periapical ▽
       tissues

K04.99 Other diseases of pulp and periapical tissues

✓4th K05 Gingivitis and periodontal diseases

Use additional code to identify:
   alcohol abuse and dependence (F10.-)
   exposure to environmental tobacco smoke (Z77.22)
   exposure to tobacco smoke in the perinatal period (P96.81)
   history of tobacco dependence (Z87.891)
   occupational exposure to environmental tobacco smoke (Z57.31)
   tobacco dependence (F17.-)
   tobacco use (Z72.0)

✓5th K05.0 Acute gingivitis
   EXCLUDES 1   acute necrotizing ulcerative gingivitis (A69.1)
       herpesviral [herpes simplex] gingivostomatitis (B00.2)

K05.00 Acute gingivitis, plaque induced
   Acute gingivitis NOS
   Plaque induced gingival disease

K05.01 Acute gingivitis, non-plaque induced

✓5th K05.1 Chronic gingivitis
   Desquamative gingivitis (chronic)
   Gingivitis (chronic) NOS
   Hyperplastic gingivitis (chronic)
   Pregnancy associated gingivitis
   Simple marginal gingivitis (chronic)
   Ulcerative gingivitis (chronic)
   Code first, if applicable, diseases of the digestive system
       complicating pregnancy (O99.61-)

K05.10 Chronic gingivitis, plaque induced
   Chronic gingivitis NOS
   Gingivitis NOS

K05.11 Chronic gingivitis, non-plaque induced

✓5th K05.2 Aggressive periodontitis
   Acute pericoronitis
   EXCLUDES 1   acute apical periodontitis (K04.4)
       periapical abscess (K04.7)
       periapical abscess with sinus (K04.6)

K05.20 Aggressive periodontitis, unspecified ▽

✓6th K05.21 Aggressive periodontitis, localized
   Periodontal abscess

K05.211 Aggressive periodontitis, localized, slight

K05.212 Aggressive periodontitis, localized, moderate

K05.213 Aggressive periodontitis, localized, severe

K05.219 Aggressive periodontitis, localized, ▽
       unspecified severity

✓6th K05.22 Aggressive periodontitis, generalized

K05.221 Aggressive periodontitis, generalized, slight

K05.222 Aggressive periodontitis, generalized, moderate

K05.223 Aggressive periodontitis, generalized, severe

K05.229 Aggressive periodontitis, generalized, ▽
       unspecified severity

✓5th K05.3 Chronic periodontitis
   Chronic pericoronitis
   Complex periodontitis
   Periodontitis NOS
   Simplex periodontitis
   EXCLUDES 1   chronic apical periodontitis (K04.5)

K05.30 Chronic periodontitis, unspecified ▽

✓6th K05.31 Chronic periodontitis, localized

K05.311 Chronic periodontitis, localized, slight

K05.312 Chronic periodontitis, localized, moderate

☑ Additional Character Req   ✓x7th Placeholder Alert   Manifestation   HCC CMS-HCC Condition   ▽ Unspecified Code   ▶◀ Revised Text   ● New Code   ▲ Revised Code Title

ICD-10-CM 2018   673

K05.313   **Chronic periodontitis, localized, severe**

K05.319   **Chronic periodontitis, localized, unspecified severity** ▽

✓6th   **K05.32 Chronic periodontitis, generalized**

K05.321   **Chronic periodontitis, generalized, slight**

K05.322   **Chronic periodontitis, generalized, moderate**

K05.323   **Chronic periodontitis, generalized, severe**

K05.329   **Chronic periodontitis, generalized, unspecified severity** ▽

K05.4 Periodontosis
Juvenile periodontosis

K05.5 Other periodontal diseases
Combined periodontic-endodontic lesion
Narrow gingival width (of periodontal soft tissue)
EXCLUDES 2 *leukoplakia of gingiva (K13.21)*

K05.6 Periodontal disease, unspecified ▽

✓4th **K06 Other disorders of gingiva and edentulous alveolar ridge**
EXCLUDES 2 *acute gingivitis (K05.0)*
atrophy of edentulous alveolar ridge (K08.2)
chronic gingivitis (K05.1)
gingivitis NOS (K05.1)

✓5th **K06.0 Gingival recession**
▶Gingival recession (postinfective) (postprocedural)◀

•   ✓6th **K06.01 Gingival recession, localized**
•

K06.010   **Localized gingival recession, unspecified** ▽
Localized gingival recession, NOS

•   K06.011   **Localized gingival recession, minimal**
•   K06.012   **Localized gingival recession, moderate**
•   K06.013   **Localized gingival recession, severe**

•   ✓6th **K06.02 Gingival recession, generalized**
•

K06.020   **Generalized gingival recession, unspecified** ▽
Generalized gingival recession, NOS

•   K06.021   **Generalized gingival recession, minimal**
•   K06.022   **Generalized gingival recession, moderate**
•   K06.023   **Generalized gingival recession, severe**

K06.1 Gingival enlargement
Gingival fibromatosis

K06.2 Gingival and edentulous alveolar ridge lesions associated with trauma
Irritative hyperplasia of edentulous ridge [denture hyperplasia]
Use additional code (Chapter 20) to identify external cause or denture status (Z97.2)

K06.3 Horizontal alveolar bone loss

K06.8 Other specified disorders of gingiva and edentulous alveolar ridge
Fibrous epulis
Flabby alveolar ridge
Giant cell epulis
Peripheral giant cell granuloma of gingiva
Pyogenic granuloma of gingiva
Vertical ridge deficiency
EXCLUDES 2 *gingival cyst (K09.0)*

K06.9 Disorder of gingiva and edentulous alveolar ridge, unspecified ▽

✓4th **K08 Other disorders of teeth and supporting structures**
EXCLUDES 2 *dentofacial anomalies [including malocclusion] (M26.-)*
disorders of jaw (M27.-)

K08.0 Exfoliation of teeth due to systemic causes
Code also underlying systemic condition

✓5th **K08.1 Complete loss of teeth**
Acquired loss of teeth, complete
EXCLUDES 1 *congenital absence of teeth (K00.0)*
exfoliation of teeth due to systemic causes (K08.0)
partial loss of teeth (K08.4-)

✓6th **K08.10 Complete loss of teeth, unspecified cause**

K08.101   **Complete loss of teeth, unspecified cause, class I** ▽

K08.102   **Complete loss of teeth, unspecified cause, class II** ▽

K08.103   **Complete loss of teeth, unspecified cause, class III** ▽

K08.104   **Complete loss of teeth, unspecified cause, class IV** ▽

K08.109   **Complete loss of teeth, unspecified cause, unspecified class** ▽
Edentulism NOS

✓6th **K08.11 Complete loss of teeth due to trauma**

K08.111   **Complete loss of teeth due to trauma, class I**

K08.112   **Complete loss of teeth due to trauma, class II**

K08.113   **Complete loss of teeth due to trauma, class III**

K08.114   **Complete loss of teeth due to trauma, class IV**

K08.119   **Complete loss of teeth due to trauma, unspecified class** ▽

✓6th **K08.12 Complete loss of teeth due to periodontal diseases**

K08.121   **Complete loss of teeth due to periodontal diseases, class I**

K08.122   **Complete loss of teeth due to periodontal diseases, class II**

K08.123   **Complete loss of teeth due to periodontal diseases, class III**

K08.124   **Complete loss of teeth due to periodontal diseases, class IV**

K08.129   **Complete loss of teeth due to periodontal diseases, unspecified class** ▽

✓6th **K08.13 Complete loss of teeth due to caries**

K08.131   **Complete loss of teeth due to caries, class I**

K08.132   **Complete loss of teeth due to caries, class II**

K08.133   **Complete loss of teeth due to caries, class III**

K08.134   **Complete loss of teeth due to caries, class IV**

K08.139   **Complete loss of teeth due to caries, unspecified class** ▽

✓6th **K08.19 Complete loss of teeth due to other specified cause**

K08.191   **Complete loss of teeth due to other specified cause, class I**

K08.192   **Complete loss of teeth due to other specified cause, class II**

K08.193   **Complete loss of teeth due to other specified cause, class III**

K08.194   **Complete loss of teeth due to other specified cause, class IV**

K08.199   **Complete loss of teeth due to other specified cause, unspecified class** ▽

✓5th **K08.2 Atrophy of edentulous alveolar ridge**

K08.20   **Unspecified atrophy of edentulous alveolar ridge** ▽
Atrophy of the mandible NOS
Atrophy of the maxilla NOS

K08.21   **Minimal atrophy of the mandible**
Minimal atrophy of the edentulous mandible

K08.22   **Moderate atrophy of the mandible**
Moderate atrophy of the edentulous mandible

K08.23   **Severe atrophy of the mandible**
Severe atrophy of the edentulous mandible

K08.24   **Minimal atrophy of maxilla**
Minimal atrophy of the edentulous maxilla

K08.25   **Moderate atrophy of maxilla**
Moderate atrophy of the edentulous maxilla

K08.26   **Severe atrophy of maxilla**
Severe atrophy of the edentulous maxilla

K08.3 Retained dental root

✓5th **K08.4 Partial loss of teeth**
Acquired loss of teeth, partial
EXCLUDES 1 *complete loss of teeth (K08.1-)*
congenital absence of teeth (K00.0)
EXCLUDES 2 *exfoliation of teeth due to systemic causes (K08.0)*

✓6th **K08.40 Partial loss of teeth, unspecified cause**

K08.401   **Partial loss of teeth, unspecified cause, class I** ▽

K08.402   **Partial loss of teeth, unspecified cause, class II** ▽

K08.403   **Partial loss of teeth, unspecified cause, class III** ▽

EXCLUDES 1 Not coded here   EXCLUDES 2 Not included here   N Newborn Age: 0   P Pediatric Age: 0-17   M Maternity Age: 12-55   A Adult Age: 15-124

674   ICD-10-CM 2018

K08.404 Partial loss of teeth, unspecified cause, ▽
class IV

K08.409 Partial loss of teeth, unspecified ▽
cause, unspecified class
Tooth extraction status NOS

✓6ᵗʰ **K08.41** Partial loss of teeth due to trauma

K08.411 Partial loss of teeth due to trauma, class I

K08.412 Partial loss of teeth due to trauma, class II

K08.413 Partial loss of teeth due to trauma, class III

K08.414 Partial loss of teeth due to trauma, class IV

K08.419 Partial loss of teeth due to trauma, ▽
unspecified class

✓6ᵗʰ **K08.42** Partial loss of teeth due to periodontal diseases

K08.421 Partial loss of teeth due to periodontal
diseases, class I

K08.422 Partial loss of teeth due to periodontal
diseases, class II

K08.423 Partial loss of teeth due to periodontal
diseases, class III

K08.424 Partial loss of teeth due to periodontal
diseases, class IV

K08.429 Partial loss of teeth due to periodontal ▽
diseases, unspecified class

✓6ᵗʰ **K08.43** Partial loss of teeth due to caries

K08.431 Partial loss of teeth due to caries, class I

K08.432 Partial loss of teeth due to caries, class II

K08.433 Partial loss of teeth due to caries, class III

K08.434 Partial loss of teeth due to caries, class IV

K08.439 Partial loss of teeth due to caries, ▽
unspecified class

✓6ᵗʰ **K08.49** Partial loss of teeth due to other specified cause

K08.491 Partial loss of teeth due to other specified
cause, class I

K08.492 Partial loss of teeth due to other specified
cause, class II

K08.493 Partial loss of teeth due to other specified
cause, class III

K08.494 Partial loss of teeth due to other specified
cause, class IV

K08.499 Partial loss of teeth due to other ▽
specified cause, unspecified class

✓5ᵗʰ **K08.5** Unsatisfactory restoration of tooth
Defective bridge, crown, filling
Defective dental restoration
EXCLUDES 1   dental restoration status (Z98.811)
EXCLUDES 2   endosseous dental implant failure (M27.6-)
unsatisfactory endodontic treatment (M27.5-)

K08.50 Unsatisfactory restoration of tooth, unspecified ▽
Defective dental restoration NOS

K08.51 Open restoration margins of tooth
Dental restoration failure of marginal integrity
Open margin on tooth restoration
Poor gingival margin to tooth restoration

K08.52 Unrepairable overhanging of dental restorative
materials
Overhanging of tooth restoration

✓6ᵗʰ **K08.53** Fractured dental restorative material
EXCLUDES 1   cracked tooth (K03.81)
traumatic fracture of tooth (S02.5)

K08.530 Fractured dental restorative material
without loss of material

K08.531 Fractured dental restorative material with
loss of material

K08.539 Fractured dental restorative material, ▽
unspecified

K08.54 Contour of existing restoration of tooth biologically
incompatible with oral health
Dental restoration failure of periodontal anatomical
integrity
Unacceptable contours of existing restoration of tooth
Unacceptable morphology of existing restoration of
tooth

K08.55 Allergy to existing dental restorative material
Use additional code to identify the specific type of
allergy

K08.56 Poor aesthetic of existing restoration of tooth
Dental restoration aesthetically inadequate or
displeasing

K08.59 Other unsatisfactory restoration of tooth
Other defective dental restoration

✓5ᵗʰ **K08.8** Other specified disorders of teeth and supporting structures

K08.81 Primary occlusal trauma

K08.82 Secondary occlusal trauma

K08.89 Other specified disorders of teeth and supporting
structures
Enlargement of alveolar ridge NOS
Insufficient anatomic crown height
Insufficient clinical crown length
Irregular alveolar process
Toothache NOS

K08.9 Disorder of teeth and supporting structures, unspecified ▽

✓4ᵗʰ **K09** Cysts of oral region, not elsewhere classified
INCLUDES   lesions showing histological features both of aneurysmal cyst
and of another fibro-osseous lesion
EXCLUDES 2   cysts of jaw (M27.0-, M27.4-)
radicular cyst (K04.8)

K09.0 Developmental odontogenic cysts
Dentigerous cyst
Eruption cyst
Follicular cyst
Gingival cyst
Lateral periodontal cyst
Primordial cyst
EXCLUDES 2   keratocysts (D16.4, D16.5)
odontogenic keratocystic tumors (D16.4, D16.5)

K09.1 Developmental (nonodontogenic) cysts of oral region
Cyst (of) incisive canal
Cyst (of) palatine of papilla
Globulomaxillary cyst
Median palatal cyst
Nasoalveolar cyst
Nasolabial cyst
Nasopalatine duct cyst

K09.8 Other cysts of oral region, not elsewhere classified
Dermoid cyst
Epidermoid cyst
Lymphoepithelial cyst
Epstein's pearl

K09.9 Cyst of oral region, unspecified ▽

✓4ᵗʰ **K11** Diseases of salivary glands
Use additional code to identify:
alcohol abuse and dependence (F10.-)
exposure to environmental tobacco smoke (Z77.22)
exposure to tobacco smoke in the perinatal period (P96.81)
history of tobacco dependence (Z87.891)
occupational exposure to environmental tobacco smoke (Z57.31)
tobacco dependence (F17.-)
tobacco use (Z72.0)

K11.0 Atrophy of salivary gland

K11.1 Hypertrophy of salivary gland
DEF: Overgrowth of or enlarged salivary gland tissue; caused by
infection, salivary duct blockage, autoimmune diseases, and
benign and malignant tumors.

✓5ᵗʰ **K11.2** Sialoadenitis
Parotitis
EXCLUDES 1   epidemic parotitis (B26.-)
mumps (B26.-)
uveoparotid fever [Heerfordt] (D86.89)

K11.20 Sialoadenitis, unspecified ▽

K11.21 Acute sialoadenitis
EXCLUDES 1   acute recurrent sialoadenitis (K11.22)

K11.22 Acute recurrent sialoadenitis

K11.23 Chronic sialoadenitis

K11.3 Abscess of salivary gland

K11.4 Fistula of salivary gland
EXCLUDES 1   congenital fistula of salivary gland (Q38.4)

K11.5 Sialolithiasis
Calculus of salivary gland or duct
Stone of salivary gland or duct

K11.6 Mucocele of salivary gland
Mucous extravasation cyst of salivary gland
Mucous retention cyst of salivary gland
Ranula

✓ Additional Character Req   ✓x7ᵗʰ Placeholder Alert   Manifestation   HCC CMS-HCC Condition   ▽ Unspecified Code   ►◄ Revised Text   ● New Code   ▲ Revised Code Title

ICD-10-CM 2018   **675**

K11.7 Disturbances of salivary secretion
Hypoptyalism
Ptyalism
Xerostomia
EXCLUDES 2   dry mouth NOS (R68.2)

K11.8 Other diseases of salivary glands
Benign lymphoepithelial lesion of salivary gland
Mikulicz' disease
Necrotizing sialometaplasia
Sialectasia
Stenosis of salivary duct
Stricture of salivary duct
EXCLUDES 1   sicca syndrome [Sjögren] (M35.0-)

K11.9 Disease of salivary gland, unspecified   ▽
Sialoadenopathy NOS

✓4ᵗʰ K12 Stomatitis and related lesions
Use additional code to identify:
alcohol abuse and dependence (F10.-)
exposure to environmental tobacco smoke (Z77.22)
exposure to tobacco smoke in the perinatal period (P96.81)
history of tobacco dependence (Z87.891)
occupational exposure to environmental tobacco smoke (Z57.31)
tobacco dependence (F17.-)
tobacco use (Z72.0)
EXCLUDES 1   cancrum oris (A69.0)
        cheilitis (K13.0)
        gangrenous stomatitis (A69.0)
        herpesviral [herpes simplex] gingivostomatitis (B00.2)
        noma (A69.0)

K12.0 Recurrent oral aphthae
Aphthous stomatitis (major) (minor)
Bednar's aphthae
Periadenitis mucosa necrotica recurrens
Recurrent aphthous ulcer
Stomatitis herpetiformis
DEF: Disorder of unknown etiology with small oval or round painful ulcers of the mouth marked by a grayish exudate and a red halo effect.

K12.1 Other forms of stomatitis
Stomatitis NOS   Ulcerative stomatitis
Denture stomatitis   Vesicular stomatitis
EXCLUDES 1   acute necrotizing ulcerative stomatitis (A69.1)
        Vincent's stomatitis (A69.1)

K12.2 Cellulitis and abscess of mouth
Cellulitis of mouth (floor)
Submandibular abscess
EXCLUDES 2   abscess of salivary gland (K11.3)
        abscess of tongue (K14.0)
        periapical abscess (K04.6-K04.7)
        periodontal abscess (K05.21)
        peritonsillar abscess (J36)

✓5ᵗʰ K12.3 Oral mucositis (ulcerative)
Mucositis (oral) (oropharyneal)
EXCLUDES 2   gastrointestinal mucositis (ulcerative) (K92.81)
        mucositis (ulcerative) of vagina and vulva (N76.81)
        nasal mucositis (ulcerative) (J34.81)

K12.30 Oral mucositis (ulcerative), unspecified ▽
K12.31 Oral mucositis (ulcerative) due to antineoplastic therapy
Use additional code for adverse effect, if applicable, to identify antineoplastic and immunosuppressive drugs (T45.1X5)
Use additional code for other antineoplastic therapy, such as:
radiological procedure and radiotherapy (Y84.2)

K12.32 Oral mucositis (ulcerative) due to other drugs
Use additional code for adverse effect, if applicable, to identify drug (T36-T50 with fifth or sixth character 5)

K12.33 Oral mucositis (ulcerative) due to radiation
Use additional external cause code (W88-W90, X39.0-) to identify cause

K12.39 Other oral mucositis (ulcerative)
Viral oral mucositis (ulcerative)

✓4ᵗʰ K13 Other diseases of lip and oral mucosa
INCLUDES epithelial disturbances of tongue
Use additional code to identify:
alcohol abuse and dependence (F10.-)
exposure to environmental tobacco smoke (Z77.22)
exposure to tobacco smoke in the perinatal period (P96.81)
history of tobacco dependence (Z87.891)
occupational exposure to environmental tobacco smoke (Z57.31)
tobacco dependence (F17.-)
tobacco use (Z72.0)
EXCLUDES 2   certain disorders of gingiva and edentulous alveolar ridge (K05-K06)
        cysts of oral region (K09.-)
        diseases of tongue (K14.-)
        stomatitis and related lesions (K12.-)

K13.0 Diseases of lips
Abscess of lips   Exfoliative cheilitis
Angular cheilitis   Fistula of lips
Cellulitis of lips   Glandular cheilitis
Cheilitis NOS   Hypertrophy of lips
Cheilodynia   Perlèche NEC
Cheilosis
EXCLUDES 1   ariboflavinosis (E53.0)
        cheilitis due to radiation-related disorders (L55-L59)
        congenital fistula of lips (Q38.0)
        congenital hypertrophy of lips (Q18.6)
        Perlèche due to candidiasis (B37.83)
        Perlèche due to riboflavin deficiency (E53.0)

K13.1 Cheek and lip biting

✓5ᵗʰ K13.2 Leukoplakia and other disturbances of oral epithelium, including tongue
EXCLUDES 1   carcinoma in situ of oral epithelium (D00.0-)
        hairy leukoplakia (K13.3)

K13.21 Leukoplakia of oral mucosa, including tongue
Leukokeratosis of oral mucosa
Leukoplakia of gingiva, lips, tongue
EXCLUDES 1   hairy leukoplakia (K13.3)
        leukokeratosis nicotina palati (K13.24)

K13.22 Minimal keratinized residual ridge mucosa
Minimal keratinization of alveolar ridge mucosa

K13.23 Excessive keratinized residual ridge mucosa
Excessive keratinization of alveolar ridge mucosa

K13.24 Leukokeratosis nicotina palati
Smoker's palate

K13.29 Other disturbances of oral epithelium, including tongue
Erythroplakia of mouth or tongue
Focal epithelial hyperplasia of mouth or tongue
Leukoedema of mouth or tongue
Other oral epithelium disturbances

K13.3 Hairy leukoplakia

K13.4 Granuloma and granuloma-like lesions of oral mucosa
Eosinophilic granuloma
Granuloma pyogenicum
Verrucous xanthoma

K13.5 Oral submucous fibrosis
Submucous fibrosis of tongue

K13.6 Irritative hyperplasia of oral mucosa
EXCLUDES 2   irritative hyperplasia of edentulous ridge [denture hyperplasia] (K06.2)

✓5ᵗʰ K13.7 Other and unspecified lesions of oral mucosa
K13.70 Unspecified lesions of oral mucosa   ▽
K13.79 Other lesions of oral mucosa
Focal oral mucinosis

Chapter 11. Diseases of the Digestive System

✓4ᵗʰ **K14 Diseases of tongue**

Use additional code to identify:
alcohol abuse and dependence (F10.-)
exposure to environmental tobacco smoke (Z77.22)
history of tobacco dependence (Z87.891)
occupational exposure to environmental tobacco smoke (Z57.31)
tobacco dependence (F17.-)
tobacco use (Z72.0)

EXCLUDES 2 erythroplakia (K13.29)
focal epithelial hyperplasia (K13.29)
leukedema of tongue (K13.29)
leukoplakia of tongue (K13.21)
hairy leukoplakia (K13.3)
macroglossia (congenital) (Q38.2)
submucous fibrosis of tongue (K13.5)

K14.0 Glossitis
Abscess of tongue
Ulceration (traumatic) of tongue
EXCLUDES 1 atrophic glossitis (K14.4)

K14.1 Geographic tongue
Benign migratory glossitis
Glossitis areata exfoliativa

K14.2 Median rhomboid glossitis

K14.3 Hypertrophy of tongue papillae
Black hairy tongue
Coated tongue
Hypertrophy of foliate papillae
Lingua villosa nigra

K14.4 Atrophy of tongue papillae
Atrophic glossitis

K14.5 Plicated tongue
Fissured tongue
Furrowed tongue
Scrotal tongue
EXCLUDES 1 fissured tongue, congenital (Q38.3)

K14.6 Glossodynia
Glossopyrosis
Painful tongue

K14.8 Other diseases of tongue
Atrophy of tongue   Glossocele
Crenated tongue   Glossoptosis
Enlargement of tongue   Hypertrophy of tongue

K14.9 Disease of tongue, unspecified   ▽
Glossopathy NOS

Diseases of esophagus, stomach and duodenum (K20-K31)

EXCLUDES 2 hiatus hernia (K44.-)

✓4ᵗʰ **K20 Esophagitis**

Use additional code to identify:
alcohol abuse and dependence (F10.-)
EXCLUDES 1 erosion of esophagus (K22.1-)
esophagitis with gastro-esophageal reflux disease (K21.0)
reflux esophagitis (K21.0)
ulcerative esophagitis (K22.1-)
EXCLUDES 2 eosinophilic gastritis or gastroenteritis (K52.81)

K20.0 Eosinophilic esophagitis

K20.8 Other esophagitis
Abscess of esophagus

K20.9 Esophagitis, unspecified   ▽
Esophagitis NOS

✓4ᵗʰ **K21 Gastro-esophageal reflux disease**
EXCLUDES 1 newborn esophageal reflux (P78.83)

K21.0 Gastro-esophageal reflux disease with esophagitis
Reflux esophagitis

K21.9 Gastro-esophageal reflux disease without esophagitis
Esophageal reflux NOS
AHA: 2016, 1Q, 18

✓4ᵗʰ **K22 Other diseases of esophagus**
EXCLUDES 2 esophageal varices (I85.-)

K22.0 Achalasia of cardia
Achalasia NOS
Cardiospasm
EXCLUDES 1 congenital cardiospasm (Q39.5)
DEF: Esophageal motility disorder; caused by absence of
esophageal peristalsis and impaired relaxation of lower
esophageal sphincter; characterized by dysphagia, regurgitation,
and heartburn.

✓5ᵗʰ **K22.1 Ulcer of esophagus**
Barrett's ulcer
Erosion of esophagus
Fungal ulcer of esophagus
Peptic ulcer of esophagus
Ulcer of esophagus due to ingestion of chemicals
Ulcer of esophagus due to ingestion of drugs and medicaments
Ulcerative esophagitis
Code first poisoning due to drug or toxin, if applicable (T36-T65
with fifth or sixth character 1-4 or 6)
Use additional code for adverse effect, if applicable, to identify
drug (T36-T50 with fifth or sixth character 5)
EXCLUDES 2 Barrett's esophagus (K22.7-)

K22.10 Ulcer of esophagus without bleeding
Ulcer of esophagus NOS

K22.11 Ulcer of esophagus with bleeding
EXCLUDES 2 bleeding esophageal varices (I85.01, I85.11)

K22.2 Esophageal obstruction
Compression of esophagus
Constriction of esophagus
Stenosis of esophagus
Stricture of esophagus
EXCLUDES 1 congenital stenosis or stricture of esophagus (Q39.3)

K22.3 Perforation of esophagus
Rupture of esophagus
EXCLUDES 1 traumatic perforation of (thoracic) esophagus (S27.8-)

K22.4 Dyskinesia of esophagus
Corkscrew esophagus
Diffuse esophageal spasm
Spasm of esophagus
EXCLUDES 1 cardiospasm (K22.0)

K22.5 Diverticulum of esophagus, acquired
Esophageal pouch, acquired
EXCLUDES 1 diverticulum of esophagus (congenital) (Q39.6)

K22.6 Gastro-esophageal laceration-hemorrhage syndrome
Mallory-Weiss syndrome

✓5ᵗʰ **K22.7 Barrett's esophagus**
Barrett's disease
Barrett's syndrome
EXCLUDES 1 Barrett's ulcer (K22.1)
malignant neoplasm of esophagus (C15.-)
DEF: A metaplastic disorder in which specialized columnar
epithelial cells replace the normal squamous epithelial cells;
secondary to chronic gastroesophageal reflux damage to the
mucosa; increases risk of developing adenocarcinoma.

K22.70 Barrett's esophagus without dysplasia
Barrett's esophagus NOS

✓6ᵗʰ **K22.71 Barrett's esophagus with dysplasia**
K22.710 Barrett's esophagus with low grade dysplasia
K22.711 Barrett's esophagus with high grade dysplasia
K22.719 Barrett's esophagus with dysplasia, unspecified   ▽

K22.8 Other specified diseases of esophagus
Hemorrhage of esophagus NOS
EXCLUDES 2 esophageal varices (I85.-)
Paterson-Kelly syndrome (D50.1)

K22.9 Disease of esophagus, unspecified   ▽

K23 Disorders of esophagus in diseases classified elsewhere
Code first underlying disease, such as:
congenital syphilis (A50.5)
EXCLUDES 1 late syphilis (A52.79)
megaesophagus due to Chagas' disease (B57.31)
tuberculosis (A18.83)

✓4ᵗʰ **K25 Gastric ulcer**
INCLUDES erosion (acute) of stomach
pylorus ulcer (peptic)
stomach ulcer (peptic)
Use additional code to identify:
alcohol abuse and dependence (F10.-)
EXCLUDES 1 acute gastritis (K29.0-)
peptic ulcer NOS (K27.-)

K25.0 Acute gastric ulcer with hemorrhage
K25.1 Acute gastric ulcer with perforation   HCC
K25.2 Acute gastric ulcer with both hemorrhage and perforation   HCC
K25.3 Acute gastric ulcer without hemorrhage or perforation

✓ Additional Character Req   ✓x7ᵗʰ Placeholder Alert   **Manifestation**   HCC CMS-HCC Condition   ▽ Unspecified Code   ▶◀ Revised Text   ● New Code   ▲ Revised Code Title

Gastrointestinal Ulcers

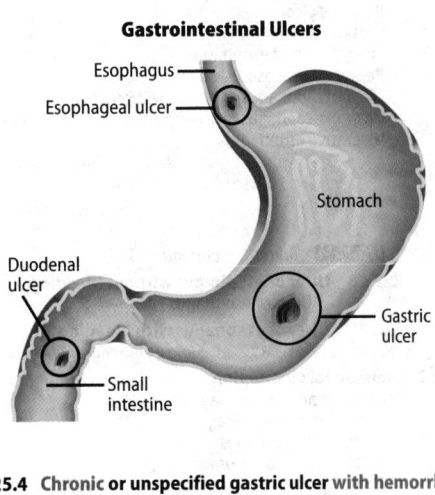

Esophagus
Esophageal ulcer
Stomach
Duodenal ulcer
Gastric ulcer
Small intestine

K25.4 Chronic or unspecified gastric ulcer with hemorrhage

K25.5 Chronic or unspecified gastric ulcer with perforation `HCC`

K25.6 Chronic or unspecified gastric ulcer with both hemorrhage and perforation `HCC`

K25.7 Chronic gastric ulcer without hemorrhage or perforation

K25.9 Gastric ulcer, unspecified as acute or chronic, without hemorrhage or perforation ▽

☑4ᵗʰ **K26 Duodenal ulcer**
> INCLUDES   erosion (acute) of duodenum
> duodenum ulcer (peptic)
> postpyloric ulcer (peptic)
> Use additional code to identify:
> alcohol abuse and dependence (F1Ø.-)
> EXCLUDES 1   peptic ulcer NOS (K27.-)

K26.Ø Acute duodenal ulcer with hemorrhage

K26.1 Acute duodenal ulcer with perforation `HCC`

K26.2 Acute duodenal ulcer with both hemorrhage and perforation `HCC`

K26.3 Acute duodenal ulcer without hemorrhage or perforation

K26.4 Chronic or unspecified duodenal ulcer with hemorrhage
> AHA: 2016, 1Q, 14

K26.5 Chronic or unspecified duodenal ulcer with perforation `HCC`

K26.6 Chronic or unspecified duodenal ulcer with both hemorrhage and perforation `HCC`

K26.7 Chronic duodenal ulcer without hemorrhage or perforation

K26.9 Duodenal ulcer, unspecified as acute or chronic, without hemorrhage or perforation ▽

☑4ᵗʰ **K27 Peptic ulcer, site unspecified**
> INCLUDES   gastroduodenal ulcer NOS
> peptic ulcer NOS
> Use additional code to identify:
> alcohol abuse and dependence (F1Ø.-)
> EXCLUDES 1   peptic ulcer of newborn (P78.82)

K27.Ø Acute peptic ulcer, site unspecified, with hemorrhage

K27.1 Acute peptic ulcer, site unspecified, with perforation `HCC`

K27.2 Acute peptic ulcer, site unspecified, with both hemorrhage and perforation `HCC`

K27.3 Acute peptic ulcer, site unspecified, without hemorrhage or perforation

K27.4 Chronic or unspecified peptic ulcer, site unspecified, with hemorrhage

K27.5 Chronic or unspecified peptic ulcer, site unspecified, with perforation `HCC`

K27.6 Chronic or unspecified peptic ulcer, site unspecified, with both hemorrhage and perforation `HCC`

K27.7 Chronic peptic ulcer, site unspecified, without hemorrhage or perforation

K27.9 Peptic ulcer, site unspecified, unspecified as acute or chronic, without hemorrhage or perforation ▽

☑4ᵗʰ **K28 Gastrojejunal ulcer**
> INCLUDES   anastomotic ulcer (peptic) or erosion
> gastrocolic ulcer (peptic) or erosion
> gastrointestinal ulcer (peptic) or erosion
> gastrojejunal ulcer (peptic) or erosion
> jejunal ulcer (peptic) or erosion
> marginal ulcer (peptic) or erosion
> stomal ulcer (peptic) or erosion
> Use additional code to identify:
> alcohol abuse and dependence (F1Ø.-)
> EXCLUDES 1   primary ulcer of small intestine (K63.3)

K28.Ø Acute gastrojejunal ulcer with hemorrhage

K28.1 Acute gastrojejunal ulcer with perforation `HCC`

K28.2 Acute gastrojejunal ulcer with both hemorrhage and perforation `HCC`

K28.3 Acute gastrojejunal ulcer without hemorrhage or perforation

K28.4 Chronic or unspecified gastrojejunal ulcer with hemorrhage

K28.5 Chronic or unspecified gastrojejunal ulcer with perforation `HCC`

K28.6 Chronic or unspecified gastrojejunal ulcer with both hemorrhage and perforation `HCC`

K28.7 Chronic gastrojejunal ulcer without hemorrhage or perforation

K28.9 Gastrojejunal ulcer, unspecified as acute or chronic, without hemorrhage or perforation ▽

☑4ᵗʰ **K29 Gastritis and duodenitis**
> EXCLUDES 1   eosinophilic gastritis or gastroenteritis (K52.81)
> Zollinger-Ellison syndrome (E16.4)

☑5ᵗʰ **K29.Ø** Acute gastritis
> Use additional code to identify:
> alcohol abuse and dependence (F1Ø.-)
> EXCLUDES 1   erosion (acute) of stomach (K25.-)

K29.ØØ Acute gastritis without bleeding

K29.Ø1 Acute gastritis with bleeding

☑5ᵗʰ **K29.2** Alcoholic gastritis
> Use additional code to identify:
> alcohol abuse and dependence (F1Ø.-)

K29.2Ø Alcoholic gastritis without bleeding

K29.21 Alcoholic gastritis with bleeding

☑5ᵗʰ **K29.3** Chronic superficial gastritis

K29.3Ø Chronic superficial gastritis without bleeding

K29.31 Chronic superficial gastritis with bleeding

☑5ᵗʰ **K29.4** Chronic atrophic gastritis
> Gastric atrophy

K29.4Ø Chronic atrophic gastritis without bleeding

K29.41 Chronic atrophic gastritis with bleeding

☑5ᵗʰ **K29.5** Unspecified chronic gastritis
> Chronic antral gastritis
> Chronic fundal gastritis

K29.5Ø Unspecified chronic gastritis without bleeding ▽

K29.51 Unspecified chronic gastritis with bleeding ▽

☑5ᵗʰ **K29.6** Other gastritis
> Giant hypertrophic gastritis
> Granulomatous gastritis
> Ménétrier's disease

K29.6Ø Other gastritis without bleeding

K29.61 Other gastritis with bleeding

☑5ᵗʰ **K29.7** Gastritis, unspecified

K29.7Ø Gastritis, unspecified, without bleeding ▽

K29.71 Gastritis, unspecified, with bleeding ▽

☑5ᵗʰ **K29.8** Duodenitis

K29.8Ø Duodenitis without bleeding

K29.81 Duodenitis with bleeding

☑5ᵗʰ **K29.9** Gastroduodenitis, unspecified

K29.9Ø Gastroduodenitis, unspecified, without bleeding ▽

K29.91 Gastroduodenitis, unspecified, with bleeding ▽

K3Ø Functional dyspepsia
> Indigestion
> EXCLUDES 1   dyspepsia NOS (R1Ø.13)
> heartburn (R12)
> nervous dyspepsia (F45.8)
> neurotic dyspepsia (F45.8)
> psychogenic dyspepsia (F45.8)

EXCLUDES 1 Not coded here   EXCLUDES 2 Not included here   N Newborn Age: 0   P Pediatric Age: 0-17   M Maternity Age: 12-55   A Adult Age: 15-124

678   ICD-10-CM 2018

✓4ᵗʰ K31 Other diseases of stomach and duodenum
INCLUDES functional disorders of stomach
EXCLUDES 2 diabetic gastroparesis (E08.43, E09.43, E10.43, E11.43, E13.43)
diverticulum of duodenum (K57.00-K57.13)

K31.0 Acute dilatation of stomach
Acute distention of stomach

K31.1 Adult hypertrophic pyloric stenosis 🅰
Pyloric stenosis NOS
EXCLUDES 1 congenital or infantile pyloric stenosis (Q40.0)

K31.2 Hourglass stricture and stenosis of stomach
EXCLUDES 1 congenital hourglass stomach (Q40.2)
hourglass contraction of stomach (K31.89)

K31.3 Pylorospasm, not elsewhere classified
EXCLUDES 1 congenital or infantile pylorospasm (Q40.0)
neurotic pylorospasm (F45.8)
psychogenic pylorospasm (F45.8)

K31.4 Gastric diverticulum
EXCLUDES 1 congenital diverticulum of stomach (Q40.2)

K31.5 Obstruction of duodenum
Constriction of duodenum
Duodenal ileus (chronic)
Stenosis of duodenum
Stricture of duodenum
Volvulus of duodenum
EXCLUDES 1 congenital stenosis of duodenum (Q41.0)

K31.6 Fistula of stomach and duodenum
Gastrocolic fistula
Gastrojejunocolic fistula

K31.7 Polyp of stomach and duodenum
EXCLUDES 1 adenomatous polyp of stomach (D13.1)

✓5ᵗʰ K31.8 Other specified diseases of stomach and duodenum
✓6ᵗʰ K31.81 Angiodysplasia of stomach and duodenum
K31.811 Angiodysplasia of stomach and duodenum with bleeding
K31.819 Angiodysplasia of stomach and duodenum without bleeding
Angiodysplasia of stomach and duodenum NOS

K31.82 Dieulafoy lesion (hemorrhagic) of stomach and duodenum
EXCLUDES 2 Dieulafoy lesion of intestine (K63.81)

K31.83 Achlorhydria
DEF: Absence of hydrochloric acid in gastric secretions due to gastric mucosa atrophy; unresponsive to histamines; also known as gastric anacidity.

K31.84 Gastroparesis
Gastroparalysis
Code first underlying disease, if known, such as:
anorexia nervosa (F50.0-)
diabetes mellitus (E08.43, E09.43, E10.43, E11.43, E13.43)
scleroderma (M34.-)
AHA: 2013, 4Q, 114

K31.89 Other diseases of stomach and duodenum
AHA: 2017, 1Q, 28

K31.9 Disease of stomach and duodenum, unspecified ▽

Diseases of appendix (K35-K38)

✓4ᵗʰ K35 Acute appendicitis
K35.2 Acute appendicitis with generalized peritonitis
Appendicitis (acute) with generalized (diffuse) peritonitis following rupture or perforation of appendix
Perforated appendix NOS
Ruptured appendix NOS

K35.3 Acute appendicitis with localized peritonitis
Acute appendicitis with or without perforation or rupture with peritonitis NOS
Acute appendicitis with or without perforation or rupture with localized peritonitis
Acute appendicitis with peritoneal abscess

✓5ᵗʰ K35.8 Other and unspecified acute appendicitis
K35.80 Unspecified acute appendicitis ▽
Acute appendicitis NOS
Acute appendicitis without (localized) (generalized) peritonitis

K35.89 Other acute appendicitis

K36 Other appendicitis
Chronic appendicitis
Recurrent appendicitis

K37 Unspecified appendicitis ▽
EXCLUDES 1 unspecified appendicitis with peritonitis (K35.2-K35.3)

✓4ᵗʰ K38 Other diseases of appendix
K38.0 Hyperplasia of appendix

K38.1 Appendicular concretions
Fecalith of appendix
Stercolith of appendix

K38.2 Diverticulum of appendix

K38.3 Fistula of appendix

K38.8 Other specified diseases of appendix
Intussusception of appendix

K38.9 Disease of appendix, unspecified ▽

Hernia (K40-K46)
NOTE Hernia with both gangrene and obstruction is classified to hernia with gangrene.
INCLUDES acquired hernia
congenital [except diaphragmatic or hiatus] hernia
recurrent hernia

✓4ᵗʰ K40 Inguinal hernia
INCLUDES bubonocele
direct inguinal hernia
double inguinal hernia
indirect inguinal hernia
inguinal hernia NOS
oblique inguinal hernia
scrotal hernia

✓5ᵗʰ K40.0 Bilateral inguinal hernia, with obstruction, without gangrene
Inguinal hernia (bilateral) causing obstruction without gangrene
Incarcerated inguinal hernia (bilateral) without gangrene
Irreducible inguinal hernia (bilateral) without gangrene
Strangulated inguinal hernia (bilateral) without gangrene

K40.00 Bilateral inguinal hernia, with obstruction, without gangrene, not specified as recurrent
Bilateral inguinal hernia, with obstruction, without gangrene NOS

K40.01 Bilateral inguinal hernia, with obstruction, without gangrene, recurrent

✓5ᵗʰ K40.1 Bilateral inguinal hernia, with gangrene
K40.10 Bilateral inguinal hernia, with gangrene, not specified as recurrent
Bilateral inguinal hernia, with gangrene NOS
K40.11 Bilateral inguinal hernia, with gangrene, recurrent

✓5ᵗʰ K40.2 Bilateral inguinal hernia, without obstruction or gangrene
K40.20 Bilateral inguinal hernia, without obstruction or gangrene, not specified as recurrent
Bilateral inguinal hernia NOS
K40.21 Bilateral inguinal hernia, without obstruction or gangrene, recurrent

✓5ᵗʰ K40.3 Unilateral inguinal hernia, with obstruction, without gangrene
Inguinal hernia (unilateral) causing obstruction without gangrene
Incarcerated inguinal hernia (unilateral) without gangrene
Irreducible inguinal hernia (unilateral) without gangrene
Strangulated inguinal hernia (unilateral) without gangrene

K40.30 Unilateral inguinal hernia, with obstruction, without gangrene, not specified as recurrent
Inguinal hernia, with obstruction NOS
Unilateral inguinal hernia, with obstruction, without gangrene NOS

K40.31 Unilateral inguinal hernia, with obstruction, without gangrene, recurrent

✓5ᵗʰ K40.4 Unilateral inguinal hernia, with gangrene
K40.40 Unilateral inguinal hernia, with gangrene, not specified as recurrent
Inguinal hernia with gangrene NOS
Unilateral inguinal hernia with gangrene NOS
K40.41 Unilateral inguinal hernia, with gangrene, recurrent

✓5ᵗʰ K40.9 Unilateral inguinal hernia, without obstruction or gangrene
K40.90 Unilateral inguinal hernia, without obstruction or gangrene, not specified as recurrent
Inguinal hernia NOS
Unilateral inguinal hernia NOS
K40.91 Unilateral inguinal hernia, without obstruction or gangrene, recurrent

Hernia Sites

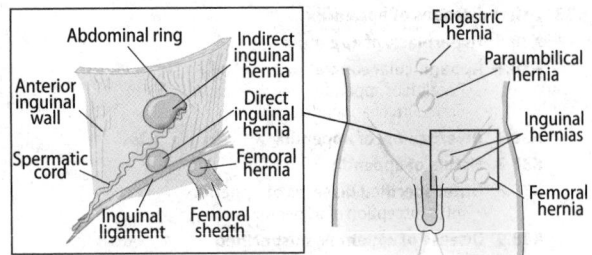

✓4ᵗʰ K41   Femoral **hernia**

✓5ᵗʰ K41.0   Bilateral femoral hernia, with obstruction, without gangrene
Femoral hernia (bilateral) causing obstruction, without gangrene
Incarcerated femoral hernia (bilateral), without gangrene
Irreducible femoral hernia (bilateral), without gangrene
Strangulated femoral hernia (bilateral), without gangrene

     K41.00   Bilateral femoral hernia, with obstruction, without gangrene, not specified as recurrent
Bilateral femoral hernia, with obstruction, without gangrene NOS

     K41.01   Bilateral femoral hernia, with obstruction, without gangrene, recurrent

✓5ᵗʰ K41.1   Bilateral femoral hernia, with gangrene

     K41.10   Bilateral femoral hernia, with gangrene, not specified as recurrent
Bilateral femoral hernia, with gangrene NOS

     K41.11   Bilateral femoral hernia, with gangrene, recurrent

✓5ᵗʰ K41.2   Bilateral femoral hernia, without obstruction or gangrene

     K41.20   Bilateral femoral hernia, without obstruction or gangrene, not specified as recurrent
Bilateral femoral hernia NOS

     K41.21   Bilateral femoral hernia, without obstruction or gangrene, recurrent

✓5ᵗʰ K41.3   Unilateral femoral hernia, with obstruction, without gangrene
Femoral hernia (unilateral) causing obstruction, without gangrene
Incarcerated femoral hernia (unilateral), without gangrene
Irreducible femoral hernia (unilateral), without gangrene
Strangulated femoral hernia (unilateral), without gangrene

     K41.30   Unilateral femoral hernia, with obstruction, without gangrene, not specified as recurrent
Femoral hernia, with obstruction NOS
Unilateral femoral hernia, with obstruction NOS

     K41.31   Unilateral femoral hernia, with obstruction, without gangrene, recurrent

✓5ᵗʰ K41.4   Unilateral femoral hernia, with gangrene

     K41.40   Unilateral femoral hernia, with gangrene, not specified as recurrent
Femoral hernia, with gangrene NOS
Unilateral femoral hernia, with gangrene NOS

     K41.41   Unilateral femoral hernia, with gangrene, recurrent

✓5ᵗʰ K41.9   Unilateral femoral hernia, without obstruction or gangrene

     K41.90   Unilateral femoral hernia, without obstruction or gangrene, not specified as recurrent
Femoral hernia NOS
Unilateral femoral hernia NOS

     K41.91   Unilateral femoral hernia, without obstruction or gangrene, recurrent

✓4ᵗʰ K42   Umbilical **hernia**
     INCLUDES   paraumbilical hernia
     EXCLUDES 1   *omphalocele (Q79.2)*

K42.0   Umbilical hernia with obstruction, without gangrene
Umbilical hernia causing obstruction, without gangrene
Incarcerated umbilical hernia, without gangrene
Irreducible umbilical hernia, without gangrene
Strangulated umbilical hernia, without gangrene

K42.1   Umbilical hernia with gangrene
Gangrenous umbilical hernia

K42.9   Umbilical hernia without obstruction or gangrene
Umbilical hernia NOS

✓4ᵗʰ K43   Ventral **hernia**

K43.0   Incisional hernia with obstruction, without gangrene
Incisional hernia causing obstruction, without gangrene
Incarcerated incisional hernia, without gangrene
Irreducible incisional hernia, without gangrene
Strangulated incisional hernia, without gangrene

K43.1   Incisional hernia with gangrene
Gangrenous incisional hernia

K43.2   Incisional hernia without obstruction or gangrene
Incisional hernia NOS

K43.3   Parastomal hernia with obstruction, without gangrene
Incarcerated parastomal hernia, without gangrene
Irreducible parastomal hernia, without gangrene
Parastomal hernia causing obstruction, without gangrene
Strangulated parastomal hernia, without gangrene

K43.4   Parastomal hernia with gangrene
Gangrenous parastomal hernia

K43.5   Parastomal hernia without obstruction or gangrene
Parastomal hernia NOS

K43.6   Other and unspecified ventral hernia with obstruction, without gangrene   ▽
Epigastric hernia causing obstruction, without gangrene
Hypogastric hernia causing obstruction, without gangrene
Incarcerated epigastric hernia without gangrene
Incarcerated hypogastric hernia without gangrene
Incarcerated midline hernia without gangrene
Incarcerated spigelian hernia without gangrene
Incarcerated subxiphoid hernia without gangrene
Irreducible epigastric hernia without gangrene
Irreducible hypogastric hernia without gangrene
Irreducible midline hernia without gangrene
Irreducible spigelian hernia without gangrene
Irreducible subxiphoid hernia without gangrene
Midline hernia causing obstruction, without gangrene
Spigelian hernia causing obstruction, without gangrene
Strangulated epigastric hernia without gangrene
Strangulated hypogastric hernia without gangrene
Strangulated midline hernia without gangrene
Strangulated spigelian hernia without gangrene
Strangulated subxiphoid hernia without gangrene
Subxiphoid hernia causing obstruction, without gangrene

K43.7   Other and unspecified ventral hernia with gangrene   ▽
Any condition listed under K43.6 specified as gangrenous

K43.9   Ventral hernia without obstruction or gangrene   ▽
Epigastric hernia
Ventral hernia NOS

✓4ᵗʰ K44   Diaphragmatic **hernia**
     INCLUDES   hiatus hernia (esophageal) (sliding)
             paraesophageal hernia
     EXCLUDES 1   *congenital diaphragmatic hernia (Q79.0)*
               congenital hiatus hernia (Q40.1)

K44.0   Diaphragmatic hernia with obstruction, without gangrene
Diaphragmatic hernia causing obstruction
Incarcerated diaphragmatic hernia
Irreducible diaphragmatic hernia
Strangulated diaphragmatic hernia

K44.1   Diaphragmatic hernia with gangrene
Gangrenous diaphragmatic hernia

Hiatal Hernia

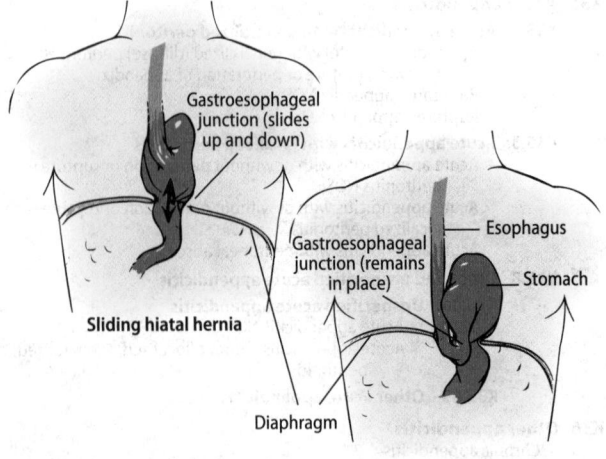

Sliding hiatal hernia

Gastroesophageal junction (slides up and down)

Gastroesophageal junction (remains in place)

Esophagus

Stomach

Diaphragm

Paraesophageal hiatal hernia

EXCLUDES 1 Not coded here   **EXCLUDES 2** Not included here   **N** Newborn Age: 0   **P** Pediatric Age: 0-17   **M** Maternity Age: 12-55   **A** Adult Age: 15-124

680   ICD-10-CM 2018

K44.9 Diaphragmatic hernia without obstruction or gangrene
Diaphragmatic hernia NOS

✓4ᵗʰ **K45 Other abdominal hernia**
INCLUDES abdominal hernia, specified site NEC
lumbar hernia
obturator hernia
pudendal hernia
retroperitoneal hernia
sciatic hernia

K45.0 Other specified abdominal hernia with obstruction, without gangrene
Other specified abdominal hernia causing obstruction
Other specified incarcerated abdominal hernia
Other specified irreducible abdominal hernia
Other specified strangulated abdominal hernia

K45.1 Other specified abdominal hernia with gangrene
Any condition listed under K45 specified as gangrenous

K45.8 Other specified abdominal hernia without obstruction or gangrene

✓4ᵗʰ **K46 Unspecified abdominal hernia**
INCLUDES enterocele
epiplocele
hernia NOS
interstitial hernia
intestinal hernia
intra-abdominal hernia
EXCLUDES 1 vaginal enterocele (N81.5)

K46.0 Unspecified abdominal hernia with obstruction, without gangrene ▽
Unspecified abdominal hernia causing obstruction
Unspecified incarcerated abdominal hernia
Unspecified irreducible abdominal hernia
Unspecified strangulated abdominal hernia

K46.1 Unspecified abdominal hernia with gangrene ▽
Any condition listed under K46 specified as gangrenous

K46.9 Unspecified abdominal hernia without obstruction or gangrene ▽
Abdominal hernia NOS

Noninfective enteritis and colitis (K50-K52)

INCLUDES noninfective inflammatory bowel disease
EXCLUDES 1 irritable bowel syndrome (K58.-)
megacolon (K59.3-)

✓4ᵗʰ **K50 Crohn's disease [regional enteritis]**
INCLUDES granulomatous enteritis
Use additional code to identify manifestations, such as:
pyoderma gangrenosum (L88)
EXCLUDES 1 ulcerative colitis (K51.-)
AHA: 2012, 4Q, 104

✓5ᵗʰ **K50.0 Crohn's disease of** small intestine
Crohn's disease [regional enteritis] of duodenum
Crohn's disease [regional enteritis] of ileum
Crohn's disease [regional enteritis] of jejunum
Regional ileitis
Terminal ileitis
EXCLUDES 1 Crohn's disease of both small and large intestine (K50.8-)

K50.00 Crohn's disease of small intestine without complications HCC

✓6ᵗʰ **K50.01 Crohn's disease of small intestine** with complications
K50.011 Crohn's disease of small intestine with rectal bleeding HCC
K50.012 Crohn's disease of small intestine with intestinal obstruction HCC
K50.013 Crohn's disease of small intestine with fistula HCC
K50.014 Crohn's disease of small intestine with abscess HCC
    AHA: 2012, 4Q, 104
K50.018 Crohn's disease of small intestine with other complication HCC
K50.019 Crohn's disease of small intestine with unspecified complications HCC ▽

✓5ᵗʰ **K50.1 Crohn's disease of** large intestine
Crohn's disease [regional enteritis] of colon
Crohn's disease [regional enteritis] of large bowel
Crohn's disease [regional enteritis] of rectum
Granulomatous colitis
Regional colitis
EXCLUDES 1 Crohn's disease of both small and large intestine (K50.8)

K50.10 Crohn's disease of large intestine without complications HCC

✓6ᵗʰ **K50.11 Crohn's disease of large intestine** with complications
K50.111 Crohn's disease of large intestine with rectal bleeding HCC
K50.112 Crohn's disease of large intestine with intestinal obstruction HCC
K50.113 Crohn's disease of large intestine with fistula HCC
K50.114 Crohn's disease of large intestine with abscess HCC
K50.118 Crohn's disease of large intestine with other complication HCC
K50.119 Crohn's disease of large intestine with unspecified complications HCC ▽

✓5ᵗʰ **K50.8 Crohn's disease of** both small and large intestine
K50.80 Crohn's disease of both small and large intestine without complications HCC

✓6ᵗʰ **K50.81 Crohn's disease of both small and large intestine** with complications
K50.811 Crohn's disease of both small and large intestine with rectal bleeding HCC
K50.812 Crohn's disease of both small and large intestine with intestinal obstruction HCC
K50.813 Crohn's disease of both small and large intestine with fistula HCC
K50.814 Crohn's disease of both small and large intestine with abscess HCC
K50.818 Crohn's disease of both small and large intestine with other complication HCC
K50.819 Crohn's disease of both small and large intestine with unspecified complications HCC ▽

✓5ᵗʰ **K50.9 Crohn's disease, unspecified**
K50.90 Crohn's disease, unspecified, without complications HCC ▽
Crohn's disease NOS
Regional enteritis NOS

✓6ᵗʰ **K50.91 Crohn's disease, unspecified,** with complications
K50.911 Crohn's disease, unspecified, with rectal bleeding HCC ▽
K50.912 Crohn's disease, unspecified, with intestinal obstruction HCC ▽
K50.913 Crohn's disease, unspecified, with fistula HCC ▽
K50.914 Crohn's disease, unspecified, with abscess HCC ▽
K50.918 Crohn's disease, unspecified, with other complication HCC ▽
K50.919 Crohn's disease, unspecified, with unspecified complications HCC ▽

✓4ᵗʰ **K51 Ulcerative colitis**
Use additional code to identify manifestations, such as:
pyoderma gangrenosum (L88)
EXCLUDES 1 Crohn's disease [regional enteritis] (K50.-)

✓5ᵗʰ **K51.0 Ulcerative (chronic) pancolitis**
Backwash ileitis
K51.00 Ulcerative (chronic) pancolitis without complications HCC
Ulcerative (chronic) pancolitis NOS

✓6ᵗʰ **K51.01 Ulcerative (chronic) pancolitis** with complications
K51.011 Ulcerative (chronic) pancolitis with rectal bleeding HCC
K51.012 Ulcerative (chronic) pancolitis with intestinal obstruction HCC
K51.013 Ulcerative (chronic) pancolitis with fistula HCC
K51.014 Ulcerative (chronic) pancolitis with abscess HCC

         K51.Ø18   **Ulcerative (chronic) pancolitis with other complication**   HCC

         K51.Ø19   **Ulcerative (chronic) pancolitis with unspecified complications**   HCC ▽

✓5ᵗʰ   **K51.2**   **Ulcerative (chronic) proctitis**

     K51.2Ø   **Ulcerative (chronic) proctitis without complications**   HCC
         Ulcerative (chronic) proctitis NOS

   ✓6ᵗʰ   **K51.21**   **Ulcerative (chronic) proctitis with complications**

         K51.211   **Ulcerative (chronic) proctitis with rectal bleeding**   HCC

         K51.212   **Ulcerative (chronic) proctitis with intestinal obstruction**   HCC

         K51.213   **Ulcerative (chronic) proctitis with fistula**   HCC

         K51.214   **Ulcerative (chronic) proctitis with abscess**   HCC

         K51.218   **Ulcerative (chronic) proctitis with other complication**   HCC

         K51.219   **Ulcerative (chronic) proctitis with unspecified complications**   HCC ▽

✓5ᵗʰ   **K51.3**   **Ulcerative (chronic) rectosigmoiditis**

     K51.3Ø   **Ulcerative (chronic) rectosigmoiditis without complications**   HCC
         Ulcerative (chronic) rectosigmoiditis NOS

   ✓6ᵗʰ   **K51.31**   **Ulcerative (chronic) rectosigmoiditis with complications**

         K51.311   **Ulcerative (chronic) rectosigmoiditis with rectal bleeding**   HCC

         K51.312   **Ulcerative (chronic) rectosigmoiditis with intestinal obstruction**   HCC

         K51.313   **Ulcerative (chronic) rectosigmoiditis with fistula**   HCC

         K51.314   **Ulcerative (chronic) rectosigmoiditis with abscess**   HCC

         K51.318   **Ulcerative (chronic) rectosigmoiditis with other complication**   HCC

         K51.319   **Ulcerative (chronic) rectosigmoiditis with unspecified complications**   HCC ▽

✓5ᵗʰ   **K51.4**   **Inflammatory polyps of colon**
       EXCLUDES 1   *adenomatous polyp of colon (D12.6)*
                    polyposis of colon (D12.6)
                    polyps of colon NOS (K63.5)

     K51.4Ø   **Inflammatory polyps of colon without complications**   HCC
         Inflammatory polyps of colon NOS

   ✓6ᵗʰ   **K51.41**   **Inflammatory polyps of colon with complications**

         K51.411   **Inflammatory polyps of colon with rectal bleeding**   HCC

         K51.412   **Inflammatory polyps of colon with intestinal obstruction**   HCC

         K51.413   **Inflammatory polyps of colon with fistula**   HCC

         K51.414   **Inflammatory polyps of colon with abscess**   HCC

         K51.418   **Inflammatory polyps of colon with other complication**   HCC

         K51.419   **Inflammatory polyps of colon with unspecified complications**   HCC ▽

✓5ᵗʰ   **K51.5**   **Left sided colitis**
         Left hemicolitis

     K51.5Ø   **Left sided colitis without complications**   HCC
         Left sided colitis NOS

   ✓6ᵗʰ   **K51.51**   **Left sided colitis with complications**

         K51.511   **Left sided colitis with rectal bleeding**   HCC

         K51.512   **Left sided colitis with intestinal obstruction**   HCC

         K51.513   **Left sided colitis with fistula**   HCC

         K51.514   **Left sided colitis with abscess**   HCC

         K51.518   **Left sided colitis with other complication**   HCC

         K51.519   **Left sided colitis with unspecified complications**   HCC ▽

✓5ᵗʰ   **K51.8**   **Other ulcerative colitis**

     K51.8Ø   **Other ulcerative colitis without complications**   HCC

   ✓6ᵗʰ   **K51.81**   **Other ulcerative colitis with complications**

         K51.811   **Other ulcerative colitis with rectal bleeding**   HCC

         K51.812   **Other ulcerative colitis with intestinal obstruction**   HCC

         K51.813   **Other ulcerative colitis with fistula**   HCC

         K51.814   **Other ulcerative colitis with abscess**   HCC

         K51.818   **Other ulcerative colitis with other complication**   HCC

         K51.819   **Other ulcerative colitis with unspecified complications**   HCC ▽

✓5ᵗʰ   **K51.9**   **Ulcerative colitis, unspecified**

     K51.9Ø   **Ulcerative colitis, unspecified, without complications**   HCC

   ✓6ᵗʰ   **K51.91**   **Ulcerative colitis, unspecified, with complications**

         K51.911   **Ulcerative colitis, unspecified with rectal bleeding**   HCC ▽

         K51.912   **Ulcerative colitis, unspecified with intestinal obstruction**   HCC ▽

         K51.913   **Ulcerative colitis, unspecified with fistula**   HCC ▽

         K51.914   **Ulcerative colitis, unspecified with abscess**   HCC ▽

         K51.918   **Ulcerative colitis, unspecified with other complication**   HCC ▽

         K51.919   **Ulcerative colitis, unspecified with unspecified complications**   HCC ▽

✓4ᵗʰ   **K52**   **Other and unspecified noninfective gastroenteritis and colitis**

     K52.Ø   **Gastroenteritis and colitis due to radiation**

     K52.1   **Toxic gastroenteritis and colitis**
         Drug-induced gastroenteritis and colitis
         Code first (T51-T65) to identify toxic agent
         Use additional code for adverse effect, if applicable, to identify drug (T36-T5Ø with fifth or sixth character 5)

✓5ᵗʰ   **K52.2**   **Allergic and dietetic gastroenteritis and colitis**
         Food hypersensitivity gastroenteritis or colitis
         Use additional code to identify type of food allergy (Z91.Ø1-, Z91.Ø2-)
       EXCLUDES 2   *allergic eosinophilic colitis (K52.82)*
                   allergic eosinophilic esophagitis (K2Ø.Ø)
                   allergic eosinophilic gastritis (K52.81)
                   allergic eosinophilic gastroenteritis (K52.81)
                   food protein-induced proctocolitis (K52.82)
         DEF: True immunoglobulin E (IgE)-mediated allergic reaction of the lining of the stomach, intestines, or colon to food proteins; causes nausea, vomiting, diarrhea, and abdominal cramping.

     K52.21   **Food protein-induced enterocolitis syndrome**
         Use additional code for hypovolemic shock, if present (R57.1)

     K52.22   **Food protein-induced enteropathy**

     K52.29   **Other allergic and dietetic gastroenteritis and colitis**
         Food hypersensitivity gastroenteritis or colitis
         Immediate gastrointestinal hypersensitivity

     K52.3   **Indeterminate colitis**
         Colonic inflammatory bowel disease unclassified (IBDU)
       EXCLUDES 1 *unspecified colitis (K52.9)*

✓5ᵗʰ   **K52.8**   **Other specified noninfective gastroenteritis and colitis**

     K52.81   **Eosinophilic gastritis or gastroenteritis**
         Eosinophilic enteritis
       EXCLUDES 2   *eosinophilic esophagitis (K2Ø.Ø)*

     K52.82   **Eosinophilic colitis**
         Allergic proctocolitis
         Food-induced eosinophilic proctocolitis
         Food protein-induced proctocolitis
         Milk protein-induced proctocolitis

   ✓6ᵗʰ   **K52.83**   **Microscopic colitis**

         K52.831   **Collagenous colitis**

         K52.832   **Lymphocytic colitis**

         K52.838   **Other microscopic colitis**

         K52.839   **Microscopic colitis, unspecified**   ▽

     K52.89   **Other specified noninfective gastroenteritis and colitis**

EXCLUDES 1 Not coded here   EXCLUDES 2 Not included here   N Newborn Age: 0   P Pediatric Age: 0-17   M Maternity Age: 12-55   A Adult Age: 15-124

682   ICD-10-CM 2018

K52.9 **Noninfective gastroenteritis and colitis, unspecified** ▽
Colitis NOS   Ileitis NOS
Enteritis NOS   Jejunitis NOS
Gastroenteritis NOS   Sigmoiditis NOS
> **EXCLUDES 1** diarrhea NOS (R19.7)
> functional diarrhea (K59.1)
> infectious gastroenteritis and colitis NOS (A09)
> neonatal diarrhea (noninfective) (P78.3)
> psychogenic diarrhea (F45.8)

Other diseases of intestines (K55-K64)

✓4th **K55** **Vascular disorders of intestine**
> **EXCLUDES 1** necrotizing enterocolitis of newborn (P77.-)

✓5th **K55.0** **Acute vascular disorders of intestine**   HCC
Infarction of appendices epiploicae
Mesenteric (artery) (vein) embolism
Mesenteric (artery) (vein) infarction
Mesenteric (artery) (vein) thrombosis

✓6th **K55.01** **Acute (reversible) ischemia of small intestine**

> **K55.011** **Focal (segmental) acute (reversible)** HCC
> **ischemia of small intestine**

> **K55.012** **Diffuse acute (reversible) ischemia of** HCC
> **small intestine**

> **K55.019** **Acute (reversible) ischemia of small** HCC ▽
> **intestine, extent unspecified**

✓6th **K55.02** **Acute infarction of small intestine**
Gangrene of small intestine
Necrosis of small intestine

> **K55.021** **Focal (segmental) acute infarction of** HCC
> **small intestine**

> **K55.022** **Diffuse acute infarction of small** HCC
> **intestine**

> **K55.029** **Acute infarction of small intestine,** HCC ▽
> **extent unspecified**

✓6th **K55.03** **Acute (reversible) ischemia of large intestine**
Acute fulminant ischemic colitis
Subacute ischemic colitis

> **K55.031** **Focal (segmental) acute (reversible)** HCC
> **ischemia of large intestine**

> **K55.032** **Diffuse acute (reversible) ischemia of** HCC
> **large intestine**

> **K55.039** **Acute (reversible) ischemia of large** HCC ▽
> **intestine, extent unspecified**

✓6th **K55.04** **Acute infarction of large intestine**
Gangrene of small intestine
Necrosis of small intestine

> **K55.041** **Focal (segmental) acute infarction of** HCC
> **large intestine**

> **K55.042** **Diffuse acute infarction of large** HCC
> **intestine**

> **K55.049** **Acute infarction of large intestine,** HCC ▽
> **extent unspecified**

✓6th **K55.05** **Acute (reversible) ischemia of intestine, part unspecified**

> **K55.051** **Focal (segmental) acute (reversible)** HCC ▽
> **ischemia of intestine, part unspecified**

> **K55.052** **Diffuse acute (reversible) ischemia** HCC ▽
> **of intestine, part unspecified**

> **K55.059** **Acute (reversible) ischemia of** HCC ▽
> **intestine, part and extent unspecified**

✓6th **K55.06** **Acute infarction of intestine, part unspecified**
Acute intestinal infarction
Gangrene of intestine
Necrosis of intestine

> **K55.061** **Focal (segmental) acute infarction** HCC ▽
> **of intestine, part unspecified**

> **K55.062** **Diffuse acute infarction of** HCC ▽
> **intestine, part unspecified**

> **K55.069** **Acute infarction of intestine, part** HCC ▽
> **and extent unspecified**

K55.1 **Chronic vascular disorders of intestine**   HCC
Chronic ischemic colitis   Mesenteric atherosclerosis
Chronic ischemic enteritis   Mesenteric vascular
Chronic ischemic enterocolitis   insufficiency
Ischemic stricture of intestine

✓5th **K55.2** **Angiodysplasia of colon**

> **K55.20** **Angiodysplasia of colon without hemorrhage**

> **K55.21** **Angiodysplasia of colon with hemorrhage**
> **DEF:** Small vascular abnormalities due to fragile blood
> vessels in the colon; results in blood loss from the
> gastrointestinal (GI) tract.

✓5th **K55.3** **Necrotizing enterocolitis**
> **EXCLUDES 1** necrotizing enterocolitis of newborn (P77.-)
> **EXCLUDES 2** necrotizing enterocolitis due to Clostridium difficile
> ▶(A04.7-)◀

> **K55.30** **Necrotizing enterocolitis, unspecified**   HCC ▽
> Necrotizing enterocolitis, NOS

> **K55.31** **Stage 1 necrotizing enterocolitis**   HCC
> Necrotizing enterocolitis without pneumatosis,
> without perforation

> **K55.32** **Stage 2 necrotizing enterocolitis**   HCC
> Necrotizing enterocolitis with pneumatosis, without
> perforation

> **K55.33** **Stage 3 necrotizing enterocolitis**   HCC
> Necrotizing enterocolitis with perforation
> Necrotizing enterocolitis with pneumatosis and
> perforation

K55.8 **Other vascular disorders of intestine**   HCC

K55.9 **Vascular disorder of intestine, unspecified**   HCC ▽
Ischemic colitis   Ischemic enterocolitis
Ischemic enteritis

✓4th **K56** **Paralytic ileus and intestinal obstruction without hernia**
> **EXCLUDES 1** congenital stricture or stenosis of intestine (Q41-Q42)
> cystic fibrosis with meconium ileus (E84.11)
> ~~intestinal obstruction with hernia (K40-K46)~~
> ischemic stricture of intestine (K55.1)
> meconium ileus NOS (P76.0)
> neonatal intestinal obstructions classifiable to P76-
> obstruction of duodenum (K31.5)
> postprocedural intestinal obstruction ▶(K91.3-)◀
> stenosis of anus or rectum (K62.4)

K56.0 **Paralytic ileus**   HCC
Paralysis of bowel   Paralysis of intestine
Paralysis of colon
> **EXCLUDES 1** gallstone ileus (K56.3)
> ileus NOS (K56.7)
> obstructive ileus NOS ▶(K56.69-)◀

K56.1 **Intussusception**   HCC
Intussusception or invagination of bowel
Intussusception or invagination of colon
Intussusception or invagination of intestine
Intussusception or invagination of rectum
> **EXCLUDES 2** intussusception of appendix (K38.8)
> **DEF:** Intestinal obstruction due to prolapse of a bowel section into
> adjacent section; occurs primarily in children; symptoms include
> acute abdominal pain, vomiting, and passage of blood and mucus
> from rectum.

K56.2 **Volvulus**   HCC
Strangulation of colon or intestine
Torsion of colon or intestine
Twist of colon or intestine
> **EXCLUDES 2** volvulus of duodenum (K31.5)

Volvulus

Knotted
intestine
(volvulus)

K56.3 **Gallstone ileus** `HCC`
Obstruction of intestine by gallstone

✓5ᵗʰ **K56.4** **Other impaction of intestine**

    K56.41 **Fecal impaction** `HCC`
        EXCLUDES 1   constipation (K59.0-)
                    incomplete defecation (R15.0)

    K56.49 **Other impaction of intestine** `HCC`

▲ ✓5ᵗʰ **K56.5** **Intestinal adhesions [bands] with obstruction (postinfection)**
Abdominal hernia due to adhesions with obstruction
▶Peritoneal adhesions [bands] with intestinal obstruction (postinfection)◀

●   **K56.50** **Intestinal adhesions [bands], unspecified as to partial versus complete obstruction** ▽
        Intestinal adhesions with obstruction NOS

●   **K56.51** **Intestinal adhesions [bands], with partial obstruction**
        Intestinal adhesions with incomplete obstruction

●   **K56.52** **Intestinal adhesions [bands] with complete obstruction**

✓5ᵗʰ **K56.6** **Other and unspecified intestinal obstruction**
    AHA: 2017, 2Q, 12

  ✓6ᵗʰ **K56.60** **Unspecified intestinal obstruction**
    Intestinal obstruction NOS
        EXCLUDES 1   intestinal obstruction due to specified condition—code to condition

●   **K56.600** **Partial intestinal obstruction, unspecified as to cause** ▽
        Incomplete intestinal obstruction, NOS

●   **K56.601** **Complete intestinal obstruction, unspecified as to cause** ▽

●   **K56.609** **Unspecified intestinal obstruction, unspecified as to partial versus complete obstruction** ▽
        Intestinal obstruction NOS

  ✓6ᵗʰ **K56.69** **Other intestinal obstruction**
    Enterostenosis NOS
    Obstructive ileus NOS
    Occlusion of colon or intestine NOS
    Stenosis of colon or intestine NOS
    Stricture of colon or intestine NOS
        EXCLUDES 1   intestinal obstruction due to specified condition—code to condition

●   **K56.690** **Other partial intestinal obstruction**
        Other incomplete intestinal obstruction

●   **K56.691** **Other complete intestinal obstruction**

●   **K56.699** **Other intestinal obstruction unspecified as to partial versus complete obstruction** ▽
        Other intestinal obstruction, NEC

K56.7 **Ileus, unspecified** `HCC` ▽
    EXCLUDES 1   obstructive ileus ▶(K56.69-)◀
    EXCLUDES 2 ▶intestinal obstruction with hernia (K40-K46)◀
    AHA: 2017, 1Q, 40

✓4ᵗʰ **K57** **Diverticular disease of intestine**
    EXCLUDES 1   congenital diverticulum of intestine (Q43.8)
                  Meckel's diverticulum (Q43.0)
    EXCLUDES 2   diverticulum of appendix (K38.2)

✓5ᵗʰ **K57.0** **Diverticulitis of small intestine with perforation and abscess**
Diverticulitis of small intestine with peritonitis
    EXCLUDES 1   diverticulitis of both small and large intestine with perforation and abscess (K57.4-)

    K57.00 **Diverticulitis of small intestine with perforation and abscess without bleeding**

    K57.01 **Diverticulitis of small intestine with perforation and abscess with bleeding**

✓5ᵗʰ **K57.1** **Diverticular disease of small intestine without perforation or abscess**
    EXCLUDES 1   diverticular disease of both small and large intestine without perforation or abscess (K57.5-)

    K57.10 **Diverticulosis of small intestine without perforation or abscess without bleeding**
        Diverticular disease of small intestine NOS

    K57.11 **Diverticulosis of small intestine without perforation or abscess with bleeding**

    K57.12 **Diverticulitis of small intestine without perforation or abscess without bleeding**

    K57.13 **Diverticulitis of small intestine without perforation or abscess with bleeding**

✓5ᵗʰ **K57.2** **Diverticulitis of large intestine with perforation and abscess**
Diverticulitis of colon with peritonitis
    EXCLUDES 1   diverticulitis of both small and large intestine with perforation and abscess (K57.4-)

    K57.20 **Diverticulitis of large intestine with perforation and abscess without bleeding**

    K57.21 **Diverticulitis of large intestine with perforation and abscess with bleeding**

✓5ᵗʰ **K57.3** **Diverticular disease of large intestine without perforation or abscess**
    EXCLUDES 1   diverticular disease of both small and large intestine without perforation or abscess (K57.5-)

    K57.30 **Diverticulosis of large intestine without perforation or abscess without bleeding**
        Diverticular disease of colon NOS

    K57.31 **Diverticulosis of large intestine without perforation or abscess with bleeding**

    K57.32 **Diverticulitis of large intestine without perforation or abscess without bleeding**

    K57.33 **Diverticulitis of large intestine without perforation or abscess with bleeding**

✓5ᵗʰ **K57.4** **Diverticulitis of both small and large intestine with perforation and abscess**
Diverticulitis of both small and large intestine with peritonitis

    K57.40 **Diverticulitis of both small and large intestine with perforation and abscess without bleeding**

    K57.41 **Diverticulitis of both small and large intestine with perforation and abscess with bleeding**

✓5ᵗʰ **K57.5** **Diverticular disease of both small and large intestine without perforation or abscess**

    K57.50 **Diverticulosis of both small and large intestine without perforation or abscess without bleeding**
        Diverticular disease of both small and large intestine NOS

    K57.51 **Diverticulosis of both small and large intestine without perforation or abscess with bleeding**

    K57.52 **Diverticulitis of both small and large intestine without perforation or abscess without bleeding**

    K57.53 **Diverticulitis of both small and large intestine without perforation or abscess with bleeding**

✓5ᵗʰ **K57.8** **Diverticulitis of intestine, part unspecified, with perforation and abscess**
Diverticulitis of intestine NOS with peritonitis

    K57.80 **Diverticulitis of intestine, part unspecified, with perforation and abscess without bleeding** ▽

    K57.81 **Diverticulitis of intestine, part unspecified, with perforation and abscess with bleeding** ▽

✓5ᵗʰ **K57.9** **Diverticular disease of intestine, part unspecified, without perforation or abscess**

    K57.90 **Diverticulosis of intestine, part unspecified, without perforation or abscess without bleeding** ▽
        Diverticular disease of intestine NOS

    K57.91 **Diverticulosis of intestine, part unspecified, without perforation or abscess with bleeding** ▽

    K57.92 **Diverticulitis of intestine, part unspecified, without perforation or abscess without bleeding** ▽

    K57.93 **Diverticulitis of intestine, part unspecified, without perforation or abscess with bleeding** ▽

✓4ᵗʰ **K58** **Irritable bowel syndrome**
    INCLUDES   irritable colon
                  spastic colon

    K58.0 **Irritable bowel syndrome with diarrhea**

    K58.1 **Irritable bowel syndrome with constipation**

    K58.2 **Mixed irritable bowel syndrome**

    K58.8 **Other irritable bowel syndrome**

    K58.9 **Irritable bowel syndrome without diarrhea**
        Irritable bowel syndrome NOS

EXCLUDES 1 Not coded here   EXCLUDES 2 Not included here   N Newborn Age: 0   P Pediatric Age: 0-17   M Maternity Age: 12-55   A Adult Age: 15-124

ICD-10-CM 2018

684

K59   Other functional intestinal disorders
EXCLUDES 1   *change in bowel habit NOS (R19.4)*
intestinal malabsorption (K90.-)
psychogenic intestinal disorders (F45.8)
EXCLUDES 2   *functional disorders of stomach (K31.-)*

K59.0   Constipation
Use additional code for adverse effect, if applicable, to identify drug (T36-T50 with fifth or sixth character 5)
EXCLUDES 1   *fecal impaction (K56.41)*
incomplete defecation (R15.0)

K59.00   **Constipation, unspecified**   ▽

K59.01   **Slow transit constipation**
DEF: Delay in the transit of fecal material through the colon secondary to smooth muscle dysfunction or decreased peristaltic contractions along the colon: also called colonic inertia or delayed transit.

K59.02   **Outlet dysfunction constipation**

K59.03   **Drug induced constipation**
Use additional code for adverse effect, if applicable, to identify drug (T36-T50 with fifth or sixth character 5)

K59.04   **Chronic idiopathic constipation**
Functional constipation

K59.09   **Other constipation**
Chronic constipation

K59.1   Functional diarrhea
EXCLUDES 1   *diarrhea NOS (R19.7)*
irritable bowel syndrome with diarrhea (K58.0)

K59.2   Neurogenic bowel, not elsewhere classified
DEF: Disorder of bowel due to spinal cord lesion due to injury or as a complication of conditions such as multiple sclerosis (MS) or spina bifida; loss of bowel control is the primary symptom, manifested as constipation or bowel incontinence.

K59.3   Megacolon, not elsewhere classified
Dilatation of colon
Code first, if applicable (T51-T65) to identify toxic agent
EXCLUDES 1   *congenital megacolon (aganglionic) (Q43.1)*
megacolon (due to) (in) Chagas' disease (B57.32)
megacolon (due to) (in) Clostridium difficile
   ▶*(A04.7-)*◀
megacolon (due to) (in) Hirschsprung's disease (Q43.1)

K59.31   **Toxic megacolon**   HCC

K59.39   **Other megacolon**
Megacolon NOS

K59.4   Anal spasm
Proctalgia fugax

K59.8   Other specified functional intestinal disorders
Atony of colon
Pseudo-obstruction (acute) (chronic) of intestine

K59.9   Functional intestinal disorder, unspecified   ▽

K60   Fissure and fistula of anal and rectal regions
EXCLUDES 1   *fissure and fistula of anal and rectal regions with abscess or cellulitis (K61.-)*
EXCLUDES 2   *anal sphincter tear (healed) (nontraumatic) (old) (K62.81)*

K60.0   Acute anal fissure

K60.1   Chronic anal fissure

K60.2   Anal fissure, unspecified   ▽

K60.3   Anal fistula

K60.4   Rectal fistula
Fistula of rectum to skin
EXCLUDES 1   *rectovaginal fistula (N82.3)*
vesicorectal fistual (N32.1)

K60.5   Anorectal fistula

K61   Abscess of anal and rectal regions
INCLUDES   abscess of anal and rectal regions
cellulitis of anal and rectal regions

K61.0   Anal abscess
Perianal abscess
EXCLUDES 1   *intrasphincteric abscess (K61.4)*

K61.1   Rectal abscess
Perirectal abscess
EXCLUDES 1   *ischiorectal abscess (K61.3)*
AHA: 2012, 4Q, 104

K61.2   Anorectal abscess

K61.3   Ischiorectal abscess
Abscess of ischiorectal fossa

K61.4   Intrasphincteric abscess

K62   Other diseases of anus and rectum
INCLUDES   anal canal
EXCLUDES 2   *colostomy and enterostomy malfunction (K94.0-, K94.1-)*
fecal incontinence (R15.-)
hemorrhoids (K64.-)

K62.0   Anal polyp

K62.1   Rectal polyp
EXCLUDES 1   *adenomatous polyp (D12.8)*

K62.2   Anal prolapse
Prolapse of anal canal

K62.3   Rectal prolapse
Prolapse of rectal mucosa

K62.4   Stenosis of anus and rectum
Stricture of anus (sphincter)

K62.5   Hemorrhage of anus and rectum
EXCLUDES 1   *gastrointestinal bleeding NOS (K92.2)*
melena (K92.1)
neonatal rectal hemorrhage (P54.2)

K62.6   Ulcer of anus and rectum
Solitary ulcer of anus and rectum
Stercoral ulcer of anus and rectum
EXCLUDES 1   *fissure and fistula of anus and rectum (K60.-)*
ulcerative colitis (K51.-)

K62.7   Radiation proctitis
Use additional code to identify the type of radiation (W90.-)

K62.8   Other specified diseases of anus and rectum
EXCLUDES 2   *ulcerative proctitis (K51.2)*

K62.81   **Anal sphincter tear (healed) (nontraumatic) (old)**
Tear of anus, nontraumatic
Use additional code for any associated fecal incontinence (R15.-)
EXCLUDES 2   *anal fissure (K60.-)*
anal sphincter tear (healed) (old) complicating delivery (O34.7-)
traumatic tear of anal sphincter (S31.831)

K62.82   **Dysplasia of anus**
Anal intraepithelial neoplasia I and II (AIN I and II) (histologically confirmed)
Dysplasia of anus NOS
Mild and moderate dysplasia of anus (histologically confirmed)
EXCLUDES 1   *abnormal results from anal cytologic examination without histologic confirmation (R85.61-)*
anal intraepithelial neoplasia III (D01.3)
carcinoma in situ of anus (D01.3)
HGSIL of anus (R85.613)
severe dysplasia of anus (D01.3)

K62.89   **Other specified diseases of anus and rectum**
Proctitis NOS
Use additional code for any associated fecal incontinence (R15.-)

K62.9   Disease of anus and rectum, unspecified   ▽

K63   Other diseases of intestine

K63.0   Abscess of intestine
EXCLUDES 1   *abscess of intestine with Crohn's disease (K50.014, K50.114, K50.814, K50.914)*
abscess of intestine with diverticular disease (K57.0, K57.2, K57.4, K57.8)
abscess of intestine with ulcerative colitis (K51.014, K51.214, K51.314, K51.414, K51.514, K51.814, K51.914)
EXCLUDES 2   *abscess of anal and rectal regions (K61.-)*
abscess of appendix (K35.3)

K63.1   Perforation of intestine (nontraumatic)   HCC
Perforation (nontraumatic) of rectum
EXCLUDES 1   *perforation (nontraumatic) of duodenum (K26.-)*
perforation (nontraumatic) of intestine with diverticular disease (K57.0, K57.2, K57.4, K57.8)
EXCLUDES 2   *perforation (nontraumatic) of appendix (K35.2, K35.3)*

☑ Additional Character Req   ✓x7ᵗʰ Placeholder Alert   **Manifestation**   HCC CMS-HCC Condition   ▽ Unspecified Code   ▶◀ Revised Text   ● New Code   ▲ Revised Code Title

K63.2 Fistula of intestine
> EXCLUDES 1 fistula of duodenum (K31.6)
> fistula of intestine with Crohn's disease (K50.013,
> K50.113, K50.813, K50.913)
> fistula of intestine with ulcerative colitis (K51.013,
> K51.213, K51.313, K51.413, K51.513, K51.813,
> K51.913)
> EXCLUDES 2 fistula of anal and rectal regions (K60.-)
> fistula of appendix (K38.3)
> intestinal-genital fistula, female (N82.2-N82.4)
> vesicointestinal fistula (N32.1)

K63.3 Ulcer of intestine
Primary ulcer of small intestine
> EXCLUDES 1 duodenal ulcer (K26.-)
> gastrointestinal ulcer (K28.-)
> gastrojejunal ulcer (K28.-)
> jejunal ulcer (K28.-)
> peptic ulcer, site unspecified (K27.-)
> ulcer of intestine with perforation (K63.1)
> ulcer of anus or rectum (K62.6)
> ulcerative colitis (K51.-)

K63.4 Enteroptosis

K63.5 Polyp of colon
> EXCLUDES 1 adenomatous polyp of colon (D12.6)
> inflammatory polyp of colon (K51.4-)
> polyposis of colon (D12.6)
> AHA: 2017, 1Q, 15; 2015, 2Q, 14

✓5th K63.8 Other specified diseases of intestine

   K63.81 Dieulafoy lesion of intestine
> EXCLUDES 2 Dieulafoy lesion of stomach and duodenum
> (K31.82)

   K63.89 Other specified diseases of intestine
> AHA: 2013, 2Q, 31

K63.9 Disease of intestine, unspecified ▽

✓4th K64 Hemorrhoids and perianal venous thrombosis
> INCLUDES piles
> EXCLUDES 1 hemorrhoids complicating childbirth and the puerperium
> (O87.2)
> hemorrhoids complicating pregnancy (O22.4)

K64.0 First degree hemorrhoids
Grade/stage I hemorrhoids
Hemorrhoids (bleeding) without prolapse outside of anal canal

K64.1 Second degree hemorrhoids
Grade/stage II hemorrhoids
Hemorrhoids (bleeding) that prolapse with straining, but retract
spontaneously

K64.2 Third degree hemorrhoids
Grade/stage III hemorrhoids
Hemorrhoids (bleeding) that prolapse with straining and require
manual replacement back inside anal cana

K64.3 Fourth degree hemorrhoids
Grade/stage IV hemorrhoids
Hemorrhoids (bleeding) with prolapsed tissue that cannot be
manually replaced

K64.4 Residual hemorrhoidal skin tags
External hemorrhoids, NOS
Skin tags of anus

Hemorrhoids

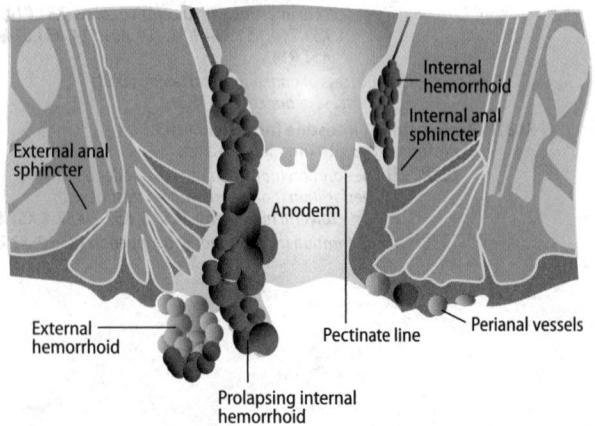

External anal sphincter
Internal hemorrhoid
Internal anal sphincter
Anoderm
Perianal vessels
External anal sphincter
External hemorrhoid
Pectinate line
Prolapsing internal hemorrhoid

K64.5 Perianal venous thrombosis
External hemorrhoids with thrombosis
Perianal hematoma
Thrombosed hemorrhoids NOS

K64.8 Other hemorrhoids
Internal hemorrhoids, without mention of degree
Prolapsed hemorrhoids, degree not specified

K64.9 Unspecified hemorrhoids ▽
Hemorrhoids (bleeding) NOS
Hemorrhoids (bleeding) without mention of degree

Diseases of peritoneum and retroperitoneum (K65-K68)

✓4th K65 Peritonitis
> Use additional code (B95-B97), to identify infectious agent
> EXCLUDES 1 acute appendicitis with generalized peritonitis (K35.2)
> aseptic peritonitis (T81.6)
> benign paroxysmal peritonitis (E85.0)
> chemical peritonitis (T81.6)
> diverticulitis of both small and large intestine with peritonitis
> (K57.4-)
> diverticulitis of colon with peritonitis (K57.2-)
> diverticulitis of intestine, NOS, with peritonitis (K57.8-)
> diverticulitis of small intestine with peritonitis (K57.0-)
> gonococcal peritonitis (A54.85)
> neonatal peritonitis (P78.0-P78.1)
> pelvic peritonitis, female (N73.3-N73.5)
> periodic familial peritonitis (E85.0)
> peritonitis due to talc or other foreign substance (T81.6)
> peritonitis in chlamydia (A74.81)
> peritonitis in diphtheria (A36.89)
> peritonitis in syphilis (late) (A52.74)
> peritonitis in tuberculosis (A18.31)
> peritonitis with or following abortion or ectopic or molar
> pregnancy (O00-O07, O08.0)
> peritonitis with or following appendicitis (K35.-)
> peritonitis with or following diverticular disease of intestine
> (K57.-)
> puerperal peritonitis (O85)
> retroperitoneal infections (K68.-)

K65.0 Generalized (acute) peritonitis HCC
Pelvic peritonitis (acute), male
Subphrenic peritonitis (acute)
Suppurative peritonitis (acute)

K65.1 Peritoneal abscess HCC
Abdominopelvic abscess   Subdiaphragmatic abscess
Abscess (of) omentum   Subhepatic abscess
Abscess (of) peritoneum   Subphrenic abscess
Mesenteric abscess
Retrocecal abscess

K65.2 Spontaneous bacterial peritonitis HCC
> EXCLUDES 1 bacterial peritonitis NOS (K65.9)

K65.3 Choleperitonitis HCC
Peritonitis due to bile
DEF: Inflammation of the peritoneum due to leakage of bile into
the peritoneal cavity resulting from rupture of the bile passages or
gallbladder.

K65.4 Sclerosing mesenteritis HCC
Fat necrosis of peritoneum
(Idiopathic) sclerosing mesenteric fibrosis
Mesenteric lipodystrophy
Mesenteric panniculitis
Retractile mesenteritis

K65.8 Other peritonitis HCC
Chronic proliferative peritonitis
Peritonitis due to urine

K65.9 Peritonitis, unspecified HCC ▽
Bacterial peritonitis NOS
AHA: 2013, 2Q, 31

✓4th K66 Other disorders of peritoneum
> EXCLUDES 2 ascites (R18.-)
> peritoneal effusion (chronic) (R18.8)

K66.0 Peritoneal adhesions (postprocedural) (postinfection)
Adhesions (of) abdominal (wall)   Adhesions (of) omentum
Adhesions (of) diaphragm   Adhesions (of) stomach
Adhesions (of) intestine   Adhesive bands
Adhesions (of) male pelvis   Mesenteric adhesions
> EXCLUDES 1 female pelvic adhesions [bands] (N73.6)
> peritoneal adhesions with intestinal obstruction
> ▶(K56.5-)◀

K66.1   Hemoperitoneum
> **EXCLUDES 1**   traumatic hemoperitoneum (S36.8-)

K66.8   Other specified disorders of peritoneum

K66.9   Disorder of peritoneum, unspecified   ▽

K67   *Disorders of peritoneum in infectious diseases classified elsewhere*   HCC
> Code first underlying disease, such as:
>   congenital syphilis (A50.0)
>   helminthiasis (B65.0-B83.9)
> **EXCLUDES 1**   peritonitis in chlamydia (A74.81)
>   peritonitis in diphtheria (A36.89)
>   peritonitis in gonococcal (A54.85)
>   peritonitis in syphilis (late) (A52.74)
>   peritonitis in tuberculosis (A18.31)

✓4ᵗʰ **K68**   **Disorders of retroperitoneum**

   ✓5ᵗʰ **K68.1**   **Retroperitoneal abscess**

     K68.11   **Postprocedural** retroperitoneal abscess

     K68.12   **Psoas muscle** abscess   HCC

     K68.19   **Other** retroperitoneal abscess   HCC

   K68.9   **Other disorders of retroperitoneum**

Diseases of liver (K70-K77)

> **EXCLUDES 1**   jaundice NOS (R17)
> **EXCLUDES 2**   hemochromatosis (E83.11-)
>   Reye's syndrome (G93.7)
>   viral hepatitis (B15-B19)
>   Wilson's disease (E83.0)

✓4ᵗʰ **K70**   **Alcoholic liver disease**
> Use additional code to identify:
>   alcohol abuse and dependence (F10.-)

   K70.0   **Alcoholic fatty liver**   A

   ✓5ᵗʰ **K70.1**   **Alcoholic hepatitis**   A

     K70.10   **Alcoholic hepatitis without ascites**   A

     K70.11   **Alcoholic hepatitis with ascites**   A

   K70.2   **Alcoholic fibrosis and sclerosis of liver**   A

   ✓5ᵗʰ **K70.3**   **Alcoholic cirrhosis of liver**
> Alcoholic cirrhosis NOS

     K70.30   **Alcoholic cirrhosis of liver without ascites**   HCC A

     K70.31   **Alcoholic cirrhosis of liver with ascites**   HCC A

   ✓5ᵗʰ **K70.4**   **Alcoholic hepatic failure**
> Acute alcoholic hepatic failure
> Alcoholic hepatic failure NOS
> Chronic alcoholic hepatic failure
> Subacute alcoholic hepatic failure

     K70.40   **Alcoholic hepatic failure without coma**   HCC A

     K70.41   **Alcoholic hepatic failure with coma**   HCC A

   K70.9   **Alcoholic liver disease, unspecified**   HCC A ▽

✓4ᵗʰ **K71**   **Toxic liver disease**
> **INCLUDES**   drug-induced idiosyncratic (unpredictable) liver disease
>   drug-induced toxic (predictable) liver disease
> Code first poisoning due to drug or toxin, if applicable (T36-T65 with fifth or sixth character 1-4 or 6)
> Use additional code for adverse effect, if applicable, to identify drug (T36-T50 with fifth or sixth character 5)
> **EXCLUDES 2**   alcoholic liver disease (K70.-)
>   Budd-Chiari syndrome (I82.0)

   K71.0   **Toxic liver disease with cholestasis**
> Cholestasis with hepatocyte injury
> "Pure" cholestasis

   ✓5ᵗʰ **K71.1**   **Toxic liver disease with hepatic necrosis**
> Hepatic failure (acute) (chronic) due to drugs

     K71.10   **Toxic liver disease with hepatic necrosis, without coma**

     K71.11   **Toxic liver disease with hepatic necrosis, with coma**   HCC

   K71.2   **Toxic liver disease with acute hepatitis**

   K71.3   **Toxic liver disease with chronic persistent hepatitis**

   K71.4   **Toxic liver disease with chronic lobular hepatitis**

   ✓5ᵗʰ **K71.5**   **Toxic liver disease with chronic active hepatitis**
> Toxic liver disease with lupoid hepatitis

     K71.50   **Toxic liver disease with chronic active hepatitis without ascites**

     K71.51   **Toxic liver disease with chronic active hepatitis with ascites**

K71.6   **Toxic liver disease with hepatitis, not elsewhere classified**

K71.7   **Toxic liver disease with fibrosis and cirrhosis of liver**

K71.8   **Toxic liver disease with other disorders of liver**
> Toxic liver disease with focal nodular hyperplasia
> Toxic liver disease with hepatic granulomas
> Toxic liver disease with peliosis hepatis
> Toxic liver disease with veno-occlusive disease of liver

K71.9   **Toxic liver disease, unspecified**   ▽

✓4ᵗʰ **K72**   **Hepatic failure, not elsewhere classified**
> **INCLUDES**   fulminant hepatitis NEC, with hepatic failure
>   hepatic encephalopathy NOS
>   liver (cell) necrosis with hepatic failure
>   malignant hepatitis NEC, with hepatic failure
>   yellow liver atrophy or dystrophy
> **EXCLUDES 1**   alcoholic hepatic failure (K70.4)
>   hepatic failure with toxic liver disease (K71.1-)
>   icterus of newborn (P55-P59)
>   postprocedural hepatic failure (K91.82)
> **EXCLUDES 2**   hepatic failure complicating abortion or ectopic or molar pregnancy (O00-O07, O08.8)
>   hepatic failure complicating pregnancy, childbirth and the puerperium (O26.6-)
>   viral hepatitis with hepatic coma (B15-B19)
> **AHA:** 2017, 1Q, 41

   ✓5ᵗʰ **K72.0**   **Acute and subacute hepatic failure**
> Acute non-viral hepatitis NOS
> **AHA:** 2015, 2Q, 17; 2014, 2Q, 13

     K72.00   **Acute and subacute hepatic failure without coma**

     K72.01   **Acute and subacute hepatic failure with coma**   HCC

   ✓5ᵗʰ **K72.1**   **Chronic hepatic failure**

     K72.10   **Chronic hepatic failure without coma**   HCC

     K72.11   **Chronic hepatic failure with coma**   HCC

   ✓5ᵗʰ **K72.9**   **Hepatic failure, unspecified**

     K72.90   **Hepatic failure, unspecified without coma**   HCC ▽
> **AHA:** 2016, 2Q, 35

     K72.91   **Hepatic failure, unspecified with coma**   HCC ▽
> Hepatic coma NOS

✓4ᵗʰ **K73**   **Chronic hepatitis, not elsewhere classified**
> **EXCLUDES 1**   alcoholic hepatitis (chronic) (K70.1-)
>   drug-induced hepatitis (chronic) (K71.-)
>   granulomatous hepatitis (chronic) NEC (K75.3)
>   reactive, nonspecific hepatitis (chronic) (K75.2)
>   viral hepatitis (chronic) (B15-B19)

   K73.0   **Chronic persistent hepatitis, not elsewhere classified**   HCC

   K73.1   **Chronic lobular hepatitis, not elsewhere classified**   HCC

   K73.2   **Chronic active hepatitis, not elsewhere classified**   HCC

   K73.8   **Other chronic hepatitis, not elsewhere classified**   HCC

   K73.9   **Chronic hepatitis, unspecified**   HCC ▽

✓4ᵗʰ **K74**   **Fibrosis and cirrhosis of liver**
> Code also, if applicable, viral hepatitis (acute) (chronic) (B15-B19)
> **EXCLUDES 1**   alcoholic cirrhosis (of liver) (K70.3)
>   alcoholic fibrosis of liver (K70.2)
>   cardiac sclerosis of liver (K76.1)
>   cirrhosis (of liver) with toxic liver disease (K71.7)
>   congenital cirrhosis (of liver) (P78.81)
>   pigmentary cirrhosis (of liver) (E83.110)

   K74.0   **Hepatic fibrosis**

   K74.1   **Hepatic sclerosis**

   K74.2   **Hepatic fibrosis with hepatic sclerosis**

   K74.3   **Primary biliary cirrhosis**   HCC
> Chronic nonsuppurative destructive cholangitis

   K74.4   **Secondary biliary cirrhosis**   HCC

   K74.5   **Biliary cirrhosis, unspecified**   HCC ▽

   ✓5ᵗʰ **K74.6**   **Other and unspecified cirrhosis of liver**

     K74.60   **Unspecified cirrhosis of liver**   HCC ▽
> Cirrhosis (of liver) NOS

     K74.69   **Other cirrhosis of liver**   HCC
> Cryptogenic cirrhosis (of liver)
> Macronodular cirrhosis (of liver)
> Micronodular cirrhosis (of liver)
> Mixed type cirrhosis (of liver)
> Portal cirrhosis (of liver)
> Postnecrotic cirrhosis (of liver)

☑ Additional Character Req   ✓x7ᵗʰ Placeholder Alert   Manifestation   HCC CMS-HCC Condition   ▽ Unspecified Code   ►◄ Revised Text   ● New Code   ▲ Revised Code Title

√4th K75 Other inflammatory liver diseases

EXCLUDES 2 *toxic liver disease (K71.-)*

K75.0 Abscess of liver
Cholangitic hepatic abscess
Hematogenic hepatic abscess
Hepatic abscess NOS
Lymphogenic hepatic abscess
Pylephlebitic hepatic abscess

EXCLUDES 1 *amebic liver abscess (A06.4)*
cholangitis without liver abscess (K83.0)
pylephlebitis without liver abscess (K75.1)

EXCLUDES 2 *acute or subacute hepatitis NOS (B17.9)*
acute or subacute non-viral hepatitis (K72.0)
chronic hepatitis NEC (K73.8)

K75.1 Phlebitis of portal vein
Pylephlebitis

EXCLUDES 1 *pylephlebitic liver abscess (K75.0)*

DEF: Inflammation of portal vein or branches; may be due to diverticulitis, perforated appendicitis, or peritonitis; symptoms include fever, chills, jaundice, sweating, and abscess in various body parts.

K75.2 Nonspecific reactive hepatitis
EXCLUDES 1 *acute or subacute hepatitis (K72.0-)*
chronic hepatitis NEC (K73.-)
viral hepatitis (B15-B19)

K75.3 Granulomatous hepatitis, not elsewhere classified
EXCLUDES 1 *acute or subacute hepatitis (K72.0-)*
chronic hepatitis NEC (K73.-)
viral hepatitis (B15-B19)

K75.4 Autoimmune hepatitis   HCC
Lupoid hepatitis NEC

√5th K75.8 Other specified inflammatory liver diseases
K75.81 Nonalcoholic steatohepatitis (NASH)

K75.89 Other specified inflammatory liver diseases

K75.9 Inflammatory liver disease, unspecified   ▽
Hepatitis NOS

EXCLUDES 1 *acute or subacute hepatitis (K72.0-)*
chronic hepatitis NEC (K73.-)
viral hepatitis (B15-B19)

AHA: 2015, 2Q, 17

√4th K76 Other diseases of liver

EXCLUDES 2 *alcoholic liver disease (K70.-)*
amyloid degeneration of liver (E85.-)
cystic disease of liver (congenital) (Q44.6)
hepatic vein thrombosis (I82.0)
hepatomegaly NOS (R16.0)
pigmentary cirrhosis (of liver) (E83.110)
portal vein thrombosis (I81)
toxic liver disease (K71.-)

K76.0 Fatty (change of) liver, not elsewhere classified
Nonalcoholic fatty liver disease (NAFLD)

EXCLUDES 1 *nonalcoholic steatohepatitis (NASH) (K75.81)*

K76.1 Chronic passive congestion of liver
Cardiac cirrhosis
Cardiac sclerosis

K76.2 Central hemorrhagic necrosis of liver
EXCLUDES 1 *liver necrosis with hepatic failure (K72.-)*

K76.3 Infarction of liver

K76.4 Peliosis hepatis
Hepatic angiomatosis

K76.5 Hepatic veno-occlusive disease
EXCLUDES 1 *Budd-Chiari syndrome (I82.0)*

K76.6 Portal hypertension   HCC
Use additional code for any associated complications, such as:
portal hypertensive gastropathy (K31.89)

K76.7 Hepatorenal syndrome   HCC
EXCLUDES 1 *hepatorenal syndrome following labor and delivery (O90.4)*
postprocedural hepatorenal syndrome (K91.83)

√5th K76.8 Other specified diseases of liver
K76.81 Hepatopulmonary syndrome   HCC
Code first underlying liver disease, such as:
alcoholic cirrhosis of liver (K70.3-)
cirrhosis of liver without mention of alcohol (K74.6-)

K76.89 Other specified diseases of liver
Cyst (simple) of liver
Focal nodular hyperplasia of liver
Hepatoptosis

K76.9 Liver disease, unspecified   ▽

K77 *Liver disorders in diseases classified elsewhere*
Code first underlying disease, such as:
amyloidosis (E85.-)
congenital syphilis (A50.0, A50.5)
congenital toxoplasmosis (P37.1)
schistosomiasis (B65.0-B65.9)

EXCLUDES 1 *alcoholic hepatitis (K70.1-)*
alcoholic liver disease (K70-.)
cytomegaloviral hepatitis (B25.1)
herpesviral [herpes simplex] hepatitis (B00.81)
infectious mononucleosis with liver disease (B27.0-B27.9 with .9)
mumps hepatitis (B26.81)
sarcoidosis with liver disease (D86.89)
secondary syphilis with liver disease (A51.45)
syphilis (late) with liver disease (A52.74)
toxoplasmosis (acquired) hepatitis (B58.1)
tuberculosis with liver disease (A18.83)

Disorders of gallbladder, biliary tract and pancreas (K80-K87)

√4th K80 Cholelithiasis
EXCLUDES 1 *retained cholelithiasis following cholecystectomy (K91.86)*

√5th K80.0 Calculus of gallbladder with acute cholecystitis
Any condition listed in K80.2 with acute cholecystitis

K80.00 Calculus of gallbladder with acute cholecystitis without obstruction

K80.01 Calculus of gallbladder with acute cholecystitis with obstruction

√5th K80.1 Calculus of gallbladder with other cholecystitis
K80.10 Calculus of gallbladder with chronic cholecystitis without obstruction
Cholelithiasis with cholecystitis NOS

K80.11 Calculus of gallbladder with chronic cholecystitis with obstruction

K80.12 Calculus of gallbladder with acute and chronic cholecystitis without obstruction

K80.13 Calculus of gallbladder with acute and chronic cholecystitis with obstruction

K80.18 Calculus of gallbladder with other cholecystitis without obstruction

K80.19 Calculus of gallbladder with other cholecystitis with obstruction

√5th K80.2 Calculus of gallbladder without cholecystitis
Cholecystolithiasis without cholecystitis
Cholelithiasis (without cholecystitis)
Colic (recurrent) of gallbladder (without cholecystitis)
Gallstone (impacted) of cystic duct (without cholecystitis)
Gallstone (impacted) of gallbladder (without cholecystitis)

K80.20 Calculus of gallbladder without cholecystitis without obstruction

K80.21 Calculus of gallbladder without cholecystitis with obstruction

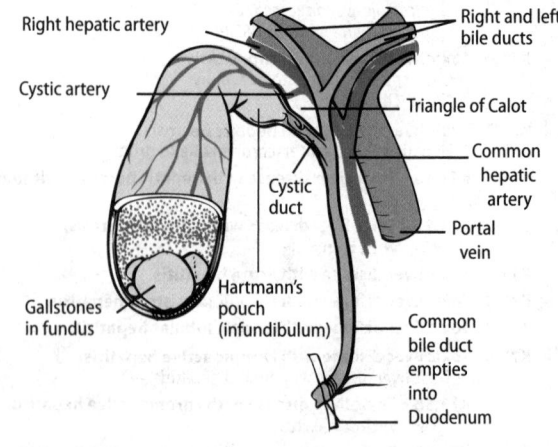

Cholelithiasis

Right hepatic artery
Cystic artery
Right and left bile ducts
Triangle of Calot
Common hepatic artery
Cystic duct
Portal vein
Gallstones in fundus
Hartmann's pouch (infundibulum)
Common bile duct empties into Duodenum

EXCLUDES 1 Not coded here   EXCLUDES 2 Not included here   N Newborn Age: 0   P Pediatric Age: 0-17   M Maternity Age: 12-55   A Adult Age: 15-124

688   ICD-10-CM 2018

✓5ᵗʰ **K80.3 Calculus of** bile duct with cholangitis
    Any condition listed in K80.5 with cholangitis

  K80.30 Calculus of bile duct with cholangitis, ▽
    unspecified, without obstruction

  K80.31 Calculus of bile duct with cholangitis, ▽
    unspecified, with obstruction

  K80.32 Calculus of bile duct with acute cholangitis without
    obstruction

  K80.33 Calculus of bile duct with acute cholangitis with
    obstruction

  K80.34 Calculus of bile duct with chronic cholangitis
    without obstruction

  K80.35 Calculus of bile duct with chronic cholangitis with
    obstruction

  K80.36 Calculus of bile duct with acute and chronic
    cholangitis without obstruction

  K80.37 Calculus of bile duct with acute and chronic
    cholangitis with obstruction

✓5ᵗʰ **K80.4 Calculus of** bile duct with cholecystitis
    Any condition listed in K80.5 with cholecystitis (with cholangitis)

  K80.40 Calculus of bile duct with cholecystitis, ▽
    unspecified, without obstruction

  K80.41 Calculus of bile duct with cholecystitis, ▽
    unspecified, with obstruction

  K80.42 Calculus of bile duct with acute cholecystitis without
    obstruction

  K80.43 Calculus of bile duct with acute cholecystitis with
    obstruction

  K80.44 Calculus of bile duct with chronic cholecystitis
    without obstruction

  K80.45 Calculus of bile duct with chronic cholecystitis with
    obstruction

  K80.46 Calculus of bile duct with acute and chronic
    cholecystitis without obstruction

  K80.47 Calculus of bile duct with acute and chronic
    cholecystitis with obstruction

✓5ᵗʰ **K80.5 Calculus of** bile duct without cholangitis or cholecystitis
    Choledocholithiasis (without cholangitis or cholecystitis)
    Gallstone (impacted) of bile duct NOS (without cholangitis or
      cholecystitis)
    Gallstone (impacted) of common duct (without cholangitis or
      cholecystitis)
    Gallstone (impacted) of hepatic duct (without cholangitis or
      cholecystitis)
    Hepatic cholelithiasis (without cholangitis or cholecystitis)
    Hepatic colic (recurrent) (without cholangitis or cholecystitis)

  K80.50 Calculus of bile duct without cholangitis or
    cholecystitis without obstruction

  K80.51 Calculus of bile duct without cholangitis or
    cholecystitis with obstruction

✓5ᵗʰ **K80.6 Calculus of** gallbladder and bile duct with cholecystitis

  K80.60 Calculus of gallbladder and bile duct with ▽
    cholecystitis, unspecified, without obstruction

  K80.61 Calculus of gallbladder and bile duct with ▽
    cholecystitis, unspecified, with obstruction

  K80.62 Calculus of gallbladder and bile duct with acute
    cholecystitis without obstruction

  K80.63 Calculus of gallbladder and bile duct with acute
    cholecystitis with obstruction

  K80.64 Calculus of gallbladder and bile duct with chronic
    cholecystitis without obstruction

  K80.65 Calculus of gallbladder and bile duct with chronic
    cholecystitis with obstruction

  K80.66 Calculus of gallbladder and bile duct with acute and
    chronic cholecystitis without obstruction

  K80.67 Calculus of gallbladder and bile duct with acute and
    chronic cholecystitis with obstruction

✓5ᵗʰ **K80.7 Calculus of** gallbladder and bile duct without cholecystitis

  K80.70 Calculus of gallbladder and bile duct without
    cholecystitis without obstruction

  K80.71 Calculus of gallbladder and bile duct without
    cholecystitis with obstruction

✓5ᵗʰ **K80.8 Other cholelithiasis**

  K80.80 Other cholelithiasis without obstruction

  K80.81 Other cholelithiasis with obstruction

✓4ᵗʰ **K81 Cholecystitis**
    EXCLUDES 1 cholecystitis with cholelithiasis (K80.-)

K81.0 Acute cholecystitis
    Abscess of gallbladder
    Angiocholecystitis
    Emphysematous (acute) cholecystitis
    Empyema of gallbladder
    Gangrene of gallbladder
    Gangrenous cholecystitis
    Suppurative cholecystitis

K81.1 Chronic cholecystitis

K81.2 Acute cholecystitis with chronic cholecystitis

K81.9 Cholecystitis, unspecified ▽

✓4ᵗʰ **K82 Other diseases of gallbladder**
    EXCLUDES 1 nonvisualization of gallbladder (R93.2)
         postcholecystectomy syndrome (K91.5)

K82.0 Obstruction of gallbladder
    Occlusion of cystic duct or gallbladder without cholelithiasis
    Stenosis of cystic duct or gallbladder without cholelithiasis
    Stricture of cystic duct or gallbladder without cholelithiasis
    EXCLUDES 1 obstruction of gallbladder with cholelithiasis (K80.-)

K82.1 Hydrops of gallbladder
    Mucocele of gallbladder

K82.2 Perforation of gallbladder
    Rupture of cystic duct or gallbladder

K82.3 Fistula of gallbladder
    Cholecystocolic fistula
    Cholecystoduodenal fistula

K82.4 Cholesterolosis of gallbladder
    Strawberry gallbladder
    EXCLUDES 1 cholesterolosis of gallbladder with cholecystitis (K81.-)
         cholesterolosis of gallbladder with cholelithiasis (K80.-)

K82.8 Other specified diseases of gallbladder
    Adhesions of cystic duct or gallbladder
    Atrophy of cystic duct or gallbladder
    Cyst of cystic duct or gallbladder
    Dyskinesia of cystic duct or gallbladder
    Hypertrophy of cystic duct or gallbladder
    Nonfunctioning of cystic duct or gallbladder
    Ulcer of cystic duct or gallbladder

K82.9 Disease of gallbladder, unspecified ▽

✓4ᵗʰ **K83 Other diseases of biliary tract**
    EXCLUDES 1 postcholecystectomy syndrome (K91.5)
    EXCLUDES 2 conditions involving the gallbladder (K81-K82)
         conditions involving the cystic duct (K81-K82)

K83.0 Cholangitis
    Ascending cholangitis
    Cholangitis NOS
    Primary cholangitis
    Recurrent cholangitis
    Sclerosing cholangitis
    Secondary cholangitis
    Stenosing cholangitis
    Suppurative cholangitis
    EXCLUDES 1 cholangitic liver abscess (K75.0)
         cholangitis with choledocholithiasis (K80.3-, K80.4-)
         chronic nonsuppurative destructive cholangitis (K74.3)

K83.1 Obstruction of bile duct
    Occlusion of bile duct without cholelithiasis
    Stenosis of bile duct without cholelithiasis
    Stricture of bile duct without cholelithiasis
    EXCLUDES 1 congenital obstruction of bile duct (Q44.3)
         obstruction of bile duct with cholelithiasis (K80.-)
    AHA: 2016, 1Q, 18

K83.2 Perforation of bile duct
    Rupture of bile duct

K83.3 Fistula of bile duct
    Choledochoduodenal fistula

K83.4 Spasm of sphincter of Oddi

K83.5 Biliary cyst

K83.8 Other specified diseases of biliary tract
    Adhesions of biliary tract
    Atrophy of biliary tract
    Hypertrophy of biliary tract
    Ulcer of biliary tract

K83.9 Disease of biliary tract, unspecified ▽

✓ Additional Character Req   ✗7ᵗʰ Placeholder Alert   Manifestation   HCC CMS-HCC Condition   ▽ Unspecified Code   ▶◀ Revised Text   ● New Code   ▲ Revised Code Title

✓4th K85 Acute pancreatitis
INCLUDES acute (recurrent) pancreatitis
subacute pancreatitis

✓5th K85.0 Idiopathic acute pancreatitis

K85.00 **Idiopathic acute pancreatitis without necrosis or infection**

K85.01 **Idiopathic acute pancreatitis with uninfected necrosis**

K85.02 **Idiopathic acute pancreatitis with infected necrosis**

✓5th K85.1 Biliary acute pancreatitis
Gallstone pancreatitis

K85.10 **Biliary acute pancreatitis without necrosis or infection**

K85.11 **Biliary acute pancreatitis with uninfected necrosis**

K85.12 **Biliary acute pancreatitis with infected necrosis**

✓5th K85.2 Alcohol induced acute pancreatitis
EXCLUDES 2 alcohol induced chronic pancreatitis (K86.0)

K85.20 **Alcohol induced acute pancreatitis without necrosis or infection**

K85.21 **Alcohol induced acute pancreatitis with uninfected necrosis**

K85.22 **Alcohol induced acute pancreatitis with infected necrosis**

✓5th K85.3 Drug induced acute pancreatitis
Use additional code for adverse effect, if applicable, to identify drug (T36-T50 with fifth or sixth character 5)
Use additional code to identify drug abuse and dependence (F11. – F17.-)

K85.30 **Drug induced acute pancreatitis without necrosis or infection**

K85.31 **Drug induced acute pancreatitis with uninfected necrosis**

K85.32 **Drug induced acute pancreatitis with infected necrosis**

✓5th K85.8 Other acute pancreatitis

K85.80 **Other acute pancreatitis without necrosis or infection**

K85.81 **Other acute pancreatitis with uninfected necrosis**

K85.82 **Other acute pancreatitis with infected necrosis**

✓5th K85.9 Acute pancreatitis, unspecified
Pancreatitis NOS

K85.90 **Acute pancreatitis without necrosis or infection, unspecified** ▽

K85.91 **Acute pancreatitis with uninfected necrosis, unspecified** ▽

K85.92 **Acute pancreatitis with infected necrosis, unspecified** ▽

✓4th K86 Other diseases of pancreas
EXCLUDES 2 fibrocystic disease of pancreas (E84.-)
islet cell tumor (of pancreas) (D13.7)
pancreatic steatorrhea (K90.3)

K86.0 **Alcohol-induced chronic pancreatitis** HCC
Use additional code to identify:
alcohol abuse and dependence (F10.-)
Code also exocrine pancreatic insufficiency (K86.81)
EXCLUDES 2 alcohol induced acute pancreatitis (K85.2-)

K86.1 **Other chronic pancreatitis** HCC
Chronic pancreatitis NOS
Infectious chronic pancreatitis
Recurrent chronic pancreatitis
Relapsing chronic pancreatitis
Code also exocrine pancreatic insufficiency (K86.81)

K86.2 **Cyst of pancreas**

K86.3 **Pseudocyst of pancreas**

✓5th K86.8 Other specified diseases of pancreas

K86.81 **Exocrine pancreatic insufficiency**

K86.89 **Other specified diseases of pancreas**
Aseptic pancreatic necrosis, unrelated to acute pancreatitis
Atrophy of pancreas
Calculus of pancreas
Cirrhosis of pancreas
Fibrosis of pancreas
Pancreatic fat necrosis, unrelated to acute pancreatitis
Pancreatic infantilism
Pancreatic necrosis NOS, unrelated to acute pancreatitis

K86.9 **Disease of pancreas, unspecified** ▽

K87 *Disorders of gallbladder, biliary tract and pancreas in diseases classified elsewhere*
Code first underlying disease
EXCLUDES 1 cytomegaloviral pancreatitis (B25.2)
mumps pancreatitis (B26.3)
syphilitic gallbladder (A52.74)
syphilitic pancreas (A52.74)
tuberculosis of gallbladder (A18.83)
tuberculosis of pancreas (A18.83)

Other diseases of the digestive system (K90-K95)

✓4th K90 Intestinal malabsorption
EXCLUDES 1 intestinal malabsorption following gastrointestinal surgery (K91.2)

K90.0 **Celiac disease**
Celiac disease with steatorrhea
►Celiac gluten-sensitive enteropathy◄
Nontropical sprue
Use additional code for associated disorders including:
dermatitis herpetiformis (L13.0)
gluten ataxia (G32.81)
Code also exocrine pancreatic insufficiency (K86.81)
DEF: Malabsorption syndrome due to gluten consumption; symptoms include fetid, bulky, frothy, oily stools, distended abdomen, gas, asthenia, electrolyte depletion, and vitamin B, D, and K deficiency.

K90.1 **Tropical sprue**
Sprue NOS
Tropical steatorrhea

K90.2 **Blind loop syndrome, not elsewhere classified**
Blind loop syndrome NOS
EXCLUDES 1 congenital blind loop syndrome (Q43.8)
postsurgical blind loop syndrome (K91.2)

K90.3 **Pancreatic steatorrhea**

✓5th K90.4 Other malabsorption due to intolerance
EXCLUDES 2 ►celiac gluten-sensitive enteropathy◄ (K90.0)
lactose intolerance (E73.-)

K90.41 **Non-celiac gluten sensitivity**
Gluten sensitivity NOS
Non-celiac gluten sensitive enteropathy

K90.49 **Malabsorption due to intolerance, not elsewhere classified**
Malabsorption due to intolerance to carbohydrate
Malabsorption due to intolerance to fat
Malabsorption due to intolerance to protein
Malabsorption due to intolerance to starch

✓5th K90.8 Other intestinal malabsorption

K90.81 **Whipple's disease**

K90.89 **Other intestinal malabsorption**

K90.9 **Intestinal malabsorption, unspecified** ▽

✓4th K91 Intraoperative and postprocedural complications and disorders of digestive system, not elsewhere classified
EXCLUDES 2 complications of artificial opening of digestive system (K94.-)
complications of bariatric procedures (K95.-)
gastrojejunal ulcer (K28.-)
postprocedural (radiation) retroperitoneal abscess (K68.11)
radiation colitis (K52.0)
radiation gastroenteritis (K52.0)
radiation proctitis (K62.7)

K91.0 **Vomiting following gastrointestinal surgery**

K91.1 **Postgastric surgery syndromes**
Dumping syndrome
Postgastrectomy syndrome
Postvagotomy syndrome

K91.2 **Postsurgical malabsorption, not elsewhere classified**
Postsurgical blind loop syndrome
EXCLUDES 1 malabsorption osteomalacia in adults (M83.2)
malabsorption osteoporosis, postsurgical (M80.8-, M81.8)

✓5th K91.3 Postprocedural intestinal obstruction
AHA: 2017, 1Q, 40

● K91.30 **Postprocedural intestinal obstruction, unspecified as to partial versus complete** ▽
Postprocedural intestinal obstruction NOS

● K91.31 **Postprocedural partial intestinal obstruction**
Postprocedural incomplete intestinal obstruction

● K91.32 **Postprocedural complete intestinal obstruction**

K91.5   **Postcholecystectomy syndrome**

✓5ʰ **K91.6**   **Intraoperative hemorrhage and hematoma** of a digestive system organ or structure complicating a procedure

> *EXCLUDES 1*   *intraoperative hemorrhage and hematoma of a digestive system organ or structure due to accidental puncture and laceration during a procedure (K91.7-)*

     K91.61   **Intraoperative hemorrhage and hematoma of a digestive system organ or structure complicating a** digestive system procedure

     K91.62   **Intraoperative hemorrhage and hematoma of a digestive system organ or structure complicating** other procedure

✓5ʰ **K91.7**   **Accidental puncture and laceration** of a digestive system organ or structure during a procedure

     K91.71   **Accidental puncture and laceration of a digestive system organ or structure during a** digestive system procedure

     K91.72   **Accidental puncture and laceration of a digestive system organ or structure during** other procedure

✓5ʰ **K91.8**   **Other intraoperative and postprocedural complications and disorders of digestive system**

     K91.81   **Other intraoperative complications of digestive system**

     K91.82   **Postprocedural** hepatic failure

     K91.83   **Postprocedural** hepatorenal syndrome

   ✓6ʰ **K91.84**   **Postprocedural** hemorrhage of a digestive system organ or structure following a procedure

       K91.840   **Postprocedural hemorrhage of a digestive system organ or structure following a** digestive system procedure
> **AHA:** 2016, 1Q, 15

       K91.841   **Postprocedural hemorrhage of a digestive system organ or structure following** other procedure

   ✓6ʰ **K91.85**   **Complications of** intestinal pouch

       K91.850   **Pouchitis**   HCC
> Inflammation of internal ileoanal pouch
> **DEF:** Inflammatory complication of an existing surgically created ileoanal pouch, resulting in multiple GI complaints, including diarrhea, abdominal pain, rectal bleeding, fecal urgency, or incontinence.

       K91.858   **Other complications of intestinal pouch**   HCC

     K91.86   **Retained cholelithiasis** following cholecystectomy

   ✓6ʰ **K91.87**   **Postprocedural hematoma and seroma** of a digestive system organ or structure following a procedure

       K91.870   **Postprocedural** hematoma **of a digestive system organ or structure following a** digestive system procedure

       K91.871   **Postprocedural** hematoma **of a digestive system organ or structure following** other procedure

       K91.872   **Postprocedural** seroma **of a digestive system organ or structure following a** digestive system procedure

       K91.873   **Postprocedural** seroma **of a digestive system organ or structure following** other procedure

     K91.89   **Other postprocedural complications and disorders of digestive system**
> Use additional code, if applicable, to further specify disorder
> *EXCLUDES 2*   *postprocedural retroperitoneal abscess (K68.11)*
> **AHA:** 2017, 1Q, 40

✓4ʰ **K92**   **Other diseases of digestive system**
> *EXCLUDES 1*   *neonatal gastrointestinal hemorrhage (P54.0-P54.3)*

K92.0   **Hematemesis**

K92.1   **Melena**
> *EXCLUDES 1*   *occult blood in feces (R19.5)*

K92.2   **Gastrointestinal hemorrhage, unspecified**   ▽
> Gastric hemorrhage NOS
> Intestinal hemorrhage NOS
> *EXCLUDES 1*   *acute hemorrhagic gastritis (K29.01)*
> *hemorrhage of anus and rectum (K62.5)*
> *angiodysplasia of stomach with hemorrhage (K31.811)*
> *diverticular disease with hemorrhage (K57.-)*
> *gastritis and duodenitis with hemorrhage (K29.-)*
> *peptic ulcer with hemorrhage (K25-K28)*

✓5ʰ **K92.8**   **Other specified diseases of the digestive system**

     K92.81   **Gastrointestinal mucositis (ulcerative)**
> Code also type of associated therapy, such as:
> antineoplastic and immunosuppressive drugs (T45.1X-)
> radiological procedure and radiotherapy (Y84.2)
> *EXCLUDES 2*   *mucositis (ulcerative) of vagina and vulva (N76.81)*
> *nasal mucositis (ulcerative) (J34.81)*
> *oral mucositis (ulcerative) (K12.3-)*

     K92.89   **Other specified diseases of the digestive system**

K92.9   **Disease of digestive system, unspecified**   ▽

✓4ʰ **K94**   **Complications of artificial openings of the digestive system**

✓5ʰ **K94.0**   **Colostomy** complications

     K94.00   **Colostomy complication, unspecified**   HCC ▽

     K94.01   **Colostomy** hemorrhage   HCC

     K94.02   **Colostomy** infection   HCC
> Use additional code to specify type of infection, such as:
> cellulitis of abdominal wall (L03.311)
> sepsis (A40-, A41-)

     K94.03   **Colostomy** malfunction   HCC
> Mechanical complication of colostomy

     K94.09   **Other complications of colostomy**   HCC

✓5ʰ **K94.1**   **Enterostomy** complications

     K94.10   **Enterostomy complication, unspecified**   HCC ▽

     K94.11   **Enterostomy** hemorrhage   HCC

     K94.12   **Enterostomy** infection   HCC
> Use additional code to specify type of infection, such as:
> cellulitis of abdominal wall (L03.311)
> sepsis (A40-, A41-)

     K94.13   **Enterostomy** malfunction   HCC
> Mechanical complication of enterostomy

     K94.19   **Other complications of enterostomy**   HCC

✓5ʰ **K94.2**   **Gastrostomy** complications

     K94.20   **Gastrostomy complication, unspecified**   HCC ▽

     K94.21   **Gastrostomy** hemorrhage   HCC

     K94.22   **Gastrostomy** infection   HCC
> Use additional code to specify type of infection, such as:
> cellulitis of abdominal wall (L03.311)
> sepsis (A40-, A41-)

     K94.23   **Gastrostomy** malfunction   HCC
> Mechanical complication of gastrostomy

     K94.29   **Other complications of gastrostomy**   HCC

✓5ʰ **K94.3**   **Esophagostomy** complications

     K94.30   **Esophagostomy complications, unspecified**   HCC ▽

     K94.31   **Esophagostomy** hemorrhage   HCC

     K94.32   **Esophagostomy** infection   HCC
> Use additional code to identify the infection

     K94.33   **Esophagostomy** malfunction   HCC
> Mechanical complication of esophagostomy

     K94.39   **Other complications of esophagostomy**   HCC

✓4ʰ **K95**   **Complications of bariatric procedures**

✓5ʰ **K95.0**   **Complications of** gastric band procedure

     K95.01   **Infection due to gastric band procedure**
> Use additional code to specify type of infection or organism, such as:
> bacterial and viral infectious agents (B95.-, B96.-)
> cellulitis of abdominal wall (L03.311)
> sepsis (A40.-, A41.-)

     K95.09   **Other complications of gastric band procedure**
> Use additional code, if applicable, to further specify complication

---

✅ Additional Character Req   ✓x7ʰ Placeholder Alert   Manifestation   HCC CMS-HCC Condition   ▽ Unspecified Code   ▶◀ Revised Text   ● New Code   ▲ Revised Code Title

ICD-10-CM 2018   **691**

✓5ᵗʰ **K95.8** **Complications of other bariatric procedure**

> EXCLUDES 1 *complications of gastric band surgery (K95.Ø-)*

K95.81 **Infection due to other bariatric procedure**
> Use additional code to specify type of infection or organism, such as:
> bacterial and viral infectious agents (B95.-, B96.-)
> cellulitis of abdominal wall (LØ3.311)
> sepsis (A4Ø.-, A41.-)

K95.89 **Other complications of other bariatric procedure**
> Use additional code, if applicable, to further specify complication

EXCLUDES 1 Not coded here   EXCLUDES 2 Not included here   N Newborn Age: 0   P Pediatric Age: 0-17   M Maternity Age: 12-55   A Adult Age: 15-124

692   ICD-10-CM 2018

Chapter 12. Diseases of the Skin and Subcutaneous Tissue (L00–L99)

Chapter Specific Guidelines with Coding Examples

The chapter specific guidelines from the ICD-10-CM Official Guidelines for Coding and Reporting have been provided below. Along with these guidelines are coding examples, contained in the shaded boxes, that have been developed to help illustrate the coding and/or sequencing guidance found in these guidelines.

a. Pressure ulcer stage codes

1) Pressure ulcer stages

Codes from category L89, Pressure ulcer, identify the site of the pressure ulcer as well as the stage of the ulcer.

The ICD-10-CM classifies pressure ulcer stages based on severity, which is designated by stages 1-4, unspecified stage and unstageable.

Assign as many codes from category L89 as needed to identify all the pressure ulcers the patient has, if applicable.

> Stage 3 pressure ulcer left ankle, 6 x 7 cm that invades the fascia; stage 2 pressure ulcer of left hip
>
> **L89.523**   **Pressure ulcer of left ankle, stage 3**
>
> **L89.222**   **Pressure ulcer of left hip, stage 2**
>
> *Explanation:* Patient has a left ankle pressure ulcer documented as stage 3 and a left hip pressure ulcer documented as stage 2. Combination codes from category L89 Pressure ulcer, identify the site of the pressure ulcer as well as the stage. Assign as many codes from category L89 as needed to identify all the pressure ulcers the patient has.

2) Unstageable pressure ulcers

Assignment of the code for unstageable pressure ulcer (L89.--0) should be based on the clinical documentation. These codes are used for pressure ulcers whose stage cannot be clinically determined (e.g., the ulcer is covered by eschar or has been treated with a skin or muscle graft) and pressure ulcers that are documented as deep tissue injury but not documented as due to trauma. This code should not be confused with the codes for unspecified stage (L89.--9). When there is no documentation regarding the stage of the pressure ulcer, assign the appropriate code for unspecified stage (L89.--9).

> Pressure ulcer of the right lower back documented as unstageable due to the presence of thick eschar covering the ulcer
>
> **L89.130**   **Pressure ulcer of right lower back, unstageable**
>
> *Explanation:* Codes for unstageable pressure ulcers are assigned when the stage cannot be clinically determined (e.g., the ulcer is covered by eschar or has been treated with a skin or muscle graft).

3) Documented pressure ulcer stage

Assignment of the pressure ulcer stage code should be guided by clinical documentation of the stage or documentation of the terms found in the Alphabetic Index. For clinical terms describing the stage that are not found in the Alphabetic Index, and there is no documentation of the stage, the provider should be queried.

> Left heel pressure ulcer with partial thickness skin loss involving the dermis
>
> **L89.622**   **Pressure ulcer of left heel, stage 2**
>
> *Explanation:* Code assignment for the pressure ulcer stage should be guided by either the clinical documentation of the stage or the documentation of terms found in the Alphabetic Index. The clinical documentation describing the left heel pressure ulcer "partial thickness skin loss involving the dermis" matches the ICD-10-CM index parenthetical description for stage 2 "(abrasion, blister, partial thickness skin loss involving epidermis and/or dermis)."

4) Patients admitted with pressure ulcers documented as healed

No code is assigned if the documentation states that the pressure ulcer is completely healed.

> Patient receiving follow-up examination of a completely healed pressure ulcer of the foot
>
> **Z09**   **Encounter for follow-up examination after completed treatment for conditions other than malignant neoplasm**
>
> **Z87.2**   **Personal history of diseases of the skin and subcutaneous tissue**
>
> *Explanation:* Assign only codes for the reason for the encounter and the personal history of the pressure ulcer. Personal history code Z87.2 includes conditions classifiable to L00–L99 such as pressure ulcer. No code is assigned for a pressure ulcer documented as completely healed.

5) Patients admitted with pressure ulcers documented as healing

Pressure ulcers described as healing should be assigned the appropriate pressure ulcer stage code based on the documentation in the medical record. If the documentation does not provide information about the stage of the healing pressure ulcer, assign the appropriate code for unspecified stage.

If the documentation is unclear as to whether the patient has a current (new) pressure ulcer or if the patient is being treated for a healing pressure ulcer, query the provider.

For ulcers that were present on admission but healed at the time of discharge, assign the code for the site and stage of the pressure ulcer at the time of admission.

6) Patient admitted with pressure ulcer evolving into another stage during the admission

If a patient is admitted **to an inpatient hospital** with a pressure ulcer at one stage and it progresses to a higher stage, two separate codes should be assigned: one code for the site and stage of the ulcer on admission and a second code for the same ulcer site and the highest stage reported during the stay.

b. Non-pressure chronic ulcers

1) Patients admitted with non-pressure ulcers documented as healed

No code is assigned if the documentation states that the non-pressure ulcer is completely healed.

2) Patients admitted with non-pressure ulcers documented as healing

Non-pressure ulcers described as healing should be assigned the appropriate non-pressure ulcer code based on the documentation in the medical record. If the documentation does not provide information about the severity of the healing non-pressure ulcer, assign the appropriate code for unspecified severity.

If the documentation is unclear as to whether the patient has a current (new) non-pressure ulcer or if the patient is being treated for a healing non-pressure ulcer, query the provider.

For ulcers that were present on admission but healed at the time of discharge, assign the code for the site and severity of the non-pressure ulcer at the time of admission.

3) Patient admitted with non-pressure ulcer that progresses to another severity level during the admission

If a patient is admitted to an inpatient hospital with a non-pressure ulcer at one severity level and it progresses to a higher severity level, two separate codes should be assigned: one code for the site and severity level of the ulcer on admission and a second code for the same ulcer site and the highest severity level reported during the stay.

Chapter 12. Diseases of the Skin and Subcutaneous Tissue (L00-L99)

EXCLUDES 2 *certain conditions originating in the perinatal period (P04-P96)*
certain infectious and parasitic diseases (A00-B99)
complications of pregnancy, childbirth and the puerperium (O00-O9A)
congenital malformations, deformations, and chromosomal abnormalities (Q00-Q99)
endocrine, nutritional and metabolic diseases (E00-E88)
lipomelanotic reticulosis (I89.8)
neoplasms (C00-D49)
symptoms, signs and abnormal clinical and laboratory findings, not elsewhere classified (R00-R94)
systemic connective tissue disorders (M30-M36)
viral warts (B07.-)

This chapter contains the following blocks:

L00-L08 Infections of the skin and subcutaneous tissue
L10-L14 Bullous disorders
L20-L30 Dermatitis and eczema
L40-L45 Papulosquamous disorders
L49-L54 Urticaria and erythema
L55-L59 Radiation-related disorders of the skin and subcutaneous tissue
L60-L75 Disorders of skin appendages
L76 Intraoperative and postprocedural complications of skin and subcutaneous tissue
L80-L99 Other disorders of the skin and subcutaneous tissue

Infections of the skin and subcutaneous tissue (L00-L08)

Use additional code (B95-B97) to identify infectious agent
EXCLUDES 2 *hordeolum (H00.0)*
infective dermatitis (L30.3)
local infections of skin classified in Chapter 1
lupus panniculitis (L93.2)
panniculitis NOS (M79.3)
panniculitis of neck and back (M54.0-)
perlèche NOS (K13.0)
perlèche due to candidiasis (B37.0)
perlèche due to riboflavin deficiency (E53.0)
pyogenic granuloma (L98.0)
relapsing panniculitis [Weber-Christian] (M35.6)
viral warts (B07.-)
zoster (B02.-)

L00 Staphylococcal scalded skin syndrome
Ritter's disease
Use additional code to identify percentage of skin exfoliation (L49.-)
EXCLUDES 1 *bullous impetigo (L01.03)*
pemphigus neonatorum (L01.03)
toxic epidermal necrolysis [Lyell] (L51.2)
DEF: Infectious skin disease of children younger than 5 years marked by eruptions ranging from a few localized blisters to widespread, easily ruptured, fine vesicles and bullae affecting almost the entire body; results in exfoliation of large planes of skin and leaves raw areas.

✓4ᵗʰ **L01 Impetigo**
EXCLUDES 1 *impetigo herpetiformis (L40.1)*

✓5ᵗʰ **L01.0 Impetigo**
Impetigo contagiosa
Impetigo vulgaris

L01.00 Impetigo, unspecified ▽
Impetigo NOS

L01.01 Non-bullous impetigo

L01.02 Bockhart's impetigo
Impetigo follicularis
Perifolliculitis NOS
Superficial pustular perifolliculitis

L01.03 Bullous impetigo
Impetigo neonatorum
Pemphigus neonatorum

L01.09 Other impetigo
Ulcerative impetigo

L01.1 Impetiginization of other dermatoses

✓4ᵗʰ **L02 Cutaneous abscess, furuncle and carbuncle**
Use additional code to identify organism (B95-B96)
EXCLUDES 2 *abscess of anus and rectal regions (K61.-)*
abscess of female genital organs (external) (N76.4)
abscess of male genital organs (external) (N48.2, N49-)

✓5ᵗʰ **L02.0 Cutaneous abscess, furuncle and carbuncle of face**
EXCLUDES 2 *abscess of ear, external (H60.0)*
abscess of eyelid (H00.0)
abscess of head [any part, except face] (L02.8)
abscess of lacrimal gland (H04.0)
abscess of lacrimal passages (H04.3)
abscess of mouth (K12.2)
abscess of nose (J34.0)
abscess of orbit (H05.0)
submandibular abscess (K12.2)

L02.01 Cutaneous abscess of face

L02.02 Furuncle of face
Boil of face
Folliculitis of face

L02.03 Carbuncle of face

✓5ᵗʰ **L02.1 Cutaneous abscess, furuncle and carbuncle of neck**

L02.11 Cutaneous abscess of neck

L02.12 Furuncle of neck
Boil of neck
Folliculitis of neck

L02.13 Carbuncle of neck

✓5ᵗʰ **L02.2 Cutaneous abscess, furuncle and carbuncle of trunk**
EXCLUDES 1 *non-newborn omphalitis (L08.82)*
omphalitis of newborn (P38.-)
EXCLUDES 2 *abscess of breast (N61.1)*
abscess of buttocks (L02.3)
abscess of female external genital organs (N76.4)
abscess of hip (L02.4)
abscess of male external genital organs (N48.2, N49-)

✓6ᵗʰ **L02.21 Cutaneous abscess of trunk**

L02.211 Cutaneous abscess of abdominal wall
L02.212 Cutaneous abscess of back [any part, except buttock]
L02.213 Cutaneous abscess of chest wall
L02.214 Cutaneous abscess of groin
L02.215 Cutaneous abscess of perineum
L02.216 Cutaneous abscess of umbilicus
L02.219 Cutaneous abscess of trunk, unspecified ▽

✓6ᵗʰ **L02.22 Furuncle of trunk**
Boil of trunk
Folliculitis of trunk

L02.221 Furuncle of abdominal wall
L02.222 Furuncle of back [any part, except buttock]
L02.223 Furuncle of chest wall
L02.224 Furuncle of groin
L02.225 Furuncle of perineum
L02.226 Furuncle of umbilicus
L02.229 Furuncle of trunk, unspecified ▽

✓6ᵗʰ **L02.23 Carbuncle of trunk**

L02.231 Carbuncle of abdominal wall
L02.232 Carbuncle of back [any part, except buttock]
L02.233 Carbuncle of chest wall
L02.234 Carbuncle of groin
L02.235 Carbuncle of perineum
L02.236 Carbuncle of umbilicus
L02.239 Carbuncle of trunk, unspecified ▽

✓5ᵗʰ **L02.3 Cutaneous abscess, furuncle and carbuncle of buttock**
EXCLUDES 1 *pilonidal cyst with abscess (L05.01)*

L02.31 Cutaneous abscess of buttock
Cutaneous abscess of gluteal region

L02.32 Furuncle of buttock
Boil of buttock
Folliculitis of buttock
Furuncle of gluteal region

L02.33 Carbuncle of buttock
Carbuncle of gluteal region

EXCLUDES 1 Not coded here   EXCLUDES 2 Not included here   N Newborn Age: 0   P Pediatric Age: 0-17   M Maternity Age: 12-55   A Adult Age: 15-124

694   ICD-10-CM 2018

✓5th **L02.4** **Cutaneous abscess, furuncle and carbuncle of limb**
    EXCLUDES 2   *cutaneous abscess, furuncle and carbuncle of groin (L02.214, L02.224, L02.234)*
      cutaneous abscess, furuncle and carbuncle of hand (L02.5-)
      cutaneous abscess, furuncle and carbuncle of foot (L02.6-)

   ✓6th **L02.41** **Cutaneous abscess of limb**
     L02.411 **Cutaneous abscess of right axilla**
     L02.412 **Cutaneous abscess of left axilla**
     L02.413 **Cutaneous abscess of right upper limb**
     L02.414 **Cutaneous abscess of left upper limb**
     L02.415 **Cutaneous abscess of right lower limb**
     L02.416 **Cutaneous abscess of left lower limb**
     L02.419 **Cutaneous abscess of limb, unspecified** ▽

   ✓6th **L02.42** **Furuncle of limb**
     Boil of limb
     Folliculitis of limb
     L02.421 **Furuncle of right axilla**
     L02.422 **Furuncle of left axilla**
     L02.423 **Furuncle of right upper limb**
     L02.424 **Furuncle of left upper limb**
     L02.425 **Furuncle of right lower limb**
     L02. **Furuncle of left lower limb**
     L02.429 **Furuncle of limb, unspecified** ▽

   ✓6th **L02.43** **Carbuncle of limb**
     L02.431 **Carbuncle of right axilla**
     L02.432 **Carbuncle of left axilla**
     L02.433 **Carbuncle of right upper limb**
     L02.434 **Carbuncle of left upper limb**
     L02.435 **Carbuncle of right lower limb**
     L02.436 **Carbuncle of left lower limb**
     L02.439 **Carbuncle of limb, unspecified** ▽

✓5th **L02.5** **Cutaneous abscess, furuncle and carbuncle of hand**
   ✓6th **L02.51** **Cutaneous abscess of hand**
     L02.511 **Cutaneous abscess of right hand**
     L02.512 **Cutaneous abscess of left hand**
     L02.519 **Cutaneous abscess of unspecified hand** ▽

   ✓6th **L02.52** **Furuncle hand**
     Boil of hand
     Folliculitis of hand
     L02.521 **Furuncle right hand**
     L02.522 **Furuncle left hand**
     L02.529 **Furuncle unspecified hand** ▽

   ✓6th **L02.53** **Carbuncle of hand**
     L02.531 **Carbuncle of right hand**
     L02.532 **Carbuncle of left hand**
     L02.539 **Carbuncle of unspecified hand** ▽

✓5th **L02.6** **Cutaneous abscess, furuncle and carbuncle of foot**
   ✓6th **L02.61** **Cutaneous abscess of foot**
     L02.611 **Cutaneous abscess of right foot**
     L02.612 **Cutaneous abscess of left foot**
     L02.619 **Cutaneous abscess of unspecified foot** ▽

   ✓6th **L02.62** **Furuncle of foot**
     Boil of foot
     Folliculitis of foot
     L02.621 **Furuncle of right foot**
     L02.622 **Furuncle of left foot**
     L02.629 **Furuncle of unspecified foot** ▽

   ✓6th **L02.63** **Carbuncle of foot**
     L02.631 **Carbuncle of right foot**
     L02.632 **Carbuncle of left foot**
     L02.639 **Carbuncle of unspecified foot** ▽

✓5th **L02.8** **Cutaneous abscess, furuncle and carbuncle of other sites**
   ✓6th **L02.81** **Cutaneous abscess of other sites**
     L02.811 **Cutaneous abscess of head [any part, except face]**
     L02.818 **Cutaneous abscess of other sites**

   ✓6th **L02.82** **Furuncle of other sites**
     Boil of other sites
     Folliculitis of other sites
     L02.821 **Furuncle of head [any part, except face]**
     L02.828 **Furuncle of other sites**

   ✓6th **L02.83** **Carbuncle of other sites**
     L02.831 **Carbuncle of head [any part, except face]**
     L02.838 **Carbuncle of other sites**

✓5th **L02.9** **Cutaneous abscess, furuncle and carbuncle, unspecified**
     L02.91 **Cutaneous abscess, unspecified** ▽
     L02.92 **Furuncle, unspecified** ▽
      Boil NOS
      Furunculosis NOS
     L02.93 **Carbuncle, unspecified** ▽

✓4th **L03** **Cellulitis and acute lymphangitis**
    EXCLUDES 2   *cellulitis of anal and rectal region (K61.-)*
      cellulitis of external auditory canal (H60.1)
      cellulitis of eyelid (H00.03-)
      cellulitis of female external genital organs (N76.4)
      cellulitis of lacrimal apparatus (H04.3)
      cellulitis of male external genital organs (N48.2, N49-)
      cellulitis of mouth (K12.2)
      cellulitis of nose (J34.0)
      eosinophilic cellulitis [Wells] (L98.3)
      febrile neutrophilic dermatosis [Sweet] (L98.2)
      lymphangitis (chronic) (subacute) (I89.1)

   ✓5th **L03.0** **Cellulitis and acute lymphangitis of finger and toe**
     Infection of nail
     Onychia
     Paronychia
     Perionychia

    ✓6th **L03.01** **Cellulitis of finger**
     Felon
     Whitlow
     EXCLUDES 1   *herpetic whitlow (B00.89)*
     DEF: Felon: Superficial bacterial skin infection at the tip of the finger.
     L03.011 **Cellulitis of right finger**
     L03.012 **Cellulitis of left finger**
     L03.019 **Cellulitis of unspecified finger** ▽

    ✓6th **L03.02** **Acute lymphangitis of finger**
     Hangnail with lymphangitis of finger
     L03.021 **Acute lymphangitis of right finger**
     L03.022 **Acute lymphangitis of left finger**
     L03.029 **Acute lymphangitis of unspecified finger** ▽

    ✓6th **L03.03** **Cellulitis of toe**
     L03.031 **Cellulitis of right toe**
     L03.032 **Cellulitis of left toe**
     L03.039 **Cellulitis of unspecified toe** ▽

    ✓6th **L03.04** **Acute lymphangitis of toe**
     Hangnail with lymphangitis of toe
     L03.041 **Acute lymphangitis of right toe**
     L03.042 **Acute lymphangitis of left toe**
     L03.049 **Acute lymphangitis of unspecified toe** ▽

   ✓5th **L03.1** **Cellulitis and acute lymphangitis of other parts of limb**
    ✓6th **L03.11** **Cellulitis of other parts of limb**
     EXCLUDES 2   *cellulitis of fingers (L03.01-)*
      cellulitis of toes (L03.03-)
      groin (L03.314)
     L03.111 **Cellulitis of right axilla**
     L03.112 **Cellulitis of left axilla**
     L03.113 **Cellulitis of right upper limb**
     L03.114 **Cellulitis of left upper limb**
     L03.115 **Cellulitis of right lower limb**
     L03.116 **Cellulitis of left lower limb**
     L03.119 **Cellulitis of unspecified part of limb** ▽

    ✓6th **L03.12** **Acute lymphangitis of other parts of limb**
     EXCLUDES 2   *acute lymphangitis of fingers (L03.02-)*
      acute lymphangitis of groin (L03.324)
      acute lymphangitis of toes (L03.04-)
     L03.121 **Acute lymphangitis of right axilla**
     L03.122 **Acute lymphangitis of left axilla**
     L03.123 **Acute lymphangitis of right upper limb**
     L03.124 **Acute lymphangitis of left upper limb**
     L03.125 **Acute lymphangitis of right lower limb**
     L03.126 **Acute lymphangitis of left lower limb**
     L03.129 **Acute lymphangitis of unspecified part of limb** ▽

✓ Additional Character Req   ✓x7th Placeholder Alert   Manifestation   HCC CMS-HCC Condition   ▽ Unspecified Code   ▶◀ Revised Text   ● New Code   ▲ Revised Code Title

✓5ᵗʰ **L03.2 Cellulitis and acute lymphangitis of face and neck**

  ✓6ᵗʰ **L03.21 Cellulitis and acute lymphangitis of face**

    L03.211 Cellulitis of face

      EXCLUDES 2   *abscess of orbit (H05.01-)*
          cellulitis of ear (H60.1-)
          cellulitis of eyelid (H00.03-)
          cellulitis of head (L03.811)
          cellulitis of lacrimal apparatus (H04.3)
          cellulitis of lip (K13.0)
          cellulitis of mouth (K12.2)
          cellulitis of nose (internal) (J34.0)
          cellulitis of orbit (H05.01-)
          cellulitis of scalp (L03.811)

      AHA: 2013, 4Q, 123

    L03.212 Acute lymphangitis of face

    L03.213 Periorbital cellulitis
       Preseptal cellulitis

  ✓6ᵗʰ **L03.22 Cellulitis and acute lymphangitis of neck**

    L03.221 Cellulitis of neck

    L03.222 Acute lymphangitis of neck

✓5ᵗʰ **L03.3 Cellulitis and acute lymphangitis of trunk**

  ✓6ᵗʰ **L03.31 Cellulitis of trunk**

    EXCLUDES 2   *cellulitis of anal and rectal regions (K61.-)*
       cellulitis of breast NOS (N61.0)
       cellulitis of female external genital organs (N76.4)
       cellulitis of male external genital organs (N48.2, N49-)
       omphalitis of newborn (P38.-)
       puerperal cellulitis of breast (O91.2)

    L03.311 Cellulitis of abdominal wall
      EXCLUDES 2   *cellulitis of umbilicus (L03.316)*
          cellulitis of groin (L03.314)

    L03.312 Cellulitis of back [any part except buttock]

    L03.313 Cellulitis of chest wall

    L03.314 Cellulitis of groin

    L03.315 Cellulitis of perineum

    L03.316 Cellulitis of umbilicus

    L03.317 Cellulitis of buttock

    L03.319 Cellulitis of trunk, unspecified ▽

  ✓6ᵗʰ **L03.32 Acute lymphangitis of trunk**

    L03.321 Acute lymphangitis of abdominal wall

    L03.322 Acute lymphangitis of back [any part except buttock]

    L03.323 Acute lymphangitis of chest wall

    L03.324 Acute lymphangitis of groin

    L03.325 Acute lymphangitis of perineum

    L03.326 Acute lymphangitis of umbilicus

    L03.327 Acute lymphangitis of buttock

    L03.329 Acute lymphangitis of trunk, unspecified ▽

✓5ᵗʰ **L03.8 Cellulitis and acute lymphangitis of other sites**

  ✓6ᵗʰ **L03.81 Cellulitis of other sites**

    L03.811 Cellulitis of head [any part, except face]
       Cellulitis of scalp
      EXCLUDES 2   *cellulitis of face (L03.211)*

    L03.818 Cellulitis of other sites

  ✓6ᵗʰ **L03.89 Acute lymphangitis of other sites**

    L03.891 Acute lymphangitis of head [any part, except face]

    L03.898 Acute lymphangitis of other sites

✓5ᵗʰ **L03.9 Cellulitis and acute lymphangitis, unspecified**

  L03.90 Cellulitis, unspecified ▽

  L03.91 Acute lymphangitis, unspecified ▽
    EXCLUDES 1   *lymphangitis NOS (I89.1)*

✓4ᵗʰ **L04 Acute lymphadenitis**

  INCLUDES   abscess (acute) of lymph nodes, except mesenteric
     acute lymphadenitis, except mesenteric

  EXCLUDES 1   *chronic or subacute lymphadenitis, except mesenteric (I88.1)*
     enlarged lymph nodes (R59.-)
     human immunodeficiency virus [HIV] disease resulting in generalized lymphadenopathy (B20)
     lymphadenitis NOS (I88.9)
     nonspecific mesenteric lymphadenitis (I88.0)

  L04.0 Acute lymphadenitis of face, head and neck

Pilonidal Cyst

  — Skin
  — Fistula
  — Pilonidal cyst
  — Fat
  — Bone

L04.1 Acute lymphadenitis of trunk

L04.2 Acute lymphadenitis of upper limb
   Acute lymphadenitis of axilla
   Acute lymphadenitis of shoulder

L04.3 Acute lymphadenitis of lower limb
   Acute lymphadenitis of hip
  EXCLUDES 2   *acute lymphadenitis of groin (L04.1)*

L04.8 Acute lymphadenitis of other sites

L04.9 Acute lymphadenitis, unspecified ▽

✓4ᵗʰ **L05 Pilonidal cyst and sinus**

  ✓5ᵗʰ **L05.0 Pilonidal cyst and sinus with abscess**

    L05.01 Pilonidal cyst with abscess
       Pilonidal abscess
       Pilonidal dimple with abscess
       Postanal dimple with abscess
      EXCLUDES 2   *congenital sacral dimple (Q82.6)*
          parasacral dimple (Q82.6)

    L05.02 Pilonidal sinus with abscess
       Coccygeal fistula with abscess
       Coccygeal sinus with abscess
       Pilonidal fistula with abscess

  ✓5ᵗʰ **L05.9 Pilonidal cyst and sinus without abscess**

    L05.91 Pilonidal cyst without abscess
       Pilonidal dimple
       Postanal dimple
       Pilonidal cyst NOS
      EXCLUDES 2   *congenital sacral dimple (Q82.6)*
          parasacral dimple (Q82.6)

    L05.92 Pilonidal sinus without abscess
       Coccygeal fistula
       Coccygeal sinus without abscess
       Pilonidal fistula

✓4ᵗʰ **L08 Other local infections of skin and subcutaneous tissue**

  L08.0 Pyoderma
     Dermatitis gangrenosa
     Purulent dermatitis
     Septic dermatitis
     Suppurative dermatitis
    EXCLUDES 1   *pyoderma gangrenosum (L88)*
       pyoderma vegetans (L08.81)

  L08.1 Erythrasma

  ✓5ᵗʰ **L08.8 Other specified local infections of the skin and subcutaneous tissue**

    L08.81 Pyoderma vegetans
      EXCLUDES 1   *pyoderma gangrenosum (L88)*
          pyoderma NOS (L08.0)

    L08.82 Omphalitis not of newborn
      EXCLUDES 1   *omphalitis of newborn (P38.-)*

    L08.89 Other specified local infections of the skin and subcutaneous tissue

  L08.9 Local infection of the skin and subcutaneous tissue, unspecified ▽

EXCLUDES 1 Not coded here   EXCLUDES 2 Not included here   N Newborn Age: 0   P Pediatric Age: 0-17   M Maternity Age: 12-55   A Adult Age: 15-124

696   ICD-10-CM 2018

Bullous disorders (L10-L14)

EXCLUDES 1   *benign familial pemphigus [Hailey-Hailey] (Q82.8)*
staphylococcal scalded skin syndrome (L00)
toxic epidermal necrolysis [Lyell] (L51.2)

✓4th L10   Pemphigus
EXCLUDES 1   *pemphigus neonatorum (L01.03)*

L10.0   **Pemphigus** vulgaris

L10.1   **Pemphigus** vegetans

L10.2   **Pemphigus** foliaceous

L10.3   **Brazilian pemphigus [fogo selvagem]**

L10.4   **Pemphigus** erythematosus
Senear-Usher syndrome

L10.5   **Drug-induced pemphigus**
Use additional code for adverse effect, if applicable, to identify drug (T36-T50 with fifth or sixth character 5)

✓5th **L10.8**   **Other pemphigus**

    L10.81   **Paraneoplastic pemphigus**

    L10.89   **Other pemphigus**

L10.9   **Pemphigus, unspecified**   ▽

✓4th L11   Other acantholytic disorders

L11.0   **Acquired keratosis follicularis**
EXCLUDES 1   *keratosis follicularis (congenital) [Darier-White] (Q82.8)*

L11.1   **Transient acantholytic dermatosis [Grover]**

L11.8   **Other specified acantholytic disorders**

L11.9   **Acantholytic disorder, unspecified**   ▽

✓4th L12   Pemphigoid
EXCLUDES 1   *herpes gestationis (O26.4-)*
impetigo herpetiformis (L40.1)

L12.0   **Bullous pemphigoid**

L12.1   **Cicatricial pemphigoid**
Benign mucous membrane pemphigoid
DEF: Chronic autoimmune disease characterized by subepidermal blistering lesions of mucosa, including the conjunctiva; seen predominantly in the elderly; produces adhesions and scarring.

L12.2   **Chronic bullous disease of childhood**   P
Juvenile dermatitis herpetiformis

✓5th **L12.3**   **Acquired epidermolysis bullosa**
EXCLUDES 1   *epidermolysis bullosa (congenital) (Q81.-)*

    L12.30   **Acquired epidermolysis bullosa, unspecified**   HCC ▽

    L12.31   **Epidermolysis bullosa due to drug**   HCC
Use additional code for adverse effect, if applicable, to identify drug (T36-T50 with fifth or sixth character 5)

    L12.35   **Other acquired epidermolysis bullosa**   HCC

L12.8   **Other pemphigoid**

L12.9   **Pemphigoid, unspecified**   ▽

✓4th L13   Other bullous disorders

L13.0   **Dermatitis herpetiformis**
Duhring's disease
Hydroa herpetiformis
EXCLUDES 1   *juvenile dermatitis herpetiformis (L12.2)*
senile dermatitis herpetiformis (L12.0)
DEF: Skin disease to which people are genetically predisposed resulting from an immunological response to gluten; seen as an extremely pruritic eruption of various lesions that frequently heal, leaving hyperpigmentation or hypopigmentation and occasionally scarring; usually associated with an asymptomatic gluten-sensitive enteropathy.

L13.1   **Subcorneal pustular dermatitis**
Sneddon-Wilkinson disease

L13.8   **Other specified bullous disorders**

L13.9   **Bullous disorder, unspecified**   ▽

L14   *Bullous disorders in diseases classified elsewhere*
Code first underlying disease

Dermatitis and eczema (L20-L30)

NOTE   In this block the terms dermatitis and eczema are used synonymously and interchangeably.

EXCLUDES 2   *chronic (childhood) granulomatous disease (D71)*
dermatitis gangrenosa (L08.0)
dermatitis herpetiformis (L13.0)
dry skin dermatitis (L85.3)
factitial dermatitis (L98.1)
perioral dermatitis (L71.0)
radiation-related disorders of the skin and subcutaneous tissue (L55-L59)
stasis dermatitis (I87.2)

✓4th L20   Atopic dermatitis

L20.0   **Besnier's prurigo**

✓5th **L20.8**   **Other atopic dermatitis**
EXCLUDES 2   *circumscribed neurodermatitis (L28.0)*

    L20.81   **Atopic neurodermatitis**
Diffuse neurodermatitis

    L20.82   **Flexural eczema**

    L20.83   **Infantile (acute) (chronic) eczema**   P

    L20.84   **Intrinsic (allergic) eczema**

    L20.89   **Other atopic dermatitis**

L20.9   **Atopic dermatitis, unspecified**   ▽

✓4th L21   Seborrheic dermatitis
EXCLUDES 2   *infective dermatitis (L30.3)*
seborrheic keratosis (L82.-)

L21.0   **Seborrhea capitis**   P
Cradle cap

L21.1   **Seborrheic infantile dermatitis**   P

L21.8   **Other seborrheic dermatitis**

L21.9   **Seborrheic dermatitis, unspecified**   ▽
Seborrhea NOS

L22   Diaper dermatitis
Diaper erythema
Diaper rash
Psoriasiform diaper rash

✓4th L23   Allergic contact dermatitis
EXCLUDES 1   *allergy NOS (T78.40)*
contact dermatitis NOS (L25.9)
dermatitis NOS (L30.9)

EXCLUDES 2   *dermatitis due to substances taken internally (L27.-)*
dermatitis of eyelid (H01.1-)
diaper dermatitis (L22)
eczema of external ear (H60.5-)
irritant contact dermatitis (L24.-)
perioral dermatitis (L71.0)
radiation-related disorders of the skin and subcutaneous tissue (L55-L59)

L23.0   **Allergic contact dermatitis due to metals**
Allergic contact dermatitis due to chromium
Allergic contact dermatitis due to nickel

L23.1   **Allergic contact dermatitis due to adhesives**

L23.2   **Allergic contact dermatitis due to cosmetics**

L23.3   **Allergic contact dermatitis due to drugs in contact with skin**
Use additional code for adverse effect, if applicable, to identify drug (T36-T50 with fifth or sixth character 5)
EXCLUDES 2   *dermatitis due to ingested drugs and medicaments (L27.0-L27.1)*

L23.4   **Allergic contact dermatitis due to dyes**

L23.5   **Allergic contact dermatitis due to other chemical products**
Allergic contact dermatitis due to cement
Allergic contact dermatitis due to insecticide
Allergic contact dermatitis due to plastic
Allergic contact dermatitis due to rubber

L23.6   **Allergic contact dermatitis due to food in contact with the skin**
EXCLUDES 2   *dermatitis due to ingested food (L27.2)*

L23.7   **Allergic contact dermatitis due to plants, except food**
EXCLUDES 2   *allergy NOS due to pollen (J30.1)*

✓5th **L23.8**   **Allergic contact dermatitis due to other agents**

    L23.81   **Allergic contact dermatitis due to animal (cat) (dog) dander**
Allergic contact dermatitis due to animal (cat) (dog) hair

    L23.89   **Allergic contact dermatitis due to other agents**

☑ Additional Character Req   ✓x7th Placeholder Alert   **Manifestation**   HCC CMS-HCC Condition   ▽ Unspecified Code   ►◄ Revised Text   ● New Code   ▲ Revised Code Title

ICD-10-CM 2018   697

L10–L23.89

L23.9   Allergic contact dermatitis, unspecified cause ▽
Allergic contact eczema NOS

✓4ᵗʰ L24   Irritant contact dermatitis
> EXCLUDES 1   allergy NOS (T78.40)
> contact dermatitis NOS (L25.9)
> dermatitis NOS (L30.9)
> EXCLUDES 2   allergic contact dermatitis (L23.-)
> dermatitis due to substances taken internally (L27.-)
> dermatitis of eyelid (H01.1-)
> diaper dermatitis (L22)
> eczema of external ear (H60.5-)
> perioral dermatitis (L71.0)
> radiation-related disorders of the skin and subcutaneous tissue (L55-L59)

L24.0   Irritant contact dermatitis due to detergents

L24.1   Irritant contact dermatitis due to oils and greases

L24.2   Irritant contact dermatitis due to solvents
Irritant contact dermatitis due to chlorocompound
Irritant contact dermatitis due to cyclohexane
Irritant contact dermatitis due to ester
Irritant contact dermatitis due to glycol
Irritant contact dermatitis due to hydrocarbon
Irritant contact dermatitis due to ketone

L24.3   Irritant contact dermatitis due to cosmetics

L24.4   Irritant contact dermatitis due to drugs in contact with skin
Use additional code for adverse effect, if applicable, to identify drug (T36-T50 with fifth or sixth character 5)

L24.5   Irritant contact dermatitis due to other chemical products
Irritant contact dermatitis due to cement
Irritant contact dermatitis due to insecticide
Irritant contact dermatitis due to plastic
Irritant contact dermatitis due to rubber

L24.6   Irritant contact dermatitis due to food in contact with skin
> EXCLUDES 2   dermatitis due to ingested food (L27.2)

L24.7   Irritant contact dermatitis due to plants, except food
> EXCLUDES 2   allergy NOS to pollen (J30.1)

✓5ᵗʰ L24.8   Irritant contact dermatitis due to other agents
> **L24.81   Irritant contact dermatitis due to metals**
> Irritant contact dermatitis due to chromium
> Irritant contact dermatitis due to nickel
>
> **L24.89   Irritant contact dermatitis due to other agents**
> Irritant contact dermatitis due to dyes

L24.9   Irritant contact dermatitis, unspecified cause ▽
Irritant contact eczema NOS

✓4ᵗʰ L25   Unspecified contact dermatitis
> EXCLUDES 1   allergic contact dermatitis (L23.-)
> allergy NOS (T78.40)
> dermatitis NOS (L30.9)
> irritant contact dermatitis (L24.-)
> EXCLUDES 2   dermatitis due to ingested substances (L27.-)
> dermatitis of eyelid (H01.1-)
> eczema of external ear (H60.5-)
> perioral dermatitis (L71.0)
> radiation-related disorders of the skin and subcutaneous tissue (L55-L59)

L25.0   Unspecified contact dermatitis due to cosmetics ▽

L25.1   Unspecified contact dermatitis due to drugs in contact with skin ▽
Use additional code for adverse effect, if applicable, to identify drug (T36-T50 with fifth or sixth character 5)
> EXCLUDES 2   dermatitis due to ingested drugs and medicaments (L27.0-L27.1)

L25.2   Unspecified contact dermatitis due to dyes ▽

L25.3   Unspecified contact dermatitis due to other chemical products ▽
Unspecified contact dermatitis due to cement
Unspecified contact dermatitis due to insecticide

L25.4   Unspecified contact dermatitis due to food in contact with skin ▽
> EXCLUDES 2   dermatitis due to ingested food (L27.2)

L25.5   Unspecified contact dermatitis due to plants, except food ▽
> EXCLUDES 1   nettle rash (L50.9)
> EXCLUDES 2   allergy NOS due to pollen (J30.1)

L25.8   Unspecified contact dermatitis due to other agents ▽

L25.9   Unspecified contact dermatitis, unspecified cause ▽
Contact dermatitis (occupational) NOS
Contact eczema (occupational) NOS

L26   Exfoliative dermatitis
Hebra's pityriasis
> EXCLUDES 1   Ritter's disease (L00)

✓4ᵗʰ L27   Dermatitis due to substances taken internally
> EXCLUDES 1   allergy NOS (T78.40)
> EXCLUDES 2   adverse food reaction, except dermatitis (T78.0-T78.1)
> contact dermatitis (L23-L25)
> drug photoallergic response (L56.1)
> drug phototoxic response (L56.0)
> urticaria (L50.-)

L27.0   Generalized skin eruption due to drugs and medicaments taken internally
Use additional code for adverse effect, if applicable, to identify drug (T36-T50 with fifth or sixth character 5)

L27.1   Localized skin eruption due to drugs and medicaments taken internally
Use additional code for adverse effect, if applicable, to identify drug (T36-T50 with fifth or sixth character 5)

L27.2   Dermatitis due to ingested food
> EXCLUDES 2   dermatitis due to food in contact with skin (L23.6, L24.6, L25.4)

L27.8   Dermatitis due to other substances taken internally

L27.9   Dermatitis due to unspecified substance taken internally ▽

✓4ᵗʰ L28   Lichen simplex chronicus and prurigo
> **L28.0   Lichen simplex chronicus**
> Circumscribed neurodermatitis
> Lichen NOS
>
> **L28.1   Prurigo nodularis**
>
> **L28.2   Other prurigo**
> Prurigo NOS
> Prurigo Hebra
> Prurigo mitis
> Urticaria papulosa

✓4ᵗʰ L29   Pruritus
> EXCLUDES 1   neurotic excoriation (L98.1)
> psychogenic pruritus (F45.8)

L29.0   Pruritus ani

L29.1   Pruritus scroti ♂

L29.2   Pruritus vulvae ♀

L29.3   Anogenital pruritus, unspecified ▽

L29.8   Other pruritus

L29.9   Pruritus, unspecified ▽
Itch NOS

✓4ᵗʰ L30   Other and unspecified dermatitis
> EXCLUDES 2   contact dermatitis (L23-L25)
> dry skin dermatitis (L85.3)
> small plaque parapsoriasis (L41.3)
> stasis dermatitis (I87.2)

L30.0   Nummular dermatitis

L30.1   Dyshidrosis [pompholyx]

L30.2   Cutaneous autosensitization
Candidid [levurid]
Dermatophytid
Eczematid

L30.3   Infective dermatitis
Infectious eczematoid dermatitis

L30.4   Erythema intertrigo

L30.5   Pityriasis alba

L30.8   Other specified dermatitis

L30.9   Dermatitis, unspecified ▽
Eczema NOS

Papulosquamous disorders (L40-L45)

✓4ᵗʰ L40   Psoriasis
> **L40.0   Psoriasis vulgaris**
> Nummular psoriasis
> Plaque psoriasis
>
> **L40.1   Generalized pustular psoriasis**
> Impetigo herpetiformis
> Von Zumbusch's disease
>
> **L40.2   Acrodermatitis continua**
>
> **L40.3   Pustulosis palmaris et plantaris**
>
> **L40.4   Guttate psoriasis**

EXCLUDES 1 Not coded here   EXCLUDES 2 Not included here   N Newborn Age: 0   P Pediatric Age: 0-17   M Maternity Age: 12-55   A Adult Age: 15-124

698   ICD-10-CM 2018

☑5ᵗʰ **L40.5 Arthropathic psoriasis**

    L40.50 Arthropathic psoriasis, unspecified HCC ▽

    L40.51 Distal interphalangeal psoriatic arthropathy HCC

    L40.52 Psoriatic arthritis mutilans HCC

    L40.53 Psoriatic spondylitis HCC

    L40.54 Psoriatic juvenile arthropathy HCC

    L40.59 Other psoriatic arthropathy HCC

L40.8 Other psoriasis
    Flexural psoriasis

L40.9 Psoriasis, unspecified ▽

☑4ᵗʰ **L41 Parapsoriasis**

    EXCLUDES 1 *poikiloderma vasculare atrophicans (L94.5)*

L41.0 Pityriasis lichenoides et varioliformis acuta
    Mucha-Habermann disease

L41.1 Pityriasis lichenoides chronica

L41.3 Small plaque parapsoriasis

L41.4 Large plaque parapsoriasis

L41.5 Retiform parapsoriasis

L41.8 Other parapsoriasis

L41.9 Parapsoriasis, unspecified ▽

L42 Pityriasis rosea

☑4ᵗʰ **L43 Lichen planus**

    EXCLUDES 1 *lichen planopilaris (L66.1)*

L43.0 Hypertrophic lichen planus

L43.1 Bullous lichen planus

L43.2 Lichenoid drug reaction
    Use additional code for adverse effect, if applicable, to identify drug (T36-T50 with fifth or sixth character 5)

L43.3 Subacute (active) lichen planus
    Lichen planus tropicus

L43.8 Other lichen planus

L43.9 Lichen planus, unspecified ▽

☑4ᵗʰ **L44 Other papulosquamous disorders**

L44.0 Pityriasis rubra pilaris

L44.1 Lichen nitidus
    DEF: Chronic, inflammatory, asymptomatic skin disorder, characterized by numerous glistening, flat-topped, discrete, skin-colored micropapules, most often on the penis, lower abdomen, inner thighs, wrists, forearms, breasts and buttocks.

L44.2 Lichen striatus

L44.3 Lichen ruber moniliformis

L44.4 Infantile papular acrodermatitis [Gianotti-Crosti] P

L44.8 Other specified papulosquamous disorders

L44.9 Papulosquamous disorder, unspecified ▽

L45 Papulosquamous disorders in diseases classified elsewhere
    Code first underlying disease

Urticaria and erythema (L49-L54)

EXCLUDES 1 *Lyme disease (A69.2-)*
    rosacea (L71.-)

☑4ᵗʰ **L49 Exfoliation due to erythematous conditions according to extent of body surface involved**
    Code first erythematous condition causing exfoliation, such as:
    Ritter's disease (L00)
    (Staphylococcal) scalded skin syndrom (L00)
    Stevens-Johnson syndrome (L51.1)
    Stevens-Johnson syndrome-toxic epidermal necrolysis overlap syndrome (L51.3)
    toxic epidermal necrolysis (L51.2)

L49.0 Exfoliation due to erythematous condition involving less than 10 percent of body surface
    Exfoliation due to erythematous condition NOS

L49.1 Exfoliation due to erythematous condition involving 10-19 percent of body surface

L49.2 Exfoliation due to erythematous condition involving 20-29 percent of body surface

L49.3 Exfoliation due to erythematous condition involving 30-39 percent of body surface

L49.4 Exfoliation due to erythematous condition involving 40-49 percent of body surface

L49.5 Exfoliation due to erythematous condition involving 50-59 percent of body surface

L49.6 Exfoliation due to erythematous condition involving 60-69 percent of body surface

L49.7 Exfoliation due to erythematous condition involving 70-79 percent of body surface

L49.8 Exfoliation due to erythematous condition involving 80-89 percent of body surface

L49.9 Exfoliation due to erythematous condition involving 90 or more percent of body surface

☑4ᵗʰ **L50 Urticaria**

    EXCLUDES 1 *allergic contact dermatitis (L23.-)*
    angioneurotic edema (T78.3)
    giant urticaria (T78.3)
    hereditary angio-edema (D84.1)
    Quincke's edema (T78.3)
    serum urticaria (T80.6-)
    solar urticaria (L56.3)
    urticaria neonatorum (P83.8)
    urticaria papulosa (L28.2)
    urticaria pigmentosa (Q82.2)

L50.0 Allergic urticaria

L50.1 Idiopathic urticaria

L50.2 Urticaria due to cold and heat
    EXCLUDES 2 *familial cold urticaria (M04.2)*

L50.3 Dermatographic urticaria

L50.4 Vibratory urticaria

L50.5 Cholinergic urticaria

L50.6 Contact urticaria

L50.8 Other urticaria
    Chronic urticaria
    Recurrent periodic urticaria

L50.9 Urticaria, unspecified ▽

☑4ᵗʰ **L51 Erythema multiforme**
    Use additional code for adverse effect, if applicable, to identify drug (T36-T50 with fifth or sixth character 5)
    Use additional code to identify associated manifestations, such as:
    arthropathy associated with dermatological disorders (M14.8-)
    conjunctival edema (H11.42)
    conjunctivitis (H10.22-)
    corneal scars and opacities (H17.-)
    corneal ulcer (H16.0-)
    edema of eyelid (H02.84)
    inflammation of eyelid (H01.8)
    keratoconjunctivitis sicca (H16.22-)
    mechanical lagophthalmos (H02.22-)
    stomatitis (K12.-)
    symblepharon (H11.23-)
    Use additional code to identify percentage of skin exfoliation (L49.-)
    EXCLUDES 1 *staphylococcal scalded skin syndrome (L00)*
    Ritter's disease (L00)

L51.0 Nonbullous erythema multiforme

L51.1 Stevens-Johnson syndrome HCC

L51.2 Toxic epidermal necrolysis [Lyell] HCC

L51.3 Stevens-Johnson syndrome-toxic epidermal necrolysis overlap syndrome HCC
    SJS-TEN overlap syndrome

L51.8 Other erythema multiforme

L51.9 Erythema multiforme, unspecified ▽
    Erythema iris
    Erythema multiforme major NOS
    Erythema multiforme minor NOS
    Herpes iris

L52 Erythema nodosum
    EXCLUDES 1 *tuberculous erythema nodosum (A18.4)*
    DEF: A form of panniculitis (inflammation of the fat layer beneath the skin) of particularly women, usually seen as a hypersensitivity reaction to infections, drugs, sarcoidosis, and specific enteropathies; the acute stage is associated with fever, malaise, and arthralgia; the lesions are pink to blue in color as tender nodules and are found on the front of the legs below the knees.

☑4ᵗʰ **L53 Other erythematous conditions**
    EXCLUDES 1 *erythema ab igne (L59.0)*
    erythema due to external agents in contact with skin (L23-L25)
    erythema intertrigo (L30.4)

L53.0 Toxic erythema
    Code first poisoning due to drug or toxin, if applicable (T36-T65 with fifth or sixth character 1-4 or 6)
    Use additional code for adverse effect, if applicable, to identify drug (T36-T50 with fifth or sixth character 5)
    EXCLUDES 1 *neonatal erythema toxicum (P83.1)*

☑ Additional Character Req   x7ᵗʰ Placeholder Alert   Manifestation   HCC CMS-HCC Condition   ▽ Unspecified Code   ▶◀ Revised Text   ● New Code   ▲ Revised Code Title

L53.1 Erythema annulare centrifugum

L53.2 Erythema marginatum

L53.3 Other chronic figurate erythema

L53.8 Other specified erythematous conditions

L53.9 Erythematous condition, unspecified ▽
Erythema NOS
Erythroderma NOS

L54 Erythema in diseases classified elsewhere
Code first underlying disease

Radiation-related disorders of the skin and subcutaneous tissue (L55-L59)

✓4ᵗʰ **L55 Sunburn**

L55.Ø Sunburn of first degree

L55.1 Sunburn of second degree

L55.2 Sunburn of third degree

L55.9 Sunburn, unspecified ▽

✓4ᵗʰ **L56 Other acute skin changes due to ultraviolet radiation**
Use additional code to identify the source of the ultraviolet radiation (W89, X32)

L56.Ø Drug phototoxic response
Use additional code for adverse effect, if applicable, to identify drug (T36-T5Ø with fifth or sixth character 5)

L56.1 Drug photoallergic response
Use additional code for adverse effect, if applicable, to identify drug (T36-T5Ø with fifth or sixth character 5)

L56.2 Photocontact dermatitis [berloque dermatitis]

L56.3 Solar urticaria

L56.4 Polymorphous light eruption

L56.5 Disseminated superficial actinic porokeratosis (DSAP)
DEF: Autosomal dominant skin condition occurring in sun-exposed areas of the skin (particularly the arms and legs); characterized by superficial annular, keratotic, brownish-red spots or thickenings with depressed centers and sharp, ridged borders; may evolve into squamous cell carcinoma.

L56.8 Other specified acute skin changes due to ultraviolet radiation

L56.9 Acute skin change due to ultraviolet radiation, unspecified ▽

✓4ᵗʰ **L57 Skin changes due to chronic exposure to nonionizing radiation**
Use additional code to identify the source of the ultraviolet radiation ▶(W89)◀

L57.Ø Actinic keratosis
Keratosis NOS
Senile keratosis
Solar keratosis

L57.1 Actinic reticuloid

L57.2 Cutis rhomboidalis nuchae

L57.3 Poikiloderma of Civatte

L57.4 Cutis laxa senilis
Elastosis senilis

L57.5 Actinic granuloma

L57.8 Other skin changes due to chronic exposure to nonionizing radiation
Farmer's skin
Sailor's skin
Solar dermatitis

L57.9 Skin changes due to chronic exposure to nonionizing radiation, unspecified ▽

✓4ᵗʰ **L58 Radiodermatitis**
Use additional code to identify the source of the radiation (W88, W9Ø)

L58.Ø Acute radiodermatitis

L58.1 Chronic radiodermatitis

L58.9 Radiodermatitis, unspecified ▽

✓4ᵗʰ **L59 Other disorders of skin and subcutaneous tissue related to radiation**

L59.Ø Erythema ab igne [dermatitis ab igne]

L59.8 Other specified disorders of the skin and subcutaneous tissue related to radiation
AHA: 2017, 1Q, 33

L59.9 Disorder of the skin and subcutaneous tissue related to radiation, unspecified ▽

Nail Disorders

Normal

Koilonychia

Beau's Lines

Disorders of skin appendages (L6Ø-L75)

EXCLUDES 1 congenital malformations of integument (Q84.-)

✓4ᵗʰ **L6Ø Nail disorders**
EXCLUDES 2 clubbing of nails (R68.3)
onychia and paronychia (LØ3.Ø-)

L6Ø.Ø Ingrowing nail

L6Ø.1 Onycholysis

L6Ø.2 Onychogryphosis

L6Ø.3 Nail dystrophy

L6Ø.4 Beau's lines

L6Ø.5 Yellow nail syndrome

L6Ø.8 Other nail disorders

L6Ø.9 Nail disorder, unspecified ▽

L62 Nail disorders in diseases classified elsewhere
Code first underlying disease, such as:
pachydermoperiostosis (M89.4-)

✓4ᵗʰ **L63 Alopecia areata**

L63.Ø Alopecia (capitis) totalis

L63.1 Alopecia universalis

L63.2 Ophiasis

L63.8 Other alopecia areata

L63.9 Alopecia areata, unspecified ▽

✓4ᵗʰ **L64 Androgenic alopecia**
INCLUDES male-pattern baldness

L64.Ø Drug-induced androgenic alopecia
Use additional code for adverse effect, if applicable, to identify drug (T36-T5Ø with fifth or sixth character 5)

L64.8 Other androgenic alopecia

L64.9 Androgenic alopecia, unspecified ▽

✓4ᵗʰ **L65 Other nonscarring hair loss**
Use additional code for adverse effect, if applicable, to identify drug (T36-T5Ø with fifth or sixth character 5)
EXCLUDES 1 trichotillomania (F63.3)

L65.Ø Telogen effluvium
DEF: A form of nonscarring alopecia characterized by shedding of hair from premature telogen development in follicles due to stress, including shock, childbirth, surgery, drugs, or weight loss.

L65.1 Anagen effluvium

L65.2 Alopecia mucinosa

L65.8 Other specified nonscarring hair loss

L65.9 Nonscarring hair loss, unspecified ▽
Alopecia NOS

✓4ᵗʰ **L66 Cicatricial alopecia [scarring hair loss]**

L66.Ø Pseudopelade

L66.1 Lichen planopilaris
Follicular lichen planus

L66.2 Folliculitis decalvans

L66.3 Perifolliculitis capitis abscedens

L66.4 Folliculitis ulerythematosa reticulata

L66.8 Other cicatricial alopecia
AHA: 2015, 1Q, 19

L66.9 Cicatricial alopecia, unspecified ▽

✓4th L67 Hair color and hair shaft abnormalities
     EXCLUDES 1   monilethrix (Q84.1)
                 pili annulati (Q84.1)
                 telogen effluvium (L65.0)

     L67.0 Trichorrhexis nodosa

     L67.1 Variations in hair color
         Canities
         Greyness, hair (premature)
         Heterochromia of hair
         Poliosis circumscripta, acquired
         Poliosis NOS

     L67.8 Other hair color and hair shaft abnormalities
         Fragilitas crinium

     L67.9 Hair color and hair shaft abnormality, unspecified ▽

✓4th L68 Hypertrichosis
     INCLUDES   excess hair
     EXCLUDES 1   congenital hypertrichosis (Q84.2)
                 persistent lanugo (Q84.2)

     L68.0 Hirsutism
     L68.1 Acquired hypertrichosis lanuginosa
     L68.2 Localized hypertrichosis
     L68.3 Polytrichia
     L68.8 Other hypertrichosis
     L68.9 Hypertrichosis, unspecified ▽

✓4th L70 Acne
     EXCLUDES 2   acne keloid (L73.0)

     L70.0 Acne vulgaris
     L70.1 Acne conglobata
     L70.2 Acne varioliformis
         Acne necrotica miliaris
         DEF: Rare form of acne characterized by development of
         persistent brown papulo-pustules followed by scar formation;
         usually on the brow and temporoparietal part of the scalp.

     L70.3 Acne tropica
     L70.4 Infantile acne P
     L70.5 Acné excoriée
         Acné excoriée des jeunes filles
         Picker's acne

     L70.8 Other acne
     L70.9 Acne, unspecified ▽

✓4th L71 Rosacea
     Use additional code for adverse effect, if applicable, to identify drug
     (T36-T50 with fifth or sixth character 5)

     L71.0 Perioral dermatitis
     L71.1 Rhinophyma
     L71.8 Other rosacea
     L71.9 Rosacea, unspecified ▽

✓4th L72 Follicular cysts of skin and subcutaneous tissue
     L72.0 Epidermal cyst
     ✓5th L72.1 Pilar and trichodermal cyst
         L72.11 Pilar cyst
         L72.12 Trichodermal cyst
             Trichilemmal (proliferating) cyst

     L72.2 Steatocystoma multiplex
     L72.3 Sebaceous cyst
         EXCLUDES 2   pilar cyst (L72.11)
                  trichilemmal (proliferating) cyst (L72.12)

     L72.8 Other follicular cysts of the skin and subcutaneous tissue
     L72.9 Follicular cyst of the skin and subcutaneous tissue, unspecified ▽

✓4th L73 Other follicular disorders
     L73.0 Acne keloid
     L73.1 Pseudofolliculitis barbae
     L73.2 Hidradenitis suppurativa
     L73.8 Other specified follicular disorders
         Sycosis barbae
     L73.9 Follicular disorder, unspecified ▽

✓4th L74 Eccrine sweat disorders
     EXCLUDES 2   generalized hyperhidrosis (R61)

     L74.0 Miliaria rubra
     L74.1 Miliaria crystallina
     L74.2 Miliaria profunda
         Miliaria tropicalis

     L74.3 Miliaria, unspecified ▽
     L74.4 Anhidrosis
         Hypohidrosis

     ✓5th L74.5 Focal hyperhidrosis
         ✓6th L74.51 Primary focal hyperhidrosis
               L74.510 Primary focal hyperhidrosis, axilla
               L74.511 Primary focal hyperhidrosis, face
               L74.512 Primary focal hyperhidrosis, palms
               L74.513 Primary focal hyperhidrosis, soles
               L74.519 Primary focal hyperhidrosis, unspecified ▽

         L74.52 Secondary focal hyperhidrosis
            Frey's syndrome

     L74.8 Other eccrine sweat disorders
     L74.9 Eccrine sweat disorder, unspecified ▽
         Sweat gland disorder NOS

✓4th L75 Apocrine sweat disorders
     EXCLUDES 1   dyshidrosis (L30.1)
                 hidradenitis suppurativa (L73.2)

     L75.0 Bromhidrosis
     L75.1 Chromhidrosis
     L75.2 Apocrine miliaria
         Fox-Fordyce disease
         DEF: Chronic, usually pruritic disease evidenced by small follicular
         papular eruptions, especially in the axillary and pubic areas;
         develops from the closure and rupture of the affected apocrine
         glands' intraepidermal portion of the ducts.

     L75.8 Other apocrine sweat disorders
     L75.9 Apocrine sweat disorder, unspecified ▽

Intraoperative and postprocedural complications of skin and subcutaneous tissue (L76)

✓4th L76 Intraoperative and postprocedural complications of skin and subcutaneous tissue
     ✓5th L76.0 Intraoperative hemorrhage and hematoma of skin and subcutaneous tissue complicating a procedure
         EXCLUDES 1   intraoperative hemorrhage and hematoma of skin and
                 subcutaneous tissue due to accidental puncture
                 and laceration during a procedure (L76.1-)

         L76.01 Intraoperative hemorrhage and hematoma of skin and subcutaneous tissue complicating a dermatologic procedure
         L76.02 Intraoperative hemorrhage and hematoma of skin and subcutaneous tissue complicating other procedure

     ✓5th L76.1 Accidental puncture and laceration of skin and subcutaneous tissue during a procedure
         L76.11 Accidental puncture and laceration of skin and subcutaneous tissue during a dermatologic procedure
         L76.12 Accidental puncture and laceration of skin and subcutaneous tissue during other procedure

     ✓5th L76.2 Postprocedural hemorrhage of skin and subcutaneous tissue following a procedure
         L76.21 Postprocedural hemorrhage of skin and subcutaneous tissue following a dermatologic procedure
         L76.22 Postprocedural hemorrhage of skin and subcutaneous tissue following other procedure

     ✓5th L76.3 Postprocedural hematoma and seroma of skin and subcutaneous tissue following a procedure
         L76.31 Postprocedural hematoma of skin and subcutaneous tissue following a dermatologic procedure
         L76.32 Postprocedural hematoma of skin and subcutaneous tissue following other procedure
         L76.33 Postprocedural seroma of skin and subcutaneous tissue following a dermatologic procedure
         L76.34 Postprocedural seroma of skin and subcutaneous tissue following other procedure

     ✓5th L76.8 Other intraoperative and postprocedural complications of skin and subcutaneous tissue
         Use additional code, if applicable, to further specify disorder
         L76.81 Other intraoperative complications of skin and subcutaneous tissue
         L76.82 Other postprocedural complications of skin and subcutaneous tissue

---

✓ Additional Character Req   ✓x7th Placeholder Alert   Manifestation   HCC CMS-HCC Condition   ▽ Unspecified Code   ►◄ Revised Text   ● New Code   ▲ Revised Code Title

Chapter 12. Diseases of the Skin and Subcutaneous Tissue

Other disorders of the skin and subcutaneous tissue (L80-L99)

L80 **Vitiligo**
> *EXCLUDES 2*   vitiligo of eyelids (H02.73-)
>   vitiligo of vulva (N90.89)
> **DEF:** Persistent, progressive development of nonpigmented white patches on otherwise normal skin.

✓4ᵗʰ **L81** **Other disorders of pigmentation**
> *EXCLUDES 1*   birthmark NOS (Q82.5)
>   Peutz-Jeghers syndrome (Q85.8)
> *EXCLUDES 2*   nevus—see Alphabetical Index

L81.0   **Postinflammatory hyperpigmentation**

L81.1   **Chloasma**

L81.2   **Freckles**

L81.3   **Café au lait spots**

L81.4   **Other melanin hyperpigmentation**
> Lentigo

L81.5   **Leukoderma, not elsewhere classified**

L81.6   **Other disorders of diminished melanin formation**

L81.7   **Pigmented purpuric dermatosis**
> Angioma serpiginosum

L81.8   **Other specified disorders of pigmentation**
> Iron pigmentation
> Tattoo pigmentation

L81.9   **Disorder of pigmentation, unspecified**   ▽

✓4ᵗʰ **L82** **Seborrheic keratosis**
> *INCLUDES*   basal cell papilloma
>   dermatosis papulosa nigra
>   Leser-Trélat disease
> *EXCLUDES 2*   seborrheic dermatitis (L21.-)

L82.0   **Inflamed seborrheic keratosis**

L82.1   **Other seborrheic keratosis**
> Seborrheic keratosis NOS

L83 **Acanthosis nigricans**
> Confluent and reticulated papillomatosis
> **DEF:** Diffuse, velvety hyperplasia of the spinous skin layer of the axilla and other body folds marked by gray, brown, or black pigmentation; in adult form often associated with malignant acanthosis nigricans in a benign, nevoid form relatively generalized.

L84 **Corns and callosities**
> Callus
> Clavus

✓4ᵗʰ **L85** **Other epidermal thickening**
> *EXCLUDES 2*   hypertrophic disorders of the skin (L91.-)

L85.0   **Acquired ichthyosis**
> *EXCLUDES 1*   congenital ichthyosis (Q80.-)

L85.1   **Acquired keratosis [keratoderma] palmaris et plantaris**
> *EXCLUDES 1*   inherited keratosis palmaris et plantaris (Q82.8)

L85.2   **Keratosis punctata (palmaris et plantaris)**

L85.3   **Xerosis cutis**
> Dry skin dermatitis

L85.8   **Other specified epidermal thickening**
> Cutaneous horn

L85.9   **Epidermal thickening, unspecified**   ▽

L86 ***Keratoderma in diseases classified elsewhere***
> Code first underlying disease, such as:
>   Reiter's disease (M02.3-)
> *EXCLUDES 1*   gonococcal keratoderma (A54.89)
>   gonococcal keratosis (A54.89)
>   keratoderma due to vitamin A deficiency (E50.8)
>   keratosis due to vitamin A deficiency (E50.8)
>   xeroderma due to vitamin A deficiency (E50.8)

✓4ᵗʰ **L87** **Transepidermal elimination disorders**
> *EXCLUDES 1*   granuloma annulare (perforating) (L92.0)

L87.0   **Keratosis follicularis et parafollicularis in cutem penetrans**
> Hyperkeratosis follicularis penetrans
> Kyrle disease

L87.1   **Reactive perforating collagenosis**

L87.2   **Elastosis perforans serpiginosa**

L87.8   **Other transepidermal elimination disorders**

L87.9   **Transepidermal elimination disorder, unspecified**   ▽

L88 **Pyoderma gangrenosum**
> Phagedenic pyoderma
> *EXCLUDES 1*   dermatitis gangrenosa (L08.0)
> **DEF:** Persistent debilitating skin disease characterized by irregular, boggy, blue-red ulcerations, with central healing and undermined edges.

Four Stages of Pressure Ulcer

Stage 1
Persistent focal erythema

Stage 2
Abrasion, blister, partial thickness skin loss involving epidermis and/or dermis

Stage 3
Full thickness skin loss involving damage or necrosis of subcutaneous tissue

Stage 4
Necrosis of soft tissues through to underlying muscle, tendon, or bone

✓4ᵗʰ **L89** **Pressure ulcer**
> *INCLUDES*   bed sore
>   decubitus ulcer
>   plaster ulcer
>   pressure area
>   pressure sore
> Code first any associated gangrene (I96)
> *EXCLUDES 2*   decubitus (trophic) ulcer of cervix (uteri) (N86)
>   diabetic ulcers (E08.621, E08.622, E09.621, E09.622, E10.621, E10.622, E11.621, E11.622, E13.621, E13.622)
>   non-pressure chronic ulcer of skin (L97.-)
>   skin infections (L00-L08)
>   varicose ulcer (I83.0, I83.2)
> **AHA:** 2017, 1Q, 49; 2016, 4Q, 143

✓5ᵗʰ **L89.0**   **Pressure ulcer of elbow**

✓6ᵗʰ   **L89.00**   **Pressure ulcer of unspecified elbow**

L89.000   **Pressure ulcer of unspecified elbow,** ᴴᶜᶜ ▽ **unstageable**

L89.001   **Pressure ulcer of unspecified elbow,** ▽ **stage 1**
> Healing pressure ulcer of unspecified elbow, stage 1
> Pressure pre-ulcer skin changes limited to persistent focal edema, unspecified elbow

L89.002   **Pressure ulcer of unspecified elbow,** ▽ **stage 2**
> Healing pressure ulcer of unspecified elbow, stage 2
> Pressure ulcer with abrasion, blister, partial thickness skin loss involving epidermis and/or dermis, unspecified elbow

L89.003   **Pressure ulcer of unspecified** ᴴᶜᶜ ▽ **elbow, stage 3**
> Healing pressure ulcer of unspecified elbow, stage 3
> Pressure ulcer with full thickness skin loss involving damage or necrosis of subcutaneous tissue, unspecified elbow

L89.004   **Pressure ulcer of unspecified** ᴴᶜᶜ **elbow, stage 4**
> Healing pressure ulcer of unspecified elbow, stage 4
> Pressure ulcer with necrosis of soft tissues through to underlying muscle, tendon, or bone, unspecified elbow

L89.009   **Pressure ulcer of unspecified elbow,** ▽ **unspecified stage**
> Healing pressure ulcer of elbow NOS
> Healing pressure ulcer of unspecified elbow, unspecified stage

✓6ᵗʰ   **L89.01**   **Pressure ulcer of right elbow**

L89.010   **Pressure ulcer of right elbow,** ᴴᶜᶜ **unstageable**

EXCLUDES 1 Not coded here   *EXCLUDES 2* Not included here   N Newborn Age: 0   P Pediatric Age: 0-17   M Maternity Age: 12-55   A Adult Age: 15-124

702   ICD-10-CM 2018

L89.011 **Pressure ulcer of right elbow, stage 1**
Healing pressure ulcer of right elbow, stage 1
Pressure pre-ulcer skin changes limited to persistent focal edema, right elbow

L89.012 **Pressure ulcer of right elbow, stage 2**
Healing pressure ulcer of right elbow, stage 2
Pressure ulcer with abrasion, blister, partial thickness skin loss involving epidermis and/or dermis, right elbow

L89.013 **Pressure ulcer of right elbow, stage 3** HCC
Healing pressure ulcer of right elbow, stage 3
Pressure ulcer with full thickness skin loss involving damage or necrosis of subcutaneous tissue, right elbow

L89.014 **Pressure ulcer of right elbow, stage 4** HCC
Healing pressure ulcer of right elbow, stage 4
Pressure ulcer with necrosis of soft tissues through to underlying muscle, tendon, or bone, right elbow

L89.019 **Pressure ulcer of right elbow, unspecified stage** ▽
Healing pressure right of elbow NOS
▶Healing pressure ulcer of right elbow, unspecified stage◀

✓6th L89.02 **Pressure ulcer of left elbow**

L89.020 **Pressure ulcer of left elbow, unstageable** HCC

L89.021 **Pressure ulcer of left elbow, stage 1**
Healing pressure ulcer of left elbow, stage 1
Pressure pre-ulcer skin changes limited to persistent focal edema, left elbow

L89.022 **Pressure ulcer of left elbow, stage 2**
Healing pressure ulcer of left elbow, stage 2
Pressure ulcer with abrasion, blister, partial thickness skin loss involving epidermis and/or dermis, left elbow

L89.023 **Pressure ulcer of left elbow, stage 3** HCC
Healing pressure ulcer of left elbow, stage 3
Pressure ulcer with full thickness skin loss involving damage or necrosis of subcutaneous tissue, left elbow

L89.024 **Pressure ulcer of left elbow, stage 4** HCC
Healing pressure ulcer of left elbow, stage 4
Pressure ulcer with necrosis of soft tissues through to underlying muscle, tendon, or bone, left elbow

L89.029 **Pressure ulcer of left elbow, unspecified stage** ▽
Healing pressure ulcer of left of elbow NOS
▶Healing pressure ulcer of left elbow, unspecified stage◀

✓5th L89.1 **Pressure ulcer of back**

✓6th L89.10 **Pressure ulcer of unspecified part of back**

L89.100 **Pressure ulcer of unspecified part of back, unstageable** HCC ▽

L89.101 **Pressure ulcer of unspecified part of back, stage 1** ▽
Healing pressure ulcer of unspecified part of back, stage 1
Pressure pre-ulcer skin changes limited to persistent focal edema, unspecified part of back

L89.102 **Pressure ulcer of unspecified part of back, stage 2** ▽
Healing pressure ulcer of unspecified part of back, stage 2
Pressure ulcer with abrasion, blister, partial thickness skin loss involving epidermis and/or dermis, unspecified part of back

L89.103 **Pressure ulcer of unspecified part of back, stage 3** HCC ▽
Healing pressure ulcer of unspecified part of back, stage 3
Pressure ulcer with full thickness skin loss involving damage or necrosis of subcutaneous tissue, unspecified part of back

L89.104 **Pressure ulcer of unspecified part of back, stage 4** HCC ▽
Healing pressure ulcer of unspecified part of back, stage 4
Pressure ulcer with necrosis of soft tissues through to underlying muscle, tendon, or bone, unspecified part of back

L89.109 **Pressure ulcer of unspecified part of back, unspecified stage** ▽
Healing pressure ulcer of unspecified part of back NOS
Healing pressure ulcer of unspecified part of back, unspecified stage

✓6th L89.11 **Pressure ulcer of right upper back**
Pressure ulcer of right shoulder blade

L89.110 **Pressure ulcer of right upper back, unstageable** HCC

L89.111 **Pressure ulcer of right upper back, stage 1**
Healing pressure ulcer of right upper back, stage 1
Pressure pre-ulcer skin changes limited to persistent focal edema, right upper back

L89.112 **Pressure ulcer of right upper back, stage 2**
Healing pressure ulcer of right upper back, stage 2
Pressure ulcer with abrasion, blister, partial thickness skin loss involving epidermis and/or dermis, right upper back

L89.113 **Pressure ulcer of right upper back, stage 3** HCC
Healing pressure ulcer of right upper back, stage 3
Pressure ulcer with full thickness skin loss involving damage or necrosis of subcutaneous tissue, right upper back

L89.114 **Pressure ulcer of right upper back, stage 4** HCC
Healing pressure ulcer of right upper back, stage 4
Pressure ulcer with necrosis of soft tissues through to underlying muscle, tendon, or bone, right upper back

L89.119 **Pressure ulcer of right upper back, unspecified stage** ▽
Healing pressure ulcer of right upper back NOS
Healing pressure ulcer of right upper back, unspecified stage

✓6th L89.12 **Pressure ulcer of left upper back**
Pressure ulcer of left shoulder blade

L89.120 **Pressure ulcer of left upper back, unstageable** HCC

L89.121 **Pressure ulcer of left upper back, stage 1**
Healing pressure ulcer of left upper back, stage 1
Pressure pre-ulcer skin changes limited to persistent focal edema, left upper back

L89.122 **Pressure ulcer of left upper back, stage 2**
Healing pressure ulcer of left upper back, stage 2
Pressure ulcer with abrasion, blister, partial thickness skin loss involving epidermis and/or dermis, left upper back

L89.123 **Pressure ulcer of left upper back, stage 3** HCC
Healing pressure ulcer of left upper back, stage 3
Pressure ulcer with full thickness skin loss involving damage or necrosis of subcutaneous tissue, left upper back

L89.124 **Pressure ulcer of left upper back, stage 4** HCC
Healing pressure ulcer of left upper back, stage 4
Pressure ulcer with necrosis of soft tissues through to underlying muscle, tendon, or bone, left upper back

---

☑ Additional Character Req   ✓x7th Placeholder Alert   Manifestation   HCC CMS-HCC Condition   ▽ Unspecified Code   ▶◀ Revised Text   ● New Code   ▲ Revised Code Title

Chapter 12. Diseases of the Skin and Subcutaneous Tissue

L89.129–L89.213

        L89.129   **Pressure ulcer of left upper back,**   ▽
              unspecified stage
                 Healing pressure ulcer of left upper back
                    NOS
                 Healing pressure ulcer of left upper back,
                    unspecified stage

    ✓6ᵗʰ   **L89.13**   **Pressure ulcer of right lower back**

        L89.130   **Pressure ulcer of right lower back,**   HCC
              unstageable

        L89.131   **Pressure ulcer of right lower back, stage 1**
                 Healing pressure ulcer of right lower back,
                    stage 1
                 Pressure pre-ulcer skin changes limited to
                    persistent focal edema, right lower
                    back

        L89.132   **Pressure ulcer of right lower back, stage 2**
                 Healing pressure ulcer of right lower back,
                    stage 2
                 Pressure ulcer with abrasion, blister, partial
                    thickness skin loss involving epidermis
                    and/or dermis, right lower back

        L89.133   **Pressure ulcer of right lower back,**   HCC
              stage 3
                 Healing pressure ulcer of right lower back,
                    stage 3
                 Pressure ulcer with full thickness skin loss
                    involving damage or necrosis of
                    subcutaneous tissue, right lower back

        L89.134   **Pressure ulcer of right lower back,**   HCC
              stage 4
                 Healing pressure ulcer of right lower back,
                    stage 4
                 Pressure ulcer with necrosis of soft tissues
                    through to underlying muscle,
                    tendon, or bone, right lower back

        L89.139   **Pressure ulcer of right lower back,**   ▽
              unspecified stage
                 Healing pressure ulcer of right lower back
                    NOS
                 Healing pressure ulcer of right lower back,
                    unspecified stage

    ✓6ᵗʰ   **L89.14**   **Pressure ulcer of left lower back**

        L89.140   **Pressure ulcer of left lower back,**   HCC
              unstageable

        L89.141   **Pressure ulcer of left lower back, stage 1**
                 Healing pressure ulcer of left lower back,
                    stage 1
                 Pressure pre-ulcer skin changes limited to
                    persistent focal edema, left lower back

        L89.142   **Pressure ulcer of left lower back, stage 2**
                 Healing pressure ulcer of left lower back,
                    stage 2
                 Pressure ulcer with abrasion, blister, partial
                    thickness skin loss involving epidermis
                    and/or dermis, left lower back

        L89.143   **Pressure ulcer of left lower back,**   HCC
              stage 3
                 Healing pressure ulcer of left lower back,
                    stage 3
                 Pressure ulcer with full thickness skin loss
                    involving damage or necrosis of
                    subcutaneous tissue, left lower back

        L89.144   **Pressure ulcer of left lower back,**   HCC
              stage 4
                 Healing pressure ulcer of left lower back,
                    stage 4
                 Pressure ulcer with necrosis of soft tissues
                    through to underlying muscle,
                    tendon, or bone, left lower back

        L89.149   **Pressure ulcer of left lower back,**   ▽
              unspecified stage
                 Healing pressure ulcer of left lower back
                    NOS
                 Healing pressure ulcer of left lower back,
                    unspecified stage

    ✓6ᵗʰ   **L89.15**   **Pressure ulcer of sacral region**
                 Pressure ulcer of coccyx
                 Pressure ulcer of tailbone

        L89.150   **Pressure ulcer of sacral region,**   HCC
              unstageable

        L89.151   **Pressure ulcer of sacral region, stage 1**
                 Healing pressure ulcer of sacral region,
                    stage 1
                 Pressure pre-ulcer skin changes limited to
                    persistent focal edema, sacral region

        L89.152   **Pressure ulcer of sacral region, stage 2**
                 Healing pressure ulcer of sacral region,
                    stage 2
                 Pressure ulcer with abrasion, blister, partial
                    thickness skin loss involving epidermis
                    and/or dermis, sacral region

        L89.153   **Pressure ulcer of sacral region, stage 3**   HCC
                 Healing pressure ulcer of sacral region,
                    stage 3
                 Pressure ulcer with full thickness skin loss
                    involving damage or necrosis of
                    subcutaneous tissue, sacral region

        L89.154   **Pressure ulcer of sacral region, stage 4**   HCC
                 Healing pressure ulcer of sacral region,
                    stage 4
                 Pressure ulcer with necrosis of soft tissues
                    through to underlying muscle,
                    tendon, or bone, sacral region

        L89.159   **Pressure ulcer of sacral region,**   ▽
              unspecified stage
                 Healing pressure ulcer of sacral region NOS
                 Healing pressure ulcer of sacral region,
                    unspecified stage

  ✓5ᵗʰ   **L89.2**   **Pressure ulcer of hip**

    ✓6ᵗʰ   **L89.20**   **Pressure ulcer of unspecified hip**

        L89.200   **Pressure ulcer of unspecified hip,**   HCC ▽
              unstageable

        L89.201   **Pressure ulcer of unspecified hip,**   ▽
              stage 1
                 Healing pressure ulcer of unspecified hip,
                    stage 1
                 Pressure pre-ulcer skin changes limited to
                    persistent focal edema, unspecified
                    hip

        L89.202   **Pressure ulcer of unspecified hip,**   ▽
              stage 2
                 Healing pressure ulcer of unspecified hip,
                    stage 2
                 Pressure ulcer with abrasion, blister, partial
                    thickness skin loss involving epidermis
                    and/or dermis, unspecified hip

        L89.203   **Pressure ulcer of unspecified hip,**   HCC ▽
              stage 3
                 Healing pressure ulcer of unspecified hip,
                    stage 3
                 Pressure ulcer with full thickness skin loss
                    involving damage or necrosis of
                    subcutaneous tissue, unspecified hip

        L89.204   **Pressure ulcer of unspecified hip,**   HCC ▽
              stage 4
                 Healing pressure ulcer of unspecified hip,
                    stage 4
                 Pressure ulcer with necrosis of soft tissues
                    through to underlying muscle,
                    tendon, or bone, unspecified hip

        L89.209   **Pressure ulcer of unspecified hip,**   ▽
              unspecified stage
                 Healing pressure ulcer of unspecified hip
                    NOS
                 Healing pressure ulcer of unspecified hip,
                    unspecified stage

    ✓6ᵗʰ   **L89.21**   **Pressure ulcer of right hip**

        L89.210   **Pressure ulcer of right hip,**   HCC
              unstageable

        L89.211   **Pressure ulcer of right hip, stage 1**
                 Healing pressure ulcer of right hip, stage 1
                 Pressure pre-ulcer skin changes limited to
                    persistent focal edema, right hip

        L89.212   **Pressure ulcer of right hip, stage 2**
                 Healing pressure ulcer of right hip, stage 2
                 Pressure ulcer with abrasion, blister, partial
                    thickness skin loss involving epidermis
                    and/or dermis, right hip

        L89.213   **Pressure ulcer of right hip, stage 3**   HCC
                 Healing pressure ulcer of right hip, stage 3
                 Pressure ulcer with full thickness skin loss
                    involving damage or necrosis of
                    subcutaneous tissue, right hip

EXCLUDES 1 Not coded here   EXCLUDES 2 Not included here   N Newborn Age: 0   P Pediatric Age: 0-17   M Maternity Age: 12-55   A Adult Age: 15-124

704   ICD-10-CM 2018

L89.214 Pressure ulcer of right hip, stage 4 HCC
  Healing pressure ulcer of right hip, stage 4
  Pressure ulcer with necrosis of soft tissues through to underlying muscle, tendon, or bone, right hip

L89.219 Pressure ulcer of right hip, unspecified stage ▽
  Healing pressure ulcer of right hip NOS
  Healing pressure ulcer of right hip, unspecified stage

✓6th **L89.22 Pressure ulcer of left hip**

L89.220 Pressure ulcer of left hip, unstageable HCC

L89.221 Pressure ulcer of left hip, stage 1
  Healing pressure ulcer of left hip, stage 1
  Pressure pre-ulcer skin changes limited to persistent focal edema, left hip

L89.222 Pressure ulcer of left hip, stage 2
  Healing pressure ulcer of left hip, stage 2
  Pressure ulcer with abrasion, blister, partial thickness skin loss involving epidermis and/or dermis, left hip

L89.223 Pressure ulcer of left hip, stage 3 HCC
  Healing pressure ulcer of left hip, stage 3
  Pressure ulcer with full thickness skin loss involving damage or necrosis of subcutaneous tissue, left hip

L89.224 Pressure ulcer of left hip, stage 4 HCC
  Healing pressure ulcer of left hip, stage 4
  Pressure ulcer with necrosis of soft tissues through to underlying muscle, tendon, or bone, left hip

L89.229 Pressure ulcer of left hip, unspecified stage ▽
  Healing pressure ulcer of left hip NOS
  Healing pressure ulcer of left hip, unspecified stage

✓5th **L89.3 Pressure ulcer of buttock**

✓6th **L89.30 Pressure ulcer of unspecified buttock**

L89.300 Pressure ulcer of unspecified buttock, unstageable HCC ▽

L89.301 Pressure ulcer of unspecified buttock, stage 1 ▽
  Healing pressure ulcer of unspecified buttock, stage 1
  Pressure pre-ulcer skin changes limited to persistent focal edema, unspecified buttock

L89.302 Pressure ulcer of unspecified buttock, stage 2 ▽
  Healing pressure ulcer of unspecified buttock, stage 2
  Pressure ulcer with abrasion, blister, partial thickness skin loss involving epidermis and/or dermis, unspecified buttock

L89.303 Pressure ulcer of unspecified buttock, stage 3 HCC ▽
  Healing pressure ulcer of unspecified buttock, stage 3
  Pressure ulcer with full thickness skin loss involving damage or necrosis of subcutaneous tissue, unspecified buttock

L89.304 Pressure ulcer of unspecified buttock, stage 4 HCC ▽
  Healing pressure ulcer of unspecified buttock, stage 4
  Pressure ulcer with necrosis of soft tissues through to underlying muscle, tendon, or bone, unspecified buttock

L89.309 Pressure ulcer of unspecified buttock, unspecified stage ▽
  Healing pressure ulcer of unspecified buttock NOS
  Healing pressure ulcer of unspecified buttock, unspecified stage

✓6th **L89.31 Pressure ulcer of right buttock**

L89.310 Pressure ulcer of right buttock, unstageable HCC

L89.311 Pressure ulcer of right buttock, stage 1
  Healing pressure ulcer of right buttock, stage 1
  Pressure pre-ulcer skin changes limited to persistent focal edema, right buttock

L89.312 Pressure ulcer of right buttock, stage 2
  Healing pressure ulcer of right buttock, stage 2
  Pressure ulcer with abrasion, blister, partial thickness skin loss involving epidermis and/or dermis, right buttock

L89.313 Pressure ulcer of right buttock, stage 3 HCC
  Healing pressure ulcer of right buttock, stage 3
  Pressure ulcer with full thickness skin loss involving damage or necrosis of subcutaneous tissue, right buttock

L89.314 Pressure ulcer of right buttock, stage 4 HCC
  Healing pressure ulcer of right buttock, stage 4
  Pressure ulcer with necrosis of soft tissues through to underlying muscle, tendon, or bone, right buttock

L89.319 Pressure ulcer of right buttock, unspecified stage ▽
  Healing pressure ulcer of right buttock NOS
  Healing pressure ulcer of right buttock, unspecified stage

✓6th **L89.32 Pressure ulcer of left buttock**

L89.320 Pressure ulcer of left buttock, unstageable HCC

L89.321 Pressure ulcer of left buttock, stage 1
  Healing pressure ulcer of left buttock, stage 1
  Pressure pre-ulcer skin changes limited to persistent focal edema, left buttock

L89.322 Pressure ulcer of left buttock, stage 2
  Healing pressure ulcer of left buttock, stage 2
  Pressure ulcer with abrasion, blister, partial thickness skin loss involving epidermis and/or dermis, left buttock

L89.323 Pressure ulcer of left buttock, stage 3 HCC
  Healing pressure ulcer of left buttock, stage 3
  Pressure ulcer with full thickness skin loss involving damage or necrosis of subcutaneous tissue, left buttock

L89.324 Pressure ulcer of left buttock, stage 4 HCC
  Healing pressure ulcer of left buttock, stage 4
  Pressure ulcer with necrosis of soft tissues through to underlying muscle, tendon, or bone, left buttock

L89.329 Pressure ulcer of left buttock, unspecified stage ▽
  Healing pressure ulcer of left buttock NOS
  Healing pressure ulcer of left buttock, unspecified stage

✓5th **L89.4 Pressure ulcer of contiguous site of back, buttock and hip**

L89.40 Pressure ulcer of contiguous site of back, buttock and hip, unspecified stage ▽
  Healing pressure ulcer of contiguous site of back, buttock and hip NOS
  Healing pressure ulcer of contiguous site of back, buttock and hip, unspecified stage

L89.41 Pressure ulcer of contiguous site of back, buttock and hip, stage 1
  Healing pressure ulcer of contiguous site of back, buttock and hip, stage 1
  Pressure pre-ulcer skin changes limited to persistent focal edema, contiguous site of back, buttock and hip

L89.42 Pressure ulcer of contiguous site of back, buttock and hip, stage 2
  Healing pressure ulcer of contiguous site of back, buttock and hip, stage 2
  Pressure ulcer with abrasion, blister, partial thickness skin loss involving epidermis and/or dermis, contiguous site of back, buttock and hip

---

☑ Additional Character Req   ✓x7th Placeholder Alert   Manifestation   HCC CMS-HCC Condition   ▽ Unspecified Code   ▶◀ Revised Text   ● New Code   ▲ Revised Code Title

ICD-10-CM 2018   705

L89.43 Pressure ulcer of contiguous site of back, buttock and hip, stage 3 `HCC`
Healing pressure ulcer of contiguous site of back, buttock and hip, stage 3
Pressure ulcer with full thickness skin loss involving damage or necrosis of subcutaneous tissue, contiguous site of back, buttock and hip

L89.44 Pressure ulcer of contiguous site of back, buttock and hip, stage 4 `HCC`
Healing pressure ulcer of contiguous site of back, buttock and hip, stage 4
Pressure ulcer with necrosis of soft tissues through to underlying muscle, tendon, or bone, contiguous site of back, buttock and hip

L89.45 Pressure ulcer of contiguous site of back, buttock and hip, unstageable `HCC`

√5ᵗʰ **L89.5 Pressure ulcer of ankle**

√6ᵗʰ **L89.50 Pressure ulcer of unspecified ankle**

L89.500 Pressure ulcer of unspecified ankle, unstageable `HCC` ▽

L89.501 Pressure ulcer of unspecified ankle, stage 1 ▽
Healing pressure ulcer of unspecified ankle, stage 1
Pressure pre-ulcer skin changes limited to persistent focal edema, unspecified ankle

L89.502 Pressure ulcer of unspecified ankle, stage 2 ▽
Healing pressure ulcer of unspecified ankle, stage 2
Pressure ulcer with abrasion, blister, partial thickness skin loss involving epidermis and/or dermis, unspecified ankle

L89.503 Pressure ulcer of unspecified ankle, stage 3 `HCC` ▽
Healing pressure ulcer of unspecified ankle, stage 3
Pressure ulcer with full thickness skin loss involving damage or necrosis of subcutaneous tissue, unspecified ankle

L89.504 Pressure ulcer of unspecified ankle, stage 4 `HCC` ▽
Healing pressure ulcer of unspecified ankle, stage 4
Pressure ulcer with necrosis of soft tissues through to underlying muscle, tendon, or bone, unspecified ankle

L89.509 Pressure ulcer of unspecified ankle, unspecified stage ▽
Healing pressure ulcer of unspecified ankle NOS
Healing pressure ulcer of unspecified ankle, unspecified stage

√6ᵗʰ **L89.51 Pressure ulcer of right ankle**

L89.510 Pressure ulcer of right ankle, unstageable `HCC`

L89.511 Pressure ulcer of right ankle, stage 1
Healing pressure ulcer of right ankle, stage 1
Pressure pre-ulcer skin changes limited to persistent focal edema, right ankle

L89.512 Pressure ulcer of right ankle, stage 2
Healing pressure ulcer of right ankle, stage 2
Pressure ulcer with abrasion, blister, partial thickness skin loss involving epidermis and/or dermis, right ankle

L89.513 Pressure ulcer of right ankle, stage 3 `HCC`
Healing pressure ulcer of right ankle, stage 3
Pressure ulcer with full thickness skin loss involving damage or necrosis of subcutaneous tissue, right ankle

L89.514 Pressure ulcer of right ankle, stage 4 `HCC`
Healing pressure ulcer of right ankle, stage 4
Pressure ulcer with necrosis of soft tissues through to underlying muscle, tendon, or bone, right ankle

L89.519 Pressure ulcer of right ankle, unspecified stage ▽
Healing pressure ulcer of right ankle NOS
Healing pressure ulcer of right ankle, unspecified stage

√6ᵗʰ **L89.52 Pressure ulcer of left ankle**

L89.520 Pressure ulcer of left ankle, unstageable `HCC`

L89.521 Pressure ulcer of left ankle, stage 1
Healing pressure ulcer of left ankle, stage 1
Pressure pre-ulcer skin changes limited to persistent focal edema, left ankle

L89.522 Pressure ulcer of left ankle, stage 2
Healing pressure ulcer of left ankle, stage 2
Pressure ulcer with abrasion, blister, partial thickness skin loss involving epidermis and/or dermis, left ankle

L89.523 Pressure ulcer of left ankle, stage 3 `HCC`
Healing pressure ulcer of left ankle, stage 3
Pressure ulcer with full thickness skin loss involving damage or necrosis of subcutaneous tissue, left ankle

L89.524 Pressure ulcer of left ankle, stage 4 `HCC`
Healing pressure ulcer of left ankle, stage 4
Pressure ulcer with necrosis of soft tissues through to underlying muscle, tendon, or bone, left ankle

L89.529 Pressure ulcer of left ankle, unspecified stage ▽
Healing pressure ulcer of left ankle NOS
Healing pressure ulcer of left ankle, unspecified stage

√5ᵗʰ **L89.6 Pressure ulcer of heel**

√6ᵗʰ **L89.60 Pressure ulcer of unspecified heel**

L89.600 Pressure ulcer of unspecified heel, unstageable `HCC` ▽

L89.601 Pressure ulcer of unspecified heel, stage 1 ▽
Healing pressure ulcer of unspecified heel, stage 1
Pressure pre-ulcer skin changes limited to persistent focal edema, unspecified heel

L89.602 Pressure ulcer of unspecified heel, stage 2 ▽
Healing pressure ulcer of unspecified heel, stage 2
Pressure ulcer with abrasion, blister, partial thickness skin loss involving epidermis and/or dermis, unspecified heel

L89.603 Pressure ulcer of unspecified heel, stage 3 `HCC` ▽
Healing pressure ulcer of unspecified heel, stage 3
Pressure ulcer with full thickness skin loss involving damage or necrosis of subcutaneous tissue, unspecified heel

L89.604 Pressure ulcer of unspecified heel, stage 4 `HCC` ▽
Healing pressure ulcer of unspecified heel, stage 4
Pressure ulcer with necrosis of soft tissues through to underlying muscle, tendon, or bone, unspecified heel

L89.609 Pressure ulcer of unspecified heel, unspecified stage ▽
Healing pressure ulcer of unspecified heel NOS
Healing pressure ulcer of unspecified heel, unspecified stage

√6ᵗʰ **L89.61 Pressure ulcer of right heel**

L89.610 Pressure ulcer of right heel, unstageable `HCC`

L89.611 Pressure ulcer of right heel, stage 1
Healing pressure ulcer of right heel, stage 1
Pressure pre-ulcer skin changes limited to persistent focal edema, right heel

EXCLUDES 1 Not coded here **EXCLUDES 2** Not included here N Newborn Age: 0 P Pediatric Age: 0-17 M Maternity Age: 12-55 A Adult Age: 15-124

706 ICD-10-CM 2018

L89.612 **Pressure ulcer of right heel, stage 2**
Healing pressure ulcer of right heel, stage 2
Pressure ulcer with abrasion, blister, partial thickness skin loss involving epidermis and/or dermis, right heel

L89.613 **Pressure ulcer of right heel, stage 3** HCC
Healing pressure ulcer of right heel, stage 3
Pressure ulcer with full thickness skin loss involving damage or necrosis of subcutaneous tissue, right heel

L89.614 **Pressure ulcer of right heel, stage 4** HCC
Healing pressure ulcer of right heel, stage 4
Pressure ulcer with necrosis of soft tissues through to underlying muscle, tendon, or bone, right heel

L89.619 **Pressure ulcer of right heel, unspecified stage** ▽
Healing pressure ulcer of right heel NOS
▶Healing pressure ulcer of right heel, unspecified stage◀

✓6th **L89.62 Pressure ulcer of left heel**

L89.620 **Pressure ulcer of left heel, unstageable** HCC

L89.621 **Pressure ulcer of left heel, stage 1**
Healing pressure ulcer of left heel, stage 1
Pressure pre-ulcer skin changes limited to persistent focal edema, left heel

L89.622 **Pressure ulcer of left heel, stage 2**
Healing pressure ulcer of left heel, stage 2
Pressure ulcer with abrasion, blister, partial thickness skin loss involving epidermis and/or dermis, left heel

L89.623 **Pressure ulcer of left heel, stage 3** HCC
Healing pressure ulcer of left heel, stage 3
Pressure ulcer with full thickness skin loss involving damage or necrosis of subcutaneous tissue, left heel

L89.624 **Pressure ulcer of left heel, stage 4** HCC
Healing pressure ulcer of left heel, stage 4
Pressure ulcer with necrosis of soft tissues through to underlying muscle, tendon, or bone, left heel

L89.629 **Pressure ulcer of left heel, unspecified stage** ▽
Healing pressure ulcer of left heel NOS
Healing pressure ulcer of left heel, unspecified stage

✓5th **L89.8 Pressure ulcer of other site**

✓6th **L89.81 Pressure ulcer of head**
Pressure ulcer of face

L89.810 **Pressure ulcer of head, unstageable** HCC

L89.811 **Pressure ulcer of head, stage 1**
Healing pressure ulcer of head, stage 1
Pressure pre-ulcer skin changes limited to persistent focal edema, head

L89.812 **Pressure ulcer of head, stage 2**
Healing pressure ulcer of head, stage 2
Pressure ulcer with abrasion, blister, partial thickness skin loss involving epidermis and/or dermis, head

L89.813 **Pressure ulcer of head, stage 3** HCC
Healing pressure ulcer of head, stage 3
Pressure ulcer with full thickness skin loss involving damage or necrosis of subcutaneous tissue, head

L89.814 **Pressure ulcer of head, stage 4** HCC
Healing pressure ulcer of head, stage 4
Pressure ulcer with necrosis of soft tissues through to underlying muscle, tendon, or bone, head

L89.819 **Pressure ulcer of head, unspecified stage** ▽
Healing pressure ulcer of head NOS
Healing pressure ulcer of head, unspecified stage

✓6th **L89.89 Pressure ulcer of other site**

L89.890 **Pressure ulcer of other site, unstageable** HCC

L89.891 **Pressure ulcer of other site, stage 1**
Healing pressure ulcer of other site, stage 1
Pressure pre-ulcer skin changes limited to persistent focal edema, other site

L89.892 **Pressure ulcer of other site, stage 2**
Healing pressure ulcer of other site, stage 2
Pressure ulcer with abrasion, blister, partial thickness skin loss involving epidermis and/or dermis, other site

L89.893 **Pressure ulcer of other site, stage 3** HCC
Healing pressure ulcer of other site, stage 3
Pressure ulcer with full thickness skin loss involving damage or necrosis of subcutaneous tissue, other site

L89.894 **Pressure ulcer of other site, stage 4** HCC
Healing pressure ulcer of other site, stage 4
Pressure ulcer with necrosis of soft tissues through to underlying muscle, tendon, or bone, other site

L89.899 **Pressure ulcer of other site, unspecified stage** ▽
Healing pressure ulcer of other site NOS
Healing pressure ulcer of other site, unspecified stage

✓5th **L89.9 Pressure ulcer of unspecified site**

L89.90 **Pressure ulcer of unspecified site, unspecified stage** ▽
Healing pressure ulcer of unspecified site NOS
Healing pressure ulcer of unspecified site, unspecified stage

L89.91 **Pressure ulcer of unspecified site, stage 1** ▽
Healing pressure ulcer of unspecified site, stage 1
Pressure pre-ulcer skin changes limited to persistent focal edema, unspecified site

L89.92 **Pressure ulcer of unspecified site, stage 2** ▽
Healing pressure ulcer of unspecified site, stage 2
Pressure ulcer with abrasion, blister, partial thickness skin loss involving epidermis and/or dermis, unspecified site

L89.93 **Pressure ulcer of unspecified site, stage 3** HCC ▽
Healing pressure ulcer of unspecified site, stage 3
Pressure ulcer with full thickness skin loss involving damage or necrosis of subcutaneous tissue, unspecified site

L89.94 **Pressure ulcer of unspecified site, stage 4** HCC ▽
Healing pressure ulcer of unspecified site, stage 4
Pressure ulcer with necrosis of soft tissues through to underlying muscle, tendon, or bone, unspecified site

L89.95 **Pressure ulcer of unspecified site, unstageable** HCC ▽

✓4th **L90 Atrophic disorders of skin**

L90.0 **Lichen sclerosus et atrophicus**
EXCLUDES 2 *lichen sclerosus of external female genital organs (N90.4)*
lichen sclerosus of external male genital organs (N48.0)

L90.1 **Anetoderma of Schweninger-Buzzi**

L90.2 **Anetoderma of Jadassohn-Pellizzari**

L90.3 **Atrophoderma of Pasini and Pierini**

L90.4 **Acrodermatitis chronica atrophicans**

L90.5 **Scar conditions and fibrosis of skin**
Adherent scar (skin)
Cicatrix
Disfigurement of skin due to scar
Fibrosis of skin NOS
Scar NOS
EXCLUDES 2 *hypertrophic scar (L91.0)*
keloid scar (L91.0)
AHA: 2016, 2Q, 5; 2015, 1Q, 19

L90.6 **Striae atrophicae**

L90.8 **Other atrophic disorders of skin**

L90.9 **Atrophic disorder of skin, unspecified** ▽

✓ Additional Character Req   ✓x7th Placeholder Alert   Manifestation   HCC CMS-HCC Condition   ▽ Unspecified Code   ▶◀ Revised Text   ● New Code   ▲ Revised Code Title

ICD-10-CM 2018   707

✓4th **L91   Hypertrophic disorders of skin**

L91.0   **Hypertrophic scar**
Keloid
Keloid scar
EXCLUDES 2   *acne keloid (L73.0)*
scar NOS (L90.5)
DEF: Overgrowth of scar tissue due to excess amounts of collagen during connective tissue repair; occurs mainly on upper trunk, face.

L91.8   **Other hypertrophic disorders of the skin**

L91.9   **Hypertrophic disorder of the skin, unspecified**   ▽

✓4th **L92   Granulomatous disorders of skin and subcutaneous tissue**
EXCLUDES 2   *actinic granuloma (L57.5)*

L92.0   **Granuloma annulare**
Perforating granuloma annulare

L92.1   **Necrobiosis lipoidica, not elsewhere classified**
EXCLUDES 1   *necrobiosis lipoidica associated with diabetes mellitus (E08-E13 with .620)*

L92.2   **Granuloma faciale [eosinophilic granuloma of skin]**

L92.3   **Foreign body granuloma of the skin and subcutaneous tissue**
Use additional code to identify the type of retained foreign body (Z18.-)

L92.8   **Other granulomatous disorders of the skin and subcutaneous tissue**

L92.9   **Granulomatous disorder of the skin and subcutaneous**   ▽
tissue, unspecified
EXCLUDES 2   ▶*umbilical granuloma (P83.81)*◀

✓4th **L93   Lupus erythematosus**
Use additional code for adverse effect, if applicable, to identify drug (T36-T50 with fifth or sixth character 5)
EXCLUDES 1   *lupus exedens (A18.4)*
lupus vulgaris (A18.4)
scleroderma (M34.-)
systemic lupus erythematosus (M32.-)

L93.0   **Discoid lupus erythematosus**
Lupus erythematosus NOS

L93.1   **Subacute cutaneous lupus erythematosus**

L93.2   **Other local lupus erythematosus**
Lupus erythematosus profundus
Lupus panniculitis

✓4th **L94   Other localized connective tissue disorders**
EXCLUDES 1   *systemic connective tissue disorders (M30-M36)*

L94.0   **Localized scleroderma [morphea]**
Circumscribed scleroderma

L94.1   **Linear scleroderma**
En coup de sabre lesion

L94.2   **Calcinosis cutis**

L94.3   **Sclerodactyly**

L94.4   **Gottron's papules**

L94.5   **Poikiloderma vasculare atrophicans**

L94.6   **Ainhum**

L94.8   **Other specified localized connective tissue disorders**

L94.9   **Localized connective tissue disorder, unspecified**   ▽

✓4th **L95   Vasculitis limited to skin, not elsewhere classified**
EXCLUDES 1   *angioma serpiginosum (L81.7)*
Henoch(-Schönlein) purpura (D69.0)
hypersensitivity angiitis (M31.0)
lupus panniculitis (L93.2)
panniculitis NOS (M79.3)
panniculitis of neck and back (M54.0-)
polyarteritis nodosa (M30.0)
relapsing panniculitis (M35.6)
rheumatoid vasculitis (M05.2)
serum sickness (T80.6-)
urticaria (L50.-)
Wegener's granulomatosis (M31.3-)

L95.0   **Livedoid vasculitis**
Atrophie blanche (en plaque)

L95.1   **Erythema elevatum diutinum**

L95.8   **Other vasculitis limited to the skin**

L95.9   **Vasculitis limited to the skin, unspecified**   ▽

✓4th **L97   Non-pressure chronic ulcer of lower limb, not elsewhere classified**
INCLUDES   chronic ulcer of skin of lower limb NOS
non-healing ulcer of skin
non-infected sinus of skin
trophic ulcer NOS
tropical ulcer NOS
ulcer of skin of lower limb NOS
Code first any associated underlying condition, such as:
any associated gangrene (I96)
atherosclerosis of the lower extremities (I70.23-, I70.24-, I70.33-, I70.34-, I70.43-, I70.44-, I70.53-, I70.54-, I70.63-, I70.64-, I70.73-, I70.74-)
chronic venous hypertension (I87.31-, I87.33-)
diabetic ulcers (E08.621, E08.622, E09.621, E09.622, E10.621, E10.622, E11.621, E11.622, E13.621, E13.622)
postphlebitic syndrome (I87.01-, I87.03-)
postthrombotic syndrome (I87.01-, I87.03-)
varicose ulcer (I83.0-, I83.2-)
EXCLUDES 2   *pressure ulcer (pressure area) (L89.-)*
skin infections (L00-L08)
specific infections classified to A00-B99

✓5th **L97.1   Non-pressure chronic ulcer of thigh**

✓6th **L97.10   Non-pressure chronic ulcer of unspecified thigh**

L97.101   **Non-pressure chronic ulcer of**   HCC ▽
unspecified thigh limited to breakdown of skin

L97.102   **Non-pressure chronic ulcer of**   HCC ▽
unspecified thigh with fat layer exposed

L97.103   **Non-pressure chronic ulcer of**   HCC ▽
unspecified thigh with necrosis of muscle

L97.104   **Non-pressure chronic ulcer of**   HCC ▽
unspecified thigh with necrosis of bone

● L97.105   **Non-pressure chronic ulcer of**   ▽
unspecified thigh with muscle involvement without evidence of necrosis

● L97.106   **Non-pressure chronic ulcer of**   ▽
unspecified thigh with bone involvement without evidence of necrosis

● L97.108   **Non-pressure chronic ulcer of**   ▽
unspecified thigh with other specified severity

L97.109   **Non-pressure chronic ulcer of**   HCC ▽
unspecified thigh with unspecified severity

✓6th **L97.11   Non-pressure chronic ulcer of right thigh**

L97.111   **Non-pressure chronic ulcer of right**   HCC
thigh limited to breakdown of skin

L97.112   **Non-pressure chronic ulcer of right**   HCC
thigh with fat layer exposed

L97.113   **Non-pressure chronic ulcer of right**   HCC
high with necrosis of muscle

L97.114   **Non-pressure chronic ulcer of right**   HCC
thigh with necrosis of bone

● L97.115   **Non-pressure chronic ulcer of right thigh with muscle involvement without evidence of necrosis**

● L97.116   **Non-pressure chronic ulcer of right thigh with bone involvement without evidence of necrosis**

● L97.118   **Non-pressure chronic ulcer of right thigh with other specified severity**

L97.119   **Non-pressure chronic ulcer of right**   HCC ▽
thigh with unspecified severity

✓6th **L97.12   Non-pressure chronic ulcer of left thigh**

L97.121   **Non-pressure chronic ulcer of left**   HCC
thigh limited to breakdown of skin

L97.122   **Non-pressure chronic ulcer of left**   HCC
thigh with fat layer exposed

L97.123   **Non-pressure chronic ulcer of left**   HCC
thigh with necrosis of muscle

L97.124   **Non-pressure chronic ulcer of left**   HCC
thigh with necrosis of bone

● L97.125   **Non-pressure chronic ulcer of left thigh with muscle involvement without evidence of necrosis**

L97.126 Non-pressure chronic ulcer of left thigh with bone involvement without evidence of necrosis

● **L97.128** Non-pressure chronic ulcer of left thigh with other specified severity

L97.129 Non-pressure chronic ulcer of left thigh with unspecified severity 〔HCC〕▽

✓5ᵗʰ **L97.2** Non-pressure chronic ulcer of calf

✓6ᵗʰ **L97.20** Non-pressure chronic ulcer of unspecified calf

L97.201 Non-pressure chronic ulcer of unspecified calf limited to breakdown of skin 〔HCC〕▽

L97.202 Non-pressure chronic ulcer of unspecified calf with fat layer exposed 〔HCC〕▽

L97.203 Non-pressure chronic ulcer of unspecified calf with necrosis of muscle 〔HCC〕▽

L97.204 Non-pressure chronic ulcer of unspecified calf with necrosis of bone 〔HCC〕▽

● **L97.205** Non-pressure chronic ulcer of unspecified calf with muscle involvement without evidence of necrosis ▽

● **L97.206** Non-pressure chronic ulcer of unspecified calf with bone involvement without evidence of necrosis ▽

● **L97.208** Non-pressure chronic ulcer of unspecified calf with other specified severity ▽

L97.209 Non-pressure chronic ulcer of unspecified calf with unspecified severity 〔HCC〕▽

✓6ᵗʰ **L97.21** Non-pressure chronic ulcer of right calf

L97.211 Non-pressure chronic ulcer of right calf limited to breakdown of skin 〔HCC〕

L97.212 Non-pressure chronic ulcer of right calf with fat layer exposed 〔HCC〕

L97.213 Non-pressure chronic ulcer of right calf with necrosis of muscle 〔HCC〕

L97.214 Non-pressure chronic ulcer of right calf with necrosis of bone 〔HCC〕

● **L97.215** Non-pressure chronic ulcer of right calf with muscle involvement without evidence of necrosis

● **L97.216** Non-pressure chronic ulcer of right calf with bone involvement without evidence of necrosis

● **L97.218** Non-pressure chronic ulcer of right calf with other specified severity

L97.219 Non-pressure chronic ulcer of right calf with unspecified severity 〔HCC〕▽

✓6ᵗʰ **L97.22** Non-pressure chronic ulcer of left calf

L97.221 Non-pressure chronic ulcer of left calf limited to breakdown of skin 〔HCC〕

L97.222 Non-pressure chronic ulcer of left calf with fat layer exposed 〔HCC〕

L97.223 Non-pressure chronic ulcer of left calf with necrosis of muscle 〔HCC〕

L97.224 Non-pressure chronic ulcer of left calf with necrosis of bone 〔HCC〕

● **L97.225** Non-pressure chronic ulcer of left calf with muscle involvement without evidence of necrosis

● **L97.226** Non-pressure chronic ulcer of left calf with bone involvement without evidence of necrosis

● **L97.228** Non-pressure chronic ulcer of left calf with other specified severity

L97.229 Non-pressure chronic ulcer of left calf with unspecified severity 〔HCC〕▽

✓5ᵗʰ **L97.3** Non-pressure chronic ulcer of ankle

✓6ᵗʰ **L97.30** Non-pressure chronic ulcer of unspecified ankle

L97.301 Non-pressure chronic ulcer of unspecified ankle limited to breakdown of skin 〔HCC〕▽

L97.302 Non-pressure chronic ulcer of unspecified ankle with fat layer exposed 〔HCC〕▽

L97.303 Non-pressure chronic ulcer of unspecified ankle with necrosis of muscle 〔HCC〕▽

L97.304 Non-pressure chronic ulcer of unspecified ankle with necrosis of bone 〔HCC〕▽

● **L97.305** Non-pressure chronic ulcer of unspecified ankle with muscle involvement without evidence of necrosis ▽

● **L97.306** Non-pressure chronic ulcer of unspecified ankle with bone involvement without evidence of necrosis ▽

● **L97.308** Non-pressure chronic ulcer of unspecified ankle with other specified severity ▽

L97.309 Non-pressure chronic ulcer of unspecified ankle with unspecified severity 〔HCC〕▽

✓6ᵗʰ **L97.31** Non-pressure chronic ulcer of right ankle

L97.311 Non-pressure chronic ulcer of right ankle limited to breakdown of skin 〔HCC〕

L97.312 Non-pressure chronic ulcer of right ankle with fat layer exposed 〔HCC〕

L97.313 Non-pressure chronic ulcer of right ankle with necrosis of muscle 〔HCC〕

L97.314 Non-pressure chronic ulcer of right ankle with necrosis of bone 〔HCC〕

● **L97.315** Non-pressure chronic ulcer of right ankle with muscle involvement without evidence of necrosis

● **L97.316** Non-pressure chronic ulcer of right ankle with bone involvement without evidence of necrosis

● **L97.318** Non-pressure chronic ulcer of right ankle with other specified severity

L97.319 Non-pressure chronic ulcer of right ankle with unspecified severity 〔HCC〕▽

✓6ᵗʰ **L97.32** Non-pressure chronic ulcer of left ankle

L97.321 Non-pressure chronic ulcer of left ankle limited to breakdown of skin 〔HCC〕

L97.322 Non-pressure chronic ulcer of left ankle with fat layer exposed 〔HCC〕

L97.323 Non-pressure chronic ulcer of left ankle with necrosis of muscle 〔HCC〕

L97.324 Non-pressure chronic ulcer of left ankle with necrosis of bone 〔HCC〕

● **L97.325** Non-pressure chronic ulcer of left ankle with muscle involvement without evidence of necrosis

● **L97.326** Non-pressure chronic ulcer of left ankle with bone involvement without evidence of necrosis

● **L97.328** Non-pressure chronic ulcer of left ankle with other specified severity

L97.329 Non-pressure chronic ulcer of left ankle with unspecified severity 〔HCC〕▽

✓5ᵗʰ **L97.4** Non-pressure chronic ulcer of heel and midfoot
Non-pressure chronic ulcer of plantar surface of midfoot

✓6ᵗʰ **L97.40** Non-pressure chronic ulcer of unspecified heel and midfoot

L97.401 Non-pressure chronic ulcer of unspecified heel and midfoot limited to breakdown of skin 〔HCC〕▽

L97.402 Non-pressure chronic ulcer of unspecified heel and midfoot with fat layer exposed 〔HCC〕▽

L97.403 Non-pressure chronic ulcer of unspecified heel and midfoot with necrosis of muscle 〔HCC〕▽

L97.404 Non-pressure chronic ulcer of unspecified heel and midfoot with necrosis of bone 〔HCC〕▽

● **L97.405** Non-pressure chronic ulcer of unspecified heel and midfoot with muscle involvement without evidence of necrosis ▽

● **L97.406** Non-pressure chronic ulcer of unspecified heel and midfoot with bone involvement without evidence of necrosis ▽

☑ Additional Character Req   ✓ₓ7ᵗʰ Placeholder Alert   Manifestation   〔HCC〕 CMS-HCC Condition   ▽ Unspecified Code   ▶◀ Revised Text   ● New Code   ▲ Revised Code Title

Chapter 12. Diseases of the Skin and Subcutaneous Tissue

L97.408–L97.812

● L97.408　Non-pressure chronic ulcer of unspecified heel and midfoot with other specified severity ▽

L97.409　Non-pressure chronic ulcer of unspecified heel and midfoot with unspecified severity HCC ▽

✓6ᵗʰ L97.41　Non-pressure chronic ulcer of right heel and midfoot

L97.411　Non-pressure chronic ulcer of right heel and midfoot limited to breakdown of skin HCC

L97.412　Non-pressure chronic ulcer of right heel and midfoot with fat layer exposed HCC

L97.413　Non-pressure chronic ulcer of right heel and midfoot with necrosis of muscle HCC

L97.414　Non-pressure chronic ulcer of right heel and midfoot with necrosis of bone HCC

● L97.415　Non-pressure chronic ulcer of right heel and midfoot with muscle involvement without evidence of necrosis

● L97.416　Non-pressure chronic ulcer of right heel and midfoot with bone involvement without evidence of necrosis

● L97.418　Non-pressure chronic ulcer of right heel and midfoot with other specified severity

● L97.419　Non-pressure chronic ulcer of right heel and midfoot with unspecified severity HCC ▽

✓6ᵗʰ L97.42　Non-pressure chronic ulcer of left heel and midfoot

L97.421　Non-pressure chronic ulcer of left heel and midfoot limited to breakdown of skin HCC
　　　　　AHA: 2016, 1Q, 12

L97.422　Non-pressure chronic ulcer of left heel and midfoot with fat layer exposed HCC

L97.423　Non-pressure chronic ulcer of left heel and midfoot with necrosis of muscle HCC

L97.424　Non-pressure chronic ulcer of left heel and midfoot with necrosis of bone HCC

● L97.425　Non-pressure chronic ulcer of left heel and midfoot with muscle involvement without evidence of necrosis

● L97.426　Non-pressure chronic ulcer of left heel and midfoot with bone involvement without evidence of necrosis

● L97.428　Non-pressure chronic ulcer of left heel and midfoot with other specified severity

● L97.429　Non-pressure chronic ulcer of left heel and midfoot with unspecified severity HCC ▽

✓5ᵗʰ L97.5　Non-pressure chronic ulcer of other part of foot
　　　　Non-pressure chronic ulcer of toe

✓6ᵗʰ L97.50　Non-pressure chronic ulcer of other part of unspecified foot

L97.501　Non-pressure chronic ulcer of other part of unspecified foot limited to breakdown of skin HCC ▽

L97.502　Non-pressure chronic ulcer of other part of unspecified foot with fat layer exposed HCC ▽

L97.503　Non-pressure chronic ulcer of other part of unspecified foot with necrosis of muscle HCC ▽

L97.504　Non-pressure chronic ulcer of other part of unspecified foot with necrosis of bone HCC ▽

● L97.505　Non-pressure chronic ulcer of other part of unspecified foot with muscle involvement without evidence of necrosis ▽

● L97.506　Non-pressure chronic ulcer of other part of unspecified foot with bone involvement without evidence of necrosis ▽

● L97.508　Non-pressure chronic ulcer of other part of unspecified foot with other specified severity ▽

L97.509　Non-pressure chronic ulcer of other part of unspecified foot with unspecified severity HCC ▽

✓6ᵗʰ L97.51　Non-pressure chronic ulcer of other part of right foot

L97.511　Non-pressure chronic ulcer of other part of right foot limited to breakdown of skin HCC

L97.512　Non-pressure chronic ulcer of other part of right foot with fat layer exposed HCC

L97.513　Non-pressure chronic ulcer of other part of right foot with necrosis of muscle HCC

L97.514　Non-pressure chronic ulcer of other part of right foot with necrosis of bone HCC

● L97.515　Non-pressure chronic ulcer of other part of right foot with muscle involvement without evidence of necrosis

● L97.516　Non-pressure chronic ulcer of other part of right foot with bone involvement without evidence of necrosis

● L97.518　Non-pressure chronic ulcer of other part of right foot with other specified severity

L97.519　Non-pressure chronic ulcer of other part of right foot with unspecified severity HCC ▽

✓6ᵗʰ L97.52　Non-pressure chronic ulcer of other part of left foot

L97.521　Non-pressure chronic ulcer of other part of left foot limited to breakdown of skin HCC

L97.522　Non-pressure chronic ulcer of other part of left foot with fat layer exposed HCC

L97.523　Non-pressure chronic ulcer of other part of left foot with necrosis of muscle HCC

L97.524　Non-pressure chronic ulcer of other part of left foot with necrosis of bone HCC

● L97.525　Non-pressure chronic ulcer of other part of left foot with muscle involvement without evidence of necrosis

● L97.526　Non-pressure chronic ulcer of other part of left foot with bone involvement without evidence of necrosis

● L97.528　Non-pressure chronic ulcer of other part of left foot with other specified severity

L97.529　Non-pressure chronic ulcer of other part of left foot with unspecified severity HCC ▽

✓5ᵗʰ L97.8　Non-pressure chronic ulcer of other part of lower leg

✓6ᵗʰ L97.80　Non-pressure chronic ulcer of other part of unspecified lower leg

L97.801　Non-pressure chronic ulcer of other part of unspecified lower leg limited to breakdown of skin HCC ▽

L97.802　Non-pressure chronic ulcer of other part of unspecified lower leg with fat layer exposed HCC ▽

L97.803　Non-pressure chronic ulcer of other part of unspecified lower leg with necrosis of muscle HCC ▽

L97.804　Non-pressure chronic ulcer of other part of unspecified lower leg with necrosis of bone HCC ▽

● L97.805　Non-pressure chronic ulcer of other part of unspecified lower leg with muscle involvement without evidence of necrosis ▽

● L97.806　Non-pressure chronic ulcer of other part of unspecified lower leg with bone involvement without evidence of necrosis ▽

● L97.808　Non-pressure chronic ulcer of other part of unspecified lower leg with other specified severity ▽

L97.809　Non-pressure chronic ulcer of other part of unspecified lower leg with unspecified severity HCC ▽

✓6ᵗʰ L97.81　Non-pressure chronic ulcer of other part of right lower leg

L97.811　Non-pressure chronic ulcer of other part of right lower leg limited to breakdown of skin HCC

L97.812　Non-pressure chronic ulcer of other part of right lower leg with fat layer exposed HCC

L97.813 **Non-pressure chronic ulcer of other part of right lower leg with necrosis of muscle** HCC

L97.814 **Non-pressure chronic ulcer of other part of right lower leg with necrosis of bone** HCC

● L97.815 **Non-pressure chronic ulcer of other part of right lower leg** with muscle involvement without evidence of necrosis

● L97.816 **Non-pressure chronic ulcer of other part of right lower leg** with bone involvement without evidence of necrosis

● L97.818 **Non-pressure chronic ulcer of other part of right lower leg** with other specified severity

L97.819 **Non-pressure chronic ulcer of other part of right lower leg with unspecified severity** HCC ▽

√6ᵗʰ **L97.82** **Non-pressure chronic ulcer of other part of left lower leg**

L97.821 **Non-pressure chronic ulcer of other part of left lower leg** limited to breakdown of skin HCC

L97.822 **Non-pressure chronic ulcer of other part of left lower leg** with fat layer exposed HCC

L97.823 **Non-pressure chronic ulcer of other part of left lower leg** with necrosis of muscle HCC

L97.824 **Non-pressure chronic ulcer of other part of left lower leg** with necrosis of bone HCC

● L97.825 **Non-pressure chronic ulcer of other part of left lower leg** with muscle involvement without evidence of necrosis

● L97.826 **Non-pressure chronic ulcer of other part of left lower leg** with bone involvement without evidence of necrosis

● L97.828 **Non-pressure chronic ulcer of other part of left lower leg** with other specified severity

L97.829 **Non-pressure chronic ulcer of other part of left lower leg with unspecified severity** HCC ▽

√5ᵗʰ **L97.9** **Non-pressure chronic ulcer of unspecified part of** lower leg

√6ᵗʰ **L97.90** **Non-pressure chronic ulcer of unspecified part of unspecified lower leg**

L97.901 **Non-pressure chronic ulcer of unspecified part of unspecified lower leg** limited to breakdown of skin HCC ▽

L97.902 **Non-pressure chronic ulcer of unspecified part of unspecified lower leg** with fat layer exposed HCC ▽

L97.903 **Non-pressure chronic ulcer of unspecified part of unspecified lower leg** with necrosis of muscle HCC ▽

L97.904 **Non-pressure chronic ulcer of unspecified part of unspecified lower leg** with necrosis of bone HCC ▽

● L97.905 **Non-pressure chronic ulcer of unspecified part of unspecified lower leg** with muscle involvement without evidence of necrosis ▽

● L97.906 **Non-pressure chronic ulcer of unspecified part of unspecified lower leg** with bone involvement without evidence of necrosis ▽

● L97.908 **Non-pressure chronic ulcer of unspecified part of unspecified lower leg** with other specified severity ▽

L97.909 **Non-pressure chronic ulcer of unspecified part of unspecified lower leg** with unspecified severity HCC ▽

√6ᵗʰ **L97.91** **Non-pressure chronic ulcer of unspecified part of right lower leg**

L97.911 **Non-pressure chronic ulcer of unspecified part of right lower leg** limited to breakdown of skin HCC ▽

L97.912 **Non-pressure chronic ulcer of unspecified part of right lower leg** with fat layer exposed HCC ▽

L97.913 **Non-pressure chronic ulcer of unspecified part of right lower leg** with necrosis of muscle HCC ▽

L97.914 **Non-pressure chronic ulcer of unspecified part of right lower leg** with necrosis of bone HCC ▽

● L97.915 **Non-pressure chronic ulcer of unspecified part of right lower leg** with muscle involvement without evidence of necrosis ▽

● L97.916 **Non-pressure chronic ulcer of unspecified part of right lower leg** with bone involvement without evidence of necrosis ▽

● L97.918 **Non-pressure chronic ulcer of unspecified part of right lower leg with other specified severity** ▽

L97.919 **Non-pressure chronic ulcer of unspecified part of right lower leg with unspecified severity** HCC ▽

√6ᵗʰ **L97.92** **Non-pressure chronic ulcer of unspecified part of left lower leg**

L97.921 **Non-pressure chronic ulcer of unspecified part of left lower leg limited to breakdown of skin** HCC ▽

L97.922 **Non-pressure chronic ulcer of unspecified part of left lower leg with fat layer exposed** HCC ▽

L97.923 **Non-pressure chronic ulcer of unspecified part of left lower leg with necrosis of muscle** HCC ▽

L97.924 **Non-pressure chronic ulcer of unspecified part of left lower leg with necrosis of bone** HCC ▽

● L97.925 **Non-pressure chronic ulcer of unspecified part of left lower leg** with muscle involvement without evidence of necrosis ▽

● L97.926 **Non-pressure chronic ulcer of unspecified part of left lower leg** with bone involvement without evidence of necrosis ▽

● L97.928 **Non-pressure chronic ulcer of unspecified part of left lower leg** with other specified severity ▽

L97.929 **Non-pressure chronic ulcer of unspecified part of left lower leg with unspecified severity** HCC ▽

√4ᵗʰ **L98** **Other disorders of skin and subcutaneous tissue, not elsewhere classified**

L98.0 Pyogenic granuloma

EXCLUDES 2 *pyogenic granuloma of gingiva (K06.8)*
pyogenic granuloma of maxillary alveolar ridge (K04.5)
pyogenic granuloma of oral mucosa (K13.4)

DEF: Solitary polypoid capillary hemangioma often associated with local irritation, trauma, and superimposed inflammation; located on the skin and gingival or oral mucosa; they bleed easily and may ulcerate and form crusted sores.

L98.1 Factitial dermatitis
Neurotic excoriation

EXCLUDES 1 *excoriation (skin-picking) disorder (F42.4)*

DEF: Self-inflicted skin lesions to satisfy an unconscious psychological or emotional need; methods used to injure the skin include deep excoriations with a sharp instrument, scarification with a knife, or the application of caustic chemicals and burning, sometimes with a cigarette.

L98.2 Febrile neutrophilic dermatosis [Sweet]

L98.3 Eosinophilic cellulitis [Wells]

√5ᵗʰ **L98.4** **Non-pressure chronic ulcer of skin, not elsewhere classified**
Chronic ulcer of skin NOS
Tropical ulcer NOS
Ulcer of skin NOS

EXCLUDES 2 *pressure ulcer (pressure area) (L89.-)*
gangrene (I96)
skin infections (L00-L08)
specific infections classified to A00-B99
ulcer of lower limb NEC (L97.-)
varicose ulcer (I83.0-I82.2)

√6ᵗʰ **L98.41** **Non-pressure chronic ulcer of buttock**

L98.411 **Non-pressure chronic ulcer of buttock** HCC **limited to breakdown of skin**

☑ Additional Character Req   ✓x7ᵗʰ Placeholder Alert   Manifestation   HCC CMS-HCC Condition   ▽ Unspecified Code   ►◄ Revised Text   ● New Code   ▲ Revised Code Title

ICD-10-CM 2018   **711**

L98.412 Non-pressure chronic ulcer of buttock HCC
with fat layer exposed

L98.413 Non-pressure chronic ulcer of buttock HCC
with necrosis of muscle

L98.414 Non-pressure chronic ulcer of buttock HCC
with necrosis of bone

● **L98.415 Non-pressure chronic ulcer of buttock**
with muscle involvement without
evidence of necrosis

● **L98.416 Non-pressure chronic ulcer of buttock**
with bone involvement without evidence
of necrosis

● **L98.418 Non-pressure chronic ulcer of buttock**
with other specified severity

L98.419 Non-pressure chronic ulcer of HCC ▽
buttock with unspecified severity

✓6ᵗʰ **L98.42 Non-pressure chronic ulcer of back**

L98.421 Non-pressure chronic ulcer of back HCC
limited to breakdown of skin

L98.422 Non-pressure chronic ulcer of back HCC
with fat layer exposed

L98.423 Non-pressure chronic ulcer of back HCC
with necrosis of muscle

L98.424 Non-pressure chronic ulcer of back HCC
with necrosis of bone

● **L98.425 Non-pressure chronic ulcer of back** with
muscle involvement without evidence of
necrosis

● **L98.426 Non-pressure chronic ulcer of back** with
bone involvement without evidence of
necrosis

● **L98.428 Non-pressure chronic ulcer of back** with
other specified severity

L98.429 Non-pressure chronic ulcer of back HCC ▽
with unspecified severity

✓6ᵗʰ **L98.49 Non-pressure chronic ulcer of skin of other sites**
Non-pressure chronic ulcer of skin NOS

L98.491 Non-pressure chronic ulcer of skin of HCC
other sites limited to breakdown of skin

L98.492 Non-pressure chronic ulcer of skin of HCC
other sites with fat layer exposed

L98.493 Non-pressure chronic ulcer of skin of HCC
other sites with necrosis of muscle

L98.494 Non-pressure chronic ulcer of skin of HCC
other sites with necrosis of bone

● **L98.495 Non-pressure chronic ulcer of other sites**
with muscle involvement without
evidence of necrosis

● **L98.496 Non-pressure chronic ulcer of other sites**
with bone involvement without evidence
of necrosis

● **L98.498 Non-pressure chronic ulcer of other sites**
with other specified severity

L98.499 Non-pressure chronic ulcer of skin HCC ▽
of other sites with unspecified severity

L98.5 Mucinosis of the skin
Focal mucinosis
Lichen myxedematosus
Reticular erythematous mucinosis
EXCLUDES 1 *focal oral mucinosis (K13.79)*
myxedema (E03.9)

**L98.6 Other infiltrative disorders of the skin and subcutaneous
tissue**
EXCLUDES 1 *hyalinosis cutis et mucosae (E78.89)*

L98.7 Excessive and redundant skin and subcutaneous tissue
Loose or sagging skin following bariatric surgery weight loss
Loose or sagging skin following dietary weight loss
Loose or sagging skin, NOS
EXCLUDES 2 *acquired excess or redundant skin of eyelid (H02.3-)*
congenital excess or redundant skin of eyelid (Q10.3)
*skin changes due to chronic exposure to nonionizing
radiation (L57.-)*

L98.8 Other specified disorders of the skin and subcutaneous tissue
AHA: 2013, 2Q, 32

L98.9 Disorder of the skin and subcutaneous tissue, unspecified ▽

**L99 *Other disorders of skin and subcutaneous tissue in diseases
classified elsewhere***
Code first underlying disease, such as:
amyloidosis (E85.-)
EXCLUDES 1 *skin disorders in diabetes (E08-E13 with .62)*
skin disorders in gonorrhea (A54.89)
skin disorders in syphilis (A51.31, A52.79)

EXCLUDES 1 Not coded here   EXCLUDES 2 Not included here   N Newborn Age: 0   P Pediatric Age: 0-17   M Maternity Age: 12-55   A Adult Age: 15-124

712   ICD-10-CM 2018

Chapter 13. Diseases of the Musculoskeletal System and Connective Tissue (M00–M99)

Chapter Specific Guidelines with Coding Examples

The chapter specific guidelines from the ICD-10-CM Official Guidelines for Coding and Reporting have been provided below. Along with these guidelines are coding examples, contained in the shaded boxes, that have been developed to help illustrate the coding and/or sequencing guidance found in these guidelines.

a. Site and laterality

Most of the codes within Chapter 13 have site and laterality designations. The site represents the bone, joint or the muscle involved. For some conditions where more than one bone, joint or muscle is usually involved, such as osteoarthritis, there is a "multiple sites" code available. For categories where no multiple site code is provided and more than one bone, joint or muscle is involved, multiple codes should be used to indicate the different sites involved.

Olecranon bursitis of the left elbow

M70.22   Olecranon bursitis, left elbow

Explanation: Most of the codes within chapter 13 have site and laterality designations. The site represents the bone, joint, or the muscle involved.

Rheumatoid arthritis of multiple sites without rheumatoid factor

M06.09   Rheumatoid arthritis without rheumatoid factor, multiple sites

Explanation: For some conditions where more than one bone, joint or muscle is usually involved, such as osteoarthritis, there is a "multiple sites" code available.

Adolescent scoliosis in the upper thoracic region and the lumbar vertebrae

M41.124   Adolescent idiopathic scoliosis, thoracic region

M41.126   Adolescent idiopathic scoliosis, lumbar region

Explanation: For categories without a multiple site code and more than one bone, joint, or muscle is involved, multiple codes should be used to indicate the different sites involved.

---

1) Bone versus joint

For certain conditions, the bone may be affected at the upper or lower end, (e.g., avascular necrosis of bone, M87, Osteoporosis, M80, M81). Though the portion of the bone affected may be at the joint, the site designation will be the bone, not the joint.

Idiopathic avascular necrosis of the femoral head of the left hip joint

M87.052   Idiopathic aseptic necrosis of left femur

Explanation: For certain conditions such as avascular necrosis, the bone may be affected at the joint, but the site designation is the bone, not the joint.

---

b. Acute traumatic versus chronic or recurrent musculoskeletal conditions

Many musculoskeletal conditions are a result of previous injury or trauma to a site, or are recurrent conditions. Bone, joint or muscle conditions that are the result of a healed injury are usually found in chapter 13. Recurrent bone, joint or muscle conditions are also usually found in chapter 13. Any current, acute injury should be coded to the appropriate injury code from chapter 19. Chronic or recurrent conditions should generally be coded with a code from chapter 13. If it is difficult to determine from the documentation in the record which code is best to describe a condition, query the provider.

Acute traumatic bucket handle tear of right medial meniscus

S83.211A   Bucket-handle tear of medial meniscus, current injury, right knee, initial encounter

Explanation: Any current, acute injury is not coded in chapter 13. It should instead be coded to the appropriate injury code from chapter 19.

Old bucket handle tear of right medial meniscus

M23.203   Derangement of unspecified medial meniscus due to old tear or injury, right knee

Explanation: Chronic or recurrent conditions should generally be coded with a code from chapter 13.

---

c. Coding of Pathologic Fractures

7th character A is for use as long as the patient is receiving active treatment for the fracture. Examples of active treatment are: surgical treatment, emergency department encounter, evaluation and continuing treatment by the same or a different physician. While the patient may be seen by a new or different provider over the course of treatment for a pathological fracture, assignment of the 7th character is based on whether the patient is undergoing active treatment and not whether the provider is seeing the patient for the first time.

Pathologic fracture of left foot, unknown cause, currently under active treatment by a follow-up provider

M84.475A   Pathological fracture, left foot, initial encounter for fracture

Explanation: Seventh character A is for use as long as the patient is receiving active treatment for a pathologic fracture. Examples of active treatment are surgical treatment, emergency department encounter, evaluation, and continuing treatment by the same or a different physician.

The seventh character is based on whether the patient is undergoing active treatment and not whether the provider is seeing the patient for the first time.

7th character D is to be used for encounters after the patient has completed active treatment **for the fracture and is receiving routine care for the fracture during the healing or recovery phase.** The other 7th characters, listed under each subcategory in the Tabular List, are to be used for subsequent encounters for treatment of problems associated with the healing, such as malunions, nonunions, and sequelae.

Care for complications of surgical treatment for fracture repairs during the healing or recovery phase should be coded with the appropriate complication codes.

See Section I.C.19. Coding of traumatic fractures.

d. Osteoporosis

Osteoporosis is a systemic condition, meaning that all bones of the musculoskeletal system are affected. Therefore, site is not a component of the codes under category M81, Osteoporosis without current pathological fracture. The site codes under category M80, Osteoporosis with current pathological fracture, identify the site of the fracture, not the osteoporosis.

1) Osteoporosis without pathological fracture

Category M81, Osteoporosis without current pathological fracture, is for use for patients with osteoporosis who do not currently have a pathologic fracture due to the osteoporosis, even if they have had a fracture in the past. For patients with a history of osteoporosis fractures, status code Z87.310, Personal history of (healed) osteoporosis fracture, should follow the code from M81.

Age-related osteoporosis with healed osteoporotic fracture of the lumbar vertebra

M81.0   Age-related osteoporosis without current pathological fracture

Z87.310   Personal history of (healed) osteoporosis fracture

Explanation: Category M81 is used for patients with osteoporosis who do not currently have a pathologic fracture due to the osteoporosis. To report a previous (healed) fracture, status code Z87.310 Personal history of (healed) osteoporosis fracture, should follow the code from M81.

---

2) Osteoporosis with current pathological fracture

Category M80, Osteoporosis with current pathological fracture, is for patients who have a current pathologic fracture at the time of an encounter. The codes under M80 identify the site of the fracture. A code from category M80, not a traumatic fracture code, should be used for any patient with known osteoporosis who suffers a fracture, even if the patient had a minor fall or trauma, if that fall or trauma would not usually break a normal, healthy bone.

Disuse osteoporosis with current fracture of right shoulder sustained lifting a grocery bag, initial encounter

M80.811A   Other osteoporosis with current pathological fracture, right shoulder, initial encounter for fracture

Explanation: A code from category M80, not a traumatic fracture code, should be used for any patient with known osteoporosis who suffers a fracture, even if the patient had a minor fall or trauma, if that fall or trauma would not usually break a normal, healthy bone.

Muscle/Tendon Table

ICD-10-CM categorizes certain muscles and tendons in the upper and lower extremities by their action (e.g., extension, flexion), their anatomical location (e.g., posterior, anterior), and/or whether they are intrinsic or extrinsic to a certain anatomical area. The Muscle/Tendon Table is provided at the beginning of chapters 13 and 19 as a resource to help users when code selection depends on one or more of these characteristics. A **TIP** has been placed at those categories and/or subcategories that relate to this table. Please note that this table is not all-inclusive, and proper code assignment should be based on the provider's documentation.

Body Region	Muscle	Extensor Tendon	Flexor Tendon	Other Tendon
Shoulder				
	Deltoid	Posterior deltoid	Anterior deltoid	
	Rotator cuff			
	Infraspinatus			Infraspinatus
	Subscapularis			Subscapularis
	Supraspinatus			Supraspinatus
	Teres minor			Teres minor
	Teres major	Teres major		
Upper arm				
	Anterior muscles			
	Biceps brachii — long head		Biceps brachii — long head	
	Biceps brachii — short head		Biceps brachii — short head	
	Brachialis		Brachialis	
	Coracobrachialis		Coracobrachialis	
	Posterior muscles			
	Triceps brachii	Triceps brachii		
Forearm				
	Anterior muscles			
	Flexors			
	Deep			
	Flexor digitorum profundus		Flexor digitorum profundus	
	Flexor pollicis longus		Flexor pollicis longus	
	Intermediate			
	Flexor digitorum superficialis		Flexor digitorum superficialis	
	Superficial			
	Flexor carpi radialis		Flexor carpi radialis	
	Flexor carpi ulnaris		Flexor carpi ulnaris	
	Palmaris longus		Palmaris longus	
	Pronators			
	Pronator quadratus			Pronator quadratus
	Pronator teres			Pronator teres
	Posterior muscles			
	Extensors			
	Deep			
	Abductor pollicis longus			Abductor pollicis longus
	Extensor indicis	Extensor indicis		
	Extensor pollicis brevis	Extensor pollicis brevis		
	Extensor pollicis longus	Extensor pollicis longus		
	Superficial			
	Brachioradialis			Brachioradialis
	Extensor carpi radialis brevis	Extensor carpi radialis brevis		
	Extensor carpi radialis longus	Extensor carpi radialis longus		
	Extensor carpi ulnaris	Extensor carpi ulnaris		
	Extensor digiti minimi	Extensor digiti minimi		
	Extensor digitorum	Extensor digitorum		
	Anconeus	Anconeus		
	Supinator			Supinator

Body Region	Muscle	Extensor Tendon	Flexor Tendon	Other Tendon
Hand				
Extrinsic — attach to a site in the forearm as well as a site in the hand with action related to hand movement at the wrist				
	Extensor carpi radialis brevis	Extensor carpi radialis brevis		
	Extensor carpi radialis longus	Extensor carpie radialis longus		
	Extensor carpi ulnaris	Extensor carpi ulnaris		
	Flexor carpi radialis		Flexor carpi radialis	
	Flexor carpi ulnaris		Flexor carpi ulnaris	
	Flexor digitorum superficialis		Flexor digitorum superficialis	
	Palmaris longus		Palmaris longus	
Extrinsic — attach to a site in the forearm as well as a site in the hand with action in the hand related to finger movement				
	Adductor pollicis longus			Adductor pollicis longus
	Extensor digiti minimi	Extensor digiti minimi		
	Extensor digitorum	Extensor digitorum		
	Extensor indicis	Extensor indicis		
	Flexor digitorum profundus		Flexor digitorum profundus	
	Flexor digitorum superficialis		Flexor digitorum superficialis	
Extrinsic — attach to a site in the forearm as well as a site in the hand with action in the hand related to thumb movement				
	Extensor pollicis brevis	Extensor pollicis brevis		
	Extensor pollicis longus	Extensor pollicis longus		
	Flexor pollicis longus		Flexor pollicis longus	
Intrinsic — found within the hand only				
	Adductor pollicis			Adductor pollicis
	Dorsal interossei	Dorsal interossei	Dorsal interossei	
	Lumbricals	Lumbricals	Lumbricals	
	Palmaris brevis			Palmaris brevis
	Palmar interossei	Palmar interossei	Palmar interossei	
	Hypothenar muscles			
	Abductor digiti minimi			Abductor digiti minimi
	Flexor digiti minimi brevis		Flexor digiti minimi brevis	
	Oppenens digiti minimi		Oppenens digiti minimi	
	Thenar muscles			
	Abductor pollicis brevis			Abductor pollicis brevis
	Flexor pollicis brevis		Flexor pollicis brevis	
	Oppenens pollicis		Oppenens pollicis	
Thigh				
	Anterior muscles			
	Iliopsoas		Iliopsoas	
	Pectineus		Pectineus	
	Quadriceps	Quadriceps		
	Rectus femoris	Rectus femoris — Extends knee	Rectus femoris — Flexes hip	
	Vastus intermedius	Vastus intermedius		
	Vastus lateralis	Vastus lateralis		
	Vastus medialis	Vastus medialis		
	Sartorius		Sartorius	
	Medial muscles			
	Adductor brevis			Adductor brevis
	Adductor longus			Adductor longus
	Adductor magnus			Adductor magnus
	Gracilis			Gracilis
	Obturator externus			Obturator externus
	Posterior muscles			
	Hamstring	Hamstring — Extends hip	Hamstring — Flexes knee	
	Biceps femoris	Biceps femoris	Biceps femoris	
	Semimembranosus	Semimembranosus	Semimembranosus	
	Semitendinosus	Semitendinosus	Semitendinosus	

Chapter 13. Diseases of the Musculoskeletal System and Connective Tissue

Body Region	Muscle	Extensor Tendon	Flexor Tendon	Other Tendon
Lower leg				
	Anterior muscles			
	Extensor digitorum longus	Extensor digitorum longus		
	Extensor hallucis longus	Extensor hallucis longus		
	Fibularis (peroneus) tertius	Fibularis (peroneus) tertius		
	Tibialis anterior	Tibialis anterior		Tibialis anterior
	Lateral muscles			
	Fibularis (peroneus) brevis		Fibularis (peroneus) brevis	
	Fibularis (peroneus) longus		Fibularis (peroneus) longus	
	Posterior muscles			
	Deep			
	Flexor digitorum longus		Flexor digitorum longus	
	Flexor hallucis longus		Flexor hallucis longus	
	Popliteus		Popliteus	
	Tibialis posterior		Tibialis posterior	
	Superficial			
	Gastrocnemius		Gastrocnemius	
	Plantaris		Plantaris	
	Soleus		Soleus	
				Calcaneal (Achilles)
Ankle/Foot				
Extrinsic — attach to a site in the lower leg as well as a site in the foot with action related to foot movement at the ankle				
	Plantaris		Plantaris	
	Soleus		Soleus	
	Tibialis anterior	Tibialis anterior		
	Tibialis posterior		Tibialis posterior	
Extrinsic — attach to a site in the lower leg as well as a site in the foot with action in the foot related to toe movement				
	Extensor digitorum longus	Extensor digitorum longus		
	Extensor hallucis longus	Extensor hallucis longus		
	Flexor digitorum longus		Flexor digitorum longus	
	Flexor hallucis longus		Flexor hallucis longus	
Intrinsic — found within the ankle/foot only				
	Dorsal muscles			
	Extensor digitorum brevis	Extensor digitorum brevis		
	Extensor hallucis brevis	Extensor hallucis brevis		
	Plantar muscles			
	Abductor digiti minimi		Abductor digiti minimi	
	Abductor hallucis		Abductor hallucis	
	Dorsal interossei	Dorsal interossei	Dorsal interossei	
	Flexor digiti minimi brevis		Flexor digiti minimi brevis	
	Flexor digitorum brevis		Flexor digitorum brevis	
	Flexor hallucis brevis		Flexor hallucis brevis	
	Lumbricals	Lumbricals	Lumbricals	
	Quadratus plantae		Quadratus plantae	
	Plantar interossei	Plantar interossei	Plantar interossei	

Chapter 13. Diseases of the Musculoskeletal System and Connective Tissue (M00-M99)

NOTE Use an external cause code following the code for the musculoskeletal condition, if applicable, to identify the cause of the musculoskeletal condition.

EXCLUDES 2 *arthropathic psoriasis (L40.5-)*
certain conditions originating in the perinatal period (P04-P96)
certain infectious and parasitic diseases (A00-B99)
compartment syndrome (traumatic) (T79.A-)
complications of pregnancy, childbirth and the puerperium (O00-O9A)
congenital malformations, deformations, and chromosomal abnormalities (Q00-Q99)
endocrine, nutritional and metabolic diseases (E00-E88)
injury, poisoning and certain other consequences of external causes (S00-T88)
neoplasms (C00-D49)
symptoms, signs and abnormal clinical and laboratory findings, not elsewhere classified (R00-R94)

This chapter contains the following blocks:

M00-M02	Infectious arthropathies
M04	~~Autoinflammatory syndromes~~
M05-M14	Inflammatory polyarthropathies
M15-M19	Osteoarthritis
M20-M25	Other joint disorders
M26-M27	Dentofacial anomalies [including malocclusion] and other disorders of jaw
M30-M36	Systemic connective tissue disorders
M40-M43	Deforming dorsopathies
M45-M49	Spondylopathies
M50-M54	Other dorsopathies
M60-M63	Disorders of muscles
M65-M67	Disorders of synovium and tendon
M70-M79	Other soft tissue disorders
M80-M85	Disorders of bone density and structure
M86-M90	Other osteopathies
M91-M94	Chondropathies
M95	Other disorders of the musculoskeletal system and connective tissue
M96	Intraoperative and postprocedural complications and disorders of musculoskeletal system, not elsewhere classified
M97	~~Periprosthetic fracture around internal prosthetic joint~~
M99	Biomechanical lesions, not elsewhere classified

ARTHROPATHIES (M00-M25)

INCLUDES disorders affecting predominantly peripheral (limb) joints

Infectious arthropathies (M00-M02)

NOTE This block comprises arthropathies due to microbiological agents. Distinction is made between the following types of etiological relationship:

a) direct infection of joint, where organisms invade synovial tissue and microbial antigen is present in the joint;

b) indirect infection, which may be of two types: a reactive arthropathy, where microbial infection of the body is established but neither organisms nor antigens can be identified in the joint, and a postinfective arthropathy, where microbial antigen is present but recovery of an organism is inconstant and evidence of local multiplication is lacking.

✓4ᵗʰ **M00 Pyogenic arthritis**

   ✓5ᵗʰ **M00.0 Staphylococcal arthritis and polyarthritis**

      Use additional code (B95.61-B95.8) to identify bacterial agent

        EXCLUDES 2 *infection and inflammatory reaction due to internal joint prosthesis (T84.5-)*

      M00.00 Staphylococcal arthritis, unspecified joint HCC ▽

      ✓6ᵗʰ **M00.01 Staphylococcal arthritis,** shoulder

          M00.011 Staphylococcal arthritis, right shoulder HCC

          M00.012 Staphylococcal arthritis, left shoulder HCC

          M00.019 Staphylococcal arthritis, unspecified shoulder HCC ▽

      ✓6ᵗʰ **M00.02 Staphylococcal arthritis,** elbow

          M00.021 Staphylococcal arthritis, right elbow HCC

          M00.022 Staphylococcal arthritis, left elbow HCC

          M00.029 Staphylococcal arthritis, unspecified elbow HCC ▽

✓6ᵗʰ **M00.03 Staphylococcal arthritis,** wrist
     Staphylococcal arthritis of carpal bones

      M00.031 Staphylococcal arthritis, right wrist HCC

      M00.032 Staphylococcal arthritis, left wrist HCC

      M00.039 Staphylococcal arthritis, unspecified wrist HCC ▽

✓6ᵗʰ **M00.04 Staphylococcal arthritis,** hand
     Staphylococcal arthritis of metacarpus and phalanges

      M00.041 Staphylococcal arthritis, right hand HCC

      M00.042 Staphylococcal arthritis, left hand HCC

      M00.049 Staphylococcal arthritis, unspecified hand HCC ▽

✓6ᵗʰ **M00.05 Staphylococcal arthritis,** hip

      M00.051 Staphylococcal arthritis, right hip HCC

      M00.052 Staphylococcal arthritis, left hip HCC

      M00.059 Staphylococcal arthritis, unspecified hip HCC ▽

✓6ᵗʰ **M00.06 Staphylococcal arthritis,** knee

      M00.061 Staphylococcal arthritis, right knee HCC

      M00.062 Staphylococcal arthritis, left knee HCC

      M00.069 Staphylococcal arthritis, unspecified knee HCC ▽

✓6ᵗʰ **M00.07 Staphylococcal arthritis,** ankle and foot
     Staphylococcal arthritis, tarsus, metatarsus and phalanges

      M00.071 Staphylococcal arthritis, right ankle and foot HCC

      M00.072 Staphylococcal arthritis, left ankle and foot HCC

      M00.079 Staphylococcal arthritis, unspecified ankle and foot HCC ▽

    M00.08 Staphylococcal arthritis, vertebrae HCC

    M00.09 Staphylococcal polyarthritis HCC

✓5ᵗʰ **M00.1 Pneumococcal arthritis and polyarthritis**

    M00.10 Pneumococcal arthritis, unspecified joint HCC ▽

✓6ᵗʰ **M00.11 Pneumococcal arthritis,** shoulder

      M00.111 Pneumococcal arthritis, right shoulder HCC

      M00.112 Pneumococcal arthritis, left shoulder HCC

      M00.119 Pneumococcal arthritis, unspecified shoulder HCC ▽

✓6ᵗʰ **M00.12 Pneumococcal arthritis,** elbow

      M00.121 Pneumococcal arthritis, right elbow HCC

      M00.122 Pneumococcal arthritis, left elbow HCC

      M00.129 Pneumococcal arthritis, unspecified elbow HCC ▽

✓6ᵗʰ **M00.13 Pneumococcal arthritis,** wrist
     Pneumococcal arthritis of carpal bones

      M00.131 Pneumococcal arthritis, right wrist HCC

      M00.132 Pneumococcal arthritis, left wrist HCC

      M00.139 Pneumococcal arthritis, unspecified wrist HCC ▽

✓6ᵗʰ **M00.14 Pneumococcal arthritis,** hand
     Pneumococcal arthritis of metacarpus and phalanges

      M00.141 Pneumococcal arthritis, right hand HCC

      M00.142 Pneumococcal arthritis, left hand HCC

      M00.149 Pneumococcal arthritis, unspecified hand HCC ▽

✓6ᵗʰ **M00.15 Pneumococcal arthritis,** hip

      M00.151 Pneumococcal arthritis, right hip HCC

      M00.152 Pneumococcal arthritis, left hip HCC

      M00.159 Pneumococcal arthritis, unspecified hip HCC ▽

✓6ᵗʰ **M00.16 Pneumococcal arthritis,** knee

      M00.161 Pneumococcal arthritis, right knee HCC

      M00.162 Pneumococcal arthritis, left knee HCC

      M00.169 Pneumococcal arthritis, unspecified knee HCC ▽

✓6ᵗʰ **M00.17 Pneumococcal arthritis,** ankle and foot
     Pneumococcal arthritis, tarsus, metatarsus and phalanges

      M00.171 Pneumococcal arthritis, right ankle and foot HCC

      M00.172 Pneumococcal arthritis, left ankle and foot HCC

✓ Additional Character Req   ✓x7ᵗʰ Placeholder Alert   Manifestation   HCC CMS-HCC Condition   ▽ Unspecified Code   ▶◀ Revised Text   ● New Code   ▲ Revised Code Title

ICD-10-CM 2018   717

M00.179   **Pneumococcal arthritis, unspecified ankle and foot** HCC ▽

M00.18   **Pneumococcal arthritis, vertebrae** HCC

M00.19   **Pneumococcal polyarthritis** HCC

✓5ᵗʰ M00.2   **Other streptococcal arthritis and polyarthritis**
Use additional code (B95.0-B95.2, B95.4-B95.5) to identify bacterial agent

M00.20   **Other streptococcal arthritis, unspecified joint** HCC ▽

✓6ᵗʰ M00.21   **Other streptococcal arthritis, shoulder**

M00.211   **Other streptococcal arthritis, right shoulder** HCC

M00.212   **Other streptococcal arthritis, left shoulder** HCC

M00.219   **Other streptococcal arthritis, unspecified shoulder** HCC ▽

✓6ᵗʰ M00.22   **Other streptococcal arthritis, elbow**

M00.221   **Other streptococcal arthritis, right elbow** HCC

M00.222   **Other streptococcal arthritis, left elbow** HCC

M00.229   **Other streptococcal arthritis, unspecified elbow** HCC ▽

✓6ᵗʰ M00.23   **Other streptococcal arthritis, wrist**
Other streptococcal arthritis of carpal bones

M00.231   **Other streptococcal arthritis, right wrist** HCC

M00.232   **Other streptococcal arthritis, left wrist** HCC

M00.239   **Other streptococcal arthritis, unspecified wrist** HCC ▽

✓6ᵗʰ M00.24   **Other streptococcal arthritis, hand**
Other streptococcal arthritis metacarpus and phalanges

M00.241   **Other streptococcal arthritis, right hand** HCC

M00.242   **Other streptococcal arthritis, left hand** HCC

M00.249   **Other streptococcal arthritis, unspecified hand** HCC ▽

✓6ᵗʰ M00.25   **Other streptococcal arthritis, hip**

M00.251   **Other streptococcal arthritis, right hip** HCC

M00.252   **Other streptococcal arthritis, left hip** HCC

M00.259   **Other streptococcal arthritis, unspecified hip** HCC ▽

✓6ᵗʰ M00.26   **Other streptococcal arthritis, knee**

M00.261   **Other streptococcal arthritis, right knee** HCC

M00.262   **Other streptococcal arthritis, left knee** HCC

M00.269   **Other streptococcal arthritis, unspecified knee** HCC ▽

✓6ᵗʰ M00.27   **Other streptococcal arthritis, ankle and foot**
Other streptococcal arthritis, tarsus, metatarsus and phalanges

M00.271   **Other streptococcal arthritis, right ankle and foot** HCC

M00.272   **Other streptococcal arthritis, left ankle and foot** HCC

M00.279   **Other streptococcal arthritis, unspecified ankle and foot** HCC ▽

M00.28   **Other streptococcal arthritis, vertebrae** HCC

M00.29   **Other streptococcal polyarthritis** HCC

✓5ᵗʰ M00.8   **Arthritis and polyarthritis due to other bacteria**
Use additional code (B96) to identify bacteria

M00.80   **Arthritis due to other bacteria, unspecified joint** HCC ▽

✓6ᵗʰ M00.81   **Arthritis due to other bacteria, shoulder**

M00.811   **Arthritis due to other bacteria, right shoulder** HCC

M00.812   **Arthritis due to other bacteria, left shoulder** HCC

M00.819   **Arthritis due to other bacteria, unspecified shoulder** HCC ▽

✓6ᵗʰ M00.82   **Arthritis due to other bacteria, elbow**

M00.821   **Arthritis due to other bacteria, right elbow** HCC

M00.822   **Arthritis due to other bacteria, left elbow** HCC

M00.829   **Arthritis due to other bacteria, unspecified elbow** HCC ▽

✓6ᵗʰ M00.83   **Arthritis due to other bacteria, wrist**
Arthritis due to other bacteria, carpal bones

M00.831   **Arthritis due to other bacteria, right wrist** HCC

M00.832   **Arthritis due to other bacteria, left wrist** HCC

M00.839   **Arthritis due to other bacteria, unspecified wrist** HCC ▽

✓6ᵗʰ M00.84   **Arthritis due to other bacteria, hand**
Arthritis due to other bacteria, metacarpus and phalanges

M00.841   **Arthritis due to other bacteria, right hand** HCC

M00.842   **Arthritis due to other bacteria, left hand** HCC

M00.849   **Arthritis due to other bacteria, unspecified hand** HCC ▽

✓6ᵗʰ M00.85   **Arthritis due to other bacteria, hip**

M00.851   **Arthritis due to other bacteria, right hip** HCC

M00.852   **Arthritis due to other bacteria, left hip** HCC

M00.859   **Arthritis due to other bacteria, unspecified hip** HCC ▽

✓6ᵗʰ M00.86   **Arthritis due to other bacteria, knee**

M00.861   **Arthritis due to other bacteria, right knee** HCC

M00.862   **Arthritis due to other bacteria, left knee** HCC

M00.869   **Arthritis due to other bacteria, unspecified knee** HCC ▽

✓6ᵗʰ M00.87   **Arthritis due to other bacteria, ankle and foot**
Arthritis due to other bacteria, tarsus, metatarsus, and phalanges

M00.871   **Arthritis due to other bacteria, right ankle and foot** HCC

M00.872   **Arthritis due to other bacteria, left ankle and foot** HCC

M00.879   **Arthritis due to other bacteria, unspecified ankle and foot** HCC ▽

M00.88   **Arthritis due to other bacteria, vertebrae** HCC

M00.89   **Polyarthritis due to other bacteria** HCC

M00.9   **Pyogenic arthritis, unspecified** HCC ▽
Infective arthritis NOS

✓4ᵗʰ **M01   Direct infections of joint in infectious and parasitic diseases classified elsewhere**
Code first underlying disease, such as:
leprosy [Hansen's disease] (A30.-)
mycoses (B35-B49)
O'nyong-nyong fever (A92.1)
paratyphoid fever (A01.1-A01.4)

EXCLUDES 1   arthropathy in Lyme disease (A69.23)
gonococcal arthritis (A54.42)
meningococcal arthritis (A39.83)
mumps arthritis (B26.85)
postinfective arthropathy (M02.-)
postmeningococcal arthritis (A39.84)
reactive arthritis (M02.3)
rubella arthritis (B06.82)
sarcoidosis arthritis (D86.86)
typhoid fever arthritis (A01.04)
tuberculosis arthritis (A18.01-A18.02)

✓5ᵗʰ **M01.X   Direct infection of joint in infectious and parasitic diseases classified elsewhere**

M01.X0   *Direct infection of unspecified joint in infectious and parasitic diseases classified elsewhere* HCC ▽

✓6ᵗʰ M01.X1   **Direct infection of shoulder joint in infectious and parasitic diseases classified elsewhere**

M01.X11   *Direct infection of right shoulder in infectious and parasitic diseases classified elsewhere* HCC

EXCLUDES 1 Not coded here   EXCLUDES 2 Not included here   Ⓝ Newborn Age: 0   Ⓟ Pediatric Age: 0-17   Ⓜ Maternity Age: 12-55   Ⓐ Adult Age: 15-124

718   ICD-10-CM 2018

M01.X12 Direct infection of left shoulder in infectious and parasitic diseases classified elsewhere HCC

M01.X19 Direct infection of unspecified shoulder in infectious and parasitic diseases classified elsewhere HCC ▽

✓6ᵗʰ **M01.X2** Direct infection of elbow in infectious and parasitic diseases classified elsewhere

M01.X21 Direct infection of right elbow in infectious and parasitic diseases classified elsewhere HCC

M01.X22 Direct infection of left elbow in infectious and parasitic diseases classified elsewhere HCC

M01.X29 Direct infection of unspecified elbow in infectious and parasitic diseases classified elsewhere HCC ▽

✓6ᵗʰ **M01.X3** Direct infection of wrist in infectious and parasitic diseases classified elsewhere
Direct infection of carpal bones in infectious and parasitic diseases classified elsewhere

M01.X31 Direct infection of right wrist in infectious and parasitic diseases classified elsewhere HCC

M01.X32 Direct infection of left wrist in infectious and parasitic diseases classified elsewhere HCC

M01.X39 Direct infection of unspecified wrist in infectious and parasitic diseases classified elsewhere HCC ▽

✓6ᵗʰ **M01.X4** Direct infection of hand in infectious and parasitic diseases classified elsewhere
Direct infection of metacarpus and phalanges in infectious and parasitic diseases classified elsewhere

M01.X41 Direct infection of right hand in infectious and parasitic diseases classified elsewhere HCC

M01.X42 Direct infection of left hand in infectious and parasitic diseases classified elsewhere HCC

M01.X49 Direct infection of unspecified hand in infectious and parasitic diseases classified elsewhere HCC ▽

✓6ᵗʰ **M01.X5** Direct infection of hip in infectious and parasitic diseases classified elsewhere

M01.X51 Direct infection of right hip in infectious and parasitic diseases classified elsewhere HCC

M01.X52 Direct infection of left hip in infectious and parasitic diseases classified elsewhere HCC

M01.X59 Direct infection of unspecified hip in infectious and parasitic diseases classified elsewhere HCC ▽

✓6ᵗʰ **M01.X6** Direct infection of knee in infectious and parasitic diseases classified elsewhere

M01.X61 Direct infection of right knee in infectious and parasitic diseases classified elsewhere HCC

M01.X62 Direct infection of left knee in infectious and parasitic diseases classified elsewhere HCC

M01.X69 Direct infection of unspecified knee in infectious and parasitic diseases classified elsewhere HCC ▽

✓6ᵗʰ **M01.X7** Direct infection of ankle and foot in infectious and parasitic diseases classified elsewhere
Direct infection of tarsus, metatarsus and phalanges in infectious and parasitic diseases classified elsewhere

M01.X71 Direct infection of right ankle and foot in infectious and parasitic diseases classified elsewhere HCC

M01.X72 Direct infection of left ankle and foot in infectious and parasitic diseases classified elsewhere HCC

M01.X79 Direct infection of unspecified ankle and foot in infectious and parasitic diseases classified elsewhere HCC ▽

M01.X8 Direct infection of vertebrae in infectious and parasitic diseases classified elsewhere HCC

M01.X9 Direct infection of multiple joints in infectious and parasitic diseases classified elsewhere HCC

✓4ᵗʰ **M02 Postinfective and reactive arthropathies**
Code first underlying disease, such as:
  congenital syphilis [Clutton's joints] (A50.5)
  enteritis due to Yersinia enterocolitica (A04.6)
  infective endocarditis (I33.0)
  viral hepatitis (B15-B19)

EXCLUDES 1 Behçet's disease (M35.2)
    direct infections of joint in infectious and parasitic diseases classified elsewhere (M01.-)
    postmeningococcal arthritis (A39.84)
    mumps arthritis (B26.85)
    rheumatic fever (I00)
    rubella arthritis (B06.82)
    syphilis arthritis (late) (A52.77)
    tabetic arthropathy [Charcôt's] (A52.16)

✓5ᵗʰ **M02.0 Arthropathy following intestinal bypass**

M02.00 Arthropathy following intestinal bypass, unspecified site ▽

✓6ᵗʰ **M02.01** Arthropathy following intestinal bypass, shoulder

M02.011 Arthropathy following intestinal bypass, right shoulder

M02.012 Arthropathy following intestinal bypass, left shoulder

M02.019 Arthropathy following intestinal bypass, unspecified shoulder ▽

✓6ᵗʰ **M02.02** Arthropathy following intestinal bypass, elbow

M02.021 Arthropathy following intestinal bypass, right elbow

M02.022 Arthropathy following intestinal bypass, left elbow

M02.029 Arthropathy following intestinal bypass, unspecified elbow ▽

✓6ᵗʰ **M02.03** Arthropathy following intestinal bypass, wrist
Arthropathy following intestinal bypass, carpal bones

M02.031 Arthropathy following intestinal bypass, right wrist

M02.032 Arthropathy following intestinal bypass, left wrist

M02.039 Arthropathy following intestinal bypass, unspecified wrist ▽

✓6ᵗʰ **M02.04** Arthropathy following intestinal bypass, hand
Arthropathy following intestinal bypass, metacarpals and phalanges

M02.041 Arthropathy following intestinal bypass, right hand

M02.042 Arthropathy following intestinal bypass, left hand

M02.049 Arthropathy following intestinal bypass, unspecified hand ▽

✓6ᵗʰ **M02.05** Arthropathy following intestinal bypass, hip

M02.051 Arthropathy following intestinal bypass, right hip

M02.052 Arthropathy following intestinal bypass, left hip

M02.059 Arthropathy following intestinal bypass, unspecified hip ▽

✓6ᵗʰ **M02.06** Arthropathy following intestinal bypass, knee

M02.061 Arthropathy following intestinal bypass, right knee

M02.062 Arthropathy following intestinal bypass, left knee

M02.069 Arthropathy following intestinal bypass, unspecified knee ▽

✓6ᵗʰ **M02.07** Arthropathy following intestinal bypass, ankle and foot
Arthropathy following intestinal bypass, tarsus, metatarsus and phalanges

M02.071 Arthropathy following intestinal bypass, right ankle and foot

M02.072 Arthropathy following intestinal bypass, left ankle and foot

M02.079 Arthropathy following intestinal bypass, unspecified ankle and foot ▽

M02.08 Arthropathy following intestinal bypass, vertebrae

✓ Additional Character Req   x7ᵗʰ Placeholder Alert   Manifestation   HCC CMS-HCC Condition   ▽ Unspecified Code   ►◄ Revised Text   ● New Code   ▲ Revised Code Title

Chapter 13. Diseases of the Musculoskeletal System and Connective Tissue

M02.09–M02.38

M02.09   **Arthropathy following intestinal bypass, multiple sites**

✓5ᵗʰ **M02.1**   **Postdysenteric arthropathy**

    M02.10   Postdysenteric arthropathy, unspecified site   HCC ▽

✓6ᵗʰ **M02.11**   Postdysenteric arthropathy, shoulder
     M02.111   Postdysenteric arthropathy, right shoulder   HCC
     M02.112   Postdysenteric arthropathy, left shoulder   HCC
     M02.119   Postdysenteric arthropathy, unspecified shoulder   HCC ▽

✓6ᵗʰ **M02.12**   Postdysenteric arthropathy, elbow
     M02.121   Postdysenteric arthropathy, right elbow   HCC
     M02.122   Postdysenteric arthropathy, left elbow   HCC
     M02.129   Postdysenteric arthropathy, unspecified elbow   HCC ▽

✓6ᵗʰ **M02.13**   Postdysenteric arthropathy, wrist
     Postdysenteric arthropathy, carpal bones
     M02.131   Postdysenteric arthropathy, right wrist   HCC
     M02.132   Postdysenteric arthropathy, left wrist   HCC
     M02.139   Postdysenteric arthropathy, unspecified wrist   HCC ▽

✓6ᵗʰ **M02.14**   Postdysenteric arthropathy, hand
     Postdysenteric arthropathy, metacarpus and phalanges
     M02.141   Postdysenteric arthropathy, right hand   HCC
     M02.142   Postdysenteric arthropathy, left hand   HCC
     M02.149   Postdysenteric arthropathy, unspecified hand   HCC ▽

✓6ᵗʰ **M02.15**   Postdysenteric arthropathy, hip
     M02.151   Postdysenteric arthropathy, right hip   HCC
     M02.152   Postdysenteric arthropathy, left hip   HCC
     M02.159   Postdysenteric arthropathy, unspecified hip   HCC ▽

✓6ᵗʰ **M02.16**   Postdysenteric arthropathy, knee
     M02.161   Postdysenteric arthropathy, right knee   HCC
     M02.162   Postdysenteric arthropathy, left knee   HCC
     M02.169   Postdysenteric arthropathy, unspecified knee   HCC ▽

✓6ᵗʰ **M02.17**   Postdysenteric arthropathy, ankle and foot
     Postdysenteric arthropathy, tarsus, metatarsus and phalanges
     M02.171   Postdysenteric arthropathy, right ankle and foot   HCC
     M02.172   Postdysenteric arthropathy, left ankle and foot   HCC
     M02.179   Postdysenteric arthropathy, unspecified ankle and foot   HCC ▽

    M02.18   Postdysenteric arthropathy, vertebrae   HCC
    M02.19   Postdysenteric arthropathy, multiple sites   HCC

✓5ᵗʰ **M02.2**   **Postimmunization arthropathy**

    M02.20   Postimmunization arthropathy, unspecified site   ▽

✓6ᵗʰ **M02.21**   Postimmunization arthropathy, shoulder
     M02.211   Postimmunization arthropathy, right shoulder
     M02.212   Postimmunization arthropathy, left shoulder
     M02.219   Postimmunization arthropathy, unspecified shoulder   ▽

✓6ᵗʰ **M02.22**   Postimmunization arthropathy, elbow
     M02.221   Postimmunization arthropathy, right elbow
     M02.222   Postimmunization arthropathy, left elbow
     M02.229   Postimmunization arthropathy, unspecified elbow   ▽

✓6ᵗʰ **M02.23**   Postimmunization arthropathy, wrist
     Postimmunization arthropathy, carpal bones
     M02.231   Postimmunization arthropathy, right wrist
     M02.232   Postimmunization arthropathy, left wrist
     M02.239   Postimmunization arthropathy, unspecified wrist   ▽

✓6ᵗʰ **M02.24**   Postimmunization arthropathy, hand
     Postimmunization arthropathy, metacarpus and phalanges
     M02.241   Postimmunization arthropathy, right hand
     M02.242   Postimmunization arthropathy, left hand
     M02.249   Postimmunization arthropathy, unspecified hand   ▽

✓6ᵗʰ **M02.25**   Postimmunization arthropathy, hip
     M02.251   Postimmunization arthropathy, right hip
     M02.252   Postimmunization arthropathy, left hip
     M02.259   Postimmunization arthropathy, unspecified hip   ▽

✓6ᵗʰ **M02.26**   Postimmunization arthropathy, knee
     M02.261   Postimmunization arthropathy, right knee
     M02.262   Postimmunization arthropathy, left knee
     M02.269   Postimmunization arthropathy, unspecified knee   ▽

✓6ᵗʰ **M02.27**   Postimmunization arthropathy, ankle and foot
     Postimmunization arthropathy, tarsus, metatarsus and phalanges
     M02.271   Postimmunization arthropathy, right ankle and foot
     M02.272   Postimmunization arthropathy, left ankle and foot
     M02.279   Postimmunization arthropathy, unspecified ankle and foot   ▽

    M02.28   Postimmunization arthropathy, vertebrae
    M02.29   Postimmunization arthropathy, multiple sites

✓5ᵗʰ **M02.3**   **Reiter's disease**
    Reactive arthritis

    M02.30   Reiter's disease, unspecified site   HCC ▽

✓6ᵗʰ **M02.31**   Reiter's disease, shoulder
     M02.311   Reiter's disease, right shoulder   HCC
     M02.312   Reiter's disease, left shoulder   HCC
     M02.319   Reiter's disease, unspecified shoulder   HCC ▽

✓6ᵗʰ **M02.32**   Reiter's disease, elbow
     M02.321   Reiter's disease, right elbow   HCC
     M02.322   Reiter's disease, left elbow   HCC
     M02.329   Reiter's disease, unspecified elbow   HCC

✓6ᵗʰ **M02.33**   Reiter's disease, wrist
     Reiter's disease, carpal bones
     M02.331   Reiter's disease, right wrist   HCC
     M02.332   Reiter's disease, left wrist   HCC
     M02.339   Reiter's disease, unspecified wrist   HCC ▽

✓6ᵗʰ **M02.34**   Reiter's disease, hand
     Reiter's disease, metacarpus and phalanges
     M02.341   Reiter's disease, right hand   HCC
     M02.342   Reiter's disease, left hand   HCC
     M02.349   Reiter's disease, unspecified hand   HCC ▽

✓6ᵗʰ **M02.35**   Reiter's disease, hip
     M02.351   Reiter's disease, right hip   HCC
     M02.352   Reiter's disease, left hip   HCC
     M02.359   Reiter's disease, unspecified hip   HCC ▽

✓6ᵗʰ **M02.36**   Reiter's disease, knee
     M02.361   Reiter's disease, right knee   HCC
     M02.362   Reiter's disease, left knee   HCC
     M02.369   Reiter's disease, unspecified knee   HCC ▽

✓6ᵗʰ **M02.37**   Reiter's disease, ankle and foot
     Reiter's disease, tarsus, metatarsus and phalanges
     M02.371   Reiter's disease, right ankle and foot   HCC
     M02.372   Reiter's disease, left ankle and foot   HCC
     M02.379   Reiter's disease, unspecified ankle and foot   HCC ▽

    M02.38   Reiter's disease, vertebrae   HCC

EXCLUDES 1 Not coded here   EXCLUDES 2 Not included here   N Newborn Age: 0   P Pediatric Age: 0-17   M Maternity Age: 12-55   A Adult Age: 15-124

720   ICD-10-CM 2018

M02.39 Reiter's disease, multiple sites ☐HCC

✓5th **M02.8 Other reactive arthropathies**

   M02.80 Other reactive arthropathies, unspecified site HCC ▽

   ✓6th **M02.81 Other reactive arthropathies, shoulder**

     M02.811 Other reactive arthropathies, right shoulder HCC

     M02.812 Other reactive arthropathies, left shoulder HCC

     M02.819 Other reactive arthropathies, unspecified shoulder HCC ▽

   ✓6th **M02.82 Other reactive arthropathies, elbow**

     M02.821 Other reactive arthropathies, right elbow HCC

     M02.822 Other reactive arthropathies, left elbow HCC

     M02.829 Other reactive arthropathies, unspecified elbow HCC ▽

   ✓6th **M02.83 Other reactive arthropathies, wrist**

     Other reactive arthropathies, carpal bones

     M02.831 Other reactive arthropathies, right wrist HCC

     M02.832 Other reactive arthropathies, left wrist HCC

     M02.839 Other reactive arthropathies, unspecified wrist HCC ▽

   ✓6th **M02.84 Other reactive arthropathies, hand**

     Other reactive arthropathies, metacarpus and phalanges

     M02.841 Other reactive arthropathies, right hand HCC

     M02.842 Other reactive arthropathies, left hand HCC

     M02.849 Other reactive arthropathies, unspecified hand HCC ▽

   ✓6th **M02.85 Other reactive arthropathies, hip**

     M02.851 Other reactive arthropathies, right hip HCC

     M02.852 Other reactive arthropathies, left hip HCC

     M02.859 Other reactive arthropathies, unspecified hip HCC ▽

   ✓6th **M02.86 Other reactive arthropathies, knee**

     M02.861 Other reactive arthropathies, right knee HCC

     M02.862 Other reactive arthropathies, left knee HCC

     M02.869 Other reactive arthropathies, unspecified knee HCC ▽

   ✓6th **M02.87 Other reactive arthropathies, ankle and foot**

     Other reactive arthropathies, tarsus, metatarsus and phalanges

     M02.871 Other reactive arthropathies, right ankle and foot HCC

     M02.872 Other reactive arthropathies, left ankle and foot HCC

     M02.879 Other reactive arthropathies, unspecified ankle and foot HCC ▽

   M02.88 Other reactive arthropathies, vertebrae HCC

   M02.89 Other reactive arthropathies, multiple sites HCC

 M02.9 Reactive arthropathy, unspecified HCC ▽

Autoinflammatory syndromes (M04)

✓4th **M04 Autoinflammatory syndromes**

  EXCLUDES 2 *Crohn's disease (K50.-)*

 M04.1 Periodic fever syndromes HCC

    Familial Mediterranean fever

    Hyperimmunoglobin D syndrome

    Mevalonate kinase deficiency

    Tumor necrosis factor receptor associated periodic syndrome [TRAPS]

 M04.2 Cryopyrin-associated periodic syndromes HCC

    Chronic infantile neurological, cutaneous and articular syndrome [CINCA]

    Familial cold autoinflammatory syndrome

    Familial cold urticaria

    Muckle-Wells syndrome

    Neonatal onset multisystemic inflammatory disorder [NOMID]

 M04.8 Other autoinflammatory syndromes HCC

    Blau syndrome

    Deficiency of interleukin 1 receptor antagonist [DIRA]

    Majeed syndrome

    Periodic fever, aphthous stomatitis, pharyngitis, and adenopathy syndrome [PFAPA]

    Pyogenic arthritis, pyoderma gangrenosum, and acne syndrome [PAPA]

 M04.9 Autoinflammatory syndrome, unspecified HCC ▽

Inflammatory polyarthropathies (M05-M14)

✓4th **M05 Rheumatoid arthritis with rheumatoid factor**

  EXCLUDES 1 *rheumatic fever (I00)*

           juvenile rheumatoid arthritis (M08.-)

           rheumatoid arthritis of spine (M45.-)

  DEF: Autoimmune systemic disease that causes chronic inflammation of joints and other areas of the body, manifested by inflammatory changes in articular structures and synovial membranes, atrophy, and loss in bone density.

 ✓5th **M05.0 Felty's syndrome**

    Rheumatoid arthritis with splenoadenomegaly and leukopenia

   M05.00 Felty's syndrome, unspecified site HCC ▽

   ✓6th **M05.01 Felty's syndrome, shoulder**

     M05.011 Felty's syndrome, right shoulder HCC

     M05.012 Felty's syndrome, left shoulder HCC

     M05.019 Felty's syndrome, unspecified shoulder HCC ▽

   ✓6th **M05.02 Felty's syndrome, elbow**

     M05.021 Felty's syndrome, right elbow HCC

     M05.022 Felty's syndrome, left elbow HCC

     M05.029 Felty's syndrome, unspecified elbow HCC ▽

   ✓6th **M05.03 Felty's syndrome, wrist**

     Felty's syndrome, carpal bones

     M05.031 Felty's syndrome, right wrist HCC

     M05.032 Felty's syndrome, left wrist HCC

     M05.039 Felty's syndrome, unspecified wrist HCC ▽

   ✓6th **M05.04 Felty's syndrome, hand**

     Felty's syndrome, metacarpus and phalanges

     M05.041 Felty's syndrome, right hand HCC

     M05.042 Felty's syndrome, left hand HCC

     M05.049 Felty's syndrome, unspecified hand HCC ▽

   ✓6th **M05.05 Felty's syndrome, hip**

     M05.051 Felty's syndrome, right hip HCC

     M05.052 Felty's syndrome, left hip HCC

     M05.059 Felty's syndrome, unspecified hip HCC ▽

   ✓6th **M05.06 Felty's syndrome, knee**

     M05.061 Felty's syndrome, right knee HCC

     M05.062 Felty's syndrome, left knee HCC

     M05.069 Felty's syndrome, unspecified knee HCC ▽

   ✓6th **M05.07 Felty's syndrome, ankle and foot**

     Felty's syndrome, tarsus, metatarsus and phalanges

     M05.071 Felty's syndrome, right ankle and foot HCC

     M05.072 Felty's syndrome, left ankle and foot HCC

     M05.079 Felty's syndrome, unspecified ankle and foot HCC ▽

   M05.09 Felty's syndrome, multiple sites HCC

 ✓5th **M05.1 Rheumatoid lung disease with rheumatoid arthritis**

    DEF: Lung disorders associated with rheumatoid arthritis.

   M05.10 Rheumatoid lung disease with rheumatoid arthritis of unspecified site HCC ▽

   ✓6th **M05.11 Rheumatoid lung disease with rheumatoid arthritis of shoulder**

     M05.111 Rheumatoid lung disease with rheumatoid arthritis of right shoulder HCC

     M05.112 Rheumatoid lung disease with rheumatoid arthritis of left shoulder HCC

     M05.119 Rheumatoid lung disease with rheumatoid arthritis of unspecified shoulder HCC ▽

✓ Additional Character Req   ✓x7th Placeholder Alert   Manifestation   HCC CMS-HCC Condition   ▽ Unspecified Code   ►◄ Revised Text   ● New Code   ▲ Revised Code Title

ICD-10-CM 2018   721

Chapter 13. Diseases of the Musculoskeletal System and Connective Tissue

M05.12–M05.319

✓6ᵗʰ **M05.12 Rheumatoid lung disease with rheumatoid arthritis of elbow**
    M05.121 Rheumatoid lung disease with rheumatoid arthritis of right elbow `HCC`
    M05.122 Rheumatoid lung disease with rheumatoid arthritis of left elbow `HCC`
    M05.129 Rheumatoid lung disease with rheumatoid arthritis of unspecified elbow `HCC` ▽

✓6ᵗʰ **M05.13 Rheumatoid lung disease with rheumatoid arthritis of wrist**
    Rheumatoid lung disease with rheumatoid arthritis, carpal bones
    M05.131 Rheumatoid lung disease with rheumatoid arthritis of right wrist `HCC`
    M05.132 Rheumatoid lung disease with rheumatoid arthritis of left wrist `HCC`
    M05.139 Rheumatoid lung disease with rheumatoid arthritis of unspecified wrist `HCC` ▽

✓6ᵗʰ **M05.14 Rheumatoid lung disease with rheumatoid arthritis of hand**
    Rheumatoid lung disease with rheumatoid arthritis, metacarpus and phalanges
    M05.141 Rheumatoid lung disease with rheumatoid arthritis of right hand `HCC`
    M05.142 Rheumatoid lung disease with rheumatoid arthritis of left hand `HCC`
    M05.149 Rheumatoid lung disease with rheumatoid arthritis of unspecified hand `HCC` ▽

✓6ᵗʰ **M05.15 Rheumatoid lung disease with rheumatoid arthritis of hip**
    M05.151 Rheumatoid lung disease with rheumatoid arthritis of right hip `HCC`
    M05.152 Rheumatoid lung disease with rheumatoid arthritis of left hip `HCC`
    M05.159 Rheumatoid lung disease with rheumatoid arthritis of unspecified hip `HCC` ▽

✓6ᵗʰ **M05.16 Rheumatoid lung disease with rheumatoid arthritis of knee**
    M05.161 Rheumatoid lung disease with rheumatoid arthritis of right knee `HCC`
    M05.162 Rheumatoid lung disease with rheumatoid arthritis of left knee `HCC`
    M05.169 Rheumatoid lung disease with rheumatoid arthritis of unspecified knee `HCC` ▽

✓6ᵗʰ **M05.17 Rheumatoid lung disease with rheumatoid arthritis of ankle and foot**
    Rheumatoid lung disease with rheumatoid arthritis, tarsus, metatarsus and phalanges
    M05.171 Rheumatoid lung disease with rheumatoid arthritis of right ankle and foot `HCC`
    M05.172 Rheumatoid lung disease with rheumatoid arthritis of left ankle and foot `HCC`
    M05.179 Rheumatoid lung disease with rheumatoid arthritis of unspecified ankle and foot `HCC` ▽

M05.19 Rheumatoid lung disease with rheumatoid arthritis of multiple sites `HCC`

✓5ᵗʰ **M05.2 Rheumatoid vasculitis with rheumatoid arthritis**
    M05.20 Rheumatoid vasculitis with rheumatoid arthritis of unspecified site `HCC` ▽

✓6ᵗʰ **M05.21 Rheumatoid vasculitis with rheumatoid arthritis of shoulder**
    M05.211 Rheumatoid vasculitis with rheumatoid arthritis of right shoulder `HCC`
    M05.212 Rheumatoid vasculitis with rheumatoid arthritis of left shoulder `HCC`
    M05.219 Rheumatoid vasculitis with rheumatoid arthritis of unspecified shoulder `HCC` ▽

✓6ᵗʰ **M05.22 Rheumatoid vasculitis with rheumatoid arthritis of elbow**
    M05.221 Rheumatoid vasculitis with rheumatoid arthritis of right elbow `HCC`
    M05.222 Rheumatoid vasculitis with rheumatoid arthritis of left elbow `HCC`
    M05.229 Rheumatoid vasculitis with rheumatoid arthritis of unspecified elbow `HCC` ▽

✓6ᵗʰ **M05.23 Rheumatoid vasculitis with rheumatoid arthritis of wrist**
    Rheumatoid vasculitis with rheumatoid arthritis, carpal bones
    M05.231 Rheumatoid vasculitis with rheumatoid arthritis of right wrist `HCC`
    M05.232 Rheumatoid vasculitis with rheumatoid arthritis of left wrist `HCC`
    M05.239 Rheumatoid vasculitis with rheumatoid arthritis of unspecified wrist `HCC` ▽

✓6ᵗʰ **M05.24 Rheumatoid vasculitis with rheumatoid arthritis of hand**
    Rheumatoid vasculitis with rheumatoid arthritis, metacarpus and phalanges
    M05.241 Rheumatoid vasculitis with rheumatoid arthritis of right hand `HCC`
    M05.242 Rheumatoid vasculitis with rheumatoid arthritis of left hand `HCC`
    M05.249 Rheumatoid vasculitis with rheumatoid arthritis of unspecified hand `HCC` ▽

✓6ᵗʰ **M05.25 Rheumatoid vasculitis with rheumatoid arthritis of hip**
    M05.251 Rheumatoid vasculitis with rheumatoid arthritis of right hip `HCC`
    M05.252 Rheumatoid vasculitis with rheumatoid arthritis of left hip `HCC`
    M05.259 Rheumatoid vasculitis with rheumatoid arthritis of unspecified hip `HCC` ▽

✓6ᵗʰ **M05.26 Rheumatoid vasculitis with rheumatoid arthritis of knee**
    M05.261 Rheumatoid vasculitis with rheumatoid arthritis of right knee `HCC`
    M05.262 Rheumatoid vasculitis with rheumatoid arthritis of left knee `HCC`
    M05.269 Rheumatoid vasculitis with rheumatoid arthritis of unspecified knee `HCC` ▽

✓6ᵗʰ **M05.27 Rheumatoid vasculitis with rheumatoid arthritis of ankle and foot**
    Rheumatoid vasculitis with rheumatoid arthritis, tarsus, metatarsus and phalanges
    M05.271 Rheumatoid vasculitis with rheumatoid arthritis of right ankle and foot `HCC`
    M05.272 Rheumatoid vasculitis with rheumatoid arthritis of left ankle and foot `HCC`
    M05.279 Rheumatoid vasculitis with rheumatoid arthritis of unspecified ankle and foot `HCC` ▽

M05.29 Rheumatoid vasculitis with rheumatoid arthritis of multiple sites `HCC`

✓5ᵗʰ **M05.3 Rheumatoid heart disease with rheumatoid arthritis**
    Rheumatoid carditis   Rheumatoid myocarditis
    Rheumatoid endocarditis   Rheumatoid pericarditis
    M05.30 Rheumatoid heart disease with rheumatoid arthritis of unspecified site `HCC` ▽

✓6ᵗʰ **M05.31 Rheumatoid heart disease with rheumatoid arthritis of shoulder**
    M05.311 Rheumatoid heart disease with rheumatoid arthritis of right shoulder `HCC`
    M05.312 Rheumatoid heart disease with rheumatoid arthritis of left shoulder `HCC`
    M05.319 Rheumatoid heart disease with rheumatoid arthritis of unspecified shoulder `HCC` ▽

EXCLUDES1 Not coded here   **EXCLUDES2** Not included here   N Newborn Age: 0   P Pediatric Age: 0-17   M Maternity Age: 12-55   A Adult Age: 15-124

722   ICD-10-CM 2018

√6ᵗʰ **M05.32 Rheumatoid heart disease with rheumatoid arthritis of elbow**

     M05.321 Rheumatoid heart disease with rheumatoid arthritis of right elbow `HCC`

     M05.322 Rheumatoid heart disease with rheumatoid arthritis of left elbow `HCC`

     M05.329 Rheumatoid heart disease with rheumatoid arthritis of unspecified elbow `HCC` ▽

√6ᵗʰ **M05.33 Rheumatoid heart disease with rheumatoid arthritis of wrist**
     Rheumatoid heart disease with rheumatoid arthritis, carpal bones

     M05.331 Rheumatoid heart disease with rheumatoid arthritis of right wrist `HCC`

     M05.332 Rheumatoid heart disease with rheumatoid arthritis of left wrist `HCC`

     M05.339 Rheumatoid heart disease with rheumatoid arthritis of unspecified wrist `HCC` ▽

√6ᵗʰ **M05.34 Rheumatoid heart disease with rheumatoid arthritis of hand**
     Rheumatoid heart disease with rheumatoid arthritis, metacarpus and phalanges

     M05.341 Rheumatoid heart disease with rheumatoid arthritis of right hand `HCC`

     M05.342 Rheumatoid heart disease with rheumatoid arthritis of left hand `HCC`

     M05.349 Rheumatoid heart disease with rheumatoid arthritis of unspecified hand `HCC` ▽

√6ᵗʰ **M05.35 Rheumatoid heart disease with rheumatoid arthritis of hip**

     M05.351 Rheumatoid heart disease with rheumatoid arthritis of right hip `HCC`

     M05.352 Rheumatoid heart disease with rheumatoid arthritis of left hip `HCC`

     M05.359 Rheumatoid heart disease with rheumatoid arthritis of unspecified hip `HCC` ▽

√6ᵗʰ **M05.36 Rheumatoid heart disease with rheumatoid arthritis of knee**

     M05.361 Rheumatoid heart disease with rheumatoid arthritis of right knee `HCC`

     M05.362 Rheumatoid heart disease with rheumatoid arthritis of left knee `HCC`

     M05.369 Rheumatoid heart disease with rheumatoid arthritis of unspecified knee `HCC` ▽

√6ᵗʰ **M05.37 Rheumatoid heart disease with rheumatoid arthritis of ankle and foot**
     Rheumatoid heart disease with rheumatoid arthritis, tarsus, metatarsus and phalanges

     M05.371 Rheumatoid heart disease with rheumatoid arthritis of right ankle and foot `HCC`

     M05.372 Rheumatoid heart disease with rheumatoid arthritis of left ankle and foot `HCC`

     M05.379 Rheumatoid heart disease with rheumatoid arthritis of unspecified ankle and foot `HCC` ▽

     M05.39 Rheumatoid heart disease with rheumatoid arthritis of multiple sites `HCC`

√5ᵗʰ **M05.4 Rheumatoid myopathy with rheumatoid arthritis**

     M05.40 Rheumatoid myopathy with rheumatoid arthritis of unspecified site `HCC` ▽

√6ᵗʰ **M05.41 Rheumatoid myopathy with rheumatoid arthritis of shoulder**

     M05.411 Rheumatoid myopathy with rheumatoid arthritis of right shoulder `HCC`

     M05.412 Rheumatoid myopathy with rheumatoid arthritis of left shoulder `HCC`

     M05.419 Rheumatoid myopathy with rheumatoid arthritis of unspecified shoulder `HCC` ▽

√6ᵗʰ **M05.42 Rheumatoid myopathy with rheumatoid arthritis of elbow**

     M05.421 Rheumatoid myopathy with rheumatoid arthritis of right elbow `HCC`

     M05.422 Rheumatoid myopathy with rheumatoid arthritis of left elbow `HCC`

     M05.429 Rheumatoid myopathy with rheumatoid arthritis of unspecified elbow `HCC` ▽

√6ᵗʰ **M05.43 Rheumatoid myopathy with rheumatoid arthritis of wrist**
     Rheumatoid myopathy with rheumatoid arthritis, carpal bones

     M05.431 Rheumatoid myopathy with rheumatoid arthritis of right wrist `HCC`

     M05.432 Rheumatoid myopathy with rheumatoid arthritis of left wrist `HCC`

     M05.439 Rheumatoid myopathy with rheumatoid arthritis of unspecified wrist `HCC` ▽

√6ᵗʰ **M05.44 Rheumatoid myopathy with rheumatoid arthritis of hand**
     Rheumatoid myopathy with rheumatoid arthritis, metacarpus and phalanges

     M05.441 Rheumatoid myopathy with rheumatoid arthritis of right hand `HCC`

     M05.442 Rheumatoid myopathy with rheumatoid arthritis of left hand `HCC`

     M05.449 Rheumatoid myopathy with rheumatoid arthritis of unspecified hand `HCC` ▽

√6ᵗʰ **M05.45 Rheumatoid myopathy with rheumatoid arthritis of hip**

     M05.451 Rheumatoid myopathy with rheumatoid arthritis of right hip `HCC`

     M05.452 Rheumatoid myopathy with rheumatoid arthritis of left hip `HCC`

     M05.459 Rheumatoid myopathy with rheumatoid arthritis of unspecified hip `HCC` ▽

√6ᵗʰ **M05.46 Rheumatoid myopathy with rheumatoid arthritis of knee**

     M05.461 Rheumatoid myopathy with rheumatoid arthritis of right knee `HCC`

     M05.462 Rheumatoid myopathy with rheumatoid arthritis of left knee `HCC`

     M05.469 Rheumatoid myopathy with rheumatoid arthritis of unspecified knee `HCC` ▽

√6ᵗʰ **M05.47 Rheumatoid myopathy with rheumatoid arthritis of ankle and foot**
     Rheumatoid myopathy with rheumatoid arthritis, tarsus, metatarsus and phalanges

     M05.471 Rheumatoid myopathy with rheumatoid arthritis of right ankle and foot `HCC`

     M05.472 Rheumatoid myopathy with rheumatoid arthritis of left ankle and foot `HCC`

     M05.479 Rheumatoid myopathy with rheumatoid arthritis of unspecified ankle and foot `HCC` ▽

     M05.49 Rheumatoid myopathy with rheumatoid arthritis of multiple sites `HCC`

√5ᵗʰ **M05.5 Rheumatoid polyneuropathy with rheumatoid arthritis**

     M05.50 Rheumatoid polyneuropathy with rheumatoid arthritis of unspecified site `HCC` ▽

√6ᵗʰ **M05.51 Rheumatoid polyneuropathy with rheumatoid arthritis of shoulder**

     M05.511 Rheumatoid polyneuropathy with rheumatoid arthritis of right shoulder `HCC`

     M05.512 Rheumatoid polyneuropathy with rheumatoid arthritis of left shoulder `HCC`

     M05.519 Rheumatoid polyneuropathy with rheumatoid arthritis of unspecified shoulder `HCC` ▽

☑ Additional Character Req   ⑦ Placeholder Alert   Manifestation   `HCC` CMS-HCC Condition   ▽ Unspecified Code   ►◄ Revised Text   ● New Code   ▲ Revised Code Title

✓6th **M05.52 Rheumatoid polyneuropathy with rheumatoid arthritis of elbow**

    M05.521 Rheumatoid polyneuropathy with rheumatoid arthritis of right elbow HCC

    M05.522 Rheumatoid polyneuropathy with rheumatoid arthritis of left elbow HCC

    M05.529 Rheumatoid polyneuropathy with rheumatoid arthritis of unspecified elbow HCC ▽

✓6th **M05.53 Rheumatoid polyneuropathy with rheumatoid arthritis of wrist**

Rheumatoid polyneuropathy with rheumatoid arthritis, carpal bones

    M05.531 Rheumatoid polyneuropathy with rheumatoid arthritis of right wrist HCC

    M05.532 Rheumatoid polyneuropathy with rheumatoid arthritis of left wrist HCC

    M05.539 Rheumatoid polyneuropathy with rheumatoid arthritis of unspecified wrist HCC ▽

✓6th **M05.54 Rheumatoid polyneuropathy with rheumatoid arthritis of hand**

Rheumatoid polyneuropathy with rheumatoid arthritis, metacarpus and phalanges

    M05.541 Rheumatoid polyneuropathy with rheumatoid arthritis of right hand HCC

    M05.542 Rheumatoid polyneuropathy with rheumatoid arthritis of left hand HCC

    M05.549 Rheumatoid polyneuropathy with rheumatoid arthritis of unspecified hand HCC ▽

✓6th **M05.55 Rheumatoid polyneuropathy with rheumatoid arthritis of hip**

    M05.551 Rheumatoid polyneuropathy with rheumatoid arthritis of right hip HCC

    M05.552 Rheumatoid polyneuropathy with rheumatoid arthritis of left hip HCC

    M05.559 Rheumatoid polyneuropathy with rheumatoid arthritis of unspecified hip HCC ▽

✓6th **M05.56 Rheumatoid polyneuropathy with rheumatoid arthritis of knee**

    M05.561 Rheumatoid polyneuropathy with rheumatoid arthritis of right knee HCC

    M05.562 Rheumatoid polyneuropathy with rheumatoid arthritis of left knee HCC

    M05.569 Rheumatoid polyneuropathy with rheumatoid arthritis of unspecified knee HCC ▽

✓6th **M05.57 Rheumatoid polyneuropathy with rheumatoid arthritis of ankle and foot**

Rheumatoid polyneuropathy with rheumatoid arthritis, tarsus, metatarsus and phalanges

    M05.571 Rheumatoid polyneuropathy with rheumatoid arthritis of right ankle and foot HCC

    M05.572 Rheumatoid polyneuropathy with rheumatoid arthritis of left ankle and foot HCC

    M05.579 Rheumatoid polyneuropathy with rheumatoid arthritis of unspecified ankle and foot HCC ▽

    M05.59 Rheumatoid polyneuropathy with rheumatoid arthritis of multiple sites HCC

✓5th **M05.6 Rheumatoid arthritis with involvement of other organs and systems**

    M05.60 Rheumatoid arthritis of unspecified site with involvement of other organs and systems HCC ▽

✓6th **M05.61 Rheumatoid arthritis of shoulder with involvement of other organs and systems**

    M05.611 Rheumatoid arthritis of right shoulder with involvement of other organs and systems HCC

    M05.612 Rheumatoid arthritis of left shoulder with involvement of other organs and systems HCC

    M05.619 Rheumatoid arthritis of unspecified shoulder with involvement of other organs and systems HCC ▽

✓6th **M05.62 Rheumatoid arthritis of elbow with involvement of other organs and systems**

    M05.621 Rheumatoid arthritis of right elbow with involvement of other organs and systems HCC

    M05.622 Rheumatoid arthritis of left elbow with involvement of other organs and systems HCC

    M05.629 Rheumatoid arthritis of unspecified elbow with involvement of other organs and systems HCC ▽

✓6th **M05.63 Rheumatoid arthritis of wrist with involvement of other organs and systems**

Rheumatoid arthritis of carpal bones with involvement of other organs and systems

    M05.631 Rheumatoid arthritis of right wrist with involvement of other organs and systems HCC

    M05.632 Rheumatoid arthritis of left wrist with involvement of other organs and systems HCC

    M05.639 Rheumatoid arthritis of unspecified wrist with involvement of other organs and systems HCC ▽

✓6th **M05.64 Rheumatoid arthritis of hand with involvement of other organs and systems**

Rheumatoid arthritis of metacarpus and phalanges with involvement of other organs and systems

    M05.641 Rheumatoid arthritis of right hand with involvement of other organs and systems HCC

    M05.642 Rheumatoid arthritis of left hand with involvement of other organs and systems HCC

    M05.649 Rheumatoid arthritis of unspecified hand with involvement of other organs and systems HCC ▽

✓6th **M05.65 Rheumatoid arthritis of hip with involvement of other organs and systems**

    M05.651 Rheumatoid arthritis of right hip with involvement of other organs and systems HCC

    M05.652 Rheumatoid arthritis of left hip with involvement of other organs and systems HCC

    M05.659 Rheumatoid arthritis of unspecified hip with involvement of other organs and systems HCC ▽

✓6th **M05.66 Rheumatoid arthritis of knee with involvement of other organs and systems**

    M05.661 Rheumatoid arthritis of right knee with involvement of other organs and systems HCC

    M05.662 Rheumatoid arthritis of left knee with involvement of other organs and systems HCC

    M05.669 Rheumatoid arthritis of unspecified knee with involvement of other organs and systems HCC ▽

✓6th **M05.67 Rheumatoid arthritis of ankle and foot with involvement of other organs and systems**

Rheumatoid arthritis of tarsus, metatarsus and phalanges with involvement of other organs and systems

    M05.671 Rheumatoid arthritis of right ankle and foot with involvement of other organs and systems HCC

    M05.672 Rheumatoid arthritis of left ankle and foot with involvement of other organs and systems HCC

    M05.679 Rheumatoid arthritis of unspecified ankle and foot with involvement of other organs and systems HCC ▽

    M05.69 Rheumatoid arthritis of multiple sites with involvement of other organs and systems HCC

✓5th **M05.7 Rheumatoid arthritis with rheumatoid factor without organ or systems involvement**

    M05.70 Rheumatoid arthritis with rheumatoid factor of unspecified site without organ or systems involvement HCC ▽

EXCLUDES 1 Not coded here   EXCLUDES 2 Not included here   N Newborn Age: 0   P Pediatric Age: 0-17   M Maternity Age: 12-55   A Adult Age: 15-124

✓6ᵗʰ **M05.71** Rheumatoid arthritis with rheumatoid factor of shoulder without organ or systems involvement

M05.711 Rheumatoid arthritis with rheumatoid factor of right shoulder without organ or systems involvement   HCC

M05.712 Rheumatoid arthritis with rheumatoid factor of left shoulder without organ or systems involvement   HCC

M05.719 Rheumatoid arthritis with rheumatoid factor of unspecified shoulder without organ or systems involvement   HCC ▽

✓6ᵗʰ **M05.72** Rheumatoid arthritis with rheumatoid factor of elbow without organ or systems involvement

M05.721 Rheumatoid arthritis with rheumatoid factor of right elbow without organ or systems involvement   HCC

M05.722 Rheumatoid arthritis with rheumatoid factor of left elbow without organ or systems involvement   HCC

M05.729 Rheumatoid arthritis with rheumatoid factor of unspecified elbow without organ or systems involvement   HCC ▽

✓6ᵗʰ **M05.73** Rheumatoid arthritis with rheumatoid factor of wrist without organ or systems involvement

M05.731 Rheumatoid arthritis with rheumatoid factor of right wrist without organ or systems involvement   HCC

M05.732 Rheumatoid arthritis with rheumatoid factor of left wrist without organ or systems involvement   HCC

M05.739 Rheumatoid arthritis with rheumatoid factor of unspecified wrist without organ or systems involvement   HCC ▽

✓6ᵗʰ **M05.74** Rheumatoid arthritis with rheumatoid factor of hand without organ or systems involvement

M05.741 Rheumatoid arthritis with rheumatoid factor of right hand without organ or systems involvement   HCC

M05.742 Rheumatoid arthritis with rheumatoid factor of left hand without organ or systems involvement   HCC

M05.749 Rheumatoid arthritis with factor of rheumatoid unspecified hand without organ or systems involvement   HCC ▽

✓6ᵗʰ **M05.75** Rheumatoid arthritis with rheumatoid factor of hip without organ or systems involvement

M05.751 Rheumatoid arthritis with rheumatoid factor of right hip without organ or systems involvement   HCC

M05.752 Rheumatoid arthritis with rheumatoid factor of left hip without organ or systems involvement   HCC

M05.759 Rheumatoid arthritis with rheumatoid factor of unspecified hip without organ or systems involvement   HCC ▽

✓6ᵗʰ **M05.76** Rheumatoid arthritis with rheumatoid factor of knee without organ or systems involvement

M05.761 Rheumatoid arthritis with rheumatoid factor of right knee without organ or systems involvement   HCC

M05.762 Rheumatoid arthritis with rheumatoid factor of left knee without organ or systems involvement   HCC

M05.769 Rheumatoid arthritis with rheumatoidfactor of unspecified knee without organ or systems involvement   HCC ▽

✓6ᵗʰ **M05.77** Rheumatoid arthritis with rheumatoid factor of ankle and foot without organ or systems involvement

M05.771 Rheumatoid arthritis with rheumatoid factor of right ankle and foot without organ or systems involvement   HCC

M05.772 Rheumatoid arthritis with rheumatoid factor of left ankle and foot without organ or systems involvement   HCC

M05.779 Rheumatoid arthritis with rheumatoid factor of unspecified ankle and foot without organ or systems involvement   HCC ▽

M05.79 Rheumatoid arthritis with rheumatoid factor of multiple sites without organ or systems involvement   HCC

✓5ᵗʰ **M05.8** Other rheumatoid arthritis with rheumatoid factor

M05.80 Other rheumatoid arthritis with rheumatoid factor of unspecified site   HCC ▽

✓6ᵗʰ **M05.81** Other rheumatoid arthritis with rheumatoid factor of shoulder

M05.811 Other rheumatoid arthritis with rheumatoid factor of right shoulder   HCC

M05.812 Other rheumatoid arthritis with rheumatoid factor of left shoulder   HCC

M05.819 Other rheumatoid arthritis with rheumatoid factor of unspecified shoulder   HCC ▽

✓6ᵗʰ **M05.82** Other rheumatoid arthritis with rheumatoid factor of elbow

M05.821 Other rheumatoid arthritis with rheumatoid factor of right elbow   HCC

M05.822 Other rheumatoid arthritis with rheumatoid factor of left elbow   HCC

M05.829 Other rheumatoid arthritis with rheumatoid factor of unspecified elbow   HCC ▽

✓6ᵗʰ **M05.83** Other rheumatoid arthritis with rheumatoid factor of wrist

M05.831 Other rheumatoid arthritis with rheumatoid factor of right wrist   HCC

M05.832 Other rheumatoid arthritis with rheumatoid factor of left wrist   HCC

M05.839 Other rheumatoid arthritis with rheumatoid factor of unspecified wrist   HCC ▽

✓6ᵗʰ **M05.84** Other rheumatoid arthritis with rheumatoid factor of hand

M05.841 Other rheumatoid arthritis with rheumatoid factor of right hand   HCC

M05.842 Other rheumatoid arthritis with rheumatoid factor of left hand   HCC

M05.849 Other rheumatoid arthritis with rheumatoid factor of unspecified hand   HCC ▽

✓6ᵗʰ **M05.85** Other rheumatoid arthritis with rheumatoid factor of hip

M05.851 Other rheumatoid arthritis with rheumatoid factor of right hip   HCC

M05.852 Other rheumatoid arthritis with rheumatoid factor of left hip   HCC

M05.859 Other rheumatoid arthritis with rheumatoid factor of unspecified hip   HCC ▽

✓6ᵗʰ **M05.86** Other rheumatoid arthritis with rheumatoid factor of knee

M05.861 Other rheumatoid arthritis with rheumatoid factor of right knee   HCC

M05.862 Other rheumatoid arthritis with rheumatoid factor of left knee   HCC

M05.869 Other rheumatoid arthritis with rheumatoid factor of unspecified knee   HCC ▽

✓6ᵗʰ **M05.87** Other rheumatoid arthritis with rheumatoid factor of ankle and foot

M05.871 Other rheumatoid arthritis with rheumatoid factor of right ankle and foot   HCC

M05.872 Other rheumatoid arthritis with rheumatoid factor of left ankle and foot   HCC

M05.879 Other rheumatoid arthritis with rheumatoid factor of unspecified ankle and foot   HCC ▽

M05.89 Other rheumatoid arthritis with rheumatoid factor of multiple sites   HCC

M05.9 Rheumatoid arthritis with rheumatoid factor, unspecified   HCC ▽

✓4ᵗʰ **M06** **Other rheumatoid arthritis**

DEF: Autoimmune systemic disease that causes chronic inflammation of joints and other areas of the body, manifested by inflammatory changes in articular structures and synovial membranes, atrophy, and loss in bone density.

✓5ᵗʰ **M06.0** Rheumatoid arthritis without rheumatoid factor

M06.00 Rheumatoid arthritis without rheumatoid factor, unspecified site   HCC ▽

✓ Additional Character Req   ✓x7ᵗʰ Placeholder Alert   Manifestation   HCC CMS-HCC Condition   ▽ Unspecified Code   ▶◀ Revised Text   ● New Code   ▲ Revised Code Title

ICD-10-CM 2018   725

✓6ᵗʰ **M06.01 Rheumatoid arthritis without rheumatoid factor, shoulder**
- **M06.011 Rheumatoid arthritis without rheumatoid factor, right shoulder** HCC
- **M06.012 Rheumatoid arthritis without rheumatoid factor, left shoulder** HCC
- **M06.019 Rheumatoid arthritis without rheumatoid factor, unspecified shoulder** HCC ▽

✓6ᵗʰ **M06.02 Rheumatoid arthritis without rheumatoid factor, elbow**
- **M06.021 Rheumatoid arthritis without rheumatoid factor, right elbow** HCC
- **M06.022 Rheumatoid arthritis without rheumatoid factor, left elbow** HCC
- **M06.029 Rheumatoid arthritis without rheumatoid factor, unspecified elbow** HCC ▽

✓6ᵗʰ **M06.03 Rheumatoid arthritis without rheumatoid factor, wrist**
- **M06.031 Rheumatoid arthritis without rheumatoid factor, right wrist** HCC
- **M06.032 Rheumatoid arthritis without rheumatoid factor, left wrist** HCC
- **M06.039 Rheumatoid arthritis without rheumatoid factor, unspecified wrist** HCC ▽

✓6ᵗʰ **M06.04 Rheumatoid arthritis without rheumatoid factor, hand**
- **M06.041 Rheumatoid arthritis without rheumatoid factor, right hand** HCC
- **M06.042 Rheumatoid arthritis without rheumatoid factor, left hand** HCC
- **M06.049 Rheumatoid arthritis without rheumatoid factor, unspecified hand** HCC ▽

✓6ᵗʰ **M06.05 Rheumatoid arthritis without rheumatoid factor, hip**
- **M06.051 Rheumatoid arthritis without rheumatoid factor, right hip** HCC
- **M06.052 Rheumatoid arthritis without rheumatoid factor, left hip** HCC
- **M06.059 Rheumatoid arthritis without rheumatoid factor, unspecified hip** HCC ▽

✓6ᵗʰ **M06.06 Rheumatoid arthritis without rheumatoid factor, knee**
- **M06.061 Rheumatoid arthritis without rheumatoid factor, right knee** HCC
- **M06.062 Rheumatoid arthritis without rheumatoid factor, left knee** HCC
- **M06.069 Rheumatoid arthritis without rheumatoid factor, unspecified knee** HCC ▽

✓6ᵗʰ **M06.07 Rheumatoid arthritis without rheumatoid factor, ankle and foot**
- **M06.071 Rheumatoid arthritis without rheumatoid factor, right ankle and foot** HCC
- **M06.072 Rheumatoid arthritis without rheumatoid factor, left ankle and foot** HCC
- **M06.079 Rheumatoid arthritis without rheumatoid factor, unspecified ankle and foot** HCC ▽

M06.08 Rheumatoid arthritis without rheumatoid factor, vertebrae HCC

M06.09 Rheumatoid arthritis without rheumatoid factor, multiple sites HCC

M06.1 Adult-onset Still's disease HCC Ⓐ
> *EXCLUDES 1*   Still's disease NOS (M08.2-)

✓5ᵗʰ **M06.2 Rheumatoid bursitis**
- **M06.20 Rheumatoid bursitis, unspecified site** HCC ▽
- ✓6ᵗʰ **M06.21 Rheumatoid bursitis, shoulder**
  - **M06.211 Rheumatoid bursitis, right shoulder** HCC
  - **M06.212 Rheumatoid bursitis, left shoulder** HCC
  - **M06.219 Rheumatoid bursitis, unspecified shoulder** HCC ▽
- ✓6ᵗʰ **M06.22 Rheumatoid bursitis, elbow**
  - **M06.221 Rheumatoid bursitis, right elbow** HCC
  - **M06.222 Rheumatoid bursitis, left elbow** HCC
  - **M06.229 Rheumatoid bursitis, unspecified elbow** HCC ▽

✓6ᵗʰ **M06.23 Rheumatoid bursitis, wrist**
- **M06.231 Rheumatoid bursitis, right wrist** HCC
- **M06.232 Rheumatoid bursitis, left wrist** HCC
- **M06.239 Rheumatoid bursitis, unspecified wrist** HCC ▽

✓6ᵗʰ **M06.24 Rheumatoid bursitis, hand**
- **M06.241 Rheumatoid bursitis, right hand** HCC
- **M06.242 Rheumatoid bursitis, left hand** HCC
- **M06.249 Rheumatoid bursitis, unspecified hand** HCC ▽

✓6ᵗʰ **M06.25 Rheumatoid bursitis, hip**
- **M06.251 Rheumatoid bursitis, right hip** HCC
- **M06.252 Rheumatoid bursitis, left hip** HCC
- **M06.259 Rheumatoid bursitis, unspecified hip** HCC ▽

✓6ᵗʰ **M06.26 Rheumatoid bursitis, knee**
- **M06.261 Rheumatoid bursitis, right knee** HCC
- **M06.262 Rheumatoid bursitis, left knee** HCC
- **M06.269 Rheumatoid bursitis, unspecified knee** HCC ▽

✓6ᵗʰ **M06.27 Rheumatoid bursitis, ankle and foot**
- **M06.271 Rheumatoid bursitis, right ankle and foot** HCC
- **M06.272 Rheumatoid bursitis, left ankle and foot** HCC
- **M06.279 Rheumatoid bursitis, unspecified ankle and foot** HCC ▽

M06.28 Rheumatoid bursitis, vertebrae HCC

M06.29 Rheumatoid bursitis, multiple sites HCC

✓5ᵗʰ **M06.3 Rheumatoid nodule**
- **M06.30 Rheumatoid nodule, unspecified site** HCC ▽
- ✓6ᵗʰ **M06.31 Rheumatoid nodule, shoulder**
  - **M06.311 Rheumatoid nodule, right shoulder** HCC
  - **M06.312 Rheumatoid nodule, left shoulder** HCC
  - **M06.319 Rheumatoid nodule, unspecified shoulder** HCC ▽
- ✓6ᵗʰ **M06.32 Rheumatoid nodule, elbow**
  - **M06.321 Rheumatoid nodule, right elbow** HCC
  - **M06.322 Rheumatoid nodule, left elbow** HCC
  - **M06.329 Rheumatoid nodule, unspecified elbow** HCC ▽
- ✓6ᵗʰ **M06.33 Rheumatoid nodule, wrist**
  - **M06.331 Rheumatoid nodule, right wrist** HCC
  - **M06.332 Rheumatoid nodule, left wrist** HCC
  - **M06.339 Rheumatoid nodule, unspecified wrist** HCC ▽
- ✓6ᵗʰ **M06.34 Rheumatoid nodule, hand**
  - **M06.341 Rheumatoid nodule, right hand** HCC
  - **M06.342 Rheumatoid nodule, left hand** HCC
  - **M06.349 Rheumatoid nodule, unspecified hand** HCC ▽
- ✓6ᵗʰ **M06.35 Rheumatoid nodule, hip**
  - **M06.351 Rheumatoid nodule, right hip** HCC
  - **M06.352 Rheumatoid nodule, left hip** HCC
  - **M06.359 Rheumatoid nodule, unspecified hip** HCC ▽
- ✓6ᵗʰ **M06.36 Rheumatoid nodule, knee**
  - **M06.361 Rheumatoid nodule, right knee** HCC
  - **M06.362 Rheumatoid nodule, left knee** HCC
  - **M06.369 Rheumatoid nodule, unspecified knee** HCC ▽
- ✓6ᵗʰ **M06.37 Rheumatoid nodule, ankle and foot**
  - **M06.371 Rheumatoid nodule, right ankle and foot** HCC
  - **M06.372 Rheumatoid nodule, left ankle and foot** HCC
  - **M06.379 Rheumatoid nodule, unspecified and ankle foot** HCC ▽

M06.38 Rheumatoid nodule, vertebrae HCC

M06.39 Rheumatoid nodule, multiple sites HCC

M06.4 Inflammatory polyarthropathy
> *EXCLUDES 1*   polyarthritis NOS (M13.0)

EXCLUDES 1 Not coded here   *EXCLUDES 2* Not included here   Ⓝ Newborn Age: 0   Ⓟ Pediatric Age: 0-17   Ⓜ Maternity Age: 12-55   Ⓐ Adult Age: 15-124

726   ICD-10-CM 2018

✓5th **M06.8 Other specified rheumatoid arthritis**

    M06.80 Other specified rheumatoid arthritis, unspecified site HCC ▽

    ✓6th **M06.81 Other specified rheumatoid arthritis, shoulder**

       M06.811 Other specified rheumatoid arthritis, right shoulder HCC

       M06.812 Other specified rheumatoid arthritis, left shoulder HCC

       M06.819 Other specified rheumatoid arthritis, unspecified shoulder HCC ▽

    ✓6th **M06.82 Other specified rheumatoid arthritis, elbow**

       M06.821 Other specified rheumatoid arthritis, right elbow HCC

       M06.822 Other specified rheumatoid arthritis, left elbow HCC

       M06.829 Other specified rheumatoid arthritis, unspecified elbow HCC ▽

    ✓6th **M06.83 Other specified rheumatoid arthritis, wrist**

       M06.831 Other specified rheumatoid arthritis, right wrist HCC

       M06.832 Other specified rheumatoid arthritis, left wrist HCC

       M06.839 Other specified rheumatoid arthritis, unspecified wrist HCC ▽

    ✓6th **M06.84 Other specified rheumatoid arthritis, hand**

       M06.841 Other specified rheumatoid arthritis, right hand HCC

       M06.842 Other specified rheumatoid arthritis, left hand HCC

       M06.849 Other specified rheumatoid arthritis, unspecified hand HCC ▽

    ✓6th **M06.85 Other specified rheumatoid arthritis, hip**

       M06.851 Other specified rheumatoid arthritis, right hip HCC

       M06.852 Other specified rheumatoid arthritis, left hip HCC

       M06.859 Other specified rheumatoid arthritis, unspecified hip HCC ▽

    ✓6th **M06.86 Other specified rheumatoid arthritis, knee**

       M06.861 Other specified rheumatoid arthritis, right knee HCC

       M06.862 Other specified rheumatoid arthritis, left knee HCC

       M06.869 Other specified rheumatoid arthritis, unspecified knee HCC ▽

    ✓6th **M06.87 Other specified rheumatoid arthritis, ankle and foot**

       M06.871 Other specified rheumatoid arthritis, right ankle and foot HCC

       M06.872 Other specified rheumatoid arthritis, left ankle and foot HCC

       M06.879 Other specified rheumatoid arthritis, unspecified ankle and foot HCC ▽

    M06.88 Other specified rheumatoid arthritis, vertebrae HCC

    M06.89 Other specified rheumatoid arthritis, multiple sites HCC

M06.9 Rheumatoid arthritis, unspecified HCC ▽

DEF: Autoimmune systemic disease that causes chronic inflammation of joints and other areas of the body, manifested by inflammatory changes in articular structures and synovial membranes, atrophy, and loss in bone density.

✓4th **M07 Enteropathic arthropathies**

Code also associated enteropathy, such as:
    regional enteritis [Crohn's disease] (K50.-)
    ulcerative colitis (K51.-)
    EXCLUDES 1   psoriatic arthropathies (L40.5-)

✓5th **M07.6 Enteropathic arthropathies**

    M07.60 Enteropathic arthropathies, unspecified site ▽

    ✓6th **M07.61 Enteropathic arthropathies, shoulder**

       M07.611 Enteropathic arthropathies, right shoulder

       M07.612 Enteropathic arthropathies, left shoulder

       M07.619 Enteropathic arthropathies, unspecified shoulder ▽

    ✓6th **M07.62 Enteropathic arthropathies, elbow**

       M07.621 Enteropathic arthropathies, right elbow

       M07.622 Enteropathic arthropathies, left elbow

       M07.629 Enteropathic arthropathies, unspecified elbow ▽

    ✓6th **M07.63 Enteropathic arthropathies, wrist**

       M07.631 Enteropathic arthropathies, right wrist

       M07.632 Enteropathic arthropathies, left wrist

       M07.639 Enteropathic arthropathies, unspecified wrist ▽

    ✓6th **M07.64 Enteropathic arthropathies, hand**

       M07.641 Enteropathic arthropathies, right hand

       M07.642 Enteropathic arthropathies, left hand

       M07.649 Enteropathic arthropathies, unspecified hand ▽

    ✓6th **M07.65 Enteropathic arthropathies, hip**

       M07.651 Enteropathic arthropathies, right hip

       M07.652 Enteropathic arthropathies, left hip

       M07.659 Enteropathic arthropathies, unspecified hip ▽

    ✓6th **M07.66 Enteropathic arthropathies, knee**

       M07.661 Enteropathic arthropathies, right knee

       M07.662 Enteropathic arthropathies, left knee

       M07.669 Enteropathic arthropathies, unspecified knee ▽

    ✓6th **M07.67 Enteropathic arthropathies, ankle and foot**

       M07.671 Enteropathic arthropathies, right ankle and foot

       M07.672 Enteropathic arthropathies, left ankle and foot

       M07.679 Enteropathic arthropathies, unspecified ankle and foot ▽

    M07.68 Enteropathic arthropathies, vertebrae

    M07.69 Enteropathic arthropathies, multiple sites

✓4th **M08 Juvenile arthritis**

Code also any associated underlying condition, such as:
    regional enteritis [Crohn's disease] (K50.-)
    ulcerative colitis (K51.-)
    EXCLUDES 1   arthropathy in Whipple's disease (M14.8)
           Felty's syndrome (M05.0)
           juvenile dermatomyositis (M33.0-)
           psoriatic juvenile arthropathy (L40.54)

✓5th **M08.0 Unspecified juvenile rheumatoid arthritis**

Juvenile rheumatoid arthritis with or without rheumatoid factor

    M08.00 Unspecified juvenile rheumatoid arthritis of unspecified site HCC ▽

    ✓6th **M08.01 Unspecified juvenile rheumatoid arthritis, shoulder**

       M08.011 Unspecified juvenile rheumatoid arthritis, right shoulder HCC ▽

       M08.012 Unspecified juvenile rheumatoid arthritis, left shoulder HCC ▽

       M08.019 Unspecified juvenile rheumatoid arthritis, unspecified shoulder HCC ▽

    ✓6th **M08.02 Unspecified juvenile rheumatoid arthritis of elbow**

       M08.021 Unspecified juvenile rheumatoid arthritis, right elbow HCC ▽

       M08.022 Unspecified juvenile rheumatoid arthritis, left elbow HCC ▽

       M08.029 Unspecified juvenile rheumatoid arthritis, unspecified elbow HCC ▽

    ✓6th **M08.03 Unspecified juvenile rheumatoid arthritis, wrist**

       M08.031 Unspecified juvenile rheumatoid arthritis, right wrist HCC ▽

       M08.032 Unspecified juvenile rheumatoid arthritis, left wrist HCC ▽

       M08.039 Unspecified juvenile rheumatoid arthritis, unspecified wrist HCC ▽

    ✓6th **M08.04 Unspecified juvenile rheumatoid arthritis, hand**

       M08.041 Unspecified juvenile rheumatoid arthritis, right hand HCC ▽

       M08.042 Unspecified juvenile rheumatoid arthritis, left hand HCC ▽

       M08.049 Unspecified juvenile rheumatoid arthritis, unspecified hand HCC ▽

    ✓6th **M08.05 Unspecified juvenile rheumatoid arthritis, hip**

       M08.051 Unspecified juvenile rheumatoid arthritis, right hip HCC ▽

✓ Additional Character Req   ✓x7th Placeholder Alert   Manifestation   HCC CMS-HCC Condition   ▽ Unspecified Code   ▶◀ Revised Text   ● New Code   ▲ Revised Code Title

ICD-10-CM 2018   727

M08.052 Unspecified juvenile rheumatoid arthritis, left hip HCC ▽

M08.059 Unspecified juvenile rheumatoid arthritis, unspecified hip HCC ▽

✓6ᵗʰ M08.06 Unspecified juvenile rheumatoid arthritis, knee

M08.061 Unspecified juvenile rheumatoid arthritis, right knee HCC ▽

M08.062 Unspecified juvenile rheumatoid arthritis, left knee HCC ▽

M08.069 Unspecified juvenile rheumatoid arthritis, unspecified knee HCC ▽

✓6ᵗʰ M08.07 Unspecified juvenile rheumatoid arthritis, ankle and foot

M08.071 Unspecified juvenile rheumatoid arthritis, right ankle and foot HCC ▽

M08.072 Unspecified juvenile rheumatoid arthritis, left ankle and foot HCC ▽

M08.079 Unspecified juvenile rheumatoid arthritis, unspecified ankle and foot HCC ▽

M08.08 Unspecified juvenile rheumatoid arthritis, vertebrae HCC ▽

M08.09 Unspecified juvenile rheumatoid arthritis, multiple sites HCC ▽

M08.1 Juvenile ankylosing spondylitis HCC

> EXCLUDES 1 ankylosing spondylitis in adults (M45.0-)

✓5ᵗʰ M08.2 Juvenile rheumatoid arthritis with systemic onset

Still's disease NOS

> EXCLUDES 1 adult-onset Still's disease (M06.1-)

M08.20 Juvenile rheumatoid arthritis with systemic onset, unspecified site HCC ▽

✓6ᵗʰ M08.21 Juvenile rheumatoid arthritis with systemic onset, shoulder

M08.211 Juvenile rheumatoid arthritis with systemic onset, right shoulder HCC

M08.212 Juvenile rheumatoid arthritis with systemic onset, left shoulder HCC

M08.219 Juvenile rheumatoid arthritis with systemic onset, unspecified shoulder HCC ▽

✓6ᵗʰ M08.22 Juvenile rheumatoid arthritis with systemic onset, elbow

M08.221 Juvenile rheumatoid arthritis with systemic onset, right elbow HCC

M08.222 Juvenile rheumatoid arthritis with systemic onset, left elbow HCC

M08.229 Juvenile rheumatoid arthritis with systemic onset, unspecified elbow HCC ▽

✓6ᵗʰ M08.23 Juvenile rheumatoid arthritis with systemic onset, wrist

M08.231 Juvenile rheumatoid arthritis with systemic onset, right wrist HCC

M08.232 Juvenile rheumatoid arthritis with systemic onset, left wrist HCC

M08.239 Juvenile rheumatoid arthritis with systemic onset, unspecified wrist HCC ▽

✓6ᵗʰ M08.24 Juvenile rheumatoid arthritis with systemic onset, hand

M08.241 Juvenile rheumatoid arthritis with systemic onset, right hand HCC

M08.242 Juvenile rheumatoid arthritis with systemic onset, left hand HCC

M08.249 Juvenile rheumatoid arthritis with systemic onset, unspecified hand HCC ▽

✓6ᵗʰ M08.25 Juvenile rheumatoid arthritis with systemic onset, hip

M08.251 Juvenile rheumatoid arthritis with systemic onset, right hip HCC

M08.252 Juvenile rheumatoid arthritis with systemic onset, left hip HCC

M08.259 Juvenile rheumatoid arthritis with systemic onset, unspecified hip HCC ▽

✓6ᵗʰ M08.26 Juvenile rheumatoid arthritis with systemic onset, knee

M08.261 Juvenile rheumatoid arthritis with systemic onset, right knee HCC

M08.262 Juvenile rheumatoid arthritis with systemic onset, left knee HCC

M08.269 Juvenile rheumatoid arthritis with systemic onset, unspecified knee HCC ▽

✓6ᵗʰ M08.27 Juvenile rheumatoid arthritis with systemic onset, ankle and foot

M08.271 Juvenile rheumatoid arthritis with systemic onset, right ankle and foot HCC

M08.272 Juvenile rheumatoid arthritis with systemic onset, left ankle and foot HCC

M08.279 Juvenile rheumatoid arthritis with systemic onset, unspecified ankle and foot HCC ▽

M08.28 Juvenile rheumatoid arthritis with systemic onset, vertebrae HCC

M08.29 Juvenile rheumatoid arthritis with systemic onset, multiple sites HCC

M08.3 Juvenile rheumatoid polyarthritis (seronegative) HCC

✓5ᵗʰ M08.4 Pauciarticular juvenile rheumatoid arthritis

M08.40 Pauciarticular juvenile rheumatoid arthritis, unspecified site HCC ▽

✓6ᵗʰ M08.41 Pauciarticular juvenile rheumatoid arthritis, shoulder

M08.411 Pauciarticular juvenile rheumatoid arthritis, right shoulder HCC

M08.412 Pauciarticular juvenile rheumatoid arthritis, left shoulder HCC

M08.419 Pauciarticular juvenile rheumatoid arthritis, unspecified shoulder HCC ▽

✓6ᵗʰ M08.42 Pauciarticular juvenile rheumatoid arthritis, elbow

M08.421 Pauciarticular juvenile rheumatoid arthritis, right elbow HCC

M08.422 Pauciarticular juvenile rheumatoid arthritis, left elbow HCC

M08.429 Pauciarticular juvenile rheumatoid arthritis, unspecified elbow HCC ▽

✓6ᵗʰ M08.43 Pauciarticular juvenile rheumatoid arthritis, wrist

M08.431 Pauciarticular juvenile rheumatoid arthritis, right wrist HCC

M08.432 Pauciarticular juvenile rheumatoid arthritis, left wrist HCC

M08.439 Pauciarticular juvenile rheumatoid arthritis, unspecified wrist HCC ▽

✓6ᵗʰ M08.44 Pauciarticular juvenile rheumatoid arthritis, hand

M08.441 Pauciarticular juvenile rheumatoid arthritis, right hand HCC

M08.442 Pauciarticular juvenile rheumatoid arthritis, left hand HCC

M08.449 Pauciarticular juvenile rheumatoid arthritis, unspecified hand HCC ▽

✓6ᵗʰ M08.45 Pauciarticular juvenile rheumatoid arthritis, hip

M08.451 Pauciarticular juvenile rheumatoid arthritis, right hip HCC

M08.452 Pauciarticular juvenile rheumatoid arthritis, left hip HCC

M08.459 Pauciarticular juvenile rheumatoid arthritis, unspecified hip HCC ▽

✓6ᵗʰ M08.46 Pauciarticular juvenile rheumatoid arthritis, knee

M08.461 Pauciarticular juvenile rheumatoid arthritis, right knee HCC

M08.462 Pauciarticular juvenile rheumatoid arthritis, left knee HCC

M08.469 Pauciarticular juvenile rheumatoid arthritis, unspecified knee HCC ▽

✓6ᵗʰ M08.47 Pauciarticular juvenile rheumatoid arthritis, ankle and foot

M08.471 Pauciarticular juvenile rheumatoid arthritis, right ankle and foot HCC

M08.472 Pauciarticular juvenile rheumatoid arthritis, left ankle and foot HCC

M08.479 Pauciarticular juvenile rheumatoid arthritis, unspecified ankle and foot HCC ▽

M08.48 Pauciarticular juvenile rheumatoid arthritis, vertebrae HCC

✓5ᵗʰ M08.8 Other juvenile arthritis

M08.80 Other juvenile arthritis, unspecified site HCC ▽

✓6ᵗʰ M08.81 Other juvenile arthritis, shoulder

M08.811 Other juvenile arthritis, right shoulder HCC

M08.812 Other juvenile arthritis, left shoulder HCC

M08.819 Other juvenile arthritis, unspecified shoulder HCC ▽

EXCLUDES 1 Not coded here   EXCLUDES 2 Not included here   N Newborn Age: 0   P Pediatric Age: 0-17   M Maternity Age: 12-55   A Adult Age: 15-124

728   ICD-10-CM 2018

✓6ᵗʰ **M08.82 Other juvenile arthritis, elbow**
    M08.821 Other juvenile arthritis, right elbow   HCC
    M08.822 Other juvenile arthritis, left elbow   HCC
    M08.829 Other juvenile arthritis, unspecified   HCC ▽
         elbow

✓6ᵗʰ **M08.83 Other juvenile arthritis, wrist**
    M08.831 Other juvenile arthritis, right wrist   HCC
    M08.832 Other juvenile arthritis, left wrist   HCC
    M08.839 Other juvenile arthritis, unspecified   HCC ▽
         wrist

✓6ᵗʰ **M08.84 Other juvenile arthritis, hand**
    M08.841 Other juvenile arthritis, right hand   HCC
    M08.842 Other juvenile arthritis, left hand   HCC
    M08.849 Other juvenile arthritis, unspecified   HCC ▽
         hand

✓6ᵗʰ **M08.85 Other juvenile arthritis, hip**
    M08.851 Other juvenile arthritis, right hip   HCC
    M08.852 Other juvenile arthritis, left hip   HCC
    M08.859 Other juvenile arthritis,   HCC ▽
         unspecified hip

✓6ᵗʰ **M08.86 Other juvenile arthritis, knee**
    M08.861 Other juvenile arthritis, right knee   HCC
    M08.862 Other juvenile arthritis, left knee   HCC
    M08.869 Other juvenile arthritis,   HCC ▽
         unspecified knee

✓6ᵗʰ **M08.87 Other juvenile arthritis, ankle and foot**
    M08.871 Other juvenile arthritis, right ankle   HCC
         and foot
    M08.872 Other juvenile arthritis, left ankle   HCC
         and foot
    M08.879 Other juvenile arthritis,   HCC ▽
         unspecified ankle and foot

    M08.88 Other juvenile arthritis, other specified site   HCC
         Other juvenile arthritis, vertebrae

    M08.89 Other juvenile arthritis, multiple sites   HCC

✓5ᵗʰ **M08.9 Juvenile arthritis, unspecified**
    EXCLUDES 1   juvenile rheumatoid arthritis, unspecified (M08.0-)

    M08.90 Juvenile arthritis, unspecified,   HCC ▽
         unspecified site

✓6ᵗʰ **M08.91 Juvenile arthritis, unspecified, shoulder**
    M08.911 Juvenile arthritis, unspecified, right   HCC ▽
         shoulder
    M08.912 Juvenile arthritis, unspecified, left   HCC ▽
         shoulder
    M08.919 Juvenile arthritis, unspecified,   HCC ▽
         unspecified shoulder

✓6ᵗʰ **M08.92 Juvenile arthritis, unspecified, elbow**
    M08.921 Juvenile arthritis, unspecified,   HCC ▽
         right elbow
    M08.922 Juvenile arthritis, unspecified,   HCC ▽
         left elbow
    M08.929 Juvenile arthritis, unspecified,   HCC ▽
         unspecified elbow

✓6ᵗʰ **M08.93 Juvenile arthritis, unspecified, wrist**
    M08.931 Juvenile arthritis, unspecified,   HCC ▽
         right wrist
    M08.932 Juvenile arthritis, unspecified,   HCC ▽
         left wrist
    M08.939 Juvenile arthritis, unspecified,   HCC ▽
         unspecified wrist

✓6ᵗʰ **M08.94 Juvenile arthritis, unspecified, hand**
    M08.941 Juvenile arthritis, unspecified,   HCC ▽
         right hand
    M08.942 Juvenile arthritis, unspecified,   HCC ▽
         left hand
    M08.949 Juvenile arthritis, unspecified,   HCC ▽
         unspecified hand

✓6ᵗʰ **M08.95 Juvenile arthritis, unspecified, hip**
    M08.951 Juvenile arthritis, unspecified,   HCC ▽
         right hip
    M08.952 Juvenile arthritis, unspecified,   HCC ▽
         left hip
    M08.959 Juvenile arthritis, unspecified,   HCC ▽
         unspecified hip

✓6ᵗʰ **M08.96 Juvenile arthritis, unspecified, knee**
    M08.961 Juvenile arthritis, unspecified,   HCC ▽
         right knee
    M08.962 Juvenile arthritis, unspecified,   HCC ▽
         left knee
    M08.969 Juvenile arthritis, unspecified,   HCC ▽
         unspecified knee

✓6ᵗʰ **M08.97 Juvenile arthritis, unspecified, ankle and foot**
    M08.971 Juvenile arthritis, unspecified,   HCC ▽
         right ankle and foot
    M08.972 Juvenile arthritis, unspecified,   HCC ▽
         left ankle and foot
    M08.979 Juvenile arthritis, unspecified,   HCC ▽
         unspecified ankle and foot

    M08.98 Juvenile arthritis, unspecified, vertebrae   HCC ▽

    M08.99 Juvenile arthritis, unspecified, multiple sites   HCC ▽

✓4ᵗʰ **M1A Chronic gout**
     Use additional code to identify:
         autonomic neuropathy in diseases classified elsewhere (G99.0)
         calculus of urinary tract in diseases classified elsewhere (N22)
         cardiomyopathy in diseases classified elsewhere (I43)
         disorders of external ear in diseases classified elsewhere (H61.1-,
           H62.8-)
         disorders of iris and ciliary body in diseases classified elsewhere (H22)
         glomerular disorders in diseases classified elsewhere (N08)
    EXCLUDES 1   gout NOS (M10.-)
    EXCLUDES 2   acute gout (M10.-)

     The appropriate 7th character is to be added to each code
     from category M1A.
     0   without tophus (tophi)
     1   with tophus (tophi)

✓5ᵗʰ **M1A.0 Idiopathic chronic gout**
     Chronic gouty bursitis   Primary chronic gout

    ✓x7ᵗʰ **M1A.00 Idiopathic chronic gout, unspecified site** ▽

    ✓6ᵗʰ **M1A.01 Idiopathic chronic gout, shoulder**
        ✓7ᵗʰ **M1A.011** Idiopathic chronic gout, right shoulder
        ✓7ᵗʰ **M1A.012** Idiopathic chronic gout, left shoulder
        ✓7ᵗʰ **M1A.019** Idiopathic chronic gout, unspecified ▽
             shoulder

    ✓6ᵗʰ **M1A.02 Idiopathic chronic gout, elbow**
        ✓7ᵗʰ **M1A.021** Idiopathic chronic gout, right elbow
        ✓7ᵗʰ **M1A.022** Idiopathic chronic gout, left elbow
        ✓7ᵗʰ **M1A.029** Idiopathic chronic gout, unspecified ▽
             elbow

    ✓6ᵗʰ **M1A.03 Idiopathic chronic gout, wrist**
        ✓7ᵗʰ **M1A.031** Idiopathic chronic gout, right wrist
        ✓7ᵗʰ **M1A.032** Idiopathic chronic gout, left wrist
        ✓7ᵗʰ **M1A.039** Idiopathic chronic gout, unspecified ▽
             wrist

    ✓6ᵗʰ **M1A.04 Idiopathic chronic gout, hand**
        ✓7ᵗʰ **M1A.041** Idiopathic chronic gout, right hand
        ✓7ᵗʰ **M1A.042** Idiopathic chronic gout, left hand
        ✓7ᵗʰ **M1A.049** Idiopathic chronic gout, unspecified ▽
             hand

    ✓6ᵗʰ **M1A.05 Idiopathic chronic gout, hip**
        ✓7ᵗʰ **M1A.051** Idiopathic chronic gout, right hip
        ✓7ᵗʰ **M1A.052** Idiopathic chronic gout, left hip
        ✓7ᵗʰ **M1A.059** Idiopathic chronic gout, unspecified hip ▽

    ✓6ᵗʰ **M1A.06 Idiopathic chronic gout, knee**
        ✓7ᵗʰ **M1A.061** Idiopathic chronic gout, right knee
        ✓7ᵗʰ **M1A.062** Idiopathic chronic gout, left knee
        ✓7ᵗʰ **M1A.069** Idiopathic chronic gout, unspecified ▽
             knee

    ✓6ᵗʰ **M1A.07 Idiopathic chronic gout, ankle and foot**
        ✓7ᵗʰ **M1A.071** Idiopathic chronic gout, right ankle and
             foot
        ✓7ᵗʰ **M1A.072** Idiopathic chronic gout, left ankle and
             foot
        ✓7ᵗʰ **M1A.079** Idiopathic chronic gout, unspecified ▽
             ankle and foot

    ✓x7ᵗʰ **M1A.08 Idiopathic chronic gout, vertebrae**
    ✓x7ᵗʰ **M1A.09 Idiopathic chronic gout, multiple sites**

✓ Additional Character Req   ✓x7ᵗʰ Placeholder Alert   Manifestation   HCC CMS-HCC Condition   ▽ Unspecified Code   ►◄ Revised Text   ● New Code   ▲ Revised Code Title

√5ᵗʰ **M1A.1 Lead-induced chronic gout**
Code first toxic effects of lead and its compounds (T56.0-)

√x7ᵗʰ **M1A.10** Lead-induced chronic gout, unspecified site ▽

√6ᵗʰ **M1A.11** Lead-induced chronic gout, **shoulder**
  √7ᵗʰ **M1A.111** Lead-induced chronic gout, **right** shoulder
  √7ᵗʰ **M1A.112** Lead-induced chronic gout, **left** shoulder
  √7ᵗʰ **M1A.119** Lead-induced chronic gout, unspecified shoulder ▽

√6ᵗʰ **M1A.12** Lead-induced chronic gout, **elbow**
  √7ᵗʰ **M1A.121** Lead-induced chronic gout, **right** elbow
  √7ᵗʰ **M1A.122** Lead-induced chronic gout, **left** elbow
  √7ᵗʰ **M1A.129** Lead-induced chronic gout, unspecified elbow ▽

√6ᵗʰ **M1A.13** Lead-induced chronic gout, **wrist**
  √7ᵗʰ **M1A.131** Lead-induced chronic gout, **right** wrist
  √7ᵗʰ **M1A.132** Lead-induced chronic gout, **left** wrist
  √7ᵗʰ **M1A.139** Lead-induced chronic gout, unspecified wrist ▽

√6ᵗʰ **M1A.14** Lead-induced chronic gout, **hand**
  √7ᵗʰ **M1A.141** Lead-induced chronic gout, **right** hand
  √7ᵗʰ **M1A.142** Lead-induced chronic gout, **left** hand
  √7ᵗʰ **M1A.149** Lead-induced chronic gout, unspecified hand ▽

√6ᵗʰ **M1A.15** Lead-induced chronic gout, **hip**
  √7ᵗʰ **M1A.151** Lead-induced chronic gout, **right** hip
  √7ᵗʰ **M1A.152** Lead-induced chronic gout, **left** hip
  √7ᵗʰ **M1A.159** Lead-induced chronic gout, unspecified hip ▽

√6ᵗʰ **M1A.16** Lead-induced chronic gout, **knee**
  √7ᵗʰ **M1A.161** Lead-induced chronic gout, **right** knee
  √7ᵗʰ **M1A.162** Lead-induced chronic gout, **left** knee
  √7ᵗʰ **M1A.169** Lead-induced chronic gout, unspecified knee ▽

√6ᵗʰ **M1A.17** Lead-induced chronic gout, **ankle and foot**
  √7ᵗʰ **M1A.171** Lead-induced chronic gout, **right** ankle and foot
  √7ᵗʰ **M1A.172** Lead-induced chronic gout, **left** ankle and foot
  √7ᵗʰ **M1A.179** Lead-induced chronic gout, unspecified ankle and foot ▽

√x7ᵗʰ **M1A.18** Lead-induced chronic gout, **vertebrae**

√x7ᵗʰ **M1A.19** Lead-induced chronic gout, **multiple sites**

√5ᵗʰ **M1A.2 Drug-induced chronic gout**
Use additional code for adverse effect, if applicable, to identify drug (T36-T50 with fifth or sixth character 5)

√x7ᵗʰ **M1A.20** Drug-induced chronic gout, unspecified site ▽

√6ᵗʰ **M1A.21** Drug-induced chronic gout, **shoulder**
  √7ᵗʰ **M1A.211** Drug-induced chronic gout, **right** shoulder
  √7ᵗʰ **M1A.212** Drug-induced chronic gout, **left** shoulder
  √7ᵗʰ **M1A.219** Drug-induced chronic gout, unspecified shoulder ▽

√6ᵗʰ **M1A.22** Drug-induced chronic gout, **elbow**
  √7ᵗʰ **M1A.221** Drug-induced chronic gout, **right** elbow
  √7ᵗʰ **M1A.222** Drug-induced chronic gout, **left** elbow
  √7ᵗʰ **M1A.229** Drug-induced chronic gout, unspecified elbow ▽

√6ᵗʰ **M1A.23** Drug-induced chronic gout, **wrist**
  √7ᵗʰ **M1A.231** Drug-induced chronic gout, **right** wrist
  √7ᵗʰ **M1A.232** Drug-induced chronic gout, **left** wrist
  √7ᵗʰ **M1A.239** Drug-induced chronic gout, unspecified wrist ▽

√6ᵗʰ **M1A.24** Drug-induced chronic gout, **hand**
  √7ᵗʰ **M1A.241** Drug-induced chronic gout, **right** hand
  √7ᵗʰ **M1A.242** Drug-induced chronic gout, **left** hand
  √7ᵗʰ **M1A.249** Drug-induced chronic gout, unspecified hand ▽

√6ᵗʰ **M1A.25** Drug-induced chronic gout, **hip**
  √7ᵗʰ **M1A.251** Drug-induced chronic gout, **right** hip
  √7ᵗʰ **M1A.252** Drug-induced chronic gout, **left** hip

√7ᵗʰ **M1A.259** Drug-induced chronic gout, unspecified hip ▽

√6ᵗʰ **M1A.26** Drug-induced chronic gout, **knee**
  √7ᵗʰ **M1A.261** Drug-induced chronic gout, **right** knee
  √7ᵗʰ **M1A.262** Drug-induced chronic gout, **left** knee
  √7ᵗʰ **M1A.269** Drug-induced chronic gout, unspecified knee ▽

√6ᵗʰ **M1A.27** Drug-induced chronic gout, **ankle and foot**
  √7ᵗʰ **M1A.271** Drug-induced chronic gout, **right** ankle and foot
  √7ᵗʰ **M1A.272** Drug-induced chronic gout, **left** ankle and foot
  √7ᵗʰ **M1A.279** Drug-induced chronic gout, unspecified ankle and foot ▽

√x7ᵗʰ **M1A.28** Drug-induced chronic gout, **vertebrae**

√x7ᵗʰ **M1A.29** Drug-induced chronic gout, **multiple sites**

√5ᵗʰ **M1A.3 Chronic gout due to renal impairment**
Code first associated renal disease

√x7ᵗʰ **M1A.30** Chronic gout due to renal impairment, unspecified site ▽

√6ᵗʰ **M1A.31** Chronic gout due to renal impairment, **shoulder**
  √7ᵗʰ **M1A.311** Chronic gout due to renal impairment, **right** shoulder
  √7ᵗʰ **M1A.312** Chronic gout due to renal impairment, **left** shoulder
  √7ᵗʰ **M1A.319** Chronic gout due to renal impairment, unspecified shoulder ▽

√6ᵗʰ **M1A.32** Chronic gout due to renal impairment, **elbow**
  √7ᵗʰ **M1A.321** Chronic gout due to renal impairment, **right** elbow
  √7ᵗʰ **M1A.322** Chronic gout due to renal impairment, **left** elbow
  √7ᵗʰ **M1A.329** Chronic gout due to renal impairment, unspecified elbow ▽

√6ᵗʰ **M1A.33** Chronic gout due to renal impairment, **wrist**
  √7ᵗʰ **M1A.331** Chronic gout due to renal impairment, **right** wrist
  √7ᵗʰ **M1A.332** Chronic gout due to renal impairment, **left** wrist
  √7ᵗʰ **M1A.339** Chronic gout due to renal impairment, unspecified wrist ▽

√6ᵗʰ **M1A.34** Chronic gout due to renal impairment, **hand**
  √7ᵗʰ **M1A.341** Chronic gout due to renal impairment, **right** hand
  √7ᵗʰ **M1A.342** Chronic gout due to renal impairment, **left** hand
  √7ᵗʰ **M1A.349** Chronic gout due to renal impairment, unspecified hand ▽

√6ᵗʰ **M1A.35** Chronic gout due to renal impairment, **hip**
  √7ᵗʰ **M1A.351** Chronic gout due to renal impairment, **right** hip
  √7ᵗʰ **M1A.352** Chronic gout due to renal impairment, **left** hip
  √7ᵗʰ **M1A.359** Chronic gout due to renal impairment, unspecified hip ▽

√6ᵗʰ **M1A.36** Chronic gout due to renal impairment, **knee**
  √7ᵗʰ **M1A.361** Chronic gout due to renal impairment, **right** knee
  √7ᵗʰ **M1A.362** Chronic gout due to renal impairment, **left** knee
  √7ᵗʰ **M1A.369** Chronic gout due to renal impairment, unspecified knee ▽

√6ᵗʰ **M1A.37** Chronic gout due to renal impairment, **ankle and foot**
  √7ᵗʰ **M1A.371** Chronic gout due to renal impairment, **right** ankle and foot
  √7ᵗʰ **M1A.372** Chronic gout due to renal impairment, **left** ankle and foot
  √7ᵗʰ **M1A.379** Chronic gout due to renal impairment, unspecified ankle and foot ▽

√x7ᵗʰ **M1A.38** Chronic gout due to renal impairment, **vertebrae**

√x7ᵗʰ **M1A.39** Chronic gout due to renal impairment, **multiple sites**

EXCLUDES 1 Not coded here   EXCLUDES 2 Not included here   N Newborn Age: 0   P Pediatric Age: 0-17   M Maternity Age: 12-55   A Adult Age: 15-124

√5ᵗʰ **M1A.4 Other** secondary chronic gout
    Code first associated condition
    √x7ᵗʰ **M1A.40 Other** secondary chronic gout, unspecified site ▽
    √6ᵗʰ **M1A.41 Other** secondary chronic gout, shoulder
       √7ᵗʰ **M1A.411 Other** secondary chronic gout, right shoulder
       √7ᵗʰ **M1A.412 Other** secondary chronic gout, left shoulder
       √7ᵗʰ **M1A.419 Other** secondary chronic gout, unspecified shoulder ▽
    √6ᵗʰ **M1A.42 Other** secondary chronic gout, elbow
       √7ᵗʰ **M1A.421 Other** secondary chronic gout, right elbow
       √7ᵗʰ **M1A.422 Other** secondary chronic gout, left elbow
       √7ᵗʰ **M1A.429 Other** secondary chronic gout, unspecified elbow ▽
    √6ᵗʰ **M1A.43 Other** secondary chronic gout, wrist
       √7ᵗʰ **M1A.431 Other** secondary chronic gout, right wrist
       √7ᵗʰ **M1A.432 Other** secondary chronic gout, left wrist
       √7ᵗʰ **M1A.439 Other** secondary chronic gout, unspecified wrist ▽
    √6ᵗʰ **M1A.44 Other** secondary chronic gout, hand
       √7ᵗʰ **M1A.441 Other** secondary chronic gout, right hand
       √7ᵗʰ **M1A.442 Other** secondary chronic gout, left hand
       √7ᵗʰ **M1A.449 Other** secondary chronic gout, unspecified hand ▽
    √6ᵗʰ **M1A.45 Other** secondary chronic gout, hip
       √7ᵗʰ **M1A.451 Other** secondary chronic gout, right hip
       √7ᵗʰ **M1A.452 Other** secondary chronic gout, left hip
       √7ᵗʰ **M1A.459 Other** secondary chronic gout, unspecified hip ▽
    √6ᵗʰ **M1A.46 Other** secondary chronic gout, knee
       √7ᵗʰ **M1A.461 Other** secondary chronic gout, right knee
       √7ᵗʰ **M1A.462 Other** secondary chronic gout, left knee
       √7ᵗʰ **M1A.469 Other** secondary chronic gout, unspecified knee ▽
    √6ᵗʰ **M1A.47 Other** secondary chronic gout, ankle and foot
       √7ᵗʰ **M1A.471 Other** secondary chronic gout, right ankle and foot
       √7ᵗʰ **M1A.472 Other** secondary chronic gout, left ankle and foot
       √7ᵗʰ **M1A.479 Other** secondary chronic gout, unspecified ankle and foot ▽
    √x7ᵗʰ **M1A.48 Other** secondary chronic gout, vertebrae
    √x7ᵗʰ **M1A.49 Other** secondary chronic gout, multiple sites
√x7ᵗʰ **M1A.9 Chronic gout, unspecified** ▽

√4ᵗʰ **M10 Gout**
    Acute gout   Gout flare
    Gout attack   Podagra
    Use additional code to identify:
       autonomic neuropathy in diseases classified elsewhere (G99.0)
       calculus of urinary tract in diseases classified elsewhere (N22)
       cardiomyopathy in diseases classified elsewhere (I43)
       disorders of external ear in diseases classified elsewhere (H61.1-, H62.8-)
       disorders of iris and ciliary body in diseases classified elsewhere (H22)
       glomerular disorders in diseases classified elsewhere (N08)
    EXCLUDES 2   chronic gout (M1A.-)
    DEF: Purine and pyrimidine metabolic disorders; manifested by hyperuricemia and recurrent acute inflammatory arthritis; monosodium urate or monohydrate crystals may be deposited in and around the joints, leading to joint destruction and severe crippling.
    √5ᵗʰ **M10.0 Idiopathic gout**
       Gouty bursitis
       Primary gout
       M10.00 Idiopathic gout, unspecified site ▽
       √6ᵗʰ **M10.01 Idiopathic gout, shoulder**
          M10.011 Idiopathic gout, right shoulder
          M10.012 Idiopathic gout, left shoulder
          M10.019 Idiopathic gout, unspecified shoulder ▽
       √6ᵗʰ **M10.02 Idiopathic gout, elbow**
          M10.021 Idiopathic gout, right elbow
          M10.022 Idiopathic gout, left elbow
          M10.029 Idiopathic gout, unspecified elbow ▽

√6ᵗʰ **M10.03 Idiopathic gout, wrist**
    M10.031 Idiopathic gout, right wrist
    M10.032 Idiopathic gout, left wrist
    M10.039 Idiopathic gout, unspecified wrist ▽
√6ᵗʰ **M10.04 Idiopathic gout, hand**
    M10.041 Idiopathic gout, right hand
    M10.042 Idiopathic gout, left hand
    M10.049 Idiopathic gout, unspecified hand ▽
√6ᵗʰ **M10.05 Idiopathic gout, hip**
    M10.051 Idiopathic gout, right hip
    M10.052 Idiopathic gout, left hip
    M10.059 Idiopathic gout, unspecified hip ▽
√6ᵗʰ **M10.06 Idiopathic gout, knee**
    M10.061 Idiopathic gout, right knee
    M10.062 Idiopathic gout, left knee
    M10.069 Idiopathic gout, unspecified knee ▽
√6ᵗʰ **M10.07 Idiopathic gout, ankle and foot**
    M10.071 Idiopathic gout, right ankle and foot
    M10.072 Idiopathic gout, left ankle and foot
    M10.079 Idiopathic gout, unspecified ankle and foot ▽
M10.08 Idiopathic gout, vertebrae
M10.09 Idiopathic gout, multiple sites
√5ᵗʰ **M10.1 Lead-induced gout**
    Code first toxic effects of lead and its compounds (T56.0-)
    M10.10 Lead-induced gout, unspecified site ▽
    √6ᵗʰ **M10.11 Lead-induced gout, shoulder**
       M10.111 Lead-induced gout, right shoulder
       M10.112 Lead-induced gout, left shoulder
       M10.119 Lead-induced gout, unspecified shoulder ▽
    √6ᵗʰ **M10.12 Lead-induced gout, elbow**
       M10.121 Lead-induced gout, right elbow
       M10.122 Lead-induced gout, left elbow
       M10.129 Lead-induced gout, unspecified elbow ▽
    √6ᵗʰ **M10.13 Lead-induced gout, wrist**
       M10.131 Lead-induced gout, right wrist
       M10.132 Lead-induced gout, left wrist
       M10.139 Lead-induced gout, unspecified wrist ▽
    √6ᵗʰ **M10.14 Lead-induced gout, hand**
       M10.141 Lead-induced gout, right hand
       M10.142 Lead-induced gout, left hand
       M10.149 Lead-induced gout, unspecified hand ▽
    √6ᵗʰ **M10.15 Lead-induced gout, hip**
       M10.151 Lead-induced gout, right hip
       M10.152 Lead-induced gout, left hip
       M10.159 Lead-induced gout, unspecified hip ▽
    √6ᵗʰ **M10.16 Lead-induced gout, knee**
       M10.161 Lead-induced gout, right knee
       M10.162 Lead-induced gout, left knee
       M10.169 Lead-induced gout, unspecified knee ▽
    √6ᵗʰ **M10.17 Lead-induced gout, ankle and foot**
       M10.171 Lead-induced gout, right ankle and foot
       M10.172 Lead-induced gout, left ankle and foot
       M10.179 Lead-induced gout, unspecified ankle and foot ▽
    M10.18 Lead-induced gout, vertebrae
    M10.19 Lead-induced gout, multiple sites
√5ᵗʰ **M10.2 Drug-induced gout**
    Use additional code for adverse effect, if applicable, to identify drug (T36-T50 with fifth or sixth character 5)
    M10.20 Drug-induced gout, unspecified site ▽
    √6ᵗʰ **M10.21 Drug-induced gout, shoulder**
       M10.211 Drug-induced gout, right shoulder
       M10.212 Drug-induced gout, left shoulder
       M10.219 Drug-induced gout, unspecified shoulder ▽
    √6ᵗʰ **M10.22 Drug-induced gout, elbow**
       M10.221 Drug-induced gout, right elbow
       M10.222 Drug-induced gout, left elbow
       M10.229 Drug-induced gout, unspecified elbow ▽

☑ Additional Character Req   √x7ᵗʰ Placeholder Alert   Manifestation   HCC CMS-HCC Condition   ▽ Unspecified Code   ►◄ Revised Text   ● New Code   ▲ Revised Code Title

ICD-10-CM 2018   731

✓6th **M10.23 Drug-induced gout, wrist**
  M10.231 Drug-induced gout, right wrist
  M10.232 Drug-induced gout, left wrist
  M10.239 Drug-induced gout, unspecified wrist ▽

✓6th **M10.24 Drug-induced gout, hand**
  M10.241 Drug-induced gout, right hand
  M10.242 Drug-induced gout, left hand
  M10.249 Drug-induced gout, unspecified hand ▽

✓6th **M10.25 Drug-induced gout, hip**
  M10.251 Drug-induced gout, right hip
  M10.252 Drug-induced gout, left hip
  M10.259 Drug-induced gout, unspecified hip ▽

✓6th **M10.26 Drug-induced gout, knee**
  M10.261 Drug-induced gout, right knee
  M10.262 Drug-induced gout, left knee
  M10.269 Drug-induced gout, unspecified knee ▽

✓6th **M10.27 Drug-induced gout, ankle and foot**
  M10.271 Drug-induced gout, right ankle and foot
  M10.272 Drug-induced gout, left ankle and foot
  M10.279 Drug-induced gout, unspecified ankle and foot ▽

  M10.28 Drug-induced gout, vertebrae
  M10.29 Drug-induced gout, multiple sites

✓5th **M10.3 Gout due to renal impairment**
  Code first associated renal disease
  M10.30 Gout due to renal impairment, unspecified site ▽

✓6th **M10.31 Gout due to renal impairment, shoulder**
  M10.311 Gout due to renal impairment, right shoulder
  M10.312 Gout due to renal impairment, left shoulder
  M10.319 Gout due to renal impairment, unspecified shoulder ▽

✓6th **M10.32 Gout due to renal impairment, elbow**
  M10.321 Gout due to renal impairment, right elbow
  M10.322 Gout due to renal impairment, left elbow
  M10.329 Gout due to renal impairment, unspecified elbow ▽

✓6th **M10.33 Gout due to renal impairment, wrist**
  M10.331 Gout due to renal impairment, right wrist
  M10.332 Gout due to renal impairment, left wrist
  M10.339 Gout due to renal impairment, unspecified wrist ▽

✓6th **M10.34 Gout due to renal impairment, hand**
  M10.341 Gout due to renal impairment, right hand
  M10.342 Gout due to renal impairment, left hand
  M10.349 Gout due to renal impairment, unspecified hand ▽

✓6th **M10.35 Gout due to renal impairment, hip**
  M10.351 Gout due to renal impairment, right hip
  M10.352 Gout due to renal impairment, left hip
  M10.359 Gout due to renal impairment, unspecified hip ▽

✓6th **M10.36 Gout due to renal impairment, knee**
  M10.361 Gout due to renal impairment, right knee
  M10.362 Gout due to renal impairment, left knee
  M10.369 Gout due to renal impairment, unspecified knee ▽

✓6th **M10.37 Gout due to renal impairment, ankle and foot**
  M10.371 Gout due to renal impairment, right ankle and foot
  M10.372 Gout due to renal impairment, left ankle and foot
  M10.379 Gout due to renal impairment, unspecified ankle and foot ▽

  M10.38 Gout due to renal impairment, vertebrae
  M10.39 Gout due to renal impairment, multiple sites

✓5th **M10.4 Other secondary gout**
  Code first associated condition
  M10.40 Other secondary gout, unspecified site ▽

✓6th **M10.41 Other secondary gout, shoulder**
  M10.411 Other secondary gout, right shoulder
  M10.412 Other secondary gout, left shoulder

  M10.419 Other secondary gout, unspecified shoulder ▽

✓6th **M10.42 Other secondary gout, elbow**
  M10.421 Other secondary gout, right elbow
  M10.422 Other secondary gout, left elbow
  M10.429 Other secondary gout, unspecified elbow ▽

✓6th **M10.43 Other secondary gout, wrist**
  M10.431 Other secondary gout, right wrist
  M10.432 Other secondary gout, left wrist
  M10.439 Other secondary gout, unspecified wrist ▽

✓6th **M10.44 Other secondary gout, hand**
  M10.441 Other secondary gout, right hand
  M10.442 Other secondary gout, left hand
  M10.449 Other secondary gout, unspecified hand ▽

✓6th **M10.45 Other secondary gout, hip**
  M10.451 Other secondary gout, right hip
  M10.452 Other secondary gout, left hip
  M10.459 Other secondary gout, unspecified hip ▽

✓6th **M10.46 Other secondary gout, knee**
  M10.461 Other secondary gout, right knee
  M10.462 Other secondary gout, left knee
  M10.469 Other secondary gout, unspecified knee ▽

✓6th **M10.47 Other secondary gout, ankle and foot**
  M10.471 Other secondary gout, right ankle and foot
  M10.472 Other secondary gout, left ankle and foot
  M10.479 Other secondary gout, unspecified ankle and foot ▽

  M10.48 Other secondary gout, vertebrae
  M10.49 Other secondary gout, multiple sites

M10.9 Gout, unspecified ▽
  Gout NOS

✓4th **M11 Other crystal arthropathies**

✓5th **M11.0 Hydroxyapatite deposition disease**
  M11.00 Hydroxyapatite deposition disease, unspecified site ▽

✓6th **M11.01 Hydroxyapatite deposition disease, shoulder**
  M11.011 Hydroxyapatite deposition disease, right shoulder
  M11.012 Hydroxyapatite deposition disease, left shoulder
  M11.019 Hydroxyapatite deposition disease, unspecified shoulder ▽

✓6th **M11.02 Hydroxyapatite deposition disease, elbow**
  M11.021 Hydroxyapatite deposition disease, right elbow
  M11.022 Hydroxyapatite deposition disease, left elbow
  M11.029 Hydroxyapatite deposition disease, unspecified elbow ▽

✓6th **M11.03 Hydroxyapatite deposition disease, wrist**
  M11.031 Hydroxyapatite deposition disease, right wrist
  M11.032 Hydroxyapatite deposition disease, left wrist
  M11.039 Hydroxyapatite deposition disease, unspecified wrist ▽

✓6th **M11.04 Hydroxyapatite deposition disease, hand**
  M11.041 Hydroxyapatite deposition disease, right hand
  M11.042 Hydroxyapatite deposition disease, left hand
  M11.049 Hydroxyapatite deposition disease, unspecified hand ▽

✓6th **M11.05 Hydroxyapatite deposition disease, hip**
  M11.051 Hydroxyapatite deposition disease, right hip
  M11.052 Hydroxyapatite deposition disease, left hip
  M11.059 Hydroxyapatite deposition disease, unspecified hip ▽

✓6ᵗʰ **M11.06 Hydroxyapatite deposition disease,** knee
     M11.061 Hydroxyapatite deposition disease, right knee
     M11.062 Hydroxyapatite deposition disease, left knee
     M11.069 Hydroxyapatite deposition disease, unspecified knee ▽

✓6ᵗʰ **M11.07 Hydroxyapatite deposition disease,** ankle and foot
     M11.071 Hydroxyapatite deposition disease, right ankle and foot
     M11.072 Hydroxyapatite deposition disease, left ankle and foot
     M11.079 Hydroxyapatite deposition disease, unspecified ankle and foot ▽

     M11.08 Hydroxyapatite deposition disease, vertebrae
     M11.09 Hydroxyapatite deposition disease, multiple sites

✓5ᵗʰ **M11.1 Familial chondrocalcinosis**
     M11.10 Familial chondrocalcinosis, unspecified site ▽

✓6ᵗʰ **M11.11 Familial chondrocalcinosis,** shoulder
     M11.111 Familial chondrocalcinosis, right shoulder
     M11.112 Familial chondrocalcinosis, left shoulder
     M11.119 Familial chondrocalcinosis, unspecified shoulder ▽

✓6ᵗʰ **M11.12 Familial chondrocalcinosis,** elbow
     M11.121 Familial chondrocalcinosis, right elbow
     M11.122 Familial chondrocalcinosis, left elbow
     M11.129 Familial chondrocalcinosis, unspecified elbow ▽

✓6ᵗʰ **M11.13 Familial chondrocalcinosis,** wrist
     M11.131 Familial chondrocalcinosis, right wrist
     M11.132 Familial chondrocalcinosis, left wrist
     M11.139 Familial chondrocalcinosis, unspecified wrist ▽

✓6ᵗʰ **M11.14 Familial chondrocalcinosis,** hand
     M11.141 Familial chondrocalcinosis, right hand
     M11.142 Familial chondrocalcinosis, left hand
     M11.149 Familial chondrocalcinosis, unspecified hand ▽

✓6ᵗʰ **M11.15 Familial chondrocalcinosis,** hip
     M11.151 Familial chondrocalcinosis, right hip
     M11.152 Familial chondrocalcinosis, left hip
     M11.159 Familial chondrocalcinosis, unspecified hip ▽

✓6ᵗʰ **M11.16 Familial chondrocalcinosis,** knee
     M11.161 Familial chondrocalcinosis, right knee
     M11.162 Familial chondrocalcinosis, left knee
     M11.169 Familial chondrocalcinosis, unspecified knee ▽

✓6ᵗʰ **M11.17 Familial chondrocalcinosis,** ankle and foot
     M11.171 Familial chondrocalcinosis, right ankle and foot
     M11.172 Familial chondrocalcinosis, left ankle and foot
     M11.179 Familial chondrocalcinosis, unspecified ankle and foot ▽

     M11.18 Familial chondrocalcinosis, vertebrae
     M11.19 Familial chondrocalcinosis, multiple sites

✓5ᵗʰ **M11.2 Other chondrocalcinosis**
     Chondrocalcinosis NOS
     M11.20 Other chondrocalcinosis, unspecified site ▽

✓6ᵗʰ **M11.21 Other chondrocalcinosis,** shoulder
     M11.211 Other chondrocalcinosis, right shoulder
     M11.212 Other chondrocalcinosis, left shoulder
     M11.219 Other chondrocalcinosis, unspecified shoulder ▽

✓6ᵗʰ **M11.22 Other chondrocalcinosis,** elbow
     M11.221 Other chondrocalcinosis, right elbow
     M11.222 Other chondrocalcinosis, left elbow
     M11.229 Other chondrocalcinosis, unspecified elbow ▽

✓6ᵗʰ **M11.23 Other chondrocalcinosis,** wrist
     M11.231 Other chondrocalcinosis, right wrist
     M11.232 Other chondrocalcinosis, left wrist

     M11.239 Other chondrocalcinosis, unspecified wrist ▽

✓6ᵗʰ **M11.24 Other chondrocalcinosis,** hand
     M11.241 Other chondrocalcinosis, right hand
     M11.242 Other chondrocalcinosis, left hand
     M11.249 Other chondrocalcinosis, unspecified hand ▽

✓6ᵗʰ **M11.25 Other chondrocalcinosis,** hip
     M11.251 Other chondrocalcinosis, right hip
     M11.252 Other chondrocalcinosis, left hip
     M11.259 Other chondrocalcinosis, unspecified hip ▽

✓6ᵗʰ **M11.26 Other chondrocalcinosis,** knee
     M11.261 Other chondrocalcinosis, right knee
     M11.262 Other chondrocalcinosis, left knee
     M11.269 Other chondrocalcinosis, unspecified knee ▽

✓6ᵗʰ **M11.27 Other chondrocalcinosis,** ankle and foot
     M11.271 Other chondrocalcinosis, right ankle and foot
     M11.272 Other chondrocalcinosis, left ankle and foot
     M11.279 Other chondrocalcinosis, unspecified ankle and foot ▽

     M11.28 Other chondrocalcinosis, vertebrae
     M11.29 Other chondrocalcinosis, multiple sites

✓5ᵗʰ **M11.8 Other specified crystal arthropathies**
     M11.80 Other specified crystal arthropathies, unspecified site ▽

✓6ᵗʰ **M11.81 Other specified crystal arthropathies,** shoulder
     M11.811 Other specified crystal arthropathies, right shoulder
     M11.812 Other specified crystal arthropathies, left shoulder
     M11.819 Other specified crystal arthropathies, unspecified shoulder ▽

✓6ᵗʰ **M11.82 Other specified crystal arthropathies,** elbow
     M11.821 Other specified crystal arthropathies, right elbow
     M11.822 Other specified crystal arthropathies, left elbow
     M11.829 Other specified crystal arthropathies, unspecified elbow ▽

✓6ᵗʰ **M11.83 Other specified crystal arthropathies,** wrist
     M11.831 Other specified crystal arthropathies, right wrist
     M11.832 Other specified crystal arthropathies, left wrist
     M11.839 Other specified crystal arthropathies, unspecified wrist ▽

✓6ᵗʰ **M11.84 Other specified crystal arthropathies,** hand
     M11.841 Other specified crystal arthropathies, right hand
     M11.842 Other specified crystal arthropathies, left hand
     M11.849 Other specified crystal arthropathies, unspecified hand ▽

✓6ᵗʰ **M11.85 Other specified crystal arthropathies,** hip
     M11.851 Other specified crystal arthropathies, right hip
     M11.852 Other specified crystal arthropathies, left hip
     M11.859 Other specified crystal arthropathies, unspecified hip ▽

✓6ᵗʰ **M11.86 Other specified crystal arthropathies,** knee
     M11.861 Other specified crystal arthropathies, right knee
     M11.862 Other specified crystal arthropathies, left knee
     M11.869 Other specified crystal arthropathies, unspecified knee ▽

✓6ᵗʰ **M11.87 Other specified crystal arthropathies,** ankle and foot
     M11.871 Other specified crystal arthropathies, right ankle and foot
     M11.872 Other specified crystal arthropathies, left ankle and foot

---

✓ Additional Character Req   ✗7ᵗʰ Placeholder Alert   Manifestation   HCC CMS-HCC Condition   ▽ Unspecified Code   ▶◀ Revised Text   ● New Code   ▲ Revised Code Title

M11.879 Other specified crystal arthropathies, ▽
unspecified ankle and foot

M11.88 Other specified crystal arthropathies, vertebrae

M11.89 Other specified crystal arthropathies, multiple sites

M11.9 Crystal arthropathy, unspecified ▽

✓4th **M12** **Other and unspecified arthropathy**

> **EXCLUDES 1** arthrosis (M15-M19)
> cricoarytenoid arthropathy (J38.7)

✓5th **M12.0** Chronic postrheumatic arthropathy [Jaccoud]

M12.00 Chronic postrheumatic arthropathy [Jaccoud], HCC ▽
unspecified site

✓6th **M12.01** Chronic postrheumatic arthropathy [Jaccoud],
shoulder

M12.011 Chronic postrheumatic arthropathy HCC
[Jaccoud], right shoulder

M12.012 Chronic postrheumatic arthropathy HCC
[Jaccoud], left shoulder

M12.019 Chronic postrheumatic arthropathy HCC ▽
[Jaccoud], unspecified shoulder

✓6th **M12.02** Chronic postrheumatic arthropathy [Jaccoud], elbow

M12.021 Chronic postrheumatic arthropathy HCC
[Jaccoud], right elbow

M12.022 Chronic postrheumatic arthropathy HCC
[Jaccoud], left elbow

M12.029 Chronic postrheumatic arthropathy HCC ▽
[Jaccoud], unspecified elbow

✓6th **M12.03** Chronic postrheumatic arthropathy [Jaccoud], wrist

M12.031 Chronic postrheumatic arthropathy HCC
[Jaccoud], right wrist

M12.032 Chronic postrheumatic arthropathy HCC
[Jaccoud], left wrist

M12.039 Chronic postrheumatic arthropathy HCC ▽
[Jaccoud], unspecified wrist

✓6th **M12.04** Chronic postrheumatic arthropathy [Jaccoud], hand

M12.041 Chronic postrheumatic arthropathy HCC
[Jaccoud], right hand

M12.042 Chronic postrheumatic arthropathy HCC
[Jaccoud], left hand

M12.049 Chronic postrheumatic arthropathy HCC ▽
[Jaccoud], unspecified hand

✓6th **M12.05** Chronic postrheumatic arthropathy [Jaccoud], hip

M12.051 Chronic postrheumatic arthropathy HCC
[Jaccoud], right hip

M12.052 Chronic postrheumatic arthropathy HCC
[Jaccoud], left hip

M12.059 Chronic postrheumatic arthropathy HCC ▽
[Jaccoud], unspecified hip

✓6th **M12.06** Chronic postrheumatic arthropathy [Jaccoud], knee

M12.061 Chronic postrheumatic arthropathy HCC
[Jaccoud], right knee

M12.062 Chronic postrheumatic arthropathy HCC
[Jaccoud], left knee

M12.069 Chronic postrheumatic arthropathy HCC ▽
[Jaccoud], unspecified knee

✓6th **M12.07** Chronic postrheumatic arthropathy [Jaccoud],
ankle and foot

M12.071 Chronic postrheumatic arthropathy HCC
[Jaccoud], right ankle and foot

M12.072 Chronic postrheumatic arthropathy HCC
[Jaccoud], left ankle and foot

M12.079 Chronic postrheumatic arthropathy HCC ▽
[Jaccoud], unspecified ankle and foot

M12.08 Chronic postrheumatic arthropathy [Jaccoud], HCC
other specified site
Chronic postrheumatic arthropathy [Jaccoud],
vertebrae

M12.09 Chronic postrheumatic arthropathy [Jaccoud], HCC
multiple sites

✓5th **M12.1** Kaschin-Beck disease
Osteochondroarthrosis deformans endemica

M12.10 Kaschin-Beck disease, unspecified site ▽

✓6th **M12.11** Kaschin-Beck disease, shoulder

M12.111 Kaschin-Beck disease, right shoulder

M12.112 Kaschin-Beck disease, left shoulder

M12.119 Kaschin-Beck disease, unspecified ▽
shoulder

✓6th **M12.12** Kaschin-Beck disease, elbow

M12.121 Kaschin-Beck disease, right elbow

M12.122 Kaschin-Beck disease, left elbow

M12.129 Kaschin-Beck disease, unspecified ▽
elbow

✓6th **M12.13** Kaschin-Beck disease, wrist

M12.131 Kaschin-Beck disease, right wrist

M12.132 Kaschin-Beck disease, left wrist

M12.139 Kaschin-Beck disease, unspecified wrist ▽

✓6th **M12.14** Kaschin-Beck disease, hand

M12.141 Kaschin-Beck disease, right hand

M12.142 Kaschin-Beck disease, left hand

M12.149 Kaschin-Beck disease, unspecified hand ▽

✓6th **M12.15** Kaschin-Beck disease, hip

M12.151 Kaschin-Beck disease, right hip

M12.152 Kaschin-Beck disease, left hip

M12.159 Kaschin-Beck disease, unspecified hip ▽

✓6th **M12.16** Kaschin-Beck disease, knee

M12.161 Kaschin-Beck disease, right knee

M12.162 Kaschin-Beck disease, left knee

M12.169 Kaschin-Beck disease, unspecified ▽
knee

✓6th **M12.17** Kaschin-Beck disease, ankle and foot

M12.171 Kaschin-Beck disease, right ankle and foot

M12.172 Kaschin-Beck disease, left ankle and foot

M12.179 Kaschin-Beck disease, unspecified a ▽
nkle and foot

M12.18 Kaschin-Beck disease, vertebrae

M12.19 Kaschin-Beck disease, multiple sites

✓5th **M12.2** Villonodular synovitis (pigmented)

M12.20 Villonodular synovitis (pigmented), unspecified ▽
site

✓6th **M12.21** Villonodular synovitis (pigmented), shoulder

M12.211 Villonodular synovitis (pigmented), right
shoulder

M12.212 Villonodular synovitis (pigmented), left
shoulder

M12.219 Villonodular synovitis (pigmented), ▽
unspecified shoulder

✓6th **M12.22** Villonodular synovitis (pigmented), elbow

M12.221 Villonodular synovitis (pigmented), right
elbow

M12.222 Villonodular synovitis (pigmented), left
elbow

M12.229 Villonodular synovitis (pigmented), ▽
unspecified elbow

✓6th **M12.23** Villonodular synovitis (pigmented), wrist

M12.231 Villonodular synovitis (pigmented), right
wrist

M12.232 Villonodular synovitis (pigmented), left
wrist

M12.239 Villonodular synovitis (pigmented), ▽
unspecified wrist

✓6th **M12.24** Villonodular synovitis (pigmented), hand

M12.241 Villonodular synovitis (pigmented), right
hand

M12.242 Villonodular synovitis (pigmented), left
hand

M12.249 Villonodular synovitis (pigmented), ▽
unspecified hand

✓6th **M12.25** Villonodular synovitis (pigmented), hip

M12.251 Villonodular synovitis (pigmented), right
hip

M12.252 Villonodular synovitis (pigmented), left
hip

M12.259 Villonodular synovitis (pigmented), ▽
unspecified hip

✓6th **M12.26** Villonodular synovitis (pigmented), knee

M12.261 Villonodular synovitis (pigmented), right
knee

M12.262 Villonodular synovitis (pigmented), left
knee

M12.269 Villonodular synovitis (pigmented), ▽
unspecified knee

EXCLUDES 1 Not coded here   **EXCLUDES 2** Not included here   N Newborn Age: 0   P Pediatric Age: 0-17   M Maternity Age: 12-55   A Adult Age: 15-124

734   ICD-10-CM 2018

✓6ᵗʰ **M12.27** Villonodular synovitis (pigmented), ankle and foot
     M12.271 Villonodular synovitis (pigmented), right ankle and foot
     M12.272 Villonodular synovitis (pigmented), left ankle and foot
     M12.279 Villonodular synovitis (pigmented), unspecified ankle and foot ▽
   M12.28 Villonodular synovitis (pigmented), other specified site
      Villonodular synovitis (pigmented), vertebrae
   M12.29 Villonodular synovitis (pigmented), multiple sites

✓5ᵗʰ **M12.3** Palindromic rheumatism
   M12.30 Palindromic rheumatism, unspecified site ▽
  ✓6ᵗʰ **M12.31** Palindromic rheumatism, shoulder
     M12.311 Palindromic rheumatism, right shoulder
     M12.312 Palindromic rheumatism, left shoulder
     M12.319 Palindromic rheumatism, unspecified shoulder ▽
  ✓6ᵗʰ **M12.32** Palindromic rheumatism, elbow
     M12.321 Palindromic rheumatism, right elbow
     M12.322 Palindromic rheumatism, left elbow
     M12.329 Palindromic rheumatism, unspecified elbow ▽
  ✓6ᵗʰ **M12.33** Palindromic rheumatism, wrist
     M12.331 Palindromic rheumatism, right wrist
     M12.332 Palindromic rheumatism, left wrist
     M12.339 Palindromic rheumatism, unspecified wrist ▽
  ✓6ᵗʰ **M12.34** Palindromic rheumatism, hand
     M12.341 Palindromic rheumatism, right hand
     M12.342 Palindromic rheumatism, left hand
     M12.349 Palindromic rheumatism, unspecified hand ▽
  ✓6ᵗʰ **M12.35** Palindromic rheumatism, hip
     M12.351 Palindromic rheumatism, right hip
     M12.352 Palindromic rheumatism, left hip
     M12.359 Palindromic rheumatism, unspecified hip ▽
  ✓6ᵗʰ **M12.36** Palindromic rheumatism, knee
     M12.361 Palindromic rheumatism, right knee
     M12.362 Palindromic rheumatism, left knee
     M12.369 Palindromic rheumatism, unspecified knee ▽
  ✓6ᵗʰ **M12.37** Palindromic rheumatism, ankle and foot
     M12.371 Palindromic rheumatism, right ankle and foot
     M12.372 Palindromic rheumatism, left ankle and foot
     M12.379 Palindromic rheumatism, unspecified ankle and foot ▽
   M12.38 Palindromic rheumatism, other specified site
      Palindromic rheumatism, vertebrae
   M12.39 Palindromic rheumatism, multiple sites

✓5ᵗʰ **M12.4** Intermittent hydrarthrosis
   M12.40 Intermittent hydrarthrosis, unspecified site ▽
  ✓6ᵗʰ **M12.41** Intermittent hydrarthrosis, shoulder
     M12.411 Intermittent hydrarthrosis, right shoulder
     M12.412 Intermittent hydrarthrosis, left shoulder
     M12.419 Intermittent hydrarthrosis, unspecified shoulder ▽
  ✓6ᵗʰ **M12.42** Intermittent hydrarthrosis, elbow
     M12.421 Intermittent hydrarthrosis, right elbow
     M12.422 Intermittent hydrarthrosis, left elbow
     M12.429 Intermittent hydrarthrosis, unspecified elbow ▽
  ✓6ᵗʰ **M12.43** Intermittent hydrarthrosis, wrist
     M12.431 Intermittent hydrarthrosis, right wrist
     M12.432 Intermittent hydrarthrosis, left wrist
     M12.439 Intermittent hydrarthrosis, unspecified wrist ▽
  ✓6ᵗʰ **M12.44** Intermittent hydrarthrosis, hand
     M12.441 Intermittent hydrarthrosis, right hand
     M12.442 Intermittent hydrarthrosis, left hand

     M12.449 Intermittent hydrarthrosis, unspecified hand ▽
  ✓6ᵗʰ **M12.45** Intermittent hydrarthrosis, hip
     M12.451 Intermittent hydrarthrosis, right hip
     M12.452 Intermittent hydrarthrosis, left hip
     M12.459 Intermittent hydrarthrosis, unspecified hip ▽
  ✓6ᵗʰ **M12.46** Intermittent hydrarthrosis, knee
     M12.461 Intermittent hydrarthrosis, right knee
     M12.462 Intermittent hydrarthrosis, left knee
     M12.469 Intermittent hydrarthrosis, unspecified knee ▽
  ✓6ᵗʰ **M12.47** Intermittent hydrarthrosis, ankle and foot
     M12.471 Intermittent hydrarthrosis, right ankle and foot
     M12.472 Intermittent hydrarthrosis, left ankle and foot
     M12.479 Intermittent hydrarthrosis, unspecified ankle and foot ▽
   M12.48 Intermittent hydrarthrosis, other site
   M12.49 Intermittent hydrarthrosis, multiple sites

✓5ᵗʰ **M12.5** Traumatic arthropathy
    EXCLUDES 1   *current injury-see Alphabetic Index*
       post-traumatic osteoarthritis NOS (M19.1-)
       post-traumatic osteoarthritis of first carpometacarpal joint (M18.2-M18.3)
       post-traumatic osteoarthritis of hip (M16.4-M16.5)
       post-traumatic osteoarthritis of knee (M17.2-M17.3)
       post-traumatic osteoarthritis of other single joints (M19.1-)
    AHA: 2015, 1Q, 17
   M12.50 Traumatic arthropathy, unspecified site ▽
  ✓6ᵗʰ **M12.51** Traumatic arthropathy, shoulder
     M12.511 Traumatic arthropathy, right shoulder
     M12.512 Traumatic arthropathy, left shoulder
     M12.519 Traumatic arthropathy, unspecified shoulder ▽
  ✓6ᵗʰ **M12.52** Traumatic arthropathy, elbow
     M12.521 Traumatic arthropathy, right elbow
     M12.522 Traumatic arthropathy, left elbow
     M12.529 Traumatic arthropathy, unspecified elbow ▽
  ✓6ᵗʰ **M12.53** Traumatic arthropathy, wrist
     M12.531 Traumatic arthropathy, right wrist
     M12.532 Traumatic arthropathy, left wrist
     M12.539 Traumatic arthropathy, unspecified wrist ▽
  ✓6ᵗʰ **M12.54** Traumatic arthropathy, hand
     M12.541 Traumatic arthropathy, right hand
     M12.542 Traumatic arthropathy, left hand
     M12.549 Traumatic arthropathy, unspecified hand ▽
  ✓6ᵗʰ **M12.55** Traumatic arthropathy, hip
     M12.551 Traumatic arthropathy, right hip
     M12.552 Traumatic arthropathy, left hip
     M12.559 Traumatic arthropathy, unspecified hip ▽
  ✓6ᵗʰ **M12.56** Traumatic arthropathy, knee
     M12.561 Traumatic arthropathy, right knee
     M12.562 Traumatic arthropathy, left knee
     M12.569 Traumatic arthropathy, unspecified knee ▽
  ✓6ᵗʰ **M12.57** Traumatic arthropathy, ankle and foot
     M12.571 Traumatic arthropathy, right ankle and foot
     M12.572 Traumatic arthropathy, left ankle and foot
     M12.579 Traumatic arthropathy, unspecified ankle and foot ▽
   M12.58 Traumatic arthropathy, other specified site
      Traumatic arthropathy, vertebrae
   M12.59 Traumatic arthropathy, multiple sites

✓5ᵗʰ **M12.8** Other specific arthropathies, not elsewhere classified
      Transient arthropathy
   M12.80 Other specific arthropathies, not elsewhere classified, unspecified site ▽

✓ Additional Character Req   ✓7ᵗʰ Placeholder Alert   Manifestation   HCC CMS-HCC Condition   ▽ Unspecified Code   ►◄ Revised Text   ● New Code   ▲ Revised Code Title

ICD-10-CM 2018   **735**

✓6ᵗʰ **M12.81** **Other specific arthropathies, not elsewhere classified, shoulder**
     M12.811 Other specific arthropathies, not elsewhere classified, right shoulder
     M12.812 Other specific arthropathies, not elsewhere classified, left shoulder
     M12.819 Other specific arthropathies, not elsewhere classified, unspecified shoulder ▽

✓6ᵗʰ **M12.82** **Other specific arthropathies, not elsewhere classified, elbow**
     M12.821 Other specific arthropathies, not elsewhere classified, right elbow
     M12.822 Other specific arthropathies, not elsewhere classified, left elbow
     M12.829 Other specific arthropathies, not elsewhere classified, unspecified elbow ▽

✓6ᵗʰ **M12.83** **Other specific arthropathies, not elsewhere classified, wrist**
     M12.831 Other specific arthropathies, not elsewhere classified, right wrist
     M12.832 Other specific arthropathies, not elsewhere classified, left wrist
     M12.839 Other specific arthropathies, not elsewhere classified, unspecified wrist ▽

✓6ᵗʰ **M12.84** **Other specific arthropathies, not elsewhere classified, hand**
     M12.841 Other specific arthropathies, not elsewhere classified, right hand
     M12.842 Other specific arthropathies, not elsewhere classified, left hand
     M12.849 Other specific arthropathies, not elsewhere classified, unspecified hand ▽

✓6ᵗʰ **M12.85** **Other specific arthropathies, not elsewhere classified, hip**
     M12.851 Other specific arthropathies, not elsewhere classified, right hip
     M12.852 Other specific arthropathies, not elsewhere classified, left hip
     M12.859 Other specific arthropathies, not elsewhere classified, unspecified hip ▽

✓6ᵗʰ **M12.86** **Other specific arthropathies, not elsewhere classified, knee**
     M12.861 Other specific arthropathies, not elsewhere classified, right knee
     M12.862 Other specific arthropathies, not elsewhere classified, left knee
     M12.869 Other specific arthropathies, not elsewhere classified, unspecified knee ▽

✓6ᵗʰ **M12.87** **Other specific arthropathies, not elsewhere classified, ankle and foot**
     M12.871 Other specific arthropathies, not elsewhere classified, right ankle and foot
     M12.872 Other specific arthropathies, not elsewhere classified, left ankle and foot
     M12.879 Other specific arthropathies, not elsewhere classified, unspecified ankle and foot ▽

     M12.88 **Other specific arthropathies, not elsewhere classified, other specified site**
         Other specific arthropathies, not elsewhere classified, vertebrae

     M12.89 **Other specific arthropathies, not elsewhere classified, multiple sites**

     M12.9 **Arthropathy, unspecified** ▽

✓4ᵗʰ **M13** **Other arthritis**
     EXCLUDES 1   arthrosis (M15-M19)
               osteoarthritis (M15-M19)

     M13.0 **Polyarthritis, unspecified** ▽

✓5ᵗʰ **M13.1** **Monoarthritis, not elsewhere classified**
     M13.10 Monoarthritis, not elsewhere classified, unspecified site ▽

✓6ᵗʰ **M13.11** **Monoarthritis, not elsewhere classified, shoulder**
     M13.111 Monoarthritis, not elsewhere classified, right shoulder
     M13.112 Monoarthritis, not elsewhere classified, left shoulder
     M13.119 Monoarthritis, not elsewhere classified, unspecified shoulder ▽

✓6ᵗʰ **M13.12** **Monoarthritis, not elsewhere classified, elbow**
     M13.121 Monoarthritis, not elsewhere classified, right elbow
     M13.122 Monoarthritis, not elsewhere classified, left elbow
     M13.129 Monoarthritis, not elsewhere classified, unspecified elbow ▽

✓6ᵗʰ **M13.13** **Monoarthritis, not elsewhere classified, wrist**
     M13.131 Monoarthritis, not elsewhere classified, right wrist
     M13.132 Monoarthritis, not elsewhere classified, left wrist
     M13.139 Monoarthritis, not elsewhere classified, unspecified wrist ▽

✓6ᵗʰ **M13.14** **Monoarthritis, not elsewhere classified, hand**
     M13.141 Monoarthritis, not elsewhere classified, right hand
     M13.142 Monoarthritis, not elsewhere classified, left hand
     M13.149 Monoarthritis, not elsewhere classified, unspecified hand ▽

✓6ᵗʰ **M13.15** **Monoarthritis, not elsewhere classified, hip**
     M13.151 Monoarthritis, not elsewhere classified, right hip
     M13.152 Monoarthritis, not elsewhere classified, left hip
     M13.159 Monoarthritis, not elsewhere classified, unspecified hip ▽

✓6ᵗʰ **M13.16** **Monoarthritis, not elsewhere classified, knee**
     M13.161 Monoarthritis, not elsewhere classified, right knee
     M13.162 Monoarthritis, not elsewhere classified, left knee
     M13.169 Monoarthritis, not elsewhere classified, unspecified knee ▽

✓6ᵗʰ **M13.17** **Monoarthritis, not elsewhere classified, ankle and foot**
     M13.171 Monoarthritis, not elsewhere classified, right ankle and foot
     M13.172 Monoarthritis, not elsewhere classified, left ankle and foot
     M13.179 Monoarthritis, not elsewhere classified, unspecified ankle and foot ▽

✓5ᵗʰ **M13.8** **Other specified arthritis**
     Allergic arthritis
     EXCLUDES 1   osteoarthritis (M15-M19)
     M13.80 Other specified arthritis, unspecified site ▽

✓6ᵗʰ **M13.81** **Other specified arthritis, shoulder**
     M13.811 Other specified arthritis, right shoulder
     M13.812 Other specified arthritis, left shoulder
     M13.819 Other specified arthritis, unspecified shoulder ▽

✓6ᵗʰ **M13.82** **Other specified arthritis, elbow**
     M13.821 Other specified arthritis, right elbow
     M13.822 Other specified arthritis, left elbow
     M13.829 Other specified arthritis, unspecified elbow ▽

✓6ᵗʰ **M13.83** **Other specified arthritis, wrist**
     M13.831 Other specified arthritis, right wrist
     M13.832 Other specified arthritis, left wrist
     M13.839 Other specified arthritis, unspecified wrist ▽

✓6ᵗʰ **M13.84** **Other specified arthritis, hand**
     M13.841 Other specified arthritis, right hand
     M13.842 Other specified arthritis, left hand
     M13.849 Other specified arthritis, unspecified hand ▽

✓6ᵗʰ **M13.85** **Other specified arthritis, hip**
     M13.851 Other specified arthritis, right hip
     M13.852 Other specified arthritis, left hip
     M13.859 Other specified arthritis, unspecified hip ▽

EXCLUDES 1 Not coded here   *EXCLUDES 2* Not included here   N Newborn Age: 0   P Pediatric Age: 0-17   M Maternity Age: 12-55   A Adult Age: 15-124

736   ICD-10-CM 2018

√6ᵗʰ **M13.86 Other specified arthritis,** knee
- **M13.861 Other specified arthritis,** right **knee**
- **M13.862 Other specified arthritis,** left **knee**
- **M13.869 Other specified arthritis, unspecified** ▽
  knee

√6ᵗʰ **M13.87 Other specified arthritis,** ankle and foot
- **M13.871 Other specified arthritis,** right **ankle and foot**
- **M13.872 Other specified arthritis,** left **ankle and foot**
- **M13.879 Other specified arthritis, unspecified** ▽
  ankle and foot

M13.88 Other specified arthritis, other site

M13.89 Other specified arthritis, multiple sites

√4ᵗʰ **M14 Arthropathies in other diseases classified elsewhere**

> **EXCLUDES 1**   *arthropathy in:*
> *diabetes mellitus (E08-E13 with .61-)*
> *hematological disorders (M36.2-M36.3)*
> *hypersensitivity reactions (M36.4)*
> *neoplastic disease (M36.1)*
> *neurosyphillis (A52.16)*
> *sarcoidosis (D86.86)*
> *enteropathic arthropathies (M07.-)*
> *juvenile psoriatic arthropathy (L40.54)*
> *lipoid dermatoarthritis (E78.81)*

√5ᵗʰ **M14.6 Charcôt's joint**

> Neuropathic arthropathy
>
> **EXCLUDES 1**   *Charcôt's joint in diabetes mellitus (E08-E13 with .610)*
> *Charcôt's joint in tabes dorsalis (A52.16)*

M14.60 Charcôt's joint, unspecified site   ▽

√6ᵗʰ **M14.61 Charcôt's joint,** shoulder
- **M14.611 Charcôt's joint,** right **shoulder**
- **M14.612 Charcôt's joint,** left **shoulder**
- **M14.619 Charcôt's joint, unspecified shoulder**   ▽

√6ᵗʰ **M14.62 Charcôt's joint,** elbow
- **M14.621 Charcôt's joint,** right **elbow**
- **M14.622 Charcôt's joint,** left **elbow**
- **M14.629 Charcôt's joint, unspecified elbow**   ▽

√6ᵗʰ **M14.63 Charcôt's joint,** wrist
- **M14.631 Charcôt's joint,** right **wrist**
- **M14.632 Charcôt's joint,** left **wrist**
- **M14.639 Charcôt's joint, unspecified wrist**   ▽

√6ᵗʰ **M14.64 Charcôt's joint,** hand
- **M14.641 Charcôt's joint,** right **hand**
- **M14.642 Charcôt's joint,** left **hand**
- **M14.649 Charcôt's joint, unspecified hand**   ▽

√6ᵗʰ **M14.65 Charcôt's joint,** hip
- **M14.651 Charcôt's joint,** right **hip**
- **M14.652 Charcôt's joint,** left **hip**
- **M14.659 Charcôt's joint, unspecified hip**   ▽

√6ᵗʰ **M14.66 Charcôt's joint,** knee
- **M14.661 Charcôt's joint,** right **knee**
- **M14.662 Charcôt's joint,** left **knee**
- **M14.669 Charcôt's joint, unspecified knee**   ▽

√6ᵗʰ **M14.67 Charcôt's joint,** ankle and foot
- **M14.671 Charcôt's joint,** right **ankle and foot**
- **M14.672 Charcôt's joint,** left **ankle and foot**
- **M14.679 Charcôt's joint, unspecified ankle**   ▽
  and foot

M14.68 Charcôt's joint, vertebrae

M14.69 Charcôt's joint, multiple sites

√5ᵗʰ **M14.8 Arthropathies in other specified diseases classified elsewhere**

> Code first underlying disease, such as:
> amyloidosis (E85.-)
> erythema multiforme (L51.-)
> erythema nodosum (L52)
> hemochromatosis (E83.11-)
> hyperparathyroidism (E21.-)
> hypothyroidism (E00-E03)
> sickle-cell disorders (D57.-)
> thyrotoxicosis [hyperthyroidism] (E05.-)
> Whipple's disease (K90.81)

M14.80 Arthropathies in other specified diseases   ▽
classified elsewhere, unspecified site

√6ᵗʰ **M14.81 Arthropathies in other specified diseases classified elsewhere,** shoulder
- *M14.811 Arthropathies in other specified diseases classified elsewhere, right shoulder*
- *M14.812 Arthropathies in other specified diseases classified elsewhere, left shoulder*
- *M14.819 Arthropathies in other specified diseases* ▽
  classified elsewhere, unspecified shoulder

√6ᵗʰ **M14.82 Arthropathies in other specified diseases classified elsewhere,** elbow
- *M14.821 Arthropathies in other specified diseases classified elsewhere, right elbow*
- *M14.822 Arthropathies in other specified diseases classified elsewhere, left elbow*
- *M14.829 Arthropathies in other specified diseases* ▽
  classified elsewhere, unspecified elbow

√6ᵗʰ **M14.83 Arthropathies in other specified diseases classified elsewhere,** wrist
- *M14.831 Arthropathies in other specified diseases classified elsewhere, right wrist*
- *M14.832 Arthropathies in other specified diseases classified elsewhere, left wrist*
- *M14.839 Arthropathies in other specified diseases* ▽
  classified elsewhere, unspecified wrist

√6ᵗʰ **M14.84 Arthropathies in other specified diseases classified elsewhere,** hand
- *M14.841 Arthropathies in other specified diseases classified elsewhere, right hand*
- *M14.842 Arthropathies in other specified diseases classified elsewhere, left hand*
- *M14.849 Arthropathies in other specified diseases* ▽
  classified elsewhere, unspecified hand

√6ᵗʰ **M14.85 Arthropathies in other specified diseases classified elsewhere,** hip
- *M14.851 Arthropathies in other specified diseases classified elsewhere, right hip*
- *M14.852 Arthropathies in other specified diseases classified elsewhere, left hip*
- *M14.859 Arthropathies in other specified diseases* ▽
  classified elsewhere, unspecified hip

√6ᵗʰ **M14.86 Arthropathies in other specified diseases classified elsewhere,** knee
- *M14.861 Arthropathies in other specified diseases classified elsewhere, right knee*
- *M14.862 Arthropathies in other specified diseases classified elsewhere, left knee*
- *M14.869 Arthropathies in other specified diseases* ▽
  classified elsewhere, unspecified knee

√6ᵗʰ **M14.87 Arthropathies in other specified diseases classified elsewhere,** ankle and foot
- *M14.871 Arthropathies in other specified diseases classified elsewhere, right ankle and foot*
- *M14.872 Arthropathies in other specified diseases classified elsewhere, left ankle and foot*
- *M14.879 Arthropathies in other specified diseases* ▽
  classified elsewhere, unspecified ankle and foot

M14.88 Arthropathies in other specified diseases elsewhere, vertebrae

M14.89 Arthropathies in other specified diseases elsewhere, multiple sites

Osteoarthritis (M15-M19)

> **EXCLUDES 2**   *osteoarthritis of spine (M47.-)*

√4ᵗʰ **M15 Polyosteoarthritis**

> **INCLUDES**   arthritis of multiple sites
> **EXCLUDES 1**   *bilateral involvement of single joint (M16-M19)*

M15.0 Primary generalized (osteo)arthritis

M15.1 Heberden's nodes (with arthropathy)
> Interphalangeal distal osteoarthritis

M15.2 Bouchard's nodes (with arthropathy)
> Juxtaphalangeal distal osteoarthritis

M15.3 Secondary multiple arthritis
> Post-traumatic polyosteoarthritis

M15.4 Erosive (osteo)arthritis

M15.8 Other polyosteoarthritis

☑ Additional Character Req   √x7ᵗʰ Placeholder Alert   Manifestation   **HCC** CMS-HCC Condition   ▽ Unspecified Code   ►◄ Revised Text   ● New Code   ▲ Revised Code Title

Chapter 13. Diseases of the Musculoskeletal System and Connective Tissue

M15.9   **Polyosteoarthritis, unspecified**
    Generalized osteoarthritis NOS

✓4ᵗʰ **M16**   **Osteoarthritis of hip**
    AHA: 2016, 4Q, 146

    M16.0   **Bilateral primary osteoarthritis of hip**

✓5ᵗʰ   **M16.1**   **Unilateral primary osteoarthritis of hip**
      Primary osteoarthritis of hip NOS

      M16.10   **Unilateral primary osteoarthritis, unspecified hip** ▽
      M16.11   **Unilateral primary osteoarthritis, right hip**
      M16.12   **Unilateral primary osteoarthritis, left hip**

    M16.2   **Bilateral osteoarthritis resulting from hip dysplasia**

✓5ᵗʰ   **M16.3**   **Unilateral osteoarthritis resulting from hip dysplasia**
      Dysplastic osteoarthritis of hip NOS

      M16.30   **Unilateral osteoarthritis resulting from hip dysplasia, unspecified hip** ▽
      M16.31   **Unilateral osteoarthritis resulting from hip dysplasia, right hip**
      M16.32   **Unilateral osteoarthritis resulting from hip dysplasia, left hip**

    M16.4   **Bilateral post-traumatic osteoarthritis of hip**

✓5ᵗʰ   **M16.5**   **Unilateral post-traumatic osteoarthritis of hip**
      Post-traumatic osteoarthritis of hip NOS

      M16.50   **Unilateral post-traumatic osteoarthritis, unspecified hip** ▽
      M16.51   **Unilateral post-traumatic osteoarthritis, right hip**
      M16.52   **Unilateral post-traumatic osteoarthritis, left hip**

    M16.6   **Other bilateral secondary osteoarthritis of hip**

    M16.7   **Other unilateral secondary osteoarthritis of hip**
      Secondary osteoarthritis of hip NOS

    M16.9   **Osteoarthritis of hip, unspecified** ▽

✓4ᵗʰ **M17**   **Osteoarthritis of knee**
    AHA: 2016, 4Q, 146-147

    M17.0   **Bilateral primary osteoarthritis of knee**

✓5ᵗʰ   **M17.1**   **Unilateral primary osteoarthritis of knee**
      Primary osteoarthritis of knee NOS

      M17.10   **Unilateral primary osteoarthritis, unspecified knee** ▽
      M17.11   **Unilateral primary osteoarthritis, right knee**
      M17.12   **Unilateral primary osteoarthritis, left knee**

    M17.2   **Bilateral post-traumatic osteoarthritis of knee**

✓5ᵗʰ   **M17.3**   **Unilateral post-traumatic osteoarthritis of knee**
      Post-traumatic osteoarthritis of knee NOS

      M17.30   **Unilateral post-traumatic osteoarthritis, unspecified knee** ▽
      M17.31   **Unilateral post-traumatic osteoarthritis, right knee**
      M17.32   **Unilateral post-traumatic osteoarthritis, left knee**

    M17.4   **Other bilateral secondary osteoarthritis of knee**

    M17.5   **Other unilateral secondary osteoarthritis of knee**
      Secondary osteoarthritis of knee NOS

    M17.9   **Osteoarthritis of knee, unspecified** ▽

✓4ᵗʰ **M18**   **Osteoarthritis of first carpometacarpal joint**

    M18.0   **Bilateral primary osteoarthritis of first carpometacarpal joints**

✓5ᵗʰ   **M18.1**   **Unilateral primary osteoarthritis of first carpometacarpal joint**
      Primary osteoarthritis of first carpometacarpal joint NOS

      M18.10   **Unilateral primary osteoarthritis of first carpometacarpal joint, unspecified hand** ▽
      M18.11   **Unilateral primary osteoarthritis of first carpometacarpal joint, right hand**
      M18.12   **Unilateral primary osteoarthritis of first carpometacarpal joint, left hand**

    M18.2   **Bilateral post-traumatic osteoarthritis of first carpometacarpal joints**

✓5ᵗʰ   **M18.3**   **Unilateral post-traumatic osteoarthritis of first carpometacarpal joint**
      Post-traumatic osteoarthritis of first carpometacarpal joint NOS

      M18.30   **Unilateral post-traumatic osteoarthritis of first carpometacarpal joint, unspecified hand** ▽
      M18.31   **Unilateral post-traumatic osteoarthritis of first carpometacarpal joint, right hand**
      M18.32   **Unilateral post-traumatic osteoarthritis of first carpometacarpal joint, left hand**

    M18.4   **Other bilateral secondary osteoarthritis of first carpometacarpal joints**

✓5ᵗʰ   **M18.5**   **Other unilateral secondary osteoarthritis of first carpometacarpal joint**
      Secondary osteoarthritis of first carpometacarpal joint NOS

      M18.50   **Other unilateral secondary osteoarthritis of first carpometacarpal joint, unspecified hand** ▽
      M18.51   **Other unilateral secondary osteoarthritis of first carpometacarpal joint, right hand**
      M18.52   **Other unilateral secondary osteoarthritis of first carpometacarpal joint, left hand**

    M18.9   **Osteoarthritis of first carpometacarpal joint, unspecified** ▽

✓4ᵗʰ **M19**   **Other and unspecified osteoarthritis**
    EXCLUDES 1   polyarthritis (M15.-)
    EXCLUDES 2   arthrosis of spine (M47.-)
            hallux rigidus (M20.2)
            osteoarthritis of spine (M47.-)

✓5ᵗʰ   **M19.0**   **Primary osteoarthritis of other joints**
      AHA: 2016, 4Q, 145

✓6ᵗʰ   **M19.01**   **Primary osteoarthritis, shoulder**
        M19.011   **Primary osteoarthritis, right shoulder**
        M19.012   **Primary osteoarthritis, left shoulder**
        M19.019   **Primary osteoarthritis, unspecified shoulder** ▽

✓6ᵗʰ   **M19.02**   **Primary osteoarthritis, elbow**
        M19.021   **Primary osteoarthritis, right elbow**
        M19.022   **Primary osteoarthritis, left elbow**
        M19.029   **Primary osteoarthritis, unspecified elbow** ▽

✓6ᵗʰ   **M19.03**   **Primary osteoarthritis, wrist**
        M19.031   **Primary osteoarthritis, right wrist**
        M19.032   **Primary osteoarthritis, left wrist**
        M19.039   **Primary osteoarthritis, unspecified wrist** ▽

✓6ᵗʰ   **M19.04**   **Primary osteoarthritis, hand**
        EXCLUDES 2   primary osteoarthritis of first carpometacarpal joint (M18.0-, M18.1-)
        M19.041   **Primary osteoarthritis, right hand**
        M19.042   **Primary osteoarthritis, left hand**
        M19.049   **Primary osteoarthritis, unspecified hand** ▽

✓6ᵗʰ   **M19.07**   **Primary osteoarthritis ankle and foot**
        M19.071   **Primary osteoarthritis, right ankle and foot**
        M19.072   **Primary osteoarthritis, left ankle and foot**
        M19.079   **Primary osteoarthritis, unspecified ankle and foot** ▽

✓5ᵗʰ   **M19.1**   **Post-traumatic osteoarthritis of other joints**

✓6ᵗʰ   **M19.11**   **Post-traumatic osteoarthritis, shoulder**
        M19.111   **Post-traumatic osteoarthritis, right shoulder**
        M19.112   **Post-traumatic osteoarthritis, left shoulder**
        M19.119   **Post-traumatic osteoarthritis, unspecified shoulder** ▽

✓6ᵗʰ   **M19.12**   **Post-traumatic osteoarthritis, elbow**
        M19.121   **Post-traumatic osteoarthritis, right elbow**
        M19.122   **Post-traumatic osteoarthritis, left elbow**
        M19.129   **Post-traumatic osteoarthritis, unspecified elbow** ▽

✓6ᵗʰ   **M19.13**   **Post-traumatic osteoarthritis, wrist**
        M19.131   **Post-traumatic osteoarthritis, right wrist**
        M19.132   **Post-traumatic osteoarthritis, left wrist**
        M19.139   **Post-traumatic osteoarthritis, unspecified wrist** ▽

✓6ᵗʰ   **M19.14**   **Post-traumatic osteoarthritis, hand**
        EXCLUDES 2   post-traumatic osteoarthritis of first carpometacarpal joint (M18.2-, M18.3-)
        M19.141   **Post-traumatic osteoarthritis, right hand**
        M19.142   **Post-traumatic osteoarthritis, left hand**
        M19.149   **Post-traumatic osteoarthritis, unspecified hand** ▽

EXCLUDES 1 Not coded here   EXCLUDES 2 Not included here   N Newborn Age: 0   P Pediatric Age: 0-17   M Maternity Age: 12-55   A Adult Age: 15-124

738   ICD-10-CM 2018

☑6ᵗʰ **M19.17 Post-traumatic osteoarthritis, ankle and foot**
     M19.171 Post-traumatic osteoarthritis, right ankle and foot
     M19.172 Post-traumatic osteoarthritis, left ankle and foot
     M19.179 Post-traumatic osteoarthritis, unspecified ankle and foot ▽

☑5ᵗʰ **M19.2 Secondary osteoarthritis of other joints**

☑6ᵗʰ **M19.21 Secondary osteoarthritis, shoulder**
     M19.211 Secondary osteoarthritis, right shoulder
     M19.212 Secondary osteoarthritis, left shoulder
     M19.219 Secondary osteoarthritis, unspecified shoulder ▽

☑6ᵗʰ **M19.22 Secondary osteoarthritis, elbow**
     M19.221 Secondary osteoarthritis, right elbow
     M19.222 Secondary osteoarthritis, left elbow
     M19.229 Secondary osteoarthritis, unspecified elbow ▽

☑6ᵗʰ **M19.23 Secondary osteoarthritis, wrist**
     M19.231 Secondary osteoarthritis, right wrist
     M19.232 Secondary osteoarthritis, left wrist
     M19.239 Secondary osteoarthritis, unspecified wrist ▽

☑6ᵗʰ **M19.24 Secondary osteoarthritis, hand**
     M19.241 Secondary osteoarthritis, right hand
     M19.242 Secondary osteoarthritis, left hand
     M19.249 Secondary osteoarthritis, unspecified hand ▽

☑6ᵗʰ **M19.27 Secondary osteoarthritis, ankle and foot**
     M19.271 Secondary osteoarthritis, right ankle and foot
     M19.272 Secondary osteoarthritis, left ankle and foot
     M19.279 Secondary osteoarthritis, unspecified ankle and foot ▽

☑5ᵗʰ **M19.9 Osteoarthritis, unspecified site**
     M19.90 Unspecified osteoarthritis, unspecified site ▽
       Arthrosis NOS Osteoarthritis NOS
       Arthritis NOS
       AHA: 2016, 4Q, 147
     M19.91 Primary osteoarthritis, unspecified site ▽
       Primary osteoarthritis NOS
     M19.92 Post-traumatic osteoarthritis, unspecified site ▽
       Post-traumatic osteoarthritis NOS
     M19.93 Secondary osteoarthritis, unspecified site ▽
       Secondary osteoarthritis NOS

Other joint disorders (M20-M25)

EXCLUDES 2   joints of the spine (M40-M54)

☑4ᵗʰ **M20 Acquired deformities of fingers and toes**
     EXCLUDES 1   acquired absence of fingers and toes (Z89.-)
       congenital absence of fingers and toes (Q71.3-, Q72.3-)
       congenital deformities and malformations of fingers and toes (Q66-, Q68-Q70, Q74-)

☑5ᵗʰ **M20.0 Deformity of finger(s)**
     EXCLUDES 1   clubbing of fingers (R68.3)
       palmar fascial fibromatosis [Dupuytren] (M72.0)
       trigger finger (M65.3)

☑6ᵗʰ **M20.00 Unspecified deformity of finger(s)**
     M20.001 Unspecified deformity of right finger(s) ▽
     M20.002 Unspecified deformity of left finger(s) ▽
     M20.009 Unspecified deformity of unspecified finger(s) ▽

☑6ᵗʰ **M20.01 Mallet finger**
     M20.011 Mallet finger of right finger(s)
     M20.012 Mallet finger of left finger(s)
     M20.019 Mallet finger of unspecified finger(s) ▽

☑6ᵗʰ **M20.02 Boutonnière deformity**
     DEF: A deformity of the finger caused by flexion of the proximal interphalangeal joint and hyperextension of the distal joint; results from rheumatoid arthritis, osteoarthritis, or injury; also called buttonhole deformity.
     M20.021 Boutonnière deformity of right finger(s)
     M20.022 Boutonnière deformity of left finger(s)

     M20.029 Boutonnière deformity of unspecified finger(s) ▽

☑6ᵗʰ **M20.03 Swan-neck deformity**
     DEF: Flexed distal and hyperextended proximal interphalangeal joint; most commonly caused by rheumatoid arthritis.
     M20.031 Swan-neck deformity of right finger(s)
     M20.032 Swan-neck deformity of left finger(s)
     M20.039 Swan-neck deformity of unspecified finger(s) ▽

☑6ᵗʰ **M20.09 Other deformity of finger(s)**
     M20.091 Other deformity of right finger(s)
     M20.092 Other deformity of left finger(s)
     M20.099 Other deformity of finger(s), unspecified finger(s) ▽

☑5ᵗʰ **M20.1 Hallux valgus (acquired)**
     EXCLUDES 2   bunion (M21.6-)
     M20.10 Hallux valgus (acquired), unspecified foot ▽
     M20.11 Hallux valgus (acquired), right foot
     M20.12 Hallux valgus (acquired), left foot

☑5ᵗʰ **M20.2 Hallux rigidus**
     M20.20 Hallux rigidus, unspecified foot ▽
     M20.21 Hallux rigidus, right foot
     M20.22 Hallux rigidus, left foot

☑5ᵗʰ **M20.3 Hallux varus (acquired)**
     M20.30 Hallux varus (acquired), unspecified foot ▽
     M20.31 Hallux varus (acquired), right foot
     M20.32 Hallux varus (acquired), left foot

☑5ᵗʰ **M20.4 Other hammer toe(s) (acquired)**
     M20.40 Other hammer toe(s) (acquired), unspecified foot ▽
     M20.41 Other hammer toe(s) (acquired), right foot
     M20.42 Other hammer toe(s) (acquired), left foot

☑5ᵗʰ **M20.5 Other deformities of toe(s) (acquired)**
     ☑6ᵗʰ **M20.5X Other deformities of toe(s) (acquired)**
       M20.5X1 Other deformities of toe(s) (acquired), right foot
       M20.5X2 Other deformities of toe(s) (acquired), left foot
       M20.5X9 Other deformities of toe(s) (acquired), unspecified foot ▽

☑5ᵗʰ **M20.6 Acquired deformities of toe(s), unspecified**
     M20.60 Acquired deformities of toe(s), unspecified, unspecified foot ▽
     M20.61 Acquired deformities of toe(s), unspecified, right foot ▽
     M20.62 Acquired deformities of toe(s), unspecified, left foot ▽

Hallux Valgus

Hallux valgus

Medial eminence of metatarsal bone

Right foot

Genu Valga (knock-knee)

Genu Varus (bowleg)

✓4th **M21   Other acquired deformities of limbs**

> EXCLUDES 1   *acquired absence of limb (Z89.-)*
> *congenital absence of limbs (Q71-Q73)*
> *congenital deformities and malformations of limbs (Q65-Q66, Q68-Q74)*
>
> EXCLUDES 2   *acquired deformities of fingers or toes (M20.-)*
> *coxa plana (M91.2)*

✓5th **M21.0   Valgus deformity, not elsewhere classified**

> EXCLUDES 1   *metatarsus valgus (Q66.6)*
> *talipes calcaneovalgus (Q66.4)*

     M21.00   Valgus deformity, not elsewhere classified, unspecified site ▽

✓6th   **M21.02   Valgus deformity, not elsewhere classified, elbow**
          Cubitus valgus

          M21.021   Valgus deformity, not elsewhere classified, right elbow

          M21.022   Valgus deformity, not elsewhere classified, left elbow

          M21.029   Valgus deformity, not elsewhere classified, unspecified elbow ▽

✓6th   **M21.05   Valgus deformity, not elsewhere classified, hip**

          M21.051   Valgus deformity, not elsewhere classified, right hip

          M21.052   Valgus deformity, not elsewhere classified, left hip

          M21.059   Valgus deformity, not elsewhere classified, unspecified hip ▽

✓6th   **M21.06   Valgus deformity, not elsewhere classified, knee**
          Genu valgum
          Knock knee

          M21.061   Valgus deformity, not elsewhere classified, right knee

          M21.062   Valgus deformity, not elsewhere classified, left knee

          M21.069   Valgus deformity, not elsewhere classified, unspecified knee ▽

✓6th   **M21.07   Valgus deformity, not elsewhere classified, ankle**

          M21.071   Valgus deformity, not elsewhere classified, right ankle

          M21.072   Valgus deformity, not elsewhere classified, left ankle

          M21.079   Valgus deformity, not elsewhere classified, unspecified ankle ▽

✓5th **M21.1   Varus deformity, not elsewhere classified**

> EXCLUDES 1   *metatarsus varus (Q66.22)*
> *tibia vara (M92.5)*

     M21.10   Varus deformity, not elsewhere classified, unspecified site ▽

✓6th   **M21.12   Varus deformity, not elsewhere classified, elbow**
          Cubitus varus, elbow

          M21.121   Varus deformity, not elsewhere classified, right elbow

          M21.122   Varus deformity, not elsewhere classified, left elbow

          M21.129   Varus deformity, not elsewhere classified, unspecified elbow ▽

✓6th   **M21.15   Varus deformity, not elsewhere classified, hip**

          M21.151   Varus deformity, not elsewhere classified, right hip

          M21.152   Varus deformity, not elsewhere classified, left hip

          M21.159   Varus deformity, not elsewhere classified, unspecified ▽

✓6th   **M21.16   Varus deformity, not elsewhere classified, knee**
          Bow leg
          Genu varum

          M21.161   Varus deformity, not elsewhere classified, right knee

          M21.162   Varus deformity, not elsewhere classified, left knee

          M21.169   Varus deformity, not elsewhere classified, unspecified knee ▽

✓6th   **M21.17   Varus deformity, not elsewhere classified, ankle**

          M21.171   Varus deformity, not elsewhere classified, right ankle

          M21.172   Varus deformity, not elsewhere classified, left ankle

          M21.179   Varus deformity, not elsewhere classified, unspecified ankle ▽

✓5th **M21.2   Flexion deformity**

     M21.20   Flexion deformity, unspecified site ▽

✓6th   **M21.21   Flexion deformity, shoulder**

          M21.211   Flexion deformity, right shoulder

          M21.212   Flexion deformity, left shoulder

          M21.219   Flexion deformity, unspecified shoulder ▽

✓6th   **M21.22   Flexion deformity, elbow**

          M21.221   Flexion deformity, right elbow

          M21.222   Flexion deformity, left elbow

          M21.229   Flexion deformity, unspecified elbow ▽

✓6th   **M21.23   Flexion deformity, wrist**

          M21.231   Flexion deformity, right wrist

          M21.232   Flexion deformity, left wrist

          M21.239   Flexion deformity, unspecified wrist ▽

✓6th   **M21.24   Flexion deformity, finger joints**

          M21.241   Flexion deformity, right finger joints

          M21.242   Flexion deformity, left finger joints

          M21.249   Flexion deformity, unspecified finger joints ▽

✓6th   **M21.25   Flexion deformity, hip**

          M21.251   Flexion deformity, right hip

          M21.252   Flexion deformity, left hip

          M21.259   Flexion deformity, unspecified hip ▽

EXCLUDES 1 Not coded here   EXCLUDES 2 Not included here   N Newborn Age: 0   P Pediatric Age: 0-17   M Maternity Age: 12-55   A Adult Age: 15-124

☑6ᵗʰ **M21.26 Flexion deformity,** knee
    M21.261 Flexion deformity, right **knee**
    M21.262 Flexion deformity, left **knee**
    M21.269 Flexion deformity, unspecified knee ▽

☑6ᵗʰ **M21.27 Flexion deformity,** ankle and toes
    M21.271 Flexion deformity, right **ankle and toes**
    M21.272 Flexion deformity, left **ankle and toes**
    M21.279 Flexion deformity, unspecified ankle and toes ▽

☑5ᵗʰ **M21.3 Wrist or foot drop (acquired)**

☑6ᵗʰ **M21.33 Wrist drop (acquired)**
    M21.331 Wrist drop, right **wrist**
    M21.332 Wrist drop, left **wrist**
    M21.339 Wrist drop, unspecified wrist ▽

☑6ᵗʰ **M21.37 Foot drop (acquired)**
    M21.371 Foot drop, right **foot**
    M21.372 Foot drop, left **foot**
    M21.379 Foot drop, unspecified foot ▽

☑5ᵗʰ **M21.4 Flat foot [pes planus] (acquired)**
    EXCLUDES 1 *congenital pes planus (Q66.5-)*
    M21.40 Flat foot [pes planus] (acquired), unspecified foot ▽
    M21.41 Flat foot [pes planus] (acquired), right **foot**
    M21.42 Flat foot [pes planus] (acquired), left **foot**

☑5ᵗʰ **M21.5 Acquired** clawhand, clubhand, clawfoot and clubfoot
    EXCLUDES 1 *clubfoot, not specified as acquired (Q66.89)*

☑6ᵗʰ **M21.51 Acquired** clawhand
    M21.511 Acquired clawhand, right **hand**
    M21.512 Acquired clawhand, left **hand**
    M21.519 Acquired clawhand, unspecified hand ▽

☑6ᵗʰ **M21.52 Acquired** clubhand
    M21.521 Acquired clubhand, right **hand**
    M21.522 Acquired clubhand, left **hand**
    M21.529 Acquired clubhand, unspecified hand ▽

☑6ᵗʰ **M21.53 Acquired** clawfoot
    DEF: High foot arch with hyperextended toes at metatarsophalangeal joint and flexed toes at distal joints.
    M21.531 Acquired clawfoot, right **foot**
    M21.532 Acquired clawfoot, left **foot**
    M21.539 Acquired clawfoot, unspecified foot ▽

☑6ᵗʰ **M21.54 Acquired** clubfoot
    M21.541 Acquired clubfoot, right **foot**
    M21.542 Acquired clubfoot, left **foot**
    M21.549 Acquired clubfoot, unspecified foot ▽

☑5ᵗʰ **M21.6 Other acquired deformities of foot**
    EXCLUDES 2 *deformities of toe (acquired) (M20.1-M20.6-)*

☑6ᵗʰ **M21.61 Bunion**
    M21.611 Bunion of right **foot**
    M21.612 Bunion of left **foot**
    M21.619 Bunion of unspecified foot ▽

☑6ᵗʰ **M21.62 Bunionette**
    M21.621 Bunionette of right **foot**
    M21.622 Bunionette of left **foot**
    M21.629 Bunionette of unspecified foot ▽

☑6ᵗʰ **M21.6X Other acquired deformities of** foot
    M21.6X1 Other acquired deformities of right **foot**
    M21.6X2 Other acquired deformities of left **foot**
    M21.6X9 Other acquired deformities of unspecified foot ▽

☑5ᵗʰ **M21.7 Unequal limb length (acquired)**
    NOTE The site used should correspond to the shorter limb.
    M21.70 Unequal limb length (acquired), unspecified site ▽

☑6ᵗʰ **M21.72 Unequal limb length (acquired),** humerus
    M21.721 Unequal limb length (acquired), right **humerus**
    M21.722 Unequal limb length (acquired), left **humerus**
    M21.729 Unequal limb length (acquired), unspecified humerus ▽

☑6ᵗʰ **M21.73 Unequal limb length (acquired), ulna and radius**
    M21.731 Unequal limb length (acquired), right **ulna**
    M21.732 Unequal limb length (acquired), left **ulna**

    M21.733 Unequal limb length (acquired), right **radius**
    M21.734 Unequal limb length (acquired), left **radius**
    M21.739 Unequal limb length (acquired), unspecified ulna and radius ▽

☑6ᵗʰ **M21.75 Unequal limb length (acquired),** femur
    M21.751 Unequal limb length (acquired), right **femur**
    M21.752 Unequal limb length (acquired), left **femur**
    M21.759 Unequal limb length (acquired), unspecified femur ▽

☑6ᵗʰ **M21.76 Unequal limb length (acquired),** tibia and fibula
    M21.761 Unequal limb length (acquired), right **tibia**
    M21.762 Unequal limb length (acquired), left **tibia**
    M21.763 Unequal limb length (acquired), right **fibula**
    M21.764 Unequal limb length (acquired), left **fibula**
    M21.769 Unequal limb length (acquired), unspecified tibia and fibula ▽

☑5ᵗʰ **M21.8 Other specified acquired deformities of limbs**
    EXCLUDES 2 *coxa plana (M91.2)*
    M21.80 Other specified acquired deformities of unspecified limb ▽

☑6ᵗʰ **M21.82 Other specified acquired deformities of** upper arm
    M21.821 Other specified acquired deformities of right upper arm
    M21.822 Other specified acquired deformities of left upper arm
    M21.829 Other specified acquired deformities of unspecified upper arm ▽

☑6ᵗʰ **M21.83 Other specified acquired deformities of** forearm
    M21.831 Other specified acquired deformities of right forearm
    M21.832 Other specified acquired deformities of left forearm
    M21.839 Other specified acquired deformities of unspecified forearm ▽

☑6ᵗʰ **M21.85 Other specified acquired deformities of** thigh
    M21.851 Other specified acquired deformities of right thigh
    M21.852 Other specified acquired deformities of left thigh
    M21.859 Other specified acquired deformities of unspecified thigh ▽

☑6ᵗʰ **M21.86 Other specified acquired deformities of** lower leg
    M21.861 Other specified acquired deformities of right lower leg
    M21.862 Other specified acquired deformities of left lower leg
    M21.869 Other specified acquired deformities of unspecified lower leg ▽

☑5ᵗʰ **M21.9 Unspecified acquired deformity of** limb and hand
    M21.90 Unspecified acquired deformity of unspecified limb ▽

☑6ᵗʰ **M21.92 Unspecified acquired deformity of** upper arm
    M21.921 Unspecified acquired deformity of right upper arm ▽
    M21.922 Unspecified acquired deformity of left upper arm ▽
    M21.929 Unspecified acquired deformity of unspecified upper arm ▽

☑6ᵗʰ **M21.93 Unspecified acquired deformity of** forearm
    M21.931 Unspecified acquired deformity of right forearm ▽
    M21.932 Unspecified acquired deformity of left forearm ▽
    M21.939 Unspecified acquired deformity of unspecified forearm ▽

☑6ᵗʰ **M21.94 Unspecified acquired deformity of** hand
    M21.941 Unspecified acquired deformity of hand, right **hand** ▽
    M21.942 Unspecified acquired deformity of hand, left **hand** ▽
    M21.949 Unspecified acquired deformity of hand, unspecified hand ▽

☑ Additional Character Req   ᵛˣ⁷ᵗʰ Placeholder Alert   Manifestation   ᴴᶜᶜ CMS-HCC Condition   ▽ Unspecified Code   ▶◀ Revised Text   ● New Code   ▲ Revised Code Title

✓6ᵗʰ **M21.95 Unspecified acquired deformity of** thigh
    M21.951 Unspecified acquired deformity of right thigh ▽
    M21.952 Unspecified acquired deformity of left thigh ▽
    M21.959 Unspecified acquired deformity of unspecified thigh ▽

✓6ᵗʰ **M21.96 Unspecified acquired deformity of** lower leg
    M21.961 Unspecified acquired deformity of right lower leg ▽
    M21.962 Unspecified acquired deformity of left lower leg ▽
    M21.969 Unspecified acquired deformity of unspecified lower leg ▽

✓4ᵗʰ **M22 Disorder of** patella
    EXCLUDES 1   *traumatic dislocation of patella (S83.0-)*

✓5ᵗʰ **M22.0 Recurrent dislocation of patella**
    M22.00 Recurrent dislocation of patella, unspecified knee ▽
    M22.01 Recurrent dislocation of patella, right knee
    M22.02 Recurrent dislocation of patella, left knee

✓5ᵗʰ **M22.1 Recurrent subluxation of patella**
    Incomplete dislocation of patella
    M22.10 Recurrent subluxation of patella, unspecified knee ▽
    M22.11 Recurrent subluxation of patella, right knee
    M22.12 Recurrent subluxation of patella, left knee

✓5ᵗʰ **M22.2 Patellofemoral disorders**
    ✓6ᵗʰ **M22.2X Patellofemoral disorders**
      M22.2X1 Patellofemoral disorders, right knee
      M22.2X2 Patellofemoral disorders, left knee
      M22.2X9 Patellofemoral disorders, unspecified knee ▽

✓5ᵗʰ **M22.3 Other derangements of patella**
    ✓6ᵗʰ **M22.3X Other derangements of patella**
      M22.3X1 Other derangements of patella, right knee
      M22.3X2 Other derangements of patella, left knee
      M22.3X9 Other derangements of patella, unspecified knee ▽

✓5ᵗʰ **M22.4 Chondromalacia patellae**
    M22.40 Chondromalacia patellae, unspecified knee ▽
    M22.41 Chondromalacia patellae, right knee
    M22.42 Chondromalacia patellae, left knee

✓5ᵗʰ **M22.8 Other disorders of patella**
    ✓6ᵗʰ **M22.8X Other disorders of patella**
      M22.8X1 Other disorders of patella, right knee
      M22.8X2 Other disorders of patella, left knee
      M22.8X9 Other disorders of patella, unspecified knee ▽

✓5ᵗʰ **M22.9 Unspecified disorder of patella**
    M22.90 Unspecified disorder of patella, unspecified knee ▽
    M22.91 Unspecified disorder of patella, right knee ▽
    M22.92 Unspecified disorder of patella, left knee ▽

✓4ᵗʰ **M23 Internal derangement of knee**
    EXCLUDES 1   *ankylosis (M24.66)*
         current injury—see injury of knee and lower leg (S80-S89)
         deformity of knee (M21.-)
         osteochondritis dissecans (M93.2)
         recurrent dislocation or subluxation of joints (M24.4)
         recurrent dislocation or subluxation of patella (M22.0-M22.1)

✓5ᵗʰ **M23.0 Cystic meniscus**
    ✓6ᵗʰ **M23.00 Cystic meniscus, unspecified meniscus**
      Cystic meniscus, unspecified lateral meniscus
      Cystic meniscus, unspecified medial meniscus
      M23.000 Cystic meniscus, unspecified lateral meniscus, right knee
      M23.001 Cystic meniscus, unspecified lateral meniscus, left knee
      M23.002 Cystic meniscus, unspecified lateral meniscus, unspecified knee ▽
      M23.003 Cystic meniscus, unspecified medial meniscus, right knee
      M23.004 Cystic meniscus, unspecified medial meniscus, left knee

      M23.005 Cystic meniscus, unspecified medial **meniscus, unspecified knee** ▽
      M23.006 Cystic meniscus, unspecified meniscus, right knee
      M23.007 Cystic meniscus, unspecified meniscus, left knee
      M23.009 Cystic meniscus, unspecified meniscus, unspecified knee ▽

✓6ᵗʰ **M23.01 Cystic meniscus,** anterior horn of medial **meniscus**
    M23.011 Cystic meniscus, anterior horn of medial meniscus, right knee
    M23.012 Cystic meniscus, anterior horn of medial meniscus, left knee
    M23.019 Cystic meniscus, anterior horn of medial meniscus, unspecified knee ▽

✓6ᵗʰ **M23.02 Cystic meniscus,** posterior horn of medial **meniscus**
    M23.021 Cystic meniscus, posterior horn of medial meniscus, right knee
    M23.022 Cystic meniscus, posterior horn of medial meniscus, left knee
    M23.029 Cystic meniscus, posterior horn of medial meniscus, unspecified knee ▽

✓6ᵗʰ **M23.03 Cystic meniscus,** other medial **meniscus**
    M23.031 Cystic meniscus, other medial meniscus, right knee
    M23.032 Cystic meniscus, other medial meniscus, left knee
    M23.039 Cystic meniscus, other medial meniscus, unspecified knee ▽

✓6ᵗʰ **M23.04 Cystic meniscus,** anterior horn of lateral **meniscus**
    M23.041 Cystic meniscus, anterior horn of lateral meniscus, right knee
    M23.042 Cystic meniscus, anterior horn of lateral meniscus, left knee
    M23.049 Cystic meniscus, anterior horn of lateral meniscus, unspecified knee ▽

✓6ᵗʰ **M23.05 Cystic meniscus,** posterior horn of lateral **meniscus**
    M23.051 Cystic meniscus, posterior horn of lateral meniscus, right knee
    M23.052 Cystic meniscus, posterior horn of lateral meniscus, left knee
    M23.059 Cystic meniscus, posterior horn of lateral meniscus, unspecified knee ▽

✓6ᵗʰ **M23.06 Cystic meniscus,** other lateral **meniscus**
    M23.061 Cystic meniscus, other lateral meniscus, right knee
    M23.062 Cystic meniscus, other lateral meniscus, left knee
    M23.069 Cystic meniscus, other lateral meniscus, unspecified knee ▽

✓5ᵗʰ **M23.2 Derangement of meniscus due to old tear or injury**
    Old bucket-handle tear
    ✓6ᵗʰ **M23.20 Derangement of unspecified meniscus due to old tear or injury**
      Derangement of unspecified lateral meniscus due to old tear or injury
      Derangement of unspecified medial meniscus due to old tear or injury
      M23.200 Derangement of unspecified lateral meniscus due to old tear or injury, right knee ▽
      M23.201 Derangement of unspecified lateral meniscus due to old tear or injury, left knee ▽
      M23.202 Derangement of unspecified lateral meniscus due to old tear or injury, unspecified knee ▽
      M23.203 Derangement of unspecified medial meniscus due to old tear or injury, right knee ▽
      M23.204 Derangement of unspecified medial meniscus due to old tear or injury, left knee ▽

EXCLUDES 1   Not coded here   EXCLUDES 2   Not included here   N Newborn Age: 0   P Pediatric Age: 0-17   M Maternity Age: 12-55   A Adult Age: 15-124

742   ICD-10-CM 2018

Derangement of Meniscus

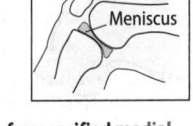

Bucket handle tear

Radial tear

Meniscus

Overhead view of right knee

M23.205 Derangement of unspecified medial meniscus due to old tear or injury, unspecified knee ▽

M23.206 Derangement of unspecified meniscus due to old tear or injury, right knee ▽

M23.207 Derangement of unspecified meniscus due to old tear or injury, left knee ▽

M23.209 Derangement of unspecified meniscus due to old tear or injury, unspecified knee ▽

✓6ᵗʰ **M23.21** Derangement of anterior horn of medial meniscus due to old tear or injury

   M23.211 Derangement of anterior horn of medial meniscus due to old tear or injury, right knee

   M23.212 Derangement of anterior horn of medial meniscus due to old tear or injury, left knee

   M23.219 Derangement of anterior horn of medial meniscus due to old tear or injury, unspecified knee ▽

✓6ᵗʰ **M23.22** Derangement of posterior horn of medial meniscus due to old tear or injury

   M23.221 Derangement of posterior horn of medial meniscus due to old tear or injury, right knee

   M23.222 Derangement of posterior horn of medial meniscus due to old tear or injury, left knee

   M23.229 Derangement of posterior horn of medial meniscus due to old tear or injury, unspecified knee ▽

✓6ᵗʰ **M23.23** Derangement of other medial meniscus due to old tear or injury

   M23.231 Derangement of other medial meniscus due to old tear or injury, right knee

   M23.232 Derangement of other medial meniscus due to old tear or injury, left knee

   M23.239 Derangement of other medial meniscus due to old tear or injury, unspecified knee ▽

✓6ᵗʰ **M23.24** Derangement of anterior horn of lateral meniscus due to old tear or injury

   M23.241 Derangement of anterior horn of lateral meniscus due to old tear or injury, right knee

   M23.242 Derangement of anterior horn of lateral meniscus due to old tear or injury, left knee

   M23.249 Derangement of anterior horn of lateral meniscus due to old tear or injury, unspecified knee ▽

✓6ᵗʰ **M23.25** Derangement of posterior horn of lateral meniscus due to old tear or injury

   M23.251 Derangement of posterior horn of lateral meniscus due to old tear or injury, right knee

   M23.252 Derangement of posterior horn of lateral meniscus due to old tear or injury, left knee

   M23.259 Derangement of posterior horn of lateral meniscus due to old tear or injury, unspecified knee ▽

✓6ᵗʰ **M23.26** Derangement of other lateral meniscus due to old tear or injury

   M23.261 Derangement of other lateral meniscus due to old tear or injury, right knee

   M23.262 Derangement of other lateral meniscus due to old tear or injury, left knee

   M23.269 Derangement of other lateral meniscus due to old tear or injury, unspecified knee ▽

✓5ᵗʰ **M23.3** **Other meniscus derangements**
   Degenerate meniscus
   Detached meniscus
   Retained meniscus

✓6ᵗʰ **M23.30** Other meniscus derangements, unspecified meniscus
   Other meniscus derangements, unspecified lateral meniscus
   Other meniscus derangements, unspecified medial meniscus

   M23.300 Other meniscus derangements, unspecified lateral meniscus, right knee ▽

   M23.301 Other meniscus derangements, unspecified lateral meniscus, left knee

   M23.302 Other meniscus derangements, unspecified lateral meniscus, unspecified knee ▽

   M23.303 Other meniscus derangements, unspecified medial meniscus, right knee ▽

   M23.304 Other meniscus derangements, unspecified medial meniscus, left knee ▽

   M23.305 Other meniscus derangements, unspecified medial meniscus, unspecified knee ▽

   M23.306 Other meniscus derangements, unspecified meniscus, right knee ▽

   M23.307 Other meniscus derangements, unspecified meniscus, left knee ▽

   M23.309 Other meniscus derangements, unspecified meniscus, unspecified knee ▽

✓6ᵗʰ **M23.31** Other meniscus derangements, anterior horn of medial meniscus

   M23.311 Other meniscus derangements, anterior horn of medial meniscus, right knee

   M23.312 Other meniscus derangements, anterior horn of medial meniscus, left knee

   M23.319 Other meniscus derangements, anterior horn of medial meniscus, unspecified knee ▽

✓6ᵗʰ **M23.32** Other meniscus derangements, posterior horn of medial meniscus

   M23.321 Other meniscus derangements, posterior horn of medial meniscus, right knee

   M23.322 Other meniscus derangements, posterior horn of medial meniscus, left knee

   M23.329 Other meniscus derangements, posterior horn of medial meniscus, unspecified knee ▽

✓6ᵗʰ **M23.33** Other meniscus derangements, other medial meniscus

   M23.331 Other meniscus derangements, other medial meniscus, right knee

   M23.332 Other meniscus derangements, other medial meniscus, left knee

   M23.339 Other meniscus derangements, other medial meniscus, unspecified knee ▽

✓6ᵗʰ **M23.34** Other meniscus derangements, anterior horn of lateral meniscus

   M23.341 Other meniscus derangements, anterior horn of lateral meniscus, right knee

☑ Additional Character Req   ✓x7ᵗʰ Placeholder Alert   Manifestation   HCC CMS-HCC Condition   ▽ Unspecified Code   ▶◀ Revised Text   ● New Code   ▲ Revised Code Title

ICD-10-CM 2018   **743**

M23.342   Other meniscus derangements, anterior horn of lateral meniscus, **left** knee

M23.349   Other meniscus derangements, anterior ▽ horn of lateral meniscus, unspecified knee

✓6ᵗʰ **M23.35**   Other meniscus derangements, **posterior horn of lateral meniscus**

M23.351   Other meniscus derangements, posterior horn of lateral meniscus, **right** knee

M23.352   Other meniscus derangements, posterior horn of lateral meniscus, **left** knee

M23.359   Other meniscus derangements, ▽ posterior horn of lateral meniscus, unspecified knee

✓6ᵗʰ **M23.36**   Other meniscus derangements, **other lateral meniscus**

M23.361   Other meniscus derangements, other lateral meniscus, **right** knee

M23.362   Other meniscus derangements, other lateral meniscus, **left** knee

M23.369   Other meniscus derangements, other ▽ lateral meniscus, unspecified knee

✓5ᵗʰ **M23.4**   **Loose body in knee**

M23.40   Loose body in knee, unspecified knee ▽

M23.41   Loose body in knee, **right** knee

M23.42   Loose body in knee, **left** knee

✓5ᵗʰ **M23.5**   **Chronic instability of knee**

M23.50   Chronic instability of knee, unspecified knee ▽

M23.51   Chronic instability of knee, **right** knee

M23.52   Chronic instability of knee, **left** knee

✓5ᵗʰ **M23.6**   **Other spontaneous disruption of ligament(s) of knee**

✓6ᵗʰ **M23.60**   Other spontaneous disruption of unspecified ligament of knee

M23.601   Other spontaneous disruption of ▽ unspecified ligament of **right** knee

M23.602   Other spontaneous disruption of ▽ unspecified ligament of **left** knee

M23.609   Other spontaneous disruption of ▽ unspecified ligament of unspecified knee

✓6ᵗʰ **M23.61**   Other spontaneous disruption of **anterior cruciate** ligament of knee

M23.611   Other spontaneous disruption of anterior cruciate ligament of **right** knee

M23.612   Other spontaneous disruption of anterior cruciate ligament of **left** knee

M23.619   Other spontaneous disruption of ▽ anterior cruciate ligament of unspecified knee

✓6ᵗʰ **M23.62**   Other spontaneous disruption of **posterior cruciate** ligament of knee

M23.621   Other spontaneous disruption of posterior cruciate ligament of **right** knee

M23.622   Other spontaneous disruption of posterior cruciate ligament of **left** knee

M23.629   Other spontaneous disruption of ▽ posterior cruciate ligament of unspecified knee

✓6ᵗʰ **M23.63**   Other spontaneous disruption of **medial collateral** ligament of knee

M23.631   Other spontaneous disruption of medial collateral ligament of **right** knee

M23.632   Other spontaneous disruption of medial collateral ligament of **left** knee

M23.639   Other spontaneous disruption of ▽ medial collateral ligament of unspecified knee

✓6ᵗʰ **M23.64**   Other spontaneous disruption of **lateral collateral** ligament of knee

M23.641   Other spontaneous disruption of lateral collateral ligament of **right** knee

M23.642   Other spontaneous disruption of lateral collateral ligament of **left** knee

M23.649   Other spontaneous disruption of ▽ lateral collateral ligament of unspecified knee

✓6ᵗʰ **M23.67**   Other spontaneous disruption of **capsular** ligament of knee

M23.671   Other spontaneous disruption of capsular ligament of **right** knee

M23.672   Other spontaneous disruption of capsular ligament of **left** knee

M23.679   Other spontaneous disruption of ▽ capsular ligament of unspecified knee

✓5ᵗʰ **M23.8**   **Other internal derangements of knee**

Laxity of ligament of knee

Snapping knee

✓6ᵗʰ **M23.8X**   Other internal derangements of knee

M23.8X1   Other internal derangements of **right** knee

M23.8X2   Other internal derangements of **left** knee

M23.8X9   Other internal derangements of ▽ unspecified knee

✓5ᵗʰ **M23.9**   **Unspecified internal derangement of knee**

M23.90   Unspecified internal derangement of unspecified ▽ knee

M23.91   Unspecified internal derangement of **right** knee ▽

M23.92   Unspecified internal derangement of **left** knee ▽

✓4ᵗʰ **M24**   **Other specific joint derangements**

EXCLUDES 1   current injury—see injury of joint by body region

EXCLUDES 2   ganglion (M67.4)

snapping knee (M23.8-)

temporomandibular joint disorders (M26.6-)

✓5ᵗʰ **M24.0**   **Loose body in joint**

EXCLUDES 2   loose body in knee (M23.4)

M24.00   Loose body in unspecified joint ▽

✓6ᵗʰ **M24.01**   Loose body in **shoulder**

M24.011   Loose body in **right** shoulder

M24.012   Loose body in **left** shoulder

M24.019   Loose body in unspecified shoulder ▽

✓6ᵗʰ **M24.02**   Loose body in **elbow**

M24.021   Loose body in **right** elbow

M24.022   Loose body in **left** elbow

M24.029   Loose body in unspecified elbow ▽

✓6ᵗʰ **M24.03**   Loose body in **wrist**

M24.031   Loose body in **right** wrist

M24.032   Loose body in **left** wrist

M24.039   Loose body in unspecified wrist ▽

✓6ᵗʰ **M24.04**   Loose body in **finger joints**

M24.041   Loose body in **right** finger joint(s)

M24.042   Loose body in **left** finger joint(s)

M24.049   Loose body in unspecified finger ▽ joint(s)

✓6ᵗʰ **M24.05**   Loose body in **hip**

M24.051   Loose body in **right** hip

M24.052   Loose body in **left** hip

M24.059   Loose body in unspecified hip ▽

✓6ᵗʰ **M24.07**   Loose body in **ankle and toe joints**

M24.071   Loose body in **right** ankle

M24.072   Loose body in **left** ankle

M24.073   Loose body in unspecified ankle ▽

M24.074   Loose body in **right** toe joint(s)

M24.075   Loose body in **left** toe joint(s)

M24.076   Loose body in unspecified toe joints ▽

M24.08   Loose body, other site

✓5ᵗʰ **M24.1**   **Other articular cartilage disorders**

EXCLUDES 2   chondrocalcinosis (M11.1, M11.2-)

internal derangement of knee (M23.-)

metastatic calcification (E83.5)

ochronosis (E70.2)

M24.10   Other articular cartilage disorders, unspecified ▽ site

✓6ᵗʰ **M24.11**   Other articular cartilage disorders, **shoulder**

M24.111   Other articular cartilage disorders, **right** shoulder

M24.112   Other articular cartilage disorders, **left** shoulder

M24.119   Other articular cartilage disorders, ▽ unspecified shoulder

EXCLUDES 1 Not coded here   *EXCLUDES 2* Not included here   N Newborn Age: 0   P Pediatric Age: 0-17   M Maternity Age: 12-55   A Adult Age: 15-124

744   ICD-10-CM 2018

✓6ᵗʰ **M24.12** Other articular cartilage disorders, elbow
    M24.121 Other articular cartilage disorders, right elbow
    M24.122 Other articular cartilage disorders, left elbow
    M24.129 Other articular cartilage disorders, unspecified elbow ▽

✓6ᵗʰ **M24.13** Other articular cartilage disorders, wrist
    M24.131 Other articular cartilage disorders, right wrist
    M24.132 Other articular cartilage disorders, left wrist
    M24.139 Other articular cartilage disorders, unspecified wrist ▽

✓6ᵗʰ **M24.14** Other articular cartilage disorders, hand
    M24.141 Other articular cartilage disorders, right hand
    M24.142 Other articular cartilage disorders, left hand
    M24.149 Other articular cartilage disorders, unspecified hand ▽

✓6ᵗʰ **M24.15** Other articular cartilage disorders, hip
    M24.151 Other articular cartilage disorders, right hip
    M24.152 Other articular cartilage disorders, left hip
    M24.159 Other articular cartilage disorders, unspecified hip ▽

✓6ᵗʰ **M24.17** Other articular cartilage disorders, ankle and foot
    M24.171 Other articular cartilage disorders, right ankle
    M24.172 Other articular cartilage disorders, left ankle
    M24.173 Other articular cartilage disorders, unspecified ankle ▽
    M24.174 Other articular cartilage disorders, right foot
    M24.175 Other articular cartilage disorders, left foot
    M24.176 Other articular cartilage disorders, unspecified foot ▽

✓5ᵗʰ **M24.2 Disorder of ligament**
Instability secondary to old ligament injury
Ligamentous laxity NOS
  EXCLUDES 1   familial ligamentous laxity (M35.7)
  EXCLUDES 2   internal derangement of knee (M23.5-M23.89)
    M24.20 Disorder of ligament, unspecified site ▽

✓6ᵗʰ **M24.21** Disorder of ligament, shoulder
    M24.211 Disorder of ligament, right shoulder
    M24.212 Disorder of ligament, left shoulder
    M24.219 Disorder of ligament, unspecified shoulder ▽

✓6ᵗʰ **M24.22** Disorder of ligament, elbow
    M24.221 Disorder of ligament, right elbow
    M24.222 Disorder of ligament, left elbow
    M24.229 Disorder of ligament, unspecified elbow ▽

✓6ᵗʰ **M24.23** Disorder of ligament, wrist
    M24.231 Disorder of ligament, right wrist
    M24.232 Disorder of ligament, left wrist
    M24.239 Disorder of ligament, unspecified wrist ▽

✓6ᵗʰ **M24.24** Disorder of ligament, hand
    M24.241 Disorder of ligament, right hand
    M24.242 Disorder of ligament, left hand
    M24.249 Disorder of ligament, unspecified hand ▽

✓6ᵗʰ **M24.25** Disorder of ligament, hip
    M24.251 Disorder of ligament, right hip
    M24.252 Disorder of ligament, left hip
    M24.259 Disorder of ligament, unspecified hip ▽

✓6ᵗʰ **M24.27** Disorder of ligament, ankle and foot
    M24.271 Disorder of ligament, right ankle
    M24.272 Disorder of ligament, left ankle
    M24.273 Disorder of ligament, unspecified ankle ▽
    M24.274 Disorder of ligament, right foot
    M24.275 Disorder of ligament, left foot
    M24.276 Disorder of ligament, unspecified foot ▽

M24.28 Disorder of ligament, vertebrae

✓5ᵗʰ **M24.3 Pathological dislocation of joint, not elsewhere classified**
  EXCLUDES 1   congenital dislocation or displacement of joint—see congenital malformations and deformations of the musculoskeletal system (Q65-Q79)
            current injury—see injury of joints and ligaments by body region
            recurrent dislocation of joint (M24.4-)
    M24.30 Pathological dislocation of unspecified joint, not elsewhere classified ▽

✓6ᵗʰ **M24.31** Pathological dislocation of shoulder, not elsewhere classified
    M24.311 Pathological dislocation of right shoulder, not elsewhere classified
    M24.312 Pathological dislocation of left shoulder, not elsewhere classified
    M24.319 Pathological dislocation of unspecified shoulder, not elsewhere classified ▽

✓6ᵗʰ **M24.32** Pathological dislocation of elbow, not elsewhere classified
    M24.321 Pathological dislocation of right elbow, not elsewhere classified
    M24.322 Pathological dislocation of left elbow, not elsewhere classified
    M24.329 Pathological dislocation of unspecified elbow, not elsewhere classified ▽

✓6ᵗʰ **M24.33** Pathological dislocation of wrist, not elsewhere classified
    M24.331 Pathological dislocation of right wrist, not elsewhere classified
    M24.332 Pathological dislocation of left wrist, not elsewhere classified
    M24.339 Pathological dislocation of unspecified wrist, not elsewhere classified ▽

✓6ᵗʰ **M24.34** Pathological dislocation of hand, not elsewhere classified
    M24.341 Pathological dislocation of right hand, not elsewhere classified
    M24.342 Pathological dislocation of left hand, not elsewhere classified
    M24.349 Pathological dislocation of unspecified hand, not elsewhere classified ▽

✓6ᵗʰ **M24.35** Pathological dislocation of hip, not elsewhere classified
    M24.351 Pathological dislocation of right hip, not elsewhere classified
    M24.352 Pathological dislocation of left hip, not elsewhere classified
    M24.359 Pathological dislocation of unspecified hip, not elsewhere classified ▽

✓6ᵗʰ **M24.36** Pathological dislocation of knee, not elsewhere classified
    M24.361 Pathological dislocation of right knee, not elsewhere classified
    M24.362 Pathological dislocation of left knee, not elsewhere classified
    M24.369 Pathological dislocation of unspecified knee, not elsewhere classified ▽

✓6ᵗʰ **M24.37** Pathological dislocation of ankle and foot, not elsewhere classified
    M24.371 Pathological dislocation of right ankle, not elsewhere classified
    M24.372 Pathological dislocation of left ankle, not elsewhere classified
    M24.373 Pathological dislocation of unspecified ankle, not elsewhere classified ▽
    M24.374 Pathological dislocation of right foot, not elsewhere classified
    M24.375 Pathological dislocation of left foot, not elsewhere classified
    M24.376 Pathological dislocation of unspecified foot, not elsewhere classified ▽

✓ Additional Character Req   ✓x7ᵗʰ Placeholder Alert   Manifestation   HCC CMS-HCC Condition   ▽ Unspecified Code   ►◄ Revised Text   ● New Code   ▲ Revised Code Title

ICD-10-CM 2018   745

Chapter 13. Diseases of the Musculoskeletal System and Connective Tissue

M24.4–M24.829

✓5ᵗʰ **M24.4 Recurrent dislocation of joint**
Recurrent subluxation of joint
> EXCLUDES 2   recurrent dislocation of patella (M22.0-M22.1)
> recurrent vertebral dislocation (M43.3-, M43.4, M43.5-)

M24.40 Recurrent dislocation, unspecified joint ▽

✓6ᵗʰ **M24.41 Recurrent dislocation, shoulder**
M24.411 Recurrent dislocation, right shoulder
M24.412 Recurrent dislocation, left shoulder
M24.419 Recurrent dislocation, unspecified shoulder ▽

✓6ᵗʰ **M24.42 Recurrent dislocation, elbow**
M24.421 Recurrent dislocation, right elbow
M24.422 Recurrent dislocation, left elbow
M24.429 Recurrent dislocation, unspecified elbow ▽

✓6ᵗʰ **M24.43 Recurrent dislocation, wrist**
M24.431 Recurrent dislocation, right wrist
M24.432 Recurrent dislocation, left wrist
M24.439 Recurrent dislocation, unspecified wrist ▽

✓6ᵗʰ **M24.44 Recurrent dislocation, hand and finger(s)**
M24.441 Recurrent dislocation, right hand
M24.442 Recurrent dislocation, left hand
M24.443 Recurrent dislocation, unspecified hand ▽
M24.444 Recurrent dislocation, right finger
M24.445 Recurrent dislocation, left finger
M24.446 Recurrent dislocation, unspecified finger ▽

✓6ᵗʰ **M24.45 Recurrent dislocation, hip**
M24.451 Recurrent dislocation, right hip
M24.452 Recurrent dislocation, left hip
M24.459 Recurrent dislocation, unspecified hip ▽

✓6ᵗʰ **M24.46 Recurrent dislocation, knee**
M24.461 Recurrent dislocation, right knee
M24.462 Recurrent dislocation, left knee
M24.469 Recurrent dislocation, unspecified knee ▽

✓6ᵗʰ **M24.47 Recurrent dislocation, ankle, foot and toes**
M24.471 Recurrent dislocation, right ankle
M24.472 Recurrent dislocation, left ankle
M24.473 Recurrent dislocation, unspecified ankle ▽
M24.474 Recurrent dislocation, right foot
M24.475 Recurrent dislocation, left foot
M24.476 Recurrent dislocation, unspecified foot ▽
M24.477 Recurrent dislocation, right toe(s)
M24.478 Recurrent dislocation, left toe(s)
M24.479 Recurrent dislocation, unspecified toe(s) ▽

✓5ᵗʰ **M24.5 Contracture of joint**
> EXCLUDES 1   contracture of muscle without contracture of joint (M62.4-)
> contracture of tendon (sheath) without contracture of joint (M62.4-)
> Dupuytren's contracture (M72.0)
> EXCLUDES 2   acquired deformities of limbs (M20-M21)
> AHA: 2016, 2Q, 6

M24.50 Contracture, unspecified joint ▽

✓6ᵗʰ **M24.51 Contracture, shoulder**
M24.511 Contracture, right shoulder
M24.512 Contracture, left shoulder
M24.519 Contracture, unspecified shoulder ▽

✓6ᵗʰ **M24.52 Contracture, elbow**
M24.521 Contracture, right elbow
M24.522 Contracture, left elbow
M24.529 Contracture, unspecified elbow ▽

✓6ᵗʰ **M24.53 Contracture, wrist**
M24.531 Contracture, right wrist
M24.532 Contracture, left wrist
M24.539 Contracture, unspecified wrist ▽

✓6ᵗʰ **M24.54 Contracture, hand**
M24.541 Contracture, right hand
M24.542 Contracture, left hand
M24.549 Contracture, unspecified hand ▽

✓6ᵗʰ **M24.55 Contracture, hip**
M24.551 Contracture, right hip
M24.552 Contracture, left hip
M24.559 Contracture, unspecified hip ▽

✓6ᵗʰ **M24.56 Contracture, knee**
M24.561 Contracture, right knee
M24.562 Contracture, left knee
M24.569 Contracture, unspecified knee ▽

✓6ᵗʰ **M24.57 Contracture, ankle and foot**
M24.571 Contracture, right ankle
M24.572 Contracture, left ankle
M24.573 Contracture, unspecified ankle ▽
M24.574 Contracture, right foot
M24.575 Contracture, left foot
M24.576 Contracture, unspecified foot ▽

✓5ᵗʰ **M24.6 Ankylosis of joint**
> EXCLUDES 1   stiffness of joint without ankylosis (M25.6-)
> EXCLUDES 2   spine (M43.2-)

M24.60 Ankylosis, unspecified joint ▽

✓6ᵗʰ **M24.61 Ankylosis, shoulder**
M24.611 Ankylosis, right shoulder
M24.612 Ankylosis, left shoulder
M24.619 Ankylosis, unspecified shoulder ▽

✓6ᵗʰ **M24.62 Ankylosis, elbow**
M24.621 Ankylosis, right elbow
M24.622 Ankylosis, left elbow
M24.629 Ankylosis, unspecified elbow ▽

✓6ᵗʰ **M24.63 Ankylosis, wrist**
M24.631 Ankylosis, right wrist
M24.632 Ankylosis, left wrist
M24.639 Ankylosis, unspecified wrist ▽

✓6ᵗʰ **M24.64 Ankylosis, hand**
M24.641 Ankylosis, right hand
M24.642 Ankylosis, left hand
M24.649 Ankylosis, unspecified hand ▽

✓6ᵗʰ **M24.65 Ankylosis, hip**
M24.651 Ankylosis, right hip
M24.652 Ankylosis, left hip
M24.659 Ankylosis, unspecified hip ▽

✓6ᵗʰ **M24.66 Ankylosis, knee**
M24.661 Ankylosis, right knee
M24.662 Ankylosis, left knee
M24.669 Ankylosis, unspecified knee ▽

✓6ᵗʰ **M24.67 Ankylosis, ankle and foot**
M24.671 Ankylosis, right ankle
M24.672 Ankylosis, left ankle
M24.673 Ankylosis, unspecified ankle ▽
M24.674 Ankylosis, right foot
M24.675 Ankylosis, left foot
M24.676 Ankylosis, unspecified foot ▽

M24.7 Protrusio acetabuli

✓5ᵗʰ **M24.8 Other specific joint derangements, not elsewhere classified**
> EXCLUDES 2   iliotibial band syndrome (M76.3)

M24.80 Other specific joint derangements of unspecified joint, not elsewhere classified ▽

✓6ᵗʰ **M24.81 Other specific joint derangements of shoulder, not elsewhere classified**
M24.811 Other specific joint derangements of right shoulder, not elsewhere classified
M24.812 Other specific joint derangements of left shoulder, not elsewhere classified
M24.819 Other specific joint derangements of unspecified shoulder, not elsewhere classified ▽

✓6ᵗʰ **M24.82 Other specific joint derangements of elbow, not elsewhere classified**
M24.821 Other specific joint derangements of right elbow, not elsewhere classified
M24.822 Other specific joint derangements of left elbow, not elsewhere classified
M24.829 Other specific joint derangements of unspecified elbow, not elsewhere classified ▽

✓6ᵗʰ **M24.83** Other specific joint derangements of wrist, not elsewhere classified
     M24.831 Other specific joint derangements of right wrist, not elsewhere classified
     M24.832 Other specific joint derangements of left wrist, not elsewhere classified
     M24.839 Other specific joint derangements of unspecified wrist, not elsewhere classified ▽

✓6ᵗʰ **M24.84** Other specific joint derangements of hand, not elsewhere classified
     M24.841 Other specific joint derangements of right hand, not elsewhere classified
     M24.842 Other specific joint derangements of left hand, not elsewhere classified
     M24.849 Other specific joint derangements of unspecified hand, not elsewhere classified ▽

✓6ᵗʰ **M24.85** Other specific joint derangements of hip, not elsewhere classified
     Irritable hip
     M24.851 Other specific joint derangements of right hip, not elsewhere classified
     M24.852 Other specific joint derangements of left hip, not elsewhere classified
     M24.859 Other specific joint derangements of unspecified hip, not elsewhere classified ▽

✓6ᵗʰ **M24.87** Other specific joint derangements of ankle and foot, not elsewhere classified
     M24.871 Other specific joint derangements of right ankle, not elsewhere classified
     M24.872 Other specific joint derangements of left ankle, not elsewhere classified
     M24.873 Other specific joint derangements of unspecified ankle, not elsewhere classified ▽
     M24.874 Other specific joint derangements of right foot, not elsewhere classified
     M24.875 Other specific joint derangements left foot, not elsewhere classified
     M24.876 Other specific joint derangements of unspecified foot, not elsewhere classified ▽

M24.9 Joint derangement, unspecified ▽

✓4ᵗʰ **M25** Other joint disorder, not elsewhere classified
     EXCLUDES 2   abnormality of gait and mobility (R26.-)
               acquired deformities of limb (M20-M21)
               calcification of bursa (M71.4-)
               calcification of shoulder (joint) (M75.3)
               calcification of tendon (M65.2-)
               difficulty in walking (R26.2)
               temporomandibular joint disorder (M26.6-)

✓5ᵗʰ **M25.0** Hemarthrosis
     EXCLUDES 1   current injury—see injury of joint by body region
               hemophilic arthropathy (M36.2)
     M25.00 Hemarthrosis, unspecified joint ▽

✓6ᵗʰ **M25.01** Hemarthrosis, shoulder
     M25.011 Hemarthrosis, right shoulder
     M25.012 Hemarthrosis, left shoulder
     M25.019 Hemarthrosis, unspecified shoulder ▽

✓6ᵗʰ **M25.02** Hemarthrosis, elbow
     M25.021 Hemarthrosis, right elbow
     M25.022 Hemarthrosis, left elbow
     M25.029 Hemarthrosis, unspecified elbow ▽

✓6ᵗʰ **M25.03** Hemarthrosis, wrist
     M25.031 Hemarthrosis, right wrist
     M25.032 Hemarthrosis, left wrist
     M25.039 Hemarthrosis, unspecified wrist ▽

✓6ᵗʰ **M25.04** Hemarthrosis, hand
     M25.041 Hemarthrosis, right hand
     M25.042 Hemarthrosis, left hand
     M25.049 Hemarthrosis, unspecified hand ▽

✓6ᵗʰ **M25.05** Hemarthrosis, hip
     M25.051 Hemarthrosis, right hip
     M25.052 Hemarthrosis, left hip
     M25.059 Hemarthrosis, unspecified hip ▽

✓6ᵗʰ **M25.06** Hemarthrosis, knee
     M25.061 Hemarthrosis, right knee
     M25.062 Hemarthrosis, left knee

     M25.069 Hemarthrosis, unspecified knee ▽

✓6ᵗʰ **M25.07** Hemarthrosis, ankle and foot
     M25.071 Hemarthrosis, right ankle
     M25.072 Hemarthrosis, left ankle
     M25.073 Hemarthrosis, unspecified ankle ▽
     M25.074 Hemarthrosis, right foot
     M25.075 Hemarthrosis, left foot
     M25.076 Hemarthrosis, unspecified foot ▽

M25.08 Hemarthrosis, other specified site
     Hemarthrosis, vertebrae

✓5ᵗʰ **M25.1** Fistula of joint
     M25.10 Fistula, unspecified joint ▽

✓6ᵗʰ **M25.11** Fistula, shoulder
     M25.111 Fistula, right shoulder
     M25.112 Fistula, left shoulder
     M25.119 Fistula, unspecified shoulder ▽

✓6ᵗʰ **M25.12** Fistula, elbow
     M25.121 Fistula, right elbow
     M25.122 Fistula, left elbow
     M25.129 Fistula, unspecified elbow ▽

✓6ᵗʰ **M25.13** Fistula, wrist
     M25.131 Fistula, right wrist
     M25.132 Fistula, left wrist
     M25.139 Fistula, unspecified wrist ▽

✓6ᵗʰ **M25.14** Fistula, hand
     M25.141 Fistula, right hand
     M25.142 Fistula, left hand
     M25.149 Fistula, unspecified hand ▽

✓6ᵗʰ **M25.15** Fistula, hip
     M25.151 Fistula, right hip
     M25.152 Fistula, left hip
     M25.159 Fistula, unspecified hip ▽

✓6ᵗʰ **M25.16** Fistula, knee
     M25.161 Fistula, right knee
     M25.162 Fistula, left knee
     M25.169 Fistula, unspecified knee ▽

✓6ᵗʰ **M25.17** Fistula, ankle and foot
     M25.171 Fistula, right ankle
     M25.172 Fistula, left ankle
     M25.173 Fistula, unspecified ankle ▽
     M25.174 Fistula, right foot
     M25.175 Fistula, left foot
     M25.176 Fistula, unspecified foot ▽

M25.18 Fistula, other specified site
     Fistula, vertebrae

✓5ᵗʰ **M25.2** Flail joint
     M25.20 Flail joint, unspecified joint ▽

✓6ᵗʰ **M25.21** Flail joint, shoulder
     M25.211 Flail joint, right shoulder
     M25.212 Flail joint, left shoulder
     M25.219 Flail joint, unspecified shoulder ▽

✓6ᵗʰ **M25.22** Flail joint, elbow
     M25.221 Flail joint, right elbow
     M25.222 Flail joint, left elbow
     M25.229 Flail joint, unspecified elbow ▽

✓6ᵗʰ **M25.23** Flail joint, wrist
     M25.231 Flail joint, right wrist
     M25.232 Flail joint, left wrist
     M25.239 Flail joint, unspecified wrist ▽

✓6ᵗʰ **M25.24** Flail joint, hand
     M25.241 Flail joint, right hand
     M25.242 Flail joint, left hand
     M25.249 Flail joint, unspecified hand ▽

✓6ᵗʰ **M25.25** Flail joint, hip
     M25.251 Flail joint, right hip
     M25.252 Flail joint, left hip
     M25.259 Flail joint, unspecified hip ▽

✓6ᵗʰ **M25.26** Flail joint, knee
     M25.261 Flail joint, right knee
     M25.262 Flail joint, left knee
     M25.269 Flail joint, unspecified knee ▽

✓ Additional Character Req   ✓ˣ7ᵗʰ Placeholder Alert   Manifestation   HCC CMS-HCC Condition   ▽ Unspecified Code   ►◄ Revised Text   ● New Code   ▲ Revised Code Title

✓6ᵗʰ **M25.27 Flail joint, ankle and foot**
    M25.271 Flail joint, right ankle and foot
    M25.272 Flail joint, left ankle and foot
    M25.279 Flail joint, unspecified ankle and foot ▽
    M25.28 Flail joint, other site

✓5ᵗʰ **M25.3 Other instability of joint**
    EXCLUDES 1   instability of joint secondary to old ligament injury (M24.2-)
        instability of joint secondary to removal of joint prosthesis (M96.8-)
    EXCLUDES 2   spinal instabilities (M53.2-)
    M25.30 Other instability, unspecified joint ▽
✓6ᵗʰ **M25.31 Other instability, shoulder**
    M25.311 Other instability, right shoulder
    M25.312 Other instability, left shoulder
    M25.319 Other instability, unspecified shoulder ▽
✓6ᵗʰ **M25.32 Other instability, elbow**
    M25.321 Other instability, right elbow
    M25.322 Other instability, left elbow
    M25.329 Other instability, unspecified elbow ▽
✓6ᵗʰ **M25.33 Other instability, wrist**
    M25.331 Other instability, right wrist
    M25.332 Other instability, left wrist
    M25.339 Other instability, unspecified wrist ▽
✓6ᵗʰ **M25.34 Other instability, hand**
    M25.341 Other instability, right hand
    M25.342 Other instability, left hand
    M25.349 Other instability, unspecified hand ▽
✓6ᵗʰ **M25.35 Other instability, hip**
    M25.351 Other instability, right hip
    M25.352 Other instability, left hip
    M25.359 Other instability, unspecified hip ▽
✓6ᵗʰ **M25.36 Other instability, knee**
    M25.361 Other instability, right knee
    M25.362 Other instability, left knee
    M25.369 Other instability, unspecified knee ▽
✓6ᵗʰ **M25.37 Other instability, ankle and foot**
    M25.371 Other instability, right ankle
    M25.372 Other instability, left ankle
    M25.373 Other instability, unspecified ankle ▽
    M25.374 Other instability, right foot
    M25.375 Other instability, left foot
    M25.376 Other instability, unspecified foot ▽

✓5ᵗʰ **M25.4 Effusion of joint**
    EXCLUDES 1   hydrarthrosis in yaws (A66.6)
        intermittent hydrarthrosis (M12.4-)
        other infective (teno)synovitis (M65.1-)
    M25.40 Effusion, unspecified joint ▽
✓6ᵗʰ **M25.41 Effusion, shoulder**
    M25.411 Effusion, right shoulder
    M25.412 Effusion, left shoulder
    M25.419 Effusion, unspecified shoulder ▽
✓6ᵗʰ **M25.42 Effusion, elbow**
    M25.421 Effusion, right elbow
    M25.422 Effusion, left elbow
    M25.429 Effusion, unspecified elbow ▽
✓6ᵗʰ **M25.43 Effusion, wrist**
    M25.431 Effusion, right wrist
    M25.432 Effusion, left wrist
    M25.439 Effusion, unspecified wrist ▽
✓6ᵗʰ **M25.44 Effusion, hand**
    M25.441 Effusion, right hand
    M25.442 Effusion, left hand
    M25.449 Effusion, unspecified hand ▽
✓6ᵗʰ **M25.45 Effusion, hip**
    M25.451 Effusion, right hip
    M25.452 Effusion, left hip
    M25.459 Effusion, unspecified hip ▽
✓6ᵗʰ **M25.46 Effusion, knee**
    M25.461 Effusion, right knee
    M25.462 Effusion, left knee
    M25.469 Effusion, unspecified knee

✓6ᵗʰ **M25.47 Effusion, ankle and foot**
    M25.471 Effusion, right ankle
    M25.472 Effusion, left ankle
    M25.473 Effusion, unspecified ankle ▽
    M25.474 Effusion, right foot
    M25.475 Effusion, left foot
    M25.476 Effusion, unspecified foot ▽
    M25.48 Effusion, other site

✓5ᵗʰ **M25.5 Pain in joint**
    EXCLUDES 2   pain in hand (M79.64-)
        pain in fingers (M79.64-)
        pain in foot (M79.67-)
        pain in limb (M79.6-)
        pain in toes (M79.67-)
    M25.50 Pain in unspecified joint ▽
✓6ᵗʰ **M25.51 Pain in shoulder**
    M25.511 Pain in right shoulder
    M25.512 Pain in left shoulder
    M25.519 Pain in unspecified shoulder ▽
✓6ᵗʰ **M25.52 Pain in elbow**
    M25.521 Pain in right elbow
    M25.522 Pain in left elbow
    M25.529 Pain in unspecified elbow ▽
✓6ᵗʰ **M25.53 Pain in wrist**
    M25.531 Pain in right wrist
    M25.532 Pain in left wrist
    M25.539 Pain in unspecified wrist ▽
✓6ᵗʰ **M25.54 Pain in joints of hand**
    M25.541 Pain in joints of right hand
    M25.542 Pain in joints of left hand
    M25.549 Pain in joints of unspecified hand ▽
        Pain in joints of hand NOS
✓6ᵗʰ **M25.55 Pain in hip**
    M25.551 Pain in right hip
    M25.552 Pain in left hip
    M25.559 Pain in unspecified hip ▽
✓6ᵗʰ **M25.56 Pain in knee**
    M25.561 Pain in right knee
    M25.562 Pain in left knee
    M25.569 Pain in unspecified knee ▽
✓6ᵗʰ **M25.57 Pain in ankle and joints of foot**
    M25.571 Pain in right ankle and joints of right foot
    M25.572 Pain in left ankle and joints of left foot
    M25.579 Pain in unspecified ankle and joints of unspecified foot ▽

✓5ᵗʰ **M25.6 Stiffness of joint, not elsewhere classified**
    EXCLUDES 1   ankylosis of joint (M24.6-)
        contracture of joint (M24.5-)
    M25.60 Stiffness of unspecified joint, not elsewhere classified ▽
✓6ᵗʰ **M25.61 Stiffness of shoulder, not elsewhere classified**
    M25.611 Stiffness of right shoulder, not elsewhere classified
    M25.612 Stiffness of left shoulder, not elsewhere classified
    M25.619 Stiffness of unspecified shoulder, not elsewhere classified ▽
✓6ᵗʰ **M25.62 Stiffness of elbow, not elsewhere classified**
    M25.621 Stiffness of right elbow, not elsewhere classified
    M25.622 Stiffness of left elbow, not elsewhere classified
    M25.629 Stiffness of unspecified elbow, not elsewhere classified ▽
✓6ᵗʰ **M25.63 Stiffness of wrist, not elsewhere classified**
    M25.631 Stiffness of right wrist, not elsewhere classified
    M25.632 Stiffness of left wrist, not elsewhere classified
    M25.639 Stiffness of unspecified wrist, not elsewhere classified ▽

EXCLUDES 1 Not coded here   EXCLUDES 2 Not included here   N Newborn Age: 0   P Pediatric Age: 0-17   M Maternity Age: 12-55   A Adult Age: 15-124

748   ICD-10-CM 2018

✓6ᵗʰ **M25.64 Stiffness of hand, not elsewhere classified**
    M25.641 Stiffness of right hand, not elsewhere classified
    M25.642 Stiffness of left hand, not elsewhere classified
    M25.649 Stiffness of unspecified hand, not elsewhere classified ▽

✓6ᵗʰ **M25.65 Stiffness of hip, not elsewhere classified**
    M25.651 Stiffness of right hip, not elsewhere classified
    M25.652 Stiffness of left hip, not elsewhere classified
    M25.659 Stiffness of unspecified hip, not elsewhere classified ▽

✓6ᵗʰ **M25.66 Stiffness of knee, not elsewhere classified**
    M25.661 Stiffness of right knee, not elsewhere classified
    M25.662 Stiffness of left knee, not elsewhere classified
    M25.669 Stiffness of unspecified knee, not elsewhere classified ▽

✓6ᵗʰ **M25.67 Stiffness of ankle and foot, not elsewhere classified**
    M25.671 Stiffness of right ankle, not elsewhere classified
    M25.672 Stiffness of left ankle, not elsewhere classified
    M25.673 Stiffness of unspecified ankle, not elsewhere classified ▽
    M25.674 Stiffness of right foot, not elsewhere classified
    M25.675 Stiffness of left foot, not elsewhere classified
    M25.676 Stiffness of unspecified foot, not elsewhere classified ▽

✓5ᵗʰ **M25.7 Osteophyte**
    M25.70 Osteophyte, unspecified joint ▽

✓6ᵗʰ **M25.71 Osteophyte, shoulder**
    M25.711 Osteophyte, right shoulder
    M25.712 Osteophyte, left shoulder
    M25.719 Osteophyte, unspecified shoulder ▽

✓6ᵗʰ **M25.72 Osteophyte, elbow**
    M25.721 Osteophyte, right elbow
    M25.722 Osteophyte, left elbow
    M25.729 Osteophyte, unspecified elbow ▽

✓6ᵗʰ **M25.73 Osteophyte, wrist**
    M25.731 Osteophyte, right wrist
    M25.732 Osteophyte, left wrist
    M25.739 Osteophyte, unspecified wrist ▽

✓6ᵗʰ **M25.74 Osteophyte, hand**
    M25.741 Osteophyte, right hand
    M25.742 Osteophyte, left hand
    M25.749 Osteophyte, unspecified hand ▽

✓6ᵗʰ **M25.75 Osteophyte, hip**
    M25.751 Osteophyte, right hip
    M25.752 Osteophyte, left hip
    M25.759 Osteophyte, unspecified hip ▽

✓6ᵗʰ **M25.76 Osteophyte, knee**
    M25.761 Osteophyte, right knee
    M25.762 Osteophyte, left knee
    M25.769 Osteophyte, unspecified knee ▽

✓6ᵗʰ **M25.77 Osteophyte, ankle and foot**
    M25.771 Osteophyte, right ankle
    M25.772 Osteophyte, left ankle
    M25.773 Osteophyte, unspecified ankle ▽
    M25.774 Osteophyte, right foot
    M25.775 Osteophyte, left foot
    M25.776 Osteophyte, unspecified foot ▽
    M25.78 Osteophyte, vertebrae

✓5ᵗʰ **M25.8 Other specified joint disorders**
    M25.80 Other specified joint disorders, unspecified joint ▽

✓6ᵗʰ **M25.81 Other specified joint disorders, shoulder**
    M25.811 Other specified joint disorders, right shoulder

    M25.812 Other specified joint disorders, left shoulder
    M25.819 Other specified joint disorders, unspecified shoulder ▽

✓6ᵗʰ **M25.82 Other specified joint disorders, elbow**
    M25.821 Other specified joint disorders, right elbow
    M25.822 Other specified joint disorders, left elbow
    M25.829 Other specified joint disorders, unspecified elbow ▽

✓6ᵗʰ **M25.83 Other specified joint disorders, wrist**
    M25.831 Other specified joint disorders, right wrist
    M25.832 Other specified joint disorders, left wrist
    M25.839 Other specified joint disorders, unspecifiedwrist ▽

✓6ᵗʰ **M25.84 Other specified joint disorders, hand**
    M25.841 Other specified joint disorders, right hand
    M25.842 Other specified joint disorders, left hand
    M25.849 Other specified joint disorders, unspecified hand ▽

✓6ᵗʰ **M25.85 Other specified joint disorders, hip**
    AHA: 2014, 4Q, 25
    M25.851 Other specified joint disorders, right hip
    M25.852 Other specified joint disorders, left hip
    M25.859 Other specified joint disorders, unspecified hip ▽

✓6ᵗʰ **M25.86 Other specified joint disorders, knee**
    M25.861 Other specified joint disorders, right knee
    M25.862 Other specified joint disorders, left knee
    M25.869 Other specified joint disorders, unspecified knee ▽

✓6ᵗʰ **M25.87 Other specified joint disorders, ankle and foot**
    M25.871 Other specified joint disorders, right ankle and foot
    M25.872 Other specified joint disorders, left ankle and foot
    M25.879 Other specified joint disorders, unspecified ankle and foot ▽

M25.9 Joint disorder, unspecified ▽

Dentofacial anomalies [including malocclusion] and other disorders of jaw (M26-M27)

EXCLUDES 1   *hemifacial atrophy or hypertrophy (Q67.4)*
         unilateral condylar hyperplasia or hypoplasia (M27.8)

✓4ᵗʰ **M26 Dentofacial anomalies [including malocclusion]**

✓5ᵗʰ **M26.0 Major anomalies of jaw size**
    EXCLUDES 1   *acromegaly (E22.0)*
             Robin's syndrome (Q87.0)
    M26.00 Unspecified anomaly of jaw size ▽
    M26.01 Maxillary hyperplasia
    M26.02 Maxillary hypoplasia
        AHA: 2014, 3Q, 23
    M26.03 Mandibular hyperplasia
    M26.04 Mandibular hypoplasia
    M26.05 Macrogenia
    M26.06 Microgenia
    M26.07 Excessive tuberosity of jaw
        Entire maxillary tuberosity
    M26.09 Other specified anomalies of jaw size

✓5ᵗʰ **M26.1 Anomalies of jaw-cranial base relationship**
    M26.10 Unspecified anomaly of jaw-cranial base relationship ▽
    M26.11 Maxillary asymmetry
    M26.12 Other jaw asymmetry
    M26.19 Other specified anomalies of jaw-cranial base relationship

✓5ᵗʰ **M26.2 Anomalies of dental arch relationship**
    M26.20 Unspecified anomaly of dental arch relationship ▽

✓6ᵗʰ **M26.21 Malocclusion, Angle's class**
    M26.211 Malocclusion, Angle's class I
        Neutro-occlusion
    M26.212 Malocclusion, Angle's class II
        Disto-occlusion Division I
        Disto-occlusion Division II

☑ Additional Character Req   ✓x7ᵗʰ Placeholder Alert   Manifestation   HCC CMS-HCC Condition   ▽ Unspecified Code   ▶◀ Revised Text   ● New Code   ▲ Revised Code Title

ICD-10-CM 2018   749

M26.213   **Malocclusion, Angle's class III**
     Mesio-occlusion

M26.219   **Malocclusion, Angle's class, unspecified** ▽

✓6th **M26.22**   **Open occlusal relationship**

     M26.220   **Open anterior occlusal relationship**
         Anterior openbite

     M26.221   **Open posterior occlusal relationship**
         Posterior openbite

     M26.23   **Excessive horizontal overlap**
         Excessive horizontal overjet

     M26.24   **Reverse articulation**
         Crossbite (anterior) (posterior)

     M26.25   **Anomalies of interarch distance**

     M26.29   **Other anomalies of dental arch relationship**
         Midline deviation of dental arch
         Overbite (excessive) deep
         Overbite (excessive) horizontal
         Overbite (excessive) vertical
         Posterior lingual occlusion of mandibular teeth

✓5th **M26.3**   **Anomalies of tooth position of fully erupted tooth or teeth**
     EXCLUDES 2   *embedded and impacted teeth (K01.-)*

     M26.30   **Unspecified anomaly of tooth position of fully** ▽ **erupted tooth or teeth**
         Abnormal spacing of fully erupted tooth or teeth NOS
         Displacement of fully erupted tooth or teeth NOS
         Transposition of fully erupted tooth or teeth NOS

     M26.31   **Crowding of fully erupted teeth**

     M26.32   **Excessive spacing of fully erupted teeth**
         Diastema of fully erupted tooth or teeth NOS

     M26.33   **Horizontal displacement of fully erupted tooth or teeth**
         Tipped tooth or teeth
         Tipping of fully erupted tooth

     M26.34   **Vertical displacement of fully erupted tooth or teeth**
         Extruded tooth
         Infraeruption of tooth or teeth
         Supraeruption of tooth or teeth

     M26.35   **Rotation of fully erupted tooth or teeth**

     M26.36   **Insufficient interocclusal distance of fully erupted teeth (ridge)**
         Lack of adequate intermaxillary vertical dimension of fully erupted teeth

     M26.37   **Excessive interocclusal distance of fully erupted teeth**
         Excessive intermaxillary vertical dimension of fully erupted teeth
         Loss of occlusal vertical dimension of fully erupted teeth

     M26.39   **Other anomalies of tooth position of fully erupted tooth or teeth**

M26.4   **Malocclusion, unspecified** ▽

✓5th **M26.5**   **Dentofacial functional abnormalities**
     EXCLUDES 1   *bruxism (F45.8)*
             teeth-grinding NOS (F45.8)

     M26.50   **Dentofacial functional abnormalities, unspecified** ▽

     M26.51   **Abnormal jaw closure**

     M26.52   **Limited mandibular range of motion**

     M26.53   **Deviation in opening and closing of the mandible**

     M26.54   **Insufficient anterior guidance**
         Insufficient anterior occlusal guidance

     M26.55   **Centric occlusion maximum intercuspation discrepancy**
         EXCLUDES 1   *centric occlusion NOS (M26.59)*

     M26.56   **Non-working side interference**
         Balancing side interference

     M26.57   **Lack of posterior occlusal support**

     M26.59   **Other dentofacial functional abnormalities**
         Centric occlusion (of teeth) NOS
         Malocclusion due to abnormal swallowing
         Malocclusion due to mouth breathing
         Malocclusion due to tongue, lip or finger habits

Temporomandibular Joint

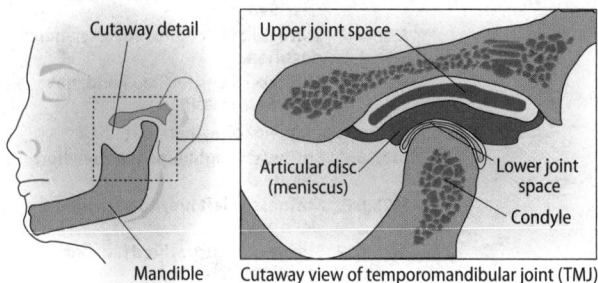

Cutaway detail   Upper joint space

Articular disc (meniscus)   Lower joint space

Condyle

Mandible   Cutaway view of temporomandibular joint (TMJ)

✓5th **M26.6**   **Temporomandibular joint disorders**
     EXCLUDES 2   *current temporomandibular joint dislocation (S03.0)*
             current temporomandibular joint sprain (S03.4)

     ✓6th **M26.60**   **Temporomandibular joint disorder, unspecified**

         M26.601   **Right temporomandibular joint** ▽ **disorder, unspecified**

         M26.602   **Left temporomandibular joint** ▽ **disorder, unspecified**

         M26.603   **Bilateral temporomandibular joint** ▽ **disorder, unspecified**

         M26.609   **Unspecified temporomandibular joint** ▽ **disorder, unspecified side**
             Temporomandibular joint disorder NOS

     ✓6th **M26.61**   **Adhesions and ankylosis of temporomandibular joint**

         M26.611   **Adhesions and ankylosis of right temporomandibular joint**

         M26.612   **Adhesions and ankylosis of left temporomandibular joint**

         M26.613   **Adhesions and ankylosis of bilateral temporomandibular joint**

         M26.619   **Adhesions and ankylosis of** ▽ **temporomandibular joint, unspecified side**

     ✓6th **M26.62**   **Arthralgia of temporomandibular joint**

         M26.621   **Arthralgia of right temporomandibular joint**

         M26.622   **Arthralgia of left temporomandibular joint**

         M26.623   **Arthralgia of bilateral temporomandibular joint**

         M26.629   **Arthralgia of temporomandibular** ▽ **joint, unspecified side**

     ✓6th **M26.63**   **Articular disc disorder of temporomandibular joint**

         M26.631   **Articular disc disorder of right temporomandibular joint**

         M26.632   **Articular disc disorder of left temporomandibular joint**

         M26.633   **Articular disc disorder of bilateral temporomandibular joint**

         M26.639   **Articular disc disorder of** ▽ **temporomandibular joint, unspecified side**

     M26.69   **Other specified disorders of temporomandibular joint**

✓5th **M26.7**   **Dental alveolar anomalies**

     M26.70   **Unspecified alveolar anomaly** ▽

     M26.71   **Alveolar maxillary hyperplasia**

     M26.72   **Alveolar mandibular hyperplasia**

     M26.73   **Alveolar maxillary hypoplasia**

     M26.74   **Alveolar mandibular hypoplasia**

     M26.79   **Other specified alveolar anomalies**

✓5th **M26.8**   **Other dentofacial anomalies**

     M26.81   **Anterior soft tissue impingement**
         Anterior soft tissue impingement on teeth

     M26.82   **Posterior soft tissue impingement**
         Posterior soft tissue impingement on teeth

     M26.89   **Other dentofacial anomalies**

M26.9   **Dentofacial anomaly, unspecified** ▽

EXCLUDES 1 Not coded here   *EXCLUDES 2* Not included here   N Newborn Age: 0   P Pediatric Age: 0-17   M Maternity Age: 12-55   A Adult Age: 15-124

750   ICD-10-CM 2018

☑4ᵗʰ **M27 Other diseases of jaws**

M27.0 Developmental disorders of jaws
Latent bone cyst of jaw   Torus mandibularis
Stafne's cyst   Torus palatinus

M27.1 Giant cell granuloma, central
Giant cell granuloma NOS
EXCLUDES 1 peripheral giant cell granuloma (K06.8)

M27.2 Inflammatory conditions of jaws
Osteitis of jaw(s)   Periostitis jaw(s)
Osteomyelitis (neonatal) jaw(s)   Sequestrum of jaw bone
Osteoradionecrosis jaw(s)
Use additional code (W88-W90, X39.0) to identify radiation, if radiation-induced
EXCLUDES 2 osteonecrosis of jaw due to drug (M87.180)

M27.3 Alveolitis of jaws
Alveolar osteitis   Dry socket

☑5ᵗʰ **M27.4 Other and unspecified cysts of jaw**
EXCLUDES 1 cysts of oral region (K09.-)
latent bone cyst of jaw (M27.0)
Stafne's cyst (M27.0)

M27.40 Unspecified cyst of jaw ▽
Cyst of jaw NOS

M27.49 Other cysts of jaw
Aneurysmal cyst of jaw
Hemorrhagic cyst of jaw
Traumatic cyst of jaw

☑5ᵗʰ **M27.5 Periradicular pathology associated with previous endodontic treatment**

M27.51 Perforation of root canal space due to endodontic treatment

M27.52 Endodontic overfill

M27.53 Endodontic underfill

M27.59 Other periradicular pathology associated with previous endodontic treatment

☑5ᵗʰ **M27.6 Endosseous dental implant failure**

M27.61 Osseointegration failure of dental implant
Hemorrhagic complications of dental implant placement
Iatrogenic osseointegration failure of dental implant
Osseointegration failure of dental implant due to complications of systemic disease
Osseointegration failure of dental implant due to poor bone quality
Pre-integration failure of dental implant NOS
Pre-osseointegration failure of dental implant

M27.62 Post-osseointegration biological failure of dental implant
Failure of dental implant due to lack of attached gingiva
Failure of dental implant due to occlusal trauma (caused by poor prosthetic design)
Failure of dental implant due to parafunctional habits
Failure of dental implant due to periodontal infection (peri-implantitis)
Failure of dental implant due to poor oral hygiene
Iatrogenic post-osseointegration failure of dental implant
Post-osseointegration failure of dental implant due to complications of systemic disease

M27.63 Post-osseointegration mechanical failure of dental implant
Failure of dental prosthesis causing loss of dental implant
Fracture of dental implant
EXCLUDES 2 cracked tooth (K03.81)
fractured dental restorative material with loss of material (K08.531)
fractured dental restorative material without loss of material (K08.530)
fractured tooth (S02.5)

M27.69 Other endosseous dental implant failure
Dental implant failure NOS

M27.8 Other specified diseases of jaws
Cherubism   Unilateral condylar hyperplasia
Exostosis   Unilateral condylar hypoplasia
Fibrous dysplasia
EXCLUDES 1 jaw pain (R68.84)

M27.9 Disease of jaws, unspecified ▽

Systemic connective tissue disorders (M30-M36)

INCLUDES autoimmune disease NOS
collagen (vascular) disease NOS
systemic autoimmune disease
systemic collagen (vascular) disease
EXCLUDES 1 autoimmune disease, single organ or single cell-type—code to relevant condition category

☑4ᵗʰ **M30 Polyarteritis nodosa and related conditions**
EXCLUDES 1 microscopic polyarteritis (M31.7)

M30.0 Polyarteritis nodosa HCC

M30.1 Polyarteritis with lung involvement [Churg-Strauss] HCC
Allergic granulomatous angiitis

M30.2 Juvenile polyarteritis HCC

M30.3 Mucocutaneous lymph node syndrome [Kawasaki] HCC

M30.8 Other conditions related to polyarteritis nodosa HCC
Polyangiitis overlap syndrome

☑4ᵗʰ **M31 Other necrotizing vasculopathies**

M31.0 Hypersensitivity angiitis HCC
Goodpasture's syndrome

M31.1 Thrombotic microangiopathy HCC
Thrombotic thrombocytopenic purpura

M31.2 Lethal midline granuloma HCC

☑5ᵗʰ **M31.3 Wegener's granulomatosis**
Necrotizing respiratory granulomatosis

M31.30 Wegener's granulomatosis without renal involvement HCC
Wegener's granulomatosis NOS

M31.31 Wegener's granulomatosis with renal involvement HCC

M31.4 Aortic arch syndrome [Takayasu] HCC

M31.5 Giant cell arteritis with polymyalgia rheumatica HCC

M31.6 Other giant cell arteritis HCC

M31.7 Microscopic polyangiitis HCC
Microscopic polyarteritis
EXCLUDES 1 polyarteritis nodosa (M30.0)

M31.8 Other specified necrotizing vasculopathies HCC
Hypocomplementemic vasculitis
Septic vasculitis

M31.9 Necrotizing vasculopathy, unspecified HCC ▽

☑4ᵗʰ **M32 Systemic lupus erythematosus (SLE)**
EXCLUDES 1 lupus erythematosus (discoid) (NOS) (L93.0)

M32.0 Drug-induced systemic lupus erythematosus HCC
Use additional code for adverse effect, if applicable, to identify drug (T36-T50 with fifth or sixth character 5)

☑5ᵗʰ **M32.1 Systemic lupus erythematosus with organ or system involvement**

M32.10 Systemic lupus erythematosus, organ or system involvement unspecified HCC ▽

M32.11 Endocarditis in systemic lupus erythematosus HCC
Libman-Sacks disease

M32.12 Pericarditis in systemic lupus erythematosus HCC
Lupus pericarditis

M32.13 Lung involvement in systemic lupus erythematosus HCC
Pleural effusion due to systemic lupus erythematosus

M32.14 Glomerular disease in systemic lupus erythematosus HCC
Lupus renal disease NOS
AHA: 2013, 4Q, 125

M32.15 Tubulo-interstitial nephropathy in systemic lupus erythematosus HCC

M32.19 Other organ or system involvement in systemic lupus erythematosus HCC

M32.8 Other forms of systemic lupus erythematosus HCC

M32.9 Systemic lupus erythematosus, unspecified HCC ▽
SLE NOS
Systemic lupus erythematosus NOS
Systemic lupus erythematosus without organ involvement

☑4ᵗʰ **M33 Dermatopolymyositis**

▲ ☑5ᵗʰ **M33.0 Juvenile dermatomyositis**

▲ **M33.00 Juvenile dermatomyositis, organ involvement** HCC ▽
unspecified

▲ **M33.01 Juvenile dermatomyositis with respiratory involvement** HCC

▲ **M33.02 Juvenile dermatomyositis with myopathy** HCC

☑ Additional Character Req   ☑x7ᵗʰ Placeholder Alert   Manifestation   HCC CMS-HCC Condition   ▽ Unspecified Code   ▶◀ Revised Text   ● New Code   ▲ Revised Code Title

●   **M33.Ø3 Juvenile dermatomyositis without myopathy**

▲   **M33.Ø9 Juvenile dermatomyositis with other organ** HCC
           involvement

▲   ✓5th **M33.1 Other dermatomyositis**
         ▶Adult dermatomyositis◀

▲   **M33.1Ø Other dermatomyositis, organ involvement** HCC ▽
           unspecified

▲   **M33.11 Other dermatomyositis with respiratory** HCC
           involvement

▲   **M33.12 Other dermatomyositis with myopathy** HCC

●   **M33.13 Other dermatomyositis without myopathy**
           Dermatomyositis NOS

▲   **M33.19 Other dermatomyositis with other organ** HCC
           involvement

  ✓5th **M33.2 Polymyositis**

     M33.2Ø Polymyositis, organ involvement unspecified HCC ▽

     M33.21 Polymyositis with respiratory involvement HCC

     M33.22 Polymyositis with myopathy HCC

     M33.29 Polymyositis with other organ involvement HCC

  ✓5th **M33.9 Dermatopolymyositis, unspecified**

     M33.9Ø Dermatopolymyositis, unspecified, organ HCC ▽
           involvement unspecified

     M33.91 Dermatopolymyositis, unspecified with HCC ▽
           respiratory involvement

     M33.92 Dermatopolymyositis, unspecified with HCC ▽
           myopathy

●   **M33.93 Dermatopolymyositis, unspecified without** ▽
           myopathy

     M33.99 Dermatopolymyositis, unspecified with HCC ▽
           other organ involvement

✓4th **M34 Systemic sclerosis [scleroderma]**
     EXCLUDES 1   circumscribed scleroderma (L94.Ø)
                  neonatal scleroderma (P83.8)

     M34.Ø Progressive systemic sclerosis HCC

     M34.1 CR(E)ST syndrome HCC
         Combination of calcinosis, Raynaud's phenomenon,
         esophageal dysfunction, sclerodactyly, telangiectasia

     M34.2 Systemic sclerosis induced by drug and chemical HCC
         Code first poisoning due to drug or toxin, if applicable (T36-T65
             with fifth or sixth character 1-4 or 6)
         Use additional code for adverse effect, if applicable, to identify
             drug (T36-T5Ø with fifth or sixth character 5)

  ✓5th **M34.8 Other forms of systemic sclerosis**

     M34.81 Systemic sclerosis with lung involvement HCC

     M34.82 Systemic sclerosis with myopathy HCC

     M34.83 Systemic sclerosis with polyneuropathy HCC

     M34.89 Other systemic sclerosis HCC

     M34.9 Systemic sclerosis, unspecified HCC ▽

✓4th **M35 Other systemic involvement of connective tissue**
     EXCLUDES 1   reactive perforating collagenosis (L87.1)

  ✓5th **M35.Ø Sicca syndrome [Sjögren]**
         DEF: Autoimmune disease; associated with keratoconjunctivitis,
         laryngopharyngitis, rhinitis, dry mouth, enlarged parotid gland,
         and chronic polyarthritis.

     M35.ØØ Sicca syndrome, unspecified HCC ▽

     M35.Ø1 Sicca syndrome with keratoconjunctivitis HCC

     M35.Ø2 Sicca syndrome with lung involvement HCC

     M35.Ø3 Sicca syndrome with myopathy HCC

     M35.Ø4 Sicca syndrome with tubulo-interstitial HCC
           nephropathy
             Renal tubular acidosis in sicca syndrome

     M35.Ø9 Sicca syndrome with other organ involvement HCC

     M35.1 Other overlap syndromes HCC
         Mixed connective tissue disease
         EXCLUDES 1   polyangiitis overlap syndrome (M3Ø.8)

     M35.2 Behçet's disease HCC

     M35.3 Polymyalgia rheumatica HCC
         EXCLUDES 1   polymyalgia rheumatica with giant cell arteritis
                  (M31.5)

     M35.4 Diffuse (eosinophilic) fasciitis

     M35.5 Multifocal fibrosclerosis HCC

     M35.6 Relapsing panniculitis [Weber-Christian]
         EXCLUDES 1   lupus panniculitis (L93.2)
                  panniculitis NOS (M79.3-)

     M35.7 Hypermobility syndrome
         Familial ligamentous laxity
         EXCLUDES 1   Ehlers-Danlos syndrome (Q79.6)
                  ligamentous laxity, NOS (M24.2-)

     M35.8 Other specified systemic involvement of connective HCC
         tissue

     M35.9 Systemic involvement of connective tissue, HCC ▽
         unspecified
         Autoimmune disease (systemic) NOS
         Collagen (vascular) disease NOS

✓4th **M36 Systemic disorders of connective tissue in diseases classified**
     elsewhere
     EXCLUDES 2   arthropathies in diseases classified elsewhere (M14.-)

     M36.Ø Dermato(poly)myositis in neoplastic disease HCC
         Code first underlying neoplasm (CØØ-D49)

     M36.1 Arthropathy in neoplastic disease
         Code first underlying neoplasm, such as:
           leukemia (C91-C95)
           malignant histiocytosis (C96.A)
           multiple myeloma (C9Ø.Ø)

     M36.2 Hemophilic arthropathy
         Hemarthrosis in hemophilic arthropathy
         Code first underlying disease, such as:
           factor VIII deficiency (D66)
             with vascular defect (D68.Ø)
           factor IX deficiency (D67)
           hemophilia (classical) (D66)
           hemophilia B (D67)
           hemophilia C (D68.1)

     M36.3 Arthropathy in other blood disorders

     M36.4 Arthropathy in hypersensitivity reactions classified elsewhere
         Code first underlying disease, such as:
           Henoch (-Schönlein) purpura (D69.Ø)
           serum sickness (T8Ø.6-)

     M36.8 Systemic disorders of connective tissue in other diseases HCC
         classified elsewhere
         Code first underlying disease, such as:
           alkaptonuria (E7Ø.2)
           hypogammaglobulinemia (D8Ø.-)
           ochronosis (E7Ø.2)

Dorsopathies (M4Ø-M54)

Deforming dorsopathies (M4Ø-M43)

✓4th **M4Ø Kyphosis and lordosis**
     EXCLUDES 1   congenital kyphosis and lordosis (Q76.4)
                  kyphoscoliosis (M41.-)
                  postprocedural kyphosis and lordosis (M96.-)

  ✓5th **M4Ø.Ø Postural kyphosis**
         EXCLUDES 1   osteochondrosis of spine (M42.-)

     M4Ø.ØØ Postural kyphosis, site unspecified ▽

     M4Ø.Ø3 Postural kyphosis, cervicothoracic region

     M4Ø.Ø4 Postural kyphosis, thoracic region

     M4Ø.Ø5 Postural kyphosis, thoracolumbar region

  ✓5th **M4Ø.1 Other secondary kyphosis**

     M4Ø.1Ø Other secondary kyphosis, site unspecified ▽

     M4Ø.12 Other secondary kyphosis, cervical region

     M4Ø.13 Other secondary kyphosis, cervicothoracic region

     M4Ø.14 Other secondary kyphosis, thoracic region

     M4Ø.15 Other secondary kyphosis, thoracolumbar region

  ✓5th **M4Ø.2 Other and unspecified kyphosis**

   ✓6th **M4Ø.2Ø Unspecified kyphosis**

         M4Ø.2Ø2 Unspecified kyphosis, cervical region ▽

         M4Ø.2Ø3 Unspecified kyphosis, cervicothoracic ▽
               region

         M4Ø.2Ø4 Unspecified kyphosis, thoracic region ▽

         M4Ø.2Ø5 Unspecified kyphosis, thoracolumbar ▽
               region

         M4Ø.2Ø9 Unspecified kyphosis, site unspecified ▽

   ✓6th **M4Ø.29 Other kyphosis**

         M4Ø.292 Other kyphosis, cervical region

         M4Ø.293 Other kyphosis, cervicothoracic region

         M4Ø.294 Other kyphosis, thoracic region

         M4Ø.295 Other kyphosis, thoracolumbar region

         M4Ø.299 Other kyphosis, site unspecified ▽

EXCLUDES 1 Not coded here   EXCLUDES 2 Not included here   N Newborn Age: 0   P Pediatric Age: 0-17   M Maternity Age: 12-55   A Adult Age: 15-124

752   ICD-10-CM 2018

Kyphosis and Lordosis

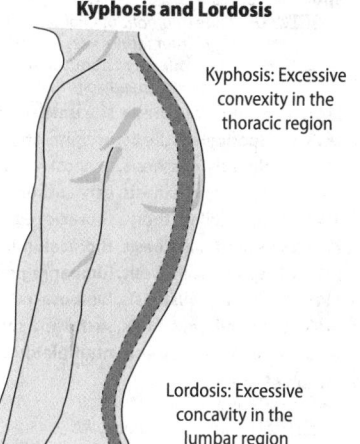

Kyphosis: Excessive convexity in the thoracic region

Lordosis: Excessive concavity in the lumbar region

✓5ᵗʰ **M40.3 Flatback syndrome**
  M40.30 Flatback syndrome, site unspecified ▽
  M40.35 Flatback syndrome, thoracolumbar region
  M40.36 Flatback syndrome, lumbar region
  M40.37 Flatback syndrome, lumbosacral region

✓5ᵗʰ **M40.4 Postural lordosis**
  Acquired lordosis
  M40.40 Postural lordosis, site unspecified ▽
  M40.45 Postural lordosis, thoracolumbar region
  M40.46 Postural lordosis, lumbar region
  M40.47 Postural lordosis, lumbosacral region

✓5ᵗʰ **M40.5 Lordosis, unspecified**
  M40.50 Lordosis, unspecified, site unspecified ▽
  M40.55 Lordosis, unspecified, thoracolumbar region
  M40.56 Lordosis, unspecified, lumbar region
  M40.57 Lordosis, unspecified, lumbosacral region

✓4ᵗʰ **M41 Scoliosis**
  INCLUDES kyphoscoliosis
  EXCLUDES 1 congenital scoliosis due to bony malformation (Q76.3)
    congenital scoliosis NOS (Q67.5)
    kyphoscoliotic heart disease (I27.1)
    postprocedural scoliosis (M96.-)
    postural congenital scoliosis (Q67.5)

✓5ᵗʰ **M41.0 Infantile idiopathic scoliosis**
  AHA: 2014, 4Q, 26
  M41.00 Infantile idiopathic scoliosis, site unspecified ▽
  M41.02 Infantile idiopathic scoliosis, cervical region
  M41.03 Infantile idiopathic scoliosis, cervicothoracic region
  M41.04 Infantile idiopathic scoliosis, thoracic region
  M41.05 Infantile idiopathic scoliosis, thoracolumbar region
  M41.06 Infantile idiopathic scoliosis, lumbar region
  M41.07 Infantile idiopathic scoliosis, lumbosacral region
  M41.08 Infantile idiopathic scoliosis, sacral and sacrococcygeal region

✓5ᵗʰ **M41.1 Juvenile and adolescent idiopathic scoliosis**
  ✓6ᵗʰ **M41.11 Juvenile idiopathic scoliosis**
    AHA: 2014, 4Q, 28
    M41.112 Juvenile idiopathic scoliosis, cervical region
    M41.113 Juvenile idiopathic scoliosis, cervicothoracic region
    M41.114 Juvenile idiopathic scoliosis, thoracic region
    M41.115 Juvenile idiopathic scoliosis, thoracolumbar region
    M41.116 Juvenile idiopathic scoliosis, lumbar region
    M41.117 Juvenile idiopathic scoliosis, lumbosacral region
    M41.119 Juvenile idiopathic scoliosis, site unspecified ▽

Scoliosis

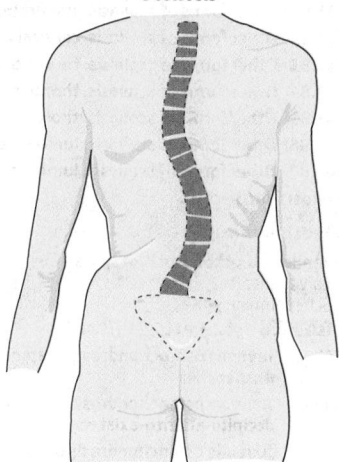

Lateral curvature of spine

✓6ᵗʰ **M41.12 Adolescent scoliosis**
    M41.122 Adolescent idiopathic scoliosis, cervical region
    M41.123 Adolescent idiopathic scoliosis, cervicothoracic region
    M41.124 Adolescent idiopathic scoliosis, thoracic region
    M41.125 Adolescent idiopathic scoliosis, thoracolumbar region
    M41.126 Adolescent idiopathic scoliosis, lumbar region
    M41.127 Adolescent idiopathic scoliosis, lumbosacral region
    M41.129 Adolescent idiopathic scoliosis, site unspecified ▽

✓5ᵗʰ **M41.2 Other idiopathic scoliosis**
  M41.20 Other idiopathic scoliosis, site unspecified ▽
  M41.22 Other idiopathic scoliosis, cervical region
  M41.23 Other idiopathic scoliosis, cervicothoracic region
  M41.24 Other idiopathic scoliosis, thoracic region
  M41.25 Other idiopathic scoliosis, thoracolumbar region
  M41.26 Other idiopathic scoliosis, lumbar region
  M41.27 Other idiopathic scoliosis, lumbosacral region

✓5ᵗʰ **M41.3 Thoracogenic scoliosis**
  M41.30 Thoracogenic scoliosis, site unspecified ▽
  M41.34 Thoracogenic scoliosis, thoracic region
  M41.35 Thoracogenic scoliosis, thoracolumbar region

✓5ᵗʰ **M41.4 Neuromuscular scoliosis**
  Scoliosis secondary to cerebral palsy, Friedreich's ataxia, poliomyelitis and other neuromuscular disorders
  Code also underlying condition
  AHA: 2014, 4Q, 27
  M41.40 Neuromuscular scoliosis, site unspecified ▽
  M41.41 Neuromuscular scoliosis, occipito-atlanto-axial region
  M41.42 Neuromuscular scoliosis, cervical region
  M41.43 Neuromuscular scoliosis, cervicothoracic region
  M41.44 Neuromuscular scoliosis, thoracic region
  M41.45 Neuromuscular scoliosis, thoracolumbar region
  M41.46 Neuromuscular scoliosis, lumbar region
  M41.47 Neuromuscular scoliosis, lumbosacral region

✓5ᵗʰ **M41.5 Other secondary scoliosis**
  M41.50 Other secondary scoliosis, site unspecified ▽
  M41.52 Other secondary scoliosis, cervical region
  M41.53 Other secondary scoliosis, cervicothoracic region
  M41.54 Other secondary scoliosis, thoracic region
  M41.55 Other secondary scoliosis, thoracolumbar region
  M41.56 Other secondary scoliosis, lumbar region
  M41.57 Other secondary scoliosis, lumbosacral region

√5ᵗʰ **M41.8** **Other forms of scoliosis**

     M41.80 **Other forms of scoliosis, site unspecified** ▽

     M41.82 **Other forms of scoliosis, cervical region**

     M41.83 **Other forms of scoliosis, cervicothoracic region**

     M41.84 **Other forms of scoliosis, thoracic region**

     M41.85 **Other forms of scoliosis, thoracolumbar region**

     M41.86 **Other forms of scoliosis, lumbar region**

     M41.87 **Other forms of scoliosis, lumbosacral region**

M41.9 **Scoliosis, unspecified** ▽

√4ᵗʰ **M42** **Spinal osteochondrosis**

√5ᵗʰ **M42.0** **Juvenile osteochondrosis of spine**

     Calvé's disease

     Scheuermann's disease

     EXCLUDES 1   *postural kyphosis (M40.0)*

     M42.00 **Juvenile osteochondrosis of spine, site unspecified** ▽

     M42.01 **Juvenile osteochondrosis of spine, occipito-atlanto-axial region**

     M42.02 **Juvenile osteochondrosis of spine, cervical region**

     M42.03 **Juvenile osteochondrosis of spine, cervicothoracic region**

     M42.04 **Juvenile osteochondrosis of spine, thoracic region**

     M42.05 **Juvenile osteochondrosis of spine, thoracolumbar region**

     M42.06 **Juvenile osteochondrosis of spine, lumbar region**

     M42.07 **Juvenile osteochondrosis of spine, lumbosacral region**

     M42.08 **Juvenile osteochondrosis of spine, sacral and sacrococcygeal region**

     M42.09 **Juvenile osteochondrosis of spine, multiple sites in spine**

√5ᵗʰ **M42.1** **Adult osteochondrosis of spine**

     M42.10 **Adult osteochondrosis of spine, site unspecified** A ▽

     M42.11 **Adult osteochondrosis of spine, occipito-atlanto-axial region** A

     M42.12 **Adult osteochondrosis of spine, cervical region** A

     M42.13 **Adult osteochondrosis of spine, cervicothoracic region** A

     M42.14 **Adult osteochondrosis of spine, thoracic region** A

     M42.15 **Adult osteochondrosis of spine, thoracolumbar region** A

     M42.16 **Adult osteochondrosis of spine, lumbar region** A

     M42.17 **Adult osteochondrosis of spine, lumbosacral region** A

     M42.18 **Adult osteochondrosis of spine, sacral and sacrococcygeal region** A

     M42.19 **Adult osteochondrosis of spine, multiple sites in spine** A

M42.9 **Spinal osteochondrosis, unspecified** ▽

√4ᵗʰ **M43** **Other deforming dorsopathies**

     EXCLUDES 1   *congenital spondylolysis and spondylolisthesis (Q76.2)*
               hemivertebra (Q76.3-Q76.4)
               Klippel-Feil syndrome (Q76.1)
               lumbarization and sacralization (Q76.4)
               platyspondylisis (Q76.4)
               spina bifida occulta (Q76.0)
               spinal curvature in osteoporosis (M80.-)
               spinal curvature in Paget's disease of bone [osteitis deformans] (M88.-)

√5ᵗʰ **M43.0** **Spondylolysis**

     EXCLUDES 1   *congenital spondylolysis (Q76.2)*
               spondylolisthesis (M43.1)

     M43.00 **Spondylolysis, site unspecified** ▽

     M43.01 **Spondylolysis, occipito-atlanto-axial region**

     M43.02 **Spondylolysis, cervical region**

     M43.03 **Spondylolysis, cervicothoracic region**

     M43.04 **Spondylolysis, thoracic region**

     M43.05 **Spondylolysis, thoracolumbar region**

     M43.06 **Spondylolysis, lumbar region**

     M43.07 **Spondylolysis, lumbosacral region**

     M43.08 **Spondylolysis, sacral and sacrococcygeal region**

     M43.09 **Spondylolysis, multiple sites in spine**

√5ᵗʰ **M43.1** **Spondylolisthesis**

     EXCLUDES 1   *acute traumatic of lumbosacral region (S33.1)*
               acute traumatic of sites other than lumbosacral—
               code to Fracture, vertebra, by region
               congenital spondylolisthesis (Q76.2)

     M43.10 **Spondylolisthesis, site unspecified** ▽

     M43.11 **Spondylolisthesis, occipito-atlanto-axial region**

     M43.12 **Spondylolisthesis, cervical region**

     M43.13 **Spondylolisthesis, cervicothoracic region**

     M43.14 **Spondylolisthesis, thoracic region**

     M43.15 **Spondylolisthesis, thoracolumbar region**

     M43.16 **Spondylolisthesis, lumbar region**

     M43.17 **Spondylolisthesis, lumbosacral region**

     M43.18 **Spondylolisthesis, sacral and sacrococcygeal region**

     M43.19 **Spondylolisthesis, multiple sites in spine**

√5ᵗʰ **M43.2** **Fusion of spine**

     Ankylosis of spinal joint

     EXCLUDES 1   *ankylosing spondylitis (M45.0-)*
               congenital fusion of spine (Q76.4)

     EXCLUDES 2   *arthrodesis status (Z98.1)*
               pseudoarthrosis after fusion or arthrodesis (M96.0)

     M43.20 **Fusion of spine, site unspecified** ▽

     M43.21 **Fusion of spine, occipito-atlanto-axial region**

     M43.22 **Fusion of spine, cervical region**

     M43.23 **Fusion of spine, cervicothoracic region**

     M43.24 **Fusion of spine, thoracic region**

     M43.25 **Fusion of spine, thoracolumbar region**

     M43.26 **Fusion of spine, lumbar region**

     M43.27 **Fusion of spine, lumbosacral region**

     M43.28 **Fusion of spine, sacral and sacrococcygeal region**

M43.3 **Recurrent atlantoaxial dislocation with myelopathy**

M43.4 **Other recurrent atlantoaxial dislocation**

√5ᵗʰ **M43.5** **Other recurrent vertebral dislocation**

     EXCLUDES 1   *biomechanical lesions NEC (M99.-)*

     √6ᵗʰ **M43.5X** **Other recurrent vertebral dislocation**

         M43.5X2 **Other recurrent vertebral dislocation, cervical region**

         M43.5X3 **Other recurrent vertebral dislocation, cervicothoracic region**

         M43.5X4 **Other recurrent vertebral dislocation, thoracic region**

         M43.5X5 **Other recurrent vertebral dislocation, thoracolumbar region**

         M43.5X6 **Other recurrent vertebral dislocation, lumbar region**

         M43.5X7 **Other recurrent vertebral dislocation, lumbosacral region**

         M43.5X8 **Other recurrent vertebral dislocation, sacral and sacrococcygeal region**

         M43.5X9 **Other recurrent vertebral dislocation, site unspecified** ▽

M43.6 **Torticollis**

     EXCLUDES 1   *congenital (sternomastoid) torticollis (Q68.0)*
               current injury—see Injury, of spine, by body region
               ocular torticollis (R29.891)
               psychogenic torticollis (F45.8)
               spasmodic torticollis (G24.3)
               torticollis due to birth injury (P15.2)

√5ᵗʰ **M43.8** **Other specified deforming dorsopathies**

     EXCLUDES 2   *kyphosis and lordosis (M40.-)*
               scoliosis (M41.-)

     √6ᵗʰ **M43.8X** **Other specified deforming dorsopathies**

         M43.8X1 **Other specified deforming dorsopathies, occipito-atlanto-axial region**

         M43.8X2 **Other specified deforming dorsopathies, cervical region**

         M43.8X3 **Other specified deforming dorsopathies, cervicothoracic region**

         M43.8X4 **Other specified deforming dorsopathies, thoracic region**

         M43.8X5 **Other specified deforming dorsopathies, thoracolumbar region**

         M43.8X6 **Other specified deforming dorsopathies, lumbar region**

         M43.8X7 **Other specified deforming dorsopathies, lumbosacral region**

EXCLUDES 1 Not coded here   *EXCLUDES 2* Not included here   N Newborn Age: 0   P Pediatric Age: 0-17   M Maternity Age: 12-55   A Adult Age: 15-124

754   ICD-10-CM 2018

M43.8X8 **Other specified deforming dorsopathies,** **sacral and sacrococcygeal** region

M43.8X9 **Other specified deforming** **dorsopathies, site unspecified** ▽

M43.9 **Deforming dorsopathy, unspecified** ▽
Curvature of spine NOS

Spondylopathies (M45-M49)

✓4ᵗʰ **M45 Ankylosing spondylitis**
Rheumatoid arthritis of spine
EXCLUDES 1 *arthropathy in Reiter's disease (M02.3-)*
juvenile (ankylosing) spondylitis (M08.1)
EXCLUDES 2 *Behçet's disease (M35.2)*

M45.0 **Ankylosing spondylitis of multiple sites in spine** HCC

M45.1 **Ankylosing spondylitis of occipito-atlanto-axial region** HCC

M45.2 **Ankylosing spondylitis of cervical region** HCC

M45.3 **Ankylosing spondylitis of cervicothoracic region** HCC

M45.4 **Ankylosing spondylitis of thoracic region** HCC

M45.5 **Ankylosing spondylitis of thoracolumbar region** HCC

M45.6 **Ankylosing spondylitis lumbar region** HCC

M45.7 **Ankylosing spondylitis of lumbosacral region** HCC

M45.8 **Ankylosing spondylitis sacral and sacrococcygeal region** HCC

M45.9 **Ankylosing spondylitis of unspecified sites in spine** HCC ▽

✓4ᵗʰ **M46 Other inflammatory spondylopathies**

✓5ᵗʰ M46.0 **Spinal enthesopathy**
Disorder of ligamentous or muscular attachments of spine

M46.00 **Spinal enthesopathy, site unspecified** HCC ▽

M46.01 **Spinal enthesopathy, occipito-atlanto-axial region** HCC

M46.02 **Spinal enthesopathy, cervical region** HCC

M46.03 **Spinal enthesopathy, cervicothoracic region** HCC

M46.04 **Spinal enthesopathy, thoracic region** HCC

M46.05 **Spinal enthesopathy, thoracolumbar region** HCC

M46.06 **Spinal enthesopathy, lumbar region** HCC

M46.07 **Spinal enthesopathy, lumbosacral region** HCC

M46.08 **Spinal enthesopathy, sacral and sacrococcygeal region** HCC

M46.09 **Spinal enthesopathy, multiple sites in spine** HCC

M46.1 **Sacroiliitis, not elsewhere classified** HCC
DEF: Inflammation of sacroiliac joint (situated at juncture of sacrum and hip); characterized by pain in buttocks or lower back that can extend down one or both legs.

✓5ᵗʰ M46.2 **Osteomyelitis of vertebra**

M46.20 **Osteomyelitis of vertebra, site unspecified** HCC ▽

M46.21 **Osteomyelitis of vertebra, occipito-atlanto-axial region** HCC

M46.22 **Osteomyelitis of vertebra, cervical region** HCC

M46.23 **Osteomyelitis of vertebra, cervicothoracic region** HCC

M46.24 **Osteomyelitis of vertebra, thoracic region** HCC

M46.25 **Osteomyelitis of vertebra, thoracolumbar region** HCC

M46.26 **Osteomyelitis of vertebra, lumbar region** HCC

M46.27 **Osteomyelitis of vertebra, lumbosacral region** HCC

M46.28 **Osteomyelitis of vertebra, sacral and sacrococcygeal region** HCC

✓5ᵗʰ M46.3 **Infection of intervertebral disc (pyogenic)**
Use additional code (B95-B97) to identify infectious agent

M46.30 **Infection of intervertebral disc (pyogenic), site unspecified** HCC ▽

M46.31 **Infection of intervertebral disc (pyogenic), occipito-atlanto-axial region** HCC

M46.32 **Infection of intervertebral disc (pyogenic), cervical region** HCC

M46.33 **Infection of intervertebral disc (pyogenic), cervicothoracic region** HCC

M46.34 **Infection of intervertebral disc (pyogenic), thoracic region** HCC

M46.35 **Infection of intervertebral disc (pyogenic), thoracolumbar region** HCC

M46.36 **Infection of intervertebral disc (pyogenic), lumbar region** HCC

M46.37 **Infection of intervertebral disc (pyogenic), lumbosacral region** HCC

M46.38 **Infection of intervertebral disc (pyogenic), sacral and sacrococcygeal region** HCC

M46.39 **Infection of intervertebral disc (pyogenic), multiple sites in spine** HCC

✓5ᵗʰ M46.4 **Discitis, unspecified**

M46.40 **Discitis, unspecified, site unspecified** ▽

M46.41 **Discitis, unspecified, occipito-atlanto-axial region** ▽

M46.42 **Discitis, unspecified, cervical region** ▽

M46.43 **Discitis, unspecified, cervicothoracic region** ▽

M46.44 **Discitis, unspecified, thoracic region** ▽

M46.45 **Discitis, unspecified, thoracolumbar region** ▽

M46.46 **Discitis, unspecified, lumbar region** ▽

M46.47 **Discitis, unspecified, lumbosacral region** ▽

M46.48 **Discitis, unspecified, sacral and sacrococcygeal region** ▽

M46.49 **Discitis, unspecified, multiple sites in spine** ▽

✓5ᵗʰ M46.5 **Other infective spondylopathies**

M46.50 **Other infective spondylopathies, site unspecified** HCC ▽

M46.51 **Other infective spondylopathies, occipito-atlanto-axial region** HCC

M46.52 **Other infective spondylopathies, cervical region** HCC

M46.53 **Other infective spondylopathies, cervicothoracic region** HCC

M46.54 **Other infective spondylopathies, thoracic region** HCC

M46.55 **Other infective spondylopathies, thoracolumbar region** HCC

M46.56 **Other infective spondylopathies, lumbar region** HCC

M46.57 **Other infective spondylopathies, lumbosacral region** HCC

M46.58 **Other infective spondylopathies, sacral and sacrococcygeal region** HCC

M46.59 **Other infective spondylopathies, multiple sites in spine** HCC

✓5ᵗʰ M46.8 **Other specified inflammatory spondylopathies**

M46.80 **Other specified inflammatory spondylopathies, site unspecified** HCC ▽

M46.81 **Other specified inflammatory spondylopathies, occipito-atlanto-axial region** HCC

M46.82 **Other specified inflammatory spondylopathies, cervical region** HCC

M46.83 **Other specified inflammatory spondylopathies, cervicothoracic region** HCC

M46.84 **Other specified inflammatory spondylopathies, thoracic region** HCC

M46.85 **Other specified inflammatory spondylopathies, thoracolumbar region** HCC

M46.86 **Other specified inflammatory spondylopathies, lumbar region** HCC

M46.87 **Other specified inflammatory spondylopathies, lumbosacral region** HCC

M46.88 **Other specified inflammatory spondylopathies, sacral and sacrococcygeal region** HCC

M46.89 **Other specified inflammatory spondylopathies, multiple sites in spine** HCC

✓5ᵗʰ M46.9 **Unspecified inflammatory spondylopathy**

M46.90 **Unspecified inflammatory spondylopathy, site unspecified** HCC ▽

M46.91 **Unspecified inflammatory spondylopathy, occipito-atlanto-axial region** HCC ▽

M46.92 **Unspecified inflammatory spondylopathy, cervical region** HCC ▽

M46.93 **Unspecified inflammatory spondylopathy, cervicothoracic region** HCC ▽

M46.94 **Unspecified inflammatory spondylopathy, thoracic region** HCC ▽

M46.95 **Unspecified inflammatory spondylopathy, thoracolumbar region** HCC ▽

M46.96 **Unspecified inflammatory spondylopathy, lumbar region** HCC ▽

M46.97 **Unspecified inflammatory spondylopathy, lumbosacral region** HCC ▽

☑ Additional Character Req   ✓x7ᵗʰ Placeholder Alert   Manifestation   HCC CMS-HCC Condition   ▽ Unspecified Code   ▶◀ Revised Text   ● New Code   ▲ Revised Code Title

M46.98 Unspecified inflammatory spondylopathy, sacral and sacrococcygeal region HCC ▽

M46.99 Unspecified inflammatory spondylopathy, multiple sites in spine HCC ▽

✓4ᵗʰ **M47 Spondylosis**
INCLUDES arthrosis or osteoarthritis of spine
degeneration of facet joints

✓5ᵗʰ **M47.0 Anterior spinal and vertebral artery compression syndromes**

✓6ᵗʰ **M47.01 Anterior spinal artery compression syndromes**

M47.011 Anterior spinal artery compression syndromes, occipito-atlanto-axial region

M47.012 Anterior spinal artery compression syndromes, cervical region

M47.013 Anterior spinal artery compression syndromes, cervicothoracic region

M47.014 Anterior spinal artery compression syndromes, thoracic region

M47.015 Anterior spinal artery compression syndromes, thoracolumbar region

M47.016 Anterior spinal artery compression syndromes, lumbar region

M47.019 Anterior spinal artery compression syndromes, site unspecified ▽

✓6ᵗʰ **M47.02 Vertebral artery compression syndromes**

M47.021 Vertebral artery compression syndromes, occipito-atlanto-axial region

M47.022 Vertebral artery compression syndromes, cervical region

M47.029 Vertebral artery compression syndromes, site unspecified ▽

✓5ᵗʰ **M47.1 Other spondylosis with myelopathy**
Spondylogenic compression of spinal cord
EXCLUDES 1 vertebral subluxation (M43.3-M43.5X9)

M47.10 Other spondylosis with myelopathy, site unspecified ▽

M47.11 Other spondylosis with myelopathy, occipito-atlanto-axial region

M47.12 Other spondylosis with myelopathy, cervical region

M47.13 Other spondylosis with myelopathy, cervicothoracic region

M47.14 Other spondylosis with myelopathy, thoracic region

M47.15 Other spondylosis with myelopathy, thoracolumbar region

M47.16 Other spondylosis with myelopathy, lumbar region

✓5ᵗʰ **M47.2 Other spondylosis with radiculopathy**

M47.20 Other spondylosis with radiculopathy, site unspecified ▽

M47.21 Other spondylosis with radiculopathy, occipito-atlanto-axial region

M47.22 Other spondylosis with radiculopathy, cervical region

M47.23 Other spondylosis with radiculopathy, cervicothoracic region

M47.24 Other spondylosis with radiculopathy, thoracic region

M47.25 Other spondylosis with radiculopathy, thoracolumbar region

M47.26 Other spondylosis with radiculopathy, lumbar region

M47.27 Other spondylosis with radiculopathy, lumbosacral region

M47.28 Other spondylosis with radiculopathy, sacral and sacrococcygeal region

✓5ᵗʰ **M47.8 Other spondylosis**

✓6ᵗʰ **M47.81 Spondylosis without myelopathy or radiculopathy**

M47.811 Spondylosis without myelopathy or radiculopathy, occipito-atlanto-axial region

M47.812 Spondylosis without myelopathy or radiculopathy, cervical region

M47.813 Spondylosis without myelopathy or radiculopathy, cervicothoracic region

M47.814 Spondylosis without myelopathy or radiculopathy, thoracic region

M47.815 Spondylosis without myelopathy or radiculopathy, thoracolumbar region

M47.816 Spondylosis without myelopathy or radiculopathy, lumbar region

M47.817 Spondylosis without myelopathy or radiculopathy, lumbosacral region

M47.818 Spondylosis without myelopathy or radiculopathy, sacral and sacrococcygeal region

M47.819 Spondylosis without myelopathy or radiculopathy, site unspecified ▽

✓6ᵗʰ **M47.89 Other spondylosis**

M47.891 Other spondylosis, occipito-atlanto- axial region

M47.892 Other spondylosis, cervical region

M47.893 Other spondylosis, cervicothoracic region

M47.894 Other spondylosis, thoracic region

M47.895 Other spondylosis, thoracolumbar region

M47.896 Other spondylosis, lumbar region

M47.897 Other spondylosis, lumbosacral region

M47.898 Other spondylosis, sacral and sacrococcygeal region

M47.899 Other spondylosis, site unspecified ▽

M47.9 Spondylosis, unspecified ▽

✓4ᵗʰ **M48 Other spondylopathies**

✓5ᵗʰ **M48.0 Spinal stenosis**
Caudal stenosis

M48.00 Spinal stenosis, site unspecified ▽

M48.01 Spinal stenosis, occipito-atlanto-axial region

M48.02 Spinal stenosis, cervical region

M48.03 Spinal stenosis, cervicothoracic region

M48.04 Spinal stenosis, thoracic region

M48.05 Spinal stenosis, thoracolumbar region

✓6ᵗʰ **M48.06 Spinal stenosis, lumbar region**
DEF: Spinal canal narrowing in the lumbar area with nerve root compression, causing muscle pain, fatigue, and weakness during extension of the lumbar spine; pain is relieved by sitting or bending.

● **M48.061** Spinal stenosis, lumbar region without neurogenic claudication
Spinal stenosis, lumbar region NOS

● **M48.062** Spinal stenosis, lumbar region with neurogenic claudication

M48.07 Spinal stenosis, lumbosacral region

M48.08 Spinal stenosis, sacral and sacrococcygeal region

✓5ᵗʰ **M48.1 Ankylosing hyperostosis [Forestier]**
Diffuse idiopathic skeletal hyperostosis [DISH]

M48.10 Ankylosing hyperostosis [Forestier], site unspecified ▽

M48.11 Ankylosing hyperostosis [Forestier], occipito-atlanto-axial region

M48.12 Ankylosing hyperostosis [Forestier], cervical region

M48.13 Ankylosing hyperostosis [Forestier], cervicothoracic region

M48.14 Ankylosing hyperostosis [Forestier], thoracic region

M48.15 Ankylosing hyperostosis [Forestier], thoracolumbar region

M48.16 Ankylosing hyperostosis [Forestier], lumbar region

M48.17 Ankylosing hyperostosis [Forestier], lumbosacral region

M48.18 Ankylosing hyperostosis [Forestier], sacral and sacrococcygeal region

M48.19 Ankylosing hyperostosis [Forestier], multiple sites in spine

✓5ᵗʰ **M48.2 Kissing spine**

M48.20 Kissing spine, site unspecified ▽

M48.21 Kissing spine, occipito-atlanto-axial region

M48.22 Kissing spine, cervical region

M48.23 Kissing spine, cervicothoracic region

M48.24 Kissing spine, thoracic region

M48.25 Kissing spine, thoracolumbar region

M48.26 Kissing spine, lumbar region

M48.27 Kissing spine, lumbosacral region

EXCLUDES 1 Not coded here   EXCLUDES 2 Not included here   N Newborn Age: 0   P Pediatric Age: 0-17   M Maternity Age: 12-55   A Adult Age: 15-124

756   ICD-10-CM 2018

✓5ᵗʰ **M48.3 Traumatic spondylopathy**

    M48.30 Traumatic spondylopathy, site unspecified ▽

    M48.31 Traumatic spondylopathy, occipito-atlanto-axial region

    M48.32 Traumatic spondylopathy, cervical region

    M48.33 Traumatic spondylopathy, cervicothoracic region

    M48.34 Traumatic spondylopathy, thoracic region

    M48.35 Traumatic spondylopathy, thoracolumbar region

    M48.36 Traumatic spondylopathy, lumbar region

    M48.37 Traumatic spondylopathy, lumbosacral region

    M48.38 Traumatic spondylopathy, sacral and sacrococcygeal region

✓5ᵗʰ **M48.4 Fatigue fracture of vertebra**
    Stress fracture of vertebra

    EXCLUDES 1 *pathological fracture NOS (M84.4-)*
         pathological fracture of vertebra due to neoplasm (M84.58)
         pathological fracture of vertebra due to other diagnosis (M84.68)
         pathological fracture of vertebra due to osteoporosis (M80.-)
         traumatic fracture of vertebrae (S12.0-S12.3-, S22.0-, S32.0-)

> The appropriate 7th character is to be added to each code from subcategory M48.4.
> A   initial encounter for fracture
> D   subsequent encounter for fracture with routine healing
> G   subsequent encounter for fracture with delayed healing
> S   sequela of fracture

  ✓×7ᵗʰ **M48.40** Fatigue fracture of vertebra, site unspecified ▽

  ✓×7ᵗʰ **M48.41** Fatigue fracture of vertebra, occipito-atlanto-axial region

  ✓×7ᵗʰ **M48.42** Fatigue fracture of vertebra, cervical region

  ✓×7ᵗʰ **M48.43** Fatigue fracture of vertebra, cervicothoracic region

  ✓×7ᵗʰ **M48.44** Fatigue fracture of vertebra, thoracic region

  ✓×7ᵗʰ **M48.45** Fatigue fracture of vertebra, thoracolumbar region

  ✓×7ᵗʰ **M48.46** Fatigue fracture of vertebra, lumbar region

  ✓×7ᵗʰ **M48.47** Fatigue fracture of vertebra, lumbosacral region

  ✓×7ᵗʰ **M48.48** Fatigue fracture of vertebra, sacral and sacrococcygeal region

✓5ᵗʰ **M48.5 Collapsed vertebra, not elsewhere classified**
    Collapsed vertebra NOS
    Compression fracture of vertebra NOS
    Wedging of vertebra NOS

    EXCLUDES 1 *current injury—see Injury of spine, by body region*
         fatigue fracture of vertebra (M48.4)
         pathological fracture of vertebra due to neoplasm (M84.58)
         pathological fracture of vertebra due to other diagnosis (M84.68)
         pathological fracture of vertebra due to osteoporosis (M80.-)
         pathological fracture NOS (M84.4-)
         stress fracture of vertebra (M48.4-)
         traumatic fracture of vertebra (S12-, S22-, S32-)

> The appropriate 7th character is to be added to each code from subcategory M48.5.
> A   initial encounter for fracture
> D   subsequent encounter for fracture with routine healing
> G   subsequent encounter for fracture with delayed healing
> S   sequela of fracture

[1] ✓×7ᵗʰ **M48.50** Collapsed vertebra, not elsewhere classified, site unspecified HCC ▽

[1] ✓×7ᵗʰ **M48.51** Collapsed vertebra, not elsewhere classified, occipito-atlanto-axial region HCC

[1] ✓×7ᵗʰ **M48.52** Collapsed vertebra, not elsewhere classified, cervical region HCC

[1] ✓×7ᵗʰ **M48.53** Collapsed vertebra, not elsewhere classified, cervicothoracic region HCC

[1] ✓×7ᵗʰ **M48.54** Collapsed vertebra, not elsewhere classified, thoracic region HCC

[1] ✓×7ᵗʰ **M48.55** Collapsed vertebra, not elsewhere classified, thoracolumbar region HCC

[1] ✓×7ᵗʰ **M48.56** Collapsed vertebra, not elsewhere classified, lumbar region HCC

[1] ✓×7ᵗʰ **M48.57** Collapsed vertebra, not elsewhere classified, lumbosacral region HCC

[1] ✓×7ᵗʰ **M48.58** Collapsed vertebra, not elsewhere classified, sacral and sacrococcygeal region HCC

✓5ᵗʰ **M48.8 Other specified spondylopathies**
    Ossification of posterior longitudinal ligament

  ✓6ᵗʰ **M48.8X** Other specified spondylopathies

    M48.8X1 Other specified spondylopathies, occipito-atlanto-axial region HCC

    M48.8X2 Other specified spondylopathies, cervical region HCC

    M48.8X3 Other specified spondylopathies, cervicothoracic region HCC

    M48.8X4 Other specified spondylopathies, thoracic region HCC

    M48.8X5 Other specified spondylopathies, thoracolumbar region HCC

    M48.8X6 Other specified spondylopathies, lumbar region HCC

    M48.8X7 Other specified spondylopathies, lumbosacral region HCC

    M48.8X8 Other specified spondylopathies, sacral and sacrococcygeal region HCC

    M48.8X9 Other specified spondylopathies, site unspecified HCC ▽

  M48.9 Spondylopathy, unspecified ▽

✓4ᵗʰ **M49 Spondylopathies in diseases classified elsewhere**
    INCLUDES curvature of spine in diseases classified elsewhere
         deformity of spine in diseases classified elsewhere
         kyphosis in diseases classified elsewhere
         scoliosis in diseases classified elsewhere
         spondylopathy in diseases classified elsewhere

    Code first underlying disease, such as:
      brucellosis (A23.-)
      Charcôt-Marie-Tooth disease (G60.0)
      enterobacterial infections (A01-A04)
      osteitis fibrosa cystica (E21.0)

    EXCLUDES 1 *curvature of spine in tuberculosis [Pott's] (A18.01)*
         enteropathic arthropathies (M07.-)
         gonococcal spondylitis (A54.41)
         neuropathic [tabes dorsalis] spondylitis (A52.11)
         neuropathic spondylopathy in syringomyelia (G95.0)
         neuropathic spondylopathy in tabes dorsalis (A52.11)
         nonsyphilitic neuropathic spondylopathy NEC (G98.0)
         spondylitis in syphilis (acquired) (A52.77)
         tuberculous spondylitis (A18.01)
         typhoid fever spondylitis (A01.05)

  ✓5ᵗʰ **M49.8 Spondylopathy in diseases classified elsewhere**

    M49.80 *Spondylopathy in diseases classified elsewhere, site unspecified* HCC ▽

    M49.81 *Spondylopathy in diseases classified elsewhere, occipito-atlanto-axial region* HCC

    M49.82 *Spondylopathy in diseases classified elsewhere, cervical region* HCC

    M49.83 *Spondylopathy in diseases classified elsewhere, cervicothoracic region* HCC

    M49.84 *Spondylopathy in diseases classified elsewhere, thoracic region* HCC

    M49.85 *Spondylopathy in diseases classified elsewhere, thoracolumbar region* HCC

    M49.86 *Spondylopathy in diseases classified elsewhere, lumbar region* HCC

    M49.87 *Spondylopathy in diseases classified elsewhere, lumbosacral region* HCC

    M49.88 *Spondylopathy in diseases classified elsewhere, sacral and sacrococcygeal region* HCC

    M49.89 *Spondylopathy in diseases classified elsewhere, multiple sites in spine* HCC

---

[1] HCC with 7th character indicating initial encounter (A, B or C - specific to category).

✓ Additional Character Req   ✓×7ᵗʰ Placeholder Alert   Manifestation   HCC CMS-HCC Condition   ▽ Unspecified Code   ▶◀ Revised Text   ● New Code   ▲ Revised Code Title

ICD-10-CM 2018   757

Other dorsopathies (M50-M54)

EXCLUDES 1 current injury—see injury of spine by body region
discitis NOS (M46.4-)

✓4th M50 Cervical disc disorders
NOTE Code to the most superior level of disorder.
INCLUDES cervicothoracic disc disorders with cervicalgia
cervicothoracic disc disorders
AHA: 2016, 1Q, 17

✓5th M50.0 Cervical disc disorder with myelopathy
M50.00 Cervical disc disorder with myelopathy, unspecified cervical region   ▽

M50.01 Cervical disc disorder with myelopathy, high cervical region
C2-C3 disc disorder with myelopathy
C3-C4 disc disorder with myelopathy

✓6th M50.02 Cervical disc disorder with myelopathy, mid-cervical region
M50.020 Cervical disc disorder with myelopathy, mid-cervical region, unspecified level   ▽

M50.021 Cervical disc disorder at C4-C5 level with myelopathy
C4-C5 disc disorder with myelopathy

M50.022 Cervical disc disorder at C5-C6 level with myelopathy
C5-C6 disc disorder with myelopathy

M50.023 Cervical disc disorder at C6-C7 level with myelopathy
C6-C7 disc disorder with myelopathy

M50.03 Cervical disc disorder with myelopathy, cervicothoracic region
C7-T1 disc disorder with myelopathy

✓5th M50.1 Cervical disc disorder with radiculopathy
EXCLUDES 2 brachial radiculitis NOS (M54.13)

M50.10 Cervical disc disorder with radiculopathy, unspecified cervical region   ▽

M50.11 Cervical disc disorder with radiculopathy, high cervical region
C2-C3 disc disorder with radiculopathy
C3 radiculopathy due to disc disorder
C3-C4 disc disorder with radiculopathy
C4 radiculopathy due to disc disorder

✓6th M50.12 Cervical disc disorder with radiculopathy, mid-cervical region
M50.120 Mid-cervical disc disorder, unspecified   ▽

M50.121 Cervical disc disorder at C4-C5 level with radiculopathy
C4-C5 disc disorder with radiculopathy
C5 radiculopathy due to disc disorder

M50.122 Cervical disc disorder at C5-C6 level with radiculopathy
C5-C6 disc disorder with radiculopathy
C6 radiculopathy due to disc disorder

M50.123 Cervical disc disorder at C6-C7 level with radiculopathy
C6-C7 disc disorder with radiculopathy
C7 radiculopathy due to disc disorder

M50.13 Cervical disc disorder with radiculopathy, cervicothoracic region
C7-T1 disc disorder with radiculopathy
C8 radiculopathy due to disc disorder

✓5th M50.2 Other cervical disc displacement
M50.20 Other cervical disc displacement, unspecified cervical region   ▽

M50.21 Other cervical disc displacement, high cervical region
Other C2-C3 cervical disc displacement
Other C3-C4 cervical disc displacement

✓6th M50.22 Other cervical disc displacement, mid-cervical region
M50.220 Other cervical disc displacement, mid-cervical region, unspecified level   ▽

M50.221 Other cervical disc displacement at C4-C5 level
Other C4-C5 cervical disc displacement

M50.222 Other cervical disc displacement at C5-C6 level
Other C5-C6 cervical disc displacement

M50.223 Other cervical disc displacement at C6-C7 level
Other C6-C7 cervical disc displacement

M50.23 Other cervical disc displacement, cervicothoracic region
Other C7-T1 cervical disc displacement

✓5th M50.3 Other cervical disc degeneration
M50.30 Other cervical disc degeneration, unspecified cervical region   ▽

M50.31 Other cervical disc degeneration, high cervical region
Other C2-C3 cervical disc degeneration
Other C3-C4 cervical disc degeneration

✓6th M50.32 Other cervical disc degeneration, mid-cervical region
M50.320 Other cervical disc degeneration, mid-cervical region, unspecified level   ▽

M50.321 Other cervical disc degeneration at C4-C5 level
Other C4-C5 cervical disc degeneration

M50.322 Other cervical disc degeneration at C5-C6 level
Other C5-C6 cervical disc degeneration

M50.323 Other cervical disc degeneration at C6-C7 level
Other C6-C7 cervical disc degeneration

M50.33 Other cervical disc degeneration, cervicothoracic region
Other C7-T1 cervical disc degeneration

✓5th M50.8 Other cervical disc disorders
M50.80 Other cervical disc disorders, unspecified cervical region   ▽

M50.81 Other cervical disc disorders, high cervical region
Other C2-C3 cervical disc disorders
Other C3-C4 cervical disc disorders

✓6th M50.82 Other cervical disc disorders, mid-cervical region
M50.820 Other cervical disc disorders, mid-cervical region, unspecified level   ▽

M50.821 Other cervical disc disorders at C4-C5 level
Other C4-C5 cervical disc disorders

M50.822 Other cervical disc disorders at C5-C6 level
Other C5-C6 cervical disc disorders

M50.823 Other cervical disc disorders at C6-C7 level
Other C6-C7 cervical disc disorders

M50.83 Other cervical disc disorders, cervicothoracic region
Other C7-T1 cervical disc disorders

✓5th M50.9 Cervical disc disorder, unspecified
M50.90 Cervical disc disorder, unspecified, unspecified cervical region   ▽

M50.91 Cervical disc disorder, unspecified, high cervical region   ▽
C2-C3 cervical disc disorder, unspecified
C3-C4 cervical disc disorder, unspecified

✓6th M50.92 Cervical disc disorder, unspecified, mid-cervical region
M50.920 Unspecified cervical disc disorder, mid-cervical region, unspecified level   ▽

M50.921 Unspecified cervical disc disorder at C4-C5 level   ▽
Unspecified C4-C5 cervical disc disorder

M50.922 Unspecified cervical disc disorder at C5-C6 level   ▽
Unspecified C5-C6 cervical disc disorder

M50.923 Unspecified cervical disc disorder at C6-C7 level   ▽
Unspecified C6-C7 cervical disc disorder

M50.93 Cervical disc disorder, unspecified, cervicothoracic region   ▽
C7-T1 cervical disc disorder, unspecified

✓4th M51 Thoracic, thoracolumbar, and lumbosacral intervertebral disc disorders
EXCLUDES 2 cervical and cervicothoracic disc disorders (M50.-)
sacral and sacrococcygeal disorders (M53.3)

✓5th M51.0 Thoracic, thoracolumbar and lumbosacral intervertebral disc disorders with myelopathy
M51.04 Intervertebral disc disorders with myelopathy, thoracic region

EXCLUDES 1 Not coded here   **EXCLUDES 2** Not included here   N Newborn Age: 0   P Pediatric Age: 0-17   M Maternity Age: 12-55   A Adult Age: 15-124

758   ICD-10-CM 2018

M50–M51.04

M51.Ø5 Intervertebral disc disorders with myelopathy, thoracolumbar region

M51.Ø6 Intervertebral disc disorders with myelopathy, lumbar region

√5ᵗʰ **M51.1** **Thoracic, thoracolumbar and lumbosacral intervertebral disc disorders with radiculopathy**
Sciatica due to intervertebral disc disorder
> **EXCLUDES 1** *lumbar radiculitis NOS (M54.16)*
> *sciatica NOS (M54.3)*

M51.14 Intervertebral disc disorders with radiculopathy, thoracic region

M51.15 Intervertebral disc disorders with radiculopathy, thoracolumbar region

M51.16 Intervertebral disc disorders with radiculopathy, lumbar region

M51.17 Intervertebral disc disorders with radiculopathy, lumbosacral region

√5ᵗʰ **M51.2** **Other thoracic, thoracolumbar and lumbosacral intervertebral disc displacement**
Lumbago due to displacement of intervertebral disc

M51.24 Other intervertebral disc displacement, thoracic region

M51.25 Other intervertebral disc displacement, thoracolumbar region

M51.26 Other intervertebral disc displacement, lumbar region

M51.27 Other intervertebral disc displacement, lumbosacral region

√5ᵗʰ **M51.3** **Other thoracic, thoracolumbar and lumbosacral intervertebral disc degeneration**
AHA: 2013, 3Q, 22

M51.34 Other intervertebral disc degeneration, thoracic region

M51.35 Other intervertebral disc degeneration, thoracolumbar region

M51.36 Other intervertebral disc degeneration, lumbar region

M51.37 Other intervertebral disc degeneration, lumbosacral region

√5ᵗʰ **M51.4** **Schmorl's nodes**
DEF: Irregular bone defect in the margin of the vertebral body; causes herniation into end plate of vertebral body.

M51.44 Schmorl's nodes, thoracic region

M51.45 Schmorl's nodes, thoracolumbar region

M51.46 Schmorl's nodes, lumbar region

M51.47 Schmorl's nodes, lumbosacral region

√5ᵗʰ **M51.8** **Other thoracic, thoracolumbar and lumbosacral intervertebral disc disorders**

M51.84 Other intervertebral disc disorders, thoracic region

M51.85 Other intervertebral disc disorders, thoracolumbar region

M51.86 Other intervertebral disc disorders, lumbar region

M51.87 Other intervertebral disc disorders, lumbosacral region

M51.9 Unspecified thoracic, thoracolumbar and lumbosacral intervertebral disc disorder ▽

√4ᵗʰ **M53** **Other and unspecified dorsopathies, not elsewhere classified**

M53.Ø **Cervicocranial syndrome**
Posterior cervical sympathetic syndrome

M53.1 **Cervicobrachial syndrome**
> **EXCLUDES 2** *cervical disc disorder (M5Ø.-)*
> *thoracic outlet syndrome (G54.Ø)*

√5ᵗʰ **M53.2** **Spinal instabilities**

√6ᵗʰ **M53.2X** Spinal instabilities

M53.2X1 Spinal instabilities, occipito-atlanto-axial region

M53.2X2 Spinal instabilities, cervical region

M53.2X3 Spinal instabilities, cervicothoracic region

M53.2X4 Spinal instabilities, thoracic region

M53.2X5 Spinal instabilities, thoracolumbar region

M53.2X6 Spinal instabilities, lumbar region

M53.2X7 Spinal instabilities, lumbosacral region

M53.2X8 Spinal instabilities, sacral and sacrococcygeal region

Displacement Intervertebral Disc

Normal Top View   Herniated Top View

Lamina · Ligamentum flavum · Nucleus pulposus · Spinal cord · Spinal nerve · Herniates through annulus · Disc annulus · Nucleus pulposus

M53.2X9 Spinal instabilities, site unspecified ▽

M53.3 **Sacrococcygeal disorders, not elsewhere classified**
Coccygodynia

√5ᵗʰ **M53.8** **Other specified dorsopathies**

M53.8Ø Other specified dorsopathies, site unspecified ▽

M53.81 Other specified dorsopathies, occipito-atlanto-axial region

M53.82 Other specified dorsopathies, cervical region

M53.83 Other specified dorsopathies, cervicothoracic region

M53.84 Other specified dorsopathies, thoracic region

M53.85 Other specified dorsopathies, thoracolumbar region

M53.86 Other specified dorsopathies, lumbar region

M53.87 Other specified dorsopathies, lumbosacral region

M53.88 Other specified dorsopathies, sacral and sacrococcygeal region

M53.9 Dorsopathy, unspecified ▽

√4ᵗʰ **M54** **Dorsalgia**
> **EXCLUDES 1** *psychogenic dorsalgia (F45.41)*

√5ᵗʰ **M54.Ø** **Panniculitis affecting regions of neck and back**
> **EXCLUDES 1** *lupus panniculitis (L93.2)*
> *panniculitis NOS (M79.3)*
> *relapsing [Weber-Christian] panniculitis (M35.6)*

M54.ØØ Panniculitis affecting regions of neck and back, site unspecified ▽

M54.Ø1 Panniculitis affecting regions of neck and back, occipito-atlanto-axial region

M54.Ø2 Panniculitis affecting regions of neck and back, cervical region

M54.Ø3 Panniculitis affecting regions of neck and back, cervicothoracic region

M54.Ø4 Panniculitis affecting regions of neck and back, thoracic region

M54.Ø5 Panniculitis affecting regions of neck and back, thoracolumbar region

M54.Ø6 Panniculitis affecting regions of neck and back, lumbar region

M54.Ø7 Panniculitis affecting regions of neck and back, lumbosacral region

M54.Ø8 Panniculitis affecting regions of neck and back, sacral and sacrococcygeal region

M54.Ø9 Panniculitis affecting regions, neck and back, multiple sites in spine

√5ᵗʰ **M54.1** **Radiculopathy**
Brachial neuritis or radiculitis NOS
Lumbar neuritis or radiculitis NOS
Lumbosacral neuritis or radiculitis NOS
Thoracic neuritis or radiculitis NOS
Radiculitis NOS
> **EXCLUDES 1** *neuralgia and neuritis NOS (M79.2)*
> *radiculopathy with cervical disc disorder (M5Ø.1)*
> *radiculopathy with lumbar and other intervertebral disc disorder (M51.1-)*
> *radiculopathy with spondylosis (M47.2-)*

M54.1Ø Radiculopathy, site unspecified ▽

M54.11 Radiculopathy, occipito-atlanto-axial region

M54.12 Radiculopathy, cervical region

M54.13 Radiculopathy, cervicothoracic region

M54.14 Radiculopathy, thoracic region

☑ Additional Character Req   ✓x7ᵗʰ Placeholder Alert   Manifestation   HCC CMS-HCC Condition   ▽ Unspecified Code   ▶◀ Revised Text   ● New Code   ▲ Revised Code Title

ICD-10-CM 2018   759

M54.15   Radiculopathy, **thoracolumbar** region
M54.16   Radiculopathy, **lumbar** region
M54.17   Radiculopathy, **lumbosacral** region
M54.18   Radiculopathy, **sacral and sacrococcygeal** region

M54.2 Cervicalgia
> EXCLUDES 1   *cervicalgia due to intervertebral cervical disc disorder (M50.-)*

✓5th **M54.3 Sciatica**
> EXCLUDES 1   *lesion of sciatic nerve (G57.0)*
> *sciatica due to intervertebral disc disorder (M51.1-)*
> *sciatica with lumbago (M54.4-)*

M54.30   Sciatica, **unspecified side** ▽
M54.31   Sciatica, **right** side
M54.32   Sciatica, **left** side

✓5th **M54.4 Lumbago with sciatica**
> EXCLUDES 1   *lumbago with sciatica due to intervertebral disc disorder (M51.1-)*
>
> **AHA:** 2016, 2Q, 7

M54.40   Lumbago with sciatica, **unspecified side** ▽
M54.41   Lumbago with sciatica, **right** side
M54.42   Lumbago with sciatica, **left** side

M54.5 Low back pain
> Loin pain
> Lumbago NOS
> EXCLUDES 1   *low back strain (S39.012)*
> *lumbago due to intervertebral disc displacement (M51.2-)*
> *lumbago with sciatica (M54.4-)*

M54.6 Pain in thoracic spine
> EXCLUDES 1   *pain in thoracic spine due to intervertebral disc disorder (M51.-)*

✓5th **M54.8 Other dorsalgia**
> EXCLUDES 1   *dorsalgia in thoracic region (M54.6)*
> *low back pain (M54.5)*

M54.81   **Occipital neuralgia**
M54.89   **Other dorsalgia**
M54.9   **Dorsalgia, unspecified** ▽
> Backache NOS   Back pain NOS

SOFT TISSUE DISORDERS (M60-M79)

Disorders of muscles (M60-M63)

> EXCLUDES 1   *dermatopolymyositis (M33.-)*
> *muscular dystrophies and myopathies (G71-G72)*
> *myopathy in amyloidosis (E85.-)*
> *myopathy in polyarteritis nodosa (M30.0)*
> *myopathy in rheumatoid arthritis (M05.32)*
> *myopathy in scleroderma (M34.-)*
> *myopathy in Sjögren's syndrome (M35.03)*
> *myopathy in systemic lupus erythematosus (M32.-)*

✓4th **M60 Myositis**
> EXCLUDES 2   *inclusion body myositis [IBM] (G72.41)*

✓5th **M60.0 Infective myositis**
> Tropical pyomyositis
> Use additional code (B95-B97) to identify infectious agent

✓6th   **M60.00 Infective myositis, unspecified site**
M60.000   Infective myositis, unspecified **right** arm
> Infective myositis, right upper limb NOS
M60.001   Infective myositis, unspecified **left** arm
> Infective myositis, left upper limb NOS
M60.002   Infective myositis, unspecified **arm** ▽
> Infective myositis, upper limb NOS
M60.003   Infective myositis, unspecified **right** leg
> Infective myositis, right lower limb NOS
M60.004   Infective myositis, unspecified **left** leg
> Infective myositis, left lower limb NOS
M60.005   Infective myositis, unspecified **leg** ▽
> Infective myositis, lower limb NOS
M60.009   Infective myositis, unspecified **site** ▽

✓6th   **M60.01 Infective myositis, shoulder**
M60.011   Infective myositis, **right** shoulder
M60.012   Infective myositis, **left** shoulder
M60.019   Infective myositis, **unspecified** shoulder ▽

✓6th   **M60.02 Infective myositis, upper arm**
M60.021   Infective myositis, **right** upper arm

M60.022   Infective myositis, **left** upper arm
M60.029   Infective myositis, **unspecified** upper arm ▽

✓6th   **M60.03 Infective myositis, forearm**
M60.031   Infective myositis, **right** forearm
M60.032   Infective myositis, **left** forearm
M60.039   Infective myositis, **unspecified** forearm ▽

✓6th   **M60.04 Infective myositis, hand and fingers**
M60.041   Infective myositis, **right** hand
M60.042   Infective myositis, **left** hand
M60.043   Infective myositis, **unspecified** hand ▽
M60.044   Infective myositis, **right** finger(s)
M60.045   Infective myositis, **left** finger(s)
M60.046   Infective myositis, **unspecified** finger(s) ▽

✓6th   **M60.05 Infective myositis, thigh**
M60.051   Infective myositis, **right** thigh
M60.052   Infective myositis, **left** thigh
M60.059   Infective myositis, **unspecified** thigh ▽

✓6th   **M60.06 Infective myositis, lower leg**
M60.061   Infective myositis, **right** lower leg
M60.062   Infective myositis, **left** lower leg
M60.069   Infective myositis, **unspecified** lower leg ▽

✓6th   **M60.07 Infective myositis, ankle, foot and toes**
M60.070   Infective myositis, **right** ankle
M60.071   Infective myositis, **left** ankle
M60.072   Infective myositis, **unspecified** ankle ▽
M60.073   Infective myositis, **right** foot
M60.074   Infective myositis, **left** foot
M60.075   Infective myositis, **unspecified** foot ▽
M60.076   Infective myositis, **right** toe(s)
M60.077   Infective myositis, **left** toe(s)
M60.078   Infective myositis, **unspecified** toe(s) ▽

M60.08   Infective myositis, **other site**
M60.09   Infective myositis, **multiple sites**

✓5th **M60.1 Interstitial myositis**
M60.10   Interstitial myositis of **unspecified site** ▽

✓6th   **M60.11 Interstitial myositis, shoulder**
M60.111   Interstitial myositis, **right** shoulder
M60.112   Interstitial myositis, **left** shoulder
M60.119   Interstitial myositis, **unspecified** shoulder ▽

✓6th   **M60.12 Interstitial myositis, upper arm**
M60.121   Interstitial myositis, **right** upper arm
M60.122   Interstitial myositis, **left** upper arm
M60.129   Interstitial myositis, **unspecified** upper arm ▽

✓6th   **M60.13 Interstitial myositis, forearm**
M60.131   Interstitial myositis, **right** forearm
M60.132   Interstitial myositis, **left** forearm
M60.139   Interstitial myositis, **unspecified** forearm ▽

✓6th   **M60.14 Interstitial myositis, hand**
M60.141   Interstitial myositis, **right** hand
M60.142   Interstitial myositis, **left** hand
M60.149   Interstitial myositis, **unspecified** hand ▽

✓6th   **M60.15 Interstitial myositis, thigh**
M60.151   Interstitial myositis, **right** thigh
M60.152   Interstitial myositis, **left** thigh
M60.159   Interstitial myositis, **unspecified** thigh ▽

✓6th   **M60.16 Interstitial myositis, lower leg**
M60.161   Interstitial myositis, **right** lower leg
M60.162   Interstitial myositis, **left** lower leg
M60.169   Interstitial myositis, **unspecified** lower leg ▽

✓6th   **M60.17 Interstitial myositis, ankle and foot**
M60.171   Interstitial myositis, **right** ankle and foot
M60.172   Interstitial myositis, **left** ankle and foot
M60.179   Interstitial myositis, **unspecified** ankle and foot ▽

M60.18   Interstitial myositis, **other site**
M60.19   Interstitial myositis, **multiple sites**

✓5ᵗʰ **M60.2 Foreign body granuloma of soft tissue, not elsewhere classified**

Use additional code to identify the type of retained foreign body (Z18.-)

EXCLUDES 1 *foreign body granuloma of skin and subcutaneous tissue (L92.3)*

M60.20 Foreign body granuloma of soft tissue, not elsewhere classified, unspecified site ▽

✓6ᵗʰ **M60.21** Foreign body granuloma of soft tissue, not elsewhere classified, shoulder

M60.211 Foreign body granuloma of soft tissue, not elsewhere classified, right shoulder

M60.212 Foreign body granuloma of soft tissue, not elsewhere classified, left shoulder

M60.219 Foreign body granuloma of soft tissue, not elsewhere classified, unspecified shoulder ▽

✓6ᵗʰ **M60.22** Foreign body granuloma of soft tissue, not elsewhere classified, upper arm

M60.221 Foreign body granuloma of soft tissue, not elsewhere classified, right upper arm

M60.222 Foreign body granuloma of soft tissue, not elsewhere classified, left upper arm

M60.229 Foreign body granuloma of soft tissue, not elsewhere classified, unspecified upper arm ▽

✓6ᵗʰ **M60.23** Foreign body granuloma of soft tissue, not elsewhere classified, forearm

M60.231 Foreign body granuloma of soft tissue, not elsewhere classified, right forearm

M60.232 Foreign body granuloma of soft tissue, not elsewhere classified, left forearm

M60.239 Foreign body granuloma of soft tissue, not elsewhere classified, unspecified forearm ▽

✓6ᵗʰ **M60.24** Foreign body granuloma of soft tissue, not elsewhere classified, hand

M60.241 Foreign body granuloma of soft tissue, not elsewhere classified, right hand

M60.242 Foreign body granuloma of soft tissue, not elsewhere classified, left hand

M60.249 Foreign body granuloma of soft tissue, not elsewhere classified, unspecified hand ▽

✓6ᵗʰ **M60.25** Foreign body granuloma of soft tissue, not elsewhere classified, thigh

M60.251 Foreign body granuloma of soft tissue, not elsewhere classified, right thigh

M60.252 Foreign body granuloma of soft tissue, not elsewhere classified, left thigh

M60.259 Foreign body granuloma of soft tissue, not elsewhere classified, unspecified thigh ▽

✓6ᵗʰ **M60.26** Foreign body granuloma of soft tissue, not elsewhere classified, lower leg

M60.261 Foreign body granuloma of soft tissue, not elsewhere classified, right lower leg

M60.262 Foreign body granuloma of soft tissue, not elsewhere classified, left lower leg

M60.269 Foreign body granuloma of soft tissue, not elsewhere classified, unspecified lower leg ▽

✓6ᵗʰ **M60.27** Foreign body granuloma of soft tissue, not elsewhere classified, ankle and foot

M60.271 Foreign body granuloma of soft tissue, not elsewhere classified, right ankle and foot

M60.272 Foreign body granuloma of soft tissue, not elsewhere classified, left ankle and foot

M60.279 Foreign body granuloma of soft tissue, not elsewhere classified, unspecified ankle and foot ▽

M60.28 Foreign body granuloma of soft tissue, not elsewhere classified, other site

✓5ᵗʰ **M60.8 Other myositis**

M60.80 Other myositis, unspecified site ▽

✓6ᵗʰ **M60.81** Other myositis shoulder

M60.811 Other myositis, right shoulder

M60.812 Other myositis, left shoulder

M60.819 Other myositis, unspecified shoulder ▽

✓6ᵗʰ **M60.82** Other myositis, upper arm

M60.821 Other myositis, right upper arm

M60.822 Other myositis, left upper arm

M60.829 Other myositis, unspecified upper arm ▽

✓6ᵗʰ **M60.83** Other myositis, forearm

M60.831 Other myositis, right forearm

M60.832 Other myositis, left forearm

M60.839 Other myositis, unspecified forearm ▽

✓6ᵗʰ **M60.84** Other myositis, hand

M60.841 Other myositis, right hand

M60.842 Other myositis, left hand

M60.849 Other myositis, unspecified hand ▽

✓6ᵗʰ **M60.85** Other myositis, thigh

M60.851 Other myositis, right thigh

M60.852 Other myositis, left thigh

M60.859 Other myositis, unspecified thigh ▽

✓6ᵗʰ **M60.86** Other myositis, lower leg

M60.861 Other myositis, right lower leg

M60.862 Other myositis, left lower leg

M60.869 Other myositis, unspecified lower leg ▽

✓6ᵗʰ **M60.87** Other myositis, ankle and foot

M60.871 Other myositis, right ankle and foot

M60.872 Other myositis, left ankle and foot

M60.879 Other myositis, unspecified ankle and foot ▽

M60.88 Other myositis, other site

M60.89 Other myositis, multiple sites

M60.9 Myositis, unspecified ▽

✓4ᵗʰ **M61 Calcification and ossification of muscle**

✓5ᵗʰ **M61.0 Myositis ossificans traumatica**

M61.00 Myositis ossificans traumatica, unspecified site ▽

✓6ᵗʰ **M61.01** Myositis ossificans traumatica, shoulder

M61.011 Myositis ossificans traumatica, right shoulder

M61.012 Myositis ossificans traumatica, left shoulder

M61.019 Myositis ossificans traumatica, unspecified shoulder ▽

✓6ᵗʰ **M61.02** Myositis ossificans traumatica, upper arm

M61.021 Myositis ossificans traumatica, right upper arm

M61.022 Myositis ossificans traumatica, left upper arm

M61.029 Myositis ossificans traumatica, unspecified upper arm ▽

✓6ᵗʰ **M61.03** Myositis ossificans traumatica, forearm

M61.031 Myositis ossificans traumatica, right forearm

M61.032 Myositis ossificans traumatica, left forearm

M61.039 Myositis ossificans traumatica, unspecified forearm ▽

✓6ᵗʰ **M61.04** Myositis ossificans traumatica, hand

M61.041 Myositis ossificans traumatica, right hand

M61.042 Myositis ossificans traumatica, left hand

M61.049 Myositis ossificans traumatica, unspecified hand ▽

✓6ᵗʰ **M61.05** Myositis ossificans traumatica, thigh

M61.051 Myositis ossificans traumatica, right thigh

M61.052 Myositis ossificans traumatica, left thigh

M61.059 Myositis ossificans traumatica, unspecified thigh ▽

✓6ᵗʰ **M61.06** Myositis ossificans traumatica, lower leg

M61.061 Myositis ossificans traumatica, right lower leg

M61.062 Myositis ossificans traumatica, left lower leg

M61.069 Myositis ossificans traumatica, unspecified lower leg ▽

✓6ᵗʰ **M61.07** Myositis ossificans traumatica, ankle and foot

M61.071 Myositis ossificans traumatica, right ankle and foot

✓ Additional Character Req   ✓ₓ7ᵗʰ Placeholder Alert   Manifestation   HCC CMS-HCC Condition   ▽ Unspecified Code   ▶◀ Revised Text   ● New Code   ▲ Revised Code Title

ICD-10-CM 2018   761

M61.072 Myositis ossificans traumatica, left ankle and foot

M61.079 Myositis ossificans traumatica, unspecified ankle and foot ▽

M61.08 Myositis ossificans traumatica, other site

M61.09 Myositis ossificans traumatica, multiple sites

✓5ᵗʰ **M61.1** Myositis ossificans progressiva
Fibrodysplasia ossificans progressiva

M61.10 Myositis ossificans progressiva, unspecified site ▽

✓6ᵗʰ **M61.11** Myositis ossificans progressiva, shoulder

M61.111 Myositis ossificans progressiva, right shoulder

M61.112 Myositis ossificans progressiva, left shoulder

M61.119 Myositis ossificans progressiva, unspecified shoulder ▽

✓6ᵗʰ **M61.12** Myositis ossificans progressiva, upper arm

M61.121 Myositis ossificans progressiva, right upper arm

M61.122 Myositis ossificans progressiva, left upper arm

M61.129 Myositis ossificans progressiva, unspecified arm ▽

✓6ᵗʰ **M61.13** Myositis ossificans progressiva, forearm

M61.131 Myositis ossificans progressiva, right forearm

M61.132 Myositis ossificans progressiva, left forearm

M61.139 Myositis ossificans progressiva, unspecified forearm ▽

✓6ᵗʰ **M61.14** Myositis ossificans progressiva, hand and finger(s)

M61.141 Myositis ossificans progressiva, right hand

M61.142 Myositis ossificans progressiva, left hand

M61.143 Myositis ossificans progressiva, unspecified hand ▽

M61.144 Myositis ossificans progressiva, right finger(s)

M61.145 Myositis ossificans progressiva, left finger(s)

M61.146 Myositis ossificans progressiva, unspecified finger(s) ▽

✓6ᵗʰ **M61.15** Myositis ossificans progressiva, thigh

M61.151 Myositis ossificans progressiva, right thigh

M61.152 Myositis ossificans progressiva, left thigh

M61.159 Myositis ossificans progressiva, unspecified thigh ▽

✓6ᵗʰ **M61.16** Myositis ossificans progressiva, lower leg

M61.161 Myositis ossificans progressiva, right lower leg

M61.162 Myositis ossificans progressiva, left lower leg

M61.169 Myositis ossificans progressiva, unspecified lower leg ▽

✓6ᵗʰ **M61.17** Myositis ossificans progressiva, ankle, foot and toe(s)

M61.171 Myositis ossificans progressiva, right ankle

M61.172 Myositis ossificans progressiva, left ankle

M61.173 Myositis ossificans progressiva, unspecified ankle ▽

M61.174 Myositis ossificans progressiva, right foot

M61.175 Myositis ossificans progressiva, left foot

M61.176 Myositis ossificans progressiva, unspecified foot ▽

M61.177 Myositis ossificans progressiva, right toe(s)

M61.178 Myositis ossificans progressiva, left toe(s)

M61.179 Myositis ossificans progressiva, unspecified toe(s) ▽

M61.18 Myositis ossificans progressiva, other site

M61.19 Myositis ossificans progressiva, multiple sites

✓5ᵗʰ **M61.2** Paralytic calcification and ossification of muscle
Myositis ossificans associated with quadriplegia or paraplegia

M61.20 Paralytic calcification and ossification of muscle, unspecified site ▽

✓6ᵗʰ **M61.21** Paralytic calcification and ossification of muscle, shoulder

M61.211 Paralytic calcification and ossification of muscle, right shoulder

M61.212 Paralytic calcification and ossification of muscle, left shoulder

M61.219 Paralytic calcification and ossification of muscle, unspecified shoulder ▽

✓6ᵗʰ **M61.22** Paralytic calcification and ossification of muscle, upper arm

M61.221 Paralytic calcification and ossification of muscle, right upper arm

M61.222 Paralytic calcification and ossification of muscle, left upper arm

M61.229 Paralytic calcification and ossification of muscle, unspecified upper arm ▽

✓6ᵗʰ **M61.23** Paralytic calcification and ossification of muscle, forearm

M61.231 Paralytic calcification and ossification of muscle, right forearm

M61.232 Paralytic calcification and ossification of muscle, left forearm

M61.239 Paralytic calcification and ossification of muscle, unspecified forearm ▽

✓6ᵗʰ **M61.24** Paralytic calcification and ossification of muscle, hand

M61.241 Paralytic calcification and ossification of muscle, right hand

M61.242 Paralytic calcification and ossification of muscle, left hand

M61.249 Paralytic calcification and ossification of muscle, unspecified hand ▽

✓6ᵗʰ **M61.25** Paralytic calcification and ossification of muscle, thigh

M61.251 Paralytic calcification and ossification of muscle, right thigh

M61.252 Paralytic calcification and ossification of muscle, left thigh

M61.259 Paralytic calcification and ossification of muscle, unspecified thigh ▽

✓6ᵗʰ **M61.26** Paralytic calcification and ossification of muscle, lower leg

M61.261 Paralytic calcification and ossification of muscle, right lower leg

M61.262 Paralytic calcification and ossification of muscle, left lower leg

M61.269 Paralytic calcification and ossification of muscle, unspecified lower leg ▽

✓6ᵗʰ **M61.27** Paralytic calcification and ossification of muscle, ankle and foot

M61.271 Paralytic calcification and ossification of muscle, right ankle and foot

M61.272 Paralytic calcification and ossification of muscle, left ankle and foot

M61.279 Paralytic calcification and ossification of muscle, unspecified ankle and foot ▽

M61.28 Paralytic calcification and ossification of muscle, other site

M61.29 Paralytic calcification and ossification of muscle, multiple sites

✓5ᵗʰ **M61.3** Calcification and ossification of muscles associated with burns
Myositis ossificans associated with burns

M61.30 Calcification and ossification of muscles associated with burns, unspecified site ▽

✓6ᵗʰ **M61.31** Calcification and ossification of muscles associated with burns, shoulder

M61.311 Calcification and ossification of muscles associated with burns, right shoulder

M61.312 Calcification and ossification of muscles associated with burns, left shoulder

M61.319 Calcification and ossification of muscles associated with burns, unspecified shoulder ▽

✓6ᵗʰ **M61.32** Calcification and ossification of muscles associated with burns, upper arm

M61.321 Calcification and ossification of muscles associated with burns, right upper arm

EXCLUDES 1 Not coded here   EXCLUDES 2 Not included here   Ⓝ Newborn Age: 0   Ⓟ Pediatric Age: 0-17   Ⓜ Maternity Age: 12-55   Ⓐ Adult Age: 15-124

762   ICD-10-CM 2018

M61.322   Calcification and ossification of muscles associated with burns, **left upper arm**

M61.329   Calcification and ossification of muscles associated with burns, unspecified upper arm   ▽

✓6ᵗʰ **M61.33**   Calcification and ossification of muscles associated with burns, **forearm**

    M61.331   Calcification and ossification of muscles associated with burns, **right forearm**

    M61.332   Calcification and ossification of muscles associated with burns, **left forearm**

    M61.339   Calcification and ossification of muscles associated with burns, unspecified forearm   ▽

✓6ᵗʰ **M61.34**   Calcification and ossification of muscles associated with burns, **hand**

    M61.341   Calcification and ossification of muscles associated with burns, **right hand**

    M61.342   Calcification and ossification of muscles associated with burns, **left hand**

    M61.349   Calcification and ossification of muscles associated with burns, unspecified hand   ▽

✓6ᵗʰ **M61.35**   Calcification and ossification of muscles associated with burns, **thigh**

    M61.351   Calcification and ossification of muscles associated with burns, **right thigh**

    M61.352   Calcification and ossification of muscles associated with burns, **left thigh**

    M61.359   Calcification and ossification of muscles associated with burns, unspecified thigh   ▽

✓6ᵗʰ **M61.36**   Calcification and ossification of muscles associated with burns, **lower leg**

    M61.361   Calcification and ossification of muscles associated with burns, **right lower leg**

    M61.362   Calcification and ossification of muscles associated with burns, **left lower leg**

    M61.369   Calcification and ossification of muscles associated with burns, unspecified lower leg   ▽

✓6ᵗʰ **M61.37**   Calcification and ossification of muscles associated with burns, **ankle and foot**

    M61.371   Calcification and ossification of muscles associated with burns, **right ankle and foot**

    M61.372   Calcification and ossification of muscles associated with burns, **left ankle and foot**

    M61.379   Calcification and ossification of muscles associated with burns, unspecified ankle and foot   ▽

M61.38   Calcification and ossification of muscles associated with burns, **other site**

M61.39   Calcification and ossification of muscles associated with burns, **multiple sites**

✓5ᵗʰ **M61.4**   Other **calcification** of muscle

    EXCLUDES 1   calcific tendinitis NOS (M65.2-)
               calcific tendinitis of shoulder (M75.3)

    M61.40   Other calcification of muscle, unspecified site   ▽

✓6ᵗʰ **M61.41**   Other calcification of muscle, **shoulder**

    M61.411   Other calcification of muscle, **right shoulder**

    M61.412   Other calcification of muscle, **left shoulder**

    M61.419   Other calcification of muscle, unspecified shoulder   ▽

✓6ᵗʰ **M61.42**   Other calcification of muscle, **upper arm**

    M61.421   Other calcification of muscle, **right upper arm**

    M61.422   Other calcification of muscle, **left upper arm**

    M61.429   Other calcification of muscle, unspecified upper arm   ▽

✓6ᵗʰ **M61.43**   Other calcification of muscle, **forearm**

    M61.431   Other calcification of muscle, **right forearm**

    M61.432   Other calcification of muscle, **left forearm**

    M61.439   Other calcification of muscle, unspecified forearm   ▽

✓6ᵗʰ **M61.44**   Other calcification of muscle, **hand**

    M61.441   Other calcification of muscle, **right hand**

    M61.442   Other calcification of muscle, **left hand**

    M61.449   Other calcification of muscle, unspecified hand   ▽

✓6ᵗʰ **M61.45**   Other calcification of muscle, **thigh**

    M61.451   Other calcification of muscle, **right thigh**

    M61.452   Other calcification of muscle, **left thigh**

    M61.459   Other calcification of muscle, unspecified thigh   ▽

✓6ᵗʰ **M61.46**   Other calcification of muscle, **lower leg**

    M61.461   Other calcification of muscle, **right lower leg**

    M61.462   Other calcification of muscle, **left lower leg**

    M61.469   Other calcification of muscle, unspecified lower leg   ▽

✓6ᵗʰ **M61.47**   Other calcification of muscle, **ankle and foot**

    M61.471   Other calcification of muscle, **right ankle and foot**

    M61.472   Other calcification of muscle, **left ankle and foot**

    M61.479   Other calcification of muscle, unspecified ankle and foot   ▽

M61.48   Other calcification of muscle, **other site**

M61.49   Other calcification of muscle, **multiple sites**

✓5ᵗʰ **M61.5**   Other **ossification** of muscle

    M61.50   Other ossification of muscle, unspecified site   ▽

✓6ᵗʰ **M61.51**   Other ossification of muscle, **shoulder**

    M61.511   Other ossification of muscle, **right shoulder**

    M61.512   Other ossification of muscle, **left shoulder**

    M61.519   Other ossification of muscle, unspecified shoulder   ▽

✓6ᵗʰ **M61.52**   Other ossification of muscle, **upper arm**

    M61.521   Other ossification of muscle, **right upper arm**

    M61.522   Other ossification of muscle, **left upper arm**

    M61.529   Other ossification of muscle, unspecified upper arm   ▽

✓6ᵗʰ **M61.53**   Other ossification of muscle, **forearm**

    M61.531   Other ossification of muscle, **right forearm**

    M61.532   Other ossification of muscle, **left forearm**

    M61.539   Other ossification of muscle, unspecified forearm   ▽

✓6ᵗʰ **M61.54**   Other ossification of muscle, **hand**

    M61.541   Other ossification of muscle, **right hand**

    M61.542   Other ossification of muscle, **left hand**

    M61.549   Other ossification of muscle, unspecified hand   ▽

✓6ᵗʰ **M61.55**   Other ossification of muscle, **thigh**

    M61.551   Other ossification of muscle, **right thigh**

    M61.552   Other ossification of muscle, **left thigh**

    M61.559   Other ossification of muscle, unspecified thigh   ▽

✓6ᵗʰ **M61.56**   Other ossification of muscle, **lower leg**

    M61.561   Other ossification of muscle, **right lower leg**

    M61.562   Other ossification of muscle, **left lower leg**

    M61.569   Other ossification of muscle, unspecified lower leg   ▽

✓6ᵗʰ **M61.57**   Other ossification of muscle, **ankle and foot**

    M61.571   Other ossification of muscle, **right ankle and foot**

    M61.572   Other ossification of muscle, **left ankle and foot**

    M61.579   Other ossification of muscle, unspecified ankle and foot   ▽

M61.58   Other ossification of muscle, **other site**

M61.59   Other ossification of muscle, **multiple sites**

M61.9   Calcification and ossification of muscle, unspecified   ▽

✓ Additional Character Req   ✓7ᵗʰ Placeholder Alert   Manifestation   HCC CMS-HCC Condition   ▽ Unspecified Code   ►◄ Revised Text   ● New Code   ▲ Revised Code Title

ICD-10-CM 2018   **763**

√4th **M62 Other disorders of muscle**
  EXCLUDES1   *alcoholic myopathy (G72.1)*
    cramp and spasm (R25.2)
    drug-induced myopathy (G72.0)
    myalgia (M79.1)
    stiff-man syndrome (G25.82)
  EXCLUDES2   *nontraumatic hematoma of muscle (M79.81)*

√5th **M62.0 Separation of muscle (nontraumatic)**
  Diastasis of muscle
  EXCLUDES1   *diastasis recti complicating pregnancy, labor and delivery (O71.8)*
    traumatic separation of muscle—see strain of muscle by body region

M62.00 Separation of muscle (nontraumatic), unspecified site ▽

√6th **M62.01** Separation of muscle (nontraumatic), shoulder
  M62.011 Separation of muscle (nontraumatic), right shoulder
  M62.012 Separation of muscle (nontraumatic), left shoulder
  M62.019 Separation of muscle (nontraumatic), unspecified shoulder ▽

√6th **M62.02** Separation of muscle (nontraumatic), upper arm
  M62.021 Separation of muscle (nontraumatic), right upper arm
  M62.022 Separation of muscle (nontraumatic), left upper arm
  M62.029 Separation of muscle (nontraumatic), unspecified upper arm ▽

√6th **M62.03** Separation of muscle (nontraumatic), forearm
  M62.031 Separation of muscle (nontraumatic), right forearm
  M62.032 Separation of muscle (nontraumatic), left forearm
  M62.039 Separation of muscle (nontraumatic), unspecified forearm ▽

√6th **M62.04** Separation of muscle (nontraumatic), hand
  M62.041 Separation of muscle (nontraumatic), right hand
  M62.042 Separation of muscle (nontraumatic), left hand
  M62.049 Separation of muscle (nontraumatic), unspecified hand ▽

√6th **M62.05** Separation of muscle (nontraumatic), thigh
  M62.051 Separation of muscle (nontraumatic), right thigh
  M62.052 Separation of muscle (nontraumatic), left thigh
  M62.059 Separation of muscle (nontraumatic), unspecified thigh ▽

√6th **M62.06** Separation of muscle (nontraumatic), lower leg
  M62.061 Separation of muscle (nontraumatic), right lower leg
  M62.062 Separation of muscle (nontraumatic), left lower leg
  M62.069 Separation of muscle (nontraumatic), unspecified lower leg ▽

√6th **M62.07** Separation of muscle (nontraumatic), ankle and foot
  M62.071 Separation of muscle (nontraumatic), right ankle and foot
  M62.072 Separation of muscle (nontraumatic), left ankle and foot
  M62.079 Separation of muscle (nontraumatic), unspecified ankle and foot ▽

M62.08 Separation of muscle (nontraumatic), other site

√5th **M62.1 Other rupture of muscle (nontraumatic)**
  EXCLUDES1   *traumatic rupture of muscle—see strain of muscle by body region*
  EXCLUDES2   *rupture of tendon (M66.-)*

M62.10 Other rupture of muscle (nontraumatic), unspecified site ▽

√6th **M62.11** Other rupture of muscle (nontraumatic), shoulder
  M62.111 Other rupture of muscle (nontraumatic), right shoulder
  M62.112 Other rupture of muscle (nontraumatic), left shoulder

M62.119 Other rupture of muscle (nontraumatic), unspecified shoulder ▽

√6th **M62.12** Other rupture of muscle (nontraumatic), upper arm
  M62.121 Other rupture of muscle (nontraumatic), right upper arm
  M62.122 Other rupture of muscle (nontraumatic), left upper arm
  M62.129 Other rupture of muscle (nontraumatic), unspecified upper arm ▽

√6th **M62.13** Other rupture of muscle (nontraumatic), forearm
  M62.131 Other rupture of muscle (nontraumatic), right forearm
  M62.132 Other rupture of muscle (nontraumatic), left forearm
  M62.139 Other rupture of muscle (nontraumatic), unspecified forearm ▽

√6th **M62.14** Other rupture of muscle (nontraumatic), hand
  M62.141 Other rupture of muscle (nontraumatic), right hand
  M62.142 Other rupture of muscle (nontraumatic), left hand
  M62.149 Other rupture of muscle (nontraumatic), unspecified hand ▽

√6th **M62.15** Other rupture of muscle (nontraumatic), thigh
  M62.151 Other rupture of muscle (nontraumatic), right thigh
  M62.152 Other rupture of muscle (nontraumatic), left thigh
  M62.159 Other rupture of muscle (nontraumatic), unspecified thigh ▽

√6th **M62.16** Other rupture of muscle (nontraumatic), lower leg
  M62.161 Other rupture of muscle (nontraumatic), right lower leg
  M62.162 Other rupture of muscle (nontraumatic), left lower leg
  M62.169 Other rupture of muscle (nontraumatic), unspecified lower leg ▽

√6th **M62.17** Other rupture of muscle (nontraumatic), ankle and foot
  M62.171 Other rupture of muscle (nontraumatic), right ankle and foot
  M62.172 Other rupture of muscle (nontraumatic), left ankle and foot
  M62.179 Other rupture of muscle (nontraumatic), unspecified ankle and foot ▽

M62.18 Other rupture of muscle (nontraumatic), other site

√5th **M62.2 Nontraumatic ischemic infarction of muscle**
  EXCLUDES1   *compartment syndrome (traumatic) (T79.A-)*
    nontraumatic compartment syndrome (M79.A-)
    rhabdomyolysis (M62.82)
    traumatic ischemia of muscle (T79.6)
    Volkmann's ischemic contracture (T79.6)

M62.20 Nontraumatic ischemic infarction of muscle, unspecified site ▽

√6th **M62.21** Nontraumatic ischemic infarction of muscle, shoulder
  M62.211 Nontraumatic ischemic infarction of muscle, right shoulder
  M62.212 Nontraumatic ischemic infarction of muscle, left shoulder
  M62.219 Nontraumatic ischemic infarction of muscle, unspecified shoulder ▽

√6th **M62.22** Nontraumatic ischemic infarction of muscle, upper arm
  M62.221 Nontraumatic ischemic infarction of muscle, right upper arm
  M62.222 Nontraumatic ischemic infarction of muscle, left upper arm
  M62.229 Nontraumatic ischemic infarction of muscle, unspecified upper arm ▽

√6th **M62.23** Nontraumatic ischemic infarction of muscle, forearm
  M62.231 Nontraumatic ischemic infarction of muscle, right forearm
  M62.232 Nontraumatic ischemic infarction of muscle, left forearm
  M62.239 Nontraumatic ischemic infarction of muscle, unspecified forearm ▽

EXCLUDES1 Not coded here   EXCLUDES2 Not included here   N Newborn Age: 0   P Pediatric Age: 0-17   M Maternity Age: 12-55   A Adult Age: 15-124

764   ICD-10-CM 2018

✓6ᵗʰ **M62.24** **Nontraumatic ischemic infarction of muscle, hand**

     M62.241 **Nontraumatic ischemic infarction of muscle, right hand**

     M62.242 **Nontraumatic ischemic infarction of muscle, left hand**

     M62.249 **Nontraumatic ischemic infarction of muscle, unspecified hand** ▽

✓6ᵗʰ **M62.25** **Nontraumatic ischemic infarction of muscle, thigh**

     M62.251 **Nontraumatic ischemic infarction of muscle, right thigh**

     M62.252 **Nontraumatic ischemic infarction of muscle, left thigh**

     M62.259 **Nontraumatic ischemic infarction of muscle, unspecified thigh** ▽

✓6ᵗʰ **M62.26** **Nontraumatic ischemic infarction of muscle, lower leg**

     M62.261 **Nontraumatic ischemic infarction of muscle, right lower leg**

     M62.262 **Nontraumatic ischemic infarction of muscle, left lower leg**

     M62.269 **Nontraumatic ischemic infarction of muscle, unspecified lower leg** ▽

✓6ᵗʰ **M62.27** **Nontraumatic ischemic infarction of muscle, ankle and foot**

     M62.271 **Nontraumatic ischemic infarction of muscle, right ankle and foot**

     M62.272 **Nontraumatic ischemic infarction of muscle, left ankle and foot**

     M62.279 **Nontraumatic ischemic infarction of muscle, unspecified ankle and foot** ▽

     M62.28 **Nontraumatic ischemic infarction of muscle, other site**

     M62.3 **Immobility syndrome (paraplegic)**

✓5ᵗʰ **M62.4** **Contracture of muscle**

     Contracture of tendon (sheath)

     EXCLUDES 1   contracture of joint (M24.5-)

     M62.40 **Contracture of muscle, unspecified site** ▽

✓6ᵗʰ **M62.41** **Contracture of muscle, shoulder**

     M62.411 **Contracture of muscle, right shoulder**

     M62.412 **Contracture of muscle, left shoulder**

     M62.419 **Contracture of muscle, unspecified shoulder** ▽

✓6ᵗʰ **M62.42** **Contracture of muscle, upper arm**

     M62.421 **Contracture of muscle, right upper arm**

     M62.422 **Contracture of muscle, left upper arm**

     M62.429 **Contracture of muscle, unspecified upper arm** ▽

✓6ᵗʰ **M62.43** **Contracture of muscle, forearm**

     M62.431 **Contracture of muscle, right forearm**

     M62.432 **Contracture of muscle, left forearm**

     M62.439 **Contracture of muscle, unspecified forearm** ▽

✓6ᵗʰ **M62.44** **Contracture of muscle, hand**

     M62.441 **Contracture of muscle, right hand**

     M62.442 **Contracture of muscle, left hand**

     M62.449 **Contracture of muscle, unspecified hand** ▽

✓6ᵗʰ **M62.45** **Contracture of muscle, thigh**

     M62.451 **Contracture of muscle, right thigh**

     M62.452 **Contracture of muscle, left thigh**

     M62.459 **Contracture of muscle, unspecified thigh** ▽

✓6ᵗʰ **M62.46** **Contracture of muscle, lower leg**

     M62.461 **Contracture of muscle, right lower leg**

     M62.462 **Contracture of muscle, left lower leg**

     M62.469 **Contracture of muscle, unspecified lower leg** ▽

✓6ᵗʰ **M62.47** **Contracture of muscle, ankle and foot**

     M62.471 **Contracture of muscle, right ankle and foot**

     M62.472 **Contracture of muscle, left ankle and foot**

     M62.479 **Contracture of muscle, unspecified ankle and foot** ▽

     M62.48 **Contracture of muscle, other site**

     M62.49 **Contracture of muscle, multiple sites**

✓5ᵗʰ **M62.5** **Muscle wasting and atrophy, not elsewhere classified**

     Disuse atrophy NEC

     EXCLUDES 1   neuralgic amyotrophy (G54.5)

         progressive muscular atrophy ▶(G12.21)◀

         sarcopenia (M62.84)

     EXCLUDES 2   pelvic muscle wasting (N81.84)

     M62.50 **Muscle wasting and atrophy, not elsewhere classified, unspecified site** ▽

✓6ᵗʰ **M62.51** **Muscle wasting and atrophy, not elsewhere classified, shoulder**

     M62.511 **Muscle wasting and atrophy, not elsewhere classified, right shoulder**

     M62.512 **Muscle wasting and atrophy, not elsewhere classified, left shoulder**

     M62.519 **Muscle wasting and atrophy, not elsewhere classified, unspecified shoulder** ▽

✓6ᵗʰ **M62.52** **Muscle wasting and atrophy, not elsewhere classified, upper arm**

     M62.521 **Muscle wasting and atrophy, not elsewhere classified, right upper arm**

     M62.522 **Muscle wasting and atrophy, not elsewhere classified, left upper arm**

     M62.529 **Muscle wasting and atrophy, not elsewhere classified, unspecified upper arm** ▽

✓6ᵗʰ **M62.53** **Muscle wasting and atrophy, not elsewhere classified, forearm**

     M62.531 **Muscle wasting and atrophy, not elsewhere classified, right forearm**

     M62.532 **Muscle wasting and atrophy, not elsewhere classified, left forearm**

     M62.539 **Muscle wasting and atrophy, not elsewhere classified, unspecified forearm** ▽

✓6ᵗʰ **M62.54** **Muscle wasting and atrophy, not elsewhere classified, hand**

     M62.541 **Muscle wasting and atrophy, not elsewhere classified, right hand**

     M62.542 **Muscle wasting and atrophy, not elsewhere classified, left hand**

     M62.549 **Muscle wasting and atrophy, not elsewhere classified, unspecified hand** ▽

✓6ᵗʰ **M62.55** **Muscle wasting and atrophy, not elsewhere classified, thigh**

     M62.551 **Muscle wasting and atrophy, not elsewhere classified, right thigh**

     M62.552 **Muscle wasting and atrophy, not elsewhere classified, left thigh**

     M62.559 **Muscle wasting and atrophy, not elsewhere classified, unspecified thigh** ▽

✓6ᵗʰ **M62.56** **Muscle wasting and atrophy, not elsewhere classified, lower leg**

     M62.561 **Muscle wasting and atrophy, not elsewhere classified, right lower leg**

     M62.562 **Muscle wasting and atrophy, not elsewhere classified, left lower leg**

     M62.569 **Muscle wasting and atrophy, not elsewhere classified, unspecified lower leg** ▽

✓6ᵗʰ **M62.57** **Muscle wasting and atrophy, not elsewhere classified, ankle and foot**

     M62.571 **Muscle wasting and atrophy, not elsewhere classified, right ankle and foot**

     M62.572 **Muscle wasting and atrophy, not elsewhere classified, left ankle and foot**

     M62.579 **Muscle wasting and atrophy, not elsewhere classified, unspecified ankle and foot** ▽

     M62.58 **Muscle wasting and atrophy, not elsewhere classified, other site**

     M62.59 **Muscle wasting and atrophy, not elsewhere classified, multiple sites**

✓5ᵗʰ **M62.8** **Other specified disorders of muscle**

     EXCLUDES 2   nontraumatic hematoma of muscle (M79.81)

     M62.81 **Muscle weakness (generalized)**

         EXCLUDES 1   muscle weakness in sarcopenia (M62.84)

✓ Additional Character Req   ✓x7ᵗʰ Placeholder Alert   Manifestation   HCC CMS-HCC Condition   ▽ Unspecified Code   ▶◀ Revised Text   ● New Code   ▲ Revised Code Title

M62.82 Rhabdomyolysis
> **EXCLUDES 1**   *traumatic rhabdomyolysis (T79.6)*
> **DEF:** Rapid disintegration or destruction of skeletal muscle caused by direct or indirect injury; resulting in the excretion of muscle protein myoglobin into the urine.

✓6ᵗʰ **M62.83 Muscle spasm**
> **M62.830 Muscle spasm of back**
> **M62.831 Muscle spasm of calf**
> > Charley-horse
> **M62.838 Other muscle spasm**

M62.84 Sarcopenia
> Age-related sarcopenia
> Code first underlying disease, if applicable, such as:
> > disorders of myoneural junction and muscle disease in diseases classified elsewhere (G73.-)
> > other and unspecified myopathies (G72.-)
> > primary disorders of muscles (G71.-)

M62.89 Other specified disorders of muscle
> Muscle (sheath) hernia

M62.9 Disorder of muscle, unspecified   ▽

✓4ᵗʰ **M63 Disorders of muscle in diseases classified elsewhere**
> Code first underlying disease, such as:
> > leprosy (A30.-)
> > neoplasm (C49-, C79.89, D21-, D48.1)
> > schistosomiasis (B65.-)
> > trichinellosis (B75)
>
> **EXCLUDES 1**   *myopathy in cysticercosis (B69.81)*
> > *myopathy in endocrine diseases (G73.7)*
> > *myopathy in metabolic diseases (G73.7)*
> > *myopathy in sarcoidosis (D86.87)*
> > *myopathy in secondary syphilis (A51.49)*
> > *myopathy in syphilis (late) (A52.78)*
> > *myopathy in toxoplasmosis (B58.82)*
> > *myopathy in tuberculosis (A18.09)*

✓5ᵗʰ **M63.8 Disorders of muscle in diseases classified elsewhere**
> *M63.80*   *Disorders of muscle in diseases classified elsewhere, unspecified site*   ▽

✓6ᵗʰ **M63.81 Disorders of muscle in diseases classified elsewhere, shoulder**
> *M63.811*   *Disorders of muscle in diseases classified elsewhere, right shoulder*
> *M63.812*   *Disorders of muscle in diseases classified elsewhere, left shoulder*
> *M63.819*   *Disorders of muscle in diseases classified elsewhere, unspecified shoulder*   ▽

✓6ᵗʰ **M63.82 Disorders of muscle in diseases classified elsewhere, upper arm**
> *M63.821*   *Disorders of muscle in diseases classified elsewhere, right upper arm*
> *M63.822*   *Disorders of muscle in diseases classified elsewhere, left upper arm*
> *M63.829*   *Disorders of muscle in diseases classified elsewhere, unspecified upper arm*   ▽

✓6ᵗʰ **M63.83 Disorders of muscle in diseases classified elsewhere, forearm**
> *M63.831*   *Disorders of muscle in diseases classified elsewhere, right forearm*
> *M63.832*   *Disorders of muscle in diseases classified elsewhere, left forearm*
> *M63.839*   *Disorders of muscle in diseases classified elsewhere, unspecified forearm*   ▽

✓6ᵗʰ **M63.84 Disorders of muscle in diseases classified elsewhere, hand**
> *M63.841*   *Disorders of muscle in diseases classified elsewhere, right hand*
> *M63.842*   *Disorders of muscle in diseases classified elsewhere, left hand*
> *M63.849*   *Disorders of muscle in diseases classified elsewhere, unspecified hand*   ▽

✓6ᵗʰ **M63.85 Disorders of muscle in diseases classified elsewhere, thigh**
> *M63.851*   *Disorders of muscle in diseases classified elsewhere, right thigh*
> *M63.852*   *Disorders of muscle in diseases classified elsewhere, left thigh*
> *M63.859*   *Disorders of muscle in diseases classified elsewhere, unspecified thigh*   ▽

✓6ᵗʰ **M63.86 Disorders of muscle in diseases classified elsewhere, lower leg**
> *M63.861*   *Disorders of muscle in diseases classified elsewhere, right lower leg*
> *M63.862*   *Disorders of muscle in diseases classified elsewhere, left lower leg*
> *M63.869*   *Disorders of muscle in diseases classified elsewhere, unspecified lower leg*   ▽

✓6ᵗʰ **M63.87 Disorders of muscle in diseases classified elsewhere, ankle and foot**
> *M63.871*   *Disorders of muscle in diseases classified elsewhere, right ankle and foot*
> *M63.872*   *Disorders of muscle in diseases classified elsewhere, left ankle and foot*
> *M63.879*   *Disorders of muscle in diseases classified elsewhere, unspecified ankle and foot*   ▽

M63.88   *Disorders of muscle in diseases classified elsewhere, other site*

M63.89   *Disorders of muscle in diseases classified elsewhere, multiple sites*

Disorders of synovium and tendon (M65-M67)

✓4ᵗʰ **M65 Synovitis and tenosynovitis**
> **EXCLUDES 1**   *chronic crepitant synovitis of hand and wrist (M70.0-)*
> > *current injury—see injury of ligament or tendon by body region*
> > *soft tissue disorders related to use, overuse and pressure (M70.-)*

✓5ᵗʰ **M65.0 Abscess of tendon sheath**
> Use additional code (B95-B96) to identify bacterial agent.
> **M65.00 Abscess of tendon sheath, unspecified site**   ▽

✓6ᵗʰ **M65.01 Abscess of tendon sheath, shoulder**
> **M65.011 Abscess of tendon sheath, right shoulder**
> **M65.012 Abscess of tendon sheath, left shoulder**
> **M65.019 Abscess of tendon sheath, unspecified shoulder**   ▽

✓6ᵗʰ **M65.02 Abscess of tendon sheath, upper arm**
> **M65.021 Abscess of tendon sheath, right upper arm**
> **M65.022 Abscess of tendon sheath, left upper arm**
> **M65.029 Abscess of tendon sheath, unspecified upper arm**   ▽

✓6ᵗʰ **M65.03 Abscess of tendon sheath, forearm**
> **M65.031 Abscess of tendon sheath, right forearm**
> **M65.032 Abscess of tendon sheath, left forearm**
> **M65.039 Abscess of tendon sheath, unspecified forearm**   ▽

✓6ᵗʰ **M65.04 Abscess of tendon sheath, hand**
> **M65.041 Abscess of tendon sheath, right hand**
> **M65.042 Abscess of tendon sheath, left hand**
> **M65.049 Abscess of tendon sheath, unspecified hand**   ▽

✓6ᵗʰ **M65.05 Abscess of tendon sheath, thigh**
> **M65.051 Abscess of tendon sheath, right thigh**
> **M65.052 Abscess of tendon sheath, left thigh**
> **M65.059 Abscess of tendon sheath, unspecified thigh**   ▽

✓6ᵗʰ **M65.06 Abscess of tendon sheath, lower leg**
> **M65.061 Abscess of tendon sheath, right lower leg**
> **M65.062 Abscess of tendon sheath, left lower leg**
> **M65.069 Abscess of tendon sheath, unspecified lower leg**   ▽

✓6ᵗʰ **M65.07 Abscess of tendon sheath, ankle and foot**
> **M65.071 Abscess of tendon sheath, right ankle and foot**
> **M65.072 Abscess of tendon sheath, left ankle and foot**
> **M65.079 Abscess of tendon sheath, unspecified ankle and foot**   ▽

M65.08 Abscess of tendon sheath, other site

✓5ᵗʰ **M65.1 Other infective (teno)synovitis**
> **M65.10 Other infective (teno)synovitis, unspecified site**   ▽

✓6ᵗʰ **M65.11 Other infective (teno)synovitis, shoulder**
> **M65.111 Other infective (teno)synovitis, right shoulder**
> **M65.112 Other infective (teno)synovitis, left shoulder**

EXCLUDES 1 Not coded here   **EXCLUDES 2** Not included here   N Newborn Age: 0   P Pediatric Age: 0-17   M Maternity Age: 12-55   A Adult Age: 15-124

766   ICD-10-CM 2018

M65.119   Other infective (teno)synovitis, unspecified shoulder ▽

✓6th M65.12   Other infective (teno)synovitis, elbow
    M65.121   Other infective (teno)synovitis, right elbow
    M65.122   Other infective (teno)synovitis, left elbow
    M65.129   Other infective (teno)synovitis, unspecified elbow ▽

✓6th M65.13   Other infective (teno)synovitis, wrist
    M65.131   Other infective (teno)synovitis, right wrist
    M65.132   Other infective (teno)synovitis, left wrist
    M65.139   Other infective (teno)synovitis, unspecified wrist

✓6th M65.14   Other infective (teno)synovitis, hand
    M65.141   Other infective (teno)synovitis, right hand
    M65.142   Other infective (teno)synovitis, left hand
    M65.149   Other infective (teno)synovitis, unspecified hand ▽

✓6th M65.15   Other infective (teno)synovitis, hip
    M65.151   Other infective (teno)synovitis, right hip
    M65.152   Other infective (teno)synovitis, left hip
    M65.159   Other infective (teno)synovitis, unspecified hip ▽

✓6th M65.16   Other infective (teno)synovitis, knee
    M65.161   Other infective (teno)synovitis, right knee
    M65.162   Other infective (teno)synovitis, left knee
    M65.169   Other infective (teno)synovitis, unspecified knee ▽

✓6th M65.17   Other infective (teno)synovitis, ankle and foot
    M65.171   Other infective (teno)synovitis, right ankle and foot
    M65.172   Other infective (teno)synovitis, left ankle and foot
    M65.179   Other infective (teno)synovitis, unspecified ankle and foot ▽

    M65.18   Other infective (teno)synovitis, other site
    M65.19   Other infective (teno)synovitis, multiple sites

✓5th M65.2   Calcific tendinitis
    EXCLUDES 1   tendinitis as classified in M75-M77
          calcified tendinitis of shoulder (M75.3)
    M65.20   Calcific tendinitis, unspecified site ▽

✓6th M65.22   Calcific tendinitis, upper arm
    M65.221   Calcific tendinitis, right upper arm
    M65.222   Calcific tendinitis, left upper arm
    M65.229   Calcific tendinitis, unspecified upper arm ▽

✓6th M65.23   Calcific tendinitis, forearm
    M65.231   Calcific tendinitis, right forearm
    M65.232   Calcific tendinitis, left forearm
    M65.239   Calcific tendinitis, unspecified forearm ▽

✓6th M65.24   Calcific tendinitis, hand
    M65.241   Calcific tendinitis, right hand
    M65.242   Calcific tendinitis, left hand
    M65.249   Calcific tendinitis, unspecified hand ▽

✓6th M65.25   Calcific tendinitis, thigh
    M65.251   Calcific tendinitis, right thigh
    M65.252   Calcific tendinitis, left thigh
    M65.259   Calcific tendinitis, unspecified thigh ▽

✓6th M65.26   Calcific tendinitis, lower leg
    M65.261   Calcific tendinitis, right lower leg
    M65.262   Calcific tendinitis, left lower leg
    M65.269   Calcific tendinitis, unspecified lower leg ▽

✓6th M65.27   Calcific tendinitis, ankle and foot
    M65.271   Calcific tendinitis, right ankle and foot
    M65.272   Calcific tendinitis, left ankle and foot
    M65.279   Calcific tendinitis, unspecified ankle and foot ▽

    M65.28   Calcific tendinitis, other site
    M65.29   Calcific tendinitis, multiple sites

✓5th M65.3   Trigger finger
    Nodular tendinous disease
    M65.30   Trigger finger, unspecified finger ▽

✓6th M65.31   Trigger thumb
    M65.311   Trigger thumb, right thumb
    M65.312   Trigger thumb, left thumb
    M65.319   Trigger thumb, unspecified thumb ▽

✓6th M65.32   Trigger finger, index finger
    M65.321   Trigger finger, right index finger
    M65.322   Trigger finger, left index finger
    M65.329   Trigger finger, unspecified index finger ▽

✓6th M65.33   Trigger finger, middle finger
    M65.331   Trigger finger, right middle finger
    M65.332   Trigger finger, left middle finger
    M65.339   Trigger finger, unspecified middle finger ▽

✓6th M65.34   Trigger finger, ring finger
    M65.341   Trigger finger, right ring finger
    M65.342   Trigger finger, left ring finger
    M65.349   Trigger finger, unspecified ring finger ▽

✓6th M65.35   Trigger finger, little finger
    M65.351   Trigger finger, right little finger
    M65.352   Trigger finger, left little finger
    M65.359   Trigger finger, unspecified little finger ▽

M65.4   Radial styloid tenosynovitis [de Quervain]

✓5th M65.8   Other synovitis and tenosynovitis
    M65.80   Other synovitis and tenosynovitis, unspecified site ▽

✓6th M65.81   Other synovitis and tenosynovitis, shoulder
    M65.811   Other synovitis and tenosynovitis, right shoulder
    M65.812   Other synovitis and tenosynovitis, left shoulder
    M65.819   Other synovitis and tenosynovitis, unspecified shoulder ▽

✓6th M65.82   Other synovitis and tenosynovitis, upper arm
    M65.821   Other synovitis and tenosynovitis, right upper arm
    M65.822   Other synovitis and tenosynovitis, left upper arm
    M65.829   Other synovitis and tenosynovitis, unspecified upper arm ▽

✓6th M65.83   Other synovitis and tenosynovitis, forearm
    M65.831   Other synovitis and tenosynovitis, right forearm
    M65.832   Other synovitis and tenosynovitis, left forearm
    M65.839   Other synovitis and tenosynovitis, unspecified forearm ▽

✓6th M65.84   Other synovitis and tenosynovitis, hand
    M65.841   Other synovitis and tenosynovitis, right hand
    M65.842   Other synovitis and tenosynovitis, left hand
    M65.849   Other synovitis and tenosynovitis, unspecified hand ▽

✓6th M65.85   Other synovitis and tenosynovitis, thigh
    M65.851   Other synovitis and tenosynovitis, right thigh
    M65.852   Other synovitis and tenosynovitis, left thigh
    M65.859   Other synovitis and tenosynovitis, unspecified thigh ▽

✓6th M65.86   Other synovitis and tenosynovitis, lower leg
    M65.861   Other synovitis and tenosynovitis, right lower leg
    M65.862   Other synovitis and tenosynovitis, left lower leg
    M65.869   Other synovitis and tenosynovitis, unspecified lower leg ▽

✓6th M65.87   Other synovitis and tenosynovitis, ankle and foot
    M65.871   Other synovitis and tenosynovitis, right ankle and foot
    M65.872   Other synovitis and tenosynovitis, left ankle and foot
    M65.879   Other synovitis and tenosynovitis, unspecified ankle and foot ▽

✓ Additional Character Req   ✓x7th Placeholder Alert   Manifestation   HCC CMS-HCC Condition   ▽ Unspecified Code   ▶◀ Revised Text   ● New Code   ▲ Revised Code Title

M65.88 Other synovitis and tenosynovitis, other site
M65.89 Other synovitis and tenosynovitis, multiple sites
M65.9 Synovitis and tenosynovitis, unspecified ▽

✓4ᵗʰ M66 Spontaneous rupture of synovium and tendon
  INCLUDES rupture that occurs when a normal force is applied to tissues that are inferred to have less than normal strength
  EXCLUDES 2 rotator cuff syndrome (M75.1-)
   rupture where an abnormal force is applied to normal tissue—see injury of tendon by body region

M66.0 Rupture of popliteal cyst
✓5ᵗʰ M66.1 Rupture of synovium
  Rupture of synovial cyst
  EXCLUDES 2 rupture of popliteal cyst (M66.0)
  M66.10 Rupture of synovium, unspecified joint ▽
  ✓6ᵗʰ M66.11 Rupture of synovium, shoulder
   M66.111 Rupture of synovium, right shoulder
   M66.112 Rupture of synovium, left shoulder
   M66.119 Rupture of synovium, unspecified shoulder ▽
  ✓6ᵗʰ M66.12 Rupture of synovium, elbow
   M66.121 Rupture of synovium, right elbow
   M66.122 Rupture of synovium, left elbow
   M66.129 Rupture of synovium, unspecified elbow ▽
  ✓6ᵗʰ M66.13 Rupture of synovium, wrist
   M66.131 Rupture of synovium, right wrist
   M66.132 Rupture of synovium, left wrist
   M66.139 Rupture of synovium, unspecified wrist ▽
  ✓6ᵗʰ M66.14 Rupture of synovium, hand and fingers
   M66.141 Rupture of synovium, right hand
   M66.142 Rupture of synovium, left hand
   M66.143 Rupture of synovium, unspecified hand ▽
   M66.144 Rupture of synovium, right finger(s)
   M66.145 Rupture of synovium, left finger(s)
   M66.146 Rupture of synovium, unspecified finger(s) ▽
  ✓6ᵗʰ M66.15 Rupture of synovium, hip
   M66.151 Rupture of synovium, right hip
   M66.152 Rupture of synovium, left hip
   M66.159 Rupture of synovium, unspecified hip ▽
  ✓6ᵗʰ M66.17 Rupture of synovium, ankle, foot and toes
   M66.171 Rupture of synovium, right ankle
   M66.172 Rupture of synovium, left ankle
   M66.173 Rupture of synovium, unspecified ankle ▽
   M66.174 Rupture of synovium, right foot
   M66.175 Rupture of synovium, left foot
   M66.176 Rupture of synovium, unspecified foot ▽
   M66.177 Rupture of synovium, right toe(s)
   M66.178 Rupture of synovium, left toe(s)
   M66.179 Rupture of synovium, unspecified toe(s) ▽
  M66.18 Rupture of synovium, other site
✓5ᵗʰ M66.2 Spontaneous rupture of extensor tendons
  TIP: Refer to the Muscle/Tendon table at the beginning of this chapter.
  M66.20 Spontaneous rupture of extensor tendons, unspecified site ▽
  ✓6ᵗʰ M66.21 Spontaneous rupture of extensor tendons, shoulder
   M66.211 Spontaneous rupture of extensor tendons, right shoulder
   M66.212 Spontaneous rupture of extensor tendons, left shoulder
   M66.219 Spontaneous rupture of extensor tendons, unspecified shoulder ▽
  ✓6ᵗʰ M66.22 Spontaneous rupture of extensor tendons, upper arm
   M66.221 Spontaneous rupture of extensor tendons, right upper arm
   M66.222 Spontaneous rupture of extensor tendons, left upper arm
   M66.229 Spontaneous rupture of extensor tendons, unspecified upper arm ▽

✓6ᵗʰ M66.23 Spontaneous rupture of extensor tendons, forearm
  M66.231 Spontaneous rupture of extensor tendons, right forearm
  M66.232 Spontaneous rupture of extensor tendons, left forearm
  M66.239 Spontaneous rupture of extensor tendons, unspecified forearm ▽
✓6ᵗʰ M66.24 Spontaneous rupture of extensor tendons, hand
  M66.241 Spontaneous rupture of extensor tendons, right hand
  M66.242 Spontaneous rupture of extensor tendons, left hand
  M66.249 Spontaneous rupture of extensor tendons, unspecified hand ▽
✓6ᵗʰ M66.25 Spontaneous rupture of extensor tendons, thigh
  M66.251 Spontaneous rupture of extensor tendons, right thigh
  M66.252 Spontaneous rupture of extensor tendons, left thigh
  M66.259 Spontaneous rupture of extensor tendons, unspecified thigh ▽
✓6ᵗʰ M66.26 Spontaneous rupture of extensor tendons, lower leg
  M66.261 Spontaneous rupture of extensor tendons, right lower leg
  M66.262 Spontaneous rupture of extensor tendons, left lower leg
  M66.269 Spontaneous rupture of extensor tendons, unspecified lower leg ▽
✓6ᵗʰ M66.27 Spontaneous rupture of extensor tendons, ankle and foot
  M66.271 Spontaneous rupture of extensor tendons, right ankle and foot
  M66.272 Spontaneous rupture of extensor tendons, left ankle and foot
  M66.279 Spontaneous rupture of extensor tendons, unspecified ankle and foot ▽
M66.28 Spontaneous rupture of extensor tendons, other site
M66.29 Spontaneous rupture of extensor tendons, multiple sites
✓5ᵗʰ M66.3 Spontaneous rupture of flexor tendons
  TIP: Refer to the Muscle/Tendon table at the beginning of this chapter.
  M66.30 Spontaneous rupture of flexor tendons, unspecified site ▽
  ✓6ᵗʰ M66.31 Spontaneous rupture of flexor tendons, shoulder
   M66.311 Spontaneous rupture of flexor tendons, right shoulder
   M66.312 Spontaneous rupture of flexor tendons, left shoulder
   M66.319 Spontaneous rupture of flexor tendons, unspecified shoulder ▽
  ✓6ᵗʰ M66.32 Spontaneous rupture of flexor tendons, upper arm
   M66.321 Spontaneous rupture of flexor tendons, right upper arm
   M66.322 Spontaneous rupture of flexor tendons, left upper arm
   M66.329 Spontaneous rupture of flexor tendons, unspecified upper arm ▽
  ✓6ᵗʰ M66.33 Spontaneous rupture of flexor tendons, forearm
   M66.331 Spontaneous rupture of flexor tendons, right forearm
   M66.332 Spontaneous rupture of flexor tendons, left forearm
   M66.339 Spontaneous rupture of flexor tendons, unspecified forearm ▽
  ✓6ᵗʰ M66.34 Spontaneous rupture of flexor tendons, hand
   M66.341 Spontaneous rupture of flexor tendons, right hand
   M66.342 Spontaneous rupture of flexor tendons, left hand
   M66.349 Spontaneous rupture of flexor tendons, unspecified hand ▽
  ✓6ᵗʰ M66.35 Spontaneous rupture of flexor tendons, thigh
   M66.351 Spontaneous rupture of flexor tendons, right thigh
   M66.352 Spontaneous rupture of flexor tendons, left thigh

M66.359   Spontaneous rupture of flexor tendons, unspecified thigh ▽

✓6ᵗʰ **M66.36**   **Spontaneous rupture of flexor tendons, lower leg**

M66.361   Spontaneous rupture of flexor tendons, right lower leg

M66.362   Spontaneous rupture of flexor tendons, left lower leg

M66.369   Spontaneous rupture of flexor tendons, unspecified lower leg ▽

✓6ᵗʰ **M66.37**   **Spontaneous rupture of flexor tendons, ankle and foot**

M66.371   Spontaneous rupture of flexor tendons, right ankle and foot

M66.372   Spontaneous rupture of flexor tendons, left ankle and foot

M66.379   Spontaneous rupture of flexor tendons, unspecified ankle and foot ▽

M66.38   Spontaneous rupture of flexor tendons, other site

M66.39   Spontaneous rupture of flexor tendons, multiple sites

✓5ᵗʰ **M66.8**   **Spontaneous rupture of other tendons**
     TIP: Refer to the Muscle/Tendon table at the beginning of this chapter.

M66.80   Spontaneous rupture of other tendons, unspecified site ▽

✓6ᵗʰ **M66.81**   **Spontaneous rupture of other tendons, shoulder**

M66.811   Spontaneous rupture of other tendons, right shoulder

M66.812   Spontaneous rupture of other tendons, left shoulder

M66.819   Spontaneous rupture of other tendons, unspecified shoulder ▽

✓6ᵗʰ **M66.82**   **Spontaneous rupture of other tendons, upper arm**

M66.821   Spontaneous rupture of other tendons, right upper arm

M66.822   Spontaneous rupture of other tendons, left upper arm

M66.829   Spontaneous rupture of other tendons, unspecified upper arm ▽

✓6ᵗʰ **M66.83**   **Spontaneous rupture of other tendons, forearm**

M66.831   Spontaneous rupture of other tendons, right forearm

M66.832   Spontaneous rupture of other tendons, left forearm

M66.839   Spontaneous rupture of other tendons, unspecified forearm ▽

✓6ᵗʰ **M66.84**   **Spontaneous rupture of other tendons, hand**

M66.841   Spontaneous rupture of other tendons, right hand

M66.842   Spontaneous rupture of other tendons, left hand

M66.849   Spontaneous rupture of other tendons, unspecified hand ▽

✓6ᵗʰ **M66.85**   **Spontaneous rupture of other tendons, thigh**

M66.851   Spontaneous rupture of other tendons, right thigh

M66.852   Spontaneous rupture of other tendons, left thigh

M66.859   Spontaneous rupture of other tendons, unspecified thigh ▽

✓6ᵗʰ **M66.86**   **Spontaneous rupture of other tendons, lower leg**

M66.861   Spontaneous rupture of other tendons, right lower leg

M66.862   Spontaneous rupture of other tendons, left lower leg

M66.869   Spontaneous rupture of other tendons, unspecified lower leg ▽

✓6ᵗʰ **M66.87**   **Spontaneous rupture of other tendons, ankle and foot**

M66.871   Spontaneous rupture of other tendons, right ankle and foot

M66.872   Spontaneous rupture of other tendons, left ankle and foot

M66.879   Spontaneous rupture of other tendons, unspecified ankle and foot ▽

M66.88   Spontaneous rupture of other tendons, other

M66.89   Spontaneous rupture of other tendons, multiple sites

M66.9   **Spontaneous rupture of unspecified tendon** ▽
     Rupture at musculotendinous junction, nontraumatic

✓4ᵗʰ **M67**   **Other disorders of synovium and tendon**
     EXCLUDES 1   palmar fascial fibromatosis [Dupuytren] (M72.0)
           tendinitis NOS (M77.9-)
           xanthomatosis localized to tendons (E78.2)

✓5ᵗʰ **M67.0**   **Short Achilles tendon (acquired)**

M67.00   Short Achilles tendon (acquired), unspecified ankle ▽

M67.01   Short Achilles tendon (acquired), right ankle

M67.02   Short Achilles tendon (acquired), left ankle

✓5ᵗʰ **M67.2**   **Synovial hypertrophy, not elsewhere classified**
     EXCLUDES 1   villonodular synovitis (pigmented) (M12.2-)

M67.20   Synovial hypertrophy, not elsewhere classified, unspecified site ▽

✓6ᵗʰ **M67.21**   **Synovial hypertrophy, not elsewhere classified, shoulder**

M67.211   Synovial hypertrophy, not elsewhere classified, right shoulder

M67.212   Synovial hypertrophy, not elsewhere classified, left shoulder

M67.219   Synovial hypertrophy, not elsewhere classified, unspecified shoulder ▽

✓6ᵗʰ **M67.22**   **Synovial hypertrophy, not elsewhere classified, upper arm**

M67.221   Synovial hypertrophy, not elsewhere classified, right upper arm

M67.222   Synovial hypertrophy, not elsewhere classified, left upper arm

M67.229   Synovial hypertrophy, not elsewhere classified, unspecified upper arm ▽

✓6ᵗʰ **M67.23**   **Synovial hypertrophy, not elsewhere classified, forearm**

M67.231   Synovial hypertrophy, not elsewhere classified, right forearm

M67.232   Synovial hypertrophy, not elsewhere classified, left forearm

M67.239   Synovial hypertrophy, not elsewhere classified, unspecified forearm ▽

✓6ᵗʰ **M67.24**   **Synovial hypertrophy, not elsewhere classified, hand**

M67.241   Synovial hypertrophy, not elsewhere classified, right hand

M67.242   Synovial hypertrophy, not elsewhere classified, left hand

M67.249   Synovial hypertrophy, not elsewhere classified, unspecified hand ▽

✓6ᵗʰ **M67.25**   **Synovial hypertrophy, not elsewhere classified, thigh**

M67.251   Synovial hypertrophy, not elsewhere classified, right thigh

M67.252   Synovial hypertrophy, not elsewhere classified, left thigh

M67.259   Synovial hypertrophy, not elsewhere classified, unspecified thigh ▽

✓6ᵗʰ **M67.26**   **Synovial hypertrophy, not elsewhere classified, lower leg**

M67.261   Synovial hypertrophy, not elsewhere classified, right lower leg

M67.262   Synovial hypertrophy, not elsewhere classified, left lower leg

M67.269   Synovial hypertrophy, not elsewhere classified, unspecified lower leg ▽

✓6ᵗʰ **M67.27**   **Synovial hypertrophy, not elsewhere classified, ankle and foot**

M67.271   Synovial hypertrophy, not elsewhere classified, right ankle and foot

M67.272   Synovial hypertrophy, not elsewhere classified, left ankle and foot

M67.279   Synovial hypertrophy, not elsewhere classified, unspecified ankle and foot ▽

M67.28   Synovial hypertrophy, not elsewhere classified, other site

M67.29   Synovial hypertrophy, not elsewhere classified, multiple sites

---

☑ Additional Character Req   ✓ˣ7ᵗʰ Placeholder Alert   Manifestation   HCC CMS-HCC Condition   ▽ Unspecified Code   ▶◀ Revised Text   ● New Code   ▲ Revised Code Title

ICD-10-CM 2018   769

✓5ᵗʰ M67.3 Transient synovitis
   Toxic synovitis
   EXCLUDES 1 *palindromic rheumatism (M12.3-)*
   M67.30 Transient synovitis, unspecified site ▽
   ✓6ᵗʰ M67.31 Transient synovitis, shoulder
      M67.311 Transient synovitis, right shoulder
      M67.312 Transient synovitis, left shoulder
      M67.319 Transient synovitis, unspecified ▽
         shoulder
   ✓6ᵗʰ M67.32 Transient synovitis, elbow
      M67.321 Transient synovitis, right elbow
      M67.322 Transient synovitis, left elbow
      M67.329 Transient synovitis, unspecified elbow ▽
   ✓6ᵗʰ M67.33 Transient synovitis, wrist
      M67.331 Transient synovitis, right wrist
      M67.332 Transient synovitis, left wrist
      M67.339 Transient synovitis, unspecified wrist ▽
   ✓6ᵗʰ M67.34 Transient synovitis, hand
      M67.341 Transient synovitis, right hand
      M67.342 Transient synovitis, left hand
      M67.349 Transient synovitis, unspecified hand ▽
   ✓6ᵗʰ M67.35 Transient synovitis, hip
      M67.351 Transient synovitis, right hip
      M67.352 Transient synovitis, left hip
      M67.359 Transient synovitis, unspecified hip ▽
   ✓6ᵗʰ M67.36 Transient synovitis, knee
      M67.361 Transient synovitis, right knee
      M67.362 Transient synovitis, left knee
      M67.369 Transient synovitis, unspecified knee ▽
   ✓6ᵗʰ M67.37 Transient synovitis, ankle and foot
      M67.371 Transient synovitis, right ankle and foot
      M67.372 Transient synovitis, left ankle and foot
      M67.379 Transient synovitis, unspecified ▽
         ankle and foot
   M67.38 Transient synovitis, other site
   M67.39 Transient synovitis, multiple sites
✓5ᵗʰ M67.4 Ganglion
   Ganglion of joint or tendon (sheath)
   EXCLUDES 1 *ganglion in yaws (A66.6)*
   EXCLUDES 2 *cyst of bursa (M71.2-M71.3)*
         cyst of synovium (M71.2-M71.3)
   M67.40 Ganglion, unspecified site ▽
   ✓6ᵗʰ M67.41 Ganglion, shoulder
      M67.411 Ganglion, right shoulder
      M67.412 Ganglion, left shoulder
      M67.419 Ganglion, unspecified shoulder ▽
   ✓6ᵗʰ M67.42 Ganglion, elbow
      M67.421 Ganglion, right elbow
      M67.422 Ganglion, left elbow
      M67.429 Ganglion, unspecified elbow ▽
   ✓6ᵗʰ M67.43 Ganglion, wrist
      M67.431 Ganglion, right wrist
      M67.432 Ganglion, left wrist
      M67.439 Ganglion, unspecified wrist ▽
   ✓6ᵗʰ M67.44 Ganglion, hand
      M67.441 Ganglion, right hand
      M67.442 Ganglion, left hand
      M67.449 Ganglion, unspecified hand ▽
   ✓6ᵗʰ M67.45 Ganglion, hip
      M67.451 Ganglion, right hip
      M67.452 Ganglion, left hip
      M67.459 Ganglion, unspecified hip ▽
   ✓6ᵗʰ M67.46 Ganglion, knee
      M67.461 Ganglion, right knee
      M67.462 Ganglion, left knee
      M67.469 Ganglion, unspecified knee ▽

Ganglion of Wrist

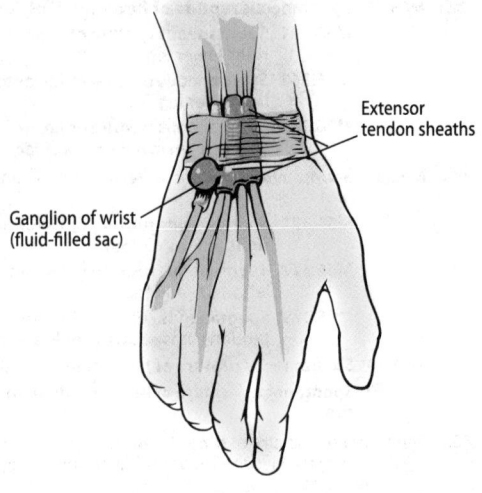

Extensor tendon sheaths

Ganglion of wrist (fluid-filled sac)

   ✓6ᵗʰ M67.47 Ganglion, ankle and foot
      M67.471 Ganglion, right ankle and foot
      M67.472 Ganglion, left ankle and foot
      M67.479 Ganglion, unspecified ankle and foot ▽
   M67.48 Ganglion, other site
   M67.49 Ganglion, multiple sites
✓5ᵗʰ M67.5 Plica syndrome
   Plica knee
   M67.50 Plica syndrome, unspecified knee ▽
   M67.51 Plica syndrome, right knee
   M67.52 Plica syndrome, left knee
✓5ᵗʰ M67.8 Other specified disorders of synovium and tendon
   M67.80 Other specified disorders of synovium and ▽
      tendon, unspecified site
   ✓6ᵗʰ M67.81 Other specified disorders of synovium and tendon, shoulder
      M67.811 Other specified disorders of synovium, right shoulder
      M67.812 Other specified disorders of synovium, left shoulder
      M67.813 Other specified disorders of tendon, right shoulder
      M67.814 Other specified disorders of tendon, left shoulder
      M67.819 Other specified disorders of synovium ▽
         and tendon, unspecified shoulder
   ✓6ᵗʰ M67.82 Other specified disorders of synovium and tendon, elbow
      M67.821 Other specified disorders of synovium, right elbow
      M67.822 Other specified disorders of synovium, left elbow
      M67.823 Other specified disorders of tendon, right elbow
      M67.824 Other specified disorders of tendon, left elbow
      M67.829 Other specified disorders of synovium ▽
         and tendon, unspecified elbow
   ✓6ᵗʰ M67.83 Other specified disorders of synovium and tendon, wrist
      M67.831 Other specified disorders of synovium, right wrist
      M67.832 Other specified disorders of synovium, left wrist
      M67.833 Other specified disorders of tendon, right wrist
      M67.834 Other specified disorders of tendon, left wrist
      M67.839 Other specified disorders of synovium ▽
         and tendon, unspecified forearm

☑6ᵗʰ **M67.84** Other specified disorders of synovium and tendon, hand

　　　M67.841 Other specified disorders of synovium, right hand

　　　M67.842 Other specified disorders of synovium, left hand

　　　M67.843 Other specified disorders of tendon, right hand

　　　M67.844 Other specified disorders of tendon, left hand

　　　M67.849 Other specified disorders of synovium and tendon, unspecified hand　▽

☑6ᵗʰ **M67.85** Other specified disorders of synovium and tendon, hip

　　　M67.851 Other specified disorders of synovium, right hip

　　　M67.852 Other specified disorders of synovium, left hip

　　　M67.853 Other specified disorders of tendon, right hip

　　　M67.854 Other specified disorders of tendon, left hip

　　　M67.859 Other specified disorders of synovium and tendon, unspecified hip　▽

☑6ᵗʰ **M67.86** Other specified disorders of synovium and tendon, knee

　　　M67.861 Other specified disorders of synovium, right knee

　　　M67.862 Other specified disorders of synovium, left knee

　　　M67.863 Other specified disorders of tendon, right knee

　　　M67.864 Other specified disorders of tendon, left knee

　　　M67.869 Other specified disorders of synovium and tendon, unspecified knee　▽

☑6ᵗʰ **M67.87** Other specified disorders of synovium and tendon, ankle and foot

　　　M67.871 Other specified disorders of synovium, right ankle and foot

　　　M67.872 Other specified disorders of synovium, left ankle and foot

　　　M67.873 Other specified disorders of tendon, right ankle and foot

　　　M67.874 Other specified disorders of tendon, left ankle and foot

　　　M67.879 Other specified disorders of synovium and tendon, unspecified ankle and foot　▽

　　M67.88 Other specified disorders of synovium and tendon, other site

　　M67.89 Other specified disorders of synovium and tendon, multiple sites

☑5ᵗʰ **M67.9** Unspecified disorder of synovium and tendon

　　M67.90 Unspecified disorder of synovium and tendon, unspecified site　▽

☑6ᵗʰ **M67.91** Unspecified disorder of synovium and tendon, shoulder

　　　M67.911 Unspecified disorder of synovium and tendon, right shoulder　▽

　　　M67.912 Unspecified disorder of synovium and tendon, left shoulder　▽

　　　M67.919 Unspecified disorder of synovium and tendon, unspecified shoulder　▽

☑6ᵗʰ **M67.92** Unspecified disorder of synovium and tendon, upper arm

　　　M67.921 Unspecified disorder of synovium and tendon, right upper arm　▽

　　　M67.922 Unspecified disorder of synovium and tendon, left upper arm　▽

　　　M67.929 Unspecified disorder of synovium and tendon, unspecified upper arm　▽

☑6ᵗʰ **M67.93** Unspecified disorder of synovium and tendon, forearm

　　　M67.931 Unspecified disorder of synovium and tendon, right forearm　▽

　　　M67.932 Unspecified disorder of synovium and tendon, left forearm　▽

　　　M67.939 Unspecified disorder of synovium and tendon, unspecified forearm　▽

☑6ᵗʰ **M67.94** Unspecified disorder of synovium and tendon, hand

　　　M67.941 Unspecified disorder of synovium and tendon, right hand　▽

　　　M67.942 Unspecified disorder of synovium and tendon, left hand　▽

　　　M67.949 Unspecified disorder of synovium and tendon, unspecified hand　▽

☑6ᵗʰ **M67.95** Unspecified disorder of synovium and tendon, thigh

　　　M67.951 Unspecified disorder of synovium and tendon, right thigh　▽

　　　M67.952 Unspecified disorder of synovium and tendon, left thigh　▽

　　　M67.959 Unspecified disorder of synovium and tendon, unspecified thigh　▽

☑6ᵗʰ **M67.96** Unspecified disorder of synovium and tendon, lower leg

　　　M67.961 Unspecified disorder of synovium and tendon, right lower leg　▽

　　　M67.962 Unspecified disorder of synovium and tendon, left lower leg　▽

　　　M67.969 Unspecified disorder of synovium and tendon, unspecified lower leg　▽

☑6ᵗʰ **M67.97** Unspecified disorder of synovium and tendon, ankle and foot

　　　M67.971 Unspecified disorder of synovium and tendon, right ankle and foot　▽

　　　M67.972 Unspecified disorder of synovium and tendon, left ankle and foot　▽

　　　M67.979 Unspecified disorder of synovium and tendon, unspecified ankle and foot　▽

　　M67.98 Unspecified disorder of synovium and tendon, other site　▽

　　M67.99 Unspecified disorder of synovium and tendon, multiple sites　▽

Other soft tissue disorders (M70-M79)

☑4ᵗʰ **M70 Soft tissue disorders related to use, overuse and pressure**

　　INCLUDES soft tissue disorders of occupational origin

　　Use additional external cause code to identify activity causing disorder (Y93.-)

　　EXCLUDES 1 bursitis NOS (M71.9-)

　　EXCLUDES 2 bursitis of shoulder (M75.5)
　　　　enthesopathies (M76-M77)
　　　　pressure ulcer (pressure area) (L89.-)

☑5ᵗʰ **M70.0** Crepitant synovitis (acute) (chronic) of hand and wrist

☑6ᵗʰ **M70.03** Crepitant synovitis (acute) (chronic), wrist

　　　M70.031 Crepitant synovitis (acute) (chronic), right wrist

　　　M70.032 Crepitant synovitis (acute) (chronic), left wrist

　　　M70.039 Crepitant synovitis (acute) (chronic), unspecified wrist　▽

☑6ᵗʰ **M70.04** Crepitant synovitis (acute) (chronic), hand

　　　M70.041 Crepitant synovitis (acute) (chronic), right hand

　　　M70.042 Crepitant synovitis (acute) (chronic), left hand

　　　M70.049 Crepitant synovitis (acute) (chronic), unspecified hand　▽

☑5ᵗʰ **M70.1** Bursitis of hand

　　M70.10 Bursitis, unspecified hand　▽

　　M70.11 Bursitis, right hand

　　M70.12 Bursitis, left hand

☑5ᵗʰ **M70.2** Olecranon bursitis

　　M70.20 Olecranon bursitis, unspecified elbow　▽

　　M70.21 Olecranon bursitis, right elbow

　　M70.22 Olecranon bursitis, left elbow

☑5ᵗʰ **M70.3** Other bursitis of elbow

　　M70.30 Other bursitis of elbow, unspecified elbow　▽

　　M70.31 Other bursitis of elbow, right elbow

　　M70.32 Other bursitis of elbow, left elbow

☑ Additional Character Req　　ᵛˣ⁷ᵗʰ Placeholder Alert　　Manifestation　　HCC CMS-HCC Condition　　▽ Unspecified Code　　▶◀ Revised Text　　● New Code　　▲ Revised Code Title

ICD-10-CM 2018　　　　　　　　　　　　　　　　　　　　　　　　　　　　　　　　**771**

√5th **M70.4 Prepatellar bursitis**
    M70.40 Prepatellar bursitis, unspecified knee ▽
    M70.41 Prepatellar bursitis, right knee
    M70.42 Prepatellar bursitis, left knee

√5th **M70.5 Other bursitis of knee**
    M70.50 Other bursitis of knee, unspecified knee ▽
    M70.51 Other bursitis of knee, right knee
    M70.52 Other bursitis of knee, left knee

√5th **M70.6 Trochanteric bursitis**
    Trochanteric tendinitis
    M70.60 Trochanteric bursitis, unspecified hip ▽
    M70.61 Trochanteric bursitis, right hip
    M70.62 Trochanteric bursitis, left hip

√5th **M70.7 Other bursitis of hip**
    Ischial bursitis
    M70.70 Other bursitis of hip, unspecified hip ▽
    M70.71 Other bursitis of hip, right hip
    M70.72 Other bursitis of hip, left hip

√5th **M70.8 Other soft tissue disorders related to use, overuse and pressure**
    M70.80 Other soft tissue disorders related to use, overuse and pressure of unspecified site ▽
  √6th **M70.81 Other soft tissue disorders related to use, overuse and pressure of shoulder**
    M70.811 Other soft tissue disorders related to use, overuse and pressure, right shoulder
    M70.812 Other soft tissue disorders related to use, overuse and pressure, left shoulder
    M70.819 Other soft tissue disorders related to use, overuse and pressure, unspecified shoulder ▽
  √6th **M70.82 Other soft tissue disorders related to use, overuse and pressure of upper arm**
    M70.821 Other soft tissue disorders related to use, overuse and pressure, right upper arm
    M70.822 Other soft tissue disorders related to use, overuse and pressure, left upper arm
    M70.829 Other soft tissue disorders related to use, overuse and pressure, unspecified upper arms ▽
  √6th **M70.83 Other soft tissue disorders related to use, overuse and pressure of forearm**
    M70.831 Other soft tissue disorders related to use, overuse and pressure, right forearm
    M70.832 Other soft tissue disorders related to use, overuse and pressure, left forearm
    M70.839 Other soft tissue disorders related to use, overuse and pressure, unspecified forearm ▽
  √6th **M70.84 Other soft tissue disorders related to use, overuse and pressure of hand**
    M70.841 Other soft tissue disorders related to use, overuse and pressure, right hand
    M70.842 Other soft tissue disorders related to use, overuse and pressure, left hand
    M70.849 Other soft tissue disorders related to use, overuse and pressure, unspecified hand ▽
  √6th **M70.85 Other soft tissue disorders related to use, overuse and pressure of thigh**
    M70.851 Other soft tissue disorders related to use, overuse and pressure, right thigh
    M70.852 Other soft tissue disorders related to use, overuse and pressure, left thigh
    M70.859 Other soft tissue disorders related to use, overuse and pressure, unspecified thigh ▽
  √6th **M70.86 Other soft tissue disorders related to use, overuse and pressure lower leg**
    M70.861 Other soft tissue disorders related to use, overuse and pressure, right lower leg
    M70.862 Other soft tissue disorders related to use, overuse and pressure, left lower leg
    M70.869 Other soft tissue disorders related to use, overuse and pressure, unspecified leg ▽

  √6th **M70.87 Other soft tissue disorders related to use, overuse and pressure of ankle and foot**
    M70.871 Other soft tissue disorders related to use, overuse and pressure, right ankle and foot
    M70.872 Other soft tissue disorders related to use, overuse and pressure, left ankle and foot
    M70.879 Other soft tissue disorders related to use, overuse and pressure, unspecified ankle and foot ▽
    M70.88 Other soft tissue disorders related to use, overuse and pressure other site
    M70.89 Other soft tissue disorders related to use, overuse and pressure multiple sites

√5th **M70.9 Unspecified soft tissue disorder related to use, overuse and pressure**
    M70.90 Unspecified soft tissue disorder related to use, overuse and pressure of unspecified site ▽
  √6th **M70.91 Unspecified soft tissue disorder related to use, overuse and pressure of shoulder**
    M70.911 Unspecified soft tissue disorder related to use, overuse and pressure, right shoulder ▽
    M70.912 Unspecified soft tissue disorder related to use, overuse and pressure, left shoulder ▽
    M70.919 Unspecified soft tissue disorder related to use, overuse and pressure, unspecified shoulder ▽
  √6th **M70.92 Unspecified soft tissue disorder related to use, overuse and pressure of upper arm**
    M70.921 Unspecified soft tissue disorder related to use, overuse and pressure, right upper arm ▽
    M70.922 Unspecified soft tissue disorder related to use, overuse and pressure, left upper arm ▽
    M70.929 Unspecified soft tissue disorder related to use, overuse and pressure, unspecified upper arm ▽
  √6th **M70.93 Unspecified soft tissue disorder related to use, overuse and pressure of forearm**
    M70.931 Unspecified soft tissue disorder related to use, overuse and pressure, right forearm ▽
    M70.932 Unspecified soft tissue disorder related to use, overuse and pressure, left forearm ▽
    M70.939 Unspecified soft tissue disorder related to use, overuse and pressure, unspecified forearm ▽
  √6th **M70.94 Unspecified soft tissue disorder related to use, overuse and pressure of hand**
    M70.941 Unspecified soft tissue disorder related to use, overuse and pressure, right hand ▽
    M70.942 Unspecified soft tissue disorder related to use, overuse and pressure, left hand ▽
    M70.949 Unspecified soft tissue disorder related to use, overuse and pressure, unspecified hand ▽
  √6th **M70.95 Unspecified soft tissue disorder related to use, overuse and pressure of thigh**
    M70.951 Unspecified soft tissue disorder related to use, overuse and pressure, right thigh ▽
    M70.952 Unspecified soft tissue disorder related to use, overuse and pressure, left thigh ▽
    M70.959 Unspecified soft tissue disorder related to use, overuse and pressure, unspecified thigh ▽
  √6th **M70.96 Unspecified soft tissue disorder related to use, overuse and pressure lower leg**
    M70.961 Unspecified soft tissue disorder related to use, overuse and pressure, right lower leg ▽
    M70.962 Unspecified soft tissue disorder related to use, overuse and pressure, left lower leg ▽
    M70.969 Unspecified soft tissue disorder related to use, overuse and pressure, unspecified lower leg ▽

EXCLUDES 1 Not coded here　　**EXCLUDES 2** Not included here　　N Newborn Age: 0　　P Pediatric Age: 0-17　　M Maternity Age: 12-55　　A Adult Age: 15-124

772　　ICD-10-CM 2018

✓6ᵗʰ **M70.97 Unspecified soft tissue disorder related to use, overuse and pressure of** ankle and foot

    M70.971 Unspecified soft tissue disorder related ▽ **to use, overuse and pressure,** right **ankle and foot**

    M70.972 Unspecified soft tissue disorder related ▽ **to use, overuse and pressure,** left **ankle and foot**

    M70.979 Unspecified soft tissue disorder related to use, overuse and pressure, unspecified ankle and foot

   M70.98 Unspecified soft tissue disorder related to use, ▽ **overuse and pressure other**

   M70.99 Unspecified soft tissue disorder related to use, ▽ **overuse and pressure** multiple sites

✓4ᵗʰ **M71 Other bursopathies**

    EXCLUDES 1   bunion (M20.1)
              bursitis related to use, overuse or pressure (M70.-)
              enthesopathies (M76-M77)

✓5ᵗʰ **M71.0 Abscess of bursa**

    Use additional code (B95.-, B96.-) to identify causative organism

   M71.00 Abscess of bursa, unspecified site ▽

  ✓6ᵗʰ **M71.01 Abscess of bursa,** shoulder

    M71.011 Abscess of bursa, right **shoulder**
    M71.012 Abscess of bursa, left **shoulder**
    M71.019 Abscess of bursa, unspecified shoulder ▽

  ✓6ᵗʰ **M71.02 Abscess of bursa,** elbow

    M71.021 Abscess of bursa, right **elbow**
    M71.022 Abscess of bursa, left **elbow**
    M71.029 Abscess of bursa, unspecified elbow ▽

  ✓6ᵗʰ **M71.03 Abscess of bursa,** wrist

    M71.031 Abscess of bursa, right **wrist**
    M71.032 Abscess of bursa, left **wrist**
    M71.039 Abscess of bursa, unspecified wrist ▽

  ✓6ᵗʰ **M71.04 Abscess of bursa,** hand

    M71.041 Abscess of bursa, right **hand**
    M71.042 Abscess of bursa, left **hand**
    M71.049 Abscess of bursa, unspecified hand ▽

  ✓6ᵗʰ **M71.05 Abscess of bursa,** hip

    M71.051 Abscess of bursa, right **hip**
    M71.052 Abscess of bursa, left **hip**
    M71.059 Abscess of bursa, unspecified hip ▽

  ✓6ᵗʰ **M71.06 Abscess of bursa,** knee

    M71.061 Abscess of bursa, right **knee**
    M71.062 Abscess of bursa, left **knee**
    M71.069 Abscess of bursa, unspecified knee ▽

  ✓6ᵗʰ **M71.07 Abscess of bursa,** ankle and foot

    M71.071 Abscess of bursa, right **ankle and foot**
    M71.072 Abscess of bursa, left **ankle and foot**
    M71.079 Abscess of bursa, unspecified ankle ▽ **and foot**

   M71.08 Abscess of bursa, other site

   M71.09 Abscess of bursa, multiple sites

✓5ᵗʰ **M71.1 Other infective bursitis**

    Use additional code (B95.-, B96.-) to identify causative organism

   M71.10 Other infective bursitis, unspecified site ▽

  ✓6ᵗʰ **M71.11 Other infective bursitis,** shoulder

    M71.111 Other infective bursitis, right **shoulder**
    M71.112 Other infective bursitis, left **shoulder**
    M71.119 Other infective bursitis, unspecified ▽ **shoulder**

  ✓6ᵗʰ **M71.12 Other infective bursitis,** elbow

    M71.121 Other infective bursitis, right **elbow**
    M71.122 Other infective bursitis, left **elbow**
    M71.129 Other infective bursitis, unspecified ▽ **elbow**

  ✓6ᵗʰ **M71.13 Other infective bursitis,** wrist

    M71.131 Other infective bursitis, right **wrist**
    M71.132 Other infective bursitis, left **wrist**
    M71.139 Other infective bursitis, unspecified ▽ **wrist**

✓6ᵗʰ **M71.14 Other infective bursitis,** hand

    M71.141 Other infective bursitis, right **hand**
    M71.142 Other infective bursitis, left **hand**
    M71.149 Other infective bursitis, unspecified ▽ **hand**

✓6ᵗʰ **M71.15 Other infective bursitis,** hip

    M71.151 Other infective bursitis, right **hip**
    M71.152 Other infective bursitis, left **hip**
    M71.159 Other infective bursitis, unspecified hip ▽

✓6ᵗʰ **M71.16 Other infective bursitis,** knee

    M71.161 Other infective bursitis, right **knee**
    M71.162 Other infective bursitis, left **knee**
    M71.169 Other infective bursitis, unspecified ▽ **knee**

✓6ᵗʰ **M71.17 Other infective bursitis,** ankle and foot

    M71.171 Other infective bursitis, right **ankle and foot**
    M71.172 Other infective bursitis, left **ankle and foot**
    M71.179 Other infective bursitis, unspecified ▽ **ankle and foot**

   M71.18 Other infective bursitis, other site

   M71.19 Other infective bursitis, multiple sites

✓5ᵗʰ **M71.2 Synovial cyst of popliteal space [Baker]**

    EXCLUDES 1   synovial cyst of popliteal space with rupture (M66.0)

   M71.20 Synovial cyst of popliteal space [Baker], ▽ **unspecified knee**

   M71.21 Synovial cyst of popliteal space [Baker], right **knee**

   M71.22 Synovial cyst of popliteal space [Baker], left **knee**

✓5ᵗʰ **M71.3 Other bursal cyst**

    Synovial cyst NOS

    EXCLUDES 1   synovial cyst with rupture (M66.1-)

   M71.30 Other bursal cyst, unspecified site ▽

  ✓6ᵗʰ **M71.31 Other bursal cyst,** shoulder

    M71.311 Other bursal cyst, right **shoulder**
    M71.312 Other bursal cyst, left **shoulder**
    M71.319 Other bursal cyst, unspecified shoulder ▽

  ✓6ᵗʰ **M71.32 Other bursal cyst,** elbow

    M71.321 Other bursal cyst, right **elbow**
    M71.322 Other bursal cyst, left **elbow**
    M71.329 Other bursal cyst, unspecified elbow ▽

  ✓6ᵗʰ **M71.33 Other bursal cyst,** wrist

    M71.331 Other bursal cyst, right **wrist**
    M71.332 Other bursal cyst, left **wrist**
    M71.339 Other bursal cyst, unspecified wrist ▽

  ✓6ᵗʰ **M71.34 Other bursal cyst,** hand

    M71.341 Other bursal cyst, right **hand**
    M71.342 Other bursal cyst, left **hand**
    M71.349 Other bursal cyst, unspecified hand ▽

Baker's Cyst

Baker's cyst connected to knee joint synovial cavity

✓6ᵗʰ **M71.35 Other bursal cyst, hip**
　　M71.351 Other bursal cyst, right hip
　　M71.352 Other bursal cyst, left hip
　　M71.359 Other bursal cyst, unspecified hip ▽

✓6ᵗʰ **M71.37 Other bursal cyst, ankle and foot**
　　M71.371 Other bursal cyst, right ankle and foot
　　M71.372 Other bursal cyst, left ankle and foot
　　M71.379 Other bursal cyst, unspecified ankle and foot ▽

　M71.38 Other bursal cyst, other site
　M71.39 Other bursal cyst, multiple sites

✓5ᵗʰ **M71.4 Calcium deposit in bursa**
　　EXCLUDES 2　calcium deposit in bursa of shoulder (M75.3)
　M71.40 Calcium deposit in bursa, unspecified site ▽

✓6ᵗʰ **M71.42 Calcium deposit in bursa, elbow**
　　M71.421 Calcium deposit in bursa, right elbow
　　M71.422 Calcium deposit in bursa, left elbow
　　M71.429 Calcium deposit in bursa, unspecified elbow ▽

✓6ᵗʰ **M71.43 Calcium deposit in bursa, wrist**
　　M71.431 Calcium deposit in bursa, right wrist
　　M71.432 Calcium deposit in bursa, left wrist
　　M71.439 Calcium deposit in bursa, unspecified wrist ▽

✓6ᵗʰ **M71.44 Calcium deposit in bursa, hand**
　　M71.441 Calcium deposit in bursa, right hand
　　M71.442 Calcium deposit in bursa, left hand
　　M71.449 Calcium deposit in bursa, unspecified hand ▽

✓6ᵗʰ **M71.45 Calcium deposit in bursa, hip**
　　M71.451 Calcium deposit in bursa, right hip
　　M71.452 Calcium deposit in bursa, left hip
　　M71.459 Calcium deposit in bursa, unspecified hip ▽

✓6ᵗʰ **M71.46 Calcium deposit in bursa, knee**
　　M71.461 Calcium deposit in bursa, right knee
　　M71.462 Calcium deposit in bursa, left knee
　　M71.469 Calcium deposit in bursa, unspecified knee ▽

✓6ᵗʰ **M71.47 Calcium deposit in bursa, ankle and foot**
　　M71.471 Calcium deposit in bursa, right ankle and foot
　　M71.472 Calcium deposit in bursa, left ankle and foot
　　M71.479 Calcium deposit in bursa, unspecified ankle and foot ▽

　M71.48 Calcium deposit in bursa, other site
　M71.49 Calcium deposit in bursa, multiple sites

✓5ᵗʰ **M71.5 Other bursitis, not elsewhere classified**
　　EXCLUDES 1　bursitis NOS (M71.9-)
　　EXCLUDES 2　bursitis of shoulder (M75.5)
　　　　　　　bursitis of tibial collateral [Pellegrini-Stieda] (M76.4-)
　M71.50 Other bursitis, not elsewhere classified, unspecified site ▽

✓6ᵗʰ **M71.52 Other bursitis, not elsewhere classified, elbow**
　　M71.521 Other bursitis, not elsewhere classified, right elbow
　　M71.522 Other bursitis, not elsewhere classified, left elbow
　　M71.529 Other bursitis, not elsewhere classified, unspecified elbow ▽

✓6ᵗʰ **M71.53 Other bursitis, not elsewhere classified, wrist**
　　M71.531 Other bursitis, not elsewhere classified, right wrist
　　M71.532 Other bursitis, not elsewhere classified, left wrist
　　M71.539 Other bursitis, not elsewhere classified, unspecified wrist ▽

✓6ᵗʰ **M71.54 Other bursitis, not elsewhere classified, hand**
　　M71.541 Other bursitis, not elsewhere classified, right hand
　　M71.542 Other bursitis, not elsewhere classified, left hand

　　M71.549 Other bursitis, not elsewhere classified, unspecified hand ▽

✓6ᵗʰ **M71.55 Other bursitis, not elsewhere classified, hip**
　　M71.551 Other bursitis, not elsewhere classified, right hip
　　M71.552 Other bursitis, not elsewhere classified, left hip
　　M71.559 Other bursitis, not elsewhere classified, unspecified hip ▽

✓6ᵗʰ **M71.56 Other bursitis, not elsewhere classified, knee**
　　M71.561 Other bursitis, not elsewhere classified, right knee
　　M71.562 Other bursitis, not elsewhere classified, left knee
　　M71.569 Other bursitis, not elsewhere classified, unspecified knee ▽

✓6ᵗʰ **M71.57 Other bursitis, not elsewhere classified, ankle and foot**
　　M71.571 Other bursitis, not elsewhere classified, right ankle and foot
　　M71.572 Other bursitis, not elsewhere classified, left ankle and foot
　　M71.579 Other bursitis, not elsewhere classified, unspecified ankle and foot ▽

　M71.58 Other bursitis, not elsewhere classified, other site

✓5ᵗʰ **M71.8 Other specified bursopathies**
　M71.80 Other specified bursopathies, unspecified site ▽

✓6ᵗʰ **M71.81 Other specified bursopathies, shoulder**
　　M71.811 Other specified bursopathies, right shoulder
　　M71.812 Other specified bursopathies, left shoulder
　　M71.819 Other specified bursopathies, unspecified shoulder ▽

✓6ᵗʰ **M71.82 Other specified bursopathies, elbow**
　　M71.821 Other specified bursopathies, right elbow
　　M71.822 Other specified bursopathies, left elbow
　　M71.829 Other specified bursopathies, unspecified elbow ▽

✓6ᵗʰ **M71.83 Other specified bursopathies, wrist**
　　M71.831 Other specified bursopathies, right wrist
　　M71.832 Other specified bursopathies, left wrist
　　M71.839 Other specified bursopathies, unspecified wrist ▽

✓6ᵗʰ **M71.84 Other specified bursopathies, hand**
　　M71.841 Other specified bursopathies, right hand
　　M71.842 Other specified bursopathies, left hand
　　M71.849 Other specified bursopathies, unspecified hand ▽

✓6ᵗʰ **M71.85 Other specified bursopathies, hip**
　　M71.851 Other specified bursopathies, right hip
　　M71.852 Other specified bursopathies, left hip
　　M71.859 Other specified bursopathies, unspecified hip ▽

✓6ᵗʰ **M71.86 Other specified bursopathies, knee**
　　M71.861 Other specified bursopathies, right knee
　　M71.862 Other specified bursopathies, left knee
　　M71.869 Other specified bursopathies, unspecified knee ▽

✓6ᵗʰ **M71.87 Other specified bursopathies, ankle and foot**
　　M71.871 Other specified bursopathies, right ankle and foot
　　M71.872 Other specified bursopathies, left ankle and foot
　　M71.879 Other specified bursopathies, unspecified ankle and foot ▽

　M71.88 Other specified bursopathies, other site
　M71.89 Other specified bursopathies, multiple sites

M71.9 Bursopathy, unspecified ▽
　Bursitis NOS

EXCLUDES 1 Not coded here　　EXCLUDES 2 Not included here　　N Newborn Age: 0　　P Pediatric Age: 0-17　　M Maternity Age: 12-55　　A Adult Age: 15-124

774　　ICD-10-CM 2018

✓4ᵗʰ **M72 Fibroblastic disorders**

    EXCLUDES 2   *retroperitoneal fibromatosis (D48.3)*

  M72.0 Palmar fascial fibromatosis [Dupuytren]   A

    DEF: Dupuytren's contracture: Flexion deformity of finger, due to shortened, thickened fibrosing of palmar fascia; cause unknown; associated with long-standing epilepsy.

  M72.1 Knuckle pads

  M72.2 Plantar fascial fibromatosis

    Plantar fasciitis

    DEF: Rapid-growing and multiplanar nodular swellings and pain in the foot; not associated with contractures.

  M72.4 Pseudosarcomatous fibromatosis

    Nodular fasciitis

  M72.6 Necrotizing fasciitis   HCC

    Use additional code (B95.-, B96.-) to identify causative organism

  M72.8 Other fibroblastic disorders

    Abscess of fascia

    Fasciitis NEC

    Other infective fasciitis

    Use additional code to (B95.-, B96.-) identify causative organism

    EXCLUDES 1   *diffuse (eosinophilic) fasciitis (M35.4)*
           necrotizing fasciitis (M72.6)
           nodular fasciitis (M72.4)
           perirenal fasciitis NOS (N13.5)
           perirenal fasciitis with infection (N13.6)
           plantar fasciitis (M72.2)

  M72.9 Fibroblastic disorder, unspecified   ▽

    Fasciitis NOS

    Fibromatosis NOS

✓4ᵗʰ **M75 Shoulder lesions**

    EXCLUDES 2   *shoulder-hand syndrome (M89.0-)*

  ✓5ᵗʰ **M75.0 Adhesive capsulitis of shoulder**

    Frozen shoulder

    Periarthritis of shoulder

    AHA: 2015, 2Q, 23

    M75.00 Adhesive capsulitis of unspecified shoulder   ▽

    M75.01 Adhesive capsulitis of right shoulder

    M75.02 Adhesive capsulitis of left shoulder

  ✓5ᵗʰ **M75.1 Rotator cuff tear or rupture, not specified as traumatic**

    Rotator cuff syndrome

    Supraspinatus syndrome

    Supraspinatus tear or rupture, not specified as traumatic

    EXCLUDES 1   *tear of rotator cuff, traumatic (S46.01-)*

    ✓6ᵗʰ **M75.10 Unspecified rotator cuff tear or rupture, not specified as traumatic**

      M75.100 Unspecified rotator cuff tear or rupture ▽ **of unspecified shoulder, not specified as traumatic**

      M75.101 Unspecified rotator cuff tear or rupture ▽ **of right shoulder, not specified as traumatic**

      M75.102 Unspecified rotator cuff tear or rupture ▽ **of left shoulder, not specified as traumatic**

    ✓6ᵗʰ **M75.11 Incomplete rotator cuff tear or rupture not specified as traumatic**

      M75.110 Incomplete rotator cuff tear or rupture ▽ **of unspecified shoulder, not specified as traumatic**

      M75.111 Incomplete rotator cuff tear or rupture of right shoulder, not specified as traumatic

      M75.112 Incomplete rotator cuff tear or rupture of left shoulder, not specified as traumatic

    ✓6ᵗʰ **M75.12 Complete rotator cuff tear or rupture not specified as traumatic**

      M75.120 Complete rotator cuff tear or rupture ▽ **of unspecified shoulder, not specified as traumatic**

      M75.121 Complete rotator cuff tear or rupture of right shoulder, not specified as traumatic

      M75.122 Complete rotator cuff tear or rupture of left shoulder, not specified as traumatic

  ✓5ᵗʰ **M75.2 Bicipital tendinitis**

    M75.20 Bicipital tendinitis, unspecified shoulder   ▽

    M75.21 Bicipital tendinitis, right shoulder

    M75.22 Bicipital tendinitis, left shoulder

  ✓5ᵗʰ **M75.3 Calcific tendinitis of shoulder**

    Calcified bursa of shoulder

    M75.30 Calcific tendinitis of unspecified shoulder   ▽

    M75.31 Calcific tendinitis of right shoulder

    M75.32 Calcific tendinitis of left shoulder

  ✓5ᵗʰ **M75.4 Impingement syndrome of shoulder**

    M75.40 Impingement syndrome of unspecified shoulder ▽

    M75.41 Impingement syndrome of right shoulder

    M75.42 Impingement syndrome of left shoulder

  ✓5ᵗʰ **M75.5 Bursitis of shoulder**

    M75.50 Bursitis of unspecified shoulder   ▽

    M75.51 Bursitis of right shoulder

    M75.52 Bursitis of left shoulder

  ✓5ᵗʰ **M75.8 Other shoulder lesions**

    M75.80 Other shoulder lesions, unspecified shoulder   ▽

    M75.81 Other shoulder lesions, right shoulder

    M75.82 Other shoulder lesions, left shoulder

  ✓5ᵗʰ **M75.9 Shoulder lesion, unspecified**

    M75.90 Shoulder lesion, unspecified, unspecified ▽ **shoulder**

    M75.91 Shoulder lesion, unspecified, right shoulder ▽

    M75.92 Shoulder lesion, unspecified, left shoulder ▽

✓4ᵗʰ **M76 Enthesopathies, lower limb, excluding foot**

    EXCLUDES 2   *bursitis due to use, overuse and pressure (M70.-)*
           enthesopathies of ankle and foot (M77.5-)

  ✓5ᵗʰ **M76.0 Gluteal tendinitis**

    M76.00 Gluteal tendinitis, unspecified hip   ▽

    M76.01 Gluteal tendinitis, right hip

    M76.02 Gluteal tendinitis, left hip

  ✓5ᵗʰ **M76.1 Psoas tendinitis**

    M76.10 Psoas tendinitis, unspecified hip   ▽

    M76.11 Psoas tendinitis, right hip

    M76.12 Psoas tendinitis, left hip

  ✓5ᵗʰ **M76.2 Iliac crest spur**

    M76.20 Iliac crest spur, unspecified hip   ▽

    M76.21 Iliac crest spur, right hip

    M76.22 Iliac crest spur, left hip

  ✓5ᵗʰ **M76.3 Iliotibial band syndrome**

    M76.30 Iliotibial band syndrome, unspecified leg   ▽

    M76.31 Iliotibial band syndrome, right leg

    M76.32 Iliotibial band syndrome, left leg

  ✓5ᵗʰ **M76.4 Tibial collateral bursitis [Pellegrini-Stieda]**

    M76.40 Tibial collateral bursitis [Pellegrini-Stieda], unspecified leg   ▽

    M76.41 Tibial collateral bursitis [Pellegrini-Stieda], right leg

    M76.42 Tibial collateral bursitis [Pellegrini-Stieda], left leg

  ✓5ᵗʰ **M76.5 Patellar tendinitis**

    M76.50 Patellar tendinitis, unspecified knee   ▽

    M76.51 Patellar tendinitis, right knee

    M76.52 Patellar tendinitis, left knee

  ✓5ᵗʰ **M76.6 Achilles tendinitis**

    Achilles bursitis

    M76.60 Achilles tendinitis, unspecified leg   ▽

    M76.61 Achilles tendinitis, right leg

    M76.62 Achilles tendinitis, left leg

  ✓5ᵗʰ **M76.7 Peroneal tendinitis**

    M76.70 Peroneal tendinitis, unspecified leg   ▽

    M76.71 Peroneal tendinitis, right leg

    M76.72 Peroneal tendinitis, left leg

  ✓5ᵗʰ **M76.8 Other specified enthesopathies of lower limb, excluding foot**

    ✓6ᵗʰ **M76.81 Anterior tibial syndrome**

      M76.811 Anterior tibial syndrome, right leg

      M76.812 Anterior tibial syndrome, left leg

      M76.819 Anterior tibial syndrome, unspecified ▽ **leg**

    ✓6ᵗʰ **M76.82 Posterior tibial tendinitis**

      M76.821 Posterior tibial tendinitis, right leg

      M76.822 Posterior tibial tendinitis, left leg

      M76.829 Posterior tibial tendinitis, unspecified ▽ **leg**

✓ Additional Character Req   x7ᵗʰ Placeholder Alert   Manifestation   HCC CMS-HCC Condition   ▽ Unspecified Code   ▶◀ Revised Text   ● New Code   ▲ Revised Code Title

ICD-10-CM 2018   **775**

✓6ᵗʰ **M76.89** **Other specified enthesopathies of lower limb, excluding foot**

   M76.891 Other specified enthesopathies of right lower limb, excluding foot

   M76.892 Other specified enthesopathies of left lower limb, excluding foot

   M76.899 Other specified enthesopathies of unspecified lower limb, excluding foot ▽

M76.9 Unspecified enthesopathy, lower limb, excluding foot ▽

✓4ᵗʰ **M77 Other enthesopathies**

  EXCLUDES 1   bursitis NOS (M71.9-)

  EXCLUDES 2   bursitis due to use, overuse and pressure (M70.-)

          osteophyte (M25.7)

          spinal enthesopathy (M46.0-)

✓5ᵗʰ **M77.0 Medial epicondylitis**

   M77.00 Medial epicondylitis, unspecified elbow ▽

   M77.01 Medial epicondylitis, right elbow

   M77.02 Medial epicondylitis, left elbow

✓5ᵗʰ **M77.1 Lateral epicondylitis**

   Tennis elbow

   M77.10 Lateral epicondylitis, unspecified elbow ▽

   M77.11 Lateral epicondylitis, right elbow

   M77.12 Lateral epicondylitis, left elbow

✓5ᵗʰ **M77.2 Periarthritis of wrist**

   M77.20 Periarthritis, unspecified wrist ▽

   M77.21 Periarthritis, right wrist

   M77.22 Periarthritis, left wrist

✓5ᵗʰ **M77.3 Calcaneal spur**

   DEF: Overgrowth of calcaneus bone on underside of the heel; causes pain on walking; due to chronic avulsion injury of plantar fascia from calcaneus.

   M77.30 Calcaneal spur, unspecified foot ▽

   M77.31 Calcaneal spur, right foot

   M77.32 Calcaneal spur, left foot

✓5ᵗʰ **M77.4 Metatarsalgia**

  EXCLUDES 1   Morton's metatarsalgia (G57.6)

   M77.40 Metatarsalgia, unspecified foot ▽

   M77.41 Metatarsalgia, right foot

   M77.42 Metatarsalgia, left foot

✓5ᵗʰ **M77.5 Other enthesopathy of foot**

   M77.50 Other enthesopathy of unspecified foot ▽

   M77.51 Other enthesopathy of right foot

   M77.52 Other enthesopathy of left foot

M77.8 Other enthesopathies, not elsewhere classified

M77.9 Enthesopathy, unspecified ▽

   Bone spur NOS   Periarthritis NOS

   Capsulitis NOS   Tendinitis NOS

✓4ᵗʰ **M79 Other and unspecified soft tissue disorders, not elsewhere classified**

  EXCLUDES 1   psychogenic rheumatism (F45.8)

          soft tissue pain, psychogenic (F45.41)

M79.0 Rheumatism, unspecified ▽

  EXCLUDES 1   fibromyalgia (M79.7)

          palindromic rheumatism (M12.3-)

M79.1 Myalgia

   Myofascial pain syndrome

  EXCLUDES 1   fibromyalgia (M79.7)

          myositis (M60.-)

M79.2 Neuralgia and neuritis, unspecified ▽

  EXCLUDES 1   brachial radiculitis NOS (M54.1)

          lumbosacral radiculitis NOS (M54.1)

          mononeuropathies (G56-G58)

          radiculitis NOS (M54.1)

          sciatica (M54.3-M54.4)

M79.3 Panniculitis, unspecified ▽

  EXCLUDES 1   lupus panniculitis (L93.2)

          neck and back panniculitis (M54.0-)

          relapsing [Weber-Christian] panniculitis (M35.6)

M79.4 Hypertrophy of (infrapatellar) fat pad

M79.5 Residual foreign body in soft tissue

  EXCLUDES 1   foreign body granuloma of skin and subcutaneous tissue (L92.3)

          foreign body granuloma of soft tissue (M60.2-)

✓5ᵗʰ **M79.6 Pain in limb, hand, foot, fingers and toes**

  EXCLUDES 2   pain in joint (M25.5-)

✓6ᵗʰ **M79.60 Pain in limb, unspecified**

   M79.601 Pain in right arm

         Pain in right upper limb NOS

   M79.602 Pain in left arm

         Pain in left upper limb NOS

   M79.603 Pain in arm, unspecified ▽

         Pain in upper limb NOS

   M79.604 Pain in right leg

         Pain in right lower limb NOS

   M79.605 Pain in left leg

         Pain in left lower limb NOS

   M79.606 Pain in leg, unspecified ▽

         Pain in lower limb NOS

   M79.609 Pain in unspecified limb ▽

         Pain in limb NOS

✓6ᵗʰ **M79.62 Pain in upper arm**

   Pain in axillary region

   M79.621 Pain in right upper arm

   M79.622 Pain in left upper arm

   M79.629 Pain in unspecified upper arm ▽

✓6ᵗʰ **M79.63 Pain in forearm**

   M79.631 Pain in right forearm

   M79.632 Pain in left forearm

   M79.639 Pain in unspecified forearm ▽

✓6ᵗʰ **M79.64 Pain in hand and fingers**

   M79.641 Pain in right hand

   M79.642 Pain in left hand

   M79.643 Pain in unspecified hand ▽

   M79.644 Pain in right finger(s)

   M79.645 Pain in left finger(s)

   M79.646 Pain in unspecified finger(s) ▽

✓6ᵗʰ **M79.65 Pain in thigh**

   M79.651 Pain in right thigh

   M79.652 Pain in left thigh

   M79.659 Pain in unspecified thigh ▽

✓6ᵗʰ **M79.66 Pain in lower leg**

   M79.661 Pain in right lower leg

   M79.662 Pain in left lower leg

   M79.669 Pain in unspecified lower leg ▽

✓6ᵗʰ **M79.67 Pain in foot and toes**

   M79.671 Pain in right foot

   M79.672 Pain in left foot

   M79.673 Pain in unspecified foot ▽

   M79.674 Pain in right toe(s)

   M79.675 Pain in left toe(s)

   M79.676 Pain in unspecified toe(s) ▽

M79.7 Fibromyalgia

   Fibromyositis   Myofibrositis

   Fibrositis

✓5ᵗʰ **M79.A Nontraumatic compartment syndrome**

   Code first, if applicable, associated postprocedural complication

  EXCLUDES 1   compartment syndrome NOS (T79.A-)

          fibromyalgia (M79.7)

          nontraumatic ischemic infarction of muscle (M62.2-)

          traumatic compartment syndrome (T79.A-)

✓6ᵗʰ **M79.A1 Nontraumatic compartment syndrome of upper extremity**

   Nontraumatic compartment syndrome of shoulder, arm, forearm, wrist, hand, and fingers

   M79.A11 Nontraumatic compartment syndrome of right upper extremity

   M79.A12 Nontraumatic compartment syndrome of left upper extremity

   M79.A19 Nontraumatic compartment syndrome ▽ of unspecified upper extremity

✓6ᵗʰ **M79.A2 Nontraumatic compartment syndrome of lower extremity**

   Nontraumatic compartment syndrome of hip, buttock, thigh, leg, foot, and toes

   M79.A21 Nontraumatic compartment syndrome of right lower extremity

   M79.A22 Nontraumatic compartment syndrome of left lower extremity

---

EXCLUDES 1 Not coded here   *EXCLUDES 2* Not included here   N Newborn Age: 0   P Pediatric Age: 0-17   M Maternity Age: 12-55   A Adult Age: 15-124

776   ICD-10-CM 2018

M79.A29 Nontraumatic compartment syndrome ▽
of unspecified lower extremity

M79.A3 Nontraumatic compartment syndrome of abdomen

M79.A9 Nontraumatic compartment syndrome of other sites

✓5ᵗʰ **M79.8** Other specified soft tissue disorders

M79.81 Nontraumatic hematoma of soft tissue
Nontraumatic hematoma of muscle
Nontraumatic seroma of muscle and soft tissue

M79.89 Other specified soft tissue disorders
Polyalgia

M79.9 Soft tissue disorder, unspecified ▽

OSTEOPATHIES AND CHONDROPATHIES (M80-M94)

Disorders of bone density and structure (M80-M85)

✓4ᵗʰ **M80** Osteoporosis with current pathological fracture

INCLUDES osteoporosis with current fragility fracture

Use additional code to identify major osseous defect, if applicable (M89.7-)

EXCLUDES 1 collapsed vertebra NOS (M48.5)
pathological fracture NOS (M84.4)
wedging of vertebra NOS (M48.5)

EXCLUDES 2 personal history of (healed) osteoporosis fracture (Z87.310)

The appropriate 7th character is to be added to each code from category M80.
A   initial encounter for fracture
D   subsequent encounter for fracture with routine healing
G   subsequent encounter for fracture with delayed healing
K   subsequent encounter for fracture with nonunion
P   subsequent encounter for fracture with malunion
S   sequela

✓5ᵗʰ **M80.0** Age-related osteoporosis with current pathological fracture
Involutional osteoporosis with current pathological fracture
Osteoporosis NOS with current pathological fracture
Postmenopausal osteoporosis with current pathological fracture
Senile osteoporosis with current pathological fracture

✓x7ᵗʰ **M80.00** Age-related osteoporosis with current ⒜ ▽
pathological fracture, unspecified site

✓6ᵗʰ **M80.01** Age-related osteoporosis with current pathological fracture, shoulder

✓7ᵗʰ **M80.011** Age-related osteoporosis with current ⒜
pathological fracture, right shoulder

✓7ᵗʰ **M80.012** Age-related osteoporosis with current ⒜
pathological fracture, left shoulder

✓7ᵗʰ **M80.019** Age-related osteoporosis with ⒜ ▽
current pathological fracture,
unspecified shoulder

✓6ᵗʰ **M80.02** Age-related osteoporosis with current pathological fracture, humerus

✓7ᵗʰ **M80.021** Age-related osteoporosis with current ⒜
pathological fracture, right humerus

✓7ᵗʰ **M80.022** Age-related osteoporosis with current ⒜
pathological fracture, left humerus

✓7ᵗʰ **M80.029** Age-related osteoporosis with ⒜ ▽
current pathological fracture,
unspecified humerus

✓6ᵗʰ **M80.03** Age-related osteoporosis with current pathological fracture, forearm
Age-related osteoporosis with current pathological fracture of wrist

✓7ᵗʰ **M80.031** Age-related osteoporosis with current ⒜
pathological fracture, right forearm

✓7ᵗʰ **M80.032** Age-related osteoporosis with current ⒜
pathological fracture, left forearm

✓7ᵗʰ **M80.039** Age-related osteoporosis with ⒜ ▽
current pathological fracture,
unspecified forearm

✓6ᵗʰ **M80.04** Age-related osteoporosis with current pathological fracture, hand

✓7ᵗʰ **M80.041** Age-related osteoporosis with current ⒜
pathological fracture, right hand

✓7ᵗʰ **M80.042** Age-related osteoporosis with current ⒜
pathological fracture, left hand

✓7ᵗʰ **M80.049** Age-related osteoporosis with ⒜ ▽
current pathological fracture,
unspecified hand

✓6ᵗʰ **M80.05** Age-related osteoporosis with current pathological fracture, femur
Age-related osteoporosis with current pathological fracture of hip

[1] ✓7ᵗʰ **M80.051** Age-related osteoporosis with HCC ⒜
current pathological fracture,
right femur

[1] ✓7ᵗʰ **M80.052** Age-related osteoporosis with HCC ⒜
current pathological fracture,
left femur

[1] ✓7ᵗʰ **M80.059** Age-related osteoporosis with HCC ⒜ ▽
current pathological fracture,
unspecified femur

✓6ᵗʰ **M80.06** Age-related osteoporosis with current pathological fracture, lower leg

✓7ᵗʰ **M80.061** Age-related osteoporosis with current ⒜
pathological fracture, right lower leg

✓7ᵗʰ **M80.062** Age-related osteoporosis with current ⒜
pathological fracture, left lower leg

✓7ᵗʰ **M80.069** Age-related osteoporosis with ⒜ ▽
current pathological fracture,
unspecified lower leg

✓6ᵗʰ **M80.07** Age-related osteoporosis with current pathological fracture, ankle and foot

✓7ᵗʰ **M80.071** Age-related osteoporosis with current ⒜
pathological fracture, right ankle and foot

✓7ᵗʰ **M80.072** Age-related osteoporosis with current ⒜
pathological fracture, left ankle and foot

✓7ᵗʰ **M80.079** Age-related osteoporosis with ⒜ ▽
current pathological fracture,
unspecified ankle and foot

[1] ✓x7ᵗʰ **M80.08** Age-related osteoporosis with current HCC ⒜
pathological fracture, vertebra(e)

✓5ᵗʰ **M80.8** Other osteoporosis with current pathological fracture
Drug-induced osteoporosis with current pathological fracture
Idiopathic osteoporosis with current pathological fracture
Osteoporosis of disuse with current pathological fracture
Postoophorectomy osteoporosis with current pathological fracture
Postsurgical malabsorption osteoporosis with current pathological fracture
Post-traumatic osteoporosis with current pathological fracture
Use additional code for adverse effect, if applicable, to identify drug (T36-T50 with fifth or sixth character 5)

✓x7ᵗʰ **M80.80** Other osteoporosis with current pathological ▽
fracture, unspecified site

✓6ᵗʰ **M80.81** Other osteoporosis with pathological fracture, shoulder

✓7ᵗʰ **M80.811** Other osteoporosis with current
pathological fracture, right shoulder

✓7ᵗʰ **M80.812** Other osteoporosis with current
pathological fracture, left shoulder

✓7ᵗʰ **M80.819** Other osteoporosis with current ▽
pathological fracture, unspecified
shoulder

✓6ᵗʰ **M80.82** Other osteoporosis with current pathological fracture, humerus

✓7ᵗʰ **M80.821** Other osteoporosis with current
pathological fracture, right humerus

✓7ᵗʰ **M80.822** Other osteoporosis with current
pathological fracture, left humerus

✓7ᵗʰ **M80.829** Other osteoporosis with current ▽
pathological fracture, unspecified
humerus

✓6ᵗʰ **M80.83** Other osteoporosis with current pathological fracture, forearm
Other osteoporosis with current pathological fracture of wrist

✓7ᵗʰ **M80.831** Other osteoporosis with current
pathological fracture, right forearm

✓7ᵗʰ **M80.832** Other osteoporosis with current
pathological fracture, left forearm

✓7ᵗʰ **M80.839** Other osteoporosis with current ▽
pathological fracture, unspecified forearm

---

[1] HCC with 7th character indicating initial encounter (A, B or C - specific to category).

☑ Additional Character Req   ✓x7ᵗʰ Placeholder Alert   Manifestation   HCC CMS-HCC Condition   ▽ Unspecified Code   ▶◀ Revised Text   ● New Code   ▲ Revised Code Title

Chapter 13. Diseases of the Musculoskeletal System and Connective Tissue

M80.84–M84.369

✓6th **M80.84 Other osteoporosis with current pathological fracture, hand**

    ✓7th **M80.841 Other osteoporosis with current pathological fracture, right hand**

    ✓7th **M80.842 Other osteoporosis with current pathological fracture, left hand**

    ✓7th **M80.849 Other osteoporosis with current pathological fracture, unspecified hand** ▽

✓6th **M80.85 Other osteoporosis with current pathological fracture, femur**

    Other osteoporosis with current pathological fracture of hip

    1 ✓7th **M80.851 Other osteoporosis with current pathological fracture, right femur** HCC

    1 ✓7th **M80.852 Other osteoporosis with current pathological fracture, left femur** HCC

    1 ✓7th **M80.859 Other osteoporosis with current pathological fracture, unspecified femur** HCC ▽

✓6th **M80.86 Other osteoporosis with current pathological fracture, lower leg**

    ✓7th **M80.861 Other osteoporosis with current pathological fracture, right lower leg**

    ✓7th **M80.862 Other osteoporosis with current pathological fracture, left lower leg**

    ✓7th **M80.869 Other osteoporosis with current pathological fracture, unspecified lower leg** ▽

✓6th **M80.87 Other osteoporosis with current pathological fracture, ankle and foot**

    ✓7th **M80.871 Other osteoporosis with current pathological fracture, right ankle and foot**

    ✓7th **M80.872 Other osteoporosis with current pathological fracture, left ankle and foot**

    ✓7th **M80.879 Other osteoporosis with current pathological fracture, unspecified ankle and foot** ▽

1 ✓x7th **M80.88 Other osteoporosis with current pathological fracture, vertebra(e)** HCC

✓4th **M81 Osteoporosis without current pathological fracture**

    Use additional code to identify:
    major osseous defect, if applicable (M89.7-)
    personal history of (healed) osteoporosis fracture, if applicable (Z87.310)

    EXCLUDES 1   osteoporosis with current pathological fracture (M80.-)
         Sudeck's atrophy (M89.0)

M81.0 Age-related osteoporosis without current pathological fracture Ⓐ

    Involutional osteoporosis without current pathological fracture
    Osteoporosis NOS
    Postmenopausal osteoporosis without current pathological fracture
    Senile osteoporosis without current pathological fracture

M81.6 Localized osteoporosis [Lequesne]

    EXCLUDES 1   Sudeck's atrophy (M89.0)

M81.8 Other osteoporosis without current pathological fracture

    Drug-induced osteoporosis without current pathological fracture
    Idiopathic osteoporosis without current pathological fracture
    Osteoporosis of disuse without current pathological fracture
    Postoophorectomy osteoporosis without current pathological fracture
    Postsurgical malabsorption osteoporosis without current pathological fracture
    Post-traumatic osteoporosis without current pathological fracture

    Use additional code for adverse effect, if applicable, to identify drug (T36-T50 with fifth or sixth character 5)

✓4th **M83 Adult osteomalacia**

    EXCLUDES 1   infantile and juvenile osteomalacia (E55.0)
         renal osteodystrophy (N25.0)
         rickets (active) (E55.0)
         rickets (active) sequelae (E64.3)
         vitamin D-resistant osteomalacia (E83.3)
         vitamin D-resistant rickets (active) (E83.3)

M83.0 Puerperal osteomalacia Ⓜ♀

M83.1 Senile osteomalacia Ⓐ

M83.2 Adult osteomalacia due to malabsorption Ⓐ

    Postsurgical malabsorption osteomalacia in adults

M83.3 Adult osteomalacia due to malnutrition Ⓐ

M83.4 Aluminum bone disease

M83.5 Other drug-induced osteomalacia in adults Ⓐ

    Use additional code for adverse effect, if applicable, to identify drug (T36-T50 with fifth or sixth character 5)

M83.8 Other adult osteomalacia Ⓐ

M83.9 Adult osteomalacia, unspecified Ⓐ▽

✓4th **M84 Disorder of continuity of bone**

    EXCLUDES 2   traumatic fracture of bone-see fracture, by site

✓5th **M84.3 Stress fracture**

    Fatigue fracture   Stress fracture NOS
    March fracture   Stress reaction
    Use additional external cause code(s) to identify the cause of the stress fracture

    EXCLUDES 1   pathological fracture NOS (M84.4-)
         pathological fracture due to osteoporosis (M80.-)
         traumatic fracture (S12-, S22-, S32-, S42-, S52-, S62-, S72-, S82-, S92-)

    EXCLUDES 2   personal history of (healed) stress (fatigue) fracture (Z87.312)
         stress fracture of vertebra (M48.4-)

    The appropriate 7th character is to be added to each code from subcategory M84.3.
    A   initial encounter for fracture
    D   subsequent encounter for fracture with routine healing
    G   subsequent encounter for fracture with delayed healing
    K   subsequent encounter for fracture with nonunion
    P   subsequent encounter for fracture with malunion
    S   sequela

    ✓x7th **M84.30 Stress fracture, unspecified site** ▽

    ✓6th **M84.31 Stress fracture, shoulder**

       ✓7th **M84.311 Stress fracture, right shoulder**

       ✓7th **M84.312 Stress fracture, left shoulder**

       ✓7th **M84.319 Stress fracture, unspecified shoulder** ▽

    ✓6th **M84.32 Stress fracture, humerus**

       ✓7th **M84.321 Stress fracture, right humerus**

       ✓7th **M84.322 Stress fracture, left humerus**

       ✓7th **M84.329 Stress fracture, unspecified humerus** ▽

    ✓6th **M84.33 Stress fracture, ulna and radius**

       ✓7th **M84.331 Stress fracture, right ulna**

       ✓7th **M84.332 Stress fracture, left ulna**

       ✓7th **M84.333 Stress fracture, right radius**

       ✓7th **M84.334 Stress fracture, left radius**

       ✓7th **M84.339 Stress fracture, unspecified ulna and radius** ▽

    ✓6th **M84.34 Stress fracture, hand and fingers**

       ✓7th **M84.341 Stress fracture, right hand**

       ✓7th **M84.342 Stress fracture, left hand**

       ✓7th **M84.343 Stress fracture, unspecified hand** ▽

       ✓7th **M84.344 Stress fracture, right finger(s)**

       ✓7th **M84.345 Stress fracture, left finger(s)**

       ✓7th **M84.346 Stress fracture, unspecified finger(s)** ▽

    ✓6th **M84.35 Stress fracture, pelvis and femur**

       Stress fracture, hip

       ✓7th **M84.350 Stress fracture, pelvis**

       ✓7th **M84.351 Stress fracture, right femur**

       ✓7th **M84.352 Stress fracture, left femur**

       ✓7th **M84.353 Stress fracture, unspecified femur** ▽

       ✓7th **M84.359 Stress fracture, hip, unspecified** ▽

    ✓6th **M84.36 Stress fracture, tibia and fibula**

       ✓7th **M84.361 Stress fracture, right tibia**

       ✓7th **M84.362 Stress fracture, left tibia**

       ✓7th **M84.363 Stress fracture, right fibula**

       ✓7th **M84.364 Stress fracture, left fibula**

       ✓7th **M84.369 Stress fracture, unspecified tibia and fibula** ▽

---

1   HCC with 7th character indicating initial encounter (A, B or C - specific to category).

EXCLUDES 1 Not coded here   EXCLUDES 2 Not included here   Ⓝ Newborn Age: 0   Ⓟ Pediatric Age: 0-17   Ⓜ Maternity Age: 12-55   Ⓐ Adult Age: 15-124

778   ICD-10-CM 2018

√6ᵗʰ **M84.37** Stress fracture, ankle, foot and toes
- √7ᵗʰ **M84.371** Stress fracture, right ankle
- √7ᵗʰ **M84.372** Stress fracture, left ankle
- √7ᵗʰ **M84.373** Stress fracture, unspecified ankle ▽
- √7ᵗʰ **M84.374** Stress fracture, right foot
- √7ᵗʰ **M84.375** Stress fracture, left foot
- √7ᵗʰ **M84.376** Stress fracture, unspecified foot ▽
- √7ᵗʰ **M84.377** Stress fracture, right toe(s)
- √7ᵗʰ **M84.378** Stress fracture, left toe(s)
- √7ᵗʰ **M84.379** Stress fracture, unspecified toe(s) ▽

√x7ᵗʰ **M84.38** Stress fracture, other site
- *EXCLUDES 2*   stress fracture of vertebra (M48.4-)

√5ᵗʰ **M84.4** Pathological fracture, not elsewhere classified
Chronic fracture
Pathological fracture NOS
- *EXCLUDES 1*   collapsed vertebra NEC (M48.5)
pathological fracture in neoplastic disease (M84.5-)
pathological fracture in osteoporosis (M80.-)
pathological fracture in other disease (M84.6-)
stress fracture (M84.3-)
traumatic fracture (S12.-, S22.-, S32.-, S42.-, S52.-, S62.-, S72.-, S82.-, S92.-)
- *EXCLUDES 2*   personal history of (healed) pathological fracture (Z87.311)

The appropriate 7th character is to be added to each code from subcategory M84.4.
A   initial encounter for fracture
D   subsequent encounter for fracture with routine healing
G   subsequent encounter for fracture with delayed healing
K   subsequent encounter for fracture with nonunion
P   subsequent encounter for fracture with malunion
S   sequela

√x7ᵗʰ **M84.40** Pathological fracture, unspecified site ▽

√6ᵗʰ **M84.41** Pathological fracture, shoulder
- √7ᵗʰ **M84.411** Pathological fracture, right shoulder
- √7ᵗʰ **M84.412** Pathological fracture, left shoulder
- √7ᵗʰ **M84.419** Pathological fracture, unspecified shoulder ▽

√6ᵗʰ **M84.42** Pathological fracture, humerus
- √7ᵗʰ **M84.421** Pathological fracture, right humerus
- √7ᵗʰ **M84.422** Pathological fracture, left humerus
- √7ᵗʰ **M84.429** Pathological fracture, unspecified humerus ▽

√6ᵗʰ **M84.43** Pathological fracture, ulna and radius
- √7ᵗʰ **M84.431** Pathological fracture, right ulna
- √7ᵗʰ **M84.432** Pathological fracture, left ulna
- √7ᵗʰ **M84.433** Pathological fracture, right radius
- √7ᵗʰ **M84.434** Pathological fracture, left radius
- √7ᵗʰ **M84.439** Pathological fracture, unspecified ulna and radius ▽

√6ᵗʰ **M84.44** Pathological fracture, hand and fingers
- √7ᵗʰ **M84.441** Pathological fracture, right hand
- √7ᵗʰ **M84.442** Pathological fracture, left hand
- √7ᵗʰ **M84.443** Pathological fracture, unspecified hand ▽
- √7ᵗʰ **M84.444** Pathological fracture, right finger(s)
- √7ᵗʰ **M84.445** Pathological fracture, left finger(s)
- √7ᵗʰ **M84.446** Pathological fracture, unspecified finger(s) ▽

√6ᵗʰ **M84.45** Pathological fracture, femur and pelvis
- 1 √7ᵗʰ **M84.451** Pathological fracture, right femur `HCC`
- 1 √7ᵗʰ **M84.452** Pathological fracture, left femur `HCC`
- 1 √7ᵗʰ **M84.453** Pathological fracture, unspecified femur `HCC` ▽
- √7ᵗʰ **M84.454** Pathological fracture, pelvis
- 1 √7ᵗʰ **M84.459** Pathological fracture, hip, unspecified `HCC` ▽

√6ᵗʰ **M84.46** Pathological fracture, tibia and fibula
- √7ᵗʰ **M84.461** Pathological fracture, right tibia
- √7ᵗʰ **M84.462** Pathological fracture, left tibia
- √7ᵗʰ **M84.463** Pathological fracture, right fibula
- √7ᵗʰ **M84.464** Pathological fracture, left fibula

- √7ᵗʰ **M84.469** Pathological fracture, unspecified tibia and fibula ▽

√6ᵗʰ **M84.47** Pathological fracture, ankle, foot and toes
- √7ᵗʰ **M84.471** Pathological fracture, right ankle
- √7ᵗʰ **M84.472** Pathological fracture, left ankle
- √7ᵗʰ **M84.473** Pathological fracture, unspecified ankle ▽
- √7ᵗʰ **M84.474** Pathological fracture, right foot
- √7ᵗʰ **M84.475** Pathological fracture, left foot
- √7ᵗʰ **M84.476** Pathological fracture, unspecified foot ▽
- √7ᵗʰ **M84.477** Pathological fracture, right toe(s)
- √7ᵗʰ **M84.478** Pathological fracture, left toe(s)
- √7ᵗʰ **M84.479** Pathological fracture, unspecified toe(s) ▽

√x7ᵗʰ **M84.48** Pathological fracture, other site

√5ᵗʰ **M84.5** Pathological fracture in neoplastic disease
Code also underlying neoplasm

The appropriate 7th character is to be added to each code from subcategory M84.5.
A   initial encounter for fracture
D   subsequent encounter for fracture with routine healing
G   subsequent encounter for fracture with delayed healing
K   subsequent encounter for fracture with nonunion
P   subsequent encounter for fracture with malunion
S   sequela

√x7ᵗʰ **M84.50** Pathological fracture in neoplastic disease, unspecified site ▽

√6ᵗʰ **M84.51** Pathological fracture in neoplastic disease, shoulder
- √7ᵗʰ **M84.511** Pathological fracture in neoplastic disease, right shoulder
- √7ᵗʰ **M84.512** Pathological fracture in neoplastic disease, left shoulder
- √7ᵗʰ **M84.519** Pathological fracture in neoplastic disease, unspecified shoulder ▽

√6ᵗʰ **M84.52** Pathological fracture in neoplastic disease, humerus
- √7ᵗʰ **M84.521** Pathological fracture in neoplastic disease, right humerus
- √7ᵗʰ **M84.522** Pathological fracture in neoplastic disease, left humerus
- √7ᵗʰ **M84.529** Pathological fracture in neoplastic disease, unspecified humerus ▽

√6ᵗʰ **M84.53** Pathological fracture in neoplastic disease, ulna and radius
- √7ᵗʰ **M84.531** Pathological fracture in neoplastic disease, right ulna
- √7ᵗʰ **M84.532** Pathological fracture in neoplastic disease, left ulna
- √7ᵗʰ **M84.533** Pathological fracture in neoplastic disease, right radius
- √7ᵗʰ **M84.534** Pathological fracture in neoplastic disease, left radius
- √7ᵗʰ **M84.539** Pathological fracture in neoplastic disease, unspecified ulna and radius ▽

√6ᵗʰ **M84.54** Pathological fracture in neoplastic disease, hand
- √7ᵗʰ **M84.541** Pathological fracture in neoplastic disease, right hand
- √7ᵗʰ **M84.542** Pathological fracture in neoplastic disease, left hand
- √7ᵗʰ **M84.549** Pathological fracture in neoplastic disease, unspecified hand ▽

√6ᵗʰ **M84.55** Pathological fracture in neoplastic disease, pelvis and femur
- √7ᵗʰ **M84.550** Pathological fracture in neoplastic disease, pelvis
- 1 √7ᵗʰ **M84.551** Pathological fracture in neoplastic disease, right femur `HCC`
- 1 √7ᵗʰ **M84.552** Pathological fracture in neoplastic disease, left femur `HCC`
- 1 √7ᵗʰ **M84.553** Pathological fracture in neoplastic disease, unspecified femur `HCC` ▽
- 1 √7ᵗʰ **M84.559** Pathological fracture in neoplastic disease, hip, unspecified `HCC` ▽

---

1   HCC with 7th character indicating initial encounter (A, B or C - specific to category).

☑ Additional Character Req   √x7ᵗʰ Placeholder Alert   Manifestation   `HCC` CMS-HCC Condition   ▽ Unspecified Code   ►◄ Revised Text   ● New Code   ▲ Revised Code Title

Chapter 13. Diseases of the Musculoskeletal System and Connective Tissue

✓6ᵗʰ **M84.56** **Pathological fracture in neoplastic disease,** tibia and fibula

    ✓7ᵗʰ **M84.561** **Pathological fracture in neoplastic disease,** right tibia

    ✓7ᵗʰ **M84.562** **Pathological fracture in neoplastic disease,** left tibia

    ✓7ᵗʰ **M84.563** **Pathological fracture in neoplastic disease,** right fibula

    ✓7ᵗʰ **M84.564** **Pathological fracture in neoplastic disease,** left fibula

    ✓7ᵗʰ **M84.569** **Pathological fracture in neoplastic disease,** unspecified tibia and fibula ▽

✓6ᵗʰ **M84.57** **Pathological fracture in neoplastic disease,** ankle and foot

    ✓7ᵗʰ **M84.571** **Pathological fracture in neoplastic disease,** right ankle

    ✓7ᵗʰ **M84.572** **Pathological fracture in neoplastic disease,** left ankle

    ✓7ᵗʰ **M84.573** **Pathological fracture in neoplastic disease,** unspecified ankle ▽

    ✓7ᵗʰ **M84.574** **Pathological fracture in neoplastic disease,** right foot

    ✓7ᵗʰ **M84.575** **Pathological fracture in neoplastic disease,** left foot

    ✓7ᵗʰ **M84.576** **Pathological fracture in neoplastic disease,** unspecified foot ▽

✓x7ᵗʰ **M84.58** **Pathological fracture in neoplastic disease, other specified site**
         Pathological fracture in neoplastic disease, vertebrae

✓5ᵗʰ **M84.6** **Pathological fracture in other disease**
    Code also underlying condition
    EXCLUDES 1   *pathological fracture in osteoporosis (M80.-)*

> The appropriate 7th character is to be added to each code from subcategory M84.6.
> A   initial encounter for fracture
> D   subsequent encounter for fracture with routine healing
> G   subsequent encounter for fracture with delayed healing
> K   subsequent encounter for fracture with nonunion
> P   subsequent encounter for fracture with malunion
> S   sequela

✓x7ᵗʰ **M84.60** **Pathological fracture in other disease, unspecified site** ▽

✓6ᵗʰ **M84.61** **Pathological fracture in other disease,** shoulder

    ✓7ᵗʰ **M84.611** **Pathological fracture in other disease,** right shoulder

    ✓7ᵗʰ **M84.612** **Pathological fracture in other disease,** left shoulder

    ✓7ᵗʰ **M84.619** **Pathological fracture in other disease,** unspecified shoulder ▽

✓6ᵗʰ **M84.62** **Pathological fracture in other disease,** humerus

    ✓7ᵗʰ **M84.621** **Pathological fracture in other disease,** right humerus

    ✓7ᵗʰ **M84.622** **Pathological fracture in other disease,** left humerus

    ✓7ᵗʰ **M84.629** **Pathological fracture in other disease,** unspecified humerus ▽

✓6ᵗʰ **M84.63** **Pathological fracture in other disease,** ulna and radius

    ✓7ᵗʰ **M84.631** **Pathological fracture in other disease,** right ulna

    ✓7ᵗʰ **M84.632** **Pathological fracture in other disease,** left ulna

    ✓7ᵗʰ **M84.633** **Pathological fracture in other disease,** right radius

    ✓7ᵗʰ **M84.634** **Pathological fracture in other disease,** left radius

    ✓7ᵗʰ **M84.639** **Pathological fracture in other disease,** unspecified ulna and radius ▽

✓6ᵗʰ **M84.64** **Pathological fracture in other disease,** hand

    ✓7ᵗʰ **M84.641** **Pathological fracture in other disease,** right hand

    ✓7ᵗʰ **M84.642** **Pathological fracture in other disease,** left hand

    ✓7ᵗʰ **M84.649** **Pathological fracture in other disease,** unspecified hand ▽

✓6ᵗʰ **M84.65** **Pathological fracture in other disease,** pelvis and femur

    ✓7ᵗʰ **M84.650** **Pathological fracture in other disease,** pelvis

    1 ✓7ᵗʰ **M84.651** **Pathological fracture in other disease,** right femur   HCC

    1 ✓7ᵗʰ **M84.652** **Pathological fracture in other disease,** left femur   HCC

    1 ✓7ᵗʰ **M84.653** **Pathological fracture in other disease,** unspecified femur   HCC ▽

    1 ✓7ᵗʰ **M84.659** **Pathological fracture in other disease, hip, unspecified**   HCC ▽

✓6ᵗʰ **M84.66** **Pathological fracture in other disease,** tibia and fibula

    ✓7ᵗʰ **M84.661** **Pathological fracture in other disease,** right tibia

    ✓7ᵗʰ **M84.662** **Pathological fracture in other disease,** left tibia

    ✓7ᵗʰ **M84.663** **Pathological fracture in other disease,** right fibula

    ✓7ᵗʰ **M84.664** **Pathological fracture in other disease,** left fibula

    ✓7ᵗʰ **M84.669** **Pathological fracture in other disease,** unspecified tibia and fibula ▽

✓6ᵗʰ **M84.67** **Pathological fracture in other disease,** ankle and foot

    ✓7ᵗʰ **M84.671** **Pathological fracture in other disease,** right ankle

    ✓7ᵗʰ **M84.672** **Pathological fracture in other disease,** left ankle

    ✓7ᵗʰ **M84.673** **Pathological fracture in other disease,** unspecified ankle ▽

    ✓7ᵗʰ **M84.674** **Pathological fracture in other disease,** right foot

    ✓7ᵗʰ **M84.675** **Pathological fracture in other disease,** left foot

    ✓7ᵗʰ **M84.676** **Pathological fracture in other disease,** unspecified foot ▽

✓x7ᵗʰ **M84.68** **Pathological fracture in other disease, other site**

✓5ᵗʰ **M84.7** **Nontraumatic fracture, not elsewhere classified**

✓6ᵗʰ **M84.75** **Atypical** femoral fracture

> The appropriate 7th character is to be added to each code from subcategory M84.75.
> A   initial encounter for fracture
> D   subsequent encounter for fracture with routine healing
> G   subsequent encounter for fracture with delayed healing
> K   subsequent encounter for fracture with nonunion
> P   subsequent encounter for fracture with malunion
> S   sequela

    ✓7ᵗʰ **M84.750** **Atypical femoral fracture, unspecified** ▽

    ✓7ᵗʰ **M84.751** **Incomplete atypical femoral fracture,** right leg

    ✓7ᵗʰ **M84.752** **Incomplete atypical femoral fracture,** left leg

    ✓7ᵗʰ **M84.753** **Incomplete atypical femoral fracture,** unspecified leg ▽

    1 ✓7ᵗʰ **M84.754** **Complete transverse atypical femoral fracture,** right leg   HCC

    1 ✓7ᵗʰ **M84.755** **Complete transverse atypical femoral fracture,** left leg   HCC

    1 ✓7ᵗʰ **M84.756** **Complete transverse atypical femoral fracture, unspecified leg**   HCC ▽

    1 ✓7ᵗʰ **M84.757** **Complete oblique atypical femoral fracture,** right leg   HCC

    1 ✓7ᵗʰ **M84.758** **Complete oblique atypical femoral fracture,** left leg   HCC

    1 ✓7ᵗʰ **M84.759** **Complete oblique atypical femoral fracture, unspecified leg**   HCC ▽

---

1   HCC with 7th character indicating initial encounter (A, B or C - specific to category).

EXCLUDES 1 Not coded here   **EXCLUDES 2** Not included here   N Newborn Age: 0   P Pediatric Age: 0-17   M Maternity Age: 12-55   A Adult Age: 15-124

780   ICD-10-CM 2018

✓5ᵗʰ **M84.8 Other disorders of continuity of bone**

     M84.80 Other disorders of continuity of bone, unspecified site ▽

     ✓6ᵗʰ **M84.81 Other disorders of continuity of bone, shoulder**

       M84.811 Other disorders of continuity of bone, right shoulder

       M84.812 Other disorders of continuity of bone, left shoulder

       M84.819 Other disorders of continuity of bone, unspecified shoulder ▽

     ✓6ᵗʰ **M84.82 Other disorders of continuity of bone, humerus**

       M84.821 Other disorders of continuity of bone, right humerus

       M84.822 Other disorders of continuity of bone, left humerus

       M84.829 Other disorders of continuity of bone, unspecified humerus ▽

     ✓6ᵗʰ **M84.83 Other disorders of continuity of bone, ulna and radius**

       M84.831 Other disorders of continuity of bone, right ulna

       M84.832 Other disorders of continuity of bone, left ulna

       M84.833 Other disorders of continuity of bone, right radius

       M84.834 Other disorders of continuity of bone, left radius

       M84.839 Other disorders of continuity of bone, unspecified ulna and radius ▽

     ✓6ᵗʰ **M84.84 Other disorders of continuity of bone, hand**

       M84.841 Other disorders of continuity of bone, right hand

       M84.842 Other disorders of continuity of bone, left hand

       M84.849 Other disorders of continuity of bone, unspecified hand ▽

     ✓6ᵗʰ **M84.85 Other disorders of continuity of bone, pelvic region and thigh**

       M84.851 Other disorders of continuity of bone, right pelvic region and thigh

       M84.852 Other disorders of continuity of bone, left pelvic region and thigh

       M84.859 Other disorders of continuity of bone, unspecified pelvic region and thigh ▽

     ✓6ᵗʰ **M84.86 Other disorders of continuity of bone, tibia and fibula**

       M84.861 Other disorders of continuity of bone, right tibia

       M84.862 Other disorders of continuity of bone, left tibia

       M84.863 Other disorders of continuity of bone, right fibula

       M84.864 Other disorders of continuity of bone, left fibula

       M84.869 Other disorders of continuity of bone, unspecified tibia and fibula ▽

     ✓6ᵗʰ **M84.87 Other disorders of continuity of bone, ankle and foot**

       M84.871 Other disorders of continuity of bone, right ankle and foot

       M84.872 Other disorders of continuity of bone, left ankle and foot

       M84.879 Other disorders of continuity of bone, unspecified ankle and foot ▽

     M84.88 Other disorders of continuity of bone, other site

   M84.9 Disorder of continuity of bone, unspecified ▽

✓4ᵗʰ **M85 Other disorders of bone density and structure**

     EXCLUDES 1   osteogenesis imperfecta (Q78.0)
                 osteopetrosis (Q78.2)
                 osteopoikilosis (Q78.8)
                 polyostotic fibrous dysplasia (Q78.1)

   ✓5ᵗʰ **M85.0 Fibrous dysplasia (monostotic)**

     EXCLUDES 2   fibrous dysplasia of jaw (M27.8)

     M85.00 Fibrous dysplasia (monostotic), unspecified site ▽

     ✓6ᵗʰ **M85.01 Fibrous dysplasia (monostotic), shoulder**

       M85.011 Fibrous dysplasia (monostotic), right shoulder

       M85.012 Fibrous dysplasia (monostotic), left shoulder

       M85.019 Fibrous dysplasia (monostotic), unspecified shoulder ▽

     ✓6ᵗʰ **M85.02 Fibrous dysplasia (monostotic), upper arm**

       M85.021 Fibrous dysplasia (monostotic), right upper arm

       M85.022 Fibrous dysplasia (monostotic), left upper arm

       M85.029 Fibrous dysplasia (monostotic), unspecified upper arm ▽

     ✓6ᵗʰ **M85.03 Fibrous dysplasia (monostotic), forearm**

       M85.031 Fibrous dysplasia (monostotic), right forearm

       M85.032 Fibrous dysplasia (monostotic), left forearm

       M85.039 Fibrous dysplasia (monostotic), unspecified forearm ▽

     ✓6ᵗʰ **M85.04 Fibrous dysplasia (monostotic), hand**

       M85.041 Fibrous dysplasia (monostotic), right hand

       M85.042 Fibrous dysplasia (monostotic), left hand

       M85.049 Fibrous dysplasia (monostotic), unspecified hand ▽

     ✓6ᵗʰ **M85.05 Fibrous dysplasia (monostotic), thigh**

       M85.051 Fibrous dysplasia (monostotic), right thigh

       M85.052 Fibrous dysplasia (monostotic), left thigh

       M85.059 Fibrous dysplasia (monostotic), unspecified thigh ▽

     ✓6ᵗʰ **M85.06 Fibrous dysplasia (monostotic), lower leg**

       M85.061 Fibrous dysplasia (monostotic), right lower leg

       M85.062 Fibrous dysplasia (monostotic), left lower leg

       M85.069 Fibrous dysplasia (monostotic), unspecified lower leg ▽

     ✓6ᵗʰ **M85.07 Fibrous dysplasia (monostotic), ankle and foot**

       M85.071 Fibrous dysplasia (monostotic), right ankle and foot

       M85.072 Fibrous dysplasia (monostotic), left ankle and foot

       M85.079 Fibrous dysplasia (monostotic), unspecified ankle and foot ▽

     M85.08 Fibrous dysplasia (monostotic), other site

     M85.09 Fibrous dysplasia (monostotic), multiple sites

   ✓5ᵗʰ **M85.1 Skeletal fluorosis**

     M85.10 Skeletal fluorosis, unspecified site ▽

     ✓6ᵗʰ **M85.11 Skeletal fluorosis, shoulder**

       M85.111 Skeletal fluorosis, right shoulder

       M85.112 Skeletal fluorosis, left shoulder

       M85.119 Skeletal fluorosis, unspecified shoulder ▽

     ✓6ᵗʰ **M85.12 Skeletal fluorosis, upper arm**

       M85.121 Skeletal fluorosis, right upper arm

       M85.122 Skeletal fluorosis, left upper arm

       M85.129 Skeletal fluorosis, unspecified upper arm ▽

     ✓6ᵗʰ **M85.13 Skeletal fluorosis, forearm**

       M85.131 Skeletal fluorosis, right forearm

       M85.132 Skeletal fluorosis, left forearm

       M85.139 Skeletal fluorosis, unspecified forearm ▽

     ✓6ᵗʰ **M85.14 Skeletal fluorosis, hand**

       M85.141 Skeletal fluorosis, right hand

       M85.142 Skeletal fluorosis, left hand

       M85.149 Skeletal fluorosis, unspecified hand ▽

     ✓6ᵗʰ **M85.15 Skeletal fluorosis, thigh**

       M85.151 Skeletal fluorosis, right thigh

       M85.152 Skeletal fluorosis, left thigh

       M85.159 Skeletal fluorosis, unspecified thigh ▽

     ✓6ᵗʰ **M85.16 Skeletal fluorosis, lower leg**

       M85.161 Skeletal fluorosis, right lower leg

       M85.162 Skeletal fluorosis, left lower leg

       M85.169 Skeletal fluorosis, unspecified lower leg ▽

☑ Additional Character Req   ✓×7ᵗʰ Placeholder Alert   Manifestation   HCC CMS-HCC Condition   ▽ Unspecified Code   ▶◀ Revised Text   ● New Code   ▲ Revised Code Title

✓6ᵗʰ **M85.17 Skeletal fluorosis,** ankle and foot
     M85.171 Skeletal fluorosis, right ankle and foot
     M85.172 Skeletal fluorosis, left ankle and foot
     M85.179 Skeletal fluorosis, unspecified ankle and foot ▽
     M85.18 Skeletal fluorosis, other site
     M85.19 Skeletal fluorosis, multiple sites

M85.2 Hyperostosis of skull
     DEF: Abnormal bone growth on inner aspect of cranial bones.

✓5ᵗʰ **M85.3 Osteitis condensans**
     M85.30 Osteitis condensans, unspecified site ▽

✓6ᵗʰ **M85.31 Osteitis condensans,** shoulder
     M85.311 Osteitis condensans, right shoulder
     M85.312 Osteitis condensans, left shoulder
     M85.319 Osteitis condensans, unspecified shoulder ▽

✓6ᵗʰ **M85.32 Osteitis condensans,** upper arm
     M85.321 Osteitis condensans, right upper arm
     M85.322 Osteitis condensans, left upper arm
     M85.329 Osteitis condensans, unspecified upper arm ▽

✓6ᵗʰ **M85.33 Osteitis condensans,** forearm
     M85.331 Osteitis condensans, right forearm
     M85.332 Osteitis condensans, left forearm
     M85.339 Osteitis condensans, unspecified forearm ▽

✓6ᵗʰ **M85.34 Osteitis condensans,** hand
     M85.341 Osteitis condensans, right hand
     M85.342 Osteitis condensans, left hand
     M85.349 Osteitis condensans, unspecified hand ▽

✓6ᵗʰ **M85.35 Osteitis condensans,** thigh
     M85.351 Osteitis condensans, right thigh
     M85.352 Osteitis condensans, left thigh
     M85.359 Osteitis condensans, unspecified thigh ▽

✓6ᵗʰ **M85.36 Osteitis condensans,** lower leg
     M85.361 Osteitis condensans, right lower leg
     M85.362 Osteitis condensans, left lower leg
     M85.369 Osteitis condensans, unspecified lower leg ▽

✓6ᵗʰ **M85.37 Osteitis condensans,** ankle and foot
     M85.371 Osteitis condensans, right ankle and foot
     M85.372 Osteitis condensans, left ankle and foot
     M85.379 Osteitis condensans, unspecified ankle and foot ▽
     M85.38 Osteitis condensans, other site
     M85.39 Osteitis condensans, multiple sites

✓5ᵗʰ **M85.4 Solitary bone cyst**
     EXCLUDES 2   solitary cyst of jaw (M27.4)
     M85.40 Solitary bone cyst, unspecified site ▽

✓6ᵗʰ **M85.41 Solitary bone cyst,** shoulder
     M85.411 Solitary bone cyst, right shoulder
     M85.412 Solitary bone cyst, left shoulder
     M85.419 Solitary bone cyst, unspecified shoulder ▽

✓6ᵗʰ **M85.42 Solitary bone cyst,** humerus
     M85.421 Solitary bone cyst, right humerus
     M85.422 Solitary bone cyst, left humerus
     M85.429 Solitary bone cyst, unspecified humerus ▽

✓6ᵗʰ **M85.43 Solitary bone cyst,** ulna and radius
     M85.431 Solitary bone cyst, right ulna and radius
     M85.432 Solitary bone cyst, left ulna and radius
     M85.439 Solitary bone cyst, unspecified ulna and radius ▽

✓6ᵗʰ **M85.44 Solitary bone cyst,** hand
     M85.441 Solitary bone cyst, right hand
     M85.442 Solitary bone cyst, left hand
     M85.449 Solitary bone cyst, unspecified hand ▽

✓6ᵗʰ **M85.45 Solitary bone cyst,** pelvis
     M85.451 Solitary bone cyst, right pelvis
     M85.452 Solitary bone cyst, left pelvis
     M85.459 Solitary bone cyst, unspecified pelvis ▽

✓6ᵗʰ **M85.46 Solitary bone cyst,** tibia and fibula
     M85.461 Solitary bone cyst, right tibia and fibula
     M85.462 Solitary bone cyst, left tibia and fibula
     M85.469 Solitary bone cyst, unspecified tibia and fibula ▽

✓6ᵗʰ **M85.47 Solitary bone cyst,** ankle and foot
     M85.471 Solitary bone cyst, right ankle and foot
     M85.472 Solitary bone cyst, left ankle and foot
     M85.479 Solitary bone cyst, unspecified ankle and foot ▽
     M85.48 Solitary bone cyst, other site

✓5ᵗʰ **M85.5 Aneurysmal bone cyst**
     EXCLUDES 2   aneurysmal cyst of jaw (M27.4)
     DEF: Solitary bone lesion, bulges into periosteum; marked by calcified rim.
     M85.50 Aneurysmal bone cyst, unspecified site ▽

✓6ᵗʰ **M85.51 Aneurysmal bone cyst,** shoulder
     M85.511 Aneurysmal bone cyst, right shoulder
     M85.512 Aneurysmal bone cyst, left shoulder
     M85.519 Aneurysmal bone cyst, unspecified shoulder ▽

✓6ᵗʰ **M85.52 Aneurysmal bone cyst,** upper arm
     M85.521 Aneurysmal bone cyst, right upper arm
     M85.522 Aneurysmal bone cyst, left upper arm
     M85.529 Aneurysmal bone cyst, unspecified upper arm ▽

✓6ᵗʰ **M85.53 Aneurysmal bone cyst,** forearm
     M85.531 Aneurysmal bone cyst, right forearm
     M85.532 Aneurysmal bone cyst, left forearm
     M85.539 Aneurysmal bone cyst, unspecified forearm ▽

✓6ᵗʰ **M85.54 Aneurysmal bone cyst,** hand
     M85.541 Aneurysmal bone cyst, right hand
     M85.542 Aneurysmal bone cyst, left hand
     M85.549 Aneurysmal bone cyst, unspecified hand ▽

✓6ᵗʰ **M85.55 Aneurysmal bone cyst,** thigh
     M85.551 Aneurysmal bone cyst, right thigh
     M85.552 Aneurysmal bone cyst, left thigh
     M85.559 Aneurysmal bone cyst, unspecified thigh ▽

✓6ᵗʰ **M85.56 Aneurysmal bone cyst,** lower leg
     M85.561 Aneurysmal bone cyst, right lower leg
     M85.562 Aneurysmal bone cyst, left lower leg
     M85.569 Aneurysmal bone cyst, unspecified lower leg ▽

✓6ᵗʰ **M85.57 Aneurysmal bone cyst,** ankle and foot
     M85.571 Aneurysmal bone cyst, right ankle and foot
     M85.572 Aneurysmal bone cyst, left ankle and foot
     M85.579 Aneurysmal bone cyst, unspecified ankle and foot ▽
     M85.58 Aneurysmal bone cyst, other site
     M85.59 Aneurysmal bone cyst, multiple sites

✓5ᵗʰ **M85.6 Other cyst of bone**
     EXCLUDES 1   cyst of jaw NEC (M27.4)
             osteitis fibrosa cystica generalisata [von Recklinghausen's disease of bone] (E21.0)
     M85.60 Other cyst of bone, unspecified site ▽

✓6ᵗʰ **M85.61 Other cyst of bone,** shoulder
     M85.611 Other cyst of bone, right shoulder
     M85.612 Other cyst of bone, left shoulder
     M85.619 Other cyst of bone, unspecified shoulder ▽

✓6ᵗʰ **M85.62 Other cyst of bone,** upper arm
     M85.621 Other cyst of bone, right upper arm
     M85.622 Other cyst of bone, left upper arm
     M85.629 Other cyst of bone, unspecified upper arm ▽

✓6ᵗʰ **M85.63 Other cyst of bone,** forearm
     M85.631 Other cyst of bone, right forearm
     M85.632 Other cyst of bone, left forearm
     M85.639 Other cyst of bone, unspecified forearm ▽

EXCLUDES 1 Not coded here   **EXCLUDES 2** Not included here   N Newborn Age: 0   P Pediatric Age: 0-17   M Maternity Age: 12-55   A Adult Age: 15-124

782   ICD-10-CM 2018

✓6ᵗʰ **M85.64** Other cyst of bone, hand
     M85.641 Other cyst of bone, right hand
     M85.642 Other cyst of bone, left hand
     M85.649 Other cyst of bone, unspecified hand ▽

✓6ᵗʰ **M85.65** Other cyst of bone, thigh
     M85.651 Other cyst of bone, right thigh
     M85.652 Other cyst of bone, left thigh
     M85.659 Other cyst of bone, unspecified thigh ▽

✓6ᵗʰ **M85.66** Other cyst of bone, lower leg
     M85.661 Other cyst of bone, right lower leg
     M85.662 Other cyst of bone, left lower leg
     M85.669 Other cyst of bone, unspecified lower leg ▽

✓6ᵗʰ **M85.67** Other cyst of bone, ankle and foot
     M85.671 Other cyst of bone, right ankle and foot
     M85.672 Other cyst of bone, left ankle and foot
     M85.679 Other cyst of bone, unspecified ankle and foot ▽

     M85.68 Other cyst of bone, other site

     M85.69 Other cyst of bone, multiple sites

✓5ᵗʰ **M85.8** Other specified disorders of bone density and structure
     Hyperostosis of bones, except skull
     Osteosclerosis, acquired
     EXCLUDES 1   *diffuse idiopathic skeletal hyperostosis [DISH] (M48.1)*
                 osteosclerosis congenita (Q77.4)
                 osteosclerosis fragilitas (generalista) (Q78.2)
                 osteosclerosis myelofibrosis (D75.81)

     M85.80 Other specified disorders of bone density and structure, unspecified site ▽

✓6ᵗʰ **M85.81** Other specified disorders of bone density and structure, shoulder
     M85.811 Other specified disorders of bone density and structure, right shoulder
     M85.812 Other specified disorders of bone density and structure, left shoulder
     M85.819 Other specified disorders of bone density and structure, unspecified shoulder ▽

✓6ᵗʰ **M85.82** Other specified disorders of bone density and structure, upper arm
     M85.821 Other specified disorders of bone density and structure, right upper arm
     M85.822 Other specified disorders of bone density and structure, left upper arm
     M85.829 Other specified disorders of bone density and structure, unspecified upper arm ▽

✓6ᵗʰ **M85.83** Other specified disorders of bone density and structure, forearm
     M85.831 Other specified disorders of bone density and structure, right forearm
     M85.832 Other specified disorders of bone density and structure, left forearm
     M85.839 Other specified disorders of bone density and structure, unspecified forearm ▽

✓6ᵗʰ **M85.84** Other specified disorders of bone density and structure, hand
     M85.841 Other specified disorders of bone density and structure, right hand
     M85.842 Other specified disorders of bone density and structure, left hand
     M85.849 Other specified disorders of bone density and structure, unspecified hand ▽

✓6ᵗʰ **M85.85** Other specified disorders of bone density and structure, thigh
     M85.851 Other specified disorders of bone density and structure, right thigh
     M85.852 Other specified disorders of bone density and structure, left thigh
     M85.859 Other specified disorders of bone density and structure, unspecified thigh ▽

✓6ᵗʰ **M85.86** Other specified disorders of bone density and structure, lower leg
     M85.861 Other specified disorders of bone density and structure, right lower leg

     M85.862 Other specified disorders of bone density and structure, left lower leg
     M85.869 Other specified disorders of bone density and structure, unspecified lower leg ▽

✓6ᵗʰ **M85.87** Other specified disorders of bone density and structure, ankle and foot
     M85.871 Other specified disorders of bone density and structure, right ankle and foot
     M85.872 Other specified disorders of bone density and structure, left ankle and foot
     M85.879 Other specified disorders of bone density and structure, unspecified ankle and foot ▽

     M85.88 Other specified disorders of bone density and structure, other site

     M85.89 Other specified disorders of bone density and structure, multiple sites

     M85.9 Disorder of bone density and structure, unspecified ▽

Other osteopathies (M86–M90)

EXCLUDES 1   *postprocedural osteopathies (M96.-)*

✓4ᵗʰ **M86 Osteomyelitis**
     Use additional code (B95-B97) to identify infectious agent
     Use additional code to identify major osseous defect, if applicable (M89.7-)
     EXCLUDES 1   *osteomyelitis due to:*
                 echinococcus (B67.2)
                 gonococcus (A54.43)
                 salmonella (A02.24)
     EXCLUDES 2   *ostemyelitis of:*
                  orbit (H05.0-)
                  petrous bone (H70.2-)
                  vertebra (M46.2-)

✓5ᵗʰ **M86.0** Acute hematogenous osteomyelitis
     M86.00 Acute hematogenous osteomyelitis, unspecified site   HCC ▽

✓6ᵗʰ **M86.01** Acute hematogenous osteomyelitis, shoulder
     M86.011 Acute hematogenous osteomyelitis, right shoulder   HCC
     M86.012 Acute hematogenous osteomyelitis, left shoulder   HCC
     M86.019 Acute hematogenous osteomyelitis, unspecified shoulder   HCC ▽

✓6ᵗʰ **M86.02** Acute hematogenous osteomyelitis, humerus
     M86.021 Acute hematogenous osteomyelitis, right humerus   HCC
     M86.022 Acute hematogenous osteomyelitis, left humerus   HCC
     M86.029 Acute hematogenous osteomyelitis, unspecified humerus   HCC ▽

✓6ᵗʰ **M86.03** Acute hematogenous osteomyelitis, radius and ulna
     M86.031 Acute hematogenous osteomyelitis, right radius and ulna   HCC
     M86.032 Acute hematogenous osteomyelitis, left radius and ulna   HCC
     M86.039 Acute hematogenous osteomyelitis, unspecified radius and ulna   HCC ▽

✓6ᵗʰ **M86.04** Acute hematogenous osteomyelitis, hand
     M86.041 Acute hematogenous osteomyelitis, right hand   HCC
     M86.042 Acute hematogenous osteomyelitis, left hand   HCC
     M86.049 Acute hematogenous osteomyelitis, unspecified hand   HCC ▽

✓6ᵗʰ **M86.05** Acute hematogenous osteomyelitis, femur
     M86.051 Acute hematogenous osteomyelitis, right femur   HCC
     M86.052 Acute hematogenous osteomyelitis, left femur   HCC
     M86.059 Acute hematogenous osteomyelitis, unspecified femur   HCC ▽

✓ Additional Character Req   ✓x7ᵗʰ Placeholder Alert   Manifestation   HCC CMS-HCC Condition   ▽ Unspecified Code   ▶◀ Revised Text   ● New Code   ▲ Revised Code Title

ICD-10-CM 2018   **783**

Chapter 13. Diseases of the Musculoskeletal System and Connective Tissue

M86.06–M86.349

✓6th **M86.06 Acute hematogenous osteomyelitis, tibia and fibula**
     M86.061 Acute hematogenous osteomyelitis, right tibia and fibula   HCC
     M86.062 Acute hematogenous osteomyelitis, left tibia and fibula   HCC
     M86.069 Acute hematogenous osteomyelitis, unspecified tibia and fibula   HCC ▽

✓6th **M86.07 Acute hematogenous osteomyelitis, ankle and foot**
     M86.071 Acute hematogenous osteomyelitis, right ankle and foot   HCC
     M86.072 Acute hematogenous osteomyelitis, left ankle and foot   HCC
     M86.079 Acute hematogenous osteomyelitis, unspecified ankle and foot   HCC ▽

     M86.08 Acute hematogenous osteomyelitis, other sites   HCC
     M86.09 Acute hematogenous osteomyelitis, multiple sites   HCC

✓5th **M86.1 Other acute osteomyelitis**
     M86.10 Other acute osteomyelitis, unspecified site   HCC ▽

✓6th **M86.11 Other acute osteomyelitis, shoulder**
     M86.111 Other acute osteomyelitis, right shoulder   HCC
     M86.112 Other acute osteomyelitis, left shoulder   HCC
     M86.119 Other acute osteomyelitis, unspecified shoulder   HCC ▽

✓6th **M86.12 Other acute osteomyelitis, humerus**
     M86.121 Other acute osteomyelitis, right humerus   HCC
     M86.122 Other acute osteomyelitis, left humerus   HCC
     M86.129 Other acute osteomyelitis, unspecified humerus   HCC ▽

✓6th **M86.13 Other acute osteomyelitis, radius and ulna**
     M86.131 Other acute osteomyelitis, right radius and ulna   HCC
     M86.132 Other acute osteomyelitis, left radius and ulna   HCC
     M86.139 Other acute osteomyelitis, unspecified radius and ulna   HCC ▽

✓6th **M86.14 Other acute osteomyelitis, hand**
     M86.141 Other acute osteomyelitis, right hand   HCC
     M86.142 Other acute osteomyelitis, left hand   HCC
     M86.149 Other acute osteomyelitis, unspecified hand   HCC ▽

✓6th **M86.15 Other acute osteomyelitis, femur**
     M86.151 Other acute osteomyelitis, right femur   HCC
     M86.152 Other acute osteomyelitis, left femur   HCC
     M86.159 Other acute osteomyelitis, unspecified femur   HCC ▽

✓6th **M86.16 Other acute osteomyelitis, tibia and fibula**
     M86.161 Other acute osteomyelitis, right tibia and fibula   HCC
     M86.162 Other acute osteomyelitis, left tibia and fibula   HCC
     M86.169 Other acute osteomyelitis, unspecified tibia and fibula   HCC ▽

✓6th **M86.17 Other acute osteomyelitis, ankle and foot**
     M86.171 Other acute osteomyelitis, right ankle and foot   HCC
     M86.172 Other acute osteomyelitis, left ankle and foot   HCC
     M86.179 Other acute osteomyelitis, unspecified ankle and foot   HCC ▽

     M86.18 Other acute osteomyelitis, other site   HCC
     M86.19 Other acute osteomyelitis, multiple sites   HCC

✓5th **M86.2 Subacute osteomyelitis**
     M86.20 Subacute osteomyelitis, unspecified site   HCC ▽

✓6th **M86.21 Subacute osteomyelitis, shoulder**
     M86.211 Subacute osteomyelitis, right shoulder   HCC
     M86.212 Subacute osteomyelitis, left shoulder   HCC
     M86.219 Subacute osteomyelitis, unspecified shoulder   HCC ▽

✓6th **M86.22 Subacute osteomyelitis, humerus**
     M86.221 Subacute osteomyelitis, right humerus   HCC
     M86.222 Subacute osteomyelitis, left humerus   HCC
     M86.229 Subacute osteomyelitis, unspecified humerus   HCC ▽

✓6th **M86.23 Subacute osteomyelitis, radius and ulna**
     M86.231 Subacute osteomyelitis, right radius and ulna   HCC
     M86.232 Subacute osteomyelitis, left radius and ulna   HCC
     M86.239 Subacute osteomyelitis, unspecified radius and ulna   HCC ▽

✓6th **M86.24 Subacute osteomyelitis, hand**
     M86.241 Subacute osteomyelitis, right hand   HCC
     M86.242 Subacute osteomyelitis, left hand   HCC
     M86.249 Subacute osteomyelitis, unspecified hand   HCC ▽

✓6th **M86.25 Subacute osteomyelitis, femur**
     M86.251 Subacute osteomyelitis, right femur   HCC
     M86.252 Subacute osteomyelitis, left femur   HCC
     M86.259 Subacute osteomyelitis, unspecified femur   HCC ▽

✓6th **M86.26 Subacute osteomyelitis, tibia and fibula**
     M86.261 Subacute osteomyelitis, right tibia and fibula   HCC
     M86.262 Subacute osteomyelitis, left tibia and fibula   HCC
     M86.269 Subacute osteomyelitis, unspecified tibia and fibula   HCC ▽

✓6th **M86.27 Subacute osteomyelitis, ankle and foot**
     M86.271 Subacute osteomyelitis, right ankle and foot   HCC
     M86.272 Subacute osteomyelitis, left ankle and foot   HCC
     M86.279 Subacute osteomyelitis, unspecified ankle and foot   HCC ▽

     M86.28 Subacute osteomyelitis, other site   HCC
     M86.29 Subacute osteomyelitis, multiple sites   HCC

✓5th **M86.3 Chronic multifocal osteomyelitis**
     M86.30 Chronic multifocal osteomyelitis, unspecified site   HCC ▽

✓6th **M86.31 Chronic multifocal osteomyelitis, shoulder**
     M86.311 Chronic multifocal osteomyelitis, right shoulder   HCC
     M86.312 Chronic multifocal osteomyelitis, left shoulder   HCC
     M86.319 Chronic multifocal osteomyelitis, unspecified shoulder   HCC ▽

✓6th **M86.32 Chronic multifocal osteomyelitis, humerus**
     M86.321 Chronic multifocal osteomyelitis, right humerus   HCC
     M86.322 Chronic multifocal osteomyelitis, left humerus   HCC
     M86.329 Chronic multifocal osteomyelitis, unspecified humerus   HCC ▽

✓6th **M86.33 Chronic multifocal osteomyelitis, radius and ulna**
     M86.331 Chronic multifocal osteomyelitis, right radius and ulna   HCC
     M86.332 Chronic multifocal osteomyelitis, left radius and ulna   HCC
     M86.339 Chronic multifocal osteomyelitis, unspecified radius and ulna   HCC ▽

✓6th **M86.34 Chronic multifocal osteomyelitis, hand**
     M86.341 Chronic multifocal osteomyelitis, right hand   HCC
     M86.342 Chronic multifocal osteomyelitis, left hand   HCC
     M86.349 Chronic multifocal osteomyelitis, unspecified hand   HCC ▽

EXCLUDES 1 Not coded here   EXCLUDES 2 Not included here   N Newborn Age: 0   P Pediatric Age: 0-17   M Maternity Age: 12-55   A Adult Age: 15-124

784   ICD-10-CM 2018

√6ᵗʰ **M86.35 Chronic multifocal osteomyelitis, femur**
     M86.351 **Chronic multifocal osteomyelitis, right femur** `HCC`
     M86.352 **Chronic multifocal osteomyelitis, left femur** `HCC`
     M86.359 **Chronic multifocal osteomyelitis, unspecified femur** `HCC` ▽

√6ᵗʰ **M86.36 Chronic multifocal osteomyelitis, tibia and fibula**
     M86.361 **Chronic multifocal osteomyelitis, right tibia and fibula** `HCC`
     M86.362 **Chronic multifocal osteomyelitis, left tibia and fibula** `HCC`
     M86.369 **Chronic multifocal osteomyelitis, unspecified tibia and fibula** `HCC` ▽

√6ᵗʰ **M86.37 Chronic multifocal osteomyelitis, ankle and foot**
     M86.371 **Chronic multifocal osteomyelitis, right ankle and foot** `HCC`
     M86.372 **Chronic multifocal osteomyelitis, left ankle and foot** `HCC`
     M86.379 **Chronic multifocal osteomyelitis, unspecified ankle and foot** `HCC` ▽

     M86.38 **Chronic multifocal osteomyelitis, other site** `HCC`
     M86.39 **Chronic multifocal osteomyelitis, multiple sites** `HCC`

√5ᵗʰ **M86.4 Chronic osteomyelitis with draining sinus**
     M86.40 **Chronic osteomyelitis with draining sinus, unspecified site** `HCC` ▽

√6ᵗʰ **M86.41 Chronic osteomyelitis with draining sinus, shoulder**
     M86.411 **Chronic osteomyelitis with draining sinus, right shoulder** `HCC`
     M86.412 **Chronic osteomyelitis with draining sinus, left shoulder** `HCC`
     M86.419 **Chronic osteomyelitis with draining sinus, unspecified shoulder** `HCC` ▽

√6ᵗʰ **M86.42 Chronic osteomyelitis with draining sinus, humerus**
     M86.421 **Chronic osteomyelitis with draining sinus, right humerus** `HCC`
     M86.422 **Chronic osteomyelitis with draining sinus, left humerus** `HCC`
     M86.429 **Chronic osteomyelitis with draining sinus, unspecified humerus** `HCC` ▽

√6ᵗʰ **M86.43 Chronic osteomyelitis with draining sinus, radius and ulna**
     M86.431 **Chronic osteomyelitis with draining sinus, right radius and ulna** `HCC`
     M86.432 **Chronic osteomyelitis with draining sinus, left radius and ulna** `HCC`
     M86.439 **Chronic osteomyelitis with draining sinus, unspecified radius and ulna** `HCC` ▽

√6ᵗʰ **M86.44 Chronic osteomyelitis with draining sinus, hand**
     M86.441 **Chronic osteomyelitis with draining sinus, right hand** `HCC`
     M86.442 **Chronic osteomyelitis with draining sinus, left hand** `HCC`
     M86.449 **Chronic osteomyelitis with draining sinus, unspecified hand** `HCC` ▽

√6ᵗʰ **M86.45 Chronic osteomyelitis with draining sinus, femur**
     M86.451 **Chronic osteomyelitis with draining sinus, right femur** `HCC`
     M86.452 **Chronic osteomyelitis with draining sinus, left femur** `HCC`
     M86.459 **Chronic osteomyelitis with draining sinus, unspecified femur** `HCC` ▽

√6ᵗʰ **M86.46 Chronic osteomyelitis with draining sinus, tibia and fibula**
     M86.461 **Chronic osteomyelitis with draining sinus, right tibia and fibula** `HCC`
     M86.462 **Chronic osteomyelitis with draining sinus, left tibia and fibula** `HCC`
     M86.469 **Chronic osteomyelitis with draining sinus, unspecified tibia and fibula** `HCC` ▽

√6ᵗʰ **M86.47 Chronic osteomyelitis with draining sinus, ankle and foot**
     M86.471 **Chronic osteomyelitis with draining sinus, right ankle and foot** `HCC`
     M86.472 **Chronic osteomyelitis with draining sinus, left ankle and foot** `HCC`
     M86.479 **Chronic osteomyelitis with draining sinus, unspecified ankle and foot** `HCC` ▽

     M86.48 **Chronic osteomyelitis with draining sinus, other site** `HCC`
     M86.49 **Chronic osteomyelitis with draining sinus, multiple sites** `HCC`

√5ᵗʰ **M86.5 Other chronic hematogenous osteomyelitis**
     M86.50 **Other chronic hematogenous osteomyelitis, unspecified site** `HCC` ▽

√6ᵗʰ **M86.51 Other chronic hematogenous osteomyelitis, shoulder**
     M86.511 **Other chronic hematogenous osteomyelitis, right shoulder** `HCC`
     M86.512 **Other chronic hematogenous osteomyelitis, left shoulder** `HCC`
     M86.519 **Other chronic hematogenous osteomyelitis, unspecified shoulder** `HCC` ▽

√6ᵗʰ **M86.52 Other chronic hematogenous osteomyelitis, humerus**
     M86.521 **Other chronic hematogenous osteomyelitis, right humerus** `HCC`
     M86.522 **Other chronic hematogenous osteomyelitis, left humerus** `HCC`
     M86.529 **Other chronic hematogenous osteomyelitis, unspecified humerus** `HCC` ▽

√6ᵗʰ **M86.53 Other chronic hematogenous osteomyelitis, radius and ulna**
     M86.531 **Other chronic hematogenous osteomyelitis, right radius and ulna** `HCC`
     M86.532 **Other chronic hematogenous osteomyelitis, left radius and ulna** `HCC`
     M86.539 **Other chronic hematogenous osteomyelitis, unspecified radius and ulna** `HCC` ▽

√6ᵗʰ **M86.54 Other chronic hematogenous osteomyelitis, hand**
     M86.541 **Other chronic hematogenous osteomyelitis, right hand** `HCC`
     M86.542 **Other chronic hematogenous osteomyelitis, left hand** `HCC`
     M86.549 **Other chronic hematogenous osteomyelitis, unspecified hand** `HCC` ▽

√6ᵗʰ **M86.55 Other chronic hematogenous osteomyelitis, femur**
     M86.551 **Other chronic hematogenous osteomyelitis, right femur** `HCC`
     M86.552 **Other chronic hematogenous osteomyelitis, left femur** `HCC`
     M86.559 **Other chronic hematogenous osteomyelitis, unspecified femur** `HCC` ▽

√6ᵗʰ **M86.56 Other chronic hematogenous osteomyelitis, tibia and fibula**
     M86.561 **Other chronic hematogenous osteomyelitis, right tibia and fibula** `HCC`
     M86.562 **Other chronic hematogenous osteomyelitis, left tibia and fibula** `HCC`
     M86.569 **Other chronic hematogenous osteomyelitis, unspecified tibia and fibula** `HCC` ▽

√6ᵗʰ **M86.57 Other chronic hematogenous osteomyelitis, ankle and foot**
     M86.571 **Other chronic hematogenous osteomyelitis, right ankle and foot** `HCC`
     M86.572 **Other chronic hematogenous osteomyelitis, left ankle and foot** `HCC`
     M86.579 **Other chronic hematogenous osteomyelitis, unspecified ankle and foot** `HCC` ▽

     M86.58 **Other chronic hematogenous osteomyelitis, other site** `HCC`
     M86.59 **Other chronic hematogenous osteomyelitis, multiple sites** `HCC`

√5ᵗʰ **M86.6 Other chronic osteomyelitis**
     M86.60 **Other chronic osteomyelitis, unspecified site** `HCC` ▽

√6ᵗʰ **M86.61 Other chronic osteomyelitis, shoulder**
     M86.611 **Other chronic osteomyelitis, right shoulder** `HCC`
     M86.612 **Other chronic osteomyelitis, left shoulder** `HCC`
     M86.619 **Other chronic osteomyelitis, unspecified shoulder** `HCC` ▽

✓ Additional Character Req   ✓x7ᵗʰ Placeholder Alert   Manifestation   `HCC` CMS-HCC Condition   ▽ Unspecified Code   ▶◀ Revised Text   ● New Code   ▲ Revised Code Title

√6ᵗʰ M86.62 Other chronic osteomyelitis, humerus
     M86.621 Other chronic osteomyelitis, right humerus   `HCC`
     M86.622 Other chronic osteomyelitis, left humerus   `HCC`
     M86.629 Other chronic osteomyelitis, unspecified humerus   `HCC` ▽

√6ᵗʰ M86.63 Other chronic osteomyelitis, radius and ulna
     M86.631 Other chronic osteomyelitis, right radius and ulna   `HCC`
     M86.632 Other chronic osteomyelitis, left radius and ulna   `HCC`
     M86.639 Other chronic osteomyelitis, unspecified radius and ulna   `HCC` ▽

√6ᵗʰ M86.64 Other chronic osteomyelitis, hand
     M86.641 Other chronic osteomyelitis, right hand   `HCC`
     M86.642 Other chronic osteomyelitis, left hand   `HCC`
     M86.649 Other chronic osteomyelitis, unspecified hand   `HCC` ▽

√6ᵗʰ M86.65 Other chronic osteomyelitis, thigh
     M86.651 Other chronic osteomyelitis, right thigh   `HCC`
     M86.652 Other chronic osteomyelitis, left thigh   `HCC`
     M86.659 Other chronic osteomyelitis, unspecified thigh   `HCC` ▽

√6ᵗʰ M86.66 Other chronic osteomyelitis, tibia and fibula
     M86.661 Other chronic osteomyelitis, right tibia and fibula   `HCC`
     M86.662 Other chronic osteomyelitis, left tibia and fibula   `HCC`
     M86.669 Other chronic osteomyelitis, unspecified tibia and fibula   `HCC` ▽

√6ᵗʰ M86.67 Other chronic osteomyelitis, ankle and foot
     M86.671 Other chronic osteomyelitis, right ankle and foot   `HCC`
         AHA: 2016, 1Q, 13
     M86.672 Other chronic osteomyelitis, left ankle and foot   `HCC`
     M86.679 Other chronic osteomyelitis, unspecified ankle and foot   `HCC` ▽

     M86.68 Other chronic osteomyelitis, other site   `HCC`
     M86.69 Other chronic osteomyelitis, multiple sites   `HCC`

√5ᵗʰ M86.8 Other osteomyelitis
     Brodie's abscess

     √6ᵗʰ M86.8X Other osteomyelitis
         M86.8X0 Other osteomyelitis, multiple sites   `HCC`
         M86.8X1 Other osteomyelitis, shoulder   `HCC`
         M86.8X2 Other osteomyelitis, upper arm   `HCC`
         M86.8X3 Other osteomyelitis, forearm   `HCC`
         M86.8X4 Other osteomyelitis, hand   `HCC`
         M86.8X5 Other osteomyelitis, thigh   `HCC`
         M86.8X6 Other osteomyelitis, lower leg   `HCC`
         M86.8X7 Other osteomyelitis, ankle and foot   `HCC`
         M86.8X8 Other osteomyelitis, other site   `HCC`
         M86.8X9 Other osteomyelitis, unspecified sites   `HCC` ▽

     M86.9 Osteomyelitis, unspecified   `HCC` ▽
         Infection of bone NOS
         Periostitis without osteomyelitis

√4ᵗʰ M87 Osteonecrosis
     `INCLUDES` avascular necrosis of bone
     Use additional code to identify major osseous defect, if applicable (M89.7-)
     `EXCLUDES 1` juvenile osteonecrosis (M91-M92)
                 osteochondropathies (M90-M93)

√5ᵗʰ M87.0 Idiopathic aseptic necrosis of bone
     M87.00 Idiopathic aseptic necrosis of unspecified bone   `HCC` ▽

     √6ᵗʰ M87.01 Idiopathic aseptic necrosis of shoulder
         Idiopathic aseptic necrosis of clavicle and scapula
         M87.011 Idiopathic aseptic necrosis of right shoulder   `HCC`

         M87.012 Idiopathic aseptic necrosis of left shoulder   `HCC`
         M87.019 Idiopathic aseptic necrosis of unspecified shoulder   `HCC` ▽

√6ᵗʰ M87.02 Idiopathic aseptic necrosis of humerus
     M87.021 Idiopathic aseptic necrosis of right humerus   `HCC`
     M87.022 Idiopathic aseptic necrosis of left humerus   `HCC`
     M87.029 Idiopathic aseptic necrosis of unspecified humerus   `HCC` ▽

√6ᵗʰ M87.03 Idiopathic aseptic necrosis of radius, ulna and carpus
     M87.031 Idiopathic aseptic necrosis of right radius   `HCC`
     M87.032 Idiopathic aseptic necrosis of left radius   `HCC`
     M87.033 Idiopathic aseptic necrosis of unspecified radius   `HCC` ▽
     M87.034 Idiopathic aseptic necrosis of right ulna   `HCC`
     M87.035 Idiopathic aseptic necrosis of left ulna   `HCC`
     M87.036 Idiopathic aseptic necrosis of unspecified ulna   `HCC` ▽
     M87.037 Idiopathic aseptic necrosis of right carpus   `HCC`
     M87.038 Idiopathic aseptic necrosis of left carpus   `HCC`
     M87.039 Idiopathic aseptic necrosis of unspecified carpus   `HCC` ▽

√6ᵗʰ M87.04 Idiopathic aseptic necrosis of hand and fingers
     Idiopathic aseptic necrosis of metacarpals and phalanges of hands
     M87.041 Idiopathic aseptic necrosis of right hand   `HCC`
     M87.042 Idiopathic aseptic necrosis of left hand   `HCC`
     M87.043 Idiopathic aseptic necrosis of unspecified hand   `HCC` ▽
     M87.044 Idiopathic aseptic necrosis of right finger(s)   `HCC`
     M87.045 Idiopathic aseptic necrosis of left finger(s)   `HCC`
     M87.046 Idiopathic aseptic necrosis of unspecified finger(s)   `HCC` ▽

√6ᵗʰ M87.05 Idiopathic aseptic necrosis of pelvis and femur
     M87.050 Idiopathic aseptic necrosis of pelvis   `HCC`
     M87.051 Idiopathic aseptic necrosis of right femur   `HCC`
     M87.052 Idiopathic aseptic necrosis of left femur   `HCC`
     M87.059 Idiopathic aseptic necrosis of unspecified femur   `HCC` ▽
         Idiopathic aseptic necrosis of hip NOS

√6ᵗʰ M87.06 Idiopathic aseptic necrosis of tibia and fibula
     M87.061 Idiopathic aseptic necrosis of right tibia   `HCC`
     M87.062 Idiopathic aseptic necrosis of left tibia   `HCC`
     M87.063 Idiopathic aseptic necrosis of unspecified tibia   `HCC` ▽
     M87.064 Idiopathic aseptic necrosis of right fibula   `HCC`
     M87.065 Idiopathic aseptic necrosis of left fibula   `HCC`
     M87.066 Idiopathic aseptic necrosis of unspecified fibula   `HCC` ▽

√6ᵗʰ M87.07 Idiopathic aseptic necrosis of ankle, foot and toes
     Idiopathic aseptic necrosis of metatarsus, tarsus, and phalanges of toes
     M87.071 Idiopathic aseptic necrosis of right ankle   `HCC`
     M87.072 Idiopathic aseptic necrosis of left ankle   `HCC`
     M87.073 Idiopathic aseptic necrosis of unspecified ankle   `HCC` ▽
     M87.074 Idiopathic aseptic necrosis of right foot   `HCC`

`EXCLUDES 1` Not coded here   `EXCLUDES 2` Not included here   N Newborn Age: 0   P Pediatric Age: 0-17   M Maternity Age: 12-55   A Adult Age: 15-124

ICD-10-CM 2018

M87.075 **Idiopathic aseptic necrosis of left foot** `HCC`

M87.076 **Idiopathic aseptic necrosis of unspecified foot** `HCC` ▽

M87.077 **Idiopathic aseptic necrosis of right toe(s)** `HCC`

M87.078 **Idiopathic aseptic necrosis of left toe(s)** `HCC`

M87.079 **Idiopathic aseptic necrosis of unspecified toe(s)** `HCC` ▽

M87.08 **Idiopathic aseptic necrosis of bone, other site'** `HCC`

M87.09 **Idiopathic aseptic necrosis of bone, multiple sites** `HCC`

✓5ᵗʰ **M87.1 Osteonecrosis** due to drugs

    Use additional code for adverse effect, if applicable, to identify drug (T36-T50 with fifth or sixth character 5)

M87.10 **Osteonecrosis due to drugs, unspecified bone** `HCC` ▽

✓6ᵗʰ **M87.11 Osteonecrosis due to drugs, shoulder**

M87.111 **Osteonecrosis due to drugs, right shoulder** `HCC`

M87.112 **Osteonecrosis due to drugs, left shoulder** `HCC`

M87.119 **Osteonecrosis due to drugs, unspecified shoulder** `HCC` ▽

✓6ᵗʰ **M87.12 Osteonecrosis due to drugs, humerus**

M87.121 **Osteonecrosis due to drugs, right humerus** `HCC`

M87.122 **Osteonecrosis due to drugs, left humerus** `HCC`

M87.129 **Osteonecrosis due to drugs, unspecified humerus** `HCC` ▽

✓6ᵗʰ **M87.13 Osteonecrosis due to drugs of radius, ulna and carpus**

M87.131 **Osteonecrosis due to drugs of right radius** `HCC`

M87.132 **Osteonecrosis due to drugs of left radius** `HCC`

M87.133 **Osteonecrosis due to drugs of unspecified radius** `HCC` ▽

M87.134 **Osteonecrosis due to drugs of right ulna** `HCC`

M87.135 **Osteonecrosis due to drugs of left ulna** `HCC`

M87.136 **Osteonecrosis due to drugs of unspecified ulna** `HCC` ▽

M87.137 **Osteonecrosis due to drugs of right carpus** `HCC`

M87.138 **Osteonecrosis due to drugs of left carpus** `HCC`

M87.139 **Osteonecrosis due to drugs of unspecified carpus** `HCC` ▽

✓6ᵗʰ **M87.14 Osteonecrosis due to drugs, hand and fingers**

M87.141 **Osteonecrosis due to drugs, right hand** `HCC`

M87.142 **Osteonecrosis due to drugs, left hand** `HCC`

M87.143 **Osteonecrosis due to drugs, unspecified hand** `HCC` ▽

M87.144 **Osteonecrosis due to drugs, right finger(s)** `HCC`

M87.145 **Osteonecrosis due to drugs, left finger(s)** `HCC`

M87.146 **Osteonecrosis due to drugs, unspecified finger(s)** `HCC` ▽

✓6ᵗʰ **M87.15 Osteonecrosis due to drugs, pelvis and femur**

M87.150 **Osteonecrosis due to drugs, pelvis** `HCC`

M87.151 **Osteonecrosis due to drugs, right femur** `HCC`

M87.152 **Osteonecrosis due to drugs, left femur** `HCC`

M87.159 **Osteonecrosis due to drugs, unspecified femur** `HCC` ▽

✓6ᵗʰ **M87.16 Osteonecrosis due to drugs, tibia and fibula**

M87.161 **Osteonecrosis due to drugs, right tibia** `HCC`

M87.162 **Osteonecrosis due to drugs, left tibia** `HCC`

M87.163 **Osteonecrosis due to drugs, unspecified tibia** `HCC` ▽

M87.164 **Osteonecrosis due to drugs, right fibula** `HCC`

M87.165 **Osteonecrosis due to drugs, left fibula** `HCC`

M87.166 **Osteonecrosis due to drugs, unspecified fibula** `HCC` ▽

✓6ᵗʰ **M87.17 Osteonecrosis due to drugs, ankle, foot and toes**

M87.171 **Osteonecrosis due to drugs, right ankle** `HCC`

M87.172 **Osteonecrosis due to drugs, left ankle** `HCC`

M87.173 **Osteonecrosis due to drugs, unspecified ankle** `HCC` ▽

M87.174 **Osteonecrosis due to drugs, right foot** `HCC`

M87.175 **Osteonecrosis due to drugs, left foot** `HCC`

M87.176 **Osteonecrosis due to drugs, unspecified foot** `HCC` ▽

M87.177 **Osteonecrosis due to drugs, right toe(s)** `HCC`

M87.178 **Osteonecrosis due to drugs, left toe(s)** `HCC`

M87.179 **Osteonecrosis due to drugs, unspecified toe(s)** `HCC` ▽

✓6ᵗʰ **M87.18 Osteonecrosis due to drugs, other site**

M87.180 **Osteonecrosis due to drugs, jaw** `HCC`

M87.188 **Osteonecrosis due to drugs, other site** `HCC`

M87.19 **Osteonecrosis due to drugs, multiple sites** `HCC`

✓5ᵗʰ **M87.2 Osteonecrosis** due to previous trauma

M87.20 **Osteonecrosis due to previous trauma, unspecified bone** `HCC` ▽

✓6ᵗʰ **M87.21 Osteonecrosis due to previous trauma, shoulder**

M87.211 **Osteonecrosis due to previous trauma, right shoulder** `HCC`

M87.212 **Osteonecrosis due to previous trauma, left shoulder** `HCC`

M87.219 **Osteonecrosis due to previous trauma, unspecified shoulder** `HCC` ▽

✓6ᵗʰ **M87.22 Osteonecrosis due to previous trauma, humerus**

M87.221 **Osteonecrosis due to previous trauma, right humerus** `HCC`

M87.222 **Osteonecrosis due to previous trauma, left humerus** `HCC`

M87.229 **Osteonecrosis due to previous trauma, unspecified humerus** `HCC` ▽

✓6ᵗʰ **M87.23 Osteonecrosis due to previous trauma of radius, ulna and carpus**

M87.231 **Osteonecrosis due to previous trauma of right radius** `HCC`

M87.232 **Osteonecrosis due to previous trauma of left radius** `HCC`

M87.233 **Osteonecrosis due to previous trauma of unspecified radius** `HCC` ▽

M87.234 **Osteonecrosis due to previous trauma of right ulna** `HCC`

M87.235 **Osteonecrosis due to previous trauma of left ulna** `HCC`

M87.236 **Osteonecrosis due to previous trauma of unspecified ulna** `HCC` ▽

M87.237 **Osteonecrosis due to previous trauma of right carpus** `HCC`

M87.238 **Osteonecrosis due to previous trauma of left carpus** `HCC`

M87.239 **Osteonecrosis due to previous trauma of unspecified carpus** `HCC` ▽

✓6ᵗʰ **M87.24 Osteonecrosis due to previous trauma, hand and fingers**

M87.241 **Osteonecrosis due to previous trauma, right hand** `HCC`

M87.242 **Osteonecrosis due to previous trauma, left hand** `HCC`

M87.243 **Osteonecrosis due to previous trauma, unspecified hand** `HCC` ▽

✓ Additional Character Req   ✓x7ᵗʰ Placeholder Alert   Manifestation   `HCC` CMS-HCC Condition   ▽ Unspecified Code   ►◄ Revised Text   ● New Code   ▲ Revised Code Title

ICD-10-CM 2018   787

M87.075–M87.243

M87.244 Osteonecrosis due to previous trauma, right finger(s) `HCC`

M87.245 Osteonecrosis due to previous trauma, left finger(s) `HCC`

M87.246 Osteonecrosis due to previous trauma, unspecified finger(s) `HCC` ▽

✓6ᵗʰ M87.25 Osteonecrosis due to previous trauma, pelvis and femur

  M87.250 Osteonecrosis due to previous trauma, pelvis `HCC`

  M87.251 Osteonecrosis due to previous trauma, right femur `HCC`

  M87.252 Osteonecrosis due to previous trauma, left femur `HCC`

  M87.256 Osteonecrosis due to previous trauma, unspecified femur `HCC` ▽

✓6ᵗʰ M87.26 Osteonecrosis due to previous trauma, tibia and fibula

  M87.261 Osteonecrosis due to previous trauma, right tibia `HCC`

  M87.262 Osteonecrosis due to previous trauma, left tibia `HCC`

  M87.263 Osteonecrosis due to previous trauma, unspecified tibia `HCC` ▽

  M87.264 Osteonecrosis due to previous trauma, right fibula `HCC`

  M87.265 Osteonecrosis due to previous trauma, left fibula `HCC`

  M87.266 Osteonecrosis due to previous trauma, unspecified fibula `HCC` ▽

✓6ᵗʰ M87.27 Osteonecrosis due to previous trauma, ankle, foot and toes

  M87.271 Osteonecrosis due to previous trauma, right ankle `HCC`

  M87.272 Osteonecrosis due to previous trauma, left ankle `HCC`

  M87.273 Osteonecrosis due to previous trauma, unspecified ankle `HCC` ▽

  M87.274 Osteonecrosis due to previous trauma, right foot `HCC`

  M87.275 Osteonecrosis due to previous trauma, left foot `HCC`

  M87.276 Osteonecrosis due to previous trauma, unspecified foot `HCC` ▽

  M87.277 Osteonecrosis due to previous trauma, right toe(s) `HCC`

  M87.278 Osteonecrosis due to previous trauma, left toe(s) `HCC`

  M87.279 Osteonecrosis due to previous trauma, unspecified toe(s) `HCC` ▽

M87.28 Osteonecrosis due to previous trauma, other site `HCC`

M87.29 Osteonecrosis due to previous trauma, multiple sites `HCC`

✓5ᵗʰ M87.3 Other secondary osteonecrosis

M87.30 Other secondary osteonecrosis, unspecified bone `HCC` ▽

✓6ᵗʰ M87.31 Other secondary osteonecrosis, shoulder

  M87.311 Other secondary osteonecrosis, right shoulder `HCC`

  M87.312 Other secondary osteonecrosis, left shoulder `HCC`

  M87.319 Other secondary osteonecrosis, unspecified shoulder `HCC` ▽

✓6ᵗʰ M87.32 Other secondary osteonecrosis, humerus

  M87.321 Other secondary osteonecrosis, right humerus `HCC`

  M87.322 Other secondary osteonecrosis, left humerus `HCC`

  M87.329 Other secondary osteonecrosis, unspecified humerus `HCC` ▽

✓6ᵗʰ M87.33 Other secondary osteonecrosis of radius, ulna and carpus

  M87.331 Other secondary osteonecrosis of right radius `HCC`

  M87.332 Other secondary osteonecrosis of left radius `HCC`

M87.333 Other secondary osteonecrosis of unspecified radius `HCC` ▽

M87.334 Other secondary osteonecrosis of right ulna `HCC`

M87.335 Other secondary osteonecrosis of left ulna `HCC`

M87.336 Other secondary osteonecrosis of unspecified ulna `HCC` ▽

M87.337 Other secondary osteonecrosis of right carpus `HCC`

M87.338 Other secondary osteonecrosis of left carpus `HCC`

M87.339 Other secondary osteonecrosis of unspecified carpus `HCC` ▽

✓6ᵗʰ M87.34 Other secondary osteonecrosis, hand and fingers

  M87.341 Other secondary osteonecrosis, right hand `HCC`

  M87.342 Other secondary osteonecrosis, left hand `HCC`

  M87.343 Other secondary osteonecrosis, unspecified hand `HCC` ▽

  M87.344 Other secondary osteonecrosis, right finger(s) `HCC`

  M87.345 Other secondary osteonecrosis, left finger(s) `HCC`

  M87.346 Other secondary osteonecrosis, unspecified finger(s) `HCC` ▽

✓6ᵗʰ M87.35 Other secondary osteonecrosis, pelvis and femur

  M87.350 Other secondary osteonecrosis, pelvis `HCC`

  M87.351 Other secondary osteonecrosis, right femur `HCC`

  M87.352 Other secondary osteonecrosis, left femur `HCC`

  M87.353 Other secondary osteonecrosis, unspecified femur `HCC` ▽

✓6ᵗʰ M87.36 Other secondary osteonecrosis, tibia and fibula

  M87.361 Other secondary osteonecrosis, right tibia `HCC`

  M87.362 Other secondary osteonecrosis, left tibia `HCC`

  M87.363 Other secondary osteonecrosis, unspecified tibia `HCC` ▽

  M87.364 Other secondary osteonecrosis, right fibula `HCC`

  M87.365 Other secondary osteonecrosis, left fibula `HCC`

  M87.366 Other secondary osteonecrosis, unspecified fibula `HCC` ▽

✓6ᵗʰ M87.37 Other secondary osteonecrosis, ankle and foot

  M87.371 Other secondary osteonecrosis, right ankle `HCC`

  M87.372 Other secondary osteonecrosis, left ankle `HCC`

  M87.373 Other secondary osteonecrosis, unspecified ankle `HCC` ▽

  M87.374 Other secondary osteonecrosis, right foot `HCC`

  M87.375 Other secondary osteonecrosis, left foot `HCC`

  M87.376 Other secondary osteonecrosis, unspecified foot `HCC` ▽

  M87.377 Other secondary osteonecrosis, right toe(s) `HCC`

  M87.378 Other secondary osteonecrosis, left toe(s) `HCC`

  M87.379 Other secondary osteonecrosis, unspecified toe(s) `HCC` ▽

M87.38 Other secondary osteonecrosis, other site `HCC`

M87.39 Other secondary osteonecrosis, multiple sites `HCC`

✓5ᵗʰ M87.8 Other osteonecrosis

M87.80 Other osteonecrosis, unspecified bone `HCC` ▽

✓6ᵗʰ M87.81 Other osteonecrosis, shoulder

  M87.811 Other osteonecrosis, right shoulder `HCC`

  M87.812 Other osteonecrosis, left shoulder `HCC`

  M87.819 Other osteonecrosis, unspecified shoulder `HCC` ▽

EXCLUDES 1 Not coded here   *EXCLUDES 2* Not included here   N Newborn Age: 0   P Pediatric Age: 0-17   M Maternity Age: 12-55   A Adult Age: 15-124

788   ICD-10-CM 2018

√6th M87.82 Other osteonecrosis, humerus
  M87.821 Other osteonecrosis, right humerus HCC
  M87.822 Other osteonecrosis, left humerus HCC
  M87.829 Other osteonecrosis, unspecified humerus HCC ▽

√6th M87.83 Other osteonecrosis of radius, ulna and carpus
  M87.831 Other osteonecrosis of right radius HCC
  M87.832 Other osteonecrosis of left radius HCC
  M87.833 Other osteonecrosis of unspecified radius HCC ▽
  M87.834 Other osteonecrosis of right ulna HCC
  M87.835 Other osteonecrosis of left ulna HCC
  M87.836 Other osteonecrosis of unspecified ulna HCC ▽
  M87.837 Other osteonecrosis of right carpus HCC
  M87.838 Other osteonecrosis of left carpus HCC
  M87.839 Other osteonecrosis of unspecified carpus HCC ▽

√6th M87.84 Other osteonecrosis, hand and fingers
  M87.841 Other osteonecrosis, right hand HCC
  M87.842 Other osteonecrosis, left hand HCC
  M87.843 Other osteonecrosis, unspecified hand HCC ▽
  M87.844 Other osteonecrosis, right finger(s) HCC
  M87.845 Other osteonecrosis, left finger(s) HCC
  M87.849 Other osteonecrosis, unspecified finger(s) HCC ▽

√6th M87.85 Other osteonecrosis, pelvis and femur
  M87.850 Other osteonecrosis, pelvis HCC
  M87.851 Other osteonecrosis, right femur HCC
  M87.852 Other osteonecrosis, left femur HCC
  M87.859 Other osteonecrosis, unspecified femur HCC ▽

√6th M87.86 Other osteonecrosis, tibia and fibula
  M87.861 Other osteonecrosis, right tibia HCC
  M87.862 Other osteonecrosis, left tibia HCC
  M87.863 Other osteonecrosis, unspecified tibia HCC ▽
  M87.864 Other osteonecrosis, right fibula HCC
  M87.865 Other osteonecrosis, left fibula HCC
  M87.869 Other osteonecrosis, unspecified fibula HCC ▽

√6th M87.87 Other osteonecrosis, ankle, foot and toes
  M87.871 Other osteonecrosis, right ankle HCC
  M87.872 Other osteonecrosis, left ankle HCC
  M87.873 Other osteonecrosis, unspecified ankle HCC ▽
  M87.874 Other osteonecrosis, right foot HCC
  M87.875 Other osteonecrosis, left foot HCC
  M87.876 Other osteonecrosis, unspecified foot HCC ▽
  M87.877 Other osteonecrosis, right toe(s) HCC
  M87.878 Other osteonecrosis, left toe(s) HCC
  M87.879 Other osteonecrosis, unspecified toe(s) HCC ▽

M87.88 Other osteonecrosis, other site HCC
M87.89 Other osteonecrosis, multiple sites HCC
M87.9 Osteonecrosis, unspecified HCC ▽
  Necrosis of bone NOS

√4th M88 Osteitis deformans [Paget's disease of bone]
  EXCLUDES 1 osteitis deformans in neoplastic disease (M90.6)
M88.0 Osteitis deformans of skull
M88.1 Osteitis deformans of vertebrae
√5th M88.8 Osteitis deformans of other bones
  √6th M88.81 Osteitis deformans of shoulder
    M88.811 Osteitis deformans of right shoulder
    M88.812 Osteitis deformans of left shoulder
    M88.819 Osteitis deformans of unspecified shoulder ▽
  √6th M88.82 Osteitis deformans of upper arm
    M88.821 Osteitis deformans of right upper arm
    M88.822 Osteitis deformans of left upper arm
    M88.829 Osteitis deformans of unspecified upper arm ▽

√6th M88.83 Osteitis deformans of forearm
  M88.831 Osteitis deformans of right forearm
  M88.832 Osteitis deformans of left forearm
  M88.839 Osteitis deformans of unspecified forearm ▽
√6th M88.84 Osteitis deformans of hand
  M88.841 Osteitis deformans of right hand
  M88.842 Osteitis deformans of left hand
  M88.849 Osteitis deformans of unspecified hand ▽
√6th M88.85 Osteitis deformans of thigh
  M88.851 Osteitis deformans of right thigh
  M88.852 Osteitis deformans of left thigh
  M88.859 Osteitis deformans of unspecified thigh ▽
√6th M88.86 Osteitis deformans of lower leg
  M88.861 Osteitis deformans of right lower leg
  M88.862 Osteitis deformans of left lower leg
  M88.869 Osteitis deformans of unspecified lower leg ▽
√6th M88.87 Osteitis deformans of ankle and foot
  M88.871 Osteitis deformans of right ankle and foot
  M88.872 Osteitis deformans of left ankle and foot
  M88.879 Osteitis deformans of unspecified ankle and foot ▽
M88.88 Osteitis deformans of other bones
  EXCLUDES 2 osteitis deformans of skull (M88.0)
    osteitis deformans of vertebrae (M88.1)
M88.89 Osteitis deformans of multiple sites
M88.9 Osteitis deformans of unspecified bone ▽

√4th M89 Other disorders of bone
 √5th M89.0 Algoneurodystrophy
  Shoulder-hand syndrome
  Sudeck's atrophy
  EXCLUDES 1 causalgia, lower limb (G57.7-)
    causalgia, upper limb (G56.4-)
    complex regional pain syndrome II, lower limb (G57.7-)
    complex regional pain syndrome II, upper limb (G56.4-)
    reflex sympathetic dystrophy (G90.5-)
  M89.00 Algoneurodystrophy, unspecified site ▽
  √6th M89.01 Algoneurodystrophy, shoulder
    M89.011 Algoneurodystrophy, right shoulder
    M89.012 Algoneurodystrophy, left shoulder
    M89.019 Algoneurodystrophy, unspecified shoulder ▽
  √6th M89.02 Algoneurodystrophy, upper arm
    M89.021 Algoneurodystrophy, right upper arm
    M89.022 Algoneurodystrophy, left upper arm
    M89.029 Algoneurodystrophy, unspecified upper arm ▽
  √6th M89.03 Algoneurodystrophy, forearm
    M89.031 Algoneurodystrophy, right forearm
    M89.032 Algoneurodystrophy, left forearm
    M89.039 Algoneurodystrophy, unspecified forearm ▽
  √6th M89.04 Algoneurodystrophy, hand
    M89.041 Algoneurodystrophy, right hand
    M89.042 Algoneurodystrophy, left hand
    M89.049 Algoneurodystrophy, unspecified hand ▽
  √6th M89.05 Algoneurodystrophy, thigh
    M89.051 Algoneurodystrophy, right thigh
    M89.052 Algoneurodystrophy, left thigh
    M89.059 Algoneurodystrophy, unspecified thigh ▽
  √6th M89.06 Algoneurodystrophy, lower leg
    M89.061 Algoneurodystrophy, right lower leg
    M89.062 Algoneurodystrophy, left lower leg
    M89.069 Algoneurodystrophy, unspecified lower leg ▽
  √6th M89.07 Algoneurodystrophy, ankle and foot
    M89.071 Algoneurodystrophy, right ankle and foot
    M89.072 Algoneurodystrophy, left ankle and foot
    M89.079 Algoneurodystrophy, unspecified ankle and foot ▽
  M89.08 Algoneurodystrophy, other site
  M89.09 Algoneurodystrophy, multiple sites

✓ Additional Character Req ✓7th Placeholder Alert Manifestation HCC CMS-HCC Condition ▽ Unspecified Code ►◄ Revised Text ● New Code ▲ Revised Code Title

Chapter 13. Diseases of the Musculoskeletal System and Connective Tissue

✓5ᵗʰ **M89.1 Physeal arrest**
Arrest of growth plate   Growth plate arrest
Epiphyseal arrest

✓6ᵗʰ **M89.12 Physeal arrest, humerus**
- **M89.121** Complete physeal arrest, right proximal humerus
- **M89.122** Complete physeal arrest, left proximal humerus
- **M89.123** Partial physeal arrest, right proximal humerus
- **M89.124** Partial physeal arrest, left proximal humerus
- **M89.125** Complete physeal arrest, right distal humerus
- **M89.126** Complete physeal arrest, left distal humerus
- **M89.127** Partial physeal arrest, right distal humerus
- **M89.128** Partial physeal arrest, left distal humerus
- **M89.129** Physeal arrest, humerus, unspecified ▽

✓6ᵗʰ **M89.13 Physeal arrest, forearm**
- **M89.131** Complete physeal arrest, right distal radius
- **M89.132** Complete physeal arrest, left distal radius
- **M89.133** Partial physeal arrest, right distal radius
- **M89.134** Partial physeal arrest, left distal radius
- **M89.138** Other physeal arrest of forearm
- **M89.139** Physeal arrest, forearm, unspecified ▽

✓6ᵗʰ **M89.15 Physeal arrest, femur**
- **M89.151** Complete physeal arrest, right proximal femur
- **M89.152** Complete physeal arrest, left proximal femur
- **M89.153** Partial physeal arrest, right proximal femur
- **M89.154** Partial physeal arrest, left proximal femur
- **M89.155** Complete physeal arrest, right distal femur
- **M89.156** Complete physeal arrest, left distal femur
- **M89.157** Partial physeal arrest, right distal femur
- **M89.158** Partial physeal arrest, left distal femur
- **M89.159** Physeal arrest, femur, unspecified ▽

✓6ᵗʰ **M89.16 Physeal arrest, lower leg**
- **M89.160** Complete physeal arrest, right proximal tibia
- **M89.161** Complete physeal arrest, left proximal tibia
- **M89.162** Partial physeal arrest, right proximal tibia
- **M89.163** Partial physeal arrest, left proximal tibia
- **M89.164** Complete physeal arrest, right distal tibia
- **M89.165** Complete physeal arrest, left distal tibia
- **M89.166** Partial physeal arrest, right distal tibia
- **M89.167** Partial physeal arrest, left distal tibia
- **M89.168** Other physeal arrest of lower leg
- **M89.169** Physeal arrest, lower leg, unspecified ▽

M89.18 Physeal arrest, other site

✓5ᵗʰ **M89.2 Other disorders of bone development and growth**
- **M89.20** Other disorders of bone development and growth, unspecified site ▽

✓6ᵗʰ **M89.21 Other disorders of bone development and growth, shoulder**
- **M89.211** Other disorders of bone development and growth, right shoulder
- **M89.212** Other disorders of bone development and growth, left shoulder
- **M89.219** Other disorders of bone development and growth, unspecified shoulder ▽

✓6ᵗʰ **M89.22 Other disorders of bone development and growth, humerus**
- **M89.221** Other disorders of bone development and growth, right humerus
- **M89.222** Other disorders of bone development and growth, left humerus
- **M89.229** Other disorders of bone development and growth, unspecified humerus ▽

✓6ᵗʰ **M89.23 Other disorders of bone development and growth, ulna and radius**
- **M89.231** Other disorders of bone development and growth, right ulna
- **M89.232** Other disorders of bone development and growth, left ulna
- **M89.233** Other disorders of bone development and growth, right radius
- **M89.234** Other disorders of bone development and growth, left radius
- **M89.239** Other disorders of bone development and growth, unspecified ulna and radius ▽

✓6ᵗʰ **M89.24 Other disorders of bone development and growth, hand**
- **M89.241** Other disorders of bone development and growth, right hand
- **M89.242** Other disorders of bone development and growth, left hand
- **M89.249** Other disorders of bone development and growth, unspecified hand ▽

✓6ᵗʰ **M89.25 Other disorders of bone development and growth, femur**
- **M89.251** Other disorders of bone development and growth, right femur
- **M89.252** Other disorders of bone development and growth, left femur
- **M89.259** Other disorders of bone development and growth, unspecified femur ▽

✓6ᵗʰ **M89.26 Other disorders of bone development and growth, tibia and fibula**
- **M89.261** Other disorders of bone development and growth, right tibia
- **M89.262** Other disorders of bone development and growth, left tibia
- **M89.263** Other disorders of bone development and growth, right fibula
- **M89.264** Other disorders of bone development and growth, left fibula
- **M89.269** Other disorders of bone development and growth, unspecified lower leg ▽

✓6ᵗʰ **M89.27 Other disorders of bone development and growth, ankle and foot**
- **M89.271** Other disorders of bone development and growth, right ankle and foot
- **M89.272** Other disorders of bone development and growth, left ankle and foot
- **M89.279** Other disorders of bone development and growth, unspecified ankle and foot ▽

M89.28 Other disorders of bone development and growth, other site

M89.29 Other disorders of bone development and growth, multiple sites

✓5ᵗʰ **M89.3 Hypertrophy of bone**
- **M89.30** Hypertrophy of bone, unspecified site ▽

✓6ᵗʰ **M89.31 Hypertrophy of bone, shoulder**
- **M89.311** Hypertrophy of bone, right shoulder
- **M89.312** Hypertrophy of bone, left shoulder
- **M89.319** Hypertrophy of bone, unspecified shoulder ▽

✓6ᵗʰ **M89.32 Hypertrophy of bone, humerus**
- **M89.321** Hypertrophy of bone, right humerus
- **M89.322** Hypertrophy of bone, left humerus
- **M89.329** Hypertrophy of bone, unspecified humerus ▽

✓6ᵗʰ **M89.33 Hypertrophy of bone, ulna and radius**
- **M89.331** Hypertrophy of bone, right ulna
- **M89.332** Hypertrophy of bone, left ulna
- **M89.333** Hypertrophy of bone, right radius
- **M89.334** Hypertrophy of bone, left radius
- **M89.339** Hypertrophy of bone, unspecified ulna and radius ▽

✓6ᵗʰ **M89.34 Hypertrophy of bone, hand**
- **M89.341** Hypertrophy of bone, right hand
- **M89.342** Hypertrophy of bone, left hand
- **M89.349** Hypertrophy of bone, unspecified hand ▽

EXCLUDES 1 Not coded here   EXCLUDES 2 Not included here   N Newborn Age: 0   P Pediatric Age: 0-17   M Maternity Age: 12-55   A Adult Age: 15-124

790   ICD-10-CM 2018

✓6ᵗʰ **M89.35 Hypertrophy of bone, femur**
    M89.351 Hypertrophy of bone, right femur
    M89.352 Hypertrophy of bone, left femur
    M89.359 Hypertrophy of bone, unspecified ▽
        femur

✓6ᵗʰ **M89.36 Hypertrophy of bone, tibia and fibula**
    M89.361 Hypertrophy of bone, right tibia
    M89.362 Hypertrophy of bone, left tibia
    M89.363 Hypertrophy of bone, right fibula
    M89.364 Hypertrophy of bone, left fibula
    M89.369 Hypertrophy of bone, unspecified ▽
        tibia and fibula

✓6ᵗʰ **M89.37 Hypertrophy of bone, ankle and foot**
    M89.371 Hypertrophy of bone, right ankle and foot
    M89.372 Hypertrophy of bone, left ankle and foot
    M89.379 Hypertrophy of bone, unspecified ▽
        ankle and foot

    M89.38 Hypertrophy of bone, other site
    M89.39 Hypertrophy of bone, multiple sites

✓5ᵗʰ **M89.4 Other hypertrophic osteoarthropathy**
    Marie-Bamberger disease   Pachydermoperiostosis
    M89.40 Other hypertrophic osteoarthropathy, ▽
        unspecified site

✓6ᵗʰ **M89.41 Other hypertrophic osteoarthropathy, shoulder**
    M89.411 Other hypertrophic osteoarthropathy,
        right shoulder
    M89.412 Other hypertrophic osteoarthropathy,
        left shoulder
    M89.419 Other hypertrophic osteoarthropathy, ▽
        unspecified shoulder

✓6ᵗʰ **M89.42 Other hypertrophic osteoarthropathy, upper arm**
    M89.421 Other hypertrophic osteoarthropathy,
        right upper arm
    M89.422 Other hypertrophic osteoarthropathy,
        left upper arm
    M89.429 Other hypertrophic osteoarthropathy, ▽
        unspecified upper arm

✓6ᵗʰ **M89.43 Other hypertrophic osteoarthropathy, forearm**
    M89.431 Other hypertrophic osteoarthropathy,
        right forearm
    M89.432 Other hypertrophic osteoarthropathy,
        left forearm
    M89.439 Other hypertrophic osteoarthropathy, ▽
        unspecified forearm

✓6ᵗʰ **M89.44 Other hypertrophic osteoarthropathy, hand**
    M89.441 Other hypertrophic osteoarthropathy,
        right hand
    M89.442 Other hypertrophic osteoarthropathy,
        left hand
    M89.449 Other hypertrophic osteoarthropathy, ▽
        unspecified hand

✓6ᵗʰ **M89.45 Other hypertrophic osteoarthropathy, thigh**
    M89.451 Other hypertrophic osteoarthropathy,
        right thigh
    M89.452 Other hypertrophic osteoarthropathy,
        left thigh
    M89.459 Other hypertrophic osteoarthropathy, ▽
        unspecified thigh

✓6ᵗʰ **M89.46 Other hypertrophic osteoarthropathy, lower leg**
    M89.461 Other hypertrophic osteoarthropathy,
        right lower leg
    M89.462 Other hypertrophic osteoarthropathy,
        left lower leg
    M89.469 Other hypertrophic osteoarthropathy, ▽
        unspecified lower leg

✓6ᵗʰ **M89.47 Other hypertrophic osteoarthropathy, ankle and**
    foot
    M89.471 Other hypertrophic osteoarthropathy,
        right ankle and foot
    M89.472 Other hypertrophic osteoarthropathy,
        left ankle and foot
    M89.479 Other hypertrophic osteoarthropathy, ▽
        unspecified ankle and foot

    M89.48 Other hypertrophic osteoarthropathy, other site
    M89.49 Other hypertrophic osteoarthropathy, multiple sites

✓5ᵗʰ **M89.5 Osteolysis**
    Use additional code to identify major osseous defect, if
    applicable (M89.7-)
    EXCLUDES 2   periprosthetic osteolysis of internal prosthetic joint
         (T84.05-)
    M89.50 Osteolysis, unspecified site ▽

✓6ᵗʰ **M89.51 Osteolysis, shoulder**
    M89.511 Osteolysis, right shoulder
    M89.512 Osteolysis, left shoulder
    M89.519 Osteolysis, unspecified shoulder ▽

✓6ᵗʰ **M89.52 Osteolysis, upper arm**
    M89.521 Osteolysis, right upper arm
    M89.522 Osteolysis, left upper arm
    M89.529 Osteolysis, unspecified upper arm ▽

✓6ᵗʰ **M89.53 Osteolysis, forearm**
    M89.531 Osteolysis, right forearm
    M89.532 Osteolysis, left forearm
    M89.539 Osteolysis, unspecified forearm ▽

✓6ᵗʰ **M89.54 Osteolysis, hand**
    M89.541 Osteolysis, right hand
    M89.542 Osteolysis, left hand
    M89.549 Osteolysis, unspecified hand ▽

✓6ᵗʰ **M89.55 Osteolysis, thigh**
    M89.551 Osteolysis, right thigh
    M89.552 Osteolysis, left thigh
    M89.559 Osteolysis, unspecified thigh ▽

✓6ᵗʰ **M89.56 Osteolysis, lower leg**
    M89.561 Osteolysis, right lower leg
    M89.562 Osteolysis, left lower leg
    M89.569 Osteolysis, unspecified lower leg ▽

✓6ᵗʰ **M89.57 Osteolysis, ankle and foot**
    M89.571 Osteolysis, right ankle and foot
    M89.572 Osteolysis, left ankle and foot
    M89.579 Osteolysis, unspecified ankle and foot ▽

    M89.58 Osteolysis, other site
    M89.59 Osteolysis, multiple sites

✓5ᵗʰ **M89.6 Osteopathy after poliomyelitis**
    Use additional code (B91) to identify previous poliomyelitis
    EXCLUDES 1   postpolio syndrome (G14)
    M89.60 Osteopathy after poliomyelitis, unspecified HCC ▽
        site

✓6ᵗʰ **M89.61 Osteopathy after poliomyelitis, shoulder**
    M89.611 Osteopathy after poliomyelitis, right HCC
        shoulder
    M89.612 Osteopathy after poliomyelitis, left HCC
        shoulder
    M89.619 Osteopathy after poliomyelitis, HCC ▽
        unspecified shoulder

✓6ᵗʰ **M89.62 Osteopathy after poliomyelitis, upper arm**
    M89.621 Osteopathy after poliomyelitis, right HCC
        upper arm
    M89.622 Osteopathy after poliomyelitis, left HCC
        upper arm
    M89.629 Osteopathy after poliomyelitis, HCC ▽
        unspecified upper arm

✓6ᵗʰ **M89.63 Osteopathy after poliomyelitis, forearm**
    M89.631 Osteopathy after poliomyelitis, right HCC
        forearm
    M89.632 Osteopathy after poliomyelitis, left HCC
        forearm
    M89.639 Osteopathy after poliomyelitis, HCC ▽
        unspecified forearm

✓6ᵗʰ **M89.64 Osteopathy after poliomyelitis, hand**
    M89.641 Osteopathy after poliomyelitis, HCC
        right hand
    M89.642 Osteopathy after poliomyelitis, HCC
        left hand
    M89.649 Osteopathy after poliomyelitis, HCC ▽
        unspecified hand

✓6ᵗʰ **M89.65 Osteopathy after poliomyelitis, thigh**
    M89.651 Osteopathy after poliomyelitis, HCC
        right thigh
    M89.652 Osteopathy after poliomyelitis, HCC
        left thigh

☑ Additional Character Req   ✓x7ᵗʰ Placeholder Alert   Manifestation   HCC CMS-HCC Condition   ▽ Unspecified Code   ►◄ Revised Text   ● New Code   ▲ Revised Code Title

M89.659   **Osteopathy after poliomyelitis,** HCC ▽
unspecified thigh

✓6ᵗʰ   **M89.66**   **Osteopathy after poliomyelitis,** lower leg

M89.661   **Osteopathy after poliomyelitis,** right HCC
lower leg

M89.662   **Osteopathy after poliomyelitis,** left HCC
lower leg

M89.669   **Osteopathy after poliomyelitis,** HCC ▽
unspecified lower leg

✓6ᵗʰ   **M89.67**   **Osteopathy after poliomyelitis,** ankle and foot

M89.671   **Osteopathy after poliomyelitis,** right HCC
ankle and foot

M89.672   **Osteopathy after poliomyelitis,** left HCC
ankle and foot

M89.679   **Osteopathy after poliomyelitis,** HCC ▽
unspecified ankle and foot

M89.68   **Osteopathy after poliomyelitis, other site** HCC

M89.69   **Osteopathy after poliomyelitis,** multiple sites HCC

✓5ᵗʰ   **M89.7**   **Major osseous defect**

Code first underlying disease, if known, such as:
aseptic necrosis of bone (M87.-)
malignant neoplasm of bone (C40.-)
osteolysis (M89.5)
osteomyelitis (M86.-)
osteonecrosis (M87.-)
osteoporosis (M80.-, M81.-)
periprosthetic osteolysis (T84.05-)

M89.70   **Major osseous defect, unspecified site** ▽

✓6ᵗʰ   **M89.71**   **Major osseous defect,** shoulder region
Major osseous defect clavicle or scapula

M89.711   **Major osseous defect,** right shoulder
region

M89.712   **Major osseous defect,** left shoulder region

M89.719   **Major osseous defect,** unspecified ▽
shoulder region

✓6ᵗʰ   **M89.72**   **Major osseous defect,** humerus

M89.721   **Major osseous defect,** right humerus

M89.722   **Major osseous defect,** left humerus

M89.729   **Major osseous defect,** unspecified ▽
humerus

✓6ᵗʰ   **M89.73**   **Major osseous defect,** forearm
Major osseous defect of radius and ulna

M89.731   **Major osseous defect,** right forearm

M89.732   **Major osseous defect,** left forearm

M89.739   **Major osseous defect,** unspecified ▽
forearm

✓6ᵗʰ   **M89.74**   **Major osseous defect,** hand
Major osseous defect of carpus, fingers, metacarpus

M89.741   **Major osseous defect,** right hand

M89.742   **Major osseous defect,** left hand

M89.749   **Major osseous defect,** unspecified hand ▽

✓6ᵗʰ   **M89.75**   **Major osseous defect,** pelvic region and thigh
Major osseous defect of femur and pelvis

M89.751   **Major osseous defect,** right pelvic region
and thigh

M89.752   **Major osseous defect,** left pelvic region
and thigh

M89.759   **Major osseous defect,** unspecified ▽
pelvic region and thigh

✓6ᵗʰ   **M89.76**   **Major osseous defect,** lower leg
Major osseous defect of fibula and tibia

M89.761   **Major osseous defect,** right lower leg

M89.762   **Major osseous defect,** left lower leg

M89.769   **Major osseous defect,** unspecified ▽
lower leg

✓6ᵗʰ   **M89.77**   **Major osseous defect,** ankle and foot
Major osseous defect of metatarsus, tarsus, toes

M89.771   **Major osseous defect,** right ankle and foot

M89.772   **Major osseous defect,** left ankle and foot

M89.779   **Major osseous defect,** unspecified ▽
ankle and foot

M89.78   **Major osseous defect, other site**

M89.79   **Major osseous defect,** multiple sites

✓5ᵗʰ   **M89.8**   **Other specified disorders of bone**
Infantile cortical hyperostoses
Post-traumatic subperiosteal ossification

✓6ᵗʰ   **M89.8X**   **Other specified disorders of bone**

M89.8X0   **Other specified disorders of bone,**
multiple sites

M89.8X1   **Other specified disorders of bone,**
shoulder

M89.8X2   **Other specified disorders of bone,** upper
arm

M89.8X3   **Other specified disorders of bone,** forearm

M89.8X4   **Other specified disorders of bone,** hand

M89.8X5   **Other specified disorders of bone,** thigh

M89.8X6   **Other specified disorders of bone,** lower
leg

M89.8X7   **Other specified disorders of bone,** ankle
and foot

M89.8X8   **Other specified disorders of bone, other**
site

M89.8X9   **Other specified disorders of bone,** ▽
unspecified site

M89.9   **Disorder of bone, unspecified** ▽

✓4ᵗʰ   **M90**   **Osteopathies in diseases classified elsewhere**

EXCLUDES 1   osteochondritis, osteomyelitis, and osteopathy (in):
cryptococcosis (B45.3)
diabetes mellitus (E08-E13 with .69-)
gonococcal (A54.43)
neurogenic syphilis (A52.11)
renal osteodystrophy (N25.0)
salmonellosis (A02.24)
secondary syphilis (A51.46)
syphilis (late) (A52.77)

✓5ᵗʰ   **M90.5**   **Osteonecrosis in diseases classified elsewhere**

Code first underlying disease, such as:
caisson disease (T70.3)
hemoglobinopathy (D50-D64)

M90.50   **Osteonecrosis in diseases classified elsewhere,** HCC ▽
unspecified site

✓6ᵗʰ   **M90.51**   **Osteonecrosis in diseases classified elsewhere,**
shoulder

M90.511   **Osteonecrosis in diseases classified** HCC
elsewhere, right shoulder

M90.512   **Osteonecrosis in diseases classified** HCC
elsewhere, left shoulder

M90.519   **Osteonecrosis in diseases classified** HCC ▽
elsewhere, unspecified shoulder

✓6ᵗʰ   **M90.52**   **Osteonecrosis in diseases classified elsewhere,**
upper arm

M90.521   **Osteonecrosis in diseases classified** HCC
elsewhere, right upper arm

M90.522   **Osteonecrosis in diseases classified** HCC
elsewhere, left upper arm

M90.529   **Osteonecrosis in diseases classified** HCC ▽
elsewhere, unspecified upper arm

✓6ᵗʰ   **M90.53**   **Osteonecrosis in diseases classified elsewhere,**
forearm

M90.531   **Osteonecrosis in diseases classified** HCC
elsewhere, right forearm

M90.532   **Osteonecrosis in diseases classified** HCC
elsewhere, left forearm

M90.539   **Osteonecrosis in diseases classified** HCC ▽
elsewhere, unspecified forearm

✓6ᵗʰ   **M90.54**   **Osteonecrosis in diseases classified elsewhere,** hand

M90.541   **Osteonecrosis in diseases classified** HCC
elsewhere, right hand

M90.542   **Osteonecrosis in diseases classified** HCC
elsewhere, left hand

M90.549   **Osteonecrosis in diseases classified** HCC ▽
elsewhere, unspecified hand

✓6ᵗʰ   **M90.55**   **Osteonecrosis in diseases classified elsewhere,** thigh

M90.551   **Osteonecrosis in diseases classified** HCC
elsewhere, right thigh

M90.552   **Osteonecrosis in diseases classified** HCC
elsewhere, left thigh

M90.559   **Osteonecrosis in diseases classified** HCC ▽
elsewhere, unspecified thigh

EXCLUDES 1 Not coded here   *EXCLUDES 2* Not included here   N Newborn Age: 0   P Pediatric Age: 0-17   M Maternity Age: 12-55   A Adult Age: 15-124

792   ICD-10-CM 2018

☑6ᵗʰ **M90.56** Osteonecrosis in diseases classified elsewhere, lower leg

    M90.561 Osteonecrosis in diseases classified elsewhere, *right* lower leg   HCC

    M90.562 Osteonecrosis in diseases classified elsewhere, *left* lower leg   HCC

    M90.569 Osteonecrosis in diseases classified elsewhere, unspecified lower leg   HCC ▽

☑6ᵗʰ **M90.57** Osteonecrosis in diseases classified elsewhere, ankle and foot

    M90.571 Osteonecrosis in diseases classified elsewhere, *right* ankle and foot   HCC

    M90.572 Osteonecrosis in diseases classified elsewhere, *left* ankle and foot   HCC

    M90.579 Osteonecrosis in diseases classified elsewhere, unspecified ankle and foot   HCC ▽

   M90.58 Osteonecrosis in diseases classified elsewhere, other site   HCC

   M90.59 Osteonecrosis in diseases classified elsewhere, multiple sites   HCC

☑5ᵗʰ **M90.6** Osteitis deformans in neoplastic diseases

    Osteitis deformans in malignant neoplasm of bone

    Code first the neoplasm (C40-, C41-)

    EXCLUDES 1   osteitis deformans [Paget's disease of bone] (M88.-)

   M90.60 Osteitis deformans in neoplastic diseases, unspecified site ▽

☑6ᵗʰ **M90.61** Osteitis deformans in neoplastic diseases, shoulder

    M90.611 Osteitis deformans in neoplastic diseases, *right* shoulder

    M90.612 Osteitis deformans in neoplastic diseases, *left* shoulder

    M90.619 Osteitis deformans in neoplastic diseases, unspecified shoulder ▽

☑6ᵗʰ **M90.62** Osteitis deformans in neoplastic diseases, upper arm

    M90.621 Osteitis deformans in neoplastic diseases, *right* upper arm

    M90.622 Osteitis deformans in neoplastic diseases, *left* upper arm

    M90.629 Osteitis deformans in neoplastic diseases, unspecified upper arm ▽

☑6ᵗʰ **M90.63** Osteitis deformans in neoplastic diseases, forearm

    M90.631 Osteitis deformans in neoplastic diseases, *right* forearm

    M90.632 Osteitis deformans in neoplastic diseases, *left* forearm

    M90.639 Osteitis deformans in neoplastic diseases, unspecified forearm ▽

☑6ᵗʰ **M90.64** Osteitis deformans in neoplastic diseases, hand

    M90.641 Osteitis deformans in neoplastic diseases, *right* hand

    M90.642 Osteitis deformans in neoplastic diseases, *left* hand

    M90.649 Osteitis deformans in neoplastic diseases, unspecified hand ▽

☑6ᵗʰ **M90.65** Osteitis deformans in neoplastic diseases, thigh

    M90.651 Osteitis deformans in neoplastic diseases, *right* thigh

    M90.652 Osteitis deformans in neoplastic diseases, *left* thigh

    M90.659 Osteitis deformans in neoplastic diseases, unspecified thigh ▽

☑6ᵗʰ **M90.66** Osteitis deformans in neoplastic diseases, lower leg

    M90.661 Osteitis deformans in neoplastic diseases, *right* lower leg

    M90.662 Osteitis deformans in neoplastic diseases, *left* lower leg

    M90.669 Osteitis deformans in neoplastic diseases, unspecified lower leg ▽

☑6ᵗʰ **M90.67** Osteitis deformans in neoplastic diseases, ankle and foot

    M90.671 Osteitis deformans in neoplastic diseases, *right* ankle and foot

    M90.672 Osteitis deformans in neoplastic diseases, *left* ankle and foot

    M90.679 Osteitis deformans in neoplastic diseases, unspecified ankle and foot ▽

   M90.68 Osteitis deformans in neoplastic diseases, other site

   M90.69 Osteitis deformans in neoplastic diseases, multiple sites

☑5ᵗʰ **M90.8** Osteopathy in diseases classified elsewhere

    Code first underlying disease, such as:

     rickets (E55.0)

     vitamin-D-resistant rickets (E83.3)

   M90.80 Osteopathy in diseases classified elsewhere, unspecified site ▽

☑6ᵗʰ **M90.81** Osteopathy in diseases classified elsewhere, shoulder

    M90.811 Osteopathy in diseases classified elsewhere, *right* shoulder

    M90.812 Osteopathy in diseases classified elsewhere, *left* shoulder

    M90.819 Osteopathy in diseases classified elsewhere, unspecified shoulder ▽

☑6ᵗʰ **M90.82** Osteopathy in diseases classified elsewhere, upper arm

    M90.821 Osteopathy in diseases classified elsewhere, *right* upper arm

    M90.822 Osteopathy in diseases classified elsewhere, *left* upper arm

    M90.829 Osteopathy in diseases classified elsewhere, unspecified upper arm ▽

☑6ᵗʰ **M90.83** Osteopathy in diseases classified elsewhere, forearm

    M90.831 Osteopathy in diseases classified elsewhere, *right* forearm

    M90.832 Osteopathy in diseases classified elsewhere, *left* forearm

    M90.839 Osteopathy in diseases classified elsewhere, unspecified forearm ▽

☑6ᵗʰ **M90.84** Osteopathy in diseases classified elsewhere, hand

    M90.841 Osteopathy in diseases classified elsewhere, *right* hand

    M90.842 Osteopathy in diseases classified elsewhere, *left* hand

    M90.849 Osteopathy in diseases classified elsewhere, unspecified hand ▽

☑6ᵗʰ **M90.85** Osteopathy in diseases classified elsewhere, thigh

    M90.851 Osteopathy in diseases classified elsewhere, *right* thigh

    M90.852 Osteopathy in diseases classified elsewhere, *left* thigh

    M90.859 Osteopathy in diseases classified elsewhere, unspecified thigh ▽

☑6ᵗʰ **M90.86** Osteopathy in diseases classified elsewhere, lower leg

    M90.861 Osteopathy in diseases classified elsewhere, *right* lower leg

    M90.862 Osteopathy in diseases classified elsewhere, *left* lower leg

    M90.869 Osteopathy in diseases classified elsewhere, unspecified lower leg ▽

☑6ᵗʰ **M90.87** Osteopathy in diseases classified elsewhere, ankle and foot

    M90.871 Osteopathy in diseases classified elsewhere, *right* ankle and foot

    M90.872 Osteopathy in diseases classified elsewhere, *left* ankle and foot

    M90.879 Osteopathy in diseases classified elsewhere, unspecified ankle and foot ▽

   M90.88 Osteopathy in diseases classified elsewhere, other site

   M90.89 Osteopathy in diseases classified elsewhere, multiple sites

Chondropathies (M91-M94)

   EXCLUDES 1   postprocedural chondropathies (M96.-)

☑4ᵗʰ **M91** Juvenile osteochondrosis of hip and pelvis

    EXCLUDES 1   slipped upper femoral epiphysis (nontraumatic) (M93.0)

   M91.0 Juvenile osteochondrosis of pelvis

    Osteochondrosis (juvenile) of acetabulum

    Osteochondrosis (juvenile) of iliac crest [Buchanan]

    Osteochondrosis (juvenile) of ischiopubic synchondrosis [van Neck]

    Osteochondrosis (juvenile) of symphysis pubis [Pierson]

☑ Additional Character Req   ☑7ᵗʰ Placeholder Alert   Manifestation   HCC CMS-HCC Condition   ▽ Unspecified Code   ▶◀ Revised Text   ● New Code   ▲ Revised Code Title

√5ᵗʰ **M91.1** Juvenile osteochondrosis of head of femur [Legg-Calvé-Perthes]

    M91.10 Juvenile osteochondrosis of head of femur [Legg-Calvé-Perthes], unspecified leg ▽

    M91.11 Juvenile osteochondrosis of head of femur [Legg-Calvé-Perthes], right leg

    M91.12 Juvenile osteochondrosis of head of femur [Legg-Calvé-Perthes], left leg

√5ᵗʰ **M91.2** Coxa plana
    Hip deformity due to previous juvenile osteochondrosis

    M91.20 Coxa plana, unspecified hip ▽

    M91.21 Coxa plana, right hip

    M91.22 Coxa plana, left hip

√5ᵗʰ **M91.3** Pseudocoxalgia

    M91.30 Pseudocoxalgia, unspecified hip ▽

    M91.31 Pseudocoxalgia, right hip

    M91.32 Pseudocoxalgia, left hip

√5ᵗʰ **M91.4** Coxa magna

    M91.40 Coxa magna, unspecified hip ▽

    M91.41 Coxa magna, right hip

    M91.42 Coxa magna, left hip

√5ᵗʰ **M91.8** Other juvenile osteochondrosis of hip and pelvis
    Juvenile osteochondrosis after reduction of congenital dislocation of hip

    M91.80 Other juvenile osteochondrosis of hip and pelvis, unspecified leg ▽

    M91.81 Other juvenile osteochondrosis of hip and pelvis, right leg

    M91.82 Other juvenile osteochondrosis of hip and pelvis, left leg

√5ᵗʰ **M91.9** Juvenile osteochondrosis of hip and pelvis, unspecified

    M91.90 Juvenile osteochondrosis of hip and pelvis, unspecified, unspecified leg ▽

    M91.91 Juvenile osteochondrosis of hip and pelvis, unspecified, right leg ▽

    M91.92 Juvenile osteochondrosis of hip and pelvis, unspecified, left leg ▽

√4ᵗʰ **M92** Other juvenile osteochondrosis

√5ᵗʰ **M92.0** Juvenile osteochondrosis of humerus
    Osteochondrosis (juvenile) of capitulum of humerus [Panner]
    Osteochondrosis (juvenile) of head of humerus [Haas]

    M92.00 Juvenile osteochondrosis of humerus, unspecified arm ▽

    M92.01 Juvenile osteochondrosis of humerus, right arm

    M92.02 Juvenile osteochondrosis of humerus, left arm

√5ᵗʰ **M92.1** Juvenile osteochondrosis of radius and ulna
    Osteochondrosis (juvenile) of lower ulna [Burns]
    Osteochondrosis (juvenile) of radial head [Brailsford]

    M92.10 Juvenile osteochondrosis of radius and ulna, unspecified arm ▽

    M92.11 Juvenile osteochondrosis of radius and ulna, right arm

    M92.12 Juvenile osteochondrosis of radius and ulna, left arm

√5ᵗʰ **M92.2** Juvenile osteochondrosis, hand

    √6ᵗʰ **M92.20** Unspecified juvenile osteochondrosis, hand

      M92.201 Unspecified juvenile osteochondrosis, right hand ▽

      M92.202 Unspecified juvenile osteochondrosis, left hand ▽

      M92.209 Unspecified juvenile osteochondrosis, unspecified hand ▽

    √6ᵗʰ **M92.21** Osteochondrosis (juvenile) of carpal lunate [Kienböck]

      M92.211 Osteochondrosis (juvenile) of carpal lunate [Kienböck], right hand

      M92.212 Osteochondrosis (juvenile) of carpal lunate [Kienböck], left hand

      M92.219 Osteochondrosis (juvenile) of carpal lunate [Kienböck], unspecified hand ▽

    √6ᵗʰ **M92.22** Osteochondrosis (juvenile) of metacarpal heads [Mauclaire]

      M92.221 Osteochondrosis (juvenile) of metacarpal heads [Mauclaire], right hand

      M92.222 Osteochondrosis (juvenile) of metacarpal heads [Mauclaire], left hand

      M92.229 Osteochondrosis (juvenile) of metacarpal heads [Mauclaire], unspecified hand ▽

    √6ᵗʰ **M92.29** Other juvenile osteochondrosis, hand

      M92.291 Other juvenile osteochondrosis, right hand

      M92.292 Other juvenile osteochondrosis, left hand

      M92.299 Other juvenile osteochondrosis, unspecified hand ▽

√5ᵗʰ **M92.3** Other juvenile osteochondrosis, upper limb

    M92.30 Other juvenile osteochondrosis, unspecified upper limb ▽

    M92.31 Other juvenile osteochondrosis, right upper limb

    M92.32 Other juvenile osteochondrosis, left upper limb

√5ᵗʰ **M92.4** Juvenile osteochondrosis of patella
    Osteochondrosis (juvenile) of primary patellar center [Köhler]
    Osteochondrosis (juvenile) of secondary patellar centre [Sinding Larsen]

    M92.40 Juvenile osteochondrosis of patella, unspecified knee ▽

    M92.41 Juvenile osteochondrosis of patella, right knee

    M92.42 Juvenile osteochondrosis of patella, left knee

√5ᵗʰ **M92.5** Juvenile osteochondrosis of tibia and fibula
    Osteochondrosis (juvenile) of proximal tibia [Blount]
    Osteochondrosis (juvenile) of tibial tubercle [Osgood-Schlatter]
    Tibia vara

    M92.50 Juvenile osteochondrosis of tibia and fibula, unspecified leg ▽

    M92.51 Juvenile osteochondrosis of tibia and fibula, right leg

    M92.52 Juvenile osteochondrosis of tibia and fibula, left leg

√5ᵗʰ **M92.6** Juvenile osteochondrosis of tarsus
    Osteochondrosis (juvenile) of calcaneum [Sever]
    Osteochondrosis (juvenile) of os tibiale externum [Haglund]
    Osteochondrosis (juvenile) of talus [Diaz]
    Osteochondrosis (juvenile) of tarsal navicular [Köhler]

    M92.60 Juvenile osteochondrosis of tarsus, unspecified ankle ▽

    M92.61 Juvenile osteochondrosis of tarsus, right ankle

    M92.62 Juvenile osteochondrosis of tarsus, left ankle

√5ᵗʰ **M92.7** Juvenile osteochondrosis of metatarsus
    Osteochondrosis (juvenile) of fifth metatarsus [Iselin]
    Osteochondrosis (juvenile) of second metatarsus [Freiberg]

    M92.70 Juvenile osteochondrosis of metatarsus, unspecified foot ▽

    M92.71 Juvenile osteochondrosis of metatarsus, right foot

    M92.72 Juvenile osteochondrosis of metatarsus, left foot

M92.8 Other specified juvenile osteochondrosis
    Calcaneal apophysitis

M92.9 Juvenile osteochondrosis, unspecified ▽
    Juvenile apophysitis NOS
    Juvenile epiphysitis NOS
    Juvenile osteochondritis NOS
    Juvenile osteochondrosis NOS

√4ᵗʰ **M93** Other osteochondropathies
    EXCLUDES 2   osteochondrosis of spine (M42.-)

√5ᵗʰ **M93.0** Slipped upper femoral epiphysis (nontraumatic)
    Use additional code for associated chondrolysis (M94.3)

    √6ᵗʰ **M93.00** Unspecified slipped upper femoral epiphysis (nontraumatic)

      M93.001 Unspecified slipped upper femoral epiphysis (nontraumatic), right hip ▽

      M93.002 Unspecified slipped upper femoral epiphysis (nontraumatic), left hip ▽

      M93.003 Unspecified slipped upper femoral epiphysis (nontraumatic), unspecified hip ▽

    √6ᵗʰ **M93.01** Acute slipped upper femoral epiphysis (nontraumatic)

      M93.011 Acute slipped upper femoral epiphysis (nontraumatic), right hip

      M93.012 Acute slipped upper femoral epiphysis (nontraumatic), left hip

      M93.013 Acute slipped upper femoral epiphysis (nontraumatic), unspecified hip ▽

EXCLUDES 1 Not coded here   *EXCLUDES 2* Not included here   N Newborn Age: 0   P Pediatric Age: 0-17   M Maternity Age: 12-55   A Adult Age: 15-124

✓6ᵗʰ **M93.02 Chronic slipped upper femoral epiphysis (nontraumatic)**
    M93.021 Chronic slipped upper femoral epiphysis (nontraumatic), right hip
    M93.022 Chronic slipped upper femoral epiphysis (nontraumatic), left hip
    M93.023 Chronic slipped upper femoral epiphysis (nontraumatic), unspecified hip ▽

✓6ᵗʰ **M93.03 Acute on chronic slipped upper femoral epiphysis (nontraumatic)**
    M93.031 Acute on chronic slipped upper femoral epiphysis (nontraumatic), right hip
    M93.032 Acute on chronic slipped upper femoral epiphysis (nontraumatic), left hip
    M93.033 Acute on chronic slipped upper femoral epiphysis (nontraumatic), unspecified hip ▽

M93.1 Kienböck's disease of adults Ⓐ
    Adult osteochondrosis of carpal lunates

✓5ᵗʰ **M93.2 Osteochondritis dissecans**
    M93.20 Osteochondritis dissecans of unspecified site ▽

✓6ᵗʰ **M93.21 Osteochondritis dissecans of shoulder**
    M93.211 Osteochondritis dissecans, right shoulder
    M93.212 Osteochondritis dissecans, left shoulder
    M93.219 Osteochondritis dissecans, unspecified shoulder ▽

✓6ᵗʰ **M93.22 Osteochondritis dissecans of elbow**
    M93.221 Osteochondritis dissecans, right elbow
    M93.222 Osteochondritis dissecans, left elbow
    M93.229 Osteochondritis dissecans, unspecified elbow ▽

✓6ᵗʰ **M93.23 Osteochondritis dissecans of wrist**
    M93.231 Osteochondritis dissecans, right wrist
    M93.232 Osteochondritis dissecans, left wrist
    M93.239 Osteochondritis dissecans, unspecified wrist ▽

✓6ᵗʰ **M93.24 Osteochondritis dissecans of joints of hand**
    M93.241 Osteochondritis dissecans, joints of right hand
    M93.242 Osteochondritis dissecans, joints of left hand
    M93.249 Osteochondritis dissecans, joints of unspecified hand ▽

✓6ᵗʰ **M93.25 Osteochondritis dissecans of hip**
    M93.251 Osteochondritis dissecans, right hip
    M93.252 Osteochondritis dissecans, left hip
    M93.259 Osteochondritis dissecans, unspecified hip ▽

✓6ᵗʰ **M93.26 Osteochondritis dissecans knee**
    M93.261 Osteochondritis dissecans, right knee
    M93.262 Osteochondritis dissecans, left knee
    M93.269 Osteochondritis dissecans, unspecified knee ▽

✓6ᵗʰ **M93.27 Osteochondritis dissecans of ankle and joints of foot**
    M93.271 Osteochondritis dissecans, right ankle and joints of right foot
    M93.272 Osteochondritis dissecans, left ankle and joints of left foot
    M93.279 Osteochondritis dissecans, unspecified ankle and joints of foot ▽

    M93.28 Osteochondritis dissecans other site
    M93.29 Osteochondritis dissecans multiple sites

✓5ᵗʰ **M93.8 Other specified osteochondropathies**
    M93.80 Other specified osteochondropathies of unspecified site ▽

✓6ᵗʰ **M93.81 Other specified osteochondropathies of shoulder**
    M93.811 Other specified osteochondropathies, right shoulder
    M93.812 Other specified osteochondropathies, left shoulder
    M93.819 Other specified osteochondropathies, unspecified shoulder ▽

✓6ᵗʰ **M93.82 Other specified osteochondropathies of upper arm**
    M93.821 Other specified osteochondropathies, right upper arm
    M93.822 Other specified osteochondropathies, left upper arm
    M93.829 Other specified osteochondropathies, unspecified upper arm ▽

✓6ᵗʰ **M93.83 Other specified osteochondropathies of forearm**
    M93.831 Other specified osteochondropathies, right forearm
    M93.832 Other specified osteochondropathies, left forearm
    M93.839 Other specified osteochondropathies, unspecified forearm ▽

✓6ᵗʰ **M93.84 Other specified osteochondropathies of hand**
    M93.841 Other specified osteochondropathies, right hand
    M93.842 Other specified osteochondropathies, left hand
    M93.849 Other specified osteochondropathies, unspecified hand ▽

✓6ᵗʰ **M93.85 Other specified osteochondropathies of thigh**
    M93.851 Other specified osteochondropathies, right thigh
    M93.852 Other specified osteochondropathies, left thigh
    M93.859 Other specified osteochondropathies, unspecified thigh ▽

✓6ᵗʰ **M93.86 Other specified osteochondropathies lower leg**
    M93.861 Other specified osteochondropathies, right lower leg
    M93.862 Other specified osteochondropathies, left lower leg
    M93.869 Other specified osteochondropathies, unspecified lower leg ▽

✓6ᵗʰ **M93.87 Other specified osteochondropathies of ankle and foot**
    M93.871 Other specified osteochondropathies, right ankle and foot
    M93.872 Other specified osteochondropathies, left ankle and foot
    M93.879 Other specified osteochondropathies, unspecified ankle and foot ▽

    M93.88 Other specified osteochondropathies other site
    M93.89 Other specified osteochondropathies multiple sites

✓5ᵗʰ **M93.9 Osteochondropathy, unspecified**
    Apophysitis NOS   Osteochondritis NOS
    Epiphysitis NOS   Osteochondrosis NOS
    M93.90 Osteochondropathy, unspecified of unspecified site ▽

✓6ᵗʰ **M93.91 Osteochondropathy, unspecified of shoulder**
    M93.911 Osteochondropathy, unspecified, right shoulder ▽
    M93.912 Osteochondropathy, unspecified, left shoulder ▽
    M93.919 Osteochondropathy, unspecified, unspecified shoulder ▽

✓6ᵗʰ **M93.92 Osteochondropathy, unspecified of upper arm**
    M93.921 Osteochondropathy, unspecified, right upper arm ▽
    M93.922 Osteochondropathy, unspecified, left upper arm ▽
    M93.929 Osteochondropathy, unspecified, unspecified upper arm ▽

✓6ᵗʰ **M93.93 Osteochondropathy, unspecified of forearm**
    M93.931 Osteochondropathy, unspecified, right forearm ▽
    M93.932 Osteochondropathy, unspecified, left forearm ▽
    M93.939 Osteochondropathy, unspecified, unspecified forearm ▽

✓6ᵗʰ **M93.94 Osteochondropathy, unspecified of hand**
    M93.941 Osteochondropathy, unspecified, right hand ▽
    M93.942 Osteochondropathy, unspecified, left hand ▽
    M93.949 Osteochondropathy, unspecified, unspecified hand ▽

✓ Additional Character Req   ✗7ᵗʰ Placeholder Alert   Manifestation   ᴴᶜᶜ CMS-HCC Condition   ▽ Unspecified Code   ▶◀ Revised Text   ● New Code   ▲ Revised Code Title

ICD-10-CM 2018   795

✓6ᵗʰ M93.95 Osteochondropathy, unspecified of thigh
- M93.951 Osteochondropathy, unspecified, right thigh ▽
- M93.952 Osteochondropathy, unspecified, left thigh ▽
- M93.959 Osteochondropathy, unspecified, unspecified thigh ▽

✓6ᵗʰ M93.96 Osteochondropathy, unspecified lower leg
- M93.961 Osteochondropathy, unspecified, right lower leg ▽
- M93.962 Osteochondropathy, unspecified, left lower leg ▽
- M93.969 Osteochondropathy, unspecified, unspecified lower leg ▽

✓6ᵗʰ M93.97 Osteochondropathy, unspecified of ankle and foot
- M93.971 Osteochondropathy, unspecified, right ankle and foot ▽
- M93.972 Osteochondropathy, unspecified, left ankle and foot ▽
- M93.979 Osteochondropathy, unspecified, unspecified ankle and foot ▽

M93.98 Osteochondropathy, unspecified other site ▽
M93.99 Osteochondropathy, unspecified multiple sites ▽

✓4ᵗʰ M94 Other disorders of cartilage

M94.0 Chondrocostal junction syndrome [Tietze]
  Costochondritis

M94.1 Relapsing polychondritis

✓5ᵗʰ M94.2 Chondromalacia
  EXCLUDES 1   chondromalacia patellae (M22.4)
- **M94.20 Chondromalacia, unspecified site** ▽
- **✓6ᵗʰ M94.21 Chondromalacia, shoulder**
  - M94.211 Chondromalacia, right shoulder
  - M94.212 Chondromalacia, left shoulder
  - M94.219 Chondromalacia, unspecified shoulder ▽
- **✓6ᵗʰ M94.22 Chondromalacia, elbow**
  - M94.221 Chondromalacia, right elbow
  - M94.222 Chondromalacia, left elbow
  - M94.229 Chondromalacia, unspecified elbow ▽
- **✓6ᵗʰ M94.23 Chondromalacia, wrist**
  - M94.231 Chondromalacia, right wrist
  - M94.232 Chondromalacia, left wrist
  - M94.239 Chondromalacia, unspecified wrist ▽
- **✓6ᵗʰ M94.24 Chondromalacia, joints of hand**
  - M94.241 Chondromalacia, joints of right hand
  - M94.242 Chondromalacia, joints of left hand
  - M94.249 Chondromalacia, joints of unspecified hand ▽
- **✓6ᵗʰ M94.25 Chondromalacia, hip**
  - M94.251 Chondromalacia, right hip
  - M94.252 Chondromalacia, left hip
  - M94.259 Chondromalacia, unspecified hip ▽
- **✓6ᵗʰ M94.26 Chondromalacia, knee**
  - M94.261 Chondromalacia, right knee
  - M94.262 Chondromalacia, left knee
  - M94.269 Chondromalacia, unspecified knee ▽
- **✓6ᵗʰ M94.27 Chondromalacia, ankle and joints of foot**
  - M94.271 Chondromalacia, right ankle and joints of right foot
  - M94.272 Chondromalacia, left ankle and joints of left foot
  - M94.279 Chondromalacia, unspecified ankle and joints of foot ▽
- **M94.28 Chondromalacia, other site**
- **M94.29 Chondromalacia, multiple sites**

✓5ᵗʰ M94.3 Chondrolysis
  Code first any associated slipped upper femoral epiphysis (nontraumatic) (M93.0-)
- **✓6ᵗʰ M94.35 Chondrolysis, hip**
  - M94.351 Chondrolysis, right hip
  - M94.352 Chondrolysis, left hip
  - M94.359 Chondrolysis, unspecified hip ▽

✓5ᵗʰ M94.8 Other specified disorders of cartilage
- **✓6ᵗʰ M94.8X Other specified disorders of cartilage**
  - M94.8X0 Other specified disorders of cartilage, multiple sites
  - M94.8X1 Other specified disorders of cartilage, shoulder
  - M94.8X2 Other specified disorders of cartilage, upper arm
  - M94.8X3 Other specified disorders of cartilage, forearm
  - M94.8X4 Other specified disorders of cartilage, hand
  - M94.8X5 Other specified disorders of cartilage, thigh
  - M94.8X6 Other specified disorders of cartilage, lower leg
  - M94.8X7 Other specified disorders of cartilage, ankle and foot
  - M94.8X8 Other specified disorders of cartilage, other site
  - M94.8X9 Other specified disorders of cartilage, unspecified sites ▽

M94.9 Disorder of cartilage, unspecified ▽

Other disorders of the musculoskeletal system and connective tissue (M95)

✓4ᵗʰ M95 Other acquired deformities of musculoskeletal system and connective tissue
  EXCLUDES 2   acquired absence of limbs and organs (Z89-Z90)
        acquired deformities of limbs (M20-M21)
        congenital malformations and deformations of the musculoskeletal system (Q65-Q79)
        deforming dorsopathies (M40-M43)
        dentofacial anomalies [including malocclusion] (M26.-)
        postprocedural musculoskeletal disorders (M96.-)

M95.0 Acquired deformity of nose
  EXCLUDES 2   deviated nasal septum (J34.2)

✓5ᵗʰ M95.1 Cauliflower ear
  EXCLUDES 2   other acquired deformities of ear (H61.1)
  DEF: Acquired deformity of the external ear; due to injury, subsequent perichondritis.
- **M95.10 Cauliflower ear, unspecified ear** ▽
- **M95.11 Cauliflower ear, right ear**
- **M95.12 Cauliflower ear, left ear**

M95.2 Other acquired deformity of head
M95.3 Acquired deformity of neck
M95.4 Acquired deformity of chest and rib
  AHA: 2014, 4Q, 26-27
M95.5 Acquired deformity of pelvis
  EXCLUDES 1   maternal care for known or suspected disproportion (O33.-)
M95.8 Other specified acquired deformities of musculoskeletal system
M95.9 Acquired deformity of musculoskeletal system, unspecified ▽

Intraoperative and postprocedural complications and disorders of musculoskeletal system, not elsewhere classified (M96)

✓4ᵗʰ M96 Intraoperative and postprocedural complications and disorders of musculoskeletal system, not elsewhere classified
  EXCLUDES 2   arthropathy following intestinal bypass (M02.0-)
        complications of internal orthopedic prosthetic devices, implants and grafts (T84.-)
        disorders associated with osteoporosis (M80)
        periprosthetic fracture around internal prosthetic joint (M97.-)
        presence of functional implants and other devices (Z96-Z97)

M96.0 Pseudarthrosis after fusion or arthrodesis
M96.1 Postlaminectomy syndrome, not elsewhere classified
M96.2 Postradiation kyphosis
M96.3 Postlaminectomy kyphosis
M96.4 Postsurgical lordosis
M96.5 Postradiation scoliosis

EXCLUDES 1 Not coded here   EXCLUDES 2 Not included here   N Newborn Age: 0   P Pediatric Age: 0-17   M Maternity Age: 12-55   A Adult Age: 15-124

796   ICD-10-CM 2018

✓5ᵗʰ **M96.6 Fracture of bone following insertion of orthopedic implant, joint prosthesis, or bone plate**
Intraoperative fracture of bone during insertion of orthopedic implant, joint prosthesis, or bone plate
EXCLUDES 2   *complication of internal orthopedic devices, implants or grafts (T84.-)*

✓6ᵗʰ **M96.62 Fracture of humerus following insertion of orthopedic implant, joint prosthesis, or bone plate**
M96.621   Fracture of humerus following insertion of orthopedic implant, joint prosthesis, or bone plate, **right arm**   HCC
M96.622   Fracture of humerus following insertion of orthopedic implant, joint prosthesis, or bone plate, **left arm**   HCC
M96.629   Fracture of humerus following insertion of orthopedic implant, joint prosthesis, or bone plate, **unspecified arm**   HCC ▽

✓6ᵗʰ **M96.63 Fracture of radius or ulna following insertion of orthopedic implant, joint prosthesis, or bone plate**
M96.631   Fracture of radius or ulna following insertion of orthopedic implant, joint prosthesis, or bone plate, **right arm**   HCC
M96.632   Fracture of radius or ulna following insertion of orthopedic implant, joint prosthesis, or bone plate, **left arm**   HCC
M96.639   Fracture of radius or ulna following insertion of orthopedic implant, joint prosthesis, or bone plate, **unspecified arm**   HCC ▽

M96.65 Fracture of pelvis following insertion of orthopedic implant, joint prosthesis, or bone plate   HCC

✓6ᵗʰ **M96.66 Fracture of femur following insertion of orthopedic implant, joint prosthesis, or bone plate**
M96.661   Fracture of femur following insertion of orthopedic implant, joint prosthesis, or bone plate, **right leg**   HCC
M96.662   Fracture of femur following insertion of orthopedic implant, joint prosthesis, or bone plate, **left leg**   HCC
M96.669   Fracture of femur following insertion of orthopedic implant, joint prosthesis, or bone plate, **unspecified leg**   HCC ▽

✓6ᵗʰ **M96.67 Fracture of tibia or fibula following insertion of orthopedic implant, joint prosthesis, or bone plate**
M96.671   Fracture of tibia or fibula following insertion of orthopedic implant, joint prosthesis, or bone plate, **right leg**   HCC
M96.672   Fracture of tibia or fibula following insertion of orthopedic implant, joint prosthesis, or bone plate, **left leg**   HCC
M96.679   Fracture of tibia or fibula following insertion of orthopedic implant, joint prosthesis, or bone plate, **unspecified leg**   HCC ▽

M96.69 Fracture of other bone following insertion of orthopedic implant, joint prosthesis, or bone plate   HCC

✓5ᵗʰ **M96.8 Other intraoperative and postprocedural complications and disorders of musculoskeletal system, not elsewhere classified**

✓6ᵗʰ **M96.81 Intraoperative hemorrhage and hematoma of a musculoskeletal structure complicating a procedure**
EXCLUDES 1   *intraoperative hemorrhage and hematoma of a musculoskeletal structure due to accidental puncture and laceration during a procedure (M96.82-)*
M96.810   Intraoperative hemorrhage and hematoma of a musculoskeletal structure complicating a **musculoskeletal system procedure**
M96.811   Intraoperative hemorrhage and hematoma of a musculoskeletal structure complicating **other procedure**

✓6ᵗʰ **M96.82 Accidental puncture and laceration of a musculoskeletal structure during a procedure**
M96.820   Accidental puncture and laceration of a musculoskeletal structure during a **musculoskeletal system procedure**
M96.821   Accidental puncture and laceration of a musculoskeletal structure during **other procedure**

✓6ᵗʰ **M96.83 Postprocedural hemorrhage of a musculoskeletal structure following a procedure**
M96.830   Postprocedural hemorrhage of a musculoskeletal structure following a **musculoskeletal system procedure**
M96.831   Postprocedural hemorrhage of a musculoskeletal structure following **other procedure**

✓6ᵗʰ **M96.84 Postprocedural hematoma and seroma of a musculoskeletal structure following a procedure**
M96.840   Postprocedural hematoma of a musculoskeletal structure following a **musculoskeletal system procedure**
M96.841   Postprocedural hematoma of a musculoskeletal structure following **other procedure**
M96.842   Postprocedural seroma of a musculoskeletal structure following a **musculoskeletal system procedure**
M96.843   Postprocedural seroma of a musculoskeletal structure following **other procedure**

M96.89 Other intraoperative and postprocedural complications and disorders of the musculoskeletal system
Instability of joint secondary to removal of joint prosthesis
Use additional code, if applicable, to further specify disorder

Periprosthetic fracture around internal prosthetic joint (M97)

✓4ᵗʰ **M97 Periprosthetic fracture around internal prosthetic joint**
EXCLUDES 2   *breakage (fracture) of prosthetic joint (T84.01-)*
fracture of bone following insertion of orthopedic implant, joint prosthesis or bone plate (M96.6-)

The appropriate 7th character is to be added to each code from category M97.
A   initial encounter
D   subsequent encounter
S   sequela

✓5ᵗʰ **M97.0 Periprosthetic fracture around internal prosthetic hip joint**
[1] ✓x7ᵗʰ **M97.01**   Periprosthetic fracture around internal prosthetic **right hip joint**   HCC
[1] ✓x7ᵗʰ **M97.02**   Periprosthetic fracture around internal prosthetic **left hip joint**   HCC

✓5ᵗʰ **M97.1 Periprosthetic fracture around internal prosthetic knee joint**
✓x7ᵗʰ **M97.11**   Periprosthetic fracture around internal prosthetic **right knee joint**
✓x7ᵗʰ **M97.12**   Periprosthetic fracture around internal prosthetic **left knee joint**

✓5ᵗʰ **M97.2 Periprosthetic fracture around internal prosthetic ankle joint**
✓x7ᵗʰ **M97.21**   Periprosthetic fracture around internal prosthetic **right ankle joint**
✓x7ᵗʰ **M97.22**   Periprosthetic fracture around internal prosthetic **left ankle joint**

✓5ᵗʰ **M97.3 Periprosthetic fracture around internal prosthetic shoulder joint**
✓x7ᵗʰ **M97.31**   Periprosthetic fracture around internal prosthetic **right shoulder joint**
✓x7ᵗʰ **M97.32**   Periprosthetic fracture around internal prosthetic **left shoulder joint**

✓5ᵗʰ **M97.4 Periprosthetic fracture around internal prosthetic elbow joint**
✓x7ᵗʰ **M97.41**   Periprosthetic fracture around internal prosthetic **right elbow joint**
✓x7ᵗʰ **M97.42**   Periprosthetic fracture around internal prosthetic **left elbow joint**

✓x7ᵗʰ **M97.8 Periprosthetic fracture around other internal prosthetic joint**
Periprosthetic fracture around internal prosthetic finger joint
Periprosthetic fracture around internal prosthetic spinal joint
Periprosthetic fracture around internal prosthetic toe joint
Periprosthetic fracture around internal prosthetic wrist joint
Use additional code to identify the joint (Z96.6-)

✓x7ᵗʰ **M97.9 Periprosthetic fracture around unspecified internal prosthetic joint**   ▽

---

[1]   HCC with 7th character indicating initial encounter (A, B or C - specific to category).

Biomechanical lesions, not elsewhere classified (M99)

✓4ᵗʰ M99 Biomechanical lesions, not elsewhere classified
> **NOTE** This category should not be used if the condition can be classified elsewhere.

✓5ᵗʰ M99.0 Segmental and somatic dysfunction
- M99.00 Segmental and somatic dysfunction of head region
- M99.01 Segmental and somatic dysfunction of cervical region
- M99.02 Segmental and somatic dysfunction of thoracic region
- M99.03 Segmental and somatic dysfunction of lumbar region
- M99.04 Segmental and somatic dysfunction of sacral region
- M99.05 Segmental and somatic dysfunction of pelvic region
- M99.06 Segmental and somatic dysfunction of lower extremity
- M99.07 Segmental and somatic dysfunction of upper extremity
- M99.08 Segmental and somatic dysfunction of rib cage
- M99.09 Segmental and somatic dysfunction of abdomen and other regions

✓5ᵗʰ M99.1 Subluxation complex (vertebral)
- M99.10 Subluxation complex (vertebral) of head region
- M99.11 Subluxation complex (vertebral) of cervical region
- M99.12 Subluxation complex (vertebral) of thoracic region
- M99.13 Subluxation complex (vertebral) of lumbar region
- M99.14 Subluxation complex (vertebral) of sacral region
- M99.15 Subluxation complex (vertebral) of pelvic region
- M99.16 Subluxation complex (vertebral) of lower extremity
- M99.17 Subluxation complex (vertebral) of upper extremity
- M99.18 Subluxation complex (vertebral) of rib cage
- M99.19 Subluxation complex (vertebral) of abdomen and other regions

✓5ᵗʰ M99.2 Subluxation stenosis of neural canal
- M99.20 Subluxation stenosis of neural canal of head region
- M99.21 Subluxation stenosis of neural canal of cervical region
- M99.22 Subluxation stenosis of neural canal of thoracic region
- M99.23 Subluxation stenosis of neural canal of lumbar region
- M99.24 Subluxation stenosis of neural canal of sacral region
- M99.25 Subluxation stenosis of neural canal of pelvic region
- M99.26 Subluxation stenosis of neural canal of lower extremity
- M99.27 Subluxation stenosis of neural canal of upper extremity
- M99.28 Subluxation stenosis of neural canal of rib cage
- M99.29 Subluxation stenosis of neural canal of abdomen and other regions

✓5ᵗʰ M99.3 Osseous stenosis of neural canal
- M99.30 Osseous stenosis of neural canal of head region
- M99.31 Osseous stenosis of neural canal of cervical region
- M99.32 Osseous stenosis of neural canal of thoracic region
- M99.33 Osseous stenosis of neural canal of lumbar region
- M99.34 Osseous stenosis of neural canal of sacral region
- M99.35 Osseous stenosis of neural canal of pelvic region
- M99.36 Osseous stenosis of neural canal of lower extremity
- M99.37 Osseous stenosis of neural canal of upper extremity
- M99.38 Osseous stenosis of neural canal of rib cage
- M99.39 Osseous stenosis of neural canal of abdomen and other regions

✓5ᵗʰ M99.4 Connective tissue stenosis of neural canal
- M99.40 Connective tissue stenosis of neural canal of head region
- M99.41 Connective tissue stenosis of neural canal of cervical region
- M99.42 Connective tissue stenosis of neural canal of thoracic region
- M99.43 Connective tissue stenosis of neural canal of lumbar region
- M99.44 Connective tissue stenosis of neural canal of sacral region
- M99.45 Connective tissue stenosis of neural canal of pelvic region
- M99.46 Connective tissue stenosis of neural canal of lower extremity
- M99.47 Connective tissue stenosis of neural canal of upper extremity
- M99.48 Connective tissue stenosis of neural canal of rib cage
- M99.49 Connective tissue stenosis of neural canal of abdomen and other regions

✓5ᵗʰ M99.5 Intervertebral disc stenosis of neural canal
- M99.50 Intervertebral disc stenosis of neural canal of head region
- M99.51 Intervertebral disc stenosis of neural canal of cervical region
- M99.52 Intervertebral disc stenosis of neural canal of thoracic region
- M99.53 Intervertebral disc stenosis of neural canal of lumbar region
- M99.54 Intervertebral disc stenosis of neural canal of sacral region
- M99.55 Intervertebral disc stenosis of neural canal of pelvic region
- M99.56 Intervertebral disc stenosis of neural canal of lower extremity
- M99.57 Intervertebral disc stenosis of neural canal of upper extremity
- M99.58 Intervertebral disc stenosis of neural canal of rib cage
- M99.59 Intervertebral disc stenosis of neural canal of abdomen and other regions

✓5ᵗʰ M99.6 Osseous and subluxation stenosis of intervertebral foramina
- M99.60 Osseous and subluxation stenosis of intervertebral foramina of head region
- M99.61 Osseous and subluxation stenosis of intervertebral foramina of cervical region
- M99.62 Osseous and subluxation stenosis of intervertebral foramina of thoracic region
- M99.63 Osseous and subluxation stenosis of intervertebral foramina of lumbar region
- M99.64 Osseous and subluxation stenosis of intervertebral foramina of sacral region
- M99.65 Osseous and subluxation stenosis of intervertebral foramina of pelvic region
- M99.66 Osseous and subluxation stenosis of intervertebral foramina of lower extremity
- M99.67 Osseous and subluxation stenosis of intervertebral foramina of upper extremity
- M99.68 Osseous and subluxation stenosis of intervertebral foramina of rib cage
- M99.69 Osseous and subluxation stenosis of intervertebral foramina of abdomen and other regions

✓5ᵗʰ M99.7 Connective tissue and disc stenosis of intervertebral foramina
- M99.70 Connective tissue and disc stenosis of intervertebral foramina of head region
- M99.71 Connective tissue and disc stenosis of intervertebral foramina of cervical region
- M99.72 Connective tissue and disc stenosis of intervertebral foramina of thoracic region
- M99.73 Connective tissue and disc stenosis of intervertebral foramina of lumbar region
- M99.74 Connective tissue and disc stenosis of intervertebral foramina of sacral region
- M99.75 Connective tissue and disc stenosis of intervertebral foramina of pelvic region

M99.76 **Connective tissue and disc stenosis of intervertebral foramina of** lower extremity

M99.77 **Connective tissue and disc stenosis of intervertebral foramina of** upper extremity

M99.78 **Connective tissue and disc stenosis of intervertebral foramina of** rib cage

M99.79 **Connective tissue and disc stenosis of intervertebral foramina of** abdomen and other regions

 M99.8 Other biomechanical lesions

M99.80 **Other biomechanical lesions of** head **region**

M99.81 **Other biomechanical lesions of** cervical **region**

M99.82 **Other biomechanical lesions of** thoracic **region**

M99.83 **Other biomechanical lesions of** lumbar **region**

M99.84 **Other biomechanical lesions of** sacral **region**

M99.85 **Other biomechanical lesions of** pelvic **region**

M99.86 **Other biomechanical lesions of** lower extremity

M99.87 **Other biomechanical lesions of** upper extremity

M99.88 **Other biomechanical lesions of** rib cage

M99.89 **Other biomechanical lesions of** abdomen and other regions

M99.9 Biomechanical lesion, unspecified   ▽

☑ Additional Character Req   ⓥₓ⁷ᵗʰ Placeholder Alert   Manifestation   ᴴᶜᶜ CMS-HCC Condition   ▽ Unspecified Code   ►◄ Revised Text   ● New Code   ▲ Revised Code Title

Chapter 14. Diseases of Genitourinary System (N00–N99)

Chapter Specific Guidelines with Coding Examples

The chapter specific guidelines from the ICD-10-CM Official Guidelines for Coding and Reporting have been provided below. Along with these guidelines are coding examples, contained in the shaded boxes, that have been developed to help illustrate the coding and/or sequencing guidance found in these guidelines.

a. Chronic kidney disease

1) Stages of chronic kidney disease (CKD)

The ICD-10-CM classifies CKD based on severity. The severity of CKD is designated by stages 1-5. Stage 2, code N18.2, equates to mild CKD; stage 3, code N18.3, equates to moderate CKD; and stage 4, code N18.4, equates to severe CKD. Code N18.6, End stage renal disease (ESRD), is assigned when the provider has documented end-stage-renal disease (ESRD).

If both a stage of CKD and ESRD are documented, assign code N18.6 only.

> **Stage 5 chronic kidney disease with ESRD requiring chronic dialysis**
>
> **N18.6**   **End stage renal disease**
>
> **Z99.2**   **Dependence on renal dialysis**
>
> *Explanation:* The diagnostic statement indicates the patient has chronic kidney disease, documented both as stage 5 and as ESRD requiring chronic dialysis. Code N18.6 End stage renal disease (ESRD), is assigned when the provider has documented end-stage-renal disease (ESRD). If both a stage of CKD and ESRD are documented, assign code N18.6 only.

2) Chronic kidney disease and kidney transplant status

Patients who have undergone kidney transplant may still have some form of chronic kidney disease (CKD) because the kidney transplant may not fully restore kidney function. Therefore, the presence of CKD alone does not constitute a transplant complication. Assign the appropriate N18 code for the patient's stage of CKD and code Z94.0, Kidney transplant status. If a transplant complication such as failure or rejection or other transplant complication is documented, see section I.C.19.g for information on coding complications of a kidney transplant. If the documentation is unclear as to whether the patient has a complication of the transplant, query the provider.

> **Patient with residual chronic kidney disease stage 1 after kidney transplant**
>
> **N18.1**   **Chronic kidney disease, stage 1**
>
> **Z94.0**   **Kidney transplant status**
>
> *Explanation:* Patients who have undergone kidney transplant may still have some form of chronic kidney disease (CKD) because the kidney transplant may not fully restore kidney function. The presence of CKD alone does not constitute a transplant complication. Assign the appropriate N18 code for the patient's stage of CKD and code Z94.0 Kidney transplant status.

3) Chronic kidney disease with other conditions

Patients with CKD may also suffer from other serious conditions, most commonly diabetes mellitus and hypertension. The sequencing of the CKD code in relationship to codes for other contributing conditions is based on the conventions in the Tabular List.

See I.C.9. Hypertensive chronic kidney disease.

See I.C.19. Chronic kidney disease and kidney transplant complications.

> **Type 1 diabetic chronic kidney disease, stage 2**
>
> **E10.22**   **Type 1 diabetes mellitus with diabetic chronic kidney disease**
>
> **N18.2**   **Chronic kidney disease, stage 2 (mild)**
>
> *Explanation:* Patients with CKD may also suffer from other serious conditions such as diabetes mellitus. The sequencing of the CKD code in relationship to codes for other contributing conditions is based on the conventions in the Tabular List. Diabetic CKD code E10.22 includes an instructional note to "Use additional code to identify stage of chronic kidney disease (N18.1–N18.6)," thus providing sequencing direction.

Chapter 14. Diseases of the Genitourinary System (N00-N99)

EXCLUDES 2
certain conditions originating in the perinatal period (P04-P96)
certain infectious and parasitic diseases (A00-B99)
complications of pregnancy, childbirth and the puerperium (O00-O9A)
congenital malformations, deformations and chromosomal abnormalities (Q00-Q99)
endocrine, nutritional and metabolic diseases (E00-E88)
injury, poisoning and certain other consequences of external causes (S00-T88)
neoplasms (C00-D49)
symptoms, signs and abnormal clinical and laboratory findings, not elsewhere classified (R00-R94)

This chapter contains the following blocks:

N00-N08	Glomerular diseases
N10-N16	Renal tubulo-interstitial diseases
N17-N19	Acute kidney failure and chronic kidney disease
N20-N23	Urolithiasis
N25-N29	Other disorders of kidney and ureter
N30-N39	Other diseases of the urinary system
N40-N53	Diseases of male genital organs
N60-N65	Disorders of breast
N70-N77	Inflammatory diseases of female pelvic organs
N80-N98	Noninflammatory disorders of female genital tract
N99	Intraoperative and postprocedural complications and disorders of genitourinary system, not elsewhere classified

Glomerular diseases (N00-N08)

Code also any associated kidney failure (N17-N19)

EXCLUDES 1 hypertensive chronic kidney disease (I12.-)

✓4ᵗʰ **N00 Acute nephritic syndrome**

INCLUDES acute glomerular disease
acute glomerulonephritis
acute nephritis

EXCLUDES 1 acute tubulo-interstitial nephritis (N10)
nephritic syndrome NOS (N05.-)

N00.0 Acute nephritic syndrome with minor glomerular abnormality
Acute nephritic syndrome with minimal change lesion

N00.1 Acute nephritic syndrome with focal and segmental glomerular lesions
Acute nephritic syndrome with focal and segmental hyalinosis
Acute nephritic syndrome with focal and segmental sclerosis
Acute nephritic syndrome with focal glomerulonephritis

N00.2 Acute nephritic syndrome with diffuse membranous glomerulonephritis

N00.3 Acute nephritic syndrome with diffuse mesangial proliferative glomerulonephritis

N00.4 Acute nephritic syndrome with diffuse endocapillary proliferative glomerulonephritis

N00.5 Acute nephritic syndrome with diffuse mesangiocapillary glomerulonephritis
Acute nephritic syndrome with membranoproliferative glomerulonephritis, types 1 and 3, or NOS

N00.6 Acute nephritic syndrome with dense deposit disease
Acute nephritic syndrome with membranoproliferative glomerulonephritis, type 2

N00.7 Acute nephritic syndrome with diffuse crescentic glomerulonephritis
Acute nephritic syndrome with extracapillary glomerulonephritis

N00.8 Acute nephritic syndrome with other morphologic changes
Acute nephritic syndrome with proliferative glomerulonephritis NOS

N00.9 Acute nephritic syndrome with unspecified morphologic changes ▽

✓4ᵗʰ **N01 Rapidly progressive nephritic syndrome**

INCLUDES rapidly progressive glomerular disease
rapidly progressive glomerulonephritis
rapidly progressive nephritis

EXCLUDES 1 nephritic syndrome NOS (N05.-)

N01.0 Rapidly progressive nephritic syndrome with minor glomerular abnormality
Rapidly progressive nephritic syndrome with minimal change lesion

N01.1 Rapidly progressive nephritic syndrome with focal and segmental glomerular lesions
Rapidly progressive nephritic syndrome with focal and segmental hyalinosis
Rapidly progressive nephritic syndrome with focal and segmental sclerosis
Rapidly progressive nephritic syndrome with focal glomerulonephritis

N01.2 Rapidly progressive nephritic syndrome with diffuse membranous glomerulonephritis

N01.3 Rapidly progressive nephritic syndrome with diffuse mesangial proliferative glomerulonephritis

N01.4 Rapidly progressive nephritic syndrome with diffuse endocapillary proliferative glomerulonephritis

N01.5 Rapidly progressive nephritic syndrome with diffuse mesangiocapillary glomerulonephritis
Rapidly progressive nephritic syndrome with membranoproliferative glomerulonephritis, types 1 and 3, or NOS

N01.6 Rapidly progressive nephritic syndrome with dense deposit disease
Rapidly progressive nephritic syndrome with membranoproliferative glomerulonephritis, type 2

N01.7 Rapidly progressive nephritic syndrome with diffuse crescentic glomerulonephritis
Rapidly progressive nephritic syndrome with extracapillary glomerulonephritis

N01.8 Rapidly progressive nephritic syndrome with other morphologic changes
Rapidly progressive nephritic syndrome with proliferative glomerulonephritis NOS

N01.9 Rapidly progressive nephritic syndrome with unspecified morphologic changes ▽

✓4ᵗʰ **N02 Recurrent and persistent hematuria**

EXCLUDES 1 acute cystitis with hematuria (N30.01)
hematuria NOS (R31.9)
hematuria not associated with specified morphologic lesions (R31.-)

N02.0 Recurrent and persistent hematuria with minor glomerular abnormality
Recurrent and persistent hematuria with minimal change lesion

N02.1 Recurrent and persistent hematuria with focal and segmental glomerular lesions
Recurrent and persistent hematuria with focal and segmental hyalinosis
Recurrent and persistent hematuria with focal and segmental sclerosis
Recurrent and persistent hematuria with focal glomerulonephritis

N02.2 Recurrent and persistent hematuria with diffuse membranous glomerulonephritis

N02.3 Recurrent and persistent hematuria with diffuse mesangial proliferative glomerulonephritis

N02.4 Recurrent and persistent hematuria with diffuse endocapillary proliferative glomerulonephritis

N02.5 Recurrent and persistent hematuria with diffuse mesangiocapillary glomerulonephritis
Recurrent and persistent hematuria with membranoproliferative glomerulonephritis, types 1 and 3, or NOS

N02.6 Recurrent and persistent hematuria with dense deposit disease
Recurrent and persistent hematuria with membranoproliferative glomerulonephritis, type 2

N02.7 Recurrent and persistent hematuria with diffuse crescentic glomerulonephritis
Recurrent and persistent hematuria with extracapillary glomerulonephritis

N02.8 Recurrent and persistent hematuria with other morphologic changes
Recurrent and persistent hematuria with proliferative glomerulonephritis NOS

N02.9 Recurrent and persistent hematuria with unspecified morphologic changes ▽
AHA: 2017, 2Q, 5

EXCLUDES 1 Not coded here   **EXCLUDES 2** Not included here   N Newborn Age: 0   P Pediatric Age: 0-17   M Maternity Age: 12-55   A Adult Age: 15-124

802   ICD-10-CM 2018

✓4ᵗʰ **N03 Chronic nephritic syndrome**

    INCLUDES chronic glomerular disease
                  chronic glomerulonephritis
                  chronic nephritis

    EXCLUDES 1 *chronic tubulo-interstitial nephritis (N11.-)*
                 diffuse sclerosing glomerulonephritis (N05.8-)
                 nephritic syndrome NOS (N05.-)

    DEF: Slow, progressive type of nephritis characterized by inflammation of the capillary loops in the glomeruli of the kidney, which leads to renal failure.

N03.0 Chronic nephritic syndrome with minor glomerular abnormality
    Chronic nephritic syndrome with minimal change lesion

N03.1 Chronic nephritic syndrome with focal and segmental glomerular lesions
    Chronic nephritic syndrome with focal and segmental hyalinosis
    Chronic nephritic syndrome with focal and segmental sclerosis
    Chronic nephritic syndrome with focal glomerulonephritis

N03.2 Chronic nephritic syndrome with diffuse membranous glomerulonephritis

N03.3 Chronic nephritic syndrome with diffuse mesangial proliferative glomerulonephritis

N03.4 Chronic nephritic syndrome with diffuse endocapillary proliferative glomerulonephritis

N03.5 Chronic nephritic syndrome with diffuse mesangiocapillary glomerulonephritis
    Chronic nephritic syndrome with membranoproliferative glomerulonephritis, types 1 and 3, or NOS

N03.6 Chronic nephritic syndrome with dense deposit disease
    Chronic nephritic syndrome with membranoproliferative glomerulonephritis, type 2

N03.7 Chronic nephritic syndrome with diffuse crescentic glomerulonephritis
    Chronic nephritic syndrome with extracapillary glomerulonephritis

N03.8 Chronic nephritic syndrome with other morphologic changes
    Chronic nephritic syndrome with proliferative glomerulonephritis NOS

N03.9 Chronic nephritic syndrome with unspecified morphologic changes ▽

✓4ᵗʰ **N04 Nephrotic syndrome**

    INCLUDES congenital nephrotic syndrome
                  lipoid nephrosis

N04.0 Nephrotic syndrome with minor glomerular abnormality
    Nephrotic syndrome with minimal change lesion

N04.1 Nephrotic syndrome with focal and segmental glomerular lesions
    Nephrotic syndrome with focal and segmental hyalinosis
    Nephrotic syndrome with focal and segmental sclerosis
    Nephrotic syndrome with focal glomerulonephritis

N04.2 Nephrotic syndrome with diffuse membranous glomerulonephritis

N04.3 Nephrotic syndrome with diffuse mesangial proliferative glomerulonephritis

N04.4 Nephrotic syndrome with diffuse endocapillary proliferative glomerulonephritis

N04.5 Nephrotic syndrome with diffuse mesangiocapillary glomerulonephritis
    Nephrotic syndrome with membranoproliferative glomerulonephritis, types 1 and 3, or NOS

N04.6 Nephrotic syndrome with dense deposit disease
    Nephrotic syndrome with membranoproliferative glomerulonephritis, type 2

N04.7 Nephrotic syndrome with diffuse crescentic glomerulonephritis
    Nephrotic syndrome with extracapillary glomerulonephritis

N04.8 Nephrotic syndrome with other morphologic changes
    Nephrotic syndrome with proliferative glomerulonephritis NOS

N04.9 Nephrotic syndrome with unspecified morphologic changes ▽

✓4ᵗʰ **N05 Unspecified nephritic syndrome**

    INCLUDES glomerular disease NOS
                  glomerulonephritis NOS
                  nephritis NOS
                  nephropathy NOS and renal disease NOS with morphological lesion specified in .0-.8

    EXCLUDES 1 *nephropathy NOS with no stated morphological lesion (N28.9)*
                 renal disease NOS with no stated morphological lesion (N28.9)
                 tubulo-interstitial nephritis NOS (N12)

N05.0 Unspecified nephritic syndrome with minor glomerular abnormality ▽
    Unspecified nephritic syndrome with minimal change lesion

N05.1 Unspecified nephritic syndrome with focal and segmental glomerular lesions ▽
    Unspecified nephritic syndrome with focal and segmental hyalinosis
    Unspecified nephritic syndrome with focal and segmental sclerosis
    Unspecified nephritic syndrome with focal glomerulonephritis

N05.2 Unspecified nephritic syndrome with diffuse membranous glomerulonephritis ▽

N05.3 Unspecified nephritic syndrome with diffuse mesangial proliferative glomerulonephritis ▽

N05.4 Unspecified nephritic syndrome with diffuse endocapillary proliferative glomerulonephritis ▽

N05.5 Unspecified nephritic syndrome with diffuse mesangiocapillary glomerulonephritis ▽
    Unspecified nephritic syndrome with membranoproliferative glomerulonephritis, types 1 and 3, or NOS

N05.6 Unspecified nephritic syndrome with dense deposit disease ▽
    Unspecified nephritic syndrome with membranoproliferative glomerulonephritis, type 2

N05.7 Unspecified nephritic syndrome with diffuse crescentic glomerulonephritis ▽
    Unspecified nephritic syndrome with extracapillary glomerulonephritis

N05.8 Unspecified nephritic syndrome with other morphologic changes ▽
    Unspecified nephritic syndrome with proliferative glomerulonephritis NOS

N05.9 Unspecified nephritic syndrome with unspecified morphologic changes ▽

✓4ᵗʰ **N06 Isolated proteinuria with specified morphological lesion**

    EXCLUDES 1 *proteinuria not associated with specific morphologic lesions (R80.0)*

N06.0 Isolated proteinuria with minor glomerular abnormality
    Isolated proteinuria with minimal change lesion

N06.1 Isolated proteinuria with focal and segmental glomerular lesions
    Isolated proteinuria with focal and segmental hyalinosis
    Isolated proteinuria with focal and segmental sclerosis
    Isolated proteinuria with focal glomerulonephritis

N06.2 Isolated proteinuria with diffuse membranous glomerulonephritis

N06.3 Isolated proteinuria with diffuse mesangial proliferative glomerulonephritis

N06.4 Isolated proteinuria with diffuse endocapillary proliferative glomerulonephritis

N06.5 Isolated proteinuria with diffuse mesangiocapillary glomerulonephritis
    Isolated proteinuria with membranoproliferative glomerulonephritis, types 1 and 3, or NOS

N06.6 Isolated proteinuria with dense deposit disease
    Isolated proteinuria with membranoproliferative glomerulonephritis, type 2

N06.7 Isolated proteinuria with diffuse crescentic glomerulonephritis
    Isolated proteinuria with extracapillary glomerulonephritis

N06.8 Isolated proteinuria with other morphologic lesion
    Isolated proteinuria with proliferative glomerulonephritis NOS

N06.9 Isolated proteinuria with unspecified morphologic lesion ▽

☑ Additional Character Req   ✓ₓ7ᵗʰ Placeholder Alert   Manifestation   HCC CMS-HCC Condition   ▽ Unspecified Code   ►◄ Revised Text   ● New Code   ▲ Revised Code Title

✓4ᵗʰ N07 Hereditary nephropathy, not elsewhere classified

EXCLUDES 2   *Alport's syndrome (Q87.81-)*
hereditary amyloid nephropathy (E85.-)
nail patella syndrome (Q87.2)
non-neuropathic heredofamilial amyloidosis (E85.-)

N07.0 Hereditary nephropathy, not elsewhere classified with minor glomerular abnormality
Hereditary nephropathy, not elsewhere classified with minimal change lesion

N07.1 Hereditary nephropathy, not elsewhere classified with focal and segmental glomerular lesions
Hereditary nephropathy, not elsewhere classified with focal and segmental hyalinosis
Hereditary nephropathy, not elsewhere classified with focal and segmental sclerosis
Hereditary nephropathy, not elsewhere classified with focal glomerulonephritis

N07.2 Hereditary nephropathy, not elsewhere classified with diffuse membranous glomerulonephritis

N07.3 Hereditary nephropathy, not elsewhere classified with diffuse mesangial proliferative glomerulonephritis

N07.4 Hereditary nephropathy, not elsewhere classified with diffuse endocapillary proliferative glomerulonephritis

N07.5 Hereditary nephropathy, not elsewhere classified with diffuse mesangiocapillary glomerulonephritis
Hereditary nephropathy, not elsewhere classified with membranoproliferative glomerulonephritis, types 1 and 3, or NOS

N07.6 Hereditary nephropathy, not elsewhere classified with dense deposit disease
Hereditary nephropathy, not elsewhere classified with membranoproliferative glomerulonephritis, type 2

N07.7 Hereditary nephropathy, not elsewhere classified with diffuse crescentic glomerulonephritis
Hereditary nephropathy, not elsewhere classified with extracapillary glomerulonephritis

N07.8 Hereditary nephropathy, not elsewhere classified with other morphologic lesions
Hereditary nephropathy, not elsewhere classified with proliferative glomerulonephritis NOS

N07.9 Hereditary nephropathy, not elsewhere classified with unspecified morphologic lesions ▽

N08 *Glomerular disorders in diseases classified elsewhere*

Glomerulonephritis
Nephritis
Nephropathy
Code first underlying disease, such as:
amyloidosis (E85.-)
congenital syphilis (A50.5)
cryoglobulinemia (D89.1)
disseminated intravascular coagulation (D65)
gout (M1A.-, M10.-)
microscopic polyangiitis (M31.7)
multiple myeloma (C90.0-)
sepsis (A40.0-A41.9)
sickle-cell disease (D57.0-D57.8)

EXCLUDES 1   *glomerulonephritis, nephritis and nephropathy (in):*
antiglomerular basement membrane disease (M31.0)
diabetes (E08-E13 with .21)
gonococcal (A54.21)
Goodpasture's syndrome (M31.0)
hemolytic-uremic syndrome (D59.3)
lupus (M32.14)
mumps (B26.83)
syphilis (A52.75)
systemic lupus erythematosus (M32.14)
Wegener's granulomatosis (M31.31)
pyelonephritis in diseases classified elsewhere (N16)
renal tubulo-interstitial disorders classified elsewhere (N16)

Renal tubulo-interstitial diseases (N10-N16)

INCLUDES   pyelonephritis
EXCLUDES 1   *pyeloureteritis cystica (N28.85)*

N10 Acute pyelonephritis

Acute infectious interstitial nephritis
Acute pyelitis
Acute tubulo-interstitial nephritis
Hemoglobin nephrosis
Myoglobin nephrosis
Use additional code (B95-B97), to identify infectious agent

✓4ᵗʰ N11 Chronic tubulo-interstitial nephritis

INCLUDES   chronic infectious interstitial nephritis
chronic pyelitis
chronic pyelonephritis
Use additional code (B95-B97), to identify infectious agent

N11.0 Nonobstructive reflux-associated chronic pyelonephritis
Pyelonephritis (chronic) associated with (vesicoureteral) reflux
EXCLUDES 1   *vesicoureteral reflux NOS (N13.70)*

N11.1 Chronic obstructive pyelonephritis
Pyelonephritis (chronic) associated with anomaly of pelviureteric junction
Pyelonephritis (chronic) associated with anomaly of pyeloureteric junction
Pyelonephritis (chronic) associated with crossing of vessel
Pyelonephritis (chronic) associated with kinking of ureter
Pyelonephritis (chronic) associated with obstruction of ureter
Pyelonephritis (chronic) associated with stricture of pelviureteric junction
Pyelonephritis (chronic) associated with stricture of ureter
EXCLUDES 1   *calculus pyelonephritis (N20.9)*
obstructive uropathy (N13.-)

N11.8 Other chronic tubulo-interstitial nephritis
Nonobstructive chronic pyelonephritis NOS

N11.9 Chronic tubulo-interstitial nephritis, unspecified ▽
Chronic interstitial nephritis NOS
Chronic pyelitis NOS
Chronic pyelonephritis NOS

N12 Tubulo-interstitial nephritis, not specified as acute or chronic

Interstitial nephritis NOS
Pyelitis NOS
Pyelonephritis NOS
EXCLUDES 1   *calculous pyelonephritis (N20.9)*

✓4ᵗʰ N13 Obstructive and reflux uropathy

EXCLUDES 2   *calculus of kidney and ureter without hydronephrosis (N20.-)*
congenital obstructive defects of renal pelvis and ureter (Q62.0-Q62.3)
hydronephrosis with ureteropelvic junction obstruction ▶(Q62.11)◀
obstructive pyelonephritis (N11.1)

N13.0 Hydronephrosis with ureteropelvic junction obstruction
Hydronephrosis due to acquired occlusion of ureteropelvic junction
EXCLUDES 2   *hydronephrosis with ureteropelvic junction obstruction due to calculus (N13.2)*

N13.1 Hydronephrosis with ureteral stricture, not elsewhere classified
EXCLUDES 1   *hydronephrosis with ureteral stricture with infection (N13.6)*

N13.2 Hydronephrosis with renal and ureteral calculous obstruction
EXCLUDES 1   *hydronephrosis with renal and ureteral calculous obstruction with infection (N13.6)*

Hydronephrosis/UPJ Obstruction

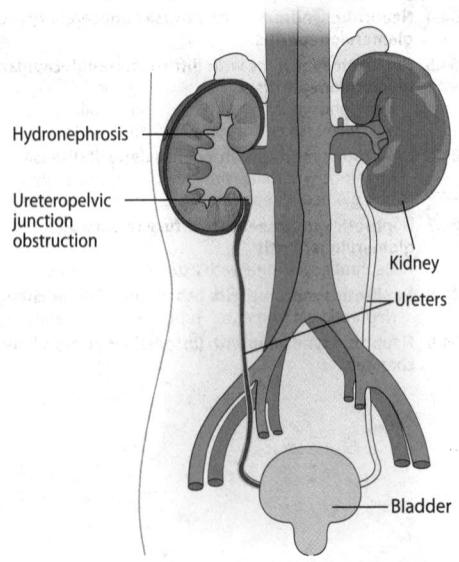

Hydronephrosis
Ureteropelvic junction obstruction
Kidney
Ureters
Bladder

EXCLUDES 1 Not coded here   EXCLUDES 2 Not included here   N Newborn Age: 0   P Pediatric Age: 0-17   M Maternity Age: 12-55   A Adult Age: 15-124

804   ICD-10-CM 2018

N07–N13.2

Chapter 14. Diseases of Genitourinary System

Vesicoureteral Reflux

Kidneys

Ureters

Bladder

Normal flow of urine   Urine flowing the wrong way (VUR)

☑5ᵗʰ **N13.3** **Other and unspecified hydronephrosis**
     EXCLUDES 1   hydronephrosis with infection (N13.6)

     N13.30 **Unspecified hydronephrosis** ▽

     N13.39 **Other hydronephrosis**

N13.4 **Hydroureter**
     EXCLUDES 1   congenital hydroureter (Q62.3-)
          hydroureter with infection (N13.6)
          vesicoureteral-reflux with hydroureter (N13.73-)

N13.5 **Crossing vessel and stricture of ureter without hydronephrosis**
     Kinking and stricture of ureter without hydronephrosis
     EXCLUDES 1   crossing vessel and stricture of ureter without
          hydronephrosis with infection (N13.6)

N13.6 **Pyonephrosis**
     Conditions in N13.0-N13.5 with infection
     Obstructive uropathy with infection
     Use additional code (B95-B97), to identify infectious agent

☑5ᵗʰ **N13.7** **Vesicoureteral-reflux**
     EXCLUDES 1   reflux-associated pyelonephritis (N11.0)

     N13.70 **Vesicoureteral-reflux, unspecified** ▽
          Vesicoureteral-reflux NOS

     N13.71 **Vesicoureteral-reflux** without reflux nephropathy

☑6ᵗʰ   **N13.72** **Vesicoureteral-reflux** with reflux nephropathy without hydroureter

         N13.721 **Vesicoureteral-reflux with reflux nephropathy without hydroureter, unilateral**

         N13.722 **Vesicoureteral-reflux with reflux nephropathy without hydroureter, bilateral**

         N13.729 **Vesicoureteral-reflux with reflux nephropathy without hydroureter, unspecified** ▽

☑6ᵗʰ   **N13.73** **Vesicoureteral-reflux** with reflux nephropathy with hydroureter

         N13.731 **Vesicoureteral-reflux with reflux nephropathy with hydroureter, unilateral**

         N13.732 **Vesicoureteral-reflux with reflux nephropathy with hydroureter, bilateral**

         N13.739 **Vesicoureteral-reflux with reflux nephropathy with hydroureter, unspecified** ▽

N13.8 **Other obstructive and reflux uropathy**
     Urinary tract obstruction due to specified cause
     Code first, if applicable, any causal condition, such as:
         enlarged prostate (N40.1)

N13.9 **Obstructive and reflux uropathy, unspecified** ▽
     Urinary tract obstruction NOS

☑4ᵗʰ **N14** **Drug- and heavy-metal-induced tubulo-interstitial and tubular conditions**
     Code first poisoning due to drug or toxin, if applicable (T36-T65 with
         fifth or sixth character 1-4 or 6)
     Use additional code for adverse effect, if applicable, to identify drug
         (T36-T50 with fifth or sixth character 5)

N14.0 **Analgesic nephropathy**

N14.1 **Nephropathy induced by other drugs, medicaments and biological substances**

N14.2 **Nephropathy induced by unspecified drug, medicament or biological substance** ▽

N14.3 **Nephropathy induced by heavy metals**

N14.4 **Toxic nephropathy, not elsewhere classified**

☑4ᵗʰ **N15** **Other renal tubulo-interstitial diseases**

     N15.0 **Balkan nephropathy**
         Balkan endemic nephropathy

     N15.1 **Renal and perinephric abscess**

     N15.8 **Other specified renal tubulo-interstitial diseases**

     N15.9 **Renal tubulo-interstitial disease, unspecified** ▽
         Infection of kidney NOS
         EXCLUDES 1   urinary tract infection NOS (N39.0)

N16 *Renal tubulo-interstitial disorders in diseases classified elsewhere*
     Pyelonephritis
     Tubulo-interstitial nephritis
     Code first underlying disease, such as:
         brucellosis (A23.0-A23.9)
         cryoglobulinemia (D89.1)
         glycogen storage disease (E74.0)
         leukemia (C91-C95)
         lymphoma (C81.0-C85.9, C96.0-C96.9)
         multiple myeloma (C90.0-)
         sepsis (A40.0-A41.9)
         Wilson's disease (E83.0)
     EXCLUDES 1   diphtheritic pyelonephritis and tubulo-interstitial nephritis
         (A36.84)
         pyelonephritis and tubulo-interstitial nephritis in candidiasis
         (B37.49)
         pyelonephritis and tubulo-interstitial nephritis in cystinosis
         (E72.04)
         pyelonephritis and tubulo-interstitial nephritis in salmonella
         infection (A02.25)
         pyelonephritis and tubulo-interstitial nephritis in sarcoidosis
         (D86.84)
         pyelonephritis and tubulo-interstitial nephritis in sicca
         syndrome [Sjogren's] (M35.04)
         pyelonephritis and tubulo-interstitial nephritis in systemic lupus
         erythematosus (M32.15)
         pyelonephritis and tubulo-interstitial nephritis in toxoplasmosis
         (B58.83)
         renal tubular degeneration in diabetes (E08-E13 with .29)
         syphilitic pyelonephritis and tubulo-interstitial nephritis
         (A52.75)

Acute kidney failure and chronic kidney disease (N17-N19)
     EXCLUDES 2   congenital renal failure (P96.0)
         drug- and heavy-metal-induced tubulo-interstitial and tubular
            conditions (N14.-)
         extrarenal uremia (R39.2)
         hemolytic-uremic syndrome (D59.3)
         hepatorenal syndrome (K76.7)
         postpartum hepatorenal syndrome (O90.4)
         posttraumatic renal failure (T79.5)
         prerenal uremia (R39.2)
         renal failure complicating abortion or ectopic or molar pregnancy
            (O00-O07, O08.4)
         renal failure following labor and delivery (O90.4)
         renal failure postprocedural (N99.0)

☑4ᵗʰ **N17** **Acute kidney failure**
     Code also associated underlying condition
     EXCLUDES 1   posttraumatic renal failure (T79.5)
     AHA: 2013, 4Q, 124

     N17.0 **Acute kidney failure with tubular necrosis**   HCC
         Acute tubular necrosis
         Renal tubular necrosis
         Tubular necrosis NOS

     N17.1 **Acute kidney failure with acute cortical necrosis**   HCC
         Acute cortical necrosis
         Cortical necrosis NOS
         Renal cortical necrosis

     N17.2 **Acute kidney failure with medullary necrosis**   HCC
         Medullary [papillary] necrosis NOS
         Acute medullary [papillary] necrosis
         Renal medullary [papillary] necrosis

     N17.8 **Other acute kidney failure**   HCC

     N17.9 **Acute kidney failure, unspecified**   HCC ▽
         Acute kidney injury (nontraumatic)
         EXCLUDES 2   traumatic kidney injury (S37.0-)

☑ Additional Character Req   ☑7ᵗʰ Placeholder Alert   Manifestation   HCC CMS-HCC Condition   ▽ Unspecified Code   ►◄ Revised Text   ● New Code   ▲ Revised Code Title

✓4ᵗʰ **N18 Chronic kidney disease (CKD)**
Code first any associated:
     diabetic chronic kidney disease (E08.22, E09.22, E10.22, E11.22, E13.22)
     hypertensive chronic kidney disease (I12-, I13-)
Use additional code to identify kidney transplant status, if applicable, (Z94.0)
     AHA: 2013, 1Q, 24

     N18.1 Chronic kidney disease, stage 1

     N18.2 Chronic kidney disease, stage 2 (mild)

     N18.3 Chronic kidney disease, stage 3 (moderate)

     N18.4 Chronic kidney disease, stage 4 (severe)   HCC

     N18.5 Chronic kidney disease, stage 5   HCC
         EXCLUDES 1   *chronic kidney disease, stage 5 requiring chronic dialysis (N18.6)*
         DEF: End-stage renal disease (ESRD) with GFR value of 15 ml/min or less not yet requiring chronic dialysis.

     N18.6 End stage renal disease   HCC
         Chronic kidney disease requiring chronic dialysis
         Use additional code to identify dialysis status (Z99.2)
         AHA: 2016, 3Q, 22; 2016, 1Q, 12; 2013, 4Q, 124-125

     N18.9 Chronic kidney disease, unspecified ▽
         Chronic renal disease
         Chronic renal failure NOS
         Chronic renal insufficiency
         ▶Chronic uremia NOS
         Diffuse sclerosing glomerulonephritis NOS◀

N19 Unspecified kidney failure ▽
     Uremia NOS
     EXCLUDES 1   *acute kidney failure (N17.-)*
                chronic kidney disease (N18.-)
                chronic uremia (N18.9)
                extrarenal uremia (R39.2)
                prerenal uremia (R39.2)
                renal insufficiency (acute) (N28.9)
                uremia of newborn (P96.0)

Urolithiasis (N20-N23)

AHA: 2017, 1Q, 5; 2015, 2Q, 8

✓4ᵗʰ **N20 Calculus of kidney and ureter**
     Calculous pyelonephritis
     EXCLUDES 1   *nephrocalcinosis (E83.5)*
                that with hydronephrosis (N13.2)

     N20.0 Calculus of kidney
         Nephrolithiasis NOS
         Renal calculus
         Renal stone
         Staghorn calculus
         Stone in kidney

     N20.1 Calculus of ureter
         Ureteric stone
         AHA: 2016, 3Q, 22

     N20.2 Calculus of kidney with calculus of ureter

     N20.9 Urinary calculus, unspecified ▽

✓4ᵗʰ **N21 Calculus of lower urinary tract**
     Calculus of lower urinary tract with cystitis and urethritis

     N21.0 Calculus in bladder
         Calculus in diverticulum of bladder
         Urinary bladder stone
         EXCLUDES 2   *staghorn calculus (N20.0)*

     N21.1 Calculus in urethra
         EXCLUDES 2   *calculus of prostate (N42.0)*

     N21.8 Other lower urinary tract calculus

     N21.9 Calculus of lower urinary tract, unspecified ▽
         EXCLUDES 1   *calculus of urinary tract NOS (N20.9)*

N22   *Calculus of urinary tract in diseases classified elsewhere*
     Code first underlying disease, such as:
         gout (M1A.-, M10.-)
         schistosomiasis (B65.0-B65.9)

N23 Unspecified renal colic ▽

Other disorders of kidney and ureter (N25-N29)

EXCLUDES 2   *disorders of kidney and ureter with urolithiasis (N20-N23)*

✓4ᵗʰ **N25 Disorders resulting from impaired renal tubular function**
     EXCLUDES 1   *metabolic disorders classifiable to E70-E88*

     N25.0 Renal osteodystrophy
         Azotemic osteodystrophy
         Phosphate-losing tubular disorders
         Renal rickets
         Renal short stature
         EXCLUDES 2   ▶*metabolic disorders classifiable to E70-E88*◀

     N25.1 Nephrogenic diabetes insipidus   HCC
         EXCLUDES 1   *diabetes insipidus NOS (E23.2)*
         DEF: Type of diabetes due to inability of renal tubules to reabsorb water back into the body; not responsive to vasopressin (antidiuretic hormone); characterized by excessive thirst and excessive urine production; may develop into chronic renal insufficiency.

✓5ᵗʰ   **N25.8 Other disorders resulting from impaired renal tubular function**

         N25.81 Secondary hyperparathyroidism of renal origin   HCC
             EXCLUDES 1   *secondary hyperparathyroidism, non-renal (E21.1)*
             EXCLUDES 2   ▶*metabolic disorders classifiable to E70-E88*◀
             DEF: Parathyroid dysfunction caused by chronic renal failure; phosphate clearance is impaired, phosphate is released from bone, vitamin D is not produced, intestinal calcium absorption is low, and blood levels of calcium are lowered, causing excessive production of parathyroid hormone.

         N25.89 Other disorders resulting from impaired renal tubular function
             Hypokalemic nephropathy
             Lightwood-Albright syndrome
             Renal tubular acidosis NOS

     N25.9 Disorder resulting from impaired renal tubular function, unspecified ▽

✓4ᵗʰ **N26 Unspecified contracted kidney**
     EXCLUDES 1   *contracted kidney due to hypertension (I12.-)*
                diffuse sclerosing glomerulonephritis (N05.8-)
                hypertensive nephrosclerosis (arteriolar) (arteriosclerotic) (I12.-)
                small kidney of unknown cause (N27.-)

     N26.1 Atrophy of kidney (terminal)

     N26.2 Page kidney

     N26.9 Renal sclerosis, unspecified ▽

✓4ᵗʰ **N27 Small kidney of unknown cause**
     INCLUDES   oligonephronia

     N27.0 Small kidney, unilateral

     N27.1 Small kidney, bilateral

     N27.9 Small kidney, unspecified ▽

✓4ᵗʰ **N28 Other disorders of kidney and ureter, not elsewhere classified**

     N28.0 Ischemia and infarction of kidney   HCC
         Renal artery embolism   Renal artery thrombosis
         Renal artery obstruction   Renal infarct
         Renal artery occlusion
         EXCLUDES 1   *atherosclerosis of renal artery (extrarenal part) (I70.1)*
             congenital stenosis of renal artery (Q27.1)
             Goldblatt's kidney (I70.1)

     N28.1 Cyst of kidney, acquired
         ▶Cyst (multiple) (solitary) of kidney (acquired)◀
         EXCLUDES 1   *cystic kidney disease (congenital) (Q61.-)*

✓5ᵗʰ   **N28.8 Other specified disorders of kidney and ureter**
         EXCLUDES 1   *hydroureter (N13.4)*
             ureteric stricture with hydronephrosis (N13.1)
             ureteric stricture without hydronephrosis (N13.5)

         N28.81 Hypertrophy of kidney

         N28.82 Megaloureter

         N28.83 Nephroptosis

         N28.84 Pyelitis cystica

         N28.85 Pyeloureteritis cystica

         N28.86 Ureteritis cystica

         N28.89 Other specified disorders of kidney and ureter

N28.9 Disorder of kidney and ureter, unspecified ▽
Nephropathy NOS
Renal disease (acute) NOS
Renal insufficiency (acute)
  EXCLUDES 1   *chronic renal insufficiency (N18.9)*
       unspecified nephritic syndrome (N05.-)
  AHA: 2016, 1Q, 13

N29 *Other disorders of kidney and ureter in diseases classified elsewhere*
Code first underlying disease, such as:
  amyloidosis (E85.-)
  nephrocalcinosis (E83.5)
  schistosomiasis (B65.0-B65.9)
  EXCLUDES 1   *disorders of kidney and ureter in:*
       cystinosis (E72.0)
       gonorrhea (A54.21)
       syphilis (A52.75)
       tuberculosis (A18.11)

Other diseases of the urinary system (N30-N39)

  EXCLUDES 1   *urinary infection (complicating):*
       abortion or ectopic or molar pregnancy (-O07, O08.8)
       pregnancy, childbirth and the puerperium (O23-, O75.3, O86.2-)

✓4th N30 Cystitis
Use additional code to identify infectious agent (B95-B97)
  EXCLUDES 1   *prostatocystitis (N41.3)*
  AHA: 2017, 1Q, 6

  ✓5th N30.0 Acute cystitis
    EXCLUDES 1   *irradiation cystitis (N30.4-)*
         trigonitis (N30.3-)
    N30.00 Acute cystitis without hematuria
    N30.01 Acute cystitis with hematuria

  ✓5th N30.1 Interstitial cystitis (chronic)
    N30.10 Interstitial cystitis (chronic) without hematuria
    N30.11 Interstitial cystitis (chronic) with hematuria

  ✓5th N30.2 Other chronic cystitis
    N30.20 Other chronic cystitis without hematuria
    N30.21 Other chronic cystitis with hematuria

  ✓5th N30.3 Trigonitis
    Urethrotrigonitis
    N30.30 Trigonitis without hematuria
    N30.31 Trigonitis with hematuria

  ✓5th N30.4 Irradiation cystitis
    N30.40 Irradiation cystitis without hematuria
    N30.41 Irradiation cystitis with hematuria

  ✓5th N30.8 Other cystitis
    Abscess of bladder
    N30.80 Other cystitis without hematuria
    N30.81 Other cystitis with hematuria

  ✓5th N30.9 Cystitis, unspecified
    N30.90 Cystitis, unspecified without hematuria ▽
    N30.91 Cystitis, unspecified with hematuria ▽

✓4th N31 Neuromuscular dysfunction of bladder, not elsewhere classified
Use additional code to identify any associated urinary incontinence (N39.3-N39.4-)
  EXCLUDES 1   *cord bladder NOS (G95.89)*
       neurogenic bladder due to cauda equina syndrome (G83.4)
       neuromuscular dysfunction due to spinal cord lesion (G95.89)

  N31.0 Uninhibited neuropathic bladder, not elsewhere classified
  N31.1 Reflex neuropathic bladder, not elsewhere classified
  N31.2 Flaccid neuropathic bladder, not elsewhere classified
    Atonic (motor) (sensory) neuropathic bladder
    Autonomous neuropathic bladder
    Nonreflex neuropathic bladder
  N31.8 Other neuromuscular dysfunction of bladder
  N31.9 Neuromuscular dysfunction of bladder, unspecified ▽
    Neurogenic bladder dysfunction NOS

✓4th N32 Other disorders of bladder
  EXCLUDES 2   *calculus of bladder (N21.0)*
       cystocele (N81.1-)
       hernia or prolapse of bladder, female (N81.1-)

N32.0 Bladder-neck obstruction
Bladder-neck stenosis (acquired)
  EXCLUDES 1   *congenital bladder-neck obstruction (Q64.3-)*
  DEF: Bladder outlet and vesicourethral obstruction; occurs as a consequence of benign prostatic hypertrophy or prostatic cancer; may also occur in either sex due to strictures, radiation, cystoscopy, catheterization, injury, infection, blood clots, bladder cancer, impaction, or other disease that compresses the bladder neck.

N32.1 Vesicointestinal fistula
Vesicorectal fistula

N32.2 Vesical fistula, not elsewhere classified
  EXCLUDES 1   *fistula between bladder and female genital tract (N82.0-N82.1)*

N32.3 Diverticulum of bladder
  EXCLUDES 1   *congenital diverticulum of bladder (Q64.6)*
       diverticulitis of bladder (N30.8-)

✓5th N32.8 Other specified disorders of bladder
  N32.81 Overactive bladder
    Detrusor muscle hyperactivity
    EXCLUDES 1   *frequent urination due to specified bladder condition—code to condition*
    DEF: Sudden involuntary contractions of the muscular wall of bladder; results in sudden, strong urge to urinate.

  N32.89 Other specified disorders of bladder
    Bladder hemorrhage
    Bladder hypertrophy
    Calcified bladder
    Contracted bladder

N32.9 Bladder disorder, unspecified ▽

N33 *Bladder disorders in diseases classified elsewhere*
Code first underlying disease, such as:
  schistosomiasis (B65.0-B65.9)
  EXCLUDES 1   *bladder disorder in syphilis (A52.76)*
       bladder disorder in tuberculosis (A18.12)
       candidal cystitis (B37.41)
       chlamydial cystitis (A56.01)
       cystitis in gonorrhea (A54.01)
       cystitis in neurogenic bladder (N31.-)
       diphtheritic cystitis (A36.85)
       neurogenic bladder (N31.-)
       syphilitic cystitis (A52.76)
       trichomonal cystitis (A59.03)

✓4th N34 Urethritis and urethral syndrome
Use additional code (B95-B97), to identify infectious agent
  EXCLUDES 2   *Reiter's disease (M02.3-)*
       urethritis in diseases with a predominantly sexual mode of transmission (A50-A64)
       urethrotrigonitis (N30.3-)
  AHA: 2017, 1Q, 6

  N34.0 Urethral abscess
    Abscess (of) Cowper's gland
    Abscess (of) Littrés gland
    Abscess (of) urethral (gland)
    Periurethral abscess
    EXCLUDES 1   *urethral caruncle (N36.2)*

  N34.1 Nonspecific urethritis
    Nongonococcal urethritis
    Nonvenereal urethritis

  N34.2 Other urethritis
    Meatitis, urethral
    Postmenopausal urethritis
    Ulcer of urethra (meatus)
    Urethritis NOS

  N34.3 Urethral syndrome, unspecified ▽

✓4th N35 Urethral stricture
  EXCLUDES 1   *congenital urethral stricture (Q64.3-)*
       postprocedural urethral stricture (N99.1-)

  ✓5th N35.0 Post-traumatic urethral stricture
    Urethral stricture due to injury
    EXCLUDES 1   *postprocedural urethral stricture (N99.1-)*

    ✓6th N35.01 Post-traumatic urethral stricture, male
      N35.010 Post-traumatic urethral stricture, male, meatal ♂
      N35.011 Post-traumatic bulbous urethral stricture
      N35.012 Post-traumatic membranous urethral stricture
      N35.013 Post-traumatic anterior urethral stricture

✓ Additional Character Req   ✓x7th Placeholder Alert   Manifestation   HCC CMS-HCC Condition   ▽ Unspecified Code   ►◄ Revised Text   ● New Code   ▲ Revised Code Title

ICD-10-CM 2018   807

N35.Ø14   **Post-traumatic urethral stricture, male, unspecified** ♂▽

√6ᵗʰ **N35.Ø2**   **Post-traumatic urethral stricture, female**

    N35.Ø21   **Urethral stricture due to childbirth** ♀

    N35.Ø28   **Other post-traumatic urethral stricture, female** ♀

√5ᵗʰ **N35.1**   **Postinfective urethral stricture, not elsewhere classified**
> EXCLUDES 1   urethral stricture associated with schistosomiasis (B65-, N29)
> gonococcal urethral stricture (A54.Ø1)
> syphilitic urethral stricture (A52.76)

√6ᵗʰ **N35.11**   **Postinfective urethral stricture, not elsewhere classified, male**

    N35.111   **Postinfective urethral stricture, not elsewhere classified, male, meatal** ♂

▲   **N35.112**   **Postinfective bulbous urethral stricture, not elsewhere classified, male**

▲   **N35.113**   **Postinfective membranous urethral stricture, not elsewhere classified, male**

▲   **N35.114**   **Postinfective anterior urethral stricture, not elsewhere classified, male**

    N35.119   **Postinfective urethral stricture, not elsewhere classified, male, unspecified** ♂▽

    N35.12   **Postinfective urethral stricture, not elsewhere classified, female** ♀

N35.8   **Other urethral stricture**
> EXCLUDES 1   postprocedural urethral stricture (N99.1-)

N35.9   **Urethral stricture, unspecified** ▽

√4ᵗʰ **N36**   **Other disorders of urethra**

N36.Ø   **Urethral fistula**
Urethroperineal fistula
Urethrorectal fistula
Urinary fistula NOS
> EXCLUDES 1   urethroscrotal fistula (N5Ø.89)
> urethrovaginal fistula (N82.1)
> urethrovesicovaginal fistula (N82.1)

N36.1   **Urethral diverticulum**

N36.2   **Urethral caruncle**

√5ᵗʰ **N36.4**   **Urethral functional and muscular disorders**
Use additional code to identify associated urinary stress incontinence (N39.3)

    N36.41   **Hypermobility of urethra**

    N36.42   **Intrinsic sphincter deficiency (ISD)**

    N36.43   **Combined hypermobility of urethra and intrinsic sphincter deficiency**

    N36.44   **Muscular disorders of urethra**
Bladder sphincter dyssynergy

N36.5   **Urethral false passage**

N36.8   **Other specified disorders of urethra**
> EXCLUDES 1   congenital urethrocele (Q64.7)
> female urethrocele (N81.Ø)

N36.9   **Urethral disorder, unspecified** ▽

N37   *Urethral disorders in diseases classified elsewhere*
Code first underlying disease
> EXCLUDES 1   urethritis (in):
> candidal infection (B37.41)
> chlamydial (A56.Ø1)
> gonorrhea (A54.Ø1)
> syphilis (A52.76)
> trichomonal infection (A59.Ø3)
> tuberculosis (A18.13)

√4ᵗʰ **N39**   **Other disorders of urinary system**
> EXCLUDES 2   hematuria NOS (R31.-)
> recurrent or persistent hematuria (NØ2.-)
> recurrent or persistent hematuria with specified morphological lesion (NØ2.-)
> proteinuria NOS (R8Ø.-)

N39.Ø   **Urinary tract infection, site not specified** ▽
Use additional code (B95-B97), to identify infectious agent
> EXCLUDES 1   candidiasis of urinary tract (B37.4-)
> neonatal urinary tract infection (P39.3)
> urinary tract infection of specified site, such as:
> cystitis (N3Ø.-)
> urethritis (N34.-)

AHA: 2017, 1Q, 6; 2012, 4Q, 94

N39.3   **Stress incontinence (female) (male)**
Code also any associated overactive bladder (N32.81)
> EXCLUDES 1   mixed incontinence (N39.46)

√5ᵗʰ **N39.4**   **Other specified urinary incontinence**
Code also any associated overactive bladder (N32.81)
> EXCLUDES 1   enuresis NOS (R32)
> functional urinary incontinence (R39.81)
> urinary incontinence associated with cognitive impairment (R39.81)
> urinary incontinence NOS (R32)
> urinary incontinence of nonorganic origin (F98.Ø)

    N39.41   **Urge incontinence**
> EXCLUDES 1   mixed incontinence (N39.46)

    N39.42   **Incontinence without sensory awareness**
Insensible (urinary) incontinence

    N39.43   **Post-void dribbling**

    N39.44   **Nocturnal enuresis**

    N39.45   **Continuous leakage**

    N39.46   **Mixed incontinence**
Urge and stress incontinence

√6ᵗʰ **N39.49**   **Other specified urinary incontinence**

    N39.49Ø   **Overflow incontinence**

    N39.491   **Coital incontinence**

    N39.492   **Postural (urinary) incontinence**

    N39.498   **Other specified urinary incontinence**
Reflex incontinence
Total incontinence

N39.8   **Other specified disorders of urinary system**

N39.9   **Disorder of urinary system, unspecified** ▽

Diseases of male genital organs (N4Ø-N53)

√4ᵗʰ **N4Ø**   **Benign prostatic hyperplasia**
> INCLUDES   adenofibromatous hypertrophy of prostate
> benign hypertrophy of the prostate
> benign prostatic hypertrophy
> BPH
> enlarged prostate
> nodular prostate
> polyp of prostate
> EXCLUDES 1   benign neoplasms of prostate (adenoma, benign) (fibroadenoma) (fibroma) (myoma) (D29.1)
> EXCLUDES 2   malignant neoplasm of prostate (C61)

N4Ø.Ø   **Benign prostatic hyperplasia without lower urinary tract symptoms** A♂
Enlarged prostate NOS
Enlarged prostate without LUTS

N4Ø.1   **Benign prostatic hyperplasia with lower urinary tract symptoms** A♂
Enlarged prostate with LUTS
Use additional code for associated symptoms, when specified:
incomplete bladder emptying (R39.14)
nocturia (R35.1)
straining on urination (R39.16)
urinary frequency (R35.Ø)
urinary hesitancy (R39.11)
urinary incontinence (N39.4-)
urinary obstruction (N13.8)
urinary retention (R33.8)
urinary urgency (R39.15)
weak urinary stream (R39.12)

N4Ø.2   **Nodular prostate without lower urinary tract symptoms** A♂
Nodular prostate without LUTS

N4Ø.3   **Nodular prostate with lower urinary tract symptoms** A♂
Use additional code for associated symptoms, when specified:
incomplete bladder emptying (R39.14)
nocturia (R35.1)
straining on urination (R39.16)
urinary frequency (R35.Ø)
urinary hesitancy (R39.11)
urinary incontinence (N39.4-)
urinary obstruction (N13.8)
urinary retention (R33.8)
urinary urgency (R39.15)
weak urinary stream (R39.12)

√4ᵗʰ **N41**   **Inflammatory diseases of prostate**
Use additional code (B95-B97), to identify infectious agent

N41.Ø   **Acute prostatitis** A♂

N41.1   **Chronic prostatitis** A♂

EXCLUDES 1 Not coded here   EXCLUDES 2 Not included here   N Newborn Age: 0   P Pediatric Age: 0-17   M Maternity Age: 12-55   A Adult Age: 15-124

N41.2 **Abscess of prostate**   Ⓐ♂

N41.3 **Prostatocystitis**   Ⓐ♂

N41.4 **Granulomatous prostatitis**   Ⓐ♂

N41.8 **Other inflammatory diseases of prostate**   Ⓐ♂

N41.9 **Inflammatory disease of prostate, unspecified**   Ⓐ♂▽
Prostatitis NOS

✓4ᵗʰ **N42** **Other and unspecified disorders of prostate**

N42.0 **Calculus of prostate**   Ⓐ♂
Prostatic stone
DEF: Formation of small, solid stone often composed of calcium carbonate or calcium phosphate in the prostate gland.

N42.1 **Congestion and hemorrhage of prostate**   Ⓐ♂
EXCLUDES 1   enlarged prostate (N40.-)
hematuria (R31.-)
hyperplasia of prostate (N40.-)
inflammatory diseases of prostate (N41.-)

✓5ᵗʰ **N42.3** **Dysplasia of prostate**

N42.30 **Unspecified dysplasia of prostate**   ♂▽

N42.31 **Prostatic intraepithelial neoplasia**   ♂
PIN
Prostatic intraepithelial neoplasia I (PIN I)
Prostatic intraepithelial neoplasia II (PIN II)
EXCLUDES 1   prostatic intraepithelial neoplasia III (PIN III) (D07.5)
DEF: Abnormality of shape and size of the intraepithelial tissues of the prostate; premalignant condition characterized by stalks and absence of a basilar cell layer; synonyms are intraductal dysplasia, large acinar atypical hyperplasia, atypical primary hyperplasia, hyperplasia with malignant changes, marked atypia, or duct-acinar dysplasia.

N42.32 **Atypical small acinar proliferation of prostate**   ♂

N42.39 **Other dysplasia of prostate**   ♂

✓5ᵗʰ **N42.8** **Other specified disorders of prostate**

N42.81 **Prostatodynia syndrome**   Ⓐ♂
Painful prostate syndrome

N42.82 **Prostatosis syndrome**   Ⓐ♂

N42.83 **Cyst of prostate**   Ⓐ♂

N42.89 **Other specified disorders of prostate**   Ⓐ♂

N42.9 **Disorder of prostate, unspecified**   Ⓐ♂▽

✓4ᵗʰ **N43** **Hydrocele and spermatocele**
INCLUDES   hydrocele of spermatic cord, testis or tunica vaginalis
EXCLUDES 1   congenital hydrocele (P83.5)

N43.0 **Encysted hydrocele**   ♂

N43.1 **Infected hydrocele**   ♂
Use additional code (B95-B97), to identify infectious agent

N43.2 **Other hydrocele**   ♂

N43.3 **Hydrocele, unspecified**   ♂▽

✓5ᵗʰ **N43.4** **Spermatocele of epididymis**
Spermatic cyst

N43.40 **Spermatocele of epididymis, unspecified**   ♂▽

N43.41 **Spermatocele of epididymis, single**   ♂

N43.42 **Spermatocele of epididymis, multiple**   ♂

Hydrocele

Normal   Noncommunicating hydrocele   Communicating hydrocele   Hydrocele of the cord

Testicle
Scrotum

✓4ᵗʰ **N44** **Noninflammatory disorders of testis**

✓5ᵗʰ **N44.0** **Torsion of testis**

N44.00 **Torsion of testis, unspecified**   ♂▽

N44.01 **Extravaginal torsion of spermatic cord**   ♂
DEF: Torsion of the spermatic cord just below the tunica vaginalis attachments.

N44.02 **Intravaginal torsion of spermatic cord**   ♂
Torsion of spermatic cord NOS

N44.03 **Torsion of appendix testis**   ♂

N44.04 **Torsion of appendix epididymis**   ♂

N44.1 **Cyst of tunica albuginea testis**   ♂

N44.2 **Benign cyst of testis**   ♂

N44.8 **Other noninflammatory disorders of the testis**   ♂

✓4ᵗʰ **N45** **Orchitis and epididymitis**
Use additional code (B95-B97), to identify infectious agent

N45.1 **Epididymitis**   ♂

N45.2 **Orchitis**   ♂

N45.3 **Epididymo-orchitis**   ♂

N45.4 **Abscess of epididymis or testis**   ♂

✓4ᵗʰ **N46** **Male infertility**
EXCLUDES 1   vasectomy status (Z98.52)

✓5ᵗʰ **N46.0** **Azoospermia**
Absolute male infertility
Male infertility due to germinal (cell) aplasia
Male infertility due to spermatogenic arrest (complete)

N46.01 **Organic azoospermia**   Ⓐ♂
Azoospermia NOS

✓6ᵗʰ **N46.02** **Azoospermia due to extratesticular causes**
Code also associated cause

N46.021 **Azoospermia due to drug therapy**   Ⓐ♂

N46.022 **Azoospermia due to infection**   Ⓐ♂

N46.023 **Azoospermia due to obstruction of efferent ducts**   Ⓐ♂

N46.024 **Azoospermia due to radiation**   Ⓐ♂

N46.025 **Azoospermia due to systemic disease**   Ⓐ♂

N46.029 **Azoospermia due to other extratesticular causes**   Ⓐ♂

✓5ᵗʰ **N46.1** **Oligospermia**
Male infertility due to germinal cell desquamation
Male infertility due to hypospermatogenesis
Male infertility due to incomplete spermatogenic arrest

N46.11 **Organic oligospermia**   Ⓐ♂
Oligospermia NOS

✓6ᵗʰ **N46.12** **Oligospermia due to extratesticular causes**
Code also associated cause

N46.121 **Oligospermia due to drug therapy**   Ⓐ♂

N46.122 **Oligospermia due to infection**   Ⓐ♂

N46.123 **Oligospermia due to obstruction of efferent ducts**   Ⓐ♂

N46.124 **Oligospermia due to radiation**   Ⓐ♂

N46.125 **Oligospermia due to systemic disease**   Ⓐ♂

N46.129 **Oligospermia due to other extratesticular causes**   Ⓐ♂

N46.8 **Other male infertility**   Ⓐ♂

N46.9 **Male infertility, unspecified**   Ⓐ♂▽

✓4ᵗʰ **N47** **Disorders of prepuce**

N47.0 **Adherent prepuce, newborn**   Ⓝ♂

N47.1 **Phimosis**   ♂

N47.2 **Paraphimosis**   ♂

N47.3 **Deficient foreskin**   ♂

N47.4 **Benign cyst of prepuce**   ♂

N47.5 **Adhesions of prepuce and glans penis**   ♂

N47.6 **Balanoposthitis**   ♂
Use additional code (B95-B97), to identify infectious agent
EXCLUDES 1   balanitis (N48.1)

N47.7 **Other inflammatory diseases of prepuce**   ♂
Use additional code (B95-B97), to identify infectious agent

N47.8 **Other disorders of prepuce**   ♂

Chapter 14. Diseases of Genitourinary System

✓4ᵗʰ **N48** **Other disorders of penis**

N48.0 **Leukoplakia of penis**   ♂
     Balanitis xerotica obliterans
     Kraurosis of penis
     Lichen sclerosus of external male genital organs
     EXCLUDES 1   *carcinoma in situ of penis (D07.4)*

N48.1 **Balanitis**   ♂
     Use additional code (B95-B97), to identify infectious agent
     EXCLUDES 1   *amebic balanitis (A06.8)*
         balanitis xerotica obliterans (N48.0)
         candidal balanitis (B37.42)
         gonococcal balanitis (A54.23)
         herpesviral [herpes simplex] balanitis (A60.01)

✓5ᵗʰ **N48.2** **Other inflammatory disorders of penis**
     Use additional code (B95-B97), to identify infectious agent
     EXCLUDES 1   *balanitis (N48.1)*
         balanitis xerotica obliterans (N48.0)
         balanoposthitis (N47.6)

     N48.21   **Abscess of corpus cavernosum and penis**   ♂
     N48.22   **Cellulitis of corpus cavernosum and penis**   ♂
     N48.29   **Other inflammatory disorders of penis**   ♂

✓5ᵗʰ **N48.3** **Priapism**
     Painful erection
     Code first underlying cause

     N48.30   **Priapism, unspecified**   ♂ ▽
     N48.31   **Priapism** due to trauma   ♂
     N48.32   *Priapism due to disease classified elsewhere*   ♂
     N48.33   **Priapism,** drug-induced   ♂
     N48.39   **Other priapism**   ♂

N48.5 **Ulcer of penis**   ♂

N48.6 **Induration penis plastica**   ♂
     Peyronie's disease
     Plastic induration of penis

✓5ᵗʰ **N48.8** **Other specified disorders of penis**

     N48.81   **Thrombosis of superficial vein of penis**   ♂
     N48.82   **Acquired torsion of penis**   ♂
         Acquired torsion of penis NOS
         EXCLUDES 1   *congenital torsion of penis (Q55.63)*
     N48.83   **Acquired buried penis**   ♂
         EXCLUDES 1   *congenital hidden penis (Q55.64)*
     N48.89   **Other specified disorders of penis**   ♂

N48.9 **Disorder of penis, unspecified**   ♂ ▽

✓4ᵗʰ **N49** **Inflammatory disorders of male genital organs, not elsewhere classified**
     Use additional code (B95-B97), to identify infectious agent
     EXCLUDES 1   *inflammation of penis (N48.1, N48.2-)*
         orchitis and epididymitis (N45.-)

N49.0 **Inflammatory disorders of** seminal vesicle   ♂
     Vesiculitis NOS

N49.1 **Inflammatory disorders of** spermatic cord, tunica   ♂
vaginalis and vas deferens
     Vasitis

N49.2 **Inflammatory disorders of** scrotum   ♂

N49.3 **Fournier gangrene**   ♂

N49.8 **Inflammatory disorders of other specified male genital**   ♂
organs
     Inflammation of multiple sites in male genital organs

N49.9 **Inflammatory disorder of unspecified male genital**   ♂ ▽
organ
     Abscess of unspecified male genital organ
     Boil of unspecified male genital organ
     Carbuncle of unspecified male genital organ
     Cellulitis of unspecified male genital organ

✓4ᵗʰ **N50** **Other and unspecified disorders of male genital organs**
     EXCLUDES 2   *torsion of testis (N44.0-)*

N50.0 **Atrophy of testis**   ♂

N50.1 **Vascular disorders of male genital organs**   ♂
     Hematocele, NOS, of male genital organs
     Hemorrhage of male genital organs
     Thrombosis of male genital organs

N50.3 **Cyst of epididymis**   ♂

✓5ᵗʰ **N50.8** **Other specified disorders of male genital organs**

     ✓6ᵗʰ **N50.81**   **Testicular pain**
         N50.811   **Right testicular pain**   ♂
         N50.812   **Left testicular pain**   ♂

         N50.819   **Testicular pain, unspecified**   ♂ ▽
     N50.82   **Scrotal pain**   ♂
     N50.89   **Other specified disorders of the male genital**   ♂
         organs
         Atrophy of scrotum, seminal vesicle, spermatic cord, tunica vaginalis and vas deferens
         Chylocele, tunica vaginalis (nonfilarial) NOS
         Edema of scrotum, seminal vesicle, spermatic cord, testis, tunica vaginalis and vas deferens
         Hypertrophy of scrotum, seminal vesicle, spermatic cord, testis, tunica vaginalis and vas deferens
         Stricture of spermatic cord, tunica vaginalis, and vas deferens
         Ulcer of scrotum, seminal vesicle, spermatic cord, testis, tunica vaginalis and vas deferens
         Urethroscrotal fistula

N50.9 **Disorder of male genital organs, unspecified**   ♂ ▽

N51   *Disorders of male genital organs in diseases classified*   ♂
elsewhere
     Code first underlying disease, such as:
         filariasis (B74.0-B74.9)
     EXCLUDES 1   *amebic balanitis (A06.8)*
         candidal balanitis (B37.42)
         gonococcal balanitis (A54.23)
         gonococcal prostatitis (A54.22)
         herpesviral [herpes simplex] balanitis (A60.01)
         trichomonal prostatitis (A59.02)
         tuberculous prostatitis (A18.14)

✓4ᵗʰ **N52** **Male erectile dysfunction**
     EXCLUDES 1   *psychogenic impotence (F52.21)*

✓5ᵗʰ **N52.0** **Vasculogenic erectile dysfunction**

     N52.01   **Erectile dysfunction due to** arterial insufficiency   Ⓐ ♂
     N52.02   **Corporo-venous occlusive** erectile dysfunction   Ⓐ ♂
     N52.03   **Combined arterial insufficiency and**   Ⓐ ♂
         corporo-venous occlusive erectile dysfunction

N52.1   *Erectile dysfunction due to diseases classified elsewhere*   Ⓐ ♂
     Code first underlying disease

N52.2 **Drug-induced** erectile dysfunction   Ⓐ ♂

✓5ᵗʰ **N52.3** **Postprocedural** erectile dysfunction

     N52.31   **Erectile dysfunction following** radical   Ⓐ ♂
         prostatectomy
     N52.32   **Erectile dysfunction following** radical   Ⓐ ♂
         cystectomy
     N52.33   **Erectile dysfunction following** urethral surgery   Ⓐ ♂
     N52.34   **Erectile dysfunction following** simple   Ⓐ ♂
         prostatectomy
     N52.35   **Erectile dysfunction following** radiation   Ⓐ ♂
         therapy
     N52.36   **Erectile dysfunction following** interstitial   Ⓐ ♂
         seed therapy
     N52.37   **Erectile dysfunction following** prostate   Ⓐ ♂
         ablative therapy
         Erectile dysfunction following cryotherapy
         Erectile dysfunction following other prostate ablative therapies
         Erectile dysfunction following ultrasound ablative therapies
     N52.39   **Other and unspecified postprocedural**   Ⓐ ♂ ▽
         erectile dysfunction

N52.8 **Other male erectile dysfunction**   Ⓐ ♂

N52.9 **Male erectile dysfunction, unspecified**   Ⓐ ♂ ▽
     Impotence NOS

✓4ᵗʰ **N53** **Other male sexual dysfunction**
     EXCLUDES 1   *psychogenic sexual dysfunction (F52.-)*

✓5ᵗʰ **N53.1** **Ejaculatory dysfunction**
     EXCLUDES 1   *premature ejaculation (F52.4)*

     N53.11   **Retarded ejaculation**   ♂
     N53.12   **Painful ejaculation**   ♂
     N53.13   **Anejaculatory orgasm**   ♂
     N53.14   **Retrograde ejaculation**   ♂
         DEF: A form of male sexual dysfunction in which the semen enters the bladder instead of going out through the urethra during ejaculation.
     N53.19   **Other ejaculatory dysfunction**   ♂
         Ejaculatory dysfunction NOS

N53.8 **Other male sexual dysfunction**   ♂

N53.9 **Unspecified male sexual dysfunction**   ♂ ▽

EXCLUDES 1 Not coded here   *EXCLUDES 2* Not included here   Ⓝ Newborn Age: 0   Ⓟ Pediatric Age: 0-17   Ⓜ Maternity Age: 12-55   Ⓐ Adult Age: 15-124

810   ICD-10-CM 2018

Disorders of breast (N60-N65)

EXCLUDES 1   *disorders of breast associated with childbirth (O91-O92)*

✓4ᵗʰ **N60 Benign mammary dysplasia**
     INCLUDES   fibrocystic mastopathy

✓5ᵗʰ **N60.0 Solitary cyst of breast**
     Cyst of breast
- **N60.01 Solitary cyst of right breast**
- **N60.02 Solitary cyst of left breast**
- **N60.09 Solitary cyst of unspecified breast** ▽

✓5ᵗʰ **N60.1 Diffuse cystic mastopathy**
     Cystic breast
     Fibrocystic disease of breast
     EXCLUDES 1   *diffuse cystic mastopathy with epithelial proliferation (N60.3-)*
- **N60.11 Diffuse cystic mastopathy of right breast** Ⓐ
- **N60.12 Diffuse cystic mastopathy of left breast** Ⓐ
- **N60.19 Diffuse cystic mastopathy of unspecified breast** Ⓐ▽

✓5ᵗʰ **N60.2 Fibroadenosis of breast**
     Adenofibrosis of breast
     EXCLUDES 2   *fibroadenoma of breast (D24.-)*
- **N60.21 Fibroadenosis of right breast**
- **N60.22 Fibroadenosis of left breast**
- **N60.29 Fibroadenosis of unspecified breast** ▽

✓5ᵗʰ **N60.3 Fibrosclerosis of breast**
     Cystic mastopathy with epithelial proliferation
- **N60.31 Fibrosclerosis of right breast**
- **N60.32 Fibrosclerosis of left breast**
- **N60.39 Fibrosclerosis of unspecified breast** ▽

✓5ᵗʰ **N60.4 Mammary duct ectasia**
- **N60.41 Mammary duct ectasia of right breast**
- **N60.42 Mammary duct ectasia of left breast**
- **N60.49 Mammary duct ectasia of unspecified breast** ▽

✓5ᵗʰ **N60.8 Other benign mammary dysplasias**
- **N60.81 Other benign mammary dysplasias of right breast**
- **N60.82 Other benign mammary dysplasias of left breast**
- **N60.89 Other benign mammary dysplasias of unspecified breast** ▽

✓5ᵗʰ **N60.9 Unspecified benign mammary dysplasia**
- **N60.91 Unspecified benign mammary dysplasia of right breast** ▽
- **N60.92 Unspecified benign mammary dysplasia of left breast** ▽
- **N60.99 Unspecified benign mammary dysplasia of unspecified breast** ▽

✓4ᵗʰ **N61 Inflammatory disorders of breast**
     EXCLUDES 1   *inflammatory carcinoma of breast (C50.9)*
         inflammatory disorder of breast associated with childbirth (O91.-)
         neonatal infective mastitis (P39.0)
         thrombophlebitis of breast [Mondor's disease] (I80.8)

N61.0 Mastitis without abscess
     Infective mastitis (acute) (nonpuerperal) (subacute)
     Mastitis (acute) (nonpuerperal) (subacute) NOS
     Cellulitis (acute) (nonpuerperal) (subacute) of breast NOS
     Cellulitis (acute) (nonpuerperal) (subacute) of nipple NOS

N61.1 Abscess of the breast and nipple
     Abscess (acute) (chronic) (nonpuerperal) of areola
     Abscess (acute) (chronic) (nonpuerperal) of breast
     Carbuncle of breast
     Mastitis with abscess

N62 Hypertrophy of breast
     Gynecomastia
     Hypertrophy of breast NOS
     Massive pubertal hypertrophy of breast
     EXCLUDES 1   *breast engorgement of newborn (P83.4)*
         disproportion of reconstructed breast (N65.1)

✓4ᵗʰ **N63 Unspecified lump in breast**
     Nodule(s) NOS in breast
- **N63.0 Unspecified lump in unspecified breast** ▽
- ✓5ᵗʰ **N63.1 Unspecified lump in the right breast**
  - **N63.10 Unspecified lump in the right breast, unspecified quadrant** ▽
  - **N63.11 Unspecified lump in the right breast, upper outer quadrant** ▽
  - **N63.12 Unspecified lump in the right breast, upper inner quadrant** ▽
  - **N63.13 Unspecified lump in the right breast, lower outer quadrant** ▽
  - **N63.14 Unspecified lump in the right breast, lower inner quadrant** ▽
- ✓5ᵗʰ **N63.2 Unspecified lump in the left breast**
  - **N63.20 Unspecified lump in the left breast, unspecified quadrant** ▽
  - **N63.21 Unspecified lump in the left breast, upper outer quadrant** ▽
  - **N63.22 Unspecified lump in the left breast, upper inner quadrant** ▽
  - **N63.23 Unspecified lump in the left breast, lower outer quadrant** ▽
  - **N63.24 Unspecified lump in the left breast, lower inner quadrant** ▽
- ✓5ᵗʰ **N63.3 Unspecified lump in axillary tail**
  - **N63.31 Unspecified lump in axillary tail of the right breast** ▽
  - **N63.32 Unspecified lump in axillary tail of the left breast** ▽
- ✓5ᵗʰ **N63.4 Unspecified lump in breast, subareolar**
  - **N63.41 Unspecified lump in right breast, subareolar** ▽
  - **N63.42 Unspecified lump in left breast, subareolar** ▽

✓4ᵗʰ **N64 Other disorders of breast**
     EXCLUDES 2   *mechanical complication of breast prosthesis and implant (T85.4-)*

N64.0 Fissure and fistula of nipple

N64.1 Fat necrosis of breast
     Fat necrosis (segmental) of breast
     Code first breast necrosis due to breast graft (T85.898)

N64.2 Atrophy of breast

N64.3 Galactorrhea not associated with childbirth

N64.4 Mastodynia

✓5ᵗʰ **N64.5 Other signs and symptoms in breast**
     EXCLUDES 2   *abnormal findings on diagnostic imaging of breast (R92.-)*
- **N64.51 Induration of breast**
- **N64.52 Nipple discharge**
     EXCLUDES 1   *abnormal findings in nipple discharge (R89.-)*
- **N64.53 Retraction of nipple**
- **N64.59 Other signs and symptoms in breast**

✓5ᵗʰ **N64.8 Other specified disorders of breast**
- **N64.81 Ptosis of breast** Ⓐ
     EXCLUDES 1   *ptosis of native breast in relation to reconstructed breast (N65.1)*
- **N64.82 Hypoplasia of breast** Ⓐ
     Micromastia
     EXCLUDES 1   *congenital absence of breast (Q83.0)*
         hypoplasia of native breast in relation to reconstructed breast (N65.1)
- **N64.89 Other specified disorders of breast**
     Galactocele
     Subinvolution of breast (postlactational)

N64.9 Disorder of breast, unspecified ▽

✓4ᵗʰ **N65 Deformity and disproportion of reconstructed breast**

N65.0 Deformity of reconstructed breast Ⓐ
     Contour irregularity in reconstructed breast
     Excess tissue in reconstructed breast
     Misshapen reconstructed breast

N65.1 Disproportion of reconstructed breast Ⓐ
     Breast asymmetry between native breast and reconstructed breast
     Disproportion between native breast and reconstructed breast

---

✓ Additional Character Req   ✓x7ᵗʰ Placeholder Alert   Manifestation   HCC CMS-HCC Condition   ▽ Unspecified Code   ►◄ Revised Text   ● New Code   ▲ Revised Code Title

Chapter 14. Diseases of Genitourinary System

Inflammatory diseases of female pelvic organs (N70-N77)

> **EXCLUDES 1**   inflammatory diseases of female pelvic organs complicating:
> abortion or ectopic or molar pregnancy (O00-O07, O08.0)
> pregnancy, childbirth and the puerperium (O23-, O75.3, O85, O86-)

✓4ᵗʰ N70 Salpingitis and oophoritis

> **INCLUDES**   abscess (of) fallopian tube
> abscess (of) ovary
> pyosalpinx
> salpingo-oophoritis
> tubo-ovarian abscess
> tubo-ovarian inflammatory disease

Use additional code (B95-B97), to identify infectious agent

> **EXCLUDES 1**   gonococcal infection (A54.24)
> tuberculous infection (A18.17)

✓5ᵗʰ N70.0 Acute salpingitis and oophoritis

N70.01	Acute salpingitis	♀
N70.02	Acute oophoritis	♀
N70.03	Acute salpingitis and oophoritis	♀

✓5ᵗʰ N70.1 Chronic salpingitis and oophoritis
Hydrosalpinx

N70.11	Chronic salpingitis	♀
N70.12	Chronic oophoritis	♀
N70.13	Chronic salpingitis and oophoritis	♀

✓5ᵗʰ N70.9 Salpingitis and oophoritis, unspecified

N70.91	Salpingitis, unspecified	♀ ▽
N70.92	Oophoritis, unspecified	♀▽
N70.93	Salpingitis and oophoritis, unspecified	♀ ▽

✓4ᵗʰ N71 Inflammatory disease of uterus, except cervix

> **INCLUDES**   endo (myo) metritis   pyometra
> metritis   uterine abscess
> myometritis

Use additional code (B95-B97), to identify infectious agent

> **EXCLUDES 1**   hyperplastic endometritis (N85.0-)
> infection of uterus following delivery (O85, O86.-)

N71.0	Acute inflammatory disease of uterus	♀
N71.1	Chronic inflammatory disease of uterus	♀
N71.9	Inflammatory disease of uterus, unspecified	♀ ▽

N72 Inflammatory disease of cervix uteri   ♀

> **INCLUDES**   cervicitis (with or without erosion or ectropion)
> endocervicitis (with or without erosion or ectropion)
> exocervicitis (with or without erosion or ectropion)

Use additional code (B95-B97), to identify infectious agent

> **EXCLUDES 1**   erosion and ectropion of cervix without cervicitis (N86)

✓4ᵗʰ N73 Other female pelvic inflammatory diseases

Use additional code (B95-B97), to identify infectious agent

N73.0 Acute parametritis and pelvic cellulitis   ♀
Abscess of broad ligament
Abscess of parametrium
Pelvic cellulitis, female
DEF: Parametritis: Inflammation of the parametrium; pelvic
cellulitis is a synonym for parametritis.

N73.1 Chronic parametritis and pelvic cellulitis   ♀
Any condition in N73.0 specified as chronic
> **EXCLUDES 1**   tuberculous parametritis and pelvic cellultis (A18.17)

N73.2 Unspecified parametritis and pelvic cellulitis   ♀ ▽
Any condition in N73.0 unspecified whether acute or chronic

N73.3	Female acute pelvic peritonitis	♀
N73.4	Female chronic pelvic peritonitis	♀

> **EXCLUDES 1**   tuberculous pelvic (female) peritonitis (A18.17)

N73.5 Female pelvic peritonitis, unspecified   ♀▽

N73.6 Female pelvic peritoneal adhesions (postinfective)   ♀
> **EXCLUDES 2**   postprocedural pelvic peritoneal adhesions (N99.4)
AHA: 2014, 1Q, 6

N73.8	Other specified female pelvic inflammatory diseases	♀
N73.9	Female pelvic inflammatory disease, unspecified	♀ ▽

Female pelvic infection or inflammation NOS

N74 Female pelvic inflammatory disorders in diseases classified   ♀ elsewhere

Code first underlying disease

> **EXCLUDES 1**   chlamydial cervicitis (A56.02)
> chlamydial pelvic inflammatory disease (A56.11)
> gonococcal cervicitis (A54.03)
> gonococcal pelvic inflammatory disease (A54.24)
> herpesviral [herpes simplex] cervicitis (A60.03)
> herpesviral [herpes simplex] pelvic inflammatory disease
> (A60.09)
> syphilitic cervicitis (A52.76)
> syphilitic pelvic inflammatory disease (A52.76)
> trichomonal cervicitis (A59.09)
> tuberculous cervicitis (A18.16)
> tuberculous pelvic inflammatory disease (A18.17)

✓4ᵗʰ N75 Diseases of Bartholin's gland

N75.0	Cyst of Bartholin's gland	♀
N75.1	Abscess of Bartholin's gland	♀
N75.8	Other diseases of Bartholin's gland	♀

Bartholinitis

N75.9	Disease of Bartholin's gland, unspecified	♀ ▽

✓4ᵗʰ N76 Other inflammation of vagina and vulva

Use additional code (B95-B97), to identify infectious agent

> **EXCLUDES 2**   senile (atrophic) vaginitis (N95.2)
> vulvar vestibulitis (N94.810)

N76.0 Acute vaginitis   ♀
Acute vulvovaginitis
Vaginitis NOS
Vulvovaginitis NOS

N76.1 Subacute and chronic vaginitis   ♀
Chronic vulvovaginitis
Subacute vulvovaginitis

N76.2 Acute vulvitis   ♀
Vulvitis NOS

N76.3	Subacute and chronic vulvitis	♀

N76.4 Abscess of vulva   ♀
Furuncle of vulva

N76.5	Ulceration of vagina	♀
N76.6	Ulceration of vulva	♀

✓5ᵗʰ N76.8 Other specified inflammation of vagina and vulva

N76.81 Mucositis (ulcerative) of vagina and vulva   ♀
Code also type of associated therapy, such as:
antineoplastic and immunosuppressive drugs
(T45.1X-)
radiological procedure and radiotherapy (Y84.2)
> **EXCLUDES 2**   gastrointestinal mucositis (ulcerative)
> (K92.81)
> nasal mucositis (ulcerative) (J34.81)
> oral mucositis (ulcerative) (K12.3-)

N76.89 Other specified inflammation of vagina and vulva   ♀

✓4ᵗʰ N77 Vulvovaginal ulceration and inflammation in diseases classified elsewhere

N77.0 *Ulceration of vulva in diseases classified elsewhere*   ♀
Code first underlying disease, such as:
Behçet's disease (M35.2)
> **EXCLUDES 1**   ulceration of vulva in gonococcal infection (A54.02)
> ulceration of vulva in herpesviral [herpes simplex]
> infection (A60.04)
> ulceration of vulva in syphilis (A51.0)
> ulceration of vulva in tuberculosis (A18.18)

N77.1 *Vaginitis, vulvitis and vulvovaginitis in diseases classified*   ♀ ***elsewhere***
Code first underlying disease, such as:
pinworm (B80)
> **EXCLUDES 1**   candidal vulvovaginitis (B37.3)
> chlamydial vulvovaginitis (A56.02)
> gonococcal vulvovaginitis (A54.02)
> herpesviral [herpes simplex] vulvovaginitis (A60.04)
> trichomonal vulvovaginitis (A59.01)
> tuberculous vulvovaginitis (A18.18)
> vulvovaginitis in early syphilis (A51.0)
> vulvovaginitis in late syphilis (A52.76)

EXCLUDES 1 Not coded here   **EXCLUDES 2** Not included here   **N** Newborn Age: 0   **P** Pediatric Age: 0-17   **M** Maternity Age: 12-55   **A** Adult Age: 15-124

812   **ICD-10-CM 2018**

N70–N77.1

Types of Pelvic Organ Prolapse

Urethrocele

Cystocele

Rectocele

Enterocele

Noninflammatory disorders of female genital tract (N80-N98)

☑4ᵗʰ N80 Endometriosis

N80.0 Endometriosis of uterus ♀
Adenomyosis
EXCLUDES 1 *stromal endometriosis (D39.0)*

N80.1 Endometriosis of ovary ♀

N80.2 Endometriosis of fallopian tube ♀

N80.3 Endometriosis of pelvic peritoneum ♀

N80.4 Endometriosis of rectovaginal septum and vagina ♀

N80.5 Endometriosis of intestine ♀

N80.6 Endometriosis in cutaneous scar ♀

N80.8 Other endometriosis ♀
▶Endometriosis of thorax◀

N80.9 Endometriosis, unspecified ♀ ▽

☑4ᵗʰ N81 Female genital prolapse
EXCLUDES 1 *genital prolapse complicating pregnancy, labor or delivery (O34.5-)*
prolapse and hernia of ovary and fallopian tube (N83.4-)
prolapse of vaginal vault after hysterectomy (N99.3)

N81.0 Urethrocele ♀
EXCLUDES 1 *urethrocele with cystocele (N81.1-)*
urethrocele with prolapse of uterus (N81.2-N81.4)

☑5ᵗʰ N81.1 Cystocele
Cystocele with urethrocele
Cystourethrocele
EXCLUDES 1 *cystocele with prolapse of uterus (N81.2-N81.4)*

N81.10 Cystocele, unspecified ♀ ▽
Prolapse of (anterior) vaginal wall NOS

N81.11 Cystocele, midline ♀

N81.12 Cystocele, lateral ♀
Paravaginal cystocele
DEF: Detachment of the lateral support connections of the vagina at the arcus tendineus fasciae pelvis (ATFP) results in bladder drop; bladder herniates into the vagina laterally.

N81.2 Incomplete uterovaginal prolapse ♀
First degree uterine prolapse
Prolapse of cervix NOS
Second degree uterine prolapse
EXCLUDES 1 ▶cervical stump prolapse◀ (N81.85)

N81.3 Complete uterovaginal prolapse ♀
Procidentia (uteri) NOS
Third degree uterine prolapse

N81.4 Uterovaginal prolapse, unspecified ♀ ▽
Prolapse of uterus NOS

N81.5 Vaginal enterocele ♀
EXCLUDES 1 *enterocele with prolapse of uterus (N81.2-N81.4)*

N81.6 Rectocele ♀
Prolapse of posterior vaginal wall
Use additional code for any associated fecal incontinence, if applicable (R15.-)
EXCLUDES 2 *perineocele (N81.81)*
rectal prolapse (K62.3)
rectocele with prolapse of uterus (N81.2-N81.4)

☑5ᵗʰ N81.8 Other female genital prolapse

N81.81 Perineocele ♀

N81.82 Incompetence or weakening of pubocervical tissue ♀

N81.83 Incompetence or weakening of rectovaginal tissue ♀

N81.84 Pelvic muscle wasting ♀
Disuse atrophy of pelvic muscles and anal sphincter

N81.85 Cervical stump prolapse ♀

N81.89 Other female genital prolapse ♀
Deficient perineum
Old laceration of muscles of pelvic floor

N81.9 Female genital prolapse, unspecified ♀ ▽

☑4ᵗʰ N82 Fistulae involving female genital tract
EXCLUDES 1 *vesicointestinal fistulae (N32.1)*

N82.0 Vesicovaginal fistula ♀

N82.1 Other female urinary-genital tract fistulae ♀
Cervicovesical fistula
Ureterovaginal fistula
Urethrovaginal fistula
Uteroureteric fistula
Uterovesical fistula

N82.2 Fistula of vagina to small intestine ♀

N82.3 Fistula of vagina to large intestine ♀
Rectovaginal fistula

N82.4 Other female intestinal-genital tract fistulae ♀
Intestinouterine fistula

N82.5 Female genital tract-skin fistulae ♀
Uterus to abdominal wall fistula
Vaginoperineal fistula

N82.8 Other female genital tract fistulae ♀

N82.9 Female genital tract fistula, unspecified ♀ ▽

☑4ᵗʰ N83 Noninflammatory disorders of ovary, fallopian tube and broad ligament
EXCLUDES 2 *hydrosalpinx (N70.1-)*

☑5ᵗʰ N83.0 Follicular cyst of ovary
Cyst of graafian follicle
Hemorrhagic follicular cyst (of ovary)

N83.00 Follicular cyst of ovary, unspecified side ♀ ▽

N83.01 Follicular cyst of right ovary ♀

N83.02 Follicular cyst of left ovary ♀

☑5ᵗʰ N83.1 Corpus luteum cyst
Hemorrhagic corpus luteum cyst

N83.10 Corpus luteum cyst of ovary, unspecified side ♀ ▽

N83.11 Corpus luteum cyst of right ovary ♀

N83.12 Corpus luteum cyst of left ovary ♀

☑5ᵗʰ N83.2 Other and unspecified ovarian cysts
EXCLUDES 1 *developmental ovarian cyst (Q50.1)*
neoplastic ovarian cyst (D27.-)
polycystic ovarian syndrome (E28.2)
Stein-Leventhal syndrome (E28.2)

☑6ᵗʰ N83.20 Unspecified ovarian cysts

N83.201 Unspecified ovarian cyst, right side ♀ ▽

N83.202 Unspecified ovarian cyst, left side ♀ ▽

N83.209 Unspecified ovarian cyst, unspecified side ♀ ▽
Ovarian cyst, NOS

☑6ᵗʰ N83.29 Other ovarian cysts
Retention cyst of ovary
Simple cyst of ovary

N83.291 Other ovarian cyst, right side ♀

N83.292 Other ovarian cyst, left side ♀

N83.299 Other ovarian cyst, unspecified side ♀ ▽

☑5ᵗʰ N83.3 Acquired atrophy of ovary and fallopian tube

☑6ᵗʰ N83.31 Acquired atrophy of ovary

N83.311 Acquired atrophy of right ovary ♀

N83.312 Acquired atrophy of left ovary ♀

☑ Additional Character Req   ☑✗7ᵗʰ Placeholder Alert   Manifestation   HCC CMS-HCC Condition   ▽ Unspecified Code   ▶◀ Revised Text   ● New Code   ▲ Revised Code Title

N83.319 **Acquired atrophy of ovary,** ♀▽
unspecified side
Acquired atrophy of ovary, NOS

✓6th **N83.32** **Acquired atrophy of fallopian tube**

N83.321 **Acquired atrophy of right fallopian** ♀
tube

N83.322 **Acquired atrophy of left fallopian tube** ♀

N83.329 **Acquired atrophy of fallopian tube,** ♀▽
unspecified side
Acquired atrophy of fallopian tube, NOS

✓6th **N83.33** **Acquired atrophy of ovary and fallopian tube**

N83.331 **Acquired atrophy of right ovary and** ♀
fallopian tube

N83.332 **Acquired atrophy of left ovary and** ♀
fallopian tube

N83.339 **Acquired atrophy of ovary and** ♀▽
fallopian tube, unspecified side
Acquired atrophy of ovary and fallopian
tube, NOS

✓5th **N83.4** **Prolapse and hernia of ovary and fallopian tube**

N83.40 **Prolapse and hernia of ovary and fallopian** ♀▽
tube, unspecified side
Prolapse and hernia of ovary and fallopian tube, NOS

N83.41 **Prolapse and hernia of right ovary and** ♀
fallopian tube

N83.42 **Prolapse and hernia of left ovary and** ♀
fallopian tube

✓5th **N83.5** **Torsion of ovary, ovarian pedicle and fallopian tube**
Torsion of accessory tube

✓6th **N83.51** **Torsion of ovary and ovarian pedicle**

N83.511 **Torsion of right ovary and ovarian** ♀
pedicle

N83.512 **Torsion of left ovary and ovarian** ♀
pedicle

N83.519 **Torsion of ovary and ovarian pedicle,** ♀▽
unspecified side
Torsion of ovary and ovarian pedicle, NOS

✓6th **N83.52** **Torsion of fallopian tube**
Torsion of hydatid of Morgagni

N83.521 **Torsion of right fallopian tube** ♀

N83.522 **Torsion of left fallopian tube** ♀

N83.529 **Torsion of fallopian tube, unspecified** ♀▽
side
Torsion of fallopian tube, NOS

N83.53 **Torsion of ovary, ovarian pedicle and fallopian** ♀
tube

N83.6 **Hematosalpinx** ♀
EXCLUDES 1　hematosalpinx (with) (in):
hematocolpos (N89.7)
hematometra (N85.7)
tubal pregnancy (O00.1-)

N83.7 **Hematoma of broad ligament** ♀

N83.8 **Other noninflammatory disorders of ovary, fallopian** ♀
tube and broad ligament
Broad ligament laceration syndrome [Allen-Masters]

N83.9 **Noninflammatory disorder of ovary, fallopian tube** ♀▽
and broad ligament, unspecified

✓4th **N84** **Polyp of female genital tract**
EXCLUDES 1　adenomatous polyp (D28.-)
placental polyp (O90.89)

N84.0 **Polyp of corpus uteri** ♀
Polyp of endometrium
Polyp of uterus NOS
EXCLUDES 1　polypoid endometrial hyperplasia (N85.0-)

N84.1 **Polyp of cervix uteri** ♀
Mucous polyp of cervix

N84.2 **Polyp of vagina** ♀

N84.3 **Polyp of vulva** ♀
Polyp of labia

N84.8 **Polyp of other parts of female genital tract** ♀

N84.9 **Polyp of female genital tract, unspecified** ♀▽

Inversion of Uterus

Uterus

✓4th **N85** **Other noninflammatory disorders of uterus, except cervix**
EXCLUDES 1　endometriosis (N80.-)
inflammatory diseases of uterus (N71.-)
noninflammatory disorders of cervix, except malposition
(N86-N88)
polyp of corpus uteri (N84.0)
uterine prolapse (N81.-)

✓5th **N85.0** **Endometrial hyperplasia**

N85.00 **Endometrial hyperplasia, unspecified** ♀▽
Hyperplasia (adenomatous) (cystic) (glandular) of
endometrium
Hyperplastic endometritis

N85.01 **Benign endometrial hyperplasia** ♀
Endometrial hyperplasia (complex) (simple) without
atypia

N85.02 **Endometrial intraepithelial neoplasia [EIN]** ♀
Endometrial hyperplasia with atypia
EXCLUDES 1　malignant neoplasm of endometrium (with
endometrial intraepithelial neoplasia
[EIN]) (C54.1)

N85.2 **Hypertrophy of uterus** ♀
Bulky or enlarged uterus
EXCLUDES 1　puerperal hypertrophy of uterus (O90.89)

N85.3 **Subinvolution of uterus** ♀
EXCLUDES 1　puerperal subinvolution of uterus (O90.89)

N85.4 **Malposition of uterus** ♀
Anteversion of uterus　　　Retroversion of uterus
Retroflexion of uterus
EXCLUDES 1　malposition of uterus complicating pregnancy, labor
or delivery (O34.5-, O65.5)

N85.5 **Inversion of uterus** ♀
EXCLUDES 1　current obstetric trauma (O71.2)
postpartum inversion of uterus (O71.2)

N85.6 **Intrauterine synechiae** ♀

N85.7 **Hematometra** ♀
Hematosalpinx with hematometra
EXCLUDES 1　hematometra with hematocolpos (N89.7)
DEF: Accumulation of blood within the uterus.

N85.8 **Other specified noninflammatory disorders of uterus** ♀
Atrophy of uterus, acquired
Fibrosis of uterus NOS

N85.9 **Noninflammatory disorder of uterus, unspecified** ♀▽
Disorder of uterus NOS

N86 **Erosion and ectropion of cervix uteri** ♀
Decubitus (trophic) ulcer of cervix
Eversion of cervix
EXCLUDES 1　erosion and ectropion of cervix with cervicitis (N72)

✓4th **N87** **Dysplasia of cervix uteri**
EXCLUDES 1　abnormal results from cervical cytologic examination without
histologic confirmation (R87.61-)
carcinoma in situ of cervix uteri (D06.-)
cervical intraepithelial neoplasia III [CIN III] (D06.-)
HGSIL of cervix (R87.613)
severe dysplasia of cervix uteri (D06.-)

N87.0 **Mild cervical dysplasia** ♀
Cervical intraepithelial neoplasia I [CIN I]

N87.1 **Moderate cervical dysplasia** ♀
Cervical intraepithelial neoplasia II [CIN II]

N87.9 **Dysplasia of cervix uteri, unspecified** ♀▽
Anaplasia of cervix　　　Cervical dysplasia NOS
Cervical atypism

EXCLUDES 1 Not coded here　　EXCLUDES 2 Not included here　　N Newborn Age: 0　　P Pediatric Age: 0-17　　M Maternity Age: 12-55　　A Adult Age: 15-124

814　　ICD-10-CM 2018

✓4ᵗʰ N88 Other noninflammatory disorders of cervix uteri

EXCLUDES 2   inflammatory disease of cervix (N72)
polyp of cervix (N84.1)

N88.0 Leukoplakia of cervix uteri ♀

N88.1 Old laceration of cervix uteri ♀
Adhesions of cervix
EXCLUDES 1   current obstetric trauma (O71.3)

N88.2 Stricture and stenosis of cervix uteri ♀
EXCLUDES 1   stricture and stenosis of cervix uteri complicating labor
(O65.5)

N88.3 Incompetence of cervix uteri ♀
Investigation and management of (suspected) cervical
incompetence in a nonpregnant woman
EXCLUDES 1   cervical incompetence complicating pregnancy
(O34.3-)

N88.4 Hypertrophic elongation of cervix uteri ♀

N88.8 Other specified noninflammatory disorders of cervix uteri ♀
EXCLUDES 1   current obstetric trauma (O71.3)

N88.9 Noninflammatory disorder of cervix uteri, unspecified ♀ ▽

✓4ᵗʰ N89 Other noninflammatory disorders of vagina

EXCLUDES 1   abnormal results from vaginal cytologic examination without
histologic confirmation (R87.62-)
carcinoma in situ of vagina (D07.2)
HGSIL of vagina (R87.623)
inflammation of vagina (N76.-)
senile (atrophic) vaginitis (N95.2)
severe dysplasia of vagina (D07.2)
trichomonal leukorrhea (A59.00)
vaginal intraepithelial neoplasia [VAIN], grade III (D07.2)

N89.0 Mild vaginal dysplasia ♀
Vaginal intraepithelial neoplasia [VAIN], grade I

N89.1 Moderate vaginal dysplasia ♀
Vaginal intraepithelial neoplasia [VAIN], grade II

N89.3 Dysplasia of vagina, unspecified ♀ ▽

N89.4 Leukoplakia of vagina ♀

N89.5 Stricture and atresia of vagina ♀
Vaginal adhesions
Vaginal stenosis
EXCLUDES 1   congenital atresia or stricture (Q52.4)
postprocedural adhesions of vagina (N99.2)

N89.6 Tight hymenal ring ♀
Rigid hymen
Tight introitus
EXCLUDES 1   imperforate hymen (Q52.3)

N89.7 Hematocolpos ♀
Hematocolpos with hematometra or hematosalpinx

N89.8 Other specified noninflammatory disorders of vagina ♀
Leukorrhea NOS
Old vaginal laceration
Pessary ulcer of vagina
EXCLUDES 1   current obstetric trauma (O70-, O71.4, O71.7-O71.8)
old laceration involving muscles of pelvic floor (N81.8)

N89.9 Noninflammatory disorder of vagina, unspecified ♀ ▽

✓4ᵗʰ N90 Other noninflammatory disorders of vulva and perineum

EXCLUDES 1   anogenital (venereal) warts (A63.0)
carcinoma in situ of vulva (D07.1)
condyloma acuminatum (A63.0)
current obstetric trauma (O70-, O71.7-O71.8)
inflammation of vulva (N76.-)
severe dysplasia of vulva (D07.1)
vulvar intraepithelial neoplasm III [VIN III] (D07.1)

N90.0 Mild vulvar dysplasia ♀
Vulvar intraepithelial neoplasia [VIN], grade I

N90.1 Moderate vulvar dysplasia ♀
Vulvar intraepithelial neoplasia [VIN], grade II

N90.3 Dysplasia of vulva, unspecified ♀ ▽

N90.4 Leukoplakia of vulva ♀
Dystrophy of vulva
Kraurosis of vulva
Lichen sclerosus of external female genital organs

N90.5 Atrophy of vulva ♀
Stenosis of vulva

✓5ᵗʰ N90.6 Hypertrophy of vulva ♀

N90.60 Unspecified hypertrophy of vulva ♀ ▽
Unspecified hypertrophy of labia

N90.61 Childhood asymmetric labium majus enlargement ♀
CALME

N90.69 Other specified hypertrophy of vulva ♀
Other specified hypertrophy of labia

N90.7 Vulvar cyst ♀

✓5ᵗʰ N90.8 Other specified noninflammatory disorders of vulva and perineum

✓6ᵗʰ N90.81 Female genital mutilation status
Female genital cutting status

N90.810 Female genital mutilation status, unspecified ♀ ▽
Female genital cutting status, unspecified
Female genital mutilation status NOS

N90.811 Female genital mutilation Type I status ♀
Clitorectomy status
Female genital cutting Type I status

N90.812 Female genital mutilation Type II status ♀
Clitorectomy with excision of labia minora
status
Female genital cutting Type II status

N90.813 Female genital mutilation Type III status ♀
Female genital cutting Type III status
Infibulation status

N90.818 Other female genital mutilation status ♀
Female genital cutting Type IV status
Female genital mutilation Type IV status
Other female genital cutting status

N90.89 Other specified noninflammatory disorders of vulva and perineum ♀
Adhesions of vulva   Hypertrophy of clitoris

N90.9 Noninflammatory disorder of vulva and perineum, unspecified ♀ ▽

✓4ᵗʰ N91 Absent, scanty and rare menstruation

EXCLUDES 1   ovarian dysfunction (E28.-)

N91.0 Primary amenorrhea ♀

N91.1 Secondary amenorrhea ♀

N91.2 Amenorrhea, unspecified ♀ ▽

N91.3 Primary oligomenorrhea ♀

N91.4 Secondary oligomenorrhea ♀

N91.5 Oligomenorrhea, unspecified ♀ ▽
Hypomenorrhea NOS

✓4ᵗʰ N92 Excessive, frequent and irregular menstruation

EXCLUDES 1   postmenopausal bleeding (N95.0)
precocious puberty (menstruation) (E30.1)

N92.0 Excessive and frequent menstruation with regular cycle ♀
Heavy periods NOS
Menorrhagia NOS
Polymenorrhea

N92.1 Excessive and frequent menstruation with irregular cycle ♀
Irregular intermenstrual bleeding
Irregular, shortened intervals between menstrual bleeding
Menometrorrhagia
Metrorrhagia

N92.2 Excessive menstruation at puberty Ⓟ♀
Excessive bleeding associated with onset of menstrual periods
Pubertal menorrhagia
Puberty bleeding

N92.3 Ovulation bleeding ♀
Regular intermenstrual bleeding

N92.4 Excessive bleeding in the premenopausal period ♀
Climacteric menorrhagia or metrorrhagia
Menopausal menorrhagia or metrorrhagia
Preclimacteric menorrhagia or metrorrhagia
Premenopausal menorrhagia or metrorrhagia

N92.5 Other specified irregular menstruation ♀

N92.6 Irregular menstruation, unspecified ♀ ▽
Irregular bleeding NOS
Irregular periods NOS
EXCLUDES 1   irregular menstruation with:
lengthened intervals or scanty bleeding
(N91.3-N91.5)
shortened intervals or excessive bleeding (N92.1)

☑ Additional Character Req   ✕7ᵗʰ Placeholder Alert   Manifestation   ʜᴄᴄ CMS-HCC Condition   ▽ Unspecified Code   ▶◀ Revised Text   ● New Code   ▲ Revised Code Title

ICD-10-CM 2018   815

Chapter 14. Diseases of Genitourinary System

N93–N99.4

✓4ᵗʰ **N93 Other abnormal uterine and vaginal bleeding**
     EXCLUDES 1   *neonatal vaginal hemorrhage (P54.6)*
                precocious puberty (menstruation) (E30.1)
                pseudomenses (P54.6)

    N93.0 Postcoital and contact bleeding ♀

    N93.1 Pre-pubertal vaginal bleeding ♀

    N93.8 Other specified abnormal uterine and vaginal bleeding ♀
       Dysfunctional or functional uterine or vaginal bleeding NOS

    N93.9 Abnormal uterine and vaginal bleeding, unspecified ♀▽

✓4ᵗʰ **N94 Pain and other conditions associated with female genital organs and menstrual cycle**

    N94.0 Mittelschmerz ♀
       DEF: One-sided, lower abdominal pain occurring between menstrual periods; associated with ovulation.

   ✓5ᵗʰ **N94.1 Dyspareunia**
       EXCLUDES 1   *psychogenic dyspareunia (F52.6)*

      N94.10 Unspecified dyspareunia ♀▽

      N94.11 Superficial (introital) dyspareunia ♀

      N94.12 Deep dyspareunia ♀

      N94.19 Other specified dyspareunia ♀

    N94.2 Vaginismus ♀
       EXCLUDES 1   *psychogenic vaginismus (F52.5)*

    N94.3 Premenstrual tension syndrome ♀
       ~~Premenstrual dysphoric disorder~~
       Code also associated menstrual migraine (G43.82-, G43.83-)
       EXCLUDES 1   *premenstrual dysphoric disorder (F32.81)*

    N94.4 Primary dysmenorrhea ♀

    N94.5 Secondary dysmenorrhea ♀

    N94.6 Dysmenorrhea, unspecified ♀▽
       EXCLUDES 1   *psychogenic dysmenorrhea (F45.8)*

   ✓5ᵗʰ **N94.8 Other specified conditions associated with female genital organs and menstrual cycle**

     ✓6ᵗʰ **N94.81 Vulvodynia**

         N94.810 Vulvar vestibulitis ♀

         N94.818 Other vulvodynia ♀

         N94.819 Vulvodynia, unspecified ♀▽
           Vulvodynia NOS

      N94.89 Other specified conditions associated with female genital organs and menstrual cycle ♀

    N94.9 Unspecified condition associated with female genital organs and menstrual cycle ♀▽

✓4ᵗʰ **N95 Menopausal and other perimenopausal disorders**
       Menopausal and other perimenopausal disorders due to naturally occurring (age-related) menopause and perimenopause
       EXCLUDES 1   *excessive bleeding in the premenopausal period (N92.4)*
                menopausal and perimenopausal disorders due to artificial or premature menopause (E89.4-, E28.31-)
                premature menopause (E28.31-)
       EXCLUDES 2   *postmenopausal osteoporosis (M81.0-)*
                postmenopausal osteoporosis with current pathological fracture (M80.0-)
                postmenopausal urethritis (N34.2)

    N95.0 Postmenopausal bleeding ♀

    N95.1 Menopausal and female climacteric states ♀
       Symptoms such as flushing, sleeplessness, headache, lack of concentration, associated with natural (age-related) menopause
       Use additional code for associated symptoms
       EXCLUDES 1   *asymptomatic menopausal state (Z78.0)*
                symptoms associated with artificial menopause (E89.41)
                symptoms associated with premature menopause (E28.310)

    N95.2 Postmenopausal atrophic vaginitis ♀
       Senile (atrophic) vaginitis

    N95.8 Other specified menopausal and perimenopausal disorders ♀

    N95.9 Unspecified menopausal and perimenopausal disorder ♀▽

N96 Recurrent pregnancy loss ♀
       Investigation or care in a nonpregnant woman with history of recurrent pregnancy loss
       EXCLUDES 1   *recurrent pregnancy loss with current pregnancy (O26.2-)*

✓4ᵗʰ **N97 Female infertility**
     INCLUDES   inability to achieve a pregnancy
              sterility, female NOS
     EXCLUDES 1   *female infertility associated with:*
                hypopituitarism (E23.0)
                Stein-Leventhal syndrome (E28.2)
     EXCLUDES 2   *incompetence of cervix uteri (N88.3)*
     DEF: Infertility: Inability to conceive for at least one year with regular intercourse.
     DEF: Primary infertility: Infertility occurring in patients who have never conceived.
     DEF: Secondary infertility: Infertility occurring in patients who have previously conceived.

    N97.0 Female infertility associated with anovulation ♀

    N97.1 Female infertility of tubal origin ♀
       Female infertility associated with congenital anomaly of tube
       Female infertility due to tubal block
       Female infertility due to tubal occlusion
       Female infertility due to tubal stenosis

    N97.2 Female infertility of uterine origin ♀
       Female infertility associated with congenital anomaly of uterus
       Female infertility due to nonimplantation of ovum

    N97.8 Female infertility of other origin ♀

    N97.9 Female infertility, unspecified ♀▽

✓4ᵗʰ **N98 Complications associated with artificial fertilization**

    N98.0 Infection associated with artificial insemination ♀

    N98.1 Hyperstimulation of ovaries ♀
       Hyperstimulation of ovaries NOS
       Hyperstimulation of ovaries associated with induced ovulation

    N98.2 Complications of attempted introduction of fertilized ovum following in vitro fertilization ♀

    N98.3 Complications of attempted introduction of embryo in embryo transfer ♀

    N98.8 Other complications associated with artificial fertilization ♀

    N98.9 Complication associated with artificial fertilization, unspecified ♀▽

Intraoperative and postprocedural complications and disorders of genitourinary system, not elsewhere classified (N99)

✓4ᵗʰ **N99 Intraoperative and postprocedural complications and disorders of genitourinary system, not elsewhere classified**
       EXCLUDES 2   *irradiation cystitis (N30.4-)*
                postoophorectomy osteoporosis with current pathological fracture (M80.8-)
                postoophorectomy osteoporosis without current pathological fracture (M81.8)

    N99.0 Postprocedural (acute) (chronic) kidney failure
       Use additional code to type of kidney disease

   ✓5ᵗʰ **N99.1 Postprocedural urethral stricture**
       Postcatheterization urethral stricture

     ✓6ᵗʰ **N99.11 Postprocedural urethral stricture, male**

         N99.110 Postprocedural urethral stricture, male, meatal ♂

   ▲   **N99.111 Postprocedural bulbous urethral stricture, male** ♂

   ▲   **N99.112 Postprocedural membranous urethral stricture, male** ♂

   ▲   **N99.113 Postprocedural anterior bulbous urethral stricture, male** ♂

         N99.114 Postprocedural urethral stricture, male, unspecified ♂▽

         N99.115 Postprocedural fossa navicularis urethral stricture ♂

     N99.12 Postprocedural urethral stricture, female ♀

    N99.2 Postprocedural adhesions of vagina ♀

    N99.3 Prolapse of vaginal vault after hysterectomy ♀

    N99.4 Postprocedural pelvic peritoneal adhesions
       EXCLUDES 2   *pelvic peritoneal adhesions NOS (N73.6)*
                postinfective pelvic peritoneal adhesions (N73.6)

EXCLUDES 1 Not coded here   EXCLUDES 2 Not included here   N Newborn Age: 0   P Pediatric Age: 0-17   M Maternity Age: 12-55   A Adult Age: 15-124

816   ICD-10-CM 2018

✓5ᵗʰ **N99.5 Complications of stoma of urinary tract**
   EXCLUDES 2   mechanical complication of urinary catheter (T83.Ø-)

✓6ᵗʰ **N99.51 Complication of** cystostomy
   N99.51Ø Cystostomy hemorrhage   HCC
   N99.511 Cystostomy infection   HCC
   N99.512 Cystostomy malfunction   HCC
   N99.518 Other cystostomy complication   HCC

✓6ᵗʰ **N99.52 Complication of** incontinent external stoma **of urinary tract**
   N99.52Ø Hemorrhage **of incontinent external stoma of urinary tract**   HCC
   N99.521 Infection **of incontinent external stoma of urinary tract**   HCC
   N99.522 Malfunction **of incontinent external stoma of urinary tract**   HCC
   N99.523 Herniation **of incontinent stoma of urinary tract**   HCC
   N99.524 Stenosis **of incontinent stoma of urinary tract**   HCC
   N99.528 Other complication of incontinent external stoma of urinary tract   HCC

✓6ᵗʰ **N99.53 Complication of** continent stoma **of urinary tract**
   N99.53Ø Hemorrhage **of continent stoma of urinary tract**   HCC
   N99.531 Infection **of continent stoma of urinary tract**   HCC
   N99.532 Malfunction **of continent stoma of urinary tract**   HCC
   N99.533 Herniation **of continent stoma of urinary tract**   HCC
   N99.534 Stenosis **of continent stoma of urinary tract**   HCC
   N99.538 Other complication of continent stoma of urinary tract   HCC

✓5ᵗʰ **N99.6** Intraoperative hemorrhage and hematoma **of a genitourinary system organ or structure complicating a procedure**
   EXCLUDES 1   intraoperative hemorrhage and hematoma of a genitourinary system organ or structure due to accidental puncture or laceration during a procedure (N99.7-)
   N99.61 Intraoperative hemorrhage and hematoma of a genitourinary system organ or structure complicating a genitourinary system procedure
   N99.62 Intraoperative hemorrhage and hematoma of a genitourinary system organ or structure complicating other procedure

✓5ᵗʰ **N99.7** Accidental puncture and laceration **of a genitourinary system organ or structure during a procedure**
   N99.71 Accidental puncture and laceration of a genitourinary system organ or structure during a genitourinary system procedure
   N99.72 Accidental puncture and laceration of a genitourinary system organ or structure during other procedure

✓5ᵗʰ **N99.8 Other intraoperative and postprocedural complications and disorders of genitourinary system**
   N99.81 Other intraoperative complications **of genitourinary system**
✓6ᵗʰ **N99.82** Postprocedural hemorrhage **of a genitourinary system organ or structure following a procedure**
   N99.82Ø Postprocedural hemorrhage of a genitourinary system organ or structure following a genitourinary system procedure
   N99.821 Postprocedural hemorrhage of a genitourinary system organ or structure following other procedure
   N99.83 Residual ovary syndrome   ♀
✓6ᵗʰ **N99.84** Postprocedural hematoma and seroma **of a genitourinary system organ or structure following a procedure**
   N99.84Ø Postprocedural hematoma **of a genitourinary system organ or structure following a** genitourinary system procedure
   N99.841 Postprocedural hematoma **of a genitourinary system organ or structure following** other procedure
   N99.842 Postprocedural seroma **of a genitourinary system organ or structure following a** genitourinary system procedure
   N99.843 Postprocedural seroma **of a genitourinary system organ or structure following** other procedure
   N99.89 Other postprocedural complications and disorders of genitourinary system

Chapter 15. Pregnancy, Childbirth, and the Puerperium (O00–O9A)

Chapter Specific Guidelines with Coding Examples

The chapter specific guidelines from the ICD-10-CM Official Guidelines for Coding and Reporting have been provided below. Along with these guidelines are coding examples, contained in the shaded boxes, that have been developed to help illustrate the coding and/or sequencing guidance found in these guidelines.

a. General rules for obstetric cases

1) Codes from Chapter 15 and sequencing priority

Obstetric cases require codes from chapter 15, codes in the range O00-O9A, Pregnancy, Childbirth, and the Puerperium. Chapter 15 codes have sequencing priority over codes from other chapters. Additional codes from other chapters may be used in conjunction with chapter 15 codes to further specify conditions. Should the provider document that the pregnancy is incidental to the encounter, then code Z33.1, Pregnant state, incidental, should be used in place of any chapter 15 codes. It is the provider's responsibility to state that the condition being treated is not affecting the pregnancy.

> Bladder abscess in pregnant patient at 25 weeks' gestation
>
> **O23.12**   **Infections of bladder in pregnancy, second trimester**
>
> **N30.80**   **Other cystitis without hematuria**
>
> **Z3A.25**   **25 weeks gestation of pregnancy**
>
> *Explanation:* The documentation does not indicate that the pregnancy is incidental or in any way unaffected by the bladder abscess; therefore, an obstetrics code should be sequenced first. An additional code was provided to identify the specific bladder condition as this information is not called out specifically in the obstetrics code.

2) Chapter 15 codes used only on the maternal record

Chapter 15 codes are to be used only on the maternal record, never on the record of the newborn.

3) Final character for trimester

The majority of codes in Chapter 15 have a final character indicating the trimester of pregnancy. The timeframes for the trimesters are indicated at the beginning of the chapter. If trimester is not a component of a code, it is because the condition always occurs in a specific trimester, or the concept of trimester of pregnancy is not applicable. Certain codes have characters for only certain trimesters because the condition does not occur in all trimesters, but it may occur in more than just one. Assignment of the final character for the trimester should be based on the provider's documentation of the trimester (or number of weeks) for the current admission/encounter. This applies to the assignment of trimester for pre-existing conditions as well as those that develop during or are due to the pregnancy. The provider's documentation of the number of weeks may be used to assign the appropriate code identifying the trimester.

Whenever delivery occurs during the current admission, and there is an "in childbirth" option for the obstetric complication being coded, the "in childbirth" code should be assigned.

> Pregnant patient at 21 weeks' gestation admitted with excessive vomiting
>
> **O21.2**   **Late vomiting of pregnancy**
>
> **Z3A.21**   **21 weeks gestation of pregnancy**
>
> *Explanation:* Category O21 classifies vomiting in pregnancy. Although code selection is based on whether the vomiting is before or after 20 completed weeks, these codes are not further classified by trimester. If vomiting only in the second trimester was documented, the provider should be queried for the specific week of gestation, as this will affect code selection.

4) Selection of trimester for inpatient admissions that encompass more than one trimester

In instances when a patient is admitted to a hospital for complications of pregnancy during one trimester and remains in the hospital into a subsequent trimester, the trimester character for the antepartum complication code should be assigned on the basis of the trimester when the complication developed, not the trimester of the discharge. If the condition developed prior to the current admission/encounter or represents a pre-existing condition, the trimester character for the trimester at the time of the admission/encounter should be assigned.

5) Unspecified trimester

Each category that includes codes for trimester has a code for "unspecified trimester." The "unspecified trimester" code should rarely be used, such as when the documentation in the record is insufficient to determine the trimester and it is not possible to obtain clarification.

6) 7th character for fetus identification

Where applicable, a 7th character is to be assigned for certain categories (O31, O32, O33.3 - O33.6, O35, O36, O40, O41, O60.1, O60.2, O64, and O69) to identify the fetus for which the complication code applies.

Assign 7th character "0":

- For single gestations
- When the documentation in the record is insufficient to determine the fetus affected and it is not possible to obtain clarification.
- When it is not possible to clinically determine which fetus is affected.

> Maternal patient with twin gestations is seen after ultrasound identifies fetus B to be in breech presentation
>
> **O32.1XX2**   **Maternal care for breech presentation, fetus 2**
>
> *Explanation:* The documentation indicates that although there are two fetuses, only one fetus is determined to be in breech presentation. Whether fetus 2 or fetus B is used, the coder can assign the seventh character of 2 to identify the second fetus as the one in breech.

b. Selection of OB principal or first-listed diagnosis

1) Routine outpatient prenatal visits

For routine outpatient prenatal visits when no complications are present, a code from category Z34, Encounter for supervision of normal pregnancy, should be used as the first-listed diagnosis. These codes should not be used in conjunction with chapter 15 codes.

2) Supervision of high-risk pregnancy

Codes from category O09, Supervision of high-risk pregnancy, are intended for use only during the prenatal period. For complications during the labor or delivery episode as a result of a high-risk pregnancy, assign the applicable complication codes from Chapter 15. If there are no complications during the labor or delivery episode, assign code O80, Encounter for full-term uncomplicated delivery.

For routine prenatal outpatient visits for patients with high-risk pregnancies, a code from category O09, Supervision of high-risk pregnancy, should be used as the first-listed diagnosis. Secondary chapter 15 codes may be used in conjunction with these codes if appropriate.

> 36-year-old seen in labor with second child at 39 weeks' gestation, delivered a healthy baby, delivery complicated by tear of fourchette that was repaired
>
> **O70.0**   **First degree perineal laceration during delivery**
>
> **Z3A.39**   **39 weeks gestation of pregnancy**
>
> **Z37.0**   **Single live birth**
>
> Explanation: Although this patient is over 35 and having her second child (elderly multigravida), do not append a code from subcategory O09.52-. A code describing the tear of the fourchette, which complicated the delivery, should be used in addition to the applicable Z codes.

3) Episodes when no delivery occurs

In episodes when no delivery occurs, the principal diagnosis should correspond to the principal complication of the pregnancy which necessitated the encounter. Should more than one complication exist, all of which are treated or monitored, any of the complications codes may be sequenced first.

4) When a delivery occurs

When an obstetric patient is admitted and delivers during that admission, the condition that prompted the admission should be sequenced as the principal diagnosis. If multiple conditions prompted the admission, sequence the one most related to the delivery as the principal diagnosis. A code for any complication of the delivery should be assigned as an additional diagnosis. In cases of cesarean delivery, if the patient was admitted with a condition that resulted in the performance of a cesarean procedure, that condition should be selected as the principal diagnosis. If the reason for the admission was unrelated to the condition resulting in the cesarean delivery, the condition related to the reason for the admission should be selected as the principal diagnosis.

Maternal patient with diet-controlled gestational diabetes was seen at 38 weeks' gestation in obstructed labor due to footling presentation; cesarean performed for the malpresentation	
O64.8XX0	Obstructed labor due to other malposition and malpresentation, not applicable or unspecified
O24.420	Gestational diabetes mellitus in childbirth, diet controlled
Z3A.38	38 weeks gestation of pregnancy
Z37.0	Single live birth

Explanation: The obstructed labor necessitated the cesarean procedure.

5) Outcome of delivery

A code from category Z37, Outcome of delivery, should be included on every maternal record when a delivery has occurred. These codes are not to be used on subsequent records or on the newborn record.

c. Pre-existing conditions versus conditions due to the pregnancy

Certain categories in Chapter 15 distinguish between conditions of the mother that existed prior to pregnancy (pre-existing) and those that are a direct result of pregnancy. When assigning codes from Chapter 15, it is important to assess if a condition was pre-existing prior to pregnancy or developed during or due to the pregnancy in order to assign the correct code.

Categories that do not distinguish between pre-existing and pregnancy-related conditions may be used for either. It is acceptable to use codes specifically for the puerperium with codes complicating pregnancy and childbirth if a condition arises postpartum during the delivery encounter.

d. Pre-existing hypertension in pregnancy

Category O10, Pre-existing hypertension complicating pregnancy, childbirth and the puerperium, includes codes for hypertensive heart and hypertensive chronic kidney disease. When assigning one of the O10 codes that includes hypertensive heart disease or hypertensive chronic kidney disease, it is necessary to add a secondary code from the appropriate hypertension category to specify the type of heart failure or chronic kidney disease.

See Section I.C.9. Hypertension.

e. Fetal conditions affecting the management of the mother

1) Codes from categories O35 and O36

Codes from categories O35, Maternal care for known or suspected fetal abnormality and damage, and O36, Maternal care for other fetal problems, are assigned only when the fetal condition is actually responsible for modifying the management of the mother, i.e., by requiring diagnostic studies, additional observation, special care, or termination of pregnancy. The fact that the fetal condition exists does not justify assigning a code from this series to the mother's record.

A patient with twin gestation is seen for spotting 15 weeks into her pregnancy; the doctors also suspect fetal hydrocephalus. Patient is instructed to return in one week for additional diagnostic testing, sooner if the problem worsens.	
O35.0XX0	Maternal care for (suspected) central nervous system malformation in fetus, not applicable or unspecified
O26.852	Spotting complicating pregnancy, second trimester
Z3A.15	15 weeks gestation of pregnancy

Explanation: Whether the fetal hydrocephalus was suspected or confirmed, an additional code is warranted for this condition since documentation indicates the patient is to return sooner than her routine visit for further testing.

2) In utero surgery

In cases when surgery is performed on the fetus, a diagnosis code from category O35, Maternal care for known or suspected fetal abnormality and damage, should be assigned identifying the fetal condition. Assign the appropriate procedure code for the procedure performed.

No code from Chapter 16, the perinatal codes, should be used on the mother's record to identify fetal conditions. Surgery performed in utero on a fetus is still to be coded as an obstetric encounter.

f. HIV infection in pregnancy, childbirth and the puerperium

During pregnancy, childbirth or the puerperium, a patient admitted because of an HIV-related illness should receive a principal diagnosis from subcategory O98.7-, Human immunodeficiency [HIV] disease complicating pregnancy, childbirth and the puerperium, followed by the code(s) for the HIV-related illness(es).

Patients with asymptomatic HIV infection status admitted during pregnancy, childbirth, or the puerperium should receive codes of O98.7- and Z21, Asymptomatic human immunodeficiency virus [HIV] infection status.

A previously asymptomatic HIV patient who is 13 weeks pregnant is evaluated for HIV-related candidal bronchitis	
O98.711	Human immunodeficiency virus [HIV] disease complicating pregnancy, first trimester
B20	Human immunodeficiency virus [HIV] disease
B37.1	Candidal bronchitis
Z3A.13	13 weeks gestation of pregnancy

Explanation: Because candidal bronchitis is an AIDS-related condition, this patient is now considered to have HIV disease. An obstetrics code indicating that HIV is complicating the pregnancy is coded first, followed by B20 for HIV disease as well as a code for the candidal bronchitis.

g. Diabetes mellitus in pregnancy

Diabetes mellitus is a significant complicating factor in pregnancy. Pregnant women who are diabetic should be assigned a code from category O24, Diabetes mellitus in pregnancy, childbirth, and the puerperium, first, followed by the appropriate diabetes code(s) (E08-E13) from Chapter 4.

h. Long term use of insulin and oral hypoglycemics

See section I.C.4.a.3 for information on the long term use of insulin and oral hypoglycemic.

i. Gestational (pregnancy induced) diabetes

Gestational (pregnancy induced) diabetes can occur during the second and third trimester of pregnancy in women who were not diabetic prior to pregnancy. Gestational diabetes can cause complications in the pregnancy similar to those of pre-existing diabetes mellitus. It also puts the woman at greater risk of developing diabetes after the pregnancy. Codes for gestational diabetes are in subcategory O24.4, Gestational diabetes mellitus. No other code from category O24, Diabetes mellitus in pregnancy, childbirth, and the puerperium, should be used with a code from O24.4.

The codes under subcategory O24.4 include diet controlled, insulin controlled, and controlled by oral hypoglycemic drugs. If a patient with gestational diabetes is treated with both diet and insulin, only the code for insulin-controlled is required. If a patient with gestational diabetes is treated with both diet and oral hypoglycemic medications, only the code for "controlled by oral hypoglycemic drugs" is required. Code Z79.4, Long-term (current) use of insulin or code Z79.84, Long-term (current) use of oral hypoglycemic drugs, should not be assigned with codes from subcategory O24.4.

An abnormal glucose tolerance in pregnancy is assigned a code from subcategory O99.81, Abnormal glucose complicating pregnancy, childbirth, and the puerperium.

j. Sepsis and septic shock complicating abortion, pregnancy, childbirth and the puerperium

When assigning a chapter 15 code for sepsis complicating abortion, pregnancy, childbirth, and the puerperium, a code for the specific type of infection should be assigned as an additional diagnosis. If severe sepsis is present, a code from subcategory R65.2, Severe sepsis, and code(s) for associated organ dysfunction(s) should also be assigned as additional diagnoses.

Patient is seen several days after a miscarriage with sepsis; cultures return MSSA

O03.87	**Sepsis following complete or unspecified spontaneous abortion**
B95.61	**Methicillin susceptible Staphylococcus aureus infection as the cause of diseases classified elsewhere**

Explanation: The type of infection that caused this patient to become septic was methicillin susceptible *Staphylococcus aureus* (MSSA), which as a secondary code helps capture all aspects related to this patient's septic condition.

k. Puerperal sepsis

Code O85, Puerperal sepsis, should be assigned with a secondary code to identify the causal organism (e.g., for a bacterial infection, assign a code from category B95-B96, Bacterial infections in conditions classified elsewhere). A code from category A40, Streptococcal sepsis, or A41, Other sepsis, should not be used for puerperal sepsis. If applicable, use additional codes to identify severe sepsis (R65.2-) and any associated acute organ dysfunction.

l. Alcohol and tobacco use during pregnancy, childbirth and the puerperium

1) Alcohol use during pregnancy, childbirth and the puerperium

Codes under subcategory O99.31, Alcohol use complicating pregnancy, childbirth, and the puerperium, should be assigned for any pregnancy case when a mother uses alcohol during the pregnancy or postpartum. A secondary code from category F10, Alcohol related disorders, should also be assigned to identify manifestations of the alcohol use.

2) Tobacco use during pregnancy, childbirth and the puerperium

Codes under subcategory O99.33, Smoking (tobacco) complicating pregnancy, childbirth, and the puerperium, should be assigned for any pregnancy case when a mother uses any type of tobacco product during the pregnancy or postpartum. A secondary code from category F17, Nicotine dependence, should also be assigned to identify the type of nicotine dependence.

m. Poisoning, toxic effects, adverse effects and underdosing in a pregnant patient

A code from subcategory O9A.2, Injury, poisoning and certain other consequences of external causes complicating pregnancy, childbirth, and the puerperium, should be sequenced first, followed by the appropriate injury, poisoning, toxic effect, adverse effect or underdosing code, and then the additional code(s) that specifies the condition caused by the poisoning, toxic effect, adverse effect or underdosing.

See Section I.C.19. Adverse effects, poisoning, underdosing and toxic effects.

Patient treated for accidental carbon monoxide poisoning from a gas heating implement; the patient is 18 weeks' pregnant

O9A.212	**Injury, poisoning and certain other consequences of external causes complicating pregnancy, second trimester**
T58.11XA	**Toxic effect of carbon monoxide from utility gas, accidental (unintentional), initial encounter**
Z3A.18	**18 weeks gestation of pregnancy**

Explanation: Although the carbon monoxide poisoning is the reason for the encounter, a code from the obstetrics chapter must be sequenced first. Chapter 15 codes have sequencing priority over codes from other chapters.

n. Normal delivery, code O80

1) Encounter for full term uncomplicated delivery

Code O80 should be assigned when a woman is admitted for a full-term normal delivery and delivers a single, healthy infant without any complications antepartum, during the delivery, or postpartum during the delivery episode. Code O80 is always a principal diagnosis. It is not to be used if any other code from chapter 15 is needed to describe a current complication of the antenatal, delivery, or perinatal period. Additional codes from other chapters may be used with code O80 if they are not related to or are in any way complicating the pregnancy.

2) Uncomplicated delivery with resolved antepartum complication

Code O80 may be used if the patient had a complication at some point during the pregnancy, but the complication is not present at the time of the admission for delivery.

Patient presents in labor at 39 weeks' gestation and delivers a healthy newborn; patient had abnormal glucose levels in her first trimester, which have since resolved

O80	**Encounter for full-term uncomplicated delivery**
Z37.0	**Single live birth**

Explanation: The abnormal glucose levels during the first trimester cannot be coded if they are not affecting the patient's current trimester. Without additional complications associated with the pregnancy, fetus, or mother, code O80 is appropriate.

3) Outcome of delivery for O80

Z37.0, Single live birth, is the only outcome of delivery code appropriate for use with O80.

o. The peripartum and postpartum periods

1) Peripartum and postpartum periods

The postpartum period begins immediately after delivery and continues for six weeks following delivery. The peripartum period is defined as the last month of pregnancy to five months postpartum.

2) Peripartum and postpartum complication

A postpartum complication is any complication occurring within the six-week period.

3) Pregnancy-related complications after 6 week period

Chapter 15 codes may also be used to describe pregnancy-related complications after the peripartum or postpartum period if the provider documents that a condition is pregnancy related.

Patient referred for varicose veins. She had a baby boy three months ago; the varicose veins started to appear one month ago. The doctor attributes the patient's pregnancy as the cause of the varicose veins, which continue to be painful and bother the patient. She is seeking surgical relief.

O87.4	**Varicose veins of the lower extremity in the puerperium**

Explanation: Although the varicose veins occurred several months after the delivery of the newborn, the doctor attributed the varicose veins to pregnancy and therefore a code from chapter 15 is appropriate.

4) Admission for routine postpartum care following delivery outside hospital

When the mother delivers outside the hospital prior to admission and is admitted for routine postpartum care and no complications are noted, code Z39.0, Encounter for care and examination of mother immediately after delivery, should be assigned as the principal diagnosis.

5) Pregnancy associated cardiomyopathy

Pregnancy associated cardiomyopathy, code O90.3, is unique in that it may be diagnosed in the third trimester of pregnancy but may continue to progress months after delivery. For this reason, it is referred to as peripartum cardiomyopathy. Code O90.3 is only for use when the cardiomyopathy develops as a result of pregnancy in a woman who did not have pre-existing heart disease.

p. Code O94, Sequelae of complication of pregnancy, childbirth, and the puerperium

1) Code O94

Code O94, Sequelae of complication of pregnancy, childbirth, and the puerperium, is for use in those cases when an initial complication of a pregnancy develops a sequelae requiring care or treatment at a future date.

2) After the initial postpartum period

This code may be used at any time after the initial postpartum period.

3) Sequencing of code O94

This code, like all sequela codes, is to be sequenced following the code describing the sequelae of the complication.

q. Termination of pregnancy and spontaneous abortions

1) Abortion with Liveborn Fetus

When an attempted termination of pregnancy results in a liveborn fetus, assign code Z33.2, Encounter for elective termination of pregnancy and a code from category Z37, Outcome of Delivery.

2) Retained Products of Conception following an abortion

Subsequent encounters for retained products of conception following a spontaneous abortion or elective termination of pregnancy, **without complications** are assigned O03.4, **Incomplete spontaneous,** abortion **without complication**, or codes O07.4, Failed attempted termination of pregnancy without complication. This advice is appropriate even when the patient was discharged previously with a discharge diagnosis of complete abortion. **If the patient has a specific complication associated with the spontaneous abortion or elective termination of pregnancy in addition to retained products of conception, assign the appropriate complication in category O03 or O07 instead of code O03.4 or O07.4**

Patient was seen two days ago for complete spontaneous abortion but returns today for urinary tract infection (UTI) with ultrasound showing retained products of conception

O03.38   Urinary tract infection following incomplete spontaneous abortion

Explanation: Although the diagnosis from the patient's previous stay indicated that the patient had a complete abortion, it is now determined that there were actually retained products of conception (POC). An abortion with retained POC is considered incomplete and in this case resulted in the patient developing a UTI.

3) Complications leading to abortion

Codes from Chapter 15 may be used as additional codes to identify any documented complications of the pregnancy in conjunction with codes in categories in **O04,** O07 and O08.

r. Abuse in a pregnant patient

For suspected or confirmed cases of abuse of a pregnant patient, a code(s) from subcategories O9A.3, Physical abuse complicating pregnancy, childbirth, and the puerperium, O9A.4, Sexual abuse complicating pregnancy, childbirth, and the puerperium, and O9A.5, Psychological abuse complicating pregnancy, childbirth, and the puerperium, should be sequenced first, followed by the appropriate codes (if applicable) to identify any associated current injury due to physical abuse, sexual abuse, and the perpetrator of abuse.

See Section I.C.19. Adult and child abuse, neglect and other maltreatment.

Chapter 15. Pregnancy, Childbirth and the Puerperium (O00-O9A)

NOTE CODES FROM THIS CHAPTER ARE FOR USE ONLY ON MATERNAL RECORDS, NEVER ON NEWBORN RECORDS.

Codes from this chapter are for use for conditions related to or aggravated by the pregnancy, childbirth, or by the puerperium (maternal causes or obstetric causes).

NOTE Trimesters are counted from the first day of the last menstrual period. They are defined as follows:

   1st trimester- less than 14 weeks Ø days
   2nd trimester- 14 weeks Ø days to less than 28 weeks Ø days
   3rd trimester- 28 weeks Ø days until delivery.

Use additional code from category Z3A, Weeks of gestation, to identify the specific week of the pregnancy, if known

EXCLUDES 1 *supervision of normal pregnancy (Z34.-)*
EXCLUDES 2 *mental and behavioral disorders associated with the puerperium (F53)*
   obstetrical tetanus (A34)
   postpartum necrosis of pituitary gland (E23.Ø)
   puerperal osteomalacia (M83.Ø)
AHA: 2016, 1Q, 3-5; 2014, 3Q, 17

This chapter contains the following blocks:

O00-O08	Pregnancy with abortive outcome
O09	Supervision of high risk pregnancy
O10-O16	Edema, proteinuria and hypertensive disorders in pregnancy, childbirth and the puerperium
O20-O29	Other maternal disorders predominantly related to pregnancy
O30-O48	Maternal care related to the fetus and amniotic cavity and possible delivery problems
O60-O77	Complications of labor and delivery
O80, O82	Encounter for delivery
O85-O92	Complications predominantly related to the puerperium
O94-O9A	Other obstetric conditions, not elsewhere classified

Pregnancy with abortive outcome (O00-O08)

EXCLUDES 1 *continuing pregnancy in multiple gestation after abortion of one fetus or more (O31.1-, O31.3-)*

✓4ᵗʰ **O00   Ectopic pregnancy**
   INCLUDES ruptured ectopic pregnancy
   Use additional code from category O08 to identify any associated complication
   AHA: 2014, 3Q, 17
   DEF: Implantation of fertilized egg outside the uterus, usually in fallopian tube or abdomen; requires emergency treatment.

✓5ᵗʰ **O00.Ø** Abdominal **pregnancy**
      EXCLUDES 1 *maternal care for viable fetus in abdominal pregnancy (O36.7-)*

   O00.00   Abdominal pregnancy without intrauterine   M♀
            pregnancy
            Abdominal pregnancy NOS

   O00.01   Abdominal pregnancy with intrauterine   M♀
            pregnancy

✓5ᵗʰ **O00.1** Tubal **pregnancy**
            Fallopian pregnancy
            Rupture of (fallopian) tube due to pregnancy
            Tubal abortion

   ✓6ᵗʰ **O00.10   Tubal pregnancy** without intrauterine pregnancy
               Tubal pregnancy NOS

      ● **O00.101   Right tubal pregnancy without**
                  intrauterine pregnancy

      ● **O00.102   Left tubal pregnancy without intrauterine**
                  pregnancy

      ● **O00.109   Unspecified tubal pregnancy without**   ▽
                  intrauterine pregnancy

   ✓6ᵗʰ **O00.11   Tubal pregnancy** with intrauterine pregnancy

      ● **O00.111   Right tubal pregnancy with intrauterine**
                  pregnancy

      ● **O00.112   Left tubal pregnancy with intrauterine**
                  pregnancy

      ● **O00.119   Unspecified tubal pregnancy with**   ▽
                  intrauterine pregnancy

✓5ᵗʰ **O00.2** Ovarian **pregnancy**

   ✓6ᵗʰ **O00.20   Ovarian pregnancy** without intrauterine pregnancy
               Ovarian pregnancy NOS

      ● **O00.201   Right ovarian pregnancy without**
                  intrauterine pregnancy

      ● **O00.202   Left ovarian pregnancy without**
                  intrauterine pregnancy

Ectopic Pregnancy

Cornual/interstitial · Isthmic · Ampullar · Tubal (fallopian) · Infundibular · Ovarian · Intraligamentous · Abdominal · Intramural/mural · Cervical

      ● **O00.209   Unspecified ovarian pregnancy**   ▽
                  without intrauterine pregnancy

   ✓6ᵗʰ **O00.21   Ovarian pregnancy** with intrauterine pregnancy

      ● **O00.211   Right ovarian pregnancy with intrauterine**
                  pregnancy

      ● **O00.212   Left ovarian pregnancy with intrauterine**
                  pregnancy

      ● **O00.219   Unspecified ovarian pregnancy with**   ▽
                  intrauterine pregnancy

✓5ᵗʰ **O00.8   Other ectopic pregnancy**
            Cervical pregnancy
            Cornual pregnancy
            Intraligamentous pregnancy
            Mural pregnancy

   O00.80   Other ectopic pregnancy without intrauterine   M♀
            pregnancy
            Other ectopic pregnancy NOS

   O00.81   Other ectopic pregnancy with intrauterine   M♀
            pregnancy

✓5ᵗʰ **O00.9   Ectopic pregnancy, unspecified**

   O00.90   Unspecified ectopic pregnancy without   M♀▽
            intrauterine pregnancy
            Ectopic pregnancy NOS

   O00.91   Unspecified ectopic pregnancy with   M♀▽
            intrauterine pregnancy

✓4ᵗʰ **O01   Hydatidiform mole**
      Use additional code from category O08 to identify any associated complication
      EXCLUDES 1 *chorioadenoma (destruens) (D39.2)*
            malignant hydatidiform mole (D39.2)
      AHA: 2014, 3Q, 17
      DEF: Abnormal product of pregnancy; marked by mass of cysts resembling bunch of grapes due to chorionic villi proliferation and dissolution; must be surgically removed.

   O01.0   Classical hydatidiform mole   M♀
            Complete hydatidiform mole

   O01.1   Incomplete and partial hydatidiform mole   M♀

   O01.9   Hydatidiform mole, unspecified   M♀▽
            Trophoblastic disease NOS
            Vesicular mole NOS

✓4ᵗʰ **O02   Other abnormal products of conception**
      Use additional code from category O08 to identify any associated complication
      EXCLUDES 1 *papyraceous fetus (O31.0-)*
      AHA: 2014, 3Q, 17

   O02.0   Blighted ovum and nonhydatidiform mole   M♀
            Carneous mole
            Fleshy mole
            Intrauterine mole NOS
            Molar pregnancy NEC
            Pathological ovum

✓ Additional Character Req   ✓x7ᵗʰ Placeholder Alert   Manifestation   HCC CMS-HCC Condition   ▽ Unspecified Code   ▶◀ Revised Text   ● New Code   ▲ Revised Code Title

Chapter 15. Pregnancy, Childbirth, and the Puerperium

O02.1 Missed abortion   Ⓜ♀

Early fetal death, before completion of 20 weeks of gestation, with retention of dead fetus

EXCLUDES 1   *failed induced abortion (O07.-)*
fetal death (intrauterine) (late) (O36.4)
missed abortion with blighted ovum (O02.0)
missed abortion with hydatidiform mole (O01.-)
missed abortion with nonhydatidiform (O02.0)
missed abortion with other abnormal products of conception (O02.8-)
missed delivery (O36.4)
stillbirth (P95)

✓5ᵗʰ **O02.8 Other specified abnormal products of conception**

EXCLUDES 1   *abnormal products of conception with blighted ovum (O02.0)*
abnormal products of conception with hydatidiform mole (O01.-)
abnormal products of conception with nonhydatidiform mole (O02.0)

O02.81 Inappropriate change in quantitative human chorionic gonadotropin (hCG) in early pregnancy   Ⓜ♀

Biochemical pregnancy
Chemical pregnancy
Inappropriate level of quantitative human chorionic gonadotropin (hCG) for gestational age in early pregnancy

O02.89 Other abnormal products of conception   Ⓜ♀

O02.9 Abnormal product of conception, unspecified   Ⓜ♀▽

✓4ᵗʰ **O03 Spontaneous abortion**

NOTE   Incomplete abortion includes retained products of conception following spontaneous abortion

INCLUDES   miscarriage

O03.0 Genital tract and pelvic infection following incomplete spontaneous abortion   Ⓜ♀

Endometritis following incomplete spontaneous abortion
Oophoritis following incomplete spontaneous abortion
Parametritis following incomplete spontaneous abortion
Pelvic peritonitis following incomplete spontaneous abortion
Salpingitis following incomplete spontaneous abortion
Salpingo-oophoritis following incomplete spontaneous abortion

EXCLUDES 1   *sepsis following incomplete spontaneous abortion (O03.37)*
urinary tract infection following incomplete spontaneous abortion (O03.38)

O03.1 Delayed or excessive hemorrhage following incomplete spontaneous abortion   Ⓜ♀

Afibrinogenemia following incomplete spontaneous abortion
Defibrination syndrome following incomplete spontaneous abortion
Hemolysis following incomplete spontaneous abortion
Intravascular coagulation following incomplete spontaneous abortion

O03.2 Embolism following incomplete spontaneous abortion   Ⓜ♀

Air embolism following incomplete spontaneous abortion
Amniotic fluid embolism following incomplete spontaneous abortion
Blood-clot embolism following incomplete spontaneous abortion
Embolism NOS following incomplete spontaneous abortion
Fat embolism following incomplete spontaneous abortion
Pulmonary embolism following incomplete spontaneous abortion
Pyemic embolism following incomplete spontaneous abortion
Septic or septicopyemic embolism following incomplete spontaneous abortion
Soap embolism following incomplete spontaneous abortion

✓5ᵗʰ **O03.3 Other and unspecified complications following incomplete spontaneous abortion**

O03.30 Unspecified complication following incomplete spontaneous abortion   Ⓜ♀▽

O03.31 Shock following incomplete spontaneous abortion   Ⓜ♀

Circulatory collapse following incomplete spontaneous abortion
Shock (postprocedural) following incomplete spontaneous abortion

EXCLUDES 1   *shock due to infection following incomplete spontaneous abortion (O03.37)*

O03.32 Renal failure following incomplete spontaneous abortion   Ⓜ♀

Kidney failure (acute) following incomplete spontaneous abortion
Oliguria following incomplete spontaneous abortion
Renal shutdown following incomplete spontaneous abortion
Renal tubular necrosis following incomplete spontaneous abortion
Uremia following incomplete spontaneous abortion

O03.33 Metabolic disorder following incomplete spontaneous abortion   Ⓜ♀

O03.34 Damage to pelvic organs following incomplete spontaneous abortion   Ⓜ♀

Laceration, perforation, tear or chemical damage of bladder following incomplete spontaneous abortion
Laceration, perforation, tear or chemical damage of bowel following incomplete spontaneous abortion
Laceration, perforation, tear or chemical damage of broad ligament following incomplete spontaneous abortion
Laceration, perforation, tear or chemical damage of cervix following incomplete spontaneous abortion
Laceration, perforation, tear or chemical damage of periurethral tissue following incomplete spontaneous abortion
Laceration, perforation, tear or chemical damage of uterus following incomplete spontaneous abortion
Laceration, perforation, tear or chemical damage of vagina following incomplete spontaneous abortion

O03.35 Other venous complications following incomplete spontaneous abortion   Ⓜ♀

O03.36 Cardiac arrest following incomplete spontaneousabortion   Ⓜ♀

O03.37 Sepsis following incomplete spontaneous abortion   Ⓜ♀

Use additional code to identify infectious agent (B95-B97)
Use additional code to identify severe sepsis, if applicable (R65.2-)

EXCLUDES 1   *septic or septicopyemic embolism following incomplete spontaneous abortion (O03.2)*

O03.38 Urinary tract infection following incomplete spontaneous abortion   Ⓜ♀

Cystitis following incomplete spontaneous abortion

O03.39 Incomplete spontaneous abortion with other complications   Ⓜ♀

O03.4 Incomplete spontaneous abortion without complication   Ⓜ♀

O03.5 Genital tract and pelvic infection following complete or unspecified spontaneous abortion   Ⓜ♀

Endometritis following complete or unspecified spontaneous abortion
Oophoritis following complete or unspecified spontaneous abortion
Parametritis following complete or unspecified spontaneous abortion
Pelvic peritonitis following complete or unspecified spontaneous abortion
Salpingitis following complete or unspecified spontaneous abortion
Salpingo-oophoritis following complete or unspecified spontaneous abortion

EXCLUDES 1   *sepsis following complete or unspecified spontaneous abortion (O03.87)*
urinary tract infection following complete or unspecified spontaneous abortion (O03.88)

O03.6 Delayed or excessive hemorrhage following complete or unspecified spontaneous abortion   Ⓜ♀

Afibrinogenemia following complete or unspecified spontaneous abortion
Defibrination syndrome following complete or unspecified spontaneous abortion
Hemolysis following complete or unspecified spontaneous abortion
Intravascular coagulation following complete or unspecified spontaneous abortion

EXCLUDES 1 Not coded here   EXCLUDES 2 Not included here   Ⓝ Newborn Age: 0   Ⓟ Pediatric Age: 0-17   Ⓜ Maternity Age: 12-55   Ⓐ Adult Age: 15-124

O02.1–O03.6

824   ICD-10-CM 2018

O03.7 **Embolism** **following** **complete or unspecified**   Ⓜ♀
spontaneous abortion
Air embolism following complete or unspecified spontaneous abortion
Amniotic fluid embolism following complete or unspecified spontaneous abortion
Blood-clot embolism following complete or unspecified spontaneous abortion
Embolism NOS following complete or unspecified spontaneous abortion
Fat embolism following complete or unspecified spontaneous abortion
Pulmonary embolism following complete or unspecified spontaneous abortion
Pyemic embolism following complete or unspecified spontaneous abortion
Septic or septicopyemic embolism following complete or unspecified spontaneous abortion
Soap embolism following complete or unspecified spontaneous abortion

✓5ᵗʰ **O03.8** **Other and unspecified complications following complete or unspecified spontaneous abortion**

  O03.80 **Unspecified complication following**   Ⓜ♀▽
complete or unspecified spontaneous abortion

  O03.81 **Shock** **following** **complete or unspecified**   Ⓜ♀
spontaneous abortion
Circulatory collapse following complete or unspecified spontaneous abortion
Shock (postprocedural) following complete or unspecified spontaneous abortion
EXCLUDES 1   *shock due to infection following complete or unspecified spontaneous abortion (O03.87)*

  O03.82 **Renal failure** **following** **complete or unspecified**   Ⓜ♀
spontaneous abortion
Kidney failure (acute) following complete or unspecified spontaneous abortion
Oliguria following complete or unspecified spontaneous abortion
Renal shutdown following complete or unspecified spontaneous abortion
Renal tubular necrosis following complete or unspecified spontaneous abortion
Uremia following complete or unspecified spontaneous abortion

  O03.83 **Metabolic** **disorder following** **complete or**   Ⓜ♀
unspecified spontaneous abortion

  O03.84 **Damage to pelvic organs** **following** **complete or**   Ⓜ♀
unspecified spontaneous abortion
Laceration, perforation, tear or chemical damage of bladder following complete or unspecified spontaneous abortion
Laceration, perforation, tear or chemical damage of bowel following complete or unspecified spontaneous abortion
Laceration, perforation, tear or chemical damage of broad ligament following complete or unspecified spontaneous abortion
Laceration, perforation, tear or chemical damage of cervix following complete or unspecified spontaneous abortion
Laceration, perforation, tear or chemical damage of periurethral tissue following complete or unspecified spontaneous abortion
Laceration, perforation, tear or chemical damage of uterus following complete or unspecified spontaneous abortion
Laceration, perforation, tear or chemical damage of vagina following complete or unspecified spontaneous abortion

  O03.85 **Other venous complications following complete**   Ⓜ♀
or unspecified spontaneous abortion

  O03.86 **Cardiac arrest** **following** **complete or unspecified**   Ⓜ♀
spontaneous abortion

  O03.87 **Sepsis** **following** **complete or unspecified**   Ⓜ♀
spontaneous abortion
Use additional code to identify infectious agent (B95-B97)
Use additional code to identify severe sepsis, if applicable (R65.2-)
EXCLUDES 1   *septic or septicopyemic embolism following complete or unspecified spontaneous abortion (O03.7)*

  O03.88 **Urinary tract infection following complete or**   Ⓜ♀
unspecified spontaneous abortion
Cystitis following complete or unspecified spontaneous abortion

  O03.89 **Complete or unspecified spontaneous abortion**   Ⓜ♀
with other complications

O03.9 **Complete or unspecified spontaneous abortion**   Ⓜ♀▽
without complication
Miscarriage NOS
Spontaneous abortion NOS

✓4ᵗʰ **O04** **Complications** **following (induced) termination of pregnancy**
INCLUDES   complications following (induced) termination of pregnancy
EXCLUDES 1   *encounter for elective termination of pregnancy, uncomplicated (Z33.2)*
failed attempted termination of pregnancy (O07.-)

O04.5 **Genital tract and pelvic infection** **following (induced)**   Ⓜ♀
termination of pregnancy
Endometritis following (induced) termination of pregnancy
Oophoritis following (induced) termination of pregnancy
Parametritis following (induced) termination of pregnancy
Pelvic peritonitis following (induced) termination of pregnancy
Salpingitis following (induced) termination of pregnancy
Salpingo-oophoritis following (induced) termination of pregnancy
EXCLUDES 1   *sepsis following (induced) termination of pregnancy (O04.87)*
urinary tract infection following (induced) termination of pregnancy (O04.88)

O04.6 **Delayed or excessive hemorrhage** **following (induced)**   Ⓜ♀
termination of pregnancy
Afibrinogenemia following (induced) termination of pregnancy
Defibrination syndrome following (induced) termination of pregnancy
Hemolysis following (induced) termination of pregnancy
Intravascular coagulation following (induced) termination of pregnancy

O04.7 **Embolism** **following (induced) termination of pregnancy**   Ⓜ♀
Air embolism following (induced) termination of pregnancy
Amniotic fluid embolism following (induced) termination of pregnancy
Blood-clot embolism following (induced) termination of pregnancy
Embolism NOS following (induced) termination of pregnancy
Fat embolism following (induced) termination of pregnancy
Pulmonary embolism following (induced) termination of pregnancy
Pyemic embolism following (induced) termination of pregnancy
Septic or septicopyemic embolism following (induced) termination of pregnancy
Soap embolism following (induced) termination of pregnancy

✓5ᵗʰ **O04.8** **(Induced) termination of pregnancy with other and unspecified complications**

  O04.80 **(Induced) termination of pregnancy with**   Ⓜ♀▽
unspecified complications

  O04.81 **Shock** **following (induced) termination of**   Ⓜ♀
pregnancy
Circulatory collapse following (induced) termination of pregnancy
Shock (postprocedural) following (induced) termination of pregnancy
EXCLUDES 1   *shock due to infection following (induced) termination of pregnancy (O04.87)*

  O04.82 **Renal failure** **following (induced) termination**   Ⓜ♀
of pregnancy
Kidney failure (acute) following (induced) termination of pregnancy
Oliguria following (induced) termination of pregnancy
Renal shutdown following (induced) termination of pregnancy
Renal tubular necrosis following (induced) termination of pregnancy
Uremia following (induced) termination of pregnancy

  O04.83 **Metabolic disorder following (induced)**   Ⓜ♀
termination of pregnancy

✓ Additional Character Req   ✓×7ᵗʰ Placeholder Alert   Manifestation   HCC CMS-HCC Condition   ▽ Unspecified Code   ►◄ Revised Text   ● New Code   ▲ Revised Code Title

ICD-10-CM 2018   825

O04.84   **Damage to pelvic organs following (induced) termination of pregnancy**   Ⓜ♀
Laceration, perforation, tear or chemical damage of bladder following (induced) termination of pregnancy
Laceration, perforation, tear or chemical damage of bowel following (induced) termination of pregnancy
Laceration, perforation, tear or chemical damage of broad ligament following (induced) termination of pregnancy
Laceration, perforation, tear or chemical damage of cervix following (induced) termination of pregnancy
Laceration, perforation, tear or chemical damage of periurethral tissue following (induced) termination of pregnancy
Laceration, perforation, tear or chemical damage of uterus following (induced) termination of pregnancy
Laceration, perforation, tear or chemical damage of vagina following (induced) termination of pregnancy

O04.85   **Other venous complications following (induced) termination of pregnancy**   Ⓜ♀

O04.86   **Cardiac arrest following (induced) termination of pregnancy**   Ⓜ♀

O04.87   **Sepsis following (induced) termination of pregnancy**   Ⓜ♀
Use additional code to identify infectious agent (B95-B97)
Use additional code to identify severe sepsis, if applicable (R65.2-)
> **EXCLUDES 1**   *septic or septicopyemic embolism following (induced) termination of pregnancy (O04.7)*

O04.88   **Urinary tract infection following (induced) termination of pregnancy**   Ⓜ♀
Cystitis following (induced) termination of pregnancy

O04.89   **(Induced) termination of pregnancy with other complications**   Ⓜ♀

√4ᵗʰ **O07**   **Failed attempted termination of pregnancy**
> **INCLUDES**   failure of attempted induction of pregnancy
> incomplete elective abortion
> **EXCLUDES 1**   *incomplete spontaneous abortion (O03.0-)*

O07.0   **Genital tract and pelvic infection following failed attempted termination of pregnancy**   Ⓜ♀
Endometritis following failed attempted termination of pregnancy
Oophoritis following failed attempted termination of pregnancy
Parametritis following failed attempted termination of pregnancy
Pelvic peritonitis following failed attempted termination of pregnancy
Salpingitis following failed attempted termination of pregnancy
Salpingo-oophoritis following failed attempted termination of pregnancy
> **EXCLUDES 1**   *sepsis following failed attempted termination of pregnancy (O07.37)*
> *urinary tract infection following failed attempted termination of pregnancy (O07.38)*

O07.1   **Delayed or excessive hemorrhage following failed attempted termination of pregnancy**   Ⓜ♀
Afibrinogenemia following failed attempted termination of pregnancy
Defibrination syndrome following failed attempted termination of pregnancy
Hemolysis following failed attempted termination of pregnancy
Intravascular coagulation following failed attempted termination of pregnancy

O07.2   **Embolism following failed attempted termination of pregnancy**   Ⓜ♀
Air embolism following failed attempted termination of pregnancy
Amniotic fluid embolism following failed attempted termination of pregnancy
Blood-clot embolism following failed attempted termination of pregnancy
Embolism NOS following failed attempted termination of pregnancy
Fat embolism following failed attempted termination of pregnancy
Pulmonary embolism following failed attempted termination of pregnancy
Pyemic embolism following failed attempted termination of pregnancy
Septic or septicopyemic embolism following failed attempted termination of pregnancy
Soap embolism following failed attempted termination of pregnancy

√5ᵗʰ **O07.3**   **Failed attempted termination of pregnancy with other and unspecified complications**

O07.30   **Failed attempted termination of pregnancy with unspecified complications**   Ⓜ♀▽

O07.31   **Shock following failed attempted termination of pregnancy**   Ⓜ♀
Circulatory collapse following failed attempted termination of pregnancy
Shock (postprocedural) following failed attempted termination of pregnancy
> **EXCLUDES 1**   *shock due to infection following failed attempted termination of pregnancy (O07.37)*

O07.32   **Renal failure following failed attempted termination of pregnancy**   Ⓜ♀
Kidney failure (acute) following failed attempted termination of pregnancy
Oliguria following failed attempted termination of pregnancy
Renal shutdown following failed attempted termination of pregnancy
Renal tubular necrosis following failed attempted termination of pregnancy
Uremia following failed attempted termination of pregnancy

O07.33   **Metabolic disorder following failed attempted termination of pregnancy**   Ⓜ♀

O07.34   **Damage to pelvic organs following failed attempted termination of pregnancy**   Ⓜ♀
Laceration, perforation, tear or chemical damage of bladder following failed attempted termination of pregnancy
Laceration, perforation, tear or chemical damage of bowel following failed attempted termination of pregnancy
Laceration, perforation, tear or chemical damage of broad ligament following failed attempted termination of pregnancy
Laceration, perforation, tear or chemical damage of cervix following failed attempted termination of pregnancy
Laceration, perforation, tear or chemical damage of periurethral tissue following failed attempted termination of pregnancy
Laceration, perforation, tear or chemical damage of uterus following failed attempted termination of pregnancy
Laceration, perforation, tear or chemical damage of vagina following failed attempted termination of pregnancy

O07.35   **Other venous complications following failed attempted termination of pregnancy**   Ⓜ♀

O07.36   **Cardiac arrest following failed attempted termination of pregnancy**   Ⓜ♀

O07.37   **Sepsis following failed attempted termination of pregnancy**   Ⓜ♀
Use additional code to identify infectious agent (B95-B97)
Use additional code to identify severe sepsis, if applicable (R65.2-)
> **EXCLUDES 1**   *septic or septicopyemic embolism following failed attempted termination of pregnancy (O07.2)*

EXCLUDES 1 Not coded here   **EXCLUDES 2** Not included here   Ⓝ Newborn Age: 0   Ⓟ Pediatric Age: 0-17   Ⓜ Maternity Age: 12-55   Ⓐ Adult Age: 15-124

826   ICD-10-CM 2018

O07.38 Urinary tract infection following failed attempted termination of pregnancy ⓜ♀
Cystitis following failed attempted termination of pregnancy

O07.39 Failed attempted termination of pregnancy with other complications ⓜ♀

O07.4 Failed attempted termination of pregnancy without complication ⓜ♀

✓4ᵗʰ **O08 Complications following ectopic and molar pregnancy**
This category is for use with categories O00-O02 to identify any associated complications

O08.0 Genital tract and pelvic infection following ectopic and molar pregnancy ⓜ♀
Endometritis following ectopic and molar pregnancy
Oophoritis following ectopic and molar pregnancy
Parametritis following ectopic and molar pregnancy
Pelvic peritonitis following ectopic and molar pregnancy
Salpingitis following ectopic and molar pregnancy
Salpingo-oophoritis following ectopic and molar pregnancy
EXCLUDES 1   *sepsis following ectopic and molar pregnancy (O08.82)*
urinary tract infection (O08.83)

O08.1 Delayed or excessive hemorrhage following ectopic and molar pregnancy ⓜ♀
Afibrinogenemia following ectopic and molar pregnancy
Defibrination syndrome following ectopic and molar pregnancy
Hemolysis following ectopic and molar pregnancy
Intravascular coagulation following ectopic and molar pregnancy
EXCLUDES 1   *delayed or excessive hemorrhage due to incomplete abortion (O03.1)*

O08.2 Embolism following ectopic and molar pregnancy ⓜ♀
Air embolism following ectopic and molar pregnancy
Amniotic fluid embolism following ectopic and molar pregnancy
Blood-clot embolism following ectopic and molar pregnancy
Embolism NOS following ectopic and molar pregnancy
Fat embolism following ectopic and molar pregnancy
Pulmonary embolism following ectopic and molar pregnancy
Pyemic embolism following ectopic and molar pregnancy
Septic or septicopyemic embolism following ectopic and molar pregnancy
Soap embolism following ectopic and molar pregnancy

O08.3 Shock following ectopic and molar pregnancy ⓜ♀
Circulatory collapse following ectopic and molar pregnancy
Shock (postprocedural) following ectopic and molar pregnancy
EXCLUDES 1   *shock due to infection following ectopic and molar pregnancy (O08.82)*

O08.4 Renal failure following ectopic and molar pregnancy ⓜ♀
Kidney failure (acute) following ectopic and molar pregnancy
Oliguria following ectopic and molar pregnancy
Renal shutdown following ectopic and molar pregnancy
Renal tubular necrosis following ectopic and molar pregnancy
Uremia following ectopic and molar pregnancy

O08.5 Metabolic disorders following an ectopic and molar pregnancy ⓜ♀

O08.6 Damage to pelvic organs and tissues following an ectopic and molar pregnancy ⓜ♀
Laceration, perforation, tear or chemical damage of bladder following an ectopic and molar pregnancy
Laceration, perforation, tear or chemical damage of bowel following an ectopic and molar pregnancy
Laceration, perforation, tear or chemical damage of broad ligament following an ectopic and molar pregnancy
Laceration, perforation, tear or chemical damage of cervix following an ectopic and molar pregnancy
Laceration, perforation, tear or chemical damage of periurethral tissue following an ectopic and molar pregnancy
Laceration, perforation, tear or chemical damage of uterus following an ectopic and molar pregnancy
Laceration, perforation, tear or chemical damage of vagina following an ectopic and molar pregnancy

O08.7 Other venous complications following an ectopic and molar pregnancy ⓜ♀

✓5ᵗʰ **O08.8 Other complications following an ectopic and molar pregnancy**
O08.81 Cardiac arrest following an ectopic and molar pregnancy ⓜ♀
O08.82 Sepsis following ectopic and molar pregnancy ⓜ♀
Use additional code to identify infectious agent (B95-B97)
Use additional code to identify severe sepsis, if applicable (R65.2-)
EXCLUDES 1   *septic or septicopyemic embolism following ectopic and molar pregnancy (O08.2)*

O08.83 Urinary tract infection following an ectopic and molar pregnancy ⓜ♀
Cystitis following an ectopic and molar pregnancy

O08.89 Other complications following an ectopic and molar pregnancy ⓜ♀

O08.9 Unspecified complication following an ectopic and molar pregnancy ⓜ♀▽

Supervision of high risk pregnancy (O09)

✓4ᵗʰ **O09 Supervision of high risk pregnancy**
AHA: 2016, 4Q, 150

✓5ᵗʰ **O09.0 Supervision of pregnancy with history of infertility**
O09.00 Supervision of pregnancy with history of infertility, unspecified trimester ⓜ♀▽
O09.01 Supervision of pregnancy with history of infertility, first trimester ⓜ♀
O09.02 Supervision of pregnancy with history of infertility, second trimester ⓜ♀
O09.03 Supervision of pregnancy with history of infertility, third trimester ⓜ♀

✓5ᵗʰ **O09.1 Supervision of pregnancy with history of ectopic pregnancy**
O09.10 Supervision of pregnancy with history of ectopic pregnancy, unspecified trimester ⓜ♀▽
O09.11 Supervision of pregnancy with history of ectopic pregnancy, first trimester ⓜ♀
O09.12 Supervision of pregnancy with history of ectopic pregnancy, second trimester ⓜ♀
O09.13 Supervision of pregnancy with history of ectopic pregnancy, third trimester ⓜ♀

✓5ᵗʰ **O09.A Supervision of pregnancy with history of molar pregnancy**
O09.A0 Supervision of pregnancy with history of molar pregnancy, unspecified trimester ⓜ♀▽
O09.A1 Supervision of pregnancy with history of molar pregnancy, first trimester ⓜ♀
O09.A2 Supervision of pregnancy with history of molar pregnancy, second trimester ⓜ♀
O09.A3 Supervision of pregnancy with history of molar pregnancy, third trimester ⓜ♀

✓5ᵗʰ **O09.2 Supervision of pregnancy with other poor reproductive or obstetric history**
EXCLUDES 2   *pregnancy care for patient with history of recurrent pregnancy loss (O26.2-)*

✓6ᵗʰ **O09.21 Supervision of pregnancy with history of pre-term labor**
O09.211 Supervision of pregnancy with history of pre-term labor, first trimester ⓜ♀
O09.212 Supervision of pregnancy with history of pre-term labor, second trimester ⓜ♀
O09.213 Supervision of pregnancy with history of pre-term labor, third trimester ⓜ♀
O09.219 Supervision of pregnancy with history of pre-term labor, unspecified trimester ⓜ♀▽

✓6ᵗʰ **O09.29 Supervision of pregnancy with other poor reproductive or obstetric history**
Supervision of pregnancy with history of neonatal death
Supervision of pregnancy with history of stillbirth
O09.291 Supervision of pregnancy with other poor reproductive or obstetric history, first trimester ⓜ♀
O09.292 Supervision of pregnancy with other poor reproductive or obstetric history, second trimester ⓜ♀
O09.293 Supervision of pregnancy with other poor reproductive or obstetric history, third trimester ⓜ♀
O09.299 Supervision of pregnancy with other poor reproductive or obstetric history, unspecified trimester ⓜ♀▽

✓5ᵗʰ **O09.3 Supervision of pregnancy with insufficient antenatal care**
Supervision of concealed pregnancy
Supervision of hidden pregnancy
O09.30 Supervision of pregnancy with insufficient antenatal care, unspecified trimester ⓜ♀▽
O09.31 Supervision of pregnancy with insufficient antenatal care, first trimester ⓜ♀

Chapter 15. Pregnancy, Childbirth, and the Puerperium

O09.32–O10.03

O09.32 Supervision of pregnancy with insufficient antenatal care, second trimester Ⓜ♀

O09.33 Supervision of pregnancy with insufficient antenatal care, third trimester Ⓜ♀

✓5ᵗʰ **O09.4 Supervision of pregnancy with** grand multiparity

O09.40 Supervision of pregnancy with grand multiparity, unspecified trimester Ⓜ♀▽

O09.41 Supervision of pregnancy with grand multiparity, first trimester Ⓜ♀

O09.42 Supervision of pregnancy with grand multiparity, second trimester Ⓜ♀

O09.43 Supervision of pregnancy with grand multiparity, third trimester Ⓜ♀

✓5ᵗʰ **O09.5 Supervision of** elderly primigravida and multigravida
Pregnancy for a female 35 years and older at expected date of delivery

✓6ᵗʰ **O09.51 Supervision of** elderly primigravida

O09.511 Supervision of elderly primigravida, first trimester Ⓜ♀

O09.512 Supervision of elderly primigravida, second trimester Ⓜ♀

O09.513 Supervision of elderly primigravida, third trimester Ⓜ♀

O09.519 Supervision of elderly primigravida, unspecified trimester Ⓜ♀▽

✓6ᵗʰ **O09.52 Supervision of** elderly multigravida

O09.521 Supervision of elderly multigravida, first trimester Ⓜ♀

O09.522 Supervision of elderly multigravida, second trimester Ⓜ♀

O09.523 Supervision of elderly multigravida, third trimester Ⓜ♀

O09.529 Supervision of elderly multigravida, unspecified trimester Ⓜ♀▽

✓5ᵗʰ **O09.6 Supervision of** young primigravida and multigravida
Supervision of pregnancy for a female less than 16 years old at expected date of delivery

✓6ᵗʰ **O09.61 Supervision of** young primigravida

O09.611 Supervision of young primigravida, first trimester Ⓜ♀

O09.612 Supervision of young primigravida, second trimester Ⓜ♀

O09.613 Supervision of young primigravida, third trimester Ⓜ♀

O09.619 Supervision of young primigravida, unspecified trimester Ⓜ♀▽

✓6ᵗʰ **O09.62 Supervision of** young multigravida

O09.621 Supervision of young multigravida, first trimester Ⓜ♀

O09.622 Supervision of young multigravida, second trimester Ⓜ♀

O09.623 Supervision of young multigravida, third trimester Ⓜ♀

O09.629 Supervision of young multigravida, unspecified trimester Ⓜ♀▽

✓5ᵗʰ **O09.7 Supervision of high risk pregnancy due to** social problems

O09.70 Supervision of high risk pregnancy due to social problems, unspecified trimester Ⓜ♀▽

O09.71 Supervision of high risk pregnancy due to social problems, first trimester Ⓜ♀

O09.72 Supervision of high risk pregnancy due to social problems, second trimester Ⓜ♀

O09.73 Supervision of high risk pregnancy due to social problems, third trimester Ⓜ♀

✓5ᵗʰ **O09.8 Supervision of other high risk pregnancies**

✓6ᵗʰ **O09.81 Supervision of pregnancy** resulting from assisted reproductive technology
Supervision of pregnancy resulting from in-vitro fertilization
EXCLUDES 2 gestational carrier status (Z33.3)

O09.811 Supervision of pregnancy resulting from assisted reproductive technology, first trimester Ⓜ♀

O09.812 Supervision of pregnancy resulting from assisted reproductive technology, second trimester Ⓜ♀

O09.813 Supervision of pregnancy resulting from assisted reproductive technology, third trimester Ⓜ♀

O09.819 Supervision of pregnancy resulting from assisted reproductive technology, unspecified trimester Ⓜ♀▽

✓6ᵗʰ **O09.82 Supervision of pregnancy with** history of in utero procedure during previous pregnancy

O09.821 Supervision of pregnancy with history of in utero procedure during previous pregnancy, first trimester Ⓜ♀

O09.822 Supervision of pregnancy with history of in utero procedure during previous pregnancy, second trimester Ⓜ♀

O09.823 Supervision of pregnancy with history of in utero procedure during previous pregnancy, third trimester Ⓜ♀

O09.829 Supervision of pregnancy with history of in utero procedure during previous pregnancy, unspecified trimester Ⓜ♀▽
EXCLUDES 1 supervision of pregnancy affected by in utero procedure during current pregnancy (O35.7)

✓6ᵗʰ **O09.89 Supervision of other high risk pregnancies**

O09.891 Supervision of other high risk pregnancies, first trimester Ⓜ♀

O09.892 Supervision of other high risk pregnancies, second trimester Ⓜ♀

O09.893 Supervision of other high risk pregnancies, third trimester Ⓜ♀

O09.899 Supervision of other high risk pregnancies, unspecified trimester Ⓜ♀

✓5ᵗʰ **O09.9 Supervision of high risk pregnancy, unspecified**

O09.90 Supervision of high risk pregnancy, unspecified, unspecified trimester Ⓜ♀▽

O09.91 Supervision of high risk pregnancy, unspecified, first trimester Ⓜ♀▽

O09.92 Supervision of high risk pregnancy, unspecified, second trimester Ⓜ♀▽

O09.93 Supervision of high risk pregnancy, unspecified, third trimester Ⓜ♀▽

Edema, proteinuria and hypertensive disorders in pregnancy, childbirth and the puerperium (O10-O16)

✓4ᵗʰ **O10 Pre-existing hypertension complicating pregnancy, childbirth and the puerperium**
Pre-existing hypertension with pre-existing proteinuria complicating pregnancy, childbirth and the puerperium
EXCLUDES 2 pre-existing hypertension with superimposed pre-eclampsia complicating pregnancy, childbirth and the puerperium (O11.-)

✓5ᵗʰ **O10.0 Pre-existing** essential **hypertension complicating pregnancy, childbirth and the puerperium**
Any condition in I10 specified as a reason for obstetric care during pregnancy, childbirth or the puerperium

✓6ᵗʰ **O10.01 Pre-existing essential hypertension complicating** pregnancy

O10.011 Pre-existing essential hypertension complicating pregnancy, first trimester Ⓜ♀

O10.012 Pre-existing essential hypertension complicating pregnancy, second trimester Ⓜ♀

O10.013 Pre-existing essential hypertension complicating pregnancy, third trimester Ⓜ♀

O10.019 Pre-existing essential hypertension complicating pregnancy, unspecified trimester Ⓜ♀▽

O10.02 Pre-existing essential hypertension complicating childbirth Ⓜ♀

O10.03 Pre-existing essential hypertension complicating the puerperium Ⓜ♀

EXCLUDES 1 Not coded here   *EXCLUDES 2* Not included here   Ⓝ Newborn Age: 0   Ⓟ Pediatric Age: 0-17   Ⓜ Maternity Age: 12-55   Ⓐ Adult Age: 15-124

828   ICD-10-CM 2018

Chapter 15. Pregnancy, Childbirth, and the Puerperium

☑5ᵗʰ **O10.1** **Pre-existing hypertensive** heart disease **complicating pregnancy, childbirth and the puerperium**
Any condition in I11 specified as a reason for obstetric care during pregnancy, childbirth or the puerperium
Use additional code from I11 to identify the type of hypertensive heart disease

     ☑6ᵗʰ **O10.11** **Pre-existing hypertensive heart disease complicating** pregnancy

         O10.111 **Pre-existing hypertensive heart disease complicating pregnancy, first trimester** Ⓜ♀

         O10.112 **Pre-existing hypertensive heart disease complicating pregnancy, second trimester** Ⓜ♀

         O10.113 **Pre-existing hypertensive heart disease complicating pregnancy, third trimester** Ⓜ♀

         O10.119 **Pre-existing hypertensive heart disease complicating pregnancy, unspecified trimester** Ⓜ♀▽

     O10.12 **Pre-existing hypertensive heart disease complicating** childbirth Ⓜ♀

     O10.13 **Pre-existing hypertensive heart disease complicating the** puerperium Ⓜ♀

☑5ᵗʰ **O10.2** **Pre-existing hypertensive** chronic kidney disease **complicating pregnancy, childbirth and the puerperium**
Any condition in I12 specified as a reason for obstetric care during pregnancy, childbirth or the puerperium
Use additional code from I12 to identify the type of hypertensive chronic kidney disease

     ☑6ᵗʰ **O10.21** **Pre-existing hypertensive chronic kidney disease complicating** pregnancy

         O10.211 **Pre-existing hypertensive chronic kidney disease complicating pregnancy, first trimester** Ⓜ♀

         O10.212 **Pre-existing hypertensive chronic kidney disease complicating pregnancy, second trimester** Ⓜ♀

         O10.213 **Pre-existing hypertensive chronic kidney disease complicating pregnancy, third trimester** Ⓜ♀

         O10.219 **Pre-existing hypertensive chronic kidney disease complicating pregnancy, unspecified trimester** Ⓜ♀▽

     O10.22 **Pre-existing hypertensive chronic kidney disease complicating** childbirth Ⓜ♀

     O10.23 **Pre-existing hypertensive chronic kidney disease complicating the** puerperium Ⓜ♀

☑5ᵗʰ **O10.3** **Pre-existing hypertensive** heart and chronic kidney disease **complicating pregnancy, childbirth and the puerperium**
Any condition in I13 specified as a reason for obstetric care during pregnancy, childbirth or the puerperium
Use additional code from I13 to identify the type of hypertensive heart and chronic kidney disease

     ☑6ᵗʰ **O10.31** **Pre-existing hypertensive heart and chronic kidney disease complicating** pregnancy

         O10.311 **Pre-existing hypertensive heart and chronic kidney disease complicating pregnancy, first trimester** Ⓜ♀

         O10.312 **Pre-existing hypertensive heart and chronic kidney disease complicating pregnancy, second trimester** Ⓜ♀

         O10.313 **Pre-existing hypertensive heart and chronic kidney disease complicating pregnancy, third trimester** Ⓜ♀

         O10.319 **Pre-existing hypertensive heart and** Ⓜ♀▽ **chronic kidney disease complicating pregnancy, unspecified trimester**

     O10.32 **Pre-existing hypertensive heart and chronic kidney disease complicating** childbirth Ⓜ♀

     O10.33 **Pre-existing hypertensive heart and chronic kidney disease complicating the** puerperium Ⓜ♀

☑5ᵗʰ **O10.4** **Pre-existing** secondary **hypertension complicating pregnancy, childbirth and the puerperium**
Any condition in I15 specified as a reason for obstetric care during pregnancy, childbirth or the puerperium
Use additional code from I15 to identify the type of secondary hypertension

     ☑6ᵗʰ **O10.41** **Pre-existing secondary hypertension complicating** pregnancy

         O10.411 **Pre-existing secondary hypertension complicating pregnancy, first trimester** Ⓜ♀

         O10.412 **Pre-existing secondary hypertension complicating pregnancy, second trimester** Ⓜ♀

         O10.413 **Pre-existing secondary hypertension complicating pregnancy, third trimester** Ⓜ♀

         O10.419 **Pre-existing secondary hypertension complicating pregnancy, unspecified trimester** Ⓜ♀▽

     O10.42 **Pre-existing secondary hypertension complicating** childbirth Ⓜ♀

     O10.43 **Pre-existing secondary hypertension complicating the** puerperium Ⓜ♀

☑5ᵗʰ **O10.9** **Unspecified pre-existing hypertension complicating pregnancy, childbirth and the puerperium**

     ☑6ᵗʰ **O10.91** **Unspecified pre-existing hypertension complicating** pregnancy

         O10.911 **Unspecified pre-existing hypertension complicating pregnancy, first trimester** Ⓜ♀▽

         O10.912 **Unspecified pre-existing hypertension complicating pregnancy, second trimester** Ⓜ♀▽

         O10.913 **Unspecified pre-existing hypertension complicating pregnancy, third trimester** Ⓜ♀▽

         O10.919 **Unspecified pre-existing hypertension complicating pregnancy, unspecified trimester** Ⓜ♀▽

     O10.92 **Unspecified pre-existing hypertension complicating** childbirth Ⓜ♀▽

     O10.93 **Unspecified pre-existing hypertension complicating the** puerperium Ⓜ♀▽

☑4ᵗʰ **O11** Pre-existing **hypertension** with pre-eclampsia
[INCLUDES] conditions in O10 complicated by pre-eclampsia
pre-eclampsia superimposed pre-existing hypertension
Use additional code from O10 to identify the type of hypertension

     O11.1 **Pre-existing hypertension with pre-eclampsia, first trimester** Ⓜ♀

     O11.2 **Pre-existing hypertension with pre-eclampsia, second trimester** Ⓜ♀

     O11.3 **Pre-existing hypertension with pre-eclampsia, third trimester** Ⓜ♀

     O11.4 **Pre-existing hypertension with pre-eclampsia, complicating** childbirth Ⓜ♀

     O11.5 **Pre-existing hypertension with pre-eclampsia, complicating the** puerperium Ⓜ♀

     O11.9 **Pre-existing hypertension with pre-eclampsia, unspecified trimester** Ⓜ♀▽

☑4ᵗʰ **O12** Gestational **[pregnancy-induced] edema and proteinuria** without hypertension

     ☑5ᵗʰ **O12.0** **Gestational** edema

         O12.00 **Gestational edema, unspecified trimester** Ⓜ♀▽

         O12.01 **Gestational edema,** first trimester Ⓜ♀

         O12.02 **Gestational edema,** second trimester Ⓜ♀

         O12.03 **Gestational edema,** third trimester Ⓜ♀

         O12.04 **Gestational edema, complicating** childbirth Ⓜ♀

         O12.05 **Gestational edema, complicating the** puerperium Ⓜ♀

     ☑5ᵗʰ **O12.1** **Gestational** proteinuria

         O12.10 **Gestational proteinuria, unspecified trimester** Ⓜ♀▽

         O12.11 **Gestational proteinuria,** first trimester Ⓜ♀

         O12.12 **Gestational proteinuria,** second trimester Ⓜ♀

         O12.13 **Gestational proteinuria,** third trimester Ⓜ♀

         O12.14 **Gestational proteinuria, complicating** childbirth Ⓜ♀

☑ Additional Character Req   ☑x7ᵗʰ Placeholder Alert   **Manifestation**   [HCC] CMS-HCC Condition   ▽ Unspecified Code   ►◄ Revised Text   ● New Code   ▲ Revised Code Title

O12.15   **Gestational proteinuria, complicating the puerperium**   Ⓜ♀

✓5ᵗʰ **O12.2 Gestational edema with proteinuria**

O12.20   **Gestational edema with proteinuria, unspecified trimester**   Ⓜ♀▽

O12.21   **Gestational edema with proteinuria, first trimester**   Ⓜ♀

O12.22   **Gestational edema with proteinuria, second trimester**   Ⓜ♀

O12.23   **Gestational edema with proteinuria, third trimester**   Ⓜ♀

O12.24   **Gestational edema with proteinuria, complicating childbirth**   Ⓜ♀

O12.25   **Gestational edema with proteinuria, complicating the puerperium**   Ⓜ♀

✓4ᵗʰ **O13 Gestational [pregnancy-induced] hypertension without significant proteinuria**

INCLUDES   gestational hypertension NOS
transient hypertension of pregnancy

AHA: 2016, 1Q, 5

O13.1   **Gestational [pregnancy-induced] hypertension without significant proteinuria, first trimester**   Ⓜ♀

O13.2   **Gestational [pregnancy-induced] hypertension without significant proteinuria, second trimester**   Ⓜ♀

O13.3   **Gestational [pregnancy-induced] hypertension without significant proteinuria, third trimester**   Ⓜ♀

O13.4   **Gestational [pregnancy-induced] hypertension without significant proteinuria, complicating childbirth**   Ⓜ♀

O13.5   **Gestational [pregnancy-induced] hypertension without significant proteinuria, complicating the puerperium**   Ⓜ♀

O13.9   **Gestational [pregnancy-induced] hypertension without significant proteinuria, unspecified trimester**   Ⓜ♀▽

✓4ᵗʰ **O14 Pre-eclampsia**

EXCLUDES 1   pre-existing hypertension with pre-eclampsia (O11)

✓5ᵗʰ **O14.0 Mild to moderate pre-eclampsia**

O14.00   **Mild to moderate pre-eclampsia, unspecified trimester**   Ⓜ♀▽

O14.02   **Mild to moderate pre-eclampsia, second trimester**   Ⓜ♀

O14.03   **Mild to moderate pre-eclampsia, third trimester**   Ⓜ♀

O14.04   **Mild to moderate pre-eclampsia, complicating childbirth**   Ⓜ♀

O14.05   **Mild to moderate pre-eclampsia, complicating the puerperium**   Ⓜ♀

✓5ᵗʰ **O14.1 Severe pre-eclampsia**

EXCLUDES 1   HELLP syndrome (O14.2-)

O14.10   **Severe pre-eclampsia, unspecified trimester**   Ⓜ♀▽

O14.12   **Severe pre-eclampsia, second trimester**   Ⓜ♀

O14.13   **Severe pre-eclampsia, third trimester**   Ⓜ♀

O14.14   **Severe pre-eclampsia complicating childbirth**   Ⓜ♀

O14.15   **Severe pre-eclampsia, complicating the puerperium**   Ⓜ♀

✓5ᵗʰ **O14.2 HELLP syndrome**

Severe pre-eclampsia with hemolysis, elevated liver enzymes and low platelet count (HELLP)

O14.20   **HELLP syndrome (HELLP), unspecified trimester**   Ⓜ♀▽

O14.22   **HELLP syndrome (HELLP), second trimester**   Ⓜ♀

O14.23   **HELLP syndrome (HELLP), third trimester**   Ⓜ♀

O14.24   **HELLP syndrome, complicating childbirth**   Ⓜ♀

O14.25   **HELLP syndrome, complicating the puerperium**   Ⓜ♀

✓5ᵗʰ **O14.9 Unspecified pre-eclampsia**

O14.90   **Unspecified pre-eclampsia, unspecified trimester**   Ⓜ♀▽

O14.92   **Unspecified pre-eclampsia, second trimester**   Ⓜ♀▽

O14.93   **Unspecified pre-eclampsia, third trimester**   Ⓜ♀▽

O14.94   **Unspecified pre-eclampsia, complicating childbirth**   Ⓜ♀▽

O14.95   **Unspecified pre-eclampsia, complicating the puerperium**   Ⓜ♀▽

✓4ᵗʰ **O15 Eclampsia**

INCLUDES   convulsions following conditions in O10-O14 and O16

✓5ᵗʰ **O15.0 Eclampsia complicating pregnancy**

O15.00   **Eclampsia complicating pregnancy, unspecified trimester**   Ⓜ♀▽

O15.02   **Eclampsia complicating pregnancy, second trimester**   Ⓜ♀

O15.03   **Eclampsia complicating pregnancy, third trimester**   Ⓜ♀

O15.1   **Eclampsia complicating labor**   Ⓜ♀

O15.2   **Eclampsia complicating the puerperium**   Ⓜ♀

O15.9   **Eclampsia, unspecified as to time period**   Ⓜ♀▽
Eclampsia NOS

✓4ᵗʰ **O16 Unspecified maternal hypertension**

O16.1   **Unspecified maternal hypertension, first trimester**   Ⓜ♀▽

O16.2   **Unspecified maternal hypertension, second trimester**   Ⓜ♀▽

O16.3   **Unspecified maternal hypertension, third trimester**   Ⓜ♀▽

O16.4   **Unspecified maternal hypertension, complicating childbirth**   Ⓜ♀▽

O16.5   **Unspecified maternal hypertension, complicating the puerperium**   Ⓜ♀▽

O16.9   **Unspecified maternal hypertension, unspecified trimester**   Ⓜ♀▽

Other maternal disorders predominantly related to pregnancy (O20-O29)

EXCLUDES 2   maternal care related to the fetus and amniotic cavity and possible delivery problems (O30-O48)
maternal diseases classifiable elsewhere but complicating pregnancy, labor and delivery, and the puerperium (O98-O99)

✓4ᵗʰ **O20 Hemorrhage in early pregnancy**

INCLUDES   hemorrhage before completion of 20 weeks gestation

EXCLUDES 1   pregnancy with abortive outcome (O00-O08)

O20.0   **Threatened abortion**   Ⓜ♀
Hemorrhage specified as due to threatened abortion
DEF: Bloody discharge during pregnancy; cervix may be dilated and pregnancy threatened, but the pregnancy is not terminated.

O20.8   **Other hemorrhage in early pregnancy**   Ⓜ♀

O20.9   **Hemorrhage in early pregnancy, unspecified**   Ⓜ♀▽

✓4ᵗʰ **O21 Excessive vomiting in pregnancy**

O21.0   **Mild hyperemesis gravidarum**   Ⓜ♀
Hyperemesis gravidarum, mild or unspecified, starting before the end of the 20th week of gestation

O21.1   **Hyperemesis gravidarum with metabolic disturbance**   Ⓜ♀
Hyperemesis gravidarum, starting before the end of the 20th week of gestation, with metabolic disturbance such as carbohydrate depletion
Hyperemesis gravidarum, starting before the end of the 20th week of gestation, with metabolic disturbance such as dehydration
Hyperemesis gravidarum, starting before the end of the 20th week of gestation, with metabolic disturbance such as electrolyte imbalance

O21.2   **Late vomiting of pregnancy**   Ⓜ♀
Excessive vomiting starting after 20 completed weeks of gestation

O21.8   **Other vomiting complicating pregnancy**   Ⓜ♀
Vomiting due to diseases classified elsewhere, complicating pregnancy
Use additional code, to identify cause

O21.9   **Vomiting of pregnancy, unspecified**   Ⓜ♀▽

✓4ᵗʰ **O22 Venous complications and hemorrhoids in pregnancy**

EXCLUDES 1   venous complications of:
abortion NOS (O03.9)
ectopic or molar pregnancy (O08.7)
failed attempted abortion (O07.35)
induced abortion (O04.85)
spontaneous abortion (O03.89)

EXCLUDES 2   obstetric pulmonary embolism (O88.-)
venous complications and hemorrhoids of childbirth and the puerperium (O87.-)

✓5ᵗʰ **O22.0 Varicose veins of lower extremity in pregnancy**
Varicose veins NOS in pregnancy
DEF: Distended, tortuous veins of lower extremities associated with pregnancy.

O22.00   **Varicose veins of lower extremity in pregnancy, unspecified trimester**   Ⓜ♀▽

EXCLUDES 1 Not coded here   EXCLUDES 2 Not included here   Ⓝ Newborn Age: 0   Ⓟ Pediatric Age: 0-17   Ⓜ Maternity Age: 12-55   Ⓐ Adult Age: 15-124

830   ICD-10-CM 2018

O22.01   **Varicose veins of lower extremity in pregnancy,** Ⓜ♀
     first trimester

O22.02   **Varicose veins of lower extremity in pregnancy,** Ⓜ♀
     second trimester

O22.03   **Varicose veins of lower extremity in pregnancy,** Ⓜ♀
     third trimester

√5ᵗʰ **O22.1**   **Genital varices in pregnancy**
     Perineal varices in pregnancy
     Vaginal varices in pregnancy
     Vulval varices in pregnancy

   O22.10   **Genital varices in pregnancy, unspecified** Ⓜ♀▽
     trimester

   O22.11   **Genital varices in pregnancy, first trimester** Ⓜ♀

   O22.12   **Genital varices in pregnancy, second trimester** Ⓜ♀

   O22.13   **Genital varices in pregnancy, third trimester** Ⓜ♀

√5ᵗʰ **O22.2**   **Superficial thrombophlebitis in pregnancy**
     Phlebitis in pregnancy NOS
     Thrombophlebitis of legs in pregnancy
     Thrombosis in pregnancy NOS
     Use additional code to identify the superficial thrombophlebitis
     (I80.0-)

   O22.20   **Superficial thrombophlebitis in pregnancy,** Ⓜ♀▽
     unspecified trimester

   O22.21   **Superficial thrombophlebitis in pregnancy,** Ⓜ♀
     first trimester

   O22.22   **Superficial thrombophlebitis in pregnancy,** Ⓜ♀
     second trimester

   O22.23   **Superficial thrombophlebitis in pregnancy,** Ⓜ♀
     third trimester

√5ᵗʰ **O22.3**   **Deep phlebothrombosis in pregnancy**
     Deep vein thrombosis, antepartum
     Use additional code to identify the deep vein thrombosis (I82.4-,
     I82.5-, I82.62-. I82.72-)
     Use additional code, if applicable, for associated long-term
     (current) use of anticoagulants (Z79.01)

   O22.30   **Deep phlebothrombosis in pregnancy,** Ⓜ♀▽
     unspecified trimester

   O22.31   **Deep phlebothrombosis in pregnancy,** Ⓜ♀
     first trimester

   O22.32   **Deep phlebothrombosis in pregnancy,** Ⓜ♀
     second trimester

   O22.33   **Deep phlebothrombosis in pregnancy,** Ⓜ♀
     third trimester

√5ᵗʰ **O22.4**   **Hemorrhoids in pregnancy**

   O22.40   **Hemorrhoids in pregnancy, unspecified** Ⓜ♀▽
     trimester

   O22.41   **Hemorrhoids in pregnancy, first trimester** Ⓜ♀

   O22.42   **Hemorrhoids in pregnancy, second trimester** Ⓜ♀

   O22.43   **Hemorrhoids in pregnancy, third trimester** Ⓜ♀

√5ᵗʰ **O22.5**   **Cerebral venous thrombosis in pregnancy**
     Cerebrovenous sinus thrombosis in pregnancy

   O22.50   **Cerebral venous thrombosis in pregnancy,** Ⓜ♀▽
     unspecified trimester

   O22.51   **Cerebral venous thrombosis in pregnancy,** Ⓜ♀
     first trimester

   O22.52   **Cerebral venous thrombosis in pregnancy,** Ⓜ♀
     second trimester

   O22.53   **Cerebral venous thrombosis in pregnancy,** Ⓜ♀
     third trimester

√5ᵗʰ **O22.8**   **Other venous complications in pregnancy**

   √6ᵗʰ **O22.8X**   **Other venous complications in pregnancy**

     O22.8X1   **Other venous complications in** Ⓜ♀
       pregnancy, first trimester

     O22.8X2   **Other venous complications in** Ⓜ♀
       pregnancy, second trimester

     O22.8X3   **Other venous complications in** Ⓜ♀
       pregnancy, third trimester

     O22.8X9   **Other venous complications in** Ⓜ♀▽
       pregnancy, unspecified trimester

√5ᵗʰ **O22.9**   **Venous complication in pregnancy, unspecified**
     Gestational phlebitis NOS
     Gestational phlebopathy NOS
     Gestational thrombosis NOS

   O22.90   **Venous complication in pregnancy,** Ⓜ♀ ▽
     unspecified,unspecified trimester

   O22.91   **Venous complication in pregnancy,** Ⓜ♀▽
     unspecified, first trimester

   O22.92   **Venous complication in pregnancy,** Ⓜ♀▽
     unspecified, second trimester

   O22.93   **Venous complication in pregnancy,** Ⓜ♀▽
     unspecified, third trimester

√4ᵗʰ **O23**   **Infections of genitourinary tract in pregnancy**
     Use additional code to identify organism (B95.-, B96.-)
     EXCLUDES 2   gonococcal infections complicating pregnancy, childbirth and
       the puerperium (O98.2)
       infections with a predominantly sexual mode of transmission
       NOS complicating pregnancy, childbirth and the
       puerperium (O98.3)
       syphilis complicating pregnancy, childbirth and the puerperium
       (O98.1)
       tuberculosis of genitourinary system complicating pregnancy,
       childbirth and the puerperium (O98.0)
       venereal disease NOS complicating pregnancy, childbirth and
       the puerperium (O98.3)

√5ᵗʰ **O23.0**   **Infections of kidney in pregnancy**
     Pyelonephritis in pregnancy

   O23.00   **Infections of kidney in pregnancy, unspecified** Ⓜ♀▽
     trimester

   O23.01   **Infections of kidney in pregnancy, first trimester** Ⓜ♀

   O23.02   **Infections of kidney in pregnancy, second** Ⓜ♀
     trimester

   O23.03   **Infections of kidney in pregnancy, third** Ⓜ♀
     trimester

√5ᵗʰ **O23.1**   **Infections of bladder in pregnancy**

   O23.10   **Infections of bladder in pregnancy,** Ⓜ♀▽
     unspecified trimester

   O23.11   **Infections of bladder in pregnancy,** Ⓜ♀
     first trimester

   O23.12   **Infections of bladder in pregnancy,** Ⓜ♀
     second trimester

   O23.13   **Infections of bladder in pregnancy,** Ⓜ♀
     third trimester

√5ᵗʰ **O23.2**   **Infections of urethra in pregnancy**

   O23.20   **Infections of urethra in pregnancy,** Ⓜ♀▽
     unspecified trimester

   O23.21   **Infections of urethra in pregnancy,** Ⓜ♀
     first trimester

   O23.22   **Infections of urethra in pregnancy,** Ⓜ♀
     second trimester

   O23.23   **Infections of urethra in pregnancy,** Ⓜ♀
     third trimester

√5ᵗʰ **O23.3**   **Infections of other parts of urinary tract in pregnancy**

   O23.30   **Infections of other parts of urinary tract in** Ⓜ♀▽
     pregnancy, unspecified trimester

   O23.31   **Infections of other parts of urinary tract in** Ⓜ♀
     pregnancy, first trimester

   O23.32   **Infections of other parts of urinary tract in** Ⓜ♀
     pregnancy, second trimester

   O23.33   **Infections of other parts of urinary tract in** Ⓜ♀
     pregnancy, third trimester

√5ᵗʰ **O23.4**   **Unspecified infection of urinary tract in pregnancy**

   O23.40   **Unspecified infection of urinary tract in** Ⓜ♀▽
     pregnancy, unspecified trimester

   O23.41   **Unspecified infection of urinary tract in** Ⓜ♀▽
     pregnancy, first trimester

   O23.42   **Unspecified infection of urinary tract in** Ⓜ♀▽
     pregnancy, second trimester

   O23.43   **Unspecified infection of urinary tract in** Ⓜ♀▽
     pregnancy, third trimester

√5ᵗʰ **O23.5**   **Infections of the genital tract in pregnancy**

   √6ᵗʰ **O23.51**   **Infection of cervix in pregnancy**

     O23.511   **Infections of cervix in pregnancy,** Ⓜ♀
       first trimester

     O23.512   **Infections of cervix in pregnancy,** Ⓜ♀
       second trimester

     O23.513   **Infections of cervix in pregnancy,** Ⓜ♀
       third trimester

     O23.519   **Infections of cervix in pregnancy,** Ⓜ♀▽
       unspecified trimester

☑ Additional Character Req   ✓x7ᵗʰ Placeholder Alert   Manifestation   HCC CMS-HCC Condition   ▽ Unspecified Code   ►◄ Revised Text   ● New Code   ▲ Revised Code Title

ICD-10-CM 2018   **831**

√6ᵗʰ **O23.52 Salpingo-oophoritis in pregnancy**
Oophoritis in pregnancy
Salpingitis in pregnancy

     O23.521 Salpingo-oophoritis in pregnancy, first trimester Ⓜ♀

     O23.522 Salpingo-oophoritis in pregnancy, second trimester Ⓜ♀

     O23.523 Salpingo-oophoritis in pregnancy, third trimester Ⓜ♀

     O23.529 Salpingo-oophoritis in pregnancy, unspecified trimester Ⓜ♀▽

√6ᵗʰ **O23.59 Infection of other part of genital tract in pregnancy**

     O23.591 Infection of other part of genital tract in pregnancy, first trimester Ⓜ♀

     O23.592 Infection of other part of genital tract in pregnancy, second trimester Ⓜ♀

     O23.593 Infection of other part of genital tract in pregnancy, third trimester Ⓜ♀

     O23.599 Infection of other part of genital tract in pregnancy, unspecified trimester Ⓜ♀▽

√5ᵗʰ **O23.9 Unspecified genitourinary tract infection in pregnancy**
Genitourinary tract infection in pregnancy NOS

     O23.90 Unspecified genitourinary tract infection in pregnancy, unspecified trimester Ⓜ♀▽

     O23.91 Unspecified genitourinary tract infection in pregnancy, first trimester Ⓜ♀▽

     O23.92 Unspecified genitourinary tract infection in pregnancy, second trimester Ⓜ♀▽

     O23.93 Unspecified genitourinary tract infection in pregnancy, third trimester Ⓜ♀▽

√4ᵗʰ **O24 Diabetes mellitus in pregnancy, childbirth and the puerperium**

√5ᵗʰ **O24.0 Pre-existing type 1 diabetes mellitus, in pregnancy, childbirth and the puerperium**
Juvenile onset diabetes mellitus, in pregnancy, childbirth and the puerperium
Ketosis-prone diabetes mellitus in pregnancy, childbirth and the puerperium
Use additional code from category E10 to further identify any manifestations

√6ᵗʰ **O24.01 Pre-existing type 1 diabetes mellitus, in pregnancy**

     O24.011 Pre-existing type 1 diabetes mellitus, in pregnancy, first trimester Ⓜ♀

     O24.012 Pre-existing type 1 diabetes mellitus, in pregnancy, second trimester Ⓜ♀

     O24.013 Pre-existing type 1 diabetes mellitus, in pregnancy, third trimester Ⓜ♀

     O24.019 Pre-existing type 1 diabetes mellitus, in pregnancy, unspecified trimester Ⓜ♀▽

     O24.02 Pre-existing type 1 diabetes mellitus, in childbirth Ⓜ♀

     O24.03 Pre-existing type 1 diabetes mellitus, in the puerperium Ⓜ♀

√5ᵗʰ **O24.1 Pre-existing type 2 diabetes mellitus, in pregnancy, childbirth and the puerperium**
Insulin-resistant diabetes mellitus in pregnancy, childbirth and the puerperium
Use additional code (for):
from category E11 to further identify any manifestations
long-term (current) use of insulin (Z79.4)

√6ᵗʰ **O24.11 Pre-existing type 2 diabetes mellitus, in pregnancy**

     O24.111 Pre-existing type 2 diabetes mellitus, in pregnancy, first trimester Ⓜ♀

     O24.112 Pre-existing type 2 diabetes mellitus, in pregnancy, second trimester Ⓜ♀

     O24.113 Pre-existing type 2 diabetes mellitus, in pregnancy, third trimester Ⓜ♀

     O24.119 Pre-existing type 2 diabetes mellitus, in pregnancy, unspecified trimester Ⓜ♀▽

     O24.12 Pre-existing type 2 diabetes mellitus, in childbirth Ⓜ♀

     O24.13 Pre-existing type 2 diabetes mellitus, in the puerperium Ⓜ♀

√5ᵗʰ **O24.3 Unspecified pre-existing diabetes mellitus in pregnancy, childbirth and the puerperium**
Use additional code (for):
from category E11 to further identify any manifestation
long-term (current) use of insulin (Z79.4)

√6ᵗʰ **O24.31 Unspecified pre-existing diabetes mellitus in pregnancy**

     O24.311 Unspecified pre-existing diabetes mellitus in pregnancy, first trimester Ⓜ♀▽

     O24.312 Unspecified pre-existing diabetes mellitus in pregnancy, second trimester Ⓜ♀▽

     O24.313 Unspecified pre-existing diabetes mellitus in pregnancy, third trimester Ⓜ♀▽

     O24.319 Unspecified pre-existing diabetes mellitus in pregnancy, unspecified trimester Ⓜ♀▽

     O24.32 Unspecified pre-existing diabetes mellitus in childbirth Ⓜ♀▽

     O24.33 Unspecified pre-existing diabetes mellitus in the puerperium Ⓜ♀▽

√5ᵗʰ **O24.4 Gestational diabetes mellitus**
Diabetes mellitus arising in pregnancy
Gestational diabetes mellitus NOS

√6ᵗʰ **O24.41 Gestational diabetes mellitus in pregnancy**

     O24.410 Gestational diabetes mellitus in pregnancy, diet controlled Ⓜ♀

     O24.414 Gestational diabetes mellitus in pregnancy, insulin controlled Ⓜ♀

     O24.415 Gestational diabetes mellitus in pregnancy, controlled by oral hypoglycemic drugs Ⓜ♀
Gestational diabetes mellitus in pregnancy, controlled by oral antidiabetic drugs

     O24.419 Gestational diabetes mellitus in pregnancy, unspecified control Ⓜ♀▽
AHA: 2015, 4Q, 34

√6ᵗʰ **O24.42 Gestational diabetes mellitus in childbirth**
AHA: 2016, 1Q, 5

     O24.420 Gestational diabetes mellitus in childbirth, diet controlled Ⓜ♀

     O24.424 Gestational diabetes mellitus in childbirth, insulin controlled Ⓜ♀

     O24.425 Gestational diabetes mellitus in childbirth, controlled by oral hypoglycemic drugs Ⓜ♀
Gestational diabetes mellitus in childbirth, controlled by oral antidiabetic drugs

     O24.429 Gestational diabetes mellitus in childbirth, unspecified control Ⓜ♀▽
AHA: 2015, 4Q, 34

√6ᵗʰ **O24.43 Gestational diabetes mellitus in the puerperium**

     O24.430 Gestational diabetes mellitus in the puerperium, diet controlled Ⓜ♀

     O24.434 Gestational diabetes mellitus in the puerperium, insulin controlled Ⓜ♀

     O24.435 Gestational diabetes mellitus in puerperium, controlled by oral hypoglycemic drugs Ⓜ♀
Gestational diabetes mellitus in puerperium, controlled by oral antidiabetic drugs

     O24.439 Gestational diabetes mellitus in the puerperium, unspecified control Ⓜ♀▽
AHA: 2015, 4Q, 34

√5ᵗʰ **O24.8 Other pre-existing diabetes mellitus in pregnancy, childbirth, and the puerperium**
Use additional code (for):
from categories E08, E09 and E13 to further identify any manifestation
long-term (current) use of insulin (Z79.4)

√6ᵗʰ **O24.81 Other pre-existing diabetes mellitus in pregnancy**

     O24.811 Other pre-existing diabetes mellitus in pregnancy, first trimester Ⓜ♀

     O24.812 Other pre-existing diabetes mellitus in pregnancy, second trimester Ⓜ♀

     O24.813 Other pre-existing diabetes mellitus in pregnancy, third trimester Ⓜ♀

     O24.819 Other pre-existing diabetes mellitus in pregnancy, unspecified trimester Ⓜ♀▽

EXCLUDES 1 Not coded here   **EXCLUDES 2** Not included here   Ⓝ Newborn Age: 0   Ⓟ Pediatric Age: 0-17   Ⓜ Maternity Age: 12-55   Ⓐ Adult Age: 15-124

832   ICD-10-CM 2018

O24.82 Other pre-existing diabetes mellitus in childbirth Ⓜ♀

O24.83 Other pre-existing diabetes mellitus in the puerperium Ⓜ♀

✓5ᵗʰ **O24.9** Unspecified diabetes mellitus in pregnancy, childbirth and the puerperium
> Use additional code for long-term (current) use of insulin (Z79.4)

  ✓6ᵗʰ **O24.91** Unspecified diabetes mellitus in pregnancy

    O24.911 Unspecified diabetes mellitus in pregnancy, first trimester Ⓜ♀▽

    O24.912 Unspecified diabetes mellitus in pregnancy, second trimester Ⓜ♀▽

    O24.913 Unspecified diabetes mellitus in pregnancy, third trimester Ⓜ♀▽

    O24.919 Unspecified diabetes mellitus in pregnancy, unspecified trimester Ⓜ♀▽

  O24.92 Unspecified diabetes mellitus in childbirth Ⓜ♀▽

  O24.93 Unspecified diabetes mellitus in the puerperium Ⓜ♀▽

✓4ᵗʰ **O25** Malnutrition in pregnancy, childbirth and the puerperium

  ✓5ᵗʰ **O25.1** Malnutrition in pregnancy

    O25.10 Malnutrition in pregnancy, unspecified trimester Ⓜ♀▽

    O25.11 Malnutrition in pregnancy, first trimester Ⓜ♀

    O25.12 Malnutrition in pregnancy, second trimester Ⓜ♀

    O25.13 Malnutrition in pregnancy, third trimester Ⓜ♀

  O25.2 Malnutrition in childbirth Ⓜ♀

  O25.3 Malnutrition in the puerperium Ⓜ♀

✓4ᵗʰ **O26** Maternal care for other conditions predominantly related to pregnancy

  ✓5ᵗʰ **O26.0** Excessive weight gain in pregnancy
> EXCLUDES 2   gestational edema (O12.0, O12.2)

    O26.00 Excessive weight gain in pregnancy, unspecified trimester Ⓜ♀▽

    O26.01 Excessive weight gain in pregnancy, first trimester Ⓜ♀

    O26.02 Excessive weight gain in pregnancy, second trimester Ⓜ♀

    O26.03 Excessive weight gain in pregnancy, third trimester Ⓜ♀

  ✓5ᵗʰ **O26.1** Low weight gain in pregnancy

    O26.10 Low weight gain in pregnancy, unspecified trimester Ⓜ♀▽

    O26.11 Low weight gain in pregnancy, first trimester Ⓜ♀

    O26.12 Low weight gain in pregnancy, second trimester Ⓜ♀

    O26.13 Low weight gain in pregnancy, third trimester Ⓜ♀

  ✓5ᵗʰ **O26.2** Pregnancy care for patient with recurrent pregnancy loss

    O26.20 Pregnancy care for patient with recurrent pregnancy loss, unspecified trimester Ⓜ♀▽

    O26.21 Pregnancy care for patient with recurrent pregnancy loss, first trimester Ⓜ♀

    O26.22 Pregnancy care for patient with recurrent pregnancy loss, second trimester Ⓜ♀

    O26.23 Pregnancy care for patient with recurrent pregnancy loss, third trimester Ⓜ♀

  ✓5ᵗʰ **O26.3** Retained intrauterine contraceptive device in pregnancy

    O26.30 Retained intrauterine contraceptive device in pregnancy, unspecified trimester Ⓜ♀▽

    O26.31 Retained intrauterine contraceptive device in pregnancy, first trimester Ⓜ♀

    O26.32 Retained intrauterine contraceptive device in pregnancy, second trimester Ⓜ♀

    O26.33 Retained intrauterine contraceptive device in pregnancy, third trimester Ⓜ♀

  ✓5ᵗʰ **O26.4** Herpes gestationis

    O26.40 Herpes gestationis, unspecified trimester Ⓜ♀▽

    O26.41 Herpes gestationis, first trimester Ⓜ♀

    O26.42 Herpes gestationis, second trimester Ⓜ♀

    O26.43 Herpes gestationis, third trimester Ⓜ♀

✓5ᵗʰ **O26.5** Maternal hypotension syndrome
> Supine hypotensive syndrome

  O26.50 Maternal hypotension syndrome, unspecified trimester Ⓜ♀▽

  O26.51 Maternal hypotension syndrome, first trimester Ⓜ♀

  O26.52 Maternal hypotension syndrome, second trimester Ⓜ♀

  O26.53 Maternal hypotension syndrome, third trimester Ⓜ♀

✓5ᵗʰ **O26.6** Liver and biliary tract disorders in pregnancy, childbirth and the puerperium
> Use additional code to identify the specific disorder
> EXCLUDES 2   hepatorenal syndrome following labor and delivery (O90.4)

  ✓6ᵗʰ **O26.61** Liver and biliary tract disorders in pregnancy

    O26.611 Liver and biliary tract disorders in pregnancy, first trimester Ⓜ♀

    O26.612 Liver and biliary tract disorders in pregnancy, second trimester Ⓜ♀

    O26.613 Liver and biliary tract disorders in pregnancy, third trimester Ⓜ♀

    O26.619 Liver and biliary tract disorders in pregnancy, unspecified trimester Ⓜ♀▽

  O26.62 Liver and biliary tract disorders in childbirth Ⓜ♀

  O26.63 Liver and biliary tract disorders in the puerperium Ⓜ♀

✓5ᵗʰ **O26.7** Subluxation of symphysis (pubis) in pregnancy, childbirth and the puerperium
> EXCLUDES 1   traumatic separation of symphysis (pubis) during childbirth (O71.6)

  ✓6ᵗʰ **O26.71** Subluxation of symphysis (pubis) in pregnancy

    O26.711 Subluxation of symphysis (pubis) in pregnancy, first trimester Ⓜ♀

    O26.712 Subluxation of symphysis (pubis) in pregnancy, second trimester Ⓜ♀

    O26.713 Subluxation of symphysis (pubis) in pregnancy, third trimester Ⓜ♀

    O26.719 Subluxation of symphysis (pubis) in pregnancy, unspecified trimester Ⓜ♀▽

  O26.72 Subluxation of symphysis (pubis) in childbirth Ⓜ♀

  O26.73 Subluxation of symphysis (pubis) in the puerperium Ⓜ♀

✓5ᵗʰ **O26.8** Other specified pregnancy related conditions

  ✓6ᵗʰ **O26.81** Pregnancy related exhaustion and fatigue

    O26.811 Pregnancy related exhaustion and fatigue, first trimester Ⓜ♀

    O26.812 Pregnancy related exhaustion and fatigue, second trimester Ⓜ♀

    O26.813 Pregnancy related exhaustion and fatigue, third trimester Ⓜ♀

    O26.819 Pregnancy related exhaustion and fatigue, unspecified trimester Ⓜ♀▽

  ✓6ᵗʰ **O26.82** Pregnancy related peripheral neuritis

    O26.821 Pregnancy related peripheral neuritis, first trimester Ⓜ♀

    O26.822 Pregnancy related peripheral neuritis, second trimester Ⓜ♀

    O26.823 Pregnancy related peripheral neuritis, third trimester Ⓜ♀

    O26.829 Pregnancy related peripheral neuritis, unspecified trimester Ⓜ♀▽

  ✓6ᵗʰ **O26.83** Pregnancy related renal disease
> Use additional code to identify the specific disorder

    O26.831 Pregnancy related renal disease, first trimester Ⓜ♀

    O26.832 Pregnancy related renal disease, second trimester Ⓜ♀

    O26.833 Pregnancy related renal disease, third trimester Ⓜ♀

    O26.839 Pregnancy related renal disease, unspecified trimester Ⓜ♀▽

☑ Additional Character Req   ✓ 7ᵗʰ Placeholder Alert   Manifestation   HCC CMS-HCC Condition   ▽ Unspecified Code   ►◄ Revised Text   ● New Code   ▲ Revised Code Title

ICD-10-CM 2018   833

Chapter 15. Pregnancy, Childbirth, and the Puerperium

✓6ᵗʰ **O26.84 Uterine size-date discrepancy complicating pregnancy**
- EXCLUDES 1   *encounter for suspected problem with fetal growth ruled out (Z03.74)*
  - **O26.841 Uterine size-date discrepancy, first trimester** Ⓜ♀
  - **O26.842 Uterine size-date discrepancy, second trimester** Ⓜ♀
  - **O26.843 Uterine size-date discrepancy, third trimester** Ⓜ♀
  - **O26.849 Uterine size-date discrepancy, unspecified trimester** Ⓜ♀▽

✓6ᵗʰ **O26.85 Spotting complicating pregnancy**
  - **O26.851 Spotting complicating pregnancy, first trimester** Ⓜ♀
  - **O26.852 Spotting complicating pregnancy, second trimester** Ⓜ♀
  - **O26.853 Spotting complicating pregnancy, third trimester** Ⓜ♀
  - **O26.859 Spotting complicating pregnancy, unspecified trimester** Ⓜ♀▽

O26.86 Pruritic urticarial papules and plaques of pregnancy (PUPPP) Ⓜ♀
    Polymorphic eruption of pregnancy

✓6ᵗʰ **O26.87 Cervical shortening**
- EXCLUDES 1   *encounter for suspected cervical shortening ruled out (Z03.75)*
- **DEF:** A cervix that has shortened to < 25 mm before the 24th week of pregnancy; warning sign for impending premature delivery; treated by cervical cerclage placement or progesterone.
  - **O26.872 Cervical shortening, second trimester** Ⓜ♀
  - **O26.873 Cervical shortening, third trimester** Ⓜ♀
  - **O26.879 Cervical shortening, unspecified trimester** Ⓜ♀▽

✓6ᵗʰ **O26.89 Other specified pregnancy related conditions**
- AHA: 2015, 3Q, 40
  - **O26.891 Other specified pregnancy related conditions, first trimester** Ⓜ♀
  - **O26.892 Other specified pregnancy related conditions, second trimester** Ⓜ♀
  - **O26.893 Other specified pregnancy related conditions, third trimester** Ⓜ♀
  - **O26.899 Other specified pregnancy related conditions, unspecified trimester** Ⓜ♀▽

✓5ᵗʰ **O26.9 Pregnancy related conditions, unspecified**
  - **O26.90 Pregnancy related conditions, unspecified, unspecified trimester** Ⓜ♀▽
  - **O26.91 Pregnancy related conditions, unspecified, first trimester** Ⓜ♀▽
  - **O26.92 Pregnancy related conditions, unspecified, second trimester** Ⓜ♀▽
  - **O26.93 Pregnancy related conditions, unspecified, third trimester** Ⓜ♀▽

✓4ᵗʰ **O28 Abnormal findings on antenatal screening of mother**
- EXCLUDES 1   *diagnostic findings classified elsewhere—see Alphabetical Index*
  - **O28.0 Abnormal hematological finding on antenatal screening of mother** Ⓜ♀
  - **O28.1 Abnormal biochemical finding on antenatal screening of mother** Ⓜ♀
  - **O28.2 Abnormal cytological finding on antenatal screening of mother** Ⓜ♀
  - **O28.3 Abnormal ultrasonic finding on antenatal screening of mother** Ⓜ♀
  - **O28.4 Abnormal radiological finding on antenatal screening of mother** Ⓜ♀
  - **O28.5 Abnormal chromosomal and genetic finding on antenatal screening of mother** Ⓜ♀
  - **O28.8 Other abnormal findings on antenatal screening of mother** Ⓜ♀
  - **O28.9 Unspecified abnormal findings on antenatal screening of mother** Ⓜ♀▽

✓4ᵗʰ **O29 Complications of anesthesia during pregnancy**
- INCLUDES   maternal complications arising from the administration of a general, regional or local anesthetic, analgesic or other sedation during pregnancy
- Use additional code, if necessary, to identify the complication
- EXCLUDES 2   *complications of anesthesia during labor and delivery (O74.-)*
    complications of anesthesia during the puerperium (O89.-)

✓5ᵗʰ **O29.0 Pulmonary complications of anesthesia during pregnancy**
- ✓6ᵗʰ **O29.01 Aspiration pneumonitis due to anesthesia during pregnancy**
  - Inhalation of stomach contents or secretions NOS due to anesthesia during pregnancy
  - Mendelson's syndrome due to anesthesia during pregnancy
  - **O29.011 Aspiration pneumonitis due to anesthesia during pregnancy, first trimester** Ⓜ♀
  - **O29.012 Aspiration pneumonitis due to anesthesia during pregnancy, second trimester** Ⓜ♀
  - **O29.013 Aspiration pneumonitis due to anesthesia during pregnancy, third trimester** Ⓜ♀
  - **O29.019 Aspiration pneumonitis due to anesthesia during pregnancy, unspecified trimester** Ⓜ♀▽
- ✓6ᵗʰ **O29.02 Pressure collapse of lung due to anesthesia during pregnancy**
  - **O29.021 Pressure collapse of lung due to anesthesia during pregnancy, first trimester** Ⓜ♀
  - **O29.022 Pressure collapse of lung due to anesthesia during pregnancy, second trimester** Ⓜ♀
  - **O29.023 Pressure collapse of lung due to anesthesia during pregnancy, third trimester** Ⓜ♀
  - **O29.029 Pressure collapse of lung due to anesthesia during pregnancy, unspecified trimester** Ⓜ♀▽
- ✓6ᵗʰ **O29.09 Other pulmonary complications of anesthesia during pregnancy**
  - **O29.091 Other pulmonary complications of anesthesia during pregnancy, first trimester** Ⓜ♀
  - **O29.092 Other pulmonary complications of anesthesia during pregnancy, second trimester** Ⓜ♀
  - **O29.093 Other pulmonary complications of anesthesia during pregnancy, third trimester** Ⓜ♀
  - **O29.099 Other pulmonary complications of anesthesia during pregnancy, unspecified trimester** Ⓜ♀▽

✓5ᵗʰ **O29.1 Cardiac complications of anesthesia during pregnancy**
- ✓6ᵗʰ **O29.11 Cardiac arrest due to anesthesia during pregnancy**
  - **O29.111 Cardiac arrest due to anesthesia during pregnancy, first trimester** Ⓜ♀
  - **O29.112 Cardiac arrest due to anesthesia during pregnancy, second trimester** Ⓜ♀
  - **O29.113 Cardiac arrest due to anesthesia during pregnancy, third trimester** Ⓜ♀
  - **O29.119 Cardiac arrest due to anesthesia during pregnancy, unspecified trimester** Ⓜ♀▽
- ✓6ᵗʰ **O29.12 Cardiac failure due to anesthesia during pregnancy**
  - **O29.121 Cardiac failure due to anesthesia during pregnancy, first trimester** Ⓜ♀
  - **O29.122 Cardiac failure due to anesthesia during pregnancy, second trimester** Ⓜ♀
  - **O29.123 Cardiac failure due to anesthesia during pregnancy, third trimester** Ⓜ♀
  - **O29.129 Cardiac failure due to anesthesia during pregnancy, unspecified trimester** Ⓜ♀▽

EXCLUDES 1 Not coded here   EXCLUDES 2 Not included here   Ⓝ Newborn Age: 0   Ⓟ Pediatric Age: 0-17   Ⓜ Maternity Age: 12-55   Ⓐ Adult Age: 15-124

834   ICD-10-CM 2018

✓6ᵗʰ O29.19 Other cardiac complications of anesthesia during pregnancy

    O29.191 Other cardiac complications of anesthesia during pregnancy, first trimester Ⓜ♀

    O29.192 Other cardiac complications of anesthesia during pregnancy, second trimester Ⓜ♀

    O29.193 Other cardiac complications of anesthesia during pregnancy, third trimester Ⓜ♀

    O29.199 Other cardiac complications of anesthesia during pregnancy, unspecified trimester Ⓜ♀▽

✓5ᵗʰ O29.2 Central nervous system complications of anesthesia during pregnancy

  ✓6ᵗʰ O29.21 Cerebral anoxia due to anesthesia during pregnancy

    O29.211 Cerebral anoxia due to anesthesia during pregnancy, first trimester Ⓜ♀

    O29.212 Cerebral anoxia due to anesthesia during pregnancy, second trimester Ⓜ♀

    O29.213 Cerebral anoxia due to anesthesia during pregnancy, third trimester Ⓜ♀

    O29.219 Cerebral anoxia due to anesthesia during pregnancy, unspecified trimester Ⓜ♀▽

  ✓6ᵗʰ O29.29 Other central nervous system complications of anesthesia during pregnancy

    O29.291 Other central nervous system complications of anesthesia during pregnancy, first trimester Ⓜ♀

    O29.292 Other central nervous system complications of anesthesia during pregnancy, second trimester Ⓜ♀

    O29.293 Other central nervous system complications of anesthesia during pregnancy, third trimester Ⓜ♀

    O29.299 Other central nervous system complications of anesthesia during pregnancy, unspecified trimester Ⓜ♀▽

✓5ᵗʰ O29.3 Toxic reaction to local anesthesia during pregnancy

  ✓6ᵗʰ O29.3X Toxic reaction to local anesthesia during pregnancy

    O29.3X1 Toxic reaction to local anesthesia during pregnancy, first trimester Ⓜ♀

    O29.3X2 Toxic reaction to local anesthesia during pregnancy, second trimester Ⓜ♀

    O29.3X3 Toxic reaction to local anesthesia during pregnancy, third trimester Ⓜ♀

    O29.3X9 Toxic reaction to local anesthesia during pregnancy, unspecified trimester Ⓜ♀▽

✓5ᵗʰ O29.4 Spinal and epidural anesthesia induced headache during pregnancy

    O29.40 Spinal and epidural anesthesia induced headache during pregnancy, unspecified trimester Ⓜ♀▽

    O29.41 Spinal and epidural anesthesia induced headache during pregnancy, first trimester Ⓜ♀

    O29.42 Spinal and epidural anesthesia induced headache during pregnancy, second trimester Ⓜ♀

    O29.43 Spinal and epidural anesthesia induced headache during pregnancy, third trimester Ⓜ♀

✓5ᵗʰ O29.5 Other complications of spinal and epidural anesthesia during pregnancy

  ✓6ᵗʰ O29.5X Other complications of spinal and epidural anesthesia during pregnancy

    O29.5X1 Other complications of spinal and epidural anesthesia during pregnancy, first trimester Ⓜ♀

    O29.5X2 Other complications of spinal and epidural anesthesia during pregnancy, second trimester Ⓜ♀

    O29.5X3 Other complications of spinal and epidural anesthesia during pregnancy, third trimester Ⓜ♀

    O29.5X9 Other complications of spinal and epidural anesthesia during pregnancy, unspecified trimester Ⓜ♀▽

✓5ᵗʰ O29.6 Failed or difficult intubation for anesthesia during pregnancy

    O29.60 Failed or difficult intubation for anesthesia during pregnancy, unspecified trimester Ⓜ♀▽

    O29.61 Failed or difficult intubation for anesthesia during pregnancy, first trimester Ⓜ♀

    O29.62 Failed or difficult intubation for anesthesia during pregnancy, second trimester Ⓜ♀

    O29.63 Failed or difficult intubation for anesthesia during pregnancy, third trimester Ⓜ♀

✓5ᵗʰ O29.8 Other complications of anesthesia during pregnancy

  ✓6ᵗʰ O29.8X Other complications of anesthesia during pregnancy

    O29.8X1 Other complications of anesthesia during pregnancy, first trimester Ⓜ♀

    O29.8X2 Other complications of anesthesia during pregnancy, second trimester Ⓜ♀

    O29.8X3 Other complications of anesthesia during pregnancy, third trimester Ⓜ♀

    O29.8X9 Other complications of anesthesia during pregnancy, unspecified trimester Ⓜ♀▽

✓5ᵗʰ O29.9 Unspecified complication of anesthesia during pregnancy

    O29.90 Unspecified complication of anesthesia during pregnancy, unspecified trimester Ⓜ♀▽

    O29.91 Unspecified complication of anesthesia during pregnancy, first trimester Ⓜ♀▽

    O29.92 Unspecified complication of anesthesia during pregnancy, second trimester Ⓜ♀▽

    O29.93 Unspecified complication of anesthesia during pregnancy, third trimester Ⓜ♀▽

Maternal care related to the fetus and amniotic cavity and possible delivery problems (O30-O48)

✓4ᵗʰ O30 Multiple gestation

Code also any complications specific to multiple gestation

✓5ᵗʰ O30.0 Twin pregnancy

  ✓6ᵗʰ O30.00 Twin pregnancy, unspecified number of placenta and unspecified number of amniotic sacs

    O30.001 Twin pregnancy, unspecified number of placenta and unspecified number of amniotic sacs, first trimester Ⓜ♀▽

    O30.002 Twin pregnancy, unspecified number of placenta and unspecified number of amniotic sacs, second trimester Ⓜ♀▽

    O30.003 Twin pregnancy, unspecified number of placenta and unspecified number of amniotic sacs, third trimester Ⓜ♀▽

    O30.009 Twin pregnancy, unspecified number of placenta and unspecified number of amniotic sacs, unspecified trimester Ⓜ♀▽

  ✓6ᵗʰ O30.01 Twin pregnancy, monochorionic/monoamniotic

Twin pregnancy, one placenta, one amniotic sac

EXCLUDES 1   conjoined twins (O30.02-)

    O30.011 Twin pregnancy, monochorionic/monoamniotic, first trimester Ⓜ♀

    O30.012 Twin pregnancy, monochorionic/monoamniotic, second trimester Ⓜ♀

    O30.013 Twin pregnancy, monochorionic/monoamniotic, third trimester Ⓜ♀

    O30.019 Twin pregnancy, monochorionic/monoamniotic, unspecified trimester Ⓜ♀▽

Twin Gestation – Monochorionic/Monoamniotic

- 1 Chorionic sac
- 1 Amniotic sac
- 2 Fetuses
- 2 Umbilical cords
- 1 Placenta

☑ Additional Character Req   ✓ׂₓ₇ᵗʰ Placeholder Alert   Manifestation   Ⓗᴄᴄ CMS-HCC Condition   ▽ Unspecified Code   ►◄ Revised Text   ● New Code   ▲ Revised Code Title

ICD-10-CM 2018   835

Twin Gestation – Monochorionic/Diamniotic

- 1 Chorionic sac
- 2 Amniotic sacs
- 2 Fetuses
- 2 Umbilical cords
- 1 Placenta

Twin Gestation – Dichorionic/Diamniotic

- 2 Chorionic sacs
- 2 Amniotic sacs
- 2 Fetuses
- 2 Umbilical cords
- 2 Placentas

✓6th **O30.02** Conjoined twin pregnancy

O30.021 Conjoined twin pregnancy, **first** trimester   Ⓜ♀

O30.022 Conjoined twin pregnancy, **second** trimester   Ⓜ♀

O30.023 Conjoined twin pregnancy, **third** trimester   Ⓜ♀

O30.029 Conjoined twin pregnancy, **unspecified trimester**   Ⓜ♀▽

✓6th **O30.03** Twin pregnancy, **monochorionic/diamniotic**
Twin pregnancy, one placenta, two amniotic sacs

O30.031 Twin pregnancy, monochorionic/ diamniotic, **first trimester**   Ⓜ♀

O30.032 Twin pregnancy, monochorionic/ diamniotic, **second trimester**   Ⓜ♀

O30.033 Twin pregnancy, monochorionic/ diamniotic, **third trimester**   Ⓜ♀

O30.039 Twin pregnancy, monochorionic/ diamniotic, **unspecified trimester**   Ⓜ♀▽

✓6th **O30.04** Twin pregnancy, **dichorionic/diamniotic**
Twin pregnancy, two placentae, two amniotic sacs

O30.041 Twin pregnancy, dichorionic/ diamniotic, **first trimester**   Ⓜ♀

O30.042 Twin pregnancy, dichorionic/ diamniotic, **second trimester**   Ⓜ♀

O30.043 Twin pregnancy, dichorionic/ diamniotic, **third trimester**   Ⓜ♀

O30.049 Twin pregnancy, dichorionic/ diamniotic, **unspecified trimester**   Ⓜ♀▽

✓6th **O30.09** Twin pregnancy, **unable to determine number of placenta and number of amniotic sacs**

O30.091 Twin pregnancy, unable to determine number of placenta and number of amniotic sacs, **first trimester**   Ⓜ♀

O30.092 Twin pregnancy, unable to determine number of placenta and number of amniotic sacs, **second trimester**   Ⓜ♀

O30.093 Twin pregnancy, unable to determine number of placenta and number of amniotic sacs, **third trimester**   Ⓜ♀

O30.099 Twin pregnancy, unable to determine number of placenta and number of amniotic sacs, **unspecified trimester**   Ⓜ♀▽

✓5th **O30.1** Triplet pregnancy

✓6th **O30.10** Triplet pregnancy, unspecified number of placenta and unspecified number of amniotic sacs
    AHA: 2016, 2Q, 8

O30.101 Triplet pregnancy, unspecified number of placenta and unspecified number of amniotic sacs, **first trimester**   Ⓜ♀▽

O30.102 Triplet pregnancy, unspecified number of placenta and unspecified number of amniotic sacs, **second trimester**   Ⓜ♀▽

O30.103 Triplet pregnancy, unspecified number of placenta and unspecified number of amniotic sacs, **third trimester**   Ⓜ♀▽

O30.109 Triplet pregnancy, unspecified number of placenta and unspecified number of amniotic sacs, **unspecified trimester**   Ⓜ♀▽

✓6th **O30.11** Triplet pregnancy with **two or more monochorionic fetuses**

O30.111 Triplet pregnancy with two or more monochorionic fetuses, **first trimester**   Ⓜ♀

O30.112 Triplet pregnancy with two or more monochorionic fetuses, **second trimester**   Ⓜ♀

O30.113 Triplet pregnancy with two or more monochorionic fetuses, **third trimester**   Ⓜ♀

O30.119 Triplet pregnancy with two or more monochorionic fetuses, **unspecified trimester**   Ⓜ♀▽

✓6th **O30.12** Triplet pregnancy with **two or more monoamniotic fetuses**

O30.121 Triplet pregnancy with two or more monoamniotic fetuses, **first trimester**   Ⓜ♀

O30.122 Triplet pregnancy with two or more monoamniotic fetuses, **second trimester**   Ⓜ♀

O30.123 Triplet pregnancy with two or more monoamniotic fetuses, **third trimester**   Ⓜ♀

O30.129 Triplet pregnancy with two or more monoamniotic fetuses, **unspecified trimester**   Ⓜ♀▽

✓6th **O30.19** Triplet pregnancy, **unable to determine number of placenta and number of amniotic sacs**

O30.191 Triplet pregnancy, unable to determine number of placenta and number of amniotic sacs, **first trimester**   Ⓜ♀

O30.192 Triplet pregnancy, unable to determine number of placenta and number of amniotic sacs, **second trimester**   Ⓜ♀

O30.193 Triplet pregnancy, unable to determine number of placenta and number of amniotic sacs, **third trimester**   Ⓜ♀

O30.199 Triplet pregnancy, unable to determine number of placenta and number of amniotic sacs, **unspecified trimester**   Ⓜ♀▽

✓5th **O30.2** Quadruplet pregnancy

✓6th **O30.20** Quadruplet pregnancy, unspecified number of placenta and unspecified number of amniotic sacs

O30.201 Quadruplet pregnancy, unspecified number of placenta and unspecified number of amniotic sacs, **first trimester**   Ⓜ♀▽

O30.202 Quadruplet pregnancy, unspecified number of placenta and unspecified number of amniotic sacs, **second trimester**   Ⓜ♀▽

EXCLUDES 1 Not coded here   EXCLUDES 2 Not included here   Ⓝ Newborn Age: 0   Ⓟ Pediatric Age: 0-17   Ⓜ Maternity Age: 12-55   🅰 Adult Age: 15-124

836   ICD-10-CM 2018

O30.203 Quadruplet pregnancy, unspecified Ⓜ♀▽
number of placenta and unspecified
number of amniotic sacs, third trimester

O30.209 Quadruplet pregnancy, unspecified Ⓜ♀▽
number of placenta and unspecified
number of amniotic sacs, unspecified
trimester

✓6ᵗʰ **O30.21** Quadruplet pregnancy with two or more
monochorionic fetuses

O30.211 Quadruplet pregnancy with two or Ⓜ♀
more monochorionic fetuses, first
trimester

O30.212 Quadruplet pregnancy with two or Ⓜ♀
more monochorionic fetuses, second
trimester

O30.213 Quadruplet pregnancy with two or Ⓜ♀
more monochorionic fetuses, third
trimester

O30.219 Quadruplet pregnancy with two or Ⓜ♀▽
more monochorionic fetuses,
unspecified trimester

✓6ᵗʰ **O30.22** Quadruplet pregnancy with two or more
monoamniotic fetuses

O30.221 Quadruplet pregnancy with two or Ⓜ♀
more monoamniotic fetuses, first
trimester

O30.222 Quadruplet pregnancy with two or Ⓜ♀
more monoamniotic fetuses, second
trimester

O30.223 Quadruplet pregnancy with two or Ⓜ♀
more monoamniotic fetuses, third
trimester

O30.229 Quadruplet pregnancy with two or Ⓜ♀▽
more monoamniotic fetuses,
unspecified trimester

✓6ᵗʰ **O30.29** Quadruplet pregnancy, unable to determine number
of placenta and number of amniotic sacs

O30.291 Quadruplet pregnancy, unable to Ⓜ♀
determine number of placenta and
number of amniotic sacs, first
trimester

O30.292 Quadruplet pregnancy, unable to Ⓜ♀
determine number of placenta and
number of amniotic sacs, second
trimester

O30.293 Quadruplet pregnancy, unable to Ⓜ♀
determine number of placenta and
number of amniotic sacs, third
trimester

O30.299 Quadruplet pregnancy, unable to Ⓜ♀▽
determine number of placenta and
number of amniotic sacs, unspecified

✓5ᵗʰ **O30.8** Other specified multiple gestation
Multiple gestation pregnancy greater than quadruplets

✓6ᵗʰ **O30.80** Other specified multiple gestation, unspecified
number of placenta and unspecified number of
amniotic sacs

O30.801 Other specified multiple gestation, Ⓜ♀▽
unspecified number of placenta and
unspecified number of amniotic sacs,
first trimester

O30.802 Other specified multiple gestation, Ⓜ♀▽
unspecified number of placenta and
unspecified number of amniotic sacs,
second trimester

O30.803 Other specified multiple gestation, Ⓜ♀▽
unspecified number of placenta and
unspecified number of amniotic sacs,
third trimester

O30.809 Other specified multiple Ⓜ♀▽
gestation,unspecified number of placenta
and unspecified number of amniotic sacs,
unspecified trimester

✓6ᵗʰ **O30.81** Other specified multiple gestation with two or more
monochorionic fetuses

O30.811 Other specified multiple gestation Ⓜ♀
with two or more monochorionic
fetuses, first trimester

O30.812 Other specified multiple gestation Ⓜ♀
with two or more monochorionic
fetuses, second trimester

O30.813 Other specified multiple gestation Ⓜ♀
with two or more monochorionic
fetuses, third trimester

O30.819 Other specified multiple gestation Ⓜ♀
with two or more monochorionic
fetuses, unspecified trimester

✓6ᵗʰ **O30.82** Other specified multiple gestation with two or more
monoamniotic fetuses

O30.821 Other specified multiple gestation Ⓜ♀
with two or more monoamniotic
fetuses, first trimester

O30.822 Other specified multiple gestation Ⓜ♀
with two or more monoamniotic
fetuses, second trimester

O30.823 Other specified multiple gestation Ⓜ♀
with two or more monoamniotic
fetuses, third trimester

O30.829 Other specified multiple gestation Ⓜ♀▽
with two or more monoamniotic
fetuses, unspecified trimester

✓6ᵗʰ **O30.89** Other specified multiple gestation, unable to
determine number of placenta and number of
amniotic sacs

O30.891 Other specified multiple gestation, Ⓜ♀
unable to determine number of
placenta and number of amniotic sacs,
first trimester

O30.892 Other specified multiple gestation, Ⓜ♀
unable to determine number of placenta
and number of amniotic sacs, second
trimester

O30.893 Other specified multiple gestation, Ⓜ♀
unable to determine number of placenta
and number of amniotic sacs, third
trimester

O30.899 Other specified multiple gestation, Ⓜ♀▽
unable to determine number of
placenta and number of amniotic
sacs, unspecified trimester

✓5ᵗʰ **O30.9** Multiple gestation, unspecified
Multiple pregnancy NOS

O30.90 Multiple gestation, unspecified, unspecified Ⓜ♀▽
trimester

O30.91 Multiple gestation, unspecified, first trimester Ⓜ♀▽

O30.92 Multiple gestation, unspecified, second Ⓜ♀▽
trimester

O30.93 Multiple gestation, unspecified, third Ⓜ♀▽
trimester

✓4ᵗʰ **O31** **Complications specific to multiple gestation**
EXCLUDES 2   delayed delivery of second twin, triplet, etc. (O63.2)
     malpresentation of one fetus or more (O32.9)
     placental transfusion syndromes (O43.0-)
AHA: 2012, 4Q, 107

One of the following 7th characters is to be assigned to each code
under category O31. 7th character 0 is for single gestations and
multiple gestations where the fetus is unspecified. 7th characters 1
through 9 are for cases of multiple gestations to identify the fetus for
which the code applies. The appropriate code from category O30,
Multiple gestation, must also be assigned when assigning a code
from category O31 that has a 7th character of 1 through 9.

0	not applicable or unspecified	4	fetus 4
1	fetus 1	5	fetus 5
2	fetus 2	9	other fetus
3	fetus 3		

✓5ᵗʰ **O31.0** Papyraceous fetus
Fetus compressus

✓x7ᵗʰ **O31.00** Papyraceous fetus, unspecified trimester Ⓜ♀▽

✓x7ᵗʰ **O31.01** Papyraceous fetus, first trimester Ⓜ♀

✓x7ᵗʰ **O31.02** Papyraceous fetus, second trimester Ⓜ♀

✓x7ᵗʰ **O31.03** Papyraceous fetus, third trimester Ⓜ♀

✓5ᵗʰ **O31.1** Continuing pregnancy after spontaneous abortion of one
fetus or more

✓x7ᵗʰ **O31.10** Continuing pregnancy after spontaneous Ⓜ♀▽
abortion of one fetus or more, unspecified
trimester

✓x7ᵗʰ **O31.11** Continuing pregnancy after spontaneous Ⓜ♀
abortion of one fetus or more, first trimester

✓ Additional Character Req   x7ᵗʰ Placeholder Alert   Manifestation   ᴴᶜᶜ CMS-HCC Condition   ▽ Unspecified Code   ►◄ Revised Text   ● New Code   ▲ Revised Code Title

ICD-10-CM 2018   837

√x7ᵗʰ **O31.12** **Continuing pregnancy after spontaneous abortion of one fetus or more, second trimester** Ⓜ♀

√x7ᵗʰ **O31.13** **Continuing pregnancy after spontaneous abortion of one fetus or more, third trimester** Ⓜ♀

√5ᵗʰ **O31.2** **Continuing pregnancy** after intrauterine death **of one fetus or more**

√x7ᵗʰ **O31.20** **Continuing pregnancy after intrauterine death of one fetus or more, unspecified trimester** Ⓜ♀▽

√x7ᵗʰ **O31.21** **Continuing pregnancy after intrauterine death of one fetus or more, first trimester** Ⓜ♀

√x7ᵗʰ **O31.22** **Continuing pregnancy after intrauterine death of one fetus or more, second trimester** Ⓜ♀

√x7ᵗʰ **O31.23** **Continuing pregnancy after intrauterine death of one fetus or more, third trimester** Ⓜ♀

√5ᵗʰ **O31.3** **Continuing pregnancy after** elective fetal reduction **of one fetus or more**
    Continuing pregnancy after selective termination of one fetus or more

√x7ᵗʰ **O31.30** **Continuing pregnancy after elective fetal reduction of one fetus or more, unspecified trimester** Ⓜ♀▽

√x7ᵗʰ **O31.31** **Continuing pregnancy after elective fetal reduction of one fetus or more, first trimester** Ⓜ♀

√x7ᵗʰ **O31.32** **Continuing pregnancy after elective fetal reduction of one fetus or more, second trimester** Ⓜ♀

√x7ᵗʰ **O31.33** **Continuing pregnancy after elective fetal reduction of one fetus or more, third trimester** Ⓜ♀

√5ᵗʰ **O31.8** **Other complications specific to multiple gestation**

√6ᵗʰ **O31.8X** **Other complications specific to multiple gestation**

√7ᵗʰ **O31.8X1** **Other complications specific to multiple gestation, first trimester** Ⓜ♀

√7ᵗʰ **O31.8X2** **Other complications specific to multiple gestation, second trimester** Ⓜ♀

√7ᵗʰ **O31.8X3** **Other complications specific to multiple gestation, third trimester** Ⓜ♀

√7ᵗʰ **O31.8X9** **Other complications specific to multiple gestation, unspecified trimester** Ⓜ♀▽

√4ᵗʰ **O32** **Maternal care for malpresentation of fetus**
    INCLUDES the listed conditions as a reason for observation, hospitalization or other obstetric care of the mother, or for cesarean delivery before onset of labor
    EXCLUDES 1 *malpresentation of fetus with obstructed labor (O64.-)*
    AHA: 2012, 4Q, 107

One of the following 7th characters is to be assigned to each code under category O32. 7th character 0 is for single gestations and multiple gestations where the fetus is unspecified. 7th characters 1 through 9 are for cases of multiple gestations to identify the fetus for which the code applies. The appropriate code from category O30, Multiple gestation, must also be assigned when assigning a code from category O32 that has a 7th character of 1 through 9.
0	not applicable or unspecified	4	fetus 4
1	fetus 1	5	fetus 5
2	fetus 2	9	other fetus
3	fetus 3		

Fetal Malpresentation

Breech

Shoulder (arm prolapse)

Mother's pelvis

Compound (extremity together with head)

Face (mentum)

Oblique

√x7ᵗʰ **O32.0** **Maternal care for** unstable lie Ⓜ♀

√x7ᵗʰ **O32.1** **Maternal care for** breech presentation Ⓜ♀
    Maternal care for buttocks presentation
    Maternal care for complete breech
    Maternal care for frank breech
    EXCLUDES 1 *footling presentation (O32.8)*
       incomplete breech (O32.8)
    DEF: Fetus presentation in a longitudinal lie with the buttocks or feet closest to birth canal; may require external cephalic version or cesarean delivery.

√x7ᵗʰ **O32.2** **Maternal care for** transverse and oblique lie Ⓜ♀
    Maternal care for oblique presentation
    Maternal care for transverse presentation

√x7ᵗʰ **O32.3** **Maternal care for** face, brow and chin presentation Ⓜ♀

√x7ᵗʰ **O32.4** **Maternal care for** high head at term Ⓜ♀
    Maternal care for failure of head to enter pelvic brim

√x7ᵗʰ **O32.6** **Maternal care for** compound presentation Ⓜ♀

√x7ᵗʰ **O32.8** **Maternal care for other** malpresentation of fetus Ⓜ♀
    Maternal care for footling presentation
    Maternal care for incomplete breech

√x7ᵗʰ **O32.9** **Maternal care for malpresentation of fetus, unspecified** Ⓜ♀▽

√4ᵗʰ **O33** **Maternal care for disproportion**
    INCLUDES the listed conditions as a reason for observation, hospitalization or other obstetric care of the mother, or for cesarean delivery before onset of labor
    EXCLUDES 1 *disproportion with obstructed labor (O65-O66)*

O33.0 **Maternal care for disproportion due to** deformity of maternal pelvic bones Ⓜ♀
    Maternal care for disproportion due to pelvic deformity causing disproportion NOS

O33.1 **Maternal care for disproportion due to** generally contracted pelvis Ⓜ♀
    Maternal care for disproportion due to contracted pelvis NOS causing disproportion

O33.2 **Maternal care for disproportion due to** inlet contraction of pelvis Ⓜ♀
    Maternal care for disproportion due to inlet contraction (pelvis) causing disproportion

√x7ᵗʰ **O33.3** **Maternal care for disproportion due to** outlet contraction of pelvis Ⓜ♀
    Maternal care for disproportion due to mid-cavity contraction (pelvis)
    Maternal care for disproportion due to outlet contraction (pelvis)

One of the following 7th characters is to be assigned to code O33.3. 7th character 0 is for single gestations and multiple gestations where the fetus is unspecified. 7th characters 1 through 9 are for cases of multiple gestations to identify the fetus for which the code applies. The appropriate code from category O30, Multiple gestation, must also be assigned when assigning code O33.3 with a 7th character of 1 through 9.
0	not applicable or unspecified	4	fetus 4
1	fetus 1	5	fetus 5
2	fetus 2	9	other fetus
3	fetus 3		

√x7ᵗʰ **O33.4** **Maternal care for disproportion of mixed maternal and fetal origin** Ⓜ♀

One of the following 7th characters is to be assigned to code O33.4. 7th character 0 is for single gestations and multiple gestations where the fetus is unspecified. 7th characters 1 through 9 are for cases of multiple gestations to identify the fetus for which the code applies. The appropriate code from category O30, Multiple gestation, must also be assigned when assigning code O33.4 with a 7th character of 1 through 9.
0	not applicable or unspecified	4	fetus 4
1	fetus 1	5	fetus 5
2	fetus 2	9	other fetus
3	fetus 3		

EXCLUDES 1 Not coded here   **EXCLUDES 2** Not included here   Ⓝ Newborn Age: 0   Ⓟ Pediatric Age: 0-17   Ⓜ Maternity Age: 12-55   Ⓐ Adult Age: 15-124

838   ICD-10-CM 2018

✓x7ᵗʰ **O33.5** **Maternal care for disproportion due to unusually large** Ⓜ♀
fetus
Maternal care for disproportion due to disproportion of fetal
origin with normally formed fetus
Maternal care for disproportion due to fetal disproportion NOS

> One of the following 7th characters is to be assigned to code
> O33.5. 7th character Ø is for single gestations and multiple
> gestations where the fetus is unspecified. 7th characters 1
> through 9 are for cases of multiple gestations to identify the
> fetus for which the code applies. The appropriate code from
> category O3Ø, Multiple gestation, must also be assigned when
> assigning code O33.5 with a 7th character of 1 through 9.
> Ø   not applicable or unspecified   4   fetus 4
> 1   fetus 1   5   fetus 5
> 2   fetus 2   9   other fetus
> 3   fetus 3

✓x7ᵗʰ **O33.6** **Maternal care for disproportion due to hydrocephalic** Ⓜ♀
fetus

> One of the following 7th characters is to be assigned to code
> O33.6. 7th character Ø is for single gestations and multiple
> gestations where the fetus is unspecified. 7th characters 1
> through 9 are for cases of multiple gestations to identify the
> fetus for which the code applies. The appropriate code from
> category O3Ø, Multiple gestation, must also be assigned when
> assigning code O33.6 with a 7th character of 1 through 9.
> Ø   not applicable or unspecified   4   fetus 4
> 1   fetus 1   5   fetus 5
> 2   fetus 2   9   other fetus
> 3   fetus 3

✓x7ᵗʰ **O33.7** **Maternal care for disproportion due to other fetal** Ⓜ♀
deformities
Maternal care for disproportion due to fetal ascites
Maternal care for disproportion due to fetal hydrops
Maternal care for disproportion due to fetal meningomyelocele
Maternal care for disproportion due to fetal sacral teratoma
Maternal care for disproportion due to fetal tumor
EXCLUDES 1   obstructed labor due to other fetal deformities (O66.3)

> One of the following 7th characters is to be assigned to code
> O33.7. 7th character Ø is for single gestations and multiple
> gestations where the fetus is unspecified. 7th characters 1
> through 9 are for cases of multiple gestations to identify the
> fetus for which the code applies. The appropriate code from
> category O3Ø, Multiple gestation, must also be assigned when
> assigning code O33.7 with a 7th character of 1 through 9.
> Ø   not applicable or unspecified   4   fetus 4
> 1   fetus 1   5   fetus 5
> 2   fetus 2   9   other fetus
> 3   fetus 3

O33.8 **Maternal care for disproportion of other origin** Ⓜ♀

O33.9 **Maternal care for disproportion, unspecified** Ⓜ♀▽
Maternal care for disproportion due to cephalopelvic
disproportion NOS
Maternal care for disproportion due to fetopelvic disproportion
NOS

✓4ᵗʰ **O34** **Maternal care for abnormality of pelvic organs**
INCLUDES   the listed conditions as a reason for hospitalization or other
obstetric care of the mother, or for cesarean delivery
before onset of labor
Code first any associated obstructed labor (O65.5)
Use additional code for specific condition

✓5ᵗʰ **O34.0** **Maternal care for congenital malformation of uterus**
Maternal care for double uterus
Maternal care for uterus bicornis
    O34.00 **Maternal care for unspecified congenital** Ⓜ♀▽
malformation of uterus, unspecified trimester
    O34.01 **Maternal care for unspecified congenital** Ⓜ♀▽
malformation of uterus, first trimester
    O34.02 **Maternal care for unspecified congenital** Ⓜ♀▽
malformation of uterus, second trimester
    O34.03 **Maternal care for unspecified congenital** Ⓜ♀▽
malformation of uterus, third trimester

✓5ᵗʰ **O34.1** **Maternal care for benign tumor of corpus uteri**
EXCLUDES 2   maternal care for benign tumor of cervix (O34.4-)
maternal care for malignant neoplasm of uterus
(O9A.1-)
    O34.10 **Maternal care for benign tumor of corpus** Ⓜ♀▽
uteri, unspecified trimester
    O34.11 **Maternal care for benign tumor of corpus uteri,** Ⓜ♀
first trimester

    O34.12 **Maternal care for benign tumor of corpus uteri,** Ⓜ♀
second trimester
    O34.13 **Maternal care for benign tumor of corpus uteri,** Ⓜ♀
third trimester

✓5ᵗʰ **O34.2** **Maternal care due to uterine scar from previous surgery**
✓6ᵗʰ   **O34.21** **Maternal care for scar from previous cesarean**
delivery
    O34.211 **Maternal care for low transverse scar** Ⓜ♀
from previous cesarean delivery
    O34.212 **Maternal care for vertical scar from** Ⓜ♀
previous cesarean delivery
Maternal care for classical scar from
previous cesarean delivery
    O34.219 **Maternal care for unspecified type** Ⓜ♀▽
scar from previous cesarean delivery
Maternal care due to uterine scar from
other transmural uterine incision
    O34.29 **Maternal care due to uterine scar from other** Ⓜ♀
previous surgery
Maternal care due to uterine scar from other
transmural uterine incision

✓5ᵗʰ **O34.3** **Maternal care for cervical incompetence**
Maternal care for cerclage with or without cervical
incompetence
Maternal care for Shirodkar suture with or without cervical
incompetence
DEF: Inadequate functioning of cervix marked by abnormal
widening during pregnancy and causing premature birth or
miscarriage.
    O34.30 **Maternal care for cervical incompetence,** Ⓜ♀▽
unspecified trimester
    O34.31 **Maternal care for cervical incompetence, first** Ⓜ♀
trimester
    O34.32 **Maternal care for cervical incompetence, second** Ⓜ♀
trimester
    O34.33 **Maternal care for cervical incompetence, third** Ⓜ♀
trimester

✓5ᵗʰ **O34.4** **Maternal care for other abnormalities of cervix**
    O34.40 **Maternal care for other abnormalities of** Ⓜ♀▽
cervix, unspecified trimester
    O34.41 **Maternal care for other abnormalities of cervix,** Ⓜ♀
first trimester
    O34.42 **Maternal care for other abnormalities of cervix,** Ⓜ♀
second trimester
    O34.43 **Maternal care for other abnormalities of cervix,** Ⓜ♀
third trimester

✓5ᵗʰ **O34.5** **Maternal care for other abnormalities of gravid uterus**
✓6ᵗʰ   **O34.51** **Maternal care for incarceration of gravid uterus**
    O34.511 **Maternal care for incarceration of** Ⓜ♀
gravid uterus, first trimester
    O34.512 **Maternal care for incarceration of** Ⓜ♀
gravid uterus, second trimester
    O34.513 **Maternal care for incarceration of** Ⓜ♀
gravid uterus, third trimester
    O34.519 **Maternal care for incarceration of** Ⓜ♀▽
gravid uterus, unspecified trimester
✓6ᵗʰ   **O34.52** **Maternal care for prolapse of gravid uterus**
    O34.521 **Maternal care for prolapse of gravid** Ⓜ♀
uterus, first trimester
    O34.522 **Maternal care for prolapse of gravid** Ⓜ♀
uterus, second trimester
    O34.523 **Maternal care for prolapse of gravid** Ⓜ♀
uterus, third trimester
    O34.529 **Maternal care for prolapse of gravid** Ⓜ♀▽
uterus, unspecified trimester
✓6ᵗʰ   **O34.53** **Maternal care for retroversion of gravid uterus**
    O34.531 **Maternal care for retroversion of** Ⓜ♀
gravid uterus, first trimester
    O34.532 **Maternal care for retroversion of** Ⓜ♀
gravid uterus, second trimester
    O34.533 **Maternal care for retroversion of** Ⓜ♀
gravid uterus, third trimester
    O34.539 **Maternal care for retroversion of** Ⓜ♀▽
gravid uterus, unspecified trimester
✓6ᵗʰ   **O34.59** **Maternal care for other abnormalities of gravid**
uterus
    O34.591 **Maternal care for other abnormalities** Ⓜ♀
of gravid uterus, first trimester

✓ Additional Character Req   ✓x7ᵗʰ Placeholder Alert   Manifestation   HCC CMS-HCC Condition   ▽ Unspecified Code   ▶◀ Revised Text   ● New Code   ▲ Revised Code Title

O34.592   Maternal care for other abnormalities of gravid uterus, second trimester Ⓜ♀

O34.593   Maternal care for other abnormalities of gravid uterus, third trimester Ⓜ♀

O34.599   Maternal care for other abnormalities of gravid uterus, unspecified trimester Ⓜ♀▽

✓5th **O34.6**   **Maternal care for** abnormality of vagina
> EXCLUDES 2   maternal care for vaginal varices in pregnancy (O22.1-)

O34.60   Maternal care for abnormality of vagina, unspecified trimester Ⓜ♀▽

O34.61   Maternal care for abnormality of vagina, first trimester Ⓜ♀

O34.62   Maternal care for abnormality of vagina, second trimester Ⓜ♀

O34.63   Maternal care for abnormality of vagina, third trimester Ⓜ♀

✓5th **O34.7**   **Maternal care for** abnormality of vulva and perineum
> EXCLUDES 2   maternal care for perineal and vulval varices in pregnancy (O22.1-)

O34.70   Maternal care for abnormality of vulva and perineum, unspecified trimester Ⓜ♀▽

O34.71   Maternal care for abnormality of vulva and perineum, first trimester Ⓜ♀

O34.72   Maternal care for abnormality of vulva and perineum, second trimester Ⓜ♀

O34.73   Maternal care for abnormality of vulva and perineum, third trimester Ⓜ♀

✓5th **O34.8**   **Maternal care for other** abnormalities of pelvic organs

O34.80   Maternal care for other abnormalities of pelvic organs, unspecified trimester Ⓜ♀▽

O34.81   Maternal care for other abnormalities of pelvic organs, first trimester Ⓜ♀

O34.82   Maternal care for other abnormalities of pelvic organs, second trimester Ⓜ♀

O34.83   Maternal care for other abnormalities of pelvic organs, third trimester Ⓜ♀

✓5th **O34.9**   **Maternal care for abnormality of pelvic organ, unspecified**

O34.90   Maternal care for abnormality of pelvic organ, unspecified, unspecified trimester Ⓜ♀▽

O34.91   Maternal care for abnormality of pelvic organ, unspecified, first trimester Ⓜ♀▽

O34.92   Maternal care for abnormality of pelvic organ, unspecified, second trimester Ⓜ♀▽

O34.93   Maternal care for abnormality of pelvic organ, unspecified, third trimester Ⓜ♀▽

✓4th **O35**   **Maternal care for known or suspected fetal abnormality and damage**
> INCLUDES   the listed conditions in the fetus as a reason for hospitalization or other obstetric care to the mother, or for termination of pregnancy

Code also any associated maternal condition
> EXCLUDES 1   encounter for suspected maternal and fetal conditions ruled out (Z03.7-)

> One of the following 7th characters is to be assigned to each code under category O35. 7th character Ø is for single gestations and multiple gestations where the fetus is unspecified. 7th characters 1 through 9 are for cases of multiple gestations to identify the fetus for which the code applies. The appropriate code from category O30, Multiple gestation, must also be assigned when assigning a code from category O35 that has a 7th character of 1 through 9.
> | | | | |
> |---|---|---|---|
> | Ø | not applicable or unspecified | 4 | fetus 4 |
> | 1 | fetus 1 | 5 | fetus 5 |
> | 2 | fetus 2 | 9 | other fetus |
> | 3 | fetus 3 | | |

✓x7th **O35.0**   **Maternal care for (suspected)** central nervous system malformation in fetus Ⓜ♀
> Maternal care for fetal anencephaly
> Maternal care for fetal hydrocephalus
> Maternal care for fetal spina bifida
> > EXCLUDES 2   chromosomal abnormality in fetus (O35.1)

✓x7th **O35.1**   **Maternal care for (suspected)** chromosomal abnormality in fetus Ⓜ♀

✓x7th **O35.2**   **Maternal care for (suspected)** hereditary disease in fetus Ⓜ♀
> > EXCLUDES 2   chromosomal abnormality in fetus (O35.1)

✓x7th **O35.3**   **Maternal care for (suspected)** damage to fetus from viral disease in mother Ⓜ♀
> Maternal care for damage to fetus from maternal cytomegalovirus infection
> Maternal care for damage to fetus from maternal rubella

✓x7th **O35.4**   **Maternal care for (suspected)** damage to fetus from alcohol Ⓜ♀

✓x7th **O35.5**   **Maternal care for (suspected)** damage to fetus by drugs Ⓜ♀
> Maternal care for damage to fetus from drug addiction

✓x7th **O35.6**   **Maternal care for (suspected)** damage to fetus by radiation Ⓜ♀

✓x7th **O35.7**   **Maternal care for (suspected)** damage to fetus by other medical procedures Ⓜ♀
> Maternal care for damage to fetus by amniocentesis
> Maternal care for damage to fetus by biopsy procedures
> Maternal care for damage to fetus by hematological investigation
> Maternal care for damage to fetus by intrauterine contraceptive device
> Maternal care for damage to fetus by intrauterine surgery

✓x7th **O35.8**   **Maternal care for other (suspected) fetal abnormality and damage** Ⓜ♀
> Maternal care for damage to fetus from maternal listeriosis
> Maternal care for damage to fetus from maternal toxoplasmosis

✓x7th **O35.9**   **Maternal care for (suspected) fetal abnormality and damage, unspecified** Ⓜ♀▽

✓4th **O36**   **Maternal care for other fetal problems**
> INCLUDES   the listed conditions in the fetus as a reason for hospitalization or other obstetric care of the mother, or for termination of pregnancy
> EXCLUDES 1   encounter for suspected maternal and fetal conditions ruled out (Z03.7-)
>   placental transfusion syndromes (O43.0-)
> EXCLUDES 2   labor and delivery complicated by fetal stress (O77.-)
> AHA: 2015, 3Q, 40

> One of the following 7th characters is to be assigned to each code under category O36. 7th character Ø is for single gestations and multiple gestations where the fetus is unspecified. 7th characters 1 through 9 are for cases of multiple gestations to identify the fetus for which the code applies. The appropriate code from category O30, Multiple gestation, must also be assigned when assigning a code from category O36 that has a 7th character of 1 through 9.
> | | | | |
> |---|---|---|---|
> | Ø | not applicable or unspecified | 4 | fetus 4 |
> | 1 | fetus 1 | 5 | fetus 5 |
> | 2 | fetus 2 | 9 | other fetus |
> | 3 | fetus 3 | | |

✓5th **O36.0**   **Maternal care for rhesus isoimmunization**
> Maternal care for Rh incompatibility (with hydrops fetalis)

✓6th **O36.01**   **Maternal care for** anti-D [Rh] antibodies
> AHA: 2014, 4Q, 17

✓7th **O36.011**   Maternal care for anti-D [Rh] antibodies, first trimester Ⓜ♀

✓7th **O36.012**   Maternal care for anti-D [Rh] antibodies, second trimester Ⓜ♀

✓7th **O36.013**   Maternal care for anti-D [Rh] antibodies, third trimester Ⓜ♀

✓7th **O36.019**   Maternal care for anti-D [Rh] antibodies, unspecified trimester Ⓜ♀▽

✓6th **O36.09**   **Maternal care for other rhesus isoimmunization**

✓7th **O36.091**   Maternal care for other rhesus isoimmunization, first trimester Ⓜ♀

✓7th **O36.092**   Maternal care for other rhesus isoimmunization, second trimester Ⓜ♀

✓7th **O36.093**   Maternal care for other rhesus isoimmunization, third trimester Ⓜ♀

✓7th **O36.099**   Maternal care for other rhesus isoimmunization, unspecified trimester Ⓜ♀▽

✓5th **O36.1**   **Maternal care for other isoimmunization**
> Maternal care for ABO isoimmunization

✓6th **O36.11**   **Maternal care for** Anti-A sensitization
> Maternal care for isoimmunization NOS (with hydrops fetalis)

✓7th **O36.111**   Maternal care for Anti-A sensitization, first trimester Ⓜ♀

✓7th **O36.112**   Maternal care for Anti-A sensitization, second trimester Ⓜ♀

✓7th **O36.113**   Maternal care for Anti-A sensitization, third trimester Ⓜ♀

EXCLUDES 1 Not coded here   EXCLUDES 2 Not included here   Ⓝ Newborn Age: 0   Ⓟ Pediatric Age: 0-17   Ⓜ Maternity Age: 12-55   Ⓐ Adult Age: 15-124

840   ICD-10-CM 2018

√7ᵗʰ **O36.119** **Maternal care for Anti-A**   Ⓜ♀▽
     sensitization, unspecified trimester

√6ᵗʰ **O36.19** **Maternal care for other isoimmunization**
     Maternal care for Anti-B sensitization

√7ᵗʰ **O36.191** **Maternal care for other**   Ⓜ♀
     isoimmunization, first trimester

√7ᵗʰ **O36.192** **Maternal care for other**   Ⓜ♀
     isoimmunization, second trimester

√7ᵗʰ **O36.193** **Maternal care for other**   Ⓜ♀
     isoimmunization, third trimester

√7ᵗʰ **O36.199** **Maternal care for other**   Ⓜ♀▽
     isoimmunization, unspecified trimester

√5ᵗʰ **O36.2** **Maternal care for hydrops fetalis**
     Maternal care for hydrops fetalis NOS
     Maternal care for hydrops fetalis not associated with isoimmunization
     EXCLUDES 1   hydrops fetalis associated with ABO isoimmunization (O36.1-)
        hydrops fetalis associated with rhesus isoimmunization (O36.0-)

√x7ᵗʰ **O36.20** **Maternal care for hydrops fetalis,** unspecified   Ⓜ♀▽
     trimester

√x7ᵗʰ **O36.21** **Maternal care for hydrops fetalis,** first   Ⓜ♀
     trimester

√x7ᵗʰ **O36.22** **Maternal care for hydrops fetalis,** second   Ⓜ♀
     trimester

√x7ᵗʰ **O36.23** **Maternal care for hydrops fetalis,** third   Ⓜ♀
     trimester

√x7ᵗʰ **O36.4** **Maternal care for intrauterine death**   Ⓜ♀
     Maternal care for intrauterine fetal death NOS
     Maternal care for intrauterine fetal death after completion of 20 weeks of gestation
     Maternal care for late fetal death
     Maternal care for missed delivery
     EXCLUDES 1   missed abortion (O02.1)
        stillbirth (P95)

√5ᵗʰ **O36.5** **Maternal care for known or suspected poor fetal growth**

√6ᵗʰ **O36.51** **Maternal care for known or suspected placental insufficiency**

√7ᵗʰ **O36.511** **Maternal care for known or suspected**   Ⓜ♀
     placental insufficiency, first trimester

√7ᵗʰ **O36.512** **Maternal care for known or suspected**   Ⓜ♀
     placental insufficiency, second trimester

√7ᵗʰ **O36.513** **Maternal care for known or suspected**   Ⓜ♀
     placental insufficiency, third trimester

√7ᵗʰ **O36.519** **Maternal care for known or**   Ⓜ♀▽
     suspected placental insufficiency, unspecified trimester

√6ᵗʰ **O36.59** **Maternal care for other known or suspected poor fetal growth**
     Maternal care for known or suspected light-for-dates NOS
     Maternal care for known or suspected small-for-dates NOS

√7ᵗʰ **O36.591** **Maternal care for other known or**   Ⓜ♀
     suspected poor fetal growth, first trimester

√7ᵗʰ **O36.592** **Maternal care for other known or**   Ⓜ♀
     suspected poor fetal growth, second trimester

√7ᵗʰ **O36.593** **Maternal care for other known or**   Ⓜ♀
     suspected poor fetal growth, third trimester

√7ᵗʰ **O36.599** **Maternal care for other known or**   Ⓜ♀▽
     suspected poor fetal growth, unspecified trimester

√5ᵗʰ **O36.6** **Maternal care for excessive fetal growth**
     Maternal care for known or suspected large-for-dates

√x7ᵗʰ **O36.60** **Maternal care for excessive fetal growth,**   Ⓜ♀▽
     unspecified trimester

√x7ᵗʰ **O36.61** **Maternal care for excessive fetal growth,**   Ⓜ♀
     first trimester

√x7ᵗʰ **O36.62** **Maternal care for excessive fetal growth,**   Ⓜ♀
     second trimester

√x7ᵗʰ **O36.63** **Maternal care for excessive fetal growth,**   Ⓜ♀
     third trimester

√5ᵗʰ **O36.7** **Maternal care for viable fetus in abdominal pregnancy**

√x7ᵗʰ **O36.70** **Maternal care for viable fetus in abdominal**   Ⓜ♀▽
     pregnancy, unspecified trimester

√x7ᵗʰ **O36.71** **Maternal care for viable fetus in abdominal**   Ⓜ♀
     pregnancy, first trimester

√x7ᵗʰ **O36.72** **Maternal care for viable fetus in abdominal**   Ⓜ♀
     pregnancy, second trimester

√x7ᵗʰ **O36.73** **Maternal care for viable fetus in abdominal**   Ⓜ♀
     pregnancy, third trimester

√5ᵗʰ **O36.8** **Maternal care for other specified fetal problems**

√x7ᵗʰ **O36.80** **Pregnancy with inconclusive fetal viability**   Ⓜ♀
     Encounter to determine fetal viability of pregnancy

√6ᵗʰ **O36.81** **Decreased fetal movements**

√7ᵗʰ **O36.812** **Decreased fetal movements,** second   Ⓜ♀
     trimester

√7ᵗʰ **O36.813** **Decreased fetal movements,** third   Ⓜ♀
     trimester

√7ᵗʰ **O36.819** **Decreased fetal movements,**   Ⓜ♀▽
     unspecified trimester

√6ᵗʰ **O36.82** **Fetal anemia and thrombocytopenia**

√7ᵗʰ **O36.821** **Fetal anemia and thrombocytopenia,**   Ⓜ♀
     first trimester

√7ᵗʰ **O36.822** **Fetal anemia and thrombocytopenia,**   Ⓜ♀
     second trimester

√7ᵗʰ **O36.823** **Fetal anemia and thrombocytopenia,**   Ⓜ♀
     third trimester

√7ᵗʰ **O36.829** **Fetal anemia and**   Ⓜ♀▽
     thrombocytopenia, unspecified trimester

√6ᵗʰ **O36.83** **Maternal care for abnormalities of the fetal heart rate or rhythm**

√7ᵗʰ **O36.831** **Maternal care for abnormalities of the**
     fetal heart rate or rhythm, first trimester

√7ᵗʰ **O36.832** **Maternal care for abnormalities of the**
     fetal heart rate or rhythm, second trimester

√7ᵗʰ **O36.833** **Maternal care for abnormalities of the**
     fetal heart rate or rhythm, third trimester

√7ᵗʰ **O36.839** **Maternal care for abnormalities of the**   ▽
     fetal heart rate or rhythm, unspecified trimester

√6ᵗʰ **O36.89** **Maternal care for other specified fetal problems**

√7ᵗʰ **O36.891** **Maternal care for other specified fetal**   Ⓜ♀
     problems, first trimester

√7ᵗʰ **O36.892** **Maternal care for other specified fetal**   Ⓜ♀
     problems, second trimester

√7ᵗʰ **O36.893** **Maternal care for other specified fetal**   Ⓜ♀
     problems, third trimester

√7ᵗʰ **O36.899** **Maternal care for other specified**   Ⓜ♀▽
     fetal problems, unspecified trimester

√5ᵗʰ **O36.9** **Maternal care for fetal problem, unspecified**

√x7ᵗʰ **O36.90** **Maternal care for fetal problem, unspecified,**   Ⓜ♀▽
     unspecified trimester

√x7ᵗʰ **O36.91** **Maternal care for fetal problem, unspecified,**   Ⓜ♀▽
     first trimester

√x7ᵗʰ **O36.92** **Maternal care for fetal problem, unspecified,**   Ⓜ♀▽
     second trimester

√x7ᵗʰ **O36.93** **Maternal care for fetal problem, unspecified,**   Ⓜ♀▽
     third trimester

√4ᵗʰ **O40** **Polyhydramnios**
     Hydramnios
     EXCLUDES 1   encounter for suspected maternal and fetal conditions ruled out (Z03.7-)
     AHA: 2016, 1Q, 4

> One of the following 7th characters is to be assigned to each code under category O40. 7th character 0 is for single gestations and multiple gestations where the fetus is unspecified. 7th characters 1 through 9 are for cases of multiple gestations to identify the fetus for which the code applies. The appropriate code from category O30, Multiple gestation, must also be assigned when assigning a code from category O40 that has a 7th character of 1 through 9.
>
> 0   not applicable or unspecified   4   fetus 4
> 1   fetus 1   5   fetus 5
> 2   fetus 2   9   other fetus
> 3   fetus 3

√x7ᵗʰ **O40.1** **Polyhydramnios,** first trimester   Ⓜ♀

☑ Additional Character Req   √x7ᵗʰ Placeholder Alert   Manifestation   ᴴᶜᶜ CMS-HCC Condition   ▽ Unspecified Code   ▶◀ Revised Text   ● New Code   ▲ Revised Code Title

ICD-10-CM 2018   841

√x7ᵗʰ **O40.2** **Polyhydramnios,** second trimester   Ⓜ♀

√x7ᵗʰ **O40.3** **Polyhydramnios,** third trimester   Ⓜ♀

√x7ᵗʰ **O40.9** **Polyhydramnios,** unspecified trimester   Ⓜ♀▽

√4ᵗʰ **O41** **Other disorders of amniotic fluid and membranes**

     EXCLUDES 1   *encounter for suspected maternal and fetal conditions ruled out (Z03.7-)*

> One of the following 7th characters is to be assigned to each code under category O41. 7th character Ø is for single gestations and multiple gestations where the fetus is unspecified. 7th characters 1 through 9 are for cases of multiple gestations to identify the fetus for which the code applies. The appropriate code from category O30, Multiple gestation, must also be assigned when assigning a code from category O41 that has a 7th character of 1 through 9.
>
> | | | | |
> |---|---|---|---|
> | Ø | not applicable or unspecified | 4 | fetus 4 |
> | 1 | fetus 1 | 5 | fetus 5 |
> | 2 | fetus 2 | 9 | other fetus |
> | 3 | fetus 3 | | |

√5ᵗʰ **O41.0** **Oligohydramnios**

     Oligohydramnios without rupture of membranes

√x7ᵗʰ **O41.00** **Oligohydramnios,** unspecified trimester   Ⓜ♀▽

√x7ᵗʰ **O41.01** **Oligohydramnios,** first trimester   Ⓜ♀

√x7ᵗʰ **O41.02** **Oligohydramnios,** second trimester   Ⓜ♀

√x7ᵗʰ **O41.03** **Oligohydramnios,** third trimester   Ⓜ♀

√5ᵗʰ **O41.1** **Infection of amniotic sac and membranes**

√6ᵗʰ **O41.10** **Infection of amniotic sac and membranes, unspecified**

√7ᵗʰ **O41.101** **Infection of amniotic sac and membranes, unspecified, first trimester**   Ⓜ♀▽

√7ᵗʰ **O41.102** **Infection of amniotic sac and membranes, unspecified, second trimester**   Ⓜ♀▽

√7ᵗʰ **O41.103** **Infection of amniotic sac and membranes, unspecified, third trimester**   Ⓜ♀▽

√7ᵗʰ **O41.109** **Infection of amniotic sac and membranes, unspecified, unspecified trimester**   Ⓜ♀▽

√6ᵗʰ **O41.12** **Chorioamnionitis**

√7ᵗʰ **O41.121** **Chorioamnionitis,** first trimester   Ⓜ♀

√7ᵗʰ **O41.122** **Chorioamnionitis,** second trimester   Ⓜ♀

√7ᵗʰ **O41.123** **Chorioamnionitis,** third trimester   Ⓜ♀

√7ᵗʰ **O41.129** **Chorioamnionitis,** unspecified trimester   Ⓜ♀▽

√6ᵗʰ **O41.14** **Placentitis**

√7ᵗʰ **O41.141** **Placentitis,** first trimester   Ⓜ♀

√7ᵗʰ **O41.142** **Placentitis,** second trimester   Ⓜ♀

√7ᵗʰ **O41.143** **Placentitis,** third trimester   Ⓜ♀

√7ᵗʰ **O41.149** **Placentitis,** unspecified trimester   Ⓜ♀▽

√5ᵗʰ **O41.8** **Other specified disorders of amniotic fluid and membranes**

√6ᵗʰ **O41.8X** **Other specified disorders of amniotic fluid and membranes**

√7ᵗʰ **O41.8X1** **Other specified disorders of amniotic fluid and membranes,** first trimester   Ⓜ♀

√7ᵗʰ **O41.8X2** **Other specified disorders of amniotic fluid and membranes,** second trimester   Ⓜ♀

√7ᵗʰ **O41.8X3** **Other specified disorders of amniotic fluid and membranes,** third trimester   Ⓜ♀

√7ᵗʰ **O41.8X9** **Other specified disorders of amniotic fluid and membranes, unspecified trimester**   Ⓜ♀▽

√5ᵗʰ **O41.9** **Disorder of amniotic fluid and membranes, unspecified**

√x7ᵗʰ **O41.90** **Disorder of amniotic fluid and membranes, unspecified, unspecified trimester**   Ⓜ♀▽

√x7ᵗʰ **O41.91** **Disorder of amniotic fluid and membranes, unspecified,** first trimester   Ⓜ♀▽

√x7ᵗʰ **O41.92** **Disorder of amniotic fluid and membranes, unspecified,** second trimester   Ⓜ♀▽

√x7ᵗʰ **O41.93** **Disorder of amniotic fluid and membranes, unspecified,** third trimester   Ⓜ♀▽

√4ᵗʰ **O42** **Premature rupture of membranes**

     AHA: 2016, 1Q, 3

√5ᵗʰ **O42.0** **Premature rupture of membranes,** onset of labor within 24 hours of rupture

O42.00 **Premature rupture of membranes, onset of labor within 24 hours of rupture, unspecified weeks of gestation**   Ⓜ♀▽

√6ᵗʰ **O42.01** **Preterm premature rupture of membranes, onset of labor within 24 hours of rupture**

     Premature rupture of membranes before 37 completed weeks of gestation

O42.011 **Preterm premature rupture of membranes, onset of labor within 24 hours of rupture,** first trimester   Ⓜ♀

O42.012 **Preterm premature rupture of membranes, onset of labor within 24 hours of rupture,** second trimester   Ⓜ♀

O42.013 **Preterm premature rupture of membranes, onset of labor within 24 hours of rupture,** third trimester   Ⓜ♀

O42.019 **Preterm premature rupture of membranes, onset of labor within 24 hours of rupture,** unspecified trimester   Ⓜ♀▽

O42.02 **Full-term** premature rupture of membranes, onset of labor within 24 hours of rupture   Ⓜ♀

     Premature rupture of membranes at or after 37 completed weeks of gestation, onset of labor within 24 hours of rupture

√5ᵗʰ **O42.1** **Premature rupture of membranes,** onset of labor more than 24 hours following rupture

     AHA: 2016, 1Q, 5

O42.10 **Premature rupture of membranes, onset of labor more than 24 hours following rupture, unspecified weeks of gestation**   Ⓜ♀▽

√6ᵗʰ **O42.11** **Preterm** premature rupture of membranes, onset of labor more than 24 hours following rupture

     Premature rupture of membranes before 37 completed weeks of gestation

O42.111 **Preterm premature rupture of membranes, onset of labor more than 24 hours following rupture,** first trimester   Ⓜ♀

O42.112 **Preterm premature rupture of membranes, onset of labor more than 24 hours following rupture,** second trimester   Ⓜ♀

O42.113 **Preterm premature rupture of membranes, onset of labor more than 24 hours following rupture,** third trimester   Ⓜ♀

O42.119 **Preterm premature rupture of membranes, onset of labor more than 24 hours following rupture, unspecified trimester**   Ⓜ♀▽

O42.12 **Full-term** premature rupture of membranes, onset of labor more than 24 hours following rupture   Ⓜ♀

     Premature rupture of membranes at or after 37 completed weeks of gestation, onset of labor within 24 hours of rupture

√5ᵗʰ **O42.9** **Premature rupture of membranes,** unspecified as to length of time between rupture and onset of labor

O42.90 **Premature rupture of membranes, unspecified as to length of time between rupture and onset of labor, unspecified weeks of gestation**   Ⓜ♀▽

√6ᵗʰ **O42.91** **Preterm** premature rupture of membranes, unspecified as to length of time between rupture and onset of labor

     Premature rupture of membranes before 37 completed weeks of gestation

O42.911 **Preterm premature rupture of membranes, unspecified as to length of time between rupture and onset of labor,** first trimester   Ⓜ♀▽

O42.912 **Preterm premature rupture of membranes, unspecified as to length of time between rupture and onset of labor,** second trimester   Ⓜ♀

O42.913 **Preterm premature rupture of membranes, unspecified as to length of time between rupture and onset of labor,** third trimester   Ⓜ♀▽

EXCLUDES 1 Not coded here   EXCLUDES 2 Not included here   Ⓝ Newborn Age: 0   Ⓟ Pediatric Age: 0-17   Ⓜ Maternity Age: 12-55   Ⓐ Adult Age: 15-124

842   ICD-10-CM 2018

Twin to Twin Transfusion Syndrome (TTTS)

Healthy twins   Twins with TTTS

O42.919 **Preterm premature rupture of** Ⓜ♀▽
membranes, unspecified as to length
of time between rupture and onset of
labor, unspecified trimester

O42.92 **Full-term** premature rupture of membranes, Ⓜ♀▽
unspecified as to length of time between
rupture and onset of labor
Premature rupture of membranes at or after 37
completed weeks of gestation, unspecified as to
length of time between rupture and onset of
labor

✅4ᵗʰ **O43** **Placental disorders**
EXCLUDES 2 *maternal care for poor fetal growth due to placental*
insufficiency (O36.5-)
placenta previa (O44.-)
placental polyp (O90.89)
placentitis (O41.14-)
premature separation of placenta [abruptio placentae] (O45.-)

✅5ᵗʰ **O43.0** **Placental transfusion syndromes**

✅6ᵗʰ **O43.01** **Fetomaternal** placental transfusion syndrome
Maternofetal placental transfusion syndrome

O43.011 **Fetomaternal placental transfusion** Ⓜ♀
syndrome, first trimester

O43.012 **Fetomaternal placental transfusion** Ⓜ♀
syndrome, second trimester

O43.013 **Fetomaternal placental transfusion** Ⓜ♀
syndrome, third trimester

O43.019 **Fetomaternal placental transfusion** Ⓜ♀▽
syndrome, unspecified trimester

✅6ᵗʰ **O43.02** **Fetus-to-fetus** placental transfusion syndrome

O43.021 **Fetus-to-fetus placental transfusion** Ⓜ♀
syndrome, first trimester

O43.022 **Fetus-to-fetus placental transfusion** Ⓜ♀
syndrome, second trimester

O43.023 **Fetus-to-fetus placental transfusion** Ⓜ♀
syndrome, third trimester

O43.029 **Fetus-to-fetus placental transfusion** Ⓜ♀▽
syndrome, unspecified trimester

✅5ᵗʰ **O43.1** **Malformation of placenta**

✅6ᵗʰ **O43.10** **Malformation of placenta, unspecified**
Abnormal placenta NOS

O43.101 **Malformation of placenta,** Ⓜ♀▽
unspecified, first trimester

O43.102 **Malformation of placenta,** Ⓜ♀▽
unspecified, second trimester

O43.103 **Malformation of placenta,** Ⓜ♀▽
unspecified, third trimester

O43.109 **Malformation of placenta,** Ⓜ♀▽
unspecified, unspecified trimester

✅6ᵗʰ **O43.11** **Circumvallate** placenta

O43.111 **Circumvallate placenta,** first trimester Ⓜ♀

O43.112 **Circumvallate placenta,** second Ⓜ♀
trimester

O43.113 **Circumvallate placenta,** third Ⓜ♀
trimester

O43.119 **Circumvallate placenta, unspecified** Ⓜ♀▽
trimester

✅6ᵗʰ **O43.12** **Velamentous insertion of umbilical cord**

O43.121 **Velamentous insertion of umbilical** Ⓜ♀
cord, first trimester

O43.122 **Velamentous insertion of umbilical** Ⓜ♀
cord, second trimester

O43.123 **Velamentous insertion of umbilical** Ⓜ♀
cord, third trimester

O43.129 **Velamentous insertion of umbilical** Ⓜ♀▽
cord, unspecified trimester

✅6ᵗʰ **O43.19** **Other malformation of placenta**

O43.191 **Other malformation of placenta,** Ⓜ♀
first trimester

O43.192 **Other malformation of placenta,** Ⓜ♀
second trimester

O43.193 **Other malformation of placenta,** Ⓜ♀
third trimester

O43.199 **Other malformation of placenta,** Ⓜ♀▽
unspecified trimester

✅5ᵗʰ **O43.2** **Morbidly adherent placenta**
Code also associated third stage postpartum hemorrhage, if
applicable (O72.0)
EXCLUDES 1 *retained placenta (O73.-)*

✅6ᵗʰ **O43.21** **Placenta** accreta

O43.211 **Placenta accreta,** first trimester Ⓜ♀

O43.212 **Placenta accreta,** second trimester Ⓜ♀

O43.213 **Placenta accreta,** third trimester Ⓜ♀

O43.219 **Placenta accreta, unspecified** Ⓜ♀▽
trimester

✅6ᵗʰ **O43.22** **Placenta** increta

O43.221 **Placenta increta,** first trimester Ⓜ♀

O43.222 **Placenta increta,** second trimester Ⓜ♀

O43.223 **Placenta increta,** third trimester Ⓜ♀

O43.229 **Placenta increta, unspecified** Ⓜ♀▽
trimester

✅6ᵗʰ **O43.23** **Placenta** percreta

O43.231 **Placenta percreta,** first trimester Ⓜ♀

O43.232 **Placenta percreta,** second trimester Ⓜ♀

O43.233 **Placenta percreta,** third trimester Ⓜ♀

O43.239 **Placenta percreta, unspecified** Ⓜ♀▽
trimester

✅5ᵗʰ **O43.8** **Other placental disorders**

✅6ᵗʰ **O43.81** **Placental infarction**

O43.811 **Placental infarction,** first trimester Ⓜ♀

O43.812 **Placental infarction,** second trimester Ⓜ♀

O43.813 **Placental infarction,** third trimester Ⓜ♀

O43.819 **Placental infarction,** unspecified Ⓜ♀▽
trimester

✅6ᵗʰ **O43.89** **Other placental disorders**
Placental dysfunction

O43.891 **Other placental disorders,** first Ⓜ♀
trimester

O43.892 **Other placental disorders,** second Ⓜ♀
trimester

O43.893 **Other placental disorders,** third Ⓜ♀
trimester

O43.899 **Other placental disorders,** Ⓜ♀▽
unspecified trimester

✅5ᵗʰ **O43.9** **Unspecified placental disorder**

O43.90 **Unspecified placental disorder,** unspecified Ⓜ♀▽
trimester

O43.91 **Unspecified placental disorder,** first trimester Ⓜ♀▽

O43.92 **Unspecified placental disorder,** second Ⓜ♀▽
trimester

O43.93 **Unspecified placental disorder,** third Ⓜ♀▽
trimester

✅4ᵗʰ **O44** **Placenta previa**
DEF: Placenta implanted in lower segment of uterus; commonly causes
hemorrhage in the last trimester of pregnancy.

✅5ᵗʰ **O44.0** **Complete** placenta previa NOS or without hemorrhage
Placenta previa NOS

O44.00 **Complete placenta previa NOS or without** Ⓜ♀▽
hemorrhage, unspecified trimester

O44.01 **Complete placenta previa NOS or without** Ⓜ♀
hemorrhage, first trimester

✅ Additional Character Req   ✓7ᵗʰ Placeholder Alert   Manifestation   HCC CMS-HCC Condition   ▽Unspecified Code   ▶◀ Revised Text   ● New Code   ▲ Revised Code Title

ICD-10-CM 2018   **843**

O44.02   Complete placenta previa NOS or without hemorrhage, second trimester   M♀

O44.03   Complete placenta previa NOS or without hemorrhage, third trimester   M♀

✓5th **O44.1** Complete **placenta previa** with hemorrhage
> EXCLUDES 1   labor and delivery complicated by hemorrhage from vasa previa (O69.4)

O44.10   Complete placenta previa with hemorrhage, unspecified trimester   M♀▽

O44.11   Complete placenta previa with hemorrhage, first trimester   M♀

O44.12   Complete placenta previa with hemorrhage, second trimester   M♀

O44.13   Complete placenta previa with hemorrhage, third trimester   M♀

✓5th **O44.2** Partial **placenta previa** without hemorrhage
> Marginal placenta previa, NOS or without hemorrhage

O44.20   Partial placenta previa NOS or without hemorrhage, unspecified trimester   M♀▽

O44.21   Partial placenta previa NOS or without hemorrhage, first trimester   M♀

O44.22   Partial placenta previa NOS or without hemorrhage, second trimester   M♀

O44.23   Partial placenta previa NOS or without hemorrhage, third trimester   M♀

✓5th **O44.3** Partial **placenta previa** with hemorrhage
> Marginal placenta previa with hemorrhage

O44.30   Partial placenta previa with hemorrhage, unspecified trimester   M♀▽

O44.31   Partial placenta previa with hemorrhage, first trimester   M♀

O44.32   Partial placenta previa with hemorrhage, second trimester   M♀

O44.33   Partial placenta previa with hemorrhage, third trimester   M♀

✓5th **O44.4** Low lying **placenta NOS** or without hemorrhage
> Low implantation of placenta NOS or without hemorrhage

O44.40   Low lying placenta NOS or without hemorrhage, unspecified trimester   M♀▽

O44.41   Low lying placenta NOS or without hemorrhage, first trimester   M♀

O44.42   Low lying placenta NOS or without hemorrhage, second trimester   M♀

O44.43   Low lying placenta NOS or without hemorrhage, third trimester   M♀

✓5th **O44.5** Low lying **placenta** with hemorrhage
> Low implantation of placenta with hemorrhage

O44.50   Low lying placenta with hemorrhage, unspecified trimester   M♀▽

O44.51   Low lying placenta with hemorrhage, first trimester   M♀

O44.52   Low lying placenta with hemorrhage, second trimester   M♀

O44.53   Low lying placenta with hemorrhage, third trimester   M♀

✓4th **O45** Premature separation of placenta [abruptio placentae]

✓5th **O45.0** Premature separation of placenta with coagulation defect

✓6th **O45.00** Premature separation of placenta with coagulation defect, unspecified

O45.001   Premature separation of placenta with coagulation defect, unspecified, first trimester   M♀▽

O45.002   Premature separation of placenta with coagulation defect, unspecified, second trimester   M♀▽

O45.003   Premature separation of placenta with coagulation defect, unspecified, third trimester   M♀▽

O45.009   Premature separation of placenta with coagulation defect, unspecified, unspecified trimester   M♀▽

✓6th **O45.01** Premature separation of placenta with afibrinogenemia
> Premature separation of placenta with hypofibrinogenemia

O45.011   Premature separation of placenta with afibrinogenemia, first trimester   M♀

O45.012   Premature separation of placenta with afibrinogenemia, second trimester   M♀

O45.013   Premature separation of placenta with afibrinogenemia, third trimester   M♀

O45.019   Premature separation of placenta with afibrinogenemia, unspecified trimester   M♀▽

✓6th **O45.02** Premature separation of placenta with disseminated intravascular coagulation

O45.021   Premature separation of placenta with disseminated intravascular coagulation, first trimester   M♀

O45.022   Premature separation of placenta with disseminated intravascular coagulation, second trimester   M♀

O45.023   Premature separation of placenta with disseminated intravascular coagulation, third trimester   M♀

O45.029   Premature separation of placenta with disseminated intravascular coagulation, unspecified trimester   M♀▽

✓6th **O45.09** Premature separation of placenta with other coagulation defect

O45.091   Premature separation of placenta with other coagulation defect, first trimester   M♀

O45.092   Premature separation of placenta with other coagulation defect, second trimester   M♀

O45.093   Premature separation of placenta with other coagulation defect, third trimester   M♀

O45.099   Premature separation of placenta with other coagulation defect, unspecified trimester   M♀▽

✓5th **O45.8** Other premature separation of placenta

✓6th **O45.8X** Other premature separation of placenta

O45.8X1   Other premature separation of placenta, first trimester   M♀

O45.8X2   Other premature separation of placenta, second trimester   M♀

O45.8X3   Other premature separation of placenta, third trimester   M♀

O45.8X9   Other premature separation of placenta, unspecified trimester   M♀▽

✓5th **O45.9** Premature separation of placenta, unspecified
> Abruptio placentae NOS

O45.90   Premature separation of placenta, unspecified, unspecified trimester   M♀▽

O45.91   Premature separation of placenta, unspecified, first trimester   M♀▽

O45.92   Premature separation of placenta, unspecified, second trimester   M♀▽

O45.93   Premature separation of placenta, unspecified, third trimester   M♀▽

✓4th **O46** Antepartum hemorrhage, not elsewhere classified
> EXCLUDES 1   hemorrhage in early pregnancy (O20.-)
> intrapartum hemorrhage NEC (O67.-)
> placenta previa (O44.-)
> premature separation of placenta [abruptio placentae] (O45.-)
> **DEF:** Uterine hemorrhage prior to delivery; not related to placenta previa or abruptio placentae.

✓5th **O46.0** Antepartum hemorrhage with coagulation defect

✓6th **O46.00** Antepartum hemorrhage with coagulation defect, unspecified

O46.001   Antepartum hemorrhage with coagulation defect, unspecified, first trimester   M♀▽

O46.002   Antepartum hemorrhage with coagulation defect, unspecified, second trimester   M♀▽

O46.003   Antepartum hemorrhage with coagulation defect, unspecified, third trimester   M♀▽

O46.009   Antepartum hemorrhage with coagulation defect, unspecified, unspecified trimester   M♀▽

EXCLUDES 1 Not coded here   EXCLUDES 2 Not included here   N Newborn Age: 0   P Pediatric Age: 0-17   M Maternity Age: 12-55   A Adult Age: 15-124

844   ICD-10-CM 2018

√6ᵗʰ **O46.01 Antepartum hemorrhage** with afibrinogenemia
Antepartum hemorrhage with hypofibrinogenemia

    O46.011 Antepartum hemorrhage with Ⓜ♀
afibrinogenemia, **first trimester**

    O46.012 Antepartum hemorrhage with Ⓜ♀
afibrinogenemia, **second trimester**

    O46.013 Antepartum hemorrhage with Ⓜ♀
afibrinogenemia, **third trimester**

    O46.019 Antepartum hemorrhage with Ⓜ♀▽
afibrinogenemia, **unspecified trimester**

√6ᵗʰ **O46.02 Antepartum hemorrhage** with disseminated intravascular coagulation

    O46.021 Antepartum hemorrhage with Ⓜ♀
disseminated intravascular coagulation, **first trimester**

    O46.022 Antepartum hemorrhage with Ⓜ♀
disseminated intravascular coagulation, **second trimester**

    O46.023 Antepartum hemorrhage with Ⓜ♀
disseminated intravascular coagulation, **third trimester**

    O46.029 Antepartum hemorrhage with Ⓜ♀▽
disseminated intravascular coagulation, **unspecified trimester**

√6ᵗʰ **O46.09 Antepartum hemorrhage with other coagulation** defect

    O46.091 Antepartum hemorrhage with other Ⓜ♀
coagulation defect, **first trimester**

    O46.092 Antepartum hemorrhage with other Ⓜ♀
coagulation defect, **second trimester**

    O46.093 Antepartum hemorrhage with other Ⓜ♀
coagulation defect, **third trimester**

    O46.099 Antepartum hemorrhage with other Ⓜ♀▽
coagulation defect, **unspecified trimester**

√5ᵗʰ **O46.8 Other antepartum hemorrhage**

√6ᵗʰ **O46.8X Other antepartum hemorrhage**

    O46.8X1 Other antepartum hemorrhage, Ⓜ♀
first trimester

    O46.8X2 Other antepartum hemorrhage, Ⓜ♀
second trimester

    O46.8X3 Other antepartum hemorrhage, Ⓜ♀
third trimester

    O46.8X9 Other antepartum hemorrhage, Ⓜ♀▽
unspecified trimester

√5ᵗʰ **O46.9 Antepartum hemorrhage, unspecified**

    O46.90 Antepartum hemorrhage, unspecified, Ⓜ♀▽
unspecified trimester

    O46.91 Antepartum hemorrhage, unspecified, Ⓜ♀▽
first trimester

    O46.92 Antepartum hemorrhage, unspecified, Ⓜ♀▽
second trimester

    O46.93 Antepartum hemorrhage, unspecified, Ⓜ♀▽
third trimester

√4ᵗʰ **O47 False labor**
INCLUDES Braxton Hicks contractions
threatened labor
EXCLUDES 1 preterm labor (O60.-)

√5ᵗʰ **O47.0 False labor** before 37 completed weeks of gestation

    O47.00 False labor before 37 completed weeks of Ⓜ♀▽
gestation, **unspecified trimester**

    O47.02 False labor before 37 completed weeks of Ⓜ♀
gestation, **second trimester**

    O47.03 False labor before 37 completed weeks of Ⓜ♀
gestation, **third trimester**

    O47.1 False labor at or after 37 completed weeks of gestation Ⓜ♀

    O47.9 False labor, unspecified Ⓜ♀▽

√4ᵗʰ **O48 Late pregnancy**

    O48.0 Post-term pregnancy Ⓜ♀
Pregnancy over 40 completed weeks to 42 completed weeks gestation

    O48.1 Prolonged pregnancy Ⓜ♀
Pregnancy which has advanced beyond 42 completed weeks gestation
AHA: 2016, 1Q, 5

Complications of labor and delivery (O60-O77)

√4ᵗʰ **O60 Preterm labor**
INCLUDES onset (spontaneous) of labor before 37 completed weeks of gestation
EXCLUDES 1 false labor (O47.0-)
threatened labor NOS (O47.0-)

√5ᵗʰ **O60.0 Preterm labor** without delivery

    O60.00 Preterm labor without delivery, unspecified Ⓜ♀▽
trimester

    O60.02 Preterm labor without delivery, second Ⓜ♀
trimester

    O60.03 Preterm labor without delivery, third trimester Ⓜ♀

√5ᵗʰ **O60.1 Preterm labor** with preterm delivery
AHA: 2016, 2Q, 10

> One of the following 7th characters is to be assigned to each code under subcategory O60.1. 7th character 0 is for single gestations and multiple gestations where the fetus is unspecified. 7th characters 1 through 9 are for cases of multiple gestations to identify the fetus for which the code applies. The appropriate code from category O30, Multiple gestation, must also be assigned when assigning a code from subcategory O60.1 that has a 7th character of 1 through 9.
> | | | | |
> |---|---|---|---|
> | 0 | not applicable or unspecified | 4 | fetus 4 |
> | 1 | fetus 1 | 5 | fetus 5 |
> | 2 | fetus 2 | 9 | other fetus |
> | 3 | fetus 3 | | |

√x7ᵗʰ **O60.10 Preterm labor with preterm delivery,** Ⓜ♀▽
unspecified trimester
Preterm labor with delivery NOS

√x7ᵗʰ **O60.12 Preterm labor** second trimester **with preterm** Ⓜ♀
delivery second trimester

√x7ᵗʰ **O60.13 Preterm labor** second trimester **with preterm** Ⓜ♀
delivery third trimester

√x7ᵗʰ **O60.14 Preterm labor** third trimester **with preterm** Ⓜ♀
delivery third trimester

√5ᵗʰ **O60.2 Term delivery with preterm labor**

> One of the following 7th characters is to be assigned to each code under subcategory O60.2. 7th character 0 is for single gestations and multiple gestations where the fetus is unspecified. 7th characters 1 through 9 are for cases of multiple gestations to identify the fetus for which the code applies. The appropriate code from category O30, Multiple gestation, must also be assigned when assigning a code from subcategory O60.2 that has a 7th character of 1 through 9.
> | | | | |
> |---|---|---|---|
> | 0 | not applicable or unspecified | 4 | fetus 4 |
> | 1 | fetus 1 | 5 | fetus 5 |
> | 2 | fetus 2 | 9 | other fetus |
> | 3 | fetus 3 | | |

√x7ᵗʰ **O60.20 Term delivery with preterm labor, unspecified** Ⓜ♀▽
trimester

√x7ᵗʰ **O60.22 Term delivery with preterm labor, second** Ⓜ♀
trimester

√x7ᵗʰ **O60.23 Term delivery with preterm labor, third** Ⓜ♀
trimester

√4ᵗʰ **O61 Failed induction of labor**

    O61.0 Failed medical **induction of labor** Ⓜ♀
Failed induction (of labor) by oxytocin
Failed induction (of labor) by prostaglandins

    O61.1 Failed instrumental **induction of labor** Ⓜ♀
Failed mechanical induction (of labor)
Failed surgical induction (of labor)

    O61.8 Other failed induction of labor Ⓜ♀

    O61.9 Failed induction of labor, unspecified Ⓜ♀▽

√4ᵗʰ **O62 Abnormalities of forces of labor**

    O62.0 Primary inadequate contractions Ⓜ♀
Failure of cervical dilatation
Primary hypotonic uterine dysfunction
Uterine inertia during latent phase of labor

    O62.1 Secondary uterine inertia Ⓜ♀
Arrested active phase of labor
Secondary hypotonic uterine dysfunction

☑ Additional Character Req   √x7ᵗʰ Placeholder Alert   Manifestation   HCC CMS-HCC Condition   ▽ Unspecified Code   ►◄ Revised Text   ● New Code   ▲ Revised Code Title

ICD-10-CM 2018   845

Fetal Malposition

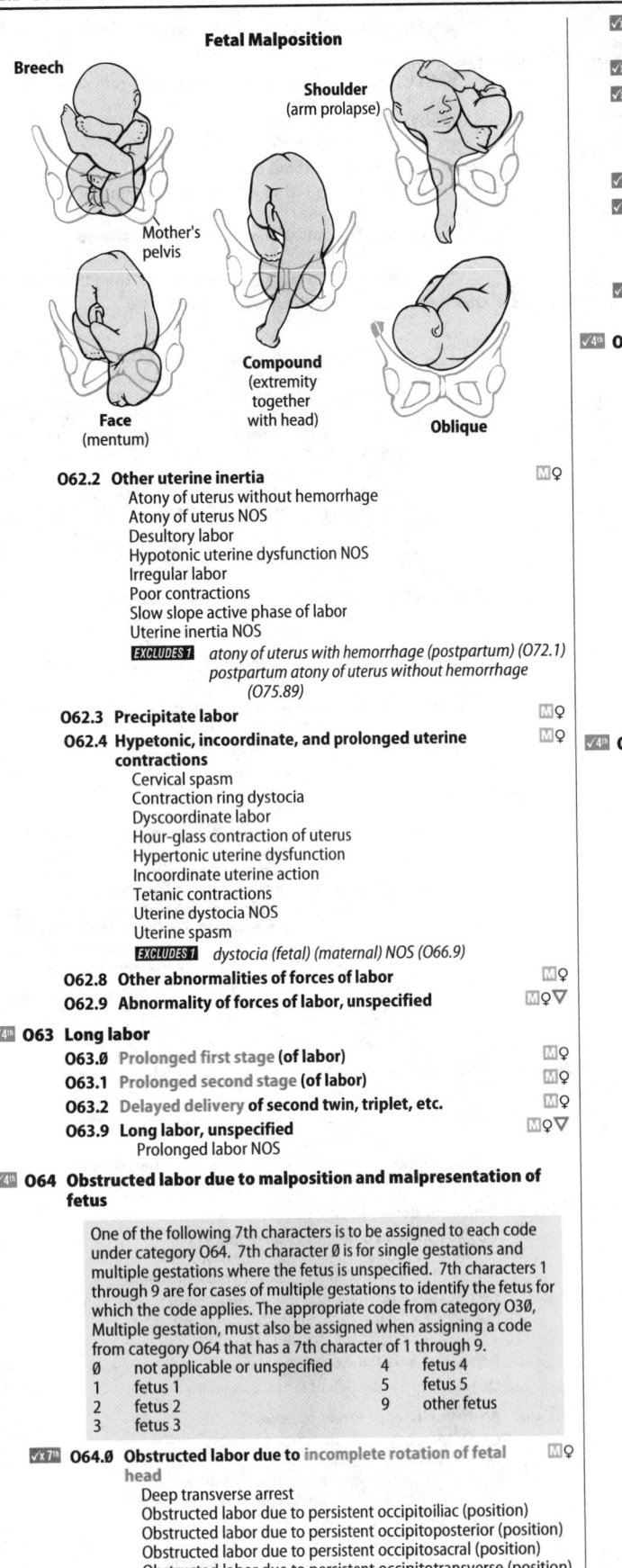

Breech

Shoulder
(arm prolapse)

Mother's
pelvis

Compound
(extremity
together
with head)

Face
(mentum)

Oblique

O62.2 Other uterine inertia   Ⓜ♀
     Atony of uterus without hemorrhage
     Atony of uterus NOS
     Desultory labor
     Hypotonic uterine dysfunction NOS
     Irregular labor
     Poor contractions
     Slow slope active phase of labor
     Uterine inertia NOS
     EXCLUDES 1   *atony of uterus with hemorrhage (postpartum) (O72.1)*
           postpartum atony of uterus without hemorrhage (O75.89)

O62.3 Precipitate labor   Ⓜ♀

O62.4 Hypetonic, incoordinate, and prolonged uterine   Ⓜ♀
     contractions
     Cervical spasm
     Contraction ring dystocia
     Dyscoordinate labor
     Hour-glass contraction of uterus
     Hypertonic uterine dysfunction
     Incoordinate uterine action
     Tetanic contractions
     Uterine dystocia NOS
     Uterine spasm
     EXCLUDES 1   *dystocia (fetal) (maternal) NOS (O66.9)*

O62.8 Other abnormalities of forces of labor   Ⓜ♀

O62.9 Abnormality of forces of labor, unspecified   Ⓜ♀▽

✓4ᵗʰ **O63 Long labor**

O63.0 Prolonged first stage (of labor)   Ⓜ♀

O63.1 Prolonged second stage (of labor)   Ⓜ♀

O63.2 Delayed delivery of second twin, triplet, etc.   Ⓜ♀

O63.9 Long labor, unspecified   Ⓜ♀▽
     Prolonged labor NOS

✓4ᵗʰ **O64 Obstructed labor due to malposition and malpresentation of fetus**

> One of the following 7th characters is to be assigned to each code under category O64. 7th character 0 is for single gestations and multiple gestations where the fetus is unspecified. 7th characters 1 through 9 are for cases of multiple gestations to identify the fetus for which the code applies. The appropriate code from category O30, Multiple gestation, must also be assigned when assigning a code from category O64 that has a 7th character of 1 through 9.
> 0   not applicable or unspecified   4   fetus 4
> 1   fetus 1   5   fetus 5
> 2   fetus 2   9   other fetus
> 3   fetus 3

✓x7ᵗʰ **O64.0 Obstructed labor due to incomplete rotation of fetal**   Ⓜ♀
     head
     Deep transverse arrest
     Obstructed labor due to persistent occipitoiliac (position)
     Obstructed labor due to persistent occipitoposterior (position)
     Obstructed labor due to persistent occipitosacral (position)
     Obstructed labor due to persistent occipitotransverse (position)

✓x7ᵗʰ **O64.1 Obstructed labor due to breech presentation**   Ⓜ♀
     Obstructed labor due to buttocks presentation
     Obstructed labor due to complete breech presentation
     Obstructed labor due to frank breech presentation

✓x7ᵗʰ **O64.2 Obstructed labor due to face presentation**   Ⓜ♀
     Obstructed labor due to chin presentation

✓x7ᵗʰ **O64.3 Obstructed labor due to brow presentation**   Ⓜ♀

✓x7ᵗʰ **O64.4 Obstructed labor due to shoulder presentation**   Ⓜ♀
     Prolapsed arm
     EXCLUDES 1   *impacted shoulders (O66.0)*
                  shoulder dystocia (O66.0)

✓x7ᵗʰ **O64.5 Obstructed labor due to compound presentation**   Ⓜ♀

✓x7ᵗʰ **O64.8 Obstructed labor due to other malposition and**   Ⓜ♀
     malpresentation
     Obstructed labor due to footling presentation
     Obstructed labor due to incomplete breech presentation

✓x7ᵗʰ **O64.9 Obstructed labor due to malposition and**   Ⓜ♀▽
     malpresentation, unspecified

✓4ᵗʰ **O65 Obstructed labor due to maternal pelvic abnormality**

O65.0 Obstructed labor due to deformed pelvis   Ⓜ♀

O65.1 Obstructed labor due to generally contracted pelvis   Ⓜ♀

O65.2 Obstructed labor due to pelvic inlet contraction   Ⓜ♀

O65.3 Obstructed labor due to pelvic outlet and mid-cavity   Ⓜ♀
     contraction

O65.4 Obstructed labor due to fetopelvic disproportion,   Ⓜ♀▽
     unspecified
     EXCLUDES 1   *dystocia due to abnormality of fetus (O66.2-O66.3)*

O65.5 Obstructed labor due to abnormality of maternal   Ⓜ♀
     pelvic organs
     Obstructed labor due to conditions listed in O34-
     Use additional code to identify abnormality of pelvic organs
     (O34.-)

O65.8 Obstructed labor due to other maternal pelvic   Ⓜ♀
     abnormalities

O65.9 Obstructed labor due to maternal pelvic abnormality,   Ⓜ♀▽
     unspecified

✓4ᵗʰ **O66 Other obstructed labor**

O66.0 Obstructed labor due to shoulder dystocia   Ⓜ♀
     Impacted shoulders
     DEF: Obstructed labor due to impacted fetal shoulders;
     emergency condition that may require cesarean section, forceps
     delivery, vacuum extraction, or simphysiotomy.

O66.1 Obstructed labor due to locked twins   Ⓜ♀

O66.2 Obstructed labor due to unusually large fetus   Ⓜ♀

O66.3 Obstructed labor due to other abnormalities of fetus   Ⓜ♀
     Dystocia due to fetal ascites
     Dystocia due to fetal hydrops
     Dystocia due to fetal meningomyelocele
     Dystocia due to fetal sacral teratoma
     Dystocia due to fetal tumor
     Dystocia due to hydrocephalic fetus
     Use additional code to identify cause of obstruction

✓5ᵗʰ **O66.4 Failed trial of labor**

     O66.40 Failed trial of labor, unspecified   Ⓜ♀▽

     O66.41 Failed attempted vaginal birth after previous   Ⓜ♀
               cesarean delivery
               Code first rupture of uterus, if applicable (O71.0-,
               O71.1)

O66.5 Attempted application of vacuum extractor and forceps   Ⓜ♀
     Attempted application of vacuum or forceps, with subsequent
     delivery by forceps or cesarean delivery

O66.6 Obstructed labor due to other multiple fetuses   Ⓜ♀

O66.8 Other specified obstructed labor   Ⓜ♀
     Use additional code to identify cause of obstruction

O66.9 Obstructed labor, unspecified   Ⓜ♀▽
     Dystocia NOS
     Fetal dystocia NOS
     Maternal dystocia NOS

EXCLUDES 1 Not coded here   **EXCLUDES 2** Not included here   Ⓝ Newborn Age: 0   Ⓟ Pediatric Age: 0-17   Ⓜ Maternity Age: 12-55   Ⓐ Adult Age: 15-124

846   ICD-10-CM 2018

☑4ᵗʰ O67 Labor and delivery complicated by intrapartum hemorrhage, not elsewhere classified
> EXCLUDES 1   antepartum hemorrhage NEC (O46.-)
> placenta previa (O44.-)
> premature separation of placenta [abruptio placentae] (O45.-)
> EXCLUDES 2   postpartum hemorrhage (O72.-)

O67.0 Intrapartum hemorrhage with coagulation defect   M♀
> Intrapartum hemorrhage (excessive) associated with afibrinogenemia
> Intrapartum hemorrhage (excessive) associated with disseminated intravascular coagulation
> Intrapartum hemorrhage (excessive) associated with hyperfibrinolysis
> Intrapartum hemorrhage (excessive) associated with hypofibrinogenemia

O67.8 Other intrapartum hemorrhage   M♀
> Excessive intrapartum hemorrhage

O67.9 Intrapartum hemorrhage, unspecified   M♀▽

O68 Labor and delivery complicated by abnormality of fetal acid-base balance   M♀
> Fetal acidemia complicating labor and delivery
> Fetal acidosis complicating labor and delivery
> Fetal alkalosis complicating labor and delivery
> Fetal metabolic acidemia complicating labor and delivery
> EXCLUDES 1   fetal stress NOS (O77.9)
> labor and delivery complicated by electrocardiographic evidence of fetal stress (O77.8)
> labor and delivery complicated by ultrasonic evidence of fetal stress (O77.8)
> EXCLUDES 2   abnormality in fetal heart rate or rhythm (O76)
> labor and delivery complicated by meconium in amniotic fluid (O77.0)

☑4ᵗʰ O69 Labor and delivery complicated by umbilical cord complications
> AHA: 2016, 1Q, 5

> One of the following 7th characters is to be assigned to each code under category O69. 7th character 0 is for single gestations and multiple gestations where the fetus is unspecified. 7th characters 1 through 9 are for cases of multiple gestations to identify the fetus for which the code applies. The appropriate code from category O30, Multiple gestation, must also be assigned when assigning a code from category O69 that has a 7th character of 1 through 9.
> | | | | |
> |---|---|---|---|
> | 0 | not applicable or unspecified | 4 | fetus 4 |
> | 1 | fetus 1 | 5 | fetus 5 |
> | 2 | fetus 2 | 9 | other fetus |
> | 3 | fetus 3 | | |

√x7ᵗʰ O69.0 Labor and delivery complicated by prolapse of cord   M♀
> DEF: Abnormal presentation of fetus; marked by protruding umbilical cord during labor; can cause fetal death.

√x7ᵗʰ O69.1 Labor and delivery complicated by cord around neck, with compression   M♀
> EXCLUDES 1   labor and delivery complicated by cord around neck, without compression (O69.81)

√x7ᵗʰ O69.2 Labor and delivery complicated by other cord entanglement, with compression   M♀
> Labor and delivery complicated by compression of cord NOS
> Labor and delivery complicated by entanglement of cords of twins in monoamniotic sac
> Labor and delivery complicated by knot in cord
> EXCLUDES 1   labor and delivery complicated by other cord entanglement, without compression (O69.82)

√x7ᵗʰ O69.3 Labor and delivery complicated by short cord   M♀

√x7ᵗʰ O69.4 Labor and delivery complicated by vasa previa   M♀
> Labor and delivery complicated by hemorrhage from vasa previa

√x7ᵗʰ O69.5 Labor and delivery complicated by vascular lesion of cord   M♀
> Labor and delivery complicated by cord bruising
> Labor and delivery complicated by cord hematoma
> Labor and delivery complicated by thrombosis of umbilical vessels

√5ᵗʰ O69.8 Labor and delivery complicated by other cord complications

√x7ᵗʰ O69.81 Labor and delivery complicated by cord around neck, without compression   M♀
> AHA: 2016, 1Q, 5

√x7ᵗʰ O69.82 Labor and delivery complicated by other cord entanglement, without compression   M♀

√x7ᵗʰ O69.89 Labor and delivery complicated by other cord complications   M♀

√x7ᵗʰ O69.9 Labor and delivery complicated by cord complication, unspecified   M♀▽

☑4ᵗʰ O70 Perineal laceration during delivery
> Episiotomy extended by laceration
> EXCLUDES 1   obstetric high vaginal laceration alone (O71.4)
> AHA: 2016, 2Q, 34; 2016, 1Q, 3-4, 5

O70.0 First degree perineal laceration during delivery   M♀
> Perineal laceration, rupture or tear involving fourchette during delivery
> Perineal laceration, rupture or tear involving labia during delivery
> Perineal laceration, rupture or tear involving skin during delivery
> Perineal laceration, rupture or tear involving vagina during delivery
> Perineal laceration, rupture or tear involving vulva during delivery
> Slight perineal laceration, rupture or tear during delivery

O70.1 Second degree perineal laceration during delivery   M♀
> Perineal laceration, rupture or tear during delivery as in O70.0, also involving pelvic floor
> Perineal laceration, rupture or tear during delivery as in O70.0, also involving perineal muscles
> Perineal laceration, rupture or tear during delivery as in O70.0, also involving vaginal muscles
> EXCLUDES 1   perineal laceration involving anal sphincter (O70.2)

√5ᵗʰ O70.2 Third degree perineal laceration during delivery
> Perineal laceration, rupture or tear during delivery as in O70.1, also involving anal sphincter
> Perineal laceration, rupture or tear during delivery as in O70.1, also involving rectovaginal septum
> Perineal laceration, rupture or tear during delivery as in O70.1, also involving sphincter NOS
> EXCLUDES 1   anal sphincter tear during delivery without third degree perineal laceration (O70.4)
> perineal laceration involving anal or rectal mucosa (O70.3)

O70.20 Third degree perineal laceration during delivery, unspecified   M♀▽

O70.21 Third degree perineal laceration during delivery, IIIa   M♀
> Third degree perineal laceration during delivery with less than 50% of external anal sphincter (EAS) thickness torn

O70.22 Third degree perineal laceration during delivery, IIIb   M♀
> Third degree perineal laceration during delivery with more than 50% external anal sphincter (EAS) thickness torn

O70.23 Third degree perineal laceration during delivery, IIIc   M♀
> Third degree perineal laceration during delivery with both external anal sphincter (EAS) and internal anal sphincter (IAS) torn

O70.3 Fourth degree perineal laceration during delivery   M♀
> Perineal laceration, rupture or tear during delivery as in O70.2, also involving anal mucosa
> Perineal laceration, rupture or tear during delivery as in O70.2, also involving rectal mucosa

O70.4 Anal sphincter tear complicating delivery, not associated with third degree laceration   M♀
> EXCLUDES 1   anal sphincter tear with third degree perineal laceration (O70.2)

O70.9 Perineal laceration during delivery, unspecified   M♀▽

☑4ᵗʰ O71 Other obstetric trauma
> INCLUDES   obstetric damage from instruments

√5ᵗʰ O71.0 Rupture of uterus (spontaneous) before onset of labor
> EXCLUDES 1   disruption of (current) cesarean delivery wound (O90.0)
> laceration of uterus, NEC (O71.81)

O71.00 Rupture of uterus before onset of labor, unspecified trimester   M♀▽

O71.02 Rupture of uterus before onset of labor, second trimester   M♀

O71.03 Rupture of uterus before onset of labor, third trimester   M♀

O71.1 Rupture of uterus during labor   M♀
> Rupture of uterus not stated as occurring before onset of labor
> EXCLUDES 1   disruption of cesarean delivery wound (O90.0)
> laceration of uterus, NEC (O71.81)

O71.2 Postpartum inversion of uterus   M♀

O71.3 Obstetric laceration of cervix   M♀
> Annular detachment of cervix

☑ Additional Character Req   √x7ᵗʰ Placeholder Alert   Manifestation   HCC CMS-HCC Condition   ▽ Unspecified Code   ►◄ Revised Text   ● New Code   ▲ Revised Code Title

O71.4 Obstetric high vaginal laceration alone Ⓜ♀
Laceration of vaginal wall without perineal laceration
EXCLUDES 1   obstetric high vaginal laceration with perineal laceration (O70.-)
AHA: 2016, 1Q, 5

O71.5 Other obstetric injury to pelvic organs Ⓜ♀
Obstetric injury to bladder
Obstetric injury to urethra
EXCLUDES 2   obstetric periurethral trauma (O71.82)
AHA: 2014, 4Q, 18

O71.6 Obstetric damage to pelvic joints and ligaments Ⓜ♀
Obstetric avulsion of inner symphyseal cartilage
Obstetric damage to coccyx
Obstetric traumatic separation of symphysis (pubis)

O71.7 Obstetric hematoma of pelvis Ⓜ♀
Obstetric hematoma of perineum
Obstetric hematoma of vagina
Obstetric hematoma of vulva

✓5ᵗʰ O71.8 Other specified obstetric trauma
   O71.81 Laceration of uterus, not elsewhere classified Ⓜ♀
   O71.82 Other specified trauma to perineum and vulva Ⓜ♀
      Obstetric periurethral trauma
      AHA: 2016, 1Q, 4; 2014, 4Q, 18
   O71.89 Other specified obstetric trauma Ⓜ♀

O71.9 Obstetric trauma, unspecified Ⓜ♀▽

✓4ᵗʰ O72 Postpartum hemorrhage
INCLUDES   hemorrhage after delivery of fetus or infant

O72.0 Third-stage hemorrhage Ⓜ♀
Hemorrhage associated with retained, trapped or adherent placenta
Retained placenta NOS
Code also type of adherent placenta (O43.2-)

O72.1 Other immediate postpartum hemorrhage Ⓜ♀
Hemorrhage following delivery of placenta
Postpartum hemorrhage (atonic) NOS
Uterine atony with hemorrhage
EXCLUDES 1   uterine atony NOS (O62.2)
       uterine atony without hemorrhage (O62.2)
       postpartum atony of uterus without hemorrhage (O75.89)
AHA: 2016, 1Q, 4

O72.2 Delayed and secondary postpartum hemorrhage Ⓜ♀
Hemorrhage associated with retained portions of placenta or membranes after the first 24 hours following delivery of placenta
Retained products of conception NOS, following delivery

O72.3 Postpartum coagulation defects Ⓜ♀
Postpartum afibrinogenemia
Postpartum fibrinolysis

✓4ᵗʰ O73 Retained placenta and membranes, without hemorrhage
EXCLUDES 1   placenta accreta (O43.21-)
       placenta increta (O43.22-)
       placenta percreta (O43.23-)
DEF: Postpartum condition resulting from failure to expel placental membrane tissues due to failed contractions of uterine wall.

O73.0 Retained placenta without hemorrhage Ⓜ♀
Adherent placenta, without hemorrhage
Trapped placenta without hemorrhage

O73.1 Retained portions of placenta and membranes, without hemorrhage Ⓜ♀
Retained products of conception following delivery, without hemorrhage

✓4ᵗʰ O74 Complications of anesthesia during labor and delivery
INCLUDES   maternal complications arising from the administration of a general, regional or local anesthetic, analgesic or other sedation during labor and delivery
Use additional code, if applicable, to identify specific complication

O74.0 Aspiration pneumonitis due to anesthesia during labor and delivery Ⓜ♀
Inhalation of stomach contents or secretions NOS due to anesthesia during labor and delivery
Mendelson's syndrome due to anesthesia during labor and delivery

O74.1 Other pulmonary complications of anesthesia during labor and delivery Ⓜ♀

O74.2 Cardiac complications of anesthesia during labor and delivery Ⓜ♀

O74.3 Central nervous system complications of anesthesia during labor and delivery Ⓜ♀

O74.4 Toxic reaction to local anesthesia during labor and delivery Ⓜ♀

O74.5 Spinal and epidural anesthesia-induced headache during labor and delivery Ⓜ♀

O74.6 Other complications of spinal and epidural anesthesia during labor and delivery Ⓜ♀

O74.7 Failed or difficult intubation for anesthesia during labor and delivery Ⓜ♀

O74.8 Other complications of anesthesia during labor and delivery Ⓜ♀

O74.9 Complication of anesthesia during labor and delivery, unspecified Ⓜ♀▽

✓4ᵗʰ O75 Other complications of labor and delivery, not elsewhere classified
EXCLUDES 2   puerperal (postpartum) infection (O86.-)
       puerperal (postpartum) sepsis (O85)

O75.0 Maternal distress during labor and delivery Ⓜ♀

O75.1 Shock during or following labor and delivery Ⓜ♀
Obstetric shock following labor and delivery

O75.2 Pyrexia during labor, not elsewhere classified Ⓜ♀

O75.3 Other infection during labor Ⓜ♀
Sepsis during labor
Use additional code (B95-B97), to identify infectious agent

O75.4 Other complications of obstetric surgery and procedures Ⓜ♀
Cardiac arrest following obstetric surgery or procedures
Cardiac failure following obstetric surgery or procedures
Cerebral anoxia following obstetric surgery or procedures
Pulmonary edema following obstetric surgery or procedures
Use additional code to identify specific complication
EXCLUDES 2   complications of anesthesia during labor and delivery (O74.-)
       disruption of obstetrical (surgical) wound (O90.0-O90.1)
       hematoma of obstetrical (surgical) wound (O90.2)
       infection of obstetrical (surgical) wound (O86.0)

O75.5 Delayed delivery after artificial rupture of membranes Ⓜ♀

✓5ᵗʰ O75.8 Other specified complications of labor and delivery
   O75.81 Maternal exhaustion complicating labor and delivery Ⓜ♀
   O75.82 Onset (spontaneous) of labor after 37 completed weeks of gestation but before 39 completed weeks gestation, with delivery by (planned) cesarean section Ⓜ♀
      Delivery by (planned) cesarean section occurring after 37 completed weeks of gestation but before 39 completed weeks gestation due to (spontaneous) onset of labor
      Code first to specify reason for planned cesarean section such as:
      cephalopelvic disproportion (normally formed fetus) (O33.9)
      previous cesarean delivery (O34.21)
   O75.89 Other specified complications of labor and delivery Ⓜ♀

O75.9 Complication of labor and delivery, unspecified Ⓜ♀▽

O76 Abnormality in fetal heart rate and rhythm complicating labor and delivery Ⓜ♀
Depressed fetal heart rate tones complicating labor and delivery
Fetal bradycardia complicating labor and delivery
Fetal heart rate abnormal variability complicating labor and delivery
Fetal heart rate decelerations complicating labor and delivery
Fetal heart rate irregularity complicating labor and delivery
Fetal tachycardia complicating labor and delivery
Non-reassuring fetal heart rate or rhythm complicating labor and delivery
EXCLUDES 1   fetal stress NOS (O77.9)
       labor and delivery complicated by electrocardiographic evidence of fetal stress (O77.8)
       labor and delivery complicated by ultrasonic evidence of fetal stress (O77.8)
EXCLUDES 2   fetal metabolic acidemia (O68)
       other fetal stress (O77.0-O77.1)
AHA: 2013, 4Q, 118

✓4ᵗʰ O77 Other fetal stress complicating labor and delivery
   O77.0 Labor and delivery complicated by meconium in amniotic fluid Ⓜ♀
      AHA: 2013, 4Q, 117-118
   O77.1 Fetal stress in labor or delivery due to drug administration Ⓜ♀

O77.8 **Labor and delivery complicated by other evidence of fetal stress**   Ⓜ♀

Labor and delivery complicated by electrocardiographic evidence of fetal stress

Labor and delivery complicated by ultrasonic evidence of fetal stress

> *EXCLUDES 1*   abnormality in fetal heart rate or rhythm (O76)
> abnormality of fetal acid-base balance (O68)
> fetal metabolic acidemia (O68)

O77.9 **Labor and delivery complicated by fetal stress, unspecified**   Ⓜ♀▽

> *EXCLUDES 1*   abnormality in fetal heart rate or rhythm (O76)
> abnormality of fetal acid-base balance (O68)
> fetal metabolic acidemia (O68)

Encounter for delivery (O80, O82)

O80 **Encounter for full-term uncomplicated delivery**   Ⓜ♀

> *NOTE*   Delivery requiring minimal or no assistance, with or without episiotomy, without fetal manipulation [e.g., rotation version] or instrumentation [forceps] of a spontaneous, cephalic, vaginal, full-term, single, live-born infant. This code is for use as a single diagnosis code and is not to be used with any other code from chapter 15.
> Use additional code to indicate outcome of delivery (Z37.0)
> **AHA:** 2016, 4Q, 150; 2014, 2Q, 9

O82 **Encounter for cesarean delivery without indication**   Ⓜ♀

> Use additional code to indicate outcome of delivery (Z37.0)

Complications predominantly related to the puerperium (O85-O92)

> *EXCLUDES 2*   mental and behavioral disorders associated with the puerperium (F53)
> obstetrical tetanus (A34)
> puerperal osteomalacia (M83.0)

O85 **Puerperal sepsis**   Ⓜ♀

Postpartum sepsis
Puerperal peritonitis
Puerperal pyemia

> Use additional code (B95-B97), to identify infectious agent
> Use additional code (R65.2-) to identify severe sepsis, if applicable
> *EXCLUDES 1*   fever of unknown origin following delivery (O86.4)
> genital tract infection following delivery (O86.1-)
> obstetric pyemic and septic embolism (O88.3-)
> puerperal septic thrombophlebitis (O86.81)
> urinary tract infection following delivery (O86.2-)
> *EXCLUDES 2*   sepsis during labor (O75.3)

✓4ᵗʰ O86 **Other puerperal infections**

> Use additional code (B95-B97), to identify infectious agent
> *EXCLUDES 2*   infection during labor (O75.3)
> obstetrical tetanus (A34)

O86.0 **Infection of obstetric surgical wound**   Ⓜ♀

Infected cesarean delivery wound following delivery
Infected perineal repair following delivery

✓5ᵗʰ O86.1 **Other infection of genital tract following delivery**

  O86.11 **Cervicitis following delivery**   Ⓜ♀

  O86.12 **Endometritis following delivery**   Ⓜ♀

  O86.13 **Vaginitis following delivery**   Ⓜ♀

  O86.19 **Other infection of genital tract following delivery**   Ⓜ♀

✓5ᵗʰ O86.2 **Urinary tract infection following delivery**

  O86.20 **Urinary tract infection following delivery, unspecified**   Ⓜ♀▽

    Puerperal urinary tract infection NOS

  O86.21 **Infection of kidney following delivery**   Ⓜ♀

  O86.22 **Infection of bladder following delivery**   Ⓜ♀

    Infection of urethra following delivery

  O86.29 **Other urinary tract infection following delivery**   Ⓜ♀

O86.4 **Pyrexia of unknown origin following delivery**   Ⓜ♀

Puerperal infection NOS following delivery
Puerperal pyrexia NOS following delivery

> *EXCLUDES 2*   pyrexia during labor (O75.2)
> **DEF:** Fever of unknown origin experienced by the mother after childbirth.

✓5ᵗʰ O86.8 **Other specified puerperal infections**

  O86.81 **Puerperal septic thrombophlebitis**   Ⓜ♀

  O86.89 **Other specified puerperal infections**   Ⓜ♀

✓4ᵗʰ O87 **Venous complications and hemorrhoids in the puerperium**

> *INCLUDES*   venous complications in labor, delivery and the puerperium
> *EXCLUDES 2*   obstetric embolism (O88.-)
> puerperal septic thrombophlebitis (O86.81)
> venous complications in pregnancy (O22.-)

O87.0 **Superficial thrombophlebitis in the puerperium**   Ⓜ♀

Puerperal phlebitis NOS
Puerperal thrombosis NOS

O87.1 **Deep phlebothrombosis in the puerperium**   Ⓜ♀

Deep vein thrombosis, postpartum
Pelvic thrombophlebitis, postpartum

> Use additional code to identify the deep vein thrombosis (I82.4-, I82.5-, I82.62-. I82.72-)
> Use additional code, if applicable, for associated long-term (current) use of anticoagulants (Z79.01)

O87.2 **Hemorrhoids in the puerperium**   Ⓜ♀

O87.3 **Cerebral venous thrombosis in the puerperium**   Ⓜ♀

Cerebrovenous sinus thrombosis in the puerperium

O87.4 **Varicose veins of lower extremity in the puerperium**   Ⓜ♀

O87.8 **Other venous complications in the puerperium**   Ⓜ♀

Genital varices in the puerperium

O87.9 **Venous complication in the puerperium, unspecified**   Ⓜ♀▽

Puerperal phlebopathy NOS

✓4ᵗʰ O88 **Obstetric embolism**

> *EXCLUDES 1*   embolism complicating abortion NOS (O03.2)
> embolism complicating ectopic or molar pregnancy (O08.2)
> embolism complicating failed attempted abortion (O07.2)
> embolism complicating induced abortion (O04.7)
> embolism complicating spontaneous abortion (O03.2, O03.7)

✓5ᵗʰ O88.0 **Obstetric air embolism**

> **DEF:** Sudden blocking of pulmonary artery or right ventricle with air or nitrogen bubbles.

✓6ᵗʰ O88.01 **Obstetric air embolism in pregnancy**

  O88.011 **Air embolism in pregnancy, first trimester**   Ⓜ♀

  O88.012 **Air embolism in pregnancy, second trimester**   Ⓜ♀

  O88.013 **Air embolism in pregnancy, third trimester**   Ⓜ♀

  O88.019 **Air embolism in pregnancy, unspecified trimester**   Ⓜ♀▽

O88.02 **Air embolism in childbirth**   Ⓜ♀

O88.03 **Air embolism in the puerperium**   Ⓜ♀

✓5ᵗʰ O88.1 **Amniotic fluid embolism**

Anaphylactoid syndrome in pregnancy

✓6ᵗʰ O88.11 **Amniotic fluid embolism in pregnancy**

  O88.111 **Amniotic fluid embolism in pregnancy, first trimester**   Ⓜ♀

  O88.112 **Amniotic fluid embolism in pregnancy, second trimester**   Ⓜ♀

  O88.113 **Amniotic fluid embolism in pregnancy, third trimester**   Ⓜ♀

  O88.119 **Amniotic fluid embolism in pregnancy, unspecified trimester**   Ⓜ♀▽

O88.12 **Amniotic fluid embolism in childbirth**   Ⓜ♀

O88.13 **Amniotic fluid embolism in the puerperium**   Ⓜ♀

✓5ᵗʰ O88.2 **Obstetric thromboembolism**

✓6ᵗʰ O88.21 **Thromboembolism in pregnancy**

Obstetric (pulmonary) embolism NOS

  O88.211 **Thromboembolism in pregnancy, first trimester**   Ⓜ♀

  O88.212 **Thromboembolism in pregnancy, second trimester**   Ⓜ♀

  O88.213 **Thromboembolism in pregnancy, third trimester**   Ⓜ♀

  O88.219 **Thromboembolism in pregnancy, unspecified trimester**   Ⓜ♀▽

O88.22 **Thromboembolism in childbirth**   Ⓜ♀

O88.23 **Thromboembolism in the puerperium**   Ⓜ♀

Puerperal (pulmonary) embolism NOS

✓5ᵗʰ O88.3 **Obstetric pyemic and septic embolism**

✓6ᵗʰ O88.31 **Pyemic and septic embolism in pregnancy**

  O88.311 **Pyemic and septic embolism in pregnancy, first trimester**   Ⓜ♀

  O88.312 **Pyemic and septic embolism in pregnancy, second trimester**   Ⓜ♀

☑ Additional Character Req   ⁷ˣ⁷ Placeholder Alert   Manifestation   ᴴᶜᶜ CMS-HCC Condition   ▽ Unspecified Code   ▶◀ Revised Text   ● New Code   ▲ Revised Code Title

Chapter 15. Pregnancy, Childbirth, and the Puerperium

O88.313–O91.23

           O88.313   Pyemic and septic embolism in pregnancy, **third trimester**   Ⓜ♀

           O88.319   Pyemic and septic embolism in pregnancy, **unspecified trimester**   Ⓜ♀▽

      O88.32   Pyemic and septic embolism in **childbirth**   Ⓜ♀

      O88.33   Pyemic and septic embolism in the **puerperium**   Ⓜ♀

✓5ᵗʰ   **O88.8**   **Other obstetric embolism**
       Obstetric fat embolism

      ✓6ᵗʰ   **O88.81**   **Other embolism in** pregnancy

           O88.811   Other embolism in pregnancy, **first trimester**   Ⓜ♀

           O88.812   Other embolism in pregnancy, **second trimester**   Ⓜ♀

           O88.813   Other embolism in pregnancy, **third trimester**   Ⓜ♀

           O88.819   Other embolism in pregnancy, **unspecified trimester**   Ⓜ♀▽

      O88.82   Other embolism in **childbirth**   Ⓜ♀

      O88.83   Other embolism in the **puerperium**   Ⓜ♀

✓4ᵗʰ   **O89**   **Complications of anesthesia during the puerperium**

    INCLUDES   maternal complications arising from the administration of a general, regional or local anesthetic, analgesic or other sedation during the puerperium

    Use additional code, if applicable, to identify specific complication

    ✓5ᵗʰ   **O89.0**   **Pulmonary complications of anesthesia during the puerperium**

      O89.01   **Aspiration pneumonitis due to anesthesia during the puerperium**   Ⓜ♀
         Inhalation of stomach contents or secretions NOS due to anesthesia during the puerperium
         Mendelson's syndrome due to anesthesia during the puerperium

      O89.09   **Other pulmonary complications of anesthesia during the puerperium**   Ⓜ♀

    O89.1   **Cardiac complications of anesthesia during the puerperium**   Ⓜ♀

    O89.2   **Central nervous system complications of anesthesia during the puerperium**   Ⓜ♀

    O89.3   **Toxic reaction to local anesthesia during the puerperium**   Ⓜ♀

    O89.4   **Spinal and epidural anesthesia-induced headache during the puerperium**   Ⓜ♀

    O89.5   **Other complications of spinal and epidural anesthesia during the puerperium**   Ⓜ♀

    O89.6   **Failed or difficult intubation for anesthesia during the puerperium**   Ⓜ♀

    O89.8   **Other complications of anesthesia during the puerperium**   Ⓜ♀

    O89.9   **Complication of anesthesia during the puerperium, unspecified**   Ⓜ♀▽

✓4ᵗʰ   **O90**   **Complications of the puerperium, not elsewhere classified**

    O90.0   **Disruption of cesarean delivery wound**   Ⓜ♀
      Dehiscence of cesarean delivery wound
      EXCLUDES 1   *rupture of uterus (spontaneous) before onset of labor (O71.0-)*
          rupture of uterus during labor (O71.1)

    O90.1   **Disruption of perineal obstetric wound**   Ⓜ♀
      Disruption of wound of episiotomy
      Disruption of wound of perineal laceration
      Secondary perineal tear

    O90.2   **Hematoma of obstetric wound**   Ⓜ♀

    O90.3   **Peripartum cardiomyopathy**   Ⓜ♀
      Conditions in I42- arising during pregnancy and the puerperium
      EXCLUDES 1   *pre-existing heart disease complicating pregnancy and the puerperium (O99.4-)*
      DEF: Any structural or functional abnormality of the ventricular myocardium, noninflammatory disease of obscure or unknown etiology with onset during the postpartum period.

    O90.4   **Postpartum acute kidney failure**   Ⓜ♀
      Hepatorenal syndrome following labor and delivery

    O90.5   **Postpartum thyroiditis**   Ⓜ♀

    O90.6   **Postpartum mood disturbance**   Ⓜ♀
      Postpartum blues
      Postpartum dysphoria
      Postpartum sadness
      EXCLUDES 1   *postpartum depression (F53)*
          puerperal psychosis (F53)

    ✓5ᵗʰ   **O90.8**   **Other complications of the puerperium, not elsewhere classified**

      O90.81   **Anemia of the puerperium**   Ⓜ♀
         Postpartum anemia NOS
         EXCLUDES 1   *pre-existing anemia complicating the puerperium (O99.03)*

      O90.89   **Other complications of the puerperium, not elsewhere classified**   Ⓜ♀
         Placental polyp

    O90.9   **Complication of the puerperium, unspecified**   Ⓜ♀▽

✓4ᵗʰ   **O91**   **Infections of breast associated with pregnancy, the puerperium and lactation**

    Use additional code to identify infection

    ✓5ᵗʰ   **O91.0**   **Infection of nipple associated with pregnancy, the puerperium and lactation**

      ✓6ᵗʰ   **O91.01**   **Infection of nipple associated with** pregnancy
         Gestational abscess of nipple

           O91.011   **Infection of nipple associated with pregnancy, first trimester**   Ⓜ♀

           O91.012   **Infection of nipple associated with pregnancy, second trimester**   Ⓜ♀

           O91.013   **Infection of nipple associated with pregnancy, third trimester**   Ⓜ♀

           O91.019   **Infection of nipple associated with pregnancy, unspecified trimester**   Ⓜ♀▽

      O91.02   **Infection of nipple associated with the puerperium**   Ⓜ♀
         Puerperal abscess of nipple

      O91.03   **Infection of nipple associated with lactation**   Ⓜ♀
         Abscess of nipple associated with lactation

    ✓5ᵗʰ   **O91.1**   **Abscess of breast associated with pregnancy, the puerperium and lactation**

      ✓6ᵗʰ   **O91.11**   **Abscess of breast associated with** pregnancy
         Gestational mammary abscess
         Gestational purulent mastitis
         Gestational subareolar abscess

           O91.111   **Abscess of breast associated with pregnancy, first trimester**   Ⓜ♀

           O91.112   **Abscess of breast associated with pregnancy, second trimester**   Ⓜ♀

           O91.113   **Abscess of breast associated with pregnancy, third trimester**   Ⓜ♀

           O91.119   **Abscess of breast associated with pregnancy, unspecified trimester**   Ⓜ♀▽

      O91.12   **Abscess of breast associated with the puerperium**   Ⓜ♀
         Puerperal mammary abscess
         Puerperal purulent mastitis
         Puerperal subareolar abscess

      O91.13   **Abscess of breast associated with lactation**   Ⓜ♀
         Mammary abscess associated with lactation
         Purulent mastitis associated with lactation
         Subareolar abscess associated with lactation

    ✓5ᵗʰ   **O91.2**   **Nonpurulent mastitis associated with pregnancy, the puerperium and lactation**

      ✓6ᵗʰ   **O91.21**   **Nonpurulent mastitis associated with** pregnancy
         Gestational interstitial mastitis
         Gestational lymphangitis of breast
         Gestational mastitis NOS
         Gestational parenchymatous mastitis

           O91.211   **Nonpurulent mastitis associated with pregnancy, first trimester**   Ⓜ♀

           O91.212   **Nonpurulent mastitis associated with pregnancy, second trimester**   Ⓜ♀

           O91.213   **Nonpurulent mastitis associated with pregnancy, third trimester**   Ⓜ♀

           O91.219   **Nonpurulent mastitis associated with pregnancy, unspecified trimester**   Ⓜ♀▽

      O91.22   **Nonpurulent mastitis associated with the puerperium**   Ⓜ♀
         Puerperal interstitial mastitis
         Puerperal lymphangitis of breast
         Puerperal mastitis NOS
         Puerperal parenchymatous mastitis

      O91.23   **Nonpurulent mastitis associated with lactation**   Ⓜ♀
         Interstitial mastitis associated with lactation
         Lymphangitis of breast associated with lactation
         Mastitis NOS associated with lactation
         Parenchymatous mastitis associated with lactation

EXCLUDES 1 Not coded here   EXCLUDES 2 Not included here   Ⓝ Newborn Age: 0   Ⓟ Pediatric Age: 0-17   Ⓜ Maternity Age: 12-55   Ⓐ Adult Age: 15-124

850   ICD-10-CM 2018

√4ᵗʰ **O92 Other disorders of breast and disorders of lactation associated with pregnancy and the puerperium**

  √5ᵗʰ **O92.0 Retracted nipple associated with pregnancy, the puerperium, and lactation**

    √6ᵗʰ **O92.01 Retracted nipple associated with pregnancy**

       O92.011 Retracted nipple associated with pregnancy, first trimester   M♀

       O92.012 Retracted nipple associated with pregnancy, second trimester   M♀

       O92.013 Retracted nipple associated with pregnancy, third trimester   M♀

       O92.019 Retracted nipple associated with pregnancy, unspecified trimester   M♀▽

     O92.02 Retracted nipple associated with the puerperium   M♀

     O92.03 Retracted nipple associated with lactation   M♀

  √5ᵗʰ **O92.1 Cracked nipple associated with pregnancy, the puerperium, and lactation**
       Fissure of nipple, gestational or puerperal

    √6ᵗʰ **O92.11 Cracked nipple associated with pregnancy**

       O92.111 Cracked nipple associated with pregnancy, first trimester   M♀

       O92.112 Cracked nipple associated with pregnancy, second trimester   M♀

       O92.113 Cracked nipple associated with pregnancy, third trimester   M♀

       O92.119 Cracked nipple associated with pregnancy, unspecified trimester   M♀▽

     O92.12 Cracked nipple associated with the puerperium   M♀

     O92.13 Cracked nipple associated with lactation   M♀

  √5ᵗʰ **O92.2 Other and unspecified disorders of breast associated with pregnancy and the puerperium**

     O92.20 Unspecified disorder of breast associated with pregnancy and the puerperium   M♀▽

     O92.29 Other disorders of breast associated with pregnancy and the puerperium   M♀

   O92.3 Agalactia   M♀
     Primary agalactia
     EXCLUDES 1   elective agalactia (O92.5)
         secondary agalactia (O92.5)
         therapeutic agalactia (O92.5)
     DEF: Absence of milk secretion in a female after delivery.

   O92.4 Hypogalactia   M♀

   O92.5 Suppressed lactation   M♀
     Elective agalactia
     Secondary agalactia
     Therapeutic agalactia
     EXCLUDES 1   primary agalactia (O92.3)

   O92.6 Galactorrhea   M♀
     DEF: Excessive or persistent milk secretion by breast; may occur in absence of nursing.

  √5ᵗʰ **O92.7 Other and unspecified disorders of lactation**

     O92.70 Unspecified disorders of lactation   M♀▽

     O92.79 Other disorders of lactation   M♀
       Puerperal galactocele

Other obstetric conditions, not elsewhere classified (O94-O9A)

O94 Sequelae of complication of pregnancy, childbirth, and the puerperium   M♀
   NOTE   This category is to be used to indicate conditions in O00-O77.-, O85-O94 and O98-O9A.- as the cause of late effects. The sequelae include conditions specified as such, or as late effects, which may occur at any time after the puerperium.
   Code first condition resulting from (sequela) of complication of pregnancy, childbirth, and the puerperium

√4ᵗʰ **O98 Maternal infectious and parasitic diseases classifiable elsewhere but complicating pregnancy, childbirth and the puerperium**
   INCLUDES   the listed conditions when complicating the pregnant state, when aggravated by the pregnancy, or as a reason for obstetric care
   Use additional code (Chapter 1), to identify specific infectious or parasitic disease
   EXCLUDES 2   herpes gestationis (O26.4-)
         infectious carrier state (O99.82-, O99.83-)
         obstetrical tetanus (A34)
         puerperal infection (O86.-)
         puerperal sepsis (O85)
         when the reason for maternal care is that the disease is known or suspected to have affected the fetus (O35-O36)

  √5ᵗʰ **O98.0 Tuberculosis complicating pregnancy, childbirth and the puerperium**
     Conditions in A15-A19

    √6ᵗʰ **O98.01 Tuberculosis complicating pregnancy**

       O98.011 Tuberculosis complicating pregnancy, first trimester   M♀

       O98.012 Tuberculosis complicating pregnancy, second trimester   M♀

       O98.013 Tuberculosis complicating pregnancy, third trimester   M♀

       O98.019 Tuberculosis complicating pregnancy, unspecified trimester   M♀▽

     O98.02 Tuberculosis complicating childbirth   M♀

     O98.03 Tuberculosis complicating the puerperium   M♀

  √5ᵗʰ **O98.1 Syphilis complicating pregnancy, childbirth and the puerperium**
     Conditions in A50-A53

    √6ᵗʰ **O98.11 Syphilis complicating pregnancy**

       O98.111 Syphilis complicating pregnancy, first trimester   M♀

       O98.112 Syphilis complicating pregnancy, second trimester   M♀

       O98.113 Syphilis complicating pregnancy, third trimester   M♀

       O98.119 Syphilis complicating pregnancy, unspecified trimester   M♀▽

     O98.12 Syphilis complicating childbirth   M♀

     O98.13 Syphilis complicating the puerperium   M♀

  √5ᵗʰ **O98.2 Gonorrhea complicating pregnancy, childbirth and the puerperium**
     Conditions in A54-

    √6ᵗʰ **O98.21 Gonorrhea complicating pregnancy**

       O98.211 Gonorrhea complicating pregnancy, first trimester   M♀

       O98.212 Gonorrhea complicating pregnancy, second trimester   M♀

       O98.213 Gonorrhea complicating pregnancy, third trimester   M♀

       O98.219 Gonorrhea complicating pregnancy, ▽ unspecified trimester   M♀

     O98.22 Gonorrhea complicating childbirth   M♀

     O98.23 Gonorrhea complicating the puerperium   M♀

  √5ᵗʰ **O98.3 Other infections with a predominantly sexual mode of transmission complicating pregnancy, childbirth and the puerperium**
     Conditions in A55-A64

    √6ᵗʰ **O98.31 Other infections with a predominantly sexual mode of transmission complicating pregnancy**

       O98.311 Other infections with a predominantly sexual mode of transmission complicating pregnancy, first trimester   M♀

       O98.312 Other infections with a predominantly sexual mode of transmission complicating pregnancy, second trimester   M♀

       O98.313 Other infections with a predominantly sexual mode of transmission complicating pregnancy, third trimester   M♀

       O98.319 Other infections with a predominantly sexual mode of transmission complicating pregnancy, unspecified trimester   M♀▽

O98.32 Other infections with a predominantly sexual mode of transmission complicating childbirth Ⓜ♀

O98.33 Other infections with a predominantly sexual mode of transmission complicating the puerperium Ⓜ♀

O98.4 Viral hepatitis complicating pregnancy, childbirth and the puerperium
Conditions in B15-B19

  O98.41 Viral hepatitis complicating pregnancy
    O98.411 Viral hepatitis complicating pregnancy, first trimester Ⓜ♀
    O98.412 Viral hepatitis complicating pregnancy, second trimester Ⓜ♀
    O98.413 Viral hepatitis complicating pregnancy, third trimester Ⓜ♀
    O98.419 Viral hepatitis complicating pregnancy, unspecified trimester Ⓜ♀▽

  O98.42 Viral hepatitis complicating childbirth Ⓜ♀
  O98.43 Viral hepatitis complicating the puerperium Ⓜ♀

O98.5 Other viral diseases complicating pregnancy, childbirth and the puerperium
Conditions in A80-B09, B25-B34, R87.81-, R87.82-
EXCLUDES 1   human immunodeficiency virus [HIV] disease complicating pregnancy, childbirth and the puerperium (O98.7-)

  O98.51 Other viral diseases complicating pregnancy
    O98.511 Other viral diseases complicating pregnancy, first trimester Ⓜ♀
    O98.512 Other viral diseases complicating pregnancy, second trimester Ⓜ♀
    O98.513 Other viral diseases complicating pregnancy, third trimester Ⓜ♀
    O98.519 Other viral diseases complicating pregnancy, unspecified trimester Ⓜ♀▽

  O98.52 Other viral diseases complicating childbirth Ⓜ♀
  O98.53 Other viral diseases complicating the puerperium Ⓜ♀

O98.6 Protozoal diseases complicating pregnancy, childbirth and the puerperium
Conditions in B50-B64

  O98.61 Protozoal diseases complicating pregnancy
    O98.611 Protozoal diseases complicating pregnancy, first trimester Ⓜ♀
    O98.612 Protozoal diseases complicating pregnancy, second trimester Ⓜ♀
    O98.613 Protozoal diseases complicating pregnancy, third trimester Ⓜ♀
    O98.619 Protozoal diseases complicating pregnancy, unspecified trimester Ⓜ♀▽

  O98.62 Protozoal diseases complicating childbirth Ⓜ♀
  O98.63 Protozoal diseases complicating the puerperium Ⓜ♀

O98.7 Human immunodeficiency virus [HIV] disease complicating pregnancy, childbirth and the puerperium
Use additional code to identify the type of HIV disease:
acquired immune deficiency syndrome (AIDS) (B20)
asymptomatic HIV status (Z21)
HIV positive NOS (Z21)
symptomatic HIV disease (B20)

  O98.71 Human immunodeficiency virus [HIV] disease complicating pregnancy
    O98.711 Human immunodeficiency virus [HIV] disease complicating pregnancy, first trimester Ⓜ♀
    O98.712 Human immunodeficiency virus [HIV] disease complicating pregnancy, second trimester Ⓜ♀
    O98.713 Human immunodeficiency virus [HIV] disease complicating pregnancy, third trimester Ⓜ♀
    O98.719 Human immunodeficiency virus [HIV] disease complicating pregnancy, unspecified trimester Ⓜ♀▽

  O98.72 Human immunodeficiency virus [HIV] disease complicating childbirth Ⓜ♀
  O98.73 Human immunodeficiency virus [HIV] disease complicating the puerperium Ⓜ♀

O98.8 Other maternal infectious and parasitic diseases complicating pregnancy, childbirth and the puerperium

  O98.81 Other maternal infectious and parasitic diseases complicating pregnancy
    O98.811 Other maternal infectious and parasitic diseases complicating pregnancy, first trimester Ⓜ♀
    O98.812 Other maternal infectious and parasitic diseases complicating pregnancy, second trimester Ⓜ♀
    O98.813 Other maternal infectious and parasitic diseases complicating pregnancy, third trimester Ⓜ♀
    O98.819 Other maternal infectious and parasitic diseases complicating pregnancy, unspecified trimester Ⓜ♀▽

  O98.82 Other maternal infectious and parasitic diseases complicating childbirth Ⓜ♀
  O98.83 Other maternal infectious and parasitic diseases complicating the puerperium Ⓜ♀

O98.9 Unspecified maternal infectious and parasitic disease complicating pregnancy, childbirth and the puerperium

  O98.91 Unspecified maternal infectious and parasitic disease complicating pregnancy
    O98.911 Unspecified maternal infectious and parasitic disease complicating pregnancy, first trimester Ⓜ♀▽
    O98.912 Unspecified maternal infectious and parasitic disease complicating pregnancy, second trimester Ⓜ♀▽
    O98.913 Unspecified maternal infectious and parasitic disease complicating pregnancy, third trimester Ⓜ♀▽
    O98.919 Unspecified maternal infectious and parasitic disease complicating pregnancy, unspecified trimester Ⓜ♀▽

  O98.92 Unspecified maternal infectious and parasitic disease complicating childbirth Ⓜ♀▽
  O98.93 Unspecified maternal infectious and parasitic disease complicating the puerperium Ⓜ♀▽

O99 Other maternal diseases classifiable elsewhere but complicating pregnancy, childbirth and the puerperium
INCLUDES   conditions which complicate the pregnant state, are aggravated by the pregnancy or are a main reason for obstetric care
Use additional code to identify specific condition
EXCLUDES 2   when the reason for maternal care is that the condition is known or suspected to have affected the fetus (O35-O36)

O99.0 Anemia complicating pregnancy, childbirth and the puerperium
Conditions in D50-D64
EXCLUDES 1   anemia arising in the puerperium (O90.81)
postpartum anemia NOS (O90.81)

  O99.01 Anemia complicating pregnancy
AHA: 2016, 1Q, 4
    O99.011 Anemia complicating pregnancy, first trimester Ⓜ♀
    O99.012 Anemia complicating pregnancy, second trimester Ⓜ♀
    O99.013 Anemia complicating pregnancy, third trimester Ⓜ♀
    O99.019 Anemia complicating pregnancy, unspecified trimester Ⓜ♀▽

  O99.02 Anemia complicating childbirth Ⓜ♀
  O99.03 Anemia complicating the puerperium Ⓜ♀
    EXCLUDES 1   postpartum anemia not pre-existing prior to delivery (O90.81)

O99.1 Other diseases of the blood and blood-forming organs and certain disorders involving the immune mechanism complicating pregnancy, childbirth and the puerperium
Conditions in D65-D89
EXCLUDES 1 ▶ hemorrhage with coagulation defects (O45.-, O46.0-, O67.0, O72.3) ◀
EXCLUDES 2   ~~hemorrhage with coagulation defects (O45.-, O46.0-, O67.0, O72.3)~~

EXCLUDES 1 Not coded here   EXCLUDES 2 Not included here   Ⓝ Newborn Age: 0   Ⓟ Pediatric Age: 0-17   Ⓜ Maternity Age: 12-55   Ⓐ Adult Age: 15-124

852   ICD-10-CM 2018

✓6ᵗʰ **O99.11 Other diseases of the blood and blood-forming organs and certain disorders involving the immune mechanism complicating** pregnancy

    O99.111 Other diseases of the blood and blood-forming organs and certain disorders involving the immune mechanism complicating pregnancy, first trimester   Ⓜ♀

    O99.112 Other diseases of the blood and blood-forming organs and certain disorders involving the immune mechanism complicating pregnancy, second trimester   Ⓜ♀

    O99.113 Other diseases of the blood and blood-forming organs and certain disorders involving the immune mechanism complicating pregnancy, third trimester   Ⓜ♀

    O99.119 Other diseases of the blood and blood-forming organs and certain disorders involving the immune mechanism complicating pregnancy, unspecified trimester   Ⓜ♀▽

O99.12 Other diseases of the blood and blood-forming organs and certain disorders involving the immune mechanism complicating childbirth   Ⓜ♀

O99.13 Other diseases of the blood and blood-forming organs and certain disorders involving the immune mechanism complicating the puerperium   Ⓜ♀

✓5ᵗʰ **O99.2 Endocrine, nutritional and metabolic diseases complicating pregnancy, childbirth and the puerperium**
    Conditions in E00-E88
    EXCLUDES 2   diabetes mellitus (O24.-)
        malnutrition (O25.-)
        postpartum thyroiditis (O90.5)

✓6ᵗʰ **O99.21 Obesity complicating pregnancy, childbirth, and the puerperium**
    Use additional code to identify the type of obesity (E66.-)

    O99.210 Obesity complicating pregnancy, unspecified trimester   Ⓜ♀▽

    O99.211 Obesity complicating pregnancy, first trimester   Ⓜ♀

    O99.212 Obesity complicating pregnancy, second trimester   Ⓜ♀

    O99.213 Obesity complicating pregnancy, third trimester   Ⓜ♀

    O99.214 Obesity complicating childbirth   Ⓜ♀

    O99.215 Obesity complicating the puerperium   Ⓜ♀

✓6ᵗʰ **O99.28 Other endocrine, nutritional and metabolic diseases complicating pregnancy, childbirth and the puerperium**

    O99.280 Endocrine, nutritional and metabolic diseases complicating pregnancy, unspecified trimester   Ⓜ♀▽

    O99.281 Endocrine, nutritional and metabolic diseases complicating pregnancy, first trimester   Ⓜ♀

    O99.282 Endocrine, nutritional and metabolic diseases complicating pregnancy, second trimester   Ⓜ♀

    O99.283 Endocrine, nutritional and metabolic diseases complicating pregnancy, third trimester   Ⓜ♀

    O99.284 Endocrine, nutritional and metabolic diseases complicating childbirth   Ⓜ♀

    O99.285 Endocrine, nutritional and metabolic diseases complicating the puerperium   Ⓜ♀

✓5ᵗʰ **O99.3 Mental disorders and diseases of the nervous system complicating pregnancy, childbirth and the puerperium**

✓6ᵗʰ **O99.31 Alcohol use complicating pregnancy, childbirth, and the puerperium**
    Use additional code(s) from F10 to identify manifestations of the alcohol use

    O99.310 Alcohol use complicating pregnancy, unspecified trimester   Ⓜ♀▽

    O99.311 Alcohol use complicating pregnancy, first trimester   Ⓜ♀

    O99.312 Alcohol use complicating pregnancy, second trimester   Ⓜ♀

    O99.313 Alcohol use complicating pregnancy, third trimester   Ⓜ♀

    O99.314 Alcohol use complicating childbirth   Ⓜ♀

    O99.315 Alcohol use complicating the puerperium   Ⓜ♀

✓6ᵗʰ **O99.32 Drug use complicating pregnancy, childbirth, and the puerperium**
    Use additional code(s) from F11-F16 and F18-F19 to identify manifestations of the drug use

    O99.320 Drug use complicating pregnancy, unspecified trimester   Ⓜ♀▽

    O99.321 Drug use complicating pregnancy, first trimester   Ⓜ♀

    O99.322 Drug use complicating pregnancy, second trimester   Ⓜ♀

    O99.323 Drug use complicating pregnancy, third trimester   Ⓜ♀

    O99.324 Drug use complicating childbirth   Ⓜ♀

    O99.325 Drug use complicating the puerperium   Ⓜ♀

✓6ᵗʰ **O99.33 Tobacco use disorder complicating pregnancy, childbirth, and the puerperium**
    Smoking complicating pregnancy, childbirth, and the puerperium
    Use additional code from category F17 to identify type of tobacco nicotine dependence

    O99.330 Smoking (tobacco) complicating pregnancy, unspecified trimester   Ⓜ♀▽

    O99.331 Smoking (tobacco) complicating pregnancy, first trimester   Ⓜ♀

    O99.332 Smoking (tobacco) complicating pregnancy, second trimester   Ⓜ♀

    O99.333 Smoking (tobacco) complicating pregnancy, third trimester   Ⓜ♀

    O99.334 Smoking (tobacco) complicating childbirth   Ⓜ♀

    O99.335 Smoking (tobacco) complicating the puerperium   Ⓜ♀

✓6ᵗʰ **O99.34 Other mental disorders complicating pregnancy, childbirth, and the puerperium**
    Conditions in F01-F09 and F20-F99
    EXCLUDES 2   postpartum mood disturbance (O90.6)
        postnatal psychosis (F53)
        puerperal psychosis (F53)

    O99.340 Other mental disorders complicating pregnancy, unspecified trimester   Ⓜ♀▽

    O99.341 Other mental disorders complicating pregnancy, first trimester   Ⓜ♀

    O99.342 Other mental disorders complicating pregnancy, second trimester   Ⓜ♀

    O99.343 Other mental disorders complicating pregnancy, third trimester   Ⓜ♀

    O99.344 Other mental disorders complicating childbirth   Ⓜ♀

    O99.345 Other mental disorders complicating the puerperium   Ⓜ♀

✓6ᵗʰ **O99.35 Diseases of the nervous system complicating pregnancy, childbirth, and the puerperium**
    Conditions in G00-G99
    EXCLUDES 2   pregnancy related peripheral neuritis (O26.8-)

    O99.350 Diseases of the nervous system complicating pregnancy, unspecified trimester   Ⓜ♀▽

    O99.351 Diseases of the nervous system complicating pregnancy, first trimester   Ⓜ♀

    O99.352 Diseases of the nervous system complicating pregnancy, second trimester   Ⓜ♀

    O99.353 Diseases of the nervous system complicating pregnancy, third trimester   Ⓜ♀

    O99.354 Diseases of the nervous system complicating childbirth   Ⓜ♀

    O99.355 Diseases of the nervous system complicating the puerperium   Ⓜ♀

☑ Additional Character Req   ✓x7ᵗʰ Placeholder Alert   Manifestation   HCC CMS-HCC Condition   ▽ Unspecified Code   ►◄ Revised Text   ● New Code   ▲ Revised Code Title

Chapter 15. Pregnancy, Childbirth, and the Puerperium

O99.4–O99.842

✓5ᵗʰ **O99.4 Diseases of the circulatory system complicating pregnancy, childbirth and the puerperium**
Conditions in I00-I99
> EXCLUDES 1   peripartum cardiomyopathy (O90.3)
> EXCLUDES 2   hypertensive disorders (O10-O16)
> obstetric embolism (O88.-)
> venous complications and cerebrovenous sinus thrombosis in labor, childbirth and the puerperium (O87.-)
> venous complications and cerebrovenous sinus thrombosis in pregnancy (O22.-)

AHA: 2016, 2Q, 8

✓6ᵗʰ **O99.41 Diseases of the circulatory system complicating pregnancy**
- **O99.411 Diseases of the circulatory system complicating pregnancy, first trimester**   M♀
- **O99.412 Diseases of the circulatory system complicating pregnancy, second trimester**   M♀
- **O99.413 Diseases of the circulatory system complicating pregnancy, third trimester**   M♀
- **O99.419 Diseases of the circulatory system complicating pregnancy, unspecified trimester**   M♀▽

- **O99.42 Diseases of the circulatory system complicating childbirth**   M♀
- **O99.43 Diseases of the circulatory system complicating the puerperium**   M♀

✓5ᵗʰ **O99.5 Diseases of the respiratory system complicating pregnancy, childbirth and the puerperium**
Conditions in J00-J99

✓6ᵗʰ **O99.51 Diseases of the respiratory system complicating pregnancy**
- **O99.511 Diseases of the respiratory system complicating pregnancy, first trimester**   M♀
- **O99.512 Diseases of the respiratory system complicating pregnancy, second trimester**   M♀
- **O99.513 Diseases of the respiratory system complicating pregnancy, third trimester**   M♀
- **O99.519 Diseases of the respiratory system complicating pregnancy, unspecified trimester**   M♀▽

- **O99.52 Diseases of the respiratory system complicating childbirth**   M♀
- **O99.53 Diseases of the respiratory system complicating the puerperium**   M♀

✓5ᵗʰ **O99.6 Diseases of the digestive system complicating pregnancy, childbirth and the puerperium**
Conditions in K00-K93
> EXCLUDES 2   hemorrhoids in pregnancy (O22.4-)
> liver and biliary tract disorders in pregnancy, childbirth and the puerperium (O26.6-)

✓6ᵗʰ **O99.61 Diseases of the digestive system complicating pregnancy**
AHA: 2016, 1Q, 4
- **O99.611 Diseases of the digestive system complicating pregnancy, first trimester**   M♀
- **O99.612 Diseases of the digestive system complicating pregnancy, second trimester**   M♀
- **O99.613 Diseases of the digestive system complicating pregnancy, third trimester**   M♀
- **O99.619 Diseases of the digestive system complicating pregnancy, unspecified trimester**   M♀▽

- **O99.62 Diseases of the digestive system complicating childbirth**   M♀
- **O99.63 Diseases of the digestive system complicating the puerperium**   M♀

✓5ᵗʰ **O99.7 Diseases of the skin and subcutaneous tissue complicating pregnancy, childbirth and the puerperium**
Conditions in L00-L99
> EXCLUDES 2   herpes gestationis (O26.4)
> pruritic urticarial papules and plaques of pregnancy (PUPPP) (O26.86)

✓6ᵗʰ **O99.71 Diseases of the skin and subcutaneous tissue complicating pregnancy**
- **O99.711 Diseases of the skin and subcutaneous tissue complicating pregnancy, first trimester**   M♀
- **O99.712 Diseases of the skin and subcutaneous tissue complicating pregnancy, second trimester**   M♀
- **O99.713 Diseases of the skin and subcutaneous tissue complicating pregnancy, third trimester**   M♀
- **O99.719 Diseases of the skin and subcutaneous tissue complicating pregnancy, unspecified trimester**   M♀▽

- **O99.72 Diseases of the skin and subcutaneous tissue complicating childbirth**   M♀
- **O99.73 Diseases of the skin and subcutaneous tissue complicating the puerperium**   M♀

✓5ᵗʰ **O99.8 Other specified diseases and conditions complicating pregnancy, childbirth and the puerperium**
Conditions in D00-D48, H00-H95, M00-N99, and Q00-Q99
Use additional code to identify condition
> EXCLUDES 2   genitourinary infections in pregnancy (O23.-)
> infection of genitourinary tract following delivery (O86.1-O86.3)
> malignant neoplasm complicating pregnancy, childbirth and the puerperium (O9A.1-)
> maternal care for known or suspected abnormality of maternal pelvic organs (O34.-)
> postpartum acute kidney failure (O90.4)
> traumatic injuries in pregnancy (O9A.2)

✓6ᵗʰ **O99.81 Abnormal glucose complicating pregnancy, childbirth and the puerperium**
> EXCLUDES 1   gestational diabetes (O24.4-)
- **O99.810 Abnormal glucose complicating pregnancy**   M♀
- **O99.814 Abnormal glucose complicating childbirth**   M♀
- **O99.815 Abnormal glucose complicating the puerperium**   M♀

✓6ᵗʰ **O99.82 Streptococcus B carrier state complicating pregnancy, childbirth and the puerperium**
> EXCLUDES 1   carrier of streptococcus group B (GBS) in a nonpregnant woman (Z22.330)
- **O99.820 Streptococcus B carrier state complicating pregnancy**   M♀
- **O99.824 Streptococcus B carrier state complicating childbirth**   M♀
- **O99.825 Streptococcus B carrier state complicating the puerperium**   M♀

✓6ᵗʰ **O99.83 Other infection carrier state complicating pregnancy, childbirth and the puerperium**
Use additional code to identify the carrier state (Z22.-)
- **O99.830 Other infection carrier state complicating pregnancy**   M♀
- **O99.834 Other infection carrier state complicating childbirth**   M♀
- **O99.835 Other infection carrier state complicating the puerperium**   M♀

✓6ᵗʰ **O99.84 Bariatric surgery status complicating pregnancy, childbirth and the puerperium**
Gastric banding status complicating pregnancy, childbirth and the puerperium
Gastric bypass status for obesity complicating pregnancy, childbirth and the puerperium
Obesity surgery status complicating pregnancy, childbirth and the puerperium
- **O99.840 Bariatric surgery status complicating pregnancy, unspecified trimester**   M♀▽
- **O99.841 Bariatric surgery status complicating pregnancy, first trimester**   M♀
- **O99.842 Bariatric surgery status complicating pregnancy, second trimester**   M♀

EXCLUDES 1 Not coded here   EXCLUDES 2 Not included here   N Newborn Age: 0   P Pediatric Age: 0-17   M Maternity Age: 12-55   A Adult Age: 15-124

854   ICD-10-CM 2018

O99.843 **Bariatric surgery status complicating** Ⓜ♀
pregnancy, third trimester

O99.844 **Bariatric surgery status complicating** Ⓜ♀
childbirth

O99.845 **Bariatric surgery status complicating** Ⓜ♀
the puerperium

O99.89 **Other specified diseases and conditions** Ⓜ♀
complicating pregnancy, childbirth and the
puerperium

☑4ᵗʰ **O9A Maternal malignant neoplasms, traumatic injuries and abuse**
classifiable elsewhere but complicating pregnancy, childbirth
and the puerperium

☑5ᵗʰ **O9A.1 Malignant neoplasm complicating pregnancy, childbirth and**
the puerperium
Conditions in C00-C96
Use additional code to identify neoplasm
EXCLUDES 2 *maternal care for benign tumor of corpus uteri (O34.1-)*
maternal care for benign tumor of cervix (O34.4-)
AHA: 2015, 3Q, 19

☑6ᵗʰ **O9A.11 Malignant neoplasm complicating pregnancy**

O9A.111 **Malignant neoplasm complicating** Ⓜ♀
pregnancy, first trimester

O9A.112 **Malignant neoplasm complicating** Ⓜ♀
pregnancy, second trimester

O9A.113 **Malignant neoplasm complicating** Ⓜ♀
pregnancy, third trimester

O9A.119 **Malignant neoplasm complicating** Ⓜ♀▽
pregnancy, unspecified trimester

O9A.12 **Malignant neoplasm complicating childbirth** Ⓜ♀

O9A.13 **Malignant neoplasm complicating the** Ⓜ♀
puerperium

☑5ᵗʰ **O9A.2 Injury, poisoning and certain other consequences of external**
causes complicating pregnancy, childbirth and the
puerperium
Conditions in S00-T88, except T74 and T76
Use additional code(s) to identify the injury or poisoning
EXCLUDES 2 *physical, sexual and psychological abuse complicating*
pregnancy, childbirth and the puerperium
(O9A.3-, O9A.4-, O9A.5-)

☑6ᵗʰ **O9A.21 Injury, poisoning and certain other consequences of**
external causes complicating pregnancy

O9A.211 **Injury, poisoning and certain other** Ⓜ♀
consequences of external causes
complicating pregnancy, first
trimester

O9A.212 **Injury, poisoning and certain other** Ⓜ♀
consequences of external causes
complicating pregnancy, second
trimester

O9A.213 **Injury, poisoning and certain other** Ⓜ♀
consequences of external causes
complicating pregnancy, third
trimester

O9A.219 **Injury, poisoning and certain other** Ⓜ♀▽
consequences of external causes
complicating pregnancy, unspecified
trimester

O9A.22 **Injury, poisoning and certain other** Ⓜ♀
consequences of external causes complicating
childbirth

O9A.23 **Injury, poisoning and certain other** Ⓜ♀
consequencesof external causes complicating the
puerperium

☑5ᵗʰ **O9A.3 Physical abuse complicating pregnancy, childbirth and the**
puerperium
Conditions in T74.11 or T76.11
Use additional code (if applicable):
to identify any associated current injury due to physical abuse
to identify the perpetrator of abuse (Y07.-)
EXCLUDES 2 *sexual abuse complicating pregnancy, childbirth and*
the puerperium (O9A.4)

☑6ᵗʰ **O9A.31 Physical abuse complicating pregnancy**

O9A.311 **Physical abuse complicating** Ⓜ♀
pregnancy, first trimester

O9A.312 **Physical abuse complicating** Ⓜ♀
pregnancy,second trimester

O9A.313 **Physical abuse complicating** Ⓜ♀
pregnancy, third trimester

O9A.319 **Physical abuse complicating** Ⓜ♀▽
pregnancy,unspecified trimester

O9A.32 **Physical abuse complicating childbirth** Ⓜ♀

O9A.33 **Physical abuse complicating the puerperium** Ⓜ♀

☑5ᵗʰ **O9A.4 Sexual abuse complicating pregnancy, childbirth and the**
puerperium
Conditions in T74.21 or T76.21
Use additional code (if applicable):
to identify any associated current injury due to sexual abuse
to identify the perpetrator of abuse (Y07.-)

☑6ᵗʰ **O9A.41 Sexual abuse complicating pregnancy**

O9A.411 **Sexual abuse complicating** Ⓜ♀
pregnancy, first trimester

O9A.412 **Sexual abuse complicating pregnancy,** Ⓜ♀
second trimester

O9A.413 **Sexual abuse complicating** Ⓜ♀
pregnancy, third trimester

O9A.419 **Sexual abuse complicating** Ⓜ♀▽
pregnancy, unspecified trimester

O9A.42 **Sexual abuse complicating childbirth** Ⓜ♀

O9A.43 **Sexual abuse complicating the puerperium** Ⓜ♀

☑5ᵗʰ **O9A.5 Psychological abuse complicating pregnancy, childbirth and**
the puerperium
Conditions in T74.31 or T76.31
Use additional code to identify the perpetrator of abuse (Y07.-)

☑6ᵗʰ **O9A.51 Psychological abuse complicating pregnancy**

O9A.511 **Psychological abuse complicating** Ⓜ♀
pregnancy, first trimester

O9A.512 **Psychological abuse complicating** Ⓜ♀
pregnancy, second trimester

O9A.513 **Psychological abuse complicating** Ⓜ♀
pregnancy, third trimester

O9A.519 **Psychological abuse complicating** Ⓜ♀▽
pregnancy, unspecified trimester

O9A.52 **Psychological abuse complicating childbirth** Ⓜ♀

O9A.53 **Psychological abuse complicating the** Ⓜ♀
puerperium

Chapter 16. Certain Conditions Originating in the Perinatal Period (P00–P96)

Chapter Specific Guidelines with Coding Examples

The chapter specific guidelines from the ICD-10-CM Official Guidelines for Coding and Reporting have been provided below. Along with these guidelines are coding examples, contained in the shaded boxes, that have been developed to help illustrate the coding and/or sequencing guidance found in these guidelines.

For coding and reporting purposes the perinatal period is defined as before birth through the 28th day following birth. The following guidelines are provided for reporting purposes

a. General perinatal rules

1) Use of Chapter 16 codes

Codes in this chapter are <u>never</u> for use on the maternal record. Codes from Chapter 15, the obstetric chapter, are never permitted on the newborn record. Chapter 16 codes may be used throughout the life of the patient if the condition is still present.

2) Principal diagnosis for birth record

When coding the birth episode in a newborn record, assign a code from category Z38, Liveborn infants according to place of birth and type of delivery, as the principal diagnosis. A code from category Z38 is assigned only once, to a newborn at the time of birth. If a newborn is transferred to another institution, a code from category Z38 should not be used at the receiving hospital.

A code from category Z38 is used only on the newborn record, not on the mother's record.

3) Use of codes from other chapters with codes from Chapter 16

Codes from other chapters may be used with codes from chapter 16 if the codes from the other chapters provide more specific detail. Codes for signs and symptoms may be assigned when a definitive diagnosis has not been established. If the reason for the encounter is a perinatal condition, the code from chapter 16 should be sequenced first.

4) Use of Chapter 16 codes after the perinatal period

Should a condition originate in the perinatal period, and continue throughout the life of the patient, the perinatal code should continue to be used regardless of the patient's age.

> A 7-year-old patient with history of birth injury that resulted in Erb's palsy is seen for subscapularis release
>
> **P14.0**   **Erb's paralysis due to birth injury**
>
> *Explanation:* Although in this instance Erb's palsy is specifically related to a birth injury, it has not resolved and continues to be a health concern. A perinatal code is appropriate even though this patient is beyond the perinatal period.

5) Birth process or community acquired conditions

If a newborn has a condition that may be either due to the birth process or community acquired and the documentation does not indicate which it is, the default is due to the birth process and the code from Chapter 16 should be used. If the condition is community-acquired, a code from Chapter 16 should not be assigned.

6) Code all clinically significant conditions

All clinically significant conditions noted on routine newborn examination should be coded. A condition is clinically significant if it requires:

clinical evaluation; or

therapeutic treatment; or

diagnostic procedures; or

extended length of hospital stay; or

increased nursing care and/or monitoring; or

has implications for future health care needs

Note: The perinatal guidelines listed above are the same as the general coding guidelines for "additional diagnoses", except for the final point regarding implications for future health care needs. Codes should be assigned for conditions that have been specified by the provider as having implications for future health care needs.

b. Observation and evaluation of newborns for suspected conditions not found

1) Use of Z05 codes

Assign a code from category Z05, Observation and evaluation of newborns and infants for suspected conditions ruled out, to identify those instances when a healthy newborn is evaluated for a suspected condition that is determined after study not to be present. Do not use a code from category Z05 when the patient has identified signs or symptoms of a suspected problem; in such cases code the sign or symptom.

2) Z05 on other than the birth record

A code from category Z05 may also be assigned as a principal or first-listed code for readmissions or encounters when the code from category Z38 code no longer applies. Codes from category Z05 are for use only for healthy newborns and infants for which no condition after study is found to be present.

3) Z05 on a birth record

A code from category Z05 is to be used as a secondary code after the code from category Z38, Liveborn infants according to place of birth and type of delivery.

> Newborn delivered via vaginal delivery; previous ultrasounds showed what appeared to be an abnormality of the right kidney. Kidney function tests were performed and ultrasounds taken and any genitourinary conditions ruled out.
>
> **Z38.00**   **Single liveborn infant, delivered vaginally**
>
> **Z05.6**   **Observation and evaluation of newborn for suspected genitourinary condition ruled out**
>
> Explanation: The newborn had no signs or symptoms of kidney or other genitourinary condition but was evaluated after delivery due to the abnormal prenatal ultrasound findings. A Z code describing the type and place of birth should be coded first, followed by a Z05 category code for the work performed to rule out a suspected genitourinary condition.

c. Coding additional perinatal diagnoses

1) Assigning codes for conditions that require treatment

Assign codes for conditions that require treatment or further investigation, prolong the length of stay, or require resource utilization.

2) Codes for conditions specified as having implications for future health care needs

Assign codes for conditions that have been specified by the provider as having implications for future health care needs.

Note: This guideline should not be used for adult patients.

> An abnormal noise was heard in the left hip of a post-term newborn during a physical examination. The pediatrician would like to follow the patient after discharge as a hip click can be an early sign of hip dysplasia. The newborn was delivered via cesarean at 41 weeks.
>
> **Z38.01**   **Single liveborn infant, delivered by cesarean**
>
> **P08.21**   **Post-term newborn**
>
> **R29.4**   **Clicking hip**
>
> *Explanation:* The abnormal hip noise or click is appended as a secondary diagnosis not only because it is an abnormal finding upon examination, but also due to its potential to be part of a bigger health issue. The hip dysplasia has not yet been diagnosed and does not warrant a code at this time.

d. Prematurity and fetal growth retardation

Providers utilize different criteria in determining prematurity. A code for prematurity should not be assigned unless it is documented. Assignment of codes in categories P05, Disorders of newborn related to slow fetal growth and fetal malnutrition, and P07, Disorders of newborn related to short gestation and low birth weight, not elsewhere classified, should be based on the recorded birth weight and estimated gestational age.

When both birth weight and gestational age are available, two codes from category P07 should be assigned, with the code for birth weight sequenced before the code for gestational age.

Chapter 16. Certain Conditions Originating in the Perinatal Period

e. Low birth weight and immaturity status

Codes from category P07, Disorders of newborn related to short gestation and low birth weight, not elsewhere classified, are for use for a child or adult who was premature or had a low birth weight as a newborn and this is affecting the patient's current health status.

See Section I.C.21. Factors influencing health status and contact with health services, Status.

A 35-year-old patient, who weighed 659 grams at birth, is seen for heart disease documented as being a consequence of the low birth weight

I51.9	**Heart disease, unspecified**
P07.02	**Extremely low birth weight newborn, 500–749 grams**

Explanation: A code from subcategories P07.0- and P07.1- is appropriate, regardless of the age of the patient, as long as the documentation provides a clear link between the patient's current illness and the low birth weight.

---

f. Bacterial sepsis of newborn

Category P36, Bacterial sepsis of newborn, includes congenital sepsis. If a perinate is documented as having sepsis without documentation of congenital or community acquired, the default is congenital and a code from category P36 should be assigned. If the P36 code includes the causal organism, an additional code from category B95, Streptococcus, Staphylococcus, and Enterococcus as the cause of diseases classified elsewhere, or B96, Other bacterial agents as the cause of diseases classified elsewhere, should not be assigned. If the P36 code does not include the causal organism, assign an additional code from category B96. If applicable, use additional codes to identify severe sepsis (R65.2-) and any associated acute organ dysfunction.

A full-term infant develops severe sepsis 24 hours after discharge from the hospital and is readmitted; cultures identified *E. coli* as the infective agent

P36.4	**Sepsis of newborn due to Escherichia coli**
R65.20	**Severe sepsis without septic shock**

Explanation: Even though this newborn was discharged and could have acquired *E. coli* from his/her external environment, due to the lack of documentation specifying specifically how this pathogen was acquired, the default is to code the *E. coli* sepsis as congenital. A code from chapter 1, "Certain Infectious and Parasitic Diseases," is not required because the perinatal sepsis code identifies both the sepsis and the bacteria causing the sepsis.

---

g. Stillbirth

Code P95, Stillbirth, is only for use in institutions that maintain separate records for stillbirths. No other code should be used with P95. Code P95 should not be used on the mother's record.

Chapter 16. Certain Conditions Originating in the Perinatal Period (P00-P96)

NOTE   Codes from this chapter are for use on newborn records only, never on maternal records.

INCLUDES   conditions that have their origin in the fetal or perinatal period (before birth through the first 28 days after birth) even if morbidity occurs later

EXCLUDES 2   congenital malformations, deformations and chromosomal abnormalities (Q00-Q99)
endocrine, nutritional and metabolic diseases (E00-E88)
injury, poisoning and certain other consequences of external causes (S00-T88)
neoplasms (C00-D49)
tetanus neonatorum (A33)

This chapter contains the following blocks:

P00-P04	Newborn affected by maternal factors and by complications of pregnancy, labor, and delivery
P05-P08	Disorders of newborn related to length of gestation and fetal growth
P09	Abnormal findings on neonatal screening
P10-P15	Birth trauma
P19-P29	Respiratory and cardiovascular disorders specific to the perinatal period
P35-P39	Infections specific to the perinatal period
P50-P61	Hemorrhagic and hematological disorders of newborn
P70-P74	Transitory endocrine and metabolic disorders specific to newborn
P76-P78	Digestive system disorders of newborn
P80-P83	Conditions involving the integument and temperature regulation of newborn
P84	Other problems with newborn
P90-P96	Other disorders originating in the perinatal period

Newborn affected by maternal factors and by complications of pregnancy, labor, and delivery (P00-P04)

NOTE   These codes are for use when the listed maternal conditions are specified as the cause of confirmed morbidity or potential morbidity which have their origin in the perinatal period (before birth through the first 28 days after birth).

√4ᵗʰ **P00**   **Newborn affected by** maternal conditions **that may be unrelated to present pregnancy**

Code first any current condition in newborn

EXCLUDES 2   encounter for observation of newborn for suspected diseases and conditions ruled out (Z05.-)
newborn affected by maternal complications of pregnancy (P01.-)
newborn affected by maternal endocrine and metabolic disorders (P70-P74)
newborn affected by noxious substances transmitted via placenta or breast milk (P04.-)

P00.0   **Newborn affected by maternal** hypertensive **disorders**
Newborn affected by maternal conditions classifiable to O10-O11, O13-O16

P00.1   **Newborn affected by maternal** renal and urinary tract **diseases**
Newborn affected by maternal conditions classifiable to N00-N39

P00.2   **Newborn affected by maternal** infectious and parasitic **diseases**
Newborn affected by maternal infectious disease classifiable to A00-B99, J09 and J10
EXCLUDES 1   ~~infections specific to the perinatal period (P35-P39)~~
maternal genital tract or other localized infections (P00.8)
EXCLUDES 2 ▶ infections specific to the perinatal period (P35-P39) ◀
AHA: 2015, 3Q, 20

P00.3   **Newborn affected by other maternal** circulatory and respiratory **diseases**
Newborn affected by maternal conditions classifiable to I00-I99, J00-J99, Q20-Q34 and not included in P00.0, P00.2

P00.4   **Newborn affected by maternal** nutritional **disorders**
Newborn affected by maternal disorders classifiable to E40-E64
Maternal malnutrition NOS

P00.5   **Newborn affected by maternal** injury
Newborn affected by maternal conditions classifiable to O9A.2-

P00.6   **Newborn affected by** surgical procedure on mother
Newborn affected by amniocentesis
EXCLUDES 1   Cesarean delivery for present delivery (P03.4)
damage to placenta from amniocentesis, Cesarean delivery or surgical induction (P02.1)
previous surgery to uterus or pelvic organs (P03.89)
EXCLUDES 2   newborn affected by complication of (fetal) intrauterine procedure (P96.5)

P00.7   **Newborn affected by other medical procedures on mother, not elsewhere classified**
Newborn affected by radiation to mother
EXCLUDES 1   damage to placenta from amniocentesis, cesarean delivery or surgical induction (P02.1)
newborn affected by other complications of labor and delivery (P03.-)

√5ᵗʰ **P00.8**   **Newborn affected by other maternal conditions**

     P00.81   **Newborn affected by** periodontal disease **in mother**

     P00.89   **Newborn affected by other maternal conditions**
Newborn affected by conditions classifiable to T80-T88
Newborn affected by maternal genital tract or other localized infections
Newborn affected by maternal systemic lupus erythematosus

P00.9   **Newborn affected by unspecified maternal condition** ▽

√4ᵗʰ **P01**   **Newborn affected by** maternal complications of pregnancy
Code first any current condition in newborn
EXCLUDES 2   encounter for observation of newborn for suspected diseases and conditions ruled out (Z05.-)

P01.0   **Newborn affected by** incompetent cervix

P01.1   **Newborn affected by** premature rupture of membranes

P01.2   **Newborn affected by** oligohydramnios
EXCLUDES 1   oligohydramnios due to premature rupture of membranes (P01.1)
DEF: Low amniotic fluid level, resulting in underdeveloped organs in the fetus.

P01.3   **Newborn affected by** polyhydramnios
Newborn affected by hydramnios

P01.4   **Newborn affected by** ectopic pregnancy
Newborn affected by abdominal pregnancy

P01.5   **Newborn affected by** multiple pregnancy
Newborn affected by triplet (pregnancy)
Newborn affected by twin (pregnancy)

P01.6   **Newborn affected by** maternal death

P01.7   **Newborn affected by** malpresentation before labor
Newborn affected by breech presentation before labor
Newborn affected by external version before labor
Newborn affected by face presentation before labor
Newborn affected by transverse lie before labor
Newborn affected by unstable lie before labor

P01.8   **Newborn affected by other maternal complications of pregnancy**

P01.9   **Newborn affected by maternal complication of pregnancy, unspecified** ▽

√4ᵗʰ **P02**   **Newborn affected by complications of** placenta, cord and membranes
Code first any current condition in newborn
EXCLUDES 2   encounter for observation of newborn for suspected diseases and conditions ruled out (Z05.-)

P02.0   **Newborn affected by** placenta previa
DEF: Placenta developed in lower segment of uterus; can cause hemorrhaging leading to preterm delivery.

P02.1   **Newborn affected by other forms of placental** separation and hemorrhage
Newborn affected by abruptio placenta
Newborn affected by accidental hemorrhage
Newborn affected by antepartum hemorrhage
Newborn affected by damage to placenta from amniocentesis, cesarean delivery or surgical induction
Newborn affected by maternal blood loss
Newborn affected by premature separation of placenta

√5ᵗʰ **P02.2**   **Newborn affected by other and unspecified** morphological and functional abnormalities **of placenta**

     P02.20   **Newborn affected by unspecified morphological** ▽ **and functional abnormalities of placenta**

Chapter 16. Certain Conditions Originating in the Perinatal Period

P02.29 Newborn affected by other morphological and functional abnormalities of placenta
Newborn affected by placental dysfunction
Newborn affected by placental infarction
Newborn affected by placental insufficiency

P02.3 Newborn affected by placental transfusion syndromes
Newborn affected by placental and cord abnormalities resulting in twin-to-twin or other transplacental transfusion

P02.4 Newborn affected by prolapsed cord

P02.5 Newborn affected by other compression of umbilical cord
Newborn affected by umbilical cord (tightly) around neck
Newborn affected by entanglement of umbilical cord
Newborn affected by knot in umbilical cord

√5ᵗʰ **P02.6 Newborn affected by other and unspecified conditions of umbilical cord**

     P02.60 Newborn affected by unspecified conditions of umbilical cord ▽

     P02.69 Newborn affected by other conditions of umbilical cord
Newborn affected by short umbilical cord
Newborn affected by vasa previa
EXCLUDES 1   newborn affected by single umbilical artery (Q27.0)

P02.7 Newborn affected by chorioamnionitis
Newborn affected by amnionitis
Newborn affected by membranitis
Newborn affected by placentitis
DEF: Inflammation of the fetal membranes due to maternal infection; characterized by fetal tachycardia, respiratory distress, apnea, weak cries, and poor sucking.

P02.8 Newborn affected by other abnormalities of membranes

P02.9 Newborn affected by abnormality of membranes, unspecified ▽

√4ᵗʰ **P03 Newborn affected by other complications of labor and delivery**
Code first any current condition in newborn
EXCLUDES 2   encounter for observation of newborn for suspected diseases and conditions ruled out (Z05.-)

P03.0 Newborn affected by breech delivery and extraction

P03.1 Newborn affected by other malpresentation, malposition and disproportion during labor and delivery
Newborn affected by contracted pelvis
Newborn affected by conditions classifiable to O64-O66
Newborn affected by persistent occipitoposterior
Newborn affected by transverse lie

Forceps Assisted Birth

Forceps extractor

Vacuum Assisted Birth

Vacuum extractor

P03.2 Newborn affected by forceps delivery

P03.3 Newborn affected by delivery by vacuum extractor [ventouse]

P03.4 Newborn affected by Cesarean delivery

P03.5 Newborn affected by precipitate delivery
Newborn affected by rapid second stage

P03.6 Newborn affected by abnormal uterine contractions
Newborn affected by conditions classifiable to O62-, except O62.3
Newborn affected by hypertonic labor
Newborn affected by uterine inertia

√5ᵗʰ **P03.8 Newborn affected by other specified complications of labor and delivery**

√6ᵗʰ   **P03.81 Newborn affected by abnormality in fetal (intrauterine) heart rate or rhythm**
EXCLUDES 1   neonatal cardiac dysrhythmia (P29.1-)

     P03.810 Newborn affected by abnormality in fetal (intrauterine) heart rate or rhythm before the onset of labor

     P03.811 Newborn affected by abnormality in fetal (intrauterine) heart rate or rhythm during labor

     P03.819 Newborn affected by abnormality in fetal (intrauterine) heart rate or rhythm, unspecified as to time of onset ▽

   P03.82 Meconium passage during delivery
EXCLUDES 1   meconium aspiration (P24.00, P24.01) meconium staining (P96.83)
DEF: Fetal intestinal activity that increases in response to a fetomaternal distressed state during delivery; the anal sphincter relaxes, and meconium is passed into the amniotic fluid.

   P03.89 Newborn affected by other specified complications of labor and delivery
Newborn affected by abnormality of maternal soft tissues
Newborn affected by conditions classifiable to O60-O75 and by procedures used in labor and delivery not included in P02.- and P03.0-P03.6
Newborn affected by induction of labor

P03.9 Newborn affected by complication of labor and delivery, unspecified ▽

√4ᵗʰ **P04 Newborn affected by noxious substances transmitted via placenta or breast milk**
INCLUDES   nonteratogenic effects of substances transmitted via placenta
EXCLUDES 2   congenital malformations (Q00-Q99)
encounter for observation of newborn for suspected diseases and conditions ruled out (Z05.-)
neonatal jaundice from excessive hemolysis due to drugs or toxins transmitted from mother (P58.4)
newborn in contact with and (suspected) exposures hazardous to health not transmitted via placenta or breast milk (Z77.-)

P04.0 Newborn affected by maternal anesthesia and analgesia in pregnancy, labor and delivery
Newborn affected by reactions and intoxications from maternal opiates and tranquilizers administered during labor and delivery

P04.1 Newborn affected by other maternal medication
Newborn affected by cancer chemotherapy
Newborn affected by cytotoxic drugs
EXCLUDES 1   dysmorphism due to warfarin (Q86.2)
fetal hydantoin syndrome (Q86.1)
maternal use of drugs of addiction (P04.4-)

P04.2 Newborn affected by maternal use of tobacco
Newborn affected by exposure in utero to tobacco smoke
EXCLUDES 2   newborn exposure to environmental tobacco smoke (P96.81)

P04.3 Newborn affected by maternal use of alcohol
EXCLUDES 1   fetal alcohol syndrome (Q86.0)

√5ᵗʰ **P04.4 Newborn affected by maternal use of drugs of addiction**

     P04.41 Newborn affected by maternal use of cocaine
"Crack baby"

     P04.49 Newborn affected by maternal use of other drugs of addiction
EXCLUDES 2   newborn affected by maternal anesthesia and analgesia (P04.0)
withdrawal symptoms from maternal use of drugs of addiction (P96.1)

EXCLUDES 1 Not coded here   **EXCLUDES 2** Not included here   **N** Newborn Age: 0   **P** Pediatric Age: 0-17   **M** Maternity Age: 12-55   **A** Adult Age: 15-124

860   ICD-10-CM 2018

P04.5   Newborn affected by maternal use of nutritional chemical substances

P04.6   Newborn affected by maternal exposure to environmental chemical substances

P04.8   Newborn affected by other maternal noxious substances

P04.9   Newborn affected by maternal noxious substance, unspecified   ▽

Disorders of newborn related to length of gestation and fetal growth (P05-P08)

✓4ᵗʰ P05   **Disorders of newborn related to slow fetal growth and fetal malnutrition**

   ✓5ᵗʰ P05.0   **Newborn light for gestational age**
Newborn light-for-dates
Weight below but length above 10th percentile for gestational age

     P05.00   **Newborn light for gestational age, unspecified weight**   ▽

     P05.01   **Newborn light for gestational age,** less than 500 grams

     P05.02   **Newborn light for gestational age,** 500-749 grams

     P05.03   **Newborn light for gestational age,** 750-999 grams

     P05.04   **Newborn light for gestational age,** 1000-1249 grams

     P05.05   **Newborn light for gestational age,** 1250-1499 grams

     P05.06   **Newborn light for gestational age,** 1500-1749 grams

     P05.07   **Newborn light for gestational age,** 1750-1999 grams

     P05.08   **Newborn light for gestational age,** 2000-2499 grams

     P05.09   **Newborn light for gestational age,** 2500 grams and over
Newborn light for gestational age, other

   ✓5ᵗʰ P05.1   **Newborn small for gestational age**
Newborn small-and-light-for-dates
Newborn small-for-dates
Weight and length below 10th percentile for gestational age

     P05.10   **Newborn small for gestational age, unspecified weight**   ▽

     P05.11   **Newborn small for gestational age,** less than 500 grams

     P05.12   **Newborn small for gestational age,** 500-749 grams

     P05.13   **Newborn small for gestational age,** 750-999 grams

     P05.14   **Newborn small for gestational age,** 1000-1249 grams

     P05.15   **Newborn small for gestational age,** 1250-1499 grams

     P05.16   **Newborn small for gestational age,** 1500-1749 grams

     P05.17   **Newborn small for gestational age,** 1750-1999 grams

     P05.18   **Newborn small for gestational age,** 2000-2499 grams

     P05.19   **Newborn small for gestational age, other**
Newborn small for gestational age, 2500 grams and over

   P05.2   **Newborn affected by fetal (intrauterine) malnutrition not light or small for gestational age**
Infant, not light or small for gestational age, showing signs of fetal malnutrition, such as dry, peeling skin and loss of subcutaneous tissue
     EXCLUDES 1   newborn affected by fetal malnutrition with light for gestational age (P05.0-)
newborn affected by fetal malnutrition with small for gestational age (P05.1-)

   P05.9   **Newborn affected by slow intrauterine growth, unspecified**   ▽
Newborn affected by fetal growth retardation NOS

✓4ᵗʰ P07   **Disorders of newborn related to short gestation and low birth weight, not elsewhere classified**
     NOTE   When both birth weight and gestational age of the newborn are available, both should be coded with birth weight sequenced before gestational age
     INCLUDES   the listed conditions, without further specification, as the cause of morbidity or additional care, in newborn

   ✓5ᵗʰ P07.0   **Extremely low birth weight newborn**
Newborn birth weight 999 g. or less
     EXCLUDES 1   low birth weight due to slow fetal growth and fetal malnutrition (P05.-)

     P07.00   **Extremely low birth weight newborn, unspecified weight**   ▽

     P07.01   **Extremely low birth weight newborn,** less than 500 grams

     P07.02   **Extremely low birth weight newborn,** 500-749 grams

     P07.03   **Extremely low birth weight newborn,** 750-999 grams

   ✓5ᵗʰ P07.1   **Other low birth weight newborn**
Newborn birth weight 1000-2499 g.
     EXCLUDES 1   low birth weight due to slow fetal growth and fetal malnutrition (P05.-)

     P07.10   **Other low birth weight newborn, unspecified weight**   ▽

     P07.14   **Other low birth weight newborn,** 1000-1249 grams

     P07.15   **Other low birth weight newborn,** 1250-1499 grams

     P07.16   **Other low birth weight newborn,** 1500-1749 grams

     P07.17   **Other low birth weight newborn,** 1750-1999 grams

     P07.18   **Other low birth weight newborn,** 2000-2499 grams

   ✓5ᵗʰ P07.2   **Extreme immaturity of newborn**
Less than 28 completed weeks (less than 196 completed days) of gestation.

     P07.20   **Extreme immaturity of newborn, unspecified weeks of gestation**   ▽
Gestational age less than 28 completed weeks NOS

     P07.21   **Extreme immaturity of newborn, gestational age less than 23 completed weeks**
Extreme immaturity of newborn, gestational age less than 23 weeks, 0 days

     P07.22   **Extreme immaturity of newborn, gestational age 23 completed weeks**
Extreme immaturity of newborn, gestational age 23 weeks, 0 days through 23 weeks, 6 days

     P07.23   **Extreme immaturity of newborn, gestational age 24 completed weeks**
Extreme immaturity of newborn, gestational age 24 weeks, 0 days through 24 weeks, 6 days

     P07.24   **Extreme immaturity of newborn, gestational age 25 completed weeks**
Extreme immaturity of newborn, gestational age 25 weeks, 0 days through 25 weeks, 6 days

     P07.25   **Extreme immaturity of newborn, gestational age 26 completed weeks**
Extreme immaturity of newborn, gestational age 26 weeks, 0 days through 26 weeks, 6 days

     P07.26   **Extreme immaturity of newborn, gestational age 27 completed weeks**
Extreme immaturity of newborn, gestational age 27 weeks, 0 days through 27 weeks, 6 days

   ✓5ᵗʰ P07.3   **Preterm [premature] newborn [other]**
28 completed weeks or more but less than 37 completed weeks (196 completed days but less than 259 completed days) of gestation
Prematurity NOS

     P07.30   **Preterm newborn, unspecified weeks of gestation**   ▽

     P07.31   **Preterm newborn, gestational age** 28 completed weeks
Preterm newborn, gestational age 28 weeks, 0 days through 28 weeks, 6 days

     P07.32   **Preterm newborn, gestational age** 29 completed weeks
Preterm newborn, gestational age 29 weeks, 0 days through 29 weeks, 6 days

     P07.33   **Preterm newborn, gestational age** 30 completed weeks
Preterm newborn, gestational age 30 weeks, 0 days through 30 weeks, 6 days

---

☑ Additional Character Req   ✓x7ᵗʰ Placeholder Alert   Manifestation   HCC CMS-HCC Condition   ▽ Unspecified Code   ►◄ Revised Text   ● New Code   ▲ Revised Code Title

P07.34   **Preterm newborn, gestational age** 31 completed weeks
> Preterm newborn, gestational age 31 weeks, 0 days through 31 weeks, 6 days

P07.35   **Preterm newborn, gestational age** 32 completed weeks
> Preterm newborn, gestational age 32 weeks, 0 days through 32 weeks, 6 days

P07.36   **Preterm newborn, gestational age** 33 completed weeks
> Preterm newborn, gestational age 33 weeks, 0 days through 33 weeks, 6 days

P07.37   **Preterm newborn, gestational age** 34 completed weeks
> Preterm newborn, gestational age 34 weeks, 0 days through 34 weeks, 6 days

P07.38   **Preterm newborn, gestational age** 35 completed weeks
> Preterm newborn, gestational age 35 weeks, 0 days through 35 weeks, 6 days

P07.39   **Preterm newborn, gestational age** 36 completed weeks
> Preterm newborn, gestational age 36 weeks, 0 days through 36 weeks, 6 days

✓4ᵗʰ **P08**   **Disorders of newborn related to long gestation and high birth weight**
> NOTE   When both birth weight and gestational age of the newborn are available, priority of assignment should be given to birth weight
> INCLUDES   the listed conditions, without further specification, as causes of morbidity or additional care, in newborn

P08.0   **Exceptionally large newborn baby**
> Usually implies a birth weight of 4500 g. or more
> EXCLUDES 1   *syndrome of infant of diabetic mother (P70.1)*
> *syndrome of infant of mother with gestational diabetes (P70.0)*

P08.1   **Other heavy for gestational age newborn**
> Other newborn heavy- or large-for-dates regardless of period of gestation
> Usually implies a birth weight of 4000 g. to 4499 g.
> EXCLUDES 1   *newborn with a birth weight of 4500 or more (P08.0)*
> *syndrome of infant of diabetic mother (P70.1)*
> *syndrome of infant of mother with gestational diabetes (P70.0).*

✓5ᵗʰ **P08.2**   **Late newborn, not heavy for gestational age**
> AHA: 2014, 1Q, 14

P08.21   **Post-term newborn**
> Newborn with gestation period over 40 completed weeks to 42 completed weeks

P08.22   **Prolonged gestation of newborn**
> Newborn with gestation period over 42 completed weeks (294 days or more), not heavy- or large-for-dates.
> Postmaturity NOS

Abnormal findings on neonatal screening (P09)

P09   **Abnormal findings on neonatal screening**
> Use additional code to identify signs, symptoms and conditions associated with the screening
> EXCLUDES 2   *nonspecific serologic evidence of human immunodeficiency virus [HIV] (R75)*

Birth trauma (P10-P15)

✓4ᵗʰ **P10**   **Intracranial laceration and hemorrhage due to birth injury**
> EXCLUDES 1   *intracranial hemorrhage of newborn NOS (P52.9)*
> *intracranial hemorrhage of newborn due to anoxia or hypoxia (P52.-)*
> *nontraumatic intracranial hemorrhage of newborn (P52.-)*

P10.0   **Subdural hemorrhage due to birth injury**
> Subdural hematoma (localized) due to birth injury
> EXCLUDES 1   *subdural hemorrhage accompanying tentorial tear (P10.4)*

P10.1   **Cerebral hemorrhage due to birth injury**

P10.2   **Intraventricular hemorrhage due to birth injury**

P10.3   **Subarachnoid hemorrhage due to birth injury**

P10.4   **Tentorial tear due to birth injury**

P10.8   **Other intracranial lacerations and hemorrhages due to birth injury**

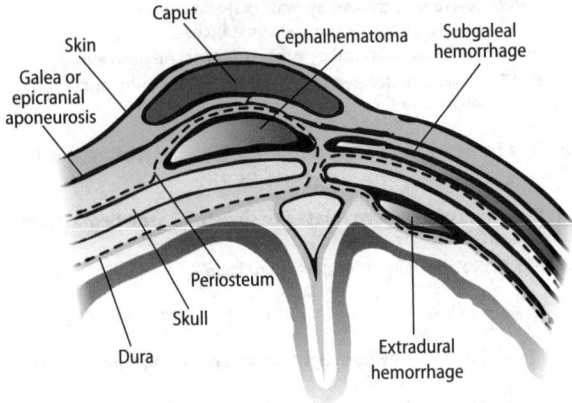

Birth Injuries to Scalp

P10.9   **Unspecified intracranial laceration and hemorrhage due to birth injury** ▽

✓4ᵗʰ **P11**   **Other birth injuries to central nervous system**

P11.0   **Cerebral edema due to birth injury**

P11.1   **Other specified brain damage due to birth injury**

P11.2   **Unspecified brain damage due to birth injury** ▽

P11.3   **Birth injury to facial nerve**
> Facial palsy due to birth injury

P11.4   **Birth injury to other cranial nerves**

P11.5   **Birth injury to spine and spinal cord**
> Fracture of spine due to birth injury

P11.9   **Birth injury to central nervous system, unspecified** ▽

✓4ᵗʰ **P12**   **Birth injury to scalp**

P12.0   **Cephalhematoma due to birth injury**

P12.1   **Chignon (from vacuum extraction) due to birth injury**

P12.2   **Epicranial subaponeurotic hemorrhage due to birth injury**
> Subgaleal hemorrhage

P12.3   **Bruising of scalp due to birth injury**

P12.4   **Injury of scalp of newborn due to monitoring equipment**
> Sampling incision of scalp of newborn
> Scalp clip (electrode) injury of newborn

✓5ᵗʰ **P12.8**   **Other birth injuries to scalp**

P12.81   **Caput succedaneum**

P12.89   **Other birth injuries to scalp**

P12.9   **Birth injury to scalp, unspecified** ▽

✓4ᵗʰ **P13**   **Birth injury to skeleton**
> EXCLUDES 2   *birth injury to spine (P11.5)*

P13.0   **Fracture of skull due to birth injury**

P13.1   **Other birth injuries to skull**
> EXCLUDES 1   *cephalhematoma (P12.0)*

P13.2   **Birth injury to femur**

P13.3   **Birth injury to other long bones**

P13.4   **Fracture of clavicle due to birth injury**

P13.8   **Birth injuries to other parts of skeleton**

P13.9   **Birth injury to skeleton, unspecified** ▽

✓4ᵗʰ **P14**   **Birth injury to peripheral nervous system**

P14.0   **Erb's paralysis due to birth injury**

P14.1   **Klumpke's paralysis due to birth injury**

P14.2   **Phrenic nerve paralysis due to birth injury**

P14.3   **Other brachial plexus birth injuries**

P14.8   **Birth injuries to other parts of peripheral nervous system**

P14.9   **Birth injury to peripheral nervous system, unspecified** ▽

✓4ᵗʰ **P15**   **Other birth injuries**

P15.0   **Birth injury to liver**
> Rupture of liver due to birth injury

P15.1   **Birth injury to spleen**
> Rupture of spleen due to birth injury

P15.2   **Sternomastoid injury due to birth injury**

P15.3   **Birth injury to eye**
> Subconjunctival hemorrhage due to birth injury
> Traumatic glaucoma due to birth injury

EXCLUDES 1 Not coded here   EXCLUDES 2 Not included here   N Newborn Age: 0   P Pediatric Age: 0-17   M Maternity Age: 12-55   A Adult Age: 15-124

P15.4 Birth injury to face
Facial congestion due to birth injury

P15.5 Birth injury to external genitalia

P15.6 Subcutaneous fat necrosis due to birth injury

P15.8 Other specified birth injuries
TIP: Use for any injury of newborn from scalpel.

P15.9 Birth injury, unspecified   ▽

Respiratory and cardiovascular disorders specific to the perinatal period (P19-P29)

P19 Metabolic acidemia in newborn
INCLUDES metabolic acidemia in newborn

P19.0 Metabolic acidemia in newborn first noted before onset of labor

P19.1 Metabolic acidemia in newborn first noted during labor

P19.2 Metabolic acidemia noted at birth

P19.9 Metabolic acidemia, unspecified   ▽

P22 Respiratory distress of newborn
EXCLUDES 1 respiratory arrest of newborn (P28.81)
respiratory failure of newborn NOS (P28.5)

P22.0 Respiratory distress syndrome of newborn
Cardiorespiratory distress syndrome of newborn
Hyaline membrane disease
Idiopathic respiratory distress syndrome [IRDS or RDS] of newborn
Pulmonary hypoperfusion syndrome
Respiratory distress syndrome, type I
DEF: Severe chest contractions upon air intake and expiratory grunting; infant appears blue due to oxygen deficiency and has rapid respiratory rate; formerly called hyaline membrane disease.

P22.1 Transient tachypnea of newborn
Idiopathic tachypnea of newborn
Respiratory distress syndrome, type II
Wet lung syndrome
DEF: Rapid, labored breathing of newborn; short-term problem that begins after birth and lasts about three days.

P22.8 Other respiratory distress of newborn

P22.9 Respiratory distress of newborn, unspecified   ▽

P23 Congenital pneumonia
INCLUDES infective pneumonia acquired in utero or during birth
EXCLUDES 1 neonatal pneumonia resulting from aspiration (P24.-)

P23.0 Congenital pneumonia due to viral agent
Use additional code (B97) to identify organism
EXCLUDES 1 congenital rubella pneumonitis (P35.0)

P23.1 Congenital pneumonia due to Chlamydia

P23.2 Congenital pneumonia due to staphylococcus

P23.3 Congenital pneumonia due to streptococcus, group B

P23.4 Congenital pneumonia due to Escherichia coli

P23.5 Congenital pneumonia due to Pseudomonas

P23.6 Congenital pneumonia due to other bacterial agents
Congenital pneumonia due to Hemophilus influenzae
Congenital pneumonia due to Klebsiella pneumoniae
Congenital pneumonia due to Mycoplasma
Congenital pneumonia due to Streptococcus, except group B
Use additional code (B95-B96) to identify organism

P23.8 Congenital pneumonia due to other organisms

P23.9 Congenital pneumonia, unspecified   ▽

P24 Neonatal aspiration
INCLUDES aspiration in utero and during delivery

P24.0 Meconium aspiration
EXCLUDES 1 meconium passage (without aspiration) during delivery (P03.82)
meconium staining (P96.83)

P24.00 Meconium aspiration without respiratory symptoms
Meconium aspiration NOS

P24.01 Meconium aspiration with respiratory symptoms
Meconium aspiration pneumonia
Meconium aspiration pneumonitis
Meconium aspiration syndrome NOS
Use additional code to identify any secondary pulmonary hypertension, if applicable ▶(I27.2-)◀
DEF: Aspiration of fetal intestinal material during or prior to delivery; usually a complication of placental insufficiency, causing pneumonitis and bronchial obstruction (inflammatory reaction of lungs).

P24.1 Neonatal aspiration of (clear) amniotic fluid and mucus
Neonatal aspiration of liquor (amnii)

P24.10 Neonatal aspiration of (clear) amniotic fluid and mucus without respiratory symptoms
Neonatal aspiration of amniotic fluid and mucus NOS

P24.11 Neonatal aspiration of (clear) amniotic fluid and mucus with respiratory symptoms
Neonatal aspiration of amniotic fluid and mucus with pneumonia
Neonatal aspiration of amniotic fluid and mucus with pneumonitis
Use additional code to identify any secondary pulmonary hypertension, if applicable ▶(I27.2-)◀

P24.2 Neonatal aspiration of blood

P24.20 Neonatal aspiration of blood without respiratory symptoms
Neonatal aspiration of blood NOS

P24.21 Neonatal aspiration of blood with respiratory symptoms
Neonatal aspiration of blood with pneumonia
Neonatal aspiration of blood with pneumonitis
Use additional code to identify any secondary pulmonary hypertension, if applicable ▶(I27.2-)◀

P24.3 Neonatal aspiration of milk and regurgitated food
Neonatal aspiration of stomach contents

P24.30 Neonatal aspiration of milk and regurgitated food without respiratory symptoms
Neonatal aspiration of milk and regurgitated food NOS

P24.31 Neonatal aspiration of milk and regurgitated food with respiratory symptoms
Neonatal aspiration of milk and regurgitated food with pneumonia
Neonatal aspiration of milk and regurgitated food with pneumonitis
Use additional code to identify any secondary pulmonary hypertension, if applicable ▶(I27.2-)◀

P24.8 Other neonatal aspiration

P24.80 Other neonatal aspiration without respiratory symptoms
Neonatal aspiration NEC

P24.81 Other neonatal aspiration with respiratory symptoms
Neonatal aspiration pneumonia NEC
Neonatal aspiration with pneumonitis NEC
Neonatal aspiration with pneumonia NOS
Neonatal aspiration with pneumonitis NOS
Use additional code to identify any secondary pulmonary hypertension, if applicable ▶(I27.2-)◀

P24.9 Neonatal aspiration, unspecified   ▽

P25 Interstitial emphysema and related conditions originating in the perinatal period

P25.0 Interstitial emphysema originating in the perinatal period

P25.1 Pneumothorax originating in the perinatal period

P25.2 Pneumomediastinum originating in the perinatal period

P25.3 Pneumopericardium originating in the perinatal period

P25.8 Other conditions related to interstitial emphysema originating in the perinatal period

P26 Pulmonary hemorrhage originating in the perinatal period
EXCLUDES 1 acute idiopathic hemorrhage in infants over 28 days old (R04.81)

P26.0 Tracheobronchial hemorrhage originating in the perinatal period

P26.1 Massive pulmonary hemorrhage originating in the perinatal period

P26.8 Other pulmonary hemorrhages originating in the perinatal period

P26.9 Unspecified pulmonary hemorrhage originating in the perinatal period   ▽

P27 Chronic respiratory disease originating in the perinatal period
EXCLUDES 1 respiratory distress of newborn (P22.0-P22.9)
EXCLUDES 2 ▶respiratory distress of newborn (P22.0-P22.9)◀

P27.0 Wilson-Mikity syndrome
Pulmonary dysmaturity

P27.1 Bronchopulmonary dysplasia originating in the perinatal period

---

✓ Additional Character Req   ✓x7th Placeholder Alert   Manifestation   HCC CMS-HCC Condition   ▽ Unspecified Code   ▶◀ Revised Text   ● New Code   ▲ Revised Code Title

P27.8 **Other chronic respiratory diseases originating in the perinatal period**
Congenital pulmonary fibrosis
Ventilator lung in newborn

P27.9 **Unspecified chronic respiratory disease originating in the perinatal period** ▽

✓4th **P28** **Other respiratory conditions originating in the perinatal period**
EXCLUDES 1   congenital malformations of the respiratory system (Q30-Q34)

P28.0 **Primary atelectasis of newborn**
Primary failure to expand terminal respiratory units
Pulmonary hypoplasia associated with short gestation
Pulmonary immaturity NOS

✓5th **P28.1** **Other and unspecified atelectasis of newborn**

P28.10 **Unspecified atelectasis of newborn** ▽
Atelectasis of newborn NOS

P28.11 **Resorption atelectasis without respiratory distress syndrome**
EXCLUDES 1   resorption atelectasis with respiratory distress syndrome (P22.0)

P28.19 **Other atelectasis of newborn**
Partial atelectasis of newborn
Secondary atelectasis of newborn

P28.2 **Cyanotic attacks of newborn**
EXCLUDES 1   apnea of newborn (P28.3-P28.4)

P28.3 **Primary sleep apnea of newborn**
Central sleep apnea of newborn
Obstructive sleep apnea of newborn
Sleep apnea of newborn NOS
DEF: Unexplained cessation of breathing when a neonate makes no respiratory effort for 20 seconds or longer, or when neonate's breathing cessation is accompanied by cyanosis, bradycardia, or hypotonia.

P28.4 **Other apnea of newborn**
Apnea of prematurity
Obstructive apnea of newborn
EXCLUDES 1   obstructive sleep apnea of newborn (P28.3)

P28.5 **Respiratory failure of newborn**
EXCLUDES 1   respiratory arrest of newborn (P28.81)
respiratory distress of newborn (P22.0-)

✓5th **P28.8** **Other specified respiratory conditions of newborn**

P28.81 **Respiratory arrest of newborn**

P28.89 **Other specified respiratory conditions of newborn**
Congenital laryngeal stridor
Sniffles in newborn
Snuffles in newborn
EXCLUDES 1   early congenital syphilitic rhinitis (A50.05)

P28.9 **Respiratory condition of newborn, unspecified** ▽
Respiratory depression in newborn

✓4th **P29** **Cardiovascular disorders originating in the perinatal period**
EXCLUDES 1   congenital malformations of the circulatory system (Q20-Q28)

P29.0 **Neonatal cardiac failure**

✓5th **P29.1** **Neonatal cardiac dysrhythmia**

P29.11 **Neonatal tachycardia**

P29.12 **Neonatal bradycardia**

P29.2 **Neonatal hypertension**

✓5th **P29.3** **Persistent fetal circulation**
Delayed closure of ductus arteriosus
(Persistent) pulmonary hypertension of newborn

P29.30 **Pulmonary hypertension of newborn**
Persistent pulmonary hypertension of newborn

P29.38 **Other persistent fetal circulation**
Delayed closure of ductus arteriosus

P29.4 **Transient myocardial ischemia in newborn**

✓5th **P29.8** **Other cardiovascular disorders originating in the perinatal period**

P29.81 **Cardiac arrest of newborn**

P29.89 **Other cardiovascular disorders originating in the perinatal period**
AHA: 2014, 4Q, 23

P29.9 **Cardiovascular disorder originating in the perinatal period, unspecified** ▽

Infections specific to the perinatal period (P35-P39)

Infections acquired in utero, during birth via the umbilicus, or during the first 28 days after birth
EXCLUDES 2   asymptomatic human immunodeficiency virus [HIV] infection status (Z21)
congenital gonococcal infection (A54.-)
congenital pneumonia (P23.-)
congenital syphilis (A50.-)
human immunodeficiency virus [HIV] disease (B20)
infant botulism (A48.51)
infectious diseases not specific to the perinatal period (A00-B99, J09, J10-)
intestinal infectious disease (A00-A09)
laboratory evidence of human immunodeficiency virus [HIV] (R75)
tetanus neonatorum (A33)

✓4th **P35** **Congenital viral diseases**
INCLUDES   infections acquired in utero or during birth

P35.0 **Congenital rubella syndrome**
Congenital rubella pneumonitis

P35.1 **Congenital cytomegalovirus infection**

P35.2 **Congenital herpesviral [herpes simplex] infection**

P35.3 **Congenital viral hepatitis**

P35.8 **Other congenital viral diseases**
Congenital varicella [chickenpox]

P35.9 **Congenital viral disease, unspecified** ▽

✓4th **P36** **Bacterial sepsis of newborn**
INCLUDES   congenital sepsis
Use additional code(s), if applicable, to identify severe sepsis (R65.2-) and associated acute organ dysfunction(s)

P36.0 **Sepsis of newborn due to streptococcus, group B** HCC

✓5th **P36.1** **Sepsis of newborn due to other and unspecified streptococci**

P36.10 **Sepsis of newborn due to unspecified streptococci** HCC ▽

P36.19 **Sepsis of newborn due to other streptococci** HCC

P36.2 **Sepsis of newborn due to Staphylococcus aureus** HCC

✓5th **P36.3** **Sepsis of newborn due to other and unspecified staphylococci**

P36.30 **Sepsis of newborn due to unspecified staphylococci** HCC ▽

P36.39 **Sepsis of newborn due to other staphylococci** HCC

P36.4 **Sepsis of newborn due to Escherichia coli** HCC

P36.5 **Sepsis of newborn due to anaerobes** HCC

P36.8 **Other bacterial sepsis of newborn** HCC
Use additional code from category B96 to identify organism

P36.9 **Bacterial sepsis of newborn, unspecified** HCC ▽

✓4th **P37** **Other congenital infectious and parasitic diseases**
EXCLUDES 2   congenital syphilis (A50.-)
infectious neonatal diarrhea (A00-A09)
necrotizing enterocolitis in newborn (P77.-)
noninfectious neonatal diarrhea (P78.3)
ophthalmia neonatorum due to gonococcus (A54.31)
tetanus neonatorum (A33)

P37.0 **Congenital tuberculosis**

P37.1 **Congenital toxoplasmosis**
Hydrocephalus due to congenital toxoplasmosis

P37.2 **Neonatal (disseminated) listeriosis**

P37.3 **Congenital falciparum malaria**

P37.4 **Other congenital malaria**

P37.5 **Neonatal candidiasis**

P37.8 **Other specified congenital infectious and parasitic diseases**

P37.9 **Congenital infectious or parasitic disease, unspecified** ▽

✓4th **P38** **Omphalitis of newborn**
EXCLUDES 1   omphalitis not of newborn (L08.82)
tetanus omphalitis (A33)
umbilical hemorrhage of newborn (P51.-)

P38.1 **Omphalitis with mild hemorrhage**

P38.9 **Omphalitis without hemorrhage**
Omphalitis of newborn NOS

✓4ᵗʰ **P39   Other infections specific to the perinatal period**
    Use additional code to identify organism or specific infection

P39.0   Neonatal infective mastitis
    EXCLUDES 1   breast engorgement of newborn (P83.4)
               noninfective mastitis of newborn (P83.4)

P39.1   Neonatal conjunctivitis and dacryocystitis
    Neonatal chlamydial conjunctivitis
    Ophthalmia neonatorum NOS
    EXCLUDES 1   gonococcal conjunctivitis (A54.31)

P39.2   Intra-amniotic infection affecting newborn, not elsewhere classified

P39.3   Neonatal urinary tract infection

P39.4   Neonatal skin infection
    Neonatal pyoderma
    EXCLUDES 1   pemphigus neonatorum (L00)
               staphylococcal scalded skin syndrome (L00)

P39.8   Other specified infections specific to the perinatal period

P39.9   Infection specific to the perinatal period, unspecified   ▽

Hemorrhagic and hematological disorders of newborn (P50-P61)

EXCLUDES 1   congenital stenosis and stricture of bile ducts (Q44.3)
               Crigler-Najjar syndrome (E80.5)
               Dubin-Johnson syndrome (E80.6)
               Gilbert syndrome (E80.4)
               hereditary hemolytic anemias (D55-D58)

✓4ᵗʰ **P50   Newborn affected by intrauterine (fetal)** blood loss
    EXCLUDES 1   congenital anemia from intrauterine (fetal) blood loss (P61.3)

P50.0   Newborn affected by intrauterine (fetal) blood loss from vasa previa

P50.1   Newborn affected by intrauterine (fetal) blood loss from ruptured cord

P50.2   Newborn affected by intrauterine (fetal) blood loss from placenta

P50.3   Newborn affected by hemorrhage into co-twin

P50.4   Newborn affected by hemorrhage into maternal circulation

P50.5   Newborn affected by intrauterine (fetal) blood loss from cut end of co-twin's cord

P50.8   Newborn affected by other intrauterine (fetal) blood loss

P50.9   Newborn affected by intrauterine (fetal) blood loss, unspecified   ▽
    Newborn affected by fetal hemorrhage NOS

✓4ᵗʰ **P51   Umbilical** hemorrhage of newborn
    EXCLUDES 1   omphalitis with mild hemorrhage (P38.1)
               umbilical hemorrhage from cut end of co-twins cord (P50.5)

P51.0   Massive umbilical hemorrhage of newborn

P51.8   Other umbilical hemorrhages of newborn
    Slipped umbilical ligature NOS

P51.9   Umbilical hemorrhage of newborn, unspecified   ▽

✓4ᵗʰ **P52   Intracranial nontraumatic hemorrhage** of newborn
    INCLUDES   intracranial hemorrhage due to anoxia or hypoxia
    EXCLUDES 1   intracranial hemorrhage due to birth injury (P10.-)
               intracranial hemorrhage due to other injury (S06.-)

P52.0   Intraventricular (nontraumatic) hemorrhage, grade 1, **of newborn**
    Subependymal hemorrhage (without intraventricular extension)
    Bleeding into germinal matrix

P52.1   Intraventricular (nontraumatic) hemorrhage, grade 2, **of newborn**
    Subependymal hemorrhage with intraventricular extension
    Bleeding into ventricle

✓5ᵗʰ **P52.2   Intraventricular (nontraumatic) hemorrhage, grade 3 and grade 4, of newborn**

    P52.21   Intraventricular (nontraumatic) hemorrhage, grade 3, of newborn
        Subependymal hemorrhage with intraventricular extension with enlargement of ventricle

    P52.22   Intraventricular (nontraumatic) hemorrhage, grade 4, of newborn
        Bleeding into cerebral cortex
        Subependymal hemorrhage with intracerebral extension

P52.3   Unspecified intraventricular (nontraumatic) hemorrhage of newborn   ▽

P52.4   Intracerebral (nontraumatic) hemorrhage of newborn

P52.5   Subarachnoid (nontraumatic) hemorrhage of newborn

P52.6   Cerebellar (nontraumatic) and posterior fossa hemorrhage of newborn

P52.8   Other intracranial (nontraumatic) hemorrhages of newborn

P52.9   Intracranial (nontraumatic) hemorrhage of newborn, unspecified   ▽

P53   Hemorrhagic disease of newborn
    Vitamin K deficiency of newborn

✓4ᵗʰ **P54   Other neonatal hemorrhages**
    EXCLUDES 1   newborn affected by (intrauterine) blood loss (P50.-)
               pulmonary hemorrhage originating in the perinatal period (P26.-)

P54.0   Neonatal hematemesis
    EXCLUDES 1   neonatal hematemesis due to swallowed maternal blood (P78.2)

P54.1   Neonatal melena
    EXCLUDES 1   neonatal melena due to swallowed maternal blood (P78.2)

P54.2   Neonatal rectal hemorrhage

P54.3   Other neonatal gastrointestinal hemorrhage

P54.4   Neonatal adrenal hemorrhage

P54.5   Neonatal cutaneous hemorrhage
    Neonatal bruising
    Neonatal ecchymoses
    Neonatal petechiae
    Neonatal superficial hematoma
    EXCLUDES 2   bruising of scalp due to birth injury (P12.3)
               cephalhematoma due to birth injury (P12.0)

P54.6   Neonatal vaginal hemorrhage   ♀
    Neonatal pseudomenses

P54.8   Other specified neonatal hemorrhages

P54.9   Neonatal hemorrhage, unspecified   ▽

✓4ᵗʰ **P55   Hemolytic disease of newborn**

P55.0   Rh isoimmunization of newborn
    DEF: Incompatible Rh fetal-maternal blood grouping; prematurely destroys red blood cells; characterized by jaundice, asphyxia, pulmonary hypertension, edema, respiratory distress, kernicterus, and coagulopathies; detected by Coombs test.

P55.1   ABO isoimmunization of newborn
    AHA: 2015, 3Q, 20

P55.8   Other hemolytic diseases of newborn

P55.9   Hemolytic disease of newborn, unspecified   ▽

✓4ᵗʰ **P56   Hydrops fetalis due to hemolytic disease**
    EXCLUDES 1   hydrops fetalis NOS (P83.2)

P56.0   Hydrops fetalis due to isoimmunization

✓5ᵗʰ **P56.9   Hydrops fetalis due to other and unspecified hemolytic disease**

    P56.90   Hydrops fetalis due to unspecified hemolytic disease   ▽

    P56.99   Hydrops fetalis due to other hemolytic disease

✓4ᵗʰ **P57   Kernicterus**

P57.0   Kernicterus due to isoimmunization
    DEF: Complication of erythroblastosis fetalis associated with severe neural symptoms, high blood bilirubin levels and nerve cell destruction; results in bilirubin-pigmented gray matter of central nervous system.

P57.8   Other specified kernicterus
    EXCLUDES 1   Crigler-Najjar syndrome (E80.5)

P57.9   Kernicterus, unspecified   ▽

✓4ᵗʰ **P58   Neonatal jaundice due to other excessive hemolysis**
    EXCLUDES 1   jaundice due to isoimmunization (P55-P57)

P58.0   Neonatal jaundice due to bruising

P58.1   Neonatal jaundice due to bleeding

P58.2   Neonatal jaundice due to infection

P58.3   Neonatal jaundice due to polycythemia

✓5ᵗʰ **P58.4   Neonatal jaundice due to drugs or toxins transmitted from mother or given to newborn**
    Code first poisoning due to drug or toxin, if applicable (T36-T65 with fifth or sixth character 1-4 or 6)
    Use additional code for adverse effect, if applicable, to identify drug (T36-T50 with fifth or sixth character 5)

    P58.41   Neonatal jaundice due to drugs or toxins transmitted from mother

    P58.42   Neonatal jaundice due to drugs or toxins given to newborn

Chapter 16. Certain Conditions Originating in the Perinatal Period

P58.5   **Neonatal jaundice due to** swallowed maternal blood

P58.8   **Neonatal jaundice due to other specified excessive hemolysis**

P58.9   **Neonatal jaundice due to excessive hemolysis, unspecified** ▽

✓4ᵗʰ **P59**   **Neonatal jaundice from other and unspecified causes**
> EXCLUDES 1   *jaundice due to inborn errors of metabolism (E70-E88)*
> *kernicterus (P57.-)*

P59.0   **Neonatal jaundice associated with** preterm delivery
Hyperbilirubinemia of prematurity
Jaundice due to delayed conjugation associated with preterm delivery

P59.1   Inspissated bile syndrome

✓5ᵗʰ **P59.2**   **Neonatal jaundice from other and unspecified** hepatocellular damage
> EXCLUDES 1   *congenital viral hepatitis (P35.3)*

> **P59.20**   **Neonatal jaundice from unspecified hepatocellular damage** ▽

> **P59.29**   **Neonatal jaundice from other hepatocellular damage**
> Neonatal giant cell hepatitis
> Neonatal (idiopathic) hepatitis

P59.3   **Neonatal jaundice from** breast milk inhibitor

P59.8   **Neonatal jaundice from other specified causes**

P59.9   **Neonatal jaundice, unspecified** ▽
Neonatal physiological jaundice (intense)(prolonged) NOS
AHA: 2015, 3Q, 20

P60   **Disseminated intravascular coagulation of newborn**
Defibrination syndrome of newborn

✓4ᵗʰ **P61**   **Other perinatal hematological disorders**
> EXCLUDES 1   *transient hypogammaglobulinemia of infancy (D80.7)*

P61.0   **Transient neonatal thrombocytopenia**
Neonatal thrombocytopenia due to exchange transfusion
Neonatal thrombocytopenia due to idiopathic maternal thrombocytopenia
Neonatal thrombocytopenia due to isoimmunization
DEF: Temporary decrease in blood platelets of newborn; secondary to placental insufficiency.

P61.1   **Polycythemia neonatorum**
DEF: Abnormal increase of total red blood cells of newborn; results in hyperviscosity, which slows the flow of blood through small blood vessels.

P61.2   **Anemia of prematurity**

P61.3   **Congenital anemia from fetal blood loss**

P61.4   **Other congenital anemias, not elsewhere classified**
Congenital anemia NOS

P61.5   **Transient neonatal neutropenia**
> EXCLUDES 1   *congenital neutropenia (nontransient) (D70.0)*
DEF: Low blood neutrophil counts of newborn; occurs due to maternal hypertension, sepsis, twin-twin transfusion, alloimmunization, and hemolytic disease.

P61.6   **Other transient neonatal disorders of coagulation**

P61.8   **Other specified perinatal hematological disorders**

P61.9   **Perinatal hematological disorder, unspecified** ▽

Transitory endocrine and metabolic disorders specific to newborn (P70-P74)

> INCLUDES   transitory endocrine and metabolic disturbances caused by the infant's response to maternal endocrine and metabolic factors, or its adjustment to extrauterine environment

✓4ᵗʰ **P70**   **Transitory disorders of** carbohydrate metabolism **specific to newborn**

P70.0   **Syndrome of infant of mother with** gestational diabetes
Newborn (with hypoglycemia) affected by maternal gestational diabetes
> EXCLUDES 1   *newborn (with hypoglycemia) affected by maternal (pre-existing) diabetes mellitus (P70.1)*
> *syndrome of infant of a diabetic mother (P70.1)*

P70.1   **Syndrome of infant of a** diabetic mother
Newborn (with hypoglycemia) affected by maternal (pre-existing) diabetes mellitus
> EXCLUDES 1   *newborn (with hypoglycemia) affected by maternal gestational diabetes (P70.0)*
> *syndrome of infant of mother with gestational diabetes (P70.0)*

P70.2   **Neonatal** diabetes mellitus

P70.3   Iatrogenic **neonatal** hypoglycemia

P70.4   **Other neonatal hypoglycemia**
Transitory neonatal hypoglycemia

P70.8   **Other transitory disorders of carbohydrate metabolism of newborn**

P70.9   **Transitory disorder of carbohydrate metabolism of newborn, unspecified** ▽

✓4ᵗʰ **P71**   **Transitory neonatal disorders of** calcium and magnesium metabolism

P71.0   **Cow's milk hypocalcemia in newborn**

P71.1   **Other neonatal hypocalcemia**
> EXCLUDES 1   *neonatal hypoparathyroidism (P71.4)*

P71.2   **Neonatal** hypomagnesemia

P71.3   **Neonatal** tetany without calcium or magnesium deficiency
Neonatal tetany NOS

P71.4   **Transitory neonatal** hypoparathyroidism

P71.8   **Other transitory neonatal disorders of calcium and magnesium metabolism**

P71.9   **Transitory neonatal disorder of calcium and magnesium metabolism, unspecified** ▽

✓4ᵗʰ **P72**   **Other transitory neonatal** endocrine disorders
> EXCLUDES 1   *congenital hypothyroidism with or without goiter (E03.0-E03.1)*
> *dyshormogenetic goiter (E07.1)*
> *Pendred's syndrome (E07.1)*

P72.0   **Neonatal goiter, not elsewhere classified**
Transitory congenital goiter with normal functioning

P72.1   **Transitory neonatal** hyperthyroidism
Neonatal thyrotoxicosis

P72.2   **Other transitory neonatal disorders of** thyroid function, **not elsewhere classified**
Transitory neonatal hypothyroidism

P72.8   **Other specified transitory neonatal endocrine disorders**

P72.9   **Transitory neonatal endocrine disorder, unspecified** ▽

✓4ᵗʰ **P74**   **Other transitory neonatal** electrolyte and metabolic disturbances

P74.0   Late metabolic acidosis of newborn
> EXCLUDES 1   *(fetal) metabolic acidosis of newborn (P19)*

P74.1   Dehydration of newborn

P74.2   **Disturbances of** sodium balance of newborn

P74.3   **Disturbances of** potassium balance of newborn

P74.4   **Other transitory electrolyte disturbances of newborn**

P74.5   **Transitory** tyrosinemia of newborn

P74.6   **Transitory** hyperammonemia of newborn

P74.8   **Other transitory metabolic disturbances of newborn**
Amino-acid metabolic disorders described as transitory

P74.9   **Transitory metabolic disturbance of newborn, unspecified** ▽

Digestive system disorders of newborn (P76-P78)

✓4ᵗʰ **P76**   **Other intestinal obstruction of newborn**

P76.0   **Meconium plug syndrome**
Meconium ileus NOS
> EXCLUDES 1   *meconium ileus in cystic fibrosis (E84.11)*

P76.1   **Transitory ileus of newborn**
> EXCLUDES 1   *Hirschsprung's disease (Q43.1)*

P76.2   **Intestinal obstruction due to inspissated milk**

P76.8   **Other specified intestinal obstruction of newborn**
> EXCLUDES 1   *intestinal obstruction classifiable to K56-*

P76.9   **Intestinal obstruction of newborn, unspecified** ▽

✓4ᵗʰ **P77**   **Necrotizing enterocolitis of newborn**
DEF: Serious intestinal infection and inflammation in preterm infants; severity is measured by stages and may progress to life-threatening perforation or peritonitis; resection surgical treatment may be necessary.

P77.1   Stage 1 **necrotizing enterocolitis in newborn**
Necrotizing enterocolitis without pneumatosis, without perforation
DEF: Broad-spectrum symptoms with nonspecific signs, including feeding intolerance, abdominal distention, bradycardia, and metabolic abnormalities.

P77.2   Stage 2 **necrotizing enterocolitis in newborn**
Necrotizing enterocolitis with pneumatosis, without perforation
DEF: Radiographic confirmation of necrotizing enterocolitis showing intestinal dilatation, fixed loops of bowels, pneumatosis intestinalis, metabolic acidosis, and thrombocytopenia.

EXCLUDES 1 Not coded here   EXCLUDES 2 Not included here   N Newborn Age: 0   P Pediatric Age: 0-17   M Maternity Age: 12-55   A Adult Age: 15-124

866   ICD-10-CM 2018

P77.3   Stage 3 necrotizing enterocolitis in newborn
Necrotizing enterocolitis with perforation
Necrotizing enterocolitis with pneumatosis and perforation
DEF: Advanced stage in which infant demonstrates signs of bowel perforation, septic shock, metabolic acidosis, ascites, disseminated intravascular coagulopathy, neutropenia.

P77.9   **Necrotizing enterocolitis in newborn, unspecified** ▽
Necrotizing enterocolitis in newborn, NOS

✓4ᵗʰ **P78**   **Other perinatal digestive system disorders**
    EXCLUDES 1   cystic fibrosis (E84.0-E84.9)
            neonatal gastrointestinal hemorrhages (P54.0-P54.3)

P78.0   **Perinatal intestinal perforation**
Meconium peritonitis

P78.1   **Other neonatal peritonitis**
Neonatal peritonitis NOS

P78.2   **Neonatal hematemesis and melena due to swallowed maternal blood**

P78.3   **Noninfective neonatal diarrhea**
Neonatal diarrhea NOS

✓5ᵗʰ **P78.8**   **Other specified perinatal digestive system disorders**

   P78.81   **Congenital cirrhosis (of liver)**

   P78.82   **Peptic ulcer of newborn**

   P78.83   **Newborn esophageal reflux**
        Neonatal esophageal reflux

   ● **P78.84**   **Gestational alloimmune liver disease**
        GALD
        Neonatal hemochromatosis
        EXCLUDES 1   hemochromatosis (E83.11-)

   P78.89   **Other specified perinatal digestive system disorders**

P78.9   **Perinatal digestive system disorder, unspecified** ▽

Conditions involving the integument and temperature regulation of newborn (P80-P83)

✓4ᵗʰ **P80**   **Hypothermia of newborn**

P80.0   **Cold injury syndrome**
Severe and usually chronic hypothermia associated with a pink flushed appearance, edema and neurological and biochemical abnormalities.
EXCLUDES 1   mild hypothermia of newborn (P80.8)

P80.8   **Other hypothermia of newborn**
Mild hypothermia of newborn

P80.9   **Hypothermia of newborn, unspecified** ▽

✓4ᵗʰ **P81**   **Other disturbances of temperature regulation of newborn**

P81.0   **Environmental hyperthermia of newborn**

P81.8   **Other specified disturbances of temperature regulation of newborn**

P81.9   **Disturbance of temperature regulation of newborn, unspecified** ▽
Fever of newborn NOS

✓4ᵗʰ **P83**   **Other conditions of integument specific to newborn**
    EXCLUDES 1   congenital malformations of skin and integument (Q80-Q84)
            hydrops fetalis due to hemolytic disease (P56.-)
            neonatal skin infection (P39.4)
            staphylococcal scalded skin syndrome (L00)
    EXCLUDES 2   cradle cap (L21.0)
            diaper [napkin] dermatitis (L22)

P83.0   **Sclerema neonatorum**
DEF: Diffuse, rapidly progressing white, waxy, nonpitting hardening of tissue, usually of legs and feet that is life-threatening; found in preterm or debilitated infants; unknown etiology.

P83.1   **Neonatal erythema toxicum**

P83.2   **Hydrops fetalis not due to hemolytic disease**
Hydrops fetalis NOS
DEF: Severe, life-threatening problem of newborn characterized by severe edema of entire body; unrelated to immune response.

✓5ᵗʰ **P83.3**   **Other and unspecified edema specific to newborn**

   P83.30   **Unspecified edema specific to newborn** ▽

   P83.39   **Other edema specific to newborn**

P83.4   **Breast engorgement of newborn**
Noninfective mastitis of newborn

P83.5   **Congenital hydrocele** ♂

P83.6   **Umbilical polyp of newborn**

✓5ᵗʰ **P83.8**   **Other specified conditions of integument specific to newborn**
~~Bronze baby syndrome~~
~~Neonatal scleroderma~~
~~Urticaria neonatorum~~

   ● **P83.81**   **Umbilical granuloma**
        EXCLUDES 2   granulomatous disorder of the skin and subcutaneous tissue, unspecified (L92.9)

   ● **P83.88**   **Other specified conditions of integument specific to newborn**
        Bronze baby syndrome
        Neonatal scleroderma
        Urticaria neonatorum

P83.9   **Condition of the integument specific to newborn, unspecified** ▽

Other problems with newborn (P84)

P84   **Other problems with newborn**
Acidemia of newborn
Acidosis of newborn
Anoxia of newborn NOS
Asphyxia of newborn NOS
Hypercapnia of newborn
Hypoxemia of newborn
Hypoxia of newborn NOS
Mixed metabolic and respiratory acidosis of newborn
    EXCLUDES 1   intracranial hemorrhage due to anoxia or hypoxia (P52.-)
            hypoxic ischemic encephalopathy [HIE] (P91.6-)
            late metabolic acidosis of newborn (P74.0)

Other disorders originating in the perinatal period (P90-P96)

P90   **Convulsions of newborn**
    EXCLUDES 1   benign myoclonic epilepsy in infancy (G40.3-)
            benign neonatal convulsions (familial) (G40.3-)

✓4ᵗʰ **P91**   **Other disturbances of cerebral status of newborn**

P91.0   **Neonatal cerebral ischemia**

P91.1   **Acquired periventricular cysts of newborn**

P91.2   **Neonatal cerebral leukomalacia**
Periventricular leukomalacia

P91.3   **Neonatal cerebral irritability**

P91.4   **Neonatal cerebral depression**

P91.5   **Neonatal coma**

✓5ᵗʰ **P91.6**   **Hypoxic ischemic encephalopathy [HIE]**
    EXCLUDES 1 ▶ neonatal cerebral depression (P91.4)
            neonatal cerebral irritability (P91.3)
            neonatal coma (P91.5)◀

   P91.60   **Hypoxic ischemic encephalopathy [HIE], unspecified** ▽

   P91.61   **Mild hypoxic ischemic encephalopathy [HIE]**

   P91.62   **Moderate hypoxic ischemic encephalopathy [HIE]**

   P91.63   **Severe hypoxic ischemic encephalopathy [HIE]**

✓5ᵗʰ **P91.8**   **Other specified disturbances of cerebral status of newborn**

   ● ✓6ᵗʰ **P91.81**   **Neonatal encephalopathy**

     P91.811   **Neonatal encephalopathy in diseases classified elsewhere**
        Code first underlying condition, if known, such as:
        congenital cirrhosis (of liver) (P78.71)
        intracranial nontraumatic hemorrhage of newborn (P52.-)
        kernicterus (P57.-)

   ●   **P91.819**   **Neonatal encephalopathy, unspecified** ▽

   ● **P91.88**   **Other specified disturbances of cerebral status of newborn**

P91.9   **Disturbance of cerebral status of newborn, unspecified** ▽

✓4ᵗʰ **P92**   **Feeding problems of newborn**
    EXCLUDES 1 ▶ eating disorders (F50.-)◀
            feeding problems in child over 28 days old (R63.3)
    AHA: 2016, 3Q, 19

✓5ᵗʰ **P92.0**   **Vomiting of newborn**
    EXCLUDES 1   vomiting of child over 28 days old (R11.-)

   P92.01   **Bilious vomiting of newborn**
        EXCLUDES 1   bilious vomiting in child over 28 days old (R11.14)

   P92.09   **Other vomiting of newborn**
        EXCLUDES 1   regurgitation of food in newborn (P92.1)

☑ Additional Character Req   ✓x7ᵗʰ Placeholder Alert   **Manifestation**   HCC CMS-HCC Condition   ▽ Unspecified Code   ▶◀ Revised Text   ● New Code   ▲ Revised Code Title

ICD-10-CM 2018   867

Chapter 16. Certain Conditions Originating in the Perinatal Period

P92.1   **Regurgitation and rumination** of newborn

P92.2   **Slow feeding** of newborn

P92.3   **Underfeeding** of newborn

P92.4   **Overfeeding** of newborn

P92.5   **Neonatal difficulty in feeding at breast**
     AHA: 2017, 1Q, 28

P92.6   **Failure to thrive** in newborn
     EXCLUDES 1   *failure to thrive in child over 28 days old (R62.51)*

P92.8   **Other feeding problems of newborn**

P92.9   **Feeding problem of newborn, unspecified**   ▽

✓4ᵗʰ   **P93**   **Reactions and intoxications due to drugs administered to newborn**
     INCLUDES   reactions and intoxications due to drugs administered to fetus affecting newborn
     EXCLUDES 1   *jaundice due to drugs or toxins transmitted from mother or given to newborn (P58.4-)*
         reactions and intoxications from maternal opiates, tranquilizers and other medication (P04.0-P04.1, P04.4)
         withdrawal symptoms from maternal use of drugs of addiction (P96.1)
         withdrawal symptoms from therapeutic use of drugs in newborn (P96.2)

P93.0   **Grey baby syndrome**
     Grey syndrome from chloramphenicol administration in newborn

P93.8   **Other reactions and intoxications due to drugs administered to newborn**
     Use additional code for adverse effect, if applicable, to identify drug (T36-T50 with fifth or sixth character 5)

✓4ᵗʰ   **P94**   **Disorders of muscle tone of newborn**

P94.0   **Transient neonatal myasthenia gravis**
     EXCLUDES 1   *myasthenia gravis (G70.0)*

P94.1   **Congenital hypertonia**

P94.2   **Congenital hypotonia**
     Floppy baby syndrome, unspecified

P94.8   **Other disorders of muscle tone of newborn**

P94.9   **Disorder of muscle tone of newborn, unspecified**   ▽

P95   **Stillbirth**
     Deadborn fetus NOS
     Fetal death of unspecified cause
     Stillbirth NOS
     EXCLUDES 1   *maternal care for intrauterine death (O36.4)*
         missed abortion (O02.1)
         outcome of delivery, stillbirth (Z37.1, Z37.3, Z37.4, Z37.7)

✓4ᵗʰ   **P96**   **Other conditions originating in the perinatal period**

P96.0   **Congenital renal failure**
     Uremia of newborn

P96.1   **Neonatal withdrawal symptoms from maternal use of drugs of addiction**
     Drug withdrawal syndrome in infant of dependent mother
     Neonatal abstinence syndrome
     EXCLUDES 1   *reactions and intoxications from maternal opiates and tranquilizers administered during labor and delivery (P04.0)*

P96.2   **Withdrawal symptoms from therapeutic use of drugs in newborn**

P96.3   **Wide cranial sutures of newborn**
     Neonatal craniotabes

P96.5   **Complication to newborn due to (fetal) intrauterine procedure**
     EXCLUDES 2   *newborn affected by amniocentesis (P00.6)*

✓5ᵗʰ   **P96.8**   **Other specified conditions originating in the perinatal period**

P96.81   **Exposure to (parental) (environmental) tobacco smoke in the perinatal period**
     EXCLUDES 2   *newborn affected by in utero exposure to tobacco (P04.2)*
         exposure to environmental tobacco smoke after the perinatal period (Z77.22)

P96.82   **Delayed separation of umbilical cord**

P96.83   **Meconium staining**
     EXCLUDES 1   *meconium aspiration (P24.00, P24.01)*
         meconium passage during delivery (P03.82)

P96.89   **Other specified conditions originating in the perinatal period**
     Use additional code to specify condition

P96.9   **Condition originating in the perinatal period, unspecified**   ▽
     Congenital debility NOS

EXCLUDES 1 Not coded here   **EXCLUDES 2** Not included here   **N** Newborn Age: 0   **P** Pediatric Age: 0-17   **M** Maternity Age: 12-55   **A** Adult Age: 15-124

868   ICD-10-CM 2018

Chapter 17. Congenital Malformations, Deformations, and Chromosomal Abnormalities (Q00–Q99)

Chapter Specific Guidelines with Coding Examples

The chapter specific guidelines from the ICD-10-CM Official Guidelines for Coding and Reporting have been provided below. Along with these guidelines are coding examples, contained in the shaded boxes, that have been developed to help illustrate the coding and/or sequencing guidance found in these guidelines.

Assign an appropriate code(s) from categories Q00-Q99, Congenital malformations, deformations, and chromosomal abnormalities when a malformation/deformation or chromosomal abnormality is documented. A malformation/deformation/or chromosomal abnormality may be the principal/first-listed diagnosis on a record or a secondary diagnosis.

When a malformation/deformation/or chromosomal abnormality does not have a unique code assignment, assign additional code(s) for any manifestations that may be present.

When the code assignment specifically identifies the malformation/deformation/or chromosomal abnormality, manifestations that are an inherent component of the anomaly should not be coded separately. Additional codes should be assigned for manifestations that are not an inherent component.

8-day-old infant with tetralogy of Fallot and pulmonary stenosis

Q21.3　　Tetralogy of Fallot

Explanation: Pulmonary stenosis is inherent in the disease process of tetralogy of Fallot. When the code assignment specifically identifies the malformation/deformation/or chromosomal abnormality, manifestations that are inherent components of the anomaly should not be coded separately.

7-month-old infant with Down syndrome and common atrioventricular canal

Q90.9　　Down syndrome, unspecified

Q21.2　　Atrioventricular septal defect

Explanation: While a common atrioventricular canal is often associated with patients with Down syndrome, this manifestation is not an inherent component and may be reported separately. When the code assignment specifically identifies the anomaly, manifestations that are inherent components of the condition should not be coded separately. Additional codes should be assigned for manifestations that are not inherent components.

Codes from Chapter 17 may be used throughout the life of the patient. If a congenital malformation or deformity has been corrected, a personal history code should be used to identify the history of the malformation or deformity. Although present at birth, malformation/deformation/or chromosomal abnormality may not be identified until later in life. Whenever the condition is diagnosed by the physician, it is appropriate to assign a code from codes Q00-Q99. For the birth admission, the appropriate code from category Z38, Liveborn infants, according to place of birth and type of delivery, should be sequenced as the principal diagnosis, followed by any congenital anomaly codes, Q00- Q99.

Three-year-old with history of corrected ventricular septal defect

Z87.74　　Personal history of (corrected) congenital malformations of heart and circulatory system

Explanation: If a congenital malformation or deformity has been corrected, a personal history code should be used to identify the history of the malformation or deformity.

Forty-year-old man with headaches diagnosed with congenital arteriovenous malformation by brain scan

Q28.2　　Arteriovenous malformation of cerebral vessels

Explanation: Although present at birth, malformations may not be identified until later in life. Whenever the condition is diagnosed by the physician, it is appropriate to assign a code from the range Q00–Q99.

Newborn with anencephaly delivered vaginally in hospital

Z38.00　　Single liveborn infant, delivered vaginally

Q00.0　　Anencephaly

Explanation: For the birth admission, the appropriate code from category Z38 Liveborn infants, according to place of birth and type of delivery, should be sequenced as the principal diagnosis, followed by any congenital anomaly codes, Q00–Q99.

Chapter 17. Congenital Malformations, Deformations and Chromosomal Abnormalities(Q00-Q99)

NOTE   Codes from this chapter are not for use on maternal or fetal records.

EXCLUDES 2   *inborn errors of metabolism (E70-E88)*

This chapter contains the following blocks:

Q00-Q07   Congenital malformations of the nervous system
Q10-Q18   Congenital malformations of eye, ear, face and neck
Q20-Q28   Congenital malformations of the circulatory system
Q30-Q34   Congenital malformations of the respiratory system
Q35-Q37   Cleft lip and cleft palate
Q38-Q45   Other congenital malformations of the digestive system
Q50-Q56   Congenital malformations of genital organs
Q60-Q64   Congenital malformations of the urinary system
Q65-Q79   Congenital malformations and deformations of the musculoskeletal system
Q80-Q89   Other congenital malformations
Q90-Q99   Chromosomal abnormalities, not elsewhere classified

Congenital malformations of the nervous system (Q00-Q07)

✓4ᵗʰ **Q00   Anencephaly and similar malformations**

     Q00.0   Anencephaly   HCC
         Acephaly
         Acrania
         Amyelencephaly
         Hemianencephaly
         Hemicephaly

     Q00.1   Craniorachischisis   HCC

     Q00.2   Iniencephaly   HCC

✓4ᵗʰ **Q01   Encephalocele**
     INCLUDES   Arnold-Chiari syndrome, type III
                 encephalocystocele
                 encephalomyelocele
                 hydroencephalocele
                 hydromeningocele, cranial
                 meningocele, cerebral
                 meningoencephalocele
     EXCLUDES 1   *Meckel-Gruber syndrome (Q61.9)*

     Q01.0   Frontal encephalocele   HCC

     Q01.1   Nasofrontal encephalocele   HCC

     Q01.2   Occipital encephalocele   HCC

     Q01.8   Encephalocele of other sites   HCC

     Q01.9   Encephalocele, unspecified   HCC ▽

     Q02   Microcephaly   HCC
     INCLUDES   hydromicrocephaly
                 micrencephalon
     EXCLUDES 1   *Meckel-Gruber syndrome (Q61.9)*

✓4ᵗʰ **Q03   Congenital hydrocephalus**
     INCLUDES   hydrocephalus in newborn
     EXCLUDES 1   *Arnold-Chiari syndrome, type II (Q07.0-)*
                   acquired hydrocephalus (G91.-)
                   hydrocephalus due to congenital toxoplasmosis (P37.1)
                   hydrocephalus with spina bifida (Q05.0-Q05.4)

     Q03.0   Malformations of aqueduct of Sylvius   HCC
         Anomaly of aqueduct of Sylvius
         Obstruction of aqueduct of Sylvius, congenital
         Stenosis of aqueduct of Sylvius

     Q03.1   Atresia of foramina of Magendie and Luschkaq   HCC
         Dandy-Walker syndrome

Congenital Hydrocephalus

Normal ventricles   Hydrocephalic ventricles

     Q03.8   Other congenital hydrocephalus   HCC
     Q03.9   Congenital hydrocephalus, unspecified   HCC ▽

✓4ᵗʰ **Q04   Other congenital malformations of brain**
     EXCLUDES 1   *cyclopia (Q87.0)*
                   macrocephaly (Q75.3)

     Q04.0   Congenital malformations of corpus callosum   HCC
         Agenesis of corpus callosum

     Q04.1   Arhinencephaly   HCC

     Q04.2   Holoprosencephaly   HCC

     Q04.3   Other reduction deformities of brain   HCC
         Absence of part of brain
         Agenesis of part of brain
         Agyria
         Aplasia of part of brain
         Hydranencephaly
         Hypoplasia of part of brain
         Lissencephaly
         Microgyria
         Pachygyria
     EXCLUDES 1   *congenital malformations of corpus callosum (Q04.0)*

     Q04.4   Septo-optic dysplasia of brain   HCC

     Q04.5   Megalencephaly   HCC

     Q04.6   Congenital cerebral cysts   HCC
         Porencephaly
         Schizencephaly
     EXCLUDES 1   *acquired porencephalic cyst (G93.0)*

     Q04.8   Other specified congenital malformations of brain   HCC
         Arnold-Chiari syndrome, type IV
         Macrogyria

     Q04.9   Congenital malformation of brain, unspecified   HCC ▽
         Congenital anomaly NOS of brain
         Congenital deformity NOS of brain
         Congenital disease or lesion NOS of brain
         Multiple anomalies NOS of brain, congenital

✓4ᵗʰ **Q05   Spina bifida**
     INCLUDES   hydromeningocele (spinal)
                 meningocele (spinal)
                 meningomyelocele
                 myelocele
                 myelomeningocele
                 rachischisis
                 spina bifida (aperta)(cystica)
                 syringomyelocele
     Use additional code for any associated paraplegia (paraparesis) (G82.2-)
     EXCLUDES 1   *Arnold-Chiari syndrome, type II (Q07.0-)*
                   spina bifida occulta (Q76.0)

     Q05.0   Cervical spina bifida with hydrocephalus   HCC

     Q05.1   Thoracic spina bifida with hydrocephalus   HCC
         Dorsal spina bifida with hydrocephalus
         Thoracolumbar spina bifida with hydrocephalus

     Q05.2   Lumbar spina bifida with hydrocephalus   HCC
         Lumbosacral spina bifida with hydrocephalus

     Q05.3   Sacral spina bifida with hydrocephalus   HCC

     Q05.4   Unspecified spina bifida with hydrocephalus   HCC ▽

     Q05.5   Cervical spina bifida without hydrocephalus   HCC

     Q05.6   Thoracic spina bifida without hydrocephalus   HCC
         Dorsal spina bifida NOS
         Thoracolumbar spina bifida NOS

     Q05.7   Lumbar spina bifida without hydrocephalus   HCC
         Lumbosacral spina bifida NOS

     Q05.8   Sacral spina bifida without hydrocephalus   HCC

     Q05.9   Spina bifida, unspecified   HCC ▽

Spina Bifida

Spina bifida occulta   Meningocele   Myelomeningocele

EXCLUDES 1 Not coded here   **EXCLUDES 2** Not included here   **N** Newborn Age: 0   **P** Pediatric Age: 0-17   **M** Maternity Age: 12-55   **A** Adult Age: 15-124

✓4th **Q06 Other congenital malformations of spinal cord**

Q06.0 Amyelia   HCC

Q06.1 Hypoplasia and dysplasia of spinal cord   HCC
Atelomyelia
Myelatelia
Myelodysplasia of spinal cord

Q06.2 Diastematomyelia   HCC
DEF: Rare congenital anomaly often associated with spina bifida; the spinal cord is separated into longitudinal halves by a bony, cartilaginous or fibrous septum, each half surrounded by a dural sac.

Q06.3 Other congenital cauda equina malformations   HCC

Q06.4 Hydromyelia   HCC
Hydrorachis

Q06.8 Other specified congenital malformations of spinal cord   HCC

Q06.9 Congenital malformation of spinal cord, unspecified   HCC ▽
Congenital anomaly NOS of spinal cord
Congenital deformity NOS of spinal cord
Congenital disease or lesion NOS of spinal cord

✓4th **Q07 Other congenital malformations of nervous system**

EXCLUDES 2   *congenital central alveolar hypoventilation syndrome (G47.35)*
familial dysautonomia [Riley-Day] (G90.1)
neurofibromatosis (nonmalignant) (Q85.0-)

✓5th **Q07.0 Arnold-Chiari syndrome**
Arnold-Chiari syndrome, type II
EXCLUDES 1   *Arnold-Chiari syndrome, type III (Q01.-)*
Arnold-Chiari syndrome, type IV (Q04.8)

Q07.00 Arnold-Chiari syndrome without spina bifida or   HCC
hydrocephalus

Q07.01 Arnold-Chiari syndrome with spina bifida   HCC

Q07.02 Arnold-Chiari syndrome with hydrocephalus   HCC

Q07.03 Arnold-Chiari syndrome with spina bifida and   HCC
hydrocephalus

Q07.8 Other specified congenital malformations of nervous   HCC
system
Agenesis of nerve
Displacement of brachial plexus
Jaw-winking syndrome
Marcus Gunn's syndrome

Q07.9 Congenital malformation of nervous system,   HCC ▽
unspecified
Congenital anomaly NOS of nervous system
Congenital deformity NOS of nervous system
Congenital disease or lesion NOS of nervous system

Congenital malformations of eye, ear, face and neck (Q10-Q18)

EXCLUDES 2   *cleft lip and cleft palate (Q35-Q37)*
congenital malformation of cervical spine (Q05.0, Q05.5, Q67.5, Q76.0-Q76.4)
congenital malformation of larynx (Q31.-)
congenital malformation of lip NEC (Q38.0)
congenital malformation of nose (Q30.-)
congenital malformation of parathyroid gland (Q89.2)
congenital malformation of thyroid gland (Q89.2)

✓4th **Q10 Congenital malformations of eyelid, lacrimal apparatus and orbit**

EXCLUDES 1   *cryptophthalmos NOS (Q11.2)*
cryptophthalmos syndrome (Q87.0)

Q10.0 Congenital ptosis
DEF: Congenital drooping of eyelid; mostly idiopathic, but may occur genetically.

Q10.1 Congenital ectropion

Q10.2 Congenital entropion

Q10.3 Other congenital malformations of eyelid
Ablepharon
Blepharophimosis, congenital
Coloboma of eyelid
Congenital absence or agenesis of cilia
Congenital absence or agenesis of eyelid
Congenital accessory eyelid
Congenital accessory eye muscle
Congenital malformation of eyelid NOS

Q10.4 Absence and agenesis of lacrimal apparatus
Congenital absence of punctum lacrimale

Q10.5 Congenital stenosis and stricture of lacrimal duct

Q10.6 Other congenital malformations of lacrimal apparatus
Congenital malformation of lacrimal apparatus NOS

Q10.7 Congenital malformation of orbit

Coloboma of Lens

Coloboma

✓4th **Q11 Anophthalmos, microphthalmos and macrophthalmos**

Q11.0 Cystic eyeball

Q11.1 Other anophthalmos
Anophthalmos NOS
Agenesis of eye
Aplasia of eye

Q11.2 Microphthalmos
Cryptophthalmos NOS
Dysplasia of eye
Hypoplasia of eye
Rudimentary eye
EXCLUDES 1   *cryptophthalmos syndrome (Q87.0)*

Q11.3 Macrophthalmos
EXCLUDES 1   *macrophthalmos in congenital glaucoma (Q15.0)*

✓4th **Q12 Congenital lens malformations**

Q12.0 Congenital cataract

Q12.1 Congenital displaced lens

Q12.2 Coloboma of lens

Q12.3 Congenital aphakia

Q12.4 Spherophakia

Q12.8 Other congenital lens malformations
Microphakia

Q12.9 Congenital lens malformation, unspecified   ▽

✓4th **Q13 Congenital malformations of anterior segment of eye**

Q13.0 Coloboma of iris
Coloboma NOS

Q13.1 Absence of iris
Aniridia
Use additional code for associated glaucoma (H42)
DEF: Incompletely formed or absent iris; affects both eyes; dominant trait.

Q13.2 Other congenital malformations of iris
Anisocoria, congenital
Atresia of pupil
Congenital malformation of iris NOS
Corectopia

Q13.3 Congenital corneal opacity

Q13.4 Other congenital corneal malformations
Congenital malformation of cornea NOS
Microcornea
Peter's anomaly

Q13.5 Blue sclera

✓5th **Q13.8 Other congenital malformations of anterior segment of eye**

Q13.81 Rieger's anomaly
Use additional code for associated glaucoma (H42)

Q13.89 Other congenital malformations of anterior segment of eye

Q13.9 Congenital malformation of anterior segment of eye,   ▽
unspecified

✓4th **Q14 Congenital malformations of posterior segment of eye**
EXCLUDES 2   *optic nerve hypoplasia (H47.03-)*

Q14.0 Congenital malformation of vitreous humor
Congenital vitreous opacity

Q14.1 Congenital malformation of retina
Congenital retinal aneurysm

Q14.2 Congenital malformation of optic disc
Coloboma of optic disc

Q14.3 Congenital malformation of choroid

Q14.8 Other congenital malformations of posterior segment of eye
Coloboma of the fundus

Q14.9 Congenital malformation of posterior segment of eye, unspecified ▽

✓4ᵗʰ Q15 Other congenital malformations of eye
  EXCLUDES 1   *congenital nystagmus (H55.01)*
              ocular albinism (E70.31-)
              optic nerve hypoplasia (H47.03-)
              retinitis pigmentosa (H35.52)

Q15.0 Congenital glaucoma
  Axenfeld's anomaly
  Buphthalmos
  Glaucoma of childhood
  Glaucoma of newborn
  Hydrophthalmos
  Keratoglobus, congenital, with glaucoma
  Macrocornea with glaucoma
  Macrophthalmos in congenital glaucoma
  Megalocornea with glaucoma

Q15.8 Other specified congenital malformations of eye

Q15.9 Congenital malformation of eye, unspecified ▽
  Congenital anomaly of eye
  Congenital deformity of eye

✓4ᵗʰ Q16 Congenital malformations of ear causing impairment of hearing
  EXCLUDES 1   *congenital deafness (H90.-)*

Q16.0 Congenital absence of (ear) auricle

Q16.1 Congenital absence, atresia and stricture of auditory canal (external)
  Congenital atresia or stricture of osseous meatus

Q16.2 Absence of eustachian tube

Q16.3 Congenital malformation of ear ossicles
  Congenital fusion of ear ossicles

Q16.4 Other congenital malformations of middle ear
  Congenital malformation of middle ear NOS

Q16.5 Congenital malformation of inner ear
  Congenital anomaly of membranous labyrinth
  Congenital anomaly of organ of Corti

Q16.9 Congenital malformation of ear causing impairment of hearing, unspecified ▽
  Congenital absence of ear NOS

✓4ᵗʰ Q17 Other congenital malformations of ear
  EXCLUDES 1   *congenital malformations of ear with impairment of hearing (Q16.0- Q16.9)*
              preauricular sinus (Q18.1)

Q17.0 Accessory auricle
  Accessory tragus
  Polyotia
  Preauricular appendage or tag
  Supernumerary ear
  Supernumerary lobule

Q17.1 Macrotia
  DEF: Birth defect characterized by abnormal enlargement of the pinna of the ear.

Q17.2 Microtia

Q17.3 Other misshapen ear
  Pointed ear

Q17.4 Misplaced ear
  Low-set ears
  EXCLUDES 1   *cervical auricle (Q18.2)*

Q17.5 Prominent ear
  Bat ear

Q17.8 Other specified congenital malformations of ear
  Congenital absence of lobe of ear

Q17.9 Congenital malformation of ear, unspecified ▽
  Congenital anomaly of ear NOS

✓4ᵗʰ Q18 Other congenital malformations of face and neck
  EXCLUDES 1   *cleft lip and cleft palate (Q35-Q37)*
              conditions classified to Q67.0-Q67.4
              congenital malformations of skull and face bones (Q75.-)
              cyclopia (Q87.0)
              dentofacial anomalies [including malocclusion] (M26.-)
              malformation syndromes affecting facial appearance (Q87.0)
              persistent thyroglossal duct (Q89.2)

Q18.0 Sinus, fistula and cyst of branchial cleft
  Branchial vestige

Q18.1 Preauricular sinus and cyst
  Fistula of auricle, congenital
  Cervicoaural fistula

Q18.2 Other branchial cleft malformations
  Branchial cleft malformation NOS
  Cervical auricle
  Otocephaly

Q18.3 Webbing of neck
  Pterygium colli
  DEF: Congenital malformation characterized by thick, triangular skinfold that stretches from the lateral side of the neck across the shoulder; associated with genetic conditions Turner's and Noonan's syndromes.

Q18.4 Macrostomia
  DEF: Rare congenital craniofacial bilateral or unilateral anomaly of mouth due to malformed maxillary and mandibular processes; results in abnormally large mouth extending towards ear.

Q18.5 Microstomia

Q18.6 Macrocheilia
  Hypertrophy of lip, congenital

Q18.7 Microcheilia

Q18.8 Other specified congenital malformations of face and neck
  Medial cyst of face and neck
  Medial fistula of face and neck
  Medial sinus of face and neck

Q18.9 Congenital malformation of face and neck, unspecified ▽
  Congenital anomaly NOS of face and neck

Congenital malformations of the circulatory system (Q20-Q28)

✓4ᵗʰ Q20 Congenital malformations of cardiac chambers and connections
  EXCLUDES 1   *dextrocardia with situs inversus (Q89.3)*
              mirror-image atrial arrangement with situs inversus (Q89.3)

Q20.0 Common arterial trunk
  Persistent truncus arteriosus
  EXCLUDES 1   *aortic septal defect (Q21.4)*

Q20.1 Double outlet right ventricle
  Taussig-Bing syndrome

Q20.2 Double outlet left ventricle

Q20.3 Discordant ventriculoarterial connection
  Dextrotransposition of aorta
  Transposition of great vessels (complete)

Q20.4 Double inlet ventricle
  Common ventricle
  Cor triloculare biatriatum
  Single ventricle

Q20.5 Discordant atrioventricular connection
  Corrected transposition
  Levotransposition
  Ventricular inversion

Q20.6 Isomerism of atrial appendages
  Isomerism of atrial appendages with asplenia or polysplenia

Q20.8 Other congenital malformations of cardiac chambers and connections
  Cor binoculare

Q20.9 Congenital malformation of cardiac chambers and connections, unspecified ▽

✓4ᵗʰ Q21 Congenital malformations of cardiac septa
  EXCLUDES 1   *acquired cardiac septal defect (I51.0)*

Q21.0 Ventricular septal defect
  Roger's disease

Ventricular Septal Defect

EXCLUDES 1 Not coded here   EXCLUDES 2 Not included here   N Newborn Age: 0   P Pediatric Age: 0-17   M Maternity Age: 12-55   A Adult Age: 15-124

872   ICD-10-CM 2018

Atrial Septal Defect

Atrioventricular Septal Defect

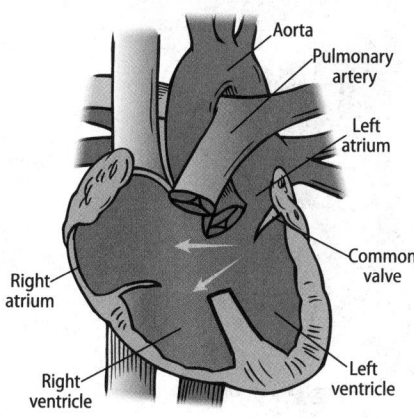

Q21.1 Atrial septal defect
Coronary sinus defect
Patent or persistent foramen ovale
Patent or persistent ostium secundum defect (type II)
Patent or persistent sinus venosus defect

Q21.2 Atrioventricular septal defect
Common atrioventricular canal
Endocardial cushion defect
Ostium primum atrial septal defect (type I)

Q21.3 Tetralogy of Fallot
Ventricular septal defect with pulmonary stenosis or atresia, dextroposition of aorta and hypertrophy of right ventricle.
AHA: 2014, 3Q, 16

Q21.4 Aortopulmonary septal defect
Aortic septal defect   Aortopulmonary window

Q21.8 Other congenital malformations of cardiac septa
Eisenmenger's defect
Pentalogy of Fallot
▶Code also if applicable:
Eisenmenger's complex (I27.83)
Eisenmenger's syndrome (I27.83)◀
EXCLUDES 1   *Eisenmenger's complex (I27.8)*
                    Eisenmenger's syndrome (I27.8)

Q21.9 Congenital malformation of cardiac septum, unspecified ▽
Septal (heart) defect NOS

✓4ᵗʰ **Q22 Congenital malformations of pulmonary and tricuspid valves**

Q22.Ø Pulmonary valve atresia

Q22.1 Congenital pulmonary valve stenosis
DEF: Stenosis of opening between pulmonary artery and right ventricle; causes obstructed blood outflow from right ventricle.

Q22.2 Congenital pulmonary valve insufficiency
Congenital pulmonary valve regurgitation

Q22.3 Other congenital malformations of pulmonary valve
Congenital malformation of pulmonary valve NOS
Supernumerary cusps of pulmonary valve

Q22.4 Congenital tricuspid stenosis
Congenital tricuspid atresia

Q22.5 Ebstein's anomaly
DEF: Malformation of the tricuspid valve characterized by septal and posterior leaflets attaching to the wall of the right ventricle; causes the right ventricle to fuse with the atrium into a large right atrium and a small ventricle; leads to heart failure and abnormal cardiac rhythm.

Q22.6 Hypoplastic right heart syndrome

Q22.8 Other congenital malformations of tricuspid valve

Q22.9 Congenital malformation of tricuspid valve, unspecified ▽

✓4ᵗʰ **Q23 Congenital malformations of aortic and mitral valves**

Q23.Ø Congenital stenosis of aortic valve
Congenital aortic atresia
Congenital aortic stenosis NOS
EXCLUDES 1   *congenital stenosis of aortic valve in hypoplastic left*
                    heart syndrome (Q23.4)
                    congenital subaortic stenosis (Q24.4)
                    supravalvular aortic stenosis (congenital) (Q25.3)

Q23.1 Congenital insufficiency of aortic valve
Bicuspid aortic valve
Congenital aortic insufficiency

Q23.2 Congenital mitral stenosis
Congenital mitral atresia
DEF: Congenital stenosis of mitral valve orifice between left atrium and ventricle; at the supravalvular, valvular, or subvalvular levels; causes obstruction to left ventricular filling.

Q23.3 Congenital mitral insufficiency

Q23.4 Hypoplastic left heart syndrome

Q23.8 Other congenital malformations of aortic and mitral valves

Q23.9 Congenital malformation of aortic and mitral valves, unspecified ▽

✓4ᵗʰ **Q24 Other congenital malformations of heart**
EXCLUDES 1   endocardial fibroelastosis (I42.4)

Q24.Ø Dextrocardia
EXCLUDES 1   *dextrocardia with situs inversus (Q89.3)*
                    isomerism of atrial appendages (with asplenia or
                    polysplenia) (Q20.6)
                    mirror-image atrial arrangement with situs inversus
                    (Q89.3)

Q24.1 Levocardia

Q24.2 Cor triatriatum

Q24.3 Pulmonary infundibular stenosis
Subvalvular pulmonic stenosis

Q24.4 Congenital subaortic stenosis
DEF: Congenital heart defect characterized by stenosis of left ventricular outflow tract due to fibrous tissue ring or septal hypertrophy below aortic valve.

Q24.5 Malformation of coronary vessels
Congenital coronary (artery) aneurysm

Q24.6 Congenital heart block

Q24.8 Other specified congenital malformations of heart
Congenital diverticulum of left ventricle
Congenital malformation of myocardium
Congenital malformation of pericardium
Malposition of heart
Uhl's disease

Q24.9 Congenital malformation of heart, unspecified ▽
Congenital anomaly of heart
Congenital disease of heart

✓4ᵗʰ **Q25 Congenital malformations of great arteries**

Q25.Ø Patent ductus arteriosus
Patent ductus Botallo   Persistent ductus arteriosus

Q25.1 Coarctation of aorta
Coarctation of aorta (preductal) (postductal)
Stenosis of Aorta

✓5ᵗʰ **Q25.2 Atresia of aorta**

Q25.21 Interruption of Aortic Arch
Atresia of aortic arch

Q25.29 Other atresia of aorta
Atresia of aorta

Q25.3 Supravalvular aortic stenosis
EXCLUDES 1   *congenital aortic stenosis NOS (Q23.Ø)*
                    congenital stenosis of aortic valve (Q23.Ø)

✓ Additional Character Req   ✓ₓ7ᵗʰ Placeholder Alert   Manifestation   HCC CMS-HCC Condition   ▽ Unspecified Code   ▶◀ Revised Text   ● New Code   ▲ Revised Code Title

ICD-10-CM 2018   873

Patent Ductus Arteriosus

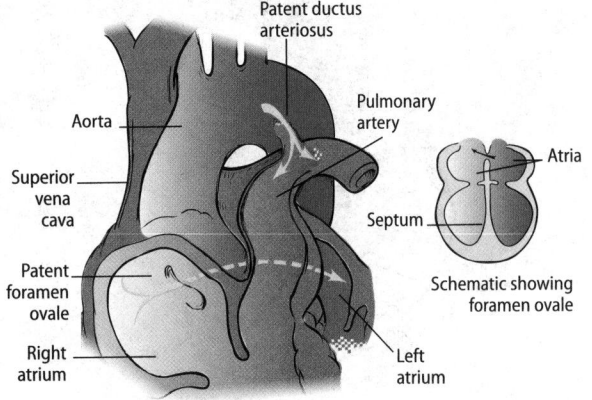

Patent ductus arteriosus
Pulmonary artery
Aorta
Superior vena cava
Patent foramen ovale
Right atrium
Left atrium
Atria
Septum
Schematic showing foramen ovale

Aortic Arch Anomalies

Esophagus
Trachea
Aortic arch

Normal aortic arch

Double aortic arch

Right aortic arch

✓5ᵗʰ **Q25.4 Other congenital malformations of aorta**
> EXCLUDES 1 *hypoplasia of aorta in hypoplastic left heart syndrome (Q23.4)*

Q25.40 Congenital malformation of aorta unspecified ▽

Q25.41 Absence and aplasia of aorta

Q25.42 Hypoplasia of aorta

Q25.43 Congenital aneurysm of aorta
Congenital aneurysm of aortic root
Congenital aneurysm of aortic sinus

Q25.44 Congenital dilation of aorta

Q25.45 Double aortic arch
Vascular ring of aorta

Q25.46 Tortuous aortic arch
Persistent convolutions of aortic arch

Q25.47 Right aortic arch
Persistent right aortic arch

Q25.48 Anomalous origin of subclavian artery

Q25.49 Other congenital malformations of aorta
▶Aortic arch
Bovine arch◀

Q25.5 Atresia of pulmonary artery

Q25.6 Stenosis of pulmonary artery
Supravalvular pulmonary stenosis

✓5ᵗʰ **Q25.7 Other congenital malformations of pulmonary artery**

Q25.71 Coarctation of pulmonary artery

Q25.72 Congenital pulmonary arteriovenous malformation
Congenital pulmonary arteriovenous aneurysm

Q25.79 Other congenital malformations of pulmonary artery
Aberrant pulmonary artery
Agenesis of pulmonary artery
Congenital aneurysm of pulmonary artery
Congenital anomaly of pulmonary artery
Hypoplasia of pulmonary artery

Q25.8 Other congenital malformations of other great arteries

Q25.9 Congenital malformation of great arteries, unspecified ▽

✓4ᵗʰ **Q26 Congenital malformations of great veins**

Q26.0 Congenital stenosis of vena cava
Congenital stenosis of vena cava (inferior)(superior)

Q26.1 Persistent left superior vena cava

Q26.2 Total anomalous pulmonary venous connection
Total anomalous pulmonary venous return [TAPVR], subdiaphragmatic
Total anomalous pulmonary venous return [TAPVR], supradiaphragmatic

Q26.3 Partial anomalous pulmonary venous connection
Partial anomalous pulmonary venous return

Q26.4 Anomalous pulmonary venous connection, unspecified ▽

Q26.5 Anomalous portal venous connection

Q26.6 Portal vein-hepatic artery fistula

Q26.8 Other congenital malformations of great veins
Absence of vena cava (inferior) (superior)
Azygos continuation of inferior vena cava
Persistent left posterior cardinal vein
Scimitar syndrome

Q26.9 Congenital malformation of great vein, unspecified ▽
Congenital anomaly of vena cava (inferior) (superior) NOS

✓4ᵗʰ **Q27 Other congenital malformations of peripheral vascular system**
> EXCLUDES 2 *anomalies of cerebral and precerebral vessels (Q28.0-Q28.3)*
> *anomalies of coronary vessels (Q24.5)*
> *anomalies of pulmonary artery (Q25.5-Q25.7)*
> *congenital retinal aneurysm (Q14.1)*
> *hemangioma and lymphangioma (D18.-)*

Q27.0 Congenital absence and hypoplasia of umbilical artery
Single umbilical artery

Q27.1 Congenital renal artery stenosis

Q27.2 Other congenital malformations of renal artery
Congenital malformation of renal artery NOS
Multiple renal arteries

✓5ᵗʰ **Q27.3 Arteriovenous malformation (peripheral)**
Arteriovenous aneurysm
> EXCLUDES 1 *acquired arteriovenous aneurysm (I77.0)*
> EXCLUDES 2 *arteriovenous malformation of cerebral vessels (Q28.2)*
> *arteriovenous malformation of precerebral vessels (Q28.0)*

Q27.30 Arteriovenous malformation, site unspecified ▽

Q27.31 Arteriovenous malformation of vessel of upper limb

Q27.32 Arteriovenous malformation of vessel of lower limb

Q27.33 Arteriovenous malformation of digestive system vessel

Q27.34 Arteriovenous malformation of renal vessel

Q27.39 Arteriovenous malformation, other site

Q27.4 Congenital phlebectasia

Q27.8 Other specified congenital malformations of peripheral vascular system
Absence of peripheral vascular system
Atresia of peripheral vascular system
Congenital aneurysm (peripheral)
Congenital stricture, artery
Congenital varix
> EXCLUDES 1 *arteriovenous malformation (Q27.3-)*

Q27.9 Congenital malformation of peripheral vascular system, unspecified ▽
Anomaly of artery or vein NOS

EXCLUDES 1 Not coded here   EXCLUDES 2 Not included here   N Newborn Age: 0   P Pediatric Age: 0-17   M Maternity Age: 12-55   A Adult Age: 15-124

874   ICD-10-CM 2018

Q25.4–Q27.9

✓4ᵗʰ **Q28 Other congenital malformations of circulatory system**
  EXCLUDES 1 *congenital aneurysm NOS (Q27.8)*
  congenital coronary aneurysm (Q24.5)
  ruptured cerebral arteriovenous malformation (I60.8)
  ruptured malformation of precerebral vessels (I72.0)
  EXCLUDES 2 *congenital peripheral aneurysm (Q27.8)*
  congenital pulmonary aneurysm (Q25.79)
  congenital retinal aneurysm (Q14.1)

Q28.0 Arteriovenous malformation of precerebral vessels
  Congenital arteriovenous precerebral aneurysm (nonruptured)

Q28.1 Other malformations of precerebral vessels
  Congenital malformation of precerebral vessels NOS
  Congenital precerebral aneurysm (nonruptured)

Q28.2 Arteriovenous malformation of cerebral vessels
  Arteriovenous malformation of brain NOS
  Congenital arteriovenous cerebral aneurysm (nonruptured)

Q28.3 Other malformations of cerebral vessels
  Congenital cerebral aneurysm (nonruptured)
  Congenital malformation of cerebral vessels NOS
  Developmental venous anomaly

Q28.8 Other specified congenital malformations of circulatory system
  Congenital aneurysm, specified site NEC
  Spinal vessel anomaly

Q28.9 Congenital malformation of circulatory system, unspecified ▽

Congenital malformations of the respiratory system (Q30-Q34)

✓4ᵗʰ **Q30 Congenital malformations of nose**
  EXCLUDES 1 *congenital deviation of nasal septum (Q67.4)*

Q30.0 Choanal atresia
  Atresia of nares (anterior) (posterior)
  Congenital stenosis of nares (anterior) (posterior)

Q30.1 Agenesis and underdevelopment of nose
  Congenital absent of nose

Q30.2 Fissured, notched and cleft nose

Q30.3 Congenital perforated nasal septum

Q30.8 Other congenital malformations of nose
  Accessory nose
  Congenital anomaly of nasal sinus wall

Q30.9 Congenital malformation of nose, unspecified ▽

✓4ᵗʰ **Q31 Congenital malformations of larynx**
  EXCLUDES 1 *congenital laryngeal stridor NOS (P28.89)*

Q31.0 Web of larynx
  Glottic web of larynx
  Subglottic web of larynx
  Web of larynx NOS
  DEF: Congenital malformation of larynx; marked by thin, translucent, or thick, fibrotic membrane-like structure between vocal folds; characterized by shortness of breath, and stridor.

Q31.1 Congenital subglottic stenosis

Q31.2 Laryngeal hypoplasia

Q31.3 Laryngocele

Q31.5 Congenital laryngomalacia

Q31.8 Other congenital malformations of larynx
  Absence of larynx
  Agenesis of larynx
  Atresia of larynx
  Congenital cleft thyroid cartilage
  Congenital fissure of epiglottis
  Congenital stenosis of larynx NEC
  Posterior cleft of cricoid cartilage

Q31.9 Congenital malformation of larynx, unspecified ▽

✓4ᵗʰ **Q32 Congenital malformations of trachea and bronchus**
  EXCLUDES 1 *congenital bronchiectasis (Q33.4)*

Q32.0 Congenital tracheomalacia

Q32.1 Other congenital malformations of trachea
  Atresia of trachea
  Congenital anomaly of tracheal cartilage
  Congenital dilatation of trachea
  Congenital malformation of trachea
  Congenital stenosis of trachea
  Congenital tracheocele

Q32.2 Congenital bronchomalacia

Q32.3 Congenital stenosis of bronchus

Q32.4 Other congenital malformations of bronchus
  Absence of bronchus
  Agenesis of bronchus
  Atresia of bronchus
  Congenital diverticulum of bronchus
  Congenital malformation of bronchus NOS

✓4ᵗʰ **Q33 Congenital malformations of lung**

Q33.0 Congenital cystic lung
  Congenital cystic lung disease
  Congenital honeycomb lung
  Congenital polycystic lung disease
  EXCLUDES 1 *cystic fibrosis (E84.0)*
  cystic lung disease, acquired or unspecified (J98.4)

Q33.1 Accessory lobe of lung
  Azygos lobe (fissured), lung

Q33.2 Sequestration of lung

Q33.3 Agenesis of lung
  Congenital absence of lung (lobe)

Q33.4 Congenital bronchiectasis

Q33.5 Ectopic tissue in lung

Q33.6 Congenital hypoplasia and dysplasia of lung
  EXCLUDES 1 *pulmonary hypoplasia associated with short gestation (P28.0)*

Q33.8 Other congenital malformations of lung

Q33.9 Congenital malformation of lung, unspecified ▽

✓4ᵗʰ **Q34 Other congenital malformations of respiratory system**
  EXCLUDES 2 *congenital central alveolar hypoventilation syndrome (G47.35)*

Q34.0 Anomaly of pleura

Q34.1 Congenital cyst of mediastinum

Q34.8 Other specified congenital malformations of respiratory system
  Atresia of nasopharynx

Q34.9 Congenital malformation of respiratory system, unspecified ▽
  Congenital absence of respiratory system
  Congenital anomaly of respiratory system NOS

Cleft lip and cleft palate (Q35-Q37)

Use additional code to identify associated malformation of the nose (Q30.2)
  EXCLUDES 1 *Robin's syndrome (Q87.0)*

✓4ᵗʰ **Q35 Cleft palate**
  INCLUDES fissure of palate
  palatoschisis
  EXCLUDES 1 *cleft palate with cleft lip (Q37.-)*

Q35.1 Cleft hard palate

Q35.3 Cleft soft palate

Q35.5 Cleft hard palate with cleft soft palate

Q35.7 Cleft uvula

Q35.9 Cleft palate, unspecified ▽
  Cleft palate NOS

✓4ᵗʰ **Q36 Cleft lip**
  INCLUDES cheiloschisis
  congenital fissure of lip
  harelip
  labium leporinum
  EXCLUDES 1 *cleft lip with cleft palate (Q37.-)*

Q36.0 Cleft lip, bilateral

Q36.1 Cleft lip, median

Q36.9 Cleft lip, unilateral
  Cleft lip NOS

Cleft Palate

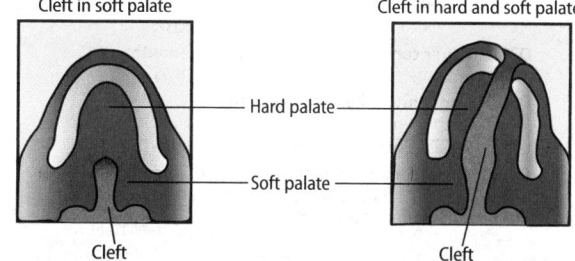

Cleft in soft palate · Cleft in hard and soft palate · Hard palate · Soft palate · Cleft · Cleft

Cleft Lip

Unilateral incomplete   Unilateral complete   Bilateral complete

✓4ᵗʰ Q37   Cleft palate with cleft lip
INCLUDES   cheilopalatoschisis

Q37.0   Cleft hard palate with bilateral cleft lip

Q37.1   Cleft hard palate with unilateral cleft lip
Cleft hard palate with cleft lip NOS

Q37.2   Cleft soft palate with bilateral cleft lip

Q37.3   Cleft soft palate with unilateral cleft lip
Cleft soft palate with cleft lip NOS

Q37.4   Cleft hard and soft palate with bilateral cleft lip

Q37.5   Cleft hard and soft palate with unilateral cleft lip
Cleft hard and soft palate with cleft lip NOS

Q37.8   Unspecified cleft palate with bilateral cleft lip   ▽

Q37.9   Unspecified cleft palate with unilateral cleft lip   ▽
Cleft palate with cleft lip NOS

Other congenital malformations of the digestive system (Q38-Q45)

✓4ᵗʰ Q38   Other congenital malformations of tongue, mouth and pharynx
EXCLUDES 1   *dentofacial anomalies (M26.-)*
macrostomia (Q18.4)
microstomia (Q18.5)

Q38.0   Congenital malformations of lips, not elsewhere classified
Congenital fistula of lip
Congenital malformation of lip NOS
Van der Woude's syndrome
EXCLUDES 1   *cleft lip (Q36.-)*
cleft lip with cleft palate (Q37.-)
macrocheilia (Q18.6)
microcheilia (Q18.7)

Q38.1   Ankyloglossia
Tongue tie

Q38.2   Macroglossia
Congenital hypertrophy of tongue

Q38.3   Other congenital malformations of tongue
Aglossia
Bifid tongue
Congenital adhesion of tongue
Congenital fissure of tongue
Congenital malformation of tongue NOS
Double tongue
Hypoglossia
Hypoplasia of tongue
Microglossia

Q38.4   Congenital malformations of salivary glands and ducts
Atresia of salivary glands and ducts
Congenital absence of salivary glands and ducts
Congenital accessory salivary glands and ducts
Congenital fistula of salivary gland

Q38.5   Congenital malformations of palate, not elsewhere classified
Congenital absence of uvula
Congenital malformation of palate NOS
Congenital high arched palate
EXCLUDES 1   *cleft palate (Q35.-)*
cleft palate with cleft lip (Q37.-)

Q38.6   Other congenital malformations of mouth
Congenital malformation of mouth NOS

Q38.7   Congenital pharyngeal pouch
Congenital diverticulum of pharynx
EXCLUDES 1   *pharyngeal pouch syndrome (D82.1)*

Q38.8   Other congenital malformations of pharynx
Congenital malformation of pharynx NOS
Imperforate pharynx

✓4ᵗʰ Q39   Congenital malformations of esophagus

Q39.0   Atresia of esophagus without fistula
Atresia of esophagus NOS

Q39.1   Atresia of esophagus with tracheo-esophageal fistula
Atresia of esophagus with broncho-esophageal fistula

Q39.2   Congenital tracheo-esophageal fistula without atresia
Congenital tracheo-esophageal fistula NOS

Q39.3   Congenital stenosis and stricture of esophagus

Q39.4   Esophageal web

Q39.5   Congenital dilatation of esophagus
Congenital cardiospasm

Q39.6   Congenital diverticulum of esophagus
Congenital esophageal pouch

Q39.8   Other congenital malformations of esophagus
Congenital absence of esophagus
Congenital displacement of esophagus
Congenital duplication of esophagus

Q39.9   Congenital malformation of esophagus, unspecified   ▽

✓4ᵗʰ Q40   Other congenital malformations of upper alimentary tract

Q40.0   Congenital hypertrophic pyloric stenosis
Congenital or infantile constriction
Congenital or infantile hypertrophy
Congenital or infantile spasm
Congenital or infantile stenosis
Congenital or infantile stricture

Q40.1   Congenital hiatus hernia
Congenital displacement of cardia through esophageal hiatus
EXCLUDES 1   *congenital diaphragmatic hernia (Q79.0)*

Q40.2   Other specified congenital malformations of stomach
Congenital displacement of stomach
Congenital diverticulum of stomach
Congenital hourglass stomach
Congenital duplication of stomach
Megalogastria
Microgastria

Q40.3   Congenital malformation of stomach, unspecified   ▽

Q40.8   Other specified congenital malformations of upper alimentary tract

Q40.9   Congenital malformation of upper alimentary tract, unspecified   ▽
Congenital anomaly of upper alimentary tract
Congenital deformity of upper alimentary tract

✓4ᵗʰ Q41   Congenital absence, atresia and stenosis of small intestine
INCLUDES   congenital obstruction, occlusion or stricture of small intestine or intestine NOS
EXCLUDES 1   *cystic fibrosis with intestinal manifestation (E84.11)*
meconium ileus NOS (without cystic fibrosis) (P76.0)

Q41.0   Congenital absence, atresia and stenosis of duodenum

Q41.1   Congenital absence, atresia and stenosis of jejunum
Apple peel syndrome
Imperforate jejunum

Q41.2   Congenital absence, atresia and stenosis of ileum

Q41.8   Congenital absence, atresia and stenosis of other specified parts of small intestine

Q41.9   Congenital absence, atresia and stenosis of small intestine, part unspecified   ▽
Congenital absence, atresia and stenosis of intestine NOS

✓4ᵗʰ Q42   Congenital absence, atresia and stenosis of large intestine
INCLUDES   congenital obstruction, occlusion and stricture of large intestine

Q42.0   Congenital absence, atresia and stenosis of rectum with fistula

Q42.1   Congenital absence, atresia and stenosis of rectum without fistula
Imperforate rectum

Q42.2   Congenital absence, atresia and stenosis of anus with fistula

Q42.3   Congenital absence, atresia and stenosis of anus without fistula
Imperforate anus

Q42.8   Congenital absence, atresia and stenosis of other parts of large intestine

Q42.9   Congenital absence, atresia and stenosis of large intestine, part unspecified   ▽

EXCLUDES 1 Not coded here   EXCLUDES 2 Not included here   N Newborn Age: 0   P Pediatric Age: 0-17   M Maternity Age: 12-55   A Adult Age: 15-124

876   ICD-10-CM 2018

☑4ᵗʰ **Q43** **Other congenital malformations of intestine**

Q43.0 **Meckel's diverticulum (displaced) (hypertrophic)**
Persistent omphalomesenteric duct
Persistent vitelline duct

Q43.1 **Hirschsprung's disease**
Aganglionosis
Congenital (aganglionic) megacolon

Q43.2 **Other congenital functional disorders of colon**
Congenital dilatation of colon

Q43.3 **Congenital malformations of intestinal fixation**
Congenital omental, anomalous adhesions [bands]
Congenital peritoneal adhesions [bands]
Incomplete rotation of cecum and colon
Insufficient rotation of cecum and colon
Jackson's membrane
Malrotation of colon
Rotation failure of cecum and colon
Universal mesentery

Q43.4 **Duplication of intestine**

Q43.5 **Ectopic anus**

Q43.6 **Congenital fistula of rectum and anus**
EXCLUDES 1   *congenital fistula of anus with absence, atresia and*
stenosis (Q42.2)
congenital fistula of rectum with absence, atresia and
stenosis (Q42.0)
congenital rectovaginal fistula (Q52.2)
congenital urethrorectal fistula (Q64.73)
pilonidal fistula or sinus (L05.-)

Q43.7 **Persistent cloaca**
Cloaca NOS

Q43.8 **Other specified congenital malformations of intestine**
Congenital blind loop syndrome
Congenital diverticulitis, colon
Congenital diverticulum, intestine
Dolichocolon
Megaloappendix
Megaloduodenum
Microcolon
Transposition of appendix
Transposition of colon
Transposition of intestine
AHA: 2013, 2Q, 31

Q43.9 **Congenital malformation of intestine, unspecified**   ▽

☑4ᵗʰ **Q44** **Congenital malformations of gallbladder, bile ducts and liver**

Q44.0 **Agenesis, aplasia and hypoplasia of gallbladder**
Congenital absence of gallbladder

Q44.1 **Other congenital malformations of gallbladder**
Congenital malformation of gallbladder NOS
Intrahepatic gallbladder

Q44.2 **Atresia of bile ducts**

Q44.3 **Congenital stenosis and stricture of bile ducts**

Q44.4 **Choledochal cyst**

Q44.5 **Other congenital malformations of bile ducts**
Accessory hepatic duct
Biliary duct duplication
Congenital malformation of bile duct NOS
Cystic duct duplication

Q44.6 **Cystic disease of liver**
Fibrocystic disease of liver

Q44.7 **Other congenital malformations of liver**
Accessory liver
Alagille's syndrome
Congenital absence of liver
Congenital hepatomegaly
Congenital malformation of liver NOS

☑4ᵗʰ **Q45** **Other congenital malformations of digestive system**
EXCLUDES 2   *congenital diaphragmatic hernia (Q79.0)*
congenital hiatus hernia (Q40.1)

Q45.0 **Agenesis, aplasia and hypoplasia of pancreas**
Congenital absence of pancreas

Q45.1 **Annular pancreas**

Q45.2 **Congenital pancreatic cyst**

Q45.3 **Other congenital malformations of pancreas and pancreatic duct**
Accessory pancreas
Congenital malformation of pancreas or pancreatic duct NOS
EXCLUDES 1   *congenital diabetes mellitus (E10.-)*
cystic fibrosis (E84.0-E84.9)
fibrocystic disease of pancreas (E84.-)
neonatal diabetes mellitus (P70.2)

Q45.8 **Other specified congenital malformations of digestive system**
Absence (complete) (partial) of alimentary tract NOS
Duplication of digestive system
Malposition, congenital of digestive system

Q45.9 **Congenital malformation of digestive system, unspecified** ▽
Congenital anomaly of digestive system
Congenital deformity of digestive system

Congenital malformations of genital organs (Q50-Q56)

EXCLUDES 1   *androgen insensitivity syndrome (E34.5-)*
syndromes associated with anomalies in the number and form of
chromosomes (Q90-Q99)

☑4ᵗʰ **Q50** **Congenital malformations of ovaries, fallopian tubes and broad ligaments**

☑5ᵗʰ **Q50.0** **Congenital absence of ovary**
EXCLUDES 1   *Turner's syndrome (Q96.-)*

    Q50.01 **Congenital absence of ovary, unilateral**   ♀

    Q50.02 **Congenital absence of ovary, bilateral**   ♀

Q50.1 **Developmental ovarian cyst**   ♀

Q50.2 **Congenital torsion of ovary**   ♀

☑5ᵗʰ **Q50.3** **Other congenital malformations of ovary**

    Q50.31 **Accessory ovary**   ♀

    Q50.32 **Ovarian streak**   ♀
46, XX with streak gonads

    Q50.39 **Other congenital malformation of ovary**   ♀
Congenital malformation of ovary NOS

Q50.4 **Embryonic cyst of fallopian tube**   ♀
Fimbrial cyst

Q50.5 **Embryonic cyst of broad ligament**   ♀
Epoophoron cyst
Parovarian cyst

Q50.6 **Other congenital malformations of fallopian tube and broad ligament**   ♀
Absence of fallopian tube and broad ligament
Accessory fallopian tube and broad ligament
Atresia of fallopian tube and broad ligament
Congenital malformation of fallopian tube or broad ligament NOS

☑4ᵗʰ **Q51** **Congenital malformations of uterus and cervix**

Q51.0 **Agenesis and aplasia of uterus**   ♀
Congenital absence of uterus

☑5ᵗʰ **Q51.1** **Doubling of uterus with doubling of cervix and vagina**

    Q51.10 **Doubling of uterus with doubling of cervix and vagina without obstruction**   ♀
Doubling of uterus with doubling of cervix and vagina NOS

    Q51.11 **Doubling of uterus with doubling of cervix and vagina with obstruction**   ♀

Q51.2 **Other doubling of uterus**   ♀
Doubling of uterus NOS
Septate uterus, complete or partial

Q51.3 **Bicornate uterus**   ♀
Bicornate uterus, complete or partial

Q51.4 **Unicornate uterus**   ♀
Unicornate uterus with or without a separate uterine horn
Uterus with only one functioning horn

Q51.5 **Agenesis and aplasia of cervix**   ♀
Congenital absence of cervix

Q51.6 **Embryonic cyst of cervix**   ♀

Q51.7 **Congenital fistulae between uterus and digestive and urinary tracts**   ♀

☑5ᵗʰ **Q51.8** **Other congenital malformations of uterus and cervix**

   ☑6ᵗʰ **Q51.81** **Other congenital malformations of uterus**

     Q51.810 **Arcuate uterus**   ♀
Arcuatus uterus

     Q51.811 **Hypoplasia of uterus**   ♀

     Q51.818 **Other congenital malformations of uterus**   ♀
Müllerian anomaly of uterus NEC

   ☑6ᵗʰ **Q51.82** **Other congenital malformations of cervix**

     Q51.820 **Cervical duplication**   ♀

     Q51.821 **Hypoplasia of cervix**   ♀

     Q51.828 **Other congenital malformations of cervix**   ♀

Q51.9 **Congenital malformation of uterus and cervix, unspecified**   ♀▽

Chapter 17. Congenital Malformations, Deformations, and Chromosomal Abnormalities   **Q43–Q51.9**

☑ Additional Character Req   ✓x7ᵗʰ Placeholder Alert   Manifestation   HCC CMS-HCC Condition   ▽ Unspecified Code   ▶◀ Revised Text   ● New Code   ▲ Revised Code Title

✓4ᵗʰ **Q52　Other congenital malformations of female genitalia**

Q52.0　Congenital absence of vagina　♀
Vaginal agenesis, total or partial

✓5ᵗʰ **Q52.1　Doubling of vagina**
EXCLUDES 1　doubling of vagina with doubling of uterus and cervix (Q51.1-)

Q52.10　Doubling of vagina, unspecified　♀▽
Septate vagina NOS

Q52.11　Transverse vaginal septum　♀

✓6ᵗʰ **Q52.12　Longitudinal vaginal septum**

Q52.120　Longitudinal vaginal septum, nonobstructing　♀

Q52.121　Longitudinal vaginal septum, obstructing, right side　♀

Q52.122　Longitudinal vaginal septum, obstructing, left side　♀

Q52.123　Longitudinal vaginal septum, microperforate, right side　♀

Q52.124　Longitudinal vaginal septum, microperforate, left side　♀

Q52.129　Other and unspecified longitudinal vaginal septum　♀▽

Q52.2　Congenital rectovaginal fistula　♀
EXCLUDES 1　cloaca (Q43.7)

Q52.3　Imperforate hymen
DEF: Obstructive anomaly of vagina, characterized by complete closure of membranous fold around external opening of vagina, obstructing the vaginal introitus.

Q52.4　Other congenital malformations of vagina　♀
Canal of Nuck cyst, congenital
Congenital malformation of vagina NOS
Embryonic vaginal cyst
Gartner's duct cyst

Q52.5　Fusion of labia　♀

Q52.6　Congenital malformation of clitoris　♀

✓5ᵗʰ **Q52.7　Other and unspecified congenital malformations of vulva**

Q52.70　Unspecified congenital malformations of vulva　♀▽
Congenital malformation of vulva NOS

Q52.71　Congenital absence of vulva　♀

Q52.79　Other congenital malformations of vulva　♀
Congenital cyst of vulva

Q52.8　Other specified congenital malformations of female genitalia　♀

Q52.9　Congenital malformation of female genitalia, unspecified　♀▽

✓4ᵗʰ **Q53　Undescended and ectopic testicle**

✓5ᵗʰ **Q53.0　Ectopic testis**

Q53.00　Ectopic testis, unspecified　♂▽

Q53.01　Ectopic testis, unilateral　♂

Q53.02　Ectopic testes, bilateral　♂

✓5ᵗʰ **Q53.1　Undescended testicle, unilateral**

Q53.10　Unspecified undescended testicle, unilateral　♂▽

✓6ᵗʰ **Q53.11　Abdominal testis, unilateral**

● 　　**Q53.111　Unilateral intraabdominal testis**

● 　　**Q53.112　Unilateral inguinal testis**

Q53.12　Ectopic perineal testis, unilateral　♂

● **Q53.13　Unilateral high scrotal testis**

✓5ᵗʰ **Q53.2　Undescended testicle, bilateral**

Q53.20　Undescended testicle, unspecified, bilateral　♂▽

✓6ᵗʰ **Q53.21　Abdominal testis, bilateral**

● 　　**Q53.211　Bilateral intraabdominal testes**

● 　　**Q53.212　Bilateral inguinal testes**

Q53.22　Ectopic perineal testis, bilateral　♂

● **Q53.23　Bilateral high scrotal testes**

Q53.9　Undescended testicle, unspecified　♂▽
Cryptorchism NOS

✓4ᵗʰ **Q54　Hypospadias**
EXCLUDES 1　epispadias (Q64.0)
DEF: Abnormal opening of urethra on the ventral (underside) surface of the penis.

Q54.0　Hypospadias, balanic　♂
Hypospadias, coronal
Hypospadias, glandular

Q54.1　Hypospadias, penile　♂

Hypospadias and Epispadias

Balanic (glanular, coronal) hypospadias
Subcoronal hypospadias
Penile hypospadias
Scrotal hypospadias
Scrotum
Penile raphe
Penoscrotal hypospadius
Scrotal raphe
Perineal hypospadias
Hypospadias (ventral view)

Normal external urethral orifice
Glans penis
Foreskin (retracted)
Epispadias
Epispadias (dorsal view)

Q54.2　Hypospadias, penoscrotal　♂

Q54.3　Hypospadias, perineal　♂

Q54.4　Congenital chordee　♂
Chordee without hypospadias

Q54.8　Other hypospadias　♂
Hypospadias with intersex state

Q54.9　Hypospadias, unspecified　♂▽

✓4ᵗʰ **Q55　Other congenital malformations of male genital organs**
EXCLUDES 1　congenital hydrocele (P83.5)
hypospadias (Q54.-)

Q55.0　Absence and aplasia of testis　♂
Monorchism

Q55.1　Hypoplasia of testis and scrotum　♂
Fusion of testes

✓5ᵗʰ **Q55.2　Other and unspecified congenital malformations of testis and scrotum**

Q55.20　Unspecified congenital malformations of testis and scrotum　♂▽
Congenital malformation of testis or scrotum NOS

Q55.21　Polyorchism　♂

Q55.22　Retractile testis　♂

Q55.23　Scrotal transposition　♂

Q55.29　Other congenital malformations of testis and scrotum　♂

Q55.3　Atresia of vas deferens　♂
Code first any associated cystic fibrosis (E84.-)

Q55.4　Other congenital malformations of vas deferens, epididymis, seminal vesicles and prostate　♂
Absence or aplasia of prostate
Absence or aplasia of spermatic cord
Congenital malformation of vas deferens, epididymis, seminal vesicles or prostate NOS

Q55.5　Congenital absence and aplasia of penis　♂

✓5ᵗʰ **Q55.6　Other congenital malformations of penis**

Q55.61　Curvature of penis (lateral)　♂

Q55.62　Hypoplasia of penis　♂
Micropenis

Q55.63　Congenital torsion of penis　♂
EXCLUDES 1　acquired torsion of penis (N48.82)

Q55.64　Hidden penis　♂
Buried penis
Concealed penis
EXCLUDES 1　acquired buried penis (N48.83)

Q55.69　Other congenital malformation of penis　♂
Congenital malformation of penis NOS

Q55.7　Congenital vasocutaneous fistula　♂

Q55.8　Other specified congenital malformations of male genital organs　♂

Q55.9　Congenital malformation of male genital organ, unspecified　♂▽
Congenital anomaly of male genital organ
Congenital deformity of male genital organ

EXCLUDES 1　Not coded here　　EXCLUDES 2　Not included here　　N Newborn Age: 0　　P Pediatric Age: 0-17　　M Maternity Age: 12-55　　A Adult Age: 15-124

878

ICD-10-CM 2018

Q52–Q55.9

☑️4ᵗʰ **Q56 Indeterminate sex and pseudohermaphroditism**
> **EXCLUDES 1** *46, XX true hermaphrodite (Q99.1)*
> *androgen insensitivity syndrome (E34.5-)*
> *chimera 46, XX/46, XY true hermaphrodite (Q99.0)*
> *female pseudohermaphroditism with adrenocortical disorder (E25.-)*
> *pseudohermaphroditism with specified chromosomal anomaly (Q96-Q99)*
> *pure gonadal dysgenesis (Q99.1)*

Q56.0 Hermaphroditism, not elsewhere classified
Ovotestis

Q56.1 Male pseudohermaphroditism, not elsewhere classified ♂
46, XY with streak gonads
Male pseudohermaphroditism NOS

Q56.2 Female pseudohermaphroditism, not elsewhere classified ♀
Female pseudohermaphroditism NOS

Q56.3 Pseudohermaphroditism, unspecified ▽

Q56.4 Indeterminate sex, unspecified ▽
Ambiguous genitalia

Congenital malformations of the urinary system (Q60-Q64)

☑️4ᵗʰ **Q60 Renal agenesis and other reduction defects of kidney**
> **INCLUDES** congenital absence of kidney
> congenital atrophy of kidney
> infantile atrophy of kidney

Q60.0 Renal agenesis, unilateral

Q60.1 Renal agenesis, bilateral

Q60.2 Renal agenesis, unspecified ▽

Q60.3 Renal hypoplasia, unilateral

Q60.4 Renal hypoplasia, bilateral

Q60.5 Renal hypoplasia, unspecified ▽

Q60.6 Potter's syndrome

☑️4ᵗʰ **Q61 Cystic kidney disease**
> **EXCLUDES 1** *acquired cyst of kidney (N28.1)*
> *Potter's syndrome (Q60.6)*

☑️5ᵗʰ **Q61.0 Congenital renal cyst**

  Q61.00 Congenital renal cyst, unspecified ▽
    Cyst of kidney NOS (congenital)

  Q61.01 Congenital single renal cyst

  Q61.02 Congenital multiple renal cysts

☑️5ᵗʰ **Q61.1 Polycystic kidney, infantile type**
Polycystic kidney, autosomal recessive

  Q61.11 Cystic dilatation of collecting ducts

  Q61.19 Other polycystic kidney, infantile type

Q61.2 Polycystic kidney, adult type
Polycystic kidney, autosomal dominant

Q61.3 Polycystic kidney, unspecified ▽
AHA: 2016, 3Q, 22

Q61.4 Renal dysplasia
Multicystic dysplastic kidney
Multicystic kidney (development)
Multicystic kidney disease
Multicystic renal dysplasia
> **EXCLUDES 1** *polycystic kidney disease (Q61.11-Q61.3)*

Q61.5 Medullary cystic kidney
Nephronopthisis
Sponge kidney NOS
DEF: Sponge kidney: Dilated collecting tubules; usually asymptomatic but calcinosis in tubules may cause renal insufficiency.

Q61.8 Other cystic kidney diseases
Fibrocystic kidney
Fibrocystic renal degeneration or disease

Q61.9 Cystic kidney disease, unspecified ▽
Meckel-Gruber syndrome

☑️4ᵗʰ **Q62 Congenital obstructive defects of renal pelvis and congenital malformations of ureter**

Q62.0 Congenital hydronephrosis

☑️5ᵗʰ **Q62.1 Congenital occlusion of ureter**
Atresia and stenosis of ureter

  Q62.10 Congenital occlusion of ureter, unspecified ▽

  Q62.11 Congenital occlusion of ureteropelvic junction

  Q62.12 Congenital occlusion of ureterovesical orifice

Q62.2 Congenital megaureter
Congenital dilatation of ureter

☑️5ᵗʰ **Q62.3 Other obstructive defects of renal pelvis and ureter**

  Q62.31 Congenital ureterocele, orthotopic

  Q62.32 Cecoureterocele
    Ectopic ureterocele

  Q62.39 Other obstructive defects of renal pelvis and ureter
    Ureteropelvic junction obstruction NOS

Q62.4 Agenesis of ureter
Congenital absence ureter

Q62.5 Duplication of ureter
Accessory ureter
Double ureter

☑️5ᵗʰ **Q62.6 Malposition of ureter**

  Q62.60 Malposition of ureter, unspecified ▽

  Q62.61 Deviation of ureter

  Q62.62 Displacement of ureter

  Q62.63 Anomalous implantation of ureter
    Ectopia of ureter
    Ectopic ureter

  Q62.69 Other malposition of ureter

Q62.7 Congenital vesico-uretero-renal reflux

Q62.8 Other congenital malformations of ureter
Anomaly of ureter NOS

☑️4ᵗʰ **Q63 Other congenital malformations of kidney**
> **EXCLUDES 1** *congenital nephrotic syndrome (N04.-)*

Q63.0 Accessory kidney

Q63.1 Lobulated, fused and horseshoe kidney

Q63.2 Ectopic kidney
Congenital displaced kidney
Malrotation of kidney

Q63.3 Hyperplastic and giant kidney
Compensatory hypertrophy of kidney

Q63.8 Other specified congenital malformations of kidney
Congenital renal calculi

Q63.9 Congenital malformation of kidney, unspecified ▽

☑️4ᵗʰ **Q64 Other congenital malformations of urinary system**

Q64.0 Epispadias ♂
> **EXCLUDES 1** *hypospadias (Q54.-)*

☑️5ᵗʰ **Q64.1 Exstrophy of urinary bladder**

  Q64.10 Exstrophy of urinary bladder, unspecified ▽
    Ectopia vesicae

  Q64.11 Supravesical fissure of urinary bladder

▲   **Q64.12 Cloacal exstrophy of urinary bladder**

  Q64.19 Other exstrophy of urinary bladder
    Extroversion of bladder

Q64.2 Congenital posterior urethral valves

☑️5ᵗʰ **Q64.3 Other atresia and stenosis of urethra and bladder neck**

  Q64.31 Congenital bladder neck obstruction
    Congenital obstruction of vesicourethral orifice

  Q64.32 Congenital stricture of urethra

  Q64.33 Congenital stricture of urinary meatus

  Q64.39 Other atresia and stenosis of urethra and bladder neck
    Atresia and stenosis of urethra and bladder neck NOS

Q64.4 Malformation of urachus
Cyst of urachus
Patent urachus
Prolapse of urachus

Q64.5 Congenital absence of bladder and urethra

Q64.6 Congenital diverticulum of bladder

☑️5ᵗʰ **Q64.7 Other and unspecified congenital malformations of bladder and urethra**
> **EXCLUDES 1** *congenital prolapse of bladder (mucosa) (Q79.4)*

  Q64.70 Unspecified congenital malformation of bladder and urethra ▽
    Malformation of bladder or urethra NOS

  Q64.71 Congenital prolapse of urethra

  Q64.72 Congenital prolapse of urinary meatus

  Q64.73 Congenital urethrorectal fistula

  Q64.74 Double urethra

  Q64.75 Double urinary meatus

  Q64.79 Other congenital malformations of bladder and urethra

Q64.8 Other specified congenital malformations of urinary system

---

☑️ Additional Character Req   ✔️x7ᵗʰ Placeholder Alert   Manifestation   HCC CMS-HCC Condition   ▽ Unspecified Code   ►◄ Revised Text   ● New Code   ▲ Revised Code Title

Q64.9 Congenital malformation of urinary system, unspecified ▽
     Congenital anomaly NOS of urinary system
     Congenital deformity NOS of urinary system

Congenital malformations and deformations of the musculoskeletal system (Q65-Q79)

✓4ᵗʰ **Q65 Congenital deformities of hip**
     EXCLUDES 1   clicking hip (R29.4)

  ✓5ᵗʰ **Q65.0 Congenital dislocation of hip, unilateral**
     Q65.00 Congenital dislocation of unspecified hip, unilateral ▽
     Q65.01 Congenital dislocation of right hip, unilateral
     Q65.02 Congenital dislocation of left hip, unilateral

  Q65.1 Congenital dislocation of hip, bilateral
  Q65.2 Congenital dislocation of hip, unspecified ▽

  ✓5ᵗʰ **Q65.3 Congenital partial dislocation of hip, unilateral**
     Q65.30 Congenital partial dislocation of unspecified hip, unilateral ▽
     Q65.31 Congenital partial dislocation of right hip, unilateral
     Q65.32 Congenital partial dislocation of left hip, unilateral

  Q65.4 Congenital partial dislocation of hip, bilateral
  Q65.5 Congenital partial dislocation of hip, unspecified ▽
  Q65.6 Congenital unstable hip
     Congenital dislocatable hip

  ✓5ᵗʰ **Q65.8 Other congenital deformities of hip**
     Q65.81 Congenital coxa valga
     Q65.82 Congenital coxa vara
     Q65.89 Other specified congenital deformities of hip
       Anteversion of femoral neck
       Congenital acetabular dysplasia

  Q65.9 Congenital deformity of hip, unspecified ▽

✓4ᵗʰ **Q66 Congenital deformities of feet**
     EXCLUDES 1   reduction defects of feet (Q72.-)
         valgus deformities (acquired) (M21.0-)
         varus deformities (acquired) (M21.1-)

  Q66.0 Congenital talipes equinovarus
  Q66.1 Congenital talipes calcaneovarus

  ✓5ᵗʰ **Q66.2 Congenital metatarsus (primus) varus**
     Q66.21 Congenital metatarsus primus varus
     Q66.22 Congenital metatarsus adductus
       Congenital metatarsus varus

  Q66.3 Other congenital varus deformities of feet
     Hallux varus, congenital
  Q66.4 Congenital talipes calcaneovalgus

  ✓5ᵗʰ **Q66.5 Congenital pes planus**
     Congenital flat foot
     Congenital rigid flat foot
     Congenital spastic (everted) flat foot
     EXCLUDES 1   pes planus, acquired (M21.4)
     Q66.50 Congenital pes planus, unspecified foot ▽
     Q66.51 Congenital pes planus, right foot
     Q66.52 Congenital pes planus, left foot

  Q66.6 Other congenital valgus deformities of feet
     Congenital metatarsus valgus
  Q66.7 Congenital pes cavus

  ✓5ᵗʰ **Q66.8 Other congenital deformities of feet**
     Q66.80 Congenital vertical talus deformity, unspecified foot ▽
     Q66.81 Congenital vertical talus deformity, right foot
     Q66.82 Congenital vertical talus deformity, left foot
     Q66.89 Other specified congenital deformities of feet
       Congenital asymmetric talipes
       Congenital clubfoot NOS
       Congenital talipes NOS
       Congenital tarsal coalition
       Hammer toe, congenital

  Q66.9 Congenital deformity of feet, unspecified ▽

✓4ᵗʰ **Q67 Congenital musculoskeletal deformities of head, face, spine and chest**
     EXCLUDES 1   congenital malformation syndromes classified to Q87-
         Potter's syndrome (Q60.6)

  Q67.0 Congenital facial asymmetry
  Q67.1 Congenital compression facies

Q67.2 Dolichocephaly
Q67.3 Plagiocephaly
Q67.4 Other congenital deformities of skull, face and jaw
     Congenital depressions in skull
     Congenital hemifacial atrophy or hypertrophy
     Deviation of nasal septum, congenital
     Squashed or bent nose, congenital
     EXCLUDES 1   dentofacial anomalies [including malocclusion] (M26.-)
         syphilitic saddle nose (A50.5)

Q67.5 Congenital deformity of spine
     Congenital postural scoliosis
     Congenital scoliosis NOS
     EXCLUDES 1   infantile idiopathic scoliosis (M41.0)
         scoliosis due to congenital bony malformation (Q76.3
     AHA: 2014, 4Q, 26

Q67.6 Pectus excavatum
     Congenital funnel chest
Q67.7 Pectus carinatum
     Congenital pigeon chest
Q67.8 Other congenital deformities of chest
     Congenital deformity of chest wall NOS

✓4ᵗʰ **Q68 Other congenital musculoskeletal deformities**
     EXCLUDES 1   reduction defects of limb(s) (Q71-Q73)
     EXCLUDES 2   congenital myotonic chondrodystrophy (G71.13)

  Q68.0 Congenital deformity of sternocleidomastoid muscle
     Congenital contracture of sternocleidomastoid (muscle)
     Congenital (sternomastoid) torticollis
     Sternomastoid tumor (congenital)

  Q68.1 Congenital deformity of finger(s) and hand
     Congenital clubfinger
     Spade-like hand (congenital)

  Q68.2 Congenital deformity of knee
     Congenital dislocation of knee
     Congenital genu recurvatum

  Q68.3 Congenital bowing of femur
     EXCLUDES 1   anteversion of femur (neck) (Q65.89)

  Q68.4 Congenital bowing of tibia and fibula
  Q68.5 Congenital bowing of long bones of leg, unspecified ▽
  Q68.6 Discoid meniscus
  Q68.8 Other specified congenital musculoskeletal deformities
     Congenital deformity of clavicle
     Congenital deformity of elbow
     Congenital deformity of forearm
     Congenital deformity of scapula
     Congenital deformity of wrist
     Congenital dislocation of elbow
     Congenital dislocation of shoulder
     Congenital dislocation of wrist

✓4ᵗʰ **Q69 Polydactyly**
  Q69.0 Accessory finger(s)
  Q69.1 Accessory thumb(s)
  Q69.2 Accessory toe(s)
     Accessory hallux
  Q69.9 Polydactyly, unspecified ▽
     Supernumerary digit(s) NOS

✓4ᵗʰ **Q70 Syndactyly**
  ✓5ᵗʰ **Q70.0 Fused fingers**
     Complex syndactyly of fingers with synostosis
     Q70.00 Fused fingers, unspecified hand ▽
     Q70.01 Fused fingers, right hand
     Q70.02 Fused fingers, left hand
     Q70.03 Fused fingers, bilateral

  ✓5ᵗʰ **Q70.1 Webbed fingers**
     Simple syndactyly of fingers without synostosis
     Q70.10 Webbed fingers, unspecified hand ▽
     Q70.11 Webbed fingers, right hand
     Q70.12 Webbed fingers, left hand
     Q70.13 Webbed fingers, bilateral

  ✓5ᵗʰ **Q70.2 Fused toes**
     Complex syndactyly of toes with synostosis
     Q70.20 Fused toes, unspecified foot ▽
     Q70.21 Fused toes, right foot
     Q70.22 Fused toes, left foot
     Q70.23 Fused toes, bilateral

EXCLUDES 1 Not coded here   *EXCLUDES 2* Not included here   Ⓝ Newborn Age: 0   Ⓟ Pediatric Age: 0-17   Ⓜ Maternity Age: 12-55   Ⓐ Adult Age: 15-124

880   ICD-10-CM 2018

✓5ᵗʰ **Q70.3** Webbed toes
     Simple syndactyly of toes without synostosis
     Q70.30 Webbed toes, unspecified foot ▽
     Q70.31 Webbed toes, right foot
     Q70.32 Webbed toes, left foot
     Q70.33 Webbed toes, bilateral

Q70.4 Polysyndactyly, unspecified ▽
     EXCLUDES 1   specified syndactyly of hand and feet—code to specified conditions (Q70.0-Q70.3-)

Q70.9 Syndactyly, unspecified ▽
     Symphalangy NOS

✓4ᵗʰ **Q71 Reduction defects of upper limb**

✓5ᵗʰ **Q71.0** Congenital complete absence of upper limb
     Q71.00 Congenital complete absence of unspecified upper limb ▽
     Q71.01 Congenital complete absence of right upper limb
     Q71.02 Congenital complete absence of left upper limb
     Q71.03 Congenital complete absence of upper limb, bilateral

✓5ᵗʰ **Q71.1** Congenital absence of upper arm and forearm with hand present
     Q71.10 Congenital absence of unspecified upper arm and forearm with hand present ▽
     Q71.11 Congenital absence of right upper arm and forearm with hand present
     Q71.12 Congenital absence of left upper arm and forearm with hand present
     Q71.13 Congenital absence of upper arm and forearm with hand present, bilateral

✓5ᵗʰ **Q71.2** Congenital absence of both forearm and hand
     Q71.20 Congenital absence of both forearm and hand, unspecified upper limb ▽
     Q71.21 Congenital absence of both forearm and hand, right upper limb
     Q71.22 Congenital absence of both forearm and hand, left upper limb
     Q71.23 Congenital absence of both forearm and hand, bilateral

✓5ᵗʰ **Q71.3** Congenital absence of hand and finger
     Q71.30 Congenital absence of unspecified hand and finger ▽
     Q71.31 Congenital absence of right hand and finger
     Q71.32 Congenital absence of left hand and finger
     Q71.33 Congenital absence of hand and finger, bilateral

✓5ᵗʰ **Q71.4** Longitudinal reduction defect of radius
     Clubhand (congenital)
     Radial clubhand
     Q71.40 Longitudinal reduction defect of unspecified radius ▽
     Q71.41 Longitudinal reduction defect of right radius
     Q71.42 Longitudinal reduction defect of left radius
     Q71.43 Longitudinal reduction defect of radius, bilateral

✓5ᵗʰ **Q71.5** Longitudinal reduction defect of ulna
     Q71.50 Longitudinal reduction defect of unspecified ulna ▽
     Q71.51 Longitudinal reduction defect of right ulna
     Q71.52 Longitudinal reduction defect of left ulna
     Q71.53 Longitudinal reduction defect of ulna, bilateral

✓5ᵗʰ **Q71.6** Lobster-claw hand
     Q71.60 Lobster-claw hand, unspecified hand ▽
     Q71.61 Lobster-claw right hand
     Q71.62 Lobster-claw left hand
     Q71.63 Lobster-claw hand, bilateral

✓5ᵗʰ **Q71.8** Other reduction defects of upper limb
     ✓6ᵗʰ **Q71.81 Congenital shortening of upper limb**
         Q71.811 Congenital shortening of right upper limb
         Q71.812 Congenital shortening of left upper limb
         Q71.813 Congenital shortening of upper limb, bilateral
         Q71.819 Congenital shortening of unspecified upper limb ▽

✓6ᵗʰ **Q71.89** Other reduction defects of upper limb
     Q71.891 Other reduction defects of right upper limb
     Q71.892 Other reduction defects of left upper limb
     Q71.893 Other reduction defects of upper limb, bilateral
     Q71.899 Other reduction defects of unspecified upper limb ▽

✓5ᵗʰ **Q71.9** Unspecified reduction defect of upper limb
     Q71.90 Unspecified reduction defect of unspecified upper limb ▽
     Q71.91 Unspecified reduction defect of right upper limb ▽
     Q71.92 Unspecified reduction defect of left upper limb ▽
     Q71.93 Unspecified reduction defect of upper limb, bilateral ▽

✓4ᵗʰ **Q72 Reduction defects of lower limb**

✓5ᵗʰ **Q72.0** Congenital complete absence of lower limb
     Q72.00 Congenital complete absence of unspecified lower limb ▽
     Q72.01 Congenital complete absence of right lower limb
     Q72.02 Congenital complete absence of left lower limb
     Q72.03 Congenital complete absence of lower limb, bilateral

✓5ᵗʰ **Q72.1** Congenital absence of thigh and lower leg with foot present
     Q72.10 Congenital absence of unspecified thigh and lower leg with foot present ▽
     Q72.11 Congenital absence of right thigh and lower leg with foot present
     Q72.12 Congenital absence of left thigh and lower leg with foot present
     Q72.13 Congenital absence of thigh and lower leg with foot present, bilateral

✓5ᵗʰ **Q72.2** Congenital absence of both lower leg and foot
     Q72.20 Congenital absence of both lower leg and foot, unspecified lower limb ▽
     Q72.21 Congenital absence of both lower leg and foot, right lower limb
     Q72.22 Congenital absence of both lower leg and foot, left lower limb
     Q72.23 Congenital absence of both lower leg and foot, bilateral

✓5ᵗʰ **Q72.3** Congenital absence of foot and toe(s)
     Q72.30 Congenital absence of unspecified foot and toe(s) ▽
     Q72.31 Congenital absence of right foot and toe(s)
     Q72.32 Congenital absence of left foot and toe(s)
     Q72.33 Congenital absence of foot and toe(s), bilateral

✓5ᵗʰ **Q72.4** Longitudinal reduction defect of femur
     Proximal femoral focal deficiency
     Q72.40 Longitudinal reduction defect of unspecified femur ▽
     Q72.41 Longitudinal reduction defect of right femur
     Q72.42 Longitudinal reduction defect of left femur
     Q72.43 Longitudinal reduction defect of femur, bilateral

✓5ᵗʰ **Q72.5** Longitudinal reduction defect of tibia
     Q72.50 Longitudinal reduction defect of unspecified tibia ▽
     Q72.51 Longitudinal reduction defect of right tibia
     Q72.52 Longitudinal reduction defect of left tibia
     Q72.53 Longitudinal reduction defect of tibia, bilateral

✓5ᵗʰ **Q72.6** Longitudinal reduction defect of fibula
     Q72.60 Longitudinal reduction defect of unspecified fibula ▽
     Q72.61 Longitudinal reduction defect of right fibula
     Q72.62 Longitudinal reduction defect of left fibula
     Q72.63 Longitudinal reduction defect of fibula, bilateral

✓5ᵗʰ **Q72.7** Split foot
     Q72.70 Split foot, unspecified lower limb ▽
     Q72.71 Split foot, right lower limb
     Q72.72 Split foot, left lower limb
     Q72.73 Split foot, bilateral

✓5ᵗʰ **Q72.8** Other reduction defects of lower limb
     ✓6ᵗʰ **Q72.81 Congenital shortening of lower limb**
         Q72.811 Congenital shortening of right lower limb
         Q72.812 Congenital shortening of left lower limb

✓ Additional Character Req   ✗x7ᵗʰ Placeholder Alert   Manifestation   HCC CMS-HCC Condition   ▽ Unspecified Code   ▶◀ Revised Text   ● New Code   ▲ Revised Code Title

ICD-10-CM 2018   881

Chapter 17. Congenital Malformations, Deformations, and Chromosomal Abnormalities

Q70.3–Q72.812

Q72.813 **Congenital shortening of lower limb, bilateral**

Q72.819 **Congenital shortening of unspecified lower limb** ▽

✓6ᵗʰ Q72.89 **Other reduction defects of lower limb**

Q72.891 **Other reduction defects of right lower limb**

Q72.892 **Other reduction defects of left lower limb**

Q72.893 **Other reduction defects of lower limb, bilateral**

Q72.899 **Other reduction defects of unspecified lower limb** ▽

✓5ᵗʰ Q72.9 **Unspecified reduction defect of lower limb**

Q72.90 **Unspecified reduction defect of unspecified lower limb** ▽

Q72.91 **Unspecified reduction defect of right lower limb** ▽

Q72.92 **Unspecified reduction defect of left lower limb** ▽

Q72.93 **Unspecified reduction defect of lower limb, bilateral** ▽

✓4ᵗʰ **Q73 Reduction defects of unspecified limb**

Q73.0 **Congenital absence of unspecified limb(s)** ▽
Amelia NOS

Q73.1 **Phocomelia, unspecified limb(s)** ▽
Phocomelia NOS

Q73.8 **Other reduction defects of unspecified limb(s)** ▽
Longitudinal reduction deformity of unspecified limb(s)
Ectromelia of limb NOS
Hemimelia of limb NOS
Reduction defect of limb NOS

✓4ᵗʰ **Q74 Other congenital malformations of limb(s)**
EXCLUDES 1   polydactyly (Q69.-)
reduction defect of limb (Q71-Q73)
syndactyly (Q70.-)

Q74.0 **Other congenital malformations of upper limb(s), including shoulder girdle**
Accessory carpal bones
Cleidocranial dysostosis
Congenital pseudarthrosis of clavicle
Macrodactylia (fingers)
Madelung's deformity
Radioulnar synostosis
Sprengel's deformity
Triphalangeal thumb

Q74.1 **Congenital malformation of knee**
Congenital absence of patella
Congenital dislocation of patella
Congenital genu valgum
Congenital genu varum
Rudimentary patella
EXCLUDES 1   congenital dislocation of knee (Q68.2)
congenital genu recurvatum (Q68.2)
nail patella syndrome (Q87.2)

Q74.2 **Other congenital malformations of lower limb(s), including pelvic girdle**
Congenital fusion of sacroiliac joint
Congenital malformation of ankle joint
Congenital malformation of sacroiliac joint
EXCLUDES 1   anteversion of femur (neck) (Q65.89)

Q74.3 **Arthrogryposis multiplex congenita**

Q74.8 **Other specified congenital malformations of limb(s)**

Q74.9 **Unspecified congenital malformation of limb(s)** ▽
Congenital anomaly of limb(s) NOS

✓4ᵗʰ **Q75 Other congenital malformations of skull and face bones**
EXCLUDES 1   congenital malformation of face NOS (Q18.-)
congenital malformation syndromes classified to Q87.-
dentofacial anomalies [including malocclusion] (M26.-)
musculoskeletal deformities of head and face (Q67.0-Q67.4)
skull defects associated with congenital anomalies of brain such as:
anencephaly (Q00.0)
encephalocele (Q01.-)
hydrocephalus (Q03.-)
microcephaly (Q02)

Q75.0 **Craniosynostosis**
Acrocephaly
Imperfect fusion of skull
Oxycephaly
Trigonocephaly

Q75.1 **Craniofacial dysostosis**
Crouzon's disease

Q75.2 **Hypertelorism**

Q75.3 **Macrocephaly**

Q75.4 **Mandibulofacial dysostosis**
Franceschetti syndrome
Treacher Collins syndrome

Q75.5 **Oculomandibular dysostosis**

Q75.8 **Other specified congenital malformations of skull and face bones**
Absence of skull bone, congenital
Congenital deformity of forehead
Platybasia

Q75.9 **Congenital malformation of skull and face bones, unspecified** ▽
Congenital anomaly of face bones NOS
Congenital anomaly of skull NOS

✓4ᵗʰ **Q76 Congenital malformations of spine and bony thorax**
EXCLUDES 1   congenital musculoskeletal deformities of spine and chest (Q67.5-Q67.8)

Q76.0 **Spina bifida occulta**
EXCLUDES 1   meningocele (spinal) (Q05.-)
spina bifida (aperta) (cystica) (Q05.-)

Q76.1 **Klippel-Feil syndrome**
Cervical fusion syndrome

Q76.2 **Congenital spondylolisthesis**
Congenital spondylolysis
EXCLUDES 1   spondylolisthesis (acquired) (M43.1-)
spondylolysis (acquired) (M43.0-)

Q76.3 **Congenital scoliosis due to congenital bony malformation**
Hemivertebra fusion or failure of segmentation with scoliosis

✓5ᵗʰ Q76.4 **Other congenital malformations of spine, not associated with scoliosis**

✓6ᵗʰ Q76.41 **Congenital kyphosis**

Q76.411 **Congenital kyphosis, occipito-atlanto-axial region**

Q76.412 **Congenital kyphosis, cervical region**

Q76.413 **Congenital kyphosis, cervicothoracic region**

Q76.414 **Congenital kyphosis, thoracic region**

Q76.415 **Congenital kyphosis, thoracolumbar region**

Q76.419 **Congenital kyphosis, unspecified region** ▽

✓6ᵗʰ Q76.42 **Congenital lordosis**

Q76.425 **Congenital lordosis, thoracolumbar region**

Q76.426 **Congenital lordosis, lumbar region**

Q76.427 **Congenital lordosis, lumbosacral region**

Q76.428 **Congenital lordosis, sacral and sacrococcygeal region**

Q76.429 **Congenital lordosis, unspecified region** ▽

Q76.49 **Other congenital malformations of spine, not associated with scoliosis**
Congenital absence of vertebra NOS
Congenital fusion of spine NOS
Congenital malformation of lumbosacral (joint) (region) NOS
Congenital malformation of spine NOS
Hemivertebra NOS
Malformation of spine NOS
Platyspondylisis NOS
Supernumerary vertebra NOS

Q76.5 **Cervical rib**
Supernumerary rib in cervical region

Q76.6 **Other congenital malformations of ribs**
Accessory rib
Congenital absence of rib
Congenital fusion of ribs
Congenital malformation of ribs NOS
EXCLUDES 1   short rib syndrome (Q77.2)

Q76.7 **Congenital malformation of sternum**
Congenital absence of sternum
Sternum bifidum

Q76.8 **Other congenital malformations of bony thorax**

Q76.9 **Congenital malformation of bony thorax, unspecified** ▽

EXCLUDES 1 Not coded here   EXCLUDES 2 Not included here   N Newborn Age: 0   P Pediatric Age: 0-17   M Maternity Age: 12-55   A Adult Age: 15-124

882   ICD-10-CM 2018

☑️4ᵗʰ **Q77 Osteochondrodysplasia with defects of growth of tubular bones and spine**
> EXCLUDES 1 *mucopolysaccharidosis (E76.0-E76.3)*
> EXCLUDES 2 *congenital myotonic chondrodystrophy (G71.13)*

Q77.0 Achondrogenesis
Hypochondrogenesis

Q77.1 Thanatophoric short stature

Q77.2 Short rib syndrome
Asphyxiating thoracic dysplasia [Jeune]

Q77.3 Chondrodysplasia punctata
> EXCLUDES 1 *Rhizomelic chondrodysplasia punctata (E71.43)*

Q77.4 Achondroplasia
Hypochondroplasia
Osteosclerosis congenita

Q77.5 Diastrophic dysplasia

Q77.6 Chondroectodermal dysplasia
Ellis-van Creveld syndrome

Q77.7 Spondyloepiphyseal dysplasia

Q77.8 Other osteochondrodysplasia with defects of growth of tubular bones and spine

Q77.9 Osteochondrodysplasia with defects of growth of tubular bones and spine, unspecified ▽

☑️4ᵗʰ **Q78 Other osteochondrodysplasias**
> EXCLUDES 2 *congenital myotonic chondrodystrophy (G71.13)*

Q78.0 Osteogenesis imperfecta
Fragilitas ossium
Osteopsathyrosis

Q78.1 Polyostotic fibrous dysplasia
Albright(-McCune)(-Sternberg) syndrome

Q78.2 Osteopetrosis
Albers-Schönberg syndrome
Osteosclerosis NOS

Q78.3 Progressive diaphyseal dysplasia
Camurati-Engelmann syndrome

Q78.4 Enchondromatosis
Maffucci's syndrome
Ollier's disease

Q78.5 Metaphyseal dysplasia
Pyle's syndrome

Q78.6 Multiple congenital exostoses
Diaphyseal aclasis

Q78.8 Other specified osteochondrodysplasias
Osteopoikilosis

Q78.9 Osteochondrodysplasia, unspecified ▽
Chondrodystrophy NOS
Osteodystrophy NOS

☑️4ᵗʰ **Q79 Congenital malformations of musculoskeletal system, not elsewhere classified**
> EXCLUDES 2 *congenital (sternomastoid) torticollis (Q68.0)*

Q79.0 Congenital diaphragmatic hernia
> EXCLUDES 1 *congenital hiatus hernia (Q40.1)*

Q79.1 Other congenital malformations of diaphragm
Absence of diaphragm
Congenital malformation of diaphragm NOS
Eventration of diaphragm

Q79.2 Exomphalos
Omphalocele
> EXCLUDES 1 *umbilical hernia (K42.-)*

Q79.3 Gastroschisis

Q79.4 Prune belly syndrome
Congenital prolapse of bladder mucosa
Eagle-Barrett syndrome

☑️5ᵗʰ **Q79.5 Other congenital malformations of abdominal wall**
> EXCLUDES 1 *umbilical hernia (K42.-)*

Q79.51 Congenital hernia of bladder

Q79.59 Other congenital malformations of abdominal wall

Q79.6 Ehlers-Danlos syndrome
DEF: Connective tissue disorder that causes hyperextended skin and joints; results in fragile blood vessels with bleeding, poor wound healing, and subcutaneous pseudotumors.

Gastroschisis
Herniated small bowel (gastroschisis)
Rectus abdominus m.
Umbilicus
skin
distal
proximal
Defect

Q79.8 Other congenital malformations of musculoskeletal system
Absence of muscle
Absence of tendon
Accessory muscle
Amyotrophia congenita
Congenital constricting bands
Congenital shortening of tendon
Poland syndrome

Q79.9 Congenital malformation of musculoskeletal system, unspecified ▽
Congenital anomaly of musculoskeletal system NOS
Congenital deformity of musculoskeletal system NOS

Other congenital malformations (Q80-Q89)

☑️4ᵗʰ **Q80 Congenital ichthyosis**
> EXCLUDES 1 *Refsum's disease (G60.1)*

Q80.0 Ichthyosis vulgaris

Q80.1 X-linked ichthyosis

Q80.2 Lamellar ichthyosis
Collodion baby

Q80.3 Congenital bullous ichthyosiform erythroderma

Q80.4 Harlequin fetus

Q80.8 Other congenital ichthyosis

Q80.9 Congenital ichthyosis, unspecified ▽

☑️4ᵗʰ **Q81 Epidermolysis bullosa**

Q81.0 Epidermolysis bullosa simplex
> EXCLUDES 1 *Cockayne's syndrome (Q87.1)*

Q81.1 Epidermolysis bullosa letalis
Herlitz' syndrome

Q81.2 Epidermolysis bullosa dystrophica

Q81.8 Other epidermolysis bullosa

Q81.9 Epidermolysis bullosa, unspecified ▽

☑️4ᵗʰ **Q82 Other congenital malformations of skin**
> EXCLUDES 1 *acrodermatitis enteropathica (E83.2)*
> *congenital erythropoietic porphyria (E80.0)*
> *pilonidal cyst or sinus (L05.-)*
> *Sturge-Weber (-Dimitri) syndrome (Q85.8)*

Q82.0 Hereditary lymphedema

Q82.1 Xeroderma pigmentosum

▲ **Q82.2 Congenital cutaneous mastocytosis**
▶Congenital diffuse cutaneous mastocytosis
Congenital maculopapular cutaneous mastocytosis
Congenital urticaria pigmentosa◀
Urticaria pigmentosa
> EXCLUDES 1 ▶*cutaneous mastocytosis NOS (D47.01)*
> *diffuse cutaneous mastocytosis (with onset after newborn period) (D47.01)*◀
> *malignant mastocytosis* ▶*(C96.2-)*◀
> ▶*systemic mastocytosis (D47.02)*
> *urticaria pigmentosa (non-congenital) (with onset after newborn period) (D47.01)*◀

Q82.3 Incontinentia pigmenti

Q82.4 Ectodermal dysplasia (anhidrotic)
> EXCLUDES 1 *Ellis-van Creveld syndrome (Q77.6)*

☑️ Additional Character Req   ✗ˣ⁷ᵗʰ Placeholder Alert   Manifestation   HCC CMS-HCC Condition   ▽ Unspecified Code   ▶◀ Revised Text   ● New Code   ▲ Revised Code Title

Q82.5 Congenital non-neoplastic nevus

Birthmark NOS	Strawberry Nevus
Flammeus Nevus	Vascular Nevus NOS
Portwine Nevus	Verrucous Nevus
Sanguineous Nevus	

EXCLUDES 2 *araneus nevus (I78.1)*
café au lait spots (L81.3)
lentigo (L81.4)
melanocytic nevus (D22.-)
nevus NOS (D22.-)
pigmented nevus (D22.-)
spider nevus (I78.1)
stellar nevus (I78.1)

Q82.6 Congenital sacral dimple
Parasacral dimple
EXCLUDES 2 *pilonidal cyst with abscess (L05.01)*
pilonidal cyst without abscess (L05.91)

Q82.8 Other specified congenital malformations of skin
Abnormal palmar creases
Accessory skin tags
Benign familial pemphigus [Hailey-Hailey]
Congenital poikiloderma
Cutis laxa (hyperelastica)
Dermatoglyphic anomalies
Inherited keratosis palmaris et plantaris
Keratosis follicularis [Darier-White]
EXCLUDES 1 *Ehlers-Danlos syndrome (Q79.6)*
AHA: 2016, 1Q, 17

Q82.9 Congenital malformation of skin, unspecified ▽

✓4ᵗʰ Q83 Congenital malformations of breast
EXCLUDES 2 *absence of pectoral muscle (Q79.8)*
hypoplasia of breast (N64.82)
micromastia (N64.82)

Q83.0 Congenital absence of breast with absent nipple

Q83.1 Accessory breast
Supernumerary breast

Q83.2 Absent nipple

Q83.3 Accessory nipple
Supernumerary nipple

Q83.8 Other congenital malformations of breast

Q83.9 Congenital malformation of breast, unspecified ▽

✓4ᵗʰ Q84 Other congenital malformations of integument

Q84.0 Congenital alopecia
Congenital atrichosis

Q84.1 Congenital morphological disturbances of hair, not elsewhere classified
Beaded hair
Monilethrix
Pili annulati
EXCLUDES 1 *Menkes' kinky hair syndrome (E83.0)*

Q84.2 Other congenital malformations of hair
Congenital hypertrichosis
Congenital malformation of hair NOS
Persistent lanugo

Q84.3 Anonychia
EXCLUDES 1 *nail patella syndrome (Q87.2)*

Q84.4 Congenital leukonychia

Q84.5 Enlarged and hypertrophic nails
Congenital onychauxis
Pachyonychia

Q84.6 Other congenital malformations of nails
Congenital clubnail
Congenital koilonychia
Congenital malformation of nail NOS

Q84.8 Other specified congenital malformations of integument
Aplasia cutis congenita

Q84.9 Congenital malformation of integument, unspecified ▽
Congenital anomaly of integument NOS
Congenital deformity of integument NOS

✓4ᵗʰ Q85 Phakomatoses, not elsewhere classified
EXCLUDES 1 *ataxia telangiectasia [Louis-Bar] (G11.3)*
familial dysautonomia [Riley-Day] (G90.1)

✓5ᵗʰ Q85.0 Neurofibromatosis (nonmalignant)

Q85.00 Neurofibromatosis, unspecified HCC ▽

Q85.01 Neurofibromatosis, type 1 HCC
Von Recklinghausen disease

Q85.02 Neurofibromatosis, type 2 HCC
Acoustic neurofibromatosis
DEF: Inherited condition with cutaneous lesions, benign tumors of peripheral nerves, and bilateral 8th nerve masses.

Q85.03 Schwannomatosis HCC
DEF: A genetic mutation (SMARCB1/INI1) causing multiple benign tumors along nerve pathways; characterized by the exception of 8th cranial nerve involvement.

Q85.09 Other neurofibromatosis HCC

Q85.1 Tuberous sclerosis HCC
Bourneville's disease
Epiloia

Q85.8 Other phakomatoses, not elsewhere classified HCC
Peutz-Jeghers Syndrome
Sturge-Weber(-Dimitri) syndrome
von Hippel-Lindau syndrome
EXCLUDES 1 *Meckel-Gruber syndrome (Q61.9)*

Q85.9 Phakomatosis, unspecified HCC ▽
Hamartosis NOS

✓4ᵗʰ Q86 Congenital malformation syndromes due to known exogenous causes, not elsewhere classified
EXCLUDES 2 *iodine-deficiency-related hypothyroidism (E00-E02)*
nonteratogenic effects of substances transmitted via placenta or breast milk (P04.-)

Q86.0 Fetal alcohol syndrome (dysmorphic)

Q86.1 Fetal hydantoin syndrome
Meadow's syndrome

Q86.2 Dysmorphism due to warfarin

Q86.8 Other congenital malformation syndromes due to known exogenous causes

✓4ᵗʰ Q87 Other specified congenital malformation syndromes affecting multiple systems
Use additional code(s) to identify all associated manifestations

Q87.0 Congenital malformation syndromes predominantly affecting facial appearance

Acrocephalopolysyndactyly	Moebius syndrome
Acrocephalosyndactyly [Apert] syndrome	Oro-facial-digital
Cryptophthalmos syndrome	Robin syndrome
Cyclopia	Whistling face
Goldenhar syndrome	

Q87.1 Congenital malformation syndromes predominantly associated with short stature

Aarskog syndrome	Robinow-Silverman-Smith
Cockayne syndrome	syndrome
De Lange syndrome	Russell-Silver syndrome
Dubowitz syndrome	Seckel syndrome
Noonan syndrome	
Prader-Willi syndrome	

EXCLUDES 1 *Ellis-van Creveld syndrome (Q77.6)*
Smith-Lemli-Opitz syndrome (E78.72)

Q87.2 Congenital malformation syndromes predominantly involving limbs
Holt-Oram syndrome
Klippel-Trenaunay-Weber syndrome
Nail patella syndrome
Rubinstein-Taybi syndrome
Sirenomelia syndrome
Thrombocytopenia with absent radius [TAR] syndrome
VATER syndrome

Q87.3 Congenital malformation syndromes involving early overgrowth
Beckwith-Wiedemann syndrome
Sotos syndrome
Weaver syndrome

✓5ᵗʰ Q87.4 Marfan's syndrome

Q87.40 Marfan's syndrome, unspecified ▽

✓6ᵗʰ Q87.41 Marfan's syndrome with cardiovascular manifestations

Q87.410 Marfan's syndrome with aortic dilation

Q87.418 Marfan's syndrome with other cardiovascular manifestations

Q87.42 Marfan's syndrome with ocular manifestations

Q87.43 Marfan's syndrome with skeletal manifestation

Q87.5 Other congenital malformation syndromes with other skeletal changes

✓5ᵗʰ **Q87.8** **Other specified congenital malformation syndromes, not elsewhere classified**
  EXCLUDES 1 *Zellweger syndrome (E71.510)*

Q87.81 **Alport syndrome**
  Use additional code to identify stage of chronic kidney disease (N18.1-N18.6)

Q87.82 **Arterial tortuosity syndrome**

Q87.89 **Other specified congenital malformation syndromes, not elsewhere classified**
  Laurence-Moon (-Bardet)-Biedl syndrome

✓4ᵗʰ **Q89** **Other congenital malformations, not elsewhere classified**

  ✓5ᵗʰ **Q89.0** **Congenital absence and malformations of spleen**
    EXCLUDES 1 *isomerism of atrial appendages (with asplenia or polysplenia) (Q20.6)*

  Q89.01 **Asplenia (congenital)**

  Q89.09 **Congenital malformations of spleen**
    Congenital splenomegaly

  Q89.1 **Congenital malformations of adrenal gland**
    EXCLUDES 1 *adrenogenital disorders (E25.-)*
    congenital adrenal hyperplasia (E25.0)

  Q89.2 **Congenital malformations of other endocrine glands**
    Congenital malformation of parathyroid or thyroid gland
    Persistent thyroglossal duct
    Thyroglossal cyst
    EXCLUDES 1 *congenital goiter (E03.0)*
    congenital hypothyroidism (E03.1)

  Q89.3 **Situs inversus**
    Dextrocardia with situs inversus
    Mirror-image atrial arrangement with situs inversus
    Situs inversus or transversus abdominalis
    Situs inversus or transversus thoracis
    Transposition of abdominal viscera
    Transposition of thoracic viscera
    EXCLUDES 1 *dextrocardia NOS (Q24.0)*

  Q89.4 **Conjoined twins**
    Craniopagus   Pygopagus
    Dicephalus   Thoracopagus

  Q89.7 **Multiple congenital malformations, not elsewhere classified**
    Multiple congenital anomalies NOS
    Multiple congenital deformities NOS
    EXCLUDES 1 *congenital malformation syndromes affecting multiple systems (Q87.-)*

  Q89.8 **Other specified congenital malformations**
    Use additional code(s) to identify all associated manifestations

  Q89.9 **Congenital malformation, unspecified**   ▽
    Congenital anomaly NOS
    Congenital deformity NOS

Chromosomal abnormalities, not elsewhere classified (Q90-Q99)
  EXCLUDES 2 *mitochondrial metabolic disorders (E88.4-)*

✓4ᵗʰ **Q90** **Down syndrome**
  Use additional code(s) to identify any associated physical conditions and degree of intellectual disabilities (F70-F79)

  Q90.0 **Trisomy 21, nonmosaicism (meiotic nondisjunction)**

  Q90.1 **Trisomy 21, mosaicism (mitotic nondisjunction)**

  Q90.2 **Trisomy 21, translocation**

  Q90.9 **Down syndrome, unspecified**   ▽
    Trisomy 21 NOS

✓4ᵗʰ **Q91** **Trisomy 18 and Trisomy 13**

  Q91.0 **Trisomy 18, nonmosaicism (meiotic nondisjunction)**

  Q91.1 **Trisomy 18, mosaicism (mitotic nondisjunction)**

  Q91.2 **Trisomy 18, translocation**

  Q91.3 **Trisomy 18, unspecified**   ▽

  Q91.4 **Trisomy 13, nonmosaicism (meiotic nondisjunction)**

  Q91.5 **Trisomy 13, mosaicism (mitotic nondisjunction)**

  Q91.6 **Trisomy 13, translocation**

  Q91.7 **Trisomy 13, unspecified**   ▽

✓4ᵗʰ **Q92** **Other trisomies and partial trisomies of the autosomes, not elsewhere classified**
  INCLUDES unbalanced translocations and insertions
  EXCLUDES 1 *trisomies of chromosomes 13, 18, 21 (Q90-Q91)*

  Q92.0 **Whole chromosome trisomy, nonmosaicism (meiotic nondisjunction)**

  Q92.1 **Whole chromosome trisomy, mosaicism (mitotic nondisjunction)**

Q92.2 **Partial trisomy**
  Less than whole arm duplicated
  Whole arm or more duplicated
  EXCLUDES 1 *partial trisomy due to unbalanced translocation (Q92.5)*

Q92.5 **Duplications with other complex rearrangements**
  Partial trisomy due to unbalanced translocations
  Code also any associated deletions due to unbalanced translocations, inversions and insertions (Q93.7)

✓5ᵗʰ **Q92.6** **Marker chromosomes**
  Trisomies due to dicentrics
  Trisomies due to extra rings
  Trisomies due to isochromosomes
  Individual with marker heterochromatin

  Q92.61 **Marker chromosomes in normal individual**

  Q92.62 **Marker chromosomes in abnormal individual**

Q92.7 **Triploidy and polyploidy**

Q92.8 **Other specified trisomies and partial trisomies of autosomes**
  Duplications identified by fluorescence in situ hybridization (FISH)
  Duplications identified by in situ hybridization (ISH)
  Duplications seen only at prometaphase

Q92.9 **Trisomy and partial trisomy of autosomes, unspecified**   ▽

✓4ᵗʰ **Q93** **Monosomies and deletions from the autosomes, not elsewhere classified**

  Q93.0 **Whole chromosome monosomy, nonmosaicism (meiotic nondisjunction)**

  Q93.1 **Whole chromosome monosomy, mosaicism (mitotic nondisjunction)**

  Q93.2 **Chromosome replaced with ring, dicentric or isochromosome**

  Q93.3 **Deletion of short arm of chromosome 4**
    Wolff-Hirschorn syndrome

  Q93.4 **Deletion of short arm of chromosome 5**
    Cri-du-chat syndrome

  Q93.5 **Other deletions of part of a chromosome**
    Angelman syndrome

  Q93.7 **Deletions with other complex rearrangements**
    Deletions due to unbalanced translocations, inversions and insertions
    Code also any associated duplications due to unbalanced translocations, inversions and insertions (Q92.5)

  ✓5ᵗʰ **Q93.8** **Other deletions from the autosomes**

    Q93.81 **Velo-cardio-facial syndrome**
      Deletion 22q11.2
      DEF: Microdeletion syndrome affecting multiple organs; characteristic cleft palate, heart defects, elongated face with almond-shaped eyes, wide nose, small ears, weak immune system, weak musculature, hypothyroidism, short stature, and scoliosis; deletion at q11.2 on the long arm of the chromosome 22.

    Q93.88 **Other microdeletions**
      Miller-Dieker syndrome
      Smith-Magenis syndrome

    Q93.89 **Other deletions from the autosomes**
      Deletions identified by fluorescence in situ hybridization (FISH)
      Deletions identified by in situ hybridization (ISH)
      Deletions seen only at prometaphase

  Q93.9 **Deletion from autosomes, unspecified**   ▽

✓4ᵗʰ **Q95** **Balanced rearrangements and structural markers, not elsewhere classified**
  INCLUDES Robertsonian and balanced reciprocal translocations and insertions

  Q95.0 **Balanced translocation and insertion in normal individual**

  Q95.1 **Chromosome inversion in normal individual**

  Q95.2 **Balanced autosomal rearrangement in abnormal individual**

  Q95.3 **Balanced sex/autosomal rearrangement in abnormal individual**

  Q95.5 **Individual with autosomal fragile site**

  Q95.8 **Other balanced rearrangements and structural markers**

  Q95.9 **Balanced rearrangement and structural marker, unspecified**   ▽

✓4ᵗʰ **Q96** **Turner's syndrome**
  EXCLUDES 1 *Noonan syndrome (Q87.1)*

  Q96.0 **Karyotype 45, X**   ♀

  Q96.1 **Karyotype 46, X iso (Xq)**   ♀
    Karyotype 46, isochromosome Xq

✓ Additional Character Req   ✓7ᵗʰ Placeholder Alert   Manifestation   HCC CMS-HCC Condition   ▽ Unspecified Code   ▶◀ Revised Text   ● New Code   ▲ Revised Code Title

Q96.2 **Karyotype 46, X with abnormal sex chromosome, except iso (Xq)** ♀

     Karyotype 46, X with abnormal sex chromosome, except isochromosome Xq

Q96.3 **Mosaicism, 45, X/46, XX or XY** ♀

Q96.4 **Mosaicism, 45, X/other cell line(s) with abnormal sex chromosome** ♀

Q96.8 **Other variants of Turner's syndrome** ♀

Q96.9 **Turner's syndrome, unspecified** ♀▽

✓4ᵗʰ **Q97   Other sex chromosome abnormalities, female phenotype, not elsewhere classified**

     EXCLUDES 1   Turner's syndrome (Q96.-)

Q97.0 **Karyotype 47, XXX** ♀

Q97.1 **Female with more than three X chromosomes** ♀

Q97.2 **Mosaicism, lines with various numbers of X chromosomes** ♀

Q97.3 **Female with 46, XY karyotype** ♀

Q97.8 **Other specified sex chromosome abnormalities, female phenotype** ♀

Q97.9 **Sex chromosome abnormality, female phenotype, unspecified** ♀▽

✓4ᵗʰ **Q98   Other sex chromosome abnormalities, male phenotype, not elsewhere classified**

Q98.0 **Klinefelter syndrome karyotype 47, XXY** ♂

Q98.1 **Klinefelter syndrome, male with more than two X chromosomes** ♂

Q98.3 **Other male with 46, XX karyotype** ♂

Q98.4 **Klinefelter syndrome, unspecified** ♂▽

Q98.5 **Karyotype 47, XYY**

Q98.6 **Male with structurally abnormal sex chromosome** ♂

Q98.7 **Male with sex chromosome mosaicism** ♂

Q98.8 **Other specified sex chromosome abnormalities, male phenotype** ♂

Q98.9 **Sex chromosome abnormality, male phenotype, unspecified** ♂▽

✓4ᵗʰ **Q99   Other chromosome abnormalities, not elsewhere classified**

Q99.0 **Chimera 46, XX/46, XY**

     Chimera 46, XX/46, XY true hermaphrodite

Q99.1 **46, XX true hermaphrodite**

     46, XX with streak gonads   Pure gonadal dysgenesis

     46, XY with streak gonads

Q99.2 **Fragile X chromosome**

     Fragile X syndrome

Q99.8 **Other specified chromosome abnormalities**

Q99.9 **Chromosomal abnormality, unspecified** ▽

EXCLUDES 1 Not coded here   **EXCLUDES 2** Not included here   N Newborn Age: 0   P Pediatric Age: 0-17   M Maternity Age: 12-55   A Adult Age: 15-124

886   ICD-10-CM 2018

Chapter 18. Symptoms, Signs, and Abnormal Clinical and Laboratory Findings, Not Elsewhere Classified (R00–R99)

Chapter Specific Guidelines with Coding Examples

The chapter specific guidelines from the ICD-10-CM Official Guidelines for Coding and Reporting have been provided below. Along with these guidelines are coding examples, contained in the shaded boxes, that have been developed to help illustrate the coding and/or sequencing guidance found in these guidelines.

Chapter 18 includes symptoms, signs, abnormal results of clinical or other investigative procedures, and ill-defined conditions regarding which no diagnosis classifiable elsewhere is recorded. Signs and symptoms that point to a specific diagnosis have been assigned to a category in other chapters of the classification.

a. Use of symptom codes

Codes that describe symptoms and signs are acceptable for reporting purposes when a related definitive diagnosis has not been established (confirmed) by the provider.

> Tenderness and localized pain in the right upper quadrant; based on presentation, probable gallstones
>
> **R10.11**   **Right upper quadrant pain**
>
> **R10.811**   **Right upper quadrant abdominal tenderness**
>
> *Explanation:* Codes that describe symptoms such as abdominal pain are acceptable for reporting purposes when the provider has not established (confirmed) a definitive diagnosis.

b. Use of a symptom code with a definitive diagnosis code

Codes for signs and symptoms may be reported in addition to a related definitive diagnosis when the sign or symptom is not routinely associated with that diagnosis, such as the various signs and symptoms associated with complex syndromes. The definitive diagnosis code should be sequenced before the symptom code.

Signs or symptoms that are associated routinely with a disease process should not be assigned as additional codes, unless otherwise instructed by the classification.

> Pneumonia with hemoptysis
>
> **J18.9**   **Pneumonia, unspecified organism**
>
> **R04.2**   **Hemoptysis**
>
> *Explanation:* Codes for signs and symptoms may be reported in addition to a related definitive diagnosis when the sign or symptom is not routinely associated with that diagnosis.

> Abdominal pain due to acute appendicitis
>
> **K35.80**   **Unspecified acute appendicitis**
>
> *Explanation:* Codes for signs or symptoms routinely associated with a disease process should not be assigned unless the classification instructs otherwise.

c. Combination codes that include symptoms

ICD-10-CM contains a number of combination codes that identify both the definitive diagnosis and common symptoms of that diagnosis. When using one of these combination codes, an additional code should not be assigned for the symptom.

> IBS with diarrhea
>
> **K58.0**   **Irritable bowel syndrome, with diarrhea**
>
> *Explanation:* When a combination code identifies both the definitive diagnosis and the symptom, an additional code should not be assigned for the symptom.

d. Repeated falls

Code R29.6, Repeated falls, is for use for encounters when a patient has recently fallen and the reason for the fall is being investigated.

Code Z91.81, History of falling, is for use when a patient has fallen in the past and is at risk for future falls. When appropriate, both codes R29.6 and Z91.81 may be assigned together.

e. Coma scale

The coma scale codes (R40.2-) can be used in conjunction with traumatic brain injury codes, acute cerebrovascular disease or sequelae of cerebrovascular disease codes. These codes are primarily for use by trauma registries, but they may be used in any setting where this information is collected. The coma scale may also be used to assess the status of the central nervous system for other non-trauma conditions, such as monitoring patients in the intensive care unit regardless of medical condition. The coma scale codes should be sequenced after the diagnosis code(s).

These codes, one from each subcategory, are needed to complete the scale. The 7th character indicates when the scale was recorded. The 7th character should match for all three codes.

At a minimum, report the initial score documented on presentation at your facility. This may be a score from the emergency medicine technician (EMT) or in the emergency department. If desired, a facility may choose to capture multiple coma scale scores.

Assign code R40.24, Glasgow coma scale, total score, when only the total score is documented in the medical record and not the individual score(s).

> 36-year-old man found down after unknown injury with skull fracture and with concussion and loss of consciousness of unknown duration. Upon hospital admission, the patient was evaluated with the following Glasgow coma scores:
>
> Eye-opening response—3: eyes open to speech
>
> Verbal response—3: random speech with no conversational exchange
>
> Motor response—4: pulls limb away from painful stimulus
>
> **S02.0XXA**   **Fracture of vault of skull, initial encounter for closed fracture**
>
> **S06.0X9A**   **Concussion with loss of consciousness of unspecified duration, initial encounter**
>
> **R40.2133**   **Coma scale, eyes open, to sound, at hospital admission**
>
> **R40.2233**   **Coma scale, best verbal response, inappropriate words, at hospital admission**
>
> **R40.2343**   **Coma scale, best motor response, flexion withdrawal, at hospital admission**
>
> *Explanation:* When individual scores for the Glasgow coma scale are documented, one code from each category is needed to complete the scale. The seventh character indicates when the scale was recorded and should match for all three codes. Assign a code from subcategory R40.24- Glasgow coma scale, total score, when only the total and not the individual score(s) is documented.

f. Functional quadriplegia

GUIDELINE HAS BEEN DELETED EFFECTIVE OCTOBER 1, 2017

g. SIRS due to non-infectious process

The systemic inflammatory response syndrome (SIRS) can develop as a result of certain non-infectious disease processes, such as trauma, malignant neoplasm, or pancreatitis. When SIRS is documented with a noninfectious condition, and no subsequent infection is documented, the code for the underlying condition, such as an injury, should be assigned, followed by code R65.10, Systemic inflammatory response syndrome (SIRS) of non-infectious origin without acute organ dysfunction, or code R65.11, Systemic inflammatory response syndrome (SIRS) of non-infectious origin with acute organ dysfunction. If an associated acute organ dysfunction is documented, the appropriate code(s) for the specific type of organ dysfunction(s) should be assigned in addition to code R65.11. If acute organ dysfunction is documented, but it cannot be determined if the acute organ dysfunction is associated with SIRS or due to another condition (e.g., directly due to the trauma), the provider should be queried.

Systemic inflammatory response syndrome (SIRS) due to acute gallstone pancreatitis

K85.1Ø   **Biliary acute pancreatitis without necrosis or infection**

R65.1Ø   **Systemic inflammatory response syndrome (SIRS) of noninfectious origin without acute organ dysfunction**

Explanation: When SIRS is documented with a noninfectious condition without subsequent infection documented, the code for the underlying condition such as pancreatitis should be assigned followed by the appropriate code for SIRS of noninfectious origin, either with or without associated organ dysfunction.

h. Death NOS

Code R99, Ill-defined and unknown cause of mortality, is only for use in the very limited circumstance when a patient who has already died is brought into an emergency department or other healthcare facility and is pronounced dead upon arrival. It does not represent the discharge disposition of death.

i. NIHSS stroke scale

The NIH stroke scale (NIHSS) codes (R29.7- -) can be used in conjunction with acute stroke codes (I63) to identify the patient's neurological status and the severity of the stroke. The stroke scale codes should be sequenced after the acute stroke diagnosis code(s).

At a minimum, report the initial score documented. If desired, a facility may choose to capture multiple stroke scale scores.

See Section I.B.14. for information concerning the medical record documentation that may be used for assignment of the NIHSS codes.

Chapter 18. Symptoms, Signs and Abnormal Clinical and Laboratory Findings, Not Elsewhere Classified (R00-R99)

NOTE This chapter includes symptoms, signs, abnormal results of clinical or other investigative procedures, and ill-defined conditions regarding which no diagnosis classifiable elsewhere is recorded.

Signs and symptoms that point rather definitely to a given diagnosis have been assigned to a category in other chapters of the classification. In general, categories in this chapter include the less well-defined conditions and symptoms that, without the necessary study of the case to establish a final diagnosis, point perhaps equally to two or more diseases or to two or more systems of the body. Practically all categories in the chapter could be designated "not otherwise specified", "unknown etiology" or "transient". The Alphabetical Index should be consulted to determine which symptoms and signs are to be allocated here and which to other chapters. The residual subcategories, numbered .8, are generally provided for other relevant symptoms that cannot be allocated elsewhere in the classification.

The conditions and signs or symptoms included in categories R00-R94 consist of:

(a)   cases for which no more specific diagnosis can be made even after all the facts bearing on the case have been investigated;

(b)   signs or symptoms existing at the time of initial encounter that proved to be transient and whose causes could not be determined;

(c)   provisional diagnosis in a patient who failed to return for further investigation or care;

(d)   cases referred elsewhere for investigation or treatment before the diagnosis was made;

(e)   cases in which a more precise diagnosis was not available for any other reason;

(f)   certain symptoms, for which supplementary information is provided, that represent important problems in medical care in their own right.

EXCLUDES 2 abnormal findings on antenatal screening of mother (O28.-)
certain conditions originating in the perinatal period (P04-P96)
signs and symptoms classified in the body system chapters
signs and symptoms of breast (N63, N64.5)

AHA: 2017, 1Q, 6, 7

This chapter contains the following blocks:

R00-R09	Symptoms and signs involving the circulatory and respiratory systems
R10-R19	Symptoms and signs involving the digestive system and abdomen
R20-R23	Symptoms and signs involving the skin and subcutaneous tissue
R25-R29	Symptoms and signs involving the nervous and musculoskeletal systems
R30-R39	Symptoms and signs involving the genitourinary system
R40-R46	Symptoms and signs involving cognition, perception, emotional state and behavior
R47-R49	Symptoms and signs involving speech and voice
R50-R69	General symptoms and signs
R70-R79	Abnormal findings on examination of blood, without diagnosis
R80-R82	Abnormal findings on examination of urine, without diagnosis
R83-R89	Abnormal findings on examination of other body fluids, substances and tissues, without diagnosis
R90-R94	Abnormal findings on diagnostic imaging and in function studies, without diagnosis
R97	Abnormal tumor markers
R99	Ill-defined and unknown cause of mortality

Symptoms and signs involving the circulatory and respiratory systems (R00-R09)

✓4ᵗʰ R00 Abnormalities of heart beat
EXCLUDES 1 abnormalities originating in the perinatal period (P29.1-)
EXCLUDES 2 specified arrhythmias (I47-I49)

R00.0 Tachycardia, unspecified   ▽
Rapid heart beat
Sinoauricular tachycardia NOS
Sinus [sinusal] tachycardia NOS
EXCLUDES 1 neonatal tachycardia (P29.11)
paroxysmal tachycardia (I47.-)
DEF: Excessively rapid heart rate of more than 100 beats per minute.

R00.1 Bradycardia, unspecified   ▽
Sinoatrial bradycardia
Sinus bradycardia
Slow heart beat
Vagal bradycardia
Use additional code for adverse effect, if applicable, to identify drug (T36-T50 with fifth or sixth character 5)
EXCLUDES 1 neonatal bradycardia (P29.12)

R00.2 Palpitations
Awareness of heart beat

R00.8 Other abnormalities of heart beat

R00.9 Unspecified abnormalities of heart beat   ▽

✓4ᵗʰ R01 Cardiac murmurs and other cardiac sounds
EXCLUDES 1 cardiac murmurs and sounds originating in the perinatal period (P29.8)

R01.0 Benign and innocent cardiac murmurs
Functional cardiac murmur

R01.1 Cardiac murmur, unspecified   ▽
Cardiac bruit NOS
Heart murmur NOS
Systolic murmur NOS

R01.2 Other cardiac sounds
Cardiac dullness, increased or decreased
Precordial friction

✓4ᵗʰ R03 Abnormal blood-pressure reading, without diagnosis

R03.0 Elevated blood-pressure reading, without diagnosis of hypertension
NOTE This category is to be used to record an episode of elevated blood pressure in a patient in whom no formal diagnosis of hypertension has been made, or as an isolated incidental finding.

R03.1 Nonspecific low blood-pressure reading
EXCLUDES 1 hypotension (I95.-)
maternal hypotension syndrome (O26.5-)
neurogenic orthostatic hypotension (G90.3)

✓4ᵗʰ R04 Hemorrhage from respiratory passages

R04.0 Epistaxis
Hemorrhage from nose
Nosebleed

R04.1 Hemorrhage from throat
EXCLUDES 2 hemoptysis (R04.2)

R04.2 Hemoptysis
Blood-stained sputum
Cough with hemorrhage
AHA: 2013, 4Q, 118

✓5ᵗʰ R04.8 Hemorrhage from other sites in respiratory passages

R04.81 Acute idiopathic pulmonary hemorrhage in infants   🅟
AIPHI
Acute idiopathic hemorrhage in infants over 28 days old
EXCLUDES 1 perinatal pulmonary hemorrhage (P26.-)
von Willebrand's disease (D68.0)

R04.89 Hemorrhage from other sites in respiratory passages
Pulmonary hemorrhage NOS

R04.9 Hemorrhage from respiratory passages, unspecified   ▽

R05 Cough
EXCLUDES 1 cough with hemorrhage (R04.2)
smoker's cough (J41.0)
AHA: 2016, 2Q, 33

✓4ᵗʰ R06 Abnormalities of breathing
EXCLUDES 1 acute respiratory distress syndrome (J80)
respiratory arrest (R09.2)
respiratory arrest of newborn (P28.81)
respiratory distress syndrome of newborn (P22.-)
respiratory failure (J96.-)
respiratory failure of newborn (P28.5)

✓5ᵗʰ R06.0 Dyspnea
EXCLUDES 1 tachypnea NOS (R06.82)
transient tachypnea of newborn (P22.1)

R06.00 Dyspnea, unspecified   ▽
AHA: 2017, 1Q, 26

R06.01 Orthopnea

R06.02 Shortness of breath

● **R06.03 Acute respiratory distress**

R06.09 Other forms of dyspnea

✓ Additional Character Req   ✓⁷ᵗʰ Placeholder Alert   **Manifestation**   HCC CMS-HCC Condition   ▽ Unspecified Code   ►◄ Revised Text   ● New Code   ▲ Revised Code Title

ICD-10-CM 2018   **889**

Chapter 18. Symptoms, Signs, and Abnormal Clinical and Laboratory Findings, Not Elsewhere Classified

R06.1–R10.0

R06.1 Stridor
> EXCLUDES 1   *congenital laryngeal stridor (P28.89)*
> *laryngismus (stridulus) (J38.5)*

R06.2 Wheezing
> EXCLUDES 1   *asthma (J45.-)*
> AHA: 2016, 2Q, 33
> DEF: High-pitched whistling sound during breathing due to stenosis of respiratory passageway; associated with asthma, sleep apnea, bronchiectasis, bronchiolitis, COPD, and pleural effusion.

R06.3 Periodic breathing
> Cheyne-Stokes breathing

R06.4 Hyperventilation
> EXCLUDES 1   *psychogenic hyperventilation (F45.8)*

R06.5 Mouth breathing
> EXCLUDES 2   *dry mouth NOS (R68.2)*

R06.6 Hiccough
> EXCLUDES 1   *psychogenic hiccough (F45.8)*

R06.7 Sneezing

✓5ᵗʰ **R06.8 Other abnormalities of breathing**

> **R06.81 Apnea, not elsewhere classified**
> Apnea NOS
> EXCLUDES 1   *apnea (of) newborn (P28.4)*
> *sleep apnea (G47.3-)*
> *sleep apnea of newborn (primary) (P28.3)*

> **R06.82 Tachypnea, not elsewhere classified**
> Tachypnea NOS
> EXCLUDES 1   *transitory tachypnea of newborn (P22.1)*

> **R06.83 Snoring**

> **R06.89 Other abnormalities of breathing**
> Breath-holding (spells)
> Sighing

R06.9 Unspecified abnormalities of breathing ▽

✓4ᵗʰ **R07 Pain in throat and chest**
> EXCLUDES 1   *epidemic myalgia (B33.0)*
> EXCLUDES 2   *jaw pain (R68.84)*
> *pain in breast (N64.4)*

R07.0 Pain in throat
> EXCLUDES 1   *chronic sore throat (J31.2)*
> *sore throat (acute) NOS (J02.9)*
> EXCLUDES 2   *dysphagia (R13.1-)*
> *pain in neck (M54.2)*

R07.1 Chest pain on breathing
> Painful respiration

R07.2 Precordial pain

✓5ᵗʰ **R07.8 Other chest pain**

> **R07.81 Pleurodynia**
> Pleurodynia NOS
> EXCLUDES 1   *epidemic pleurodynia (B33.0)*

> **R07.82 Intercostal pain**

> **R07.89 Other chest pain**
> Anterior chest-wall pain NOS

R07.9 Chest pain, unspecified ▽

✓4ᵗʰ **R09 Other symptoms and signs involving the circulatory and respiratory system**
> EXCLUDES 1   *acute respiratory distress syndrome (J80)*
> *respiratory arrest of newborn (P28.81)*
> *respiratory distress syndrome of newborn (P22.0)*
> *respiratory failure (J96.-)*
> *respiratory failure of newborn (P28.5)*

✓5ᵗʰ **R09.0 Asphyxia and hypoxemia**
> EXCLUDES 1   *asphyxia due to carbon monoxide (T58.-)*
> *asphyxia due to foreign body in respiratory tract (T17.-)*
> *birth (intrauterine) asphyxia (P84)*
> ~~*hypercapnia (R06.4)*~~
> *hyperventilation (R06.4)*
> *traumatic asphyxia (T71.-)*
> EXCLUDES 2   ▶*hypercapnia (R06.89)*◀

> **R09.01 Asphyxia**

> **R09.02 Hypoxemia**

R09.1 Pleurisy
> EXCLUDES 1   *pleurisy with effusion (J90)*

R09.2 Respiratory arrest   HCC
> Cardiorespiratory failure
> EXCLUDES 1   *cardiac arrest (I46.-)*
> *respiratory arrest of newborn (P28.81)*
> *respiratory distress of newborn (P22.0)*
> *respiratory failure (J96.-)*
> *respiratory failure of newborn (P28.5)*
> *respiratory insufficiency (R06.89)*
> *respiratory insufficiency of newborn (P28.5)*

R09.3 Abnormal sputum
> Abnormal amount of sputum
> Abnormal color of sputum
> Abnormal odor of sputum
> Excessive sputum
> EXCLUDES 1   *blood-stained sputum (R04.2)*

✓5ᵗʰ **R09.8 Other specified symptoms and signs involving the circulatory and respiratory systems**

> **R09.81 Nasal congestion**

> **R09.82 Postnasal drip**

> **R09.89 Other specified symptoms and signs involving the circulatory and respiratory systems**
> Abnormal chest percussion
> Bruit (arterial)
> Chest tympany
> Choking sensation
> Feeling of foreign body in throat
> Friction sounds in chest
> Rales
> Weak pulse
> EXCLUDES 2   *foreign body in throat (T17.2-)*
> *wheezing (R06.2)*

Symptoms and signs involving the digestive system and abdomen (R10-R19)

> EXCLUDES 2   *congenital or infantile pylorospasm (Q40.0)*
> *gastrointestinal hemorrhage (K92.0-K92.2)*
> *intestinal obstruction (K56.-)*
> *newborn gastrointestinal hemorrhage (P54.0-P54.3)*
> *newborn intestinal obstruction (P76.-)*
> *pylorospasm (K31.3)*
> *signs and symptoms involving the urinary system (R30-R39)*
> *symptoms referable to female genital organs (N94.-)*
> *symptoms referable to male genital organs (N48-N50)*

✓4ᵗʰ **R10 Abdominal and pelvic pain**
> EXCLUDES 1   *renal colic (N23)*
> EXCLUDES 2   *dorsalgia (M54.-)*
> *flatulence and related conditions (R14.-)*

R10.0 Acute abdomen
> Severe abdominal pain (generalized) (with abdominal rigidity)
> EXCLUDES 1   *abdominal rigidity NOS (R19.3)*
> *generalized abdominal pain NOS (R10.84)*
> *localized abdominal pain (R10.1-R10.3-)*

Abdominal Pain

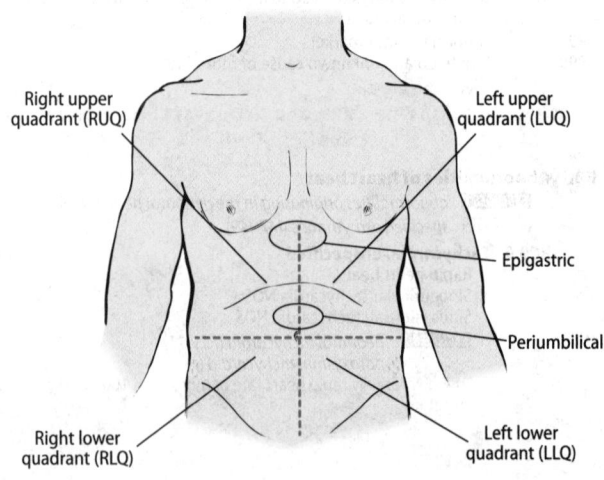

Right upper quadrant (RUQ)

Left upper quadrant (LUQ)

Epigastric

Periumbilical

Right lower quadrant (RLQ)

Left lower quadrant (LLQ)

EXCLUDES 1 Not coded here   EXCLUDES 2 Not included here   N Newborn Age: 0   P Pediatric Age: 0-17   M Maternity Age: 12-55   A Adult Age: 15-124

890   ICD-10-CM 2018

√5ᵗʰ **R10.1   Pain localized to upper abdomen**   ▽
    R10.10   Upper abdominal pain, unspecified
    R10.11   Right upper quadrant pain
    R10.12   Left upper quadrant pain
    R10.13   Epigastric pain
        Dyspepsia
        EXCLUDES 1   *functional dyspepsia (K30)*

R10.2   Pelvic and perineal pain
    EXCLUDES 1   *vulvodynia (N94.81)*

√5ᵗʰ **R10.3   Pain localized to other parts of lower abdomen**   ▽
    R10.30   Lower abdominal pain, unspecified
    R10.31   Right lower quadrant pain
    R10.32   Left lower quadrant pain
    R10.33   Periumbilical pain

√5ᵗʰ **R10.8   Other abdominal pain**
  √6ᵗʰ **R10.81   Abdominal tenderness**
        Abdominal tenderness NOS
      R10.811   Right upper quadrant abdominal tenderness
      R10.812   Left upper quadrant abdominal tenderness
      R10.813   Right lower quadrant abdominal tenderness
      R10.814   Left lower quadrant abdominal tenderness
      R10.815   Periumbilic abdominal tenderness
      R10.816   Epigastric abdominal tenderness
      R10.817   Generalized abdominal tenderness
      R10.819   Abdominal tenderness, unspecified site ▽
  √6ᵗʰ **R10.82   Rebound abdominal tenderness**
      R10.821   Right upper quadrant rebound abdominal tenderness
      R10.822   Left upper quadrant rebound abdominal tenderness
      R10.823   Right lower quadrant rebound abdominal tenderness
      R10.824   Left lower quadrant rebound abdominal tenderness
      R10.825   Periumbilic rebound abdominal tenderness
      R10.826   Epigastric rebound abdominal tenderness
      R10.827   Generalized rebound abdominal tenderness
      R10.829   Rebound abdominal tenderness, unspecified site ▽
  R10.83   Colic   P
      Colic NOS
      Infantile colic
      EXCLUDES 1   *colic in adult and child over 12 months old (R10.84)*
      DEF: Inconsolable crying in an otherwise well-fed and healthy infant for more than three hours a day, three days a week, for more than three weeks.
  R10.84   Generalized abdominal pain
      EXCLUDES 1   *generalized abdominal pain associated with acute abdomen (R10.0)*

R10.9   Unspecified abdominal pain   ▽

√4ᵗʰ **R11   Nausea and vomiting**
  EXCLUDES 1   *cyclical vomiting associated with migraine (G43.A-)*
        excessive vomiting in pregnancy (O21.-)
        hematemesis (K92.0)
        neonatal hematemesis (P54.0)
        newborn vomiting (P92.0-)
        psychogenic vomiting (F50.89)
        vomiting associated with bulimia nervosa (F50.2)
        vomiting following gastrointestinal surgery (K91.0)
  AHA: 2017, 1Q, 28
  R11.0   Nausea
      Nausea NOS
      Nausea without vomiting
  √5ᵗʰ **R11.1   Vomiting**
    R11.10   Vomiting, unspecified   ▽
        Vomiting NOS
    R11.11   Vomiting without nausea
    R11.12   Projectile vomiting
    R11.13   Vomiting of fecal matter

Swallowing Function

Oral phase

Oropharyngeal phase

Pharyngeal phase

Pharyngoesophageal phase

    R11.14   Bilious vomiting
        Bilious emesis
  R11.2   Nausea with vomiting, unspecified   ▽
      Persistent nausea with vomiting NOS

R12   Heartburn
  EXCLUDES 1   *dyspepsia NOS (R10.13)*
        functional dyspepsia (K30)

√4ᵗʰ **R13   Aphagia and dysphagia**
  R13.0   Aphagia
      Inability to swallow
      EXCLUDES 1   *psychogenic aphagia (F50.9)*
  √5ᵗʰ **R13.1   Dysphagia**
      Code first, if applicable, dysphagia following cerebrovascular disease (I69. with final characters -91)
      EXCLUDES 1   *psychogenic dysphagia (F45.8)*
    R13.10   Dysphagia, unspecified   ▽
        Difficulty in swallowing NOS
    R13.11   Dysphagia, oral phase
    R13.12   Dysphagia, oropharyngeal phase
    R13.13   Dysphagia, pharyngeal phase
    R13.14   Dysphagia, pharyngoesophageal phase
    R13.19   Other dysphagia
        Cervical dysphagia
        Neurogenic dysphagia

√4ᵗʰ **R14   Flatulence and related conditions**
  EXCLUDES 1   *psychogenic aerophagy (F45.8)*
  R14.0   Abdominal distension (gaseous)
      Bloating
      Tympanites (abdominal) (intestinal)
  R14.1   Gas pain
  R14.2   Eructation
  R14.3   Flatulence

√4ᵗʰ **R15   Fecal incontinence**
  INCLUDES   encopresis NOS
  EXCLUDES 1   *fecal incontinence of nonorganic origin (F98.1)*
  R15.0   Incomplete defecation
      EXCLUDES 1   *constipation (K59.0-)*
                 fecal impaction (K56.41)
  R15.1   Fecal smearing
      Fecal soiling
  R15.2   Fecal urgency
  R15.9   Full incontinence of feces
      Fecal incontinence NOS

√4ᵗʰ **R16   Hepatomegaly and splenomegaly, not elsewhere classified**
  R16.0   Hepatomegaly, not elsewhere classified
      Hepatomegaly NOS
  R16.1   Splenomegaly, not elsewhere classified
      Splenomegaly NOS
  R16.2   Hepatomegaly with splenomegaly, not elsewhere classified
      Hepatosplenomegaly NOS

R17   Unspecified jaundice   ▽
  EXCLUDES 1   *neonatal jaundice (P55, P57-P59)*

☑ Additional Character Req   √x7ᵗʰ Placeholder Alert   Manifestation   HCC CMS-HCC Condition   ▽ Unspecified Code   ▶◀ Revised Text   ● New Code   ▲ Revised Code Title

ICD-10-CM 2018   891

☑4ᵗʰ R18 Ascites
> **INCLUDES** fluid in peritoneal cavity
> **EXCLUDES 1** *ascites in alcoholic cirrhosis (K70.31)*
> *ascites in alcoholic hepatitis (K70.11)*
> *ascites in toxic liver disease with chronic active hepatitis (K71.51)*

R18.0 Malignant ascites
> Code first malignancy, such as:
> malignant neoplasm of ovary (C56.-)
> secondary malignant neoplasm of retroperitoneum and peritoneum (C78.6)

R18.8 Other ascites
> Ascites NOS
> Peritoneal effusion (chronic)

☑4ᵗʰ R19 Other symptoms and signs involving the digestive system and abdomen
> **EXCLUDES 1** *acute abdomen (R10.0)*

☑5ᵗʰ R19.0 Intra-abdominal and pelvic swelling, mass and lump
> **EXCLUDES 1** *abdominal distension (gaseous) (R14.-)*
> *ascites (R18.-)*

R19.00 Intra-abdominal and pelvic swelling, mass and lump, unspecified site ▽

R19.01 Right upper quadrant abdominal swelling, mass and lump

R19.02 Left upper quadrant abdominal swelling, mass and lump

R19.03 Right lower quadrant abdominal swelling, mass and lump

R19.04 Left lower quadrant abdominal swelling, mass and lump

R19.05 Periumbilic swelling, mass or lump
> Diffuse or generalized umbilical swelling or mass

R19.06 Epigastric swelling, mass or lump

R19.07 Generalized intra-abdominal and pelvic swelling, mass and lump
> Diffuse or generalized intra-abdominal swelling or mass NOS
> Diffuse or generalized pelvic swelling or mass NOS

R19.09 Other intra-abdominal and pelvic swelling, mass and lump

☑5ᵗʰ R19.1 Abnormal bowel sounds

R19.11 Absent bowel sounds

R19.12 Hyperactive bowel sounds

R19.15 Other abnormal bowel sounds
> Abnormal bowel sounds NOS

R19.2 Visible peristalsis
> Hyperperistalsis
> **DEF:** Visible movements of muscular attempts to move food through the digestive tract; due to pyloric obstruction, stomach obstruction, or intestinal obstruction.

☑5ᵗʰ R19.3 Abdominal rigidity
> **EXCLUDES 1** *abdominal rigidity with severe abdominal pain (R10.0)*

R19.30 Abdominal rigidity, unspecified site ▽

R19.31 Right upper quadrant abdominal rigidity

R19.32 Left upper quadrant abdominal rigidity

R19.33 Right lower quadrant abdominal rigidity

R19.34 Left lower quadrant abdominal rigidity

R19.35 Periumbilic abdominal rigidity

R19.36 Epigastric abdominal rigidity

R19.37 Generalized abdominal rigidity

R19.4 Change in bowel habit
> **EXCLUDES 1** *constipation (K59.0-)*
> *functional diarrhea (K59.1)*

R19.5 Other fecal abnormalities
> Abnormal stool color
> Bulky stools
> Mucus in stools
> Occult blood in feces
> Occult blood in stools
> **EXCLUDES 1** *melena (K92.1)*
> *neonatal melena (P54.1)*

R19.6 Halitosis

R19.7 Diarrhea, unspecified ▽
> Diarrhea NOS
> **EXCLUDES 1** *functional diarrhea (K59.1)*
> *neonatal diarrhea (P78.3)*
> *psychogenic diarrhea (F45.8)*

R19.8 Other specified symptoms and signs involving the digestive system and abdomen

Symptoms and signs involving the skin and subcutaneous tissue (R20-R23)
> **EXCLUDES 2** *symptoms relating to breast (N64.4-N64.5)*

☑4ᵗʰ R20 Disturbances of skin sensation
> **EXCLUDES 1** *dissociative anesthesia and sensory loss (F44.6)*
> *psychogenic disturbances (F45.8)*

R20.0 Anesthesia of skin

R20.1 Hypoesthesia of skin

R20.2 Paresthesia of skin
> Formication
> Pins and needles
> Tingling skin
> **EXCLUDES 1** *acroparesthesia (I73.8)*

R20.3 Hyperesthesia

R20.8 Other disturbances of skin sensation

R20.9 Unspecified disturbances of skin sensation ▽

R21 Rash and other nonspecific skin eruption
> **INCLUDES** rash NOS
> **EXCLUDES 1** *specified type of rash—code to condition*
> *vesicular eruption (R23.8)*

☑4ᵗʰ R22 Localized swelling, mass and lump of skin and subcutaneous tissue
> **INCLUDES** subcutaneous nodules (localized)(superficial)
> **EXCLUDES 1** *abnormal findings on diagnostic imaging (R90-R93)*
> *edema (R60.-)*
> *enlarged lymph nodes (R59.-)*
> *localized adiposity (E65)*
> *swelling of joint (M25.4-)*

R22.0 Localized swelling, mass and lump, head

R22.1 Localized swelling, mass and lump, neck

R22.2 Localized swelling, mass and lump, trunk
> **EXCLUDES 1** *intra-abdominal or pelvic mass and lump (R19.0-)*
> *intra-abdominal or pelvic swelling (R19.0-)*
> **EXCLUDES 2** *breast mass and lump (N63)*

☑5ᵗʰ R22.3 Localized swelling, mass and lump, upper limb

R22.30 Localized swelling, mass and lump, unspecified upper limb ▽

R22.31 Localized swelling, mass and lump, right upper limb

R22.32 Localized swelling, mass and lump, left upper limb

R22.33 Localized swelling, mass and lump, upper limb, bilateral

☑5ᵗʰ R22.4 Localized swelling, mass and lump, lower limb

R22.40 Localized swelling, mass and lump, unspecified lower limb ▽

R22.41 Localized swelling, mass and lump, right lower limb

R22.42 Localized swelling, mass and lump, left lower limb

R22.43 Localized swelling, mass and lump, lower limb, bilateral

R22.9 Localized swelling, mass and lump, unspecified ▽

☑4ᵗʰ R23 Other skin changes

R23.0 Cyanosis
> **EXCLUDES 1** *acrocyanosis (I73.8)*
> *cyanotic attacks of newborn (P28.2)*
> **DEF:** Bluish or purplish discoloration of the skin due to inadequate oxygen level of blood.

R23.1 Pallor
> Clammy skin

R23.2 Flushing
> Excessive blushing
> Code first, if applicable, menopausal and female climacteric states (N95.1)

R23.3 Spontaneous ecchymoses
> Petechiae
> **EXCLUDES 1** *ecchymoses of newborn (P54.5)*
> *purpura (D69.-)*

R23.4 Changes in skin texture
> Desquamation of skin
> Induration of skin
> Scaling of skin
> **EXCLUDES 1** *epidermal thickening NOS (L85.9)*

R23.8 Other skin changes

R23.9 Unspecified skin changes ▽

EXCLUDES 1 Not coded here   **EXCLUDES 2** Not included here   N Newborn Age: 0   P Pediatric Age: 0-17   M Maternity Age: 12-55   A Adult Age: 15-124

892   ICD-10-CM 2018

Symptoms and signs involving the nervous and musculoskeletal systems (R25-R29)

✓4th **R25 Abnormal involuntary movements**
    EXCLUDES 1 *specific movement disorders (G20-G26)*
          stereotyped movement disorders (F98.4)
          tic disorders (F95.-)

  R25.0 Abnormal head movements

  R25.1 Tremor, unspecified ▽
      EXCLUDES 1 *chorea NOS (G25.5)*
           essential tremor (G25.0)
           hysterical tremor (F44.4)
           intention tremor (G25.2)

  R25.2 Cramp and spasm
      EXCLUDES 2 *carpopedal spasm (R29.0)*
           charley-horse (M62.831)
           infantile spasms (G40.4-)
           muscle spasm of back (M62.830)
           muscle spasm of calf (M62.831)

  R25.3 Fasciculation
      Twitching NOS

  R25.8 Other abnormal involuntary movements

  R25.9 Unspecified abnormal involuntary movements ▽

✓4th **R26 Abnormalities of gait and mobility**
    EXCLUDES 1 *ataxia NOS (R27.0)*
          hereditary ataxia (G11.-)
          locomotor (syphilitic) ataxia (A52.11)
          immobility syndrome (paraplegic) (M62.3)

  R26.0 Ataxic gait
      Staggering gait

  R26.1 Paralytic gait
      Spastic gait

  R26.2 Difficulty in walking, not elsewhere classified
      EXCLUDES 1 *falling (R29.6)*
           unsteadiness on feet (R26.81)
      AHA: 2016, 2Q, 7

✓5th **R26.8 Other abnormalities of gait and mobility**
      R26.81 Unsteadiness on feet
      R26.89 Other abnormalities of gait and mobility

  R26.9 Unspecified abnormalities of gait and mobility ▽

✓4th **R27 Other lack of coordination**
    EXCLUDES 1 *ataxic gait (R26.0)*
          hereditary ataxia (G11.-)
          vertigo NOS (R42)

  R27.0 Ataxia, unspecified ▽
      EXCLUDES 1 *ataxia following cerebrovascular disease (I69. with final characters -93)*

  R27.8 Other lack of coordination

  R27.9 Unspecified lack of coordination ▽

✓4th **R29 Other symptoms and signs involving the nervous and musculoskeletal systems**

  R29.0 Tetany
      Carpopedal spasm
      EXCLUDES 1 *hysterical tetany (F44.5)*
           neonatal tetany (P71.3)
           parathyroid tetany (E20.9)
           post-thyroidectomy tetany (E89.2)

  R29.1 Meningismus

  R29.2 Abnormal reflex
      EXCLUDES 2 *abnormal pupillary reflex (H57.0)*
           hyperactive gag reflex (J39.2)
           vasovagal reaction or syncope (R55)

  R29.3 Abnormal posture

  R29.4 Clicking hip
      EXCLUDES 1 *congenital deformities of hip (Q65.-)*

  R29.5 Transient paralysis
      Code first any associated spinal cord injury (S14.0, S14.1-, S24.0, S24.1-, S34.0-, S34.1-)
      EXCLUDES 1 *transient ischemic attack (G45.9)*

  R29.6 Repeated falls
      Falling
      Tendency to fall
      EXCLUDES 2 *at risk for falling (Z91.81)*
           history of falling (Z91.81)
      AHA: 2016, 2Q, 6

✓5th **R29.7 National Institutes of Health Stroke Scale (NIHSS) Score**
      Code first the type of cerebral infarction (I63.-)

  ✓6th **R29.70 NIHSS score 0-9**
      R29.700 NIHSS score 0
      R29.701 NIHSS score 1
      R29.702 NIHSS score 2
      R29.703 NIHSS score 3
      R29.704 NIHSS score 4
      R29.705 NIHSS score 5
      R29.706 NIHSS score 6
      R29.707 NIHSS score 7
      R29.708 NIHSS score 8
      R29.709 NIHSS score 9

  ✓6th **R29.71 NIHSS score 10-19**
      R29.710 NIHSS score 10
      R29.711 NIHSS score 11
      R29.712 NIHSS score 12
      R29.713 NIHSS score 13
      R29.714 NIHSS score 14
      R29.715 NIHSS score 15
      R29.716 NIHSS score 16
      R29.717 NIHSS score 17
      R29.718 NIHSS score 18
      R29.719 NIHSS score 19

  ✓6th **R29.72 NIHSS score 20-29**
      R29.720 NIHSS score 20
      R29.721 NIHSS score 21
      R29.722 NIHSS score 22
      R29.723 NIHSS score 23
      R29.724 NIHSS score 24
      R29.725 NIHSS score 25
      R29.726 NIHSS score 26
      R29.727 NIHSS score 27
      R29.728 NIHSS score 28
      R29.729 NIHSS score 29

  ✓6th **R29.73 NIHSS score 30-39**
      R29.730 NIHSS score 30
      R29.731 NIHSS score 31
      R29.732 NIHSS score 32
      R29.733 NIHSS score 33
      R29.734 NIHSS score 34
      R29.735 NIHSS score 35
      R29.736 NIHSS score 36
      R29.737 NIHSS score 37
      R29.738 NIHSS score 38
      R29.739 NIHSS score 39

  ✓6th **R29.74 NIHSS score 40-42**
      R29.740 NIHSS score 40
      R29.741 NIHSS score 41
      R29.742 NIHSS score 42

✓5th **R29.8 Other symptoms and signs involving the nervous and musculoskeletal systems**

  ✓6th **R29.81 Other symptoms and signs involving the nervous system**
      R29.810 Facial weakness
           Facial droop
           EXCLUDES 1 *Bell's palsy (G51.0)*
                  facial weakness following cerebrovascular disease (I69. with final characters -92)
      R29.818 Other symptoms and signs involving the nervous system

  ✓6th **R29.89 Other symptoms and signs involving the musculoskeletal system**
      EXCLUDES 2 *pain in limb (M79.6-)*
      R29.890 Loss of height
           EXCLUDES 1 *osteoporosis (M80-M81)*

✓ Additional Character Req   ✓x7th Placeholder Alert   Manifestation   HCC CMS-HCC Condition   ▽ Unspecified Code   ▶◀ Revised Text   ● New Code   ▲ Revised Code Title

Chapter 18. Symptoms, Signs, and Abnormal Clinical and Laboratory Findings, Not Elsewhere Classified

R29.891   Ocular torticollis
> EXCLUDES 1   congenital (sternomastoid) torticollis Q68.0
> psychogenic torticollis (F45.8)
> spasmodic torticollis (G24.3)
> torticollis due to birth injury (P15.8)
> torticollis NOS M43.6
>
> **DEF:** Abnormal head posture as a result of a contracted state of cervical muscles to correct a visual disturbance, either double vision or a visual field defect.

R29.898   Other symptoms and signs involving the musculoskeletal system

✓5ᵗʰ **R29.9   Unspecified symptoms and signs involving the nervous and musculoskeletal systems**

R29.90   Unspecified symptoms and signs involving the nervous system ▽

R29.91   Unspecified symptoms and signs involving the musculoskeletal system ▽

Symptoms and signs involving the genitourinary system (R30-R39)

✓4ᵗʰ **R30   Pain associated with micturition**
> EXCLUDES 1   psychogenic pain associated with micturition (F45.8)

R30.0   Dysuria
> Strangury

R30.1   Vesical tenesmus

R30.9   Painful micturition, unspecified ▽
> Painful urination NOS

✓4ᵗʰ **R31   Hematuria**
> EXCLUDES 1   hematuria included with underlying conditions, such as:
> acute cystitis with hematuria (N30.01)
> recurrent and persistent hematuria in glomerular diseases (N02.-)
>
> **AHA:** 2017, 1Q, 17

R31.0   Gross hematuria

R31.1   Benign essential microscopic hematuria

✓5ᵗʰ **R31.2   Other microscopic hematuria**

R31.21   Asymptomatic microscopic hematuria
> AMH

R31.29   Other microscopic hematuria

R31.9   Hematuria, unspecified ▽

R32   Unspecified urinary incontinence ▽
> Enuresis NOS
> EXCLUDES 1   functional urinary incontinence (R39.81)
> nonorganic enuresis (F98.0)
> stress incontinence and other specified urinary incontinence (N39.3-N39.4-)
> urinary incontinence associated with cognitive impairment (R39.81)

✓4ᵗʰ **R33   Retention of urine**
> EXCLUDES 1   psychogenic retention of urine (F45.8)

R33.0   Drug induced retention of urine
> Use additional code for adverse effect, if applicable, to identify drug (T36-T50 with fifth or sixth character 5)

R33.8   Other retention of urine
> Code first, if applicable, any causal condition, such as:
> enlarged prostate (N40.1)

R33.9   Retention of urine, unspecified ▽

R34   Anuria and oliguria
> EXCLUDES 1   anuria and oliguria complicating abortion or ectopic or molar pregnancy (O00-O07, O08.4)
> anuria and oliguria complicating pregnancy (O26.83-)
> anuria and oliguria complicating the puerperium (O90.4)

✓4ᵗʰ **R35   Polyuria**
> Code first, if applicable, any causal condition, such as:
> enlarged prostate (N40.1)
> EXCLUDES 1   psychogenic polyuria (F45.8)

R35.0   Frequency of micturition

R35.1   Nocturia

R35.8   Other polyuria
> Polyuria NOS

✓4ᵗʰ **R36   Urethral discharge**

R36.0   Urethral discharge without blood

R36.1   Hematospermia ♂

R36.9   Urethral discharge, unspecified ▽
> Penile discharge NOS
> Urethrorrhea

R37   Sexual dysfunction, unspecified ▽

✓4ᵗʰ **R39   Other and unspecified symptoms and signs involving the genitourinary system**

R39.0   Extravasation of urine

✓5ᵗʰ **R39.1   Other difficulties with micturition**
> Code first, if applicable, any causal condition, such as:
> enlarged prostate (N40.1)

R39.11   Hesitancy of micturition

R39.12   Poor urinary stream
> Weak urinary steam

R39.13   Splitting of urinary stream

R39.14   Feeling of incomplete bladder emptying

R39.15   Urgency of urination
> EXCLUDES 1   urge incontinence (N39.41, N39.46)

R39.16   Straining to void

✓6ᵗʰ **R39.19   Other difficulties with micturition**

R39.191   Need to immediately re-void

R39.192   Position dependent micturition

R39.198   Other difficulties with micturition

R39.2   Extrarenal uremia
> Prerenal uremia
> EXCLUDES 1   uremia NOS (N19)

✓5ᵗʰ **R39.8   Other symptoms and signs involving the genitourinary system**

R39.81   Functional urinary incontinence
> Urinary incontinence due to cognitive impairment, or severe physical disability or immobility
> EXCLUDES 1   stress incontinence and other specified urinary incontinence (N39.3-N39.4-)
> urinary incontinence NOS (R32)

R39.82   Chronic bladder pain

● **R39.83   Unilateral non-palpable testicle**

● **R39.84   Bilateral non-palpable testicles**

R39.89   Other symptoms and signs involving the genitourinary system

R39.9   Unspecified symptoms and signs involving the genitourinary system ▽

Symptoms and signs involving cognition, perception, emotional state and behavior (R40-R46)

> EXCLUDES 2   symptoms and signs constituting part of a pattern of mental disorder (F01-F99)

✓4ᵗʰ **R40   Somnolence, stupor and coma**
> EXCLUDES 1   neonatal coma (P91.5)
> somnolence, stupor and coma in diabetes (E08-E13)
> somnolence, stupor and coma in hepatic failure (K72.-)
> somnolence, stupor and coma in hypoglycemia (nondiabetic) (E15)

R40.0   Somnolence
> Drowsiness
> EXCLUDES 1   coma (R40.2-)

R40.1   Stupor
> Catatonic stupor
> Semicoma
> EXCLUDES 1   catatonic schizophrenia (F20.2)
> coma (R40.2-)
> depressive stupor (F31-F33)
> dissociative stupor (F44.2)
> manic stupor (F30.2)

✓5ᵗʰ **R40.2   Coma**
> Code first any associated:
> fracture of skull (S02.-)
> intracranial injury (S06.-)
> **NOTE**   One code from each subcategory, R40.21-R40.23, is required to complete the coma scale
> **AHA:** 2015, 2Q, 17; 2014, 1Q, 19

R40.20   Unspecified coma HCC
> Coma NOS
> Unconsciousness NOS

EXCLUDES 1 Not coded here   EXCLUDES 2 Not included here   N Newborn Age: 0   P Pediatric Age: 0-17   M Maternity Age: 12-55   A Adult Age: 15-124

R29.891–R40.20

894   ICD-10-CM 2018

✓6ᵗʰ **R40.21   Coma scale, eyes open**

> The following appropriate 7th character is to be
> added to subcategories R40.21-, R40.22-,
> R40.23-, and R40.24-.
> Ø   unspecified time
> 1   in the field [EMT or ambulance]
> 2   at arrival to emergency department
> 3   at hospital admission
> 4   24 hours or more after hospital admission

  ✓7ᵗʰ **R40.211   Coma scale, eyes open, never**   HCC
  ✓7ᵗʰ **R40.212   Coma scale, eyes open, to pain**   HCC
  ✓7ᵗʰ **R40.213   Coma scale, eyes open, to sound**
  ✓7ᵗʰ **R40.214   Coma scale, eyes open, spontaneous**

✓6ᵗʰ **R40.22   Coma scale, best verbal response**

  ✓7ᵗʰ **R40.221   Coma scale, best verbal response,
           none**   HCC
  ✓7ᵗʰ **R40.222   Coma scale, best verbal response,
           incomprehensible words**   HCC
           ▶Incomprehensible sounds
              (2-5 years of age)
           Moans/grunts to pain; restless
              (< 2 years old)◀
  ✓7ᵗʰ **R40.223   Coma scale, best verbal response,
           inappropriate words**
           ▶Inappropriate crying or screaming
              (< 2 years of age)
           Screaming (2-5 years of age)
  ✓7ᵗʰ **R40.224   Coma scale, best verbal response,
           confused conversation**
           ▶Inappropriate words (2-5 years of age)
           Irritable cries (< 2 years of age)◀
  ✓7ᵗʰ **R40.225   Coma scale, best verbal response,
           oriented**
           ▶Cooing or babbling or crying appropriately
              (< 2 years of age)
           Uses appropriate words (2- 5 years of age)◀

✓6ᵗʰ **R40.23   Coma scale, best motor response**

  ✓7ᵗʰ **R40.231   Coma scale, best motor response,
           none**   HCC
  ✓7ᵗʰ **R40.232   Coma scale, best motor response,
           extension**   HCC
           ▶Abnormal extensor posturing to pain or
              noxious stimuli (< 2 years of age)
           Extensor posturing to pain or noxious
              stimuli (2-5 years of age)◀
  ✓7ᵗʰ **R40.233   Coma scale, best motor response,
           abnormal**
           ▶Abnormal flexure posturing to pain or
              noxious stimuli (Ø-5 years of age)
           Flexion/decorticate posturing (< 2 years of
              age)◀
  ✓7ᵗʰ **R40.234   Coma scale, best motor response,
           flexion withdrawal**   HCC
           ▶Withdraws from pain or noxious stimuli
              (Ø-5 years of age)◀
  ✓7ᵗʰ **R40.235   Coma scale, best motor response,
           localizes pain**
           ▶Localizes pain (2-5 years of age)
           Withdraws to touch (< 2 years of age)◀
  ✓7ᵗʰ **R40.236   Coma scale, best motor response,
           obeys commands**
           ▶Normal or spontaneous movement (< 2
              years of age)
           Obeys commands (2-5 years of age)◀

✓6ᵗʰ **R40.24   Glasgow coma scale, total score**
           NOTE   Assign a code from subcategory R40.24,
                    when only the total coma score is
                    documented

  ✓7ᵗʰ **R40.241   Glasgow coma scale score 13-15**
  ✓7ᵗʰ **R40.242   Glasgow coma scale score 9-12**
  ✓7ᵗʰ **R40.243   Glasgow coma scale score 3-8**   HCC
  ✓7ᵗʰ **R40.244   Other coma, without documented
           Glasgow coma scale score, or with
           partial score reported**   HCC

R40.3   Persistent vegetative state   HCC
           DEF: Persistent wakefulness without consciousness due to
           nonfunctioning cerebral cortex.

R40.4   Transient alteration of awareness

✓4ᵗʰ **R41   Other symptoms and signs involving cognitive functions and
         awareness**
         EXCLUDES 1   *dissociative [conversion] disorders (F44.-)*
                       mild cognitive impairment, so stated (G31.84)

  R41.Ø   Disorientation, unspecified   ▽
           Confusion NOS
           Delirium NOS

  R41.1   Anterograde amnesia
  R41.2   Retrograde amnesia
  R41.3   Other amnesia
           Amnesia NOS
           Memory loss NOS
           EXCLUDES 1   *amnestic disorder due to known physiologic condition
                         (FØ4)*
                         *amnestic syndrome due to psychoactive substance use
                         (F1Ø-F19 with 5th character .6)*
                         *mild memory disturbance due to known physiological
                         condition (FØ6.8)*
                         transient global amnesia (G45.4)

  R41.4   Neurologic neglect syndrome
           Asomatognosia
           Hemi-akinesia
           Hemi-inattention
           Hemispatial neglect
           Left-sided neglect
           Sensory neglect
           Visuospatial neglect
           EXCLUDES 1   *visuospatial deficit (R41.842)*

✓5ᵗʰ **R41.8   Other symptoms and signs involving cognitive functions and
         awareness**

  R41.81   Age-related cognitive decline   A
           Senility NOS

  R41.82   Altered mental status, unspecified   ▽
           Change in mental status NOS
           EXCLUDES 1   *altered level of consciousness (R4Ø.-)*
                         *altered mental status due to known
                         condition—code to condition
                         delirium NOS (R41.Ø)*
           AHA: 2012, 4Q, 97

  R41.83   Borderline intellectual functioning
           IQ level 71 to 84
           EXCLUDES 1   *intellectual disabilities (F7Ø-F79)*

  ✓6ᵗʰ **R41.84   Other specified cognitive deficit**
           EXCLUDES 1   *cognitive deficits as sequelae of
                         cerebrovascular disease (I69.Ø1-,
                         I69.11-, I69.21-, I69.31-, I69.81-,
                         I69.91-)*

           R41.84Ø   Attention and concentration deficit
                    EXCLUDES 1   *attention-deficit hyperactivity
                                  disorders (F9Ø.-)*
           R41.841   Cognitive communication deficit
           R41.842   Visuospatial deficit
           R41.843   Psychomotor deficit
           R41.844   Frontal lobe and executive function deficit

  **R41.89   Other symptoms and signs involving cognitive
           functions and awareness**
           Anosognosia

  **R41.9   Unspecified symptoms and signs involving cognitive
           functions and awareness**   ▽
           ▶Unspecified neurocognitive disorder◀

R42   Dizziness and giddiness
           Light-headedness
           Vertigo NOS
           EXCLUDES 1   *vertiginous syndromes (H81.-)*
                         vertigo from infrasound (T75.23)

✓4ᵗʰ **R43   Disturbances of smell and taste**
  R43.Ø   Anosmia
  R43.1   Parosmia
  R43.2   Parageusia
  R43.8   Other disturbances of smell and taste
           Mixed disturbance of smell and taste
  R43.9   Unspecified disturbances of smell and taste   ▽

✓ Additional Character Req   ✓7ᵗʰ Placeholder Alert   Manifestation   HCC CMS-HCC Condition   ▽ Unspecified Code   ▶◀ Revised Text   ● New Code   ▲ Revised Code Title

Chapter 18. Symptoms, Signs, and Abnormal Clinical and Laboratory Findings, Not Elsewhere Classified

☑4ᵗʰ R44 Other symptoms and signs involving general sensations and perceptions

> EXCLUDES 1   alcoholic hallucinations (F1.5)
> hallucinations in drug psychosis (F11-F19 with .5)
> hallucinations in mood disorders with psychotic symptoms (F30.2, F31.5, F32.3, F33.3)
> hallucinations in schizophrenia, schizotypal and delusional disorders (F20-F29)
>
> EXCLUDES 2   disturbances of skin sensation (R20.-)

- **R44.0 Auditory hallucinations**
- **R44.1 Visual hallucinations**
- **R44.2 Other hallucinations**
- **R44.3 Hallucinations, unspecified** ▽
- **R44.8 Other symptoms and signs involving general sensations and perceptions**
- **R44.9 Unspecified symptoms and signs involving general sensations and perceptions** ▽

☑4ᵗʰ R45 Symptoms and signs involving emotional state

- **R45.0 Nervousness**
  - Nervous tension
- **R45.1 Restlessness and agitation**
- **R45.2 Unhappiness**
- **R45.3 Demoralization and apathy**
  - EXCLUDES 1   anhedonia (R45.84)
- **R45.4 Irritability and anger**
- **R45.5 Hostility**
- **R45.6 Violent behavior**
- **R45.7 State of emotional shock and stress, unspecified** ▽
- **☑5ᵗʰ R45.8 Other symptoms and signs involving emotional state**
  - **R45.81 Low self-esteem**
  - **R45.82 Worries**
  - **R45.83 Excessive crying of child, adolescent or adult**
    - EXCLUDES 1   excessive crying of infant (baby) R68.11
  - **R45.84 Anhedonia**
  - **☑6ᵗʰ R45.85 Homicidal and suicidal ideations**
    - EXCLUDES 1   suicide attempt (T14.91)
    - **R45.850 Homicidal ideations**
    - **R45.851 Suicidal ideations**
      - **DEF:** Thoughts of committing suicide; no actual attempt of suicide has been made.
  - **R45.86 Emotional lability**
  - **R45.87 Impulsiveness**
  - **R45.89 Other symptoms and signs involving emotional state**

☑4ᵗʰ R46 Symptoms and signs involving appearance and behavior

> EXCLUDES 1   appearance and behavior in schizophrenia, schizotypal and delusional disorders (F20-F29)
> mental and behavioral disorders (F01-F99)

- **R46.0 Very low level of personal hygiene**
- **R46.1 Bizarre personal appearance**
- **R46.2 Strange and inexplicable behavior**
- **R46.3 Overactivity**
- **R46.4 Slowness and poor responsiveness**
  - EXCLUDES 1   stupor (R40.1)
- **R46.5 Suspiciousness and marked evasiveness**
- **R46.6 Undue concern and preoccupation with stressful events**
- **R46.7 Verbosity and circumstantial detail obscuring reason for contact**
- **☑5ᵗʰ R46.8 Other symptoms and signs involving appearance and behavior**
  - **R46.81 Obsessive-compulsive behavior**
    - EXCLUDES 1   obsessive-compulsive disorder (F42-)
  - **R46.89 Other symptoms and signs involving appearance and behavior**

Symptoms and signs involving speech and voice (R47-R49)

☑4ᵗʰ R47 Speech disturbances, not elsewhere classified

> EXCLUDES 1   autism (F84.0)
> cluttering (F80.81)
> specific developmental disorders of speech and language (F80.-)
> stuttering (F80.81)

- **☑5ᵗʰ R47.0 Dysphasia and aphasia**
  - **R47.01 Aphasia**
    - EXCLUDES 1   aphasia following cerebrovascular disease (I69. with final characters -20)
    - progressive isolated aphasia (G31.01)
  - **R47.02 Dysphasia**
    - EXCLUDES 1   dysphasia following cerebrovascular disease (I69. with final characters -21)
- **R47.1 Dysarthria and anarthria**
  - EXCLUDES 1   dysarthria following cerebrovascular disease (I69. with final characters -22)
- **☑5ᵗʰ R47.8 Other speech disturbances**
  - EXCLUDES 1   dysarthria following cerebrovascular disease (I69. with final characters -28)
  - **R47.81 Slurred speech**
  - **R47.82 Fluency disorder in conditions classified elsewhere**
    - Stuttering in conditions classified elsewhere
    - Code first underlying disease or condition, such as:
    - Parkinson's disease (G20)
    - EXCLUDES 1   adult onset fluency disorder (F98.5)
    - childhood onset fluency disorder (F80.81)
    - fluency disorder (stuttering) following cerebrovascular disease (I69. with final characters-23)
  - **R47.89 Other speech disturbances**
- **R47.9 Unspecified speech disturbances** ▽

☑4ᵗʰ R48 Dyslexia and other symbolic dysfunctions, not elsewhere classified

> EXCLUDES 1   specific developmental disorders of scholastic skills (F81.-)

- **R48.0 Dyslexia and alexia**
- **R48.1 Agnosia**
  - Astereognosia (astereognosis)
  - Autotopagnosia
  - EXCLUDES 1   visual object agnosia (R48.3)
- **R48.2 Apraxia**
  - EXCLUDES 1   apraxia following cerebrovascular disease (I69. with final characters -90)
- **R48.3 Visual agnosia**
  - Prosopagnosia
  - Simultanagnosia (asimultagnosia)
- **R48.8 Other symbolic dysfunctions**
  - Acalculia
  - Agraphia
  - **AHA:** 2017, 1Q, 27
- **R48.9 Unspecified symbolic dysfunctions** ▽

☑4ᵗʰ R49 Voice and resonance disorders

> EXCLUDES 1   psychogenic voice and resonance disorders (F44.4)

- **R49.0 Dysphonia**
  - Hoarseness
- **R49.1 Aphonia**
  - Loss of voice
- **☑5ᵗʰ R49.2 Hypernasality and hyponasality**
  - **R49.21 Hypernasality**
  - **R49.22 Hyponasality**
- **R49.8 Other voice and resonance disorders**
- **R49.9 Unspecified voice and resonance disorder** ▽
  - Change in voice NOS
  - Resonance disorder NOS

EXCLUDES 1 Not coded here   EXCLUDES 2 Not included here   N Newborn Age: 0   P Pediatric Age: 0-17   M Maternity Age: 12-55   A Adult Age: 15-124

896   ICD-10-CM 2018

General symptoms and signs (R50-R69)

✅4ᵗʰ R50 Fever of other and unknown origin

EXCLUDES 1   chills without fever (R68.83)
febrile convulsions (R56.0-)
fever of unknown origin during labor (O75.2)
fever of unknown origin in newborn (P81.9)
hypothermia due to illness (R68.0)
malignant hyperthermia due to anesthesia (T88.3)
puerperal pyrexia NOS (O86.4)

R50.2 Drug induced fever
Use additional code for adverse effect, if applicable, to identify drug (T36-T50 with fifth or sixth character 5)

EXCLUDES 1   postvaccination (postimmunization) fever (R50.83)

✅5ᵗʰ R50.8 Other specified fever

R50.81 Fever presenting with conditions classified elsewhere
Code first underlying condition when associated fever is present, such as with:
leukemia (C91-C95)
neutropenia (D70.-)
sickle-cell disease (D57.-)
AHA: 2014, 4Q, 22

R50.82 Postprocedural fever
EXCLUDES 1   postprocedural infection (T81.4-)
posttransfusion fever (R50.84)
postvaccination (postimmunization) fever (R50.83)

R50.83 Postvaccination fever
Postimmunization fever

R50.84 Febrile nonhemolytic transfusion reaction
FNHTR
Posttransfusion fever

R50.9 Fever, unspecified   ▽
Fever NOS
Fever of unknown origin [FUO]
Fever with chills
Fever with rigors
Hyperpyrexia NOS
Persistent fever
Pyrexia NOS

R51 Headache
Facial pain NOS

EXCLUDES 1   atypical face pain (G50.1)
migraine and other headache syndromes (G43-G44)
trigeminal neuralgia (G50.0)

R52 Pain, unspecified   ▽
Acute pain NOS
Generalized pain NOS
Pain NOS

EXCLUDES 1   acute and chronic pain, not elsewhere classified (G89.-)
localized pain, unspecified type—code to pain by site, such as:
abdomen pain (R10.-)
back pain (M54.9)
breast pain (N64.4)
chest pain (R07.1-R07.9)
ear pain (H92.0-)
eye pain (H57.1)
headache (R51)
joint pain (M25.5-)
limb pain (M79.6-)
lumbar region pain (M54.5)
pelvic and perineal pain (R10.2)
renal colic (N23)
shoulder pain (M25.51-)
spine pain (M54.-)
throat pain (R07.0)
tongue pain (K14.6)
tooth pain (K08.8)
pain disorders exclusively related to psychological factors (F45.41)

✅4ᵗʰ R53 Malaise and fatigue

R53.0 Neoplastic (malignant) related fatigue
Code first associated neoplasm

R53.1 Weakness
Asthenia NOS

EXCLUDES 1   age-related weakness (R54)
muscle weakness (M62.8-)
sarcopenia (M62.84)
senile asthenia (R54)
AHA: 2017, 1Q, 7; 2015, 1Q, 25

R53.2 Functional quadriplegia   HCC
Complete immobility due to severe physical disability or frailty

EXCLUDES 1   frailty NOS (R54)
hysterical paralysis (F44.4)
immobility syndrome (M62.3)
neurologic quadriplegia (G82.5-)
quadriplegia (G82.50)

AHA: 2016, 2Q, 6
DEF: Inability to move due to a nonphysiological condition, such as dementia; no mental ability to move independently; typically found in severely demented patients.

✅5ᵗʰ R53.8 Other malaise and fatigue

EXCLUDES 1   combat exhaustion and fatigue (F43.0)
congenital debility (P96.9)
~~exhaustion and fatigue due to depressive episode (F32.-)~~
exhaustion and fatigue due to excessive exertion (T73.3)
exhaustion and fatigue due to exposure (T73.2)
exhaustion and fatigue due to heat (T67.-)
exhaustion and fatigue due to pregnancy (O26.8-)
exhaustion and fatigue due to recurrent depressive episode (F33)
exhaustion and fatigue due to senile debility (R54)

R53.81 Other malaise
Chronic debility
Debility NOS
General physical deterioration
Malaise NOS
Nervous debility

EXCLUDES 1   age-related physical debility (R54)

R53.82 Chronic fatigue, unspecified   ▽
Chronic fatigue syndrome NOS

EXCLUDES 1   postviral fatigue syndrome (G93.3)

R53.83 Other fatigue
Fatigue NOS
Lack of energy
Lethargy
Tiredness

EXCLUDES 2   ▶exhaustion and fatigue due to depressive episode (F32.-)◀

R54 Age-related physical debility   Ⓐ
Frailty
Old age
Senescence
Senile asthenia
Senile debility

EXCLUDES 1   age-related cognitive decline (R41.81)
sarcopenia (M62.84)
senile psychosis (F03)
senility NOS (R41.81)

R55 Syncope and collapse
Blackout
Fainting
Vasovagal attack

EXCLUDES 1   cardiogenic shock (R57.0)
carotid sinus syncope (G90.01)
heat syncope (T67.1)
neurocirculatory asthenia (F45.8)
neurogenic orthostatic hypotension (G90.3)
orthostatic hypotension (I95.1)
postprocedural shock (T81.1-)
psychogenic syncope (F48.8)
shock NOS (R57.9)
shock complicating or following abortion or ectopic or molar pregnancy (O00-O07, O08.3)
shock complicating or following labor and delivery (O75.1)
Stokes-Adams attack (I45.9)
unconsciousness NOS (R40.2-)

✅4ᵗʰ R56 Convulsions, not elsewhere classified

EXCLUDES 1   dissociative convulsions and seizures (F44.5)
epileptic convulsions and seizures (G40.-)
newborn convulsions and seizures (P90)

✅5ᵗʰ R56.0 Febrile convulsions

R56.00 Simple febrile convulsions   HCC
Febrile convulsion NOS
Febrile seizure NOS

R56.01 Complex febrile convulsions   HCC
Atypical febrile seizure
Complex febrile seizure
Complicated febrile seizure

EXCLUDES 1   status epilepticus (G40.901)

✅ Additional Character Req   ✅7ᵗʰ Placeholder Alert   Manifestation   HCC CMS-HCC Condition   ▽ Unspecified Code   ▶◀ Revised Text   ● New Code   ▲ Revised Code Title

ICD-10-CM 2018   897

Chapter 18. Symptoms, Signs, and Abnormal Clinical and Laboratory Findings, Not Elsewhere Classified

R50–R56.01

R56.1 Post traumatic seizures HCC
> *EXCLUDES 1* *post traumatic epilepsy (G40.-)*

R56.9 Unspecified convulsions HCC ▽
Convulsion disorder
Fit NOS
Recurrent convulsions
Seizure(s) (convulsive) NOS

✓4th **R57 Shock, not elsewhere classified**
> *EXCLUDES 1* *anaphylactic shock NOS (T78.2)*
> *anaphylactic reaction or shock due to adverse food reaction (T78.0-)*
> *anaphylactic shock due to adverse effect of correct drug or medicament properly administered (T88.6)*
> *anaphylactic shock due to serum (T80.5-)*
> *anesthetic shock (T88.3)*
> *electric shock (T75.4)*
> *obstetric shock (O75.1)*
> *postprocedural shock (T81.1-)*
> *psychic shock (F43.0)*
> ~~*septic shock (R65.21)*~~
> *shock complicating or following ectopic or molar pregnancy (O00-O07, O08.3)*
> *shock due to lightning (T75.01)*
> *traumatic shock (T79.4)*
> *toxic shock syndrome (A48.3)*

R57.0 Cardiogenic shock HCC
> *EXCLUDES 2* ▶*septic shock (R65.21)*◀

DEF: Associated with myocardial infarction, cardiac tamponade, and massive pulmonary embolism; symptoms include mental confusion, reduced blood pressure, tachycardia, pallor, and cold, clammy skin.

R57.1 Hypovolemic shock HCC

R57.8 Other shock HCC

R57.9 Shock, unspecified HCC ▽
Failure of peripheral circulation NOS

R58 Hemorrhage, not elsewhere classified
Hemorrhage NOS
> *EXCLUDES 1* *hemorrhage included with underlying conditions, such as:*
> *acute duodenal ulcer with hemorrhage (K26.0)*
> *acute gastritis with bleeding (K29.01)*
> *ulcerative enterocolitis with rectal bleeding (K51.01)*

✓4th **R59 Enlarged lymph nodes**
> *INCLUDES* swollen glands
> *EXCLUDES 1* *acute lymphadenitis (L04.-)*
> *chronic lymphadenitis (I88.1)*
> *lymphadenitis NOS (I88.9)*
> *mesenteric (acute) (chronic) lymphadenitis (I88.0)*

R59.0 Localized enlarged lymph nodes

R59.1 Generalized enlarged lymph nodes
Lymphadenopathy NOS

R59.9 Enlarged lymph nodes, unspecified ▽

✓4th **R60 Edema, not elsewhere classified**
> *EXCLUDES 1* *angioneurotic edema (T78.3)*
> *ascites (R18.-)*
> *cerebral edema (G93.6)*
> *cerebral edema due to birth injury (P11.0)*
> *edema of larynx (J38.4)*
> *edema of nasopharynx (J39.2)*
> *edema of pharynx (J39.2)*
> *gestational edema (O12.0-)*
> *hereditary edema (Q82.0)*
> *hydrops fetalis NOS (P83.2)*
> *hydrothorax (J94.8)*
> ~~*nutritional edema (E40-E46)*~~
> *hydrops fetalis NOS (P83.2)*
> *newborn edema (P83.3)*
> *pulmonary edema (J81.-)*

R60.0 Localized edema

R60.1 Generalized edema
> *EXCLUDES 2* ▶*nutritional edema (E40-E46)*◀

R60.9 Edema, unspecified ▽
Fluid retention NOS

R61 Generalized hyperhidrosis
Excessive sweating
Night sweats
Secondary hyperhidrosis
Code first, if applicable, menopausal and female climacteric states (N95.1)
> *EXCLUDES 1* *focal (primary) (secondary) hyperhidrosis (L74.5-)*
> *Frey's syndrome (L74.52)*
> *localized (primary) (secondary) hyperhidrosis (L74.5-)*

✓4th **R62 Lack of expected normal physiological development in childhood and adults**
> *EXCLUDES 1* *delayed puberty (E30.0)*
> *gonadal dysgenesis (Q99.1)*
> *hypopituitarism (E23.0)*

R62.0 Delayed milestone in childhood P
Delayed attainment of expected physiological developmental stage
Late talker
Late walker

✓5th **R62.5 Other and unspecified lack of expected normal physiological development in childhood**
> *EXCLUDES 1* *HIV disease resulting in failure to thrive (B20)*
> *physical retardation due to malnutrition (E45)*

R62.50 Unspecified lack of expected normal physiological development in childhood ▽
Infantilism NOS

R62.51 Failure to thrive (child) P
Failure to gain weight
> *EXCLUDES 1* *failure to thrive in child under 28 days old (P92.6)*

DEF: Organic failure to thrive (FTT): Acute or chronic illness that interferes with nutritional intake, absorption, metabolism excretion, and energy requirements; nonorganic FTT is a symptom of neglect or abuse.

R62.52 Short stature (child)
Lack of growth
Physical retardation
Short stature NOS
> *EXCLUDES 1* *short stature due to endocrine disorder (E34.3)*

R62.59 Other lack of expected normal physiological development in childhood

R62.7 Adult failure to thrive A

✓4th **R63 Symptoms and signs concerning food and fluid intake**
> *EXCLUDES 1* *bulimia NOS (F50.2)*
> *eating disorders of nonorganic origin (F50.-)*
> *malnutrition (E40-E46)*

R63.0 Anorexia
Loss of appetite
> *EXCLUDES 1* *anorexia nervosa (F50.0-)*
> *loss of appetite of nonorganic origin (F50.89)*

R63.1 Polydipsia
Excessive thirst

R63.2 Polyphagia
Excessive eating
Hyperalimentation NOS

R63.3 Feeding difficulties
Feeding problem (elderly) (infant) NOS
▶Picky eater◀
> *EXCLUDES 1* ▶*eating disorders (F50.-)*◀
> *feeding problems of newborn (P92.-)*
> *infant feeding disorder of nonorganic origin (F98.2-)*
AHA: 2017, 1Q, 28; 2016, 3Q, 19

R63.4 Abnormal weight loss

R63.5 Abnormal weight gain
> *EXCLUDES 1* *excessive weight gain in pregnancy (O26.0-)*
> *obesity (E66.-)*

R63.6 Underweight
Use additional code to identify body mass index (BMI), if known (Z68.-)
> *EXCLUDES 1* *abnormal weight loss (R63.4)*
> *anorexia nervosa (F50.0-)*
> *malnutrition (E40-E46)*

R63.8 Other symptoms and signs concerning food and fluid intake

R64 Cachexia HCC
Wasting syndrome
Code first underlying condition, if known
> *EXCLUDES 1* *abnormal weight loss (R63.4)*
> *nutritional marasmus (E41)*

EXCLUDES 1 Not coded here   *EXCLUDES 2* Not included here   N Newborn Age: 0   P Pediatric Age: 0-17   M Maternity Age: 12-55   A Adult Age: 15-124

898   ICD-10-CM 2018

☑4ᵗʰ R65 Symptoms and signs specifically associated with systemic inflammation and infection

☑5ᵗʰ R65.1 Systemic inflammatory response syndrome [SIRS] of non-infectious origin
Code first underlying condition, such as:
   heatstroke (T67.0)
   injury and trauma (S00-T88)
   EXCLUDES 1   sepsis—code to infection
        severe sepsis (R65.2)

R65.10 Systemic inflammatory response syndrome   **HCC**
[SIRS] of non-infectious origin without acute organ dysfunction
Systemic inflammatory response syndrome (SIRS) NOS

R65.11 Systemic inflammatory response syndrome   **HCC**
[SIRS] of non-infectious origin with acute organ dysfunction
Use additional code to identify specific acute organ dysfunction, such as:
   acute kidney failure (N17.-)
   acute respiratory failure (J96.0-)
   critical illness myopathy (G72.81)
   critical illness polyneuropathy (G62.81)
   disseminated intravascular coagulopathy [DIC] (D65)
   encephalopathy (metabolic) (septic) (G93.41)
   hepatic failure (K72.0-)

☑5ᵗʰ R65.2 Severe sepsis
Infection with associated acute organ dysfunction
Sepsis with acute organ dysfunction
Sepsis with multiple organ dysfunction
Systemic inflammatory response syndrome due to infectious process with acute organ dysfunction
Code first underlying infection, such as:
   infection following a procedure (T81.4-)
   infections following infusion, transfusion and therapeutic injection (T80.2-)
   puerperal sepsis (O85)
   sepsis following complete or unspecified spontaneous abortion (O03.87)
   sepsis following ectopic and molar pregnancy (O08.82)
   sepsis following incomplete spontaneous abortion (O03.37)
   sepsis following (induced) termination of pregnancy (O04.87)
   sepsis NOS (A41.9)
Use additional code to identify specific acute organ dysfunction, such as:
   acute kidney failure (N17.-)
   acute respiratory failure (J96.0-)
   critical illness myopathy (G72.81)
   critical illness polyneuropathy (G62.81)
   disseminated intravascular coagulopathy [DIC] (D65)
   encephalopathy (metabolic) (septic) (G93.41)
   hepatic failure (K72.0-)
AHA: 2016, 3Q, 8

R65.20 Severe sepsis without septic shock   **HCC**
Severe sepsis NOS
AHA: 2016, 3Q, 14; 2013, 4Q, 119

R65.21 Severe sepsis with septic shock   **HCC**

☑4ᵗʰ R68 Other general symptoms and signs

R68.0 Hypothermia, not associated with low environmental temperature
   EXCLUDES 1   hypothermia NOS (accidental) (T68)
        hypothermia due to anesthesia (T88.51)
        hypothermia due to low environmental temperature (T68)
        newborn hypothermia (P80.-)

☑5ᵗʰ R68.1 Nonspecific symptoms peculiar to infancy
   EXCLUDES 1   colic, infantile (R10.83)
        neonatal cerebral irritability (P91.3)
        teething syndrome (K00.7)

R68.11 Excessive crying of infant (baby)   **P**
   EXCLUDES 1   excessive crying of child, adolescent, or adult (R45.83)

R68.12 Fussy infant (baby)   **P**
Irritable infant

R68.13 Apparent life threatening event in infant (ALTE)   **P**
Apparent life threatening event in newborn
►Brief resolved unexplained event (BRUE)◄
Code first confirmed diagnosis, if known
Use additional code(s) for associated signs and symptoms if no confirmed diagnosis established, or if signs and symptoms are not associated routinely with confirmed diagnosis, or provide additional information for cause of ALTE

R68.19 Other nonspecific symptoms peculiar to infancy   **P**

R68.2 Dry mouth, unspecified   **▽**
   EXCLUDES 1   dry mouth due to dehydration (E86.0)
        dry mouth due to sicca syndrome [Sjögren] (M35.0-)
        salivary gland hyposecretion (K11.7)

R68.3 Clubbing of fingers
Clubbing of nails
DEF: Enlarged soft tissue of distal fingers; usually occurs in heart and lung diseases.
   EXCLUDES 1   congenital clubfinger (Q68.1)

☑5ᵗʰ R68.8 Other general symptoms and signs

R68.81 Early satiety
DEF: The premature feeling of being full after eating only a small amount of food; mechanism of satiety is multifactorial.

R68.82 Decreased libido   **A**
Decreased sexual desire

R68.83 Chills (without fever)
Chills NOS
   EXCLUDES 1   chills with fever (R50.9)

R68.84 Jaw pain
Mandibular pain
Maxilla pain
   EXCLUDES 1   temporomandibular joint arthralgia (M26.62-)

R68.89 Other general symptoms and signs

R69 Illness, unspecified   **▽**
Unknown and unspecified cases of morbidity

Abnormal findings on examination of blood, without diagnosis (R70-R79)

   EXCLUDES 2   abnormal findings on antenatal screening of mother (O28.-)
        abnormalities of lipids (E78.-)
        abnormalities of platelets and thrombocytes (D69.-)
        abnormalities of white blood cells classified elsewhere (D70-D72)
        coagulation hemorrhagic disorders (D65-D68)
        diagnostic abnormal findings classified elsewhere—see Alphabetical Index
        hemorrhagic and hematological disorders of newborn (P50-P61)

☑4ᵗʰ R70 Elevated erythrocyte sedimentation rate and abnormality of plasma viscosity

R70.0 Elevated erythrocyte sedimentation rate

R70.1 Abnormal plasma viscosity

☑4ᵗʰ R71 Abnormality of red blood cells
   EXCLUDES 1   anemias (D50-D64)
        anemia of premature infant (P61.2)
        benign (familial) polycythemia (D75.0)
        congenital anemias (P61.2-P61.4)
        newborn anemia due to isoimmunization (P55.-)
        polycythemia neonatorum (P61.1)
        polycythemia NOS (D75.1)
        polycythemia vera (D45)
        secondary polycythemia (D75.1)

R71.0 Precipitous drop in hematocrit
Drop (precipitous) in hemoglobin
Drop in hematocrit

R71.8 Other abnormality of red blood cells
Abnormal red-cell morphology NOS
Abnormal red-cell volume NOS
Anisocytosis
Poikilocytosis

☑ Additional Character Req   ☑x7ᵗʰ Placeholder Alert   **Manifestation**   **HCC** CMS-HCC Condition   ▽ Unspecified Code   ►◄ Revised Text   ● New Code   ▲ Revised Code Title

ICD-10-CM 2018   899

√4th R73 Elevated blood glucose level
> *EXCLUDES 1*   diabetes mellitus (E08-E13)
> diabetes mellitus in pregnancy, childbirth and the puerperium (O24.-)
> neonatal disorders (P70.0-P70.2)
> postsurgical hypoinsulinemia (E89.1)

   √5th R73.0 Abnormal glucose
> *EXCLUDES 1*   abnormal glucose in pregnancy (O99.81-)
> diabetes mellitus (E08-E13)
> dysmetabolic syndrome X (E88.81)
> gestational diabetes (O24.4-)
> glycosuria (R81)
> hypoglycemia (E16.2)

     R73.01 Impaired fasting glucose
       Elevated fasting glucose

     R73.02 Impaired glucose tolerance (oral)
       Elevated glucose tolerance

     R73.03 Prediabetes
       Latent diabetes

     R73.09 Other abnormal glucose
       Abnormal glucose NOS
       Abnormal non-fasting glucose tolerance

   R73.9 Hyperglycemia, unspecified ▽

√4th R74 Abnormal serum enzyme levels
   R74.0 Nonspecific elevation of levels of transaminase and lactic acid dehydrogenase [LDH]

   R74.8 Abnormal levels of other serum enzymes
     Abnormal level of acid phosphatase
     Abnormal level of alkaline phosphatase
     Abnormal level of amylase
     Abnormal level of lipase [triacylglycerol lipase]

   R74.9 Abnormal serum enzyme level, unspecified ▽

R75 Inconclusive laboratory evidence of human immunodeficiency virus [HIV]
   Nonconclusive HIV-test finding in infants
> *EXCLUDES 1*   asymptomatic human immunodeficiency virus [HIV] infection status (Z21)
> human immunodeficiency virus [HIV] disease (B20)

√4th R76 Other abnormal immunological findings in serum
   R76.0 Raised antibody titer
> *EXCLUDES 1*   isoimmunization in pregnancy (O36.0-O36.1)
> isoimmunization affecting newborn (P55.-)

   √5th R76.1 Nonspecific reaction to test for tuberculosis
     R76.11 Nonspecific reaction to tuberculin skin test without active tuberculosis
       Abnormal result of Mantoux test
       PPD positive
       Tuberculin (skin test) positive
       Tuberculin (skin test) reactor
> *EXCLUDES 1*   nonspecific reaction to cell mediated immunity measurement of gamma interferon antigen response without active tuberculosis (R76.12)

     R76.12 Nonspecific reaction to cell mediated immunity measurement of gamma interferon antigen response without active tuberculosis
       Nonspecific reaction to QuantiFERON-TB test (QFT) without active tuberculosis
> *EXCLUDES 1*   nonspecific reaction to tuberculin skin test without active tuberculosis (R76.11)
> positive tuberculin skin test (R76.11)

   R76.8 Other specified abnormal immunological findings in serum
     Raised level of immunoglobulins NOS

   R76.9 Abnormal immunological finding in serum, unspecified ▽

√4th R77 Other abnormalities of plasma proteins
> *EXCLUDES 1*   disorders of plasma-protein metabolism (E88.0)

   R77.0 Abnormality of albumin
   R77.1 Abnormality of globulin
     Hyperglobulinemia NOS
   R77.2 Abnormality of alphafetoprotein
   R77.8 Other specified abnormalities of plasma proteins
   R77.9 Abnormality of plasma protein, unspecified ▽

√4th R78 Findings of drugs and other substances, not normally found in blood
   Use additional code to identify any retained foreign body, if applicable (Z18.-)
> *EXCLUDES 1*   mental or behavioral disorders due to psychoactive substance use (F10-F19)

   R78.0 Finding of alcohol in blood
     Use additional external cause code (Y90.-), for detail regarding alcohol level

   R78.1 Finding of opiate drug in blood
   R78.2 Finding of cocaine in blood
   R78.3 Finding of hallucinogen in blood
   R78.4 Finding of other drugs of addictive potential in blood
   R78.5 Finding of other psychotropic drug in blood
   R78.6 Finding of steroid agent in blood

   √5th R78.7 Finding of abnormal level of heavy metals in blood
     R78.71 Abnormal lead level in blood
> *EXCLUDES 1*   lead poisoning (T56.0-)

     R78.79 Finding of abnormal level of heavy metals in blood

   √5th R78.8 Finding of other specified substances, not normally found in blood
     R78.81 Bacteremia
> *EXCLUDES 1*   sepsis—code to specified infection
> **DEF:** Laboratory finding of bacteria in the blood in the absence of two or more signs of sepsis; transient in nature, it progresses to septicemia with severe infectious process.

     R78.89 Finding of other specified substances, not normally found in blood
       Finding of abnormal level of lithium in blood

   R78.9 Finding of unspecified substance, not normally found in blood ▽

√4th R79 Other abnormal findings of blood chemistry
   Use additional code to identify any retained foreign body, if applicable (Z18.-)
> *EXCLUDES 1*   ~~abnormality of fluid, electrolyte or acid-base balance (E86-E87)~~
> asymptomatic hyperuricemia (E79.0)
> hyperglycemia NOS (R73.9)
> hypoglycemia NOS (E16.2)
> neonatal hypoglycemia (P70.3-P70.4)
> specific findings indicating disorder of amino-acid metabolism (E70-E72)
> specific findings indicating disorder of carbohydrate metabolism (E73-E74)
> specific findings indicating disorder of lipid metabolism (E75.-)

   R79.0 Abnormal level of blood mineral
     Abnormal blood level of cobalt
     Abnormal blood level of copper
     Abnormal blood level of iron
     Abnormal blood level of magnesium
     Abnormal blood level of mineral NEC
     Abnormal blood level of zinc
> *EXCLUDES 1*   abnormal level of lithium (R78.89)
> disorders of mineral metabolism (E83.-)
> neonatal hypomagnesemia (P71.2)
> nutritional mineral deficiency (E58-E61)

   R79.1 Abnormal coagulation profile
     Abnormal or prolonged bleeding time
     Abnormal or prolonged coagulation time
     Abnormal or prolonged partial thromboplastin time [PTT]
     Abnormal or prolonged prothrombin time [PT]
> *EXCLUDES 1*   coagulation defects (D68.-)
> *EXCLUDES 2*   ▶abnormality of fluid, electrolyte or acid-base balance (E86-E87)◀

   √5th R79.8 Other specified abnormal findings of blood chemistry
     R79.81 Abnormal blood-gas level
     R79.82 Elevated C-reactive protein [CRP]
     R79.89 Other specified abnormal findings of blood chemistry

   R79.9 Abnormal finding of blood chemistry, unspecified ▽

Abnormal findings on examination of urine, without diagnosis (R80-R82)

EXCLUDES 1   *abnormal findings on antenatal screening of mother (O28.-)*
diagnostic abnormal findings classified elsewhere—see Alphabetical Index
specific findings indicating disorder of amino-acid metabolism (E70-E72)
specific findings indicating disorder of carbohydrate metabolism (E73-E74)

✓4ᵗʰ R80   Proteinuria

EXCLUDES 1   *gestational proteinuria (O12.1-)*

R80.0   Isolated proteinuria
Idiopathic proteinuria
EXCLUDES 1   *isolated proteinuria with specific morphological lesion (N06.-)*

R80.1   Persistent proteinuria, unspecified ▽

R80.2   Orthostatic proteinuria, unspecified ▽
Postural proteinuria

R80.3   Bence Jones proteinuria

R80.8   Other proteinuria

R80.9   Proteinuria, unspecified ▽
Albuminuria NOS

R81   Glycosuria

EXCLUDES 1   *renal glycosuria (E74.8)*

✓4ᵗʰ R82   Other and unspecified abnormal findings in urine

INCLUDES   chromoabnormalities in urine
Use additional code to identify any retained foreign body, if applicable (Z18.-)
EXCLUDES 2   *hematuria (R31.-)*

R82.0   Chyluria
EXCLUDES 1   *filarial chyluria (B74.-)*

R82.1   Myoglobinuria

R82.2   Biliuria

R82.3   Hemoglobinuria
EXCLUDES 1   *hemoglobinuria due to hemolysis from external causes NEC (D59.6)*
hemoglobinuria due to paroxysmal nocturnal [Marchiafava-Micheli] (D59.5)
DEF: Free hemoglobin in blood due to rapid hemolysis of red blood cells; causes include burns, crushed injury, sickle cell anemia, thalassemia, parasitic infections, or kidney infections.

R82.4   Acetonuria
Ketonuria
DEF: Excessive excretion of acetone in urine; commonly occurs in diabetic acidosis.

R82.5   Elevated urine levels of drugs, medicaments and biological substances
Elevated urine levels of catecholamines
Elevated urine levels of indoleacetic acid
Elevated urine levels of 17-ketosteroids
Elevated urine levels of steroids

R82.6   Abnormal urine levels of substances chiefly nonmedicinal as to source
Abnormal urine level of heavy metals

✓5ᵗʰ R82.7   Abnormal findings on microbiological examination of urine
EXCLUDES 1   *colonization status (Z22.-)*

R82.71   Bacteriuria

R82.79   Other abnormal findings on microbiological examination of urine
Positive culture findings of urine

R82.8   Abnormal findings on cytological and histological examination of urine

✓5ᵗʰ R82.9   Other and unspecified abnormal findings in urine

R82.90   Unspecified abnormal findings in urine ▽

R82.91   Other chromoabnormalities of urine
Chromoconversion (dipstick)
Idiopathic dipstick converts positive for blood with no cellular forms in sediment
EXCLUDES 1   *hemoglobinuria (R82.3)*
myoglobinuria (R82.1)

R82.99   Other abnormal findings in urine
Cells and casts in urine
Crystalluria
Melanuria

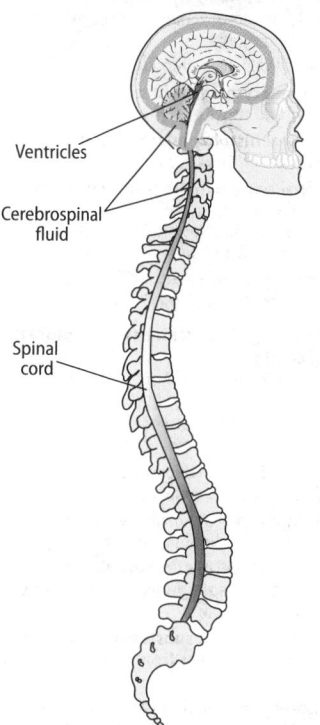

Cerebrospinal Fluid

Ventricles

Cerebrospinal fluid

Spinal cord

Abnormal findings on examination of other body fluids, substances and tissues, without diagnosis (R83-R89)

EXCLUDES 1   *abnormal findings on antenatal screening of mother (O28.-)*
diagnostic abnormal findings classified elsewhere—see Alphabetical Index
EXCLUDES 2   *abnormal findings on examination of blood, without diagnosis (R70-R79)*
abnormal findings on examination of urine, without diagnosis (R80-R82)
abnormal tumor markers (R97.-)

R83.3   Abnormal level of substances chiefly nonmedicinal as to source in cerebrospinal fluid

✓4ᵗʰ R83   Abnormal findings in cerebrospinal fluid

R83.0   Abnormal level of enzymes in cerebrospinal fluid

R83.1   Abnormal level of hormones in cerebrospinal fluid

R83.2   Abnormal level of other drugs, medicaments and biological substances in cerebrospinal fluid

R83.4   Abnormal immunological findings in cerebrospinal fluid

R83.5   Abnormal microbiological findings in cerebrospinal fluid
Positive culture findings in cerebrospinal fluid
EXCLUDES 1   *colonization status (Z22.-)*

R83.6   Abnormal cytological findings in cerebrospinal fluid

R83.8   Other abnormal findings in cerebrospinal fluid
Abnormal chromosomal findings in cerebrospinal fluid

R83.9   Unspecified abnormal finding in cerebrospinal fluid ▽

✓4ᵗʰ R84   Abnormal findings in specimens from respiratory organs and thorax

INCLUDES   abnormal findings in bronchial washings
abnormal findings in nasal secretions
abnormal findings in pleural fluid
abnormal findings in sputum
abnormal findings in throat scrapings
EXCLUDES 1   *blood-stained sputum (R04.2)*

R84.0   Abnormal level of enzymes in specimens from respiratory organs and thorax

R84.1   Abnormal level of hormones in specimens from respiratory organs and thorax

R84.2   Abnormal level of other drugs, medicaments and biological substances in specimens from respiratory organs and thorax

R84.3   Abnormal level of substances chiefly nonmedicinal as to source in specimens from respiratory organs and thorax

R84.4   Abnormal immunological findings in specimens from respiratory organs and thorax

R84.5 **Abnormal microbiological findings in specimens from respiratory organs and thorax**
> Positive culture findings in specimens from respiratory organs and thorax
>> EXCLUDES 1   *colonization status (Z22.-)*

R84.6 **Abnormal cytological findings in specimens from respiratory organs and thorax**

R84.7 **Abnormal histological findings in specimens from respiratory organs and thorax**

R84.8 **Other abnormal findings in specimens from respiratory organs and thorax**
> Abnormal chromosomal findings in specimens from respiratory organs and thorax

R84.9 **Unspecified abnormal finding in specimens from respiratory organs and thorax**   ▽

✓4ᵗʰ **R85** **Abnormal findings in specimens from digestive organs and abdominal cavity**
> INCLUDES   abnormal findings in peritoneal fluid
> abnormal findings in saliva
>> EXCLUDES 1   *cloudy peritoneal dialysis effluent (R88.0)*
>> *fecal abnormalities (R19.5)*

R85.0 **Abnormal level of enzymes in specimens from digestive organs and abdominal cavity**

R85.1 **Abnormal level of hormones in specimens from digestive organs and abdominal cavity**

R85.2 **Abnormal level of other drugs, medicaments and biological substances in specimens from digestive organs and abdominal cavity**

R85.3 **Abnormal level of substances chiefly nonmedicinal as to source in specimens from digestive organs and abdominal cavity**

R85.4 **Abnormal immunological findings in specimens from digestive organs and abdominal cavity**

R85.5 **Abnormal microbiological findings in specimens from digestive organs and abdominal cavity**
> Positive culture findings in specimens from digestive organs and abdominal cavity
>> EXCLUDES 1   *colonization status (Z22.-)*

✓5ᵗʰ **R85.6** **Abnormal cytological findings in specimens from digestive organs and abdominal cavity**

✓6ᵗʰ **R85.61** **Abnormal cytologic smear of anus**
>> EXCLUDES 1   *abnormal cytological findings in specimens from other digestive organs and abdominal cavity (R85.69)*
>> *anal intraepithelial neoplasia I [AIN I] (K62.82)*
>> *anal intraepithelial neoplasia II [AIN II] (K62.82)*
>> *anal intraepithelial neoplasia III [AIN III] (D01.3)*
>> *carcinoma in situ of anus (histologically confirmed) (D01.3)*
>> *dysplasia (mild) (moderate) of anus (histologically confirmed) (K62.82)*
>> *severe dysplasia of anus (histologically confirmed) (D01.3)*
>> EXCLUDES 2   *anal high risk human papillomavirus (HPV) DNA test positive (R85.81)*
>> *anal low risk human papillomavirus (HPV) DNA test positive (R85.82)*

R85.610 **Atypical squamous cells of undetermined significance on cytologic smear of anus [ASC-US]**

R85.611 **Atypical squamous cells cannot exclude high grade squamous intraepithelial lesion on cytologic smear of anus [ASC-H]**

R85.612 **Low grade squamous intraepithelial lesion on cytologic smear of anus [LGSIL]**

R85.613 **High grade squamous intraepithelial lesion on cytologic smear of anus [HGSIL]**

R85.614 **Cytologic evidence of malignancy on smear of anus**

R85.615 **Unsatisfactory cytologic smear of anus**
> Inadequate sample of cytologic smear of anus

R85.616 **Satisfactory anal smear but lacking transformation zone**

R85.618 **Other abnormal cytological findings on specimens from anus**

R85.619 **Unspecified abnormal cytological findings in specimens from anus**   ▽
> Abnormal anal cytology NOS
> Atypical glandular cells of anus NOS

R85.69 **Abnormal cytological findings in specimens from other digestive organs and abdominal cavity**

R85.7 **Abnormal histological findings in specimens from digestive organs and abdominal cavity**

✓5ᵗʰ **R85.8** **Other abnormal findings in specimens from digestive organs and abdominal cavity**

R85.81 **Anal high risk human papillomavirus [HPV] DNA test positive**
>> EXCLUDES 1   *anogenital warts due to human papillomavirus (HPV) (A63.0)*
>> *condyloma acuminatum (A63.0)*

R85.82 **Anal low risk human papillomavirus [HPV] DNA test positive**
> Use additional code for associated human papillomavirus (B97.7)

R85.89 **Other abnormal findings in specimens from digestive organs and abdominal cavity**
> Abnormal chromosomal findings in specimens from digestive organs and abdominal cavity

R85.9 **Unspecified abnormal finding in specimens from digestive organs and abdominal cavity**   ▽

✓4ᵗʰ **R86** **Abnormal findings in specimens from male genital organs**
> INCLUDES   abnormal findings in prostatic secretions
> abnormal findings in semen, seminal fluid
> abnormal spermatozoa
>> EXCLUDES 1   *azoospermia (N46.0-)*
>> *oligospermia (N46.1-)*

R86.0 **Abnormal level of enzymes in specimens from male genital organs**   ♂

R86.1 **Abnormal level of hormones in specimens from male genital organs**   ♂

R86.2 **Abnormal level of other drugs, medicaments and biological substances in specimens from male genital organs**   ♂

R86.3 **Abnormal level of substances chiefly nonmedicinal as to source in specimens from male genital organs**   ♂

R86.4 **Abnormal immunological findings in specimens from male genital organs**   ♂

R86.5 **Abnormal microbiological findings in specimens from male genital organs**   ♂
> Positive culture findings in specimens from male genital organs
>> EXCLUDES 1   *colonization status (Z22.-)*

R86.6 **Abnormal cytological findings in specimens from male genital organs**   ♂

R86.7 **Abnormal histological findings in specimens from male genital organs**   ♂

R86.8 **Other abnormal findings in specimens from male genital organs**   ♂
> Abnormal chromosomal findings in specimens from male genital organs

R86.9 **Unspecified abnormal finding in specimens from male genital organs**   ♂▽

✓4ᵗʰ **R87** **Abnormal findings in specimens from female genital organs**
> INCLUDES   abnormal findings in secretion and smears from cervix uteri
> abnormal findings in secretion and smears from vagina
> abnormal findings in secretion and smears from vulva

R87.0 **Abnormal level of enzymes in specimens from female genital organs**   ♀

R87.1 **Abnormal level of hormones in specimens from female genital organs**   ♀

R87.2 **Abnormal level of other drugs, medicaments and biological substances in specimens from female genital organs**   ♀

R87.3 **Abnormal level of substances chiefly nonmedicinal as to source in specimens from female genital organs**   ♀

R87.4 **Abnormal immunological findings in specimens from female genital organs**   ♀

R87.5 **Abnormal microbiological findings in specimens from female genital organs**   ♀
> Positive culture findings in specimens from female genital organs
>> EXCLUDES 1   *colonization status (Z22.-)*

☑5ᵗʰ **R87.6** **Abnormal cytological findings in specimens from female genital organs**

☑6ᵗʰ **R87.61** **Abnormal cytological findings in specimens from cervix uteri**

EXCLUDES 1 abnormal cytological findings in specimens from other female genital organs (R87.69)
abnormal cytological findings in specimens from vagina (R87.62-)
carcinoma in situ of cervix uteri (histologically confirmed) (D06.-)
cervical intraepithelial neoplasia I [CIN I] (N87.0)
cervical intraepithelial neoplasia II [CIN II] (N87.1)
cervical intraepithelial neoplasia III [CIN III] (D06.-)
dysplasia (mild) (moderate) of cervix uteri (histologically confirmed) (N87.-)
severe dysplasia of cervix uteri (histologically confirmed) (D06.-)

EXCLUDES 2 cervical high risk human papillomavirus (HPV) DNA test positive (R87.810)
cervical low risk human papillomavirus (HPV) DNA test positive (R87.820)

R87.610 **Atypical squamous cells of undetermined significance on cytologic smear of cervix [ASC-US]** ♀

R87.611 **Atypical squamous cells cannot exclude high grade squamous intraepithelial lesion on cytologic smear of cervix [ASC-H]** ♀

R87.612 **Low grade squamous intraepithelial lesion on cytologic smear of cervix [LGSIL]** ♀

R87.613 **High grade squamous intraepithelial lesion on cytologic smear of cervix [HGSIL]** ♀

R87.614 **Cytologic evidence of malignancy on smear of cervix** ♀

R87.615 **Unsatisfactory cytologic smear of cervix** ♀
Inadequate sample of cytologic smear of cervix

R87.616 **Satisfactory cervical smear but lacking transformation zone** ♀

R87.618 **Other abnormal cytological findings on specimens from cervix uteri** ♀

R87.619 **Unspecified abnormal cytological findings in specimens from cervix uteri** ♀ ▽
Abnormal cervical cytology NOS
Abnormal Papanicolaou smear of cervix NOS
Abnormal thin preparation smear of cervix NOS
Atypical endocervial cells of cervix NOS
Atypical endometrial cells of cervix NOS
Atypical glandular cells of cervix NOS

☑6ᵗʰ **R87.62** **Abnormal cytological findings in specimens from vagina**
Use additional code to identify acquired absence of uterus and cervix, if applicable (Z90.71-)

EXCLUDES 1 abnormal cytological findings in specimens from cervix uteri (R87.61-)
abnormal cytological findings in specimens from other female genital organs (R87.69)
carcinoma in situ of vagina (histologically confirmed) (D07.2)
dysplasia (mild) (moderate) of vagina (histologically confirmed) (N89.-)
severe dysplasia of vagina (histologically confirmed) (D07.2)
vaginal intraepithelial neoplasia I [VAIN I] (N89.0)
vaginal intraepithelial neoplasia II [VAIN II] (N89.1)
vaginal intraepithelial neoplasia III [VAIN III] (D07.2)

EXCLUDES 2 vaginal high risk human papillomavirus (HPV) DNA test positive (R87.811)
vaginal low risk human papillomavirus (HPV) DNA test positive (R87.821)

R87.620 **Atypical squamous cells of undetermined significance on cytologic smear of vagina [ASC-US]** ♀

R87.621 **Atypical squamous cells cannot exclude high grade squamous intraepithelial lesion on cytologic smear of vagina [ASC-H]** ♀

R87.622 **Low grade squamous intraepithelial lesion on cytologic smear of vagina [LGSIL]** ♀

R87.623 **High grade squamous intraepithelial lesion on cytologic smear of vagina [HGSIL]** ♀

R87.624 **Cytologic evidence of malignancy on smear of vagina** ♀

R87.625 **Unsatisfactory cytologic smear of vagina** ♀
Inadequate sample of cytologic smear of vagina

R87.628 **Other abnormal cytological findings on specimens from vagina** ♀

R87.629 **Unspecified abnormal cytological findings in specimens from vagina** ♀ ▽
Abnormal Papanicolaou smear of vagina NOS
Abnormal thin preparation smear of vagina NOS
Abnormal vaginal cytology NOS
Atypical endocervical cells of vagina NOS
Atypical endometrial cells of vagina NOS
Atypical glandular cells of vagina NOS

R87.69 **Abnormal cytological findings in specimens from other female genital organs** ♀
Abnormal cytological findings in specimens from female genital organs NOS

EXCLUDES 1 dysplasia of vulva (histologically confirmed) (N90.0-N90.3)

R87.7 **Abnormal histological findings in specimens from female genital organs** ♀

EXCLUDES 1 carcinoma in situ (histologically confirmed) of female genital organs (D06-D07.3)
cervical intraepithelial neoplasia I [CIN I] (N87.0)
cervical intraepithelial neoplasia II [CIN II] (N87.1)
cervical intraepithelial neoplasia III [CIN III] (D06.-)
dysplasia (mild) (moderate) of cervix uteri (histologically confirmed) (N87.-)
dysplasia (mild) (moderate) of vagina (histologically confirmed) (N89.-)
severe dysplasia of cervix uteri (histologically confirmed) (D06.-)
severe dysplasia of vagina (histologically confirmed) (D07.2)
vaginal intraepithelial neoplasia I [VAIN I] (N89.0)
vaginal intraepithelial neoplasia II [VAIN II] (N89.1)
vaginal intraepithelial neoplasia III [VAIN III] (D07.2)

☑5ᵗʰ **R87.8** **Other abnormal findings in specimens from female genital organs**

☑6ᵗʰ **R87.81** **High risk human papillomavirus [HPV] DNA test positive from female genital organs**

EXCLUDES 1 anogenital warts due to human papillomavirus (HPV) (A63.0)
condyloma acuminatum (A63.0)

R87.810 **Cervical high risk human papillomavirus [HPV] DNA test positive** ♀

R87.811 **Vaginal high risk human papillomavirus [HPV] DNA test positive** ♀

☑6ᵗʰ **R87.82** **Low risk human papillomavirus [HPV] DNA test positive from female genital organs**
Use additional code for associated human papillomavirus (B97.7)

R87.820 **Cervical low risk human papillomavirus [HPV] DNA test positive** ♀

R87.821 **Vaginal low risk human papillomavirus [HPV] DNA test positive** ♀

R87.89 **Other abnormal findings in specimens from female genital organs** ♀
Abnormal chromosomal findings in specimens from female genital organs

R87.9 **Unspecified abnormal finding in specimens from female genital organs** ♀ ▽

✓4ᵗʰ **R88** **Abnormal findings in other body fluids and substances**

     R88.0 **Cloudy (hemodialysis) (peritoneal) dialysis effluent**

     R88.8 **Abnormal findings in other body fluids and substances**

✓4ᵗʰ **R89** **Abnormal findings in specimens from other organs, systems and tissues**

     INCLUDES   abnormal findings in nipple discharge
                        abnormal findings in synovial fluid
                        abnormal findings in wound secretions

     R89.0 **Abnormal level of enzymes in specimens from other organs, systems and tissues**

     R89.1 **Abnormal level of hormones in specimens from other organs, systems and tissues**

     R89.2 **Abnormal level of other drugs, medicaments and biological substances in specimens from other organs, systems and tissues**

     R89.3 **Abnormal level of substances chiefly nonmedicinal as to source in specimens from other organs, systems and tissues**

     R89.4 **Abnormal immunological findings in specimens from other organs, systems and tissues**

     R89.5 **Abnormal microbiological findings in specimens from other organs, systems and tissues**
         Positive culture findings in specimens from other organs, systems and tissues
         EXCLUDES 1   colonization status (Z22.-)

     R89.6 **Abnormal cytological findings in specimens from other organs, systems and tissues**

     R89.7 **Abnormal histological findings in specimens from other organs, systems and tissues**

     R89.8 **Other abnormal findings in specimens from other organs, systems and tissues**
         Abnormal chromosomal findings in specimens from other organs, systems and tissues

     R89.9 **Unspecified abnormal finding in specimens from other organs, systems and tissues** ▽

Abnormal findings on diagnostic imaging and in function studies, without diagnosis (R90-R94)

     INCLUDES   nonspecific abnormal findings on diagnostic imaging by computerized axial tomography [CAT scan]
                       nonspecific abnormal findings on diagnostic imaging by magnetic resonance imaging [MRI][NMR]
                       nonspecific abnormal findings on diagnostic imaging by positron emission tomography [PET scan]
                       nonspecific abnormal findings on diagnostic imaging by thermography
                       nonspecific abnormal findings on diagnostic imaging by ultrasound [echogram]
                       nonspecific abnormal findings on diagnostic imaging by X-ray examination
     EXCLUDES 1   abnormal findings on antenatal screening of mother (O28.-)
                       diagnostic abnormal findings classified elsewhere—see Alphabetical Index

✓4ᵗʰ **R90** **Abnormal findings on diagnostic imaging of central nervous system**

     R90.0 **Intracranial space-occupying lesion found on diagnostic imaging of central nervous system**

     ✓5ᵗʰ **R90.8** **Other abnormal findings on diagnostic imaging of central nervous system**

         R90.81 **Abnormal echoencephalogram**

         R90.82 **White matter disease, unspecified** ▽

         R90.89 **Other abnormal findings on diagnostic imaging of central nervous system**
                 Other cerebrovascular abnormality found on diagnostic imaging of central nervous system

✓4ᵗʰ **R91** **Abnormal findings on diagnostic imaging of lung**

     R91.1 **Solitary pulmonary nodule**
         Coin lesion lung
         Solitary pulmonary nodule, subsegmental branch of the bronchial tree

     R91.8 **Other nonspecific abnormal finding of lung field**
         Lung mass NOS found on diagnostic imaging of lung
         Pulmonary infiltrate NOS
         Shadow, lung

✓4ᵗʰ **R92** **Abnormal and inconclusive findings on diagnostic imaging of breast**

     R92.0 **Mammographic microcalcification found on diagnostic imaging of breast**
         EXCLUDES 2   mammographic calcification (calculus) found on diagnostic imaging of breast (R92.1)
         DEF: Calcium and cellular debris deposits in the breast that cannot be felt but can be detected on a mammogram; can be a sign of cancer, benign conditions, or changes in the breast tissue as a result of inflammation, injury, or obstructed duct.

     R92.1 **Mammographic calcification found on diagnostic imaging of breast**
         Mammographic calculus found on diagnostic imaging of breast

     R92.2 **Inconclusive mammogram**
         Dense breasts NOS
         Inconclusive mammogram NEC
         Inconclusive mammography due to dense breasts
         Inconclusive mammography NEC
         AHA: 2015, 1Q, 24

     R92.8 **Other abnormal and inconclusive findings on diagnostic imaging of breast**

✓4ᵗʰ **R93** **Abnormal findings on diagnostic imaging of other body structures**

     R93.0 **Abnormal findings on diagnostic imaging of skull and head, not elsewhere classified**
         EXCLUDES 1   intracranial space-occupying lesion found on diagnostic imaging (R90.0)

     R93.1 **Abnormal findings on diagnostic imaging of heart and coronary circulation**
         Abnormal echocardiogram NOS
         Abnormal heart shadow

     R93.2 **Abnormal findings on diagnostic imaging of liver and biliary tract**
         Nonvisualization of gallbladder

     R93.3 **Abnormal findings on diagnostic imaging of other parts of digestive tract**

     ✓5ᵗʰ **R93.4** **Abnormal findings on diagnostic imaging of urinary organs**
         EXCLUDES 2   hypertrophy of kidney (N28.81)

         R93.41 **Abnormal radiologic findings on diagnostic imaging of renal pelvis, ureter, or bladder**
                 Filling defect of bladder found on diagnostic imaging
                 Filling defect of renal pelvis found on diagnostic imaging
                 Filling defect of ureter found on diagnostic imaging

         ✓6ᵗʰ **R93.42** **Abnormal radiologic findings on diagnositic imaging of kidney**

             R93.421 **Abnormal radiologic findings on diagnositic imaging of right kidney**

             R93.422 **Abnormal radiologic findings on diagnositic imaging of left kidney**

             R93.429 **Abnormal radiologic findings on diagnositic imaging of unspecified kidney** ▽

         R93.49 **Abnormal radiologic findings on diagnositic imaging of other urinary organs**

     R93.5 **Abnormal findings on diagnostic imaging of other abdominal regions, including retroperitoneum**

     R93.6 **Abnormal findings on diagnostic imaging of limbs**
         EXCLUDES 2   abnormal finding in skin and subcutaneous tissue (R93.8)

     R93.7 **Abnormal findings on diagnostic imaging of other parts of musculoskeletal system**
         EXCLUDES 2   abnormal findings on diagnostic imaging of skull (R93.0)

     R93.8 **Abnormal findings on diagnostic imaging of other specified body structures**
         Abnormal finding by radioisotope localization of placenta
         Abnormal radiological finding in skin and subcutaneous tissue
         Mediastinal shift

     R93.9 **Diagnostic imaging inconclusive due to excess body fat of patient**

✓4ᵗʰ **R94** **Abnormal results of function studies**
     INCLUDES   abnormal results of radionuclide [radioisotope] uptake studies
                       abnormal results of scintigraphy

     ✓5ᵗʰ **R94.0** **Abnormal results of function studies of central nervous system**

         R94.01 **Abnormal electroencephalogram [EEG]**

         R94.02 **Abnormal brain scan**

EXCLUDES 1 Not coded here   EXCLUDES 2 Not included here   N Newborn Age: 0   P Pediatric Age: 0-17   M Maternity Age: 12-55   A Adult Age: 15-124

904   ICD-10-CM 2018

R94.09   **Abnormal results of other function studies of central nervous system**

☑5ᵗʰ **R94.1** **Abnormal results of function studies of peripheral nervous system and special senses**

     ☑6ᵗʰ **R94.11** **Abnormal results of function studies of eye**

         R94.110   **Abnormal electro-oculogram [EOG]**

         R94.111   **Abnormal electroretinogram [ERG]**
             Abnormal retinal function study

         R94.112   **Abnormal visually evoked potential [VEP]**

         R94.113   **Abnormal oculomotor study**

         R94.118   **Abnormal results of other function studies of eye**

     ☑6ᵗʰ **R94.12** **Abnormal results of function studies of ear and other special senses**
          AHA: 2016, 3Q, 17

         R94.120   **Abnormal auditory function study**

         R94.121   **Abnormal vestibular function study**

         R94.128   **Abnormal results of other function studies of ear and other special senses**

     ☑6ᵗʰ **R94.13** **Abnormal results of function studies of peripheral nervous system**

         R94.130   **Abnormal response to nerve stimulation, unspecified** ▽

         R94.131   **Abnormal electromyogram [EMG]**
             EXCLUDES 1   *electromyogram of eye (R94.113)*

         R94.138   **Abnormal results of other function studies of peripheral nervous system**

R94.2   **Abnormal results of pulmonary function studies**
     Reduced ventilatory capacity
     Reduced vital capacity

☑5ᵗʰ **R94.3** **Abnormal results of cardiovascular function studies**

     R94.30   **Abnormal result of cardiovascular function study, unspecified** ▽

     R94.31   **Abnormal electrocardiogram [ECG] [EKG]**
         EXCLUDES 1   *long QT syndrome (I45.81)*

     R94.39   **Abnormal result of other cardiovascular function study**
         Abnormal electrophysiological intracardiac studies
         Abnormal phonocardiogram
         Abnormal vectorcardiogram

R94.4   **Abnormal results of kidney function studies**
     Abnormal renal function test

R94.5   **Abnormal results of liver function studies**

R94.6   **Abnormal results of thyroid function studies**

R94.7   **Abnormal results of other endocrine function studies**
     EXCLUDES 2   *abnormal glucose (R73.0-)*

R94.8   **Abnormal results of function studies of other organs and systems**
     Abnormal basal metabolic rate [BMR]
     Abnormal bladder function test
     Abnormal splenic function test

Abnormal tumor markers (R97)

☑4ᵗʰ **R97** **Abnormal tumor markers**
     Elevated tumor associated antigens [TAA]
     Elevated tumor specific antigens [TSA]

     R97.0   **Elevated carcinoembryonic antigen [CEA]**

     R97.1   **Elevated cancer antigen 125 [CA 125]**   ♀

     ☑5ᵗʰ **R97.2** **Elevated prostate specific antigen [PSA]**

         R97.20   **Elevated prostate specific antigen [PSA]**   Ⓐ♂

         R97.21   **Rising PSA following treatment for malignant neoplasm of prostate**   Ⓐ♂

     R97.8   **Other abnormal tumor markers**

Ill-defined and unknown cause of mortality (R99)

R99   **Ill-defined and unknown cause of mortality** ▽
     Death (unexplained) NOS
     Unspecified cause of mortality

Chapter 19. Injury, Poisoning, and Certain Other Consequences of External Causes (S00–T88)

Chapter Specific Guidelines with Coding Examples

The chapter specific guidelines from the ICD-10-CM Official Guidelines for Coding and Reporting have been provided below. Along with these guidelines are coding examples, contained in the shaded boxes, that have been developed to help illustrate the coding and/or sequencing guidance found in these guidelines.

a. Application of 7th characters in Chapter 19

Most categories in chapter 19 have a 7th character requirement for each applicable code. Most categories in this chapter have three 7th character values (with the exception of fractures): A, initial encounter, D, subsequent encounter and S, sequela. Categories for traumatic fractures have additional 7th character values. While the patient may be seen by a new or different provider over the course of treatment for an injury, assignment of the 7th character is based on whether the patient is undergoing active treatment and not whether the provider is seeing the patient for the first time.

For complication codes, active treatment refers to treatment for the condition described by the code, even though it may be related to an earlier precipitating problem. For example, code T84.50XA, Infection and inflammatory reaction due to unspecified internal joint prosthesis, initial encounter, is used when active treatment is provided for the infection, even though the condition relates to the prosthetic device, implant or graft that was placed at a previous encounter.

7th character "A", initial encounter is used for each encounter where the patient is receiving active treatment for the condition.

> Patient evaluated after fall from a skateboard onto the sidewalk, x-rays identify a nondisplaced fracture to the distal pole of the right scaphoid bone. The patient is placed in a cast.
>
> | | |
> |---|---|
> | S62.014A | Nondisplaced fracture of distal pole of navicular [scaphoid] bone of right wrist, initial encounter for closed fracture |
> | V00.131A | Fall from skateboard, initial encounter |
> | Y93.51 | Activity, roller skating (inline) and skateboarding |
> | Y92.480 | Sidewalk as the place of occurrence of the external cause |
> | Y99.8 | Other external cause status |
>
> *Explanation:* This fracture would be coded with a seventh character A for initial encounter because the patient received x-rays to identify the site of the fracture and treatment was rendered; this would be considered active treatment.

7th character "D" subsequent encounter is used for encounters after the patient has completed active treatment of the condition and is receiving routine care for the condition during the healing or recovery phase.

> Patient seen in follow-up after fall from a skateboard onto the sidewalk resulted in casting of the right arm. X-rays are taken to evaluate how well the nondisplaced fracture to the distal pole of the right scaphoid bone is healing. The physician feels the fracture is healing appropriately; no adjustments to the cast are made.
>
> | | |
> |---|---|
> | S62.014D | Nondisplaced fracture of distal pole of navicular [scaphoid] bone of right wrist, subsequent encounter for fracture with routine healing |
> | V00.131D | Fall from skateboard, subsequent encounter |
>
> *Explanation:* This fracture would be coded with a seventh character D for subsequent encounter, whether the same physician who provided the initial cast application or a different physician is now seeing the patient. Although the patient received x-rays, the intent of the x-rays was to assess how the fracture was healing. There was no active treatment rendered and the visit is therefore considered a subsequent encounter.

The aftercare Z codes should not be used for aftercare for conditions such as injuries or poisonings, where 7th characters are provided to identify subsequent care. For example, for aftercare of an injury, assign the acute injury code with the 7th character "D" (subsequent encounter).

7th character "S", sequela, is for use for complications or conditions that arise as a direct result of a condition, such as scar formation after a burn.

The scars are sequelae of the burn. When using 7th character "S", it is necessary to use both the injury code that precipitated the sequela and the code for the sequela itself. The "S" is added only to the injury code, not the sequela code. The 7th character "S" identifies the injury responsible for the sequela. The specific type of sequela (e.g. scar) is sequenced first, followed by the injury code.

See Section I.B.10 Sequelae, (Late Effects)

> Patient with a history of a nondisplaced fracture to the distal pole of the right scaphoid bone due to a fall from a skateboard is seen for evaluation of arthritis to the right wrist that has developed as a consequence of the traumatic fracture.
>
> | | |
> |---|---|
> | M12.531 | Traumatic arthropathy, right wrist |
> | S62.014S | Nondisplaced fracture of distal pole of navicular [scaphoid] bone of right wrist, sequela |
> | V00.131S | Fall from skateboard, sequela |
>
> *Explanation:* The code identifying the specific sequela condition (traumatic arthritis) should be coded first followed by the injury that instigated the development of the sequela (fracture). The scaphoid fracture injury code is given a 7th character S for sequela to represent its role as the inciting injury. The fracture has healed and is not being managed or treated on this admit and therefore is not applicable as a first listed or principal diagnosis. However, it is directly related to the development of the arthritis and should be appended as a secondary code to signify this cause and effect relationship.

b. Coding of injuries

When coding injuries, assign separate codes for each injury unless a combination code is provided, in which case the combination code is assigned. **Codes from category** T07, Unspecified multiple injuries should not be assigned in the inpatient setting unless information for a more specific code is not available. Traumatic injury codes (S00-T14.9) are not to be used for normal, healing surgical wounds or to identify complications of surgical wounds.

> 11-year-old girl fell from her horse, resulting in a laceration to her right forearm with several large pieces of wooden fragments embedded in the wound as well as abrasions to her right ear; in addition, her right shoulder was dislocated
>
> | | |
> |---|---|
> | S43.004A | Unspecified dislocation of right shoulder joint, initial encounter |
> | S51.821A | Laceration with foreign body of right forearm, initial encounter |
> | S00.411A | Abrasion of right ear, initial encounter |
> | V80.010A | Animal-rider injured by fall from or being thrown from horse in noncollision accident, initial encounter |
> | Y93.52 | Activity, horseback riding |
>
> *Explanation:* Each separate injury should be reported. The patient's injury to the forearm is reported with one combination code that captures both the laceration and the foreign body.

The code for the most serious injury, as determined by the provider and the focus of treatment, is sequenced first.

1) Superficial injuries

Superficial injuries such as abrasions or contusions are not coded when associated with more severe injuries of the same site.

2) Primary injury with damage to nerves/blood vessels

When a primary injury results in minor damage to peripheral nerves or blood vessels, the primary injury is sequenced first with additional code(s) for injuries to nerves and spinal cord (such as category S04), and/or injury to blood vessels (such as category S15). When the primary injury is to the blood vessels or nerves, that injury should be sequenced first.

c. Coding of traumatic fractures

The principles of multiple coding of injuries should be followed in coding fractures. Fractures of specified sites are coded individually by site in accordance with both the provisions within categories S02, S12, S22, S32, S42, S49, S52, S59, S62, S72, S79, S82, S89, S92 and the level of detail furnished by medical record content.

A fracture not indicated as open or closed should be coded to closed. A fracture not indicated whether displaced or not displaced should be coded to displaced.

More specific guidelines are as follows:

1) Initial vs. subsequent encounter for fractures

Traumatic fractures are coded using the appropriate 7th character for initial encounter (A, B, C) for each encounter where the patient is receiving active treatment for the fracture. The appropriate 7th character for initial encounter should also be assigned for a patient who delayed seeking treatment for the fracture or nonunion.

Fractures are coded using the appropriate 7th character for subsequent care for encounters after the patient has completed active treatment of the fracture and is receiving routine care for the fracture during the healing or recovery phase.

Care for complications of surgical treatment for fracture repairs during the healing or recovery phase should be coded with the appropriate complication codes.

Care of complications of fractures, such as malunion and nonunion, should be reported with the appropriate 7th character for subsequent care with nonunion (K, M, N,) or subsequent care with malunion (P, Q, R).

Malunion/nonunion: The appropriate 7th character for initial encounter should also be assigned for a patient who delayed seeking treatment for the fracture or nonunion.

Female patient fell during a forest hiking excursion almost six months ago and until recently did not feel she needed to seek medical attention for her left ankle pain; x-rays show nonunion of lateral malleolus and surgery has been scheduled

S82.62XA	Displaced fracture of lateral malleolus of left fibula, initial encounter for closed fracture
W01.0XXA	Fall on same level from slipping, tripping and stumbling without subsequent striking against object, initial encounter
Y92.821	Forest as place of occurrence of the external cause
Y93.01	Activity, walking, marching and hiking
Y99.8	Other external cause status

Explanation: A seventh character of A is used for the lateral malleolus nonunion fracture to signify that the fracture is receiving active treatment. The delayed care for the fracture has resulted in a nonunion, but capturing the nonunion in the seventh character is trumped by the provision of active care.

The open fracture designations in the assignment of the 7th character for fractures of the forearm, femur and lower leg, including ankle are based on the Gustilo open fracture classification. When the Gustilo classification type is not specified for an open fracture, the 7th character for open fracture type I or II should be assigned (B, E, H, M, Q).

A code from category M80, not a traumatic fracture code, should be used for any patient with known osteoporosis who suffers a fracture, even if the patient had a minor fall or trauma, if that fall or trauma would not usually break a normal, healthy bone.

See Section I.C.13. Osteoporosis.

The aftercare Z codes should not be used for aftercare for traumatic fractures. For aftercare of a traumatic fracture, assign the acute fracture code with the appropriate 7th character.

2) Multiple fractures sequencing

Multiple fractures are sequenced in accordance with the severity of the fracture.

d. Coding of burns and corrosions

The ICD-10-CM makes a distinction between burns and corrosions. The burn codes are for thermal burns, except sunburns, that come from a heat source, such as a fire or hot appliance. The burn codes are also for burns resulting from electricity and radiation. Corrosions are burns due to chemicals. The guidelines are the same for burns and corrosions.

Current burns (T20-T25) are classified by depth, extent and by agent (X code). Burns are classified by depth as first degree (erythema), second degree (blistering), and third degree (full-thickness involvement). Burns of the eye and internal organs (T26-T28) are classified by site, but not by degree.

1) Sequencing of burn and related condition codes

Sequence first the code that reflects the highest degree of burn when more than one burn is present.

a. When the reason for the admission or encounter is for treatment of external multiple burns, sequence first the code that reflects the burn of the highest degree.

b. When a patient has both internal and external burns, the circumstances of admission govern the selection of the principal diagnosis or first-listed diagnosis.

c. When a patient is admitted for burn injuries and other related conditions such as smoke inhalation and/or respiratory failure, the circumstances of admission govern the selection of the principal or first-listed diagnosis.

Patient referred for minor first-degree burns to multiple sites of her right and left hands as well as severe smoke inhalation. While she was sleeping at home, a candle on her dresser lit the bedroom curtains on fire.

T59.811A	Toxic effect of smoke, accidental (unintentional), initial encounter
J70.5	Respiratory conditions due to smoke inhalation
T23.191A	Burn of first degree of multiple sites of right wrist and hand, initial encounter
T23.192A	Burn of first degree of multiple sites of left wrist and hand, initial encounter
X08.8XXA	Exposure to other specified smoke, fire and flames, initial encounter
Y99.8	Other exteranl cause status
Y92.003	Bedroom of unspecified non-institutional (private) residence as the place of occurrence of the external cause
Y93.84	Activity, sleeping

Explanation: Based on the documentation, the inhalation injury is more severe than the first-degree burns and is sequenced first. The burns to the hands are appended as secondary diagnoses.

2) Burns of the same local site

Classify burns of the same local site (three-character category level, T20-T28) but of different degrees to the subcategory identifying the highest degree recorded in the diagnosis.

10-year-old male patient is treated for third-degree burns of his right palm and second-degree burns of multiple right fingers; right thumb not affected

| T23.351A | Burn of third degree of right palm, initial encounter |

Explanation: Although there is a code for second-degree burns of multiple fingers, not including the thumb (T23.131-), this code falls in the same three-digit category that the third-degree burn of the right palm falls under, category T23. Only the subcategory identifying the highest degree is captured when different burn degrees are classified to a single category.

Patient is treated for third-degree burns of the scalp as well as second-degree burns to the back of the right hand

| T20.35XA | Burn of third degree of scalp [any part], initial encounter |
| T23.261A | Burn of second degree of back of right hand, initial encounter |

Explanation: Since burns to the hand and scalp are classified to two different three-digit categories, both burns may be reported as they represent distinct sites.

3) Non-healing burns

Non-healing burns are coded as acute burns.

Necrosis of burned skin should be coded as a non-healed burn.

4) Infected burn

For any documented infected burn site, use an additional code for the infection.

5) Assign separate codes for each burn site

When coding burns, assign separate codes for each burn site. Category T30, Burn and corrosion, body region unspecified is extremely vague and should rarely be used.

6) Burns and corrosions classified according to extent of body surface involved

Assign codes from category T31, Burns classified according to extent of body surface involved, or T32, Corrosions classified according to extent of body surface involved, when the site of the burn is not specified or when there is a need for additional data. It is advisable to use category T31 as additional coding when needed to provide data for evaluating burn mortality, such as that needed by burn units. It is also advisable to use category T31 as an additional code for reporting purposes when there is mention of a third-degree burn involving 20 percent or more of the body surface.

Categories T31 and T32 are based on the classic "rule of nines" in estimating body surface involved: head and neck are assigned nine percent, each arm nine percent, each leg 18 percent, the anterior trunk 18 percent, posterior trunk 18 percent, and genitalia one percent. Providers may change these percentage assignments where necessary to accommodate infants and children who have proportionately larger heads than adults, and patients who have large buttocks, thighs, or abdomen that involve burns.

Patient seen for dressing change after he accidentally spilled acetic acid on himself two days ago. The second-degree burns to his right thigh, covering about 3 percent of his body surface, are healing appropriately.

T54.2X1D	**Toxic effect of corrosive acids and acid-like substances, accidental (unintentional), subsequent encounter**
T24.611D	**Corrosion of second degree of right thigh, subsequent encounter**
T32.0	**Corrosions involving less than 10% of body surface**

Explanation: Code T32.0 provides additional information as to how much of the patient's body was affected by the corrosive substance.

7) Encounters for treatment of sequela of burns

Encounters for the treatment of the late effects of burns or corrosions (i.e., scars or joint contractures) should be coded with a burn or corrosion code with the 7th character "S" for sequela.

8) Sequelae with a late effect code and current burn

When appropriate, both a code for a current burn or corrosion with 7th character "A" or "D" and a burn or corrosion code with 7th character "S" may be assigned on the same record (when both a current burn and sequelae of an old burn exist). Burns and corrosions do not heal at the same rate and a current healing wound may still exist with sequela of a healed burn or corrosion.

See Section I.B.10 Sequela (Late Effects)

Female patient seen for second-degree burn to the left ear; she also has significant scarring on her left elbow from a third-degree burn from childhood

T20.212A	**Burn of second degree of left ear [any part, except ear drum], initial encounter**
L90.5	**Scar conditions and fibrosis of skin**
T22.322S	**Burn of third degree of left elbow, sequela**

Explanation: The patient is being seen for management of a current second-degree burn, which is reflected in the code by appending the seventh character of A, indicating active treatment or management of this burn. The elbow scarring is a sequela of a previous third-degree burn. The sequela condition precedes the original burn injury, which is appended with a seventh character of S.

9) Use of an external cause code with burns and corrosions

An external cause code should be used with burns and corrosions to identify the source and intent of the burn, as well as the place where it occurred.

e. Adverse effects, poisoning, underdosing and toxic effects

Codes in categories T36-T65 are combination codes that include the substance that was taken as well as the intent. No additional external cause code is required for poisonings, toxic effects, adverse effects and underdosing codes.

1) Do not code directly from the Table of Drugs

Do not code directly from the Table of Drugs and Chemicals. Always refer back to the Tabular List.

2) Use as many codes as necessary to describe

Use as many codes as necessary to describe completely all drugs, medicinal or biological substances.

3) If the same code would describe the causative agent

If the same code would describe the causative agent for more than one adverse reaction, poisoning, toxic effect or underdosing, assign the code only once.

4) If two or more drugs, medicinal or biological substances

If two or more drugs, medicinal or biological substances are reported, code each individually unless a combination code is listed in the Table of Drugs and Chemicals.

5) The occurrence of drug toxicity is classified in ICD-10-CM as follows:

(a) Adverse effect

When coding an adverse effect of a drug that has been correctly prescribed and properly administered, assign the appropriate code for the nature of the adverse effect followed by the appropriate code for the adverse effect of the drug (T36-T50). The code for the drug should have a 5th or 6th character "5" (for example T36.0X5-) Examples of the nature of an adverse effect are tachycardia, delirium, gastrointestinal hemorrhaging, vomiting, hypokalemia, hepatitis, renal failure, or respiratory failure.

Patient seen for stomach pain and jaundice, indicated by physician as possible side-effects of Inderal, recently started for hypertension. Inderal was discontinued and the patient switched to Atenolol instead.

R10.9	**Unspecified abdominal pain**
R17	**Unspecified jaundice**
T44.7X5A	**Adverse effect of beta-adrenoreceptor antagonists, initial encounter**
I10	**Essential (primary) hypertension**

Explanation: The side-effects caused by the drug are listed first, followed by the code for the adverse effect of the drug to capture the specific drug that was used.

(b) Poisoning

When coding a poisoning or reaction to the improper use of a medication (e.g., overdose, wrong substance given or taken in error, wrong route of administration), first assign the appropriate code from categories T36-T50. The poisoning codes have an associated intent as their 5th or 6th character (accidental, intentional self-harm, assault and undetermined. If the intent of the poisoning is unknown or unspecified, code the intent as accidental intent. The undetermined intent is only for use if the documentation in the record specifies that the intent cannot be determined. Use additional code(s) for all manifestations of poisonings.

If there is also a diagnosis of abuse or dependence of the substance, the abuse or dependence is assigned as an additional code.

Examples of poisoning include:

(i)   Error was made in drug prescription

Errors made in drug prescription or in the administration of the drug by provider, nurse, patient, or other person.

(ii)   Overdose of a drug intentionally taken

If an overdose of a drug was intentionally taken or administered and resulted in drug toxicity, it would be coded as a poisoning.

(iii)   Nonprescribed drug taken with correctly prescribed and properly administered drug

If a nonprescribed drug or medicinal agent was taken in combination with a correctly prescribed and properly administered drug, any drug toxicity or other reaction resulting from the interaction of the two drugs would be classified as a poisoning.

(iv)   Interaction of drug(s) and alcohol

When a reaction results from the interaction of a drug(s) and alcohol, this would be classified as poisoning.

See Section I.C.4. if poisoning is the result of insulin pump malfunctions.

(c) Underdosing

Underdosing refers to taking less of a medication than is prescribed by a provider or a manufacturer's instruction. For underdosing, assign the code from categories T36-T50 (fifth or sixth character "6").

Codes for underdosing should never be assigned as principal or first-listed codes. If a patient has a relapse or exacerbation of the medical

Chapter 19. Injury, Poisoning, and Certain Other Consequences of External Causes

condition for which the drug is prescribed because of the reduction in dose, then the medical condition itself should be coded.

Noncompliance (Z91.12-, Z91.13-) or complication of care (Y63.6-Y63.9) codes are to be used with an underdosing code to indicate intent, if known.

> Patient referred for atrial fibrillation with history of chronic atrial fibrillation for which she is prescribed amiodarone. Financial concerns have left the patient unable to pay for her prescriptions and she has been skipping her amiodarone dose every other day to offset the cost.
>
> **I48.2**   **Chronic atrial fibrillation**
>
> **T46.2X6A**   **Underdosing of other antidysrhythmic drugs, initial encounter**
>
> **Z91.120**   **Patient's intentional underdosing of medication regimen due to financial hardship**
>
> *Explanation:* By skipping her amiodarone pill every other day, the patient's atrial fibrillation returned. The condition for which the drug was being taken is reported first, followed by an underdosing code to show that the patient was not adhering to her prescription regiment. The Z code helps elaborate on the patient's social and/or economic circumstances that led to the patient taking less then what she was prescribed.

(d) Toxic effects

When a harmful substance is ingested or comes in contact with a person, this is classified as a toxic effect. The toxic effect codes are in categories T51-T65.

Toxic effect codes have an associated intent: accidental, intentional self-harm, assault and undetermined.

f. Adult and child abuse, neglect and other maltreatment

Sequence first the appropriate code from categories T74.- (Adult and child abuse, neglect and other maltreatment, confirmed) or T76.- (Adult and child abuse, neglect and other maltreatment, suspected) for abuse, neglect and other maltreatment, followed by any accompanying mental health or injury code(s).

If the documentation in the medical record states abuse or neglect it is coded as confirmed (T74.-). It is coded as suspected if it is documented as suspected (T76.-).

For cases of confirmed abuse or neglect an external cause code from the assault section (X92-Y09) should be added to identify the cause of any physical injuries. A perpetrator code (Y07) should be added when the perpetrator of the abuse is known. For suspected cases of abuse or neglect, do not report external cause or perpetrator code.

If a suspected case of abuse, neglect or mistreatment is ruled out during an encounter code Z04.71, Encounter for examination and observation following alleged physical adult abuse, ruled out, or code Z04.72, Encounter for examination and observation following alleged child physical abuse, ruled out, should be used, not a code from T76.

If a suspected case of alleged rape or sexual abuse is ruled out during an encounter code Z04.41, Encounter for examination and observation following alleged adult rape or code Z04.42, Encounter for examination and observation following alleged child rape, should be used, not a code from T76.

See Section I.C.15. Abuse in a pregnant patient.

g. Complications of care

1) General guidelines for complications of care

(a) Documentation of complications of care

> *See Section I.B.16. for information on documentation of complications of care.*

2) Pain due to medical devices

Pain associated with devices, implants or grafts left in a surgical site (for example painful hip prosthesis) is assigned to the appropriate code(s) found in Chapter 19, Injury, poisoning, and certain other consequences of external causes. Specific codes for pain due to medical devices are found in the T code section of the ICD-10-CM. Use additional code(s) from category G89 to identify acute or chronic pain due to presence of the device, implant or graft (G89.18 or G89.28).

> Chronic left breast pain secondary to breast implant
>
> **T85.848A**   **Pain due to other internal prosthetic devices, implants and grafts, initial encounter**
>
> **N64.4**   **Mastodynia**
>
> **G89.28**   **Other chronic postprocedural pain**
>
> *Explanation:* As the pain is a complication related to the breast implant, the complication code is sequenced first. The T code does not describe the site or type of pain, so additional codes may be appended to indicate that the patient is experiencing chronic pain in the breast.

3) Transplant complications

(a) Transplant complications other than kidney

Codes under category T86, Complications of transplanted organs and tissues, are for use for both complications and rejection of transplanted organs. A transplant complication code is only assigned if the complication affects the function of the transplanted organ. Two codes are required to fully describe a transplant complication: the appropriate code from category T86 and a secondary code that identifies the complication.

Pre-existing conditions or conditions that develop after the transplant are not coded as complications unless they affect the function of the transplanted organs.

See I.C.21. for transplant organ removal status

See I.C.2. for malignant neoplasm associated with transplanted organ.

(b) Kidney transplant complications

Patients who have undergone kidney transplant may still have some form of chronic kidney disease (CKD) because the kidney transplant may not fully restore kidney function. Code T86.1- should be assigned for documented complications of a kidney transplant, such as transplant failure or rejection or other transplant complication. Code T86.1- should not be assigned for post kidney transplant patients who have chronic kidney (CKD) unless a transplant complication such as transplant failure or rejection is documented. If the documentation is unclear as to whether the patient has a complication of the transplant, query the provider.

Conditions that affect the function of the transplanted kidney, other than CKD, should be assigned a code from subcategory T86.1, Complications of transplanted organ, Kidney, and a secondary code that identifies the complication.

For patients with CKD following a kidney transplant, but who do not have a complication such as failure or rejection, *see section I.C.14. Chronic kidney disease and kidney transplant status.*

> Patient seen for chronic kidney disease stage 2; history of successful kidney transplant with no complications identified
>
> **N18.2**   **Chronic kidney disease, stage 2 (mild)**
>
> **Z94.0**   **Kidney transplant status**
>
> *Explanation:* This patient's stage 2 CKD is not indicated as being due to the transplanted kidney but instead is just the residual disease the patient had prior to the transplant.

4) Complication codes that include the external cause

As with certain other T codes, some of the complications of care codes have the external cause included in the code. The code includes the nature of the complication as well as the type of procedure that caused the complication. No external cause code indicating the type of procedure is necessary for these codes.

5) Complications of care codes within the body system chapters

Intraoperative and postprocedural complication codes are found within the body system chapters with codes specific to the organs and structures of that body system. These codes should be sequenced first, followed by a code(s) for the specific complication, if applicable.

> During a spinal fusion procedure, the surgeon inadvertently punctured the dura. The midline durotomy was repaired, and the fusion procedure was completed.
>
> **G97.41**   **Accidental puncture or laceration of dura during a procedure**
>
> *Explanation:* The accidental durotomy is not coded to an injury code in chapter 19 but instead is categorized to the nervous system chapter.

Muscle/Tendon Table

ICD-10-CM categorizes certain muscles and tendons in the upper and lower extremities by their action (e.g., extension, flexion), their anatomical location (e.g., posterior, anterior), and/or whether they are intrinsic or extrinsic to a certain anatomical area. The Muscle/Tendon Table is provided at the beginning of chapters 13 and 19 as a resource to help users when code selection depends on one or more of these characteristics. A **TIP** has been placed at those categories and/or subcategories that relate to this table. Please note that this table is not all-inclusive, and proper code assignment should be based on the provider's documentation.

Body Region	Muscle	Extensor Tendon	Flexor Tendon	Other Tendon
Shoulder				
	Deltoid	Posterior deltoid	Anterior deltoid	
	Rotator cuff			
	Infraspinatus			Infraspinatus
	Subscapularis			Subscapularis
	Supraspinatus			Supraspinatus
	Teres minor			Teres minor
	Teres major	Teres major		
Upper arm				
	Anterior muscles			
	Biceps brachii — long head		Biceps brachii — long head	
	Biceps brachii — short head		Biceps brachii — short head	
	Brachialis		Brachialis	
	Coracobrachialis		Coracobrachialis	
	Posterior muscles			
	Triceps brachii	Triceps brachii		
Forearm				
	Anterior muscles			
	Flexors			
	Deep			
	Flexor digitorum profundus		Flexor digitorum profundus	
	Flexor pollicis longus		Flexor pollicis longus	
	Intermediate			
	Flexor digitorum superficialis		Flexor digitorum superficialis	
	Superficial			
	Flexor carpi radialis		Flexor carpi radialis	
	Flexor carpi ulnaris		Flexor carpi ulnaris	
	Palmaris longus		Palmaris longus	
	Pronators			
	Pronator quadratus			Pronator quadratus
	Pronator teres			Pronator teres
	Posterior muscles			
	Extensors			
	Deep			
	Abductor pollicis longus			Abductor pollicis longus
	Extensor indicis	Extensor indicis		
	Extensor pollicis brevis	Extensor pollicis brevis		
	Extensor pollicis longus	Extensor pollicis longus		
	Superficial			
	Brachioradialis			Brachioradialis
	Extensor carpi radialis brevis	Extensor carpi radialis brevis		
	Extensor carpi radialis longus	Extensor carpi radialis longus		
	Extensor carpi ulnaris	Extensor carpi ulnaris		
	Extensor digiti minimi	Extensor digiti minimi		
	Extensor digitorum	Extensor digitorum		
	Anconeus	Anconeus		
	Supinator			Supinator

Body Region	Muscle	Extensor Tendon	Flexor Tendon	Other Tendon
Hand				
Extrinsic — attach to a site in the forearm as well as a site in the hand with action related to hand movement at the wrist				
	Extensor carpi radialis brevis	Extensor carpi radialis brevis		
	Extensor carpi radialis longus	Extensor carpie radialis longus		
	Extensor carpi ulnaris	Extensor carpi ulnaris		
	Flexor carpi radialis		Flexor carpi radialis	
	Flexor carpi ulnaris		Flexor carpi ulnaris	
	Flexor digitorum superficialis		Flexor digitorum superficialis	
	Palmaris longus		Palmaris longus	
Extrinsic — attach to a site in the forearm as well as a site in the hand with action in the hand related to finger movement				
	Adductor pollicis longus			Adductor pollicis longus
	Extensor digiti minimi	Extensor digiti minimi		
	Extensor digitorum	Extensor digitorum		
	Extensor indicis	Extensor indicis		
	Flexor digitorum profundus		Flexor digitorum profundus	
	Flexor digitorum superficialis		Flexor digitorum superficialis	
Extrinsic — attach to a site in the forearm as well as a site in the hand with action in the hand related to thumb movement				
	Extensor pollicis brevis	Extensor pollicis brevis		
	Extensor pollicis longus	Extensor pollicis longus		
	Flexor pollicis longus		Flexor pollicis longus	
Intrinsic — found within the hand only				
	Adductor pollicis			Adductor pollicis
	Dorsal interossei	Dorsal interossei	Dorsal interossei	
	Lumbricals	Lumbricals	Lumbricals	
	Palmaris brevis			Palmaris brevis
	Palmar interossei	Palmar interossei	Palmar interossei	
	Hypothenar muscles			
	Abductor digiti minimi			Abductor digiti minimi
	Flexor digiti minimi brevis		Flexor digiti minimi brevis	
	Oppenens digiti minimi		Oppenens digiti minimi	
	Thenar muscles			
	Abductor pollicis brevis			Abductor pollicis brevis
	Flexor pollicis brevis		Flexor pollicis brevis	
	Oppenens pollicis		Oppenens pollicis	
Thigh				
	Anterior muscles			
	Iliopsoas		Iliopsoas	
	Pectineus		Pectineus	
	Quadriceps	Quadriceps		
	Rectus femoris	Rectus femoris — Extends knee	Rectus femoris — Flexes hip	
	Vastus intermedius	Vastus intermedius		
	Vastus lateralis	Vastus lateralis		
	Vastus medialis	Vastus medialis		
	Sartorius		Sartorius	
	Medial muscles			
	Adductor brevis			Adductor brevis
	Adductor longus			Adductor longus
	Adductor magnus			Adductor magnus
	Gracilis			Gracilis
	Obturator externus			Obturator externus
	Posterior muscles			
	Hamstring	Hamstring — Extends hip	Hamstring — Flexes knee	
	Biceps femoris	Biceps femoris	Biceps femoris	
	Semimembranosus	Semimembranosus	Semimembranosus	
	Semitendinosus	Semitendinosus	Semitendinosus	

Body Region	Muscle	Extensor Tendon	Flexor Tendon	Other Tendon
Lower leg				
	Anterior muscles			
	Extensor digitorum longus	Extensor digitorum longus		
	Extensor hallucis longus	Extensor hallucis longus		
	Fibularis (peroneus) tertius	Fibularis (peroneus) tertius		
	Tibialis anterior	Tibialis anterior		Tibialis anterior
	Lateral muscles			
	Fibularis (peroneus) brevis		Fibularis (peroneus) brevis	
	Fibularis (peroneus) longus		Fibularis (peroneus) longus	
	Posterior muscles			
	Deep			
	Flexor digitorum longus		Flexor digitorum longus	
	Flexor hallucis longus		Flexor hallucis longus	
	Popliteus		Popliteus	
	Tibialis posterior		Tibialis posterior	
	Superficial			
	Gastrocnemius		Gastrocnemius	
	Plantaris		Plantaris	
	Soleus		Soleus	
				Calcaneal (Achilles)
Ankle/Foot				
Extrinsic — attach to a site in the lower leg as well as a site in the foot with action related to foot movement at the ankle				
	Plantaris		Plantaris	
	Soleus		Soleus	
	Tibialis anterior	Tibialis anterior		
	Tibialis posterior		Tibialis posterior	
Extrinsic — attach to a site in the lower leg as well as a site in the foot with action in the foot related to toe movement				
	Extensor digitorum longus	Extensor digitorum longus		
	Extensor hallicus longus	Extensor hallicus longus		
	Flexor digitorum longus		Flexor digitorum longus	
	Flexor hallucis longus		Flexor hallucis longus	
Intrinsic — found within the ankle/foot only				
	Dorsal muscles			
	Extensor digitorum brevis	Extensor digitorum brevis		
	Extensor hallucis brevis	Extensor hallucis brevis		
	Plantar muscles			
	Abductor digiti minimi		Abductor digiti minimi	
	Abductor hallucis		Abductor hallucis	
	Dorsal interossei	Dorsal interossei	Dorsal interossei	
	Flexor digiti minimi brevis		Flexor digiti minimi brevis	
	Flexor digitorum brevis		Flexor digitorum brevis	
	Flexor hallucis brevis		Flexor hallucis brevis	
	Lumbricals	Lumbricals	Lumbricals	
	Quadratus plantae		Quadratus plantae	
	Plantar interossei	Plantar interossei	Plantar interossei	

Chapter 19. Injury, Poisoning and Certain Other Consequences of External Causes (S00-T88)

> **NOTE** Use secondary code(s) from Chapter 20, External causes of morbidity, to indicate cause of injury. Codes within the T section that include the external cause do not require an additional external cause code.
>
> Use additional code to identify any retained foreign body, if applicable (Z18.-)
>
> **EXCLUDES 1** birth trauma (P10-P15)
> obstetric trauma (O70-O71)
>
> **NOTE** The chapter uses the S-section for coding different types of injuries related to single body regions and the T-section to cover injuries to unspecified body regions as well as poisoning and certain other consequences of external causes.
>
> **AHA:** 2016, 2Q, 3-7; 2015, 4Q, 35-38; 2015, 3Q, 37-39, 40; 2015, 2Q, 6; 2015, 1Q, 3-21

This chapter contains the following blocks:

S00-S09	Injuries to the head
S10-S19	Injuries to the neck
S20-S29	Injuries to the thorax
S30-S39	Injuries to the abdomen, lower back, lumbar spine, pelvis and external genitals
S40-S49	Injuries to the shoulder and upper arm
S50-S59	Injuries to the elbow and forearm
S60-S69	Injuries to the wrist, hand and fingers
S70-S79	Injuries to the hip and thigh
S80-S89	Injuries to the knee and lower leg
S90-S99	Injuries to the ankle and foot
T07	Injuries involving multiple body regions
T14	Injury of unspecified body region
T15-T19	Effects of foreign body entering through natural orifice
T20-T25	Burns and corrosions of external body surface, specified by site
T26-T28	Burns and corrosions confined to eye and internal organs
T30-T32	Burns and corrosions of multiple and unspecified body regions
T33-T34	Frostbite
T36-T50	Poisoning by, adverse effect of and underdosing of drugs, medicaments and biological substances
T51-T65	Toxic effects of substances chiefly nonmedicinal as to source
T66-T78	Other and unspecified effects of external causes
T79	Certain early complications of trauma
T80-T88	Complications of surgical and medical care, not elsewhere classified

Injuries to the head (S00-S09)

INCLUDES injuries of ear
injuries of eye
injuries of face [any part]
injuries of gum
injuries of jaw
injuries of oral cavity
injuries of palate
injuries of periocular area
injuries of scalp
injuries of temporomandibular joint area
injuries of tongue
injuries of tooth

Code also for any associated infection

EXCLUDES 2 burns and corrosions (T20-T32)
effects of foreign body in ear (T16)
effects of foreign body in larynx (T17.3)
effects of foreign body in mouth NOS (T18.0)
effects of foreign body in nose (T17.0-T17.1)
effects of foreign body in pharynx (T17.2)
effects of foreign body on external eye (T15.-)
frostbite (T33-T34)
insect bite or sting, venomous (T63.4)

√4ᵗʰ **S00 Superficial injury of head**

> **EXCLUDES 1** diffuse cerebral contusion (S06.2-)
> focal cerebral contusion (S06.3-)
> injury of eye and orbit (S05.-)
> open wound of head (S01.-)

The appropriate 7th character is to be added to each code from category S00.
A   initial encounter
D   subsequent encounter
S   sequela

√5ᵗʰ **S00.0 Superficial injury of scalp**

√x7ᵗʰ   **S00.00 Unspecified superficial injury of scalp** ▽

√x7ᵗʰ   **S00.01 Abrasion of scalp**

√x7ᵗʰ   **S00.02 Blister (nonthermal) of scalp**

√x7ᵗʰ   **S00.03 Contusion of scalp**
Bruise of scalp
Hematoma of scalp

√x7ᵗʰ   **S00.04 External constriction of part of scalp**

√x7ᵗʰ   **S00.05 Superficial foreign body of scalp**
Splinter in the scalp

√x7ᵗʰ   **S00.06 Insect bite (nonvenomous) of scalp**

√x7ᵗʰ   **S00.07 Other superficial bite of scalp**
> **EXCLUDES 1** open bite of scalp (S01.05)

√5ᵗʰ **S00.1 Contusion of eyelid and periocular area**
Black eye
> **EXCLUDES 2** contusion of eyeball and orbital tissues (S05.1)

√x7ᵗʰ   **S00.10 Contusion of unspecified eyelid and periocular area** ▽

√x7ᵗʰ   **S00.11 Contusion of right eyelid and periocular area**

√x7ᵗʰ   **S00.12 Contusion of left eyelid and periocular area**

√5ᵗʰ **S00.2 Other and unspecified superficial injuries of eyelid and periocular area**
> **EXCLUDES 2** superficial injury of conjunctiva and cornea (S05.0-)

√6ᵗʰ   **S00.20 Unspecified superficial injury of eyelid and periocular area**

√7ᵗʰ   **S00.201 Unspecified superficial injury of right eyelid and periocular area** ▽

√7ᵗʰ   **S00.202 Unspecified superficial injury of left eyelid and periocular area** ▽

√7ᵗʰ   **S00.209 Unspecified superficial injury of unspecified eyelid and periocular area** ▽

√6ᵗʰ   **S00.21 Abrasion of eyelid and periocular area**

√7ᵗʰ   **S00.211 Abrasion of right eyelid and periocular area**

√7ᵗʰ   **S00.212 Abrasion of left eyelid and periocular area**

√7ᵗʰ   **S00.219 Abrasion of unspecified eyelid and periocular area** ▽

√6ᵗʰ   **S00.22 Blister (nonthermal) of eyelid and periocular area**

√7ᵗʰ   **S00.221 Blister (nonthermal) of right eyelid and periocular area**

√7ᵗʰ   **S00.222 Blister (nonthermal) of left eyelid and periocular area**

√7ᵗʰ   **S00.229 Blister (nonthermal) of unspecified eyelid and periocular area** ▽

√6ᵗʰ   **S00.24 External constriction of eyelid and periocular area**

√7ᵗʰ   **S00.241 External constriction of right eyelid and periocular area**

√7ᵗʰ   **S00.242 External constriction of left eyelid and periocular area**

√7ᵗʰ   **S00.249 External constriction of unspecified eyelid and periocular area** ▽

√6ᵗʰ   **S00.25 Superficial foreign body of eyelid and periocular area**
Splinter of eyelid and periocular area
> **EXCLUDES 2** retained foreign body in eyelid (H02.81-)

√7ᵗʰ   **S00.251 Superficial foreign body of right eyelid and periocular area**

√7ᵗʰ   **S00.252 Superficial foreign body of left eyelid and periocular area**

√7ᵗʰ   **S00.259 Superficial foreign body of unspecified eyelid and periocular area** ▽

√6ᵗʰ   **S00.26 Insect bite (nonvenomous) of eyelid and periocular area**

√7ᵗʰ   **S00.261 Insect bite (nonvenomous) of right eyelid and periocular area**

√7ᵗʰ   **S00.262 Insect bite (nonvenomous) of left eyelid and periocular area**

√7ᵗʰ   **S00.269 Insect bite (nonvenomous) of unspecified eyelid and periocular area** ▽

√6ᵗʰ   **S00.27 Other superficial bite of eyelid and periocular area**
> **EXCLUDES 1** open bite of eyelid and periocular area (S01.15)

√7ᵗʰ   **S00.271 Other superficial bite of right eyelid and periocular area**

√7ᵗʰ   **S00.272 Other superficial bite of left eyelid and periocular area**

√7ᵗʰ   **S00.279 Other superficial bite of unspecified eyelid and periocular area** ▽

EXCLUDES 1 Not coded here   **EXCLUDES 2** Not included here   N Newborn Age: 0   P Pediatric Age: 0-17   M Maternity Age: 12-55   A Adult Age: 15-124

914   ICD-10-CM 2018

✓5ᵗʰ **S00.3 Superficial injury of** nose

   ✓x7ᵗʰ **S00.30 Unspecified superficial injury of nose** ▽

   ✓x7ᵗʰ **S00.31 Abrasion of nose**

   ✓x7ᵗʰ **S00.32 Blister (nonthermal) of nose**

   ✓x7ᵗʰ **S00.33 Contusion of nose**
       Bruise of nose
       Hematoma of nose

   ✓x7ᵗʰ **S00.34 External constriction of nose**

   ✓x7ᵗʰ **S00.35 Superficial foreign body of nose**
       Splinter in the nose

   ✓x7ᵗʰ **S00.36 Insect bite (nonvenomous) of nose**

   ✓x7ᵗʰ **S00.37 Other superficial bite of nose**
       EXCLUDES 1   *open bite of nose (S01.25)*

✓5ᵗʰ **S00.4 Superficial injury of** ear

  ✓6ᵗʰ **S00.40 Unspecified superficial injury of ear**

    ✓7ᵗʰ **S00.401 Unspecified superficial injury of right ear** ▽

    ✓7ᵗʰ **S00.402 Unspecified superficial injury of left ear** ▽

    ✓7ᵗʰ **S00.409 Unspecified superficial injury of unspecified ear** ▽

  ✓6ᵗʰ **S00.41 Abrasion of ear**

    ✓7ᵗʰ **S00.411 Abrasion of right ear**

    ✓7ᵗʰ **S00.412 Abrasion of left ear**

    ✓7ᵗʰ **S00.419 Abrasion of unspecified ear** ▽

  ✓6ᵗʰ **S00.42 Blister (nonthermal) of ear**

    ✓7ᵗʰ **S00.421 Blister (nonthermal) of right ear**

    ✓7ᵗʰ **S00.422 Blister (nonthermal) of left ear**

    ✓7ᵗʰ **S00.429 Blister (nonthermal) of unspecified ear** ▽

  ✓6ᵗʰ **S00.43 Contusion of ear**
      Bruise of ear
      Hematoma of ear

    ✓7ᵗʰ **S00.431 Contusion of right ear**

    ✓7ᵗʰ **S00.432 Contusion of left ear**

    ✓7ᵗʰ **S00.439 Contusion of unspecified ear** ▽

  ✓6ᵗʰ **S00.44 External constriction of ear**

    ✓7ᵗʰ **S00.441 External constriction of right ear**

    ✓7ᵗʰ **S00.442 External constriction of left ear**

    ✓7ᵗʰ **S00.449 External constriction of unspecified ear** ▽

  ✓6ᵗʰ **S00.45 Superficial foreign body of ear**
      Splinter in the ear

    ✓7ᵗʰ **S00.451 Superficial foreign body of right ear**

    ✓7ᵗʰ **S00.452 Superficial foreign body of left ear**

    ✓7ᵗʰ **S00.459 Superficial foreign body of unspecified ear** ▽

  ✓6ᵗʰ **S00.46 Insect bite (nonvenomous) of ear**

    ✓7ᵗʰ **S00.461 Insect bite (nonvenomous) of right ear**

    ✓7ᵗʰ **S00.462 Insect bite (nonvenomous) of left ear**

    ✓7ᵗʰ **S00.469 Insect bite (nonvenomous) of unspecified ear** ▽

  ✓6ᵗʰ **S00.47 Other superficial bite of ear**
      EXCLUDES 1   *open bite of ear (S01.35)*

    ✓7ᵗʰ **S00.471 Other superficial bite of right ear**

    ✓7ᵗʰ **S00.472 Other superficial bite of left ear**

    ✓7ᵗʰ **S00.479 Other superficial bite of unspecified ear** ▽

✓5ᵗʰ **S00.5 Superficial injury of** lip and oral cavity

  ✓6ᵗʰ **S00.50 Unspecified superficial injury of lip and oral cavity**

    ✓7ᵗʰ **S00.501 Unspecified superficial injury of lip** ▽

    ✓7ᵗʰ **S00.502 Unspecified superficial injury of oral cavity** ▽

  ✓6ᵗʰ **S00.51 Abrasion of lip and oral cavity**

    ✓7ᵗʰ **S00.511 Abrasion of lip**

    ✓7ᵗʰ **S00.512 Abrasion of oral cavity**

  ✓6ᵗʰ **S00.52 Blister (nonthermal) of lip and oral cavity**

    ✓7ᵗʰ **S00.521 Blister (nonthermal) of lip**

    ✓7ᵗʰ **S00.522 Blister (nonthermal) of oral cavity**

  ✓6ᵗʰ **S00.53 Contusion of lip and oral cavity**

    ✓7ᵗʰ **S00.531 Contusion of lip**
      Bruise of lip
      ►Hematoma of lip◄

    ✓7ᵗʰ **S00.532 Contusion of oral cavity**
      ►Bruise of oral cavity◄
      Hematoma of oral cavity

  ✓6ᵗʰ **S00.54 External constriction of lip and oral cavity**

    ✓7ᵗʰ **S00.541 External constriction of lip**

    ✓7ᵗʰ **S00.542 External constriction of oral cavity**

  ✓6ᵗʰ **S00.55 Superficial foreign body of lip and oral cavity**

    ✓7ᵗʰ **S00.551 Superficial foreign body of lip**
      Splinter of lip and oral cavity

    ✓7ᵗʰ **S00.552 Superficial foreign body of oral cavity**
      Splinter of lip and oral cavity

  ✓6ᵗʰ **S00.56 Insect bite (nonvenomous) of lip and oral cavity**

    ✓7ᵗʰ **S00.561 Insect bite (nonvenomous) of lip**

    ✓7ᵗʰ **S00.562 Insect bite (nonvenomous) of oral cavity**

  ✓6ᵗʰ **S00.57 Other superficial bite of lip and oral cavity**

    ✓7ᵗʰ **S00.571 Other superficial bite of lip**
      EXCLUDES 1   *open bite of lip (S01.551)*

    ✓7ᵗʰ **S00.572 Other superficial bite of oral cavity**
      EXCLUDES 1   *open bite of oral cavity (S01.552)*

✓5ᵗʰ **S00.8 Superficial injury of other parts of head**
   Superficial injuries of face [any part]

  ✓x7ᵗʰ **S00.80 Unspecified superficial injury of other part of head** ▽

  ✓x7ᵗʰ **S00.81 Abrasion of other part of head**

  ✓x7ᵗʰ **S00.82 Blister (nonthermal) of other part of head**

  ✓x7ᵗʰ **S00.83 Contusion of other part of head**
     Bruise of other part of head
     Hematoma of other part of head

  ✓x7ᵗʰ **S00.84 External constriction of other part of head**

  ✓x7ᵗʰ **S00.85 Superficial foreign body of other part of head**
     Splinter in other part of head

  ✓x7ᵗʰ **S00.86 Insect bite (nonvenomous) of other part of head**

  ✓x7ᵗʰ **S00.87 Other superficial bite of other part of head**
     EXCLUDES 1   *open bite of other part of head (S01.85)*

✓5ᵗʰ **S00.9 Superficial injury of unspecified part of head**

  ✓x7ᵗʰ **S00.90 Unspecified superficial injury of unspecified part of head** ▽

  ✓x7ᵗʰ **S00.91 Abrasion of unspecified part of head** ▽

  ✓x7ᵗʰ **S00.92 Blister (nonthermal) of unspecified part of head** ▽

  ✓x7ᵗʰ **S00.93 Contusion of unspecified part of head** ▽
     Bruise of head
     Hematoma of head

  ✓x7ᵗʰ **S00.94 External constriction of unspecified part of head** ▽

  ✓x7ᵗʰ **S00.95 Superficial foreign body of unspecified part of head** ▽
     Splinter of head

  ✓x7ᵗʰ **S00.96 Insect bite (nonvenomous) of unspecified part of head** ▽

  ✓x7ᵗʰ **S00.97 Other superficial bite of unspecified part of head** ▽
     EXCLUDES 1   *open bite of head (S01.95)*

✓4ᵗʰ **S01 Open wound of head**
   Code also any associated:
    injury of cranial nerve (S04.-)
    injury of muscle and tendon of head (S09.1-)
    intracranial injury (S06.-)
    wound infection
   EXCLUDES 1   *open skull fracture (S02- with 7th character B)*
   EXCLUDES 2   *injury of eye and orbit (S05.-)*
          traumatic amputation of part of head (S08.-)

   The appropriate 7th character is to be added to each code from category S01.
   A   initial encounter
   D   subsequent encounter
   S   sequela

  ✓5ᵗʰ **S01.0 Open wound of scalp**
    EXCLUDES 1   *avulsion of scalp (S08.0)*

   ✓x7ᵗʰ **S01.00 Unspecified open wound of scalp** ▽

   ✓x7ᵗʰ **S01.01 Laceration without foreign body of scalp**

✓ Additional Character Req   ✓x7ᵗʰ Placeholder Alert   Manifestation   HCC CMS-HCC Condition   ▽ Unspecified Code   ►◄ Revised Text   ● New Code   ▲ Revised Code Title

ICD-10-CM 2018   915

Chapter 19. Injury, Poisoning, and Certain Other Consequences of External Causes

S00.3–S01.01

√x7ᵗʰ **S01.02** Laceration with foreign body of scalp

√x7ᵗʰ **S01.03** Puncture wound without foreign body of scalp

√x7ᵗʰ **S01.04** Puncture wound with foreign body of scalp

√x7ᵗʰ **S01.05** Open bite of scalp
Bite of scalp NOS
EXCLUDES 1 *superficial bite of scalp (S00.06, S00.07-)*

√5ᵗʰ **S01.1** Open wound of eyelid and periocular area
Open wound of eyelid and periocular area with or without involvement of lacrimal passages

√6ᵗʰ **S01.10** Unspecified open wound of eyelid and periocular area

√7ᵗʰ **S01.101** Unspecified open wound of right eyelid and periocular area ▽

√7ᵗʰ **S01.102** Unspecified open wound of left eyelid and periocular area ▽

√7ᵗʰ **S01.109** Unspecified open wound of unspecified eyelid and periocular area ▽

√6ᵗʰ **S01.11** Laceration without foreign body of eyelid and periocular area

√7ᵗʰ **S01.111** Laceration without foreign body of right eyelid and periocular area

√7ᵗʰ **S01.112** Laceration without foreign body of left eyelid and periocular area

√7ᵗʰ **S01.119** Laceration without foreign body of unspecified eyelid and periocular area ▽

√6ᵗʰ **S01.12** Laceration with foreign body of eyelid and periocular area

√7ᵗʰ **S01.121** Laceration with foreign body of right eyelid and periocular area

√7ᵗʰ **S01.122** Laceration with foreign body of left eyelid and periocular area

√7ᵗʰ **S01.129** Laceration with foreign body of unspecified eyelid and periocular area ▽

√6ᵗʰ **S01.13** Puncture wound without foreign body of eyelid and periocular area

√7ᵗʰ **S01.131** Puncture wound without foreign body of right eyelid and periocular area

√7ᵗʰ **S01.132** Puncture wound without foreign body of left eyelid and periocular area

√7ᵗʰ **S01.139** Puncture wound without foreign body of unspecified eyelid and periocular area ▽

√6ᵗʰ **S01.14** Puncture wound with foreign body of eyelid and periocular area

√7ᵗʰ **S01.141** Puncture wound with foreign body of right eyelid and periocular area

√7ᵗʰ **S01.142** Puncture wound with foreign body of left eyelid and periocular area

√7ᵗʰ **S01.149** Puncture wound with foreign body of unspecified eyelid and periocular area ▽

√6ᵗʰ **S01.15** Open bite of eyelid and periocular area
Bite of eyelid and periocular area NOS
EXCLUDES 1 *superficial bite of eyelid and periocular area (S00.26, S00.27)*

√7ᵗʰ **S01.151** Open bite of right eyelid and periocular area

√7ᵗʰ **S01.152** Open bite of left eyelid and periocular area

√7ᵗʰ **S01.159** Open bite of unspecified eyelid and periocular area ▽

√5ᵗʰ **S01.2** Open wound of nose

√x7ᵗʰ **S01.20** Unspecified open wound of nose ▽

√x7ᵗʰ **S01.21** Laceration without foreign body of nose

√x7ᵗʰ **S01.22** Laceration with foreign body of nose

√x7ᵗʰ **S01.23** Puncture wound without foreign body of nose

√x7ᵗʰ **S01.24** Puncture wound with foreign body of nose

√x7ᵗʰ **S01.25** Open bite of nose
Bite of nose NOS
EXCLUDES 1 *superficial bite of nose (S00.36, S00.37)*

√5ᵗʰ **S01.3** Open wound of ear

√6ᵗʰ **S01.30** Unspecified open wound of ear

√7ᵗʰ **S01.301** Unspecified open wound of right ear ▽

√7ᵗʰ **S01.302** Unspecified open wound of left ear ▽

√7ᵗʰ **S01.309** Unspecified open wound of unspecified ear ▽

√6ᵗʰ **S01.31** Laceration without foreign body of ear

√7ᵗʰ **S01.311** Laceration without foreign body of right ear

√7ᵗʰ **S01.312** Laceration without foreign body of left ear

√7ᵗʰ **S01.319** Laceration without foreign body of unspecified ear ▽

√6ᵗʰ **S01.32** Laceration with foreign body of ear

√7ᵗʰ **S01.321** Laceration with foreign body of right ear

√7ᵗʰ **S01.322** Laceration with foreign body of left ear

√7ᵗʰ **S01.329** Laceration with foreign body of unspecified ear ▽

√6ᵗʰ **S01.33** Puncture wound without foreign body of ear

√7ᵗʰ **S01.331** Puncture wound without foreign body of right ear

√7ᵗʰ **S01.332** Puncture wound without foreign body of left ear

√7ᵗʰ **S01.339** Puncture wound without foreign body of unspecified ear ▽

√6ᵗʰ **S01.34** Puncture wound with foreign body of ear

√7ᵗʰ **S01.341** Puncture wound with foreign body of right ear

√7ᵗʰ **S01.342** Puncture wound with foreign body of left ear

√7ᵗʰ **S01.349** Puncture wound with foreign body of unspecified ear ▽

√6ᵗʰ **S01.35** Open bite of ear
Bite of ear NOS
EXCLUDES 1 *superficial bite of ear (S00.46, S00.47)*

√7ᵗʰ **S01.351** Open bite of right ear

√7ᵗʰ **S01.352** Open bite of left ear

√7ᵗʰ **S01.359** Open bite of unspecified ear ▽

√5ᵗʰ **S01.4** Open wound of cheek and temporomandibular area

√6ᵗʰ **S01.40** Unspecified open wound of cheek and temporomandibular area

√7ᵗʰ **S01.401** Unspecified open wound of right cheek and temporomandibular area ▽

√7ᵗʰ **S01.402** Unspecified open wound of left cheek and temporomandibular area ▽

√7ᵗʰ **S01.409** Unspecified open wound of unspecified cheek and temporomandibular area ▽

√6ᵗʰ **S01.41** Laceration without foreign body of cheek and temporomandibular area

√7ᵗʰ **S01.411** Laceration without foreign body of right cheek and temporomandibular area

√7ᵗʰ **S01.412** Laceration without foreign body of left cheek and temporomandibular area

√7ᵗʰ **S01.419** Laceration without foreign body of unspecified cheek and temporomandibular area ▽

√6ᵗʰ **S01.42** Laceration with foreign body of cheek and temporomandibular area

√7ᵗʰ **S01.421** Laceration with foreign body of right cheek and temporomandibular area

√7ᵗʰ **S01.422** Laceration with foreign body of left cheek and temporomandibular area

√7ᵗʰ **S01.429** Laceration with foreign body of unspecified cheek and temporomandibular area ▽

√6ᵗʰ **S01.43** Puncture wound without foreign body of cheek and temporomandibular area

√7ᵗʰ **S01.431** Puncture wound without foreign body of right cheek and temporomandibular area

√7ᵗʰ **S01.432** Puncture wound without foreign body of left cheek and temporomandibular area

√7ᵗʰ **S01.439** Puncture wound without foreign body of unspecified cheek and temporomandibular area ▽

√6ᵗʰ **S01.44** Puncture wound with foreign body of cheek and temporomandibular area

√7ᵗʰ **S01.441** Puncture wound with foreign body of right cheek and temporomandibular area

---

EXCLUDES 1 Not coded here   **EXCLUDES 2** Not included here   N Newborn Age: 0   P Pediatric Age: 0-17   M Maternity Age: 12-55   A Adult Age: 15-124

916   ICD-10-CM 2018

√7ᵗʰ **S01.442** Puncture wound with foreign body of left cheek and temporomandibular area

√7ᵗʰ **S01.449** Puncture wound with foreign body of unspecified cheek and temporomandibular area ▽

√6ᵗʰ **S01.45** Open bite of cheek and temporomandibular area
     Bite of cheek and temporomandibular area NOS
     EXCLUDES 2   superficial bite of cheek and temporomandibular area (S00.86, S00.87)

√7ᵗʰ **S01.451** Open bite of right cheek and temporomandibular area

√7ᵗʰ **S01.452** Open bite of left cheek and temporomandibular area

√7ᵗʰ **S01.459** Open bite of unspecified cheek and temporomandibular area ▽

√5ᵗʰ **S01.5** Open wound of lip and oral cavity
     EXCLUDES 2   tooth dislocation (S03.2)
                  tooth fracture (S02.5)

√6ᵗʰ **S01.50** Unspecified open wound of lip and oral cavity

√7ᵗʰ **S01.501** Unspecified open wound of lip ▽

√7ᵗʰ **S01.502** Unspecified open wound of oral cavity ▽

√6ᵗʰ **S01.51** Laceration of lip and oral cavity without foreign body

√7ᵗʰ **S01.511** Laceration without foreign body of lip

√7ᵗʰ **S01.512** Laceration without foreign body of oral cavity

√6ᵗʰ **S01.52** Laceration of lip and oral cavity with foreign body

√7ᵗʰ **S01.521** Laceration with foreign body of lip

√7ᵗʰ **S01.522** Laceration with foreign body of oral cavity

√6ᵗʰ **S01.53** Puncture wound of lip and oral cavity without foreign body

√7ᵗʰ **S01.531** Puncture wound without foreign body of lip

√7ᵗʰ **S01.532** Puncture wound without foreign body of oral cavity

√6ᵗʰ **S01.54** Puncture wound of lip and oral cavity with foreign body

√7ᵗʰ **S01.541** Puncture wound with foreign body of lip

√7ᵗʰ **S01.542** Puncture wound with foreign body of oral cavity

√6ᵗʰ **S01.55** Open bite of lip and oral cavity

√7ᵗʰ **S01.551** Open bite of lip
     Bite of lip NOS
     EXCLUDES 1   superficial bite of lip (S00.571)

√7ᵗʰ **S01.552** Open bite of oral cavity
     Bite of oral cavity NOS
     EXCLUDES 1   superficial bite of oral cavity (S00.572)

√5ᵗʰ **S01.8** Open wound of other parts of head

√x7ᵗʰ **S01.80** Unspecified open wound of other part of head ▽

√x7ᵗʰ **S01.81** Laceration without foreign body of other part of head

√x7ᵗʰ **S01.82** Laceration with foreign body of other part of head

√x7ᵗʰ **S01.83** Puncture wound without foreign body of other part of head

√x7ᵗʰ **S01.84** Puncture wound with foreign body of other part of head

√x7ᵗʰ **S01.85** Open bite of other part of head
     Bite of other part of head NOS
     EXCLUDES 1   superficial bite of other part of head ►(S00.87)◄

√5ᵗʰ **S01.9** Open wound of unspecified part of head

√x7ᵗʰ **S01.90** Unspecified open wound of unspecified part of head ▽

√x7ᵗʰ **S01.91** Laceration without foreign body of unspecified part of head ▽

√x7ᵗʰ **S01.92** Laceration with foreign body of unspecified part of head ▽

√x7ᵗʰ **S01.93** Puncture wound without foreign body of unspecified part of head ▽

√x7ᵗʰ **S01.94** Puncture wound with foreign body of unspecified part of head ▽

√x7ᵗʰ **S01.95** Open bite of unspecified part of head ▽
     Bite of head NOS
     EXCLUDES 1   superficial bite of head NOS (S00.97)

√4ᵗʰ **S02** Fracture of skull and facial bones
     NOTE   A fracture not indicated as open or closed should be coded to closed.
     Code also any associated intracranial injury (S06.-).
     AHA: 2017, 1Q, 42

     The appropriate 7th character is to be added to each code from category S02.
     A   initial encounter for closed fracture
     B   initial encounter for open fracture
     D   subsequent encounter for fracture with routine healing
     G   subsequent encounter for fracture with delayed healing
     K   subsequent encounter for fracture with nonunion
     S   sequela

² √x7ᵗʰ **S02.0** Fracture of vault of skull   HCC
     Fracture of frontal bone
     Fracture of parietal bone

√5ᵗʰ **S02.1** Fracture of base of skull
     EXCLUDES 1   orbit NOS (S02.8)
     EXCLUDES 2   orbital floor (S02.3-)

√6ᵗʰ **S02.10** Unspecified fracture of base of skull

² √7ᵗʰ **S02.101** Fracture of base of skull, right side   HCC

² √7ᵗʰ **S02.102** Fracture of base of skull, left side   HCC

² √7ᵗʰ **S02.109** Fracture of base of skull, unspecified side   HCC ▽

√6ᵗʰ **S02.11** Fracture of occiput

² √7ᵗʰ **S02.110** Type I occipital condyle fracture, unspecified side   HCC ▽

² √7ᵗʰ **S02.111** Type II occipital condyle fracture, unspecified side   HCC ▽

² √7ᵗʰ **S02.112** Type III occipital condyle fracture, unspecified side   HCC ▽

² √7ᵗʰ **S02.113** Unspecified occipital condyle fracture   HCC ▽

² √7ᵗʰ **S02.118** Other fracture of occiput, unspecified side   HCC ▽

² √7ᵗʰ **S02.119** Unspecified fracture of occiput   HCC ▽

² √7ᵗʰ **S02.11A** Type I occipital condyle fracture, right side   HCC

² √7ᵗʰ **S02.11B** Type I occipital condyle fracture, left side   HCC

² √7ᵗʰ **S02.11C** Type II occipital condyle fracture, right side   HCC

² √7ᵗʰ **S02.11D** Type II occipital condyle fracture, left side   HCC

² √7ᵗʰ **S02.11E** Type III occipital condyle fracture, right side   HCC

² √7ᵗʰ **S02.11F** Type III occipital condyle fracture, left side   HCC

² √7ᵗʰ **S02.11G** Other fracture of occiput, right side   HCC

² √7ᵗʰ **S02.11H** Other fracture of occiput, left side   HCC

² √x7ᵗʰ **S02.19** Other fracture of base of skull   HCC
     Fracture of anterior fossa of base of skull
     Fracture of ethmoid sinus
     Fracture of frontal sinus
     Fracture of middle fossa of base of skull
     Fracture of orbital roof
     Fracture of posterior fossa of base of skull
     Fracture of sphenoid
     Fracture of temporal bone

√x7ᵗʰ **S02.2** Fracture of nasal bones

√5ᵗʰ **S02.3** Fracture of orbital floor
     EXCLUDES 1   orbit NOS (S02.8)
     EXCLUDES 2   orbital roof (S02.1-)

² √x7ᵗʰ **S02.30** Fracture of orbital floor, unspecified side   HCC ▽

² √x7ᵗʰ **S02.31** Fracture of orbital floor, right side   HCC

² √x7ᵗʰ **S02.32** Fracture of orbital floor, left side   HCC

---

²   HCC with 7th character indicating initial encounter (A or B - specific to category) OR sequela.

☑ Additional Character Req   √x7ᵗʰ Placeholder Alert   Manifestation   HCC CMS-HCC Condition   ▽ Unspecified Code   ►◄ Revised Text   ● New Code   ▲ Revised Code Title

Chapter 19. Injury, Poisoning, and Certain Other Consequences of External Causes

S02.4–S03.9

LeFort Fracture Types

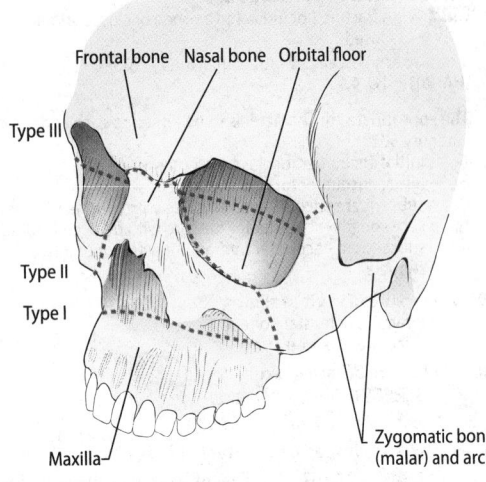

Frontal bone   Nasal bone   Orbital floor

Type III

Type II

Type I

Maxilla

Zygomatic bone (malar) and arch

✓5ᵗʰ **S02.4** **Fracture of malar, maxillary and zygoma bones**
Fracture of superior maxilla
Fracture of upper jaw (bone)
Fracture of zygomatic process of temporal bone

    ✓6ᵗʰ **S02.40** **Fracture of malar, maxillary and zygoma bones, unspecified**

      2   ✓7ᵗʰ   **S02.400**   Malar fracture, unspecified side   HCC ▽
      2   ✓7ᵗʰ   **S02.401**   Maxillary fracture, unspecified side   HCC ▽
      2   ✓7ᵗʰ   **S02.402**   Zygomatic fracture, unspecified side   HCC ▽
      2   ✓7ᵗʰ   **S02.40A**   Malar fracture, right side   HCC
      2   ✓7ᵗʰ   **S02.40B**   Malar fracture, left side   HCC
      2   ✓7ᵗʰ   **S02.40C**   Maxillary fracture, right side   HCC
      2   ✓7ᵗʰ   **S02.40D**   Maxillary fracture, left side   HCC
      2   ✓7ᵗʰ   **S02.40E**   Zygomatic fracture, right side   HCC
      2   ✓7ᵗʰ   **S02.40F**   Zygomatic fracture, left side   HCC

    ✓6ᵗʰ **S02.41** **LeFort fracture**
      2   ✓7ᵗʰ   **S02.411**   LeFort I fracture   HCC
      2   ✓7ᵗʰ   **S02.412**   LeFort II fracture   HCC
      2   ✓7ᵗʰ   **S02.413**   LeFort III fracture   HCC

    2   ✓x7ᵗʰ   **S02.42** **Fracture of alveolus of maxilla**   HCC

✓x7ᵗʰ **S02.5** **Fracture of tooth (traumatic)**
Broken tooth
    EXCLUDES 1   cracked tooth (nontraumatic) (K03.81)

✓5ᵗʰ **S02.6** **Fracture of mandible**
Fracture of lower jaw (bone)

    ✓6ᵗʰ **S02.60** **Fracture of mandible, unspecified**
      2   ✓7ᵗʰ   **S02.600**   Fracture of unspecified part of body of mandible, unspecified side   HCC ▽
      2   ✓7ᵗʰ   **S02.601**   Fracture of unspecified part of body of right mandible   HCC ▽
      2   ✓7ᵗʰ   **S02.602**   Fracture of unspecified part of body of left mandible   HCC ▽
      2   ✓7ᵗʰ   **S02.609**   Fracture of mandible, unspecified   HCC ▽

    ✓6ᵗʰ **S02.61** **Fracture of condylar process of mandible**
      2   ✓7ᵗʰ   **S02.610**   Fracture of condylar process of mandible, unspecified side   HCC ▽
      2   ✓7ᵗʰ   **S02.611**   Fracture of condylar process of right mandible   HCC
      2   ✓7ᵗʰ   **S02.612**   Fracture of condylar process of left mandible   HCC

    ✓6ᵗʰ **S02.62** **Fracture of subcondylar process of mandible**
      2   ✓7ᵗʰ   **S02.620**   Fracture of subcondylar process of mandible, unspecified side   HCC ▽
      2   ✓7ᵗʰ   **S02.621**   Fracture of subcondylar process of right mandible   HCC
      2   ✓7ᵗʰ   **S02.622**   Fracture of subcondylar process of left mandible   HCC

    ✓6ᵗʰ **S02.63** **Fracture of coronoid process of mandible**
      2   ✓7ᵗʰ   **S02.630**   Fracture of coronoid process of mandible, unspecified side   HCC ▽
      2   ✓7ᵗʰ   **S02.631**   Fracture of coronoid process of right mandible   HCC
      2   ✓7ᵗʰ   **S02.632**   Fracture of coronoid process of left mandible   HCC

    ✓6ᵗʰ **S02.64** **Fracture of ramus of mandible**
      2   ✓7ᵗʰ   **S02.640**   Fracture of ramus of mandible, unspecified side   HCC ▽
      2   ✓7ᵗʰ   **S02.641**   Fracture of ramus of right mandible   HCC
      2   ✓7ᵗʰ   **S02.642**   Fracture of ramus of left mandible   HCC

    ✓6ᵗʰ **S02.65** **Fracture of angle of mandible**
      2   ✓7ᵗʰ   **S02.650**   Fracture of angle of mandible, unspecified side   HCC ▽
      2   ✓7ᵗʰ   **S02.651**   Fracture of angle of right mandible   HCC
      2   ✓7ᵗʰ   **S02.652**   Fracture of angle of left mandible   HCC

    2   ✓x7ᵗʰ   **S02.66** **Fracture of symphysis of mandible**   HCC

    ✓6ᵗʰ **S02.67** **Fracture of alveolus of mandible**
      2   ✓7ᵗʰ   **S02.670**   Fracture of alveolus of mandible, unspecified side   HCC ▽
      2   ✓7ᵗʰ   **S02.671**   Fracture of alveolus of right mandible   HCC
      2   ✓7ᵗʰ   **S02.672**   Fracture of alveolus of left mandible   HCC

    2   ✓x7ᵗʰ   **S02.69** **Fracture of mandible of other specified site**   HCC

✓5ᵗʰ **S02.8** **Fractures of other specified skull and facial bones**
Fracture of orbit NOS
Fracture of palate
    EXCLUDES 1   fracture of orbital floor (S02.3-)
              fracture of orbital roof (S02.1-)

    2   ✓x7ᵗʰ   **S02.80**   Fracture of other specified skull and facial bones, unspecified side   HCC ▽
    2   ✓x7ᵗʰ   **S02.81**   Fracture of other specified skull and facial bones, right side   HCC
    2   ✓x7ᵗʰ   **S02.82**   Fracture of other specified skull and facial bones, left side   HCC

✓5ᵗʰ **S02.9** **Fracture of unspecified skull and facial bones**
    2   ✓x7ᵗʰ   **S02.91**   Unspecified fracture of skull   HCC ▽
    2   ✓x7ᵗʰ   **S02.92**   Unspecified fracture of facial bones   HCC ▽

✓4ᵗʰ **S03** **Dislocation and sprain of joints and ligaments of head**
    INCLUDES   avulsion of joint (capsule) or ligament of head
              laceration of cartilage, joint (capsule) or ligament of head
              sprain of cartilage, joint (capsule) or ligament of head
              traumatic hemarthrosis of joint or ligament of head
              traumatic rupture of joint or ligament of head
              traumatic subluxation of joint or ligament of head
              traumatic tear of joint or ligament of head
    Code also any associated open wound
    EXCLUDES 2   strain of muscle or tendon of head (S09.1)

    The appropriate 7th character is to be added to each code from category S03.
    A   initial encounter
    D   subsequent encounter
    S   sequela

✓5ᵗʰ **S03.0** **Dislocation of jaw**
Dislocation of jaw (cartilage) (meniscus)
Dislocation of mandible
Dislocation of temporomandibular (joint)

    ✓7ᵗʰ   **S03.00**   Dislocation of jaw, unspecified side   ▽
    ✓7ᵗʰ   **S03.01**   Dislocation of jaw, right side
    ✓7ᵗʰ   **S03.02**   Dislocation of jaw, left side
    ✓7ᵗʰ   **S03.03**   Dislocation of jaw, bilateral

✓x7ᵗʰ **S03.1** **Dislocation of septal cartilage of nose**

✓x7ᵗʰ **S03.2** **Dislocation of tooth**

✓5ᵗʰ **S03.4** **Sprain of jaw**
Sprain of temporomandibular (joint) (ligament)

    ✓7ᵗʰ   **S03.40**   Sprain of jaw, unspecified side   ▽
    ✓7ᵗʰ   **S03.41**   Sprain of jaw, right side
    ✓7ᵗʰ   **S03.42**   Sprain of jaw, left side
    ✓7ᵗʰ   **S03.43**   Sprain of jaw, bilateral

✓x7ᵗʰ **S03.8** **Sprain of joints and ligaments of other parts of head**

✓x7ᵗʰ **S03.9** **Sprain of joints and ligaments of unspecified parts of head**   ▽

---

2   HCC with 7th character indicating initial encounter (A or B - specific to category) OR sequela.

EXCLUDES 1 Not coded here   *EXCLUDES 2* Not included here   N Newborn Age: 0   P Pediatric Age: 0-17   M Maternity Age: 12-55   A Adult Age: 15-124

918   ICD-10-CM 2018

✓4th **S04 Injury of cranial nerve**

The selection of side should be based on the side of the body being affected

Codes first any associated intracranial injury (S06.-)

Code also any associated:
open wound of head (S01.-)
skull fracture (S02.-)

The appropriate 7th character is to be added to each code from category S04.
A   initial encounter
D   subsequent encounter
S   sequela

✓5th **S04.0 Injury of optic nerve and pathways**

Use additional code to identify any visual field defect or blindness ▶(H53.4-, H54.-)◀

✓6th **S04.01 Injury of optic nerve**
Injury of 2nd cranial nerve

  ✓7th **S04.011 Injury of optic nerve, right eye**

  ✓7th **S04.012 Injury of optic nerve, left eye**

  ✓7th **S04.019 Injury of optic nerve, unspecified eye** ▽
Injury of optic nerve NOS

✓x7th **S04.02 Injury of optic chiasm**

✓6th **S04.03 Injury of optic tract and pathways**
Injury of optic radiation

▲   ✓7th **S04.031 Injury of optic tract and pathways, right side**

▲   ✓7th **S04.032 Injury of optic tract and pathways, left side**

▲   ✓7th **S04.039 Injury of optic tract and pathways, unspecified side** ▽
Injury of optic tract and pathways NOS

✓6th **S04.04 Injury of visual cortex**

▲   ✓7th **S04.041 Injury of visual cortex, right side**

▲   ✓7th **S04.042 Injury of visual cortex, left side**

▲   ✓7th **S04.049 Injury of visual cortex, unspecified side** ▽
Injury of visual cortex NOS

✓5th **S04.1 Injury of oculomotor nerve**
Injury of 3rd cranial nerve

 ✓x7th **S04.10 Injury of oculomotor nerve, unspecified side** ▽

 ✓x7th **S04.11 Injury of oculomotor nerve, right side**

 ✓x7th **S04.12 Injury of oculomotor nerve, left side**

✓5th **S04.2 Injury of trochlear nerve**
Injury of 4th cranial nerve

 ✓x7th **S04.20 Injury of trochlear nerve, unspecified side** ▽

 ✓x7th **S04.21 Injury of trochlear nerve, right side**

 ✓x7th **S04.22 Injury of trochlear nerve, left side**

✓5th **S04.3 Injury of trigeminal nerve**
Injury of 5th cranial nerve

 ✓x7th **S04.30 Injury of trigeminal nerve, unspecified side** ▽

 ✓x7th **S04.31 Injury of trigeminal nerve, right side**

 ✓x7th **S04.32 Injury of trigeminal nerve, left side**

✓5th **S04.4 Injury of abducent nerve**
Injury of 6th cranial nerve

 ✓x7th **S04.40 Injury of abducent nerve, unspecified side** ▽

 ✓x7th **S04.41 Injury of abducent nerve, right side**

 ✓x7th **S04.42 Injury of abducent nerve, left side**

✓5th **S04.5 Injury of facial nerve**
Injury of 7th cranial nerve

 ✓x7th **S04.50 Injury of facial nerve, unspecified side** ▽

 ✓x7th **S04.51 Injury of facial nerve, right side**

 ✓x7th **S04.52 Injury of facial nerve, left side**

✓5th **S04.6 Injury of acoustic nerve**
Injury of auditory nerve
Injury of 8th cranial nerve

 ✓x7th **S04.60 Injury of acoustic nerve, unspecified side** ▽

 ✓x7th **S04.61 Injury of acoustic nerve, right side**

 ✓x7th **S04.62 Injury of acoustic nerve, left side**

✓5th **S04.7 Injury of accessory nerve**
Injury of 11th cranial nerve

 ✓x7th **S04.70 Injury of accessory nerve, unspecified side** ▽

 ✓x7th **S04.71 Injury of accessory nerve, right side**

 ✓x7th **S04.72 Injury of accessory nerve, left side**

✓5th **S04.8 Injury of other cranial nerves**

✓6th **S04.81 Injury of olfactory [1st] nerve**

 ✓7th **S04.811 Injury of olfactory [1st] nerve, right side**

 ✓7th **S04.812 Injury of olfactory [1st] nerve, left side**

 ✓7th **S04.819 Injury of olfactory [1st] nerve, unspecified side** ▽

✓6th **S04.89 Injury of other cranial nerves**
Injury of vagus [10th] nerve

 ✓7th **S04.891 Injury of other cranial nerves, right side**

 ✓7th **S04.892 Injury of other cranial nerves, left side**

 ✓7th **S04.899 Injury of other cranial nerves, unspecified side** ▽

✓x7th **S04.9 Injury of unspecified cranial nerve** ▽

✓4th **S05 Injury of eye and orbit**

INCLUDES open wound of eye and orbit

EXCLUDES 2 2nd cranial [optic] nerve injury (S04.0-)
3rd cranial [oculomotor] nerve injury (S04.1-)
open wound of eyelid and periocular area (S01.1-)
orbital bone fracture (S02.1-, S02.3-, S02.8-)
superficial injury of eyelid (S00.1-S00.2)

The appropriate 7th character is to be added to each code from category S05.
A   initial encounter
D   subsequent encounter
S   sequela

✓5th **S05.0 Injury of conjunctiva and corneal abrasion without foreign body**

EXCLUDES 1 foreign body in conjunctival sac (T15.1)
foreign body in cornea (T15.0)

 ✓x7th **S05.00 Injury of conjunctiva and corneal abrasion without foreign body, unspecified eye** ▽

 ✓x7th **S05.01 Injury of conjunctiva and corneal abrasion without foreign body, right eye**

 ✓x7th **S05.02 Injury of conjunctiva and corneal abrasion without foreign body, left eye**

✓5th **S05.1 Contusion of eyeball and orbital tissues**
Traumatic hyphema

EXCLUDES 2 black eye NOS (S00.1)
contusion of eyelid and periocular area (S00.1)

 ✓x7th **S05.10 Contusion of eyeball and orbital tissues, unspecified eye** ▽

 ✓x7th **S05.11 Contusion of eyeball and orbital tissues, right eye**

 ✓x7th **S05.12 Contusion of eyeball and orbital tissues, left eye**

✓5th **S05.2 Ocular laceration and rupture with prolapse or loss of intraocular tissue**

 ✓x7th **S05.20 Ocular laceration and rupture with prolapse or loss of intraocular tissue, unspecified eye** ▽

 ✓x7th **S05.21 Ocular laceration and rupture with prolapse or loss of intraocular tissue, right eye**

 ✓x7th **S05.22 Ocular laceration and rupture with prolapse or loss of intraocular tissue, left eye**

✓5th **S05.3 Ocular laceration without prolapse or loss of intraocular tissue**
Laceration of eye NOS
DEF: Tear in ocular tissue without displacing structures; due to blunt trauma; characterized by pain, redness, and decreased vision.

 ✓x7th **S05.30 Ocular laceration without prolapse or loss of intraocular tissue, unspecified eye** ▽

 ✓x7th **S05.31 Ocular laceration without prolapse or loss of intraocular tissue, right eye**

 ✓x7th **S05.32 Ocular laceration without prolapse or loss of intraocular tissue, left eye**

✓5th **S05.4 Penetrating wound of orbit with or without foreign body**

EXCLUDES 2 retained (old) foreign body following penetrating wound in orbit (H05.5-)

 ✓x7th **S05.40 Penetrating wound of orbit with or without foreign body, unspecified eye** ▽

 ✓x7th **S05.41 Penetrating wound of orbit with or without foreign body, right eye**

 ✓x7th **S05.42 Penetrating wound of orbit with or without foreign body, left eye**

✓ Additional Character Req   ✓x7th Placeholder Alert   Manifestation   HCC CMS-HCC Condition   ▽ Unspecified Code   ▶◀ Revised Text   ● New Code   ▲ Revised Code Title

ICD-10-CM 2018   919

Chapter 19. Injury, Poisoning, and Certain Other Consequences of External Causes *(side margin)*

S05.5 Penetrating wound with foreign body of eyeball
EXCLUDES 2 retained (old) intraocular foreign body (H44.6-, H44.7)

S05.50 Penetrating wound with foreign body of unspecified eyeball ▽

S05.51 Penetrating wound with foreign body of right eyeball

S05.52 Penetrating wound with foreign body of left eyeball

S05.6 Penetrating wound without foreign body of eyeball
Ocular penetration NOS

S05.60 Penetrating wound without foreign body of unspecified eyeball ▽

S05.61 Penetrating wound without foreign body of right eyeball

S05.62 Penetrating wound without foreign body of left eyeball

S05.7 Avulsion of eye
Traumatic enucleation

S05.70 Avulsion of unspecified eye ▽

S05.71 Avulsion of right eye

S05.72 Avulsion of left eye

S05.8 Other injuries of eye and orbit
Lacrimal duct injury

S05.8X Other injuries of eye and orbit

S05.8X1 Other injuries of right eye and orbit

S05.8X2 Other injuries of left eye and orbit

S05.8X9 Other injuries of unspecified eye and orbit ▽

S05.9 Unspecified injury of eye and orbit
Injury of eye NOS

S05.90 Unspecified injury of unspecified eye and orbit ▽

S05.91 Unspecified injury of right eye and orbit ▽

S05.92 Unspecified injury of left eye and orbit ▽

S06 Intracranial injury
NOTE ▶7th characters D and S do not apply to codes in category S06 with 6th character 7 – death due to brain injury prior to regaining consciousness, or 8 – death due to other cause prior to regaining consciousness◀
INCLUDES traumatic brain injury
Code also any associated:
 open wound of head (S01.-)
 skull fracture (S02.-)
EXCLUDES 1 head injury NOS (S09.90)
AHA: 2017, 1Q, 42; 2015, 3Q, 37

The appropriate 7th character is to be added to each code from category S06.
A initial encounter
D subsequent encounter
S sequela

S06.0 Concussion
Commotio cerebri
EXCLUDES 1 concussion with intracranial injuries classified in subcategories S06.1- to S06.6-, S06.81-, S06.82- code to specified intracranial injury

S06.0X Concussion

S06.0X0 Concussion without loss of consciousness HCC

S06.0X1 Concussion with loss of consciousness of 30 minutes or less HCC

S06.0X9 Concussion with loss of consciousness of unspecified duration HCC ▽
Concussion NOS

S06.1 Traumatic cerebral edema
Diffuse traumatic cerebral edema
Focal traumatic cerebral edema

S06.1X Traumatic cerebral edema

S06.1X0 Traumatic cerebral edema without loss of consciousness HCC

S06.1X1 Traumatic cerebral edema with loss of consciousness of 30 minutes or less HCC

S06.1X2 Traumatic cerebral edema with loss of consciousness of 31 minutes to 59 minutes HCC

S06.1X3 Traumatic cerebral edema with loss of consciousness of 1 hour to 5 hours 59 minutes HCC

S06.1X4 Traumatic cerebral edema with loss of consciousness of 6 hours to 24 hours HCC

S06.1X5 Traumatic cerebral edema with loss of consciousness greater than 24 hours with return to pre-existing conscious level HCC

S06.1X6 Traumatic cerebral edema with loss of consciousness greater than 24 hours without return to pre-existing conscious level with patient surviving HCC

S06.1X7 Traumatic cerebral edema with loss of consciousness of any duration with death due to brain injury prior to regaining consciousness

S06.1X8 Traumatic cerebral edema with loss of consciousness of any duration with death due to other cause prior to regaining consciousness

S06.1X9 Traumatic cerebral edema with loss of consciousness of unspecified duration HCC ▽
Traumatic cerebral edema NOS

S06.2 Diffuse traumatic brain injury
Diffuse axonal brain injury
EXCLUDES 1 traumatic diffuse cerebral edema (S06.1X-)

S06.2X Diffuse traumatic brain injury

S06.2X0 Diffuse traumatic brain injury without loss of consciousness HCC

S06.2X1 Diffuse traumatic brain injury with loss of consciousness of 30 minutes or less HCC

S06.2X2 Diffuse traumatic brain injury with loss of consciousness of 31 minutes to 59 minutes HCC

S06.2X3 Diffuse traumatic brain injury with loss of consciousness of 1 hour to 5 hours 59 minutes HCC

S06.2X4 Diffuse traumatic brain injury with loss of consciousness of 6 hours to 24 hours HCC

S06.2X5 Diffuse traumatic brain injury with loss of consciousness greater than 24 hours with return to pre-existing conscious levels HCC

S06.2X6 Diffuse traumatic brain injury with loss of consciousness greater than 24 hours without return to pre-existing conscious level with patient surviving HCC

S06.2X7 Diffuse traumatic brain injury with loss of consciousness of any duration with death due to brain injury prior to regaining consciousness

S06.2X8 Diffuse traumatic brain injury with loss of consciousness of any duration with death due to other cause prior to regaining consciousness

S06.2X9 Diffuse traumatic brain injury with loss of consciousness of unspecified duration HCC ▽
Diffuse traumatic brain injury NOS

S06.3 Focal traumatic brain injury
EXCLUDES 1 any condition classifiable to S06.4-S06.6
focal cerebral edema (S06.1)

S06.30 Unspecified focal traumatic brain injury

S06.300 Unspecified focal traumatic brain injury without loss of consciousness HCC ▽

S06.301 Unspecified focal traumatic brain injury with loss of consciousness of 30 minutes or less HCC ▽

S06.302 Unspecified focal traumatic brain injury with loss of consciousness of 31 minutes to 59 minutes HCC ▽

S06.303 Unspecified focal traumatic brain injury with loss of consciousness of 1 hour to 5 hours 59 minutes HCC ▽

2 HCC with 7th character indicating initial encounter (A or B - specific to category) OR sequela.
3 HCC with 7th character indicating sequela.

² ✓7ᵗʰ **S06.304 Unspecified focal traumatic brain** HCC ▽
**injury with loss of consciousness
of** 6 hours to 24 hours

² ✓7ᵗʰ **S06.305 Unspecified focal traumatic brain** HCC ▽
injury with loss of consciousness
greater than 24 hours with return
to pre-existing conscious level

² ✓7ᵗʰ **S06.306 Unspecified focal traumatic brain** HCC ▽
injury with loss of consciousness
greater than 24 hours without return to
pre-existing conscious level with patient
surviving

✓7ᵗʰ **S06.307 Unspecified focal traumatic brain** ▽
injury with loss of consciousness of any
duration with death due to brain injury
prior to regaining consciousness

✓7ᵗʰ **S06.308 Unspecified focal traumatic brain** ▽
injury with loss of consciousness of any
duration with death due to other cause
prior to regaining consciousness

² ✓7ᵗʰ **S06.309 Unspecified focal traumatic brain** HCC ▽
**injury with loss of consciousness of
unspecified duration**
Unspecified focal traumatic brain injury
NOS

✓6ᵗʰ **S06.31 Contusion and laceration of** right cerebrum

² ✓7ᵗʰ **S06.310 Contusion and laceration of right** HCC
cerebrum without loss of consciousness

² ✓7ᵗʰ **S06.311 Contusion and laceration of right** HCC
cerebrum with loss of consciousness of
30 minutes or less

² ✓7ᵗʰ **S06.312 Contusion and laceration of right** HCC
cerebrum with loss of consciousness of
31 minutes to 59 minutes

² ✓7ᵗʰ **S06.313 Contusion and laceration of right** HCC
cerebrum with loss of consciousness of
1 hour to 5 hours 59 minutes

² ✓7ᵗʰ **S06.314 Contusion and laceration of right** HCC
cerebrum with loss of consciousness of
6 hours to 24 hours

² ✓7ᵗʰ **S06.315 Contusion and laceration of right** HCC
cerebrum with loss of consciousness
greater than 24 hours with return to
pre-existing conscious level

² ✓7ᵗʰ **S06.316 Contusion and laceration of right** HCC
cerebrum with loss of consciousness
greater than 24 hours without return to
pre-existing conscious level with patient
surviving

✓7ᵗʰ **S06.317 Contusion and laceration of right**
cerebrum with loss of consciousness of
any duration with death due to brain
injury prior to regaining consciousness

✓7ᵗʰ **S06.318 Contusion and laceration of right**
cerebrum with loss of consciousness of
any duration with death due to other
cause prior to regaining consciousness

² ✓7ᵗʰ **S06.319 Contusion and laceration of right** HCC ▽
**cerebrum with loss of consciousness
of unspecified duration**
Contusion and laceration of right cerebrum
NOS

✓6ᵗʰ **S06.32 Contusion and laceration of** left cerebrum

² ✓7ᵗʰ **S06.320 Contusion and laceration of left** HCC
cerebrum without loss of consciousness

² ✓7ᵗʰ **S06.321 Contusion and laceration of left** HCC
**cerebrum with loss of consciousness
of** 30 minutes or less

² ✓7ᵗʰ **S06.322 Contusion and laceration of left** HCC
**cerebrum with loss of consciousness
of** 31 minutes to 59 minutes

² ✓7ᵗʰ **S06.323 Contusion and laceration of left** HCC
**cerebrum with loss of consciousness
of** 1 hour to 5 hours 59 minutes

² ✓7ᵗʰ **S06.324 Contusion and laceration of left** HCC
**cerebrum with loss of consciousness
of** 6 hours to 24 hours

² ✓7ᵗʰ **S06.325 Contusion and laceration of left** HCC
cerebrum with loss of consciousness
greater than 24 hours with return
to pre-existing conscious level

² ✓7ᵗʰ **S06.326 Contusion and laceration of left** HCC
cerebrum with loss of consciousness
greater than 24 hours without return
to pre-existing conscious level with
patient surviving

✓7ᵗʰ **S06.327 Contusion and laceration of left cerebrum**
with loss of consciousness of any duration
with death due to brain injury prior to
regaining consciousness

✓7ᵗʰ **S06.328 Contusion and laceration of left cerebrum**
with loss of consciousness of any duration
with death due to other cause prior to
regaining consciousness

² ✓7ᵗʰ **S06.329 Contusion and laceration of left** HCC ▽
**cerebrum with loss of consciousness of
unspecified duration**
Contusion and laceration of left cerebrum
NOS

✓6ᵗʰ **S06.33 Contusion and laceration of** cerebrum, unspecified

² ✓7ᵗʰ **S06.330 Contusion and laceration of** HCC ▽
**cerebrum, unspecified, without loss
of consciousness**

² ✓7ᵗʰ **S06.331 Contusion and laceration of** HCC ▽
**cerebrum, unspecified, with loss of
consciousness of** 30 minutes or less

² ✓7ᵗʰ **S06.332 Contusion and laceration of** HCC ▽
**cerebrum, unspecified, with loss of
consciousness of** 31 minutes to
59 minutes

² ✓7ᵗʰ **S06.333 Contusion and laceration of** HCC ▽
**cerebrum, unspecified, with loss of
consciousness of** 1 hour to 5 hours
59 minutes

² ✓7ᵗʰ **S06.334 Contusion and laceration of** HCC ▽
**cerebrum, unspecified, with loss of
consciousness of** 6 hours to 24 hours

² ✓7ᵗʰ **S06.335 Contusion and laceration of** HCC ▽
**cerebrum, unspecified, with loss of
consciousness** greater than 24 hours with
return to pre-existing conscious level

² ✓7ᵗʰ **S06.336 Contusion and laceration of** HCC ▽
**cerebrum, unspecified, with loss of
consciousness** greater than 24 hours
without return to pre-existing conscious
level with patient surviving

✓7ᵗʰ **S06.337 Contusion and laceration of cerebrum,** ▽
unspecified, with loss of consciousness of
any duration with death due to brain
injury prior to regaining consciousness

✓7ᵗʰ **S06.338 Contusion and laceration of cerebrum,** ▽
unspecified, with loss of consciousness of
any duration with death due to other
cause prior to regaining consciousness

² ✓7ᵗʰ **S06.339 Contusion and laceration of** HCC ▽
**cerebrum, unspecified, with loss of
consciousness of unspecified duration**
Contusion and laceration of cerebrum NOS

✓6ᵗʰ **S06.34 Traumatic hemorrhage of** right cerebrum
Traumatic intracerebral hemorrhage and hematoma
of right cerebrum

² ✓7ᵗʰ **S06.340 Traumatic hemorrhage of right** HCC
cerebrum without loss of consciousness

² ✓7ᵗʰ **S06.341 Traumatic hemorrhage of right** HCC
**cerebrum with loss of consciousness
of** 30 minutes or less

² ✓7ᵗʰ **S06.342 Traumatic hemorrhage of right** HCC
**cerebrum with loss of consciousness
of** 31 minutes to 59 minutes

² ✓7ᵗʰ **S06.343 Traumatic hemorrhage of right** HCC
**cerebrum with loss of consciousness
of** 1 hours to 5 hours 59 minutes

² ✓7ᵗʰ **S06.344 Traumatic hemorrhage of right** HCC
**cerebrum with loss of consciousness
of** 6 hours to 24 hours

---

² HCC with 7th character indicating initial encounter (A or B - specific to category) OR sequela.

✓ Additional Character Req   ✓x7ᵗʰ Placeholder Alert   Manifestation   HCC CMS-HCC Condition   ▽ Unspecified Code   ▶◀ Revised Text   ● New Code   ▲ Revised Code Title

2 ✓7ᵗʰ S06.345 Traumatic hemorrhage of right cerebrum with loss of consciousness greater than 24 hours with return to pre-existing conscious level   HCC

2 ✓7ᵗʰ S06.346 Traumatic hemorrhage of right cerebrum with loss of consciousness greater than 24 hours without return to pre-existing conscious level with patient surviving   HCC

✓7ᵗʰ S06.347 Traumatic hemorrhage of right cerebrum with loss of consciousness of any duration with death due to brain injury prior to regaining consciousness

✓7ᵗʰ S06.348 Traumatic hemorrhage of right cerebrum with loss of consciousness of any duration with death due to other cause prior to regaining consciousness

2 ✓7ᵗʰ S06.349 Traumatic hemorrhage of right cerebrum with loss of consciousness of unspecified duration   HCC ▽
Traumatic hemorrhage of right cerebrum NOS

✓6ᵗʰ S06.35 Traumatic hemorrhage of left cerebrum
Traumatic intracerebral hemorrhage and hematoma of left cerebrum

2 ✓7ᵗʰ S06.350 Traumatic hemorrhage of left cerebrum without loss of consciousness   HCC

2 ✓7ᵗʰ S06.351 Traumatic hemorrhage of left cerebrum with loss of consciousness of 30 minutes or less   HCC

2 ✓7ᵗʰ S06.352 Traumatic hemorrhage of left cerebrum with loss of consciousness of 31 minutes to 59 minutes   HCC

2 ✓7ᵗʰ S06.353 Traumatic hemorrhage of left cerebrum with loss of consciousness of 1 hours to 5 hours 59 minutes   HCC

2 ✓7ᵗʰ S06.354 Traumatic hemorrhage of left cerebrum with loss of consciousness of 6 hours to 24 hours   HCC

2 ✓7ᵗʰ S06.355 Traumatic hemorrhage of left cerebrum with loss of consciousness greater than 24 hours with return to pre-existing conscious level   HCC

2 ✓7ᵗʰ S06.356 Traumatic hemorrhage of left cerebrum with loss of consciousness greater than 24 hours without return to pre-existing conscious level with patient surviving   HCC

✓7ᵗʰ S06.357 Traumatic hemorrhage of left cerebrum with loss of consciousness of any duration with death due to brain injury prior to regaining consciousness

✓7ᵗʰ S06.358 Traumatic hemorrhage of left cerebrum with loss of consciousness of any duration with death due to other cause prior to regaining consciousness

2 ✓7ᵗʰ S06.359 Traumatic hemorrhage of left cerebrum with loss of consciousness of unspecified duration   HCC ▽
Traumatic hemorrhage of left cerebrum NOS

✓6ᵗʰ S06.36 Traumatic hemorrhage of cerebrum, unspecified
Traumatic intracerebral hemorrhage and hematoma, unspecified

2 ✓7ᵗʰ S06.360 Traumatic hemorrhage of cerebrum, unspecified, without loss of consciousness   HCC ▽

2 ✓7ᵗʰ S06.361 Traumatic hemorrhage of cerebrum, unspecified, with loss of consciousness of 30 minutes or less   HCC ▽

2 ✓7ᵗʰ S06.362 Traumatic hemorrhage of cerebrum, unspecified, with loss of consciousness of 31 minutes to 59 minutes   HCC ▽

2 ✓7ᵗʰ S06.363 Traumatic hemorrhage of cerebrum, unspecified, with loss of consciousness of 1 hours to 5 hours 59 minutes   HCC ▽

2 ✓7ᵗʰ S06.364 Traumatic hemorrhage of cerebrum, unspecified, with loss of consciousness of 6 hours to 24 hours   HCC ▽

2 ✓7ᵗʰ S06.365 Traumatic hemorrhage of cerebrum, unspecified, with loss of consciousness greater than 24 hours with return to pre-existing conscious level   HCC ▽

2 ✓7ᵗʰ S06.366 Traumatic hemorrhage of cerebrum, unspecified, with loss of consciousness greater than 24 hours without return to pre-existing conscious level with patient surviving   HCC ▽

✓7ᵗʰ S06.367 Traumatic hemorrhage of cerebrum, unspecified, with loss of consciousness of any duration with death due to brain injury prior to regaining consciousness   ▽

✓7ᵗʰ S06.368 Traumatic hemorrhage of cerebrum, unspecified, with loss of consciousness of any duration with death due to other cause prior to regaining consciousness   ▽

2 ✓7ᵗʰ S06.369 Traumatic hemorrhage of cerebrum, unspecified, with loss of consciousness of unspecified duration   HCC ▽
Traumatic hemorrhage of cerebrum NOS

✓6ᵗʰ S06.37 Contusion, laceration, and hemorrhage of cerebellum

2 ✓7ᵗʰ S06.370 Contusion, laceration, and hemorrhage of cerebellum without loss of consciousness   HCC

2 ✓7ᵗʰ S06.371 Contusion, laceration, and hemorrhage of cerebellum with loss of consciousness of 30 minutes or less   HCC

2 ✓7ᵗʰ S06.372 Contusion, laceration, and hemorrhage of cerebellum with loss of consciousness of 31 minutes to 59 minutes   HCC

2 ✓7ᵗʰ S06.373 Contusion, laceration, and hemorrhage of cerebellum with loss of consciousness of 1 hour to 5 hours 59 minutes   HCC

2 ✓7ᵗʰ S06.374 Contusion, laceration, and hemorrhage of cerebellum with loss of consciousness of 6 hours to 24 hours   HCC

2 ✓7ᵗʰ S06.375 Contusion, laceration, and hemorrhage of cerebellum with loss of consciousness greater than 24 hours with return to pre-existing conscious level   HCC

2 ✓7ᵗʰ S06.376 Contusion, laceration, and hemorrhage of cerebellum with loss of consciousness greater than 24 hours without return to pre-existing conscious level with patient surviving   HCC

✓7ᵗʰ S06.377 Contusion, laceration, and hemorrhage of cerebellum with loss of consciousness of any duration with death due to brain injury prior to regaining consciousness

✓7ᵗʰ S06.378 Contusion, laceration, and hemorrhage of cerebellum with loss of consciousness of any duration with death due to other cause prior to regaining consciousness

2 ✓7ᵗʰ S06.379 Contusion, laceration, and hemorrhage of cerebellum with loss of consciousness of unspecified duration   HCC ▽
Contusion, laceration, and hemorrhage of cerebellum NOS

✓6ᵗʰ S06.38 Contusion, laceration, and hemorrhage of brainstem

2 ✓7ᵗʰ S06.380 Contusion, laceration, and hemorrhage of brainstem without loss of consciousness   HCC

2 ✓7ᵗʰ S06.381 Contusion, laceration, and hemorrhage of brainstem with loss of consciousness of 30 minutes or less   HCC

2 ✓7ᵗʰ S06.382 Contusion, laceration, and hemorrhage of brainstem with loss of consciousness of 31 minutes to 59 minutes   HCC

---

2 HCC with 7th character indicating initial encounter (A or B - specific to category) OR sequela.

EXCLUDES 1 Not coded here   EXCLUDES 2 Not included here   N Newborn Age: 0   P Pediatric Age: 0-17   M Maternity Age: 12-55   A Adult Age: 15-124

922   ICD-10-CM 2018

2 ✓7th **S06.383** Contusion, laceration, and hemorrhage of brainstem with loss of consciousness of 1 hour to 5 hours 59 minutes `HCC`

2 ✓7th **S06.384** Contusion, laceration, and hemorrhage of brainstem with loss of consciousness of 6 hours to 24 hours `HCC`

2 ✓7th **S06.385** Contusion, laceration, and hemorrhage of brainstem with loss of consciousness greater than 24 hours with return to pre-existing conscious level `HCC`

2 ✓7th **S06.386** Contusion, laceration, and hemorrhage of brainstem with loss of consciousness greater than 24 hours without return to pre-existing conscious level with patient surviving `HCC`

✓7th **S06.387** Contusion, laceration, and hemorrhage of brainstem with loss of consciousness of any duration with death due to brain injury prior to regaining consciousness

✓7th **S06.388** Contusion, laceration, and hemorrhage of brainstem with loss of consciousness of any duration with death due to other cause prior to regaining consciousness

2 ✓7th **S06.389** Contusion, laceration, and hemorrhage of brainstem with loss of consciousness of unspecified duration `HCC` ▽
  Contusion, laceration, and hemorrhage of brainstem NOS

✓5th **S06.4** Epidural hemorrhage
  Extradural hemorrhage NOS
  Extradural hemorrhage (traumatic)

✓6th **S06.4X** Epidural hemorrhage

2 ✓7th **S06.4X0** Epidural hemorrhage without loss of consciousness `HCC`

2 ✓7th **S06.4X1** Epidural hemorrhage with loss of consciousness of 30 minutes or less `HCC`

2 ✓7th **S06.4X2** Epidural hemorrhage with loss of consciousness of 31 minutes to 59 minutes `HCC`

2 ✓7th **S06.4X3** Epidural hemorrhage with loss of consciousness of 1 hour to 5 hours 59 minutes `HCC`

2 ✓7th **S06.4X4** Epidural hemorrhage with loss of consciousness of 6 hours to 24 hours `HCC`

2 ✓7th **S06.4X5** Epidural hemorrhage with loss of consciousness greater than 24 hours with return to pre-existing conscious level `HCC`

2 ✓7th **S06.4X6** Epidural hemorrhage with loss of consciousness greater than 24 hours without return to pre-existing conscious level with patient surviving `HCC`

✓7th **S06.4X7** Epidural hemorrhage with loss of consciousness of any duration with death due to brain injury prior to regaining consciousness

✓7th **S06.4X8** Epidural hemorrhage with loss of consciousness of any duration with death due to other causes prior to regaining consciousness

2 ✓7th **S06.4X9** Epidural hemorrhage with loss of consciousness of unspecified duration `HCC` ▽
  Epidural hemorrhage NOS

✓5th **S06.5** Traumatic subdural hemorrhage

✓6th **S06.5X** Traumatic subdural hemorrhage

2 ✓7th **S06.5X0** Traumatic subdural hemorrhage without loss of consciousness `HCC`

2 ✓7th **S06.5X1** Traumatic subdural hemorrhage with loss of consciousness of 30 minutes or less `HCC`

2 ✓7th **S06.5X2** Traumatic subdural hemorrhage with loss of consciousness of 31 minutes to 59 minutes `HCC`

2 ✓7th **S06.5X3** Traumatic subdural hemorrhage with loss of consciousness of 1 hour to 5 hours 59 minutes `HCC`

2 ✓7th **S06.5X4** Traumatic subdural hemorrhage with loss of consciousness of 6 hours to 24 hours `HCC`

2 ✓7th **S06.5X5** Traumatic subdural hemorrhage with loss of consciousness greater than 24 hours with return to pre-existing conscious level `HCC`

2 ✓7th **S06.5X6** Traumatic subdural hemorrhage with loss of consciousness greater than 24 hours without return to pre-existing conscious level with patient surviving `HCC`

✓7th **S06.5X7** Traumatic subdural hemorrhage with loss of consciousness of any duration with death due to brain injury before regaining consciousness

✓7th **S06.5X8** Traumatic subdural hemorrhage with loss of consciousness of any duration with death due to other cause before regaining consciousness

2 ✓7th **S06.5X9** Traumatic subdural hemorrhage with loss of consciousness of unspecified duration `HCC` ▽
  Traumatic subdural hemorrhage NOS

✓5th **S06.6** Traumatic subarachnoid hemorrhage

✓6th **S06.6X** Traumatic subarachnoid hemorrhage

2 ✓7th **S06.6X0** Traumatic subarachnoid hemorrhage without loss of consciousness `HCC`

2 ✓7th **S06.6X1** Traumatic subarachnoid hemorrhage with loss of consciousness of 30 minutes or less `HCC`

2 ✓7th **S06.6X2** Traumatic subarachnoid hemorrhage with loss of consciousness of 31 minutes to 59 minutes `HCC`

2 ✓7th **S06.6X3** Traumatic subarachnoid hemorrhage with loss of consciousness of 1 hour to 5 hours 59 minutes `HCC`

2 ✓7th **S06.6X4** Traumatic subarachnoid hemorrhage with loss of consciousness of 6 hours to 24 hours `HCC`

2 ✓7th **S06.6X5** Traumatic subarachnoid hemorrhage with loss of consciousness greater than 24 hours with return to pre-existing conscious level `HCC`

2 ✓7th **S06.6X6** Traumatic subarachnoid hemorrhage with loss of consciousness greater than 24 hours without return to pre-existing conscious level with patient surviving `HCC`

✓7th **S06.6X7** Traumatic subarachnoid hemorrhage with loss of consciousness of any duration with death due to brain injury prior to regaining consciousness

✓7th **S06.6X8** Traumatic subarachnoid hemorrhage with loss of consciousness of any duration with death due to other cause prior to regaining consciousness

2 ✓7th **S06.6X9** Traumatic subarachnoid hemorrhage with loss of consciousness of unspecified duration `HCC` ▽
  Traumatic subarachnoid hemorrhage NOS

✓5th **S06.8** Other specified intracranial injuries

✓6th **S06.81** Injury of right internal carotid artery, intracranial portion, not elsewhere classified

2 ✓7th **S06.810** Injury of right internal carotid artery, intracranial portion, not elsewhere classified without loss of consciousness `HCC`

2 ✓7th **S06.811** Injury of right internal carotid artery, intracranial portion, not elsewhere classified with loss of consciousness of 30 minutes or less `HCC`

2 ✓7th **S06.812** Injury of right internal carotid artery, intracranial portion, not elsewhere classified with loss of consciousness of 31 minutes to 59 minutes `HCC`

2 ✓7th **S06.813** Injury of right internal carotid artery, intracranial portion, not elsewhere classified with loss of consciousness of 1 hour to 5 hours 59 minutes `HCC`

2 HCC with 7th character indicating initial encounter (A or B - specific to category) OR sequela.

✓ Additional Character Req ✓7th Placeholder Alert Manifestation `HCC` CMS-HCC Condition ▽ Unspecified Code ►◄ Revised Text ● New Code ▲ Revised Code Title

2 ✓7ᵗʰ **S06.814** **Injury of right internal carotid artery, intracranial portion, not elsewhere classified with loss of consciousness of 6 hours to 24 hours** ᴴᶜᶜ

2 ✓7ᵗʰ **S06.815** **Injury of right internal carotid artery, intracranial portion, not elsewhere classified with loss of consciousness greater than 24 hours with return to pre-existing conscious level** ᴴᶜᶜ

2 ✓7ᵗʰ **S06.816** **Injury of right internal carotid artery, intracranial portion, not elsewhere classified with loss of consciousness greater than 24 hours without return to pre-existing conscious level with patient surviving** ᴴᶜᶜ

✓7ᵗʰ **S06.817** **Injury of right internal carotid artery, intracranial portion, not elsewhere classified with loss of consciousness of any duration with death due to brain injury prior to regaining consciousness**

✓7ᵗʰ **S06.818** **Injury of right internal carotid artery, intracranial portion, not elsewhere classified with loss of consciousness of any duration with death due to other cause prior to regaining consciousness**

2 ✓7ᵗʰ **S06.819** **Injury of right internal carotid artery, intracranial portion, not elsewhere classified with loss of consciousness of unspecified duration** ᴴᶜᶜ ▽
Injury of right internal carotid artery, intracranial portion, not elsewhere classified NOS

✓6ᵗʰ **S06.82** **Injury of left internal carotid artery, intracranial portion, not elsewhere classified**

2 ✓7ᵗʰ **S06.820** **Injury of left internal carotid artery, intracranial portion, not elsewhere classified without loss of consciousness** ᴴᶜᶜ

2 ✓7ᵗʰ **S06.821** **Injury of left internal carotid artery, intracranial portion, not elsewhere classified with loss of consciousness of 30 minutes or less** ᴴᶜᶜ

2 ✓7ᵗʰ **S06.822** **Injury of left internal carotid artery, intracranial portion, not elsewhere classified with loss of consciousness of 31 minutes to 59 minutes** ᴴᶜᶜ

2 ✓7ᵗʰ **S06.823** **Injury of left internal carotid artery, intracranial portion, not elsewhere classified with loss of consciousness of 1 hour to 5 hours 59 minutes** ᴴᶜᶜ

2 ✓7ᵗʰ **S06.824** **Injury of left internal carotid artery, intracranial portion, not elsewhere classified with loss of consciousness of 6 hours to 24 hours** ᴴᶜᶜ

2 ✓7ᵗʰ **S06.825** **Injury of left internal carotid artery, intracranial portion, not elsewhere classified with loss of consciousness greater than 24 hours with return to pre-existing conscious level** ᴴᶜᶜ

2 ✓7ᵗʰ **S06.826** **Injury of left internal carotid artery, intracranial portion, not elsewhere classified with loss of consciousness greater than 24 hours without return to pre-existing conscious level with patient surviving** ᴴᶜᶜ

✓7ᵗʰ **S06.827** **Injury of left internal carotid artery, intracranial portion, not elsewhere classified with loss of consciousness of any duration with death due to brain injury prior to regaining consciousness**

✓7ᵗʰ **S06.828** **Injury of left internal carotid artery, intracranial portion, not elsewhere classified with loss of consciousness of any duration with death due to other cause prior to regaining consciousness**

2 ✓7ᵗʰ **S06.829** **Injury of left internal carotid artery, intracranial portion, not elsewhere classified with loss of consciousness of unspecified duration** ᴴᶜᶜ ▽
Injury of left internal carotid artery, intracranial portion, not elsewhere classified NOS

✓6ᵗʰ **S06.89** **Other specified intracranial injury**
EXCLUDES 1   concussion (S06.0X-)

2 ✓7ᵗʰ **S06.890** **Other specified intracranial injury without loss of consciousness** ᴴᶜᶜ

2 ✓7ᵗʰ **S06.891** **Other specified intracranial injury with loss of consciousness of 30 minutes or less** ᴴᶜᶜ

2 ✓7ᵗʰ **S06.892** **Other specified intracranial injury with loss of consciousness of 31 minutes to 59 minutes** ᴴᶜᶜ

2 ✓7ᵗʰ **S06.893** **Other specified intracranial injury with loss of consciousness of 1 hour to 5 hours 59 minutes** ᴴᶜᶜ

2 ✓7ᵗʰ **S06.894** **Other specified intracranial injury with loss of consciousness of 6 hours to 24 hours** ᴴᶜᶜ

2 ✓7ᵗʰ **S06.895** **Other specified intracranial injury with loss of consciousness greater than 24 hours with return to pre-existing conscious level** ᴴᶜᶜ

2 ✓7ᵗʰ **S06.896** **Other specified intracranial injury with loss of consciousness greater than 24 hours without return to pre-existing conscious level with patient surviving** ᴴᶜᶜ

✓7ᵗʰ **S06.897** **Other specified intracranial injury with loss of consciousness of any duration with death due to brain injury prior to regaining consciousness**

✓7ᵗʰ **S06.898** **Other specified intracranial injury with loss of consciousness of any duration with death due to other cause prior to regaining consciousness**

2 ✓7ᵗʰ **S06.899** **Other specified intracranial injury with loss of consciousness of unspecified duration** ᴴᶜᶜ ▽

✓5ᵗʰ **S06.9** **Unspecified intracranial injury**
Brain injury NOS
Head injury NOS with loss of consciousness
Traumatic brain injury NOS
EXCLUDES 1   conditions classifiable to S06.0- to S06.8- code to specified intracranial injury
head injury NOS (S09.90)

✓6ᵗʰ **S06.9X** **Unspecified intracranial injury**

2 ✓7ᵗʰ **S06.9X0** **Unspecified intracranial injury without loss of consciousness** ᴴᶜᶜ ▽

2 ✓7ᵗʰ **S06.9X1** **Unspecified intracranial injury with loss of consciousness of 30 minutes or less** ᴴᶜᶜ ▽

2 ✓7ᵗʰ **S06.9X2** **Unspecified intracranial injury with loss of consciousness of 31 minutes to 59 minutes** ᴴᶜᶜ ▽

2 ✓7ᵗʰ **S06.9X3** **Unspecified intracranial injury with loss of consciousness of 1 hour to 5 hours 59 minutes** ᴴᶜᶜ ▽

2 ✓7ᵗʰ **S06.9X4** **Unspecified intracranial injury with loss of consciousness of 6 hours to 24 hours** ᴴᶜᶜ ▽

2 ✓7ᵗʰ **S06.9X5** **Unspecified intracranial injury with loss of consciousness greater than 24 hours with return to pre-existing conscious level** ᴴᶜᶜ ▽

2 ✓7ᵗʰ **S06.9X6** **Unspecified intracranial injury with loss of consciousness greater than 24 hours without return to pre-existing conscious level with patient surviving** ᴴᶜᶜ ▽

✓7ᵗʰ **S06.9X7** **Unspecified intracranial injury with loss of consciousness of any duration with death due to brain injury prior to regaining consciousness** ▽

✓7ᵗʰ **S06.9X8** **Unspecified intracranial injury with loss of consciousness of any duration with death due to other cause prior to regaining consciousness** ▽

2 ✓7ᵗʰ **S06.9X9** **Unspecified intracranial injury with loss of consciousness of unspecified duration** ᴴᶜᶜ ▽

---

2   HCC with 7th character indicating initial encounter (A or B - specific to category) OR sequela.

EXCLUDES 1 Not coded here   **EXCLUDES 2** Not included here   N Newborn Age: 0   P Pediatric Age: 0-17   M Maternity Age: 12-55   A Adult Age: 15-124

ICD-10-CM 2018

924

√4ᵗʰ **S07   Crushing injury of head**

Use additional code for all associated injuries, such as:
intracranial injuries (S06.-)
skull fractures (S02.-)

The appropriate 7th character is to be added to each code from category S07.
A   initial encounter
D   subsequent encounter
S   sequela

√x7ᵗʰ **S07.0   Crushing injury of face**

√x7ᵗʰ **S07.1   Crushing injury of skull**

√x7ᵗʰ **S07.8   Crushing injury of other parts of head**

√x7ᵗʰ **S07.9   Crushing injury of head, part unspecified**   ▽

√4ᵗʰ **S08   Avulsion and traumatic amputation of part of head**

An amputation not identified as partial or complete should be coded to complete

The appropriate 7th character is to be added to each code from category S08.
A   initial encounter
D   subsequent encounter
S   sequela

√x7ᵗʰ **S08.0   Avulsion of scalp**

√5ᵗʰ **S08.1   Traumatic amputation of ear**

√6ᵗʰ **S08.11   Complete traumatic amputation of ear**

√7ᵗʰ **S08.111   Complete traumatic amputation of right ear**

√7ᵗʰ **S08.112   Complete traumatic amputation of left ear**

√7ᵗʰ **S08.119   Complete traumatic amputation of unspecified ear**   ▽

√6ᵗʰ **S08.12   Partial traumatic amputation of ear**

√7ᵗʰ **S08.121   Partial traumatic amputation of right ear**

√7ᵗʰ **S08.122   Partial traumatic amputation of left ear**

√7ᵗʰ **S08.129   Partial traumatic amputation of unspecified ear**   ▽

√5ᵗʰ **S08.8   Traumatic amputation of other parts of head**

√6ᵗʰ **S08.81   Traumatic amputation of nose**

√7ᵗʰ **S08.811   Complete traumatic amputation of nose**

√7ᵗʰ **S08.812   Partial traumatic amputation of nose**

√x7ᵗʰ **S08.89   Traumatic amputation of other parts of head**

√4ᵗʰ **S09   Other and unspecified injuries of head**

The appropriate 7th character is to be added to each code from category S09.
A   initial encounter
D   subsequent encounter
S   sequela

√x7ᵗʰ **S09.0   Injury of blood vessels of head, not elsewhere classified**

EXCLUDES 1   injury of cerebral blood vessels (S06.-)
injury of precerebral blood vessels (S15.-)

√5ᵗʰ **S09.1   Injury of muscle and tendon of head**

Code also any associated open wound (S01.-)
EXCLUDES 2   sprain to joints and ligament of head (S03.9)

√x7ᵗʰ **S09.10   Unspecified injury of muscle and tendon of head**   ▽
Injury of muscle and tendon of head NOS

√x7ᵗʰ **S09.11   Strain of muscle and tendon of head**

√x7ᵗʰ **S09.12   Laceration of muscle and tendon of head**

√x7ᵗʰ **S09.19   Other specified injury of muscle and tendon of head**

√5ᵗʰ **S09.2   Traumatic rupture of ear drum**

EXCLUDES 1   traumatic rupture of ear drum due to blast injury (S09.31-)

√x7ᵗʰ **S09.20   Traumatic rupture of unspecified ear drum**   ▽

√x7ᵗʰ **S09.21   Traumatic rupture of right ear drum**

√x7ᵗʰ **S09.22   Traumatic rupture of left ear drum**

√5ᵗʰ **S09.3   Other specified and unspecified injury of middle and inner ear**

EXCLUDES 1   injury to ear NOS (S09.91-)
EXCLUDES 2   injury to external ear (S00.4-, S01.3-, S08.1-)

√6ᵗʰ **S09.30   Unspecified injury of middle and inner ear**

√7ᵗʰ **S09.301   Unspecified injury of right middle and inner ear**   ▽

√7ᵗʰ **S09.302   Unspecified injury of left middle and inner ear**   ▽

√7ᵗʰ **S09.309   Unspecified injury of unspecified middle and inner ear**   ▽

√6ᵗʰ **S09.31   Primary blast injury of ear**
Blast injury of ear NOS

√7ᵗʰ **S09.311   Primary blast injury of right ear**

√7ᵗʰ **S09.312   Primary blast injury of left ear**

√7ᵗʰ **S09.313   Primary blast injury of ear, bilateral**

√7ᵗʰ **S09.319   Primary blast injury of unspecified ear**   ▽

√6ᵗʰ **S09.39   Other specified injury of middle and inner ear**
Secondary blast injury to ear

√7ᵗʰ **S09.391   Other specified injury of right middle and inner ear**

√7ᵗʰ **S09.392   Other specified injury of left middle and inner ear**

√7ᵗʰ **S09.399   Other specified injury of unspecified middle and inner ear**   ▽

√x7ᵗʰ **S09.8   Other specified injuries of head**

√5ᵗʰ **S09.9   Unspecified injury of face and head**

√x7ᵗʰ **S09.90   Unspecified injury of head**   ▽
Head injury NOS
EXCLUDES 1   brain injury NOS (S06.9-)
head injury NOS with loss of consciousness (S06.9-)
intracranial injury NOS (S06.9-)

√x7ᵗʰ **S09.91   Unspecified injury of ear**   ▽
Injury of ear NOS

√x7ᵗʰ **S09.92   Unspecified injury of nose**   ▽
Injury of nose NOS

√x7ᵗʰ **S09.93   Unspecified injury of face**   ▽
Injury of face NOS

Injuries to the neck (S10-S19)

INCLUDES   injuries of nape
injuries of supraclavicular region
injuries of throat
EXCLUDES 2   burns and corrosions (T20-T32)
effects of foreign body in esophagus (T18.1)
effects of foreign body in larynx (T17.3)
effects of foreign body in pharynx (T17.2)
effects of foreign body in trachea (T17.4)
frostbite (T33-T34)
insect bite or sting, venomous (T63.4)

√4ᵗʰ **S10   Superficial injury of neck**

The appropriate 7th character is to be added to each code from category S10.
A   initial encounter
D   subsequent encounter
S   sequela

√x7ᵗʰ **S10.0   Contusion of throat**
Contusion of cervical esophagus
Contusion of larynx
Contusion of pharynx
Contusion of trachea

√5ᵗʰ **S10.1   Other and unspecified superficial injuries of throat**

√x7ᵗʰ **S10.10   Unspecified superficial injuries of throat**   ▽

√x7ᵗʰ **S10.11   Abrasion of throat**

√x7ᵗʰ **S10.12   Blister (nonthermal) of throat**

√x7ᵗʰ **S10.14   External constriction of part of throat**

√x7ᵗʰ **S10.15   Superficial foreign body of throat**
Splinter in the throat

√x7ᵗʰ **S10.16   Insect bite (nonvenomous) of throat**

√x7ᵗʰ **S10.17   Other superficial bite of throat**
EXCLUDES 1   open bite of throat (S11.85)

√5ᵗʰ **S10.8   Superficial injury of other specified parts of neck**

√x7ᵗʰ **S10.80   Unspecified superficial injury of other specified part of neck**   ▽

√x7ᵗʰ **S10.81   Abrasion of other specified part of neck**

√x7ᵗʰ **S10.82   Blister (nonthermal) of other specified part of neck**

√x7ᵗʰ **S10.83   Contusion of other specified part of neck**

√x7ᵗʰ **S10.84   External constriction of other specified part of neck**

☑ Additional Character Req   √x7ᵗʰ Placeholder Alert   Manifestation   HCC CMS-HCC Condition   ▽ Unspecified Code   ►◄ Revised Text   ● New Code   ▲ Revised Code Title

ICD-10-CM 2018   925

√x7ᵗʰ **S10.85** **Superficial foreign body** of other specified part of neck
> Splinter in other specified part of neck

√x7ᵗʰ **S10.86** **Insect bite** of other specified part of neck

√x7ᵗʰ **S10.87** **Other superficial bite** of other specified part of neck
> EXCLUDES 1   open bite of other specified parts of neck (S11.85)

√5ᵗʰ **S10.9** **Superficial injury of unspecified part of neck**

√x7ᵗʰ **S10.90** **Unspecified superficial injury** of unspecified part of neck ▽

√x7ᵗʰ **S10.91** **Abrasion** of unspecified part of neck ▽

√x7ᵗʰ **S10.92** **Blister (nonthermal)** of unspecified part of neck ▽

√x7ᵗʰ **S10.93** **Contusion** of unspecified part of neck ▽

√x7ᵗʰ **S10.94** **External constriction** of unspecified part of neck ▽

√x7ᵗʰ **S10.95** **Superficial foreign body** of unspecified part of neck ▽

√x7ᵗʰ **S10.96** **Insect bite** of unspecified part of neck ▽

√x7ᵗʰ **S10.97** **Other superficial bite** of unspecified part of neck ▽

√4ᵗʰ **S11** **Open wound of neck**
> Code also any associated:
>   spinal cord injury (S14.0, S14.1-)
>   wound infection
> EXCLUDES 2   open fracture of vertebra (S12- with 7th character B)

> The appropriate 7th character is to be added to each code from category S11.
> A   initial encounter
> D   subsequent encounter
> S   sequela

√5ᵗʰ **S11.0** **Open wound of larynx and trachea**

√6ᵗʰ **S11.01** **Open wound of larynx**
> EXCLUDES 2   open wound of vocal cord (S11.03)

√7ᵗʰ **S11.011** **Laceration without foreign body of larynx**

√7ᵗʰ **S11.012** **Laceration with foreign body of larynx**

√7ᵗʰ **S11.013** **Puncture wound without foreign body of larynx**

√7ᵗʰ **S11.014** **Puncture wound with foreign body of larynx**

√7ᵗʰ **S11.015** **Open bite of larynx**
> Bite of larynx NOS

√7ᵗʰ **S11.019** **Unspecified open wound of larynx** ▽

√6ᵗʰ **S11.02** **Open wound of trachea**
> Open wound of cervical trachea
> Open wound of trachea NOS
> EXCLUDES 2   open wound of thoracic trachea (S27.5-)

√7ᵗʰ **S11.021** **Laceration without foreign body of trachea**

√7ᵗʰ **S11.022** **Laceration with foreign body of trachea**

√7ᵗʰ **S11.023** **Puncture wound without foreign body of trachea**

√7ᵗʰ **S11.024** **Puncture wound with foreign body of trachea**

√7ᵗʰ **S11.025** **Open bite of trachea**
> Bite of trachea NOS

√7ᵗʰ **S11.029** **Unspecified open wound of trachea** ▽

√6ᵗʰ **S11.03** **Open wound of vocal cord**

√7ᵗʰ **S11.031** **Laceration without foreign body of vocal cord**

√7ᵗʰ **S11.032** **Laceration with foreign body of vocal cord**

√7ᵗʰ **S11.033** **Puncture wound without foreign body of vocal cord**

√7ᵗʰ **S11.034** **Puncture wound with foreign body of vocal cord**

√7ᵗʰ **S11.035** **Open bite of vocal cord**
> Bite of vocal cord NOS

√7ᵗʰ **S11.039** **Unspecified open wound of vocal cord** ▽

√5ᵗʰ **S11.1** **Open wound of thyroid gland**

√x7ᵗʰ **S11.10** **Unspecified open wound of thyroid gland** ▽

√x7ᵗʰ **S11.11** **Laceration without foreign body of thyroid gland**

√x7ᵗʰ **S11.12** **Laceration with foreign body of thyroid gland**

√x7ᵗʰ **S11.13** **Puncture wound without foreign body of thyroid gland**

√x7ᵗʰ **S11.14** **Puncture wound with foreign body of thyroid gland**

√x7ᵗʰ **S11.15** **Open bite of thyroid gland**
> Bite of thyroid gland NOS

√5ᵗʰ **S11.2** **Open wound of pharynx and cervical esophagus**
> EXCLUDES 1   open wound of esophagus NOS (S27.8-)

√x7ᵗʰ **S11.20** **Unspecified open wound of pharynx and cervical esophagus** ▽

√x7ᵗʰ **S11.21** **Laceration without foreign body of pharynx and cervical esophagus**

√x7ᵗʰ **S11.22** **Laceration with foreign body of pharynx and cervical esophagus**

√x7ᵗʰ **S11.23** **Puncture wound without foreign body of pharynx and cervical esophagus**

√x7ᵗʰ **S11.24** **Puncture wound with foreign body of pharynx and cervical esophagus**

√x7ᵗʰ **S11.25** **Open bite of pharynx and cervical esophagus**
> Bite of pharynx and cervical esophagus NOS

√5ᵗʰ **S11.8** **Open wound of other specified parts of neck**

√x7ᵗʰ **S11.80** **Unspecified open wound of other specified part of neck** ▽

√x7ᵗʰ **S11.81** **Laceration without foreign body of other specified part of neck**

√x7ᵗʰ **S11.82** **Laceration with foreign body of other specified part of neck**

√x7ᵗʰ **S11.83** **Puncture wound without foreign body of other specified part of neck**

√x7ᵗʰ **S11.84** **Puncture wound with foreign body of other specified part of neck**

√x7ᵗʰ **S11.85** **Open bite of other specified part of neck**
> Bite of other specified part of neck NOS
> EXCLUDES 1   superficial bite of other specified part of neck (S10.87)

√x7ᵗʰ **S11.89** **Other open wound of other specified part of neck**

√5ᵗʰ **S11.9** **Open wound of unspecified part of neck**

√x7ᵗʰ **S11.90** **Unspecified open wound of unspecified part of neck** ▽

√x7ᵗʰ **S11.91** **Laceration without foreign body of unspecified part of neck** ▽

√x7ᵗʰ **S11.92** **Laceration with foreign body of unspecified part of neck** ▽

√x7ᵗʰ **S11.93** **Puncture wound without foreign body of unspecified part of neck** ▽

√x7ᵗʰ **S11.94** **Puncture wound with foreign body of unspecified part of neck** ▽

√x7ᵗʰ **S11.95** **Open bite of unspecified part of neck** ▽
> Bite of neck NOS
> EXCLUDES 1   superficial bite of neck (S10.97)

√4ᵗʰ **S12** **Fracture of cervical vertebra and other parts of neck**
> NOTE   A fracture not indicated as nondisplaced or displaced should be coded to displaced.
> A fracture not indicated as open or closed should be coded to closed.
> INCLUDES   fracture of cervical neural arch
>   fracture of cervical spine
>   fracture of cervical spinous process
>   fracture of cervical transverse process
>   fracture of cervical vertebral arch
>   fracture of neck
> Code first any associated cervical spinal cord injury (S14.0, S14.1-)
> AHA: 2015, 3Q, 37-39

> The appropriate 7th character is to be added to all codes from subcategories S12.0-S12.6.
> A   initial encounter for closed fracture
> B   initial encounter for open fracture
> D   subsequent encounter for fracture with routine healing
> G   subsequent encounter for fracture with delayed healing
> K   subsequent encounter for fracture with nonunion
> S   sequela

√5ᵗʰ **S12.0** **Fracture of first cervical vertebra**
> Atlas

√6ᵗʰ **S12.00** **Unspecified fracture of first cervical vertebra**

[1] √7ᵗʰ **S12.000** **Unspecified displaced fracture of first cervical vertebra** HCC ▽

---

[1]   HCC with 7th character indicating initial encounter (A, B or C - specific to category).

EXCLUDES 1 Not coded here   EXCLUDES 2 Not included here   N Newborn Age: 0   P Pediatric Age: 0-17   M Maternity Age: 12-55   A Adult Age: 15-124

926   ICD-10-CM 2018

1 √7ᵗʰ **S12.001** Unspecified nondisplaced fracture of first cervical vertebra **HCC** ▽

1 √x7ᵗʰ **S12.01** Stable burst fracture of first cervical vertebra **HCC**

1 √x7ᵗʰ **S12.02** Unstable burst fracture of first cervical vertebra **HCC**

√6ᵗʰ **S12.03** Posterior arch fracture of first cervical vertebra

    1 √7ᵗʰ **S12.030** Displaced posterior arch fracture of first cervical vertebra **HCC**

    1 √7ᵗʰ **S12.031** Nondisplaced posterior arch fracture of first cervical vertebra **HCC**

√6ᵗʰ **S12.04** Lateral mass fracture of first cervical vertebra

    1 √7ᵗʰ **S12.040** Displaced lateral mass fracture of first cervical vertebra **HCC**

    1 √7ᵗʰ **S12.041** Nondisplaced lateral mass fracture of first cervical vertebra **HCC**

√6ᵗʰ **S12.09** Other fracture of first cervical vertebra

    1 √7ᵗʰ **S12.090** Other displaced fracture of first cervical vertebra **HCC**

    1 √7ᵗʰ **S12.091** Other nondisplaced fracture of first cervical vertebra **HCC**

√5ᵗʰ **S12.1** Fracture of second cervical vertebra
     Axis

√6ᵗʰ **S12.10** Unspecified fracture of second cervical vertebra

    1 √7ᵗʰ **S12.100** Unspecified displaced fracture of second cervical vertebra **HCC** ▽

    1 √7ᵗʰ **S12.101** Unspecified nondisplaced fracture of second cervical vertebra **HCC** ▽

√6ᵗʰ **S12.11** Type II dens fracture

    1 √7ᵗʰ **S12.110** Anterior displaced Type II dens fracture **HCC**

    1 √7ᵗʰ **S12.111** Posterior displaced Type II dens fracture **HCC**

    1 √7ᵗʰ **S12.112** Nondisplaced Type II dens fracture **HCC**

√6ᵗʰ **S12.12** Other dens fracture

    1 √7ᵗʰ **S12.120** Other displaced dens fracture **HCC**

    1 √7ᵗʰ **S12.121** Other nondisplaced dens fracture **HCC**

√6ᵗʰ **S12.13** Unspecified traumatic spondylolisthesis of second cervical vertebra

    1 √7ᵗʰ **S12.130** Unspecified traumatic displaced spondylolisthesis of second cervical vertebra **HCC** ▽

    1 √7ᵗʰ **S12.131** Unspecified traumatic nondisplaced spondylolisthesis of second cervical vertebra **HCC** ▽

1 √x7ᵗʰ **S12.14** Type III traumatic spondylolisthesis of second cervical vertebra **HCC**

√6ᵗʰ **S12.15** Other traumatic spondylolisthesis of second cervical vertebra

    1 √7ᵗʰ **S12.150** Other traumatic displaced spondylolisthesis of second cervical vertebra **HCC**

    1 √7ᵗʰ **S12.151** Other traumatic nondisplaced spondylolisthesis of second cervical vertebra **HCC**

√6ᵗʰ **S12.19** Other fracture of second cervical vertebra

    1 √7ᵗʰ **S12.190** Other displaced fracture of second cervical vertebra **HCC**

    1 √7ᵗʰ **S12.191** Other nondisplaced fracture of second cervical vertebra **HCC**

√5ᵗʰ **S12.2** Fracture of third cervical vertebra

√6ᵗʰ **S12.20** Unspecified fracture of third cervical vertebra

    1 √7ᵗʰ **S12.200** Unspecified displaced fracture of third cervical vertebra **HCC** ▽

    1 √7ᵗʰ **S12.201** Unspecified nondisplaced fracture of third cervical vertebra **HCC** ▽

√6ᵗʰ **S12.23** Unspecified traumatic spondylolisthesis of third cervical vertebra

    1 √7ᵗʰ **S12.230** Unspecified traumatic displaced spondylolisthesis of third cervical vertebra **HCC** ▽

    1 √7ᵗʰ **S12.231** Unspecified traumatic nondisplaced spondylolisthesis of third cervical vertebra **HCC** ▽

1 √x7ᵗʰ **S12.24** Type III traumatic spondylolisthesis of third cervical vertebra **HCC**

√6ᵗʰ **S12.25** Other traumatic spondylolisthesis of third cervical vertebra

    1 √7ᵗʰ **S12.250** Other traumatic displaced spondylolisthesis of third cervical vertebra **HCC**

    1 √7ᵗʰ **S12.251** Other traumatic nondisplaced spondylolisthesis of third cervical vertebra **HCC**

√6ᵗʰ **S12.29** Other fracture of third cervical vertebra

    1 √7ᵗʰ **S12.290** Other displaced fracture of third cervical vertebra **HCC**

    1 √7ᵗʰ **S12.291** Other nondisplaced fracture of third cervical vertebra **HCC**

√5ᵗʰ **S12.3** Fracture of fourth cervical vertebra

√6ᵗʰ **S12.30** Unspecified fracture of fourth cervical vertebra

    1 √7ᵗʰ **S12.300** Unspecified displaced fracture of fourth cervical vertebra **HCC** ▽

    1 √7ᵗʰ **S12.301** Unspecified nondisplaced fracture of fourth cervical vertebra **HCC** ▽

√6ᵗʰ **S12.33** Unspecified traumatic spondylolisthesis of fourth cervical vertebra

    1 √7ᵗʰ **S12.330** Unspecified traumatic displaced spondylolisthesis of fourth cervical vertebra **HCC** ▽

    1 √7ᵗʰ **S12.331** Unspecified traumatic nondisplaced spondylolisthesis of fourth cervical vertebra **HCC** ▽

1 √x7ᵗʰ **S12.34** Type III traumatic spondylolisthesis of fourth cervical vertebra **HCC**

√6ᵗʰ **S12.35** Other traumatic spondylolisthesis of fourth cervical vertebra

    1 √7ᵗʰ **S12.350** Other traumatic displaced spondylolisthesis of fourth cervical vertebra **HCC**

    1 √7ᵗʰ **S12.351** Other traumatic nondisplaced spondylolisthesis of fourth cervical vertebra **HCC**

√6ᵗʰ **S12.39** Other fracture of fourth cervical vertebra

    1 √7ᵗʰ **S12.390** Other displaced fracture of fourth cervical vertebra **HCC**

    1 √7ᵗʰ **S12.391** Other nondisplaced fracture of fourth cervical vertebra **HCC**

√5ᵗʰ **S12.4** Fracture of fifth cervical vertebra

√6ᵗʰ **S12.40** Unspecified fracture of fifth cervical vertebra

    1 √7ᵗʰ **S12.400** Unspecified displaced fracture of fifth cervical vertebra **HCC** ▽

    1 √7ᵗʰ **S12.401** Unspecified nondisplaced fracture of fifth cervical vertebra **HCC** ▽

√6ᵗʰ **S12.43** Unspecified traumatic spondylolisthesis of fifth cervical vertebra

    1 √7ᵗʰ **S12.430** Unspecified traumatic displaced spondylolisthesis of fifth cervical vertebra **HCC** ▽

    1 √7ᵗʰ **S12.431** Unspecified traumatic nondisplaced spondylolisthesis of fifth cervical vertebra **HCC** ▽

1 √x7ᵗʰ **S12.44** Type III traumatic spondylolisthesis of fifth cervical vertebra **HCC**

√6ᵗʰ **S12.45** Other traumatic spondylolisthesis of fifth cervical vertebra

    1 √7ᵗʰ **S12.450** Other traumatic displaced spondylolisthesis of fifth cervical vertebra **HCC**

    1 √7ᵗʰ **S12.451** Other traumatic nondisplaced spondylolisthesis of fifth cervical vertebra **HCC**

√6ᵗʰ **S12.49** Other fracture of fifth cervical vertebra

    1 √7ᵗʰ **S12.490** Other displaced fracture of fifth cervical vertebra **HCC**

    1 √7ᵗʰ **S12.491** Other nondisplaced fracture of fifth cervical vertebra **HCC**

---

1   HCC with 7th character indicating initial encounter (A, B or C - specific to category).

☑ Additional Character Req   √x7ᵗʰ Placeholder Alert   Manifestation   **HCC** CMS-HCC Condition   ▽ Unspecified Code   ▶◀ Revised Text   ● New Code   ▲ Revised Code Title

√5th S12.5 Fracture of sixth cervical vertebra

  √6th **S12.50 Unspecified fracture of sixth cervical vertebra**

    1 √7th **S12.500 Unspecified displaced fracture of sixth cervical vertebra** HCC ▽

    1 √7th **S12.501 Unspecified nondisplaced fracture of sixth cervical vertebra** HCC ▽

  √6th **S12.53 Unspecified traumatic spondylolisthesis of sixth cervical vertebra**

    1 √7th **S12.530 Unspecified traumatic displaced spondylolisthesis of sixth cervical vertebra** HCC ▽

    1 √7th **S12.531 Unspecified traumatic nondisplaced spondylolisthesis of sixth cervical vertebra** HCC ▽

  1 √x7th **S12.54 Type III traumatic spondylolisthesis of sixth cervical vertebra** HCC

  √6th **S12.55 Other traumatic spondylolisthesis of sixth cervical vertebra**

    1 √7th **S12.550 Other traumatic displaced spondylolisthesis of sixth cervical vertebra** HCC

    1 √7th **S12.551 Other traumatic nondisplaced spondylolisthesis of sixth cervical vertebra** HCC

  √6th **S12.59 Other fracture of sixth cervical vertebra**

    1 √7th **S12.590 Other displaced fracture of sixth cervical vertebra** HCC

    1 √7th **S12.591 Other nondisplaced fracture of sixth cervical vertebra** HCC

√5th S12.6 Fracture of seventh cervical vertebra

  √6th **S12.60 Unspecified fracture of seventh cervical vertebra**

    1 √7th **S12.600 Unspecified displaced fracture of seventh cervical vertebra** HCC ▽

    1 √7th **S12.601 Unspecified nondisplaced fracture of seventh cervical vertebra** HCC ▽

  √6th **S12.63 Unspecified traumatic spondylolisthesis of seventh cervical vertebra**

    1 √7th **S12.630 Unspecified traumatic displaced spondylolisthesis of seventh cervical vertebra** HCC ▽

    1 √7th **S12.631 Unspecified traumatic nondisplaced spondylolisthesis of seventh cervical vertebra** HCC ▽

  1 √x7th **S12.64 Type III traumatic spondylolisthesis of seventh cervical vertebra** HCC

  √6th **S12.65 Other traumatic spondylolisthesis of seventh cervical vertebra**

    1 √7th **S12.650 Other traumatic displaced spondylolisthesis of seventh cervical vertebra** HCC

    1 √7th **S12.651 Other traumatic nondisplaced spondylolisthesis of seventh cervical vertebra** HCC

  √6th **S12.69 Other fracture of seventh cervical vertebra**

    1 √7th **S12.690 Other displaced fracture of seventh cervical vertebra** HCC

    1 √7th **S12.691 Other nondisplaced fracture of | seventh cervical vertebra** HCC

1 √x7th **S12.8 Fracture of other parts of neck** HCC

  Hyoid bone   Thyroid cartilage
  Larynx   Trachea

The appropriate 7th character is to be added to code S12.8.
A   initial encounter
D   subsequent encounter
S   sequela

1 √x7th **S12.9 Fracture of neck, unspecified** HCC ▽

  Fracture of cervical spine NOS
  Fracture of cervical vertebra NOS
  Fracture of neck NOS

The appropriate 7th character is to be added to code S12.9.
A   initial encounter
D   subsequent encounter
S   sequela

√4th S13 Dislocation and sprain of joints and ligaments at neck level

  INCLUDES   avulsion of joint or ligament at neck level
    laceration of cartilage, joint or ligament at neck level
    sprain of cartilage, joint or ligament at neck level
    traumatic hemarthrosis of joint or ligament at neck level
    traumatic rupture of joint or ligament at neck level
    traumatic subluxation of joint or ligament at neck level
    traumatic tear of joint or ligament at neck level

Code also any associated open wound

EXCLUDES 2   strain of muscle or tendon at neck level (S16.1)

The appropriate 7th character is to be added to each code from category S13.
A   initial encounter
D   subsequent encounter
S   sequela

√x7th **S13.0 Traumatic rupture of cervical intervertebral disc**

  EXCLUDES 1   rupture or displacement (nontraumatic) of cervical intervertebral disc NOS (M50.-)

√5th **S13.1 Subluxation and dislocation of cervical vertebrae**

  Code also any associated:
    open wound of neck (S11.-)
    spinal cord injury (S14.1-)

  EXCLUDES 2   fracture of cervical vertebrae (S12.0--S12.3-)

  √6th **S13.10 Subluxation and dislocation of unspecified cervical vertebrae**

    √7th **S13.100 Subluxation of unspecified cervical vertebrae** ▽

    √7th **S13.101 Dislocation of unspecified cervical vertebrae** ▽

  √6th **S13.11 Subluxation and dislocation of C0/C1 cervical vertebrae**

    Subluxation and dislocation of atlantooccipital joint
    Subluxation and dislocation of atloidooccipital joint
    Subluxation and dislocation of occipitoatloid joint

    √7th **S13.110 Subluxation of C0/C1 cervical vertebrae**

    √7th **S13.111 Dislocation of C0/C1 cervical vertebrae**

  √6th **S13.12 Subluxation and dislocation of C1/C2 cervical vertebrae**

    Subluxation and dislocation of atlantoaxial joint

    √7th **S13.120 Subluxation of C1/C2 cervical vertebrae**

    √7th **S13.121 Dislocation of C1/C2 cervical vertebrae**

  √6th **S13.13 Subluxation and dislocation of C2/C3 cervical vertebrae**

    √7th **S13.130 Subluxation of C2/C3 cervical vertebrae**

    √7th **S13.131 Dislocation of C2/C3 cervical vertebrae**

  √6th **S13.14 Subluxation and dislocation of C3/C4 cervical vertebrae**

    √7th **S13.140 Subluxation of C3/C4 cervical vertebrae**

    √7th **S13.141 Dislocation of C3/C4 cervical vertebrae**

  √6th **S13.15 Subluxation and dislocation of C4/C5 cervical vertebrae**

    √7th **S13.150 Subluxation of C4/C5 cervical vertebrae**

    √7th **S13.151 Dislocation of C4/C5 cervical vertebrae**

  √6th **S13.16 Subluxation and dislocation of C5/C6 cervical vertebrae**

    √7th **S13.160 Subluxation of C5/C6 cervical vertebrae**

    √7th **S13.161 Dislocation of C5/C6 cervical vertebrae**

  √6th **S13.17 Subluxation and dislocation of C6/C7 cervical vertebrae**

    √7th **S13.170 Subluxation of C6/C7 cervical vertebrae**

    √7th **S13.171 Dislocation of C6/C7 cervical vertebrae**

  √6th **S13.18 Subluxation and dislocation of C7/T1 cervical vertebrae**

    √7th **S13.180 Subluxation of C7/T1 cervical vertebrae**

    √7th **S13.181 Dislocation of C7/T1 cervical vertebrae**

√5th **S13.2 Dislocation of other and unspecified parts of neck**

  √x7th **S13.20 Dislocation of unspecified parts of neck** ▽

  √x7th **S13.29 Dislocation of other parts of neck**

√x7th **S13.4 Sprain of ligaments of cervical spine**

  Sprain of anterior longitudinal (ligament), cervical
  Sprain of atlanto-axial (joints)
  Sprain of atlanto-occipital (joints)
  Whiplash injury of cervical spine

---

1   HCC with 7th character indicating initial encounter (A, B or C - specific to category).

EXCLUDES 1 Not coded here   EXCLUDES 2 Not included here   N Newborn Age: 0   P Pediatric Age: 0-17   M Maternity Age: 12-55   A Adult Age: 15-124

928   ICD-10-CM 2018

√x7ᵗʰ **S13.5** **Sprain of thyroid region**
     Sprain of cricoarytenoid (joint) (ligament)
     Sprain of cricothyroid (joint) (ligament)
     Sprain of thyroid cartilage

√x7ᵗʰ **S13.8** **Sprain of joints and ligaments of other parts of neck**

√x7ᵗʰ **S13.9** **Sprain of joints and ligaments of unspecified parts of neck** ▽

√4ᵗʰ **S14** **Injury of nerves and spinal cord at neck level**
     NOTE   Code to highest level of cervical cord injury.
     Code also any associated:
       fracture of cervical vertebra (S12.0- -S12.6-)
       open wound of neck (S11.-)
       transient paralysis (R29.5)

> The appropriate 7th character is to be added to each code from category S14.
> A   initial encounter
> D   subsequent encounter
> S   sequela

√x7ᵗʰ **S14.0** **Concussion and edema of cervical spinal cord**   HCC

√5ᵗʰ **S14.1** **Other and unspecified injuries of cervical spinal cord**

    √6ᵗʰ **S14.10** **Unspecified injury of cervical spinal cord**

       √7ᵗʰ **S14.101** **Unspecified injury at** C1 level **of cervical spinal cord**   HCC ▽

       √7ᵗʰ **S14.102** **Unspecified injury at** C2 level **of cervical spinal cord**   HCC ▽

       √7ᵗʰ **S14.103** **Unspecified injury at** C3 level **of cervical spinal cord**   HCC ▽

       √7ᵗʰ **S14.104** **Unspecified injury at** C4 level **of cervical spinal cord**   HCC ▽

       √7ᵗʰ **S14.105** **Unspecified injury at** C5 level **of cervical spinal cord**   HCC ▽

       √7ᵗʰ **S14.106** **Unspecified injury at** C6 level **of cervical spinal cord**   HCC ▽

       √7ᵗʰ **S14.107** **Unspecified injury at** C7 level **of cervical spinal cord**   HCC ▽

       √7ᵗʰ **S14.108** **Unspecified injury at** C8 level **of cervical spinal cord**   HCC ▽

       √7ᵗʰ **S14.109** **Unspecified injury at unspecified level of cervical spinal cord**   HCC ▽
         Injury of cervical spinal cord NOS

    √6ᵗʰ **S14.11** **Complete lesion of cervical spinal cord**

       √7ᵗʰ **S14.111** **Complete lesion at** C1 level **of cervical spinal cord**   HCC

       √7ᵗʰ **S14.112** **Complete lesion at** C2 level **of cervical spinal cord**   HCC

       √7ᵗʰ **S14.113** **Complete lesion at** C3 level **of cervical spinal cord**   HCC

       √7ᵗʰ **S14.114** **Complete lesion at** C4 level **of cervical spinal cord**   HCC

       √7ᵗʰ **S14.115** **Complete lesion at** C5 level **of cervical spinal cord**   HCC

       √7ᵗʰ **S14.116** **Complete lesion at** C6 level **of cervical spinal cord**   HCC

       √7ᵗʰ **S14.117** **Complete lesion at** C7 level **of cervical spinal cord**   HCC

       √7ᵗʰ **S14.118** **Complete lesion at** C8 level **of cervical spinal cord**   HCC

       √7ᵗʰ **S14.119** **Complete lesion at unspecified level of cervical spinal cord**   HCC ▽

    √6ᵗʰ **S14.12** **Central cord syndrome of cervical spinal cord**

       √7ᵗʰ **S14.121** **Central cord syndrome at** C1 level **of cervical spinal cord**   HCC

       √7ᵗʰ **S14.122** **Central cord syndrome at** C2 level **of cervical spinal cord**   HCC

       √7ᵗʰ **S14.123** **Central cord syndrome at** C3 level **of cervical spinal cord**   HCC

       √7ᵗʰ **S14.124** **Central cord syndrome at** C4 level **of cervical spinal cord**   HCC

       √7ᵗʰ **S14.125** **Central cord syndrome at** C5 level **of cervical spinal cord**   HCC

       √7ᵗʰ **S14.126** **Central cord syndrome at** C6 level **of cervical spinal cord**   HCC

       √7ᵗʰ **S14.127** **Central cord syndrome at** C7 level **of cervical spinal cord**   HCC

       √7ᵗʰ **S14.128** **Central cord syndrome at** C8 level **of cervical spinal cord**   HCC

       √7ᵗʰ **S14.129** **Central cord syndrome at unspecified level of cervical spinal cord**   HCC ▽

    √6ᵗʰ **S14.13** **Anterior cord syndrome of cervical spinal cord**

       √7ᵗʰ **S14.131** **Anterior cord syndrome at** C1 level **of cervical spinal cord**   HCC

       √7ᵗʰ **S14.132** **Anterior cord syndrome at** C2 level **of cervical spinal cord**   HCC

       √7ᵗʰ **S14.133** **Anterior cord syndrome at** C3 level **of cervical spinal cord**   HCC

       √7ᵗʰ **S14.134** **Anterior cord syndrome at** C4 level **of cervical spinal cord**   HCC

       √7ᵗʰ **S14.135** **Anterior cord syndrome at** C5 level **of cervical spinal cord**   HCC

       √7ᵗʰ **S14.136** **Anterior cord syndrome at** C6 level **of cervical spinal cord**   HCC

       √7ᵗʰ **S14.137** **Anterior cord syndrome at** C7 level **of cervical spinal cord**   HCC

       √7ᵗʰ **S14.138** **Anterior cord syndrome at** C8 level **of cervical spinal cord**   HCC

       √7ᵗʰ **S14.139** **Anterior cord syndrome at unspecified level of cervical spinal cord**   HCC ▽

    √6ᵗʰ **S14.14** **Brown-Séquard syndrome of cervical spinal cord**

       √7ᵗʰ **S14.141** **Brown-Séquard syndrome at** C1 level **of cervical spinal cord**   HCC

       √7ᵗʰ **S14.142** **Brown-Séquard syndrome at** C2 level **of cervical spinal cord**   HCC

       √7ᵗʰ **S14.143** **Brown-Séquard syndrome at** C3 level **of cervical spinal cord**   HCC

       √7ᵗʰ **S14.144** **Brown-Séquard syndrome at** C4 level **of cervical spinal cord**   HCC

       √7ᵗʰ **S14.145** **Brown-Séquard syndrome at** C5 level **of cervical spinal cord**   HCC

       √7ᵗʰ **S14.146** **Brown-Séquard syndrome at** C6 level **of cervical spinal cord**   HCC

       √7ᵗʰ **S14.147** **Brown-Séquard syndrome at** C7 level **of cervical spinal cord**   HCC

       √7ᵗʰ **S14.148** **Brown-Séquard syndrome at** C8 level **of cervical spinal cord**   HCC

       √7ᵗʰ **S14.149** **Brown-Séquard syndrome at unspecified level of cervical spinal cord**   HCC ▽

    √6ᵗʰ **S14.15** **Other incomplete lesions of cervical spinal cord**
       Incomplete lesion of cervical spinal cord NOS
       Posterior cord syndrome of cervical spinal cord

       √7ᵗʰ **S14.151** **Other incomplete lesion at** C1 level **of cervical spinal cord**   HCC

       √7ᵗʰ **S14.152** **Other incomplete lesion at** C2 level **of cervical spinal cord**   HCC

       √7ᵗʰ **S14.153** **Other incomplete lesion at** C3 level **of cervical spinal cord**   HCC

       √7ᵗʰ **S14.154** **Other incomplete lesion at** C4 level **of cervical spinal cord**   HCC

       √7ᵗʰ **S14.155** **Other incomplete lesion at** C5 level **of cervical spinal cord**   HCC

       √7ᵗʰ **S14.156** **Other incomplete lesion at** C6 level **of cervical spinal cord**   HCC

       √7ᵗʰ **S14.157** **Other incomplete lesion at** C7 level **of cervical spinal cord**   HCC

       √7ᵗʰ **S14.158** **Other incomplete lesion at** C8 level **of cervical spinal cord**   HCC

       √7ᵗʰ **S14.159** **Other incomplete lesion at unspecified level of cervical spinal cord**   HCC ▽

√x7ᵗʰ **S14.2** **Injury of** nerve root of cervical spine

√x7ᵗʰ **S14.3** **Injury of** brachial plexus

√x7ᵗʰ **S14.4** **Injury of** peripheral nerves of neck

√x7ᵗʰ **S14.5** **Injury of** cervical sympathetic nerves

√x7ᵗʰ **S14.8** **Injury of other specified nerves of neck**

√x7ᵗʰ **S14.9** **Injury of unspecified nerves of neck**   ▽

☑ Additional Character Req   √x7ᵗʰ Placeholder Alert   Manifestation   HCC CMS-HCC Condition   ▽ Unspecified Code   ►◄ Revised Text   ● New Code   ▲ Revised Code Title

S15 Injury of blood vessels at neck level
Code also any associated open wound (S11.-)

The appropriate 7th character is to be added to each code from category S15.
A   initial encounter
D   subsequent encounter
S   sequela

S15.0 Injury of carotid artery of neck
Injury of carotid artery (common) (external) (internal, extracranial portion)
Injury of carotid artery NOS
EXCLUDES 1   injury of internal carotid artery, intracranial portion (S06.8)

   S15.00 Unspecified injury of carotid artery
     S15.001   Unspecified injury of right carotid artery ▽
     S15.002   Unspecified injury of left carotid artery ▽
     S15.009   Unspecified injury of unspecified carotid artery ▽

   S15.01 Minor laceration of carotid artery
Incomplete transection of carotid artery
Laceration of carotid artery NOS
Superficial laceration of carotid artery
     S15.011   Minor laceration of right carotid artery
     S15.012   Minor laceration of left carotid artery
     S15.019   Minor laceration of unspecified carotid artery ▽

   S15.02 Major laceration of carotid artery
Complete transection of carotid artery
Traumatic rupture of carotid artery
     S15.021   Major laceration of right carotid artery
     S15.022   Major laceration of left carotid artery
     S15.029   Major laceration of unspecified carotid artery ▽

   S15.09 Other specified injury of carotid artery
     S15.091   Other specified injury of right carotid artery
     S15.092   Other specified injury of left carotid artery
     S15.099   Other specified injury of unspecified carotid artery ▽

S15.1 Injury of vertebral artery
   S15.10 Unspecified injury of vertebral artery
     S15.101   Unspecified injury of right vertebral artery ▽
     S15.102   Unspecified injury of left vertebral artery ▽
     S15.109   Unspecified injury of unspecified vertebral artery ▽

   S15.11 Minor laceration of vertebral artery
Incomplete transection of vertebral artery
Laceration of vertebral artery NOS
Superficial laceration of vertebral artery
     S15.111   Minor laceration of right vertebral artery
     S15.112   Minor laceration of left vertebral artery
     S15.119   Minor laceration of unspecified vertebral artery ▽

   S15.12 Major laceration of vertebral artery
Complete transection of vertebral artery
Traumatic rupture of vertebral artery
     S15.121   Major laceration of right vertebral artery
     S15.122   Major laceration of left vertebral artery
     S15.129   Major laceration of unspecified vertebral artery ▽

   S15.19 Other specified injury of vertebral artery
     S15.191   Other specified injury of right vertebral artery
     S15.192   Other specified injury of left vertebral artery
     S15.199   Other specified injury of unspecified vertebral artery ▽

S15.2 Injury of external jugular vein
   S15.20 Unspecified injury of external jugular vein
     S15.201   Unspecified injury of right external jugular vein ▽
     S15.202   Unspecified injury of left external jugular vein ▽
     S15.209   Unspecified injury of unspecified external jugular vein ▽

   S15.21 Minor laceration of external jugular vein
Incomplete transection of external jugular vein
Laceration of external jugular vein NOS
Superficial laceration of external jugular vein
     S15.211   Minor laceration of right external jugular vein
     S15.212   Minor laceration of left external jugular vein
     S15.219   Minor laceration of unspecified external jugular vein ▽

   S15.22 Major laceration of external jugular vein
Complete transection of external jugular vein
Traumatic rupture of external jugular vein
     S15.221   Major laceration of right external jugular vein
     S15.222   Major laceration of left external jugular vein
     S15.229   Major laceration of unspecified external jugular vein ▽

   S15.29 Other specified injury of external jugular vein
     S15.291   Other specified injury of right external jugular vein
     S15.292   Other specified injury of left external jugular vein
     S15.299   Other specified injury of unspecified external jugular vein

S15.3 Injury of internal jugular vein
   S15.30 Unspecified injury of internal jugular vein
     S15.301   Unspecified injury of right internal jugular vein ▽
     S15.302   Unspecified injury of left internal jugular vein ▽
     S15.309   Unspecified injury of unspecified internal jugular vein ▽

   S15.31 Minor laceration of internal jugular vein
Incomplete transection of internal jugular vein
Laceration of internal jugular vein NOS
Superficial laceration of internal jugular vein
     S15.311   Minor laceration of right internal jugular vein
     S15.312   Minor laceration of left internal jugular vein
     S15.319   Minor laceration of unspecified internal jugular vein ▽

   S15.32 Major laceration of internal jugular vein
Complete transection of internal jugular vein
Traumatic rupture of internal jugular vein
     S15.321   Major laceration of right internal jugular vein
     S15.322   Major laceration of left internal jugular vein
     S15.329   Major laceration of unspecified internal jugular vein ▽

   S15.39 Other specified injury of internal jugular vein
     S15.391   Other specified injury of right internal jugular vein
     S15.392   Other specified injury of left internal jugular vein
     S15.399   Other specified injury of unspecified internal jugular vein ▽

S15.8 Injury of other specified blood vessels at neck level
S15.9 Injury of unspecified blood vessel at neck level ▽

EXCLUDES 1 Not coded here   *EXCLUDES 2* Not included here   N Newborn Age: 0   P Pediatric Age: 0-17   M Maternity Age: 12-55   A Adult Age: 15-124

930   ICD-10-CM 2018

✓4ᵗʰ **S16 Injury of muscle, fascia and tendon at neck level**

Code also any associated open wound (S11.-)

EXCLUDES 2 *sprain of joint or ligament at neck level (S13.9)*

The appropriate 7th character is to be added to each code from category S16.
A   initial encounter
D   subsequent encounter
S   sequela

✓x7ᵗʰ **S16.1** Strain of muscle, fascia and tendon at neck level

✓x7ᵗʰ **S16.2** Laceration of muscle, fascia and tendon at neck level

✓x7ᵗʰ **S16.8** Other specified injury of muscle, fascia and tendon at neck level

✓x7ᵗʰ **S16.9** Unspecified injury of muscle, fascia and tendon at ▽ neck level

✓4ᵗʰ **S17 Crushing injury of neck**

Use additional code for all associated injuries, such as:
injury of blood vessels (S15.-)
open wound of neck (S11.-)
spinal cord injury (S14.0, S14.1-)
vertebral fracture (S12.0- -S12.3-)

The appropriate 7th character is to be added to each code from category S17.
A   initial encounter
D   subsequent encounter
S   sequela

✓x7ᵗʰ **S17.0** Crushing injury of larynx and trachea

✓x7ᵗʰ **S17.8** Crushing injury of other specified parts of neck

✓x7ᵗʰ **S17.9** Crushing injury of neck, part unspecified ▽

✓4ᵗʰ **S19 Other specified and unspecified injuries of neck**

The appropriate 7th character is to be added to each code from category S19.
A   initial encounter
D   subsequent encounter
S   sequela

✓5ᵗʰ **S19.8** Other specified injuries of neck

✓x7ᵗʰ **S19.80** Other specified injuries of unspecified ▽ part of neck

✓x7ᵗʰ **S19.81** Other specified injuries of larynx

✓x7ᵗʰ **S19.82** Other specified injuries of cervical trachea

EXCLUDES 2 *other specified injury of thoracic trachea (S27.5-)*

✓x7ᵗʰ **S19.83** Other specified injuries of vocal cord

✓x7ᵗʰ **S19.84** Other specified injuries of thyroid gland

✓x7ᵗʰ **S19.85** Other specified injuries of pharynx and cervical esophagus

✓x7ᵗʰ **S19.89** Other specified injuries of other specified part of neck

✓x7ᵗʰ **S19.9** Unspecified injury of neck ▽

Injuries to the thorax (S20-S29)

INCLUDES   injuries of breast
injuries of chest (wall)
injuries of interscapular area
EXCLUDES 2   *burns and corrosions (T20-T32)*
effects of foreign body in bronchus (T17.5)
effects of foreign body in esophagus (T18.1)
effects of foreign body in lung (T17.8)
effects of foreign body in trachea (T17.4)
frostbite (T33-T34)
injuries of axilla
injuries of clavicle
injuries of scapular region
injuries of shoulder
insect bite or sting, venomous (T63.4)

✓4ᵗʰ **S20 Superficial injury of thorax**

The appropriate 7th character is to be added to each code from category S20.
A   initial encounter
D   subsequent encounter
S   sequela

✓5ᵗʰ **S20.0** Contusion of breast

✓x7ᵗʰ **S20.00** Contusion of breast, unspecified breast ▽

✓x7ᵗʰ **S20.01** Contusion of right breast

✓x7ᵗʰ **S20.02** Contusion of left breast

✓5ᵗʰ **S20.1** Other and unspecified superficial injuries of breast

✓6ᵗʰ **S20.10** Unspecified superficial injuries of breast

✓7ᵗʰ **S20.101** Unspecified superficial injuries of ▽ breast, right breast

✓7ᵗʰ **S20.102** Unspecified superficial injuries of ▽ breast, left breast

✓7ᵗʰ **S20.109** Unspecified superficial injuries of ▽ breast, unspecified breast

✓6ᵗʰ **S20.11** Abrasion of breast

✓7ᵗʰ **S20.111** Abrasion of breast, right breast

✓7ᵗʰ **S20.112** Abrasion of breast, left breast

✓7ᵗʰ **S20.119** Abrasion of breast, unspecified breast ▽

✓6ᵗʰ **S20.12** Blister (nonthermal) of breast

✓7ᵗʰ **S20.121** Blister (nonthermal) of breast, right breast

✓7ᵗʰ **S20.122** Blister (nonthermal) of breast, left breast

✓7ᵗʰ **S20.129** Blister (nonthermal) of breast, ▽ unspecified breast

✓6ᵗʰ **S20.14** External constriction of part of breast

✓7ᵗʰ **S20.141** External constriction of part of breast, right breast

✓7ᵗʰ **S20.142** External constriction of part of breast, left breast

✓7ᵗʰ **S20.149** External constriction of part of breast, ▽ unspecified breast

✓6ᵗʰ **S20.15** Superficial foreign body of breast

Splinter in the breast

✓7ᵗʰ **S20.151** Superficial foreign body of breast, right breast

✓7ᵗʰ **S20.152** Superficial foreign body of breast, left breast

✓7ᵗʰ **S20.159** Superficial foreign body of breast, ▽ unspecified breast

✓6ᵗʰ **S20.16** Insect bite (nonvenomous) of breast

✓7ᵗʰ **S20.161** Insect bite (nonvenomous) of breast, right breast

✓7ᵗʰ **S20.162** Insect bite (nonvenomous) of breast, left breast

✓7ᵗʰ **S20.169** Insect bite (nonvenomous) of breast, ▽ unspecified breast

✓6ᵗʰ **S20.17** Other superficial bite of breast

EXCLUDES 1 *open bite of breast (S21.05-)*

✓7ᵗʰ **S20.171** Other superficial bite of breast, right breast

✓7ᵗʰ **S20.172** Other superficial bite of breast, left breast

✓7ᵗʰ **S20.179** Other superficial bite of breast, ▽ unspecified breast

✓5ᵗʰ **S20.2** Contusion of thorax

✓x7ᵗʰ **S20.20** Contusion of thorax, unspecified ▽

✓6ᵗʰ **S20.21** Contusion of front wall of thorax

✓7ᵗʰ **S20.211** Contusion of right front wall of thorax

✓7ᵗʰ **S20.212** Contusion of left front wall of thorax

✓7ᵗʰ **S20.219** Contusion of unspecified front wall ▽ of thorax

✓6ᵗʰ **S20.22** Contusion of back wall of thorax

✓7ᵗʰ **S20.221** Contusion of right back wall of thorax

✓7ᵗʰ **S20.222** Contusion of left back wall of thorax

✓7ᵗʰ **S20.229** Contusion of unspecified back wall ▽ of thorax

✓5ᵗʰ **S20.3** Other and unspecified superficial injuries of front wall of thorax

✓6ᵗʰ **S20.30** Unspecified superficial injuries of front wall of thorax

✓7ᵗʰ **S20.301** Unspecified superficial injuries of ▽ right front wall of thorax

✓7ᵗʰ **S20.302** Unspecified superficial injuries of ▽ left front wall of thorax

✓7ᵗʰ **S20.309** Unspecified superficial injuries of ▽ unspecified front wall of thorax

✓6ᵗʰ **S20.31** Abrasion of front wall of thorax

✓7ᵗʰ **S20.311** Abrasion of right front wall of thorax

✓7ᵗʰ **S20.312** Abrasion of left front wall of thorax

☑ Additional Character Req   ✓x7ᵗʰ Placeholder Alert   Manifestation   HCC CMS-HCC Condition   ▽ Unspecified Code   ▶◀ Revised Text   ● New Code   ▲ Revised Code Title

ICD-10-CM 2018   931

√7th **S20.319** **Abrasion of unspecified front wall of thorax** ▽

√6th **S20.32** Blister (nonthermal) of front wall of thorax

√7th **S20.321** **Blister (nonthermal) of right front wall of thorax**

√7th **S20.322** **Blister (nonthermal) of left front wall of thorax**

√7th **S20.329** **Blister (nonthermal) of unspecified front wall of thorax** ▽

√6th **S20.34** External constriction of front wall of thorax

√7th **S20.341** **External constriction of right front wall of thorax**

√7th **S20.342** **External constriction of left front wall of thorax**

√7th **S20.349** **External constriction of unspecified front wall of thorax** ▽

√6th **S20.35** Superficial foreign body of front wall of thorax
Splinter in front wall of thorax

√7th **S20.351** **Superficial foreign body of right front wall of thorax**

√7th **S20.352** **Superficial foreign body of left front wall of thorax**

√7th **S20.359** **Superficial foreign body of unspecified front wall of thorax** ▽

√6th **S20.36** Insect bite (nonvenomous) of front wall of thorax

√7th **S20.361** **Insect bite (nonvenomous) of right front wall of thorax**

√7th **S20.362** **Insect bite (nonvenomous) of left front wall of thorax**

√7th **S20.369** **Insect bite (nonvenomous) of unspecified front wall of thorax** ▽

√6th **S20.37** Other superficial bite of front wall of thorax
EXCLUDES 1 open bite of front wall of thorax (S21.14)

√7th **S20.371** **Other superficial bite of right front wall of thorax**

√7th **S20.372** **Other superficial bite of left front wall of thorax**

√7th **S20.379** **Other superficial bite of unspecified front wall of thorax** ▽

√5th **S20.4** Other and unspecified superficial injuries of back wall of thorax

√6th **S20.40** Unspecified superficial injuries of back wall of thorax

√7th **S20.401** **Unspecified superficial injuries of right back wall of thorax** ▽

√7th **S20.402** **Unspecified superficial injuries of left back wall of thorax** ▽

√7th **S20.409** **Unspecified superficial injuries of unspecified back wall of thorax** ▽

√6th **S20.41** Abrasion of back wall of thorax

√7th **S20.411** **Abrasion of right back wall of thorax**

√7th **S20.412** **Abrasion of left back wall of thorax**

√7th **S20.419** **Abrasion of unspecified back wall of thorax** ▽

√6th **S20.42** Blister (nonthermal) of back wall of thorax

√7th **S20.421** **Blister (nonthermal) of right back wall of thorax**

√7th **S20.422** **Blister (nonthermal) of left back wall of thorax**

√7th **S20.429** **Blister (nonthermal) of unspecified back wall of thorax** ▽

√6th **S20.44** External constriction of back wall of thorax

√7th **S20.441** **External constriction of right back wall of thorax**

√7th **S20.442** **External constriction of left back wall of thorax**

√7th **S20.449** **External constriction of unspecified back wall of thorax** ▽

√6th **S20.45** Superficial foreign body of back wall of thorax
Splinter of back wall of thorax

√7th **S20.451** **Superficial foreign body of right back wall of thorax**

√7th **S20.452** **Superficial foreign body of left back wall of thorax**

√7th **S20.459** **Superficial foreign body of unspecified back wall of thorax** ▽

√6th **S20.46** Insect bite (nonvenomous) of back wall of thorax

√7th **S20.461** **Insect bite (nonvenomous) of right back wall of thorax**

√7th **S20.462** **Insect bite (nonvenomous) of left back wall of thorax**

√7th **S20.469** **Insect bite (nonvenomous) of unspecified back wall of thorax** ▽

√6th **S20.47** Other superficial bite of back wall of thorax
EXCLUDES 1 open bite of back wall of thorax (S21.24)

√7th **S20.471** **Other superficial bite of right back wall of thorax**

√7th **S20.472** **Other superficial bite of left back wall of thorax**

√7th **S20.479** **Other superficial bite of unspecified back wall of thorax** ▽

√5th **S20.9** Superficial injury of unspecified parts of thorax
EXCLUDES 1 contusion of thorax NOS (S20.20)

√x7th **S20.90** **Unspecified superficial injury of unspecified parts of thorax** ▽
Superficial injury of thoracic wall NOS

√x7th **S20.91** **Abrasion of unspecified parts of thorax** ▽

√x7th **S20.92** **Blister (nonthermal) of unspecified parts of thorax** ▽

√x7th **S20.94** **External constriction of unspecified parts of thorax** ▽

√x7th **S20.95** **Superficial foreign body of unspecified parts of thorax** ▽
Splinter in thorax NOS

√x7th **S20.96** **Insect bite (nonvenomous) of unspecified parts of thorax** ▽

√x7th **S20.97** **Other superficial bite of unspecified parts of thorax** ▽
EXCLUDES 1 open bite of thorax NOS (S21.95)

√4th **S21** **Open wound of thorax**
Code also any associated injury, such as:
injury of heart (S26.-)
injury of intrathoracic organs (S27.-)
rib fracture (S22.3-, S22.4-)
spinal cord injury (S24.0-, S24.1-)
traumatic hemopneumothorax (S27.3)
traumatic hemothorax (S27.1)
traumatic pneumothorax (S27.0)
wound infection
EXCLUDES 1 traumatic amputation (partial) of thorax (S28.1)

The appropriate 7th character is to be added to each code from category S21.
A   initial encounter
D   subsequent encounter
S   sequela

√5th **S21.0** Open wound of breast

√6th **S21.00** Unspecified open wound of breast

√7th **S21.001** **Unspecified open wound of right breast** ▽

√7th **S21.002** **Unspecified open wound of left breast** ▽

√7th **S21.009** **Unspecified open wound of unspecified breast** ▽

√6th **S21.01** Laceration without foreign body of breast

√7th **S21.011** **Laceration without foreign body of right breast**

√7th **S21.012** **Laceration without foreign body of left breast**

√7th **S21.019** **Laceration without foreign body of unspecified breast** ▽

√6th **S21.02** Laceration with foreign body of breast

√7th **S21.021** **Laceration with foreign body of right breast**

√7th **S21.022** **Laceration with foreign body of left breast**

√7th **S21.029** **Laceration with foreign body of unspecified breast** ▽

EXCLUDES 1 Not coded here   EXCLUDES 2 Not included here   N Newborn Age: 0   P Pediatric Age: 0-17   M Maternity Age: 12-55   A Adult Age: 15-124

932   ICD-10-CM 2018

√6ᵗʰ **S21.03** Puncture wound without foreign body of breast
　√7ᵗʰ **S21.031** Puncture wound without foreign body of right breast
　√7ᵗʰ **S21.032** Puncture wound without foreign body of left breast
　√7ᵗʰ **S21.039** Puncture wound without foreign body of unspecified breast ▽

√6ᵗʰ **S21.04** Puncture wound with foreign body of breast
　√7ᵗʰ **S21.041** Puncture wound with foreign body of right breast
　√7ᵗʰ **S21.042** Puncture wound with foreign body of left breast
　√7ᵗʰ **S21.049** Puncture wound with foreign body of unspecified breast ▽

√6ᵗʰ **S21.05** Open bite of breast
　Bite of breast NOS
　EXCLUDES 1 *superficial bite of breast (S20.17)*
　√7ᵗʰ **S21.051** Open bite of right breast
　√7ᵗʰ **S21.052** Open bite of left breast
　√7ᵗʰ **S21.059** Open bite of unspecified breast ▽

√5ᵗʰ **S21.1** Open wound of front wall of thorax without penetration into thoracic cavity
　Open wound of chest without penetration into thoracic cavity

√6ᵗʰ **S21.10** Unspecified open wound of front wall of thorax without penetration into thoracic cavity
　√7ᵗʰ **S21.101** Unspecified open wound of right front wall of thorax without penetration into thoracic cavity ▽
　√7ᵗʰ **S21.102** Unspecified open wound of left front wall of thorax without penetration into thoracic cavity ▽
　√7ᵗʰ **S21.109** Unspecified open wound of unspecified front wall of thorax without penetration into thoracic cavity ▽

√6ᵗʰ **S21.11** Laceration without foreign body of front wall of thorax without penetration into thoracic cavity
　√7ᵗʰ **S21.111** Laceration without foreign body of right front wall of thorax without penetration into thoracic cavity
　√7ᵗʰ **S21.112** Laceration without foreign body of left front wall of thorax without penetration into thoracic cavity
　√7ᵗʰ **S21.119** Laceration without foreign body of unspecified front wall of thorax without penetration into thoracic cavity ▽

√6ᵗʰ **S21.12** Laceration with foreign body of front wall of thorax without penetration into thoracic cavity
　√7ᵗʰ **S21.121** Laceration with foreign body of right front wall of thorax without penetration into thoracic cavity
　√7ᵗʰ **S21.122** Laceration with foreign body of left front wall of thorax without penetration into thoracic cavity
　√7ᵗʰ **S21.129** Laceration with foreign body of unspecified front wall of thorax without penetration into thoracic cavity ▽

√6ᵗʰ **S21.13** Puncture wound without foreign body of front wall of thorax without penetration into thoracic cavity
　√7ᵗʰ **S21.131** Puncture wound without foreign body of right front wall of thorax without penetration into thoracic cavity
　√7ᵗʰ **S21.132** Puncture wound without foreign body of left front wall of thorax without penetration into thoracic cavity
　√7ᵗʰ **S21.139** Puncture wound without foreign body of unspecified front wall of thorax without penetration into thoracic cavity ▽

√6ᵗʰ **S21.14** Puncture wound with foreign body of front wall of thorax without penetration into thoracic cavity
　√7ᵗʰ **S21.141** Puncture wound with foreign body of right front wall of thorax without penetration into thoracic cavity
　√7ᵗʰ **S21.142** Puncture wound with foreign body of left front wall of thorax without penetration into thoracic cavity

　√7ᵗʰ **S21.149** Puncture wound with foreign body of unspecified front wall of thorax without penetration into thoracic cavity ▽

√6ᵗʰ **S21.15** Open bite of front wall of thorax without penetration into thoracic cavity
　Bite of front wall of thorax NOS
　EXCLUDES 1 *superficial bite of front wall of thorax (S20.37)*
　√7ᵗʰ **S21.151** Open bite of right front wall of thorax without penetration into thoracic cavity
　√7ᵗʰ **S21.152** Open bite of left front wall of thorax without penetration into thoracic cavity
　√7ᵗʰ **S21.159** Open bite of unspecified front wall of thorax without penetration into thoracic cavity ▽

√5ᵗʰ **S21.2** Open wound of back wall of thorax without penetration into thoracic cavity

√6ᵗʰ **S21.20** Unspecified open wound of back wall of thorax without penetration into thoracic cavity
　√7ᵗʰ **S21.201** Unspecified open wound of right back wall of thorax without penetration into thoracic cavity ▽
　√7ᵗʰ **S21.202** Unspecified open wound of left back wall of thorax without penetration into thoracic cavity ▽
　√7ᵗʰ **S21.209** Unspecified open wound of unspecified back wall of thorax without penetration into thoracic cavity ▽

√6ᵗʰ **S21.21** Laceration without foreign body of back wall of thorax without penetration into thoracic cavity
　√7ᵗʰ **S21.211** Laceration without foreign body of right back wall of thorax without penetration into thoracic cavity
　√7ᵗʰ **S21.212** Laceration without foreign body of left back wall of thorax without penetration into thoracic cavity
　√7ᵗʰ **S21.219** Laceration without foreign body of unspecified back wall of thorax without penetration into thoracic cavity ▽

√6ᵗʰ **S21.22** Laceration with foreign body of back wall of thorax without penetration into thoracic cavity
　√7ᵗʰ **S21.221** Laceration with foreign body of right back wall of thorax without penetration into thoracic cavity
　√7ᵗʰ **S21.222** Laceration with foreign body of left back wall of thorax without penetration into thoracic cavity
　√7ᵗʰ **S21.229** Laceration with foreign body of unspecified back wall of thorax without penetration into thoracic cavity ▽

√6ᵗʰ **S21.23** Puncture wound without foreign body of back wall of thorax without penetration into thoracic cavity
　√7ᵗʰ **S21.231** Puncture wound without foreign body of right back wall of thorax without penetration into thoracic cavity
　√7ᵗʰ **S21.232** Puncture wound without foreign body of left back wall of thorax without penetration into thoracic cavity
　√7ᵗʰ **S21.239** Puncture wound without foreign body of unspecified back wall of thorax without penetration into thoracic cavity ▽

√6ᵗʰ **S21.24** Puncture wound with foreign body of back wall of thorax without penetration into thoracic cavity
　√7ᵗʰ **S21.241** Puncture wound with foreign body of right back wall of thorax without penetration into thoracic cavity
　√7ᵗʰ **S21.242** Puncture wound with foreign body of left back wall of thorax without penetration into thoracic cavity
　√7ᵗʰ **S21.249** Puncture wound with foreign body of unspecified back wall of thorax without penetration into thoracic cavity ▽

√ Additional Character Req　√x7ᵗʰ Placeholder Alert　Manifestation　**HCC** CMS-HCC Condition　▽ Unspecified Code　►◄ Revised Text　● New Code　▲ Revised Code Title

√6ᵗʰ S21.25 Open bite of back wall of thorax without penetration into thoracic cavity
Bite of back wall of thorax NOS
EXCLUDES 1 superficial bite of back wall of thorax (S20.47)

√7ᵗʰ S21.251 Open bite of right back wall of thorax without penetration into thoracic cavity

√7ᵗʰ S21.252 Open bite of left back wall of thorax without penetration into thoracic cavity

√7ᵗʰ S21.259 Open bite of unspecified back wall of thorax without penetration into thoracic cavity ▽

√5ᵗʰ S21.3 Open wound of front wall of thorax with penetration into thoracic cavity
Open wound of chest with penetration into thoracic cavity

√6ᵗʰ S21.30 Unspecified open wound of front wall of thorax with penetration into thoracic cavity

√7ᵗʰ S21.301 Unspecified open wound of right front wall of thorax with penetration into thoracic cavity ▽

√7ᵗʰ S21.302 Unspecified open wound of left front wall of thorax with penetration into thoracic cavity ▽

√7ᵗʰ S21.309 Unspecified open wound of unspecified front wall of thorax with penetration into thoracic cavity ▽

√6ᵗʰ S21.31 Laceration without foreign body of front wall of thorax with penetration into thoracic cavity

√7ᵗʰ S21.311 Laceration without foreign body of right front wall of thorax with penetration into thoracic cavity

√7ᵗʰ S21.312 Laceration without foreign body of left front wall of thorax with penetration into thoracic cavity

√7ᵗʰ S21.319 Laceration without foreign body of unspecified front wall of thorax with penetration into thoracic cavity ▽

√6ᵗʰ S21.32 Laceration with foreign body of front wall of thorax with penetration into thoracic cavity

√7ᵗʰ S21.321 Laceration with foreign body of right front wall of thorax with penetration into thoracic cavity

√7ᵗʰ S21.322 Laceration with foreign body of left front wall of thorax with penetration into thoracic cavity

√7ᵗʰ S21.329 Laceration with foreign body of unspecified front wall of thorax with penetration into thoracic cavity ▽

√6ᵗʰ S21.33 Puncture wound without foreign body of front wall of thorax with penetration into thoracic cavity

√7ᵗʰ S21.331 Puncture wound without foreign body of right front wall of thorax with penetration into thoracic cavity

√7ᵗʰ S21.332 Puncture wound without foreign body of left front wall of thorax with penetration into thoracic cavity

√7ᵗʰ S21.339 Puncture wound without foreign body of unspecified front wall of thorax with penetration into thoracic cavity ▽

√6ᵗʰ S21.34 Puncture wound with foreign body of front wall of thorax with penetration into thoracic cavity

√7ᵗʰ S21.341 Puncture wound with foreign body of right front wall of thorax with penetration into thoracic cavity

√7ᵗʰ S21.342 Puncture wound with foreign body of left front wall of thorax with penetration into thoracic cavity

√7ᵗʰ S21.349 Puncture wound with foreign body of unspecified front wall of thorax with penetration into thoracic cavity ▽

√6ᵗʰ S21.35 Open bite of front wall of thorax with penetration into thoracic cavity
EXCLUDES 1 superficial bite of front wall of thorax (S20.37)

√7ᵗʰ S21.351 Open bite of right front wall of thorax with penetration into thoracic cavity

√7ᵗʰ S21.352 Open bite of left front wall of thorax with penetration into thoracic cavity

√7ᵗʰ S21.359 Open bite of unspecified front wall of thorax with penetration into thoracic cavity ▽

√5ᵗʰ S21.4 Open wound of back wall of thorax with penetration into thoracic cavity

√6ᵗʰ S21.40 Unspecified open wound of back wall of thorax with penetration into thoracic cavity

√7ᵗʰ S21.401 Unspecified open wound of right back wall of thorax with penetration into thoracic cavity ▽

√7ᵗʰ S21.402 Unspecified open wound of left back wall of thorax with penetration into thoracic cavity ▽

√7ᵗʰ S21.409 Unspecified open wound of unspecified back wall of thorax with penetration into thoracic cavity ▽

√6ᵗʰ S21.41 Laceration without foreign body of back wall of thorax with penetration into thoracic cavity

√7ᵗʰ S21.411 Laceration without foreign body of right back wall of thorax with penetration into thoracic cavity

√7ᵗʰ S21.412 Laceration without foreign body of left back wall of thorax with penetration into thoracic cavity

√7ᵗʰ S21.419 Laceration without foreign body of unspecified back wall of thorax with penetration into thoracic cavity ▽

√6ᵗʰ S21.42 Laceration with foreign body of back wall of thorax with penetration into thoracic cavity

√7ᵗʰ S21.421 Laceration with foreign body of right back wall of thorax with penetration into thoracic cavity

√7ᵗʰ S21.422 Laceration with foreign body of left back wall of thorax with penetration into thoracic cavity

√7ᵗʰ S21.429 Laceration with foreign body of unspecified back wall of thorax with penetration into thoracic cavity ▽

√6ᵗʰ S21.43 Puncture wound without foreign body of back wall of thorax with penetration into thoracic cavity

√7ᵗʰ S21.431 Puncture wound without foreign body of right back wall of thorax with penetration into thoracic cavity

√7ᵗʰ S21.432 Puncture wound without foreign body of left back wall of thorax with penetration into thoracic cavity

√7ᵗʰ S21.439 Puncture wound without foreign body of unspecified back wall of thorax with penetration into thoracic cavity ▽

√6ᵗʰ S21.44 Puncture wound with foreign body of back wall of thorax with penetration into thoracic cavity

√7ᵗʰ S21.441 Puncture wound with foreign body of right back wall of thorax with penetration into thoracic cavity

√7ᵗʰ S21.442 Puncture wound with foreign body of left back wall of thorax with penetration into thoracic cavity

√7ᵗʰ S21.449 Puncture wound with foreign body of unspecified back wall of thorax with penetration into thoracic cavity ▽

√6ᵗʰ S21.45 Open bite of back wall of thorax with penetration into thoracic cavity
Bite of back wall of thorax NOS
EXCLUDES 1 superficial bite of back wall of thorax (S20.47)

√7ᵗʰ S21.451 Open bite of right back wall of thorax with penetration into thoracic cavity

√7ᵗʰ S21.452 Open bite of left back wall of thorax with penetration into thoracic cavity

√7ᵗʰ S21.459 Open bite of unspecified back wall of thorax with penetration into thoracic cavity ▽

√5ᵗʰ S21.9 Open wound of unspecified part of thorax
Open wound of thoracic wall NOS

√x7ᵗʰ S21.90 Unspecified open wound of unspecified part of thorax ▽

√x7ᵗʰ S21.91 Laceration without foreign body of unspecified part of thorax ▽

✓x7th **S21.92** Laceration with foreign body of unspecified part of thorax ▽

✓x7th **S21.93** Puncture wound without foreign body of unspecified part of thorax ▽

✓x7th **S21.94** Puncture wound with foreign body of unspecified part of thorax ▽

✓x7th **S21.95** Open bite of unspecified part of thorax ▽
     EXCLUDES 1   *superficial bite of thorax (S20.97)*

✓4th **S22 Fracture of rib(s), sternum and thoracic spine**

   NOTE   A fracture not indicated as nondisplaced or displaced should be coded to displaced.
         A fracture not indicated as open or closed should be coded to closed.

   INCLUDES   fracture of thoracic neural arch
         fracture of thoracic spinous process
         fracture of thoracic transverse process
         fracture of thoracic vertebra
         fracture of thoracic vertebral arch

Code first any associated:
    injury of intrathoracic organ (S27.-)
    spinal cord injury (S24.0-, S24.1-)
   EXCLUDES 1   *transection of thorax (S28.1)*
   EXCLUDES 2   *fracture of clavicle (S42.0-)*
            fracture of scapula (S42.1-)
   AHA: 2015, 3Q, 37-39

> The appropriate 7th character is to be added to each code from category S22.
> A   initial encounter for closed fracture
> B   initial encounter for open fracture
> D   subsequent encounter for fracture with routine healing
> G   subsequent encounter for fracture with delayed healing
> K   subsequent encounter for fracture with nonunion
> S   sequela

✓5th **S22.0 Fracture of thoracic vertebra**

   ✓6th **S22.00 Fracture of unspecified thoracic vertebra**

     1 ✓7th **S22.000** Wedge compression fracture of unspecified thoracic vertebra HCC ▽

     1 ✓7th **S22.001** Stable burst fracture of unspecified thoracic vertebra HCC ▽

     1 ✓7th **S22.002** Unstable burst fracture of unspecified thoracic vertebra HCC ▽

     1 ✓7th **S22.008** Other fracture of unspecified thoracic vertebra HCC ▽

     1 ✓7th **S22.009** Unspecified fracture of unspecified thoracic vertebra HCC ▽

   ✓6th **S22.01 Fracture of first thoracic vertebra**

     1 ✓7th **S22.010** Wedge compression fracture of first thoracic vertebra HCC

     1 ✓7th **S22.011** Stable burst fracture of first thoracic vertebra HCC

     1 ✓7th **S22.012** Unstable burst fracture of first thoracic vertebra HCC

     1 ✓7th **S22.018** Other fracture of first thoracic vertebra HCC

     1 ✓7th **S22.019** Unspecified fracture of first thoracic vertebra HCC ▽

   ✓6th **S22.02 Fracture of second thoracic vertebra**

     1 ✓7th **S22.020** Wedge compression fracture of second thoracic vertebra HCC

     1 ✓7th **S22.021** Stable burst fracture of second thoracic vertebra HCC

     1 ✓7th **S22.022** Unstable burst fracture of second thoracic vertebra HCC

     1 ✓7th **S22.028** Other fracture of second thoracic vertebra HCC

     1 ✓7th **S22.029** Unspecified fracture of second thoracic vertebra HCC ▽

   ✓6th **S22.03 Fracture of third thoracic vertebra**

     1 ✓7th **S22.030** Wedge compression fracture of third thoracic vertebra HCC

     1 ✓7th **S22.031** Stable burst fracture of third thoracic vertebra HCC

     1 ✓7th **S22.032** Unstable burst fracture of third thoracic vertebra HCC

     1 ✓7th **S22.038** Other fracture of third thoracic vertebra HCC

     1 ✓7th **S22.039** Unspecified fracture of third thoracic vertebra HCC ▽

   ✓6th **S22.04 Fracture of fourth thoracic vertebra**

     1 ✓7th **S22.040** Wedge compression fracture of fourth thoracic vertebra HCC

     1 ✓7th **S22.041** Stable burst fracture of fourth thoracic vertebra HCC

     1 ✓7th **S22.042** Unstable burst fracture of fourth thoracic vertebra HCC

     1 ✓7th **S22.048** Other fracture of fourth thoracic vertebra HCC

     1 ✓7th **S22.049** Unspecified fracture of fourth thoracic vertebra HCC ▽

   ✓6th **S22.05 Fracture of T5-T6 vertebra**

     1 ✓7th **S22.050** Wedge compression fracture of T5-T6 vertebra HCC

     1 ✓7th **S22.051** Stable burst fracture of T5-T6 vertebra HCC

     1 ✓7th **S22.052** Unstable burst fracture of T5-T6 vertebra HCC

     1 ✓7th **S22.058** Other fracture of T5-T6 vertebra HCC

     1 ✓7th **S22.059** Unspecified fracture of T5-T6 vertebra HCC ▽

   ✓6th **S22.06 Fracture of T7-T8 vertebra**

     1 ✓7th **S22.060** Wedge compression fracture of T7-T8 vertebra HCC

     1 ✓7th **S22.061** Stable burst fracture of T7-T8 vertebra HCC

     1 ✓7th **S22.062** Unstable burst fracture of T7-T8 vertebra HCC

     1 ✓7th **S22.068** Other fracture of T7-T8 thoracic vertebra HCC

     1 ✓7th **S22.069** Unspecified fracture of T7-T8 vertebra HCC ▽

   ✓6th **S22.07 Fracture of T9-T10 vertebra**

     1 ✓7th **S22.070** Wedge compression fracture of T9-T10 vertebra HCC

     1 ✓7th **S22.071** Stable burst fracture of T9-T10 vertebra HCC

     1 ✓7th **S22.072** Unstable burst fracture of T9-T10 vertebra HCC

     1 ✓7th **S22.078** Other fracture of T9-T10 vertebra HCC

     1 ✓7th **S22.079** Unspecified fracture of T9-T10 vertebra HCC ▽

   ✓6th **S22.08 Fracture of T11-T12 vertebra**

     1 ✓7th **S22.080** Wedge compression fracture of T11-T12 vertebra HCC

     1 ✓7th **S22.081** Stable burst fracture of T11-T12 vertebra HCC

     1 ✓7th **S22.082** Unstable burst fracture of T11-T12 vertebra HCC

     1 ✓7th **S22.088** Other fracture of T11-T12 vertebra HCC

     1 ✓7th **S22.089** Unspecified fracture of T11-T12 vertebra HCC ▽

✓5th **S22.2 Fracture of sternum**
    DEF: Break in flat bone (breast bone) in anterior thorax; caused by blunt trauma to anterior chest.

   ✓x7th **S22.20** Unspecified fracture of sternum ▽

   ✓x7th **S22.21** Fracture of manubrium

   ✓x7th **S22.22** Fracture of body of sternum

   ✓x7th **S22.23** Sternal manubrial dissociation

   ✓x7th **S22.24** Fracture of xiphoid process

✓5th **S22.3 Fracture of one rib**

   ✓x7th **S22.31** Fracture of one rib, right side

   ✓x7th **S22.32** Fracture of one rib, left side

   ✓x7th **S22.39** Fracture of one rib, unspecified side ▽

✓5th **S22.4 Multiple fractures of ribs**
    Fractures of two or more ribs
     EXCLUDES 1   *flail chest (S22.5-)*

   ✓x7th **S22.41** Multiple fractures of ribs, right side

---

1   HCC with 7th character indicating initial encounter (A, B or C - specific to category).

☑ Additional Character Req   ✓x7th Placeholder Alert   Manifestation   HCC CMS-HCC Condition   ▽ Unspecified Code   ▶◀ Revised Text   ● New Code   ▲ Revised Code Title

ICD-10-CM 2018   935

✓x7ᵗʰ **S22.42**   **Multiple fractures of ribs, left side**

✓x7ᵗʰ **S22.43**   **Multiple fractures of ribs, bilateral**

✓x7ᵗʰ **S22.49**   **Multiple fractures of ribs, unspecified side**   ▽

✓x7ᵗʰ **S22.5**   **Flail chest**

✓x7ᵗʰ **S22.9**   **Fracture of bony thorax, part unspecified**   ▽

✓4ᵗʰ **S23**   **Dislocation and sprain of joints and ligaments of thorax**

   INCLUDES   avulsion of joint or ligament of thorax
      laceration of cartilage, joint or ligament of thorax
      sprain of cartilage, joint or ligament of thorax
      traumatic hemarthrosis of joint or ligament of thorax
      traumatic rupture of joint or ligament of thorax
      traumatic subluxation of joint or ligament of thorax
      traumatic tear of joint or ligament of thorax

   Code also any associated open wound

   EXCLUDES 2   *dislocation, sprain of sternoclavicular joint (S43.2, S43.6)*
      strain of muscle or tendon of thorax (S29.01-)

> The appropriate 7th character is to be added to each code from category S23.
> A   initial encounter
> D   subsequent encounter
> S   sequela

✓x7ᵗʰ **S23.0**   **Traumatic rupture of thoracic intervertebral disc**

   EXCLUDES 1   *rupture or displacement (nontraumatic) of thoracic intervertebral disc NOS (M51- with fifth character 4)*

✓5ᵗʰ **S23.1**   **Subluxation and dislocation of thoracic vertebra**

   Code also any associated
     open wound of thorax (S21.-)
     spinal cord injury (S24.0-, S24.1-)

   EXCLUDES 2   *fracture of thoracic vertebrae (S22.0-)*

   ✓6ᵗʰ **S23.10**   **Subluxation and dislocation of unspecified thoracic vertebra**

     ✓7ᵗʰ **S23.100**   Subluxation of unspecified thoracic vertebra   ▽

     ✓7ᵗʰ **S23.101**   Dislocation of unspecified thoracic vertebra   ▽

   ✓6ᵗʰ **S23.11**   **Subluxation and dislocation of T1/T2 thoracic vertebra**

     ✓7ᵗʰ **S23.110**   Subluxation of T1/T2 thoracic vertebra

     ✓7ᵗʰ **S23.111**   Dislocation of T1/T2 thoracic vertebra

   ✓6ᵗʰ **S23.12**   **Subluxation and dislocation of T2/T3-T3/T4 thoracic vertebra**

     ✓7ᵗʰ **S23.120**   Subluxation of T2/T3 thoracic vertebra

     ✓7ᵗʰ **S23.121**   Dislocation of T2/T3 thoracic vertebra

     ✓7ᵗʰ **S23.122**   Subluxation of T3/T4 thoracic vertebra

     ✓7ᵗʰ **S23.123**   Dislocation of T3/T4 thoracic vertebra

   ✓6ᵗʰ **S23.13**   **Subluxation and dislocation of T4/T5-T5/T6 thoracic vertebra**

     ✓7ᵗʰ **S23.130**   Subluxation of T4/T5 thoracic vertebra

     ✓7ᵗʰ **S23.131**   Dislocation of T4/T5 thoracic vertebra

     ✓7ᵗʰ **S23.132**   Subluxation of T5/T6 thoracic vertebra

     ✓7ᵗʰ **S23.133**   Dislocation of T5/T6 thoracic vertebra

   ✓6ᵗʰ **S23.14**   **Subluxation and dislocation of T6/T7-T7/T8 thoracic vertebra**

     ✓7ᵗʰ **S23.140**   Subluxation of T6/T7 thoracic vertebra

     ✓7ᵗʰ **S23.141**   Dislocation of T6/T7 thoracic vertebra

     ✓7ᵗʰ **S23.142**   Subluxation of T7/T8 thoracic vertebra

     ✓7ᵗʰ **S23.143**   Dislocation of T7/T8 thoracic vertebra

   ✓6ᵗʰ **S23.15**   **Subluxation and dislocation of T8/T9-T9/T10 thoracic vertebra**

     ✓7ᵗʰ **S23.150**   Subluxation of T8/T9 thoracic vertebra

     ✓7ᵗʰ **S23.151**   Dislocation of T8/T9 thoracic vertebra

     ✓7ᵗʰ **S23.152**   Subluxation of T9/T10 thoracic vertebra

     ✓7ᵗʰ **S23.153**   Dislocation of T9/T10 thoracic vertebra

   ✓6ᵗʰ **S23.16**   **Subluxation and dislocation of T10/T11-T11/T12 thoracic vertebra**

     ✓7ᵗʰ **S23.160**   Subluxation of T10/T11 thoracic vertebra

     ✓7ᵗʰ **S23.161**   Dislocation of T10/T11 thoracic vertebra

     ✓7ᵗʰ **S23.162**   Subluxation of T11/T12 thoracic vertebra

     ✓7ᵗʰ **S23.163**   Dislocation of T11/T12 thoracic vertebra

   ✓6ᵗʰ **S23.17**   **Subluxation and dislocation of T12/L1 thoracic vertebra**

     ✓7ᵗʰ **S23.170**   Subluxation of T12/L1 thoracic vertebra

     ✓7ᵗʰ **S23.171**   Dislocation of T12/L1 thoracic vertebra

✓5ᵗʰ **S23.2**   **Dislocation of other and unspecified parts of thorax**

   ✓x7ᵗʰ **S23.20**   **Dislocation of unspecified part of thorax**   ▽

   ✓x7ᵗʰ **S23.29**   **Dislocation of other parts of thorax**

✓x7ᵗʰ **S23.3**   **Sprain of ligaments of thoracic spine**

✓5ᵗʰ **S23.4**   **Sprain of ribs and sternum**

   ✓x7ᵗʰ **S23.41**   **Sprain of ribs**

   ✓6ᵗʰ **S23.42**   **Sprain of sternum**

     ✓7ᵗʰ **S23.420**   Sprain of sternoclavicular (joint) (ligament)

     ✓7ᵗʰ **S23.421**   Sprain of chondrosternal joint

     ✓7ᵗʰ **S23.428**   Other sprain of sternum

     ✓7ᵗʰ **S23.429**   Unspecified sprain of sternum   ▽

✓x7ᵗʰ **S23.8**   **Sprain of other specified parts of thorax**   ▽

✓x7ᵗʰ **S23.9**   **Sprain of unspecified parts of thorax**   ▽

✓4ᵗʰ **S24**   **Injury of nerves and spinal cord at thorax level**

   NOTE   Code to highest level of thoracic spinal cord injury. Injuries to the spinal cord (S24.0 and S24.1) refer to the cord level and not bone level injury, and can affect nerve roots at and below the level given.

   Code also any associated:
     fracture of thoracic vertebra (S22.0-)
     open wound of thorax (S21.-)
     transient paralysis (R29.5)

   EXCLUDES 2   *injury of brachial plexus (S14.3)*

> The appropriate 7th character is to be added to each code from category S24.
> A   initial encounter
> D   subsequent encounter
> S   sequela

✓x7ᵗʰ **S24.0**   **Concussion and edema of thoracic spinal cord**   HCC

✓5ᵗʰ **S24.1**   **Other and unspecified injuries of thoracic spinal cord**

   ✓6ᵗʰ **S24.10**   **Unspecified injury of thoracic spinal cord**

     ✓7ᵗʰ **S24.101**   Unspecified injury at T1 level of thoracic spinal cord   HCC ▽

     ✓7ᵗʰ **S24.102**   Unspecified injury at T2-T6 level of thoracic spinal cord   HCC ▽

     ✓7ᵗʰ **S24.103**   Unspecified injury at T7-T10 level of thoracic spinal cord   HCC ▽

     ✓7ᵗʰ **S24.104**   Unspecified injury at T11-T12 level of thoracic spinal cord   HCC ▽

     ✓7ᵗʰ **S24.109**   Unspecified injury at unspecified level of thoracic spinal cord   HCC ▽
       Injury of thoracic spinal cord NOS

   ✓6ᵗʰ **S24.11**   **Complete lesion of thoracic spinal cord**

     ✓7ᵗʰ **S24.111**   Complete lesion at T1 level of thoracic spinal cord   HCC

     ✓7ᵗʰ **S24.112**   Complete lesion at T2-T6 level of thoracic spinal cord   HCC

     ✓7ᵗʰ **S24.113**   Complete lesion at T7-T10 level of thoracic spinal cord   HCC

     ✓7ᵗʰ **S24.114**   Complete lesion at T11-T12 level of thoracic spinal cord   HCC

     ✓7ᵗʰ **S24.119**   Complete lesion at unspecified level of thoracic spinal cord   HCC ▽

   ✓6ᵗʰ **S24.13**   **Anterior cord syndrome of thoracic spinal cord**

     ✓7ᵗʰ **S24.131**   Anterior cord syndrome at T1 level of thoracic spinal cord   HCC

     ✓7ᵗʰ **S24.132**   Anterior cord syndrome at T2-T6 level of thoracic spinal cord   HCC

     ✓7ᵗʰ **S24.133**   Anterior cord syndrome at T7-T10 level of thoracic spinal cord   HCC

     ✓7ᵗʰ **S24.134**   Anterior cord syndrome at T11-T12 level of thoracic spinal cord   HCC

     ✓7ᵗʰ **S24.139**   Anterior cord syndrome at unspecified level of thoracic spinal cord   HCC ▽

   ✓6ᵗʰ **S24.14**   **Brown-Séquard syndrome of thoracic spinal cord**

     ✓7ᵗʰ **S24.141**   Brown-Séquard syndrome at T1 level of thoracic spinal cord   HCC

EXCLUDES 1 Not coded here   EXCLUDES 2 Not included here   N Newborn Age: 0   P Pediatric Age: 0-17   M Maternity Age: 12-55   A Adult Age: 15-124

936

ICD-10-CM 2018

√7ᵗʰ **S24.142** **Brown-Séquard syndrome at T2-T6 level of thoracic spinal cord** HCC

√7ᵗʰ **S24.143** **Brown-Séquard syndrome at T7-T10 level of thoracic spinal cord** HCC

√7ᵗʰ **S24.144** **Brown-Séquard syndrome at T11-T12 level of thoracic spinal cord** HCC

√7ᵗʰ **S24.149** **Brown-Séquard syndrome at unspecified level of thoracic spinal cord** HCC ▽

√6ᵗʰ **S24.15** **Other incomplete lesions of thoracic spinal cord**
Incomplete lesion of thoracic spinal cord NOS
Posterior cord syndrome of thoracic spinal cord

√7ᵗʰ **S24.151** **Other incomplete lesion at T1 level of thoracic spinal cord** HCC

√7ᵗʰ **S24.152** **Other incomplete lesion at T2-T6 level of thoracic spinal cord** HCC

√7ᵗʰ **S24.153** **Other incomplete lesion at T7-T10 level of thoracic spinal cord** HCC

√7ᵗʰ **S24.154** **Other incomplete lesion at T11-T12 level of thoracic spinal cord** HCC

√7ᵗʰ **S24.159** **Other incomplete lesion at unspecified level of thoracic spinal cord** HCC ▽

√x7ᵗʰ **S24.2** **Injury of nerve root of thoracic spine**

√x7ᵗʰ **S24.3** **Injury of peripheral nerves of thorax**

√x7ᵗʰ **S24.4** **Injury of thoracic sympathetic nervous system**
Injury of cardiac plexus
Injury of esophageal plexus
Injury of pulmonary plexus
Injury of stellate ganglion
Injury of thoracic sympathetic ganglion

√x7ᵗʰ **S24.8** **Injury of other specified nerves of thorax**

√x7ᵗʰ **S24.9** **Injury of unspecified nerve of thorax** ▽

√4ᵗʰ **S25** **Injury of blood vessels of thorax**
Code also any associated open wound (S21.-)

The appropriate 7th character is to be added to each code from category S25.
A   initial encounter
D   subsequent encounter
S   sequela

√5ᵗʰ **S25.0** **Injury of thoracic aorta**
Injury of aorta NOS

√x7ᵗʰ **S25.00** **Unspecified injury of thoracic aorta** ▽

√x7ᵗʰ **S25.01** **Minor laceration of thoracic aorta**
Incomplete transection of thoracic aorta
Laceration of thoracic aorta NOS
Superficial laceration of thoracic aorta

√x7ᵗʰ **S25.02** **Major laceration of thoracic aorta**
Complete transection of thoracic aorta
Traumatic rupture of thoracic aorta

√x7ᵗʰ **S25.09** **Other specified injury of thoracic aorta**

√5ᵗʰ **S25.1** **Injury of innominate or subclavian artery**

√6ᵗʰ **S25.10** **Unspecified injury of innominate or subclavian artery**

√7ᵗʰ **S25.101** **Unspecified injury of right innominate or subclavian artery** ▽

√7ᵗʰ **S25.102** **Unspecified injury of left innominate or subclavian artery** ▽

√7ᵗʰ **S25.109** **Unspecified injury of unspecified innominate or subclavian artery** ▽

√6ᵗʰ **S25.11** **Minor laceration of innominate or subclavian artery**
Incomplete transection of innominate or subclavian artery
Laceration of innominate or subclavian artery NOS
Superficial laceration of innominate or subclavian artery

√7ᵗʰ **S25.111** **Minor laceration of right innominate or subclavian artery**

√7ᵗʰ **S25.112** **Minor laceration of left innominate or subclavian artery**

√7ᵗʰ **S25.119** **Minor laceration of unspecified innominate or subclavian artery** ▽

√6ᵗʰ **S25.12** **Major laceration of innominate or subclavian artery**
Complete transection of innominate or subclavian artery
Traumatic rupture of innominate or subclavian artery

√7ᵗʰ **S25.121** **Major laceration of right innominate or subclavian artery**

√7ᵗʰ **S25.122** **Major laceration of left innominate or subclavian artery**

√7ᵗʰ **S25.129** **Major laceration of unspecified innominate or subclavian artery** ▽

√6ᵗʰ **S25.19** **Other specified injury of innominate or subclavian artery**

√7ᵗʰ **S25.191** **Other specified injury of right innominate or subclavian artery**

√7ᵗʰ **S25.192** **Other specified injury of left innominate or subclavian artery**

√7ᵗʰ **S25.199** **Other specified injury of unspecified innominate or subclavian artery** ▽

√5ᵗʰ **S25.2** **Injury of superior vena cava**
Injury of vena cava NOS

√x7ᵗʰ **S25.20** **Unspecified injury of superior vena cava** ▽

√x7ᵗʰ **S25.21** **Minor laceration of superior vena cava**
Incomplete transection of superior vena cava
Laceration of superior vena cava NOS
Superficial laceration of superior vena cava

√x7ᵗʰ **S25.22** **Major laceration of superior vena cava**
Complete transection of superior vena cava
Traumatic rupture of superior vena cava

√x7ᵗʰ **S25.29** **Other specified injury of superior vena cava**

√5ᵗʰ **S25.3** **Injury of innominate or subclavian vein**

√6ᵗʰ **S25.30** **Unspecified injury of innominate or subclavian vein**

√7ᵗʰ **S25.301** **Unspecified injury of right innominate or subclavian vein** ▽

√7ᵗʰ **S25.302** **Unspecified injury of left innominate or subclavian vein** ▽

√7ᵗʰ **S25.309** **Unspecified injury of unspecified innominate or subclavian vein** ▽

√6ᵗʰ **S25.31** **Minor laceration of innominate or subclavian vein**
Incomplete transection of innominate or subclavian vein
Laceration of innominate or subclavian vein NOS
Superficial laceration of innominate or subclavian vein

√7ᵗʰ **S25.311** **Minor laceration of right innominate or subclavian vein**

√7ᵗʰ **S25.312** **Minor laceration of left innominate or subclavian vein**

√7ᵗʰ **S25.319** **Minor laceration of unspecified innominate or subclavian vein** ▽

√6ᵗʰ **S25.32** **Major laceration of innominate or subclavian vein**
Complete transection of innominate or subclavian vein
Traumatic rupture of innominate or subclavian vein

√7ᵗʰ **S25.321** **Major laceration of right innominate or subclavian vein**

√7ᵗʰ **S25.322** **Major laceration of left innominate or subclavian vein**

√7ᵗʰ **S25.329** **Major laceration of unspecified innominate or subclavian vein** ▽

√6ᵗʰ **S25.39** **Other specified injury of innominate or subclavian vein**

√7ᵗʰ **S25.391** **Other specified injury of right innominate or subclavian vein**

√7ᵗʰ **S25.392** **Other specified injury of left innominate or subclavian vein**

√7ᵗʰ **S25.399** **Other specified injury of unspecified innominate or subclavian vein** ▽

√5ᵗʰ **S25.4** **Injury of pulmonary blood vessels**

√6ᵗʰ **S25.40** **Unspecified injury of pulmonary blood vessels**

√7ᵗʰ **S25.401** **Unspecified injury of right pulmonary blood vessels** ▽

√7ᵗʰ **S25.402** **Unspecified injury of left pulmonary blood vessels** ▽

√7ᵗʰ **S25.409** **Unspecified injury of unspecified pulmonary blood vessels** ▽

☑ Additional Character Req   √x7ᵗʰ Placeholder Alert   Manifestation   HCC CMS-HCC Condition   ▽ Unspecified Code   ►◄ Revised Text   ● New Code   ▲ Revised Code Title

ICD-10-CM 2018   937

√6ᵗʰ **S25.41** **Minor laceration of pulmonary blood vessels**
Incomplete transection of pulmonary blood vessels
Laceration of pulmonary blood vessels NOS
Superficial laceration of pulmonary blood vessels
- √7ᵗʰ **S25.411** **Minor laceration of right pulmonary blood vessels**
- √7ᵗʰ **S25.412** **Minor laceration of left pulmonary blood vessels**
- √7ᵗʰ **S25.419** **Minor laceration of unspecified pulmonary blood vessels** ▽

√6ᵗʰ **S25.42** **Major laceration of pulmonary blood vessels**
Complete transection of pulmonary blood vessels
Traumatic rupture of pulmonary blood vessels
- √7ᵗʰ **S25.421** **Major laceration of right pulmonary blood vessels**
- √7ᵗʰ **S25.422** **Major laceration of left pulmonary blood vessels**
- √7ᵗʰ **S25.429** **Major laceration of unspecified pulmonary blood vessels** ▽

√6ᵗʰ **S25.49** **Other specified injury of pulmonary blood vessels**
- √7ᵗʰ **S25.491** **Other specified injury of right pulmonary blood vessels**
- √7ᵗʰ **S25.492** **Other specified injury of left pulmonary blood vessels**
- √7ᵗʰ **S25.499** **Other specified injury of unspecified pulmonary blood vessels** ▽

√5ᵗʰ **S25.5** **Injury of intercostal blood vessels**
√6ᵗʰ **S25.50** **Unspecified injury of intercostal blood vessels**
- √7ᵗʰ **S25.501** **Unspecified injury of intercostal blood vessels, right side** ▽
- √7ᵗʰ **S25.502** **Unspecified injury of intercostal blood vessels, left side** ▽
- √7ᵗʰ **S25.509** **Unspecified injury of intercostal blood vessels, unspecified side** ▽

√6ᵗʰ **S25.51** **Laceration of intercostal blood vessels**
- √7ᵗʰ **S25.511** **Laceration of intercostal blood vessels, right side**
- √7ᵗʰ **S25.512** **Laceration of intercostal blood vessels, left side**
- √7ᵗʰ **S25.519** **Laceration of intercostal blood vessels, unspecified side** ▽

√6ᵗʰ **S25.59** **Other specified injury of intercostal blood vessels**
- √7ᵗʰ **S25.591** **Other specified injury of intercostal blood vessels, right side**
- √7ᵗʰ **S25.592** **Other specified injury of intercostal blood vessels, left side**
- √7ᵗʰ **S25.599** **Other specified injury of intercostal blood vessels, unspecified side** ▽

√5ᵗʰ **S25.8** **Injury of other blood vessels of thorax**
Injury of azygos vein
Injury of mammary artery or vein
√6ᵗʰ **S25.80** **Unspecified injury of other blood vessels of thorax**
- √7ᵗʰ **S25.801** **Unspecified injury of other blood vessels of thorax, right side** ▽
- √7ᵗʰ **S25.802** **Unspecified injury of other blood vessels of thorax, left side** ▽
- √7ᵗʰ **S25.809** **Unspecified injury of other blood vessels of thorax, unspecified side** ▽

√6ᵗʰ **S25.81** **Laceration of other blood vessels of thorax**
- √7ᵗʰ **S25.811** **Laceration of other blood vessels of thorax, right side**
- √7ᵗʰ **S25.812** **Laceration of other blood vessels of thorax, left side**
- √7ᵗʰ **S25.819** **Laceration of other blood vessels of thorax, unspecified side** ▽

√6ᵗʰ **S25.89** **Other specified injury of other blood vessels of thorax**
- √7ᵗʰ **S25.891** **Other specified injury of other blood vessels of thorax, right side**
- √7ᵗʰ **S25.892** **Other specified injury of other blood vessels of thorax, left side**
- √7ᵗʰ **S25.899** **Other specified injury of other blood vessels of thorax, unspecified side** ▽

√5ᵗʰ **S25.9** **Injury of unspecified blood vessel of thorax**
- √x7ᵗʰ **S25.90** **Unspecified injury of unspecified blood vessel of thorax** ▽
- √x7ᵗʰ **S25.91** **Laceration of unspecified blood vessel of thorax** ▽
- √x7ᵗʰ **S25.99** **Other specified injury of unspecified blood vessel of thorax** ▽

√4ᵗʰ **S26** **Injury of heart**
Code also any associated:
open wound of thorax (S21.-)
traumatic hemopneumothorax (S27.2)
traumatic hemothorax (S27.1)
traumatic pneumothorax (S27.0)

The appropriate 7th character is to be added to each code from category S26.
A initial encounter
D subsequent encounter
S sequela

√5ᵗʰ **S26.0** **Injury of heart with hemopericardium**
- √x7ᵗʰ **S26.00** **Unspecified injury of heart with hemopericardium** ▽
- √x7ᵗʰ **S26.01** **Contusion of heart with hemopericardium**
- √6ᵗʰ **S26.02** **Laceration of heart with hemopericardium**
  - √7ᵗʰ **S26.020** **Mild laceration of heart with hemopericardium**
    Laceration of heart without penetration of heart chamber
  - √7ᵗʰ **S26.021** **Moderate laceration of heart with hemopericardium**
    Laceration of heart with penetration of heart chamber
  - √7ᵗʰ **S26.022** **Major laceration of heart with hemopericardium**
    Laceration of heart with penetration of multiple heart chambers
- √x7ᵗʰ **S26.09** **Other injury of heart with hemopericardium**

√5ᵗʰ **S26.1** **Injury of heart without hemopericardium**
- √x7ᵗʰ **S26.10** **Unspecified injury of heart without hemopericardium** ▽
- √x7ᵗʰ **S26.11** **Contusion of heart without hemopericardium**
- √x7ᵗʰ **S26.12** **Laceration of heart without hemopericardium**
- √x7ᵗʰ **S26.19** **Other injury of heart without hemopericardium**

√5ᵗʰ **S26.9** **Injury of heart, unspecified with or without hemopericardium**
- √x7ᵗʰ **S26.90** **Unspecified injury of heart, unspecified with or without hemopericardium** ▽
- √x7ᵗʰ **S26.91** **Contusion of heart, unspecified with or without hemopericardium**
  DEF: Bruising within the heart muscle with no mention of open wound; usually caused by blunt chest trauma in motor vehicle accidents, falling from great heights, or receiving CPR.
- √x7ᵗʰ **S26.92** **Laceration of heart, unspecified with or without hemopericardium** ▽
  Laceration of heart NOS
- √x7ᵗʰ **S26.99** **Other injury of heart, unspecified with or without hemopericardium** ▽

√4ᵗʰ **S27** **Injury of other and unspecified intrathoracic organs**
Code also any associated open wound of thorax (S21.-)
EXCLUDES 2 injury of cervical esophagus (S10-S19)
injury of trachea (cervical) (S10-S19)

The appropriate 7th character is to be added to each code from category S27.
A initial encounter
D subsequent encounter
S sequela

√x7ᵗʰ **S27.0** **Traumatic pneumothorax**
EXCLUDES 1 spontaneous pneumothorax (J93.-)
√x7ᵗʰ **S27.1** **Traumatic hemothorax**
√x7ᵗʰ **S27.2** **Traumatic hemopneumothorax**
√5ᵗʰ **S27.3** **Other and unspecified injuries of lung**
√6ᵗʰ **S27.30** **Unspecified injury of lung**
- √7ᵗʰ **S27.301** **Unspecified injury of lung, unilateral** ▽
- √7ᵗʰ **S27.302** **Unspecified injury of lung, bilateral** ▽
- √7ᵗʰ **S27.309** **Unspecified injury of lung, unspecified** ▽

√6ᵗʰ **S27.31** Primary blast injury of lung
    Blast injury of lung NOS

√7ᵗʰ **S27.311** Primary blast injury of lung, unilateral

√7ᵗʰ **S27.312** Primary blast injury of lung, bilateral

√7ᵗʰ **S27.319** Primary blast injury of lung, unspecified ▽

√6ᵗʰ **S27.32** Contusion of lung
    DEF: Bruising of lung without mention of open wound.

√7ᵗʰ **S27.321** Contusion of lung, unilateral

√7ᵗʰ **S27.322** Contusion of lung, bilateral

√7ᵗʰ **S27.329** Contusion of lung, unspecified ▽

√6ᵗʰ **S27.33** Laceration of lung

√7ᵗʰ **S27.331** Laceration of lung, unilateral

√7ᵗʰ **S27.332** Laceration of lung, bilateral

√7ᵗʰ **S27.339** Laceration of lung, unspecified ▽

√6ᵗʰ **S27.39** Other injuries of lung
    Secondary blast injury of lung

√7ᵗʰ **S27.391** Other injuries of lung, unilateral

√7ᵗʰ **S27.392** Other injuries of lung, bilateral

√7ᵗʰ **S27.399** Other injuries of lung, unspecified ▽

√5ᵗʰ **S27.4** Injury of bronchus

√6ᵗʰ **S27.40** Unspecified injury of bronchus

√7ᵗʰ **S27.401** Unspecified injury of bronchus, unilateral ▽

√7ᵗʰ **S27.402** Unspecified injury of bronchus, bilateral ▽

√7ᵗʰ **S27.409** Unspecified injury of bronchus, unspecified ▽

√6ᵗʰ **S27.41** Primary blast injury of bronchus
    Blast injury of bronchus NOS

√7ᵗʰ **S27.411** Primary blast injury of bronchus, unilateral

√7ᵗʰ **S27.412** Primary blast injury of bronchus, bilateral

√7ᵗʰ **S27.419** Primary blast injury of bronchus, unspecified ▽

√6ᵗʰ **S27.42** Contusion of bronchus

√7ᵗʰ **S27.421** Contusion of bronchus, unilateral

√7ᵗʰ **S27.422** Contusion of bronchus, bilateral

√7ᵗʰ **S27.429** Contusion of bronchus, unspecified ▽

√6ᵗʰ **S27.43** Laceration of bronchus

√7ᵗʰ **S27.431** Laceration of bronchus, unilateral

√7ᵗʰ **S27.432** Laceration of bronchus, bilateral

√7ᵗʰ **S27.439** Laceration of bronchus, unspecified ▽

√6ᵗʰ **S27.49** Other injury of bronchus
    Secondary blast injury of bronchus

√7ᵗʰ **S27.491** Other injury of bronchus, unilateral

√7ᵗʰ **S27.492** Other injury of bronchus, bilateral

√7ᵗʰ **S27.499** Other injury of bronchus, unspecified ▽

√5ᵗʰ **S27.5** Injury of thoracic trachea

√x7ᵗʰ **S27.50** Unspecified injury of thoracic trachea ▽

√x7ᵗʰ **S27.51** Primary blast injury of thoracic trachea
    Blast injury of thoracic trachea NOS

√x7ᵗʰ **S27.52** Contusion of thoracic trachea

√x7ᵗʰ **S27.53** Laceration of thoracic trachea

√x7ᵗʰ **S27.59** Other injury of thoracic trachea
    Secondary blast injury of thoracic trachea

√5ᵗʰ **S27.6** Injury of pleura

√x7ᵗʰ **S27.60** Unspecified injury of pleura ▽

√x7ᵗʰ **S27.63** Laceration of pleura

√x7ᵗʰ **S27.69** Other injury of pleura

√5ᵗʰ **S27.8** Injury of other specified intrathoracic organs

√6ᵗʰ **S27.80** Injury of diaphragm

√7ᵗʰ **S27.802** Contusion of diaphragm

√7ᵗʰ **S27.803** Laceration of diaphragm

√7ᵗʰ **S27.808** Other injury of diaphragm

√7ᵗʰ **S27.809** Unspecified injury of diaphragm ▽

√6ᵗʰ **S27.81** Injury of esophagus (thoracic part)

√7ᵗʰ **S27.812** Contusion of esophagus (thoracic part)

√7ᵗʰ **S27.813** Laceration of esophagus (thoracic part)

√7ᵗʰ **S27.818** Other injury of esophagus (thoracic part)

√7ᵗʰ **S27.819** Unspecified injury of esophagus (thoracic part) ▽

√6ᵗʰ **S27.89** Injury of other specified intrathoracic organs
    Injury of lymphatic thoracic duct
    Injury of thymus gland

√7ᵗʰ **S27.892** Contusion of other specified intrathoracic organs

√7ᵗʰ **S27.893** Laceration of other specified intrathoracic organs

√7ᵗʰ **S27.898** Other injury of other specified intrathoracic organs

√7ᵗʰ **S27.899** Unspecified injury of other specified intrathoracic organs ▽

√x7ᵗʰ **S27.9** Injury of unspecified intrathoracic organ ▽

√4ᵗʰ **S28** Crushing injury of thorax, and traumatic amputation of part of thorax

The appropriate 7th character is to be added to each code from category S28.
A   initial encounter
D   subsequent encounter
S   sequela

√x7ᵗʰ **S28.0** Crushed chest
    Use additional code for all associated injuries
    EXCLUDES 1   *flail chest (S22.5)*

√x7ᵗʰ **S28.1** Traumatic amputation (partial) of part of thorax, except breast

√5ᵗʰ **S28.2** Traumatic amputation of breast

√6ᵗʰ **S28.21** Complete traumatic amputation of breast
    Traumatic amputation of breast NOS

√7ᵗʰ **S28.211** Complete traumatic amputation of right breast

√7ᵗʰ **S28.212** Complete traumatic amputation of left breast

√7ᵗʰ **S28.219** Complete traumatic amputation of unspecified breast ▽

√6ᵗʰ **S28.22** Partial traumatic amputation of breast

√7ᵗʰ **S28.221** Partial traumatic amputation of right breast

√7ᵗʰ **S28.222** Partial traumatic amputation of left breast

√7ᵗʰ **S28.229** Partial traumatic amputation of unspecified breast ▽

√4ᵗʰ **S29** Other and unspecified injuries of thorax
    Code also any associated open wound (S21.-)

The appropriate 7th character is to be added to each code from category S29.
A   initial encounter
D   subsequent encounter
S   sequela

√5ᵗʰ **S29.0** Injury of muscle and tendon at thorax level

√6ᵗʰ **S29.00** Unspecified injury of muscle and tendon of thorax

√7ᵗʰ **S29.001** Unspecified injury of muscle and tendon of front wall of thorax ▽

√7ᵗʰ **S29.002** Unspecified injury of muscle and tendon of back wall of thorax ▽

√7ᵗʰ **S29.009** Unspecified injury of muscle and tendon of unspecified wall of thorax ▽

√6ᵗʰ **S29.01** Strain of muscle and tendon of thorax

√7ᵗʰ **S29.011** Strain of muscle and tendon of front wall of thorax

√7ᵗʰ **S29.012** Strain of muscle and tendon of back wall of thorax

√7ᵗʰ **S29.019** Strain of muscle and tendon of unspecified wall of thorax ▽

√6ᵗʰ **S29.02** Laceration of muscle and tendon of thorax

√7ᵗʰ **S29.021** Laceration of muscle and tendon of front wall of thorax

√7ᵗʰ **S29.022** Laceration of muscle and tendon of back wall of thorax

√7ᵗʰ **S29.029** Laceration of muscle and tendon of unspecified wall of thorax ▽

☑ Additional Character Req   √x7ᵗʰ Placeholder Alert   Manifestation   HCC CMS-HCC Condition   ▽ Unspecified Code   ▶◀ Revised Text   ● New Code   ▲ Revised Code Title

ICD-10-CM 2018   939

√6ᵗʰ **S29.09**   **Other injury of muscle and tendon of thorax**

     √7ᵗʰ **S29.091**   **Other injury of muscle and tendon of** front wall of thorax

     √7ᵗʰ **S29.092**   **Other injury of muscle and tendon of** back wall of thorax

     √7ᵗʰ **S29.099**   **Other injury of muscle and tendon of unspecified wall of thorax**   ▽

√x7ᵗʰ **S29.8**   **Other specified injuries of thorax**

√x7ᵗʰ **S29.9**   **Unspecified injury of thorax**   ▽

Injuries to the abdomen, lower back, lumbar spine, pelvis and external genitals (S30-S39)

INCLUDES   injuries to the abdominal wall
           injuries to the anus
           injuries to the buttock
           injuries to the external genitalia
           injuries to the flank
           injuries to the groin

EXCLUDES 2   *burns and corrosions (T20-T32)*
           effects of foreign body in anus and rectum (T18.5)
           effects of foreign body in genitourinary tract (T19.-)
           effects of foreign body in stomach, small intestine and colon (T18.2-T18.4)
           frostbite (T33-T34)
           insect bite or sting, venomous (T63.4)

√4ᵗʰ **S30**   **Superficial injury of abdomen, lower back, pelvis and external genitals**

     EXCLUDES 2   *superficial injury of hip (S70.-)*

     The appropriate 7th character is to be added to each code from category S30.
     A   initial encounter
     D   subsequent encounter
     S   sequela

√x7ᵗʰ **S30.0**   **Contusion of lower back and pelvis**
     Contusion of buttock

√x7ᵗʰ **S30.1**   **Contusion of abdominal wall**
     Contusion of flank   Contusion of groin

√5ᵗʰ **S30.2**   **Contusion of external genital organs**

     √6ᵗʰ **S30.20**   **Contusion of unspecified external genital organ**

         √7ᵗʰ **S30.201**   **Contusion of unspecified external genital organ, male**   ♂▽

         √7ᵗʰ **S30.202**   **Contusion of unspecified external genital organ, female**   ♀▽

     √x7ᵗʰ **S30.21**   **Contusion of penis**   ♂

     √x7ᵗʰ **S30.22**   **Contusion of scrotum and testes**   ♂

     √x7ᵗʰ **S30.23**   **Contusion of vagina and vulva**   ♀

√x7ᵗʰ **S30.3**   **Contusion of anus**

√5ᵗʰ **S30.8**   **Other superficial injuries of abdomen, lower back, pelvis and external genitals**

     √6ᵗʰ **S30.81**   **Abrasion of abdomen, lower back, pelvis and external genitals**

         √7ᵗʰ **S30.810**   **Abrasion of** lower back and pelvis

         √7ᵗʰ **S30.811**   **Abrasion of** abdominal wall

         √7ᵗʰ **S30.812**   **Abrasion of** penis   ♂

         √7ᵗʰ **S30.813**   **Abrasion of** scrotum and testes   ♂

         √7ᵗʰ **S30.814**   **Abrasion of** vagina and vulva   ♀

         √7ᵗʰ **S30.815**   **Abrasion of unspecified** external genital organs, male   ♂▽

         √7ᵗʰ **S30.816**   **Abrasion of unspecified** external genital organs, female   ♀▽

         √7ᵗʰ **S30.817**   **Abrasion of** anus

     √6ᵗʰ **S30.82**   **Blister (nonthermal) of abdomen, lower back, pelvis and external genitals**

         √7ᵗʰ **S30.820**   **Blister (nonthermal) of** lower back and pelvis

         √7ᵗʰ **S30.821**   **Blister (nonthermal) of** abdominal wall

         √7ᵗʰ **S30.822**   **Blister (nonthermal) of** penis   ♂

         √7ᵗʰ **S30.823**   **Blister (nonthermal) of** scrotum and testes   ♂

         √7ᵗʰ **S30.824**   **Blister (nonthermal) of** vagina and vulva   ♀

         √7ᵗʰ **S30.825**   **Blister (nonthermal) of unspecified external genital organs, male**   ♂▽

√7ᵗʰ **S30.826**   **Blister (nonthermal) of unspecified external genital organs, female**   ♀▽

√7ᵗʰ **S30.827**   **Blister (nonthermal) of** anus

√6ᵗʰ **S30.84**   **External constriction of abdomen, lower back, pelvis and external genitals**

     √7ᵗʰ **S30.840**   **External constriction of** lower back and pelvis

     √7ᵗʰ **S30.841**   **External constriction of** abdominal wall

     √7ᵗʰ **S30.842**   **External constriction of** penis   ♂
         Hair tourniquet syndrome of penis
         Use additional cause code to identify the constricting item (W49.0-)

     √7ᵗʰ **S30.843**   **External constriction of** scrotum and testes   ♂

     √7ᵗʰ **S30.844**   **External constriction of** vagina and vulva   ♀

     √7ᵗʰ **S30.845**   **External constriction of unspecified** external genital organs, male   ♂▽

     √7ᵗʰ **S30.846**   **External constriction of unspecified** external genital organs, female   ♀▽

√6ᵗʰ **S30.85**   **Superficial foreign body of abdomen, lower back, pelvis and external genitals**
     Splinter in the abdomen, lower back, pelvis and external genitals

     √7ᵗʰ **S30.850**   **Superficial foreign body of** lower back and pelvis

     √7ᵗʰ **S30.851**   **Superficial foreign body of** abdominal wall

     √7ᵗʰ **S30.852**   **Superficial foreign body of** penis   ♂

     √7ᵗʰ **S30.853**   **Superficial foreign body of** scrotum and testes   ♂

     √7ᵗʰ **S30.854**   **Superficial foreign body of** vagina and vulva   ♀

     √7ᵗʰ **S30.855**   **Superficial foreign body of unspecified** external genital organs, male   ♂▽

     √7ᵗʰ **S30.856**   **Superficial foreign body of unspecified** external genital organs, female   ♀▽

     √7ᵗʰ **S30.857**   **Superficial foreign body of** anus

√6ᵗʰ **S30.86**   **Insect bite (nonvenomous) of abdomen, lower back, pelvis and external genitals**

     √7ᵗʰ **S30.860**   **Insect bite (nonvenomous) of** lower back and pelvis

     √7ᵗʰ **S30.861**   **Insect bite (nonvenomous) of** abdominal wall

     √7ᵗʰ **S30.862**   **Insect bite (nonvenomous) of** penis   ♂

     √7ᵗʰ **S30.863**   **Insect bite (nonvenomous) of** scrotum and testes   ♂

     √7ᵗʰ **S30.864**   **Insect bite (nonvenomous) of** vagina and vulva   ♀

     √7ᵗʰ **S30.865**   **Insect bite (nonvenomous) of unspecified** external genital organs, male   ♂▽

     √7ᵗʰ **S30.866**   **Insect bite (nonvenomous) of unspecified** external genital organs, female   ♀▽

     √7ᵗʰ **S30.867**   **Insect bite (nonvenomous) of** anus

√6ᵗʰ **S30.87**   **Other superficial bite of abdomen, lower back, pelvis and external genitals**

     EXCLUDES 1   *open bite of abdomen, lower back, pelvis and external genitals (S31.05, S31.15, S31.25, S31.35, S31.45, S31.55)*

     √7ᵗʰ **S30.870**   **Other superficial bite of** lower back and pelvis

     √7ᵗʰ **S30.871**   **Other superficial bite of** abdominal wall

     √7ᵗʰ **S30.872**   **Other superficial bite of** penis   ♂

     √7ᵗʰ **S30.873**   **Other superficial bite of** scrotum and testes   ♂

     √7ᵗʰ **S30.874**   **Other superficial bite of** vagina and vulva   ♀

     √7ᵗʰ **S30.875**   **Other superficial bite of unspecified** external genital organs, male   ♂▽

     √7ᵗʰ **S30.876**   **Other superficial bite of unspecified** external genital organs, female   ♀▽

     √7ᵗʰ **S30.877**   **Other superficial bite of** anus

EXCLUDES 1 Not coded here   **EXCLUDES 2** Not included here   N Newborn Age: 0   P Pediatric Age: 0-17   M Maternity Age: 12-55   A Adult Age: 15-124

940   ICD-10-CM 2018

✓5ᵗʰ **S30.9** **Unspecified superficial injury of abdomen, lower back, pelvis and external genitals**

     ✓x7ᵗʰ **S30.91** **Unspecified superficial injury of** lower back and pelvis ▽

     ✓x7ᵗʰ **S30.92** **Unspecified superficial injury of** abdominal wall ▽

     ✓x7ᵗʰ **S30.93** **Unspecified superficial injury of** penis ♂▽

     ✓x7ᵗʰ **S30.94** **Unspecified superficial injury of** scrotum and testes ♂▽

     ✓x7ᵗʰ **S30.95** **Unspecified superficial injury of** vagina and vulva ♀▽

     ✓x7ᵗʰ **S30.96** **Unspecified superficial injury of** unspecified external genital organs, male ♂▽

     ✓x7ᵗʰ **S30.97** **Unspecified superficial injury of** unspecified external genital organs, female ♀▽

     ✓x7ᵗʰ **S30.98** **Unspecified superficial injury of** anus ▽

✓4ᵗʰ **S31** **Open wound of abdomen, lower back, pelvis and external genitals**

     Code also any associated:
     spinal cord injury (S24.0, S24.1-, S34.0-, S34.1-)
     wound infection

     EXCLUDES 1 *traumatic amputation of part of abdomen, lower back and pelvis (S38.2-, S38.3)*

     EXCLUDES 2 *open wound of hip (S71.00-S71.02)*
           open fracture of pelvis (S32.1- -S32.9 with 7th character B)

     The appropriate 7th character is to be added to each code from category S31.
     A   initial encounter
     D   subsequent encounter
     S   sequela

   ✓5ᵗʰ **S31.0** **Open wound of** lower back and pelvis

     ✓6ᵗʰ **S31.00** **Unspecified open wound of lower back and pelvis**

       ✓7ᵗʰ **S31.000** **Unspecified open wound of lower back** ▽ **and pelvis** without penetration into retroperitoneum
           Unspecified open wound of lower back and pelvis NOS

       ✓7ᵗʰ **S31.001** **Unspecified open wound of lower back** ▽ **and pelvis** with penetration into retroperitoneum

     ✓6ᵗʰ **S31.01** **Laceration without foreign body of lower back and pelvis**

       ✓7ᵗʰ **S31.010** **Laceration without foreign body of lower back and pelvis** without penetration into retroperitoneum
           Laceration without foreign body of lower back and pelvis NOS

       ✓7ᵗʰ **S31.011** **Laceration without foreign body of lower back and pelvis** with penetration into retroperitoneum

     ✓6ᵗʰ **S31.02** **Laceration with foreign body of lower back and pelvis**

       ✓7ᵗʰ **S31.020** **Laceration with foreign body of lower back and pelvis** without penetration into retroperitoneum
           Laceration with foreign body of lower back and pelvis NOS

       ✓7ᵗʰ **S31.021** **Laceration with foreign body of lower back and pelvis** with penetration into retroperitoneum

     ✓6ᵗʰ **S31.03** **Puncture wound without foreign body of lower back and pelvis**

       ✓7ᵗʰ **S31.030** **Puncture wound without foreign body of lower back and pelvis** without penetration into retroperitoneum
           Puncture wound without foreign body of lower back and pelvis NOS

       ✓7ᵗʰ **S31.031** **Puncture wound without foreign body of lower back and pelvis** with penetration into retroperitoneum

     ✓6ᵗʰ **S31.04** **Puncture wound with foreign body of lower back and pelvis**

       ✓7ᵗʰ **S31.040** **Puncture wound with foreign body of lower back and pelvis** without penetration into retroperitoneum
           Puncture wound with foreign body of lower back and pelvis NOS

       ✓7ᵗʰ **S31.041** **Puncture wound with foreign body of lower back and pelvis** with penetration into retroperitoneum

     ✓6ᵗʰ **S31.05** **Open bite of lower back and pelvis**
           Bite of lower back and pelvis NOS

       EXCLUDES 1 *superficial bite of lower back and pelvis (S30.860, S30.870)*

       ✓7ᵗʰ **S31.050** **Open bite of lower back and pelvis** without penetration into retroperitoneum
           Open bite of lower back and pelvis NOS

       ✓7ᵗʰ **S31.051** **Open bite of lower back and pelvis** with penetration into retroperitoneum

   ✓5ᵗʰ **S31.1** **Open wound of abdominal wall without penetration into peritoneal cavity**
     Open wound of abdominal wall NOS

     EXCLUDES 2 *open wound of abdominal wall with penetration into peritoneal cavity (S31.6-)*

     ✓6ᵗʰ **S31.10** **Unspecified open wound of abdominal wall without penetration into peritoneal cavity**

       ✓7ᵗʰ **S31.100** **Unspecified open wound of abdominal** ▽ **wall,** right upper quadrant without penetration into peritoneal cavity

       ✓7ᵗʰ **S31.101** **Unspecified open wound of abdominal** ▽ **wall,** left upper quadrant without penetration into peritoneal cavity

       ✓7ᵗʰ **S31.102** **Unspecified open wound of abdominal** ▽ **wall,** epigastric region without penetration into peritoneal cavity

       ✓7ᵗʰ **S31.103** **Unspecified open wound of abdominal** ▽ **wall,** right lower quadrant without penetration into peritoneal cavity

       ✓7ᵗʰ **S31.104** **Unspecified open wound of abdominal** ▽ **wall,** left lower quadrant without penetration into peritoneal cavity

       ✓7ᵗʰ **S31.105** **Unspecified open wound of abdominal** ▽ **wall,** periumbilic region without penetration into peritoneal cavity

       ✓7ᵗʰ **S31.109** **Unspecified open wound of abdominal** ▽ **wall,** unspecified quadrant without penetration into peritoneal cavity
           Unspecified open wound of abdominal wall NOS

     ✓6ᵗʰ **S31.11** **Laceration without foreign body of abdominal wall without penetration into peritoneal cavity**

       ✓7ᵗʰ **S31.110** **Laceration without foreign body of abdominal wall,** right upper quadrant without penetration into peritoneal cavity

       ✓7ᵗʰ **S31.111** **Laceration without foreign body of abdominal wall,** left upper quadrant without penetration into peritoneal cavity

       ✓7ᵗʰ **S31.112** **Laceration without foreign body of abdominal wall,** epigastric region without penetration into peritoneal cavity

       ✓7ᵗʰ **S31.113** **Laceration without foreign body of abdominal wall,** right lower quadrant without penetration into peritoneal cavity

       ✓7ᵗʰ **S31.114** **Laceration without foreign body of abdominal wall,** left lower quadrant without penetration into peritoneal cavity

       ✓7ᵗʰ **S31.115** **Laceration without foreign body of abdominal wall,** periumbilic region without penetration into peritoneal cavity

       ✓7ᵗʰ **S31.119** **Laceration without foreign body of** ▽ **abdominal wall,** unspecified quadrant without penetration into peritoneal cavity

     ✓6ᵗʰ **S31.12** **Laceration with foreign body of abdominal wall without penetration into peritoneal cavity**

       ✓7ᵗʰ **S31.120** **Laceration of abdominal wall with foreign body,** right upper quadrant without penetration into peritoneal cavity

       ✓7ᵗʰ **S31.121** **Laceration of abdominal wall with foreign body,** left upper quadrant without penetration into peritoneal cavity

       ✓7ᵗʰ **S31.122** **Laceration of abdominal wall with foreign body,** epigastric region without penetration into peritoneal cavity

       ✓7ᵗʰ **S31.123** **Laceration of abdominal wall with foreign body,** right lower quadrant without penetration into peritoneal cavity

---

☑ Additional Character Req   ✓x7ᵗʰ Placeholder Alert   Manifestation   HCC CMS-HCC Condition   ▽ Unspecified Code   ▶◀ Revised Text   ● New Code   ▲ Revised Code Title

ICD-10-CM 2018   941

√7ᵗʰ S31.124 Laceration of abdominal wall with foreign body, left lower quadrant without penetration into peritoneal cavity

√7ᵗʰ S31.125 Laceration of abdominal wall with foreign body, periumbilic region without penetration into peritoneal cavity

√7ᵗʰ S31.129 Laceration of abdominal wall with foreign body, unspecified quadrant without penetration into peritoneal cavity ▽

√6ᵗʰ S31.13 Puncture wound of abdominal wall without foreign body without penetration into peritoneal cavity

√7ᵗʰ S31.130 Puncture wound of abdominal wall without foreign body, right upper quadrant without penetration into peritoneal cavity

√7ᵗʰ S31.131 Puncture wound of abdominal wall without foreign body, left upper quadrant without penetration into peritoneal cavity

√7ᵗʰ S31.132 Puncture wound of abdominal wall without foreign body, epigastric region without penetration into peritoneal cavity

√7ᵗʰ S31.133 Puncture wound of abdominal wall without foreign body, right lower quadrant without penetration into peritoneal cavity

√7ᵗʰ S31.134 Puncture wound of abdominal wall without foreign body, left lower quadrant without penetration into peritoneal cavity

√7ᵗʰ S31.135 Puncture wound of abdominal wall without foreign body, periumbilic region without penetration into peritoneal cavity

√7ᵗʰ S31.139 Puncture wound of abdominal wall without foreign body, unspecified quadrant without penetration into peritoneal cavity ▽

√6ᵗʰ S31.14 Puncture wound of abdominal wall with foreign body without penetration into peritoneal cavity

√7ᵗʰ S31.140 Puncture wound of abdominal wall with foreign body, right upper quadrant without penetration into peritoneal cavity

√7ᵗʰ S31.141 Puncture wound of abdominal wall with foreign body, left upper quadrant without penetration into peritoneal cavity

√7ᵗʰ S31.142 Puncture wound of abdominal wall with foreign body, epigastric region without penetration into peritoneal cavity

√7ᵗʰ S31.143 Puncture wound of abdominal wall with foreign body, right lower quadrant without penetration into peritoneal cavity

√7ᵗʰ S31.144 Puncture wound of abdominal wall with foreign body, left lower quadrant without penetration into peritoneal cavity

√7ᵗʰ S31.145 Puncture wound of abdominal wall with foreign body, periumbilic region without penetration into peritoneal cavity

√7ᵗʰ S31.149 Puncture wound of abdominal wall with foreign body, unspecified quadrant without penetration into peritoneal cavity ▽

√6ᵗʰ S31.15 Open bite of abdominal wall without penetration into peritoneal cavity
Bite of abdominal wall NOS
EXCLUDES 1   superficial bite of abdominal wall (S30.871)

√7ᵗʰ S31.150 Open bite of abdominal wall, right upper quadrant without penetration into peritoneal cavity

√7ᵗʰ S31.151 Open bite of abdominal wall, left upper quadrant without penetration into peritoneal cavity

√7ᵗʰ S31.152 Open bite of abdominal wall, epigastric region without penetration into peritoneal cavity

√7ᵗʰ S31.153 Open bite of abdominal wall, right lower quadrant without penetration into peritoneal cavity

√7ᵗʰ S31.154 Open bite of abdominal wall, left lower quadrant without penetration into peritoneal cavity

√7ᵗʰ S31.155 Open bite of abdominal wall, periumbilic region without penetration into peritoneal cavity

√7ᵗʰ S31.159 Open bite of abdominal wall, unspecified quadrant without penetration into peritoneal cavity ▽

√5ᵗʰ S31.2 Open wound of penis

√x7ᵗʰ S31.20 Unspecified open wound of penis ♂▽

√x7ᵗʰ S31.21 Laceration without foreign body of penis ♂

√x7ᵗʰ S31.22 Laceration with foreign body of penis ♂

√x7ᵗʰ S31.23 Puncture wound without foreign body of penis ♂

√x7ᵗʰ S31.24 Puncture wound with foreign body of penis ♂

√x7ᵗʰ S31.25 Open bite of penis ♂
Bite of penis NOS
EXCLUDES 1   superficial bite of penis (S30.862, S30.872)

√5ᵗʰ S31.3 Open wound of scrotum and testes

√x7ᵗʰ S31.30 Unspecified open wound of scrotum and testes ♂▽

√x7ᵗʰ S31.31 Laceration without foreign body of scrotum and testes ♂

√x7ᵗʰ S31.32 Laceration with foreign body of scrotum and testes ♂

√x7ᵗʰ S31.33 Puncture wound without foreign body of scrotum and testes ♂

√x7ᵗʰ S31.34 Puncture wound with foreign body of scrotum and testes ♂

√x7ᵗʰ S31.35 Open bite of scrotum and testes ♂
Bite of scrotum and testes NOS
EXCLUDES 1   superficial bite of scrotum and testes (S30.863, S30.873)

√5ᵗʰ S31.4 Open wound of vagina and vulva
EXCLUDES 1   injury to vagina and vulva during delivery (O70-, O71.4)

√x7ᵗʰ S31.40 Unspecified open wound of vagina and vulva ♀▽

√x7ᵗʰ S31.41 Laceration without foreign body of vagina and vulva ♀

√x7ᵗʰ S31.42 Laceration with foreign body of vagina and vulva ♀

√x7ᵗʰ S31.43 Puncture wound without foreign body of vagina and vulva ♀

√x7ᵗʰ S31.44 Puncture wound with foreign body of vagina and vulva ♀

√x7ᵗʰ S31.45 Open bite of vagina and vulva ♀
Bite of vagina and vulva NOS
EXCLUDES 1   superficial bite of vagina and vulva (S30.864, S30.874)

√5ᵗʰ S31.5 Open wound of unspecified external genital organs
EXCLUDES 1   traumatic amputation of external genital organs (S38.21, S38.22)

√6ᵗʰ S31.50 Unspecified open wound of unspecified external genital organs

√7ᵗʰ S31.501 Unspecified open wound of unspecified external genital organs, male ♂▽

√7ᵗʰ S31.502 Unspecified open wound of unspecified external genital organs, female ♀▽

√6ᵗʰ S31.51 Laceration without foreign body of unspecified external genital organs

√7ᵗʰ S31.511 Laceration without foreign body of unspecified external genital organs, male ♂▽

√7ᵗʰ S31.512 Laceration without foreign body of unspecified external genital organs, female ♀▽

√6ᵗʰ S31.52 Laceration with foreign body of unspecified external genital organs

√7ᵗʰ S31.521 Laceration with foreign body of unspecified external genital organs, male ♂▽

√7ᵗʰ S31.522 Laceration with foreign body of unspecified external genital organs, female ♀▽

EXCLUDES 1 Not coded here   *EXCLUDES 2* Not included here   Ⓝ Newborn Age: 0   Ⓟ Pediatric Age: 0-17   Ⓜ Maternity Age: 12-55   Ⓐ Adult Age: 15-124

942   ICD-10-CM 2018

✓6ᵗʰ **S31.53** Puncture wound without foreign body of unspecified external genital organs

     ✓7ᵗʰ **S31.531** Puncture wound without foreign body of unspecified external genital organs, male ♂▽

     ✓7ᵗʰ **S31.532** Puncture wound without foreign body of unspecified external genital organs, female ♀▽

✓6ᵗʰ **S31.54** Puncture wound with foreign body of unspecified external genital organs

     ✓7ᵗʰ **S31.541** Puncture wound with foreign body of unspecified external genital organs, male ♂▽

     ✓7ᵗʰ **S31.542** Puncture wound with foreign body of unspecified external genital organs, female ♀▽

✓6ᵗʰ **S31.55** Open bite of unspecified external genital organs
     Bite of unspecified external genital organs NOS
     EXCLUDES 1 *superficial bite of unspecified external genital organs (S30.865, S30.866, S30.875, S30.876)*

     ✓7ᵗʰ **S31.551** Open bite of unspecified external genital organs, male ♂▽

     ✓7ᵗʰ **S31.552** Open bite of unspecified external genital organs, female ♀▽

✓5ᵗʰ **S31.6** Open wound of abdominal wall with penetration into peritoneal cavity

✓6ᵗʰ **S31.60** Unspecified open wound of abdominal wall with penetration into peritoneal cavity

     ✓7ᵗʰ **S31.600** Unspecified open wound of abdominal wall, right upper quadrant with penetration into peritoneal cavity ▽

     ✓7ᵗʰ **S31.601** Unspecified open wound of abdominal wall, left upper quadrant with penetration into peritoneal cavity ▽

     ✓7ᵗʰ **S31.602** Unspecified open wound of abdominal wall, epigastric region with penetration into peritoneal cavity ▽

     ✓7ᵗʰ **S31.603** Unspecified open wound of abdominal wall, right lower quadrant with penetration into peritoneal cavity ▽

     ✓7ᵗʰ **S31.604** Unspecified open wound of abdominal wall, left lower quadrant with penetration into peritoneal cavity ▽

     ✓7ᵗʰ **S31.605** Unspecified open wound of abdominal wall, periumbilic region with penetration into peritoneal cavity ▽

     ✓7ᵗʰ **S31.609** Unspecified open wound of abdominal wall, unspecified quadrant with penetration into peritoneal cavity ▽

✓6ᵗʰ **S31.61** Laceration without foreign body of abdominal wall with penetration into peritoneal cavity

     ✓7ᵗʰ **S31.610** Laceration without foreign body of abdominal wall, right upper quadrant with penetration into peritoneal cavity

     ✓7ᵗʰ **S31.611** Laceration without foreign body of abdominal wall, left upper quadrant with penetration into peritoneal cavity

     ✓7ᵗʰ **S31.612** Laceration without foreign body of abdominal wall, epigastric region with penetration into peritoneal cavity

     ✓7ᵗʰ **S31.613** Laceration without foreign body of abdominal wall, right lower quadrant with penetration into peritoneal cavity

     ✓7ᵗʰ **S31.614** Laceration without foreign body of abdominal wall, left lower quadrant with penetration into peritoneal cavity

     ✓7ᵗʰ **S31.615** Laceration without foreign body of abdominal wall, periumbilic region with penetration into peritoneal cavity

     ✓7ᵗʰ **S31.619** Laceration without foreign body of abdominal wall, unspecified quadrant with penetration into peritoneal cavity ▽

✓6ᵗʰ **S31.62** Laceration with foreign body of abdominal wall with penetration into peritoneal cavity

     ✓7ᵗʰ **S31.620** Laceration with foreign body of abdominal wall, right upper quadrant with penetration into peritoneal cavity

     ✓7ᵗʰ **S31.621** Laceration with foreign body of abdominal wall, left upper quadrant with penetration into peritoneal cavity

     ✓7ᵗʰ **S31.622** Laceration with foreign body of abdominal wall, epigastric region with penetration into peritoneal cavity

     ✓7ᵗʰ **S31.623** Laceration with foreign body of abdominal wall, right lower quadrant with penetration into peritoneal cavity

     ✓7ᵗʰ **S31.624** Laceration with foreign body of abdominal wall, left lower quadrant with penetration into peritoneal cavity

     ✓7ᵗʰ **S31.625** Laceration with foreign body of abdominal wall, periumbilic region with penetration into peritoneal cavity

     ✓7ᵗʰ **S31.629** Laceration with foreign body of abdominal wall, unspecified quadrant with penetration into peritoneal cavity ▽

✓6ᵗʰ **S31.63** Puncture wound without foreign body of abdominal wall with penetration into peritoneal cavity

     ✓7ᵗʰ **S31.630** Puncture wound without foreign body of abdominal wall, right upper quadrant with penetration into peritoneal cavity

     ✓7ᵗʰ **S31.631** Puncture wound without foreign body of abdominal wall, left upper quadrant with penetration into peritoneal cavity

     ✓7ᵗʰ **S31.632** Puncture wound without foreign body of abdominal wall, epigastric region with penetration into peritoneal cavity

     ✓7ᵗʰ **S31.633** Puncture wound without foreign body of abdominal wall, right lower quadrant with penetration into peritoneal cavity

     ✓7ᵗʰ **S31.634** Puncture wound without foreign body of abdominal wall, left lower quadrant with penetration into peritoneal cavity

     ✓7ᵗʰ **S31.635** Puncture wound without foreign body of abdominal wall, periumbilic region with penetration into peritoneal cavity

     ✓7ᵗʰ **S31.639** Puncture wound without foreign body of abdominal wall, unspecified quadrant with penetration into peritoneal cavity ▽

✓6ᵗʰ **S31.64** Puncture wound with foreign body of abdominal wall with penetration into peritoneal cavity

     ✓7ᵗʰ **S31.640** Puncture wound with foreign body of abdominal wall, right upper quadrant with penetration into peritoneal cavity

     ✓7ᵗʰ **S31.641** Puncture wound with foreign body of abdominal wall, left upper quadrant with penetration into peritoneal cavity

     ✓7ᵗʰ **S31.642** Puncture wound with foreign body of abdominal wall, epigastric region with penetration into peritoneal cavity

     ✓7ᵗʰ **S31.643** Puncture wound with foreign body of abdominal wall, right lower quadrant with penetration into peritoneal cavity

     ✓7ᵗʰ **S31.644** Puncture wound with foreign body of abdominal wall, left lower quadrant with penetration into peritoneal cavity

     ✓7ᵗʰ **S31.645** Puncture wound with foreign body of abdominal wall, periumbilic region with penetration into peritoneal cavity

     ✓7ᵗʰ **S31.649** Puncture wound with foreign body of abdominal wall, unspecified quadrant with penetration into peritoneal cavity ▽

✓6ᵗʰ **S31.65** Open bite of abdominal wall with penetration into peritoneal cavity
     EXCLUDES 1 *superficial bite of abdominal wall (S30.861, S30.871)*

     ✓7ᵗʰ **S31.650** Open bite of abdominal wall, right upper quadrant with penetration into peritoneal cavity

     ✓7ᵗʰ **S31.651** Open bite of abdominal wall, left upper quadrant with penetration into peritoneal cavity

     ✓7ᵗʰ **S31.652** Open bite of abdominal wall, epigastric region with penetration into peritoneal cavity

☑ Additional Character Req   ✓×7ᵗʰ Placeholder Alert   Manifestation   ℍℂℂ CMS-HCC Condition   ▽ Unspecified Code   ▶◀ Revised Text   ● New Code   ▲ Revised Code Title

ICD-10-CM 2018   **943**

☑7ᵗʰ **S31.653** **Open bite of abdominal wall, right lower quadrant with penetration into peritoneal cavity**

☑7ᵗʰ **S31.654** **Open bite of abdominal wall, left lower quadrant with penetration into peritoneal cavity**

☑7ᵗʰ **S31.655** **Open bite of abdominal wall, periumbilic region with penetration into peritoneal cavity**

☑7ᵗʰ **S31.659** **Open bite of abdominal wall, unspecified quadrant with penetration into peritoneal cavity** ▽

☑5ᵗʰ **S31.8** **Open wound of other parts of abdomen, lower back and pelvis**

   ☑6ᵗʰ **S31.80** **Open wound of unspecified buttock**

      ☑7ᵗʰ **S31.801** **Laceration without foreign body of unspecified buttock** ▽

      ☑7ᵗʰ **S31.802** **Laceration with foreign body of unspecified buttock** ▽

      ☑7ᵗʰ **S31.803** **Puncture wound without foreign body of unspecified buttock** ▽

      ☑7ᵗʰ **S31.804** **Puncture wound with foreign body of unspecified buttock** ▽

      ☑7ᵗʰ **S31.805** **Open bite of unspecified buttock** ▽
         Bite of buttock NOS
         EXCLUDES 1 *superficial bite of buttock (S30.870)*

      ☑7ᵗʰ **S31.809** **Unspecified open wound of unspecified buttock** ▽

   ☑6ᵗʰ **S31.81** **Open wound of right buttock**

      ☑7ᵗʰ **S31.811** **Laceration without foreign body of right buttock**

      ☑7ᵗʰ **S31.812** **Laceration with foreign body of right buttock**

      ☑7ᵗʰ **S31.813** **Puncture wound without foreign body of right buttock**

      ☑7ᵗʰ **S31.814** **Puncture wound with foreign body of right buttock**

      ☑7ᵗʰ **S31.815** **Open bite of right buttock**
         Bite of right buttock NOS
         EXCLUDES 1 *superficial bite of buttock (S30.870)*

      ☑7ᵗʰ **S31.819** **Unspecified open wound of right buttock** ▽

   ☑6ᵗʰ **S31.82** **Open wound of left buttock**

      ☑7ᵗʰ **S31.821** **Laceration without foreign body of left buttock**

      ☑7ᵗʰ **S31.822** **Laceration with foreign body of left buttock**

      ☑7ᵗʰ **S31.823** **Puncture wound without foreign body of left buttock**

      ☑7ᵗʰ **S31.824** **Puncture wound with foreign body of left buttock**

      ☑7ᵗʰ **S31.825** **Open bite of left buttock**
         Bite of left buttock NOS
         EXCLUDES 1 *superficial bite of buttock (S30.870)*

      ☑7ᵗʰ **S31.829** **Unspecified open wound of left buttock** ▽

   ☑6ᵗʰ **S31.83** **Open wound of anus**

      ☑7ᵗʰ **S31.831** **Laceration without foreign body of anus**

      ☑7ᵗʰ **S31.832** **Laceration with foreign body of anus**

      ☑7ᵗʰ **S31.833** **Puncture wound without foreign body of anus**

      ☑7ᵗʰ **S31.834** **Puncture wound with foreign body of anus**

      ☑7ᵗʰ **S31.835** **Open bite of anus**
         Bite of anus NOS
         EXCLUDES 1 *superficial bite of anus (S30.877)*

      ☑7ᵗʰ **S31.839** **Unspecified open wound of anus** ▽

☑4ᵗʰ **S32** **Fracture of lumbar spine and pelvis**

   NOTE A fracture not indicated as displaced or nondisplaced should be coded to displaced.
        A fracture not indicated as opened or closed should be coded to closed.

   INCLUDES fracture of lumbosacral neural arch
        fracture of lumbosacral spinous process
        fracture of lumbosacral transverse process
        fracture of lumbosacral vertebra
        fracture of lumbosacral vertebral arch

   Code first any associated spinal cord and spinal nerve injury (S34.-)
   EXCLUDES 1 *transection of abdomen (S38.3)*
   EXCLUDES 2 *fracture of hip NOS (S72.0-)*
   AHA: 2015, 3Q, 37-39; 2012, 4Q, 93

   The appropriate 7th character is to be added to each code from category S32.
   A   initial encounter for closed fracture
   B   initial encounter for open fracture
   D   subsequent encounter for fracture with routine healing
   G   subsequent encounter for fracture with delayed healing
   K   subsequent encounter for fracture with nonunion
   S   sequela

☑5ᵗʰ **S32.0** **Fracture of lumbar vertebra**
   Fracture of lumbar spine NOS

   ☑6ᵗʰ **S32.00** **Fracture of unspecified lumbar vertebra**

      [1] ☑7ᵗʰ **S32.000** **Wedge compression fracture of unspecified lumbar vertebra** HCC ▽

      [1] ☑7ᵗʰ **S32.001** **Stable burst fracture of unspecified lumbar vertebra** HCC ▽

      [1] ☑7ᵗʰ **S32.002** **Unstable burst fracture of unspecified lumbar vertebra** HCC

      [1] ☑7ᵗʰ **S32.008** **Other fracture of unspecified lumbar vertebra** HCC ▽

      [1] ☑7ᵗʰ **S32.009** **Unspecified fracture of unspecified lumbar vertebra** HCC ▽

   ☑6ᵗʰ **S32.01** **Fracture of first lumbar vertebra**

      [1] ☑7ᵗʰ **S32.010** **Wedge compression fracture of first lumbar vertebra** HCC

      [1] ☑7ᵗʰ **S32.011** **Stable burst fracture of first lumbar vertebra** HCC

      [1] ☑7ᵗʰ **S32.012** **Unstable burst fracture of first lumbar vertebra** HCC

      [1] ☑7ᵗʰ **S32.018** **Other fracture of first lumbar vertebra** HCC

      [1] ☑7ᵗʰ **S32.019** **Unspecified fracture of first lumbar vertebra** HCC ▽

   ☑6ᵗʰ **S32.02** **Fracture of second lumbar vertebra**

      [1] ☑7ᵗʰ **S32.020** **Wedge compression fracture of second lumbar vertebra** HCC

      [1] ☑7ᵗʰ **S32.021** **Stable burst fracture of second lumbar vertebra** HCC

      [1] ☑7ᵗʰ **S32.022** **Unstable burst fracture of second lumbar vertebra** HCC

      [1] ☑7ᵗʰ **S32.028** **Other fracture of second lumbar vertebra** HCC

      [1] ☑7ᵗʰ **S32.029** **Unspecified fracture of second lumbar vertebra** HCC ▽

   ☑6ᵗʰ **S32.03** **Fracture of third lumbar vertebra**

      [1] ☑7ᵗʰ **S32.030** **Wedge compression fracture of third lumbar vertebra** HCC

      [1] ☑7ᵗʰ **S32.031** **Stable burst fracture of third lumbar vertebra** HCC

      [1] ☑7ᵗʰ **S32.032** **Unstable burst fracture of third lumbar vertebra** HCC

      [1] ☑7ᵗʰ **S32.038** **Other fracture of third lumbar vertebra** HCC

      [1] ☑7ᵗʰ **S32.039** **Unspecified fracture of third lumbar vertebra** HCC ▽

   ☑6ᵗʰ **S32.04** **Fracture of fourth lumbar vertebra**

      [1] ☑7ᵗʰ **S32.040** **Wedge compression fracture of fourth lumbar vertebra** HCC

      [1] ☑7ᵗʰ **S32.041** **Stable burst fracture of fourth lumbar vertebra** HCC

      [1] ☑7ᵗʰ **S32.042** **Unstable burst fracture of fourth lumbar vertebra** HCC

---

[1] HCC with 7th character indicating initial encounter (A, B or C - specific to category).

EXCLUDES 1 Not coded here   *EXCLUDES 2* Not included here   N Newborn Age: 0   P Pediatric Age: 0-17   M Maternity Age: 12-55   A Adult Age: 15-124

944   ICD-10-CM 2018

¹ ☑7ᵗʰ **S32.048** Other fracture of fourth lumbar vertebra ᴴᶜᶜ

¹ ☑7ᵗʰ **S32.049** Unspecified fracture of fourth lumbar vertebra ᴴᶜᶜ ▽

☑6ᵗʰ **S32.05** Fracture of fifth lumbar vertebra

    ¹ ☑7ᵗʰ **S32.050** Wedge compression **fracture of fifth lumbar vertebra** ᴴᶜᶜ

    ¹ ☑7ᵗʰ **S32.051** Stable burst **fracture of fifth lumbar vertebra** ᴴᶜᶜ

    ¹ ☑7ᵗʰ **S32.052** Unstable burst **fracture of fifth lumbar vertebra** ᴴᶜᶜ

    ¹ ☑7ᵗʰ **S32.058** Other fracture of fifth lumbar vertebra ᴴᶜᶜ

    ¹ ☑7ᵗʰ **S32.059** Unspecified fracture of fifth lumbar vertebra ᴴᶜᶜ ▽

☑5ᵗʰ **S32.1 Fracture of sacrum**

    NOTE For vertical fractures, code to most medial fracture extension.

    Use two codes if both a vertical and transverse fracture are present.

    Code also any associated fracture of pelvic ring (S32.8-)

¹ ☑x7ᵗʰ **S32.10** Unspecified fracture of sacrum ᴴᶜᶜ ▽

☑6ᵗʰ **S32.11** Zone I fracture of sacrum

    Vertical sacral ala fracture of sacrum

    ¹ ☑7ᵗʰ **S32.110** Nondisplaced **Zone I fracture of sacrum** ᴴᶜᶜ

    ¹ ☑7ᵗʰ **S32.111** Minimally displaced **Zone I fracture of sacrum** ᴴᶜᶜ

    ¹ ☑7ᵗʰ **S32.112** Severely displaced **Zone I fracture of sacrum** ᴴᶜᶜ

    ¹ ☑7ᵗʰ **S32.119** Unspecified **Zone I fracture of sacrum** ᴴᶜᶜ ▽

☑6ᵗʰ **S32.12** Zone II fracture of sacrum

    Vertical foraminal region fracture of sacrum

    ¹ ☑7ᵗʰ **S32.120** Nondisplaced **Zone II fracture of sacrum** ᴴᶜᶜ

    ¹ ☑7ᵗʰ **S32.121** Minimally displaced **Zone II fracture of sacrum** ᴴᶜᶜ

    ¹ ☑7ᵗʰ **S32.122** Severely displaced **Zone II fracture of sacrum** ᴴᶜᶜ

    ¹ ☑7ᵗʰ **S32.129** Unspecified **Zone II fracture of sacrum** ᴴᶜᶜ ▽

Vertical Sacral Fracture Zones

Zones: ① ② ③

Transverse Sacral Fracture Types

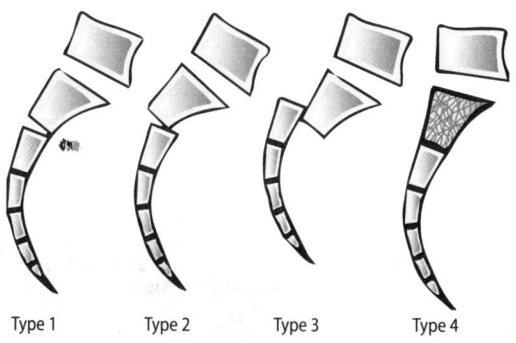

Type 1   Type 2   Type 3   Type 4

☑6ᵗʰ **S32.13** Zone III fracture of sacrum

    Vertical fracture into spinal canal region of sacrum

    ¹ ☑7ᵗʰ **S32.130** Nondisplaced **Zone III fracture of sacrum** ᴴᶜᶜ

    ¹ ☑7ᵗʰ **S32.131** Minimally displaced **Zone III fracture of sacrum** ᴴᶜᶜ

    ¹ ☑7ᵗʰ **S32.132** Severely displaced **Zone III fracture of sacrum** ᴴᶜᶜ

    ¹ ☑7ᵗʰ **S32.139** Unspecified **Zone III fracture of sacrum** ᴴᶜᶜ ▽

¹ ☑x7ᵗʰ **S32.14** Type 1 **fracture of sacrum** ᴴᶜᶜ

    Transverse flexion fracture of sacrum without displacement

¹ ☑x7ᵗʰ **S32.15** Type 2 **fracture of sacrum** ᴴᶜᶜ

    Transverse flexion fracture of sacrum with posterior displacement

¹ ☑x7ᵗʰ **S32.16** Type 3 **fracture of sacrum** ᴴᶜᶜ

    Transverse extension fracture of sacrum with anterior displacement

¹ ☑x7ᵗʰ **S32.17** Type 4 **fracture of sacrum** ᴴᶜᶜ

    Transverse segmental comminution of upper sacrum

¹ ☑x7ᵗʰ **S32.19** Other fracture of sacrum ᴴᶜᶜ

¹ ☑x7ᵗʰ **S32.2 Fracture of coccyx** ᴴᶜᶜ

☑5ᵗʰ **S32.3 Fracture of ilium**

    EXCLUDES 1 *fracture of ilium with associated disruption of pelvic ring (S32.8-)*

☑6ᵗʰ **S32.30** Unspecified fracture of ilium

    ¹ ☑7ᵗʰ **S32.301** Unspecified fracture of right ilium ᴴᶜᶜ ▽

    ¹ ☑7ᵗʰ **S32.302** Unspecified fracture of left ilium ᴴᶜᶜ ▽

    ¹ ☑7ᵗʰ **S32.309** Unspecified fracture of unspecified ilium ᴴᶜᶜ ▽

☑6ᵗʰ **S32.31** Avulsion fracture of ilium

    ¹ ☑7ᵗʰ **S32.311** Displaced avulsion **fracture of right ilium** ᴴᶜᶜ

    ¹ ☑7ᵗʰ **S32.312** Displaced avulsion **fracture of left ilium** ᴴᶜᶜ

    ¹ ☑7ᵗʰ **S32.313** Displaced avulsion **fracture of unspecified ilium** ᴴᶜᶜ ▽

    ¹ ☑7ᵗʰ **S32.314** Nondisplaced avulsion **fracture of right ilium** ᴴᶜᶜ

    ¹ ☑7ᵗʰ **S32.315** Nondisplaced avulsion **fracture of left ilium** ᴴᶜᶜ

    ¹ ☑7ᵗʰ **S32.316** Nondisplaced avulsion **fracture of unspecified ilium** ᴴᶜᶜ ▽

☑6ᵗʰ **S32.39** Other fracture of ilium

    ¹ ☑7ᵗʰ **S32.391** Other fracture of right ilium ᴴᶜᶜ

    ¹ ☑7ᵗʰ **S32.392** Other fracture of left ilium ᴴᶜᶜ

    ¹ ☑7ᵗʰ **S32.399** Other fracture of unspecified ilium ᴴᶜᶜ ▽

☑5ᵗʰ **S32.4 Fracture of acetabulum**

    Code also any associated fracture of pelvic ring (S32.8-)

    AHA: 2016, 3Q, 16

☑6ᵗʰ **S32.40** Unspecified fracture of acetabulum

    ¹ ☑7ᵗʰ **S32.401** Unspecified fracture of right acetabulum ᴴᶜᶜ ▽

    ¹ ☑7ᵗʰ **S32.402** Unspecified fracture of left acetabulum ᴴᶜᶜ ▽

    ¹ ☑7ᵗʰ **S32.409** Unspecified fracture of unspecified acetabulum ᴴᶜᶜ ▽

☑6ᵗʰ **S32.41** Fracture of anterior wall of acetabulum

    ¹ ☑7ᵗʰ **S32.411** Displaced fracture of anterior wall of right acetabulum ᴴᶜᶜ

    ¹ ☑7ᵗʰ **S32.412** Displaced fracture of anterior wall of left acetabulum ᴴᶜᶜ

    ¹ ☑7ᵗʰ **S32.413** Displaced fracture of anterior wall of unspecified acetabulum ᴴᶜᶜ ▽

    ¹ ☑7ᵗʰ **S32.414** Nondisplaced fracture of anterior wall of right acetabulum ᴴᶜᶜ

    ¹ ☑7ᵗʰ **S32.415** Nondisplaced fracture of anterior wall of left acetabulum ᴴᶜᶜ

    ¹ ☑7ᵗʰ **S32.416** Nondisplaced fracture of anterior wall of unspecified acetabulum ᴴᶜᶜ ▽

---

¹ HCC with 7th character indicating initial encounter (A, B or C - specific to category).

☑ Additional Character Req   ☑x7ᵗʰ Placeholder Alert   Manifestation   ᴴᶜᶜ CMS-HCC Condition   ▽ Unspecified Code   ▶◀ Revised Text   ● New Code   ▲ Revised Code Title

ICD-10-CM 2018   945

√6th **S32.42** Fracture of posterior wall of acetabulum

- 1 √7th **S32.421** Displaced fracture of posterior wall of right acetabulum   HCC
- 1 √7th **S32.422** Displaced fracture of posterior wall of left acetabulum   HCC
- 1 √7th **S32.423** Displaced fracture of posterior wall of unspecified acetabulum   HCC ▽
- 1 √7th **S32.424** Nondisplaced fracture of posterior wall of right acetabulum   HCC
- 1 √7th **S32.425** Nondisplaced fracture of posterior wall of left acetabulum   HCC
- 1 √7th **S32.426** Nondisplaced fracture of posterior wall of unspecified acetabulum   HCC ▽

√6th **S32.43** Fracture of anterior column [iliopubic] of acetabulum

- 1 √7th **S32.431** Displaced fracture of anterior column [iliopubic] of right acetabulum   HCC
- 1 √7th **S32.432** Displaced fracture of anterior column [iliopubic] of left acetabulum   HCC
- 1 √7th **S32.433** Displaced fracture of anterior column [iliopubic] of unspecified acetabulum   HCC ▽
- 1 √7th **S32.434** Nondisplaced fracture of anterior column [iliopubic] of right acetabulum   HCC
- 1 √7th **S32.435** Nondisplaced fracture of anterior column [iliopubic] of left acetabulum   HCC
- 1 √7th **S32.436** Nondisplaced fracture of anterior column [iliopubic] of unspecified acetabulum   HCC ▽

√6th **S32.44** Fracture of posterior column [ilioischial] of acetabulum

- 1 √7th **S32.441** Displaced fracture of posterior column [ilioischial] of right acetabulum   HCC
- 1 √7th **S32.442** Displaced fracture of posterior column [ilioischial] of left acetabulum   HCC
- 1 √7th **S32.443** Displaced fracture of posterior column [ilioischial] of unspecified acetabulum   HCC ▽
- 1 √7th **S32.444** Nondisplaced fracture of posterior column [ilioischial] of right acetabulum   HCC
- 1 √7th **S32.445** Nondisplaced fracture of posterior column [ilioischial] of left acetabulum   HCC
- 1 √7th **S32.446** Nondisplaced fracture of posterior column [ilioischial] of unspecified acetabulum   HCC ▽

√6th **S32.45** Transverse fracture of acetabulum

- 1 √7th **S32.451** Displaced transverse fracture of right acetabulum   HCC
- 1 √7th **S32.452** Displaced transverse fracture of left acetabulum   HCC
- 1 √7th **S32.453** Displaced transverse fracture of unspecified acetabulum   HCC ▽
- 1 √7th **S32.454** Nondisplaced transverse fracture of right acetabulum   HCC
- 1 √7th **S32.455** Nondisplaced transverse fracture of left acetabulum   HCC
- 1 √7th **S32.456** Nondisplaced transverse fracture of unspecified acetabulum   HCC ▽

√6th **S32.46** Associated transverse-posterior fracture of acetabulum

- 1 √7th **S32.461** Displaced associated transverse-posterior fracture of right acetabulum   HCC
- 1 √7th **S32.462** Displaced associated transverse-posterior fracture of left acetabulum   HCC
- 1 √7th **S32.463** Displaced associated transverse-posterior fracture of unspecified acetabulum   HCC ▽
- 1 √7th **S32.464** Nondisplaced associated transverse posterior fracture of right acetabulum   HCC
- 1 √7th **S32.465** Nondisplaced associated transverse-posterior fracture of left acetabulum   HCC
- 1 √7th **S32.466** Nondisplaced associated transverse-posterior fracture of unspecified acetabulum   HCC ▽

√6th **S32.47** Fracture of medial wall of acetabulum

- 1 √7th **S32.471** Displaced fracture of medial wall of right acetabulum   HCC
- 1 √7th **S32.472** Displaced fracture of medial wall of left acetabulum   HCC
- 1 √7th **S32.473** Displaced fracture of medial wall of unspecified acetabulum   HCC ▽
- 1 √7th **S32.474** Nondisplaced fracture of medial wall of right acetabulum   HCC
- 1 √7th **S32.475** Nondisplaced fracture of medial wall of left acetabulum   HCC
- 1 √7th **S32.476** Nondisplaced fracture of medial wall of unspecified acetabulum   HCC ▽

√6th **S32.48** Dome fracture of acetabulum

- 1 √7th **S32.481** Displaced dome fracture of right acetabulum   HCC
- 1 √7th **S32.482** Displaced dome fracture of left acetabulum   HCC
- 1 √7th **S32.483** Displaced dome fracture of unspecified acetabulum   HCC ▽
- 1 √7th **S32.484** Nondisplaced dome fracture of right acetabulum   HCC
- 1 √7th **S32.485** Nondisplaced dome fracture of left acetabulum   HCC
- 1 √7th **S32.486** Nondisplaced dome fracture of unspecified acetabulum   HCC ▽

√6th **S32.49** Other specified fracture of acetabulum

- 1 √7th **S32.491** Other specified fracture of right acetabulum   HCC
- 1 √7th **S32.492** Other specified fracture of left acetabulum   HCC
- 1 √7th **S32.499** Other specified fracture of unspecified acetabulum   HCC ▽

√5th **S32.5** Fracture of pubis

> **EXCLUDES 1**   fracture of pubis with associated disruption of pelvic ring (S32.8-)

√6th **S32.50** Unspecified fracture of pubis

- 1 √7th **S32.501** Unspecified fracture of right pubis   HCC ▽
- 1 √7th **S32.502** Unspecified fracture of left pubis   HCC ▽
- 1 √7th **S32.509** Unspecified fracture of unspecified pubis   HCC ▽

√6th **S32.51** Fracture of superior rim of pubis

- 1 √7th **S32.511** Fracture of superior rim of right pubis   HCC
- 1 √7th **S32.512** Fracture of superior rim of left pubis   HCC
- 1 √7th **S32.519** Fracture of superior rim of unspecified pubis   HCC ▽

√6th **S32.59** Other specified fracture of pubis

- 1 √7th **S32.591** Other specified fracture of right pubis   HCC
- 1 √7th **S32.592** Other specified fracture of left pubis   HCC
- 1 √7th **S32.599** Other specified fracture of unspecified pubis   HCC ▽

√5th **S32.6** Fracture of ischium

> **EXCLUDES 1**   fracture of ischium with associated disruption of pelvic ring (S32.8-)

√6th **S32.60** Unspecified fracture of ischium

- 1 √7th **S32.601** Unspecified fracture of right ischium   HCC ▽
- 1 √7th **S32.602** Unspecified fracture of left ischium   HCC ▽
- 1 √7th **S32.609** Unspecified fracture of unspecified ischium   HCC ▽

√6th **S32.61** Avulsion fracture of ischium

- 1 √7th **S32.611** Displaced avulsion fracture of right ischium   HCC
- 1 √7th **S32.612** Displaced avulsion fracture of left ischium   HCC
- 1 √7th **S32.613** Displaced avulsion fracture of unspecified ischium   HCC ▽

---

1   HCC with 7th character indicating initial encounter (A, B or C - specific to category).

EXCLUDES 1 Not coded here   **EXCLUDES 2** Not included here   N Newborn Age: 0   P Pediatric Age: 0-17   M Maternity Age: 12-55   A Adult Age: 15-124

946   ICD-10-CM 2018

1 ☑7ᵗʰ **S32.614** **Nondisplaced** avulsion fracture of **right ischium**   HCC

1 ☑7ᵗʰ **S32.615** **Nondisplaced** avulsion fracture of **left ischium**   HCC

1 ☑7ᵗʰ **S32.616** **Nondisplaced** avulsion fracture of **unspecified ischium**   HCC ▽

☑6ᵗʰ **S32.69** **Other specified fracture of ischium**

1 ☑7ᵗʰ **S32.691** **Other specified fracture of right ischium**   HCC

1 ☑7ᵗʰ **S32.692** **Other specified fracture of left ischium**   HCC

1 ☑7ᵗʰ **S32.699** **Other specified fracture of unspecified ischium**   HCC ▽

☑5ᵗʰ **S32.8** **Fracture of other parts of pelvis**

Code also any associated:
fracture of acetabulum (S32.4-)
sacral fracture (S32.1-)

☑6ᵗʰ **S32.81** **Multiple fractures of pelvis with disruption of pelvic ring**

Multiple pelvic fractures with disruption of pelvic circle

1 ☑7ᵗʰ **S32.810** **Multiple fractures of pelvis with stable disruption of pelvic ring**   HCC

1 ☑7ᵗʰ **S32.811** **Multiple fractures of pelvis with unstable disruption of pelvic ring**   HCC

1 ☑x7ᵗʰ **S32.82** **Multiple fractures of pelvis without disruption of pelvic ring**   HCC

Multiple pelvic fractures without disruption of pelvic circle

1 ☑x7ᵗʰ **S32.89** **Fracture of other parts of pelvis**   HCC

1 ☑x7ᵗʰ **S32.9** **Fracture of unspecified parts of lumbosacral spine and pelvis**   HCC ▽

Fracture of lumbosacral spine NOS
Fracture of pelvis NOS
AHA: 2012, 4Q, 93

Fractures Disrupting Pelvic Circle

Pelvic circle
Stable

Unstable
(two-place fracture)

Iliac crest
Anterior superior iliac spine
Ischial spine
Acetabulum
Femur
Ischium

Ilium
L5

Pelvic Bones

Sacrum
Coccyx
Pubis
Pubic symphysis

☑4ᵗʰ **S33** **Dislocation and sprain of joints and ligaments of lumbar spine and pelvis**

INCLUDES   avulsion of joint or ligament of lumbar spine and pelvis
laceration of cartilage, joint or ligament of lumbar spine and pelvis
sprain of cartilage, joint or ligament of lumbar spine and pelvis
traumatic hemarthrosis of joint or ligament of lumbar spine and pelvis
traumatic rupture of joint or ligament of lumbar spine and pelvis
traumatic subluxation of joint or ligament of lumbar spine and pelvis
traumatic tear of joint or ligament of lumbar spine and pelvis

Code also any associated open wound

EXCLUDES 1   nontraumatic rupture or displacement of lumbar intervertebral disc NOS (M51.-)
obstetric damage to pelvic joints and ligaments (O71.6)

EXCLUDES 2   dislocation and sprain of joints and ligaments of hip (S73.-)
strain of muscle of lower back and pelvis (S39.01-)

The appropriate 7th character is to be added to each code from category S33.
A   initial encounter
D   subsequent encounter
S   sequela

☑x7ᵗʰ **S33.0** **Traumatic rupture of lumbar intervertebral disc**

EXCLUDES 1   rupture or displacement (nontraumatic) of lumbar intervertebral disc NOS (M51- with fifth character 6)

☑5ᵗʰ **S33.1** **Subluxation and dislocation of lumbar vertebra**

Code also any associated:
open wound of abdomen, lower back and pelvis (S31)
spinal cord injury (S24.0, S24.1-, S34.0-, S34.1-)

EXCLUDES 2   fracture of lumbar vertebrae (S32.0-)

☑6ᵗʰ **S33.10** **Subluxation and dislocation of unspecified lumbar vertebra**

☑7ᵗʰ **S33.100** **Subluxation of unspecified lumbar vertebra** ▽

☑7ᵗʰ **S33.101** **Dislocation of unspecified lumbar vertebra** ▽

☑6ᵗʰ **S33.11** **Subluxation and dislocation of L1/L2 lumbar vertebra**

☑7ᵗʰ **S33.110** **Subluxation of L1/L2 lumbar vertebra**

☑7ᵗʰ **S33.111** **Dislocation of L1/L2 lumbar vertebra**

☑6ᵗʰ **S33.12** **Subluxation and dislocation of L2/L3 lumbar vertebra**

☑7ᵗʰ **S33.120** **Subluxation of L2/L3 lumbar vertebra**

☑7ᵗʰ **S33.121** **Dislocation of L2/L3 lumbar vertebra**

☑6ᵗʰ **S33.13** **Subluxation and dislocation of L3/L4 lumbar vertebra**

☑7ᵗʰ **S33.130** **Subluxation of L3/L4 lumbar vertebra**

☑7ᵗʰ **S33.131** **Dislocation of L3/L4 lumbar vertebra**

☑6ᵗʰ **S33.14** **Subluxation and dislocation of L4/L5 lumbar vertebra**

☑7ᵗʰ **S33.140** **Subluxation of L4/L5 lumbar vertebra**

☑7ᵗʰ **S33.141** **Dislocation of L4/L5 lumbar vertebra**

☑x7ᵗʰ **S33.2** **Dislocation of sacroiliac and sacrococcygeal joint**

☑5ᵗʰ **S33.3** **Dislocation of other and unspecified parts of lumbar spine and pelvis**

☑x7ᵗʰ **S33.30** **Dislocation of unspecified parts of lumbar spine and pelvis** ▽

☑x7ᵗʰ **S33.39** **Dislocation of other parts of lumbar spine and pelvis**

☑x7ᵗʰ **S33.4** **Traumatic rupture of symphysis pubis**

☑x7ᵗʰ **S33.5** **Sprain of ligaments of lumbar spine**

☑x7ᵗʰ **S33.6** **Sprain of sacroiliac joint**

☑x7ᵗʰ **S33.8** **Sprain of other parts of lumbar spine and pelvis**

☑x7ᵗʰ **S33.9** **Sprain of unspecified parts of lumbar spine and pelvis** ▽

---

1   HCC with 7th character indicating initial encounter (A, B or C - specific to category).

☑ Additional Character Req   ☑x7ᵗʰ Placeholder Alert   Manifestation   HCC CMS-HCC Condition   ▽ Unspecified Code   ▶◀ Revised Text   ● New Code   ▲ Revised Code Title

✓4ᵗʰ **S34 Injury of lumbar and sacral spinal cord and nerves at abdomen, lower back and pelvis level**

> **NOTE** Code to highest level of lumbar cord injury.
> Injuries to the spinal cord (S34.0 and S34.1) refer to the cord level and not bone level injury, and can affect nerve roots at and below the level given.

Code also any associated:
   fracture of vertebra (S22.0-, S32.0-)
   open wound of abdomen, lower back and pelvis (S31.-)
   transient paralysis (R29.5)

> The appropriate 7th character is to be added to each code from category S34.
> A   initial encounter
> D   subsequent encounter
> S   sequela

✓5ᵗʰ **S34.0 Concussion and edema of lumbar and sacral spinal cord**

✓x7ᵗʰ **S34.01 Concussion and edema of lumbar spinal cord** HCC

✓x7ᵗʰ **S34.02 Concussion and edema of sacral spinal cord** HCC
   Concussion and edema of conus medullaris

✓5ᵗʰ **S34.1 Other and unspecified injury of lumbar and sacral spinal cord**

✓6ᵗʰ **S34.10 Unspecified injury to lumbar spinal cord**

✓7ᵗʰ **S34.101 Unspecified injury to L1 level of lumbar spinal cord** HCC ▽
   Unspecified injury to lumbar spinal cord level 1

✓7ᵗʰ **S34.102 Unspecified injury to L2 level of lumbar spinal cord** HCC ▽
   Unspecified injury to lumbar spinal cord level 2

✓7ᵗʰ **S34.103 Unspecified injury to L3 level of lumbar spinal cord** HCC ▽
   Unspecified injury to lumbar spinal cord level 3

✓7ᵗʰ **S34.104 Unspecified injury to L4 level of lumbar spinal cord** HCC ▽
   Unspecified injury to lumbar spinal cord level 4

✓7ᵗʰ **S34.105 Unspecified injury to L5 level of lumbar spinal cord** HCC ▽
   Unspecified injury to lumbar spinal cord level 5

✓7ᵗʰ **S34.109 Unspecified injury to unspecified level of lumbar spinal cord** HCC ▽

✓6ᵗʰ **S34.11 Complete lesion of lumbar spinal cord**

✓7ᵗʰ **S34.111 Complete lesion of L1 level of lumbar spinal cord** HCC
   Complete lesion of lumbar spinal cord level 1

✓7ᵗʰ **S34.112 Complete lesion of L2 level of lumbar spinal cord** HCC
   Complete lesion of lumbar spinal cord level 2

✓7ᵗʰ **S34.113 Complete lesion of L3 level of lumbar spinal cord** HCC
   Complete lesion of lumbar spinal cord level 3

✓7ᵗʰ **S34.114 Complete lesion of L4 level of lumbar spinal cord** HCC
   Complete lesion of lumbar spinal cord level 4

✓7ᵗʰ **S34.115 Complete lesion of L5 level of lumbar spinal cord** HCC
   Complete lesion of lumbar spinal cord level 5

✓7ᵗʰ **S34.119 Complete lesion of unspecified level of lumbar spinal cord** HCC ▽

✓6ᵗʰ **S34.12 Incomplete lesion of lumbar spinal cord**

✓7ᵗʰ **S34.121 Incomplete lesion of L1 level of lumbar spinal cord** HCC
   Incomplete lesion of lumbar spinal cord level 1

✓7ᵗʰ **S34.122 Incomplete lesion of L2 level of lumbar spinal cord** HCC
   Incomplete lesion of lumbar spinal cord level 2

✓7ᵗʰ **S34.123 Incomplete lesion of L3 level of lumbar spinal cord** HCC
   Incomplete lesion of lumbar spinal cord level 3

✓7ᵗʰ **S34.124 Incomplete lesion of L4 level of lumbar spinal cord** HCC
   Incomplete lesion of lumbar spinal cord level 4

✓7ᵗʰ **S34.125 Incomplete lesion of L5 level of lumbar spinal cord** HCC
   Incomplete lesion of lumbar spinal cord level 5

✓7ᵗʰ **S34.129 Incomplete lesion of unspecified level of lumbar spinal cord** HCC ▽

✓6ᵗʰ **S34.13 Other and unspecified injury to sacral spinal cord**
   Other injury to conus medullaris

✓7ᵗʰ **S34.131 Complete lesion of sacral spinal cord** HCC
   Complete lesion of conus medullaris

✓7ᵗʰ **S34.132 Incomplete lesion of sacral spinal cord** HCC
   Incomplete lesion of conus medullaris

✓7ᵗʰ **S34.139 Unspecified injury to sacral spinal cord** HCC ▽
   Unspecified injury of conus medullaris

✓5ᵗʰ **S34.2 Injury of nerve root of lumbar and sacral spine**

✓x7ᵗʰ **S34.21 Injury of nerve root of lumbar spine**

✓x7ᵗʰ **S34.22 Injury of nerve root of sacral spine**

¹ ✓x7ᵗʰ **S34.3 Injury of cauda equina** HCC

✓x7ᵗʰ **S34.4 Injury of lumbosacral plexus**

✓x7ᵗʰ **S34.5 Injury of lumbar, sacral and pelvic sympathetic nerves**
   Injury of celiac ganglion or plexus
   Injury of hypogastric plexus
   Injury of mesenteric plexus (inferior) (superior)
   Injury of splanchnic nerve

✓x7ᵗʰ **S34.6 Injury of peripheral nerve(s) at abdomen, lower back and pelvis level**

✓x7ᵗʰ **S34.8 Injury of other nerves at abdomen, lower back and pelvis level**

✓x7ᵗʰ **S34.9 Injury of unspecified nerves at abdomen, lower back and pelvis level** ▽

✓4ᵗʰ **S35 Injury of blood vessels at abdomen, lower back and pelvis level**
   Code also any associated open wound (S31.-)

> The appropriate 7th character is to be added to each code from category S35.
> A   initial encounter
> D   subsequent encounter
> S   sequela

✓5ᵗʰ **S35.0 Injury of abdominal aorta**
   EXCLUDES 1 *injury of aorta NOS (S25.0)*

✓x7ᵗʰ **S35.00 Unspecified injury of abdominal aorta** ▽

✓x7ᵗʰ **S35.01 Minor laceration of abdominal aorta**
   Incomplete transection of abdominal aorta
   Laceration of abdominal aorta NOS
   Superficial laceration of abdominal aorta

✓x7ᵗʰ **S35.02 Major laceration of abdominal aorta**
   Complete transection of abdominal aorta
   Traumatic rupture of abdominal aorta

✓x7ᵗʰ **S35.09 Other injury of abdominal aorta**

✓5ᵗʰ **S35.1 Injury of inferior vena cava**
   Injury of hepatic vein
   EXCLUDES 1 *injury of vena cava NOS (S25.2)*

✓x7ᵗʰ **S35.10 Unspecified injury of inferior vena cava** ▽

✓x7ᵗʰ **S35.11 Minor laceration of inferior vena cava**
   Incomplete transection of inferior vena cava
   Laceration of inferior vena cava NOS
   Superficial laceration of inferior vena cava

✓x7ᵗʰ **S35.12 Major laceration of inferior vena cava**
   Complete transection of inferior vena cava
   Traumatic rupture of inferior vena cava

✓x7ᵗʰ **S35.19 Other injury of inferior vena cava**

---

¹ HCC with 7th character indicating initial encounter (A, B or C - specific to category).

✓5ᵗʰ **S35.2 Injury of celiac or mesenteric artery and branches**

  ✓6ᵗʰ **S35.21 Injury of celiac artery**

    ✓7ᵗʰ **S35.211 Minor laceration of celiac artery**
         Incomplete transection of celiac artery
         Laceration of celiac artery NOS
         Superficial laceration of celiac artery

    ✓7ᵗʰ **S35.212 Major laceration of celiac artery**
         Complete transection of celiac artery
         Traumatic rupture of celiac artery

    ✓7ᵗʰ **S35.218 Other injury of celiac artery**

    ✓7ᵗʰ **S35.219 Unspecified injury of celiac artery** ▽

  ✓6ᵗʰ **S35.22 Injury of superior mesenteric artery**

    ✓7ᵗʰ **S35.221 Minor laceration of superior mesenteric artery**
         Incomplete transection of superior mesenteric artery
         Laceration of superior mesenteric artery NOS
         Superficial laceration of superior mesenteric artery

    ✓7ᵗʰ **S35.222 Major laceration of superior mesenteric artery**
         Complete transection of superior mesenteric artery
         Traumatic rupture of superior mesenteric artery

    ✓7ᵗʰ **S35.228 Other injury of superior mesenteric artery**

    ✓7ᵗʰ **S35.229 Unspecified injury of superior mesenteric artery** ▽

  ✓6ᵗʰ **S35.23 Injury of inferior mesenteric artery**

    ✓7ᵗʰ **S35.231 Minor laceration of inferior mesenteric artery**
         Incomplete transection of inferior mesenteric artery
         Laceration of inferior mesenteric artery NOS
         Superficial laceration of inferior mesenteric artery

    ✓7ᵗʰ **S35.232 Major laceration of inferior mesenteric artery**
         Complete transection of inferior mesenteric artery
         Traumatic rupture of inferior mesenteric artery

    ✓7ᵗʰ **S35.238 Other injury of inferior mesenteric artery**

    ✓7ᵗʰ **S35.239 Unspecified injury of inferior mesenteric artery** ▽

  ✓6ᵗʰ **S35.29 Injury of branches of celiac and mesenteric artery**
      Injury of gastric artery
      Injury of gastroduodenal artery
      Injury of hepatic artery
      Injury of splenic artery

    ✓7ᵗʰ **S35.291 Minor laceration of branches of celiac and mesenteric artery**
         Incomplete transection of branches of celiac and mesenteric artery
         Laceration of branches of celiac and mesenteric artery NOS
         Superficial laceration of branches of celiac and mesenteric artery

    ✓7ᵗʰ **S35.292 Major laceration of branches of celiac and mesenteric artery**
         Complete transection of branches of celiac and mesenteric artery
         Traumatic rupture of branches of celiac and mesenteric artery

    ✓7ᵗʰ **S35.298 Other injury of branches of celiac and mesenteric artery**

    ✓7ᵗʰ **S35.299 Unspecified injury of branches of celiac and mesenteric artery** ▽

✓5ᵗʰ **S35.3 Injury of portal or splenic vein and branches**

  ✓6ᵗʰ **S35.31 Injury of portal vein**

    ✓7ᵗʰ **S35.311 Laceration of portal vein**

    ✓7ᵗʰ **S35.318 Other specified injury of portal vein**

    ✓7ᵗʰ **S35.319 Unspecified injury of portal vein** ▽

  ✓6ᵗʰ **S35.32 Injury of splenic vein**

    ✓7ᵗʰ **S35.321 Laceration of splenic vein**

    ✓7ᵗʰ **S35.328 Other specified injury of splenic vein**

    ✓7ᵗʰ **S35.329 Unspecified injury of splenic vein** ▽

  ✓6ᵗʰ **S35.33 Injury of superior mesenteric vein**

    ✓7ᵗʰ **S35.331 Laceration of superior mesenteric vein**

    ✓7ᵗʰ **S35.338 Other specified injury of superior mesenteric vein**

    ✓7ᵗʰ **S35.339 Unspecified injury of superior mesenteric vein** ▽

  ✓6ᵗʰ **S35.34 Injury of inferior mesenteric vein**

    ✓7ᵗʰ **S35.341 Laceration of inferior mesenteric vein**

    ✓7ᵗʰ **S35.348 Other specified injury of inferior mesenteric vein**

    ✓7ᵗʰ **S35.349 Unspecified injury of inferior mesenteric vein** ▽

✓5ᵗʰ **S35.4 Injury of renal blood vessels**

  ✓6ᵗʰ **S35.40 Unspecified injury of renal blood vessel**

    ✓7ᵗʰ **S35.401 Unspecified injury of right renal artery** ▽

    ✓7ᵗʰ **S35.402 Unspecified injury of left renal artery** ▽

    ✓7ᵗʰ **S35.403 Unspecified injury of unspecified renal artery** ▽

    ✓7ᵗʰ **S35.404 Unspecified injury of right renal vein** ▽

    ✓7ᵗʰ **S35.405 Unspecified injury of left renal vein** ▽

    ✓7ᵗʰ **S35.406 Unspecified injury of unspecified renal vein** ▽

  ✓6ᵗʰ **S35.41 Laceration of renal blood vessel**

    ✓7ᵗʰ **S35.411 Laceration of right renal artery**

    ✓7ᵗʰ **S35.412 Laceration of left renal artery**

    ✓7ᵗʰ **S35.413 Laceration of unspecified renal artery** ▽

    ✓7ᵗʰ **S35.414 Laceration of right renal vein**

    ✓7ᵗʰ **S35.415 Laceration of left renal vein**

    ✓7ᵗʰ **S35.416 Laceration of unspecified renal vein** ▽

  ✓6ᵗʰ **S35.49 Other specified injury of renal blood vessel**

    ✓7ᵗʰ **S35.491 Other specified injury of right renal artery**

    ✓7ᵗʰ **S35.492 Other specified injury of left renal artery**

    ✓7ᵗʰ **S35.493 Other specified injury of unspecified renal artery** ▽

    ✓7ᵗʰ **S35.494 Other specified injury of right renal vein**

    ✓7ᵗʰ **S35.495 Other specified injury of left renal vein**

    ✓7ᵗʰ **S35.496 Other specified injury of unspecified renal vein** ▽

✓5ᵗʰ **S35.5 Injury of iliac blood vessels**

  ✓x7ᵗʰ **S35.50 Injury of unspecified iliac blood vessel(s)** ▽

  ✓6ᵗʰ **S35.51 Injury of iliac artery or vein**
      Injury of hypogastric artery or vein

    ✓7ᵗʰ **S35.511 Injury of right iliac artery**

    ✓7ᵗʰ **S35.512 Injury of left iliac artery**

    ✓7ᵗʰ **S35.513 Injury of unspecified iliac artery** ▽

    ✓7ᵗʰ **S35.514 Injury of right iliac vein**

    ✓7ᵗʰ **S35.515 Injury of left iliac vein**

    ✓7ᵗʰ **S35.516 Injury of unspecified iliac vein** ▽

  ✓6ᵗʰ **S35.53 Injury of uterine artery or vein**

    ✓7ᵗʰ **S35.531 Injury of right uterine artery** ♀

    ✓7ᵗʰ **S35.532 Injury of left uterine artery** ♀

    ✓7ᵗʰ **S35.533 Injury of unspecified uterine artery** ♀▽

    ✓7ᵗʰ **S35.534 Injury of right uterine vein** ♀

    ✓7ᵗʰ **S35.535 Injury of left uterine vein** ♀

    ✓7ᵗʰ **S35.536 Injury of unspecified uterine vein** ♀▽

  ✓x7ᵗʰ **S35.59 Injury of other iliac blood vessels**

✓5ᵗʰ **S35.8 Injury of other blood vessels at abdomen, lower back and pelvis level**
      Injury of ovarian artery or vein

  ✓6ᵗʰ **S35.8X Injury of other blood vessels at abdomen, lower back and pelvis level**

    ✓7ᵗʰ **S35.8X1 Laceration of other blood vessels at abdomen, lower back and pelvis level**

    ✓7ᵗʰ **S35.8X8 Other specified injury of other blood vessels at abdomen, lower back and pelvis level**

    ✓7ᵗʰ **S35.8X9 Unspecified injury of other blood vessels at abdomen, lower back and pelvis level** ▽

☑ Additional Character Req   ✓x7ᵗʰ Placeholder Alert   Manifestation   HCC CMS-HCC Condition   ▽ Unspecified Code   ►◄ Revised Text   ● New Code   ▲ Revised Code Title

ICD-10-CM 2018   949

✓5ᵗʰ **S35.9 Injury of unspecified blood vessel at abdomen, lower back and pelvis level**

    ✓x7ᵗʰ **S35.90 Unspecified injury of unspecified blood vessel at abdomen, lower back and pelvis level** ▽

    ✓x7ᵗʰ **S35.91 Laceration of unspecified blood vessel at abdomen, lower back and pelvis level** ▽

    ✓x7ᵗʰ **S35.99 Other specified injury of unspecified blood vessel at abdomen, lower back and pelvis level** ▽

✓4ᵗʰ **S36 Injury of intra-abdominal organs**

    Code also any associated open wound (S31.-)

> The appropriate 7th character is to be added to each code from category S36.
> A   initial encounter
> D   subsequent encounter
> S   sequela

✓5ᵗʰ **S36.0 Injury of spleen**
    AHA: 2015, 2Q, 36; 2015, 1Q, 10

    ✓x7ᵗʰ **S36.00 Unspecified injury of spleen** ▽

    ✓6ᵗʰ **S36.02 Contusion of spleen**

       ✓7ᵗʰ **S36.020 Minor contusion of spleen**
         Contusion of spleen less than 2 cm

       ✓7ᵗʰ **S36.021 Major contusion of spleen**
         Contusion of spleen greater than 2 cm

       ✓7ᵗʰ **S36.029 Unspecified contusion of spleen** ▽

    ✓6ᵗʰ **S36.03 Laceration of spleen**

       ✓7ᵗʰ **S36.030 Superficial (capsular) laceration of spleen**
         Laceration of spleen less than 1cm
         Minor laceration of spleen

       ✓7ᵗʰ **S36.031 Moderate laceration of spleen**
         Laceration of spleen 1 to 3 cm

       ✓7ᵗʰ **S36.032 Major laceration of spleen**
         Avulsion of spleen
         Laceration of spleen greater than 3 cm
         Massive laceration of spleen
         Multiple moderate lacerations of spleen
         Stellate laceration of spleen

       ✓7ᵗʰ **S36.039 Unspecified laceration of spleen** ▽

    ✓x7ᵗʰ **S36.09 Other injury of spleen**

✓5ᵗʰ **S36.1 Injury of liver and gallbladder and bile duct**

    ✓6ᵗʰ **S36.11 Injury of liver**

       ✓7ᵗʰ **S36.112 Contusion of liver**

       ✓7ᵗʰ **S36.113 Laceration of liver, unspecified degree** ▽

       ✓7ᵗʰ **S36.114 Minor laceration of liver**
         Laceration involving capsule only, or, without significant involvement of hepatic parenchyma [i.e., less than 1cm deep]

       ✓7ᵗʰ **S36.115 Moderate laceration of liver**
         Laceration involving parenchyma but without major disruption of parenchyma [i.e., less than 10 cm long and less than 3 cm deep]

       ✓7ᵗʰ **S36.116 Major laceration of liver**
         Laceration with significant disruption of hepatic parenchyma [i.e., greater than 10 cm long and 3 cm deep]
         Multiple moderate lacerations, with or without hematoma
         Stellate laceration of liver

       ✓7ᵗʰ **S36.118 Other injury of liver**

       ✓7ᵗʰ **S36.119 Unspecified injury of liver** ▽

    ✓6ᵗʰ **S36.12 Injury of gallbladder**

       ✓7ᵗʰ **S36.122 Contusion of gallbladder**

       ✓7ᵗʰ **S36.123 Laceration of gallbladder**

       ✓7ᵗʰ **S36.128 Other injury of gallbladder**

       ✓7ᵗʰ **S36.129 Unspecified injury of gallbladder** ▽

    ✓x7ᵗʰ **S36.13 Injury of bile duct**

✓5ᵗʰ **S36.2 Injury of pancreas**

    ✓6ᵗʰ **S36.20 Unspecified injury of pancreas**

       ✓7ᵗʰ **S36.200 Unspecified injury of head of pancreas** ▽

       ✓7ᵗʰ **S36.201 Unspecified injury of body of pancreas** ▽

       ✓7ᵗʰ **S36.202 Unspecified injury of tail of pancreas** ▽

       ✓7ᵗʰ **S36.209 Unspecified injury of unspecified part of pancreas** ▽

    ✓6ᵗʰ **S36.22 Contusion of pancreas**

       ✓7ᵗʰ **S36.220 Contusion of head of pancreas**

       ✓7ᵗʰ **S36.221 Contusion of body of pancreas**

       ✓7ᵗʰ **S36.222 Contusion of tail of pancreas**

       ✓7ᵗʰ **S36.229 Contusion of unspecified part of pancreas** ▽

    ✓6ᵗʰ **S36.23 Laceration of pancreas, unspecified degree**

       ✓7ᵗʰ **S36.230 Laceration of head of pancreas, unspecified degree** ▽

       ✓7ᵗʰ **S36.231 Laceration of body of pancreas, unspecified degree** ▽

       ✓7ᵗʰ **S36.232 Laceration of tail of pancreas, unspecified degree** ▽

       ✓7ᵗʰ **S36.239 Laceration of unspecified part of pancreas, unspecified degree** ▽

    ✓6ᵗʰ **S36.24 Minor laceration of pancreas**

       ✓7ᵗʰ **S36.240 Minor laceration of head of pancreas**

       ✓7ᵗʰ **S36.241 Minor laceration of body of pancreas**

       ✓7ᵗʰ **S36.242 Minor laceration of tail of pancreas**

       ✓7ᵗʰ **S36.249 Minor laceration of unspecified part of pancreas** ▽

    ✓6ᵗʰ **S36.25 Moderate laceration of pancreas**

       ✓7ᵗʰ **S36.250 Moderate laceration of head of pancreas**

       ✓7ᵗʰ **S36.251 Moderate laceration of body of pancreas**

       ✓7ᵗʰ **S36.252 Moderate laceration of tail of pancreas**

       ✓7ᵗʰ **S36.259 Moderate laceration of unspecified part of pancreas** ▽

    ✓6ᵗʰ **S36.26 Major laceration of pancreas**

       ✓7ᵗʰ **S36.260 Major laceration of head of pancreas**

       ✓7ᵗʰ **S36.261 Major laceration of body of pancreas**

       ✓7ᵗʰ **S36.262 Major laceration of tail of pancreas**

       ✓7ᵗʰ **S36.269 Major laceration of unspecified part of pancreas** ▽

    ✓6ᵗʰ **S36.29 Other injury of pancreas**

       ✓7ᵗʰ **S36.290 Other injury of head of pancreas**

       ✓7ᵗʰ **S36.291 Other injury of body of pancreas**

       ✓7ᵗʰ **S36.292 Other injury of tail of pancreas**

       ✓7ᵗʰ **S36.299 Other injury of unspecified part of pancreas** ▽

✓5ᵗʰ **S36.3 Injury of stomach**

    ✓x7ᵗʰ **S36.30 Unspecified injury of stomach** ▽

    ✓x7ᵗʰ **S36.32 Contusion of stomach**

    ✓x7ᵗʰ **S36.33 Laceration of stomach**

    ✓x7ᵗʰ **S36.39 Other injury of stomach**

✓5ᵗʰ **S36.4 Injury of small intestine**

    ✓6ᵗʰ **S36.40 Unspecified injury of small intestine**

       ✓7ᵗʰ **S36.400 Unspecified injury of duodenum** ▽

       ✓7ᵗʰ **S36.408 Unspecified injury of other part of small intestine** ▽

       ✓7ᵗʰ **S36.409 Unspecified injury of unspecified part of small intestine** ▽

    ✓6ᵗʰ **S36.41 Primary blast injury of small intestine**
       Blast injury of small intestine NOS

       ✓7ᵗʰ **S36.410 Primary blast injury of duodenum**

       ✓7ᵗʰ **S36.418 Primary blast injury of other part of small intestine**

       ✓7ᵗʰ **S36.419 Primary blast injury of unspecified part of small intestine** ▽

    ✓6ᵗʰ **S36.42 Contusion of small intestine**

       ✓7ᵗʰ **S36.420 Contusion of duodenum**

       ✓7ᵗʰ **S36.428 Contusion of other part of small intestine**

       ✓7ᵗʰ **S36.429 Contusion of unspecified part of small intestine** ▽

    ✓6ᵗʰ **S36.43 Laceration of small intestine**

       ✓7ᵗʰ **S36.430 Laceration of duodenum**

       ✓7ᵗʰ **S36.438 Laceration of other part of small intestine**

       ✓7ᵗʰ **S36.439 Laceration of unspecified part of small intestine** ▽

EXCLUDES 1 Not coded here   EXCLUDES 2 Not included here   N Newborn Age: 0   P Pediatric Age: 0-17   M Maternity Age: 12-55   A Adult Age: 15-124

√6ᵗʰ **S36.49 Other injury of small intestine**

  √7ᵗʰ **S36.490 Other injury of** duodenum

  √7ᵗʰ **S36.498 Other injury of other part of small intestine**

  √7ᵗʰ **S36.499 Other injury of unspecified part of small intestine** ▽

√5ᵗʰ **S36.5 Injury of** colon

  EXCLUDES 2   *injury of rectum (S36.6-)*

  √6ᵗʰ **S36.50 Unspecified injury of colon**

    √7ᵗʰ **S36.500 Unspecified injury of** ascending [right] colon ▽

    √7ᵗʰ **S36.501 Unspecified injury of** transverse colon ▽

    √7ᵗʰ **S36.502 Unspecified injury of** descending [left] colon ▽

    √7ᵗʰ **S36.503 Unspecified injury of** sigmoid colon ▽

    √7ᵗʰ **S36.508 Unspecified injury of other part of colon** ▽

    √7ᵗʰ **S36.509 Unspecified injury of unspecified part of colon** ▽

  √6ᵗʰ **S36.51 Primary blast injury of colon**
    Blast injury of colon NOS

    √7ᵗʰ **S36.510 Primary blast injury of** ascending [right] colon

    √7ᵗʰ **S36.511 Primary blast injury of** transverse colon

    √7ᵗʰ **S36.512 Primary blast injury of** descending [left] colon

    √7ᵗʰ **S36.513 Primary blast injury of** sigmoid colon

    √7ᵗʰ **S36.518 Primary blast injury of other part of colon**

    √7ᵗʰ **S36.519 Primary blast injury of unspecified part of colon** ▽

  √6ᵗʰ **S36.52 Contusion of colon**

    √7ᵗʰ **S36.520 Contusion of** ascending [right] colon

    √7ᵗʰ **S36.521 Contusion of** transverse colon

    √7ᵗʰ **S36.522 Contusion of** descending [left] colon

    √7ᵗʰ **S36.523 Contusion of** sigmoid colon

    √7ᵗʰ **S36.528 Contusion of other part of colon**

    √7ᵗʰ **S36.529 Contusion of unspecified part of colon** ▽

  √6ᵗʰ **S36.53 Laceration of colon**

    √7ᵗʰ **S36.530 Laceration of** ascending [right] colon

    √7ᵗʰ **S36.531 Laceration of** transverse colon

    √7ᵗʰ **S36.532 Laceration of** descending [left] colon

    √7ᵗʰ **S36.533 Laceration of** sigmoid colon

    √7ᵗʰ **S36.538 Laceration of other part of colon**

    √7ᵗʰ **S36.539 Laceration of unspecified part of colon** ▽

  √6ᵗʰ **S36.59 Other injury of colon**
    Secondary blast injury of colon

    √7ᵗʰ **S36.590 Other injury of** ascending [right] colon

    √7ᵗʰ **S36.591 Other injury of** transverse colon

    √7ᵗʰ **S36.592 Other injury of** descending [left] colon

    √7ᵗʰ **S36.593 Other injury of** sigmoid colon

    √7ᵗʰ **S36.598 Other injury of other part of colon**

    √7ᵗʰ **S36.599 Other injury of unspecified part of colon** ▽

√5ᵗʰ **S36.6 Injury of** rectum

  √x7ᵗʰ **S36.60 Unspecified injury of rectum** ▽

  √x7ᵗʰ **S36.61 Primary blast injury of rectum**
    Blast injury of rectum NOS

  √x7ᵗʰ **S36.62 Contusion of rectum**

  √x7ᵗʰ **S36.63 Laceration of rectum**

  √x7ᵗʰ **S36.69 Other injury of rectum**
    Secondary blast injury of rectum

√5ᵗʰ **S36.8 Injury of other intra-abdominal organs**

  √x7ᵗʰ **S36.81 Injury of** peritoneum

  √6ᵗʰ **S36.89 Injury of other intra-abdominal organs**
    Injury of retroperitoneum

    √7ᵗʰ **S36.892 Contusion of other intra-abdominal organs**

    √7ᵗʰ **S36.893 Laceration of other intra-abdominal organs**

    √7ᵗʰ **S36.898 Other injury of other intra-abdominal organs**

    √7ᵗʰ **S36.899 Unspecified injury of other intra-abdominal organs** ▽

√5ᵗʰ **S36.9 Injury of unspecified intra-abdominal organ**

  √x7ᵗʰ **S36.90 Unspecified injury of unspecified intra-abdominal organ** ▽

  √x7ᵗʰ **S36.92 Contusion of unspecified intra-abdominal organ** ▽

  √x7ᵗʰ **S36.93 Laceration of unspecified intra-abdominal organ** ▽

  √x7ᵗʰ **S36.99 Other injury of unspecified intra-abdominal organ** ▽

√4ᵗʰ **S37 Injury of urinary and pelvic organs**

  Code also any associated open wound (S31.-)

  EXCLUDES 1   *obstetric trauma to pelvic organs (O71.-)*

  EXCLUDES 2   *injury of peritoneum (S36.81)*
    injury of retroperitoneum (S36.89-)

  The appropriate 7th character is to be added to each code from category S37.
  A   initial encounter
  D   subsequent encounter
  S   sequela

√5ᵗʰ **S37.0 Injury of kidney**

  EXCLUDES 2   *acute kidney injury (nontraumatic) (N17.9)*

  √6ᵗʰ **S37.00 Unspecified injury of kidney**

    √x7ᵗʰ **S37.001 Unspecified injury of** right kidney ▽

    √x7ᵗʰ **S37.002 Unspecified injury of** left kidney ▽

    √x7ᵗʰ **S37.009 Unspecified injury of unspecified kidney** ▽

  √6ᵗʰ **S37.01 Minor contusion of kidney**
    Contusion of kidney less than 2 cm
    Contusion of kidney NOS

    √7ᵗʰ **S37.011 Minor contusion of** right kidney

    √7ᵗʰ **S37.012 Minor contusion of** left kidney

    √7ᵗʰ **S37.019 Minor contusion of unspecified kidney** ▽

  √6ᵗʰ **S37.02 Major contusion of kidney**
    Contusion of kidney greater than 2 cm

    √7ᵗʰ **S37.021 Major contusion of** right kidney

    √7ᵗʰ **S37.022 Major contusion of** left kidney

    √7ᵗʰ **S37.029 Major contusion of unspecified kidney** ▽

  √6ᵗʰ **S37.03 Laceration of kidney, unspecified degree**

    √7ᵗʰ **S37.031 Laceration of** right kidney, unspecified degree ▽

    √7ᵗʰ **S37.032 Laceration of** left kidney, unspecified degree ▽

    √7ᵗʰ **S37.039 Laceration of unspecified kidney, unspecified degree** ▽

  √6ᵗʰ **S37.04 Minor laceration of kidney**
    Laceration of kidney less than 1 cm

    √7ᵗʰ **S37.041 Minor laceration of** right kidney

    √7ᵗʰ **S37.042 Minor laceration of** left kidney

    √7ᵗʰ **S37.049 Minor laceration of unspecified kidney** ▽

  √6ᵗʰ **S37.05 Moderate laceration of kidney**
    Laceration of kidney 1 to 3 cm

    √7ᵗʰ **S37.051 Moderate laceration of** right kidney

    √7ᵗʰ **S37.052 Moderate laceration of** left kidney

    √7ᵗʰ **S37.059 Moderate laceration of unspecified kidney** ▽

  √6ᵗʰ **S37.06 Major laceration of kidney**
    Avulsion of kidney
    Laceration of kidney greater than 3 cm
    Massive laceration of kidney
    Multiple moderate lacerations of kidney
    Stellate laceration of kidney

    √7ᵗʰ **S37.061 Major laceration of** right kidney

    √7ᵗʰ **S37.062 Major laceration of** left kidney

    √7ᵗʰ **S37.069 Major laceration of unspecified kidney** ▽

  √6ᵗʰ **S37.09 Other injury of kidney**

    √7ᵗʰ **S37.091 Other injury of** right kidney

    √7ᵗʰ **S37.092 Other injury of** left kidney

    √7ᵗʰ **S37.099 Other injury of unspecified kidney** ▽

√5ᵗʰ **S37.1 Injury of ureter**

  √x7ᵗʰ **S37.10 Unspecified injury of ureter** ▽

  √x7ᵗʰ **S37.12 Contusion of ureter**

  √x7ᵗʰ **S37.13 Laceration of ureter**

☑ Additional Character Req   √x7ᵗʰ Placeholder Alert   Manifestation   HCC CMS-HCC Condition   ▽ Unspecified Code   ►◄ Revised Text   ● New Code   ▲ Revised Code Title

√x7ᵗʰ **S37.19** **Other injury of ureter**

√5ᵗʰ **S37.2** **Injury of bladder**

√x7ᵗʰ **S37.20** **Unspecified injury of bladder** ▽

√x7ᵗʰ **S37.22** **Contusion of bladder**

√x7ᵗʰ **S37.23** **Laceration of bladder**

√x7ᵗʰ **S37.29** **Other injury of bladder**

√5ᵗʰ **S37.3** **Injury of urethra**

√x7ᵗʰ **S37.30** **Unspecified injury of urethra** ▽

√x7ᵗʰ **S37.32** **Contusion of urethra**

√x7ᵗʰ **S37.33** **Laceration of urethra**

√x7ᵗʰ **S37.39** **Other injury of urethra**

√5ᵗʰ **S37.4** **Injury of ovary**

√6ᵗʰ **S37.40** **Unspecified injury of ovary**

√7ᵗʰ **S37.401** **Unspecified injury of ovary, unilateral** ♀▽

√7ᵗʰ **S37.402** **Unspecified injury of ovary, bilateral** ♀▽

√7ᵗʰ **S37.409** **Unspecified injury of ovary, unspecified** ♀▽

√6ᵗʰ **S37.42** **Contusion of ovary**

√7ᵗʰ **S37.421** **Contusion of ovary, unilateral** ♀

√7ᵗʰ **S37.422** **Contusion of ovary, bilateral** ♀

√7ᵗʰ **S37.429** **Contusion of ovary, unspecified** ♀▽

√6ᵗʰ **S37.43** **Laceration of ovary**

√7ᵗʰ **S37.431** **Laceration of ovary, unilateral** ♀

√7ᵗʰ **S37.432** **Laceration of ovary, bilateral** ♀

√7ᵗʰ **S37.439** **Laceration of ovary, unspecified** ♀▽

√6ᵗʰ **S37.49** **Other injury of ovary**

√7ᵗʰ **S37.491** **Other injury of ovary, unilateral** ♀

√7ᵗʰ **S37.492** **Other injury of ovary, bilateral** ♀

√7ᵗʰ **S37.499** **Other injury of ovary, unspecified** ♀▽

√5ᵗʰ **S37.5** **Injury of fallopian tube**

√6ᵗʰ **S37.50** **Unspecified injury of fallopian tube**

√7ᵗʰ **S37.501** **Unspecified injury of fallopian tube, unilateral** ♀▽

√7ᵗʰ **S37.502** **Unspecified injury of fallopian tube, bilateral** ♀▽

√7ᵗʰ **S37.509** **Unspecified injury of fallopian tube, unspecified** ♀▽

√6ᵗʰ **S37.51** **Primary blast injury of fallopian tube**
Blast injury of fallopian tube NOS

√7ᵗʰ **S37.511** **Primary blast injury of fallopian tube, unilateral** ♀

√7ᵗʰ **S37.512** **Primary blast injury of fallopian tube, bilateral** ♀

√7ᵗʰ **S37.519** **Primary blast injury of fallopian tube, unspecified** ♀▽

√6ᵗʰ **S37.52** **Contusion of fallopian tube**

√7ᵗʰ **S37.521** **Contusion of fallopian tube, unilateral** ♀

√7ᵗʰ **S37.522** **Contusion of fallopian tube, bilateral** ♀

√7ᵗʰ **S37.529** **Contusion of fallopian tube, unspecified** ♀▽

√6ᵗʰ **S37.53** **Laceration of fallopian tube**

√7ᵗʰ **S37.531** **Laceration of fallopian tube, unilateral** ♀

√7ᵗʰ **S37.532** **Laceration of fallopian tube, bilateral** ♀

√7ᵗʰ **S37.539** **Laceration of fallopian tube, unspecified** ♀▽

√6ᵗʰ **S37.59** **Other injury of fallopian tube**
Secondary blast injury of fallopian tube

√7ᵗʰ **S37.591** **Other injury of fallopian tube, unilateral** ♀

√7ᵗʰ **S37.592** **Other injury of fallopian tube, bilateral** ♀

√7ᵗʰ **S37.599** **Other injury of fallopian tube, unspecified** ♀▽

√5ᵗʰ **S37.6** **Injury of uterus**
EXCLUDES 1 *injury to gravid uterus (O9A.2-)*
injury to uterus during delivery (O71.-)

√x7ᵗʰ **S37.60** **Unspecified injury of uterus** ♀▽

√x7ᵗʰ **S37.62** **Contusion of uterus** ♀

√x7ᵗʰ **S37.63** **Laceration of uterus** ♀

√x7ᵗʰ **S37.69** **Other injury of uterus** ♀

√5ᵗʰ **S37.8** **Injury of other urinary and pelvic organs**

√6ᵗʰ **S37.81** **Injury of adrenal gland**

√7ᵗʰ **S37.812** **Contusion of adrenal gland**

√7ᵗʰ **S37.813** **Laceration of adrenal gland**

√7ᵗʰ **S37.818** **Other injury of adrenal gland**

√7ᵗʰ **S37.819** **Unspecified injury of adrenal gland** ▽

√6ᵗʰ **S37.82** **Injury of prostate**

√7ᵗʰ **S37.822** **Contusion of prostate** ♂

√7ᵗʰ **S37.823** **Laceration of prostate** ♂

√7ᵗʰ **S37.828** **Other injury of prostate** ♂

√7ᵗʰ **S37.829** **Unspecified injury of prostate** ♂▽

√6ᵗʰ **S37.89** **Injury of other urinary and pelvic organ**

√7ᵗʰ **S37.892** **Contusion of other urinary and pelvic organ**

√7ᵗʰ **S37.893** **Laceration of other urinary and pelvic organ**

√7ᵗʰ **S37.898** **Other injury of other urinary and pelvic organ**

√7ᵗʰ **S37.899** **Unspecified injury of other urinary and pelvic organ** ▽

√5ᵗʰ **S37.9** **Injury of unspecified urinary and pelvic organ**

√x7ᵗʰ **S37.90** **Unspecified injury of unspecified urinary and pelvic organ** ▽

√x7ᵗʰ **S37.92** **Contusion of unspecified urinary and pelvic organ** ▽

√x7ᵗʰ **S37.93** **Laceration of unspecified urinary and pelvic organ** ▽

√x7ᵗʰ **S37.99** **Other injury of unspecified urinary and pelvic organ** ▽

√4ᵗʰ **S38** **Crushing injury and traumatic amputation of abdomen, lower back, pelvis and external genitals**
An amputation not identified as partial or complete should be coded to complete.

The appropriate 7th character is to be added to each code from category S38.
A   initial encounter
D   subsequent encounter
S   sequela

√5ᵗʰ **S38.0** **Crushing injury of external genital organs**
Use additional code for any associated injuries

√6ᵗʰ **S38.00** **Crushing injury of unspecified external genital organs**

√7ᵗʰ **S38.001** **Crushing injury of unspecified external genital organs, male** ♂▽

√7ᵗʰ **S38.002** **Crushing injury of unspecified external genital organs, female** ♀▽

√x7ᵗʰ **S38.01** **Crushing injury of penis** ♂

√x7ᵗʰ **S38.02** **Crushing injury of scrotum and testis** ♂

√x7ᵗʰ **S38.03** **Crushing injury of vulva** ♀

√x7ᵗʰ **S38.1** **Crushing injury of abdomen, lower back, and pelvis**
Use additional code for all associated injuries, such as:
fracture of thoracic or lumbar spine and pelvis (S22.0-, S32-)
injury to intra-abdominal organs (S36.-)
injury to urinary and pelvic organs (S37.-)
open wound of abdominal wall (S31.-)
spinal cord injury (S34.0, S34.1-)
EXCLUDES 2 *crushing injury of external genital organs (S38.0-)*

√5ᵗʰ **S38.2** **Traumatic amputation of external genital organs**

√6ᵗʰ **S38.21** **Traumatic amputation of female external genital organs**
Traumatic amputation of clitoris
Traumatic amputation of labium (majus) (minus)
Traumatic amputation of vulva

√7ᵗʰ **S38.211** **Complete traumatic amputation of female external genital organs** ♀

√7ᵗʰ **S38.212** **Partial traumatic amputation of female external genital organs** ♀

√6ᵗʰ **S38.22** **Traumatic amputation of penis**

√7ᵗʰ **S38.221** **Complete traumatic amputation of penis** ♂

√7ᵗʰ **S38.222** **Partial traumatic amputation of penis** ♂

✓6ᵗʰ **S38.23**   **Traumatic amputation of** scrotum and testis

    ✓7ᵗʰ **S38.231**   **Complete traumatic amputation of**   ♂
       scrotum and testis

    ✓7ᵗʰ **S38.232**   **Partial traumatic amputation of**   ♂
       scrotum and testis

✓x7ᵗʰ **S38.3**   **Transection (partial) of abdomen**

✓4ᵗʰ **S39**   **Other and unspecified injuries of abdomen, lower back, pelvis and external genitals**

  Code also any associated open wound (S31.-)

  EXCLUDES 2   *sprain of joints and ligaments of lumbar spine and pelvis (S33.-)*

  The appropriate 7th character is to be added to each code from category S39.
  A   initial encounter
  D   subsequent encounter
  S   sequela

✓5ᵗʰ **S39.0**   **Injury of muscle, fascia and tendon of abdomen, lower back and pelvis**

  ✓6ᵗʰ **S39.00**   **Unspecified injury of muscle, fascia and tendon of abdomen, lower back and pelvis**

    ✓7ᵗʰ **S39.001**   **Unspecified injury of muscle, fascia**   ▽
       and tendon of abdomen

    ✓7ᵗʰ **S39.002**   **Unspecified injury of muscle, fascia**   ▽
       and tendon of lower back

    ✓7ᵗʰ **S39.003**   **Unspecified injury of muscle, fascia**   ▽
       and tendon of pelvis

  ✓6ᵗʰ **S39.01**   **Strain** of muscle, fascia and tendon of abdomen, lower back and pelvis

    ✓7ᵗʰ **S39.011**   **Strain of muscle, fascia and tendon of**
       abdomen

    ✓7ᵗʰ **S39.012**   **Strain of muscle, fascia and tendon of**
       lower back

    ✓7ᵗʰ **S39.013**   **Strain of muscle, fascia and tendon of**
       pelvis

  ✓6ᵗʰ **S39.02**   **Laceration** of muscle, fascia and tendon of abdomen, lower back and pelvis

    ✓7ᵗʰ **S39.021**   **Laceration of muscle, fascia and tendon of**
       abdomen

    ✓7ᵗʰ **S39.022**   **Laceration of muscle, fascia and tendon of**
       lower back

    ✓7ᵗʰ **S39.023**   **Laceration of muscle, fascia and tendon of**
       pelvis

  ✓6ᵗʰ **S39.09**   **Other injury of muscle, fascia and tendon of abdomen, lower back and pelvis**

    ✓7ᵗʰ **S39.091**   **Other injury of muscle, fascia and tendon of** abdomen

    ✓7ᵗʰ **S39.092**   **Other injury of muscle, fascia and tendon of** lower back

    ✓7ᵗʰ **S39.093**   **Other injury of muscle, fascia and tendon of** pelvis

✓5ᵗʰ **S39.8**   **Other specified injuries of abdomen, lower back, pelvis and external genitals**

  ✓x7ᵗʰ **S39.81**   **Other specified injuries of** abdomen

  ✓x7ᵗʰ **S39.82**   **Other specified injuries of** lower back

  ✓x7ᵗʰ **S39.83**   **Other specified injuries of** pelvis

  ✓6ᵗʰ **S39.84**   **Other specified injuries of** external genitals

    ✓7ᵗʰ **S39.840**   **Fracture of** corpus cavernosum penis   ♂

    ✓7ᵗʰ **S39.848**   **Other specified injuries of external genitals**

✓5ᵗʰ **S39.9**   **Unspecified injury of abdomen, lower back, pelvis and external genitals**

  ✓x7ᵗʰ **S39.91**   **Unspecified injury of** abdomen   ▽

  ✓x7ᵗʰ **S39.92**   **Unspecified injury of** lower back   ▽

  ✓x7ᵗʰ **S39.93**   **Unspecified injury of** pelvis   ▽

  ✓x7ᵗʰ **S39.94**   **Unspecified injury of** external genitals   ▽

Injuries to the shoulder and upper arm (S40-S49)

INCLUDES   injuries of axilla
        injuries of scapular region

EXCLUDES 2   *burns and corrosions (T20-T32)*
      frostbite (T33-T34)
      injuries of elbow (S50-S59)
      insect bite or sting, venomous (T63.4)

✓4ᵗʰ **S40**   **Superficial injury of shoulder and upper arm**

  The appropriate 7th character is to be added to each code from category S40.
  A   initial encounter
  D   subsequent encounter
  S   sequela

✓5ᵗʰ **S40.0**   **Contusion of shoulder and upper arm**

  ✓6ᵗʰ **S40.01**   **Contusion of** shoulder

    ✓7ᵗʰ **S40.011**   **Contusion of** right **shoulder**

    ✓7ᵗʰ **S40.012**   **Contusion of** left **shoulder**

    ✓7ᵗʰ **S40.019**   **Contusion of unspecified shoulder**   ▽

  ✓6ᵗʰ **S40.02**   **Contusion of** upper arm

    ✓7ᵗʰ **S40.021**   **Contusion of** right **upper arm**

    ✓7ᵗʰ **S40.022**   **Contusion of** left **upper arm**

    ✓7ᵗʰ **S40.029**   **Contusion of unspecified upper arm**   ▽

✓5ᵗʰ **S40.2**   **Other superficial injuries of** shoulder

  ✓6ᵗʰ **S40.21**   **Abrasion** of shoulder

    ✓7ᵗʰ **S40.211**   **Abrasion of** right **shoulder**

    ✓7ᵗʰ **S40.212**   **Abrasion of** left **shoulder**

    ✓7ᵗʰ **S40.219**   **Abrasion of unspecified shoulder**   ▽

  ✓6ᵗʰ **S40.22**   **Blister (nonthermal) of** shoulder

    ✓7ᵗʰ **S40.221**   **Blister (nonthermal) of** right **shoulder**

    ✓7ᵗʰ **S40.222**   **Blister (nonthermal) of** left **shoulder**

    ✓7ᵗʰ **S40.229**   **Blister (nonthermal) of unspecified**   ▽
       shoulder

  ✓6ᵗʰ **S40.24**   **External constriction** of shoulder

    ✓7ᵗʰ **S40.241**   **External constriction of** right **shoulder**

    ✓7ᵗʰ **S40.242**   **External constriction of** left **shoulder**

    ✓7ᵗʰ **S40.249**   **External constriction of unspecified**   ▽
       shoulder

  ✓6ᵗʰ **S40.25**   **Superficial foreign body of shoulder**
    Splinter in the shoulder

    ✓7ᵗʰ **S40.251**   **Superficial foreign body of** right **shoulder**

    ✓7ᵗʰ **S40.252**   **Superficial foreign body of** left **shoulder**

    ✓7ᵗʰ **S40.259**   **Superficial foreign body of**   ▽
       unspecified shoulder

  ✓6ᵗʰ **S40.26**   **Insect bite (nonvenomous) of** shoulder

    ✓7ᵗʰ **S40.261**   **Insect bite (nonvenomous) of** right
       shoulder

    ✓7ᵗʰ **S40.262**   **Insect bite (nonvenomous) of** left **shoulder**

    ✓7ᵗʰ **S40.269**   **Insect bite (nonvenomous) of**   ▽
       unspecified shoulder

  ✓6ᵗʰ **S40.27**   **Other superficial bite of** shoulder
    EXCLUDES 1   *open bite of shoulder (S41.05)*

    ✓7ᵗʰ **S40.271**   **Other superficial bite of** right **shoulder**

    ✓7ᵗʰ **S40.272**   **Other superficial bite of** left **shoulder**

    ✓7ᵗʰ **S40.279**   **Other superficial bite of unspecified**   ▽
       shoulder

✓5ᵗʰ **S40.8**   **Other superficial injuries of** upper arm

  ✓6ᵗʰ **S40.81**   **Abrasion** of upper arm

    ✓7ᵗʰ **S40.811**   **Abrasion of** right **upper arm**

    ✓7ᵗʰ **S40.812**   **Abrasion of** left **upper arm**

    ✓7ᵗʰ **S40.819**   **Abrasion of unspecified upper arm**   ▽

  ✓6ᵗʰ **S40.82**   **Blister (nonthermal) of** upper arm

    ✓7ᵗʰ **S40.821**   **Blister (nonthermal) of** right **upper arm**

    ✓7ᵗʰ **S40.822**   **Blister (nonthermal) of** left **upper arm**

    ✓7ᵗʰ **S40.829**   **Blister (nonthermal) of unspecified**   ▽
       upper arm

  ✓6ᵗʰ **S40.84**   **External constriction** of upper arm

    ✓7ᵗʰ **S40.841**   **External constriction of** right **upper arm**

    ✓7ᵗʰ **S40.842**   **External constriction of** left **upper arm**

    ✓7ᵗʰ **S40.849**   **External constriction of unspecified**   ▽
       upper arm

☑ Additional Character Req   ✓x7ᵗʰ Placeholder Alert   Manifestation   ᴴᶜᶜ CMS-HCC Condition   ▽ Unspecified Code   ►◄ Revised Text   ● New Code   ▲ Revised Code Title

ICD-10-CM 2018   **953**

√6ᵗʰ S40.85 Superficial foreign body of upper arm
Splinter in the upper arm

- **√7ᵗʰ S40.851 Superficial foreign body of right upper arm**
- **√7ᵗʰ S40.852 Superficial foreign body of left upper arm**
- **√7ᵗʰ S40.859 Superficial foreign body of unspecified upper arm** ▽

√6ᵗʰ S40.86 Insect bite (nonvenomous) of upper arm

- **√7ᵗʰ S40.861 Insect bite (nonvenomous) of right upper arm**
- **√7ᵗʰ S40.862 Insect bite (nonvenomous) of left upper arm**
- **√7ᵗʰ S40.869 Insect bite (nonvenomous) of unspecified upper arm** ▽

√6ᵗʰ S40.87 Other superficial bite of upper arm
> **EXCLUDES 1** open bite of upper arm (S41.14)
> **EXCLUDES 2** other superficial bite of shoulder (S40.27-)

- **√7ᵗʰ S40.871 Other superficial bite of right upper arm**
- **√7ᵗʰ S40.872 Other superficial bite of left upper arm**
- **√7ᵗʰ S40.879 Other superficial bite of unspecified upper arm** ▽

√5ᵗʰ S40.9 Unspecified superficial injury of shoulder and upper arm

√6ᵗʰ S40.91 Unspecified superficial injury of shoulder

- **√7ᵗʰ S40.911 Unspecified superficial injury of right shoulder** ▽
- **√7ᵗʰ S40.912 Unspecified superficial injury of left shoulder** ▽
- **√7ᵗʰ S40.919 Unspecified superficial injury of unspecified shoulder** ▽

√6ᵗʰ S40.92 Unspecified superficial injury of upper arm

- **√7ᵗʰ S40.921 Unspecified superficial injury of right upper arm** ▽
- **√7ᵗʰ S40.922 Unspecified superficial injury of left upper arm** ▽
- **√7ᵗʰ S40.929 Unspecified superficial injury of unspecified upper arm** ▽

√4ᵗʰ S41 Open wound of shoulder and upper arm
Code also any associated wound infection
> **EXCLUDES 1** traumatic amputation of shoulder and upper arm (S48.-)
> **EXCLUDES 2** open fracture of shoulder and upper arm (S42.- with 7th character B or C)

The appropriate 7th character is to be added to each code from category S41.
A initial encounter
D subsequent encounter
S sequela

√5ᵗʰ S41.0 Open wound of shoulder

√6ᵗʰ S41.00 Unspecified open wound of shoulder

- **√7ᵗʰ S41.001 Unspecified open wound of right shoulder** ▽
- **√7ᵗʰ S41.002 Unspecified open wound of left shoulder** ▽
- **√7ᵗʰ S41.009 Unspecified open wound of unspecified shoulder** ▽

√6ᵗʰ S41.01 Laceration without foreign body of shoulder

- **√7ᵗʰ S41.011 Laceration without foreign body of right shoulder**
- **√7ᵗʰ S41.012 Laceration without foreign body of left shoulder**
- **√7ᵗʰ S41.019 Laceration without foreign body of unspecified shoulder** ▽

√6ᵗʰ S41.02 Laceration with foreign body of shoulder

- **√7ᵗʰ S41.021 Laceration with foreign body of right shoulder**
- **√7ᵗʰ S41.022 Laceration with foreign body of left shoulder**
- **√7ᵗʰ S41.029 Laceration with foreign body of unspecified shoulder** ▽

√6ᵗʰ S41.03 Puncture wound without foreign body of shoulder

- **√7ᵗʰ S41.031 Puncture wound without foreign body of right shoulder**
- **√7ᵗʰ S41.032 Puncture wound without foreign body of left shoulder**

- **√7ᵗʰ S41.039 Puncture wound without foreign body of unspecified shoulder** ▽

√6ᵗʰ S41.04 Puncture wound with foreign body of shoulder

- **√7ᵗʰ S41.041 Puncture wound with foreign body of right shoulder**
- **√7ᵗʰ S41.042 Puncture wound with foreign body of left shoulder**
- **√7ᵗʰ S41.049 Puncture wound with foreign body of unspecified shoulder** ▽

√6ᵗʰ S41.05 Open bite of shoulder
Bite of shoulder NOS
> **EXCLUDES 1** superficial bite of shoulder (S40.27)

- **√7ᵗʰ S41.051 Open bite of right shoulder**
- **√7ᵗʰ S41.052 Open bite of left shoulder**
- **√7ᵗʰ S41.059 Open bite of unspecified shoulder** ▽

√5ᵗʰ S41.1 Open wound of upper arm

√6ᵗʰ S41.10 Unspecified open wound of upper arm
AHA: 2016, 3Q, 24

- **√7ᵗʰ S41.101 Unspecified open wound of right upper arm** ▽
- **√7ᵗʰ S41.102 Unspecified open wound of left upper arm** ▽
- **√7ᵗʰ S41.109 Unspecified open wound of unspecified upper arm** ▽

√6ᵗʰ S41.11 Laceration without foreign body of upper arm

- **√7ᵗʰ S41.111 Laceration without foreign body of right upper arm**
- **√7ᵗʰ S41.112 Laceration without foreign body of left upper arm**
- **√7ᵗʰ S41.119 Laceration without foreign body of unspecified upper arm** ▽

√6ᵗʰ S41.12 Laceration with foreign body of upper arm

- **√7ᵗʰ S41.121 Laceration with foreign body of right upper arm**
- **√7ᵗʰ S41.122 Laceration with foreign body of left upper arm**
- **√7ᵗʰ S41.129 Laceration with foreign body of unspecified upper arm** ▽

√6ᵗʰ S41.13 Puncture wound without foreign body of upper arm
AHA: 2016, 3Q, 24

- **√7ᵗʰ S41.131 Puncture wound without foreign body of right upper arm**
- **√7ᵗʰ S41.132 Puncture wound without foreign body of left upper arm**
- **√7ᵗʰ S41.139 Puncture wound without foreign body of unspecified upper arm** ▽

√6ᵗʰ S41.14 Puncture wound with foreign body of upper arm
AHA: 2016, 3Q, 24

- **√7ᵗʰ S41.141 Puncture wound with foreign body of right upper arm**
- **√7ᵗʰ S41.142 Puncture wound with foreign body of left upper arm**
- **√7ᵗʰ S41.149 Puncture wound with foreign body of unspecified upper arm** ▽

√6ᵗʰ S41.15 Open bite of upper arm
Bite of upper arm NOS
> **EXCLUDES 1** superficial bite of upper arm (S40.87)

- **√7ᵗʰ S41.151 Open bite of right upper arm**
- **√7ᵗʰ S41.152 Open bite of left upper arm**
- **√7ᵗʰ S41.159 Open bite of unspecified upper arm** ▽

✓4ᵗʰ **S42** **Fracture of shoulder and upper arm**

> **NOTE**   A fracture not indicated as displaced or nondisplaced should be coded to displaced.
> A fracture not indicated as open or closed should be coded to closed.

> **EXCLUDES 1**   *traumatic amputation of shoulder and upper arm (S48.-)*
> **AHA:** 2015, 3Q, 37-39

> The appropriate 7th character is to be added to all codes from category S42 [unless otherwise indicated].
> A   initial encounter for closed fracture
> B   initial encounter for open fracture
> D   subsequent encounter for fracture with routine healing
> G   subsequent encounter for fracture with delayed healing
> K   subsequent encounter for fracture with nonunion
> P   subsequent encounter for fracture with malunion
> S   sequela

✓5ᵗʰ **S42.0** **Fracture of** clavicle

   ✓6ᵗʰ **S42.00** **Fracture of unspecified part of clavicle**

     ✓7ᵗʰ **S42.001** **Fracture of unspecified part of** right **clavicle** ▽

     ✓7ᵗʰ **S42.002** **Fracture of unspecified part of** left **clavicle** ▽

     ✓7ᵗʰ **S42.009** **Fracture of unspecified part of unspecified clavicle** ▽
       AHA: 2012, 4Q, 93

   ✓6ᵗʰ **S42.01** **Fracture of** sternal end **of clavicle**

     ✓7ᵗʰ **S42.011** **Anterior displaced fracture of sternal end of** right **clavicle**

     ✓7ᵗʰ **S42.012** **Anterior displaced fracture of sternal end of** left **clavicle**

     ✓7ᵗʰ **S42.013** **Anterior displaced fracture of sternal end of unspecified clavicle** ▽
       Displaced fracture of sternal end of clavicle NOS

     ✓7ᵗʰ **S42.014** **Posterior displaced fracture of sternal end of** right **clavicle**

     ✓7ᵗʰ **S42.015** **Posterior displaced fracture of sternal end of** left **clavicle**

     ✓7ᵗʰ **S42.016** **Posterior displaced fracture of sternal end of unspecified clavicle** ▽

     ✓7ᵗʰ **S42.017** **Nondisplaced fracture of sternal end of** right **clavicle**

     ✓7ᵗʰ **S42.018** **Nondisplaced fracture of sternal end of** left **clavicle**

     ✓7ᵗʰ **S42.019** **Nondisplaced fracture of sternal end of unspecified clavicle** ▽

   ✓6ᵗʰ **S42.02** **Fracture of** shaft **of clavicle**

     ✓7ᵗʰ **S42.021** **Displaced fracture of shaft of** right **clavicle**

     ✓7ᵗʰ **S42.022** **Displaced fracture of shaft of** left **clavicle**

     ✓7ᵗʰ **S42.023** **Displaced fracture of shaft of unspecified clavicle** ▽

     ✓7ᵗʰ **S42.024** **Nondisplaced fracture of shaft of** right **clavicle**

     ✓7ᵗʰ **S42.025** **Nondisplaced fracture of shaft of** left **clavicle**

     ✓7ᵗʰ **S42.026** **Nondisplaced fracture of shaft of unspecified clavicle** ▽

   ✓6ᵗʰ **S42.03** **Fracture of** lateral end **of clavicle**
     Fracture of acromial end of clavicle

     ✓7ᵗʰ **S42.031** **Displaced fracture of lateral end of** right **clavicle**

     ✓7ᵗʰ **S42.032** **Displaced fracture of lateral end of** left **clavicle**

     ✓7ᵗʰ **S42.033** **Displaced fracture of lateral end of unspecified clavicle** ▽

     ✓7ᵗʰ **S42.034** **Nondisplaced fracture of lateral end of** right **clavicle**

     ✓7ᵗʰ **S42.035** **Nondisplaced fracture of lateral end of** left **clavicle**

     ✓7ᵗʰ **S42.036** **Nondisplaced fracture of lateral end of unspecified clavicle** ▽

✓5ᵗʰ **S42.1** **Fracture of** scapula

   ✓6ᵗʰ **S42.10** **Fracture of unspecified part of scapula**

     ✓7ᵗʰ **S42.101** **Fracture of unspecified part of scapula,** right **shoulder** ▽

     ✓7ᵗʰ **S42.102** **Fracture of unspecified part of scapula,** left **shoulder** ▽

     ✓7ᵗʰ **S42.109** **Fracture of unspecified part of scapula, unspecified shoulder** ▽

   ✓6ᵗʰ **S42.11** **Fracture of** body of scapula

     ✓7ᵗʰ **S42.111** **Displaced fracture of body of scapula, right shoulder**

     ✓7ᵗʰ **S42.112** **Displaced fracture of body of scapula, left shoulder**

     ✓7ᵗʰ **S42.113** **Displaced fracture of body of scapula, unspecified shoulder** ▽

     ✓7ᵗʰ **S42.114** **Nondisplaced fracture of body of scapula, right shoulder**

     ✓7ᵗʰ **S42.115** **Nondisplaced fracture of body of scapula, left shoulder**

     ✓7ᵗʰ **S42.116** **Nondisplaced fracture of body of scapula, unspecified shoulder** ▽

   ✓6ᵗʰ **S42.12** **Fracture of** acromial process

     ✓7ᵗʰ **S42.121** **Displaced fracture of acromial process, right shoulder**

     ✓7ᵗʰ **S42.122** **Displaced fracture of acromial process,** left **shoulder**

     ✓7ᵗʰ **S42.123** **Displaced fracture of acromial process, unspecified shoulder** ▽

     ✓7ᵗʰ **S42.124** **Nondisplaced fracture of acromial process, right shoulder**

     ✓7ᵗʰ **S42.125** **Nondisplaced fracture of acromial process,** left **shoulder**

     ✓7ᵗʰ **S42.126** **Nondisplaced fracture of acromial process, unspecified shoulder** ▽

   ✓6ᵗʰ **S42.13** **Fracture of** coracoid process

     ✓7ᵗʰ **S42.131** **Displaced fracture of coracoid process, right shoulder**

     ✓7ᵗʰ **S42.132** **Displaced fracture of coracoid process, left shoulder**

     ✓7ᵗʰ **S42.133** **Displaced fracture of coracoid process, unspecified shoulder** ▽

     ✓7ᵗʰ **S42.134** **Nondisplaced fracture of coracoid process, right shoulder**

     ✓7ᵗʰ **S42.135** **Nondisplaced fracture of coracoid process, left shoulder**

     ✓7ᵗʰ **S42.136** **Nondisplaced fracture of coracoid process, unspecified shoulder** ▽

   ✓6ᵗʰ **S42.14** **Fracture of** glenoid cavity of scapula

     ✓7ᵗʰ **S42.141** **Displaced fracture of glenoid cavity of scapula, right shoulder**

     ✓7ᵗʰ **S42.142** **Displaced fracture of glenoid cavity of scapula, left shoulder**

     ✓7ᵗʰ **S42.143** **Displaced fracture of glenoid cavity of scapula, unspecified shoulder** ▽

     ✓7ᵗʰ **S42.144** **Nondisplaced fracture of glenoid cavity of scapula, right shoulder**

     ✓7ᵗʰ **S42.145** **Nondisplaced fracture of glenoid cavity of scapula, left shoulder**

     ✓7ᵗʰ **S42.146** **Nondisplaced fracture of glenoid cavity of scapula, unspecified shoulder** ▽

   ✓6ᵗʰ **S42.15** **Fracture of** neck of scapula

     ✓7ᵗʰ **S42.151** **Displaced fracture of neck of scapula,** right **shoulder**

     ✓7ᵗʰ **S42.152** **Displaced fracture of neck of scapula,** left **shoulder**

     ✓7ᵗʰ **S42.153** **Displaced fracture of neck of scapula, unspecified shoulder** ▽

     ✓7ᵗʰ **S42.154** **Nondisplaced fracture of neck of scapula, right shoulder**

     ✓7ᵗʰ **S42.155** **Nondisplaced fracture of neck of scapula, left shoulder**

     ✓7ᵗʰ **S42.156** **Nondisplaced fracture of neck of scapula, unspecified shoulder** ▽

   ✓6ᵗʰ **S42.19** **Fracture of other part of scapula**

     ✓7ᵗʰ **S42.191** **Fracture of other part of scapula,** right **shoulder**

     ✓7ᵗʰ **S42.192** **Fracture of other part of scapula,** left **shoulder**

☑ Additional Character Req   ✓x7ᵗʰ Placeholder Alert   Manifestation   **HCC** CMS-HCC Condition   ▽ Unspecified Code   ▶◀ Revised Text   ● New Code   ▲ Revised Code Title

ICD-10-CM 2018   **955**

✓7ᵗʰ **S42.199　Fracture of other part of scapula, unspecified shoulder** ▽

✓5ᵗʰ **S42.2　Fracture of upper end of humerus**
Fracture of proximal end of humerus
EXCLUDES 2　*fracture of shaft of humerus (S42.3-)*
physeal fracture of upper end of humerus (S49.0-)

✓6ᵗʰ **S42.20　Unspecified fracture of upper end of humerus**

✓7ᵗʰ **S42.201　Unspecified fracture of upper end of right humerus** ▽

✓7ᵗʰ **S42.202　Unspecified fracture of upper end of left humerus** ▽

✓7ᵗʰ **S42.209　Unspecified fracture of upper end of unspecified humerus** ▽

✓6ᵗʰ **S42.21　Unspecified fracture of surgical neck of humerus**
Fracture of neck of humerus NOS

✓7ᵗʰ **S42.211　Unspecified displaced fracture of surgical neck of right humerus** ▽

✓7ᵗʰ **S42.212　Unspecified displaced fracture of surgical neck of left humerus** ▽

✓7ᵗʰ **S42.213　Unspecified displaced fracture of surgical neck of unspecified humerus** ▽

✓7ᵗʰ **S42.214　Unspecified nondisplaced fracture of surgical neck of right humerus** ▽

✓7ᵗʰ **S42.215　Unspecified nondisplaced fracture of surgical neck of left humerus** ▽

✓7ᵗʰ **S42.216　Unspecified nondisplaced fracture of surgical neck of unspecified humerus** ▽

✓6ᵗʰ **S42.22　2-part fracture of surgical neck of humerus**

✓7ᵗʰ **S42.221　2-part displaced fracture of surgical neck of right humerus**

✓7ᵗʰ **S42.222　2-part displaced fracture of surgical neck of left humerus**

✓7ᵗʰ **S42.223　2-part displaced fracture of surgical neck of unspecified humerus** ▽

✓7ᵗʰ **S42.224　2-part nondisplaced fracture of surgical neck of right humerus**

✓7ᵗʰ **S42.225　2-part nondisplaced fracture of surgical neck of left humerus**

✓7ᵗʰ **S42.226　2-part nondisplaced fracture of surgical neck of unspecified humerus** ▽

✓6ᵗʰ **S42.23　3-part fracture of surgical neck of humerus**

✓7ᵗʰ **S42.231　3-part fracture of surgical neck of right humerus**

✓7ᵗʰ **S42.232　3-part fracture of surgical neck of left humerus**

✓7ᵗʰ **S42.239　3-part fracture of surgical neck of unspecified humerus** ▽

✓6ᵗʰ **S42.24　4-part fracture of surgical neck of humerus**

✓7ᵗʰ **S42.241　4-part fracture of surgical neck of right humerus**

✓7ᵗʰ **S42.242　4-part fracture of surgical neck of left humerus**

✓7ᵗʰ **S42.249　4-part fracture of surgical neck of unspecified humerus** ▽

✓6ᵗʰ **S42.25　Fracture of greater tuberosity of humerus**

✓7ᵗʰ **S42.251　Displaced fracture of greater tuberosity of right humerus**

✓7ᵗʰ **S42.252　Displaced fracture of greater tuberosity of left humerus**

✓7ᵗʰ **S42.253　Displaced fracture of greater tuberosity of unspecified humerus** ▽

✓7ᵗʰ **S42.254　Nondisplaced fracture of greater tuberosity of right humerus**

✓7ᵗʰ **S42.255　Nondisplaced fracture of greater tuberosity of left humerus**

✓7ᵗʰ **S42.256　Nondisplaced fracture of greater tuberosity of unspecified humerus** ▽

✓6ᵗʰ **S42.26　Fracture of lesser tuberosity of humerus**

✓7ᵗʰ **S42.261　Displaced fracture of lesser tuberosity of right humerus**

✓7ᵗʰ **S42.262　Displaced fracture of lesser tuberosity of left humerus**

✓7ᵗʰ **S42.263　Displaced fracture of lesser tuberosity of unspecified humerus** ▽

✓7ᵗʰ **S42.264　Nondisplaced fracture of lesser tuberosity of right humerus**

✓7ᵗʰ **S42.265　Nondisplaced fracture of lesser tuberosity of left humerus**

✓7ᵗʰ **S42.266　Nondisplaced fracture of lesser tuberosity of unspecified humerus** ▽

✓6ᵗʰ **S42.27　Torus fracture of upper end of humerus**

> The appropriate 7th character is to be added to all codes in subcategory S42.27.
> A　initial encounter for closed fracture
> D　subsequent encounter for fracture with routine healing
> G　subsequent encounter for fracture with delayed healing
> K　subsequent encounter for fracture with nonunion
> P　subsequent encounter for fracture with malunion
> S　sequela

✓7ᵗʰ **S42.271　Torus fracture of upper end of right humerus**

✓7ᵗʰ **S42.272　Torus fracture of upper end of left humerus**

✓7ᵗʰ **S42.279　Torus fracture of upper end of unspecified humerus** ▽

✓6ᵗʰ **S42.29　Other fracture of upper end of humerus**
Fracture of anatomical neck of humerus
Fracture of articular head of humerus

✓7ᵗʰ **S42.291　Other displaced fracture of upper end of right humerus**

✓7ᵗʰ **S42.292　Other displaced fracture of upper end of left humerus**

✓7ᵗʰ **S42.293　Other displaced fracture of upper end of unspecified humerus** ▽

✓7ᵗʰ **S42.294　Other nondisplaced fracture of upper end of right humerus**

✓7ᵗʰ **S42.295　Other nondisplaced fracture of upper end of left humerus**

✓7ᵗʰ **S42.296　Other nondisplaced fracture of upper end of unspecified humerus** ▽

✓5ᵗʰ **S42.3　Fracture of shaft of humerus**
Fracture of humerus NOS
Fracture of upper arm NOS
EXCLUDES 2　*physeal fractures of upper end of humerus (S49.0-)*
physeal fractures of lower end of humerus (S49.1-)

✓6ᵗʰ **S42.30　Unspecified fracture of shaft of humerus**

✓7ᵗʰ **S42.301　Unspecified fracture of shaft of humerus, right arm** ▽

✓7ᵗʰ **S42.302　Unspecified fracture of shaft of humerus, left arm** ▽

✓7ᵗʰ **S42.309　Unspecified fracture of shaft of humerus, unspecified arm** ▽

✓6ᵗʰ **S42.31　Greenstick fracture of shaft of humerus**

> The appropriate 7th character is to be added to all codes in subcategory S42.31.
> A　initial encounter for closed fracture
> D　subsequent encounter for fracture with routine healing
> G　subsequent encounter for fracture with delayed healing
> K　subsequent encounter for fracture with nonunion
> P　subsequent encounter for fracture with malunion
> S　sequela

✓7ᵗʰ **S42.311　Greenstick fracture of shaft of humerus, right arm**

✓7ᵗʰ **S42.312　Greenstick fracture of shaft of humerus, left arm**

✓7ᵗʰ **S42.319　Greenstick fracture of shaft of humerus, unspecified arm** ▽

✓6ᵗʰ **S42.32　Transverse fracture of shaft of humerus**

✓7ᵗʰ **S42.321　Displaced transverse fracture of shaft of humerus, right arm**

✓7ᵗʰ **S42.322　Displaced transverse fracture of shaft of humerus, left arm**

√7ᵗʰ **S42.323** Displaced **transverse fracture of shaft of humerus, unspecified arm** ▽

√7ᵗʰ **S42.324** Nondisplaced **transverse fracture of shaft of humerus, right arm**

√7ᵗʰ **S42.325** Nondisplaced **transverse fracture of shaft of humerus, left arm**

√7ᵗʰ **S42.326** Nondisplaced **transverse fracture of shaft of humerus, unspecified arm** ▽

√6ᵗʰ **S42.33** Oblique **fracture of shaft of humerus**

√7ᵗʰ **S42.331** Displaced **oblique fracture of shaft of humerus, right arm**

√7ᵗʰ **S42.332** Displaced **oblique fracture of shaft of humerus, left arm**

√7ᵗʰ **S42.333** Displaced **oblique fracture of shaft of humerus, unspecified arm** ▽

√7ᵗʰ **S42.334** Nondisplaced **oblique fracture of shaft of humerus, right arm**

√7ᵗʰ **S42.335** Nondisplaced **oblique fracture of shaft of humerus, left arm**

√7ᵗʰ **S42.336** Nondisplaced **oblique fracture of shaft of humerus, unspecified arm** ▽

√6ᵗʰ **S42.34** Spiral **fracture of shaft of humerus**

√7ᵗʰ **S42.341** Displaced **spiral fracture of shaft of humerus, right arm**

√7ᵗʰ **S42.342** Displaced **spiral fracture of shaft of humerus, left arm**

√7ᵗʰ **S42.343** Displaced **spiral fracture of shaft of humerus, unspecified arm** ▽

√7ᵗʰ **S42.344** Nondisplaced **spiral fracture of shaft of humerus, right arm**

√7ᵗʰ **S42.345** Nondisplaced **spiral fracture of shaft of humerus, left arm**

√7ᵗʰ **S42.346** Nondisplaced **spiral fracture of shaft of humerus, unspecified arm** ▽

√6ᵗʰ **S42.35** Comminuted **fracture of shaft of humerus**

√7ᵗʰ **S42.351** Displaced **comminuted fracture of shaft of humerus, right arm**

√7ᵗʰ **S42.352** Displaced **comminuted fracture of shaft of humerus, left arm**

√7ᵗʰ **S42.353** Displaced **comminuted fracture of shaft of humerus, unspecified arm** ▽

√7ᵗʰ **S42.354** Nondisplaced **comminuted fracture of shaft of humerus, right arm**

√7ᵗʰ **S42.355** Nondisplaced **comminuted fracture of shaft of humerus, left arm**

√7ᵗʰ **S42.356** Nondisplaced **comminuted fracture of shaft of humerus, unspecified arm** ▽

√6ᵗʰ **S42.36** Segmental **fracture of shaft of humerus**

√7ᵗʰ **S42.361** Displaced **segmental fracture of shaft of humerus, right arm**

√7ᵗʰ **S42.362** Displaced **segmental fracture of shaft of humerus, left arm**

√7ᵗʰ **S42.363** Displaced **segmental fracture of shaft of humerus, unspecified arm** ▽

√7ᵗʰ **S42.364** Nondisplaced **segmental fracture of shaft of humerus, right arm**

√7ᵗʰ **S42.365** Nondisplaced **segmental fracture of shaft of humerus, left arm**

√7ᵗʰ **S42.366** Nondisplaced **segmental fracture of shaft of humerus, unspecified arm** ▽

√6ᵗʰ **S42.39** Other **fracture of shaft of humerus**

√7ᵗʰ **S42.391** Other **fracture of shaft of right humerus**

√7ᵗʰ **S42.392** Other **fracture of shaft of left humerus**

√7ᵗʰ **S42.399** Other **fracture of shaft of unspecified humerus** ▽

√5ᵗʰ **S42.4** Fracture of lower end of humerus
Fracture of distal end of humerus
EXCLUDES 2 *fracture of shaft of humerus (S42.3-)*
physeal fracture of lower end of humerus (S49.1-)

√6ᵗʰ **S42.40** Unspecified fracture of lower end of humerus
Fracture of elbow NOS

√7ᵗʰ **S42.401** Unspecified fracture of lower end of right humerus ▽

√7ᵗʰ **S42.402** Unspecified fracture of lower end of left humerus ▽

√7ᵗʰ **S42.409** Unspecified fracture of lower end of unspecified humerus ▽

√6ᵗʰ **S42.41** Simple supracondylar **fracture without intercondylar fracture of humerus**

√7ᵗʰ **S42.411** Displaced **simple supracondylar fracture without intercondylar fracture of right humerus**

√7ᵗʰ **S42.412** Displaced **simple supracondylar fracture without intercondylar fracture of left humerus**

√7ᵗʰ **S42.413** Displaced **simple supracondylar fracture without intercondylar fracture of unspecified humerus** ▽

√7ᵗʰ **S42.414** Nondisplaced **simple supracondylar fracture without intercondylar fracture of right humerus**

√7ᵗʰ **S42.415** Nondisplaced **simple supracondylar fracture without intercondylar fracture of left humerus**

√7ᵗʰ **S42.416** Nondisplaced **simple supracondylar fracture without intercondylar fracture of unspecified humerus** ▽

√6ᵗʰ **S42.42** Comminuted supracondylar **fracture without intercondylar fracture of humerus**

√7ᵗʰ **S42.421** Displaced **comminuted supracondylar fracture without intercondylar fracture of right humerus**

√7ᵗʰ **S42.422** Displaced **comminuted supracondylar fracture without intercondylar fracture of left humerus**

√7ᵗʰ **S42.423** Displaced **comminuted supracondylar fracture without intercondylar fracture of unspecified humerus** ▽

√7ᵗʰ **S42.424** Nondisplaced **comminuted supracondylar fracture without intercondylar fracture of right humerus**

√7ᵗʰ **S42.425** Nondisplaced **comminuted supracondylar fracture without intercondylar fracture of left humerus**

√7ᵗʰ **S42.426** Nondisplaced **comminuted supracondylar fracture without intercondylar fracture of unspecified humerus** ▽

√6ᵗʰ **S42.43** Fracture (avulsion) of lateral epicondyle of humerus

√7ᵗʰ **S42.431** Displaced **fracture (avulsion) of lateral epicondyle of right humerus**

√7ᵗʰ **S42.432** Displaced **fracture (avulsion) of lateral epicondyle of left humerus**

√7ᵗʰ **S42.433** Displaced **fracture (avulsion) of lateral epicondyle of unspecified humerus** ▽

√7ᵗʰ **S42.434** Nondisplaced **fracture (avulsion) of lateral epicondyle of right humerus**

√7ᵗʰ **S42.435** Nondisplaced **fracture (avulsion) of lateral epicondyle of left humerus**

√7ᵗʰ **S42.436** Nondisplaced **fracture (avulsion) of lateral epicondyle of unspecified humerus** ▽

√6ᵗʰ **S42.44** Fracture (avulsion) of medial epicondyle of humerus

S42.441 Displaced **fracture (avulsion) of medial epicondyle of right humerus**

√7ᵗʰ **S42.442** Displaced **fracture (avulsion) of medial epicondyle of left humerus**

√7ᵗʰ **S42.443** Displaced **fracture (avulsion) of medial epicondyle of unspecified humerus** ▽

√7ᵗʰ **S42.444** Nondisplaced **fracture (avulsion) of medial epicondyle of right humerus**

√7ᵗʰ **S42.445** Nondisplaced **fracture (avulsion) of medial epicondyle of left humerus**

√7ᵗʰ **S42.446** Nondisplaced **fracture (avulsion) of medial epicondyle of unspecified humerus** ▽

√7ᵗʰ **S42.447** Incarcerated **fracture (avulsion) of medial epicondyle of right humerus**

√7ᵗʰ **S42.448** Incarcerated **fracture (avulsion) of medial epicondyle of left humerus**

√7ᵗʰ **S42.449** Incarcerated **fracture (avulsion) of medial epicondyle of unspecified humerus** ▽

☑ Additional Character Req ✓ˣ7ᵗʰ Placeholder Alert ▪ Manifestation ᴴᶜᶜ CMS-HCC Condition ▽ Unspecified Code ▶◀ Revised Text ● New Code ▲ Revised Code Title

✓6ᵗʰ **S42.45** **Fracture of lateral condyle of humerus**
Fracture of capitellum of humerus

✓7ᵗʰ   **S42.451**   **Displaced fracture of lateral condyle of right humerus**

✓7ᵗʰ   **S42.452**   **Displaced fracture of lateral condyle of left humerus**

✓7ᵗʰ   **S42.453**   **Displaced fracture of lateral condyle of unspecified humerus** ▽

✓7ᵗʰ   **S42.454**   **Nondisplaced fracture of lateral condyle of right humerus**

✓7ᵗʰ   **S42.455**   **Nondisplaced fracture of lateral condyle of left humerus**

✓7ᵗʰ   **S42.456**   **Nondisplaced fracture of lateral condyle of unspecified humerus** ▽

✓6ᵗʰ **S42.46** **Fracture of medial condyle of humerus**
Trochlea fracture of humerus

✓7ᵗʰ   **S42.461**   **Displaced fracture of medial condyle of right humerus**

✓7ᵗʰ   **S42.462**   **Displaced fracture of medial condyle of left humerus**

✓7ᵗʰ   **S42.463**   **Displaced fracture of medial condyle of unspecified humerus** ▽

✓7ᵗʰ   **S42.464**   **Nondisplaced fracture of medial condyle of right humerus**

✓7ᵗʰ   **S42.465**   **Nondisplaced fracture of medial condyle of left humerus**

✓7ᵗʰ   **S42.466**   **Nondisplaced fracture of medial condyle of unspecified humerus** ▽

✓6ᵗʰ **S42.47** **Transcondylar fracture of humerus**

✓7ᵗʰ   **S42.471**   **Displaced transcondylar fracture of right humerus**

✓7ᵗʰ   **S42.472**   **Displaced transcondylar fracture of left humerus**

✓7ᵗʰ   **S42.473**   **Displaced transcondylar fracture of unspecified humerus** ▽

✓7ᵗʰ   **S42.474**   **Nondisplaced transcondylar fracture of right humerus**

✓7ᵗʰ   **S42.475**   **Nondisplaced transcondylar fracture of left humerus**

✓7ᵗʰ   **S42.476**   **Nondisplaced transcondylar fracture of unspecified humerus** ▽

✓6ᵗʰ **S42.48** **Torus fracture of lower end of humerus**

> The appropriate 7th character is to be added to all codes in subcategory S42.48.
> A   initial encounter for closed fracture
> D   subsequent encounter for fracture with routine healing
> G   subsequent encounter for fracture with delayed healing
> K   subsequent encounter for fracture with nonunion
> P   subsequent encounter for fracture with malunion
> S   sequela

✓7ᵗʰ   **S42.481**   **Torus fracture of lower end of right humerus**

✓7ᵗʰ   **S42.482**   **Torus fracture of lower end of left humerus**

✓7ᵗʰ   **S42.489**   **Torus fracture of lower end of unspecified humerus** ▽

✓6ᵗʰ **S42.49** **Other fracture of lower end of humerus**

✓7ᵗʰ   **S42.491**   **Other displaced fracture of lower end of right humerus**

✓7ᵗʰ   **S42.492**   **Other displaced fracture of lower end of left humerus**

✓7ᵗʰ   **S42.493**   **Other displaced fracture of lower end of unspecified humerus** ▽

✓7ᵗʰ   **S42.494**   **Other nondisplaced fracture of lower end of right humerus**

✓7ᵗʰ   **S42.495**   **Other nondisplaced fracture of lower end of left humerus**

✓7ᵗʰ   **S42.496**   **Other nondisplaced fracture of lower end of unspecified humerus** ▽

✓5ᵗʰ **S42.9** **Fracture of shoulder girdle, part unspecified**
Fracture of shoulder NOS

✓x7ᵗʰ   **S42.90**   **Fracture of unspecified shoulder girdle, part unspecified** ▽

✓x7ᵗʰ   **S42.91**   **Fracture of right shoulder girdle, part unspecified** ▽

✓x7ᵗʰ   **S42.92**   **Fracture of left shoulder girdle, part unspecified** ▽

✓4ᵗʰ **S43** **Dislocation and sprain of joints and ligaments of shoulder girdle**
INCLUDES   avulsion of joint or ligament of shoulder girdle
laceration of cartilage, joint or ligament of shoulder girdle
sprain of cartilage, joint or ligament of shoulder girdle
traumatic hemarthrosis of joint or ligament of shoulder girdle
traumatic rupture of joint or ligament of shoulder girdle
traumatic subluxation of joint or ligament of shoulder girdle
traumatic tear of joint or ligament of shoulder girdle

Code also any associated open wound

EXCLUDES 2   *strain of muscle, fascia and tendon of shoulder and upper arm (S46.-)*

> The appropriate 7th character is to be added to each code from category S43.
> A   initial encounter
> D   subsequent encounter
> S   sequela

✓5ᵗʰ **S43.0** **Subluxation and dislocation of shoulder joint**
Dislocation of glenohumeral joint
Subluxation of glenohumeral joint

✓6ᵗʰ **S43.00** **Unspecified subluxation and dislocation of shoulder joint**
Dislocation of humerus NOS
Subluxation of humerus NOS

✓7ᵗʰ   **S43.001**   **Unspecified subluxation of right shoulder joint** ▽

✓7ᵗʰ   **S43.002**   **Unspecified subluxation of left shoulder joint** ▽

✓7ᵗʰ   **S43.003**   **Unspecified subluxation of unspecified shoulder joint** ▽

✓7ᵗʰ   **S43.004**   **Unspecified dislocation of right shoulder joint** ▽

✓7ᵗʰ   **S43.005**   **Unspecified dislocation of left shoulder joint** ▽

✓7ᵗʰ   **S43.006**   **Unspecified dislocation of unspecified shoulder joint** ▽

✓6ᵗʰ **S43.01** **Anterior subluxation and dislocation of humerus**

✓7ᵗʰ   **S43.011**   **Anterior subluxation of right humerus**

✓7ᵗʰ   **S43.012**   **Anterior subluxation of left humerus**

✓7ᵗʰ   **S43.013**   **Anterior subluxation of unspecified humerus**

✓7ᵗʰ   **S43.014**   **Anterior dislocation of right humerus**

✓7ᵗʰ   **S43.015**   **Anterior dislocation of left humerus**

✓7ᵗʰ   **S43.016**   **Anterior dislocation of unspecified humerus** ▽

✓6ᵗʰ **S43.02** **Posterior subluxation and dislocation of humerus**

✓7ᵗʰ   **S43.021**   **Posterior subluxation of right humerus**

✓7ᵗʰ   **S43.022**   **Posterior subluxation of left humerus**

✓7ᵗʰ   **S43.023**   **Posterior subluxation of unspecified humerus** ▽

✓7ᵗʰ   **S43.024**   **Posterior dislocation of right humerus**

✓7ᵗʰ   **S43.025**   **Posterior dislocation of left humerus**

✓7ᵗʰ   **S43.026**   **Posterior dislocation of unspecified humerus** ▽

✓6ᵗʰ **S43.03** **Inferior subluxation and dislocation of humerus**

✓7ᵗʰ   **S43.031**   **Inferior subluxation of right humerus**

✓7ᵗʰ   **S43.032**   **Inferior subluxation of left humerus**

✓7ᵗʰ   **S43.033**   **Inferior subluxation of unspecified humerus** ▽

✓7ᵗʰ   **S43.034**   **Inferior dislocation of right humerus**

✓7ᵗʰ   **S43.035**   **Inferior dislocation of left humerus**

✓7ᵗʰ   **S43.036**   **Inferior dislocation of unspecified humerus** ▽

✓6ᵗʰ **S43.08** **Other subluxation and dislocation of shoulder joint**

✓7ᵗʰ   **S43.081**   **Other subluxation of right shoulder joint**

✓7ᵗʰ   **S43.082**   **Other subluxation of left shoulder joint**

✓7ᵗʰ   **S43.083**   **Other subluxation of unspecified shoulder joint** ▽

EXCLUDES 1 Not coded here   EXCLUDES 2 Not included here   N Newborn Age: 0   P Pediatric Age: 0-17   M Maternity Age: 12-55   A Adult Age: 15-124

958   ICD-10-CM 2018

✓7ᵗʰ **S43.084** Other dislocation of right shoulder joint

✓7ᵗʰ **S43.085** Other dislocation of left shoulder joint

✓7ᵗʰ **S43.086** Other dislocation of unspecified shoulder joint ▽

✓5ᵗʰ **S43.1 Subluxation and dislocation of acromioclavicular joint**

  ✓6ᵗʰ **S43.10 Unspecified dislocation of acromioclavicular joint**

    ✓7ᵗʰ **S43.101** Unspecified dislocation of right acromioclavicular joint ▽

    ✓7ᵗʰ **S43.102** Unspecified dislocation of left acromioclavicular joint ▽

    ✓7ᵗʰ **S43.109** Unspecified dislocation of unspecified acromioclavicular joint ▽

  ✓6ᵗʰ **S43.11 Subluxation of acromioclavicular joint**

    ✓7ᵗʰ **S43.111** Subluxation of right acromioclavicular joint

    ✓7ᵗʰ **S43.112** Subluxation of left acromioclavicular joint

    ✓7ᵗʰ **S43.119** Subluxation of unspecified acromioclavicular joint ▽

  ✓6ᵗʰ **S43.12 Dislocation of acromioclavicular joint, 100%-200% displacement**

    ✓7ᵗʰ **S43.121** Dislocation of right acromioclavicular joint, 100%-200% displacement

    ✓7ᵗʰ **S43.122** Dislocation of left acromioclavicular joint, 100%-200% displacement

    ✓7ᵗʰ **S43.129** Dislocation of unspecified acromioclavicular joint, 100%-200% displacement ▽

  ✓6ᵗʰ **S43.13 Dislocation of acromioclavicular joint, greater than 200% displacement**

    ✓7ᵗʰ **S43.131** Dislocation of right acromioclavicular joint, greater than 200% displacement

    ✓7ᵗʰ **S43.132** Dislocation of left acromioclavicular joint, greater than 200% displacement

    ✓7ᵗʰ **S43.139** Dislocation of unspecified acromioclavicular joint, greater than 200% displacement ▽

  ✓6ᵗʰ **S43.14 Inferior dislocation of acromioclavicular joint**

    ✓7ᵗʰ **S43.141** Inferior dislocation of right acromioclavicular joint

    ✓7ᵗʰ **S43.142** Inferior dislocation of left acromioclavicular joint

    ✓7ᵗʰ **S43.149** Inferior dislocation of unspecified acromioclavicular joint ▽

  ✓6ᵗʰ **S43.15 Posterior dislocation of acromioclavicular joint**

    ✓7ᵗʰ **S43.151** Posterior dislocation of right acromioclavicular joint

    ✓7ᵗʰ **S43.152** Posterior dislocation of left acromioclavicular joint

    ✓7ᵗʰ **S43.159** Posterior dislocation of unspecified acromioclavicular joint ▽

✓5ᵗʰ **S43.2 Subluxation and dislocation of sternoclavicular joint**

  ✓6ᵗʰ **S43.20 Unspecified subluxation and dislocation of sternoclavicular joint**

    ✓7ᵗʰ **S43.201** Unspecified subluxation of right sternoclavicular joint ▽

    ✓7ᵗʰ **S43.202** Unspecified subluxation of left sternoclavicular joint ▽

    ✓7ᵗʰ **S43.203** Unspecified subluxation of unspecified sternoclavicular joint ▽

    ✓7ᵗʰ **S43.204** Unspecified dislocation of right sternoclavicular joint ▽

    ✓7ᵗʰ **S43.205** Unspecified dislocation of left sternoclavicular joint ▽

    ✓7ᵗʰ **S43.206** Unspecified dislocation of unspecified sternoclavicular joint ▽

  ✓6ᵗʰ **S43.21 Anterior subluxation and dislocation of sternoclavicular joint**

    ✓7ᵗʰ **S43.211** Anterior subluxation of right sternoclavicular joint

    ✓7ᵗʰ **S43.212** Anterior subluxation of left sternoclavicular joint

    ✓7ᵗʰ **S43.213** Anterior subluxation of unspecified sternoclavicular joint ▽

    ✓7ᵗʰ **S43.214** Anterior dislocation of right sternoclavicular joint

    ✓7ᵗʰ **S43.215** Anterior dislocation of left sternoclavicular joint

    ✓7ᵗʰ **S43.216** Anterior dislocation of unspecified sternoclavicular joint ▽

  ✓6ᵗʰ **S43.22 Posterior subluxation and dislocation of sternoclavicular joint**

    ✓7ᵗʰ **S43.221** Posterior subluxation of right sternoclavicular joint

    ✓7ᵗʰ **S43.222** Posterior subluxation of left sternoclavicular joint

    ✓7ᵗʰ **S43.223** Posterior subluxation of unspecified sternoclavicular joint ▽

    ✓7ᵗʰ **S43.224** Posterior dislocation of right sternoclavicular joint

    ✓7ᵗʰ **S43.225** Posterior dislocation of left sternoclavicular joint

    ✓7ᵗʰ **S43.226** Posterior dislocation of unspecified sternoclavicular joint ▽

✓5ᵗʰ **S43.3 Subluxation and dislocation of other and unspecified parts of shoulder girdle**

  ✓6ᵗʰ **S43.30 Subluxation and dislocation of unspecified parts of shoulder girdle**

    Dislocation of shoulder girdle NOS

    Subluxation of shoulder girdle NOS

    ✓7ᵗʰ **S43.301** Subluxation of unspecified parts of right shoulder girdle ▽

    ✓7ᵗʰ **S43.302** Subluxation of unspecified parts of left shoulder girdle ▽

    ✓7ᵗʰ **S43.303** Subluxation of unspecified parts of unspecified shoulder girdle ▽

    ✓7ᵗʰ **S43.304** Dislocation of unspecified parts of right shoulder girdle ▽

    ✓7ᵗʰ **S43.305** Dislocation of unspecified parts of left shoulder girdle ▽

    ✓7ᵗʰ **S43.306** Dislocation of unspecified parts of unspecified shoulder girdle ▽

  ✓6ᵗʰ **S43.31 Subluxation and dislocation of scapula**

    ✓7ᵗʰ **S43.311** Subluxation of right scapula

    ✓7ᵗʰ **S43.312** Subluxation of left scapula

    ✓7ᵗʰ **S43.313** Subluxation of unspecified scapula ▽

    ✓7ᵗʰ **S43.314** Dislocation of right scapula

    ✓7ᵗʰ **S43.315** Dislocation of left scapula

    ✓7ᵗʰ **S43.316** Dislocation of unspecified scapula ▽

  ✓6ᵗʰ **S43.39 Subluxation and dislocation of other parts of shoulder girdle**

    ✓7ᵗʰ **S43.391** Subluxation of other parts of right shoulder girdle

    ✓7ᵗʰ **S43.392** Subluxation of other parts of left shoulder girdle

    ✓7ᵗʰ **S43.393** Subluxation of other parts of unspecified shoulder girdle ▽

    ✓7ᵗʰ **S43.394** Dislocation of other parts of right shoulder girdle

    ✓7ᵗʰ **S43.395** Dislocation of other parts of left shoulder girdle

    ✓7ᵗʰ **S43.396** Dislocation of other parts of unspecified shoulder girdle ▽

✓5ᵗʰ **S43.4 Sprain of shoulder joint**

  ✓6ᵗʰ **S43.40 Unspecified sprain of shoulder joint**

    ✓7ᵗʰ **S43.401** Unspecified sprain of right shoulder joint ▽

    ✓7ᵗʰ **S43.402** Unspecified sprain of left shoulder joint ▽

    ✓7ᵗʰ **S43.409** Unspecified sprain of unspecified shoulder joint ▽

  ✓6ᵗʰ **S43.41 Sprain of coracohumeral (ligament)**

    ✓7ᵗʰ **S43.411** Sprain of right coracohumeral (ligament)

    ✓7ᵗʰ **S43.412** Sprain of left coracohumeral (ligament)

    ✓7ᵗʰ **S43.419** Sprain of unspecified coracohumeral (ligament) ▽

☑ Additional Character Req   ✓7ᵗʰ Placeholder Alert   Manifestation   HCC CMS-HCC Condition   ▽ Unspecified Code   ▶◀ Revised Text   ● New Code   ▲ Revised Code Title

ICD-10-CM 2018   **959**

√6ᵗʰ **S43.42** Sprain of **rotator cuff capsule**
   EXCLUDES 1 *rotator cuff syndrome (complete) (incomplete), not specified as traumatic (M75.1-)*
   EXCLUDES 2 *injury of tendon of rotator cuff (S46.0-)*
  √7ᵗʰ **S43.421** Sprain of **right** rotator cuff capsule
  √7ᵗʰ **S43.422** Sprain of **left** rotator cuff capsule
  √7ᵗʰ **S43.429** Sprain of unspecified rotator cuff capsule ▽

√6ᵗʰ **S43.43** **Superior glenoid labrum lesion**
   SLAP lesion
   DEF: Detachment injury of the superior aspect of the glenoid labrum, which is the ring of fibrocartilage attached to the rim of the glenoid cavity of the scapula.
  √7ᵗʰ **S43.431** Superior glenoid labrum lesion of **right** shoulder
  √7ᵗʰ **S43.432** Superior glenoid labrum lesion of **left** shoulder
  √7ᵗʰ **S43.439** Superior glenoid labrum lesion of unspecified shoulder ▽

√6ᵗʰ **S43.49** Other sprain of shoulder joint
  √7ᵗʰ **S43.491** Other sprain of **right** shoulder joint
  √7ᵗʰ **S43.492** Other sprain of **left** shoulder joint
  √7ᵗʰ **S43.499** Other sprain of unspecified shoulder joint ▽

√5ᵗʰ **S43.5** Sprain of **acromioclavicular** joint
  Sprain of acromioclavicular ligament
  √x7ᵗʰ **S43.50** Sprain of unspecified acromioclavicular joint ▽
  √x7ᵗʰ **S43.51** Sprain of **right** acromioclavicular joint
  √x7ᵗʰ **S43.52** Sprain of **left** acromioclavicular joint

√5ᵗʰ **S43.6** Sprain of **sternoclavicular** joint
  √x7ᵗʰ **S43.60** Sprain of unspecified sternoclavicular joint ▽
  √x7ᵗʰ **S43.61** Sprain of **right** sternoclavicular joint
  √x7ᵗʰ **S43.62** Sprain of **left** sternoclavicular joint

√5ᵗʰ **S43.8** Sprain of other specified parts of shoulder girdle
  √x7ᵗʰ **S43.80** Sprain of other specified parts of unspecified shoulder girdle ▽
  √x7ᵗʰ **S43.81** Sprain of other specified parts of **right** shoulder girdle
  √x7ᵗʰ **S43.82** Sprain of other specified parts of **left** shoulder girdle

√5ᵗʰ **S43.9** Sprain of unspecified parts of shoulder girdle
  √x7ᵗʰ **S43.90** Sprain of unspecified parts of unspecified shoulder girdle ▽
   Sprain of shoulder girdle NOS
  √x7ᵗʰ **S43.91** Sprain of unspecified parts of **right** shoulder girdle ▽
  √x7ᵗʰ **S43.92** Sprain of unspecified parts of **left** shoulder girdle ▽

√4ᵗʰ **S44** **Injury of nerves at shoulder and upper arm level**
  Code also any associated open wound (S41.-)
  EXCLUDES 2 *injury of brachial plexus (S14.3-)*

  The appropriate 7th character is to be added to each code from category S44.
  A   initial encounter
  D   subsequent encounter
  S   sequela

√5ᵗʰ **S44.0** Injury of **ulnar nerve** at upper arm level
   EXCLUDES 1 *ulnar nerve NOS (S54.0)*
  √x7ᵗʰ **S44.00** Injury of ulnar nerve at upper arm level, unspecified arm ▽
  √x7ᵗʰ **S44.01** Injury of ulnar nerve at upper arm level, **right** arm
  √x7ᵗʰ **S44.02** Injury of ulnar nerve at upper arm level, **left** arm

√5ᵗʰ **S44.1** Injury of **median nerve** at upper arm level
   EXCLUDES 1 *median nerve NOS (S54.1)*
  √x7ᵗʰ **S44.10** Injury of median nerve at upper arm level, unspecified arm ▽
  √x7ᵗʰ **S44.11** Injury of median nerve at upper arm level, **right** arm
  √x7ᵗʰ **S44.12** Injury of median nerve at upper arm level, **left** arm

√5ᵗʰ **S44.2** Injury of **radial nerve** at upper arm level
   EXCLUDES 1 *radial nerve NOS (S54.2)*
  √x7ᵗʰ **S44.20** Injury of radial nerve at upper arm level, unspecified arm ▽
  √x7ᵗʰ **S44.21** Injury of radial nerve at upper arm level, **right** arm

√x7ᵗʰ **S44.22** Injury of radial nerve at upper arm level, **left** arm

√5ᵗʰ **S44.3** Injury of **axillary nerve**
  √x7ᵗʰ **S44.30** Injury of axillary nerve, unspecified arm ▽
  √x7ᵗʰ **S44.31** Injury of axillary nerve, **right** arm
  √x7ᵗʰ **S44.32** Injury of axillary nerve, **left** arm

√5ᵗʰ **S44.4** Injury of **musculocutaneous nerve**
  √x7ᵗʰ **S44.40** Injury of musculocutaneous nerve, unspecified arm ▽
  √x7ᵗʰ **S44.41** Injury of musculocutaneous nerve, **right** arm
  √x7ᵗʰ **S44.42** Injury of musculocutaneous nerve, **left** arm

√5ᵗʰ **S44.5** Injury of **cutaneous sensory nerve** at shoulder and upper arm level
  √x7ᵗʰ **S44.50** Injury of cutaneous sensory nerve at shoulder and upper arm level, unspecified arm ▽
  √x7ᵗʰ **S44.51** Injury of cutaneous sensory nerve at shoulder and upper arm level, **right** arm
  √x7ᵗʰ **S44.52** Injury of cutaneous sensory nerve at shoulder and upper arm level, **left** arm

√5ᵗʰ **S44.8** Injury of other nerves at shoulder and upper arm level
  √6ᵗʰ **S44.8X** Injury of other nerves at shoulder and upper arm level
    √7ᵗʰ **S44.8X1** Injury of other nerves at shoulder and upper arm level, **right** arm
    √7ᵗʰ **S44.8X2** Injury of other nerves at shoulder and upper arm level, **left** arm
    √7ᵗʰ **S44.8X9** Injury of other nerves at shoulder and upper arm level, unspecified arm ▽

√5ᵗʰ **S44.9** Injury of unspecified nerve at shoulder and upper arm level
  √x7ᵗʰ **S44.90** Injury of unspecified nerve at shoulder and upper arm level, unspecified arm ▽
  √x7ᵗʰ **S44.91** Injury of unspecified nerve at shoulder and upper arm level, **right** arm ▽
  √x7ᵗʰ **S44.92** Injury of unspecified nerve at shoulder and upper arm level, **left** arm ▽

√4ᵗʰ **S45** **Injury of blood vessels at shoulder and upper arm level**
  Code also any associated open wound (S41.-)
  EXCLUDES 2 *injury of subclavian artery (S25.1)*
      injury of subclavian vein (S25.3)

  The appropriate 7th character is to be added to each code from category S45.
  A   initial encounter
  D   subsequent encounter
  S   sequela

√5ᵗʰ **S45.0** Injury of **axillary artery**
  √6ᵗʰ **S45.00** Unspecified injury of axillary artery
    √7ᵗʰ **S45.001** Unspecified injury of axillary artery, **right** side ▽
    √7ᵗʰ **S45.002** Unspecified injury of axillary artery, **left** side ▽
    √7ᵗʰ **S45.009** Unspecified injury of axillary artery, unspecified side ▽
  √6ᵗʰ **S45.01** **Laceration** of axillary artery
    √7ᵗʰ **S45.011** Laceration of axillary artery, **right** side
    √7ᵗʰ **S45.012** Laceration of axillary artery, **left** side
    √7ᵗʰ **S45.019** Laceration of axillary artery, unspecified side ▽
  √6ᵗʰ **S45.09** Other specified injury of axillary artery
    √7ᵗʰ **S45.091** Other specified injury of axillary artery, **right** side
    √7ᵗʰ **S45.092** Other specified injury of axillary artery, **left** side
    √7ᵗʰ **S45.099** Other specified injury of axillary artery, unspecified side ▽

√5ᵗʰ **S45.1** Injury of **brachial artery**
  √6ᵗʰ **S45.10** Unspecified injury of brachial artery
    √7ᵗʰ **S45.101** Unspecified injury of brachial artery, **right** side ▽
    √7ᵗʰ **S45.102** Unspecified injury of brachial artery, **left** side ▽
    √7ᵗʰ **S45.109** Unspecified injury of brachial artery, unspecified side ▽

√6ᵗʰ **S45.11** Laceration of brachial artery
     √7ᵗʰ **S45.111** Laceration of brachial artery, right side
     √7ᵗʰ **S45.112** Laceration of brachial artery, left side
     √7ᵗʰ **S45.119** Laceration of brachial artery, unspecified side ▽

√6ᵗʰ **S45.19** Other specified injury of brachial artery
     √7ᵗʰ **S45.191** Other specified injury of brachial artery, right side
     √7ᵗʰ **S45.192** Other specified injury of brachial artery, left side
     √7ᵗʰ **S45.199** Other specified injury of brachial artery, unspecified side ▽

√5ᵗʰ **S45.2** Injury of axillary or brachial vein

√6ᵗʰ **S45.20** Unspecified injury of axillary or brachial vein
     √7ᵗʰ **S45.201** Unspecified injury of axillary or brachial vein, right side ▽
     √7ᵗʰ **S45.202** Unspecified injury of axillary or brachial vein, left side ▽
     √7ᵗʰ **S45.209** Unspecified injury of axillary or brachial vein, unspecified side ▽

√6ᵗʰ **S45.21** Laceration of axillary or brachial vein
     √7ᵗʰ **S45.211** Laceration of axillary or brachial vein, right side
     √7ᵗʰ **S45.212** Laceration of axillary or brachial vein, left side
     √7ᵗʰ **S45.219** Laceration of axillary or brachial vein, unspecified side ▽

√6ᵗʰ **S45.29** Other specified injury of axillary or brachial vein
     √7ᵗʰ **S45.291** Other specified injury of axillary or brachial vein, right side
     √7ᵗʰ **S45.292** Other specified injury of axillary or brachial vein, left side
     √7ᵗʰ **S45.299** Other specified injury of axillary or brachial vein, unspecified side ▽

√5ᵗʰ **S45.3** Injury of superficial vein at shoulder and upper arm level

√6ᵗʰ **S45.30** Unspecified injury of superficial vein at shoulder and upper arm level
     √7ᵗʰ **S45.301** Unspecified injury of superficial vein at shoulder and upper arm level, right arm ▽
     √7ᵗʰ **S45.302** Unspecified injury of superficial vein at shoulder and upper arm level, left arm ▽
     √7ᵗʰ **S45.309** Unspecified injury of superficial vein at shoulder and upper arm level, unspecified arm ▽

√6ᵗʰ **S45.31** Laceration of superficial vein at shoulder and upper arm level
     √7ᵗʰ **S45.311** Laceration of superficial vein at shoulder and upper arm level, right arm
     √7ᵗʰ **S45.312** Laceration of superficial vein at shoulder and upper arm level, left arm
     √7ᵗʰ **S45.319** Laceration of superficial vein at shoulder and upper arm level, unspecified arm ▽

√6ᵗʰ **S45.39** Other specified injury of superficial vein at shoulder and upper arm level
     √7ᵗʰ **S45.391** Other specified injury of superficial vein at shoulder and upper arm level, right arm
     √7ᵗʰ **S45.392** Other specified injury of superficial vein at shoulder and upper arm level, left arm
     √7ᵗʰ **S45.399** Other specified injury of superficial vein at shoulder and upper arm level, unspecified arm ▽

√5ᵗʰ **S45.8** Injury of other specified blood vessels at shoulder and upper arm level

√6ᵗʰ **S45.80** Unspecified injury of other specified blood vessels at shoulder and upper arm level
     √7ᵗʰ **S45.801** Unspecified injury of other specified blood vessels at shoulder and upper arm level, right arm ▽
     √7ᵗʰ **S45.802** Unspecified injury of other specified blood vessels at shoulder and upper arm level, left arm ▽

     √7ᵗʰ **S45.809** Unspecified injury of other specified blood vessels at shoulder and upper arm level, unspecified arm ▽

√6ᵗʰ **S45.81** Laceration of other specified blood vessels at shoulder and upper arm level
     √7ᵗʰ **S45.811** Laceration of other specified blood vessels at shoulder and upper arm level, right arm
     √7ᵗʰ **S45.812** Laceration of other specified blood vessels at shoulder and upper arm level, left arm
     √7ᵗʰ **S45.819** Laceration of other specified blood vessels at shoulder and upper arm level, unspecified arm ▽

√6ᵗʰ **S45.89** Other specified injury of other specified blood vessels at shoulder and upper arm level
     √7ᵗʰ **S45.891** Other specified injury of other specified blood vessels at shoulder and upper arm level, right arm
     √7ᵗʰ **S45.892** Other specified injury of other specified blood vessels at shoulder and upper arm level, left arm
     √7ᵗʰ **S45.899** Other specified injury of other specified blood vessels at shoulder and upper arm level, unspecified arm ▽

√5ᵗʰ **S45.9** Injury of unspecified blood vessel at shoulder and upper arm level

√6ᵗʰ **S45.90** Unspecified injury of unspecified blood vessel at shoulder and upper arm level
     √7ᵗʰ **S45.901** Unspecified injury of unspecified blood vessel at shoulder and upper arm level, right arm ▽
     √7ᵗʰ **S45.902** Unspecified injury of unspecified blood vessel at shoulder and upper arm level, left arm ▽
     √7ᵗʰ **S45.909** Unspecified injury of unspecified blood vessel at shoulder and upper arm level, unspecified arm ▽

√6ᵗʰ **S45.91** Laceration of unspecified blood vessel at shoulder and upper arm level
     √7ᵗʰ **S45.911** Laceration of unspecified blood vessel at shoulder and upper arm level, right arm ▽
     √7ᵗʰ **S45.912** Laceration of unspecified blood vessel at shoulder and upper arm level, left arm ▽
     √7ᵗʰ **S45.919** Laceration of unspecified blood vessel at shoulder and upper arm level, unspecified arm ▽

√6ᵗʰ **S45.99** Other specified injury of unspecified blood vessel at shoulder and upper arm level
     √7ᵗʰ **S45.991** Other specified injury of unspecified blood vessel at shoulder and upper arm level, right arm ▽
     √7ᵗʰ **S45.992** Other specified injury of unspecified blood vessel at shoulder and upper arm level, left arm ▽
     √7ᵗʰ **S45.999** Other specified injury of unspecified blood vessel at shoulder and upper arm level, unspecified arm ▽

√4ᵗʰ **S46** Injury of muscle, fascia and tendon at shoulder and upper arm level
    Code also any associated open wound (S41.-)
    EXCLUDES 2 injury of muscle, fascia and tendon at elbow (S56.-)
           sprain of joints and ligaments of shoulder girdle (S43.9)
    TIP: Refer to the Muscle/Tendon table at the beginning of this chapter.

    The appropriate 7th character is to be added to each code from category S46.
    A   initial encounter
    D   subsequent encounter
    S   sequela

√5ᵗʰ **S46.0** Injury of muscle(s) and tendon(s) of the rotator cuff of shoulder

√6ᵗʰ **S46.00** Unspecified injury of muscle(s) and tendon(s) of the rotator cuff of shoulder
     √7ᵗʰ **S46.001** Unspecified injury of muscle(s) and tendon(s) of the rotator cuff of right shoulder ▽
     √7ᵗʰ **S46.002** Unspecified injury of muscle(s) and tendon(s) of the rotator cuff of left shoulder ▽

√ Additional Character Req   √x7ᵗʰ Placeholder Alert   Manifestation   ℍℂℂ CMS-HCC Condition   ▽ Unspecified Code   ▶◀ Revised Text   ● New Code   ▲ Revised Code Title

✓7ᵗʰ **S46.009** Unspecified injury of muscle(s) and tendon(s) of the rotator cuff of unspecified shoulder ▽

✓6ᵗʰ **S46.01** Strain of muscle(s) and tendon(s) of the rotator cuff of shoulder

✓7ᵗʰ **S46.011** Strain of muscle(s) and tendon(s) of the rotator cuff of right shoulder

✓7ᵗʰ **S46.012** Strain of muscle(s) and tendon(s) of the rotator cuff of left shoulder

✓7ᵗʰ **S46.019** Strain of muscle(s) and tendon(s) of the rotator cuff of unspecified shoulder ▽

✓6ᵗʰ **S46.02** Laceration of muscle(s) and tendon(s) of the rotator cuff of shoulder

✓7ᵗʰ **S46.021** Laceration of muscle(s) and tendon(s) of the rotator cuff of right shoulder

✓7ᵗʰ **S46.022** Laceration of muscle(s) and tendon(s) of the rotator cuff of left shoulder

✓7ᵗʰ **S46.029** Laceration of muscle(s) and tendon(s) of the rotator cuff of unspecified shoulder ▽

✓6ᵗʰ **S46.09** Other injury of muscle(s) and tendon(s) of the rotator cuff of shoulder

✓7ᵗʰ **S46.091** Other injury of muscle(s) and tendon(s) of the rotator cuff of right shoulder

✓7ᵗʰ **S46.092** Other injury of muscle(s) and tendon(s) of the rotator cuff of left shoulder

✓7ᵗʰ **S46.099** Other injury of muscle(s) and tendon(s) of the rotator cuff of unspecified shoulder ▽

✓5ᵗʰ **S46.1** Injury of muscle, fascia and tendon of long head of biceps

✓6ᵗʰ **S46.10** Unspecified injury of muscle, fascia and tendon of long head of biceps

✓7ᵗʰ **S46.101** Unspecified injury of muscle, fascia and tendon of long head of biceps, right arm ▽

✓7ᵗʰ **S46.102** Unspecified injury of muscle, fascia and tendon of long head of biceps, left arm ▽

✓7ᵗʰ **S46.109** Unspecified injury of muscle, fascia and tendon of long head of biceps, unspecified arm ▽

✓6ᵗʰ **S46.11** Strain of muscle, fascia and tendon of long head of biceps

✓7ᵗʰ **S46.111** Strain of muscle, fascia and tendon of long head of biceps, right arm

✓7ᵗʰ **S46.112** Strain of muscle, fascia and tendon of long head of biceps, left arm

✓7ᵗʰ **S46.119** Strain of muscle, fascia and tendon of long head of biceps, unspecified arm ▽

✓6ᵗʰ **S46.12** Laceration of muscle, fascia and tendon of long head of biceps

✓7ᵗʰ **S46.121** Laceration of muscle, fascia and tendon of long head of biceps, right arm

✓7ᵗʰ **S46.122** Laceration of muscle, fascia and tendon of long head of biceps, left arm

✓7ᵗʰ **S46.129** Laceration of muscle, fascia and tendon of long head of biceps, unspecified arm ▽

✓6ᵗʰ **S46.19** Other injury of muscle, fascia and tendon of long head of biceps

✓7ᵗʰ **S46.191** Other injury of muscle, fascia and tendon of long head of biceps, right arm

✓7ᵗʰ **S46.192** Other injury of muscle, fascia and tendon of long head of biceps, left arm

✓7ᵗʰ **S46.199** Other injury of muscle, fascia and tendon of long head of biceps, unspecified arm ▽

✓5ᵗʰ **S46.2** Injury of muscle, fascia and tendon of other parts of biceps

✓6ᵗʰ **S46.20** Unspecified injury of muscle, fascia and tendon of other parts of biceps

✓7ᵗʰ **S46.201** Unspecified injury of muscle, fascia and tendon of other parts of biceps, right arm ▽

✓7ᵗʰ **S46.202** Unspecified injury of muscle, fascia and tendon of other parts of biceps, left arm ▽

✓7ᵗʰ **S46.209** Unspecified injury of muscle, fascia and tendon of other parts of biceps, unspecified arm ▽

✓6ᵗʰ **S46.21** Strain of muscle, fascia and tendon of other parts of biceps

✓7ᵗʰ **S46.211** Strain of muscle, fascia and tendon of other parts of biceps, right arm

✓7ᵗʰ **S46.212** Strain of muscle, fascia and tendon of other parts of biceps, left arm

✓7ᵗʰ **S46.219** Strain of muscle, fascia and tendon of other parts of biceps, unspecified arm ▽

✓6ᵗʰ **S46.22** Laceration of muscle, fascia and tendon of other parts of biceps

✓7ᵗʰ **S46.221** Laceration of muscle, fascia and tendon of other parts of biceps, right arm

✓7ᵗʰ **S46.222** Laceration of muscle, fascia and tendon of other parts of biceps, left arm

✓7ᵗʰ **S46.229** Laceration of muscle, fascia and tendon of other parts of biceps, unspecified arm ▽

✓6ᵗʰ **S46.29** Other injury of muscle, fascia and tendon of other parts of biceps

✓7ᵗʰ **S46.291** Other injury of muscle, fascia and tendon of other parts of biceps, right arm

✓7ᵗʰ **S46.292** Other injury of muscle, fascia and tendon of other parts of biceps, left arm

✓7ᵗʰ **S46.299** Other injury of muscle, fascia and tendon of other parts of biceps, unspecified arm ▽

✓5ᵗʰ **S46.3** Injury of muscle, fascia and tendon of triceps

✓6ᵗʰ **S46.30** Unspecified injury of muscle, fascia and tendon of triceps

✓7ᵗʰ **S46.301** Unspecified injury of muscle, fascia and tendon of triceps, right arm ▽

✓7ᵗʰ **S46.302** Unspecified injury of muscle, fascia and tendon of triceps, left arm ▽

✓7ᵗʰ **S46.309** Unspecified injury of muscle, fascia and tendon of triceps, unspecified arm ▽

✓6ᵗʰ **S46.31** Strain of muscle, fascia and tendon of triceps

✓7ᵗʰ **S46.311** Strain of muscle, fascia and tendon of triceps, right arm

✓7ᵗʰ **S46.312** Strain of muscle, fascia and tendon of triceps, left arm

✓7ᵗʰ **S46.319** Strain of muscle, fascia and tendon of triceps, unspecified arm ▽

✓6ᵗʰ **S46.32** Laceration of muscle, fascia and tendon of triceps

✓7ᵗʰ **S46.321** Laceration of muscle, fascia and tendon of triceps, right arm

✓7ᵗʰ **S46.322** Laceration of muscle, fascia and tendon of triceps, left arm

✓7ᵗʰ **S46.329** Laceration of muscle, fascia and tendon of triceps, unspecified arm ▽

✓6ᵗʰ **S46.39** Other injury of muscle, fascia and tendon of triceps

✓7ᵗʰ **S46.391** Other injury of muscle, fascia and tendon of triceps, right arm

✓7ᵗʰ **S46.392** Other injury of muscle, fascia and tendon of triceps, left arm

✓7ᵗʰ **S46.399** Other injury of muscle, fascia and tendon of triceps, unspecified arm ▽

✓5ᵗʰ **S46.8** Injury of other muscles, fascia and tendons at shoulder and upper arm level

✓6ᵗʰ **S46.80** Unspecified injury of other muscles, fascia and tendons at shoulder and upper arm level

✓7ᵗʰ **S46.801** Unspecified injury of other muscles, fascia and tendons at shoulder and upper arm level, right arm ▽

✓7ᵗʰ **S46.802** Unspecified injury of other muscles, fascia and tendons at shoulder and upper arm level, left arm ▽

✓7ᵗʰ **S46.809** Unspecified injury of other muscles, fascia and tendons at shoulder and upper arm level, unspecified arm ▽

✓6ᵗʰ **S46.81** Strain of other muscles, fascia and tendons at shoulder and upper arm level

✓7ᵗʰ **S46.811** Strain of other muscles, fascia and tendons at shoulder and upper arm level, right arm

✓7ᵗʰ **S46.812** Strain of other muscles, fascia and tendons at shoulder and upper arm level, left arm

EXCLUDES 1 Not coded here   **EXCLUDES 2** Not included here   N Newborn Age: 0   P Pediatric Age: 0-17   M Maternity Age: 12-55   A Adult Age: 15-124

962   ICD-10-CM 2018

✓7ᵗʰ **S46.819** Strain of other muscles, fascia and tendons at shoulder and upper arm level, unspecified arm ▽

✓6ᵗʰ **S46.82** Laceration of other muscles, fascia and tendons at shoulder and upper arm level

     ✓7ᵗʰ **S46.821** Laceration of other muscles, fascia and tendons at shoulder and upper arm level, right arm

     ✓7ᵗʰ **S46.822** Laceration of other muscles, fascia and tendons at shoulder and upper arm level, left arm

     ✓7ᵗʰ **S46.829** Laceration of other muscles, fascia and tendons at shoulder and upper arm level, unspecified arm ▽

✓6ᵗʰ **S46.89** Other injury of other muscles, fascia and tendons at shoulder and upper arm level

     ✓7ᵗʰ **S46.891** Other injury of other muscles, fascia and tendons at shoulder and upper arm level, right arm

     ✓7ᵗʰ **S46.892** Other injury of other muscles, fascia and tendons at shoulder and upper arm level, left arm

     ✓7ᵗʰ **S46.899** Other injury of other muscles, fascia and tendons at shoulder and upper arm level, unspecified arm ▽

✓5ᵗʰ **S46.9** Injury of unspecified muscle, fascia and tendon at shoulder and upper arm level

✓6ᵗʰ **S46.90** Unspecified injury of unspecified muscle, fascia and tendon at shoulder and upper arm level

     ✓7ᵗʰ **S46.901** Unspecified injury of unspecified muscle, fascia and tendon at shoulder and upper arm level, right arm ▽

     ✓7ᵗʰ **S46.902** Unspecified injury of unspecified muscle, fascia and tendon at shoulder and upper arm level, left arm ▽

     ✓7ᵗʰ **S46.909** Unspecified injury of unspecified muscle, fascia and tendon at shoulder and upper arm level, unspecified arm ▽

✓6ᵗʰ **S46.91** Strain of unspecified muscle, fascia and tendon at shoulder and upper arm level

     ✓7ᵗʰ **S46.911** Strain of unspecified muscle, fascia and tendon at shoulder and upper arm level, right arm ▽

     ✓7ᵗʰ **S46.912** Strain of unspecified muscle, fascia and tendon at shoulder and upper arm level, left arm ▽

     ✓7ᵗʰ **S46.919** Strain of unspecified muscle, fascia and tendon at shoulder and upper arm level, unspecified arm ▽

✓6ᵗʰ **S46.92** Laceration of unspecified muscle, fascia and tendon at shoulder and upper arm level

     ✓7ᵗʰ **S46.921** Laceration of unspecified muscle, fascia and tendon at shoulder and upper arm level, right arm ▽

     ✓7ᵗʰ **S46.922** Laceration of unspecified muscle, fascia and tendon at shoulder and upper arm level, left arm ▽

     ✓7ᵗʰ **S46.929** Laceration of unspecified muscle, fascia and tendon at shoulder and upper arm level, unspecified arm ▽

✓6ᵗʰ **S46.99** Other injury of unspecified muscle, fascia and tendon at shoulder and upper arm level

     ✓7ᵗʰ **S46.991** Other injury of unspecified muscle, fascia and tendon at shoulder and upper arm level, right arm ▽

     ✓7ᵗʰ **S46.992** Other injury of unspecified muscle, fascia and tendon at shoulder and upper arm level, left arm ▽

     ✓7ᵗʰ **S46.999** Other injury of unspecified muscle, fascia and tendon at shoulder and upper arm level, unspecified arm ▽

✓4ᵗʰ **S47 Crushing injury of shoulder and upper arm**
Use additional code for all associated injuries
EXCLUDES 2 crushing injury of elbow (S57.0-)

> The appropriate 7th character is to be added to each code from category S47.
> A   initial encounter
> D   subsequent encounter
> S   sequela

✓ₓ7ᵗʰ **S47.1** Crushing injury of right shoulder and upper arm

✓ₓ7ᵗʰ **S47.2** Crushing injury of left shoulder and upper arm

✓ₓ7ᵗʰ **S47.9** Crushing injury of shoulder and upper arm, unspecified arm ▽

✓4ᵗʰ **S48 Traumatic amputation of shoulder and upper arm**
An amputation not identified as partial or complete should be coded to complete.
EXCLUDES 1 traumatic amputation at elbow level (S58.0)

> The appropriate 7th character is to be added to each code from category S48.
> A   initial encounter
> D   subsequent encounter
> S   sequela

✓5ᵗʰ **S48.0** Traumatic amputation at shoulder joint

✓6ᵗʰ **S48.01** Complete traumatic amputation at shoulder joint

     2 ✓7ᵗʰ **S48.011** Complete traumatic amputation at right shoulder joint   HCC

     2 ✓7ᵗʰ **S48.012** Complete traumatic amputation at left shoulder joint   HCC

     2 ✓7ᵗʰ **S48.019** Complete traumatic amputation at unspecified shoulder joint   HCC ▽

✓6ᵗʰ **S48.02** Partial traumatic amputation at shoulder joint

     2 ✓7ᵗʰ **S48.021** Partial traumatic amputation at right shoulder joint   HCC

     2 ✓7ᵗʰ **S48.022** Partial traumatic amputation at left shoulder joint   HCC

     2 ✓7ᵗʰ **S48.029** Partial traumatic amputation at unspecified shoulder joint   HCC ▽

✓5ᵗʰ **S48.1** Traumatic amputation at level between shoulder and elbow

✓6ᵗʰ **S48.11** Complete traumatic amputation at level between shoulder and elbow

     2 ✓7ᵗʰ **S48.111** Complete traumatic amputation at level between right shoulder and elbow   HCC

     2 ✓7ᵗʰ **S48.112** Complete traumatic amputation at level between left shoulder and elbow   HCC

     2 ✓7ᵗʰ **S48.119** Complete traumatic amputation at level between unspecified shoulder and elbow   HCC ▽

✓6ᵗʰ **S48.12** Partial traumatic amputation at level between shoulder and elbow

     2 ✓7ᵗʰ **S48.121** Partial traumatic amputation at level between right shoulder and elbow   HCC

     2 ✓7ᵗʰ **S48.122** Partial traumatic amputation at level between left shoulder and elbow   HCC

     2 ✓7ᵗʰ **S48.129** Partial traumatic amputation at level between unspecified shoulder and elbow   HCC ▽

✓5ᵗʰ **S48.9** Traumatic amputation of shoulder and upper arm, level unspecified

✓6ᵗʰ **S48.91** Complete traumatic amputation of shoulder and upper arm, level unspecified

     2 ✓7ᵗʰ **S48.911** Complete traumatic amputation of right shoulder and upper arm, level unspecified   HCC ▽

     2 ✓7ᵗʰ **S48.912** Complete traumatic amputation of left shoulder and upper arm, level unspecified   HCC ▽

     2 ✓7ᵗʰ **S48.919** Complete traumatic amputation of unspecified shoulder and upper arm, level unspecified   HCC ▽

✓6ᵗʰ **S48.92** Partial traumatic amputation of shoulder and upper arm, level unspecified

     2 ✓7ᵗʰ **S48.921** Partial traumatic amputation of right shoulder and upper arm, level unspecified   HCC ▽

---

2   HCC with 7th character indicating initial encounter (A or B - specific to category) OR sequela.

✓ Additional Character Req   ✓ₓ7ᵗʰ Placeholder Alert   Manifestation   HCC CMS-HCC Condition   ▽ Unspecified Code   ▶◀ Revised Text   ● New Code   ▲ Revised Code Title

ICD-10-CM 2018   963

2 ✓7ᵗʰ **S48.922** **Partial traumatic amputation of left shoulder and upper arm, level unspecified** HCC ▽

2 ✓7ᵗʰ **S48.929** **Partial traumatic amputation of unspecified shoulder and upper arm, level unspecified** HCC ▽

✓4ᵗʰ **S49** **Other and unspecified injuries of shoulder and upper arm**

> The appropriate 7th character is to be added to each code from subcategories S49.0 and S49.1.
> A initial encounter for closed fracture
> D subsequent encounter for fracture with routine healing
> G subsequent encounter for fracture with delayed healing
> K subsequent encounter for fracture with nonunion
> P subsequent encounter for fracture with malunion
> S sequela

✓5ᵗʰ **S49.0** **Physeal fracture of upper end of humerus**

✓6ᵗʰ **S49.00** **Unspecified physeal fracture of upper end of humerus**

✓7ᵗʰ **S49.001** **Unspecified physeal fracture of upper end of humerus, right arm** ▽

✓7ᵗʰ **S49.002** **Unspecified physeal fracture of upper end of humerus, left arm** ▽

✓7ᵗʰ **S49.009** **Unspecified physeal fracture of upper end of humerus, unspecified arm** ▽

✓6ᵗʰ **S49.01** **Salter-Harris Type I physeal fracture of upper end of humerus**

✓7ᵗʰ **S49.011** **Salter-Harris Type I physeal fracture of upper end of humerus, right arm**

✓7ᵗʰ **S49.012** **Salter-Harris Type I physeal fracture of upper end of humerus, left arm**

✓7ᵗʰ **S49.019** **Salter-Harris Type I physeal fracture of upper end of humerus, unspecified arm** ▽

✓6ᵗʰ **S49.02** **Salter-Harris Type II physeal fracture of upper end of humerus**

✓7ᵗʰ **S49.021** **Salter-Harris Type II physeal fracture of upper end of humerus, right arm**

✓7ᵗʰ **S49.022** **Salter-Harris Type II physeal fracture of upper end of humerus, left arm**

✓7ᵗʰ **S49.029** **Salter-Harris Type II physeal fracture of upper end of humerus, unspecified arm** ▽

✓6ᵗʰ **S49.03** **Salter-Harris Type III physeal fracture of upper end of humerus**

✓7ᵗʰ **S49.031** **Salter-Harris Type III physeal fracture of upper end of humerus, right arm**

✓7ᵗʰ **S49.032** **Salter-Harris Type III physeal fracture of upper end of humerus, left arm**

✓7ᵗʰ **S49.039** **Salter-Harris Type III physeal fracture of upper end of humerus, unspecified arm** ▽

✓6ᵗʰ **S49.04** **Salter-Harris Type IV physeal fracture of upper end of humerus**

✓7ᵗʰ **S49.041** **Salter-Harris Type IV physeal fracture of upper end of humerus, right arm**

✓7ᵗʰ **S49.042** **Salter-Harris Type IV physeal fracture of upper end of humerus, left arm**

✓7ᵗʰ **S49.049** **Salter-Harris Type IV physeal fracture of upper end of humerus, unspecified arm** ▽

✓6ᵗʰ **S49.09** **Other physeal fracture of upper end of humerus**

✓7ᵗʰ **S49.091** **Other physeal fracture of upper end of humerus, right arm**

✓7ᵗʰ **S49.092** **Other physeal fracture of upper end of humerus, left arm**

✓7ᵗʰ **S49.099** **Other physeal fracture of upper end of humerus, unspecified arm** ▽

✓5ᵗʰ **S49.1** **Physeal fracture of lower end of humerus**

✓6ᵗʰ **S49.10** **Unspecified physeal fracture of lower end of humerus**

✓7ᵗʰ **S49.101** **Unspecified physeal fracture of lower end of humerus, right arm** ▽

✓7ᵗʰ **S49.102** **Unspecified physeal fracture of lower end of humerus, left arm** ▽

✓7ᵗʰ **S49.109** **Unspecified physeal fracture of lower end of humerus, unspecified arm** ▽

✓6ᵗʰ **S49.11** **Salter-Harris Type I physeal fracture of lower end of humerus**

✓7ᵗʰ **S49.111** **Salter-Harris Type I physeal fracture of lower end of humerus, right arm**

✓7ᵗʰ **S49.112** **Salter-Harris Type I physeal fracture of lower end of humerus, left arm**

✓7ᵗʰ **S49.119** **Salter-Harris Type I physeal fracture of lower end of humerus, unspecified arm** ▽

✓6ᵗʰ **S49.12** **Salter-Harris Type II physeal fracture of lower end of humerus**

✓7ᵗʰ **S49.121** **Salter-Harris Type II physeal fracture of lower end of humerus, right arm**

✓7ᵗʰ **S49.122** **Salter-Harris Type II physeal fracture of lower end of humerus, left arm**

✓7ᵗʰ **S49.129** **Salter-Harris Type II physeal fracture of lower end of humerus, unspecified arm** ▽

✓6ᵗʰ **S49.13** **Salter Harris Type III physeal fracture of lower end of humerus**

✓7ᵗʰ **S49.131** **Salter-Harris Type III physeal fracture of lower end of humerus, right arm**

✓7ᵗʰ **S49.132** **Salter-Harris Type III physeal fracture of lower end of humerus, left arm**

✓7ᵗʰ **S49.139** **Salter-Harris Type III physeal fracture of lower end of humerus, unspecified arm** ▽

✓6ᵗʰ **S49.14** **Salter-Harris Type IV physeal fracture of lower end of humerus**

✓7ᵗʰ **S49.141** **Salter-Harris Type IV physeal fracture of lower end of humerus, right arm**

✓7ᵗʰ **S49.142** **Salter-Harris Type IV physeal fracture of lower end of humerus, left arm**

✓7ᵗʰ **S49.149** **Salter-Harris Type IV physeal fracture of lower end of humerus, unspecified arm** ▽

✓6ᵗʰ **S49.19** **Other physeal fracture of lower end of humerus**

✓7ᵗʰ **S49.191** **Other physeal fracture of lower end of humerus, right arm**

✓7ᵗʰ **S49.192** **Other physeal fracture of lower end of humerus, left arm**

✓7ᵗʰ **S49.199** **Other physeal fracture of lower end of humerus, unspecified arm** ▽

✓5ᵗʰ **S49.8** **Other specified injuries of shoulder and upper arm**

> The appropriate 7th character is to be added to each code in subcategory S49.8.
> A initial encounter
> D subsequent encounter
> S sequela

✓x7ᵗʰ **S49.80** **Other specified injuries of shoulder and upper arm, unspecified arm** ▽

✓x7ᵗʰ **S49.81** **Other specified injuries of right shoulder and upper arm**

✓x7ᵗʰ **S49.82** **Other specified injuries of left shoulder and upper arm**

✓5ᵗʰ **S49.9** **Unspecified injury of shoulder and upper arm**

> The appropriate 7th character is to be added to each code in subcategory S49.9.
> A initial encounter
> D subsequent encounter
> S sequela

✓x7ᵗʰ **S49.90** **Unspecified injury of shoulder and upper arm, unspecified arm** ▽

✓x7ᵗʰ **S49.91** **Unspecified injury of right shoulder and upper arm** ▽

✓x7ᵗʰ **S49.92** **Unspecified injury of left shoulder and upper arm** ▽

---

2 HCC with 7th character indicating initial encounter (A or B - specific to category) OR sequela.

EXCLUDES 1 Not coded here   EXCLUDES 2 Not included here   N Newborn Age: 0   P Pediatric Age: 0-17   M Maternity Age: 12-55   A Adult Age: 15-124

Injuries to the elbow and forearm (S50-S59)

EXCLUDES 2 burns and corrosions (T20-T32)
   frostbite (T33-T34)
   injuries of wrist and hand (S60-S69)
   insect bite or sting, venomous (T63.4)

√4th **S50   Superficial injury of elbow and forearm**
   EXCLUDES 2   superficial injury of wrist and hand (S60.-)

   The appropriate 7th character is to be added to each code from
   category S50.
   A   initial encounter
   D   subsequent encounter
   S   sequela

√5th **S50.0   Contusion of elbow**
   √x7th **S50.00   Contusion of unspecified elbow**   ▽
   √x7th **S50.01   Contusion of right elbow**
   √x7th **S50.02   Contusion of left elbow**

√5th **S50.1   Contusion of forearm**
   √x7th **S50.10   Contusion of unspecified forearm**   ▽
   √x7th **S50.11   Contusion of right forearm**
   √x7th **S50.12   Contusion of left forearm**

√5th **S50.3   Other superficial injuries of elbow**
   √6th **S50.31   Abrasion of elbow**
      √7th **S50.311   Abrasion of right elbow**
      √7th **S50.312   Abrasion of left elbow**
      √7th **S50.319   Abrasion of unspecified elbow**   ▽
   √6th **S50.32   Blister (nonthermal) of elbow**
      √7th **S50.321   Blister (nonthermal) of right elbow**
      √7th **S50.322   Blister (nonthermal) of left elbow**
      √7th **S50.329   Blister (nonthermal) of unspecified   ▽
         elbow**
   √6th **S50.34   External constriction of elbow**
      √7th **S50.341   External constriction of right elbow**
      √7th **S50.342   External constriction of left elbow**
      √7th **S50.349   External constriction of unspecified   ▽
         elbow**
   √6th **S50.35   Superficial foreign body of elbow**
         Splinter in the elbow
      √7th **S50.351   Superficial foreign body of right elbow**
      √7th **S50.352   Superficial foreign body of left elbow**
      √7th **S50.359   Superficial foreign body of unspecified   ▽
         elbow**
   √6th **S50.36   Insect bite (nonvenomous) of elbow**
      √7th **S50.361   Insect bite (nonvenomous) of right elbow**
      √7th **S50.362   Insect bite (nonvenomous) of left elbow**
      √7th **S50.369   Insect bite (nonvenomous) of   ▽
         unspecified elbow**
   √6th **S50.37   Other superficial bite of elbow**
         EXCLUDES 1   open bite of elbow (S51.05)
      √7th **S50.371   Other superficial bite of right elbow**
      √7th **S50.372   Other superficial bite of left elbow**
      √7th **S50.379   Other superficial bite of unspecified   ▽
         elbow**

√5th **S50.8   Other superficial injuries of forearm**
   √6th **S50.81   Abrasion of forearm**
      √7th **S50.811   Abrasion of right forearm**
      √7th **S50.812   Abrasion of left forearm**
      √7th **S50.819   Abrasion of unspecified forearm**   ▽
   √6th **S50.82   Blister (nonthermal) of forearm**
      √7th **S50.821   Blister (nonthermal) of right forearm**
      √7th **S50.822   Blister (nonthermal) of left forearm**
      √7th **S50.829   Blister (nonthermal) of unspecified   ▽
         forearm**
   √6th **S50.84   External constriction of forearm**
      √7th **S50.841   External constriction of right forearm**
      √7th **S50.842   External constriction of left forearm**
      √7th **S50.849   External constriction of unspecified   ▽
         forearm**

   √6th **S50.85   Superficial foreign body of forearm**
         Splinter in the forearm
      √7th **S50.851   Superficial foreign body of right forearm**
      √7th **S50.852   Superficial foreign body of left forearm**
      √7th **S50.859   Superficial foreign body of unspecified   ▽
         forearm**
   √6th **S50.86   Insect bite (nonvenomous) of forearm**
      √7th **S50.861   Insect bite (nonvenomous) of right
         forearm**
      √7th **S50.862   Insect bite (nonvenomous) of left forearm**
      √7th **S50.869   Insect bite (nonvenomous) of   ▽
         unspecified forearm**
   √6th **S50.87   Other superficial bite of forearm**
         EXCLUDES 1   open bite of forearm (S51.85)
      √7th **S50.871   Other superficial bite of right forearm**
      √7th **S50.872   Other superficial bite of left forearm**
      √7th **S50.879   Other superficial bite of unspecified   ▽
         forearm**

√5th **S50.9   Unspecified superficial injury of elbow and forearm**
   √6th **S50.90   Unspecified superficial injury of elbow**
      √7th **S50.901   Unspecified superficial injury of right   ▽
         elbow**
      √7th **S50.902   Unspecified superficial injury of left   ▽
         elbow**
      √7th **S50.909   Unspecified superficial injury of   ▽
         unspecified elbow**
   √6th **S50.91   Unspecified superficial injury of forearm**
      √7th **S50.911   Unspecified superficial injury of right   ▽
         forearm**
      √7th **S50.912   Unspecified superficial injury of left   ▽
         forearm**
      √7th **S50.919   Unspecified superficial injury of   ▽
         unspecified forearm**

√4th **S51   Open wound of elbow and forearm**
   Code also any associated wound infection
   EXCLUDES 1   open fracture of elbow and forearm (S52- with open fracture 7th
      character)
      traumatic amputation of elbow and forearm (S58.-)
   EXCLUDES 2   open wound of wrist and hand (S61.-)

   The appropriate 7th character is to be added to each code from
   category S51.
   A   initial encounter
   D   subsequent encounter
   S   sequela

√5th **S51.0   Open wound of elbow**
   √6th **S51.00   Unspecified open wound of elbow**
      √7th **S51.001   Unspecified open wound of right elbow** ▽
         AHA: 2012, 4Q, 108
      √7th **S51.002   Unspecified open wound of left elbow**   ▽
      √7th **S51.009   Unspecified open wound of   ▽
         unspecified elbow**
         Open wound of elbow NOS
   √6th **S51.01   Laceration without foreign body of elbow**
      √7th **S51.011   Laceration without foreign body of right
         elbow**
      √7th **S51.012   Laceration without foreign body of left
         elbow**
      √7th **S51.019   Laceration without foreign body of   ▽
         unspecified elbow**
   √6th **S51.02   Laceration with foreign body of elbow**
      √7th **S51.021   Laceration with foreign body of right
         elbow**
      √7th **S51.022   Laceration with foreign body of left elbow**
      √7th **S51.029   Laceration with foreign body of   ▽
         unspecified elbow**
   √6th **S51.03   Puncture wound without foreign body of elbow**
      √7th **S51.031   Puncture wound without foreign body of
         right elbow**
      √7th **S51.032   Puncture wound without foreign body of
         left elbow**
      √7th **S51.039   Puncture wound without foreign   ▽
         body of unspecified elbow**

✓6ᵗʰ S51.04 Puncture wound with foreign body of elbow
- **✓7ᵗʰ S51.041** Puncture wound with foreign body of right elbow
- **✓7ᵗʰ S51.042** Puncture wound with foreign body of left elbow
- **✓7ᵗʰ S51.049** Puncture wound with foreign body of unspecified elbow ▽

✓6ᵗʰ S51.05 Open bite of elbow
Bite of elbow NOS
EXCLUDES 1   superficial bite of elbow (S50.36, S50.37)
- **✓7ᵗʰ S51.051** Open bite, right elbow
- **✓7ᵗʰ S51.052** Open bite, left elbow
- **✓7ᵗʰ S51.059** Open bite, unspecified elbow ▽

✓5ᵗʰ S51.8 Open wound of forearm
EXCLUDES 2   open wound of elbow (S51.0-)

✓6ᵗʰ S51.80 Unspecified open wound of forearm
AHA: 2016, 3Q, 24
- **✓7ᵗʰ S51.801** Unspecified open wound of right forearm ▽
- **✓7ᵗʰ S51.802** Unspecified open wound of left forearm ▽
- **✓7ᵗʰ S51.809** Unspecified open wound of unspecified forearm ▽
  Open wound of forearm NOS

✓6ᵗʰ S51.81 Laceration without foreign body of forearm
- **✓7ᵗʰ S51.811** Laceration without foreign body of right forearm
- **✓7ᵗʰ S51.812** Laceration without foreign body of left forearm
- **✓7ᵗʰ S51.819** Laceration without foreign body of unspecified forearm ▽

✓6ᵗʰ S51.82 Laceration with foreign body of forearm
- **✓7ᵗʰ S51.821** Laceration with foreign body of right forearm
- **✓7ᵗʰ S51.822** Laceration with foreign body of left forearm
- **✓7ᵗʰ S51.829** Laceration with foreign body of unspecified forearm ▽

✓6ᵗʰ S51.83 Puncture wound without foreign body of forearm
AHA: 2016, 3Q, 24
- **✓7ᵗʰ S51.831** Puncture wound without foreign body of right forearm
- **✓7ᵗʰ S51.832** Puncture wound without foreign body of left forearm
- **✓7ᵗʰ S51.839** Puncture wound without foreign body of unspecified forearm ▽

✓6ᵗʰ S51.84 Puncture wound with foreign body of forearm
AHA: 2016, 3Q, 24
- **✓7ᵗʰ S51.841** Puncture wound with foreign body of right forearm
- **✓7ᵗʰ S51.842** Puncture wound with foreign body of left forearm
- **✓7ᵗʰ S51.849** Puncture wound with foreign body of unspecified forearm ▽

✓6ᵗʰ S51.85 Open bite of forearm
Bite of forearm NOS
EXCLUDES 1   superficial bite of forearm (S50.86, S50.87)
- **✓7ᵗʰ S51.851** Open bite of right forearm
- **✓7ᵗʰ S51.852** Open bite of left forearm
- **✓7ᵗʰ S51.859** Open bite of unspecified forearm ▽

✓4ᵗʰ S52 Fracture of forearm
NOTE   A fracture not indicated as displaced or nondisplaced should be coded to displaced.
A fracture not indicated as open or closed should be coded to closed.
The open fracture designations are based on the Gustilo open fracture classification.
EXCLUDES 1   traumatic amputation of forearm (S58.-)
EXCLUDES 2   fracture at wrist and hand level (S62.-)
AHA: 2016, 1Q, 33; 2015, 3Q, 37-39

The appropriate 7th character is to be added to all codes from category S52 [unless otherwise indicated].
A   initial encounter for closed fracture
B   initial encounter for open fracture type I or II
    initial encounter for open fracture NOS
C   initial encounter for open fracture type IIIA, IIIB, or IIIC
D   subsequent encounter for closed fracture with routine healing
E   subsequent encounter for open fracture type I or II with routine healing
F   subsequent encounter for open fracture type IIIA, IIIB, or IIIC with routine healing
G   subsequent encounter for closed fracture with delayed healing
H   subsequent encounter for open fracture type I or II with delayed healing
J   subsequent encounter for open fracture type IIIA, IIIB, or IIIC with delayed healing
K   subsequent encounter for closed fracture with nonunion
M   subsequent encounter for open fracture type I or II with nonunion
N   subsequent encounter for open fracture type IIIA, IIIB, or IIIC with nonunion
P   subsequent encounter for closed fracture with malunion
Q   subsequent encounter for open fracture type I or II with malunion
R   subsequent encounter for open fracture type IIIA, IIIB, or IIIC with malunion
S   sequela

✓5ᵗʰ S52.0 Fracture of upper end of ulna
Fracture of proximal end of ulna
EXCLUDES 2   fracture of elbow NOS (S42.40-)
    fractures of shaft of ulna (S52.2-)

✓6ᵗʰ S52.00 Unspecified fracture of upper end of ulna
- **✓7ᵗʰ S52.001** Unspecified fracture of upper end of right ulna ▽
- **✓7ᵗʰ S52.002** Unspecified fracture of upper end of left ulna ▽
- **✓7ᵗʰ S52.009** Unspecified fracture of upper end of unspecified ulna ▽

✓6ᵗʰ S52.01 Torus fracture of upper end of ulna

The appropriate 7th character is to be added to all codes in subcategory S52.01.
A   initial encounter for closed fracture
D   subsequent encounter for fracture with routine healing
G   subsequent encounter for fracture with delayed healing
K   subsequent encounter for fracture with nonunion
P   subsequent encounter for fracture with malunion
S   sequela

- **✓7ᵗʰ S52.011** Torus fracture of upper end of right ulna
- **✓7ᵗʰ S52.012** Torus fracture of upper end of left ulna
- **✓7ᵗʰ S52.019** Torus fracture of upper end of unspecified ulna ▽

✓6ᵗʰ S52.02 Fracture of olecranon process without intraarticular extension of ulna
- **✓7ᵗʰ S52.021** Displaced fracture of olecranon process without intraarticular extension of right ulna
- **✓7ᵗʰ S52.022** Displaced fracture of olecranon process without intraarticular extension of left ulna
- **✓7ᵗʰ S52.023** Displaced fracture of olecranon process without intraarticular extension of unspecified ulna ▽

√7ᵗʰ **S52.024** Nondisplaced fracture of olecranon process without intraarticular extension of right ulna

√7ᵗʰ **S52.025** Nondisplaced fracture of olecranon process without intraarticular extension of left ulna

√7ᵗʰ **S52.026** Nondisplaced fracture of olecranon ▽ process without intraarticular extension of unspecified ulna

√6ᵗʰ **S52.03** Fracture of olecranon process with intraarticular extension of ulna

√7ᵗʰ **S52.031** Displaced fracture of olecranon process with intraarticular extension of right ulna

√7ᵗʰ **S52.032** Displaced fracture of olecranon process with intraarticular extension of left ulna

√7ᵗʰ **S52.033** Displaced fracture of olecranon ▽ process with intraarticular extension of unspecified ulna

√7ᵗʰ **S52.034** Nondisplaced fracture of olecranon process with intraarticular extension of right ulna

√7ᵗʰ **S52.035** Nondisplaced fracture of olecranon process with intraarticular extension of left ulna

√7ᵗʰ **S52.036** Nondisplaced fracture of olecranon ▽ process with intraarticular extension of unspecified ulna

√6ᵗʰ **S52.04** Fracture of coronoid process of ulna

√7ᵗʰ **S52.041** Displaced fracture of coronoid process of right ulna

√7ᵗʰ **S52.042** Displaced fracture of coronoid process of left ulna

√7ᵗʰ **S52.043** Displaced fracture of coronoid process ▽ of unspecified ulna

√7ᵗʰ **S52.044** Nondisplaced fracture of coronoid process of right ulna

√7ᵗʰ **S52.045** Nondisplaced fracture of coronoid process of left ulna

√7ᵗʰ **S52.046** Nondisplaced fracture of coronoid ▽ process of unspecified ulna

√6ᵗʰ **S52.09** Other fracture of upper end of ulna

√7ᵗʰ **S52.091** Other fracture of upper end of right ulna

√7ᵗʰ **S52.092** Other fracture of upper end of left ulna

√7ᵗʰ **S52.099** Other fracture of upper end of ▽ unspecified ulna

√5ᵗʰ **S52.1** Fracture of upper end of radius
Fracture of proximal end of radius
EXCLUDES 2 *physeal fractures of upper end of radius (S59.2-)*
fracture of shaft of radius (S52.3-)

√6ᵗʰ **S52.10** Unspecified fracture of upper end of radius

√7ᵗʰ **S52.101** Unspecified fracture of upper end of ▽ right radius

√7ᵗʰ **S52.102** Unspecified fracture of upper end of ▽ left radius

√7ᵗʰ **S52.109** Unspecified fracture of upper end of ▽ unspecified radius

√6ᵗʰ **S52.11** Torus fracture of upper end of radius

The appropriate 7th character is to be added to all codes in subcategory S52.11.
A   initial encounter for closed fracture
D   subsequent encounter for fracture with routine healing
G   subsequent encounter for fracture with delayed healing
K   subsequent encounter for fracture with nonunion
P   subsequent encounter for fracture with malunion
S   sequela

√7ᵗʰ **S52.111** Torus fracture of upper end of right radius

√7ᵗʰ **S52.112** Torus fracture of upper end of left radius

√7ᵗʰ **S52.119** Torus fracture of upper end of ▽ unspecified radius

√6ᵗʰ **S52.12** Fracture of head of radius

√7ᵗʰ **S52.121** Displaced fracture of head of right radius

√7ᵗʰ **S52.122** Displaced fracture of head of left radius

√7ᵗʰ **S52.123** Displaced fracture of head of ▽ unspecified radius

√7ᵗʰ **S52.124** Nondisplaced fracture of head of right radius

√7ᵗʰ **S52.125** Nondisplaced fracture of head of left radius

√7ᵗʰ **S52.126** Nondisplaced fracture of head of ▽ unspecified radius

√6ᵗʰ **S52.13** Fracture of neck of radius

√7ᵗʰ **S52.131** Displaced fracture of neck of right radius

√7ᵗʰ **S52.132** Displaced fracture of neck of left radius

√7ᵗʰ **S52.133** Displaced fracture of neck of ▽ unspecified radius

√7ᵗʰ **S52.134** Nondisplaced fracture of neck of right radius

√7ᵗʰ **S52.135** Nondisplaced fracture of neck of left radius

√7ᵗʰ **S52.136** Nondisplaced fracture of neck of ▽ unspecified radius

√6ᵗʰ **S52.18** Other fracture of upper end of radius

√7ᵗʰ **S52.181** Other fracture of upper end of right radius

√7ᵗʰ **S52.182** Other fracture of upper end of left radius

√7ᵗʰ **S52.189** Other fracture of upper end of ▽ unspecified radius

√5ᵗʰ **S52.2** Fracture of shaft of ulna

√6ᵗʰ **S52.20** Unspecified fracture of shaft of ulna
Fracture of ulna NOS

√7ᵗʰ **S52.201** Unspecified fracture of shaft of right ▽ ulna

√7ᵗʰ **S52.202** Unspecified fracture of shaft of left ▽ ulna

√7ᵗʰ **S52.209** Unspecified fracture of shaft of ▽ unspecified ulna

√6ᵗʰ **S52.21** Greenstick fracture of shaft of ulna

The appropriate 7th character is to be added to all codes in subcategory S52.21.
A   initial encounter for closed fracture
D   subsequent encounter for fracture with routine healing
G   subsequent encounter for fracture with delayed healing
K   subsequent encounter for fracture with nonunion
P   subsequent encounter for fracture with malunion
S   sequela

√7ᵗʰ **S52.211** Greenstick fracture of shaft of right ulna

√7ᵗʰ **S52.212** Greenstick fracture of shaft of left ulna

√7ᵗʰ **S52.219** Greenstick fracture of shaft of ▽ unspecified ulna

√6ᵗʰ **S52.22** Transverse fracture of shaft of ulna

√7ᵗʰ **S52.221** Displaced transverse fracture of shaft of right ulna

√7ᵗʰ **S52.222** Displaced transverse fracture of shaft of left ulna

√7ᵗʰ **S52.223** Displaced transverse fracture of shaft ▽ of unspecified ulna

√7ᵗʰ **S52.224** Nondisplaced transverse fracture of shaft of right ulna

√7ᵗʰ **S52.225** Nondisplaced transverse fracture of shaft of left ulna

√7ᵗʰ **S52.226** Nondisplaced transverse fracture of ▽ shaft of unspecified ulna

√6ᵗʰ **S52.23** Oblique fracture of shaft of ulna

√7ᵗʰ **S52.231** Displaced oblique fracture of shaft of right ulna

√7ᵗʰ **S52.232** Displaced oblique fracture of shaft of left ulna

√7ᵗʰ **S52.233** Displaced oblique fracture of shaft of ▽ unspecified ulna

√7ᵗʰ **S52.234** Nondisplaced oblique fracture of shaft of right ulna

√7ᵗʰ **S52.235** Nondisplaced oblique fracture of shaft of left ulna

√7ᵗʰ **S52.236** Nondisplaced oblique fracture of shaft ▽ of unspecified ulna

√6ᵗʰ **S52.24** Spiral fracture of shaft of ulna

  √7ᵗʰ **S52.241** Displaced spiral fracture of shaft of ulna, right arm

  √7ᵗʰ **S52.242** Displaced spiral fracture of shaft of ulna, left arm

  √7ᵗʰ **S52.243** Displaced spiral fracture of shaft of ▽ ulna, unspecified arm

  √7ᵗʰ **S52.244** Nondisplaced spiral fracture of shaft of ulna, right arm

  √7ᵗʰ **S52.245** Nondisplaced spiral fracture of shaft of ulna, left arm

  √7ᵗʰ **S52.246** Nondisplaced spiral fracture of shaft ▽ of ulna, unspecified arm

√6ᵗʰ **S52.25** Comminuted fracture of shaft of ulna

  √7ᵗʰ **S52.251** Displaced comminuted fracture of shaft of ulna, right arm

  √7ᵗʰ **S52.252** Displaced comminuted fracture of shaft of ulna, left arm

  √7ᵗʰ **S52.253** Displaced comminuted fracture of ▽ shaft of ulna, unspecified arm

  √7ᵗʰ **S52.254** Nondisplaced comminuted fracture of shaft of ulna, right arm

  √7ᵗʰ **S52.255** Nondisplaced comminuted fracture of shaft of ulna, left arm

  √7ᵗʰ **S52.256** Nondisplaced comminuted fracture of ▽ shaft of ulna, unspecified arm

√6ᵗʰ **S52.26** Segmental fracture of shaft of ulna

  √7ᵗʰ **S52.261** Displaced segmental fracture of shaft of ulna, right arm

  √7ᵗʰ **S52.262** Displaced segmental fracture of shaft of ulna, left arm

  √7ᵗʰ **S52.263** Displaced segmental fracture of shaft ▽ of ulna, unspecified arm

  √7ᵗʰ **S52.264** Nondisplaced segmental fracture of shaft of ulna, right arm

  √7ᵗʰ **S52.265** Nondisplaced segmental fracture of shaft of ulna, left arm

  √7ᵗʰ **S52.266** Nondisplaced segmental fracture of ▽ shaft of ulna, unspecified arm

√6ᵗʰ **S52.27** Monteggia's fracture of ulna
    Fracture of upper shaft of ulna with dislocation of radial head

  √7ᵗʰ **S52.271** Monteggia's fracture of right ulna

  √7ᵗʰ **S52.272** Monteggia's fracture of left ulna

  √7ᵗʰ **S52.279** Monteggia's fracture of unspecified ▽ ulna

√6ᵗʰ **S52.28** Bent bone of ulna

  √7ᵗʰ **S52.281** Bent bone of right ulna

  √7ᵗʰ **S52.282** Bent bone of left ulna

  √7ᵗʰ **S52.283** Bent bone of unspecified ulna ▽

√6ᵗʰ **S52.29** Other fracture of shaft of ulna

  √7ᵗʰ **S52.291** Other fracture of shaft of right ulna

  √7ᵗʰ **S52.292** Other fracture of shaft of left ulna

  √7ᵗʰ **S52.299** Other fracture of shaft of unspecified ▽ ulna

√5ᵗʰ **S52.3** Fracture of shaft of radius

  √6ᵗʰ **S52.30** Unspecified fracture of shaft of radius

    √7ᵗʰ **S52.301** Unspecified fracture of shaft of right ▽ radius

    √7ᵗʰ **S52.302** Unspecified fracture of shaft of left ▽ radius

    √7ᵗʰ **S52.309** Unspecified fracture of shaft of ▽ unspecified radius

√6ᵗʰ **S52.31** Greenstick fracture of shaft of radius

> The appropriate 7th character is to be added to all codes in subcategory S52.31.
> A   initial encounter for closed fracture
> D   subsequent encounter for fracture with routine healing
> G   subsequent encounter for fracture with delayed healing
> K   subsequent encounter for fracture with nonunion
> P   subsequent encounter for fracture with malunion
> S   sequela

  √7ᵗʰ **S52.311** Greenstick fracture of shaft of radius, right arm

  √7ᵗʰ **S52.312** Greenstick fracture of shaft of radius, left arm

  √7ᵗʰ **S52.319** Greenstick fracture of shaft of radius, ▽ unspecified arm

√6ᵗʰ **S52.32** Transverse fracture of shaft of radius

  √7ᵗʰ **S52.321** Displaced transverse fracture of shaft of right radius

  √7ᵗʰ **S52.322** Displaced transverse fracture of shaft of left radius

  √7ᵗʰ **S52.323** Displaced transverse fracture of shaft ▽ of unspecified radius

  √7ᵗʰ **S52.324** Nondisplaced transverse fracture of shaft of right radius

  √7ᵗʰ **S52.325** Nondisplaced transverse fracture of shaft of left radius

  √7ᵗʰ **S52.326** Nondisplaced transverse fracture of ▽ shaft of unspecified radius

√6ᵗʰ **S52.33** Oblique fracture of shaft of radius

  √7ᵗʰ **S52.331** Displaced oblique fracture of shaft of right radius

  √7ᵗʰ **S52.332** Displaced oblique fracture of shaft of left radius

  √7ᵗʰ **S52.333** Displaced oblique fracture of shaft of ▽ unspecified radius

  √7ᵗʰ **S52.334** Nondisplaced oblique fracture of shaft of right radius

  √7ᵗʰ **S52.335** Nondisplaced oblique fracture of shaft of left radius

  √7ᵗʰ **S52.336** Nondisplaced oblique fracture of shaft ▽ of unspecified radius

√6ᵗʰ **S52.34** Spiral fracture of shaft of radius

  √7ᵗʰ **S52.341** Displaced spiral fracture of shaft of radius, right arm

  √7ᵗʰ **S52.342** Displaced spiral fracture of shaft of radius, left arm

  √7ᵗʰ **S52.343** Displaced spiral fracture of shaft of ▽ radius, unspecified arm

  √7ᵗʰ **S52.344** Nondisplaced spiral fracture of shaft of radius, right arm

  √7ᵗʰ **S52.345** Nondisplaced spiral fracture of shaft of radius, left arm

  √7ᵗʰ **S52.346** Nondisplaced spiral fracture of shaft ▽ of radius, unspecified arm

√6ᵗʰ **S52.35** Comminuted fracture of shaft of radius

  √7ᵗʰ **S52.351** Displaced comminuted fracture of shaft of radius, right arm

  √7ᵗʰ **S52.352** Displaced comminuted fracture of shaft of radius, left arm

  √7ᵗʰ **S52.353** Displaced comminuted fracture of ▽ shaft of radius, unspecified arm

  √7ᵗʰ **S52.354** Nondisplaced comminuted fracture of shaft of radius, right arm

  √7ᵗʰ **S52.355** Nondisplaced comminuted fracture of shaft of radius, left arm

  √7ᵗʰ **S52.356** Nondisplaced comminuted fracture ▽ of shaft of radius, unspecified arm

√6ᵗʰ **S52.36** Segmental fracture of shaft of radius

  √7ᵗʰ **S52.361** Displaced segmental fracture of shaft of radius, right arm

EXCLUDES 1 Not coded here   EXCLUDES 2 Not included here   N Newborn Age: 0   P Pediatric Age: 0-17   M Maternity Age: 12-55   A Adult Age: 15-124

968   ICD-10-CM 2018

☑7ᵗʰ **S52.362** Displaced segmental fracture of shaft of radius, left arm

☑7ᵗʰ **S52.363** Displaced segmental fracture of shaft of radius, unspecified arm ▽

☑7ᵗʰ **S52.364** Nondisplaced segmental fracture of shaft of radius, right arm

☑7ᵗʰ **S52.365** Nondisplaced segmental fracture of shaft of radius, left arm

☑7ᵗʰ **S52.366** Nondisplaced segmental fracture of shaft of radius, unspecified arm ▽

☑6ᵗʰ **S52.37** Galeazzi's fracture
Fracture of lower shaft of radius with radioulnar joint dislocation

☑7ᵗʰ **S52.371** Galeazzi's fracture of right radius

☑7ᵗʰ **S52.372** Galeazzi's fracture of left radius

☑7ᵗʰ **S52.379** Galeazzi's fracture of unspecified radius ▽

☑6ᵗʰ **S52.38** Bent bone of radius

☑7ᵗʰ **S52.381** Bent bone of right radius

☑7ᵗʰ **S52.382** Bent bone of left radius

☑7ᵗʰ **S52.389** Bent bone of unspecified radius ▽

☑6ᵗʰ **S52.39** Other fracture of shaft of radius

☑7ᵗʰ **S52.391** Other fracture of shaft of radius, right arm

☑7ᵗʰ **S52.392** Other fracture of shaft of radius, left arm

☑7ᵗʰ **S52.399** Other fracture of shaft of radius, unspecified arm ▽

☑5ᵗʰ **S52.5** Fracture of lower end of radius
Fracture of distal end of radius

     EXCLUDES 2   physeal fractures of lower end of radius (S59.2-)
       DEF: Fracture of distal end of radius above the wrist; most commonly caused by fall onto an outstretched hand.

☑6ᵗʰ **S52.50** Unspecified fracture of the lower end of radius

☑7ᵗʰ **S52.501** Unspecified fracture of the lower end of right radius ▽

☑7ᵗʰ **S52.502** Unspecified fracture of the lower end of left radius ▽

☑7ᵗʰ **S52.509** Unspecified fracture of the lower end of unspecified radius ▽

☑6ᵗʰ **S52.51** Fracture of radial styloid process

☑7ᵗʰ **S52.511** Displaced fracture of right radial styloid process

☑7ᵗʰ **S52.512** Displaced fracture of left radial styloid process

☑7ᵗʰ **S52.513** Displaced fracture of unspecified radial styloid process ▽

☑7ᵗʰ **S52.514** Nondisplaced fracture of right radial styloid process

☑7ᵗʰ **S52.515** Nondisplaced fracture of left radial styloid process

☑7ᵗʰ **S52.516** Nondisplaced fracture of unspecified radial styloid process ▽

☑6ᵗʰ **S52.52** Torus fracture of lower end of radius

The appropriate 7th character is to be added to all codes in subcategory S52.52.
A   initial encounter for closed fracture
D   subsequent encounter for fracture with routine healing
G   subsequent encounter for fracture with delayed healing
K   subsequent encounter for fracture with nonunion
P   subsequent encounter for fracture with malunion
S   sequela

☑7ᵗʰ **S52.521** Torus fracture of lower end of right radius

☑7ᵗʰ **S52.522** Torus fracture of lower end of left radius

☑7ᵗʰ **S52.529** Torus fracture of lower end of unspecified radius ▽

☑6ᵗʰ **S52.53** Colles' fracture
AHA: 2016, 2Q, 4

☑7ᵗʰ **S52.531** Colles' fracture of right radius

☑7ᵗʰ **S52.532** Colles' fracture of left radius

☑7ᵗʰ **S52.539** Colles' fracture of unspecified radius ▽

☑6ᵗʰ **S52.54** Smith's fracture

☑7ᵗʰ **S52.541** Smith's fracture of right radius

☑7ᵗʰ **S52.542** Smith's fracture of left radius

☑7ᵗʰ **S52.549** Smith's fracture of unspecified radius ▽

☑6ᵗʰ **S52.55** Other extraarticular fracture of lower end of radius

☑7ᵗʰ **S52.551** Other extraarticular fracture of lower end of right radius

☑7ᵗʰ **S52.552** Other extraarticular fracture of lower end of left radius

☑7ᵗʰ **S52.559** Other extraarticular fracture of lower end of unspecified radius ▽

☑6ᵗʰ **S52.56** Barton's fracture

☑7ᵗʰ **S52.561** Barton's fracture of right radius

☑7ᵗʰ **S52.562** Barton's fracture of left radius

☑7ᵗʰ **S52.569** Barton's fracture of unspecified radius ▽

☑6ᵗʰ **S52.57** Other intraarticular fracture of lower end of radius

☑7ᵗʰ **S52.571** Other intraarticular fracture of lower end of right radius

☑7ᵗʰ **S52.572** Other intraarticular fracture of lower end of left radius

☑7ᵗʰ **S52.579** Other intraarticular fracture of lower end of unspecified radius ▽

☑6ᵗʰ **S52.59** Other fractures of lower end of radius

☑7ᵗʰ **S52.591** Other fractures of lower end of right radius

☑7ᵗʰ **S52.592** Other fractures of lower end of left radius

☑7ᵗʰ **S52.599** Other fractures of lower end of unspecified radius ▽

☑5ᵗʰ **S52.6** Fracture of lower end of ulna

☑6ᵗʰ **S52.60** Unspecified fracture of lower end of ulna

☑7ᵗʰ **S52.601** Unspecified fracture of lower end of right ulna ▽

☑7ᵗʰ **S52.602** Unspecified fracture of lower end of left ulna ▽

☑7ᵗʰ **S52.609** Unspecified fracture of lower end of unspecified ulna ▽

☑6ᵗʰ **S52.61** Fracture of ulna styloid process

☑7ᵗʰ **S52.611** Displaced fracture of right ulna styloid process

☑7ᵗʰ **S52.612** Displaced fracture of left ulna styloid process

☑7ᵗʰ **S52.613** Displaced fracture of unspecified ulna styloid process ▽

☑7ᵗʰ **S52.614** Nondisplaced fracture of right ulna styloid process

☑7ᵗʰ **S52.615** Nondisplaced fracture of left ulna styloid process

☑7ᵗʰ **S52.616** Nondisplaced fracture of unspecified ulna styloid process ▽

☑6ᵗʰ **S52.62** Torus fracture of lower end of ulna

The appropriate 7th character is to be added to all codes in subcategory S52.62.
A   initial encounter for closed fracture
D   subsequent encounter for fracture with routine healing
G   subsequent encounter for fracture with delayed healing
K   subsequent encounter for fracture with nonunion
P   subsequent encounter for fracture with malunion
S   sequela

☑7ᵗʰ **S52.621** Torus fracture of lower end of right ulna

☑7ᵗʰ **S52.622** Torus fracture of lower end of left ulna

☑7ᵗʰ **S52.629** Torus fracture of lower end of unspecified ulna ▽

☑6ᵗʰ **S52.69** Other fracture of lower end of ulna

☑7ᵗʰ **S52.691** Other fracture of lower end of right ulna

☑7ᵗʰ **S52.692** Other fracture of lower end of left ulna

☑7ᵗʰ **S52.699** Other fracture of lower end of unspecified ulna ▽

☑ Additional Character Req   ☑7ᵗʰ Placeholder Alert   Manifestation   **HCC** CMS-HCC Condition   ▽ Unspecified Code   ▶◀ Revised Text   ● New Code   ▲ Revised Code Title

✓5ᵗʰ **S52.9** Unspecified fracture of forearm

 ✓x7ᵗʰ **S52.90** Unspecified fracture of unspecified forearm ▽

 ✓x7ᵗʰ **S52.91** Unspecified fracture of right forearm ▽

 ✓x7ᵗʰ **S52.92** Unspecified fracture of left forearm ▽

✓4ᵗʰ **S53** Dislocation and sprain of joints and ligaments of elbow

 INCLUDES avulsion of joint or ligament of elbow
laceration of cartilage, joint or ligament of elbow
sprain of cartilage, joint or ligament of elbow
traumatic hemarthrosis of joint or ligament of elbow
traumatic rupture of joint or ligament of elbow
traumatic subluxation of joint or ligament of elbow
traumatic tear of joint or ligament of elbow

Code also any associated open wound

EXCLUDES 2 *strain of muscle, fascia and tendon at forearm level (S56.-)*

The appropriate 7th character is to be added to each code from category S53.
A initial encounter
D subsequent encounter
S sequela

✓5ᵗʰ **S53.0** Subluxation and dislocation of radial head

 Dislocation of radiohumeral joint
 Subluxation of radiohumeral joint

 EXCLUDES 1 *Monteggia's fracture-dislocation (S52.27-)*

 ✓6ᵗʰ **S53.00** Unspecified subluxation and dislocation of radial head

  ✓7ᵗʰ **S53.001** Unspecified subluxation of right radial head ▽

  ✓7ᵗʰ **S53.002** Unspecified subluxation of left radial head ▽

  ✓7ᵗʰ **S53.003** Unspecified subluxation of unspecified radial head ▽

  ✓7ᵗʰ **S53.004** Unspecified dislocation of right radial head ▽

  ✓7ᵗʰ **S53.005** Unspecified dislocation of left radial head ▽

  ✓7ᵗʰ **S53.006** Unspecified dislocation of unspecified radial head ▽

 ✓6ᵗʰ **S53.01** Anterior subluxation and dislocation of radial head
  Anteriomedial subluxation and dislocation of radial head

  ✓7ᵗʰ **S53.011** Anterior subluxation of right radial head

  ✓7ᵗʰ **S53.012** Anterior subluxation of left radial head

  ✓7ᵗʰ **S53.013** Anterior subluxation of unspecified radial head ▽

  ✓7ᵗʰ **S53.014** Anterior dislocation of right radial head

  ✓7ᵗʰ **S53.015** Anterior dislocation of left radial head

  ✓7ᵗʰ **S53.016** Anterior dislocation of unspecified radial head ▽

 ✓6ᵗʰ **S53.02** Posterior subluxation and dislocation of radial head
  Posteriolateral subluxation and dislocation of radial head

  ✓7ᵗʰ **S53.021** Posterior subluxation of right radial head

  ✓7ᵗʰ **S53.022** Posterior subluxation of left radial head

  ✓7ᵗʰ **S53.023** Posterior subluxation of unspecified radial head ▽

  ✓7ᵗʰ **S53.024** Posterior dislocation of right radial head

  ✓7ᵗʰ **S53.025** Posterior dislocation of left radial head

  ✓7ᵗʰ **S53.026** Posterior dislocation of unspecified radial head ▽

 ✓6ᵗʰ **S53.03** Nursemaid's elbow

  ✓7ᵗʰ **S53.031** Nursemaid's elbow, right elbow

  ✓7ᵗʰ **S53.032** Nursemaid's elbow, left elbow

  ✓7ᵗʰ **S53.033** Nursemaid's elbow, unspecified elbow ▽

 ✓6ᵗʰ **S53.09** Other subluxation and dislocation of radial head

  ✓7ᵗʰ **S53.091** Other subluxation of right radial head

  ✓7ᵗʰ **S53.092** Other subluxation of left radial head

  ✓7ᵗʰ **S53.093** Other subluxation of unspecified radial head ▽

  ✓7ᵗʰ **S53.094** Other dislocation of right radial head

  ✓7ᵗʰ **S53.095** Other dislocation of left radial head

  ✓7ᵗʰ **S53.096** Other dislocation of unspecified radial head ▽

✓5ᵗʰ **S53.1** Subluxation and dislocation of ulnohumeral joint

 Subluxation and dislocation of elbow NOS

 EXCLUDES 1 *dislocation of radial head alone (S53.0-)*

 ✓6ᵗʰ **S53.10** Unspecified subluxation and dislocation of ulnohumeral joint

  ✓7ᵗʰ **S53.101** Unspecified subluxation of right ulnohumeral joint ▽

  ✓7ᵗʰ **S53.102** Unspecified subluxation of left ulnohumeral joint ▽

  ✓7ᵗʰ **S53.103** Unspecified subluxation of unspecified ulnohumeral joint ▽

  ✓7ᵗʰ **S53.104** Unspecified dislocation of right ulnohumeral joint ▽

  ✓7ᵗʰ **S53.105** Unspecified dislocation of left ulnohumeral joint ▽

  ✓7ᵗʰ **S53.106** Unspecified dislocation of unspecified ulnohumeral joint ▽

 ✓6ᵗʰ **S53.11** Anterior subluxation and dislocation of ulnohumeral joint

  ✓7ᵗʰ **S53.111** Anterior subluxation of right ulnohumeral joint

  ✓7ᵗʰ **S53.112** Anterior subluxation of left ulnohumeral joint

  ✓7ᵗʰ **S53.113** Anterior subluxation of unspecified ulnohumeral joint ▽

  ✓7ᵗʰ **S53.114** Anterior dislocation of right ulnohumeral joint
   AHA: 2012, 4Q, 108

  ✓7ᵗʰ **S53.115** Anterior dislocation of left ulnohumeral joint

  ✓7ᵗʰ **S53.116** Anterior dislocation of unspecified ulnohumeral joint ▽

 ✓6ᵗʰ **S53.12** Posterior subluxation and dislocation of ulnohumeral joint

  ✓7ᵗʰ **S53.121** Posterior subluxation of right ulnohumeral joint

  ✓7ᵗʰ **S53.122** Posterior subluxation of left ulnohumeral joint

  ✓7ᵗʰ **S53.123** Posterior subluxation of unspecified ulnohumeral joint ▽

  ✓7ᵗʰ **S53.124** Posterior dislocation of right ulnohumeral joint

  ✓7ᵗʰ **S53.125** Posterior dislocation of left ulnohumeral joint

  ✓7ᵗʰ **S53.126** Posterior dislocation of unspecified ulnohumeral joint ▽

 ✓6ᵗʰ **S53.13** Medial subluxation and dislocation of ulnohumeral joint

  ✓7ᵗʰ **S53.131** Medial subluxation of right ulnohumeral joint

  ✓7ᵗʰ **S53.132** Medial subluxation of left ulnohumeral joint

  ✓7ᵗʰ **S53.133** Medial subluxation of unspecified ulnohumeral joint ▽

  ✓7ᵗʰ **S53.134** Medial dislocation of right ulnohumeral joint

  ✓7ᵗʰ **S53.135** Medial dislocation of left ulnohumeral joint

  ✓7ᵗʰ **S53.136** Medial dislocation of unspecified ulnohumeral joint ▽

 ✓6ᵗʰ **S53.14** Lateral subluxation and dislocation of ulnohumeral joint

  ✓7ᵗʰ **S53.141** Lateral subluxation of right ulnohumeral joint

  ✓7ᵗʰ **S53.142** Lateral subluxation of left ulnohumeral joint

  ✓7ᵗʰ **S53.143** Lateral subluxation of unspecified ulnohumeral joint ▽

  ✓7ᵗʰ **S53.144** Lateral dislocation of right ulnohumeral joint

  ✓7ᵗʰ **S53.145** Lateral dislocation of left ulnohumeral joint

  ✓7ᵗʰ **S53.146** Lateral dislocation of unspecified ulnohumeral joint ▽

EXCLUDES 1 Not coded here EXCLUDES 2 Not included here N Newborn Age: 0 P Pediatric Age: 0-17 M Maternity Age: 12-55 A Adult Age: 15-124

970   ICD-10-CM 2018

√6ᵗʰ **S53.19** **Other subluxation and dislocation of ulnohumeral joint**

√7ᵗʰ **S53.191** Other subluxation of right ulnohumeral joint

√7ᵗʰ **S53.192** Other subluxation of left ulnohumeral joint

√7ᵗʰ **S53.193** Other subluxation of unspecified ▽ ulnohumeral joint

√7ᵗʰ **S53.194** Other dislocation of right ulnohumeral joint

√7ᵗʰ **S53.195** Other dislocation of left ulnohumeral joint

√7ᵗʰ **S53.196** Other dislocation of unspecified ▽ ulnohumeral joint

√5ᵗʰ **S53.2** **Traumatic rupture of radial collateral ligament**

     EXCLUDES 1   sprain of radial collateral ligament NOS (S53.43-)

√x7ᵗʰ **S53.20** Traumatic rupture of unspecified radial ▽ collateral ligament

√x7ᵗʰ **S53.21** Traumatic rupture of right radial collateral ligament

√x7ᵗʰ **S53.22** Traumatic rupture of left radial collateral ligament

√5ᵗʰ **S53.3** **Traumatic rupture of ulnar collateral ligament**

     EXCLUDES 1   sprain of ulnar collateral ligament (S53.44-)

√x7ᵗʰ **S53.30** Traumatic rupture of unspecified ulnar ▽ collateral ligament

√x7ᵗʰ **S53.31** Traumatic rupture of right ulnar collateral ligament

√x7ᵗʰ **S53.32** Traumatic rupture of left ulnar collateral ligament

√5ᵗʰ **S53.4** **Sprain of elbow**

     EXCLUDES 2   traumatic rupture of radial collateral ligament (S53.2-)
                  traumatic rupture of ulnar collateral ligament (S53.3-)

√6ᵗʰ **S53.40** **Unspecified sprain of elbow**

√7ᵗʰ **S53.401** Unspecified sprain of right elbow ▽

√7ᵗʰ **S53.402** Unspecified sprain of left elbow ▽

√7ᵗʰ **S53.409** Unspecified sprain of unspecified elbow ▽
           Sprain of elbow NOS

√6ᵗʰ **S53.41** **Radiohumeral (joint) sprain**

√7ᵗʰ **S53.411** Radiohumeral (joint) sprain of right elbow

√7ᵗʰ **S53.412** Radiohumeral (joint) sprain of left elbow

√7ᵗʰ **S53.419** Radiohumeral (joint) sprain of ▽ unspecified elbow

√6ᵗʰ **S53.42** **Ulnohumeral (joint) sprain**

√7ᵗʰ **S53.421** Ulnohumeral (joint) sprain of right elbow

√7ᵗʰ **S53.422** Ulnohumeral (joint) sprain of left elbow

√7ᵗʰ **S53.429** Ulnohumeral (joint) sprain of ▽ unspecified elbow

√6ᵗʰ **S53.43** **Radial collateral ligament sprain**

√7ᵗʰ **S53.431** Radial collateral ligament sprain of right elbow

√7ᵗʰ **S53.432** Radial collateral ligament sprain of left elbow

√7ᵗʰ **S53.439** Radial collateral ligament sprain of ▽ unspecified elbow

√6ᵗʰ **S53.44** **Ulnar collateral ligament sprain**

√7ᵗʰ **S53.441** Ulnar collateral ligament sprain of right elbow

√7ᵗʰ **S53.442** Ulnar collateral ligament sprain of left elbow

√7ᵗʰ **S53.449** Ulnar collateral ligament sprain of ▽ unspecified elbow

√6ᵗʰ **S53.49** **Other sprain of elbow**

√7ᵗʰ **S53.491** Other sprain of right elbow

√7ᵗʰ **S53.492** Other sprain of left elbow

√7ᵗʰ **S53.499** Other sprain of unspecified elbow ▽

√4ᵗʰ **S54** **Injury of nerves at forearm level**

     Code also any associated open wound (S51.-)

     EXCLUDES 2   injury of nerves at wrist and hand level (S64.-)

The appropriate 7th character is to be added to each code from category S54.
A   initial encounter
D   subsequent encounter
S   sequela

√5ᵗʰ **S54.0** **Injury of ulnar nerve at forearm level**
     Injury of ulnar nerve NOS

√x7ᵗʰ **S54.00** Injury of ulnar nerve at forearm level, ▽ unspecified arm

√x7ᵗʰ **S54.01** Injury of ulnar nerve at forearm level, right arm

√x7ᵗʰ **S54.02** Injury of ulnar nerve at forearm level, left arm

√5ᵗʰ **S54.1** **Injury of median nerve at forearm level**
     Injury of median nerve NOS

√x7ᵗʰ **S54.10** Injury of median nerve at forearm level, ▽ unspecified arm

√x7ᵗʰ **S54.11** Injury of median nerve at forearm level, right arm

√x7ᵗʰ **S54.12** Injury of median nerve at forearm level, left arm

√5ᵗʰ **S54.2** **Injury of radial nerve at forearm level**
     Injury of radial nerve NOS

√x7ᵗʰ **S54.20** Injury of radial nerve at forearm level, ▽ unspecified arm

√x7ᵗʰ **S54.21** Injury of radial nerve at forearm level, right arm

√x7ᵗʰ **S54.22** Injury of radial nerve at forearm level, left arm

√5ᵗʰ **S54.3** **Injury of cutaneous sensory nerve at forearm level**

√x7ᵗʰ **S54.30** Injury of cutaneous sensory nerve at forearm ▽ level, unspecified arm

√x7ᵗʰ **S54.31** Injury of cutaneous sensory nerve at forearm level, right arm

√x7ᵗʰ **S54.32** Injury of cutaneous sensory nerve at forearm level, left arm

√5ᵗʰ **S54.8** **Injury of other nerves at forearm level**

√6ᵗʰ **S54.8X** **Injury of other nerves at forearm level**

√7ᵗʰ **S54.8X1** Injury of other nerves at forearm level, right arm

√7ᵗʰ **S54.8X2** Injury of other nerves at forearm level, left arm

√7ᵗʰ **S54.8X9** Injury of other nerves at forearm level, ▽ unspecified arm

√5ᵗʰ **S54.9** **Injury of unspecified nerve at forearm level**

√x7ᵗʰ **S54.90** Injury of unspecified nerve at forearm level, ▽ unspecified arm

√x7ᵗʰ **S54.91** Injury of unspecified nerve at forearm level, ▽ right arm

√x7ᵗʰ **S54.92** Injury of unspecified nerve at forearm level, ▽ left arm

√4ᵗʰ **S55** **Injury of blood vessels at forearm level**

     Code also any associated open wound (S51.-)

     EXCLUDES 2   injury of blood vessels at wrist and hand level (S65.-)
                  injury of brachial vessels (S45.1-S45.2)

The appropriate 7th character is to be added to each code from category S55.
A   initial encounter
D   subsequent encounter
S   sequela

√5ᵗʰ **S55.0** **Injury of ulnar artery at forearm level**

√6ᵗʰ **S55.00** **Unspecified injury of ulnar artery at forearm level**

√7ᵗʰ **S55.001** Unspecified injury of ulnar artery at ▽ forearm level, right arm

√7ᵗʰ **S55.002** Unspecified injury of ulnar artery at ▽ forearm level, left arm

√7ᵗʰ **S55.009** Unspecified injury of ulnar artery at ▽ forearm level, unspecified arm

√6ᵗʰ **S55.01** **Laceration of ulnar artery at forearm level**

√7ᵗʰ **S55.011** Laceration of ulnar artery at forearm level, right arm

√7ᵗʰ **S55.012** Laceration of ulnar artery at forearm level, left arm

√7ᵗʰ **S55.019** Laceration of ulnar artery at forearm ▽ level, unspecified arm

☑ Additional Character Req   √x7ᵗʰ Placeholder Alert   Manifestation   HCC CMS-HCC Condition   ▽ Unspecified Code   ►◄ Revised Text   ● New Code   ▲ Revised Code Title

ICD-10-CM 2018   971

✓6th **S55.09** **Other specified injury of ulnar artery at forearm level**

✓7th **S55.091** Other specified injury of ulnar artery at forearm level, **right arm**

✓7th **S55.092** Other specified injury of ulnar artery at forearm level, **left arm**

✓7th **S55.099** Other specified injury of ulnar artery at forearm level, unspecified arm ▽

✓5th **S55.1** **Injury of radial artery at forearm level**

✓6th **S55.10** **Unspecified injury of radial artery at forearm level**

✓7th **S55.101** Unspecified injury of radial artery at forearm level, **right arm** ▽

✓7th **S55.102** Unspecified injury of radial artery at forearm level, **left arm** ▽

✓7th **S55.109** Unspecified injury of radial artery at forearm level, unspecified arm ▽

✓6th **S55.11** **Laceration of radial artery at forearm level**

✓7th **S55.111** Laceration of radial artery at forearm level, **right arm**

✓7th **S55.112** Laceration of radial artery at forearm level, **left arm**

✓7th **S55.119** Laceration of radial artery at forearm level, unspecified arm ▽

✓6th **S55.19** **Other specified injury of radial artery at forearm level**

✓7th **S55.191** Other specified injury of radial artery at forearm level, **right arm**

✓7th **S55.192** Other specified injury of radial artery at forearm level, **left arm**

✓7th **S55.199** Other specified injury of radial artery at forearm level, unspecified arm ▽

✓5th **S55.2** **Injury of vein at forearm level**

✓6th **S55.20** **Unspecified injury of vein at forearm level**

✓7th **S55.201** Unspecified injury of vein at forearm level, **right arm** ▽

✓7th **S55.202** Unspecified injury of vein at forearm level, **left arm** ▽

✓7th **S55.209** Unspecified injury of vein at forearm level, unspecified arm ▽

✓6th **S55.21** **Laceration of vein at forearm level**

✓7th **S55.211** Laceration of vein at forearm level, **right arm**

✓7th **S55.212** Laceration of vein at forearm level, **left arm**

✓7th **S55.219** Laceration of vein at forearm level, unspecified arm ▽

✓6th **S55.29** **Other specified injury of vein at forearm level**

✓7th **S55.291** Other specified injury of vein at forearm level, **right arm**

✓7th **S55.292** Other specified injury of vein at forearm level, **left arm**

✓7th **S55.299** Other specified injury of vein at forearm level, unspecified arm ▽

✓5th **S55.8** **Injury of other blood vessels at forearm level**

✓6th **S55.80** **Unspecified injury of other blood vessels at forearm level**

✓7th **S55.801** Unspecified injury of other blood vessels at forearm level, **right arm** ▽

✓7th **S55.802** Unspecified injury of other blood vessels at forearm level, **left arm** ▽

✓7th **S55.809** Unspecified injury of other blood vessels at forearm level, unspecified arm ▽

✓6th **S55.81** **Laceration of other blood vessels at forearm level**

✓7th **S55.811** Laceration of other blood vessels at forearm level, **right arm**

✓7th **S55.812** Laceration of other blood vessels at forearm level, **left arm**

✓7th **S55.819** Laceration of other blood vessels at forearm level, unspecified arm ▽

✓6th **S55.89** **Other specified injury of other blood vessels at forearm level**

✓7th **S55.891** Other specified injury of other blood vessels at forearm level, **right arm**

✓7th **S55.892** Other specified injury of other blood vessels at forearm level, **left arm**

✓7th **S55.899** Other specified injury of other blood vessels at forearm level, unspecified arm ▽

✓5th **S55.9** **Injury of unspecified blood vessel at forearm level**

✓6th **S55.90** **Unspecified injury of unspecified blood vessel at forearm level**

✓7th **S55.901** Unspecified injury of unspecified blood vessel at forearm level, **right arm** ▽

✓7th **S55.902** Unspecified injury of unspecified blood vessel at forearm level, **left arm** ▽

✓7th **S55.909** Unspecified injury of unspecified blood vessel at forearm level, unspecified arm ▽

✓6th **S55.91** **Laceration of unspecified blood vessel at forearm level**

✓7th **S55.911** Laceration of unspecified blood vessel at forearm level, **right arm** ▽

✓7th **S55.912** Laceration of unspecified blood vessel at forearm level, **left arm** ▽

✓7th **S55.919** Laceration of unspecified blood vessel at forearm level, unspecified arm ▽

✓6th **S55.99** **Other specified injury of unspecified blood vessel at forearm level**

✓7th **S55.991** Other specified injury of unspecified blood vessel at forearm level, **right arm** ▽

✓7th **S55.992** Other specified injury of unspecified blood vessel at forearm level, **left arm** ▽

✓7th **S55.999** Other specified injury of unspecified blood vessel at forearm level, unspecified arm ▽

✓4th **S56** **Injury of muscle, fascia and tendon at forearm level**

Code also any associated open wound (S51.-)

EXCLUDES 2 injury of muscle, fascia and tendon at or below wrist (S66.-)
sprain of joints and ligaments of elbow (S53.4-)

TIP: Refer to the Muscle/Tendon table at the beginning of this chapter.

The appropriate 7th character is to be added to each code from category S56.
A   initial encounter
D   subsequent encounter
S   sequela

✓5th **S56.0** **Injury of flexor muscle, fascia and tendon of thumb at forearm level**

✓6th **S56.00** **Unspecified injury of flexor muscle, fascia and tendon of thumb at forearm level**

✓7th **S56.001** Unspecified injury of flexor muscle, fascia and tendon of **right thumb** at forearm level ▽

✓7th **S56.002** Unspecified injury of flexor muscle, fascia and tendon of **left thumb** at forearm level ▽

✓7th **S56.009** Unspecified injury of flexor muscle, fascia and tendon of unspecified thumb at forearm level ▽

✓6th **S56.01** **Strain of flexor muscle, fascia and tendon of thumb at forearm level**

✓7th **S56.011** Strain of flexor muscle, fascia and tendon of **right thumb** at forearm level

✓7th **S56.012** Strain of flexor muscle, fascia and tendon of **left thumb** at forearm level

✓7th **S56.019** Strain of flexor muscle, fascia and tendon of unspecified thumb at forearm level ▽

✓6th **S56.02** **Laceration of flexor muscle, fascia and tendon of thumb at forearm level**

✓7th **S56.021** Laceration of flexor muscle, fascia and tendon of **right thumb** at forearm level

✓7th **S56.022** Laceration of flexor muscle, fascia and tendon of **left thumb** at forearm level

✓7th **S56.029** Laceration of flexor muscle, fascia and tendon of unspecified thumb at forearm level ▽

✓6th **S56.09** **Other injury of flexor muscle, fascia and tendon of thumb at forearm level**

✓7th **S56.091** Other injury of flexor muscle, fascia and tendon of **right thumb** at forearm level

EXCLUDES 1 Not coded here   *EXCLUDES 2* Not included here   N Newborn Age: 0   P Pediatric Age: 0-17   M Maternity Age: 12-55   A Adult Age: 15-124

972   ICD-10-CM 2018

√7ᵗʰ **S56.092** Other injury of flexor muscle, fascia and tendon of left thumb at forearm level

√7ᵗʰ **S56.099** Other injury of flexor muscle, fascia and tendon of unspecified thumb at forearm level ▽

√5ᵗʰ **S56.1** Injury of flexor muscle, fascia and tendon of other and unspecified finger at forearm level

√6ᵗʰ **S56.10** Unspecified injury of flexor muscle, fascia and tendon of other and unspecified finger at forearm level

√7ᵗʰ **S56.101** Unspecified injury of flexor muscle, fascia and tendon of right index finger at forearm level ▽

√7ᵗʰ **S56.102** Unspecified injury of flexor muscle, fascia and tendon of left index finger at forearm level ▽

√7ᵗʰ **S56.103** Unspecified injury of flexor muscle, fascia and tendon of right middle finger at forearm level ▽

√7ᵗʰ **S56.104** Unspecified injury of flexor muscle, fascia and tendon of left middle finger at forearm level ▽

√7ᵗʰ **S56.105** Unspecified injury of flexor muscle, fascia and tendon of right ring finger at forearm level ▽

√7ᵗʰ **S56.106** Unspecified injury of flexor muscle, fascia and tendon of left ring finger at forearm level ▽

√7ᵗʰ **S56.107** Unspecified injury of flexor muscle, fascia and tendon of right little finger at forearm level ▽

√7ᵗʰ **S56.108** Unspecified injury of flexor muscle, fascia and tendon of left little finger at forearm level ▽

√7ᵗʰ **S56.109** Unspecified injury of flexor muscle, fascia and tendon of unspecified finger at forearm level ▽

√6ᵗʰ **S56.11** Strain of flexor muscle, fascia and tendon of other and unspecified finger at forearm level

√7ᵗʰ **S56.111** Strain of flexor muscle, fascia and tendon of right index finger at forearm level

√7ᵗʰ **S56.112** Strain of flexor muscle, fascia and tendon of left index finger at forearm level

√7ᵗʰ **S56.113** Strain of flexor muscle, fascia and tendon of right middle finger at forearm level

√7ᵗʰ **S56.114** Strain of flexor muscle, fascia and tendon of left middle finger at forearm level

√7ᵗʰ **S56.115** Strain of flexor muscle, fascia and tendon of right ring finger at forearm level

√7ᵗʰ **S56.116** Strain of flexor muscle, fascia and tendon of left ring finger at forearm level

√7ᵗʰ **S56.117** Strain of flexor muscle, fascia and tendon of right little finger at forearm level

√7ᵗʰ **S56.118** Strain of flexor muscle, fascia and tendon of left little finger at forearm level

√7ᵗʰ **S56.119** Strain of flexor muscle, fascia and tendon of finger of unspecified finger at forearm level ▽

√6ᵗʰ **S56.12** Laceration of flexor muscle, fascia and tendon of other and unspecified finger at forearm level

√7ᵗʰ **S56.121** Laceration of flexor muscle, fascia and tendon of right index finger at forearm level

√7ᵗʰ **S56.122** Laceration of flexor muscle, fascia and tendon of left index finger at forearm level

√7ᵗʰ **S56.123** Laceration of flexor muscle, fascia and tendon of right middle finger at forearm level

√7ᵗʰ **S56.124** Laceration of flexor muscle, fascia and tendon of left middle finger at forearm level

√7ᵗʰ **S56.125** Laceration of flexor muscle, fascia and tendon of right ring finger at forearm level

√7ᵗʰ **S56.126** Laceration of flexor muscle, fascia and tendon of left ring finger at forearm level

√7ᵗʰ **S56.127** Laceration of flexor muscle, fascia and tendon of right little finger at forearm level

√7ᵗʰ **S56.128** Laceration of flexor muscle, fascia and tendon of left little finger at forearm level

√7ᵗʰ **S56.129** Laceration of flexor muscle, fascia and tendon of unspecified finger at forearm level ▽

√6ᵗʰ **S56.19** Other injury of flexor muscle, fascia and tendon of other and unspecified finger at forearm level

√7ᵗʰ **S56.191** Other injury of flexor muscle, fascia and tendon of right index finger at forearm level

√7ᵗʰ **S56.192** Other injury of flexor muscle, fascia and tendon of left index finger at forearm level

√7ᵗʰ **S56.193** Other injury of flexor muscle, fascia and tendon of right middle finger at forearm level

√7ᵗʰ **S56.194** Other injury of flexor muscle, fascia and tendon of left middle finger at forearm level

√7ᵗʰ **S56.195** Other injury of flexor muscle, fascia and tendon of right ring finger at forearm level

√7ᵗʰ **S56.196** Other injury of flexor muscle, fascia and tendon of left ring finger at forearm level

√7ᵗʰ **S56.197** Other injury of flexor muscle, fascia and tendon of right little finger at forearm level

√7ᵗʰ **S56.198** Other injury of flexor muscle, fascia and tendon of left little finger at forearm level

√7ᵗʰ **S56.199** Other injury of flexor muscle, fascia and tendon of unspecified finger at forearm level ▽

√5ᵗʰ **S56.2** Injury of other flexor muscle, fascia and tendon at forearm level

√6ᵗʰ **S56.20** Unspecified injury of other flexor muscle, fascia and tendon at forearm level

√7ᵗʰ **S56.201** Unspecified injury of other flexor muscle, fascia and tendon at forearm level, right arm ▽

√7ᵗʰ **S56.202** Unspecified injury of other flexor muscle, fascia and tendon at forearm level, left arm ▽

√7ᵗʰ **S56.209** Unspecified injury of other flexor muscle, fascia and tendon at forearm level, unspecified arm ▽

√6ᵗʰ **S56.21** Strain of other flexor muscle, fascia and tendon at forearm level

√7ᵗʰ **S56.211** Strain of other flexor muscle, fascia and tendon at forearm level, right arm

√7ᵗʰ **S56.212** Strain of other flexor muscle, fascia and tendon at forearm level, left arm

√7ᵗʰ **S56.219** Strain of other flexor muscle, fascia and tendon at forearm level, unspecified arm ▽

√6ᵗʰ **S56.22** Laceration of other flexor muscle, fascia and tendon at forearm level

√7ᵗʰ **S56.221** Laceration of other flexor muscle, fascia and tendon at forearm level, right arm

√7ᵗʰ **S56.222** Laceration of other flexor muscle, fascia and tendon at forearm level, left arm

√7ᵗʰ **S56.229** Laceration of other flexor muscle, fascia and tendon at forearm level, unspecified arm ▽

√6ᵗʰ **S56.29** Other injury of other flexor muscle, fascia and tendon at forearm level

√7ᵗʰ **S56.291** Other injury of other flexor muscle, fascia and tendon at forearm level, right arm

√7ᵗʰ **S56.292** Other injury of other flexor muscle, fascia and tendon at forearm level, left arm

√7ᵗʰ **S56.299** Other injury of other flexor muscle, fascia and tendon at forearm level, unspecified arm ▽

☑ Additional Character Req   √x7ᵗʰ Placeholder Alert   Manifestation   HCC CMS-HCC Condition   ▽ Unspecified Code   ►◄ Revised Text   ● New Code   ▲ Revised Code Title

ICD-10-CM 2018   973

✓5ᵗʰ S56.3 Injury of extensor or abductor muscles, fascia and tendons of thumb at forearm level

    ✓6ᵗʰ S56.30 Unspecified injury of extensor or abductor muscles, fascia and tendons of thumb at forearm level

        ✓7ᵗʰ S56.301 Unspecified injury of extensor or abductor muscles, fascia and tendons of right thumb at forearm level ▽

        ✓7ᵗʰ S56.302 Unspecified injury of extensor or abductor muscles, fascia and tendons of left thumb at forearm level ▽

        ✓7ᵗʰ S56.309 Unspecified injury of extensor or abductor muscles, fascia and tendons of unspecified thumb at forearm level ▽

    ✓6ᵗʰ S56.31 Strain of extensor or abductor muscles, fascia and tendons of thumb at forearm level

        ✓7ᵗʰ S56.311 Strain of extensor or abductor muscles, fascia and tendons of right thumb at forearm level

        ✓7ᵗʰ S56.312 Strain of extensor or abductor muscles, fascia and tendons of left thumb at forearm level

        ✓7ᵗʰ S56.319 Strain of extensor or abductor muscles, fascia and tendons of unspecified thumb at forearm level ▽

    ✓6ᵗʰ S56.32 Laceration of extensor or abductor muscles, fascia and tendons of thumb at forearm level

        ✓7ᵗʰ S56.321 Laceration of extensor or abductor muscles, fascia and tendons of right thumb at forearm level

        ✓7ᵗʰ S56.322 Laceration of extensor or abductor muscles, fascia and tendons of left thumb at forearm level

        ✓7ᵗʰ S56.329 Laceration of extensor or abductor muscles, fascia and tendons of unspecified thumb at forearm level ▽

    ✓6ᵗʰ S56.39 Other injury of extensor or abductor muscles, fascia and tendons of thumb at forearm level

        ✓7ᵗʰ S56.391 Other injury of extensor or abductor muscles, fascia and tendons of right thumb at forearm level

        ✓7ᵗʰ S56.392 Other injury of extensor or abductor muscles, fascia and tendons of left thumb at forearm level

        ✓7ᵗʰ S56.399 Other injury of extensor or abductor muscles, fascia and tendons of unspecified thumb at forearm level ▽

✓5ᵗʰ S56.4 Injury of extensor muscle, fascia and tendon of other and unspecified finger at forearm level

    ✓6ᵗʰ S56.40 Unspecified injury of extensor muscle, fascia and tendon of other and unspecified finger at forearm level

        ✓7ᵗʰ S56.401 Unspecified injury of extensor muscle, fascia and tendon of right index finger at forearm level ▽

        ✓7ᵗʰ S56.402 Unspecified injury of extensor muscle, fascia and tendon of left index finger at forearm level ▽

        ✓7ᵗʰ S56.403 Unspecified injury of extensor muscle, fascia and tendon of right middle finger at forearm level ▽

        ✓7ᵗʰ S56.404 Unspecified injury of extensor muscle, fascia and tendon of left middle finger at forearm level ▽

        ✓7ᵗʰ S56.405 Unspecified injury of extensor muscle, fascia and tendon of right ring finger at forearm level ▽

        ✓7ᵗʰ S56.406 Unspecified injury of extensor muscle, fascia and tendon of left ring finger at forearm level ▽

        ✓7ᵗʰ S56.407 Unspecified injury of extensor muscle, fascia and tendon of right little finger at forearm level ▽

        ✓7ᵗʰ S56.408 Unspecified injury of extensor muscle, fascia and tendon of left little finger at forearm level ▽

        ✓7ᵗʰ S56.409 Unspecified injury of extensor muscle, fascia and tendon of unspecified finger at forearm level ▽

✓6ᵗʰ S56.41 Strain of extensor muscle, fascia and tendon of other and unspecified finger at forearm level

    ✓7ᵗʰ S56.411 Strain of extensor muscle, fascia and tendon of right index finger at forearm level

    ✓7ᵗʰ S56.412 Strain of extensor muscle, fascia and tendon of left index finger at forearm level

    ✓7ᵗʰ S56.413 Strain of extensor muscle, fascia and tendon of right middle finger at forearm level

    ✓7ᵗʰ S56.414 Strain of extensor muscle, fascia and tendon of left middle finger at forearm level

    ✓7ᵗʰ S56.415 Strain of extensor muscle, fascia and tendon of right ring finger at forearm level

    ✓7ᵗʰ S56.416 Strain of extensor muscle, fascia and tendon of left ring finger at forearm level

    ✓7ᵗʰ S56.417 Strain of extensor muscle, fascia and tendon of right little finger at forearm level

    ✓7ᵗʰ S56.418 Strain of extensor muscle, fascia and tendon of left little finger at forearm level

    ✓7ᵗʰ S56.419 Strain of extensor muscle, fascia and tendon of finger, unspecified finger at forearm level ▽

✓6ᵗʰ S56.42 Laceration of extensor muscle, fascia and tendon of other and unspecified finger at forearm level

    ✓7ᵗʰ S56.421 Laceration of extensor muscle, fascia and tendon of right index finger at forearm level

    ✓7ᵗʰ S56.422 Laceration of extensor muscle, fascia and tendon of left index finger at forearm level

    ✓7ᵗʰ S56.423 Laceration of extensor muscle, fascia and tendon of right middle finger at forearm level

    ✓7ᵗʰ S56.424 Laceration of extensor muscle, fascia and tendon of left middle finger at forearm level

    ✓7ᵗʰ S56.425 Laceration of extensor muscle, fascia and tendon of right ring finger at forearm level

    ✓7ᵗʰ S56.426 Laceration of extensor muscle, fascia and tendon of left ring finger at forearm level

    ✓7ᵗʰ S56.427 Laceration of extensor muscle, fascia and tendon of right little finger at forearm level

    ✓7ᵗʰ S56.428 Laceration of extensor muscle, fascia and tendon of left little finger at forearm level

    ✓7ᵗʰ S56.429 Laceration of extensor muscle, fascia and tendon of unspecified finger at forearm level ▽

✓6ᵗʰ S56.49 Other injury of extensor muscle, fascia and tendon of other and unspecified finger at forearm level

    ✓7ᵗʰ S56.491 Other injury of extensor muscle, fascia and tendon of right index finger at forearm level

    ✓7ᵗʰ S56.492 Other injury of extensor muscle, fascia and tendon of left index finger at forearm level

    ✓7ᵗʰ S56.493 Other injury of extensor muscle, fascia and tendon of right middle finger at forearm level

    ✓7ᵗʰ S56.494 Other injury of extensor muscle, fascia and tendon of left middle finger at forearm level

    ✓7ᵗʰ S56.495 Other injury of extensor muscle, fascia and tendon of right ring finger at forearm level

    ✓7ᵗʰ S56.496 Other injury of extensor muscle, fascia and tendon of left ring finger at forearm level

    ✓7ᵗʰ S56.497 Other injury of extensor muscle, fascia and tendon of right little finger at forearm level

    ✓7ᵗʰ S56.498 Other injury of extensor muscle, fascia and tendon of left little finger at forearm level

    ✓7ᵗʰ S56.499 Other injury of extensor muscle, fascia and tendon of unspecified finger at forearm level ▽

EXCLUDES 1 Not coded here   **EXCLUDES 2** Not included here   **N** Newborn Age: 0   **P** Pediatric Age: 0-17   **M** Maternity Age: 12-55   **A** Adult Age: 15-124

974   ICD-10-CM 2018

√5ᵗʰ **S56.5** **Injury of other extensor muscle, fascia and tendon at** forearm **level**

√6ᵗʰ **S56.50** **Unspecified injury of other extensor muscle, fascia and tendon at forearm level**

√7ᵗʰ **S56.501** Unspecified injury of other extensor muscle, fascia and tendon at forearm level, right arm ▽

√7ᵗʰ **S56.502** Unspecified injury of other extensor muscle, fascia and tendon at forearm level, left arm ▽

√7ᵗʰ **S56.509** Unspecified injury of other extensor muscle, fascia and tendon at forearm level, unspecified arm ▽

√6ᵗʰ **S56.51** Strain **of other extensor muscle, fascia and tendon at forearm level**

√7ᵗʰ **S56.511** Strain of other extensor muscle, fascia and tendon at forearm level, right arm

√7ᵗʰ **S56.512** Strain of other extensor muscle, fascia and tendon at forearm level, left arm

√7ᵗʰ **S56.519** Strain of other extensor muscle, fascia and tendon at forearm level, unspecified arm ▽

√6ᵗʰ **S56.52** Laceration **of other extensor muscle, fascia and tendon at forearm level**

√7ᵗʰ **S56.521** Laceration of other extensor muscle, fascia and tendon at forearm level, right arm

√7ᵗʰ **S56.522** Laceration of other extensor muscle, fascia and tendon at forearm level, left arm

√7ᵗʰ **S56.529** Laceration of other extensor muscle, fascia and tendon at forearm level, unspecified arm ▽

√6ᵗʰ **S56.59** **Other injury of other extensor muscle, fascia and tendon at forearm level**

√7ᵗʰ **S56.591** Other injury of other extensor muscle, fascia and tendon at forearm level, right arm

√7ᵗʰ **S56.592** Other injury of other extensor muscle, fascia and tendon at forearm level, left arm

√7ᵗʰ **S56.599** Other injury of other extensor muscle, fascia and tendon at forearm level, unspecified arm ▽

√5ᵗʰ **S56.8** **Injury of other muscles, fascia and tendons at forearm level**

√6ᵗʰ **S56.80** **Unspecified injury of other muscles, fascia and tendons at forearm level**

√7ᵗʰ **S56.801** Unspecified injury of other muscles, fascia and tendons at forearm level, right arm ▽

√7ᵗʰ **S56.802** Unspecified injury of other muscles, fascia and tendons at forearm level, left arm ▽

√7ᵗʰ **S56.809** Unspecified injury of other muscles, fascia and tendons at forearm level, unspecified arm ▽

√6ᵗʰ **S56.81** Strain **of other muscles, fascia and tendons at forearm level**

√7ᵗʰ **S56.811** Strain of other muscles, fascia and tendons at forearm level, right arm

√7ᵗʰ **S56.812** Strain of other muscles, fascia and tendons at forearm level, left arm

√7ᵗʰ **S56.819** Strain of other muscles, fascia and tendons at forearm level, unspecified arm ▽

√6ᵗʰ **S56.82** Laceration **of other muscles, fascia and tendons at forearm level**

√7ᵗʰ **S56.821** Laceration of other muscles, fascia and tendons at forearm level, right arm

√7ᵗʰ **S56.822** Laceration of other muscles, fascia and tendons at forearm level, left arm

√7ᵗʰ **S56.829** Laceration of other muscles, fascia and tendons at forearm level, unspecified arm ▽

√6ᵗʰ **S56.89** **Other injury of other muscles, fascia and tendons at forearm level**

√7ᵗʰ **S56.891** Other injury of other muscles, fascia and tendons at forearm level, right arm

√7ᵗʰ **S56.892** Other injury of other muscles, fascia and tendons at forearm level, left arm

√7ᵗʰ **S56.899** Other injury of other muscles, fascia and tendons at forearm level, unspecified arm ▽

√5ᵗʰ **S56.9** **Injury of unspecified muscles, fascia and tendons at** forearm **level**

√6ᵗʰ **S56.90** **Unspecified injury of unspecified muscles, fascia and tendons at forearm level**

√7ᵗʰ **S56.901** Unspecified injury of unspecified muscles, fascia and tendons at forearm level, right arm ▽

√7ᵗʰ **S56.902** Unspecified injury of unspecified muscles, fascia and tendons at forearm level, left arm ▽

√7ᵗʰ **S56.909** Unspecified injury of unspecified muscles, fascia and tendons at forearm level, unspecified arm ▽

√6ᵗʰ **S56.91** Strain **of unspecified muscles, fascia and tendons at forearm level**

√7ᵗʰ **S56.911** Strain of unspecified muscles, fascia and tendons at forearm level, right arm ▽

√7ᵗʰ **S56.912** Strain of unspecified muscles, fascia and tendons at forearm level, left arm ▽

√7ᵗʰ **S56.919** Strain of unspecified muscles, fascia and tendons at forearm level, unspecified arm ▽

√6ᵗʰ **S56.92** Laceration **of unspecified muscles, fascia and tendons at forearm level**

√7ᵗʰ **S56.921** Laceration of unspecified muscles, fascia and tendons at forearm level, right arm ▽

√7ᵗʰ **S56.922** Laceration of unspecified muscles, fascia and tendons at forearm level, left arm ▽

√7ᵗʰ **S56.929** Laceration of unspecified muscles, fascia and tendons at forearm level, unspecified arm ▽

√6ᵗʰ **S56.99** **Other injury of unspecified muscles, fascia and tendons at forearm level**

√7ᵗʰ **S56.991** Other injury of unspecified muscles, fascia and tendons at forearm level, right arm ▽

√7ᵗʰ **S56.992** Other injury of unspecified muscles, fascia and tendons at forearm level, left arm ▽

√7ᵗʰ **S56.999** Other injury of unspecified muscles, fascia and tendons at forearm level, unspecified arm ▽

√4ᵗʰ **S57** **Crushing injury of elbow and forearm**

Use additional code(s) for all associated injuries

EXCLUDES 2   crushing injury of wrist and hand (S67.-)

The appropriate 7th character is to be added to each code from category S57.
A   initial encounter
D   subsequent encounter
S   sequela

√5ᵗʰ **S57.0** **Crushing injury of** elbow

√x7ᵗʰ **S57.00** **Crushing injury of unspecified elbow** ▽

√x7ᵗʰ **S57.01** **Crushing injury of** right **elbow**

√x7ᵗʰ **S57.02** **Crushing injury of** left **elbow**

√5ᵗʰ **S57.8** **Crushing injury of** forearm

√x7ᵗʰ **S57.80** **Crushing injury of unspecified forearm** ▽

√x7ᵗʰ **S57.81** **Crushing injury of** right **forearm**

√x7ᵗʰ **S57.82** **Crushing injury of** left **forearm**

☑ Additional Character Req   √x7ᵗʰ Placeholder Alert   Manifestation   ᴴᶜᶜ CMS-HCC Condition   ▽ Unspecified Code   ▶◀ Revised Text   ● New Code   ▲ Revised Code Title

✓4th S58 Traumatic amputation of elbow and forearm

An amputation not identified as partial or complete should be coded to complete.

EXCLUDES 1   traumatic amputation of wrist and hand (S68.-)

The appropriate 7th character is to be added to each code from category S58.
A   initial encounter
D   subsequent encounter
S   sequela

✓5th S58.0 Traumatic amputation at elbow level

✓6th S58.01 Complete traumatic amputation at elbow level

2 ✓7th **S58.011** Complete traumatic amputation at elbow level, right arm   HCC

2 ✓7th **S58.012** Complete traumatic amputation at elbow level, left arm   HCC

2 ✓7th **S58.019** Complete traumatic amputation at elbow level, unspecified arm   HCC ▽

✓6th S58.02 Partial traumatic amputation at elbow level

2 ✓7th **S58.021** Partial traumatic amputation at elbow level, right arm   HCC

2 ✓7th **S58.022** Partial traumatic amputation at elbow level, left arm   HCC

2 ✓7th **S58.029** Partial traumatic amputation at elbow level, unspecified arm   HCC ▽

✓5th S58.1 Traumatic amputation at level between elbow and wrist

✓6th S58.11 Complete traumatic amputation at level between elbow and wrist

2 ✓7th **S58.111** Complete traumatic amputation at level between elbow and wrist, right arm   HCC

2 ✓7th **S58.112** Complete traumatic amputation at level between elbow and wrist, left arm   HCC

2 ✓7th **S58.119** Complete traumatic amputation at level between elbow and wrist, unspecified arm   HCC ▽

✓6th S58.12 Partial traumatic amputation at level between elbow and wrist

2 ✓7th **S58.121** Partial traumatic amputation at level between elbow and wrist, right arm   HCC

2 ✓7th **S58.122** Partial traumatic amputation at level between elbow and wrist, left arm   HCC

2 ✓7th **S58.129** Partial traumatic amputation at level between elbow and wrist, unspecified arm   HCC ▽

✓5th S58.9 Traumatic amputation of forearm, level unspecified

EXCLUDES 1   traumatic amputation of wrist (S68.-)

✓6th S58.91 Complete traumatic amputation of forearm, level unspecified

2 ✓7th **S58.911** Complete traumatic amputation of right forearm, level unspecified   HCC ▽

2 ✓7th **S58.912** Complete traumatic amputation of left forearm, level unspecified   HCC ▽

2 ✓7th **S58.919** Complete traumatic amputation of unspecified forearm, level unspecified   HCC ▽

✓6th S58.92 Partial traumatic amputation of forearm, level unspecified

2 ✓7th **S58.921** Partial traumatic amputation of right forearm, level unspecified   HCC ▽

2 ✓7th **S58.922** Partial traumatic amputation of left forearm, level unspecified   HCC ▽

2 ✓7th **S58.929** Partial traumatic amputation of unspecified forearm, level unspecified   HCC ▽

✓4th S59 Other and unspecified injuries of elbow and forearm

EXCLUDES 2   other and unspecified injuries of wrist and hand (S69.-)

AHA: 2015, 3Q, 37-39

The appropriate 7th character is to be added to each code from subcategories S59.0, S59.1, and S59.2.
A   initial encounter for closed fracture
D   subsequent encounter for fracture with routine healing
G   subsequent encounter for fracture with delayed healing
K   subsequent encounter for fracture with nonunion
P   subsequent encounter for fracture with malunion
S   sequela

✓5th S59.0 Physeal fracture of lower end of ulna

✓6th S59.00 Unspecified physeal fracture of lower end of ulna

✓7th **S59.001** Unspecified physeal fracture of lower end of ulna, right arm ▽

✓7th **S59.002** Unspecified physeal fracture of lower end of ulna, left arm ▽

✓7th **S59.009** Unspecified physeal fracture of lower end of ulna, unspecified arm ▽

✓6th S59.01 Salter-Harris Type I physeal fracture of lower end of ulna

✓7th **S59.011** Salter-Harris Type I physeal fracture of lower end of ulna, right arm

✓7th **S59.012** Salter-Harris Type I physeal fracture of lower end of ulna, left arm

✓7th **S59.019** Salter-Harris Type I physeal fracture of lower end of ulna, unspecified arm ▽

✓6th S59.02 Salter-Harris Type II physeal fracture of lower end of ulna

✓7th **S59.021** Salter-Harris Type II physeal fracture of lower end of ulna, right arm

✓7th **S59.022** Salter-Harris Type II physeal fracture of lower end of ulna, left arm

✓7th **S59.029** Salter-Harris Type II physeal fracture of lower end of ulna, unspecified arm ▽

✓6th S59.03 Salter-Harris Type III physeal fracture of lower end of ulna

✓7th **S59.031** Salter-Harris Type III physeal fracture of lower end of ulna, right arm

✓7th **S59.032** Salter-Harris Type III physeal fracture of lower end of ulna, left arm

✓7th **S59.039** Salter-Harris Type III physeal fracture of lower end of ulna, unspecified arm ▽

✓6th S59.04 Salter-Harris Type IV physeal fracture of lower end of ulna

✓7th **S59.041** Salter-Harris Type IV physeal fracture of lower end of ulna, right arm

✓7th **S59.042** Salter-Harris Type IV physeal fracture of lower end of ulna, left arm

✓7th **S59.049** Salter-Harris Type IV physeal fracture of lower end of ulna, unspecified arm ▽

✓6th S59.09 Other physeal fracture of lower end of ulna

✓7th **S59.091** Other physeal fracture of lower end of ulna, right arm

✓7th **S59.092** Other physeal fracture of lower end of ulna, left arm

✓7th **S59.099** Other physeal fracture of lower end of ulna, unspecified arm ▽

✓5th S59.1 Physeal fracture of upper end of radius

✓6th S59.10 Unspecified physeal fracture of upper end of radius

✓7th **S59.101** Unspecified physeal fracture of upper end of radius, right arm ▽

✓7th **S59.102** Unspecified physeal fracture of upper end of radius, left arm ▽

✓7th **S59.109** Unspecified physeal fracture of upper end of radius, unspecified arm ▽

✓6th S59.11 Salter-Harris Type I physeal fracture of upper end of radius

✓7th **S59.111** Salter-Harris Type I physeal fracture of upper end of radius, right arm

✓7th **S59.112** Salter-Harris Type I physeal fracture of upper end of radius, left arm

✓7th **S59.119** Salter-Harris Type I physeal fracture of upper end of radius, unspecified arm ▽

---

2   HCC with 7th character indicating initial encounter (A or B - specific to category) OR sequela.

EXCLUDES 1 Not coded here   EXCLUDES 2 Not included here   N Newborn Age: 0   P Pediatric Age: 0-17   M Maternity Age: 12-55   A Adult Age: 15-124

976   ICD-10-CM 2018

S58–S59.119

✓6ᵗʰ **S59.12** Salter-Harris Type II physeal fracture of upper end of radius

   ✓7ᵗʰ **S59.121** Salter-Harris Type II physeal fracture of upper end of radius, right arm

   ✓7ᵗʰ **S59.122** Salter-Harris Type II physeal fracture of upper end of radius, left arm

   ✓7ᵗʰ **S59.129** Salter-Harris Type II physeal fracture of upper end of radius, unspecified arm ▽

✓6ᵗʰ **S59.13** Salter-Harris Type III physeal fracture of upper end of radius

   ✓7ᵗʰ **S59.131** Salter-Harris Type III physeal fracture of upper end of radius, right arm

   ✓7ᵗʰ **S59.132** Salter-Harris Type III physeal fracture of upper end of radius, left arm

   ✓7ᵗʰ **S59.139** Salter-Harris Type III physeal fracture of upper end of radius, unspecified arm ▽

✓6ᵗʰ **S59.14** Salter-Harris Type IV physeal fracture of upper end of radius

   ✓7ᵗʰ **S59.141** Salter-Harris Type IV physeal fracture of upper end of radius, right arm

   ✓7ᵗʰ **S59.142** Salter-Harris Type IV physeal fracture of upper end of radius, left arm

   ✓7ᵗʰ **S59.149** Salter-Harris Type IV physeal fracture of upper end of radius, unspecified arm ▽

✓6ᵗʰ **S59.19** Other physeal fracture of upper end of radius

   ✓7ᵗʰ **S59.191** Other physeal fracture of upper end of radius, right arm

   ✓7ᵗʰ **S59.192** Other physeal fracture of upper end of radius, left arm

   ✓7ᵗʰ **S59.199** Other physeal fracture of upper end of radius, unspecified arm ▽

✓5ᵗʰ **S59.2** Physeal fracture of lower end of radius

✓6ᵗʰ **S59.20** Unspecified physeal fracture of lower end of radius

   ✓7ᵗʰ **S59.201** Unspecified physeal fracture of lower end of radius, right arm ▽

   ✓7ᵗʰ **S59.202** Unspecified physeal fracture of lower end of radius, left arm ▽

   ✓7ᵗʰ **S59.209** Unspecified physeal fracture of lower end of radius, unspecified arm ▽

✓6ᵗʰ **S59.21** Salter-Harris Type I physeal fracture of lower end of radius

   ✓7ᵗʰ **S59.211** Salter-Harris Type I physeal fracture of lower end of radius, right arm

   ✓7ᵗʰ **S59.212** Salter-Harris Type I physeal fracture of lower end of radius, left arm

   ✓7ᵗʰ **S59.219** Salter-Harris Type I physeal fracture of lower end of radius, unspecified arm ▽

✓6ᵗʰ **S59.22** Salter-Harris Type II physeal fracture of lower end of radius

   ✓7ᵗʰ **S59.221** Salter-Harris Type II physeal fracture of lower end of radius, right arm

   ✓7ᵗʰ **S59.222** Salter-Harris Type II physeal fracture of lower end of radius, left arm

   ✓7ᵗʰ **S59.229** Salter-Harris Type II physeal fracture of lower end of radius, unspecified arm ▽

✓6ᵗʰ **S59.23** Salter-Harris Type III physeal fracture of lower end of radius

   ✓7ᵗʰ **S59.231** Salter-Harris Type III physeal fracture of lower end of radius, right arm

   ✓7ᵗʰ **S59.232** Salter-Harris Type III physeal fracture of lower end of radius, left arm

   ✓7ᵗʰ **S59.239** Salter-Harris Type III physeal fracture of lower end of radius, unspecified arm ▽

✓6ᵗʰ **S59.24** Salter-Harris Type IV physeal fracture of lower end of radius

   ✓7ᵗʰ **S59.241** Salter-Harris Type IV physeal fracture of lower end of radius, right arm

   ✓7ᵗʰ **S59.242** Salter-Harris Type IV physeal fracture of lower end of radius, left arm

   ✓7ᵗʰ **S59.249** Salter-Harris Type IV physeal fracture of lower end of radius, unspecified arm ▽

✓6ᵗʰ **S59.29** Other physeal fracture of lower end of radius

   ✓7ᵗʰ **S59.291** Other physeal fracture of lower end of radius, right arm

   ✓7ᵗʰ **S59.292** Other physeal fracture of lower end of radius, left arm

   ✓7ᵗʰ **S59.299** Other physeal fracture of lower end of radius, unspecified arm ▽

✓5ᵗʰ **S59.8** Other specified injuries of elbow and forearm

> The appropriate 7th character is to be added to each code in subcategory S59.8.
> A   initial encounter
> D   subsequent encounter
> S   sequela

✓6ᵗʰ **S59.80** Other specified injuries of elbow

   ✓7ᵗʰ **S59.801** Other specified injuries of right elbow

   ✓7ᵗʰ **S59.802** Other specified injuries of left elbow

   ✓7ᵗʰ **S59.809** Other specified injuries of unspecified elbow

✓6ᵗʰ **S59.81** Other specified injuries of forearm

   ✓7ᵗʰ **S59.811** Other specified injuries right forearm

   ✓7ᵗʰ **S59.812** Other specified injuries left forearm

   ✓7ᵗʰ **S59.819** Other specified injuries unspecified forearm ▽

✓5ᵗʰ **S59.9** Unspecified injury of elbow and forearm

> The appropriate 7th character is to be added to each code in subcategory S59.9.
> A   initial encounter
> D   subsequent encounter
> S   sequela

✓6ᵗʰ **S59.90** Unspecified injury of elbow

   ✓7ᵗʰ **S59.901** Unspecified injury of right elbow ▽

   ✓7ᵗʰ **S59.902** Unspecified injury of left elbow ▽

   ✓7ᵗʰ **S59.909** Unspecified injury of unspecified elbow ▽

✓6ᵗʰ **S59.91** Unspecified injury of forearm

   ✓7ᵗʰ **S59.911** Unspecified injury of right forearm ▽

   ✓7ᵗʰ **S59.912** Unspecified injury of left forearm ▽

   ✓7ᵗʰ **S59.919** Unspecified injury of unspecified forearm ▽

Injuries to the wrist, hand and fingers (S60-S69)

EXCLUDES 2 burns and corrosions (T20-T32)
     frostbite (T33-T34)
     insect bite or sting, venomous (T63.4)

✓4ᵗʰ **S60** Superficial injury of wrist, hand and fingers

> The appropriate 7th character is to be added to each code from category S60.
> A   initial encounter
> D   subsequent encounter
> S   sequela

✓5ᵗʰ **S60.0** Contusion of finger without damage to nail

   EXCLUDES 1 contusion involving nail (matrix) (S60.1)

✓x7ᵗʰ **S60.00** Contusion of unspecified finger without damage to nail ▽
   Contusion of finger(s) NOS

✓6ᵗʰ **S60.01** Contusion of thumb without damage to nail

   ✓7ᵗʰ **S60.011** Contusion of right thumb without damage to nail

   ✓7ᵗʰ **S60.012** Contusion of left thumb without damage to nail

   ✓7ᵗʰ **S60.019** Contusion of unspecified thumb without damage to nail ▽

✓6ᵗʰ **S60.02** Contusion of index finger without damage to nail

   ✓7ᵗʰ **S60.021** Contusion of right index finger without damage to nail

   ✓7ᵗʰ **S60.022** Contusion of left index finger without damage to nail

   ✓7ᵗʰ **S60.029** Contusion of unspecified index finger without damage to nail ▽

✓6ᵗʰ **S60.03** Contusion of middle finger without damage to nail

   ✓7ᵗʰ **S60.031** Contusion of right middle finger without damage to nail

   ✓7ᵗʰ **S60.032** Contusion of left middle finger without damage to nail

✓ Additional Character Req   ✓x7ᵗʰ Placeholder Alert   Manifestation   HCC CMS-HCC Condition   ▽ Unspecified Code   ►◄ Revised Text   ● New Code   ▲ Revised Code Title

ICD-10-CM 2018   977

Chapter 19. Injury, Poisoning, and Certain Other Consequences of External Causes

✓7ᵗʰ **S60.039** **Contusion of unspecified middle finger without damage to nail** ▽

✓6ᵗʰ **S60.04** **Contusion of ring finger without damage to nail**

✓7ᵗʰ **S60.041** **Contusion of right ring finger without damage to nail**

✓7ᵗʰ **S60.042** **Contusion of left ring finger without damage to nail**

✓7ᵗʰ **S60.049** **Contusion of unspecified ring finger without damage to nail** ▽

✓6ᵗʰ **S60.05** **Contusion of little finger without damage to nail**

✓7ᵗʰ **S60.051** **Contusion of right little finger without damage to nail**

✓7ᵗʰ **S60.052** **Contusion of left little finger without damage to nail**

✓7ᵗʰ **S60.059** **Contusion of unspecified little finger without damage to nail** ▽

✓5ᵗʰ **S60.1** **Contusion of finger with damage to nail**

✓x7ᵗʰ **S60.10** **Contusion of unspecified finger with damage to nail** ▽

✓6ᵗʰ **S60.11** **Contusion of thumb with damage to nail**

✓7ᵗʰ **S60.111** **Contusion of right thumb with damage to nail**

✓7ᵗʰ **S60.112** **Contusion of left thumb with damage to nail**

✓7ᵗʰ **S60.119** **Contusion of unspecified thumb with damage to nail** ▽

✓6ᵗʰ **S60.12** **Contusion of index finger with damage to nail**

✓7ᵗʰ **S60.121** **Contusion of right index finger with damage to nail**

✓7ᵗʰ **S60.122** **Contusion of left index finger with damage to nail**

✓7ᵗʰ **S60.129** **Contusion of unspecified index finger with damage to nail** ▽

✓6ᵗʰ **S60.13** **Contusion of middle finger with damage to nail**

✓7ᵗʰ **S60.131** **Contusion of right middle finger with damage to nail**

✓7ᵗʰ **S60.132** **Contusion of left middle finger with damage to nail**

✓7ᵗʰ **S60.139** **Contusion of unspecified middle finger with damage to nail** ▽

✓6ᵗʰ **S60.14** **Contusion of ring finger with damage to nail**

✓7ᵗʰ **S60.141** **Contusion of right ring finger with damage to nail**

✓7ᵗʰ **S60.142** **Contusion of left ring finger with damage to nail**

✓7ᵗʰ **S60.149** **Contusion of unspecified ring finger with damage to nail** ▽

✓6ᵗʰ **S60.15** **Contusion of little finger with damage to nail**

✓7ᵗʰ **S60.151** **Contusion of right little finger with damage to nail**

✓7ᵗʰ **S60.152** **Contusion of left little finger with damage to nail**

✓7ᵗʰ **S60.159** **Contusion of unspecified little finger with damage to nail** ▽

✓5ᵗʰ **S60.2** **Contusion of wrist and hand**

     EXCLUDES 2   contusion of fingers (S60.0-, S60.1-)

✓6ᵗʰ **S60.21** **Contusion of wrist**

✓7ᵗʰ **S60.211** **Contusion of right wrist**

✓7ᵗʰ **S60.212** **Contusion of left wrist**

✓7ᵗʰ **S60.219** **Contusion of unspecified wrist** ▽

✓6ᵗʰ **S60.22** **Contusion of hand**

✓7ᵗʰ **S60.221** **Contusion of right hand**

✓7ᵗʰ **S60.222** **Contusion of left hand**

✓7ᵗʰ **S60.229** **Contusion of unspecified hand** ▽

✓5ᵗʰ **S60.3** **Other superficial injuries of thumb**

✓6ᵗʰ **S60.31** **Abrasion of thumb**

✓7ᵗʰ **S60.311** **Abrasion of right thumb**

✓7ᵗʰ **S60.312** **Abrasion of left thumb**

✓7ᵗʰ **S60.319** **Abrasion of unspecified thumb** ▽

✓6ᵗʰ **S60.32** **Blister (nonthermal) of thumb**

✓7ᵗʰ **S60.321** **Blister (nonthermal) of right thumb**

✓7ᵗʰ **S60.322** **Blister (nonthermal) of left thumb**

✓7ᵗʰ **S60.329** **Blister (nonthermal) of unspecified thumb** ▽

✓6ᵗʰ **S60.34** **External constriction of thumb**

     Hair tourniquet syndrome of thumb

     Use additional cause code to identify the constricting item (W49.0-)

✓7ᵗʰ **S60.341** **External constriction of right thumb**

✓7ᵗʰ **S60.342** **External constriction of left thumb**

✓7ᵗʰ **S60.349** **External constriction of unspecified thumb** ▽

✓6ᵗʰ **S60.35** **Superficial foreign body of thumb**

     Splinter in the thumb

✓7ᵗʰ **S60.351** **Superficial foreign body of right thumb**

✓7ᵗʰ **S60.352** **Superficial foreign body of left thumb**

✓7ᵗʰ **S60.359** **Superficial foreign body of unspecified thumb** ▽

✓6ᵗʰ **S60.36** **Insect bite (nonvenomous) of thumb**

✓7ᵗʰ **S60.361** **Insect bite (nonvenomous) of right thumb**

✓7ᵗʰ **S60.362** **Insect bite (nonvenomous) of left thumb**

✓7ᵗʰ **S60.369** **Insect bite (nonvenomous) of unspecified thumb** ▽

✓6ᵗʰ **S60.37** **Other superficial bite of thumb**

     EXCLUDES 1   open bite of thumb (S61.05-, S61.15-)

✓7ᵗʰ **S60.371** **Other superficial bite of right thumb**

✓7ᵗʰ **S60.372** **Other superficial bite of left thumb**

✓7ᵗʰ **S60.379** **Other superficial bite of unspecified thumb** ▽

✓6ᵗʰ **S60.39** **Other superficial injuries of thumb**

✓7ᵗʰ **S60.391** **Other superficial injuries of right thumb**

✓7ᵗʰ **S60.392** **Other superficial injuries of left thumb**

✓7ᵗʰ **S60.399** **Other superficial injuries of unspecified thumb** ▽

✓5ᵗʰ **S60.4** **Other superficial injuries of other fingers**

✓6ᵗʰ **S60.41** **Abrasion of fingers**

✓7ᵗʰ **S60.410** **Abrasion of right index finger**

✓7ᵗʰ **S60.411** **Abrasion of left index finger**

✓7ᵗʰ **S60.412** **Abrasion of right middle finger**

✓7ᵗʰ **S60.413** **Abrasion of left middle finger**

✓7ᵗʰ **S60.414** **Abrasion of right ring finger**

✓7ᵗʰ **S60.415** **Abrasion of left ring finger**

✓7ᵗʰ **S60.416** **Abrasion of right little finger**

✓7ᵗʰ **S60.417** **Abrasion of left little finger**

✓7ᵗʰ **S60.418** **Abrasion of other finger**

     Abrasion of specified finger with unspecified laterality

✓7ᵗʰ **S60.419** **Abrasion of unspecified finger** ▽

✓6ᵗʰ **S60.42** **Blister (nonthermal) of fingers**

✓7ᵗʰ **S60.420** **Blister (nonthermal) of right index finger**

✓7ᵗʰ **S60.421** **Blister (nonthermal) of left index finger**

✓7ᵗʰ **S60.422** **Blister (nonthermal) of right middle finger**

✓7ᵗʰ **S60.423** **Blister (nonthermal) of left middle finger**

✓7ᵗʰ **S60.424** **Blister (nonthermal) of right ring finger**

✓7ᵗʰ **S60.425** **Blister (nonthermal) of left ring finger**

✓7ᵗʰ **S60.426** **Blister (nonthermal) of right little finger**

✓7ᵗʰ **S60.427** **Blister (nonthermal) of left little finger**

✓7ᵗʰ **S60.428** **Blister (nonthermal) of other finger**

     Blister (nonthermal) of specified finger with unspecified laterality

✓7ᵗʰ **S60.429** **Blister (nonthermal) of unspecified finger** ▽

✓6ᵗʰ **S60.44** **External constriction of fingers**

     Hair tourniquet syndrome of finger

     Use additional cause code to identify the constricting item (W49.0-)

✓7ᵗʰ **S60.440** **External constriction of right index finger**

✓7ᵗʰ **S60.441** **External constriction of left index finger**

✓7ᵗʰ **S60.442** **External constriction of right middle finger**

✓7ᵗʰ **S60.443** **External constriction of left middle finger**

✓7ᵗʰ **S60.444** **External constriction of right ring finger**

✓7ᵗʰ **S60.445** **External constriction of left ring finger**

EXCLUDES 1 Not coded here   *EXCLUDES 2* Not included here   N Newborn Age: 0   P Pediatric Age: 0-17   M Maternity Age: 12-55   A Adult Age: 15-124

978   ICD-10-CM 2018

S60.039–S60.445

✓7ᵗʰ **S60.446** External constriction of right little finger

✓7ᵗʰ **S60.447** External constriction of left little finger

✓7ᵗʰ **S60.448** External constriction of other finger
External constriction of specified finger with unspecified laterality

✓7ᵗʰ **S60.449** External constriction of unspecified finger ▽

✓6ᵗʰ **S60.45** Superficial foreign body of fingers
Splinter in the finger(s)

✓7ᵗʰ **S60.450** Superficial foreign body of right index finger

✓7ᵗʰ **S60.451** Superficial foreign body of left index finger

✓7ᵗʰ **S60.452** Superficial foreign body of right middle finger

✓7ᵗʰ **S60.453** Superficial foreign body of left middle finger

✓7ᵗʰ **S60.454** Superficial foreign body of right ring finger

✓7ᵗʰ **S60.455** Superficial foreign body of left ring finger

✓7ᵗʰ **S60.456** Superficial foreign body of right little finger

✓7ᵗʰ **S60.457** Superficial foreign body of left little finger

✓7ᵗʰ **S60.458** Superficial foreign body of other finger
Superficial foreign body of specified finger with unspecified laterality

✓7ᵗʰ **S60.459** Superficial foreign body of unspecified finger ▽

✓6ᵗʰ **S60.46** Insect bite (nonvenomous) of fingers

✓7ᵗʰ **S60.460** Insect bite (nonvenomous) of right index finger

✓7ᵗʰ **S60.461** Insect bite (nonvenomous) of left index finger

✓7ᵗʰ **S60.462** Insect bite (nonvenomous) of right middle finger

✓7ᵗʰ **S60.463** Insect bite (nonvenomous) of left middle finger

✓7ᵗʰ **S60.464** Insect bite (nonvenomous) of right ring finger

✓7ᵗʰ **S60.465** Insect bite (nonvenomous) of left ring finger

✓7ᵗʰ **S60.466** Insect bite (nonvenomous) of right little finger

✓7ᵗʰ **S60.467** Insect bite (nonvenomous) of left little finger

✓7ᵗʰ **S60.468** Insect bite (nonvenomous) of other finger
Insect bite (nonvenomous) of specified finger with unspecified laterality

✓7ᵗʰ **S60.469** Insect bite (nonvenomous) of unspecified finger ▽

✓6ᵗʰ **S60.47** Other superficial bite of fingers
EXCLUDES 1   open bite of fingers (S61.25-, S61.35-)

✓7ᵗʰ **S60.470** Other superficial bite of right index finger

✓7ᵗʰ **S60.471** Other superficial bite of left index finger

✓7ᵗʰ **S60.472** Other superficial bite of right middle finger

✓7ᵗʰ **S60.473** Other superficial bite of left middle finger

✓7ᵗʰ **S60.474** Other superficial bite of right ring finger

✓7ᵗʰ **S60.475** Other superficial bite of left ring finger

✓7ᵗʰ **S60.476** Other superficial bite of right little finger

✓7ᵗʰ **S60.477** Other superficial bite of left little finger

✓7ᵗʰ **S60.478** Other superficial bite of other finger
Other superficial bite of specified finger with unspecified laterality

✓7ᵗʰ **S60.479** Other superficial bite of unspecified finger ▽

✓5ᵗʰ **S60.5** Other superficial injuries of hand
EXCLUDES 2   superficial injuries of fingers (S60.3-, S60.4-)

✓6ᵗʰ **S60.51** Abrasion of hand

✓7ᵗʰ **S60.511** Abrasion of right hand

✓7ᵗʰ **S60.512** Abrasion of left hand

✓7ᵗʰ **S60.519** Abrasion of unspecified hand ▽

✓6ᵗʰ **S60.52** Blister (nonthermal) of hand

✓7ᵗʰ **S60.521** Blister (nonthermal) of right hand

✓7ᵗʰ **S60.522** Blister (nonthermal) of left hand

✓7ᵗʰ **S60.529** Blister (nonthermal) of unspecified hand ▽

✓6ᵗʰ **S60.54** External constriction of hand

✓7ᵗʰ **S60.541** External constriction of right hand

✓7ᵗʰ **S60.542** External constriction of left hand

✓7ᵗʰ **S60.549** External constriction of unspecified hand ▽

✓6ᵗʰ **S60.55** Superficial foreign body of hand
Splinter in the hand

✓7ᵗʰ **S60.551** Superficial foreign body of right hand

✓7ᵗʰ **S60.552** Superficial foreign body of left hand

✓7ᵗʰ **S60.559** Superficial foreign body of unspecified hand ▽

✓6ᵗʰ **S60.56** Insect bite (nonvenomous) of hand

✓7ᵗʰ **S60.561** Insect bite (nonvenomous) of right hand

✓7ᵗʰ **S60.562** Insect bite (nonvenomous) of left hand

✓7ᵗʰ **S60.569** Insect bite (nonvenomous) of unspecified hand ▽

✓6ᵗʰ **S60.57** Other superficial bite of hand
EXCLUDES 1   open bite of hand (S61.45-)

✓7ᵗʰ **S60.571** Other superficial bite of hand of right hand

✓7ᵗʰ **S60.572** Other superficial bite of hand of left hand

✓7ᵗʰ **S60.579** Other superficial bite of hand of unspecified hand ▽

✓5ᵗʰ **S60.8** Other superficial injuries of wrist

✓6ᵗʰ **S60.81** Abrasion of wrist

✓7ᵗʰ **S60.811** Abrasion of right wrist

✓7ᵗʰ **S60.812** Abrasion of left wrist

✓7ᵗʰ **S60.819** Abrasion of unspecified wrist ▽

✓6ᵗʰ **S60.82** Blister (nonthermal) of wrist

✓7ᵗʰ **S60.821** Blister (nonthermal) of right wrist

✓7ᵗʰ **S60.822** Blister (nonthermal) of left wrist

✓7ᵗʰ **S60.829** Blister (nonthermal) of unspecified wrist ▽

✓6ᵗʰ **S60.84** External constriction of wrist

✓7ᵗʰ **S60.841** External constriction of right wrist

✓7ᵗʰ **S60.842** External constriction of left wrist

✓7ᵗʰ **S60.849** External constriction of unspecified wrist ▽

✓6ᵗʰ **S60.85** Superficial foreign body of wrist
Splinter in the wrist

✓7ᵗʰ **S60.851** Superficial foreign body of right wrist

✓7ᵗʰ **S60.852** Superficial foreign body of left wrist

✓7ᵗʰ **S60.859** Superficial foreign body of unspecified wrist ▽

✓6ᵗʰ **S60.86** Insect bite (nonvenomous) of wrist

✓7ᵗʰ **S60.861** Insect bite (nonvenomous) of right wrist

✓7ᵗʰ **S60.862** Insect bite (nonvenomous) of left wrist

✓7ᵗʰ **S60.869** Insect bite (nonvenomous) of unspecified wrist ▽

✓6ᵗʰ **S60.87** Other superficial bite of wrist
EXCLUDES 1   open bite of wrist (S61.55)

✓7ᵗʰ **S60.871** Other superficial bite of right wrist

✓7ᵗʰ **S60.872** Other superficial bite of left wrist

✓7ᵗʰ **S60.879** Other superficial bite of unspecified wrist ▽

✓5ᵗʰ **S60.9** Unspecified superficial injury of wrist, hand and fingers

✓6ᵗʰ **S60.91** Unspecified superficial injury of wrist

✓7ᵗʰ **S60.911** Unspecified superficial injury of right wrist ▽

✓7ᵗʰ **S60.912** Unspecified superficial injury of left wrist ▽

✓7ᵗʰ **S60.919** Unspecified superficial injury of unspecified wrist ▽

✓6ᵗʰ **S60.92** Unspecified superficial injury of hand

✓7ᵗʰ **S60.921** Unspecified superficial injury of right hand ▽

☑ Additional Character Req   ✓7ᵗʰ Placeholder Alert   Manifestation   HCC CMS-HCC Condition   ▽ Unspecified Code   ►◄ Revised Text   ● New Code   ▲ Revised Code Title

ICD-10-CM 2018

979

S60.922 Unspecified superficial injury of left hand

S60.929 Unspecified superficial injury of unspecified hand

√6ᵗʰ **S60.93** Unspecified superficial injury of thumb

    √7ᵗʰ **S60.931** Unspecified superficial injury of right thumb

    √7ᵗʰ **S60.932** Unspecified superficial injury of left thumb

    √7ᵗʰ **S60.939** Unspecified superficial injury of unspecified thumb

√6ᵗʰ **S60.94** Unspecified superficial injury of other fingers

    √7ᵗʰ **S60.940** Unspecified superficial injury of right index finger

    √7ᵗʰ **S60.941** Unspecified superficial injury of left index finger

    √7ᵗʰ **S60.942** Unspecified superficial injury of right middle finger

    √7ᵗʰ **S60.943** Unspecified superficial injury of left middle finger

    √7ᵗʰ **S60.944** Unspecified superficial injury of right ring finger

    √7ᵗʰ **S60.945** Unspecified superficial injury of left ring finger

    √7ᵗʰ **S60.946** Unspecified superficial injury of right little finger

    √7ᵗʰ **S60.947** Unspecified superficial injury of left little finger

    √7ᵗʰ **S60.948** Unspecified superficial injury of other finger
       Unspecified superficial injury of specified finger with unspecified laterality

    √7ᵗʰ **S60.949** Unspecified superficial injury of unspecified finger

√4ᵗʰ **S61** Open wound of wrist, hand and fingers
    Code also any associated wound infection
    EXCLUDES 1 open fracture of wrist, hand and finger (S62- with 7th character B)
       traumatic amputation of wrist and hand (S68.-)

> The appropriate 7th character is to be added to each code from category S61.
> A   initial encounter
> D   subsequent encounter
> S   sequela

√5ᵗʰ **S61.0** Open wound of thumb without damage to nail
    EXCLUDES 1 open wound of thumb with damage to nail (S61.1-)

    √6ᵗʰ **S61.00** Unspecified open wound of thumb without damage to nail

       √7ᵗʰ **S61.001** Unspecified open wound of right thumb without damage to nail

       √7ᵗʰ **S61.002** Unspecified open wound of left thumb without damage to nail

       √7ᵗʰ **S61.009** Unspecified open wound of unspecified thumb without damage to nail

    √6ᵗʰ **S61.01** Laceration without foreign body of thumb without damage to nail

       √7ᵗʰ **S61.011** Laceration without foreign body of right thumb without damage to nail

       √7ᵗʰ **S61.012** Laceration without foreign body of left thumb without damage to nail

       √7ᵗʰ **S61.019** Laceration without foreign body of unspecified thumb without damage to nail

    √6ᵗʰ **S61.02** Laceration with foreign body of thumb without damage to nail

       √7ᵗʰ **S61.021** Laceration with foreign body of right thumb without damage to nail

       √7ᵗʰ **S61.022** Laceration with foreign body of left thumb without damage to nail

       √7ᵗʰ **S61.029** Laceration with foreign body of unspecified thumb without damage to nail

√6ᵗʰ **S61.03** Puncture wound without foreign body of thumb without damage to nail

    √7ᵗʰ **S61.031** Puncture wound without foreign body of right thumb without damage to nail

    √7ᵗʰ **S61.032** Puncture wound without foreign body of left thumb without damage to nail

    √7ᵗʰ **S61.039** Puncture wound without foreign body of unspecified thumb without damage to nail

√6ᵗʰ **S61.04** Puncture wound with foreign body of thumb without damage to nail

    √7ᵗʰ **S61.041** Puncture wound with foreign body of right thumb without damage to nail

    √7ᵗʰ **S61.042** Puncture wound with foreign body of left thumb without damage to nail

    √7ᵗʰ **S61.049** Puncture wound with foreign body of unspecified thumb without damage to nail

√6ᵗʰ **S61.05** Open bite of thumb without damage to nail
    Bite of thumb NOS
    EXCLUDES 1 superficial bite of thumb (S60.36-, S60.37-)

    √7ᵗʰ **S61.051** Open bite of right thumb without damage to nail

    √7ᵗʰ **S61.052** Open bite of left thumb without damage to nail

    √7ᵗʰ **S61.059** Open bite of unspecified thumb without damage to nail

√5ᵗʰ **S61.1** Open wound of thumb with damage to nail

    √6ᵗʰ **S61.10** Unspecified open wound of thumb with damage to nail

       √7ᵗʰ **S61.101** Unspecified open wound of right thumb with damage to nail

       √7ᵗʰ **S61.102** Unspecified open wound of left thumb with damage to nail

       √7ᵗʰ **S61.109** Unspecified open wound of unspecified thumb with damage to nail

    √6ᵗʰ **S61.11** Laceration without foreign body of thumb with damage to nail

       √7ᵗʰ **S61.111** Laceration without foreign body of right thumb with damage to nail

       √7ᵗʰ **S61.112** Laceration without foreign body of left thumb with damage to nail

       √7ᵗʰ **S61.119** Laceration without foreign body of unspecified thumb with damage to nail

    √6ᵗʰ **S61.12** Laceration with foreign body of thumb with damage to nail

       √7ᵗʰ **S61.121** Laceration with foreign body of right thumb with damage to nail

       √7ᵗʰ **S61.122** Laceration with foreign body of left thumb with damage to nail

       √7ᵗʰ **S61.129** Laceration with foreign body of unspecified thumb with damage to nail

    √6ᵗʰ **S61.13** Puncture wound without foreign body of thumb with damage to nail

       √7ᵗʰ **S61.131** Puncture wound without foreign body of right thumb with damage to nail

       √7ᵗʰ **S61.132** Puncture wound without foreign body of left thumb with damage to nail

       √7ᵗʰ **S61.139** Puncture wound without foreign body of unspecified thumb with damage to nail

    √6ᵗʰ **S61.14** Puncture wound with foreign body of thumb with damage to nail

       √7ᵗʰ **S61.141** Puncture wound with foreign body of right thumb with damage to nail

       √7ᵗʰ **S61.142** Puncture wound with foreign body of left thumb with damage to nail

       √7ᵗʰ **S61.149** Puncture wound with foreign body of unspecified thumb with damage to nail

    √6ᵗʰ **S61.15** Open bite of thumb with damage to nail
       Bite of thumb with damage to nail NOS
       EXCLUDES 1 superficial bite of thumb (S60.36-, S60.37-)

       √7ᵗʰ **S61.151** Open bite of right thumb with damage to nail

       √7ᵗʰ **S61.152** Open bite of left thumb with damage to nail

EXCLUDES 1 Not coded here   *EXCLUDES 2* Not included here   N Newborn Age: 0   P Pediatric Age: 0-17   M Maternity Age: 12-55   A Adult Age: 15-124

980   ICD-10-CM 2018

√7ᵗʰ **S61.159** Open bite of unspecified thumb with damage to nail ▽

√5ᵗʰ **S61.2** **Open wound of other** finger without damage to nail

     EXCLUDES 1   open wound of finger involving nail (matrix) (S61.3-)
     EXCLUDES 2   open wound of thumb without damage to nail (S61.0-)

√6ᵗʰ **S61.20** **Unspecified open wound of other finger without damage to nail**

   √7ᵗʰ **S61.200** Unspecified open wound of right index finger without damage to nail ▽

   √7ᵗʰ **S61.201** Unspecified open wound of left index finger without damage to nail ▽

   √7ᵗʰ **S61.202** Unspecified open wound of right middle finger without damage to nail ▽

   √7ᵗʰ **S61.203** Unspecified open wound of left middle finger without damage to nail ▽

   √7ᵗʰ **S61.204** Unspecified open wound of right ring finger without damage to nail ▽

   √7ᵗʰ **S61.205** Unspecified open wound of left ring finger without damage to nail ▽

   √7ᵗʰ **S61.206** Unspecified open wound of right little finger without damage to nail ▽

   √7ᵗʰ **S61.207** Unspecified open wound of left little finger without damage to nail ▽

   √7ᵗʰ **S61.208** Unspecified open wound of other finger without damage to nail ▽
     Unspecified open wound of specified finger with unspecified laterality without damage to nail

   √7ᵗʰ **S61.209** Unspecified open wound of unspecified finger without damage to nail ▽

√6ᵗʰ **S61.21** **Laceration without foreign body** of finger without damage to nail

   √7ᵗʰ **S61.210** Laceration without foreign body of right index finger without damage to nail

   √7ᵗʰ **S61.211** Laceration without foreign body of left index finger without damage to nail

   √7ᵗʰ **S61.212** Laceration without foreign body of right middle finger without damage to nail

   √7ᵗʰ **S61.213** Laceration without foreign body of left middle finger without damage to nail

   √7ᵗʰ **S61.214** Laceration without foreign body of right ring finger without damage to nail

   √7ᵗʰ **S61.215** Laceration without foreign body of left ring finger without damage to nail

   √7ᵗʰ **S61.216** Laceration without foreign body of right little finger without damage to nail

   √7ᵗʰ **S61.217** Laceration without foreign body of left little finger without damage to nail

   √7ᵗʰ **S61.218** Laceration without foreign body of other finger without damage to nail
     Laceration without foreign body of specified finger with unspecified laterality without damage to nail

   √7ᵗʰ **S61.219** Laceration without foreign body of unspecified finger without damage to nail ▽

√6ᵗʰ **S61.22** **Laceration with foreign body** of finger without damage to nail

   √7ᵗʰ **S61.220** Laceration with foreign body of right index finger without damage to nail

   √7ᵗʰ **S61.221** Laceration with foreign body of left index finger without damage to nail

   √7ᵗʰ **S61.222** Laceration with foreign body of right middle finger without damage to nail

   √7ᵗʰ **S61.223** Laceration with foreign body of left middle finger without damage to nail

   √7ᵗʰ **S61.224** Laceration with foreign body of right ring finger without damage to nail

   √7ᵗʰ **S61.225** Laceration with foreign body of left ring finger without damage to nail

   √7ᵗʰ **S61.226** Laceration with foreign body of right little finger without damage to nail

   √7ᵗʰ **S61.227** Laceration with foreign body of left little finger without damage to nail

   √7ᵗʰ **S61.228** Laceration with foreign body of other finger without damage to nail
     Laceration with foreign body of specified finger with unspecified laterality without damage to nail

   √7ᵗʰ **S61.229** Laceration with foreign body of unspecified finger without damage to nail ▽

√6ᵗʰ **S61.23** **Puncture wound without foreign body** of finger without damage to nail

   √7ᵗʰ **S61.230** Puncture wound without foreign body of right index finger without damage to nail

   √7ᵗʰ **S61.231** Puncture wound without foreign body of left index finger without damage to nail

   √7ᵗʰ **S61.232** Puncture wound without foreign body of right middle finger without damage to nail

   √7ᵗʰ **S61.233** Puncture wound without foreign body of left middle finger without damage to nail

   √7ᵗʰ **S61.234** Puncture wound without foreign body of right ring finger without damage to nail

   √7ᵗʰ **S61.235** Puncture wound without foreign body of left ring finger without damage to nail

   √7ᵗʰ **S61.236** Puncture wound without foreign body of right little finger without damage to nail

   √7ᵗʰ **S61.237** Puncture wound without foreign body of left little finger without damage to nail

   √7ᵗʰ **S61.238** Puncture wound without foreign body of other finger without damage to nail
     Puncture wound without foreign body of specified finger with unspecified laterality without damage to nail

   √7ᵗʰ **S61.239** Puncture wound without foreign body of unspecified finger without damage to nail ▽

√6ᵗʰ **S61.24** **Puncture wound with foreign body** of finger without damage to nail

   √7ᵗʰ **S61.240** Puncture wound with foreign body of right index finger without damage to nail

   √7ᵗʰ **S61.241** Puncture wound with foreign body of left index finger without damage to nail

   √7ᵗʰ **S61.242** Puncture wound with foreign body of right middle finger without damage to nail

   √7ᵗʰ **S61.243** Puncture wound with foreign body of left middle finger without damage to nail

   √7ᵗʰ **S61.244** Puncture wound with foreign body of right ring finger without damage to nail

   √7ᵗʰ **S61.245** Puncture wound with foreign body of left ring finger without damage to nail

   √7ᵗʰ **S61.246** Puncture wound with foreign body of right little finger without damage to nail

   √7ᵗʰ **S61.247** Puncture wound with foreign body of left little finger without damage to nail

   √7ᵗʰ **S61.248** Puncture wound with foreign body of other finger without damage to nail
     Puncture wound with foreign body of specified finger with unspecified laterality without damage to nail

   √7ᵗʰ **S61.249** Puncture wound with foreign body of unspecified finger without damage to nail ▽

√6ᵗʰ **S61.25** **Open bite** of finger without damage to nail
     Bite of finger without damage to nail NOS
     EXCLUDES 1   superficial bite of finger (S60.46-, S60.47-)

   √7ᵗʰ **S61.250** Open bite of right index finger without damage to nail

   √7ᵗʰ **S61.251** Open bite of left index finger without damage to nail

   √7ᵗʰ **S61.252** Open bite of right middle finger without damage to nail

   √7ᵗʰ **S61.253** Open bite of left middle finger without damage to nail

   √7ᵗʰ **S61.254** Open bite of right ring finger without damage to nail

   √7ᵗʰ **S61.255** Open bite of left ring finger without damage to nail

---

√ Additional Character Req   √x7ᵗʰ Placeholder Alert   Manifestation   HCC CMS-HCC Condition   ▽ Unspecified Code   ▶◀ Revised Text   ● New Code   ▲ Revised Code Title

✓7ᵗʰ **S61.256 Open bite of right little finger without damage to nail**

✓7ᵗʰ **S61.257 Open bite of left little finger without damage to nail**

✓7ᵗʰ **S61.258 Open bite of other finger without damage to nail**
Open bite of specified finger with unspecified laterality without damage to nail

✓7ᵗʰ **S61.259 Open bite of unspecified finger without damage to nail** ▽

✓5ᵗʰ **S61.3 Open wound of other finger with damage to nail**

　✓6ᵗʰ **S61.30 Unspecified open wound of finger with damage to nail**

　　✓7ᵗʰ **S61.300 Unspecified open wound of right index finger with damage to nail** ▽

　　✓7ᵗʰ **S61.301 Unspecified open wound of left index finger with damage to nail** ▽

　　✓7ᵗʰ **S61.302 Unspecified open wound of right middle finger with damage to nail** ▽

　　✓7ᵗʰ **S61.303 Unspecified open wound of left middle finger with damage to nail** ▽

　　✓7ᵗʰ **S61.304 Unspecified open wound of right ring finger with damage to nail** ▽

　　✓7ᵗʰ **S61.305 Unspecified open wound of left ring finger with damage to nail** ▽

　　✓7ᵗʰ **S61.306 Unspecified open wound of right little finger with damage to nail** ▽

　　✓7ᵗʰ **S61.307 Unspecified open wound of left little finger with damage to nail** ▽

　　✓7ᵗʰ **S61.308 Unspecified open wound of other finger with damage to nail** ▽
Unspecified open wound of specified finger with unspecified laterality with damage to nail

　　✓7ᵗʰ **S61.309 Unspecified open wound of unspecified finger with damage to nail** ▽

　✓6ᵗʰ **S61.31 Laceration without foreign body of finger with damage to nail**

　　✓7ᵗʰ **S61.310 Laceration without foreign body of right index finger with damage to nail**

　　✓7ᵗʰ **S61.311 Laceration without foreign body of left index finger with damage to nail**

　　✓7ᵗʰ **S61.312 Laceration without foreign body of right middle finger with damage to nail**

　　✓7ᵗʰ **S61.313 Laceration without foreign body of left middle finger with damage to nail**

　　✓7ᵗʰ **S61.314 Laceration without foreign body of right ring finger with damage to nail**

　　✓7ᵗʰ **S61.315 Laceration without foreign body of left ring finger with damage to nail**

　　✓7ᵗʰ **S61.316 Laceration without foreign body of right little finger with damage to nail**

　　✓7ᵗʰ **S61.317 Laceration without foreign body of left little finger with damage to nail**

　　✓7ᵗʰ **S61.318 Laceration without foreign body of other finger with damage to nail**
Laceration without foreign body of specified finger with unspecified laterality with damage to nail

　　✓7ᵗʰ **S61.319 Laceration without foreign body of unspecified finger with damage to nail** ▽

　✓6ᵗʰ **S61.32 Laceration with foreign body of finger with damage to nail**

　　✓7ᵗʰ **S61.320 Laceration with foreign body of right index finger with damage to nail**

　　✓7ᵗʰ **S61.321 Laceration with foreign body of left index finger with damage to nail**

　　✓7ᵗʰ **S61.322 Laceration with foreign body of right middle finger with damage to nail**

　　✓7ᵗʰ **S61.323 Laceration with foreign body of left middle finger with damage to nail**

　　✓7ᵗʰ **S61.324 Laceration with foreign body of right ring finger with damage to nail**

　　✓7ᵗʰ **S61.325 Laceration with foreign body of left ring finger with damage to nail**

　　✓7ᵗʰ **S61.326 Laceration with foreign body of right little finger with damage to nail**

　　✓7ᵗʰ **S61.327 Laceration with foreign body of left little finger with damage to nail**

　　✓7ᵗʰ **S61.328 Laceration with foreign body of other finger with damage to nail**
Laceration with foreign body of specified finger with unspecified laterality with damage to nail

　　✓7ᵗʰ **S61.329 Laceration with foreign body of unspecified finger with damage to nail** ▽

　✓6ᵗʰ **S61.33 Puncture wound without foreign body of finger with damage to nail**

　　✓7ᵗʰ **S61.330 Puncture wound without foreign body of right index finger with damage to nail**

　　✓7ᵗʰ **S61.331 Puncture wound without foreign body of left index finger with damage to nail**

　　✓7ᵗʰ **S61.332 Puncture wound without foreign body of right middle finger with damage to nail**

　　✓7ᵗʰ **S61.333 Puncture wound without foreign body of left middle finger with damage to nail**

　　✓7ᵗʰ **S61.334 Puncture wound without foreign body of right ring finger with damage to nail**

　　✓7ᵗʰ **S61.335 Puncture wound without foreign body of left ring finger with damage to nail**

　　✓7ᵗʰ **S61.336 Puncture wound without foreign body of right little finger with damage to nail**

　　✓7ᵗʰ **S61.337 Puncture wound without foreign body of left little finger with damage to nail**

　　✓7ᵗʰ **S61.338 Puncture wound without foreign body of other finger with damage to nail**
Puncture wound without foreign body of specified finger with unspecified laterality with damage to nail

　　✓7ᵗʰ **S61.339 Puncture wound without foreign body of unspecified finger with damage to nail** ▽

　✓6ᵗʰ **S61.34 Puncture wound with foreign body of finger with damage to nail**

　　✓7ᵗʰ **S61.340 Puncture wound with foreign body of right index finger with damage to nail**

　　✓7ᵗʰ **S61.341 Puncture wound with foreign body of left index finger with damage to nail**

　　✓7ᵗʰ **S61.342 Puncture wound with foreign body of right middle finger with damage to nail**

　　✓7ᵗʰ **S61.343 Puncture wound with foreign body of left middle finger with damage to nail**

　　✓7ᵗʰ **S61.344 Puncture wound with foreign body of right ring finger with damage to nail**

　　✓7ᵗʰ **S61.345 Puncture wound with foreign body of left ring finger with damage to nail**

　　✓7ᵗʰ **S61.346 Puncture wound with foreign body of right little finger with damage to nail**

　　✓7ᵗʰ **S61.347 Puncture wound with foreign body of left little finger with damage to nail**

　　✓7ᵗʰ **S61.348 Puncture wound with foreign body of other finger with damage to nail**
Puncture wound with foreign body of specified finger with unspecified laterality with damage to nail

　　✓7ᵗʰ **S61.349 Puncture wound with foreign body of unspecified finger with damage to nail** ▽

　✓6ᵗʰ **S61.35 Open bite of finger with damage to nail**
Bite of finger with damage to nail NOS
　EXCLUDES 1 superficial bite of finger (S60.46-, S60.47-)

　　✓7ᵗʰ **S61.350 Open bite of right index finger with damage to nail**

　　✓7ᵗʰ **S61.351 Open bite of left index finger with damage to nail**

　　✓7ᵗʰ **S61.352 Open bite of right middle finger with damage to nail**

　　✓7ᵗʰ **S61.353 Open bite of left middle finger with damage to nail**

　　✓7ᵗʰ **S61.354 Open bite of right ring finger with damage to nail**

　　✓7ᵗʰ **S61.355 Open bite of left ring finger with damage to nail**

✓7ᵗʰ **S61.356** Open bite of right little finger with damage to nail

✓7ᵗʰ **S61.357** Open bite of left little finger with damage to nail

✓7ᵗʰ **S61.358** Open bite of other finger with damage to nail

     Open bite of specified finger with unspecified laterality with damage to nail

✓7ᵗʰ **S61.359** Open bite of unspecified finger with damage to nail ▽

✓5ᵗʰ **S61.4**   **Open wound of hand**

   ✓6ᵗʰ **S61.40**   Unspecified open wound of hand

     ✓7ᵗʰ **S61.401** Unspecified open wound of right hand ▽

     ✓7ᵗʰ **S61.402** Unspecified open wound of left hand ▽

     ✓7ᵗʰ **S61.409** Unspecified open wound of unspecified hand ▽

   ✓6ᵗʰ **S61.41**   Laceration without foreign body of hand

     ✓7ᵗʰ **S61.411** Laceration without foreign body of right hand

     ✓7ᵗʰ **S61.412** Laceration without foreign body of left hand

     ✓7ᵗʰ **S61.419** Laceration without foreign body of unspecified hand ▽

   ✓6ᵗʰ **S61.42**   Laceration with foreign body of hand

     ✓7ᵗʰ **S61.421** Laceration with foreign body of right hand

     ✓7ᵗʰ **S61.422** Laceration with foreign body of left hand

     ✓7ᵗʰ **S61.429** Laceration with foreign body of unspecified hand ▽

   ✓6ᵗʰ **S61.43**   Puncture wound without foreign body of hand

     ✓7ᵗʰ **S61.431** Puncture wound without foreign body of right hand

     ✓7ᵗʰ **S61.432** Puncture wound without foreign body of left hand

     ✓7ᵗʰ **S61.439** Puncture wound without foreign body of unspecified hand ▽

   ✓6ᵗʰ **S61.44**   Puncture wound with foreign body of hand

     ✓7ᵗʰ **S61.441** Puncture wound with foreign body of right hand

     ✓7ᵗʰ **S61.442** Puncture wound with foreign body of left hand

     ✓7ᵗʰ **S61.449** Puncture wound with foreign body of unspecified hand ▽

   ✓6ᵗʰ **S61.45**   Open bite of hand

     Bite of hand NOS

     EXCLUDES 1 superficial bite of hand (S60.56-, S60.57-)

     ✓7ᵗʰ **S61.451** Open bite of right hand

     ✓7ᵗʰ **S61.452** Open bite of left hand

     ✓7ᵗʰ **S61.459** Open bite of unspecified hand ▽

✓5ᵗʰ **S61.5**   **Open wound of wrist**

   ✓6ᵗʰ **S61.50**   Unspecified open wound of wrist

     ✓7ᵗʰ **S61.501** Unspecified open wound of right wrist ▽

     ✓7ᵗʰ **S61.502** Unspecified open wound of left wrist ▽

     ✓7ᵗʰ **S61.509** Unspecified open wound of unspecified wrist ▽

   ✓6ᵗʰ **S61.51**   Laceration without foreign body of wrist

     ✓7ᵗʰ **S61.511** Laceration without foreign body of right wrist

     ✓7ᵗʰ **S61.512** Laceration without foreign body of left wrist

     ✓7ᵗʰ **S61.519** Laceration without foreign body of unspecified wrist ▽

   ✓6ᵗʰ **S61.52**   Laceration with foreign body of wrist

     ✓7ᵗʰ **S61.521** Laceration with foreign body of right wrist

     ✓7ᵗʰ **S61.522** Laceration with foreign body of left wrist

     ✓7ᵗʰ **S61.529** Laceration with foreign body of unspecified wrist ▽

   ✓6ᵗʰ **S61.53**   Puncture wound without foreign body of wrist

     ✓7ᵗʰ **S61.531** Puncture wound without foreign body of right wrist

     ✓7ᵗʰ **S61.532** Puncture wound without foreign body of left wrist

---

     ✓7ᵗʰ **S61.539** Puncture wound without foreign body ▽ of unspecified wrist

   ✓6ᵗʰ **S61.54**   Puncture wound with foreign body of wrist

     ✓7ᵗʰ **S61.541** Puncture wound with foreign body of right wrist

     ✓7ᵗʰ **S61.542** Puncture wound with foreign body of left wrist

     ✓7ᵗʰ **S61.549** Puncture wound with foreign body of ▽ unspecified wrist

   ✓6ᵗʰ **S61.55**   Open bite of wrist

     Bite of wrist NOS

     EXCLUDES 1 superficial bite of wrist (S60.86-, S60.87-)

     ✓7ᵗʰ **S61.551** Open bite of right wrist

     ✓7ᵗʰ **S61.552** Open bite of left wrist

     ✓7ᵗʰ **S61.559** Open bite of unspecified wrist ▽

✓4ᵗʰ **S62**   **Fracture at wrist and hand level**

   NOTE   A fracture not indicated as displaced or nondisplaced should be coded to displaced.

     A fracture not indicated as open or closed should be coded to closed.

   EXCLUDES 1 traumatic amputation of wrist and hand (S68.-)

   EXCLUDES 2 fracture of distal parts of ulna and radius (S52.-)

   AHA: 2015, 3Q, 37-39

   The appropriate 7th character is to be added to each code from category S62.

   A   initial encounter for closed fracture

   B   initial encounter for open fracture

   D   subsequent encounter for fracture with routine healing

   G   subsequent encounter for fracture with delayed healing

   K   subsequent encounter for fracture with nonunion

   P   subsequent encounter for fracture with malunion

   S   sequela

✓5ᵗʰ **S62.0**   **Fracture of navicular [scaphoid] bone of wrist**

   ✓6ᵗʰ **S62.00**   Unspecified fracture of navicular [scaphoid] bone of wrist

     ✓7ᵗʰ **S62.001** Unspecified fracture of navicular ▽ [scaphoid] bone of right wrist

     ✓7ᵗʰ **S62.002** Unspecified fracture of navicular ▽ [scaphoid] bone of left wrist

       AHA: 2012, 4Q, 106

     ✓7ᵗʰ **S62.009** Unspecified fracture of navicular ▽ [scaphoid] bone of unspecified wrist

   ✓6ᵗʰ **S62.01**   Fracture of distal pole of navicular [scaphoid] bone of wrist

     Fracture of volar tuberosity of navicular [scaphoid] bone of wrist

     ✓7ᵗʰ **S62.011** Displaced fracture of distal pole of navicular [scaphoid] bone of right wrist

     ✓7ᵗʰ **S62.012** Displaced fracture of distal pole of navicular [scaphoid] bone of left wrist

     ✓7ᵗʰ **S62.013** Displaced fracture of distal pole of ▽ navicular [scaphoid] bone of unspecified wrist

     ✓7ᵗʰ **S62.014** Nondisplaced fracture of distal pole of navicular [scaphoid] bone of right wrist

     ✓7ᵗʰ **S62.015** Nondisplaced fracture of distal pole of navicular [scaphoid] bone of left wrist

     ✓7ᵗʰ **S62.016** Nondisplaced fracture of distal pole ▽ of navicular [scaphoid] bone of unspecified wrist

   ✓6ᵗʰ **S62.02**   Fracture of middle third of navicular [scaphoid] bone of wrist

     ✓7ᵗʰ **S62.021** Displaced fracture of middle third of navicular [scaphoid] bone of right wrist

     ✓7ᵗʰ **S62.022** Displaced fracture of middle third of navicular [scaphoid] bone of left wrist

     ✓7ᵗʰ **S62.023** Displaced fracture of middle third of ▽ navicular [scaphoid] bone of unspecified wrist

     ✓7ᵗʰ **S62.024** Nondisplaced fracture of middle third of navicular [scaphoid] bone of right wrist

     ✓7ᵗʰ **S62.025** Nondisplaced fracture of middle third of navicular [scaphoid] bone of left wrist

     ✓7ᵗʰ **S62.026** Nondisplaced fracture of middle third ▽ of navicular [scaphoid] bone of unspecified wrist

---

✓ Additional Character Req   ✓x7ᵗʰ Placeholder Alert   Manifestation   HCC CMS-HCC Condition   ▽ Unspecified Code   ►◄ Revised Text   ● New Code   ▲ Revised Code Title

ICD-10-CM 2018   983

✓6ᵗʰ **S62.03 Fracture of proximal third of navicular [scaphoid] bone of wrist**

   ✓7ᵗʰ **S62.031 Displaced fracture of proximal third of navicular [scaphoid] bone of right wrist**

   ✓7ᵗʰ **S62.032 Displaced fracture of proximal third of navicular [scaphoid] bone of left wrist**

   ✓7ᵗʰ **S62.033 Displaced fracture of proximal third of navicular [scaphoid] bone of unspecified wrist** ▽

   ✓7ᵗʰ **S62.034 Nondisplaced fracture of proximal third of navicular [scaphoid] bone of right wrist**

   ✓7ᵗʰ **S62.035 Nondisplaced fracture of proximal third of navicular [scaphoid] bone of left wrist**

   ✓7ᵗʰ **S62.036 Nondisplaced fracture of proximal third of navicular [scaphoid] bone of unspecified wrist** ▽

✓5ᵗʰ **S62.1 Fracture of other and unspecified carpal bone(s)**
    EXCLUDES 2 *fracture of scaphoid of wrist (S62.0-)*

  ✓6ᵗʰ **S62.10 Fracture of unspecified carpal bone**
       Fracture of wrist NOS

   ✓7ᵗʰ **S62.101 Fracture of unspecified carpal bone, right wrist** ▽

   ✓7ᵗʰ **S62.102 Fracture of unspecified carpal bone, left wrist** ▽
         AHA: 2012, 4Q, 95

   ✓7ᵗʰ **S62.109 Fracture of unspecified carpal bone, unspecified wrist** ▽

  ✓6ᵗʰ **S62.11 Fracture of triquetrum [cuneiform] bone of wrist**

   ✓7ᵗʰ **S62.111 Displaced fracture of triquetrum [cuneiform] bone, right wrist**

   ✓7ᵗʰ **S62.112 Displaced fracture of triquetrum [cuneiform] bone, left wrist**

   ✓7ᵗʰ **S62.113 Displaced fracture of triquetrum [cuneiform] bone, unspecified wrist** ▽

   ✓7ᵗʰ **S62.114 Nondisplaced fracture of triquetrum [cuneiform] bone, right wrist**

   ✓7ᵗʰ **S62.115 Nondisplaced fracture of triquetrum [cuneiform] bone, left wrist**

   ✓7ᵗʰ **S62.116 Nondisplaced fracture of triquetrum [cuneiform] bone, unspecified wrist** ▽

  ✓6ᵗʰ **S62.12 Fracture of lunate [semilunar]**

   ✓7ᵗʰ **S62.121 Displaced fracture of lunate [semilunar], right wrist**

   ✓7ᵗʰ **S62.122 Displaced fracture of lunate [semilunar], left wrist**

   ✓7ᵗʰ **S62.123 Displaced fracture of lunate [semilunar], unspecified wrist** ▽

   ✓7ᵗʰ **S62.124 Nondisplaced fracture of lunate [semilunar], right wrist**

   ✓7ᵗʰ **S62.125 Nondisplaced fracture of lunate [semilunar], left wrist**

   ✓7ᵗʰ **S62.126 Nondisplaced fracture of lunate [semilunar], unspecified wrist** ▽

  ✓6ᵗʰ **S62.13 Fracture of capitate [os magnum] bone**

   ✓7ᵗʰ **S62.131 Displaced fracture of capitate [os magnum] bone, right wrist**

   ✓7ᵗʰ **S62.132 Displaced fracture of capitate [os magnum] bone, left wrist**

   ✓7ᵗʰ **S62.133 Displaced fracture of capitate [os magnum] bone, unspecified wrist** ▽

   ✓7ᵗʰ **S62.134 Nondisplaced fracture of capitate [os magnum] bone, right wrist**

   ✓7ᵗʰ **S62.135 Nondisplaced fracture of capitate [os magnum] bone, left wrist**

   ✓7ᵗʰ **S62.136 Nondisplaced fracture of capitate [os magnum] bone, unspecified wrist** ▽

  ✓6ᵗʰ **S62.14 Fracture of body of hamate [unciform] bone**
       Fracture of hamate [unciform] bone NOS

   ✓7ᵗʰ **S62.141 Displaced fracture of body of hamate [unciform] bone, right wrist**

   ✓7ᵗʰ **S62.142 Displaced fracture of body of hamate [unciform] bone, left wrist**

   ✓7ᵗʰ **S62.143 Displaced fracture of body of hamate [unciform] bone, unspecified wrist** ▽

   ✓7ᵗʰ **S62.144 Nondisplaced fracture of body of hamate [unciform] bone, right wrist**

   ✓7ᵗʰ **S62.145 Nondisplaced fracture of body of hamate [unciform] bone, left wrist**

   ✓7ᵗʰ **S62.146 Nondisplaced fracture of body of hamate [unciform] bone, unspecified wrist** ▽

  ✓6ᵗʰ **S62.15 Fracture of hook process of hamate [unciform] bone**
       Fracture of unciform process of hamate [unciform] bone

   ✓7ᵗʰ **S62.151 Displaced fracture of hook process of hamate [unciform] bone, right wrist**

   ✓7ᵗʰ **S62.152 Displaced fracture of hook process of hamate [unciform] bone, left wrist**

   ✓7ᵗʰ **S62.153 Displaced fracture of hook process of hamate [unciform] bone, unspecified wrist** ▽

   ✓7ᵗʰ **S62.154 Nondisplaced fracture of hook process of hamate [unciform] bone, right wrist**

   ✓7ᵗʰ **S62.155 Nondisplaced fracture of hook process of hamate [unciform] bone, left wrist**

   ✓7ᵗʰ **S62.156 Nondisplaced fracture of hook process of hamate [unciform] bone, unspecified wrist** ▽

  ✓6ᵗʰ **S62.16 Fracture of pisiform**

   ✓7ᵗʰ **S62.161 Displaced fracture of pisiform, right wrist**

   ✓7ᵗʰ **S62.162 Displaced fracture of pisiform, left wrist**

   ✓7ᵗʰ **S62.163 Displaced fracture of pisiform, unspecified wrist** ▽

   ✓7ᵗʰ **S62.164 Nondisplaced fracture of pisiform, right wrist**

   ✓7ᵗʰ **S62.165 Nondisplaced fracture of pisiform, left wrist**

   ✓7ᵗʰ **S62.166 Nondisplaced fracture of pisiform, unspecified wrist** ▽

  ✓6ᵗʰ **S62.17 Fracture of trapezium [larger multangular]**

   ✓7ᵗʰ **S62.171 Displaced fracture of trapezium [larger multangular], right wrist**

   ✓7ᵗʰ **S62.172 Displaced fracture of trapezium [larger multangular], left wrist**

   ✓7ᵗʰ **S62.173 Displaced fracture of trapezium [larger multangular], unspecified wrist** ▽

   ✓7ᵗʰ **S62.174 Nondisplaced fracture of trapezium [larger multangular], right wrist**

   ✓7ᵗʰ **S62.175 Nondisplaced fracture of trapezium [larger multangular], left wrist**

   ✓7ᵗʰ **S62.176 Nondisplaced fracture of trapezium [larger multangular], unspecified wrist** ▽

  ✓6ᵗʰ **S62.18 Fracture of trapezoid [smaller multangular]**

   ✓7ᵗʰ **S62.181 Displaced fracture of trapezoid [smaller multangular], right wrist**

   ✓7ᵗʰ **S62.182 Displaced fracture of trapezoid [smaller multangular], left wrist**

   ✓7ᵗʰ **S62.183 Displaced fracture of trapezoid [smaller multangular], unspecified wrist** ▽

   ✓7ᵗʰ **S62.184 Nondisplaced fracture of trapezoid [smaller multangular], right wrist**

   ✓7ᵗʰ **S62.185 Nondisplaced fracture of trapezoid [smaller multangular], left wrist**

   ✓7ᵗʰ **S62.186 Nondisplaced fracture of trapezoid [smaller multangular], unspecified wrist** ▽

✓5ᵗʰ **S62.2 Fracture of first metacarpal bone**

  ✓6ᵗʰ **S62.20 Unspecified fracture of first metacarpal bone**

   ✓7ᵗʰ **S62.201 Unspecified fracture of first metacarpal bone, right hand** ▽

   ✓7ᵗʰ **S62.202 Unspecified fracture of first metacarpal bone, left hand** ▽

   ✓7ᵗʰ **S62.209 Unspecified fracture of first metacarpal bone, unspecified hand** ▽

  ✓6ᵗʰ **S62.21 Bennett's fracture**

   ✓7ᵗʰ **S62.211 Bennett's fracture, right hand**

   ✓7ᵗʰ **S62.212 Bennett's fracture, left hand**

   ✓7ᵗʰ **S62.213 Bennett's fracture, unspecified hand** ▽

EXCLUDES 1 Not coded here   EXCLUDES 2 Not included here   N Newborn Age: 0   P Pediatric Age: 0-17   M Maternity Age: 12-55   A Adult Age: 15-124

984   ICD-10-CM 2018

✓6th **S62.22**   Rolando's fracture

    ✓7th **S62.221**   Displaced Rolando's fracture, right hand

    ✓7th **S62.222**   Displaced Rolando's fracture, left hand

    ✓7th **S62.223**   Displaced Rolando's fracture, unspecified hand ▽

    ✓7th **S62.224**   Nondisplaced Rolando's fracture, right hand

    ✓7th **S62.225**   Nondisplaced Rolando's fracture, left hand

    ✓7th **S62.226**   Nondisplaced Rolando's fracture, unspecified hand ▽

✓6th **S62.23**   Other fracture of base of first metacarpal bone

    ✓7th **S62.231**   Other displaced fracture of base of first metacarpal bone, right hand

    ✓7th **S62.232**   Other displaced fracture of base of first metacarpal bone, left hand

    ✓7th **S62.233**   Other displaced fracture of base of first metacarpal bone, unspecified hand ▽

    ✓7th **S62.234**   Other nondisplaced fracture of base of first metacarpal bone, right hand

    ✓7th **S62.235**   Other nondisplaced fracture of base of first metacarpal bone, left hand

    ✓7th **S62.236**   Other nondisplaced fracture of base of first metacarpal bone, unspecified hand ▽

✓6th **S62.24**   Fracture of shaft of first metacarpal bone ▲

    ✓7th **S62.241**   Displaced fracture of shaft of first metacarpal bone, right hand

    ✓7th **S62.242**   Displaced fracture of shaft of first metacarpal bone, left hand

    ✓7th **S62.243**   Displaced fracture of shaft of first metacarpal bone, unspecified hand ▽

    ✓7th **S62.244**   Nondisplaced fracture of shaft of first metacarpal bone, right hand

    ✓7th **S62.245**   Nondisplaced fracture of shaft of first metacarpal bone, left hand

    ✓7th **S62.246**   Nondisplaced fracture of shaft of first metacarpal bone, unspecified hand ▽

✓6th **S62.25**   Fracture of neck of first metacarpal bone

    ✓7th **S62.251**   Displaced fracture of neck of first metacarpal bone, right hand

    ✓7th **S62.252**   Displaced fracture of neck of first metacarpal bone, left hand

    ✓7th **S62.253**   Displaced fracture of neck of first metacarpal bone, unspecified hand ▽

    ✓7th **S62.254**   Nondisplaced fracture of neck of first metacarpal bone, right hand

    ✓7th **S62.255**   Nondisplaced fracture of neck of first metacarpal bone, left hand

    ✓7th **S62.256**   Nondisplaced fracture of neck of first metacarpal bone, unspecified hand ▽

✓6th **S62.29**   Other fracture of first metacarpal bone

    ✓7th **S62.291**   Other fracture of first metacarpal bone, right hand

    ✓7th **S62.292**   Other fracture of first metacarpal bone, left hand

    ✓7th **S62.299**   Other fracture of first metacarpal bone, unspecified hand ▽

✓5th **S62.3**   Fracture of other and unspecified metacarpal bone

    EXCLUDES 2   *fracture of first metacarpal bone (S62.2-)*

   ✓6th **S62.30**   Unspecified fracture of other metacarpal bone

    ✓7th **S62.300**   Unspecified fracture of second metacarpal bone, right hand ▽

    ✓7th **S62.301**   Unspecified fracture of second metacarpal bone, left hand ▽

    ✓7th **S62.302**   Unspecified fracture of third metacarpal bone, right hand ▽

    ✓7th **S62.303**   Unspecified fracture of third metacarpal bone, left hand ▽

    ✓7th **S62.304**   Unspecified fracture of fourth metacarpal bone, right hand ▽

    ✓7th **S62.305**   Unspecified fracture of fourth metacarpal bone, left hand ▽

    ✓7th **S62.306**   Unspecified fracture of fifth metacarpal bone, right hand ▽

    ✓7th **S62.307**   Unspecified fracture of fifth metacarpal bone, left hand ▽

    ✓7th **S62.308**   Unspecified fracture of other metacarpal bone ▽
      Unspecified fracture of specified metacarpal bone with unspecified laterality

    ✓7th **S62.309**   Unspecified fracture of unspecified metacarpal bone ▽

   ✓6th **S62.31**   Displaced fracture of base of other metacarpal bone

    ✓7th **S62.310**   Displaced fracture of base of second metacarpal bone, right hand

    ✓7th **S62.311**   Displaced fracture of base of second metacarpal bone, left hand

    ✓7th **S62.312**   Displaced fracture of base of third metacarpal bone, right hand

    ✓7th **S62.313**   Displaced fracture of base of third metacarpal bone, left hand

    ✓7th **S62.314**   Displaced fracture of base of fourth metacarpal bone, right hand

    ✓7th **S62.315**   Displaced fracture of base of fourth metacarpal bone, left hand

    ✓7th **S62.316**   Displaced fracture of base of fifth metacarpal bone, right hand

    ✓7th **S62.317**   Displaced fracture of base of fifth metacarpal bone, left hand

    ✓7th **S62.318**   Displaced fracture of base of other metacarpal bone
      Displaced fracture of base of specified metacarpal bone with unspecified laterality

    ✓7th **S62.319**   Displaced fracture of base of unspecified metacarpal bone ▽

   ✓6th **S62.32**   Displaced fracture of shaft of other metacarpal bone

    ✓7th **S62.320**   Displaced fracture of shaft of second metacarpal bone, right hand

    ✓7th **S62.321**   Displaced fracture of shaft of second metacarpal bone, left hand

    ✓7th **S62.322**   Displaced fracture of shaft of third metacarpal bone, right hand

    ✓7th **S62.323**   Displaced fracture of shaft of third metacarpal bone, left hand

    ✓7th **S62.324**   Displaced fracture of shaft of fourth metacarpal bone, right hand

    ✓7th **S62.325**   Displaced fracture of shaft of fourth metacarpal bone, left hand

    ✓7th **S62.326**   Displaced fracture of shaft of fifth metacarpal bone, right hand

    ✓7th **S62.327**   Displaced fracture of shaft of fifth metacarpal bone, left hand

    ✓7th **S62.328**   Displaced fracture of shaft of other metacarpal bone
      Displaced fracture of shaft of specified metacarpal bone with unspecified laterality

    ✓7th **S62.329**   Displaced fracture of shaft of unspecified metacarpal bone ▽

   ✓6th **S62.33**   Displaced fracture of neck of other metacarpal bone

    ✓7th **S62.330**   Displaced fracture of neck of second metacarpal bone, right hand

    ✓7th **S62.331**   Displaced fracture of neck of second metacarpal bone, left hand

    ✓7th **S62.332**   Displaced fracture of neck of third metacarpal bone, right hand

    ✓7th **S62.333**   Displaced fracture of neck of third metacarpal bone, left hand

    ✓7th **S62.334**   Displaced fracture of neck of fourth metacarpal bone, right hand

    ✓7th **S62.335**   Displaced fracture of neck of fourth metacarpal bone, left hand

    ✓7th **S62.336**   Displaced fracture of neck of fifth metacarpal bone, right hand

    ✓7th **S62.337**   Displaced fracture of neck of fifth metacarpal bone, left hand

✔ Additional Character Req   ✓x7th Placeholder Alert   Manifestation   HCC CMS-HCC Condition   ▽ Unspecified Code   ►◄ Revised Text   ● New Code   ▲ Revised Code Title

ICD-10-CM 2018   985

Chapter 19. Injury, Poisoning, and Certain Other Consequences of External Causes

✓7ᵗʰ **S62.338 Displaced fracture of neck of other metacarpal bone**
　　Displaced fracture of neck of specified metacarpal bone with unspecified laterality

✓7ᵗʰ **S62.339 Displaced fracture of neck of unspecified metacarpal bone** ▽

✓6ᵗʰ **S62.34 Nondisplaced fracture of base of other metacarpal bone**

✓7ᵗʰ **S62.340 Nondisplaced fracture of base of second metacarpal bone, right hand**

✓7ᵗʰ **S62.341 Nondisplaced fracture of base of second metacarpal bone, left hand**

✓7ᵗʰ **S62.342 Nondisplaced fracture of base of third metacarpal bone, right hand**

✓7ᵗʰ **S62.343 Nondisplaced fracture of base of third metacarpal bone, left hand**

✓7ᵗʰ **S62.344 Nondisplaced fracture of base of fourth metacarpal bone, right hand**

✓7ᵗʰ **S62.345 Nondisplaced fracture of base of fourth metacarpal bone, left hand**

✓7ᵗʰ **S62.346 Nondisplaced fracture of base of fifth metacarpal bone, right hand**

✓7ᵗʰ **S62.347 Nondisplaced fracture of base of fifth metacarpal bone, left hand**

✓7ᵗʰ **S62.348 Nondisplaced fracture of base of other metacarpal bone**
　　Nondisplaced fracture of base of specified metacarpal bone with unspecified laterality

✓7ᵗʰ **S62.349 Nondisplaced fracture of base of unspecified metacarpal bone** ▽

✓6ᵗʰ **S62.35 Nondisplaced fracture of shaft of other metacarpal bone**

✓7ᵗʰ **S62.350 Nondisplaced fracture of shaft of second metacarpal bone, right hand**

✓7ᵗʰ **S62.351 Nondisplaced fracture of shaft of second metacarpal bone, left hand**

✓7ᵗʰ **S62.352 Nondisplaced fracture of shaft of third metacarpal bone, right hand**

✓7ᵗʰ **S62.353 Nondisplaced fracture of shaft of third metacarpal bone, left hand**

✓7ᵗʰ **S62.354 Nondisplaced fracture of shaft of fourth metacarpal bone, right hand**

✓7ᵗʰ **S62.355 Nondisplaced fracture of shaft of fourth metacarpal bone, left hand**

✓7ᵗʰ **S62.356 Nondisplaced fracture of shaft of fifth metacarpal bone, right hand**

✓7ᵗʰ **S62.357 Nondisplaced fracture of shaft of fifth metacarpal bone, left hand**

✓7ᵗʰ **S62.358 Nondisplaced fracture of shaft of other metacarpal bone**
　　Nondisplaced fracture of shaft of specified metacarpal bone with unspecified laterality

✓7ᵗʰ **S62.359 Nondisplaced fracture of shaft of unspecified metacarpal bone** ▽

✓6ᵗʰ **S62.36 Nondisplaced fracture of neck of other metacarpal bone**

✓7ᵗʰ **S62.360 Nondisplaced fracture of neck of second metacarpal bone, right hand**

✓7ᵗʰ **S62.361 Nondisplaced fracture of neck of second metacarpal bone, left hand**

✓7ᵗʰ **S62.362 Nondisplaced fracture of neck of third metacarpal bone, right hand**

✓7ᵗʰ **S62.363 Nondisplaced fracture of neck of third metacarpal bone, left hand**

✓7ᵗʰ **S62.364 Nondisplaced fracture of neck of fourth metacarpal bone, right hand**

✓7ᵗʰ **S62.365 Nondisplaced fracture of neck of fourth metacarpal bone, left hand**

✓7ᵗʰ **S62.366 Nondisplaced fracture of neck of fifth metacarpal bone, right hand**

✓7ᵗʰ **S62.367 Nondisplaced fracture of neck of fifth metacarpal bone, left hand**

✓7ᵗʰ **S62.368 Nondisplaced fracture of neck of other metacarpal bone**
　　Nondisplaced fracture of neck of specified metacarpal bone with unspecified laterality

✓7ᵗʰ **S62.369 Nondisplaced fracture of neck of unspecified metacarpal bone** ▽

✓6ᵗʰ **S62.39 Other fracture of other metacarpal bone**

✓7ᵗʰ **S62.390 Other fracture of second metacarpal bone, right hand**

✓7ᵗʰ **S62.391 Other fracture of second metacarpal bone, left hand**

✓7ᵗʰ **S62.392 Other fracture of third metacarpal bone, right hand**

✓7ᵗʰ **S62.393 Other fracture of third metacarpal bone, left hand**

✓7ᵗʰ **S62.394 Other fracture of fourth metacarpal bone, right hand**

✓7ᵗʰ **S62.395 Other fracture of fourth metacarpal bone, left hand**

✓7ᵗʰ **S62.396 Other fracture of fifth metacarpal bone, right hand**

✓7ᵗʰ **S62.397 Other fracture of fifth metacarpal bone, left hand**

✓7ᵗʰ **S62.398 Other fracture of other metacarpal bone**
　　Other fracture of specified metacarpal bone with unspecified laterality

✓7ᵗʰ **S62.399 Other fracture of unspecified metacarpal bone** ▽

✓5ᵗʰ **S62.5 Fracture of thumb**

✓6ᵗʰ **S62.50 Fracture of unspecified phalanx of thumb**

✓7ᵗʰ **S62.501 Fracture of unspecified phalanx of right thumb** ▽

✓7ᵗʰ **S62.502 Fracture of unspecified phalanx of left thumb**

✓7ᵗʰ **S62.509 Fracture of unspecified phalanx of unspecified thumb** ▽

✓6ᵗʰ **S62.51 Fracture of proximal phalanx of thumb**

✓7ᵗʰ **S62.511 Displaced fracture of proximal phalanx of right thumb**

✓7ᵗʰ **S62.512 Displaced fracture of proximal phalanx of left thumb**

✓7ᵗʰ **S62.513 Displaced fracture of proximal phalanx of unspecified thumb** ▽

✓7ᵗʰ **S62.514 Nondisplaced fracture of proximal phalanx of right thumb**

✓7ᵗʰ **S62.515 Nondisplaced fracture of proximal phalanx of left thumb**

✓7ᵗʰ **S62.516 Nondisplaced fracture of proximal phalanx of unspecified thumb** ▽

✓6ᵗʰ **S62.52 Fracture of distal phalanx of thumb**

✓7ᵗʰ **S62.521 Displaced fracture of distal phalanx of right thumb**

✓7ᵗʰ **S62.522 Displaced fracture of distal phalanx of left thumb**

✓7ᵗʰ **S62.523 Displaced fracture of distal phalanx of unspecified thumb** ▽

✓7ᵗʰ **S62.524 Nondisplaced fracture of distal phalanx of right thumb**

✓7ᵗʰ **S62.525 Nondisplaced fracture of distal phalanx of left thumb**

✓7ᵗʰ **S62.526 Nondisplaced fracture of distal phalanx of unspecified thumb** ▽

✓5ᵗʰ **S62.6 Fracture of other and unspecified finger(s)**
　EXCLUDES 2   fracture of thumb (S62.5-)

✓6ᵗʰ **S62.60 Fracture of unspecified phalanx of finger**

✓7ᵗʰ **S62.600 Fracture of unspecified phalanx of right index finger** ▽

✓7ᵗʰ **S62.601 Fracture of unspecified phalanx of left index finger** ▽

✓7ᵗʰ **S62.602 Fracture of unspecified phalanx of right middle finger** ▽

✓7ᵗʰ **S62.603 Fracture of unspecified phalanx of left middle finger** ▽

EXCLUDES 1 Not coded here   *EXCLUDES 2* Not included here   N Newborn Age: 0   P Pediatric Age: 0-17   M Maternity Age: 12-55   A Adult Age: 15-124

986   ICD-10-CM 2018

√7ᵗʰ **S62.604** Fracture of unspecified phalanx of right ring finger ▽

√7ᵗʰ **S62.605** Fracture of unspecified phalanx of left ring finger ▽

√7ᵗʰ **S62.606** Fracture of unspecified phalanx of right little finger ▽

√7ᵗʰ **S62.607** Fracture of unspecified phalanx of left little finger ▽

√7ᵗʰ **S62.608** Fracture of unspecified phalanx of other finger ▽
     Fracture of unspecified phalanx of specified finger with unspecified laterality

√7ᵗʰ **S62.609** Fracture of unspecified phalanx of unspecified finger ▽

√6ᵗʰ **S62.61** Displaced fracture of proximal phalanx of finger

√7ᵗʰ **S62.610** Displaced fracture of proximal phalanx of right index finger

√7ᵗʰ **S62.611** Displaced fracture of proximal phalanx of left index finger

√7ᵗʰ **S62.612** Displaced fracture of proximal phalanx of right middle finger

√7ᵗʰ **S62.613** Displaced fracture of proximal phalanx of left middle finger

√7ᵗʰ **S62.614** Displaced fracture of proximal phalanx of right ring finger

√7ᵗʰ **S62.615** Displaced fracture of proximal phalanx of left ring finger

√7ᵗʰ **S62.616** Displaced fracture of proximal phalanx of right little finger

√7ᵗʰ **S62.617** Displaced fracture of proximal phalanx of left little finger

√7ᵗʰ **S62.618** Displaced fracture of proximal phalanx of other finger
     Displaced fracture of proximal phalanx of specified finger with unspecified laterality

√7ᵗʰ **S62.619** Displaced fracture of proximal phalanx ▽ of unspecified finger

▲ √6ᵗʰ **S62.62** Displaced fracture of middle phalanx of finger

▲ √7ᵗʰ **S62.620** Displaced fracture of middle phalanx of right index finger

▲ √7ᵗʰ **S62.621** Displaced fracture of middle phalanx of left index finger

▲ √7ᵗʰ **S62.622** Displaced fracture of middle phalanx of right middle finger

▲ √7ᵗʰ **S62.623** Displaced fracture of middle phalanx of left middle finger

▲ √7ᵗʰ **S62.624** Displaced fracture of middle phalanx of right ring finger

▲ √7ᵗʰ **S62.625** Displaced fracture of middle phalanx of left ring finger

√7ᵗʰ **S62.626** Displaced fracture of medial phalanx of right little finger

√7ᵗʰ **S62.627** Displaced fracture of medial phalanx of left little finger

√7ᵗʰ **S62.628** Displaced fracture of medial phalanx of other finger
     Displaced fracture of medial phalanx of specified finger with unspecified laterality

√7ᵗʰ **S62.629** Displaced fracture of medial phalanx ▽ of unspecified finger

√6ᵗʰ **S62.63** Displaced fracture of distal phalanx of finger

√7ᵗʰ **S62.630** Displaced fracture of distal phalanx of right index finger

√7ᵗʰ **S62.631** Displaced fracture of distal phalanx of left index finger

√7ᵗʰ **S62.632** Displaced fracture of distal phalanx of right middle finger

√7ᵗʰ **S62.633** Displaced fracture of distal phalanx of left middle finger

√7ᵗʰ **S62.634** Displaced fracture of distal phalanx of right ring finger

√7ᵗʰ **S62.635** Displaced fracture of distal phalanx of left ring finger

√7ᵗʰ **S62.636** Displaced fracture of distal phalanx of right little finger

√7ᵗʰ **S62.637** Displaced fracture of distal phalanx of left little finger

√7ᵗʰ **S62.638** Displaced fracture of distal phalanx of other finger
     Displaced fracture of distal phalanx of specified finger with unspecified laterality

√7ᵗʰ **S62.639** Displaced fracture of distal phalanx of ▽ unspecified finger

√6ᵗʰ **S62.64** Nondisplaced fracture of proximal phalanx of finger

√7ᵗʰ **S62.640** Nondisplaced fracture of proximal phalanx of right index finger

√7ᵗʰ **S62.641** Nondisplaced fracture of proximal phalanx of left index finger

√7ᵗʰ **S62.642** Nondisplaced fracture of proximal phalanx of right middle finger

√7ᵗʰ **S62.643** Nondisplaced fracture of proximal phalanx of left middle finger

√7ᵗʰ **S62.644** Nondisplaced fracture of proximal phalanx of right ring finger

√7ᵗʰ **S62.645** Nondisplaced fracture of proximal phalanx of left ring finger

√7ᵗʰ **S62.646** Nondisplaced fracture of proximal phalanx of right little finger

√7ᵗʰ **S62.647** Nondisplaced fracture of proximal phalanx of left little finger

√7ᵗʰ **S62.648** Nondisplaced fracture of proximal phalanx of other finger
     Nondisplaced fracture of proximal phalanx of specified finger with unspecified laterality

√7ᵗʰ **S62.649** Nondisplaced fracture of proximal ▽ phalanx of unspecified finger

√6ᵗʰ **S62.65** Nondisplaced fracture of middle phalanx of finger

√7ᵗʰ **S62.650** Nondisplaced fracture of middle phalanx of right index finger

√7ᵗʰ **S62.651** Nondisplaced fracture of middle phalanx of left index finger

√7ᵗʰ **S62.652** Nondisplaced fracture of middle phalanx of right middle finger

√7ᵗʰ **S62.653** Nondisplaced fracture of middle phalanx of left middle finger

√7ᵗʰ **S62.654** Nondisplaced fracture of medial phalanx of right ring finger

√7ᵗʰ **S62.655** Nondisplaced fracture of medial phalanx of left ring finger

√7ᵗʰ **S62.656** Nondisplaced fracture of medial phalanx of right little finger

√7ᵗʰ **S62.657** Nondisplaced fracture of medial phalanx of left little finger

√7ᵗʰ **S62.658** Nondisplaced fracture of medial phalanx of other finger
     Nondisplaced fracture of medial phalanx of specified finger with unspecified laterality

√7ᵗʰ **S62.659** Nondisplaced fracture of medial ▽ phalanx of unspecified finger

√6ᵗʰ **S62.66** Nondisplaced fracture of distal phalanx of finger

√7ᵗʰ **S62.660** Nondisplaced fracture of distal phalanx of right index finger

√7ᵗʰ **S62.661** Nondisplaced fracture of distal phalanx of left index finger

√7ᵗʰ **S62.662** Nondisplaced fracture of distal phalanx of right middle finger

√7ᵗʰ **S62.663** Nondisplaced fracture of distal phalanx of left middle finger

√7ᵗʰ **S62.664** Nondisplaced fracture of distal phalanx of right ring finger

√7ᵗʰ **S62.665** Nondisplaced fracture of distal phalanx of left ring finger

√7ᵗʰ **S62.666** Nondisplaced fracture of distal phalanx of right little finger

√7ᵗʰ **S62.667** Nondisplaced fracture of distal phalanx of left little finger

☑ Additional Character Req   √×7ᵗʰ Placeholder Alert   Manifestation   HCC CMS-HCC Condition   ▽ Unspecified Code   ▶◀ Revised Text   ● New Code   ▲ Revised Code Title

ICD-10-CM 2018   987

✓7ᵗʰ S62.668 Nondisplaced fracture of distal phalanx of other finger
Nondisplaced fracture of distal phalanx of specified finger with unspecified laterality

✓7ᵗʰ S62.669 Nondisplaced fracture of distal phalanx ▽ **of unspecified finger**

✓5ᵗʰ S62.9 Unspecified fracture of wrist and hand

✓x7ᵗʰ S62.90 Unspecified fracture of unspecified wrist and ▽ **hand**

✓x7ᵗʰ S62.91 Unspecified fracture of right wrist and hand ▽

✓x7ᵗʰ S62.92 Unspecified fracture of left wrist and hand ▽

✓4ᵗʰ S63 Dislocation and sprain of joints and ligaments at wrist and hand level

INCLUDES   avulsion of joint or ligament at wrist and hand level
laceration of cartilage, joint or ligament at wrist and hand level
sprain of cartilage, joint or ligament at wrist and hand level
traumatic hemarthrosis of joint or ligament at wrist and hand level
traumatic rupture of joint or ligament at wrist and hand level
traumatic subluxation of joint or ligament at wrist and hand level
traumatic tear of joint or ligament at wrist and hand level

Code also any associated open wound
EXCLUDES 2   strain of muscle, fascia and tendon of wrist and hand (S66.-)

The appropriate 7th character is to be added to each code from category S63.
A   initial encounter
D   subsequent encounter
S   sequela

✓5ᵗʰ S63.0 Subluxation and dislocation of wrist and hand joints

✓6ᵗʰ S63.00 Unspecified subluxation and dislocation of wrist and hand
Dislocation of carpal bone NOS
Dislocation of distal end of radius NOS
Subluxation of carpal bone NOS
Subluxation of distal end of radius NOS

✓7ᵗʰ S63.001 Unspecified subluxation of right wrist ▽ **and hand**

✓7ᵗʰ S63.002 Unspecified subluxation of left wrist ▽ **and hand**

✓7ᵗʰ S63.003 Unspecified subluxation of unspecified ▽ **wrist and hand**

✓7ᵗʰ S63.004 Unspecified dislocation of right wrist ▽ **and hand**

✓7ᵗʰ S63.005 Unspecified dislocation of left wrist ▽ **and hand**

✓7ᵗʰ S63.006 Unspecified dislocation of unspecified ▽ **wrist and hand**

✓6ᵗʰ S63.01 Subluxation and dislocation of distal radioulnar joint

✓7ᵗʰ S63.011 Subluxation of distal radioulnar joint of right wrist

✓7ᵗʰ S63.012 Subluxation of distal radioulnar joint of left wrist

✓7ᵗʰ S63.013 Subluxation of distal radioulnar joint ▽ **of unspecified wrist**

✓7ᵗʰ S63.014 Dislocation of distal radioulnar joint of right wrist

✓7ᵗʰ S63.015 Dislocation of distal radioulnar joint of left wrist

✓7ᵗʰ S63.016 Dislocation of distal radioulnar joint ▽ **of unspecified wrist**

✓6ᵗʰ S63.02 Subluxation and dislocation of radiocarpal joint

✓7ᵗʰ S63.021 Subluxation of radiocarpal joint of right wrist

✓7ᵗʰ S63.022 Subluxation of radiocarpal joint of left wrist

✓7ᵗʰ S63.023 Subluxation of radiocarpal joint of ▽ **unspecified wrist**

✓7ᵗʰ S63.024 Dislocation of radiocarpal joint of right wrist

✓7ᵗʰ S63.025 Dislocation of radiocarpal joint of left wrist

✓7ᵗʰ S63.026 Dislocation of radiocarpal joint of ▽ **unspecified wrist**

✓6ᵗʰ S63.03 Subluxation and dislocation of midcarpal joint

✓7ᵗʰ S63.031 Subluxation of midcarpal joint of right wrist

✓7ᵗʰ S63.032 Subluxation of midcarpal joint of left wrist

✓7ᵗʰ S63.033 Subluxation of midcarpal joint of ▽ **unspecified wrist**

✓7ᵗʰ S63.034 Dislocation of midcarpal joint of right wrist

✓7ᵗʰ S63.035 Dislocation of midcarpal joint of left wrist

✓7ᵗʰ S63.036 Dislocation of midcarpal joint of ▽ **unspecified wrist**

✓6ᵗʰ S63.04 Subluxation and dislocation of carpometacarpal joint of thumb
EXCLUDES 2   interphalangeal subluxation and dislocation of thumb (S63.1-)

✓7ᵗʰ S63.041 Subluxation of carpometacarpal joint of right thumb

✓7ᵗʰ S63.042 Subluxation of carpometacarpal joint of left thumb

✓7ᵗʰ S63.043 Subluxation of carpometacarpal joint ▽ **of unspecified thumb**

✓7ᵗʰ S63.044 Dislocation of carpometacarpal joint of right thumb

✓7ᵗʰ S63.045 Dislocation of carpometacarpal joint of left thumb

✓7ᵗʰ S63.046 Dislocation of carpometacarpal joint ▽ **of unspecified thumb**

✓6ᵗʰ S63.05 Subluxation and dislocation of other carpometacarpal joint
EXCLUDES 2   subluxation and dislocation of carpometacarpal joint of thumb (S63.04-)

✓7ᵗʰ S63.051 Subluxation of other carpometacarpal joint of right hand

✓7ᵗʰ S63.052 Subluxation of other carpometacarpal joint of left hand

✓7ᵗʰ S63.053 Subluxation of other carpometacarpal ▽ **joint of unspecified hand**

✓7ᵗʰ S63.054 Dislocation of other carpometacarpal joint of right hand

✓7ᵗʰ S63.055 Dislocation of other carpometacarpal joint of left hand

✓7ᵗʰ S63.056 Dislocation of other carpometacarpal ▽ **joint of unspecified hand**

✓6ᵗʰ S63.06 Subluxation and dislocation of metacarpal (bone), proximal end

✓7ᵗʰ S63.061 Subluxation of metacarpal (bone), proximal end of right hand

✓7ᵗʰ S63.062 Subluxation of metacarpal (bone), proximal end of left hand

✓7ᵗʰ S63.063 Subluxation of metacarpal (bone), ▽ **proximal end of unspecified hand**

✓7ᵗʰ S63.064 Dislocation of metacarpal (bone), proximal end of right hand

✓7ᵗʰ S63.065 Dislocation of metacarpal (bone), proximal end of left hand

✓7ᵗʰ S63.066 Dislocation of metacarpal (bone), ▽ **proximal end of unspecified hand**

✓6ᵗʰ S63.07 Subluxation and dislocation of distal end of ulna

✓7ᵗʰ S63.071 Subluxation of distal end of right ulna

✓7ᵗʰ S63.072 Subluxation of distal end of left ulna

✓7ᵗʰ S63.073 Subluxation of distal end of unspecified ▽ **ulna**

✓7ᵗʰ S63.074 Dislocation of distal end of right ulna

✓7ᵗʰ S63.075 Dislocation of distal end of left ulna

✓7ᵗʰ S63.076 Dislocation of distal end of unspecified ▽ **ulna**

✓6ᵗʰ S63.09 Other subluxation and dislocation of wrist and hand

✓7ᵗʰ S63.091 Other subluxation of right wrist and hand

✓7ᵗʰ S63.092 Other subluxation of left wrist and hand

✓7ᵗʰ S63.093 Other subluxation of unspecified wrist ▽ **and hand**

✓7ᵗʰ S63.094 Other dislocation of right wrist and hand

EXCLUDES 1 Not coded here   EXCLUDES 2 Not included here   N Newborn Age: 0   P Pediatric Age: 0-17   M Maternity Age: 12-55   A Adult Age: 15-124

988

ICD-10-CM 2018

S62.668–S63.094

✓7ᵗʰ **S63.095** **Other** dislocation of left wrist and hand

✓7ᵗʰ **S63.096** **Other** dislocation of unspecified wrist ▽
and hand

✓5ᵗʰ **S63.1** **Subluxation and dislocation of** thumb

✓6ᵗʰ **S63.10** **Unspecified subluxation and dislocation of thumb**

✓7ᵗʰ **S63.101** **Unspecified** subluxation of right thumb ▽

✓7ᵗʰ **S63.102** **Unspecified** subluxation of left thumb ▽

✓7ᵗʰ **S63.103** **Unspecified** subluxation of unspecified ▽
thumb

✓7ᵗʰ **S63.104** **Unspecified** dislocation of right thumb ▽

✓7ᵗʰ **S63.105** **Unspecified** dislocation of left thumb ▽

✓7ᵗʰ **S63.106** **Unspecified** dislocation of unspecified ▽
thumb

✓6ᵗʰ **S63.11** **Subluxation and dislocation of**
metacarpophalangeal joint of thumb

✓7ᵗʰ **S63.111** Subluxation of metacarpophalangeal
joint of right thumb

✓7ᵗʰ **S63.112** Subluxation of metacarpophalangeal
joint of left thumb

✓7ᵗʰ **S63.113** Subluxation of metacarpophalangeal ▽
joint of unspecified thumb

✓7ᵗʰ **S63.114** Dislocation of metacarpophalangeal joint
of right thumb

✓7ᵗʰ **S63.115** Dislocation of metacarpophalangeal joint
of left thumb

✓7ᵗʰ **S63.116** Dislocation of metacarpophalangeal ▽
joint of unspecified thumb

▲ ✓6ᵗʰ **S63.12** **Subluxation and dislocation of** interphalangeal joint
of thumb

▲ ✓7ᵗʰ **S63.121** Subluxation of interphalangeal joint of
right thumb

▲ ✓7ᵗʰ **S63.122** Subluxation of interphalangeal joint of
left thumb

▲ ✓7ᵗʰ **S63.123** Subluxation of interphalangeal joint ▽
of unspecified thumb

▲ ✓7ᵗʰ **S63.124** Dislocation of interphalangeal joint of
right thumb

▲ ✓7ᵗʰ **S63.125** Dislocation of interphalangeal joint of left
thumb

▲ ✓7ᵗʰ **S63.126** Dislocation of interphalangeal joint ▽
of unspecified thumb

✓6ᵗʰ ~~**S63.13**~~ ~~**Subluxation and dislocation of proximal**~~
~~**interphalangeal joint of thumb**~~

✓7ᵗʰ ~~**S63.131**~~ ~~Subluxation of proximal interphalangeal~~
~~joint of right thumb~~

✓7ᵗʰ ~~**S63.132**~~ ~~Subluxation of proximal interphalangeal~~
~~joint of left thumb~~

✓7ᵗʰ ~~**S63.133**~~ ~~Subluxation of proximal interphalangeal~~
~~joint of unspecified thumb~~

✓7ᵗʰ ~~**S63.134**~~ ~~Dislocation of proximal interphalangeal~~
~~joint of right thumb~~

✓7ᵗʰ ~~**S63.135**~~ ~~Dislocation of proximal interphalangeal~~
~~joint of left thumb~~

✓7ᵗʰ ~~**S63.136**~~ ~~Dislocation of proximal interphalangeal~~
~~joint of unspecified thumb~~

✓6ᵗʰ ~~**S63.14**~~ ~~**Subluxation and dislocation of distal**~~
~~**interphalangeal joint of thumb**~~

✓7ᵗʰ ~~**S63.141**~~ ~~Subluxation of distal interphalangeal~~
~~joint of right thumb~~

✓7ᵗʰ ~~**S63.142**~~ ~~Subluxation of distal interphalangeal~~
~~joint of left thumb~~

✓7ᵗʰ ~~**S63.143**~~ ~~Subluxation of distal interphalangeal~~
~~joint of unspecified thumb~~

✓7ᵗʰ ~~**S63.144**~~ ~~Dislocation of distal interphalangeal joint~~
~~of right thumb~~

✓7ᵗʰ ~~**S63.145**~~ ~~Dislocation of distal interphalangeal joint~~
~~of left thumb~~

✓7ᵗʰ ~~**S63.146**~~ ~~Dislocation of distal interphalangeal joint~~
~~of unspecified thumb~~

✓5ᵗʰ **S63.2** **Subluxation and dislocation of other finger(s)**

EXCLUDES 2   *subluxation and dislocation of thumb (S63.1-)*

✓6ᵗʰ **S63.20** **Unspecified subluxation of other finger**

✓7ᵗʰ **S63.200** **Unspecified subluxation of** right index ▽
finger

✓7ᵗʰ **S63.201** **Unspecified subluxation of** left index ▽
finger

✓7ᵗʰ **S63.202** **Unspecified subluxation of** right ▽
middle finger

✓7ᵗʰ **S63.203** **Unspecified subluxation of** left middle ▽
finger

✓7ᵗʰ **S63.204** **Unspecified subluxation of** right ring ▽
finger

✓7ᵗʰ **S63.205** **Unspecified subluxation of** left ring ▽
finger

✓7ᵗʰ **S63.206** **Unspecified subluxation of** right little ▽
finger

✓7ᵗʰ **S63.207** **Unspecified subluxation of** left little ▽
finger

✓7ᵗʰ **S63.208** **Unspecified subluxation of other finger** ▽
Unspecified subluxation of specified finger
with unspecified laterality

✓7ᵗʰ **S63.209** **Unspecified subluxation of unspecified** ▽
finger

✓6ᵗʰ **S63.21** **Subluxation of** metacarpophalangeal joint of finger

✓7ᵗʰ **S63.210** **Subluxation of metacarpophalangeal**
joint of right index finger

✓7ᵗʰ **S63.211** **Subluxation of metacarpophalangeal**
joint of left index finger

✓7ᵗʰ **S63.212** **Subluxation of metacarpophalangeal**
joint of right middle finger

✓7ᵗʰ **S63.213** **Subluxation of metacarpophalangeal**
joint of left middle finger

✓7ᵗʰ **S63.214** **Subluxation of metacarpophalangeal**
joint of right ring finger

✓7ᵗʰ **S63.215** **Subluxation of metacarpophalangeal**
joint of left ring finger

✓7ᵗʰ **S63.216** **Subluxation of metacarpophalangeal**
joint of right little finger

✓7ᵗʰ **S63.217** **Subluxation of metacarpophalangeal**
joint of left little finger

✓7ᵗʰ **S63.218** **Subluxation of metacarpophalangeal**
joint of other finger
Subluxation of metacarpophalangeal joint
of specified finger with unspecified
laterality

✓7ᵗʰ **S63.219** **Subluxation of metacarpophalangeal** ▽
joint of unspecified finger

✓6ᵗʰ **S63.22** **Subluxation of unspecified** interphalangeal joint of
finger

✓7ᵗʰ **S63.220** **Subluxation of unspecified** ▽
interphalangeal joint of right index finger

✓7ᵗʰ **S63.221** **Subluxation of unspecified** ▽
interphalangeal joint of left index finger

✓7ᵗʰ **S63.222** **Subluxation of unspecified** ▽
interphalangeal joint of right middle
finger

✓7ᵗʰ **S63.223** **Subluxation of unspecified** ▽
interphalangeal joint of left middle finger

✓7ᵗʰ **S63.224** **Subluxation of unspecified** ▽
interphalangeal joint of right ring finger

✓7ᵗʰ **S63.225** **Subluxation of unspecified** ▽
interphalangeal joint of left ring finger

✓7ᵗʰ **S63.226** **Subluxation of unspecified** ▽
interphalangeal joint of right little finger

✓7ᵗʰ **S63.227** **Subluxation of unspecified** ▽
interphalangeal joint of left little finger

✓7ᵗʰ **S63.228** **Subluxation of unspecified** ▽
interphalangeal joint of other finger
Subluxation of unspecified interphalangeal
joint of specified finger with
unspecified laterality

✓7ᵗʰ **S63.229** **Subluxation of unspecified inter-** ▽
phalangeal joint of unspecified finger

✓ Additional Character Req   ✓x7ᵗʰ Placeholder Alert   Manifestation   HCC CMS-HCC Condition   ▽ Unspecified Code   ►◄ Revised Text   ● New Code   ▲ Revised Code Title

√6ᵗʰ **S63.23** **Subluxation of proximal interphalangeal joint of finger**

√7ᵗʰ   **S63.230** **Subluxation of proximal interphalangeal joint of right index finger**

√7ᵗʰ   **S63.231** **Subluxation of proximal interphalangeal joint of left index finger**

√7ᵗʰ   **S63.232** **Subluxation of proximal interphalangeal joint of right middle finger**

√7ᵗʰ   **S63.233** **Subluxation of proximal interphalangeal joint of left middle finger**

√7ᵗʰ   **S63.234** **Subluxation of proximal interphalangeal joint of right ring finger**

√7ᵗʰ   **S63.235** **Subluxation of proximal interphalangeal joint of left ring finger**

√7ᵗʰ   **S63.236** **Subluxation of proximal interphalangeal joint of right little finger**

√7ᵗʰ   **S63.237** **Subluxation of proximal interphalangeal joint of left little finger**

√7ᵗʰ   **S63.238** **Subluxation of proximal interphalangeal joint of other finger**
Subluxation of proximal interphalangeal joint of specified finger with unspecified laterality

√7ᵗʰ   **S63.239** **Subluxation of proximal inter-phalangeal joint of unspecified finger** ▽

√6ᵗʰ **S63.24** **Subluxation of distal interphalangeal joint of finger**

√7ᵗʰ   **S63.240** **Subluxation of distal interphalangeal joint of right index finger**

√7ᵗʰ   **S63.241** **Subluxation of distal interphalangeal joint of left index finger**

√7ᵗʰ   **S63.242** **Subluxation of distal interphalangeal joint of right middle finger**

√7ᵗʰ   **S63.243** **Subluxation of distal interphalangeal joint of left middle finger**

√7ᵗʰ   **S63.244** **Subluxation of distal interphalangeal joint of right ring finger**

√7ᵗʰ   **S63.245** **Subluxation of distal interphalangeal joint of left ring finger**

√7ᵗʰ   **S63.246** **Subluxation of distal interphalangeal joint of right little finger**

√7ᵗʰ   **S63.247** **Subluxation of distal interphalangeal joint of left little finger**

√7ᵗʰ   **S63.248** **Subluxation of distal interphalangeal joint of other finger**
Subluxation of distal interphalangeal joint of specified finger with unspecified laterality

√7ᵗʰ   **S63.249** **Subluxation of distal interphalangeal joint of unspecified finger** ▽

√6ᵗʰ **S63.25** **Unspecified dislocation of other finger**

√7ᵗʰ   **S63.250** **Unspecified dislocation of right index finger** ▽

√7ᵗʰ   **S63.251** **Unspecified dislocation of left index finger** ▽

√7ᵗʰ   **S63.252** **Unspecified dislocation of right middle finger** ▽

√7ᵗʰ   **S63.253** **Unspecified dislocation of left middle finger** ▽

√7ᵗʰ   **S63.254** **Unspecified dislocation of right ring finger** ▽

√7ᵗʰ   **S63.255** **Unspecified dislocation of left ring finger** ▽

√7ᵗʰ   **S63.256** **Unspecified dislocation of right little finger** ▽

√7ᵗʰ   **S63.257** **Unspecified dislocation of left little finger** ▽

√7ᵗʰ   **S63.258** **Unspecified dislocation of other finger** ▽
Unspecified dislocation of specified finger with unspecified laterality

√7ᵗʰ   **S63.259** **Unspecified dislocation of unspecified finger** ▽
▶Unspecified dislocation of unspecified finger with unspecified laterality◀

√6ᵗʰ **S63.26** **Dislocation of metacarpophalangeal joint of finger**

√7ᵗʰ   **S63.260** **Dislocation of metacarpophalangeal joint of right index finger**

√7ᵗʰ   **S63.261** **Dislocation of metacarpophalangeal joint of left index finger**

√7ᵗʰ   **S63.262** **Dislocation of metacarpophalangeal joint of right middle finger**

√7ᵗʰ   **S63.263** **Dislocation of metacarpophalangeal joint of left middle finger**

√7ᵗʰ   **S63.264** **Dislocation of metacarpophalangeal joint of right ring finger**

√7ᵗʰ   **S63.265** **Dislocation of metacarpophalangeal joint of left ring finger**

√7ᵗʰ   **S63.266** **Dislocation of metacarpophalangeal joint of right little finger**

√7ᵗʰ   **S63.267** **Dislocation of metacarpophalangeal joint of left little finger**

√7ᵗʰ   **S63.268** **Dislocation of metacarpophalangeal joint of other finger**
Dislocation of metacarpophalangeal joint of specified finger with unspecified laterality

√7ᵗʰ   **S63.269** **Dislocation of metacarpophalangeal joint of unspecified finger** ▽

√6ᵗʰ **S63.27** **Dislocation of unspecified interphalangeal joint of finger**

√7ᵗʰ   **S63.270** **Dislocation of unspecified interphalangeal joint of right index finger** ▽

√7ᵗʰ   **S63.271** **Dislocation of unspecified interphalangeal joint of left index finger** ▽

√7ᵗʰ   **S63.272** **Dislocation of unspecified interphalangeal joint of right middle finger** ▽

√7ᵗʰ   **S63.273** **Dislocation of unspecified interphalangeal joint of left middle finger** ▽

√7ᵗʰ   **S63.274** **Dislocation of unspecified interphalangeal joint of right ring finger** ▽

√7ᵗʰ   **S63.275** **Dislocation of unspecified interphalangeal joint of left ring finger** ▽

√7ᵗʰ   **S63.276** **Dislocation of unspecified interphalangeal joint of right little finger** ▽

√7ᵗʰ   **S63.277** **Dislocation of unspecified interphalangeal joint of left little finger** ▽

√7ᵗʰ   **S63.278** **Dislocation of unspecified interphalangeal joint of other finger** ▽
Dislocation of unspecified interphalangeal joint of specified finger with unspecified laterality

√7ᵗʰ   **S63.279** **Dislocation of unspecified interphalangeal joint of unspecified finger** ▽
▶Dislocation of unspecified interphalangeal joint of unspecified finger without specified laterality◀

√6ᵗʰ **S63.28** **Dislocation of proximal interphalangeal joint of finger**

√7ᵗʰ   **S63.280** **Dislocation of proximal interphalangeal joint of right index finger**

√7ᵗʰ   **S63.281** **Dislocation of proximal interphalangeal joint of left index finger**

√7ᵗʰ   **S63.282** **Dislocation of proximal interphalangeal joint of right middle finger**

√7ᵗʰ   **S63.283** **Dislocation of proximal interphalangeal joint of left middle finger**

√7ᵗʰ   **S63.284** **Dislocation of proximal interphalangeal joint of right ring finger**

√7ᵗʰ   **S63.285** **Dislocation of proximal interphalangeal joint of left ring finger**

√7ᵗʰ   **S63.286** **Dislocation of proximal interphalangeal joint of right little finger**

√7ᵗʰ   **S63.287** **Dislocation of proximal interphalangeal joint of left little finger**

√7ᵗʰ   **S63.288** **Dislocation of proximal interphalangeal joint of other finger**
Dislocation of proximal interphalangeal joint of specified finger with unspecified laterality

√7ᵗʰ   **S63.289** **Dislocation of proximal inter-phalangeal joint of unspecified finger** ▽

EXCLUDES 1 Not coded here   _EXCLUDES 2_ Not included here   N Newborn Age: 0   P Pediatric Age: 0-17   M Maternity Age: 12-55   A Adult Age: 15-124

990   ICD-10-CM 2018

√6ᵗʰ **S63.29 Dislocation of distal interphalangeal joint of finger**

√7ᵗʰ **S63.290 Dislocation of distal interphalangeal joint of right index finger**

√7ᵗʰ **S63.291 Dislocation of distal interphalangeal joint of left index finger**

√7ᵗʰ **S63.292 Dislocation of distal interphalangeal joint of right middle finger**

√7ᵗʰ **S63.293 Dislocation of distal interphalangeal joint of left middle finger**

√7ᵗʰ **S63.294 Dislocation of distal interphalangeal joint of right ring finger**

√7ᵗʰ **S63.295 Dislocation of distal interphalangeal joint of left ring finger**

√7ᵗʰ **S63.296 Dislocation of distal interphalangeal joint of right little finger**

√7ᵗʰ **S63.297 Dislocation of distal interphalangeal joint of left little finger**

√7ᵗʰ **S63.298 Dislocation of distal interphalangeal joint of other finger**
    Dislocation of distal interphalangeal joint of specified finger with unspecified laterality

√7ᵗʰ **S63.299 Dislocation of distal interphalangeal joint of unspecified finger** ▽

√5ᵗʰ **S63.3 Traumatic rupture of ligament of wrist**

√6ᵗʰ **S63.30 Traumatic rupture of unspecified ligament of wrist**

√7ᵗʰ **S63.301 Traumatic rupture of unspecified ligament of right wrist** ▽

√7ᵗʰ **S63.302 Traumatic rupture of unspecified ligament of left wrist** ▽

√7ᵗʰ **S63.309 Traumatic rupture of unspecified ligament of unspecified wrist** ▽

√6ᵗʰ **S63.31 Traumatic rupture of collateral ligament of wrist**

√7ᵗʰ **S63.311 Traumatic rupture of collateral ligament of right wrist**

√7ᵗʰ **S63.312 Traumatic rupture of collateral ligament of left wrist**

√7ᵗʰ **S63.319 Traumatic rupture of collateral ligament of unspecified wrist** ▽

√6ᵗʰ **S63.32 Traumatic rupture of radiocarpal ligament**

√7ᵗʰ **S63.321 Traumatic rupture of right radiocarpal ligament**

√7ᵗʰ **S63.322 Traumatic rupture of left radiocarpal ligament**

√7ᵗʰ **S63.329 Traumatic rupture of unspecified radiocarpal ligament** ▽

√6ᵗʰ **S63.33 Traumatic rupture of ulnocarpal (palmar) ligament**

√7ᵗʰ **S63.331 Traumatic rupture of right ulnocarpal (palmar) ligament**

√7ᵗʰ **S63.332 Traumatic rupture of left ulnocarpal (palmar) ligament**

√7ᵗʰ **S63.339 Traumatic rupture of unspecified ulnocarpal (palmar) ligament** ▽

√6ᵗʰ **S63.39 Traumatic rupture of other ligament of wrist**

√7ᵗʰ **S63.391 Traumatic rupture of other ligament of right wrist**

√7ᵗʰ **S63.392 Traumatic rupture of other ligament of left wrist**

√7ᵗʰ **S63.399 Traumatic rupture of other ligament of unspecified wrist** ▽

√5ᵗʰ **S63.4 Traumatic rupture of ligament of finger at metacarpophalangeal and interphalangeal joint(s)**

√6ᵗʰ **S63.40 Traumatic rupture of unspecified ligament of finger at metacarpophalangeal and interphalangeal joint**

√7ᵗʰ **S63.400 Traumatic rupture of unspecified ligament of right index finger at metacarpo- phalangeal and interphalangeal joint** ▽

√7ᵗʰ **S63.401 Traumatic rupture of unspecified ligament of left index finger at metacarpophalangeal and interphalangeal joint** ▽

√7ᵗʰ **S63.402 Traumatic rupture of unspecified ligament of right middle finger at metacarpophalangeal and interphalangeal joint** ▽

√7ᵗʰ **S63.403 Traumatic rupture of unspecified ligament of left middle finger at metacarpo- phalangeal and interphalangeal joint** ▽

√7ᵗʰ **S63.404 Traumatic rupture of unspecified ligament of right ring finger at metacarpophalangeal and interphalangeal joint** ▽

√7ᵗʰ **S63.405 Traumatic rupture of unspecified ligament of left ring finger at metacarpophalangeal and interphalangeal joint** ▽

√7ᵗʰ **S63.406 Traumatic rupture of unspecified ligament of right little finger at metacarpophalangeal and interphalangeal joint** ▽

√7ᵗʰ **S63.407 Traumatic rupture of unspecified ligament of left little finger at metacarpophalangeal and interphalangeal joint** ▽

√7ᵗʰ **S63.408 Traumatic rupture of unspecified ligament of other finger at metacarpophalangeal and interphalangeal joint** ▽
    Traumatic rupture of unspecified ligament of specified finger with unspecified laterality at metacarpophalangeal and interphalangeal joint

√7ᵗʰ **S63.409 Traumatic rupture of unspecified ligament of unspecified finger at metacarpophalangeal and interphalangeal joint** ▽

√6ᵗʰ **S63.41 Traumatic rupture of collateral ligament of finger at metacarpophalangeal and interphalangeal joint**

√7ᵗʰ **S63.410 Traumatic rupture of collateral ligament of right index finger at metacarpo- phalangeal and interphalangeal joint**

√7ᵗʰ **S63.411 Traumatic rupture of collateral ligament of left index finger at metacarpo- phalangeal and interphalangeal joint**

√7ᵗʰ **S63.412 Traumatic rupture of collateral ligament of right middle finger at metacarpo- phalangeal and interphalangeal joint**

√7ᵗʰ **S63.413 Traumatic rupture of collateral ligament of left middle finger at metacarpo- phalangeal and interphalangeal joint**

√7ᵗʰ **S63.414 Traumatic rupture of collateral ligament of right ring finger at metacarpo- phalangeal and interphalangeal joint**

√7ᵗʰ **S63.415 Traumatic rupture of collateral ligament of left ring finger at metacarpophalangeal and interphalangeal joint**

√7ᵗʰ **S63.416 Traumatic rupture of collateral ligament of right little finger at metacarpo- phalangeal and interphalangeal joint**

√7ᵗʰ **S63.417 Traumatic rupture of collateral ligament of left little finger at metacarpo- phalangeal and interphalangeal joint**

√7ᵗʰ **S63.418 Traumatic rupture of collateral ligament of other finger at metacarpophalangeal and interphalangeal joint**
    Traumatic rupture of collateral ligament of specified finger with unspecified laterality at metacarpophalangeal and interphalangeal joint

√7ᵗʰ **S63.419 Traumatic rupture of collateral ligament of unspecified finger at metacarpophalangeal and interphalangeal joint** ▽

√6ᵗʰ **S63.42 Traumatic rupture of palmar ligament of finger at metacarpophalangeal and interphalangeal joint**

√7ᵗʰ **S63.420 Traumatic rupture of palmar ligament of right index finger at metacarpo- phalangeal and interphalangeal joint**

√7ᵗʰ **S63.421 Traumatic rupture of palmar ligament of left index finger at metacarpophalangeal and interphalangeal joint**

√7ᵗʰ **S63.422 Traumatic rupture of palmar ligament of right middle finger at metacarpo- phalangeal and interphalangeal joint**

☑ Additional Character Req   √ₓ7ᵗʰ Placeholder Alert   Manifestation   ᴴᶜᶜ CMS-HCC Condition   ▽ Unspecified Code   ►◄ Revised Text   ● New Code   ▲ Revised Code Title

√7ᵗʰ **S63.423** **Traumatic rupture of palmar ligament of left middle finger at metacarpophalangeal and interphalangeal joint**

√7ᵗʰ **S63.424** **Traumatic rupture of palmar ligament of right ring finger at metacarpophalangeal and interphalangeal joint**

√7ᵗʰ **S63.425** **Traumatic rupture of palmar ligament of left ring finger at metacarpophalangeal and interphalangeal joint**

√7ᵗʰ **S63.426** **Traumatic rupture of palmar ligament of right little finger at metacarpophalangeal and interphalangeal joint**

√7ᵗʰ **S63.427** **Traumatic rupture of palmar ligament of left little finger at metacarpophalangeal and interphalangeal joint**

√7ᵗʰ **S63.428** **Traumatic rupture of palmar ligament of other finger at metacarpophalangeal and interphalangeal joint**
Traumatic rupture of palmar ligament of specified finger with unspecified laterality at metacarpophalangeal and interphalangeal joint

√7ᵗʰ **S63.429** **Traumatic rupture of palmar ligament of unspecified finger at metacarpophalangeal and interphalangeal joint** ▽

√6ᵗʰ **S63.43** **Traumatic rupture of volar plate of finger at metacarpophalangeal and interphalangeal joint**

√7ᵗʰ **S63.430** **Traumatic rupture of volar plate of right index finger at metacarpophalangeal and interphalangeal joint**

√7ᵗʰ **S63.431** **Traumatic rupture of volar plate of left index finger at metacarpophalangeal and interphalangeal joint**

√7ᵗʰ **S63.432** **Traumatic rupture of volar plate of right middle finger at metacarpophalangeal and interphalangeal joint**

√7ᵗʰ **S63.433** **Traumatic rupture of volar plate of left middle finger at metacarpophalangeal and interphalangeal joint**

√7ᵗʰ **S63.434** **Traumatic rupture of volar plate of right ring finger at metacarpophalangeal and interphalangeal joint**

√7ᵗʰ **S63.435** **Traumatic rupture of volar plate of left ring finger at metacarpophalangeal and interphalangeal joint**

√7ᵗʰ **S63.436** **Traumatic rupture of volar plate of right little finger at metacarpophalangeal and interphalangeal joint**

√7ᵗʰ **S63.437** **Traumatic rupture of volar plate of left little finger at metacarpophalangeal and interphalangeal joint**

√7ᵗʰ **S63.438** **Traumatic rupture of volar plate of other finger at metacarpophalangeal and interphalangeal joint**
Traumatic rupture of volar plate of specified finger with unspecified laterality at metacarpophalangeal and interphalangeal joint

√7ᵗʰ **S63.439** **Traumatic rupture of volar plate of unspecified finger at metacarpophalangeal and interphalangeal joint** ▽

√6ᵗʰ **S63.49** **Traumatic rupture of other ligament of finger at metacarpophalangeal and interphalangeal joint**

√7ᵗʰ **S63.490** **Traumatic rupture of other ligament of right index finger at metacarpophalangeal and interphalangeal joint**

√7ᵗʰ **S63.491** **Traumatic rupture of other ligament of left index finger at metacarpophalangeal and interphalangeal joint**

√7ᵗʰ **S63.492** **Traumatic rupture of other ligament of right middle finger at metacarpophalangeal and interphalangeal joint**

√7ᵗʰ **S63.493** **Traumatic rupture of other ligament of left middle finger at metacarpophalangeal and interphalangeal joint**

√7ᵗʰ **S63.494** **Traumatic rupture of other ligament of right ring finger at metacarpophalangeal and interphalangeal joint**

√7ᵗʰ **S63.495** **Traumatic rupture of other ligament of left ring finger at metacarpophalangeal and interphalangeal joint**

√7ᵗʰ **S63.496** **Traumatic rupture of other ligament of right little finger at metacarpophalangeal and interphalangeal joint**

√7ᵗʰ **S63.497** **Traumatic rupture of other ligament of left little finger at metacarpophalangeal and interphalangeal joint**

√7ᵗʰ **S63.498** **Traumatic rupture of other ligament of other finger at metacarpophalangeal and interphalangeal joint**
Traumatic rupture of ligament of specified finger with unspecified laterality at metacarpophalangeal and interphalangeal joint

√7ᵗʰ **S63.499** **Traumatic rupture of other ligament of unspecified finger at metacarpophalangeal and interphalangeal joint** ▽

√5ᵗʰ **S63.5** **Other and unspecified sprain of wrist**

√6ᵗʰ **S63.50** **Unspecified sprain of wrist**

√7ᵗʰ **S63.501** **Unspecified sprain of right wrist** ▽

√7ᵗʰ **S63.502** **Unspecified sprain of left wrist** ▽

√7ᵗʰ **S63.509** **Unspecified sprain of unspecified wrist** ▽

√6ᵗʰ **S63.51** **Sprain of carpal (joint)**

√7ᵗʰ **S63.511** **Sprain of carpal joint of right wrist**

√7ᵗʰ **S63.512** **Sprain of carpal joint of left wrist**

√7ᵗʰ **S63.519** **Sprain of carpal joint of unspecified wrist** ▽

√6ᵗʰ **S63.52** **Sprain of radiocarpal joint**
EXCLUDES 1 *traumatic rupture of radiocarpal ligament (S63.32-)*

√7ᵗʰ **S63.521** **Sprain of radiocarpal joint of right wrist**

√7ᵗʰ **S63.522** **Sprain of radiocarpal joint of left wrist**

√7ᵗʰ **S63.529** **Sprain of radiocarpal joint of unspecified wrist** ▽

√6ᵗʰ **S63.59** **Other specified sprain of wrist**

√7ᵗʰ **S63.591** **Other specified sprain of right wrist**

√7ᵗʰ **S63.592** **Other specified sprain of left wrist**

√7ᵗʰ **S63.599** **Other specified sprain of unspecified wrist** ▽

√5ᵗʰ **S63.6** **Other and unspecified sprain of finger(s)**
EXCLUDES 1 *traumatic rupture of ligament of finger at metacarpophalangeal and interphalangeal joint(s) (S63.4-)*

√6ᵗʰ **S63.60** **Unspecified sprain of thumb**

√7ᵗʰ **S63.601** **Unspecified sprain of right thumb** ▽

√7ᵗʰ **S63.602** **Unspecified sprain of left thumb** ▽

√7ᵗʰ **S63.609** **Unspecified sprain of unspecified thumb** ▽

√6ᵗʰ **S63.61** **Unspecified sprain of other and unspecified finger(s)**

√7ᵗʰ **S63.610** **Unspecified sprain of right index finger** ▽

√7ᵗʰ **S63.611** **Unspecified sprain of left index finger** ▽

√7ᵗʰ **S63.612** **Unspecified sprain of right middle finger** ▽

√7ᵗʰ **S63.613** **Unspecified sprain of left middle finger** ▽

√7ᵗʰ **S63.614** **Unspecified sprain of right ring finger** ▽

√7ᵗʰ **S63.615** **Unspecified sprain of left ring finger** ▽

√7ᵗʰ **S63.616** **Unspecified sprain of right little finger** ▽

√7ᵗʰ **S63.617** **Unspecified sprain of left little finger** ▽

√7ᵗʰ **S63.618** **Unspecified sprain of other finger** ▽
Unspecified sprain of specified finger with unspecified laterality

√7ᵗʰ **S63.619** **Unspecified sprain of unspecified finger** ▽

√6ᵗʰ **S63.62** **Sprain of interphalangeal joint of thumb**

√7ᵗʰ **S63.621** **Sprain of interphalangeal joint of right thumb**

EXCLUDES 1 Not coded here   **EXCLUDES 2** Not included here   N Newborn Age: 0   P Pediatric Age: 0-17   M Maternity Age: 12-55   A Adult Age: 15-124

992   ICD-10-CM 2018

✓7ᵗʰ **S63.622**	**Sprain of interphalangeal joint of** left thumb
✓7ᵗʰ **S63.629**	**Sprain of interphalangeal joint of** unspecified thumb ▽
✓6ᵗʰ **S63.63**	**Sprain of** interphalangeal joint **of other and unspecified** finger(s)
✓7ᵗʰ **S63.630**	**Sprain of interphalangeal joint of** right index finger
✓7ᵗʰ **S63.631**	**Sprain of interphalangeal joint of** left index finger
✓7ᵗʰ **S63.632**	**Sprain of interphalangeal joint of** right middle finger
✓7ᵗʰ **S63.633**	**Sprain of interphalangeal joint of** left middle finger
✓7ᵗʰ **S63.634**	**Sprain of interphalangeal joint of** right ring finger
✓7ᵗʰ **S63.635**	**Sprain of interphalangeal joint of** left ring finger
✓7ᵗʰ **S63.636**	**Sprain of interphalangeal joint of** right little finger
✓7ᵗʰ **S63.637**	**Sprain of interphalangeal joint of** left little finger
✓7ᵗʰ **S63.638**	**Sprain of interphalangeal joint of other** finger
✓7ᵗʰ **S63.639**	**Sprain of interphalangeal joint of** unspecified finger ▽
✓6ᵗʰ **S63.64**	**Sprain of** metacarpophalangeal joint of thumb
✓7ᵗʰ **S63.641**	**Sprain of metacarpophalangeal joint of** right thumb
✓7ᵗʰ **S63.642**	**Sprain of metacarpophalangeal joint of** left thumb
✓7ᵗʰ **S63.649**	**Sprain of metacarpophalangeal joint of unspecified thumb** ▽
✓6ᵗʰ **S63.65**	**Sprain of** metacarpophalangeal joint **of other and unspecified** finger(s)
✓7ᵗʰ **S63.650**	**Sprain of metacarpophalangeal joint of** right index finger
✓7ᵗʰ **S63.651**	**Sprain of metacarpophalangeal joint of** left index finger
✓7ᵗʰ **S63.652**	**Sprain of metacarpophalangeal joint of** right middle finger
✓7ᵗʰ **S63.653**	**Sprain of metacarpophalangeal joint of** left middle finger
✓7ᵗʰ **S63.654**	**Sprain of metacarpophalangeal joint of** right ring finger
✓7ᵗʰ **S63.655**	**Sprain of metacarpophalangeal joint of** left ring finger
✓7ᵗʰ **S63.656**	**Sprain of metacarpophalangeal joint of** right little finger
✓7ᵗʰ **S63.657**	**Sprain of metacarpophalangeal joint of** left little finger
✓7ᵗʰ **S63.658**	**Sprain of metacarpophalangeal joint of other** finger
	Sprain of metacarpophalangeal joint of specified finger with unspecified laterality
✓7ᵗʰ **S63.659**	**Sprain of metacarpophalangeal joint of** unspecified finger ▽
✓6ᵗʰ **S63.68**	**Other sprain of** thumb
✓7ᵗʰ **S63.681**	**Other sprain of** right thumb
✓7ᵗʰ **S63.682**	**Other sprain of** left thumb
✓7ᵗʰ **S63.689**	**Other sprain of** unspecified thumb ▽
✓6ᵗʰ **S63.69**	**Other sprain of other and unspecified** finger(s)
✓7ᵗʰ **S63.690**	**Other sprain of** right index finger
✓7ᵗʰ **S63.691**	**Other sprain of** left index finger
✓7ᵗʰ **S63.692**	**Other sprain of** right middle finger
✓7ᵗʰ **S63.693**	**Other sprain of** left middle finger
✓7ᵗʰ **S63.694**	**Other sprain of** right ring finger
✓7ᵗʰ **S63.695**	**Other sprain of** left ring finger
✓7ᵗʰ **S63.696**	**Other sprain of** right little finger
✓7ᵗʰ **S63.697**	**Other sprain of** left little finger
✓7ᵗʰ **S63.698**	**Other sprain of other** finger
	Other sprain of specified finger with unspecified laterality

✓7ᵗʰ **S63.699**	**Other sprain of unspecified finger** ▽
✓5ᵗʰ **S63.8**	**Sprain of other part of wrist and hand**
✓6ᵗʰ **S63.8X**	**Sprain of other part of wrist and hand**
✓7ᵗʰ **S63.8X1**	**Sprain of other part of** right wrist and hand
✓7ᵗʰ **S63.8X2**	**Sprain of other part of** left wrist and hand
✓7ᵗʰ **S63.8X9**	**Sprain of other part of unspecified wrist and hand** ▽
✓5ᵗʰ **S63.9**	**Sprain of unspecified part of wrist and hand**
✓x7ᵗʰ **S63.90**	**Sprain of unspecified part of unspecified wrist and hand** ▽
✓x7ᵗʰ **S63.91**	**Sprain of unspecified part of** right wrist and hand ▽
✓x7ᵗʰ **S63.92**	**Sprain of unspecified part of** left wrist and hand ▽

✓4ᵗʰ S64 Injury of nerves at wrist and hand level
Code also any associated open wound (S61.-)

The appropriate 7th character is to be added to each code from category S64.
A   initial encounter
D   subsequent encounter
S   sequela

✓5ᵗʰ **S64.0**	**Injury of** ulnar nerve at wrist and hand level
✓x7ᵗʰ **S64.00**	**Injury of ulnar nerve at wrist and hand level of** unspecified arm ▽
✓x7ᵗʰ **S64.01**	**Injury of ulnar nerve at wrist and hand level of** right arm
✓x7ᵗʰ **S64.02**	**Injury of ulnar nerve at wrist and hand level of** left arm
✓5ᵗʰ **S64.1**	**Injury of** median nerve at wrist and hand level
✓x7ᵗʰ **S64.10**	**Injury of median nerve at wrist and hand level of** unspecified arm ▽
✓x7ᵗʰ **S64.11**	**Injury of median nerve at wrist and hand level of** right arm
✓x7ᵗʰ **S64.12**	**Injury of median nerve at wrist and hand level of** left arm
✓5ᵗʰ **S64.2**	**Injury of** radial nerve at wrist and hand level
✓x7ᵗʰ **S64.20**	**Injury of radial nerve at wrist and hand level of** unspecified arm ▽
✓x7ᵗʰ **S64.21**	**Injury of radial nerve at wrist and hand level of** right arm
✓x7ᵗʰ **S64.22**	**Injury of radial nerve at wrist and hand level of** left arm
✓5ᵗʰ **S64.3**	**Injury of** digital nerve of thumb
✓x7ᵗʰ **S64.30**	**Injury of digital nerve of unspecified thumb** ▽
✓x7ᵗʰ **S64.31**	**Injury of digital nerve of** right thumb
✓x7ᵗʰ **S64.32**	**Injury of digital nerve of** left thumb
✓5ᵗʰ **S64.4**	**Injury of** digital nerve of other and unspecified finger
✓x7ᵗʰ **S64.40**	**Injury of digital nerve of unspecified finger** ▽
✓6ᵗʰ **S64.49**	**Injury of digital nerve of other finger**
✓7ᵗʰ **S64.490**	**Injury of digital nerve of** right index finger
✓7ᵗʰ **S64.491**	**Injury of digital nerve of** left index finger
✓7ᵗʰ **S64.492**	**Injury of digital nerve of** right middle finger
✓7ᵗʰ **S64.493**	**Injury of digital nerve of** left middle finger
✓7ᵗʰ **S64.494**	**Injury of digital nerve of** right ring finger
✓7ᵗʰ **S64.495**	**Injury of digital nerve of** left ring finger
✓7ᵗʰ **S64.496**	**Injury of digital nerve of** right little finger
✓7ᵗʰ **S64.497**	**Injury of digital nerve of** left little finger
✓7ᵗʰ **S64.498**	**Injury of digital nerve of other** finger
	Injury of digital nerve of specified finger with unspecified laterality
✓5ᵗʰ **S64.8**	**Injury of other nerves at wrist and hand level**
✓6ᵗʰ **S64.8X**	**Injury of other nerves at wrist and hand level**
✓7ᵗʰ **S64.8X1**	**Injury of other nerves at wrist and hand level of** right arm
✓7ᵗʰ **S64.8X2**	**Injury of other nerves at wrist and hand level of** left arm
✓7ᵗʰ **S64.8X9**	**Injury of other nerves at wrist and hand level of unspecified arm** ▽

√5ᵗʰ **S64.9　Injury of unspecified nerve at wrist and hand level**

√x7ᵗʰ **S64.90　Injury of unspecified nerve at wrist and hand level of unspecified arm**　▽

√x7ᵗʰ **S64.91　Injury of unspecified nerve at wrist and hand level of right arm**　▽

√x7ᵗʰ **S64.92　Injury of unspecified nerve at wrist and hand level of left arm**　▽

√4ᵗʰ **S65　Injury of blood vessels at wrist and hand level**

Code also any associated open wound (S61.-)

The appropriate 7th character is to be added to each code from category S65.
A　initial encounter
D　subsequent encounter
S　sequela

√5ᵗʰ **S65.0　Injury of ulnar artery at wrist and hand level**

√6ᵗʰ **S65.00　Unspecified injury of ulnar artery at wrist and hand level**

√7ᵗʰ **S65.001　Unspecified injury of ulnar artery at wrist and hand level of right arm**　▽

√7ᵗʰ **S65.002　Unspecified injury of ulnar artery at wrist and hand level of left arm**　▽

√7ᵗʰ **S65.009　Unspecified injury of ulnar artery at wrist and hand level of unspecified arm**　▽

√6ᵗʰ **S65.01　Laceration of ulnar artery at wrist and hand level**

√7ᵗʰ **S65.011　Laceration of ulnar artery at wrist and hand level of right arm**

√7ᵗʰ **S65.012　Laceration of ulnar artery at wrist and hand level of left arm**

√7ᵗʰ **S65.019　Laceration of ulnar artery at wrist and hand level of unspecified arm**　▽

√6ᵗʰ **S65.09　Other specified injury of ulnar artery at wrist and hand level**

√7ᵗʰ **S65.091　Other specified injury of ulnar artery at wrist and hand level of right arm**

√7ᵗʰ **S65.092　Other specified injury of ulnar artery at wrist and hand level of left arm**

√7ᵗʰ **S65.099　Other specified injury of ulnar artery at wrist and hand level of unspecified arm**　▽

√5ᵗʰ **S65.1　Injury of radial artery at wrist and hand level**

√6ᵗʰ **S65.10　Unspecified injury of radial artery at wrist and hand level**

√7ᵗʰ **S65.101　Unspecified injury of radial artery at wrist and hand level of right arm**　▽

√7ᵗʰ **S65.102　Unspecified injury of radial artery at wrist and hand level of left arm**　▽

√7ᵗʰ **S65.109　Unspecified injury of radial artery at wrist and hand level of unspecified arm**　▽

√6ᵗʰ **S65.11　Laceration of radial artery at wrist and hand level**

√7ᵗʰ **S65.111　Laceration of radial artery at wrist and hand level of right arm**

√7ᵗʰ **S65.112　Laceration of radial artery at wrist and hand level of left arm**

√7ᵗʰ **S65.119　Laceration of radial artery at wrist and hand level of unspecified arm**　▽

√6ᵗʰ **S65.19　Other specified injury of radial artery at wrist and hand level**

√7ᵗʰ **S65.191　Other specified injury of radial artery at wrist and hand level of right arm**

√7ᵗʰ **S65.192　Other specified injury of radial artery at wrist and hand level of left arm**

√7ᵗʰ **S65.199　Other specified injury of radial artery at wrist and hand level of unspecified arm**　▽

√5ᵗʰ **S65.2　Injury of superficial palmar arch**

√6ᵗʰ **S65.20　Unspecified injury of superficial palmar arch**

√7ᵗʰ **S65.201　Unspecified injury of superficial palmar arch of right hand**　▽

√7ᵗʰ **S65.202　Unspecified injury of superficial palmar arch of left hand**　▽

√7ᵗʰ **S65.209　Unspecified injury of superficial palmar arch of unspecified hand**　▽

√6ᵗʰ **S65.21　Laceration of superficial palmar arch**

√7ᵗʰ **S65.211　Laceration of superficial palmar arch of right hand**

√7ᵗʰ **S65.212　Laceration of superficial palmar arch of left hand**

√7ᵗʰ **S65.219　Laceration of superficial palmar arch of unspecified hand**　▽

√6ᵗʰ **S65.29　Other specified injury of superficial palmar arch**

√7ᵗʰ **S65.291　Other specified injury of superficial palmar arch of right hand**

√7ᵗʰ **S65.292　Other specified injury of superficial palmar arch of left hand**

√7ᵗʰ **S65.299　Other specified injury of superficial palmar arch of unspecified hand**　▽

√5ᵗʰ **S65.3　Injury of deep palmar arch**

√6ᵗʰ **S65.30　Unspecified injury of deep palmar arch**

√7ᵗʰ **S65.301　Unspecified injury of deep palmar arch of right hand**　▽

√7ᵗʰ **S65.302　Unspecified injury of deep palmar arch of left hand**　▽

√7ᵗʰ **S65.309　Unspecified injury of deep palmar arch of unspecified hand**　▽

√6ᵗʰ **S65.31　Laceration of deep palmar arch**

√7ᵗʰ **S65.311　Laceration of deep palmar arch of right hand**

√7ᵗʰ **S65.312　Laceration of deep palmar arch of left hand**

√7ᵗʰ **S65.319　Laceration of deep palmar arch of unspecified hand**　▽

√6ᵗʰ **S65.39　Other specified injury of deep palmar arch**

√7ᵗʰ **S65.391　Other specified injury of deep palmar arch of right hand**

√7ᵗʰ **S65.392　Other specified injury of deep palmar arch of left hand**

√7ᵗʰ **S65.399　Other specified injury of deep palmar arch of unspecified hand**　▽

√5ᵗʰ **S65.4　Injury of blood vessel of thumb**

√6ᵗʰ **S65.40　Unspecified injury of blood vessel of thumb**

√7ᵗʰ **S65.401　Unspecified injury of blood vessel of right thumb**　▽

√7ᵗʰ **S65.402　Unspecified injury of blood vessel of left thumb**　▽

√7ᵗʰ **S65.409　Unspecified injury of blood vessel of unspecified thumb**　▽

√6ᵗʰ **S65.41　Laceration of blood vessel of thumb**

√7ᵗʰ **S65.411　Laceration of blood vessel of right thumb**

√7ᵗʰ **S65.412　Laceration of blood vessel of left thumb**

√7ᵗʰ **S65.419　Laceration of blood vessel of unspecified thumb**　▽

√6ᵗʰ **S65.49　Other specified injury of blood vessel of thumb**

√7ᵗʰ **S65.491　Other specified injury of blood vessel of right thumb**

√7ᵗʰ **S65.492　Other specified injury of blood vessel of left thumb**

√7ᵗʰ **S65.499　Other specified injury of blood vessel of unspecified thumb**　▽

√5ᵗʰ **S65.5　Injury of blood vessel of other and unspecified finger**

√6ᵗʰ **S65.50　Unspecified injury of blood vessel of other and unspecified finger**

√7ᵗʰ **S65.500　Unspecified injury of blood vessel of right index finger**　▽

√7ᵗʰ **S65.501　Unspecified injury of blood vessel of left index finger**　▽

√7ᵗʰ **S65.502　Unspecified injury of blood vessel of right middle finger**　▽

√7ᵗʰ **S65.503　Unspecified injury of blood vessel of left middle finger**　▽

√7ᵗʰ **S65.504　Unspecified injury of blood vessel of right ring finger**　▽

√7ᵗʰ **S65.505　Unspecified injury of blood vessel of left ring finger**　▽

√7ᵗʰ **S65.506　Unspecified injury of blood vessel of right little finger**　▽

√7ᵗʰ **S65.507　Unspecified injury of blood vessel of left little finger**　▽

√7ᵗʰ **S65.508** **Unspecified injury of blood vessel of other finger** ▽
Unspecified injury of blood vessel of specified finger with unspecified laterality

√7ᵗʰ **S65.509** **Unspecified injury of blood vessel of unspecified finger** ▽

√6ᵗʰ **S65.51** **Laceration** of blood vessel of other and unspecified finger

√7ᵗʰ **S65.510** **Laceration of blood vessel of right index finger**

√7ᵗʰ **S65.511** **Laceration of blood vessel of left index finger**

√7ᵗʰ **S65.512** **Laceration of blood vessel of right middle finger**

√7ᵗʰ **S65.513** **Laceration of blood vessel of left middle finger**

√7ᵗʰ **S65.514** **Laceration of blood vessel of right ring finger**

√7ᵗʰ **S65.515** **Laceration of blood vessel of left ring finger**

√7ᵗʰ **S65.516** **Laceration of blood vessel of right little finger**

√7ᵗʰ **S65.517** **Laceration of blood vessel of left little finger**

√7ᵗʰ **S65.518** **Laceration of blood vessel of other finger**
Laceration of blood vessel of specified finger with unspecified laterality

√7ᵗʰ **S65.519** **Laceration of blood vessel of unspecified finger** ▽

√6ᵗʰ **S65.59** **Other specified injury of blood vessel of other and unspecified finger**

√7ᵗʰ **S65.590** **Other specified injury of blood vessel of right index finger**

√7ᵗʰ **S65.591** **Other specified injury of blood vessel of left index finger**

√7ᵗʰ **S65.592** **Other specified injury of blood vessel of right middle finger**

√7ᵗʰ **S65.593** **Other specified injury of blood vessel of left middle finger**

√7ᵗʰ **S65.594** **Other specified injury of blood vessel of right ring finger**

√7ᵗʰ **S65.595** **Other specified injury of blood vessel of left ring finger**

√7ᵗʰ **S65.596** **Other specified injury of blood vessel of right little finger**

√7ᵗʰ **S65.597** **Other specified injury of blood vessel of left little finger**

√7ᵗʰ **S65.598** **Other specified injury of blood vessel of other finger**
Other specified injury of blood vessel of specified finger with unspecified laterality

√7ᵗʰ **S65.599** **Other specified injury of blood vessel of unspecified finger** ▽

√5ᵗʰ **S65.8** **Injury of other blood vessels at** wrist and hand level

√6ᵗʰ **S65.80** **Unspecified injury of other blood vessels at wrist and hand level**

√7ᵗʰ **S65.801** **Unspecified injury of other blood vessels at wrist and hand level of right arm** ▽

√7ᵗʰ **S65.802** **Unspecified injury of other blood vessels at wrist and hand level of left arm** ▽

√7ᵗʰ **S65.809** **Unspecified injury of other blood vessels at wrist and hand level of unspecified arm** ▽

√6ᵗʰ **S65.81** **Laceration** of other blood vessels at wrist and hand level

√7ᵗʰ **S65.811** **Laceration of other blood vessels at wrist and hand level of right arm**

√7ᵗʰ **S65.812** **Laceration of other blood vessels at wrist and hand level of left arm**

√7ᵗʰ **S65.819** **Laceration of other blood vessels at wrist and hand level of unspecified arm** ▽

√6ᵗʰ **S65.89** **Other specified injury of other blood vessels at wrist and hand level**

√7ᵗʰ **S65.891** **Other specified injury of other blood vessels at wrist and hand level of right arm**

√7ᵗʰ **S65.892** **Other specified injury of other blood vessels at wrist and hand level of left arm**

√7ᵗʰ **S65.899** **Other specified injury of other blood vessels at wrist and hand level of unspecified arm** ▽

√5ᵗʰ **S65.9** **Injury of unspecified blood vessel at** wrist and hand level

√6ᵗʰ **S65.90** **Unspecified injury of unspecified blood vessel at wrist and hand level**

√7ᵗʰ **S65.901** **Unspecified injury of unspecified blood vessel at wrist and hand level of right arm** ▽

√7ᵗʰ **S65.902** **Unspecified injury of unspecified blood vessel at wrist and hand level of left arm** ▽

√7ᵗʰ **S65.909** **Unspecified injury of unspecified blood vessel at wrist and hand level of unspecified arm** ▽

√6ᵗʰ **S65.91** **Laceration** of unspecified blood vessel at wrist and hand level

√7ᵗʰ **S65.911** **Laceration of unspecified blood vessel at wrist and hand level of right arm** ▽

√7ᵗʰ **S65.912** **Laceration of unspecified blood vessel at wrist and hand level of left arm** ▽

√7ᵗʰ **S65.919** **Laceration of unspecified blood vessel at wrist and hand level of unspecified arm** ▽

√6ᵗʰ **S65.99** **Other specified injury of unspecified blood vessel at wrist and hand level**

√7ᵗʰ **S65.991** **Other specified injury of unspecified blood vessel at wrist and hand of right arm** ▽

√7ᵗʰ **S65.992** **Other specified injury of unspecified blood vessel at wrist and hand of left arm** ▽

√7ᵗʰ **S65.999** **Other specified injury of unspecified blood vessel at wrist and hand of unspecified arm** ▽

√4ᵗʰ **S66** **Injury of muscle, fascia and tendon at wrist and hand level**
Code also any associated open wound (S61.-)
EXCLUDES 2 sprain of joints and ligaments of wrist and hand (S63.-)
TIP: Refer to the Muscle/Tendon table at the beginning of this chapter.

The appropriate 7th character is to be added to each code from category S66.
A   initial encounter
D   subsequent encounter
S   sequela

√5ᵗʰ **S66.0** **Injury of** long flexor muscle, fascia and tendon of thumb at wrist and hand level

√6ᵗʰ **S66.00** **Unspecified injury of long flexor muscle, fascia and tendon of thumb at wrist and hand level**

√7ᵗʰ **S66.001** **Unspecified injury of long flexor muscle, fascia and tendon of right thumb at wrist and hand level** ▽

√7ᵗʰ **S66.002** **Unspecified injury of long flexor muscle, fascia and tendon of left thumb at wrist and hand level** ▽

√7ᵗʰ **S66.009** **Unspecified injury of long flexor muscle, fascia and tendon of unspecified thumb at wrist and hand level** ▽

√6ᵗʰ **S66.01** **Strain** of long flexor muscle, fascia and tendon of thumb at wrist and hand level

√7ᵗʰ **S66.011** **Strain of long flexor muscle, fascia and tendon of right thumb at wrist and hand level**

√7ᵗʰ **S66.012** **Strain of long flexor muscle, fascia and tendon of left thumb at wrist and hand level**

√7ᵗʰ **S66.019** **Strain of long flexor muscle, fascia and tendon of unspecified thumb at wrist and hand level** ▽

☑ Additional Character Req   √x7ᵗʰ Placeholder Alert   Manifestation   HCC CMS-HCC Condition   ▽ Unspecified Code   ▶◀ Revised Text   ● New Code   ▲ Revised Code Title

√6ᵗʰ **S66.02** **Laceration of long flexor muscle, fascia and tendon of thumb at wrist and hand level**

√7ᵗʰ **S66.021** Laceration of long flexor muscle, fascia and tendon of right thumb at wrist and hand level

√7ᵗʰ **S66.022** Laceration of long flexor muscle, fascia and tendon of left thumb at wrist and hand level

√7ᵗʰ **S66.029** Laceration of long flexor muscle, fascia and tendon of unspecified thumb at wrist and hand level ▽

√6ᵗʰ **S66.09** **Other specified injury of long flexor muscle, fascia and tendon of thumb at wrist and hand level**

√7ᵗʰ **S66.091** Other specified injury of long flexor muscle, fascia and tendon of right thumb at wrist and hand level

√7ᵗʰ **S66.092** Other specified injury of long flexor muscle, fascia and tendon of left thumb at wrist and hand level

√7ᵗʰ **S66.099** Other specified injury of long flexor muscle, fascia and tendon of unspecified thumb at wrist and hand level ▽

√5ᵗʰ **S66.1** **Injury of flexor muscle, fascia and tendon of other and unspecified finger at wrist and hand level**

> *EXCLUDES 2* Injury of long flexor muscle, fascia and tendon of thumb at wrist and hand level (S66.0-)

√6ᵗʰ **S66.10** **Unspecified injury of flexor muscle, fascia and tendon of other and unspecified finger at wrist and hand level**

√7ᵗʰ **S66.100** Unspecified injury of flexor muscle, fascia and tendon of right index finger at wrist and hand level ▽

√7ᵗʰ **S66.101** Unspecified injury of flexor muscle, fascia and tendon of left index finger at wrist and hand level ▽

√7ᵗʰ **S66.102** Unspecified injury of flexor muscle, fascia and tendon of right middle finger at wrist and hand level ▽

√7ᵗʰ **S66.103** Unspecified injury of flexor muscle, fascia and tendon of left middle finger at wrist and hand level ▽

√7ᵗʰ **S66.104** Unspecified injury of flexor muscle, fascia and tendon of right ring finger at wrist and hand level ▽

√7ᵗʰ **S66.105** Unspecified injury of flexor muscle, fascia and tendon of left ring finger at wrist and hand level ▽

√7ᵗʰ **S66.106** Unspecified injury of flexor muscle, fascia and tendon of right little finger at wrist and hand level ▽

√7ᵗʰ **S66.107** Unspecified injury of flexor muscle, fascia and tendon of left little finger at wrist and hand level ▽

√7ᵗʰ **S66.108** Unspecified injury of flexor muscle, fascia and tendon of other finger at wrist and hand level ▽

> Unspecified injury of flexor muscle, fascia and tendon of specified finger with unspecified laterality at wrist and hand level

√7ᵗʰ **S66.109** Unspecified injury of flexor muscle, ascia and tendon of unspecified finger at wrist and hand level ▽

√6ᵗʰ **S66.11** **Strain of flexor muscle, fascia and tendon of other and unspecified finger at wrist and hand level**

√7ᵗʰ **S66.110** Strain of flexor muscle, fascia and tendon of right index finger at wrist and hand level

√7ᵗʰ **S66.111** Strain of flexor muscle, fascia and tendon of left index finger at wrist and hand level

√7ᵗʰ **S66.112** Strain of flexor muscle, fascia and tendon of right middle finger at wrist and hand level

√7ᵗʰ **S66.113** Strain of flexor muscle, fascia and tendon of left middle finger at wrist and hand level

√7ᵗʰ **S66.114** Strain of flexor muscle, fascia and tendon of right ring finger at wrist and hand level

√7ᵗʰ **S66.115** Strain of flexor muscle, fascia and tendon of left ring finger at wrist and hand level

√7ᵗʰ **S66.116** Strain of flexor muscle, fascia and tendon of right little finger at wrist and hand level

√7ᵗʰ **S66.117** Strain of flexor muscle, fascia and tendon of left little finger at wrist and hand level

√7ᵗʰ **S66.118** Strain of flexor muscle, fascia and tendon of other finger at wrist and hand level

> Strain of flexor muscle, fascia and tendon of specified finger with unspecified laterality at wrist and hand level

√7ᵗʰ **S66.119** Strain of flexor muscle, fascia and tendon of unspecified finger at wrist and hand level ▽

√6ᵗʰ **S66.12** **Laceration of flexor muscle, fascia and tendon of other and unspecified finger at wrist and hand level**

√7ᵗʰ **S66.120** Laceration of flexor muscle, fascia and tendon of right index finger at wrist and hand level

√7ᵗʰ **S66.121** Laceration of flexor muscle, fascia and tendon of left index finger at wrist and hand level

√7ᵗʰ **S66.122** Laceration of flexor muscle, fascia and tendon of right middle finger at wrist and hand level

√7ᵗʰ **S66.123** Laceration of flexor muscle, fascia and tendon of left middle finger at wrist and hand level

√7ᵗʰ **S66.124** Laceration of flexor muscle, fascia and tendon of right ring finger at wrist and hand level

√7ᵗʰ **S66.125** Laceration of flexor muscle, fascia and tendon of left ring finger at wrist and hand level

√7ᵗʰ **S66.126** Laceration of flexor muscle, fascia and tendon of right little finger at wrist and hand level

√7ᵗʰ **S66.127** Laceration of flexor muscle, fascia and tendon of left little finger at wrist and hand level

√7ᵗʰ **S66.128** Laceration of flexor muscle, fascia and tendon of other finger at wrist and hand level

> Laceration of flexor muscle, fascia and tendon of specified finger with unspecified laterality at wrist and hand level

√7ᵗʰ **S66.129** Laceration of flexor muscle, fascia and tendon of unspecified finger at wrist and hand level ▽

√6ᵗʰ **S66.19** **Other injury of flexor muscle, fascia and tendon of other and unspecified finger at wrist and hand level**

√7ᵗʰ **S66.190** Other injury of flexor muscle, fascia and tendon of right index finger at wrist and hand level

√7ᵗʰ **S66.191** Other injury of flexor muscle, fascia and tendon of left index finger at wrist and hand level

√7ᵗʰ **S66.192** Other injury of flexor muscle, fascia and tendon of right middle finger at wrist and hand level

√7ᵗʰ **S66.193** Other injury of flexor muscle, fascia and tendon of left middle finger at wrist and hand level

√7ᵗʰ **S66.194** Other injury of flexor muscle, fascia and tendon of right ring finger at wrist and hand level

√7ᵗʰ **S66.195** Other injury of flexor muscle, fascia and tendon of left ring finger at wrist and hand level

√7ᵗʰ **S66.196** Other injury of flexor muscle, fascia and tendon of right little finger at wrist and hand level

√7ᵗʰ **S66.197** Other injury of flexor muscle, fascia and tendon of left little finger at wrist and hand level

EXCLUDES 1 Not coded here   *EXCLUDES 2* Not included here   Ⓝ Newborn Age: 0   Ⓟ Pediatric Age: 0-17   Ⓜ Maternity Age: 12-55   Ⓐ Adult Age: 15-124

996   ICD-10-CM 2018

☑7th S66.198   Other injury of flexor muscle, fascia and tendon of other finger at wrist and hand level

     Other injury of flexor muscle, fascia and tendon of specified finger with unspecified laterality at wrist and hand level

☑7th S66.199   Other injury of flexor muscle, and tendon of unspecified finger at wrist and hand level ▽

☑5th S66.2   **Injury of extensor muscle, fascia and tendon of thumb at wrist and hand level**

   ☑6th S66.20   Unspecified injury of extensor muscle, fascia and tendon of thumb at wrist and hand level

     ☑7th S66.201   Unspecified injury of extensor muscle, fascia and tendon of right thumb at wrist and hand level ▽

     ☑7th S66.202   Unspecified injury of extensor muscle, fascia and tendon of left thumb at wrist and hand level ▽

     ☑7th S66.209   Unspecified injury of extensor muscle, fascia and tendon of unspecified thumb at wrist and hand level ▽

   ☑6th S66.21   Strain of extensor muscle, fascia and tendon of thumb at wrist and hand level

     ☑7th S66.211   Strain of extensor muscle, fascia and tendon of right thumb at wrist and hand level

     ☑7th S66.212   Strain of extensor muscle, fascia and tendon of left thumb at wrist and hand level

     ☑7th S66.219   Strain of extensor muscle, fascia and tendon of unspecified thumb at wrist and hand level ▽

   ☑6th S66.22   Laceration of extensor muscle, fascia and tendon of thumb at wrist and hand level

     ☑7th S66.221   Laceration of extensor muscle, fascia and tendon of right thumb at wrist and hand level

     ☑7th S66.222   Laceration of extensor muscle, fascia and tendon of left thumb at wrist and hand level

     ☑7th S66.229   Laceration of extensor muscle, and tendon of unspecified thumb at wrist and hand level ▽

   ☑6th S66.29   Other specified injury of extensor muscle, fascia and tendon of thumb at wrist and hand level

     ☑7th S66.291   Other specified injury of extensor muscle, fascia and tendon of right thumb at wrist and hand level

     ☑7th S66.292   Other specified injury of extensor muscle, fascia and tendon of left thumb at wrist and hand level

     ☑7th S66.299   Other specified injury of extensor muscle, fascia and tendon of unspecified thumb at wrist and hand level ▽

☑5th S66.3   **Injury of extensor muscle, fascia and tendon of other and unspecified finger at wrist and hand level**

     EXCLUDES 2   Injury of extensor muscle, fascia and tendon of thumb at wrist and hand level (S66.2-)

   ☑6th S66.30   Unspecified injury of extensor muscle, fascia and tendon of other and unspecified finger at wrist and hand level

     ☑7th S66.300   Unspecified injury of extensor muscle, fascia and tendon of right index finger at wrist and hand level ▽

     ☑7th S66.301   Unspecified injury of extensor muscle, fascia and tendon of left index finger at wrist and hand level ▽

     ☑7th S66.302   Unspecified injury of extensor muscle, fascia and tendon of right middle finger at wrist and hand level ▽

     ☑7th S66.303   Unspecified injury of extensor muscle, fascia and tendon of left middle finger at wrist and hand level ▽

     ☑7th S66.304   Unspecified injury of extensor muscle, fascia and tendon of right ring finger at wrist and hand level ▽

☑7th S66.305   Unspecified injury of extensor muscle, fascia and tendon of left ring finger at wrist and hand level ▽

☑7th S66.306   Unspecified injury of extensor muscle, fascia and tendon of right little finger at wrist and hand level ▽

☑7th S66.307   Unspecified injury of extensor muscle, fascia and tendon of left little finger at wrist and hand level ▽

☑7th S66.308   Unspecified injury of extensor muscle, fascia and tendon of other finger at wrist and hand level ▽

     Unspecified injury of extensor muscle, fascia and tendon of specified finger with unspecified laterality at wrist and hand level

☑7th S66.309   Unspecified injury of extensor muscle, fascia and tendon of unspecified finger at wrist and hand level ▽

   ☑6th S66.31   Strain of extensor muscle, fascia and tendon of other and unspecified finger at wrist and hand level

     ☑7th S66.310   Strain of extensor muscle, fascia and tendon of right index finger at wrist and hand level

     ☑7th S66.311   Strain of extensor muscle, fascia and tendon of left index finger at wrist and hand level

     ☑7th S66.312   Strain of extensor muscle, fascia and tendon of right middle finger at wrist and hand level

     ☑7th S66.313   Strain of extensor muscle, fascia and tendon of left middle finger at wrist and hand level

     ☑7th S66.314   Strain of extensor muscle, fascia and tendon of right ring finger at wrist and hand level

     ☑7th S66.315   Strain of extensor muscle, fascia and tendon of left ring finger at wrist and hand level

     ☑7th S66.316   Strain of extensor muscle, fascia and tendon of right little finger at wrist and hand level

     ☑7th S66.317   Strain of extensor muscle, fascia and tendon of left little finger at wrist and hand level

     ☑7th S66.318   Strain of extensor muscle, fascia and tendon of other finger at wrist and hand level

     Strain of extensor muscle, fascia and tendon of specified finger with unspecified laterality at wrist and hand level

     ☑7th S66.319   Strain of extensor muscle, fascia and tendon of unspecified finger at wrist and hand level ▽

   ☑6th S66.32   Laceration of extensor muscle, fascia and tendon of other and unspecified finger at wrist and hand level

     ☑7th S66.320   Laceration of extensor muscle, fascia and tendon of right index finger at wrist and hand level

     ☑7th S66.321   Laceration of extensor muscle, fascia and tendon of left index finger at wrist and hand level

     ☑7th S66.322   Laceration of extensor muscle, fascia and tendon of right middle finger at wrist and hand level

     ☑7th S66.323   Laceration of extensor muscle, fascia and tendon of left middle finger at wrist and hand level

     ☑7th S66.324   Laceration of extensor muscle, fascia and tendon of right ring finger at wrist and hand level

     ☑7th S66.325   Laceration of extensor muscle, fascia and tendon of left ring finger at wrist and hand level

     ☑7th S66.326   Laceration of extensor muscle, fascia and tendon of right little finger at wrist and hand level

---

☑ Additional Character Req   ☑x7th Placeholder Alert   Manifestation   HCC CMS-HCC Condition   ▽ Unspecified Code   ►◄ Revised Text   ● New Code   ▲ Revised Code Title

√7ᵗʰ **S66.327** Laceration of extensor muscle, fascia and tendon of left little finger at wrist and hand level

√7ᵗʰ **S66.328** Laceration of extensor muscle, fascia and tendon of other finger at wrist and hand level
> Laceration of extensor muscle, fascia and tendon of specified finger with unspecified laterality at wrist and hand level

√7ᵗʰ **S66.329** Laceration of extensor muscle, fascia and tendon of unspecified finger at wrist and hand level ▽

√6ᵗʰ **S66.39** Other injury of extensor muscle, fascia and tendon of other and unspecified finger at wrist and hand level

√7ᵗʰ **S66.390** Other injury of extensor muscle, fascia and tendon of right index finger at wrist and hand level

√7ᵗʰ **S66.391** Other injury of extensor muscle, fascia and tendon of left index finger at wrist and hand level

√7ᵗʰ **S66.392** Other injury of extensor muscle, fascia and tendon of right middle finger at wrist and hand level

√7ᵗʰ **S66.393** Other injury of extensor muscle, fascia and tendon of left middle finger at wrist and hand level

√7ᵗʰ **S66.394** Other injury of extensor muscle, fascia and tendon of right ring finger at wrist and hand level

√7ᵗʰ **S66.395** Other injury of extensor muscle, fascia and tendon of left ring finger at wrist and hand level

√7ᵗʰ **S66.396** Other injury of extensor muscle, fascia and tendon of right little finger at wrist and hand level

√7ᵗʰ **S66.397** Other injury of extensor muscle, fascia and tendon of left little finger at wrist and hand level

√7ᵗʰ **S66.398** Other injury of extensor muscle, fascia and tendon of other finger at wrist and hand level
> Other injury of extensor muscle, fascia and tendon of specified finger with unspecified laterality at wrist and hand level

√7ᵗʰ **S66.399** Other injury of extensor muscle, fascia and tendon of unspecified finger at wrist and hand level ▽

√5ᵗʰ **S66.4** Injury of intrinsic muscle, fascia and tendon of thumb at wrist and hand level

√6ᵗʰ **S66.40** Unspecified injury of intrinsic muscle, fascia and tendon of thumb at wrist and hand level

√7ᵗʰ **S66.401** Unspecified injury of intrinsic muscle, fascia and tendon of right thumb at wrist and hand level ▽

√7ᵗʰ **S66.402** Unspecified injury of intrinsic muscle, fascia and tendon of left thumb at wrist and hand level ▽

√7ᵗʰ **S66.409** Unspecified injury of intrinsic muscle, fascia and tendon of unspecified thumb at wrist and hand level ▽

√6ᵗʰ **S66.41** Strain of intrinsic muscle, fascia and tendon of thumb at wrist and hand level

√7ᵗʰ **S66.411** Strain of intrinsic muscle, fascia and tendon of right thumb at wrist and hand level

√7ᵗʰ **S66.412** Strain of intrinsic muscle, fascia and tendon of left thumb at wrist and hand level

√7ᵗʰ **S66.419** Strain of intrinsic muscle, fascia and tendon of unspecified thumb at wrist and hand level ▽

√6ᵗʰ **S66.42** Laceration of intrinsic muscle, fascia and tendon of thumb at wrist and hand level

√7ᵗʰ **S66.421** Laceration of intrinsic muscle, fascia and tendon of right thumb at wrist and hand level

√7ᵗʰ **S66.422** Laceration of intrinsic muscle, fascia and tendon of left thumb at wrist and hand level

√7ᵗʰ **S66.429** Laceration of intrinsic muscle, fascia and tendon of unspecified thumb at wrist and hand level ▽

√6ᵗʰ **S66.49** Other specified injury of intrinsic muscle, fascia and tendon of thumb at wrist and hand level

√7ᵗʰ **S66.491** Other specified injury of intrinsic muscle, fascia and tendon of right thumb at wrist and hand level

√7ᵗʰ **S66.492** Other specified injury of intrinsic muscle, fascia and tendon of left thumb at wrist and hand level

√7ᵗʰ **S66.499** Other specified injury of intrinsic muscle, fascia and tendon of unspecified thumb at wrist and hand level ▽

√5ᵗʰ **S66.5** Injury of intrinsic muscle, fascia and tendon of other and unspecified finger at wrist and hand level
> **EXCLUDES 2**   injury of intrinsic muscle, fascia and tendon of thumb at wrist and hand level (S66.4-)

√6ᵗʰ **S66.50** Unspecified injury of intrinsic muscle, fascia and tendon of other and unspecified finger at wrist and hand level

√7ᵗʰ **S66.500** Unspecified injury of intrinsic muscle, fascia and tendon of right index finger at wrist and hand level ▽

√7ᵗʰ **S66.501** Unspecified injury of intrinsic muscle, fascia and tendon of left index finger at wrist and hand level ▽

√7ᵗʰ **S66.502** Unspecified injury of intrinsic muscle, fascia and tendon of right middle finger at wrist and hand level ▽

√7ᵗʰ **S66.503** Unspecified injury of intrinsic muscle, fascia and tendon of left middle finger at wrist and hand level ▽

√7ᵗʰ **S66.504** Unspecified injury of intrinsic muscle, fascia and tendon of right ring finger at wrist and hand level ▽

√7ᵗʰ **S66.505** Unspecified injury of intrinsic muscle, fascia and tendon of left ring finger at wrist and hand level ▽

√7ᵗʰ **S66.506** Unspecified injury of intrinsic muscle, fascia and tendon of right little finger at wrist and hand level ▽

√7ᵗʰ **S66.507** Unspecified injury of intrinsic muscle, fascia and tendon of left little finger at wrist and hand level ▽

√7ᵗʰ **S66.508** Unspecified injury of intrinsic muscle, fascia and tendon of other finger at wrist and hand level ▽
> Unspecified injury of intrinsic muscle, fascia and tendon of specified finger with unspecified laterality at wrist and hand level

√7ᵗʰ **S66.509** Unspecified injury of intrinsic muscle, fascia and tendon of unspecified finger at wrist and hand level ▽

√6ᵗʰ **S66.51** Strain of intrinsic muscle, fascia and tendon of other and unspecified finger at wrist and hand level

√7ᵗʰ **S66.510** Strain of intrinsic muscle, fascia and tendon of right index finger at wrist and hand level

√7ᵗʰ **S66.511** Strain of intrinsic muscle, fascia and tendon of left index finger at wrist and hand level

√7ᵗʰ **S66.512** Strain of intrinsic muscle, fascia and tendon of right middle finger at wrist and hand level

√7ᵗʰ **S66.513** Strain of intrinsic muscle, fascia and tendon of left middle finger at wrist and hand level

√7ᵗʰ **S66.514** Strain of intrinsic muscle, fascia and tendon of right ring finger at wrist and hand level

√7ᵗʰ **S66.515** Strain of intrinsic muscle, fascia and tendon of left ring finger at wrist and hand level

EXCLUDES 1 Not coded here   **EXCLUDES 2** Not included here   ℕ Newborn Age: 0   ℙ Pediatric Age: 0-17   🅼 Maternity Age: 12-55   🅰 Adult Age: 15-124

998   ICD-10-CM 2018

√7ᵗʰ **S66.516** Strain of intrinsic muscle, fascia and tendon of right little finger at wrist and hand level

√7ᵗʰ **S66.517** Strain of intrinsic muscle, fascia and tendon of left little finger at wrist and hand level

√7ᵗʰ **S66.518** Strain of intrinsic muscle, fascia and tendon of other finger at wrist and hand level

     Strain of intrinsic muscle, fascia and tendon of specified finger with unspecified laterality at wrist and hand level

√7ᵗʰ **S66.519** Strain of intrinsic muscle, fascia and tendon of unspecified finger at wrist and hand level ▽

√6ᵗʰ **S66.52** Laceration of intrinsic muscle, fascia and tendon of other and unspecified finger at wrist and hand level

√7ᵗʰ **S66.520** Laceration of intrinsic muscle, fascia and tendon of right index finger at wrist and hand level

√7ᵗʰ **S66.521** Laceration of intrinsic muscle, fascia and tendon of left index finger at wrist and hand level

√7ᵗʰ **S66.522** Laceration of intrinsic muscle, fascia and tendon of right middle finger at wrist and hand level

√7ᵗʰ **S66.523** Laceration of intrinsic muscle, fascia and tendon of left middle finger at wrist and hand level

√7ᵗʰ **S66.524** Laceration of intrinsic muscle, fascia and tendon of right ring finger at wrist and hand level

√7ᵗʰ **S66.525** Laceration of intrinsic muscle, fascia and tendon of left ring finger at wrist and hand level

√7ᵗʰ **S66.526** Laceration of intrinsic muscle, fascia and tendon of right little finger at wrist and hand level

√7ᵗʰ **S66.527** Laceration of intrinsic muscle, fascia and tendon of left little finger at wrist and hand level

√7ᵗʰ **S66.528** Laceration of intrinsic muscle, fascia and tendon of other finger at wrist and hand level

     Laceration of intrinsic muscle, fascia and tendon of specified finger with unspecified laterality at wrist and hand level

√7ᵗʰ **S66.529** Laceration of intrinsic muscle, fascia and tendon of unspecified finger at wrist and hand level ▽

√6ᵗʰ **S66.59** Other injury of intrinsic muscle, fascia and tendon of other and unspecified finger at wrist and hand level

√7ᵗʰ **S66.590** Other injury of intrinsic muscle, fascia and tendon of right index finger at wrist and hand level

√7ᵗʰ **S66.591** Other injury of intrinsic muscle, fascia and tendon of left index finger at wrist and hand level

√7ᵗʰ **S66.592** Other injury of intrinsic muscle, fascia and tendon of right middle finger at wrist and hand level

√7ᵗʰ **S66.593** Other injury of intrinsic muscle, fascia and tendon of left middle finger at wrist and hand level

√7ᵗʰ **S66.594** Other injury of intrinsic muscle, fascia and tendon of right ring finger at wrist and hand level

√7ᵗʰ **S66.595** Other injury of intrinsic muscle, fascia and tendon of left ring finger at wrist and hand level

√7ᵗʰ **S66.596** Other injury of intrinsic muscle, fascia and tendon of right little finger at wrist and hand level

√7ᵗʰ **S66.597** Other injury of intrinsic muscle, fascia and tendon of left little finger at wrist and hand level

√7ᵗʰ **S66.598** Other injury of intrinsic muscle, fascia and tendon of other finger at wrist and hand level

     Other injury of intrinsic muscle, fascia and tendon of specified finger with unspecified laterality at wrist and hand level

√7ᵗʰ **S66.599** Other injury of intrinsic muscle, fascia and tendon of unspecified finger at wrist and hand level ▽

√5ᵗʰ **S66.8** Injury of other specified muscles, fascia and tendons at wrist and hand level

√6ᵗʰ **S66.80** Unspecified injury of other specified muscles, fascia and tendons at wrist and hand level

√7ᵗʰ **S66.801** Unspecified injury of other specified muscles, fascia and tendons at wrist and hand level, right hand ▽

√7ᵗʰ **S66.802** Unspecified injury of other specified muscles, fascia and tendons at wrist and hand level, left hand ▽

√7ᵗʰ **S66.809** Unspecified injury of other specified muscles, fascia and tendons at wrist and hand level, unspecified hand ▽

√6ᵗʰ **S66.81** Strain of other specified muscles, fascia and tendons at wrist and hand level

√7ᵗʰ **S66.811** Strain of other specified muscles, fascia and tendons at wrist and hand level, right hand

√7ᵗʰ **S66.812** Strain of other specified muscles, fascia and tendons at wrist and hand level, left hand

√7ᵗʰ **S66.819** Strain of other specified muscles, fascia and tendons at wrist and hand level, unspecified hand ▽

√6ᵗʰ **S66.82** Laceration of other specified muscles, fascia and tendons at wrist and hand level

√7ᵗʰ **S66.821** Laceration of other specified muscles, fascia and tendons at wrist and hand level, right hand

√7ᵗʰ **S66.822** Laceration of other specified muscles, fascia and tendons at wrist and hand level, left hand

√7ᵗʰ **S66.829** Laceration of other specified muscles, fascia and tendons at wrist and hand level, unspecified hand ▽

√6ᵗʰ **S66.89** Other injury of other specified muscles, fascia and tendons at wrist and hand level

√7ᵗʰ **S66.891** Other injury of other specified muscles, fascia and tendons at wrist and hand level, right hand

√7ᵗʰ **S66.892** Other injury of other specified muscles, fascia and tendons at wrist and hand level, left hand

√7ᵗʰ **S66.899** Other injury of other specified muscles, fascia and tendons at wrist and hand level, unspecified hand ▽

√5ᵗʰ **S66.9** Injury of unspecified muscle, fascia and tendon at wrist and hand level

√6ᵗʰ **S66.90** Unspecified injury of unspecified muscle, fascia and tendon at wrist and hand level

√7ᵗʰ **S66.901** Unspecified injury of unspecified muscle, fascia and tendon at wrist and hand level, right hand ▽

√7ᵗʰ **S66.902** Unspecified injury of unspecified muscle, fascia and tendon at wrist and hand level, left hand ▽

√7ᵗʰ **S66.909** Unspecified injury of unspecified muscle, fascia and tendon at wrist and hand level, unspecified hand ▽

√6ᵗʰ **S66.91** Strain of unspecified muscle, fascia and tendon at wrist and hand level

√7ᵗʰ **S66.911** Strain of unspecified muscle, fascia and tendon at wrist and hand level, right hand ▽

√7ᵗʰ **S66.912** Strain of unspecified muscle, fascia and tendon at wrist and hand level, left hand ▽

☑ Additional Character Req   ✓x7ᵗʰ Placeholder Alert   Manifestation   HCC CMS-HCC Condition   ▽ Unspecified Code   ►◄ Revised Text   ● New Code   ▲ Revised Code Title

ICD-10-CM 2018   999

√7ᵗʰ **S66.919** Strain of unspecified muscle, fascia ▽
and tendon at wrist and hand level,
unspecified hand

√6ᵗʰ **S66.92** Laceration of unspecified muscle, fascia and tendon
at wrist and hand level

√7ᵗʰ **S66.921** Laceration of unspecified muscle, ▽
fascia and tendon at wrist and hand
level, right hand

√7ᵗʰ **S66.922** Laceration of unspecified muscle, ▽
fascia and tendon at wrist and hand
level, left hand

√7ᵗʰ **S66.929** Laceration of unspecified muscle, ▽
fascia and tendon at wrist and hand
level, unspecified hand

√6ᵗʰ **S66.99** Other injury of unspecified muscle, fascia and
tendon at wrist and hand level

√7ᵗʰ **S66.991** Other injury of unspecified muscle, ▽
fascia and tendon at wrist and hand
level, right hand

√7ᵗʰ **S66.992** Other injury of unspecified muscle, ▽
fascia and tendon at wrist and hand
level, left hand

√7ᵗʰ **S66.999** Other injury of unspecified muscle, ▽
fascia and tendon at wrist and hand
level, unspecified hand

√4ᵗʰ **S67** Crushing injury of wrist, hand and fingers
Use additional code for all associated injuries, such as:
fracture of wrist and hand (S62.-)
open wound of wrist and hand (S61.-)

The appropriate 7th character is to be added to each code
from category S67.
A initial encounter
D subsequent encounter
S sequela

√5ᵗʰ **S67.0** Crushing injury of thumb

√x7ᵗʰ **S67.00** Crushing injury of unspecified thumb ▽

√x7ᵗʰ **S67.01** Crushing injury of right thumb

√x7ᵗʰ **S67.02** Crushing injury of left thumb

√5ᵗʰ **S67.1** Crushing injury of other and unspecified finger(s)
EXCLUDES 2 crushing injury of thumb (S67.0-)

√x7ᵗʰ **S67.10** Crushing injury of unspecified finger(s) ▽

√6ᵗʰ **S67.19** Crushing injury of other finger(s)

√7ᵗʰ **S67.190** Crushing injury of right index finger

√7ᵗʰ **S67.191** Crushing injury of left index finger

√7ᵗʰ **S67.192** Crushing injury of right middle finger

√7ᵗʰ **S67.193** Crushing injury of left middle finger

√7ᵗʰ **S67.194** Crushing injury of right ring finger

√7ᵗʰ **S67.195** Crushing injury of left ring finger

√7ᵗʰ **S67.196** Crushing injury of right little finger

√7ᵗʰ **S67.197** Crushing injury of left little finger

√7ᵗʰ **S67.198** Crushing injury of other finger
Crushing injury of specified finger with
unspecified laterality

√5ᵗʰ **S67.2** Crushing injury of hand
EXCLUDES 2 crushing injury of fingers (S67.1-)
crushing injury of thumb (S67.0-)

√x7ᵗʰ **S67.20** Crushing injury of unspecified hand ▽

√x7ᵗʰ **S67.21** Crushing injury of right hand

√x7ᵗʰ **S67.22** Crushing injury of left hand

√5ᵗʰ **S67.3** Crushing injury of wrist

√x7ᵗʰ **S67.30** Crushing injury of unspecified wrist ▽

√x7ᵗʰ **S67.31** Crushing injury of right wrist

√x7ᵗʰ **S67.32** Crushing injury of left wrist

√5ᵗʰ **S67.4** Crushing injury of wrist and hand
EXCLUDES 1 crushing injury of hand alone (S67.2-)
crushing injury of wrist alone (S67.3-)
EXCLUDES 2 crushing injury of fingers (S67.1-)
crushing injury of thumb (S67.0-)

√x7ᵗʰ **S67.40** Crushing injury of unspecified wrist and hand ▽

√x7ᵗʰ **S67.41** Crushing injury of right wrist and hand

√x7ᵗʰ **S67.42** Crushing injury of left wrist and hand

√5ᵗʰ **S67.9** Crushing injury of unspecified part(s) of wrist, hand and
fingers

√x7ᵗʰ **S67.90** Crushing injury of unspecified part(s) of ▽
unspecified wrist, hand and fingers

√x7ᵗʰ **S67.91** Crushing injury of unspecified part(s) of ▽
right wrist, hand and fingers

√x7ᵗʰ **S67.92** Crushing injury of unspecified part(s) of ▽
left wrist, hand and fingers

√4ᵗʰ **S68** Traumatic amputation of wrist, hand and fingers
An amputation not identified as partial or complete should be coded to
complete.

The appropriate 7th character is to be added to each code
from category S68.
A initial encounter
D subsequent encounter
S sequela

√5ᵗʰ **S68.0** Traumatic metacarpophalangeal amputation of thumb
Traumatic amputation of thumb NOS

√6ᵗʰ **S68.01** Complete traumatic metacarpophalangeal
amputation of thumb

³ √7ᵗʰ **S68.011** Complete traumatic metacarpo- HCC
phalangeal amputation of right thumb

³ √7ᵗʰ **S68.012** Complete traumatic metacarpo- HCC
phalangeal amputation of left thumb

³ √7ᵗʰ **S68.019** Complete traumatic metacarpo- HCC ▽
phalangeal amputation of unspecified
thumb

√6ᵗʰ **S68.02** Partial traumatic metacarpophalangeal amputation
of thumb

³ √7ᵗʰ **S68.021** Partial traumatic metacarpo- HCC
phalangeal amputation of right thumb

³ √7ᵗʰ **S68.022** Partial traumatic metacarpo- HCC
phalangeal amputation of left thumb

³ √7ᵗʰ **S68.029** Partial traumatic metacarpo- HCC ▽
phalangeal amputation of unspecified
thumb

√5ᵗʰ **S68.1** Traumatic metacarpophalangeal amputation of other and
unspecified finger
Traumatic amputation of finger NOS
EXCLUDES 2 traumatic metacarpophalangeal amputation of
thumb (S68.0-)

√6ᵗʰ **S68.11** Complete traumatic metacarpophalangeal
amputation of other and unspecified finger

³ √7ᵗʰ **S68.110** Complete traumatic metacarpo- HCC
phalangeal amputation of right index
finger

³ √7ᵗʰ **S68.111** Complete traumatic metacarpo- HCC
phalangeal amputation of left index
finger

³ √7ᵗʰ **S68.112** Complete traumatic metacarpo- HCC
phalangeal amputation of right middle
finger

³ √7ᵗʰ **S68.113** Complete traumatic metacarpo- HCC
phalangeal amputation of left middle
finger

³ √7ᵗʰ **S68.114** Complete traumatic metacarpo- HCC
phalangeal amputation of right ring
finger

³ √7ᵗʰ **S68.115** Complete traumatic metacarpo- HCC
phalangeal amputation of left ring finger

³ √7ᵗʰ **S68.116** Complete traumatic metacarpo- HCC
phalangeal amputation of right little
finger

³ √7ᵗʰ **S68.117** Complete traumatic metacarpo- HCC
phalangeal amputation of left little finger

³ √7ᵗʰ **S68.118** Complete traumatic metacarpo- HCC
phalangeal amputation of other finger
Complete traumatic metacarpophalangeal
amputation of specified finger with
unspecified laterality

³ √7ᵗʰ **S68.119** Complete traumatic metacarpo- HCC ▽
phalangeal amputation of unspecified
finger

---

³ HCC with 7th character indicating sequela.

EXCLUDES 1 Not coded here   EXCLUDES 2 Not included here   N Newborn Age: 0   P Pediatric Age: 0-17   M Maternity Age: 12-55   A Adult Age: 15-124

1000
ICD-10-CM 2018

☑6ᵗʰ **S68.12** **Partial** traumatic metacarpophalangeal amputation of other and unspecified finger

    3 ☑7ᵗʰ **S68.120** **Partial traumatic metacarpophalangeal amputation of right index finger** HCC

    3 ☑7ᵗʰ **S68.121** **Partial traumatic metacarpophalangeal amputation of left index finger** HCC

    3 ☑7ᵗʰ **S68.122** **Partial traumatic metacarpophalangeal amputation of right middle finger** HCC

    3 ☑7ᵗʰ **S68.123** **Partial traumatic metacarpophalangeal amputation of left middle finger** HCC

    3 ☑7ᵗʰ **S68.124** **Partial traumatic metacarpophalangeal amputation of right ring finger** HCC

    3 ☑7ᵗʰ **S68.125** **Partial traumatic metacarpophalangeal amputation of left ring finger** HCC

    3 ☑7ᵗʰ **S68.126** **Partial traumatic metacarpophalangeal amputation of right little finger** HCC

    3 ☑7ᵗʰ **S68.127** **Partial traumatic metacarpophalangeal amputation of left little finger** HCC

    3 ☑7ᵗʰ **S68.128** **Partial traumatic metacarpophalangeal amputation of other finger** HCC
       Partial traumatic metacarpophalangeal amputation of specified finger with unspecified laterality

    3 ☑7ᵗʰ **S68.129** **Partial traumatic metacarpophalangeal amputation of unspecified finger** HCC ▽

☑5ᵗʰ **S68.4** **Traumatic amputation of** hand at wrist level
    Traumatic amputation of hand NOS
    Traumatic amputation of wrist

    ☑6ᵗʰ **S68.41** **Complete** traumatic amputation of hand at wrist level

      2 ☑7ᵗʰ **S68.411** **Complete traumatic amputation of right hand at wrist level** HCC

      2 ☑7ᵗʰ **S68.412** **Complete traumatic amputation of left hand at wrist level** HCC

      2 ☑7ᵗʰ **S68.419** **Complete traumatic amputation of unspecified hand at wrist level** HCC ▽

    ☑6ᵗʰ **S68.42** **Partial** traumatic amputation of hand at wrist level

      2 ☑7ᵗʰ **S68.421** **Partial traumatic amputation of right hand at wrist level** HCC

      2 ☑7ᵗʰ **S68.422** **Partial traumatic amputation of left hand at wrist level** HCC

      2 ☑7ᵗʰ **S68.429** **Partial traumatic amputation of unspecified hand at wrist level** HCC ▽

☑5ᵗʰ **S68.5** **Traumatic** transphalangeal amputation of thumb
    Traumatic interphalangeal joint amputation of thumb

    ☑6ᵗʰ **S68.51** **Complete** traumatic transphalangeal amputation of thumb

      3 ☑7ᵗʰ **S68.511** **Complete traumatic transphalangeal amputation of right thumb** HCC

      3 ☑7ᵗʰ **S68.512** **Complete traumatic transphalangeal amputation of left thumb** HCC

      3 ☑7ᵗʰ **S68.519** **Complete traumatic transphalangeal amputation of unspecified thumb** HCC ▽

    ☑6ᵗʰ **S68.52** **Partial** traumatic transphalangeal amputation of thumb

      3 ☑7ᵗʰ **S68.521** **Partial traumatic transphalangeal amputation of right thumb** HCC

      3 ☑7ᵗʰ **S68.522** **Partial traumatic transphalangeal amputation of left thumb** HCC

      3 ☑7ᵗʰ **S68.529** **Partial traumatic transphalangeal amputation of unspecified thumb** HCC ▽

☑5ᵗʰ **S68.6** **Traumatic** transphalangeal amputation of other and unspecified finger

    ☑6ᵗʰ **S68.61** **Complete** traumatic transphalangeal amputation of other and unspecified finger(s)

      3 ☑7ᵗʰ **S68.610** **Complete traumatic transphalangeal amputation of right index finger** HCC

      3 ☑7ᵗʰ **S68.611** **Complete traumatic transphalangeal amputation of left index finger** HCC

      3 ☑7ᵗʰ **S68.612** **Complete traumatic transphalangeal amputation of right middle finger** HCC

      3 ☑7ᵗʰ **S68.613** **Complete traumatic transphalangeal amputation of left middle finger** HCC

      3 ☑7ᵗʰ **S68.614** **Complete traumatic transphalangeal amputation of right ring finger** HCC

      3 ☑7ᵗʰ **S68.615** **Complete traumatic transphalangeal amputation of left ring finger** HCC

      3 ☑7ᵗʰ **S68.616** **Complete traumatic transphalangeal amputation of right little finger** HCC

      3 ☑7ᵗʰ **S68.617** **Complete traumatic transphalangeal amputation of left little finger** HCC

      3 ☑7ᵗʰ **S68.618** **Complete traumatic transphalangeal amputation of other finger** HCC
       Complete traumatic transphalangeal amputation of specified finger with unspecified laterality

      3 ☑7ᵗʰ **S68.619** **Complete traumatic transphalangeal amputation of unspecified finger** HCC ▽

    ☑6ᵗʰ **S68.62** **Partial** traumatic transphalangeal amputation of other and unspecified finger

      3 ☑7ᵗʰ **S68.620** **Partial traumatic transphalangeal amputation of right index finger** HCC

      3 ☑7ᵗʰ **S68.621** **Partial traumatic transphalangeal amputation of left index finger** HCC

      3 ☑7ᵗʰ **S68.622** **Partial traumatic transphalangeal amputation of right middle finger** HCC

      3 ☑7ᵗʰ **S68.623** **Partial traumatic transphalangeal amputation of left middle finger** HCC

      3 ☑7ᵗʰ **S68.624** **Partial traumatic transphalangeal amputation of right ring finger** HCC

      3 ☑7ᵗʰ **S68.625** **Partial traumatic transphalangeal amputation of left ring finger** HCC

      3 ☑7ᵗʰ **S68.626** **Partial traumatic transphalangeal amputation of right little finger** HCC

      3 ☑7ᵗʰ **S68.627** **Partial traumatic transphalangeal amputation of left little finger** HCC

      3 ☑7ᵗʰ **S68.628** **Partial traumatic transphalangeal amputation of other finger** HCC
       Partial traumatic transphalangeal amputation of specified finger with unspecified laterality

      3 ☑7ᵗʰ **S68.629** **Partial traumatic transphalangeal amputation of unspecified finger** HCC ▽

☑5ᵗʰ **S68.7** **Traumatic** transmetacarpal amputation of hand

    ☑6ᵗʰ **S68.71** **Complete** traumatic transmetacarpal amputation of hand

      2 ☑7ᵗʰ **S68.711** **Complete traumatic transmetacarpal amputation of right hand** HCC

      2 ☑7ᵗʰ **S68.712** **Complete traumatic transmetacarpal amputation of left hand** HCC

      2 ☑7ᵗʰ **S68.719** **Complete traumatic transmetacarpal amputation of unspecified hand** HCC ▽

    ☑6ᵗʰ **S68.72** **Partial** traumatic transmetacarpal amputation of hand

      2 ☑7ᵗʰ **S68.721** **Partial traumatic transmetacarpal amputation of right hand** HCC

      2 ☑7ᵗʰ **S68.722** **Partial traumatic transmetacarpal amputation of left hand** HCC

      2 ☑7ᵗʰ **S68.729** **Partial traumatic transmetacarpal amputation of unspecified hand** HCC ▽

---

2   HCC with 7th character indicating initial encounter (A or B - specific to category) OR sequela.
3   HCC with 7th character indicating sequela.

☑ Additional Character Req   ☑×7ᵗʰ Placeholder Alert   Manifestation   HCC CMS-HCC Condition   ▽ Unspecified Code   ▶◀ Revised Text   ● New Code   ▲ Revised Code Title

✓4th S69 Other and unspecified injuries of wrist, hand and finger(s)

> The appropriate 7th character is to be added to each code from category S69.
> A   initial encounter
> D   subsequent encounter
> S   sequela

✓5th **S69.8 Other specified injuries of wrist, hand and finger(s)**

   ✓x7th **S69.80 Other specified injuries of unspecified wrist, hand and finger(s)** ▽

   ✓x7th **S69.81 Other specified injuries of right wrist, hand and finger(s)**

   ✓x7th **S69.82 Other specified injuries of left wrist, hand and finger(s)**

✓5th **S69.9 Unspecified injury of wrist, hand and finger(s)**

   ✓x7th **S69.90 Unspecified injury of unspecified wrist, hand and finger(s)** ▽

   ✓x7th **S69.91 Unspecified injury of right wrist, hand and finger(s)** ▽

   ✓x7th **S69.92 Unspecified injury of left wrist, hand and finger(s)** ▽

Injuries to the hip and thigh (S70-S79)

EXCLUDES 2   *burns and corrosions (T20-T32)*
     frostbite (T33-T34)
     snake bite (T63.0-)
     venomous insect bite or sting (T63.4-)

✓4th S70 Superficial injury of hip and thigh

> The appropriate 7th character is to be added to each code from category S70.
> A   initial encounter
> D   subsequent encounter
> S   sequela

✓5th **S70.0 Contusion of hip**

   ✓x7th **S70.00 Contusion of unspecified hip** ▽

   ✓x7th **S70.01 Contusion of right hip**

   ✓x7th **S70.02 Contusion of left hip**

✓5th **S70.1 Contusion of thigh**

   ✓x7th **S70.10 Contusion of unspecified thigh** ▽

   ✓x7th **S70.11 Contusion of right thigh**

   ✓x7th **S70.12 Contusion of left thigh**

✓5th **S70.2 Other superficial injuries of hip**

   ✓6th **S70.21 Abrasion of hip**

     ✓7th **S70.211 Abrasion, right hip**

     ✓7th **S70.212 Abrasion, left hip**

     ✓7th **S70.219 Abrasion, unspecified hip** ▽

   ✓6th **S70.22 Blister (nonthermal) of hip**

     ✓7th **S70.221 Blister (nonthermal), right hip**

     ✓7th **S70.222 Blister (nonthermal), left hip**

     ✓7th **S70.229 Blister (nonthermal), unspecified hip** ▽

   ✓6th **S70.24 External constriction of hip**

     ✓7th **S70.241 External constriction, right hip**

     ✓7th **S70.242 External constriction, left hip**

     ✓7th **S70.249 External constriction, unspecified hip** ▽

   ✓6th **S70.25 Superficial foreign body of hip**
     Splinter in the hip

     ✓7th **S70.251 Superficial foreign body, right hip**

     ✓7th **S70.252 Superficial foreign body, left hip**

     ✓7th **S70.259 Superficial foreign body, unspecified hip** ▽

   ✓6th **S70.26 Insect bite (nonvenomous) of hip**

     ✓7th **S70.261 Insect bite (nonvenomous), right hip**

     ✓7th **S70.262 Insect bite (nonvenomous), left hip**

     ✓7th **S70.269 Insect bite (nonvenomous), unspecified hip** ▽

   ✓6th **S70.27 Other superficial bite of hip**
     EXCLUDES 1   *open bite of hip (S71.05-)*

     ✓7th **S70.271 Other superficial bite of hip, right hip**

     ✓7th **S70.272 Other superficial bite of hip, left hip**

     ✓7th **S70.279 Other superficial bite of hip, unspecified hip** ▽

✓5th **S70.3 Other superficial injuries of thigh**

   ✓6th **S70.31 Abrasion of thigh**

     ✓7th **S70.311 Abrasion, right thigh**

     ✓7th **S70.312 Abrasion, left thigh**

     ✓7th **S70.319 Abrasion, unspecified thigh** ▽

   ✓6th **S70.32 Blister (nonthermal) of thigh**

     ✓7th **S70.321 Blister (nonthermal), right thigh**

     ✓7th **S70.322 Blister (nonthermal), left thigh**

     ✓7th **S70.329 Blister (nonthermal), unspecified thigh** ▽

   ✓6th **S70.34 External constriction of thigh**

     ✓7th **S70.341 External constriction, right thigh**

     ✓7th **S70.342 External constriction, left thigh**

     ✓7th **S70.349 External constriction, unspecified thigh** ▽

   ✓6th **S70.35 Superficial foreign body of thigh**
     Splinter in the thigh

     ✓7th **S70.351 Superficial foreign body, right thigh**

     ✓7th **S70.352 Superficial foreign body, left thigh**

     ✓7th **S70.359 Superficial foreign body, unspecified thigh** ▽

   ✓6th **S70.36 Insect bite (nonvenomous) of thigh**

     ✓7th **S70.361 Insect bite (nonvenomous), right thigh**

     ✓7th **S70.362 Insect bite (nonvenomous), left thigh**

     ✓7th **S70.369 Insect bite (nonvenomous), unspecified thigh** ▽

   ✓6th **S70.37 Other superficial bite of thigh**
     EXCLUDES 1   *open bite of thigh (S71.15)*

     ✓7th **S70.371 Other superficial bite of right thigh**

     ✓7th **S70.372 Other superficial bite of left thigh**

     ✓7th **S70.379 Other superficial bite of unspecified thigh** ▽

✓5th **S70.9 Unspecified superficial injury of hip and thigh**

   ✓6th **S70.91 Unspecified superficial injury of hip**

     ✓7th **S70.911 Unspecified superficial injury of right hip** ▽

     ✓7th **S70.912 Unspecified superficial injury of left hip** ▽

     ✓7th **S70.919 Unspecified superficial injury of unspecified hip** ▽

   ✓6th **S70.92 Unspecified superficial injury of thigh**

     ✓7th **S70.921 Unspecified superficial injury of right thigh** ▽

     ✓7th **S70.922 Unspecified superficial injury of left thigh** ▽

     ✓7th **S70.929 Unspecified superficial injury of unspecified thigh** ▽

✓4th S71 Open wound of hip and thigh

> Code also any associated wound infection
> EXCLUDES 1   *open fracture of hip and thigh (S72.-)*
>   *traumatic amputation of hip and thigh (S78.-)*
> EXCLUDES 2   *bite of venomous animal (T63.-)*
>   *open wound of ankle, foot and toes (S91.-)*
>   *open wound of knee and lower leg (S81.-)*

> The appropriate 7th character is to be added to each code from category S71.
> A   initial encounter
> D   subsequent encounter
> S   sequela

✓5th **S71.0 Open wound of hip**

   ✓6th **S71.00 Unspecified open wound of hip**

     ✓7th **S71.001 Unspecified open wound, right hip** ▽

     ✓7th **S71.002 Unspecified open wound, left hip** ▽

     ✓7th **S71.009 Unspecified open wound, unspecified hip** ▽

   ✓6th **S71.01 Laceration without foreign body of hip**

     ✓7th **S71.011 Laceration without foreign body, right hip**

     ✓7th **S71.012 Laceration without foreign body, left hip**

     ✓7th **S71.019 Laceration without foreign body, unspecified hip** ▽

   ✓6th **S71.02 Laceration with foreign body of hip**

     ✓7th **S71.021 Laceration with foreign body, right hip**

     ✓7th **S71.022 Laceration with foreign body, left hip**

√7ᵗʰ **S71.029** **Laceration with foreign body, unspecified hip** ▽

√6ᵗʰ **S71.03** Puncture wound without foreign body of hip

    √7ᵗʰ **S71.031** **Puncture wound without foreign body, right hip**

    √7ᵗʰ **S71.032** **Puncture wound without foreign body, left hip**

    √7ᵗʰ **S71.039** **Puncture wound without foreign body, unspecified hip** ▽

√6ᵗʰ **S71.04** Puncture wound with foreign body of hip

    √7ᵗʰ **S71.041** **Puncture wound with foreign body, right hip**

    √7ᵗʰ **S71.042** **Puncture wound with foreign body, left hip**

    √7ᵗʰ **S71.049** **Puncture wound with foreign body, unspecified hip** ▽

√6ᵗʰ **S71.05** Open bite of hip
Bite of hip NOS
    EXCLUDES 1   superficial bite of hip (S70.26, S70.27)

    √7ᵗʰ **S71.051** **Open bite, right hip**

    √7ᵗʰ **S71.052** **Open bite, left hip**

    √7ᵗʰ **S71.059** **Open bite, unspecified hip** ▽

√5ᵗʰ **S71.1** **Open wound of thigh**

√6ᵗʰ **S71.10** **Unspecified open wound of thigh**
AHA: 2016, 3Q, 24

    √7ᵗʰ **S71.101** **Unspecified open wound, right thigh** ▽

    √7ᵗʰ **S71.102** **Unspecified open wound, left thigh** ▽

    √7ᵗʰ **S71.109** **Unspecified open wound, unspecified thigh** ▽

√6ᵗʰ **S71.11** Laceration without foreign body of thigh

    √7ᵗʰ **S71.111** **Laceration without foreign body, right thigh**

    √7ᵗʰ **S71.112** **Laceration without foreign body, left thigh**

    √7ᵗʰ **S71.119** **Laceration without foreign body, unspecified thigh** ▽

√6ᵗʰ **S71.12** Laceration with foreign body of thigh

    √7ᵗʰ **S71.121** **Laceration with foreign body, right thigh**

    √7ᵗʰ **S71.122** **Laceration with foreign body, left thigh**

    √7ᵗʰ **S71.129** **Laceration with foreign body, unspecified thigh** ▽

√6ᵗʰ **S71.13** Puncture wound without foreign body of thigh
AHA: 2016, 3Q, 24

    √7ᵗʰ **S71.131** **Puncture wound without foreign body, right thigh**

    √7ᵗʰ **S71.132** **Puncture wound without foreign body, left thigh**

    √7ᵗʰ **S71.139** **Puncture wound without foreign body, unspecified thigh** ▽

√6ᵗʰ **S71.14** Puncture wound with foreign body of thigh
AHA: 2016, 3Q, 24

    √7ᵗʰ **S71.141** **Puncture wound with foreign body, right thigh**

    √7ᵗʰ **S71.142** **Puncture wound with foreign body, left thigh**

    √7ᵗʰ **S71.149** **Puncture wound with foreign body, unspecified thigh** ▽

√6ᵗʰ **S71.15** Open bite of thigh
Bite of thigh NOS
    EXCLUDES 1   superficial bite of thigh (S70.37-)

    √7ᵗʰ **S71.151** **Open bite, right thigh**

    √7ᵗʰ **S71.152** **Open bite, left thigh**

    √7ᵗʰ **S71.159** **Open bite, unspecified thigh** ▽

√4ᵗʰ **S72** **Fracture of femur**

NOTE A fracture not indicated as displaced or nondisplaced should be coded to displaced.
The open fracture designations are based on the Gustilo open fracture classification.
A fracture not indicated as open or closed should be coded to closed.

EXCLUDES 1   traumatic amputation of hip and thigh (S78.-)

EXCLUDES 2   fracture of lower leg and ankle (S82.-)
     fracture of foot (S92.-)
     periprosthetic fracture of prosthetic implant of hip ▶(M97.0-)◀

AHA: 2016, 1Q, 33; 2015, 3Q, 37-39; 2015, 1Q, 17; 2013, 4Q, 128

The appropriate 7th character is to be added to all codes from category S72 [unless otherwise indicated].
A   initial encounter for closed fracture
B   initial encounter for open fracture type I or II
     initial encounter for open fracture NOS
C   initial encounter for open fracture type IIIA, IIIB, or IIIC
D   subsequent encounter for closed fracture with routine healing
E   subsequent encounter for open fracture type I or II with routine healing
F   subsequent encounter for open fracture type IIIA, IIIB, or IIIC with routine healing
G   subsequent encounter for closed fracture with delayed healing
H   subsequent encounter for open fracture type I or II with delayed healing
J   subsequent encounter for open fracture type IIIA, IIIB, or IIIC with delayed healing
K   subsequent encounter for closed fracture with nonunion
M   subsequent encounter for open fracture type I or II with nonunion
N   subsequent encounter for open fracture type IIIA, IIIB, or IIIC with nonunion
P   subsequent encounter for closed fracture with malunion
Q   subsequent encounter for open fracture type I or II with malunion
R   subsequent encounter for open fracture type IIIA, IIIB, or IIIC with malunion
S   sequela

√5ᵗʰ **S72.0** **Fracture of head and neck of femur**
    EXCLUDES 2   physeal fracture of upper end of femur (S79.0-)
AHA: 2016, 3Q, 16

√6ᵗʰ **S72.00** **Fracture of unspecified part of neck of femur**
Fracture of hip NOS
Fracture of neck of femur NOS

    ¹ √7ᵗʰ **S72.001** **Fracture of unspecified part of neck of right femur** HCC ▽

    ¹ √7ᵗʰ **S72.002** **Fracture of unspecified part of neck of left femur** HCC ▽

    ¹ √7ᵗʰ **S72.009** **Fracture of unspecified part of neck of unspecified femur** HCC ▽

√6ᵗʰ **S72.01** **Unspecified intracapsular fracture of femur**
Subcapital fracture of femur

    ¹ √7ᵗʰ **S72.011** **Unspecified intracapsular fracture of right femur** HCC ▽

    ¹ √7ᵗʰ **S72.012** **Unspecified intracapsular fracture of left femur** HCC ▽

    ¹ √7ᵗʰ **S72.019** **Unspecified intracapsular fracture of unspecified femur** HCC ▽

√6ᵗʰ **S72.02** **Fracture of epiphysis (separation) (upper) of femur**
Transepiphyseal fracture of femur
    EXCLUDES 1   capital femoral epiphyseal fracture (pediatric) of femur (S79.01-)
         Salter-Harris Type I physeal fracture of upper end of femur (S79.01-)

    ¹ √7ᵗʰ **S72.021** **Displaced fracture of epiphysis (separation) (upper) of right femur** HCC

    ¹ √7ᵗʰ **S72.022** **Displaced fracture of epiphysis (separation) (upper) of left femur** HCC

    ¹ √7ᵗʰ **S72.023** **Displaced fracture of epiphysis (separation) (upper) of unspecified femur** HCC ▽

    ¹ √7ᵗʰ **S72.024** **Nondisplaced fracture of epiphysis (separation) (upper) of right femur** HCC

    ¹ √7ᵗʰ **S72.025** **Nondisplaced fracture of epiphysis (separation) (upper) of left femur** HCC

---

¹ HCC with 7th character indicating initial encounter (A, B or C - specific to category).

1 √7ᵗʰ **S72.026** **Nondisplaced fracture of epiphysis (separation) (upper) of unspecified femur** HCC ▽

√6ᵗʰ **S72.03** **Midcervical fracture of femur**
Transcervical fracture of femur NOS

1 √7ᵗʰ **S72.031** **Displaced midcervical fracture of right femur** HCC

1 √7ᵗʰ **S72.032** **Displaced midcervical fracture of left femur** HCC

1 √7ᵗʰ **S72.033** **Displaced midcervical fracture of unspecified femur** HCC ▽

1 √7ᵗʰ **S72.034** **Nondisplaced midcervical fracture of right femur** HCC

1 √7ᵗʰ **S72.035** **Nondisplaced midcervical fracture of left femur** HCC

1 √7ᵗʰ **S72.036** **Nondisplaced midcervical fracture of unspecified femur** HCC ▽

√6ᵗʰ **S72.04** **Fracture of base of neck of femur**
Cervicotrochanteric fracture of femur

1 √7ᵗʰ **S72.041** **Displaced fracture of base of neck of right femur** HCC

1 √7ᵗʰ **S72.042** **Displaced fracture of base of neck of left femur** HCC

1 √7ᵗʰ **S72.043** **Displaced fracture of base of neck of unspecified femur** HCC ▽

1 √7ᵗʰ **S72.044** **Nondisplaced fracture of base of neck of right femur** HCC

1 √7ᵗʰ **S72.045** **Nondisplaced fracture of base of neck of left femur** HCC

1 √7ᵗʰ **S72.046** **Nondisplaced fracture of base of neck of unspecified femur** HCC ▽

√6ᵗʰ **S72.05** **Unspecified fracture of head of femur**
Fracture of head of femur NOS

1 √7ᵗʰ **S72.051** **Unspecified fracture of head of right femur** HCC ▽

1 √7ᵗʰ **S72.052** **Unspecified fracture of head of left femur** HCC ▽

1 √7ᵗʰ **S72.059** **Unspecified fracture of head of unspecified femur** HCC ▽

√6ᵗʰ **S72.06** **Articular fracture of head of femur**

1 √7ᵗʰ **S72.061** **Displaced articular fracture of head of right femur** HCC

1 √7ᵗʰ **S72.062** **Displaced articular fracture of head of left femur** HCC

1 √7ᵗʰ **S72.063** **Displaced articular fracture of head of unspecified femur** HCC ▽

1 √7ᵗʰ **S72.064** **Nondisplaced articular fracture of head of right femur** HCC

1 √7ᵗʰ **S72.065** **Nondisplaced articular fracture of head of left femur** HCC

1 √7ᵗʰ **S72.066** **Nondisplaced articular fracture of head of unspecified femur** HCC ▽

√6ᵗʰ **S72.09** **Other fracture of head and neck of femur**

1 √7ᵗʰ **S72.091** **Other fracture of head and neck of right femur** HCC

1 √7ᵗʰ **S72.092** **Other fracture of head and neck of left femur** HCC

1 √7ᵗʰ **S72.099** **Other fracture of head and neck of unspecified femur** HCC ▽

√5ᵗʰ **S72.1** **Pertrochanteric fracture**
AHA: 2016, 3Q, 16

√6ᵗʰ **S72.10** **Unspecified trochanteric fracture of femur**
Fracture of trochanter NOS

1 √7ᵗʰ **S72.101** **Unspecified trochanteric fracture of right femur** HCC ▽

1 √7ᵗʰ **S72.102** **Unspecified trochanteric fracture of left femur** HCC ▽

1 √7ᵗʰ **S72.109** **Unspecified trochanteric fracture of unspecified femur** HCC ▽

√6ᵗʰ **S72.11** **Fracture of greater trochanter of femur**

1 √7ᵗʰ **S72.111** **Displaced fracture of greater trochanter of right femur** HCC

1 √7ᵗʰ **S72.112** **Displaced fracture of greater trochanter of left femur** HCC

1 √7ᵗʰ **S72.113** **Displaced fracture of greater trochanter of unspecified femur** HCC ▽

1 √7ᵗʰ **S72.114** **Nondisplaced fracture of greater trochanter of right femur** HCC

1 √7ᵗʰ **S72.115** **Nondisplaced fracture of greater trochanter of left femur** HCC

1 √7ᵗʰ **S72.116** **Nondisplaced fracture of greater trochanter of unspecified femur** HCC ▽

√6ᵗʰ **S72.12** **Fracture of lesser trochanter of femur**

1 √7ᵗʰ **S72.121** **Displaced fracture of lesser trochanter of right femur** HCC

1 √7ᵗʰ **S72.122** **Displaced fracture of lesser trochanter of left femur** HCC

1 √7ᵗʰ **S72.123** **Displaced fracture of lesser trochanter of unspecified femur** HCC ▽

1 √7ᵗʰ **S72.124** **Nondisplaced fracture of lesser trochanter of right femur** HCC

1 √7ᵗʰ **S72.125** **Nondisplaced fracture of lesser trochanter of left femur** HCC

1 √7ᵗʰ **S72.126** **Nondisplaced fracture of lesser trochanter of unspecified femur** HCC ▽

√6ᵗʰ **S72.13** **Apophyseal fracture of femur**
EXCLUDES 1 chronic (nontraumatic) slipped upper femoral epiphysis (M93.0-)

1 √7ᵗʰ **S72.131** **Displaced apophyseal fracture of right femur** HCC

1 √7ᵗʰ **S72.132** **Displaced apophyseal fracture of left femur** HCC

1 √7ᵗʰ **S72.133** **Displaced apophyseal fracture of unspecified femur** HCC ▽

1 √7ᵗʰ **S72.134** **Nondisplaced apophyseal fracture of right femur** HCC

1 √7ᵗʰ **S72.135** **Nondisplaced apophyseal fracture of left femur** HCC

1 √7ᵗʰ **S72.136** **Nondisplaced apophyseal fracture of unspecified femur** HCC ▽

√6ᵗʰ **S72.14** **Intertrochanteric fracture of femur**

1 √7ᵗʰ **S72.141** **Displaced intertrochanteric fracture of right femur** HCC

1 √7ᵗʰ **S72.142** **Displaced intertrochanteric fracture of left femur** HCC

1 √7ᵗʰ **S72.143** **Displaced intertrochanteric fracture of unspecified femur** HCC ▽

1 √7ᵗʰ **S72.144** **Nondisplaced intertrochanteric fracture of right femur** HCC

1 √7ᵗʰ **S72.145** **Nondisplaced intertrochanteric fracture of left femur** HCC

1 √7ᵗʰ **S72.146** **Nondisplaced intertrochanteric fracture of unspecified femur** HCC ▽

√5ᵗʰ **S72.2** **Subtrochanteric fracture of femur**

1 √x7ᵗʰ **S72.21** **Displaced subtrochanteric fracture of right femur** HCC

1 √x7ᵗʰ **S72.22** **Displaced subtrochanteric fracture of left femur** HCC

1 √x7ᵗʰ **S72.23** **Displaced subtrochanteric fracture of unspecified femur** HCC ▽

1 √x7ᵗʰ **S72.24** **Nondisplaced subtrochanteric fracture of right femur** HCC

1 √x7ᵗʰ **S72.25** **Nondisplaced subtrochanteric fracture of left femur** HCC

1 √x7ᵗʰ **S72.26** **Nondisplaced subtrochanteric fracture of unspecified femur** HCC ▽

√5ᵗʰ **S72.3** **Fracture of shaft of femur**

√6ᵗʰ **S72.30** **Unspecified fracture of shaft of femur**

1 √7ᵗʰ **S72.301** **Unspecified fracture of shaft of right femur** HCC ▽

1 √7ᵗʰ **S72.302** **Unspecified fracture of shaft of left femur** HCC ▽

1 √7ᵗʰ **S72.309** **Unspecified fracture of shaft of unspecified femur** HCC ▽

√6ᵗʰ **S72.32** **Transverse fracture of shaft of femur**

1 √7ᵗʰ **S72.321** **Displaced transverse fracture of shaft of right femur** HCC

---

1 HCC with 7th character indicating initial encounter (A, B or C - specific to category).

EXCLUDES 1 Not coded here   *EXCLUDES 2* Not included here   Ⓝ Newborn Age: 0   Ⓟ Pediatric Age: 0-17   Ⓜ Maternity Age: 12-55   Ⓐ Adult Age: 15-124

1004   ICD-10-CM 2018

[1] √7ᵗʰ **S72.322** Displaced **transverse** fracture of shaft of **left** femur   HCC

[1] √7ᵗʰ **S72.323** Displaced **transverse** fracture of shaft of **unspecified** femur   HCC ▽

[1] √7ᵗʰ **S72.324** Nondisplaced **transverse** fracture of shaft of **right** femur   HCC

[1] √7ᵗʰ **S72.325** Nondisplaced **transverse** fracture of shaft of **left** femur   HCC

[1] √7ᵗʰ **S72.326** Nondisplaced **transverse** fracture of shaft of **unspecified** femur   HCC ▽

√6ᵗʰ **S72.33** Oblique **fracture of shaft of femur**

[1] √7ᵗʰ **S72.331** Displaced **oblique** fracture of shaft of **right** femur   HCC

[1] √7ᵗʰ **S72.332** Displaced **oblique** fracture of shaft of **left** femur   HCC

[1] √7ᵗʰ **S72.333** Displaced **oblique** fracture of shaft of **unspecified** femur   HCC ▽

[1] √7ᵗʰ **S72.334** Nondisplaced **oblique** fracture of shaft of **right** femur   HCC

[1] √7ᵗʰ **S72.335** Nondisplaced **oblique** fracture of shaft of **left** femur   HCC

[1] √7ᵗʰ **S72.336** Nondisplaced **oblique** fracture of shaft of **unspecified** femur   HCC ▽

√6ᵗʰ **S72.34** Spiral **fracture of shaft of femur**

[1] √7ᵗʰ **S72.341** Displaced **spiral** fracture of shaft of **right** femur   HCC

[1] √7ᵗʰ **S72.342** Displaced **spiral** fracture of shaft of **left** femur   HCC

[1] √7ᵗʰ **S72.343** Displaced **spiral** fracture of shaft of **unspecified** femur   HCC ▽

[1] √7ᵗʰ **S72.344** Nondisplaced **spiral** fracture of shaft of **right** femur   HCC

[1] √7ᵗʰ **S72.345** Nondisplaced **spiral** fracture of shaft of **left** femur   HCC

[1] √7ᵗʰ **S72.346** Nondisplaced **spiral** fracture of shaft of **unspecified** femur   HCC ▽

√6ᵗʰ **S72.35** Comminuted **fracture of shaft of femur**

[1] √7ᵗʰ **S72.351** Displaced **comminuted** fracture of shaft of **right** femur   HCC

[1] √7ᵗʰ **S72.352** Displaced **comminuted** fracture of shaft of **left** femur   HCC

[1] √7ᵗʰ **S72.353** Displaced **comminuted** fracture of shaft of **unspecified** femur   HCC ▽

[1] √7ᵗʰ **S72.354** Nondisplaced **comminuted** fracture of shaft of **right** femur   HCC

[1] √7ᵗʰ **S72.355** Nondisplaced **comminuted** fracture of shaft of **left** femur   HCC

[1] √7ᵗʰ **S72.356** Nondisplaced **comminuted** fracture of shaft of **unspecified** femur   HCC ▽

√6ᵗʰ **S72.36** Segmental **fracture of shaft of femur**

[1] √7ᵗʰ **S72.361** Displaced **segmental** fracture of shaft of **right** femur   HCC

[1] √7ᵗʰ **S72.362** Displaced **segmental** fracture of shaft of **left** femur   HCC

[1] √7ᵗʰ **S72.363** Displaced **segmental** fracture of shaft of **unspecified** femur   HCC ▽

[1] √7ᵗʰ **S72.364** Nondisplaced **segmental** fracture of shaft of **right** femur   HCC

[1] √7ᵗʰ **S72.365** Nondisplaced **segmental** fracture of shaft of **left** femur   HCC

[1] √7ᵗʰ **S72.366** Nondisplaced **segmental** fracture of shaft of **unspecified** femur   HCC ▽

√6ᵗʰ **S72.39** Other **fracture of shaft of femur**

[1] √7ᵗʰ **S72.391** Other **fracture of shaft of right** femur   HCC

[1] √7ᵗʰ **S72.392** Other **fracture of shaft of left** femur   HCC

[1] √7ᵗʰ **S72.399** Other **fracture of shaft of unspecified** femur   HCC ▽

√5ᵗʰ **S72.4** Fracture of **lower end** of femur
Fracture of distal end of femur
EXCLUDES 2   fracture of shaft of femur (S72.3-)
physeal fracture of lower end of femur (S79.1-)

√6ᵗʰ **S72.40** Unspecified **fracture of lower end of femur**

[1] √7ᵗʰ **S72.401** Unspecified **fracture of lower end of right** femur   HCC ▽

[1] √7ᵗʰ **S72.402** Unspecified **fracture of lower end of left** femur   HCC ▽

[1] √7ᵗʰ **S72.409** Unspecified **fracture of lower end of unspecified** femur   HCC ▽

√6ᵗʰ **S72.41** Unspecified **condyle fracture of lower end of femur**
Condyle fracture of femur NOS

[1] √7ᵗʰ **S72.411** Displaced **unspecified condyle fracture of lower end of right** femur   HCC ▽

[1] √7ᵗʰ **S72.412** Displaced **unspecified condyle fracture of lower end of left** femur   HCC ▽

[1] √7ᵗʰ **S72.413** Displaced **unspecified condyle fracture of lower end of unspecified** femur   HCC ▽

[1] √7ᵗʰ **S72.414** Nondisplaced **unspecified condyle fracture of lower end of right** femur   HCC ▽

[1] √7ᵗʰ **S72.415** Nondisplaced **unspecified condyle fracture of lower end of left** femur   HCC ▽

[1] √7ᵗʰ **S72.416** Nondisplaced **unspecified condyle fracture of lower end of unspecified** femur   HCC ▽

√6ᵗʰ **S72.42** Fracture of **lateral condyle of femur**

[1] √7ᵗʰ **S72.421** Displaced **fracture of lateral condyle of right** femur   HCC

[1] √7ᵗʰ **S72.422** Displaced **fracture of lateral condyle of left** femur   HCC

[1] √7ᵗʰ **S72.423** Displaced **fracture of lateral condyle of unspecified** femur   HCC ▽

[1] √7ᵗʰ **S72.424** Nondisplaced **fracture of lateral condyle of right** femur   HCC

[1] √7ᵗʰ **S72.425** Nondisplaced **fracture of lateral condyle of left** femur   HCC

[1] √7ᵗʰ **S72.426** Nondisplaced **fracture of lateral condyle of unspecified** femur   HCC ▽

√6ᵗʰ **S72.43** Fracture of **medial condyle of femur**

[1] √7ᵗʰ **S72.431** Displaced **fracture of medial condyle of right** femur   HCC

[1] √7ᵗʰ **S72.432** Displaced **fracture of medial condyle of left** femur   HCC

[1] √7ᵗʰ **S72.433** Displaced **fracture of medial condyle of unspecified** femur   HCC ▽

[1] √7ᵗʰ **S72.434** Nondisplaced **fracture of medial condyle of right** femur   HCC

[1] √7ᵗʰ **S72.435** Nondisplaced **fracture of medial condyle of left** femur   HCC

[1] √7ᵗʰ **S72.436** Nondisplaced **fracture of medial condyle of unspecified** femur   HCC ▽

√6ᵗʰ **S72.44** Fracture of **lower epiphysis (separation) of femur**
EXCLUDES 1   Salter-Harris Type I physeal fracture of lower end of femur (S79.11-)

[1] √7ᵗʰ **S72.441** Displaced **fracture of lower epiphysis (separation) of right** femur   HCC

[1] √7ᵗʰ **S72.442** Displaced **fracture of lower epiphysis (separation) of left** femur   HCC

[1] √7ᵗʰ **S72.443** Displaced **fracture of lower epiphysis (separation) of unspecified** femur   HCC ▽

[1] √7ᵗʰ **S72.444** Nondisplaced **fracture of lower epiphysis (separation) of right** femur   HCC

[1] √7ᵗʰ **S72.445** Nondisplaced **fracture of lower epiphysis (separation) of left** femur   HCC

[1] √7ᵗʰ **S72.446** Nondisplaced **fracture of lower epiphysis (separation) of unspecified** femur   HCC ▽

√6ᵗʰ **S72.45** Supracondylar **fracture without intracondylar extension of lower end of femur**
Supracondylar fracture of lower end of femur NOS
EXCLUDES 1   supracondylar fracture with intracondylar extension of lower end of femur (S72.46-)

[1] √7ᵗʰ **S72.451** Displaced **supracondylar fracture without intracondylar extension of lower end of right** femur   HCC

[1] √7ᵗʰ **S72.452** Displaced **supracondylar fracture without intracondylar extension of lower end of left** femur   HCC

---

[1]   HCC with 7th character indicating initial encounter (A, B or C - specific to category).

☑ Additional Character Req   √×7ᵗʰ Placeholder Alert   Manifestation   HCC CMS-HCC Condition   ▽ Unspecified Code   ▶◀ Revised Text   ● New Code   ▲ Revised Code Title

1 √7ᵗʰ **S72.453 Displaced supracondylar fracture without intracondylar extension of lower end of unspecified femur** HCC ▽

1 √7ᵗʰ **S72.454 Nondisplaced supracondylar fracture without intracondylar extension of lower end of right femur** HCC

1 √7ᵗʰ **S72.455 Nondisplaced supracondylar fracture without intracondylar extension of lower end of left femur** HCC

1 √7ᵗʰ **S72.456 Nondisplaced supracondylar fracture without intracondylar extension of lower end of unspecified femur** HCC ▽

√6ᵗʰ **S72.46 Supracondylar fracture with intracondylar extension of lower end of femur**
> EXCLUDES 1 *supracondylar fracture without intracondylar extension of lower end of femur (S72.45-)*

1 √7ᵗʰ **S72.461 Displaced supracondylar fracture with intracondylar extension of lower end of right femur** HCC

1 √7ᵗʰ **S72.462 Displaced supracondylar fracture with intracondylar extension of lower end of left femur** HCC

1 √7ᵗʰ **S72.463 Displaced supracondylar fracture with intracondylar extension of lower end of unspecified femur** HCC ▽

1 √7ᵗʰ **S72.464 Nondisplaced supracondylar fracture with intracondylar extension of lower end of right femur** HCC

1 √7ᵗʰ **S72.465 Nondisplaced supracondylar fracture with intracondylar extension of lower end of left femur** HCC

1 √7ᵗʰ **S72.466 Nondisplaced supracondylar fracture with intracondylar extension of lower end of unspecified femur** HCC ▽

√6ᵗʰ **S72.47 Torus fracture of lower end of femur**

The appropriate 7th character is to be added to all codes in subcategory S72.47.
A   initial encounter for closed fracture
D   subsequent encounter for fracture with routine healing
G   subsequent encounter for fracture with delayed healing
K   subsequent encounter for fracture with nonunion
P   subsequent encounter for fracture with malunion
S   sequela

1 √7ᵗʰ **S72.471 Torus fracture of lower end of right femur** HCC

1 √7ᵗʰ **S72.472 Torus fracture of lower end of left femur** HCC

1 √7ᵗʰ **S72.479 Torus fracture of lower end of unspecified femur** HCC ▽

√6ᵗʰ **S72.49 Other fracture of lower end of femur**

1 √7ᵗʰ **S72.491 Other fracture of lower end of right femur** HCC

1 √7ᵗʰ **S72.492 Other fracture of lower end of left femur** HCC

1 √7ᵗʰ **S72.499 Other fracture of lower end of unspecified femur** HCC ▽

√5ᵗʰ **S72.8 Other fracture of femur**

√6ᵗʰ **S72.8X Other fracture of femur**

1 √7ᵗʰ **S72.8X1 Other fracture of right femur** HCC

1 √7ᵗʰ **S72.8X2 Other fracture of left femur** HCC

1 √7ᵗʰ **S72.8X9 Other fracture of unspecified femur** HCC ▽

√5ᵗʰ **S72.9 Unspecified fracture of femur**
Fracture of thigh NOS
Fracture of upper leg NOS
> EXCLUDES 1 *fracture of hip NOS (S72.00-, S72.01-)*

1 √x7ᵗʰ **S72.90 Unspecified fracture of unspecified femur** HCC ▽
AHA: 2012, 4Q, 93

1 √x7ᵗʰ **S72.91 Unspecified fracture of right femur** HCC ▽

1 √x7ᵗʰ **S72.92 Unspecified fracture of left femur** HCC ▽

√4ᵗʰ **S73 Dislocation and sprain of joint and ligaments of hip**
> INCLUDES avulsion of joint or ligament of hip
> laceration of cartilage, joint or ligament of hip
> sprain of cartilage, joint or ligament of hip
> traumatic hemarthrosis of joint or ligament of hip
> traumatic rupture of joint or ligament of hip
> traumatic subluxation of joint or ligament of hip
> traumatic tear of joint or ligament of hip

Code also any associated open wound
> EXCLUDES 2 *strain of muscle, fascia and tendon of hip and thigh (S76.-)*

The appropriate 7th character is to be added to each code from category S73.
A   initial encounter
D   subsequent encounter
S   sequela

√5ᵗʰ **S73.0 Subluxation and dislocation of hip**
> EXCLUDES 2 *dislocation and subluxation of hip prosthesis (T84.020, T84.021)*

√6ᵗʰ **S73.00 Unspecified subluxation and dislocation of hip**
Dislocation of hip NOS
Subluxation of hip NOS

1 √7ᵗʰ **S73.001 Unspecified subluxation of right hip** HCC ▽

1 √7ᵗʰ **S73.002 Unspecified subluxation of left hip** HCC ▽

1 √7ᵗʰ **S73.003 Unspecified subluxation of unspecified hip** HCC ▽

1 √7ᵗʰ **S73.004 Unspecified dislocation of right hip** HCC ▽

1 √7ᵗʰ **S73.005 Unspecified dislocation of left hip** HCC ▽

1 √7ᵗʰ **S73.006 Unspecified dislocation of unspecified hip** HCC ▽

√6ᵗʰ **S73.01 Posterior subluxation and dislocation of hip**

1 √7ᵗʰ **S73.011 Posterior subluxation of right hip** HCC

1 √7ᵗʰ **S73.012 Posterior subluxation of left hip** HCC

1 √7ᵗʰ **S73.013 Posterior subluxation of unspecified hip** HCC ▽

1 √7ᵗʰ **S73.014 Posterior dislocation of right hip** HCC

1 √7ᵗʰ **S73.015 Posterior dislocation of left hip** HCC

1 √7ᵗʰ **S73.016 Posterior dislocation of unspecified hip** HCC ▽

√6ᵗʰ **S73.02 Obturator subluxation and dislocation of hip**

1 √7ᵗʰ **S73.021 Obturator subluxation of right hip** HCC

1 √7ᵗʰ **S73.022 Obturator subluxation of left hip** HCC

1 √7ᵗʰ **S73.023 Obturator subluxation of unspecified hip** HCC ▽

1 √7ᵗʰ **S73.024 Obturator dislocation of right hip** HCC

1 √7ᵗʰ **S73.025 Obturator dislocation of left hip** HCC

1 √7ᵗʰ **S73.026 Obturator dislocation of unspecified hip** HCC ▽

▲ √6ᵗʰ **S73.03 Other anterior subluxation and dislocation of hip**

1 √7ᵗʰ **S73.031 Other anterior subluxation of right hip** HCC

1 √7ᵗʰ **S73.032 Other anterior subluxation of left hip** HCC

1 √7ᵗʰ **S73.033 Other anterior subluxation of unspecified hip** HCC ▽

1 √7ᵗʰ **S73.034 Other anterior dislocation of right hip** HCC

1 √7ᵗʰ **S73.035 Other anterior dislocation of left hip** HCC

1 √7ᵗʰ **S73.036 Other anterior dislocation of unspecified hip** HCC ▽

▲ √6ᵗʰ **S73.04 Central subluxation and dislocation of hip**

1 √7ᵗʰ **S73.041 Central subluxation of right hip** HCC

1 √7ᵗʰ **S73.042 Central subluxation of left hip** HCC

1 √7ᵗʰ **S73.043 Central subluxation of unspecified hip** HCC

---

1 HCC with 7th character indicating initial encounter (A, B or C - specific to category).

EXCLUDES 1 Not coded here   EXCLUDES 2 Not included here   N Newborn Age: 0   P Pediatric Age: 0-17   M Maternity Age: 12-55   A Adult Age: 15-124

1006   ICD-10-CM 2018

[1] ✓7th **S73.044** Central **dislocation** of **right** hip `HCC`

[1] ✓7th **S73.045** Central **dislocation** of **left** hip `HCC`

[1] ✓7th **S73.046** Central **dislocation** of unspecified hip `HCC` ▽

✓5th **S73.1** **Sprain** of hip
  AHA: 2014, 4Q, 25

✓6th **S73.10** Unspecified sprain of hip

  ✓7th **S73.101** Unspecified sprain of **right** hip ▽

  ✓7th **S73.102** Unspecified sprain of **left** hip ▽

  ✓7th **S73.109** Unspecified sprain of unspecified hip ▽

✓6th **S73.11** **Iliofemoral ligament** sprain of hip

  ✓7th **S73.111** Iliofemoral ligament sprain of **right** hip

  ✓7th **S73.112** Iliofemoral ligament sprain of **left** hip

  ✓7th **S73.119** Iliofemoral ligament sprain of unspecified hip ▽

✓6th **S73.12** **Ischiocapsular** (ligament) sprain of hip

  ✓7th **S73.121** Ischiocapsular ligament sprain of **right** hip

  ✓7th **S73.122** Ischiocapsular ligament sprain of **left** hip

  ✓7th **S73.129** Ischiocapsular ligament sprain of unspecified hip ▽

✓6th **S73.19** Other sprain of hip

  ✓7th **S73.191** Other sprain of **right** hip

  ✓7th **S73.192** Other sprain of **left** hip

  ✓7th **S73.199** Other sprain of unspecified hip ▽

✓4th **S74** **Injury of nerves at hip and thigh level**
  Code also any associated open wound (S71.-)
  EXCLUDES 2 injury of nerves at ankle and foot level (S94.-)
  injury of nerves at lower leg level (S84.-)

  The appropriate 7th character is to be added to each code from category S74.
  A initial encounter
  D subsequent encounter
  S sequela

✓5th **S74.0** Injury of **sciatic nerve** at hip and thigh level

  ✓x7th **S74.00** Injury of sciatic nerve at hip and thigh level, unspecified leg ▽

  ✓x7th **S74.01** Injury of sciatic nerve at hip and thigh level, **right** leg

  ✓x7th **S74.02** Injury of sciatic nerve at hip and thigh level, **left** leg

✓5th **S74.1** Injury of **femoral nerve** at hip and thigh level

  ✓x7th **S74.10** Injury of femoral nerve at hip and thigh level, unspecified leg ▽

  ✓x7th **S74.11** Injury of femoral nerve at hip and thigh level, **right** leg

  ✓x7th **S74.12** Injury of femoral nerve at hip and thigh level, **left** leg

✓5th **S74.2** Injury of **cutaneous sensory nerve** at hip and thigh level

  ✓x7th **S74.20** Injury of cutaneous sensory nerve at hip and thigh level, unspecified leg ▽

  ✓x7th **S74.21** Injury of cutaneous sensory nerve at hip and high level, **right** leg

  ✓x7th **S74.22** Injury of cutaneous sensory nerve at hip and thigh level, **left** leg

✓5th **S74.8** Injury of other nerves at hip and thigh level

  ✓6th **S74.8X** Injury of other nerves at hip and thigh level

  ✓7th **S74.8X1** Injury of other nerves at hip and thigh level, **right** leg

  ✓7th **S74.8X2** Injury of other nerves at hip and thigh level, **left** leg

  ✓7th **S74.8X9** Injury of other nerves at hip and thigh level, unspecified leg ▽

✓5th **S74.9** Injury of unspecified nerve at hip and thigh level

  ✓x7th **S74.90** Injury of unspecified nerve at hip and thigh level, unspecified leg ▽

  ✓x7th **S74.91** Injury of unspecified nerve at hip and thigh level, **right** leg ▽

  ✓x7th **S74.92** Injury of unspecified nerve at hip and thigh level, **left** leg ▽

✓4th **S75** **Injury of blood vessels at hip and thigh level**
  Code also any associated open wound (S71.-)
  EXCLUDES 2 injury of blood vessels at lower leg level (S85.-)
  injury of popliteal artery (S85.0)

  The appropriate 7th character is to be added to each code from category S75.
  A initial encounter
  D subsequent encounter
  S sequela

✓5th **S75.0** **Injury of femoral artery**

  ✓6th **S75.00** Unspecified injury of femoral artery

  ✓7th **S75.001** Unspecified injury of femoral artery, **right** leg ▽

  ✓7th **S75.002** Unspecified injury of femoral artery, **left** leg ▽

  ✓7th **S75.009** Unspecified injury of femoral artery, unspecified leg ▽

  ✓6th **S75.01** **Minor laceration** of femoral artery
    Incomplete transection of femoral artery
    Laceration of femoral artery NOS
    Superficial laceration of femoral artery

  ✓7th **S75.011** Minor laceration of femoral artery, **right** leg

  ✓7th **S75.012** Minor laceration of femoral artery, **left** leg

  ✓7th **S75.019** Minor laceration of femoral artery, unspecified leg ▽

  ✓6th **S75.02** **Major laceration** of femoral artery
    Complete transection of femoral artery
    Traumatic rupture of femoral artery

  ✓7th **S75.021** Major laceration of femoral artery, **right** leg

  ✓7th **S75.022** Major laceration of femoral artery, **left** leg

  ✓7th **S75.029** Major laceration of femoral artery, unspecified leg ▽

  ✓6th **S75.09** Other specified injury of femoral artery

  ✓7th **S75.091** Other specified injury of femoral artery, **right** leg

  ✓7th **S75.092** Other specified injury of femoral artery, **left** leg

  ✓7th **S75.099** Other specified injury of femoral artery, unspecified leg ▽

✓5th **S75.1** Injury of **femoral vein** at hip and thigh level

  ✓6th **S75.10** Unspecified injury of femoral vein at hip and thigh level

  ✓7th **S75.101** Unspecified injury of femoral vein at hip and thigh level, **right** leg ▽

  ✓7th **S75.102** Unspecified injury of femoral vein at hip and thigh level, **left** leg ▽

  ✓7th **S75.109** Unspecified injury of femoral vein at hip and thigh level, unspecified leg ▽

  ✓6th **S75.11** **Minor laceration** of femoral vein at hip and thigh level
    Incomplete transection of femoral vein at hip and thigh level
    Laceration of femoral vein at hip and thigh level NOS
    Superficial laceration of femoral vein at hip and thigh level

  ✓7th **S75.111** Minor laceration of femoral vein at hip and thigh level, **right** leg

  ✓7th **S75.112** Minor laceration of femoral vein at hip and thigh level, **left** leg

  ✓7th **S75.119** Minor laceration of femoral vein at hip and thigh level, unspecified leg ▽

  ✓6th **S75.12** **Major laceration** of femoral vein at hip and thigh level
    Complete transection of femoral vein at hip and thigh level
    Traumatic rupture of femoral vein at hip and thigh level

  ✓7th **S75.121** Major laceration of femoral vein at hip and thigh level, **right** leg

  ✓7th **S75.122** Major laceration of femoral vein at hip and thigh level, **left** leg

  ✓7th **S75.129** Major laceration of femoral vein at hip and thigh level, unspecified leg ▽

---

[1] HCC with 7th character indicating initial encounter (A, B or C - specific to category).

✓ Additional Character Req ✓x7th Placeholder Alert Manifestation `HCC` CMS-HCC Condition ▽ Unspecified Code ▶◀ Revised Text ● New Code ▲ Revised Code Title

ICD-10-CM 2018 **1007**

Chapter 19. Injury, Poisoning, and Certain Other Consequences of External Causes

✓6ᵗʰ **S75.19** **Other specified injury of femoral vein at hip and thigh level**

✓7ᵗʰ **S75.191** **Other specified injury of femoral vein at hip and thigh level, right leg**

✓7ᵗʰ **S75.192** **Other specified injury of femoral vein at hip and thigh level, left leg**

✓7ᵗʰ **S75.199** **Other specified injury of femoral vein at hip and thigh level, unspecified leg** ▽

✓5ᵗʰ **S75.2** **Injury of greater saphenous vein at hip and thigh level**

     EXCLUDES 1   *greater saphenous vein NOS (S85.3)*

✓6ᵗʰ **S75.20** **Unspecified injury of greater saphenous vein at hip and thigh level**

✓7ᵗʰ **S75.201** **Unspecified injury of greater saphenous vein at hip and thigh level, right leg** ▽

✓7ᵗʰ **S75.202** **Unspecified injury of greater saphenous vein at hip and thigh level, left leg** ▽

✓7ᵗʰ **S75.209** **Unspecified injury of greater saphenous vein at hip and thigh level, unspecified leg** ▽

✓6ᵗʰ **S75.21** **Minor laceration of greater saphenous vein at hip and thigh level**

     Incomplete transection of greater saphenous vein at hip and thigh level

     Laceration of greater saphenous vein at hip and thigh level NOS

     Superficial laceration of greater saphenous vein at hip and thigh level

✓7ᵗʰ **S75.211** **Minor laceration of greater saphenous vein at hip and thigh level, right leg**

✓7ᵗʰ **S75.212** **Minor laceration of greater saphenous vein at hip and thigh level, left leg**

✓7ᵗʰ **S75.219** **Minor laceration of greater saphenous vein at hip and thigh level, unspecified leg** ▽

✓6ᵗʰ **S75.22** **Major laceration of greater saphenous vein at hip and thigh level**

     Complete transection of greater saphenous vein at hip and thigh level

     Traumatic rupture of greater saphenous vein at hip and thigh level

✓7ᵗʰ **S75.221** **Major laceration of greater saphenous vein at hip and thigh level, right leg**

✓7ᵗʰ **S75.222** **Major laceration of greater saphenous vein at hip and thigh level, left leg**

✓7ᵗʰ **S75.229** **Major laceration of greater saphenous vein at hip and thigh level, unspecified leg** ▽

✓6ᵗʰ **S75.29** **Other specified injury of greater saphenous vein at hip and thigh level**

✓7ᵗʰ **S75.291** **Other specified injury of greater saphenous vein at hip and thigh level, right leg**

✓7ᵗʰ **S75.292** **Other specified injury of greater saphenous vein at hip and thigh level, left leg**

✓7ᵗʰ **S75.299** **Other specified injury of greater saphenous vein at hip and thigh level, unspecified leg** ▽

✓5ᵗʰ **S75.8** **Injury of other blood vessels at hip and thigh level**

✓6ᵗʰ **S75.80** **Unspecified injury of other blood vessels at hip and thigh level**

✓7ᵗʰ **S75.801** **Unspecified injury of other blood vessels at hip and thigh level, right leg** ▽

✓7ᵗʰ **S75.802** **Unspecified injury of other blood vessels at hip and thigh level, left leg** ▽

✓7ᵗʰ **S75.809** **Unspecified injury of other blood vessels at hip and thigh level, unspecified leg** ▽

✓6ᵗʰ **S75.81** **Laceration of other blood vessels at hip and thigh level**

✓7ᵗʰ **S75.811** **Laceration of other blood vessels at hip and thigh level, right leg**

✓7ᵗʰ **S75.812** **Laceration of other blood vessels at hip and thigh level, left leg**

✓7ᵗʰ **S75.819** **Laceration of other blood vessels at hip and thigh level, unspecified leg** ▽

✓6ᵗʰ **S75.89** **Other specified injury of other blood vessels at hip and thigh level**

✓7ᵗʰ **S75.891** **Other specified injury of other blood vessels at hip and thigh level, right leg**

✓7ᵗʰ **S75.892** **Other specified injury of other blood vessels at hip and thigh level, left leg**

✓7ᵗʰ **S75.899** **Other specified injury of other blood vessels at hip and thigh level, unspecified leg** ▽

✓5ᵗʰ **S75.9** **Injury of unspecified blood vessel at hip and thigh level**

✓6ᵗʰ **S75.90** **Unspecified injury of unspecified blood vessel at hip and thigh level**

✓7ᵗʰ **S75.901** **Unspecified injury of unspecified blood vessel at hip and thigh level, right leg** ▽

✓7ᵗʰ **S75.902** **Unspecified injury of unspecified blood vessel at hip and thigh level, left leg** ▽

✓7ᵗʰ **S75.909** **Unspecified injury of unspecified blood vessel at hip and thigh level, unspecified leg** ▽

✓6ᵗʰ **S75.91** **Laceration of unspecified blood vessel at hip and thigh level**

✓7ᵗʰ **S75.911** **Laceration of unspecified blood vessel at hip and thigh level, right leg** ▽

✓7ᵗʰ **S75.912** **Laceration of unspecified blood vessel at hip and thigh level, left leg** ▽

✓7ᵗʰ **S75.919** **Laceration of unspecified blood vessel at hip and thigh level, unspecified leg** ▽

✓6ᵗʰ **S75.99** **Other specified injury of unspecified blood vessel at hip and thigh level**

✓7ᵗʰ **S75.991** **Other specified injury of unspecified blood vessel at hip and thigh level, right leg** ▽

✓7ᵗʰ **S75.992** **Other specified injury of unspecified blood vessel at hip and thigh level, left leg** ▽

✓7ᵗʰ **S75.999** **Other specified injury of unspecified blood vessel at hip and thigh level, unspecified leg** ▽

✓4ᵗʰ **S76** **Injury of muscle, fascia and tendon at hip and thigh level**

     Code also any associated open wound (S71.-)

     EXCLUDES 2   *injury of muscle, fascia and tendon at lower leg level (S86) sprain of joint and ligament of hip (S73.1)*

     TIP: Refer to the Muscle/Tendon table at the beginning of this chapter.

     The appropriate 7th character is to be added to each code from category S76.

     A   initial encounter

     D   subsequent encounter

     S   sequela

✓5ᵗʰ **S76.0** **Injury of muscle, fascia and tendon of hip**

✓6ᵗʰ **S76.00** **Unspecified injury of muscle, fascia and tendon of hip**

✓7ᵗʰ **S76.001** **Unspecified injury of muscle, fascia and tendon of right hip** ▽

✓7ᵗʰ **S76.002** **Unspecified injury of muscle, fascia and tendon of left hip** ▽

✓7ᵗʰ **S76.009** **Unspecified injury of muscle, fascia and tendon of unspecified hip** ▽

✓6ᵗʰ **S76.01** **Strain of muscle, fascia and tendon of hip**

✓7ᵗʰ **S76.011** **Strain of muscle, fascia and tendon of right hip**

✓7ᵗʰ **S76.012** **Strain of muscle, fascia and tendon of left hip**

✓7ᵗʰ **S76.019** **Strain of muscle, fascia and tendon of unspecified hip** ▽

✓6ᵗʰ **S76.02** **Laceration of muscle, fascia and tendon of hip**

✓7ᵗʰ **S76.021** **Laceration of muscle, fascia and tendon of right hip**

✓7ᵗʰ **S76.022** **Laceration of muscle, fascia and tendon of left hip**

✓7ᵗʰ **S76.029** **Laceration of muscle, fascia and tendon of unspecified hip** ▽

EXCLUDES 1 Not coded here   **EXCLUDES 2** Not included here   N Newborn Age: 0   P Pediatric Age: 0-17   M Maternity Age: 12-55   A Adult Age: 15-124

1008   ICD-10-CM 2018

√6ᵗʰ **S76.09** **Other specified injury of muscle, fascia and tendon of hip**

√7ᵗʰ **S76.091** Other specified injury of muscle, fascia and tendon of right hip

√7ᵗʰ **S76.092** Other specified injury of muscle, fascia and tendon of left hip

√7ᵗʰ **S76.099** Other specified injury of muscle, fascia and tendon of unspecified hip ▽

√5ᵗʰ **S76.1** **Injury of quadriceps muscle, fascia and tendon**
Injury of patellar ligament (tendon)

√6ᵗʰ **S76.10** **Unspecified injury of quadriceps muscle, fascia and tendon**

√7ᵗʰ **S76.101** Unspecified injury of right quadriceps muscle, fascia and tendon ▽

√7ᵗʰ **S76.102** Unspecified injury of left quadriceps muscle, fascia and tendon ▽

√7ᵗʰ **S76.109** Unspecified injury of unspecified quadriceps muscle, fascia and tendon ▽

√6ᵗʰ **S76.11** **Strain of quadriceps muscle, fascia and tendon**

√7ᵗʰ **S76.111** Strain of right quadriceps muscle, fascia and tendon

√7ᵗʰ **S76.112** Strain of left quadriceps muscle, fascia and tendon

√7ᵗʰ **S76.119** Strain of unspecified quadriceps muscle, fascia and tendon ▽

√6ᵗʰ **S76.12** **Laceration of quadriceps muscle, fascia and tendon**

√7ᵗʰ **S76.121** Laceration of right quadriceps muscle, fascia and tendon

√7ᵗʰ **S76.122** Laceration of left quadriceps muscle, fascia and tendon

√7ᵗʰ **S76.129** Laceration of unspecified quadriceps muscle, fascia and tendon ▽

√6ᵗʰ **S76.19** **Other specified injury of quadriceps muscle, fascia and tendon**

√7ᵗʰ **S76.191** Other specified injury of right quadriceps muscle, fascia and tendon

√7ᵗʰ **S76.192** Other specified injury of left quadriceps muscle, fascia and tendon

√7ᵗʰ **S76.199** Other specified injury of unspecified quadriceps muscle, fascia and tendon ▽

√5ᵗʰ **S76.2** **Injury of adductor muscle, fascia and tendon of thigh**

√6ᵗʰ **S76.20** **Unspecified injury of adductor muscle, fascia and tendon of thigh**

√7ᵗʰ **S76.201** Unspecified injury of adductor muscle, fascia and tendon of right thigh ▽

√7ᵗʰ **S76.202** Unspecified injury of adductor muscle, fascia and tendon of left thigh ▽

√7ᵗʰ **S76.209** Unspecified injury of adductor muscle, fascia and tendon of unspecified thigh ▽

√6ᵗʰ **S76.21** **Strain of adductor muscle, fascia and tendon of thigh**

√7ᵗʰ **S76.211** Strain of adductor muscle, fascia and tendon of right thigh

√7ᵗʰ **S76.212** Strain of adductor muscle, fascia and tendon of left thigh

√7ᵗʰ **S76.219** Strain of adductor muscle, fascia and tendon of unspecified thigh ▽

√6ᵗʰ **S76.22** **Laceration of adductor muscle, fascia and tendon of thigh**

√7ᵗʰ **S76.221** Laceration of adductor muscle, fascia and tendon of right thigh

√7ᵗʰ **S76.222** Laceration of adductor muscle, fascia and tendon of left thigh

√7ᵗʰ **S76.229** Laceration of adductor muscle, fascia and tendon of unspecified thigh ▽

√6ᵗʰ **S76.29** **Other injury of adductor muscle, fascia and tendon of thigh**

√7ᵗʰ **S76.291** Other injury of adductor muscle, fascia and tendon of right thigh

√7ᵗʰ **S76.292** Other injury of adductor muscle, fascia and tendon of left thigh

√7ᵗʰ **S76.299** Other injury of adductor muscle, fascia and tendon of unspecified thigh ▽

√5ᵗʰ **S76.3** **Injury of muscle, fascia and tendon of the posterior muscle group at thigh level**

√6ᵗʰ **S76.30** **Unspecified injury of muscle, fascia and tendon of the posterior muscle group at thigh level**

√7ᵗʰ **S76.301** Unspecified injury of muscle, fascia and tendon of the posterior muscle group at thigh level, right thigh ▽

√7ᵗʰ **S76.302** Unspecified injury of muscle, fascia and tendon of the posterior muscle group at thigh level, left thigh ▽

√7ᵗʰ **S76.309** Unspecified injury of muscle, fascia and tendon of the posterior muscle group at thigh level, unspecified thigh ▽

√6ᵗʰ **S76.31** **Strain of muscle, fascia and tendon of the posterior muscle group at thigh level**

√7ᵗʰ **S76.311** Strain of muscle, fascia and tendon of the posterior muscle group at thigh level, right thigh

√7ᵗʰ **S76.312** Strain of muscle, fascia and tendon of the posterior muscle group at thigh level, left thigh

√7ᵗʰ **S76.319** Strain of muscle, fascia and tendon of the posterior muscle group at thigh level, unspecified thigh ▽

√6ᵗʰ **S76.32** **Laceration of muscle, fascia and tendon of the posterior muscle group at thigh level**

√7ᵗʰ **S76.321** Laceration of muscle, fascia and tendon of the posterior muscle group at thigh level, right thigh

√7ᵗʰ **S76.322** Laceration of muscle, fascia and tendon of the posterior muscle group at thigh level, left thigh

√7ᵗʰ **S76.329** Laceration of muscle, fascia and tendon of the posterior muscle group at thigh level, unspecified thigh ▽

√6ᵗʰ **S76.39** **Other specified injury of muscle, fascia and tendon of the posterior muscle group at thigh level**

√7ᵗʰ **S76.391** Other specified injury of muscle, fascia and tendon of the posterior muscle group at thigh level, right thigh

√7ᵗʰ **S76.392** Other specified injury of muscle, fascia and tendon of the posterior muscle group at thigh level, left thigh

√7ᵗʰ **S76.399** Other specified injury of muscle, fascia and tendon of the posterior muscle group at thigh level, unspecified thigh ▽

√5ᵗʰ **S76.8** **Injury of other specified muscles, fascia and tendons at thigh level**

√6ᵗʰ **S76.80** **Unspecified injury of other specified muscles, fascia and tendons at thigh level**

√7ᵗʰ **S76.801** Unspecified injury of other specified muscles, fascia and tendons at thigh level, right thigh ▽

√7ᵗʰ **S76.802** Unspecified injury of other specified muscles, fascia and tendons at thigh level, left thigh ▽

√7ᵗʰ **S76.809** Unspecified injury of other specified muscles, fascia and tendons at thigh level, unspecified thigh ▽

√6ᵗʰ **S76.81** **Strain of other specified muscles, fascia and tendons at thigh level**

√7ᵗʰ **S76.811** Strain of other specified muscles, fascia and tendons at thigh level, right thigh

√7ᵗʰ **S76.812** Strain of other specified muscles, fascia and tendons at thigh level, left thigh

√7ᵗʰ **S76.819** Strain of other specified muscles, fascia and tendons at thigh level, unspecified thigh ▽

√6ᵗʰ **S76.82** **Laceration of other specified muscles, fascia and tendons at thigh level**

√7ᵗʰ **S76.821** Laceration of other specified muscles, fascia and tendons at thigh level, right thigh

√7ᵗʰ **S76.822** Laceration of other specified muscles, fascia and tendons at thigh level, left thigh

☑ Additional Character Req   √x7ᵗʰ Placeholder Alert   Manifestation   HCC CMS-HCC Condition   ▽ Unspecified Code   ►◄ Revised Text   ● New Code   ▲ Revised Code Title

ICD-10-CM 2018   **1009**

√7th **S76.829** Laceration of other specified muscles, fascia and tendons at thigh level, unspecified thigh ▽

√6th **S76.89** Other injury of other specified muscles, fascia and tendons at thigh level

√7th **S76.891** Other injury of other specified muscles, fascia and tendons at thigh level, right thigh

√7th **S76.892** Other injury of other specified muscles, fascia and tendons at thigh level, left thigh

√7th **S76.899** Other injury of other specified muscles, fascia and tendons at thigh level, unspecified thigh ▽

√5th **S76.9** Injury of unspecified muscles, fascia and tendons at thigh level

√6th **S76.90** Unspecified injury of unspecified muscles, fascia and tendons at thigh level

√7th **S76.901** Unspecified injury of unspecified muscles, fascia and tendons at thigh level, right thigh ▽

√7th **S76.902** Unspecified injury of unspecified muscles, fascia and tendons at thigh level, left thigh ▽

√7th **S76.909** Unspecified injury of unspecified muscles, fascia and tendons at thigh level, unspecified thigh ▽

√6th **S76.91** Strain of unspecified muscles, fascia and tendons at thigh level

√7th **S76.911** Strain of unspecified muscles, fascia and tendons at thigh level, right thigh ▽

√7th **S76.912** Strain of unspecified muscles, fascia and tendons at thigh level, left thigh ▽

√7th **S76.919** Strain of unspecified muscles, fascia and tendons at thigh level, unspecified thigh ▽

√6th **S76.92** Laceration of unspecified muscles, fascia and tendons at thigh level

√7th **S76.921** Laceration of unspecified muscles, fascia and tendons at thigh level, right thigh ▽

√7th **S76.922** Laceration of unspecified muscles, fascia and tendons at thigh level, left thigh ▽

√7th **S76.929** Laceration of unspecified muscles, fascia and tendons at thigh level, unspecified thigh ▽

√6th **S76.99** Other specified injury of unspecified muscles, fascia and tendons at thigh level

√7th **S76.991** Other specified injury of unspecified muscles, fascia and tendons at thigh level, right thigh ▽

√7th **S76.992** Other specified injury of unspecified muscles, fascia and tendons at thigh level, left thigh ▽

√7th **S76.999** Other specified injury of unspecified muscles, fascia and tendons at thigh level, unspecified thigh ▽

√4th **S77** Crushing injury of hip and thigh
Use additional code(s) for all associated injuries
EXCLUDES 2 crushing injury of ankle and foot (S97.-)
crushing injury of lower leg (S87.-)

The appropriate 7th character is to be added to each code from category S77.
A initial encounter
D subsequent encounter
S sequela

√5th **S77.0** Crushing injury of hip
√x7th **S77.00** Crushing injury of unspecified hip ▽
√x7th **S77.01** Crushing injury of right hip
√x7th **S77.02** Crushing injury of left hip

√5th **S77.1** Crushing injury of thigh
√x7th **S77.10** Crushing injury of unspecified thigh ▽
√x7th **S77.11** Crushing injury of right thigh
√x7th **S77.12** Crushing injury of left thigh

√5th **S77.2** Crushing injury of hip with thigh
√x7th **S77.20** Crushing injury of unspecified hip with thigh ▽
√x7th **S77.21** Crushing injury of right hip with thigh
√x7th **S77.22** Crushing injury of left hip with thigh

√4th **S78** Traumatic amputation of hip and thigh
An amputation not identified as partial or complete should be coded to complete.
EXCLUDES 1 traumatic amputation of knee (S88.0-)

The appropriate 7th character is to be added to each code from category S78.
A initial encounter
D subsequent encounter
S sequela

√5th **S78.0** Traumatic amputation at hip joint
√6th **S78.01** Complete traumatic amputation at hip joint
√7th **S78.011** Complete traumatic amputation at right hip joint HCC
√7th **S78.012** Complete traumatic amputation at left hip joint HCC
√7th **S78.019** Complete traumatic amputation at unspecified hip joint HCC ▽

√6th **S78.02** Partial traumatic amputation at hip joint
√7th **S78.021** Partial traumatic amputation at right hip joint HCC
√7th **S78.022** Partial traumatic amputation at left hip joint HCC
√7th **S78.029** Partial traumatic amputation at unspecified hip joint HCC ▽

√5th **S78.1** Traumatic amputation at level between hip and knee
EXCLUDES 1 traumatic amputation of knee (S88.0-)

√6th **S78.11** Complete traumatic amputation at level between hip and knee
√7th **S78.111** Complete traumatic amputation at level between right hip and knee HCC
√7th **S78.112** Complete traumatic amputation at level between left hip and knee HCC
√7th **S78.119** Complete traumatic amputation at level between unspecified hip and knee HCC ▽

√6th **S78.12** Partial traumatic amputation at level between hip and knee
√7th **S78.121** Partial traumatic amputation at level between right hip and knee HCC
√7th **S78.122** Partial traumatic amputation at level between left hip and knee HCC
√7th **S78.129** Partial traumatic amputation at level between unspecified hip and knee HCC

√5th **S78.9** Traumatic amputation of hip and thigh, level unspecified
√6th **S78.91** Complete traumatic amputation of hip and thigh, level unspecified
√7th **S78.911** Complete traumatic amputation of right hip and thigh, level unspecified HCC ▽
√7th **S78.912** Complete traumatic amputation of left hip and thigh, level unspecified HCC ▽
√7th **S78.919** Complete traumatic amputation of unspecified hip and thigh, level unspecified HCC ▽

√6th **S78.92** Partial traumatic amputation of hip and thigh, level unspecified
√7th **S78.921** Partial traumatic amputation of right hip and thigh, level unspecified HCC ▽
√7th **S78.922** Partial traumatic amputation of left hip and thigh, level unspecified HCC ▽
√7th **S78.929** Partial traumatic amputation of unspecified hip and thigh, level unspecified HCC ▽

EXCLUDES 1 Not coded here   EXCLUDES 2 Not included here   N Newborn Age: 0   P Pediatric Age: 0-17   M Maternity Age: 12-55   A Adult Age: 15-124

1010   ICD-10-CM 2018

✓4ᵗʰ **S79** **Other and unspecified injuries of hip and thigh**

> **NOTE**   A fracture not indicated as open or closed should be coded to closed.

AHA: 2015, 3Q, 37-39

> The appropriate 7th character is to be added to each code from subcategory S79.0 and S79.1.
> A   initial encounter for closed fracture
> D   subsequent encounter for fracture with routine healing
> G   subsequent encounter for fracture with delayed healing
> K   subsequent encounter for fracture with nonunion
> P   subsequent encounter for fracture with malunion
> S   sequela

✓5ᵗʰ   **S79.0**   **Physeal fracture of upper end of femur**

> **EXCLUDES 1**   apophyseal fracture of upper end of femur (S72.13-)
> nontraumatic slipped upper femoral epiphysis (M93.0-)

   ✓6ᵗʰ   **S79.00**   **Unspecified physeal fracture of upper end of femur**

     1   ✓7ᵗʰ   **S79.001**   Unspecified physeal fracture of upper end of **right** femur   HCC ▽

     1   ✓7ᵗʰ   **S79.002**   Unspecified physeal fracture of upper end of **left** femur   HCC ▽

     1   ✓7ᵗʰ   **S79.009**   Unspecified physeal fracture of upper end of unspecified femur   HCC ▽

   ✓6ᵗʰ   **S79.01**   **Salter-Harris Type I physeal fracture of upper end of femur**

> Acute on chronic slipped capital femoral epiphysis (traumatic)
> Acute slipped capital femoral epiphysis (traumatic)
> Capital femoral epiphyseal fracture
> **EXCLUDES 1**   chronic slipped upper femoral epiphysis (nontraumatic) (M93.02-)

     1   ✓7ᵗʰ   **S79.011**   Salter-Harris Type I physeal fracture of upper end of **right** femur   HCC

     1   ✓7ᵗʰ   **S79.012**   Salter-Harris Type I physeal fracture of upper end of **left** femur   HCC

     1   ✓7ᵗʰ   **S79.019**   Salter-Harris Type I physeal fracture of upper end of unspecified femur   HCC ▽

   ✓6ᵗʰ   **S79.09**   **Other physeal fracture of upper end of femur**

     1   ✓7ᵗʰ   **S79.091**   Other physeal fracture of upper end of **right** femur   HCC

     1   ✓7ᵗʰ   **S79.092**   Other physeal fracture of upper end of **left** femur   HCC

     1   ✓7ᵗʰ   **S79.099**   Other physeal fracture of upper end of unspecified femur   HCC ▽

✓5ᵗʰ   **S79.1**   **Physeal fracture of lower end of femur**

   ✓6ᵗʰ   **S79.10**   **Unspecified physeal fracture of lower end of femur**

     1   ✓7ᵗʰ   **S79.101**   Unspecified physeal fracture of lower end of **right** femur   HCC ▽

     1   ✓7ᵗʰ   **S79.102**   Unspecified physeal fracture of lower end of **left** femur   HCC ▽

     1   ✓7ᵗʰ   **S79.109**   Unspecified physeal fracture of lower end of unspecified femur   HCC ▽

   ✓6ᵗʰ   **S79.11**   **Salter-Harris Type I physeal fracture of lower end of femur**

     1   ✓7ᵗʰ   **S79.111**   Salter-Harris Type I physeal fracture of lower end of **right** femur   HCC

     1   ✓7ᵗʰ   **S79.112**   Salter-Harris Type I physeal fracture of lower end of **left** femur   HCC

     1   ✓7ᵗʰ   **S79.119**   Salter-Harris Type I physeal fracture of lower end of unspecified femur   HCC ▽

   ✓6ᵗʰ   **S79.12**   **Salter-Harris Type II physeal fracture of lower end of femur**

     1   ✓7ᵗʰ   **S79.121**   Salter-Harris Type II physeal fracture of lower end of **right** femur   HCC

     1   ✓7ᵗʰ   **S79.122**   Salter-Harris Type II physeal fracture of lower end of **left** femur   HCC

     1   ✓7ᵗʰ   **S79.129**   Salter-Harris Type II physeal fracture of lower end of unspecified femur   HCC ▽

   ✓6ᵗʰ   **S79.13**   **Salter-Harris Type III physeal fracture of lower end of femur**

     1   ✓7ᵗʰ   **S79.131**   Salter-Harris Type III physeal fracture of lower end of **right** femur   HCC

     1   ✓7ᵗʰ   **S79.132**   Salter-Harris Type III physeal fracture of lower end of **left** femur   HCC

     1   ✓7ᵗʰ   **S79.139**   Salter-Harris Type III physeal fracture of lower end of unspecified femur   HCC ▽

   ✓6ᵗʰ   **S79.14**   **Salter-Harris Type IV physeal fracture of lower end of femur**

     1   ✓7ᵗʰ   **S79.141**   Salter-Harris Type IV physeal fracture of lower end of **right** femur   HCC

     1   ✓7ᵗʰ   **S79.142**   Salter-Harris Type IV physeal fracture of lower end of **left** femur   HCC

     1   ✓7ᵗʰ   **S79.149**   Salter-Harris Type IV physeal fracture of lower end of unspecified femur   HCC ▽

   ✓6ᵗʰ   **S79.19**   **Other physeal fracture of lower end of femur**

     1   ✓7ᵗʰ   **S79.191**   Other physeal fracture of lower end of **right** femur   HCC

     1   ✓7ᵗʰ   **S79.192**   Other physeal fracture of lower end of **left** femur   HCC

     1   ✓7ᵗʰ   **S79.199**   Other physeal fracture of lower end of unspecified femur   HCC ▽

✓5ᵗʰ   **S79.8**   **Other specified injuries of hip and thigh**

> The appropriate 7th character is to be added to each code in subcategory S79.8.
> A   initial encounter
> D   subsequent encounter
> S   sequela

   ✓6ᵗʰ   **S79.81**   **Other specified injuries of hip**

     ✓7ᵗʰ   **S79.811**   Other specified injuries of **right** hip

     ✓7ᵗʰ   **S79.812**   Other specified injuries of **left** hip

     ✓7ᵗʰ   **S79.819**   Other specified injuries of unspecified hip   ▽

   ✓6ᵗʰ   **S79.82**   **Other specified injuries of thigh**

     ✓7ᵗʰ   **S79.821**   Other specified injuries of **right** thigh

     ✓7ᵗʰ   **S79.822**   Other specified injuries of **left** thigh

     ✓7ᵗʰ   **S79.829**   Other specified injuries of unspecified thigh   ▽

✓5ᵗʰ   **S79.9**   **Unspecified injury of hip and thigh**

> The appropriate 7th character is to be added to each code in subcategory S79.9.
> A   initial encounter
> D   subsequent encounter
> S   sequela

   ✓6ᵗʰ   **S79.91**   **Unspecified injury of hip**

     ✓7ᵗʰ   **S79.911**   Unspecified injury of **right** hip   ▽

     ✓7ᵗʰ   **S79.912**   Unspecified injury of **left** hip   ▽

     ✓7ᵗʰ   **S79.919**   Unspecified injury of unspecified hip   ▽

   ✓6ᵗʰ   **S79.92**   **Unspecified injury of thigh**

     ✓7ᵗʰ   **S79.921**   Unspecified injury of **right** thigh   ▽

     ✓7ᵗʰ   **S79.922**   Unspecified injury of **left** thigh   ▽

     ✓7ᵗʰ   **S79.929**   Unspecified injury of unspecified thigh   ▽

---

1   HCC with 7th character indicating initial encounter (A, B or C - specific to category).

✓ Additional Character Req   ✓x7ᵗʰ Placeholder Alert   Manifestation   HCC CMS-HCC Condition   ▽ Unspecified Code   ▶◀ Revised Text   ● New Code   ▲ Revised Code Title

ICD-10-CM 2018   1011

Injuries to the knee and lower leg (S80-S89)

EXCLUDES 2 burns and corrosions (T20-T32)
frostbite (T33-T34)
injuries of ankle and foot, except fracture of ankle and malleolus (S90-S99)
insect bite or sting, venomous (T63.4)

✓4th **S80 Superficial injury of knee and lower leg**

EXCLUDES 2 superficial injury of ankle and foot (S90.-)

The appropriate 7th character is to be added to each code from category S80.
A   initial encounter
D   subsequent encounter
S   sequela

✓5th **S80.0 Contusion of knee**
✓x7th **S80.00 Contusion of unspecified knee** ▽
✓x7th **S80.01 Contusion of right knee**
✓x7th **S80.02 Contusion of left knee**

✓5th **S80.1 Contusion of lower leg**
✓x7th **S80.10 Contusion of unspecified lower leg** ▽
✓x7th **S80.11 Contusion of right lower leg**
✓x7th **S80.12 Contusion of left lower leg**

✓5th **S80.2 Other superficial injuries of knee**
✓6th **S80.21 Abrasion of knee**
✓7th **S80.211 Abrasion, right knee**
✓7th **S80.212 Abrasion, left knee**
✓7th **S80.219 Abrasion, unspecified knee** ▽
✓6th **S80.22 Blister (nonthermal) of knee**
✓7th **S80.221 Blister (nonthermal), right knee**
✓7th **S80.222 Blister (nonthermal), left knee**
✓7th **S80.229 Blister (nonthermal), unspecified knee** ▽
✓6th **S80.24 External constriction of knee**
✓7th **S80.241 External constriction, right knee**
✓7th **S80.242 External constriction, left knee**
✓7th **S80.249 External constriction, unspecified knee** ▽
✓6th **S80.25 Superficial foreign body of knee**
Splinter in the knee
✓7th **S80.251 Superficial foreign body, right knee**
✓7th **S80.252 Superficial foreign body, left knee**
✓7th **S80.259 Superficial foreign body, unspecified knee** ▽
✓6th **S80.26 Insect bite (nonvenomous) of knee**
✓7th **S80.261 Insect bite (nonvenomous), right knee**
✓7th **S80.262 Insect bite (nonvenomous), left knee**
✓7th **S80.269 Insect bite (nonvenomous), unspecified knee** ▽
✓6th **S80.27 Other superficial bite of knee**
EXCLUDES 1 open bite of knee (S81.05-)
✓7th **S80.271 Other superficial bite of right knee**
✓7th **S80.272 Other superficial bite of left knee**
✓7th **S80.279 Other superficial bite of unspecified knee** ▽

✓5th **S80.8 Other superficial injuries of lower leg**
✓6th **S80.81 Abrasion of lower leg**
✓7th **S80.811 Abrasion, right lower leg**
✓7th **S80.812 Abrasion, left lower leg**
✓7th **S80.819 Abrasion, unspecified lower leg** ▽
✓6th **S80.82 Blister (nonthermal) of lower leg**
✓7th **S80.821 Blister (nonthermal), right lower leg**
✓7th **S80.822 Blister (nonthermal), left lower leg**
✓7th **S80.829 Blister (nonthermal), unspecified lower leg** ▽
✓6th **S80.84 External constriction of lower leg**
✓7th **S80.841 External constriction, right lower leg**
✓7th **S80.842 External constriction, left lower leg**
✓7th **S80.849 External constriction, unspecified lower leg** ▽

✓6th **S80.85 Superficial foreign body of lower leg**
Splinter in the lower leg
✓7th **S80.851 Superficial foreign body, right lower leg**
✓7th **S80.852 Superficial foreign body, left lower leg**
✓7th **S80.859 Superficial foreign body, unspecified lower leg** ▽
✓6th **S80.86 Insect bite (nonvenomous) of lower leg**
✓7th **S80.861 Insect bite (nonvenomous), right lower leg**
✓7th **S80.862 Insect bite (nonvenomous), left lower leg**
✓7th **S80.869 Insect bite (nonvenomous), unspecified lower leg** ▽
✓6th **S80.87 Other superficial bite of lower leg**
EXCLUDES 1 open bite of lower leg (S81.85-)
✓7th **S80.871 Other superficial bite, right lower leg**
✓7th **S80.872 Other superficial bite, left lower leg**
✓7th **S80.879 Other superficial bite, unspecified lower leg** ▽

✓5th **S80.9 Unspecified superficial injury of knee and lower leg**
✓6th **S80.91 Unspecified superficial injury of knee**
✓7th **S80.911 Unspecified superficial injury of right knee** ▽
✓7th **S80.912 Unspecified superficial injury of left knee** ▽
✓7th **S80.919 Unspecified superficial injury of unspecified knee** ▽
✓6th **S80.92 Unspecified superficial injury of lower leg**
✓7th **S80.921 Unspecified superficial injury of right lower leg** ▽
✓7th **S80.922 Unspecified superficial injury of left lower leg** ▽
✓7th **S80.929 Unspecified superficial injury of unspecified lower leg** ▽

✓4th **S81 Open wound of knee and lower leg**
Code also any associated wound infection
EXCLUDES 1 open fracture of knee and lower leg (S82.-)
traumatic amputation of lower leg (S88.-)
EXCLUDES 2 open wound of ankle and foot (S91.-)

The appropriate 7th character is to be added to each code from category S81.
A   initial encounter
D   subsequent encounter
S   sequela

✓5th **S81.0 Open wound of knee**
✓6th **S81.00 Unspecified open wound of knee**
✓7th **S81.001 Unspecified open wound, right knee** ▽
✓7th **S81.002 Unspecified open wound, left knee** ▽
✓7th **S81.009 Unspecified open wound, unspecified knee** ▽
✓6th **S81.01 Laceration without foreign body of knee**
✓7th **S81.011 Laceration without foreign body, right knee**
✓7th **S81.012 Laceration without foreign body, left knee**
✓7th **S81.019 Laceration without foreign body, unspecified knee** ▽
✓6th **S81.02 Laceration with foreign body of knee**
✓7th **S81.021 Laceration with foreign body, right knee**
✓7th **S81.022 Laceration with foreign body, left knee**
✓7th **S81.029 Laceration with foreign body, unspecified knee** ▽
✓6th **S81.03 Puncture wound without foreign body of knee**
✓7th **S81.031 Puncture wound without foreign body, right knee**
✓7th **S81.032 Puncture wound without foreign body, left knee**
✓7th **S81.039 Puncture wound without foreign body, unspecified knee** ▽

☑6ᵗʰ **S81.04** Puncture wound with foreign body of knee

    ☑7ᵗʰ **S81.041** Puncture wound with foreign body, right knee

    ☑7ᵗʰ **S81.042** Puncture wound with foreign body, left knee

    ☑7ᵗʰ **S81.049** Puncture wound with foreign body, unspecified knee   ▽

☑6ᵗʰ **S81.05** Open bite of knee
    Bite of knee NOS
      EXCLUDES 1   superficial bite of knee (S80.27-)

    ☑7ᵗʰ **S81.051** Open bite, right knee

    ☑7ᵗʰ **S81.052** Open bite, left knee

    ☑7ᵗʰ **S81.059** Open bite, unspecified knee   ▽

☑5ᵗʰ **S81.8** Open wound of lower leg

   ☑6ᵗʰ **S81.80** Unspecified open wound of lower leg
      AHA: 2016, 3Q, 24

    ☑7ᵗʰ **S81.801** Unspecified open wound, right lower leg   ▽

    ☑7ᵗʰ **S81.802** Unspecified open wound, left lower leg   ▽

    ☑7ᵗʰ **S81.809** Unspecified open wound, unspecified lower leg   ▽

   ☑6ᵗʰ **S81.81** Laceration without foreign body of lower leg

    ☑7ᵗʰ **S81.811** Laceration without foreign body, right lower leg

    ☑7ᵗʰ **S81.812** Laceration without foreign body, left lower leg

    ☑7ᵗʰ **S81.819** Laceration without foreign body, unspecified lower leg   ▽

   ☑6ᵗʰ **S81.82** Laceration with foreign body of lower leg

    ☑7ᵗʰ **S81.821** Laceration with foreign body, right lower leg

    ☑7ᵗʰ **S81.822** Laceration with foreign body, left lower leg

    ☑7ᵗʰ **S81.829** Laceration with foreign body, unspecified lower leg   ▽

   ☑6ᵗʰ **S81.83** Puncture wound without foreign body of lower leg
      AHA: 2016, 3Q, 24

    ☑7ᵗʰ **S81.831** Puncture wound without foreign body, right lower leg

    ☑7ᵗʰ **S81.832** Puncture wound without foreign body, left lower leg

    ☑7ᵗʰ **S81.839** Puncture wound without foreign body, unspecified lower leg   ▽

   ☑6ᵗʰ **S81.84** Puncture wound with foreign body of lower leg
      AHA: 2016, 3Q, 24

    ☑7ᵗʰ **S81.841** Puncture wound with foreign body, right lower leg

    ☑7ᵗʰ **S81.842** Puncture wound with foreign body, left lower leg

    ☑7ᵗʰ **S81.849** Puncture wound with foreign body, unspecified lower leg   ▽

☑6ᵗʰ **S81.85** Open bite of lower leg
    Bite of lower leg NOS
      EXCLUDES 1   superficial bite of lower leg (S80.86-, S80.87-)

    ☑7ᵗʰ **S81.851** Open bite, right lower leg

    ☑7ᵗʰ **S81.852** Open bite, left lower leg

    ☑7ᵗʰ **S81.859** Open bite, unspecified lower leg   ▽

☑4ᵗʰ **S82** Fracture of lower leg, including ankle

    NOTE   A fracture not indicated as displaced or nondisplaced should be coded to displaced.
      A fracture not designated as open or closed should be coded to closed.
      The open fracture designations are based on the Gustilo open fracture classification.

    INCLUDES   fracture of malleolus

    EXCLUDES 1   traumatic amputation of lower leg (S88.-)

    EXCLUDES 2   fracture of foot, except ankle (S92.-)
      periprosthetic fracture of prosthetic implant of knee ▶(M97.0-)◀

   AHA: 2016, 1Q, 33; 2015, 3Q, 37-39

The appropriate 7th character is to be added to all codes from category S82 [unless otherwise indicated].

A   initial encounter for closed fracture
B   initial encounter for open fracture type I or II
    initial encounter for open fracture NOS
C   initial encounter for open fracture type IIIA, IIIB, or IIIC
D   subsequent encounter for closed fracture with routine healing
E   subsequent encounter for open fracture type I or II with routine healing
F   subsequent encounter for open fracture type IIIA, IIIB, or IIIC with routine healing
G   subsequent encounter for closed fracture with delayed healing
H   subsequent encounter for open fracture type I or II with delayed healing
J   subsequent encounter for open fracture type IIIA, IIIB or IIIC with delayed healing
K   subsequent encounter for closed fracture with nonunion
M   subsequent encounter for open fracture type I or II with nonunion
N   subsequent encounter for open fracture type IIIA, IIIB or IIIC with nonunion
P   subsequent encounter for closed fracture with malunion
Q   subsequent encounter for open fracture type I or II with malunion
R   subsequent encounter for open fracture type IIIA, IIIB or IIIC with malunion
S   sequela

☑5ᵗʰ **S82.0** Fracture of patella
    Knee cap

   ☑6ᵗʰ **S82.00** Unspecified fracture of patella

    ☑7ᵗʰ **S82.001** Unspecified fracture of right patella   ▽

    S82.002 Unspecified fracture of left patella   ▽

    ☑7ᵗʰ **S82.009** Unspecified fracture of unspecified patella   ▽

   ☑6ᵗʰ **S82.01** Osteochondral fracture of patella

    ☑7ᵗʰ **S82.011** Displaced osteochondral fracture of right patella

    ☑7ᵗʰ **S82.012** Displaced osteochondral fracture of left patella

    ☑7ᵗʰ **S82.013** Displaced osteochondral fracture of unspecified patella   ▽

    ☑7ᵗʰ **S82.014** Nondisplaced osteochondral fracture of right patella

    ☑7ᵗʰ **S82.015** Nondisplaced osteochondral fracture of left patella

    ☑7ᵗʰ **S82.016** Nondisplaced osteochondral fracture of unspecified patella   ▽

   ☑6ᵗʰ **S82.02** Longitudinal fracture of patella

    ☑7ᵗʰ **S82.021** Displaced longitudinal fracture of right patella

    ☑7ᵗʰ **S82.022** Displaced longitudinal fracture of left patella

    ☑7ᵗʰ **S82.023** Displaced longitudinal fracture of unspecified patella   ▽

    ☑7ᵗʰ **S82.024** Nondisplaced longitudinal fracture of right patella

    ☑7ᵗʰ **S82.025** Nondisplaced longitudinal fracture of left patella

    ☑7ᵗʰ **S82.026** Nondisplaced longitudinal fracture of unspecified patella   ▽

   ☑6ᵗʰ **S82.03** Transverse fracture of patella

    ☑7ᵗʰ **S82.031** Displaced transverse fracture of right patella

    ☑7ᵗʰ **S82.032** Displaced transverse fracture of left patella

☑ Additional Character Req   ☑x7ᵗʰ Placeholder Alert   **Manifestation**   **HCC** CMS-HCC Condition   ▽ Unspecified Code   ▶◀ Revised Text   ● New Code   ▲ Revised Code Title

ICD-10-CM 2018   **1013**

√7ᵗʰ **S82.033** Displaced **transverse** fracture of unspecified **patella** ▽

√7ᵗʰ **S82.034** Nondisplaced **transverse** fracture of **right** patella

√7ᵗʰ **S82.035** Nondisplaced **transverse** fracture of **left** patella

√7ᵗʰ **S82.036** Nondisplaced **transverse** fracture of unspecified **patella** ▽

√6ᵗʰ **S82.04** **Comminuted** fracture of patella

√7ᵗʰ **S82.041** Displaced **comminuted** fracture of **right** patella

√7ᵗʰ **S82.042** Displaced **comminuted** fracture of **left** patella

√7ᵗʰ **S82.043** Displaced **comminuted** fracture of unspecified **patella** ▽

√7ᵗʰ **S82.044** Nondisplaced **comminuted** fracture of **right** patella

√7ᵗʰ **S82.045** Nondisplaced **comminuted** fracture of **left** patella

√7ᵗʰ **S82.046** Nondisplaced **comminuted** fracture of unspecified **patella** ▽

√6ᵗʰ **S82.09** **Other** fracture of patella

√7ᵗʰ **S82.091** **Other** fracture of **right** patella

√7ᵗʰ **S82.092** **Other** fracture of **left** patella

√7ᵗʰ **S82.099** **Other** fracture of unspecified **patella** ▽

√5ᵗʰ **S82.1** Fracture of **upper end of tibia**
Fracture of proximal end of tibia
EXCLUDES 2 *fracture of shaft of tibia (S82.2-)*
physeal fracture of upper end of tibia (S89.0-)

√6ᵗʰ **S82.10** **Unspecified** fracture of upper end of tibia

√7ᵗʰ **S82.101** **Unspecified** fracture of upper end of **right tibia** ▽

√7ᵗʰ **S82.102** **Unspecified** fracture of upper end of **left tibia** ▽

√7ᵗʰ **S82.109** **Unspecified** fracture of upper end of unspecified **tibia** ▽

√6ᵗʰ **S82.11** Fracture of **tibial spine**

√7ᵗʰ **S82.111** Displaced **fracture of right tibial spine**

√7ᵗʰ **S82.112** Displaced **fracture of left tibial spine**

√7ᵗʰ **S82.113** Displaced **fracture of unspecified tibial spine** ▽

√7ᵗʰ **S82.114** Nondisplaced **fracture of right tibial spine**

√7ᵗʰ **S82.115** Nondisplaced **fracture of left tibial spine**

√7ᵗʰ **S82.116** Nondisplaced **fracture of unspecified tibial spine** ▽

√6ᵗʰ **S82.12** Fracture of **lateral condyle** of tibia

√7ᵗʰ **S82.121** Displaced **fracture of lateral condyle of right tibia**

√7ᵗʰ **S82.122** Displaced **fracture of lateral condyle of left tibia**

√7ᵗʰ **S82.123** Displaced **fracture of lateral condyle of unspecified tibia** ▽

√7ᵗʰ **S82.124** Nondisplaced **fracture of lateral condyle of right tibia**

√7ᵗʰ **S82.125** Nondisplaced **fracture of lateral condyle of left tibia**

√7ᵗʰ **S82.126** Nondisplaced **fracture of lateral condyle of unspecified tibia** ▽

√6ᵗʰ **S82.13** Fracture of **medial condyle** of tibia

√7ᵗʰ **S82.131** Displaced **fracture of medial condyle of right tibia**

√7ᵗʰ **S82.132** Displaced **fracture of medial condyle of left tibia**

√7ᵗʰ **S82.133** Displaced **fracture of medial condyle of unspecified tibia** ▽

√7ᵗʰ **S82.134** Nondisplaced **fracture of medial condyle of right tibia**

√7ᵗʰ **S82.135** Nondisplaced **fracture of medial condyle of left tibia**

√7ᵗʰ **S82.136** Nondisplaced **fracture of medial condyle of unspecified tibia** ▽

√6ᵗʰ **S82.14** **Bicondylar** fracture of tibia
Fracture of tibial plateau NOS

√7ᵗʰ **S82.141** Displaced **bicondylar** fracture of **right** tibia

√7ᵗʰ **S82.142** Displaced **bicondylar** fracture of **left** tibia

√7ᵗʰ **S82.143** Displaced **bicondylar** fracture of unspecified **tibia**

√7ᵗʰ **S82.144** Nondisplaced **bicondylar** fracture of **right** tibia

√7ᵗʰ **S82.145** Nondisplaced **bicondylar** fracture of **left** tibia

√7ᵗʰ **S82.146** Nondisplaced **bicondylar** fracture of unspecified **tibia** ▽

√6ᵗʰ **S82.15** Fracture of **tibial tuberosity**

√7ᵗʰ **S82.151** Displaced **fracture of right tibial tuberosity**

√7ᵗʰ **S82.152** Displaced **fracture of left tibial tuberosity**

√7ᵗʰ **S82.153** Displaced **fracture of unspecified tibial tuberosity** ▽

√7ᵗʰ **S82.154** Nondisplaced **fracture of right tibial tuberosity**

√7ᵗʰ **S82.155** Nondisplaced **fracture of left tibial tuberosity**

√7ᵗʰ **S82.156** Nondisplaced **fracture of unspecified tibial tuberosity** ▽

√6ᵗʰ **S82.16** **Torus** fracture of upper end of tibia

> The appropriate 7th character is to be added to all codes in subcategory S82.16.
> A   initial encounter for closed fracture
> D   subsequent encounter for fracture with routine healing
> G   subsequent encounter for fracture with delayed healing
> K   subsequent encounter for fracture with nonunion
> P   subsequent encounter for fracture with malunion
> S   sequela

√7ᵗʰ **S82.161** Torus fracture of upper end of **right tibia**

√7ᵗʰ **S82.162** Torus fracture of upper end of **left tibia**

√7ᵗʰ **S82.169** Torus fracture of upper end of unspecified **tibia** ▽

√6ᵗʰ **S82.19** **Other** fracture of upper end of tibia

√7ᵗʰ **S82.191** **Other** fracture of upper end of **right tibia**

√7ᵗʰ **S82.192** **Other** fracture of upper end of **left tibia**

√7ᵗʰ **S82.199** **Other** fracture of upper end of unspecified **tibia** ▽

√5ᵗʰ **S82.2** Fracture of **shaft of tibia**

√6ᵗʰ **S82.20** **Unspecified** fracture of shaft of tibia
Fracture of tibia NOS

√7ᵗʰ **S82.201** **Unspecified** fracture of shaft of **right tibia** ▽

√7ᵗʰ **S82.202** **Unspecified** fracture of shaft of **left tibia** ▽

√7ᵗʰ **S82.209** **Unspecified** fracture of shaft of unspecified **tibia** ▽

√6ᵗʰ **S82.22** **Transverse** fracture of shaft of tibia

√7ᵗʰ **S82.221** Displaced **transverse** fracture of shaft of **right tibia**

√7ᵗʰ **S82.222** Displaced **transverse** fracture of shaft of **left tibia**

√7ᵗʰ **S82.223** Displaced **transverse** fracture of shaft of unspecified **tibia** ▽

√7ᵗʰ **S82.224** Nondisplaced **transverse** fracture of shaft of **right tibia**

√7ᵗʰ **S82.225** Nondisplaced **transverse** fracture of shaft of **left tibia**

√7ᵗʰ **S82.226** Nondisplaced **transverse** fracture of shaft of unspecified **tibia** ▽

√6ᵗʰ **S82.23** **Oblique** fracture of shaft of tibia

√7ᵗʰ **S82.231** Displaced **oblique** fracture of shaft of **right tibia**

√7ᵗʰ **S82.232** Displaced **oblique** fracture of shaft of **left tibia**

EXCLUDES 1 Not coded here   **EXCLUDES 2** Not included here   N Newborn Age: 0   P Pediatric Age: 0-17   M Maternity Age: 12-55   A Adult Age: 15-124

1014   ICD-10-CM 2018

√7ᵗʰ **S82.233** Displaced oblique fracture of shaft of ▽
unspecified tibia

√7ᵗʰ **S82.234** Nondisplaced oblique fracture of shaft of
right tibia

√7ᵗʰ **S82.235** Nondisplaced oblique fracture of shaft of
left tibia

√7ᵗʰ **S82.236** Nondisplaced oblique fracture of shaft ▽
of unspecified tibia

√6ᵗʰ **S82.24** Spiral fracture of shaft of tibia
Toddler fracture

√7ᵗʰ **S82.241** Displaced spiral fracture of shaft of right
tibia

√7ᵗʰ **S82.242** Displaced spiral fracture of shaft of left
tibia

√7ᵗʰ **S82.243** Displaced spiral fracture of shaft of ▽
unspecified tibia

√7ᵗʰ **S82.244** Nondisplaced spiral fracture of shaft of
right tibia

√7ᵗʰ **S82.245** Nondisplaced spiral fracture of shaft of
left tibia

√7ᵗʰ **S82.246** Nondisplaced spiral fracture of shaft ▽
of unspecified tibia

√6ᵗʰ **S82.25** Comminuted fracture of shaft of tibia

√7ᵗʰ **S82.251** Displaced comminuted fracture of shaft of
right tibia

√7ᵗʰ **S82.252** Displaced comminuted fracture of shaft of
left tibia

√7ᵗʰ **S82.253** Displaced comminuted fracture of ▽
shaft of unspecified tibia

√7ᵗʰ **S82.254** Nondisplaced comminuted fracture of
shaft of right tibia

√7ᵗʰ **S82.255** Nondisplaced comminuted fracture of
shaft of left tibia

√7ᵗʰ **S82.256** Nondisplaced comminuted fracture of ▽
shaft of unspecified tibia

√6ᵗʰ **S82.26** Segmental fracture of shaft of tibia

√7ᵗʰ **S82.261** Displaced segmental fracture of shaft of
right tibia

√7ᵗʰ **S82.262** Displaced segmental fracture of shaft of
left tibia

√7ᵗʰ **S82.263** Displaced segmental fracture of shaft ▽
of unspecified tibia

√7ᵗʰ **S82.264** Nondisplaced segmental fracture of shaft
of right tibia

√7ᵗʰ **S82.265** Nondisplaced segmental fracture of shaft
of left tibia

√7ᵗʰ **S82.266** Nondisplaced segmental fracture of ▽
shaft of unspecified tibia

√6ᵗʰ **S82.29** Other fracture of shaft of tibia

√7ᵗʰ **S82.291** Other fracture of shaft of right tibia

√7ᵗʰ **S82.292** Other fracture of shaft of left tibia

√7ᵗʰ **S82.299** Other fracture of shaft of unspecified ▽
tibia

√5ᵗʰ **S82.3** Fracture of lower end of tibia

EXCLUDES 1 bimalleolar fracture of lower leg (S82.84-)
fracture of medial malleolus alone (S82.5-)
Maisonneuve's fracture (S82.86-)
pilon fracture of distal tibia (S82.87-)
trimalleolar fractures of lower leg (S82.85-)

√6ᵗʰ **S82.30** Unspecified fracture of lower end of tibia

√7ᵗʰ **S82.301** Unspecified fracture of lower end of ▽
right tibia

√7ᵗʰ **S82.302** Unspecified fracture of lower end of ▽
left tibia

√7ᵗʰ **S82.309** Unspecified fracture of lower end of ▽
unspecified tibia

√6ᵗʰ **S82.31** Torus fracture of lower end of tibia

The appropriate 7th character is to be added to all
codes in subcategory S82.31.
A   initial encounter for closed fracture
D   subsequent encounter for fracture with routine
     healing
G   subsequent encounter for fracture with
     delayed healing
K   subsequent encounter for fracture with
     nonunion
P   subsequent encounter for fracture with
     malunion
S   sequela

√7ᵗʰ **S82.311** Torus fracture of lower end of right tibia

√7ᵗʰ **S82.312** Torus fracture of lower end of left tibia

√7ᵗʰ **S82.319** Torus fracture of lower end of ▽
unspecified tibia

√6ᵗʰ **S82.39** Other fracture of lower end of tibia
AHA: 2015, 1Q, 25

√7ᵗʰ **S82.391** Other fracture of lower end of right tibia

√7ᵗʰ **S82.392** Other fracture of lower end of left tibia

√7ᵗʰ **S82.399** Other fracture of lower end of ▽
unspecified tibia

√5ᵗʰ **S82.4** Fracture of shaft of fibula

EXCLUDES 2 fracture of lateral malleolus alone (S82.6-)

√6ᵗʰ **S82.40** Unspecified fracture of shaft of fibula

√7ᵗʰ **S82.401** Unspecified fracture of shaft of right ▽
fibula

√7ᵗʰ **S82.402** Unspecified fracture of shaft of left ▽
fibula

√7ᵗʰ **S82.409** Unspecified fracture of shaft of ▽
unspecified fibula

√6ᵗʰ **S82.42** Transverse fracture of shaft of fibula

√7ᵗʰ **S82.421** Displaced transverse fracture of shaft of
right fibula

√7ᵗʰ **S82.422** Displaced transverse fracture of shaft of
left fibula

√7ᵗʰ **S82.423** Displaced transverse fracture of shaft ▽
of unspecified fibula

√7ᵗʰ **S82.424** Nondisplaced transverse fracture of shaft
of right fibula

√7ᵗʰ **S82.425** Nondisplaced transverse fracture of shaft
of left fibula

√7ᵗʰ **S82.426** Nondisplaced transverse fracture of ▽
shaft of unspecified fibula

√6ᵗʰ **S82.43** Oblique fracture of shaft of fibula

√7ᵗʰ **S82.431** Displaced oblique fracture of shaft of right
fibula

√7ᵗʰ **S82.432** Displaced oblique fracture of shaft of left
fibula

√7ᵗʰ **S82.433** Displaced oblique fracture of shaft of ▽
unspecified fibula

√7ᵗʰ **S82.434** Nondisplaced oblique fracture of shaft of
right fibula

√7ᵗʰ **S82.435** Nondisplaced oblique fracture of shaft of
left fibula

√7ᵗʰ **S82.436** Nondisplaced oblique fracture of shaft ▽
of unspecified fibula

√6ᵗʰ **S82.44** Spiral fracture of shaft of fibula

√7ᵗʰ **S82.441** Displaced spiral fracture of shaft of right
fibula

√7ᵗʰ **S82.442** Displaced spiral fracture of shaft of left
fibula

√7ᵗʰ **S82.443** Displaced spiral fracture of shaft of ▽
unspecified fibula

√7ᵗʰ **S82.444** Nondisplaced spiral fracture of shaft of
right fibula

√7ᵗʰ **S82.445** Nondisplaced spiral fracture of shaft of
left fibula

√7ᵗʰ **S82.446** Nondisplaced spiral fracture of shaft of ▽
unspecified fibula

√6ᵗʰ **S82.45** Comminuted fracture of shaft of fibula

√7ᵗʰ **S82.451** Displaced comminuted fracture of shaft of
right fibula

Chapter 19. Injury, Poisoning, and Certain Other Consequences of External Causes

☑7ᵗʰ **S82.452** Displaced **comminuted fracture of shaft of left fibula**

☑7ᵗʰ **S82.453** Displaced **comminuted fracture of shaft of unspecified fibula** ▽

☑7ᵗʰ **S82.454** Nondisplaced **comminuted fracture of shaft of right fibula**

☑7ᵗʰ **S82.455** Nondisplaced **comminuted fracture of shaft of left fibula**

☑7ᵗʰ **S82.456** Nondisplaced **comminuted fracture of shaft of unspecified fibula** ▽

☑6ᵗʰ **S82.46** Segmental **fracture of shaft of fibula**

☑7ᵗʰ **S82.461** Displaced **segmental fracture of shaft of right fibula**

☑7ᵗʰ **S82.462** Displaced **segmental fracture of shaft of left fibula**

☑7ᵗʰ **S82.463** Displaced **segmental fracture of shaft of unspecified fibula** ▽

☑7ᵗʰ **S82.464** Nondisplaced **segmental fracture of shaft of right fibula**

☑7ᵗʰ **S82.465** Nondisplaced **segmental fracture of shaft of left fibula**

☑7ᵗʰ **S82.466** Nondisplaced **segmental fracture of shaft of unspecified fibula** ▽

☑6ᵗʰ **S82.49** Other fracture of shaft of fibula

☑7ᵗʰ **S82.491** Other fracture of shaft of right **fibula**

☑7ᵗʰ **S82.492** Other fracture of shaft of left **fibula**

☑7ᵗʰ **S82.499** Other fracture of shaft of unspecified **fibula** ▽

☑5ᵗʰ **S82.5** Fracture of medial malleolus

EXCLUDES 1   *pilon fracture of distal tibia (S82.87-)*
Salter-Harris type III of lower end of tibia (S89.13-)
Salter-Harris type IV of lower end of tibia (S89.14-)

☑x7ᵗʰ **S82.51** Displaced **fracture of medial malleolus of right tibia**

☑7ᵗʰ **S82.52** Displaced **fracture of medial malleolus of left tibia**

☑7ᵗʰ **S82.53** Displaced **fracture of medial malleolus of unspecified tibia** ▽

☑x7ᵗʰ **S82.54** Nondisplaced **fracture of medial malleolus of right tibia**

☑x7ᵗʰ **S82.55** Nondisplaced **fracture of medial malleolus of left tibia**

☑x7ᵗʰ **S82.56** Nondisplaced **fracture of medial malleolus of unspecified tibia** ▽

☑5ᵗʰ **S82.6** Fracture of lateral malleolus

EXCLUDES 1   *pilon fracture of distal tibia (S82.87-)*

☑x7ᵗʰ **S82.61** Displaced **fracture of lateral malleolus of right fibula**

☑x7ᵗʰ **S82.62** Displaced **fracture of lateral malleolus of left fibula**

☑x7ᵗʰ **S82.63** Displaced **fracture of lateral malleolus of unspecified fibula** ▽

☑x7ᵗʰ **S82.64** Nondisplaced **fracture of lateral malleolus of right fibula**

☑x7ᵗʰ **S82.65** Nondisplaced **fracture of lateral malleolus of left fibula**

☑x7ᵗʰ **S82.66** Nondisplaced **fracture of lateral malleolus of unspecified fibula** ▽

☑5ᵗʰ **S82.8** Other fractures of lower leg

☑6ᵗʰ **S82.81** Torus **fracture of upper end of fibula**

The appropriate 7th character is to be added to all codes in subcategory S82.81.
A   initial encounter for closed fracture
D   subsequent encounter for fracture with routine healing
G   subsequent encounter for fracture with delayed healing
K   subsequent encounter for fracture with nonunion
P   subsequent encounter for fracture with malunion
S   sequela

☑7ᵗʰ **S82.811** Torus fracture of upper end of right **fibula**

☑7ᵗʰ **S82.812** Torus fracture of upper end of left **fibula**

☑7ᵗʰ **S82.819** Torus fracture of upper end of unspecified **fibula** ▽

☑6ᵗʰ **S82.82** Torus **fracture of lower end of fibula**

The appropriate 7th character is to be added to all codes in subcategory S82.82.
A   initial encounter for closed fracture
D   subsequent encounter for fracture with routine healing
G   subsequent encounter for fracture with delayed healing
K   subsequent encounter for fracture with nonunion
P   subsequent encounter for fracture with malunion
S   sequela

☑7ᵗʰ **S82.821** Torus fracture of lower end of right **fibula**

☑7ᵗʰ **S82.822** Torus fracture of lower end of left **fibula**

☑7ᵗʰ **S82.829** Torus fracture of lower end of unspecified **fibula** ▽

☑6ᵗʰ **S82.83** Other fracture of upper and lower end of fibula
AHA: 2015, 1Q, 25

☑7ᵗʰ **S82.831** Other fracture of upper and lower end of right **fibula**

☑7ᵗʰ **S82.832** Other fracture of upper and lower end of left **fibula**

☑7ᵗʰ **S82.839** Other fracture of upper and lower end of unspecified **fibula** ▽

☑6ᵗʰ **S82.84** Bimalleolar **fracture of lower leg**

☑7ᵗʰ **S82.841** Displaced **bimalleolar fracture of right lower leg**

☑7ᵗʰ **S82.842** Displaced **bimalleolar fracture of left lower leg**

☑7ᵗʰ **S82.843** Displaced **bimalleolar fracture of unspecified lower leg** ▽

☑7ᵗʰ **S82.844** Nondisplaced **bimalleolar fracture of right lower leg**

☑7ᵗʰ **S82.845** Nondisplaced **bimalleolar fracture of left lower leg**

☑7ᵗʰ **S82.846** Nondisplaced **bimalleolar fracture of unspecified lower leg** ▽

☑6ᵗʰ **S82.85** Trimalleolar **fracture of lower leg**

☑7ᵗʰ **S82.851** Displaced **trimalleolar fracture of right lower leg**

☑7ᵗʰ **S82.852** Displaced **trimalleolar fracture of left lower leg**

☑7ᵗʰ **S82.853** Displaced **trimalleolar fracture of unspecified lower leg** ▽

Right Bimalleolar Fracture

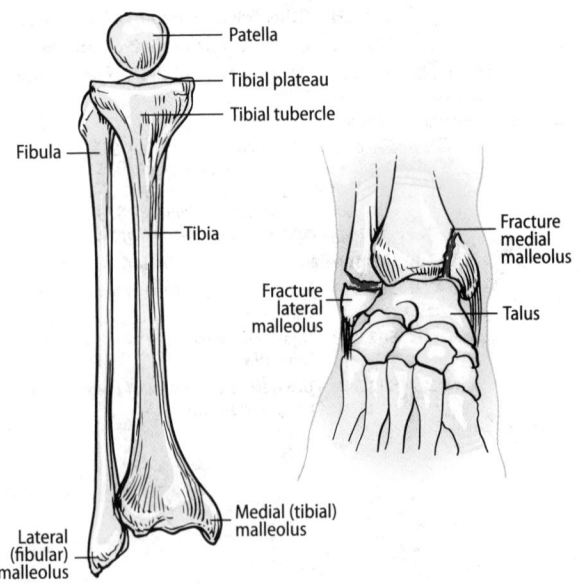

Patella
Tibial plateau
Tibial tubercle
Fibula
Tibia
Fracture medial malleolus
Fracture lateral malleolus
Talus
Medial (tibial) malleolus
Lateral (fibular) malleolus

EXCLUDES 1 Not coded here   EXCLUDES 2 Not included here   Ⓝ Newborn Age: 0   Ⓟ Pediatric Age: 0-17   Ⓜ Maternity Age: 12-55   Ⓐ Adult Age: 15-124

1016   ICD-10-CM 2018

√7ᵗʰ **S82.854** Nondisplaced **trimalleolar fracture of** right **lower leg**

√7ᵗʰ **S82.855** Nondisplaced **trimalleolar fracture of** left **lower leg**

√7ᵗʰ **S82.856** Nondisplaced **trimalleolar fracture of unspecified lower leg** ▽

√6ᵗʰ **S82.86** Maisonneuve's **fracture**

√7ᵗʰ **S82.861** Displaced **Maisonneuve's fracture of** right **leg**

√7ᵗʰ **S82.862** Displaced **Maisonneuve's fracture of** left **leg**

√7ᵗʰ **S82.863** Displaced **Maisonneuve's fracture of unspecified leg** ▽

√7ᵗʰ **S82.864** Nondisplaced **Maisonneuve's fracture of** right **leg**

√7ᵗʰ **S82.865** Nondisplaced **Maisonneuve's fracture of** left **leg**

√7ᵗʰ **S82.866** Nondisplaced **Maisonneuve's fracture of unspecified leg** ▽

√6ᵗʰ **S82.87** Pilon **fracture of tibia**

√7ᵗʰ **S82.871** Displaced **pilon fracture of** right **tibia**

√7ᵗʰ **S82.872** Displaced **pilon fracture of** left **tibia**

√7ᵗʰ **S82.873** Displaced **pilon fracture of unspecified** ▽ **tibia**

√7ᵗʰ **S82.874** Nondisplaced **pilon fracture of** right **tibia**

√7ᵗʰ **S82.875** Nondisplaced **pilon fracture of** left **tibia**

√7ᵗʰ **S82.876** Nondisplaced **pilon fracture of unspecified tibia** ▽

√6ᵗʰ **S82.89** Other fractures of lower leg
Fracture of ankle NOS

√7ᵗʰ **S82.891** Other fracture of right **lower leg**

√7ᵗʰ **S82.892** Other fracture of left **lower leg**

√7ᵗʰ **S82.899** Other fracture of unspecified lower leg ▽

√5ᵗʰ **S82.9** Unspecified fracture of lower leg

√x7ᵗʰ **S82.90** Unspecified fracture of unspecified lower leg ▽

√x7ᵗʰ **S82.91** Unspecified fracture of right **lower leg** ▽

√x7ᵗʰ **S82.92** Unspecified fracture of left **lower leg** ▽

√4ᵗʰ **S83** **Dislocation and sprain of joints and ligaments of knee**

INCLUDES   avulsion of joint or ligament of knee
laceration of cartilage, joint or ligament of knee
sprain of cartilage, joint or ligament of knee
traumatic hemarthrosis of joint or ligament of knee
traumatic rupture of joint or ligament of knee
traumatic subluxation of joint or ligament of knee
traumatic tear of joint or ligament of knee

Code also any associated open wound

EXCLUDES 1   derangement of patella (M22.0-M22.3)
injury of patellar ligament (tendon) (S76.1-)
internal derangement of knee (M23.-)
old dislocation of knee (M24.36)
pathological dislocation of knee (M24.36)
recurrent dislocation of knee (M22.0)

EXCLUDES 2   strain of muscle, fascia and tendon of lower leg (S86.-)

The appropriate 7th character is to be added to each code from category S83.
A   initial encounter
D   subsequent encounter
S   sequela

√5ᵗʰ **S83.0** Subluxation and dislocation of patella

√6ᵗʰ **S83.00** Unspecified subluxation and dislocation of patella

√7ᵗʰ **S83.001** Unspecified subluxation of right ▽ **patella**

√7ᵗʰ **S83.002** Unspecified subluxation of left **patella** ▽

√7ᵗʰ **S83.003** Unspecified subluxation of unspecified ▽ **patella**

√7ᵗʰ **S83.004** Unspecified dislocation of right **patella** ▽

√7ᵗʰ **S83.005** Unspecified dislocation of left **patella** ▽

√7ᵗʰ **S83.006** Unspecified dislocation of unspecified ▽ **patella**

√6ᵗʰ **S83.01** Lateral subluxation and dislocation of patella

√7ᵗʰ **S83.011** Lateral subluxation of right **patella**

√7ᵗʰ **S83.012** Lateral subluxation of left **patella**

√7ᵗʰ **S83.013** Lateral subluxation of unspecified ▽ **patella**

√7ᵗʰ **S83.014** Lateral dislocation of right **patella**

√7ᵗʰ **S83.015** Lateral dislocation of left **patella**

√7ᵗʰ **S83.016** Lateral dislocation of unspecified ▽ **patella**

√6ᵗʰ **S83.09** Other subluxation and dislocation of patella

√7ᵗʰ **S83.091** Other subluxation of right **patella**

√7ᵗʰ **S83.092** Other subluxation of left **patella**

√7ᵗʰ **S83.093** Other subluxation of unspecified ▽ **patella**

√7ᵗʰ **S83.094** Other dislocation of right **patella**

√7ᵗʰ **S83.095** Other dislocation of left **patella**

√7ᵗʰ **S83.096** Other dislocation of unspecified ▽ **patella**

√5ᵗʰ **S83.1** Subluxation and dislocation of knee
EXCLUDES 2   instability of knee prosthesis (T84.022, T84.023)

√6ᵗʰ **S83.10** Unspecified subluxation and dislocation of knee

√7ᵗʰ **S83.101** Unspecified subluxation of right **knee** ▽

√7ᵗʰ **S83.102** Unspecified subluxation of left **knee** ▽

√7ᵗʰ **S83.103** Unspecified subluxation of unspecified knee ▽

√7ᵗʰ **S83.104** Unspecified dislocation of right **knee** ▽

√7ᵗʰ **S83.105** Unspecified dislocation of left **knee** ▽

√7ᵗʰ **S83.106** Unspecified dislocation of unspecified knee ▽

√6ᵗʰ **S83.11** Anterior subluxation and dislocation of proximal end of tibia
Posterior subluxation and dislocation of distal end of femur

√7ᵗʰ **S83.111** Anterior subluxation of proximal end of tibia, right **knee**

√7ᵗʰ **S83.112** Anterior subluxation of proximal end of tibia, left **knee**

√7ᵗʰ **S83.113** Anterior subluxation of proximal end ▽ of tibia, unspecified **knee**

√7ᵗʰ **S83.114** Anterior dislocation of proximal end of tibia, right **knee**

√7ᵗʰ **S83.115** Anterior dislocation of proximal end of tibia, left **knee**

√7ᵗʰ **S83.116** Anterior dislocation of proximal end ▽ of tibia, unspecified **knee**

√6ᵗʰ **S83.12** Posterior subluxation and dislocation of proximal end of tibia
Anterior dislocation of distal end of femur

√7ᵗʰ **S83.121** Posterior subluxation of proximal end of tibia, right **knee**

√7ᵗʰ **S83.122** Posterior subluxation of proximal end of tibia, left **knee**

√7ᵗʰ **S83.123** Posterior subluxation of proximal end ▽ of tibia, unspecified **knee**

√7ᵗʰ **S83.124** Posterior dislocation of proximal end of tibia, right **knee**

√7ᵗʰ **S83.125** Posterior dislocation of proximal end of tibia, left **knee**

√7ᵗʰ **S83.126** Posterior dislocation of proximal end ▽ of tibia, unspecified **knee**

√6ᵗʰ **S83.13** Medial subluxation and dislocation of proximal end of tibia

√7ᵗʰ **S83.131** Medial subluxation of proximal end of tibia, right **knee**

√7ᵗʰ **S83.132** Medial subluxation of proximal end of tibia, left **knee**

√7ᵗʰ **S83.133** Medial subluxation of proximal end of ▽ tibia, unspecified **knee**

√7ᵗʰ **S83.134** Medial dislocation of proximal end of tibia, right **knee**

√7ᵗʰ **S83.135** Medial dislocation of proximal end of tibia, left **knee**

√7ᵗʰ **S83.136** Medial dislocation of proximal end of ▽ tibia, unspecified **knee**

✅ Additional Character Req   √x7ᵗʰ Placeholder Alert   Manifestation   HCC CMS-HCC Condition   ▽ Unspecified Code   ►◄ Revised Text   ● New Code   ▲ Revised Code Title

ICD-10-CM 2018   1017

✓6ᵗʰ **S83.14** **Lateral subluxation and dislocation of proximal end of tibia**

✓7ᵗʰ **S83.141** **Lateral subluxation of proximal end of tibia, right knee**

✓7ᵗʰ **S83.142** **Lateral subluxation of proximal end of tibia, left knee**

✓7ᵗʰ **S83.143** **Lateral subluxation of proximal end of tibia, unspecified knee** ▽

✓7ᵗʰ **S83.144** **Lateral dislocation of proximal end of tibia, right knee**

✓7ᵗʰ **S83.145** **Lateral dislocation of proximal end of tibia, left knee**

✓7ᵗʰ **S83.146** **Lateral dislocation of proximal end of tibia, unspecified knee** ▽

✓6ᵗʰ **S83.19** **Other subluxation and dislocation of knee**

✓7ᵗʰ **S83.191** **Other subluxation of right knee**

✓7ᵗʰ **S83.192** **Other subluxation of left knee**

✓7ᵗʰ **S83.193** **Other subluxation of unspecified knee** ▽

✓7ᵗʰ **S83.194** **Other dislocation of right knee**

✓7ᵗʰ **S83.195** **Other dislocation of left knee**

✓7ᵗʰ **S83.196** **Other dislocation of unspecified knee** ▽

✓5ᵗʰ **S83.2** **Tear of meniscus, current injury**

EXCLUDES 1 old bucket-handle tear (M23.2)

✓6ᵗʰ **S83.20** **Tear of unspecified meniscus, current injury**
Tear of meniscus of knee NOS

✓7ᵗʰ **S83.200** **Bucket-handle tear of unspecified meniscus, current injury, right knee** ▽

✓7ᵗʰ **S83.201** **Bucket-handle tear of unspecified meniscus, current injury, left knee** ▽

✓7ᵗʰ **S83.202** **Bucket-handle tear of unspecified meniscus, current injury, unspecified knee** ▽

✓7ᵗʰ **S83.203** **Other tear of unspecified meniscus, current injury, right knee** ▽

✓7ᵗʰ **S83.204** **Other tear of unspecified meniscus, current injury, left knee** ▽

✓7ᵗʰ **S83.205** **Other tear of unspecified meniscus, current injury, unspecified knee** ▽

✓7ᵗʰ **S83.206** **Unspecified tear of unspecified meniscus, current injury, right knee** ▽

✓7ᵗʰ **S83.207** **Unspecified tear of unspecified meniscus, current injury, left knee** ▽

✓7ᵗʰ **S83.209** **Unspecified tear of unspecified meniscus, current injury, unspecified knee** ▽

✓6ᵗʰ **S83.21** **Bucket-handle tear of medial meniscus, current injury**

✓7ᵗʰ **S83.211** **Bucket-handle tear of medial meniscus, current injury, right knee**

✓7ᵗʰ **S83.212** **Bucket-handle tear of medial meniscus, current injury, left knee**

✓7ᵗʰ **S83.219** **Bucket-handle tear of medial meniscus, current injury, unspecified knee** ▽

✓6ᵗʰ **S83.22** **Peripheral tear of medial meniscus, current injury**

✓7ᵗʰ **S83.221** **Peripheral tear of medial meniscus, current injury, right knee**

✓7ᵗʰ **S83.222** **Peripheral tear of medial meniscus, current injury, left knee**

✓7ᵗʰ **S83.229** **Peripheral tear of medial meniscus, current injury, unspecified knee** ▽

✓6ᵗʰ **S83.23** **Complex tear of medial meniscus, current injury**

✓7ᵗʰ **S83.231** **Complex tear of medial meniscus, current injury, right knee**

✓7ᵗʰ **S83.232** **Complex tear of medial meniscus, current injury, left knee**

✓7ᵗʰ **S83.239** **Complex tear of medial meniscus, current injury, unspecified knee** ▽

✓6ᵗʰ **S83.24** **Other tear of medial meniscus, current injury**

✓7ᵗʰ **S83.241** **Other tear of medial meniscus, current injury, right knee**

✓7ᵗʰ **S83.242** **Other tear of medial meniscus, current injury, left knee**

✓7ᵗʰ **S83.249** **Other tear of medial meniscus, current injury, unspecified knee** ▽

✓6ᵗʰ **S83.25** **Bucket-handle tear of lateral meniscus, current injury**

✓7ᵗʰ **S83.251** **Bucket-handle tear of lateral meniscus, current injury, right knee**

✓7ᵗʰ **S83.252** **Bucket-handle tear of lateral meniscus, current injury, left knee**

✓7ᵗʰ **S83.259** **Bucket-handle tear of lateral meniscus, current injury, unspecified knee** ▽

✓6ᵗʰ **S83.26** **Peripheral tear of lateral meniscus, current injury**

✓7ᵗʰ **S83.261** **Peripheral tear of lateral meniscus, current injury, right knee**

✓7ᵗʰ **S83.262** **Peripheral tear of lateral meniscus, current injury, left knee**

✓7ᵗʰ **S83.269** **Peripheral tear of lateral meniscus, current injury, unspecified knee** ▽

✓6ᵗʰ **S83.27** **Complex tear of lateral meniscus, current injury**

✓7ᵗʰ **S83.271** **Complex tear of lateral meniscus, current injury, right knee**

✓7ᵗʰ **S83.272** **Complex tear of lateral meniscus, current injury, left knee**

✓7ᵗʰ **S83.279** **Complex tear of lateral meniscus, current injury, unspecified knee** ▽

✓6ᵗʰ **S83.28** **Other tear of lateral meniscus, current injury**

✓7ᵗʰ **S83.281** **Other tear of lateral meniscus, current injury, right knee**

✓7ᵗʰ **S83.282** **Other tear of lateral meniscus, current injury, left knee**

✓7ᵗʰ **S83.289** **Other tear of lateral meniscus, current injury, unspecified knee** ▽

✓5ᵗʰ **S83.3** **Tear of articular cartilage of knee, current**

✓×7ᵗʰ **S83.30** **Tear of articular cartilage of unspecified knee, current** ▽

✓×7ᵗʰ **S83.31** **Tear of articular cartilage of right knee, current**

✓×7ᵗʰ **S83.32** **Tear of articular cartilage of left knee, current**

✓5ᵗʰ **S83.4** **Sprain of collateral ligament of knee**

✓6ᵗʰ **S83.40** **Sprain of unspecified collateral ligament of knee**

✓7ᵗʰ **S83.401** **Sprain of unspecified collateral ligament of right knee** ▽

✓7ᵗʰ **S83.402** **Sprain of unspecified collateral ligament of left knee** ▽

✓7ᵗʰ **S83.409** **Sprain of unspecified collateral ligament of unspecified knee** ▽

✓6ᵗʰ **S83.41** **Sprain of medial collateral ligament of knee**
Sprain of tibial collateral ligament

✓7ᵗʰ **S83.411** **Sprain of medial collateral ligament of right knee**

✓7ᵗʰ **S83.412** **Sprain of medial collateral ligament of left knee**

✓7ᵗʰ **S83.419** **Sprain of medial collateral ligament of unspecified knee** ▽

✓6ᵗʰ **S83.42** **Sprain of lateral collateral ligament of knee**
Sprain of fibular collateral ligament

✓7ᵗʰ **S83.421** **Sprain of lateral collateral ligament of right knee**

✓7ᵗʰ **S83.422** **Sprain of lateral collateral ligament of left knee**

✓7ᵗʰ **S83.429** **Sprain of lateral collateral ligament of unspecified knee** ▽

✓5ᵗʰ **S83.5** **Sprain of cruciate ligament of knee**
AHA: 2016, 2Q, 3

✓6ᵗʰ **S83.50** **Sprain of unspecified cruciate ligament of knee**

✓7ᵗʰ **S83.501** **Sprain of unspecified cruciate ligament of right knee** ▽

✓7ᵗʰ **S83.502** **Sprain of unspecified cruciate ligament of left knee** ▽

✓7ᵗʰ **S83.509** **Sprain of unspecified cruciate ligament of unspecified knee** ▽

✓6ᵗʰ **S83.51** **Sprain of anterior cruciate ligament of knee**

✓7ᵗʰ **S83.511** **Sprain of anterior cruciate ligament of right knee**

✓7ᵗʰ **S83.512** **Sprain of anterior cruciate ligament of left knee**

EXCLUDES 1 Not coded here   EXCLUDES 2 Not included here   N Newborn Age: 0   P Pediatric Age: 0-17   M Maternity Age: 12-55   A Adult Age: 15-124

1018   ICD-10-CM 2018

√7ᵗʰ **S83.519** Sprain of anterior cruciate ligament of unspecified knee ▽

√6ᵗʰ **S83.52** Sprain of posterior cruciate ligament of knee

     √7ᵗʰ **S83.521** Sprain of posterior cruciate ligament of right knee

     √7ᵗʰ **S83.522** Sprain of posterior cruciate ligament of left knee

     √7ᵗʰ **S83.529** Sprain of posterior cruciate ligament of unspecified knee ▽

√5ᵗʰ **S83.6** Sprain of the superior tibiofibular joint and ligament

     √x7ᵗʰ **S83.60** Sprain of the superior tibiofibular joint and ligament, unspecified knee ▽

     √x7ᵗʰ **S83.61** Sprain of the superior tibiofibular joint and ligament, right knee

     √x7ᵗʰ **S83.62** Sprain of the superior tibiofibular joint and ligament, left knee

√5ᵗʰ **S83.8** Sprain of other specified parts of knee

     √6ᵗʰ **S83.8X** Sprain of other specified parts of knee

         √7ᵗʰ **S83.8X1** Sprain of other specified parts of right knee

         √7ᵗʰ **S83.8X2** Sprain of other specified parts of left knee

         √7ᵗʰ **S83.8X9** Sprain of other specified parts of unspecified knee ▽

√5ᵗʰ **S83.9** Sprain of unspecified site of knee

     √x7ᵗʰ **S83.90** Sprain of unspecified site of unspecified knee ▽

     √x7ᵗʰ **S83.91** Sprain of unspecified site of right knee ▽

     √x7ᵗʰ **S83.92** Sprain of unspecified site of left knee ▽

√4ᵗʰ **S84** **Injury of nerves at lower leg level**

Code also any associated open wound (S81.-)

EXCLUDES 2   injury of nerves at ankle and foot level (S94.-)

The appropriate 7th character is to be added to each code from category S84.
A   initial encounter
D   subsequent encounter
S   sequela

√5ᵗʰ **S84.0** Injury of tibial nerve at lower leg level

     √x7ᵗʰ **S84.00** Injury of tibial nerve at lower leg level, unspecified leg ▽

     √x7ᵗʰ **S84.01** Injury of tibial nerve at lower leg level, right leg

     √x7ᵗʰ **S84.02** Injury of tibial nerve at lower leg level, left leg

√5ᵗʰ **S84.1** Injury of peroneal nerve at lower leg level

     √x7ᵗʰ **S84.10** Injury of peroneal nerve at lower leg level, unspecified leg ▽

     √x7ᵗʰ **S84.11** Injury of peroneal nerve at lower leg level, right leg

     √x7ᵗʰ **S84.12** Injury of peroneal nerve at lower leg level, left leg

√5ᵗʰ **S84.2** Injury of cutaneous sensory nerve at lower leg level

     √x7ᵗʰ **S84.20** Injury of cutaneous sensory nerve at lower leg level, unspecified leg ▽

     √x7ᵗʰ **S84.21** Injury of cutaneous sensory nerve at lower leg level, right leg

     √x7ᵗʰ **S84.22** Injury of cutaneous sensory nerve at lower leg level, left leg

√5ᵗʰ **S84.8** Injury of other nerves at lower leg level

     √6ᵗʰ **S84.80** Injury of other nerves at lower leg level

         √7ᵗʰ **S84.801** Injury of other nerves at lower leg level, right leg

         √7ᵗʰ **S84.802** Injury of other nerves at lower leg level, left leg

         √7ᵗʰ **S84.809** Injury of other nerves at lower leg level, unspecified leg ▽

√5ᵗʰ **S84.9** Injury of unspecified nerve at lower leg level

     √x7ᵗʰ **S84.90** Injury of unspecified nerve at lower leg level, unspecified leg ▽

     √x7ᵗʰ **S84.91** Injury of unspecified nerve at lower leg level, right leg ▽

     √x7ᵗʰ **S84.92** Injury of unspecified nerve at lower leg level, left leg ▽

√4ᵗʰ **S85** **Injury of blood vessels at lower leg level**

Code also any associated open wound (S81.-)

EXCLUDES 2   injury of blood vessels at ankle and foot level (S95.-)

The appropriate 7th character is to be added to each code from category S85.
A   initial encounter
D   subsequent encounter
S   sequela

√5ᵗʰ **S85.0** Injury of popliteal artery

     √6ᵗʰ **S85.00** Unspecified injury of popliteal artery

         √7ᵗʰ **S85.001** Unspecified injury of popliteal artery, right leg ▽

         √7ᵗʰ **S85.002** Unspecified injury of popliteal artery, left leg ▽

         √7ᵗʰ **S85.009** Unspecified injury of popliteal artery, unspecified leg ▽

     √6ᵗʰ **S85.01** Laceration of popliteal artery

         √7ᵗʰ **S85.011** Laceration of popliteal artery, right leg

         √7ᵗʰ **S85.012** Laceration of popliteal artery, left leg

         √7ᵗʰ **S85.019** Laceration of popliteal artery, unspecified leg ▽

     √6ᵗʰ **S85.09** Other specified injury of popliteal artery

         √7ᵗʰ **S85.091** Other specified injury of popliteal artery, right leg

         √7ᵗʰ **S85.092** Other specified injury of popliteal artery, left leg

         √7ᵗʰ **S85.099** Other specified injury of popliteal artery, unspecified leg ▽

√5ᵗʰ **S85.1** Injury of tibial artery

     √6ᵗʰ **S85.10** Unspecified injury of unspecified tibial artery

         Injury of tibial artery NOS

         √7ᵗʰ **S85.101** Unspecified injury of unspecified tibial artery, right leg ▽

         √7ᵗʰ **S85.102** Unspecified injury of unspecified tibial artery, left leg ▽

         √7ᵗʰ **S85.109** Unspecified injury of unspecified tibial artery, unspecified leg ▽

     √6ᵗʰ **S85.11** Laceration of unspecified tibial artery

         √7ᵗʰ **S85.111** Laceration of unspecified tibial artery, right leg ▽

         √7ᵗʰ **S85.112** Laceration of unspecified tibial artery, left leg ▽

         √7ᵗʰ **S85.119** Laceration of unspecified tibial artery, unspecified leg ▽

     √6ᵗʰ **S85.12** Other specified injury of unspecified tibial artery

         √7ᵗʰ **S85.121** Other specified injury of unspecified tibial artery, right leg ▽

         √7ᵗʰ **S85.122** Other specified injury of unspecified tibial artery, left leg ▽

         √7ᵗʰ **S85.129** Other specified injury of unspecified tibial artery, unspecified leg ▽

     √6ᵗʰ **S85.13** Unspecified injury of anterior tibial artery

         √7ᵗʰ **S85.131** Unspecified injury of anterior tibial artery, right leg ▽

         √7ᵗʰ **S85.132** Unspecified injury of anterior tibial artery, left leg ▽

         √7ᵗʰ **S85.139** Unspecified injury of anterior tibial artery, unspecified leg ▽

     √6ᵗʰ **S85.14** Laceration of anterior tibial artery

         √7ᵗʰ **S85.141** Laceration of anterior tibial artery, right leg

         √7ᵗʰ **S85.142** Laceration of anterior tibial artery, left leg

         √7ᵗʰ **S85.149** Laceration of anterior tibial artery, unspecified leg ▽

     √6ᵗʰ **S85.15** Other specified injury of anterior tibial artery

         √7ᵗʰ **S85.151** Other specified injury of anterior tibial artery, right leg

         √7ᵗʰ **S85.152** Other specified injury of anterior tibial artery, left leg

         √7ᵗʰ **S85.159** Other specified injury of anterior tibial artery, unspecified leg ▽

☑ Additional Character Req   √x7ᵗʰ Placeholder Alert   Manifestation   HCC CMS-HCC Condition   ▽ Unspecified Code   ▶◀ Revised Text   ● New Code   ▲ Revised Code Title

ICD-10-CM 2018   1019

√6ᵗʰ **S85.16 Unspecified injury of posterior tibial artery**

    √7ᵗʰ **S85.161** Unspecified injury of posterior tibial artery, **right leg** ▽

    √7ᵗʰ **S85.162** Unspecified injury of posterior tibial artery, **left leg** ▽

    √7ᵗʰ **S85.169** Unspecified injury of posterior tibial artery, unspecified leg ▽

√6ᵗʰ **S85.17 Laceration of posterior tibial artery**

    √7ᵗʰ **S85.171** Laceration of posterior tibial artery, **right leg**

    √7ᵗʰ **S85.172** Laceration of posterior tibial artery, **left leg**

    √7ᵗʰ **S85.179** Laceration of posterior tibial artery, unspecified leg ▽

√6ᵗʰ **S85.18 Other specified injury of posterior tibial artery**

    √7ᵗʰ **S85.181** Other specified injury of posterior tibial artery, **right leg**

    √7ᵗʰ **S85.182** Other specified injury of posterior tibial artery, **left leg**

    √7ᵗʰ **S85.189** Other specified injury of posterior tibial artery, unspecified leg ▽

√5ᵗʰ **S85.2 Injury of peroneal artery**

  √6ᵗʰ **S85.20 Unspecified injury of peroneal artery**

    √7ᵗʰ **S85.201** Unspecified injury of peroneal artery, **right leg** ▽

    √7ᵗʰ **S85.202** Unspecified injury of peroneal artery, **left leg** ▽

    √7ᵗʰ **S85.209** Unspecified injury of peroneal artery, unspecified leg ▽

  √6ᵗʰ **S85.21 Laceration of peroneal artery**

    √7ᵗʰ **S85.211** Laceration of peroneal artery, **right leg**

    √7ᵗʰ **S85.212** Laceration of peroneal artery, **left leg**

    √7ᵗʰ **S85.219** Laceration of peroneal artery, unspecified leg ▽

  √6ᵗʰ **S85.29 Other specified injury of peroneal artery**

    √7ᵗʰ **S85.291** Other specified injury of peroneal artery, **right leg**

    √7ᵗʰ **S85.292** Other specified injury of peroneal artery, **left leg**

    √7ᵗʰ **S85.299** Other specified injury of peroneal artery, unspecified leg ▽

√5ᵗʰ **S85.3 Injury of greater saphenous vein at lower leg level**
Injury of greater saphenous vein NOS
Injury of saphenous vein NOS

  √6ᵗʰ **S85.30 Unspecified injury of greater saphenous vein at lower leg level**

    √7ᵗʰ **S85.301** Unspecified injury of greater saphenous vein at lower leg level, **right leg** ▽

    √7ᵗʰ **S85.302** Unspecified injury of greater saphenous vein at lower leg level, **left leg** ▽

    √7ᵗʰ **S85.309** Unspecified injury of greater saphenous vein at lower leg level, unspecified leg ▽

  √6ᵗʰ **S85.31 Laceration of greater saphenous vein at lower leg level**

    √7ᵗʰ **S85.311** Laceration of greater saphenous vein at lower leg level, **right leg**

    √7ᵗʰ **S85.312** Laceration of greater saphenous vein at lower leg level, **left leg**

    √7ᵗʰ **S85.319** Laceration of greater saphenous vein at lower leg level, unspecified leg ▽

  √6ᵗʰ **S85.39 Other specified injury of greater saphenous vein at lower leg level**

    √7ᵗʰ **S85.391** Other specified injury of greater saphenous vein at lower leg level, **right leg**

    √7ᵗʰ **S85.392** Other specified injury of greater saphenous vein at lower leg level, **left leg**

    √7ᵗʰ **S85.399** Other specified injury of greater saphenous vein at lower leg level, unspecified leg ▽

√5ᵗʰ **S85.4 Injury of lesser saphenous vein at lower leg level**

  √6ᵗʰ **S85.40 Unspecified injury of lesser saphenous vein at lower leg level**

    √7ᵗʰ **S85.401** Unspecified injury of lesser saphenous vein at lower leg level, **right leg** ▽

    √7ᵗʰ **S85.402** Unspecified injury of lesser saphenous vein at lower leg level, **left leg** ▽

    √7ᵗʰ **S85.409** Unspecified injury of lesser saphenous vein at lower leg level, unspecified leg ▽

  √6ᵗʰ **S85.41 Laceration of lesser saphenous vein at lower leg level**

    √7ᵗʰ **S85.411** Laceration of lesser saphenous vein at lower leg level, **right leg**

    √7ᵗʰ **S85.412** Laceration of lesser saphenous vein at lower leg level, **left leg**

    √7ᵗʰ **S85.419** Laceration of lesser saphenous vein at lower leg level, unspecified leg ▽

  √6ᵗʰ **S85.49 Other specified injury of lesser saphenous vein at lower leg level**

    √7ᵗʰ **S85.491** Other specified injury of lesser saphenous vein at lower leg level, **right leg**

    √7ᵗʰ **S85.492** Other specified injury of lesser saphenous vein at lower leg level, **left leg**

    √7ᵗʰ **S85.499** Other specified injury of lesser saphenous vein at lower leg level, unspecified leg ▽

√5ᵗʰ **S85.5 Injury of popliteal vein**

  √6ᵗʰ **S85.50 Unspecified injury of popliteal vein**

    √7ᵗʰ **S85.501** Unspecified injury of popliteal vein, **right leg** ▽

    √7ᵗʰ **S85.502** Unspecified injury of popliteal vein, **left leg** ▽

    √7ᵗʰ **S85.509** Unspecified injury of popliteal vein, unspecified leg ▽

  √6ᵗʰ **S85.51 Laceration of popliteal vein**

    √7ᵗʰ **S85.511** Laceration of popliteal vein, **right leg**

    √7ᵗʰ **S85.512** Laceration of popliteal vein, **left leg**

    √7ᵗʰ **S85.519** Laceration of popliteal vein, unspecified leg ▽

  √6ᵗʰ **S85.59 Other specified injury of popliteal vein**

    √7ᵗʰ **S85.591** Other specified injury of popliteal vein, **right leg**

    √7ᵗʰ **S85.592** Other specified injury of popliteal vein, **left leg**

    √7ᵗʰ **S85.599** Other specified injury of popliteal vein, unspecified leg ▽

√5ᵗʰ **S85.8 Injury of other blood vessels at lower leg level**

  √6ᵗʰ **S85.80 Unspecified injury of other blood vessels at lower leg level**

    √7ᵗʰ **S85.801** Unspecified injury of other blood vessels at lower leg level, **right leg** ▽

    √7ᵗʰ **S85.802** Unspecified injury of other blood vessels at lower leg level, **left leg** ▽

    √7ᵗʰ **S85.809** Unspecified injury of other blood vessels at lower leg level, unspecified leg ▽

  √6ᵗʰ **S85.81 Laceration of other blood vessels at lower leg level**

    √7ᵗʰ **S85.811** Laceration of other blood vessels at lower leg level, **right leg**

    √7ᵗʰ **S85.812** Laceration of other blood vessels at lower leg level, **left leg**

    √7ᵗʰ **S85.819** Laceration of other blood vessels at lower leg level, unspecified leg ▽

  √6ᵗʰ **S85.89 Other specified injury of other blood vessels at lower leg level**

    √7ᵗʰ **S85.891** Other specified injury of other blood vessels at lower leg level, **right leg**

    √7ᵗʰ **S85.892** Other specified injury of other blood vessels at lower leg level, **left leg**

    √7ᵗʰ **S85.899** Other specified injury of other blood vessels at lower leg level, unspecified leg ▽

EXCLUDES 1 Not coded here   **EXCLUDES 2** Not included here   N Newborn Age: 0   P Pediatric Age: 0-17   M Maternity Age: 12-55   A Adult Age: 15-124

1020   ICD-10-CM 2018

√5ᵗʰ **S85.9**   **Injury of unspecified blood vessel at lower leg level**

    √6ᵗʰ **S85.90**   **Unspecified injury of unspecified blood vessel at lower leg level**

       √7ᵗʰ **S85.901**   Unspecified injury of unspecified blood vessel at lower leg level, right leg   ▽

       √7ᵗʰ **S85.902**   Unspecified injury of unspecified blood vessel at lower leg level, left leg   ▽

       √7ᵗʰ **S85.909**   Unspecified injury of unspecified blood vessel at lower leg level, unspecified leg   ▽

    √6ᵗʰ **S85.91**   **Laceration of unspecified blood vessel at lower leg level**

       √7ᵗʰ **S85.911**   Laceration of unspecified blood vessel at lower leg level, right leg   ▽

       √7ᵗʰ **S85.912**   Laceration of unspecified blood vessel at lower leg level, left leg   ▽

       √7ᵗʰ **S85.919**   Laceration of unspecified blood vessel at lower leg level, unspecified leg   ▽

    √6ᵗʰ **S85.99**   **Other specified injury of unspecified blood vessel at lower leg level**

       √7ᵗʰ **S85.991**   Other specified injury of unspecified blood vessel at lower leg level, right leg   ▽

       √7ᵗʰ **S85.992**   Other specified injury of unspecified blood vessel at lower leg level, left leg   ▽

       √7ᵗʰ **S85.999**   Other specified injury of unspecified blood vessel at lower leg level, unspecified leg   ▽

√4ᵗʰ **S86**   **Injury of muscle, fascia and tendon at lower leg level**

    Code also any associated open wound (S81.-)

    EXCLUDES 2   injury of muscle, fascia and tendon at ankle (S96.-)
                    injury of patellar ligament (tendon) (S76.1-)
                    sprain of joints and ligaments of knee (S83.-)

    TIP: Refer to the Muscle/Tendon table at the beginning of this chapter.

    The appropriate 7th character is to be added to each code from category S86.
    A   initial encounter
    D   subsequent encounter
    S   sequela

    √5ᵗʰ **S86.0**   **Injury of Achilles tendon**

       √6ᵗʰ **S86.00**   **Unspecified injury of Achilles tendon**

          √7ᵗʰ **S86.001**   Unspecified injury of right Achilles tendon   ▽

          √7ᵗʰ **S86.002**   Unspecified injury of left Achilles tendon   ▽

          √7ᵗʰ **S86.009**   Unspecified injury of unspecified Achilles tendon   ▽

       √6ᵗʰ **S86.01**   **Strain of Achilles tendon**

          √7ᵗʰ **S86.011**   Strain of right Achilles tendon

          √7ᵗʰ **S86.012**   Strain of left Achilles tendon

          √7ᵗʰ **S86.019**   Strain of unspecified Achilles tendon   ▽

       S86.02   **Laceration of Achilles tendon**

          √7ᵗʰ **S86.021**   Laceration of right Achilles tendon

          √7ᵗʰ **S86.022**   Laceration of left Achilles tendon

          √7ᵗʰ **S86.029**   Laceration of unspecified Achilles tendon   ▽

       √6ᵗʰ **S86.09**   **Other specified injury of Achilles tendon**

          √7ᵗʰ **S86.091**   Other specified injury of right Achilles tendon

          √7ᵗʰ **S86.092**   Other specified injury of left Achilles tendon

          √7ᵗʰ **S86.099**   Other specified injury of unspecified Achilles tendon   ▽

    √5ᵗʰ **S86.1**   **Injury of other muscle(s) and tendon(s) of posterior muscle group at lower leg level**

       √6ᵗʰ **S86.10**   **Unspecified injury of other muscle(s) and tendon(s) of posterior muscle group at lower leg level**

          √7ᵗʰ **S86.101**   Unspecified injury of other muscle(s) and tendon(s) of posterior muscle group at lower leg level, right leg   ▽

          √7ᵗʰ **S86.102**   Unspecified injury of other muscle(s) and tendon(s) of posterior muscle group at lower leg level, left leg   ▽

          √7ᵗʰ **S86.109**   Unspecified injury of other muscle(s) and tendon(s) of posterior muscle group at lower leg level, unspecified leg   ▽

       √6ᵗʰ **S86.11**   **Strain of other muscle(s) and tendon(s) of posterior muscle group at lower leg level**

          √7ᵗʰ **S86.111**   Strain of other muscle(s) and tendon(s) of posterior muscle group at lower leg level, right leg

          √7ᵗʰ **S86.112**   Strain of other muscle(s) and tendon(s) of posterior muscle group at lower leg level, left leg

          √7ᵗʰ **S86.119**   Strain of other muscle(s) and tendon(s) of posterior muscle group at lower leg level, unspecified leg   ▽

       √6ᵗʰ **S86.12**   **Laceration of other muscle(s) and tendon(s) of posterior muscle group at lower leg level**

          √7ᵗʰ **S86.121**   Laceration of other muscle(s) and tendon(s) of posterior muscle group at lower leg level, right leg

          √7ᵗʰ **S86.122**   Laceration of other muscle(s) and tendon(s) of posterior muscle group at lower leg level, left leg

          √7ᵗʰ **S86.129**   Laceration of other muscle(s) and tendon(s) of posterior muscle group at lower leg level, unspecified leg   ▽

       √6ᵗʰ **S86.19**   **Other injury of other muscle(s) and tendon(s) of posterior muscle group at lower leg level**

          √7ᵗʰ **S86.191**   Other injury of other muscle(s) and tendon(s) of posterior muscle group at lower leg level, right leg

          √7ᵗʰ **S86.192**   Other injury of other muscle(s) and tendon(s) of posterior muscle group at lower leg level, left leg

          √7ᵗʰ **S86.199**   Other injury of other muscle(s) and tendon(s) of posterior muscle group at lower leg level, unspecified leg   ▽

    √5ᵗʰ **S86.2**   **Injury of muscle(s) and tendon(s) of anterior muscle group at lower leg level**

       √6ᵗʰ **S86.20**   **Unspecified injury of muscle(s) and tendon(s) of anterior muscle group at lower leg level**

          √7ᵗʰ **S86.201**   Unspecified injury of muscle(s) and tendon(s) of anterior muscle group at lower leg level, right leg   ▽

          √7ᵗʰ **S86.202**   Unspecified injury of muscle(s) and tendon(s) of anterior muscle group at lower leg level, left leg   ▽

          √7ᵗʰ **S86.209**   Unspecified injury of muscle(s) and tendon(s) of anterior muscle group at lower leg level, unspecified leg   ▽

       √6ᵗʰ **S86.21**   **Strain of muscle(s) and tendon(s) of anterior muscle group at lower leg level**

          √7ᵗʰ **S86.211**   Strain of muscle(s) and tendon(s) of anterior muscle group at lower leg level, right leg

          √7ᵗʰ **S86.212**   Strain of muscle(s) and tendon(s) of anterior muscle group at lower leg level, left leg

          √7ᵗʰ **S86.219**   Strain of muscle(s) and tendon(s) of anterior muscle group at lower leg level, unspecified leg   ▽

       √6ᵗʰ **S86.22**   **Laceration of muscle(s) and tendon(s) of anterior muscle group at lower leg level**

          √7ᵗʰ **S86.221**   Laceration of muscle(s) and tendon(s) of anterior muscle group at lower leg level, right leg

          √7ᵗʰ **S86.222**   Laceration of muscle(s) and tendon(s) of anterior muscle group at lower leg level, left leg

          √7ᵗʰ **S86.229**   Laceration of muscle(s) and tendon(s) of anterior muscle group at lower leg level, unspecified leg   ▽

       √6ᵗʰ **S86.29**   **Other injury of muscle(s) and tendon(s) of anterior muscle group at lower leg level**

          √7ᵗʰ **S86.291**   Other injury of muscle(s) and tendon(s) of anterior muscle group at lower leg level, right leg

          √7ᵗʰ **S86.292**   Other injury of muscle(s) and tendon(s) of anterior muscle group at lower leg level, left leg

☑ Additional Character Req   √7ᵗʰ Placeholder Alert   Manifestation   HCC CMS-HCC Condition   ▽ Unspecified Code   ►◄ Revised Text   ● New Code   ▲ Revised Code Title

ICD-10-CM 2018   **1021**

- ✓7th **S86.299** Other injury of muscle(s) and tendon(s) ▽ of anterior muscle group at lower leg level, unspecified leg
- ✓5th **S86.3** Injury of muscle(s) and tendon(s) of peroneal muscle group at lower leg level
  - ✓6th **S86.30** Unspecified injury of muscle(s) and tendon(s) of peroneal muscle group at lower leg level
    - ✓7th **S86.301** Unspecified injury of muscle(s) and ▽ tendon(s) of peroneal muscle group at lower leg level, right leg
    - ✓7th **S86.302** Unspecified injury of muscle(s) and ▽ tendon(s) of peroneal muscle group at lower leg level, left leg
    - ✓7th **S86.309** Unspecified injury of muscle(s) and ▽ tendon(s) of peroneal muscle group at lower leg level, unspecified leg
  - ✓6th **S86.31** Strain of muscle(s) and tendon(s) of peroneal muscle group at lower leg level
    - ✓7th **S86.311** Strain of muscle(s) and tendon(s) of ▽ peroneal muscle group at lower leg level, right leg
    - ✓7th **S86.312** Strain of muscle(s) and tendon(s) of ▽ peroneal muscle group at lower leg level, left leg
    - ✓7th **S86.319** Strain of muscle(s) and tendon(s) of ▽ peroneal muscle group at lower leg level, unspecified leg
  - ✓6th **S86.32** Laceration of muscle(s) and tendon(s) of peroneal muscle group at lower leg level
    - ✓7th **S86.321** Laceration of muscle(s) and tendon(s) of ▽ peroneal muscle group at lower leg level, right leg
    - ✓7th **S86.322** Laceration of muscle(s) and tendon(s) of ▽ peroneal muscle group at lower leg level, left leg
    - ✓7th **S86.329** Laceration of muscle(s) and tendon(s) ▽ of peroneal muscle group at lower leg level, unspecified leg
  - ✓6th **S86.39** Other injury of muscle(s) and tendon(s) of peroneal muscle group at lower leg level
    - ✓7th **S86.391** Other injury of muscle(s) and tendon(s) of ▽ peroneal muscle group at lower leg level, right leg
    - ✓7th **S86.392** Other injury of muscle(s) and tendon(s) of ▽ peroneal muscle group at lower leg level, left leg
    - ✓7th **S86.399** Other injury of muscle(s) and tendon(s) ▽ of peroneal muscle group at lower leg level, unspecified leg
- ✓5th **S86.8** Injury of other muscles and tendons at lower leg level
  - ✓6th **S86.80** Unspecified injury of other muscles and tendons at lower leg level
    - ✓7th **S86.801** Unspecified injury of other muscle(s) ▽ and tendon(s) at lower leg level, right leg
    - ✓7th **S86.802** Unspecified injury of other muscle(s) ▽ and tendon(s) at lower leg level, left leg
    - ✓7th **S86.809** Unspecified injury of other muscle(s) ▽ and tendon(s) at lower leg level, unspecified leg
  - ✓6th **S86.81** Strain of other muscles and tendons at lower leg level
    - ✓7th **S86.811** Strain of other muscle(s) and tendon(s) at lower leg level, right leg
    - ✓7th **S86.812** Strain of other muscle(s) and tendon(s) at lower leg level, left leg
    - ✓7th **S86.819** Strain of other muscle(s) and tendon(s) ▽ at lower leg level, unspecified leg
  - ✓6th **S86.82** Laceration of other muscles and tendons at lower leg level
    - ✓7th **S86.821** Laceration of other muscle(s) and tendon(s) at lower leg level, right leg
    - ✓7th **S86.822** Laceration of other muscle(s) and tendon(s) at lower leg level, left leg
    - ✓7th **S86.829** Laceration of other muscle(s) and ▽ tendon(s) at lower leg level, unspecified leg

- ✓6th **S86.89** Other injury of other muscles and tendons at lower leg level
  - ✓7th **S86.891** Other injury of other muscle(s) and tendon(s) at lower leg level, right leg
  - ✓7th **S86.892** Other injury of other muscle(s) and tendon(s) at lower leg level, left leg
  - ✓7th **S86.899** Other injury of other muscle(s) and ▽ tendon(s) at lower leg level, unspecified leg
- ✓5th **S86.9** Injury of unspecified muscle and tendon at lower leg level
  - ✓6th **S86.90** Unspecified injury of unspecified muscle and tendon at lower leg level
    - ✓7th **S86.901** Unspecified injury of unspecified ▽ muscle(s) and tendon(s) at lower leg level, right leg
    - ✓7th **S86.902** Unspecified injury of unspecified ▽ muscle(s) and tendon(s) at lower leg level, left leg
    - ✓7th **S86.909** Unspecified injury of unspecified ▽ muscle(s) and tendon(s) at lower leg evel, unspecified leg
  - ✓6th **S86.91** Strain of unspecified muscle and tendon at lower leg level
    - ✓7th **S86.911** Strain of unspecified muscle(s) and ▽ tendon(s) at lower leg level, right leg
    - ✓7th **S86.912** Strain of unspecified muscle(s) and ▽ tendon(s) at lower leg level, left leg
    - ✓7th **S86.919** Strain of unspecified muscle(s) and ▽ tendon(s) at lower leg level, unspecified leg
  - ✓6th **S86.92** Laceration of unspecified muscle and tendon at lower leg level
    - ✓7th **S86.921** Laceration of unspecified muscle(s) ▽ and tendon(s) at lower leg level, right leg
    - ✓7th **S86.922** Laceration of unspecified muscle(s) ▽ and tendon(s) at lower leg level, left leg
    - ✓7th **S86.929** Laceration of unspecified muscle(s) ▽ and tendon(s) at lower leg level, unspecified leg
  - ✓6th **S86.99** Other injury of unspecified muscle and tendon at lower leg level
    - ✓7th **S86.991** Other injury of unspecified muscle(s) ▽ and tendon(s) at lower leg level, right leg
    - ✓7th **S86.992** Other injury of unspecified muscle(s) ▽ and tendon(s) at lower leg level, left leg
    - ✓7th **S86.999** Other injury of unspecified muscle(s) ▽ and tendon(s) at lower leg level, unspecified leg

- ✓4th **S87** Crushing injury of lower leg

  Use additional code(s) for all associated injuries
  EXCLUDES 2   *crushing injury of ankle and foot (S97.-)*

  The appropriate 7th character is to be added to each code from category S87.
  A   initial encounter
  D   subsequent encounter
  S   sequela

  - ✓5th **S87.0** Crushing injury of knee
    - ✓x7th **S87.00** Crushing injury of unspecified knee ▽
    - ✓x7th **S87.01** Crushing injury of right knee
    - ✓x7th **S87.02** Crushing injury of left knee
  - ✓5th **S87.8** Crushing injury of lower leg
    - ✓x7th **S87.80** Crushing injury of unspecified lower leg ▽
    - ✓x7th **S87.81** Crushing injury of right lower leg
    - ✓x7th **S87.82** Crushing injury of left lower leg

EXCLUDES 1 Not coded here   EXCLUDES 2 Not included here   N Newborn Age: 0   P Pediatric Age: 0-17   M Maternity Age: 12-55   A Adult Age: 15-124

1022   ICD-10-CM 2018

✓4th S88   Traumatic amputation of lower leg

An amputation not identified as partial or complete should be coded to complete.

EXCLUDES 1   *traumatic amputation of ankle and foot (S98.-)*

The appropriate 7th character is to be added to each code from category S88.
A   initial encounter
D   subsequent encounter
S   sequela

✓5th S88.0   Traumatic amputation at knee level

✓6th S88.01   Complete traumatic amputation at knee level

✓7th **S88.011**   Complete traumatic amputation at knee level, right lower leg   HCC

✓7th **S88.012**   Complete traumatic amputation at knee level, left lower leg   HCC

✓7th **S88.019**   Complete traumatic amputation at knee level, unspecified lower leg   HCC ▽

✓6th S88.02   Partial traumatic amputation at knee level

✓7th **S88.021**   Partial traumatic amputation at knee level, right lower leg   HCC

✓7th **S88.022**   Partial traumatic amputation at knee level, left lower leg   HCC

✓7th **S88.029**   Partial traumatic amputation at knee level, unspecified lower leg   HCC ▽

✓5th S88.1   Traumatic amputation at level between knee and ankle

✓6th S88.11   Complete traumatic amputation at level between knee and ankle

✓7th **S88.111**   Complete traumatic amputation at level between knee and ankle, right lower leg   HCC

✓7th **S88.112**   Complete traumatic amputation at level between knee and ankle, left lower leg   HCC

✓7th **S88.119**   Complete traumatic amputation at level between knee and ankle, unspecified lower leg   HCC ▽

✓6th S88.12   Partial traumatic amputation at level between knee and ankle

✓7th **S88.121**   Partial traumatic amputation at level between knee and ankle, right lower leg   HCC

✓7th **S88.122**   Partial traumatic amputation at level between knee and ankle, left lower leg   HCC

✓7th **S88.129**   Partial traumatic amputation at level between knee and ankle, unspecified lower leg   HCC ▽

✓5th S88.9   Traumatic amputation of lower leg, level unspecified

✓6th S88.91   Complete traumatic amputation of lower leg, level unspecified

✓7th **S88.911**   Complete traumatic amputation of right lower leg, level unspecified   HCC ▽

✓7th **S88.912**   Complete traumatic amputation of left lower leg, level unspecified   HCC ▽

✓7th **S88.919**   Complete traumatic amputation of unspecified lower leg, level unspecified   HCC ▽

✓6th S88.92   Partial traumatic amputation of lower leg, level unspecified

✓7th **S88.921**   Partial traumatic amputation of right lower leg, level unspecified   HCC ▽

✓7th **S88.922**   Partial traumatic amputation of left lower leg, level unspecified   HCC ▽

✓7th **S88.929**   Partial traumatic amputation of unspecified lower leg, level unspecified   HCC ▽

✓4th S89   Other and unspecified injuries of lower leg

NOTE   A fracture not indicated as open or closed should be coded to closed.

EXCLUDES 2   *other and unspecified injuries of ankle and foot (S99.-)*
AHA: 2015, 3Q, 37-39

The appropriate 7th character is to be added to each code from subcategories S89.0, S89.1, S89.2, and S89.3.
A   initial encounter for closed fracture
D   subsequent encounter for fracture with routine healing
G   subsequent encounter for fracture with delayed healing
K   subsequent encounter for fracture with nonunion
P   subsequent encounter for fracture with malunion
S   sequela

✓5th S89.0   Physeal fracture of upper end of tibia

✓6th S89.00   Unspecified physeal fracture of upper end of tibia

✓7th **S89.001**   Unspecified physeal fracture of upper end of right tibia   ▽

✓7th **S89.002**   Unspecified physeal fracture of upper end of left tibia   ▽

✓7th **S89.009**   Unspecified physeal fracture of upper end of unspecified tibia   ▽

✓6th S89.01   Salter-Harris Type I physeal fracture of upper end of tibia

✓7th **S89.011**   Salter-Harris Type I physeal fracture of upper end of right tibia

✓7th **S89.012**   Salter-Harris Type I physeal fracture of upper end of left tibia

✓7th **S89.019**   Salter-Harris Type I physeal fracture of upper end of unspecified tibia   ▽

✓6th S89.02   Salter-Harris Type II physeal fracture of upper end of tibia

✓7th **S89.021**   Salter-Harris Type II physeal fracture of upper end of right tibia

✓7th **S89.022**   Salter-Harris Type II physeal fracture of upper end of left tibia

✓7th **S89.029**   Salter-Harris Type II physeal fracture of upper end of unspecified tibia   ▽

✓6th S89.03   Salter-Harris Type III physeal fracture of upper end of tibia

✓7th **S89.031**   Salter-Harris Type III physeal fracture of upper end of right tibia

✓7th **S89.032**   Salter-Harris Type III physeal fracture of upper end of left tibia

✓7th **S89.039**   Salter-Harris Type III physeal fracture of upper end of unspecified tibia   ▽

✓6th S89.04   Salter-Harris Type IV physeal fracture of upper end of tibia

✓7th **S89.041**   Salter-Harris Type IV physeal fracture of upper end of right tibia

✓7th **S89.042**   Salter-Harris Type IV physeal fracture of upper end of left tibia

✓7th **S89.049**   Salter-Harris Type IV physeal fracture of upper end of unspecified tibia   ▽

✓6th S89.09   Other physeal fracture of upper end of tibia

✓7th **S89.091**   Other physeal fracture of upper end of right tibia

✓7th **S89.092**   Other physeal fracture of upper end of left tibia

✓7th **S89.099**   Other physeal fracture of upper end of unspecified tibia   ▽

✓5th S89.1   Physeal fracture of lower end of tibia

✓6th S89.10   Unspecified physeal fracture of lower end of tibia

✓7th **S89.101**   Unspecified physeal fracture of lower end of right tibia   ▽

✓7th **S89.102**   Unspecified physeal fracture of lower end of left tibia   ▽

✓7th **S89.109**   Unspecified physeal fracture of lower end of unspecified tibia   ▽

✓6th S89.11   Salter-Harris Type I physeal fracture of ower end of tibia

✓7th **S89.111**   Salter-Harris Type I physeal fracture of lower end of right tibia

✓7th **S89.112**   Salter-Harris Type I physeal fracture of lower end of left tibia

✓ Additional Character Req   ✓x7th Placeholder Alert   Manifestation   HCC CMS-HCC Condition   ▽ Unspecified Code   ▶◀ Revised Text   ● New Code   ▲ Revised Code Title

ICD-10-CM 2018   1023

S88–S89.112

√7ᵗʰ **S89.119** **Salter-Harris Type I physeal fracture of** ▽
lower end of unspecified tibia

√6ᵗʰ **S89.12** Salter-Harris Type II physeal fracture of lower end of
tibia

√7ᵗʰ **S89.121** **Salter-Harris Type II physeal fracture of**
lower end of right **tibia**

√7ᵗʰ **S89.122** **Salter-Harris Type II physeal fracture of**
lower end of left **tibia**

√7ᵗʰ **S89.129** **Salter-Harris Type II physeal fracture of** ▽
lower end of unspecified tibia

√6ᵗʰ **S89.13** Salter-Harris Type III physeal fracture of lower end of
tibia

EXCLUDES 1   *fracture of medial malleolus (adult) (S82.5-)*

√7ᵗʰ **S89.131** **Salter-Harris Type III physeal fracture of**
lower end of right **tibia**

√7ᵗʰ **S89.132** **Salter-Harris Type III physeal fracture of**
lower end of left **tibia**

√7ᵗʰ **S89.139** **Salter-Harris Type III physeal fracture** ▽
of lower end of unspecified tibia

√6ᵗʰ **S89.14** Salter-Harris Type IV physeal fracture of lower end of
tibia

EXCLUDES 1   *fracture of medial malleolus (adult) (S82.5-)*

√7ᵗʰ **S89.141** **Salter-Harris Type IV physeal fracture of**
lower end of right **tibia**

√7ᵗʰ **S89.142** **Salter-Harris Type IV physeal fracture of**
lower end of left **tibia**

√7ᵗʰ **S89.149** **Salter-Harris Type IV physeal fracture** ▽
of lower end of unspecified tibia

√6ᵗʰ **S89.19** Other physeal fracture of lower end of tibia

√7ᵗʰ **S89.191** **Other physeal fracture of lower end of**
right **tibia**

√7ᵗʰ **S89.192** **Other physeal fracture of lower end of** left
tibia

√7ᵗʰ **S89.199** **Other physeal fracture of lower end of** ▽
unspecified tibia

√5ᵗʰ **S89.2** Physeal fracture of upper end of fibula

√6ᵗʰ **S89.20** Unspecified physeal fracture of upper end of fibula

√7ᵗʰ **S89.201** **Unspecified physeal fracture of upper** ▽
end of right **fibula**

√7ᵗʰ **S89.202** **Unspecified physeal fracture of upper** ▽
end of left **fibula**

√7ᵗʰ **S89.209** **Unspecified physeal fracture of upper** ▽
end of unspecified fibula

√6ᵗʰ **S89.21** Salter-Harris Type I physeal fracture of upper end of
fibula

√7ᵗʰ **S89.211** **Salter-Harris Type I physeal fracture of**
upper end of right **fibula**

√7ᵗʰ **S89.212** **Salter-Harris Type I physeal fracture of**
upper end of left **fibula**

√7ᵗʰ **S89.219** **Salter-Harris Type I physeal fracture of** ▽
upper end of unspecified fibula

√6ᵗʰ **S89.22** Salter-Harris Type II physeal fracture of upper end of
fibula

√7ᵗʰ **S89.221** **Salter-Harris Type II physeal fracture of**
upper end of right **fibula**

√7ᵗʰ **S89.222** **Salter-Harris Type II physeal fracture of**
upper end of left **fibula**

√7ᵗʰ **S89.229** **Salter-Harris Type II physeal fracture of** ▽
upper end of unspecified fibula

√6ᵗʰ **S89.29** Other physeal fracture of upper end of fibula

√7ᵗʰ **S89.291** **Other physeal fracture of upper end of**
right **fibula**

√7ᵗʰ **S89.292** **Other physeal fracture of upper end of** left
fibula

√7ᵗʰ **S89.299** **Other physeal fracture of upper end of** ▽
unspecified fibula

√5ᵗʰ **S89.3** Physeal fracture of lower end of fibula

√6ᵗʰ **S89.30** Unspecified physeal fracture of lower end of fibula

√7ᵗʰ **S89.301** **Unspecified physeal fracture of lower** ▽
end of right **fibula**

√7ᵗʰ **S89.302** **Unspecified physeal fracture of lower** ▽
end of left **fibula**

√7ᵗʰ **S89.309** **Unspecified physeal fracture of lower** ▽
end of unspecified fibula

√6ᵗʰ **S89.31** Salter-Harris Type I physeal fracture of lower end of
fibula

√7ᵗʰ **S89.311** **Salter-Harris Type I physeal fracture of**
lower end of right **fibula**

√7ᵗʰ **S89.312** **Salter-Harris Type I physeal fracture of**
lower end of left **fibula**

√7ᵗʰ **S89.319** **Salter-Harris Type I physeal fracture of** ▽
lower end of unspecified fibula

√6ᵗʰ **S89.32** Salter-Harris Type II physeal fracture of lower end of
fibula

√7ᵗʰ **S89.321** **Salter-Harris Type II physeal fracture of**
lower end of right **fibula**

√7ᵗʰ **S89.322** **Salter-Harris Type II physeal fracture of**
lower end of left **fibula**

√7ᵗʰ **S89.329** **Salter-Harris Type II physeal fracture** ▽
of lower end of unspecified fibula

√6ᵗʰ **S89.39** Other physeal fracture of lower end of fibula

√7ᵗʰ **S89.391** **Other physeal fracture of lower end of**
right **fibula**

√7ᵗʰ **S89.392** **Other physeal fracture of lower end of** left
fibula

√7ᵗʰ **S89.399** **Other physeal fracture of lower end of** ▽
unspecified fibula

√5ᵗʰ **S89.8** **Other specified injuries of** lower leg

> The appropriate 7th character is to be added to each code
> in subcategory S89.8.
> A   initial encounter
> D   subsequent encounter
> S   sequela

√x7ᵗʰ **S89.80** **Other specified injuries of unspecified lower leg** ▽

√x7ᵗʰ **S89.81** **Other specified injuries of** right **lower leg**

√x7ᵗʰ **S89.82** **Other specified injuries of** left **lower leg**

√5ᵗʰ **S89.9** **Unspecified injury of** lower leg

> The appropriate 7th character is to be added to each code
> in subcategory S89.9.
> A   initial encounter
> D   subsequent encounter
> S   sequela

√x7ᵗʰ **S89.90** **Unspecified injury of unspecified lower leg** ▽

S89.91 **Unspecified injury of** right **lower leg** ▽

√x7ᵗʰ **S89.92** **Unspecified injury of** left **lower leg** ▽

Injuries to the ankle and foot (S90-S99)

EXCLUDES 2   *burns and corrosions (T20-T32)*
fracture of ankle and malleolus (S82.-)
frostbite (T33-T34)
insect bite or sting, venomous (T63.4)

√4ᵗʰ **S90** **Superficial injury of ankle, foot and toes**

> The appropriate 7th character is to be added to each code from
> category S90.
> A   initial encounter
> D   subsequent encounter
> S   sequela

√5ᵗʰ **S90.0** **Contusion of** ankle

√x7ᵗʰ **S90.00** **Contusion of unspecified ankle** ▽

√x7ᵗʰ **S90.01** **Contusion of** right **ankle**

√x7ᵗʰ **S90.02** **Contusion of** left **ankle**

√5ᵗʰ **S90.1** **Contusion of** toe without damage to nail

√6ᵗʰ **S90.11** Contusion of great toe without damage to nail

√7ᵗʰ **S90.111** **Contusion of** right **great toe without**
damage to nail

√7ᵗʰ **S90.112** **Contusion of** left **great toe without**
damage to nail

√7ᵗʰ **S90.119** **Contusion of unspecified great toe** ▽
without damage to nail

√6ᵗʰ **S90.12** Contusion of lesser toe without damage to nail

√7ᵗʰ **S90.121** **Contusion of** right **lesser toe(s) without**
damage to nail

√7ᵗʰ **S90.122** **Contusion of** left **lesser toe(s) without**
damage to nail

EXCLUDES 1 Not coded here   EXCLUDES 2 Not included here   N Newborn Age: 0   P Pediatric Age: 0-17   M Maternity Age: 12-55   A Adult Age: 15-124

1024   ICD-10-CM 2018

√7ᵗʰ **S90.129** **Contusion of unspecified lesser toe(s)** ▽
without damage to nail
Contusion of toe NOS

√5ᵗʰ **S90.2** **Contusion of toe with damage to nail**

√6ᵗʰ **S90.21** **Contusion of great toe with damage to nail**

√7ᵗʰ **S90.211** **Contusion of right great toe with damage to nail**

√7ᵗʰ **S90.212** **Contusion of left great toe with damage to nail**

√7ᵗʰ **S90.219** **Contusion of unspecified great toe with** ▽ **damage to nail**

√6ᵗʰ **S90.22** **Contusion of lesser toe with damage to nail**

√7ᵗʰ **S90.221** **Contusion of right lesser toe(s) with damage to nail**

√7ᵗʰ **S90.222** **Contusion of left lesser toe(s) with damage to nail**

√7ᵗʰ **S90.229** **Contusion of unspecified lesser toe(s)** ▽ **with damage to nail**

√5ᵗʰ **S90.3** **Contusion of foot**
EXCLUDES 2   contusion of toes (S90.1-, S90.2-)

√×7ᵗʰ **S90.30** **Contusion of unspecified foot** ▽
Contusion of foot NOS

√×7ᵗʰ **S90.31** **Contusion of right foot**

√×7ᵗʰ **S90.32** **Contusion of left foot**

√5ᵗʰ **S90.4** **Other superficial injuries of toe**

√6ᵗʰ **S90.41** **Abrasion of toe**

√7ᵗʰ **S90.411** **Abrasion, right great toe**

√7ᵗʰ **S90.412** **Abrasion, left great toe**

√7ᵗʰ **S90.413** **Abrasion, unspecified great toe** ▽

√7ᵗʰ **S90.414** **Abrasion, right lesser toe(s)**

√7ᵗʰ **S90.415** **Abrasion, left lesser toe(s)**

√7ᵗʰ **S90.416** **Abrasion, unspecified lesser toe(s)** ▽

√6ᵗʰ **S90.42** **Blister (nonthermal) of toe**

√7ᵗʰ **S90.421** **Blister (nonthermal), right great toe**

√7ᵗʰ **S90.422** **Blister (nonthermal), left great toe**

√7ᵗʰ **S90.423** **Blister (nonthermal), unspecified great** ▽ **toe**

√7ᵗʰ **S90.424** **Blister (nonthermal), right lesser toe(s)**

√7ᵗʰ **S90.425** **Blister (nonthermal), left lesser toe(s)**

√7ᵗʰ **S90.426** **Blister (nonthermal), unspecified lesser** ▽ **toe(s)**

√6ᵗʰ **S90.44** **External constriction of toe**
Hair tourniquet syndrome of toe

√7ᵗʰ **S90.441** **External constriction, right great toe**

√7ᵗʰ **S90.442** **External constriction, left great toe**

√7ᵗʰ **S90.443** **External constriction, unspecified** ▽ **great toe**

√7ᵗʰ **S90.444** **External constriction, right lesser toe(s)**

√7ᵗʰ **S90.445** **External constriction, left lesser toe(s)**

√7ᵗʰ **S90.446** **External constriction, unspecified** ▽ **lesser toe(s)**

√6ᵗʰ **S90.45** **Superficial foreign body of toe**
Splinter in the toe

√7ᵗʰ **S90.451** **Superficial foreign body, right great toe**

√7ᵗʰ **S90.452** **Superficial foreign body, left great toe**

√7ᵗʰ **S90.453** **Superficial foreign body, unspecified** ▽ **great toe**

√7ᵗʰ **S90.454** **Superficial foreign body, right lesser toe(s)**

√7ᵗʰ **S90.455** **Superficial foreign body, left lesser toe(s)**

√7ᵗʰ **S90.456** **Superficial foreign body, unspecified** ▽ **lesser toe(s)**

√6ᵗʰ **S90.46** **Insect bite (nonvenomous) of toe**

√7ᵗʰ **S90.461** **Insect bite (nonvenomous), right great toe**

√7ᵗʰ **S90.462** **Insect bite (nonvenomous), left great toe**

√7ᵗʰ **S90.463** **Insect bite (nonvenomous), unspecified** ▽ **great toe**

√7ᵗʰ **S90.464** **Insect bite (nonvenomous), right lesser toe(s)**

√7ᵗʰ **S90.465** **Insect bite (nonvenomous), left lesser toe(s)**

√7ᵗʰ **S90.466** **Insect bite (nonvenomous), unspecified** ▽ **lesser toe(s)**

√6ᵗʰ **S90.47** **Other superficial bite of toe**
EXCLUDES 1   open bite of toe (S91.15-, S91.25-)

√7ᵗʰ **S90.471** **Other superficial bite of right great toe**

√7ᵗʰ **S90.472** **Other superficial bite of left great toe**

√7ᵗʰ **S90.473** **Other superficial bite of unspecified** ▽ **great toe**

√7ᵗʰ **S90.474** **Other superficial bite of right lesser toe(s)**

√7ᵗʰ **S90.475** **Other superficial bite of left lesser toe(s)**

√7ᵗʰ **S90.476** **Other superficial bite of unspecified** ▽ **lesser toe(s)**

√5ᵗʰ **S90.5** **Other superficial injuries of ankle**

√6ᵗʰ **S90.51** **Abrasion of ankle**

√7ᵗʰ **S90.511** **Abrasion, right ankle**

√7ᵗʰ **S90.512** **Abrasion, left ankle**

√7ᵗʰ **S90.519** **Abrasion, unspecified ankle** ▽

√6ᵗʰ **S90.52** **Blister (nonthermal) of ankle**

√7ᵗʰ **S90.521** **Blister (nonthermal), right ankle**

√7ᵗʰ **S90.522** **Blister (nonthermal), left ankle**

√7ᵗʰ **S90.529** **Blister (nonthermal), unspecified ankle** ▽

√6ᵗʰ **S90.54** **External constriction of ankle**

√7ᵗʰ **S90.541** **External constriction, right ankle**

√7ᵗʰ **S90.542** **External constriction, left ankle**

√7ᵗʰ **S90.549** **External constriction, unspecified ankle** ▽

√6ᵗʰ **S90.55** **Superficial foreign body of ankle**
Splinter in the ankle

√7ᵗʰ **S90.551** **Superficial foreign body, right ankle**

√7ᵗʰ **S90.552** **Superficial foreign body, left ankle**

√7ᵗʰ **S90.559** **Superficial foreign body, unspecified** ▽ **ankle**

√6ᵗʰ **S90.56** **Insect bite (nonvenomous) of ankle**

√7ᵗʰ **S90.561** **Insect bite (nonvenomous), right ankle**

√7ᵗʰ **S90.562** **Insect bite (nonvenomous), left ankle**

√7ᵗʰ **S90.569** **Insect bite (nonvenomous), unspecified** ▽ **ankle**

√6ᵗʰ **S90.57** **Other superficial bite of ankle**
EXCLUDES 1   open bite of ankle (S91.05-)

√7ᵗʰ **S90.571** **Other superficial bite of ankle, right ankle**

√7ᵗʰ **S90.572** **Other superficial bite of ankle, left ankle**

√7ᵗʰ **S90.579** **Other superficial bite of ankle,** ▽ **unspecified ankle**

√5ᵗʰ **S90.8** **Other superficial injuries of foot**

√6ᵗʰ **S90.81** **Abrasion of foot**

√7ᵗʰ **S90.811** **Abrasion, right foot**

√7ᵗʰ **S90.812** **Abrasion, left foot**

√7ᵗʰ **S90.819** **Abrasion, unspecified foot** ▽

√6ᵗʰ **S90.82** **Blister (nonthermal) of foot**

√7ᵗʰ **S90.821** **Blister (nonthermal), right foot**

√7ᵗʰ **S90.822** **Blister (nonthermal), left foot**

√7ᵗʰ **S90.829** **Blister (nonthermal), unspecified foot** ▽

√6ᵗʰ **S90.84** **External constriction of foot**

√7ᵗʰ **S90.841** **External constriction, right foot**

√7ᵗʰ **S90.842** **External constriction, left foot**

√7ᵗʰ **S90.849** **External constriction, unspecified foot** ▽

√6ᵗʰ **S90.85** **Superficial foreign body of foot**
Splinter in the foot

√7ᵗʰ **S90.851** **Superficial foreign body, right foot**

√7ᵗʰ **S90.852** **Superficial foreign body, left foot**

√7ᵗʰ **S90.859** **Superficial foreign body, unspecified** ▽ **foot**

√6ᵗʰ **S90.86** **Insect bite (nonvenomous) of foot**

√7ᵗʰ **S90.861** **Insect bite (nonvenomous), right foot**

√7ᵗʰ **S90.862** **Insect bite (nonvenomous), left foot**

√7ᵗʰ **S90.869** **Insect bite (nonvenomous), unspecified** ▽ **foot**

√6ᵗʰ **S90.87** **Other superficial bite of foot**
EXCLUDES 1   open bite of foot (S91.35-)

√7ᵗʰ **S90.871** **Other superficial bite of right foot**

☑ Additional Character Req   √×7ᵗʰ Placeholder Alert   Manifestation   ᴴᶜᶜ CMS-HCC Condition   ▽ Unspecified Code   ▶◀ Revised Text   ● New Code   ▲ Revised Code Title

✓7ᵗʰ **S90.872 Other superficial bite of** left **foot**

✓7ᵗʰ **S90.879 Other superficial bite of unspecified foot** ▽

✓5ᵗʰ **S90.9 Unspecified superficial injury of ankle, foot and toe**

  ✓6ᵗʰ **S90.91 Unspecified superficial injury of** ankle

   ✓7ᵗʰ **S90.911 Unspecified superficial injury of** right **ankle** ▽

   ✓7ᵗʰ **S90.912 Unspecified superficial injury of** left **ankle** ▽

   ✓7ᵗʰ **S90.919 Unspecified superficial injury of unspecified ankle** ▽

  ✓6ᵗʰ **S90.92 Unspecified superficial injury of** foot

   ✓7ᵗʰ **S90.921 Unspecified superficial injury of** right **foot** ▽

   ✓7ᵗʰ **S90.922 Unspecified superficial injury of** left **foot** ▽

   ✓7ᵗʰ **S90.929 Unspecified superficial injury of unspecified foot** ▽

  ✓6ᵗʰ **S90.93 Unspecified superficial injury of** toes

   ✓7ᵗʰ **S90.931 Unspecified superficial injury of right great toe** ▽

   ✓7ᵗʰ **S90.932 Unspecified superficial injury of left great toe** ▽

   ✓7ᵗʰ **S90.933 Unspecified superficial injury of unspecified great toe** ▽

   ✓7ᵗʰ **S90.934 Unspecified superficial injury of right lesser toe(s)** ▽

   ✓7ᵗʰ **S90.935 Unspecified superficial injury of left lesser toe(s)** ▽

   ✓7ᵗʰ **S90.936 Unspecified superficial injury of unspecified lesser toe(s)** ▽

✓4ᵗʰ **S91 Open wound of ankle, foot and toes**

 Code also any associated wound infection

 EXCLUDES 1 open fracture of ankle, foot and toes (S92-with 7th character B)
 traumatic amputation of ankle and foot (S98.-)

 The appropriate 7th character is to be added to each code from category S91.
 A   initial encounter
 D   subsequent encounter
 S   sequela

 ✓5ᵗʰ **S91.0 Open wound of** ankle

  ✓6ᵗʰ **S91.00 Unspecified open wound of ankle**

   ✓7ᵗʰ **S91.001 Unspecified open wound,** right **ankle** ▽

   S91.002 Unspecified open wound, left **ankle** ▽

   ✓7ᵗʰ **S91.009 Unspecified open wound, unspecified ankle** ▽

  ✓6ᵗʰ **S91.01 Laceration without foreign body of ankle**

   ✓7ᵗʰ **S91.011 Laceration without foreign body,** right **ankle**

   ✓7ᵗʰ **S91.012 Laceration without foreign body,** left **ankle**

   ✓7ᵗʰ **S91.019 Laceration without foreign body, unspecified ankle** ▽

  ✓6ᵗʰ **S91.02 Laceration with foreign body of ankle**

   ✓7ᵗʰ **S91.021 Laceration with foreign body,** right **ankle**

   ✓7ᵗʰ **S91.022 Laceration with foreign body,** left **ankle**

   ✓7ᵗʰ **S91.029 Laceration with foreign body, unspecified ankle** ▽

  ✓6ᵗʰ **S91.03 Puncture wound without foreign body of ankle**

   ✓7ᵗʰ **S91.031 Puncture wound without foreign body, right ankle**

   ✓7ᵗʰ **S91.032 Puncture wound without foreign body, left ankle**

   ✓7ᵗʰ **S91.039 Puncture wound without foreign body, unspecified ankle** ▽

  ✓6ᵗʰ **S91.04 Puncture wound with foreign body of ankle**

   ✓7ᵗʰ **S91.041 Puncture wound with foreign body, right ankle**

   ✓7ᵗʰ **S91.042 Puncture wound with foreign body, left ankle**

   ✓7ᵗʰ **S91.049 Puncture wound with foreign body, unspecified ankle** ▽

✓6ᵗʰ **S91.05 Open bite of ankle**

 EXCLUDES 1 superficial bite of ankle (S90.56-, S90.57-)

 ✓7ᵗʰ **S91.051 Open bite,** right **ankle**

 ✓7ᵗʰ **S91.052 Open bite,** left **ankle**

 ✓7ᵗʰ **S91.059 Open bite, unspecified ankle** ▽

✓5ᵗʰ **S91.1 Open wound of** toe without damage to nail

  ✓6ᵗʰ **S91.10 Unspecified open wound of toe without damage to nail**

   ✓7ᵗʰ **S91.101 Unspecified open wound of** right great **toe without damage to nail** ▽

   ✓7ᵗʰ **S91.102 Unspecified open wound of** left great **toe without damage to nail** ▽

   ✓7ᵗʰ **S91.103 Unspecified open wound of unspecified great toe without damage to nail** ▽

   ✓7ᵗʰ **S91.104 Unspecified open wound of** right lesser **toe(s) without damage to nail** ▽

   ✓7ᵗʰ **S91.105 Unspecified open wound of** left lesser **toe(s) without damage to nail** ▽

   ✓7ᵗʰ **S91.106 Unspecified open wound of unspecified lesser toe(s) without damage to nail** ▽

   ✓7ᵗʰ **S91.109 Unspecified open wound of unspecified toe(s) without damage to nail** ▽

  ✓6ᵗʰ **S91.11 Laceration without foreign body of toe without damage to nail**

   ✓7ᵗʰ **S91.111 Laceration without foreign body of** right great **toe without damage to nail**

   ✓7ᵗʰ **S91.112 Laceration without foreign body of** left great **toe without damage to nail**

   ✓7ᵗʰ **S91.113 Laceration without foreign body of unspecified great toe without damage to nail** ▽

   ✓7ᵗʰ **S91.114 Laceration without foreign body of** right lesser **toe(s) without damage to nail**

   ✓7ᵗʰ **S91.115 Laceration without foreign body of** left lesser **toe(s) without damage to nail**

   ✓7ᵗʰ **S91.116 Laceration without foreign body of unspecified lesser toe(s) without damage to nail** ▽

   ✓7ᵗʰ **S91.119 Laceration without foreign body of unspecified toe without damage to nail** ▽

  ✓6ᵗʰ **S91.12 Laceration with foreign body of toe without damage to nail**

   ✓7ᵗʰ **S91.121 Laceration with foreign body of** right great **toe without damage to nail**

   ✓7ᵗʰ **S91.122 Laceration with foreign body of** left great **toe without damage to nail**

   ✓7ᵗʰ **S91.123 Laceration with foreign body of unspecified great toe without damage to nail** ▽

   ✓7ᵗʰ **S91.124 Laceration with foreign body of** right lesser **toe(s) without damage to nail**

   ✓7ᵗʰ **S91.125 Laceration with foreign body of** left lesser **toe(s) without damage to nail**

   ✓7ᵗʰ **S91.126 Laceration with foreign body of unspecified lesser toe(s) without damage to nail** ▽

   ✓7ᵗʰ **S91.129 Laceration with foreign body of unspecified toe(s) without damage to nail** ▽

  ✓6ᵗʰ **S91.13 Puncture wound without foreign body of toe without damage to nail**

   ✓7ᵗʰ **S91.131 Puncture wound without foreign body of right great toe without damage to nail**

   ✓7ᵗʰ **S91.132 Puncture wound without foreign body of left great toe without damage to nail**

   ✓7ᵗʰ **S91.133 Puncture wound without foreign body of unspecified great toe without damage to nail** ▽

   ✓7ᵗʰ **S91.134 Puncture wound without foreign body of right lesser toe(s) without damage to nail**

   ✓7ᵗʰ **S91.135 Puncture wound without foreign body of left lesser toe(s) without damage to nail**

EXCLUDES 1 Not coded here   *EXCLUDES 2* Not included here   N Newborn Age: 0   P Pediatric Age: 0-17   M Maternity Age: 12-55   A Adult Age: 15-124

1026   ICD-10-CM 2018

√7ᵗʰ **S91.136** Puncture wound without foreign body of unspecified lesser toe(s) without damage to nail ▽

√7ᵗʰ **S91.139** Puncture wound without foreign body of unspecified toe(s) without damage to nail ▽

√6ᵗʰ **S91.14** Puncture wound with foreign body of toe without damage to nail

√7ᵗʰ **S91.141** Puncture wound with foreign body of right great toe without damage to nail

√7ᵗʰ **S91.142** Puncture wound with foreign body of left great toe without damage to nail

√7ᵗʰ **S91.143** Puncture wound with foreign body of unspecified great toe without damage to nail ▽

√7ᵗʰ **S91.144** Puncture wound with foreign body of right lesser toe(s) without damage to nail

√7ᵗʰ **S91.145** Puncture wound with foreign body of left lesser toe(s) without damage to nail

√7ᵗʰ **S91.146** Puncture wound with foreign body of unspecified lesser toe(s) without damage to nail ▽

√7ᵗʰ **S91.149** Puncture wound with foreign body of unspecified toe(s) without damage to nail ▽

√6ᵗʰ **S91.15** Open bite of toe without damage to nail
Bite of toe NOS
EXCLUDES 1   *superficial bite of toe (S90.46-, S90.47-)*

√7ᵗʰ **S91.151** Open bite of right great toe without damage to nail

√7ᵗʰ **S91.152** Open bite of left great toe without damage to nail

√7ᵗʰ **S91.153** Open bite of unspecified great toe without damage to nail ▽

√7ᵗʰ **S91.154** Open bite of right lesser toe(s) without damage to nail

√7ᵗʰ **S91.155** Open bite of left lesser toe(s) without damage to nail

√7ᵗʰ **S91.156** Open bite of unspecified lesser toe(s) without damage to nail ▽

√7ᵗʰ **S91.159** Open bite of unspecified toe(s) without damage to nail ▽

√5ᵗʰ **S91.2** Open wound of toe with damage to nail

√6ᵗʰ **S91.20** Unspecified open wound of toe with damage to nail

√7ᵗʰ **S91.201** Unspecified open wound of right great toe with damage to nail ▽

√7ᵗʰ **S91.202** Unspecified open wound of left great toe with damage to nail ▽

√7ᵗʰ **S91.203** Unspecified open wound of unspecified great toe with damage to nail ▽

√7ᵗʰ **S91.204** Unspecified open wound of right lesser toe(s) with damage to nail ▽

√7ᵗʰ **S91.205** Unspecified open wound of left lesser toe(s) with damage to nail ▽

√7ᵗʰ **S91.206** Unspecified open wound of unspecified lesser toe(s) with damage to nail ▽

√7ᵗʰ **S91.209** Unspecified open wound of unspecified toe(s) with damage to nail ▽

√6ᵗʰ **S91.21** Laceration without foreign body of toe with damage to nail

√7ᵗʰ **S91.211** Laceration without foreign body of right great toe with damage to nail

√7ᵗʰ **S91.212** Laceration without foreign body of left great toe with damage to nail

√7ᵗʰ **S91.213** Laceration without foreign body of unspecified great toe with damage to nail ▽

√7ᵗʰ **S91.214** Laceration without foreign body of right lesser toe(s) with damage to nail

√7ᵗʰ **S91.215** Laceration without foreign body of left lesser toe(s) with damage to nail

√7ᵗʰ **S91.216** Laceration without foreign body of unspecified lesser toe(s) with damage to nail ▽

√7ᵗʰ **S91.219** Laceration without foreign body of unspecified toe(s) with damage to nail ▽

√6ᵗʰ **S91.22** Laceration with foreign body of toe with damage to nail

√7ᵗʰ **S91.221** Laceration with foreign body of right great toe with damage to nail

√7ᵗʰ **S91.222** Laceration with foreign body of left great toe with damage to nail

√7ᵗʰ **S91.223** Laceration with foreign body of unspecified great toe with damage to nail ▽

√7ᵗʰ **S91.224** Laceration with foreign body of right lesser toe(s) with damage to nail

√7ᵗʰ **S91.225** Laceration with foreign body of left lesser toe(s) with damage to nail

√7ᵗʰ **S91.226** Laceration with foreign body of unspecified lesser toe(s) with damage to nail ▽

√7ᵗʰ **S91.229** Laceration with foreign body of unspecified toe(s) with damage to nail ▽

√6ᵗʰ **S91.23** Puncture wound without foreign body of toe with damage to nail

√7ᵗʰ **S91.231** Puncture wound without foreign body of right great toe with damage to nail

√7ᵗʰ **S91.232** Puncture wound without foreign body of left great toe with damage to nail

√7ᵗʰ **S91.233** Puncture wound without foreign body of unspecified great toe with damage to nail ▽

√7ᵗʰ **S91.234** Puncture wound without foreign body of right lesser toe(s) with damage to nail

√7ᵗʰ **S91.235** Puncture wound without foreign body of left lesser toe(s) with damage to nail

√7ᵗʰ **S91.236** Puncture wound without foreign body of unspecified lesser toe(s) with damage to nail ▽

√7ᵗʰ **S91.239** Puncture wound without foreign body of unspecified toe(s) with damage to nail ▽

√6ᵗʰ **S91.24** Puncture wound with foreign body of toe with damage to nail

√7ᵗʰ **S91.241** Puncture wound with foreign body of right great toe with damage to nail

√7ᵗʰ **S91.242** Puncture wound with foreign body of left great toe with damage to nail

√7ᵗʰ **S91.243** Puncture wound with foreign body of unspecified great toe with damage to nail ▽

√7ᵗʰ **S91.244** Puncture wound with foreign body of right lesser toe(s) with damage to nail

√7ᵗʰ **S91.245** Puncture wound with foreign body of left lesser toe(s) with damage to nail

√7ᵗʰ **S91.246** Puncture wound with foreign body of unspecified lesser toe(s) with damage to nail ▽

√7ᵗʰ **S91.249** Puncture wound with foreign body of unspecified toe(s) with damage to nail ▽

√6ᵗʰ **S91.25** Open bite of toe with damage to nail
Bite of toe with damage to nail NOS
EXCLUDES 1   *superficial bite of toe (S90.46-, S90.47-)*

√7ᵗʰ **S91.251** Open bite of right great toe with damage to nail

√7ᵗʰ **S91.252** Open bite of left great toe with damage to nail

√7ᵗʰ **S91.253** Open bite of unspecified great toe with damage to nail ▽

√7ᵗʰ **S91.254** Open bite of right lesser toe(s) with damage to nail

√7ᵗʰ **S91.255** Open bite of left lesser toe(s) with damage to nail

√7ᵗʰ **S91.256** Open bite of unspecified lesser toe(s) with damage to nail ▽

√7ᵗʰ **S91.259** Open bite of unspecified toe(s) with damage to nail ▽

√5ᵗʰ **S91.3** Open wound of foot

√6ᵗʰ **S91.30** Unspecified open wound of foot

√7ᵗʰ **S91.301** Unspecified open wound, right foot ▽

S91.302 Unspecified open wound, left foot ▽

√7ᵗʰ **S91.309** Unspecified open wound, unspecified foot ▽

☑ Additional Character Req   √x7ᵗʰ Placeholder Alert   Manifestation   ʜᴄᴄ CMS-HCC Condition   ▽ Unspecified Code   ▶◀ Revised Text   ● New Code   ▲ Revised Code Title

√6ᵗʰ **S91.31** Laceration without foreign body **of foot**
- √7ᵗʰ **S91.311** **Laceration without foreign body, right foot**
- √7ᵗʰ **S91.312** **Laceration without foreign body, left foot**
- √7ᵗʰ **S91.319** **Laceration without foreign body, unspecified foot** ▽

√6ᵗʰ **S91.32** Laceration with foreign body **of foot**
- √7ᵗʰ **S91.321** **Laceration with foreign body, right foot**
- √7ᵗʰ **S91.322** **Laceration with foreign body, left foot**
- √7ᵗʰ **S91.329** **Laceration with foreign body, unspecified foot** ▽

√6ᵗʰ **S91.33** Puncture wound without foreign body **of foot**
- √7ᵗʰ **S91.331** **Puncture wound without foreign body, right foot**
- √7ᵗʰ **S91.332** **Puncture wound without foreign body, left foot**
- √7ᵗʰ **S91.339** **Puncture wound without foreign body, unspecified foot** ▽

√6ᵗʰ **S91.34** Puncture wound with foreign body **of foot**
- √7ᵗʰ **S91.341** **Puncture wound with foreign body, right foot**
- √7ᵗʰ **S91.342** **Puncture wound with foreign body, left foot**
- √7ᵗʰ **S91.349** **Puncture wound with foreign body, unspecified foot** ▽

√6ᵗʰ **S91.35** Open bite **of foot**
- EXCLUDES 1   *superficial bite of foot (S90.86-, S90.87-)*
- √7ᵗʰ **S91.351** **Open bite, right foot**
- √7ᵗʰ **S91.352** **Open bite, left foot**
- √7ᵗʰ **S91.359** **Open bite, unspecified foot** ▽

√4ᵗʰ **S92** **Fracture of foot and toe, except ankle**
- NOTE   A fracture not indicated as displaced or nondisplaced should be coded to displaced.
  A fracture not indicated as open or closed should be coded to closed.
- EXCLUDES 1   *traumatic amputation of ankle and foot (S98.-)*
- EXCLUDES 2   *fracture of ankle (S82.-)*
  fracture of malleolus (S82.-)
- AHA: 2015, 3Q, 37-39

The appropriate 7th character is to be added to each code from category S92.
- A   initial encounter for closed fracture
- B   initial encounter for open fracture
- D   subsequent encounter for fracture with routine healing
- G   subsequent encounter for fracture with delayed healing
- K   subsequent encounter for fracture with nonunion
- P   subsequent encounter for fracture with malunion
- S   sequela

√5ᵗʰ **S92.0** **Fracture of calcaneus**
Heel bone
Os calcis
- EXCLUDES 2   *physeal fracture of calcaneus (S99.0-)*

√6ᵗʰ **S92.00** **Unspecified fracture of calcaneus**
- √7ᵗʰ **S92.001** **Unspecified fracture of right calcaneus** ▽
- √7ᵗʰ **S92.002** **Unspecified fracture of left calcaneus** ▽
- **S92.009** **Unspecified fracture of unspecified calcaneus** ▽

√6ᵗʰ **S92.01** **Fracture of body of calcaneus**
- √7ᵗʰ **S92.011** **Displaced fracture of body of right calcaneus**
- √7ᵗʰ **S92.012** **Displaced fracture of body of left calcaneus**
- √7ᵗʰ **S92.013** **Displaced fracture of body of unspecified calcaneus** ▽
- √7ᵗʰ **S92.014** **Nondisplaced fracture of body of right calcaneus**
- √7ᵗʰ **S92.015** **Nondisplaced fracture of body of left calcaneus**
- √7ᵗʰ **S92.016** **Nondisplaced fracture of body of unspecified calcaneus** ▽

√6ᵗʰ **S92.02** **Fracture of anterior process of calcaneus**
- √7ᵗʰ **S92.021** **Displaced fracture of anterior process of right calcaneus**

- √7ᵗʰ **S92.022** **Displaced fracture of anterior process of left calcaneus**
- √7ᵗʰ **S92.023** **Displaced fracture of anterior process of unspecified calcaneus** ▽
- √7ᵗʰ **S92.024** **Nondisplaced fracture of anterior process of right calcaneus**
- √7ᵗʰ **S92.025** **Nondisplaced fracture of anterior process of left calcaneus**
- √7ᵗʰ **S92.026** **Nondisplaced fracture of anterior process of unspecified calcaneus** ▽

√6ᵗʰ **S92.03** **Avulsion fracture of tuberosity of calcaneus**
- √7ᵗʰ **S92.031** **Displaced avulsion fracture of tuberosity of right calcaneus**
- √7ᵗʰ **S92.032** **Displaced avulsion fracture of tuberosity of left calcaneus**
- √7ᵗʰ **S92.033** **Displaced avulsion fracture of tuberosity of unspecified calcaneus** ▽
- √7ᵗʰ **S92.034** **Nondisplaced avulsion fracture of tuberosity of right calcaneus**
- √7ᵗʰ **S92.035** **Nondisplaced avulsion fracture of tuberosity of left calcaneus**
- √7ᵗʰ **S92.036** **Nondisplaced avulsion fracture of tuberosity of unspecified calcaneus** ▽

√6ᵗʰ **S92.04** **Other fracture of tuberosity of calcaneus**
- √7ᵗʰ **S92.041** **Displaced other fracture of tuberosity of right calcaneus**
- √7ᵗʰ **S92.042** **Displaced other fracture of tuberosity of left calcaneus**
- √7ᵗʰ **S92.043** **Displaced other fracture of tuberosity of unspecified calcaneus** ▽
- √7ᵗʰ **S92.044** **Nondisplaced other fracture of tuberosity of right calcaneus**
- √7ᵗʰ **S92.045** **Nondisplaced other fracture of tuberosity of left calcaneus**
- √7ᵗʰ **S92.046** **Nondisplaced other fracture of tuberosity of unspecified calcaneus** ▽

√6ᵗʰ **S92.05** **Other extraarticular fracture of calcaneus**
- √7ᵗʰ **S92.051** **Displaced other extraarticular fracture of right calcaneus**
- √7ᵗʰ **S92.052** **Displaced other extraarticular fracture of left calcaneus**
- √7ᵗʰ **S92.053** **Displaced other extraarticular fracture of unspecified calcaneus** ▽
- √7ᵗʰ **S92.054** **Nondisplaced other extraarticular fracture of right calcaneus**
- √7ᵗʰ **S92.055** **Nondisplaced other extraarticular fracture of left calcaneus**
- √7ᵗʰ **S92.056** **Nondisplaced other extraarticular fracture of unspecified calcaneus** ▽

√6ᵗʰ **S92.06** **Intraarticular fracture of calcaneus**
- √7ᵗʰ **S92.061** **Displaced intraarticular fracture of right calcaneus**
- √7ᵗʰ **S92.062** **Displaced intraarticular fracture of left calcaneus**
- √7ᵗʰ **S92.063** **Displaced intraarticular fracture of unspecified calcaneus** ▽
- √7ᵗʰ **S92.064** **Nondisplaced intraarticular fracture of right calcaneus**
- √7ᵗʰ **S92.065** **Nondisplaced intraarticular fracture of left calcaneus**
- √7ᵗʰ **S92.066** **Nondisplaced intraarticular fracture of unspecified calcaneus** ▽

√5ᵗʰ **S92.1** **Fracture of talus**
Astragalus
√6ᵗʰ **S92.10** **Unspecified fracture of talus**
- √7ᵗʰ **S92.101** **Unspecified fracture of right talus** ▽
- √7ᵗʰ **S92.102** **Unspecified fracture of left talus** ▽
- **S92.109** **Unspecified fracture of unspecified talus** ▽

√6ᵗʰ **S92.11** **Fracture of neck of talus**
- √7ᵗʰ **S92.111** **Displaced fracture of neck of right talus**
- √7ᵗʰ **S92.112** **Displaced fracture of neck of left talus**
- √7ᵗʰ **S92.113** **Displaced fracture of neck of unspecified talus** ▽

EXCLUDES 1 Not coded here   EXCLUDES 2 Not included here   N Newborn Age: 0   P Pediatric Age: 0-17   M Maternity Age: 12-55   A Adult Age: 15-124

1028   ICD-10-CM 2018

S91.31–S92.113

√7ᵗʰ **S92.114** **Nondisplaced fracture of neck of** right talus

√7ᵗʰ **S92.115** **Nondisplaced fracture of neck of** left **talus**

√7ᵗʰ **S92.116** **Nondisplaced fracture of neck of** unspecified **talus** ▽

√6ᵗʰ **S92.12** **Fracture of** body **of talus**

√7ᵗʰ **S92.121** **Displaced fracture of body of** right **talus**

√7ᵗʰ **S92.122** **Displaced fracture of body of** left **talus**

√7ᵗʰ **S92.123** **Displaced fracture of body of** unspecified **talus** ▽

√7ᵗʰ **S92.124** **Nondisplaced fracture of body of** right talus

√7ᵗʰ **S92.125** **Nondisplaced fracture of body of** left **talus**

√7ᵗʰ **S92.126** **Nondisplaced fracture of body of** unspecified **talus** ▽

√6ᵗʰ **S92.13** **Fracture of** posterior process **of talus**

√7ᵗʰ **S92.131** **Displaced fracture of posterior process of** right **talus**

√7ᵗʰ **S92.132** **Displaced fracture of posterior process of** left **talus**

√7ᵗʰ **S92.133** **Displaced fracture of posterior process of unspecified talus** ▽

√7ᵗʰ **S92.134** **Nondisplaced fracture of posterior process of right talus**

√7ᵗʰ **S92.135** **Nondisplaced fracture of posterior process of left talus**

√7ᵗʰ **S92.136** **Nondisplaced fracture of posterior process of unspecified talus** ▽

√6ᵗʰ **S92.14** **Dome fracture of talus**

EXCLUDES 1   *osteochondritis dissecans (M93.2)*

√7ᵗʰ **S92.141** **Displaced dome fracture of** right **talus**

√7ᵗʰ **S92.142** **Displaced dome fracture of** left **talus**

√7ᵗʰ **S92.143** **Displaced dome fracture of** unspecified **talus** ▽

√7ᵗʰ **S92.144** **Nondisplaced dome fracture of** right **talus**

√7ᵗʰ **S92.145** **Nondisplaced dome fracture of** left **talus**

√7ᵗʰ **S92.146** **Nondisplaced dome fracture of** unspecified **talus** ▽

√6ᵗʰ **S92.15** **Avulsion fracture (chip fracture) of talus**

√7ᵗʰ **S92.151** **Displaced avulsion fracture (chip fracture) of** right **talus**

√7ᵗʰ **S92.152** **Displaced avulsion fracture (chip fracture) of** left **talus**

√7ᵗʰ **S92.153** **Displaced avulsion fracture (chip fracture) of unspecified talus** ▽

√7ᵗʰ **S92.154** **Nondisplaced avulsion fracture (chip fracture) of** right **talus**

√7ᵗʰ **S92.155** **Nondisplaced avulsion fracture (chip fracture) of** left **talus**

√7ᵗʰ **S92.156** **Nondisplaced avulsion fracture (chip fracture) of unspecified talus** ▽

√6ᵗʰ **S92.19** **Other fracture of talus**

√7ᵗʰ **S92.191** **Other fracture of** right **talus**

√7ᵗʰ **S92.192** **Other fracture of** left **talus**

√7ᵗʰ **S92.199** **Other fracture of unspecified talus** ▽

√5ᵗʰ **S92.2** **Fracture of other and unspecified tarsal bone(s)**

√6ᵗʰ **S92.20** **Fracture of unspecified tarsal bone(s)**

√7ᵗʰ **S92.201** **Fracture of unspecified tarsal bone(s) of** right **foot** ▽

√7ᵗʰ **S92.202** **Fracture of unspecified tarsal bone(s) of** left **foot** ▽

√7ᵗʰ **S92.209** **Fracture of unspecified tarsal bone(s) of unspecified foot** ▽

√6ᵗʰ **S92.21** **Fracture of** cuboid **bone**

√7ᵗʰ **S92.211** **Displaced fracture of cuboid bone of** right **foot**

√7ᵗʰ **S92.212** **Displaced fracture of cuboid bone of** left **foot**

√7ᵗʰ **S92.213** **Displaced fracture of cuboid bone of unspecified foot** ▽

√7ᵗʰ **S92.214** **Nondisplaced fracture of cuboid bone of** right **foot**

√7ᵗʰ **S92.215** **Nondisplaced fracture of cuboid bone of** left **foot**

√7ᵗʰ **S92.216** **Nondisplaced fracture of cuboid bone of unspecified foot** ▽

√6ᵗʰ **S92.22** **Fracture of lateral cuneiform**

√7ᵗʰ **S92.221** **Displaced fracture of lateral cuneiform of** right **foot**

√7ᵗʰ **S92.222** **Displaced fracture of lateral cuneiform of** left **foot**

√7ᵗʰ **S92.223** **Displaced fracture of lateral cuneiform of unspecified foot** ▽

√7ᵗʰ **S92.224** **Nondisplaced fracture of lateral cuneiform of** right **foot**

√7ᵗʰ **S92.225** **Nondisplaced fracture of lateral cuneiform of** left **foot**

√7ᵗʰ **S92.226** **Nondisplaced fracture of lateral cuneiform of unspecified foot** ▽

√6ᵗʰ **S92.23** **Fracture of intermediate cuneiform**

√7ᵗʰ **S92.231** **Displaced fracture of intermediate cuneiform of** right **foot**

√7ᵗʰ **S92.232** **Displaced fracture of intermediate cuneiform of** left **foot**

√7ᵗʰ **S92.233** **Displaced fracture of intermediate cuneiform of unspecified foot** ▽

√7ᵗʰ **S92.234** **Nondisplaced fracture of intermediate cuneiform of** right **foot**

√7ᵗʰ **S92.235** **Nondisplaced fracture of intermediate cuneiform of** left **foot**

√7ᵗʰ **S92.236** **Nondisplaced fracture of intermediate cuneiform of unspecified foot** ▽

√6ᵗʰ **S92.24** **Fracture of medial cuneiform**

√7ᵗʰ **S92.241** **Displaced fracture of medial cuneiform of** right **foot**

√7ᵗʰ **S92.242** **Displaced fracture of medial cuneiform of** left **foot**

√7ᵗʰ **S92.243** **Displaced fracture of medial cuneiform of unspecified foot** ▽

√7ᵗʰ **S92.244** **Nondisplaced fracture of medial cuneiform of** right **foot**

√7ᵗʰ **S92.245** **Nondisplaced fracture of medial cuneiform of** left **foot**

√7ᵗʰ **S92.246** **Nondisplaced fracture of medial cuneiform of unspecified foot** ▽

√6ᵗʰ **S92.25** **Fracture of** navicular [scaphoid] **of foot**

√7ᵗʰ **S92.251** **Displaced fracture of navicular [scaphoid] of** right **foot**

√7ᵗʰ **S92.252** **Displaced fracture of navicular [scaphoid] of** left **foot**

√7ᵗʰ **S92.253** **Displaced fracture of navicular [scaphoid] of unspecified foot** ▽

√7ᵗʰ **S92.254** **Nondisplaced fracture of navicular [scaphoid] of** right **foot**

√7ᵗʰ **S92.255** **Nondisplaced fracture of navicular [scaphoid] of** left **foot**

√7ᵗʰ **S92.256** **Nondisplaced fracture of navicular [scaphoid] of unspecified foot** ▽

√5ᵗʰ **S92.3** **Fracture of** metatarsal **bone(s)**

EXCLUDES 2   *physeal fracture of metatarsal (S99.1-)*

√6ᵗʰ **S92.30** **Fracture of unspecified metatarsal bone(s)**

√7ᵗʰ **S92.301** **Fracture of unspecified metatarsal bone(s),** right **foot** ▽

√7ᵗʰ **S92.302** **Fracture of unspecified metatarsal bone(s),** left **foot** ▽

√7ᵗʰ **S92.309** **Fracture of unspecified metatarsal bone(s), unspecified foot** ▽

√6ᵗʰ **S92.31** **Fracture of** first metatarsal **bone**

√7ᵗʰ **S92.311** **Displaced fracture of first metatarsal bone,** right **foot**

√7ᵗʰ **S92.312** **Displaced fracture of first metatarsal bone,** left **foot**

√7ᵗʰ **S92.313** **Displaced fracture of first metatarsal bone, unspecified foot** ▽

√7ᵗʰ **S92.314** **Nondisplaced fracture of first metatarsal bone,** right **foot**

☑ Additional Character Req   ✓1ᵀ Placeholder Alert   Manifestation   HCC CMS-HCC Condition   ▽ Unspecified Code   ►◄ Revised Text   ● New Code   ▲ Revised Code Title

ICD-10-CM 2018   1029

Chapter 19. Injury, Poisoning, and Certain Other Consequences of External Causes

√7ᵗʰ **S92.315** Nondisplaced **fracture of first metatarsal bone, left foot**

√7ᵗʰ **S92.316** Nondisplaced **fracture of first metatarsal bone, unspecified foot** ▽

√6ᵗʰ **S92.32** Fracture of **second metatarsal bone**

√7ᵗʰ **S92.321** Displaced **fracture of second metatarsal bone, right foot**

√7ᵗʰ **S92.322** Displaced **fracture of second metatarsal bone, left foot**

√7ᵗʰ **S92.323** Displaced **fracture of second metatarsal bone, unspecified foot** ▽

√7ᵗʰ **S92.324** Nondisplaced **fracture of second metatarsal bone, right foot**

√7ᵗʰ **S92.325** Nondisplaced **fracture of second metatarsal bone, left foot**

√7ᵗʰ **S92.326** Nondisplaced **fracture of second metatarsal bone, unspecified foot** ▽

√6ᵗʰ **S92.33** Fracture of **third metatarsal bone**

√7ᵗʰ **S92.331** Displaced **fracture of third metatarsal bone, right foot**

√7ᵗʰ **S92.332** Displaced **fracture of third metatarsal bone, left foot**

√7ᵗʰ **S92.333** Displaced **fracture of third metatarsal bone, unspecified foot** ▽

√7ᵗʰ **S92.334** Nondisplaced **fracture of third metatarsal bone, right foot**

√7ᵗʰ **S92.335** Nondisplaced **fracture of third metatarsal bone, left foot**

√7ᵗʰ **S92.336** Nondisplaced **fracture of third metatarsal bone, unspecified foot** ▽

√6ᵗʰ **S92.34** Fracture of **fourth metatarsal bone**

√7ᵗʰ **S92.341** Displaced **fracture of fourth metatarsal bone, right foot**

√7ᵗʰ **S92.342** Displaced **fracture of fourth metatarsal bone, left foot**

√7ᵗʰ **S92.343** Displaced **fracture of fourth metatarsal bone, unspecified foot** ▽

√7ᵗʰ **S92.344** Nondisplaced **fracture of fourth metatarsal bone, right foot**

√7ᵗʰ **S92.345** Nondisplaced **fracture of fourth metatarsal bone, left foot**

√7ᵗʰ **S92.346** Nondisplaced **fracture of fourth metatarsal bone, unspecified foot** ▽

√6ᵗʰ **S92.35** Fracture of **fifth metatarsal bone**

√7ᵗʰ **S92.351** Displaced **fracture of fifth metatarsal bone, right foot**

√7ᵗʰ **S92.352** Displaced **fracture of fifth metatarsal bone, left foot**

√7ᵗʰ **S92.353** Displaced **fracture of fifth metatarsal bone, unspecified foot** ▽

√7ᵗʰ **S92.354** Nondisplaced **fracture of fifth metatarsal bone, right foot**

√7ᵗʰ **S92.355** Nondisplaced **fracture of fifth metatarsal bone, left foot**

√7ᵗʰ **S92.356** Nondisplaced **fracture of fifth metatarsal bone, unspecified foot** ▽

√5ᵗʰ **S92.4** Fracture of **great toe**
     EXCLUDES 2   physeal fracture of phalanx of toe (S99.2-)

√6ᵗʰ **S92.40** Unspecified fracture of **great toe**

√7ᵗʰ **S92.401** Displaced **unspecified fracture of right great toe** ▽

√7ᵗʰ **S92.402** Displaced **unspecified fracture of left great toe** ▽

√7ᵗʰ **S92.403** Displaced **unspecified fracture of unspecified great toe** ▽

√7ᵗʰ **S92.404** Nondisplaced **unspecified fracture of right great toe** ▽

√7ᵗʰ **S92.405** Nondisplaced **unspecified fracture of left great toe** ▽

√7ᵗʰ **S92.406** Nondisplaced **unspecified fracture of unspecified great toe** ▽

√6ᵗʰ **S92.41** Fracture of **proximal phalanx of great toe**

√7ᵗʰ **S92.411** Displaced **fracture of proximal phalanx of right great toe**

√7ᵗʰ **S92.412** Displaced **fracture of proximal phalanx of left great toe**

√7ᵗʰ **S92.413** Displaced **fracture of proximal phalanx of unspecified great toe** ▽

√7ᵗʰ **S92.414** Nondisplaced **fracture of proximal phalanx of right great toe**

√7ᵗʰ **S92.415** Nondisplaced **fracture of proximal phalanx of left great toe**

√7ᵗʰ **S92.416** Nondisplaced **fracture of proximal phalanx of unspecified great toe** ▽

√6ᵗʰ **S92.42** Fracture of **distal phalanx of great toe**

√7ᵗʰ **S92.421** Displaced **fracture of distal phalanx of right great toe**

√7ᵗʰ **S92.422** Displaced **fracture of distal phalanx of left great toe**

√7ᵗʰ **S92.423** Displaced **fracture of distal phalanx of unspecified great toe** ▽

√7ᵗʰ **S92.424** Nondisplaced **fracture of distal phalanx of right great toe**

√7ᵗʰ **S92.425** Nondisplaced **fracture of distal phalanx of left great toe**

√7ᵗʰ **S92.426** Nondisplaced **fracture of distal phalanx of unspecified great toe** ▽

√6ᵗʰ **S92.49** Other fracture of **great toe**

√7ᵗʰ **S92.491** Other fracture of **right great toe**

√7ᵗʰ **S92.492** Other fracture of **left great toe**

√7ᵗʰ **S92.499** Other fracture of **unspecified great toe** ▽

S92.5 Fracture of **lesser toe(s)**
     EXCLUDES 2   physeal fracture of phalanx of toe (S99.2-)

√6ᵗʰ **S92.50** Unspecified fracture of **lesser toe(s)**

√7ᵗʰ **S92.501** Displaced **unspecified fracture of right lesser toe(s)** ▽

√7ᵗʰ **S92.502** Displaced **unspecified fracture of left lesser toe(s)** ▽

√7ᵗʰ **S92.503** Displaced **unspecified fracture of unspecified lesser toe(s)** ▽

√7ᵗʰ **S92.504** Nondisplaced **unspecified fracture of right lesser toe(s)** ▽

√7ᵗʰ **S92.505** Nondisplaced **unspecified fracture of left lesser toe(s)** ▽

√7ᵗʰ **S92.506** Nondisplaced **unspecified fracture of unspecified lesser toe(s)** ▽

√6ᵗʰ **S92.51** Fracture of **proximal phalanx of lesser toe(s)**

√7ᵗʰ **S92.511** Displaced **fracture of proximal phalanx of right lesser toe(s)**

√7ᵗʰ **S92.512** Displaced **fracture of proximal phalanx of left lesser toe(s)**

√7ᵗʰ **S92.513** Displaced **fracture of proximal phalanx of unspecified lesser toe(s)** ▽

√7ᵗʰ **S92.514** Nondisplaced **fracture of proximal phalanx of right lesser toe(s)**

√7ᵗʰ **S92.515** Nondisplaced **fracture of proximal phalanx of left lesser toe(s)**

√7ᵗʰ **S92.516** Nondisplaced **fracture of proximal phalanx of unspecified lesser toe(s)** ▽

▲ √6ᵗʰ **S92.52** Fracture of **middle phalanx of lesser toe(s)**

▲ √7ᵗʰ **S92.521** Displaced **fracture of middle phalanx of right lesser toe(s)**

▲ √7ᵗʰ **S92.522** Displaced **fracture of middle phalanx of left lesser toe(s)**

▲ √7ᵗʰ **S92.523** Displaced **fracture of middle phalanx of unspecified lesser toe(s)** ▽

▲ √7ᵗʰ **S92.524** Nondisplaced **fracture of middle phalanx of right lesser toe(s)**

▲ √7ᵗʰ **S92.525** Nondisplaced **fracture of middle phalanx of left lesser toe(s)**

▲ √7ᵗʰ **S92.526** Nondisplaced **fracture of middle phalanx of unspecified lesser toe(s)** ▽

√6ᵗʰ **S92.53** Fracture of **distal phalanx of lesser toe(s)**

√7ᵗʰ **S92.531** Displaced **fracture of distal phalanx of right lesser toe(s)**

√7ᵗʰ **S92.532** Displaced **fracture of distal phalanx of left lesser toe(s)**

EXCLUDES 1 Not coded here   EXCLUDES 2 Not included here   N Newborn Age: 0   P Pediatric Age: 0-17   M Maternity Age: 12-55   A Adult Age: 15-124

1030   ICD-10-CM 2018

✓7ᵗʰ **S92.533** Displaced fracture of distal phalanx of ▽
unspecified lesser toe(s)

✓7ᵗʰ **S92.534** Nondisplaced fracture of distal phalanx of
right lesser toe(s)

✓7ᵗʰ **S92.535** Nondisplaced fracture of distal phalanx of
left lesser toe(s)

✓7ᵗʰ **S92.536** Nondisplaced fracture of distal phalanx ▽
of unspecified lesser toe(s)

✓6ᵗʰ **S92.59** Other fracture of lesser toe(s)

✓7ᵗʰ **S92.591** Other fracture of right lesser toe(s)

✓7ᵗʰ **S92.592** Other fracture of left lesser toe(s)

✓7ᵗʰ **S92.599** Other fracture of unspecified lesser ▽
toe(s)

✓5ᵗʰ **S92.8** Other fracture of foot, except ankle

✓6ᵗʰ **S92.81** Other fracture of foot
Sesamoid fracture of foot

✓7ᵗʰ **S92.811** Other fracture of right foot

✓7ᵗʰ **S92.812** Other fracture of left foot

✓7ᵗʰ **S92.819** Other fracture of unspecified foot ▽

✓5ᵗʰ **S92.9** Unspecified fracture of foot and toe

✓6ᵗʰ **S92.90** Unspecified fracture of foot

✓7ᵗʰ **S92.901** Unspecified fracture of right foot ▽

✓7ᵗʰ **S92.902** Unspecified fracture of left foot ▽

✓7ᵗʰ **S92.909** Unspecified fracture of unspecified ▽
foot

✓6ᵗʰ **S92.91** Unspecified fracture of toe

✓7ᵗʰ **S92.911** Unspecified fracture of right toe(s) ▽

✓7ᵗʰ **S92.912** Unspecified fracture of left toe(s) ▽

✓7ᵗʰ **S92.919** Unspecified fracture of unspecified ▽
toe(s)

✓4ᵗʰ **S93** **Dislocation and sprain of joints and ligaments at ankle, foot and toe level**

INCLUDES   avulsion of joint or ligament of ankle, foot and toe
laceration of cartilage, joint or ligament of ankle, foot and toe
sprain of cartilage, joint or ligament of ankle, foot and toe
traumatic hemarthrosis of joint or ligament of ankle, foot and toe
traumatic rupture of joint or ligament of ankle, foot and toe
traumatic subluxation of joint or ligament of ankle, foot and toe
traumatic tear of joint or ligament of ankle, foot and toe

Code also any associated open wound

EXCLUDES 2   *strain of muscle and tendon of ankle and foot (S96.-)*

The appropriate 7th character is to be added to each code from category S93.
A   initial encounter
D   subsequent encounter
S   sequela

✓5ᵗʰ **S93.0** **Subluxation and dislocation of ankle joint**
Subluxation and dislocation of astragalus
Subluxation and dislocation of fibula, lower end
Subluxation and dislocation of talus
Subluxation and dislocation of tibia, lower end

✓x7ᵗʰ **S93.01** Subluxation of right ankle joint

✓x7ᵗʰ **S93.02** Subluxation of left ankle joint

✓x7ᵗʰ **S93.03** Subluxation of unspecified ankle joint ▽

✓x7ᵗʰ **S93.04** Dislocation of right ankle joint

✓x7ᵗʰ **S93.05** Dislocation of left ankle joint

✓x7ᵗʰ **S93.06** Dislocation of unspecified ankle joint ▽

✓5ᵗʰ **S93.1** **Subluxation and dislocation of toe**

✓6ᵗʰ **S93.10** Unspecified subluxation and dislocation of toe
Dislocation of toe NOS
Subluxation of toe NOS

✓7ᵗʰ **S93.101** Unspecified subluxation of right toe(s) ▽

✓7ᵗʰ **S93.102** Unspecified subluxation of left toe(s) ▽

✓7ᵗʰ **S93.103** Unspecified subluxation of unspecified ▽
toe(s)

✓7ᵗʰ **S93.104** Unspecified dislocation of right toe(s) ▽

✓7ᵗʰ **S93.105** Unspecified dislocation of left toe(s) ▽

✓7ᵗʰ **S93.106** Unspecified dislocation of unspecified ▽
toe(s)

✓6ᵗʰ **S93.11** Dislocation of interphalangeal joint

✓7ᵗʰ **S93.111** Dislocation of interphalangeal joint of
right great toe

✓7ᵗʰ **S93.112** Dislocation of interphalangeal joint of left
great toe

✓7ᵗʰ **S93.113** Dislocation of interphalangeal joint of ▽
unspecified great toe

✓7ᵗʰ **S93.114** Dislocation of interphalangeal joint of
right lesser toe(s)

✓7ᵗʰ **S93.115** Dislocation of interphalangeal joint of left
lesser toe(s)

✓7ᵗʰ **S93.116** Dislocation of interphalangeal joint of ▽
unspecified lesser toe(s)

✓7ᵗʰ **S93.119** Dislocation of interphalangeal joint of ▽
unspecified toe(s)

✓6ᵗʰ **S93.12** Dislocation of metatarsophalangeal joint

✓7ᵗʰ **S93.121** Dislocation of metatarsophalangeal joint
of right great toe

✓7ᵗʰ **S93.122** Dislocation of metatarsophalangeal joint
of left great toe

✓7ᵗʰ **S93.123** Dislocation of metatarsophalangeal ▽
joint of unspecified great toe

✓7ᵗʰ **S93.124** Dislocation of metatarsophalangeal joint
of right lesser toe(s)

✓7ᵗʰ **S93.125** Dislocation of metatarsophalangeal joint
of left lesser toe(s)

✓7ᵗʰ **S93.126** Dislocation of metatarsophalangeal ▽
joint of unspecified lesser toe(s)

✓7ᵗʰ **S93.129** Dislocation of metatarsophalangeal ▽
joint of unspecified toe(s)

✓6ᵗʰ **S93.13** Subluxation of interphalangeal joint

✓7ᵗʰ **S93.131** Subluxation of interphalangeal joint of
right great toe

✓7ᵗʰ **S93.132** Subluxation of interphalangeal joint of
left great toe

✓7ᵗʰ **S93.133** Subluxation of interphalangeal joint of ▽
unspecified great toe

✓7ᵗʰ **S93.134** Subluxation of interphalangeal joint of
right lesser toe(s)

✓7ᵗʰ **S93.135** Subluxation of interphalangeal joint of
left lesser toe(s)

✓7ᵗʰ **S93.136** Subluxation of interphalangeal joint of ▽
unspecified lesser toe(s)

✓7ᵗʰ **S93.139** Subluxation of interphalangeal joint of ▽
unspecified toe(s)

✓6ᵗʰ **S93.14** Subluxation of metatarsophalangeal joint

✓7ᵗʰ **S93.141** Subluxation of metatarsophalangeal joint
of right great toe

✓7ᵗʰ **S93.142** Subluxation of metatarsophalangeal joint
of left great toe

✓7ᵗʰ **S93.143** Subluxation of metatarsophalangeal ▽
joint of unspecified great toe

✓7ᵗʰ **S93.144** Subluxation of metatarsophalangeal joint
of right lesser toe(s)

✓7ᵗʰ **S93.145** Subluxation of metatarsophalangeal joint
of left lesser toe(s)

✓7ᵗʰ **S93.146** Subluxation of metatarsophalangeal ▽
joint of unspecified lesser toe(s)

✓7ᵗʰ **S93.149** Subluxation of metatarsophalangeal ▽
joint of unspecified toe(s)

✓5ᵗʰ **S93.3** **Subluxation and dislocation of foot**
EXCLUDES 2   *dislocation of toe (S93.1-)*

✓6ᵗʰ **S93.30** Unspecified subluxation and dislocation of foot
Dislocation of foot NOS
Subluxation of foot NOS

✓7ᵗʰ **S93.301** Unspecified subluxation of right foot ▽

✓7ᵗʰ **S93.302** Unspecified subluxation of left foot ▽

✓7ᵗʰ **S93.303** Unspecified subluxation of unspecified ▽
foot

✓7ᵗʰ **S93.304** Unspecified dislocation of right foot ▽

✓7ᵗʰ **S93.305** Unspecified dislocation of left foot ▽

✓7ᵗʰ **S93.306** Unspecified dislocation of unspecified ▽
foot

☑ Additional Character Req   ✓x7ᵗʰ Placeholder Alert   Manifestation   HCC CMS-HCC Condition   ▽ Unspecified Code   ►◄ Revised Text   ● New Code   ▲ Revised Code Title

ICD-10-CM 2018   1031

✓6ᵗʰ S93.31 Subluxation and dislocation of tarsal joint
- ✓7ᵗʰ **S93.311** Subluxation of tarsal joint of right foot
- ✓7ᵗʰ **S93.312** Subluxation of tarsal joint of left foot
- ✓7ᵗʰ **S93.313** Subluxation of tarsal joint of unspecified foot
- ✓7ᵗʰ **S93.314** Dislocation of tarsal joint of right foot
- ✓7ᵗʰ **S93.315** Dislocation of tarsal joint of left foot
- ✓7ᵗʰ **S93.316** Dislocation of tarsal joint of unspecified foot ▽

✓6ᵗʰ S93.32 Subluxation and dislocation of tarsometatarsal joint
- ✓7ᵗʰ **S93.321** Subluxation of tarsometatarsal joint of right foot
- ✓7ᵗʰ **S93.322** Subluxation of tarsometatarsal joint of left foot
- ✓7ᵗʰ **S93.323** Subluxation of tarsometatarsal joint of ▽ unspecified foot
- ✓7ᵗʰ **S93.324** Dislocation of tarsometatarsal joint of right foot
- ✓7ᵗʰ **S93.325** Dislocation of tarsometatarsal joint of left foot
- ✓7ᵗʰ **S93.326** Dislocation of tarsometatarsal joint of ▽ unspecified foot

✓6ᵗʰ S93.33 Other subluxation and dislocation of foot
- ✓7ᵗʰ **S93.331** Other subluxation of right foot
- ✓7ᵗʰ **S93.332** Other subluxation of left foot
- ✓7ᵗʰ **S93.333** Other subluxation of unspecified foot ▽
- ✓7ᵗʰ **S93.334** Other dislocation of right foot
- ✓7ᵗʰ **S93.335** Other dislocation of left foot
- ✓7ᵗʰ **S93.336** Other dislocation of unspecified foot ▽

✓5ᵗʰ S93.4 Sprain of ankle

     EXCLUDES 2   injury of Achilles tendon (S86.Ø-)

✓6ᵗʰ S93.4Ø Sprain of unspecified ligament of ankle
     Sprain of ankle NOS
     Sprained ankle NOS
- ✓7ᵗʰ **S93.4Ø1** Sprain of unspecified ligament of ▽ right ankle
- ✓7ᵗʰ **S93.4Ø2** Sprain of unspecified ligament of ▽ left ankle
- ✓7ᵗʰ **S93.4Ø9** Sprain of unspecified ligament of ▽ unspecified ankle

✓6ᵗʰ S93.41 Sprain of calcaneofibular ligament
- ✓7ᵗʰ **S93.411** Sprain of calcaneofibular ligament of right ankle
- ✓7ᵗʰ **S93.412** Sprain of calcaneofibular ligament of left ankle
- ✓7ᵗʰ **S93.419** Sprain of calcaneofibular ligament of ▽ unspecified ankle

✓6ᵗʰ S93.42 Sprain of deltoid ligament
- ✓7ᵗʰ **S93.421** Sprain of deltoid ligament of right ankle
- ✓7ᵗʰ **S93.422** Sprain of deltoid ligament of left ankle
- ✓7ᵗʰ **S93.429** Sprain of deltoid ligament of ▽ unspecified ankle

✓6ᵗʰ S93.43 Sprain of tibiofibular ligament
- ✓7ᵗʰ **S93.431** Sprain of tibiofibular ligament of right ankle
- ✓7ᵗʰ **S93.432** Sprain of tibiofibular ligament of left ankle
- ✓7ᵗʰ **S93.439** Sprain of tibiofibular ligament of ▽ unspecified ankle

✓6ᵗʰ S93.49 Sprain of other ligament of ankle
     Sprain of internal collateral ligament
     Sprain of talofibular ligament
- ✓7ᵗʰ **S93.491** Sprain of other ligament of right ankle
- ✓7ᵗʰ **S93.492** Sprain of other ligament of left ankle
- ✓7ᵗʰ **S93.499** Sprain of other ligament of unspecified ▽ ankle

✓5ᵗʰ S93.5 Sprain of toe

✓6ᵗʰ S93.5Ø Unspecified sprain of toe
- ✓7ᵗʰ **S93.5Ø1** Unspecified sprain of right great toe ▽
- ✓7ᵗʰ **S93.5Ø2** Unspecified sprain of left great toe ▽
- ✓7ᵗʰ **S93.5Ø3** Unspecified sprain of unspecified great ▽ toe

- ✓7ᵗʰ **S93.5Ø4** Unspecified sprain of right lesser toe(s) ▽
- ✓7ᵗʰ **S93.5Ø5** Unspecified sprain of left lesser toe(s) ▽
- ✓7ᵗʰ **S93.5Ø6** Unspecified sprain of unspecified lesser ▽ toe(s)
- ✓7ᵗʰ **S93.5Ø9** Unspecified sprain of unspecified toe(s) ▽

S93.51 Sprain of interphalangeal joint of toe
- ✓7ᵗʰ **S93.511** Sprain of interphalangeal joint of right great toe
- ✓7ᵗʰ **S93.512** Sprain of interphalangeal joint of left great toe
- ✓7ᵗʰ **S93.513** Sprain of interphalangeal joint of ▽ unspecified great toe
- ✓7ᵗʰ **S93.514** Sprain of interphalangeal joint of right lesser toe(s)
- ✓7ᵗʰ **S93.515** Sprain of interphalangeal joint of left lesser toe(s)
- ✓7ᵗʰ **S93.516** Sprain of interphalangeal joint of ▽ unspecified lesser toe(s)
- ✓7ᵗʰ **S93.519** Sprain of interphalangeal joint of ▽ unspecified toe(s)

✓6ᵗʰ S93.52 Sprain of metatarsophalangeal joint of toe
- ✓7ᵗʰ **S93.521** Sprain of metatarsophalangeal joint of right great toe
- ✓7ᵗʰ **S93.522** Sprain of metatarsophalangeal joint of left great toe
- ✓7ᵗʰ **S93.523** Sprain of metatarsophalangeal joint of ▽ unspecified great toe
- ✓7ᵗʰ **S93.524** Sprain of metatarsophalangeal joint of right lesser toe(s)
- ✓7ᵗʰ **S93.525** Sprain of metatarsophalangeal joint of left lesser toe(s)
- ✓7ᵗʰ **S93.526** Sprain of metatarsophalangeal joint of ▽ unspecified lesser toe(s)
- ✓7ᵗʰ **S93.529** Sprain of metatarsophalangeal joint of ▽ unspecified toe(s)

✓5ᵗʰ S93.6 Sprain of foot

     EXCLUDES 2   sprain of metatarsophalangeal joint of toe (S93.52-)
                     sprain of toe (S93.5-)

✓6ᵗʰ S93.6Ø Unspecified sprain of foot
- ✓7ᵗʰ **S93.6Ø1** Unspecified sprain of right foot ▽
- ✓7ᵗʰ **S93.6Ø2** Unspecified sprain of left foot ▽
- ✓7ᵗʰ **S93.6Ø9** Unspecified sprain of unspecified foot ▽

✓6ᵗʰ S93.61 Sprain of tarsal ligament of foot
- ✓7ᵗʰ **S93.611** Sprain of tarsal ligament of right foot
- ✓7ᵗʰ **S93.612** Sprain of tarsal ligament of left foot
- ✓7ᵗʰ **S93.619** Sprain of tarsal ligament of unspecified ▽ foot

✓6ᵗʰ S93.62 Sprain of tarsometatarsal ligament of foot
- ✓7ᵗʰ **S93.621** Sprain of tarsometatarsal ligament of right foot
- ✓7ᵗʰ **S93.622** Sprain of tarsometatarsal ligament of left foot
- ✓7ᵗʰ **S93.629** Sprain of tarsometatarsal ligament of ▽ unspecified foot

✓6ᵗʰ S93.69 Other sprain of foot
- ✓7ᵗʰ **S93.691** Other sprain of right foot
- ✓7ᵗʰ **S93.692** Other sprain of left foot
- ✓7ᵗʰ **S93.699** Other sprain of unspecified foot ▽

✓4ᵗʰ S94 Injury of nerves at ankle and foot level
     Code also any associated open wound (S91.-)

     The appropriate 7th character is to be added to each code from
     category S94.
     A   initial encounter
     D   subsequent encounter
     S   sequela

✓5ᵗʰ S94.Ø Injury of lateral plantar nerve
- ✓x7ᵗʰ **S94.ØØ** Injury of lateral plantar nerve, unspecified leg ▽
- ✓x7ᵗʰ **S94.Ø1** Injury of lateral plantar nerve, right leg
- ✓x7ᵗʰ **S94.Ø2** Injury of lateral plantar nerve, left leg

✓5ᵗʰ S94.1 Injury of medial plantar nerve
- ✓x7ᵗʰ **S94.1Ø** Injury of medial plantar nerve, unspecified leg ▽

EXCLUDES 1 Not coded here   *EXCLUDES 2* Not included here   N Newborn Age: 0   P Pediatric Age: 0-17   M Maternity Age: 12-55   A Adult Age: 15-124

1032   ICD-10-CM 2018

✓x7ᵗʰ **S94.11** Injury of medial plantar nerve, right leg

✓x7ᵗʰ **S94.12** Injury of medial plantar nerve, left leg

✓5ᵗʰ **S94.2** Injury of deep peroneal nerve at ankle and foot level
Injury of terminal, lateral branch of deep peroneal nerve

✓x7ᵗʰ **S94.20** Injury of deep peroneal nerve at ankle and foot ▽ level, unspecified leg

✓x7ᵗʰ **S94.21** Injury of deep peroneal nerve at ankle and foot level, right leg

✓x7ᵗʰ **S94.22** Injury of deep peroneal nerve at ankle and foot level, left leg

✓5ᵗʰ **S94.3** Injury of cutaneous sensory nerve at ankle and foot level

✓x7ᵗʰ **S94.30** Injury of cutaneous sensory nerve at ankle and ▽ foot level, unspecified leg

✓x7ᵗʰ **S94.31** Injury of cutaneous sensory nerve at ankle and foot level, right leg

✓x7ᵗʰ **S94.32** Injury of cutaneous sensory nerve at ankle and foot level, left leg

✓5ᵗʰ **S94.8** Injury of other nerves at ankle and foot level

✓6ᵗʰ **S94.8X** Injury of other nerves at ankle and foot level

✓7ᵗʰ **S94.8X1** Injury of other nerves at ankle and foot level, right leg

✓7ᵗʰ **S94.8X2** Injury of other nerves at ankle and foot level, left leg

✓7ᵗʰ **S94.8X9** Injury of other nerves at ankle and foot ▽ level, unspecified leg

✓5ᵗʰ **S94.9** Injury of unspecified nerve at ankle and foot level

✓x7ᵗʰ **S94.90** Injury of unspecified nerve at ankle and foot ▽ level, unspecified leg

✓x7ᵗʰ **S94.91** Injury of unspecified nerve at ankle and foot ▽ level, right leg

✓x7ᵗʰ **S94.92** Injury of unspecified nerve at ankle and foot ▽ level, left leg

✓4ᵗʰ **S95** Injury of blood vessels at ankle and foot level
Code also any associated open wound (S91.-)
EXCLUDES 2   *injury of posterior tibial artery and vein (S85.1-, S85.8-)*

The appropriate 7th character is to be added to each code from category S95.
A   initial encounter
D   subsequent encounter
S   sequela

✓5ᵗʰ **S95.0** Injury of dorsal artery of foot

✓6ᵗʰ **S95.00** Unspecified injury of dorsal artery of foot

✓7ᵗʰ **S95.001** Unspecified injury of dorsal artery of ▽ right foot

✓7ᵗʰ **S95.002** Unspecified injury of dorsal artery of ▽ left foot

✓7ᵗʰ **S95.009** Unspecified injury of dorsal artery of ▽ unspecified foot

✓6ᵗʰ **S95.01** Laceration of dorsal artery of foot

✓7ᵗʰ **S95.011** Laceration of dorsal artery of right foot

✓7ᵗʰ **S95.012** Laceration of dorsal artery of left foot

✓7ᵗʰ **S95.019** Laceration of dorsal artery of ▽ unspecified foot

✓6ᵗʰ **S95.09** Other specified injury of dorsal artery of foot

✓7ᵗʰ **S95.091** Other specified injury of dorsal artery of right foot

✓7ᵗʰ **S95.092** Other specified injury of dorsal artery of left foot

✓7ᵗʰ **S95.099** Other specified injury of dorsal artery ▽ of unspecified foot

✓5ᵗʰ **S95.1** Injury of plantar artery of foot

✓6ᵗʰ **S95.10** Unspecified injury of plantar artery of foot

✓7ᵗʰ **S95.101** Unspecified injury of plantar artery of ▽ right foot

✓7ᵗʰ **S95.102** Unspecified injury of plantar artery of ▽ left foot

✓7ᵗʰ **S95.109** Unspecified injury of plantar artery of ▽ unspecified foot

✓6ᵗʰ **S95.11** Laceration of plantar artery of foot

✓7ᵗʰ **S95.111** Laceration of plantar artery of right foot

✓7ᵗʰ **S95.112** Laceration of plantar artery of left foot

✓7ᵗʰ **S95.119** Laceration of plantar artery of ▽ unspecified foot

✓6ᵗʰ **S95.19** Other specified injury of plantar artery of foot

✓7ᵗʰ **S95.191** Other specified injury of plantar artery of right foot

✓7ᵗʰ **S95.192** Other specified injury of plantar artery of left foot

✓7ᵗʰ **S95.199** Other specified injury of plantar artery ▽ of unspecified foot

✓5ᵗʰ **S95.2** Injury of dorsal vein of foot

✓6ᵗʰ **S95.20** Unspecified injury of dorsal vein of foot

✓7ᵗʰ **S95.201** Unspecified injury of dorsal vein of ▽ right foot

✓7ᵗʰ **S95.202** Unspecified injury of dorsal vein of ▽ left foot

✓7ᵗʰ **S95.209** Unspecified injury of dorsal vein of ▽ unspecified foot

✓6ᵗʰ **S95.21** Laceration of dorsal vein of foot

✓7ᵗʰ **S95.211** Laceration of dorsal vein of right foot

✓7ᵗʰ **S95.212** Laceration of dorsal vein of left foot

✓7ᵗʰ **S95.219** Laceration of dorsal vein of unspecified ▽ foot

✓6ᵗʰ **S95.29** Other specified injury of dorsal vein of foot

✓7ᵗʰ **S95.291** Other specified injury of dorsal vein of right foot

✓7ᵗʰ **S95.292** Other specified injury of dorsal vein of left foot

✓7ᵗʰ **S95.299** Other specified injury of dorsal vein of ▽ unspecified foot

✓5ᵗʰ **S95.8** Injury of other blood vessels at ankle and foot level

✓6ᵗʰ **S95.80** Unspecified injury of other blood vessels at ankle and foot level

✓7ᵗʰ **S95.801** Unspecified injury of other blood ▽ vessels at ankle and foot level, right leg

✓7ᵗʰ **S95.802** Unspecified injury of other blood ▽ vessels at ankle and foot level, left leg

✓7ᵗʰ **S95.809** Unspecified injury of other blood ▽ vessels at ankle and foot level, unspecified leg

✓6ᵗʰ **S95.81** Laceration of other blood vessels at ankle and foot level

✓7ᵗʰ **S95.811** Laceration of other blood vessels at ankle and foot level, right leg

✓7ᵗʰ **S95.812** Laceration of other blood vessels at ankle and foot level, left leg

✓7ᵗʰ **S95.819** Laceration of other blood vessels at ▽ ankle and foot level, unspecified leg

✓6ᵗʰ **S95.89** Other specified injury of other blood vessels at ankle and foot level

✓7ᵗʰ **S95.891** Other specified injury of other blood vessels at ankle and foot level, right leg

✓7ᵗʰ **S95.892** Other specified injury of other blood vessels at ankle and foot level, left leg

✓7ᵗʰ **S95.899** Other specified injury of other blood ▽ vessels at ankle and foot level, unspecified leg

✓5ᵗʰ **S95.9** Injury of unspecified blood vessel at ankle and foot level

✓6ᵗʰ **S95.90** Unspecified injury of unspecified blood vessel at ankle and foot level

✓7ᵗʰ **S95.901** Unspecified injury of unspecified ▽ blood vessel at ankle and foot level, right leg

✓7ᵗʰ **S95.902** Unspecified injury of unspecified ▽ blood vessel at ankle and foot level, left leg

✓7ᵗʰ **S95.909** Unspecified injury of unspecified ▽ blood vessel at ankle and foot level, unspecified leg

✓6ᵗʰ **S95.91** Laceration of unspecified blood vessel at ankle and foot level

✓7ᵗʰ **S95.911** Laceration of unspecified blood vessel ▽ at ankle and foot level, right leg

✓7ᵗʰ **S95.912** Laceration of unspecified blood vessel ▽ at ankle and foot level, left leg

---

✓7th **S95.919** Laceration of unspecified blood vessel at ankle and foot level, unspecified leg ▽

✓6th **S95.99** Other specified injury of unspecified blood vessel at ankle and foot level

✓7th **S95.991** Other specified injury of unspecified blood vessel at ankle and foot level, right leg ▽

✓7th **S95.992** Other specified injury of unspecified blood vessel at ankle and foot level, left leg ▽

✓7th **S95.999** Other specified injury of unspecified blood vessel at ankle and foot level, unspecified leg ▽

✓4th **S96 Injury of muscle and tendon at ankle and foot level**

Code also any associated open wound (S91.-)

EXCLUDES 2 injury of Achilles tendon (S86.0-)

sprain of joints and ligaments of ankle and foot (S93.-)

TIP: Refer to the Muscle/Tendon table at the beginning of this chapter.

The appropriate 7th character is to be added to each code from category S96.

A   initial encounter

D   subsequent encounter

S   sequela

✓5th **S96.0 Injury of muscle and tendon of long flexor muscle of toe at ankle and foot level**

✓6th **S96.00** Unspecified injury of muscle and tendon of long flexor muscle of toe at ankle and foot level

✓7th **S96.001** Unspecified injury of muscle and tendon of long flexor muscle of toe at ankle and foot level, right foot ▽

✓7th **S96.002** Unspecified injury of muscle and tendon of long flexor muscle of toe at ankle and foot level, left foot ▽

✓7th **S96.009** Unspecified injury of muscle and tendon of long flexor muscle of toe at ankle and foot level, unspecified foot ▽

✓6th **S96.01** Strain of muscle and tendon of long flexor muscle of toe at ankle and foot level

✓7th **S96.011** Strain of muscle and tendon of long flexor muscle of toe at ankle and foot level, right foot

✓7th **S96.012** Strain of muscle and tendon of long flexor muscle of toe at ankle and foot level, left foot

✓7th **S96.019** Strain of muscle and tendon of long flexor muscle of toe at ankle and foot level, unspecified foot ▽

✓6th **S96.02** Laceration of muscle and tendon of long flexor muscle of toe at ankle and foot level

✓7th **S96.021** Laceration of muscle and tendon of long flexor muscle of toe at ankle and foot level, right foot

✓7th **S96.022** Laceration of muscle and tendon of long flexor muscle of toe at ankle and foot level, left foot

✓7th **S96.029** Laceration of muscle and tendon of long flexor muscle of toe at ankle and foot level, unspecified foot ▽

✓6th **S96.09** Other injury of muscle and tendon of long flexor muscle of toe at ankle and foot level

✓7th **S96.091** Other injury of muscle and tendon of long flexor muscle of toe at ankle and foot level, right foot

✓7th **S96.092** Other injury of muscle and tendon of long flexor muscle of toe at ankle and foot level, left foot

✓7th **S96.099** Other injury of muscle and tendon of long flexor muscle of toe at ankle and foot level, unspecified foot ▽

✓5th **S96.1 Injury of muscle and tendon of long extensor muscle of toe at ankle and foot level**

✓6th **S96.10** Unspecified injury of muscle and tendon of long extensor muscle of toe at ankle and foot level

✓7th **S96.101** Unspecified injury of muscle and tendon of long extensor muscle of toe at ankle and foot level, right foot ▽

✓7th **S96.102** Unspecified injury of muscle and tendon of long extensor muscle of toe at ankle and foot level, left foot ▽

✓7th **S96.109** Unspecified injury of muscle and tendon of long extensor muscle of toe at ankle and foot level, unspecified foot ▽

✓6th **S96.11** Strain of muscle and tendon of long extensor muscle of toe at ankle and foot level

✓7th **S96.111** Strain of muscle and tendon of long extensor muscle of toe at ankle and foot level, right foot

✓7th **S96.112** Strain of muscle and tendon of long extensor muscle of toe at ankle and foot level, left foot

✓7th **S96.119** Strain of muscle and tendon of long extensor muscle of toe at ankle and foot level, unspecified foot ▽

✓6th **S96.12** Laceration of muscle and tendon of long extensor muscle of toe at ankle and foot level

✓7th **S96.121** Laceration of muscle and tendon of long extensor muscle of toe at ankle and foot level, right foot

✓7th **S96.122** Laceration of muscle and tendon of long extensor muscle of toe at ankle and foot level, left foot

✓7th **S96.129** Laceration of muscle and tendon of long extensor muscle of toe at ankle and foot level, unspecified foot ▽

✓6th **S96.19** Other specified injury of muscle and tendon of long extensor muscle of toe at ankle and foot level

✓7th **S96.191** Other specified injury of muscle and tendon of long extensor muscle of toe at ankle and foot level, right foot

✓7th **S96.192** Other specified injury of muscle and tendon of long extensor muscle of toe at ankle and foot level, left foot

✓7th **S96.199** Other specified injury of muscle and tendon of long extensor muscle of toe at ankle and foot level, unspecified foot ▽

✓5th **S96.2 Injury of intrinsic muscle and tendon at ankle and foot level**

✓6th **S96.20** Unspecified injury of intrinsic muscle and tendon at ankle and foot level

✓7th **S96.201** Unspecified injury of intrinsic muscle and tendon at ankle and foot level, right foot ▽

✓7th **S96.202** Unspecified injury of intrinsic muscle and tendon at ankle and foot level, left foot ▽

✓7th **S96.209** Unspecified injury of intrinsic muscle and tendon at ankle and foot level, unspecified foot ▽

✓6th **S96.21** Strain of intrinsic muscle and tendon at ankle and foot level

✓7th **S96.211** Strain of intrinsic muscle and tendon at ankle and foot level, right foot

✓7th **S96.212** Strain of intrinsic muscle and tendon at ankle and foot level, left foot

✓7th **S96.219** Strain of intrinsic muscle and tendon at ankle and foot level, unspecified foot ▽

✓6th **S96.22** Laceration of intrinsic muscle and tendon at ankle and foot level

✓7th **S96.221** Laceration of intrinsic muscle and tendon at ankle and foot level, right foot

✓7th **S96.222** Laceration of intrinsic muscle and tendon at ankle and foot level, left foot

✓7th **S96.229** Laceration of intrinsic muscle and tendon at ankle and foot level, unspecified foot ▽

✓6th **S96.29** Other specified injury of intrinsic muscle and tendon at ankle and foot level

✓7th **S96.291** Other specified injury of intrinsic muscle and tendon at ankle and foot level, right foot

✓7th **S96.292** Other specified injury of intrinsic muscle and tendon at ankle and foot level, left foot

EXCLUDES 1 Not coded here   *EXCLUDES 2* Not included here   N Newborn Age: 0   P Pediatric Age: 0-17   M Maternity Age: 12-55   A Adult Age: 15-124

1034   ICD-10-CM 2018

√7ᵗʰ **S96.299** Other specified injury of intrinsic muscle and tendon at ankle and foot level, unspecified foot ▽

√5ᵗʰ **S96.8** **Injury of other specified muscles and tendons at ankle and foot level**

   √6ᵗʰ **S96.80** Unspecified injury of other specified muscles and tendons at ankle and foot level

     √7ᵗʰ **S96.801** Unspecified injury of other specified muscles and tendons at ankle and foot level, right foot ▽

     √7ᵗʰ **S96.802** Unspecified injury of other specified muscles and tendons at ankle and foot level, left foot ▽

     √7ᵗʰ **S96.809** Unspecified injury of other specified muscles and tendons at ankle and foot level, unspecified foot ▽

   √6ᵗʰ **S96.81** Strain of other specified muscles and tendons at ankle and foot level

     √7ᵗʰ **S96.811** Strain of other specified muscles and tendons at ankle and foot level, right foot

     √7ᵗʰ **S96.812** Strain of other specified muscles and tendons at ankle and foot level, left foot

     √7ᵗʰ **S96.819** Strain of other specified muscles and tendons at ankle and foot level, unspecified foot ▽

   √6ᵗʰ **S96.82** Laceration of other specified muscles and tendons at ankle and foot level

     √7ᵗʰ **S96.821** Laceration of other specified muscles and tendons at ankle and foot level, right foot

     √7ᵗʰ **S96.822** Laceration of other specified muscles and tendons at ankle and foot level, left foot

     √7ᵗʰ **S96.829** Laceration of other specified muscles and tendons at ankle and foot level, unspecified foot ▽

   √6ᵗʰ **S96.89** Other specified injury of other specified muscles and tendons at ankle and foot level

     √7ᵗʰ **S96.891** Other specified injury of other specified muscles and tendons at ankle and foot level, right foot

     √7ᵗʰ **S96.892** Other specified injury of other specified muscles and tendons at ankle and foot level, left foot

     √7ᵗʰ **S96.899** Other specified injury of other specified muscles and tendons at ankle and foot level, unspecified foot ▽

√5ᵗʰ **S96.9** **Injury of unspecified muscle and tendon at ankle and foot level**

   √6ᵗʰ **S96.90** Unspecified injury of unspecified muscle and tendon at ankle and foot level

     √7ᵗʰ **S96.901** Unspecified injury of unspecified muscle and tendon at ankle and foot level, right foot ▽

     √7ᵗʰ **S96.902** Unspecified injury of unspecified muscle and tendon at ankle and foot level, left foot ▽

     √7ᵗʰ **S96.909** Unspecified injury of unspecified muscle and tendon at ankle and foot level, unspecified foot ▽

   √6ᵗʰ **S96.91** Strain of unspecified muscle and tendon at ankle and foot level

     √7ᵗʰ **S96.911** Strain of unspecified muscle and tendon at ankle and foot level, right foot ▽

     √7ᵗʰ **S96.912** Strain of unspecified muscle and tendon at ankle and foot level, left foot ▽

     √7ᵗʰ **S96.919** Strain of unspecified muscle and tendon at ankle and foot level, unspecified foot ▽

   √6ᵗʰ **S96.92** Laceration of unspecified muscle and tendon at ankle and foot level

     √7ᵗʰ **S96.921** Laceration of unspecified muscle and tendon at ankle and foot level, right foot ▽

     √7ᵗʰ **S96.922** Laceration of unspecified muscle and tendon at ankle and foot level, left foot ▽

     √7ᵗʰ **S96.929** Laceration of unspecified muscle and tendon at ankle and foot level, unspecified foot ▽

√6ᵗʰ **S96.99** Other specified injury of unspecified muscle and tendon at ankle and foot level

     √7ᵗʰ **S96.991** Other specified injury of unspecified muscle and tendon at ankle and foot level, right foot ▽

     √7ᵗʰ **S96.992** Other specified injury of unspecified muscle and tendon at ankle and foot level, left foot ▽

     √7ᵗʰ **S96.999** Other specified injury of unspecified muscle and tendon at ankle and foot level, unspecified foot ▽

√4ᵗʰ **S97** **Crushing injury of ankle and foot**

Use additional code(s) for all associated injuries

> The appropriate 7th character is to be added to each code from category S97.
> A   initial encounter
> D   subsequent encounter
> S   sequela

√5ᵗʰ **S97.0** **Crushing injury of ankle**

   √x7ᵗʰ **S97.00** Crushing injury of unspecified ankle ▽

   √x7ᵗʰ **S97.01** Crushing injury of right ankle

   √x7ᵗʰ **S97.02** Crushing injury of left ankle

√5ᵗʰ **S97.1** **Crushing injury of toe**

   √6ᵗʰ **S97.10** Crushing injury of unspecified toe(s)

     √7ᵗʰ **S97.101** Crushing injury of unspecified right toe(s) ▽

     √7ᵗʰ **S97.102** Crushing injury of unspecified left toe(s) ▽

     √7ᵗʰ **S97.109** Crushing injury of unspecified toe(s)
        Crushing injury of toe NOS

   √6ᵗʰ **S97.11** Crushing injury of great toe

     √7ᵗʰ **S97.111** Crushing injury of right great toe

     √7ᵗʰ **S97.112** Crushing injury of left great toe

     √7ᵗʰ **S97.119** Crushing injury of unspecified great toe ▽

   √6ᵗʰ **S97.12** Crushing injury of lesser toe(s)

     √7ᵗʰ **S97.121** Crushing injury of right lesser toe(s)

     √7ᵗʰ **S97.122** Crushing injury of left lesser toe(s)

     √7ᵗʰ **S97.129** Crushing injury of unspecified lesser toe(s) ▽

√5ᵗʰ **S97.8** **Crushing injury of foot**

   √x7ᵗʰ **S97.80** Crushing injury of unspecified foot ▽
        Crushing injury of foot NOS

   √x7ᵗʰ **S97.81** Crushing injury of right foot

   √x7ᵗʰ **S97.82** Crushing injury of left foot

√4ᵗʰ **S98** **Traumatic amputation of ankle and foot**

An amputation not identified as partial or complete should be coded to complete

> The appropriate 7th character is to be added to each code from category S98.
> A   initial encounter
> D   subsequent encounter
> S   sequela

√5ᵗʰ **S98.0** **Traumatic amputation of foot at ankle level**

   √6ᵗʰ **S98.01** Complete traumatic amputation of foot at ankle level

     √7ᵗʰ **S98.011** Complete traumatic amputation of right foot at ankle level   HCC

     √7ᵗʰ **S98.012** Complete traumatic amputation of left foot at ankle level   HCC

     √7ᵗʰ **S98.019** Complete traumatic amputation of unspecified foot at ankle level   HCC ▽

   √6ᵗʰ **S98.02** Partial traumatic amputation of foot at ankle level

     √7ᵗʰ **S98.021** Partial traumatic amputation of right foot at ankle level   HCC

     √7ᵗʰ **S98.022** Partial traumatic amputation of left foot at ankle level   HCC

     √7ᵗʰ **S98.029** Partial traumatic amputation of unspecified foot at ankle level   HCC ▽

☑ Additional Character Req   √x7ᵗʰ Placeholder Alert   Manifestation   HCC CMS-HCC Condition   ▽ Unspecified Code   ►◄ Revised Text   ● New Code   ▲ Revised Code Title

ICD-10-CM 2018   **1035**

S98.1   Traumatic amputation of one toe
- ✓6th **S98.11**   Complete traumatic amputation of great toe
  - ✓7th **S98.111**   Complete traumatic amputation of right great toe   HCC
  - ✓7th **S98.112**   Complete traumatic amputation of left great toe   HCC
  - ✓7th **S98.119**   Complete traumatic amputation of unspecified great toe   HCC ▽
- ✓6th **S98.12**   Partial traumatic amputation of great toe
  - ✓7th **S98.121**   Partial traumatic amputation of right great toe   HCC
  - ✓7th **S98.122**   Partial traumatic amputation of left great toe   HCC
  - ✓7th **S98.129**   Partial traumatic amputation of unspecified great toe   HCC ▽
- ✓6th **S98.13**   Complete traumatic amputation of one lesser toe
  Traumatic amputation of toe NOS
  - ✓7th **S98.131**   Complete traumatic amputation of one right lesser toe   HCC
  - ✓7th **S98.132**   Complete traumatic amputation of one left lesser toe   HCC
  - ✓7th **S98.139**   Complete traumatic amputation of one unspecified lesser toe   HCC ▽
- ✓6th **S98.14**   Partial traumatic amputation of one lesser toe
  - ✓7th **S98.141**   Partial traumatic amputation of one right lesser toe   HCC
  - ✓7th **S98.142**   Partial traumatic amputation of one left lesser toe   HCC
  - ✓7th **S98.149**   Partial traumatic amputation of one unspecified lesser toe   HCC ▽

S98.2   Traumatic amputation of two or more lesser toes
- ✓6th **S98.21**   Complete traumatic amputation of two or more lesser toes
  - ✓7th **S98.211**   Complete traumatic amputation of two or more right lesser toes   HCC
  - ✓7th **S98.212**   Complete traumatic amputation of two or more left lesser toes   HCC
  - ✓7th **S98.219**   Complete traumatic amputation of two or more unspecified lesser toes   HCC ▽
- ✓6th **S98.22**   Partial traumatic amputation of two or more lesser toes
  - ✓7th **S98.221**   Partial traumatic amputation of two or more right lesser toes   HCC
  - ✓7th **S98.222**   Partial traumatic amputation of two or more left lesser toes   HCC
  - ✓7th **S98.229**   Partial traumatic amputation of two or more unspecified lesser toes   HCC ▽

S98.3   Traumatic amputation of midfoot
- ✓6th **S98.31**   Complete traumatic amputation of midfoot
  - ✓7th **S98.311**   Complete traumatic amputation of right midfoot   HCC
  - ✓7th **S98.312**   Complete traumatic amputation of left midfoot   HCC
  - ✓7th **S98.319**   Complete traumatic amputation of unspecified midfoot   HCC ▽
- ✓6th **S98.32**   Partial traumatic amputation of midfoot
  - ✓7th **S98.321**   Partial traumatic amputation of right midfoot   HCC
  - ✓7th **S98.322**   Partial traumatic amputation of left midfoot   HCC
  - ✓7th **S98.329**   Partial traumatic amputation of unspecified midfoot   HCC ▽

S98.9   Traumatic amputation of foot, level unspecified
- ✓6th **S98.91**   Complete traumatic amputation of foot, level unspecified
  - ✓7th **S98.911**   Complete traumatic amputation of right foot, level unspecified   HCC ▽
  - ✓7th **S98.912**   Complete traumatic amputation of left foot, level unspecified   HCC ▽
  - ✓7th **S98.919**   Complete traumatic amputation of unspecified foot, level unspecified   HCC ▽

- ✓6th **S98.92**   Partial traumatic amputation of foot, level unspecified
  - ✓7th **S98.921**   Partial traumatic amputation of right foot, level unspecified   HCC ▽
  - ✓7th **S98.922**   Partial traumatic amputation of left foot, level unspecified   HCC ▽
  - ✓7th **S98.929**   Partial traumatic amputation of unspecified foot, level unspecified   HCC ▽

✓4th **S99**   **Other and unspecified injuries of ankle and foot**
- ✓5th **S99.0**   Physeal fracture of calcaneus

> The appropriate 7th character is to be added to each code from subcategories S99.0.
> A   initial encounter for closed fracture
> B   initial encounter for open fracture
> D   subsequent encounter for fracture with routine healing
> G   subsequent encounter for fracture with delayed healing
> K   subsequent encounter for fracture with nonunion
> P   subsequent encounter for fracture with malunion
> S   sequela

  - ✓6th **S99.00**   Unspecified physeal fracture of calcaneus
    - ✓7th **S99.001**   Unspecified physeal fracture of right calcaneus ▽
    - ✓7th **S99.002**   Unspecified physeal fracture of left calcaneus ▽
    - ✓7th **S99.009**   Unspecified physeal fracture of unspecified calcaneus ▽
  - ✓6th **S99.01**   Salter-Harris Type I physeal fracture of calcaneus
    - ✓7th **S99.011**   Salter-Harris Type I physeal fracture of right calcaneus
    - ✓7th **S99.012**   Salter-Harris Type I physeal fracture of left calcaneus
    - ✓7th **S99.019**   Salter-Harris Type I physeal fracture of unspecified calcaneus ▽
  - ✓6th **S99.02**   Salter-Harris Type II physeal fracture of calcaneus
    - ✓7th **S99.021**   Salter-Harris Type II physeal fracture of right calcaneus
    - ✓7th **S99.022**   Salter-Harris Type II physeal fracture of left calcaneus
    - ✓7th **S99.029**   Salter-Harris Type II physeal fracture of unspecified calcaneus ▽
  - ✓6th **S99.03**   Salter-Harris Type III physeal fracture of calcaneus
    - ✓7th **S99.031**   Salter-Harris Type III physeal fracture of right calcaneus
    - ✓7th **S99.032**   Salter-Harris Type III physeal fracture of left calcaneus
    - ✓7th **S99.039**   Salter-Harris Type III physeal fracture of unspecified calcaneus ▽
  - ✓6th **S99.04**   Salter-Harris Type IV physeal fracture of calcaneus
    - ✓7th **S99.041**   Salter-Harris Type IV physeal fracture of right calcaneus
    - ✓7th **S99.042**   Salter-Harris Type IV physeal fracture of left calcaneus
    - ✓7th **S99.049**   Salter-Harris Type IV physeal fracture of unspecified calcaneus ▽
  - ✓6th **S99.09**   Other physeal fracture of calcaneus
    - ✓7th **S99.091**   Other physeal fracture of right calcaneus
    - ✓7th **S99.092**   Other physeal fracture of left calcaneus
    - ✓7th **S99.099**   Other physeal fracture of unspecified calcaneus ▽

- ✓5th **S99.1**   Physeal fracture of metatarsal

> The appropriate 7th character is to be added to each code from subcategories S99.1.
> A   initial encounter for closed fracture
> B   initial encounter for open fracture
> D   subsequent encounter for fracture with routine healing
> G   subsequent encounter for fracture with delayed healing
> K   subsequent encounter for fracture with nonunion
> P   subsequent encounter for fracture with malunion
> S   sequela

  - ✓6th **S99.10**   Unspecified physeal fracture of metatarsal
    - ✓7th **S99.101**   Unspecified physeal fracture of right metatarsal ▽

    ✓7ᵗʰ   **S99.102**   Unspecified physeal fracture of left metatarsal   ▽

    ✓7ᵗʰ   **S99.109**   Unspecified physeal fracture of unspecified metatarsal   ▽

✓6ᵗʰ   **S99.11**   Salter-Harris Type I physeal fracture of metatarsal

    ✓7ᵗʰ   **S99.111**   Salter-Harris Type I physeal fracture of right metatarsal

    ✓7ᵗʰ   **S99.112**   Salter-Harris Type I physeal fracture of left metatarsal

    ✓7ᵗʰ   **S99.119**   Salter-Harris Type I physeal fracture of unspecified metatarsal   ▽

✓6ᵗʰ   **S99.12**   Salter-Harris Type II physeal fracture of metatarsal

    ✓7ᵗʰ   **S99.121**   Salter-Harris Type II physeal fracture of right metatarsal

    ✓7ᵗʰ   **S99.122**   Salter-Harris Type II physeal fracture of left metatarsal

    ✓7ᵗʰ   **S99.129**   Salter-Harris Type II physeal fracture of unspecified metatarsal   ▽

✓6ᵗʰ   **S99.13**   Salter-Harris Type III physeal fracture of metatarsal

    ✓7ᵗʰ   **S99.131**   Salter-Harris Type III physeal fracture of right metatarsal

    ✓7ᵗʰ   **S99.132**   Salter-Harris Type III physeal fracture of left metatarsal

    ✓7ᵗʰ   **S99.139**   Salter-Harris Type III physeal fracture of unspecified metatarsal   ▽

✓6ᵗʰ   **S99.14**   Salter-Harris Type IV physeal fracture of metatarsal

    ✓7ᵗʰ   **S99.141**   Salter-Harris Type IV physeal fracture of right metatarsal

    ✓7ᵗʰ   **S99.142**   Salter-Harris Type IV physeal fracture of left metatarsal

    ✓7ᵗʰ   **S99.149**   Salter-Harris Type IV physeal fracture of unspecified metatarsal   ▽

✓6ᵗʰ   **S99.19**   Other physeal fracture of metatarsal

    ✓7ᵗʰ   **S99.191**   Other physeal fracture of right metatarsal

    ✓7ᵗʰ   **S99.192**   Other physeal fracture of left metatarsal

    ✓7ᵗʰ   **S99.199**   Other physeal fracture of unspecified metatarsal   ▽

✓5ᵗʰ   **S99.2**   Physeal fracture of phalanx of toe

> The appropriate 7th character is to be added to each code from subcategories S99.2.
> A   initial encounter for closed fracture
> B   initial encounter for open fracture
> D   subsequent encounter for fracture with routine healing
> G   subsequent encounter for fracture with delayed healing
> K   subsequent encounter for fracture with nonunion
> P   subsequent encounter for fracture with malunion
> S   sequela

✓6ᵗʰ   **S99.20**   Unspecified physeal fracture of phalanx of toe

    ✓7ᵗʰ   **S99.201**   Unspecified physeal fracture of phalanx of right toe   ▽

    ✓7ᵗʰ   **S99.202**   Unspecified physeal fracture of phalanx of left toe   ▽

    ✓7ᵗʰ   **S99.209**   Unspecified physeal fracture of phalanx of unspecified toe   ▽

✓6ᵗʰ   **S99.21**   Salter-Harris Type I physeal fracture of phalanx of toe

    ✓7ᵗʰ   **S99.211**   Salter-Harris Type I physeal fracture of phalanx of right toe

    ✓7ᵗʰ   **S99.212**   Salter-Harris Type I physeal fracture of phalanx of left toe

    ✓7ᵗʰ   **S99.219**   Salter-Harris Type I physeal fracture of phalanx of unspecified toe   ▽

✓6ᵗʰ   **S99.22**   Salter-Harris Type II physeal fracture of phalanx of toe

    ✓7ᵗʰ   **S99.221**   Salter-Harris Type II physeal fracture of phalanx of right toe

    ✓7ᵗʰ   **S99.222**   Salter-Harris Type II physeal fracture of phalanx of left toe

    ✓7ᵗʰ   **S99.229**   Salter-Harris Type II physeal fracture of phalanx of unspecified toe   ▽

✓6ᵗʰ   **S99.23**   Salter-Harris Type III physeal fracture of phalanx of toe

    ✓7ᵗʰ   **S99.231**   Salter-Harris Type III physeal fracture of phalanx of right toe

    ✓7ᵗʰ   **S99.232**   Salter-Harris Type III physeal fracture of phalanx of left toe

    ✓7ᵗʰ   **S99.239**   Salter-Harris Type III physeal fracture of phalanx of unspecified toe   ▽

✓6ᵗʰ   **S99.24**   Salter-Harris Type IV physeal fracture of phalanx of toe

    ✓7ᵗʰ   **S99.241**   Salter-Harris Type IV physeal fracture of phalanx of right toe

    ✓7ᵗʰ   **S99.242**   Salter-Harris Type IV physeal fracture of phalanx of left toe

    ✓7ᵗʰ   **S99.249**   Salter-Harris Type IV physeal fracture of phalanx of unspecified toe   ▽

✓6ᵗʰ   **S99.29**   Other physeal fracture of phalanx of toe

    ✓7ᵗʰ   **S99.291**   Other physeal fracture of phalanx of right toe

    ✓7ᵗʰ   **S99.292**   Other physeal fracture of phalanx of left toe

    ✓7ᵗʰ   **S99.299**   Other physeal fracture of phalanx of unspecified toe   ▽

✓5ᵗʰ   **S99.8**   Other specified injuries of ankle and foot

> The appropriate 7th character is to be added to each code from subcategory S99.8.
> A   initial encounter
> D   subsequent encounter
> S   sequela

✓6ᵗʰ   **S99.81**   Other specified injuries of ankle

    ✓7ᵗʰ   **S99.811**   Other specified injuries of right ankle

    ✓7ᵗʰ   **S99.812**   Other specified injuries of left ankle

    ✓7ᵗʰ   **S99.819**   Other specified injuries of unspecified ankle   ▽

✓6ᵗʰ   **S99.82**   Other specified injuries of foot

    ✓7ᵗʰ   **S99.821**   Other specified injuries of right foot

    ✓7ᵗʰ   **S99.822**   Other specified injuries of left foot

    ✓7ᵗʰ   **S99.829**   Other specified injuries of unspecified foot   ▽

✓5ᵗʰ   **S99.9**   Unspecified injury of ankle and foot

> The appropriate 7th character is to be added to each code from subcategory S99.9.
> A   initial encounter
> D   subsequent encounter
> S   sequela

✓6ᵗʰ   **S99.91**   Unspecified injury of ankle

    ✓7ᵗʰ   **S99.911**   Unspecified injury of right ankle   ▽

    ✓7ᵗʰ   **S99.912**   Unspecified injury of left ankle   ▽

    ✓7ᵗʰ   **S99.919**   Unspecified injury of unspecified ankle   ▽

✓6ᵗʰ   **S99.92**   Unspecified injury of foot

    ✓7ᵗʰ   **S99.921**   Unspecified injury of right foot   ▽

    ✓7ᵗʰ   **S99.922**   Unspecified injury of left foot   ▽

    ✓7ᵗʰ   **S99.929**   Unspecified injury of unspecified foot   ▽

Injury, Poisoning And Certain Other Consequences Of External Causes (T07-T88)

Injuries involving multiple body regions (T07)

> *EXCLUDES 1*   burns and corrosions (T20-T32)
> frostbite (T33-T34)
> insect bite or sting, venomous (T63.4)
> sunburn (L55.-)

✓x7ᵗʰ   **T07**   **Unspecified multiple injuries**   ▽
> *EXCLUDES 1*   injury NOS ▶(T14.90)◄

> The appropriate 7th character is to be added to code T07.
> A   initial encounter
> D   subsequent encounter
> S   sequela

☑ Additional Character Req   ✓x7ᵗʰ Placeholder Alert   Manifestation   HCC CMS-HCC Condition   ▽ Unspecified Code   ▶◄ Revised Text   ● New Code   ▲ Revised Code Title

ICD-10-CM 2018   1037

Injury of unspecified body region (T14)

✓4ᵗʰ **T14   Injury of unspecified body region**
> EXCLUDES 1   *multiple unspecified injuries (T07)*

> The appropriate 7th character is to be added to each code from category T14.
> A   initial encounter
> D   subsequent encounter
> S   sequela

✓x7ᵗʰ **T14.8   Other injury of unspecified body region**
> Abrasion NOS
> Contusion NOS
> Crush injury NOS
> Fracture NOS
> Skin injury NOS
> Vascular injury NOS
> ▶Wound NOS◀

✓5ᵗʰ **T14.9   Unspecified injury**

✓x7ᵗʰ **T14.90   Injury, unspecified**   ▽
> Injury NOS

✓x7ᵗʰ **T14.91   Suicide attempt**   HCC
> Attempted suicide NOS

Effects of foreign body entering through natural orifice (T15-T19)

> EXCLUDES 2   *foreign body accidentally left in operation wound (T81.5-)*
> *foreign body in penetrating wound—See open wound by body region*
> *residual foreign body in soft tissue (M79.5)*
> *splinter, without open wound—See superficial injury by body region*

✓4ᵗʰ **T15   Foreign body on external eye**
> EXCLUDES 2   *foreign body in penetrating wound of orbit and eye ball (S05.4-, S05.5-)*
> *open wound of eyelid and periocular area (S01.1-)*
> *retained foreign body in eyelid (H02.8-)*
> *retained (old) foreign body in penetrating wound of orbit and eye ball (H05.5-, H44.6-, H44.7-)*
> *superficial foreign body of eyelid and periocular area (S00.25-)*

> The appropriate 7th character is to be added to each code from category T15.
> A   initial encounter
> D   subsequent encounter
> S   sequela

✓5ᵗʰ **T15.0   Foreign body in cornea**

✓x7ᵗʰ **T15.00   Foreign body in cornea, unspecified eye**   ▽

✓x7ᵗʰ **T15.01   Foreign body in cornea, right eye**

✓x7ᵗʰ **T15.02   Foreign body in cornea, left eye**

✓5ᵗʰ **T15.1   Foreign body in conjunctival sac**

✓x7ᵗʰ **T15.10   Foreign body in conjunctival sac, unspecified eye**   ▽

✓x7ᵗʰ **T15.11   Foreign body in conjunctival sac, right eye**

✓x7ᵗʰ **T15.12   Foreign body in conjunctival sac, left eye**

✓5ᵗʰ **T15.8   Foreign body in other and multiple parts of external eye**
> Foreign body in lacrimal punctum

✓x7ᵗʰ **T15.80   Foreign body in other and multiple parts of external eye, unspecified eye**   ▽

✓x7ᵗʰ **T15.81   Foreign body in other and multiple parts of external eye, right eye**

✓x7ᵗʰ **T15.82   Foreign body in other and multiple parts of external eye, left eye**

✓5ᵗʰ **T15.9   Foreign body on external eye, part unspecified**

✓x7ᵗʰ **T15.90   Foreign body on external eye, part unspecified, unspecified eye**   ▽

✓x7ᵗʰ **T15.91   Foreign body on external eye, part unspecified, right eye**   ▽

✓x7ᵗʰ **T15.92   Foreign body on external eye, part unspecified, left eye**   ▽

✓4ᵗʰ **T16   Foreign body in ear**
> INCLUDES   foreign body in auditory canal

> The appropriate 7th character is to be added to each code from category T16.
> A   initial encounter
> D   subsequent encounter
> S   sequela

✓x7ᵗʰ **T16.1   Foreign body in right ear**

✓x7ᵗʰ **T16.2   Foreign body in left ear**

✓x7ᵗʰ **T16.9   Foreign body in ear, unspecified ear**   ▽

✓4ᵗʰ **T17   Foreign body in respiratory tract**

> The appropriate 7th character is to be added to each code from category T17.
> A   initial encounter
> D   subsequent encounter
> S   sequela

✓7ᵗʰ **T17.0   Foreign body in nasal sinus**

✓7ᵗʰ **T17.1   Foreign body in nostril**
> Foreign body in nose NOS

✓5ᵗʰ **T17.2   Foreign body in pharynx**
> Foreign body in nasopharynx
> Foreign body in throat NOS

✓6ᵗʰ **T17.20   Unspecified foreign body in pharynx**

✓7ᵗʰ **T17.200   Unspecified foreign body in pharynx causing asphyxiation**   ▽

✓7ᵗʰ **T17.208   Unspecified foreign body in pharynx causing other injury**   ▽

✓6ᵗʰ **T17.21   Gastric contents in pharynx**
> Aspiration of gastric contents into pharynx
> Vomitus in pharynx

✓7ᵗʰ **T17.210   Gastric contents in pharynx causing asphyxiation**

✓7ᵗʰ **T17.218   Gastric contents in pharynx causing other injury**

✓6ᵗʰ **T17.22   Food in pharynx**
> Bones in pharynx
> Seeds in pharynx

✓7ᵗʰ **T17.220   Food in pharynx causing asphyxiation**

✓7ᵗʰ **T17.228   Food in pharynx causing other injury**

✓6ᵗʰ **T17.29   Other foreign object in pharynx**

✓7ᵗʰ **T17.290   Other foreign object in pharynx causing asphyxiation**

✓7ᵗʰ **T17.298   Other foreign object in pharynx causing other injury**

✓5ᵗʰ **T17.3   Foreign body in larynx**

✓6ᵗʰ **T17.30   Unspecified foreign body in larynx**

✓7ᵗʰ **T17.300   Unspecified foreign body in larynx causing asphyxiation**   ▽

✓7ᵗʰ **T17.308   Unspecified foreign body in larynx causing other injury**   ▽

✓6ᵗʰ **T17.31   Gastric contents in larynx**
> Aspiration of gastric contents into larynx
> Vomitus in larynx

✓7ᵗʰ **T17.310   Gastric contents in larynx causing asphyxiation**

✓7ᵗʰ **T17.318   Gastric contents in larynx causing other injury**

✓6ᵗʰ **T17.32   Food in larynx**
> Bones in larynx
> Seeds in larynx

✓7ᵗʰ **T17.320   Food in larynx causing asphyxiation**

✓7ᵗʰ **T17.328   Food in larynx causing other injury**

✓6ᵗʰ **T17.39   Other foreign object in larynx**

✓7ᵗʰ **T17.390   Other foreign object in larynx causing asphyxiation**

✓7ᵗʰ **T17.398   Other foreign object in larynx causing other injury**

✓5ᵗʰ **T17.4   Foreign body in trachea**

✓6ᵗʰ **T17.40   Unspecified foreign body in trachea**

✓7ᵗʰ **T17.400   Unspecified foreign body in trachea causing asphyxiation**   ▽

✓7ᵗʰ **T17.408   Unspecified foreign body in trachea causing other injury**   ▽

✓6ᵗʰ **T17.41   Gastric contents in trachea**
> Aspiration of gastric contents into trachea
> Vomitus in trachea

✓7ᵗʰ **T17.410   Gastric contents in trachea causing asphyxiation**

✓7ᵗʰ **T17.418   Gastric contents in trachea causing other injury**

EXCLUDES 1   Not coded here   EXCLUDES 2   Not included here   N Newborn Age: 0   P Pediatric Age: 0-17   M Maternity Age: 12-55   A Adult Age: 15-124

1038   ICD-10-CM 2018

✓6th **T17.42** **Food** in trachea
    Bones in trachea
    Seeds in trachea
    ✓7th **T17.420** **Food in trachea** causing asphyxiation
    ✓7th **T17.428** **Food in trachea** causing other injury
✓6th **T17.49** **Other foreign object in trachea**
    ✓7th **T17.490** **Other foreign object in trachea** causing asphyxiation
    ✓7th **T17.498** **Other foreign object in trachea** causing other injury

✓5th **T17.5** **Foreign body in** bronchus
✓6th **T17.50** **Unspecified foreign body in bronchus**
    ✓7th **T17.500** **Unspecified foreign body in bronchus** causing asphyxiation ▽
    ✓7th **T17.508** **Unspecified foreign body in bronchus** causing other injury ▽
✓6th **T17.51** **Gastric contents** in bronchus
    Aspiration of gastric contents into bronchus
    Vomitus in bronchus
    ✓7th **T17.510** **Gastric contents in bronchus** causing asphyxiation
    ✓7th **T17.518** **Gastric contents in bronchus** causing other injury
✓6th **T17.52** **Food** in bronchus
    Bones in bronchus
    Seeds in bronchus
    ✓7th **T17.520** **Food in bronchus** causing asphyxiation
    ✓7th **T17.528** **Food in bronchus** causing other injury
✓6th **T17.59** **Other foreign object in bronchus**
    ✓7th **T17.590** **Other foreign object in bronchus** causing asphyxiation
    ✓7th **T17.598** **Other foreign object in bronchus** causing other injury

✓5th **T17.8** **Foreign body in other parts of respiratory tract**
    Foreign body in bronchioles
    Foreign body in lung
✓6th **T17.80** **Unspecified foreign body in other parts of respiratory tract**
    ✓7th **T17.800** **Unspecified foreign body in other parts of respiratory tract** causing asphyxiation ▽
    ✓7th **T17.808** **Unspecified foreign body in other parts of respiratory tract** causing other injury ▽
✓6th **T17.81** **Gastric contents** in other parts of respiratory tract
    Aspiration of gastric contents into other parts of respiratory tract
    Vomitus in other parts of respiratory tract
    ✓7th **T17.810** **Gastric contents in other parts of respiratory tract** causing asphyxiation
    ✓7th **T17.818** **Gastric contents in other parts of respiratory tract** causing other injury
✓6th **T17.82** **Food** in other parts of respiratory tract
    Bones in other parts of respiratory tract
    Seeds in other parts of respiratory tract
    ✓7th **T17.820** **Food in other parts of respiratory tract** causing asphyxiation
    ✓7th **T17.828** **Food in other parts of respiratory tract** causing other injury
✓6th **T17.89** **Other foreign object in other parts of respiratory tract**
    ✓7th **T17.890** **Other foreign object in other parts of respiratory tract** causing asphyxiation
    ✓7th **T17.898** **Other foreign object in other parts of respiratory tract** causing other injury

✓5th **T17.9** **Foreign body in respiratory tract, part unspecified**
✓6th **T17.90** **Unspecified foreign body in respiratory tract, part unspecified**
    ✓7th **T17.900** **Unspecified foreign body in respiratory tract, part unspecified** causing asphyxiation ▽
    ✓7th **T17.908** **Unspecified foreign body in respiratory tract, part unspecified** causing other injury

✓6th **T17.91** **Gastric contents** in respiratory tract, part unspecified
    Aspiration of gastric contents into respiratory tract, part unspecified
    Vomitus in trachea respiratory tract, part unspecified
    ✓7th **T17.910** **Gastric contents in respiratory tract, part unspecified** causing asphyxiation ▽
    ✓7th **T17.918** **Gastric contents in respiratory tract, part unspecified** causing other injury ▽
✓6th **T17.92** **Food** in respiratory tract, part unspecified
    Bones in respiratory tract, part unspecified
    Seeds in respiratory tract, part unspecified
    ✓7th **T17.920** **Food in respiratory tract, part unspecified** causing asphyxiation ▽
    ✓7th **T17.928** **Food in respiratory tract, part unspecified** causing other injury ▽
✓6th **T17.99** **Other foreign object in respiratory tract, part unspecified**
    ✓7th **T17.990** **Other foreign object in respiratory tract, part unspecified in** causing asphyxiation
    ✓7th **T17.998** **Other foreign object in respiratory tract, part unspecified** causing other injury ▽

✓4th **T18** **Foreign body in alimentary tract**
    EXCLUDES 2 foreign body in pharynx (T17.2-)

> The appropriate 7th character is to be added to each code from category T18.
> A   initial encounter
> D   subsequent encounter
> S   sequela

✓x7th **T18.0** **Foreign body in** mouth
✓5th **T18.1** **Foreign body in** esophagus
    EXCLUDES 2 foreign body in respiratory tract (T17.-)
✓6th **T18.10** **Unspecified foreign body in esophagus**
    ✓7th **T18.100** **Unspecified foreign body in esophagus** causing compression of trachea ▽
        Unspecified foreign body in esophagus causing obstruction of respiration
    ✓7th **T18.108** **Unspecified foreign body in esophagus** causing other injury ▽
✓6th **T18.11** **Gastric contents** in esophagus
    Vomitus in esophagus
    ✓7th **T18.110** **Gastric contents in esophagus** causing compression of trachea
        Gastric contents in esophagus causing obstruction of respiration
    ✓7th **T18.118** **Gastric contents in esophagus** causing other injury
✓6th **T18.12** **Food** in esophagus
    Bones in esophagus
    Seeds in esophagus
    ✓7th **T18.120** **Food in esophagus** causing compression of trachea
        Food in esophagus causing obstruction of respiration
    ✓7th **T18.128** **Food in esophagus** causing other injury
✓6th **T18.19** **Other foreign object in esophagus**
    AHA: 2015, 1Q, 23
    ✓7th **T18.190** **Other foreign object in esophagus** causing compression of trachea
        Other foreign body in esophagus causing obstruction of respiration
    ✓7th **T18.198** **Other foreign object in esophagus** causing other injury

✓x7th **T18.2** **Foreign body in** stomach
✓x7th **T18.3** **Foreign body in** small intestine
✓x7th **T18.4** **Foreign body in** colon
✓x7th **T18.5** **Foreign body in** anus and rectum
    Foreign body in rectosigmoid (junction)
✓x7th **T18.8** **Foreign body in other parts of alimentary tract**
✓x7th **T18.9** **Foreign body of alimentary tract, part unspecified** ▽
    Foreign body in digestive system NOS
    Swallowed foreign body NOS

☑4ᵗʰ **T19** **Foreign body in genitourinary tract**

EXCLUDES 2 *complications due to implanted mesh (T83.7-)*
mechanical complications of contraceptive device (intrauterine) (vaginal) (T83.3-)
presence of contraceptive device (intrauterine) (vaginal) (Z97.5)

The appropriate 7th character is to be added to each code from category T19.
A   initial encounter
D   subsequent encounter
S   sequela

☑x7ᵗʰ **T19.0** **Foreign body in urethra**

☑x7ᵗʰ **T19.1** **Foreign body in bladder**

☑x7ᵗʰ **T19.2** **Foreign body in vulva and vagina** ♀

☑x7ᵗʰ **T19.3** **Foreign body in uterus** ♀

☑x7ᵗʰ **T19.4** **Foreign body in penis** ♂

☑x7ᵗʰ **T19.8** **Foreign body in other parts of genitourinary tract**

☑x7ᵗʰ **T19.9** **Foreign body in genitourinary tract, part unspecified** ▽

Burns and corrosions (T20-T32)

INCLUDES burns (thermal) from electrical heating appliances
burns (thermal) from electricity
burns (thermal) from flame
burns (thermal) from friction
burns (thermal) from hot air and hot gases
burns (thermal) from hot objects
burns (thermal) from lightning
burns (thermal) from radiation
chemical burn [corrosion] (external) (internal)
scalds

EXCLUDES 2 *erythema [dermatitis] ab igne (L59.0)*
radiation-related disorders of the skin and subcutaneous tissue (L55-L59)
sunburn (L55.-)

AHA: 2016, 2Q, 4

Burns and corrosions of external body surface, specified by site (T20-T25)

INCLUDES burns and corrosions of first degree [erythema]
burns and corrosions of second degree [blisters] [epidermal loss]
burns and corrosions of third degree [deep necrosis of underlying tissue] [full-thickness skin loss]

Use additional code from category T31 or T32 to identify extent of body surface involved

☑4ᵗʰ **T20** **Burn and corrosion of head, face, and neck**

EXCLUDES 2 *burn and corrosion of ear drum (T28.41, T28.91)*
burn and corrosion of eye and adnexa (T26.-)
burn and corrosion of mouth and pharynx (T28.0)

AHA: 2015, 1Q, 18-19

The appropriate 7th character is to be added to each code from category T20.
A   initial encounter
D   subsequent encounter
S   sequela

☑5ᵗʰ **T20.0** **Burn of unspecified degree of head, face, and neck**

Use additional external cause code to identify the source, place and intent of the burn (X00-X19, X75-X77, X96-X98, Y92)

☑x7ᵗʰ **T20.00** **Burn of unspecified degree of head, face, and neck, unspecified site** ▽

☑6ᵗʰ **T20.01** **Burn of unspecified degree of ear [any part, except ear drum]**

EXCLUDES 2 *burn of ear drum (T28.41-)*

☑7ᵗʰ **T20.011** **Burn of unspecified degree of right ear [any part, except ear drum]** ▽

☑7ᵗʰ **T20.012** **Burn of unspecified degree of left ear [any part, except ear drum]** ▽

☑7ᵗʰ **T20.019** **Burn of unspecified degree of unspecified ear [any part, except ear drum]** ▽

☑x7ᵗʰ **T20.02** **Burn of unspecified degree of lip(s)** ▽

☑x7ᵗʰ **T20.03** **Burn of unspecified degree of chin** ▽

Rule of Nines Estimation of Total Body Surface Burned

Head and neck 9%
Each arm 9%
Anterior trunk 18%
Posterior trunk 18%
Genitalia 1%
Anterior leg 9%
Posterior leg 9%

☑x7ᵗʰ **T20.04** **Burn of unspecified degree of nose (septum)** ▽

☑x7ᵗʰ **T20.05** **Burn of unspecified degree of scalp [any part]** ▽

☑x7ᵗʰ **T20.06** **Burn of unspecified degree of forehead and cheek** ▽

☑x7ᵗʰ **T20.07** **Burn of unspecified degree of neck** ▽

☑x7ᵗʰ **T20.09** **Burn of unspecified degree of multiple sites of head, face, and neck** ▽

☑5ᵗʰ **T20.1** **Burn of first degree of head, face, and neck**

Use additional external cause code to identify the source, place and intent of the burn (X00-X19, X75-X77, X96-X98, Y92)

☑x7ᵗʰ **T20.10** **Burn of first degree of head, face, and neck, unspecified site** ▽

☑6ᵗʰ **T20.11** **Burn of first degree of ear [any part, except ear drum]**

EXCLUDES 2 *burn of ear drum (T28.41-)*

☑7ᵗʰ **T20.111** **Burn of first degree of right ear [any part, except ear drum]**

☑7ᵗʰ **T20.112** **Burn of first degree of left ear [any part, except ear drum]**

☑7ᵗʰ **T20.119** **Burn of first degree of unspecified ear [any part, except ear drum]** ▽

☑x7ᵗʰ **T20.12** **Burn of first degree of lip(s)**

☑x7ᵗʰ **T20.13** **Burn of first degree of chin**

☑x7ᵗʰ **T20.14** **Burn of first degree of nose (septum)**

☑x7ᵗʰ **T20.15** **Burn of first degree of scalp [any part]**

☑x7ᵗʰ **T20.16** **Burn of first degree of forehead and cheek**

☑x7ᵗʰ **T20.17** **Burn of first degree of neck**

☑x7ᵗʰ **T20.19** **Burn of first degree of multiple sites of head, face, and neck**

Degree of Burns

Epidermis
Dermis
Subcutaneous

Normal   First Degree Burn

Epidermis
Dermis
Subcutaneous

Second Degree Burn   Third Degree Burn

✓5ᵗʰ **T20.2** **Burn of** second degree **of head, face, and neck**
Use additional external cause code to identify the source, place and intent of the burn (X00-X19, X75-X77, X96-X98, Y92)

   ✓x7ᵗʰ **T20.20** **Burn of second degree of head, face, and neck, unspecified site** ▽

   ✓6ᵗʰ **T20.21** **Burn of second degree of** ear **[any part, except ear drum]**
EXCLUDES 2   burn of ear drum (T28.41-)

     ✓7ᵗʰ **T20.211** **Burn of second degree of** right **ear [any part, except ear drum]**

     ✓7ᵗʰ **T20.212** **Burn of second degree of** left **ear [any part, except ear drum]**

     ✓7ᵗʰ **T20.219** **Burn of second degree of unspecified ear [any part, except ear drum]** ▽

   ✓x7ᵗʰ **T20.22** **Burn of second degree of** lip(s)

   ✓x7ᵗʰ **T20.23** **Burn of second degree of** chin

   ✓x7ᵗʰ **T20.24** **Burn of second degree of** nose (septum)

   ✓x7ᵗʰ **T20.25** **Burn of second degree of** scalp [any part]

   ✓x7ᵗʰ **T20.26** **Burn of second degree of** forehead and cheek

   ✓x7ᵗʰ **T20.27** **Burn of second degree of** neck

   ✓x7ᵗʰ **T20.29** **Burn of second degree of** multiple sites **of head, face, and neck**

✓5ᵗʰ **T20.3** **Burn of** third degree **of head, face, and neck**
Use additional external cause code to identify the source, place and intent of the burn (X00-X19, X75-X77, X96-X98, Y92)

   ✓x7ᵗʰ **T20.30** **Burn of third degree of head, face, and neck, unspecified site** ▽

   ✓6ᵗʰ **T20.31** **Burn of third degree of** ear **[any part, except ear drum]**
EXCLUDES 2   burn of ear drum (T28.41-)
AHA: 2015, 1Q, 18

     ✓7ᵗʰ **T20.311** **Burn of third degree of** right **ear [any part, except ear drum]**

     ✓7ᵗʰ **T20.312** **Burn of third degree of** left **ear [any part, except ear drum]**

     ✓7ᵗʰ **T20.319** **Burn of third degree of unspecified ear [any part, except ear drum]** ▽

   ✓x7ᵗʰ **T20.32** **Burn of third degree of** lip(s)

   ✓x7ᵗʰ **T20.33** **Burn of third degree of** chin

   ✓x7ᵗʰ **T20.34** **Burn of third degree of** nose (septum)

   ✓x7ᵗʰ **T20.35** **Burn of third degree of** scalp [any part]

   ✓x7ᵗʰ **T20.36** **Burn of third degree of** forehead and cheek

   ✓x7ᵗʰ **T20.37** **Burn of third degree of** neck

   ✓x7ᵗʰ **T20.39** **Burn of third degree of** multiple sites **of head, face, and neck**

✓5ᵗʰ **T20.4** **Corrosion of unspecified degree of head, face, and neck**
Code first (T51-T65) to identify chemical and intent
Use additional external cause code to identify place (Y92)

   ✓x7ᵗʰ **T20.40** **Corrosion of unspecified degree of head, face, and neck, unspecified site** ▽

   ✓6ᵗʰ **T20.41** **Corrosion of unspecified degree of** ear **[any part, except ear drum]**
EXCLUDES 2   corrosion of ear drum (T28.91-)

     ✓7ᵗʰ **T20.411** **Corrosion of unspecified degree of** right **ear [any part, except ear drum]** ▽

     ✓7ᵗʰ **T20.412** **Corrosion of unspecified degree of** left **ear [any part, except ear drum]** ▽

     ✓7ᵗʰ **T20.419** **Corrosion of unspecified degree of unspecified ear [any part, except ear drum]** ▽

   ✓x7ᵗʰ **T20.42** **Corrosion of unspecified degree of** lip(s) ▽

   ✓x7ᵗʰ **T20.43** **Corrosion of unspecified degree of** chin ▽

   ✓x7ᵗʰ **T20.44** **Corrosion of unspecified degree of** nose (septum) ▽

   ✓x7ᵗʰ **T20.45** **Corrosion of unspecified degree of** scalp [any part] ▽

   ✓x7ᵗʰ **T20.46** **Corrosion of unspecified degree of** forehead and cheek ▽

   ✓x7ᵗʰ **T20.47** **Corrosion of unspecified degree of** neck ▽

   ✓x7ᵗʰ **T20.49** **Corrosion of unspecified degree of** multiple sites **of head, face, and neck** ▽

✓5ᵗʰ **T20.5** **Corrosion of** first degree **of head, face, and neck**
Code first (T51-T65) to identify chemical and intent
Use additional external cause code to identify place (Y92)

   ✓x7ᵗʰ **T20.50** **Corrosion of first degree of head, face, and neck, unspecified site** ▽

   ✓6ᵗʰ **T20.51** **Corrosion of first degree of** ear **[any part, except ear drum]**
EXCLUDES 2   corrosion of ear drum (T28.91-)

     ✓7ᵗʰ **T20.511** **Corrosion of first degree of** right **ear [any part, except ear drum]**

     ✓7ᵗʰ **T20.512** **Corrosion of first degree of** left **ear [any part, except ear drum]**

     ✓7ᵗʰ **T20.519** **Corrosion of first degree of unspecified ear [any part, except ear drum]** ▽

   ✓x7ᵗʰ **T20.52** **Corrosion of first degree of** lip(s)

   ✓x7ᵗʰ **T20.53** **Corrosion of first degree of** chin

   ✓x7ᵗʰ **T20.54** **Corrosion of first degree of** nose (septum)

   ✓x7ᵗʰ **T20.55** **Corrosion of first degree of** scalp [any part]

   ✓x7ᵗʰ **T20.56** **Corrosion of first degree of** forehead and cheek

   ✓x7ᵗʰ **T20.57** **Corrosion of first degree of** neck

   ✓x7ᵗʰ **T20.59** **Corrosion of first degree of** multiple sites **of head, face, and neck**

✓5ᵗʰ **T20.6** **Corrosion of** second degree **of head, face, and neck**
Code first (T51-T65) to identify chemical and intent
Use additional external cause code to identify place (Y92)

   ✓x7ᵗʰ **T20.60** **Corrosion of second degree of head, face, and neck, unspecified site** ▽

   ✓6ᵗʰ **T20.61** **Corrosion of second degree of** ear **[any part, except ear drum]**
EXCLUDES 2   corrosion of ear drum (T28.91-)

     ✓7ᵗʰ **T20.611** **Corrosion of second degree of** right **ear [any part, except ear drum]**

     ✓7ᵗʰ **T20.612** **Corrosion of second degree of** left **ear [any part, except ear drum]**

     ✓7ᵗʰ **T20.619** **Corrosion of second degree of unspecified ear [any part, except ear drum]** ▽

   ✓x7ᵗʰ **T20.62** **Corrosion of second degree of** lip(s)

   ✓x7ᵗʰ **T20.63** **Corrosion of second degree of** chin

   ✓x7ᵗʰ **T20.64** **Corrosion of second degree of** nose (septum)

   ✓x7ᵗʰ **T20.65** **Corrosion of second degree of** scalp [any part]

   ✓x7ᵗʰ **T20.66** **Corrosion of second degree of** forehead and cheek

   ✓x7ᵗʰ **T20.67** **Corrosion of second degree of** neck

   ✓x7ᵗʰ **T20.69** **Corrosion of second degree of** multiple sites **of head, face, and neck**

✓5ᵗʰ **T20.7** **Corrosion of** third degree **of head, face, and neck**
Code first (T51-T65) to identify chemical and intent
Use additional external cause code to identify place (Y92)

   ✓x7ᵗʰ **T20.70** **Corrosion of third degree of head, face, and neck, unspecified site** ▽

   ✓6ᵗʰ **T20.71** **Corrosion of third degree of** ear **[any part, except ear drum]**
EXCLUDES 2   corrosion of ear drum (T28.91-)

     ✓7ᵗʰ **T20.711** **Corrosion of third degree of** right **ear [any part, except ear drum]**

     ✓7ᵗʰ **T20.712** **Corrosion of third degree of** left **ear [any part, except ear drum]**

     ✓7ᵗʰ **T20.719** **Corrosion of third degree of unspecified ear [any part, except ear drum]** ▽

   ✓x7ᵗʰ **T20.72** **Corrosion of third degree of** lip(s)

   ✓x7ᵗʰ **T20.73** **Corrosion of third degree of** chin

   ✓x7ᵗʰ **T20.74** **Corrosion of third degree of** nose (septum)

   ✓x7ᵗʰ **T20.75** **Corrosion of third degree of** scalp [any part]

   ✓x7ᵗʰ **T20.76** **Corrosion of third degree of** forehead and cheek

   ✓x7ᵗʰ **T20.77** **Corrosion of third degree of** neck

   ✓x7ᵗʰ **T20.79** **Corrosion of third degree of** multiple sites **of head, face, and neck**

☑ Additional Character Req   ✓x7ᵗʰ Placeholder Alert   Manifestation   HCC CMS-HCC Condition   ▽ Unspecified Code   ►◄ Revised Text   ● New Code   ▲ Revised Code Title

Chapter 19. Injury, Poisoning, and Certain Other Consequences of External Causes

√4ᵗʰ **T21**   **Burn and corrosion of trunk**
  INCLUDES   burns and corrosion of hip region
  EXCLUDES 2   *burns and corrosion of axilla (T22.- with fifth character 4)*
       burns and corrosion of scapular region (T22.- with fifth character 6)
       burns and corrosion of shoulder (T22.- with fifth character 5)

  The appropriate 7th character is to be added to each code from category T21.
  A   initial encounter
  D   subsequent encounter
  S   sequela

√5ᵗʰ **T21.0**   **Burn of unspecified degree of trunk**
  Use additional external cause code to identify the source, place and intent of the burn (X00-X19, X75-X77, X96-X98, Y92)

√x7ᵗʰ **T21.00**   **Burn of unspecified degree of trunk, unspecified site**   ▽

√x7ᵗʰ **T21.01**   **Burn of unspecified degree of chest wall**   ▽
  Burn of of unspecified degree of breast

√x7ᵗʰ **T21.02**   **Burn of unspecified degree of abdominal wall**   ▽
  Burn of unspecified degree of flank
  Burn of unspecified degree of groin

√x7ᵗʰ **T21.03**   **Burn of unspecified degree of upper back**   ▽
  Burn of unspecified degree of interscapular region

√x7ᵗʰ **T21.04**   **Burn of unspecified degree of lower back**   ▽

√x7ᵗʰ **T21.05**   **Burn of unspecified degree of buttock**   ▽
  Burn of unspecified degree of anus

√x7ᵗʰ **T21.06**   **Burn of unspecified degree of male genital region**   ♂▽
  Burn of unspecified degree of penis
  Burn of unspecified degree of scrotum
  Burn of unspecified degree of testis

√x7ᵗʰ **T21.07**   **Burn of unspecified degree of female genital region**   ♀▽
  Burn of unspecified degree of labium (majus) (minus)
  Burn of unspecified degree of perineum
  Burn of unspecified degree of vulva
  EXCLUDES 2   *burn of vagina (T28.3)*

√x7ᵗʰ **T21.09**   **Burn of unspecified degree of other site of trunk**   ▽

√5ᵗʰ **T21.1**   **Burn of first degree of trunk**
  Use additional external cause code to identify the source, place and intent of the burn (X00-X19, X75-X77, X96-X98, Y92)

√x7ᵗʰ **T21.10**   **Burn of first degree of trunk, unspecified site**   ▽

√x7ᵗʰ **T21.11**   **Burn of first degree of chest wall**
  Burn of first degree of breast

√x7ᵗʰ **T21.12**   **Burn of first degree of abdominal wall**
  Burn of first degree of flank
  Burn of first degree of groin

√x7ᵗʰ **T21.13**   **Burn of first degree of upper back**
  Burn of first degree of interscapular region

√x7ᵗʰ **T21.14**   **Burn of first degree of lower back**

√x7ᵗʰ **T21.15**   **Burn of first degree of buttock**
  Burn of first degree of anus

√x7ᵗʰ **T21.16**   **Burn of first degree of male genital region**   ♂
  Burn of first degree of penis
  Burn of first degree of scrotum
  Burn of first degree of testis

√x7ᵗʰ **T21.17**   **Burn of first degree of female genital region**   ♀
  Burn of first degree of labium (majus) (minus)
  Burn of first degree of perineum
  Burn of first degree of vulva
  EXCLUDES 2   *burn of vagina (T28.3)*

√x7ᵗʰ **T21.19**   **Burn of first degree of other site of trunk**

√5ᵗʰ **T21.2**   **Burn of second degree of trunk**
  Use additional external cause code to identify the source, place and intent of the burn (X00-X19, X75-X77, X96-X98, Y92)

√x7ᵗʰ **T21.20**   **Burn of second degree of trunk, unspecified site**   ▽

√x7ᵗʰ **T21.21**   **Burn of second degree of chest wall**
  Burn of second degree of breast

√x7ᵗʰ **T21.22**   **Burn of second degree of abdominal wall**
  Burn of second degree of flank
  Burn of second degree of groin

√x7ᵗʰ **T21.23**   **Burn of second degree of upper back**
  Burn of second degree of interscapular region

√x7ᵗʰ **T21.24**   **Burn of second degree of lower back**

√x7ᵗʰ **T21.25**   **Burn of second degree of buttock**
  Burn of second degree of anus

√x7ᵗʰ **T21.26**   **Burn of second degree of male genital region**   ♂
  Burn of second degree of penis
  Burn of second degree of scrotum
  Burn of second degree of testis

√x7ᵗʰ **T21.27**   **Burn of second degree of female genital region**   ♀
  Burn of second degree of labium (majus) (minus)
  Burn of second degree of perineum
  Burn of second degree of vulva
  EXCLUDES 2   *burn of vagina (T28.3)*

√x7ᵗʰ **T21.29**   **Burn of second degree of other site of trunk**

√5ᵗʰ **T21.3**   **Burn of third degree of trunk**
  Use additional external cause code to identify the source, place and intent of the burn (X00-X19, X75-X77, X96-X98, Y92)

√x7ᵗʰ **T21.30**   **Burn of third degree of trunk, unspecified site**   ▽

√x7ᵗʰ **T21.31**   **Burn of third degree of chest wall**
  Burn of third degree of breast
  AHA: 2016, 2Q, 5

√x7ᵗʰ **T21.32**   **Burn of third degree of abdominal wall**
  Burn of third degree of flank
  Burn of third degree of groin

√x7ᵗʰ **T21.33**   **Burn of third degree of upper back**
  Burn of third degree of interscapular region

√x7ᵗʰ **T21.34**   **Burn of third degree of lower back**

√x7ᵗʰ **T21.35**   **Burn of third degree of buttock**
  Burn of third degree of anus

√x7ᵗʰ **T21.36**   **Burn of third degree of male genital region**   ♂
  Burn of third degree of penis
  Burn of third degree of scrotum
  Burn of third degree of testis

√x7ᵗʰ **T21.37**   **Burn of third degree of female genital region**   ♀
  Burn of third degree of labium (majus) (minus)
  Burn of third degree of perineum
  Burn of third degree of vulva
  EXCLUDES 2   *burn of vagina (T28.3)*

√x7ᵗʰ **T21.39**   **Burn of third degree of other site of trunk**

√5ᵗʰ **T21.4**   **Corrosion of unspecified degree of trunk**
  Code first (T51-T65) to identify chemical and intent
  Use additional external cause code to identify place (Y92)

√x7ᵗʰ **T21.40**   **Corrosion of unspecified degree of trunk, unspecified site**   ▽

√x7ᵗʰ **T21.41**   **Corrosion of unspecified degree of chest wall**   ▽
  Corrosion of unspecified degree of breast

√x7ᵗʰ **T21.42**   **Corrosion of unspecified degree of abdominal wall**   ▽
  Corrosion of unspecified degree of flank
  Corrosion of unspecified degree of groin

√x7ᵗʰ **T21.43**   **Corrosion of unspecified degree of upper back**   ▽
  Corrosion of unspecified degree of interscapular region

√x7ᵗʰ **T21.44**   **Corrosion of unspecified degree of lower back**   ▽

√x7ᵗʰ **T21.45**   **Corrosion of unspecified degree of buttock**   ▽
  Corrosion of unspecified degree of anus

√x7ᵗʰ **T21.46**   **Corrosion of unspecified degree of male genital region**   ♂▽
  Corrosion of unspecified degree of penis
  Corrosion of unspecified degree of scrotum
  Corrosion of unspecified degree of testis

√x7ᵗʰ **T21.47**   **Corrosion of unspecified degree of female genital region**   ♀▽
  Corrosion of unspecified degree of labium (majus) (minus)
  Corrosion of unspecified degree of perineum
  Corrosion of unspecified degree of vulva
  EXCLUDES 2   *corrosion of vagina (T28.8)*

√x7ᵗʰ **T21.49**   **Corrosion of unspecified degree of other site of trunk**   ▽

√5ᵗʰ **T21.5**   **Corrosion of first degree of trunk**
  Code first (T51-T65) to identify chemical and intent
  Use additional external cause code to identify place (Y92)

√x7ᵗʰ **T21.50**   **Corrosion of first degree of trunk, unspecified site**   ▽

√x7ᵗʰ **T21.51**   **Corrosion of first degree of chest wall**
  Corrosion of first degree of breast

√x7ᵗʰ **T21.52**   **Corrosion of first degree of abdominal wall**
  Corrosion of first degree of flank
  Corrosion of first degree of groin

√x7ᵗʰ **T21.53** **Corrosion of first degree of** upper back
Corrosion of first degree of interscapular region

√x7ᵗʰ **T21.54** **Corrosion of first degree of** lower back

√x7ᵗʰ **T21.55** **Corrosion of first degree of** buttock
Corrosion of first degree of anus

√x7ᵗʰ **T21.56** **Corrosion of first degree of** male genital region ♂
Corrosion of first degree of penis
Corrosion of first degree of scrotum
Corrosion of first degree of testis

√x7ᵗʰ **T21.57** **Corrosion of first degree of** female genital region ♀
Corrosion of first degree of labium (majus) (minus)
Corrosion of first degree of perineum
Corrosion of first degree of vulva
EXCLUDES 2   corrosion of vagina (T28.8)

√x7ᵗʰ **T21.59** **Corrosion of first degree of other site of trunk**

√5ᵗʰ **T21.6** **Corrosion of** second degree **of trunk**
Code first (T51-T65) to identify chemical and intent
Use additional external cause code to identify place (Y92)

√x7ᵗʰ **T21.60** **Corrosion of second degree of trunk, unspecified** ▽
site

√x7ᵗʰ **T21.61** **Corrosion of second degree of** chest wall
Corrosion of second degree of breast

√x7ᵗʰ **T21.62** **Corrosion of second degree of** abdominal wall
Corrosion of second degree of flank
Corrosion of second degree of groin

√x7ᵗʰ **T21.63** **Corrosion of second degree of** upper back
Corrosion of second degree of interscapular region

√x7ᵗʰ **T21.64** **Corrosion of second degree of** lower back

√x7ᵗʰ **T21.65** **Corrosion of second degree of** buttock
Corrosion of second degree of anus

√x7ᵗʰ **T21.66** **Corrosion of second degree of** male genital region ♂
Corrosion of second degree of penis
Corrosion of second degree of scrotum
Corrosion of second degree of testis

√x7ᵗʰ **T21.67** **Corrosion of second degree of** female genital
region ♀
Corrosion of second degree of labium (majus) (minus)
Corrosion of second degree of perineum
Corrosion of second degree of vulva
EXCLUDES 2   corrosion of vagina (T28.8)

√x7ᵗʰ **T21.69** **Corrosion of second degree of other site of trunk**

√5ᵗʰ **T21.7** **Corrosion of** third degree **of trunk**
Code first (T51-T65) to identify chemical and intent
Use additional external cause code to identify place (Y92)

√x7ᵗʰ **T21.70** **Corrosion of third degree of trunk, unspecified** ▽
site

√x7ᵗʰ **T21.71** **Corrosion of third degree of** chest wall
Corrosion of third degree of breast

√x7ᵗʰ **T21.72** **Corrosion of third degree of** abdominal wall
Corrosion of third degree of flank
Corrosion of third degree of groin

√x7ᵗʰ **T21.73** **Corrosion of third degree of** upper back
Corrosion of third degree of interscapular region

√x7ᵗʰ **T21.74** **Corrosion of third degree of** lower back

√x7ᵗʰ **T21.75** **Corrosion of third degree of** buttock
Corrosion of third degree of anus

√x7ᵗʰ **T21.76** **Corrosion of third degree of** male genital region ♂
Corrosion of third degree of penis
Corrosion of third degree of scrotum
Corrosion of third degree of testis

√x7ᵗʰ **T21.77** **Corrosion of third degree of** female genital region ♀
Corrosion of third degree of labium (majus) (minus)
Corrosion of third degree of perineum
Corrosion of third degree of vulva
EXCLUDES 2   corrosion of vagina (T28.8)

√x7ᵗʰ **T21.79** **Corrosion of third degree of other site of trunk**

√4ᵗʰ **T22** **Burn and corrosion of shoulder and upper limb, except wrist and**
hand
EXCLUDES 2   burn and corrosion of interscapular region (T21.-)
burn and corrosion of wrist and hand (T23.-)

The appropriate 7th character is to be added to each code from
category T22.
A   initial encounter
D   subsequent encounter
S   sequela

√5ᵗʰ **T22.0** **Burn of unspecified degree of shoulder and upper limb,**
except wrist and hand
Use additional external cause code to identify the source, place
and intent of the burn (X00-X19, X75-X77, X96-X98, Y92)

√x7ᵗʰ **T22.00** **Burn of unspecified degree of shoulder and** ▽
upper limb, except wrist and hand, unspecified site

√6ᵗʰ **T22.01** **Burn of unspecified degree of** forearm

√7ᵗʰ **T22.011** **Burn of unspecified degree of** right ▽
forearm

√7ᵗʰ **T22.012** **Burn of unspecified degree of** left ▽
forearm

√7ᵗʰ **T22.019** **Burn of unspecified degree of** ▽
unspecified forearm

√6ᵗʰ **T22.02** **Burn of unspecified degree of** elbow

√7ᵗʰ **T22.021** **Burn of unspecified degree of** right ▽
elbow

√7ᵗʰ **T22.022** **Burn of unspecified degree of** left ▽
elbow

√7ᵗʰ **T22.029** **Burn of unspecified degree of** ▽
unspecified elbow

√6ᵗʰ **T22.03** **Burn of unspecified degree of** upper arm

√7ᵗʰ **T22.031** **Burn of unspecified degree of** ▽
right upper arm

√7ᵗʰ **T22.032** **Burn of unspecified degree of** ▽
left upper arm

√7ᵗʰ **T22.039** **Burn of unspecified degree of** ▽
unspecified upper arm

√6ᵗʰ **T22.04** **Burn of unspecified degree of** axilla

√7ᵗʰ **T22.041** **Burn of unspecified degree of** ▽
right axilla

√7ᵗʰ **T22.042** **Burn of unspecified degree of** ▽
left axilla

√7ᵗʰ **T22.049** **Burn of unspecified degree of** ▽
unspecified axilla

√6ᵗʰ **T22.05** **Burn of unspecified degree of** shoulder

√7ᵗʰ **T22.051** **Burn of unspecified degree of** right ▽
shoulder

√7ᵗʰ **T22.052** **Burn of unspecified degree of** left ▽
shoulder

√7ᵗʰ **T22.059** **Burn of unspecified degree of** ▽
unspecified shoulder

√6ᵗʰ **T22.06** **Burn of unspecified degree of** scapular region

√7ᵗʰ **T22.061** **Burn of unspecified degree of** right ▽
scapular region

√7ᵗʰ **T22.062** **Burn of unspecified degree of** left ▽
scapular region

√7ᵗʰ **T22.069** **Burn of unspecified degree of** ▽
unspecified scapular region

√6ᵗʰ **T22.09** **Burn of unspecified degree of** multiple sites **of**
shoulder and upper limb, except wrist and hand

√7ᵗʰ **T22.091** **Burn of unspecified degree of multiple** ▽
sites of right **shoulder and upper limb,**
except wrist and hand

√7ᵗʰ **T22.092** **Burn of unspecified degree of multiple** ▽
sites of left **shoulder and upper limb,**
except wrist and hand

√7ᵗʰ **T22.099** **Burn of unspecified degree of multiple** ▽
sites of unspecified shoulder and upper
limb, except wrist and hand

√5ᵗʰ **T22.1** **Burn of** first degree **of shoulder and upper limb, except wrist**
and hand
Use additional external cause code to identify the source, place
and intent of the burn (X00-X19, X75-X77, X96-X98, Y92)

√x7ᵗʰ **T22.10** **Burn of first degree of shoulder and upper limb,** ▽
except wrist and hand, unspecified site

✅ Additional Character Req   √x7ᵗʰ Placeholder Alert   Manifestation   HCC CMS-HCC Condition   ▽ Unspecified Code   ▶◀ Revised Text   ● New Code   ▲ Revised Code Title

ICD-10-CM 2018   **1043**

✓6ᵗʰ **T22.11** **Burn of first degree of forearm**
- ✓7ᵗʰ **T22.111** Burn of first degree of right forearm
- ✓7ᵗʰ **T22.112** Burn of first degree of left forearm
- ✓7ᵗʰ **T22.119** Burn of first degree of unspecified forearm ▽

✓6ᵗʰ **T22.12** **Burn of first degree of elbow**
- ✓7ᵗʰ **T22.121** Burn of first degree of right elbow
- ✓7ᵗʰ **T22.122** Burn of first degree of left elbow
- ✓7ᵗʰ **T22.129** Burn of first degree of unspecified elbow ▽

✓6ᵗʰ **T22.13** **Burn of first degree of upper arm**
- ✓7ᵗʰ **T22.131** Burn of first degree of right upper arm
- ✓7ᵗʰ **T22.132** Burn of first degree of left upper arm
- ✓7ᵗʰ **T22.139** Burn of first degree of unspecified upper arm ▽

✓6ᵗʰ **T22.14** **Burn of first degree of axilla**
- ✓7ᵗʰ **T22.141** Burn of first degree of right axilla
- ✓7ᵗʰ **T22.142** Burn of first degree of left axilla
- ✓7ᵗʰ **T22.149** Burn of first degree of unspecified axilla ▽

✓6ᵗʰ **T22.15** **Burn of first degree of shoulder**
- ✓7ᵗʰ **T22.151** Burn of first degree of right shoulder
- ✓7ᵗʰ **T22.152** Burn of first degree of left shoulder
- ✓7ᵗʰ **T22.159** Burn of first degree of unspecified shoulder ▽

✓6ᵗʰ **T22.16** **Burn of first degree of scapular region**
- ✓7ᵗʰ **T22.161** Burn of first degree of right scapular region
- ✓7ᵗʰ **T22.162** Burn of first degree of left scapular region
- ✓7ᵗʰ **T22.169** Burn of first degree of unspecified scapular region ▽

✓6ᵗʰ **T22.19** **Burn of first degree of multiple sites of shoulder and upper limb, except wrist and hand**
- ✓7ᵗʰ **T22.191** Burn of first degree of multiple sites of right shoulder and upper limb, except wrist and hand
- ✓7ᵗʰ **T22.192** Burn of first degree of multiple sites of left shoulder and upper limb, except wrist and hand
- ✓7ᵗʰ **T22.199** Burn of first degree of multiple sites of unspecified shoulder and upper limb, except wrist and hand ▽

✓5ᵗʰ **T22.2** **Burn of second degree of shoulder and upper limb, except wrist and hand**
> Use additional external cause code to identify the source, place and intent of the burn (X00-X19, X75-X77, X96-X98, Y92)

✓×7ᵗʰ **T22.20** **Burn of second degree of shoulder and upper limb, except wrist and hand, unspecified site** ▽

✓6ᵗʰ **T22.21** **Burn of second degree of forearm**
- ✓7ᵗʰ **T22.211** Burn of second degree of right forearm
- ✓7ᵗʰ **T22.212** Burn of second degree of left forearm
- ✓7ᵗʰ **T22.219** Burn of second degree of unspecified forearm ▽

✓6ᵗʰ **T22.22** **Burn of second degree of elbow**
- ✓7ᵗʰ **T22.221** Burn of second degree of right elbow
- ✓7ᵗʰ **T22.222** Burn of second degree of left elbow
- ✓7ᵗʰ **T22.229** Burn of second degree of unspecified elbow ▽

✓6ᵗʰ **T22.23** **Burn of second degree of upper arm**
- ✓7ᵗʰ **T22.231** Burn of second degree of right upper arm
- ✓7ᵗʰ **T22.232** Burn of second degree of left upper arm
- ✓7ᵗʰ **T22.239** Burn of second degree of unspecified upper arm ▽

✓6ᵗʰ **T22.24** **Burn of second degree of axilla**
- ✓7ᵗʰ **T22.241** Burn of second degree of right axilla
- ✓7ᵗʰ **T22.242** Burn of second degree of left axilla
- ✓7ᵗʰ **T22.249** Burn of second degree of unspecified axilla ▽

✓6ᵗʰ **T22.25** **Burn of second degree of shoulder**
- ✓7ᵗʰ **T22.251** Burn of second degree of right shoulder
- ✓7ᵗʰ **T22.252** Burn of second degree of left shoulder

- ✓7ᵗʰ **T22.259** Burn of second degree of unspecified shoulder ▽

✓6ᵗʰ **T22.26** **Burn of second degree of scapular region**
- ✓7ᵗʰ **T22.261** Burn of second degree of right scapular region
- ✓7ᵗʰ **T22.262** Burn of second degree of left scapular region
- ✓7ᵗʰ **T22.269** Burn of second degree of unspecified scapular region ▽

✓6ᵗʰ **T22.29** **Burn of second degree of multiple sites of shoulder and upper limb, except wrist and hand**
- ✓7ᵗʰ **T22.291** Burn of second degree of multiple sites of right shoulder and upper limb, except wrist and hand
- ✓7ᵗʰ **T22.292** Burn of second degree of multiple sites of left shoulder and upper limb, except wrist and hand
- ✓7ᵗʰ **T22.299** Burn of second degree of multiple sites of unspecified shoulder and upper limb, except wrist and hand ▽

✓5ᵗʰ **T22.3** **Burn of third degree of shoulder and upper limb, except wrist and hand**
> Use additional external cause code to identify the source, place and intent of the burn (X00-X19, X75-X77, X96-X98, Y92)

✓×7ᵗʰ **T22.30** **Burn of third degree of shoulder and upper limb, except wrist and hand, unspecified site** ▽

✓6ᵗʰ **T22.31** **Burn of third degree of forearm**
- ✓7ᵗʰ **T22.311** Burn of third degree of right forearm
- ✓7ᵗʰ **T22.312** Burn of third degree of left forearm
- ✓7ᵗʰ **T22.319** Burn of third degree of unspecified forearm ▽

✓6ᵗʰ **T22.32** **Burn of third degree of elbow**
- ✓7ᵗʰ **T22.321** Burn of third degree of right elbow
- ✓7ᵗʰ **T22.322** Burn of third degree of left elbow
- ✓7ᵗʰ **T22.329** Burn of third degree of unspecified elbow ▽

✓6ᵗʰ **T22.33** **Burn of third degree of upper arm**
- ✓7ᵗʰ **T22.331** Burn of third degree of right upper arm
- ✓7ᵗʰ **T22.332** Burn of third degree of left upper arm
- ✓7ᵗʰ **T22.339** Burn of third degree of unspecified upper arm ▽

✓6ᵗʰ **T22.34** **Burn of third degree of axilla**
- ✓7ᵗʰ **T22.341** Burn of third degree of right axilla
- ✓7ᵗʰ **T22.342** Burn of third degree of left axilla
- ✓7ᵗʰ **T22.349** Burn of third degree of unspecified axilla ▽

✓6ᵗʰ **T22.35** **Burn of third degree of shoulder**
- ✓7ᵗʰ **T22.351** Burn of third degree of right shoulder
- ✓7ᵗʰ **T22.352** Burn of third degree of left shoulder
- ✓7ᵗʰ **T22.359** Burn of third degree of unspecified shoulder ▽

✓6ᵗʰ **T22.36** **Burn of third degree of scapular region**
- ✓7ᵗʰ **T22.361** Burn of third degree of right scapular region
- ✓7ᵗʰ **T22.362** Burn of third degree of left scapular region
- ✓7ᵗʰ **T22.369** Burn of third degree of unspecified scapular region ▽

✓6ᵗʰ **T22.39** **Burn of third degree of multiple sites of shoulder and upper limb, except wrist and hand**
- ✓7ᵗʰ **T22.391** Burn of third degree of multiple sites of right shoulder and upper limb, except wrist and hand
- ✓7ᵗʰ **T22.392** Burn of third degree of multiple sites of left shoulder and upper limb, except wrist and hand
- ✓7ᵗʰ **T22.399** Burn of third degree of multiple sites of unspecified shoulder and upper limb, except wrist and hand ▽

✓5th **T22.4** **Corrosion of unspecified degree of shoulder and upper limb, except wrist and hand**
  Code first (T51-T65) to identify chemical and intent
  Use additional external cause code to identify place (Y92)

  ✓x7th **T22.40** Corrosion of unspecified degree of shoulder and upper limb, except wrist and hand, unspecified site ▽

  ✓6th **T22.41** Corrosion of unspecified degree of forearm

   ✓7th **T22.411** Corrosion of unspecified degree of right forearm ▽

   ✓7th **T22.412** Corrosion of unspecified degree of left forearm ▽

   ✓7th **T22.419** Corrosion of unspecified degree of unspecified forearm ▽

  ✓6th **T22.42** Corrosion of unspecified degree of elbow

   ✓7th **T22.421** Corrosion of unspecified degree of right elbow ▽

   ✓7th **T22.422** Corrosion of unspecified degree of left elbow ▽

   ✓7th **T22.429** Corrosion of unspecified degree of unspecified elbow ▽

  ✓6th **T22.43** Corrosion of unspecified degree of upper arm

   ✓7th **T22.431** Corrosion of unspecified degree of right upper arm ▽

   ✓7th **T22.432** Corrosion of unspecified degree of left upper arm ▽

   ✓7th **T22.439** Corrosion of unspecified degree of unspecified upper arm ▽

  ✓6th **T22.44** Corrosion of unspecified degree of axilla

   ✓7th **T22.441** Corrosion of unspecified degree of right axilla ▽

   ✓7th **T22.442** Corrosion of unspecified degree of left axilla ▽

   ✓7th **T22.449** Corrosion of unspecified degree of unspecified axilla ▽

  ✓6th **T22.45** Corrosion of unspecified degree of shoulder

   ✓7th **T22.451** Corrosion of unspecified degree of right shoulder ▽

   ✓7th **T22.452** Corrosion of unspecified degree of left shoulder ▽

   ✓7th **T22.459** Corrosion of unspecified degree of unspecified shoulder ▽

  ✓6th **T22.46** Corrosion of unspecified degree of scapular region

   ✓7th **T22.461** Corrosion of unspecified degree of right scapular region ▽

   ✓7th **T22.462** Corrosion of unspecified degree of left scapular region ▽

   ✓7th **T22.469** Corrosion of unspecified degree of unspecified scapular region ▽

  ✓6th **T22.49** Corrosion of unspecified degree of multiple sites of shoulder and upper limb, except wrist and hand

   ✓7th **T22.491** Corrosion of unspecified degree of multiple sites of right shoulder and upper limb, except wrist and hand ▽

   ✓7th **T22.492** Corrosion of unspecified degree of multiple sites of left shoulder and upper limb, except wrist and hand ▽

   ✓7th **T22.499** Corrosion of unspecified degree of multiple sites of unspecified shoulder and upper limb, except wrist and hand ▽

✓5th **T22.5** **Corrosion of first degree of shoulder and upper limb, except wrist and hand**
  Code first (T51-T65) to identify chemical and intent
  Use additional external cause code to identify place (Y92)

  ✓x7th **T22.50** Corrosion of first degree of shoulder and upper limb, except wrist and hand unspecified site ▽

  ✓6th **T22.51** Corrosion of first degree of forearm

   ✓7th **T22.511** Corrosion of first degree of right forearm

   ✓7th **T22.512** Corrosion of first degree of left forearm

   ✓7th **T22.519** Corrosion of first degree of unspecified forearm ▽

  ✓6th **T22.52** Corrosion of first degree of elbow

   ✓7th **T22.521** Corrosion of first degree of right elbow

   ✓7th **T22.522** Corrosion of first degree of left elbow

   ✓7th **T22.529** Corrosion of first degree of unspecified elbow ▽

  ✓6th **T22.53** Corrosion of first degree of upper arm

   ✓7th **T22.531** Corrosion of first degree of right upper arm

   ✓7th **T22.532** Corrosion of first degree of left upper arm

   ✓7th **T22.539** Corrosion of first degree of unspecified upper arm ▽

  ✓6th **T22.54** Corrosion of first degree of axilla

   ✓7th **T22.541** Corrosion of first degree of right axilla

   ✓7th **T22.542** Corrosion of first degree of left axilla

   ✓7th **T22.549** Corrosion of first degree of unspecified axilla ▽

  ✓6th **T22.55** Corrosion of first degree of shoulder

   ✓7th **T22.551** Corrosion of first degree of right shoulder

   ✓7th **T22.552** Corrosion of first degree of left shoulder

   ✓7th **T22.559** Corrosion of first degree of unspecified shoulder ▽

  ✓6th **T22.56** Corrosion of first degree of scapular region

   ✓7th **T22.561** Corrosion of first degree of right scapular region

   ✓7th **T22.562** Corrosion of first degree of left scapular region

   ✓7th **T22.569** Corrosion of first degree of unspecified scapular region ▽

  ✓6th **T22.59** Corrosion of first degree of multiple sites of shoulder and upper limb, except wrist and hand

   ✓7th **T22.591** Corrosion of first degree of multiple sites of right shoulder and upper limb, except wrist and hand

   ✓7th **T22.592** Corrosion of first degree of multiple sites of left shoulder and upper limb, except wrist and hand

   ✓7th **T22.599** Corrosion of first degree of multiple sites of unspecified shoulder and upper limb, except wrist and hand ▽

✓5th **T22.6** **Corrosion of second degree of shoulder and upper limb, except wrist and hand**
  Code first (T51-T65) to identify chemical and intent
  Use additional external cause code to identify place (Y92)

  ✓x7th **T22.60** Corrosion of second degree of shoulder and upper limb, except wrist and hand, unspecified site ▽

  ✓6th **T22.61** Corrosion of second degree of forearm

   ✓7th **T22.611** Corrosion of second degree of right forearm

   ✓7th **T22.612** Corrosion of second degree of left forearm

   ✓7th **T22.619** Corrosion of second degree of unspecified forearm ▽

  ✓6th **T22.62** Corrosion of second degree of elbow

   ✓7th **T22.621** Corrosion of second degree of right elbow

   ✓7th **T22.622** Corrosion of second degree of left elbow

   ✓7th **T22.629** Corrosion of second degree of unspecified elbow ▽

  ✓6th **T22.63** Corrosion of second degree of upper arm

   ✓7th **T22.631** Corrosion of second degree of right upper arm

   ✓7th **T22.632** Corrosion of second degree of left upper arm

   ✓7th **T22.639** Corrosion of second degree of unspecified upper arm ▽

  ✓6th **T22.64** Corrosion of second degree of axilla

   ✓7th **T22.641** Corrosion of second degree of right axilla

   ✓7th **T22.642** Corrosion of second degree of left axilla

   ✓7th **T22.649** Corrosion of second degree of unspecified axilla ▽

  ✓6th **T22.65** Corrosion of second degree of shoulder

   ✓7th **T22.651** Corrosion of second degree of right shoulder

   ✓7th **T22.652** Corrosion of second degree of left shoulder

   ✓7th **T22.659** Corrosion of second degree of unspecified shoulder ▽

✓ Additional Character Req   ✓x7th Placeholder Alert   Manifestation   HCC CMS-HCC Condition   ▽ Unspecified Code   ►◄ Revised Text   ● New Code   ▲ Revised Code Title

Chapter 19. Injury, Poisoning, and Certain Other Consequences of External Causes

✓6th **T22.66** **Corrosion of second degree of** scapular region
- ✓7th **T22.661** **Corrosion of second degree of** right scapular region
- ✓7th **T22.662** **Corrosion of second degree of** left scapular region
- ✓7th **T22.669** **Corrosion of second degree of** unspecified scapular region ▽

✓6th **T22.69** **Corrosion of second degree of** multiple sites **of shoulder and upper limb, except wrist and hand**
- ✓7th **T22.691** **Corrosion of second degree of multiple sites of** right **shoulder and upper limb, except wrist and hand**
- ✓7th **T22.692** **Corrosion of second degree of multiple sites of** left **shoulder and upper limb, except wrist and hand**
- ✓7th **T22.699** **Corrosion of second degree of multiple sites of unspecified shoulder and upper limb, except wrist and hand** ▽

✓5th **T22.7** **Corrosion of** third degree **of shoulder and upper limb, except wrist and hand**
   Code first (T51-T65) to identify chemical and intent
   Use additional external cause code to identify place (Y92)

- ✓x7th **T22.70** **Corrosion of third degree of shoulder and upper limb, except wrist and hand, unspecified site** ▽

✓6th **T22.71** **Corrosion of third degree of** forearm
- ✓7th **T22.711** **Corrosion of third degree of** right **forearm**
- ✓7th **T22.712** **Corrosion of third degree of** left **forearm**
- ✓7th **T22.719** **Corrosion of third degree of unspecified forearm** ▽

✓6th **T22.72** **Corrosion of third degree of** elbow
- ✓7th **T22.721** **Corrosion of third degree of** right **elbow**
- ✓7th **T22.722** **Corrosion of third degree of** left **elbow**
- ✓7th **T22.729** **Corrosion of third degree of unspecified elbow** ▽

✓6th **T22.73** **Corrosion of third degree of** upper arm
- ✓7th **T22.731** **Corrosion of third degree of** right **upper arm**
- ✓7th **T22.732** **Corrosion of third degree of** left **upper arm**
- ✓7th **T22.739** **Corrosion of third degree of unspecified upper arm** ▽

✓6th **T22.74** **Corrosion of third degree of** axilla
- ✓7th **T22.741** **Corrosion of third degree of** right **axilla**
- ✓7th **T22.742** **Corrosion of third degree of** left **axilla**
- ✓7th **T22.749** **Corrosion of third degree of unspecified axilla** ▽

✓6th **T22.75** **Corrosion of third degree of** shoulder
- ✓7th **T22.751** **Corrosion of third degree of** right **shoulder**
- ✓7th **T22.752** **Corrosion of third degree of** left **shoulder**
- ✓7th **T22.759** **Corrosion of third degree of unspecified shoulder** ▽

✓6th **T22.76** **Corrosion of third degree of** scapular region
- ✓7th **T22.761** **Corrosion of third degree of** right **scapular region**
- ✓7th **T22.762** **Corrosion of third degree of** left **scapular region**
- ✓7th **T22.769** **Corrosion of third degree of unspecified scapular region** ▽

✓6th **T22.79** **Corrosion of third degree of** multiple sites **of shoulder and upper limb, except wrist and hand**
- ✓7th **T22.791** **Corrosion of third degree of multiple sites of** right **shoulder and upper limb, except wrist and hand**
- ✓7th **T22.792** **Corrosion of third degree of multiple sites of** left **shoulder and upper limb, except wrist and hand**
- ✓7th **T22.799** **Corrosion of third degree of multiple sites of unspecified shoulder and upper limb, except wrist and hand** ▽

✓4th **T23** **Burn and corrosion of wrist and hand**
   AHA: 2015, 1Q, 19

   The appropriate 7th character is to be added to each code from category T23.
   A   initial encounter
   D   subsequent encounter
   S   sequela

✓5th **T23.0** **Burn of unspecified degree of wrist and hand**
   Use additional external cause code to identify the source, place and intent of the burn (X00-X19, X75-X77, X96-X98, Y92)

✓6th **T23.00** **Burn of unspecified degree of hand, unspecified site**
- ✓7th **T23.001** **Burn of unspecified degree of** right **hand, unspecified site** ▽
- ✓7th **T23.002** **Burn of unspecified degree of** left **hand, unspecified site** ▽
- ✓7th **T23.009** **Burn of unspecified degree of unspecified hand, unspecified site** ▽

✓6th **T23.01** **Burn of unspecified degree of** thumb (nail)
- ✓7th **T23.011** **Burn of unspecified degree of** right **thumb (nail)** ▽
- ✓7th **T23.012** **Burn of unspecified degree of** left **thumb (nail)** ▽
- ✓7th **T23.019** **Burn of unspecified degree of unspecified thumb (nail)** ▽

✓6th **T23.02** **Burn of unspecified degree of** single finger (nail) **except thumb**
- ✓7th **T23.021** **Burn of unspecified degree of single** right **finger (nail) except thumb** ▽
- ✓7th **T23.022** **Burn of unspecified degree of single** left **finger (nail) except thumb** ▽
- ✓7th **T23.029** **Burn of unspecified degree of unspecified single finger (nail) except thumb** ▽

✓6th **T23.03** **Burn of unspecified degree of** multiple fingers (nail), not including thumb
- ✓7th **T23.031** **Burn of unspecified degree of multiple** right **fingers (nail), not including thumb** ▽
- ✓7th **T23.032** **Burn of unspecified degree of multiple** left **fingers (nail), not including thumb** ▽
- ✓7th **T23.039** **Burn of unspecified degree of unspecified multiple fingers (nail), not including thumb** ▽

✓6th **T23.04** **Burn of unspecified degree of** multiple fingers (nail), including thumb
- ✓7th **T23.041** **Burn of unspecified degree of multiple** right **fingers (nail), including thumb** ▽
- ✓7th **T23.042** **Burn of unspecified degree of multiple** left **fingers (nail), including thumb** ▽
- ✓7th **T23.049** **Burn of unspecified degree of unspecified multiple fingers (nail), including thumb** ▽

✓6th **T23.05** **Burn of unspecified degree of** palm
- ✓7th **T23.051** **Burn of unspecified degree of** right **palm** ▽
- ✓7th **T23.052** **Burn of unspecified degree of** left **palm** ▽
- ✓7th **T23.059** **Burn of unspecified degree of unspecified palm** ▽

✓6th **T23.06** **Burn of unspecified degree of** back of hand
- ✓7th **T23.061** **Burn of unspecified degree of back of** right **hand** ▽
- ✓7th **T23.062** **Burn of unspecified degree of back of** left **hand** ▽
- ✓7th **T23.069** **Burn of unspecified degree of back of unspecified hand** ▽

✓6th **T23.07** **Burn of unspecified degree of** wrist
- ✓7th **T23.071** **Burn of unspecified degree of** right **wrist** ▽
- ✓7th **T23.072** **Burn of unspecified degree of** left **wrist** ▽
- ✓7th **T23.079** **Burn of unspecified degree of unspecified wrist** ▽

EXCLUDES 1 Not coded here   EXCLUDES 2 Not included here   N Newborn Age: 0   P Pediatric Age: 0-17   M Maternity Age: 12-55   A Adult Age: 15-124

1046   ICD-10-CM 2018

✓6ᵗʰ **T23.09** Burn of unspecified degree of multiple sites of wrist and hand

    ✓7ᵗʰ **T23.091** Burn of unspecified degree of multiple sites of right wrist and hand ▽

    ✓7ᵗʰ **T23.092** Burn of unspecified degree of multiple sites of left wrist and hand ▽

    ✓7ᵗʰ **T23.099** Burn of unspecified degree of multiple sites of unspecified wrist and hand ▽

✓5ᵗʰ **T23.1** Burn of first degree of wrist and hand

    Use additional external cause code to identify the source, place and intent of the burn (X00-X19, X75-X77, X96-X98, Y92)

  ✓6ᵗʰ **T23.10** Burn of first degree of hand, unspecified site

    ✓7ᵗʰ **T23.101** Burn of first degree of right hand, unspecified site ▽

    ✓7ᵗʰ **T23.102** Burn of first degree of left hand, unspecified site ▽

    ✓7ᵗʰ **T23.109** Burn of first degree of unspecified hand, unspecified site ▽

  ✓6ᵗʰ **T23.11** Burn of first degree of thumb (nail)

    ✓7ᵗʰ **T23.111** Burn of first degree of right thumb (nail)

    ✓7ᵗʰ **T23.112** Burn of first degree of left thumb (nail)

    ✓7ᵗʰ **T23.119** Burn of first degree of unspecified thumb (nail) ▽

  ✓6ᵗʰ **T23.12** Burn of first degree of single finger (nail) except thumb

    ✓7ᵗʰ **T23.121** Burn of first degree of single right finger (nail) except thumb

    ✓7ᵗʰ **T23.122** Burn of first degree of single left finger (nail) except thumb

    ✓7ᵗʰ **T23.129** Burn of first degree of unspecified single finger (nail) except thumb ▽

  ✓6ᵗʰ **T23.13** Burn of first degree of multiple fingers (nail), not including thumb

    ✓7ᵗʰ **T23.131** Burn of first degree of multiple right fingers (nail), not including thumb

    ✓7ᵗʰ **T23.132** Burn of first degree of multiple left fingers (nail), not including thumb

    ✓7ᵗʰ **T23.139** Burn of first degree of unspecified multiple fingers (nail), not including thumb ▽

  ✓6ᵗʰ **T23.14** Burn of first degree of multiple fingers (nail), including thumb

    ✓7ᵗʰ **T23.141** Burn of first degree of multiple right fingers (nail), including thumb

    ✓7ᵗʰ **T23.142** Burn of first degree of multiple left fingers (nail), including thumb

    ✓7ᵗʰ **T23.149** Burn of first degree of unspecified multiple fingers (nail), including thumb ▽

  ✓6ᵗʰ **T23.15** Burn of first degree of palm

    ✓7ᵗʰ **T23.151** Burn of first degree of right palm

    ✓7ᵗʰ **T23.152** Burn of first degree of left palm

    ✓7ᵗʰ **T23.159** Burn of first degree of unspecified palm ▽

  ✓6ᵗʰ **T23.16** Burn of first degree of back of hand

    ✓7ᵗʰ **T23.161** Burn of first degree of back of right hand

    ✓7ᵗʰ **T23.162** Burn of first degree of back of left hand

    ✓7ᵗʰ **T23.169** Burn of first degree of back of unspecified hand ▽

  ✓6ᵗʰ **T23.17** Burn of first degree of wrist

    ✓7ᵗʰ **T23.171** Burn of first degree of right wrist

    ✓7ᵗʰ **T23.172** Burn of first degree of left wrist

    ✓7ᵗʰ **T23.179** Burn of first degree of unspecified wrist ▽

  ✓6ᵗʰ **T23.19** Burn of first degree of multiple sites of wrist and hand

    ✓7ᵗʰ **T23.191** Burn of first degree of multiple sites of right wrist and hand

    ✓7ᵗʰ **T23.192** Burn of first degree of multiple sites of left wrist and hand

    ✓7ᵗʰ **T23.199** Burn of first degree of multiple sites of unspecified wrist and hand ▽

✓5ᵗʰ **T23.2** Burn of second degree of wrist and hand

    Use additional external cause code to identify the source, place and intent of the burn (X00-X19, X75-X77, X96-X98, Y92)

  ✓6ᵗʰ **T23.20** Burn of second degree of hand, unspecified site

    ✓7ᵗʰ **T23.201** Burn of second degree of right hand, unspecified site ▽

    ✓7ᵗʰ **T23.202** Burn of second degree of left hand, unspecified site ▽

    ✓7ᵗʰ **T23.209** Burn of second degree of unspecified hand, unspecified site ▽

  ✓6ᵗʰ **T23.21** Burn of second degree of thumb (nail)

    ✓7ᵗʰ **T23.211** Burn of second degree of right thumb (nail)

    ✓7ᵗʰ **T23.212** Burn of second degree of left thumb (nail)

    ✓7ᵗʰ **T23.219** Burn of second degree of unspecified thumb (nail) ▽

  ✓6ᵗʰ **T23.22** Burn of second degree of single finger (nail) except thumb

    ✓7ᵗʰ **T23.221** Burn of second degree of single right finger (nail) except thumb

    ✓7ᵗʰ **T23.222** Burn of second degree of single left finger (nail) except thumb

    ✓7ᵗʰ **T23.229** Burn of second degree of unspecified single finger (nail) except thumb ▽

  ✓6ᵗʰ **T23.23** Burn of second degree of multiple fingers (nail), not including thumb

    ✓7ᵗʰ **T23.231** Burn of second degree of multiple right fingers (nail), not including thumb

    ✓7ᵗʰ **T23.232** Burn of second degree of multiple left fingers (nail), not including thumb

    ✓7ᵗʰ **T23.239** Burn of second degree of unspecified multiple fingers (nail), not including thumb ▽

  ✓6ᵗʰ **T23.24** Burn of second degree of multiple fingers (nail), including thumb

    ✓7ᵗʰ **T23.241** Burn of second degree of multiple right fingers (nail), including thumb

    ✓7ᵗʰ **T23.242** Burn of second degree of multiple left fingers (nail), including thumb

    ✓7ᵗʰ **T23.249** Burn of second degree of unspecified multiple fingers (nail), including thumb ▽

  ✓6ᵗʰ **T23.25** Burn of second degree of palm

    ✓7ᵗʰ **T23.251** Burn of second degree of right palm

    ✓7ᵗʰ **T23.252** Burn of second degree of left palm

    ✓7ᵗʰ **T23.259** Burn of second degree of unspecified palm ▽

  ✓6ᵗʰ **T23.26** Burn of second degree of back of hand

    ✓7ᵗʰ **T23.261** Burn of second degree of back of right hand

    ✓7ᵗʰ **T23.262** Burn of second degree of back of left hand

    ✓7ᵗʰ **T23.269** Burn of second degree of back of unspecified hand ▽

  ✓6ᵗʰ **T23.27** Burn of second degree of wrist

    ✓7ᵗʰ **T23.271** Burn of second degree of right wrist

    ✓7ᵗʰ **T23.272** Burn of second degree of left wrist

    ✓7ᵗʰ **T23.279** Burn of second degree of unspecified wrist ▽

  ✓6ᵗʰ **T23.29** Burn of second degree of multiple sites of wrist and hand

    ✓7ᵗʰ **T23.291** Burn of second degree of multiple sites of right wrist and hand

    ✓7ᵗʰ **T23.292** Burn of second degree of multiple sites of left wrist and hand

    ✓7ᵗʰ **T23.299** Burn of second degree of multiple sites of unspecified wrist and hand ▽

✓5ᵗʰ **T23.3** Burn of third degree of wrist and hand

    Use additional external cause code to identify the source, place and intent of the burn (X00-X19, X75-X77, X96-X98, Y92)

  ✓6ᵗʰ **T23.30** Burn of third degree of hand, unspecified site

    AHA: 2016, 2Q, 5

    ✓7ᵗʰ **T23.301** Burn of third degree of right hand, unspecified site ▽

✓ Additional Character Req   ✓×7ᵗʰ Placeholder Alert   Manifestation   HCC CMS-HCC Condition   ▽ Unspecified Code   ►◄ Revised Text   ● New Code   ▲ Revised Code Title

Chapter 19. Injury, Poisoning, and Certain Other Consequences of External Causes

T23.302–T23.511

☑7ᵗʰ **T23.302** **Burn of third degree of left hand, unspecified site** ▽

☑7ᵗʰ **T23.309** **Burn of third degree of unspecified hand, unspecified site** ▽

☑6ᵗʰ **T23.31** **Burn of third degree of thumb (nail)**

  ☑7ᵗʰ **T23.311** **Burn of third degree of right thumb (nail)**

  ☑7ᵗʰ **T23.312** **Burn of third degree of left thumb (nail)**

  ☑7ᵗʰ **T23.319** **Burn of third degree of unspecified thumb (nail)** ▽

☑6ᵗʰ **T23.32** **Burn of third degree of single finger (nail) except thumb**

  ☑7ᵗʰ **T23.321** **Burn of third degree of single right finger (nail) except thumb**

  ☑7ᵗʰ **T23.322** **Burn of third degree of single left finger (nail) except thumb**

  ☑7ᵗʰ **T23.329** **Burn of third degree of unspecified single finger (nail) except thumb** ▽

☑6ᵗʰ **T23.33** **Burn of third degree of multiple fingers (nail), not including thumb**

  ☑7ᵗʰ **T23.331** **Burn of third degree of multiple right fingers (nail), not including thumb**

  ☑7ᵗʰ **T23.332** **Burn of third degree of multiple left fingers (nail), not including thumb**

  ☑7ᵗʰ **T23.339** **Burn of third degree of unspecified multiple fingers (nail), not including thumb** ▽

☑6ᵗʰ **T23.34** **Burn of third degree of multiple fingers (nail), including thumb**

  ☑7ᵗʰ **T23.341** **Burn of third degree of multiple right fingers (nail), including thumb**

  ☑7ᵗʰ **T23.342** **Burn of third degree of multiple left fingers (nail), including thumb**

  ☑7ᵗʰ **T23.349** **Burn of third degree of unspecified multiple fingers (nail), including thumb** ▽

☑6ᵗʰ **T23.35** **Burn of third degree of palm**

  ☑7ᵗʰ **T23.351** **Burn of third degree of right palm**

  ☑7ᵗʰ **T23.352** **Burn of third degree of left palm**

  ☑7ᵗʰ **T23.359** **Burn of third degree of unspecified palm** ▽

☑6ᵗʰ **T23.36** **Burn of third degree of back of hand**

  ☑7ᵗʰ **T23.361** **Burn of third degree of back of right hand**

  ☑7ᵗʰ **T23.362** **Burn of third degree of back of left hand**

  ☑7ᵗʰ **T23.369** **Burn of third degree of back of unspecified hand** ▽

☑6ᵗʰ **T23.37** **Burn of third degree of wrist**

  ☑7ᵗʰ **T23.371** **Burn of third degree of right wrist**

  ☑7ᵗʰ **T23.372** **Burn of third degree of left wrist**

  ☑7ᵗʰ **T23.379** **Burn of third degree of unspecified wrist** ▽

☑6ᵗʰ **T23.39** **Burn of third degree of multiple sites of wrist and hand**

  ☑7ᵗʰ **T23.391** **Burn of third degree of multiple sites of right wrist and hand**

  ☑7ᵗʰ **T23.392** **Burn of third degree of multiple sites of left wrist and hand**

  ☑7ᵗʰ **T23.399** **Burn of third degree of multiple sites of unspecified wrist and hand** ▽

☑5ᵗʰ **T23.4** **Corrosion of unspecified degree of wrist and hand**

  Code first (T51-T65) to identify chemical and intent

  Use additional external cause code to identify place (Y92)

☑6ᵗʰ **T23.40** **Corrosion of unspecified degree of hand, unspecified site**

  ☑7ᵗʰ **T23.401** **Corrosion of unspecified degree of right hand, unspecified site** ▽

  ☑7ᵗʰ **T23.402** **Corrosion of unspecified degree of left hand, unspecified site** ▽

  ☑7ᵗʰ **T23.409** **Corrosion of unspecified degree of unspecified hand, unspecified site** ▽

☑6ᵗʰ **T23.41** **Corrosion of unspecified degree of thumb (nail)**

  ☑7ᵗʰ **T23.411** **Corrosion of unspecified degree of right thumb (nail)** ▽

  ☑7ᵗʰ **T23.412** **Corrosion of unspecified degree of left thumb (nail)** ▽

  ☑7ᵗʰ **T23.419** **Corrosion of unspecified degree of unspecified thumb (nail)** ▽

☑6ᵗʰ **T23.42** **Corrosion of unspecified degree of single finger (nail) except thumb**

  ☑7ᵗʰ **T23.421** **Corrosion of unspecified degree of single right finger (nail) except thumb** ▽

  ☑7ᵗʰ **T23.422** **Corrosion of unspecified degree of single left finger (nail) except thumb** ▽

  ☑7ᵗʰ **T23.429** **Corrosion of unspecified degree of unspecified single finger (nail) except thumb** ▽

☑6ᵗʰ **T23.43** **Corrosion of unspecified degree of multiple fingers (nail), not including thumb**

  ☑7ᵗʰ **T23.431** **Corrosion of unspecified degree of multiple right fingers (nail), not including thumb** ▽

  ☑7ᵗʰ **T23.432** **Corrosion of unspecified degree of multiple left fingers (nail), not including thumb** ▽

  ☑7ᵗʰ **T23.439** **Corrosion of unspecified degree of unspecified multiple fingers (nail), not including thumb** ▽

☑6ᵗʰ **T23.44** **Corrosion of unspecified degree of multiple fingers (nail), including thumb**

  ☑7ᵗʰ **T23.441** **Corrosion of unspecified degree of multiple right fingers (nail), including thumb** ▽

  ☑7ᵗʰ **T23.442** **Corrosion of unspecified degree of multiple left fingers (nail), including thumb** ▽

  ☑7ᵗʰ **T23.449** **Corrosion of unspecified degree of unspecified multiple fingers (nail), including thumb** ▽

☑6ᵗʰ **T23.45** **Corrosion of unspecified degree of palm**

  ☑7ᵗʰ **T23.451** **Corrosion of unspecified degree of right palm** ▽

  ☑7ᵗʰ **T23.452** **Corrosion of unspecified degree of left palm** ▽

  ☑7ᵗʰ **T23.459** **Corrosion of unspecified degree of unspecified palm** ▽

☑6ᵗʰ **T23.46** **Corrosion of unspecified degree of back of hand**

  ☑7ᵗʰ **T23.461** **Corrosion of unspecified degree of back of right hand** ▽

  ☑7ᵗʰ **T23.462** **Corrosion of unspecified degree of back of left hand** ▽

  ☑7ᵗʰ **T23.469** **Corrosion of unspecified degree of back of unspecified hand** ▽

☑6ᵗʰ **T23.47** **Corrosion of unspecified degree of wrist**

  ☑7ᵗʰ **T23.471** **Corrosion of unspecified degree of right wrist** ▽

  ☑7ᵗʰ **T23.472** **Corrosion of unspecified degree of left wrist** ▽

  ☑7ᵗʰ **T23.479** **Corrosion of unspecified degree of unspecified wrist** ▽

☑6ᵗʰ **T23.49** **Corrosion of unspecified degree of multiple sites of wrist and hand**

  ☑7ᵗʰ **T23.491** **Corrosion of unspecified degree of multiple sites of right wrist and hand** ▽

  ☑7ᵗʰ **T23.492** **Corrosion of unspecified degree of multiple sites of left wrist and hand** ▽

  ☑7ᵗʰ **T23.499** **Corrosion of unspecified degree of multiple sites of unspecified wrist and hand** ▽

☑5ᵗʰ **T23.5** **Corrosion of first degree of wrist and hand**

  Code first (T51-T65) to identify chemical and intent

  Use additional external cause code to identify place (Y92)

☑6ᵗʰ **T23.50** **Corrosion of first degree of hand, unspecified site**

  ☑7ᵗʰ **T23.501** **Corrosion of first degree of right hand, unspecified site** ▽

  ☑7ᵗʰ **T23.502** **Corrosion of first degree of left hand, unspecified site** ▽

  ☑7ᵗʰ **T23.509** **Corrosion of first degree of unspecified hand, unspecified site** ▽

☑6ᵗʰ **T23.51** **Corrosion of first degree of thumb (nail)**

  ☑7ᵗʰ **T23.511** **Corrosion of first degree of right thumb (nail)** ▽

EXCLUDES 1 Not coded here   **EXCLUDES 2** Not included here   **N** Newborn Age: 0   **P** Pediatric Age: 0-17   **M** Maternity Age: 12-55   **A** Adult Age: 15-124

1048   ICD-10-CM 2018

✓7ᵗʰ **T23.512** Corrosion of first degree of left thumb (nail)

✓7ᵗʰ **T23.519** Corrosion of first degree of unspecified ▽ thumb (nail)

✓6ᵗʰ **T23.52** Corrosion of first degree of single finger (nail) except thumb

   ✓7ᵗʰ **T23.521** Corrosion of first degree of single right finger (nail) except thumb

   ✓7ᵗʰ **T23.522** Corrosion of first degree of single left finger (nail) except thumb

   ✓7ᵗʰ **T23.529** Corrosion of first degree of unspecified ▽ single finger (nail) except thumb

✓6ᵗʰ **T23.53** Corrosion of first degree of multiple fingers (nail), not including thumb

   ✓7ᵗʰ **T23.531** Corrosion of first degree of multiple right fingers (nail), not including thumb

   ✓7ᵗʰ **T23.532** Corrosion of first degree of multiple left fingers (nail), not including thumb

   ✓7ᵗʰ **T23.539** Corrosion of first degree of unspecified ▽ multiple fingers (nail), not including thumb

✓6ᵗʰ **T23.54** Corrosion of first degree of multiple fingers (nail), including thumb

   ✓7ᵗʰ **T23.541** Corrosion of first degree of multiple right fingers (nail), including thumb

   ✓7ᵗʰ **T23.542** Corrosion of first degree of multiple left fingers (nail), including thumb

   ✓7ᵗʰ **T23.549** Corrosion of first degree of unspecified ▽ multiple fingers (nail), including thumb

✓6ᵗʰ **T23.55** Corrosion of first degree of palm

   ✓7ᵗʰ **T23.551** Corrosion of first degree of right palm

   ✓7ᵗʰ **T23.552** Corrosion of first degree of left palm

   ✓7ᵗʰ **T23.559** Corrosion of first degree of unspecified ▽ palm

✓6ᵗʰ **T23.56** Corrosion of first degree of back of hand

   ✓7ᵗʰ **T23.561** Corrosion of first degree of back of right hand

   ✓7ᵗʰ **T23.562** Corrosion of first degree of back of left hand

   ✓7ᵗʰ **T23.569** Corrosion of first degree of back of ▽ unspecified hand

✓6ᵗʰ **T23.57** Corrosion of first degree of wrist

   ✓7ᵗʰ **T23.571** Corrosion of first degree of right wrist

   ✓7ᵗʰ **T23.572** Corrosion of first degree of left wrist

   ✓7ᵗʰ **T23.579** Corrosion of first degree of unspecified ▽ wrist

✓6ᵗʰ **T23.59** Corrosion of first degree of multiple sites of wrist and hand

   ✓7ᵗʰ **T23.591** Corrosion of first degree of multiple sites of right wrist and hand

   ✓7ᵗʰ **T23.592** Corrosion of first degree of multiple sites of left wrist and hand

   ✓7ᵗʰ **T23.599** Corrosion of first degree of multiple ▽ sites of unspecified wrist and hand

✓5ᵗʰ **T23.6** Corrosion of second degree of wrist and hand

   Code first (T51-T65) to identify chemical and intent

   Use additional external cause code to identify place (Y92)

✓6ᵗʰ **T23.60** Corrosion of second degree of hand, unspecified site

   ✓7ᵗʰ **T23.601** Corrosion of second degree of right ▽ hand, unspecified site

   ✓7ᵗʰ **T23.602** Corrosion of second degree of left ▽ hand, unspecified site

   ✓7ᵗʰ **T23.609** Corrosion of second degree of ▽ unspecified hand, unspecified site

✓6ᵗʰ **T23.61** Corrosion of second degree of thumb (nail)

   ✓7ᵗʰ **T23.611** Corrosion of second degree of right thumb (nail)

   ✓7ᵗʰ **T23.612** Corrosion of second degree of left thumb (nail)

   ✓7ᵗʰ **T23.619** Corrosion of second degree of ▽ unspecified thumb (nail)

✓6ᵗʰ **T23.62** Corrosion of second degree of single finger (nail) except thumb

   ✓7ᵗʰ **T23.621** Corrosion of second degree of single right finger (nail) except thumb

   ✓7ᵗʰ **T23.622** Corrosion of second degree of single left finger (nail) except thumb

   ✓7ᵗʰ **T23.629** Corrosion of second degree of ▽ unspecified single finger (nail) except thumb

✓6ᵗʰ **T23.63** Corrosion of second degree of multiple fingers (nail), not including thumb

   ✓7ᵗʰ **T23.631** Corrosion of second degree of multiple right fingers (nail), not including thumb

   ✓7ᵗʰ **T23.632** Corrosion of second degree of multiple left fingers (nail), not including thumb

   ✓7ᵗʰ **T23.639** Corrosion of second degree of ▽ unspecified multiple fingers (nail), not including thumb

✓6ᵗʰ **T23.64** Corrosion of second degree of multiple fingers (nail), including thumb

   ✓7ᵗʰ **T23.641** Corrosion of second degree of multiple right fingers (nail), including thumb

   ✓7ᵗʰ **T23.642** Corrosion of second degree of multiple left fingers (nail), including thumb

   ✓7ᵗʰ **T23.649** Corrosion of second degree of ▽ unspecified multiple fingers (nail), including thumb

✓6ᵗʰ **T23.65** Corrosion of second degree of palm

   ✓7ᵗʰ **T23.651** Corrosion of second degree of right palm

   ✓7ᵗʰ **T23.652** Corrosion of second degree of left palm

   ✓7ᵗʰ **T23.659** Corrosion of second degree of ▽ unspecified palm

✓6ᵗʰ **T23.66** Corrosion of second degree of back of hand

   ✓7ᵗʰ **T23.661** Corrosion of second degree back of right hand

   ✓7ᵗʰ **T23.662** Corrosion of second degree back of left hand

   ✓7ᵗʰ **T23.669** Corrosion of second degree back of ▽ unspecified hand

✓6ᵗʰ **T23.67** Corrosion of second degree of wrist

   ✓7ᵗʰ **T23.671** Corrosion of second degree of right wrist

   ✓7ᵗʰ **T23.672** Corrosion of second degree of left wrist

   ✓7ᵗʰ **T23.679** Corrosion of second degree of ▽ unspecified wrist

✓6ᵗʰ **T23.69** Corrosion of second degree of multiple sites of wrist and hand

   ✓7ᵗʰ **T23.691** Corrosion of second degree of multiple sites of right wrist and hand

   ✓7ᵗʰ **T23.692** Corrosion of second degree of multiple sites of left wrist and hand

   ✓7ᵗʰ **T23.699** Corrosion of second degree of multiple ▽ sites of unspecified wrist and hand

✓5ᵗʰ **T23.7** Corrosion of third degree of wrist and hand

   Code first (T51-T65) to identify chemical and intent

   Use additional external cause code to identify place (Y92)

✓6ᵗʰ **T23.70** Corrosion of third degree of hand, unspecified site

   ✓7ᵗʰ **T23.701** Corrosion of third degree of right hand, ▽ unspecified site

   ✓7ᵗʰ **T23.702** Corrosion of third degree of left hand, ▽ unspecified site

   ✓7ᵗʰ **T23.709** Corrosion of third degree of ▽ unspecified hand, unspecified site

✓6ᵗʰ **T23.71** Corrosion of third degree of thumb (nail)

   ✓7ᵗʰ **T23.711** Corrosion of third degree of right thumb (nail)

   ✓7ᵗʰ **T23.712** Corrosion of third degree of left thumb (nail)

   ✓7ᵗʰ **T23.719** Corrosion of third degree of ▽ unspecified thumb (nail)

✓6ᵗʰ **T23.72** Corrosion of third degree of single finger (nail) except thumb

   ✓7ᵗʰ **T23.721** Corrosion of third degree of single right finger (nail) except thumb

---

✓ Additional Character Req   ✓x7ᵗʰ Placeholder Alert   Manifestation   HCC CMS-HCC Condition   ▽ Unspecified Code   ▶◀ Revised Text   ● New Code   ▲ Revised Code Title

√7ᵗʰ **T23.722** Corrosion of third degree of single left finger (nail) except thumb

√7ᵗʰ **T23.729** Corrosion of third degree of unspecified single finger (nail) except thumb ▽

√6ᵗʰ **T23.73** Corrosion of third degree of multiple fingers (nail), not including thumb

     √7ᵗʰ **T23.731** Corrosion of third degree of multiple right fingers (nail), not including thumb

     √7ᵗʰ **T23.732** Corrosion of third degree of multiple left fingers (nail), not including thumb

     √7ᵗʰ **T23.739** Corrosion of third degree of unspecified multiple fingers (nail), not including thumb ▽

√6ᵗʰ **T23.74** Corrosion of third degree of multiple fingers (nail), including thumb

     √7ᵗʰ **T23.741** Corrosion of third degree of multiple right fingers (nail), including thumb

     √7ᵗʰ **T23.742** Corrosion of third degree of multiple left fingers (nail), including thumb

     √7ᵗʰ **T23.749** Corrosion of third degree of unspecified multiple fingers (nail), including thumb ▽

√6ᵗʰ **T23.75** Corrosion of third degree of palm

     √7ᵗʰ **T23.751** Corrosion of third degree of right palm

     √7ᵗʰ **T23.752** Corrosion of third degree of left palm

     √7ᵗʰ **T23.759** Corrosion of third degree of unspecified palm ▽

√6ᵗʰ **T23.76** Corrosion of third degree of back of hand

     √7ᵗʰ **T23.761** Corrosion of third degree of back of right hand

     √7ᵗʰ **T23.762** Corrosion of third degree of back of left hand

     √7ᵗʰ **T23.769** Corrosion of third degree back of unspecified hand ▽

√6ᵗʰ **T23.77** Corrosion of third degree of wrist

     √7ᵗʰ **T23.771** Corrosion of third degree of right wrist

     √7ᵗʰ **T23.772** Corrosion of third degree of left wrist

     √7ᵗʰ **T23.779** Corrosion of third degree of unspecified wrist ▽

√6ᵗʰ **T23.79** Corrosion of third degree of multiple sites of wrist and hand

     √7ᵗʰ **T23.791** Corrosion of third degree of multiple sites of right wrist and hand

     √7ᵗʰ **T23.792** Corrosion of third degree of multiple sites of left wrist and hand

     √7ᵗʰ **T23.799** Corrosion of third degree of multiple sites of unspecified wrist and hand ▽

√4ᵗʰ **T24** **Burn and corrosion of lower limb, except ankle and foot**

     EXCLUDES 2   burn and corrosion of ankle and foot (T25.-)
                  burn and corrosion of hip region (T21.-)

> The appropriate 7th character is to be added to each code from category T24.
> A   initial encounter
> D   subsequent encounter
> S   sequela

√5ᵗʰ **T24.0** Burn of unspecified degree of lower limb, except ankle and foot

     Use additional external cause code to identify the source, place and intent of the burn (X00-X19, X75-X77, X96-X98, Y92)

     √6ᵗʰ **T24.00** Burn of unspecified degree of unspecified site of lower limb, except ankle and foot

         √7ᵗʰ **T24.001** Burn of unspecified degree of unspecified site of right lower limb, except ankle and foot ▽

         √7ᵗʰ **T24.002** Burn of unspecified degree of unspecified site of left lower limb, except ankle and foot ▽

         √7ᵗʰ **T24.009** Burn of unspecified degree of unspecified site of unspecified lower limb, except ankle and foot ▽

     √6ᵗʰ **T24.01** Burn of unspecified degree of thigh

         √7ᵗʰ **T24.011** Burn of unspecified degree of right thigh

√7ᵗʰ **T24.012** Burn of unspecified degree of left thigh ▽

√7ᵗʰ **T24.019** Burn of unspecified degree of unspecified thigh ▽

√6ᵗʰ **T24.02** Burn of unspecified degree of knee

     √7ᵗʰ **T24.021** Burn of unspecified degree of right knee ▽

     √7ᵗʰ **T24.022** Burn of unspecified degree of left knee ▽

     √7ᵗʰ **T24.029** Burn of unspecified degree of unspecified knee ▽

√6ᵗʰ **T24.03** Burn of unspecified degree of lower leg

     √7ᵗʰ **T24.031** Burn of unspecified degree of right lower leg ▽

     √7ᵗʰ **T24.032** Burn of unspecified degree of left lower leg ▽

     √7ᵗʰ **T24.039** Burn of unspecified degree of unspecified lower leg ▽

√6ᵗʰ **T24.09** Burn of unspecified degree of multiple sites of lower limb, except ankle and foot

     √7ᵗʰ **T24.091** Burn of unspecified degree of multiple sites of right lower limb, except ankle and foot ▽

     √7ᵗʰ **T24.092** Burn of unspecified degree of multiple sites of left lower limb, except ankle and foot ▽

     √7ᵗʰ **T24.099** Burn of unspecified degree of multiple sites of unspecified lower limb, except ankle and foot ▽

√5ᵗʰ **T24.1** Burn of first degree of lower limb, except ankle and foot

     Use additional external cause code to identify the source, place and intent of the burn (X00-X19, X75-X77, X96-X98, Y92)

     √6ᵗʰ **T24.10** Burn of first degree of unspecified site of lower limb, except ankle and foot

         √7ᵗʰ **T24.101** Burn of first degree of unspecified site of right lower limb, except ankle and foot ▽

         √7ᵗʰ **T24.102** Burn of first degree of unspecified site of left lower limb, except ankle and foot ▽

         √7ᵗʰ **T24.109** Burn of first degree of unspecified site of unspecified lower limb, except ankle and foot ▽

     √6ᵗʰ **T24.11** Burn of first degree of thigh

         √7ᵗʰ **T24.111** Burn of first degree of right thigh

         √7ᵗʰ **T24.112** Burn of first degree of left thigh

         √7ᵗʰ **T24.119** Burn of first degree of unspecified thigh ▽

     √6ᵗʰ **T24.12** Burn of first degree of knee

         √7ᵗʰ **T24.121** Burn of first degree of right knee

         √7ᵗʰ **T24.122** Burn of first degree of left knee

         √7ᵗʰ **T24.129** Burn of first degree of unspecified knee ▽

     √6ᵗʰ **T24.13** Burn of first degree of lower leg

         √7ᵗʰ **T24.131** Burn of first degree of right lower leg

         √7ᵗʰ **T24.132** Burn of first degree of left lower leg

         √7ᵗʰ **T24.139** Burn of first degree of unspecified lower leg ▽

     √6ᵗʰ **T24.19** Burn of first degree of multiple sites of lower limb, except ankle and foot

         √7ᵗʰ **T24.191** Burn of first degree of multiple sites of right lower limb, except ankle and foot

         √7ᵗʰ **T24.192** Burn of first degree of multiple sites of left lower limb, except ankle and foot

         √7ᵗʰ **T24.199** Burn of first degree of multiple sites of unspecified lower limb, except ankle and foot ▽

√5ᵗʰ **T24.2** Burn of second degree of lower limb, except ankle and foot

     Use additional external cause code to identify the source, place and intent of the burn (X00-X19, X75-X77, X96-X98, Y92)

     √6ᵗʰ **T24.20** Burn of second degree of unspecified site of lower limb, except ankle and foot

         √7ᵗʰ **T24.201** Burn of second degree of unspecified site of right lower limb, except ankle and foot ▽

√7ᵗʰ **T24.202** Burn of second degree of unspecified ▽
site of left lower limb, except ankle and
foot

√7ᵗʰ **T24.209** Burn of second degree of unspecified ▽
site of unspecified lower limb, except
ankle and foot

√6ᵗʰ **T24.21** Burn of second degree of thigh

√7ᵗʰ **T24.211** Burn of second degree of right thigh

√7ᵗʰ **T24.212** Burn of second degree of left thigh

√7ᵗʰ **T24.219** Burn of second degree of unspecified ▽
thigh

√6ᵗʰ **T24.22** Burn of second degree of knee

√7ᵗʰ **T24.221** Burn of second degree of right knee

√7ᵗʰ **T24.222** Burn of second degree of left knee

√7ᵗʰ **T24.229** Burn of second degree of unspecified ▽
knee

√6ᵗʰ **T24.23** Burn of second degree of lower leg

√7ᵗʰ **T24.231** Burn of second degree of right lower leg

√7ᵗʰ **T24.232** Burn of second degree of left lower leg

√7ᵗʰ **T24.239** Burn of second degree of unspecified ▽
lower leg

√6ᵗʰ **T24.29** Burn of second degree of multiple sites of lower
limb, except ankle and foot

√7ᵗʰ **T24.291** Burn of second degree of multiple sites of
right lower limb, except ankle and foot

√7ᵗʰ **T24.292** Burn of second degree of multiple sites of
left lower limb, except ankle and foot

√7ᵗʰ **T24.299** Burn of second degree of multiple ▽
sites of unspecified lower limb, except
ankle and foot

√5ᵗʰ **T24.3** Burn of third degree of lower limb, except ankle and foot
Use additional external cause code to identify the source, place
and intent of the burn (X00-X19, X75-X77, X96-X98, Y92)

√6ᵗʰ **T24.30** Burn of third degree of unspecified site of lower
limb, except ankle and foot

√7ᵗʰ **T24.301** Burn of third degree of unspecified ▽
site of right lower limb, except ankle and
foot

√7ᵗʰ **T24.302** Burn of third degree of unspecified ▽
site of left lower limb, except ankle and
foot

√7ᵗʰ **T24.309** Burn of third degree of unspecified ▽
site of unspecified lower limb, except
ankle and foot

√6ᵗʰ **T24.31** Burn of third degree of thigh

√7ᵗʰ **T24.311** Burn of third degree of right thigh

√7ᵗʰ **T24.312** Burn of third degree of left thigh

√7ᵗʰ **T24.319** Burn of third degree of unspecified ▽
thigh

√6ᵗʰ **T24.32** Burn of third degree of knee

√7ᵗʰ **T24.321** Burn of third degree of right knee

√7ᵗʰ **T24.322** Burn of third degree of left knee

√7ᵗʰ **T24.329** Burn of third degree of unspecified ▽
knee

√6ᵗʰ **T24.33** Burn of third degree of lower leg

√7ᵗʰ **T24.331** Burn of third degree of right lower leg

√7ᵗʰ **T24.332** Burn of third degree of left lower leg

√7ᵗʰ **T24.339** Burn of third degree of unspecified ▽
lower leg

√6ᵗʰ **T24.39** Burn of third degree of multiple sites of lower limb,
except ankle and foot
AHA: 2016, 2Q, 4

√7ᵗʰ **T24.391** Burn of third degree of multiple sites of
right lower limb, except ankle and foot

√7ᵗʰ **T24.392** Burn of third degree of multiple sites of
left lower limb, except ankle and foot

√7ᵗʰ **T24.399** Burn of third degree of multiple sites ▽
of unspecified lower limb, except
ankle and foot

√5ᵗʰ **T24.4** Corrosion of unspecified degree of lower limb, except ankle
and foot
Code first (T51-T65) to identify chemical and intent
Use additional external cause code to identify place (Y92)

√6ᵗʰ **T24.40** Corrosion of unspecified degree of unspecified site
of lower limb, except ankle and foot

√7ᵗʰ **T24.401** Corrosion of unspecified degree of ▽
unspecified site of right lower limb,
except ankle and foot

√7ᵗʰ **T24.402** Corrosion of unspecified degree of ▽
unspecified site of left lower limb,
except ankle and foot

√7ᵗʰ **T24.409** Corrosion of unspecified degree of ▽
unspecified site of unspecified lower l
imb, except ankle and foot

√6ᵗʰ **T24.41** Corrosion of unspecified degree of thigh

√7ᵗʰ **T24.411** Corrosion of unspecified degree of ▽
right thigh

√7ᵗʰ **T24.412** Corrosion of unspecified degree of ▽
left thigh

√7ᵗʰ **T24.419** Corrosion of unspecified degree of ▽
unspecified thigh

√6ᵗʰ **T24.42** Corrosion of unspecified degree of knee

√7ᵗʰ **T24.421** Corrosion of unspecified degree of ▽
right knee

√7ᵗʰ **T24.422** Corrosion of unspecified degree of ▽
left knee

√7ᵗʰ **T24.429** Corrosion of unspecified degree of ▽
unspecified knee

√6ᵗʰ **T24.43** Corrosion of unspecified degree of lower leg

√7ᵗʰ **T24.431** Corrosion of unspecified degree of ▽
right lower leg

√7ᵗʰ **T24.432** Corrosion of unspecified degree of ▽
left lower leg

√7ᵗʰ **T24.439** Corrosion of unspecified degree of ▽
unspecified lower leg

√6ᵗʰ **T24.49** Corrosion of unspecified degree of multiple sites of
lower limb, except ankle and foot

√7ᵗʰ **T24.491** Corrosion of unspecified degree of ▽
multiple sites of right lower limb,
except ankle and foot

√7ᵗʰ **T24.492** Corrosion of unspecified degree of ▽
multiple sites of left lower limb,
except ankle and foot

√7ᵗʰ **T24.499** Corrosion of unspecified degree of ▽
multiple sites of unspecified lower
limb, except ankle and foot

√5ᵗʰ **T24.5** Corrosion of first degree of lower limb, except ankle and foot
Code first (T51-T65) to identify chemical and intent
Use additional external cause code to identify place (Y92)

√6ᵗʰ **T24.50** Corrosion of first degree of unspecified site of lower
limb, except ankle and foot

√7ᵗʰ **T24.501** Corrosion of first degree of ▽
unspecified site of right lower limb,
except ankle and foot

√7ᵗʰ **T24.502** Corrosion of first degree of ▽
unspecified site of left lower limb,
except ankle and foot

√7ᵗʰ **T24.509** Corrosion of first degree of ▽
unspecified site of unspecified lower
limb, except ankle and foot

√6ᵗʰ **T24.51** Corrosion of first degree of thigh

√7ᵗʰ **T24.511** Corrosion of first degree of right thigh

√7ᵗʰ **T24.512** Corrosion of first degree of left thigh

√7ᵗʰ **T24.519** Corrosion of first degree of unspecified ▽
thigh

√6ᵗʰ **T24.52** Corrosion of first degree of knee

√7ᵗʰ **T24.521** Corrosion of first degree of right knee

√7ᵗʰ **T24.522** Corrosion of first degree of left knee

√7ᵗʰ **T24.529** Corrosion of first degree of unspecified ▽
knee

√6ᵗʰ **T24.53** Corrosion of first degree of lower leg

√7ᵗʰ **T24.531** Corrosion of first degree of right lower leg

√7ᵗʰ **T24.532** Corrosion of first degree of left lower leg

√7ᵗʰ **T24.539** Corrosion of first degree of unspecified ▽
lower leg

√6ᵗʰ **T24.59** Corrosion of first degree of multiple sites of lower
limb, except ankle and foot

   √7ᵗʰ **T24.591** Corrosion of first degree of multiple sites
of right lower limb, except ankle and foot

   √7ᵗʰ **T24.592** Corrosion of first degree of multiple sites
of left lower limb, except ankle and foot

   √7ᵗʰ **T24.599** Corrosion of first degree of multiple ▽
sites of unspecified lower limb, except
ankle and foot

√5ᵗʰ **T24.6** Corrosion of second degree of lower limb, except ankle and
foot

   Code first (T51-T65) to identify chemical and intent
   Use additional external cause code to identify place (Y92)

√6ᵗʰ **T24.60** Corrosion of second degree of unspecified site of
lower limb, except ankle and foot

   √7ᵗʰ **T24.601** Corrosion of second degree of ▽
unspecified site of right lower limb,
except ankle and foot

   √7ᵗʰ **T24.602** Corrosion of second degree of ▽
unspecified site of left lower limb,
except ankle and foot

   √7ᵗʰ **T24.609** Corrosion of second degree of ▽
unspecified site of unspecified lower
limb, except ankle and foot

√6ᵗʰ **T24.61** Corrosion of second degree of thigh

   √7ᵗʰ **T24.611** Corrosion of second degree of right thigh

   √7ᵗʰ **T24.612** Corrosion of second degree of left thigh

   √7ᵗʰ **T24.619** Corrosion of second degree of ▽
unspecified thigh

√6ᵗʰ **T24.62** Corrosion of second degree of knee

   √7ᵗʰ **T24.621** Corrosion of second degree of right knee

   √7ᵗʰ **T24.622** Corrosion of second degree of left knee

   √7ᵗʰ **T24.629** Corrosion of second degree of ▽
unspecified knee

√6ᵗʰ **T24.63** Corrosion of second degree of lower leg

   √7ᵗʰ **T24.631** Corrosion of second degree of right lower
leg

   √7ᵗʰ **T24.632** Corrosion of second degree of left lower
leg

   √7ᵗʰ **T24.639** Corrosion of second degree of ▽
unspecified lower leg

√6ᵗʰ **T24.69** Corrosion of second degree of multiple sites of lower
limb, except ankle and foot

   √7ᵗʰ **T24.691** Corrosion of second degree of multiple
sites of right lower limb, except ankle and
foot

   √7ᵗʰ **T24.692** Corrosion of second degree of multiple
sites of left lower limb, except ankle and
foot

   √7ᵗʰ **T24.699** Corrosion of second degree of multiple ▽
sites of unspecified lower limb, except
ankle and foot

√5ᵗʰ **T24.7** Corrosion of third degree of lower limb, except ankle and foot

   Code first (T51-T65) to identify chemical and intent
   Use additional external cause code to identify place (Y92)

√6ᵗʰ **T24.70** Corrosion of third degree of unspecified site of lower
limb, except ankle and foot

   √7ᵗʰ **T24.701** Corrosion of third degree of ▽
unspecified site of right lower limb,
except ankle and foot

   √7ᵗʰ **T24.702** Corrosion of third degree of ▽
unspecified site of left lower limb,
except ankle and foot

   √7ᵗʰ **T24.709** Corrosion of third degree of ▽
unspecified site of unspecified lower
limb, except ankle and foot

√6ᵗʰ **T24.71** Corrosion of third degree of thigh

   √7ᵗʰ **T24.711** Corrosion of third degree of right thigh

   √7ᵗʰ **T24.712** Corrosion of third degree of left thigh

   √7ᵗʰ **T24.719** Corrosion of third degree of ▽
unspecified thigh

√6ᵗʰ **T24.72** Corrosion of third degree of knee

   √7ᵗʰ **T24.721** Corrosion of third degree of right knee

   √7ᵗʰ **T24.722** Corrosion of third degree of left knee

   √7ᵗʰ **T24.729** Corrosion of third degree of ▽
unspecified knee

√6ᵗʰ **T24.73** Corrosion of third degree of lower leg

   √7ᵗʰ **T24.731** Corrosion of third degree of right lower
leg

   √7ᵗʰ **T24.732** Corrosion of third degree of left lower leg

   √7ᵗʰ **T24.739** Corrosion of third degree of ▽
unspecified lower leg

√6ᵗʰ **T24.79** Corrosion of third degree of multiple sites of lower
limb, except ankle and foot

   √7ᵗʰ **T24.791** Corrosion of third degree of multiple sites
of right lower limb, except ankle and foot

   √7ᵗʰ **T24.792** Corrosion of third degree of multiple sites
of left lower limb, except ankle and foot

   √7ᵗʰ **T24.799** Corrosion of third degree of multiple ▽
sites of unspecified lower limb, except
ankle and foot

√4ᵗʰ **T25** Burn and corrosion of ankle and foot

> The appropriate 7th character is to be added to each code from
> category T25.
> A   initial encounter
> D   subsequent encounter
> S   sequela

√5ᵗʰ **T25.0** Burn of unspecified degree of ankle and foot

   Use additional external cause code to identify the source, place
and intent of the burn (X00-X19, X75-X77, X96-X98, Y92)

√6ᵗʰ **T25.01** Burn of unspecified degree of ankle

   √7ᵗʰ **T25.011** Burn of unspecified degree of right ▽
ankle

   √7ᵗʰ **T25.012** Burn of unspecified degree of left ▽
ankle

   √7ᵗʰ **T25.019** Burn of unspecified degree of ▽
unspecified ankle

√6ᵗʰ **T25.02** Burn of unspecified degree of foot

   EXCLUDES 2   burn of unspecified degree of toe(s) (nail)
(T25.03-)

   √7ᵗʰ **T25.021** Burn of unspecified degree of right ▽
foot

   √7ᵗʰ **T25.022** Burn of unspecified degree of left ▽
foot

   √7ᵗʰ **T25.029** Burn of unspecified degree of ▽
unspecified foot

√6ᵗʰ **T25.03** Burn of unspecified degree of toe(s) (nail)

   √7ᵗʰ **T25.031** Burn of unspecified degree of right ▽
toe(s) (nail)

   √7ᵗʰ **T25.032** Burn of unspecified degree of left ▽
toe(s) (nail)

   √7ᵗʰ **T25.039** Burn of unspecified degree of ▽
unspecified toe(s) (nail)

√6ᵗʰ **T25.09** Burn of unspecified degree of multiple sites of ankle
and foot

   √7ᵗʰ **T25.091** Burn of unspecified degree of ▽
multiple sites of right ankle and foot

   √7ᵗʰ **T25.092** Burn of unspecified degree of ▽
multiple sites of left ankle and foot

   √7ᵗʰ **T25.099** Burn of unspecified degree of ▽
multiple sites of unspecified ankle
and foot

√5ᵗʰ **T25.1** Burn of first degree of ankle and foot

   Use additional external cause code to identify the source, place
and intent of the burn (X00-X19, X75-X77, X96-X98, Y92)

√6ᵗʰ **T25.11** Burn of first degree of ankle

   √7ᵗʰ **T25.111** Burn of first degree of right ankle

   √7ᵗʰ **T25.112** Burn of first degree of left ankle

   √7ᵗʰ **T25.119** Burn of first degree of unspecified ▽
ankle

√6ᵗʰ **T25.12** Burn of first degree of foot

   EXCLUDES 2   burn of first degree of toe(s) (nail) (T25.13-)

   √7ᵗʰ **T25.121** Burn of first degree of right foot

   √7ᵗʰ **T25.122** Burn of first degree of left foot

√7ᵗʰ **T25.129**   **Burn of first degree of unspecified foot** ▽

√6ᵗʰ **T25.13**   **Burn of first degree of toe(s) (nail)**

    √7ᵗʰ **T25.131**   **Burn of first degree of right toe(s) (nail)**

    √7ᵗʰ **T25.132**   **Burn of first degree of left toe(s) (nail)**

    √7ᵗʰ **T25.139**   **Burn of first degree of unspecified toe(s) (nail)** ▽

√6ᵗʰ **T25.19**   **Burn of first degree of multiple sites of ankle and foot**

    √7ᵗʰ **T25.191**   **Burn of first degree of multiple sites of right ankle and foot**

    √7ᵗʰ **T25.192**   **Burn of first degree of multiple sites of left ankle and foot**

    √7ᵗʰ **T25.199**   **Burn of first degree of multiple sites of unspecified ankle and foot** ▽

√5ᵗʰ **T25.2**   **Burn of second degree of ankle and foot**

Use additional external cause code to identify the source, place and intent of the burn (X00-X19, X75-X77, X96-X98, Y92)

√6ᵗʰ **T25.21**   **Burn of second degree of ankle**

    √7ᵗʰ **T25.211**   **Burn of second degree of right ankle**

    √7ᵗʰ **T25.212**   **Burn of second degree of left ankle**

    √7ᵗʰ **T25.219**   **Burn of second degree of unspecified ankle** ▽

√6ᵗʰ **T25.22**   **Burn of second degree of foot**

    EXCLUDES 2   *burn of second degree of toe(s) (nail) (T25.23-)*

    √7ᵗʰ **T25.221**   **Burn of second degree of right foot**

    √7ᵗʰ **T25.222**   **Burn of second degree of left foot**

    √7ᵗʰ **T25.229**   **Burn of second degree of unspecified foot** ▽

√6ᵗʰ **T25.23**   **Burn of second degree of toe(s) (nail)**

    √7ᵗʰ **T25.231**   **Burn of second degree of right toe(s) (nail)**

    √7ᵗʰ **T25.232**   **Burn of second degree of left toe(s) (nail)**

    √7ᵗʰ **T25.239**   **Burn of second degree of unspecified toe(s) (nail)** ▽

√6ᵗʰ **T25.29**   **Burn of second degree of multiple sites of ankle and foot**

    √7ᵗʰ **T25.291**   **Burn of second degree of multiple sites of right ankle and foot**

    √7ᵗʰ **T25.292**   **Burn of second degree of multiple sites of left ankle and foot**

    √7ᵗʰ **T25.299**   **Burn of second degree of multiple sites of unspecified ankle and foot** ▽

√5ᵗʰ **T25.3**   **Burn of third degree of ankle and foot**

Use additional external cause code to identify the source, place and intent of the burn (X00-X19, X75-X77, X96-X98, Y92)

√6ᵗʰ **T25.31**   **Burn of third degree of ankle**

    √7ᵗʰ **T25.311**   **Burn of third degree of right ankle**

    √7ᵗʰ **T25.312**   **Burn of third degree of left ankle**

    √7ᵗʰ **T25.319**   **Burn of third degree of unspecified ankle** ▽

√6ᵗʰ **T25.32**   **Burn of third degree of foot**

    EXCLUDES 2   *burn of third degree of toe(s) (nail) (T25.33-)*

    √7ᵗʰ **T25.321**   **Burn of third degree of right foot**

    √7ᵗʰ **T25.322**   **Burn of third degree of left foot**

    √7ᵗʰ **T25.329**   **Burn of third degree of unspecified foot** ▽

√6ᵗʰ **T25.33**   **Burn of third degree of toe(s) (nail)**

    √7ᵗʰ **T25.331**   **Burn of third degree of right toe(s) (nail)**

    √7ᵗʰ **T25.332**   **Burn of third degree of left toe(s) (nail)**

    √7ᵗʰ **T25.339**   **Burn of third degree of unspecified toe(s) (nail)** ▽

√6ᵗʰ **T25.39**   **Burn of third degree of multiple sites of ankle and foot**

    √7ᵗʰ **T25.391**   **Burn of third degree of multiple sites of right ankle and foot**

    √7ᵗʰ **T25.392**   **Burn of third degree of multiple sites of left ankle and foot**

    √7ᵗʰ **T25.399**   **Burn of third degree of multiple sites of unspecified ankle and foot** ▽

√5ᵗʰ **T25.4**   **Corrosion of unspecified degree of ankle and foot**

Code first (T51-T65) to identify chemical and intent

Use additional external cause code to identify place (Y92)

√6ᵗʰ **T25.41**   **Corrosion of unspecified degree of ankle**

    √7ᵗʰ **T25.411**   **Corrosion of unspecified degree of right ankle** ▽

    √7ᵗʰ **T25.412**   **Corrosion of unspecified degree of left ankle** ▽

    √7ᵗʰ **T25.419**   **Corrosion of unspecified degree of unspecified ankle** ▽

√6ᵗʰ **T25.42**   **Corrosion of unspecified degree of foot**

    EXCLUDES 2   *corrosion of unspecified degree of toe(s) (nail) (T25.43-)*

    √7ᵗʰ **T25.421**   **Corrosion of unspecified degree of right foot** ▽

    √7ᵗʰ **T25.422**   **Corrosion of unspecified degree of left foot** ▽

    √7ᵗʰ **T25.429**   **Corrosion of unspecified degree of unspecified foot** ▽

√6ᵗʰ **T25.43**   **Corrosion of unspecified degree of toe(s) (nail)**

    √7ᵗʰ **T25.431**   **Corrosion of unspecified degree of right toe(s) (nail)** ▽

    √7ᵗʰ **T25.432**   **Corrosion of unspecified degree of left toe(s) (nail)** ▽

    √7ᵗʰ **T25.439**   **Corrosion of unspecified degree of unspecified toe(s) (nail)** ▽

√6ᵗʰ **T25.49**   **Corrosion of unspecified degree of multiple sites of ankle and foot**

    √7ᵗʰ **T25.491**   **Corrosion of unspecified degree of multiple sites of right ankle and foot** ▽

    √7ᵗʰ **T25.492**   **Corrosion of unspecified degree of multiple sites of left ankle and foot** ▽

    √7ᵗʰ **T25.499**   **Corrosion of unspecified degree of multiple sites of unspecified ankle and foot** ▽

√5ᵗʰ **T25.5**   **Corrosion of first degree of ankle and foot**

Code first (T51-T65) to identify chemical and intent

Use additional external cause code to identify place (Y92)

√6ᵗʰ **T25.51**   **Corrosion of first degree of ankle**

    √7ᵗʰ **T25.511**   **Corrosion of first degree of right ankle**

    √7ᵗʰ **T25.512**   **Corrosion of first degree of left ankle**

    √7ᵗʰ **T25.519**   **Corrosion of first degree of unspecified ankle** ▽

√6ᵗʰ **T25.52**   **Corrosion of first degree of foot**

    EXCLUDES 2   *corrosion of first degree of toe(s) (nail) (T25.53-)*

    √7ᵗʰ **T25.521**   **Corrosion of first degree of right foot**

    √7ᵗʰ **T25.522**   **Corrosion of first degree of left foot**

    √7ᵗʰ **T25.529**   **Corrosion of first degree of unspecified foot** ▽

√6ᵗʰ **T25.53**   **Corrosion of first degree of toe(s) (nail)**

    √7ᵗʰ **T25.531**   **Corrosion of first degree of right toe(s) (nail)**

    √7ᵗʰ **T25.532**   **Corrosion of first degree of left toe(s) (nail)**

    √7ᵗʰ **T25.539**   **Corrosion of first degree of unspecified toe(s) (nail)** ▽

√6ᵗʰ **T25.59**   **Corrosion of first degree of multiple sites of ankle and foot**

    √7ᵗʰ **T25.591**   **Corrosion of first degree of multiple sites of right ankle and foot**

    √7ᵗʰ **T25.592**   **Corrosion of first degree of multiple sites of left ankle and foot**

    √7ᵗʰ **T25.599**   **Corrosion of first degree of multiple sites of unspecified ankle and foot** ▽

√5ᵗʰ **T25.6**   **Corrosion of second degree of ankle and foot**

Code first (T51-T65) to identify chemical and intent

Use additional external cause code to identify place (Y92)

√6ᵗʰ **T25.61**   **Corrosion of second degree of ankle**

    √7ᵗʰ **T25.611**   **Corrosion of second degree of right ankle**

    √7ᵗʰ **T25.612**   **Corrosion of second degree of left ankle**

    √7ᵗʰ **T25.619**   **Corrosion of second degree of unspecified ankle** ▽

☑ Additional Character Req   √x7ᵗʰ Placeholder Alert   **Manifestation**   HCC CMS-HCC Condition   ▽ Unspecified Code   ►◄ Revised Text   ● New Code   ▲ Revised Code Title

ICD-10-CM 2018   **1053**

✓6ᵗʰ T25.62 Corrosion of second degree of foot
     EXCLUDES 2   corrosion of second degree of toe(s) (nail) (T25.63-)

     ✓7ᵗʰ **T25.621** Corrosion of second degree of right foot

     ✓7ᵗʰ **T25.622** Corrosion of second degree of left foot

     ✓7ᵗʰ **T25.629** Corrosion of second degree of unspecified foot ▽

✓6ᵗʰ T25.63 Corrosion of second degree of toe(s) (nail)

     ✓7ᵗʰ **T25.631** Corrosion of second degree of right toe(s) (nail)

     ✓7ᵗʰ **T25.632** Corrosion of second degree of left toe(s) (nail)

     ✓7ᵗʰ **T25.639** Corrosion of second degree of unspecified toe(s) (nail) ▽

✓6ᵗʰ T25.69 Corrosion of second degree of multiple sites of ankle and foot

     ✓7ᵗʰ **T25.691** Corrosion of second degree of right ankle and foot

     ✓7ᵗʰ **T25.692** Corrosion of second degree of left ankle and foot

     ✓7ᵗʰ **T25.699** Corrosion of second degree of unspecified ankle and foot ▽

✓5ᵗʰ T25.7 Corrosion of third degree of ankle and foot
     Code first (T51-T65) to identify chemical and intent
     Use additional external cause code to identify place (Y92)

✓6ᵗʰ T25.71 Corrosion of third degree of ankle

     ✓7ᵗʰ **T25.711** Corrosion of third degree of right ankle

     ✓7ᵗʰ **T25.712** Corrosion of third degree of left ankle

     ✓7ᵗʰ **T25.719** Corrosion of third degree of unspecified ankle ▽

✓6ᵗʰ T25.72 Corrosion of third degree of foot
     EXCLUDES 2   corrosion of third degree of toe(s) (nail) (T25.73-)

     ✓7ᵗʰ **T25.721** Corrosion of third degree of right foot

     ✓7ᵗʰ **T25.722** Corrosion of third degree of left foot

     ✓7ᵗʰ **T25.729** Corrosion of third degree of unspecified foot ▽

✓6ᵗʰ T25.73 Corrosion of third degree of toe(s) (nail)

     ✓7ᵗʰ **T25.731** Corrosion of third degree of right toe(s) (nail)

     ✓7ᵗʰ **T25.732** Corrosion of third degree of left toe(s) (nail)

     ✓7ᵗʰ **T25.739** Corrosion of third degree of unspecified toe(s) (nail) ▽

✓6ᵗʰ T25.79 Corrosion of third degree of multiple sites of ankle and foot

     ✓7ᵗʰ **T25.791** Corrosion of third degree of multiple sites of right ankle and foot

     ✓7ᵗʰ **T25.792** Corrosion of third degree of multiple sites of left ankle and foot

     ✓7ᵗʰ **T25.799** Corrosion of third degree of multiple sites of unspecified ankle and foot ▽

Burns and corrosions confined to eye and internal organs (T26-T28)

✓4ᵗʰ T26 Burn and corrosion confined to eye and adnexa

> The appropriate 7th character is to be added to each code from category T26.
> A   initial encounter
> D   subsequent encounter
> S   sequela

✓5ᵗʰ T26.0 Burn of eyelid and periocular area
     Use additional external cause code to identify the source, place and intent of the burn (X00-X19, X75-X77, X96-X98, Y92)

     ✓x7ᵗʰ **T26.00** Burn of unspecified eyelid and periocular area ▽

     ✓x7ᵗʰ **T26.01** Burn of right eyelid and periocular area

     ✓x7ᵗʰ **T26.02** Burn of left eyelid and periocular area

✓5ᵗʰ T26.1 Burn of cornea and conjunctival sac
     Use additional external cause code to identify the source, place and intent of the burn (X00-X19, X75-X77, X96-X98, Y92)

     ✓x7ᵗʰ **T26.10** Burn of cornea and conjunctival sac, unspecified eye ▽

     ✓x7ᵗʰ **T26.11** Burn of cornea and conjunctival sac, right eye

     ✓x7ᵗʰ **T26.12** Burn of cornea and conjunctival sac, left eye

✓5ᵗʰ T26.2 Burn with resulting rupture and destruction of eyeball
     Use additional external cause code to identify the source, place and intent of the burn (X00-X19, X75-X77, X96-X98, Y92)

     ✓x7ᵗʰ **T26.20** Burn with resulting rupture and destruction of unspecified eyeball ▽

     ✓x7ᵗʰ **T26.21** Burn with resulting rupture and destruction of right eyeball

     ✓x7ᵗʰ **T26.22** Burn with resulting rupture and destruction of left eyeball

✓5ᵗʰ T26.3 Burns of other specified parts of eye and adnexa
     Use additional external cause code to identify the source, place and intent of the burn (X00-X19, X75-X77, X96-X98, Y92)

     ✓x7ᵗʰ **T26.30** Burns of other specified parts of unspecified eye and adnexa ▽

     ✓x7ᵗʰ **T26.31** Burns of other specified parts of right eye and adnexa

     ✓x7ᵗʰ **T26.32** Burns of other specified parts of left eye and adnexa

✓5ᵗʰ T26.4 Burn of eye and adnexa, part unspecified
     Use additional external cause code to identify the source, place and intent of the burn (X00-X19, X75-X77, X96-X98, Y92)

     ✓x7ᵗʰ **T26.40** Burn of unspecified eye and adnexa, part unspecified ▽

     ✓x7ᵗʰ **T26.41** Burn of right eye and adnexa, part unspecified ▽

     ✓x7ᵗʰ **T26.42** Burn of left eye and adnexa, part unspecified ▽

✓5ᵗʰ T26.5 Corrosion of eyelid and periocular area
     Code first (T51-T65) to identify chemical and intent
     Use additional external cause code to identify place (Y92)

     ✓x7ᵗʰ **T26.50** Corrosion of unspecified eyelid and periocular area ▽

     ✓x7ᵗʰ **T26.51** Corrosion of right eyelid and periocular area

     ✓x7ᵗʰ **T26.52** Corrosion of left eyelid and periocular area

✓5ᵗʰ T26.6 Corrosion of cornea and conjunctival sac
     Code first (T51-T65) to identify chemical and intent
     Use additional external cause code to identify place (Y92)

     ✓x7ᵗʰ **T26.60** Corrosion of cornea and conjunctival sac, unspecified eye ▽

     ✓x7ᵗʰ **T26.61** Corrosion of cornea and conjunctival sac, right eye

     ✓x7ᵗʰ **T26.62** Corrosion of cornea and conjunctival sac, left eye

✓5ᵗʰ T26.7 Corrosion with resulting rupture and destruction of eyeball
     Code first (T51-T65) to identify chemical and intent
     Use additional external cause code to identify place (Y92)

     ✓x7ᵗʰ **T26.70** Corrosion with resulting rupture and destruction of unspecified eyeball ▽

     ✓x7ᵗʰ **T26.71** Corrosion with resulting rupture and destruction of right eyeball

     ✓x7ᵗʰ **T26.72** Corrosion with resulting rupture and destruction of left eyeball

✓5ᵗʰ T26.8 Corrosions of other specified parts of eye and adnexa
     Code first (T51-T65) to identify chemical and intent
     Use additional external cause code to identify place (Y92)

     ✓x7ᵗʰ **T26.80** Corrosions of other specified parts of unspecified eye and adnexa ▽

     ✓x7ᵗʰ **T26.81** Corrosions of other specified parts of right eye and adnexa

     ✓x7ᵗʰ **T26.82** Corrosions of other specified parts of left eye and adnexa

✓5ᵗʰ T26.9 Corrosion of eye and adnexa, part unspecified
     Code first (T51-T65) to identify chemical and intent
     Use additional external cause code to identify place (Y92)

     ✓x7ᵗʰ **T26.90** Corrosion of unspecified eye and adnexa, part unspecified ▽

     ✓x7ᵗʰ **T26.91** Corrosion of right eye and adnexa, part unspecified ▽

     ✓x7ᵗʰ **T26.92** Corrosion of left eye and adnexa, part unspecified ▽

EXCLUDES 1 Not coded here   *EXCLUDES 2* Not included here   N Newborn Age: 0   P Pediatric Age: 0-17   M Maternity Age: 12-55   A Adult Age: 15-124

1054   ICD-10-CM 2018

✓4ᵗʰ T27 Burn and corrosion of respiratory tract

Use additional external cause code to identify the source and intent of the burn (X00-X19, X75-X77, X96-X98)

Use additional external cause code to identify place (Y92)

The appropriate 7th character is to be added to each code from category T27.
A   initial encounter
D   subsequent encounter
S   sequela

✓x7ᵗʰ **T27.0**   Burn of larynx and trachea

✓x7ᵗʰ **T27.1**   Burn involving larynx and trachea with lung

✓x7ᵗʰ **T27.2**   Burn of other parts of respiratory tract
     Burn of thoracic cavity

✓x7ᵗʰ **T27.3**   Burn of respiratory tract, part unspecified ▽
     ~~Code first (T51-T65) to identify chemical and intent for codes T27.4-T27.7~~

✓x7ᵗʰ **T27.4**   Corrosion of larynx and trachea
     ►Code first (T51-T65) to identify chemical and intent◄

✓x7ᵗʰ **T27.5**   Corrosion involving larynx and trachea with lung

✓x7ᵗʰ **T27.6**   Corrosion of other parts of respiratory tract
     ►Code first (T51-T65) to identify chemical and intent◄

✓x7ᵗʰ **T27.7**   Corrosion of respiratory tract, part unspecified ▽
     ►Code first (T51-T65) to identify chemical and intent◄

✓4ᵗʰ T28 Burn and corrosion of other internal organs

Use additional external cause code to identify the source and intent of the burn (X00- X19, X75-X77, X96-X98)

Use additional external cause code to identify place (Y92)

The appropriate 7th character is to be added to each code from category T28.
A   initial encounter
D   subsequent encounter
S   sequela

✓x7ᵗʰ **T28.0**   Burn of mouth and pharynx

✓x7ᵗʰ **T28.1**   Burn of esophagus

✓x7ᵗʰ **T28.2**   Burn of other parts of alimentary tract

✓x7ᵗʰ **T28.3**   Burn of internal genitourinary organs

✓5ᵗʰ **T28.4**   Burns of other and unspecified internal organs
     ►Code first (T51-T65) to identify chemical and intent◄

   ✓x7ᵗʰ **T28.40**   Burn of unspecified internal organ ▽

   ✓6ᵗʰ **T28.41**   Burn of ear drum

     ✓7ᵗʰ **T28.411**   Burn of right ear drum

     ✓7ᵗʰ **T28.412**   Burn of left ear drum

     ✓7ᵗʰ **T28.419**   Burn of unspecified ear drum ▽

   ✓x7ᵗʰ **T28.49**   Burn of other internal organ
     ~~Code first (T51-T65) to identify chemical and intent for T28.5-T28.9~~

✓x7ᵗʰ **T28.5**   Corrosion of mouth and pharynx
     ►Code first (T51-T65) to identify chemical and intent◄

✓x7ᵗʰ **T28.6**   Corrosion of esophagus
     ►Code first (T51-T65) to identify chemical and intent◄

✓x7ᵗʰ **T28.7**   Corrosion of other parts of alimentary tract
     ►Code first (T51-T65) to identify chemical and intent◄

✓x7ᵗʰ **T28.8**   Corrosion of internal genitourinary organs
     ►Code first (T51-T65) to identify chemical and intent◄

✓5ᵗʰ **T28.9**   Corrosions of other and unspecified internal organs
     ►Code first (T51-T65) to identify chemical and intent◄

   ✓x7ᵗʰ **T28.90**   Corrosions of unspecified internal organs ▽

   ✓6ᵗʰ **T28.91**   Corrosions of ear drum

     ✓7ᵗʰ **T28.911**   Corrosions of right ear drum

     ✓7ᵗʰ **T28.912**   Corrosions of left ear drum

     ✓7ᵗʰ **T28.919**   Corrosions of unspecified ear drum ▽

   ✓x7ᵗʰ **T28.99**   Corrosions of other internal organs

Burns and corrosions of multiple and unspecified body regions (T30-T32)

✓4ᵗʰ T30 Burn and corrosion, body region unspecified

T30.0   Burn of unspecified body region, unspecified degree ▽
     This code is not for inpatient use. Code to specified site and degree of burns.
     Burn NOS
     Multiple burns NOS

T30.4   Corrosion of unspecified body region, unspecified degree ▽
     This code is not for inpatient use. Code to specified site and degree of corrosion.
     Corrosion NOS
     Multiple corrosion NOS

✓4ᵗʰ T31 Burns classified according to extent of body surface involved

   NOTE   This category is to be used as the primary code only when the site of the burn is unspecified. It should be used as a supplementary code with categories T20-T25 when the site is specified.

T31.0   Burns involving less than 10% of body surface

✓5ᵗʰ **T31.1**   Burns involving 10-19% of body surface

   T31.10   Burns involving 10-19% of body surface with 0% to 9% third degree burns
     Burns involving 10-19% of body surface NOS

   T31.11   Burns involving 10-19% of body surface with 10-19% third degree burns   HCC

✓5ᵗʰ **T31.2**   Burns involving 20-29% of body surface

   T31.20   Burns involving 20-29% of body surface with 0% to 9% third degree burns
     Burns involving 20-29% of body surface NOS

   T31.21   Burns involving 20-29% of body surface with 10-19% third degree burns   HCC

   T31.22   Burns involving 20-29% of body surface with 20-29% third degree burns   HCC

✓5ᵗʰ **T31.3**   Burns involving 30-39% of body surface

   T31.30   Burns involving 30-39% of body surface with 0% to 9% third degree burns
     Burns involving 30-39% of body surface NOS

   T31.31   Burns involving 30-39% of body surface with 10-19% third degree burns   HCC

   T31.32   Burns involving 30-39% of body surface with 20-29% third degree burns   HCC

   T31.33   Burns involving 30-39% of body surface with 30-39% third degree burns   HCC

✓5ᵗʰ **T31.4**   Burns involving 40-49% of body surface

   T31.40   Burns involving 40-49% of body surface with 0% to 9% third degree burns
     Burns involving 40-49% of body surface NOS

   T31.41   Burns involving 40-49% of body surface with 10-19% third degree burns   HCC

   T31.42   Burns involving 40-49% of body surface with 20-29% third degree burns   HCC

   T31.43   Burns involving 40-49% of body surface with 30-39% third degree burns   HCC

   T31.44   Burns involving 40-49% of body surface with 40-49% third degree burns   HCC

✓5ᵗʰ **T31.5**   Burns involving 50-59% of body surface

   T31.50   Burns involving 50-59% of body surface with 0% to 9% third degree burns
     Burns involving 50-59% of body surface NOS

   T31.51   Burns involving 50-59% of body surface with 10-19% third degree burns   HCC

   T31.52   Burns involving 50-59% of body surface with 20-29% third degree burns   HCC

   T31.53   Burns involving 50-59% of body surface with 30-39% third degree burns   HCC

   T31.54   Burns involving 50-59% of body surface with 40-49% third degree burns   HCC

   T31.55   Burns involving 50-59% of body surface with 50-59% third degree burns   HCC

✓5ᵗʰ **T31.6**   Burns involving 60-69% of body surface

   T31.60   Burns involving 60-69% of body surface with 0% to 9% third degree burns
     Burns involving 60-69% of body surface NOS

   T31.61   Burns involving 60-69% of body surface with 10-19% third degree burns   HCC

✓ Additional Character Req   ✓x7ᵗʰ Placeholder Alert   Manifestation   HCC CMS-HCC Condition   ▽ Unspecified Code   ►◄ Revised Text   ● New Code   ▲ Revised Code Title

Chapter 19. Injury, Poisoning, and Certain Other Consequences of External Causes

T31.62 Burns involving 60-69% of body surface with 20-29% third degree burns `HCC`

T31.63 Burns involving 60-69% of body surface with 30-39% third degree burns `HCC`

T31.64 Burns involving 60-69% of body surface with 40-49% third degree burns `HCC`

T31.65 Burns involving 60-69% of body surface with 50-59% third degree burns `HCC`

T31.66 Burns involving 60-69% of body surface with 60-69% third degree burns `HCC`

✓5ᵗʰ **T31.7** Burns involving 70-79% of body surface

T31.70 Burns involving 70-79% of body surface with 0% to 9% third degree burns
Burns involving 70-79% of body surface NOS

T31.71 Burns involving 70-79% of body surface with 10-19% third degree burns `HCC`

T31.72 Burns involving 70-79% of body surface with 20-29% third degree burns `HCC`

T31.73 Burns involving 70-79% of body surface with 30-39% third degree burns `HCC`

T31.74 Burns involving 70-79% of body surface with 40-49% third degree burns `HCC`

T31.75 Burns involving 70-79% of body surface with 50-59% third degree burns `HCC`

T31.76 Burns involving 70-79% of body surface with 60-69% third degree burns `HCC`

T31.77 Burns involving 70-79% of body surface with 70-79% third degree burns `HCC`

✓5ᵗʰ **T31.8** Burns involving 80-89% of body surface

T31.80 Burns involving 80-89% of body surface with 0% to 9% third degree burns
Burns involving 80-89% of body surface NOS

T31.81 Burns involving 80-89% of body surface with 10-19% third degree burns `HCC`

T31.82 Burns involving 80-89% of body surface with 20-29% third degree burns `HCC`

T31.83 Burns involving 80-89% of body surface with 30-39% third degree burns `HCC`

T31.84 Burns involving 80-89% of body surface with 40-49% third degree burns `HCC`

T31.85 Burns involving 80-89% of body surface with 50-59% third degree burns `HCC`

T31.86 Burns involving 80-89% of body surface with 60-69% third degree burns `HCC`

T31.87 Burns involving 80-89% of body surface with 70-79% third degree burns `HCC`

T31.88 Burns involving 80-89% of body surface with 80-89% third degree burns `HCC`

✓5ᵗʰ **T31.9** Burns involving 90% or more of body surface

T31.90 Burns involving 90% or more of body surface with 0% to 9% third degree burns
Burns involving 90% or more of body surface NOS

T31.91 Burns involving 90% or more of body surface with 10-19% third degree burns `HCC`

T31.92 Burns involving 90% or more of body surface with 20-29% third degree burns `HCC`

T31.93 Burns involving 90% or more of body surface with 30-39% third degree burns `HCC`

T31.94 Burns involving 90% or more of body surface with 40-49% third degree burns `HCC`

T31.95 Burns involving 90% or more of body surface with 50-59% third degree burns `HCC`

T31.96 Burns involving 90% or more of body surface with 60-69% third degree burns `HCC`

T31.97 Burns involving 90% or more of body surface with 70-79% third degree burns `HCC`

T31.98 Burns involving 90% or more of body surface with 80-89% third degree burns `HCC`

T31.99 Burns involving 90% or more of body surface with 90% or more third degree burns `HCC`

✓4ᵗʰ **T32** Corrosions **classified** according to extent of body surface involved

NOTE   This category is to be used as the primary code only when the site of the corrosion is unspecified. It may be used as a supplementary code with categories T20-T25 when the site is specified.

T32.0 Corrosions involving less than 10% of body surface

✓5ᵗʰ **T32.1** Corrosions involving 10-19% of body surface

T32.10 Corrosions involving 10-19% of body surface with 0% to 9% third degree corrosion
Corrosions involving 10-19% of body surface NOS

T32.11 Corrosions involving 10-19% of body surface with 10-19% third degree corrosion `HCC`

✓5ᵗʰ **T32.2** Corrosions involving 20-29% of body surface

T32.20 Corrosions involving 20-29% of body surface with 0% to 9% third degree corrosion

T32.21 Corrosions involving 20-29% of body surface with 10-19% third degree corrosion `HCC`

T32.22 Corrosions involving 20-29% of body surface with 20-29% third degree corrosion `HCC`

✓5ᵗʰ **T32.3** Corrosions involving 30-39% of body surface

T32.30 Corrosions involving 30-39% of body surface with 0% to 9% third degree corrosion

T32.31 Corrosions involving 30-39% of body surface with 10-19% third degree corrosion `HCC`

T32.32 Corrosions involving 30-39% of body surface with 20-29% third degree corrosion `HCC`

T32.33 Corrosions involving 30-39% of body surface with 30-39% third degree corrosion `HCC`

✓5ᵗʰ **T32.4** Corrosions involving 40-49% of body surface

T32.40 Corrosions involving 40-49% of body surface with 0% to 9% third degree corrosion

T32.41 Corrosions involving 40-49% of body surface with 10-19% third degree corrosion `HCC`

T32.42 Corrosions involving 40-49% of body surface with 20-29% third degree corrosion `HCC`

T32.43 Corrosions involving 40-49% of body surface with 30-39% third degree corrosion `HCC`

T32.44 Corrosions involving 40-49% of body surface with 40-49% third degree corrosion `HCC`

✓5ᵗʰ **T32.5** Corrosions involving 50-59% of body surface

T32.50 Corrosions involving 50-59% of body surface with 0% to 9% third degree corrosion

T32.51 Corrosions involving 50-59% of body surface with 10-19% third degree corrosion `HCC`

T32.52 Corrosions involving 50-59% of body surface with 20-29% third degree corrosion `HCC`

T32.53 Corrosions involving 50-59% of body surface with 30-39% third degree corrosion `HCC`

T32.54 Corrosions involving 50-59% of body surface with 40-49% third degree corrosion `HCC`

T32.55 Corrosions involving 50-59% of body surface with 50-59% third degree corrosion `HCC`

✓5ᵗʰ **T32.6** Corrosions involving 60-69% of body surface

T32.60 Corrosions involving 60-69% of body surface with 0% to 9% third degree corrosion

T32.61 Corrosions involving 60-69% of body surface with 10-19% third degree corrosion `HCC`

T32.62 Corrosions involving 60-69% of body surface with 20-29% third degree corrosion `HCC`

T32.63 Corrosions involving 60-69% of body surface with 30-39% third degree corrosion `HCC`

T32.64 Corrosions involving 60-69% of body surface with 40-49% third degree corrosion `HCC`

T32.65 Corrosions involving 60-69% of body surface with 50-59% third degree corrosion `HCC`

T32.66 Corrosions involving 60-69% of body surface with 60-69% third degree corrosion `HCC`

✓5ᵗʰ **T32.7** Corrosions involving 70-79% of body surface

T32.70 Corrosions involving 70-79% of body surface with 0% to 9% third degree corrosion

T32.71 Corrosions involving 70-79% of body surface with 10-19% third degree corrosion `HCC`

T32.72 Corrosions involving 70-79% of body surface with 20-29% third degree corrosion `HCC`

EXCLUDES 1 Not coded here   EXCLUDES 2 Not included here   N Newborn Age: 0   P Pediatric Age: 0-17   M Maternity Age: 12-55   A Adult Age: 15-124

1056   ICD-10-CM 2018

T32.73 Corrosions involving 70-79% of body surface with 30-39% third degree **corrosion** `HCC`

T32.74 Corrosions involving 70-79% of body surface with 40-49% third degree **corrosion** `HCC`

T32.75 Corrosions involving 70-79% of body surface with 50-59% third degree **corrosion** `HCC`

T32.76 Corrosions involving 70-79% of body surface with 60-69% third degree **corrosion** `HCC`

T32.77 Corrosions involving 70-79% of body surface with 70-79% third degree **corrosion** `HCC`

√5ᵗʰ **T32.8 Corrosions involving 80-89% of body surface**

T32.80 Corrosions involving 80-89% of body surface with 0% to 9% third degree **corrosion**

T32.81 Corrosions involving 80-89% of body surface with 10-19% third degree **corrosion** `HCC`

T32.82 Corrosions involving 80-89% of body surface with 20-29% third degree **corrosion** `HCC`

T32.83 Corrosions involving 80-89% of body surface with 30-39% third degree **corrosion** `HCC`

T32.84 Corrosions involving 80-89% of body surface with 40-49% third degree **corrosion** `HCC`

T32.85 Corrosions involving 80-89% of body surface with 50-59% third degree **corrosion** `HCC`

T32.86 Corrosions involving 80-89% of body surface with 60-69% third degree **corrosion** `HCC`

T32.87 Corrosions involving 80-89% of body surface with 70-79% third degree **corrosion** `HCC`

T32.88 Corrosions involving 80-89% of body surface with 80-89% third degree **corrosion** `HCC`

√5ᵗʰ **T32.9 Corrosions involving 90% or more of body surface**

T32.90 Corrosions involving 90% or more of body surface with 0% to 9% third degree **corrosion**

T32.91 Corrosions involving 90% or more of body surface with 10-19% third degree **corrosion** `HCC`

T32.92 Corrosions involving 90% or more of body surface with 20-29% third degree **corrosion** `HCC`

T32.93 Corrosions involving 90% or more of body surface with 30-39% third degree **corrosion** `HCC`

T32.94 Corrosions involving 90% or more of body surface with 40-49% third degree **corrosion** `HCC`

T32.95 Corrosions involving 90% or more of body surface with 50-59% third degree **corrosion** `HCC`

T32.96 Corrosions involving 90% or more of body surface with 60-69% third degree **corrosion** `HCC`

T32.97 Corrosions involving 90% or more of body surface with 70-79% third degree **corrosion** `HCC`

T32.98 Corrosions involving 90% or more of body surface with 80-89% third degree **corrosion** `HCC`

T32.99 Corrosions involving 90% or more of body surface with 90% or more third degree **corrosion** `HCC`

Frostbite (T33-T34)

EXCLUDES 2 *hypothermia and other effects of reduced temperature (T68, T69-)*

√4ᵗʰ **T33 Superficial frostbite**

INCLUDES frostbite with partial thickness skin loss

The appropriate 7th character is to be added to each code from category T33.
A   initial encounter
D   subsequent encounter
S   sequela

√5ᵗʰ **T33.0 Superficial frostbite of head**

√6ᵗʰ **T33.01** Superficial frostbite of ear

√7ᵗʰ **T33.011** Superficial frostbite of right ear

√7ᵗʰ **T33.012** Superficial frostbite of left ear

√7ᵗʰ **T33.019** Superficial frostbite of unspecified ear ▽

√x7ᵗʰ **T33.02** Superficial frostbite of nose

√x7ᵗʰ **T33.09** Superficial frostbite of other part of head

√x7ᵗʰ **T33.1** Superficial frostbite of neck

√x7ᵗʰ **T33.2** Superficial frostbite of thorax

√x7ᵗʰ **T33.3** Superficial frostbite of abdominal wall, lower back and pelvis

√5ᵗʰ **T33.4 Superficial frostbite of arm**

EXCLUDES 2 *superficial frostbite of wrist and hand (T33.5-)*

√x7ᵗʰ **T33.40** Superficial frostbite of unspecified arm ▽

√x7ᵗʰ **T33.41** Superficial frostbite of right arm

√x7ᵗʰ **T33.42** Superficial frostbite of left arm

√5ᵗʰ **T33.5 Superficial frostbite of wrist, hand, and fingers**

√6ᵗʰ **T33.51** Superficial frostbite of wrist

√7ᵗʰ **T33.511** Superficial frostbite of right wrist

√7ᵗʰ **T33.512** Superficial frostbite of left wrist

√7ᵗʰ **T33.519** Superficial frostbite of unspecified wrist ▽

√6ᵗʰ **T33.52** Superficial frostbite of hand

EXCLUDES 2 *superficial frostbite of fingers (T33.53-)*

√7ᵗʰ **T33.521** Superficial frostbite of right hand

√7ᵗʰ **T33.522** Superficial frostbite of left hand

√7ᵗʰ **T33.529** Superficial frostbite of unspecified hand ▽

√6ᵗʰ **T33.53** Superficial frostbite of finger(s)

√7ᵗʰ **T33.531** Superficial frostbite of right finger(s)

√7ᵗʰ **T33.532** Superficial frostbite of left finger(s)

√7ᵗʰ **T33.539** Superficial frostbite of unspecified finger(s) ▽

√5ᵗʰ **T33.6 Superficial frostbite of hip and thigh**

√x7ᵗʰ **T33.60** Superficial frostbite of unspecified hip and thigh ▽

√x7ᵗʰ **T33.61** Superficial frostbite of right hip and thigh

√x7ᵗʰ **T33.62** Superficial frostbite of left hip and thigh

√5ᵗʰ **T33.7 Superficial frostbite of knee and lower leg**

EXCLUDES 2 *superficial frostbite of ankle and foot (T33.8-)*

√x7ᵗʰ **T33.70** Superficial frostbite of unspecified knee and lower leg ▽

√x7ᵗʰ **T33.71** Superficial frostbite of right knee and lower leg

√x7ᵗʰ **T33.72** Superficial frostbite of left knee and lower leg

√5ᵗʰ **T33.8 Superficial frostbite of ankle, foot, and toe(s)**

√6ᵗʰ **T33.81** Superficial frostbite of ankle

√7ᵗʰ **T33.811** Superficial frostbite of right ankle

√7ᵗʰ **T33.812** Superficial frostbite of left ankle

√7ᵗʰ **T33.819** Superficial frostbite of unspecified ankle ▽

√6ᵗʰ **T33.82** Superficial frostbite of foot

√7ᵗʰ **T33.821** Superficial frostbite of right foot

√7ᵗʰ **T33.822** Superficial frostbite of left foot

√7ᵗʰ **T33.829** Superficial frostbite of unspecified foot ▽

√6ᵗʰ **T33.83** Superficial frostbite of toe(s)

√7ᵗʰ **T33.831** Superficial frostbite of right toe(s)

√7ᵗʰ **T33.832** Superficial frostbite of left toe(s)

√7ᵗʰ **T33.839** Superficial frostbite of unspecified toe(s) ▽

√5ᵗʰ **T33.9 Superficial frostbite of other and unspecified sites**

√x7ᵗʰ **T33.90** Superficial frostbite of unspecified sites ▽
Superficial frostbite NOS

√x7ᵗʰ **T33.99** Superficial frostbite of other sites
Superficial frostbite of leg NOS
Superficial frostbite of trunk NOS

√4ᵗʰ **T34 Frostbite with tissue necrosis**

The appropriate 7th character is to be added to each code from category T34.
A   initial encounter
D   subsequent encounter
S   sequela

√5ᵗʰ **T34.0 Frostbite with tissue necrosis of head**

√6ᵗʰ **T34.01** Frostbite with tissue necrosis of ear

√7ᵗʰ **T34.011** Frostbite with tissue necrosis of right ear

√7ᵗʰ **T34.012** Frostbite with tissue necrosis of left ear

√7ᵗʰ **T34.019** Frostbite with tissue necrosis of unspecified ear ▽

√x7ᵗʰ **T34.02** Frostbite with tissue necrosis of nose

√x7ᵗʰ **T34.09** Frostbite with tissue necrosis of other part of head

√x7ᵗʰ **T34.1** Frostbite with tissue necrosis of neck

√x7ᵗʰ **T34.2** Frostbite with tissue necrosis of thorax

√x7ᵗʰ **T34.3** Frostbite with tissue necrosis of abdominal wall, lower back and pelvis

☑ Additional Character Req   √x7ᵗʰ Placeholder Alert   Manifestation   `HCC` CMS-HCC Condition   ▽ Unspecified Code   ►◄ Revised Text   ● New Code   ▲ Revised Code Title

ICD-10-CM 2018   **1057**

✓5ᵗʰ **T34.4** **Frostbite with tissue necrosis of** arm
    EXCLUDES 2 *frostbite with tissue necrosis of wrist and hand (T34.5-)*

  ✓x7ᵗʰ **T34.40** **Frostbite with tissue necrosis of unspecified arm** ▽

  ✓x7ᵗʰ **T34.41** **Frostbite with tissue necrosis of** right **arm**

  ✓x7ᵗʰ **T34.42** **Frostbite with tissue necrosis of** left **arm**

✓5ᵗʰ **T34.5** **Frostbite with tissue necrosis of** wrist, hand, and finger(s)

  ✓6ᵗʰ **T34.51** **Frostbite with tissue necrosis of** wrist

    ✓7ᵗʰ **T34.511** **Frostbite with tissue necrosis of** right **wrist**

    ✓7ᵗʰ **T34.512** **Frostbite with tissue necrosis of** left **wrist**

    ✓7ᵗʰ **T34.519** **Frostbite with tissue necrosis of unspecified wrist** ▽

  ✓6ᵗʰ **T34.52** **Frostbite with tissue necrosis of** hand
    EXCLUDES 2 *frostbite with tissue necrosis of finger(s) (T34.53-)*

    ✓7ᵗʰ **T34.521** **Frostbite with tissue necrosis of** right **hand**

    ✓7ᵗʰ **T34.522** **Frostbite with tissue necrosis of** left **hand**

    ✓7ᵗʰ **T34.529** **Frostbite with tissue necrosis of unspecified hand** ▽

  ✓6ᵗʰ **T34.53** **Frostbite with tissue necrosis of** finger(s)

    ✓7ᵗʰ **T34.531** **Frostbite with tissue necrosis of** right **finger(s)**

    ✓7ᵗʰ **T34.532** **Frostbite with tissue necrosis of** left **finger(s)**

    ✓7ᵗʰ **T34.539** **Frostbite with tissue necrosis of unspecified finger(s)** ▽

✓5ᵗʰ **T34.6** **Frostbite with tissue necrosis of** hip and thigh

  ✓x7ᵗʰ **T34.60** **Frostbite with tissue necrosis of unspecified hip and thigh** ▽

  ✓x7ᵗʰ **T34.61** **Frostbite with tissue necrosis of** right **hip and thigh**

  ✓x7ᵗʰ **T34.62** **Frostbite with tissue necrosis of** left **hip and thigh**

✓5ᵗʰ **T34.7** **Frostbite with tissue necrosis of** knee and lower leg
    EXCLUDES 2 *frostbite with tissue necrosis of ankle and foot (T34.8-)*

  ✓x7ᵗʰ **T34.70** **Frostbite with tissue necrosis of unspecified knee and lower leg** ▽

  ✓x7ᵗʰ **T34.71** **Frostbite with tissue necrosis of** right **knee and lower leg**

  ✓x7ᵗʰ **T34.72** **Frostbite with tissue necrosis of** left **knee and lower leg**

✓5ᵗʰ **T34.8** **Frostbite with tissue necrosis of** ankle, foot, and toe(s)

  ✓6ᵗʰ **T34.81** **Frostbite with tissue necrosis of** ankle

    ✓7ᵗʰ **T34.811** **Frostbite with tissue necrosis of** right **ankle**

    ✓7ᵗʰ **T34.812** **Frostbite with tissue necrosis of** left **ankle**

    ✓7ᵗʰ **T34.819** **Frostbite with tissue necrosis of unspecified ankle** ▽

  ✓6ᵗʰ **T34.82** **Frostbite with tissue necrosis of** foot

    ✓7ᵗʰ **T34.821** **Frostbite with tissue necrosis of** right **foot**

    ✓7ᵗʰ **T34.822** **Frostbite with tissue necrosis of** left **foot**

    ✓7ᵗʰ **T34.829** **Frostbite with tissue necrosis of unspecified foot** ▽

  ✓6ᵗʰ **T34.83** **Frostbite with tissue necrosis of** toe(s)

    ✓7ᵗʰ **T34.831** **Frostbite with tissue necrosis of** right **toe(s)**

    ✓7ᵗʰ **T34.832** **Frostbite with tissue necrosis of** left **toe(s)**

    ✓7ᵗʰ **T34.839** **Frostbite with tissue necrosis of unspecified toe(s)** ▽

✓5ᵗʰ **T34.9** **Frostbite with tissue necrosis of other and unspecified sites**

  ✓x7ᵗʰ **T34.90** **Frostbite with tissue necrosis of unspecified sites** ▽
    Frostbite with tissue necrosis NOS

  ✓x7ᵗʰ **T34.99** **Frostbite with tissue necrosis of other sites**
    Frostbite with tissue necrosis of leg NOS
    Frostbite with tissue necrosis of trunk NOS

Poisoning by, adverse effects of and underdosing of drugs, medicaments and biological substances (T36-T50)

INCLUDES adverse effect of correct substance properly administered
    poisoning by overdose of substance
    poisoning by wrong substance given or taken in error
    underdosing by (inadvertently) (deliberately) taking less substance than prescribed or instructed

Code first, for adverse effects, the nature of the adverse effect, such as:
  adverse effect NOS (T88.7)
  aspirin gastritis (K29.-)
  blood disorders (D56-D76)
  contact dermatitis (L23-L25)
  dermatitis due to substances taken internally (L27.-)
  nephropathy (N14.0-N14.2)

NOTE The drug giving rise to the adverse effect should be identified by use of codes from categories T36-T50 with fifth or sixth character 5.

Use additional code(s) to specify:
  manifestations of poisoning
  underdosing or failure in dosage during medical and surgical care (Y63.6, Y63.8-Y63.9)
  underdosing of medication regimen (Z91.12-, Z91.13-)

EXCLUDES 1 *toxic reaction to local anesthesia in pregnancy (O29.3-)*
EXCLUDES 2 *abuse and dependence of psychoactive substances (F10-F19)*
    abuse of non-dependence-producing substances (F55.-)
    drug reaction and poisoning affecting newborn (P00-P96)
    pathological drug intoxication (inebriation) (F10-F19)

AHA: 2016, 2Q, 8; 2015, 3Q, 22

✓4ᵗʰ **T36** **Poisoning by, adverse effect of and underdosing of systemic antibiotics**
    EXCLUDES 1 *antineoplastic antibiotics (T45.1-)*
      locally applied antibiotic NEC (T49.0)
      topically used antibiotic for ear, nose and throat (T49.6)
      topically used antibiotic for eye (T49.5)

> The appropriate 7th character is to be added to each code from category T36.
> A   initial encounter
> D   subsequent encounter
> S   sequela

  ✓5ᵗʰ **T36.0** **Poisoning by, adverse effect of and underdosing of penicillins**

    ✓6ᵗʰ **T36.0X** **Poisoning by, adverse effect of and underdosing of penicillins**

      ✓7ᵗʰ **T36.0X1** **Poisoning by penicillins, accidental (unintentional)**
        Poisoning by penicillins NOS

      2 ✓7ᵗʰ **T36.0X2** **Poisoning by penicillins, intentional self-harm** HCC

      ✓7ᵗʰ **T36.0X3** **Poisoning by penicillins, assault**

      ✓7ᵗʰ **T36.0X4** **Poisoning by penicillins, undetermined**

      ✓7ᵗʰ **T36.0X5** **Adverse effect of penicillins**

      ✓7ᵗʰ **T36.0X6** **Underdosing of penicillins**

  ✓5ᵗʰ **T36.1** **Poisoning by, adverse effect of and underdosing of cephalosporins and other beta-lactam antibiotics**

    ✓6ᵗʰ **T36.1X** **Poisoning by, adverse effect of and underdosing of cephalosporins and other beta-lactam antibiotics**

      ✓7ᵗʰ **T36.1X1** **Poisoning by cephalosporins and other beta-lactam antibiotics, accidental (unintentional)**
        Poisoning by cephalosporins and other beta-lactam antibiotics NOS

      2 ✓7ᵗʰ **T36.1X2** **Poisoning by cephalosporins and other beta-lactam antibiotics, intentional self-harm** HCC

      ✓7ᵗʰ **T36.1X3** **Poisoning by cephalosporins and other beta-lactam antibiotics, assault**

      ✓7ᵗʰ **T36.1X4** **Poisoning by cephalosporins and other beta-lactam antibiotics, undetermined**

      ✓7ᵗʰ **T36.1X5** **Adverse effect of cephalosporins and other beta-lactam antibiotics**

      ✓7ᵗʰ **T36.1X6** **Underdosing of cephalosporins and other beta-lactam antibiotics**

---

2 HCC with 7th character indicating initial encounter (A or B - specific to category) OR sequela.

EXCLUDES 1 Not coded here   *EXCLUDES 2* Not included here   N Newborn Age: 0   P Pediatric Age: 0-17   M Maternity Age: 12-55   A Adult Age: 15-124

1058   ICD-10-CM 2018

✓5ᵗʰ **T36.2** Poisoning by, adverse effect of and underdosing of chloramphenicol group

  ✓6ᵗʰ **T36.2X** Poisoning by, adverse effect of and underdosing of chloramphenicol group

    ✓7ᵗʰ **T36.2X1** Poisoning by chloramphenicol group, accidental (unintentional)
        Poisoning by chloramphenicol group NOS

    ² ✓7ᵗʰ **T36.2X2** Poisoning by chloramphenicol group, HCC intentional self-harm

    ✓7ᵗʰ **T36.2X3** Poisoning by chloramphenicol group, assault

    ✓7ᵗʰ **T36.2X4** Poisoning by chloramphenicol group, undetermined

    ✓7ᵗʰ **T36.2X5** Adverse effect of chloramphenicol group

    ✓7ᵗʰ **T36.2X6** Underdosing of chloramphenicol group

✓5ᵗʰ **T36.3** Poisoning by, adverse effect of and underdosing of macrolides

  ✓6ᵗʰ **T36.3X** Poisoning by, adverse effect of and underdosing of macrolides

    ✓7ᵗʰ **T36.3X1** Poisoning by macrolides, accidental (unintentional)
        Poisoning by macrolides NOS

    ² ✓7ᵗʰ **T36.3X2** Poisoning by macrolides, intentional self-harm HCC

    ✓7ᵗʰ **T36.3X3** Poisoning by macrolides, assault

    ✓7ᵗʰ **T36.3X4** Poisoning by macrolides, undetermined

    ✓7ᵗʰ **T36.3X5** Adverse effect of macrolides

    ✓7ᵗʰ **T36.3X6** Underdosing of macrolides

✓5ᵗʰ **T36.4** Poisoning by, adverse effect of and underdosing of tetracyclines

  ✓6ᵗʰ **T36.4X** Poisoning by, adverse effect of and underdosing of tetracyclines

    ✓7ᵗʰ **T36.4X1** Poisoning by tetracyclines, accidental (unintentional)
        Poisoning by tetracyclines NOS

    ² ✓7ᵗʰ **T36.4X2** Poisoning by tetracyclines, intentional self-harm HCC

    ✓7ᵗʰ **T36.4X3** Poisoning by tetracyclines, assault

    ✓7ᵗʰ **T36.4X4** Poisoning by tetracyclines, undetermined

    ✓7ᵗʰ **T36.4X5** Adverse effect of tetracyclines

    ✓7ᵗʰ **T36.4X6** Underdosing of tetracyclines

✓5ᵗʰ **T36.5** Poisoning by, adverse effect of and underdosing of aminoglycosides
    Poisoning by, adverse effect of and underdosing of streptomycin

  ✓6ᵗʰ **T36.5X** Poisoning by, adverse effect of and underdosing of aminoglycosides

    ✓7ᵗʰ **T36.5X1** Poisoning by aminoglycosides, accidental (unintentional)
        Poisoning by aminoglycosides NOS

    ² ✓7ᵗʰ **T36.5X2** Poisoning by aminoglycosides, intentional self-harm HCC

    ✓7ᵗʰ **T36.5X3** Poisoning by aminoglycosides, assault

    ✓7ᵗʰ **T36.5X4** Poisoning by aminoglycosides, undetermined

    ✓7ᵗʰ **T36.5X5** Adverse effect of aminoglycosides

    ✓7ᵗʰ **T36.5X6** Underdosing of aminoglycosides

✓5ᵗʰ **T36.6** Poisoning by, adverse effect of and underdosing of rifampicins

  ✓6ᵗʰ **T36.6X** Poisoning by, adverse effect of and underdosing of rifampicins

    ✓7ᵗʰ **T36.6X1** Poisoning by rifampicins, accidental (unintentional)
        Poisoning by rifampicins NOS

    ² ✓7ᵗʰ **T36.6X2** Poisoning by rifampicins, intentional self-harm HCC

    ✓7ᵗʰ **T36.6X3** Poisoning by rifampicins, assault

    ✓7ᵗʰ **T36.6X4** Poisoning by rifampicins, undetermined

    ✓7ᵗʰ **T36.6X5** Adverse effect of rifampicins

    ✓7ᵗʰ **T36.6X6** Underdosing of rifampicins

✓5ᵗʰ **T36.7** Poisoning by, adverse effect of and underdosing of antifungal antibiotics, systemically used

  ✓6ᵗʰ **T36.7X** Poisoning by, adverse effect of and underdosing of antifungal antibiotics, **systemically used**

    ✓7ᵗʰ **T36.7X1** Poisoning by antifungal antibiotics, systemically used, accidental (unintentional)
        Poisoning by antifungal antibiotics, systemically used NOS

    ² ✓7ᵗʰ **T36.7X2** Poisoning by antifungal antibiotics, systemically used, intentional self-harm HCC

    ✓7ᵗʰ **T36.7X3** Poisoning by antifungal antibiotics, systemically used, assault

    ✓7ᵗʰ **T36.7X4** Poisoning by antifungal antibiotics, systemically used, undetermined

    ✓7ᵗʰ **T36.7X5** Adverse effect of antifungal antibiotics, systemically used

    ✓7ᵗʰ **T36.7X6** Underdosing of antifungal antibiotics, systemically used

✓5ᵗʰ **T36.8** Poisoning by, adverse effect of and underdosing of other systemic antibiotics

  ✓6ᵗʰ **T36.8X** Poisoning by, adverse effect of and underdosing of other systemic antibiotics
    AHA: 2017, 1Q, 39

    ✓7ᵗʰ **T36.8X1** Poisoning by other systemic antibiotics, accidental (unintentional)
        Poisoning by other systemic antibiotics NOS

    ² ✓7ᵗʰ **T36.8X2** Poisoning by other systemic antibiotics, intentional self-harm HCC

    ✓7ᵗʰ **T36.8X3** Poisoning by other systemic antibiotics, assault

    ✓7ᵗʰ **T36.8X4** Poisoning by other systemic antibiotics, undetermined

    ✓7ᵗʰ **T36.8X5** Adverse effect of other systemic antibiotics

    ✓7ᵗʰ **T36.8X6** Underdosing of other systemic antibiotics

✓5ᵗʰ **T36.9** Poisoning by, adverse effect of and underdosing of unspecified systemic antibiotic

  ✓×7ᵗʰ **T36.91** Poisoning by unspecified systemic antibiotic, accidental (unintentional) ▽
    Poisoning by systemic antibiotic NOS

  ² ✓×7ᵗʰ **T36.92** Poisoning by unspecified systemic antibiotic, intentional self-harm HCC ▽

  ✓×7ᵗʰ **T36.93** Poisoning by unspecified systemic antibiotic, assault ▽

  ✓×7ᵗʰ **T36.94** Poisoning by unspecified systemic antibiotic, undetermined ▽

  ✓×7ᵗʰ **T36.95** Adverse effect of unspecified systemic antibiotic ▽

  ✓×7ᵗʰ **T36.96** Underdosing of unspecified systemic antibiotic ▽

✓4ᵗʰ **T37** Poisoning by, adverse effect of and underdosing of other systemic anti-infectives and antiparasitics

  EXCLUDES 1 *anti-infectives topically used for ear, nose and throat (T49.6-)*
    anti-infectives topically used for eye (T49.5-)
    locally applied anti-infectives NEC (T49.0-)

  The appropriate 7th character is to be added to each code from category T37.
  A   initial encounter
  D   subsequent encounter
  S   sequela

✓5ᵗʰ **T37.0** Poisoning by, adverse effect of and underdosing of sulfonamides

  ✓6ᵗʰ **T37.0X** Poisoning by, adverse effect of and underdosing of sulfonamides

    ✓7ᵗʰ **T37.0X1** Poisoning by sulfonamides, accidental (unintentional)
        Poisoning by sulfonamides NOS

    ² ✓7ᵗʰ **T37.0X2** Poisoning by sulfonamides, intentional self-harm HCC

    ✓7ᵗʰ **T37.0X3** Poisoning by sulfonamides, assault

    ✓7ᵗʰ **T37.0X4** Poisoning by sulfonamides, undetermined

---

² HCC with 7th character indicating initial encounter (A or B - specific to category) OR sequela.

☑ Additional Character Req   ✓×7ᵗʰ Placeholder Alert   Manifestation   HCC CMS-HCC Condition   ▽ Unspecified Code   ►◄ Revised Text   ● New Code   ▲ Revised Code Title

✓7ᵗʰ **T37.ØX5**   Adverse effect of sulfonamides

✓7ᵗʰ **T37.ØX6**   Underdosing of sulfonamides

✓5ᵗʰ **T37.1**   **Poisoning by, adverse effect of and underdosing of antimycobacterial drugs**

     EXCLUDES 1   rifampicins (T36.6-)
                    streptomycin (T36.5-)

   ✓6ᵗʰ **T37.1X**   **Poisoning by, adverse effect of and underdosing of antimycobacterial drugs**

     ✓7ᵗʰ **T37.1X1**   **Poisoning by antimycobacterial drugs, accidental (unintentional)**

         Poisoning by antimycobacterial drugs NOS

    2   ✓7ᵗʰ **T37.1X2**   **Poisoning by antimycobacterial drugs, intentional self-harm**   HCC

     ✓7ᵗʰ **T37.1X3**   **Poisoning by antimycobacterial drugs, assault**

     ✓7ᵗʰ **T37.1X4**   **Poisoning by antimycobacterial drugs, undetermined**

     ✓7ᵗʰ **T37.1X5**   **Adverse effect of antimycobacterial drugs**

     ✓7ᵗʰ **T37.1X6**   **Underdosing of antimycobacterial drugs**

✓5ᵗʰ **T37.2**   **Poisoning by, adverse effect of and underdosing of antimalarials and drugs acting on other blood protozoa**

     EXCLUDES 1   hydroxyquinoline derivatives (T37.8-)

   ✓6ᵗʰ **T37.2X**   **Poisoning by, adverse effect of and underdosing of antimalarials and drugs acting on other blood protozoa**

     ✓7ᵗʰ **T37.2X1**   **Poisoning by antimalarials and drugs acting on other blood protozoa, accidental (unintentional)**

         Poisoning by antimalarials and drugs acting on other blood protozoa NOS

    2   ✓7ᵗʰ **T37.2X2**   **Poisoning by antimalarials and drugs acting on other blood protozoa, intentional self-harm**   HCC

     ✓7ᵗʰ **T37.2X3**   **Poisoning by antimalarials and drugs acting on other blood protozoa, assault**

     ✓7ᵗʰ **T37.2X4**   **Poisoning by antimalarials and drugs acting on other blood protozoa, undetermined**

     ✓7ᵗʰ **T37.2X5**   **Adverse effect of antimalarials and drugs acting on other blood protozoa**

     ✓7ᵗʰ **T37.2X6**   **Underdosing of antimalarials and drugs acting on other blood protozoa**

✓5ᵗʰ **T37.3**   **Poisoning by, adverse effect of and underdosing of other antiprotozoal drugs**

   ✓6ᵗʰ **T37.3X**   **Poisoning by, adverse effect of and underdosing of other antiprotozoal drugs**

     ✓7ᵗʰ **T37.3X1**   **Poisoning by other antiprotozoal drugs, accidental (unintentional)**

         Poisoning by other antiprotozoal drugs NOS

    2   ✓7ᵗʰ **T37.3X2**   **Poisoning by other antiprotozoal drugs, intentional self-harm**   HCC

     ✓7ᵗʰ **T37.3X3**   **Poisoning by other antiprotozoal drugs, assault**

     ✓7ᵗʰ **T37.3X4**   **Poisoning by other antiprotozoal drugs, undetermined**

     ✓7ᵗʰ **T37.3X5**   **Adverse effect of other antiprotozoal drugs**

     ✓7ᵗʰ **T37.3X6**   **Underdosing of other antiprotozoal drugs**

✓5ᵗʰ **T37.4**   **Poisoning by, adverse effect of and underdosing of anthelminthics**

   ✓6ᵗʰ **T37.4X**   **Poisoning by, adverse effect of and underdosing of anthelminthics**

     ✓7ᵗʰ **T37.4X1**   **Poisoning by anthelminthics, accidental (unintentional)**

         Poisoning by anthelminthics NOS

    2   ✓7ᵗʰ **T37.4X2**   **Poisoning by anthelminthics, intentional self-harm**   HCC

     ✓7ᵗʰ **T37.4X3**   **Poisoning by anthelminthics, assault**

     ✓7ᵗʰ **T37.4X4**   **Poisoning by anthelminthics, undetermined**

✓7ᵗʰ **T37.4X5**   Adverse effect of anthelminthics

✓7ᵗʰ **T37.4X6**   Underdosing of anthelminthics

✓5ᵗʰ **T37.5**   **Poisoning by, adverse effect of and underdosing of antiviral drugs**

     EXCLUDES 1   amantadine (T42.8-)
                    cytarabine (T45.1-)

   ✓6ᵗʰ **T37.5X**   **Poisoning by, adverse effect of and underdosing of antiviral drugs**

     ✓7ᵗʰ **T37.5X1**   **Poisoning by antiviral drugs, accidental (unintentional)**

         Poisoning by antiviral drugs NOS

    2   ✓7ᵗʰ **T37.5X2**   **Poisoning by antiviral drugs, intentional self-harm**   HCC

     ✓7ᵗʰ **T37.5X3**   **Poisoning by antiviral drugs, assault**

     ✓7ᵗʰ **T37.5X4**   **Poisoning by antiviral drugs, undetermined**

     ✓7ᵗʰ **T37.5X5**   **Adverse effect of antiviral drugs**

     ✓7ᵗʰ **T37.5X6**   **Underdosing of antiviral drugs**

✓5ᵗʰ **T37.8**   **Poisoning by, adverse effect of and underdosing of other specified systemic anti-infectives and antiparasitics**

     Poisoning by, adverse effect of and underdosing of hydroxyquinoline derivatives

     EXCLUDES 1   antimalarial drugs (T37.2-)

   ✓6ᵗʰ **T37.8X**   **Poisoning by, adverse effect of and underdosing of other specified systemic anti-infectives and antiparasitics**

     ✓7ᵗʰ **T37.8X1**   **Poisoning by other specified systemic anti-infectives and antiparasitics, accidental (unintentional)**

         Poisoning by other specified systemic anti-infectives and antiparasitics NOS

    2   ✓7ᵗʰ **T37.8X2**   **Poisoning by other specified systemic anti-infectives and antiparasitics, intentional self-harm**   HCC

     ✓7ᵗʰ **T37.8X3**   **Poisoning by other specified systemic anti-infectives and antiparasitics, assault**

     ✓7ᵗʰ **T37.8X4**   **Poisoning by other specified systemic anti-infectives and antiparasitics, undetermined**

     ✓7ᵗʰ **T37.8X5**   **Adverse effect of other specified systemic anti-infectives and antiparasitics**

     ✓7ᵗʰ **T37.8X6**   **Underdosing of other specified systemic anti-infectives and antiparasitics**

✓5ᵗʰ **T37.9**   **Poisoning by, adverse effect of and underdosing of unspecified systemic anti-infective and antiparasitics**

   ✓x7ᵗʰ **T37.91**   **Poisoning by unspecified systemic anti-infective and antiparasitics, accidental (unintentional)**   ▽

     Poisoning by, adverse effect of and underdosing of systemic anti-infective and antiparasitics NOS

    2   ✓x7ᵗʰ **T37.92**   **Poisoning by unspecified systemic anti-infective and antiparasitics, intentional self-harm**   HCC ▽

   ✓x7ᵗʰ **T37.93**   **Poisoning by unspecified systemic anti-infective and antiparasitics, assault**   ▽

   ✓x7ᵗʰ **T37.94**   **Poisoning by unspecified systemic anti-infective and antiparasitics, undetermined**   ▽

   ✓x7ᵗʰ **T37.95**   **Adverse effect of unspecified systemic anti-infective and antiparasitic**   ▽

   ✓x7ᵗʰ **T37.96**   **Underdosing of unspecified systemic anti-infectives and antiparasitics**   ▽

---

2   HCC with 7th character indicating initial encounter (A or B - specific to category) OR sequela.

EXCLUDES 1 Not coded here   *EXCLUDES 2* Not included here   N Newborn Age: 0   P Pediatric Age: 0-17   M Maternity Age: 12-55   A Adult Age: 15-124

1060   ICD-10-CM 2018

✓4ᵗʰ **T38** **Poisoning by, adverse effect of and underdosing of hormones and their synthetic substitutes and antagonists, not elsewhere classified**

     EXCLUDES 1   mineralocorticoids and their antagonists (T50.0-)
                  oxytocic hormones (T48.0-)
                  parathyroid hormones and derivatives (T50.9-)

     The appropriate 7th character is to be added to each code from category T38.
     A   initial encounter
     D   subsequent encounter
     S   sequela

✓5ᵗʰ **T38.0** **Poisoning by, adverse effect of and underdosing of glucocorticoids and synthetic analogues**

     EXCLUDES 1   glucocorticoids, topically used (T49.-)

     ✓6ᵗʰ **T38.0X** **Poisoning by, adverse effect of and underdosing of glucocorticoids and synthetic analogues**

         ✓7ᵗʰ **T38.0X1** **Poisoning by glucocorticoids and synthetic analogues, accidental (unintentional)**
                 Poisoning by glucocorticoids and synthetic analogues NOS

         2 ✓7ᵗʰ **T38.0X2** **Poisoning by glucocorticoids and synthetic analogues, intentional self-harm**   HCC

         ✓7ᵗʰ **T38.0X3** **Poisoning by glucocorticoids and synthetic analogues, assault**

         ✓7ᵗʰ **T38.0X4** **Poisoning by glucocorticoids and synthetic analogues, undetermined**

         ✓7ᵗʰ **T38.0X5** **Adverse effect of glucocorticoids and synthetic analogues**

         ✓7ᵗʰ **T38.0X6** **Underdosing of glucocorticoids and synthetic analogues**

✓5ᵗʰ **T38.1** **Poisoning by, adverse effect of and underdosing of thyroid hormones and substitutes**

     ✓6ᵗʰ **T38.1X** **Poisoning by, adverse effect of and underdosing of thyroid hormones and substitutes**

         ✓7ᵗʰ **T38.1X1** **Poisoning by thyroid hormones and substitutes, accidental (unintentional)**
                 Poisoning by thyroid hormones and substitutes NOS

         2 ✓7ᵗʰ **T38.1X2** **Poisoning by thyroid hormones and substitutes, intentional self-harm**   HCC

         ✓7ᵗʰ **T38.1X3** **Poisoning by thyroid hormones and substitutes, assault**

         ✓7ᵗʰ **T38.1X4** **Poisoning by thyroid hormones and substitutes, undetermined**

         ✓7ᵗʰ **T38.1X5** **Adverse effect of thyroid hormones and substitutes**

         ✓7ᵗʰ **T38.1X6** **Underdosing of thyroid hormones and substitutes**

✓5ᵗʰ **T38.2** **Poisoning by, adverse effect of and underdosing of antithyroid drugs**

     ✓6ᵗʰ **T38.2X** **Poisoning by, adverse effect of and underdosing of antithyroid drugs**

         ✓7ᵗʰ **T38.2X1** **Poisoning by antithyroid drugs, accidental (unintentional)**
                 Poisoning by antithyroid drugs NOS

         2 ✓7ᵗʰ **T38.2X2** **Poisoning by antithyroid drugs, intentional self-harm**   HCC

         ✓7ᵗʰ **T38.2X3** **Poisoning by antithyroid drugs, assault**

         ✓7ᵗʰ **T38.2X4** **Poisoning by antithyroid drugs, undetermined**

         ✓7ᵗʰ **T38.2X5** **Adverse effect of antithyroid drugs**

         ✓7ᵗʰ **T38.2X6** **Underdosing of antithyroid drugs**

✓5ᵗʰ **T38.3** **Poisoning by, adverse effect of and underdosing of insulin and oral hypoglycemic [antidiabetic] drugs**

     ✓6ᵗʰ **T38.3X** **Poisoning by, adverse effect of and underdosing of insulin and oral hypoglycemic [antidiabetic] drugs**

         ✓7ᵗʰ **T38.3X1** **Poisoning by insulin and oral hypoglycemic [antidiabetic] drugs, accidental (unintentional)**
                 Poisoning by insulin and oral hypoglycemic [antidiabetic] drugs NOS

         2 ✓7ᵗʰ **T38.3X2** **Poisoning by insulin and oral hypoglycemic [antidiabetic] drugs, intentional self-harm**   HCC

         ✓7ᵗʰ **T38.3X3** **Poisoning by insulin and oral hypoglycemic [antidiabetic] drugs, assault**

         ✓7ᵗʰ **T38.3X4** **Poisoning by insulin and oral hypoglycemic [antidiabetic] drugs, undetermined**

         ✓7ᵗʰ **T38.3X5** **Adverse effect of insulin and oral hypoglycemic [antidiabetic] drugs**

         ✓7ᵗʰ **T38.3X6** **Underdosing of insulin and oral hypoglycemic [antidiabetic] drugs**

✓5ᵗʰ **T38.4** **Poisoning by, adverse effect of and underdosing of oral contraceptives**
     Poisoning by, adverse effect of and underdosing of multiple- and single-ingredient oral contraceptive preparations

     ✓6ᵗʰ **T38.4X** **Poisoning by, adverse effect of and underdosing of oral contraceptives**

         ✓7ᵗʰ **T38.4X1** **Poisoning by oral contraceptives, accidental (unintentional)**
                 Poisoning by oral contraceptives NOS

         2 ✓7ᵗʰ **T38.4X2** **Poisoning by oral contraceptives, intentional self-harm**   HCC

         ✓7ᵗʰ **T38.4X3** **Poisoning by oral contraceptives, assault**

         ✓7ᵗʰ **T38.4X4** **Poisoning by oral contraceptives, undetermined**

         ✓7ᵗʰ **T38.4X5** **Adverse effect of oral contraceptives**

         ✓7ᵗʰ **T38.4X6** **Underdosing of oral contraceptives**

✓5ᵗʰ **T38.5** **Poisoning by, adverse effect of and underdosing of other estrogens and progestogens**
     Poisoning by, adverse effect of and underdosing of estrogens and progestogens mixtures and substitutes

     ✓6ᵗʰ **T38.5X** **Poisoning by, adverse effect of and underdosing of other estrogens and progestogens**

         ✓7ᵗʰ **T38.5X1** **Poisoning by other estrogens and progestogens, accidental (unintentional)**
                 Poisoning by other estrogens and progestogens NOS

         2 ✓7ᵗʰ **T38.5X2** **Poisoning by other estrogens and progestogens, intentional self-harm**   HCC

         ✓7ᵗʰ **T38.5X3** **Poisoning by other estrogens and progestogens, assault**

         ✓7ᵗʰ **T38.5X4** **Poisoning by other estrogens and progestogens, undetermined**

         ✓7ᵗʰ **T38.5X5** **Adverse effect of other estrogens and progestogens**

         ✓7ᵗʰ **T38.5X6** **Underdosing of other estrogens and progestogens**

✓5ᵗʰ **T38.6** **Poisoning by, adverse effect of and underdosing of antigonadotrophins, antiestrogens, antiandrogens, not elsewhere classified**
     Poisoning by, adverse effect of and underdosing of tamoxifen

     ✓6ᵗʰ **T38.6X** **Poisoning by, adverse effect of and underdosing of antigonadotrophins, antiestrogens, antiandrogens, not elsewhere classified**

         ✓7ᵗʰ **T38.6X1** **Poisoning by antigonadotrophins, antiestrogens, antiandrogens, not elsewhere classified, accidental (unintentional)**
                 Poisoning by antigonadotrophins, antiestrogens, antiandrogens, not elsewhere classified NOS

         2 ✓7ᵗʰ **T38.6X2** **Poisoning by antigonadotrophins, antiestrogens, antiandrogens, not elsewhere classified, intentional self-harm**   HCC

         ✓7ᵗʰ **T38.6X3** **Poisoning by antigonadotrophins, antiestrogens, antiandrogens, not elsewhere classified, assault**

         ✓7ᵗʰ **T38.6X4** **Poisoning by antigonadotrophins, antiestrogens, antiandrogens, not elsewhere classified, undetermined**

         ✓7ᵗʰ **T38.6X5** **Adverse effect of antigonadotrophins, antiestrogens, antiandrogens, not elsewhere classified**

         ✓7ᵗʰ **T38.6X6** **Underdosing of antigonadotrophins, antiestrogens, antiandrogens, not elsewhere classified**

---

2   HCC with 7th character indicating initial encounter (A or B - specific to category) OR sequela.

☑ Additional Character Req   ✓xᵗʰ Placeholder Alert   Manifestation   HCC CMS-HCC Condition   ▽ Unspecified Code   ►◄ Revised Text   ● New Code   ▲ Revised Code Title

ICD-10-CM 2018   1061

√5ᵗʰ **T38.7** **Poisoning by, adverse effect of and underdosing of androgens and anabolic congeners**

  √6ᵗʰ **T38.7X** **Poisoning by, adverse effect of and underdosing of androgens and anabolic congeners**

    √7ᵗʰ **T38.7X1** **Poisoning by androgens and anabolic congeners, accidental (unintentional)**
      Poisoning by androgens and anabolic congeners NOS

    2 √7ᵗʰ **T38.7X2** **Poisoning by androgens and anabolic congeners, intentional self-harm** HCC

    √7ᵗʰ **T38.7X3** **Poisoning by androgens and anabolic congeners, assault**

    √7ᵗʰ **T38.7X4** **Poisoning by androgens and anabolic congeners, undetermined**

    √7ᵗʰ **T38.7X5** **Adverse effect of androgens and anabolic congeners**

    √7ᵗʰ **T38.7X6** **Underdosing of androgens and anabolic congeners**

√5ᵗʰ **T38.8** **Poisoning by, adverse effect of and underdosing of other and unspecified hormones and synthetic substitutes**

  √6ᵗʰ **T38.80** **Poisoning by, adverse effect of and underdosing of unspecified hormones and synthetic substitutes**

    √7ᵗʰ **T38.801** **Poisoning by unspecified hormones and synthetic substitutes, accidental (unintentional)** ▽
      Poisoning by unspecified hormones and synthetic substitutes NOS

    2 √7ᵗʰ **T38.802** **Poisoning by unspecified hormones and synthetic substitutes, intentional self-harm** HCC ▽

    √7ᵗʰ **T38.803** **Poisoning by unspecified hormones and synthetic substitutes, assault** ▽

    √7ᵗʰ **T38.804** **Poisoning by unspecified hormones and synthetic substitutes, undetermined** ▽

    √7ᵗʰ **T38.805** **Adverse effect of unspecified hormones and synthetic substitutes** ▽

    √7ᵗʰ **T38.806** **Underdosing of unspecified hormones and synthetic substitutes** ▽

  √6ᵗʰ **T38.81** **Poisoning by, adverse effect of and underdosing of anterior pituitary [adenohypophyseal] hormones**

    √7ᵗʰ **T38.811** **Poisoning by anterior pituitary [adenohypophyseal] hormones, accidental (unintentional)**
      Poisoning by anterior pituitary [adenohypophyseal] hormones NOS

    2 √7ᵗʰ **T38.812** **Poisoning by anterior pituitary [adenohypophyseal] hormones, intentional self-harm** HCC

    √7ᵗʰ **T38.813** **Poisoning by anterior pituitary [adenohypophyseal] hormones, assault**

    √7ᵗʰ **T38.814** **Poisoning by anterior pituitary [adenohypophyseal] hormones, undetermined**

    √7ᵗʰ **T38.815** **Adverse effect of anterior pituitary [adenohypophyseal] hormones**

    √7ᵗʰ **T38.816** **Underdosing of anterior pituitary [adenohypophyseal] hormones**

  √6ᵗʰ **T38.89** **Poisoning by, adverse effect of and underdosing of other hormones and synthetic substitutes**

    √7ᵗʰ **T38.891** **Poisoning by other hormones and synthetic substitutes, accidental (unintentional)**
      Poisoning by other hormones and synthetic substitutes NOS

    2 √7ᵗʰ **T38.892** **Poisoning by other hormones and synthetic substitutes, intentional self-harm** HCC

    √7ᵗʰ **T38.893** **Poisoning by other hormones and synthetic substitutes, assault**

    √7ᵗʰ **T38.894** **Poisoning by other hormones and synthetic substitutes, undetermined**

    √7ᵗʰ **T38.895** **Adverse effect of other hormones and synthetic substitutes**

    √7ᵗʰ **T38.896** **Underdosing of other hormones and synthetic substitutes**

√5ᵗʰ **T38.9** **Poisoning by, adverse effect of and underdosing of other and unspecified hormone antagonists**

  √6ᵗʰ **T38.90** **Poisoning by, adverse effect of and underdosing of unspecified hormone antagonists**

    √7ᵗʰ **T38.901** **Poisoning by unspecified hormone antagonists, accidental (unintentional)** ▽
      Poisoning by unspecified hormone antagonists NOS

    2 √7ᵗʰ **T38.902** **Poisoning by unspecified hormone antagonists, intentional self-harm** HCC ▽

    √7ᵗʰ **T38.903** **Poisoning by unspecified hormone antagonists, assault** ▽

    √7ᵗʰ **T38.904** **Poisoning by unspecified hormone antagonists, undetermined** ▽

    √7ᵗʰ **T38.905** **Adverse effect of unspecified hormone antagonists** ▽

    √7ᵗʰ **T38.906** **Underdosing of unspecified hormone antagonists** ▽

  √6ᵗʰ **T38.99** **Poisoning by, adverse effect of and underdosing of other hormone antagonists**

    √7ᵗʰ **T38.991** **Poisoning by other hormone antagonists, accidental (unintentional)**
      Poisoning by other hormone antagonists NOS

    2 √7ᵗʰ **T38.992** **Poisoning by other hormone antagonists, intentional self-harm** HCC

    √7ᵗʰ **T38.993** **Poisoning by other hormone antagonists, assault**

    √7ᵗʰ **T38.994** **Poisoning by other hormone antagonists, undetermined**

    √7ᵗʰ **T38.995** **Adverse effect of other hormone antagonists**

    √7ᵗʰ **T38.996** **Underdosing of other hormone antagonists**

√4ᵗʰ **T39** **Poisoning by, adverse effect of and underdosing of nonopioid analgesics, antipyretics and antirheumatics**

> The appropriate 7th character is to be added to each code from category T39.
> A   initial encounter
> D   subsequent encounter
> S   sequela

√5ᵗʰ **T39.0** **Poisoning by, adverse effect of and underdosing of salicylates**

  √6ᵗʰ **T39.01** **Poisoning by, adverse effect of and underdosing of aspirin**
    Poisoning by, adverse effect of and underdosing of acetylsalicylic acid

    √7ᵗʰ **T39.011** **Poisoning by aspirin, accidental (unintentional)**

    2 √7ᵗʰ **T39.012** **Poisoning by aspirin, intentional self-harm** HCC

    √7ᵗʰ **T39.013** **Poisoning by aspirin, assault**

    √7ᵗʰ **T39.014** **Poisoning by aspirin, undetermined**

    √7ᵗʰ **T39.015** **Adverse effect of aspirin**
      AHA: 2016, 1Q, 15

    √7ᵗʰ **T39.016** **Underdosing of aspirin**

  √6ᵗʰ **T39.09** **Poisoning by, adverse effect of and underdosing of other salicylates**

    √7ᵗʰ **T39.091** **Poisoning by salicylates, accidental (unintentional)**
      Poisoning by salicylates NOS

    2 √7ᵗʰ **T39.092** **Poisoning by salicylates, intentional self-harm** HCC

    √7ᵗʰ **T39.093** **Poisoning by salicylates, assault**

    √7ᵗʰ **T39.094** **Poisoning by salicylates, undetermined**

    √7ᵗʰ **T39.095** **Adverse effect of salicylates**

    √7ᵗʰ **T39.096** **Underdosing of salicylates**

√5ᵗʰ **T39.1** **Poisoning by, adverse effect of and underdosing of 4-Aminophenol derivatives**

  √6ᵗʰ **T39.1X** **Poisoning by, adverse effect of and underdosing of 4-Aminophenol derivatives**

    √7ᵗʰ **T39.1X1** **Poisoning by 4-Aminophenol derivatives, accidental (unintentional)**
      Poisoning by 4-Aminophenol derivatives NOS

---

2   HCC with 7th character indicating initial encounter (A or B - specific to category) OR sequela.

EXCLUDES 1 Not coded here   EXCLUDES 2 Not included here   N Newborn Age: 0   P Pediatric Age: 0-17   M Maternity Age: 12-55   A Adult Age: 15-124

1062   ICD-10-CM 2018

2 ✓7th **T39.1X2** **Poisoning by 4-Aminophenol derivatives,** intentional self-harm   HCC

✓7th **T39.1X3** **Poisoning by 4-Aminophenol derivatives,** assault

✓7th **T39.1X4** **Poisoning by 4-Aminophenol derivatives,** undetermined

✓7th **T39.1X5** Adverse effect **of 4-Aminophenol derivatives**

✓7th **T39.1X6** Underdosing **of 4-Aminophenol derivatives**

✓5th **T39.2** **Poisoning by, adverse effect of and underdosing of pyrazolone derivatives**

✓6th **T39.2X** **Poisoning by, adverse effect of and underdosing of** pyrazolone derivatives

✓7th **T39.2X1** **Poisoning by pyrazolone derivatives,** accidental **(unintentional)**
Poisoning by pyrazolone derivatives NOS

2 ✓7th **T39.2X2** **Poisoning by pyrazolone derivatives,** intentional self-harm   HCC

✓7th **T39.2X3** **Poisoning by pyrazolone derivatives,** assault

✓7th **T39.2X4** **Poisoning by pyrazolone derivatives,** undetermined

✓7th **T39.2X5** Adverse effect **of pyrazolone derivatives**

✓7th **T39.2X6** Underdosing **of pyrazolone derivatives**

✓5th **T39.3** **Poisoning by, adverse effect of and underdosing of other nonsteroidal anti-inflammatory drugs [NSAID]**

✓6th **T39.31** **Poisoning by, adverse effect of and underdosing of** propionic acid derivatives
Poisoning by, adverse effect of and underdosing of fenoprofen
Poisoning by, adverse effect of and underdosing of flurbiprofen
Poisoning by, adverse effect of and underdosing of ibuprofen
Poisoning by, adverse effect of and underdosing of ketoprofen
Poisoning by, adverse effect of and underdosing of naproxen
Poisoning by, adverse effect of and underdosing of oxaprozin

✓7th **T39.311** **Poisoning by propionic acid derivatives,** accidental **(unintentional)**

2 ✓7th **T39.312** **Poisoning by propionic acid derivatives,** intentional self-harm   HCC

✓7th **T39.313** **Poisoning by propionic acid derivatives,** assault

✓7th **T39.314** **Poisoning by propionic acid derivatives,** undetermined

✓7th **T39.315** Adverse effect **of propionic acid derivatives**

✓7th **T39.316** Underdosing **of propionic acid derivatives**

✓6th **T39.39** **Poisoning by, adverse effect of and underdosing of other nonsteroidal anti-inflammatory drugs [NSAID]**

✓7th **T39.391** **Poisoning by other nonsteroidal anti-inflammatory drugs [NSAID],** accidental **(unintentional)**
Poisoning by other nonsteroidal anti-inflammatory drugs NOS

2 ✓7th **T39.392** **Poisoning by other nonsteroidal anti-inflammatory drugs [NSAID],** intentional self-harm   HCC

✓7th **T39.393** **Poisoning by other nonsteroidal anti-inflammatory drugs [NSAID],** assault

✓7th **T39.394** **Poisoning by other nonsteroidal anti-inflammatory drugs [NSAID],** undetermined

✓7th **T39.395** Adverse effect **of other nonsteroidal anti-inflammatory drugs [NSAID]**

✓7th **T39.396** Underdosing **of other nonsteroidal anti-inflammatory drugs [NSAID]**

✓5th **T39.4** **Poisoning by, adverse effect of and underdosing of antirheumatics, not elsewhere classified**

EXCLUDES 1   poisoning by, adverse effect of and underdosing of glucocorticoids (T38.0-)
poisoning by, adverse effect of and underdosing of salicylates (T39.0-)

✓6th **T39.4X** **Poisoning by, adverse effect of and underdosing of** antirheumatics, **not elsewhere classified**

✓7th **T39.4X1** **Poisoning by antirheumatics, not elsewhere classified,** accidental **(unintentional)**
Poisoning by antirheumatics, not elsewhere classified NOS

2 ✓7th **T39.4X2** **Poisoning by antirheumatics, not elsewhere classified,** intentional self-harm   HCC

✓7th **T39.4X3** **Poisoning by antirheumatics, not elsewhere classified,** assault

✓7th **T39.4X4** **Poisoning by antirheumatics, not elsewhere classified,** undetermined

✓7th **T39.4X5** Adverse effect **of antirheumatics, not elsewhere classified**

✓7th **T39.4X6** Underdosing **of antirheumatics, not elsewhere classified**

✓5th **T39.8** **Poisoning by, adverse effect of and underdosing of other nonopioid analgesics and antipyretics, not elsewhere classified**

✓6th **T39.8X** **Poisoning by, adverse effect of and underdosing of other nonopioid analgesics and antipyretics, not elsewhere classified**

✓7th **T39.8X1** **Poisoning by other nonopioid analgesics and antipyretics, not elsewhere classified,** accidental **(unintentional)**
Poisoning by other nonopioid analgesics and antipyretics, not elsewhere classified NOS

2 ✓7th **T39.8X2** **Poisoning by other nonopioid analgesics and antipyretics, not elsewhere classified,** intentional self-harm   HCC

✓7th **T39.8X3** **Poisoning by other nonopioid analgesics and antipyretics, not elsewhere classified,** assault

✓7th **T39.8X4** **Poisoning by other nonopioid analgesics and antipyretics, not elsewhere classified,** undetermined

✓7th **T39.8X5** Adverse effect **of other nonopioid analgesics and antipyretics, not elsewhere classified**

✓7th **T39.8X6** Underdosing **of other nonopioid analgesics and antipyretics, not elsewhere classified**

✓5th **T39.9** **Poisoning by, adverse effect of and underdosing of unspecified nonopioid analgesic, antipyretic and antirheumatic**

✓x7th **T39.91** **Poisoning by unspecified nonopioid analgesic, antipyretic and antirheumatic,** accidental **(unintentional)** ▽
Poisoning by nonopioid analgesic, antipyretic and antirheumatic NOS

2 ✓x7th **T39.92** **Poisoning by unspecified nonopioid analgesic, antipyretic and antirheumatic,** intentional self-harm   HCC ▽

✓x7th **T39.93** **Poisoning by unspecified nonopioid analgesic, antipyretic and antirheumatic,** assault ▽

✓x7th **T39.94** **Poisoning by unspecified nonopioid analgesic, antipyretic and antirheumatic,** undetermined ▽

✓x7th **T39.95** Adverse effect **of unspecified nonopioid analgesic, antipyretic and antirheumatic** ▽

✓x7th **T39.96** Underdosing **of unspecified nonopioid analgesic, antipyretic and antirheumatic** ▽

---

2 HCC with 7th character indicating initial encounter (A or B - specific to category) OR sequela.

☑ Additional Character Req   ✓x7th Placeholder Alert   Manifestation   HCC CMS-HCC Condition   ▽ Unspecified Code   ►◄ Revised Text   ● New Code   ▲ Revised Code Title

ICD-10-CM 2018   1063

√4th **T40** **Poisoning by, adverse effect of and underdosing of narcotics and psychodysleptics [hallucinogens]**

EXCLUDES 2 *drug dependence and related mental and behavioral disorders due to psychoactive substance use (F10-F19-)*

The appropriate 7th character is to be added to each code from category T40.
A   initial encounter
D   subsequent encounter
S   sequela

√5th **T40.0** Poisoning by, adverse effect of and underdosing of opium

√6th **T40.0X** Poisoning by, adverse effect of and underdosing of opium

√7th **T40.0X1** Poisoning by opium, accidental (unintentional)
Poisoning by opium NOS

2 √7th **T40.0X2** Poisoning by opium, intentional self-harm HCC

√7th **T40.0X3** Poisoning by opium, assault

√7th **T40.0X4** Poisoning by opium, undetermined

√7th **T40.0X5** Adverse effect of opium

√7th **T40.0X6** Underdosing of opium

√5th **T40.1** Poisoning by and adverse effect of heroin

√6th **T40.1X** Poisoning by and adverse effect of heroin

√7th **T40.1X1** Poisoning by heroin, accidental (unintentional)
Poisoning by heroin NOS

2 √7th **T40.1X2** Poisoning by heroin, intentional self-harm HCC

√7th **T40.1X3** Poisoning by heroin, assault

√7th **T40.1X4** Poisoning by heroin, undetermined

√5th **T40.2** Poisoning by, adverse effect of and underdosing of other opioids

√6th **T40.2X** Poisoning by, adverse effect of and underdosing of other opioids

√7th **T40.2X1** Poisoning by other opioids, accidental (unintentional)
Poisoning by other opioids NOS

2 √7th **T40.2X2** Poisoning by other opioids, intentional self-harm HCC

√7th **T40.2X3** Poisoning by other opioids, assault

√7th **T40.2X4** Poisoning by other opioids, undetermined

√7th **T40.2X5** Adverse effect of other opioids

√7th **T40.2X6** Underdosing of other opioids

√5th **T40.3** Poisoning by, adverse effect of and underdosing of methadone

√6th **T40.3X** Poisoning by, adverse effect of and underdosing of methadone

√7th **T40.3X1** Poisoning by methadone, accidental (unintentional)
Poisoning by methadone NOS

2 √7th **T40.3X2** Poisoning by methadone, intentional self-harm HCC

√7th **T40.3X3** Poisoning by methadone, assault

√7th **T40.3X4** Poisoning by methadone, undetermined

√7th **T40.3X5** Adverse effect of methadone

√7th **T40.3X6** Underdosing of methadone

√5th **T40.4** Poisoning by, adverse effect of and underdosing of other synthetic narcotics

√6th **T40.4X** Poisoning by, adverse effect of and underdosing of other synthetic narcotics

√7th **T40.4X1** Poisoning by other synthetic narcotics, accidental (unintentional)
Poisoning by other synthetic narcotics NOS

2 √7th **T40.4X2** Poisoning by other synthetic narcotics, intentional self-harm HCC

√7th **T40.4X3** Poisoning by other synthetic narcotics, assault

√7th **T40.4X4** Poisoning by other synthetic narcotics, undetermined

√7th **T40.4X5** Adverse effect of other synthetic narcotics

√7th **T40.4X6** Underdosing of other synthetic narcotics

√5th **T40.5** Poisoning by, adverse effect of and underdosing of cocaine

√6th **T40.5X** Poisoning by, adverse effect of and underdosing of cocaine

√7th **T40.5X1** Poisoning by cocaine, accidental (unintentional)
Poisoning by cocaine NOS
AHA: 2016, 2Q, 8

2 √7th **T40.5X2** Poisoning by cocaine, intentional self-harm HCC

√7th **T40.5X3** Poisoning by cocaine, assault

√7th **T40.5X4** Poisoning by cocaine, undetermined

√7th **T40.5X5** Adverse effect of cocaine

√7th **T40.5X6** Underdosing of cocaine

√5th **T40.6** Poisoning by, adverse effect of and underdosing of other and unspecified narcotics

√6th **T40.60** Poisoning by, adverse effect of and underdosing of unspecified narcotics

√7th **T40.601** Poisoning by unspecified narcotics, accidental (unintentional) ▽
Poisoning by narcotics NOS

2 √7th **T40.602** Poisoning by unspecified narcotics, HCC ▽ intentional self-harm

√7th **T40.603** Poisoning by unspecified narcotics, assault ▽

√7th **T40.604** Poisoning by unspecified narcotics, undetermined ▽

√7th **T40.605** Adverse effect of unspecified narcotics ▽

√7th **T40.606** Underdosing of unspecified narcotics ▽

√6th **T40.69** Poisoning by, adverse effect of and underdosing of other narcotics

√7th **T40.691** Poisoning by other narcotics, accidental (unintentional)
Poisoning by other narcotics NOS

2 √7th **T40.692** Poisoning by other narcotics, intentional self-harm HCC

√7th **T40.693** Poisoning by other narcotics, assault

√7th **T40.694** Poisoning by other narcotics, undetermined

√7th **T40.695** Adverse effect of other narcotics

√7th **T40.696** Underdosing of other narcotics

√5th **T40.7** Poisoning by, adverse effect of and underdosing of cannabis (derivatives)

√6th **T40.7X** Poisoning by, adverse effect of and underdosing of cannabis (derivatives)

√7th **T40.7X1** Poisoning by cannabis (derivatives), accidental (unintentional)
Poisoning by cannabis NOS

2 √7th **T40.7X2** Poisoning by cannabis (derivatives), intentional self-harm HCC

√7th **T40.7X3** Poisoning by cannabis (derivatives), assault

√7th **T40.7X4** Poisoning by cannabis (derivatives), undetermined

√7th **T40.7X5** Adverse effect of cannabis (derivatives)

√7th **T40.7X6** Underdosing of cannabis (derivatives)

√5th **T40.8** Poisoning by and adverse effect of lysergide [LSD]

√6th **T40.8X** Poisoning by and adverse effect of lysergide [LSD]

√7th **T40.8X1** Poisoning by lysergide [LSD], accidental (unintentional)
Poisoning by lysergide [LSD]NOS

2 √7th **T40.8X2** Poisoning by lysergide [LSD], intentional self-harm HCC

√7th **T40.8X3** Poisoning by lysergide [LSD], assault

√7th **T40.8X4** Poisoning by lysergide [LSD], undetermined

√5th **T40.9** Poisoning by, adverse effect of and underdosing of other and unspecified psychodysleptics [hallucinogens]

√6th **T40.90** Poisoning by, adverse effect of and underdosing of unspecified psychodysleptics [hallucinogens]

√7th **T40.901** Poisoning by unspecified psychodysleptics [hallucinogens], accidental (unintentional) ▽

---

2 HCC with 7th character indicating initial encounter (A or B - specific to category) OR sequela.

EXCLUDES 1 Not coded here   EXCLUDES 2 Not included here   N Newborn Age: 0   P Pediatric Age: 0-17   M Maternity Age: 12-55   A Adult Age: 15-124

2 ✓7th **T40.902** Poisoning by unspecified psychodysleptics [hallucinogens], intentional self-harm   HCC ▽

✓7th **T40.903** Poisoning by unspecified psychodysleptics [hallucinogens], assault ▽

✓7th **T40.904** Poisoning by unspecified psychodysleptics [hallucinogens], undetermined ▽

✓7th **T40.905** Adverse effect of unspecified psychodysleptics [hallucinogens] ▽

✓7th **T40.906** Underdosing of unspecified psychodysleptics ▽

✓6th **T40.99** Poisoning by, adverse effect of and underdosing of other psychodysleptics [hallucinogens]

✓7th **T40.991** Poisoning by other psychodysleptics [hallucinogens], accidental (unintentional)
  Poisoning by other psychodysleptics [hallucinogens] NOS

2 ✓7th **T40.992** Poisoning by other psychodysleptics [hallucinogens], intentional self-harm   HCC

✓7th **T40.993** Poisoning by other psychodysleptics [hallucinogens], assault

✓7th **T40.994** Poisoning by other psychodysleptics [hallucinogens], undetermined

✓7th **T40.995** Adverse effect of other psychodysleptics [hallucinogens]

✓7th **T40.996** Underdosing of other psychodysleptics

✓4th **T41** Poisoning by, adverse effect of and underdosing of anesthetics and therapeutic gases

> EXCLUDES 1   benzodiazepines (T42.4-)
> cocaine (T40.5-)
> complications of anesthesia during labor and delivery (O74.-)
> complications of anesthesia during pregnancy (O29.-)
> complications of anesthesia during the puerperium (O89.-)
> opioids (T40.0-T40.2-)

The appropriate 7th character is to be added to each code from category T41.
A   initial encounter
D   subsequent encounter
S   sequela

✓5th **T41.0** Poisoning by, adverse effect of and underdosing of inhaled anesthetics
> EXCLUDES 1   oxygen (T41.5-)

✓6th **T41.0X** Poisoning by, adverse effect of and underdosing of inhaled anesthetics

✓7th **T41.0X1** Poisoning by inhaled anesthetics, accidental (unintentional)
  Poisoning by inhaled anesthetics NOS

2 ✓7th **T41.0X2** Poisoning by inhaled anesthetics, intentional self-harm   HCC

✓7th **T41.0X3** Poisoning by inhaled anesthetics, assault

✓7th **T41.0X4** Poisoning by inhaled anesthetics, undetermined

✓7th **T41.0X5** Adverse effect of inhaled anesthetics

✓7th **T41.0X6** Underdosing of inhaled anesthetics

✓5th **T41.1** Poisoning by, adverse effect of and underdosing of intravenous anesthetics
  Poisoning by, adverse effect of and underdosing of thiobarbiturates

✓6th **T41.1X** Poisoning by, adverse effect of and underdosing of intravenous anesthetics

✓7th **T41.1X1** Poisoning by intravenous anesthetics, accidental (unintentional)
  Poisoning by intravenous anesthetics NOS

2 ✓7th **T41.1X2** Poisoning by intravenous anesthetics, intentional self-harm   HCC

✓7th **T41.1X3** Poisoning by intravenous anesthetics, assault

✓7th **T41.1X4** Poisoning by intravenous anesthetics, undetermined

✓7th **T41.1X5** Adverse effect of intravenous anesthetics

✓7th **T41.1X6** Underdosing of intravenous anesthetics

✓5th **T41.2** Poisoning by, adverse effect of and underdosing of other and unspecified general anesthetics

✓6th **T41.20** Poisoning by, adverse effect of and underdosing of unspecified general anesthetics

✓7th **T41.201** Poisoning by unspecified general anesthetics, accidental (unintentional) ▽
  Poisoning by general anesthetics NOS

2 ✓7th **T41.202** Poisoning by unspecified general anesthetics, intentional self-harm   HCC ▽

✓7th **T41.203** Poisoning by unspecified general anesthetics, assault ▽

✓7th **T41.204** Poisoning by unspecified general anesthetics, undetermined ▽

✓7th **T41.205** Adverse effect of unspecified general anesthetics ▽

✓7th **T41.206** Underdosing of unspecified general anesthetics ▽

✓6th **T41.29** Poisoning by, adverse effect of and underdosing of other general anesthetics

✓7th **T41.291** Poisoning by other general anesthetics, accidental (unintentional)
  Poisoning by other general anesthetics NOS

2 ✓7th **T41.292** Poisoning by other general anesthetics, intentional self-harm   HCC

✓7th **T41.293** Poisoning by other general anesthetics, assault

✓7th **T41.294** Poisoning by other general anesthetics, undetermined

✓7th **T41.295** Adverse effect of other general anesthetics

✓7th **T41.296** Underdosing of other general anesthetics

✓5th **T41.3** Poisoning by, adverse effect of and underdosing of local anesthetics
  Cocaine (topical)
> EXCLUDES 2   poisoning by cocaine used as a central nervous system stimulant (T40.5X1-T40.5X4)

✓6th **T41.3X** Poisoning by, adverse effect of and underdosing of local anesthetics

✓7th **T41.3X1** Poisoning by local anesthetics, accidental (unintentional)
  Poisoning by local anesthetics NOS

2 ✓7th **T41.3X2** Poisoning by local anesthetics, intentional self-harm   HCC

✓7th **T41.3X3** Poisoning by local anesthetics, assault

✓7th **T41.3X4** Poisoning by local anesthetics, undetermined

✓7th **T41.3X5** Adverse effect of local anesthetics

✓7th **T41.3X6** Underdosing of local anesthetics

✓5th **T41.4** Poisoning by, adverse effect of and underdosing of unspecified anesthetic

✓x7th **T41.41** Poisoning by unspecified anesthetic, accidental (unintentional) ▽
  Poisoning by anesthetic NOS

2 ✓x7th **T41.42** Poisoning by unspecified anesthetic, intentional self-harm   HCC ▽

✓x7th **T41.43** Poisoning by unspecified anesthetic, assault ▽

✓x7th **T41.44** Poisoning by unspecified anesthetic, undetermined ▽

✓x7th **T41.45** Adverse effect of unspecified anesthetic ▽

✓x7th **T41.46** Underdosing of unspecified anesthetics ▽

✓5th **T41.5** Poisoning by, adverse effect of and underdosing of therapeutic gases

✓6th **T41.5X** Poisoning by, adverse effect of and underdosing of therapeutic gases

✓7th **T41.5X1** Poisoning by therapeutic gases, accidental (unintentional)
  Poisoning by therapeutic gases NOS

2 ✓7th **T41.5X2** Poisoning by therapeutic gases, intentional self-harm   HCC

✓7th **T41.5X3** Poisoning by therapeutic gases, assault

✓7th **T41.5X4** Poisoning by therapeutic gases, undetermined

✓7th **T41.5X5** Adverse effect of therapeutic gases

---

2   HCC with 7th character indicating initial encounter (A or B - specific to category) OR sequela.

✓ Additional Character Req   ✓x7th Placeholder Alert   Manifestation   HCC CMS-HCC Condition   ▽ Unspecified Code   ►◄ Revised Text   ● New Code   ▲ Revised Code Title

     ✓7th **T41.5X6**   Underdosing of therapeutic gases

✓4th **T42**   **Poisoning by, adverse effect of and underdosing of antiepileptic, sedative- hypnotic and antiparkinsonism drugs**

     EXCLUDES 2   *drug dependence and related mental and behavioral disorders due to psychoactive substance use (F10.--F19.-)*

> The appropriate 7th character is to be added to each code from category T42.
> A   initial encounter
> D   subsequent encounter
> S   sequela

   ✓5th **T42.0**   **Poisoning by, adverse effect of and underdosing of hydantoin derivatives**

     ✓6th **T42.0X**   **Poisoning by, adverse effect of and underdosing of hydantoin derivatives**

       ✓7th **T42.0X1**   **Poisoning by hydantoin derivatives, accidental (unintentional)**
            Poisoning by hydantoin derivatives NOS

       2 ✓7th **T42.0X2**   **Poisoning by hydantoin derivatives, intentional self-harm**   HCC

       ✓7th **T42.0X3**   **Poisoning by hydantoin derivatives, assault**

       ✓7th **T42.0X4**   **Poisoning by hydantoin derivatives, undetermined**

       ✓7th **T42.0X5**   **Adverse effect of hydantoin derivatives**

       ✓7th **T42.0X6**   **Underdosing of hydantoin derivatives**

   ✓5th **T42.1**   **Poisoning by, adverse effect of and underdosing of iminostilbenes**
     Poisoning by, adverse effect of and underdosing of carbamazepine

     ✓6th **T42.1X**   **Poisoning by, adverse effect of and underdosing of iminostilbenes**

       ✓7th **T42.1X1**   **Poisoning by iminostilbenes, accidental (unintentional)**
            Poisoning by iminostilbenes NOS

       2 ✓7th **T42.1X2**   **Poisoning by iminostilbenes, intentional self-harm**   HCC

       ✓7th **T42.1X3**   **Poisoning by iminostilbenes, assault**

       ✓7th **T42.1X4**   **Poisoning by iminostilbenes, undetermined**

       ✓7th **T42.1X5**   **Adverse effect of iminostilbenes**

       ✓7th **T42.1X6**   **Underdosing of iminostilbenes**

   ✓5th **T42.2**   **Poisoning by, adverse effect of and underdosing of succinimides and oxazolidinediones**

     ✓6th **T42.2X**   **Poisoning by, adverse effect of and underdosing of succinimides and oxazolidinediones**

       ✓7th **T42.2X1**   **Poisoning by succinimides and oxazolidinediones, accidental (unintentional)**
            Poisoning by succinimides and oxazolidinediones NOS

       2 ✓7th **T42.2X2**   **Poisoning by succinimides and oxazolidinediones, intentional self-harm**   HCC

       ✓7th **T42.2X3**   **Poisoning by succinimides and oxazolidinediones, assault**

       ✓7th **T42.2X4**   **Poisoning by succinimides and oxazolidinediones, undetermined**

       ✓7th **T42.2X5**   **Adverse effect of succinimides and oxazolidinediones**

       ✓7th **T42.2X6**   **Underdosing of succinimides and oxazolidinediones**

   ✓5th **T42.3**   **Poisoning by, adverse effect of and underdosing of barbiturates**
     EXCLUDES 1   *poisoning by, adverse effect of and underdosing of thiobarbiturates (T41.1-)*

     ✓6th **T42.3X**   **Poisoning by, adverse effect of and underdosing of barbiturates**

       ✓7th **T42.3X1**   **Poisoning by barbiturates, accidental (unintentional)**
            Poisoning by barbiturates NOS

       2 ✓7th **T42.3X2**   **Poisoning by barbiturates, intentional self-harm**   HCC

       ✓7th **T42.3X3**   **Poisoning by barbiturates, assault**

       ✓7th **T42.3X4**   **Poisoning by barbiturates, undetermined**

       ✓7th **T42.3X5**   **Adverse effect of barbiturates**

     ✓7th **T42.3X6**   **Underdosing of barbiturates**

   ✓5th **T42.4**   **Poisoning by, adverse effect of and underdosing of benzodiazepines**

     ✓6th **T42.4X**   **Poisoning by, adverse effect of and underdosing of benzodiazepines**

       ✓7th **T42.4X1**   **Poisoning by benzodiazepines, accidental (unintentional)**
            Poisoning by benzodiazepines NOS

       2 ✓7th **T42.4X2**   **Poisoning by benzodiazepines, intentional self-harm**   HCC

       ✓7th **T42.4X3**   **Poisoning by benzodiazepines, assault**

       ✓7th **T42.4X4**   **Poisoning by benzodiazepines, undetermined**

       ✓7th **T42.4X5**   **Adverse effect of benzodiazepines**

       ✓7th **T42.4X6**   **Underdosing of benzodiazepines**

   ✓5th **T42.5**   **Poisoning by, adverse effect of and underdosing of mixed antiepileptics**

     ✓6th **T42.5X**   **Poisoning by, adverse effect of and underdosing of antiepileptics**

       ✓7th **T42.5X1**   **Poisoning by mixed antiepileptics, accidental (unintentional)**
            Poisoning by mixed antiepileptics NOS

       2 ✓7th **T42.5X2**   **Poisoning by mixed antiepileptics, intentional self-harm**   HCC

       ✓7th **T42.5X3**   **Poisoning by mixed antiepileptics, assault**

       ✓7th **T42.5X4**   **Poisoning by mixed antiepileptics, undetermined**

       ✓7th **T42.5X5**   **Adverse effect of mixed antiepileptics**

       ✓7th **T42.5X6**   **Underdosing of mixed antiepileptics**

   ✓5th **T42.6**   **Poisoning by, adverse effect of and underdosing of other antiepileptic and sedative-hypnotic drugs**
     Poisoning by, adverse effect of and underdosing of methaqualone
     Poisoning by, adverse effect of and underdosing of valproic acid
     EXCLUDES 1   *poisoning by, adverse effect of and underdosing of carbamazepine (T42.1-)*

     ✓6th **T42.6X**   **Poisoning by, adverse effect of and underdosing of other antiepileptic and sedative-hypnotic drugs**

       ✓7th **T42.6X1**   **Poisoning by other antiepileptic and sedative-hypnotic drugs, accidental (unintentional)**
            Poisoning by other antiepileptic and sedative-hypnotic drugs NOS

       2 ✓7th **T42.6X2**   **Poisoning by other antiepileptic and sedative-hypnotic drugs, intentional self-harm**   HCC

       ✓7th **T42.6X3**   **Poisoning by other antiepileptic and sedative-hypnotic drugs, assault**

       ✓7th **T42.6X4**   **Poisoning by other antiepileptic and sedative-hypnotic drugs, undetermined**

       ✓7th **T42.6X5**   **Adverse effect of other antiepileptic and sedative-hypnotic drugs**

       ✓7th **T42.6X6**   **Underdosing of other antiepileptic and sedative-hypnotic drugs**

   ✓5th **T42.7**   **Poisoning by, adverse effect of and underdosing of unspecified antiepileptic and sedative-hypnotic drugs**

     ✓x7th **T42.71**   **Poisoning by unspecified antiepileptic and sedative-hypnotic drugs, accidental (unintentional)** ▽
       Poisoning by antiepileptic and sedative-hypnotic drugs NOS

     2 ✓x7th **T42.72**   **Poisoning by unspecified antiepileptic and sedative-hypnotic drugs, intentional self-harm**   HCC ▽

     ✓x7th **T42.73**   **Poisoning by unspecified antiepileptic and sedative-hypnotic drugs, assault** ▽

     ✓x7th **T42.74**   **Poisoning by unspecified antiepileptic and sedative-hypnotic drugs, undetermined** ▽

     ✓x7th **T42.75**   **Adverse effect of unspecified antiepileptic and sedative-hypnotic drugs** ▽

     ✓x7th **T42.76**   **Underdosing of unspecified antiepileptic and sedative-hypnotic drugs** ▽

---

2   HCC with 7th character indicating initial encounter (A or B - specific to category) OR sequela.

EXCLUDES 1 Not coded here   EXCLUDES 2 Not included here   N Newborn Age: 0   P Pediatric Age: 0-17   M Maternity Age: 12-55   A Adult Age: 15-124

1066   ICD-10-CM 2018

√5th **T42.8** **Poisoning by, adverse effect of and underdosing of antiparkinsonism drugs and other central muscle-tone depressants**
Poisoning by, adverse effect of and underdosing of amantadine

√6th **T42.8X** **Poisoning by, adverse effect of and underdosing of antiparkinsonism drugs and other central muscle-tone depressants**

√7th **T42.8X1** **Poisoning by antiparkinsonism drugs and other central muscle-tone depressants, accidental (unintentional)**
Poisoning by antiparkinsonism drugs and other central muscle-tone depressants NOS

2 √7th **T42.8X2** **Poisoning by antiparkinsonism drugs** HCC **and other central muscle-tone depressants, intentional self-harm**

√7th **T42.8X3** **Poisoning by antiparkinsonism drugs and other central muscle-tone depressants, assault**

√7th **T42.8X4** **Poisoning by antiparkinsonism drugs and other central muscle-tone depressants, undetermined**

√7th **T42.8X5** **Adverse effect of antiparkinsonism drugs and other central muscle-tone depressants**

√7th **T42.8X6** **Underdosing of antiparkinsonism drugs and other central muscle-tone depressants**

√4th **T43** **Poisoning by, adverse effect of and underdosing of psychotropic drugs, not elsewhere classified**

EXCLUDES 1 appetite depressants (T50.5-)
barbiturates (T42.3-)
benzodiazepines (T42.4-)
methaqualone (T42.6-)
psychodysleptics [hallucinogens] (T40.7-T40.9-)

EXCLUDES 2 drug dependence and related mental and behavioral disorders due to psychoactive substance use (F10.- -F19.-)

The appropriate 7th character is to be added to each code from category T43.
A initial encounter
D subsequent encounter
S sequela

√5th **T43.0** **Poisoning by, adverse effect of and underdosing of tricyclic and tetracyclic antidepressants**

√6th **T43.01** **Poisoning by, adverse effect of and underdosing of tricyclic antidepressants**

√7th **T43.011** **Poisoning by tricyclic antidepressants, accidental (unintentional)**
Poisoning by tricyclic antidepressants NOS

2 √7th **T43.012** **Poisoning by tricyclic antidepressants,** HCC **intentional self-harm**

√7th **T43.013** **Poisoning by tricyclic antidepressants, assault**

√7th **T43.014** **Poisoning by tricyclic antidepressants, undetermined**

√7th **T43.015** **Adverse effect of tricyclic antidepressants**

√7th **T43.016** **Underdosing of tricyclic antidepressants**

√6th **T43.02** **Poisoning by, adverse effect of and underdosing of tetracyclic antidepressants**

√7th **T43.021** **Poisoning by tetracyclic antidepressants, accidental (unintentional)**
Poisoning by tetracyclic antidepressants NOS

2 √7th **T43.022** **Poisoning by tetracyclic** HCC **antidepressants, intentional self-harm**

√7th **T43.023** **Poisoning by tetracyclic antidepressants, assault**

√7th **T43.024** **Poisoning by tetracyclic antidepressants, undetermined**

√7th **T43.025** **Adverse effect of tetracyclic antidepressants**

√7th **T43.026** **Underdosing of tetracyclic antidepressants**

√5th **T43.1** **Poisoning by, adverse effect of and underdosing of monoamine-oxidase-inhibitor antidepressants**

√6th **T43.1X** **Poisoning by, adverse effect of and underdosing of monoamine-oxidase-inhibitor antidepressants**

√7th **T43.1X1** **Poisoning by monoamine-oxidase-inhibitor antidepressants, accidental (unintentional)**
Poisoning by monoamine-oxidase-inhibitor antidepressants NOS

2 √7th **T43.1X2** **Poisoning by monoamine-oxidase-** HCC **inhibitor antidepressants, intentional self-harm**

√7th **T43.1X3** **Poisoning by monoamine-oxidase-inhibitor antidepressants, assault**

√7th **T43.1X4** **Poisoning by monoamine-oxidase-inhibitor antidepressants, undetermined**

√7th **T43.1X5** **Adverse effect of monoamine-oxidase-inhibitor antidepressants**

√7th **T43.1X6** **Underdosing of monoamine-oxidase-inhibitor antidepressants**

√5th **T43.2** **Poisoning by, adverse effect of and underdosing of other and unspecified antidepressants**

√6th **T43.20** **Poisoning by, adverse effect of and underdosing of unspecified antidepressants**

√7th **T43.201** **Poisoning by unspecified anti-depressants, accidental (unintentional)** ▽
Poisoning by antidepressants NOS

2 √7th **T43.202** **Poisoning by unspecified anti-** HCC ▽ **depressants, intentional self-harm**

√7th **T43.203** **Poisoning by unspecified anti-depressants, assault** ▽

√7th **T43.204** **Poisoning by unspecified anti-depressants, undetermined** ▽

√7th **T43.205** **Adverse effect of unspecified antidepressants** ▽
▶Antidepressant discontinuation syndrome◀

√7th **T43.206** **Underdosing of unspecified antidepressants** ▽

√6th **T43.21** **Poisoning by, adverse effect of and underdosing of selective serotonin and norepinephrine reuptake inhibitors**
Poisoning by, adverse effect of and underdosing of SSNRI antidepressants

√7th **T43.211** **Poisoning by selective serotonin and norepinephrine reuptake inhibitors, accidental (unintentional)**

2 √7th **T43.212** **Poisoning by selective serotonin and** HCC **norepinephrine reuptake inhibitors, intentional self-harm**

√7th **T43.213** **Poisoning by selective serotonin and norepinephrine reuptake inhibitors, assault**

√7th **T43.214** **Poisoning by selective serotonin and norepinephrine reuptake inhibitors, undetermined**

√7th **T43.215** **Adverse effect of selective serotonin and norepinephrine reuptake inhibitors**

√7th **T43.216** **Underdosing of selective serotonin and norepinephrine reuptake inhibitors**

√6th **T43.22** **Poisoning by, adverse effect of and underdosing of selective serotonin reuptake inhibitors**
Poisoning by, adverse effect of and underdosing of SSRI antidepressants

√7th **T43.221** **Poisoning by selective serotonin reuptake inhibitors, accidental (unintentional)**

2 √7th **T43.222** **Poisoning by selective serotonin** HCC **reuptake inhibitors, intentional self-harm**

√7th **T43.223** **Poisoning by selective serotonin reuptake inhibitors, assault**

√7th **T43.224** **Poisoning by selective serotonin reuptake inhibitors, undetermined**

√7th **T43.225** **Adverse effect of selective serotonin reuptake inhibitors**

√7th **T43.226** **Underdosing of selective serotonin reuptake inhibitors**

2 HCC with 7th character indicating initial encounter (A or B - specific to category) OR sequela.

☑ Additional Character Req   ✓7th Placeholder Alert   Manifestation   HCC CMS-HCC Condition   ▽ Unspecified Code   ▶◀ Revised Text   ● New Code   ▲ Revised Code Title
ICD-10-CM 2018   1067

Chapter 19. Injury, Poisoning, and Certain Other Consequences of External Causes

T42.8–T43.226

√6ᵗʰ **T43.29** **Poisoning by, adverse effect of and underdosing of other antidepressants**

　　√7ᵗʰ **T43.291** **Poisoning by other antidepressants, accidental (unintentional)**
　　　　Poisoning by other antidepressants NOS

　　² √7ᵗʰ **T43.292** **Poisoning by other antidepressants, intentional self-harm** HCC

　　√7ᵗʰ **T43.293** **Poisoning by other antidepressants, assault**

　　√7ᵗʰ **T43.294** **Poisoning by other antidepressants, undetermined**

　　√7ᵗʰ **T43.295** **Adverse effect of other antidepressants**

　　√7ᵗʰ **T43.296** **Underdosing of other antidepressants**

√5ᵗʰ **T43.3** **Poisoning by, adverse effect of and underdosing of phenothiazine antipsychotics and neuroleptics**

　√6ᵗʰ **T43.3X** **Poisoning by, adverse effect of and underdosing of phenothiazine antipsychotics and neuroleptics**

　　√7ᵗʰ **T43.3X1** **Poisoning by phenothiazine antipsychotics and neuroleptics, accidental (unintentional)**
　　　　Poisoning by phenothiazine antipsychotics and neuroleptics NOS

　　² √7ᵗʰ **T43.3X2** **Poisoning by phenothiazine antipsychotics and neuroleptics, intentional self-harm** HCC

　　√7ᵗʰ **T43.3X3** **Poisoning by phenothiazine antipsychotics and neuroleptics, assault**

　　√7ᵗʰ **T43.3X4** **Poisoning by phenothiazine antipsychotics and neuroleptics, undetermined**

　　√7ᵗʰ **T43.3X5** **Adverse effect of phenothiazine antipsychotics and neuroleptics**

　　√7ᵗʰ **T43.3X6** **Underdosing of phenothiazine antipsychotics and neuroleptics**

√5ᵗʰ **T43.4** **Poisoning by, adverse effect of and underdosing of butyrophenone and thiothixene neuroleptics**

　√6ᵗʰ **T43.4X** **Poisoning by, adverse effect of and underdosing of butyrophenone and thiothixene neuroleptics**

　　√7ᵗʰ **T43.4X1** **Poisoning by butyrophenone and thiothixene neuroleptics, accidental (unintentional)**
　　　　Poisoning by butyrophenone and thiothixene neuroleptics NOS

　　² √7ᵗʰ **T43.4X2** **Poisoning by butyrophenone and thiothixene neuroleptics, intentional self-harm** HCC

　　√7ᵗʰ **T43.4X3** **Poisoning by butyrophenone and thiothixene neuroleptics, assault**

　　√7ᵗʰ **T43.4X4** **Poisoning by butyrophenone and thiothixene neuroleptics, undetermined**

　　√7ᵗʰ **T43.4X5** **Adverse effect of butyrophenone and thiothixene neuroleptics**

　　√7ᵗʰ **T43.4X6** **Underdosing of butyrophenone and thiothixene neuroleptics**

√5ᵗʰ **T43.5** **Poisoning by, adverse effect of and underdosing of other and unspecified antipsychotics and neuroleptics**
　　EXCLUDES 1　*poisoning by, adverse effect of and underdosing of rauwolfia (T46.5-)*

　√6ᵗʰ **T43.50** **Poisoning by, adverse effect of and underdosing of unspecified antipsychotics and neuroleptics**

　　√7ᵗʰ **T43.501** **Poisoning by unspecified anti-psychotics and neuroleptics, accidental (unintentional)** ▽
　　　　Poisoning by antipsychotics and neuroleptics NOS

　　² √7ᵗʰ **T43.502** **Poisoning by unspecified anti-psychotics and neuroleptics, intentional self-harm** HCC ▽

　　√7ᵗʰ **T43.503** **Poisoning by unspecified anti-psychotics and neuroleptics, assault** ▽

　　√7ᵗʰ **T43.504** **Poisoning by unspecified anti-psychotics and neuroleptics, undetermined** ▽

　　√7ᵗʰ **T43.505** **Adverse effect of unspecified antipsychotics and neuroleptics** ▽

　　√7ᵗʰ **T43.506** **Underdosing of unspecified antipsychotics and neuroleptics** ▽

√6ᵗʰ **T43.59** **Poisoning by, adverse effect of and underdosing of other antipsychotics and neuroleptics**
　　AHA: 2017, 1Q, 40

　　√7ᵗʰ **T43.591** **Poisoning by other antipsychotics and neuroleptics, accidental (unintentional)**
　　　　Poisoning by other antipsychotics and neuroleptics NOS

　　² √7ᵗʰ **T43.592** **Poisoning by other antipsychotics and neuroleptics, intentional self-harm** HCC

　　√7ᵗʰ **T43.593** **Poisoning by other antipsychotics and neuroleptics, assault**

　　√7ᵗʰ **T43.594** **Poisoning by other antipsychotics and neuroleptics, undetermined**

　　√7ᵗʰ **T43.595** **Adverse effect of other antipsychotics and neuroleptics**

　　√7ᵗʰ **T43.596** **Underdosing of other antipsychotics and neuroleptics**

√5ᵗʰ **T43.6** **Poisoning by, adverse effect of and underdosing of psychostimulants**
　　EXCLUDES 1　*poisoning by, adverse effect of and underdosing of cocaine (T40.5-)*

　√6ᵗʰ **T43.60** **Poisoning by, adverse effect of and underdosing of unspecified psychostimulant**

　　√7ᵗʰ **T43.601** **Poisoning by unspecified psychostimulants, accidental (unintentional)** ▽
　　　　Poisoning by psychostimulants NOS

　　² √7ᵗʰ **T43.602** **Poisoning by unspecified psychostimulants, intentional self-harm** HCC ▽

　　√7ᵗʰ **T43.603** **Poisoning by unspecified psychostimulants, assault** ▽

　　√7ᵗʰ **T43.604** **Poisoning by unspecified psychostimulants, undetermined** ▽

　　√7ᵗʰ **T43.605** **Adverse effect of unspecified psychostimulants** ▽

　　√7ᵗʰ **T43.606** **Underdosing of unspecified psychostimulants** ▽

　√6ᵗʰ **T43.61** **Poisoning by, adverse effect of and underdosing of caffeine**

　　√7ᵗʰ **T43.611** **Poisoning by caffeine, accidental (unintentional)**
　　　　Poisoning by caffeine NOS

　　² √7ᵗʰ **T43.612** **Poisoning by caffeine, intentional self-harm** HCC

　　√7ᵗʰ **T43.613** **Poisoning by caffeine, assault**

　　√7ᵗʰ **T43.614** **Poisoning by caffeine, undetermined**

　　√7ᵗʰ **T43.615** **Adverse effect of caffeine**

　　√7ᵗʰ **T43.616** **Underdosing of caffeine**

　√6ᵗʰ **T43.62** **Poisoning by, adverse effect of and underdosing of amphetamines**
　　　　Poisoning by, adverse effect of and underdosing of methamphetamines

　　√7ᵗʰ **T43.621** **Poisoning by amphetamines, accidental (unintentional)**
　　　　Poisoning by amphetamines NOS

　　² √7ᵗʰ **T43.622** **Poisoning by amphetamines, intentional self-harm** HCC

　　√7ᵗʰ **T43.623** **Poisoning by amphetamines, assault**

　　√7ᵗʰ **T43.624** **Poisoning by amphetamines, undetermined**

　　√7ᵗʰ **T43.625** **Adverse effect of amphetamines**

　　√7ᵗʰ **T43.626** **Underdosing of amphetamines**

　√6ᵗʰ **T43.63** **Poisoning by, adverse effect of and underdosing of methylphenidate**

　　√7ᵗʰ **T43.631** **Poisoning by methylphenidate, accidental (unintentional)**
　　　　Poisoning by methylphenidate NOS

　　² √7ᵗʰ **T43.632** **Poisoning by methylphenidate, intentional self-harm** HCC

　　√7ᵗʰ **T43.633** **Poisoning by methylphenidate, assault**

　　√7ᵗʰ **T43.634** **Poisoning by methylphenidate, undetermined**

　　√7ᵗʰ **T43.635** **Adverse effect of methylphenidate**

---

² HCC with 7th character indicating initial encounter (A or B - specific to category) OR sequela.

EXCLUDES 1 Not coded here　　　*EXCLUDES 2* Not included here　　　N Newborn Age: 0　　　P Pediatric Age: 0-17　　　M Maternity Age: 12-55　　　A Adult Age: 15-124

ICD-10-CM 2018

1068

√7ᵗʰ **T43.636**   Underdosing of methylphenidate

√6ᵗʰ **T43.69**   **Poisoning by, adverse effect of and underdosing of other psychostimulants**

√7ᵗʰ **T43.691**   **Poisoning by other psychostimulants, accidental (unintentional)**
Poisoning by other psychostimulants NOS

2 √7ᵗʰ **T43.692**   **Poisoning by other psychostimulants, intentional self-harm** HCC

√7ᵗʰ **T43.693**   **Poisoning by other psychostimulants, assault**

√7ᵗʰ **T43.694**   **Poisoning by other psychostimulants, undetermined**

√7ᵗʰ **T43.695**   Adverse effect of other psychostimulants

√7ᵗʰ **T43.696**   Underdosing of other psychostimulants

√5ᵗʰ **T43.8**   **Poisoning by, adverse effect of and underdosing of other psychotropic drugs**

√6ᵗʰ **T43.8X**   **Poisoning by, adverse effect of and underdosing of other psychotropic drugs**

√7ᵗʰ **T43.8X1**   **Poisoning by other psychotropic drugs, accidental (unintentional)**
Poisoning by other psychotropic drugs NOS

2 √7ᵗʰ **T43.8X2**   **Poisoning by other psychotropic drugs, intentional self-harm** HCC

√7ᵗʰ **T43.8X3**   **Poisoning by other psychotropic drugs, assault**

√7ᵗʰ **T43.8X4**   **Poisoning by other psychotropic drugs, undetermined**

√7ᵗʰ **T43.8X5**   Adverse effect of other psychotropic drugs

√7ᵗʰ **T43.8X6**   Underdosing of other psychotropic drugs

√5ᵗʰ **T43.9**   **Poisoning by, adverse effect of and underdosing of unspecified psychotropic drug**

√x7ᵗʰ **T43.91**   **Poisoning by unspecified psychotropic drug, accidental (unintentional)**   ▽
Poisoning by psychotropic drug NOS

2 √x7ᵗʰ **T43.92**   **Poisoning by unspecified psychotropic drug, intentional self-harm** HCC ▽

√x7ᵗʰ **T43.93**   **Poisoning by unspecified psychotropic drug, assault**   ▽

√x7ᵗʰ **T43.94**   **Poisoning by unspecified psychotropic drug, undetermined**   ▽

√x7ᵗʰ **T43.95**   Adverse effect of unspecified psychotropic drug   ▽

√x7ᵗʰ **T43.96**   Underdosing of unspecified psychotropic drug   ▽

√4ᵗʰ **T44**   **Poisoning by, adverse effect of and underdosing of drugs primarily affecting the autonomic nervous system**

The appropriate 7th character is to be added to each code from category T44.
A   initial encounter
D   subsequent encounter
S   sequela

√5ᵗʰ **T44.0**   **Poisoning by, adverse effect of and underdosing of anticholinesterase agents**

√6ᵗʰ **T44.0X**   **Poisoning by, adverse effect of and underdosing of anticholinesterase agents**

√7ᵗʰ **T44.0X1**   **Poisoning by anticholinesterase agents, accidental (unintentional)**
Poisoning by anticholinesterase agents NOS

2 √7ᵗʰ **T44.0X2**   **Poisoning by anticholinesterase agents, intentional self-harm** HCC

√7ᵗʰ **T44.0X3**   **Poisoning by anticholinesterase agents, assault**

√7ᵗʰ **T44.0X4**   **Poisoning by anticholinesterase agents, undetermined**

√7ᵗʰ **T44.0X5**   Adverse effect of anticholinesterase agents

√7ᵗʰ **T44.0X6**   Underdosing of anticholinesterase agents

√5ᵗʰ **T44.1**   **Poisoning by, adverse effect of and underdosing of other parasympathomimetics [cholinergics]**

√6ᵗʰ **T44.1X**   **Poisoning by, adverse effect of and underdosing of other parasympathomimetics [cholinergics]**

√7ᵗʰ **T44.1X1**   **Poisoning by other parasympathomimetics [cholinergics], accidental (unintentional)**
Poisoning by other parasympathomimetics [cholinergics] NOS

2 √7ᵗʰ **T44.1X2**   **Poisoning by other parasympathomimetics [cholinergics], intentional self-harm** HCC

√7ᵗʰ **T44.1X3**   **Poisoning by other parasympathomimetics [cholinergics], assault**

√7ᵗʰ **T44.1X4**   **Poisoning by other parasympathomimetics [cholinergics], undetermined**

√7ᵗʰ **T44.1X5**   Adverse effect of other parasympathomimetics [cholinergics]

√7ᵗʰ **T44.1X6**   Underdosing of other parasympathomimetics

√5ᵗʰ **T44.2**   **Poisoning by, adverse effect of and underdosing of ganglionic blocking drugs**

√6ᵗʰ **T44.2X**   **Poisoning by, adverse effect of and underdosing of ganglionic blocking drugs**

√7ᵗʰ **T44.2X1**   **Poisoning by ganglionic blocking drugs, accidental (unintentional)**
Poisoning by ganglionic blocking drugs NOS

2 √7ᵗʰ **T44.2X2**   **Poisoning by ganglionic blocking drugs, intentional self-harm** HCC

√7ᵗʰ **T44.2X3**   **Poisoning by ganglionic blocking drugs, assault**

√7ᵗʰ **T44.2X4**   **Poisoning by ganglionic blocking drugs, undetermined**

√7ᵗʰ **T44.2X5**   Adverse effect of ganglionic blocking drugs

√7ᵗʰ **T44.2X6**   Underdosing of ganglionic blocking drugs

√5ᵗʰ **T44.3**   **Poisoning by, adverse effect of and underdosing of other parasympatholytics [anticholinergics and antimuscarinics] and spasmolytics**
Poisoning by, adverse effect of and underdosing of papaverine

√6ᵗʰ **T44.3X**   **Poisoning by, adverse effect of and underdosing of other parasympatholytics [anticholinergics and antimuscarinics] and spasmolytics**

√7ᵗʰ **T44.3X1**   **Poisoning by other parasympatholytics [anticholinergics and antimuscarinics] and spasmolytics, accidental (unintentional)**
Poisoning by other parasympatholytics [anticholinergics and antimuscarinics] and spasmolytics NOS

2 √7ᵗʰ **T44.3X2**   **Poisoning by other parasympatholytics [anticholinergics and antimuscarinics] and spasmolytics, intentional self-harm** HCC

√7ᵗʰ **T44.3X3**   **Poisoning by other parasympatholytics [anticholinergics and antimuscarinics] and spasmolytics, assault**

√7ᵗʰ **T44.3X4**   **Poisoning by other parasympatholytics [anticholinergics and antimuscarinics] and spasmolytics, undetermined**

√7ᵗʰ **T44.3X5**   Adverse effect of other parasympatholytics [anticholinergics and antimuscarinics] and spasmolytics

√7ᵗʰ **T44.3X6**   Underdosing of other parasympatholytics [anticholinergics and antimuscarinics] and spasmolytics

---

2   HCC with 7th character indicating initial encounter (A or B - specific to category) OR sequela.

✔ Additional Character Req   √x7ᵗʰ Placeholder Alert   Manifestation   HCC CMS-HCC Condition   ▽ Unspecified Code   ▶◀ Revised Text   ● New Code   ▲ Revised Code Title

√5th **T44.4** **Poisoning by, adverse effect of and underdosing of predominantly alpha-adrenoreceptor agonists**
Poisoning by, adverse effect of and underdosing of metaraminol

√6th **T44.4X** **Poisoning by, adverse effect of and underdosing of predominantly alpha-adrenoreceptor agonists**

√7th **T44.4X1** **Poisoning by predominantly alpha-adrenoreceptor agonists, accidental (unintentional)**
Poisoning by predominantly alpha-adrenoreceptor agonists NOS

2 √7th **T44.4X2** **Poisoning by predominantly alpha adrenoreceptor agonists, intentional self-harm** HCC

√7th **T44.4X3** **Poisoning by predominantly alpha-adrenoreceptor agonists, assault**

√7th **T44.4X4** **Poisoning by predominantly alpha-adrenoreceptor agonists, undetermined**

√7th **T44.4X5** **Adverse effect of predominantly alpha-adrenoreceptor agonists**

√7th **T44.4X6** **Underdosing of predominantly alpha-adrenoreceptor agonists**

√5th **T44.5** **Poisoning by, adverse effect of and underdosing of predominantly beta-adrenoreceptor agonists**

EXCLUDES 1 poisoning by, adverse effect of and underdosing of beta-adrenoreceptor agonists used in asthma therapy (T48.6-)

√6th **T44.5X** **Poisoning by, adverse effect of and underdosing of predominantly beta-adrenoreceptor agonists**

√7th **T44.5X1** **Poisoning by predominantly beta-adrenoreceptor agonists, accidental (unintentional)**
Poisoning by predominantly beta-adrenoreceptor agonists NOS

2 √7th **T44.5X2** **Poisoning by predominantly beta-adrenoreceptor agonists, intentional self-harm** HCC

√7th **T44.5X3** **Poisoning by predominantly beta-adrenoreceptor agonists, assault**

√7th **T44.5X4** **Poisoning by predominantly beta-adrenoreceptor agonists, undetermined**

√7th **T44.5X5** **Adverse effect of predominantly beta-adrenoreceptor agonists**

√7th **T44.5X6** **Underdosing of predominantly beta-adrenoreceptor agonists**

√5th **T44.6** **Poisoning by, adverse effect of and underdosing of alpha-adrenoreceptor antagonists**

EXCLUDES 1 poisoning by, adverse effect of and underdosing of ergot alkaloids (T48.0)

√6th **T44.6X** **Poisoning by, adverse effect of and underdosing of alpha-adrenoreceptor antagonists**

√7th **T44.6X1** **Poisoning by alpha-adrenoreceptor antagonists, accidental (unintentional)**
Poisoning by alpha-adrenoreceptor antagonists NOS

2 √7th **T44.6X2** **Poisoning by alpha-adrenoreceptor antagonists, intentional self-harm** HCC

√7th **T44.6X3** **Poisoning by alpha-adrenoreceptor antagonists, assault**

√7th **T44.6X4** **Poisoning by alpha-adrenoreceptor antagonists, undetermined**

√7th **T44.6X5** **Adverse effect of alpha-adrenoreceptor antagonists**

√7th **T44.6X6** **Underdosing of alpha-adrenoreceptor antagonists**

√5th **T44.7** **Poisoning by, adverse effect of and underdosing of beta-adrenoreceptor antagonists**

√6th **T44.7X** **Poisoning by, adverse effect of and underdosing of beta-adrenoreceptor antagonists**

√7th **T44.7X1** **Poisoning by beta-adrenoreceptor antagonists, accidental (unintentional)**
Poisoning by beta-adrenoreceptor antagonists NOS

2 √7th **T44.7X2** **Poisoning by beta-adrenoreceptor antagonists, intentional self-harm** HCC

√7th **T44.7X3** **Poisoning by beta-adrenoreceptor antagonists, assault**

√7th **T44.7X4** **Poisoning by beta-adrenoreceptor antagonists, undetermined**

√7th **T44.7X5** **Adverse effect of beta-adrenoreceptor antagonists**

√7th **T44.7X6** **Underdosing of beta-adrenoreceptor antagonists**

√5th **T44.8** **Poisoning by, adverse effect of and underdosing of centrally-acting and adrenergic-neuron- blocking agents**

EXCLUDES 1 poisoning by, adverse effect of and underdosing of clonidine (T46.5)
poisoning by, adverse effect of and underdosing of guanethidine (T46.5)

√6th **T44.8X** **Poisoning by, adverse effect of and underdosing of centrally-acting and adrenergic-neuron-blocking agents**

√7th **T44.8X1** **Poisoning by centrally-acting and adrenergic-neuron-blocking agents, accidental (unintentional)**
Poisoning by centrally-acting and adrenergic-neuron-blocking agents NOS

2 √7th **T44.8X2** **Poisoning by centrally-acting and adrenergic-neuron-blocking agents, intentional self-harm** HCC

√7th **T44.8X3** **Poisoning by centrally-acting and adrenergic-neuron-blocking agents, assault**

√7th **T44.8X4** **Poisoning by centrally-acting and adrenergic-neuron-blocking agents, undetermined**

√7th **T44.8X5** **Adverse effect of centrally-acting and adrenergic-neuron-blocking agents**

√7th **T44.8X6** **Underdosing of centrally-acting and adrenergic-neuron-blocking agents**

√5th **T44.9** **Poisoning by, adverse effect of and underdosing of other and unspecified drugs primarily affecting the autonomic nervous system**
Poisoning by, adverse effect of and underdosing of drug stimulating both alpha and beta-adrenoreceptors

√6th **T44.90** **Poisoning by, adverse effect of and underdosing of unspecified drugs primarily affecting the autonomic nervous system**

√7th **T44.901** **Poisoning by unspecified drugs primarily affecting the autonomic nervous system, accidental (unintentional)** ▽
Poisoning by unspecified drugs primarily affecting the autonomic nervous system NOS

2 √7th **T44.902** **Poisoning by unspecified drugs primarily affecting the autonomic nervous system, intentional self-harm** HCC ▽

√7th **T44.903** **Poisoning by unspecified drugs primarily affecting the autonomic nervous system, assault** ▽

√7th **T44.904** **Poisoning by unspecified drugs primarily affecting the autonomic nervous system, undetermined** ▽

√7th **T44.905** **Adverse effect of unspecified drugs primarily affecting the autonomic nervous system** ▽

√7th **T44.906** **Underdosing of unspecified drugs primarily affecting the autonomic nervous system** ▽

√6th **T44.99** **Poisoning by, adverse effect of and underdosing of other drugs primarily affecting the autonomic nervous system**

√7th **T44.991** **Poisoning by other drug primarily affecting the autonomic nervous system, accidental (unintentional)**
Poisoning by other drugs primarily affecting the autonomic nervous system NOS

2 √7th **T44.992** **Poisoning by other drug primarily affecting the autonomic nervous system, intentional self-harm** HCC

---

2   HCC with 7th character indicating initial encounter (A or B - specific to category) OR sequela.

EXCLUDES 1 Not coded here   **EXCLUDES 2** Not included here   N Newborn Age: 0   P Pediatric Age: 0-17   M Maternity Age: 12-55   A Adult Age: 15-124

ICD-10-CM 2018

1070

√7ᵗʰ **T44.993 Poisoning by other drug primarily affecting the autonomic nervous system, assault**

√7ᵗʰ **T44.994 Poisoning by other drug primarily affecting the autonomic nervous system, undetermined**

√7ᵗʰ **T44.995 Adverse effect of other drug primarily affecting the autonomic nervous system**

√7ᵗʰ **T44.996 Underdosing of other drug primarily affecting the autonomic nervous system**

√4ᵗʰ **T45 Poisoning by, adverse effect of and underdosing of primarily systemic and hematological agents, not elsewhere classified**

> The appropriate 7th character is to be added to each code from category T45.
> A   initial encounter
> D   subsequent encounter
> S   sequela

√5ᵗʰ **T45.0 Poisoning by, adverse effect of and underdosing of antiallergic and antiemetic drugs**
> EXCLUDES 1   poisoning by, adverse effect of and underdosing of phenothiazine-based neuroleptics (T43.3)

√6ᵗʰ **T45.0X Poisoning by, adverse effect of and underdosing of antiallergic and antiemetic drugs**

√7ᵗʰ **T45.0X1 Poisoning by antiallergic and antiemetic drugs, accidental (unintentional)**
> Poisoning by antiallergic and antiemetic drugs NOS

2 √7ᵗʰ **T45.0X2 Poisoning by antiallergic and antie metic drugs, intentional self-harm** HCC

√7ᵗʰ **T45.0X3 Poisoning by antiallergic and antiemetic drugs, assault**

√7ᵗʰ **T45.0X4 Poisoning by antiallergic and antiemetic drugs, undetermined**

√7ᵗʰ **T45.0X5 Adverse effect of antiallergic and antiemetic drugs**

√7ᵗʰ **T45.0X6 Underdosing of antiallergic and antiemetic drugs**

√5ᵗʰ **T45.1 Poisoning by, adverse effect of and underdosing of antineoplastic and immunosuppressive drugs**
> EXCLUDES 1   poisoning by, adverse effect of and underdosing of tamoxifen (T38.6)
> **AHA:** 2014, 4Q, 22

√6ᵗʰ **T45.1X Poisoning by, adverse effect of and underdosing of antineoplastic and immunosuppressive drugs**

√7ᵗʰ **T45.1X1 Poisoning by antineoplastic and immunosuppressive drugs, accidental (unintentional)**
> Poisoning by antineoplastic and immunosuppressive drugs NOS

2 √7ᵗʰ **T45.1X2 Poisoning by antineoplastic and immunosuppressive drugs, intentional self-harm** HCC

√7ᵗʰ **T45.1X3 Poisoning by antineoplastic and immunosuppressive drugs, assault**

√7ᵗʰ **T45.1X4 Poisoning by antineoplastic and immunosuppressive drugs, undetermined**

√7ᵗʰ **T45.1X5 Adverse effect of antineoplastic and immunosuppressive drugs**

√7ᵗʰ **T45.1X6 Underdosing of antineoplastic and immunosuppressive drugs**

√5ᵗʰ **T45.2 Poisoning by, adverse effect of and underdosing of vitamins**
> EXCLUDES 2   poisoning by, adverse effect of and underdosing of iron (T45.4)
> poisoning by, adverse effect of and underdosing of nicotinic acid (derivatives) (T46.7)
> poisoning by, adverse effect of and underdosing of vitamin K (T45.7)

√6ᵗʰ **T45.2X Poisoning by, adverse effect of and underdosing of vitamins**

√7ᵗʰ **T45.2X1 Poisoning by vitamins, accidental (unintentional)**
> Poisoning by vitamins NOS

2 √7ᵗʰ **T45.2X2 Poisoning by vitamins, intentional self-harm** HCC

√7ᵗʰ **T45.2X3 Poisoning by vitamins, assault**

√7ᵗʰ **T45.2X4 Poisoning by vitamins, undetermined**

√7ᵗʰ **T45.2X5 Adverse effect of vitamins**

√7ᵗʰ **T45.2X6 Underdosing of vitamins**
> EXCLUDES 1   vitamin deficiencies (E50-E56)

√5ᵗʰ **T45.3 Poisoning by, adverse effect of and underdosing of enzymes**

√6ᵗʰ **T45.3X Poisoning by, adverse effect of and underdosing of enzymes**

√7ᵗʰ **T45.3X1 Poisoning by enzymes, accidental (unintentional)**
> Poisoning by enzymes NOS

2 √7ᵗʰ **T45.3X2 Poisoning by enzymes, intentional self-harm** HCC

√7ᵗʰ **T45.3X3 Poisoning by enzymes, assault**

√7ᵗʰ **T45.3X4 Poisoning by enzymes, undetermined**

√7ᵗʰ **T45.3X5 Adverse effect of enzymes**

√7ᵗʰ **T45.3X6 Underdosing of enzymes**

√5ᵗʰ **T45.4 Poisoning by, adverse effect of and underdosing of iron and its compounds**

√6ᵗʰ **T45.4X Poisoning by, adverse effect of and underdosing of iron and its compounds**

√7ᵗʰ **T45.4X1 Poisoning by iron and its compounds, accidental (unintentional)**
> Poisoning by iron and its compounds NOS

2 √7ᵗʰ **T45.4X2 Poisoning by iron and its compounds, intentional self-harm** HCC

√7ᵗʰ **T45.4X3 Poisoning by iron and its compounds, assault**

√7ᵗʰ **T45.4X4 Poisoning by iron and its compounds, undetermined**

√7ᵗʰ **T45.4X5 Adverse effect of iron and its compounds**

√7ᵗʰ **T45.4X6 Underdosing of iron and its compounds**
> EXCLUDES 1   iron deficiency (E61.1)

√5ᵗʰ **T45.5 Poisoning by, adverse effect of and underdosing of anticoagulants and antithrombotic drugs**

√6ᵗʰ **T45.51 Poisoning by, adverse effect of and underdosing of anticoagulants**

√7ᵗʰ **T45.511 Poisoning by anticoagulants, accidental (unintentional)**
> Poisoning by anticoagulants NOS

2 √7ᵗʰ **T45.512 Poisoning by anticoagulants, intentional self-harm** HCC

√7ᵗʰ **T45.513 Poisoning by anticoagulants, assault**

√7ᵗʰ **T45.514 Poisoning by anticoagulants, undetermined**

√7ᵗʰ **T45.515 Adverse effect of anticoagulants**
> **AHA:** 2016, 1Q, 14; 2013, 2Q, 34

√7ᵗʰ **T45.516 Underdosing of anticoagulants**

√6ᵗʰ **T45.52 Poisoning by, adverse effect of and underdosing of antithrombotic drugs**
> Poisoning by, adverse effect of and underdosing of antiplatelet drugs
> EXCLUDES 2   poisoning by, adverse effect of and underdosing of aspirin (T39.01-)
> poisoning by, adverse effect of and underdosing of acetylsalicylic acid (T39.01-)

√7ᵗʰ **T45.521 Poisoning by antithrombotic drugs, accidental (unintentional)**
> Poisoning by antithrombotic drug NOS

2 √7ᵗʰ **T45.522 Poisoning by antithrombotic drugs, intentional self-harm** HCC

√7ᵗʰ **T45.523 Poisoning by antithrombotic drugs, assault**

√7ᵗʰ **T45.524 Poisoning by antithrombotic drugs, undetermined**

√7ᵗʰ **T45.525 Adverse effect of antithrombotic drugs**
> **AHA:** 2016, 1Q, 15

√7ᵗʰ **T45.526 Underdosing of antithrombotic drugs**

√5ᵗʰ **T45.6 Poisoning by, adverse effect of and underdosing of fibrinolysis-affecting drugs**

√6ᵗʰ **T45.60 Poisoning by, adverse effect of and underdosing of unspecified fibrinolysis-affecting drugs**

√7ᵗʰ **T45.601 Poisoning by unspecified fibrinolysis-affecting drugs, accidental (unintentional)** ▽
> Poisoning by fibrinolysis-affecting drug NOS

---

2   HCC with 7th character indicating initial encounter (A or B - specific to category) OR sequela.

☑ Additional Character Req   √x7ᵗʰ Placeholder Alert   Manifestation   HCC CMS-HCC Condition   ▽ Unspecified Code   ▶◀ Revised Text   ● New Code   ▲ Revised Code Title

ICD-10-CM 2018   **1071**

2 ✓7ᵗʰ **T45.602** **Poisoning by unspecified fibrinolysis-affecting drugs, intentional self-harm** `HCC` ▽

✓7ᵗʰ **T45.603** **Poisoning by unspecified fibrinolysis-affecting drugs, assault** ▽

✓7ᵗʰ **T45.604** **Poisoning by unspecified fibrinolysis-affecting drugs, undetermined** ▽

✓7ᵗʰ **T45.605** **Adverse effect of unspecified fibrinolysis- affecting drugs** ▽

✓7ᵗʰ **T45.606** **Underdosing of unspecified fibrinolysis- affecting drugs** ▽

✓6ᵗʰ **T45.61** **Poisoning by, adverse effect of and underdosing of thrombolytic drugs**

✓7ᵗʰ **T45.611** **Poisoning by thrombolytic drug, accidental (unintentional)**
Poisoning by thrombolytic drug NOS

2 ✓7ᵗʰ **T45.612** **Poisoning by thrombolytic drug, intentional self-harm** `HCC`

✓7ᵗʰ **T45.613** **Poisoning by thrombolytic drug, assault**

✓7ᵗʰ **T45.614** **Poisoning by thrombolytic drug, undetermined**

✓7ᵗʰ **T45.615** **Adverse effect of thrombolytic drugs**
AHA: 2017, 2Q, 9

✓7ᵗʰ **T45.616** **Underdosing of thrombolytic drugs**

✓6ᵗʰ **T45.62** **Poisoning by, adverse effect of and underdosing of hemostatic drugs**

✓7ᵗʰ **T45.621** **Poisoning by hemostatic drug, accidental (unintentional)**
Poisoning by hemostatic drug NOS

2 ✓7ᵗʰ **T45.622** **Poisoning by hemostatic drug, intentional self-harm** `HCC`

✓7ᵗʰ **T45.623** **Poisoning by hemostatic drug, assault**

✓7ᵗʰ **T45.624** **Poisoning by hemostatic drug, undetermined**

✓7ᵗʰ **T45.625** **Adverse effect of hemostatic drug**

✓7ᵗʰ **T45.626** **Underdosing of hemostatic drugs**

✓6ᵗʰ **T45.69** **Poisoning by, adverse effect of and underdosing of other fibrinolysis-affecting drugs**

✓7ᵗʰ **T45.691** **Poisoning by other fibrinolysis-affecting drugs, accidental (unintentional)**
Poisoning by other fibrinolysis-affecting drug NOS

2 ✓7ᵗʰ **T45.692** **Poisoning by other fibrinolysis-affecting drugs, intentional self-harm** `HCC`

✓7ᵗʰ **T45.693** **Poisoning by other fibrinolysis-affecting drugs, assault**

✓7ᵗʰ **T45.694** **Poisoning by other fibrinolysis-affecting drugs, undetermined**

✓7ᵗʰ **T45.695** **Adverse effect of other fibrinolysis-affecting drugs**

✓7ᵗʰ **T45.696** **Underdosing of other fibrinolysis-affecting drugs**

✓5ᵗʰ **T45.7** **Poisoning by, adverse effect of and underdosing of anticoagulant antagonists, vitamin K and other coagulants**

✓6ᵗʰ **T45.7X** **Poisoning by, adverse effect of and underdosing of anticoagulant antagonists, vitamin K and other coagulants**

✓7ᵗʰ **T45.7X1** **Poisoning by anticoagulant antagonists, vitamin K and other coagulants, accidental (unintentional)**
Poisoning by anticoagulant antagonists, vitamin K and other coagulants NOS

2 ✓7ᵗʰ **T45.7X2** **Poisoning by anticoagulant antagonists, vitamin K and other coagulants, intentional self-harm** `HCC`

✓7ᵗʰ **T45.7X3** **Poisoning by anticoagulant antagonists, vitamin K and other coagulants, assault**

✓7ᵗʰ **T45.7X4** **Poisoning by anticoagulant antagonists, vitamin K and other coagulants, undetermined**

✓7ᵗʰ **T45.7X5** **Adverse effect of anticoagulant antagonists, vitamin K and other coagulants**

✓7ᵗʰ **T45.7X6** **Underdosing of anticoagulant antagonist, vitamin K and other coagulants**
EXCLUDES 1 vitamin K deficiency (E56.1)

✓5ᵗʰ **T45.8** **Poisoning by, adverse effect of and underdosing of other primarily systemic and hematological agents**
Poisoning by, adverse effect of and underdosing of liver preparations and other antianemic agents
Poisoning by, adverse effect of and underdosing of natural blood and blood products
Poisoning by, adverse effect of and underdosing of plasma substitute
EXCLUDES 2   poisoning by, adverse effect of and underdosing of immunoglobulin (T50.Z1)
    poisoning by, adverse effect of and underdosing of iron (T45.4)
    transfusion reactions (T80.-)

✓6ᵗʰ **T45.8X** **Poisoning by, adverse effect of and underdosing of other primarily systemic and hematological agents**

✓7ᵗʰ **T45.8X1** **Poisoning by other primarily systemic and hematological agents, accidental (unintentional)**
Poisoning by other primarily systemic and hematological agents NOS

2 ✓7ᵗʰ **T45.8X2** **Poisoning by other primarily systemic and hematological agents, intentional self-harm** `HCC`

✓7ᵗʰ **T45.8X3** **Poisoning by other primarily systemic and hematological agents, assault**

✓7ᵗʰ **T45.8X4** **Poisoning by other primarily systemic and hematological agents, undetermined**

✓7ᵗʰ **T45.8X5** **Adverse effect of other primarily systemic and hematological agents**

✓7ᵗʰ **T45.8X6** **Underdosing of other primarily systemic and hematological agents**

✓5ᵗʰ **T45.9** **Poisoning by, adverse effect of and underdosing of unspecified primarily systemic and hematological agent**

✓x7ᵗʰ **T45.91** **Poisoning by unspecified primarily systemic and hematological agent, accidental (unintentional)** ▽
Poisoning by primarily systemic and hematological agent NOS

2 ✓x7ᵗʰ **T45.92** **Poisoning by unspecified primarily systemic and hematological agent, intentional self-harm** `HCC` ▽

✓x7ᵗʰ **T45.93** **Poisoning by unspecified primarily systemic and hematological agent, assault** ▽

✓x7ᵗʰ **T45.94** **Poisoning by unspecified primarily systemic and hematological agent, undetermined** ▽

✓x7ᵗʰ **T45.95** **Adverse effect of unspecified primarily systemic and hematological agent** ▽

✓x7ᵗʰ **T45.96** **Underdosing of unspecified primarily systemic and hematological agent** ▽

✓4ᵗʰ **T46** **Poisoning by, adverse effect of and underdosing of agents primarily affecting the cardiovascular system**
EXCLUDES 1   poisoning by, adverse effect of and underdosing of metaraminol (T44.4)

The appropriate 7th character is to be added to each code from category T46.
A   initial encounter
D   subsequent encounter
S   sequela

✓5ᵗʰ **T46.0** **Poisoning by, adverse effect of and underdosing of cardiac-stimulant glycosides and drugs of similar action**

✓6ᵗʰ **T46.0X** **Poisoning by, adverse effect of and underdosing of cardiac-stimulant glycosides and drugs of similar action**

✓7ᵗʰ **T46.0X1** **Poisoning by cardiac-stimulant glycosides and drugs of similar action, accidental (unintentional)**
Poisoning by cardiac-stimulant glycosides and drugs of similar action NOS

2 ✓7ᵗʰ **T46.0X2** **Poisoning by cardiac-stimulant glycosides and drugs of similar action, intentional self-harm** `HCC`

✓7ᵗʰ **T46.0X3** **Poisoning by cardiac-stimulant glycosides and drugs of similar action, assault**

---

2   HCC with 7th character indicating initial encounter (A or B - specific to category) OR sequela.

EXCLUDES 1 Not coded here   EXCLUDES 2 Not included here   N Newborn Age: 0   P Pediatric Age: 0-17   M Maternity Age: 12-55   A Adult Age: 15-124

☑7ᵗʰ **T46.0X4** Poisoning by cardiac-stimulant glycosides and drugs of similar action, undetermined

☑7ᵗʰ **T46.0X5** Adverse effect of cardiac-stimulant glycosides and drugs of similar action

☑7ᵗʰ **T46.0X6** Underdosing of cardiac-stimulant glycosides and drugs of similar action

☑5ᵗʰ **T46.1** Poisoning by, adverse effect of and underdosing of calcium-channel blockers

  ☑6ᵗʰ **T46.1X** Poisoning by, adverse effect of and underdosing of calcium-channel blockers

    ☑7ᵗʰ **T46.1X1** Poisoning by calcium-channel blockers, accidental (unintentional)
        Poisoning by calcium-channel blockers NOS

    2 ☑7ᵗʰ **T46.1X2** Poisoning by calcium-channel blockers, intentional self-harm   HCC

    ☑7ᵗʰ **T46.1X3** Poisoning by calcium-channel blockers, assault

    ☑7ᵗʰ **T46.1X4** Poisoning by calcium-channel blockers, undetermined

    ☑7ᵗʰ **T46.1X5** Adverse effect of calcium-channel blockers

    ☑7ᵗʰ **T46.1X6** Underdosing of calcium-channel blockers

☑5ᵗʰ **T46.2** Poisoning by, adverse effect of and underdosing of other antidysrhythmic drugs, not elsewhere classified
    EXCLUDES 1   poisoning by, adverse effect of and underdosing of beta-adrenoreceptor antagonists (T44.7-)

  ☑6ᵗʰ **T46.2X** Poisoning by, adverse effect of and underdosing of other antidysrhythmic drugs

    ☑7ᵗʰ **T46.2X1** Poisoning by other antidysrhythmic drugs, accidental (unintentional)
        Poisoning by other antidysrhythmic drugs NOS

    2 ☑7ᵗʰ **T46.2X2** Poisoning by other antidysrhythmic drugs, intentional self-harm   HCC

    ☑7ᵗʰ **T46.2X3** Poisoning by other antidysrhythmic drugs, assault

    ☑7ᵗʰ **T46.2X4** Poisoning by other antidysrhythmic drugs, undetermined

    ☑7ᵗʰ **T46.2X5** Adverse effect of other antidysrhythmic drugs

    ☑7ᵗʰ **T46.2X6** Underdosing of other antidysrhythmic drugs

☑5ᵗʰ **T46.3** Poisoning by, adverse effect of and underdosing of coronary vasodilators
    Poisoning by, adverse effect of and underdosing of dipyridamole
    EXCLUDES 1   poisoning by, adverse effect of and underdosing of calcium-channel blockers (T46.1)

  ☑6ᵗʰ **T46.3X** Poisoning by, adverse effect of and underdosing of coronary vasodilators

    ☑7ᵗʰ **T46.3X1** Poisoning by coronary vasodilators, accidental (unintentional)
        Poisoning by coronary vasodilators NOS

    2 ☑7ᵗʰ **T46.3X2** Poisoning by coronary vasodilators, intentional self-harm   HCC

    ☑7ᵗʰ **T46.3X3** Poisoning by coronary vasodilators, assault

    ☑7ᵗʰ **T46.3X4** Poisoning by coronary vasodilators, undetermined

    ☑7ᵗʰ **T46.3X5** Adverse effect of coronary vasodilators

    ☑7ᵗʰ **T46.3X6** Underdosing of coronary vasodilators

☑5ᵗʰ **T46.4** Poisoning by, adverse effect of and underdosing of angiotensin-converting-enzyme inhibitors

  ☑6ᵗʰ **T46.4X** Poisoning by, adverse effect of and underdosing of angiotensin-converting-enzyme inhibitors

    ☑7ᵗʰ **T46.4X1** Poisoning by angiotensin-converting-enzyme inhibitors, accidental (unintentional)
        Poisoning by angiotensin-converting-enzyme inhibitors NOS

    2 ☑7ᵗʰ **T46.4X2** Poisoning by angiotensin-converting- enzyme inhibitors, intentional self-harm   HCC

    ☑7ᵗʰ **T46.4X3** Poisoning by angiotensin-converting-enzyme inhibitors, assault

    ☑7ᵗʰ **T46.4X4** Poisoning by angiotensin-converting-enzyme inhibitors, undetermined

    ☑7ᵗʰ **T46.4X5** Adverse effect of angiotensin-converting-enzyme inhibitors

    ☑7ᵗʰ **T46.4X6** Underdosing of angiotensin-converting-enzyme inhibitors

☑5ᵗʰ **T46.5** Poisoning by, adverse effect of and underdosing of other antihypertensive drugs
    EXCLUDES 2   poisoning by, adverse effect of and underdosing of beta-adrenoreceptor antagonists (T44.7)
    poisoning by, adverse effect of and underdosing of calcium-channel blockers (T46.1)
    poisoning by, adverse effect of and underdosing of diuretics (T50.0-T50.2)

  ☑6ᵗʰ **T46.5X** Poisoning by, adverse effect of and underdosing of other antihypertensive drugs

    ☑7ᵗʰ **T46.5X1** Poisoning by other antihypertensive drugs, accidental (unintentional)
        Poisoning by other antihypertensive drugs NOS

    2 ☑7ᵗʰ **T46.5X2** Poisoning by other antihypertensive drugs, intentional self-harm   HCC

    ☑7ᵗʰ **T46.5X3** Poisoning by other antihypertensive drugs, assault

    ☑7ᵗʰ **T46.5X4** Poisoning by other antihypertensive drugs, undetermined

    ☑7ᵗʰ **T46.5X5** Adverse effect of other antihypertensive drugs

    ☑7ᵗʰ **T46.5X6** Underdosing of other antihypertensive drugs

☑5ᵗʰ **T46.6** Poisoning by, adverse effect of and underdosing of antihyperlipidemic and antiarteriosclerotic drugs

  ☑6ᵗʰ **T46.6X** Poisoning by, adverse effect of and underdosing of antihyperlipidemic and antiarteriosclerotic drugs

    ☑7ᵗʰ **T46.6X1** Poisoning by antihyperlipidemic and antiarteriosclerotic drugs, accidental (unintentional)
        Poisoning by antihyperlipidemic and antiarteriosclerotic drugs NOS

    2 ☑7ᵗʰ **T46.6X2** Poisoning by antihyperlipidemic and antiarteriosclerotic drugs, intentional self-harm   HCC

    ☑7ᵗʰ **T46.6X3** Poisoning by antihyperlipidemic and antiarteriosclerotic drugs, assault

    ☑7ᵗʰ **T46.6X4** Poisoning by antihyperlipidemic and antiarteriosclerotic drugs, undetermined

    ☑7ᵗʰ **T46.6X5** Adverse effect of antihyperlipidemic and antiarteriosclerotic drugs

    ☑7ᵗʰ **T46.6X6** Underdosing of antihyperlipidemic and antiarteriosclerotic drugs

☑5ᵗʰ **T46.7** Poisoning by, adverse effect of and underdosing of peripheral vasodilators
    Poisoning by, adverse effect of and underdosing of nicotinic acid (derivatives)
    EXCLUDES 1   poisoning by, adverse effect of and underdosing of papaverine (T44.3)

  ☑6ᵗʰ **T46.7X** Poisoning by, adverse effect of and underdosing of peripheral vasodilators

    ☑7ᵗʰ **T46.7X1** Poisoning by peripheral vasodilators, accidental (unintentional)
        Poisoning by peripheral vasodilators NOS

    2 ☑7ᵗʰ **T46.7X2** Poisoning by peripheral vasodilators, intentional self-harm   HCC

    ☑7ᵗʰ **T46.7X3** Poisoning by peripheral vasodilators, assault

    ☑7ᵗʰ **T46.7X4** Poisoning by peripheral vasodilators, undetermined

    ☑7ᵗʰ **T46.7X5** Adverse effect of peripheral vasodilators

    ☑7ᵗʰ **T46.7X6** Underdosing of peripheral vasodilators

---

2   HCC with 7th character indicating initial encounter (A or B - specific to category) OR sequela.

☑ Additional Character Req   ☑7ᵗʰ Placeholder Alert   Manifestation   HCC CMS-HCC Condition   ▽ Unspecified Code   ▶◀ Revised Text   ● New Code   ▲ Revised Code Title

ICD-10-CM 2018   1073

Chapter 19. Injury, Poisoning, and Certain Other Consequences of External Causes

T46.0X4–T46.7X6

Chapter 19. Injury, Poisoning, and Certain Other Consequences of External Causes

✓5ᵗʰ T46.8 Poisoning by, adverse effect of and underdosing of antivaricose drugs, including sclerosing agents

    ✓6ᵗʰ T46.8X Poisoning by, adverse effect of and underdosing of antivaricose drugs, including sclerosing agents

        ✓7ᵗʰ T46.8X1 Poisoning by antivaricose drugs, including sclerosing agents, accidental (unintentional)
            Poisoning by antivaricose drugs, including sclerosing agents NOS

        2 **✓7ᵗʰ T46.8X2 Poisoning by antivaricose drugs, including sclerosing agents, intentional self-harm** HCC

        ✓7ᵗʰ T46.8X3 Poisoning by antivaricose drugs, including sclerosing agents, assault

        ✓7ᵗʰ T46.8X4 Poisoning by antivaricose drugs, including sclerosing agents, undetermined

        ✓7ᵗʰ T46.8X5 Adverse effect of antivaricose drugs, including sclerosing agents

        ✓7ᵗʰ T46.8X6 Underdosing of antivaricose drugs, including sclerosing agents

✓5ᵗʰ T46.9 Poisoning by, adverse effect of and underdosing of other and unspecified agents primarily affecting the cardiovascular system

    ✓6ᵗʰ T46.90 Poisoning by, adverse effect of and underdosing of unspecified agents primarily affecting the cardiovascular system

        ✓7ᵗʰ T46.901 Poisoning by unspecified agents primarily affecting the cardiovascular system, accidental (unintentional) ▽

        2 **✓7ᵗʰ T46.902 Poisoning by unspecified agents primarily affecting the cardiovascular system, intentional self-harm** HCC ▽

        ✓7ᵗʰ T46.903 Poisoning by unspecified agents primarily affecting the cardiovascular system, assault ▽

        ✓7ᵗʰ T46.904 Poisoning by unspecified agents primarily affecting the cardiovascular system, undetermined ▽

        ✓7ᵗʰ T46.905 Adverse effect of unspecified agents primarily affecting the cardiovascular system ▽

        ✓7ᵗʰ T46.906 Underdosing of unspecified agents primarily affecting the cardiovascular system ▽

    ✓6ᵗʰ T46.99 Poisoning by, adverse effect of and underdosing of other agents primarily affecting the cardiovascular system

        ✓7ᵗʰ T46.991 Poisoning by other agents primarily affecting the cardiovascular system, accidental (unintentional)

        2 **✓7ᵗʰ T46.992 Poisoning by other agents primarily affecting the cardiovascular system, intentional self-harm** HCC

        ✓7ᵗʰ T46.993 Poisoning by other agents primarily affecting the cardiovascular system, assault

        ✓7ᵗʰ T46.994 Poisoning by other agents primarily affecting the cardiovascular system, undetermined

        ✓7ᵗʰ T46.995 Adverse effect of other agents primarily affecting the cardiovascular system

        ✓7ᵗʰ T46.996 Underdosing of other agents primarily affecting the cardiovascular system

✓4ᵗʰ T47 Poisoning by, adverse effect of and underdosing of agents primarily affecting the gastrointestinal system

    The appropriate 7th character is to be added to each code from category T47.
    A   initial encounter
    D   subsequent encounter
    S   sequela

✓5ᵗʰ T47.0 Poisoning by, adverse effect of and underdosing of histamine H2-receptor blockers

    ✓6ᵗʰ T47.0X Poisoning by, adverse effect of and underdosing of histamine H2-receptor blockers

        ✓7ᵗʰ T47.0X1 Poisoning by histamine H2-receptor blockers, accidental (unintentional)
            Poisoning by histamine H2-receptor blockers NOS

        2 **✓7ᵗʰ T47.0X2 Poisoning by histamine H2-receptor blockers, intentional self-harm** HCC

        ✓7ᵗʰ T47.0X3 Poisoning by histamine H2-receptor blockers, assault

        ✓7ᵗʰ T47.0X4 Poisoning by histamine H2-receptor blockers, undetermined

        ✓7ᵗʰ T47.0X5 Adverse effect of histamine H2-receptor blockers

        ✓7ᵗʰ T47.0X6 Underdosing of histamine H2-receptor blockers

✓5ᵗʰ T47.1 Poisoning by, adverse effect of and underdosing of other antacids and anti-gastric-secretion drugs

    ✓6ᵗʰ T47.1X Poisoning by, adverse effect of and underdosing of other antacids and anti-gastric-secretion drugs

        ✓7ᵗʰ T47.1X1 Poisoning by other antacids and anti-gastric-secretion drugs, accidental (unintentional)
            Poisoning by other antacids and anti-gastric-secretion drugs NOS

        2 **✓7ᵗʰ T47.1X2 Poisoning by other antacids and anti-gastric-secretion drugs, intentional self-harm** HCC

        ✓7ᵗʰ T47.1X3 Poisoning by other antacids and anti-gastric-secretion drugs, assault

        ✓7ᵗʰ T47.1X4 Poisoning by other antacids and anti-gastric-secretion drugs, undetermined

        ✓7ᵗʰ T47.1X5 Adverse effect of other antacids and anti-gastric-secretion drugs

        ✓7ᵗʰ T47.1X6 Underdosing of other antacids and anti-gastric-secretion drugs

✓5ᵗʰ T47.2 Poisoning by, adverse effect of and underdosing of stimulant laxatives

    ✓6ᵗʰ T47.2X Poisoning by, adverse effect of and underdosing of stimulant laxatives

        ✓7ᵗʰ T47.2X1 Poisoning by stimulant laxatives, accidental (unintentional)
            Poisoning by stimulant laxatives NOS

        2 **✓7ᵗʰ T47.2X2 Poisoning by stimulant laxatives, intentional self-harm** HCC

        ✓7ᵗʰ T47.2X3 Poisoning by stimulant laxatives, assault

        ✓7ᵗʰ T47.2X4 Poisoning by stimulant laxatives, undetermined

        ✓7ᵗʰ T47.2X5 Adverse effect of stimulant laxatives

        ✓7ᵗʰ T47.2X6 Underdosing of stimulant laxatives

✓5ᵗʰ T47.3 Poisoning by, adverse effect of and underdosing of saline and osmotic laxatives

    ✓6ᵗʰ T47.3X Poisoning by and adverse effect of saline and osmotic laxatives

        ✓7ᵗʰ T47.3X1 Poisoning by saline and osmotic laxatives, accidental (unintentional)
            Poisoning by saline and osmotic laxatives NOS

        2 **✓7ᵗʰ T47.3X2 Poisoning by saline and osmotic laxatives, intentional self-harm** HCC

        ✓7ᵗʰ T47.3X3 Poisoning by saline and osmotic laxatives, assault

        ✓7ᵗʰ T47.3X4 Poisoning by saline and osmotic laxatives, undetermined

        ✓7ᵗʰ T47.3X5 Adverse effect of saline and osmotic laxatives

---

2   HCC with 7th character indicating initial encounter (A or B - specific to category) OR sequela.

EXCLUDES 1 Not coded here   EXCLUDES 2 Not included here   N Newborn Age: 0   P Pediatric Age: 0-17   M Maternity Age: 12-55   A Adult Age: 15-124

1074   ICD-10-CM 2018

√7th **T47.3X6**   Underdosing of saline and osmotic laxatives

√5th **T47.4**   Poisoning by, adverse effect of and underdosing of other laxatives

√6th **T47.4X**   Poisoning by, adverse effect of and underdosing of other laxatives

√7th **T47.4X1**   **Poisoning by other laxatives,** accidental **(unintentional)**
     Poisoning by other laxatives NOS

2 √7th **T47.4X2**   **Poisoning by other laxatives, intentional self-harm**   HCC

√7th **T47.4X3**   **Poisoning by other laxatives,** assault

√7th **T47.4X4**   **Poisoning by other laxatives, undetermined**

√7th **T47.4X5**   Adverse effect of other laxatives

√7th **T47.4X6**   Underdosing of other laxatives

√5th **T47.5**   Poisoning by, adverse effect of and underdosing of digestants

√6th **T47.5X**   Poisoning by, adverse effect of and underdosing of digestants

√7th **T47.5X1**   **Poisoning by digestants,** accidental **(unintentional)**
     Poisoning by digestants NOS

2 √7th **T47.5X2**   **Poisoning by digestants, intentional self-harm**   HCC

√7th **T47.5X3**   **Poisoning by digestants,** assault

√7th **T47.5X4**   **Poisoning by digestants,** undetermined

√7th **T47.5X5**   Adverse effect of digestants

√7th **T47.5X6**   Underdosing of digestants

√5th **T47.6**   Poisoning by, adverse effect of and underdosing of antidiarrheal drugs

     EXCLUDES 2   poisoning by, adverse effect of and underdosing of systemic antibiotics and other anti-infectives (T36-T37)

√6th **T47.6X**   Poisoning by, adverse effect of and underdosing of antidiarrheal drugs

√7th **T47.6X1**   **Poisoning by antidiarrheal drugs, accidental (unintentional)**
     Poisoning by antidiarrheal drugs NOS

2 √7th **T47.6X2**   **Poisoning by antidiarrheal drugs, intentional self-harm**   HCC

√7th **T47.6X3**   **Poisoning by antidiarrheal drugs,** assault

√7th **T47.6X4**   **Poisoning by antidiarrheal drugs, undetermined**

√7th **T47.6X5**   Adverse effect of antidiarrheal drugs

√7th **T47.6X6**   Underdosing of antidiarrheal drugs

√5th **T47.7**   Poisoning by, adverse effect of and underdosing of emetics

√6th **T47.7X**   Poisoning by, adverse effect of and underdosing of emetics

√7th **T47.7X1**   **Poisoning by emetics,** accidental **(unintentional)**
     Poisoning by emetics NOS

2 √7th **T47.7X2**   **Poisoning by emetics,** intentional self-harm   HCC

√7th **T47.7X3**   **Poisoning by emetics,** assault

√7th **T47.7X4**   **Poisoning by emetics,** undetermined

√7th **T47.7X5**   Adverse effect of emetics

√7th **T47.7X6**   Underdosing of emetics

√5th **T47.8**   Poisoning by, adverse effect of and underdosing of other agents primarily affecting gastrointestinal system

√6th **T47.8X**   Poisoning by, adverse effect of and underdosing of other agents primarily affecting gastrointestinal system

√7th **T47.8X1**   **Poisoning by other agents primarily affecting gastrointestinal system,** accidental **(unintentional)**
     Poisoning by other agents primarily affecting gastrointestinal system NOS

2 √7th **T47.8X2**   **Poisoning by other agents primarily affecting gastrointestinal system, intentional self-harm**   HCC

√7th **T47.8X3**   **Poisoning by other agents primarily affecting gastrointestinal system,** assault

√7th **T47.8X4**   **Poisoning by other agents primarily affecting gastrointestinal system, undetermined**

√7th **T47.8X5**   Adverse effect of other agents primarily affecting gastrointestinal system

√7th **T47.8X6**   Underdosing of other agents primarily affecting gastrointestinal system

√5th **T47.9**   Poisoning by, adverse effect of and underdosing of unspecified agents primarily affecting the gastrointestinal system

√x7th **T47.91**   **Poisoning by unspecified agents primarily affecting the gastrointestinal system,** accidental **(unintentional)**   ▽
     Poisoning by agents primarily affecting the gastrointestinal system NOS

2 √x7th **T47.92**   **Poisoning by unspecified agents primarily affecting the gastrointestinal system, intentional self-harm**   HCC ▽

√x7th **T47.93**   **Poisoning by unspecified agents primarily affecting the gastrointestinal system,** assault   ▽

√x7th **T47.94**   **Poisoning by unspecified agents primarily affecting the gastrointestinal system,** undetermined   ▽

√x7th **T47.95**   Adverse effect of unspecified agents primarily affecting the gastrointestinal system   ▽

√x7th **T47.96**   Underdosing of unspecified agents primarily affecting the gastrointestinal system   ▽

√4th **T48**   **Poisoning by, adverse effect of and underdosing of agents primarily acting on smooth and skeletal muscles and the respiratory system**

     The appropriate 7th character is to be added to each code from category T48.
     A   initial encounter
     D   subsequent encounter
     S   sequela

√5th **T48.0**   Poisoning by, adverse effect of and underdosing of oxytocic drugs

     EXCLUDES 1   poisoning by, adverse effect of and underdosing of estrogens, progestogens and antagonists (T38.4-T38.6)

√6th **T48.0X**   Poisoning by, adverse effect of and underdosing of oxytocic drugs

√7th **T48.0X1**   **Poisoning by oxytocic drugs,** accidental **(unintentional)**
     Poisoning by oxytocic drugs NOS

2 √7th **T48.0X2**   **Poisoning by oxytocic drugs,** intentional self-harm   HCC

√7th **T48.0X3**   **Poisoning by oxytocic drugs,** assault

√7th **T48.0X4**   **Poisoning by oxytocic drugs, undetermined**

√7th **T48.0X5**   Adverse effect of oxytocic drugs

√7th **T48.0X6**   Underdosing of oxytocic drugs

√5th **T48.1**   Poisoning by, adverse effect of and underdosing of skeletal muscle relaxants [neuromuscular blocking agents]

√6th **T48.1X**   Poisoning by, adverse effect of and underdosing of skeletal muscle relaxants [neuromuscular blocking agents]

√7th **T48.1X1**   **Poisoning by skeletal muscle relaxants [neuromuscular blocking agents],** accidental **(unintentional)**
     Poisoning by skeletal muscle relaxants [neuromuscular blocking agents] NOS

2 √7th **T48.1X2**   **Poisoning by skeletal muscle relaxants [neuromuscular blocking agents], intentional self-harm**   HCC

√7th **T48.1X3**   **Poisoning by skeletal muscle relaxants [neuromuscular blocking agents],** assault

√7th **T48.1X4**   **Poisoning by skeletal muscle relaxants [neuromuscular blocking agents], undetermined**

√7th **T48.1X5**   Adverse effect of skeletal muscle relaxants [neuromuscular blocking agents]

√7th **T48.1X6**   Underdosing of skeletal muscle relaxants [neuromuscular blocking agents]

---

2   HCC with 7th character indicating initial encounter (A or B - specific to category) OR sequela.

☑ Additional Character Req   √x7th Placeholder Alert   Manifestation   HCC CMS-HCC Condition   ▽ Unspecified Code   ►◄ Revised Text   ● New Code   ▲ Revised Code Title

✓5ᵗʰ **T48.2** **Poisoning by, adverse effect of and underdosing of other and unspecified drugs acting on muscles**

     ✓6ᵗʰ **T48.20** **Poisoning by, adverse effect of and underdosing of unspecified drugs acting on muscles**

         ✓7ᵗʰ **T48.201** **Poisoning by unspecified drugs acting on muscles, accidental (unintentional)** ▽
             Poisoning by unspecified drugs acting on muscles NOS

         2 ✓7ᵗʰ **T48.202** **Poisoning by unspecified drugs acting on muscles, intentional self-harm** HCC ▽

         ✓7ᵗʰ **T48.203** **Poisoning by unspecified drugs acting on muscles, assault** ▽

         ✓7ᵗʰ **T48.204** **Poisoning by unspecified drugs acting on muscles, undetermined** ▽

         ✓7ᵗʰ **T48.205** **Adverse effect of unspecified drugs acting on muscles** ▽

         ✓7ᵗʰ **T48.206** **Underdosing of unspecified drugs acting on muscles** ▽

     ✓6ᵗʰ **T48.29** **Poisoning by, adverse effect of and underdosing of other drugs acting on muscles**

         ✓7ᵗʰ **T48.291** **Poisoning by other drugs acting on muscles, accidental (unintentional)**
             Poisoning by other drugs acting on muscles NOS

         2 ✓7ᵗʰ **T48.292** **Poisoning by other drugs acting on muscles, intentional self-harm** HCC

         ✓7ᵗʰ **T48.293** **Poisoning by other drugs acting on muscles, assault**

         ✓7ᵗʰ **T48.294** **Poisoning by other drugs acting on muscles, undetermined**

         ✓7ᵗʰ **T48.295** **Adverse effect of other drugs acting on muscles**

         ✓7ᵗʰ **T48.296** **Underdosing of other drugs acting on muscles**

✓5ᵗʰ **T48.3** **Poisoning by, adverse effect of and underdosing of antitussives**

     ✓6ᵗʰ **T48.3X** **Poisoning by, adverse effect of and underdosing of antitussives**

         ✓7ᵗʰ **T48.3X1** **Poisoning by antitussives, accidental (unintentional)**
             Poisoning by antitussives NOS

         2 ✓7ᵗʰ **T48.3X2** **Poisoning by antitussives, intentional self-harm** HCC

         ✓7ᵗʰ **T48.3X3** **Poisoning by antitussives, assault**

         ✓7ᵗʰ **T48.3X4** **Poisoning by antitussives, undetermined**

         ✓7ᵗʰ **T48.3X5** **Adverse effect of antitussives**

         ✓7ᵗʰ **T48.3X6** **Underdosing of antitussives**

✓5ᵗʰ **T48.4** **Poisoning by, adverse effect of and underdosing of expectorants**

     ✓6ᵗʰ **T48.4X** **Poisoning by, adverse effect of and underdosing of expectorants**

         ✓7ᵗʰ **T48.4X1** **Poisoning by expectorants, accidental (unintentional)**
             Poisoning by expectorants NOS

         2 ✓7ᵗʰ **T48.4X2** **Poisoning by expectorants, intentional self-harm** HCC

         ✓7ᵗʰ **T48.4X3** **Poisoning by expectorants, assault**

         ✓7ᵗʰ **T48.4X4** **Poisoning by expectorants, undetermined**

         ✓7ᵗʰ **T48.4X5** **Adverse effect of expectorants**

         ✓7ᵗʰ **T48.4X6** **Underdosing of expectorants**

✓5ᵗʰ **T48.5** **Poisoning by, adverse effect of and underdosing of other anti-common-cold drugs**
     Poisoning by, adverse effect of and underdosing of decongestants

     EXCLUDES 2 *poisoning by, adverse effect of and underdosing of antipyretics, NEC (T39.9-)*
             poisoning by, adverse effect of and underdosing of non-steroidal antiinflammatory drugs (T39.3-)
             poisoning by, adverse effect of and underdosing of salicylates (T39.0-)

     ✓6ᵗʰ **T48.5X** **Poisoning by, adverse effect of and underdosing of other anti-common-cold drugs**

         ✓7ᵗʰ **T48.5X1** **Poisoning by other anti-common-cold drugs, accidental (unintentional)**
             Poisoning by other anti-common-cold drugs NOS

         2 ✓7ᵗʰ **T48.5X2** **Poisoning by other anti-common-cold drugs, intentional self-harm** HCC

         ✓7ᵗʰ **T48.5X3** **Poisoning by other anti-common-cold drugs, assault**

         ✓7ᵗʰ **T48.5X4** **Poisoning by other anti-common-cold drugs, undetermined**

         ✓7ᵗʰ **T48.5X5** **Adverse effect of other anti-common-cold drugs**

         ✓7ᵗʰ **T48.5X6** **Underdosing of other anti-common-cold drugs**

✓5ᵗʰ **T48.6** **Poisoning by, adverse effect of and underdosing of antiasthmatics, not elsewhere classified**
     Poisoning by, adverse effect of and underdosing of beta-adrenoreceptor agonists used in asthma therapy

     EXCLUDES 1 *poisoning by, adverse effect of and underdosing of anterior pituitary [adenohypophyseal] hormones (T38.8)*
             poisoning by, adverse effect of and underdosing of beta-adrenoreceptor agonists not used in asthma therapy (T44.5)

     ✓6ᵗʰ **T48.6X** **Poisoning by, adverse effect of and underdosing of antiasthmatics**

         ✓7ᵗʰ **T48.6X1** **Poisoning by antiasthmatics, accidental (unintentional)**
             Poisoning by antiasthmatics NOS

         2 ✓7ᵗʰ **T48.6X2** **Poisoning by antiasthmatics, intentional self-harm** HCC

         ✓7ᵗʰ **T48.6X3** **Poisoning by antiasthmatics, assault**

         ✓7ᵗʰ **T48.6X4** **Poisoning by antiasthmatics, undetermined**

         ✓7ᵗʰ **T48.6X5** **Adverse effect of antiasthmatics**

         ✓7ᵗʰ **T48.6X6** **Underdosing of antiasthmatics**

✓5ᵗʰ **T48.9** **Poisoning by, adverse effect of and underdosing of other and unspecified agents primarily acting on the respiratory system**

     ✓6ᵗʰ **T48.90** **Poisoning by, adverse effect of and underdosing of unspecified agents primarily acting on the respiratory system**

         ✓7ᵗʰ **T48.901** **Poisoning by unspecified agents primarily acting on the respiratory system, accidental (unintentional)** ▽

         2 ✓7ᵗʰ **T48.902** **Poisoning by unspecified agents primarily acting on the respiratory system, intentional self-harm** HCC ▽

         ✓7ᵗʰ **T48.903** **Poisoning by unspecified agents primarily acting on the respiratory system, assault** ▽

         ✓7ᵗʰ **T48.904** **Poisoning by unspecified agents primarily acting on the respiratory system, undetermined** ▽

         ✓7ᵗʰ **T48.905** **Adverse effect of unspecified agents primarily acting on the respiratory system** ▽

         ✓7ᵗʰ **T48.906** **Underdosing of unspecified agents primarily acting on the respiratory system** ▽

     ✓6ᵗʰ **T48.99** **Poisoning by, adverse effect of and underdosing of other agents primarily acting on the respiratory system**

         ✓7ᵗʰ **T48.991** **Poisoning by other agents primarily acting on the respiratory system, accidental (unintentional)**

---

2   HCC with 7th character indicating initial encounter (A or B - specific to category) OR sequela.

EXCLUDES 1 Not coded here   EXCLUDES 2 Not included here   N Newborn Age: 0   P Pediatric Age: 0-17   M Maternity Age: 12-55   A Adult Age: 15-124

2 ☑7ᵗʰ **T48.992** **Poisoning by other agents primarily** HCC
acting on the respiratory system,
intentional self-harm

☑7ᵗʰ **T48.993** **Poisoning by other agents primarily**
acting on the respiratory system, assault

☑7ᵗʰ **T48.994** **Poisoning by other agents primarily**
acting on the respiratory system,
undetermined

☑7ᵗʰ **T48.995** Adverse effect **of other agents primarily**
acting on the respiratory system

☑7ᵗʰ **T48.996** Underdosing **of other agents primarily**
acting on the respiratory system

☑4ᵗʰ **T49** **Poisoning by, adverse effect of and underdosing of topical**
agents primarily affecting skin and mucous membrane and by
ophthalmological, otorhinolaryngological and dental drugs
   INCLUDES   poisoning by, adverse effect of and underdosing of
glucocorticoids, topically used

The appropriate 7th character is to be added to each code from
category T49.
A   initial encounter
D   subsequent encounter
S   sequela

☑5ᵗʰ **T49.0** **Poisoning by, adverse effect of and underdosing of local**
antifungal, anti-infective and anti-inflammatory drugs

☑6ᵗʰ **T49.0X** **Poisoning by, adverse effect of and underdosing of**
local antifungal, anti-infective and anti-
inflammatory **drugs**

☑7ᵗʰ **T49.0X1** **Poisoning by local antifungal, anti-**
infective and anti-inflammatory drugs,
accidental (unintentional)
Poisoning by local antifungal, anti-infective
and anti-inflammatory drugs NOS

2 ☑7ᵗʰ **T49.0X2** **Poisoning by local antifungal, anti-** HCC
infective and anti-inflammatory drugs,
intentional self-harm

☑7ᵗʰ **T49.0X3** **Poisoning by local antifungal, anti-**
infective and anti-inflammatory drugs,
assault

☑7ᵗʰ **T49.0X4** **Poisoning by local antifungal, anti-**
infective and anti-inflammatory drugs,
undetermined

☑7ᵗʰ **T49.0X5** Adverse effect **of local antifungal, anti-**
infective and anti-inflammatory drugs

☑7ᵗʰ **T49.0X6** Underdosing **of local antifungal, anti-**
infective and anti-inflammatory drugs

☑5ᵗʰ **T49.1** **Poisoning by, adverse effect of and underdosing of**
antipruritics

☑6ᵗʰ **T49.1X** **Poisoning by, adverse effect of and underdosing of**
antipruritics

☑7ᵗʰ **T49.1X1** **Poisoning by antipruritics,** accidental
(unintentional)
Poisoning by antipruritics NOS

2 ☑7ᵗʰ **T49.1X2** **Poisoning by antipruritics,** HCC
intentional self-harm

☑7ᵗʰ **T49.1X3** **Poisoning by antipruritics,** assault

☑7ᵗʰ **T49.1X4** **Poisoning by antipruritics,** undetermined

☑7ᵗʰ **T49.1X5** Adverse effect **of antipruritics**

☑7ᵗʰ **T49.1X6** Underdosing **of antipruritics**

☑5ᵗʰ **T49.2** **Poisoning by, adverse effect of and underdosing of local**
astringents and local detergents

☑6ᵗʰ **T49.2X** **Poisoning by, adverse effect of and underdosing of**
local astringents and local detergents

☑7ᵗʰ **T49.2X1** **Poisoning by local astringents and local**
detergents, accidental (unintentional)
Poisoning by local astringents and local
detergents NOS

2 ☑7ᵗʰ **T49.2X2** **Poisoning by local astringents and** HCC
local detergents, intentional self-harm

☑7ᵗʰ **T49.2X3** **Poisoning by local astringents and local**
detergents, assault

☑7ᵗʰ **T49.2X4** **Poisoning by local astringents and local**
detergents, undetermined

☑7ᵗʰ **T49.2X5** Adverse effect **of local astringents and**
local detergents

☑7ᵗʰ **T49.2X6** Underdosing **of local astringents and local**
detergents

☑5ᵗʰ **T49.3** **Poisoning by, adverse effect of and underdosing of**
emollients, demulcents and protectants

☑6ᵗʰ **T49.3X** **Poisoning by, adverse effect of and underdosing of**
emollients, demulcents and protectants

☑7ᵗʰ **T49.3X1** **Poisoning by emollients, demulcents and**
protectants, accidental (unintentional)
Poisoning by emollients, demulcents and
protectants NOS

2 ☑7ᵗʰ **T49.3X2** **Poisoning by emollients, demulcents** HCC
and protectants, intentional self-harm

☑7ᵗʰ **T49.3X3** **Poisoning by emollients, demulcents and**
protectants, assault

☑7ᵗʰ **T49.3X4** **Poisoning by emollients, demulcents and**
protectants, undetermined

☑7ᵗʰ **T49.3X5** Adverse effect **of emollients, demulcents**
and protectants

☑7ᵗʰ **T49.3X6** Underdosing **of emollients, demulcents**
and protectants

☑5ᵗʰ **T49.4** **Poisoning by, adverse effect of and underdosing of**
keratolytics, keratoplastics, and other hair treatment drugs
and preparations

☑6ᵗʰ **T49.4X** **Poisoning by, adverse effect of and underdosing of**
keratolytics, keratoplastics, and other hair
treatment drugs and preparations

☑7ᵗʰ **T49.4X1** **Poisoning by keratolytics, keratoplastics,**
and other hair treatment drugs and
preparations, accidental (unintentional)
Poisoning by keratolytics, keratoplastics,
and other hair treatment drugs and
preparations NOS

2 ☑7ᵗʰ **T49.4X2** **Poisoning by keratolytics,** HCC
keratoplastics, and other hair
treatment drugs and preparations,
intentional self-harm

☑7ᵗʰ **T49.4X3** **Poisoning by keratolytics, keratoplastics,**
and other hair treatment drugs and
preparations, assault

☑7ᵗʰ **T49.4X4** **Poisoning by keratolytics, keratoplastics,**
and other hair treatment drugs and
preparations, undetermined

☑7ᵗʰ **T49.4X5** Adverse effect **of keratolytics,**
keratoplastics, and other hair treatment
drugs and preparations

☑7ᵗʰ **T49.4X6** Underdosing **of keratolytics,**
keratoplastics, and other hair treatment
drugs and preparations

☑5ᵗʰ **T49.5** **Poisoning by, adverse effect of and underdosing of**
ophthalmological drugs and preparations

☑6ᵗʰ **T49.5X** **Poisoning by, adverse effect of and underdosing of**
ophthalmological **drugs and preparations**

☑7ᵗʰ **T49.5X1** **Poisoning by ophthalmological drugs and**
preparations, accidental (unintentional)
Poisoning by ophthalmological drugs and
preparations NOS

2 ☑7ᵗʰ **T49.5X2** **Poisoning by ophthalmological** HCC
drugs and preparations, intentional
self-harm

☑7ᵗʰ **T49.5X3** **Poisoning by ophthalmological drugs and**
preparations, assault

☑7ᵗʰ **T49.5X4** **Poisoning by ophthalmological drugs and**
preparations, undetermined

☑7ᵗʰ **T49.5X5** Adverse effect **of ophthalmological drugs**
and preparations

☑7ᵗʰ **T49.5X6** Underdosing **of ophthalmological drugs**
and preparations

☑5ᵗʰ **T49.6** **Poisoning by, adverse effect of and underdosing of**
otorhinolaryngological drugs and preparations

☑6ᵗʰ **T49.6X** **Poisoning by, adverse effect of and underdosing of**
otorhinolaryngological **drugs and preparations**

☑7ᵗʰ **T49.6X1** **Poisoning by otorhinolaryngological**
drugs and preparations, accidental
(unintentional)
Poisoning by otorhinolaryngological drugs
and preparations NOS

---

2   HCC with 7th character indicating initial encounter (A or B - specific to category) OR sequela.

☑ Additional Character Req   ☑x7ᵗʰ Placeholder Alert   Manifestation   HCC CMS-HCC Condition   ▽ Unspecified Code   ▶◀ Revised Text   ● New Code   ▲ Revised Code Title

2 ✓7th **T49.6X2** **Poisoning by otorhinolaryngological** HCC
**drugs and preparations, intentional
self-harm**

✓7th **T49.6X3** **Poisoning by otorhinolaryngological
drugs and preparations, assault**

✓7th **T49.6X4** **Poisoning by otorhinolaryngological
drugs and preparations, undetermined**

✓7th **T49.6X5** **Adverse effect of otorhinolaryngological
drugs and preparations**

✓7th **T49.6X6** **Underdosing of otorhinolaryngological
drugs and preparations**

✓5th **T49.7** **Poisoning by, adverse effect of and underdosing of dental
drugs, topically applied**

✓6th **T49.7X** **Poisoning by, adverse effect of and underdosing of
dental drugs, topically applied**

✓7th **T49.7X1** **Poisoning by dental drugs, topically
applied, accidental (unintentional)**
Poisoning by dental drugs, topically
applied NOS

2 ✓7th **T49.7X2** **Poisoning by dental drugs, topically** HCC
applied, intentional self-harm

✓7th **T49.7X3** **Poisoning by dental drugs, topically
applied, assault**

✓7th **T49.7X4** **Poisoning by dental drugs, topically
applied, undetermined**

✓7th **T49.7X5** **Adverse effect of dental drugs, topically
applied**

✓7th **T49.7X6** **Underdosing of dental drugs, topically
applied**

✓5th **T49.8** **Poisoning by, adverse effect of and underdosing of other
topical agents**
Poisoning by, adverse effect of and underdosing of spermicides

✓6th **T49.8X** **Poisoning by, adverse effect of and underdosing of
other topical agents**

✓7th **T49.8X1** **Poisoning by other topical agents,
accidental (unintentional)**
Poisoning by other topical agents NOS

2 ✓7th **T49.8X2** **Poisoning by other topical agents,** HCC
intentional self-harm

✓7th **T49.8X3** **Poisoning by other topical agents, assault**

✓7th **T49.8X4** **Poisoning by other topical agents,
undetermined**

✓7th **T49.8X5** **Adverse effect of other topical agents**

✓7th **T49.8X6** **Underdosing of other topical agents**

✓5th **T49.9** **Poisoning by, adverse effect of and underdosing of
unspecified topical agent**

✓x7th **T49.91** **Poisoning by unspecified topical agent,
accidental (unintentional)** ▽

2 ✓x7th **T49.92** **Poisoning by unspecified topical agent,
intentional self-harm** HCC ▽

✓x7th **T49.93** **Poisoning by unspecified topical agent,
assault** ▽

✓x7th **T49.94** **Poisoning by unspecified topical agent,
undetermined** ▽

✓x7th **T49.95** **Adverse effect of unspecified topical agent** ▽

✓x7th **T49.96** **Underdosing of unspecified topical agent** ▽

✓4th **T50** **Poisoning by, adverse effect of and underdosing of diuretics and
other and unspecified drugs, medicaments and biological
substances**

> The appropriate 7th character is to be added to each code from
> category T50.
> A   initial encounter
> D   subsequent encounter
> S   sequela

✓5th **T50.0** **Poisoning by, adverse effect of and underdosing of
mineralocorticoids and their antagonists**

✓6th **T50.0X** **Poisoning by, adverse effect of and underdosing of
mineralocorticoids and their antagonists**

✓7th **T50.0X1** **Poisoning by mineralocorticoids and their
antagonists, accidental (unintentional)**
Poisoning by mineralocorticoids and their
antagonists NOS

2 ✓7th **T50.0X2** **Poisoning by mineralocorticoids and** HCC
their antagonists, intentional self-harm

✓7th **T50.0X3** **Poisoning by mineralocorticoids and their
antagonists, assault**

✓7th **T50.0X4** **Poisoning by mineralocorticoids and their
antagonists, undetermined**

✓7th **T50.0X5** **Adverse effect of mineralocorticoids and
their antagonists**

✓7th **T50.0X6** **Underdosing of mineralocorticoids and
their antagonists**

✓5th **T50.1** **Poisoning by, adverse effect of and underdosing of loop
[high-ceiling] diuretics**

✓6th **T50.1X** **Poisoning by, adverse effect of and underdosing of
loop [high-ceiling] diuretics**

✓7th **T50.1X1** **Poisoning by loop [high-ceiling] diuretics,
accidental (unintentional)**
Poisoning by loop [high-ceiling] diuretics
NOS

2 ✓7th **T50.1X2** **Poisoning by loop [high-ceiling]** HCC
diuretics, intentional self-harm

✓7th **T50.1X3** **Poisoning by loop [high-ceiling]
diuretics, assault**

✓7th **T50.1X4** **Poisoning by loop [high-ceiling]
diuretics, undetermined**

✓7th **T50.1X5** **Adverse effect of loop [high-ceiling]
diuretics**

✓7th **T50.1X6** **Underdosing of loop [high-ceiling]
diuretics**

✓5th **T50.2** **Poisoning by, adverse effect of and underdosing of carbonic-
anhydrase inhibitors, benzothiadiazides and other diuretics**
Poisoning by, adverse effect of and underdosing of
acetazolamide

✓6th **T50.2X** **Poisoning by, adverse effect of and underdosing of
carbonic-anhydrase inhibitors, benzothiadiazides
and other diuretics**

✓7th **T50.2X1** **Poisoning by carbonic-anhydrase
inhibitors, benzothiadiazides and other
diuretics, accidental (unintentional)**
Poisoning by carbonic-anhydrase
inhibitors, benzothiadiazides and
other diuretics NOS

2 ✓7th **T50.2X2** **Poisoning by carbonic-anhydrase** HCC
**inhibitors, benzothiadiazides and
other diuretics, intentional self-harm**

✓7th **T50.2X3** **Poisoning by carbonic-anhydrase
inhibitors, benzothiadiazides and other
diuretics, assault**

✓7th **T50.2X4** **Poisoning by carbonic-anhydrase
inhibitors, benzothiadiazides and other
diuretics, undetermined**

✓7th **T50.2X5** **Adverse effect of carbonic-anhydrase
inhibitors, benzothiadiazides and other
diuretics**

✓7th **T50.2X6** **Underdosing of carbonic-anhydrase
inhibitors, benzothiadiazides and other
diuretics**

✓5th **T50.3** **Poisoning by, adverse effect of and underdosing of
electrolytic, caloric and water-balance agents**
Poisoning by, adverse effect of and underdosing of oral
rehydration salts

✓6th **T50.3X** **Poisoning by, adverse effect of and underdosing of
electrolytic, caloric and water-balance agents**

✓7th **T50.3X1** **Poisoning by electrolytic, caloric and
water-balance agents, accidental
(unintentional)**
Poisoning by electrolytic, caloric and water-
balance agents NOS

2 ✓7th **T50.3X2** **Poisoning by electrolytic, caloric** HCC
**and water-balance agents, intentional
self-harm**

✓7th **T50.3X3** **Poisoning by electrolytic, caloric and
water-balance agents, assault**

✓7th **T50.3X4** **Poisoning by electrolytic, caloric and
water-balance agents, undetermined**

✓7th **T50.3X5** **Adverse effect of electrolytic, caloric and
water-balance agents**

✓7th **T50.3X6** **Underdosing of electrolytic, caloric and
water-balance agents**

---

2   HCC with 7th character indicating initial encounter (A or B - specific to category) OR sequela.

EXCLUDES 1 Not coded here   **EXCLUDES 2** Not included here   N Newborn Age: 0   P Pediatric Age: 0-17   M Maternity Age: 12-55   A Adult Age: 15-124

1078   ICD-10-CM 2018

√5ᵗʰ **T50.4 Poisoning by, adverse effect of and underdosing of drugs affecting uric acid metabolism**

    √6ᵗʰ **T50.4X Poisoning by, adverse effect of and underdosing of drugs** affecting uric acid metabolism

       √7ᵗʰ **T50.4X1 Poisoning by drugs affecting uric acid metabolism, accidental (unintentional)**
          Poisoning by drugs affecting uric acid metabolism NOS

       2 √7ᵗʰ **T50.4X2 Poisoning by drugs affecting uric acid** HCC **metabolism, intentional self-harm**

       √7ᵗʰ **T50.4X3 Poisoning by drugs affecting uric acid metabolism, assault**

       √7ᵗʰ **T50.4X4 Poisoning by drugs affecting uric acid metabolism, undetermined**

       √7ᵗʰ **T50.4X5 Adverse effect of drugs affecting uric acid metabolism**

       √7ᵗʰ **T50.4X6 Underdosing of drugs affecting uric acid metabolism**

√5ᵗʰ **T50.5 Poisoning by, adverse effect of and underdosing of appetite depressants**

    √6ᵗʰ **T50.5X Poisoning by, adverse effect of and underdosing of appetite depressants**

       √7ᵗʰ **T50.5X1 Poisoning by appetite depressants, accidental (unintentional)**
          Poisoning by appetite depressants NOS

       2 √7ᵗʰ **T50.5X2 Poisoning by appetite depressants,** HCC **intentional self-harm**

       √7ᵗʰ **T50.5X3 Poisoning by appetite depressants, assault**

       √7ᵗʰ **T50.5X4 Poisoning by appetite depressants, undetermined**

       √7ᵗʰ **T50.5X5 Adverse effect of appetite depressants**

       √7ᵗʰ **T50.5X6 Underdosing of appetite depressants**

√5ᵗʰ **T50.6 Poisoning by, adverse effect of and underdosing of antidotes and chelating agents**
    Poisoning by, adverse effect of and underdosing of alcohol deterrents

    √6ᵗʰ **T50.6X Poisoning by, adverse effect of and underdosing of antidotes and chelating agents**

       √7ᵗʰ **T50.6X1 Poisoning by antidotes and chelating agents, accidental (unintentional)**
          Poisoning by antidotes and chelating agents NOS

       2 √7ᵗʰ **T50.6X2 Poisoning by antidotes and chelating** HCC **agents, intentional self-harm**

       √7ᵗʰ **T50.6X3 Poisoning by antidotes and chelating agents, assault**

       √7ᵗʰ **T50.6X4 Poisoning by antidotes and chelating agents, undetermined**

       √7ᵗʰ **T50.6X5 Adverse effect of antidotes and chelating agents**

       √7ᵗʰ **T50.6X6 Underdosing of antidotes and chelating agents**

√5ᵗʰ **T50.7 Poisoning by, adverse effect of and underdosing of analeptics and opioid receptor antagonists**

    √6ᵗʰ **T50.7X Poisoning by, adverse effect of and underdosing of analeptics and opioid receptor antagonists**

       √7ᵗʰ **T50.7X1 Poisoning by analeptics and opioid receptor antagonists, accidental (unintentional)**
          Poisoning by analeptics and opioid receptor antagonists NOS

       2 √7ᵗʰ **T50.7X2 Poisoning by analeptics and opioid** HCC **receptor antagonists, intentional self-harm**

       √7ᵗʰ **T50.7X3 Poisoning by analeptics and opioid receptor antagonists, assault**

       √7ᵗʰ **T50.7X4 Poisoning by analeptics and opioid receptor antagonists, undetermined**

       √7ᵗʰ **T50.7X5 Adverse effect of analeptics and opioid receptor antagonists**

       √7ᵗʰ **T50.7X6 Underdosing of analeptics and opioid receptor antagonists**

√5ᵗʰ **T50.8 Poisoning by, adverse effect of and underdosing of diagnostic agents**

    √6ᵗʰ **T50.8X Poisoning by, adverse effect of and underdosing of diagnostic agents**

       √7ᵗʰ **T50.8X1 Poisoning by diagnostic agents, accidental (unintentional)**
          Poisoning by diagnostic agents NOS

       2 √7ᵗʰ **T50.8X2 Poisoning by diagnostic agents,** HCC **intentional self-harm**

       √7ᵗʰ **T50.8X3 Poisoning by diagnostic agents, assault**

       √7ᵗʰ **T50.8X4 Poisoning by diagnostic agents, undetermined**

       √7ᵗʰ **T50.8X5 Adverse effect of diagnostic agents**

       √7ᵗʰ **T50.8X6 Underdosing of diagnostic agents**

√5ᵗʰ **T50.A Poisoning by, adverse effect of and underdosing of bacterial vaccines**

    √6ᵗʰ **T50.A1 Poisoning by, adverse effect of and underdosing of pertussis vaccine, including combinations with a pertussis component**

       √7ᵗʰ **T50.A11 Poisoning by pertussis vaccine, including combinations with a pertussis component, accidental (unintentional)**

       2 √7ᵗʰ **T50.A12 Poisoning by pertussis vaccine,** HCC **including combinations with a pertussis component, intentional self-harm**

       √7ᵗʰ **T50.A13 Poisoning by pertussis vaccine, including combinations with a pertussis component, assault**

       √7ᵗʰ **T50.A14 Poisoning by pertussis vaccine, including combinations with a pertussis component, undetermined**

       √7ᵗʰ **T50.A15 Adverse effect of pertussis vaccine, including combinations with a pertussis component**

       √7ᵗʰ **T50.A16 Underdosing of pertussis vaccine, including combinations with a pertussis component**

    √6ᵗʰ **T50.A2 Poisoning by, adverse effect of and underdosing of mixed bacterial vaccines without a pertussis component**

       √7ᵗʰ **T50.A21 Poisoning by mixed bacterial vaccines without a pertussis component, accidental (unintentional)**

       2 √7ᵗʰ **T50.A22 Poisoning by mixed bacterial** HCC **vaccines without a pertussis component, intentional self-harm**

       √7ᵗʰ **T50.A23 Poisoning by mixed bacterial vaccines without a pertussis component, assault**

       √7ᵗʰ **T50.A24 Poisoning by mixed bacterial vaccines without a pertussis component, undetermined**

       √7ᵗʰ **T50.A25 Adverse effect of mixed bacterial vaccines without a pertussis component**

       √7ᵗʰ **T50.A26 Underdosing of mixed bacterial vaccines without a pertussis component**

    √6ᵗʰ **T50.A9 Poisoning by, adverse effect of and underdosing of other bacterial vaccines**

       √7ᵗʰ **T50.A91 Poisoning by other bacterial vaccines, accidental (unintentional)**

       2 √7ᵗʰ **T50.A92 Poisoning by other bacterial vaccines,** HCC **intentional self-harm**

       √7ᵗʰ **T50.A93 Poisoning by other bacterial vaccines, assault**

       √7ᵗʰ **T50.A94 Poisoning by other bacterial vaccines, undetermined**

       √7ᵗʰ **T50.A95 Adverse effect of other bacterial vaccines**

       √7ᵗʰ **T50.A96 Underdosing of other bacterial vaccines**

√5ᵗʰ **T50.B Poisoning by, adverse effect of and underdosing of viral vaccines**

    √6ᵗʰ **T50.B1 Poisoning by, adverse effect of and underdosing of smallpox vaccines**

       √7ᵗʰ **T50.B11 Poisoning by smallpox vaccines, accidental (unintentional)**

       2 √7ᵗʰ **T50.B12 Poisoning by smallpox vaccines,** HCC **intentional self-harm**

---

2   HCC with 7th character indicating initial encounter (A or B - specific to category) OR sequela.

☑ Additional Character Req   ✔x7ᵗʰ Placeholder Alert   Manifestation   HCC CMS-HCC Condition   ▽ Unspecified Code   ►◄ Revised Text   ● New Code   ▲ Revised Code Title

√7ᵗʰ **T50.B13**   **Poisoning by smallpox vaccines,** assault

√7ᵗʰ **T50.B14**   **Poisoning by smallpox vaccines,** undetermined

√7ᵗʰ **T50.B15**   **Adverse effect** of smallpox vaccines

√7ᵗʰ **T50.B16**   **Underdosing** of smallpox vaccines

√6ᵗʰ **T50.B9**   **Poisoning by, adverse effect of and underdosing of other viral vaccines**

    √7ᵗʰ **T50.B91**   **Poisoning by other viral vaccines,** accidental (unintentional)

    2 √7ᵗʰ **T50.B92**   **Poisoning by other viral vaccines,** intentional self-harm   HCC

    √7ᵗʰ **T50.B93**   **Poisoning by other viral vaccines,** assault

    √7ᵗʰ **T50.B94**   **Poisoning by other viral vaccines,** undetermined

    √7ᵗʰ **T50.B95**   **Adverse effect** of other viral vaccines

    √7ᵗʰ **T50.B96**   **Underdosing** of other viral vaccines

√5ᵗʰ **T50.Z**   **Poisoning by, adverse effect of and underdosing of other vaccines and biological substances**

√6ᵗʰ **T50.Z1**   **Poisoning by, adverse effect of and underdosing of immunoglobulin**

    √7ᵗʰ **T50.Z11**   **Poisoning by immunoglobulin,** accidental (unintentional)

    2 √7ᵗʰ **T50.Z12**   **Poisoning by immunoglobulin,** intentional self-harm   HCC

    √7ᵗʰ **T50.Z13**   **Poisoning by immunoglobulin,** assault

    √7ᵗʰ **T50.Z14**   **Poisoning by immunoglobulin,** undetermined

    √7ᵗʰ **T50.Z15**   **Adverse effect** of immunoglobulin

    √7ᵗʰ **T50.Z16**   **Underdosing** of immunoglobulin

√6ᵗʰ **T50.Z9**   **Poisoning by, adverse effect of and underdosing of other vaccines and biological substances**

    √7ᵗʰ **T50.Z91**   **Poisoning by other vaccines and biological substances,** accidental (unintentional)

    2 √7ᵗʰ **T50.Z92**   **Poisoning by other vaccines and biological substances,** intentional self-harm   HCC

    √7ᵗʰ **T50.Z93**   **Poisoning by other vaccines and biological substances,** assault

    √7ᵗʰ **T50.Z94**   **Poisoning by other vaccines and biological substances,** undetermined

    √7ᵗʰ **T50.Z95**   **Adverse effect** of other vaccines and biological substances

    √7ᵗʰ **T50.Z96**   **Underdosing** of other vaccines and biological substances

√5ᵗʰ **T50.9**   **Poisoning by, adverse effect of and underdosing of other and unspecified drugs, medicaments and biological substances**
    AHA: 2016, 1Q, 38; 2015, 1Q, 21

√6ᵗʰ **T50.90**   **Poisoning by, adverse effect of and underdosing of unspecified drugs, medicaments and biological substances**

    √7ᵗʰ **T50.901**   **Poisoning by unspecified drugs, medicaments and biological substances,** accidental (unintentional) ▽

    2 √7ᵗʰ **T50.902**   **Poisoning by unspecified drugs, medicaments and biological substances,** intentional self-harm   HCC ▽

    √7ᵗʰ **T50.903**   **Poisoning by unspecified drugs, medicaments and biological substances,** assault ▽

    √7ᵗʰ **T50.904**   **Poisoning by unspecified drugs, medicaments and biological substances,** undetermined ▽

    √7ᵗʰ **T50.905**   **Adverse effect** of unspecified drugs, medicaments and biological substances ▽

    √7ᵗʰ **T50.906**   **Underdosing** of unspecified drugs, medicaments and biological substances ▽

√6ᵗʰ **T50.99**   **Poisoning by, adverse effect of and underdosing of other drugs, medicaments and biological substances**

    √7ᵗʰ **T50.991**   **Poisoning by other drugs, medicaments and biological substances,** accidental (unintentional)

    2 √7ᵗʰ **T50.992**   **Poisoning by other drugs, medicaments and biological substances,** intentional self-harm   HCC

    √7ᵗʰ **T50.993**   **Poisoning by other drugs, medicaments and biological substances,** assault

    √7ᵗʰ **T50.994**   **Poisoning by other drugs, medicaments and biological substances,** undetermined

    √7ᵗʰ **T50.995**   **Adverse effect** of other drugs, medicaments and biological substances

    √7ᵗʰ **T50.996**   **Underdosing** of other drugs, medicaments and biological substances

Toxic effects of substances chiefly nonmedicinal as to source (T51-T65)

NOTE   When no intent is indicated code to accidental. Undetermined intent is only for use when there is specific documentation in the record that the intent of the toxic effect cannot be determined.

Use additional code(s) for all associated manifestations of toxic effect, such as:
    personal history of foreign body fully removed (Z87.821)
    respiratory conditions due to external agents (J60-J70)
    to identify any retained foreign body, if applicable (Z18.-)

EXCLUDES 1   contact with and (suspected) exposure to toxic substances (Z77.-)
AHA: 2017, 1Q, 39-40

√4ᵗʰ **T51**   **Toxic effect of alcohol**

> The appropriate 7th character is to be added to each code from category T51.
> A   initial encounter
> D   subsequent encounter
> S   sequela

√5ᵗʰ **T51.0**   **Toxic effect of ethanol**
    Toxic effect of ethyl alcohol
    EXCLUDES 2   acute alcohol intoxication or 'hangover' effects (F10.129, F10.229, F10.929)
        drunkenness (F10.129, F10.229, F10.929)
        pathological alcohol intoxication (F10.129, F10.229, F10.929)

√6ᵗʰ **T51.0X**   **Toxic effect of** ethanol

    √7ᵗʰ **T51.0X1**   **Toxic effect of ethanol,** accidental (unintentional)
        Toxic effect of ethanol NOS

    2 √7ᵗʰ **T51.0X2**   **Toxic effect of ethanol,** intentional self-harm   HCC

    √7ᵗʰ **T51.0X3**   **Toxic effect of ethanol,** assault

    √7ᵗʰ **T51.0X4**   **Toxic effect of ethanol,** undetermined

√5ᵗʰ **T51.1**   **Toxic effect of methanol**
    Toxic effect of methyl alcohol

√6ᵗʰ **T51.1X**   **Toxic effect of** methanol

    √7ᵗʰ **T51.1X1**   **Toxic effect of methanol,** accidental (unintentional)
        Toxic effect of methanol NOS

    2 √7ᵗʰ **T51.1X2**   **Toxic effect of methanol,** intentional self-harm   HCC

    √7ᵗʰ **T51.1X3**   **Toxic effect of methanol,** assault

    √7ᵗʰ **T51.1X4**   **Toxic effect of methanol,** undetermined

√5ᵗʰ **T51.2**   **Toxic effect of 2-Propanol**
    Toxic effect of isopropyl alcohol

√6ᵗʰ **T51.2X**   **Toxic effect of** 2-Propanol

    √7ᵗʰ **T51.2X1**   **Toxic effect of 2-Propanol,** accidental (unintentional)
        Toxic effect of 2-Propanol NOS

    2 √7ᵗʰ **T51.2X2**   **Toxic effect of 2-Propanol,** intentional self-harm   HCC

    √7ᵗʰ **T51.2X3**   **Toxic effect of 2-Propanol,** assault

    √7ᵗʰ **T51.2X4**   **Toxic effect of 2-Propanol,** undetermined

√5ᵗʰ **T51.3**   **Toxic effect of fusel oil**
    Toxic effect of amyl alcohol
    Toxic effect of butyl [1-butanol] alcohol
    Toxic effect of propyl [1-propanol] alcohol

√6ᵗʰ **T51.3X**   **Toxic effect of** fusel oil

    √7ᵗʰ **T51.3X1**   **Toxic effect of fusel oil,** accidental (unintentional)
        Toxic effect of fusel oil NOS

    2 √7ᵗʰ **T51.3X2**   **Toxic effect of fusel oil,** intentional self-harm   HCC

    √7ᵗʰ **T51.3X3**   **Toxic effect of fusel oil,** assault

    √7ᵗʰ **T51.3X4**   **Toxic effect of fusel oil,** undetermined

---

2   HCC with 7th character indicating initial encounter (A or B - specific to category) OR sequela.

EXCLUDES 1 Not coded here   **EXCLUDES 2** Not included here   N Newborn Age: 0   P Pediatric Age: 0-17   M Maternity Age: 12-55   A Adult Age: 15-124

1080   ICD-10-CM 2018

✓5ᵗʰ **T51.8**   **Toxic effect of other alcohols**

     ✓6ᵗʰ **T51.8X**   **Toxic effect of other alcohols**

         ✓7ᵗʰ **T51.8X1**   **Toxic effect of other alcohols, accidental (unintentional)**
                 Toxic effect of other alcohols NOS

        2   ✓7ᵗʰ **T51.8X2**   **Toxic effect of other alcohols, intentional self-harm**   HCC

         ✓7ᵗʰ **T51.8X3**   **Toxic effect of other alcohols, assault**

         ✓7ᵗʰ **T51.8X4**   **Toxic effect of other alcohols, undetermined**

✓5ᵗʰ **T51.9**   **Toxic effect of unspecified alcohol**

     ✓x7ᵗʰ **T51.91**   **Toxic effect of unspecified alcohol, accidental (unintentional)**   ▽

     2   ✓x7ᵗʰ **T51.92**   **Toxic effect of unspecified alcohol, intentional self-harm**   HCC ▽

     ✓x7ᵗʰ **T51.93**   **Toxic effect of unspecified alcohol, assault**   ▽

     ✓x7ᵗʰ **T51.94**   **Toxic effect of unspecified alcohol, undetermined** ▽

✓4ᵗʰ **T52**   **Toxic effect of organic solvents**

     EXCLUDES 1   halogen derivatives of aliphatic and aromatic hydrocarbons (T53.-)

> The appropriate 7th character is to be added to each code from category T52.
> A   initial encounter
> D   subsequent encounter
> S   sequela

     ✓5ᵗʰ **T52.0**   **Toxic effects of petroleum products**
                 Toxic effects of ether petroleum
                 Toxic effects of gasoline [petrol]
                 Toxic effects of kerosene [paraffin oil]
                 Toxic effects of naphtha petroleum
                 Toxic effects of paraffin wax
                 Toxic effects of spirit petroleum

        ✓6ᵗʰ **T52.0X**   **Toxic effects of petroleum products**

           ✓7ᵗʰ **T52.0X1**   **Toxic effect of petroleum products, accidental (unintentional)**
                   Toxic effects of petroleum products NOS

         2   ✓7ᵗʰ **T52.0X2**   **Toxic effect of petroleum products, intentional self-harm**   HCC

           ✓7ᵗʰ **T52.0X3**   **Toxic effect of petroleum products, assault**

           ✓7ᵗʰ **T52.0X4**   **Toxic effect of petroleum products, undetermined**

     ✓5ᵗʰ **T52.1**   **Toxic effects of benzene**

         EXCLUDES 1   homologues of benzene (T52.2)
                     nitroderivatives and aminoderivatives of benzene and its homologues (T65.3)

        ✓6ᵗʰ **T52.1X**   **Toxic effects of benzene**

           ✓7ᵗʰ **T52.1X1**   **Toxic effect of benzene, accidental (unintentional)**
                   Toxic effects of benzene NOS

         2   ✓7ᵗʰ **T52.1X2**   **Toxic effect of benzene, intentional self-harm**   HCC

           ✓7ᵗʰ **T52.1X3**   **Toxic effect of benzene, assault**

           ✓7ᵗʰ **T52.1X4**   **Toxic effect of benzene, undetermined**

     ✓5ᵗʰ **T52.2**   **Toxic effects of homologues of benzene**
                 Toxic effects of toluene [methylbenzene]
                 Toxic effects of xylene [dimethylbenzene]

        ✓6ᵗʰ **T52.2X**   **Toxic effects of homologues of benzene**

           ✓7ᵗʰ **T52.2X1**   **Toxic effect of homologues of benzene, accidental (unintentional)**
                   Toxic effects of homologues of benzene NOS

         2   ✓7ᵗʰ **T52.2X2**   **Toxic effect of homologues of benzene, intentional self-harm**   HCC

           ✓7ᵗʰ **T52.2X3**   **Toxic effect of homologues of benzene, assault**

           ✓7ᵗʰ **T52.2X4**   **Toxic effect of homologues of benzene, undetermined**

     ✓5ᵗʰ **T52.3**   **Toxic effects of glycols**

        ✓6ᵗʰ **T52.3X**   **Toxic effects of glycols**

           ✓7ᵗʰ **T52.3X1**   **Toxic effect of glycols, accidental (unintentional)**
                   Toxic effects of glycols NOS

         2   ✓7ᵗʰ **T52.3X2**   **Toxic effect of glycols, intentional self-harm**   HCC

           ✓7ᵗʰ **T52.3X3**   **Toxic effect of glycols, assault**

           ✓7ᵗʰ **T52.3X4**   **Toxic effect of glycols, undetermined**

     ✓5ᵗʰ **T52.4**   **Toxic effects of ketones**

        ✓6ᵗʰ **T52.4X**   **Toxic effects of ketones**

           ✓7ᵗʰ **T52.4X1**   **Toxic effect of ketones, accidental (unintentional)**
                   Toxic effects of ketones NOS

         2   ✓7ᵗʰ **T52.4X2**   **Toxic effect of ketones, intentional self-harm**   HCC

           ✓7ᵗʰ **T52.4X3**   **Toxic effect of ketones, assault**

           ✓7ᵗʰ **T52.4X4**   **Toxic effect of ketones, undetermined**

     ✓5ᵗʰ **T52.8**   **Toxic effects of other organic solvents**

        ✓6ᵗʰ **T52.8X**   **Toxic effects of other organic solvents**

           ✓7ᵗʰ **T52.8X1**   **Toxic effect of other organic solvents, accidental (unintentional)**
                   Toxic effects of other organic solvents NOS

         2   ✓7ᵗʰ **T52.8X2**   **Toxic effect of other organic solvents, intentional self-harm**   HCC

           ✓7ᵗʰ **T52.8X3**   **Toxic effect of other organic solvents, assault**

           ✓7ᵗʰ **T52.8X4**   **Toxic effect of other organic solvents, undetermined**

     ✓5ᵗʰ **T52.9**   **Toxic effects of unspecified organic solvent**

        ✓x7ᵗʰ **T52.91**   **Toxic effect of unspecified organic solvent, accidental (unintentional)**   ▽

        2   ✓x7ᵗʰ **T52.92**   **Toxic effect of unspecified organic solvent, intentional self-harm**   HCC ▽

        ✓x7ᵗʰ **T52.93**   **Toxic effect of unspecified organic solvent, assault**   ▽

        ✓x7ᵗʰ **T52.94**   **Toxic effect of unspecified organic solvent, undetermined**   ▽

✓4ᵗʰ **T53**   **Toxic effect of halogen derivatives of aliphatic and aromatic hydrocarbons**

> The appropriate 7th character is to be added to each code from category T53.
> A   initial encounter
> D   subsequent encounter
> S   sequela

     ✓5ᵗʰ **T53.0**   **Toxic effects of carbon tetrachloride**
                 Toxic effects of tetrachloromethane

        ✓6ᵗʰ **T53.0X**   **Toxic effects of carbon tetrachloride**

           ✓7ᵗʰ **T53.0X1**   **Toxic effect of carbon tetrachloride, accidental (unintentional)**
                   Toxic effects of carbon tetrachloride NOS

         2   ✓7ᵗʰ **T53.0X2**   **Toxic effect of carbon tetrachloride, intentional self-harm**   HCC

           ✓7ᵗʰ **T53.0X3**   **Toxic effect of carbon tetrachloride, assault**

           ✓7ᵗʰ **T53.0X4**   **Toxic effect of carbon tetrachloride, undetermined**

     ✓5ᵗʰ **T53.1**   **Toxic effects of chloroform**
                 Toxic effects of trichloromethane

        ✓6ᵗʰ **T53.1X**   **Toxic effects of chloroform**

           ✓7ᵗʰ **T53.1X1**   **Toxic effect of chloroform, accidental (unintentional)**
                   Toxic effects of chloroform NOS

         2   ✓7ᵗʰ **T53.1X2**   **Toxic effect of chloroform, intentional self-harm**   HCC

           ✓7ᵗʰ **T53.1X3**   **Toxic effect of chloroform, assault**

           ✓7ᵗʰ **T53.1X4**   **Toxic effect of chloroform, undetermined**

     ✓5ᵗʰ **T53.2**   **Toxic effects of trichloroethylene**
                 Toxic effects of trichloroethene

        ✓6ᵗʰ **T53.2X**   **Toxic effects of trichloroethylene**

           ✓7ᵗʰ **T53.2X1**   **Toxic effect of trichloroethylene, accidental (unintentional)**
                   Toxic effects of trichloroethylene NOS

         2   ✓7ᵗʰ **T53.2X2**   **Toxic effect of trichloroethylene, intentional self-harm**   HCC

           ✓7ᵗʰ **T53.2X3**   **Toxic effect of trichloroethylene, assault**

---

2   HCC with 7th character indicating initial encounter (A or B - specific to category) OR sequela.

☑ Additional Character Req   ✓x7ᵗʰ Placeholder Alert   Manifestation   HCC CMS-HCC Condition   ▽ Unspecified Code   ▶◀ Revised Text   ● New Code   ▲ Revised Code Title

✓7ᵗʰ **T53.2X4** **Toxic effect of trichloroethylene,** undetermined

✓5ᵗʰ **T53.3** **Toxic effects of tetrachloroethylene**
Toxic effects of perchloroethylene
Toxic effect of tetrachloroethene

  ✓6ᵗʰ **T53.3X** **Toxic effects of** tetrachloroethylene

    ✓7ᵗʰ **T53.3X1** **Toxic effect of tetrachloroethylene,** accidental (unintentional)
Toxic effects of tetrachloroethylene NOS

    2 ✓7ᵗʰ **T53.3X2** **Toxic effect of tetrachloroethylene,** HCC intentional self-harm

    ✓7ᵗʰ **T53.3X3** **Toxic effect of tetrachloroethylene,** assault

    ✓7ᵗʰ **T53.3X4** **Toxic effect of tetrachloroethylene,** undetermined

✓5ᵗʰ **T53.4** **Toxic effects of dichloromethane**
Toxic effects of methylene chloride

  ✓6ᵗʰ **T53.4X** **Toxic effects of** dichloromethane

    ✓7ᵗʰ **T53.4X1** **Toxic effect of dichloromethane,** accidental (unintentional)
Toxic effects of dichloromethane NOS

    2 ✓7ᵗʰ **T53.4X2** **Toxic effect of dichloromethane,** HCC intentional self-harm

    ✓7ᵗʰ **T53.4X3** **Toxic effect of dichloromethane,** assault

    ✓7ᵗʰ **T53.4X4** **Toxic effect of dichloromethane,** undetermined

✓5ᵗʰ **T53.5** **Toxic effects of chlorofluorocarbons**

  ✓6ᵗʰ **T53.5X** **Toxic effects of** chlorofluorocarbons

    ✓7ᵗʰ **T53.5X1** **Toxic effect of chlorofluorocarbons,** accidental (unintentional)
Toxic effects of chlorofluorocarbons NOS

    2 ✓7ᵗʰ **T53.5X2** **Toxic effect of chlorofluorocarbons,** HCC intentional self-harm

    ✓7ᵗʰ **T53.5X3** **Toxic effect of chlorofluorocarbons,** assault

    ✓7ᵗʰ **T53.5X4** **Toxic effect of chlorofluorocarbons,** undetermined

✓5ᵗʰ **T53.6** **Toxic effects of other halogen derivatives of aliphatic hydrocarbons**

  ✓6ᵗʰ **T53.6X** **Toxic effects of other** halogen derivatives of aliphatic hydrocarbons

    ✓7ᵗʰ **T53.6X1** **Toxic effect of other halogen derivatives of aliphatic hydrocarbons,** accidental (unintentional)
Toxic effects of other halogen derivatives of aliphatic hydrocarbons NOS

    2 ✓7ᵗʰ **T53.6X2** **Toxic effect of other halogen** HCC **derivatives of aliphatic hydrocarbons,** intentional self-harm

    ✓7ᵗʰ **T53.6X3** **Toxic effect of other halogen derivatives of aliphatic hydrocarbons,** assault

    ✓7ᵗʰ **T53.6X4** **Toxic effect of other halogen derivatives of aliphatic hydrocarbons,** undetermined

✓5ᵗʰ **T53.7** **Toxic effects of other halogen derivatives of aromatic hydrocarbons**

  ✓6ᵗʰ **T53.7X** **Toxic effects of other** halogen derivatives of aromatic hydrocarbons

    ✓7ᵗʰ **T53.7X1** **Toxic effect of other halogen derivatives of aromatic hydrocarbons,** accidental (unintentional)
Toxic effects of other halogen derivatives of aromatic hydrocarbons NOS

    2 ✓7ᵗʰ **T53.7X2** **Toxic effect of other halogen** HCC **derivatives of aromatic hydrocarbons,** intentional self-harm

    ✓7ᵗʰ **T53.7X3** **Toxic effect of other halogen derivatives of aromatic hydrocarbons,** assault

    ✓7ᵗʰ **T53.7X4** **Toxic effect of other halogen derivatives of aromatic hydrocarbons,** undetermined

✓5ᵗʰ **T53.9** **Toxic effects of unspecified halogen derivatives of aliphatic and aromatic hydrocarbons**

  ✓x7ᵗʰ **T53.91** **Toxic effect of unspecified halogen derivatives** ▽ **of aliphatic and aromatic hydrocarbons,** accidental (unintentional)

2 ✓x7ᵗʰ **T53.92** **Toxic effect of unspecified halogen** HCC ▽ **derivatives of aliphatic and aromatic hydrocarbons,** intentional self-harm

✓x7ᵗʰ **T53.93** **Toxic effect of unspecified halogen derivatives** ▽ **of aliphatic and aromatic hydrocarbons,** assault

✓x7ᵗʰ **T53.94** **Toxic effect of unspecified halogen derivatives** ▽ **of aliphatic and aromatic hydrocarbons,** undetermined

✓4ᵗʰ **T54** **Toxic effect of corrosive substances**

> The appropriate 7th character is to be added to each code from category T54.
> A   initial encounter
> D   subsequent encounter
> S   sequela

✓5ᵗʰ **T54.0** **Toxic effects of phenol and phenol homologues**

  ✓6ᵗʰ **T54.0X** **Toxic effects of** phenol and phenol homologues

    ✓7ᵗʰ **T54.0X1** **Toxic effect of phenol and phenol homologues,** accidental (unintentional)
Toxic effects of phenol and phenol homologues NOS

    2 ✓7ᵗʰ **T54.0X2** **Toxic effect of phenol and phenol** HCC **homologues,** intentional self-harm

    ✓7ᵗʰ **T54.0X3** **Toxic effect of phenol and phenol homologues,** assault

    ✓7ᵗʰ **T54.0X4** **Toxic effect of phenol and phenol homologues,** undetermined

✓5ᵗʰ **T54.1** **Toxic effects of other corrosive organic compounds**

  ✓6ᵗʰ **T54.1X** **Toxic effects of other corrosive organic compounds**

    ✓7ᵗʰ **T54.1X1** **Toxic effect of other corrosive organic compounds,** accidental (unintentional)
Toxic effects of other corrosive organic compounds NOS

    2 ✓7ᵗʰ **T54.1X2** **Toxic effect of other corrosive organic** HCC **compounds,** intentional self-harm

    ✓7ᵗʰ **T54.1X3** **Toxic effect of other corrosive organic compounds,** assault

    ✓7ᵗʰ **T54.1X4** **Toxic effect of other corrosive organic compounds,** undetermined

✓5ᵗʰ **T54.2** **Toxic effects of corrosive acids and acid-like substances**
Toxic effects of hydrochloric acid
Toxic effects of sulfuric acid

  ✓6ᵗʰ **T54.2X** **Toxic effects of corrosive** acids and acid-like substances

    ✓7ᵗʰ **T54.2X1** **Toxic effect of corrosive acids and acid-like substances,** accidental (unintentional)
Toxic effects of corrosive acids and acid-like substances NOS

    2 ✓7ᵗʰ **T54.2X2** **Toxic effect of corrosive acids and** HCC **acid-like substances,** intentional self-harm

    ✓7ᵗʰ **T54.2X3** **Toxic effect of corrosive acids and acid-like substances,** assault

    ✓7ᵗʰ **T54.2X4** **Toxic effect of corrosive acids and acid-like substances,** undetermined

✓5ᵗʰ **T54.3** **Toxic effects of corrosive alkalis and alkali-like substances**
Toxic effects of potassium hydroxide
Toxic effects of sodium hydroxide

  ✓6ᵗʰ **T54.3X** **Toxic effects of corrosive** alkalis and alkali-like substances

    ✓7ᵗʰ **T54.3X1** **Toxic effect of corrosive alkalis and alkali-like substances,** accidental (unintentional)
Toxic effects of corrosive alkalis and alkali-like substances NOS

    2 ✓7ᵗʰ **T54.3X2** **Toxic effect of corrosive alkalis and** HCC **alkali-like substances,** intentional self-harm

    ✓7ᵗʰ **T54.3X3** **Toxic effect of corrosive alkalis and alkali-like substances,** assault

    ✓7ᵗʰ **T54.3X4** **Toxic effect of corrosive alkalis and alkali-like substances,** undetermined

✓5ᵗʰ **T54.9** **Toxic effects of unspecified corrosive substance**

  ✓x7ᵗʰ **T54.91** **Toxic effect of unspecified corrosive substance,** ▽ accidental (unintentional)

---

2   HCC with 7th character indicating initial encounter (A or B - specific to category) OR sequela.

EXCLUDES 1 Not coded here   EXCLUDES 2 Not included here   N Newborn Age: 0   P Pediatric Age: 0-17   M Maternity Age: 12-55   A Adult Age: 15-124

1082   ICD-10-CM 2018

2 ✓x7th **T54.92** **Toxic effect of unspecified corrosive** HCC ▽
substance, intentional self-harm

✓x7th **T54.93** **Toxic effect of unspecified corrosive substance,** ▽
assault

✓x7th **T54.94** **Toxic effect of unspecified corrosive substance,** ▽
undetermined

✓4th **T55** **Toxic effect of soaps and detergents**

> The appropriate 7th character is to be added to each code from
> category T55.
> A   initial encounter
> D   subsequent encounter
> S   sequela

✓5th **T55.0** **Toxic effect of soaps**

✓6th **T55.0X** **Toxic effect of soaps**

✓7th **T55.0X1** **Toxic effect of soaps, accidental**
(unintentional)
Toxic effect of soaps NOS

2 ✓7th **T55.0X2** **Toxic effect of soaps, intentional** HCC
self-harm

✓7th **T55.0X3** **Toxic effect of soaps, assault**

✓7th **T55.0X4** **Toxic effect of soaps, undetermined**

✓5th **T55.1** **Toxic effect of detergents**

✓6th **T55.1X** **Toxic effect of detergents**

✓7th **T55.1X1** **Toxic effect of detergents, accidental**
(unintentional)
Toxic effect of detergents NOS

2 ✓7th **T55.1X2** **Toxic effect of detergents, intentional** HCC
self-harm

✓7th **T55.1X3** **Toxic effect of detergents, assault**

✓7th **T55.1X4** **Toxic effect of detergents, undetermined**

✓4th **T56** **Toxic effect of metals**
INCLUDES   toxic effects of fumes and vapors of metals
toxic effects of metals from all sources, except medicinal
substances
Use additional code to identify any retained metal foreign body, if
applicable (Z18.0-, T18.1-)
EXCLUDES 1   arsenic and its compounds (T57.0)
manganese and its compounds (T57.2)

> The appropriate 7th character is to be added to each code from
> category T56.
> A   initial encounter
> D   subsequent encounter
> S   sequela

✓5th **T56.0** **Toxic effects of lead and its compounds**

✓6th **T56.0X** **Toxic effects of lead and its compounds**

✓7th **T56.0X1** **Toxic effect of lead and its compounds,**
accidental (unintentional)
Toxic effects of lead and its compounds
NOS

2 ✓7th **T56.0X2** **Toxic effect of lead and its** HCC
compounds, intentional self-harm

✓7th **T56.0X3** **Toxic effect of lead and its compounds,**
assault

✓7th **T56.0X4** **Toxic effect of lead and its compounds,**
undetermined

✓5th **T56.1** **Toxic effects of mercury and its compounds**

✓6th **T56.1X** **Toxic effects of mercury and its compounds**

✓7th **T56.1X1** **Toxic effect of mercury and its**
compounds, accidental (unintentional)
Toxic effects of mercury and its compounds
NOS

2 ✓7th **T56.1X2** **Toxic effect of mercury and its** HCC
compounds, intentional self-harm

✓7th **T56.1X3** **Toxic effect of mercury and its**
compounds, assault

✓7th **T56.1X4** **Toxic effect of mercury and its**
compounds, undetermined

✓5th **T56.2** **Toxic effects of chromium and its compounds**

✓6th **T56.2X** **Toxic effects of chromium and its compounds**

✓7th **T56.2X1** **Toxic effect of chromium and its**
compounds, accidental (unintentional)
Toxic effects of chromium and its
compounds NOS

2 ✓7th **T56.2X2** **Toxic effect of chromium and its** HCC
compounds, intentional self-harm

✓7th **T56.2X3** **Toxic effect of chromium and its**
compounds, assault

✓7th **T56.2X4** **Toxic effect of chromium and its**
compounds, undetermined

✓5th **T56.3** **Toxic effects of cadmium and its compounds**

✓6th **T56.3X** **Toxic effects of cadmium and its compounds**

✓7th **T56.3X1** **Toxic effect of cadmium and its**
compounds, accidental (unintentional)
Toxic effects of cadmium and its
compounds NOS

2 ✓7th **T56.3X2** **Toxic effect of cadmium and its** HCC
compounds, intentional self-harm

✓7th **T56.3X3** **Toxic effect of cadmium and its**
compounds, assault

✓7th **T56.3X4** **Toxic effect of cadmium and its**
compounds, undetermined

✓5th **T56.4** **Toxic effects of copper and its compounds**

✓6th **T56.4X** **Toxic effects of copper and its compounds**

✓7th **T56.4X1** **Toxic effect of copper and its compounds,**
accidental (unintentional)
Toxic effects of copper and its compounds
NOS

2 ✓7th **T56.4X2** **Toxic effect of copper and its** HCC
compounds, intentional self-harm

✓7th **T56.4X3** **Toxic effect of copper and its compounds,**
assault

✓7th **T56.4X4** **Toxic effect of copper and its compounds,**
undetermined

✓5th **T56.5** **Toxic effects of zinc and its compounds**

✓6th **T56.5X** **Toxic effects of zinc and its compounds**

✓7th **T56.5X1** **Toxic effect of zinc and its compounds,**
accidental (unintentional)
Toxic effects of zinc and its compounds
NOS

2 ✓7th **T56.5X2** **Toxic effect of zinc and its** HCC
compounds, intentional self-harm

✓7th **T56.5X3** **Toxic effect of zinc and its compounds,**
assault

✓7th **T56.5X4** **Toxic effect of zinc and its compounds,**
undetermined

✓5th **T56.6** **Toxic effects of tin and its compounds**

✓6th **T56.6X** **Toxic effects of tin and its compounds**

✓7th **T56.6X1** **Toxic effect of tin and its compounds,**
accidental (unintentional)
Toxic effects of tin and its compounds NOS

2 ✓7th **T56.6X2** **Toxic effect of tin and its** HCC
compounds, intentional self-harm

✓7th **T56.6X3** **Toxic effect of tin and its compounds,**
assault

✓7th **T56.6X4** **Toxic effect of tin and its compounds,**
undetermined

✓5th **T56.7** **Toxic effects of beryllium and its compounds**

✓6th **T56.7X** **Toxic effects of beryllium and its compounds**

✓7th **T56.7X1** **Toxic effect of beryllium and its**
compounds, accidental (unintentional)
Toxic effects of beryllium and its
compounds NOS

2 ✓7th **T56.7X2** **Toxic effect of beryllium and its** HCC
compounds, intentional self-harm

✓7th **T56.7X3** **Toxic effect of beryllium and its**
compounds, assault

✓7th **T56.7X4** **Toxic effect of beryllium and its**
compounds, undetermined

✓5th **T56.8** **Toxic effects of other metals**

✓6th **T56.81** **Toxic effect of thallium**

✓7th **T56.811** **Toxic effect of thallium, accidental**
(unintentional)
Toxic effect of thallium NOS

2 ✓7th **T56.812** **Toxic effect of thallium, intentional** HCC
self-harm

✓7th **T56.813** **Toxic effect of thallium, assault**

✓7th **T56.814** **Toxic effect of thallium, undetermined**

---

2   HCC with 7th character indicating initial encounter (A or B - specific to category) OR sequela.

✓ Additional Character Req   ✓x7th Placeholder Alert   Manifestation   HCC CMS-HCC Condition   ▽ Unspecified Code   ►◄ Revised Text   ● New Code   ▲ Revised Code Title

ICD-10-CM 2018   1083

Chapter 19. Injury, Poisoning, and Certain Other Consequences of External Causes

T54.92–T56.814

√6ᵗʰ **T56.89** **Toxic effects of other metals**

√7ᵗʰ **T56.891** **Toxic effect of other metals, accidental (unintentional)**
Toxic effects of other metals NOS

2 √7ᵗʰ **T56.892** **Toxic effect of other metals, intentional self-harm** HCC

√7ᵗʰ **T56.893** **Toxic effect of other metals, assault**

√7ᵗʰ **T56.894** **Toxic effect of other metals, undetermined**

√5ᵗʰ **T56.9** **Toxic effects of unspecified metal**

√x7ᵗʰ **T56.91** **Toxic effect of unspecified metal, accidental (unintentional)** ▽

2 √x7ᵗʰ **T56.92** **Toxic effect of unspecified metal, intentional self-harm** HCC ▽

√x7ᵗʰ **T56.93** **Toxic effect of unspecified metal, assault** ▽

√x7ᵗʰ **T56.94** **Toxic effect of unspecified metal, undetermined** ▽

√4ᵗʰ **T57** **Toxic effect of other inorganic substances**

The appropriate 7th character is to be added to each code from category T57.
A initial encounter
D subsequent encounter
S sequela

√5ᵗʰ **T57.0** **Toxic effect of arsenic and its compounds**

√6ᵗʰ **T57.0X** **Toxic effect of arsenic and its compounds**

√7ᵗʰ **T57.0X1** **Toxic effect of arsenic and its compounds, accidental (unintentional)**
Toxic effect of arsenic and its compounds NOS

2 √7ᵗʰ **T57.0X2** **Toxic effect of arsenic and its compounds, intentional self-harm** HCC

√7ᵗʰ **T57.0X3** **Toxic effect of arsenic and its compounds, assault**

√7ᵗʰ **T57.0X4** **Toxic effect of arsenic and its compounds, undetermined**

√5ᵗʰ **T57.1** **Toxic effect of phosphorus and its compounds**
EXCLUDES 1 organophosphate insecticides (T60.0)

√6ᵗʰ **T57.1X** **Toxic effect of phosphorus and its compounds**

√7ᵗʰ **T57.1X1** **Toxic effect of phosphorus and its compounds, accidental (unintentional)**
Toxic effect of phosphorus and its compounds NOS

2 √7ᵗʰ **T57.1X2** **Toxic effect of phosphorus and its compounds, intentional self-harm** HCC

√7ᵗʰ **T57.1X3** **Toxic effect of phosphorus and its compounds, assault**

√7ᵗʰ **T57.1X4** **Toxic effect of phosphorus and its compounds, undetermined**

√5ᵗʰ **T57.2** **Toxic effect of manganese and its compounds**

√6ᵗʰ **T57.2X** **Toxic effect of manganese and its compounds**

√7ᵗʰ **T57.2X1** **Toxic effect of manganese and its compounds, accidental (unintentional)**
Toxic effect of manganese and its compounds NOS

2 √7ᵗʰ **T57.2X2** **Toxic effect of manganese and its compounds, intentional self-harm** HCC

√7ᵗʰ **T57.2X3** **Toxic effect of manganese and its compounds, assault**

√7ᵗʰ **T57.2X4** **Toxic effect of manganese and its compounds, undetermined**

√5ᵗʰ **T57.3** **Toxic effect of hydrogen cyanide**

√6ᵗʰ **T57.3X** **Toxic effect of hydrogen cyanide**

√7ᵗʰ **T57.3X1** **Toxic effect of hydrogen cyanide, accidental (unintentional)**
Toxic effect of hydrogen cyanide NOS

2 √7ᵗʰ **T57.3X2** **Toxic effect of hydrogen cyanide, intentional self-harm** HCC

√7ᵗʰ **T57.3X3** **Toxic effect of hydrogen cyanide, assault**

√7ᵗʰ **T57.3X4** **Toxic effect of hydrogen cyanide, undetermined**

√5ᵗʰ **T57.8** **Toxic effect of other specified inorganic substances**

√6ᵗʰ **T57.8X** **Toxic effect of other specified inorganic substances**

√7ᵗʰ **T57.8X1** **Toxic effect of other specified inorganic substances, accidental (unintentional)**
Toxic effect of other specified inorganic substances NOS

2 √7ᵗʰ **T57.8X2** **Toxic effect of other specified inorganic substances, intentional self-harm** HCC

√7ᵗʰ **T57.8X3** **Toxic effect of other specified inorganic substances, assault**

√7ᵗʰ **T57.8X4** **Toxic effect of other specified inorganic substances, undetermined**

√5ᵗʰ **T57.9** **Toxic effect of unspecified inorganic substance**

√x7ᵗʰ **T57.91** **Toxic effect of unspecified inorganic substance, accidental (unintentional)** ▽

2 √x7ᵗʰ **T57.92** **Toxic effect of unspecified inorganic substance, intentional self-harm** HCC ▽

√x7ᵗʰ **T57.93** **Toxic effect of unspecified inorganic substance, assault** ▽

√x7ᵗʰ **T57.94** **Toxic effect of unspecified inorganic substance, undetermined** ▽

√4ᵗʰ **T58** **Toxic effect of carbon monoxide**
INCLUDES asphyxiation from carbon monoxide
toxic effect of carbon monoxide from all sources

The appropriate 7th character is to be added to each code from category T58.
A initial encounter
D subsequent encounter
S sequela

√5ᵗʰ **T58.0** **Toxic effect of carbon monoxide from motor vehicle exhaust**
Toxic effect of exhaust gas from gas engine
Toxic effect of exhaust gas from motor pump

√x7ᵗʰ **T58.01** **Toxic effect of carbon monoxide from motor vehicle exhaust, accidental (unintentional)**

2 √x7ᵗʰ **T58.02** **Toxic effect of carbon monoxide from motor vehicle exhaust, intentional self-harm** HCC

√x7ᵗʰ **T58.03** **Toxic effect of carbon monoxide from motor vehicle exhaust, assault**

√x7ᵗʰ **T58.04** **Toxic effect of carbon monoxide from motor vehicle exhaust, undetermined**

√5ᵗʰ **T58.1** **Toxic effect of carbon monoxide from utility gas**
Toxic effect of acetylene
Toxic effect of gas NOS used for lighting, heating, cooking
Toxic effect of water gas

√x7ᵗʰ **T58.11** **Toxic effect of carbon monoxide from utility gas, accidental (unintentional)**

2 √x7ᵗʰ **T58.12** **Toxic effect of carbon monoxide from utility gas, intentional self-harm** HCC

√x7ᵗʰ **T58.13** **Toxic effect of carbon monoxide from utility gas, assault**

√x7ᵗʰ **T58.14** **Toxic effect of carbon monoxide from utility gas, undetermined**

√5ᵗʰ **T58.2** **Toxic effect of carbon monoxide from incomplete combustion of other domestic fuels**
Toxic effect of carbon monoxide from incomplete combustion of coal, coke, kerosene, wood

√6ᵗʰ **T58.2X** **Toxic effect of carbon monoxide from incomplete combustion of other domestic fuels**

√7ᵗʰ **T58.2X1** **Toxic effect of carbon monoxide from incomplete combustion of other domestic fuels, accidental (unintentional)**

2 √7ᵗʰ **T58.2X2** **Toxic effect of carbon monoxide from incomplete combustion of other domestic fuels, intentional self-harm** HCC

√7ᵗʰ **T58.2X3** **Toxic effect of carbon monoxide from incomplete combustion of other domestic fuels, assault**

√7ᵗʰ **T58.2X4** **Toxic effect of carbon monoxide from incomplete combustion of other domestic fuels, undetermined**

2 HCC with 7th character indicating initial encounter (A or B - specific to category) OR sequela.

EXCLUDES 1 Not coded here   EXCLUDES 2 Not included here   N Newborn Age: 0   P Pediatric Age: 0-17   M Maternity Age: 12-55   A Adult Age: 15-124
1084   ICD-10-CM 2018

✓5th **T58.8** **Toxic effect of carbon monoxide from other source**
Toxic effect of carbon monoxide from blast furnace gas
Toxic effect of carbon monoxide from fuels in industrial use
Toxic effect of carbon monoxide from kiln vapor

   ✓6th **T58.8X** **Toxic effect of carbon monoxide from other source**

     ✓7th **T58.8X1** **Toxic effect of carbon monoxide from other source, accidental (unintentional)**

     2 ✓7th **T58.8X2** **Toxic effect of carbon monoxide from other source, intentional self-harm** HCC

     ✓7th **T58.8X3** **Toxic effect of carbon monoxide from other source, assault**

     ✓7th **T58.8X4** **Toxic effect of carbon monoxide from other source, undetermined**

✓5th **T58.9** **Toxic effect of carbon monoxide from unspecified source**

   ✓x7th **T58.91** **Toxic effect of carbon monoxide from unspecified source, accidental (unintentional)** ▽

   2 ✓x7th **T58.92** **Toxic effect of carbon monoxide from unspecified source, intentional self-harm** HCC ▽

   ✓x7th **T58.93** **Toxic effect of carbon monoxide from unspecified source, assault** ▽

   ✓x7th **T58.94** **Toxic effect of carbon monoxide from unspecified source, undetermined** ▽

✓4th **T59** **Toxic effect of other gases, fumes and vapors**
   INCLUDES   aerosol propellants
   EXCLUDES 1   *chlorofluorocarbons (T53.5)*

> The appropriate 7th character is to be added to each code from category T59.
> A   initial encounter
> D   subsequent encounter
> S   sequela

✓5th **T59.0** **Toxic effect of nitrogen oxides**

   ✓6th **T59.0X** **Toxic effect of nitrogen oxides**

     ✓7th **T59.0X1** **Toxic effect of nitrogen oxides, accidental (unintentional)**
Toxic effect of nitrogen oxides NOS

     2 ✓7th **T59.0X2** **Toxic effect of nitrogen oxides, intentional self-harm** HCC

     ✓7th **T59.0X3** **Toxic effect of nitrogen oxides, assault**

     ✓7th **T59.0X4** **Toxic effect of nitrogen oxides, undetermined**

✓5th **T59.1** **Toxic effect of sulfur dioxide**

   ✓6th **T59.1X** **Toxic effect of sulfur dioxide**

     ✓7th **T59.1X1** **Toxic effect of sulfur dioxide, accidental (unintentional)**
Toxic effect of sulfur dioxide NOS

     2 ✓7th **T59.1X2** **Toxic effect of sulfur dioxide, intentional self-harm** HCC

     ✓7th **T59.1X3** **Toxic effect of sulfur dioxide, assault**

     ✓7th **T59.1X4** **Toxic effect of sulfur dioxide, undetermined**

✓5th **T59.2** **Toxic effect of formaldehyde**

   ✓6th **T59.2X** **Toxic effect of formaldehyde**

     ✓7th **T59.2X1** **Toxic effect of formaldehyde, accidental (unintentional)**
Toxic effect of formaldehyde NOS

     2 ✓7th **T59.2X2** **Toxic effect of formaldehyde, intentional self-harm** HCC

     ✓7th **T59.2X3** **Toxic effect of formaldehyde, assault**

     ✓7th **T59.2X4** **Toxic effect of formaldehyde, undetermined**

✓5th **T59.3** **Toxic effect of lacrimogenic gas**
Toxic effect of tear gas

   ✓6th **T59.3X** **Toxic effect of lacrimogenic gas**

     ✓7th **T59.3X1** **Toxic effect of lacrimogenic gas, accidental (unintentional)**
Toxic effect of lacrimogenic gas NOS

     2 ✓7th **T59.3X2** **Toxic effect of lacrimogenic gas, intentional self-harm** HCC

     ✓7th **T59.3X3** **Toxic effect of lacrimogenic gas, assault**

     ✓7th **T59.3X4** **Toxic effect of lacrimogenic gas, undetermined**

✓5th **T59.4** **Toxic effect of chlorine gas**

   ✓6th **T59.4X** **Toxic effect of chlorine gas**

     ✓7th **T59.4X1** **Toxic effect of chlorine gas, accidental (unintentional)**
Toxic effect of chlorine gas NOS

     2 ✓7th **T59.4X2** **Toxic effect of chlorine gas, intentional self-harm** HCC

     ✓7th **T59.4X3** **Toxic effect of chlorine gas, assault**

     ✓7th **T59.4X4** **Toxic effect of chlorine gas, undetermined**

✓5th **T59.5** **Toxic effect of fluorine gas and hydrogen fluoride**

   ✓6th **T59.5X** **Toxic effect of fluorine gas and hydrogen fluoride**

     ✓7th **T59.5X1** **Toxic effect of fluorine gas and hydrogen fluoride, accidental (unintentional)**
Toxic effect of fluorine gas and hydrogen fluoride NOS

     2 ✓7th **T59.5X2** **Toxic effect of fluorine gas and hydrogen fluoride, intentional self-harm** HCC

     ✓7th **T59.5X3** **Toxic effect of fluorine gas and hydrogen fluoride, assault**

     ✓7th **T59.5X4** **Toxic effect of fluorine gas and hydrogen fluoride, undetermined**

✓5th **T59.6** **Toxic effect of hydrogen sulfide**

   ✓6th **T59.6X** **Toxic effect of hydrogen sulfide**

     ✓7th **T59.6X1** **Toxic effect of hydrogen sulfide, accidental (unintentional)**
Toxic effect of hydrogen sulfide NOS

     2 ✓7th **T59.6X2** **Toxic effect of hydrogen sulfide, intentional self-harm** HCC

     ✓7th **T59.6X3** **Toxic effect of hydrogen sulfide, assault**

     ✓7th **T59.6X4** **Toxic effect of hydrogen sulfide, undetermined**

✓5th **T59.7** **Toxic effect of carbon dioxide**

   ✓6th **T59.7X** **Toxic effect of carbon dioxide**

     ✓7th **T59.7X1** **Toxic effect of carbon dioxide, accidental (unintentional)**
Toxic effect of carbon dioxide NOS

     2 ✓7th **T59.7X2** **Toxic effect of carbon dioxide, intentional self-harm** HCC

     ✓7th **T59.7X3** **Toxic effect of carbon dioxide, assault**

     ✓7th **T59.7X4** **Toxic effect of carbon dioxide, undetermined**

✓5th **T59.8** **Toxic effect of other specified gases, fumes and vapors**

   ✓6th **T59.81** **Toxic effect of smoke**
Smoke inhalation
     EXCLUDES 2   *toxic effect of cigarette (tobacco) smoke (T65.22-)*

     ✓7th **T59.811** **Toxic effect of smoke, accidental (unintentional)**
Toxic effect of smoke NOS
AHA: 2013, 4Q, 121

     2 ✓7th **T59.812** **Toxic effect of smoke, intentional self-harm** HCC

     ✓7th **T59.813** **Toxic effect of smoke, assault**

     ✓7th **T59.814** **Toxic effect of smoke, undetermined**

   ✓6th **T59.89** **Toxic effect of other specified gases, fumes and vapors**

     ✓7th **T59.891** **Toxic effect of other specified gases, fumes and vapors, accidental (unintentional)**

     2 ✓7th **T59.892** **Toxic effect of other specified gases, fumes and vapors, intentional self-harm** HCC

     ✓7th **T59.893** **Toxic effect of other specified gases, fumes and vapors, assault**

     ✓7th **T59.894** **Toxic effect of other specified gases, fumes and vapors, undetermined**

✓5th **T59.9** **Toxic effect of unspecified gases, fumes and vapors**

   ✓x7th **T59.91** **Toxic effect of unspecified gases, fumes and vapors, accidental (unintentional)** ▽

   2 ✓x7th **T59.92** **Toxic effect of unspecified gases, fumes and vapors, intentional self-harm** HCC ▽

   ✓x7th **T59.93** **Toxic effect of unspecified gases, fumes and vapors, assault** ▽

---

2   HCC with 7th character indicating initial encounter (A or B - specific to category) OR sequela.

✓ Additional Character Req   ✓x7th Placeholder Alert   Manifestation   HCC CMS-HCC Condition   ▽ Unspecified Code   ►◄ Revised Text   ● New Code   ▲ Revised Code Title

√x7ᵗʰ **T59.94** **Toxic effect of unspecified gases, fumes and vapors,** undetermined ▽

√4ᵗʰ **T60** **Toxic effect of pesticides**
    INCLUDES   toxic effect of wood preservatives

The appropriate 7th character is to be added to each code from category T60.
A   initial encounter
D   subsequent encounter
S   sequela

√5ᵗʰ **T60.0** **Toxic effect of organophosphate and carbamate insecticides**

   √6ᵗʰ **T60.0X** **Toxic effect of** organophosphate and carbamate insecticides

     √7ᵗʰ **T60.0X1** **Toxic effect of organophosphate and carbamate insecticides,** accidental (unintentional)
       Toxic effect of organophosphate and carbamate insecticides NOS

     2 √7ᵗʰ **T60.0X2** **Toxic effect of organophosphate and carbamate insecticides,** intentional self-harm   HCC

     √7ᵗʰ **T60.0X3** **Toxic effect of organophosphate and carbamate insecticides,** assault

     √7ᵗʰ **T60.0X4** **Toxic effect of organophosphate and carbamate insecticides,** undetermined

√5ᵗʰ **T60.1** **Toxic effect of halogenated insecticides**
    EXCLUDES 1   chlorinated hydrocarbon (T53.-)

   √6ᵗʰ **T60.1X** **Toxic effect of** halogenated insecticides

     √7ᵗʰ **T60.1X1** **Toxic effect of halogenated insecticides,** accidental (unintentional)
       Toxic effect of halogenated insecticides NOS

     2 √7ᵗʰ **T60.1X2** **Toxic effect of halogenated insecticides,** intentional self-harm   HCC

     √7ᵗʰ **T60.1X3** **Toxic effect of halogenated insecticides,** assault

     √7ᵗʰ **T60.1X4** **Toxic effect of halogenated insecticides,** undetermined

√5ᵗʰ **T60.2** **Toxic effect of other insecticides**

   √6ᵗʰ **T60.2X** **Toxic effect of other insecticides**

     √7ᵗʰ **T60.2X1** **Toxic effect of other insecticides,** accidental (unintentional)
       Toxic effect of other insecticides NOS

     2 √7ᵗʰ **T60.2X2** **Toxic effect of other insecticides,** intentional self-harm   HCC

     √7ᵗʰ **T60.2X3** **Toxic effect of other insecticides,** assault

     √7ᵗʰ **T60.2X4** **Toxic effect of other insecticides,** undetermined

√5ᵗʰ **T60.3** **Toxic effect of herbicides and fungicides**

   √6ᵗʰ **T60.3X** **Toxic effect of** herbicides and fungicides

     √7ᵗʰ **T60.3X1** **Toxic effect of herbicides and fungicides,** accidental (unintentional)
       Toxic effect of herbicides and fungicides NOS

     2 √7ᵗʰ **T60.3X2** **Toxic effect of herbicides and fungicides,** intentional self-harm   HCC

     √7ᵗʰ **T60.3X3** **Toxic effect of herbicides and fungicides,** assault

     √7ᵗʰ **T60.3X4** **Toxic effect of herbicides and fungicides,** undetermined

√5ᵗʰ **T60.4** **Toxic effect of rodenticides**
    EXCLUDES 1   strychnine and its salts (T65.1)
          thallium (T56.81-)

   √6ᵗʰ **T60.4X** **Toxic effect of** rodenticides

     √7ᵗʰ **T60.4X1** **Toxic effect of rodenticides,** accidental (unintentional)
       Toxic effect of rodenticides NOS

     2 √7ᵗʰ **T60.4X2** **Toxic effect of rodenticides,** intentional self-harm   HCC

     √7ᵗʰ **T60.4X3** **Toxic effect of rodenticides,** assault

     √7ᵗʰ **T60.4X4** **Toxic effect of rodenticides,** undetermined

√5ᵗʰ **T60.8** **Toxic effect of other pesticides**

   √6ᵗʰ **T60.8X** **Toxic effect of other pesticides**

     √7ᵗʰ **T60.8X1** **Toxic effect of other pesticides,** accidental (unintentional)
       Toxic effect of other pesticides NOS

     2 √7ᵗʰ **T60.8X2** **Toxic effect of other pesticides,** intentional self-harm   HCC

     √7ᵗʰ **T60.8X3** **Toxic effect of other pesticides,** assault

     √7ᵗʰ **T60.8X4** **Toxic effect of other pesticides,** undetermined

√5ᵗʰ **T60.9** **Toxic effect of unspecified pesticide**

   √x7ᵗʰ **T60.91** **Toxic effect of unspecified pesticide,** accidental (unintentional) ▽

   2 √x7ᵗʰ **T60.92** **Toxic effect of unspecified pesticide,** intentional self-harm   HCC ▽

   √x7ᵗʰ **T60.93** **Toxic effect of unspecified pesticide,** assault ▽

   √x7ᵗʰ **T60.94** **Toxic effect of unspecified pesticide,** undetermined ▽

√4ᵗʰ **T61** **Toxic effect of noxious substances eaten as seafood**
    EXCLUDES 1   allergic reaction to food, such as:
          anaphylactic reaction or shock due to adverse food reaction (T78.0-)
          bacterial foodborne intoxications (A05.-)
          dermatitis (L23.6, L25.4, L27.2)
          food protein-induced enterocolitis syndrome (K52.21)
          food protein-induced enteropathy (K52.22)
          gastroenteritis (noninfective) (K52.29)
       toxic effect of aflatoxin and other mycotoxins (T64)
       toxic effect of cyanides (T65.0-)
       toxic effect of harmful algae bloom (T65.82-)
       toxic effect of hydrogen cyanide (T57.3-)
       toxic effect of mercury (T56.1-)
       toxic effect of red tide (T65.82-)

The appropriate 7th character is to be added to each code from category T61.
A   initial encounter
D   subsequent encounter
S   sequela

√5ᵗʰ **T61.0** **Ciguatera fish poisoning**

   √x7ᵗʰ **T61.01** **Ciguatera fish poisoning,** accidental (unintentional)

   2 √x7ᵗʰ **T61.02** **Ciguatera fish poisoning,** intentional self-harm   HCC

   √x7ᵗʰ **T61.03** **Ciguatera fish poisoning,** assault

   √x7ᵗʰ **T61.04** **Ciguatera fish poisoning,** undetermined

√5ᵗʰ **T61.1** **Scombroid fish poisoning**
    Histamine-like syndrome

   √x7ᵗʰ **T61.11** **Scombroid fish poisoning,** accidental (unintentional)

   2 √x7ᵗʰ **T61.12** **Scombroid fish poisoning,** intentional self-harm   HCC

   √x7ᵗʰ **T61.13** **Scombroid fish poisoning,** assault

   √x7ᵗʰ **T61.14** **Scombroid fish poisoning,** undetermined

√5ᵗʰ **T61.7** **Other fish and shellfish poisoning**

   √6ᵗʰ **T61.77** **Other** fish **poisoning**

     √7ᵗʰ **T61.771** **Other fish poisoning,** accidental (unintentional)

     2 √7ᵗʰ **T61.772** **Other fish poisoning,** intentional self-harm   HCC

     √7ᵗʰ **T61.773** **Other fish poisoning,** assault

     √7ᵗʰ **T61.774** **Other fish poisoning,** undetermined

   √6ᵗʰ **T61.78** **Other** shellfish **poisoning**

     √7ᵗʰ **T61.781** **Other shellfish poisoning,** accidental (unintentional)

     2 √7ᵗʰ **T61.782** **Other shellfish poisoning,** intentional self-harm   HCC

     √7ᵗʰ **T61.783** **Other shellfish poisoning,** assault

     √7ᵗʰ **T61.784** **Other shellfish poisoning,** undetermined

√5ᵗʰ **T61.8** **Toxic effect of other seafood**

   √6ᵗʰ **T61.8X** **Toxic effect of other seafood**

     √7ᵗʰ **T61.8X1** **Toxic effect of other seafood,** accidental (unintentional)

     2 √7ᵗʰ **T61.8X2** **Toxic effect of other seafood,** intentional self-harm   HCC

     √7ᵗʰ **T61.8X3** **Toxic effect of other seafood,** assault

---

2   HCC with 7th character indicating initial encounter (A or B - specific to category) OR sequela.

EXCLUDES 1 Not coded here   EXCLUDES 2 Not included here   N Newborn Age: 0   P Pediatric Age: 0-17   M Maternity Age: 12-55   A Adult Age: 15-124

1086   ICD-10-CM 2018

☑7ᵗʰ **T61.8X4   Toxic effect of other seafood,** undetermined

☑5ᵗʰ **T61.9   Toxic effect of unspecified seafood**

☑x7ᵗʰ **T61.91   Toxic effect of unspecified seafood,** accidental (unintentional) ▽

2 ☑x7ᵗʰ **T61.92   Toxic effect of unspecified seafood,** intentional self-harm HCC ▽

☑x7ᵗʰ **T61.93   Toxic effect of unspecified seafood,** assault ▽

☑x7ᵗʰ **T61.94   Toxic effect of unspecified seafood,** undetermined ▽

☑4ᵗʰ **T62   Toxic effect of other noxious substances eaten as food**

EXCLUDES 1   allergic reaction to food, such as:
  anaphylactic shock (reaction) due to adverse food reaction (T78.0-)
  bacterial food borne intoxications (A05.-)
  dermatitis (L23.6, L25.4, L27.2)
  food protein-induced enterocolitis syndrome (K52.21)
  food protein-induced enteropathy (K52.22)
  gastroenteritis (noninfective) (K52.29)
  toxic effect of aflatoxin and other mycotoxins (T64)
  toxic effect of cyanides (T65.0-)
  toxic effect of hydrogen cyanide (T57.3-)
  toxic effect of mercury (T56.1-)

The appropriate 7th character is to be added to each code from category T62.
A   initial encounter
D   subsequent encounter
S   sequela

☑5ᵗʰ **T62.0   Toxic effect of ingested mushrooms**

☑6ᵗʰ **T62.0X   Toxic effect of** ingested mushrooms

☑7ᵗʰ **T62.0X1   Toxic effect of ingested mushrooms,** accidental (unintentional)
  Toxic effect of ingested mushrooms NOS

2 ☑7ᵗʰ **T62.0X2   Toxic effect of ingested mushrooms,** intentional self-harm HCC

☑7ᵗʰ **T62.0X3   Toxic effect of ingested mushrooms,** assault

☑7ᵗʰ **T62.0X4   Toxic effect of ingested mushrooms,** undetermined

☑5ᵗʰ **T62.1   Toxic effect of ingested berries**

☑6ᵗʰ **T62.1X   Toxic effect of** ingested berries

☑7ᵗʰ **T62.1X1   Toxic effect of ingested berries,** accidental (unintentional)
  Toxic effect of ingested berries NOS

2 ☑7ᵗʰ **T62.1X2   Toxic effect of ingested berries,** intentional self-harm HCC

☑7ᵗʰ **T62.1X3   Toxic effect of ingested berries,** assault

☑7ᵗʰ **T62.1X4   Toxic effect of ingested berries,** undetermined

☑5ᵗʰ **T62.2   Toxic effect of other ingested (parts of) plant(s)**

☑6ᵗʰ **T62.2X   Toxic effect of other ingested (parts of)** plant(s)

☑7ᵗʰ **T62.2X1   Toxic effect of other ingested (parts of) plant(s),** accidental (unintentional)
  Toxic effect of other ingested (parts of) plant(s) NOS

2 ☑7ᵗʰ **T62.2X2   Toxic effect of other ingested (parts of) plant(s),** intentional self-harm HCC

☑7ᵗʰ **T62.2X3   Toxic effect of other ingested (parts of) plant(s),** assault

☑7ᵗʰ **T62.2X4   Toxic effect of other ingested (parts of) plant(s),** undetermined

☑5ᵗʰ **T62.8   Toxic effect of other specified noxious substances eaten as food**

☑6ᵗʰ **T62.8X   Toxic effect of other specified noxious substances eaten as food**

☑7ᵗʰ **T62.8X1   Toxic effect of other specified noxious substances eaten as food,** accidental (unintentional)
  Toxic effect of other specified noxious substances eaten as food NOS

2 ☑7ᵗʰ **T62.8X2   Toxic effect of other specified noxious substances eaten as food,** intentional self-harm HCC

☑7ᵗʰ **T62.8X3   Toxic effect of other specified noxious substances eaten as food,** assault

☑7ᵗʰ **T62.8X4   Toxic effect of other specified noxious substances eaten as food,** undetermined

☑5ᵗʰ **T62.9   Toxic effect of unspecified noxious substance eaten as food**

☑x7ᵗʰ **T62.91   Toxic effect of unspecified noxious substance eaten as food,** accidental (unintentional) ▽
  Toxic effect of unspecified noxious substance eaten as food NOS

2 ☑x7ᵗʰ **T62.92   Toxic effect of unspecified noxious substance eaten as food,** intentional self-harm HCC ▽

☑x7ᵗʰ **T62.93   Toxic effect of unspecified noxious substance eaten as food,** assault ▽

☑x7ᵗʰ **T62.94   Toxic effect of unspecified noxious substance eaten as food,** undetermined ▽

☑4ᵗʰ **T63   Toxic effect of contact with venomous animals and plants**

INCLUDES   bite or touch of venomous animal
  pricked or stuck by thorn or leaf
EXCLUDES 2   ingestion of toxic animal or plant (T61.-, T62.-)

The appropriate 7th character is to be added to each code from category T63.
A   initial encounter
D   subsequent encounter
S   sequela

☑5ᵗʰ **T63.0   Toxic effect of** snake venom

☑6ᵗʰ **T63.00   Toxic effect of unspecified snake venom**

☑7ᵗʰ **T63.001   Toxic effect of unspecified snake venom,** accidental (unintentional) ▽
  Toxic effect of unspecified snake venom NOS

2 ☑7ᵗʰ **T63.002   Toxic effect of unspecified snake venom,** intentional self-harm HCC ▽

☑7ᵗʰ **T63.003   Toxic effect of unspecified snake venom,** assault ▽

☑7ᵗʰ **T63.004   Toxic effect of unspecified snake venom,** undetermined ▽

☑6ᵗʰ **T63.01   Toxic effect of** rattlesnake **venom**

☑7ᵗʰ **T63.011   Toxic effect of rattlesnake venom,** accidental (unintentional)
  Toxic effect of rattlesnake venom NOS

2 ☑7ᵗʰ **T63.012   Toxic effect of rattlesnake venom,** intentional self-harm HCC

☑7ᵗʰ **T63.013   Toxic effect of rattlesnake venom,** assault

☑7ᵗʰ **T63.014   Toxic effect of rattlesnake venom,** undetermined

☑6ᵗʰ **T63.02   Toxic effect of** coral snake **venom**

☑7ᵗʰ **T63.021   Toxic effect of coral snake venom,** accidental (unintentional)
  Toxic effect of coral snake venom NOS

2 ☑7ᵗʰ **T63.022   Toxic effect of coral snake venom,** intentional self-harm HCC

☑7ᵗʰ **T63.023   Toxic effect of coral snake venom,** assault

☑7ᵗʰ **T63.024   Toxic effect of coral snake venom,** undetermined

☑6ᵗʰ **T63.03   Toxic effect of** taipan **venom**

☑7ᵗʰ **T63.031   Toxic effect of taipan venom,** accidental (unintentional)
  Toxic effect of taipan venom NOS

2 ☑7ᵗʰ **T63.032   Toxic effect of taipan venom,** intentional self-harm HCC

☑7ᵗʰ **T63.033   Toxic effect of taipan venom,** assault

☑7ᵗʰ **T63.034   Toxic effect of taipan venom,** undetermined

☑6ᵗʰ **T63.04   Toxic effect of** cobra **venom**

☑7ᵗʰ **T63.041   Toxic effect of cobra venom,** accidental (unintentional)
  Toxic effect of cobra venom NOS

2 ☑7ᵗʰ **T63.042   Toxic effect of cobra venom,** intentional self-harm HCC

☑7ᵗʰ **T63.043   Toxic effect of cobra venom,** assault

☑7ᵗʰ **T63.044   Toxic effect of cobra venom,** undetermined

---

2   HCC with 7th character indicating initial encounter (A or B - specific to category) OR sequela.

☑ Additional Character Req   ☑x7ᵗʰ Placeholder Alert   Manifestation   HCC CMS-HCC Condition   ▽ Unspecified Code   ►◄ Revised Text   ● New Code   ▲ Revised Code Title

√6ᵗʰ **T63.06** **Toxic effect of venom of other** North and South American snake

     √7ᵗʰ **T63.061** **Toxic effect of venom of other North and South American snake,** accidental (unintentional)
         Toxic effect of venom of other North and South American snake NOS

     2 √7ᵗʰ **T63.062** **Toxic effect of venom of other North and South American snake,** intentional self-harm   HCC

     √7ᵗʰ **T63.063** **Toxic effect of venom of other North and South American snake,** assault

     √7ᵗʰ **T63.064** **Toxic effect of venom of other North and South American snake,** undetermined

√6ᵗʰ **T63.07** **Toxic effect of venom of other** Australian snake

     √7ᵗʰ **T63.071** **Toxic effect of venom of other Australian snake,** accidental (unintentional)
         Toxic effect of venom of other Australian snake NOS

     2 √7ᵗʰ **T63.072** **Toxic effect of venom of other Australian snake,** intentional self-harm   HCC

     √7ᵗʰ **T63.073** **Toxic effect of venom of other Australian snake,** assault

     √7ᵗʰ **T63.074** **Toxic effect of venom of other Australian snake,** undetermined

√6ᵗʰ **T63.08** **Toxic effect of venom of other** African and Asian snake

     √7ᵗʰ **T63.081** **Toxic effect of venom of other African and Asian snake,** accidental (unintentional)
         Toxic effect of venom of other African and Asian snake NOS

     2 √7ᵗʰ **T63.082** **Toxic effect of venom of other African and Asian snake,** intentional self-harm   HCC

     √7ᵗʰ **T63.083** **Toxic effect of venom of other African and Asian snake,** assault

     √7ᵗʰ **T63.084** **Toxic effect of venom of other African and Asian snake,** undetermined

√6ᵗʰ **T63.09** **Toxic effect of venom of other snake**

     √7ᵗʰ **T63.091** **Toxic effect of venom of other snake,** accidental (unintentional)
         Toxic effect of venom of other snake NOS

     2 √7ᵗʰ **T63.092** **Toxic effect of venom of other snake,** intentional self-harm   HCC

     √7ᵗʰ **T63.093** **Toxic effect of venom of other snake,** assault

     √7ᵗʰ **T63.094** **Toxic effect of venom of other snake,** undetermined

√5ᵗʰ **T63.1** **Toxic effect of venom of other reptiles**

√6ᵗʰ **T63.11** **Toxic effect of venom of** gila monster

     √7ᵗʰ **T63.111** **Toxic effect of venom of gila monster,** accidental (unintentional)
         Toxic effect of venom of gila monster NOS

     2 √7ᵗʰ **T63.112** **Toxic effect of venom of gila monster,** intentional self-harm   HCC

     √7ᵗʰ **T63.113** **Toxic effect of venom of gila monster,** assault

     √7ᵗʰ **T63.114** **Toxic effect of venom of gila monster,** undetermined

√6ᵗʰ **T63.12** **Toxic effect of venom of other venomous lizard**

     √7ᵗʰ **T63.121** **Toxic effect of venom of other venomous lizard,** accidental (unintentional)
         Toxic effect of venom of other venomous lizard NOS

     2 √7ᵗʰ **T63.122** **Toxic effect of venom of other venomous lizard,** intentional self-harm   HCC

     √7ᵗʰ **T63.123** **Toxic effect of venom of other venomous lizard,** assault

     √7ᵗʰ **T63.124** **Toxic effect of venom of other venomous lizard,** undetermined

√6ᵗʰ **T63.19** **Toxic effect of venom of other reptiles**

     √7ᵗʰ **T63.191** **Toxic effect of venom of other reptiles,** accidental (unintentional)
         Toxic effect of venom of other reptiles NOS

     2 √7ᵗʰ **T63.192** **Toxic effect of venom of other reptiles,** intentional self-harm   HCC

     √7ᵗʰ **T63.193** **Toxic effect of venom of other reptiles,** assault

     √7ᵗʰ **T63.194** **Toxic effect of venom of other reptiles,** undetermined

√5ᵗʰ **T63.2** **Toxic effect of venom of scorpion**

√6ᵗʰ **T63.2X** **Toxic effect of venom of** scorpion

     √7ᵗʰ **T63.2X1** **Toxic effect of venom of scorpion,** accidental (unintentional)
         Toxic effect of venom of scorpion NOS

     2 √7ᵗʰ **T63.2X2** **Toxic effect of venom of scorpion,** intentional self-harm   HCC

     √7ᵗʰ **T63.2X3** **Toxic effect of venom of scorpion,** assault

     √7ᵗʰ **T63.2X4** **Toxic effect of venom of scorpion,** undetermined

√5ᵗʰ **T63.3** **Toxic effect of venom of spider**

√6ᵗʰ **T63.30** **Toxic effect of unspecified spider venom**

     √7ᵗʰ **T63.301** **Toxic effect of unspecified spider venom,** accidental (unintentional)   ▽

     2 √7ᵗʰ **T63.302** **Toxic effect of unspecified spider venom,** intentional self-harm   HCC ▽

     √7ᵗʰ **T63.303** **Toxic effect of unspecified spider venom,** assault   ▽

     √7ᵗʰ **T63.304** **Toxic effect of unspecified spider venom,** undetermined   ▽

√6ᵗʰ **T63.31** **Toxic effect of venom of** black widow **spider**

     √7ᵗʰ **T63.311** **Toxic effect of venom of black widow spider,** accidental (unintentional)

     2 √7ᵗʰ **T63.312** **Toxic effect of venom of black widow spider,** intentional self-harm   HCC

     √7ᵗʰ **T63.313** **Toxic effect of venom of black widow spider,** assault

     √7ᵗʰ **T63.314** **Toxic effect of venom of black widow spider,** undetermined

√6ᵗʰ **T63.32** **Toxic effect of venom of** tarantula

     √7ᵗʰ **T63.321** **Toxic effect of venom of tarantula,** accidental (unintentional)

     2 √7ᵗʰ **T63.322** **Toxic effect of venom of tarantula,** intentional self-harm   HCC

     √7ᵗʰ **T63.323** **Toxic effect of venom of tarantula,** assault

     √7ᵗʰ **T63.324** **Toxic effect of venom of tarantula,** undetermined

√6ᵗʰ **T63.33** **Toxic effect of venom of** brown recluse **spider**

     √7ᵗʰ **T63.331** **Toxic effect of venom of brown recluse spider,** accidental (unintentional)

     2 √7ᵗʰ **T63.332** **Toxic effect of venom of brown recluse spider,** intentional self-harm   HCC

     √7ᵗʰ **T63.333** **Toxic effect of venom of brown recluse spider,** assault

     √7ᵗʰ **T63.334** **Toxic effect of venom of brown recluse spider,** undetermined

√6ᵗʰ **T63.39** **Toxic effect of venom of other spider**

     √7ᵗʰ **T63.391** **Toxic effect of venom of other spider,** accidental (unintentional)

     2 √7ᵗʰ **T63.392** **Toxic effect of venom of other spider,** intentional self-harm   HCC

     √7ᵗʰ **T63.393** **Toxic effect of venom of other spider,** assault

     √7ᵗʰ **T63.394** **Toxic effect of venom of other spider,** undetermined

√5ᵗʰ **T63.4** **Toxic effect of venom of other arthropods**

√6ᵗʰ **T63.41** **Toxic effect of venom of** centipedes and venomous millipedes

     √7ᵗʰ **T63.411** **Toxic effect of venom of centipedes and venomous millipedes,** accidental (unintentional)

     2 √7ᵗʰ **T63.412** **Toxic effect of venom of centipedes and venomous millipedes,** intentional self-harm   HCC

     √7ᵗʰ **T63.413** **Toxic effect of venom of centipedes and venomous millipedes,** assault

---

2   HCC with 7th character indicating initial encounter (A or B - specific to category) OR sequela.

EXCLUDES 1 Not coded here   **EXCLUDES 2** Not included here   N Newborn Age: 0   P Pediatric Age: 0-17   M Maternity Age: 12-55   A Adult Age: 15-124

1088   ICD-10-CM 2018

√7ᵗʰ **T63.414** Toxic effect of venom of centipedes and venomous millipedes, undetermined

√6ᵗʰ **T63.42** Toxic effect of venom of ants

   √7ᵗʰ **T63.421** Toxic effect of venom of ants, accidental (unintentional)

   2 √7ᵗʰ **T63.422** Toxic effect of venom of ants, intentional self-harm   HCC

   √7ᵗʰ **T63.423** Toxic effect of venom of ants, assault

   √7ᵗʰ **T63.424** Toxic effect of venom of ants, undetermined

√6ᵗʰ **T63.43** Toxic effect of venom of caterpillars

   √7ᵗʰ **T63.431** Toxic effect of venom of caterpillars, accidental (unintentional)

   2 √7ᵗʰ **T63.432** Toxic effect of venom of caterpillars, intentional self-harm   HCC

   √7ᵗʰ **T63.433** Toxic effect of venom of caterpillars, assault

   √7ᵗʰ **T63.434** Toxic effect of venom of caterpillars, undetermined

√6ᵗʰ **T63.44** Toxic effect of venom of bees

   √7ᵗʰ **T63.441** Toxic effect of venom of bees, accidental (unintentional)

   2 √7ᵗʰ **T63.442** Toxic effect of venom of bees, intentional self-harm   HCC

   √7ᵗʰ **T63.443** Toxic effect of venom of bees, assault

   √7ᵗʰ **T63.444** Toxic effect of venom of bees, undetermined

√6ᵗʰ **T63.45** Toxic effect of venom of hornets

   √7ᵗʰ **T63.451** Toxic effect of venom of hornets, accidental (unintentional)

   2 √7ᵗʰ **T63.452** Toxic effect of venom of hornets, intentional self-harm   HCC

   √7ᵗʰ **T63.453** Toxic effect of venom of hornets, assault

   √7ᵗʰ **T63.454** Toxic effect of venom of hornets, undetermined

√6ᵗʰ **T63.46** Toxic effect of venom of wasps
    Toxic effect of yellow jacket

   √7ᵗʰ **T63.461** Toxic effect of venom of wasps, accidental (unintentional)

   2 √7ᵗʰ **T63.462** Toxic effect of venom of wasps, intentional self-harm   HCC

   √7ᵗʰ **T63.463** Toxic effect of venom of wasps, assault

   √7ᵗʰ **T63.464** Toxic effect of venom of wasps, undetermined

√6ᵗʰ **T63.48** Toxic effect of venom of other arthropod

   √7ᵗʰ **T63.481** Toxic effect of venom of other arthropod, accidental (unintentional)

   2 √7ᵗʰ **T63.482** Toxic effect of venom of other arthropod, intentional self-harm   HCC

   √7ᵗʰ **T63.483** Toxic effect of venom of other arthropod, assault

   √7ᵗʰ **T63.484** Toxic effect of venom of other arthropod, undetermined

√5ᵗʰ **T63.5** Toxic effect of contact with venomous fish
   EXCLUDES 2   poisoning by ingestion of fish (T61.-)

√6ᵗʰ **T63.51** Toxic effect of contact with stingray

   √7ᵗʰ **T63.511** Toxic effect of contact with stingray, accidental (unintentional)

   2 √7ᵗʰ **T63.512** Toxic effect of contact with stingray, intentional self-harm   HCC

   √7ᵗʰ **T63.513** Toxic effect of contact with stingray, assault

   √7ᵗʰ **T63.514** Toxic effect of contact with stingray, undetermined

√6ᵗʰ **T63.59** Toxic effect of contact with other venomous fish

   √7ᵗʰ **T63.591** Toxic effect of contact with other venomous fish, accidental (unintentional)

   2 √7ᵗʰ **T63.592** Toxic effect of contact with other venomous fish, intentional self-harm   HCC

   √7ᵗʰ **T63.593** Toxic effect of contact with other venomous fish, assault

   √7ᵗʰ **T63.594** Toxic effect of contact with other venomous fish, undetermined

√5ᵗʰ **T63.6** Toxic effect of contact with other venomous marine animals
   EXCLUDES 1   sea-snake venom (T63.09)
   EXCLUDES 2   poisoning by ingestion of shellfish (T61.78-)

√6ᵗʰ **T63.61** Toxic effect of contact with Portugese Man-o-war
    Toxic effect of contact with bluebottle

   √7ᵗʰ **T63.611** Toxic effect of contact with Portugese Man-o-war, accidental (unintentional)

   2 √7ᵗʰ **T63.612** Toxic effect of contact with Portugese Man-o-war, intentional self-harm   HCC

   √7ᵗʰ **T63.613** Toxic effect of contact with Portugese Man-o-war, assault

   √7ᵗʰ **T63.614** Toxic effect of contact with Portugese Man-o-war, undetermined

√6ᵗʰ **T63.62** Toxic effect of contact with other jellyfish

   √7ᵗʰ **T63.621** Toxic effect of contact with other jellyfish, accidental (unintentional)

   2 √7ᵗʰ **T63.622** Toxic effect of contact with other jellyfish, intentional self-harm   HCC

   √7ᵗʰ **T63.623** Toxic effect of contact with other jellyfish, assault

   √7ᵗʰ **T63.624** Toxic effect of contact with other jellyfish, undetermined

√6ᵗʰ **T63.63** Toxic effect of contact with sea anemone

   √7ᵗʰ **T63.631** Toxic effect of contact with sea anemone, accidental (unintentional)

   2 √7ᵗʰ **T63.632** Toxic effect of contact with sea anemone, intentional self-harm   HCC

   √7ᵗʰ **T63.633** Toxic effect of contact with sea anemone, assault

   √7ᵗʰ **T63.634** Toxic effect of contact with sea anemone, undetermined

√6ᵗʰ **T63.69** Toxic effect of contact with other venomous marine animals

   √7ᵗʰ **T63.691** Toxic effect of contact with other venomous marine animals, accidental (unintentional)

   2 √7ᵗʰ **T63.692** Toxic effect of contact with other venomous marine animals, intentional self-harm   HCC

   √7ᵗʰ **T63.693** Toxic effect of contact with other venomous marine animals, assault

   √7ᵗʰ **T63.694** Toxic effect of contact with other venomous marine animals, undetermined

√5ᵗʰ **T63.7** Toxic effect of contact with venomous plant

√6ᵗʰ **T63.71** Toxic effect of contact with venomous marine plant

   √7ᵗʰ **T63.711** Toxic effect of contact with venomous marine plant, accidental (unintentional)

   2 √7ᵗʰ **T63.712** Toxic effect of contact with venomous marine plant, intentional self-harm   HCC

   √7ᵗʰ **T63.713** Toxic effect of contact with venomous marine plant, assault

   √7ᵗʰ **T63.714** Toxic effect of contact with venomous marine plant, undetermined

√6ᵗʰ **T63.79** Toxic effect of contact with other venomous plant

   √7ᵗʰ **T63.791** Toxic effect of contact with other venomous plant, accidental (unintentional)

   2 √7ᵗʰ **T63.792** Toxic effect of contact with other venomous plant, intentional self-harm   HCC

   √7ᵗʰ **T63.793** Toxic effect of contact with other venomous plant, assault

   √7ᵗʰ **T63.794** Toxic effect of contact with other venomous plant, undetermined

√5ᵗʰ **T63.8** Toxic effect of contact with other venomous animals

√6ᵗʰ **T63.81** Toxic effect of contact with venomous frog
   EXCLUDES 1   contact with nonvenomous frog (W62.0)

   √7ᵗʰ **T63.811** Toxic effect of contact with venomous frog, accidental (unintentional)

   2 √7ᵗʰ **T63.812** Toxic effect of contact with venomous frog, intentional self-harm   HCC

   √7ᵗʰ **T63.813** Toxic effect of contact with venomous frog, assault

   √7ᵗʰ **T63.814** Toxic effect of contact with venomous frog, undetermined

---

2   HCC with 7th character indicating initial encounter (A or B - specific to category) OR sequela.

☑ Additional Character Req   √x7ᵗʰ Placeholder Alert   Manifestation   HCC CMS-HCC Condition   ▽ Unspecified Code   ►◄ Revised Text   ● New Code   ▲ Revised Code Title

Chapter 19. Injury, Poisoning, and Certain Other Consequences of External Causes *(side margin)*

✓6ᵗʰ **T63.82 Toxic effect of contact with venomous toad**
     EXCLUDES 1   contact with nonvenomous toad (W62.1)

✓7ᵗʰ **T63.821 Toxic effect of contact with venomous toad, accidental (unintentional)**

2 ✓7ᵗʰ **T63.822 Toxic effect of contact with venomous toad, intentional self-harm**   HCC

✓7ᵗʰ **T63.823 Toxic effect of contact with venomous toad, assault**

✓7ᵗʰ **T63.824 Toxic effect of contact with venomous toad, undetermined**

✓6ᵗʰ **T63.83 Toxic effect of contact with other venomous amphibian**
     EXCLUDES 1   contact with nonvenomous amphibian (W62.9)

✓7ᵗʰ **T63.831 Toxic effect of contact with other venomous amphibian, accidental (unintentional)**

2 ✓7ᵗʰ **T63.832 Toxic effect of contact with other venomous amphibian, intentional self-harm**   HCC

✓7ᵗʰ **T63.833 Toxic effect of contact with other venomous amphibian, assault**

✓7ᵗʰ **T63.834 Toxic effect of contact with other venomous amphibian, undetermined**

✓6ᵗʰ **T63.89 Toxic effect of contact with other venomous animals**

✓7ᵗʰ **T63.891 Toxic effect of contact with other venomous animals, accidental (unintentional)**

2 ✓7ᵗʰ **T63.892 Toxic effect of contact with other venomous animals, intentional self-harm**   HCC

✓7ᵗʰ **T63.893 Toxic effect of contact with other venomous animals, assault**

✓7ᵗʰ **T63.894 Toxic effect of contact with other venomous animals, undetermined**

✓5ᵗʰ **T63.9 Toxic effect of contact with unspecified venomous animal**

✓x7ᵗʰ **T63.91 Toxic effect of contact with unspecified venomous animal, accidental (unintentional)** ▽

2 ✓x7ᵗʰ **T63.92 Toxic effect of contact with unspecified venomous animal, intentional self-harm**   HCC ▽

✓x7ᵗʰ **T63.93 Toxic effect of contact with unspecified venomous animal, assault** ▽

✓x7ᵗʰ **T63.94 Toxic effect of contact with unspecified venomous animal, undetermined** ▽

✓4ᵗʰ **T64 Toxic effect of aflatoxin and other mycotoxin food contaminants**

> The appropriate 7th character is to be added to each code from category T64.
> A   initial encounter
> D   subsequent encounter
> S   sequela

✓5ᵗʰ **T64.0 Toxic effect of aflatoxin**

✓x7ᵗʰ **T64.01 Toxic effect of aflatoxin, accidental (unintentional)**

2 ✓x7ᵗʰ **T64.02 Toxic effect of aflatoxin, intentional self-harm**   HCC

✓x7ᵗʰ **T64.03 Toxic effect of aflatoxin, assault**

✓x7ᵗʰ **T64.04 Toxic effect of aflatoxin, undetermined**

✓5ᵗʰ **T64.8 Toxic effect of other mycotoxin food contaminants**

✓x7ᵗʰ **T64.81 Toxic effect of other mycotoxin food contaminants, accidental (unintentional)**

2 ✓x7ᵗʰ **T64.82 Toxic effect of other mycotoxin food contaminants, intentional self-harm**   HCC

✓x7ᵗʰ **T64.83 Toxic effect of other mycotoxin food contaminants, assault**

✓x7ᵗʰ **T64.84 Toxic effect of other mycotoxin food contaminants, undetermined**

✓4ᵗʰ **T65 Toxic effect of other and unspecified substances**

> The appropriate 7th character is to be added to each code from category T65.
> A   initial encounter
> D   subsequent encounter
> S   sequela

✓5ᵗʰ **T65.0 Toxic effect of cyanides**
     EXCLUDES 1   hydrogen cyanide (T57.3-)

✓6ᵗʰ **T65.0X Toxic effect of cyanides**

✓7ᵗʰ **T65.0X1 Toxic effect of cyanides, accidental (unintentional)**
     Toxic effect of cyanides NOS

2 ✓7ᵗʰ **T65.0X2 Toxic effect of cyanides, intentional self-harm**   HCC

✓7ᵗʰ **T65.0X3 Toxic effect of cyanides, assault**

✓7ᵗʰ **T65.0X4 Toxic effect of cyanides, undetermined**

✓5ᵗʰ **T65.1 Toxic effect of strychnine and its salts**

✓6ᵗʰ **T65.1X Toxic effect of strychnine and its salts**

✓7ᵗʰ **T65.1X1 Toxic effect of strychnine and its salts, accidental (unintentional)**
     Toxic effect of strychnine and its salts NOS

2 ✓7ᵗʰ **T65.1X2 Toxic effect of strychnine and its salts, intentional self-harm**   HCC

✓7ᵗʰ **T65.1X3 Toxic effect of strychnine and its salts, assault**

✓7ᵗʰ **T65.1X4 Toxic effect of strychnine and its salts, undetermined**

✓5ᵗʰ **T65.2 Toxic effect of tobacco and nicotine**
     EXCLUDES 2   nicotine dependence (F17.-)

✓6ᵗʰ **T65.21 Toxic effect of chewing tobacco**

✓7ᵗʰ **T65.211 Toxic effect of chewing tobacco, accidental (unintentional)**
     Toxic effect of chewing tobacco NOS

2 ✓7ᵗʰ **T65.212 Toxic effect of chewing tobacco, intentional self-harm**   HCC

✓7ᵗʰ **T65.213 Toxic effect of chewing tobacco, assault**

✓7ᵗʰ **T65.214 Toxic effect of chewing tobacco, undetermined**

✓6ᵗʰ **T65.22 Toxic effect of tobacco cigarettes**
     Toxic effect of tobacco smoke
     Use additional code for exposure to second hand tobacco smoke (Z57.31, Z77.22)

✓7ᵗʰ **T65.221 Toxic effect of tobacco cigarettes, accidental (unintentional)**
     Toxic effect of tobacco cigarettes NOS

2 ✓7ᵗʰ **T65.222 Toxic effect of tobacco cigarettes, intentional self-harm**   HCC

✓7ᵗʰ **T65.223 Toxic effect of tobacco cigarettes, assault**

✓7ᵗʰ **T65.224 Toxic effect of tobacco cigarettes, undetermined**

✓6ᵗʰ **T65.29 Toxic effect of other tobacco and nicotine**

✓7ᵗʰ **T65.291 Toxic effect of other tobacco and nicotine, accidental (unintentional)**
     Toxic effect of other tobacco and nicotine NOS

2 ✓7ᵗʰ **T65.292 Toxic effect of other tobacco and nicotine, intentional self-harm**   HCC

✓7ᵗʰ **T65.293 Toxic effect of other tobacco and nicotine, assault**

✓7ᵗʰ **T65.294 Toxic effect of other tobacco and nicotine, undetermined**

✓5ᵗʰ **T65.3 Toxic effect of nitroderivatives and aminoderivatives of benzene and its homologues**
     Toxic effect of anilin [benzenamine]
     Toxic effect of nitrobenzene
     Toxic effect of trinitrotoluene

✓6ᵗʰ **T65.3X Toxic effect of nitroderivatives and aminoderivatives of benzene and its homologues**

✓7ᵗʰ **T65.3X1 Toxic effect of nitroderivatives and aminoderivatives of benzene and its homologues, accidental (unintentional)**
     Toxic effect of nitroderivatives and aminoderivatives of benzene and its homologues NOS

---

2   HCC with 7th character indicating initial encounter (A or B - specific to category) OR sequela.

EXCLUDES 1 Not coded here   *EXCLUDES 2* Not included here   N Newborn Age: 0   P Pediatric Age: 0-17   M Maternity Age: 12-55   A Adult Age: 15-124

1090   ICD-10-CM 2018

2 ✓7ᵗʰ **T65.3X2 Toxic effect of nitroderivatives and aminoderivatives of benzene and its homologues,** intentional self-harm   HCC

✓7ᵗʰ **T65.3X3 Toxic effect of nitroderivatives and aminoderivatives of benzene and its homologues,** assault

✓7ᵗʰ **T65.3X4 Toxic effect of nitroderivatives and aminoderivatives of benzene and its homologues,** undetermined

✓5ᵗʰ **T65.4 Toxic effect of carbon disulfide**

✓6ᵗʰ **T65.4X Toxic effect of** carbon disulfide

✓7ᵗʰ **T65.4X1 Toxic effect of carbon disulfide,** accidental (unintentional)
Toxic effect of carbon disulfide NOS

2 ✓7ᵗʰ **T65.4X2 Toxic effect of carbon disulfide,** intentional self-harm   HCC

✓7ᵗʰ **T65.4X3 Toxic effect of carbon disulfide,** assault

✓7ᵗʰ **T65.4X4 Toxic effect of carbon disulfide,** undetermined

✓5ᵗʰ **T65.5 Toxic effect of nitroglycerin and other nitric acids and esters**
Toxic effect of 1,2,3-Propanetriol trinitrate

✓6ᵗʰ **T65.5X Toxic effect of** nitroglycerin and other nitric acids and esters

✓7ᵗʰ **T65.5X1 Toxic effect of nitroglycerin and other nitric acids and esters,** accidental (unintentional)
Toxic effect of nitroglycerin and other nitric acids and esters NOS

2 ✓7ᵗʰ **T65.5X2 Toxic effect of nitroglycerin and other nitric acids and esters,** intentional self-harm   HCC

✓7ᵗʰ **T65.5X3 Toxic effect of nitroglycerin and other nitric acids and esters,** assault

✓7ᵗʰ **T65.5X4 Toxic effect of nitroglycerin and other nitric acids and esters,** undetermined

✓5ᵗʰ **T65.6 Toxic effect of paints and dyes, not elsewhere classified**

✓6ᵗʰ **T65.6X Toxic effect of** paints and dyes, **not elsewhere classified**

✓7ᵗʰ **T65.6X1 Toxic effect of paints and dyes, not elsewhere classified,** accidental (unintentional)
Toxic effect of paints and dyes NOS

2 ✓7ᵗʰ **T65.6X2 Toxic effect of paints and dyes, not elsewhere classified,** intentional self-harm   HCC

✓7ᵗʰ **T65.6X3 Toxic effect of paints and dyes, not elsewhere classified,** assault

✓7ᵗʰ **T65.6X4 Toxic effect of paints and dyes, not elsewhere classified,** undetermined

✓5ᵗʰ **T65.8 Toxic effect of other specified substances**

✓6ᵗʰ **T65.81 Toxic effect of** latex

✓7ᵗʰ **T65.811 Toxic effect of latex,** accidental (unintentional)
Toxic effect of latex NOS

2 ✓7ᵗʰ **T65.812 Toxic effect of latex,** intentional self-harm   HCC

✓7ᵗʰ **T65.813 Toxic effect of latex,** assault

✓7ᵗʰ **T65.814 Toxic effect of latex,** undetermined

✓6ᵗʰ **T65.82 Toxic effect of harmful** algae **and algae toxins**
Toxic effect of (harmful) algae bloom NOS
Toxic effect of blue-green algae bloom
Toxic effect of brown tide
Toxic effect of cyanobacteria bloom
Toxic effect of Florida red tide
Toxic effect of pfiesteria piscicida
Toxic effect of red tide

✓7ᵗʰ **T65.821 Toxic effect of harmful algae and algae toxins,** accidental (unintentional)
Toxic effect of harmful algae and algae toxins NOS

2 ✓7ᵗʰ **T65.822 Toxic effect of harmful algae and algae toxins,** intentional self-harm   HCC

✓7ᵗʰ **T65.823 Toxic effect of harmful algae and algae toxins,** assault

✓7ᵗʰ **T65.824 Toxic effect of harmful algae and algae toxins,** undetermined

✓6ᵗʰ **T65.83 Toxic effect of** fiberglass

✓7ᵗʰ **T65.831 Toxic effect of fiberglass,** accidental (unintentional)
Toxic effect of fiberglass NOS

2 ✓7ᵗʰ **T65.832 Toxic effect of fiberglass,** intentional self-harm   HCC

✓7ᵗʰ **T65.833 Toxic effect of fiberglass,** assault

✓7ᵗʰ **T65.834 Toxic effect of fiberglass,** undetermined

✓6ᵗʰ **T65.89 Toxic effect of other specified substances**

✓7ᵗʰ **T65.891 Toxic effect of other specified substances,** accidental (unintentional)
Toxic effect of other specified substances NOS

2 ✓7ᵗʰ **T65.892 Toxic effect of other specified substances,** intentional self-harm   HCC

✓7ᵗʰ **T65.893 Toxic effect of other specified substances,** assault

✓7ᵗʰ **T65.894 Toxic effect of other specified substances,** undetermined

✓5ᵗʰ **T65.9 Toxic effect of unspecified substance**

✓x7ᵗʰ **T65.91 Toxic effect of unspecified substance,** accidental (unintentional)   ▽
Poisoning NOS

2 ✓x7ᵗʰ **T65.92 Toxic effect of unspecified substance,** intentional self-harm   HCC ▽

✓x7ᵗʰ **T65.93 Toxic effect of unspecified substance,** assault   ▽

✓x7ᵗʰ **T65.94 Toxic effect of unspecified substance,** undetermined   ▽

Other and unspecified effects of external causes (T66-T78)

✓x7ᵗʰ **T66 Radiation sickness, unspecified**   ▽

EXCLUDES 1   specified adverse effects of radiation, such as:
    burns (T20-T31)
    leukemia (C91-C95)
    radiation gastroenteritis and colitis (K52.0)
    radiation pneumonitis (J70.0)
    radiation related disorders of the skin and subcutaneous tissue (L55-L59)
    radiation sunburn (L55.-)

The appropriate 7th character is to be added to code T66.
A   initial encounter
D   subsequent encounter
S   sequela

✓4ᵗʰ **T67 Effects of heat and light**

EXCLUDES 1   erythema [dermatitis] ab igne (L59.0)
    malignant hyperpyrexia due to anesthesia (T88.3)
    radiation-related disorders of the skin and subcutaneous tissue (L55-L59)

EXCLUDES 2   burns (T20-T31)
    sunburn (L55.-)
    sweat disorder due to heat (L74-L75)

The appropriate 7th character is to be added to each code from category T67.
A   initial encounter
D   subsequent encounter
S   sequela

✓x7ᵗʰ **T67.0 Heatstroke and sunstroke**
Heat apoplexy   Siriasis
Heat pyrexia   Thermoplegia
Use additional code(s) to identify any associated complications of heatstroke, such as:
    coma and stupor (R40.-)
    systemic inflammatory response syndrome (R65.1-)
DEF: Headache, vertigo, cramps, and elevated body temperature due to prolonged exposure to high environmental temperatures; requires emergency intervention.

✓x7ᵗʰ **T67.1 Heat** syncope
Heat collapse

✓x7ᵗʰ **T67.2 Heat** cramp

✓x7ᵗʰ **T67.3 Heat exhaustion,** anhydrotic
Heat prostration due to water depletion
EXCLUDES 1   heat exhaustion due to salt depletion (T67.4)

✓x7ᵗʰ **T67.4 Heat exhaustion** due to salt depletion
Heat prostration due to salt (and water) depletion

---

2   HCC with 7th character indicating initial encounter (A or B - specific to category) OR sequela.

☑ Additional Character Req   ✓x7ᵗʰ Placeholder Alert   Manifestation   HCC CMS-HCC Condition   ▽ Unspecified Code   ▶◀ Revised Text   ● New Code   ▲ Revised Code Title

√x7ᵗʰ **T67.5 Heat exhaustion, unspecified** ▽
> Heat prostration NOS

√x7ᵗʰ **T67.6 Heat fatigue, transient**

√x7ᵗʰ **T67.7 Heat edema**

√x7ᵗʰ **T67.8 Other effects of heat and light**

√x7ᵗʰ **T67.9 Effect of heat and light, unspecified** ▽

√x7ᵗʰ **T68 Hypothermia**
> Accidental hypothermia
> Hypothermia NOS
> Use additional code to identify source of exposure:
> > exposure to excessive cold of man-made origin (W93)
> > exposure to excessive cold of natural origin (X31)
>
> EXCLUDES 1   *hypothermia following anesthesia (T88.51)*
> > *hypothermia not associated with low environmental*
> > *temperature (R68.0)*
> > *hypothermia of newborn (P80.-)*
>
> EXCLUDES 2   *frostbite (T33-T34)*

> The appropriate 7th character is to be added to code T68.
> A   initial encounter
> D   subsequent encounter
> S   sequela

√4ᵗʰ **T69 Other effects of reduced temperature**
> Use additional code to identify source of exposure:
> > exposure to excessive cold of man-made origin (W93)
> > exposure to excessive cold of natural origin (X31)
>
> EXCLUDES 2   *frostbite (T33-T34)*

> The appropriate 7th character is to be added to each code from
> category T69.
> A   initial encounter
> D   subsequent encounter
> S   sequela

√5ᵗʰ **T69.0 Immersion hand and foot**

√6ᵗʰ **T69.01 Immersion hand**

√7ᵗʰ **T69.011 Immersion hand, right hand**

√7ᵗʰ **T69.012 Immersion hand, left hand**

√7ᵗʰ **T69.019 Immersion hand, unspecified hand** ▽

√6ᵗʰ **T69.02 Immersion foot**
> Trench foot

√7ᵗʰ **T69.021 Immersion foot, right foot**

√7ᵗʰ **T69.022 Immersion foot, left foot**

√7ᵗʰ **T69.029 Immersion foot, unspecified foot** ▽

√x7ᵗʰ **T69.1 Chilblains**
> **DEF:** Red, swollen, itchy skin primarily affecting the fingers and
> toes, nose and ears, and legs; follows damp-cold exposure; can
> also be associated with pruritus and a burning feeling.

√x7ᵗʰ **T69.8 Other specified effects of reduced temperature**

√x7ᵗʰ **T69.9 Effect of reduced temperature, unspecified** ▽

√4ᵗʰ **T70 Effects of air pressure and water pressure**

> The appropriate 7th character is to be added to each code from
> category T70.
> A   initial encounter
> D   subsequent encounter
> S   sequela

√x7ᵗʰ **T70.0 Otitic barotrauma**
> Aero-otitis media
> Effects of change in ambient atmospheric pressure or water
> pressure on ears

√x7ᵗʰ **T70.1 Sinus barotrauma**
> Aerosinusitis
> Effects of change in ambient atmospheric pressure on sinuses

√5ᵗʰ **T70.2 Other and unspecified effects of high altitude**
> EXCLUDES 2   *polycythemia due to high altitude (D75.1)*

√x7ᵗʰ **T70.20 Unspecified effects of high altitude** ▽

√x7ᵗʰ **T70.29 Other effects of high altitude**
> Alpine sickness
> Anoxia due to high altitude
> Barotrauma NOS
> Hypobaropathy
> Mountain sickness

√x7ᵗʰ **T70.3 Caisson disease [decompression sickness]**
> Compressed-air disease
> Diver's palsy or paralysis
> **DEF:** Rapid reduction in air pressure while breathing compressed
> air; symptoms include skin lesions, joint pains, and respiratory and
> neurological problems.

√x7ᵗʰ **T70.4 Effects of high-pressure fluids**
> Hydraulic jet injection (industrial)
> Pneumatic jet injection (industrial)
> Traumatic jet injection (industrial)

√x7ᵗʰ **T70.8 Other effects of air pressure and water pressure**

√x7ᵗʰ **T70.9 Effect of air pressure and water pressure, unspecified** ▽

√4ᵗʰ **T71 Asphyxiation**
> Mechanical suffocation
> Traumatic suffocation
> EXCLUDES 1   *acute respiratory distress (syndrome) (J80)*
> > *anoxia due to high altitude (T70.2)*
> > *asphyxia NOS (R09.01)*
> > *asphyxia from carbon monoxide (T58.-)*
> > *asphyxia from inhalation of food or foreign body (T17.-)*
> > *asphyxia from other gases, fumes and vapors (T59.-)*
> > *respiratory distress (syndrome) in newborn (P22.-)*

> The appropriate 7th character is to be added to each code from
> category T71.
> A   initial encounter
> D   subsequent encounter
> S   sequela

√5ᵗʰ **T71.1 Asphyxiation due to mechanical threat to breathing**
> Suffocation due to mechanical threat to breathing

√6ᵗʰ **T71.11 Asphyxiation due to smothering under pillow**

√7ᵗʰ **T71.111 Asphyxiation due to smothering under pillow, accidental**
> Asphyxiation due to smothering under
> pillow NOS

2 √7ᵗʰ **T71.112 Asphyxiation due to smothering under pillow, intentional self-harm** `HCC`

√7ᵗʰ **T71.113 Asphyxiation due to smothering under pillow, assault**

√7ᵗʰ **T71.114 Asphyxiation due to smothering under pillow, undetermined**

√6ᵗʰ **T71.12 Asphyxiation due to plastic bag**

√7ᵗʰ **T71.121 Asphyxiation due to plastic bag, accidental**
> Asphyxiation due to plastic bag NOS

2 √7ᵗʰ **T71.122 Asphyxiation due to plastic bag, intentional self-harm** `HCC`

√7ᵗʰ **T71.123 Asphyxiation due to plastic bag, assault**

√7ᵗʰ **T71.124 Asphyxiation due to plastic bag, undetermined**

√6ᵗʰ **T71.13 Asphyxiation due to being trapped in bed linens**

√7ᵗʰ **T71.131 Asphyxiation due to being trapped in bed linens, accidental**
> Asphyxiation due to being trapped in bed
> linens NOS

2 √7ᵗʰ **T71.132 Asphyxiation due to being trapped in bed linens, intentional self-harm** `HCC`

√7ᵗʰ **T71.133 Asphyxiation due to being trapped in bed linens, assault**

√7ᵗʰ **T71.134 Asphyxiation due to being trapped in bed linens, undetermined**

√6ᵗʰ **T71.14 Asphyxiation due to smothering under another person's body (in bed)**

√7ᵗʰ **T71.141 Asphyxiation due to smothering under another person's body (in bed), accidental**
> Asphyxiation due to smothering under
> another person's body (in bed) NOS

√7ᵗʰ **T71.143 Asphyxiation due to smothering under another person's body (in bed), assault**

√7ᵗʰ **T71.144 Asphyxiation due to smothering under another person's body (in bed), undetermined**

√6ᵗʰ **T71.15 Asphyxiation due to smothering in furniture**

√7ᵗʰ **T71.151 Asphyxiation due to smothering in furniture, accidental**
> Asphyxiation due to smothering in
> furniture NOS

---

2   HCC with 7th character indicating initial encounter (A or B - specific to category) OR sequela.

EXCLUDES 1 Not coded here   EXCLUDES 2 Not included here   N Newborn Age: 0   P Pediatric Age: 0-17   M Maternity Age: 12-55   A Adult Age: 15-124

2 ✓7th **T71.152 Asphyxiation due to smothering in furniture, intentional self-harm** `HCC`

✓7th **T71.153 Asphyxiation due to smothering in furniture, assault**

✓7th **T71.154 Asphyxiation due to smothering in furniture, undetermined**

✓6th **T71.16 Asphyxiation due to hanging**
Hanging by window shade cord
Use additional code for any associated injuries, such as:
crushing injury of neck (S17.-)
fracture of cervical vertebrae (S12.0-S12.2-)
open wound of neck (S11.-)

✓7th **T71.161 Asphyxiation due to hanging, accidental**
Asphyxiation due to hanging NOS
Hanging NOS

2 ✓7th **T71.162 Asphyxiation due to hanging, intentional self-harm** `HCC`

✓7th **T71.163 Asphyxiation due to hanging, assault**

✓7th **T71.164 Asphyxiation due to hanging, undetermined**

✓6th **T71.19 Asphyxiation due to mechanical threat to breathing due to other causes**

✓7th **T71.191 Asphyxiation due to mechanical threat to breathing due to other causes, accidental**
Asphyxiation due to other causes NOS

2 ✓7th **T71.192 Asphyxiation due to mechanical threat to breathing due to other causes, intentional self-harm** `HCC`

✓7th **T71.193 Asphyxiation due to mechanical threat to breathing due to other causes, assault**

✓7th **T71.194 Asphyxiation due to mechanical threat to breathing due to other causes, undetermined**

✓5th **T71.2 Asphyxiation due to systemic oxygen deficiency due to low oxygen content in ambient air**
Suffocation due to systemic oxygen deficiency due to low oxygen content in ambient air

✓x7th **T71.20 Asphyxiation due to systemic oxygen deficiency due to low oxygen content in ambient air due to unspecified cause** ▽

✓x7th **T71.21 Asphyxiation due to cave-in or falling earth**
Use additional code for any associated cataclysm (X34-X38)

✓6th **T71.22 Asphyxiation due to being trapped in a car trunk**

✓7th **T71.221 Asphyxiation due to being trapped in a car trunk, accidental**

2 ✓7th **T71.222 Asphyxiation due to being trapped in a car trunk, intentional self-harm** `HCC`

✓7th **T71.223 Asphyxiation due to being trapped in a car trunk, assault**

✓7th **T71.224 Asphyxiation due to being trapped in a car trunk, undetermined**

✓6th **T71.23 Asphyxiation due to being trapped in a (discarded) refrigerator**

✓7th **T71.231 Asphyxiation due to being trapped in a (discarded) refrigerator, accidental**

2 ✓7th **T71.232 Asphyxiation due to being trapped in a (discarded) refrigerator, intentional self-harm** `HCC`

✓7th **T71.233 Asphyxiation due to being trapped in a (discarded) refrigerator, assault**

✓7th **T71.234 Asphyxiation due to being trapped in a (discarded) refrigerator, undetermined**

✓x7th **T71.29 Asphyxiation due to being trapped in other low oxygen environment**

✓x7th **T71.9 Asphyxiation due to unspecified cause** ▽
Suffocation (by strangulation) due to unspecified cause
Suffocation NOS
Systemic oxygen deficiency due to low oxygen content in ambient air due to unspecified cause
Systemic oxygen deficiency due to mechanical threat to breathing due to unspecified cause
Traumatic asphyxia NOS

✓4th **T73 Effects of other deprivation**

The appropriate 7th character is to be added to each code from category T73.
A   initial encounter
D   subsequent encounter
S   sequela

✓x7th **T73.0 Starvation**
Deprivation of food

✓x7th **T73.1 Deprivation of water**

✓x7th **T73.2 Exhaustion due to exposure**

✓x7th **T73.3 Exhaustion due to excessive exertion**
Exhaustion due to overexertion

✓x7th **T73.8 Other effects of deprivation**

✓x7th **T73.9 Effect of deprivation, unspecified** ▽

✓4th **T74 Adult and child abuse, neglect and other maltreatment, confirmed**
Use additional code, if applicable, to identify any associated current injury
Use additional external cause code to identify perpetrator, if known (Y07.-)
EXCLUDES 1   *abuse and maltreatment in pregnancy (O9A.3-, O9A.4-, O9A.5-)*
adult and child maltreatment, suspected (T76.-)

The appropriate 7th character is to be added to each code from category T74.
A   initial encounter
D   subsequent encounter
S   sequela

✓5th **T74.0 Neglect or abandonment, confirmed**

✓x7th **T74.01 Adult neglect or abandonment, confirmed** `A`

✓x7th **T74.02 Child neglect or abandonment, confirmed** `P`

✓5th **T74.1 Physical abuse, confirmed**
EXCLUDES 2   *sexual abuse (T74.2-)*

✓x7th **T74.11 Adult physical abuse, confirmed** `A`

✓x7th **T74.12 Child physical abuse, confirmed** `P`
EXCLUDES 2   *shaken infant syndrome (T74.4)*

✓5th **T74.2 Sexual abuse, confirmed**
Rape, confirmed
Sexual assault, confirmed

✓x7th **T74.21 Adult sexual abuse, confirmed** `A`

✓x7th **T74.22 Child sexual abuse, confirmed** `P`

✓5th **T74.3 Psychological abuse, confirmed**

✓x7th **T74.31 Adult psychological abuse, confirmed** `A`

✓x7th **T74.32 Child psychological abuse, confirmed** `P`

✓x7th **T74.4 Shaken infant syndrome** `P`

✓5th **T74.9 Unspecified maltreatment, confirmed**

✓x7th **T74.91 Unspecified adult maltreatment, confirmed** `A` ▽

✓x7th **T74.92 Unspecified child maltreatment, confirmed** `P` ▽

✓4th **T75 Other and unspecified effects of other external causes**
EXCLUDES 1   *adverse effects NEC (T78.-)*
EXCLUDES 2   *burns (electric) (T20-T31)*

The appropriate 7th character is to be added to each code from category T75.
A   initial encounter
D   subsequent encounter
S   sequela

✓5th **T75.0 Effects of lightning**
Struck by lightning

✓x7th **T75.00 Unspecified effects of lightning** ▽
Struck by lightning NOS

✓x7th **T75.01 Shock due to being struck by lightning**

✓x7th **T75.09 Other effects of lightning**
Use additional code for other effects of lightning

✓x7th **T75.1 Unspecified effects of drowning and nonfatal submersion** ▽
Immersion
EXCLUDES 1   *specified effects of drowning—code to effects*

✓5th **T75.2 Effects of vibration**

✓x7th **T75.20 Unspecified effects of vibration** ▽

✓x7th **T75.21 Pneumatic hammer syndrome**

✓x7th **T75.22 Traumatic vasospastic syndrome**

---

2   HCC with 7th character indicating initial encounter (A or B - specific to category) OR sequela.

☑ Additional Character Req   ✓x7th Placeholder Alert   Manifestation   `HCC` CMS-HCC Condition   ▽ Unspecified Code   ▶◀ Revised Text   ● New Code   ▲ Revised Code Title

ICD-10-CM 2018   **1093**

Chapter 19. Injury, Poisoning, and Certain Other Consequences of External Causes

T75.23–T79.Ø

√x7ᵗʰ **T75.23 Vertigo from infrasound**
EXCLUDES 1   *vertigo NOS (R42)*

√x7ᵗʰ **T75.29 Other effects of vibration**

√x7ᵗʰ **T75.3 Motion sickness**
Airsickness
Seasickness
Travel sickness
Use additional external cause code to identify vehicle or type of motion (Y92.81-, Y93.5-)

√x7ᵗʰ **T75.4 Electrocution**
Shock from electric current
Shock from electroshock gun (taser)

√5ᵗʰ **T75.8 Other specified effects of external causes**

√x7ᵗʰ **T75.81 Effects of abnormal gravitation [G] forces**

√x7ᵗʰ **T75.82 Effects of weightlessness**

√x7ᵗʰ **T75.89 Other specified effects of external causes**

√4ᵗʰ **T76 Adult and child abuse, neglect and other maltreatment, suspected**
Use additional code, if applicable, to identify any associated current injury
EXCLUDES 1   *adult and child maltreatment, confirmed (T74.-)*
suspected abuse and maltreatment in pregnancy (O9A.3-, O9A.4-, O9A.5-)
suspected adult physical abuse, ruled out (ZØ4.71)
suspected adult sexual abuse, ruled out (ZØ4.41)
suspected child physical abuse, ruled out (ZØ4.72)
suspected child sexual abuse, ruled out (ZØ4.42)

The appropriate 7th character is to be added to each code from category T76.
A   initial encounter
D   subsequent encounter
S   sequela

√5ᵗʰ **T76.Ø Neglect or abandonment, suspected**

√x7ᵗʰ **T76.Ø1 Adult neglect or abandonment, suspected** Ⓐ

√x7ᵗʰ **T76.Ø2 Child neglect or abandonment, suspected** Ⓟ

√5ᵗʰ **T76.1 Physical abuse, suspected**

√x7ᵗʰ **T76.11 Adult physical abuse, suspected** Ⓐ

√x7ᵗʰ **T76.12 Child physical abuse, suspected** Ⓟ

√5ᵗʰ **T76.2 Sexual abuse, suspected**
Rape, suspected
~~Sexual abuse, suspected~~
EXCLUDES 1   *alleged abuse, ruled out (ZØ4.7)*

√x7ᵗʰ **T76.21 Adult sexual abuse, suspected** Ⓐ

√x7ᵗʰ **T76.22 Child sexual abuse, suspected** Ⓟ

√5ᵗʰ **T76.3 Psychological abuse, suspected**

√x7ᵗʰ **T76.31 Adult psychological abuse, suspected** Ⓐ

√x7ᵗʰ **T76.32 Child psychological abuse, suspected** Ⓟ

√5ᵗʰ **T76.9 Unspecified maltreatment, suspected**

√x7ᵗʰ **T76.91 Unspecified adult maltreatment, suspected** Ⓐ▽

√x7ᵗʰ **T76.92 Unspecified child maltreatment, suspected** Ⓟ▽

√4ᵗʰ **T78 Adverse effects, not elsewhere classified**
EXCLUDES 2   *complications of surgical and medical care NEC (T8Ø-T88)*

The appropriate 7th character is to be added to each code from category T78.
A   initial encounter
D   subsequent encounter
S   sequela

√5ᵗʰ **T78.Ø Anaphylactic reaction due to food**
Anaphylactic reaction due to adverse food reaction
Anaphylactic shock or reaction due to nonpoisonous foods
Anaphylactoid reaction due to food

√x7ᵗʰ **T78.ØØ Anaphylactic reaction due to unspecified food** ▽

√x7ᵗʰ **T78.Ø1 Anaphylactic reaction due to peanuts**

√x7ᵗʰ **T78.Ø2 Anaphylactic reaction due to shellfish (crustaceans)**

√x7ᵗʰ **T78.Ø3 Anaphylactic reaction due to other fish**

√x7ᵗʰ **T78.Ø4 Anaphylactic reaction due to fruits and vegetables**

√x7ᵗʰ **T78.Ø5 Anaphylactic reaction due to tree nuts and seeds**
EXCLUDES 2   *anaphylactic reaction due to peanuts (T78.Ø1)*

√x7ᵗʰ **T78.Ø6 Anaphylactic reaction due to food additives**

√x7ᵗʰ **T78.Ø7 Anaphylactic reaction due to milk and dairy products**

√x7ᵗʰ **T78.Ø8 Anaphylactic reaction due to eggs**

√x7ᵗʰ **T78.Ø9 Anaphylactic reaction due to other food products**

√x7ᵗʰ **T78.1 Other adverse food reactions, not elsewhere classified**
Use additional code to identify the type of reaction, if applicable
EXCLUDES 1   *anaphylactic reaction or shock due to adverse food reaction (T78.Ø-)*
anaphylactic reaction due to food (T78.Ø-)
bacterial food borne intoxications (AØ5.-)
EXCLUDES 2   *allergic and dietetic gastroenteritis and colitis (K52.29)*
allergic rhinitis due to food (J3Ø.5)
dermatitis due to food in contact with skin (L23.6, L24.6, L25.4)
dermatitis due to ingested food (L27.2)
food protein-induced enterocolitis syndrome (K52.21)
food protein-induced enteropathy (K52.22)

√x7ᵗʰ **T78.2 Anaphylactic shock, unspecified** ▽
Allergic shock
Anaphylactic reaction
Anaphylaxis
EXCLUDES 1   *anaphylactic reaction or shock due to adverse effect of correct medicinal substance properly administered (T88.6)*
anaphylactic reaction or shock due to adverse food reaction (T78.Ø-)
anaphylactic reaction or shock due to serum (T8Ø.5-)

√x7ᵗʰ **T78.3 Angioneurotic edema**
Allergic angioedema
Giant urticaria
Quincke's edema
EXCLUDES 1   *serum urticaria (T8Ø.6-)*
urticaria (L5Ø.-)

√5ᵗʰ **T78.4 Other and unspecified allergy**
EXCLUDES 1   *specified types of allergic reaction such as:*
allergic diarrhea (K52.29)
allergic gastroenteritis and colitis (K52.29)
dermatitis (L23-L25, L27-)
food protein-induced enterocolitis syndrome (K52.21)
food protein-induced enteropathy (K52.22)
hay fever (J3Ø.1)

√x7ᵗʰ **T78.4Ø Allergy, unspecified** ▽
Allergic reaction NOS
Hypersensitivity NOS

√x7ᵗʰ **T78.41 Arthus phenomenon**
Arthus reaction

√x7ᵗʰ **T78.49 Other allergy**

√x7ᵗʰ **T78.8 Other adverse effects, not elsewhere classified**

Certain early complications of trauma (T79)

√4ᵗʰ **T79 Certain early complications of trauma, not elsewhere classified**
EXCLUDES 2   *acute respiratory distress syndrome (J8Ø)*
complications occurring during or following medical procedures (T8Ø-T88)
complications of surgical and medical care NEC (T8Ø-T88)
newborn respiratory distress syndrome (P22.Ø)

The appropriate 7th character is to be added to each code from category T79.
A   initial encounter
D   subsequent encounter
S   sequela

[1] √x7ᵗʰ **T79.Ø Air embolism (traumatic)** HCC
EXCLUDES 1   *air embolism complicating abortion or ectopic or molar pregnancy (OØØ-OØ7, OØ8.2)*
air embolism complicating pregnancy, childbirth and the puerperium (OØ8.Ø)
air embolism following infusion, transfusion, and therapeutic injection (T8Ø.Ø)
air embolism following procedure NEC (T81.7-)
DEF: Arterial or venous obstruction due to introduction of air bubbles into the blood vessels following surgery or trauma.

---

[1]   HCC with 7th character indicating initial encounter (A, B or C - specific to category).

EXCLUDES 1 Not coded here   EXCLUDES 2 Not included here   Ⓝ Newborn Age: 0   Ⓟ Pediatric Age: 0-17   Ⓜ Maternity Age: 12-55   Ⓐ Adult Age: 15-124

1094   ICD-10-CM 2018

¹ ✓x7ᵗʰ **T79.1**   **Fat embolism (traumatic)**   HCC
> EXCLUDES 1   *fat embolism complicating:*
> *abortion or ectopic or molar pregnancy (O00–O07, O08.2)*
> *pregnancy, childbirth and the puerperium (O88.8)*
> **DEF:** Arterial blockage due to the entrance of fat into the circulatory system after fracture of large bones or administration of corticosteroids.

¹ ✓x7ᵗʰ **T79.2**   **Traumatic secondary and recurrent hemorrhage and seroma**   HCC

¹ ✓x7ᵗʰ **T79.4**   **Traumatic shock**   HCC
> Shock (immediate) (delayed) following injury
> EXCLUDES 1   *anaphylactic shock due to adverse food reaction (T78.0-)*
> *anaphylactic shock due to correct medicinal substance properly administered (T88.6)*
> *anaphylactic shock due to serum (T80.5-)*
> *anaphylactic shock NOS (T78.2)*
> *anesthetic shock (T88.2)*
> *electric shock (T75.4)*
> *nontraumatic shock NEC (R57.-)*
> *obstetric shock (O75.1)*
> *postprocedural shock (T81.1-)*
> *septic shock (R65.21)*
> *shock complicating abortion or ectopic or molar pregnancy (O00–O07, O08.3)*
> *shock due to lightning (T75.01)*
> *shock NOS (R57.9)*

¹ ✓x7ᵗʰ **T79.5**   **Traumatic anuria**   HCC
> Crush syndrome
> Renal failure following crushing

¹ ✓x7ᵗʰ **T79.6**   **Traumatic ischemia of muscle**   HCC
> Traumatic rhabdomyolysis
> Volkmann's ischemic contracture
> EXCLUDES 2   *anterior tibial syndrome (M76.8)*
> *compartment syndrome (traumatic) (T79.A-)*
> *nontraumatic ischemia of muscle (M62.2-)*

¹ ✓x7ᵗʰ **T79.7**   **Traumatic subcutaneous emphysema**   HCC
> EXCLUDES 1   *emphysema NOS (J43)*
> *emphysema (subcutaneous) resulting from a procedure (T81.82)*

✓5ᵗʰ **T79.A**   **Traumatic compartment syndrome**
> EXCLUDES 1   *fibromyalgia (M79.7)*
> *nontraumatic compartment syndrome (M79.A-)*
> *traumatic ischemic infarction of muscle (T79.6)*
> **DEF:** Compression of nerves and blood vessels within an enclosed muscle space due to previous trauma, which leads to impaired blood flow and muscle and nerve damage.

¹ ✓x7ᵗʰ **T79.A0**   **Compartment syndrome, unspecified**   HCC ▽
> Compartment syndrome NOS

✓6ᵗʰ **T79.A1**   **Traumatic compartment syndrome of upper extremity**
> Traumatic compartment syndrome of shoulder, arm, forearm, wrist, hand, and fingers

     ¹ ✓7ᵗʰ **T79.A11**   **Traumatic compartment syndrome of right upper extremity**   HCC

     ¹ ✓7ᵗʰ **T79.A12**   **Traumatic compartment syndrome of left upper extremity**   HCC

     ¹ ✓7ᵗʰ **T79.A19**   **Traumatic compartment syndrome of unspecified upper extremity**   HCC ▽

✓6ᵗʰ **T79.A2**   **Traumatic compartment syndrome of lower extremity**
> Traumatic compartment syndrome of hip, buttock, thigh, leg, foot, and toes

     ¹ ✓7ᵗʰ **T79.A21**   **Traumatic compartment syndrome of right lower extremity**   HCC

     ¹ ✓7ᵗʰ **T79.A22**   **Traumatic compartment syndrome of left lower extremity**   HCC

     ¹ ✓7ᵗʰ **79.A29**   **Traumatic compartment syndrome of unspecified lower extremity**   HCC ▽

¹ ✓x7ᵗʰ **T79.A3**   **Traumatic compartment syndrome of abdomen**   HCC

¹ ✓x7ᵗʰ **T79.A9**   **Traumatic compartment syndrome of other sites**   HCC

¹ ✓x7ᵗʰ **T79.8**   **Other early complications of trauma**   HCC

¹ ✓x7ᵗʰ **T79.9**   **Unspecified early complication of trauma**   HCC ▽

Complications of surgical and medical care, not elsewhere classified (T80-T88)

Use additional code for adverse effect, if applicable, to identify drug (T36-T50 with fifth or sixth character 5)
Use additional code(s) to identify the specified condition resulting from the complication
Use additional code to identify devices involved and details of circumstances (Y62-Y82)
> EXCLUDES 2   *any encounters with medical care for postprocedural conditions in which no complications are present, such as:*
> *artificial opening status (Z93.-)*
> *closure of external stoma (Z43.-)*
> *fitting and adjustment of external prosthetic device (Z44.-)*
> *burns and corrosions from local applications and irradiation (T20-T32)*
> *complications of surgical procedures during pregnancy, childbirth and the puerperium (O00-O9A)*
> *mechanical complication of respirator [ventilator] (J95.850)*
> *poisoning and toxic effects of drugs and chemicals (T36-T65 with fifth or sixth character 1-4 or 6)*
> *postprocedural fever (R50.82)*
> *specified complications classified elsewhere, such as:*
> *cerebrospinal fluid leak from spinal puncture (G97.0)*
> *colostomy malfunction (K94.0-)*
> *disorders of fluid and electrolyte imbalance (E86-E87)*
> *functional disturbances following cardiac surgery (I97.0-I97.1)*
> *intraoperative and postprocedural complications of specified body systems (D78.-, E36.-, E89.-, G97.3-, G97.4, H59.3-, H59.-, H95.2-, H95.3, I97.4-, I97.5, J95.6-, J95.7, K91.6-, L76.-, M96.-, N99.-)*
> *ostomy complications (J95.0-, K94.-, N99.5-)*
> *postgastric surgery syndromes (K91.1)*
> *postlaminectomy syndrome NEC (M96.1)*
> *postmastectomy lymphedema syndrome (I97.2)*
> *postsurgical blind-loop syndrome (K91.2)*
> *ventilator associated pneumonia (J95.851)*

AHA: 2015, 1Q, 15

✓4ᵗʰ **T80**   **Complications following infusion, transfusion and therapeutic injection**
> INCLUDES   complications following perfusion
> EXCLUDES 2   *bone marrow transplant rejection (T86.01)*
> *febrile nonhemolytic transfusion reaction (R50.84)*
> *fluid overload due to transfusion (E87.71)*
> *posttransfusion purpura (D69.51)*
> *transfusion associated circulatory overload (TACO) (E87.71)*
> *transfusion (red blood cell) associated hemochromatosis (E83.111)*
> *transfusion related acute lung injury (TRALI) (J95.84)*

> The appropriate 7th character is to be added to each code from category T80.
> A   initial encounter
> D   subsequent encounter
> S   sequela

✓x7ᵗʰ **T80.0**   **Air embolism following infusion, transfusion and therapeutic injection**

✓x7ᵗʰ **T80.1**   **Vascular complications following infusion, transfusion and therapeutic injection**
> Use additional code to identify the vascular complication
> EXCLUDES 2   *extravasation of vesicant agent (T80.81-)*
> *infiltration of vesicant agent (T80.81-)*
> *postprocedural vascular complications (T81.7-)*
> *vascular complications specified as due to prosthetic devices, implants and grafts (T82.8-, T83.8-, T84.8-, T85.8-)*

---

¹   HCC with 7th character indicating initial encounter (A, B or C - specific to category).

✓ Additional Character Req   ✓x7ᵗʰ Placeholder Alert   Manifestation   HCC CMS-HCC Condition   ▽ Unspecified Code   ►◄ Revised Text   ● New Code   ▲ Revised Code Title

✓5th **T80.2 Infections** following infusion, transfusion and therapeutic injection

Use additional code to identify the specific infection, such as: sepsis (A41.9)

Use additional code (R65.2-) to identify severe sepsis, if applicable

EXCLUDES 2 *infections specified as due to prosthetic devices, implants and grafts (T82.6-T82.7, T83.5-T83.6, T84.5-T84.7, T85.7)*
postprocedural infections (T81.4-)

✓6th **T80.21 Infection** due to central venous catheter

Infection due to pulmonary artery catheter (Swan-Ganz catheter)

✓7th **T80.211 Bloodstream infection** due to central venous catheter

Catheter-related bloodstream infection (CRBSI) NOS

Central line-associated bloodstream infection (CLABSI)

Bloodstream infection due to Hickman catheter

Bloodstream infection due to peripherally inserted central catheter (PICC)

Bloodstream infection due to portacath (port-a-cath)

Bloodstream infection due to pulmonary artery catheter

Bloodstream infection due to triple lumen catheter

Bloodstream infection due to umbilical venous catheter

✓7th **T80.212 Local infection** due to central venous catheter

Exit or insertion site infection

Local infection due to Hickman catheter

Local infection due to peripherally inserted central catheter (PICC)

Local infection due to portacath (port-a-cath)

Local infection due to pulmonary artery catheter

Local infection due to triple lumen catheter

Local infection due to umbilical venous catheter

Port or reservoir infection

Tunnel infection

✓7th **T80.218 Other infection** due to central venous catheter

Other central line-associated infection

Other infection due to Hickman catheter

Other infection due to peripherally inserted central catheter (PICC)

Other infection due to portacath (port-a-cath)

Other infection due to pulmonary artery catheter

Other infection due to triple lumen catheter

Other infection due to umbilical venous catheter

✓7th **T80.219 Unspecified infection** due to central   ▽ venous catheter

Central line-associated infection NOS

Unspecified infection due to Hickman catheter

Unspecified infection due to peripherally inserted central catheter (PICC)

Unspecified infection due to portacath (port-a-cath)

Unspecified infection due to pulmonary artery catheter

Unspecified infection due to triple lumen catheter

Unspecified infection due to umbilical venous catheter

✓x7th **T80.22 Acute infection** following transfusion, infusion, or injection of blood and blood products

✓x7th **T80.29 Infection** following other infusion, transfusion and therapeutic injection

✓5th **T80.3 ABO incompatibility** reaction due to transfusion of blood or blood products

EXCLUDES 1 *minor blood group antigens reactions (Duffy) (E) (K(ell)) (Kidd) (Lewis) (M) (N) (P) (S) (T80.A)*

✓x7th **T80.30 ABO incompatibility** reaction due to transfusion   ▽ of blood or blood products, unspecified

ABO incompatibility blood transfusion NOS

Reaction to ABO incompatibility from transfusion NOS

✓6th **T80.31 ABO incompatibility** with hemolytic transfusion reaction

✓7th **T80.310 ABO incompatibility** with acute hemolytic transfusion reaction

ABO incompatibility with hemolytic transfusion reaction less than 24 hours after transfusion

Acute hemolytic transfusion reaction (AHTR) due to ABO incompatibility

✓7th **T80.311 ABO incompatibility** with delayed hemolytic transfusion reaction

ABO incompatibility with hemolytic transfusion reaction 24 hours or more after transfusion

Delayed hemolytic transfusion reaction (DHTR) due to ABO incompatibility

✓7th **T80.319 ABO incompatibility** with hemolytic   ▽ transfusion reaction, unspecified

ABO incompatibility with hemolytic transfusion reaction at unspecified time after transfusion

Hemolytic transfusion reaction (HTR) due to ABO incompatibility NOS

✓x7th **T80.39 Other ABO incompatibility** reaction due to transfusion of blood or blood products

Delayed serologic transfusion reaction (DSTR) from ABO incompatibility

Other ABO incompatible blood transfusion

Other reaction to ABO incompatible blood transfusion

✓5th **T80.4 Rh incompatibility** reaction due to transfusion of blood or blood products

Reaction due to incompatibility of Rh antigens (C) (c) (D) (E) (e)

✓x7th **T80.40 Rh incompatibility** reaction due to transfusion   ▽ of blood or blood products, unspecified

Reaction due to Rh factor in transfusion NOS

Rh incompatible blood transfusion NOS

✓6th **T80.41 Rh incompatibility** with hemolytic transfusion reaction

✓7th **T80.410 Rh incompatibility** with acute hemolytic transfusion reaction

Acute hemolytic transfusion reaction (AHTR) due to Rh incompatibility

Rh incompatibility with hemolytic transfusion reaction less than 24 hours after transfusion

✓7th **T80.411 Rh incompatibility** with delayed hemolytic transfusion reaction

Delayed hemolytic transfusion reaction (DHTR) due to Rh incompatibility

Rh incompatibility with hemolytic transfusion reaction 24 hours or more after transfusion

✓7th **T80.419 Rh incompatibility** with hemolytic   ▽ transfusion reaction, unspecified

Hemolytic transfusion reaction (HTR) due to Rh incompatibility NOS

Rh incompatibility with hemolytic transfusion reaction at unspecified time after transfusion

✓x7th **T80.49 Other Rh incompatibility** reaction due to transfusion of blood or blood products

Delayed serologic transfusion reaction (DSTR) from Rh incompatibility

Other reaction to Rh incompatible blood transfusion

✓5th **T80.A Non-ABO incompatibility** reaction due to transfusion of blood or blood products

Reaction due to incompatibility of minor antigens (Duffy) (Kell) (Kidd) (Lewis) (M) (N) (P) (S)

✓x7th **T80.A0 Non-ABO incompatibility** reaction due to   ▽ transfusion of blood or blood products, unspecified

Non-ABO antigen incompatibility reaction from transfusion NOS

EXCLUDES 1 Not coded here   EXCLUDES 2 Not included here   N Newborn Age: 0   P Pediatric Age: 0-17   M Maternity Age: 12-55   A Adult Age: 15-124

1096   ICD-10-CM 2018

√6ᵗʰ **T80.A1 Non-ABO incompatibility** with hemolytic transfusion reaction

√7ᵗʰ **T80.A10 Non-ABO incompatibility with** acute hemolytic transfusion reaction
Acute hemolytic transfusion reaction (AHTR) due to non-ABO incompatibility
Non-ABO incompatibility with hemolytic transfusion reaction less than 24 hours after transfusion

√7ᵗʰ **T80.A11 Non-ABO incompatibility with** delayed hemolytic transfusion reaction
Delayed hemolytic transfusion reaction (DHTR) due to non-ABO incompatibility
Non-ABO incompatibility with hemolytic transfusion reaction 24 or more hours after transfusion

√7ᵗʰ **T80.A19 Non-ABO incompatibility with hemolytic transfusion reaction, unspecified** ▽
Hemolytic transfusion reaction (HTR) due to non-ABO incompatibility NOS
Non-ABO incompatibility with hemolytic transfusion reaction at unspecified time after transfusion

√x7ᵗʰ **T80.A9 Other non-ABO incompatibility reaction due to transfusion of blood or blood products**
Delayed serologic transfusion reaction (DSTR) from non-ABO incompatibility
Other reaction to non-ABO incompatible blood transfusion

√5ᵗʰ **T80.5 Anaphylactic reaction due to serum**
Allergic shock due to serum
Anaphylactic shock due to serum
Anaphylactoid reaction due to serum
Anaphylaxis due to serum
EXCLUDES 1 *ABO incompatibility reaction due to transfusion of blood or blood products (T80.3-)*
allergic reaction or shock NOS (T78.2)
anaphylactic reaction or shock NOS (T78.2)
anaphylactic reaction or shock due to adverse effect of correct medicinal substance properly administered (T88.6)
other serum reaction (T80.6-)
DEF: Life-threatening hypersensitivity to foreign serum; causes respiratory distress, vascular collapse, and shock.

√x7ᵗʰ **T80.51 Anaphylactic reaction due to** administration of blood and blood products

√x7ᵗʰ **T80.52 Anaphylactic reaction due to** vaccination

√x7ᵗʰ **T80.59 Anaphylactic reaction due to other serum**

√5ᵗʰ **T80.6 Other serum reactions**
Intoxication by serum
Protein sickness
Serum rash
Serum sickness
Serum urticaria
EXCLUDES 2 *serum hepatitis (B16-B19)*
DEF: Serum sickness: Hypersensitivity to foreign serum; causes fever, hives, swelling, and lymphadenopathy.

√x7ᵗʰ **T80.61 Other serum reaction** due to administration of blood and blood products

√x7ᵗʰ **T80.62 Other serum reaction** due to vaccination

√x7ᵗʰ **T80.69 Other serum reaction due to other serum**
▶Code also, if applicable, arthropathy in hypersensitivity reactions classified elsewhere (M36.4)◀

√5ᵗʰ **T80.8 Other complications following infusion, transfusion and therapeutic injection**

√6ᵗʰ **T80.81 Extravasation of vesicant agent**
Infiltration of vesicant agent

√7ᵗʰ **T80.810 Extravasation of vesicant antineoplastic chemotherapy**
Infiltration of vesicant antineoplastic chemotherapy

√7ᵗʰ **T80.818 Extravasation of other vesicant agent**
Infiltration of other vesicant agent

√x7ᵗʰ **T80.89 Other complications following infusion, transfusion and therapeutic injection**
Delayed serologic transfusion reaction (DSTR), unspecified incompatibility
Use additional code to identify graft-versus-host reaction, if applicable, (D89.81-)

√5ᵗʰ **T80.9 Unspecified complication following infusion, transfusion and therapeutic injection**

√x7ᵗʰ **T80.90 Unspecified complication** following infusion and therapeutic injection ▽

√6ᵗʰ **T80.91 Hemolytic transfusion reaction, unspecified incompatibility**
EXCLUDES 1 *ABO incompatibility with hemolytic transfusion reaction (T80.31-)*
Non-ABO incompatibility with hemolytic transfusion reaction (T80.A1-)
Rh incompatibility with hemolytic transfusion reaction (T80.41-)

√7ᵗʰ **T80.910 Acute hemolytic transfusion reaction, unspecified incompatibility** ▽

√7ᵗʰ **T80.911 Delayed hemolytic transfusion reaction, unspecified incompatibility** ▽

√7ᵗʰ **T80.919 Hemolytic transfusion reaction, unspecified incompatibility, unspecified as acute or delayed** ▽
Hemolytic transfusion reaction NOS

√x7ᵗʰ **T80.92 Unspecified transfusion reaction** ▽
Transfusion reaction NOS

√4ᵗʰ **T81 Complications of procedures, not elsewhere classified**
Use additional code for adverse effect, if applicable, to identify drug (T36-T50 with fifth or sixth character 5)
EXCLUDES 2 *complications following immunization (T88.0-T88.1)*
complications following infusion, transfusion and therapeutic injection (T80.-)
complications of transplanted organs and tissue (T86.-)
specified complications classified elsewhere, such as:
complication of prosthetic devices, implants and grafts (T82-T85)
dermatitis due to drugs and medicaments (L23.3, L24.4, L25.1, L27.0-L27.1)
endosseous dental implant failure (M27.6-)
floppy iris syndrome (IFIS) (intraoperative) (H21.81)
intraoperative and postprocedural complications of specific body system (D78.-, E36.-, E89.-, G97.3-, G97.4, H59.3-, H59.-, H95.2-, H95.3, I97.4-, I97.5, J95, K91.-, L76.-, M96.-, N99.-)
ostomy complications (J95.0-, K94.-, N99.5-)
plateau iris syndrome (post-iridectomy) (postprocedural) (H21.82)
poisoning and toxic effects of drugs and chemicals (T36-T65 with fifth or sixth character 1-4 or 6)

The appropriate 7th character is to be added to each code from category T81.
A   initial encounter
D   subsequent encounter
S   sequela

√5ᵗʰ **T81.1 Postprocedural shock**
Shock during or resulting from a procedure, not elsewhere classified
EXCLUDES 1 *anaphylactic shock due to correct substance properly administered (T88.6)*
anaphylactic shock due to serum (T80.5-)
anaphylactic shock NOS (T78.2)
anesthetic shock (T88.2)
electric shock (T75.4)
obstetric shock (O75.1)
septic shock (R65.21)
shock following abortion or ectopic or molar pregnancy (O00-O07, O08.3)
traumatic shock (T79.4)

√x7ᵗʰ **T81.10 Postprocedural shock unspecified** ▽
Collapse NOS during or resulting from a procedure, not elsewhere classified
Postprocedural failure of peripheral circulation
Postprocedural shock NOS

1 √x7ᵗʰ **T81.11 Postprocedural cardiogenic shock** HCC

---

1 HCC with 7th character indicating initial encounter (A, B or C - specific to category).

Chapter 19. Injury, Poisoning, and Certain Other Consequences of External Causes *(left margin, vertical)*

T81.12–T81.524 *(left margin, vertical)*

[1] ✓x7th **T81.12 Postprocedural septic shock**   HCC
　　Postprocedural endotoxic shock resulting from a procedure, not elsewhere classified
　　Postprocedural gram-negative shock resulting from a procedure, not elsewhere classified
　　Code first underlying infection
　　Use additional code, to identify any associated acute organ dysfunction, if applicable

✓x7th **T81.19 Other postprocedural shock**
　　Postprocedural hypovolemic shock

✓5th **T81.3 Disruption of wound, not elsewhere classified**
　　Disruption of any suture materials or other closure methods
　　EXCLUDES 1　breakdown (mechanical) of permanent sutures (T85.612)
　　　　displacement of permanent sutures (T85.622)
　　　　disruption of cesarean delivery wound (O90.0)
　　　　disruption of perineal obstetric wound (O90.1)
　　　　mechanical complication of permanent sutures NEC (T85.692)
　　AHA: 2014, 1Q, 23

✓x7th **T81.30 Disruption of wound, unspecified** ▽
　　Disruption of wound NOS

✓x7th **T81.31 Disruption of external operation (surgical) wound, not elsewhere classified**
　　Dehiscence of operation wound NOS
　　Disruption of operation wound NOS
　　Disruption or dehiscence of closure of cornea
　　Disruption or dehiscence of closure of mucosa
　　Disruption or dehiscence of closure of skin and subcutaneous tissue
　　Full-thickness skin disruption or dehiscence
　　Superficial disruption or dehiscence of operation wound
　　EXCLUDES 1　dehiscence of amputation stump (T87.81)

✓x7th **T81.32 Disruption of internal operation (surgical) wound, not elsewhere classified**
　　Deep disruption or dehiscence of operation wound NOS
　　Disruption or dehiscence of closure of internal organ or other internal tissue
　　Disruption or dehiscence of closure of muscle or muscle flap
　　Disruption or dehiscence of closure of ribs or rib cage
　　Disruption or dehiscence of closure of skull or craniotomy
　　Disruption or dehiscence of closure of sternum or sternotomy
　　Disruption or dehiscence of closure of tendon or ligament
　　Disruption or dehiscence of closure of superficial or muscular fascia

✓x7th **T81.33 Disruption of traumatic injury wound repair**
　　Disruption or dehiscence of closure of traumatic laceration (external) (internal)

✓x7th **T81.4 Infection following a procedure**
　　Intra-abdominal abscess following a procedure
　　Postprocedural infection, not elsewhere classified
　　Sepsis following a procedure
　　Stitch abscess following a procedure
　　Subphrenic abscess following a procedure
　　Wound abscess following a procedure
　　Use additional code to identify infection
　　Use additional code (R65.2-) to identify severe sepsis, if applicable
　　EXCLUDES 1　obstetric surgical wound infection (O86.0)
　　　　postprocedural fever NOS (R50.82)
　　　　postprocedural retroperitoneal abscess (K68.11)
　　EXCLUDES 2　bleb associated endophthalmitis (H59.4-)
　　　　infection due to infusion, transfusion and therapeutic injection (T80.2-)
　　　　infection due to prosthetic devices, implants and grafts (T82.6-T82.7, T83.5-T83.6, T84.5-T84.7, T85.7)
　　AHA: 2014, 1Q, 23

✓5th **T81.5 Complications of foreign body accidentally left in body following procedure**
　　AHA: 2014, 4Q, 24

✓6th **T81.50 Unspecified complication of foreign body accidentally left in body following procedure**

✓7th **T81.500 Unspecified complication of foreign body accidentally left in body following surgical operation** ▽

✓7th **T81.501 Unspecified complication of foreign body accidentally left in body following infusion or transfusion** ▽

✓7th **T81.502 Unspecified complication of foreign body accidentally left in body following kidney dialysis**   HCC ▽

✓7th **T81.503 Unspecified complication of foreign body accidentally left in body following injection or immunization** ▽

✓7th **T81.504 Unspecified complication of foreign body accidentally left in body following endoscopic examination** ▽

✓7th **T81.505 Unspecified complication of foreign body accidentally left in body following heart catheterization** ▽

✓7th **T81.506 Unspecified complication of foreign body accidentally left in body following aspiration, puncture or other catheterization** ▽

✓7th **T81.507 Unspecified complication of foreign body accidentally left in body following removal of catheter or packing** ▽

✓7th **T81.508 Unspecified complication of foreign body accidentally left in body following other procedure** ▽

✓7th **T81.509 Unspecified complication of foreign body accidentally left in body following unspecified procedure** ▽

✓6th **T81.51 Adhesions due to foreign body accidentally left in body following procedure**

✓7th **T81.510 Adhesions due to foreign body accidentally left in body following surgical operation**

✓7th **T81.511 Adhesions due to foreign body accidentally left in body following infusion or transfusion**

✓7th **T81.512 Adhesions due to foreign body accidentally left in body following kidney dialysis**   HCC

✓7th **T81.513 Adhesions due to foreign body accidentally left in body following injection or immunization**

✓7th **T81.514 Adhesions due to foreign body accidentally left in body following endoscopic examination**

✓7th **T81.515 Adhesions due to foreign body accidentally left in body following heart catheterization**

✓7th **T81.516 Adhesions due to foreign body accidentally left in body following aspiration, puncture or other catheterization**

✓7th **T81.517 Adhesions due to foreign body accidentally left in body following removal of catheter or packing**

✓7th **T81.518 Adhesions due to foreign body accidentally left in body following other procedure**

✓7th **T81.519 Adhesions due to foreign body accidentally left in body following unspecified procedure** ▽

✓6th **T81.52 Obstruction due to foreign body accidentally left in body following procedure**

✓7th **T81.520 Obstruction due to foreign body accidentally left in body following surgical operation**

✓7th **T81.521 Obstruction due to foreign body accidentally left in body following infusion or transfusion**

✓7th **T81.522 Obstruction due to foreign body accidentally left in body following kidney dialysis**   HCC

✓7th **T81.523 Obstruction due to foreign body accidentally left in body following injection or immunization**

✓7th **T81.524 Obstruction due to foreign body accidentally left in body following endoscopic examination**

---

[1] HCC with 7th character indicating initial encounter (A, B or C - specific to category).

EXCLUDES 1 Not coded here   EXCLUDES 2 Not included here   N Newborn Age: 0   P Pediatric Age: 0-17   M Maternity Age: 12-55   A Adult Age: 15-124

1098   ICD-10-CM 2018

√7ᵗʰ **T81.525** **Obstruction due to foreign body accidentally left in body following** heart catheterization

√7ᵗʰ **T81.526** **Obstruction due to foreign body accidentally left in body following aspiration, puncture or other catheterization**

√7ᵗʰ **T81.527** **Obstruction due to foreign body accidentally left in body following removal of catheter or packing**

√7ᵗʰ **T81.528** **Obstruction due to foreign body accidentally left in body following other procedure**

√7ᵗʰ **T81.529** **Obstruction due to foreign body accidentally left in body following unspecified procedure** ▽

√6ᵗʰ **T81.53** Perforation **due to foreign body accidentally left in body following procedure**

√7ᵗʰ **T81.530** **Perforation due to foreign body accidentally left in body following surgical operation**

√7ᵗʰ **T81.531** **Perforation due to foreign body accidentally left in body following infusion or transfusion**

√7ᵗʰ **T81.532** **Perforation due to foreign body accidentally left in body following kidney dialysis** HCC

√7ᵗʰ **T81.533** **Perforation due to foreign body accidentally left in body following injection or immunization**

√7ᵗʰ **T81.534** **Perforation due to foreign body accidentally left in body following endoscopic examination**

√7ᵗʰ **T81.535** **Perforation due to foreign body accidentally left in body following** heart catheterization

√7ᵗʰ **T81.536** **Perforation due to foreign body accidentally left in body following aspiration, puncture or other catheterization**

√7ᵗʰ **T81.537** **Perforation due to foreign body accidentally left in body following removal of catheter or packing**

√7ᵗʰ **T81.538** **Perforation due to foreign body accidentally left in body following other procedure**

√7ᵗʰ **T81.539** **Perforation due to foreign body accidentally left in body following unspecified procedure** ▽

√6ᵗʰ **T81.59** **Other complications of foreign body accidentally left in body following procedure**

EXCLUDES 2 *obstruction or perforation due to prosthetic devices and implants intentionally left in body (T82.0-T82.5, T83.0-T83.4, T83.7, T84.0-T84.4, T85.0-T85.6)*

√7ᵗʰ **T81.590** **Other complications of foreign body accidentally left in body following surgical operation**

√7ᵗʰ **T81.591** **Other complications of foreign body accidentally left in body following infusion or transfusion**

√7ᵗʰ **T81.592** **Other complications of foreign body accidentally left in body following kidney dialysis** HCC

√7ᵗʰ **T81.593** **Other complications of foreign body accidentally left in body following injection or immunization**

√7ᵗʰ **T81.594** **Other complications of foreign body accidentally left in body following endoscopic examination**

√7ᵗʰ **T81.595** **Other complications of foreign body accidentally left in body following** heart catheterization

√7ᵗʰ **T81.596** **Other complications of foreign body accidentally left in body following aspiration, puncture or other catheterization**

√7ᵗʰ **T81.597** **Other complications of foreign body accidentally left in body following removal of catheter or packing**

√7ᵗʰ **T81.598** **Other complications of foreign body accidentally left in body following other procedure**

√7ᵗʰ **T81.599** **Other complications of foreign body accidentally left in body following unspecified procedure** ▽

√5ᵗʰ **T81.6** **Acute reaction to foreign substance accidentally left during a procedure**

EXCLUDES 2 *complications of foreign body accidentally left in body cavity or operation wound following procedure (T81.5-)*

√x7ᵗʰ **T81.60** **Unspecified acute reaction to foreign substance accidentally left during a procedure** ▽

√x7ᵗʰ **T81.61** **Aseptic peritonitis due to foreign substance accidentally left during a procedure**
Chemical peritonitis

√x7ᵗʰ **T81.69** **Other acute reaction to foreign substance accidentally left during a procedure**

√5ᵗʰ **T81.7** **Vascular complications following a procedure, not elsewhere classified**
Air embolism following procedure NEC
Phlebitis or thrombophlebitis resulting from a procedure

EXCLUDES 1 *embolism complicating abortion or ectopic or molar pregnancy (O00-O07, O08.2)*
embolism complicating pregnancy, childbirth and the puerperium (O88.-)
traumatic embolism (T79.0)

EXCLUDES 2 *embolism due to prosthetic devices, implants and grafts (T82.8-, T83.81, T84.8-, T85.81-)*
embolism following infusion, transfusion and therapeutic injection (T80.0)

√6ᵗʰ **T81.71** **Complication of artery following a procedure, not elsewhere classified**

√7ᵗʰ **T81.710** **Complication of** mesenteric **artery following a procedure, not elsewhere classified**

√7ᵗʰ **T81.711** **Complication of** renal **artery following a procedure, not elsewhere classified**

√7ᵗʰ **T81.718** **Complication of other artery following a procedure, not elsewhere classified**

√7ᵗʰ **T81.719** **Complication of unspecified artery following a procedure, not elsewhere classified** ▽

√x7ᵗʰ **T81.72** **Complication of** vein **following a procedure, not elsewhere classified**

√5ᵗʰ **T81.8** **Other complications of procedures, not elsewhere classified**

EXCLUDES 2 *hypothermia following anesthesia (T88.51)*
malignant hyperpyrexia due to anesthesia (T88.3)

√x7ᵗʰ **T81.81** **Complication of inhalation therapy**

√x7ᵗʰ **T81.82** **Emphysema (subcutaneous) resulting from a procedure**

√x7ᵗʰ **T81.83** **Persistent postprocedural fistula**

√x7ᵗʰ **T81.89** **Other complications of procedures, not elsewhere classified**
Use additional code to specify complication, such as:
postprocedural delirium (F05)
AHA: 2014, 1Q, 23

√x7ᵗʰ **T81.9** **Unspecified complication of procedure** ▽

√4ᵗʰ **T82** **Complications of cardiac and vascular prosthetic devices, implants and grafts**

EXCLUDES 2 *failure and rejection of transplanted organs and tissue (T86.-)*

The appropriate 7th character is to be added to each code from category T82.
A　　initial encounter
D　　subsequent encounter
S　　sequela

√5ᵗʰ **T82.0** **Mechanical complication of** heart valve prosthesis
Mechanical complication of artificial heart valve

EXCLUDES 1 *mechanical complication of biological heart valve graft (T82.22-)*

√x7ᵗʰ **T82.01** **Breakdown (mechanical) of heart valve prosthesis**

√x7ᵗʰ **T82.02** **Displacement of heart valve prosthesis**
Malposition of heart valve prosthesis

√x7ᵗʰ **T82.03** **Leakage of heart valve prosthesis**

☑ Additional Character Req　　√x7ᵗʰ Placeholder Alert　　Manifestation　　HCC CMS-HCC Condition　　▽ Unspecified Code　　►◄ Revised Text　　● New Code　　▲ Revised Code Title

ICD-10-CM 2018　　　　　　　　　　　　　　　　　　　　　　　　　　　　　　　　　　　1099

Chapter 19. Injury, Poisoning, and Certain Other Consequences of External Causes (side tab)

T82.09–T82.515 (side tab)

✓x7ᵗʰ **T82.09** **Other mechanical complication of heart valve prosthesis**
Obstruction (mechanical) of heart valve prosthesis
Perforation of heart valve prosthesis
Protrusion of heart valve prosthesis

✓5ᵗʰ **T82.1** **Mechanical complication of** cardiac electronic device

  ✓6ᵗʰ **T82.11** **Breakdown (mechanical) of cardiac electronic device**

    ✓7ᵗʰ **T82.110** **Breakdown (mechanical) of cardiac electrode**

    ✓7ᵗʰ **T82.111** **Breakdown (mechanical) of cardiac** pulse generator (battery)

    ✓7ᵗʰ **T82.118** **Breakdown (mechanical) of other cardiac electronic device**

    ✓7ᵗʰ **T82.119** **Breakdown (mechanical) of unspecified** ▽ **cardiac electronic device**

  ✓6ᵗʰ **T82.12** **Displacement of cardiac electronic device**
Malposition of cardiac electronic device

    ✓7ᵗʰ **T82.120** **Displacement of** cardiac electrode

    ✓7ᵗʰ **T82.121** **Displacement of cardiac** pulse generator (battery)

    ✓7ᵗʰ **T82.128** **Displacement of other cardiac electronic device**

    ✓7ᵗʰ **T82.129** **Displacement of unspecified cardiac** ▽ **electronic device**

  ✓6ᵗʰ **T82.19** **Other mechanical complication of cardiac electronic device**
Leakage of cardiac electronic device
Obstruction of cardiac electronic device
Perforation of cardiac electronic device
Protrusion of cardiac electronic device

    ✓7ᵗʰ **T82.190** **Other mechanical complication of** cardiac electrode

    ✓7ᵗʰ **T82.191** **Other mechanical complication of cardiac pulse generator (battery)**

    ✓7ᵗʰ **T82.198** **Other mechanical complication of other cardiac electronic device**

    ✓7ᵗʰ **T82.199** **Other mechanical complication of** ▽ **unspecified cardiac device**

✓5ᵗʰ **T82.2** **Mechanical complication of coronary artery bypass graft and biological heart valve graft**
    EXCLUDES 1 *mechanical complication of artificial heart valve prosthesis (T82.0-)*

  ✓6ᵗʰ **T82.21** **Mechanical complication of** coronary artery bypass graft

    ✓7ᵗʰ **T82.211** **Breakdown (mechanical) of coronary artery bypass graft**

    ✓7ᵗʰ **T82.212** **Displacement of coronary artery bypass graft**
Malposition of coronary artery bypass graft

    ✓7ᵗʰ **T82.213** **Leakage of coronary artery bypass graft**

    ✓7ᵗʰ **T82.218** **Other mechanical complication of coronary artery bypass graft**
Obstruction, mechanical of coronary artery bypass graft
Perforation of coronary artery bypass graft
Protrusion of coronary artery bypass graft

  ✓6ᵗʰ **T82.22** **Mechanical complication of** biological heart valve graft

    ✓7ᵗʰ **T82.221** **Breakdown (mechanical) of biological heart valve graft**

    ✓7ᵗʰ **T82.222** **Displacement of biological heart valve graft**
Malposition of biological heart valve graft

    ✓7ᵗʰ **T82.223** **Leakage of biological heart valve graft**

    ✓7ᵗʰ **T82.228** **Other mechanical complication of biological heart valve graft**
Obstruction of biological heart valve graft
Perforation of biological heart valve graft
Protrusion of biological heart valve graft

✓5ᵗʰ **T82.3** **Mechanical complication of other vascular grafts**

  ✓6ᵗʰ **T82.31** **Breakdown (mechanical) of other vascular grafts**

    1 ✓7ᵗʰ **T82.310** **Breakdown (mechanical) of** aortic (bifurcation) graft (replacement) HCC

    1 ✓7ᵗʰ **T82.311** **Breakdown (mechanical) of** carotid arterial graft (bypass) HCC

    1 ✓7ᵗʰ **T82.312** **Breakdown (mechanical) of** femoral arterial graft (bypass) HCC

    1 ✓7ᵗʰ **T82.318** **Breakdown (mechanical) of other vascular grafts** HCC

    1 ✓7ᵗʰ **T82.319** **Breakdown (mechanical) of unspecified vascular grafts** HCC ▽

  ✓6ᵗʰ **T82.32** **Displacement of other vascular grafts**
Malposition of other vascular grafts

    1 ✓7ᵗʰ **T82.320** **Displacement of** aortic (bifurcation) graft (replacement) HCC

    1 ✓7ᵗʰ **T82.321** **Displacement of** carotid arterial graft (bypass) HCC

    1 ✓7ᵗʰ **T82.322** **Displacement of** femoral arterial graft (bypass) HCC

    1 ✓7ᵗʰ **T82.328** **Displacement of other vascular grafts** HCC

    1 ✓7ᵗʰ **T82.329** **Displacement of unspecified vascular grafts** HCC ▽

  ✓6ᵗʰ **T82.33** **Leakage of other vascular grafts**

    1 ✓7ᵗʰ **T82.330** **Leakage of** aortic (bifurcation) graft (replacement) HCC

    1 ✓7ᵗʰ **T82.331** **Leakage of** carotid arterial graft (bypass) HCC

    1 ✓7ᵗʰ **T82.332** **Leakage of** femoral arterial graft (bypass) HCC

    1 ✓7ᵗʰ **T82.338** **Leakage of other vascular grafts** HCC

    1 ✓7ᵗʰ **T82.339** **Leakage of unspecified vascular graft** HCC ▽

  ✓6ᵗʰ **T82.39** **Other mechanical complication of other vascular grafts**
Obstruction (mechanical) of other vascular grafts
Perforation of other vascular grafts
Protrusion of other vascular grafts

    1 ✓7ᵗʰ **T82.390** **Other mechanical complication of** aortic (bifurcation) graft (replacement) HCC

    1 ✓7ᵗʰ **T82.391** **Other mechanical complication of** carotid arterial graft (bypass) HCC

    1 ✓7ᵗʰ **T82.392** **Other mechanical complication of** femoral arterial graft (bypass) HCC

    1 ✓7ᵗʰ **T82.398** **Other mechanical complication of other vascular grafts** HCC

    1 ✓7ᵗʰ **T82.399** **Other mechanical complication of unspecified vascular grafts** HCC ▽

✓5ᵗʰ **T82.4** **Mechanical complication of** vascular dialysis catheter
Mechanical complication of hemodialysis catheter
    EXCLUDES 1 *mechanical complication of intraperitoneal dialysis catheter (T85.62)*

  ✓x7ᵗʰ **T82.41** **Breakdown (mechanical) of vascular dialysis catheter** HCC

  ✓x7ᵗʰ **T82.42** **Displacement of vascular dialysis catheter** HCC
Malposition of vascular dialysis catheter

  ✓x7ᵗʰ **T82.43** **Leakage of vascular dialysis catheter** HCC

  ✓x7ᵗʰ **T82.49** **Other complication of vascular dialysis catheter** HCC
Obstruction (mechanical) of vascular dialysis catheter
Perforation of vascular dialysis catheter
Protrusion of vascular dialysis catheter

✓5ᵗʰ **T82.5** **Mechanical complication of other cardiac and vascular devices and implants**
    EXCLUDES 2 *mechanical complication of epidural and subdural infusion catheter (T85.61)*

  ✓6ᵗʰ **T82.51** **Breakdown (mechanical) of other cardiac and vascular devices and implants**

    1 ✓7ᵗʰ **T82.510** **Breakdown (mechanical) of** surgically created arteriovenous fistula HCC

    1 ✓7ᵗʰ **T82.511** **Breakdown (mechanical) of** surgically created arteriovenous shunt HCC

    ✓7ᵗʰ **T82.512** **Breakdown (mechanical) of** artificial heart

    1 ✓7ᵗʰ **T82.513** **Breakdown (mechanical) of** balloon (counterpulsation) device HCC

    1 ✓7ᵗʰ **T82.514** **Breakdown (mechanical) of** infusion catheter HCC

    1 ✓7ᵗʰ **T82.515** **Breakdown (mechanical) of** umbrella device HCC

---

1   HCC with 7th character indicating initial encounter (A, B or C - specific to category).

1 ✓7ᵗʰ	**T82.518**	**Breakdown (mechanical) of other cardiac and vascular devices and implants**	HCC
✓7ᵗʰ	**T82.519**	**Breakdown (mechanical) of unspecified cardiac and vascular devices and implants**	▽

✓6ᵗʰ **T82.52** Displacement of other cardiac and vascular devices and implants
Malposition of other cardiac and vascular devices and implants

1 ✓7ᵗʰ	**T82.520**	**Displacement of** surgically created arteriovenous fistula	HCC
1 ✓7ᵗʰ	**T82.521**	**Displacement of** surgically created arteriovenous shunt	HCC
✓7ᵗʰ	**T82.522**	**Displacement of** artificial heart	
1 ✓7ᵗʰ	**T82.523**	**Displacement of** balloon (counterpulsation) device	HCC
1 ✓7ᵗʰ	**T82.524**	**Displacement of** infusion catheter	HCC
1 ✓7ᵗʰ	**T82.525**	**Displacement of** umbrella device	HCC
1 ✓7ᵗʰ	**T82.528**	**Displacement of other cardiac and vascular devices and implants**	HCC
✓7ᵗʰ	**T82.529**	**Displacement of unspecified cardiac and vascular devices and implants**	▽

✓6ᵗʰ **T82.53** Leakage of other cardiac and vascular devices and implants

1 ✓7ᵗʰ	**T82.530**	**Leakage of** surgically created arteriovenous fistula	HCC
1 ✓7ᵗʰ	**T82.531**	**Leakage of** surgically created arteriovenous shunt	HCC
✓7ᵗʰ	**T82.532**	**Leakage of** artificial heart	
1 ✓7ᵗʰ	**T82.533**	**Leakage of** balloon (counterpulsation) device	HCC
1 ✓7ᵗʰ	**T82.534**	**Leakage of** infusion catheter	HCC
1 ✓7ᵗʰ	**T82.535**	**Leakage of** umbrella device	HCC
1 ✓7ᵗʰ	**T82.538**	**Leakage of other cardiac and vascular devices and implants**	HCC
✓7ᵗʰ	**T82.539**	**Leakage of unspecified cardiac and vascular devices and implants**	▽

✓6ᵗʰ **T82.59** Other mechanical complication of other cardiac and vascular devices and implants
Obstruction (mechanical) of other cardiac and vascular devices and implants
Perforation of other cardiac and vascular devices and implants
Protrusion of other cardiac and vascular devices and implants

1 ✓7ᵗʰ	**T82.590**	**Other mechanical complication of** surgically created arteriovenous fistula	HCC
1 ✓7ᵗʰ	**T82.591**	**Other mechanical complication of** surgically created arteriovenous shunt	HCC
✓7ᵗʰ	**T82.592**	**Other mechanical complication of** artificial heart	
1 ✓7ᵗʰ	**T82.593**	**Other mechanical complication of** balloon (counterpulsation) device	HCC
1 ✓7ᵗʰ	**T82.594**	**Other mechanical complication of** infusion catheter	HCC
1 ✓7ᵗʰ	**T82.595**	**Other mechanical complication of** umbrella device	HCC
1 ✓7ᵗʰ	**T82.598**	**Other mechanical complication of other cardiac and vascular devices and implants**	HCC
✓7ᵗʰ	**T82.599**	**Other mechanical complication of unspecified cardiac and vascular devices and implants**	▽

1 ✓x7ᵗʰ **T82.6** **Infection and inflammatory reaction due to cardiac valve prosthesis** HCC
Use additional code to identify infection

1 ✓x7ᵗʰ **T82.7** **Infection and inflammatory reaction due to other cardiac and vascular devices, implants and grafts** HCC
Use additional code to identify infection

✓5ᵗʰ **T82.8** Other specified complications of cardiac and vascular prosthetic devices, implants and grafts

✓6ᵗʰ **T82.81** Embolism due to cardiac and vascular prosthetic devices, implants and grafts

✓7ᵗʰ	**T82.817**	**Embolism due to** cardiac prosthetic devices, implants and grafts	

1 ✓7ᵗʰ	**T82.818**	**Embolism due to** vascular prosthetic devices, implants and grafts	HCC

✓6ᵗʰ **T82.82** Fibrosis due to cardiac and vascular prosthetic devices, implants and grafts

✓7ᵗʰ	**T82.827**	**Fibrosis due to** cardiac prosthetic devices, implants and grafts	
1 ✓7ᵗʰ	**T82.828**	**Fibrosis due to** vascular prosthetic devices, implants and grafts	HCC

✓6ᵗʰ **T82.83** Hemorrhage due to cardiac and vascular prosthetic devices, implants and grafts

✓7ᵗʰ	**T82.837**	**Hemorrhage due to** cardiac prosthetic devices, implants and grafts	
1 ✓7ᵗʰ	**T82.838**	**Hemorrhage due to** vascular prosthetic devices, implants and grafts	HCC

✓6ᵗʰ **T82.84** Pain due to cardiac and vascular prosthetic devices, implants and grafts

✓7ᵗʰ	**T82.847**	**Pain due to** cardiac prosthetic devices, implants and grafts	
1 ✓7ᵗʰ	**T82.848**	**Pain due to** vascular prosthetic devices, implants and grafts	HCC

✓6ᵗʰ **T82.85** Stenosis due to cardiac and vascular prosthetic devices, implants and grafts

✓7ᵗʰ	**T82.855**	**Stenosis of** coronary artery stent In-stent stenosis (restenosis) of coronary artery stent Restenosis of coronary artery stent	
1 ✓7ᵗʰ	**T82.856**	**Stenosis of** peripheral vascular stent In-stent stenosis (restenosis) of peripheral vascular stent Restenosis of peripheral vascular stent	HCC
✓7ᵗʰ	**T82.857**	**Stenosis of other** cardiac prosthetic devices, implants and grafts	
1 ✓7ᵗʰ	**T82.858**	**Stenosis of other** vascular prosthetic devices, implants and grafts	HCC

✓6ᵗʰ **T82.86** Thrombosis of cardiac and vascular prosthetic devices, implants and grafts

✓7ᵗʰ	**T82.867**	**Thrombosis due to** cardiac prosthetic devices, implants and grafts	
1 ✓7ᵗʰ	**T82.868**	**Thrombosis due to** vascular prosthetic devices, implants and grafts	HCC

✓6ᵗʰ **T82.89** Other specified complication of cardiac and vascular prosthetic devices, implants and grafts

✓7ᵗʰ	**T82.897**	**Other specified complication of** cardiac prosthetic devices, implants and grafts	
1 ✓7ᵗʰ	**T82.898**	**Other specified complication of** vascular prosthetic devices, implants and grafts	HCC

✓x7ᵗʰ **T82.9** Unspecified complication of cardiac and vascular prosthetic device, implant and graft ▽

✓4ᵗʰ **T83** **Complications of genitourinary prosthetic devices, implants and grafts**
EXCLUDES 2 failure and rejection of transplanted organs and tissue (T86.-)

The appropriate 7th character is to be added to each code from category T83.
A initial encounter
D subsequent encounter
S sequela

✓5ᵗʰ **T83.0** Mechanical complication of urinary catheter
EXCLUDES 2 complications of stoma of urinary tract (N99.5-)

✓6ᵗʰ **T83.01** Breakdown (mechanical) of urinary catheter

1 ✓7ᵗʰ	**T83.010**	**Breakdown (mechanical) of** cystostomy catheter	HCC
1 ✓7ᵗʰ	**T83.011**	**Breakdown (mechanical) of** indwelling urethral catheter	HCC
1 ✓7ᵗʰ	**T83.012**	**Breakdown (mechanical) of** nephrostomy catheter	HCC
1 ✓7ᵗʰ	**T83.018**	**Breakdown (mechanical) of other urinary catheter** Breakdown (mechanical) of Hopkins catheter Breakdown (mechanical) of ileostomy catheter Breakdown (mechanical) urostomy catheter	HCC

---

1 HCC with 7th character indicating initial encounter (A, B or C - specific to category).

✓ Additional Character Req   ✓x7ᵗʰ Placeholder Alert   Manifestation   HCC CMS-HCC Condition   ▽ Unspecified Code   ►◄ Revised Text   ● New Code   ▲ Revised Code Title

T83.02 Displacement of urinary catheter
Malposition of urinary catheter

- ✓7ᵗʰ **T83.020 Displacement of cystostomy catheter** HCC
- ✓7ᵗʰ **T83.021 Displacement of indwelling urethral catheter** HCC
- ✓7ᵗʰ **T83.022 Displacement of nephrostomy catheter** HCC
- ✓7ᵗʰ **T83.028 Displacement of other urinary catheter** HCC
  - Displacement of Hopkins catheter
  - Displacement of ileostomy catheter
  - Displacement of urostomy catheter

T83.03 Leakage of urinary catheter

- ✓7ᵗʰ **T83.030 Leakage of cystostomy catheter** HCC
- ✓7ᵗʰ **T83.031 Leakage of indwelling urethral catheter** HCC
- ✓7ᵗʰ **T83.032 Leakage of nephrostomy catheter** HCC
- ✓7ᵗʰ **T83.038 Leakage of other urinary catheter** HCC
  - Leakage of Hopkins catheter
  - Leakage of ileostomy catheter
  - Leakage of urostomy catheter

T83.09 Other mechanical complication of urinary catheter
- Obstruction (mechanical) of urinary catheter
- Perforation of urinary catheter
- Protrusion of urinary catheter

- ✓7ᵗʰ **T83.090 Other mechanical complication of cystostomy catheter** HCC
- ✓7ᵗʰ **T83.091 Other mechanical complication of indwelling urethral catheter** HCC
- ✓7ᵗʰ **T83.092 Other mechanical complication of nephrostomy catheter** HCC
- ✓7ᵗʰ **T83.098 Other mechanical complication of other urinary catheter** HCC
  - Other mechanical complication of Hopkins catheter
  - Other mechanical complication of ileostomy catheter
  - Other mechanical complication of urostomy catheter

✓5ᵗʰ **T83.1 Mechanical complication of other urinary devices and implants**

✓6ᵗʰ **T83.11 Breakdown (mechanical) of other urinary devices and implants**

- ✓7ᵗʰ **T83.110 Breakdown (mechanical) of urinary electronic stimulator device** HCC
  - *EXCLUDES 2* breakdown (mechanical) of electrode (lead) for sacral nerve neurostimulator (T85.111)
  - breakdown (mechanical) of implanted electronic sacral neurostimulator, pulse generator or receiver (T85.113)
- ✓7ᵗʰ **T83.111 Breakdown (mechanical) of implanted urinary sphincter** HCC
- ✓7ᵗʰ **T83.112 Breakdown (mechanical) of indwelling ureteral stent** HCC
- ✓7ᵗʰ **T83.113 Breakdown (mechanical) of other urinary stents** HCC
  - Breakdown (mechanical) of ileal conduit stent
  - Breakdown (mechanical) of nephroureteral stent
- ✓7ᵗʰ **T83.118 Breakdown (mechanical) of other urinary devices and implants** HCC

✓6ᵗʰ **T83.12 Displacement of other urinary devices and implants**
Malposition of other urinary devices and implants

- ✓7ᵗʰ **T83.120 Displacement of urinary electronic stimulator device** HCC
  - *EXCLUDES 2* displacement of electrode (lead) for sacral nerve neurostimulator (T85.121)
  - displacement of implanted electronic sacral neurostimulator, pulse generator or receiver (T85.123/0
- ✓7ᵗʰ **T83.121 Displacement of implanted urinary sphincter** HCC

- ✓7ᵗʰ **T83.122 Displacement of indwelling ureteral stent** HCC
- ✓7ᵗʰ **T83.123 Displacement of other urinary stents** HCC
  - Displacement of ileal conduit stent
  - Displacement of nephroureteral stent
- ✓7ᵗʰ **T83.128 Displacement of other urinary devices and implants** HCC

✓6ᵗʰ **T83.19 Other mechanical complication of other urinary devices and implants**
- Leakage of other urinary devices and implants
- Obstruction (mechanical) of other urinary devices and implants
- Perforation of other urinary devices and implants
- Protrusion of other urinary devices and implants

- ✓7ᵗʰ **T83.190 Other mechanical complication of urinary electronic stimulator device** HCC
  - *EXCLUDES 2* other mechanical complication of electrode (lead) for sacral nerve neurostimulator (T85.191)
  - other mechanical complication of implanted electronic sacral neurostimulator, pulse generator or receiver (T85.193)
- ✓7ᵗʰ **T83.191 Other mechanical complication of implanted urinary sphincter** HCC
- ✓7ᵗʰ **T83.192 Other mechanical complication of indwelling ureteral stent** HCC
- ✓7ᵗʰ **T83.193 Other mechanical complication of other urinary stent** HCC
  - Other mechanical complication of ileal conduit stent
  - Other mechanical complication of nephroureteral stent
- ✓7ᵗʰ **T83.198 Other mechanical complication of other urinary devices and implants** HCC

✓5ᵗʰ **T83.2 Mechanical complication of graft of urinary organ**

- ✓x7ᵗʰ **T83.21 Breakdown (mechanical) of graft of urinary organ** HCC
- ✓x7ᵗʰ **T83.22 Displacement of graft of urinary organ** HCC
  - Malposition of graft of urinary organ
- ✓x7ᵗʰ **T83.23 Leakage of graft of urinary organ** HCC
- ✓x7ᵗʰ **T83.24 Erosion of graft of urinary organ** HCC
- ✓x7ᵗʰ **T83.25 Exposure of graft of urinary organ** HCC
- ✓x7ᵗʰ **T83.29 Other mechanical complication of graft of urinary organ** HCC
  - Obstruction (mechanical) of graft of urinary organ
  - Perforation of graft of urinary organ
  - Protrusion of graft of urinary organ

✓5ᵗʰ **T83.3 Mechanical complication of intrauterine contraceptive device**

- ✓x7ᵗʰ **T83.31 Breakdown (mechanical) of intrauterine contraceptive device** ♀
- ✓x7ᵗʰ **T83.32 Displacement of intrauterine contraceptive device** ♀
  - Malposition of intrauterine contraceptive device
  - Missing string of intrauterine contraceptive device
- ✓x7ᵗʰ **T83.39 Other mechanical complication of intrauterine contraceptive device** ♀
  - Leakage of intrauterine contraceptive device
  - Obstruction (mechanical) of intrauterine contraceptive device
  - Perforation of intrauterine contraceptive device
  - Protrusion of intrauterine contraceptive device

✓6ᵗʰ **T83.4 Mechanical complication of other prosthetic devices, implants and grafts of genital tract**

✓6ᵗʰ **T83.41 Breakdown (mechanical) of other prosthetic devices, implants and grafts of genital tract**

- ✓7ᵗʰ **T83.410 Breakdown (mechanical) of implanted penile prosthesis** HCC ♂
  - Breakdown (mechanical) of penile prosthesis cylinder
  - Breakdown (mechanical) of penile prosthesis pump
  - Breakdown (mechanical) of penile prosthesis reservoir
- ✓7ᵗʰ **T83.411 Breakdown (mechanical) of implanted testicular prosthesis** HCC

---

1 HCC with 7th character indicating initial encounter (A, B or C - specific to category).

EXCLUDES 1 Not coded here   *EXCLUDES 2* Not included here   N Newborn Age: 0   P Pediatric Age: 0-17   M Maternity Age: 12-55   A Adult Age: 15-124

1102   ICD-10-CM 2018

[1] ✓7ᵗʰ **T83.418** **Breakdown (mechanical) of other** ᴴᶜᶜ
prosthetic devices, implants and
grafts of genital tract

✓6ᵗʰ **T83.42** Displacement of other prosthetic devices, implants
and grafts of genital tract
Malposition of other prosthetic devices, implants and
grafts of genital tract

[1] ✓7ᵗʰ **T83.420** **Displacement of** implanted penile ᴴᶜᶜ ♂
prosthesis
Displacement of penile prosthesis cylinder
Displacement of penile prosthesis pump
Displacement of penile prosthesis reservoir

[1] ✓7ᵗʰ **T83.421** **Displacement of** implanted testicular ᴴᶜᶜ
prosthesis

[1] ✓7ᵗʰ **T83.428** **Displacement of other prosthetic** ᴴᶜᶜ
devices, implants and grafts of
genital tract

✓6ᵗʰ **T83.49** **Other mechanical complication of other prosthetic**
devices, implants and grafts of genital tract
Leakage of other prosthetic devices, implants and
grafts of genital tract
Obstruction, mechanical of other prosthetic devices,
implants and grafts of genital tract
Perforation of other prosthetic devices, implants and
grafts of genital tract
Protrusion of other prosthetic devices, implants and
grafts of genital tract

[1] ✓7ᵗʰ **T83.490** **Other mechanical complication of** ᴴᶜᶜ ♂
implanted penile prosthesis
Other mechanical complication of penile
prosthesis cylinder
Other mechanical complication of penile
prosthesis pump
Other mechanical complication of penile
prosthesis reservoir

[1] ✓7ᵗʰ **T83.491** **Other mechanical complication of** ᴴᶜᶜ
implanted testicular prosthesis

[1] ✓7ᵗʰ **T83.498** **Other mechanical complication of** ᴴᶜᶜ
other prosthetic devices, implants
and grafts of genital tract

✓5ᵗʰ **T83.5** **Infection and inflammatory reaction due to prosthetic device,**
implant and graft in urinary system
Use additional code to identify infection

✓6ᵗʰ **T83.51** **Infection and inflammatory reaction due to** urinary
catheter
EXCLUDES 2 complications of stoma of urinary tract
(N99.5-)

[1] ✓7ᵗʰ **T83.510** **Infection and inflammatory reaction** ᴴᶜᶜ
due to cystostomy catheter

[1] ✓7ᵗʰ **T83.511** **Infection and inflammatory reaction** ᴴᶜᶜ
due to indwelling urethral catheter

[1] ✓7ᵗʰ **T83.512** **Infection and inflammatory reaction** ᴴᶜᶜ
due to nephrostomy catheter

[1] ✓7ᵗʰ **T83.518** **Infection and inflammatory reaction** ᴴᶜᶜ
due to other urinary catheter
Infection and inflammatory reaction due to
Hopkins catheter
Infection and inflammatory reaction due to
ileostomy catheter
Infection and inflammatory reaction due to
urostomy catheter

✓6ᵗʰ **T83.59** **Infection and inflammatory reaction due to**
prosthetic device, implant and graft **in urinary**
system

[1] ✓7ᵗʰ **T83.590** **Infection and inflammatory reaction** ᴴᶜᶜ
due to implanted urinary
neurostimulation device
EXCLUDES 2 infection and inflammatory
reaction due to electrode
lead of sacral nerve
neurostimulator (T85.732)
infection and inflammatory reaction due to pulse generator
or receiver of sacral nerve
neurostimulator (T85.734)

[1] ✓7ᵗʰ **T83.591** **Infection and inflammatory reaction** ᴴᶜᶜ
due to implanted urinary sphincter

[1] ✓7ᵗʰ **T83.592** **Infection and inflammatory reaction** ᴴᶜᶜ
due to indwelling ureteral stent

[1] ✓7ᵗʰ **T83.593** **Infection and inflammatory reaction** ᴴᶜᶜ
due to other urinary stents
Infection and inflammatory reaction due to
ileal conduit stents
Infection and inflammatory reaction due to
nephroureteral stent

[1] ✓7ᵗʰ **T83.598** **Infection and inflammatory reaction** ᴴᶜᶜ
due to other prosthetic device, implant
and graft in urinary system

✓5ᵗʰ **T83.6** **Infection and inflammatory reaction due to prosthetic device,**
implant and graft in genital tract
Use additional code to identify infection

[1] ✓x7ᵗʰ **T83.61** **Infection and inflammatory reaction due to** ᴴᶜᶜ
implanted penile prosthesis
Infection and inflammatory reaction due to penile
prosthesis cylinder
Infection and inflammatory reaction due to penile
prosthesis pump
Infection and inflammatory reaction due to penile
prosthesis reservoir

[1] ✓x7ᵗʰ **T83.62** **Infection and inflammatory reaction due to** ᴴᶜᶜ
implanted testicular prosthesis

[1] ✓x7ᵗʰ **T83.69** **Infection and inflammatory reaction due to** ᴴᶜᶜ
other prosthetic device, implant and graft in
genital tract

✓5ᵗʰ **T83.7** **Complications due to** implanted mesh and other prosthetic
materials

✓6ᵗʰ **T83.71** **Erosion of implanted mesh and other prosthetic**
materials to surrounding organ or tissue

[1] ✓7ᵗʰ **T83.711** **Erosion of implanted** vaginal mesh ᴴᶜᶜ ♀
to surrounding organ or tissue
Erosion of implanted vaginal mesh into
pelvic floor muscles

[1] ✓7ᵗʰ **T83.712** **Erosion of implanted** urethral mesh ᴴᶜᶜ
to surrounding organ or tissue
Erosion of implanted female urethral sling
Erosion of implanted male urethral sling
Erosion of implanted urethral mesh into
pelvic floor muscles

[1] ✓7ᵗʰ **T83.713** **Erosion of implanted** urethral bulking ᴴᶜᶜ
agent **to surrounding organ or tissue**

[1] ✓7ᵗʰ **T83.714** **Erosion of implanted** ureteral bulking ᴴᶜᶜ
agent **to surrounding organ or tissue**

[1] ✓7ᵗʰ **T83.718** **Erosion of other implanted mesh to** ᴴᶜᶜ
organ or tissue

[1] ✓7ᵗʰ **T83.719** **Erosion of other prosthetic materials** ᴴᶜᶜ
to surrounding organ or tissue

✓6ᵗʰ **T83.72** **Exposure of implanted mesh and other prosthetic**
materials into surrounding organ or tissue
Extrusion of implanted mesh

[1] ✓7ᵗʰ **T83.721** **Exposure of implanted** vaginal ᴴᶜᶜ ♀
mesh into vagina
Exposure of implanted vaginal mesh
through vaginal wall

[1] ✓7ᵗʰ **T83.722** **Exposure of implanted** urethral ᴴᶜᶜ
mesh into urethra
Exposure of implanted female urethral
sling
Exposure of implanted male urethral sling
Exposure of implanted urethral mesh
through urethral wall

[1] ✓7ᵗʰ **T83.723** **Exposure of implanted** urethral ᴴᶜᶜ
bulking agent **into** urethra

[1] ✓7ᵗʰ **T83.724** **Exposure of implanted** ureteral ᴴᶜᶜ
bulking agent **into** ureter

[1] ✓7ᵗʰ **T83.728** **Exposure of other implanted mesh** ᴴᶜᶜ
into organ or tissue

[1] ✓7ᵗʰ **T83.729** **Exposure of other prosthetic** ᴴᶜᶜ
materials into organ or tissue

[1] ✓x7ᵗʰ **T83.79** **Other specified complications due to other** ᴴᶜᶜ
genitourinary prosthetic materials

✓5ᵗʰ **T83.8** **Other specified complications of** genitourinary prosthetic
devices, implants and grafts

[1] ✓x7ᵗʰ **T83.81** **Embolism due to genitourinary prosthetic** ᴴᶜᶜ
devices, implants and grafts

[1] ✓x7ᵗʰ **T83.82** **Fibrosis due to genitourinary prosthetic** ᴴᶜᶜ
devices, implants and grafts

---

[1] HCC with 7th character indicating initial encounter (A, B or C - specific to category).

✓ Additional Character Req   ✓x7ᵗʰ Placeholder Alert   Manifestation   ᴴᶜᶜ CMS-HCC Condition   ▽ Unspecified Code   ▶◀ Revised Text   ● New Code   ▲ Revised Code Title

ICD-10-CM 2018   **1103**

¹ √x7ᵗʰ **T83.83** **Hemorrhage** due to genitourinary prosthetic devices, implants and grafts   `HCC`

¹ √x7ᵗʰ **T83.84** **Pain** due to genitourinary prosthetic devices, implants and grafts   `HCC`

¹ √x7ᵗʰ **T83.85** **Stenosis** due to genitourinary prosthetic devices, implants and grafts   `HCC`

¹ √x7ᵗʰ **T83.86** **Thrombosis** due to genitourinary prosthetic devices, implants and grafts   `HCC`

¹ √x7ᵗʰ **T83.89** **Other specified complication** of genitourinary prosthetic devices, implants and grafts   `HCC`

¹ √x7ᵗʰ **T83.9** **Unspecified complication** of genitourinary prosthetic device, implant and graft   `HCC` ▽

√4ᵗʰ **T84** **Complications of internal orthopedic prosthetic devices, implants and grafts**

> **EXCLUDES 2** *failure and rejection of transplanted organs and tissues (T86.-)*
> *fracture of bone following insertion of orthopedic implant, joint prosthesis or bone plate (M96.6)*

> The appropriate 7th character is to be added to each code from category T84.
> A   initial encounter
> D   subsequent encounter
> S   sequela

√5ᵗʰ **T84.0** **Mechanical complication** of **internal joint prosthesis**

√6ᵗʰ **T84.01** **Broken** internal joint prosthesis
Breakage (fracture) of prosthetic joint
Broken prosthetic joint implant
> **EXCLUDES 1** *periprosthetic joint implant fracture ▶(M97-)◀*

¹ √7ᵗʰ **T84.010** **Broken** internal **right hip** prosthesis   `HCC`

¹ √7ᵗʰ **T84.011** **Broken** internal **left hip** prosthesis   `HCC`

¹ √7ᵗʰ **T84.012** **Broken** internal **right knee** prosthesis   `HCC`

¹ √7ᵗʰ **T84.013** **Broken** internal **left knee** prosthesis   `HCC`

¹ √7ᵗʰ **T84.018** **Broken** internal joint prosthesis, other site   `HCC`
> Use additional code to identify the joint (Z96.6-)

¹ √7ᵗʰ **T84.019** **Broken** internal joint prosthesis, unspecified site   `HCC` ▽

√6ᵗʰ **T84.02** **Dislocation** of internal joint prosthesis
Instability of internal joint prosthesis
Subluxation of internal joint prosthesis

¹ √7ᵗʰ **T84.020** **Dislocation** of internal **right hip** prosthesis   `HCC`

¹ √7ᵗʰ **T84.021** **Dislocation** of internal **left hip** prosthesis   `HCC`

¹ √7ᵗʰ **T84.022** **Instability** of internal **right knee** prosthesis   `HCC`

¹ √7ᵗʰ **T84.023** **Instability** of internal **left knee** prosthesis   `HCC`

¹ √7ᵗʰ **T84.028** **Dislocation** of other internal joint prosthesis   `HCC`
> Use additional code to identify the joint (Z96.6-)

¹ √7ᵗʰ **T84.029** **Dislocation** of unspecified internal joint prosthesis   `HCC` ▽

√6ᵗʰ **T84.03** **Mechanical loosening** of internal prosthetic joint
Aseptic loosening of prosthetic joint

¹ √7ᵗʰ **T84.030** **Mechanical loosening** of internal **right hip** prosthetic joint   `HCC`

¹ √7ᵗʰ **T84.031** **Mechanical loosening** of internal **left hip** prosthetic joint   `HCC`

¹ √7ᵗʰ **T84.032** **Mechanical loosening** of internal **right knee** prosthetic joint   `HCC`

¹ √7ᵗʰ **T84.033** **Mechanical loosening** of internal **left knee** prosthetic joint   `HCC`

¹ √7ᵗʰ **T84.038** **Mechanical loosening** of other internal prosthetic joint   `HCC`
> Use additional code to identify the joint (Z96.6-)

¹ √7ᵗʰ **T84.039** **Mechanical loosening** of unspecified internal prosthetic joint   `HCC` ▽

√6ᵗʰ **T84.05** **Periprosthetic osteolysis** of internal prosthetic joint
> Use additional code to identify major osseous defect, if applicable (M89.7-)

¹ √7ᵗʰ **T84.050** **Periprosthetic osteolysis** of internal prosthetic **right hip joint**   `HCC`

¹ √7ᵗʰ **T84.051** **Periprosthetic osteolysis** of internal prosthetic **left hip joint**   `HCC`

¹ √7ᵗʰ **T84.052** **Periprosthetic osteolysis** of internal prosthetic **right knee joint**   `HCC`

¹ √7ᵗʰ **T84.053** **Periprosthetic osteolysis** of internal prosthetic **left knee joint**   `HCC`

¹ √7ᵗʰ **T84.058** **Periprosthetic osteolysis** of other internal prosthetic joint   `HCC`
> Use additional code to identify the joint (Z96.6-)

¹ √7ᵗʰ **T84.059** **Periprosthetic osteolysis** of unspecified internal prosthetic joint   `HCC` ▽

√6ᵗʰ **T84.06** **Wear of articular bearing surface** of internal prosthetic joint

¹ √7ᵗʰ **T84.060** **Wear of articular bearing surface** of internal prosthetic **right hip joint**   `HCC`

¹ √7ᵗʰ **T84.061** **Wear of articular bearing surface** of internal prosthetic **left hip joint**   `HCC`

¹ √7ᵗʰ **T84.062** **Wear of articular bearing surface** of internal prosthetic **right knee joint**   `HCC`

¹ √7ᵗʰ **T84.063** **Wear of articular bearing surface** of internal prosthetic **left knee joint**   `HCC`

¹ √7ᵗʰ **T84.068** **Wear of articular bearing surface** of other internal prosthetic joint   `HCC`
> Use additional code to identify the joint (Z96.6-)

¹ √7ᵗʰ **T84.069** **Wear of articular bearing surface** of unspecified internal prosthetic joint   `HCC` ▽

√6ᵗʰ **T84.09** **Other mechanical complication** of internal joint prosthesis
Prosthetic joint implant failure NOS

¹ √7ᵗʰ **T84.090** **Other mechanical complication** of internal **right hip** prosthesis   `HCC`

¹ √7ᵗʰ **T84.091** **Other mechanical complication** of internal **left hip** prosthesis   `HCC`

¹ √7ᵗʰ **T84.092** **Other mechanical complication** of internal **right knee** prosthesis   `HCC`

¹ √7ᵗʰ **T84.093** **Other mechanical complication** of internal **left knee** prosthesis   `HCC`

¹ √7ᵗʰ **T84.098** **Other mechanical complication** of other internal joint prosthesis   `HCC`
> Use additional code to identify the joint (Z96.6-)

¹ √7ᵗʰ **T84.099** **Other mechanical complication** of unspecified internal joint prosthesis   `HCC` ▽

√5ᵗʰ **T84.1** **Mechanical complication** of **internal fixation device** of bones of limb

> **EXCLUDES 2** *mechanical complication of internal fixation device of bones of feet (T84.2-)*
> *mechanical complication of internal fixation device of bones of fingers (T84.2-)*
> *mechanical complication of internal fixation device of bones of hands (T84.2-)*
> *mechanical complication of internal fixation device of bones of toes (T84.2-)*

√6ᵗʰ **T84.11** **Breakdown (mechanical)** of internal fixation device of bones of limb

¹ √7ᵗʰ **T84.110** **Breakdown (mechanical)** of internal fixation device of **right humerus**   `HCC`

¹ √7ᵗʰ **T84.111** **Breakdown (mechanical)** of internal fixation device of **left humerus**   `HCC`

¹ √7ᵗʰ **T84.112** **Breakdown (mechanical)** of internal fixation device of bone of **right forearm**   `HCC`

¹ √7ᵗʰ **T84.113** **Breakdown (mechanical)** of internal fixation device of bone of **left forearm**   `HCC`

¹ √7ᵗʰ **T84.114** **Breakdown (mechanical)** of internal fixation device of **right femur**   `HCC`

¹ √7ᵗʰ **T84.115** **Breakdown (mechanical)** of internal fixation device of **left femur**   `HCC`

¹ √7ᵗʰ **T84.116** **Breakdown (mechanical)** of internal fixation device of bone of **right lower leg**   `HCC`

---

¹ HCC with 7th character indicating initial encounter (A, B or C - specific to category).

EXCLUDES 1 Not coded here   **EXCLUDES 2** Not included here   ℕ Newborn Age: 0   ℙ Pediatric Age: 0-17   Ⓜ Maternity Age: 12-55   Ⓐ Adult Age: 15-124

1104   ICD-10-CM 2018

1 ✓7ᵗʰ **T84.117 Breakdown (mechanical) of internal** HCC
fixation device of bone of left lower leg

1 ✓7ᵗʰ **T84.119 Breakdown (mechanical) of** HCC ▽
internal fixation device of
unspecified bone of limb

✓6ᵗʰ **T84.12** Displacement **of internal fixation device of bones of**
limb
Malposition of internal fixation device of bones of limb

1 ✓7ᵗʰ **T84.120 Displacement of internal fixation** HCC
device of right humerus

1 ✓7ᵗʰ **T84.121 Displacement of internal fixation** HCC
device of left humerus

1 ✓7ᵗʰ **T84.122 Displacement of internal fixation** HCC
device of bone of right forearm

1 ✓7ᵗʰ **T84.123 Displacement of internal fixation** HCC
device of bone of left forearm

1 ✓7ᵗʰ **T84.124 Displacement of internal fixation** HCC
device of right femur

1 ✓7ᵗʰ **T84.125 Displacement of internal fixation** HCC
device of left femur

1 ✓7ᵗʰ **T84.126 Displacement of internal fixation** HCC
device of bone of right lower leg

1 ✓7ᵗʰ **T84.127 Displacement of internal fixation** HCC
device of bone of left lower leg

1 ✓7ᵗʰ **T84.129 Displacement of internal fixation** HCC ▽
device of unspecified bone of limb

✓6ᵗʰ **T84.19 Other mechanical complication of internal fixation**
device of bones of limb
Obstruction (mechanical) of internal fixation device of
bones of limb
Perforation of internal fixation device of bones of limb
Protrusion of internal fixation device of bones of limb

1 ✓7ᵗʰ **T84.190 Other mechanical complication of** HCC
internal fixation device of right humerus

1 ✓7ᵗʰ **T84.191 Other mechanical complication of** HCC
internal fixation device of left humerus

1 ✓7ᵗʰ **T84.192 Other mechanical complication of** HCC
internal fixation device of bone of right
forearm

1 ✓7ᵗʰ **T84.193 Other mechanical complication of** HCC
internal fixation device of bone of left
forearm

1 ✓7ᵗʰ **T84.194 Other mechanical complication of** HCC
internal fixation device of right femur

1 ✓7ᵗʰ **T84.195 Other mechanical complication of** HCC
internal fixation device of left femur

1 ✓7ᵗʰ **T84.196 Other mechanical complication of** HCC
internal fixation device of bone of right
lower leg

1 ✓7ᵗʰ **T84.197 Other mechanical complication of** HCC
internal fixation device of bone of left
lower leg

1 ✓7ᵗʰ **T84.199 Other mechanical complication of** HCC ▽
internal fixation device of unspecified
bone of limb

✓5ᵗʰ **T84.2 Mechanical complication of** internal fixation device **of other**
bones

✓6ᵗʰ **T84.21** Breakdown **(mechanical) of internal fixation device**
of other bones

1 ✓7ᵗʰ **T84.210 Breakdown (mechanical) of internal** HCC
fixation device of bones of hand and
fingers

1 ✓7ᵗʰ **T84.213 Breakdown (mechanical) of internal** HCC
fixation device of bones of foot and toes

1 ✓7ᵗʰ **T84.216 Breakdown (mechanical) of internal** HCC
fixation device of vertebrae

1 ✓7ᵗʰ **T84.218 Breakdown (mechanical) of internal** HCC
fixation device of other bones

✓6ᵗʰ **T84.22** Displacement **of internal fixation device of other**
bones
Malposition of internal fixation device of other bones

1 ✓7ᵗʰ **T84.220 Displacement of internal fixation** HCC
device of bones of hand and fingers

1 ✓7ᵗʰ **T84.223 Displacement of internal fixation** HCC
device of bones of foot and toes

1 ✓7ᵗʰ **T84.226 Displacement of internal fixation** HCC
device of vertebrae

1 ✓7ᵗʰ **T84.228 Displacement of internal fixation** HCC
device of other bones

✓6ᵗʰ **T84.29 Other mechanical complication of internal fixation**
device of other bones
Obstruction (mechanical) of internal fixation device of
other bones
Perforation of internal fixation device of other bones
Protrusion of internal fixation device of other bones

1 ✓7ᵗʰ **T84.290 Other mechanical complication of** HCC
internal fixation device of bones of
hand and fingers

1 ✓7ᵗʰ **T84.293 Other mechanical complication of** HCC
internal fixation device of bones of
foot and toes

1 ✓7ᵗʰ **T84.296 Other mechanical complication of** HCC
internal fixation device of vertebrae

1 ✓7ᵗʰ **T84.298 Other mechanical complication of** HCC
internal fixation device of other bones

✓5ᵗʰ **T84.3 Mechanical complication of other bone devices, implants and**
grafts
EXCLUDES 2   other complications of bone graft (T86.83-)

✓6ᵗʰ **T84.31** Breakdown **(mechanical) of other bone devices,**
implants and grafts

1 ✓7ᵗʰ **T84.310 Breakdown (mechanical) of** HCC
electronic bone stimulator

1 ✓7ᵗʰ **T84.318 Breakdown (mechanical) of other** HCC
bone devices, implants and grafts

✓6ᵗʰ **T84.32** Displacement **of other bone devices, implants and**
grafts
Malposition of other bone devices, implants and grafts

1 ✓7ᵗʰ **T84.320 Displacement of** electronic bone HCC
stimulator

1 ✓7ᵗʰ **T84.328 Displacement of other bone devices,** HCC
implants and grafts
AHA: 2014, 4Q, 28

✓6ᵗʰ **T84.39 Other mechanical complication of other bone**
devices, implants and grafts
Obstruction (mechanical) of other bone devices,
implants and grafts
Perforation of other bone devices, implants and grafts
Protrusion of other bone devices, implants and grafts

1 ✓7ᵗʰ **T84.390 Other mechanical complication of** HCC
electronic bone stimulator

1 ✓7ᵗʰ **T84.398 Other mechanical complication of** HCC
other bone devices, implants and grafts

✓5ᵗʰ **T84.4 Mechanical complication of other internal orthopedic**
devices, implants and grafts

✓6ᵗʰ **T84.41** Breakdown **(mechanical) of other internal**
orthopedic devices, implants and grafts

1 ✓7ᵗʰ **T84.410 Breakdown (mechanical) of** muscle HCC
and tendon graft

1 ✓7ᵗʰ **T84.418 Breakdown (mechanical) of other** HCC
internal orthopedic devices, implants
and grafts

✓6ᵗʰ **T84.42** Displacement **of other internal orthopedic devices,**
implants and grafts
Malposition of other internal orthopedic devices,
implants and grafts

1 ✓7ᵗʰ **T84.420 Displacement of** muscle and tendon HCC
graft

1 ✓7ᵗʰ **T84.428 Displacement of other internal** HCC
orthopedic devices, implants and grafts

✓6ᵗʰ **T84.49 Other mechanical complication of other internal**
orthopedic devices, implants and grafts
Mechanical complication of other internal orthopedic
devices, implants and grafts NOS
Obstruction (mechanical) of other internal orthopedic
devices, implants and grafts
Perforation of other internal orthopedic devices,
implants and grafts
Protrusion of other internal orthopedic devices,
implants and grafts

1 ✓7ᵗʰ **T84.490 Other mechanical complication of** HCC
muscle and tendon graft

1 ✓7ᵗʰ **T84.498 Other mechanical complication of** HCC
other internal orthopedic devices,
implants and grafts

---

¹ HCC with 7th character indicating initial encounter (A, B or C - specific to category).

☑ Additional Character Req   ✓ₓ7ᵗʰ Placeholder Alert   Manifestation   HCC CMS-HCC Condition   ▽ Unspecified Code   ►◄ Revised Text   ● New Code   ▲ Revised Code Title

ICD-10-CM 2018   1105

✓5ᵗʰ **T84.5** **Infection and inflammatory reaction due to** internal joint prosthesis
     Use additional code to identify infection
     AHA: 2015, 1Q, 16

1 ✓x7ᵗʰ **T84.50** **Infection and inflammatory reaction due to** unspecified internal joint prosthesis   HCC ▽

1 ✓x7ᵗʰ **T84.51** **Infection and inflammatory reaction due to** internal right hip prosthesis   HCC

1 ✓x7ᵗʰ **T84.52** **Infection and inflammatory reaction due to** internal left hip prosthesis   HCC

1 ✓x7ᵗʰ **T84.53** **Infection and inflammatory reaction due to** internal right knee prosthesis   HCC

1 ✓x7ᵗʰ **T84.54** **Infection and inflammatory reaction due to** internal left knee prosthesis   HCC

1 ✓x7ᵗʰ **T84.59** **Infection and inflammatory reaction due to** other internal joint prosthesis   HCC

✓5ᵗʰ **T84.6** **Infection and inflammatory reaction due to** internal fixation device
     Use additional code to identify infection

1 ✓x7ᵗʰ **T84.60** **Infection and inflammatory reaction due to** internal fixation device of unspecified site   HCC ▽

✓6ᵗʰ **T84.61** **Infection and inflammatory reaction due to internal fixation device of** arm

1 ✓7ᵗʰ **T84.610** **Infection and inflammatory reaction due to internal fixation device of** right humerus   HCC

1 ✓7ᵗʰ **T84.611** **Infection and inflammatory reaction due to internal fixation device of** left humerus   HCC

1 ✓7ᵗʰ **T84.612** **Infection and inflammatory reaction due to internal fixation device of** right radius   HCC

1 ✓7ᵗʰ **T84.613** **Infection and inflammatory reaction due to internal fixation device of** left radius   HCC

1 ✓7ᵗʰ **T84.614** **Infection and inflammatory reaction due to internal fixation device of** right ulna   HCC

1 ✓7ᵗʰ **T84.615** **Infection and inflammatory reaction due to internal fixation device of** left ulna   HCC

1 ✓7ᵗʰ **T84.619** **Infection and inflammatory reaction due to internal fixation device of unspecified** bone **of arm**   HCC ▽

✓6ᵗʰ **T84.62** **Infection and inflammatory reaction due to internal fixation device of** leg

1 ✓7ᵗʰ **T84.620** **Infection and inflammatory reaction due to internal fixation device of** right femur   HCC

1 ✓7ᵗʰ **T84.621** **Infection and inflammatory reaction due to internal fixation device of** left femur   HCC

1 ✓7ᵗʰ **T84.622** **Infection and inflammatory reaction due to internal fixation device of** right tibia   HCC

1 ✓7ᵗʰ **T84.623** **Infection and inflammatory reaction due to internal fixation device of** left tibia   HCC

1 ✓7ᵗʰ **T84.624** **Infection and inflammatory reaction due to internal fixation device of** right fibula   HCC

1 ✓7ᵗʰ **T84.625** **Infection and inflammatory reaction due to internal fixation device of** left fibula   HCC

1 ✓7ᵗʰ **T84.629** **Infection and inflammatory reaction due to internal fixation device of unspecified** bone **of leg**   HCC ▽

1 ✓x7ᵗʰ **T84.63** **Infection and inflammatory reaction due to internal fixation device of** spine   HCC

1 ✓x7ᵗʰ **T84.69** **Infection and inflammatory reaction due to internal fixation device of other site**   HCC

1 ✓x7ᵗʰ **T84.7** **Infection and inflammatory reaction due to other internal orthopedic prosthetic devices, implants and grafts**   HCC
     Use additional code to identify infection

✓5ᵗʰ **T84.8** **Other specified complications of internal orthopedic prosthetic devices, implants and grafts**

1 ✓x7ᵗʰ **T84.81** **Embolism due to** internal orthopedic prosthetic devices, implants and grafts   HCC

1 ✓x7ᵗʰ **T84.82** **Fibrosis due to** internal orthopedic prosthetic devices, implants and grafts   HCC

1 ✓x7ᵗʰ **T84.83** **Hemorrhage due to** internal orthopedic prosthetic devices, implants and grafts   HCC

1 ✓x7ᵗʰ **T84.84** **Pain due to** internal orthopedic prosthetic devices, implants and grafts   HCC

1 ✓x7ᵗʰ **T84.85** **Stenosis due to** internal orthopedic prosthetic devices, implants and grafts   HCC

1 ✓x7ᵗʰ **T84.86** **Thrombosis due to** internal orthopedic prosthetic devices, implants and grafts   HCC

1 ✓x7ᵗʰ **T84.89** **Other specified complication of internal orthopedic prosthetic devices, implants and grafts**   HCC

1 ✓x7ᵗʰ **T84.9** **Unspecified complication of internal orthopedic prosthetic device, implant and graft**   HCC ▽

✓4ᵗʰ **T85** **Complications of other internal prosthetic devices, implants and grafts**

     EXCLUDES 2   failure and rejection of transplanted organs and tissue (T86.-)

The appropriate 7th character is to be added to each code from category T85.
A   initial encounter
D   subsequent encounter
S   sequela

✓5ᵗʰ **T85.0** **Mechanical complication of** ventricular intracranial (communicating) shunt

1 ✓x7ᵗʰ **T85.01** **Breakdown (mechanical) of ventricular intracranial (communicating) shunt**   HCC

1 ✓x7ᵗʰ **T85.02** **Displacement of ventricular intracranial (communicating) shunt**   HCC
     Malposition of ventricular intracranial (communicating) shunt

1 ✓x7ᵗʰ **T85.03** **Leakage of ventricular intracranial (communicating) shunt**   HCC

1 ✓x7ᵗʰ **T85.09** **Other mechanical complication of ventricular intracranial (communicating) shunt**   HCC
     Obstruction (mechanical) of ventricular intracranial (communicating) shunt
     Perforation of ventricular intracranial (communicating) shunt
     Protrusion of ventricular intracranial (communicating) shunt

✓5ᵗʰ **T85.1** **Mechanical complication of** implanted electronic stimulator of nervous system

✓6ᵗʰ **T85.11** **Breakdown (mechanical) of implanted electronic stimulator of nervous system**

1 ✓7ᵗʰ **T85.110** **Breakdown (mechanical) of implanted electronic neurostimulator** of brain electrode (lead)   HCC

1 ✓7ᵗʰ **T85.111** **Breakdown (mechanical) of implanted electronic neurostimulator** of peripheral nerve electrode (lead)   HCC
     Breakdown of electrode (lead) for cranial nerve neurostimulators
     Breakdown of electrode (lead) for gastric neurostimulator
     Breakdown of electrode (lead) for sacral nerve neurostimulator
     Breakdown of electrode (lead) for vagal nerve neurostimulators

1 ✓7ᵗʰ **T85.112** **Breakdown (mechanical) of implanted electronic neurostimulator** of spinal cord electrode (lead)   HCC

1 ✓7ᵗʰ **T85.113** **Breakdown (mechanical) of implanted electronic neurostimulator,** generator   HCC
     Breakdown (mechanical) of implanted electronic neurostimuator generator, brain, peripheral, gastric, spinal
     Breakdown (mechanical) of implanted electronic sacral neurostimulator, pulse generator or receiver

---

1   HCC with 7th character indicating initial encounter (A, B or C - specific to category).

EXCLUDES 1 Not coded here   **EXCLUDES 2** Not included here   N Newborn Age: 0   P Pediatric Age: 0-17   M Maternity Age: 12-55   A Adult Age: 15-124

1106   ICD-10-CM 2018

[1] ✓7ᵗʰ **T85.118** **Breakdown (mechanical) of other** HCC
implanted electronic stimulator of
nervous system

✓6ᵗʰ **T85.12** Displacement **of implanted electronic stimulator of**
nervous system
Malposition of implanted electronic stimulator of
nervous system

[1] ✓7ᵗʰ **T85.120** **Displacement of implanted** HCC
electronic neurostimulator
of brain electrode (lead)

[1] ✓7ᵗʰ **T85.121** **Displacement of implanted** HCC
electronic neurostimulator
of peripheral nerve electrode (lead)
Displacement of electrode (lead) for cranial
nerve neurostimulators
Displacement of electrode (lead) for gastric
neurostimulator
Displacement of electrode (lead) for sacral
nerve neurostimulator
Displacement of electrode (lead) for vagal
nerve neurostimulators

[1] ✓7ᵗʰ **T85.122** **Displacement of implanted** HCC
electronic neurostimulator
of spinal cord electrode (lead)

[1] ✓7ᵗʰ **T85.123** **Displacement of implanted electronic** HCC
neurostimulator, generator
Displacement of implanted electronic
neurostimulator generator, brain,
peripheral, gastric, spinal
Displacement of implanted electronic
sacral neurostimulator, pulse
generator or receiver

[1] ✓7ᵗʰ **T85.128** **Displacement of other implanted** HCC
electronic stimulator of nervous system

✓6ᵗʰ **T85.19** **Other mechanical complication of implanted**
electronic stimulator of nervous system
Leakage of implanted electronic stimulator of nervous
system
Obstruction (mechanical) of implanted electronic
stimulator of nervous system
Perforation of implanted electronic stimulator of
nervous system
Protrusion of implanted electronic stimulator of
nervous system

[1] ✓7ᵗʰ **T85.190** **Other mechanical complication of** HCC
implanted electronic neurostimulator
of brain electrode (lead)

[1] ✓7ᵗʰ **T85.191** **Other mechanical complication of** HCC
implanted electronic neurostimulator
of peripheral nerve electrode (lead)
Other mechanical complication of
electrode (lead) for cranial nerve
neurostimulators
Other mechanical complication of
electrode (lead) for gastric
neurostimulator
Other mechanical complication of
electrode (lead) for sacral nerve
neurostimulator
Other mechanical complication of
electrode (lead) for vagal nerve
neurostimulators

[1] ✓7ᵗʰ **T85.192** **Other mechanical complication of** HCC
implanted electronic neurostimulator
of spinal cord electrode (lead)

[1] ✓7ᵗʰ **T85.193** **Other mechanical complication of** HCC
implanted electronic neurostimulator,
generator
Other mechanical complication of
implanted electronic neurostimulator
generator, brain, peripheral, gastric,
spinal
Other mechanical complication of
implanted electronic sacral
neurostimulator, pulse generator or
receiver

[1] ✓7ᵗʰ **T85.199** **Other mechanical complication of** HCC
other implanted electronic stimulator
of nervous system

✓5ᵗʰ **T85.2** **Mechanical complication of** intraocular lens

✓x7ᵗʰ **T85.21** Breakdown **(mechanical) of intraocular lens**

✓x7ᵗʰ **T85.22** **Displacement** of intraocular lens
Malposition of intraocular lens

✓x7ᵗʰ **T85.29** **Other mechanical complication of intraocular lens**
Obstruction (mechanical) of intraocular lens
Perforation of intraocular lens
Protrusion of intraocular lens

✓5ᵗʰ **T85.3** **Mechanical complication of other ocular prosthetic devices,**
implants and grafts
EXCLUDES 2   *other complications of corneal graft (T86.84-)*

✓6ᵗʰ **T85.31** **Breakdown (mechanical) of other ocular prosthetic**
devices, implants and grafts

✓7ᵗʰ **T85.310** **Breakdown (mechanical) of prosthetic**
orbit of right eye

✓7ᵗʰ **T85.311** **Breakdown (mechanical) of prosthetic**
orbit of left eye

✓7ᵗʰ **T85.318** **Breakdown (mechanical) of other ocular**
prosthetic devices, implants and grafts

✓6ᵗʰ **T85.32** **Displacement of other ocular prosthetic devices,**
implants and grafts
Malposition of other ocular prosthetic devices,
implants and grafts

✓7ᵗʰ **T85.320** **Displacement of prosthetic orbit of right**
eye

✓7ᵗʰ **T85.321** **Displacement of prosthetic orbit of left**
eye

✓7ᵗʰ **T85.328** **Displacement of other ocular prosthetic**
devices, implants and grafts

✓6ᵗʰ **T85.39** **Other mechanical complication of other ocular**
prosthetic devices, implants and grafts
Obstruction (mechanical) of other ocular prosthetic
devices, implants and grafts
Perforation of other ocular prosthetic devices,
implants and grafts
Protrusion of other ocular prosthetic devices, implants
and grafts

✓7ᵗʰ **T85.390** **Other mechanical complication of**
prosthetic orbit of right eye

✓7ᵗʰ **T85.391** **Other mechanical complication of**
prosthetic orbit of left eye

✓7ᵗʰ **T85.398** **Other mechanical complication of other**
ocular prosthetic devices, implants and
grafts

✓5ᵗʰ **T85.4** **Mechanical complication of** breast prosthesis and implant

✓x7ᵗʰ **T85.41** Breakdown **(mechanical) of breast prosthesis and**
implant

✓x7ᵗʰ **T85.42** Displacement **of breast prosthesis and implant**
Malposition of breast prosthesis and implant

✓x7ᵗʰ **T85.43** Leakage **of breast prosthesis and implant**

✓x7ᵗʰ **T85.44** Capsular contracture **of breast implant**

✓x7ᵗʰ **T85.49** **Other mechanical complication of breast prosthesis**
and implant
Obstruction (mechanical) of breast prosthesis and
implant
Perforation of breast prosthesis and implant
Protrusion of breast prosthesis and implant

✓5ᵗʰ **T85.5** **Mechanical complication of** gastrointestinal prosthetic
devices, implants and grafts

✓6ᵗʰ **T85.51** Breakdown **(mechanical) of gastrointestinal**
prosthetic devices, implants and grafts

✓7ᵗʰ **T85.510** **Breakdown (mechanical) of** bile duct
prosthesis

✓7ᵗʰ **T85.511** **Breakdown (mechanical) of** esophageal
anti-reflux **device**

✓7ᵗʰ **T85.518** **Breakdown (mechanical) of other**
gastrointestinal prosthetic devices,
implants and grafts

✓6ᵗʰ **T85.52** Displacement **of gastrointestinal prosthetic devices,**
implants and grafts
Malposition of gastrointestinal prosthetic devices,
implants and grafts

✓7ᵗʰ **T85.520** **Displacement of** bile duct **prosthesis**

✓7ᵗʰ **T85.521** **Displacement of** esophageal anti-reflux
device

✓7ᵗʰ **T85.528** **Displacement of other gastrointestinal**
prosthetic devices, implants and grafts

---

[1]   HCC with 7th character indicating initial encounter (A, B or C - specific to category).

✓ Additional Character Req   ✓x7ᵗʰ Placeholder Alert   Manifestation   HCC CMS-HCC Condition   ▽ Unspecified Code   ▶◀ Revised Text   ● New Code   ▲ Revised Code Title

√6ᵗʰ **T85.59** **Other mechanical complication of gastrointestinal prosthetic devices, implants and grafts**
     Obstruction, mechanical of gastrointestinal prosthetic devices, implants and grafts
     Perforation of gastrointestinal prosthetic devices, implants and grafts
     Protrusion of gastrointestinal prosthetic devices, implants and grafts

√7ᵗʰ **T85.590** **Other mechanical complication of bile duct prosthesis**

√7ᵗʰ **T85.591** **Other mechanical complication of esophageal anti-reflux device**

√7ᵗʰ **T85.598** **Other mechanical complication of other gastrointestinal prosthetic devices, implants and grafts**

√5ᵗʰ **T85.6** **Mechanical complication of other specified internal and external prosthetic devices, implants and grafts**

√6ᵗʰ **T85.61** **Breakdown (mechanical) of other specified internal prosthetic devices, implants and grafts**

√7ᵗʰ **T85.610** **Breakdown (mechanical) of cranial or spinal infusion catheter**
     Breakdown (mechanical) of epidural infusion catheter
     Breakdown (mechanical) of intrathecal infusion catheter
     Breakdown (mechanical) of subarachnoid infusion catheter
     Breakdown (mechanical) of subdural infusion catheter

√7ᵗʰ **T85.611** **Breakdown (mechanical) of intraperitoneal dialysis catheter** `HCC`
     EXCLUDES 1   *mechanical complication of vascular dialysis catheter (T82.4-)*

√7ᵗʰ **T85.612** **Breakdown (mechanical) of permanent sutures**
     EXCLUDES 1   *mechanical complication of permanent (wire) suture used in bone repair (T84.1-T84.2)*

√7ᵗʰ **T85.613** **Breakdown (mechanical) of artificial skin graft and decellularized allodermis**
     Failure of artificial skin graft and decellularized allodermis
     Non-adherence of artificial skin graft and decellularized allodermis
     Poor incorporation of artificial skin graft and decellularized allodermis
     Shearing of artificial skin graft and decellularized allodermis

√7ᵗʰ **T85.614** **Breakdown (mechanical) of insulin pump**

1 √7ᵗʰ **T85.615** **Breakdown (mechanical) of other nervous system device, implant or graft** `HCC`
     Breakdown (mechanical) of intrathecal infusion pump

√7ᵗʰ **T85.618** **Breakdown (mechanical) of other specified internal prosthetic devices, implants and grafts**

√6ᵗʰ **T85.62** **Displacement of other specified internal prosthetic devices, implants and grafts**
     Malposition of other specified internal prosthetic devices, implants and grafts

√7ᵗʰ **T85.620** **Displacement of cranial or spinal infusion catheter**
     Displacement of epidural infusion catheter
     Displacement of intrathecal infusion catheter
     Displacement of subarachnoid infusion catheter
     Displacement of subdural infusion catheter

√7ᵗʰ **T85.621** **Displacement of intraperitoneal dialysis catheter** `HCC`
     EXCLUDES 1   *mechanical complication of vascular dialysis catheter (T82.4-)*

√7ᵗʰ **T85.622** **Displacement of permanent sutures**
     EXCLUDES 1   *mechanical complication of permanent (wire) suture used in bone repair (T84.1-T84.2)*

√7ᵗʰ **T85.623** **Displacement of artificial skin graft and decellularized allodermis**
     Dislodgement of artificial skin graft and decellularized allodermis
     ~~Displacement of artificial skin graft and decellularized allodermis~~

√7ᵗʰ **T85.624** **Displacement of insulin pump**

1 √7ᵗʰ **T85.625** **Displacement of other nervous system device, implant or graft** `HCC`
     Displacement of intrathecal infusion pump

√7ᵗʰ **T85.628** **Displacement of other specified internal prosthetic devices, implants and grafts**

√6ᵗʰ **T85.63** **Leakage of other specified internal prosthetic devices, implants and grafts**

√7ᵗʰ **T85.630** **Leakage of cranial or spinal infusion catheter**
     Leakage of epidural infusion catheter
     Leakage of intrathecal infusion catheter
     Leakage of subdural infusion catheter
     Leakage of subarachnoid infusion catheter

√7ᵗʰ **T85.631** **Leakage of intraperitoneal dialysis catheter** `HCC`
     EXCLUDES 1   *mechanical complication of vascular dialysis catheter (T82.4)*

√7ᵗʰ **T85.633** **Leakage of insulin pump**

1 √7ᵗʰ **T85.635** **Leakage of other nervous system device, implant or graft** `HCC`
     Leakage of intrathecal infusion pump

√7ᵗʰ **T85.638** **Leakage of other specified internal prosthetic devices, implants and grafts**

√6ᵗʰ **T85.69** **Other mechanical complication of other specified internal prosthetic devices, implants and grafts**
     Obstruction, mechanical of other specified internal prosthetic devices, implants and grafts
     Perforation of other specified internal prosthetic devices, implants and grafts
     Protrusion of other specified internal prosthetic devices, implants and grafts

√7ᵗʰ **T85.690** **Other mechanical complication of cranial or spinal infusion catheter**
     Other mechanical complication of epidural infusion catheter
     Other mechanical complication of intrathecal infusion catheter
     Other mechanical complication of subarachnoid infusion catheter
     Other mechanical complication of subdural infusion catheter

√7ᵗʰ **T85.691** **Other mechanical complication of intraperitoneal dialysis catheter** `HCC`
     EXCLUDES 1   *mechanical complication of vascular dialysis catheter (T82.4)*

√7ᵗʰ **T85.692** **Other mechanical complication of permanent sutures**
     EXCLUDES 1   *mechanical complication of permanent (wire) suture used in bone repair (T84.1-T84.2)*

√7ᵗʰ **T85.693** **Other mechanical complication of artificial skin graft and decellularized allodermis**

√7ᵗʰ **T85.694** **Other mechanical complication of insulin pump**

1 √7ᵗʰ **T85.695** **Other mechanical complication of other nervous system device, implant or graft** `HCC`
     Other mechanical complication of intrathecal infusion pump

√7ᵗʰ **T85.698** **Other mechanical complication of other specified internal prosthetic devices, implants and grafts**
     Mechanical complication of nonabsorbable surgical material NOS

---

1   HCC with 7th character indicating initial encounter (A, B or C - specific to category).

EXCLUDES 1 Not coded here   *EXCLUDES 2* Not included here   N Newborn Age: 0   P Pediatric Age: 0-17   M Maternity Age: 12-55   A Adult Age: 15-124

1108   ICD-10-CM 2018

√6ᵗʰ **T85.7** Infection and inflammatory reaction due to other internal prosthetic devices, implants and grafts

     Use additional code to identify infection

   √x7ᵗʰ **T85.71** Infection and inflammatory reaction due to ~~peritoneal dialysis catheter~~ HCC

   ¹ √x7ᵗʰ **T85.72** Infection and inflammatory reaction due to insulin pump HCC

   √6ᵗʰ **T85.73** Infection and inflammatory reaction due to nervous system devices, implants and graft

     ¹ √7ᵗʰ **T85.730** Infection and inflammatory reaction due to ventricular intracranial (communicating) shunt HCC

     ¹ √7ᵗʰ **T85.731** Infection and inflammatory reaction due to implanted electronic neurostimulator of brain, electrode (lead) HCC

     ¹ √7ᵗʰ **T85.732** Infection and inflammatory reaction due to implanted electronic neurostimulator of peripheral nerve, electrode (lead) HCC

       Infection and inflammatory reaction due to electrode (lead) for cranial nerve neurostimulators

       Infection and inflammatory reaction due to electrode (lead) for gastric neurostimulator

       Infection and inflammatory reaction due to electrode (lead) for sacral nerve neurostimulator

       Infection and inflammatory reaction due to electrode (lead) for vagal nerve neurostimulators

     ¹ √7ᵗʰ **T85.733** Infection and inflammatory reaction due to implanted electronic neurostimulator of spinal cord, electrode (lead) HCC

     ¹ √7ᵗʰ **T85.734** Infection and inflammatory reaction due to implanted electronic neurostimulator, generator HCC

       Generator pocket infection

     ¹ √7ᵗʰ **T85.735** Infection and inflammatory reaction due to cranial or spinal infusion catheter HCC

       Infection and inflammatory reaction due to epidural catheter

       Infection and inflammatory reaction due to intrathecal infusion catheter

       Infection and inflammatory reaction due to subarachnoid catheter

       Infection and inflammatory reaction due to subdural catheter

     ¹ √7ᵗʰ **T85.738** Infection and inflammatory reaction due to other nervous system device, implant or graft HCC

       Infection and inflammatory reaction due to intrathecal infusion pump

   ¹ √x7ᵗʰ **T85.79** Infection and inflammatory reaction due to other internal prosthetic devices, implants and grafts HCC

√5ᵗʰ **T85.8** Other specified complications of internal prosthetic devices, implants and grafts, not elsewhere classified

   √6ᵗʰ **T85.81** Embolism due to internal prosthetic devices, implants and grafts, not elsewhere classified

     ¹ √7ᵗʰ **T85.810** Embolism due to nervous system prosthetic devices, implants and grafts HCC

     √7ᵗʰ **T85.818** Embolism due to other internal prosthetic devices, implants and grafts

   √6ᵗʰ **T85.82** Fibrosis due to internal prosthetic devices, implants and grafts, not elsewhere classified

     ¹ √7ᵗʰ **T85.820** Fibrosis due to nervous system prosthetic devices, implants and grafts HCC

     √7ᵗʰ **T85.828** Fibrosis due to other internal prosthetic devices, implants and grafts

   √6ᵗʰ **T85.83** Hemorrhage due to internal prosthetic devices, implants and grafts, not elsewhere classified

     ¹ √7ᵗʰ **T85.830** Hemorrhage due to nervous system prosthetic devices, implants and grafts HCC

     √7ᵗʰ **T85.838** Hemorrhage due to other internal prosthetic devices, implants and grafts

√6ᵗʰ **T85.84** Pain due to internal prosthetic devices, implants and grafts, not elsewhere classified

   ¹ √7ᵗʰ **T85.840** Pain due to nervous system prosthetic devices, implants and grafts HCC

   ~~√7ᵗʰ T85.848 Pain due to other internal prosthetic devices, implants and grafts~~

√6ᵗʰ **T85.85** Stenosis due to internal prosthetic devices, implants and grafts, not elsewhere classified

   ¹ √7ᵗʰ **T85.850** Stenosis due to nervous system prosthetic devices, implants and grafts HCC

   √7ᵗʰ **T85.858** Stenosis due to other internal prosthetic devices, implants and grafts

√6ᵗʰ **T85.86** Thrombosis due to internal prosthetic devices, implants and grafts, not elsewhere classified

   ¹ √7ᵗʰ **T85.860** Thrombosis due to nervous system prosthetic devices, implants and grafts HCC

   √7ᵗʰ **T85.868** Thrombosis due to other internal prosthetic devices, implants and grafts

√6ᵗʰ **T85.89** Other specified complication of internal prosthetic devices, implants and grafts, not elsewhere classified

     Erosion or breakdown of subcutaneous device pocket

   ¹ √7ᵗʰ **T85.890** Other specified complication of nervous system prosthetic devices, implants and grafts HCC

   √7ᵗʰ **T85.898** Other specified complication of other internal prosthetic devices, implants and grafts

√x7ᵗʰ **T85.9** Unspecified complication of internal prosthetic device, implant and graft ▽

     Complication of internal prosthetic device, implant and graft NOS

√4ᵗʰ **T86** Complications of transplanted organs and tissue

     Use additional code to identify other transplant complications, such as:

       graft-versus-host disease (D89.81-)

       malignancy associated with organ transplant (C80.2)

       post-transplant lymphoproliferative disorders (PTLD) (D47.Z1)

√5ᵗʰ **T86.0** Complications of bone marrow transplant

   T86.00 Unspecified complication of bone marrow transplant HCC ▽

   T86.01 Bone marrow transplant rejection HCC

   T86.02 Bone marrow transplant failure HCC

   T86.03 Bone marrow transplant infection HCC

   T86.09 Other complications of bone marrow transplant HCC

√5ᵗʰ **T86.1** Complications of kidney transplant

   T86.10 Unspecified complication of kidney transplant ▽

   T86.11 Kidney transplant rejection

   T86.12 Kidney transplant failure

     AHA: 2013, 1Q, 24

   T86.13 Kidney transplant infection

     Use additional code to specify infection

   T86.19 Other complication of kidney transplant

√5ᵗʰ **T86.2** Complications of heart transplant

   EXCLUDES 1 complication of:

       artificial heart device (T82.5)

       heart-lung transplant (T86.3)

   T86.20 Unspecified complication of heart transplant HCC ▽

   T86.21 Heart transplant rejection HCC

   T86.22 Heart transplant failure HCC

   T86.23 Heart transplant infection HCC

     Use additional code to specify infection

   √6ᵗʰ **T86.29** Other complications of heart transplant

     T86.290 Cardiac allograft vasculopathy HCC

       EXCLUDES 1 atherosclerosis of coronary arteries (I25.75-, I25.76-, I25.81-)

     T86.298 Other complications of heart transplant HCC

√5ᵗʰ **T86.3** Complications of heart-lung transplant

   T86.30 Unspecified complication of heart-lung transplant HCC ▽

   T86.31 Heart-lung transplant rejection HCC

   T86.32 Heart-lung transplant failure HCC

---

¹ HCC with 7th character indicating initial encounter (A, B or C - specific to category).

☑ Additional Character Req	√x7ᵗʰ Placeholder Alert	Manifestation	HCC CMS-HCC Condition	▽ Unspecified Code	►◄ Revised Text	● New Code	▲ Revised Code Title

T86.33   **Heart-lung transplant** infection   `HCC`
Use additional code to specify infection

T86.39   **Other complications of heart-lung transplant**   `HCC`

✓5ᵗʰ **T86.4**   **Complications of** liver **transplant**

   T86.40   **Unspecified complication of liver transplant**   `HCC` ▽

   T86.41   **Liver transplant** rejection   `HCC`

   T86.42   **Liver transplant** failure   `HCC`

   T86.43   **Liver transplant** infection   `HCC`
Use additional code to identify infection, such as:
cytomegalovirus (CMV) infection (B25.-)

   T86.49   **Other complications of liver transplant**   `HCC`

T86.5   **Complications of** stem cell **transplant**   `HCC`
Complications from stem cells from peripheral blood
Complications from stem cells from umbilical cord

✓5ᵗʰ **T86.8**   **Complications of other transplanted organs and tissues**

   ✓6ᵗʰ **T86.81**   **Complications of** lung **transplant**
     EXCLUDES 1   complication of heart-lung transplant (T86.3-)

     T86.810   **Lung transplant** rejection   `HCC`

     T86.811   **Lung transplant** failure   `HCC`

     T86.812   **Lung transplant** infection   `HCC`
Use additional code to specify infection

     T86.818   **Other complications of lung transplant**   `HCC`

     T86.819   **Unspecified complication of lung transplant**   `HCC` ▽

   ✓6ᵗʰ **T86.82**   **Complications of** skin graft (allograft) (autograft)
     EXCLUDES 2   complication of artificial skin graft (T85.693)

     T86.820   **Skin graft (allograft)** rejection

     T86.821   **Skin graft (allograft) (autograft)** failure

     T86.822   **Skin graft (allograft) (autograft)** infection
Use additional code to specify infection

     T86.828   **Other complications of skin graft (allograft) (autograft)**

     T86.829   **Unspecified complication of skin graft (allograft) (autograft)**   ▽

   ✓6ᵗʰ **T86.83**   **Complications of** bone graft
     EXCLUDES 2   mechanical complications of bone graft (T84.3-)

     T86.830   **Bone graft** rejection

     T86.831   **Bone graft** failure

     T86.832   **Bone graft** infection
Use additional code to specify infection

     T86.838   **Other complications of bone graft**

     T86.839   **Unspecified complication of bone graft**   ▽

   ✓6ᵗʰ **T86.84**   **Complications of** corneal **transplant**
     EXCLUDES 2   mechanical complications of corneal graft (T85.3-)

     T86.840   **Corneal transplant** rejection

     T86.841   **Corneal transplant** failure

     T86.842   **Corneal transplant** infection   `HCC`
Use additional code to specify infection

     T86.848   **Other complications of corneal transplant**

     T86.849   **Unspecified complication of corneal transplant**   ▽

   ✓6ᵗʰ **T86.85**   **Complication of** intestine **transplant**

     T86.850   **Intestine transplant** rejection   `HCC`

     T86.851   **Intestine transplant** failure   `HCC`

     T86.852   **Intestine transplant** infection   `HCC`
Use additional code to specify infection

     T86.858   **Other complications of intestine transplant**   `HCC`

     T86.859   **Unspecified complication of intestine transplant**   `HCC` ▽

   ✓6ᵗʰ **T86.89**   **Complications of other transplanted** tissue
Transplant failure or rejection of pancreas

     T86.890   **Other transplanted tissue** rejection

     T86.891   **Other transplanted tissue** failure

     T86.892   **Other transplanted tissue** infection
Use additional code to specify infection

     T86.898   **Other complications of other transplanted tissue**

     T86.899   **Unspecified complication of other transplanted tissue**   ▽

✓5ᵗʰ **T86.9**   **Complication of unspecified transplanted organ and tissue**

   T86.90   **Unspecified complication of unspecified transplanted organ and tissue**   ▽

   T86.91   **Unspecified transplanted organ and tissue rejection**   ▽

   T86.92   **Unspecified transplanted organ and tissue failure**   ▽

   T86.93   **Unspecified transplanted organ and tissue infection**   ▽
Use additional code to specify infection

   T86.99   **Other complications of unspecified transplanted organ and tissue**   ▽

✓4ᵗʰ **T87**   **Complications peculiar to reattachment and amputation**

   ✓5ᵗʰ **T87.0**   **Complications of reattached (part of)** upper extremity

     ✓6ᵗʰ **T87.0X**   **Complications of reattached (part of) upper extremity**

       T87.0X1   **Complications of reattached (part of)** right **upper extremity**   `HCC`

       T87.0X2   **Complications of reattached (part of)** left **upper extremity**   `HCC`

       T87.0X9   **Complications of reattached (part of) unspecified upper extremity**   `HCC` ▽

   ✓5ᵗʰ **T87.1**   **Complications of reattached (part of)** lower extremity

     ✓6ᵗʰ **T87.1X**   **Complications of reattached (part of) lower extremity**

       T87.1X1   **Complications of reattached (part of)** right **lower extremity**   `HCC`

       T87.1X2   **Complications of reattached (part of)** left **lower extremity**   `HCC`

       T87.1X9   **Complications of reattached (part of) unspecified lower extremity**   `HCC` ▽

   T87.2   **Complications of other reattached body part**   `HCC`

   ✓5ᵗʰ **T87.3**   **Neuroma of amputation stump**
DEF: Non-neoplastic tumor generated at the proximal end of severed, partially transected, or injured nerve following amputation.

     T87.30   **Neuroma of amputation stump, unspecified extremity**   `HCC` ▽

     T87.31   **Neuroma of amputation stump,** right upper **extremity**   `HCC`

     T87.32   **Neuroma of amputation stump,** left upper **extremity**   `HCC`

     T87.33   **Neuroma of amputation stump,** right lower **extremity**   `HCC`

     T87.34   **Neuroma of amputation stump,** left lower **extremity**   `HCC`

   ✓5ᵗʰ **T87.4**   **Infection of amputation stump**

     T87.40   **Infection of amputation stump, unspecified extremity**   `HCC` ▽

     T87.41   **Infection of amputation stump,** right upper **extremity**   `HCC`

     T87.42   **Infection of amputation stump,** left upper **extremity**   `HCC`

     T87.43   **Infection of amputation stump,** right lower **extremity**   `HCC`

     T87.44   **Infection of amputation stump,** left lower **extremity**   `HCC`

   ✓5ᵗʰ **T87.5**   **Necrosis of amputation stump**

     T87.50   **Necrosis of amputation stump, unspecified extremity**   `HCC` ▽

     T87.51   **Necrosis of amputation stump,** right upper **extremity**   `HCC`

     T87.52   **Necrosis of amputation stump,** left upper **extremity**   `HCC`

     T87.53   **Necrosis of amputation stump,** right lower **extremity**   `HCC`

     T87.54   **Necrosis of amputation stump,** left lower **extremity**   `HCC`

   ✓5ᵗʰ **T87.8**   **Other complications of amputation stump**

     T87.81   **Dehiscence of amputation stump**   `HCC`

EXCLUDES 1 Not coded here   *EXCLUDES 2* Not included here   Ⓝ Newborn Age: 0   Ⓟ Pediatric Age: 0-17   Ⓜ Maternity Age: 12-55   Ⓐ Adult Age: 15-124

1110   ICD-10-CM 2018

T87.89   **Other complications of amputation stump**   HCC
Amputation stump contracture
Amputation stump contracture of next proximal joint
Amputation stump flexion
Amputation stump edema
Amputation stump hematoma
    EXCLUDES 2   *phantom limb syndrome (G54.6-G54.7)*

T87.9   **Unspecified complications of amputation stump**   HCC ▽

T88   **Other complications of surgical and medical care, not elsewhere classified**
    EXCLUDES 2   *complication following infusion, transfusion and therapeutic injection (T80.-)*
complication following procedure NEC (T81.-)
complications of anesthesia in labor and delivery (O74.-)
complications of anesthesia in pregnancy (O29.-)
complications of anesthesia in puerperium (O89.-)
complications of devices, implants and grafts (T82-T85)
complications of obstetric surgery and procedure (O75.4)
dermatitis due to drugs and medicaments (L23.3, L24.4, L25.1, L27.0-L27.1)
poisoning and toxic effects of drugs and chemicals (T36-T65 with fifth or sixth character 1-4 or 6)
specified complications classified elsewhere

The appropriate 7th character is to be added to each code from category T88.
A   initial encounter
D   subsequent encounter
S   sequela

T88.0   **Infection following immunization**
Sepsis following immunization

T88.1   **Other complications following immunization, not elsewhere classified**
Generalized vaccinia
Rash following immunization
    EXCLUDES 1   *vaccinia not from vaccine (B08.011)*
    EXCLUDES 2   *anaphylactic shock due to serum (T80.5-)*
other serum reactions (T80.6-)
postimmunization arthropathy (M02.2)
postimmunization encephalitis (G04.02)
postimmunization fever (R50.83)

T88.2   **Shock due to anesthesia**
Use additional code for adverse effect, if applicable, to identify drug (T41.- with fifth or sixth character 5)
    EXCLUDES 1   *complications of anesthesia (in):*
labor and delivery (O74.-)
postprocedural shock NOS (T81.1-)
pregnancy (O29.-)
puerperium (O89.-)

T88.3   **Malignant hyperthermia due to anesthesia**
Use additional code for adverse effect, if applicable, to identify drug (T41.- with fifth or sixth character 5)

T88.4   **Failed or difficult intubation**

T88.5   **Other complications of anesthesia**
Use additional code for adverse effect, if applicable, to identify drug (T41.- with fifth or sixth character 5)

T88.51   **Hypothermia following anesthesia**

T88.52   **Failed moderate sedation during procedure**
Failed conscious sedation during procedure
    EXCLUDES 2   *personal history of failed moderate sedation (Z92.83)*

T88.53   **Unintended awareness under general anesthesia during procedure**
    EXCLUDES 2   *personal history of unintended awareness under general anesthesia (Z92.84)*

T88.59   **Other complications of anesthesia**

T88.6   **Anaphylactic reaction due to adverse effect of correct drug or medicament properly administered**
Anaphylactic shock due to adverse effect of correct drug or medicament properly administered
Anaphylactoid reaction NOS
Use additional code for adverse effect, if applicable, to identify drug (T36-T50 with fifth or sixth character 5)
    EXCLUDES 1   *anaphylactic reaction due to serum (T80.5-)*
anaphylactic shock or reaction due to adverse food reaction (T78.0-)

T88.7   **Unspecified adverse effect of drug or medicament**   ▽
Drug hypersensitivity NOS
Drug reaction NOS
Use additional code for adverse effect, if applicable, to identify drug (T36-T50 with fifth or sixth character 5)
    EXCLUDES 1   *specified adverse effects of drugs and medicaments (A00-R94 and T80-T88.6, T88.8)*

T88.8   **Other specified complications of surgical and medical care, not elsewhere classified**
Use additional code to identify the complication

T88.9   **Complication of surgical and medical care, unspecified**   ▽

Chapter 20. External Causes of Morbidity (V00–Y99)

Chapter Specific Guidelines with Coding Examples

The chapter specific guidelines from the ICD-10-CM Official Guidelines for Coding and Reporting have been provided below. Along with these guidelines are coding examples, contained in the shaded boxes, that have been developed to help illustrate the coding and/or sequencing guidance found in these guidelines.

The external causes of morbidity codes should never be sequenced as the first-listed or principal diagnosis.

External cause codes are intended to provide data for injury research and evaluation of injury prevention strategies. These codes capture how the injury or health condition happened (cause), the intent (unintentional or accidental; or intentional, such as suicide or assault), the place where the event occurred the activity of the patient at the time of the event, and the person's status (e.g., civilian, military).

There is no national requirement for mandatory ICD-10-CM external cause code reporting. Unless a provider is subject to a state-based external cause code reporting mandate or these codes are required by a particular payer, reporting of ICD-10-CM codes in Chapter 20, External Causes of Morbidity, is not required. In the absence of a mandatory reporting requirement, providers are encouraged to voluntarily report external cause codes, as they provide valuable data for injury research and evaluation of injury prevention strategies.

a. General external cause coding guidelines

1) Used with any code in the range of A00.0–T88.9, Z00–Z99

An external cause code may be used with any code in the range of A00.0–T88.9, Z00–Z99, classification that **represents** a health condition due to an external cause. Though they are most applicable to injuries, they are also valid for use with such things as infections or diseases due to an external source, and other health conditions, such as a heart attack that occurs during strenuous physical activity.

Actinic reticuloid due to tanning bed use	
L57.1	**Actinic reticuloid**
W89.1XXA	**Exposure to tanning bed, initial encounter**

Explanation: An external cause code may be used with any code in the range of A00.0–T88.9, Z00–Z99, classifications that describe health conditions due to an external cause. Code W89.1 Exposure to tanning bed requires a seventh character of A to report this initial encounter, with a placeholder X for the fifth and sixth characters.

2) External cause code used for length of treatment

Assign the external cause code, with the appropriate 7th character (initial encounter, subsequent encounter or sequela) for each encounter for which the injury or condition is being treated.

Most categories in chapter 20 have a 7th character requirement for each applicable code. Most categories in this chapter have three 7th character values: A, initial encounter, D, subsequent encounter and S, sequela. While the patient may be seen by a new or different provider over the course of treatment for an injury or condition, assignment of the 7th character for external cause should match the 7th character of the code assigned for the associated injury or condition for the encounter.

3) Use the full range of external cause codes

Use the full range of external cause codes to completely describe the cause, the intent, the place of occurrence, and if applicable, the activity of the patient at the time of the event, and the patient's status, for all injuries, and other health conditions due to an external cause.

4) Assign as many external cause codes as necessary

Assign as many external cause codes as necessary to fully explain each cause. If only one external code can be recorded, assign the code most related to the principal diagnosis.

5) The selection of the appropriate external cause code

The selection of the appropriate external cause code is guided by the Alphabetic Index of External Causes and by Inclusion and Exclusion notes in the Tabular List.

6) External cause code can never be a principal diagnosis

An external cause code can never be a principal (first-listed) diagnosis.

7) Combination external cause codes

Certain of the external cause codes are combination codes that identify sequential events that result in an injury, such as a fall which results in striking against an object. The injury may be due to either event or both.

The combination external cause code used should correspond to the sequence of events regardless of which caused the most serious injury.

Toddler tripped and fell while walking and struck his head on an end table, sustaining a scalp contusion	
S00.03XA	**Contusion of scalp, initial encounter**
W01.190A	**Fall on same level from slipping, tripping and stumbling with subsequent striking against furniture, initial encounter**

Explanation: Combination external cause codes identify sequential events that result in an injury, such as a fall resulting in striking against an object. The injury may be due to either or both events.

8) No external cause code needed in certain circumstances

No external cause code from Chapter 20 is needed if the external cause and intent are included in a code from another chapter (e.g. T36.0X1-Poisoning by penicillins, accidental (unintentional)).

b. Place of occurrence guideline

Codes from category Y92, Place of occurrence of the external cause, are secondary codes for use after other external cause codes to identify the location of the patient at the time of injury or other condition.

Generally, a place of occurrence code is assigned only once, at the initial encounter for treatment. However, in the rare instance that a new injury occurs during hospitalization, an additional place of occurrence code may be assigned. No 7th characters are used for Y92.

Do not use place of occurrence code Y92.9 if the place is not stated or is not applicable.

A farmer was working in his barn and sustained a foot contusion when the horse stepped on his left foot	
S90.32XA	**Contusion of left foot, initial encounter**
W55.19XA	**Other contact with horse, initial encounter**
Y92.71	**Barn as the place of occurrence of the external cause**

Explanation: A place-of-occurrence code from category Y92 is assigned at the initial encounter to identify the location of the patient at the time the injury occurred.

c. Activity code

Assign a code from category Y93, Activity code, to describe the activity of the patient at the time the injury or other health condition occurred.

An activity code is used only once, at the initial encounter for treatment. Only one code from Y93 should be recorded on a medical record.

The activity codes are not applicable to poisonings, adverse effects, misadventures or sequela.

Do not assign Y93.9, Unspecified activity, if the activity is not stated.

A code from category Y93 is appropriate for use with external cause and intent codes if identifying the activity provides additional information about the event.

Ranch hand who was grooming a horse sustained a foot contusion when the horse stepped on his left foot	
S90.32XA	**Contusion of left foot, initial encounter**
W55.19XA	**Other contact with horse, initial encounter**
Y93.K3	**Activity, grooming and shearing an animal**

Explanation: One activity code from category Y93 is assigned at the initial encounter only to describe the activity of the patient at the time the injury occurred.

d. Place of occurrence, activity, and status codes used with other external cause code

When applicable, place of occurrence, activity, and external cause status codes are sequenced after the main external cause code(s). Regardless of the number of external cause codes assigned, generally there should be only one place of occurrence code, one activity code, and one external cause status code assigned to an encounter. However, in the rare instance that a new injury occurs during hospitalization, an additional place of occurrence code may be assigned.

e. If the reporting format limits the number of external cause codes

If the reporting format limits the number of external cause codes that can be used in reporting clinical data, report the code for the cause/intent most related to the principal diagnosis. If the format permits capture of additional external cause codes, the cause/intent, including medical misadventures, of the additional events should be reported rather than the codes for place, activity, or external status.

f. Multiple external cause coding guidelines

More than one external cause code is required to fully describe the external cause of an illness or injury. The assignment of external cause codes should be sequenced in the following priority:

If two or more events cause separate injuries, an external cause code should be assigned for each cause. The first-listed external cause code will be selected in the following order:

External codes for child and adult abuse take priority over all other external cause codes.

See Section I.C.19., Child and Adult abuse guidelines.

External cause codes for terrorism events take priority over all other external cause codes except child and adult abuse.

External cause codes for cataclysmic events take priority over all other external cause codes except child and adult abuse and terrorism.

External cause codes for transport accidents take priority over all other external cause codes except cataclysmic events, child and adult abuse and terrorism.

Activity and external cause status codes are assigned following all causal (intent) external cause codes.

The first-listed external cause code should correspond to the cause of the most serious diagnosis due to an assault, accident, or self-harm, following the order of hierarchy listed above..

> 30-year-old man accidentally discharged his hunting rifle, sustaining an open gunshot wound, with no retained bullet fragments, to the right thigh, which caused him to fall down the stairs, resulting in closed displaced comminuted fracture of his left radial shaft
>
> **S71.131A**   **Puncture wound without foreign body, right thigh, initial encounter**
>
> **S52.352A**   **Displaced comminuted fracture of shaft of radius, left arm, initial encounter for closed fracture**
>
> **W33.02XA**   **Accidental discharge of hunting rifle, initial encounter**
>
> **W10.9XXA**   **Fall (on) (from) unspecified stairs and steps, initial encounter**
>
> *Explanation:* If two or more events cause separate injuries, an external cause code should be assigned for each cause.

g. Child and adult abuse guideline

Adult and child abuse, neglect and maltreatment are classified as assault. Any of the assault codes may be used to indicate the external cause of any injury resulting from the confirmed abuse.

For confirmed cases of abuse, neglect and maltreatment, when the perpetrator is known, a code from Y07, Perpetrator of maltreatment and neglect, should accompany any other assault codes.

See Section I.C.19. Adult and child abuse, neglect and other maltreatment

h. Unknown or undetermined intent guideline

If the intent (accident, self-harm, assault) of the cause of an injury or other condition is unknown or unspecified, code the intent as accidental intent. All transport accident categories assume accidental intent.

1) Use of undetermined intent

External cause codes for events of undetermined intent are only for use if the documentation in the record specifies that the intent cannot be determined.

i. Sequelae (late effects) of external cause guidelines

1) Sequelae external cause codes

Sequela are reported using the external cause code with the 7th character "S" for sequela. These codes should be used with any report of a late effect or sequela resulting from a previous injury.

See Section I.B.10 Sequela (Late Effects)

2) Sequela external cause code with a related current injury

A sequela external cause code should never be used with a related current nature of injury code.

3) Use of sequela external cause codes for subsequent visits

Use a late effect external cause code for subsequent visits when a late effect of the initial injury is being treated. Do not use a late effect external cause code for subsequent visits for follow-up care (e.g., to assess healing, to receive rehabilitative therapy) of the injury when no late effect of the injury has been documented.

j. Terrorism guidelines

1) Cause of injury identified by the Federal Government (FBI) as terrorism

When the cause of an injury is identified by the Federal Government (FBI) as terrorism, the first-listed external cause code should be a code from category Y38, Terrorism. The definition of terrorism employed by the FBI is found at the inclusion note at the beginning of category Y38. Use additional code for place of occurrence (Y92.-). More than one Y38 code may be assigned if the injury is the result of more than one mechanism of terrorism.

2) Cause of an injury is suspected to be the result of terrorism

When the cause of an injury is suspected to be the result of terrorism a code from category Y38 should not be assigned. Suspected cases should be classified as assault.

3) Code Y38.9, Terrorism, secondary effects

Assign code Y38.9, Terrorism, secondary effects, for conditions occurring subsequent to the terrorist event. This code should not be assigned for conditions that are due to the initial terrorist act.

It is acceptable to assign code Y38.9 with another code from Y38 if there is an injury due to the initial terrorist event and an injury that is a subsequent result of the terrorist event.

k. External cause status

A code from category Y99, External cause status, should be assigned whenever any other external cause code is assigned for an encounter, including an Activity code, except for the events noted below. Assign a code from category Y99, External cause status, to indicate the work status of the person at the time the event occurred. The status code indicates whether the event occurred during military activity, whether a non-military person was at work, whether an individual including a student or volunteer was involved in a non-work activity at the time of the causal event.

A code from Y99, External cause status, should be assigned, when applicable, with other external cause codes, such as transport accidents and falls. The external cause status codes are not applicable to poisonings, adverse effects, misadventures or late effects.

Do not assign a code from category Y99 if no other external cause codes (cause, activity) are applicable for the encounter.

An external cause status code is used only once, at the initial encounter for treatment. Only one code from Y99 should be recorded on a medical record.

Do not assign code Y99.9, Unspecified external cause status, if the status is not stated.

Chapter 20. External Causes of Morbidity (V00-Y99)

NOTE   This chapter permits the classification of environmental events and circumstances as the cause of injury, and other adverse effects. Where a code from this section is applicable, it is intended that it shall be used secondary to a code from another chapter of the Classification indicating the nature of the condition. Most often, the condition will be classifiable to Chapter 19, Injury, poisoning and certain other consequences of external causes (S00-T88). Other conditions that may be stated to be due to external causes are classified in Chapters I to XVIII. For these conditions, codes from Chapter 20 should be used to provide additional information as to the cause of the condition.

This chapter contains the following blocks:

V00-X58	Accidents
V00-V99	Transport accidents
V00-V09	Pedestrian injured in transport accident
V10-V19	Pedal cycle rider injured in transport accident
V20-V29	Motorcycle rider injured in transport accident
V30-V39	Occupant of three-wheeled motor vehicle injured in transport accident
V40-V49	Car occupant injured in transport accident
V50-V59	Occupant of pick-up truck or van injured in transport accident
V60-V69	Occupant of heavy transport vehicle injured in transport accident
V70-V79	Bus occupant injured in transport accident
V80-V89	Other land transport accidents
V90-V94	Water transport accidents
V95-V97	Air and space transport accidents
V98-V99	Other and unspecified transport accidents
W00-X58	Other external causes of accidental injury
W00-W19	Slipping, tripping, stumbling and falls
W20-W49	Exposure to inanimate mechanical forces
W50-W64	Exposure to animate mechanical forces
W65-W74	Accidental non-transport drowning and submersion
W85-W99	Exposure to electric current, radiation and extreme ambient air temperature and pressure
X00-X08	Exposure to smoke, fire and flames
X10-X19	Contact with heat and hot substances
X30-X39	Exposure to forces of nature
~~X50~~	~~Overexertion and strenuous or repetitive movements~~
X52-X58	Accidental exposure to other specified factors
X71-X83	Intentional self-harm
X92-Y09	Assault
Y21-Y33	Event of undetermined intent
Y35-Y38	Legal intervention, operations of war, military operations, and terrorism
Y62-Y84	Complications of medical and surgical care
Y62-Y69	Misadventures to patients during surgical and medical care
Y70-Y82	Medical devices associated with adverse incidents in diagnostic and therapeutic use
Y83-Y84	Surgical and other medical procedures as the cause of abnormal reaction of the patient, or of later complication, without mention of misadventure at the time of the procedure
Y90-Y99	Supplementary factors related to causes of morbidity classified elsewhere

Accidents (V00-X58)

NOTE   This section is structured in 12 groups. Those relating to land transport accidents (V00-V89) reflect the victim's mode of transport and are subdivided to identify the victim's 'counterpart' or the type of event. The vehicle of which the injured person is an occupant is identified in the first two characters since it is seen as the most important factor to identify for prevention purposes. A transport accident is one in which the vehicle involved must be moving or running or in use for transport purposes at the time of the accident.

Use additional code to identify:
   airbag injury (W22.1)
   type of street or road (Y92.4-)
   use of cellular telephone and other electronic equipment at the time of the transport accident (Y93.C-)

EXCLUDES 1   *agricultural vehicles in stationary use or maintenance (W31.-)*
   assault by crashing of motor vehicle (Y03.-)
   automobile or motor cycle in stationary use or maintenance—code to type of accident
   crashing of motor vehicle, undetermined intent (Y32)
   intentional self-harm by crashing of motor vehicle (X82)

EXCLUDES 2   *transport accidents due to cataclysm (X34-X38)*

NOTE   Definitions related to transport accidents:

(a) A transport accident (V00-V99) is any accident involving a device designed primarily for, or used at the time primarily for, conveying persons or good from one place to another.

(b) A public highway [trafficway] or street is the entire width between property lines (or other boundary lines) of land open to the public as a matter of right or custom for purposes of moving persons or property from one place to another. A roadway is that part of the public highway designed, improved and customarily used for vehicular traffic.

(c) A traffic accident is any vehicle accident occurring on the public highway [i.e. originating on, terminating on, or involving a vehicle partially on the highway]. A vehicle accident is assumed to have occurred on the public highway unless another place is specified, except in the case of accidents involving only off-road motor vehicles, which are classified as nontraffic accidents unless the contrary is stated.

(d) A nontraffic accident is any vehicle accident that occurs entirely in any place other than a public highway.

(e) A pedestrian is any person involved in an accident who was not at the time of the accident riding in or on a motor vehicle, railway train, streetcar or animal-drawn or other vehicle, or on a pedal cycle or animal. This includes, a person changing a tire, working on a parked car, or a person on foot. It also includes the user of a pedestrian conveyance such as a babystroller, ice-skates, skis, sled, roller skates, a skateboard, nonmotorized or motorized wheelchair, motorized mobility scooter, or nonmotorized scooter.

(f) A driver is an occupant of a transport vehicle who is operating or intending to operate it.

(g) A passenger is any occupant of a transport vehicle other than the driver, except a person traveling on the outside of the vehicle.

(h) A person on the outside of a vehicle is any person being transported by a vehicle but not occupying the space normally reserved for the driver or passengers, or the space intended for the transport of property. This includes a person travelling on the bodywork, bumper, fender, roof, running board or step of a vehicle, as well as, hanging on the outside of the vehicle.

(i) A pedal cycle is any land transport vehicle operated solely by nonmotorized pedals including a bicycle or tricycle.

(j) A pedal cyclist is any person riding a pedal cycle or in a sidecar or trailer attached to a pedal cycle.

(k) A motorcycle is a two-wheeled motor vehicle with one or two riding saddles and sometimes with a third wheel for the support of a sidecar. The sidecar is considered part of the motorcycle. This includes a moped, motor scooter, or motorized bicycle.

(l) A motorcycle rider is any person riding a motorcycle or in a sidecar or trailer attached to the motorcycle.

(m) A three-wheeled motor vehicle is a motorized tricycle designed primarily for on-road use. This includes a motor-driven tricycle, a motorized rickshaw, or a three-wheeled motor car.

(n) A car [automobile] is a four-wheeled motor vehicle designed primarily for carrying up to 7 persons. A trailer being towed by the car is considered part of the car. It does not include a van or minivan - see definition (o).

(o) A pick-up truck or van is a four or six-wheeled motor vehicle designed for carrying passengers as well as property or cargo weighing less than the local limit for classification as a heavy goods vehicle, and not requiring a special driver's license. This includes a minivan and a sport-utility vehicle (SUV).

(p) A heavy transport vehicle is a motor vehicle designed primarily for carrying property, meeting local criteria for classification as a heavy goods vehicle in terms of weight and requiring a special driver's license.

(q) A bus (coach) is a motor vehicle designed or adapted primarily for carrying more than 10 passengers, and requiring a special driver's license.

(r) A railway train or railway vehicle is any device, with or without freight or passenger cars couple to it, designed for traffic on a railway track. This includes subterranean (subways) or elevated trains.

(s) A streetcar, is a device designed and used primarily for transporting passengers within a municipality, running on rails, usually subject to normal traffic control signals, and operated principally on a right-of-way that forms part of the roadway. This includes a tram or trolley that runs on rails. A trailer being towed by a streetcar is considered part of the streetcar.

(t) A special vehicle mainly used on industrial premises is a motor vehicle designed primarily for use within the buildings and premises of industrial or commercial establishments. This includes battery-powered airport passenger vehicles or baggage/mail trucks, forklifts, coal-cars in a coal mine, logging cars and trucks used in mines or quarries.

(u)   A special vehicle mainly used in agriculture is a motor vehicle designed specifically for use in farming and agriculture (horticulture), to work the land, tend and harvest crops and transport materials on the farm. This includes harvesters, farm machinery and tractor and trailers.

(v)   A special construction vehicle is a motor vehicle designed specifically for use on construction and demolition sites. This includes bulldozers, diggers, earth levellers, dump trucks. backhoes, front-end loaders, pavers, and mechanical shovels.

(w)   A special all-terrain vehicle is a motor vehicle of special design to enable it to negotiate over rough or soft terrain, snow or sand. Examples of special design are high construction, special wheels and tires, tracks, and support on a cushion of air. This includes snow mobiles, All-terrain vehicles (ATV), and dune buggies. It does not include passenger vehicle designated as Sport Utility Vehicles. (SUV)

(x)   A watercraft is any device designed for transporting passengers or goods on water. This includes motor or sailboats, ships, and hovercraft.

(y)   An aircraft is any device for transporting passengers or goods in the air. This includes hot-air balloons, gliders, helicopters and airplanes.

(z)   A military vehicle is any motorized vehicle operating on a public roadway owned by the military and being operated by a member of the military

Pedestrian injured in transport accident (V00-V09)

INCLUDES   person changing tire on transport vehicle
person examining engine of vehicle broken down in (on side of) road

EXCLUDES 1 *fall due to non-transport collision with other person (W03)*
pedestrian on foot falling (slipping) on ice and snow (W00.-)
struck or bumped by another person (W51)

The appropriate 7th character is to be added to each code from categories V00-V09.
A   initial encounter
D   subsequent encounter
S   sequela

✓4th **V00   Pedestrian conveyance accident**
Use additional place of occurrence and activity external cause codes, if known (Y92-, Y93-)

EXCLUDES 1 *collision with another person without fall (W51)*
fall due to person on foot colliding with another person on foot (W03)
fall from non-moving wheelchair, nonmotorized scooter and motorized mobility scooter without collision (W05.-)
pedestrian (conveyance) collision with other land transport vehicle (V01-V09)
pedestrian on foot falling (slipping) on ice and snow (W00.-)

✓5th **V00.0   Pedestrian on foot injured in collision with pedestrian conveyance**

✓x7th   **V00.01   Pedestrian on foot injured in collision with roller-skater**

✓x7th   **V00.02   Pedestrian on foot injured in collision with skateboarder**

✓x7th   **V00.09   Pedestrian on foot injured in collision with other pedestrian conveyance**

✓5th **V00.1   Rolling-type pedestrian conveyance accident**
EXCLUDES 1 *accident with babystroller (V00.82-)*
accident with motorized mobility scooter (V00.83-)
accident with wheelchair (powered) (V00.81-)

✓6th   **V00.11   In-line roller-skate accident**

✓7th   **V00.111   Fall from in-line roller-skates**

✓7th   **V00.112   In-line roller-skater colliding with stationary object**

✓7th   **V00.118   Other in-line roller-skate accident**
EXCLUDES 1 *roller-skater collision with other land transport vehicle (V01-V09 with 5th character 1)*

✓6th   **V00.12   Non-in- line roller-skate accident**

✓7th   **V00.121   Fall from non-in-line roller-skates**

✓7th   **V00.122   Non-in-line roller-skater colliding with stationary object**

✓7th   **V00.128   Other non-in-line roller-skating accident**
EXCLUDES 1 *roller-skater collision with other land transport vehicle (V01-V09 with 5th character 1)*

✓6th **V00.13   Skateboard accident**

✓7th   **V00.131   Fall from skateboard**

✓7th   **V00.132   Skateboarder colliding with stationary object**

✓7th   **V00.138   Other skateboard accident**
EXCLUDES 1 *skateboarder collision with other land transport vehicle (V01-V09 with 5th character 2)*

✓6th **V00.14   Scooter (nonmotorized) accident**
EXCLUDES 1 *motorscooter accident (V20-V29)*

✓7th   **V00.141   Fall from scooter (nonmotorized)**

✓7th   **V00.142   Scooter (nonmotorized) colliding with stationary object**

✓7th   **V00.148   Other scooter (nonmotorized) accident**
EXCLUDES 1 *scooter (nonmotorized) collision with other land transport vehicle (V01-V09 with fifth character 9)*

✓6th **V00.15   Heelies accident**
Rolling shoe
Wheeled shoe
Wheelies accident

✓7th   **V00.151   Fall from heelies**

✓7th   **V00.152   Heelies colliding with stationary object**

✓7th   **V00.158   Other heelies accident**

✓6th **V00.18   Accident on other rolling-type pedestrian conveyance**

✓7th   **V00.181   Fall from other rolling-type pedestrian conveyance**

✓7th   **V00.182   Pedestrian on other rolling-type pedestrian conveyance colliding with stationary object**

✓7th   **V00.188   Other accident on other rolling-type pedestrian conveyance**

✓5th **V00.2   Gliding-type pedestrian conveyance accident**

✓6th   **V00.21   Ice-skates accident**

✓7th   **V00.211   Fall from ice-skates**

✓7th   **V00.212   Ice-skater colliding with stationary object**

✓7th   **V00.218   Other ice-skates accident**
EXCLUDES 1 *ice-skater collision with other land transport vehicle (V01-V09 with 5th digit 9)*

✓6th   **V00.22   Sled accident**

✓7th   **V00.221   Fall from sled**

✓7th   **V00.222   Sledder colliding with stationary object**

✓7th   **V00.228   Other sled accident**
EXCLUDES 1 *sled collision with other land transport vehicle (V01-V09 with 5th digit 9)*

✓6th   **V00.28   Other gliding-type pedestrian conveyance accident**

✓7th   **V00.281   Fall from other gliding-type pedestrian conveyance**

✓7th   **V00.282   Pedestrian on other gliding-type pedestrian conveyance colliding with stationary object**

✓7th   **V00.288   Other accident on other gliding-type pedestrian conveyance**
EXCLUDES 1 *gliding-type pedestrian conveyance collision with other land transport vehicle (V01-V09 with 5th digit 9)*

✓5th **V00.3   Flat-bottomed pedestrian conveyance accident**

✓6th   **V00.31   Snowboard accident**

✓7th   **V00.311   Fall from snowboard**

✓7th   **V00.312   Snowboarder colliding with stationary object**

✓7th   **V00.318   Other snowboard accident**
EXCLUDES 1 *snowboarder collision with other land transport vehicle (V01-V09 with 5th digit 9)*

✓6th   **V00.32   Snow-ski accident**

✓7th   **V00.321   Fall from snow-skis**

✓7th   **V00.322   Snow-skier colliding with stationary object**

EXCLUDES 1 Not coded here   EXCLUDES 2 Not included here   N Newborn Age: 0   P Pediatric Age: 0-17   M Maternity Age: 12-55   A Adult Age: 15-124

1116   ICD-10-CM 2018

✓7ᵗʰ **V00.328**   **Other snow-ski accident**
    EXCLUDES 1   snow-skier collision with other land transport vehicle (V01-V09 with 5th digit 9)

✓6ᵗʰ **V00.38**   **Other flat-bottomed pedestrian conveyance accident**

    ✓7ᵗʰ **V00.381**   **Fall from other flat-bottomed pedestrian conveyance**

    ✓7ᵗʰ **V00.382**   **Pedestrian on other flat-bottomed pedestrian conveyance colliding with stationary object**

    ✓7ᵗʰ **V00.388**   **Other accident on other flat-bottomed pedestrian conveyance**

✓5ᵗʰ **V00.8**   **Accident on other pedestrian conveyance**

   ✓6ᵗʰ **V00.81**   **Accident with wheelchair (powered)**

    ✓7ᵗʰ **V00.811**   **Fall from moving wheelchair (powered)**
      EXCLUDES 1   fall from non-moving wheelchair (W05.0)

    ✓7ᵗʰ **V00.812**   **Wheelchair (powered) colliding with stationary object**

    ✓7ᵗʰ **V00.818**   **Other accident with wheelchair (powered)**

   ✓6ᵗʰ **V00.82**   **Accident with babystroller**

    ✓7ᵗʰ **V00.821**   **Fall from babystroller**

    ✓7ᵗʰ **V00.822**   **Babystroller colliding with stationary object**

    ✓7ᵗʰ **V00.828**   **Other accident with babystroller**

   ✓6ᵗʰ **V00.83**   **Accident with motorized mobility scooter**

    V00.831   **Fall from motorized mobility scooter**
      EXCLUDES 1   fall from non-moving motorized mobility scooter (W05.2)

    V00.832   **Motorized mobility scooter colliding with stationary object**

    V00.838   **Other accident with motorized mobility scooter**

   ✓6ᵗʰ **V00.89**   **Accident on other pedestrian conveyance**

    ✓7ᵗʰ **V00.891**   **Fall from other pedestrian conveyance**

    ✓7ᵗʰ **V00.892**   **Pedestrian on other pedestrian conveyance colliding with stationary object**

    ✓7ᵗʰ **V00.898**   **Other accident on other pedestrian conveyance**
      EXCLUDES 1   other pedestrian (conveyance) collision with other land transport vehicle (V01-V09 with 5th digit 9)

✓4ᵗʰ **V01**   **Pedestrian injured in collision with pedal cycle**

   ✓5ᵗʰ **V01.0**   **Pedestrian injured in collision with pedal cycle in nontraffic accident**

    ✓x7ᵗʰ **V01.00**   **Pedestrian on foot injured in collision with pedal cycle in nontraffic accident**
      Pedestrian NOS injured in collision with pedal cycle in nontraffic accident

    ✓x7ᵗʰ **V01.01**   **Pedestrian on roller-skates injured in collision with pedal cycle in nontraffic accident**

    ✓x7ᵗʰ **V01.02**   **Pedestrian on skateboard injured in collision with pedal cycle in nontraffic accident**

    ✓x7ᵗʰ **V01.09**   **Pedestrian with other conveyance injured in collision with pedal cycle in nontraffic accident**
      Pedestrian with babystroller injured in collision with pedal cycle in nontraffic accident
      Pedestrian on ice-skates injured in collision with pedal cycle in nontraffic accident
      Pedestrian on nonmotorized scooter injured in collision with pedal cycle in nontraffic accident
      Pedestrian on sled injured in collision with pedal cycle in nontraffic accident
      Pedestrian on snowboard injured in collision with pedal cycle in nontraffic accident
      Pedestrian on snow-skis injured in collision with pedal cycle in nontraffic accident
      Pedestrian in wheelchair (powered) injured in collision with pedal cycle in nontraffic accident
      Pedestrian in motorized mobility scooter injured in collision with pedal cycle in nontraffic accident

   ✓5ᵗʰ **V01.1**   **Pedestrian injured in collision with pedal cycle in traffic accident**

    ✓x7ᵗʰ **V01.10**   **Pedestrian on foot injured in collision with pedal cycle in traffic accident**
      Pedestrian NOS injured in collision with pedal cycle in traffic accident

    ✓x7ᵗʰ **V01.11**   **Pedestrian on roller-skates injured in collision with pedal cycle in traffic accident**

    ✓x7ᵗʰ **V01.12**   **Pedestrian on skateboard injured in collision with pedal cycle in traffic accident**

    ✓x7ᵗʰ **V01.19**   **Pedestrian with other conveyance injured in collision with pedal cycle in traffic accident**
      Pedestrian with babystroller injured in collision with pedal cycle in traffic accident
      Pedestrian on ice-skates injured in collision with pedal cycle in traffic accident
      Pedestrian on nonmotorized scooter injured in collision with pedal cycle in traffic accident
      Pedestrian on sled injured in collision with pedal cycle in traffic accident
      Pedestrian on snowboard injured in collision with pedal cycle in traffic accident
      Pedestrian on snow-skis injured in collision with pedal cycle in traffic accident
      Pedestrian in wheelchair (powered) injured in collision with pedal cycle in traffic accident
      Pedestrian in motorized mobility scooter injured in collision with pedal cycle in traffic accident

   ✓5ᵗʰ **V01.9**   **Pedestrian injured in collision with pedal cycle, unspecified whether traffic or nontraffic accident**

    ✓x7ᵗʰ **V01.90**   **Pedestrian on foot injured in collision with pedal cycle, unspecified whether traffic or nontraffic accident**   ▽
      Pedestrian NOS injured in collision with pedal cycle, unspecified whether traffic or nontraffic accident

    ✓x7ᵗʰ **V01.91**   **Pedestrian on roller-skates injured in collision with pedal cycle, unspecified whether traffic or nontraffic accident**   ▽

    ✓x7ᵗʰ **V01.92**   **Pedestrian on skateboard injured in collision with pedal cycle, unspecified whether traffic or nontraffic accident**   ▽

    ✓x7ᵗʰ **V01.99**   **Pedestrian with other conveyance injured in collision with pedal cycle, unspecified whether traffic or nontraffic accident**   ▽
      Pedestrian with babystroller injured in collision with pedal cycle, unspecified whether traffic or nontraffic accident
      Pedestrian on ice-skates injured in collision with pedal cycle unspecified, whether traffic or nontraffic accident
      Pedestrian on nonmotorized scooter injured in collision with pedal cycle, unspecified whether traffic or nontraffic accident
      Pedestrian on sled injured in collision with pedal cycle unspecified, whether traffic or nontraffic accident
      Pedestrian on snowboard injured in collision with pedal cycle, unspecified whether traffic or nontraffic accident
      Pedestrian on snow-skis injured in collision with pedal cycle, unspecified whether traffic or nontraffic accident
      Pedestrian in wheelchair (powered) injured in collision with pedal cycle, unspecified whether traffic or nontraffic accident
      Pedestrian in motorized mobility scooter injured in collision with pedal cycle, unspecified whether traffic or nontraffic accident

✓4ᵗʰ **V02**   **Pedestrian injured in collision with two- or three-wheeled motor vehicle**

   ✓5ᵗʰ **V02.0**   **Pedestrian injured in collision with two- or three-wheeled motor vehicle in nontraffic accident**

    ✓x7ᵗʰ **V02.00**   **Pedestrian on foot injured in collision with two- or three-wheeled motor vehicle in nontraffic accident**
      Pedestrian NOS injured in collision with two- or three-wheeled motor vehicle in nontraffic accident

    ✓x7ᵗʰ **V02.01**   **Pedestrian on roller-skates injured in collision with two- or three-wheeled motor vehicle in nontraffic accident**

☑ Additional Character Req   ✓x7ᵗʰ Placeholder Alert   Manifestation   HCC CMS-HCC Condition   ▽ Unspecified Code   ►◄ Revised Text   ● New Code   ▲ Revised Code Title

ICD-10-CM 2018   **1117**

✓x7ᵗʰ **V02.02 Pedestrian on skateboard injured in collision with two- or three-wheeled motor vehicle in nontraffic accident**

✓x7ᵗʰ **V02.09 Pedestrian with other conveyance injured in collision with two- or three-wheeled motor vehicle in nontraffic accident**
Pedestrian with babystroller injured in collision with two- or three-wheeled motor vehicle in nontraffic accident
Pedestrian on ice-skates injured in collision with two- or three-wheeled motor vehicle in nontraffic accident
Pedestrian on nonmotorized scooter injured in collision with two- or three-wheeled motor vehicle in nontraffic accident
Pedestrian on sled injured in collision with two- or three-wheeled motor vehicle in nontraffic accident
Pedestrian on snowboard injured in collision with two- or three-wheeled motor vehicle in nontraffic accident
Pedestrian on snow-skis injured in collision with two- or three-wheeled motor vehicle in nontraffic accident
Pedestrian in wheelchair (powered) injured in collision with two- or three-wheeled motor vehicle in nontraffic accident
Pedestrian in motorized mobility scooter injured in collision with two- or three-wheeled motor vehicle in nontraffic accident

✓5ᵗʰ **V02.1 Pedestrian injured in collision with two- or three-wheeled motor vehicle in traffic accident**

✓x7ᵗʰ **V02.10 Pedestrian on foot injured in collision with two- or three-wheeled motor vehicle in traffic accident**
Pedestrian NOS injured in collision with two- or three-wheeled motor vehicle in traffic accident

✓x7ᵗʰ **V02.11 Pedestrian on roller-skates injured in collision with two- or three-wheeled motor vehicle in traffic accident**

✓x7ᵗʰ **V02.12 Pedestrian on skateboard injured in collision with two- or three-wheeled motor vehicle in traffic accident**

✓x7ᵗʰ **V02.19 Pedestrian with other conveyance injured in collision with two- or three-wheeled motor vehicle in traffic accident**
Pedestrian with babystroller injured in collision with two- or three-wheeled motor vehicle in traffic accident
Pedestrian on ice-skates injured in collision with two- or three-wheeled motor vehicle in traffic accident
Pedestrian on nonmotorized scooter injured in collision with two- or three-wheeled motor vehicle in traffic accident
Pedestrian on sled injured in collision with two- or three-wheeled motor vehicle in traffic accident
Pedestrian on snowboard injured in collision with two- or three-wheeled motor vehicle in traffic accident
Pedestrian on snow-skis injured in collision with two- or three-wheeled motor vehicle in traffic accident
Pedestrian in wheelchair (powered) injured in collision with two- or three-wheeled motor vehicle in traffic accident
Pedestrian in motorized mobility scooter injured in collision with two- or three-wheeled motor vehicle in traffic accident

✓5ᵗʰ **V02.9 Pedestrian injured in collision with two- or three-wheeled motor vehicle, unspecified whether traffic or nontraffic accident**

✓x7ᵗʰ **V02.90 Pedestrian on foot injured in collision with two- or three-wheeled motor vehicle, unspecified whether traffic or nontraffic accident** ▽
Pedestrian NOS injured in collision with two- or three-wheeled motor vehicle, unspecified whether traffic or nontraffic accident

✓x7ᵗʰ **V02.91 Pedestrian on roller-skates injured in collision with two- or three-wheeled motor vehicle, unspecified whether traffic or nontraffic accident** ▽

✓x7ᵗʰ **V02.92 Pedestrian on skateboard injured in collision with two- or three-wheeled motor vehicle, unspecified whether traffic or nontraffic accident** ▽

✓x7ᵗʰ **V02.99 Pedestrian with other conveyance injured in collision with two- or three-wheeled motor vehicle, unspecified whether traffic or nontraffic accident** ▽
Pedestrian with babystroller injured in collision with two- or three-wheeled motor vehicle, unspecified whether traffic or nontraffic accident
Pedestrian on ice-skates injured in collision with two- or three-wheeled motor vehicle, unspecified whether traffic or nontraffic accident
Pedestrian on nonmotorized scooter injured in collision with two- or three-wheeled motor vehicle, unspecified whether traffic or nontraffic accident
Pedestrian on sled injured in collision with two- or three-wheeled motor vehicle, unspecified whether traffic or nontraffic accident
Pedestrian on snowboard injured in collision with two- or three-wheeled motor vehicle, unspecified whether traffic or nontraffic accident
Pedestrian on snow-skis injured in collision with two- or three-wheeled motor vehicle, unspecified whether traffic or nontraffic accident
Pedestrian in wheelchair (powered) injured in collision with two- or three-wheeled motor vehicle, unspecified whether traffic or nontraffic accident
Pedestrian in motorized mobility scooter injured in collision with two- or three-wheeled motor vehicle, unspecified whether traffic or nontraffic accident

✓4ᵗʰ **V03 Pedestrian injured in collision with car, pick-up truck or van**

✓5ᵗʰ **V03.0 Pedestrian injured in collision with car, pick-up truck or van in nontraffic accident**

✓x7ᵗʰ **V03.00 Pedestrian on foot injured in collision with car, pick-up truck or van in nontraffic accident**
Pedestrian NOS injured in collision with car, pick-up truck or van in nontraffic accident

✓x7ᵗʰ **V03.01 Pedestrian on roller-skates injured in collision with car, pick-up truck or van in nontraffic accident**

✓x7ᵗʰ **V03.02 Pedestrian on skateboard injured in collision with car, pick-up truck or van in nontraffic accident**

✓x7ᵗʰ **V03.09 Pedestrian with other conveyance injured in collision with car, pick-up truck or van in nontraffic accident**
Pedestrian with babystroller injured in collision with car, pick-up truck or van in nontraffic accident
Pedestrian on ice-skates injured in collision with car, pick-up truck or van in nontraffic accident
Pedestrian on nonmotorized scooter injured in collision with car, pick-up truck or van in nontraffic accident
Pedestrian on sled injured in collision with car, pick-up truck or van in nontraffic accident
Pedestrian on snowboard injured in collision with car, pick-up truck or van in nontraffic accident
Pedestrian on snow-skis injured in collision with car, pick-up truck or van in nontraffic accident
Pedestrian in wheelchair (powered) injured in collision with car, pick-up truck or van in nontraffic accident
Pedestrian in motorized mobility scooter injured in collision with car, pick-up truck or van in nontraffic accident

✓5ᵗʰ **V03.1 Pedestrian injured in collision with car, pick-up truck or van in traffic accident**

✓x7ᵗʰ **V03.10 Pedestrian on foot injured in collision with car, pick-up truck or van in traffic accident**
Pedestrian NOS injured in collision with car, pick-up truck or van in traffic accident

✓x7ᵗʰ **V03.11 Pedestrian on roller-skates injured in collision with car, pick-up truck or van in traffic accident**

✓x7ᵗʰ **V03.12 Pedestrian on skateboard injured in collision with car, pick-up truck or van in traffic accident**

EXCLUDES1 Not coded here   EXCLUDES2 Not included here   N Newborn Age: 0   P Pediatric Age: 0-17   M Maternity Age: 12-55   A Adult Age: 15-124

1118   ICD-10-CM 2018

✓x7ᵗʰ **V03.19** **Pedestrian with other conveyance injured in collision with car, pick-up truck or van in traffic accident**

     Pedestrian with babystroller injured in collision with car, pick-up truck or van in traffic accident

     Pedestrian on ice-skates injured in collision with car, pick-up truck or van in traffic accident

     Pedestrian on nonmotorized scooter injured in collision with car, pick-up truck or van in traffic accident

     Pedestrian on sled injured in collision with car, pick-up truck or van in traffic accident

     Pedestrian on snowboard injured in collision with car, pick-up truck or van in traffic accident

     Pedestrian on snow-skis injured in collision with car, pick-up truck or van in traffic accident

     Pedestrian in wheelchair (powered) injured in collision with car, pick-up truck or van in traffic accident

     Pedestrian in motorized mobility scooter injured in collision with car, pick-up truck or van in traffic accident

✓5ᵗʰ **V03.9** **Pedestrian injured in collision with car, pick-up truck or van, unspecified whether traffic or nontraffic accident**

     ✓x7ᵗʰ **V03.90** **Pedestrian on foot injured in collision with car, pick-up truck or van, unspecified whether traffic or nontraffic accident** ▽

       Pedestrian NOS injured in collision with car, pick-up truck or van, unspecified whether traffic or nontraffic accident

     ✓x7ᵗʰ **V03.91** **Pedestrian on roller-skates injured in collision with car, pick-up truck or van, unspecified whether traffic or nontraffic accident** ▽

     ✓x7ᵗʰ **V03.92** **Pedestrian on skateboard injured in collision with car, pick-up truck or van, unspecified whether traffic or nontraffic accident** ▽

     ✓x7ᵗʰ **V03.99** **Pedestrian with other conveyance injured in collision with car, pick-up truck or van, unspecified whether traffic or nontraffic accident** ▽

       Pedestrian with babystroller injured in collision with car, pick-up truck or van, unspecified whether traffic or nontraffic accident

       Pedestrian on ice-skates injured in collision with car, pick-up truck or van, unspecified whether traffic or nontraffic accident

       Pedestrian on nonmotorized scooter injured in collision with car, pick-up truck or van, unspecified whether traffic or nontraffic accident

       Pedestrian on sled injured in collision with car, pick-up truck or van in nontraffic accident

       Pedestrian on snowboard injured in collision with car, pick-up truck or van, unspecified whether traffic or nontraffic accident

       Pedestrian on snow-skis injured in collision with car, pick-up truck or van, unspecified whether traffic or nontraffic accident

       Pedestrian in wheelchair (powered) injured in collision with car, pick-up truck or van, unspecified whether traffic or nontraffic accident

       Pedestrian in motorized mobility scooter injured in collision with car, pick-up truck or van, unspecified whether traffic or nontraffic accident

✓4ᵗʰ **V04** **Pedestrian injured in collision with heavy transport vehicle or bus**

     EXCLUDES 1   *pedestrian injured in collision with military vehicle (V09.01, V09.21)*

✓5ᵗʰ **V04.0** **Pedestrian injured in collision with heavy transport vehicle or bus in nontraffic accident**

     ✓x7ᵗʰ **V04.00** **Pedestrian on foot injured in collision with heavy transport vehicle or bus in nontraffic accident**

       Pedestrian NOS injured in collision with heavy transport vehicle or bus in nontraffic accident

     ✓x7ᵗʰ **V04.01** **Pedestrian on roller-skates injured in collision with heavy transport vehicle or bus in nontraffic accident**

     ✓x7ᵗʰ **V04.02** **Pedestrian on skateboard injured in collision with heavy transport vehicle or bus in nontraffic accident**

✓x7ᵗʰ **V04.09** **Pedestrian with other conveyance injured in collision with heavy transport vehicle or bus in nontraffic accident**

     Pedestrian with babystroller injured in collision with heavy transport vehicle or bus in nontraffic accident

     Pedestrian on ice-skates injured in collision with heavy transport vehicle or bus in nontraffic accident

     Pedestrian on nonmotorized scooter injured in collision with heavy transport vehicle or bus in nontraffic accident

     Pedestrian on sled injured in collision with heavy transport vehicle or bus in nontraffic accident

     Pedestrian on snowboard injured in collision with heavy transport vehicle or bus in nontraffic accident

     Pedestrian on snow-skis injured in collision with heavy transport vehicle or bus in nontraffic accident

     Pedestrian in wheelchair (powered) injured in collision with heavy transport vehicle or bus in nontraffic accident

     Pedestrian in motorized mobility scooter injured in collision with heavy transport vehicle or bus in nontraffic accident

✓5ᵗʰ **V04.1** **Pedestrian injured in collision with heavy transport vehicle or bus in traffic accident**

     ✓x7ᵗʰ **V04.10** **Pedestrian on foot injured in collision with heavy transport vehicle or bus in traffic accident**

       Pedestrian NOS injured in collision with heavy transport vehicle or bus in traffic accident

     ✓x7ᵗʰ **V04.11** **Pedestrian on roller-skates injured in collision with heavy transport vehicle or bus in traffic accident**

     ✓x7ᵗʰ **V04.12** **Pedestrian on skateboard injured in collision with heavy transport vehicle or bus in traffic accident**

     ✓x7ᵗʰ **V04.19** **Pedestrian with other conveyance injured in collision with heavy transport vehicle or bus in traffic accident**

       Pedestrian with babystroller injured in collision with heavy transport vehicle or bus in traffic accident

       Pedestrian on ice-skates injured in collision with heavy transport vehicle or bus in traffic accident

       Pedestrian on nonmotorized scooter injured in collision with heavy transport vehicle or bus in traffic accident

       Pedestrian on sled injured in collision with heavy transport vehicle or bus in traffic accident

       Pedestrian on snowboard injured in collision with heavy transport vehicle or bus in traffic accident

       Pedestrian on snow-skis injured in collision with heavy transport vehicle or bus in traffic accident

       Pedestrian in wheelchair (powered) injured in collision with heavy transport vehicle or bus in traffic accident

       Pedestrian in motorized mobility scooter injured in collision with heavy transport vehicle or bus in traffic accident

✓5ᵗʰ **V04.9** **Pedestrian injured in collision with heavy transport vehicle or bus, unspecified whether traffic or nontraffic accident**

     ✓x7ᵗʰ **V04.90** **Pedestrian on foot injured in collision with heavy transport vehicle or bus, unspecified whether traffic or nontraffic accident** ▽

       Pedestrian NOS injured in collision with heavy transport vehicle or bus, unspecified whether traffic or nontraffic accident

     ✓x7ᵗʰ **V04.91** **Pedestrian on roller-skates injured in collision with heavy transport vehicle or bus, unspecified whether traffic or nontraffic accident** ▽

     ✓x7ᵗʰ **V04.92** **Pedestrian on skateboard injured in collision with heavy transport vehicle or bus, unspecified whether traffic or nontraffic accident** ▽

☑ Additional Character Req   ✓x7ᵗʰ Placeholder Alert   Manifestation   HCC CMS-HCC Condition   ▽ Unspecified Code   ▶◀ Revised Text   ● New Code   ▲ Revised Code Title

ICD-10-CM 2018   **1119**

✓x7th **V04.99 Pedestrian with other conveyance injured in collision with heavy transport vehicle or bus, unspecified whether traffic or nontraffic accident** ▽

    Pedestrian with babystroller injured in collision with heavy transport vehicle or bus, unspecified whether traffic or nontraffic accident

    Pedestrian on ice-skates injured in collision with heavy transport vehicle or bus, unspecified whether traffic or nontraffic accident

    Pedestrian on nonmotorized scooter injured in collision with heavy transport vehicle or bus, unspecified whether traffic or nontraffic accident

    Pedestrian on sled injured in collision with heavy transport vehicle or bus, unspecified whether traffic or nontraffic accident

    Pedestrian on snowboard injured in collision with heavy transport vehicle or bus, unspecified whether traffic or nontraffic accident

    Pedestrian on snow-skis injured in collision with heavy transport vehicle or bus, unspecified whether traffic or nontraffic accident

    Pedestrian in wheelchair (powered) injured in collision with heavy transport vehicle or bus, unspecified whether traffic or nontraffic accident

    Pedestrian in motorized mobility scooter injured in collision with heavy transport vehicle or bus, unspecified whether traffic or nontraffic accident

✓4th **V05 Pedestrian injured in collision with railway train or railway vehicle**

✓5th **V05.0 Pedestrian injured in collision with railway train or railway vehicle in nontraffic accident**

  ✓x7th **V05.00 Pedestrian on foot injured in collision with railway train or railway vehicle in nontraffic accident**

    Pedestrian NOS injured in collision with railway train or railway vehicle in nontraffic accident

  ✓x7th **V05.01 Pedestrian on roller-skates injured in collision with railway train or railway vehicle in nontraffic accident**

  ✓x7th **V05.02 Pedestrian on skateboard injured in collision with railway train or railway vehicle in nontraffic accident**

  ✓x7th **V05.09 Pedestrian with other conveyance injured in collision with railway train or railway vehicle in nontraffic accident**

    Pedestrian with babystroller injured in collision with railway train or railway vehicle in nontraffic accident

    Pedestrian on ice-skates injured in collision with railway train or railway vehicle in nontraffic accident

    Pedestrian on nonmotorized scooter injured in collision with railway train or railway vehicle in nontraffic accident

    Pedestrian on sled injured in collision with railway train or railway vehicle in nontraffic accident

    Pedestrian on snowboard injured in collision with railway train or railway vehicle in nontraffic accident

    Pedestrian on snow-skis injured in collision with railway train or railway vehicle in nontraffic accident

    Pedestrian in wheelchair (powered) injured in collision with railway train or railway vehicle in nontraffic accident

    Pedestrian in motorized mobility scooter injured in collision with railway train or railway vehicle in nontraffic accident

✓5th **V05.1 Pedestrian injured in collision with railway train or railway vehicle in traffic accident**

  ✓x7th **V05.10 Pedestrian on foot injured in collision with railway train or railway vehicle in traffic accident**

    Pedestrian NOS injured in collision with railway train or railway vehicle in traffic accident

  ✓x7th **V05.11 Pedestrian on roller-skates injured in collision with railway train or railway vehicle in traffic accident**

  ✓x7th **V05.12 Pedestrian on skateboard injured in collision with railway train or railway vehicle in traffic accident**

✓x7th **V05.19 Pedestrian with other conveyance injured in collision with railway train or railway vehicle in traffic accident**

    Pedestrian with babystroller injured in collision with railway train or railway vehicle in traffic accident

    Pedestrian on ice-skates injured in collision with railway train or railway vehicle in traffic accident

    Pedestrian on nonmotorized scooter injured in collision with railway train or railway vehicle in traffic accident

    Pedestrian on sled injured in collision with railway train or railway vehicle in traffic accident

    Pedestrian on snowboard injured in collision with railway train or railway vehicle in traffic accident

    Pedestrian on snow-skis injured in collision with railway train or railway vehicle in traffic accident

    Pedestrian in wheelchair (powered) injured in collision with railway train or railway vehicle in traffic accident

    Pedestrian in motorized mobility scooter injured in collision with railway train or railway vehicle in traffic accident

✓5th **V05.9 Pedestrian injured in collision with railway train or railway vehicle, unspecified whether traffic or nontraffic accident**

  ✓x7th **V05.90 Pedestrian on foot injured in collision with railway train or railway vehicle, unspecified whether traffic or nontraffic accident** ▽

    Pedestrian NOS injured in collision with railway train or railway vehicle, unspecified whether traffic or nontraffic accident

  ✓x7th **V05.91 Pedestrian on roller-skates injured in collision with railway train or railway vehicle, unspecified whether traffic or nontraffic accident** ▽

  ✓x7th **V05.92 Pedestrian on skateboard injured in collision with railway train or railway vehicle, unspecified whether traffic or nontraffic accident** ▽

  ✓x7th **V05.99 Pedestrian with other conveyance injured in collision with railway train or railway vehicle, unspecified whether traffic or nontraffic accident** ▽

    Pedestrian with babystroller injured in collision with railway train or railway vehicle, unspecified whether traffic or nontraffic

    Pedestrian on ice-skates injured in collision with railway train or railway vehicle, unspecified whether traffic or nontraffic

    Pedestrian on nonmotorized scooter injured in collision with railway train or railway vehicle, unspecified whether traffic or nontraffic

    Pedestrian on sled injured in collision with railway train or railway vehicle, unspecified whether traffic or nontraffic

    Pedestrian on snowboard injured in collision with railway train or railway vehicle, unspecified whether traffic or nontraffic

    Pedestrian on snow-skis injured in collision with railway train or railway vehicle, unspecified whether traffic or nontraffic

    Pedestrian in wheelchair (powered) injured in collision with railway train or railway vehicle, unspecified whether traffic or nontraffic

    Pedestrian in motorized mobility scooter injured in collision with railway train or railway vehicle, unspecified whether traffic or nontraffic

✓4th **V06 Pedestrian injured in collision with other nonmotor vehicle**

  INCLUDES collision with animal-drawn vehicle, animal being ridden, nonpowered streetcar

  EXCLUDES 1 pedestrian injured in collision with pedestrian conveyance (V00.0-)

✓5th **V06.0 Pedestrian injured in collision with other nonmotor vehicle in nontraffic accident**

  ✓x7th **V06.00 Pedestrian on foot injured in collision with other nonmotor vehicle in nontraffic accident**

    Pedestrian NOS injured in collision with other nonmotor vehicle in nontraffic accident

  ✓x7th **V06.01 Pedestrian on roller-skates injured in collision with other nonmotor vehicle in nontraffic accident**

  ✓x7th **V06.02 Pedestrian on skateboard injured in collision with other nonmotor vehicle in nontraffic accident**

EXCLUDES 1 Not coded here   **EXCLUDES 2** Not included here   N Newborn Age: 0   P Pediatric Age: 0-17   M Maternity Age: 12-55   A Adult Age: 15-124

1120   ICD-10-CM 2018

Chapter 20. External Causes of Morbidity

✓x7ᵗʰ **V06.09 Pedestrian with other conveyance injured in collision with other nonmotor vehicle in nontraffic accident**
Pedestrian with babystroller injured in collision with other nonmotor vehicle in nontraffic accident
Pedestrian on ice-skates injured in collision with other nonmotor vehicle in nontraffic accident
Pedestrian on nonmotorized scooter injured in collision with other nonmotor vehicle in nontraffic accident
Pedestrian on sled injured in collision with other nonmotor vehicle in nontraffic accident
Pedestrian on snowboard injured in collision with other nonmotor vehicle in nontraffic accident
Pedestrian on snow-skis injured in collision with other nonmotor vehicle in nontraffic accident
Pedestrian in wheelchair (powered) injured in collision with other nonmotor vehicle in nontraffic accident
Pedestrian in motorized mobility scooter injured in collision with other nonmotor vehicle in nontraffic accident

✓5ᵗʰ **V06.1 Pedestrian injured in collision with other nonmotor vehicle in traffic accident**

✓x7ᵗʰ **V06.10 Pedestrian on foot injured in collision with other nonmotor vehicle in traffic accident**
Pedestrian NOS injured in collision with other nonmotor vehicle in traffic accident

✓x7ᵗʰ **V06.11 Pedestrian on roller-skates injured in collision with other nonmotor vehicle in traffic accident**

✓x7ᵗʰ **V06.12 Pedestrian on skateboard injured in collision with other nonmotor vehicle in traffic accident**

✓x7ᵗʰ **V06.19 Pedestrian with other conveyance injured in collision with other nonmotor vehicle in traffic accident**
Pedestrian with babystroller injured in collision with other nonmotor vehicle in nontraffic accident
Pedestrian on ice-skates injured in collision with other nonmotor vehicle in traffic accident
Pedestrian on nonmotorized scooter injured in collision with other nonmotor vehicle in traffic accident
Pedestrian on sled injured in collision with other nonmotor vehicle in traffic accident
Pedestrian on snowboard injured in collision with other nonmotor vehicle in traffic accident
Pedestrian on snow-skis injured in collision with other nonmotor vehicle in traffic accident
Pedestrian in wheelchair (powered) injured in collision with other nonmotor vehicle in traffic accident
Pedestrian in motorized mobility scooter injured in collision with other nonmotor vehicle in traffic accident

✓5ᵗʰ **V06.9 Pedestrian injured in collision with other nonmotor vehicle, unspecified whether traffic or nontraffic accident**

✓x7ᵗʰ **V06.90 Pedestrian on foot injured in collision with other nonmotor vehicle, unspecified whether traffic or nontraffic accident** ▽
Pedestrian NOS injured in collision with other nonmotor vehicle, unspecified whether traffic or nontraffic accident

✓x7ᵗʰ **V06.91 Pedestrian on roller-skates injured in collision with other nonmotor vehicle, unspecified whether traffic or nontraffic accident** ▽

✓x7ᵗʰ **V06.92 Pedestrian on skateboard injured in collision with other nonmotor vehicle, unspecified whether traffic or nontraffic accident** ▽

✓x7ᵗʰ **V06.99 Pedestrian with other conveyance injured in collision with other nonmotor vehicle, unspecified whether traffic or nontraffic accident** ▽
Pedestrian with babystroller injured in collision with other nonmotor vehicle, unspecified whether traffic or nontraffic accident
Pedestrian on ice-skates injured in collision with other nonmotor vehicle, unspecified whether traffic or nontraffic accident
Pedestrian on nonmotorized scooter injured in collision with other nonmotor vehicle, unspecified whether traffic or nontraffic accident
Pedestrian on sled injured in collision with other nonmotor vehicle, unspecified whether traffic or nontraffic accident
Pedestrian on snowboard injured in collision with other nonmotor vehicle, unspecified whether traffic or nontraffic accident
Pedestrian on snow-skis injured in collision with other nonmotor vehicle, unspecified whether traffic or nontraffic accident
Pedestrian in wheelchair (powered) injured in collision with other nonmotor vehicle, unspecified whether traffic or nontraffic accident
Pedestrian in motorized mobility scooter injured in collision with other nonmotor vehicle, unspecified whether traffic or nontraffic accident

✓4ᵗʰ **V09 Pedestrian injured in other and unspecified transport accidents**

✓5ᵗʰ **V09.0 Pedestrian injured in nontraffic accident involving other and unspecified motor vehicles**

✓x7ᵗʰ **V09.00 Pedestrian injured in nontraffic accident involving unspecified motor vehicles** ▽

✓x7ᵗʰ **V09.01 Pedestrian injured in nontraffic accident involving military vehicle**

✓x7ᵗʰ **V09.09 Pedestrian injured in nontraffic accident involving other motor vehicles**
Pedestrian injured in nontraffic accident by special vehicle

✓x7ᵗʰ **V09.1 Pedestrian injured in unspecified nontraffic accident** ▽

✓5ᵗʰ **V09.2 Pedestrian injured in traffic accident involving other and unspecified motor vehicles**

✓x7ᵗʰ **V09.20 Pedestrian injured in traffic accident involving unspecified motor vehicles** ▽

✓x7ᵗʰ **V09.21 Pedestrian injured in traffic accident involving military vehicle**

✓x7ᵗʰ **V09.29 Pedestrian injured in traffic accident involving other motor vehicles**

✓x7ᵗʰ **V09.3 Pedestrian injured in unspecified traffic accident** ▽

✓x7ᵗʰ **V09.9 Pedestrian injured in unspecified transport accident** ▽

Pedal cycle rider injured in transport accident (V10-V19)

INCLUDES any non-motorized vehicle, excluding an animal-drawn vehicle, or a sidecar or trailer attached to the pedal cycle
EXCLUDES 2 rupture of pedal cycle tire (W37.0)

The appropriate 7th character is to be added to each code from categories V10-V19.
A   initial encounter
D   subsequent encounter
S   sequela

✓4ᵗʰ **V10 Pedal cycle rider injured in collision with pedestrian or animal**
EXCLUDES 1 pedal cycle rider collision with animal-drawn vehicle or animal being ridden (V16.-)

✓x7ᵗʰ **V10.0 Pedal cycle driver injured in collision with pedestrian or animal in nontraffic accident**

✓x7ᵗʰ **V10.1 Pedal cycle passenger injured in collision with pedestrian or animal in nontraffic accident**

✓x7ᵗʰ **V10.2 Unspecified pedal cyclist injured in collision with pedestrian or animal in nontraffic accident** ▽

✓x7ᵗʰ **V10.3 Person boarding or alighting a pedal cycle injured in collision with pedestrian or animal**

✓x7ᵗʰ **V10.4 Pedal cycle driver injured in collision with pedestrian or animal in traffic accident**

✓x7ᵗʰ **V10.5 Pedal cycle passenger injured in collision with pedestrian or animal in traffic accident**

✓x7ᵗʰ **V10.9 Unspecified pedal cyclist injured in collision with pedestrian or animal in traffic accident** ▽

✓ Additional Character Req   ✓x7ᵗʰ Placeholder Alert   Manifestation   HCC CMS-HCC Condition   ▽ Unspecified Code   ▶◀ Revised Text   ● New Code   ▲ Revised Code Title

ICD-10-CM 2018   1121

Chapter 20. External Causes of Morbidity

✓4ᵗʰ **V11**   **Pedal cycle rider injured in collision with other pedal cycle**

✓x7ᵗʰ **V11.0**   Pedal cycle driver injured in collision with other pedal cycle in nontraffic accident

✓x7ᵗʰ **V11.1**   Pedal cycle passenger injured in collision with other pedal cycle in nontraffic accident

✓x7ᵗʰ **V11.2**   Unspecified pedal cyclist injured in collision with other pedal cycle in nontraffic accident ▽

✓x7ᵗʰ **V11.3**   Person boarding or alighting a pedal cycle injured in collision with other pedal cycle

✓x7ᵗʰ **V11.4**   Pedal cycle driver injured in collision with other pedal cycle in traffic accident

✓x7ᵗʰ **V11.5**   Pedal cycle passenger injured in collision with other pedal cycle in traffic accident

✓x7ᵗʰ **V11.9**   Unspecified pedal cyclist injured in collision with other pedal cycle in traffic accident ▽

✓4ᵗʰ **V12**   **Pedal cycle rider injured in collision with two- or three-wheeled motor vehicle**

✓x7ᵗʰ **V12.0**   Pedal cycle driver injured in collision with two- or three-wheeled motor vehicle in nontraffic accident

✓x7ᵗʰ **V12.1**   Pedal cycle passenger injured in collision with two- or three-wheeled motor vehicle in nontraffic accident

✓x7ᵗʰ **V12.2**   Unspecified pedal cyclist injured in collision with two- or three-wheeled motor vehicle in nontraffic accident ▽

✓x7ᵗʰ **V12.3**   Person boarding or alighting a pedal cycle injured in collision with two- or three-wheeled motor vehicle

✓x7ᵗʰ **V12.4**   Pedal cycle driver injured in collision with two- or three-wheeled motor vehicle in traffic accident

✓x7ᵗʰ **V12.5**   Pedal cycle passenger injured in collision with two- or three-wheeled motor vehicle in traffic accident

✓x7ᵗʰ **V12.9**   Unspecified pedal cyclist injured in collision with two- or three-wheeled motor vehicle in traffic accident ▽

✓4ᵗʰ **V13**   **Pedal cycle rider injured in collision with car, pick-up truck or van**

✓x7ᵗʰ **V13.0**   Pedal cycle driver injured in collision with car, pick-up truck or van in nontraffic accident

✓x7ᵗʰ **V13.1**   Pedal cycle passenger injured in collision with car, pick-up truck or van in nontraffic accident

✓x7ᵗʰ **V13.2**   Unspecified pedal cyclist injured in collision with car, pick-up truck or van in nontraffic accident ▽

✓x7ᵗʰ **V13.3**   Person boarding or alighting a pedal cycle injured in collision with car, pick-up truck or van

✓x7ᵗʰ **V13.4**   Pedal cycle driver injured in collision with car, pick-up truck or van in traffic accident

✓x7ᵗʰ **V13.5**   Pedal cycle passenger injured in collision with car, pick-up truck or van in traffic accident

✓x7ᵗʰ **V13.9**   Unspecified pedal cyclist injured in collision with car, pick-up truck or van in traffic accident ▽

✓4ᵗʰ **V14**   **Pedal cycle rider injured in collision with heavy transport vehicle or bus**

EXCLUDES 1   pedal cycle rider injured in collision with military vehicle (V19.81)

✓x7ᵗʰ **V14.0**   Pedal cycle driver injured in collision with heavy transport vehicle or bus in nontraffic accident

✓x7ᵗʰ **V14.1**   Pedal cycle passenger injured in collision with heavy transport vehicle or bus in nontraffic accident

✓x7ᵗʰ **V14.2**   Unspecified pedal cyclist injured in collision with heavy transport vehicle or bus in nontraffic accident ▽

✓x7ᵗʰ **V14.3**   Person boarding or alighting a pedal cycle injured in collision with heavy transport vehicle or bus

✓x7ᵗʰ **V14.4**   Pedal cycle driver injured in collision with heavy transport vehicle or bus in traffic accident

✓x7ᵗʰ **V14.5**   Pedal cycle passenger injured in collision with heavy transport vehicle or bus in traffic accident

✓x7ᵗʰ **V14.9**   Unspecified pedal cyclist injured in collision with heavy transport vehicle or bus in traffic accident ▽

✓4ᵗʰ **V15**   **Pedal cycle rider injured in collision with railway train or railway vehicle**

✓x7ᵗʰ **V15.0**   Pedal cycle driver injured in collision with railway train or railway vehicle in nontraffic accident

✓x7ᵗʰ **V15.1**   Pedal cycle passenger injured in collision with railway train or railway vehicle in nontraffic accident

✓x7ᵗʰ **V15.2**   Unspecified pedal cyclist injured in collision with railway train or railway vehicle in nontraffic accident ▽

✓x7ᵗʰ **V15.3**   Person boarding or alighting a pedal cycle injured in collision with railway train or railway vehicle

✓x7ᵗʰ **V15.4**   Pedal cycle driver injured in collision with railway train or railway vehicle in traffic accident

✓x7ᵗʰ **V15.5**   Pedal cycle passenger injured in collision with railway train or railway vehicle in traffic accident

✓x7ᵗʰ **V15.9**   Unspecified pedal cyclist injured in collision with railway train or railway vehicle in traffic accident ▽

✓4ᵗʰ **V16**   **Pedal cycle rider injured in collision with other nonmotor vehicle**

INCLUDES   collision with animal-drawn vehicle, animal being ridden, streetcar

✓x7ᵗʰ **V16.0**   Pedal cycle driver injured in collision with other nonmotor vehicle in nontraffic accident

✓x7ᵗʰ **V16.1**   Pedal cycle passenger injured in collision with other nonmotor vehicle in nontraffic accident

✓x7ᵗʰ **V16.2**   Unspecified pedal cyclist injured in collision with other nonmotor vehicle in nontraffic accident ▽

✓x7ᵗʰ **V16.3**   Person boarding or alighting a pedal cycle injured in collision with other nonmotor vehicle in nontraffic accident

✓x7ᵗʰ **V16.4**   Pedal cycle driver injured in collision with other nonmotor vehicle in traffic accident

✓x7ᵗʰ **V16.5**   Pedal cycle passenger injured in collision with other nonmotor vehicle in traffic accident

✓x7ᵗʰ **V16.9**   Unspecified pedal cyclist injured in collision with other nonmotor vehicle in traffic accident ▽

✓4ᵗʰ **V17**   **Pedal cycle rider injured in collision with fixed or stationary object**

✓x7ᵗʰ **V17.0**   Pedal cycle driver injured in collision with fixed or stationary object in nontraffic accident

✓x7ᵗʰ **V17.1**   Pedal cycle passenger injured in collision with fixed or stationary object in nontraffic accident

✓x7ᵗʰ **V17.2**   Unspecified pedal cyclist injured in collision with fixed or stationary object in nontraffic accident ▽

✓x7ᵗʰ **V17.3**   Person boarding or alighting a pedal cycle injured in collision with fixed or stationary object

✓x7ᵗʰ **V17.4**   Pedal cycle driver injured in collision with fixed or stationary object in traffic accident

✓x7ᵗʰ **V17.5**   Pedal cycle passenger injured in collision with fixed or stationary object in traffic accident

✓x7ᵗʰ **V17.9**   Unspecified pedal cyclist injured in collision with fixed or stationary object in traffic accident ▽

✓4ᵗʰ **V18**   **Pedal cycle rider injured in noncollision transport accident**

INCLUDES   fall or thrown from pedal cycle (without antecedent collision)
overturning pedal cycle NOS
overturning pedal cycle without collision

✓x7ᵗʰ **V18.0**   Pedal cycle driver injured in noncollision transport accident in nontraffic accident

✓x7ᵗʰ **V18.1**   Pedal cycle passenger injured in noncollision transport accident in nontraffic accident

✓x7ᵗʰ **V18.2**   Unspecified pedal cyclist injured in noncollision transport accident in nontraffic accident ▽

✓x7ᵗʰ **V18.3**   Person boarding or alighting a pedal cycle injured in noncollision transport accident

✓x7ᵗʰ **V18.4**   Pedal cycle driver injured in noncollision transport accident in traffic accident

✓x7ᵗʰ **V18.5**   Pedal cycle passenger injured in noncollision transport accident in traffic accident

✓x7ᵗʰ **V18.9**   Unspecified pedal cyclist injured in noncollision transport accident in traffic accident ▽

✓4ᵗʰ **V19**   **Pedal cycle rider injured in other and unspecified transport accidents**

✓5ᵗʰ **V19.0**   Pedal cycle driver injured in collision with other and unspecified motor vehicles in nontraffic accident

✓x7ᵗʰ **V19.00**   Pedal cycle driver injured in collision with unspecified motor vehicles in nontraffic accident ▽

✓x7ᵗʰ **V19.09**   Pedal cycle driver injured in collision with other motor vehicles in nontraffic accident

✓5ᵗʰ **V19.1**   Pedal cycle passenger injured in collision with other and unspecified motor vehicles in nontraffic accident

✓x7ᵗʰ **V19.10**   Pedal cycle passenger injured in collision with unspecified motor vehicles in nontraffic accident

✓x7ᵗʰ **V19.19**   Pedal cycle passenger injured in collision with other motor vehicles in nontraffic accident

EXCLUDES 1 Not coded here   EXCLUDES 2 Not included here   N Newborn Age: 0   P Pediatric Age: 0-17   M Maternity Age: 12-55   A Adult Age: 15-124

1122   ICD-10-CM 2018

✓5ᵗʰ **V19.2 Unspecified pedal cyclist injured in collision with other and unspecified motor vehicles in nontraffic accident**

     ✓x7ᵗʰ **V19.20 Unspecified pedal cyclist injured in collision with unspecified motor vehicles in nontraffic accident** ▽
        Pedal cycle collision NOS, nontraffic

     ✓x7ᵗʰ **V19.29 Unspecified pedal cyclist injured in collision with other motor vehicles in nontraffic accident** ▽

✓5ᵗʰ **V19.3 Pedal cyclist (driver) (passenger) injured in unspecified nontraffic accident** ▽
     Pedal cycle accident NOS, nontraffic
     Pedal cyclist injured in nontraffic accident NOS

✓5ᵗʰ **V19.4 Pedal cycle driver injured in collision with other and unspecified motor vehicles in traffic accident**

     ✓x7ᵗʰ **V19.40 Pedal cycle driver injured in collision with unspecified motor vehicles in traffic accident** ▽

     ✓x7ᵗʰ **V19.49 Pedal cycle driver injured in collision with other motor vehicles in traffic accident**

✓5ᵗʰ **V19.5 Pedal cycle passenger injured in collision with other and unspecified motor vehicles in traffic accident**

     ✓x7ᵗʰ **V19.50 Pedal cycle passenger injured in collision with unspecified motor vehicles in traffic accident** ▽

     ✓x7ᵗʰ **V19.59 Pedal cycle passenger injured in collision with other motor vehicles in traffic accident**

✓5ᵗʰ **V19.6 Unspecified pedal cyclist injured in collision with other and unspecified motor vehicles in traffic accident**

     ✓x7ᵗʰ **V19.60 Unspecified pedal cyclist injured in collision with unspecified motor vehicles in traffic accident** ▽
        Pedal cycle collision NOS (traffic)

     ✓x7ᵗʰ **V19.69 Unspecified pedal cyclist injured in collision with other motor vehicles in traffic accident** ▽

✓5ᵗʰ **V19.8 Pedal cyclist (driver) (passenger) injured in other specified transport accidents**

     ✓x7ᵗʰ **V19.81 Pedal cyclist (driver) (passenger) injured in transport accident with military vehicle**

     ✓x7ᵗʰ **V19.88 Pedal cyclist (driver) (passenger) injured in other specified transport accidents**

✓x7ᵗʰ **V19.9 Pedal cyclist (driver) (passenger) injured in unspecified traffic accident** ▽
     Pedal cycle accident NOS

Motorcycle rider injured in transport accident (V20-V29)

INCLUDES   moped
         motorcycle with sidecar
         motorized bicycle
         motor scooter
EXCLUDES 1   three-wheeled motor vehicle (V30-V39)

The appropriate 7th character is to be added to each code from categories V20-V29.
A   initial encounter
D   subsequent encounter
S   sequela

✓4ᵗʰ **V20 Motorcycle rider injured in collision with pedestrian or animal**
     EXCLUDES 1   motorcycle rider collision with animal-drawn vehicle or animal being ridden (V26.-)

     ✓x7ᵗʰ **V20.0 Motorcycle driver injured in collision with pedestrian or animal in nontraffic accident**

     ✓x7ᵗʰ **V20.1 Motorcycle passenger injured in collision with pedestrian or animal in nontraffic accident**

     ✓x7ᵗʰ **V20.2 Unspecified motorcycle rider injured in collision with pedestrian or animal in nontraffic accident** ▽

     ✓x7ᵗʰ **V20.3 Person boarding or alighting a motorcycle injured in collision with pedestrian or animal**

     ✓x7ᵗʰ **V20.4 Motorcycle driver injured in collision with pedestrian or animal in traffic accident**

     ✓x7ᵗʰ **V20.5 Motorcycle passenger injured in collision with pedestrian or animal in traffic accident**

     ✓x7ᵗʰ **V20.9 Unspecified motorcycle rider injured in collision with pedestrian or animal in traffic accident** ▽

✓4ᵗʰ **V21 Motorcycle rider injured in collision with pedal cycle**

     ✓x7ᵗʰ **V21.0 Motorcycle driver injured in collision with pedal cycle in nontraffic accident**

     ✓x7ᵗʰ **V21.1 Motorcycle passenger injured in collision with pedal cycle in nontraffic accident**

     ✓x7ᵗʰ **V21.2 Unspecified motorcycle rider injured in collision with pedal cycle in nontraffic accident** ▽

     ✓x7ᵗʰ **V21.3 Person boarding or alighting a motorcycle injured in collision with pedal cycle**

     ✓x7ᵗʰ **V21.4 Motorcycle driver injured in collision with pedal cycle in traffic accident**

     ✓x7ᵗʰ **V21.5 Motorcycle passenger injured in collision with pedal cycle in traffic accident**

     ✓x7ᵗʰ **V21.9 Unspecified motorcycle rider injured in collision with pedal cycle in traffic accident** ▽

✓4ᵗʰ **V22 Motorcycle rider injured in collision with two- or three-wheeled motor vehicle**

     ✓x7ᵗʰ **V22.0 Motorcycle driver injured in collision with two- or three-wheeled motor vehicle in nontraffic accident**

     ✓x7ᵗʰ **V22.1 Motorcycle passenger injured in collision with two- or three-wheeled motor vehicle in nontraffic accident**

     ✓x7ᵗʰ **V22.2 Unspecified motorcycle rider injured in collision with two- or three-wheeled motor vehicle in nontraffic accident** ▽

     ✓x7ᵗʰ **V22.3 Person boarding or alighting a motorcycle injured in collision with two- or three-wheeled motor vehicle**

     ✓x7ᵗʰ **V22.4 Motorcycle driver injured in collision with two- or three-wheeled motor vehicle in traffic accident**

     ✓x7ᵗʰ **V22.5 Motorcycle passenger injured in collision with two- or three-wheeled motor vehicle in traffic accident**

     ✓x7ᵗʰ **V22.9 Unspecified motorcycle rider injured in collision with two- or three-wheeled motor vehicle in traffic accident** ▽

✓4ᵗʰ **V23 Motorcycle rider injured in collision with car, pick-up truck or van**

     ✓x7ᵗʰ **V23.0 Motorcycle driver injured in collision with car, pick-up truck or van in nontraffic accident**

     ✓x7ᵗʰ **V23.1 Motorcycle passenger injured in collision with car, pick-up truck or van in nontraffic accident**

     ✓x7ᵗʰ **V23.2 Unspecified motorcycle rider injured in collision with car, pick-up truck or van in nontraffic accident** ▽

     ✓x7ᵗʰ **V23.3 Person boarding or alighting a motorcycle injured in collision with car, pick-up truck or van**

     ✓x7ᵗʰ **V23.4 Motorcycle driver injured in collision with car, pick-up truck or van in traffic accident**

     ✓x7ᵗʰ **V23.5 Motorcycle passenger injured in collision with car, pick-up truck or van in traffic accident**

     ✓x7ᵗʰ **V23.9 Unspecified motorcycle rider injured in collision with car, pick-up truck or van in traffic accident** ▽

✓4ᵗʰ **V24 Motorcycle rider injured in collision with heavy transport vehicle or bus**
     EXCLUDES 1   motorcycle rider injured in collision with military vehicle (V29.81)

     ✓x7ᵗʰ **V24.0 Motorcycle driver injured in collision with heavy transport vehicle or bus in nontraffic accident**

     ✓x7ᵗʰ **V24.1 Motorcycle passenger injured in collision with heavy transport vehicle or bus in nontraffic accident**

     ✓x7ᵗʰ **V24.2 Unspecified motorcycle rider injured in collision with heavy transport vehicle or bus in nontraffic accident** ▽

     ✓x7ᵗʰ **V24.3 Person boarding or alighting a motorcycle injured in collision with heavy transport vehicle or bus**

     ✓x7ᵗʰ **V24.4 Motorcycle driver injured in collision with heavy transport vehicle or bus in traffic accident**

     ✓x7ᵗʰ **V24.5 Motorcycle passenger injured in collision with heavy transport vehicle or bus in traffic accident**

     ✓x7ᵗʰ **V24.9 Unspecified motorcycle rider injured in collision with heavy transport vehicle or bus in traffic accident** ▽

✓4ᵗʰ **V25 Motorcycle rider injured in collision with railway train or railway vehicle**

     ✓x7ᵗʰ **V25.0 Motorcycle driver injured in collision with railway train or railway vehicle in nontraffic accident**

     ✓x7ᵗʰ **V25.1 Motorcycle passenger injured in collision with railway train or railway vehicle in nontraffic accident**

     ✓x7ᵗʰ **V25.2 Unspecified motorcycle rider injured in collision with railway train or railway vehicle in nontraffic accident** ▽

     ✓x7ᵗʰ **V25.3 Person boarding or alighting a motorcycle injured in collision with railway train or railway vehicle**

     ✓x7ᵗʰ **V25.4 Motorcycle driver injured in collision with railway train or railway vehicle in traffic accident**

     ✓x7ᵗʰ **V25.5 Motorcycle passenger injured in collision with railway train or railway vehicle in traffic accident**

✓ Additional Character Req   ✓x7ᵗʰ Placeholder Alert   Manifestation   HCC CMS-HCC Condition   ▽ Unspecified Code   ▶◀ Revised Text   ● New Code   ▲ Revised Code Title

✓x7ᵗʰ **V25.9　Unspecified motorcycle rider injured in collision with** ▽
railway train or railway vehicle in traffic accident

✓4ᵗʰ **V26　Motorcycle rider injured in collision with other nonmotor vehicle**
　　INCLUDES　collision with animal-drawn vehicle, animal being ridden,
　　　　　　　streetcar

✓x7ᵗʰ **V26.0　Motorcycle driver injured in collision with other nonmotor
vehicle in nontraffic accident**

✓x7ᵗʰ **V26.1　Motorcycle passenger injured in collision with other
nonmotor vehicle in nontraffic accident**

✓x7ᵗʰ **V26.2　Unspecified motorcycle rider injured in collision with** ▽
other nonmotor vehicle in nontraffic accident

✓x7ᵗʰ **V26.3　Person boarding or alighting a motorcycle injured in collision
with other nonmotor vehicle**

✓x7ᵗʰ **V26.4　Motorcycle driver injured in collision with other nonmotor
vehicle in traffic accident**

✓x7ᵗʰ **V26.5　Motorcycle passenger injured in collision with other
nonmotor vehicle in traffic accident**

✓x7ᵗʰ **V26.9　Unspecified motorcycle rider injured in collision with** ▽
other nonmotor vehicle in traffic accident

✓4ᵗʰ **V27　Motorcycle rider injured in collision with fixed or stationary
object**

✓x7ᵗʰ **V27.0　Motorcycle driver injured in collision with fixed or stationary
object in nontraffic accident**

✓x7ᵗʰ **V27.1　Motorcycle passenger injured in collision with fixed or
stationary object in nontraffic accident**

✓x7ᵗʰ **V27.2　Unspecified motorcycle rider injured in collision with** ▽
fixed or stationary object in nontraffic accident

✓x7ᵗʰ **V27.3　Person boarding or alighting a motorcycle injured in collision
with fixed or stationary object**

✓x7ᵗʰ **V27.4　Motorcycle driver injured in collision with fixed or stationary
object in traffic accident**

✓x7ᵗʰ **V27.5　Motorcycle passenger injured in collision with fixed or
stationary object in traffic accident**

✓x7ᵗʰ **V27.9　Unspecified motorcycle rider injured in collision with** ▽
fixed or stationary object in traffic accident

✓4ᵗʰ **V28　Motorcycle rider injured in noncollision transport accident**
　　INCLUDES　fall or thrown from motorcycle (without antecedent
　　　　　　　collision)
　　　　　　　overturning motorcycle NOS
　　　　　　　overturning motorcycle without collision

✓x7ᵗʰ **V28.0　Motorcycle driver injured in noncollision transport accident
in nontraffic accident**

✓x7ᵗʰ **V28.1　Motorcycle passenger injured in noncollision transport
accident in nontraffic accident**

✓x7ᵗʰ **V28.2　Unspecified motorcycle rider injured in noncollision** ▽
transport accident in nontraffic accident

✓x7ᵗʰ **V28.3　Person boarding or alighting a motorcycle injured in
noncollision transport accident**

✓x7ᵗʰ **V28.4　Motorcycle driver injured in noncollision transport accident
in traffic accident**

✓x7ᵗʰ **V28.5　Motorcycle passenger injured in noncollision transport
accident in traffic accident**

✓x7ᵗʰ **V28.9　Unspecified motorcycle rider injured in noncollision** ▽
transport accident in traffic accident

✓4ᵗʰ **V29　Motorcycle rider injured in other and unspecified transport
accidents**

✓5ᵗʰ **V29.0　Motorcycle driver injured in collision with other and
unspecified motor vehicles in nontraffic accident**

✓x7ᵗʰ **V29.00　Motorcycle driver injured in collision with** ▽
unspecified motor vehicles in nontraffic accident

✓x7ᵗʰ **V29.09　Motorcycle driver injured in collision with other
motor vehicles in nontraffic accident**

✓5ᵗʰ **V29.1　Motorcycle passenger injured in collision with other and
unspecified motor vehicles in nontraffic accident**

✓x7ᵗʰ **V29.10　Motorcycle passenger injured in collision with** ▽
unspecified motor vehicles in nontraffic accident

✓x7ᵗʰ **V29.19　Motorcycle passenger injured in collision with
other motor vehicles in nontraffic accident**

✓5ᵗʰ **V29.2　Unspecified motorcycle rider injured in collision with other
and unspecified motor vehicles in nontraffic accident**

✓x7ᵗʰ **V29.20　Unspecified motorcycle rider injured in collision** ▽
with unspecified motor vehicles in nontraffic
accident**
Motorcycle collision NOS, nontraffic

✓x7ᵗʰ **V29.29　Unspecified motorcycle rider injured in collision** ▽
with other motor vehicles in nontraffic accident

✓x7ᵗʰ **V29.3　Motorcycle rider (driver) (passenger) injured in** ▽
unspecified nontraffic accident
　　Motorcycle accident NOS, nontraffic
　　Motorcycle rider injured in nontraffic accident NOS

✓5ᵗʰ **V29.4　Motorcycle driver injured in collision with other and
unspecified motor vehicles in traffic accident**

✓x7ᵗʰ **V29.40　Motorcycle driver injured in collision with** ▽
unspecified motor vehicles in traffic accident

✓x7ᵗʰ **V29.49　Motorcycle driver injured in collision with other
motor vehicles in traffic accident**

✓5ᵗʰ **V29.5　Motorcycle passenger injured in collision with other and
unspecified motor vehicles in traffic accident**

✓x7ᵗʰ **V29.50　Motorcycle passenger injured in collision with** ▽
unspecified motor vehicles in traffic accident

✓x7ᵗʰ **V29.59　Motorcycle passenger injured in collision with other
motor vehicles in traffic accident**

✓5ᵗʰ **V29.6　Unspecified motorcycle rider injured in collision with other
and unspecified motor vehicles in traffic accident**

✓x7ᵗʰ **V29.60　Unspecified motorcycle rider injured in collision** ▽
with unspecified motor vehicles in traffic accident
　　Motorcycle collision NOS (traffic)

✓x7ᵗʰ **V29.69　Unspecified motorcycle rider injured in collision
with other motor vehicles in traffic accident**

✓5ᵗʰ **V29.8　Motorcycle rider (driver) (passenger) injured in other
specified transport accidents**

✓x7ᵗʰ **V29.81　Motorcycle rider (driver) (passenger) injured in
transport accident with military vehicle**

✓x7ᵗʰ **V29.88　Motorcycle rider (driver) (passenger) injured in
other specified transport accidents**

✓x7ᵗʰ **V29.9　Motorcycle rider (driver) (passenger) injured in** ▽
unspecified traffic accident
　　Motorcycle accident NOS

Occupant of three-wheeled motor vehicle injured in transport accident (V30-V39)

　　INCLUDES　motorized rickshaw
　　　　　　　motorized tricycle
　　　　　　　three-wheeled motor car
　　EXCLUDES 1　all-terrain vehicles (V86.-)
　　　　　　　motorcycle with sidecar (V20-V29)
　　　　　　　vehicle designed primarily for off-road use (V86.-)

The appropriate 7th character is to be added to each code from
categories V30-V39.
A　　initial encounter
D　　subsequent encounter
S　　sequela

✓4ᵗʰ **V30　Occupant of three-wheeled motor vehicle injured in collision
with pedestrian or animal**
　　EXCLUDES 1　three-wheeled motor vehicle collision with animal-drawn
　　　　　　　vehicle or animal being ridden (V36.-)

✓x7ᵗʰ **V30.0　Driver of three-wheeled motor vehicle injured in collision
with pedestrian or animal in nontraffic accident**

✓x7ᵗʰ **V30.1　Passenger in three-wheeled motor vehicle injured in collision
with pedestrian or animal in nontraffic accident**

✓x7ᵗʰ **V30.2　Person on outside of three-wheeled motor vehicle injured in
collision with pedestrian or animal in nontraffic accident**

✓x7ᵗʰ **V30.3　Unspecified occupant of three-wheeled motor vehicle** ▽
injured in collision with pedestrian or animal in
nontraffic accident

✓x7ᵗʰ **V30.4　Person boarding or alighting a three-wheeled motor vehicle
injured in collision with pedestrian or animal**

✓x7ᵗʰ **V30.5　Driver of three-wheeled motor vehicle injured in collision
with pedestrian or animal in traffic accident**

✓x7ᵗʰ **V30.6　Passenger in three-wheeled motor vehicle injured in collision
with pedestrian or animal in traffic accident**

✓x7ᵗʰ **V30.7　Person on outside of three-wheeled motor vehicle injured in
collision with pedestrian or animal in traffic accident**

✓x7ᵗʰ **V30.9　Unspecified occupant of three-wheeled motor vehicle** ▽
injured in collision with pedestrian or animal in traffic
accident

✓4ᵗʰ **V31 Occupant of three-wheeled motor vehicle injured in collision with pedal cycle**

✓x7ᵗʰ V31.0 Driver of three-wheeled motor vehicle injured in collision with pedal cycle in nontraffic accident

✓x7ᵗʰ V31.1 Passenger in three-wheeled motor vehicle injured in collision with pedal cycle in nontraffic accident

✓x7ᵗʰ V31.2 Person on outside of three-wheeled motor vehicle injured in collision with pedal cycle in nontraffic accident

✓x7ᵗʰ V31.3 Unspecified occupant of three-wheeled motor vehicle injured in collision with pedal cycle in nontraffic accident ▽

✓x7ᵗʰ V31.4 Person boarding or alighting a three-wheeled motor vehicle injured in collision with pedal cycle

✓x7ᵗʰ V31.5 Driver of three-wheeled motor vehicle injured in collision with pedal cycle in traffic accident

✓x7ᵗʰ V31.6 Passenger in three-wheeled motor vehicle injured in collision with pedal cycle in traffic accident

✓x7ᵗʰ V31.7 Person on outside of three-wheeled motor vehicle injured in collision with pedal cycle in traffic accident

✓x7ᵗʰ V31.9 Unspecified occupant of three-wheeled motor vehicle injured in collision with pedal cycle in traffic accident ▽

✓4ᵗʰ **V32 Occupant of three-wheeled motor vehicle injured in collision with two- or three-wheeled motor vehicle**

✓x7ᵗʰ V32.0 Driver of three-wheeled motor vehicle injured in collision with two- or three-wheeled motor vehicle in nontraffic accident

✓x7ᵗʰ V32.1 Passenger in three-wheeled motor vehicle injured in collision with two- or three-wheeled motor vehicle in nontraffic accident

✓x7ᵗʰ V32.2 Person on outside of three-wheeled motor vehicle injured in collision with two- or three-wheeled motor vehicle in nontraffic accident

✓x7ᵗʰ V32.3 Unspecified occupant of three-wheeled motor vehicle injured in collision with two- or three-wheeled motor vehicle in nontraffic accident ▽

✓x7ᵗʰ V32.4 Person boarding or alighting a three-wheeled motor vehicle injured in collision with two- or three-wheeled motor vehicle

✓x7ᵗʰ V32.5 Driver of three-wheeled motor vehicle injured in collision with two- or three-wheeled motor vehicle in traffic accident

✓x7ᵗʰ V32.6 Passenger in three-wheeled motor vehicle injured in collision with two- or three-wheeled motor vehicle in traffic accident

✓x7ᵗʰ V32.7 Person on outside of three-wheeled motor vehicle injured in collision with two- or three-wheeled motor vehicle in traffic accident

✓x7ᵗʰ V32.9 Unspecified occupant of three-wheeled motor vehicle injured in collision with two- or three-wheeled motor vehicle in traffic accident ▽

✓4ᵗʰ **V33 Occupant of three-wheeled motor vehicle injured in collision with car, pick-up truck or van**

✓x7ᵗʰ V33.0 Driver of three-wheeled motor vehicle injured in collision with car, pick-up truck or van in nontraffic accident

✓x7ᵗʰ V33.1 Passenger in three-wheeled motor vehicle injured in collision with car, pick-up truck or van in nontraffic accident

✓x7ᵗʰ V33.2 Person on outside of three-wheeled motor vehicle injured in collision with car, pick-up truck or van in nontraffic accident

✓x7ᵗʰ V33.3 Unspecified occupant of three-wheeled motor vehicle injured in collision with car, pick-up truck or van in nontraffic accident ▽

✓x7ᵗʰ V33.4 Person boarding or alighting a three-wheeled motor vehicle injured in collision with car, pick-up truck or van

✓x7ᵗʰ V33.5 Driver of three-wheeled motor vehicle injured in collision with car, pick-up truck or van in traffic accident

✓x7ᵗʰ V33.6 Passenger in three-wheeled motor vehicle injured in collision with car, pick-up truck or van in traffic accident

✓x7ᵗʰ V33.7 Person on outside of three-wheeled motor vehicle injured in collision with car, pick-up truck or van in traffic accident

✓x7ᵗʰ V33.9 Unspecified occupant of three-wheeled motor vehicle injured in collision with car, pick-up truck or van in traffic accident ▽

✓4ᵗʰ **V34 Occupant of three-wheeled motor vehicle injured in collision with heavy transport vehicle or bus**

EXCLUDES 1 occupant of three-wheeled motor vehicle injured in collision with military vehicle (V39.81)

✓x7ᵗʰ V34.0 Driver of three-wheeled motor vehicle injured in collision with heavy transport vehicle or bus in nontraffic accident

✓x7ᵗʰ V34.1 Passenger in three-wheeled motor vehicle injured in collision with heavy transport vehicle or bus in nontraffic accident

✓x7ᵗʰ V34.2 Person on outside of three-wheeled motor vehicle injured in collision with heavy transport vehicle or bus in nontraffic accident

✓x7ᵗʰ V34.3 Unspecified occupant of three-wheeled motor vehicle injured in collision with heavy transport vehicle or bus in nontraffic accident ▽

✓x7ᵗʰ V34.4 Person boarding or alighting a three-wheeled motor vehicle injured in collision with heavy transport vehicle or bus

✓x7ᵗʰ V34.5 Driver of three-wheeled motor vehicle injured in collision with heavy transport vehicle or bus in traffic accident

✓x7ᵗʰ V34.6 Passenger in three-wheeled motor vehicle injured in collision with heavy transport vehicle or bus in traffic accident

✓x7ᵗʰ V34.7 Person on outside of three-wheeled motor vehicle injured in collision with heavy transport vehicle or bus in traffic accident

✓x7ᵗʰ V34.9 Unspecified occupant of three-wheeled motor vehicle injured in collision with heavy transport vehicle or bus in traffic accident ▽

✓4ᵗʰ **V35 Occupant of three-wheeled motor vehicle injured in collision with railway train or railway vehicle**

✓x7ᵗʰ V35.0 Driver of three-wheeled motor vehicle injured in collision with railway train or railway vehicle in nontraffic accident

✓x7ᵗʰ V35.1 Passenger in three-wheeled motor vehicle injured in collision with railway train or railway vehicle in nontraffic accident

✓x7ᵗʰ V35.2 Person on outside of three-wheeled motor vehicle injured in collision with railway train or railway vehicle in nontraffic accident

✓x7ᵗʰ V35.3 Unspecified occupant of three-wheeled motor vehicle injured in collision with railway train or railway vehicle in nontraffic accident ▽

✓x7ᵗʰ V35.4 Person boarding or alighting a three-wheeled motor vehicle injured in collision with railway train or railway vehicle

✓x7ᵗʰ V35.5 Driver of three-wheeled motor vehicle injured in collision with railway train or railway vehicle in traffic accident

✓x7ᵗʰ V35.6 Passenger in three-wheeled motor vehicle injured in collision with railway train or railway vehicle in traffic accident

✓x7ᵗʰ V35.7 Person on outside of three-wheeled motor vehicle injured in collision with railway train or railway vehicle in traffic accident

✓x7ᵗʰ V35.9 Unspecified occupant of three-wheeled motor vehicle injured in collision with railway train or railway vehicle in traffic accident ▽

✓4ᵗʰ **V36 Occupant of three-wheeled motor vehicle injured in collision with other nonmotor vehicle**

INCLUDES collision with animal-drawn vehicle, animal being ridden, streetcar

✓x7ᵗʰ V36.0 Driver of three-wheeled motor vehicle injured in collision with other nonmotor vehicle in nontraffic accident

✓x7ᵗʰ V36.1 Passenger in three-wheeled motor vehicle injured in collision with other nonmotor vehicle in nontraffic accident

✓x7ᵗʰ V36.2 Person on outside of three-wheeled motor vehicle injured in collision with other nonmotor vehicle in nontraffic accident

✓x7ᵗʰ V36.3 Unspecified occupant of three-wheeled motor vehicle injured in collision with other nonmotor vehicle in nontraffic accident ▽

✓x7ᵗʰ V36.4 Person boarding or alighting a three-wheeled motor vehicle injured in collision with other nonmotor vehicle

✓x7ᵗʰ V36.5 Driver of three-wheeled motor vehicle injured in collision with other nonmotor vehicle in traffic accident

✓x7ᵗʰ V36.6 Passenger in three-wheeled motor vehicle injured in collision with other nonmotor vehicle in traffic accident

✓x7ᵗʰ V36.7 Person on outside of three-wheeled motor vehicle injured in collision with other nonmotor vehicle in traffic accident

✓x7ᵗʰ V36.9 Unspecified occupant of three-wheeled motor vehicle injured in collision with other nonmotor vehicle in traffic accident ▽

✓4ᵗʰ **V37 Occupant of three-wheeled motor vehicle injured in collision with fixed or stationary object**

✓x7ᵗʰ V37.0 Driver of three-wheeled motor vehicle injured in collision with fixed or stationary object in nontraffic accident

✓x7ᵗʰ V37.1 Passenger in three-wheeled motor vehicle injured in collision with fixed or stationary object in nontraffic accident

---

☑ Additional Character Req   ✓x7ᵗʰ Placeholder Alert   Manifestation   HCC CMS-HCC Condition   ▽ Unspecified Code   ▶◀ Revised Text   ● New Code   ▲ Revised Code Title

✓x 7ᵗʰ **V37.2** Person on outside of three-wheeled motor vehicle injured in collision with fixed or stationary object in nontraffic accident

✓x 7ᵗʰ **V37.3** Unspecified occupant of three-wheeled motor vehicle injured in collision with fixed or stationary object in nontraffic accident ▽

✓x 7ᵗʰ **V37.4** Person boarding or alighting a three-wheeled motor vehicle injured in collision with fixed or stationary object

✓x 7ᵗʰ **V37.5** Driver of three-wheeled motor vehicle injured in collision with fixed or stationary object in traffic accident

✓x 7ᵗʰ **V37.6** Passenger in three-wheeled motor vehicle injured in collision with fixed or stationary object in traffic accident

✓x 7ᵗʰ **V37.7** Person on outside of three-wheeled motor vehicle injured in collision with fixed or stationary object in traffic accident

✓x 7ᵗʰ **V37.9** Unspecified occupant of three-wheeled motor vehicle injured in collision with fixed or stationary object in traffic accident ▽

✓4ᵗʰ **V38** Occupant of three-wheeled motor vehicle injured in noncollision transport accident

     INCLUDES   fall or thrown from three-wheeled motor vehicle
           overturning of three-wheeled motor vehicle NOS
           overturning of three-wheeled motor vehicle without collision

✓x 7ᵗʰ **V38.0** Driver of three-wheeled motor vehicle injured in noncollision transport accident in nontraffic accident

✓x 7ᵗʰ **V38.1** Passenger in three-wheeled motor vehicle injured in noncollision transport accident in nontraffic accident

✓x 7ᵗʰ **V38.2** Person on outside of three-wheeled motor vehicle injured in noncollision transport accident in nontraffic accident

✓x 7ᵗʰ **V38.3** Unspecified occupant of three-wheeled motor vehicle injured in noncollision transport accident in nontraffic accident ▽

✓x 7ᵗʰ **V38.4** Person boarding or alighting a three-wheeled motor vehicle injured in noncollision transport accident

✓x 7ᵗʰ **V38.5** Driver of three-wheeled motor vehicle injured in noncollision transport accident in traffic accident

✓x 7ᵗʰ **V38.6** Passenger in three-wheeled motor vehicle injured in noncollision transport accident in traffic accident

✓x 7ᵗʰ **V38.7** Person on outside of three-wheeled motor vehicle injured in noncollision transport accident in traffic accident

✓x 7ᵗʰ **V38.9** Unspecified occupant of three-wheeled motor vehicle injured in noncollision transport accident in traffic accident ▽

✓4ᵗʰ **V39** Occupant of three-wheeled motor vehicle injured in other and unspecified transport accidents

✓5ᵗʰ **V39.0** Driver of three-wheeled motor vehicle injured in collision with other and unspecified motor vehicles in nontraffic accident

    ✓x 7ᵗʰ **V39.00** Driver of three-wheeled motor vehicle injured in collision with unspecified motor vehicles in nontraffic accident ▽

    ✓x 7ᵗʰ **V39.09** Driver of three-wheeled motor vehicle injured in collision with other motor vehicles in nontraffic accident

✓5ᵗʰ **V39.1** Passenger in three-wheeled motor vehicle injured in collision with other and unspecified motor vehicles in nontraffic accident

    ✓x 7ᵗʰ **V39.10** Passenger in three-wheeled motor vehicle injured in collision with unspecified motor vehicles in nontraffic accident ▽

    ✓x 7ᵗʰ **V39.19** Passenger in three-wheeled motor vehicle injured in collision with other motor vehicles in nontraffic accident

✓5ᵗʰ **V39.2** Unspecified occupant of three-wheeled motor vehicle injured in collision with other and unspecified motor vehicles in nontraffic accident

    ✓x 7ᵗʰ **V39.20** Unspecified occupant of three-wheeled motor vehicle injured in collision with unspecified motor vehicles in nontraffic accident ▽
         Collision NOS involving three-wheeled motor vehicle, nontraffic

    ✓x 7ᵗʰ **V39.29** Unspecified occupant of three-wheeled motor vehicle injured in collision with other motor vehicles in nontraffic accident ▽

✓x 7ᵗʰ **V39.3** Occupant (driver) (passenger) of three-wheeled motor vehicle injured in unspecified nontraffic accident ▽
     Accident NOS involving three-wheeled motor vehicle, nontraffic
     Occupant of three-wheeled motor vehicle injured in nontraffic accident NOS

✓5ᵗʰ **V39.4** Driver of three-wheeled motor vehicle injured in collision with other and unspecified motor vehicles in traffic accident

    ✓x 7ᵗʰ **V39.40** Driver of three-wheeled motor vehicle injured in collision with unspecified motor vehicles in traffic accident ▽

    ✓x 7ᵗʰ **V39.49** Driver of three-wheeled motor vehicle injured in collision with other motor vehicles in traffic accident

✓5ᵗʰ **V39.5** Passenger in three-wheeled motor vehicle injured in collision with other and unspecified motor vehicles in traffic accident

    ✓x 7ᵗʰ **V39.50** Passenger in three-wheeled motor vehicle injured in collision with unspecified motor vehicles in traffic accident ▽

    ✓x 7ᵗʰ **V39.59** Passenger in three-wheeled motor vehicle injured in collision with other motor vehicles in traffic accident

✓5ᵗʰ **V39.6** Unspecified occupant of three-wheeled motor vehicle injured in collision with other and unspecified motor vehicles in traffic accident

    ✓x 7ᵗʰ **V39.60** Unspecified occupant of three-wheeled motor vehicle injured in collision with unspecified motor vehicles in traffic accident ▽
         Collision NOS involving three-wheeled motor vehicle (traffic)

    ✓x 7ᵗʰ **V39.69** Unspecified occupant of three-wheeled motor vehicle injured in collision with other motor vehicles in traffic accident ▽

✓5ᵗʰ **V39.8** Occupant (driver) (passenger) of three-wheeled motor vehicle injured in other specified transport accidents

    ✓x 7ᵗʰ **V39.81** Occupant (driver) (passenger) of three-wheeled motor vehicle injured in transport accident with military vehicle

    ✓x 7ᵗʰ **V39.89** Occupant (driver) (passenger) of three-wheeled motor vehicle injured in other specified transport accidents

✓x 7ᵗʰ **V39.9** Occupant (driver) (passenger) of three-wheeled motor vehicle injured in unspecified traffic accident ▽
     Accident NOS involving three-wheeled motor vehicle

Car occupant injured in transport accident (V40-V49)

     INCLUDES   a four-wheeled motor vehicle designed primarily for carrying passengers
           automobile (pulling a trailer or camper)

     EXCLUDES 1   bus (V50-V59)
           minibus (V50-V59)
           minivan (V50-V59)
           motorcoach (V70-V79)
           pick-up truck (V50-V59)
           sport utility vehicle (SUV) (V50-V59)

> The appropriate 7th character is to be added to each code from categories V40-V49.
> A   initial encounter
> D   subsequent encounter
> S   sequela

✓4ᵗʰ **V40** Car occupant injured in collision with pedestrian or animal
     EXCLUDES 1   car collision with animal-drawn vehicle or animal being ridden (V46.-)

✓x 7ᵗʰ **V40.0** Car driver injured in collision with pedestrian or animal in nontraffic accident

✓x 7ᵗʰ **V40.1** Car passenger injured in collision with pedestrian or animal in nontraffic accident

✓x 7ᵗʰ **V40.2** Person on outside of car injured in collision with pedestrian or animal in nontraffic accident

✓x 7ᵗʰ **V40.3** Unspecified car occupant injured in collision with pedestrian or animal in nontraffic accident ▽

✓x 7ᵗʰ **V40.4** Person boarding or alighting a car injured in collision with pedestrian or animal

✓x 7ᵗʰ **V40.5** Car driver injured in collision with pedestrian or animal in traffic accident

✓x 7ᵗʰ **V40.6** Car passenger injured in collision with pedestrian or animal in traffic accident

✓x 7ᵗʰ **V40.7** Person on outside of car injured in collision with pedestrian or animal in traffic accident

EXCLUDES 1 Not coded here   EXCLUDES 2 Not included here   N Newborn Age: 0   P Pediatric Age: 0-17   M Maternity Age: 12-55   A Adult Age: 15-124

1126   ICD-10-CM 2018

√x7ᵗʰ **V40.9** Unspecified car occupant injured in collision with pedestrian or animal in traffic accident ▽

✓4ᵗʰ **V41 Car occupant injured in collision with pedal cycle**

√x7ᵗʰ **V41.0** Car driver injured in collision with pedal cycle in nontraffic accident

√x7ᵗʰ **V41.1** Car passenger injured in collision with pedal cycle in nontraffic accident

√x7ᵗʰ **V41.2** Person on outside of car injured in collision with pedal cycle in nontraffic accident

√x7ᵗʰ **V41.3** Unspecified car occupant injured in collision with pedal cycle in nontraffic accident ▽

√x7ᵗʰ **V41.4** Person boarding or alighting a car injured in collision with pedal cycle

√x7ᵗʰ **V41.5** Car driver injured in collision with pedal cycle in traffic accident

√x7ᵗʰ **V41.6** Car passenger injured in collision with pedal cycle in traffic accident

√x7ᵗʰ **V41.7** Person on outside of car injured in collision with pedal cycle in traffic accident

√x7ᵗʰ **V41.9** Unspecified car occupant injured in collision with pedal cycle in traffic accident ▽

✓4ᵗʰ **V42 Car occupant injured in collision with two- or three-wheeled motor vehicle**

√x7ᵗʰ **V42.0** Car driver injured in collision with two- or three-wheeled motor vehicle in nontraffic accident

√x7ᵗʰ **V42.1** Car passenger injured in collision with two- or three-wheeled motor vehicle in nontraffic accident

√x7ᵗʰ **V42.2** Person on outside of car injured in collision with two- or three-wheeled motor vehicle in nontraffic accident

√x7ᵗʰ **V42.3** Unspecified car occupant injured in collision with two- or three-wheeled motor vehicle in nontraffic accident ▽

√x7ᵗʰ **V42.4** Person boarding or alighting a car injured in collision with two- or three-wheeled motor vehicle

√x7ᵗʰ **V42.5** Car driver injured in collision with two- or three-wheeled motor vehicle in traffic accident

√x7ᵗʰ **V42.6** Car passenger injured in collision with two- or three-wheeled motor vehicle in traffic accident

√x7ᵗʰ **V42.7** Person on outside of car injured in collision with two- or three-wheeled motor vehicle in traffic accident

√x7ᵗʰ **V42.9** Unspecified car occupant injured in collision with two- or three-wheeled motor vehicle in traffic accident ▽

✓4ᵗʰ **V43 Car occupant injured in collision with car, pick-up truck or van**

✓5ᵗʰ **V43.0** Car driver injured in collision with car, pick-up truck or van in nontraffic accident

√x7ᵗʰ **V43.01** Car driver injured in collision with sport utility vehicle in nontraffic accident

√x7ᵗʰ **V43.02** Car driver injured in collision with other type car in nontraffic accident

√x7ᵗʰ **V43.03** Car driver injured in collision with pick-up truck in nontraffic accident

√x7ᵗʰ **V43.04** Car driver injured in collision with van in nontraffic accident

✓5ᵗʰ **V43.1** Car passenger injured in collision with car, pick-up truck or van in nontraffic accident

√x7ᵗʰ **V43.11** Car passenger injured in collision with sport utility vehicle in nontraffic accident

√x7ᵗʰ **V43.12** Car passenger injured in collision with other type car in nontraffic accident

√x7ᵗʰ **V43.13** Car passenger injured in collision with pick-up in nontraffic accident

√x7ᵗʰ **V43.14** Car passenger injured in collision with van in nontraffic accident

✓5ᵗʰ **V43.2** Person on outside of car injured in collision with car, pick-up truck or van in nontraffic accident

√x7ᵗʰ **V43.21** Person on outside of car injured in collision with sport utility vehicle in nontraffic accident

√x7ᵗʰ **V43.22** Person on outside of car injured in collision with other type car in nontraffic accident

√x7ᵗʰ **V43.23** Person on outside of car injured in collision with pick-up truck in nontraffic accident

√x7ᵗʰ **V43.24** Person on outside of car injured in collision with van in nontraffic accident

✓5ᵗʰ **V43.3** Unspecified car occupant injured in collision with car, pick-up truck or van in nontraffic accident

√x7ᵗʰ **V43.31** Unspecified car occupant injured in collision with sport utility vehicle in nontraffic accident ▽

√x7ᵗʰ **V43.32** Unspecified car occupant injured in collision with other type car in nontraffic accident ▽

√x7ᵗʰ **V43.33** Unspecified car occupant injured in collision with pick-up truck in nontraffic accident ▽

√x7ᵗʰ **V43.34** Unspecified car occupant injured in collision with van in nontraffic accident ▽

✓5ᵗʰ **V43.4** Person boarding or alighting a car injured in collision with car, pick-up truck or van

√x7ᵗʰ **V43.41** Person boarding or alighting a car injured in collision with sport utility vehicle

√x7ᵗʰ **V43.42** Person boarding or alighting a car injured in collision with other type car

√x7ᵗʰ **V43.43** Person boarding or alighting a car injured in collision with pick-up truck

√x7ᵗʰ **V43.44** Person boarding or alighting a car injured in collision with van

✓5ᵗʰ **V43.5** Car driver injured in collision with car, pick-up truck or van in traffic accident

√x7ᵗʰ **V43.51** Car driver injured in collision with sport utility vehicle in traffic accident

√x7ᵗʰ **V43.52** Car driver injured in collision with other type car in traffic accident

√x7ᵗʰ **V43.53** Car driver injured in collision with pick-up truck in traffic accident

√x7ᵗʰ **V43.54** Car driver injured in collision with van in traffic accident

✓5ᵗʰ **V43.6** Car passenger injured in collision with car, pick-up truck or van in traffic accident

√x7ᵗʰ **V43.61** Car passenger injured in collision with sport utility vehicle in traffic accident

√x7ᵗʰ **V43.62** Car passenger injured in collision with other type car in traffic accident

√x7ᵗʰ **V43.63** Car passenger injured in collision with pick-up truck in traffic accident

√x7ᵗʰ **V43.64** Car passenger injured in collision with van in traffic accident

✓5ᵗʰ **V43.7** Person on outside of car injured in collision with car, pick-up truck or van in traffic accident

√x7ᵗʰ **V43.71** Person on outside of car injured in collision with sport utility vehicle in traffic accident

√x7ᵗʰ **V43.72** Person on outside of car injured in collision with other type car in traffic accident

√x7ᵗʰ **V43.73** Person on outside of car injured in collision with pick-up truck in traffic accident

√x7ᵗʰ **V43.74** Person on outside of car injured in collision with van in traffic accident

✓5ᵗʰ **V43.9** Unspecified car occupant injured in collision with car, pick-up truck or van in traffic accident

√x7ᵗʰ **V43.91** Unspecified car occupant injured in collision with sport utility vehicle in traffic accident ▽

√x7ᵗʰ **V43.92** Unspecified car occupant injured in collision with other type car in traffic accident ▽

√x7ᵗʰ **V43.93** Unspecified car occupant injured in collision with pick-up truck in traffic accident ▽

√x7ᵗʰ **V43.94** Unspecified car occupant injured in collision with van in traffic accident ▽

✓4ᵗʰ **V44 Car occupant injured in collision with heavy transport vehicle or bus**

> **EXCLUDES 1**   car occupant injured in collision with military vehicle (V49.81)

√x7ᵗʰ **V44.0** Car driver injured in collision with heavy transport vehicle or bus in nontraffic accident

√x7ᵗʰ **V44.1** Car passenger injured in collision with heavy transport vehicle or bus in nontraffic accident

√x7ᵗʰ **V44.2** Person on outside of car injured in collision with heavy transport vehicle or bus in nontraffic accident

√x7ᵗʰ **V44.3** Unspecified car occupant injured in collision with heavy transport vehicle or bus in nontraffic accident ▽

√x7ᵗʰ **V44.4** Person boarding or alighting a car injured in collision with heavy transport vehicle or bus

---

✓ Additional Character Req   √x7ᵗʰ Placeholder Alert   Manifestation   HCC CMS-HCC Condition   ▽ Unspecified Code   ►◄ Revised Text   ● New Code   ▲ Revised Code Title

√x 7th **V44.5** Car **driver** injured in collision with heavy transport vehicle or bus in traffic accident

√x 7th **V44.6** Car **passenger** injured in collision with heavy transport vehicle or bus in traffic accident

√x 7th **V44.7** **Person on outside** of car injured in collision with heavy transport vehicle or bus in traffic accident

√x 7th **V44.9** Unspecified car occupant injured in collision with heavy ▽ transport vehicle or bus in traffic accident

√4th **V45** **Car occupant injured in collision with railway train or railway vehicle**

√x 7th **V45.0** Car **driver** injured in collision with railway train or railway vehicle in nontraffic accident

√x 7th **V45.1** Car **passenger** injured in collision with railway train or railway vehicle in nontraffic accident

√x 7th **V45.2** **Person on outside** of car injured in collision with railway train or railway vehicle in nontraffic accident

√x 7th **V45.3** Unspecified car occupant injured in collision with ▽ railway train or railway vehicle in nontraffic accident

√x 7th **V45.4** **Person boarding or alighting** a car injured in collision with railway train or railway vehicle

√x 7th **V45.5** Car **driver** injured in collision with railway train or railway vehicle in traffic accident

√x 7th **V45.6** Car **passenger** injured in collision with railway train or railway vehicle in traffic accident

√x 7th **V45.7** **Person on outside** of car injured in collision with railway train or railway vehicle in traffic accident

√x 7th **V45.9** Unspecified car occupant injured in collision with ▽ railway train or railway vehicle in traffic accident

√4th **V46** **Car occupant injured in collision with other nonmotor vehicle**
> INCLUDES   collision with animal-drawn vehicle, animal being ridden, streetcar

√x 7th **V46.0** Car **driver** injured in collision with other nonmotor vehicle in nontraffic accident

√x 7th **V46.1** Car **passenger** injured in collision with other nonmotor vehicle in nontraffic accident

√x 7th **V46.2** **Person on outside** of car injured in collision with other nonmotor vehicle in nontraffic accident

√x 7th **V46.3** Unspecified car occupant injured in collision with other ▽ nonmotor vehicle in nontraffic accident

√x 7th **V46.4** **Person boarding or alighting** a car injured in collision with other nonmotor vehicle

√x 7th **V46.5** Car **driver** injured in collision with other nonmotor vehicle in traffic accident

√x 7th **V46.6** Car **passenger** injured in collision with other nonmotor vehicle in traffic accident

√x 7th **V46.7** **Person on outside** of car injured in collision with other nonmotor vehicle in traffic accident

√x 7th **V46.9** Unspecified car occupant injured in collision with other ▽ nonmotor vehicle in traffic accident

√4th **V47** **Car occupant injured in collision with fixed or stationary object**

√x 7th **V47.0** Car **driver** injured in collision with fixed or stationary object in nontraffic accident

√x 7th **V47.1** Car **passenger** injured in collision with fixed or stationary object in nontraffic accident

√x 7th **V47.2** **Person on outside** of car injured in collision with fixed or stationary object in nontraffic accident

√x 7th **V47.3** Unspecified car occupant injured in collision with fixed ▽ or stationary object in nontraffic accident

√x 7th **V47.4** **Person boarding or alighting** a car injured in collision with fixed or stationary object

√x 7th **V47.5** Car **driver** injured in collision with fixed or stationary object in traffic accident

√x 7th **V47.6** Car **passenger** injured in collision with fixed or stationary object in traffic accident

√x 7th **V47.7** **Person on outside** of car injured in collision with fixed or stationary object in traffic accident

√x 7th **V47.9** Unspecified car occupant injured in collision with fixed or ▽ stationary object in traffic accident

√4th **V48** **Car occupant injured in noncollision transport accident**
> INCLUDES   overturning car NOS
> overturning car without collision

√x 7th **V48.0** Car **driver** injured in noncollision transport accident in nontraffic accident

√x 7th **V48.1** Car **passenger** injured in noncollision transport accident in nontraffic accident

√x 7th **V48.2** **Person on outside** of car injured in noncollision transport accident in nontraffic accident

√x 7th **V48.3** Unspecified car occupant injured in noncollision ▽ transport accident in nontraffic accident

√x 7th **V48.4** **Person boarding or alighting** a car injured in noncollision transport accident

√x 7th **V48.5** Car **driver** injured in noncollision transport accident in traffic accident

√x 7th **V48.6** Car **passenger** injured in noncollision transport accident in traffic accident

√x 7th **V48.7** **Person on outside** of car injured in noncollision transport accident in traffic accident

√x 7th **V48.9** Unspecified car occupant injured in noncollision ▽ transport accident in traffic accident

√4th **V49** **Car occupant injured in other and unspecified transport accidents**

√5th **V49.0** **Driver** injured in collision with other and unspecified motor vehicles in nontraffic accident

   √x 7th **V49.00** Driver injured in collision with unspecified motor ▽ vehicles in nontraffic accident

   √x 7th **V49.09** Driver injured in collision with other motor vehicles in nontraffic accident

√5th **V49.1** **Passenger** injured in collision with other and unspecified motor vehicles in nontraffic accident

   √x 7th **V49.10** Passenger injured in collision with unspecified ▽ motor vehicles in nontraffic accident

   √x 7th **V49.19** Passenger injured in collision with other motor vehicles in nontraffic accident

√5th **V49.2** Unspecified car occupant injured in collision with other and unspecified motor vehicles in nontraffic accident

   √x 7th **V49.20** Unspecified car occupant injured in collision with ▽ unspecified motor vehicles in nontraffic accident
       Car collision NOS, nontraffic

   √x 7th **V49.29** Unspecified car occupant injured in collision with ▽ other motor vehicles in nontraffic accident

√x 7th **V49.3** Car occupant (driver) (passenger) injured in unspecified ▽ nontraffic accident
    Car accident NOS, nontraffic
    Car occupant injured in nontraffic accident NOS

√5th **V49.4** **Driver** injured in collision with other and unspecified motor vehicles in traffic accident

   √x 7th **V49.40** Driver injured in collision with unspecified ▽ motor vehicles in traffic accident

   √x 7th **V49.49** Driver injured in collision with other motor vehicles in traffic accident

√5th **V49.5** **Passenger** injured in collision with other and unspecified motor vehicles in traffic accident

   √x 7th **V49.50** Passenger injured in collision with unspecified ▽ motor vehicles in traffic accident

   √x 7th **V49.59** Passenger injured in collision with other motor vehicles in traffic accident

√5th **V49.6** Unspecified car occupant injured in collision with other and unspecified motor vehicles in traffic accident

   √x 7th **V49.60** Unspecified car occupant injured in collision ▽ with unspecified motor vehicles in traffic accident
       Car collision NOS (traffic)

   √x 7th **V49.69** Unspecified car occupant injured in collision ▽ with other motor vehicles in traffic accident

√5th **V49.8** Car occupant (driver) (passenger) injured in other specified transport accidents

   √x 7th **V49.81** Car occupant (driver) (passenger) injured in transport accident with military vehicle

   √x 7th **V49.88** Car occupant (driver) (passenger) injured in other specified transport accidents

√x 7th **V49.9** Car occupant (driver) (passenger) injured in unspecified ▽ traffic accident
    Car accident NOS

EXCLUDES 1 Not coded here   EXCLUDES 2 Not included here   N Newborn Age: 0   P Pediatric Age: 0-17   M Maternity Age: 12-55   A Adult Age: 15-124

Occupant of pick-up truck or van injured in transport accident (V50-V59)

INCLUDES a four or six wheel motor vehicle designed primarily for carrying passengers and property but weighing less than the local limit for classification as a heavy goods vehicle

minibus
minivan
sport utility vehicle (SUV)
truck
van

EXCLUDES 1 heavy transport vehicle (V60-V69)

The appropriate 7th character is to be added to each code from categories V50-V59.
A   initial encounter
D   subsequent encounter
S   sequela

✓4th V50 Occupant of pick-up truck or van injured in collision with pedestrian or animal

EXCLUDES 1 pick-up truck or van collision with animal-drawn vehicle or animal being ridden (V56.-)

- ✓x7th **V50.0** Driver of pick-up truck or van injured in collision with pedestrian or animal in nontraffic accident
- ✓x7th **V50.1** Passenger in pick-up truck or van injured in collision with pedestrian or animal in nontraffic accident
- ✓x7th **V50.2** Person on outside of pick-up truck or van injured in collision with pedestrian or animal in nontraffic accident
- ✓x7th **V50.3** Unspecified occupant of pick-up truck or van injured in collision with pedestrian or animal in nontraffic accident ▽
- ✓x7th **V50.4** Person boarding or alighting a pick-up truck or van injured in collision with pedestrian or animal
- ✓x7th **V50.5** Driver of pick-up truck or van injured in collision with pedestrian or animal in traffic accident
- ✓x7th **V50.6** Passenger in pick-up truck or van injured in collision with pedestrian or animal in traffic accident
- ✓x7th **V50.7** Person on outside of pick-up truck or van injured in collision with pedestrian or animal in traffic accident
- ✓x7th **V50.9** Unspecified occupant of pick-up truck or van injured in collision with pedestrian or animal in traffic accident ▽

✓4th V51 Occupant of pick-up truck or van injured in collision with pedal cycle

- ✓x7th **V51.0** Driver of pick-up truck or van injured in collision with pedal cycle in nontraffic accident
- ✓x7th **V51.1** Passenger in pick-up truck or van injured in collision with pedal cycle in nontraffic accident
- ✓x7th **V51.2** Person on outside of pick-up truck or van injured in collision with pedal cycle in nontraffic accident
- ✓x7th **V51.3** Unspecified occupant of pick-up truck or van injured in collision with pedal cycle in nontraffic accident ▽
- ✓x7th **V51.4** Person boarding or alighting a pick-up truck or van injured in collision with pedal cycle
- ✓x7th **V51.5** Driver of pick-up truck or van injured in collision with pedal cycle in traffic accident
- ✓x7th **V51.6** Passenger in pick-up truck or van injured in collision with pedal cycle in traffic accident
- ✓x7th **V51.7** Person on outside of pick-up truck or van injured in collision with pedal cycle in traffic accident
- ✓x7th **V51.9** Unspecified occupant of pick-up truck or van injured in collision with pedal cycle in traffic accident ▽

✓4th V52 Occupant of pick-up truck or van injured in collision with two- or three-wheeled motor vehicle

- ✓x7th **V52.0** Driver of pick-up truck or van injured in collision with two- or three-wheeled motor vehicle in nontraffic accident
- ✓x7th **V52.1** Passenger in pick-up truck or van injured in collision with two- or three-wheeled motor vehicle in nontraffic accident
- ✓x7th **V52.2** Person on outside of pick-up truck or van injured in collision with two- or three-wheeled motor vehicle in nontraffic accident
- ✓x7th **V52.3** Unspecified occupant of pick-up truck or van injured in collision with two- or three-wheeled motor vehicle in nontraffic accident ▽
- ✓x7th **V52.4** Person boarding or alighting a pick-up truck or van injured in collision with two- or three-wheeled motor vehicle
- ✓x7th **V52.5** Driver of pick-up truck or van injured in collision with two- or three-wheeled motor vehicle in traffic accident

- ✓x7th **V52.6** Passenger in pick-up truck or van injured in collision with two- or three-wheeled motor vehicle in traffic accident
- ✓x7th **V52.7** Person on outside of pick-up truck or van injured in collision with two- or three-wheeled motor vehicle in traffic accident
- ✓x7th **V52.9** Unspecified occupant of pick-up truck or van injured in collision with two- or three-wheeled motor vehicle in traffic accident ▽

✓4th V53 Occupant of pick-up truck or van injured in collision with car, pick-up truck or van

- ✓x7th **V53.0** Driver of pick-up truck or van injured in collision with car, pick-up truck or van in nontraffic accident
- ✓x7th **V53.1** Passenger in pick-up truck or van injured in collision with car, pick-up truck or van in nontraffic accident
- ✓x7th **V53.2** Person on outside of pick-up truck or van injured in collision with car, pick-up truck or van in nontraffic accident
- ✓x7th **V53.3** Unspecified occupant of pick-up truck or van injured in collision with car, pick-up truck or van in nontraffic accident ▽
- ✓x7th **V53.4** Person boarding or alighting a pick-up truck or van injured in collision with car, pick-up truck or van
- ✓x7th **V53.5** Driver of pick-up truck or van injured in collision with car, pick-up truck or van in traffic accident
- ✓x7th **V53.6** Passenger in pick-up truck or van injured in collision with car, pick-up truck or van in traffic accident
- ✓x7th **V53.7** Person on outside of pick-up truck or van injured in collision with car, pick-up truck or van in traffic accident
- ✓x7th **V53.9** Unspecified occupant of pick-up truck or van injured in collision with car, pick-up truck or van in traffic accident ▽

✓4th V54 Occupant of pick-up truck or van injured in collision with heavy transport vehicle or bus

EXCLUDES 1 occupant of pick-up truck or van injured in collision with military vehicle (V59.81)

- ✓x7th **V54.0** Driver of pick-up truck or van injured in collision with heavy transport vehicle or bus in nontraffic accident
- ✓x7th **V54.1** Passenger in pick-up truck or van injured in collision with heavy transport vehicle or bus in nontraffic accident
- ✓x7th **V54.2** Person on outside of pick-up truck or van injured in collision with heavy transport vehicle or bus in nontraffic accident
- ✓x7th **V54.3** Unspecified occupant of pick-up truck or van injured in collision with heavy transport vehicle or bus in nontraffic accident ▽
- ✓x7th **V54.4** Person boarding or alighting a pick-up truck or van injured in collision with heavy transport vehicle or bus
- ✓x7th **V54.5** Driver of pick-up truck or van injured in collision with heavy transport vehicle or bus in traffic accident
- ✓x7th **V54.6** Passenger in pick-up truck or van injured in collision with heavy transport vehicle or bus in traffic accident
- ✓x7th **V54.7** Person on outside of pick-up truck or van injured in collision with heavy transport vehicle or bus in traffic accident
- ✓x7th **V54.9** Unspecified occupant of pick-up truck or van injured in collision with heavy transport vehicle or bus in traffic accident ▽

✓4th V55 Occupant of pick-up truck or van injured in collision with railway train or railway vehicle

- ✓x7th **V55.0** Driver of pick-up truck or van injured in collision with railway train or railway vehicle in nontraffic accident
- ✓x7th **V55.1** Passenger in pick-up truck or van injured in collision with railway train or railway vehicle in nontraffic accident
- ✓x7th **V55.2** Person on outside of pick-up truck or van injured in collision with railway train or railway vehicle in nontraffic accident
- ✓x7th **V55.3** Unspecified occupant of pick-up truck or van injured in collision with railway train or railway vehicle in nontraffic accident ▽
- ✓x7th **V55.4** Person boarding or alighting a pick-up truck or van injured in collision with railway train or railway vehicle
- ✓x7th **V55.5** Driver of pick-up truck or van injured in collision with railway train or railway vehicle in traffic accident
- ✓x7th **V55.6** Passenger in pick-up truck or van injured in collision with railway train or railway vehicle in traffic accident
- ✓x7th **V55.7** Person on outside of pick-up truck or van injured in collision with railway train or railway vehicle in traffic accident
- ✓x7th **V55.9** Unspecified occupant of pick-up truck or van injured in collision with railway train or railway vehicle in traffic accident ▽

✓ Additional Character Req ✓x7 Placeholder Alert Manifestation HCC CMS-HCC Condition ▽ Unspecified Code ▶◀ Revised Text ● New Code ▲ Revised Code Title

ICD-10-CM 2018   1129

✓4th **V56 Occupant of pick-up truck or van injured in collision with other nonmotor vehicle**
> INCLUDES   collision with animal-drawn vehicle, animal being ridden, streetcar

✓x7th **V56.0** Driver of pick-up truck or van injured in collision with other nonmotor vehicle in nontraffic accident

✓x7th **V56.1** Passenger in pick-up truck or van injured in collision with other nonmotor vehicle in nontraffic accident

✓x7th **V56.2** Person on outside of pick-up truck or van injured in collision with other nonmotor vehicle in nontraffic accident

✓x7th **V56.3** Unspecified occupant of pick-up truck or van injured in ▽ collision with other nonmotor vehicle in nontraffic accident

✓x7th **V56.4** Person boarding or alighting a pick-up truck or van injured in collision with other nonmotor vehicle

✓x7th **V56.5** Driver of pick-up truck or van injured in collision with other nonmotor vehicle in traffic accident

✓x7th **V56.6** Passenger in pick-up truck or van injured in collision with other nonmotor vehicle in traffic accident

✓x7th **V56.7** Person on outside of pick-up truck or van injured in collision with other nonmotor vehicle in traffic accident

✓x7th **V56.9** Unspecified occupant of pick-up truck or van injured in ▽ collision with other nonmotor vehicle in traffic accident

✓4th **V57 Occupant of pick-up truck or van injured in collision with fixed or stationary object**

✓x7th **V57.0** Driver of pick-up truck or van injured in collision with fixed or stationary object in nontraffic accident

✓x7th **V57.1** Passenger in pick-up truck or van injured in collision with fixed or stationary object in nontraffic accident

✓x7th **V57.2** Person on outside of pick-up truck or van injured in collision with fixed or stationary object in nontraffic accident

✓x7th **V57.3** Unspecified occupant of pick-up truck or van injured in ▽ collision with fixed or stationary object in nontraffic accident

✓x7th **V57.4** Person boarding or alighting a pick-up truck or van injured in collision with fixed or stationary object

✓x7th **V57.5** Driver of pick-up truck or van injured in collision with fixed or stationary object in traffic accident

✓x7th **V57.6** Passenger in pick-up truck or van injured in collision with fixed or stationary object in traffic accident

✓x7th **V57.7** Person on outside of pick-up truck or van injured in collision with fixed or stationary object in traffic accident

✓x7th **V57.9** Unspecified occupant of pick-up truck or van injured in ▽ collision with fixed or stationary object in traffic accident

✓4th **V58 Occupant of pick-up truck or van injured in noncollision transport accident**
> INCLUDES   overturning pick-up truck or van NOS
> overturning pick-up truck or van without collision

✓x7th **V58.0** Driver of pick-up truck or van injured in noncollision transport accident in nontraffic accident

✓x7th **V58.1** Passenger in pick-up truck or van injured in noncollision transport accident in nontraffic accident

✓x7th **V58.2** Person on outside of pick-up truck or van injured in noncollision transport accident in nontraffic accident

✓x7th **V58.3** Unspecified occupant of pick-up truck or van injured in ▽ noncollision transport accident in nontraffic accident

✓x7th **V58.4** Person boarding or alighting a pick-up truck or van injured in noncollision transport accident

✓x7th **V58.5** Driver of pick-up truck or van injured in noncollision transport accident in traffic accident

✓x7th **V58.6** Passenger in pick-up truck or van injured in noncollision transport accident in traffic accident

✓x7th **V58.7** Person on outside of pick-up truck or van injured in noncollision transport accident in traffic accident

✓x7th **V58.9** Unspecified occupant of pick-up truck or van injured in ▽ noncollision transport accident in traffic accident

✓4th **V59 Occupant of pick-up truck or van injured in other and unspecified transport accidents**

✓5th **V59.0** Driver of pick-up truck or van injured in collision with other and unspecified motor vehicles in nontraffic accident

✓x7th **V59.00** Driver of pick-up truck or van injured in collision ▽ with unspecified motor vehicles in nontraffic accident

✓x7th **V59.09** Driver of pick-up truck or van injured in collision with other motor vehicles in nontraffic accident

✓5th **V59.1** Passenger in pick-up truck or van injured in collision with other and unspecified motor vehicles in nontraffic accident

✓x7th **V59.10** Passenger in pick-up truck or van injured in ▽ collision with unspecified motor vehicles in nontraffic accident

✓x7th **V59.19** Passenger in pick-up truck or van injured in collision with other motor vehicles in nontraffic accident

✓5th **V59.2** Unspecified occupant of pick-up truck or van injured in collision with other and unspecified motor vehicles in nontraffic accident

✓x7th **V59.20** Unspecified occupant of pick-up truck or van ▽ injured in collision with unspecified motor vehicles in nontraffic accident
> Collision NOS involving pick-up truck or van, nontraffic

✓x7th **V59.29** Unspecified occupant of pick-up truck or van injured in collision with other motor vehicles in nontraffic accident

✓x7th **V59.3** Occupant (driver) (passenger) of pick-up truck or van ▽ injured in unspecified nontraffic accident
> Accident NOS involving pick-up truck or van, nontraffic
> Occupant of pick-up truck or van injured in nontraffic accident NOS

✓5th **V59.4** Driver of pick-up truck or van injured in collision with other and unspecified motor vehicles in traffic accident

✓x7th **V59.40** Driver of pick-up truck or van injured in collision ▽ with unspecified motor vehicles in traffic accident

✓x7th **V59.49** Driver of pick-up truck or van injured in collision with other motor vehicles in traffic accident

✓5th **V59.5** Passenger in pick-up truck or van injured in collision with other and unspecified motor vehicles in traffic accident

✓x7th **V59.50** Passenger in pick-up truck or van injured in ▽ collision with unspecified motor vehicles in traffic accident

✓x7th **V59.59** Passenger in pick-up truck or van injured in collision with other motor vehicles in traffic accident

✓5th **V59.6** Unspecified occupant of pick-up truck or van injured in collision with other and unspecified motor vehicles in traffic accident

✓x7th **V59.60** Unspecified occupant of pick-up truck or van ▽ injured in collision with unspecified motor vehicles in traffic accident
> Collision NOS involving pick-up truck or van (traffic)

✓x7th **V59.69** Unspecified occupant of pick-up truck or van ▽ injured in collision with other motor vehicles in traffic accident

✓5th **V59.8** Occupant (driver) (passenger) of pick-up truck or van injured in other specified transport accidents

✓x7th **V59.81** Occupant (driver) (passenger) of pick-up truck or van injured in transport accident with military vehicle

✓x7th **V59.88** Occupant (driver) (passenger) of pick-up truck or van injured in other specified transport accidents

✓x7th **V59.9** Occupant (driver) (passenger) of pick-up truck or van ▽ injured in unspecified traffic accident
> Accident NOS involving pick-up truck or van

Occupant of heavy transport vehicle injured in transport accident (V60–V69)

> INCLUDES   18 wheeler
> armored car
> panel truck
> EXCLUDES 1   bus
> motorcoach

> The appropriate 7th character is to be added to each code from categories V60–V69.
> A   initial encounter
> D   subsequent encounter
> S   sequela

✓4th **V60 Occupant of heavy transport vehicle injured in collision with pedestrian or animal**
> EXCLUDES 1   heavy transport vehicle collision with animal-drawn vehicle or animal being ridden (V66.-)

✓x7th **V60.0** Driver of heavy transport vehicle injured in collision with pedestrian or animal in nontraffic accident

✓x7th **V60.1** Passenger in heavy transport vehicle injured in collision with pedestrian or animal in nontraffic accident

EXCLUDES 1 Not coded here   EXCLUDES 2 Not included here   N Newborn Age: 0   P Pediatric Age: 0-17   M Maternity Age: 12-55   A Adult Age: 15-124

1130   ICD-10-CM 2018

✓x7ᵗʰ **V60.2** Person on outside of heavy transport vehicle injured in collision with pedestrian or animal in nontraffic accident

✓x7ᵗʰ **V60.3** Unspecified occupant of heavy transport vehicle injured in collision with pedestrian or animal in nontraffic accident ▽

✓x7ᵗʰ **V60.4** Person boarding or alighting a heavy transport vehicle injured in collision with pedestrian or animal

✓x7ᵗʰ **V60.5** Driver of heavy transport vehicle injured in collision with pedestrian or animal in traffic accident

✓x7ᵗʰ **V60.6** Passenger in heavy transport vehicle injured in collision with pedestrian or animal in traffic accident

✓x7ᵗʰ **V60.7** Person on outside of heavy transport vehicle injured in collision with pedestrian or animal in traffic accident

✓x7ᵗʰ **V60.9** Unspecified occupant of heavy transport vehicle injured in collision with pedestrian or animal in traffic accident ▽

✓4ᵗʰ **V61** **Occupant of heavy transport vehicle injured in collision with pedal cycle**

✓x7ᵗʰ **V61.0** Driver of heavy transport vehicle injured in collision with pedal cycle in nontraffic accident

✓x7ᵗʰ **V61.1** Passenger in heavy transport vehicle injured in collision with pedal cycle in nontraffic accident

✓x7ᵗʰ **V61.2** Person on outside of heavy transport vehicle injured in collision with pedal cycle in nontraffic accident

✓x7ᵗʰ **V61.3** Unspecified occupant of heavy transport vehicle injured in collision with pedal cycle in nontraffic accident ▽

✓x7ᵗʰ **V61.4** Person boarding or alighting a heavy transport vehicle injured in collision with pedal cycle while boarding or alighting

✓x7ᵗʰ **V61.5** Driver of heavy transport vehicle injured in collision with pedal cycle in traffic accident

✓x7ᵗʰ **V61.6** Passenger in heavy transport vehicle injured in collision with pedal cycle in traffic accident

✓x7ᵗʰ **V61.7** Person on outside of heavy transport vehicle injured in collision with pedal cycle in traffic accident

✓x7ᵗʰ **V61.9** Unspecified occupant of heavy transport vehicle injured in collision with pedal cycle in traffic accident ▽

✓4ᵗʰ **V62** **Occupant of heavy transport vehicle injured in collision with two- or three-wheeled motor vehicle**

✓x7ᵗʰ **V62.0** Driver of heavy transport vehicle injured in collision with two- or three-wheeled motor vehicle in nontraffic accident

✓x7ᵗʰ **V62.1** Passenger in heavy transport vehicle injured in collision with two- or three-wheeled motor vehicle in nontraffic accident

✓x7ᵗʰ **V62.2** Person on outside of heavy transport vehicle injured in collision with two- or three-wheeled motor vehicle in nontraffic accident

✓x7ᵗʰ **V62.3** Unspecified occupant of heavy transport vehicle injured in collision with two- or three-wheeled motor vehicle in nontraffic accident ▽

✓x7ᵗʰ **V62.4** Person boarding or alighting a heavy transport vehicle injured in collision with two- or three-wheeled motor vehicle

✓x7ᵗʰ **V62.5** Driver of heavy transport vehicle injured in collision with two- or three-wheeled motor vehicle in traffic accident

✓x7ᵗʰ **V62.6** Passenger in heavy transport vehicle injured in collision with two- or three-wheeled motor vehicle in traffic accident

✓x7ᵗʰ **V62.7** Person on outside of heavy transport vehicle injured in collision with two- or three-wheeled motor vehicle in traffic accident

✓x7ᵗʰ **V62.9** Unspecified occupant of heavy transport vehicle injured in collision with two- or three-wheeled motor vehicle in traffic accident ▽

✓4ᵗʰ **V63** **Occupant of heavy transport vehicle injured in collision with car, pick-up truck or van**

✓x7ᵗʰ **V63.0** Driver of heavy transport vehicle injured in collision with car, pick-up truck or van in nontraffic accident

✓x7ᵗʰ **V63.1** Passenger in heavy transport vehicle injured in collision with car, pick-up truck or van in nontraffic accident

✓x7ᵗʰ **V63.2** Person on outside of heavy transport vehicle injured in collision with car, pick-up truck or van in nontraffic accident

✓x7ᵗʰ **V63.3** Unspecified occupant of heavy transport vehicle injured in collision with car, pick-up truck or van in nontraffic accident ▽

✓x7ᵗʰ **V63.4** Person boarding or alighting a heavy transport vehicle injured in collision with car, pick-up truck or van

✓x7ᵗʰ **V63.5** Driver of heavy transport vehicle injured in collision with car, pick-up truck or van in traffic accident

✓x7ᵗʰ **V63.6** Passenger in heavy transport vehicle injured in collision with car, pick-up truck or van in traffic accident

✓x7ᵗʰ **V63.7** Person on outside of heavy transport vehicle injured in collision with car, pick-up truck or van in traffic accident

✓x7ᵗʰ **V63.9** Unspecified occupant of heavy transport vehicle injured in collision with car, pick-up truck or van in traffic accident ▽

✓4ᵗʰ **V64** **Occupant of heavy transport vehicle injured in collision with heavy transport vehicle or bus**

> **EXCLUDES 1**   occupant of heavy transport vehicle injured in collision with military vehicle (V69.81)

✓x7ᵗʰ **V64.0** Driver of heavy transport vehicle injured in collision with heavy transport vehicle or bus in nontraffic accident

✓x7ᵗʰ **V64.1** Passenger in heavy transport vehicle injured in collision with heavy transport vehicle or bus in nontraffic accident

✓x7ᵗʰ **V64.2** Person on outside of heavy transport vehicle injured in collision with heavy transport vehicle or bus in nontraffic accident

✓x7ᵗʰ **V64.3** Unspecified occupant of heavy transport vehicle injured in collision with heavy transport vehicle or bus in nontraffic accident ▽

✓x7ᵗʰ **V64.4** Person boarding or alighting a heavy transport vehicle injured in collision with heavy transport vehicle or bus while boarding or alighting

✓x7ᵗʰ **V64.5** Driver of heavy transport vehicle injured in collision with heavy transport vehicle or bus in traffic accident

✓x7ᵗʰ **V64.6** Passenger in heavy transport vehicle injured in collision with heavy transport vehicle or bus in traffic accident

✓x7ᵗʰ **V64.7** Person on outside of heavy transport vehicle injured in collision with heavy transport vehicle or bus in traffic accident

✓x7ᵗʰ **V64.9** Unspecified occupant of heavy transport vehicle injured in collision with heavy transport vehicle or bus in traffic accident ▽

✓4ᵗʰ **V65** **Occupant of heavy transport vehicle injured in collision with railway train or railway vehicle**

✓x7ᵗʰ **V65.0** Driver of heavy transport vehicle injured in collision with railway train or railway vehicle in nontraffic accident

✓x7ᵗʰ **V65.1** Passenger in heavy transport vehicle injured in collision with railway train or railway vehicle in nontraffic accident

✓x7ᵗʰ **V65.2** Person on outside of heavy transport vehicle injured in collision with railway train or railway vehicle in nontraffic accident

✓x7ᵗʰ **V65.3** Unspecified occupant of heavy transport vehicle injured in collision with railway train or railway vehicle in nontraffic accident ▽

✓x7ᵗʰ **V65.4** Person boarding or alighting a heavy transport vehicle injured in collision with railway train or railway vehicle

✓x7ᵗʰ **V65.5** Driver of heavy transport vehicle injured in collision with railway train or railway vehicle in traffic accident

✓x7ᵗʰ **V65.6** Passenger in heavy transport vehicle injured in collision with railway train or railway vehicle in traffic accident

✓x7ᵗʰ **V65.7** Person on outside of heavy transport vehicle injured in collision with railway train or railway vehicle in traffic accident

✓x7ᵗʰ **V65.9** Unspecified occupant of heavy transport vehicle injured in collision with railway train or railway vehicle in traffic accident ▽

✓4ᵗʰ **V66** **Occupant of heavy transport vehicle injured in collision with other nonmotor vehicle**

> **INCLUDES**   collision with animal-drawn vehicle, animal being ridden, streetcar

✓x7ᵗʰ **V66.0** Driver of heavy transport vehicle injured in collision with other nonmotor vehicle in nontraffic accident

✓x7ᵗʰ **V66.1** Passenger in heavy transport vehicle injured in collision with other nonmotor vehicle in nontraffic accident

✓x7ᵗʰ **V66.2** Person on outside of heavy transport vehicle injured in collision with other nonmotor vehicle in nontraffic accident

✓x7ᵗʰ **V66.3** Unspecified occupant of heavy transport vehicle injured in collision with other nonmotor vehicle in nontraffic accident ▽

✓ Additional Character Req   ✓x7ᵗʰ Placeholder Alert   Manifestation   HCC CMS-HCC Condition   ▽ Unspecified Code   ▶◀ Revised Text   ● New Code   ▲ Revised Code Title

√x7th V66.4 **Person boarding or alighting** a heavy transport vehicle injured in collision with other nonmotor vehicle

√x7th V66.5 **Driver** of heavy transport vehicle injured in collision with other nonmotor vehicle in traffic accident

√x7th V66.6 **Passenger** in heavy transport vehicle injured in collision with other nonmotor vehicle in traffic accident

√x7th V66.7 **Person on outside** of heavy transport vehicle injured in collision with other nonmotor vehicle in traffic accident

√x7th V66.9 **Unspecified occupant** of heavy transport vehicle injured ▽ in collision with other nonmotor vehicle in traffic accident

√4th V67 **Occupant of heavy transport vehicle injured in collision with fixed or stationary object**

√x7th V67.0 **Driver** of heavy transport vehicle injured in collision with fixed or stationary object in nontraffic accident

√x7th V67.1 **Passenger** in heavy transport vehicle injured in collision with fixed or stationary object in nontraffic accident

√x7th V67.2 **Person on outside** of heavy transport vehicle injured in collision with fixed or stationary object in nontraffic accident

√x7th V67.3 **Unspecified occupant** of heavy transport vehicle injured in ▽ collision with fixed or stationary object in nontraffic accident

√x7th V67.4 **Person boarding or alighting** a heavy transport vehicle injured in collision with fixed or stationary object

√x7th V67.5 **Driver** of heavy transport vehicle injured in collision with fixed or stationary object in traffic accident

√x7th V67.6 **Passenger** in heavy transport vehicle injured in collision with fixed or stationary object in traffic accident

√x7th V67.7 **Person on outside** of heavy transport vehicle injured in collision with fixed or stationary object in traffic accident

√x7th V67.9 **Unspecified occupant** of heavy transport vehicle injured ▽ in collision with fixed or stationary object in traffic accident

√4th V68 **Occupant of heavy transport vehicle injured in noncollision transport accident**

INCLUDES overturning heavy transport vehicle NOS
overturning heavy transport vehicle without collision

√x7th V68.0 **Driver** of heavy transport vehicle injured in noncollision transport accident in nontraffic accident

√x7th V68.1 **Passenger** in heavy transport vehicle injured in noncollision transport accident in nontraffic accident

√x7th V68.2 **Person on outside** of heavy transport vehicle injured in noncollision transport accident in nontraffic accident

√x7th V68.3 **Unspecified occupant** of heavy transport vehicle injured ▽ in noncollision transport accident in nontraffic accident

√x7th V68.4 **Person boarding or alighting** a heavy transport vehicle injured in noncollision transport accident

√x7th V68.5 **Driver** of heavy transport vehicle injured in noncollision transport accident in traffic accident

√x7th V68.6 **Passenger** in heavy transport vehicle injured in noncollision transport accident in traffic accident

√x7th V68.7 **Person on outside** of heavy transport vehicle injured in noncollision transport accident in traffic accident

√x7th V68.9 **Unspecified occupant** of heavy transport vehicle injured ▽ in noncollision transport accident in traffic accident

√4th V69 **Occupant of heavy transport vehicle injured in other and unspecified transport accidents**

√5th V69.0 **Driver** of heavy transport vehicle injured in collision with other and unspecified motor vehicles in nontraffic accident

√x7th V69.00 **Driver** of heavy transport vehicle injured in ▽ collision with unspecified motor vehicles in nontraffic accident

√x7th V69.09 **Driver** of heavy transport vehicle injured in collision with other motor vehicles in nontraffic accident

√5th V69.1 **Passenger** in heavy transport vehicle injured in collision with other and unspecified motor vehicles in nontraffic accident

√x7th V69.10 **Passenger** in heavy transport vehicle injured in ▽ collision with unspecified motor vehicles in nontraffic accident

√x7th V69.19 **Passenger** in heavy transport vehicle injured in collision with other motor vehicles in nontraffic accident

√5th V69.2 **Unspecified occupant** of heavy transport vehicle injured in collision with other and unspecified motor vehicles in nontraffic accident

√x7th V69.20 **Unspecified occupant** of heavy transport vehicle ▽ injured in collision with unspecified motor vehicles in nontraffic accident
Collision NOS involving heavy transport vehicle, nontraffic

√x7th V69.29 **Unspecified occupant** of heavy transport vehicle ▽ injured in collision with other motor vehicles in nontraffic accident

√x7th V69.3 **Occupant (driver) (passenger)** of heavy transport vehicle ▽ injured in unspecified nontraffic accident
Accident NOS involving heavy transport vehicle, nontraffic
Occupant of heavy transport vehicle injured in nontraffic accident NOS

√5th V69.4 **Driver** of heavy transport vehicle injured in collision with other and unspecified motor vehicles in traffic accident

√x7th V69.40 **Driver** of heavy transport vehicle injured in ▽ collision with unspecified motor vehicles in traffic accident

√x7th V69.49 **Driver** of heavy transport vehicle injured in collision with other motor vehicles in traffic accident

√5th V69.5 **Passenger** in heavy transport vehicle injured in collision with other and unspecified motor vehicles in traffic accident

√x7th V69.50 **Passenger** in heavy transport vehicle injured in ▽ collision with unspecified motor vehicles in traffic accident

√x7th V69.59 **Passenger** in heavy transport vehicle injured in collision with other motor vehicles in traffic accident

√5th V69.6 **Unspecified occupant** of heavy transport vehicle injured in collision with other and unspecified motor vehicles in traffic accident

√x7th V69.60 **Unspecified occupant** of heavy transport vehicle ▽ injured in collision with unspecified motor vehicles in traffic accident
Collision NOS involving heavy transport vehicle (traffic)

√x7th V69.69 **Unspecified occupant** of heavy transport vehicle ▽ injured in collision with other motor vehicles in traffic accident

√5th V69.8 **Occupant (driver) (passenger)** of heavy transport vehicle injured in other specified transport accidents

√x7th V69.81 **Occupant (driver) (passenger)** of heavy transport vehicle injured in transport accidents with military vehicle

√x7th V69.88 **Occupant (driver) (passenger)** of heavy transport vehicle injured in other specified transport accidents

√x7th V69.9 **Occupant (driver) (passenger)** of heavy transport vehicle ▽ injured in unspecified traffic accident
Accident NOS involving heavy transport vehicle

Bus occupant injured in transport accident (V70-V79)

INCLUDES motorcoach
EXCLUDES 1 minibus (V50-V59)

The appropriate 7th character is to be added to each code from categories V70-V79.
A   initial encounter
D   subsequent encounter
S   sequela

√4th V70 **Bus occupant injured in collision with pedestrian or animal**
EXCLUDES 1 bus collision with animal-drawn vehicle or animal being ridden (V76.-)

√x7th V70.0 **Driver** of bus injured in collision with pedestrian or animal in nontraffic accident

√x7th V70.1 **Passenger** on bus injured in collision with pedestrian or animal in nontraffic accident

√x7th V70.2 **Person on outside** of bus injured in collision with pedestrian or animal in nontraffic accident

√x7th V70.3 **Unspecified occupant** of bus injured in collision with ▽ pedestrian or animal in nontraffic accident

√x7th V70.4 **Person boarding or alighting** from bus injured in collision with pedestrian or animal

√x7th V70.5 **Driver** of bus injured in collision with pedestrian or animal in traffic accident

EXCLUDES 1 Not coded here   **EXCLUDES 2** Not included here   N Newborn Age: 0   P Pediatric Age: 0-17   M Maternity Age: 12-55   A Adult Age: 15-124

1132   ICD-10-CM 2018

√x7ᵗʰ **V70.6** Passenger on bus injured in collision with pedestrian or animal in traffic accident

√x7ᵗʰ **V70.7** Person on outside of bus injured in collision with pedestrian or animal in traffic accident

√x7ᵗʰ **V70.9** Unspecified occupant of bus injured in collision with pedestrian or animal in traffic accident ▽

√4ᵗʰ **V71 Bus occupant injured in collision with pedal cycle**

√x7ᵗʰ **V71.0** Driver of bus injured in collision with pedal cycle in nontraffic accident

√x7ᵗʰ **V71.1** Passenger on bus injured in collision with pedal cycle in nontraffic accident

√x7ᵗʰ **V71.2** Person on outside of bus injured in collision with pedal cycle in nontraffic accident

√x7ᵗʰ **V71.3** Unspecified occupant of bus injured in collision with pedal cycle in nontraffic accident ▽

√x7ᵗʰ **V71.4** Person boarding or alighting from bus injured in collision with pedal cycle

√x7ᵗʰ **V71.5** Driver of bus injured in collision with pedal cycle in traffic accident

√x7ᵗʰ **V71.6** Passenger on bus injured in collision with pedal cycle in traffic accident

√x7ᵗʰ **V71.7** Person on outside of bus injured in collision with pedal cycle in traffic accident

√x7ᵗʰ **V71.9** Unspecified occupant of bus injured in collision with pedal cycle in traffic accident ▽

√4ᵗʰ **V72 Bus occupant injured in collision with two- or three-wheeled motor vehicle**

√x7ᵗʰ **V72.0** Driver of bus injured in collision with two- or three-wheeled motor vehicle in nontraffic accident

√x7ᵗʰ **V72.1** Passenger on bus injured in collision with two- or three-wheeled motor vehicle in nontraffic accident

√x7ᵗʰ **V72.2** Person on outside of bus injured in collision with two- or three-wheeled motor vehicle in nontraffic accident

√x7ᵗʰ **V72.3** Unspecified occupant of bus injured in collision with two- or three-wheeled motor vehicle in nontraffic accident ▽

√x7ᵗʰ **V72.4** Person boarding or alighting from bus injured in collision with two- or three-wheeled motor vehicle

√x7ᵗʰ **V72.5** Driver of bus injured in collision with two- or three-wheeled motor vehicle in traffic accident

√x7ᵗʰ **V72.6** Passenger on bus injured in collision with two- or three-wheeled motor vehicle in traffic accident

√x7ᵗʰ **V72.7** Person on outside of bus injured in collision with two- or three-wheeled motor vehicle in traffic accident

√x7ᵗʰ **V72.9** Unspecified occupant of bus injured in collision with two- or three-wheeled motor vehicle in traffic accident ▽

√4ᵗʰ **V73 Bus occupant injured in collision with car, pick-up truck or van**

√x7ᵗʰ **V73.0** Driver of bus injured in collision with car, pick-up truck or van in nontraffic accident

√x7ᵗʰ **V73.1** Passenger on bus injured in collision with car, pick-up truck or van in nontraffic accident

√x7ᵗʰ **V73.2** Person on outside of bus injured in collision with car, pick-up truck or van in nontraffic accident

√x7ᵗʰ **V73.3** Unspecified occupant of bus injured in collision with car, pick-up truck or van in nontraffic accident ▽

√x7ᵗʰ **V73.4** Person boarding or alighting from bus injured in collision with car, pick-up truck or van

√x7ᵗʰ **V73.5** Driver of bus injured in collision with car, pick-up truck or van in traffic accident

√x7ᵗʰ **V73.6** Passenger on bus injured in collision with car, pick-up truck or van in traffic accident

√x7ᵗʰ **V73.7** Person on outside of bus injured in collision with car, pick-up truck or van in traffic accident

√x7ᵗʰ **V73.9** Unspecified occupant of bus injured in collision with car, pick-up truck or van in traffic accident ▽

√4ᵗʰ **V74 Bus occupant injured in collision with heavy transport vehicle or bus**

EXCLUDES 1   bus occupant injured in collision with military vehicle (V79.81)

√x7ᵗʰ **V74.0** Driver of bus injured in collision with heavy transport vehicle or bus in nontraffic accident

√x7ᵗʰ **V74.1** Passenger on bus injured in collision with heavy transport vehicle or bus in nontraffic accident

√x7ᵗʰ **V74.2** Person on outside of bus injured in collision with heavy transport vehicle or bus in nontraffic accident

√x7ᵗʰ **V74.3** Unspecified occupant of bus injured in collision with heavy transport vehicle or bus in nontraffic accident ▽

√x7ᵗʰ **V74.4** Person boarding or alighting from bus injured in collision with heavy transport vehicle or bus

√x7ᵗʰ **V74.5** Driver of bus injured in collision with heavy transport vehicle or bus in traffic accident

√x7ᵗʰ **V74.6** Passenger on bus injured in collision with heavy transport vehicle or bus in traffic accident

√x7ᵗʰ **V74.7** Person on outside of bus injured in collision with heavy transport vehicle or bus in traffic accident

√x7ᵗʰ **V74.9** Unspecified occupant of bus injured in collision with heavy transport vehicle or bus in traffic accident ▽

√4ᵗʰ **V75 Bus occupant injured in collision with railway train or railway vehicle**

√x7ᵗʰ **V75.0** Driver of bus injured in collision with railway train or railway vehicle in nontraffic accident

√x7ᵗʰ **V75.1** Passenger on bus injured in collision with railway train or railway vehicle in nontraffic accident

√x7ᵗʰ **V75.2** Person on outside of bus injured in collision with railway train or railway vehicle in nontraffic accident

√x7ᵗʰ **V75.3** Unspecified occupant of bus injured in collision with railway train or railway vehicle in nontraffic accident ▽

√x7ᵗʰ **V75.4** Person boarding or alighting from bus injured in collision with railway train or railway vehicle

√x7ᵗʰ **V75.5** Driver of bus injured in collision with railway train or railway vehicle in traffic accident

√x7ᵗʰ **V75.6** Passenger on bus injured in collision with railway train or railway vehicle in traffic accident

√x7ᵗʰ **V75.7** Person on outside of bus injured in collision with railway train or railway vehicle in traffic accident

√x7ᵗʰ **V75.9** Unspecified occupant of bus injured in collision with railway train or railway vehicle in traffic accident ▽

√4ᵗʰ **V76 Bus occupant injured in collision with other nonmotor vehicle**

INCLUDES   collision with animal-drawn vehicle, animal being ridden, streetcar

√x7ᵗʰ **V76.0** Driver of bus injured in collision with other nonmotor vehicle in nontraffic accident

√x7ᵗʰ **V76.1** Passenger on bus injured in collision with other nonmotor vehicle in nontraffic accident

√x7ᵗʰ **V76.2** Person on outside of bus injured in collision with other nonmotor vehicle in nontraffic accident

√x7ᵗʰ **V76.3** Unspecified occupant of bus injured in collision with other nonmotor vehicle in nontraffic accident ▽

√x7ᵗʰ **V76.4** Person boarding or alighting from bus injured in collision with other nonmotor vehicle

√x7ᵗʰ **V76.5** Driver of bus injured in collision with other nonmotor vehicle in traffic accident

√x7ᵗʰ **V76.6** Passenger on bus injured in collision with other nonmotor vehicle in traffic accident

√x7ᵗʰ **V76.7** Person on outside of bus injured in collision with other nonmotor vehicle in traffic accident

√x7ᵗʰ **V76.9** Unspecified occupant of bus injured in collision with other nonmotor vehicle in traffic accident ▽

√4ᵗʰ **V77 Bus occupant injured in collision with fixed or stationary object**

√x7ᵗʰ **V77.0** Driver of bus injured in collision with fixed or stationary object in nontraffic accident

√x7ᵗʰ **V77.1** Passenger on bus injured in collision with fixed or stationary object in nontraffic accident

√x7ᵗʰ **V77.2** Person on outside of bus injured in collision with fixed or stationary object in nontraffic accident

√x7ᵗʰ **V77.3** Unspecified occupant of bus injured in collision with fixed or stationary object in nontraffic accident ▽

√x7ᵗʰ **V77.4** Person boarding or alighting from bus injured in collision with fixed or stationary object

√x7ᵗʰ **V77.5** Driver of bus injured in collision with fixed or stationary object in traffic accident

√x7ᵗʰ **V77.6** Passenger on bus injured in collision with fixed or stationary object in traffic accident

√x7ᵗʰ **V77.7** Person on outside of bus injured in collision with fixed or stationary object in traffic accident

√x7ᵗʰ **V77.9** Unspecified occupant of bus injured in collision with fixed or stationary object in traffic accident ▽

✓ Additional Character Req   √x7ᵗʰ Placeholder Alert   **Manifestation**   **HCC** CMS-HCC Condition   ▽ Unspecified Code   ►◄ Revised Text   ● New Code   ▲ Revised Code Title

✓4ᵗʰ **V78 Bus occupant injured in noncollision transport accident**
INCLUDES   overturning bus NOS
overturning bus without collision

✓x7ᵗʰ **V78.0 Driver** of bus injured in noncollision transport accident in nontraffic accident

✓x7ᵗʰ **V78.1 Passenger** on bus injured in noncollision transport accident in nontraffic accident

✓x7ᵗʰ **V78.2 Person on outside** of bus injured in noncollision transport accident in nontraffic accident

✓x7ᵗʰ **V78.3 Unspecified occupant** of bus injured in noncollision transport accident in nontraffic accident ▽

✓x7ᵗʰ **V78.4 Person boarding or alighting** from bus injured in noncollision transport accident

✓x7ᵗʰ **V78.5 Driver** of bus injured in noncollision transport accident in traffic accident

✓x7ᵗʰ **V78.6 Passenger** on bus injured in noncollision transport accident in traffic accident

✓x7ᵗʰ **V78.7 Person on outside** of bus injured in noncollision transport accident in traffic accident

✓x7ᵗʰ **V78.9 Unspecified occupant** of bus injured in noncollision transport accident in traffic accident ▽

✓4ᵗʰ **V79 Bus occupant injured in other and unspecified transport accidents**

✓5ᵗʰ **V79.0 Driver** of bus injured in collision with other and unspecified motor vehicles in nontraffic accident

✓x7ᵗʰ **V79.00 Driver** of bus injured in collision with unspecified motor vehicles in nontraffic accident ▽

✓x7ᵗʰ **V79.09 Driver** of bus injured in collision with other motor vehicles in nontraffic accident

✓5ᵗʰ **V79.1 Passenger** on bus injured in collision with other and unspecified motor vehicles in nontraffic accident

✓x7ᵗʰ **V79.10 Passenger** on bus injured in collision with unspecified motor vehicles in nontraffic accident ▽

✓x7ᵗʰ **V79.19 Passenger** on bus injured in collision with other motor vehicles in nontraffic accident

✓5ᵗʰ **V79.2 Unspecified bus occupant** injured in collision with other and unspecified motor vehicles in nontraffic accident

✓x7ᵗʰ **V79.20 Unspecified bus occupant** injured in collision with unspecified motor vehicles in nontraffic accident ▽
Bus collision NOS, nontraffic

✓x7ᵗʰ **V79.29 Unspecified bus occupant** injured in collision with other motor vehicles in nontraffic accident ▽

✓x7ᵗʰ **V79.3 Bus occupant (driver) (passenger)** injured in unspecified nontraffic accident ▽
Bus accident NOS, nontraffic
Bus occupant injured in nontraffic accident NOS

✓5ᵗʰ **V79.4 Driver** of bus injured in collision with other and unspecified motor vehicles in traffic accident

✓x7ᵗʰ **V79.40 Driver** of bus injured in collision with unspecified motor vehicles in traffic accident ▽

✓x7ᵗʰ **V79.49 Driver** of bus injured in collision with other motor vehicles in traffic accident

✓5ᵗʰ **V79.5 Passenger** on bus injured in collision with other and unspecified motor vehicles in traffic accident

✓x7ᵗʰ **V79.50 Passenger** on bus injured in collision with unspecified motor vehicles in traffic accident ▽

✓x7ᵗʰ **V79.59 Passenger** on bus injured in collision with other motor vehicles in traffic accident

✓5ᵗʰ **V79.6 Unspecified bus occupant** injured in collision with other and unspecified motor vehicles in traffic accident

✓x7ᵗʰ **V79.60 Unspecified bus occupant** injured in collision with unspecified motor vehicles in traffic accident ▽
Bus collision NOS (traffic)

✓x7ᵗʰ **V79.69 Unspecified bus occupant** injured in collision with other motor vehicles in traffic accident ▽

✓5ᵗʰ **V79.8 Bus occupant (driver) (passenger)** injured in other specified transport accidents

✓x7ᵗʰ **V79.81 Bus occupant (driver) (passenger)** injured in transport accidents with military vehicle

✓x7ᵗʰ **V79.88 Bus occupant (driver) (passenger)** injured in other specified transport accidents

✓x7ᵗʰ **V79.9 Bus occupant (driver) (passenger)** injured in unspecified traffic accident ▽
Bus accident NOS

Other land transport accidents (V80-V89)

The appropriate 7th character is to be added to each code from categories V80-V89.
A   initial encounter
D   subsequent encounter
S   sequela

✓4ᵗʰ **V80 Animal-rider or occupant of animal-drawn vehicle injured in transport accident**

✓5ᵗʰ **V80.0 Animal-rider or occupant** of animal drawn vehicle injured by fall from or being thrown from animal or animal-drawn vehicle in noncollision accident

✓6ᵗʰ **V80.01 Animal-rider** injured by fall from or being thrown from animal in noncollision accident

✓7ᵗʰ **V80.010 Animal-rider** injured by fall from or being thrown from horse in noncollision accident

✓7ᵗʰ **V80.018 Animal-rider** injured by fall from or being thrown from other animal in noncollision accident

✓x7ᵗʰ **V80.02 Occupant** of animal-drawn vehicle injured by fall from or being thrown from animal-drawn vehicle in noncollision accident
Overturning animal-drawn vehicle NOS
Overturning animal-drawn vehicle without collision

✓5ᵗʰ **V80.1 Animal-rider or occupant** of animal-drawn vehicle injured in collision with pedestrian or animal
EXCLUDES 1   animal-rider or animal-drawn vehicle collision with animal-drawn vehicle or animal being ridden (V80.7)

✓x7ᵗʰ **V80.11 Animal-rider** injured in collision with pedestrian or animal

✓x7ᵗʰ **V80.12 Occupant** of animal-drawn vehicle injured in collision with pedestrian or animal

✓5ᵗʰ **V80.2 Animal-rider or occupant** of animal-drawn vehicle injured in collision with pedal cycle

✓x7ᵗʰ **V80.21 Animal-rider** injured in collision with pedal cycle

✓x7ᵗʰ **V80.22 Occupant** of animal-drawn vehicle injured in collision with pedal cycle

✓5ᵗʰ **V80.3 Animal-rider or occupant** of animal-drawn vehicle injured in collision with two- or three-wheeled motor vehicle

✓x7ᵗʰ **V80.31 Animal-rider** injured in collision with two- or three-wheeled motor vehicle

✓x7ᵗʰ **V80.32 Occupant** of animal-drawn vehicle injured in collision with two- or three-wheeled motor vehicle

✓5ᵗʰ **V80.4 Animal-rider or occupant** of animal-drawn vehicle injured in collision with car, pick-up truck, van, heavy transport vehicle or bus
EXCLUDES 1   animal-rider injured in collision with military vehicle (V80.910)
occupant of animal-drawn vehicle injured in collision with military vehicle (V80.920)

✓x7ᵗʰ **V80.41 Animal-rider** injured in collision with car, pick-up truck, van, heavy transport vehicle or bus

✓x7ᵗʰ **V80.42 Occupant** of animal-drawn vehicle injured in collision with car, pick-up truck, van, heavy transport vehicle or bus

✓5ᵗʰ **V80.5 Animal-rider or occupant** of animal-drawn vehicle injured in collision with other specified motor vehicle

✓x7ᵗʰ **V80.51 Animal-rider** injured in collision with other specified motor vehicle

✓x7ᵗʰ **V80.52 Occupant** of animal-drawn vehicle injured in collision with other specified motor vehicle

✓5ᵗʰ **V80.6 Animal-rider or occupant** of animal-drawn vehicle injured in collision with railway train or railway vehicle

✓x7ᵗʰ **V80.61 Animal-rider** injured in collision with railway train or railway vehicle

✓x7ᵗʰ **V80.62 Occupant** of animal-drawn vehicle injured in collision with railway train or railway vehicle

✓5ᵗʰ **V80.7 Animal-rider or occupant** of animal-drawn vehicle injured in collision with other nonmotor vehicles

✓6ᵗʰ **V80.71 Animal-rider or occupant** of animal-drawn vehicle injured in collision with animal being ridden

✓7ᵗʰ **V80.710 Animal-rider** injured in collision with other animal being ridden

EXCLUDES 1 Not coded here   EXCLUDES 2 Not included here   N Newborn Age: 0   P Pediatric Age: 0-17   M Maternity Age: 12-55   A Adult Age: 15-124

1134   ICD-10-CM 2018

✓7ᵗʰ **V80.711** Occupant of animal-drawn vehicle injured in collision with animal being ridden

✓6ᵗʰ **V80.72** Animal-rider or occupant of animal-drawn vehicle injured in collision with other animal-drawn vehicle

✓7ᵗʰ **V80.720** Animal-rider injured in collision with animal-drawn vehicle

✓7ᵗʰ **V80.721** Occupant of animal-drawn vehicle injured in collision with other animal-drawn vehicle

✓6ᵗʰ **V80.73** Animal-rider or occupant of animal-drawn vehicle injured in collision with streetcar

✓7ᵗʰ **V80.730** Animal-rider injured in collision with streetcar

✓7ᵗʰ **V80.731** Occupant of animal-drawn vehicle injured in collision with streetcar

✓6ᵗʰ **V80.79** Animal-rider or occupant of animal-drawn vehicle injured in collision with other nonmotor vehicles

✓7ᵗʰ **V80.790** Animal-rider injured in collision with other nonmotor vehicles

✓7ᵗʰ **V80.791** Occupant of animal-drawn vehicle injured in collision with other nonmotor vehicles

✓5ᵗʰ **V80.8** Animal-rider or occupant of animal-drawn vehicle injured in collision with fixed or stationary object

✓x7ᵗʰ **V80.81** Animal-rider injured in collision with fixed or stationary object

✓x7ᵗʰ **V80.82** Occupant of animal-drawn vehicle injured in collision with fixed or stationary object

✓5ᵗʰ **V80.9** Animal-rider or occupant of animal-drawn vehicle injured in other and unspecified transport accidents

✓6ᵗʰ **V80.91** Animal-rider injured in other and unspecified transport accidents

✓7ᵗʰ **V80.910** Animal-rider injured in transport accident with military vehicle

✓7ᵗʰ **V80.918** Animal-rider injured in other transport accident

✓7ᵗʰ **V80.919** Animal-rider injured in unspecified ▽ transport accident
     Animal rider accident NOS

✓6ᵗʰ **V80.92** Occupant of animal-drawn vehicle injured in other and unspecified transport accidents

✓7ᵗʰ **V80.920** Occupant of animal-drawn vehicle injured in transport accident with military vehicle

✓7ᵗʰ **V80.928** Occupant of animal-drawn vehicle injured in other transport accident

✓7ᵗʰ **V80.929** Occupant of animal-drawn vehicle ▽ injured in unspecified transport accident
     Animal-drawn vehicle accident NOS

✓4ᵗʰ **V81** Occupant of railway train or railway vehicle injured in transport accident

INCLUDES   derailment of railway train or railway vehicle
         person on outside of train

EXCLUDES 1   streetcar (V82.-)

✓x7ᵗʰ **V81.0** Occupant of railway train or railway vehicle injured in collision with motor vehicle in nontraffic accident

EXCLUDES 1   occupant of railway train or railway vehicle injured due to collision with military vehicle (V81.83)

✓x7ᵗʰ **V81.1** Occupant of railway train or railway vehicle injured in collision with motor vehicle in traffic accident

EXCLUDES 1   occupant of railway train or railway vehicle injured due to collision with military vehicle (V81.83)

✓x7ᵗʰ **V81.2** Occupant of railway train or railway vehicle injured in collision with or hit by rolling stock

✓x7ᵗʰ **V81.3** Occupant of railway train or railway vehicle injured in collision with other object
     Railway collision NOS

✓x7ᵗʰ **V81.4** Person injured while boarding or alighting from railway train or railway vehicle

✓x7ᵗʰ **V81.5** Occupant of railway train or railway vehicle injured by fall in railway train or railway vehicle

✓x7ᵗʰ **V81.6** Occupant of railway train or railway vehicle injured by fall from railway train or railway vehicle

✓x7ᵗʰ **V81.7** Occupant of railway train or railway vehicle injured in derailment without antecedent collision

✓5ᵗʰ **V81.8** Occupant of railway train or railway vehicle injured in other specified railway accidents

✓x7ᵗʰ **V81.81** Occupant of railway train or railway vehicle injured due to explosion or fire on train

✓x7ᵗʰ **V81.82** Occupant of railway train or railway vehicle injured due to object falling onto train
     Occupant of railway train or railway vehicle injured due to falling earth onto train
     Occupant of railway train or railway vehicle injured due to falling rocks onto train
     Occupant of railway train or railway vehicle injured due to falling snow onto train
     Occupant of railway train or railway vehicle injured due to falling trees onto train

✓x7ᵗʰ **V81.83** Occupant of railway train or railway vehicle injured due to collision with military vehicle

✓x7ᵗʰ **V81.89** Occupant of railway train or railway vehicle injured due to other specified railway accident

✓x7ᵗʰ **V81.9** Occupant of railway train or railway vehicle injured in ▽ unspecified railway accident
     Railway accident NOS

✓4ᵗʰ **V82** Occupant of powered streetcar injured in transport accident

INCLUDES   interurban electric car
         person on outside of streetcar
         tram (car)
         trolley (car)

EXCLUDES 1   bus (V70-V79)
         motorcoach (V70-V79)
         nonpowered streetcar (V76.-)
         train (V81.-)

✓x7ᵗʰ **V82.0** Occupant of streetcar injured in collision with motor vehicle in nontraffic accident

✓x7ᵗʰ **V82.1** Occupant of streetcar injured in collision with motor vehicle in traffic accident

✓x7ᵗʰ **V82.2** Occupant of streetcar injured in collision with or hit by rolling stock

✓x7ᵗʰ **V82.3** Occupant of streetcar injured in collision with other object
   EXCLUDES 1   collision with animal-drawn vehicle or animal being ridden (V82.8)

✓x7ᵗʰ **V82.4** Person injured while boarding or alighting from streetcar

✓x7ᵗʰ **V82.5** Occupant of streetcar injured by fall in streetcar
   EXCLUDES 1   fall in streetcar:
       while boarding or alighting (V82.4)
       with antecedent collision (V82.0-V82.3)

✓x7ᵗʰ **V82.6** Occupant of streetcar injured by fall from streetcar
   EXCLUDES 1   fall from streetcar:
       while boarding or alighting (V82.4)
       with antecedent collision (V82.0-V82.3)

✓x7ᵗʰ **V82.7** Occupant of streetcar injured in derailment without antecedent collision
   EXCLUDES 1   occupant of streetcar injured in derailment with antecedent collision (V82.0-V82.3)

✓x7ᵗʰ **V82.8** Occupant of streetcar injured in other specified transport accidents
     Streetcar collision with military vehicle
     Streetcar collision with train or nonmotor vehicles

✓x7ᵗʰ **V82.9** Occupant of streetcar injured in unspecified traffic ▽ accident
     Streetcar accident NOS

✓4ᵗʰ **V83** Occupant of special vehicle mainly used on industrial premises injured in transport accident

INCLUDES   battery-powered airport passenger vehicle
         battery-powered truck (baggage) (mail)
         coal-car in mine
         forklift (truck)
         logging car
         self-propelled industrial truck
         station baggage truck (powered)
         tram, truck, or tub (powered) in mine or quarry

EXCLUDES 1   special construction vehicles (V85.-)
         special industrial vehicle in stationary use or maintenance (W31.-)

✓x7ᵗʰ **V83.0** Driver of special industrial vehicle injured in traffic accident

✓x7ᵗʰ **V83.1** Passenger of special industrial vehicle injured in traffic accident

✓x7ᵗʰ **V83.2** Person on outside of special industrial vehicle injured in traffic accident

☑ Additional Character Req   ✓x7ᵗʰ Placeholder Alert   Manifestation   HCC CMS-HCC Condition   ▽ Unspecified Code   ►◄ Revised Text   ● New Code   ▲ Revised Code Title

ICD-10-CM 2018   1135

√x 7ᵗʰ **V83.3** **Unspecified occupant of special industrial vehicle injured in traffic accident** ▽

√x 7ᵗʰ **V83.4** **Person injured while boarding or alighting from special industrial vehicle**

√x 7ᵗʰ **V83.5** **Driver of special industrial vehicle injured in nontraffic accident**

√x 7ᵗʰ **V83.6** **Passenger of special industrial vehicle injured in nontraffic accident**

√x 7ᵗʰ **V83.7** **Person on outside of special industrial vehicle injured in nontraffic accident**

√x 7ᵗʰ **V83.9** **Unspecified occupant of special industrial vehicle injured in nontraffic accident** ▽
     Special-industrial-vehicle accident NOS

√ 4ᵗʰ **V84** **Occupant of special vehicle mainly used in agriculture injured in transport accident**
    INCLUDES   self-propelled farm machinery
             tractor (and trailer)
    EXCLUDES 1   animal-powered farm machinery accident (W30.8-)
             contact with combine harvester (W30.0)
             special agricultural vehicle in stationary use or maintenance (W30.-)

√x 7ᵗʰ **V84.0** **Driver of special agricultural vehicle injured in traffic accident**

√x 7ᵗʰ **V84.1** **Passenger of special agricultural vehicle injured in traffic accident**

√x 7ᵗʰ **V84.2** **Person on outside of special agricultural vehicle injured in traffic accident**

√x 7ᵗʰ **V84.3** **Unspecified occupant of special agricultural vehicle injured in traffic accident** ▽

√x 7ᵗʰ **V84.4** **Person injured while boarding or alighting from special agricultural vehicle**

√x 7ᵗʰ **V84.5** **Driver of special agricultural vehicle injured in nontraffic accident**

√x 7ᵗʰ **V84.6** **Passenger of special agricultural vehicle injured in nontraffic accident**

√x 7ᵗʰ **V84.7** **Person on outside of special agricultural vehicle injured in nontraffic accident**

√x 7ᵗʰ **V84.9** **Unspecified occupant of special agricultural vehicle injured in nontraffic accident** ▽
     Special-agricultural vehicle accident NOS

√ 4ᵗʰ **V85** **Occupant of special construction vehicle injured in transport accident**
    INCLUDES   bulldozer
             digger
             dump truck
             earth-leveller
             mechanical shovel
             road-roller
    EXCLUDES 1   special industrial vehicle (V83.-)
             special construction vehicle in stationary use or maintenance (W31.-)

√x 7ᵗʰ **V85.0** **Driver of special construction vehicle injured in traffic accident**

√x 7ᵗʰ **V85.1** **Passenger of special construction vehicle injured in traffic accident**

√x 7ᵗʰ **V85.2** **Person on outside of special construction vehicle injured in traffic accident**

√x 7ᵗʰ **V85.3** **Unspecified occupant of special construction vehicle injured in traffic accident** ▽

√x 7ᵗʰ **V85.4** **Person injured while boarding or alighting from special construction vehicle**

√x 7ᵗʰ **V85.5** **Driver of special construction vehicle injured in nontraffic accident**

√x 7ᵗʰ **V85.6** **Passenger of special construction vehicle injured in nontraffic accident**

√x 7ᵗʰ **V85.7** **Person on outside of special construction vehicle injured in nontraffic accident**

√x 7ᵗʰ **V85.9** **Unspecified occupant of special construction vehicle injured in nontraffic accident** ▽
     Special-construction-vehicle accident NOS

√ 4ᵗʰ **V86** **Occupant of special all-terrain or other off-road motor vehicle, injured in transport accident**
    EXCLUDES 1   special all-terrain vehicle in stationary use or maintenance (W31.-)
             sport-utility vehicle (V50-V59)
             three-wheeled motor vehicle designed for on-road use (V30-V39)

√ 5ᵗʰ **V86.0** **Driver of special all-terrain or other off-road motor vehicle injured in traffic accident**

√x 7ᵗʰ **V86.01** **Driver of ambulance or fire engine injured in traffic accident**

√x 7ᵗʰ **V86.02** **Driver of snowmobile injured in traffic accident**

√x 7ᵗʰ **V86.03** **Driver of dune buggy injured in traffic accident**

√x 7ᵗʰ **V86.04** **Driver of military vehicle injured in traffic accident**

● √x 7ᵗʰ **V86.05** **Driver of 3- or 4- wheeled all-terrain vehicle (ATV) injured in traffic accident**

● √x 7ᵗʰ **V86.06** **Driver of dirt bike or motor/cross bike injured in traffic accident**

√x 7ᵗʰ **V86.09** **Driver of other special all-terrain or other off-road motor vehicle injured in traffic accident**
     Driver of dirt bike in traffic accident
     Driver of go cart injured in traffic accident
     Driver of golf cart injured in traffic accident

√ 5ᵗʰ **V86.1** **Passenger of special all-terrain or other off-road motor vehicle injured in traffic accident**

√x 7ᵗʰ **V86.11** **Passenger of ambulance or fire engine injured in traffic accident**

√x 7ᵗʰ **V86.12** **Passenger of snowmobile injured in traffic accident**

√x 7ᵗʰ **V86.13** **Passenger of dune buggy injured in traffic accident**

√x 7ᵗʰ **V86.14** **Passenger of military vehicle injured in traffic accident**

● √x 7ᵗʰ **V86.15** **Passenger of 3- or 4- wheeled all-terrain vehicle (ATV) injured in traffic accident**

● √x 7ᵗʰ **V86.16** **Passenger of dirt bike or motor/cross bike injured in traffic accident**

√x 7ᵗʰ **V86.19** **Passenger of other special all-terrain or other off-road motor vehicle injured in traffic accident**
     Passenger of dirt bike injured in traffic accident
     Passenger of go cart injured in traffic accident
     Passenger of golf cart injured in traffic accident

√ 5ᵗʰ **V86.2** **Person on outside of special all-terrain or other off-road motor vehicle injured in traffic accident**

√x 7ᵗʰ **V86.21** **Person on outside of ambulance or fire engine injured in traffic accident**

√x 7ᵗʰ **V86.22** **Person on outside of snowmobile injured in traffic accident**

√x 7ᵗʰ **V86.23** **Person on outside of dune buggy injured in traffic accident**

√x 7ᵗʰ **V86.24** **Person on outside of military vehicle injured in traffic accident**

● √x 7ᵗʰ **V86.25** **Person on outside of 3- or 4- wheeled all-terrain vehicle (ATV) injured in traffic accident**

● √x 7ᵗʰ **V86.26** **Person on outside of dirt bike or motor/cross bike injured in traffic accident**

√x 7ᵗʰ **V86.29** **Person on outside of other special all-terrain or other off-road motor vehicle injured in traffic accident**
     Person on outside of dirt bike injured in traffic accident
     Person on outside of go cart in traffic accident
     Person on outside of golf cart injured in traffic accident

√ 5ᵗʰ **V86.3** **Unspecified occupant of special all-terrain or other off-road motor vehicle injured in traffic accident**

√x 7ᵗʰ **V86.31** **Unspecified occupant of ambulance or fire engine injured in traffic accident** ▽

√x 7ᵗʰ **V86.32** **Unspecified occupant of snowmobile injured in traffic accident** ▽

√x 7ᵗʰ **V86.33** **Unspecified occupant of dune buggy injured in traffic accident** ▽

√x 7ᵗʰ **V86.34** **Unspecified occupant of military vehicle injured in traffic accident** ▽

● √x 7ᵗʰ **V86.35** **Unspecified occupant of 3- or 4- wheeled all-terrain vehicle (ATV) injured in traffic accident** ▽

● √x 7ᵗʰ **V86.36** **Unspecified occupant of dirt bike or motor/cross bike injured in traffic accident** ▽

EXCLUDES 1 Not coded here   EXCLUDES 2 Not included here   N Newborn Age: 0   P Pediatric Age: 0-17   M Maternity Age: 12-55   A Adult Age: 15-124

1136   ICD-10-CM 2018

☑x7ᵗʰ **V86.39** Unspecified occupant of other special all-terrain ▽
or other off-road motor vehicle injured in traffic
accident
    Unspecified occupant of dirt bike injured in traffic
      accident
    Unspecified occupant of go cart injured in traffic
      accident
    Unspecified occupant of golf cart injured in traffic
      accident

☑5ᵗʰ **V86.4** Person injured while boarding or alighting from special
all-terrain or other off-road motor vehicle

   ☑x7ᵗʰ **V86.41** Person injured while boarding or alighting from
ambulance or fire engine

   ☑x7ᵗʰ **V86.42** Person injured while boarding or alighting from
snowmobile

   ☑x7ᵗʰ **V86.43** Person injured while boarding or alighting from
dune buggy

   ☑x7ᵗʰ **V86.44** Person injured while boarding or alighting from
military vehicle

●   ☑x7ᵗʰ **V86.45** Person injured while boarding or alighting from a 3-
or 4- wheeled all-terrain vehicle (ATV)

●   ☑x7ᵗʰ **V86.46** Person injured while boarding or alighting from a
dirt bike or motor/cross bike

   ☑x7ᵗʰ **V86.49** Person injured while boarding or alighting from
other special all-terrain or other off-road motor
vehicle
    Person injured while boarding or alighting from dirt
      bike
    Person injured while boarding or alighting from go
      cart
    Person injured while boarding or alighting from golf
      cart

☑5ᵗʰ **V86.5** Driver of special all-terrain or other off-road motor vehicle
injured in nontraffic accident

   ☑x7ᵗʰ **V86.51** Driver of ambulance or fire engine injured in
nontraffic accident

   ☑x7ᵗʰ **V86.52** Driver of snowmobile injured in nontraffic accident

   ☑x7ᵗʰ **V86.53** Driver of dune buggy injured in nontraffic accident

   ☑x7ᵗʰ **V86.54** Driver of military vehicle injured in nontraffic
accident

●   ☑x7ᵗʰ **V86.55** Driver of 3- or 4- wheeled all-terrain vehicle (ATV)
injured in nontraffic accident

●   ☑x7ᵗʰ **V86.56** Driver of dirt bike or motor/cross bike injured in
nontraffic accident

   ☑x7ᵗʰ **V86.59** Driver of other special all-terrain or other off-road
motor vehicle injured in nontraffic accident
    Driver of dirt bike injured in nontraffic accident
    Driver of go cart injured in nontraffic accident
    Driver of golf cart injured in nontraffic accident

☑5ᵗʰ **V86.6** Passenger of special all-terrain or other off-road motor
vehicle injured in nontraffic accident

   ☑x7ᵗʰ **V86.61** Passenger of ambulance or fire engine injured in
nontraffic accident

   ☑x7ᵗʰ **V86.62** Passenger of snowmobile injured in nontraffic
accident

   ☑x7ᵗʰ **V86.63** Passenger of dune buggy injured in nontraffic
accident

   ☑x7ᵗʰ **V86.64** Passenger of military vehicle injured in nontraffic
accident

●   ☑x7ᵗʰ **V86.65** Passenger of 3- or 4- wheeled all-terrain vehicle
(ATV) injured in nontraffic accident

●   ☑x7ᵗʰ **V86.66** Passenger of dirt bike or motor/cross bike injured in
nontraffic accident

   ☑x7ᵗʰ **V86.69** Passenger of other special all-terrain or other
off-road motor vehicle injured in nontraffic accident
    Passenger of dirt bike injured in nontraffic accident
    Passenger of go cart injured in nontraffic accident
    Passenger of golf cart injured in nontraffic accident

☑5ᵗʰ **V86.7** Person on outside of special all-terrain or other off-road
motor vehicle injured in nontraffic accident

   ☑x7ᵗʰ **V86.71** Person on outside of ambulance or fire engine
injured in nontraffic accident

   ☑x7ᵗʰ **V86.72** Person on outside of snowmobile injured in
nontraffic accident

   ☑x7ᵗʰ **V86.73** Person on outside of dune buggy injured in
nontraffic accident

   ☑x7ᵗʰ **V86.74** Person on outside of military vehicle injured in
nontraffic accident

●   ☑x7ᵗʰ **V86.75** Person on outside of 3- or 4- wheeled all-terrain
vehicle (ATV) injured in nontraffic accident

●   ☑x7ᵗʰ ~~**V86.76** Person on outside of dirt bike or motor/cross bike~~
~~injured in nontraffic accident~~

   ☑x7ᵗʰ **V86.79** Person on outside of other special all-terrain or
other off-road motor vehicles injured in nontraffic
accident
    Person on outside of dirt bike injured in nontraffic
      accident
    Person on outside of go cart injured in nontraffic
      accident
    Person on outside of golf cart injured in nontraffic
      accident

☑5ᵗʰ **V86.9** Unspecified occupant of special all-terrain or other off-road
motor vehicle injured in nontraffic accident

   ☑x7ᵗʰ **V86.91** Unspecified occupant of ambulance or fire ▽
engine injured in nontraffic accident

   ☑x7ᵗʰ **V86.92** Unspecified occupant of snowmobile injured in ▽
nontraffic accident

   ☑x7ᵗʰ **V86.93** Unspecified occupant of dune buggy injured in ▽
nontraffic accident

   ☑x7ᵗʰ **V86.94** Unspecified occupant of military vehicle injured ▽
in nontraffic accident

●   ☑x7ᵗʰ **V86.95** Unspecified occupant of 3- or 4- wheeled all- ▽
terrain vehicle (ATV) injured in nontraffic accident

●   ☑x7ᵗʰ **V86.96** Unspecified occupant of dirt bike or motor/cross ▽
bike injured in nontraffic accident

   ☑x7ᵗʰ **V86.99** Unspecified occupant of other special all-terrain ▽
or other off-road motor vehicle injured in
nontraffic accident
    ~~All-terrain motor-vehicle accident NOS~~
    Off-road motor-vehicle accident NOS
    Other motor-vehicle accident NOS
    ~~Unspecified occupant of dirt bike injured in nontraffic~~
      ~~accident~~
    Unspecified occupant of go cart injured in nontraffic
      accident
    Unspecified occupant of golf cart injured in nontraffic
      accident

☑4ᵗʰ **V87** Traffic accident of specified type but victim's mode of transport
unknown
   EXCLUDES 1   collision involving:
      pedal cycle (V10-V19)
      pedestrian (V01-V09)

   ☑x7ᵗʰ **V87.0** Person injured in collision between car and two- or
three-wheeled powered vehicle (traffic)

   ☑x7ᵗʰ **V87.1** Person injured in collision between other motor vehicle and
two- or three-wheeled motor vehicle (traffic)

   ☑x7ᵗʰ **V87.2** Person injured in collision between car and pick-up truck or
van (traffic)

   ☑x7ᵗʰ **V87.3** Person injured in collision between car and bus (traffic)

   ☑x7ᵗʰ **V87.4** Person injured in collision between car and heavy transport
vehicle (traffic)

   ☑x7ᵗʰ **V87.5** Person injured in collision between heavy transport vehicle
and bus (traffic)

   ☑x7ᵗʰ **V87.6** Person injured in collision between railway train or railway
vehicle and car (traffic)

   ☑x7ᵗʰ **V87.7** Person injured in collision between other specified motor
vehicles (traffic)

   ☑x7ᵗʰ **V87.8** Person injured in other specified noncollision transport
accidents involving motor vehicle (traffic)

   ☑x7ᵗʰ **V87.9** Person injured in other specified (collision)(noncollision)
transport accidents involving nonmotor vehicle (traffic)

☑4ᵗʰ **V88** Nontraffic accident of specified type but victim's mode of
transport unknown
   EXCLUDES 1   collision involving:
      pedal cycle (V10-V19)
      pedestrian (V01-V09)

   ☑x7ᵗʰ **V88.0** Person injured in collision between car and two- or
three-wheeled motor vehicle, nontraffic

   ☑x7ᵗʰ **V88.1** Person injured in collision between other motor vehicle and
two- or three-wheeled motor vehicle, nontraffic

   ☑x7ᵗʰ **V88.2** Person injured in collision between car and pick-up truck or
van, nontraffic

   ☑x7ᵗʰ **V88.3** Person injured in collision between car and bus, nontraffic

---

☑ Additional Character Req   ☑x7ᵗʰ Placeholder Alert   **Manifestation**   **HCC** CMS-HCC Condition   ▽ Unspecified Code   ►◄ Revised Text   ● New Code   ▲ Revised Code Title

√x7ᵗʰ **V88.4** **Person injured in collision between** car and heavy transport vehicle, **nontraffic**

√x7ᵗʰ **V88.5** **Person injured in collision between** heavy transport vehicle and bus, **nontraffic**

√x7ᵗʰ **V88.6** **Person injured in collision between** railway train or railway vehicle and car, **nontraffic**

√x7ᵗʰ **V88.7** **Person injured in collision between other specified motor vehicle, nontraffic**

√x7ᵗʰ **V88.8** **Person injured in other specified noncollision transport accidents involving** motor vehicle, **nontraffic**

√x7ᵗʰ **V88.9** **Person injured in other specified (collision)(noncollision) transport accidents involving** nonmotor vehicle, **nontraffic**

√4ᵗʰ **V89** **Motor- or nonmotor-vehicle accident, type of vehicle unspecified**

√x7ᵗʰ **V89.0** **Person injured in unspecified** motor-vehicle **accident, nontraffic** ▽
      Motor-vehicle accident NOS, nontraffic

√x7ᵗʰ **V89.1** **Person injured in unspecified** nonmotor-vehicle **accident, nontraffic** ▽
      Nonmotor-vehicle accident NOS (nontraffic)

√x7ᵗʰ **V89.2** **Person injured in unspecified** motor-vehicle **accident, traffic** ▽
      Motor-vehicle accident [MVA] NOS
      Road (traffic) accident [RTA] NOS

√x7ᵗʰ **V89.3** **Person injured in unspecified** nonmotor-vehicle **accident, traffic** ▽
      Nonmotor-vehicle traffic accident NOS

√x7ᵗʰ **V89.9** **Person injured in unspecified** vehicle accident ▽
      Collision NOS

Water transport accidents (V90-V94)

The appropriate 7th character is to be added to each code from categories V90-V94.
A   initial encounter
D   subsequent encounter
S   sequela

√4ᵗʰ **V90** **Drowning and submersion due to accident to watercraft**

> EXCLUDES 1   civilian water transport accident involving military watercraft (V94.81-)
> fall into water not from watercraft (W16.-)
> military watercraft accident in military or war operations (Y36.0-, Y37.0-)
> water-transport-related drowning or submersion without accident to watercraft (V92.-)

√5ᵗʰ **V90.0** **Drowning and submersion due to** watercraft overturning

√x7ᵗʰ **V90.00** **Drowning and submersion due to** merchant ship overturning

√x7ᵗʰ **V90.01** **Drowning and submersion due to** passenger ship overturning
      Drowning and submersion due to Ferry-boat overturning
      Drowning and submersion due to Liner overturning

√x7ᵗʰ **V90.02** **Drowning and submersion due to** fishing boat overturning

√x7ᵗʰ **V90.03** **Drowning and submersion due to other** powered watercraft overturning
      Drowning and submersion due to Hovercraft (on open water) overturning
      Drowning and submersion due to Jet ski overturning

√x7ᵗʰ **V90.04** **Drowning and submersion due to** sailboat overturning

√x7ᵗʰ **V90.05** **Drowning and submersion due to** canoe or kayak overturning

√x7ᵗʰ **V90.06** **Drowning and submersion due to** (nonpowered) inflatable craft **overturning**

√x7ᵗʰ **V90.08** **Drowning and submersion due to other** unpowered watercraft overturning
      Drowning and submersion due to windsurfer overturning

√x7ᵗʰ **V90.09** **Drowning and submersion due to unspecified** ▽ watercraft overturning
      Drowning and submersion due to boat NOS overturning
      Drowning and submersion due to ship NOS overturning
      Drowning and submersion due to watercraft NOS overturning

√5ᵗʰ **V90.1** **Drowning and submersion due to** watercraft sinking

√x7ᵗʰ **V90.10** **Drowning and submersion due to** merchant ship sinking

√x7ᵗʰ **V90.11** **Drowning and submersion due to** passenger ship sinking
      Drowning and submersion due to Ferry-boat sinking
      Drowning and submersion due to Liner sinking

√x7ᵗʰ **V90.12** **Drowning and submersion due to** fishing boat sinking

√x7ᵗʰ **V90.13** **Drowning and submersion due to other** powered watercraft sinking
      Drowning and submersion due to Hovercraft (on open water) sinking
      Drowning and submersion due to Jet ski sinking

√x7ᵗʰ **V90.14** **Drowning and submersion due to** sailboat sinking

√x7ᵗʰ **V90.15** **Drowning and submersion due to** canoe or kayak sinking

√x7ᵗʰ **V90.16** **Drowning and submersion due to** (nonpowered) inflatable craft **sinking**

√x7ᵗʰ **V90.18** **Drowning and submersion due to other** unpowered watercraft sinking

√x7ᵗʰ **V90.19** **Drowning and submersion due to unspecified** ▽ watercraft sinking
      Drowning and submersion due to boat NOS sinking
      Drowning and submersion due to ship NOS sinking
      Drowning and submersion due to watercraft NOS sinking

√5ᵗʰ **V90.2** **Drowning and submersion due to** falling or jumping from burning **watercraft**

√x7ᵗʰ **V90.20** **Drowning and submersion due to falling or jumping from burning** merchant ship

√x7ᵗʰ **V90.21** **Drowning and submersion due to falling or jumping from burning** passenger ship
      Drowning and submersion due to falling or jumping from burning Ferry-boat
      Drowning and submersion due to falling or jumping from burning Liner

√x7ᵗʰ **V90.22** **Drowning and submersion due to falling or jumping from burning** fishing boat

√x7ᵗʰ **V90.23** **Drowning and submersion due to falling or jumping from other burning** powered watercraft
      Drowning and submersion due to falling and jumping from burning Hovercraft (on open water)
      Drowning and submersion due to falling and jumping from burning Jet ski

√x7ᵗʰ **V90.24** **Drowning and submersion due to falling or jumping from burning** sailboat

√x7ᵗʰ **V90.25** **Drowning and submersion due to falling or jumping from burning** canoe or kayak

√x7ᵗʰ **V90.26** **Drowning and submersion due to falling or jumping from burning** (nonpowered) inflatable craft

√x7ᵗʰ **V90.27** **Drowning and submersion due to falling or jumping from burning** water-skis

√x7ᵗʰ **V90.28** **Drowning and submersion due to falling or jumping from other burning** unpowered **watercraft**
      Drowning and submersion due to falling and jumping from burning surf-board
      Drowning and submersion due to falling and jumping from burning windsurfer

√x7ᵗʰ **V90.29** **Drowning and submersion due to falling or jumping from unspecified burning watercraft** ▽
      Drowning and submersion due to falling or jumping from burning boat NOS
      Drowning and submersion due to falling or jumping from burning ship NOS
      Drowning and submersion due to falling or jumping from burning watercraft NOS

√5ᵗʰ **V90.3** **Drowning and submersion due to** falling or jumping from crushed watercraft

√x7ᵗʰ **V90.30** **Drowning and submersion due to falling or jumping from crushed** merchant ship

√x7ᵗʰ **V90.31** **Drowning and submersion due to falling or jumping from crushed** passenger ship
      Drowning and submersion due to falling and jumping from crushed Ferry boat
      Drowning and submersion due to falling and jumping from crushed Liner

EXCLUDES 1 Not coded here   EXCLUDES 2 Not included here   N Newborn Age: 0   P Pediatric Age: 0-17   M Maternity Age: 12-55   A Adult Age: 15-124

1138   ICD-10-CM 2018

✓x7ᵗʰ	**V90.32**	**Drowning and submersion due to falling or jumping from crushed fishing boat**
✓x7ᵗʰ	**V90.33**	**Drowning and submersion due to falling or jumping from other crushed powered watercraft**
		Drowning and submersion due to falling and jumping from crushed Hovercraft
		Drowning and submersion due to falling and jumping from crushed Jet ski
✓x7ᵗʰ	**V90.34**	**Drowning and submersion due to falling or jumping from crushed sailboat**
✓x7ᵗʰ	**V90.35**	**Drowning and submersion due to falling or jumping from crushed canoe or kayak**
✓x7ᵗʰ	**V90.36**	**Drowning and submersion due to falling or jumping from crushed (nonpowered) inflatable craft**
✓x7ᵗʰ	**V90.37**	**Drowning and submersion due to falling or jumping from crushed water-skis**
✓x7ᵗʰ	**V90.38**	**Drowning and submersion due to falling or jumping from other crushed unpowered watercraft**
		Drowning and submersion due to falling and jumping from crushed surf-board
		Drowning and submersion due to falling and jumping from crushed windsurfer
✓x7ᵗʰ	**V90.39**	**Drowning and submersion due to falling or jumping from crushed unspecified watercraft** ▽
		Drowning and submersion due to falling and jumping from crushed boat NOS
		Drowning and submersion due to falling and jumping from crushed ship NOS
		Drowning and submersion due to falling and jumping from crushed watercraft NOS

✓5ᵗʰ	**V90.8**	**Drowning and submersion due to other accident to watercraft**
✓x7ᵗʰ	**V90.80**	**Drowning and submersion due to other accident to merchant ship**
✓x7ᵗʰ	**V90.81**	**Drowning and submersion due to other accident to passenger ship**
		Drowning and submersion due to other accident to Ferry-boat
		Drowning and submersion due to other accident to Liner
✓x7ᵗʰ	**V90.82**	**Drowning and submersion due to other accident to fishing boat**
✓x7ᵗʰ	**V90.83**	**Drowning and submersion due to other accident to other powered watercraft**
		Drowning and submersion due to other accident to Hovercraft (on open water)
		Drowning and submersion due to other accident to Jet ski
✓x7ᵗʰ	**V90.84**	**Drowning and submersion due to other accident to sailboat**
✓x7ᵗʰ	**V90.85**	**Drowning and submersion due to other accident to canoe or kayak**
✓x7ᵗʰ	**V90.86**	**Drowning and submersion due to other accident to (nonpowered) inflatable craft**
✓x7ᵗʰ	**V90.87**	**Drowning and submersion due to other accident to water-skis**
✓x7ᵗʰ	**V90.88**	**Drowning and submersion due to other accident to other unpowered watercraft**
		Drowning and submersion due to other accident to surf-board
		Drowning and submersion due to other accident to windsurfer
✓x7ᵗʰ	**V90.89**	**Drowning and submersion due to other accident to unspecified watercraft** ▽
		Drowning and submersion due to other accident to boat NOS
		Drowning and submersion due to other accident to ship NOS
		Drowning and submersion due to other accident to watercraft NOS

✓4ᵗʰ	**V91**	**Other injury due to accident to watercraft**
	INCLUDES	any injury except drowning and submersion as a result of an accident to watercraft
	EXCLUDES 1	civilian water transport accident involving military watercraft (V94.81-)
		military watercraft accident in military or war operations (Y36, Y37.-)
	EXCLUDES 2	drowning and submersion due to accident to watercraft (V90.-)
✓5ᵗʰ	**V91.0**	**Burn due to watercraft on fire**
	EXCLUDES 1	burn from localized fire or explosion on board ship without accident to watercraft (V93.-)
✓x7ᵗʰ	**V91.00**	**Burn due to merchant ship on fire**
✓x7ᵗʰ	**V91.01**	**Burn due to passenger ship on fire**
		Burn due to Ferry-boat on fire
		Burn due to Liner on fire
✓x7ᵗʰ	**V91.02**	**Burn due to fishing boat on fire**
✓x7ᵗʰ	**V91.03**	**Burn due to other powered watercraft on fire**
		Burn due to Hovercraft (on open water) on fire
		Burn due to Jet ski on fire
✓x7ᵗʰ	**V91.04**	**Burn due to sailboat on fire**
✓x7ᵗʰ	**V91.05**	**Burn due to canoe or kayak on fire**
✓x7ᵗʰ	**V91.06**	**Burn due to (nonpowered) inflatable craft on fire**
✓x7ᵗʰ	**V91.07**	**Burn due to water-skis on fire**
✓x7ᵗʰ	**V91.08**	**Burn due to other unpowered watercraft on fire**
✓x7ᵗʰ	**V91.09**	**Burn due to unspecified watercraft on fire** ▽
		Burn due to boat NOS on fire
		Burn due to ship NOS on fire
		Burn due to watercraft NOS on fire

✓5ᵗʰ	**V91.1**	**Crushed between watercraft and other watercraft or other object due to collision**
		Crushed by lifeboat after abandoning ship in a collision
	NOTE	Select the specified type of watercraft that the victim was on at the time of the collision
✓x7ᵗʰ	**V91.10**	**Crushed between merchant ship and other watercraft or other object due to collision**
✓x7ᵗʰ	**V91.11**	**Crushed between passenger ship and other watercraft or other object due to collision**
		Crushed between Ferry-boat and other watercraft or other object due to collision
		Crushed between Liner and other watercraft or other object due to collision
✓x7ᵗʰ	**V91.12**	**Crushed between fishing boat and other watercraft or other object due to collision**
✓x7ᵗʰ	**V91.13**	**Crushed between other powered watercraft and other watercraft or other object due to collision**
		Crushed between Hovercraft (on open water) and other watercraft or other object due to collision
		Crushed between Jet ski and other watercraft or other object due to collision
✓x7ᵗʰ	**V91.14**	**Crushed between sailboat and other watercraft or other object due to collision**
✓x7ᵗʰ	**V91.15**	**Crushed between canoe or kayak and other watercraft or other object due to collision**
✓x7ᵗʰ	**V91.16**	**Crushed between (nonpowered) inflatable craft and other watercraft or other object due to collision**
✓x7ᵗʰ	**V91.18**	**Crushed between other unpowered watercraft and other watercraft or other object due to collision**
		Crushed between surfboard and other watercraft or other object due to collision
		Crushed between windsurfer and other watercraft or other object due to collision
✓x7ᵗʰ	**V91.19**	**Crushed between unspecified watercraft and other watercraft or other object due to collision** ▽
		Crushed between boat NOS and other watercraft or other object due to collision
		Crushed between ship NOS and other watercraft or other object due to collision
		Crushed between watercraft NOS and other watercraft or other object due to collision

☑ Additional Character Req	✓x7ᵗʰ Placeholder Alert	**Manifestation**	HCC CMS-HCC Condition	▽ Unspecified Code	►◄ Revised Text	● New Code ▲ Revised Code Title

ICD-10-CM 2018 1139

V91.2 Fall due to collision between watercraft and other watercraft or other object
Fall while remaining on watercraft after collision
NOTE Select the specified type of watercraft that the victim was on at the time of the collision.
EXCLUDES 1 crushed between watercraft and other watercraft and other object due to collision (V91.1-)
drowning and submersion due to falling from crushed watercraft (V90.3-)

V91.20 Fall due to collision between merchant ship and other watercraft or other object

V91.21 Fall due to collision between passenger ship and other watercraft or other object
Fall due to collision between Ferry-boat and other watercraft or other object
Fall due to collision between Liner and other watercraft or other object

V91.22 Fall due to collision between fishing boat and other watercraft or other object

V91.23 Fall due to collision between other powered watercraft and other watercraft or other object
Fall due to collision between Hovercraft (on open water) and other watercraft or other object
Fall due to collision between Jet ski and other watercraft or other object

V91.24 Fall due to collision between sailboat and other watercraft or other object

V91.25 Fall due to collision between canoe or kayak and other watercraft or other object

V91.26 Fall due to collision between (nonpowered) inflatable craft and other watercraft or other object

V91.29 Fall due to collision between unspecified watercraft and other watercraft or other object ▽
Fall due to collision between boat NOS and other watercraft or other object
Fall due to collision between ship NOS and other watercraft or other object
Fall due to collision between watercraft NOS and other watercraft or other object

V91.3 Hit or struck by falling object due to accident to watercraft
Hit or struck by falling object (part of damaged watercraft or other object) after falling or jumping from damaged watercraft
EXCLUDES 2 drowning or submersion due to fall or jumping from damaged watercraft (V90.2-, V90.3-)

V91.30 Hit or struck by falling object due to accident to merchant ship

V91.31 Hit or struck by falling object due to accident to passenger ship
Hit or struck by falling object due to accident to Ferry-boat
Hit or struck by falling object due to accident to Liner

V91.32 Hit or struck by falling object due to accident to fishing boat

V91.33 Hit or struck by falling object due to accident to other powered watercraft
Hit or struck by falling object due to accident to Hovercraft (on open water)
Hit or struck by falling object due to accident to Jet ski

V91.34 Hit or struck by falling object due to accident to sailboat

V91.35 Hit or struck by falling object due to accident to canoe or kayak

V91.36 Hit or struck by falling object due to accident to (nonpowered) inflatable craft

V91.37 Hit or struck by falling object due to accident to water-skis
Hit by water-skis after jumping off of waterskis

V91.38 Hit or struck by falling object due to accident to other unpowered watercraft
Hit or struck by surf-board after falling off damaged surf-board
Hit or struck by object after falling off damaged windsurfer

V91.39 Hit or struck by falling object due to accident to unspecified watercraft ▽
Hit or struck by falling object due to accident to boat NOS
Hit or struck by falling object due to accident to ship NOS
Hit or struck by falling object due to accident to watercraft NOS

V91.8 Other injury due to other accident to watercraft

V91.80 Other injury due to other accident to merchant ship

V91.81 Other injury due to other accident to passenger ship
Other injury due to other accident to Ferry-boat
Other injury due to other accident to Liner

V91.82 Other injury due to other accident to fishing boat

V91.83 Other injury due to other accident to other powered watercraft
Other injury due to other accident to Hovercraft (on open water)
Other injury due to other accident to Jet ski

V91.84 Other injury due to other accident to sailboat

V91.85 Other injury due to other accident to canoe or kayak

V91.86 Other injury due to other accident to (nonpowered) inflatable craft

V91.87 Other injury due to other accident to water-skis

V91.88 Other injury due to other accident to other unpowered watercraft
Other injury due to other accident to surf-board
Other injury due to other accident to windsurfer

V91.89 Other injury due to other accident to unspecified watercraft ▽
Other injury due to other accident to boat NOS
Other injury due to other accident to ship NOS
Other injury due to other accident to watercraft NOS

V92 Drowning and submersion due to accident on board watercraft, without accident to watercraft
EXCLUDES 1 civilian water transport accident involving military watercraft (V94.81-)
drowning or submersion due to accident to watercraft (V90-V91)
drowning or submersion of diver who voluntarily jumps from boat not involved in an accident (W16.711, W16.721)
fall into water without watercraft (W16.-)
military watercraft accident in military or war operations (Y36, Y37)

V92.0 Drowning and submersion due to fall off watercraft
Drowning and submersion due to fall from gangplank of watercraft
Drowning and submersion due to fall overboard watercraft
EXCLUDES 2 hitting head on object or bottom of body of water due to fall from watercraft (V94.0-)

V92.00 Drowning and submersion due to fall off merchant ship

V92.01 Drowning and submersion due to fall off passenger ship
Drowning and submersion due to fall off Ferry-boat
Drowning and submersion due to fall off Liner

V92.02 Drowning and submersion due to fall off fishing boat

V92.03 Drowning and submersion due to fall off other powered watercraft
Drowning and submersion due to fall off Hovercraft (on open water)
Drowning and submersion due to fall off Jet ski

V92.04 Drowning and submersion due to fall off sailboat

V92.05 Drowning and submersion due to fall off canoe or kayak

V92.06 Drowning and submersion due to fall off (nonpowered) inflatable craft

V92.07 Drowning and submersion due to fall off water-skis
EXCLUDES 1 drowning and submersion due to falling off burning water-skis (V90.27)
drowning and submersion due to falling off crushed water-skis (V90.37)
hit by boat while water-skiing NOS (V94.X)

✓x7ᵗʰ **V92.08** **Drowning and submersion due to fall off other unpowered watercraft**
    Drowning and submersion due to fall off surf-board
    Drowning and submersion due to fall off windsurfer
    EXCLUDES 1   *drowning and submersion due to fall off burning unpowered watercraft (V90.28)*
        drowning and submersion due to fall off crushed unpowered watercraft (V90.38)
        drowning and submersion due to fall off damaged unpowered watercraft (V90.88)
        drowning and submersion due to rider of nonpowered watercraft being hit by other watercraft (V94.-)
        other injury due to rider of nonpowered watercraft being hit by other watercraft (V94.-)

✓x7ᵗʰ **V92.09** **Drowning and submersion due to fall off unspecified watercraft** ▽
    Drowning and submersion due to fall off boat NOS
    Drowning and submersion due to fall off ship
    Drowning and submersion due to fall off watercraft NOS

✓5ᵗʰ **V92.1** **Drowning and submersion due to being thrown overboard by motion of watercraft**
    EXCLUDES 1   *drowning and submersion due to fall off surf-board (V92.08)*
        drowning and submersion due to fall off water-skis (V92.07)
        drowning and submersion due to fall off windsurfer (V92.08)

✓x7ᵗʰ **V92.10** **Drowning and submersion due to being thrown overboard by motion of merchant ship**

✓x7ᵗʰ **V92.11** **Drowning and submersion due to being thrown overboard by motion of passenger ship**
    Drowning and submersion due to being thrown overboard by motion of Ferry-boat
    Drowning and submersion due to being thrown overboard by motion of Liner

✓x7ᵗʰ **V92.12** **Drowning and submersion due to being thrown overboard by motion of fishing boat**

✓x7ᵗʰ **V92.13** **Drowning and submersion due to being thrown overboard by motion of other powered watercraft**
    Drowning and submersion due to being thrown overboard by motion of Hovercraft

✓x7ᵗʰ **V92.14** **Drowning and submersion due to being thrown overboard by motion of sailboat**

✓x7ᵗʰ **V92.15** **Drowning and submersion due to being thrown overboard by motion of canoe or kayak**

✓x7ᵗʰ **V92.16** **Drowning and submersion due to being thrown overboard by motion of (nonpowered) inflatable craft**

✓x7ᵗʰ **V92.19** **Drowning and submersion due to being thrown overboard by motion of unspecified watercraft** ▽
    Drowning and submersion due to being thrown overboard by motion of boat NOS
    Drowning and submersion due to being thrown overboard by motion of ship NOS
    Drowning and submersion due to being thrown overboard by motion of watercraft NOS

✓5ᵗʰ **V92.2** **Drowning and submersion due to being washed overboard from watercraft**
    Code first any associated cataclysm (X37.0-)

✓x7ᵗʰ **V92.20** **Drowning and submersion due to being washed overboard from merchant ship**

✓x7ᵗʰ **V92.21** **Drowning and submersion due to being washed overboard from passenger ship**
    Drowning and submersion due to being washed overboard from Ferry-boat
    Drowning and submersion due to being washed overboard from Liner

✓x7ᵗʰ **V92.22** **Drowning and submersion due to being washed overboard from fishing boat**

✓x7ᵗʰ **V92.23** **Drowning and submersion due to being washed overboard from other powered watercraft**
    Drowning and submersion due to being washed overboard from Hovercraft (on open water)
    Drowning and submersion due to being washed overboard from Jet ski

✓x7ᵗʰ **V92.24** **Drowning and submersion due to being washed overboard from sailboat**

✓x7ᵗʰ **V92.25** **Drowning and submersion due to being washed overboard from canoe or kayak**

✓x7ᵗʰ **V92.26** **Drowning and submersion due to being washed overboard from (nonpowered) inflatable craft**

✓x7ᵗʰ **V92.27** ~~**Drowning and submersion due to being washed overboard from water-skis**~~
    EXCLUDES 1   *drowning and submersion due to fall off water-skis (V92.07)*

✓x7ᵗʰ **V92.28** **Drowning and submersion due to being washed overboard from other unpowered watercraft**
    Drowning and submersion due to being washed overboard from surf-board
    Drowning and submersion due to being washed overboard from windsurfer

✓x7ᵗʰ **V92.29** **Drowning and submersion due to being washed overboard from unspecified watercraft** ▽
    Drowning and submersion due to being washed overboard from boat NOS
    Drowning and submersion due to being washed overboard from ship NOS
    Drowning and submersion due to being washed overboard from watercraft NOS

✓4ᵗʰ **V93** **Other injury due to accident on board watercraft, without accident to watercraft**
    EXCLUDES 1   *civilian water transport accident involving military watercraft (V94.81-)*
        other injury due to accident to watercraft (V91.-)
        military watercraft accident in military or war operations (Y36, Y37.-)
    EXCLUDES 2   *drowning and submersion due to accident on board watercraft, without accident to watercraft (V92.-)*

✓5ᵗʰ **V93.0** **Burn due to localized fire on board watercraft**
    EXCLUDES 1   *burn due to watercraft on fire (V91.0-)*

✓x7ᵗʰ **V93.00** **Burn due to localized fire on board merchant vessel**

✓x7ᵗʰ **V93.01** **Burn due to localized fire on board passenger vessel**
    Burn due to localized fire on board Ferry-boat
    Burn due to localized fire on board Liner

✓x7ᵗʰ **V93.02** **Burn due to localized fire on board fishing boat**

✓x7ᵗʰ **V93.03** **Burn due to localized fire on board other powered watercraft**
    Burn due to localized fire on board Hovercraft
    Burn due to localized fire on board Jet ski

✓x7ᵗʰ **V93.04** **Burn due to localized fire on board sailboat**

✓x7ᵗʰ **V93.09** **Burn due to localized fire on board unspecified watercraft** ▽
    Burn due to localized fire on board boat NOS
    Burn due to localized fire on board ship NOS
    Burn due to localized fire on board watercraft NOS

✓5ᵗʰ **V93.1** **Other burn on board watercraft**
    Burn due to source other than fire on board watercraft
    EXCLUDES 1   *burn due to watercraft on fire (V91.0-)*

✓x7ᵗʰ **V93.10** **Other burn on board merchant vessel**

✓x7ᵗʰ **V93.11** **Other burn on board passenger vessel**
    Other burn on board Ferry-boat
    Other burn on board Liner

✓x7ᵗʰ **V93.12** **Other burn on board fishing boat**

✓x7ᵗʰ **V93.13** **Other burn on board other powered watercraft**
    Other burn on board Hovercraft
    Other burn on board Jet ski

✓x7ᵗʰ **V93.14** **Other burn on board sailboat**

✓x7ᵗʰ **V93.19** **Other burn on board unspecified watercraft** ▽
    Other burn on board boat NOS
    Other burn on board ship NOS
    Other burn on board watercraft NOS

✓5ᵗʰ **V93.2** **Heat exposure on board watercraft**
    EXCLUDES 1   *exposure to man-made heat not aboard watercraft (W92)*
        exposure to natural heat while on board watercraft (X30)
        exposure to sunlight while on board watercraft (X32)
    EXCLUDES 2   *burn due to fire on board watercraft (V93.0-)*

✓x7ᵗʰ **V93.20** **Heat exposure on board merchant ship**

✓x7ᵗʰ **V93.21** **Heat exposure on board passenger ship**
    Heat exposure on board Ferry-boat
    Heat exposure on board Liner

✓x7ᵗʰ **V93.22** **Heat exposure on board fishing boat**

☑ Additional Character Req   ✓x7ᵗʰ Placeholder Alert   Manifestation   HCC CMS-HCC Condition   ▽ Unspecified Code   ►◄ Revised Text   ● New Code   ▲ Revised Code Title

ICD-10-CM 2018   1141

√x7ᵗʰ **V93.23 Heat exposure on board other powered watercraft**
Heat exposure on board hovercraft

√x7ᵗʰ **V93.24 Heat exposure on board sailboat**

√x7ᵗʰ **V93.29 Heat exposure on board unspecified watercraft** ▽
Heat exposure on board boat NOS
Heat exposure on board ship NOS
Heat exposure on board watercraft NOS

√5ᵗʰ **V93.3 Fall on board watercraft**
EXCLUDES 1   *fall due to collision of watercraft (V91.2-)*

√x7ᵗʰ **V93.3Ø Fall on board merchant ship**

√x7ᵗʰ **V93.31 Fall on board passenger ship**
Fall on board Ferry-boat
Fall on board Liner

√x7ᵗʰ **V93.32 Fall on board fishing boat**

√x7ᵗʰ **V93.33 Fall on board other powered watercraft**
Fall on board Hovercraft (on open water)
Fall on board Jet ski

√x7ᵗʰ **V93.34 Fall on board sailboat**

√x7ᵗʰ **V93.35 Fall on board canoe or kayak**

√x7ᵗʰ **V93.36 Fall on board (nonpowered) inflatable craft**

√x7ᵗʰ **V93.38 Fall on board other unpowered watercraft**

√x7ᵗʰ **V93.39 Fall on board unspecified watercraft** ▽
Fall on board boat NOS
Fall on board ship NOS
Fall on board watercraft NOS

√5ᵗʰ **V93.4 Struck by falling object on board watercraft**
Hit by falling object on board watercraft
EXCLUDES 1   *struck by falling object due to accident to watercraft (V91.3)*

√x7ᵗʰ **V93.4Ø Struck by falling object on merchant ship**

√x7ᵗʰ **V93.41 Struck by falling object on passenger ship**
Struck by falling object on Ferry-boat
Struck by falling object on Liner

√x7ᵗʰ **V93.42 Struck by falling object on fishing boat**

√x7ᵗʰ **V93.43 Struck by falling object on other powered watercraft**
Struck by falling object on Hovercraft

√x7ᵗʰ **V93.44 Struck by falling object on sailboat**

√x7ᵗʰ **V93.48 Struck by falling object on other unpowered watercraft**

√x7ᵗʰ **V93.49 Struck by falling object on unspecified watercraft** ▽

√5ᵗʰ **V93.5 Explosion on board watercraft**
Boiler explosion on steamship
EXCLUDES 2   *fire on board watercraft (V93.Ø-)*

√x7ᵗʰ **V93.5Ø Explosion on board merchant ship**

√x7ᵗʰ **V93.51 Explosion on board passenger ship**
Explosion on board Ferry-boat
Explosion on board Liner

√x7ᵗʰ **V93.52 Explosion on board fishing boat**

√x7ᵗʰ **V93.53 Explosion on board other powered watercraft**
Explosion on board Hovercraft
Explosion on board Jet ski

√x7ᵗʰ **V93.54 Explosion on board sailboat**

√x7ᵗʰ **V93.59 Explosion on board unspecified watercraft** ▽
Explosion on board boat NOS
Explosion on board ship NOS
Explosion on board watercraft NOS

√5ᵗʰ **V93.6 Machinery accident on board watercraft**
EXCLUDES 1   *machinery explosion on board watercraft (V93.4-)*
machinery fire on board watercraft (V93.Ø-)

√x7ᵗʰ **V93.6Ø Machinery accident on board merchant ship**

√x7ᵗʰ **V93.61 Machinery accident on board passenger ship**
Machinery accident on board Ferry-boat
Machinery accident on board Liner

√x7ᵗʰ **V93.62 Machinery accident on board fishing boat**

√x7ᵗʰ **V93.63 Machinery accident on board other powered watercraft**
Machinery accident on board Hovercraft

√x7ᵗʰ **V93.64 Machinery accident on board sailboat**

√x7ᵗʰ **V93.69 Machinery accident on board unspecified watercraft** ▽
Machinery accident on board boat NOS
Machinery accident on board ship NOS
Machinery accident on board watercraft NOS

√5ᵗʰ **V93.8 Other injury due to other accident on board watercraft**
Accidental poisoning by gases or fumes on watercraft

√x7ᵗʰ **V93.8Ø Other injury due to other accident on board merchant ship**

√x7ᵗʰ **V93.81 Other injury due to other accident on board passenger ship**
Other injury due to other accident on board Ferry-boat
Other injury due to other accident on board Liner

√x7ᵗʰ **V93.82 Other injury due to other accident on board fishing boat**

√x7ᵗʰ **V93.83 Other injury due to other accident on board other powered watercraft**
Other injury due to other accident on board Hovercraft
Other injury due to other accident on board Jet ski

√x7ᵗʰ **V93.84 Other injury due to other accident on board sailboat**

√x7ᵗʰ **V93.85 Other injury due to other accident on board canoe or kayak**

√x7ᵗʰ **V93.86 Other injury due to other accident on board (nonpowered) inflatable craft**

√x7ᵗʰ **V93.87 Other injury due to other accident on board water-skis**
Hit or struck by object while waterskiing

√x7ᵗʰ **V93.88 Other injury due to other accident on board other unpowered watercraft**
Hit or struck by object while surfing
Hit or struck by object while on board windsurfer

√x7ᵗʰ **V93.89 Other injury due to other accident on board unspecified watercraft** ▽
Other injury due to other accident on board boat NOS
Other injury due to other accident on board ship NOS
Other injury due to other accident on board watercraft NOS

√4ᵗʰ **V94 Other and unspecified water transport accidents**
EXCLUDES 1   *military watercraft accidents in military or war operations (Y36, Y37)*

√x7ᵗʰ **V94.Ø Hitting object or bottom of body of water due to fall from watercraft**
EXCLUDES 2   *drowning and submersion due to fall from watercraft (V92.Ø-)*

√5ᵗʰ **V94.1 Bather struck by watercraft**
Swimmer hit by watercraft

√x7ᵗʰ **V94.11 Bather struck by powered watercraft**

√x7ᵗʰ **V94.12 Bather struck by nonpowered watercraft**

√5ᵗʰ **V94.2 Rider of nonpowered watercraft struck by other watercraft**

√x7ᵗʰ **V94.21 Rider of nonpowered watercraft struck by other nonpowered watercraft**
Canoer hit by other nonpowered watercraft
Surfer hit by other nonpowered watercraft
Windsurfer hit by other nonpowered watercraft

√x7ᵗʰ **V94.22 Rider of nonpowered watercraft struck by powered watercraft**
Canoer hit by motorboat
Surfer hit by motorboat
Windsurfer hit by motorboat

√5ᵗʰ **V94.3 Injury to rider of (inflatable) watercraft being pulled behind other watercraft**

√x7ᵗʰ **V94.31 Injury to rider of (inflatable) recreational watercraft being pulled behind other watercraft**
Injury to rider of inner-tube pulled behind motor boat

√x7ᵗʰ **V94.32 Injury to rider of non-recreational watercraft being pulled behind other watercraft**
Injury to occupant of dingy being pulled behind boat or ship
Injury to occupant of life-raft being pulled behind boat or ship

√x7ᵗʰ **V94.4 Injury to barefoot water-skier**
Injury to person being pulled behind boat or ship

√5ᵗʰ **V94.8 Other water transport accident**

√6ᵗʰ **V94.81 Water transport accident involving military watercraft**

√7ᵗʰ **V94.81Ø Civilian watercraft involved in water transport accident with military watercraft**
Passenger on civilian watercraft injured due to accident with military watercraft

---

EXCLUDES 1 Not coded here   EXCLUDES 2 Not included here   N Newborn Age: 0   P Pediatric Age: 0-17   M Maternity Age: 12-55   A Adult Age: 15-124

1142   ICD-10-CM 2018

☑7ᵗʰ **V94.811** Civilian in water injured by military watercraft

☑7ᵗʰ **V94.818** Other water transport accident involving military watercraft

☑7ᵗʰ **V94.89** Other water transport accident

☑×7ᵗʰ **V94.9** Unspecified water transport accident ▽
Water transport accident NOS

Air and space transport accidents (V95-V97)

EXCLUDES 1   military aircraft accidents in military or war operations (Y36, Y37)

The appropriate 7th character is to be added to each code from categories V95-V97.
A   initial encounter
D   subsequent encounter
S   sequela

☑4ᵗʰ **V95** Accident to powered aircraft causing injury to occupant

☑5ᵗʰ **V95.0** Helicopter accident injuring occupant

☑×7ᵗʰ **V95.00** Unspecified helicopter accident injuring occupant ▽

☑×7ᵗʰ **V95.01** Helicopter crash injuring occupant

☑×7ᵗʰ **V95.02** Forced landing of helicopter injuring occupant

☑×7ᵗʰ **V95.03** Helicopter collision injuring occupant
Helicopter collision with any object, fixed, movable or moving

☑×7ᵗʰ **V95.04** Helicopter fire injuring occupant

☑×7ᵗʰ **V95.05** Helicopter explosion injuring occupant

☑×7ᵗʰ **V95.09** Other helicopter accident injuring occupant

☑5ᵗʰ **V95.1** Ultralight, microlight or powered-glider accident injuring occupant

☑×7ᵗʰ **V95.10** Unspecified ultralight, microlight or powered-glider accident injuring occupant ▽

☑×7ᵗʰ **V95.11** Ultralight, microlight or powered-glider crash injuring occupant

☑×7ᵗʰ **V95.12** Forced landing of ultralight, microlight or powered-glider injuring occupant

☑×7ᵗʰ **V95.13** Ultralight, microlight or powered-glider collision injuring occupant
Ultralight, microlight or powered-glider collision with any object, fixed, movable or moving

☑×7ᵗʰ **V95.14** Ultralight, microlight or powered-glider fire injuring occupant

☑×7ᵗʰ **V95.15** Ultralight, microlight or powered-glider explosion injuring occupant

☑×7ᵗʰ **V95.19** Other ultralight, microlight or powered-glider accident injuring occupant

☑5ᵗʰ **V95.2** Other private fixed-wing aircraft accident injuring occupant

☑×7ᵗʰ **V95.20** Unspecified accident to other private fixed-wing aircraft, injuring occupant ▽

☑×7ᵗʰ **V95.21** Other private fixed-wing aircraft crash injuring occupant

☑×7ᵗʰ **V95.22** Forced landing of other private fixed-wing aircraft injuring occupant

☑×7ᵗʰ **V95.23** Other private fixed-wing aircraft collision injuring occupant
Other private fixed-wing aircraft collision with any object, fixed, movable or moving

☑×7ᵗʰ **V95.24** Other private fixed-wing aircraft fire injuring occupant

☑×7ᵗʰ **V95.25** Other private fixed-wing aircraft explosion injuring occupant

☑×7ᵗʰ **V95.29** Other accident to other private fixed-wing aircraft injuring occupant

☑5ᵗʰ **V95.3** Commercial fixed-wing aircraft accident injuring occupant

☑×7ᵗʰ **V95.30** Unspecified accident to commercial fixed-wing aircraft injuring occupant ▽

☑×7ᵗʰ **V95.31** Commercial fixed-wing aircraft crash injuring occupant

☑×7ᵗʰ **V95.32** Forced landing of commercial fixed-wing aircraft injuring occupant

☑×7ᵗʰ **V95.33** Commercial fixed-wing aircraft collision injuring occupant
Commercial fixed-wing aircraft collision with any object, fixed, movable or moving

☑×7ᵗʰ **V95.34** Commercial fixed-wing aircraft fire injuring occupant

☑×7ᵗʰ **V95.35** Commercial fixed-wing aircraft explosion injuring occupant

☑×7ᵗʰ **V95.39** Other accident to commercial fixed-wing aircraft injuring occupant

☑5ᵗʰ **V95.4** Spacecraft accident injuring occupant

☑×7ᵗʰ **V95.40** Unspecified spacecraft accident injuring occupant ▽

☑×7ᵗʰ **V95.41** Spacecraft crash injuring occupant

☑×7ᵗʰ **V95.42** Forced landing of spacecraft injuring occupant

☑×7ᵗʰ **V95.43** Spacecraft collision injuring occupant
Spacecraft collision with any object, fixed, moveable or moving

☑×7ᵗʰ **V95.44** Spacecraft fire injuring occupant

☑×7ᵗʰ **V95.45** Spacecraft explosion injuring occupant

☑×7ᵗʰ **V95.49** Other spacecraft accident injuring occupant

☑×7ᵗʰ **V95.8** Other powered aircraft accidents injuring occupant

☑×7ᵗʰ **V95.9** Unspecified aircraft accident injuring occupant ▽
Aircraft accident NOS
Air transport accident NOS

☑4ᵗʰ **V96** Accident to nonpowered aircraft causing injury to occupant

☑5ᵗʰ **V96.0** Balloon accident injuring occupant

☑×7ᵗʰ **V96.00** Unspecified balloon accident injuring occupant ▽

☑×7ᵗʰ **V96.01** Balloon crash injuring occupant

☑×7ᵗʰ **V96.02** Forced landing of balloon injuring occupant

☑×7ᵗʰ **V96.03** Balloon collision injuring occupant
Balloon collision with any object, fixed, moveable or moving

☑×7ᵗʰ **V96.04** Balloon fire injuring occupant

☑×7ᵗʰ **V96.05** Balloon explosion injuring occupant

☑×7ᵗʰ **V96.09** Other balloon accident injuring occupant

☑5ᵗʰ **V96.1** Hang-glider accident injuring occupant

☑×7ᵗʰ **V96.10** Unspecified hang-glider accident injuring occupant ▽

☑×7ᵗʰ **V96.11** Hang-glider crash injuring occupant

☑×7ᵗʰ **V96.12** Forced landing of hang-glider injuring occupant

☑×7ᵗʰ **V96.13** Hang-glider collision injuring occupant
Hang-glider collision with any object, fixed, moveable or moving

☑×7ᵗʰ **V96.14** Hang-glider fire injuring occupant

☑×7ᵗʰ **V96.15** Hang-glider explosion injuring occupant

☑×7ᵗʰ **V96.19** Other hang-glider accident injuring occupant

☑5ᵗʰ **V96.2** Glider (nonpowered) accident injuring occupant

☑×7ᵗʰ **V96.20** Unspecified glider (nonpowered) accident injuring occupant ▽

☑×7ᵗʰ **V96.21** Glider (nonpowered) crash injuring occupant

☑×7ᵗʰ **V96.22** Forced landing of glider (nonpowered) injuring occupant

☑×7ᵗʰ **V96.23** Glider (nonpowered) collision injuring occupant
Glider (nonpowered) collision with any object, fixed, moveable or moving

☑×7ᵗʰ **V96.24** Glider (nonpowered) fire injuring occupant

☑×7ᵗʰ **V96.25** Glider (nonpowered) explosion injuring occupant

☑×7ᵗʰ **V96.29** Other glider (nonpowered) accident injuring occupant

☑×7ᵗʰ **V96.8** Other nonpowered-aircraft accidents injuring occupant
Kite carrying a person accident injuring occupant

☑×7ᵗʰ **V96.9** Unspecified nonpowered-aircraft accident injuring occupant ▽
Nonpowered-aircraft accident NOS

☑4ᵗʰ **V97** Other specified air transport accidents

☑×7ᵗʰ **V97.0** Occupant of aircraft injured in other specified air transport accidents
Fall in, on or from aircraft in air transport accident
EXCLUDES 1   accident while boarding or alighting aircraft (V97.1)

☑×7ᵗʰ **V97.1** Person injured while boarding or alighting from aircraft

☑5ᵗʰ **V97.2** Parachutist accident

☑×7ᵗʰ **V97.21** Parachutist entangled in object
Parachutist landing in tree

☑×7ᵗʰ **V97.22** Parachutist injured on landing

☑ Additional Character Req   ☑7ᵗʰ Placeholder Alert   Manifestation   HCC CMS-HCC Condition   ▽ Unspecified Code   ►◄ Revised Text   ● New Code   ▲ Revised Code Title

√x7ᵗʰ **V97.29 Other parachutist accident**

√5ᵗʰ **V97.3 Person on ground injured in air transport accident**

√x7ᵗʰ **V97.31 Hit by object falling from aircraft**
Hit by crashing aircraft
Injured by aircraft hitting house
Injured by aircraft hitting car

√x7ᵗʰ **V97.32 Injured by rotating propeller**

√x7ᵗʰ **V97.33 Sucked into jet engine**

√x7ᵗʰ **V97.39 Other injury to person on ground due to air transport accident**

√5ᵗʰ **V97.8 Other air transport accidents, not elsewhere classified**
EXCLUDES1 *aircraft accident NOS (V95.9)*
exposure to changes in air pressure during ascent or descent (W94.-)

√6ᵗʰ **V97.81 Air transport accident involving military aircraft**

√7ᵗʰ **V97.810 Civilian aircraft involved in air transport accident with military aircraft**
Passenger in civilian aircraft injured due to accident with military aircraft

√7ᵗʰ **V97.811 Civilian injured by military aircraft**

√7ᵗʰ **V97.818 Other air transport accident involving military aircraft**

√x7ᵗʰ **V97.89 Other air transport accidents, not elsewhere classified**
Injury from machinery on aircraft

Other and unspecified transport accidents (V98-V99)

EXCLUDES1 *vehicle accident, type of vehicle unspecified (V89.-)*

The appropriate 7th character is to be added to each code from categories V98-V99.
A   initial encounter
D   subsequent encounter
S   sequela

√4ᵗʰ **V98 Other specified transport accidents**

√x7ᵗʰ **V98.0 Accident to, on or involving cable-car, not on rails**
Caught or dragged by cable-car, not on rails
Fall or jump from cable-car, not on rails
Object thrown from or in cable-car, not on rails

√x7ᵗʰ **V98.1 Accident to, on or involving land-yacht**

√x7ᵗʰ **V98.2 Accident to, on or involving ice yacht**

√x7ᵗʰ **V98.3 Accident to, on or involving ski lift**
Accident to, on or involving ski chair-lift
Accident to, on or involving ski-lift with gondola

√x7ᵗʰ **V98.8 Other specified transport accidents**

√x7ᵗʰ **V99 Unspecified transport accident** ▽

OTHER EXTERNAL CAUSES OF ACCIDENTAL INJURY (W00-X58)

Slipping, tripping, stumbling and falls (W00-W19)

EXCLUDES1 *assault involving a fall (Y01-Y02)*
fall from animal (V80.-)
fall (in) (from) machinery (in operation) (W28-W31)
fall (in) (from) transport vehicle (V01-V99)
intentional self-harm involving a fall (X80-X81)
EXCLUDES2 *at risk for fall (history of fall) (Z91.81)*
fall (in) (from) burning building (X00.-)
fall into fire ▶(X00-X04, X08)◀

The appropriate 7th character is to be added to each code from category W00-W19.
A   initial encounter
D   subsequent encounter
S   sequela

√4ᵗʰ **W00 Fall due to ice and snow**
INCLUDES pedestrian on foot falling (slipping) on ice and snow
EXCLUDES1 *fall on (from) ice and snow involving pedestrian conveyance (V00.-)*
fall from stairs and steps not due to ice and snow (W10.-)
AHA: 2016, 2Q, 4

√x7ᵗʰ **W00.0 Fall on same level due to ice and snow**

√x7ᵗʰ **W00.1 Fall from stairs and steps due to ice and snow**

√x7ᵗʰ **W00.2 Other fall from one level to another due to ice and snow**

√x7ᵗʰ **W00.9 Unspecified fall due to ice and snow** ▽

√4ᵗʰ **W01 Fall on same level from slipping, tripping and stumbling**
INCLUDES fall on moving sidewalk
EXCLUDES1 *fall due to bumping (striking) against object (W18.0-)*
fall in shower or bathtub (W18.2-)
fall on same level NOS (W18.30)
fall on same level from slipping, tripping and stumbling due to ice or snow (W00.0)
fall off or from toilet (W18.1-)
slipping, tripping and stumbling NOS (W18.40)
slipping, tripping and stumbling without falling (W18.4-)

√x7ᵗʰ **W01.0 Fall on same level from slipping, tripping and stumbling without subsequent striking against object**
Falling over animal

√5ᵗʰ **W01.1 Fall on same level from slipping, tripping and stumbling with subsequent striking against object**

√x7ᵗʰ **W01.10 Fall on same level from slipping, tripping and stumbling with subsequent striking against unspecified object** ▽

√6ᵗʰ **W01.11 Fall on same level from slipping, tripping and stumbling with subsequent striking against sharp object**

√7ᵗʰ **W01.110 Fall on same level from slipping, tripping and stumbling with subsequent striking against sharp glass**

√7ᵗʰ **W01.111 Fall on same level from slipping, tripping and stumbling with subsequent striking against power tool or machine**

√7ᵗʰ **W01.118 Fall on same level from slipping, tripping and stumbling with subsequent striking against other sharp object**

√7ᵗʰ **W01.119 Fall on same level from slipping, tripping and stumbling with subsequent striking against unspecified sharp object** ▽

√6ᵗʰ **W01.19 Fall on same level from slipping, tripping and stumbling with subsequent striking against other object**

√7ᵗʰ **W01.190 Fall on same level from slipping, tripping and stumbling with subsequent striking against furniture**

√7ᵗʰ **W01.198 Fall on same level from slipping, tripping and stumbling with subsequent striking against other object**

√x7ᵗʰ **W03 Other fall on same level due to collision with another person**
Fall due to non-transport collision with other person
EXCLUDES1 *collision with another person without fall (W51)*
crushed or pushed by a crowd or human stampede (W52)
fall involving pedestrian conveyance (V00-V09)
fall due to ice or snow (W00)
fall on same level NOS (W18.30)
AHA: 2012, 4Q, 108

√x7ᵗʰ **W04 Fall while being carried or supported by other persons**
Accidentally dropped while being carried

√4ᵗʰ **W05 Fall from non-moving wheelchair, nonmotorized scooter and motorized mobility scooter**
EXCLUDES1 *fall from moving wheelchair (powered) (V00.811)*
fall from moving motorized mobility scooter (V00.831)
fall from nonmotorized scooter (V00.141)

√x7ᵗʰ **W05.0 Fall from non-moving wheelchair**

√x7ᵗʰ **W05.1 Fall from non-moving nonmotorized scooter**

√x7ᵗʰ **W05.2 Fall from non-moving motorized mobility scooter**

√x7ᵗʰ **W06 Fall from bed**

√x7ᵗʰ **W07 Fall from chair**

√x7ᵗʰ **W08 Fall from other furniture**

√4ᵗʰ **W09 Fall on and from playground equipment**
EXCLUDES1 *fall involving recreational machinery (W31)g*

√x7ᵗʰ **W09.0 Fall on or from playground slide**

√x7ᵗʰ **W09.1 Fall from playground swing**

√x7ᵗʰ **W09.2 Fall on or from jungle gym**

√x7ᵗʰ **W09.8 Fall on or from other playground equipment**

√4ᵗʰ **W10 Fall on and from stairs and steps**
EXCLUDES1 *Fall from stairs and steps due to ice and snow (W00.1)*

√x7ᵗʰ **W10.0 Fall (on)(from) escalator**

√x7ᵗʰ **W10.1 Fall (on)(from) sidewalk curb**

√x7ᵗʰ **W10.2 Fall (on)(from) incline**
Fall (on) (from) ramp

EXCLUDES1 Not coded here   EXCLUDES2 Not included here   N Newborn Age: 0   P Pediatric Age: 0-17   M Maternity Age: 12-55   A Adult Age: 15-124

√x7ᵗʰ **W10.8** Fall (on) (from) other stairs and steps

√x7ᵗʰ **W10.9** Fall (on) (from) unspecified stairs and steps ▽

√x7ᵗʰ **W11 Fall on and from ladder**

√x7ᵗʰ **W12 Fall on and from scaffolding**

√4ᵗʰ **W13 Fall from, out of or through building or structure**

  √x7ᵗʰ **W13.0** Fall from, out of or through balcony
       Fall from, out of or through railing

  √x7ᵗʰ **W13.1** Fall from, out of or through bridge

  √x7ᵗʰ **W13.2** Fall from, out of or through roof

  √x7ᵗʰ **W13.3** Fall through floor

  √x7ᵗʰ **W13.4** Fall from, out of or through window
       EXCLUDES 2   *fall with subsequent striking against sharp glass (W01.110)*

  √x7ᵗʰ **W13.8** Fall from, out of or through other building or structure
       Fall from, out of or through viaduct
       Fall from, out of or through wall
       Fall from, out of or through flag-pole

  √x7ᵗʰ **W13.9** Fall from, out of or through building, not otherwise specified ▽
       EXCLUDES 1   *collapse of a building or structure (W20.-)*
                 fall or jump from burning building or structure (X00.-)

√x7ᵗʰ **W14 Fall from tree**

√x7ᵗʰ **W15 Fall from cliff**

√4ᵗʰ **W16 Fall, jump or diving into water**
       EXCLUDES 1   *accidental non-watercraft drowning and submersion not involving fall (W65-W74)*
                 effects of air pressure from diving (W94.-)
                 fall into water from watercraft (V90-V94)
                 hitting an object or against bottom when falling from watercraft (V94.0)
       EXCLUDES 2   *striking or hitting diving board (W21.4)*

  √5ᵗʰ **W16.0 Fall into** swimming pool
       Fall into swimming pool NOS
       EXCLUDES 1   *fall into empty swimming pool (W17.3)*

    √6ᵗʰ **W16.01 Fall into swimming pool** striking water surface

      √7ᵗʰ **W16.011** Fall into swimming pool striking water surface causing drowning and submersion
          EXCLUDES 1   *drowning and submersion while in swimming pool without fall (W67)*

      √7ᵗʰ **W16.012** Fall into swimming pool striking water surface causing other injury

    √6ᵗʰ **W16.02 Fall into swimming pool** striking bottom

      √7ᵗʰ **W16.021** Fall into swimming pool striking bottom causing drowning and submersion
          EXCLUDES 1   *drowning and submersion while in swimming pool without fall (W67)*

      √7ᵗʰ **W16.022** Fall into swimming pool striking bottom causing other injury

    √6ᵗʰ **W16.03 Fall into swimming pool** striking wall

      √7ᵗʰ **W16.031** Fall into swimming pool striking wall causing drowning and submersion
          EXCLUDES 1   *drowning and submersion while in swimming pool without fall (W67)*

      √7ᵗʰ **W16.032** Fall into swimming pool striking wall causing other injury

  √6ᵗʰ **W16.1 Fall into** natural body of water
       Fall into lake   Fall into river
       Fall into open sea   Fall into stream

    √6ᵗʰ **W16.11 Fall into natural body of water** striking water surface

      √7ᵗʰ **W16.111** Fall into natural body of water striking water surface causing drowning and submersion
          EXCLUDES 1   *drowning and submersion while in natural body of water without fall (W69)*

      √7ᵗʰ **W16.112** Fall into natural body of water striking water surface causing other injury

    √6ᵗʰ **W16.12 Fall into natural body of water** striking bottom

      √7ᵗʰ **W16.121** Fall into natural body of water striking bottom causing drowning and submersion
          EXCLUDES 1   *drowning and submersion while in natural body of water without fall (W69)*

      √7ᵗʰ **W16.122** Fall into natural body of water striking bottom causing other injury

    √6ᵗʰ **W16.13 Fall into natural body of water** striking side

      √7ᵗʰ **W16.131** Fall into natural body of water striking side causing drowning and submersion
          EXCLUDES 1   *drowning and submersion while in natural body of water without fall (W69)*

      √7ᵗʰ **W16.132** Fall into natural body of water striking side causing other injury

  √5ᵗʰ **W16.2 Fall in (into) filled** bathtub or bucket of water

    √6ᵗʰ **W16.21 Fall in (into) filled** bathtub
       EXCLUDES 1   *fall into empty bathtub (W18.2)*

      √7ᵗʰ **W16.211** Fall in (into) filled bathtub causing drowning and submersion
          EXCLUDES 1   *drowning and submersion while in filled bathtub without fall (W65)*

      √7ᵗʰ **W16.212** Fall in (into) filled bathtub causing other injury

    √6ᵗʰ **W16.22 Fall in (into)** bucket of water

      √7ᵗʰ **W16.221** Fall in (into) bucket of water causing drowning and submersion

      √7ᵗʰ **W16.222** Fall in (into) bucket of water causing other injury

  √5ᵗʰ **W16.3 Fall into other water**
       Fall into fountain
       Fall into reservoir

    √6ᵗʰ **W16.31 Fall into other water** striking water surface

      √7ᵗʰ **W16.311** Fall into other water striking water surface causing drowning and submersion
          EXCLUDES 1   *drowning and submersion while in other water without fall (W73)*

      √7ᵗʰ **W16.312** Fall into other water striking water surface causing other injury

    √6ᵗʰ **W16.32 Fall into other water** striking bottom

      √7ᵗʰ **W16.321** Fall into other water striking bottom causing drowning and submersion
          EXCLUDES 1   *drowning and submersion while in other water without fall (W73)*

      √7ᵗʰ **W16.322** Fall into other water striking bottom causing other injury

    √6ᵗʰ **W16.33 Fall into other water** striking wall

      √7ᵗʰ **W16.331** Fall into other water striking wall causing drowning and submersion
          EXCLUDES 1   *drowning and submersion while in other water without fall (W73)*

      √7ᵗʰ **W16.332** Fall into other water striking wall causing other injury

  √5ᵗʰ **W16.4 Fall into unspecified water**

    √x7ᵗʰ **W16.41** Fall into unspecified water causing drowning and submersion ▽

    √x7ᵗʰ **W16.42** Fall into unspecified water causing other injury ▽

  √5ᵗʰ **W16.5 Jumping or diving into** swimming pool

    √6ᵗʰ **W16.51 Jumping or diving into swimming pool** striking water surface

      √7ᵗʰ **W16.511** Jumping or diving into swimming pool striking water surface causing drowning and submersion
          EXCLUDES 1   *drowning and submersion while in swimming pool without jumping or diving (W67)*

      √7ᵗʰ **W16.512** Jumping or diving into swimming pool striking water surface causing other injury

---

✓6ᵗʰ **W16.52 Jumping or diving into swimming pool** striking bottom

     ✓7ᵗʰ **W16.521 Jumping or diving into swimming pool striking bottom causing** drowning and submersion

         EXCLUDES 1   *drowning and submersion while in swimming pool without jumping or diving (W67)*

     ✓7ᵗʰ **W16.522 Jumping or diving into swimming pool striking bottom causing** other injury

✓6ᵗʰ **W16.53 Jumping or diving into swimming pool** striking wall

     ✓7ᵗʰ **W16.531 Jumping or diving into swimming pool striking wall causing** drowning and submersion

         EXCLUDES 1   *drowning and submersion while in swimming pool without jumping or diving (W67)*

     ✓7ᵗʰ **W16.532 Jumping or diving into swimming pool striking wall causing** other injury

✓5ᵗʰ **W16.6 Jumping or diving into** natural body of water
     Jumping or diving into lake
     Jumping or diving into open sea
     Jumping or diving into river
     Jumping or diving into stream

     ✓6ᵗʰ **W16.61 Jumping or diving into natural body of water striking water surface**

         ✓7ᵗʰ **W16.611 Jumping or diving into natural body of water striking water surface causing** drowning and submersion

             EXCLUDES 1   *drowning and submersion while in natural body of water without jumping or diving (W69)*

         ✓7ᵗʰ **W16.612 Jumping or diving into natural body of water striking water surface causing other injury**

     ✓6ᵗʰ **W16.62 Jumping or diving into natural body of water striking bottom**

         ✓7ᵗʰ **W16.621 Jumping or diving into natural body of water striking bottom causing** drowning and submersion

             EXCLUDES 1   *drowning and submersion while in natural body of water without jumping or diving (W69)*

         ✓7ᵗʰ **W16.622 Jumping or diving into natural body of water striking bottom causing other injury**

✓5ᵗʰ **W16.7 Jumping or diving** from boat

     EXCLUDES 1   *fall from boat into water—see watercraft accident (V90-V94)*

     ✓6ᵗʰ **W16.71 Jumping or diving from boat** striking water surface

         ✓7ᵗʰ **W16.711 Jumping or diving from boat striking water surface causing** drowning and submersion

         ✓7ᵗʰ **W16.712 Jumping or diving from boat striking water surface causing** other injury

     ✓6ᵗʰ **W16.72 Jumping or diving from boat** striking bottom

         ✓7ᵗʰ **W16.721 Jumping or diving from boat striking bottom causing** drowning and submersion

         ✓7ᵗʰ **W16.722 Jumping or diving from boat striking bottom causing** other injury

✓5ᵗʰ **W16.8 Jumping or diving into other water**
     Jumping or diving into fountain
     Jumping or diving into reservoir

     ✓6ᵗʰ **W16.81 Jumping or diving into other water** striking water surface

         ✓7ᵗʰ **W16.811 Jumping or diving into other water striking water surface causing** drowning and submersion

             EXCLUDES 1   *drowning and submersion while in other water without jumping or diving (W73)*

         ✓7ᵗʰ **W16.812 Jumping or diving into other water striking water surface causing** other injury

✓6ᵗʰ **W16.82 Jumping or diving into other water** striking bottom

     ✓7ᵗʰ **W16.821 Jumping or diving into other water striking bottom causing** drowning and submersion

         EXCLUDES 1   *drowning and submersion while in other water without jumping or diving (W73)*

     ✓7ᵗʰ **W16.822 Jumping or diving into other water striking bottom causing** other injury

✓6ᵗʰ **W16.83 Jumping or diving into other water** striking wall

     ✓7ᵗʰ **W16.831 Jumping or diving into other water striking wall causing** drowning and submersion

         EXCLUDES 1   *drowning and submersion while in other water without jumping or diving (W73)*

     ✓7ᵗʰ **W16.832 Jumping or diving into other water striking wall causing** other injury

✓5ᵗʰ **W16.9 Jumping or diving into unspecified water**

     ✓x7ᵗʰ **W16.91 Jumping or diving into unspecified water causing** drowning and submersion   ▽

     ✓x7ᵗʰ **W16.92 Jumping or diving into unspecified water causing** other injury   ▽

✓4ᵗʰ **W17 Other fall from one level to another**

     ✓x7ᵗʰ **W17.Ø Fall into well**

     ✓x7ᵗʰ **W17.1 Fall into storm drain or manhole**

     ✓x7ᵗʰ **W17.2 Fall into hole**
         Fall into pit

     ✓x7ᵗʰ **W17.3 Fall into empty swimming pool**
         EXCLUDES 1   *fall into filled swimming pool (W16.Ø-)*

     ✓x7ᵗʰ **W17.4 Fall from dock**

     ✓5ᵗʰ **W17.8 Other fall from one level to another**

         ✓x7ᵗʰ **W17.81 Fall down embankment (hill)**

         ✓x7ᵗʰ **W17.82 Fall from (out of) grocery cart**
             Fall due to grocery cart tipping over

         ✓x7ᵗʰ **W17.89 Other fall from one level to another**
             Fall from cherry picker
             Fall from lifting device
             Fall from mobile elevated work platform [MEWP]
             Fall from sky lift
             AHA: 2015, 2Q, 6

✓4ᵗʰ **W18 Other slipping, tripping and stumbling and falls**

     ✓5ᵗʰ **W18.Ø Fall due to bumping against object**
         Striking against object with subsequent fall
         EXCLUDES 1   *fall on same level due to slipping, tripping, or stumbling with subsequent striking against object (WØ1.1-)*

         ✓x7ᵗʰ **W18.ØØ Striking against unspecified object with subsequent fall**   ▽

         ✓x7ᵗʰ **W18.Ø1 Striking against** sports equipment **with subsequent fall**

         ✓x7ᵗʰ **W18.Ø2 Striking against** glass **with subsequent fall**

         ✓x7ᵗʰ **W18.Ø9 Striking against other object with subsequent fall**

     ✓5ᵗʰ **W18.1 Fall from or off toilet**

         ✓x7ᵗʰ **W18.11 Fall from or off toilet** without subsequent striking against object
             Fall from (off) toilet NOS

         ✓x7ᵗʰ **W18.12 Fall from or off toilet** with subsequent striking against object

     ✓x7ᵗʰ **W18.2 Fall in (into) shower or empty bathtub**
         EXCLUDES 1   *fall in full bathtub causing drowning or submersion (W16.21-)*

     ✓5ᵗʰ **W18.3 Other and unspecified fall on same level**

         ✓x7ᵗʰ **W18.3Ø Fall on same level, unspecified**   ▽

         ✓x7ᵗʰ **W18.31 Fall on same level due to stepping on an object**
             Fall on same level due to stepping on an animal
             EXCLUDES 1   *slipping, tripping and stumbling without fall due to stepping on animal (W18.41)*

         ✓x7ᵗʰ **W18.39 Other fall on same level**

     ✓5ᵗʰ **W18.4 Slipping, tripping and stumbling without falling**
         EXCLUDES 1   *collision with another person without fall (W51)*

         ✓x7ᵗʰ **W18.4Ø Slipping, tripping and stumbling without falling, unspecified**   ▽

EXCLUDES 1 Not coded here   EXCLUDES 2 Not included here   N Newborn Age: 0   P Pediatric Age: 0-17   M Maternity Age: 12-55   A Adult Age: 15-124

1146   ICD-10-CM 2018

√x7ᵗʰ **W18.41 Slipping, tripping and stumbling without falling due to** stepping on object
Slipping, tripping and stumbling without falling due to stepping on animal
EXCLUDES 1   *slipping, tripping and stumbling with fall due to stepping on animal (W18.31)*

√x7ᵗʰ **W18.42 Slipping, tripping and stumbling without falling due to** stepping into hole or opening

√x7ᵗʰ **W18.43 Slipping, tripping and stumbling without falling due to** stepping from one level to another

√x7ᵗʰ **W18.49 Other slipping, tripping and stumbling without falling**

√x7ᵗʰ **W19 Unspecified fall** ▽
Accidental fall NOS
AHA: 2012, 4Q, 95

Exposure to inanimate mechanical forces (W20-W49)

EXCLUDES 1   *assault (X92-Y09)*
contact or collision with animals or persons (W50-W64)
exposure to inanimate mechanical forces involving military or war operations (Y36.-, Y37.-)
intentional self-harm (X71-X83)

The appropriate 7th character is to be added to each code from categories W20-W49.
A   initial encounter
D   subsequent encounter
S   sequela

√4ᵗʰ **W20 Struck by thrown, projected or falling object**
Code first any associated:
cataclysm (X34-X39)
lightning strike (T75.00)
EXCLUDES 1   *falling object in machinery accident (W24, W28-W31)*
falling object in transport accident (V01-V99)
object set in motion by explosion (W35-W40)
object set in motion by firearm (W32-W34)
struck by thrown sports equipment (W21.-)

√x7ᵗʰ **W20.0 Struck by falling object in cave-in**
EXCLUDES 2   *asphyxiation due to cave-in (T71.21)*

√x7ᵗʰ **W20.1 Struck by object due to collapse of building**
EXCLUDES 1   *struck by object due to collapse of burning building (X00.2, X02.2)*

√x7ᵗʰ **W20.8 Other cause of strike by thrown, projected or falling object**
EXCLUDES 1   *struck by thrown sports equipment (W21.-)*

√4ᵗʰ **W21 Striking against or struck by sports equipment**
EXCLUDES 1   *assault with sports equipment (Y08.0-)*
striking against or struck by sports equipment with subsequent fall (W18.01)

√5ᵗʰ **W21.0 Struck by** hit **or** thrown ball

√x7ᵗʰ **W21.00 Struck by hit or thrown ball, unspecified type** ▽

√x7ᵗʰ **W21.01 Struck by** football

√x7ᵗʰ **W21.02 Struck by** soccer ball

√x7ᵗʰ **W21.03 Struck by** baseball

√x7ᵗʰ **W21.04 Struck by** golf ball

√x7ᵗʰ **W21.05 Struck by** basketball

√x7ᵗʰ **W21.06 Struck by** volleyball

√x7ᵗʰ **W21.07 Struck by** softball

√x7ᵗʰ **W21.09 Struck by other hit or thrown ball**

√5ᵗʰ **W21.1 Struck by** bat, racquet **or** club

√x7ᵗʰ **W21.11 Struck by** baseball bat

√x7ᵗʰ **W21.12 Struck by** tennis racquet

√x7ᵗʰ **W21.13 Struck by** golf club

√x7ᵗʰ **W21.19 Struck by other bat, racquet or club**

√5ᵗʰ **W21.2 Struck by** hockey stick **or** puck

√6ᵗʰ **W21.21 Struck by** hockey stick

√7ᵗʰ **W21.210 Struck by** ice **hockey stick**

√7ᵗʰ **W21.211 Struck by** field **hockey stick**

√6ᵗʰ **W21.22 Struck by** hockey puck

√7ᵗʰ **W21.220 Struck by** ice **hockey puck**

√7ᵗʰ **W21.221 Struck by** field **hockey puck**

√5ᵗʰ **W21.3 Struck by sports** foot wear

√x7ᵗʰ **W21.31 Struck by shoe** cleats
Stepped on by shoe cleats

√x7ᵗʰ **W21.32 Struck by skate blades**
Skated over by skate blades

√x7ᵗʰ **W21.39 Struck by other sports foot wear**

√x7ᵗʰ **W21.4 Striking against** diving board
Use additional code for subsequent falling into water, if applicable (W16.-)

√5ᵗʰ **W21.8 Striking against or struck by other sports equipment**

√x7ᵗʰ **W21.81 Striking against or struck by** football helmet

√x7ᵗʰ **W21.89 Striking against or struck by other sports equipment**

√x7ᵗʰ **W21.9 Striking against or struck by unspecified sports equipment** ▽

√4ᵗʰ **W22 Striking against or struck by other objects**
EXCLUDES 1   *striking against or struck by object with subsequent fall (W18.09)*

√5ᵗʰ **W22.0 Striking against** stationary object
EXCLUDES 1   *striking against stationary sports equipment (W21.8)*

√x7ᵗʰ **W22.01 Walked into** wall

√x7ᵗʰ **W22.02 Walked into** lamppost

√x7ᵗʰ **W22.03 Walked into** furniture

√6ᵗʰ **W22.04 Striking against wall of** swimming pool

√7ᵗʰ **W22.041 Striking against wall of swimming pool causing drowning and submersion**
EXCLUDES 1   *drowning and submersion while swimming without striking against wall (W67)*

√7ᵗʰ **W22.042 Striking against wall of swimming pool causing other injury**

√x7ᵗʰ **W22.09 Striking against other stationary object**

√5ᵗʰ **W22.1 Striking against or struck by** automobile airbag

√x7ᵗʰ **W22.10 Striking against or struck by unspecified automobile airbag** ▽

√x7ᵗʰ **W22.11 Striking against or struck by** driver side **automobile airbag**

√x7ᵗʰ **W22.12 Striking against or struck by** front passenger side **automobile airbag**

√x7ᵗʰ **W22.19 Striking against or struck by other automobile airbag**

√x7ᵗʰ **W22.8 Striking against or struck by other objects**
Striking against or struck by object NOS
EXCLUDES 1   *struck by thrown, projected or falling object (W20.-)*

√4ᵗʰ **W23 Caught, crushed, jammed or pinched in or between objects**
EXCLUDES 1   *injury caused by cutting or piercing instruments (W25-W27)*
injury caused by firearms malfunction (W32.1, W33.1-, W34.1-)
injury caused by lifting and transmission devices (W24.-)
injury caused by machinery (W28-W31)
injury caused by nonpowered hand tools (W27.-)
injury caused by transport vehicle being used as a means of transportation (V01-V99)
injury caused by struck by thrown, projected or falling object (W20.-)

√x7ᵗʰ **W23.0 Caught, crushed, jammed, or pinched between** moving **objects**

√x7ᵗʰ **W23.1 Caught, crushed, jammed, or pinched between** stationary **objects**

√4ᵗʰ **W24 Contact with lifting and transmission devices, not elsewhere classified**
EXCLUDES 1   *transport accidents (V01-V99)*

√x7ᵗʰ **W24.0 Contact with lifting devices, not elsewhere classified**
Contact with chain hoist
Contact with drive belt
Contact with pulley (block)

√x7ᵗʰ **W24.1 Contact with transmission devices, not elsewhere classified**
Contact with transmission belt or cable

√x7ᵗʰ **W25 Contact with sharp glass**
Code first any associated:
injury due to flying glass from explosion or firearm discharge (W32-W40)
transport accident (V00-V99)
EXCLUDES 1   *fall on same level due to slipping, tripping and stumbling with subsequent striking against sharp glass (W01.10)*
striking against sharp glass with subsequent fall (W18.02)
EXCLUDES 2   *glass embedded in skin (W45)*

Chapter 20. External Causes of Morbidity

W26–W31.9

✓4ᵗʰ **W26 Contact with other sharp objects**
> *EXCLUDES 2*   sharp object(s) embedded in skin (W45)

✓x7ᵗʰ **W26.0 Contact with knife**
> *EXCLUDES 1*   contact with electric knife (W29.1)

✓x7ᵗʰ **W26.1 Contact with sword or dagger**

✓x7ᵗʰ **W26.2 Contact with edge of stiff paper**
> Paper cut

✓x7ᵗʰ **W26.8 Contact with other sharp object(s), not elsewhere classified**
> Contact with tin can lid

✓x7ᵗʰ **W26.9 Contact with unspecified sharp object(s)** ▽

✓4ᵗʰ **W27 Contact with nonpowered hand tool**

✓x7ᵗʰ **W27.0 Contact with workbench tool**
> Contact with auger
> Contact with axe
> Contact with chisel
> Contact with handsaw
> Contact with screwdriver

✓x7ᵗʰ **W27.1 Contact with garden tool**
> Contact with hoe
> Contact with nonpowered lawn mower
> Contact with pitchfork
> Contact with rake

✓x7ᵗʰ **W27.2 Contact with scissors**

✓x7ᵗʰ **W27.3 Contact with needle (sewing)**
> *EXCLUDES 1*   contact with hypodermic needle (W46.-)

✓x7ᵗʰ **W27.4 Contact with kitchen utensil**
> Contact with fork
> Contact with ice-pick
> Contact with can-opener NOS

✓x7ᵗʰ **W27.5 Contact with paper-cutter**

✓x7ᵗʰ **W27.8 Contact with other nonpowered hand tool**
> Contact with nonpowered sewing machine
> Contact with shovel

✓x7ᵗʰ **W28 Contact with powered lawn mower**
> Powered lawn mower (commercial) (residential)
> *EXCLUDES 1*   contact with nonpowered lawn mower (W27.1)
> *EXCLUDES 2*   exposure to electric current (W86.-)

✓4ᵗʰ **W29 Contact with other powered hand tools and household machinery**
> *EXCLUDES 1*   contact with commercial machinery (W31.82)
>   contact with hot household appliance (X15)
>   contact with nonpowered hand tool (W27.-)
>   exposure to electric current (W86)

✓x7ᵗʰ **W29.0 Contact with powered kitchen appliance**
> Contact with blender
> Contact with can-opener
> Contact with garbage disposal
> Contact with mixer

✓x7ᵗʰ **W29.1 Contact with electric knife**

✓x7ᵗʰ **W29.2 Contact with other powered household machinery**
> Contact with electric fan
> Contact with powered dryer (clothes) (powered) (spin)
> Contact with washing-machine
> Contact with sewing machine

✓x7ᵗʰ **W29.3 Contact with powered garden and outdoor hand tools and machinery**
> Contact with chainsaw
> Contact with edger
> Contact with garden cultivator (tiller)
> Contact with hedge trimmer
> Contact with other powered garden tool
> *EXCLUDES 1*   contact with powered lawn mower (W28)

✓x7ᵗʰ **W29.4 Contact with nail gun**

▲ ✓x7ᵗʰ **W29.8 Contact with other powered hand tools and household machinery**
> Contact with do-it-yourself tool NOS

✓4ᵗʰ **W30 Contact with agricultural machinery**
> *INCLUDES*   animal-powered farm machine
> *EXCLUDES 1*   agricultural transport vehicle accident (V01-V99)
>   explosion of grain store (W40.8)
>   exposure to electric current (W86.-)

✓x7ᵗʰ **W30.0 Contact with combine harvester**
> Contact with reaper
> Contact with thresher

✓x7ᵗʰ **W30.1 Contact with power take-off devices (PTO)**

✓x7ᵗʰ **W30.2 Contact with hay derrick**

✓x7ᵗʰ **W30.3 Contact with grain storage elevator**
> *EXCLUDES 1*   explosion of grain store (W40.8)

✓5ᵗʰ **W30.8 Contact with other specified agricultural machinery**

✓x7ᵗʰ **W30.81 Contact with agricultural transport vehicle in stationary use**
> Contact with agricultural transport vehicle under repair, not on public roadway
> *EXCLUDES 1*   agricultural transport vehicle accident (V01-V99)

✓x7ᵗʰ **W30.89 Contact with other specified agricultural machinery**

✓x7ᵗʰ **W30.9 Contact with unspecified agricultural machinery** ▽
> Contact with farm machinery NOS

✓4ᵗʰ **W31 Contact with other and unspecified machinery**
> *EXCLUDES 1*   contact with agricultural machinery (W30.-)
>   contact with machinery in transport under own power or being towed by a vehicle (V01-V99)
>   exposure to electric current (W86)

✓x7ᵗʰ **W31.0 Contact with mining and earth-drilling machinery**
> Contact with bore or drill (land) (seabed)
> Contact with shaft hoist
> Contact with shaft lift
> Contact with undercutter

✓x7ᵗʰ **W31.1 Contact with metalworking machines**
> Contact with abrasive wheel
> Contact with forging machine
> Contact with lathe
> Contact with mechanical shears
> Contact with metal drilling machine
> Contact with milling machine
> Contact with power press
> Contact with rolling-mill
> Contact with metal sawing machine

✓x7ᵗʰ **W31.2 Contact with powered woodworking and forming machines**
> Contact with band saw
> Contact with bench saw
> Contact with circular saw
> Contact with molding machine
> Contact with overhead plane
> Contact with powered saw
> Contact with radial saw
> Contact with sander
> *EXCLUDES 1*   nonpowered woodworking tools (W27.0)

✓x7ᵗʰ **W31.3 Contact with prime movers**
> Contact with gas turbine
> Contact with internal combustion engine
> Contact with steam engine
> Contact with water driven turbine

✓5ᵗʰ **W31.8 Contact with other specified machinery**

✓x7ᵗʰ **W31.81 Contact with recreational machinery**
> Contact with roller coaster

✓x7ᵗʰ **W31.82 Contact with other commercial machinery**
> Contact with commercial electric fan
> Contact with commercial kitchen appliances
> Contact with commercial powered dryer (clothes) (powered) (spin)
> Contact with commercial washing-machine
> Contact with commercial sewing machine
> *EXCLUDES 1*   contact with household machinery (W29.-)
>   contact with powered lawn mower (W28)

✓x7ᵗʰ **W31.83 Contact with special construction vehicle in stationary use**
> Contact with special construction vehicle under repair, not on public roadway
> *EXCLUDES 1*   special construction vehicle accident (V01-V99)

✓x7ᵗʰ **W31.89 Contact with other specified machinery**

✓x7ᵗʰ **W31.9 Contact with unspecified machinery** ▽
> Contact with machinery NOS

EXCLUDES 1 Not coded here   *EXCLUDES 2* Not included here   N Newborn Age: 0   P Pediatric Age: 0-17   M Maternity Age: 12-55   A Adult Age: 15-124

W32 Accidental handgun discharge and malfunction

INCLUDES accidental discharge and malfunction of gun for single hand use
accidental discharge and malfunction of pistol
accidental discharge and malfunction of revolver
handgun discharge and malfunction NOS

EXCLUDES 1 accidental airgun discharge and malfunction (W34.010, W34.110)
accidental BB gun discharge and malfunction (W34.010, W34.110)
accidental pellet gun discharge and malfunction (W34.010, W34.110)
accidental shotgun discharge and malfunction (W33.01, W33.11)
assault by handgun discharge (X93)
handgun discharge involving legal intervention (Y35.0-)
handgun discharge involving military or war operations (Y36.4-)
intentional self-harm by handgun discharge (X72)
Very pistol discharge and malfunction (W34.09, W34.19)

W32.0 Accidental handgun discharge

W32.1 Accidental handgun malfunction
Injury due to explosion of handgun (parts)
Injury due to malfunction of mechanism or component of handgun
Injury due to recoil of handgun
Powder burn from handgun

W33 Accidental rifle, shotgun and larger firearm discharge and malfunction

INCLUDES rifle, shotgun and larger firearm discharge and malfunction NOS

EXCLUDES 1 accidental airgun discharge and malfunction (W34.010, W34.110)
accidental BB gun discharge and malfunction (W34.010, W34.110)
accidental handgun discharge and malfunction (W32.-)
accidental pellet gun discharge and malfunction (W34.010, W34.110)
assault by rifle, shotgun and larger firearm discharge (X94)
firearm discharge involving legal intervention (Y35.0-)
firearm discharge involving military or war operations (Y36.4-)
intentional self-harm by rifle, shotgun and larger firearm discharge (X73)

W33.0 Accidental rifle, shotgun and larger firearm discharge

W33.00 Accidental discharge of unspecified larger firearm
Discharge of unspecified larger firearm NOS

W33.01 Accidental discharge of shotgun
Discharge of shotgun NOS

W33.02 Accidental discharge of hunting rifle
Discharge of hunting rifle NOS

W33.03 Accidental discharge of machine gun
Discharge of machine gun NOS

W33.09 Accidental discharge of other larger firearm
Discharge of other larger firearm NOS

W33.1 Accidental rifle, shotgun and larger firearm malfunction
Injury due to explosion of rifle, shotgun and larger firearm (parts)
Injury due to malfunction of mechanism or component of rifle, shotgun and larger firearm
Injury due to piercing, cutting, crushing or pinching due to (by) slide trigger mechanism, scope or other gun part
Injury due to recoil of rifle, shotgun and larger firearm
Powder burn from rifle, shotgun and larger firearm

W33.10 Accidental malfunction of unspecified larger firearm
Malfunction of unspecified larger firearm NOS

W33.11 Accidental malfunction of shotgun
Malfunction of shotgun NOS

W33.12 Accidental malfunction of hunting rifle
Malfunction of hunting rifle NOS

W33.13 Accidental malfunction of machine gun
Malfunction of machine gun NOS

W33.19 Accidental malfunction of other larger firearm
Malfunction of other larger firearm NOS

W34 Accidental discharge and malfunction from other and unspecified firearms and guns

W34.0 Accidental discharge from other and unspecified firearms and guns

W34.00 Accidental discharge from unspecified firearms or gun
Discharge from firearm NOS
Gunshot wound NOS
Shot NOS

W34.01 Accidental discharge of gas, air or spring-operated guns

W34.010 Accidental discharge of airgun
Accidental discharge of BB gun
Accidental discharge of pellet gun

W34.011 Accidental discharge of paintball gun
Accidental injury due to paintball discharge

W34.018 Accidental discharge of other gas, air or spring-operated gun

W34.09 Accidental discharge from other specified firearms
Accidental discharge from Very pistol [flare]

W34.1 Accidental malfunction from other and unspecified firearms and guns

W34.10 Accidental malfunction from unspecified firearms or gun
Firearm malfunction NOS

W34.11 Accidental malfunction of gas, air or spring-operated guns

W34.110 Accidental malfunction of airgun
Accidental malfunction of BB gun
Accidental malfunction of pellet gun

W34.111 Accidental malfunction of paintball gun
Accidental injury due to paintball gun malfunction

W34.118 Accidental malfunction of other gas, air or spring-operated gun

W34.19 Accidental malfunction from other specified firearms
Accidental malfunction from Very pistol [flare]

W35 Explosion and rupture of boiler
EXCLUDES 1 explosion and rupture of boiler on watercraft (V93.4)

W36 Explosion and rupture of gas cylinder
W36.1 Explosion and rupture of aerosol can
W36.2 Explosion and rupture of air tank
W36.3 Explosion and rupture of pressurized-gas tank
W36.8 Explosion and rupture of other gas cylinder
W36.9 Explosion and rupture of unspecified gas cylinder

W37 Explosion and rupture of pressurized tire, pipe or hose
W37.0 Explosion of bicycle tire
W37.8 Explosion and rupture of other pressurized tire, pipe or hose

W38 Explosion and rupture of other specified pressurized devices

W39 Discharge of firework

W40 Explosion of other materials
EXCLUDES 1 assault by explosive material (X96)
explosion involving legal intervention (Y35.1-)
explosion involving military or war operations (Y36.0-, Y36.2-)
intentional self-harm by explosive material (X75)

W40.0 Explosion of blasting material
Explosion of blasting cap
Explosion of detonator
Explosion of dynamite
Explosion of explosive (any) used in blasting operations

W40.1 Explosion of explosive gases
Explosion of acetylene
Explosion of butane
Explosion of coal gas
Explosion in mine NOS
Explosion of explosive gas
Explosion of fire damp
Explosion of gasoline fumes
Explosion of methane
Explosion of propane

☑x7ᵗʰ W40.8 Explosion of other specified explosive materials
Explosion in dump NOS
Explosion in factory NOS
Explosion in grain store
Explosion in munitions

> *EXCLUDES 1* explosion involving legal intervention (Y35.1-)
> explosion involving military or war operations (Y36.0-, Y36.2-)

☑x7ᵗʰ W40.9 Explosion of unspecified explosive materials
Explosion NOS

☑4ᵗʰ W42 Exposure to noise

☑x7ᵗʰ W42.0 Exposure to supersonic waves

☑x7ᵗʰ W42.9 Exposure to other noise
Exposure to sound waves NOS

☑4ᵗʰ W45 Foreign body or object entering through skin

> *INCLUDES* foreign body or object embedded in skin
> nail embedded in skin

> *EXCLUDES 2* contact with hand tools (nonpowered) (powered) (W27-W29)
> contact with other sharp object(s) (W26.-)
> contact with sharp glass (W25.-)
> struck by objects (W20-W22)

☑x7ᵗʰ W45.0 Nail entering through skin

☑x7ᵗʰ W45.8 Other foreign body or object entering through skin
Splinter in skin NOS

☑4ᵗʰ W46 Contact with hypodermic needle

☑x7ᵗʰ W46.0 Contact with hypodermic needle
Hypodermic needle stick NOS

☑x7ᵗʰ W46.1 Contact with contaminated hypodermic needle

☑4ᵗʰ W49 Exposure to other inanimate mechanical forces

> *INCLUDES* exposure to abnormal gravitational [G] forces
> exposure to inanimate mechanical forces NEC

> *EXCLUDES 1* exposure to inanimate mechanical forces involving military or war operations (Y36.-, Y37.-)

☑5ᵗʰ W49.0 Item causing external constriction

☑x7ᵗʰ W49.01 Hair causing external constriction

☑x7ᵗʰ W49.02 String or thread causing external constriction

☑x7ᵗʰ W49.03 Rubber band causing external constriction

☑x7ᵗʰ W49.04 Ring or other jewelry causing external constriction

☑x7ᵗʰ W49.09 Other specified item causing external constriction

☑x7ᵗʰ W49.9 Exposure to other inanimate mechanical forces

Exposure to animate mechanical forces (W50-W64)

> *EXCLUDES 1* Toxic effect of contact with venomous animals and plants (T63.-)

> The appropriate 7th character is to be added to each code from categories W50-W64.
> A   initial encounter
> D   subsequent encounter
> S   sequela

☑4ᵗʰ W50 Accidental hit, strike, kick, twist, bite or scratch by another person

> *INCLUDES* hit, strike, kick, twist, bite, or scratch by another person NOS
> *EXCLUDES 1* assault by bodily force (Y04)
> struck by objects (W20-W22)

☑x7ᵗʰ W50.0 Accidental hit or strike by another person
Hit or strike by another person NOS

☑x7ᵗʰ W50.1 Accidental kick by another person
Kick by another person NOS

☑x7ᵗʰ W50.2 Accidental twist by another person
Twist by another person NOS

☑x7ᵗʰ W50.3 Accidental bite by another person
Human bite
Bite by another person NOS

☑x7ᵗʰ W50.4 Accidental scratch by another person
Scratch by another person NOS

☑x7ᵗʰ W51 Accidental striking against or bumped into by another person

> *EXCLUDES 1* assault by striking against or bumping into by another person (Y04.2)
> fall due to collision with another person (W03)

☑x7ᵗʰ W52 Crushed, pushed or stepped on by crowd or human stampede
Crushed, pushed or stepped on by crowd or human stampede with or without fall

☑4ᵗʰ W53 Contact with rodent

> *INCLUDES* contact with saliva, feces or urine of rodent

☑5ᵗʰ W53.0 Contact with mouse

☑x7ᵗʰ W53.01 Bitten by mouse

☑x7ᵗʰ W53.09 Other contact with mouse

☑5ᵗʰ W53.1 Contact with rat

☑x7ᵗʰ W53.11 Bitten by rat

☑x7ᵗʰ W53.19 Other contact with rat

☑5ᵗʰ W53.2 Contact with squirrel

☑x7ᵗʰ W53.21 Bitten by squirrel

☑x7ᵗʰ W53.29 Other contact with squirrel

☑5ᵗʰ W53.8 Contact with other rodent

☑x7ᵗʰ W53.81 Bitten by other rodent

☑x7ᵗʰ W53.89 Other contact with other rodent

☑4ᵗʰ W54 Contact with dog

> *INCLUDES* contact with saliva, feces or urine of dog

☑x7ᵗʰ W54.0 Bitten by dog

☑x7ᵗʰ W54.1 Struck by dog
Knocked over by dog

☑x7ᵗʰ W54.8 Other contact with dog

☑4ᵗʰ W55 Contact with other mammals

> *INCLUDES* contact with saliva, feces or urine of mammal
> *EXCLUDES 1* animal being ridden—see transport accidents
> bitten or struck by dog (W54)
> bitten or struck by rodent (W53.-)
> contact with marine mammals (W56.-)

☑5ᵗʰ W55.0 Contact with cat

☑x7ᵗʰ W55.01 Bitten by cat

☑x7ᵗʰ W55.03 Scratched by cat

☑x7ᵗʰ W55.09 Other contact with cat

☑5ᵗʰ W55.1 Contact with horse

☑x7ᵗʰ W55.11 Bitten by horse

☑x7ᵗʰ W55.12 Struck by horse

☑x7ᵗʰ W55.19 Other contact with horse

☑5ᵗʰ W55.2 Contact with cow
Contact with bull

☑x7ᵗʰ W55.21 Bitten by cow

☑x7ᵗʰ W55.22 Struck by cow
Gored by bull

☑x7ᵗʰ W55.29 Other contact with cow

☑5ᵗʰ W55.3 Contact with other hoof stock
Contact with goats
Contact with sheep

☑x7ᵗʰ W55.31 Bitten by other hoof stock

☑x7ᵗʰ W55.32 Struck by other hoof stock
Gored by goat
Gored by ram

☑x7ᵗʰ W55.39 Other contact with other hoof stock

☑5ᵗʰ W55.4 Contact with pig

☑x7ᵗʰ W55.41 Bitten by pig

☑x7ᵗʰ W55.42 Struck by pig

☑x7ᵗʰ W55.49 Other contact with pig

☑5ᵗʰ W55.5 Contact with raccoon

☑x7ᵗʰ W55.51 Bitten by raccoon

☑x7ᵗʰ W55.52 Struck by raccoon

☑x7ᵗʰ W55.59 Other contact with raccoon

☑5ᵗʰ W55.8 Contact with other mammals

☑x7ᵗʰ W55.81 Bitten by other mammals

☑x7ᵗʰ W55.82 Struck by other mammals

☑x7ᵗʰ W55.89 Other contact with other mammals

☑4ᵗʰ W56 Contact with nonvenomous marine animal

> *EXCLUDES 1* contact with venomous marine animal (T63.-)

☑5ᵗʰ W56.0 Contact with dolphin

☑x7ᵗʰ W56.01 Bitten by dolphin

☑x7ᵗʰ W56.02 Struck by dolphin

☑x7ᵗʰ W56.09 Other contact with dolphin

EXCLUDES 1 Not coded here   *EXCLUDES 2* Not included here   Ⓝ Newborn Age: 0   Ⓟ Pediatric Age: 0-17   Ⓜ Maternity Age: 12-55   Ⓐ Adult Age: 15-124

1150   ICD-10-CM 2018

✓5ᵗʰ **W56.1 Contact with** sea lion
- ✓x7ᵗʰ **W56.11** Bitten by sea lion
- ✓x7ᵗʰ **W56.12** Struck by sea lion
- ✓x7ᵗʰ **W56.19** Other contact with sea lion

✓5ᵗʰ **W56.2 Contact with** orca
    Contact with killer whale
- ✓x7ᵗʰ **W56.21** Bitten by orca
- ✓x7ᵗʰ **W56.22** Struck by orca
- ✓x7ᵗʰ **W56.29** Other contact with orca

✓5ᵗʰ **W56.3 Contact with other marine mammals**
- ✓x7ᵗʰ **W56.31** Bitten by other marine mammals
- ✓x7ᵗʰ **W56.32** Struck by other marine mammals
- ✓x7ᵗʰ **W56.39** Other contact with other marine mammals

✓5ᵗʰ **W56.4 Contact with** shark
- ✓x7ᵗʰ **W56.41** Bitten by shark
- ✓x7ᵗʰ **W56.42** Struck by shark
- ✓x7ᵗʰ **W56.49** Other contact with shark

✓5ᵗʰ **W56.5 Contact with other fish**
- ✓x7ᵗʰ **W56.51** Bitten by other fish
- ✓x7ᵗʰ **W56.52** Struck by other fish
- ✓x7ᵗʰ **W56.59** Other contact with other fish

✓5ᵗʰ **W56.8 Contact with other nonvenomous marine animals**
- ✓x7ᵗʰ **W56.81** Bitten by other nonvenomous marine animals
- ✓x7ᵗʰ **W56.82** Struck by other nonvenomous marine animals
- ✓x7ᵗʰ **W56.89** Other contact with other nonvenomous marine animals

✓x7ᵗʰ **W57 Bitten or stung by nonvenomous insect and other nonvenomous arthropods**
    EXCLUDES 1 *contact with venomous insects and arthropods (T63.2-, T63.3-, T63.4-)*

✓4ᵗʰ **W58 Contact with crocodile or alligator**

✓5ᵗʰ **W58.0 Contact with** alligator
- ✓x7ᵗʰ **W58.01** Bitten by alligator
- ✓x7ᵗʰ **W58.02** Struck by alligator
- ✓x7ᵗʰ **W58.03** Crushed by alligator
- ✓x7ᵗʰ **W58.09** Other contact with alligator

✓5ᵗʰ **W58.1 Contact with** crocodile
- ✓x7ᵗʰ **W58.11** Bitten by crocodile
- ✓x7ᵗʰ **W58.12** Struck by crocodile
- ✓x7ᵗʰ **W58.13** Crushed by crocodile
- ✓x7ᵗʰ **W58.19** Other contact with crocodile

✓4ᵗʰ **W59 Contact with other nonvenomous reptiles**
    EXCLUDES 1 *contact with venomous reptile (T63.0-, T63.1-)*

✓5ᵗʰ **W59.0 Contact with nonvenomous** lizards
- ✓x7ᵗʰ **W59.01** Bitten by nonvenomous lizards
- ✓x7ᵗʰ **W59.02** Struck by nonvenomous lizards
- ✓x7ᵗʰ **W59.09** Other contact with nonvenomous lizards
    Exposure to nonvenomous lizards

✓5ᵗʰ **W59.1 Contact with nonvenomous** snakes
- ✓x7ᵗʰ **W59.11** Bitten by nonvenomous snake
- ✓x7ᵗʰ **W59.12** Struck by nonvenomous snake
- ✓x7ᵗʰ **W59.13** Crushed by nonvenomous snake
- ✓x7ᵗʰ **W59.19** Other contact with nonvenomous snake

✓5ᵗʰ **W59.2 Contact with** turtles
    EXCLUDES 1 *contact with tortoises (W59.8-)*
- ✓x7ᵗʰ **W59.21** Bitten by turtle
- ✓x7ᵗʰ **W59.22** Struck by turtle
- ✓x7ᵗʰ **W59.29** Other contact with turtle
    Exposure to turtles

✓5ᵗʰ **W59.8 Contact with other nonvenomous reptiles**
- ✓x7ᵗʰ **W59.81** Bitten by other nonvenomous reptiles
- ✓x7ᵗʰ **W59.82** Struck by other nonvenomous reptiles
- ✓x7ᵗʰ **W59.83** Crushed by other nonvenomous reptiles
- ✓x7ᵗʰ **W59.89** Other contact with other nonvenomous reptiles

✓x7ᵗʰ **W60 Contact with nonvenomous plant thorns and spines and sharp leaves**
    EXCLUDES 1 *contact with venomous plants (T63.7-)*

✓4ᵗʰ **W61 Contact with birds (domestic) (wild)**
    INCLUDES contact with excreta of birds

✓5ᵗʰ **W61.0 Contact with** parrot
- ✓x7ᵗʰ **W61.01** Bitten by parrot
- ✓x7ᵗʰ **W61.02** Struck by parrot
- ✓x7ᵗʰ **W61.09** Other contact with parrot
    Exposure to parrots

✓5ᵗʰ **W61.1 Contact with** macaw
- ✓x7ᵗʰ **W61.11** Bitten by macaw
- ✓x7ᵗʰ **W61.12** Struck by macaw
- ✓x7ᵗʰ **W61.19** Other contact with macaw
    Exposure to macaws

✓5ᵗʰ **W61.2 Contact with other psittacines**
- ✓x7ᵗʰ **W61.21** Bitten by other psittacines
- ✓x7ᵗʰ **W61.22** Struck by other psittacines
- ✓x7ᵗʰ **W61.29** Other contact with other psittacines
    Exposure to other psittacines

✓5ᵗʰ **W61.3 Contact with** chicken
- ✓x7ᵗʰ **W61.32** Struck by chicken
- ✓x7ᵗʰ **W61.33** Pecked by chicken
- ✓x7ᵗʰ **W61.39** Other contact with chicken
    Exposure to chickens

✓5ᵗʰ **W61.4 Contact with** turkey
- ✓x7ᵗʰ **W61.42** Struck by turkey
- ✓x7ᵗʰ **W61.43** Pecked by turkey
- ✓x7ᵗʰ **W61.49** Other contact with turkey

✓5ᵗʰ **W61.5 Contact with** goose
- ✓x7ᵗʰ **W61.51** Bitten by goose
- ✓x7ᵗʰ **W61.52** Struck by goose
- ✓x7ᵗʰ **W61.59** Other contact with goose

✓5ᵗʰ **W61.6 Contact with** duck
- ✓x7ᵗʰ **W61.61** Bitten by duck
- ✓x7ᵗʰ **W61.62** Struck by duck
- ✓x7ᵗʰ **W61.69** Other contact with duck

✓5ᵗʰ **W61.9 Contact with other birds**
- ✓x7ᵗʰ **W61.91** Bitten by other birds
- ✓x7ᵗʰ **W61.92** Struck by other birds
- ✓x7ᵗʰ **W61.99** Other contact with other birds
    Contact with bird NOS

✓4ᵗʰ **W62 Contact with nonvenomous amphibians**
    EXCLUDES 1 *contact with venomous amphibians (T63.81-R63.83)*
- ✓x7ᵗʰ **W62.0 Contact with nonvenomous** frogs
- ✓x7ᵗʰ **W62.1 Contact with nonvenomous** toads
- ✓x7ᵗʰ **W62.9 Contact with other nonvenomous amphibians**

✓x7ᵗʰ **W64 Exposure to other animate mechanical forces**
    INCLUDES exposure to nonvenomous animal NOS
    EXCLUDES 1 *contact with venomous animal (T63.-)*

Accidental non-transport drowning and submersion (W65-W74)
    EXCLUDES 1 *accidental drowning and submersion due to fall into water (W16.-)*
    accidental drowning and submersion due to water transport accident (V90.-, V92.-)
    EXCLUDES 2 *accidental drowning and submersion due to cataclysm (X34-X39)*

> The appropriate 7th character is to be added to each code from categories W65-W74.
> A   initial encounter
> D   subsequent encounter
> S   sequela

✓x7ᵗʰ **W65 Accidental drowning and submersion while in** bath-tub
    EXCLUDES 1 *accidental drowning and submersion due to fall in (into) bathtub (W16.211)*

✓x7ᵗʰ **W67 Accidental drowning and submersion while in** swimming-pool
    EXCLUDES 1 *accidental drowning and submersion due to fall into swimming pool (W16.011, W16.021, W16.031)*
    accidental drowning and submersion due to striking into wall of swimming pool (W22.041)

√x7ᵗʰ **W69 Accidental drowning and submersion while in** natural water
Accidental drowning and submersion while in lake
Accidental drowning and submersion while in open sea
Accidental drowning and submersion while in river
Accidental drowning and submersion while in stream
EXCLUDES 1   *accidental drowning and submersion due to fall into natural body of water (W16.111, W16.121, W16.131)*

√x7ᵗʰ **W73 Other specified cause of accidental non-transport drowning and submersion**
Accidental drowning and submersion while in quenching tank
Accidental drowning and submersion while in reservoir
EXCLUDES 1   *accidental drowning and submersion due to fall into other water (W16.311, W16.321, W16.331)*

√x7ᵗʰ **W74 Unspecified cause of accidental drowning and submersion** ▽
Drowning NOS

Exposure to electric current, radiation and extreme ambient air temperature and pressure (W85-W99)

EXCLUDES 1   *exposure to:*
failure in dosage of radiation or temperature during surgical and medical care (Y63.2-Y63.5)
lightning (T75.0-)
natural cold (X31)
natural heat (X30)
natural radiation NOS (X39)
radiological procedure and radiotherapy (Y84.2)
sunlight (X32)

The appropriate 7th character is to be added to each code from categories W85-W99.
A   initial encounter
D   subsequent encounter
S   sequela

√x7ᵗʰ **W85 Exposure to electric transmission lines**
Broken power line

√4ᵗʰ **W86 Exposure to other specified electric current**

√x7ᵗʰ **W86.0 Exposure to domestic wiring and appliances**

√x7ᵗʰ **W86.1 Exposure to industrial wiring, appliances and electrical machinery**
Exposure to conductors
Exposure to control apparatus
Exposure to electrical equipment and machinery
Exposure to transformers

√x7ᵗʰ **W86.8 Exposure to other electric current**
Exposure to wiring and appliances in or on farm (not farmhouse)
Exposure to wiring and appliances outdoors
Exposure to wiring and appliances in or on public building
Exposure to wiring and appliances in or on residential institutions
Exposure to wiring and appliances in or on schools

√4ᵗʰ **W88 Exposure to ionizing radiation**
EXCLUDES 1   *exposure to sunlight (X32)*

√x7ᵗʰ **W88.0 Exposure to X-rays**

√x7ᵗʰ **W88.1 Exposure to radioactive isotopes**

√x7ᵗʰ **W88.8 Exposure to other ionizing radiation**

√4ᵗʰ **W89 Exposure to man-made visible and ultraviolet light**
INCLUDES   exposure to welding light (arc)
EXCLUDES 1   *exposure to sunlight (X32)*

√x7ᵗʰ **W89.0 Exposure to welding light (arc)**

√x7ᵗʰ **W89.1 Exposure to tanning bed**

√x7ᵗʰ **W89.8 Exposure to other man-made visible and ultraviolet light**

√x7ᵗʰ **W89.9 Exposure to unspecified man-made visible and** ▽
ultraviolet light

√4ᵗʰ **W90 Exposure to other nonionizing radiation**
EXCLUDES 1   *exposure to sunlight (X32)*

√x7ᵗʰ **W90.0 Exposure to radiofrequency**

√x7ᵗʰ **W90.1 Exposure to infrared radiation**

√x7ᵗʰ **W90.2 Exposure to laser radiation**

√x7ᵗʰ **W90.8 Exposure to other nonionizing radiation**

√x7ᵗʰ **W92 Exposure to excessive heat of man-made origin**

√4ᵗʰ **W93 Exposure to excessive cold of man-made origin**

√5ᵗʰ **W93.0 Contact with or inhalation of dry ice**

√x7ᵗʰ **W93.01 Contact with dry ice**

√x7ᵗʰ **W93.02 Inhalation of dry ice**

√5ᵗʰ **W93.1 Contact with or inhalation of liquid air**

√x7ᵗʰ **W93.11 Contact with liquid air**
Contact with liquid hydrogen
Contact with liquid nitrogen

√x7ᵗʰ **W93.12 Inhalation of liquid air**
Inhalation of liquid hydrogen
Inhalation of liquid nitrogen

√x7ᵗʰ **W93.2 Prolonged exposure in deep freeze unit or refrigerator**

√x7ᵗʰ **W93.8 Exposure to other excessive cold of man-made origin**

√4ᵗʰ **W94 Exposure to high and low air pressure and changes in air pressure**

√x7ᵗʰ **W94.0 Exposure to prolonged high air pressure**

√5ᵗʰ **W94.1 Exposure to prolonged low air pressure**

√x7ᵗʰ **W94.11 Exposure to residence or prolonged visit at high altitude**

√x7ᵗʰ **W94.12 Exposure to other prolonged low air pressure**

√5ᵗʰ **W94.2 Exposure to rapid changes in air pressure during ascent**

√x7ᵗʰ **W94.21 Exposure to reduction in atmospheric pressure while surfacing from deep-water diving**

√x7ᵗʰ **W94.22 Exposure to reduction in atmospheric pressure while surfacing from underground**

√x7ᵗʰ **W94.23 Exposure to sudden change in air pressure in aircraft during ascent**

√x7ᵗʰ **W94.29 Exposure to other rapid changes in air pressure during ascent**

√5ᵗʰ **W94.3 Exposure to rapid changes in air pressure during descent**

√x7ᵗʰ **W94.31 Exposure to sudden change in air pressure in aircraft during descent**

√x7ᵗʰ **W94.32 Exposure to high air pressure from rapid descent in water**

√x7ᵗʰ **W94.39 Exposure to other rapid changes in air pressure during descent**

√x7ᵗʰ **W99 Exposure to other man-made environmental factors**

Exposure to smoke, fire and flames (X00-X08)

EXCLUDES 1   *arson (X97)*
EXCLUDES 2   *explosions (W35-W40)*
lightning (T75.0-)
transport accident (V01-V99)

The appropriate 7th character is to be added to each code from categories X00-X08.
A   initial encounter
D   subsequent encounter
S   sequela

√4ᵗʰ **X00 Exposure to uncontrolled fire in building or structure**
INCLUDES   conflagration in building or structure
Code first any associated cataclysm
EXCLUDES 2   *exposure to ignition or melting of nightwear (X05)*
exposure to ignition or melting of other clothing and apparel (X06.-)
exposure to other specified smoke, fire and flames (X08.-)
AHA: 2016, 2Q, 5

√x7ᵗʰ **X00.0 Exposure to flames in uncontrolled fire in building or structure**

√x7ᵗʰ **X00.1 Exposure to smoke in uncontrolled fire in building or structure**

√x7ᵗʰ **X00.2 Injury due to collapse of burning building or structure in uncontrolled fire**
EXCLUDES 1   *injury due to collapse of building not on fire (W20.1)*

√x7ᵗʰ **X00.3 Fall from burning building or structure in uncontrolled fire**

√x7ᵗʰ **X00.4 Hit by object from burning building or structure in uncontrolled fire**

√x7ᵗʰ **X00.5 Jump from burning building or structure in uncontrolled fire**

√x7ᵗʰ **X00.8 Other exposure to uncontrolled fire in building or structure**

√4ᵗʰ **X01 Exposure to uncontrolled fire, not in building or structure**
INCLUDES   exposure to forest fire

√x7ᵗʰ **X01.0 Exposure to flames in uncontrolled fire, not in building or structure**

√x7ᵗʰ **X01.1 Exposure to smoke in uncontrolled fire, not in building or structure**

√x7ᵗʰ **X01.3 Fall due to uncontrolled fire, not in building or structure**

✓x 7ᵗʰ **X01.4 Hit by object** due to uncontrolled fire, not in building or structure

✓x 7ᵗʰ **X01.8 Other exposure** to uncontrolled fire, not in building or structure

✓4ᵗʰ **X02 Exposure to controlled fire in building or structure**
     INCLUDES   exposure to fire in fireplace
                  exposure to fire in stove

✓x 7ᵗʰ **X02.0 Exposure to flames** in controlled fire in building or structure

✓x 7ᵗʰ **X02.1 Exposure to smoke** in controlled fire in building or structure

✓x 7ᵗʰ **X02.2 Injury due to collapse** of burning building or structure in controlled fire
          EXCLUDES 1   injury due to collapse of building not on fire (W20.1)

✓x 7ᵗʰ **X02.3 Fall from** burning building or structure in controlled fire

✓x 7ᵗʰ **X02.4 Hit by object** from burning building or structure in controlled fire

✓x 7ᵗʰ **X02.5 Jump from** burning building or structure in controlled fire

✓x 7ᵗʰ **X02.8 Other exposure** to controlled fire in building or structure

✓4ᵗʰ **X03 Exposure to controlled fire, not in building or structure**
     INCLUDES   exposure to bon fire
                  exposure to camp-fire
                  exposure to trash fire

✓x 7ᵗʰ **X03.0 Exposure to flames** in controlled fire, not in building or structure

✓x 7ᵗʰ **X03.1 Exposure to smoke** in controlled fire, not in building or structure

✓x 7ᵗʰ **X03.3 Fall due to** controlled fire, not in building or structure

✓x 7ᵗʰ **X03.4 Hit by object** due to controlled fire, not in building or structure

✓x 7ᵗʰ **X03.8 Other exposure** to controlled fire, not in building or structure

✓x 7ᵗʰ **X04 Exposure to ignition of highly flammable material**
     Exposure to ignition of gasoline
     Exposure to ignition of kerosene
     Exposure to ignition of petrol
     EXCLUDES 2   exposure to ignition or melting of nightwear (X05)
                   exposure to ignition or melting of other clothing and apparel (X06)
     AHA: 2016, 2Q, 4

✓x 7ᵗʰ **X05 Exposure to ignition or melting of nightwear**
     EXCLUDES 2   exposure to uncontrolled fire in building or structure (X00.-)
                   exposure to uncontrolled fire, not in building or structure (X01.-)
                   exposure to controlled fire in building or structure (X02.-)
                   exposure to controlled fire, not in building or structure (X03.-)
                   exposure to ignition of highly flammable materials (X04.-)

✓4ᵗʰ **X06 Exposure to ignition or melting of other clothing and apparel**
     EXCLUDES 2   exposure to uncontrolled fire in building or structure (X00.-)
                   exposure to uncontrolled fire, not in building or structure (X01.-)
                   exposure to controlled fire in building or structure (X02.-)
                   exposure to controlled fire, not in building or structure (X03.-)
                   exposure to ignition of highly flammable materials (X04.-)

✓x 7ᵗʰ **X06.0 Exposure to ignition of plastic jewelry**

✓x 7ᵗʰ **X06.1 Exposure to melting of plastic jewelry**

✓x 7ᵗʰ **X06.2 Exposure to ignition of other clothing and apparel**

✓x 7ᵗʰ **X06.3 Exposure to melting of other clothing and apparel**

✓4ᵗʰ **X08 Exposure to other specified smoke, fire and flames**

✓5ᵗʰ **X08.0 Exposure to bed fire**
     Exposure to mattress fire

     ✓x 7ᵗʰ **X08.00 Exposure to bed fire** due to unspecified burning material   ▽

     ✓x 7ᵗʰ **X08.01 Exposure to bed fire** due to burning cigarette

     ✓x 7ᵗʰ **X08.09 Exposure to bed fire** due to other burning material

✓5ᵗʰ **X08.1 Exposure to sofa fire**

     ✓x 7ᵗʰ **X08.10 Exposure to sofa fire** due to unspecified burning material   ▽

     ✓x 7ᵗʰ **X08.11 Exposure to sofa fire** due to burning cigarette

     ✓x 7ᵗʰ **X08.19 Exposure to sofa fire** due to other burning material

✓5ᵗʰ **X08.2 Exposure to other furniture fire**

     ✓x 7ᵗʰ **X08.20 Exposure to other furniture fire** due to unspecified burning material   ▽

     ✓x 7ᵗʰ **X08.21 Exposure to other furniture fire** due to burning cigarette

     ✓x 7ᵗʰ **X08.29 Exposure to other furniture fire** due to other burning material

✓x 7ᵗʰ **X08.8 Exposure to other specified smoke, fire and flames**

Contact with heat and hot substances (X10-X19)

EXCLUDES 1   exposure to excessive natural heat (X30)
                  exposure to fire and flames ▶(X00-X08)◀

The appropriate 7th character is to be added to each code from categories X10-X19.
A   initial encounter
D   subsequent encounter
S   sequela

✓4ᵗʰ **X10 Contact with hot drinks, food, fats and cooking oils**

     ✓x 7ᵗʰ **X10.0 Contact with hot drinks**

     ✓x 7ᵗʰ **X10.1 Contact with hot food**

     ✓x 7ᵗʰ **X10.2 Contact with fats and cooking oils**

✓4ᵗʰ **X11 Contact with hot tap-water**
     INCLUDES   contact with boiling tap-water
                  contact with boiling water NOS
     EXCLUDES 1   contact with water heated on stove (X12)

     ✓x 7ᵗʰ **X11.0 Contact with hot water** in bath or tub
          EXCLUDES 1   contact with running hot water in bath or tub (X11.1)

     ✓x 7ᵗʰ **X11.1 Contact with running hot water**
          Contact with hot water running out of hose
          Contact with hot water running out of tap

     ✓x 7ᵗʰ **X11.8 Contact with other hot tap-water**
          Contact with hot water in bucket
          Contact with hot tap-water NOS

✓x 7ᵗʰ **X12 Contact with other hot fluids**
     Contact with water heated on stove
     EXCLUDES 1   hot (liquid) metals (X18)

✓4ᵗʰ **X13 Contact with steam and other hot vapors**

     ✓x 7ᵗʰ **X13.0 Inhalation of steam and other hot vapors**

     ✓x 7ᵗʰ **X13.1 Other contact with steam and other hot vapors**

✓4ᵗʰ **X14 Contact with hot air and other hot gases**

     ✓x 7ᵗʰ **X14.0 Inhalation of hot air and gases**

     ✓x 7ᵗʰ **X14.1 Other contact with hot air and other hot gases**

✓4ᵗʰ **X15 Contact with hot household appliances**
     EXCLUDES 1   contact with heating appliances (X16)
                  contact with powered household appliances (W29.-)
                  exposure to controlled fire in building or structure due to household appliance (X02.8)
                  exposure to household appliances electrical current (W86.0)

     ✓x 7ᵗʰ **X15.0 Contact with hot stove (kitchen)**

     ✓x 7ᵗʰ **X15.1 Contact with hot toaster**

     ✓x 7ᵗʰ **X15.2 Contact with hotplate**

     ✓x 7ᵗʰ **X15.3 Contact with hot saucepan or skillet**

     ✓x 7ᵗʰ **X15.8 Contact with other hot household appliances**
          Contact with cooker   Contact with light bulbs
          Contact with kettle

✓x 7ᵗʰ **X16 Contact with hot heating appliances, radiators and pipes**
     EXCLUDES 1   contact with powered appliances (W29.-)
                  exposure to controlled fire in building or structure due to appliance (X02.8)
                  exposure to industrial appliances electrical current (W86.1)

✓x 7ᵗʰ **X17 Contact with hot engines, machinery and tools**
     EXCLUDES 1   contact with hot heating appliances, radiators and pipes (X16)
                  contact with hot household appliances (X15)

✓x 7ᵗʰ **X18 Contact with other hot metals**
     Contact with liquid metal

✓x 7ᵗʰ **X19 Contact with other heat and hot substances**
     EXCLUDES 1   objects that are not normally hot, e.g., an object made hot by a house fire ▶(X00-X08)◀

✓ Additional Character Req   ✓x 7ᵗʰ Placeholder Alert   Manifestation   HCC CMS-HCC Condition   ▽ Unspecified Code   ▶◀ Revised Text   ● New Code   ▲ Revised Code Title

ICD-10-CM 2018   1153

X01.4–X19

Exposure to forces of nature (X30-X39)

The appropriate 7th character is to be added to each code from categories X30-X39.
A   initial encounter
D   subsequent encounter
S   sequela

✓x7ᵗʰ X30 Exposure to excessive natural heat
Exposure to excessive heat as the cause of sunstroke
Exposure to heat NOS
> **EXCLUDES1** excessive heat of man-made origin (W92)
> exposure to man-made radiation (W89)
> exposure to sunlight (X32)
> exposure to tanning bed (W89)

✓x7ᵗʰ X31 Exposure to excessive natural cold
Excessive cold as the cause of chilblains NOS
Excessive cold as the cause of immersion foot or hand
Exposure to cold NOS
Exposure to weather conditions
> **EXCLUDES1** cold of man-made origin (W93.-)
> contact with or inhalation of dry ice (W93.-)
> contact with or inhalation of liquefied gas (W93.-)

✓x7ᵗʰ X32 Exposure to sunlight
> **EXCLUDES1** man-made radiation (tanning bed) (W89)
> **EXCLUDES2** ▶radiation-related disorders of the skin and subcutaneous tissue (L55-L59)◄

✓x7ᵗʰ X34 Earthquake
> **EXCLUDES2** tidal wave (tsunami) due to earthquake (X37.41)

✓x7ᵗʰ X35 Volcanic eruption
> **EXCLUDES2** tidal wave (tsunami) due to volcanic eruption (X37.41)

✓4ᵗʰ X36 Avalanche, landslide and other earth movements
> **INCLUDES** victim of mudslide of cataclysmic nature
> **EXCLUDES1** earthquake (X34)
> **EXCLUDES2** transport accident involving collision with avalanche or landslide not in motion (V01-V99)

✓x7ᵗʰ X36.0 Collapse of dam or man-made structure causing earth movement

✓x7ᵗʰ X36.1 Avalanche, landslide, or mudslide

✓4ᵗʰ X37 Cataclysmic storm

  ✓x7ᵗʰ X37.0 Hurricane
Storm surge
Typhoon

  ✓x7ᵗʰ X37.1 Tornado
Cyclone
Twister

  ✓x7ᵗʰ X37.2 Blizzard (snow) (ice)

  ✓x7ᵗʰ X37.3 Dust storm

  ✓5ᵗʰ X37.4 Tidalwave

    ✓x7ᵗʰ X37.41 Tidal wave due to earthquake or volcanic eruption
Tidal wave NOS
Tsunami

    ✓x7ᵗʰ X37.42 Tidal wave due to storm

    ✓x7ᵗʰ X37.43 Tidal wave due to landslide

  ✓x7ᵗʰ X37.8 Other cataclysmic storms
Cloudburst
Torrential rain
> **EXCLUDES2** flood (X38)

  ✓x7ᵗʰ X37.9 Unspecified cataclysmic storm ▽
Storm NOS
> **EXCLUDES1** collapse of dam or man-made structure causing earth movement (X39.0)

✓x7ᵗʰ X38 Flood
Flood arising from remote storm
Flood of cataclysmic nature arising from melting snow
Flood resulting directly from storm
> **EXCLUDES1** collapse of dam or man-made structure causing earth movement (X39.0)
> tidal wave NOS (X37.41)
> tidal wave caused by storm (X37.2)

✓4ᵗʰ X39 Exposure to other forces of nature

  ✓5ᵗʰ X39.0 Exposure to natural radiation
> **EXCLUDES1** contact with and (suspected) exposure to radon and other naturally occuring radiation (Z77.123)
> exposure to man-made radiation (W88-W90)
> exposure to sunlight (X32)

    ✓x7ᵗʰ X39.01 Exposure to radon

    ✓x7ᵗʰ X39.08 Exposure to other natural radiation

  ✓x7ᵗʰ X39.8 Other exposure to forces of nature

Overexertion and strenuous or repetitive movements (X50)

✓4ᵗʰ X50 Overexertion and strenuous or repetitive movements

The appropriate 7th character is to be added to each code from category X50.
A   initial encounter
D   subsequent encounter
S   sequela

  ✓x7ᵗʰ X50.0 Overexertion from strenuous movement or load
Lifting heavy objects
Lifting weights

  ✓x7ᵗʰ X50.1 Overexertion from prolonged static or awkward postures
Prolonged bending
Prolonged kneeling
Prolonged reaching
Prolonged sitting
Prolonged standing
Prolonged twisting
Static bending
Static kneeling
Static reaching
Static sitting
Static standing
Static twisting

  ✓x7ᵗʰ X50.3 Overexertion from repetitive movements
Use of hand as hammer
> **EXCLUDES2** overuse from prolonged static or awkward postures (X50.1)

  ✓x7ᵗʰ X50.9 Other and unspecified overexertion or strenuous movements or postures ▽
Contact pressure
Contact stress

Accidental exposure to other specified factors (X52-X58)

The appropriate 7th character is to be added to each code from categories X52-X58.
A   initial encounter
D   subsequent encounter
S   sequela

✓x7ᵗʰ X52 Prolonged stay in weightless environment
Weightlessness in spacecraft (simulator)

✓x7ᵗʰ X58 Exposure to other specified factors
Accident NOS
Exposure NOS

Intentional self-harm (X71-X83)

Purposely self-inflicted injury
Suicide (attempted)

The appropriate 7th character is to be added to each code from categories X71-X83.
A   initial encounter
D   subsequent encounter
S   sequela

✓4ᵗʰ X71 Intentional self-harm by drowning and submersion

  ✓x7ᵗʰ X71.0 Intentional self-harm by drowning and submersion while in bathtub HCC

  ✓x7ᵗʰ X71.1 Intentional self-harm by drowning and submersion while in swimming pool HCC

  ✓x7ᵗʰ X71.2 Intentional self-harm by drowning and submersion after jump into swimming pool HCC

  ✓x7ᵗʰ X71.3 Intentional self-harm by drowning and submersion in natural water HCC

  ✓x7ᵗʰ X71.8 Other intentional self-harm by drowning and submersion HCC

  ✓x7ᵗʰ X71.9 Intentional self-harm by drowning and submersion, unspecified HCC ▽

✓x7ᵗʰ X72 Intentional self-harm by handgun discharge HCC
Intentional self-harm by gun for single hand use
Intentional self-harm by pistol
Intentional self-harm by revolver
> **EXCLUDES1** Very pistol (X74.8)

EXCLUDES1 Not coded here   **EXCLUDES2** Not included here   N Newborn Age: 0   P Pediatric Age: 0-17   M Maternity Age: 12-55   A Adult Age: 15-124

1154   ICD-10-CM 2018

✓4th X73   Intentional self-harm by rifle, shotgun and larger firearm discharge
     EXCLUDES 1   airgun (X74.01)

   ✓x7th   **X73.0**   Intentional self-harm by shotgun discharge   HCC

   ✓x7th   **X73.1**   Intentional self-harm by hunting rifle discharge   HCC

   ✓x7th   **X73.2**   Intentional self-harm by machine gun discharge   HCC

   ✓x7th   **X73.8**   Intentional self-harm by other larger firearm discharge   HCC

   ✓x7th   **X73.9**   Intentional self-harm by unspecified larger firearm discharge   HCC ▽

✓4th X74   Intentional self-harm by other and unspecified firearm and gun discharge

   ✓5th   **X74.0**   Intentional self-harm by gas, air or spring-operated guns

     ✓x7th   **X74.01**   Intentional self-harm by airgun   HCC
          Intentional self-harm by BB gun discharge
          Intentional self-harm by pellet gun discharge

     ✓x7th   **X74.02**   Intentional self-harm by paintball gun   HCC

     ✓x7th   **X74.09**   Intentional self-harm by other gas, air or spring-operated gun   HCC

   ✓x7th   **X74.8**   Intentional self-harm by other firearm discharge   HCC
         Intentional self-harm by Very pistol [flare] discharge

   ✓x7th   **X74.9**   Intentional self-harm by unspecified firearm discharge   HCC ▽

✓x7th X75   Intentional self-harm by explosive material   HCC

✓x7th X76   Intentional self-harm by smoke, fire and flames   HCC

✓4th X77   Intentional self-harm by steam, hot vapors and hot objects

   ✓x7th   **X77.0**   Intentional self-harm by steam or hot vapors   HCC

   ✓x7th   **X77.1**   Intentional self-harm by hot tap water   HCC

   ✓x7th   **X77.2**   Intentional self-harm by other hot fluids   HCC

   ✓x7th   **X77.3**   Intentional self-harm by hot household appliances   HCC

   ✓x7th   **X77.8**   Intentional self-harm by other hot objects   HCC

   ✓x7th   **X77.9**   Intentional self-harm by unspecified hot objects   HCC ▽

✓4th X78   Intentional self-harm by sharp object

   ✓x7th   **X78.0**   Intentional self-harm by sharp glass   HCC

   ✓x7th   **X78.1**   Intentional self-harm by knife   HCC

   ✓x7th   **X78.2**   Intentional self-harm by sword or dagger   HCC

   ✓x7th   **X78.8**   Intentional self-harm by other sharp object   HCC

   ✓x7th   **X78.9**   Intentional self-harm by unspecified sharp object   HCC ▽

✓x7th X79   Intentional self-harm by blunt object   HCC

✓x7th X80   Intentional self-harm by jumping from a high place   HCC
     Intentional fall from one level to another

✓4th X81   Intentional self-harm by jumping or lying in front of moving object

   ✓x7th   **X81.0**   Intentional self-harm by jumping or lying in front of motor vehicle   HCC

   ✓x7th   **X81.1**   Intentional self-harm by jumping or lying in front of (subway) train   HCC

   ✓x7th   **X81.8**   Intentional self-harm by jumping or lying in front of other moving object   HCC

✓4th X82   Intentional self-harm by crashing of motor vehicle

   ✓x7th   **X82.0**   Intentional collision of motor vehicle with other motor vehicle   HCC

   ✓x7th   **X82.1**   Intentional collision of motor vehicle with train   HCC

   ✓x7th   **X82.2**   Intentional collision of motor vehicle with tree   HCC

   ✓x7th   **X82.8**   Other intentional self-harm by crashing of motor vehicle   HCC

✓4th X83   Intentional self-harm by other specified means
     EXCLUDES 1   intentional self-harm by poisoning or contact with toxic substance—see Table of Drugs and Chemicals

   ✓x7th   **X83.0**   Intentional self-harm by crashing of aircraft   HCC

   ✓x7th   **X83.1**   Intentional self-harm by electrocution   HCC

   ✓x7th   **X83.2**   Intentional self-harm by exposure to extremes of cold   HCC

   ✓x7th   **X83.8**   Intentional self-harm by other specified means   HCC

Assault (X92-Y09)

INCLUDES   homicide
         injuries inflicted by another person with intent to injure or kill, by any means

EXCLUDES 1   injuries due to legal intervention (Y35.-)
         injuries due to operations of war (Y36.-)
         injuries due to terrorism (Y38.-)

> The appropriate 7th character is to be added to each code from categories X92-Y04 and Y08.
> A   initial encounter
> D   subsequent encounter
> S   sequela

✓4th X92   Assault by drowning and submersion

   ✓x7th   **X92.0**   Assault by drowning and submersion while in bathtub

   ✓x7th   **X92.1**   Assault by drowning and submersion while in swimming pool

   ✓x7th   **X92.2**   Assault by drowning and submersion after push into swimming pool

   ✓x7th   **X92.3**   Assault by drowning and submersion in natural water

   ✓x7th   **X92.8**   Other assault by drowning and submersion

   ✓x7th   **X92.9**   Assault by drowning and submersion, unspecified   ▽

✓x7th X93   Assault by handgun discharge
     Assault by discharge of gun for single hand use
     Assault by discharge of pistol
     Assault by discharge of revolver
     EXCLUDES 1   Very pistol (X95.8)

✓4th X94   Assault by rifle, shotgun and larger firearm discharge
     EXCLUDES 1   airgun (X95.01)

   ✓x7th   **X94.0**   Assault by shotgun

   ✓x7th   **X94.1**   Assault by hunting rifle

   ✓x7th   **X94.2**   Assault by machine gun

   ✓x7th   **X94.8**   Assault by other larger firearm discharge

   ✓x7th   **X94.9**   Assault by unspecified larger firearm discharge   ▽

✓4th X95   Assault by other and unspecified firearm and gun discharge

   ✓5th   **X95.0**   Assault by gas, air or spring-operated guns

     ✓x7th   **X95.01**   Assault by airgun discharge
          Assault by BB gun discharge
          Assault by pellet gun discharge

     ✓x7th   **X95.02**   Assault by paintball gun discharge

     ✓x7th   **X95.09**   Assault by other gas, air or spring-operated gun

   ✓x7th   **X95.8**   Assault by other firearm discharge
         Assault by Very pistol [flare] discharge

   ✓x7th   **X95.9**   Assault by unspecified firearm discharge   ▽

✓4th X96   Assault by explosive material
     EXCLUDES 1   incendiary device (X97)
         terrorism involving explosive material (Y38.2-)

   ✓x7th   **X96.0**   Assault by antipersonnel bomb
       EXCLUDES 1   antipersonnel bomb use in military or war (Y36.2-)

   ✓x7th   **X96.1**   Assault by gasoline bomb

   ✓x7th   **X96.2**   Assault by letter bomb

   ✓x7th   **X96.3**   Assault by fertilizer bomb

   ✓x7th   **X96.4**   Assault by pipe bomb

   ✓x7th   **X96.8**   Assault by other specified explosive

   ✓x7th   **X96.9**   Assault by unspecified explosive   ▽

✓x7th X97   Assault by smoke, fire and flames
     Assault by arson
     Assault by cigarettes
     Assault by incendiary device

✓4th X98   Assault by steam, hot vapors and hot objects

   ✓x7th   **X98.0**   Assault by steam or hot vapors

   ✓x7th   **X98.1**   Assault by hot tap water

   ✓x7th   **X98.2**   Assault by hot fluids

   ✓x7th   **X98.3**   Assault by hot household appliances

   ✓x7th   **X98.8**   Assault by other hot objects

   ✓x7th   **X98.9**   Assault by unspecified hot objects   ▽

✓4th X99   Assault by sharp object
     EXCLUDES 1   assault by strike by sports equipment (Y08.0-)

   ✓x7th   **X99.0**   Assault by sharp glass

   ✓x7th   **X99.1**   Assault by knife

   ✓x7th   **X99.2**   Assault by sword or dagger

✓ Additional Character Req   ✓x7th Placeholder Alert   Manifestation   HCC CMS-HCC Condition   ▽ Unspecified Code   ►◄ Revised Text   ● New Code   ▲ Revised Code Title

Chapter 20. External Causes of Morbidity *(side tab)*

√x7ᵗʰ **X99.8** **Assault by other sharp object**

√x7ᵗʰ **X99.9** **Assault by unspecified sharp object** ▽
Assault by stabbing NOS

√x7ᵗʰ **Y00** **Assault by blunt object**
     EXCLUDES 1   *assault by strike by sports equipment (Y08.0-)*

√x7ᵗʰ **Y01** **Assault by pushing from high place**

√4ᵗʰ **Y02** **Assault by pushing or placing victim in front of moving object**

√x7ᵗʰ **Y02.0** **Assault by pushing or placing victim in front of motor vehicle**

√x7ᵗʰ **Y02.1** **Assault by pushing or placing victim in front of (subway) train**

√x7ᵗʰ **Y02.8** **Assault by pushing or placing victim in front of other moving object**

√4ᵗʰ **Y03** **Assault by crashing of motor vehicle**

√x7ᵗʰ **Y03.0** **Assault by being hit or run over by motor vehicle**

√x7ᵗʰ **Y03.8** **Other assault by crashing of motor vehicle**

√4ᵗʰ **Y04** **Assault by bodily force**
     EXCLUDES 1   *assault by:*
          submersion (X92.-)
          use of weapon (X93-X95, X99, Y00)

√x7ᵗʰ **Y04.0** **Assault by unarmed brawl or fight**

√x7ᵗʰ **Y04.1** **Assault by human bite**

√x7ᵗʰ **Y04.2** **Assault by strike against or bumped into by another person**

√x7ᵗʰ **Y04.8** **Assault by other bodily force**
Assault by bodily force NOS

√4ᵗʰ **Y07** **Perpetrator of assault, maltreatment and neglect**
     NOTE   Codes from this category are for use only in cases of confirmed abuse (T74.-)
          Selection of the correct perpetrator code is based on the relationship between the perpetrator and the victim
     INCLUDES   perpetrator of abandonment
          perpetrator of emotional neglect
          perpetrator of mental cruelty
          perpetrator of physical abuse
          perpetrator of physical neglect
          perpetrator of sexual abuse
          perpetrator of torture

√5ᵗʰ **Y07.0** **Spouse or partner, perpetrator of maltreatment and neglect**
Spouse or partner, perpetrator of maltreatment and neglect against spouse or partner

Y07.01 **Husband, perpetrator of maltreatment and neglect**

Y07.02 **Wife, perpetrator of maltreatment and neglect**

Y07.03 **Male partner, perpetrator of maltreatment and neglect**

Y07.04 **Female partner, perpetrator of maltreatment and neglect**

√5ᵗʰ **Y07.1** **Parent (adoptive) (biological), perpetrator of maltreatment and neglect**

Y07.11 **Biological father, perpetrator of maltreatment and neglect**

Y07.12 **Biological mother, perpetrator of maltreatment and neglect**

Y07.13 **Adoptive father, perpetrator of maltreatment and neglect**

Y07.14 **Adoptive mother, perpetrator of maltreatment and neglect**

√5ᵗʰ **Y07.4** **Other family member, perpetrator of maltreatment and neglect**

√6ᵗʰ **Y07.41** **Sibling, perpetrator of maltreatment and neglect**
     EXCLUDES 1   *stepsibling, perpetrator of maltreatment and neglect (Y07.435, Y07.436)*

Y07.410 **Brother, perpetrator of maltreatment and neglect**

Y07.411 **Sister, perpetrator of maltreatment and neglect**

√6ᵗʰ **Y07.42** **Foster parent, perpetrator of maltreatment and neglect**

Y07.420 **Foster father, perpetrator of maltreatment and neglect**

Y07.421 **Foster mother, perpetrator of maltreatment and neglect**

√6ᵗʰ **Y07.43** **Stepparent or stepsibling, perpetrator of maltreatment and neglect**

Y07.430 **Stepfather, perpetrator of maltreatment and neglect**

Y07.432 **Male friend of parent (co-residing in household), perpetrator of maltreatment and neglect**

Y07.433 **Stepmother, perpetrator of maltreatment and neglect**

Y07.434 **Female friend of parent (co-residing in household), perpetrator of maltreatment and neglect**

Y07.435 **Stepbrother, perpetrator or maltreatment and neglect**

Y07.436 **Stepsister, perpetrator of maltreatment and neglect**

√6ᵗʰ **Y07.49** **Other family member, perpetrator of maltreatment and neglect**

Y07.490 **Male cousin, perpetrator of maltreatment and neglect**

Y07.491 **Female cousin, perpetrator of maltreatment and neglect**

Y07.499 **Other family member, perpetrator of maltreatment and neglect**

√5ᵗʰ **Y07.5** **Non-family member, perpetrator of maltreatment and neglect**

Y07.50 **Unspecified non-family member, perpetrator of maltreatment and neglect** ▽

√6ᵗʰ **Y07.51** **Daycare provider, perpetrator of maltreatment and neglect**

Y07.510 **At-home childcare provider, perpetrator of maltreatment and neglect**

Y07.511 **Daycare center childcare provider, perpetrator of maltreatment and neglect**

Y07.512 **At-home adultcare provider, perpetrator of maltreatment and neglect**

Y07.513 **Adultcare center provider, perpetrator of maltreatment and neglect**

Y07.519 **Unspecified daycare provider, perpetrator of maltreatment and neglect** ▽

√6ᵗʰ **Y07.52** **Healthcare provider, perpetrator of maltreatment and neglect**

Y07.521 **Mental health provider, perpetrator of maltreatment and neglect**

Y07.528 **Other therapist or healthcare provider, perpetrator of maltreatment and neglect**
Nurse, perpetrator of maltreatment and neglect
Occupational therapist, perpetrator of maltreatment and neglect
Physical therapist, perpetrator of maltreatment and neglect
Speech therapist, perpetrator of maltreatment and neglect

Y07.529 **Unspecified healthcare provider, perpetrator of maltreatment and neglect** ▽

Y07.53 **Teacher or instructor, perpetrator of maltreatment and neglect**
Coach, perpetrator of maltreatment and neglect

Y07.59 **Other non-family member, perpetrator of maltreatment and neglect**

Y07.9 **Unspecified perpetrator of maltreatment and neglect** ▽

√4ᵗʰ **Y08** **Assault by other specified means**

√5ᵗʰ **Y08.0** **Assault by strike by sport equipment**

√x7ᵗʰ **Y08.01** **Assault by strike by hockey stick**

√x7ᵗʰ **Y08.02** **Assault by strike by baseball bat**

√x7ᵗʰ **Y08.09** **Assault by strike by other specified type of sport equipment**

√5ᵗʰ **Y08.8** **Assault by other specified means**

√x7ᵗʰ **Y08.81** **Assault by crashing of aircraft**

√x7ᵗʰ **Y08.89** **Assault by other specified means**

Y09 **Assault by unspecified means** ▽
Assassination (attempted) NOS
Homicide (attempted) NOS
Manslaughter (attempted) NOS
Murder (attempted) NOS

EXCLUDES 1 Not coded here   EXCLUDES 2 Not included here   N Newborn Age: 0   P Pediatric Age: 0-17   M Maternity Age: 12-55   A Adult Age: 15-124

Event of undetermined intent (Y21-Y33)

Undetermined intent is only for use when there is specific documentation in the record that the intent of the injury cannot be determined. If no such documentation is present, code to accidental (unintentional).

The appropriate 7th character is to be added to each code from categories Y21-Y33.
A   initial encounter
D   subsequent encounter
S   sequela

☑4ᵗʰ **Y21** **Drowning and submersion, undetermined intent**

☑x7ᵗʰ **Y21.0** **Drowning and submersion** while in bathtub, **undetermined intent**

☑x7ᵗʰ **Y21.1** **Drowning and submersion** after fall into bathtub, **undetermined intent**

☑x7ᵗʰ **Y21.2** **Drowning and submersion** while in swimming pool, **undetermined intent**

☑x7ᵗʰ **Y21.3** **Drowning and submersion** after fall into swimming pool, **undetermined intent**

☑x7ᵗʰ **Y21.4** **Drowning and submersion** in natural water, **undetermined intent**

☑x7ᵗʰ **Y21.8** **Other drowning and submersion, undetermined intent**

☑x7ᵗʰ **Y21.9** **Unspecified drowning and submersion, undetermined intent** ▽

☑x7ᵗʰ **Y22** **Handgun discharge, undetermined intent**
Discharge of gun for single hand use, undetermined intent
Discharge of pistol, undetermined intent
Discharge of revolver, undetermined intent
EXCLUDES 2   Very pistol (Y24.8)

☑4ᵗʰ **Y23** **Rifle, shotgun and larger firearm discharge, undetermined intent**
EXCLUDES 2   airgun (Y24.0)

☑x7ᵗʰ **Y23.0** **Shotgun discharge, undetermined intent**

☑x7ᵗʰ **Y23.1** **Hunting rifle discharge, undetermined intent**

☑x7ᵗʰ **Y23.2** **Military firearm discharge, undetermined intent**

☑x7ᵗʰ **Y23.3** **Machine gun discharge, undetermined intent**

☑x7ᵗʰ **Y23.8** **Other larger firearm discharge, undetermined intent**

☑x7ᵗʰ **Y23.9** **Unspecified larger firearm discharge, undetermined intent** ▽

☑4ᵗʰ **Y24** **Other and unspecified firearm discharge, undetermined intent**

☑x7ᵗʰ **Y24.0** **Airgun discharge, undetermined intent**
BB gun discharge, undetermined intent
Pellet gun discharge, undetermined intent

☑x7ᵗʰ **Y24.8** **Other firearm discharge, undetermined intent**
Paintball gun discharge, undetermined intent
Very pistol [flare] discharge, undetermined intent

☑x7ᵗʰ **Y24.9** **Unspecified firearm discharge, undetermined intent** ▽

☑x7ᵗʰ **Y25** **Contact with explosive material, undetermined intent**

☑x7ᵗʰ **Y26** **Exposure to smoke, fire and flames, undetermined intent**

☑4ᵗʰ **Y27** **Contact with steam, hot vapors and hot objects, undetermined intent**

☑x7ᵗʰ **Y27.0** **Contact with steam and hot vapors, undetermined intent**

☑x7ᵗʰ **Y27.1** **Contact with hot tap water, undetermined intent**

☑x7ᵗʰ **Y27.2** **Contact with hot fluids, undetermined intent**

☑x7ᵗʰ **Y27.3** **Contact with hot household appliance, undetermined intent**

☑x7ᵗʰ **Y27.8** **Contact with other hot objects, undetermined intent**

☑x7ᵗʰ **Y27.9** **Contact with unspecified hot objects, undetermined intent** ▽

☑4ᵗʰ **Y28** **Contact with sharp object, undetermined intent**

☑x7ᵗʰ **Y28.0** **Contact with sharp glass, undetermined intent**

☑x7ᵗʰ **Y28.1** **Contact with knife, undetermined intent**

☑x7ᵗʰ **Y28.2** **Contact with sword or dagger, undetermined intent**

☑x7ᵗʰ **Y28.8** **Contact with other sharp object, undetermined intent**

☑x7ᵗʰ **Y28.9** **Contact with unspecified hot objects, undetermined intent** ▽

☑x7ᵗʰ **Y29** **Contact with blunt object, undetermined intent**

☑x7ᵗʰ **Y30** **Falling, jumping or pushed from a high place, undetermined intent**
Victim falling from one level to another, undetermined intent

☑x7ᵗʰ **Y31** **Falling, lying or running before or into moving object, undetermined intent**

☑x7ᵗʰ **Y32** **Crashing of motor vehicle, undetermined intent**

☑x7ᵗʰ **Y33** **Other specified events, undetermined intent**

Legal intervention, operations of war, military operations, and terrorism (Y35-Y38)

The appropriate 7th character is to be added to each code from categories Y35-Y38.
A   initial encounter
D   subsequent encounter
S   sequela

☑4ᵗʰ **Y35** **Legal intervention**
INCLUDES   any injury sustained as a result of an encounter with any law enforcement official, serving in any capacity at the time of the encounter, whether on-duty or off-duty. Includes: injury to law enforcement official, suspect and bystander

☑5ᵗʰ **Y35.0** **Legal intervention involving firearm discharge**

☑6ᵗʰ **Y35.00** **Legal intervention involving unspecified firearm discharge**
Legal intervention involving gunshot wound
Legal intervention involving shot NOS

☑7ᵗʰ **Y35.001** **Legal intervention involving unspecified firearm discharge, law enforcement official injured** ▽

☑7ᵗʰ **Y35.002** **Legal intervention involving unspecified firearm discharge, bystander injured** ▽

☑7ᵗʰ **Y35.003** **Legal intervention involving unspecified firearm discharge, suspect injured** ▽

☑6ᵗʰ **Y35.01** **Legal intervention involving injury by machine gun**

☑7ᵗʰ **Y35.011** **Legal intervention involving injury by machine gun, law enforcement official injured**

☑7ᵗʰ **Y35.012** **Legal intervention involving injury by machine gun, bystander injured**

☑7ᵗʰ **Y35.013** **Legal intervention involving injury by machine gun, suspect injured**

☑6ᵗʰ **Y35.02** **Legal intervention involving injury by handgun**

☑7ᵗʰ **Y35.021** **Legal intervention involving injury by handgun, law enforcement official injured**

☑7ᵗʰ **Y35.022** **Legal intervention involving injury by handgun, bystander injured**

☑7ᵗʰ **Y35.023** **Legal intervention involving injury by handgun, suspect injured**

☑6ᵗʰ **Y35.03** **Legal intervention involving injury by rifle pellet**

☑7ᵗʰ **Y35.031** **Legal intervention involving injury by rifle pellet, law enforcement official injured**

☑7ᵗʰ **Y35.032** **Legal intervention involving injury by rifle pellet, bystander injured**

☑7ᵗʰ **Y35.033** **Legal intervention involving injury by rifle pellet, suspect injured**

☑6ᵗʰ **Y35.04** **Legal intervention involving injury by rubber bullet**

☑7ᵗʰ **Y35.041** **Legal intervention involving injury by rubber bullet, law enforcement official injured**

☑7ᵗʰ **Y35.042** **Legal intervention involving injury by rubber bullet, bystander injured**

☑7ᵗʰ **Y35.043** **Legal intervention involving injury by rubber bullet, suspect injured**

☑6ᵗʰ **Y35.09** **Legal intervention involving other firearm discharge**

☑7ᵗʰ **Y35.091** **Legal intervention involving other firearm discharge, law enforcement official injured**

☑7ᵗʰ **Y35.092** **Legal intervention involving other firearm discharge, bystander injured**

☑7ᵗʰ **Y35.093** **Legal intervention involving other firearm discharge, suspect injured**

☑5ᵗʰ **Y35.1** **Legal intervention involving explosives**

☑6ᵗʰ **Y35.10** **Legal intervention involving unspecified explosives**

☑7ᵗʰ **Y35.101** **Legal intervention involving unspecified explosives, law enforcement official injured** ▽

☑ Additional Character Req   ☑x7ᵗʰ Placeholder Alert   Manifestation   HCC CMS-HCC Condition   ▽ Unspecified Code   ►◄ Revised Text   ● New Code   ▲ Revised Code Title

ICD-10-CM 2018   1157

☑7th **Y35.102** Legal intervention involving unspecified explosives, **bystander** injured ▽

☑7th **Y35.103** Legal intervention involving unspecified explosives, **suspect** injured

☑6th **Y35.11** Legal intervention involving injury by **dynamite**

　☑7th **Y35.111** Legal intervention involving injury by dynamite, **law enforcement official** injured

　☑7th **Y35.112** Legal intervention involving injury by dynamite, **bystander** injured

　☑7th **Y35.113** Legal intervention involving injury by dynamite, **suspect** injured

☑6th **Y35.12** Legal intervention involving injury by **explosive shell**

　☑7th **Y35.121** Legal intervention involving injury by explosive shell, **law enforcement official** injured

　☑7th **Y35.122** Legal intervention involving injury by explosive shell, **bystander** injured

　☑7th **Y35.123** Legal intervention involving injury by explosive shell, **suspect** injured

☑6th **Y35.19** Legal intervention involving other explosives
　Legal intervention involving injury by grenade
　Legal intervention involving injury by mortar bomb

　☑7th **Y35.191** Legal intervention involving other explosives, **law enforcement official** injured

　☑7th **Y35.192** Legal intervention involving other explosives, **bystander** injured

　☑7th **Y35.193** Legal intervention involving other explosives, **suspect** injured

☑5th **Y35.2** Legal intervention involving **gas**
　Legal intervention involving asphyxiation by gas
　Legal intervention involving poisoning by gas

☑6th **Y35.20** Legal intervention involving unspecified gas

　☑7th **Y35.201** Legal intervention involving unspecified gas, **law enforcement official** injured ▽

　☑7th **Y35.202** Legal intervention involving unspecified gas, **bystander** injured ▽

　☑7th **Y35.203** Legal intervention involving unspecified gas, **suspect** injured ▽

☑6th **Y35.21** Legal intervention involving injury by **tear gas**

　☑7th **Y35.211** Legal intervention involving injury by tear gas, **law enforcement official** injured

　☑7th **Y35.212** Legal intervention involving injury by tear gas, **bystander** injured

　☑7th **Y35.213** Legal intervention involving injury by tear gas, **suspect** injured

☑6th **Y35.29** Legal intervention involving other gas

　☑7th **Y35.291** Legal intervention involving other gas, **law enforcement official** injured

　☑7th **Y35.292** Legal intervention involving other gas, **bystander** injured

　☑7th **Y35.293** Legal intervention involving other gas, **suspect** injured

☑5th **Y35.3** Legal intervention involving **blunt objects**
　Legal intervention involving being hit or struck by blunt object

☑6th **Y35.30** Legal intervention involving unspecified blunt objects

　☑7th **Y35.301** Legal intervention involving unspecified blunt objects, **law enforcement official** injured ▽

　☑7th **Y35.302** Legal intervention involving unspecified blunt objects, **bystander** injured ▽

　☑7th **Y35.303** Legal intervention involving unspecified blunt objects, **suspect** injured ▽

☑6th **Y35.31** Legal intervention involving **baton**

　☑7th **Y35.311** Legal intervention involving baton, **law enforcement official** injured

　☑7th **Y35.312** Legal intervention involving baton, **bystander** injured

　☑7th **Y35.313** Legal intervention involving baton, **suspect** injured

☑6th **Y35.39** Legal intervention involving other blunt objects

　☑7th **Y35.391** Legal intervention involving other blunt objects, **law enforcement official** injured

　☑7th **Y35.392** Legal intervention involving other blunt objects, **bystander** injured

　☑7th **Y35.393** Legal intervention involving other blunt objects, **suspect** injured

☑5th **Y35.4** Legal intervention involving **sharp objects**
　Legal intervention involving being cut by sharp objects
　Legal intervention involving being stabbed by sharp objects

☑6th **Y35.40** Legal intervention involving unspecified sharp objects

　☑7th **Y35.401** Legal intervention involving unspecified sharp objects, **law enforcement official** injured ▽

　☑7th **Y35.402** Legal intervention involving unspecified sharp objects, **bystander** injured ▽

　☑7th **Y35.403** Legal intervention involving unspecified sharp objects, **suspect** injured ▽

☑6th **Y35.41** Legal intervention involving **bayonet**

　☑7th **Y35.411** Legal intervention involving bayonet, **law enforcement official** injured

　☑7th **Y35.412** Legal intervention involving bayonet, **bystander** injured

　☑7th **Y35.413** Legal intervention involving bayonet, **suspect** injured

☑6th **Y35.49** Legal intervention involving other sharp objects

　☑7th **Y35.491** Legal intervention involving other sharp objects, **law enforcement official** injured

　☑7th **Y35.492** Legal intervention involving other sharp objects, **bystander** injured

　☑7th **Y35.493** Legal intervention involving other sharp objects, **suspect** injured

☑5th **Y35.8** Legal intervention involving other specified means

☑6th **Y35.81** Legal intervention involving **manhandling**

　☑7th **Y35.811** Legal intervention involving manhandling, **law enforcement official** injured

　☑7th **Y35.812** Legal intervention involving manhandling, **bystander** injured

　☑7th **Y35.813** Legal intervention involving manhandling, **suspect** injured

☑6th **Y35.89** Legal intervention involving other specified means

　☑7th **Y35.891** Legal intervention involving other specified means, **law enforcement official** injured

　☑7th **Y35.892** Legal intervention involving other specified means, **bystander** injured

　☑7th **Y35.893** Legal intervention involving other specified means, **suspect** injured

☑5th **Y35.9** Legal intervention, means unspecified

　☑x7th **Y35.91** Legal intervention, means unspecified, **law enforcement official** injured ▽

　☑x7th **Y35.92** Legal intervention, means unspecified, **bystander** injured ▽

　☑x7th **Y35.93** Legal intervention, means unspecified, **suspect** injured ▽

☑4th **Y36** **Operations of war**

　INCLUDES　injuries to military personnel and civilians caused by war, civil insurrection, and peacekeeping missions

　EXCLUDES 1　injury to military personnel occurring during peacetime military operations (Y37.-)
　military vehicles involved in transport accidents with non-military vehicle during peacetime (V09.01, V09.21, V19.81, V29.81, V39.81, V49.81, V59.81, V69.81, V79.81)

　AHA: 2014, 3Q, 4

☑5th **Y36.0** War operations involving **explosion of marine weapons**

☑6th **Y36.00** War operations involving explosion of unspecified marine weapon
　War operations involving underwater blast NOS

　☑7th **Y36.000** War operations involving explosion of unspecified marine weapon, **military personnel** ▽

EXCLUDES 1 Not coded here　　EXCLUDES 2 Not included here　　N Newborn Age: 0　　P Pediatric Age: 0-17　　M Maternity Age: 12-55　　A Adult Age: 15-124

1158　　　　　ICD-10-CM 2018

☑7ᵗʰ **Y36.001** **War operations involving explosion of** ▽
      unspecified marine weapon, civilian

☑6ᵗʰ **Y36.01** **War operations involving explosion of** depth-charge

☑7ᵗʰ **Y36.010** **War operations involving explosion of**
      depth-charge, military personnel

☑7ᵗʰ **Y36.011** **War operations involving explosion of**
      depth-charge, civilian

☑6ᵗʰ **Y36.02** **War operations involving explosion of** marine mine
      War operations involving explosion of marine mine, at
      sea or in harbor

☑7ᵗʰ **Y36.020** **War operations involving explosion of**
      marine mine, military personnel

☑7ᵗʰ **Y36.021** **War operations involving explosion of**
      marine mine, civilian

☑6ᵗʰ **Y36.03** **War operations involving explosion of** sea-based
      artillery shell

☑7ᵗʰ **Y36.030** **War operations involving explosion of**
      sea-based artillery shell, military
      personnel

☑7ᵗʰ **Y36.031** **War operations involving explosion of**
      sea-based artillery shell, civilian

☑6ᵗʰ **Y36.04** **War operations involving explosion of** torpedo

☑7ᵗʰ **Y36.040** **War operations involving explosion of**
      torpedo, military personnel

☑7ᵗʰ **Y36.041** **War operations involving explosion of**
      torpedo, civilian

☑6ᵗʰ **Y36.05** **War operations involving** accidental detonation of
      onboard marine weapons

☑7ᵗʰ **Y36.050** **War operations involving accidental**
      detonation of onboard marine weapons,
      military personnel

☑7ᵗʰ **Y36.051** **War operations involving accidental**
      detonation of onboard marine weapons,
      civilian

☑6ᵗʰ **Y36.09** **War operations involving explosion of other marine**
      weapons

☑7ᵗʰ **Y36.090** **War operations involving explosion of**
      other marine weapons, military personnel

☑7ᵗʰ **Y36.091** **War operations involving explosion of**
      other marine weapons, civilian

☑5ᵗʰ **Y36.1** **War operations involving** destruction of aircraft

☑6ᵗʰ **Y36.10** **War operations involving unspecified destruction of**
      aircraft

☑7ᵗʰ **Y36.100** **War operations involving unspecified** ▽
      destruction of aircraft, military personnel

☑7ᵗʰ **Y36.101** **War operations involving unspecified** ▽
      destruction of aircraft, civilian

☑6ᵗʰ **Y36.11** **War operations involving destruction of aircraft due**
      to enemy fire or explosives
      War operations involving destruction of aircraft due to
      air to air missile
      War operations involving destruction of aircraft due to
      explosive placed on aircraft
      War operations involving destruction of aircraft due to
      rocket propelled grenade [RPG]
      War operations involving destruction of aircraft due to
      small arms fire
      War operations involving destruction of aircraft due to
      surface to air missile

☑7ᵗʰ **Y36.110** **War operations involving destruction of**
      aircraft due to enemy fire or explosives,
      military personnel

☑7ᵗʰ **Y36.111** **War operations involving destruction of**
      aircraft due to enemy fire or explosives,
      civilian

☑6ᵗʰ **Y36.12** **War operations involving destruction of aircraft** due
      to collision with other aircraft

☑7ᵗʰ **Y36.120** **War operations involving destruction of**
      aircraft due to collision with other aircraft,
      military personnel

☑7ᵗʰ **Y36.121** **War operations involving destruction of**
      aircraft due to collision with other aircraft,
      civilian

☑6ᵗʰ **Y36.13** **War operations involving destruction of aircraft due**
      to onboard fire

☑7ᵗʰ **Y36.130** **War operations involving destruction of**
      aircraft due to onboard fire, military
      personnel

☑7ᵗʰ **Y36.131** **War operations involving destruction of**
      aircraft due to onboard fire, civilian

☑6ᵗʰ **Y36.14** **War operations involving destruction of aircraft due**
      to accidental detonation of onboard munitions and
      explosives

☑7ᵗʰ **Y36.140** **War operations involving destruction of**
      aircraft due to accidental detonation of
      onboard munitions and explosives,
      military personnel

☑7ᵗʰ **Y36.141** **War operations involving destruction of**
      aircraft due to accidental detonation of
      onboard munitions and explosives,
      civilian

☑6ᵗʰ **Y36.19** **War operations involving other destruction of**
      aircraft

☑7ᵗʰ **Y36.190** **War operations involving other**
      destruction of aircraft, military personnel

☑7ᵗʰ **Y36.191** **War operations involving other**
      destruction of aircraft, civilian

☑5ᵗʰ **Y36.2** **War operations involving other explosions and fragments**

EXCLUDES 1 *war operations involving explosion of aircraft (Y36.1-)*
      war operations involving explosion of marine weapons
      (Y36.0-)
      war operations involving explosion of nuclear weapons
      (Y36.5-)
      war operations involving explosion occurring after
      cessation of hostilities (Y36.8-)

☑6ᵗʰ **Y36.20** **War operations involving unspecified explosion and**
      fragments
      War operations involving air blast NOS
      War operations involving blast NOS
      War operations involving blast fragments NOS
      War operations involving blast wave NOS
      War operations involving blast wind NOS
      War operations involving explosion NOS
      War operations involving explosion of bomb NOS

☑7ᵗʰ **Y36.200** **War operations involving unspecified** ▽
      explosion and fragments, military
      personnel

☑7ᵗʰ **Y36.201** **War operations involving unspecified** ▽
      explosion and fragments, civilian

☑6ᵗʰ **Y36.21** **War operations involving explosion of** aerial bomb

☑7ᵗʰ **Y36.210** **War operations involving explosion of**
      aerial bomb, military personnel

☑7ᵗʰ **Y36.211** **War operations involving explosion of**
      aerial bomb, civilian

☑6ᵗʰ **Y36.22** **War operations involving explosion of** guided
      missile

☑7ᵗʰ **Y36.220** **War operations involving explosion of**
      guided missile, military personnel

☑7ᵗʰ **Y36.221** **War operations involving explosion of**
      guided missile, civilian

☑6ᵗʰ **Y36.23** **War operations involving explosion of** improvised
      explosive device [IED]
      War operations involving explosion of person-borne
      improvised explosive device [IED]
      War operations involving explosion of vehicle-borne
      improvised explosive device [IED]
      War operations involving explosion of roadside
      improvised explosive device [IED]

☑7ᵗʰ **Y36.230** **War operations involving explosion of**
      improvised explosive device [IED], military
      personnel

☑7ᵗʰ **Y36.231** **War operations involving explosion of**
      improvised explosive device [IED], civilian

☑6ᵗʰ **Y36.24** **War operations involving explosion due to**
      accidental detonation and discharge of own
      munitions or munitions launch device

☑7ᵗʰ **Y36.240** **War operations involving explosion due to**
      accidental detonation and discharge of
      own munitions or munitions launch
      device, military personnel

☑7ᵗʰ **Y36.241** **War operations involving explosion due to**
      accidental detonation and discharge of
      own munitions or munitions launch
      device, civilian

☑ Additional Character Req   ✗7ᵗʰ Placeholder Alert   Manifestation   ᴴᶜᶜ CMS-HCC Condition   ▽ Unspecified Code   ▶◀ Revised Text   ● New Code   ▲ Revised Code Title

ICD-10-CM 2018   1159

Chapter 20. External Causes of Morbidity

✓6ᵗʰ **Y36.25** **War operations involving** fragments from munitions

    ✓7ᵗʰ **Y36.250** **War operations involving fragments from munitions,** military personnel

    ✓7ᵗʰ **Y36.251** **War operations involving fragments from munitions,** civilian

✓6ᵗʰ **Y36.26** **War operations involving** fragments of improvised explosive device [IED]

    War operations involving fragments of person-borne improvised explosive device [IED]

    War operations involving fragments of vehicle-borne improvised explosive device [IED]

    War operations involving fragments of roadside improvised explosive device [IED]

    ✓7ᵗʰ **Y36.260** **War operations involving fragments of improvised explosive device [IED],** military personnel

    ✓7ᵗʰ **Y36.261** **War operations involving fragments of improvised explosive device [IED],** civilian

✓6ᵗʰ **Y36.27** **War operations involving** fragments from weapons

    ✓7ᵗʰ **Y36.270** **War operations involving fragments from weapons,** military personnel

    ✓7ᵗʰ **Y36.271** **War operations involving fragments from weapons,** civilian

✓6ᵗʰ **Y36.29** **War operations involving other explosions and fragments**

    War operations involving explosion of grenade

    War operations involving explosions of land mine

    War operations involving shrapnel NOS

    ✓7ᵗʰ **Y36.290** **War operations involving other explosions and fragments,** military personnel

    ✓7ᵗʰ **Y36.291** **War operations involving other explosions and fragments,** civilian

✓5ᵗʰ **Y36.3** **War operations involving** fires, conflagrations and hot substances

    War operations involving smoke, fumes, and heat from fires, conflagrations and hot substances

    EXCLUDES 1 *war operations involving fires and conflagrations aboard military aircraft (Y36.1-)*

        war operations involving fires and conflagrations aboard military watercraft (Y36.0-)

        war operations involving fires and conflagrations caused indirectly by conventional weapons (Y36.2-)

        war operations involving fires and thermal effects of nuclear weapons (Y36.53-)

✓6ᵗʰ **Y36.30** **War operations involving unspecified fire, conflagration and hot substance**

    ✓7ᵗʰ **Y36.300** **War operations involving unspecified fire, conflagration and hot substance, military personnel** ▽

    ✓7ᵗʰ **Y36.301** **War operations involving unspecified fire, conflagration and hot substance, civilian** ▽

✓6ᵗʰ **Y36.31** **War operations involving** gasoline bomb

    War operations involving incendiary bomb

    War operations involving petrol bomb

    ✓7ᵗʰ **Y36.310** **War operations involving gasoline bomb, military personnel**

    ✓7ᵗʰ **Y36.311** **War operations involving gasoline bomb, civilian**

✓6ᵗʰ **Y36.32** **War operations involving** incendiary bullet

    ✓7ᵗʰ **Y36.320** **War operations involving incendiary bullet, military personnel**

    ✓7ᵗʰ **Y36.321** **War operations involving incendiary bullet, civilian**

✓6ᵗʰ **Y36.33** **War operations involving** flamethrower

    ✓7ᵗʰ **Y36.330** **War operations involving flamethrower, military personnel**

    ✓7ᵗʰ **Y36.331** **War operations involving flamethrower, civilian**

✓6ᵗʰ **Y36.39** **War operations involving other fires, conflagrations and hot substances**

    ✓7ᵗʰ **Y36.390** **War operations involving other fires, conflagrations and hot substances, military personnel**

    ✓7ᵗʰ **Y36.391** **War operations involving other fires, conflagrations and hot substances, civilian**

✓5ᵗʰ **Y36.4** **War operations involving firearm discharge and other forms of conventional warfare**

✓6ᵗʰ **Y36.41** **War operations involving** rubber bullets

    ✓7ᵗʰ **Y36.410** **War operations involving rubber bullets, military personnel**

    ✓7ᵗʰ **Y36.411** **War operations involving rubber bullets, civilian**

✓6ᵗʰ **Y36.42** **War operations involving** firearms pellets

    ✓7ᵗʰ **Y36.420** **War operations involving firearms pellets, military personnel**

    ✓7ᵗʰ **Y36.421** **War operations involving firearms pellets, civilian**

✓6ᵗʰ **Y36.43** **War operations involving other firearms discharge**

    War operations involving bullets NOS

    EXCLUDES 1 *war operations involving munitions fragments (Y36.25-)*

        war operations involving incendiary bullets (Y36.32-)

    ✓7ᵗʰ **Y36.430** **War operations involving other firearms discharge, military personnel**

    ✓7ᵗʰ **Y36.431** **War operations involving other firearms discharge, civilian**

✓6ᵗʰ **Y36.44** **War operations involving** unarmed hand to hand combat

    EXCLUDES 1 *war operations involving combat using blunt or piercing object (Y36.45-)*

        war operations involving intentional restriction of air and airway (Y36.46-)

        war operations involving unintentional restriction of air and airway (Y36.47-)

    ✓7ᵗʰ **Y36.440** **War operations involving unarmed hand to hand combat, military personnel**

    ✓7ᵗʰ **Y36.441** **War operations involving unarmed hand to hand combat, civilian**

✓6ᵗʰ **Y36.45** **War operations involving combat using** blunt or piercing object

    ✓7ᵗʰ **Y36.450** **War operations involving combat using blunt or piercing object, military personnel**

    ✓7ᵗʰ **Y36.451** **War operations involving combat using blunt or piercing object, civilian**

✓6ᵗʰ **Y36.46** **War operations involving** intentional restriction of air and airway

    ✓7ᵗʰ **Y36.460** **War operations involving intentional restriction of air and airway, military personnel**

    ✓7ᵗʰ **Y36.461** **War operations involving intentional restriction of air and airway, civilian**

✓6ᵗʰ **Y36.47** **War operations involving** unintentional restriction of air and airway

    ✓7ᵗʰ **Y36.470** **War operations involving unintentional restriction of air and airway, military personnel**

    ✓7ᵗʰ **Y36.471** **War operations involving unintentional restriction of air and airway, civilian**

✓6ᵗʰ **Y36.49** **War operations involving other forms of conventional warfare**

    ✓7ᵗʰ **Y36.490** **War operations involving other forms of conventional warfare, military personnel**

    ✓7ᵗʰ **Y36.491** **War operations involving other forms of conventional warfare, civilian**

✓5ᵗʰ **Y36.5** **War operations involving** nuclear weapons

    War operations involving dirty bomb NOS

✓6ᵗʰ **Y36.50** **War operations involving unspecified effect of nuclear weapon**

    ✓7ᵗʰ **Y36.500** **War operations involving unspecified effect of nuclear weapon, military personnel** ▽

    ✓7ᵗʰ **Y36.501** **War operations involving unspecified effect of nuclear weapon, civilian** ▽

✓6ᵗʰ **Y36.51** **War operations involving** direct blast **effect of nuclear weapon**

    War operations involving blast pressure of nuclear weapon

---

EXCLUDES 1 Not coded here   **EXCLUDES 2** Not included here   N Newborn Age: 0   P Pediatric Age: 0-17   M Maternity Age: 12-55   A Adult Age: 15-124

1160   ICD-10-CM 2018

√7ᵗʰ **Y36.510 War operations involving direct blast effect of nuclear weapon, military personnel**

√7ᵗʰ **Y36.511 War operations involving direct blast effect of nuclear weapon, civilian**

√6ᵗʰ **Y36.52 War operations involving indirect blast effect of nuclear weapon**
War operations involving being thrown by blast of nuclear weapon
War operations involving being struck or crushed by blast debris of nuclear weapon

√7ᵗʰ **Y36.520 War operations involving indirect blast effect of nuclear weapon, military personnel**

√7ᵗʰ **Y36.521 War operations involving indirect blast effect of nuclear weapon, civilian**

√6ᵗʰ **Y36.53 War operations involving thermal radiation effect of nuclear weapon**
War operations involving direct heat from nuclear weapon
War operation involving fireball effects from nuclear weapon

√7ᵗʰ **Y36.530 War operations involving thermal radiation effect of nuclear weapon, military personnel**

√7ᵗʰ **Y36.531 War operations involving thermal radiation effect of nuclear weapon, civilian**

√6ᵗʰ **Y36.54 War operation involving nuclear radiation effects of nuclear weapon**
War operation involving acute radiation exposure from nuclear weapon
War operation involving exposure to immediate ionizing radiation from nuclear weapon
War operation involving fallout exposure from nuclear weapon
War operation involving secondary effects of nuclear weapons

√7ᵗʰ **Y36.540 War operation involving nuclear radiation effects of nuclear weapon, military personnel**

√7ᵗʰ **Y36.541 War operation involving nuclear radiation effects of nuclear weapon, civilian**

√6ᵗʰ **Y36.59 War operation involving other effects of nuclear weapons**

√7ᵗʰ **Y36.590 War operation involving other effects of nuclear weapons, military personnel**

√7ᵗʰ **Y36.591 War operation involving other effects of nuclear weapons, civilian**

√5ᵗʰ **Y36.6 War operations involving biological weapons**

√6ᵗʰ **Y36.6X War operations involving biological weapons**

√7ᵗʰ **Y36.6X0 War operations involving biological weapons, military personnel**

√7ᵗʰ **Y36.6X1 War operations involving biological weapons, civilian**

√5ᵗʰ **Y36.7 War operations involving chemical weapons and other forms of unconventional warfare**
EXCLUDES 1   *war operations involving incendiary devices (Y36.3-, Y36.5-)*

√6ᵗʰ **Y36.7X War operations involving chemical weapons and other forms of unconventional warfare**

√7ᵗʰ **Y36.7X0 War operations involving chemical weapons and other forms of unconventional warfare, military personnel**

√7ᵗʰ **Y36.7X1 War operations involving chemical weapons and other forms of unconventional warfare, civilian**

√5ᵗʰ **Y36.8 War operations occurring after cessation of hostilities**
War operations classifiable to categories Y36.0-Y36.8 but occurring after cessation of hostilities

√6ᵗʰ **Y36.81 Explosion of mine placed during war operations but exploding after cessation of hostilities**

√7ᵗʰ **Y36.810 Explosion of mine placed during war operations but exploding after cessation of hostilities, military personnel**

√7ᵗʰ **Y36.811 Explosion of mine placed during war operations but exploding after cessation of hostilities, civilian**

√6ᵗʰ **Y36.82 Explosion of bomb placed during war operations but exploding after cessation of hostilities**

√7ᵗʰ **Y36.820 Explosion of bomb placed during war operations but exploding after cessation of hostilities, military personnel**

√7ᵗʰ **Y36.821 Explosion of bomb placed during war operations but exploding after cessation of hostilities, civilian**

√6ᵗʰ **Y36.88 Other war operations occurring after cessation of hostilities**

√7ᵗʰ **Y36.880 Other war operations occurring after cessation of hostilities, military personnel**

√7ᵗʰ **Y36.881 Other war operations occurring after cessation of hostilities, civilian**

√6ᵗʰ **Y36.89 Unspecified war operations occurring after cessation of hostilities**

√7ᵗʰ **Y36.890 Unspecified war operations occurring after cessation of hostilities, military personnel** ▽

√7ᵗʰ **Y36.891 Unspecified war operations occurring after cessation of hostilities, civilian** ▽

√5ᵗʰ **Y36.9 Other and unspecified war operations**

√x7ᵗʰ **Y36.90 War operations, unspecified** ▽

√x7ᵗʰ **Y36.91 War operations involving unspecified weapon of mass destruction [WMD]** ▽

√x7ᵗʰ **Y36.92 War operations involving friendly fire**

√4ᵗʰ **Y37 Military operations**
INCLUDES   injuries to military personnel and civilians occurring during peacetime on military property and during routine military exercises and operations
EXCLUDES 1   *military aircraft involved in aircraft accident with civilian aircraft (V97.81-)*
military vehicles involved in transport accident with civilian vehicle (V09.01, V09.21, V19.81, V29.81, V39.81, V49.81, V59.81, V69.81, V79.81)
military watercraft involved in water transport accident with civilian watercraft (V94.81-)
war operations (Y36.-)

√5ᵗʰ **Y37.0 Military operations involving explosion of marine weapons**

√6ᵗʰ **Y37.00 Military operations involving explosion of unspecified marine weapon**
Military operations involving underwater blast NOS

√7ᵗʰ **Y37.000 Military operations involving explosion of unspecified marine weapon, military personnel** ▽

√7ᵗʰ **Y37.001 Military operations involving explosion of unspecified marine weapon, civilian** ▽

√6ᵗʰ **Y37.01 Military operations involving explosion of depth-charge**

√7ᵗʰ **Y37.010 Military operations involving explosion of depth-charge, military personnel**

√7ᵗʰ **Y37.011 Military operations involving explosion of depth-charge, civilian**

√6ᵗʰ **Y37.02 Military operations involving explosion of marine mine**
Military operations involving explosion of marine mine, at sea or in harbor

√7ᵗʰ **Y37.020 Military operations involving explosion of marine mine, military personnel**

√7ᵗʰ **Y37.021 Military operations involving explosion of marine mine, civilian**

√6ᵗʰ **Y37.03 Military operations involving explosion of sea-based artillery shell**

√7ᵗʰ **Y37.030 Military operations involving explosion of sea-based artillery shell, military personnel**

√7ᵗʰ **Y37.031 Military operations involving explosion of sea-based artillery shell, civilian**

√6ᵗʰ **Y37.04 Military operations involving explosion of torpedo**

√7ᵗʰ **Y37.040 Military operations involving explosion of torpedo, military personnel**

√7ᵗʰ **Y37.041 Military operations involving explosion of torpedo, civilian**

√6th **Y37.05** **Military operations involving accidental detonation of onboard marine weapons**

     √7th **Y37.050** **Military operations involving accidental detonation of onboard marine weapons, military personnel**

     √7th **Y37.051** **Military operations involving accidental detonation of onboard marine weapons, civilian**

√6th **Y37.09** **Military operations involving explosion of other marine weapons**

     √7th **Y37.090** **Military operations involving explosion of other marine weapons, military personnel**

     √7th **Y37.091** **Military operations involving explosion of other marine weapons, civilian**

√5th **Y37.1** **Military operations involving destruction of aircraft**

   √6th **Y37.10** **Military operations involving unspecified destruction of aircraft**

     √7th **Y37.100** **Military operations involving unspecified destruction of aircraft, military personnel** ▽

     √7th **Y37.101** **Military operations involving unspecified destruction of aircraft, civilian** ▽

   √6th **Y37.11** **Military operations involving destruction of aircraft due to enemy fire or explosives**
Military operations involving destruction of aircraft due to air to air missile
Military operations involving destruction of aircraft due to explosive placed on aircraft
Military operations involving destruction of aircraft due to rocket propelled grenade [RPG]
Military operations involving destruction of aircraft due to small arms fire
Military operations involving destruction of aircraft due to surface to air missile

     √7th **Y37.110** **Military operations involving destruction of aircraft due to enemy fire or explosives, military personnel**

     √7th **Y37.111** **Military operations involving destruction of aircraft due to enemy fire or explosives, civilian**

   √6th **Y37.12** **Military operations involving destruction of aircraft due to collision with other aircraft**

     √7th **Y37.120** **Military operations involving destruction of aircraft due to collision with other aircraft, military personnel**

     √7th **Y37.121** **Military operations involving destruction of aircraft due to collision with other aircraft, civilian**

   √6th **Y37.13** **Military operations involving destruction of aircraft due to onboard fire**

     √7th **Y37.130** **Military operations involving destruction of aircraft due to onboard fire, military personnel**

     √7th **Y37.131** **Military operations involving destruction of aircraft due to onboard fire, civilian**

   √6th **Y37.14** **Military operations involving destruction of aircraft due to accidental detonation of onboard munitions and explosives**

     √7th **Y37.140** **Military operations involving destruction of aircraft due to accidental detonation of onboard munitions and explosives, military personnel**

     √7th **Y37.141** **Military operations involving destruction of aircraft due to accidental detonation of onboard munitions and explosives, civilian**

   √6th **Y37.19** **Military operations involving other destruction of aircraft**

     √7th **Y37.190** **Military operations involving other destruction of aircraft, military personnel**

     √7th **Y37.191** **Military operations involving other destruction of aircraft, civilian**

√5th **Y37.2** **Military operations involving other explosions and fragments**

   EXCLUDES 1   *military operations involving explosion of aircraft (Y37.1-)*
military operations involving explosion of marine weapons (Y37.0-)
military operations involving explosion of nuclear weapons (Y37.5-)

   √6th **Y37.20** **Military operations involving unspecified explosion and fragments**
Military operations involving air blast NOS
Military operations involving blast NOS
Military operations involving blast fragments NOS
Military operations involving blast wave NOS
Military operations involving blast wind NOS
Military operations involving explosion NOS
Military operations involving explosion of bomb NOS

     √7th **Y37.200** **Military operations involving unspecified explosion and fragments, military personnel** ▽

     √7th **Y37.201** **Military operations involving unspecified explosion and fragments, civilian** ▽

   √6th **Y37.21** **Military operations involving explosion of aerial bomb**

     √7th **Y37.210** **Military operations involving explosion of aerial bomb, military personnel**

     √7th **Y37.211** **Military operations involving explosion of aerial bomb, civilian**

   √6th **Y37.22** **Military operations involving explosion of guided missile**

     √7th **Y37.220** **Military operations involving explosion of guided missile, military personnel**

     √7th **Y37.221** **Military operations involving explosion of guided missile, civilian**

   √6th **Y37.23** **Military operations involving explosion of improvised explosive device [IED]**
Military operations involving explosion of person-borne improvised explosive device [IED]
Military operations involving explosion of vehicle-borne improvised explosive device [IED]
Military operations involving explosion of roadside improvised explosive device [IED]

     √7th **Y37.230** **Military operations involving explosion of improvised explosive device [IED], military personnel**

     √7th **Y37.231** **Military operations involving explosion of improvised explosive device [IED], civilian**

   √6th **Y37.24** **Military operations involving explosion due to accidental detonation and discharge of own munitions or munitions launch device**

     √7th **Y37.240** **Military operations involving explosion due to accidental detonation and discharge of own munitions or munitions launch device, military personnel**

     √7th **Y37.241** **Military operations involving explosion due to accidental detonation and discharge of own munitions or munitions launch device, civilian**

   √6th **Y37.25** **Military operations involving fragments from munitions**

     √7th **Y37.250** **Military operations involving fragments from munitions, military personnel**

     √7th **Y37.251** **Military operations involving fragments from munitions, civilian**

   √6th **Y37.26** **Military operations involving fragments of improvised explosive device [IED]**
Military operations involving fragments of person-borne improvised explosive device [IED]
Military operations involving fragments of vehicle-borne improvised explosive device [IED]
Military operations involving fragments of roadside improvised explosive device [IED]

     √7th **Y37.260** **Military operations involving fragments of improvised explosive device [IED], military personnel**

     √7th **Y37.261** **Military operations involving fragments of improvised explosive device [IED], civilian**

EXCLUDES 1 Not coded here   EXCLUDES 2 Not included here   N Newborn Age: 0   P Pediatric Age: 0-17   M Maternity Age: 12-55   A Adult Age: 15-124

1162   ICD-10-CM 2018

☑6th **Y37.27** Military operations involving fragments from weapons

     ☑7th **Y37.270** Military operations involving fragments from weapons, military personnel

     ☑7th **Y37.271** Military operations involving fragments from weapons, civilian

☑6th **Y37.29** Military operations involving other explosions and fragments

     Military operations involving explosion of grenade
     Military operations involving explosions of land mine
     Military operations involving shrapnel NOS

     ☑7th **Y37.290** Military operations involving other explosions and fragments, military personnel

     ☑7th **Y37.291** Military operations involving other explosions and fragments, civilian

☑5th **Y37.3** Military operations involving fires, conflagrations and hot substances

     Military operations involving smoke, fumes, and heat from fires, conflagrations and hot substances

     EXCLUDES 1   *military operations involving fires and conflagrations aboard military aircraft (Y37.1-)*
            military operations involving fires and conflagrations aboard military watercraft (Y37.0-)
            military operations involving fires and conflagrations caused indirectly by conventional weapons (Y37.2-)
            military operations involving fires and thermal effects of nuclear weapons (Y36.53-)

     ☑6th **Y37.30** Military operations involving unspecified fire, conflagration and hot substance

         ☑7th **Y37.300** Military operations involving unspecified fire, conflagration and hot substance, military personnel   ▽

         ☑7th **Y37.301** Military operations involving unspecified fire, conflagration and hot substance, civilian   ▽

     ☑6th **Y37.31** Military operations involving gasoline bomb

         Military operations involving incendiary bomb
         Military operations involving petrol bomb

         ☑7th **Y37.310** Military operations involving gasoline bomb, military personnel

         ☑7th **Y37.311** Military operations involving gasoline bomb, civilian

     ☑6th **Y37.32** Military operations involving incendiary bullet

         ☑7th **Y37.320** Military operations involving incendiary bullet, military personnel

         ☑7th **Y37.321** Military operations involving incendiary bullet, civilian

     ☑6th **Y37.33** Military operations involving flamethrower

         ☑7th **Y37.330** Military operations involving flamethrower, military personnel

         ☑7th **Y37.331** Military operations involving flamethrower, civilian

     ☑6th **Y37.39** Military operations involving other fires, conflagrations and hot substances

         ☑7th **Y37.390** Military operations involving other fires, conflagrations and hot substances, military personnel

         ☑7th **Y37.391** Military operations involving other fires, conflagrations and hot substances, civilian

☑5th **Y37.4** Military operations involving firearm discharge and other forms of conventional warfare

     ☑6th **Y37.41** Military operations involving rubber bullets

         ☑7th **Y37.410** Military operations involving rubber bullets, military personnel

         ☑7th **Y37.411** Military operations involving rubber bullets, civilian

     ☑6th **Y37.42** Military operations involving firearms pellets

         ☑7th **Y37.420** Military operations involving firearms pellets, military personnel

         ☑7th **Y37.421** Military operations involving firearms pellets, civilian

☑6th **Y37.43** Military operations involving other firearms discharge

     Military operations involving bullets NOS

     EXCLUDES 1   *military operations involving munitions fragments (Y37.25-)*
            military operations involving incendiary bullets (Y37.32-)

     ☑7th **Y37.430** Military operations involving other firearms discharge, military personnel

     ☑7th **Y37.431** Military operations involving other firearms discharge, civilian

☑6th **Y37.44** Military operations involving unarmed hand to hand combat

     EXCLUDES 1   *military operations involving combat using blunt or piercing object (Y37.45-)*
            military operations involving intentional restriction of air and airway (Y37.46-)
            military operations involving unintentional restriction of air and airway (Y37.47-)

     ☑7th **Y37.440** Military operations involving unarmed hand to hand combat, military personnel

     ☑7th **Y37.441** Military operations involving unarmed hand to hand combat, civilian

☑6th **Y37.45** Military operations involving combat using blunt or piercing object

     ☑7th **Y37.450** Military operations involving combat using blunt or piercing object, military personnel

     ☑7th **Y37.451** Military operations involving combat using blunt or piercing object, civilian

☑6th **Y37.46** Military operations involving intentional restriction of air and airway

     ☑7th **Y37.460** Military operations involving intentional restriction of air and airway, military personnel

     ☑7th **Y37.461** Military operations involving intentional restriction of air and airway, civilian

☑6th **Y37.47** Military operations involving unintentional restriction of air and airway

     ☑7th **Y37.470** Military operations involving unintentional restriction of air and airway, military personnel

     ☑7th **Y37.471** Military operations involving unintentional restriction of air and airway, civilian

☑6th **Y37.49** Military operations involving other forms of conventional warfare

     ☑7th **Y37.490** Military operations involving other forms of conventional warfare, military personnel

     ☑7th **Y37.491** Military operations involving other forms of conventional warfare, civilian

☑5th **Y37.5** Military operations involving nuclear weapons

     Military operation involving dirty bomb NOS

     ☑6th **Y37.50** Military operations involving unspecified effect of nuclear weapon

         ☑7th **Y37.500** Military operations involving unspecified effect of nuclear weapon, military personnel   ▽

         ☑7th **Y37.501** Military operations involving unspecified effect of nuclear weapon, civilian   ▽

     ☑6th **Y37.51** Military operations involving direct blast effect of nuclear weapon

         Military operations involving blast pressure of nuclear weapon

         ☑7th **Y37.510** Military operations involving direct blast effect of nuclear weapon, military personnel

         ☑7th **Y37.511** Military operations involving direct blast effect of nuclear weapon, civilian

---

☑ Additional Character Req   ☑x7th Placeholder Alert   Manifestation   HCC CMS-HCC Condition   ▽ Unspecified Code   ▶◀ Revised Text   ● New Code   ▲ Revised Code Title

ICD-10-CM 2018   **1163**

Chapter 20. External Causes of Morbidity (side margin)

Y37.52–Y38.3X3 (side margin)

✓6th **Y37.52 Military operations involving indirect blast effect of nuclear weapon**
Military operations involving being thrown by blast of nuclear weapon
Military operations involving being struck or crushed by blast debris of nuclear weapon

     ✓7th **Y37.520 Military operations involving indirect blast effect of nuclear weapon, military personnel**

     ✓7th **Y37.521 Military operations involving indirect blast effect of nuclear weapon, civilian**

✓6th **Y37.53 Military operations involving thermal radiation effect of nuclear weapon**
Military operations involving direct heat from nuclear weapon
Military operation involving fireball effects from nuclear weapon

     ✓7th **Y37.530 Military operations involving thermal radiation effect of nuclear weapon, military personnel**

     ✓7th **Y37.531 Military operations involving thermal radiation effect of nuclear weapon, civilian**

✓6th **Y37.54 Military operation involving nuclear radiation effects of nuclear weapon**
Military operation involving acute radiation exposure from nuclear weapon
Military operation involving exposure to immediate ionizing radiation from nuclear weapon
Military operation involving fallout exposure from nuclear weapon
Military operation involving secondary effects of nuclear weapons

     ✓7th **Y37.540 Military operation involving nuclear radiation effects of nuclear weapon, military personnel**

     ✓7th **Y37.541 Military operation involving nuclear radiation effects of nuclear weapon, civilian**

✓6th **Y37.59 Military operation involving other effects of nuclear weapons**

     ✓7th **Y37.590 Military operation involving other effects of nuclear weapons, military personnel**

     ✓7th **Y37.591 Military operation involving other effects of nuclear weapons, civilian**

✓5th **Y37.6 Military operations involving biological weapons**

     ✓6th **Y37.6X Military operations involving biological weapons**

         ✓7th **Y37.6X0 Military operations involving biological weapons, military personnel**

         ✓7th **Y37.6X1 Military operations involving biological weapons, civilian**

✓5th **Y37.7 Military operations involving chemical weapons and other forms of unconventional warfare**
     EXCLUDES 1   military operations involving incendiary devices (Y36.3-, Y36.5-)

     ✓6th **Y37.7X Military operations involving chemical weapons and other forms of unconventional warfare**

         ✓7th **Y37.7X0 Military operations involving chemical weapons and other forms of unconventional warfare, military personnel**

         ✓7th **Y37.7X1 Military operations involving chemical weapons and other forms of unconventional warfare, civilian**

✓5th **Y37.9 Other and unspecified military operations**

     ✓x7th **Y37.90 Military operations, unspecified** ▽

     ✓x7th **Y37.91 Military operations involving unspecified weapon of mass destruction [WMD]** ▽

     ✓x7th **Y37.92 Military operations involving friendly fire**

✓4th **Y38 Terrorism**
   NOTE   These codes are for use to identify injuries resulting from the unlawful use of force or violence against persons or property to intimidate or coerce a Government, the civilian population, or any segment thereof, in furtherance of political or social objective.

   Use additional code for place of occurrence (Y92.-)

✓5th **Y38.0 Terrorism involving explosion of marine weapons**
Terrorism involving depth-charge
Terrorism involving marine mine
Terrorism involving mine NOS, at sea or in harbor
Terrorism involving sea-based artillery shell
Terrorism involving torpedo
Terrorism involving underwater blast

     ✓6th **Y38.0X Terrorism involving explosion of marine weapons**

         ✓7th **Y38.0X1 Terrorism involving explosion of marine weapons, public safety official injured**

         ✓7th **Y38.0X2 Terrorism involving explosion of marine weapons, civilian injured**

         ✓7th **Y38.0X3 Terrorism involving explosion of marine weapons, terrorist injured**

✓5th **Y38.1 Terrorism involving destruction of aircraft**
Terrorism involving aircraft burned
Terrorism involving aircraft exploded
Terrorism involving aircraft being shot down
Terrorism involving aircraft used as a weapon

     ✓6th **Y38.1X Terrorism involving destruction of aircraft**

         ✓7th **Y38.1X1 Terrorism involving destruction of aircraft, public safety official injured**

         ✓7th **Y38.1X2 Terrorism involving destruction of aircraft, civilian injured**

         ✓7th **Y38.1X3 Terrorism involving destruction of aircraft, terrorist injured**

✓5th **Y38.2 Terrorism involving other explosions and fragments**
Terrorism involving antipersonnel (fragments) bomb
Terrorism involving blast NOS
Terrorism involving explosion NOS
Terrorism involving explosion of breech block
Terrorism involving explosion of cannon block
Terrorism involving explosion (fragments) of artillery shell
Terrorism involving explosion (fragments) of bomb
Terrorism involving explosion (fragments) of grenade
Terrorism involving explosion (fragments) of guided missile
Terrorism involving explosion (fragments) of land mine
Terrorism involving explosion of mortar bomb
Terrorism involving explosion of munitions
Terrorism involving explosion (fragments) of rocket
Terrorism involving explosion (fragments) of shell
Terrorism involving shrapnel
Terrorism involving mine NOS, on land
   EXCLUDES 1   terrorism involving explosion of nuclear weapon (Y38.5)
           terrorism involving suicide bomber (Y38.81)

     ✓6th **Y38.2X Terrorism involving other explosions and fragments**

         ✓7th **Y38.2X1 Terrorism involving other explosions and fragments, public safety official injured**

         ✓7th **Y38.2X2 Terrorism involving other explosions and fragments, civilian injured**

         ✓7th **Y38.2X3 Terrorism involving other explosions and fragments, terrorist injured**

✓5th **Y38.3 Terrorism involving fires, conflagration and hot substances**
Terrorism involving conflagration NOS
Terrorism involving fire NOS
Terrorism involving petrol bomb
   EXCLUDES 1   terrorism involving fire or heat of nuclear weapon (Y38.5)

     ✓6th **Y38.3X Terrorism involving fires, conflagration and hot substances**

         ✓7th **Y38.3X1 Terrorism involving fires, conflagration and hot substances, public safety official injured**

         ✓7th **Y38.3X2 Terrorism involving fires, conflagration and hot substances, civilian injured**

         ✓7th **Y38.3X3 Terrorism involving fires, conflagration and hot substances, terrorist injured**

EXCLUDES 1 Not coded here   *EXCLUDES 2* Not included here   N Newborn Age: 0   P Pediatric Age: 0-17   M Maternity Age: 12-55   A Adult Age: 15-124

1164   ICD-10-CM 2018

✓5ᵗʰ **Y38.4** **Terrorism involving firearms**
    Terrorism involving carbine bullet
    Terrorism involving machine gun bullet
    Terrorism involving pellets (shotgun)
    Terrorism involving pistol bullet
    Terrorism involving rifle bullet
    Terrorism involving rubber (rifle) bullet

  ✓6ᵗʰ **Y38.4X** **Terrorism involving** firearms

    ✓7ᵗʰ **Y38.4X1** **Terrorism involving firearms, public safety official injured**

    ✓7ᵗʰ **Y38.4X2** **Terrorism involving firearms, civilian injured**

    ✓7ᵗʰ **Y38.4X3** **Terrorism involving firearms, terrorist injured**

✓5ᵗʰ **Y38.5** **Terrorism involving nuclear weapons**
    Terrorism involving blast effects of nuclear weapon
    Terrorism involving exposure to ionizing radiation from nuclear weapon
    Terrorism involving fireball effect of nuclear weapon
    Terrorism involving heat from nuclear weapon

  ✓6ᵗʰ **Y38.5X** **Terrorism involving** nuclear weapons

    ✓7ᵗʰ **Y38.5X1** **Terrorism involving nuclear weapons, public safety official injured**

    ✓7ᵗʰ **Y38.5X2** **Terrorism involving nuclear weapons, civilian injured**

    ✓7ᵗʰ **Y38.5X3** **Terrorism involving nuclear weapons, terrorist injured**

✓5ᵗʰ **Y38.6** **Terrorism involving biological weapons**
    Terrorism involving anthrax
    Terrorism involving cholera
    Terrorism involving smallpox

  ✓6ᵗʰ **Y38.6X** **Terrorism involving** biological weapons

    ✓7ᵗʰ **Y38.6X1** **Terrorism involving biological weapons, public safety official injured**

    ✓7ᵗʰ **Y38.6X2** **Terrorism involving biological weapons, civilian injured**

    ✓7ᵗʰ **Y38.6X3** **Terrorism involving biological weapons, terrorist injured**

✓5ᵗʰ **Y38.7** **Terrorism involving chemical weapons**
    Terrorism involving gases, fumes, chemicals
    Terrorism involving hydrogen cyanide
    Terrorism involving phosgene
    Terrorism involving sarin

  ✓6ᵗʰ **Y38.7X** **Terrorism involving** chemical weapons

    ✓7ᵗʰ **Y38.7X1** **Terrorism involving chemical weapons, public safety official injured**

    ✓7ᵗʰ **Y38.7X2** **Terrorism involving chemical weapons, civilian injured**

    ✓7ᵗʰ **Y38.7X3** **Terrorism involving chemical weapons, terrorist injured**

✓5ᵗʰ **Y38.8** **Terrorism involving other and unspecified means**

  ✓x7ᵗʰ **Y38.80** **Terrorism involving unspecified means** ▽
    Terrorism NOS

  ✓6ᵗʰ **Y38.81** **Terrorism involving** suicide bomber

    ✓7ᵗʰ **Y38.811** **Terrorism involving suicide bomber, public safety official injured**

    ✓7ᵗʰ **Y38.812** **Terrorism involving suicide bomber, civilian injured**

  ✓6ᵗʰ **Y38.89** **Terrorism involving other means**
    Terrorism involving drowning and submersion
    Terrorism involving lasers
    Terrorism involving piercing or stabbing instruments

    ✓7ᵗʰ **Y38.891** **Terrorism involving other means, public safety official injured**

    ✓7ᵗʰ **Y38.892** **Terrorism involving other means, civilian injured**

    ✓7ᵗʰ **Y38.893** **Terrorism involving other means, terrorist injured**

✓5ᵗʰ **Y38.9** **Terrorism, secondary effects**
    NOTE   This code is for use to identify injuries occurring subsequent to a terrorist attack, not those that are due to the initial terrorist attack.

  ✓6ᵗʰ **Y38.9X** **Terrorism,** secondary effects

    ✓7ᵗʰ **Y38.9X1** **Terrorism, secondary effects, public safety official injured**

    ✓7ᵗʰ **Y38.9X2** **Terrorism, secondary effects, civilian injured**

Complications of medical and surgical care (Y62-Y84)

INCLUDES complications of medical devices
    surgical and medical procedures as the cause of abnormal reaction of the patient, or of later complication, without mention of misadventure at the time of the procedure

Misadventures to patients during surgical and medical care (Y62-Y69)

EXCLUDES 1 surgical and medical procedures as the cause of abnormal reaction of the patient, without mention of misadventure at the time of the procedure (Y83-Y84)
EXCLUDES 2 breakdown or malfunctioning of medical device (during procedure) (after implantation) (ongoing use) (Y70-Y82)

✓4ᵗʰ **Y62** **Failure of** sterile precautions **during surgical and medical care**

  Y62.0 **Failure of sterile precautions during** surgical operation

  Y62.1 **Failure of sterile precautions during** infusion or transfusion

  Y62.2 **Failure of sterile precautions during** kidney dialysis and other perfusion   HCC

  Y62.3 **Failure of sterile precautions during** injection or immunization

  Y62.4 **Failure of sterile precautions during** endoscopic examination

  Y62.5 **Failure of sterile precautions during** heart catheterization

  Y62.6 **Failure of sterile precautions during** aspiration, puncture and other catheterization

  Y62.8 **Failure of sterile precautions during other surgical and medical care**

  Y62.9 **Failure of sterile precautions during unspecified surgical and medical care** ▽

✓4ᵗʰ **Y63** **Failure in** dosage **during surgical and medical care**

  EXCLUDES 2 accidental overdose of drug or wrong drug given in error (T36-T50)

  Y63.0 **Excessive amount of blood or other fluid given during transfusion or infusion**

  Y63.1 **Incorrect dilution of fluid used during infusion**

  Y63.2 **Overdose of radiation given during therapy**

  Y63.3 **Inadvertent exposure of patient to radiation during medical care**

  Y63.4 **Failure in dosage in electroshock or insulin-shock therapy**

  Y63.5 **Inappropriate temperature in local application and packing**

  Y63.6 **Underdosing and nonadministration of necessary drug, medicament or biological substance**

  Y63.8 **Failure in dosage during other surgical and medical care**

  Y63.9 **Failure in dosage during unspecified surgical and medical care** ▽

✓4ᵗʰ **Y64** **Contaminated medical or biological substances**

  Y64.0 **Contaminated medical or biological substance,** transfused or infused

  Y64.1 **Contaminated medical or biological substance,** injected or used for immunization

  Y64.8 **Contaminated medical or biological substance administered by other means**

  Y64.9 **Contaminated medical or biological substance administered by unspecified means** ▽
    Administered contaminated medical or biological substance NOS

✓4ᵗʰ **Y65** **Other misadventures during surgical and medical care**

  Y65.0 **Mismatched blood in transfusion**

  Y65.1 **Wrong fluid used in infusion**

  Y65.2 **Failure in suture or ligature during surgical operation**

  Y65.3 **Endotracheal tube wrongly placed during anesthetic procedure**

  Y65.4 **Failure to introduce or to remove other tube or instrument**

  ✓5ᵗʰ **Y65.5** **Performance of** wrong procedure **(operation)**

    Y65.51 **Performance of wrong procedure (operation) on** correct patient
    Wrong device implanted into correct surgical site
    EXCLUDES 1 performance of correct procedure (operation) on wrong side or body part (Y65.53)

✓ Additional Character Req   ✓x7ᵗʰ Placeholder Alert   Manifestation   HCC CMS-HCC Condition   ▽ Unspecified Code   ►◄ Revised Text   ● New Code   ▲ Revised Code Title

Chapter 20. External Causes of Morbidity

Y65.52–Y79.2

> **Y65.52** **Performance of procedure (operation) on** patient not scheduled for surgery
> > Performance of procedure (operation) intended for another patient
> > Performance of procedure (operation) on wrong patient

> **Y65.53** **Performance of correct procedure (operation) on** wrong side or body part
> > Performance of correct procedure (operation) on wrong side
> > Performance of correct procedure (operation) on wrong site

> **Y65.8** **Other specified misadventures during surgical and medical care**

Y66 **Nonadministration of surgical and medical care**
> Premature cessation of surgical and medical care
> > **EXCLUDES 1** *DNR status (Z66)*
> > *palliative care (Z51.5)*

Y69 **Unspecified misadventure during surgical and medical care** ▽

Medical devices associated with adverse incidents in diagnostic and therapeutic use (Y70-Y82)

> **INCLUDES** breakdown or malfunction of medical devices (during use) (after implantation) (ongoing use)

> **EXCLUDES 2** breakdown or malfunctioning of medical device (after implantation) (during procedure) (ongoing use) (Y70-Y82)
> later complications following use of medical devices without breakdown or malfunctioning of device (Y83-Y84)
> misadventure to patients during surgical and medical care, classifiable to (Y62-Y69)
> surgical and other medical procedures as the cause of abnormal reaction of the patient, or of later complication, without mention of misadventure at the time of the procedure (Y83-Y84)

☑4ᵗʰ **Y70** **Anesthesiology devices associated with adverse incidents**
> **Y70.0** Diagnostic and monitoring **anesthesiology devices associated with adverse incidents**
> **Y70.1** Therapeutic (nonsurgical) and rehabilitative **anesthesiology devices associated with adverse incidents**
> **Y70.2** Prosthetic and other implants, **materials and accessory anesthesiology devices associated with adverse incidents**
> **Y70.3** Surgical instruments, materials **and anesthesiology devices (including sutures) associated with adverse incidents**
> **Y70.8** Miscellaneous **anesthesiology devices associated with adverse incidents, not elsewhere classified**

☑4ᵗʰ **Y71** **Cardiovascular devices associated with adverse incidents**
> **Y71.0** Diagnostic and monitoring **cardiovascular devices associated with adverse incidents**
> **Y71.1** Therapeutic (nonsurgical) and rehabilitative **cardiovascular devices associated with adverse incidents**
> **Y71.2** Prosthetic and other implants, **materials and accessory cardiovascular devices associated with adverse incidents**
> **Y71.3** Surgical instruments, materials **and cardiovascular devices (including sutures) associated with adverse incidents**
> **Y71.8** Miscellaneous **cardiovascular devices associated with adverse incidents, not elsewhere classified**

☑4ᵗʰ **Y72** **Otorhinolaryngological devices associated with adverse incidents**
> **Y72.0** Diagnostic and monitoring **otorhinolaryngological devices associated with adverse incidents**
> **Y72.1** Therapeutic (nonsurgical) and rehabilitative **otorhinolaryngological devices associated with adverse incidents**
> **Y72.2** Prosthetic and other implants, **materials and accessory otorhinolaryngological devices associated with adverse incidents**
> **Y72.3** Surgical instruments, materials **and otorhinolaryngological devices (including sutures) associated with adverse incidents**
> **Y72.8** Miscellaneous **otorhinolaryngological devices associated with adverse incidents, not elsewhere classified**

☑4ᵗʰ **Y73** **Gastroenterology and urology devices associated with adverse incidents**
> **Y73.0** Diagnostic and monitoring **gastroenterology and urology devices associated with adverse incidents**
> **Y73.1** Therapeutic (nonsurgical) and rehabilitative **gastroenterology and urology devices associated with adverse incidents**

> **Y73.2** Prosthetic and other implants, **materials and accessory gastroenterology and urology devices associated with adverse incidents**
> **Y73.3** Surgical instruments, materials **and gastroenterology and urology devices (including sutures) associated with adverse incidents**
> **Y73.8** Miscellaneous **gastroenterology and urology devices associated with adverse incidents, not elsewhere classified**

☑4ᵗʰ **Y74** **General hospital and personal-use devices associated with adverse incidents**
> **Y74.0** Diagnostic and monitoring **general hospital and personal-use devices associated with adverse incidents**
> **Y74.1** Therapeutic (nonsurgical) and rehabilitative **general hospital and personal-use devices associated with adverse incidents**
> **Y74.2** Prosthetic and other implants, **materials and accessory general hospital and personal-use devices associated with adverse incidents**
> **Y74.3** Surgical instruments, materials **and general hospital and personal-use devices (including sutures) associated with adverse incidents**
> **Y74.8** Miscellaneous **general hospital and personal-use devices associated with adverse incidents, not elsewhere classified**

☑4ᵗʰ **Y75** **Neurological devices associated with adverse incidents**
> **Y75.0** Diagnostic and monitoring **neurological devices associated with adverse incidents**
> **Y75.1** Therapeutic (nonsurgical) and rehabilitative **neurological devices associated with adverse incidents**
> **Y75.2** Prosthetic and other implants, **materials and neurological devices associated with adverse incidents**
> **Y75.3** Surgical instruments, materials **and neurological devices (including sutures) associated with adverse incidents**
> **Y75.8** Miscellaneous **neurological devices associated with adverse incidents, not elsewhere classified**

☑4ᵗʰ **Y76** **Obstetric and gynecological devices associated with adverse incidents**
> **Y76.0** Diagnostic and monitoring **obstetric and gynecological devices associated with adverse incidents** ♀
> **Y76.1** Therapeutic (nonsurgical) and rehabilitative **obstetric and gynecological devices associated with adverse incidents** ♀
> **Y76.2** Prosthetic and other implants, **materials and accessory obstetric and gynecological devices associated with adverse incidents** ♀
> **Y76.3** Surgical instruments, materials **and obstetric and gynecological devices (including sutures) associated with adverse incidents** ♀
> **Y76.8** Miscellaneous **obstetric and gynecological devices associated with adverse incidents, not elsewhere classified** ♀

☑4ᵗʰ **Y77** **Ophthalmic devices associated with adverse incidents**
> **Y77.0** Diagnostic and monitoring **ophthalmic devices associated with adverse incidents**
> **Y77.1** Therapeutic (nonsurgical) and rehabilitative **ophthalmic devices associated with adverse incidents**
> **Y77.2** Prosthetic and other implants, **materials and accessory ophthalmic devices associated with adverse incidents**
> **Y77.3** Surgical instruments, materials **and ophthalmic devices (including sutures) associated with adverse incidents**
> **Y77.8** Miscellaneous **ophthalmic devices associated with adverse incidents, not elsewhere classified**

☑4ᵗʰ **Y78** **Radiological devices associated with adverse incidents**
> **Y78.0** Diagnostic and monitoring **radiological devices associated with adverse incidents**
> **Y78.1** Therapeutic (nonsurgical) and rehabilitative **radiological devices associated with adverse incidents**
> **Y78.2** Prosthetic and other implants, **materials and accessory radiological devices associated with adverse incidents**
> **Y78.3** Surgical instruments, materials **and radiological devices (including sutures) associated with adverse incidents**
> **Y78.8** Miscellaneous **radiological devices associated with adverse incidents, not elsewhere classified**

☑4ᵗʰ **Y79** **Orthopedic devices associated with adverse incidents**
> **Y79.0** Diagnostic and monitoring **orthopedic devices associated with adverse incidents**
> **Y79.1** Therapeutic (nonsurgical) and rehabilitative **orthopedic devices associated with adverse incidents**
> **Y79.2** Prosthetic and other implants, **materials and accessory orthopedic devices associated with adverse incidents**

EXCLUDES 1 Not coded here   **EXCLUDES 2** Not included here   Ⓝ Newborn Age: 0   Ⓟ Pediatric Age: 0-17   Ⓜ Maternity Age: 12-55   Ⓐ Adult Age: 15-124

1166   ICD-10-CM 2018

Y79.3 Surgical instruments, materials and orthopedic devices (including sutures) associated with adverse incidents

Y79.8 Miscellaneous orthopedic devices associated with adverse incidents, not elsewhere classified

☑4ᵗʰ **Y80** Physical medicine devices associated with adverse incidents

Y80.0 Diagnostic and monitoring physical medicine devices associated with adverse incidents

Y80.1 Therapeutic (nonsurgical) and rehabilitative physical medicine devices associated with adverse incidents

Y80.2 Prosthetic and other implants, materials and accessory physical medicine devices associated with adverse incidents

Y80.3 Surgical instruments, materials and physical medicine devices (including sutures) associated with adverse incidents

Y80.8 Miscellaneous physical medicine devices associated with adverse incidents, not elsewhere classified

☑4ᵗʰ **Y81** General- and plastic-surgery devices associated with adverse incidents

Y81.0 Diagnostic and monitoring general- and plastic-surgery devices associated with adverse incidents

Y81.1 Therapeutic (nonsurgical) and rehabilitative general- and plastic-surgery devices associated with adverse incidents

Y81.2 Prosthetic and other implants, materials and accessory general- and plastic-surgery devices associated with adverse incidents

Y81.3 Surgical instruments, materials and general- and plastic-surgery devices (including sutures) associated with adverse incidents

Y81.8 Miscellaneous general- and plastic-surgery devices associated with adverse incidents, not elsewhere classified

☑4ᵗʰ **Y82** Other and unspecified medical devices associated with adverse incidents

Y82.8 Other medical devices associated with adverse incidents

Y82.9 Unspecified medical devices associated with adverse incidents ▽

Surgical and other medical procedures as the cause of abnormal reaction of the patient, or of later complication, without mention of misadventure at the time of the procedure (Y83-Y84)

EXCLUDES 1   misadventures to patients during surgical and medical care, classifiable to (Y62-Y69)

EXCLUDES 2   breakdown or malfunctioning of medical device (after implantation) (during procedure) (ongoing use) (Y70-Y82)

☑4ᵗʰ **Y83** Surgical operation and other surgical procedures as the cause of abnormal reaction of the patient, or of later complication, without mention of misadventure at the time of the procedure

Y83.0 Surgical operation with transplant of whole organ as the cause of abnormal reaction of the patient, or of later complication, without mention of misadventure at the time of the procedure

Y83.1 Surgical operation with implant of artificial internal device as the cause of abnormal reaction of the patient, or of later complication, without mention of misadventure at the time of the procedure

Y83.2 Surgical operation with anastomosis, bypass or graft as the cause of abnormal reaction of the patient, or of later complication, without mention of misadventure at the time of the procedure

Y83.3 Surgical operation with formation of external stoma as the cause of abnormal reaction of the patient, or of later complication, without mention of misadventure at the time of the procedure

Y83.4 Other reconstructive surgery as the cause of abnormal reaction of the patient, or of later complication, without mention of misadventure at the time of the procedure

Y83.5 Amputation of limb(s) as the cause of abnormal reaction of the patient, or of later complication, without mention of misadventure at the time of the procedure

Y83.6 Removal of other organ (partial) (total) as the cause of abnormal reaction of the patient, or of later complication, without mention of misadventure at the time of the procedure

Y83.8 Other surgical procedures as the cause of abnormal reaction of the patient, or of later complication, without mention of misadventure at the time of the procedure

Y83.9 Surgical procedure, unspecified as the cause of abnormal reaction of the patient, or of later complication, without mention of misadventure at the time of the procedure ▽

☑4ᵗʰ **Y84** Other medical procedures as the cause of abnormal reaction of the patient, or of later complication, without mention of misadventure at the time of the procedure

Y84.0 Cardiac catheterization as the cause of abnormal reaction of the patient, or of later complication, without mention of misadventure at the time of the procedure

Y84.1 Kidney dialysis as the cause of abnormal reaction of the patient, or of later complication, without mention of misadventure at the time of the procedure

Y84.2 Radiological procedure and radiotherapy as the cause of abnormal reaction of the patient, or of later complication, without mention of misadventure at the time of the procedure
     AHA: 2017, 1Q, 33

Y84.3 Shock therapy as the cause of abnormal reaction of the patient, or of later complication, without mention of misadventure at the time of the procedure

Y84.4 Aspiration of fluid as the cause of abnormal reaction of the patient, or of later complication, without mention of misadventure at the time of the procedure

Y84.5 Insertion of gastric or duodenal sound as the cause of abnormal reaction of the patient, or of later complication, without mention of misadventure at the time of the procedure

Y84.6 Urinary catheterization as the cause of abnormal reaction of the patient, or of later complication, without mention of misadventure at the time of the procedure

Y84.7 Blood-sampling as the cause of abnormal reaction of the patient, or of later complication, without mention of misadventure at the time of the procedure

Y84.8 Other medical procedures as the cause of abnormal reaction of the patient, or of later complication, without mention of misadventure at the time of the procedure
     AHA: 2014, 4Q, 24

Y84.9 Medical procedure, unspecified as the cause of abnormal reaction of the patient, or of later complication, without mention of misadventure at the time of the procedure ▽

Supplementary factors related to causes of morbidity classified elsewhere (Y90-Y99)

NOTE   These categories may be used to provide supplementary information concerning causes of morbidity. They are not to be used for single-condition coding.

☑4ᵗʰ **Y90** Evidence of alcohol involvement determined by blood alcohol level

Code first any associated alcohol related disorders (F10)

Y90.0 Blood alcohol level of less than 20 mg/100 ml

Y90.1 Blood alcohol level of 20-39 mg/100 ml

Y90.2 Blood alcohol level of 40-59 mg/100 ml

Y90.3 Blood alcohol level of 60-79 mg/100 ml

Y90.4 Blood alcohol level of 80-99 mg/100 ml

Y90.5 Blood alcohol level of 100-119 mg/100 ml

Y90.6 Blood alcohol level of 120-199 mg/100 ml

Y90.7 Blood alcohol level of 200-239 mg/100 ml

Y90.8 Blood alcohol level of 240 mg/100 ml or more

Y90.9 Presence of alcohol in blood, level not specified ▽

☑4ᵗʰ **Y92** Place of occurrence of the external cause

The following category is for use, when relevant, to identify the place of occurrence of the external cause. Use in conjunction with an activity code.

Place of occurrence should be recorded only at the initial encounter for treatment

☑5ᵗʰ **Y92.0** Non-institutional (private) residence as the place of occurrence of the external cause

EXCLUDES 1   abandoned or derelict house (Y92.89)
home under construction but not yet occupied (Y92.6-)
institutional place of residence (Y92.1-)

☑6ᵗʰ **Y92.00** Unspecified non-institutional (private) residence as the place of occurrence of the external cause

Y92.000 Kitchen of unspecified non-institutional ▽ (private) residence as the place of occurrence of the external cause

Y92.001 Dining room of unspecified ▽ non-institutional (private) residence as the place of occurrence of the external cause

☑ Additional Character Req   ☑7ᵗʰ Placeholder Alert   Manifestation   HCC CMS-HCC Condition   ▽ Unspecified Code   ▶◀ Revised Text   ● New Code   ▲ Revised Code Title

ICD-10-CM 2018   1167

Y92.002   **Bathroom** of unspecified non-institutional (private) residence single-family (private) house as the place of occurrence of the external cause ▽

Y92.003   **Bedroom** of unspecified non-institutional (private) residence as the place of occurrence of the external cause ▽

Y92.007   **Garden or yard** of unspecified non-institutional (private) residence as the place of occurrence of the external cause ▽

Y92.008   **Other place** in unspecified non-institutional (private) residence as the place of occurrence of the external cause ▽

Y92.009   **Unspecified place** in unspecified non-institutional (private) residence as the place of occurrence of the external cause ▽
     Home (NOS) as the place of occurrence of the external cause

✓6ᵗʰ   **Y92.01**   **Single-family** non-institutional (private) house as the place of occurrence of the external cause
     Farmhouse as the place of occurrence of the external cause
       EXCLUDES 1   *barn (Y92.71)*
             chicken coop or hen house (Y92.72)
             farm field (Y92.73)
             orchard (Y92.74)
             single family mobile home or trailer (Y92.02-)
             slaughter house (Y92.86)

Y92.010   **Kitchen** of single-family (private) house as the place of occurrence of the external cause

Y92.011   **Dining room** of single-family (private) house as the place of occurrence of the external cause

Y92.012   **Bathroom** of single-family (private) house as the place of occurrence of the external cause

Y92.013   **Bedroom** of single-family (private) house as the place of occurrence of the external cause

Y92.014   **Private driveway** to single-family (private) house as the place of occurrence of the external cause

Y92.015   **Private garage** of single-family (private) house as the place of occurrence of the external cause

Y92.016   **Swimming-pool** in single-family (private) house or garden as the place of occurrence of the external cause

Y92.017   **Garden or yard** in single-family (private) house as the place of occurrence of the external cause

Y92.018   **Other place** in single-family (private) house as the place of occurrence of the external cause

Y92.019   **Unspecified place** in single-family (private) house as the place of occurrence of the external cause ▽

✓6ᵗʰ   **Y92.02**   **Mobile home** as the place of occurrence of the external cause

Y92.020   **Kitchen** in mobile home as the place of occurrence of the external cause

Y92.021   **Dining room** in mobile home as the place of occurrence of the external cause

Y92.022   **Bathroom** in mobile home as the place of occurrence of the external cause

Y92.023   **Bedroom** in mobile home as the place of occurrence of the external cause

Y92.024   **Driveway** of mobile home as the place of occurrence of the external cause

Y92.025   **Garage** of mobile home as the place of occurrence of the external cause

Y92.026   **Swimming-pool** of mobile home as the place of occurrence of the external cause

Y92.027   **Garden or yard** of mobile home as the place of occurrence of the external cause

Y92.028   **Other place** in mobile home as the place of occurrence of the external cause

Y92.029   **Unspecified place** in mobile home as the place of occurrence of the external cause ▽

✓6ᵗʰ   **Y92.03**   **Apartment** as the place of occurrence of the external cause
     Condominium as the place of occurrence of the external cause
     Co-op apartment as the place of occurrence of the external cause

Y92.030   **Kitchen** in apartment as the place of occurrence of the external cause

Y92.031   **Bathroom** in apartment as the place of occurrence of the external cause

Y92.032   **Bedroom** in apartment as the place of occurrence of the external cause

Y92.038   **Other place** in apartment as the place of occurrence of the external cause

Y92.039   **Unspecified place** in apartment as the place of occurrence of the external cause ▽

✓6ᵗʰ   **Y92.04**   **Boarding-house** as the place of occurrence of the external cause

Y92.040   **Kitchen** in boarding-house as the place of occurrence of the external cause

Y92.041   **Bathroom** in boarding-house as the place of occurrence of the external cause

Y92.042   **Bedroom** in boarding-house as the place of occurrence of the external cause

Y92.043   **Driveway** of boarding-house as the place of occurrence of the external cause

Y92.044   **Garage** of boarding-house as the place of occurrence of the external cause

Y92.045   **Swimming-pool** of boarding-house as the place of occurrence of the external cause

Y92.046   **Garden or yard** of boarding-house as the place of occurrence of the external cause

Y92.048   **Other place** in boarding-house as the place of occurrence of the external cause

Y92.049   **Unspecified place** in boarding-house as the place of occurrence of the external cause ▽

✓6ᵗʰ   **Y92.09**   **Other non-institutional residence** as the place of occurrence of the external cause
     AHA: 2017, 2Q, 10

Y92.090   **Kitchen** in other non-institutional residence as the place of occurrence of the external cause

Y92.091   **Bathroom** in other non-institutional residence as the place of occurrence of the external cause

Y92.092   **Bedroom** in other non-institutional residence as the place of occurrence of the external cause

Y92.093   **Driveway** of other non-institutional residence as the place of occurrence of the external cause

Y92.094   **Garage** of other non-institutional residence as the place of occurrence of the external cause

Y92.095   **Swimming-pool** of other non-institutional residence as the place of occurrence of the external cause

Y92.096   **Garden or yard** of other non-institutional residence as the place of occurrence of the external cause

Y92.098   **Other place** in other non-institutional residence as the place of occurrence of the external cause

Y92.099   **Unspecified place** in other non-institutional residence as the place of occurrence of the external cause ▽

✓5ᵗʰ   **Y92.1**   **Institutional** (nonprivate) residence as the place of occurrence of the external cause

Y92.10   **Unspecified residential institution** as the place of occurrence of the external cause ▽

✓6ᵗʰ   **Y92.11**   **Children's home and orphanage** as the place of occurrence of the external cause

Y92.110   **Kitchen** in children's home and orphanage as the place of occurrence of the external cause

Y92.111   **Bathroom** in children's home and orphanage as the place of occurrence of the external cause

EXCLUDES 1 Not coded here   **EXCLUDES 2** Not included here   N Newborn Age: 0   P Pediatric Age: 0-17   M Maternity Age: 12-55   A Adult Age: 15-124

1168   ICD-10-CM 2018

Y92.112 Bedroom in children's home and orphanage as the place of occurrence of the external cause

Y92.113 Driveway of children's home and orphanage as the place of occurrence of the external cause

Y92.114 Garage of children's home and orphanage as the place of occurrence of the external cause

Y92.115 Swimming-pool of children's home and orphanage as the place of occurrence of the external cause

Y92.116 Garden or yard of children's home and orphanage as the place of occurrence of the external cause

Y92.118 Other place in children's home and orphanage as the place of occurrence of the external cause

Y92.119 Unspecified place in children's home ▽ and orphanage as the place of occurrence of the external cause

✓6ᵗʰ **Y92.12** Nursing home as the place of occurrence of the external cause
  Home for the sick as the place of occurrence of the external cause
  Hospice as the place of occurrence of the external cause
  AHA: 2017, 2Q, 10

Y92.120 Kitchen in nursing home as the place of occurrence of the external cause

Y92.121 Bathroom in nursing home as the place of occurrence of the external cause

Y92.122 Bedroom in nursing home as the place of occurrence of the external cause

Y92.123 Driveway of nursing home as the place of occurrence of the external cause

Y92.124 Garage of nursing home as the place of occurrence of the external cause

Y92.125 Swimming-pool of nursing home as the place of occurrence of the external cause

Y92.126 Garden or yard of nursing home as the place of occurrence of the external cause

Y92.128 Other place in nursing home as the place of occurrence of the external cause

Y92.129 Unspecified place in nursing home as ▽ the place of occurrence of the external cause

✓6ᵗʰ **Y92.13** Military base as the place of occurrence of the external cause
  EXCLUDES 1 military training grounds (Y92.83)

Y92.130 Kitchen on military base as the place of occurrence of the external cause

Y92.131 Mess hall on military base as the place of occurrence of the external cause

Y92.133 Barracks on military base as the place of occurrence of the external cause

Y92.135 Garage on military base as the place of occurrence of the external cause

Y92.136 Swimming-pool on military base as the place of occurrence of the external cause

Y92.137 Garden or yard on military base as the place of occurrence of the external cause

Y92.138 Other place on military base as the place of occurrence of the external cause

Y92.139 Unspecified place military base as the ▽ place of occurrence of the external cause

✓6ᵗʰ **Y92.14** Prison as the place of occurrence of the external cause

Y92.140 Kitchen in prison as the place of occurrence of the external cause

Y92.141 Dining room in prison as the place of occurrence of the external cause

Y92.142 Bathroom in prison as the place of occurrence of the external cause

Y92.143 Cell of prison as the place of occurrence of the external cause

Y92.146 Swimming-pool of prison as the place of occurrence of the external cause

Y92.147 Courtyard of prison as the place of occurrence of the external cause

Y92.148 Other place in prison as the place of occurrence of the external cause

Y92.149 Unspecified place in prison as the ▽ place of occurrence of the external cause

✓6ᵗʰ **Y92.15** Reform school as the place of occurrence of the external cause

Y92.150 Kitchen in reform school as the place of occurrence of the external cause

Y92.151 Dining room in reform school as the place of occurrence of the external cause

Y92.152 Bathroom in reform school as the place of occurrence of the external cause

Y92.153 Bedroom in reform school as the place of occurrence of the external cause

Y92.154 Driveway of reform school as the place of occurrence of the external cause

Y92.155 Garage of reform school as the place of occurrence of the external cause

Y92.156 Swimming-pool of reform school as the place of occurrence of the external cause

Y92.157 Garden or yard of reform school as the place of occurrence of the external cause

Y92.158 Other place in reform school as the place of occurrence of the external cause

Y92.159 Unspecified place in reform school as ▽ the place of occurrence of the external cause

✓6ᵗʰ **Y92.16** School dormitory as the place of occurrence of the external cause
  EXCLUDES 1 reform school as the place of occurrence of the external cause (Y92.15-)
    school buildings and grounds as the place of occurrence of the external cause (Y92.2-)
    school sports and athletic areas as the place of occurrence of the external cause (Y92.3-)

Y92.160 Kitchen in school dormitory as the place of occurrence of the external cause

Y92.161 Dining room in school dormitory as the place of occurrence of the external cause

Y92.162 Bathroom in school dormitory as the place of occurrence of the external cause

Y92.163 Bedroom in school dormitory as the place of occurrence of the external cause

Y92.168 Other place in school dormitory as the place of occurrence of the external cause

Y92.169 Unspecified place in school dormitory ▽ as the place of occurrence of the external cause

✓6ᵗʰ **Y92.19** Other specified residential institution as the place of occurrence of the external cause
  AHA: 2017, 2Q, 10

Y92.190 Kitchen in other specified residential institution as the place of occurrence of the external cause

Y92.191 Dining room in other specified residential institution as the place of occurrence of the external cause

Y92.192 Bathroom in other specified residential institution as the place of occurrence of the external cause

Y92.193 Bedroom in other specified residential institution as the place of occurrence of the external cause

Y92.194 Driveway of other specified residential institution as the place of occurrence of the external cause

Y92.195 Garage of other specified residential institution as the place of occurrence of the external cause

Y92.196 Pool of other specified residential institution as the place of occurrence of the external cause

Y92.197 Garden or yard of other specified residential institution as the place of occurrence of the external cause

Y92.198 Other place in other specified residential institution as the place of occurrence of the external cause

☑ Additional Character Req ✓x7ᵗʰ Placeholder Alert Manifestation HCC CMS-HCC Condition ▽ Unspecified Code ▶◀ Revised Text ● New Code ▲ Revised Code Title

ICD-10-CM 2018 1169

Y92.199 Unspecified place in other specified residential institution as the place of occurrence of the external cause ▽

✓5th Y92.2 School, other institution and public administrative area as the place of occurrence of the external cause
Building and adjacent grounds used by the general public or by a particular group of the public
EXCLUDES1 building under construction as the place of occurrence of the external cause (Y92.6)
residential institution as the place of occurrence of the external cause (Y92.1)
school dormitory as the place of occurrence of the external cause (Y92.16-)
sports and athletics area of schools as the place of occurrence of the external cause (Y92.3-)

✓6th Y92.21 School (private) (public) (state) as the place of occurrence of the external cause
Y92.210 Daycare center as the place of occurrence of the external cause
Y92.211 Elementary school as the place of occurrence of the external cause
Kindergarten as the place of occurrence of the external cause
Y92.212 Middle school as the place of occurrence of the external cause
Y92.213 High school as the place of occurrence of the external cause
AHA: 2012, 4Q, 108
Y92.214 College as the place of occurrence of the external cause
University as the place of occurrence of the external cause
Y92.215 Trade school as the place of occurrence of the external cause
Y92.218 Other school as the place of occurrence of the external cause
Y92.219 Unspecified school as the place of occurrence of the external cause ▽

Y92.22 Religious institution as the place of occurrence of the external cause
Church as the place of occurrence of the external cause
Mosque as the place of occurrence of the external cause
Synagogue as the place of occurrence of the external cause

✓6th Y92.23 Hospital as the place of occurrence of the external cause
EXCLUDES1 ambulatory (outpatient) health services establishments (Y92.53-)
home for the sick as the place of occurrence of the external cause (Y92.12-)
hospice as the place of occurrence of the external cause (Y92.12-)
nursing home as the place of occurrence of the external cause (Y92.12-)
Y92.230 Patient room in hospital as the place of occurrence of the external cause
Y92.231 Patient bathroom in hospital as the place of occurrence of the external cause
Y92.232 Corridor of hospital as the place of occurrence of the external cause
Y92.233 Cafeteria of hospital as the place of occurrence of the external cause
Y92.234 Operating room of hospital as the place of occurrence of the external cause
Y92.238 Other place in hospital as the place of occurrence of the external cause
Y92.239 Unspecified place in hospital as the place of occurrence of the external cause ▽

✓6th Y92.24 Public administrative building as the place of occurrence of the external cause
Y92.240 Courthouse as the place of occurrence of the external cause
Y92.241 Library as the place of occurrence of the external cause
Y92.242 Post office as the place of occurrence of the external cause
Y92.243 City hall as the place of occurrence of the external cause

Y92.248 Other public administrative building as the place of occurrence of the external cause

✓6th Y92.25 Cultural building as the place of occurrence of the external cause
Y92.250 Art Gallery as the place of occurrence of the external cause
Y92.251 Museum as the place of occurrence of the external cause
Y92.252 Music hall as the place of occurrence of the external cause
Y92.253 Opera house as the place of occurrence of the external cause
Y92.254 Theater (live) as the place of occurrence of the external cause
Y92.258 Other cultural public building as the place of occurrence of the external cause

Y92.26 Movie house or cinema as the place of occurrence of the external cause

Y92.29 Other specified public building as the place of occurrence of the external cause
Assembly hall as the place of occurrence of the external cause
Clubhouse as the place of occurrence of the external cause

✓5th Y92.3 Sports and athletics area as the place of occurrence of the external cause

✓6th Y92.31 Athletic court as the place of occurrence of the external cause
EXCLUDES1 tennis court in private home or garden (Y92.09)
Y92.310 Basketball court as the place of occurrence of the external cause
Y92.311 Squash court as the place of occurrence of the external cause
Y92.312 Tennis court as the place of occurrence of the external cause
Y92.318 Other athletic court as the place of occurrence of the external cause

✓6th Y92.32 Athletic field as the place of occurrence of the external cause
Y92.320 Baseball field as the place of occurrence of the external cause
Y92.321 Football field as the place of occurrence of the external cause
Y92.322 Soccer field as the place of occurrence of the external cause
Y92.328 Other athletic field as the place of occurrence of the external cause
Cricket field as the place of occurrence of the external cause
Hockey field as the place of occurrence of the external cause

✓6th Y92.33 Skating rink as the place of occurrence of the external cause
Y92.330 Ice skating rink (indoor) (outdoor) as the place of occurrence of the external cause
Y92.331 Roller skating rink as the place of occurrence of the external cause

Y92.34 Swimming pool (public) as the place of occurrence of the external cause
EXCLUDES1 swimming pool in private home or garden (Y92.016)

Y92.39 Other specified sports and athletic area as the place of occurrence of the external cause
Golf-course as the place of occurrence of the external cause
Gymnasium as the place of occurrence of the external cause
Riding-school as the place of occurrence of the external cause
Stadium as the place of occurrence of the external cause

☑5ᵗʰ **Y92.4** **Street, highway and other paved roadways as the place of occurrence of the external cause**
EXCLUDES1 *private driveway of residence (Y92.014, Y92.024, Y92.043, Y92.093, Y92.113, Y92.123, Y92.154, Y92.194)*

☑6ᵗʰ **Y92.41** **Street and highway as the place of occurrence of the external cause**

Y92.410 **Unspecified street and highway as the place of occurrence of the external cause** ▽
Road NOS as the place of occurrence of the external cause

Y92.411 **Interstate highway as the place of occurrence of the external cause**
Freeway as the place of occurrence of the external cause
Motorway as the place of occurrence of the external cause

Y92.412 **Parkway as the place of occurrence of the external cause**

Y92.413 **State road as the place of occurrence of the external cause**

Y92.414 **Local residential or business street as the place of occurrence of the external cause**

Y92.415 **Exit ramp or entrance ramp of street or highway as the place of occurrence of the external cause**

☑6ᵗʰ **Y92.48** **Other paved roadways as the place of occurrence of the external cause**

Y92.480 **Sidewalk as the place of occurrence of the external cause**

Y92.481 **Parking lot as the place of occurrence of the external cause**

Y92.482 **Bike path as the place of occurrence of the external cause**

Y92.488 **Other paved roadways as the place of occurrence of the external cause**

☑5ᵗʰ **Y92.5** **Trade and service area as the place of occurrence of the external cause**
EXCLUDES1 *garage in private home (Y92.015)*
schools and other public administration buildings (Y92.2-)

☑6ᵗʰ **Y92.51** **Private commercial establishments as the place of occurrence of the external cause**

Y92.510 **Bank as the place of occurrence of the external cause**

Y92.511 **Restaurant or café as the place of occurrence of the external cause**

Y92.512 **Supermarket, store or market as the place of occurrence of the external cause**

Y92.513 **Shop (commercial) as the place of occurrence of the external cause**

☑6ᵗʰ **Y92.52** **Service areas as the place of occurrence of the external cause**

Y92.520 **Airport as the place of occurrence of the external cause**

Y92.521 **Bus station as the place of occurrence of the external cause**

Y92.522 **Railway station as the place of occurrence of the external cause**

Y92.523 **Highway rest stop as the place of occurrence of the external cause**

Y92.524 **Gas station as the place of occurrence of the external cause**
Petroleum station as the place of occurrence of the external cause
Service station as the place of occurrence of the external cause

☑6ᵗʰ **Y92.53** **Ambulatory health services establishments as the place of occurrence of the external cause**

Y92.530 **Ambulatory surgery center as the place of occurrence of the external cause**
Outpatient surgery center, including that connected with a hospital as the place of occurrence of the external cause
Same day surgery center, including that connected with a hospital as the place of occurrence of the external cause

Y92.531 **Health care provider office as the place of occurrence of the external cause**
Physician office as the place of occurrence of the external cause

Y92.532 **Urgent care center as the place of occurrence of the external cause**

Y92.538 **Other ambulatory health services establishments as the place of occurrence of the external cause**

Y92.59 **Other trade areas as the place of occurrence of the external cause**
Office building as the place of occurrence of the external cause
Casino as the place of occurrence of the external cause
Garage (commercial) as the place of occurrence of the external cause
Hotel as the place of occurrence of the external cause
Radio or television station as the place of occurrence of the external cause
Shopping mall as the place of occurrence of the external cause
Warehouse as the place of occurrence of the external cause

☑5ᵗʰ **Y92.6** **Industrial and construction area as the place of occurrence of the external cause**

Y92.61 **Building [any] under construction as the place of occurrence of the external cause**

Y92.62 **Dock or shipyard as the place of occurrence of the external cause**
Dockyard as the place of occurrence of the external cause
Dry dock as the place of occurrence of the external cause
Shipyard as the place of occurrence of the external cause

Y92.63 **Factory as the place of occurrence of the external cause**
Factory building as the place of occurrence of the external cause
Factory premises as the place of occurrence of the external cause
Industrial yard as the place of occurrence of the external cause

Y92.64 **Mine or pit as the place of occurrence of the external cause**
Mine as the place of occurrence of the external cause

Y92.65 **Oil rig as the place of occurrence of the external cause**
Pit (coal) (gravel) (sand) as the place of occurrence of the external cause

Y92.69 **Other specified industrial and construction area as the place of occurrence of the external cause**
Gasworks as the place of occurrence of the external cause
Power-station (coal) (nuclear) (oil) as the place of occurrence of the external cause
Tunnel under construction as the place of occurrence of the external cause
Workshop as the place of occurrence of the external cause

☑5ᵗʰ **Y92.7** **Farm as the place of occurrence of the external cause**
Ranch as the place of occurrence of the external cause
EXCLUDES1 *farmhouse and home premises of farm (Y92.01-)*

Y92.71 **Barn as the place of occurrence of the external cause**

Y92.72 **Chicken coop as the place of occurrence of the external cause**
Hen house as the place of occurrence of the external cause

Y92.73 **Farm field as the place of occurrence of the external cause**

Y92.74 **Orchard as the place of occurrence of the external cause**

Y92.79 **Other farm location as the place of occurrence of the external cause**

☑5ᵗʰ **Y92.8** **Other places as the place of occurrence of the external cause**

☑6ᵗʰ **Y92.81** **Transport vehicle as the place of occurrence of the external cause**
EXCLUDES1 *transport accidents (V00-V99)*

Y92.810 **Car as the place of occurrence of the external cause**

☑ Additional Character Req   ✓x7ᵗʰ Placeholder Alert   Manifestation   HCC CMS-HCC Condition   ▽ Unspecified Code   ►◄ Revised Text   ● New Code   ▲ Revised Code Title

Y92.811 Bus as the place of occurrence of the external cause

Y92.812 Truck as the place of occurrence of the external cause

Y92.813 Airplane as the place of occurrence of the external cause

Y92.814 Boat as the place of occurrence of the external cause

Y92.815 Train as the place of occurrence of the external cause

Y92.816 Subway car as the place of occurrence of the external cause

Y92.818 Other transport vehicle as the place of occurrence of the external cause

✓6ᵗʰ **Y92.82 Wilderness area**

Y92.820 Desert as the place of occurrence of the external cause

Y92.821 Forest as the place of occurrence of the external cause

Y92.828 Other wilderness area as the place of occurrence of the external cause
Swamp as the place of occurrence of the external cause
Mountain as the place of occurrence of the external cause
Marsh as the place of occurrence of the external cause
Prairie as the place of occurrence of the external cause

✓6ᵗʰ **Y92.83 Recreation area** as the place of occurrence of the external cause

Y92.830 Public park as the place of occurrence of the external cause

Y92.831 Amusement park as the place of occurrence of the external cause

Y92.832 Beach as the place of occurrence of the external cause
Seashore as the place of occurrence of the external cause

Y92.833 Campsite as the place of occurrence of the external cause

Y92.834 Zoological garden (Zoo) as the place of occurrence of the external cause

Y92.838 Other recreation area as the place of occurrence of the external cause

Y92.84 Military training ground as the place of occurrence of the external cause

Y92.85 Railroad track as the place of occurrence of the external cause

Y92.86 Slaughter house as the place of occurrence of the external cause

Y92.89 Other specified places as the place of occurrence of the external cause
Derelict house as the place of occurrence of the external cause

Y92.9 Unspecified place or not applicable ▽

✓4ᵗʰ **Y93 Activity codes**

NOTE Category Y93 is provided for use to indicate the activity of the person seeking healthcare for an injury or health condition, such as a heart attack while shoveling snow, which resulted from, or was contributed to, by the activity. These codes are appropriate for use for both acute injuries, such as those from chapter 19, and conditions that are due to the long-term, cumulative effects of an activity, such as those from chapter 13. They are also appropriate for use with external cause codes for cause and intent if identifying the activity provides additional information on the event. These codes should be used in conjunction with codes for external cause status (Y99) and place of occurrence (Y92).

This section contains the following broad activity categories:

Y93.0 Activities involving walking and running
Y93.1 Activities involving water and water craft
Y93.2 Activities involving ice and snow
Y93.3 Activities involving climbing, rappelling, and jumping off
Y93.4 Activities involving dancing and other rhythmic movement
Y93.5 Activities involving other sports and athletics played individually
Y93.6 Activities involving other sports and athletics played as a team or group
Y93.7 Activities involving other specified sports and athletics
Y93.A Activities involving other cardiorespiratory exercise
Y93.B Activities involving other muscle strengthening exercises
Y93.C Activities involving computer technology and electronic devices
Y93.D Activities involving arts and handcrafts
Y93.E Activities involving personal hygiene and interior property and clothing maintenance
Y93.F Activities involving caregiving
Y93.G Activities involving food preparation, cooking and grilling
Y93.H Activities involving exterior property and land maintenance, building and construction
Y93.I Activities involving roller coasters and other types of external motion
Y93.J Activities involving playing musical instrument
Y93.K Activities involving animal care
Y93.8 Activities, other specified
Y93.9 Activity, unspecified

✓5ᵗʰ **Y93.0 Activities involving walking and running**
EXCLUDES 1 *activity, walking an animal (Y93.K1)*
activity, walking or running on a treadmill (Y93.A1)

Y93.01 Activity, walking, marching and hiking
Activity, walking, marching and hiking on level or elevated terrain
EXCLUDES 1 *activity, mountain climbing (Y93.31)*

Y93.02 Activity, running

✓5ᵗʰ **Y93.1 Activities involving water and water craft**
EXCLUDES 1 *activities involving ice (Y93.2-)*

Y93.11 Activity, swimming

Y93.12 Activity, springboard and platform diving

Y93.13 Activity, water polo

Y93.14 Activity, water aerobics and water exercise

Y93.15 Activity, underwater diving and snorkeling
Activity, SCUBA diving

Y93.16 Activity, rowing, canoeing, kayaking, rafting and tubing
Activity, canoeing, kayaking, rafting and tubing in calm and turbulent water

Y93.17 Activity, water skiing and wake boarding

Y93.18 Activity, surfing, windsurfing and boogie boarding
Activity, water sliding

Y93.19 Activity, other involving water and watercraft
Activity involving water NOS
Activity, parasailing
Activity, water survival training and testing

✓5ᵗʰ **Y93.2 Activities involving ice and snow**
EXCLUDES 1 *activity, shoveling ice and snow (Y93.H1)*

Y93.21 Activity, ice skating
Activity, figure skating (singles) (pairs)
Activity, ice dancing
EXCLUDES 1 *activity, ice hockey (Y93.22)*

Y93.22 Activity, ice hockey

Y93.23 Activity, snow (alpine) (downhill) skiing, snow boarding, sledding, tobogganing and snow tubing
EXCLUDES 1 *activity, cross country skiing (Y93.24)*

Y93.24 Activity, cross country skiing
Activity, nordic skiing

Y93.29   **Activity, other involving ice and snow**
Activity involving ice and snow NOS

✓5ᵗʰ **Y93.3**   **Activities involving climbing, rappelling and jumping off**
    EXCLUDES 1   *activity, hiking on level or elevated terrain (Y93.01)*
              activity, jumping rope (Y93.56)
              activity, trampoline jumping (Y93.44)

Y93.31   **Activity, mountain climbing, rock climbing and wall climbing**

Y93.32   **Activity, rappelling**

Y93.33   **Activity, BASE jumping**
Activity, Building, Antenna, Span, Earth jumping

Y93.34   **Activity, bungee jumping**

Y93.35   **Activity, hang gliding**

Y93.39   **Activity, other involving climbing, rappelling and jumping off**

✓5ᵗʰ **Y93.4**   **Activities involving dancing and other rhythmic movement**
    EXCLUDES 1   *activity, martial arts (Y93.75)*

Y93.41   **Activity, dancing**
AHA: 2012, 4Q, 108

Y93.42   **Activity, yoga**

Y93.43   **Activity, gymnastics**
Activity, rhythmic gymnastics
    EXCLUDES 1   *activity, trampolining (Y93.44)*

Y93.44   **Activity, trampolining**

Y93.45   **Activity, cheerleading**

Y93.49   **Activity, other involving dancing and other rhythmic movements**

✓5ᵗʰ **Y93.5**   **Activities involving other sports and athletics played individually**
    EXCLUDES 1   *activity, dancing (Y93.41)*
              activity, gymnastic (Y93.43)
              activity, trampolining (Y93.44)
              activity, yoga (Y93.42)

Y93.51   **Activity, roller skating (inline) and skateboarding**

Y93.52   **Activity, horseback riding**

Y93.53   **Activity, golf**

Y93.54   **Activity, bowling**

Y93.55   **Activity, bike riding**

Y93.56   **Activity, jumping rope**

Y93.57   **Activity, non-running track and field events**
    EXCLUDES 1   *activity, running (any form) (Y93.02)*

Y93.59   **Activity, other involving other sports and athletics played individually**
    EXCLUDES 1   *activities involving climbing, rappelling, and jumping (Y93.3-)*
              activities involving ice and snow (Y93.2-)
              activities involving walking and running (Y93.0-)
              activities involving water and watercraft (Y93.1-)

✓5ᵗʰ **Y93.6**   **Activities involving other sports and athletics played as a team or group**
    EXCLUDES 1   *activity, ice hockey (Y93.22)*
              activity, water polo (Y93.13)

Y93.61   **Activity, American tackle football**
Activity, football NOS

Y93.62   **Activity, American flag or touch football**

Y93.63   **Activity, rugby**

Y93.64   **Activity, baseball**
Activity, softball

Y93.65   **Activity, lacrosse and field hockey**

Y93.66   **Activity, soccer**

Y93.67   **Activity, basketball**

Y93.68   **Activity, volleyball (beach) (court)**

Y93.6A   **Activity, physical games generally associated with school recess, summer camp and children**
Activity, capture the flag
Activity, dodge ball
Activity, four square
Activity, kickball

Y93.69   **Activity, other involving other sports and athletics played as a team or group**
Activity, cricket

✓5ᵗʰ **Y93.7**   **Activities involving other specified sports and athletics**

Y93.71   **Activity, boxing**

Y93.72   **Activity, wrestling**

Y93.73   **Activity, racquet and hand sports**
Activity, handball
Activity, racquetball
Activity, squash
Activity, tennis

Y93.74   **Activity, frisbee**
Activity, ultimate frisbee

Y93.75   **Activity, martial arts**
Activity, combatives

Y93.79   **Activity, other specified sports and athletics**
    EXCLUDES 1   *sports and athletics activities specified in categories Y93.0-Y93.6*

✓5ᵗʰ **Y93.A**   **Activities involving other cardiorespiratory exercise**
Activities involving physical training

Y93.A1   **Activity, exercise machines primarily for cardiorespiratory conditioning**
Activity, elliptical and stepper machines
Activity, stationary bike
Activity, treadmill

Y93.A2   **Activity, calisthenics**
Activity, jumping jacks
Activity, warm up and cool down

Y93.A3   **Activity, aerobic and step exercise**

Y93.A4   **Activity, circuit training**

Y93.A5   **Activity, obstacle course**
Activity, challenge course
Activity, confidence course

Y93.A6   **Activity, grass drills**
Activity, guerilla drills

Y93.A9   **Activity, other involving cardiorespiratory exercise**
    EXCLUDES 1   *activities involving cardiorespiratory exercise specified in categories Y93.0-Y93.7*

✓5ᵗʰ **Y93.B**   **Activities involving other muscle strengthening exercises**

Y93.B1   **Activity, exercise machines primarily for muscle strengthening**

Y93.B2   **Activity, push-ups, pull-ups, sit-ups**

Y93.B3   **Activity, free weights**
Activity, barbells
Activity, dumbbells

Y93.B4   **Activity, pilates**

Y93.B9   **Activity, other involving muscle strengthening exercises**
    EXCLUDES 1   *activities involving muscle strengthening specified in categories Y93.0-Y93.A*

✓5ᵗʰ **Y93.C**   **Activities involving computer technology and electronic devices**
    EXCLUDES 1   *activity, electronic musical keyboard or instruments (Y93.J-)*

Y93.C1   **Activity, computer keyboarding**
Activity, electronic game playing using keyboard or other stationary device

Y93.C2   **Activity, hand held interactive electronic device**
Activity, cellular telephone and communication device
Activity, electronic game playing using interactive device
    EXCLUDES 1   *activity, electronic game playing using keyboard or other stationary device (Y93.C1)*

Y93.C9   **Activity, other involving computer technology and electronic devices**

✓5ᵗʰ **Y93.D**   **Activities involving arts and handcrafts**
    EXCLUDES 1   *activities involving playing musical instrument (Y93.J-)*

Y93.D1   **Activity, knitting and crocheting**

Y93.D2   **Activity, sewing**

Y93.D3   **Activity, furniture building and finishing**
Activity, furniture repair

Y93.D9   **Activity, other involving arts and handcrafts**

✓5ᵗʰ **Y93.E**   **Activities involving personal hygiene and interior property and clothing maintenance**
    EXCLUDES 1   *activities involving cooking and grilling (Y93.G-)*
              activities involving exterior property and land maintenance, building and construction (Y93.H-)
              activities involving caregiving (Y93.F-)
              activity, dishwashing (Y93.G1)
              activity, food preparation (Y93.G1)
              activity, gardening (Y93.H2)

Y93.E1   **Activity, personal bathing and showering**

Y93.E2   **Activity, laundry**

✓ Additional Character Req   ✓×7ᵗʰ Placeholder Alert   Manifestation   HCC CMS-HCC Condition   ▽ Unspecified Code   ►◄ Revised Text   ● New Code   ▲ Revised Code Title

ICD-10-CM 2018   1173

Y93.E3   **Activity, vacuuming**

Y93.E4   **Activity, ironing**

Y93.E5   **Activity, floor mopping and cleaning**

Y93.E6   **Activity, residential relocation**
Activity, packing up and unpacking involved in moving to a new residence

Y93.E8   **Activity, other personal hygiene**

Y93.E9   **Activity, other interior property and clothing maintenance**

✓5ᵗʰ **Y93.F**   **Activities involving caregiving**
Activity involving the provider of caregiving

Y93.F1   **Activity, caregiving, bathing**

Y93.F2   **Activity, caregiving, lifting**

Y93.F9   **Activity, other caregiving**

✓5ᵗʰ **Y93.G**   **Activities involving food preparation, cooking and grilling**

Y93.G1   **Activity, food preparation and clean up**
Activity, dishwashing

Y93.G2   **Activity, grilling and smoking food**

Y93.G3   **Activity, cooking and baking**
Activity, use of stove, oven and microwave oven

Y93.G9   **Activity, other involving cooking and grilling**

✓5ᵗʰ **Y93.H**   **Activities involving exterior property and land maintenance, building and construction**

Y93.H1   **Activity, digging, shoveling and raking**
Activity, dirt digging
Activity, raking leaves
Activity, snow shoveling

Y93.H2   **Activity, gardening and landscaping**
Activity, pruning, trimming shrubs, weeding

Y93.H3   **Activity, building and construction**

Y93.H9   **Activity, other involving exterior property and land maintenance, building and construction**

✓5ᵗʰ **Y93.I**   **Activities involving roller coasters and other types of external motion**

Y93.I1   **Activity, rollercoaster riding**

Y93.I9   **Activity, other involving external motion**

✓5ᵗʰ **Y93.J**   **Activities involving playing musical instrument**
Activity involving playing electric musical instrument

Y93.J1   **Activity, piano playing**
Activity, musical keyboard (electronic) playing

Y93.J2   **Activity, drum and other percussion instrument playing**

Y93.J3   **Activity, string instrument playing**

Y93.J4   **Activity, winds and brass instrument playing**

✓5ᵗʰ **Y93.K**   **Activities involving animal care**
EXCLUDES 1   activity, horseback riding (Y93.52)

Y93.K1   **Activity, walking an animal**

Y93.K2   **Activity, milking an animal**

Y93.K3   **Activity, grooming and shearing an animal**

Y93.K9   **Activity, other involving animal care**

✓5ᵗʰ **Y93.8**   **Activities, other specified**

Y93.81   **Activity, refereeing a sports activity**

Y93.82   **Activity, spectator at an event**

Y93.83   **Activity, rough housing and horseplay**

Y93.84   **Activity, sleeping**

Y93.85   **Activity, choking game**
Activity, blackout game
Activity, fainting game
Activity, pass out game

Y93.89   **Activity, other specified**

Y93.9   **Activity, unspecified**   ▽

Y95   **Nosocomial condition**
AHA: 2013, 4Q, 119

✓4ᵗʰ **Y99**   **External cause status**
NOTE   A single code from category Y99 should be used in conjunction with the external cause code(s) assigned to a record to indicate the status of the person at the time the event occurred.

Y99.0   **Civilian activity done for income or pay**
Civilian activity done for financial or other compensation
EXCLUDES 1   military activity (Y99.1)
volunteer activity (Y99.2)

Y99.1   **Military activity**
EXCLUDES 1   activity of off duty military personnel (Y99.8)

Y99.2   **Volunteer activity**
EXCLUDES 1   activity of child or other family member assisting in compensated work of other family member (Y99.8)

Y99.8   **Other external cause status**
Activity NEC
Activity of child or other family member assisting in compensated work of other family member
Hobby not done for income
Leisure activity
Off-duty activity of military personnel
Recreation or sport not for income or while a student
Student activity
EXCLUDES 1   civilian activity done for income or compensation (Y99.0)
military activity (Y99.1)
AHA: 2012, 4Q, 108

Y99.9   **Unspecified external cause status**   ▽

EXCLUDES 1 Not coded here   *EXCLUDES 2* Not included here   N Newborn Age: 0   P Pediatric Age: 0-17   M Maternity Age: 12-55   A Adult Age: 15-124

1174   ICD-10-CM 2018

Chapter 21. Factors Influencing Health Status and Contact with Health Services (Z00–Z99)

Chapter Specific Guidelines with Coding Examples

The chapter specific guidelines from the ICD-10-CM Official Guidelines for Coding and Reporting have been provided below. Along with these guidelines are coding examples, contained in the shaded boxes, that have been developed to help illustrate the coding and/or sequencing guidance found in these guidelines.

Note: The chapter specific guidelines provide additional information about the use of Z codes for specified encounters.

a. Use of Z codes in any healthcare setting

Z codes are for use in any healthcare setting. Z codes may be used as either a first-listed (principal diagnosis code in the inpatient setting) or secondary code, depending on the circumstances of the encounter. Certain Z codes may only be used as first-listed or principal diagnosis.

> Patient with middle lobe lung cancer presents for initiation of chemotherapy
>
> **Z51.11**   **Encounter for antineoplastic chemotherapy**
>
> **C34.2**   **Malignant neoplasm of middle lobe, bronchus or lung**
>
> *Explanation:* A Z code can be used as first-listed in this situation based on guidelines in this chapter as well as chapter 2, "Neoplasms."

> Patient has chronic lymphocytic leukemia for which the patient had previous chemotherapy and is now in remission
>
> **C91.11**   **Chronic lymphocytic leukemia of B-cell type in remission**
>
> **Z92.21**   **Personal history of antineoplastic chemotherapy**
>
> *Explanation:* The personal history Z code is used to describe a secondary (supplementary) diagnosis to identify that this patient has had chemotherapy in the past.

b. Z codes indicate a reason for an encounter

Z codes are not procedure codes. A corresponding procedure code must accompany a Z code to describe any procedure performed.

c. Categories of Z codes

1) Contact/exposure

Category Z20 indicates contact with, and suspected exposure to, communicable diseases. These codes are for patients who do not show any sign or symptom of a disease but are suspected to have been exposed to it by close personal contact with an infected individual or are in an area where a disease is epidemic.

Category Z77, Other contact with and (suspected) exposures hazardous to health, indicates contact with and suspected exposures hazardous to health.

Contact/exposure codes may be used as a first-listed code to explain an encounter for testing, or, more commonly, as a secondary code to identify a potential risk.

2) Inoculations and vaccinations

Code Z23 is for encounters for inoculations and vaccinations. It indicates that a patient is being seen to receive a prophylactic inoculation against a disease. Procedure codes are required to identify the actual administration of the injection and the type(s) of immunizations given. Code Z23 may be used as a secondary code if the inoculation is given as a routine part of preventive health care, such as a well-baby visit.

3) Status

Status codes indicate that a patient is either a carrier of a disease or has the sequelae or residual of a past disease or condition. This includes such things as the presence of prosthetic or mechanical devices resulting from past treatment. A status code is informative, because the status may affect the course of treatment and its outcome. A status code is distinct from a history code. The history code indicates that the patient no longer has the condition.

A status code should not be used with a diagnosis code from one of the body system chapters, if the diagnosis code includes the information provided by the status code. For example, code Z94.1, Heart transplant status, should not be used with a code from subcategory T86.2, Complications of heart transplant. The status code does not provide additional information. The complication code indicates that the patient is a heart transplant patient.

For encounters for weaning from a mechanical ventilator, assign a code from subcategory J96.1, Chronic respiratory failure, followed by code Z99.11, Dependence on respirator [ventilator] status.

The status Z codes/categories are:

Z14   Genetic carrier

Genetic carrier status indicates that a person carries a gene, associated with a particular disease, which may be passed to offspring who may develop that disease. The person does not have the disease and is not at risk of developing the disease.

Z15   Genetic susceptibility to disease

Genetic susceptibility indicates that a person has a gene that increases the risk of that person developing the disease.

Codes from category Z15 should not be used as principal or first-listed codes. If the patient has the condition to which he/she is susceptible, and that condition is the reason for the encounter, the code for the current condition should be sequenced first. If the patient is being seen for follow-up after completed treatment for this condition, and the condition no longer exists, a follow-up code should be sequenced first, followed by the appropriate personal history and genetic susceptibility codes. If the purpose of the encounter is genetic counseling associated with procreative management, code Z31.5, Encounter for genetic counseling, should be assigned as the first-listed code, followed by a code from category Z15. Additional codes should be assigned for any applicable family or personal history.

Z16   Resistance to antimicrobial drugs

This code indicates that a patient has a condition that is resistant to antimicrobial drug treatment. Sequence the infection code first.

Z17   Estrogen receptor status

Z18   Retained foreign body fragments

Z19   Hormone sensitivity malignancy status

Z21   Asymptomatic HIV infection status

This code indicates that a patient has tested positive for HIV but has manifested no signs or symptoms of the disease.

Z22   Carrier of infectious disease

Carrier status indicates that a person harbors the specific organisms of a disease without manifest symptoms and is capable of transmitting the infection.

Z28.3   Underimmunization status

Z33.1   Pregnant state, incidental

This code is a secondary code only for use when the pregnancy is in no way complicating the reason for visit. Otherwise, a code from the obstetric chapter is required.

Z66   Do not resuscitate

This code may be used when it is documented by the provider that a patient is on do not resuscitate status at any time during the stay.

Z67   Blood type

Z68   Body mass index (BMI)

As with all other secondary diagnosis codes, the BMI codes should only be assigned when they meet the definition of a reportable diagnosis (see Section III, Reporting Additional Diagnoses).

Z74.01   Bed confinement status

Z76.82   Awaiting organ transplant status

Z78   Other specified health status

Code Z78.1, Physical restraint status, may be used when it is documented by the provider that a patient has been put in restraints during the current encounter. Please note that this code should not be reported when it is documented by the provider that a patient is temporarily restrained during a procedure.

Z79   Long-term (current) drug therapy

Codes from this category indicate a patient's continuous use of a prescribed drug (including such things as aspirin therapy) for the long-term treatment of a condition or for prophylactic use. It is not for use for patients who have addictions to drugs. This subcategory is not for use of medications for detoxification or maintenance programs to prevent withdrawal symptoms in patients with drug dependence (e.g., methadone maintenance for opiate dependence). Assign the appropriate code for the drug dependence instead.

Assign a code from Z79 if the patient is receiving a medication for an extended period as a prophylactic measure (such as for the prevention of deep vein thrombosis) or as treatment of a chronic condition (such as arthritis) or a disease requiring a lengthy course of treatment (such as cancer). Do not assign a code from category Z79 for medication being administered for a brief period of time to treat an acute illness or injury (such as a course of antibiotics to treat acute bronchitis).

Z88	Allergy status to drugs, medicaments and biological substances

Except: Z88.9, Allergy status to unspecified drugs, medicaments and biological substances status

Z89	Acquired absence of limb
Z9Ø	Acquired absence of organs, not elsewhere classified
Z91.Ø-	Allergy status, other than to drugs and biological substances
Z92.82	Status post administration of tPA (rtPA) in a different facility within the last 24 hours prior to admission to a current facility

Assign code Z92.82, Status post administration of tPA (rtPA) in a different facility within the last 24 hours prior to admission to current facility, as a secondary diagnosis when a patient is received by transfer into a facility and documentation indicates they were administered tissue plasminogen activator (tPA) within the last 24 hours prior to admission to the current facility.

This guideline applies even if the patient is still receiving the tPA at the time they are received into the current facility.

The appropriate code for the condition for which the tPA was administered (such as cerebrovascular disease or myocardial infarction) should be assigned first.

Code Z92.82 is only applicable to the receiving facility record and not to the transferring facility record.

Z93	Artificial opening status
Z94	Transplanted organ and tissue status
Z95	Presence of cardiac and vascular implants and grafts
Z96	Presence of other functional implants
Z97	Presence of other devices
Z98	Other postprocedural states

Assign code Z98.85, Transplanted organ removal status, to indicate that a transplanted organ has been previously removed. This code should not be assigned for the encounter in which the transplanted organ is removed. The complication necessitating removal of the transplant organ should be assigned for that encounter.

See section I.C19. for information on the coding of organ transplant complications.

Z99	Dependence on enabling machines and devices, not elsewhere classified

Note: Categories Z89-Z9Ø and Z93-Z99 are for use only if there are no complications or malfunctions of the organ or tissue replaced, the amputation site or the equipment on which the patient is dependent.

4) History (of)

There are two types of history Z codes, personal and family. Personal history codes explain a patient's past medical condition that no longer exists and is not receiving any treatment, but that has the potential for recurrence, and therefore may require continued monitoring.

Family history codes are for use when a patient has a family member(s) who has had a particular disease that causes the patient to be at higher risk of also contracting the disease.

Personal history codes may be used in conjunction with follow-up codes and family history codes may be used in conjunction with screening codes to explain the need for a test or procedure. History codes are also acceptable on any medical record regardless of the reason for visit. A history of an illness, even if no longer present, is important information that may alter the type of treatment ordered.

The history Z code categories are:

Z8Ø	Family history of primary malignant neoplasm
Z81	Family history of mental and behavioral disorders
Z82	Family history of certain disabilities and chronic diseases (leading to disablement)
Z83	Family history of other specific disorders
Z84	Family history of other conditions
Z85	Personal history of malignant neoplasm
Z86	Personal history of certain other diseases
Z87	Personal history of other diseases and conditions
Z91.4-	Personal history of psychological trauma, not elsewhere classified
Z91.5	Personal history of self-harm
Z91.81	**History of falling**
Z91.82	**Personal history of military deployment**
Z92	Personal history of medical treatment

Except: Z92.Ø, Personal history of contraception

Except: Z92.82, Status post administration of tPA (rtPA) in a different facility within the last 24 hours prior to admission to a current facility

5) Screening

Screening is the testing for disease or disease precursors in seemingly well individuals so that early detection and treatment can be provided for those who test positive for the disease (e.g., screening mammogram).

The testing of a person to rule out or confirm a suspected diagnosis because the patient has some sign or symptom is a diagnostic examination, not a screening. In these cases, the sign or symptom is used to explain the reason for the test.

A screening code may be a first-listed code if the reason for the visit is specifically the screening exam. It may also be used as an additional code if the screening is done during an office visit for other health problems. A screening code is not necessary if the screening is inherent to a routine examination, such as a pap smear done during a routine pelvic examination.

Should a condition be discovered during the screening then the code for the condition may be assigned as an additional diagnosis.

Prostate screening of healthy 5Ø-year-old male patient; PSA noted to be elevated but normal digital rectal exam

Z12.5	**Encounter for screening for malignant neoplasm of prostate**
R97.2Ø	**Elevated prostate specific antigen [PSA]**

Explanation: The patient had no signs or symptoms of any prostate-related illness prior to coming in for the screening. The screening code is appropriately used as the first-listed code to signify that this was for routine screening. The elevated PSA is reported as a secondary diagnosis to reflect that an abnormal lab value was found as a result of the screening procedure(s).

The Z code indicates that a screening exam is planned. A procedure code is required to confirm that the screening was performed.

The screening Z codes/categories:

Z11	Encounter for screening for infectious and parasitic diseases
Z12	Encounter for screening for malignant neoplasms
Z13	Encounter for screening for other diseases and disorders

Except: Z13.9, Encounter for screening, unspecified

Z36	Encounter for antenatal screening for mother

6) Observation

There are three observation Z code categories. They are for use in very limited circumstances when a person is being observed for a suspected condition that is ruled out. The observation codes are not for use if an injury or illness or any signs or symptoms related to the suspected condition are present. In such cases the diagnosis/symptom code is used with the corresponding external cause code.

The observation codes are to be used as principal diagnosis only. The only exception to this is when the principal diagnosis is required to be a code from category Z38, Liveborn infants according to place of birth and type of delivery. Then a code from category Z05, Encounter for observation and evaluation of newborn for suspected diseases and conditions ruled out, is sequenced after the Z38 code. Additional codes may be used in addition to the observation code but only if they are unrelated to the suspected condition being observed.

Codes from subcategory Z03.7, Encounter for suspected maternal and fetal conditions ruled out, may either be used as a first-listed or as an additional code assignment depending on the case. They are for use in very limited circumstances on a maternal record when an encounter is for a suspected maternal or fetal condition that is ruled out during that encounter (for example, a maternal or fetal condition may be suspected due to an abnormal test result). These codes should not be used when the condition is confirmed. In those cases, the confirmed condition should be coded. In addition, these codes are not for use if an illness or any signs or symptoms related to the suspected condition or problem are present. In such cases the diagnosis/symptom code is used.

Additional codes may be used in addition to the code from subcategory Z03.7, but only if they are unrelated to the suspected condition being evaluated.

Codes from subcategory Z03.7 may not be used for encounters for antenatal screening of mother. *See Section I.C.21. Screening.*

For encounters for suspected fetal condition that are inconclusive following testing and evaluation, assign the appropriate code from category O35, O36, O40 or O41.

The observation Z code categories:

Z03   Encounter for medical observation for suspected diseases and conditions ruled out

Z04   Encounter for examination and observation for other reasons
      Except: Z04.9, Encounter for examination and observation for unspecified reason

Z05   Encounter for observation and evaluation of newborn for suspected diseases and conditions ruled out

7) Aftercare

Aftercare visit codes cover situations when the initial treatment of a disease has been performed and the patient requires continued care during the healing or recovery phase, or for the long-term consequences of the disease. The aftercare Z code should not be used if treatment is directed at a current, acute disease. The diagnosis code is to be used in these cases. Exceptions to this rule are codes Z51.0, Encounter for antineoplastic radiation therapy, and codes from subcategory Z51.1, Encounter for antineoplastic chemotherapy and immunotherapy. These codes are to be first-listed, followed by the diagnosis code when a patient's encounter is solely to receive radiation therapy, chemotherapy, or immunotherapy for the treatment of a neoplasm. If the reason for the encounter is more than one type of antineoplastic therapy, code Z51.0 and a code from subcategory Z51.1 may be assigned together, in which case one of these codes would be reported as a secondary diagnosis.

The aftercare Z codes should also not be used for aftercare for injuries. For aftercare of an injury, assign the acute injury code with the appropriate 7th character (for subsequent encounter).

The aftercare codes are generally first-listed to explain the specific reason for the encounter. An aftercare code may be used as an additional code when some type of aftercare is provided in addition to the reason for admission and no diagnosis code is applicable. An example of this would be the closure of a colostomy during an encounter for treatment of another condition.

Aftercare codes should be used in conjunction with other aftercare codes or diagnosis codes to provide better detail on the specifics of an aftercare encounter visit, unless otherwise directed by the classification. Should a patient receive multiple types of antineoplastic therapy during the same encounter, code Z51.0, Encounter for antineoplastic radiation therapy, and codes from subcategory Z51.1, Encounter for antineoplastic chemotherapy and immunotherapy, may be used together on a record. The sequencing of multiple aftercare codes depends on the circumstances of the encounter.

Certain aftercare Z code categories need a secondary diagnosis code to describe the resolving condition or sequelae. For others, the condition is included in the code title.

Additional Z code aftercare category terms include fitting and adjustment, and attention to artificial openings.

Status Z codes may be used with aftercare Z codes to indicate the nature of the aftercare. For example code Z95.1, Presence of aortocoronary bypass graft, may be used with code Z48.812, Encounter for surgical aftercare following surgery on the circulatory system, to indicate the surgery for which the aftercare is being performed. A status code should not be used when the aftercare code indicates the type of status, such as using Z43.0, Encounter for attention to tracheostomy, with Z93.0, Tracheostomy status.

The aftercare Z category/codes:

Z42   Encounter for plastic and reconstructive surgery following medical procedure or healed injury

Z43   Encounter for attention to artificial openings

Z44   Encounter for fitting and adjustment of external prosthetic device

Z45   Encounter for adjustment and management of implanted device

Z46   Encounter for fitting and adjustment of other devices

Z47   Orthopedic aftercare

Z48   Encounter for other postprocedural aftercare

Z49   Encounter for care involving renal dialysis

Z51   Encounter for other aftercare and medical care

8) Follow-up

The follow-up codes are used to explain continuing surveillance following completed treatment of a disease, condition, or injury. They imply that the condition has been fully treated and no longer exists. They should not be confused with aftercare codes, or injury codes with a 7th character for subsequent encounter, that explain ongoing care of a healing condition or its sequelae. Follow-up codes may be used in conjunction with history codes to provide the full picture of the healed condition and its treatment. The follow-up code is sequenced first, followed by the history code.

A follow-up code may be used to explain multiple visits. Should a condition be found to have recurred on the follow-up visit, then the diagnosis code for the condition should be assigned in place of the follow-up code.

The follow-up Z code categories:

Z08   Encounter for follow-up examination after completed treatment for malignant neoplasm

Z09   Encounter for follow-up examination after completed treatment for conditions other than malignant neoplasm

Z39   Encounter for maternal postpartum care and examination

Follow-up for patient several months after completing a regime of IV antibiotics for recurrent pneumonia; lungs are clear and pneumonia is resolved

Z09   **Encounter for follow-up examination after completed treatment for conditions other than malignant neoplasm**

Z87.01   **Personal history of pneumonia (recurrent)**

Explanation: Code Z09 identifies the follow-up visit as being unrelated to a malignant neoplasm, and code Z87 describes the condition that has now resolved.

Follow-up for patient several months after completing a regime of IV antibiotics for recurrent pneumonia; pneumonia has recurred, and a new antibiotic regimen has been prescribed

J18.9   **Pneumonia, unspecified organism**

Explanation: Since the follow-up exam for pneumonia determined that the pneumonia was not resolved or recurred, code Z09 Encounter for follow-up examination after completed treatment for conditions other than malignant neoplasm, no longer applies. Instead the first-listed code describes the pneumonia.

---

9) Donor

Codes in category Z52, Donors of organs and tissues, are used for living individuals who are donating blood or other body tissue. These codes are only for individuals donating for others, not for self-donations. They are not used to identify cadaveric donations.

10) Counseling

Counseling Z codes are used when a patient or family member receives assistance in the aftermath of an illness or injury, or when support is required in coping with family or social problems.

The counseling Z codes/categories:

Z30.0-   Encounter for general counseling and advice on contraception

Z31.5   Encounter for **procreative** genetic counseling

Z31.6-   Encounter for general counseling and advice on procreation

Z32.2   Encounter for childbirth instruction

Z32.3   Encounter for childcare instruction

Z69   Encounter for mental health services for victim and perpetrator of abuse

Z70   Counseling related to sexual attitude, behavior and orientation

Z71   Persons encountering health services for other counseling and medical advice, not elsewhere classified

Z76.81   Expectant mother prebirth pediatrician visit

11) Encounters for obstetrical and reproductive services

See Section I.C.15. Pregnancy, Childbirth, and the Puerperium, for further instruction on the use of these codes.

Z codes for pregnancy are for use in those circumstances when none of the problems or complications included in the codes from the Obstetrics chapter exist (a routine prenatal visit or postpartum care). Codes in category Z34, Encounter for supervision of normal pregnancy, are always first-listed and are not to be used with any other code from the OB chapter.

Codes in category Z3A, Weeks of gestation, may be assigned to provide additional information about the pregnancy. Category Z3A codes should not be assigned for pregnancies with abortive outcomes (categories O00-O08), elective termination of pregnancy (code **Z33.2**), nor for postpartum conditions, as category Z3A is not applicable to these conditions. The date of the admission should be used to determine weeks of gestation for inpatient admissions that encompass more than one gestational week.

The outcome of delivery, category Z37, should be included on all maternal delivery records. It is always a secondary code. Codes in category Z37 should not be used on the newborn record.

Z codes for family planning (contraceptive) or procreative management and counseling should be included on an obstetric record either during the pregnancy or the postpartum stage, if applicable.

Z codes/categories for obstetrical and reproductive services:

Z30	Encounter for contraceptive management
Z31	Encounter for procreative management
Z32.2	Encounter for childbirth instruction
Z32.3	Encounter for childcare instruction
Z33	Pregnant state
Z34	Encounter for supervision of normal pregnancy
Z36	Encounter for antenatal screening of mother
Z3A	Weeks of gestation
Z37	Outcome of delivery
Z39	Encounter for maternal postpartum care and examination
Z76.81	Expectant mother prebirth pediatrician visit

12) Newborns and infants

See Section I.C.16. Newborn (Perinatal) Guidelines, for further instruction on the use of these codes.

Newborn Z codes/categories:

Z76.1	Encounter for health supervision and care of foundling
Z00.1-	Encounter for routine child health examination
Z38	Liveborn infants according to place of birth and type of delivery

13) Routine and administrative examinations

The Z codes allow for the description of encounters for routine examinations, such as, a general check-up, or, examinations for administrative purposes, such as, a pre-employment physical. The codes are not to be used if the examination is for diagnosis of a suspected condition or for treatment purposes. In such cases the diagnosis code is used. During a routine exam, should a diagnosis or condition be discovered, it should be coded as an additional code. Pre-existing and chronic conditions and history codes may also be included as additional codes as long as the examination is for administrative purposes and not focused on any particular condition.

Some of the codes for routine health examinations distinguish between "with" and "without" abnormal findings. Code assignment depends on the information that is known at the time the encounter is being coded. For example, if no abnormal findings were found during the examination, but the encounter is being coded before test results are back, it is acceptable to assign the code for "without abnormal findings." When assigning a code for "with abnormal findings," additional code(s) should be assigned to identify the specific abnormal finding(s).

12-month-old boy presented for well-child visit; pediatrician notices some eczema on the child's scalp and back of the knees

Z00.121   **Encounter for routine child health examination with abnormal findings**

L30.9   **Dermatitis, unspecified**

Explanation: The Z code identifying that this is a routine well-child visit is reported first. Because an abnormal finding (eczema) was documented, a code for this condition may also be appended.

Pre-operative examination and pre-procedural laboratory examination Z codes are for use only in those situations when a patient is being cleared for a procedure or surgery and no treatment is given.

The Z codes/categories for routine and administrative examinations:

Z00	Encounter for general examination without complaint, suspected or reported diagnosis
Z01	Encounter for other special examination without complaint, suspected or reported diagnosis
Z02	Encounter for administrative examination
	Except: Z02.9, Encounter for administrative examinations, unspecified
Z32.0-	Encounter for pregnancy test

14) Miscellaneous Z codes

The miscellaneous Z codes capture a number of other health care encounters that do not fall into one of the other categories. Certain of these codes identify the reason for the encounter; others are for use as additional codes that provide useful information on circumstances that may affect a patient's care and treatment.

Prophylactic organ removal

For encounters specifically for prophylactic removal of an organ (such as prophylactic removal of breasts due to a genetic susceptibility to cancer or a family history of cancer), the principal or first-listed code should be a code from category Z40, Encounter for prophylactic surgery, followed by the appropriate codes to identify the associated risk factor (such as genetic susceptibility or family history).

If the patient has a malignancy of one site and is having prophylactic removal at another site to prevent either a new primary malignancy or metastatic disease, a code for the malignancy should also be assigned in addition to a code from subcategory Z40.0, Encounter for prophylactic surgery for risk factors related to malignant neoplasms. A Z40.0 code should not be assigned if the patient is having organ removal for treatment of a malignancy, such as the removal of the testes for the treatment of prostate cancer.

Miscellaneous Z codes/categories:

Z28	Immunization not carried out
	Except: Z28.3, Underimmunization status
Z29	Encounter for other prophylactic measures
Z40	Encounter for prophylactic surgery
Z41	Encounter for procedures for purposes other than remedying health state
	Except: Z41.9, Encounter for procedure for purposes other than remedying health state, unspecified
Z53	Persons encountering health services for specific procedures and treatment, not carried out
Z55	Problems related to education and literacy
Z56	Problems related to employment and unemployment
Z57	Occupational exposure to risk factors
Z58	Problems related to physical environment
Z59	Problems related to housing and economic circumstances
Z60	Problems related to social environment
Z62	Problems related to upbringing
Z63	Other problems related to primary support group, including family circumstances
Z64	Problems related to certain psychosocial circumstances
Z65	Problems related to other psychosocial circumstances
Z72	Problems related to lifestyle
	Note: These codes should be assigned only when the documentation specifies that the patient has an associated problem
Z73	Problems related to life management difficulty
Z74	Problems related to care provider dependency
	Except: Z74.01, Bed confinement status
Z75	Problems related to medical facilities and other health care
Z76.0	Encounter for issue of repeat prescription
Z76.3	Healthy person accompanying sick person
Z76.4	Other boarder to healthcare facility
Z76.5	Malingerer [conscious simulation]
Z91.1-	Patient's noncompliance with medical treatment and regimen
Z91.83	Wandering in diseases classified elsewhere
Z91.84-	**Oral health risk factors**
Z91.89	Other specified personal risk factors, not elsewhere classified

15) Nonspecific Z codes

Certain Z codes are so non-specific, or potentially redundant with other codes in the classification, that there can be little justification for their use in the inpatient setting. Their use in the outpatient setting should be limited to those instances when there is no further documentation to permit more precise coding. Otherwise, any sign or symptom or any other reason for visit that is captured in another code should be used.

Nonspecific Z codes/categories:

Z02.9   Encounter for administrative examinations, unspecified

Z04.9   Encounter for examination and observation for unspecified reason

Z13.9   Encounter for screening, unspecified

Z41.9   Encounter for procedure for purposes other than remedying health state, unspecified

Z52.9   Donor of unspecified organ or tissue

Z86.59   Personal history of other mental and behavioral disorders

Z88.9   Allergy status to unspecified drugs, medicaments and biological substances status

Z92.0   Personal history of contraception

16) Z codes that may only be principal/first-listed diagnosis

The following Z codes/categories may only be reported as the principal/first-listed diagnosis, except when there are multiple encounters on the same day and the medical records for the encounters are combined:

Z00   Encounter for general examination without complaint, suspected or reported diagnosis
  Except: Z00.6

Z01   Encounter for other special examination without complaint, suspected or reported diagnosis

Z02   Encounter for administrative examination

Z03   Encounter for medical observation for suspected diseases and conditions ruled out

Z04   Encounter for examination and observation for other reasons

Z33.2   Encounter for elective termination of pregnancy

Z31.81   Encounter for male factor infertility in female patient

Z31.83   Encounter for assisted reproductive fertility procedure cycle

Z31.84   Encounter for fertility preservation procedure

Z34   Encounter for supervision of normal pregnancy

Z39   Encounter for maternal postpartum care and examination

Z38   Liveborn infants according to place of birth and type of delivery

Z40   Encounter for prophylactic surgery

Z42   Encounter for plastic and reconstructive surgery following medical procedure or healed injury

Z51.0   Encounter for antineoplastic radiation therapy

Z51.1-   Encounter for antineoplastic chemotherapy and immunotherapy

Z52   Donors of organs and tissues
  Except: Z52.9, Donor of unspecified organ or tissue

Z76.1   Encounter for health supervision and care of foundling

Z76.2   Encounter for health supervision and care of other healthy infant and child

Z99.12   Encounter for respirator [ventilator] dependence during power failure

Female patient seen at 32 weeks' gestation to check the progress of her first pregnancy

Z34.03   Encounter for supervision of normal first pregnancy, third trimester

Z3A.32   32 weeks gestation of pregnancy

Explanation: Category Z34 is appropriate as a first-listed diagnosis. Category Z3A helps to clarify at which point in the pregnancy the patient was provided supervision.

Chapter 21. Factors Influencing Health Status and Contact With Health Services (Z00-Z99)

NOTE   Z codes represent reasons for encounters. A corresponding procedure code must accompany a Z code if a procedure is performed. Categories Z00-Z99 are provided for occasions when circumstances other than a disease, injury or external cause classifiable to categories A00-Y89 are recorded as "diagnoses" or "problems". This can arise in two main ways:

(a) When a person who may or may not be sick encounters the health services for some specific purpose, such as to receive limited care or service for a current condition, to donate an organ or tissue, to receive prophylactic vaccination (immunization), or to discuss a problem which is in itself not a disease or injury.

(b) When some circumstance or problem is present which influences the person's health status but is not in itself a current illness or injury.

This chapter contains the following blocks:

Z00-Z13   Persons encountering health services for examinations
Z14-Z15   Genetic carrier and genetic susceptibility to disease
Z16   Resistance to antimicrobial drugs
Z17   Estrogen receptor status
Z18   Retained foreign body fragments
~~Z19~~   ~~Hormone sensitivity malignancy status~~
Z20-Z29   Persons with potential health hazards related to communicable diseases
Z30-Z39   Persons encountering health services in circumstances related to reproduction
Z40-Z53   Encounters for other specific health care
Z55-Z65   Persons with potential health hazards related to socioeconomic and psychosocial circumstances
Z66   Do not resuscitate status
Z67   Blood type
Z68   Body mass index (BMI)
Z69-Z76   Persons encountering health services in other circumstances
Z77-Z99   Persons with potential health hazards related to family and personal history and certain conditions influencing health status

Persons encountering health services for examinations (Z00-Z13)

NOTE   Nonspecific abnormal findings disclosed at the time of these examinations are classified to categories R70-R94.

EXCLUDES 1   *examinations related to pregnancy and reproduction (Z30-Z36, Z39-)*

✓4th Z00   Encounter for general examination without complaint, suspected or reported diagnosis

EXCLUDES 1   *encounter for examination for administrative purposes (Z02.-)*
EXCLUDES 2   *encounter for pre-procedural examinations (Z01.81-)*
      special screening examinations (Z11-Z13)

✓5th Z00.0   Encounter for general adult medical examination
Encounter for adult periodic examination (annual) (physical) and any associated laboratory and radiologic examinations

EXCLUDES 1   *encounter for examination of sign or symptom—code to sign or symptom*
      general health check-up of infant or child (Z00.12-)

Z00.00   **Encounter for general adult medical examination without abnormal findings**   PDx A
Encounter for adult health check-up NOS
AHA: 2016, 1Q, 36

Z00.01   **Encounter for general adult medical examination with abnormal findings**   PDx A
Use additional code to identify abnormal findings
AHA: 2016, 1Q, 35-36

✓5th Z00.1   Encounter for newborn, infant and child health examinations

✓6th Z00.11   Newborn health examination
Health check for child under 29 days old
Use additional code to identify any abnormal findings

EXCLUDES 1   *health check for child over 28 days old (Z00.12-)*

Z00.110   **Health examination for newborn under 8 days old**   PDx N
Health check for newborn under 8 days old

Z00.111   **Health examination for newborn 8 to 28 days old**   PDx N
Health check for newborn 8 to 28 days old
Newborn weight check

✓6th Z00.12   Encounter for routine child health examination
Encounter for development testing of infant or child
Health check (routine) for child over 28 days old

EXCLUDES 1   *health check for child under 29 days old (Z00.11-)*
      health supervision of foundling or other healthy infant or child (Z76.1-Z76.2)
      newborn health examination (Z00.11-)

Z00.121   **Encounter for routine child health examination with abnormal findings**   PDx P
Use additional code to identify abnormal findings
AHA: 2016, 1Q, 34-35

Z00.129   **Encounter for routine child health examination without abnormal findings**   PDx P
Encounter for routine child health examination NOS
AHA: 2016, 1Q, 34

Z00.2   Encounter for examination for period of rapid growth in childhood   PDx P

Z00.3   Encounter for examination for adolescent development state   PDx P
Encounter for puberty development state

Z00.5   Encounter for examination of potential donor of organ and tissue   PDx

Z00.6   Encounter for examination for normal comparison and control in clinical research program
Examination of participant or control in clinical research program

✓5th Z00.7   Encounter for examination for period of delayed growth in childhood

Z00.70   **Encounter for examination for period of delayed growth in childhood without abnormal findings**   PDx P

Z00.71   **Encounter for examination for period of delayed growth in childhood with abnormal findings**   PDx P
Use additional code to identify abnormal findings

Z00.8   Encounter for other general examination   PDx
Encounter for health examination in population surveys

✓4th Z01   Encounter for other special examination without complaint, suspected or reported diagnosis

INCLUDES   routine examination of specific system
NOTE   Codes from category Z01 represent the reason for the encounter. A separate procedure code is required to identify any examinations or procedures performed.

EXCLUDES 1   *encounter for examination for administrative purposes (Z02.-)*
      encounter for examination for suspected conditions, proven not to exist (Z03.-)
      encounter for laboratory and radiologic examinations as a component of general medical examinations (Z00.0-)
      encounter for laboratory, radiologic and imaging examinations for sign(s) and symptom(s)—code to the sign(s) or symptom(s)
EXCLUDES 2   *screening examinations (Z11-Z13)*

✓5th Z01.0   Encounter for examination of eyes and vision

EXCLUDES 1   *examination for driving license (Z02.4)*

Z01.00   **Encounter for examination of eyes and vision without abnormal findings**   PDx
Encounter for examination of eyes and vision NOS

Z01.01   **Encounter for examination of eyes and vision with abnormal findings**   PDx
Use additional code to identify abnormal findings

✓5th Z01.1   Encounter for examination of ears and hearing

Z01.10   **Encounter for examination of ears and hearing without abnormal findings**   PDx
Encounter for examination of ears and hearing NOS
AHA: 2016, 4Q, 24

✓6th Z01.11   Encounter for examination of ears and hearing with abnormal findings
AHA: 2016, 3Q, 17-18

Z01.110   **Encounter for hearing examination following failed hearing screening**   PDx

Z01.118   **Encounter for examination of ears and hearing with other abnormal findings**   PDx
Use additional code to identify abnormal findings

Z01.12   **Encounter for hearing conservation and treatment**   PDx

---

EXCLUDES 1 Not coded here   *EXCLUDES 2* Not included here   N Newborn Age: 0   P Pediatric Age: 0-17   M Maternity Age: 12-55   A Adult Age: 15-124   PDx Primary Dx

1180   ICD-10-CM 2018

✓5ᵗʰ **Z01.2** **Encounter for** dental examination and cleaning

   Z01.20 **Encounter for dental examination and** `PDx`
      cleaning without abnormal findings
        Encounter for dental examination and cleaning NOS

   Z01.21 **Encounter for dental examination and cleaning** `PDx`
      with abnormal findings
        Use additional code to identify abnormal findings

✓5ᵗʰ **Z01.3** **Encounter for examination of** blood pressure

   Z01.30 **Encounter for examination of blood pressure** `PDx`
      without abnormal findings
        Encounter for examination of blood pressure NOS

   Z01.31 **Encounter for examination of blood pressure** `PDx`
      with abnormal findings
        Use additional code to identify abnormal findings

✓5ᵗʰ **Z01.4** **Encounter for** gynecological examination
    EXCLUDES 2 *pregnancy examination or test (Z32.0-)*
        routine examination for contraceptive maintenance
        (Z30.4-)

   ✓6ᵗʰ **Z01.41** **Encounter for** routine **gynecological examination**
      Encounter for general gynecological examination with
        or without cervical smear
      Encounter for gynecological examination (general)
        (routine) NOS
      Encounter for pelvic examination (annual) (periodic)
      Use additional code:
        for screening for human papillomavirus, if
          applicable, (Z11.51)
        for screening vaginal pap smear, if applicable
          (Z12.72)
        to identify acquired absence of uterus, if applicable
          (Z90.71-)
     EXCLUDES 1 *gynecologic examination status-post*
          hysterectomy for malignant condition
          (Z08)
          screening cervical pap smear not a part of a
          routine gynecological examination
          (Z12.4)

      Z01.411 **Encounter for gynecological** `PDx` ♀
        examination (general) (routine) with
        abnormal findings
          Use additional code to identify abnormal
            findings

      Z01.419 **Encounter for gynecological** `PDx` ♀
        examination (general) (routine) without
        abnormal findings

   Z01.42 **Encounter for** cervical smear to confirm `PDx` ♀
      findings of recent normal smear following initial
      abnormal smear

✓5ᵗʰ **Z01.8** **Encounter for other specified special examinations**

   ✓6ᵗʰ **Z01.81** **Encounter for** preprocedural **examinations**
      Encounter for preoperative examinations
      Encounter for radiological and imaging examinations
        as part of preprocedural examination

      Z01.810 **Encounter for preprocedural** `PDx`
        cardiovascular examination

      Z01.811 **Encounter for preprocedural** `PDx`
        respiratory examination

      Z01.812 **Encounter for preprocedural** `PDx`
        laboratory examination
          Blood and urine tests prior to treatment or
            procedure

      Z01.818 **Encounter for other preprocedural** `PDx`
        examination
          Encounter for preprocedural examination
            NOS
          Encounter for examinations prior to
            antineoplastic chemotherapy

   Z01.82 **Encounter for** allergy testing `PDx`
     EXCLUDES 1 *encounter for antibody response*
          examination (Z01.84)

   Z01.83 **Encounter for** blood typing `PDx`
      Encounter for Rh typing

   Z01.84 **Encounter for** antibody response examination `PDx`
      Encounter for immunity status testing
     EXCLUDES 1 *encounter for allergy testing (Z01.82)*

   Z01.89 **Encounter for other specified special** `PDx`
      examinations

✓4ᵗʰ **Z02** **Encounter for** administrative **examination**

   Z02.0 **Encounter for examination for** admission to educational `PDx`
      institution
      Encounter for examination for admission to preschool
        (education)
      Encounter for examination for re-admission to school following
        illness or medical treatment

   Z02.1 **Encounter for** pre-employment **examination** `PDx`

   Z02.2 **Encounter for examination for** admission to residential `PDx`
      institution
     EXCLUDES 1 *examination for admission to prison (Z02.89)*

   Z02.3 **Encounter for examination for** recruitment to armed `PDx`
      forces

   Z02.4 **Encounter for examination for** driving license `PDx`

   Z02.5 **Encounter for examination for** participation in sport `PDx`
     EXCLUDES 1 *blood-alcohol and blood-drug test (Z02.83)*

   Z02.6 **Encounter for examination for** insurance purposes `PDx`

   ✓5ᵗʰ **Z02.7** **Encounter for** issue of medical certificate
     EXCLUDES 1 *encounter for general medical examination (Z00-Z01,*
          Z02.0-Z02.6, Z02.8-Z02.9)

      Z02.71 **Encounter for** disability determination `PDx`
        Encounter for issue of medical certificate of incapacity
        Encounter for issue of medical certificate of invalidity

      Z02.79 **Encounter for issue of other medical certificate** `PDx`

   ✓5ᵗʰ **Z02.8** **Encounter for other administrative examinations**

      Z02.81 **Encounter for** paternity testing `PDx`

      Z02.82 **Encounter for** adoption services `PDx`

      Z02.83 **Encounter for** blood-alcohol and blood-drug `PDx`
        test
          Use additional code for findings of alcohol or drugs in
            blood (R78.-)

      Z02.89 **Encounter for other administrative** `PDx`
        examinations
          Encounter for examination for admission to prison
          Encounter for examination for admission to summer
            camp
          Encounter for immigration examination
          Encounter for naturalization examination
          Encounter for premarital examination
        EXCLUDES 1 *health supervision of foundling or other*
           healthy infant or child (Z76.1-Z76.2)

   Z02.9 **Encounter for administrative examinations,** `PDx` ▽
      unspecified

✓4ᵗʰ **Z03** **Encounter for** medical observation **for suspected diseases and**
   conditions ruled out
     NOTE   This category is to be used when a person without a
        diagnosis is suspected of having an abnormal condition,
        without signs or symptoms, which requires study, but after
        examination and observation, is ruled out. This category is
        also for use for administrative and legal observation status.
     EXCLUDES 1 *contact with and (suspected) exposures hazardous to health*
         (Z77.-)
      ▶*encounter for observation and evaluation of newborn for*
        suspected diseases and conditions ruled out (Z05.0-)◀
        ~~*newborn observation for suspected condition, ruled out*~~
         ~~*(P00-P04)*~~
        person with feared complaint in whom no diagnosis is made
         (Z71.1)
        signs or symptoms under study—code to signs or symptoms

   Z03.6 **Encounter for observation for suspected** toxic effect `PDx`
      from ingested substance ruled out
      Encounter for observation for suspected adverse effect from
        drug
      Encounter for observation for suspected poisoning

   ✓5ᵗʰ **Z03.7** **Encounter for suspected** maternal and fetal conditions **ruled**
      out
      Encounter for suspected maternal and fetal conditions not
        found
     EXCLUDES 1 *known or suspected fetal anomalies affecting*
         management of mother, not ruled out (O26-,
         O35-, O36-, O40-, O41-)

      Z03.71 **Encounter for suspected problem with** `PDx` M ♀
        amniotic cavity and membrane ruled out
          Encounter for suspected oligohydramnios ruled out
          Encounter for suspected polyhydramnios ruled out

      Z03.72 **Encounter for suspected** placental `PDx` M ♀
        problem ruled out

      Z03.73 **Encounter for suspected** fetal anomaly `PDx` M ♀
        ruled out

✓ Additional Character Req   ✓x7ᵗʰ Placeholder Alert   **Manifestation**   `HCC` CMS-HCC Condition   ▽ Unspecified Code   ▶◀ Revised Text   ● New Code   ▲ Revised Code Title

Z03.74 Encounter for suspected **problem with fetal growth** ruled out `PDx` `M♀`

Z03.75 Encounter for suspected **cervical shortening** ruled out `PDx` `M♀`

Z03.79 Encounter for other suspected **maternal and fetal conditions ruled out** `PDx` `M♀`

√5ᵗʰ **Z03.8** Encounter for **observation** for other suspected diseases and conditions ruled out

√6ᵗʰ **Z03.81** Encounter for observation for suspected **exposure to biological agents** ruled out

Z03.810 Encounter for observation for suspected exposure to **anthrax** ruled out `PDx`

Z03.818 Encounter for observation for suspected exposure to other biological agents ruled out `PDx`

Z03.89 Encounter for observation for other suspected diseases and conditions ruled out `PDx`

√4ᵗʰ **Z04** Encounter for examination and observation for other reasons

`INCLUDES` encounter for examination for medicolegal reasons

This category is to be used when a person without a diagnosis is suspected of having an abnormal condition, without signs or symptoms, which requires study, but after examination and observation, is ruled-out. This category is also for use for administrative and legal observation status.

Z04.1 Encounter for examination and observation following **transport accident** `PDx`

`EXCLUDES 1` encounter for examination and observation following work accident (Z04.2)

Z04.2 Encounter for examination and observation following **work accident** `PDx`

Z04.3 Encounter for examination and observation following **other accident** `PDx`

√5ᵗʰ **Z04.4** Encounter for examination and observation following **alleged rape**

Encounter for examination and observation of victim following alleged rape

Encounter for examination and observation of victim following alleged sexual abuse

Z04.41 Encounter for examination and observation following alleged **adult** rape `PDx` `A`

Suspected adult rape, ruled out

Suspected adult sexual abuse, ruled out

Z04.42 Encounter for examination and observation following alleged **child** rape `PDx` `P`

Suspected child rape, ruled out

Suspected child sexual abuse, ruled out

Z04.6 Encounter for **general psychiatric examination, requested by authority** `PDx`

√5ᵗʰ **Z04.7** Encounter for examination and observation following **alleged physical abuse**

Z04.71 Encounter for examination and observation following alleged **adult** physical abuse `PDx` `A`

Suspected adult physical abuse, ruled out

`EXCLUDES 1` confirmed case of adult physical abuse (T74.-)

encounter for examination and observation following alleged adult sexual abuse (Z04.41)

suspected case of adult physical abuse, not ruled out (T76.-)

Z04.72 Encounter for examination and observation following alleged **child** physical abuse `PDx` `P`

Suspected child physical abuse, ruled out

`EXCLUDES 1` confirmed case of child physical abuse (T74.-)

encounter for examination and observation following alleged child sexual abuse (Z04.42)

suspected case of child physical abuse, not ruled out (T76.-)

Z04.8 Encounter for examination and observation for other specified reasons `PDx`

Encounter for examination and observation for request for expert evidence

Z04.9 Encounter for examination and observation for unspecified reason `PDx` ▽

Encounter for observation NOS

√4ᵗʰ **Z05** Encounter for observation of newborn for suspected diseases and conditions ruled out

▶This category is to be used for newborns, within the neonatal period (the first 28 days of life), who are suspected of having an abnormal condition, but without signs or symptoms, and which, after examination and observation, is ruled out.◀

`EXCLUDES 2` *newborn observation for suspected condition, related to exposure from the mother or birth process (P00-P04)*

Z05.0 Observation and evaluation of newborn for suspected **cardiac** condition ruled out

Z05.1 Observation and evaluation of newborn for suspected **infectious** condition ruled out

Z05.2 Observation and evaluation of newborn for suspected **neurological** condition ruled out

Z05.3 Observation and evaluation of newborn for suspected **respiratory** condition ruled out

√5ᵗʰ **Z05.4** Observation and evaluation of newborn for suspected **genetic, metabolic or immunologic** condition ruled out

Z05.41 Observation and evaluation of newborn for suspected **genetic** condition ruled out

Z05.42 Observation and evaluation of newborn for suspected **metabolic** condition ruled out

Z05.43 Observation and evaluation of newborn for suspected **immunologic** condition ruled out

Z05.5 Observation and evaluation of newborn for suspected **gastrointestinal** condition ruled out

Z05.6 Observation and evaluation of newborn for suspected **genitourinary** condition ruled out

√5ᵗʰ **Z05.7** Observation and evaluation of newborn for suspected **skin, subcutaneous, musculoskeletal and connective tissue** condition ruled out

Z05.71 Observation and evaluation of newborn for suspected **skin and subcutaneous tissue** condition ruled out

Z05.72 Observation and evaluation of newborn for suspected **musculoskeletal** condition ruled out

Z05.73 Observation and evaluation of newborn for suspected **connective tissue** condition ruled out

Z05.8 Observation and evaluation of newborn for other specified suspected condition ruled out

Z05.9 Observation and evaluation of newborn for unspecified suspected condition ruled out ▽

Z08 Encounter for **follow-up examination** after completed treatment for **malignant neoplasm**

Medical surveillance following completed treatment

Use additional code to identify any acquired absence of organs (Z90.-)

Use additional code to identify the personal history of malignant neoplasm (Z85.-)

`EXCLUDES 1` *aftercare following medical care (Z43-Z49, Z51)*

Z09 Encounter for **follow-up examination** after completed treatment for conditions **other than malignant neoplasm**

Medical surveillance following completed treatment

Use additional code to identify any applicable history of disease code (Z86-, Z87-)

`EXCLUDES 1` *aftercare following medical care (Z43-Z49, Z51)*

surveillance of contraception (Z30.4-)

surveillance of prosthetic and other medical devices (Z44-Z46)

AHA: 2017, 1Q, 9; 2015, 1Q, 8

√4ᵗʰ **Z11** Encounter for **screening** for infectious and parasitic diseases

Screening is the testing for disease or disease precursors in asymptomatic individuals so that early detection and treatment can be provided for those who test positive for the disease.

`EXCLUDES 1` *encounter for diagnostic examination—code to sign or symptom*

Z11.0 Encounter for screening for **intestinal infectious diseases**

Z11.1 Encounter for screening for **respiratory tuberculosis**

Z11.2 Encounter for screening for **other bacterial diseases**

Z11.3 Encounter for screening for infections with a **predominantly sexual mode of transmission**

`EXCLUDES 2` *encounter for screening for human immunodeficiency virus [HIV] (Z11.4)*

encounter for screening for human papillomavirus (Z11.51)

Z11.4 Encounter for screening for **human immunodeficiency virus [HIV]**

`EXCLUDES 1` Not coded here　`EXCLUDES 2` Not included here　`N` Newborn Age: 0　`P` Pediatric Age: 0-17　`M` Maternity Age: 12-55　`A` Adult Age: 15-124　`PDx` Primary Dx

1182　　　ICD-10-CM 2018

✓5ᵗʰ Z11.5 Encounter for screening for other viral diseases
> EXCLUDES 2 *encounter for screening for viral intestinal disease (Z11.0)*

    Z11.51 Encounter for screening for human papillomavirus (HPV)

    Z11.59 Encounter for screening for other viral diseases

Z11.6 Encounter for screening for other protozoal diseases and helminthiases
> EXCLUDES 2 *encounter for screening for protozoal intestinal disease (Z11.0)*

Z11.8 Encounter for screening for other infectious and parasitic diseases
Encounter for screening for chlamydia
Encounter for screening for rickettsial
Encounter for screening for spirochetal
Encounter for screening for mycoses

Z11.9 Encounter for screening for infectious and parasitic diseases, unspecified ▽

✓4ᵗʰ Z12 Encounter for screening for malignant neoplasms
Screening is the testing for disease or disease precursors in asymptomatic individuals so that early detection and treatment can be provided for those who test positive for the disease.
Use additional code to identify any family history of malignant neoplasm (Z80.-)
> EXCLUDES 1 *encounter for diagnostic examination—code to sign or symptom*

Z12.0 Encounter for screening for malignant neoplasm of stomach

✓5ᵗʰ Z12.1 Encounter for screening for malignant neoplasm of intestinal tract
    AHA: 2017, 1Q, 8, 9

    Z12.10 Encounter for screening for malignant neoplasm of intestinal tract, unspecified ▽

    Z12.11 Encounter for screening for malignant neoplasm of colon
        Encounter for screening colonoscopy NOS

    Z12.12 Encounter for screening for malignant neoplasm of rectum

    Z12.13 Encounter for screening for malignant neoplasm of small intestine

Z12.2 Encounter for screening for malignant neoplasm of respiratory organs

✓5ᵗʰ Z12.3 Encounter for screening for malignant neoplasm of breast

    Z12.31 Encounter for screening mammogram for malignant neoplasm of breast
> EXCLUDES 1 *inconclusive mammogram (R92.2)*
        AHA: 2015, 1Q, 24

    Z12.39 Encounter for other screening for malignant neoplasm of breast

Z12.4 Encounter for screening for malignant neoplasm of cervix ♀
Encounter for screening pap smear for malignant neoplasm of cervix
> EXCLUDES 1 *when screening is part of general gynecological examination (Z01.4-)*
> EXCLUDES 2 *encounter for screening for human papillomavirus (Z11.51)*

Z12.5 Encounter for screening for malignant neoplasm of prostate ♂

Z12.6 Encounter for screening for malignant neoplasm of bladder

✓5ᵗʰ Z12.7 Encounter for screening for malignant neoplasm of other genitourinary organs

    Z12.71 Encounter for screening for malignant neoplasm of testis ♂

    Z12.72 Encounter for screening for malignant neoplasm of vagina ♀
        Vaginal pap smear status-post hysterectomy for non-malignant condition
        Use additional code to identify acquired absence of uterus (Z90.71-)
> EXCLUDES 1 *vaginal pap smear status-post hysterectomy for malignant conditions (Z08)*

    Z12.73 Encounter for screening for malignant neoplasm of ovary ♀

    Z12.79 Encounter for screening for malignant neoplasm of other genitourinary organs

✓5ᵗʰ Z12.8 Encounter for screening for malignant neoplasm of other sites

    Z12.81 Encounter for screening for malignant neoplasm of oral cavity

    Z12.82 Encounter for screening for malignant neoplasm of nervous system

    Z12.83 Encounter for screening for malignant neoplasm of skin

    Z12.89 Encounter for screening for malignant neoplasm of other sites

Z12.9 Encounter for screening for malignant neoplasm, site unspecified ▽

✓4ᵗʰ Z13 Encounter for screening for other diseases and disorders
Screening is the testing for disease or disease precursors in asymptomatic individuals so that early detection and treatment can be provided for those who test positive for the disease.
> EXCLUDES 1 *encounter for diagnostic examination—code to sign or symptom*

Z13.0 Encounter for screening for diseases of the blood and blood-forming organs and certain disorders involving the immune mechanism

Z13.1 Encounter for screening for diabetes mellitus

✓5ᵗʰ Z13.2 Encounter for screening for nutritional, metabolic and other endocrine disorders

    Z13.21 Encounter for screening for nutritional disorder

    ✓6ᵗʰ Z13.22 Encounter for screening for metabolic disorder

        Z13.220 Encounter for screening for lipoid disorders
            Encounter for screening for cholesterol level
            Encounter for screening for hypercholesterolemia
            Encounter for screening for hyperlipidemia

        Z13.228 Encounter for screening for other metabolic disorders

    Z13.29 Encounter for screening for other suspected endocrine disorder
> EXCLUDES 1 *encounter for screening for diabetes mellitus (Z13.1)*

Z13.4 Encounter for screening for certain developmental disorders in childhood Ⓟ
Encounter for screening for developmental handicaps in early childhood
> EXCLUDES 1 *routine development testing of infant or child (Z00.1-)*

Z13.5 Encounter for screening for eye and ear disorders
> EXCLUDES 2 *encounter for general hearing examination (Z01.1-)*
> *encounter for general vision examination (Z01.0-)*
    AHA: 2016, 3Q, 17

Z13.6 Encounter for screening for cardiovascular disorders

✓5ᵗʰ Z13.7 Encounter for screening for genetic and chromosomal anomalies
> EXCLUDES 1 *genetic testing for procreative management (Z31.4-)*

    Z13.71 Encounter for nonprocreative screening for genetic disease carrier status

    Z13.79 Encounter for other screening for genetic and chromosomal anomalies

✓5ᵗʰ Z13.8 Encounter for screening for other specified diseases and disorders
> EXCLUDES 2 *screening for malignant neoplasms (Z12.-)*

    ✓6ᵗʰ Z13.81 Encounter for screening for digestive system disorders

        Z13.810 Encounter for screening for upper gastrointestinal disorder

        Z13.811 Encounter for screening for lower gastrointestinal disorder
> EXCLUDES 1 *encounter for screening for intestinal infectious disease (Z11.0)*

        Z13.818 Encounter for screening for other digestive system disorders

    ✓6ᵗʰ Z13.82 Encounter for screening for musculoskeletal disorder

        Z13.820 Encounter for screening for osteoporosis

        Z13.828 Encounter for screening for other musculoskeletal disorder

✓ Additional Character Req   ✓x7ᵗʰ Placeholder Alert   Manifestation   HCC CMS-HCC Condition   ▽ Unspecified Code   ►◄ Revised Text   ● New Code   ▲ Revised Code Title

ICD-10-CM 2018   1183

Z13.83 **Encounter for screening for respiratory disorder NEC**
> EXCLUDES 1 *encounter for screening for respiratory tuberculosis (Z11.1)*

Z13.84 **Encounter for screening for dental disorders**

✓6th **Z13.85** **Encounter for screening for nervous system disorders**

　　Z13.850 **Encounter for screening for traumatic brain injury**

　　Z13.858 **Encounter for screening for other nervous system disorders**

Z13.88 **Encounter for screening for disorder due to exposure to contaminants**
> EXCLUDES 1 *those exposed to contaminants without suspected disorders (Z57-Z77-)*

Z13.89 **Encounter for screening for other disorder**
　Encounter for screening for genitourinary disorders

Z13.9 **Encounter for screening, unspecified** ▽

Genetic carrier and genetic susceptibility to disease (Z14-Z15)

✓4th **Z14** **Genetic carrier**
> **DEF:** Individuals carrying a gene mutation associated with a certain disease who typically do not develop the disease but are able to pass mutated gene to offspring.

✓5th **Z14.0** **Hemophilia A carrier**

　Z14.01 **Asymptomatic hemophilia A carrier**

　Z14.02 **Symptomatic hemophilia A carrier**

Z14.1 **Cystic fibrosis carrier**

Z14.8 **Genetic carrier of other disease**

✓4th **Z15** **Genetic susceptibility to disease**
> INCLUDES confirmed abnormal gene
> Use additional code, if applicable, for any associated family history of the disease (Z80-Z84)
> EXCLUDES 1 *chromosomal anomalies (Q90-Q99)*

✓5th **Z15.0** **Genetic susceptibility to malignant neoplasm**
> Code first, if applicable, any current malignant neoplasm (C00-C75, C81-C96)
> Use additional code, if applicable, for any personal history of malignant neoplasm (Z85.-)

　Z15.01 **Genetic susceptibility to malignant neoplasm of breast**

　Z15.02 **Genetic susceptibility to malignant neoplasm of ovary** ♀

　Z15.03 **Genetic susceptibility to malignant neoplasm of prostate** ♂

　Z15.04 **Genetic susceptibility to malignant neoplasm of endometrium** ♀

　Z15.09 **Genetic susceptibility to other malignant neoplasm**

✓5th **Z15.8** **Genetic susceptibility to other disease**

　Z15.81 **Genetic susceptibility to multiple endocrine neoplasia [MEN]**
> EXCLUDES 1 *multiple endocrine neoplasia [MEN] syndromes (E31.2-)*

　Z15.89 **Genetic susceptibility to other disease**

Resistance to antimicrobial drugs (Z16)

✓4th **Z16** **Resistance to antimicrobial drugs**
> NOTE The codes in this category are provided for use as additional codes to identify the resistance and non-responsiveness of a condition to antimicrobial drugs.
> Code first the infection
> EXCLUDES 1 *Methicillin resistant Staphylococcus aureus infection (A49.02)*
> ~~Methicillin resistant Staphylococcus aureus infection in diseases classified elsewhere (B95.62)~~
> *Methicillin resistant Staphylococcus aureus pneumonia (J15.212)*
> *sepsis due to Methicillin resistant Staphylococcus aureus (A41.02)*

✓5th **Z16.1** **Resistance to beta lactam antibiotics**

　Z16.10 **Resistance to unspecified beta lactam antibiotics** ▽

　Z16.11 **Resistance to penicillins**
　　Resistance to amoxicillin
　　Resistance to ampicillin

　Z16.12 **Extended spectrum beta lactamase (ESBL) resistance**
> EXCLUDES 2 ▶*Methicillin resistant Staphylococcus aureus infection in diseases classified elsewhere (B95.62)*◀

Z16.19 **Resistance to other specified beta lactam antibiotics**
　Resistance to cephalosporins

✓5th **Z16.2** **Resistance to other antibiotics**

　Z16.20 **Resistance to unspecified antibiotic** ▽
　　Resistance to antibiotics NOS

　Z16.21 **Resistance to vancomycin**

　Z16.22 **Resistance to vancomycin related antibiotics**

　Z16.23 **Resistance to quinolones and fluoroquinolones**

　Z16.24 **Resistance to multiple antibiotics**

　Z16.29 **Resistance to other single specified antibiotic**
　　Resistance to aminoglycosides
　　Resistance to macrolides
　　Resistance to sulfonamides
　　Resistance to tetracyclines

✓5th **Z16.3** **Resistance to other antimicrobial drugs**
> EXCLUDES 1 *resistance to antibiotics (Z16.1-, Z16.2-)*

　Z16.30 **Resistance to unspecified antimicrobial drugs** ▽
　　Drug resistance NOS

　Z16.31 **Resistance to antiparasitic drug(s)**
　　Resistance to quinine and related compounds

　Z16.32 **Resistance to antifungal drug(s)**

　Z16.33 **Resistance to antiviral drug(s)**

✓6th **Z16.34** **Resistance to antimycobacterial drug(s)**
　　Resistance to tuberculostatics

　　Z16.341 **Resistance to single antimycobacterial drug**
　　　Resistance to antimycobacterial drug NOS

　　Z16.342 **Resistance to multiple antimycobacterial drugs**

　Z16.35 **Resistance to multiple antimicrobial drugs**
> EXCLUDES 1 *Resistance to multiple antibiotics only (Z16.24)*

　Z16.39 **Resistance to other specified antimicrobial drug**

Estrogen receptor status (Z17)

✓4th **Z17** **Estrogen receptor status**
> Code first malignant neoplasm of breast (C50.-)

Z17.0 **Estrogen receptor positive status [ER+]**

Z17.1 **Estrogen receptor negative status [ER-]**

Retained foreign body fragment (Z18)

✓4th **Z18** **Retained foreign body fragments**
> INCLUDES embedded fragment (status)
> embedded splinter (status)
> retained foreign body status
> EXCLUDES 1 *artificial joint prosthesis status (Z96.6-)*
> *foreign body accidentally left during a procedure (T81.5-)*
> *foreign body entering through orifice (T15-T19)*
> *in situ cardiac device (Z95.-)*
> *organ or tissue replaced by means other than transplant (Z96.-, Z97.-)*
> *organ or tissue replaced by transplant (Z94.-)*
> *personal history of retained foreign body fully removed (Z87.821)*
> *superficial foreign body (non-embedded splinter)—code to superficial foreign body, by site*
> **DEF:** Embedded or retained fragment, splinter, or foreign body; natural or synthetic; can cause infection.

✓5th **Z18.0** **Retained radioactive fragments**

　Z18.01 **Retained depleted uranium fragments**

　Z18.09 **Other retained radioactive fragments**
　　Other retained depleted isotope fragments
　　Retained nontherapeutic radioactive fragments

✓5th **Z18.1** **Retained metal fragments**
> EXCLUDES 1 *retained radioactive metal fragments (Z18.01-Z18.09)*

　Z18.10 **Retained metal fragments, unspecified** ▽
　　Retained metal fragment NOS

　Z18.11 **Retained magnetic metal fragments**

　Z18.12 **Retained nonmagnetic metal fragments**

Z18.2 **Retained plastic fragments**
　Acrylics fragments
　Diethylhexylphthalates fragments
　Isocyanate fragments

✓5th **Z18.3** **Retained organic fragments**

　Z18.31 **Retained animal quills or spines**

　Z18.32 **Retained tooth**

EXCLUDES 1 Not coded here　EXCLUDES 2 Not included here　N Newborn Age: 0　P Pediatric Age: 0-17　M Maternity Age: 12-55　A Adult Age: 15-124　PDx Primary Dx

1184　ICD-10-CM 2018

Z18.33   Retained wood fragments

Z18.39   Other retained organic fragments

✓5ᵗʰ **Z18.8**   Other specified retained foreign body

Z18.81   Retained glass fragments

Z18.83   Retained stone or crystalline fragments
         Retained concrete or cement fragments

Z18.89   Other specified retained foreign body fragments

Z18.9   Retained foreign body fragments, unspecified material   ▽

Hormone sensitivity malignancy status (Z19)

✓4ᵗʰ **Z19**   Hormone sensitivity malignancy status
     Code first malignant neoplasm — see Table of Neoplasms, by site, malignant

Z19.1   Hormone sensitive malignancy status

Z19.2   Hormone resistant malignancy status
     Castrate resistant prostate malignancy status

Persons with potential health hazards related to communicable diseases (Z20-Z29)

✓4ᵗʰ **Z20**   Contact with and (suspected) exposure to communicable diseases
     EXCLUDES 1   carrier of infectious disease (Z22.-)
         diagnosed current infectious or parasitic disease—see Alphabetic Index
     EXCLUDES 2   personal history of infectious and parasitic diseases (Z86.1-)

✓5ᵗʰ **Z20.0**   Contact with and (suspected) exposure to intestinal infectious diseases

Z20.01   Contact with and (suspected) exposure to intestinal infectious diseases due to Escherichia coli (E. coli)

Z20.09   Contact with and (suspected) exposure to other intestinal infectious diseases

Z20.1   Contact with and (suspected) exposure to tuberculosis

Z20.2   Contact with and (suspected) exposure to infections with a predominantly sexual mode of transmission

Z20.3   Contact with and (suspected) exposure to rabies

Z20.4   Contact with and (suspected) exposure to rubella

Z20.5   Contact with and (suspected) exposure to viral hepatitis

Z20.6   Contact with and (suspected) exposure to human immunodeficiency virus [HIV]
     EXCLUDES 1   asymptomatic human immunodeficiency virus [HIV] HIV infection status (Z21)

Z20.7   Contact with and (suspected) exposure to pediculosis, acariasis and other infestations

✓5ᵗʰ **Z20.8**   Contact with and (suspected) exposure to other communicable diseases

✓6ᵗʰ **Z20.81**   Contact with and (suspected) exposure to other bacterial communicable diseases

Z20.810   Contact with and (suspected) exposure to anthrax

Z20.811   Contact with and (suspected) exposure to meningococcus

Z20.818   Contact with and (suspected) exposure to other bacterial communicable diseases

✓6ᵗʰ **Z20.82**   Contact with and (suspected) exposure to other viral communicable diseases

Z20.820   Contact with and (suspected) exposure to varicella

Z20.828   Contact with and (suspected) exposure to other viral communicable diseases

Z20.89   Contact with and (suspected) exposure to other communicable diseases

Z20.9   Contact with and (suspected) exposure to unspecified communicable disease   ▽

Z21   Asymptomatic human immunodeficiency virus [HIV] infection status   **HCC**
     HIV positive NOS
     Code first human immunodeficiency virus [HIV] disease complicating pregnancy, childbirth and the puerperium, if applicable (O98.7-)
     EXCLUDES 1   acquired immunodeficiency syndrome (B20)
         contact with human immunodeficiency virus [HIV] (Z20.6)
         exposure to human immunodeficiency virus [HIV] (Z20.6)
         human immunodeficiency virus [HIV] disease (B20)
         inconclusive laboratory evidence of human immunodeficiency virus [HIV] (R75)
     DEF: Phase of human immunodeficiency virus (HIV) infection with no clinical symptoms; may last for 10 years or more.

✓4ᵗʰ **Z22**   Carrier of infectious disease
     INCLUDES   colonization status
         suspected carrier
     EXCLUDES 2   carrier of viral hepatitis (B18.-)

Z22.0   Carrier of typhoid

Z22.1   Carrier of other intestinal infectious diseases

Z22.2   Carrier of diphtheria

✓5ᵗʰ **Z22.3**   Carrier of other specified bacterial diseases

Z22.31   Carrier of bacterial disease due to meningococci

✓6ᵗʰ **Z22.32**   Carrier of bacterial disease due to staphylococci

Z22.321   Carrier or suspected carrier of Methicillin susceptible Staphylococcus aureus
     MSSA colonization

Z22.322   Carrier or suspected carrier of Methicillin resistant Staphylococcus aureus
     MRSA colonization

✓6ᵗʰ **Z22.33**   Carrier of bacterial disease due to streptococci

Z22.330   Carrier of Group B streptococcus
     EXCLUDES 1   carrier of streptococcus group B (GBS) complicating pregnancy, childbirth and the puerperium (O99.82-)

Z22.338   Carrier of other streptococcus

Z22.39   Carrier of other specified bacterial diseases

Z22.4   Carrier of infections with a predominantly sexual mode of transmission

Z22.6   Carrier of human T-lymphotropic virus type-1 [HTLV-1] infection

Z22.8   Carrier of other infectious diseases

Z22.9   Carrier of infectious disease, unspecified   ▽

Z23   Encounter for immunization
     Code first any routine childhood examination
     NOTE   Procedure codes are required to identify the types of immunizations given

✓4ᵗʰ **Z28**   Immunization not carried out and underimmunization status
     INCLUDES   vaccination not carried out

✓5ᵗʰ **Z28.0**   Immunization not carried out because of contraindication

Z28.01   Immunization not carried out because of acute illness of patient

Z28.02   Immunization not carried out because of chronic illness or condition of patient

Z28.03   Immunization not carried out because of immune compromised state of patient

Z28.04   Immunization not carried out because of patient allergy to vaccine or component

Z28.09   Immunization not carried out because of other contraindication

Z28.1   Immunization not carried out because of patient decision for reasons of belief or group pressure
     Immunization not carried out because of religious belief

✓5ᵗʰ **Z28.2**   Immunization not carried out because of patient decision for other and unspecified reason

Z28.20   Immunization not carried out because of patient decision for unspecified reason ▽

Z28.21   Immunization not carried out because of patient refusal

Z28.29   Immunization not carried out because of patient decision for other reason

Z28.3   Underimmunization status
     Delinquent immunization status
     Lapsed immunization schedule status

✓5ᵗʰ **Z28.8**   Immunization not carried out for other reason

Z28.81   Immunization not carried out due to patient having had the disease

Z28.82   Immunization not carried out because of caregiver refusal
     Immunization not carried out because of guardian refusal
     Immunization not carried out because of parent refusal
     EXCLUDES 1   immunization not carried out because of caregiver refusal because of religious belief (Z28.1)

Z28.89   Immunization not carried out for other reason

Z28.9   Immunization not carried out for unspecified reason   ▽

✓ Additional Character Req   ✓7ᵗʰ Placeholder Alert   Manifestation   **HCC** CMS-HCC Condition   ▽ Unspecified Code   ▶◀ Revised Text   ● New Code   ▲ Revised Code Title

Z29 Encounter for other prophylactic measures
> EXCLUDES 1 desensitization to allergens (Z51.6)
> prophylactic surgery (Z40.-)

Z29.1 Encounter for prophylactic immunotherapy
Encounter for administration of immunoglobulin

Z29.11 Encounter for prophylactic immunotherapy for respiratory syncytial virus (RSV)

Z29.12 Encounter for prophylactic antivenin

Z29.13 Encounter for prophylactic Rho(D) immune globulin

Z29.14 Encounter for prophylactic rabies immune globin

Z29.3 Encounter for prophylactic fluoride administration

Z29.8 Encounter for other specified prophylactic measures

Z29.9 Encounter for prophylactic measures, unspecified ▽

Persons encountering health services in circumstances related to reproduction (Z30-Z39)

Z30 Encounter for contraceptive management
> DEF: Contraceptive management to prevent pregnancy; methods include oral medications, intrauterine devices, and surgical procedures for males and females (sterilization).

Z30.0 Encounter for general counseling and advice on contraception

Z30.01 Encounter for initial prescription of contraceptives
> EXCLUDES 1 encounter for surveillance of contraceptives (Z30.4-)

Z30.011 Encounter for initial prescription of contraceptive pills ♀

Z30.012 Encounter for prescription of emergency contraception ♀
Encounter for postcoital contraception

Z30.013 Encounter for initial prescription of injectable contraceptive ♀

Z30.014 Encounter for initial prescription of intrauterine contraceptive device ♀
> EXCLUDES 1 encounter for insertion of intrauterine contraceptive device (Z30.430, Z30.432)

Z30.015 Encounter for initial prescription of vaginal ring hormonal contraceptive

Z30.016 Encounter for initial prescription of transdermal patch hormonal contraceptive device

Z30.017 Encounter for initial prescription of implantable subdermal contraceptive

Z30.018 Encounter for initial prescription of other contraceptives ♀
Encounter for initial prescription of barrier contraception
Encounter for initial prescription of diaphragm

Z30.019 Encounter for initial prescription of contraceptives, unspecified ♀▽

Z30.02 Counseling and instruction in natural family planning to avoid pregnancy

Z30.09 Encounter for other general counseling and advice on contraception
Encounter for family planning advice NOS

Z30.2 Encounter for sterilization

Z30.4 Encounter for surveillance of contraceptives

Z30.40 Encounter for surveillance of contraceptives, unspecified ▽

Z30.41 Encounter for surveillance of contraceptive pills ♀
Encounter for repeat prescription for contraceptive pill

Z30.42 Encounter for surveillance of injectable contraceptive ♀

Z30.43 Encounter for surveillance of intrauterine contraceptive device

Z30.430 Encounter for insertion of intrauterine contraceptive device ♀

Z30.431 Encounter for routine checking of intrauterine contraceptive device ♀

Z30.432 Encounter for removal of intrauterine contraceptive device ♀

Z30.433 Encounter for removal and reinsertion of intrauterine contraceptive device ♀
Encounter for replacement of intrauterine contraceptive device

Z30.44 Encounter for surveillance of vaginal ring hormonal contraceptive device ♀

Z30.45 Encounter for surveillance of transdermal patch hormonal contraceptive device ♀

Z30.46 Encounter for surveillance of implantable subdermal contraceptive ♀
Encounter for checking, reinsertion or removal of implantable subdermal contraceptive

Z30.49 Encounter for surveillance of other contraceptives ♀
Encounter for surveillance of barrier contraception
Encounter for surveillance of diaphragm

Z30.8 Encounter for other contraceptive management
Encounter for postvasectomy sperm count
Encounter for routine examination for contraceptive maintenance
> EXCLUDES 1 sperm count following sterilization reversal (Z31.42)
> sperm count for fertility testing (Z31.41)

Z30.9 Encounter for contraceptive management, unspecified ▽

Z31 Encounter for procreative management
> EXCLUDES 1 complications associated with artificial fertilization (N98.-)
> female infertility (N97.-)
> male infertility (N46.-)

Z31.0 Encounter for reversal of previous sterilization

Z31.4 Encounter for procreative investigation and testing
> EXCLUDES 1 postvasectomy sperm count (Z30.8)

Z31.41 Encounter for fertility testing
Encounter for fallopian tube patency testing
Encounter for sperm count for fertility testing

Z31.42 Aftercare following sterilization reversal
Sperm count following sterilization reversal

Z31.43 Encounter for genetic testing of female for procreative management
Use additional code for recurrent pregnancy loss, if applicable (N96, O26.2-)
> EXCLUDES 1 nonprocreative genetic testing (Z13.7-)

Z31.430 Encounter of female for testing for genetic disease carrier status for procreative management ♀

Z31.438 Encounter for other genetic testing of female for procreative management ♀

Z31.44 Encounter for genetic testing of male for procreative management
> EXCLUDES 1 nonprocreative genetic testing (Z13.7-)

Z31.440 Encounter of male for testing for genetic disease carrier status for procreative management ♂

Z31.441 Encounter for testing of male partner patient with recurrent pregnancy loss A♂

Z31.448 Encounter for other genetic testing of male for procreative management A♂

Z31.49 Encounter for other procreative investigation and testing

Z31.5 Encounter for procreative genetic counseling

Z31.6 Encounter for general counseling and advice on procreation

Z31.61 Procreative counseling and advice using natural family planning

Z31.62 Encounter for fertility preservation counseling
Encounter for fertility preservation counseling prior to cancer therapy
Encounter for fertility preservation counseling prior to surgical removal of gonads

Z31.69 Encounter for other general counseling and advice on procreation

Z31.7 Encounter for procreative management and counseling for gestational carrier
> EXCLUDES 1 pregnant state, gestational carrier (Z33.3)

Z31.8 Encounter for other procreative management

Z31.81 Encounter for male factor infertility in female patient PDx ♀

Z31.82 Encounter for Rh incompatibility status ♀
AHA: 2015, 3Q, 40; 2014, 4Q, 17

Z31.83 Encounter for assisted reproductive fertility procedure cycle PDx ♀
Patient undergoing in vitro fertilization cycle
Use additional code to identify the type of infertility
> EXCLUDES 1 pre-cycle diagnosis and testing—code to reason for encounter

Z31.84 **Encounter for fertility preservation procedure** PDx
Encounter for fertility preservation procedure prior to cancer therapy
Encounter for fertility preservation procedure prior to surgical removal of gonads

Z31.89 **Encounter for other procreative management**

Z31.9 **Encounter for procreative management, unspecified** ▽

✓4th **Z32** **Encounter for pregnancy test and childbirth and childcare instruction**

✓5th **Z32.0** **Encounter for pregnancy test**

Z32.00 **Encounter for pregnancy test, result unknown** ♀
Encounter for pregnancy test NOS

Z32.01 **Encounter for pregnancy test, result positive** Ⓜ♀

Z32.02 **Encounter for pregnancy test, result negative** ♀

Z32.2 **Encounter for childbirth instruction**

Z32.3 **Encounter for childcare instruction**
Encounter for prenatal or postpartum childcare instruction

✓4th **Z33** **Pregnant state**

Z33.1 **Pregnant state, incidental** Ⓜ♀
Pregnant state NOS
EXCLUDES 1   complications of pregnancy (O00-O9A)
pregnant state, gestational carrier (Z33.3)

Z33.2 **Encounter for elective termination of pregnancy** PDx Ⓜ♀
EXCLUDES 1   early fetal death with retention of dead fetus (O02.1)
late fetal death (O36.4)
spontaneous abortion (O03)

Z33.3 **Pregnant state, gestational carrier** Ⓜ♀
EXCLUDES 1   encounter for procreative management and counseling for gestational carrier (Z31.7)

✓4th **Z34** **Encounter for supervision of normal pregnancy**
EXCLUDES 1   any complication of pregnancy (O00-O9A)
encounter for pregnancy test (Z32.0-)
encounter for supervision of high risk pregnancy (O09.-)
AHA: 2014, 4Q, 17

✓5th **Z34.0** **Encounter for supervision of normal first pregnancy**

Z34.00 **Encounter for supervision of normal first pregnancy, unspecified trimester** PDx Ⓜ♀ ▽

Z34.01 **Encounter for supervision of normal first pregnancy, first trimester** PDx Ⓜ♀

Z34.02 **Encounter for supervision of normal first pregnancy, second trimester** PDx Ⓜ♀

Z34.03 **Encounter for supervision of normal first pregnancy, third trimester** PDx Ⓜ♀

✓5th **Z34.8** **Encounter for supervision of other normal pregnancy**

Z34.80 **Encounter for supervision of other normal pregnancy, unspecified trimester** PDx Ⓜ♀ ▽

Z34.81 **Encounter for supervision of other normal pregnancy, first trimester** PDx Ⓜ♀

Z34.82 **Encounter for supervision of other normal pregnancy, second trimester** PDx Ⓜ♀

Z34.83 **Encounter for supervision of other normal pregnancy, third trimester** PDx Ⓜ♀

✓5th **Z34.9** **Encounter for supervision of normal pregnancy, unspecified**

Z34.90 **Encounter for supervision of normal pregnancy, unspecified, unspecified trimester** PDx Ⓜ♀ ▽

Z34.91 **Encounter for supervision of normal pregnancy, unspecified, first trimester** PDx Ⓜ♀ ▽

Z34.92 **Encounter for supervision of normal pregnancy, unspecified, second trimester** PDx Ⓜ♀ ▽

Z34.93 **Encounter for supervision of normal pregnancy, unspecified, third trimester** PDx Ⓜ♀ ▽

✓4th **Z36** **Encounter for antenatal screening of mother**
INCLUDES ▶encounter for placental sample (taken vaginally)
screening is the testing for disease or disease precursors in asymptomatic individuals so that early detection and treatment can be provided for those who test positive for the disease◀
EXCLUDES 1   *abnormal findings on antenatal screening of mother (O28.-)*
diagnostic examination—code to sign or symptom
encounter for suspected maternal and fetal conditions ruled out (Z03.7-)
suspected fetal condition affecting management of pregnancy—code to condition in Chapter 15
EXCLUDES 2 ▶*abnormal findings on antenatal screening of mother (O28.-)◀*
genetic counseling and testing (Z31.43-, Z31.5)
routine prenatal care (Z34)

● **Z36.0** **Encounter for antenatal screening for chromosomal anomalies**

● **Z36.1** **Encounter for antenatal screening for raised alphafetoprotein level**
Encounter for antenatal screening for elevated maternal serum alphafetoprotein level

● **Z36.2** **Encounter for other antenatal screening follow-up**
Non-visualized anatomy on a previous scan

● **Z36.3** **Encounter for antenatal screening for malformations**
Screening for a suspected anomaly

● **Z36.4** **Encounter for antenatal screening for fetal growth retardation**
Intrauterine growth restriction (IUGR)/small-for-dates

● **Z36.5** **Encounter for antenatal screening for isoimmunization**

✓5th **Z36.8** **Encounter for other antenatal screening**

● **Z36.81** **Encounter for antenatal screening for hydrops fetalis**

● **Z36.82** **Encounter for antenatal screening for nuchal translucency**

● **Z36.83** **Encounter for fetal screening for congenital cardiac abnormalities**

● **Z36.84** **Encounter for antenatal screening for fetal lung maturity**

● **Z36.85** **Encounter for antenatal screening for Streptococcus B**

● **Z36.86** **Encounter for antenatal screening for cervical length**
Screening for risk of pre-term labor

● **Z36.87** **Encounter for antenatal screening for uncertain dates**

● **Z36.88** **Encounter for antenatal screening for fetal macrosomia**
Screening for large-for-dates

● **Z36.89** **Encounter for other specified antenatal screening**

● **Z36.8A** **Encounter for antenatal screening for other genetic defects**

● **Z36.9** **Encounter for antenatal screening, unspecified** ▽

✓4th **Z3A** **Weeks of gestation**
NOTE   Codes from category Z3A are for use, only on the maternal record, to indicate the weeks of gestation of the pregnancy, if known.
Code first complications of pregnancy, childbirth and the puerperium ▶(O09-O9A)◀
AHA: 2016, 2Q, 34; 2014, 3Q, 17; 2014, 2Q, 9; 2013, 2Q, 33

✓5th **Z3A.0** **Weeks of gestation of pregnancy, unspecified or less than 10 weeks**

Z3A.00 **Weeks of gestation of pregnancy** not specified Ⓜ♀ ▽

Z3A.01 Less than 8 weeks **gestation of pregnancy** Ⓜ♀

Z3A.08 8 weeks **gestation of pregnancy** Ⓜ♀

Z3A.09 9 weeks **gestation of pregnancy** Ⓜ♀

✓5th **Z3A.1** **Weeks of gestation of pregnancy, weeks 10-19**

Z3A.10 10 weeks **gestation of pregnancy** Ⓜ♀

Z3A.11 11 weeks **gestation of pregnancy** Ⓜ♀

Z3A.12 12 weeks **gestation of pregnancy** Ⓜ♀

Z3A.13 13 weeks **gestation of pregnancy** Ⓜ♀

Z3A.14 14 weeks **gestation of pregnancy** Ⓜ♀

Z3A.15 15 weeks **gestation of pregnancy** Ⓜ♀

Z3A.16 16 weeks **gestation of pregnancy** Ⓜ♀

Z3A.17 17 weeks **gestation of pregnancy** Ⓜ♀

Z3A.18 18 weeks **gestation of pregnancy** Ⓜ♀

Z3A.19 19 weeks **gestation of pregnancy** Ⓜ♀

√5ᵗʰ **Z3A.2 Weeks of gestation of pregnancy, weeks 20-29**

     Z3A.20 20 weeks **gestation of pregnancy** Ⓜ♀

     Z3A.21 21 weeks **gestation of pregnancy** Ⓜ♀

     Z3A.22 22 weeks **gestation of pregnancy** Ⓜ♀

     Z3A.23 23 weeks **gestation of pregnancy** Ⓜ♀

     Z3A.24 24 weeks **gestation of pregnancy** Ⓜ♀

     Z3A.25 25 weeks **gestation of pregnancy** Ⓜ♀

     Z3A.26 26 weeks **gestation of pregnancy** Ⓜ♀

     Z3A.27 27 weeks **gestation of pregnancy** Ⓜ♀

     Z3A.28 28 weeks **gestation of pregnancy** Ⓜ♀

     Z3A.29 29 weeks **gestation of pregnancy** Ⓜ♀

√5ᵗʰ **Z3A.3 Weeks of gestation of pregnancy, weeks 30-39**

     Z3A.30 30 weeks **gestation of pregnancy** Ⓜ♀

     Z3A.31 31 weeks **gestation of pregnancy** Ⓜ♀

     Z3A.32 32 weeks **gestation of pregnancy** Ⓜ♀

     Z3A.33 33 weeks **gestation of pregnancy** Ⓜ♀

     Z3A.34 34 weeks **gestation of pregnancy** Ⓜ♀

     Z3A.35 35 weeks **gestation of pregnancy** Ⓜ♀

     Z3A.36 36 weeks **gestation of pregnancy** Ⓜ♀

     Z3A.37 37 weeks **gestation of pregnancy** Ⓜ♀

     Z3A.38 38 weeks **gestation of pregnancy** Ⓜ♀

     Z3A.39 39 weeks **gestation of pregnancy** Ⓜ♀

√5ᵗʰ **Z3A.4 Weeks of gestation of pregnancy, weeks 40 or greater**
     AHA: 2014, 4Q, 23

     Z3A.40 40 weeks **gestation of pregnancy** Ⓜ♀

     Z3A.41 41 weeks **gestation of pregnancy** Ⓜ♀

     Z3A.42 42 weeks **gestation of pregnancy** Ⓜ♀

     Z3A.49 Greater than 42 weeks **gestation of pregnancy** Ⓜ♀

√4ᵗʰ **Z37 Outcome of delivery**
     This category is intended for use as an additional code to identify the outcome of delivery on the mother's record. It is not for use on the newborn record.

     EXCLUDES 1   stillbirth (P95)

     Z37.0 Single live birth Ⓜ♀
         AHA: 2016, 2Q, 34; 2014, 2Q, 9

     Z37.1 Single stillbirth Ⓜ♀

     Z37.2 Twins, both liveborn Ⓜ♀

     Z37.3 Twins, one liveborn and one stillborn Ⓜ♀

     Z37.4 Twins, both stillborn Ⓜ♀

√5ᵗʰ **Z37.5 Other multiple births, all liveborn**

     Z37.50 Multiple births, unspecified, all liveborn Ⓜ♀▽

     Z37.51 Triplets, all liveborn Ⓜ♀

     Z37.52 Quadruplets, all liveborn Ⓜ♀

     Z37.53 Quintuplets, all liveborn Ⓜ♀

     Z37.54 Sextuplets, all liveborn Ⓜ♀

     Z37.59 Other multiple births, all liveborn Ⓜ♀

√5ᵗʰ **Z37.6 Other multiple births, some liveborn**

     Z37.60 Multiple births, unspecified, some liveborn Ⓜ♀▽

     Z37.61 Triplets, some liveborn Ⓜ♀

     Z37.62 Quadruplets, some liveborn Ⓜ♀

     Z37.63 Quintuplets, some liveborn Ⓜ♀

     Z37.64 Sextuplets, some liveborn Ⓜ♀

     Z37.69 Other multiple births, some liveborn Ⓜ♀

     Z37.7 Other multiple births, all stillborn Ⓜ♀

     Z37.9 Outcome of delivery, unspecified Ⓜ♀▽
         Multiple birth NOS
         Single birth NOS

√4ᵗʰ **Z38 Liveborn infants according to place of birth and type of delivery**
     This category is for use as the principal code on the initial record of a newborn baby. It is to be used for the initial birth record only. It is not to be used on the mother's record.
     AHA: 2017, 2Q, 5-7; 2016, 3Q, 18; 2015, 2Q, 15

√5ᵗʰ **Z38.0 Single liveborn infant, born in hospital**
     Single liveborn infant, born in birthing center or other health care facility

     Z38.00 Single liveborn infant, delivered vaginally ᴾᴰˣⓃ

     Z38.01 Single liveborn infant, delivered by cesarean ᴾᴰˣⓃ

     Z38.1 Single liveborn infant, born outside hospital ᴾᴰˣⓃ

     Z38.2 Single liveborn infant, unspecified as to place of birth ᴾᴰˣⓃ▽
         Single liveborn infant NOS

√5ᵗʰ **Z38.3 Twin liveborn infant, born in hospital**

     Z38.30 Twin liveborn infant, delivered vaginally ᴾᴰˣⓃ

     Z38.31 Twin liveborn infant, delivered by cesarean ᴾᴰˣⓃ

     Z38.4 Twin liveborn infant, born outside hospital ᴾᴰˣⓃ

     Z38.5 Twin liveborn infant, unspecified as to place of birth ᴾᴰˣⓃ▽

√5ᵗʰ **Z38.6 Other multiple liveborn infant, born in hospital**

     Z38.61 Triplet liveborn infant, delivered vaginally ᴾᴰˣⓃ

     Z38.62 Triplet liveborn infant, delivered by cesarean ᴾᴰˣⓃ

     Z38.63 Quadruplet liveborn infant, delivered vaginally ᴾᴰˣⓃ

     Z38.64 Quadruplet liveborn infant, delivered by cesarean

     Z38.65 Quintuplet liveborn infant, delivered vaginally ᴾᴰˣⓃ

     Z38.66 Quintuplet liveborn infant, delivered by cesarean

     Z38.68 Other multiple liveborn infant, delivered vaginally

     Z38.69 Other multiple liveborn infant, delivered by cesarean ᴾᴰˣⓃ

     Z38.7 Other multiple liveborn infant, born outside hospital ᴾᴰˣⓃ

     Z38.8 Other multiple liveborn infant, unspecified as to place of birth ᴾᴰˣⓃ▽

√4ᵗʰ **Z39 Encounter for maternal postpartum care and examination**

     Z39.0 Encounter for care and examination of mother immediately after delivery ᴾᴰˣⓂ♀
         Care and observation in uncomplicated cases when the delivery occurs outside a healthcare facility
         EXCLUDES 1   care for postpartum complication—see Alphabetic index

     Z39.1 Encounter for care and examination of lactating mother ᴾᴰˣⓂ♀
         Encounter for supervision of lactation
         EXCLUDES 1   disorders of lactation (O92.-)

     Z39.2 Encounter for routine postpartum follow-up ᴾᴰˣⓂ♀

Encounters for other specific health care (Z40–Z53)

Categories Z40-Z53 are intended for use to indicate a reason for care. They may be used for patients who have already been treated for a disease or injury, but who are receiving aftercare or prophylactic care, or care to consolidate the treatment, or to deal with a residual state.

     EXCLUDES 2   follow-up examination for medical surveillance after treatment (Z08-Z09)

√4ᵗʰ **Z40 Encounter for prophylactic surgery**
     EXCLUDES 1   organ donations (Z52.-)
            therapeutic organ removal—code to condition

√5ᵗʰ **Z40.0 Encounter for prophylactic surgery for risk factors related to malignant neoplasms**
     Admission for prophylactic organ removal
     Use additional code to identify risk factor

     Z40.00 Encounter for prophylactic removal of unspecified organ ▽

     Z40.01 Encounter for prophylactic removal of breast

     Z40.02 Encounter for prophylactic removal of ovary(s) ♀
         ▶Encounter for prophylactic removal of ovary(s) and fallopian tube(s)◀

     Z40.03 Encounter for prophylactic removal of fallopian tube(s)

     Z40.09 Encounter for prophylactic removal of other organ

     Z40.8 Encounter for other prophylactic surgery

     Z40.9 Encounter for prophylactic surgery, unspecified ▽

√4ᵗʰ **Z41 Encounter for procedures for purposes other than remedying health state**

     Z41.1 Encounter for cosmetic surgery
         Encounter for cosmetic breast implant
         Encounter for cosmetic procedure
         EXCLUDES 1   encounter for plastic and reconstructive surgery following medical procedure or healed injury (Z42.-)
               encounter for post-mastectomy breast implantation (Z42.1)

     Z41.2 Encounter for routine and ritual male circumcision ♂

     Z41.3 Encounter for ear piercing

EXCLUDES 1 Not coded here   *EXCLUDES 2* Not included here   Ⓝ Newborn Age: 0   Ⓟ Pediatric Age: 0-17   Ⓜ Maternity Age: 12-55   Ⓐ Adult Age: 15-124   ᴾᴰˣ Primary Dx

1188   ICD-10-CM 2018

Z41.8　Encounter for other procedures for purposes other than remedying health state

Z41.9　Encounter for procedure for purposes other than remedying health state, unspecified ▽

✓4ᵗʰ **Z42**　**Encounter for plastic and reconstructive surgery following medical procedure or healed injury**
>　EXCLUDES 1　encounter for cosmetic plastic surgery (Z41.1)
>　　encounter for plastic surgery for treatment of current injury—code to relevent injury

Z42.1　Encounter for breast reconstruction following mastectomy　PDx A
>　EXCLUDES 1　deformity and disproportion of reconstructed breast (N65.1-)

Z42.8　Encounter for other plastic and reconstructive surgery following medical procedure or healed injury　PDx
>　AHA: 2017, 1Q, 42

✓4ᵗʰ **Z43**　**Encounter for attention to artificial openings**
>　INCLUDES　closure of artificial openings
>　　passage of sounds or bougies through artificial openings
>　　reforming artificial openings
>　　removal of catheter from artificial openings
>　　toilet or cleansing of artificial openings
>　EXCLUDES 1　artificial opening status only, without need for care (Z93.-)
>　　complications of external stoma (J95.0-, K94.-, N99.5-)
>　EXCLUDES 2　fitting and adjustment of prosthetic and other devices (Z44-Z46)

Z43.0　Encounter for attention to tracheostomy　HCC

Z43.1　Encounter for attention to gastrostomy　HCC
>　EXCLUDES 2　▶artificial opening status only, without need for care (Z93.-)◀

Z43.2　Encounter for attention to ileostomy　HCC

Z43.3　Encounter for attention to colostomy　HCC

Z43.4　Encounter for attention to other artificial openings of digestive tract　HCC

Z43.5　Encounter for attention to cystostomy　HCC

Z43.6　Encounter for attention to other artificial openings of urinary tract　HCC
>　Encounter for attention to nephrostomy
>　Encounter for attention to ureterostomy
>　Encounter for attention to urethrostomy

Z43.7　Encounter for attention to artificial vagina

Z43.8　Encounter for attention to other artificial openings　HCC

Z43.9　Encounter for attention to unspecified artificial opening　HCC ▽

✓4ᵗʰ **Z44**　**Encounter for fitting and adjustment of external prosthetic device**
>　INCLUDES　removal or replacement of external prosthetic device
>　EXCLUDES 1　malfunction or other complications of device—see Alphabetical Index
>　　presence of prosthetic device (Z97.-)

✓5ᵗʰ **Z44.0**　Encounter for fitting and adjustment of artificial arm

✓6ᵗʰ **Z44.00**　Encounter for fitting and adjustment of unspecified artificial arm

Z44.001　Encounter for fitting and adjustment of unspecified right artificial arm ▽

Z44.002　Encounter for fitting and adjustment of unspecified left artificial arm ▽

Z44.009　Encounter for fitting and adjustment of unspecified artificial arm, unspecified arm ▽

✓6ᵗʰ **Z44.01**　Encounter for fitting and adjustment of complete artificial arm

Z44.011　Encounter for fitting and adjustment of complete right artificial arm

Z44.012　Encounter for fitting and adjustment of complete left artificial arm

Z44.019　Encounter for fitting and adjustment of complete artificial arm, unspecified arm ▽

✓6ᵗʰ **Z44.02**　Encounter for fitting and adjustment of partial artificial arm

Z44.021　Encounter for fitting and adjustment of partial artificial right arm

Z44.022　Encounter for fitting and adjustment of partial artificial left arm

Z44.029　Encounter for fitting and adjustment of partial artificial arm, unspecified arm ▽

✓5ᵗʰ **Z44.1**　Encounter for fitting and adjustment of artificial leg

✓6ᵗʰ **Z44.10**　Encounter for fitting and adjustment of unspecified artificial leg

Z44.101　Encounter for fitting and adjustment of unspecified right artificial leg　HCC

Z44.102　Encounter for fitting and adjustment of unspecified left artificial leg　HCC

Z44.109　Encounter for fitting and adjustment of unspecified artificial leg, unspecified leg　HCC ▽

✓6ᵗʰ **Z44.11**　Encounter for fitting and adjustment of complete artificial leg

Z44.111　Encounter for fitting and adjustment of complete right artificial leg　HCC

Z44.112　Encounter for fitting and adjustment of complete left artificial leg　HCC

Z44.119　Encounter for fitting and adjustment of complete artificial leg, unspecified leg　HCC ▽

✓6ᵗʰ **Z44.12**　Encounter for fitting and adjustment of partial artificial leg

Z44.121　Encounter for fitting and adjustment of partial artificial right leg　HCC

Z44.122　Encounter for fitting and adjustment of partial artificial left leg　HCC

Z44.129　Encounter for fitting and adjustment of partial artificial leg, unspecified leg　HCC ▽

✓5ᵗʰ **Z44.2**　Encounter for fitting and adjustment of artificial eye
>　EXCLUDES 1　mechanical complication of ocular prosthesis (T85.3)

Z44.20　Encounter for fitting and adjustment of artificial eye, unspecified ▽

Z44.21　Encounter for fitting and adjustment of artificial right eye

Z44.22　Encounter for fitting and adjustment of artificial left eye

✓5ᵗʰ **Z44.3**　Encounter for fitting and adjustment of external breast prosthesis
>　EXCLUDES 1　complications of breast implant (T85.4-)
>　　encounter for adjustment or removal of breast implant (Z45.81-)
>　　encounter for initial breast implant insertion for cosmetic breast augmentation (Z41.1)
>　　encounter for breast reconstruction following mastectomy (Z42.1)

Z44.30　Encounter for fitting and adjustment of external breast prosthesis, unspecified breast ▽

Z44.31　Encounter for fitting and adjustment of external right breast prosthesis

Z44.32　Encounter for fitting and adjustment of external left breast prosthesis

Z44.8　Encounter for fitting and adjustment of other external prosthetic devices

Z44.9　Encounter for fitting and adjustment of unspecified external prosthetic device ▽

✓4ᵗʰ **Z45**　**Encounter for adjustment and management of implanted device**
>　INCLUDES　removal or replacement of implanted device
>　EXCLUDES 1　malfunction or other complications of device – see Alphabetical Index
>　　presence of prosthetic and other devices (Z95-Z97)
>　EXCLUDES 2　encounter for fitting and adjustment of non-implanted device (Z46.-)

✓5ᵗʰ **Z45.0**　Encounter for adjustment and management of cardiac device

✓6ᵗʰ **Z45.01**　Encounter for adjustment and management of cardiac pacemaker
>　Encounter for adjustment and management of cardiac resynchronization therapy pacemaker (CRT-P)
>　EXCLUDES 1　encounter for adjustment and management of automatic implantable cardiac defibrillator with synchronous cardiac pacemaker (Z45.02)

Z45.010　Encounter for checking and testing of cardiac pacemaker pulse generator [battery]
>　Encounter for replacing cardiac pacemaker pulse generator [battery]

✓ Additional Character Req　　✓x7ᵗʰ Placeholder Alert　　Manifestation　　HCC CMS-HCC Condition　　▽ Unspecified Code　　▶◀ Revised Text　　● New Code　　▲ Revised Code Title

ICD-10-CM 2018　　**1189**

Z45.Ø18 Encounter for adjustment and management of other part of cardiac pacemaker
> *EXCLUDES 2* ▶*presence of prosthetic and other devices (Z95-Z97)*◀

Z45.Ø2 Encounter for adjustment and management of automatic implantable cardiac defibrillator
Encounter for adjustment and management of automatic implantable cardiac defibrillator with synchronous cardiac pacemaker
Encounter for adjustment and management of cardiac resynchronization therapy defibrillator (CRT-D)

Z45.Ø9 Encounter for adjustment and management of other cardiac device

Z45.1 Encounter for adjustment and management of infusion pump

Z45.2 Encounter for adjustment and management of vascular access device
Encounter for adjustment and management of vascular catheters
> *EXCLUDES 1* *encounter for adjustment and management of renal dialysis catheter (Z49.Ø1)*

✓5ᵗʰ **Z45.3 Encounter for adjustment and management of implanted devices of the special senses**

   Z45.31 Encounter for adjustment and management of implanted visual substitution device

   ✓6ᵗʰ **Z45.32 Encounter for adjustment and management of implanted hearing device**
> *EXCLUDES 1* *encounter for fitting and adjustment of hearing aide (Z46.1)*

      Z45.32Ø Encounter for adjustment and management of bone conduction device

      Z45.321 Encounter for adjustment and management of cochlear device

      Z45.328 Encounter for adjustment and management of other implanted hearing device

✓5ᵗʰ **Z45.4 Encounter for adjustment and management of implanted nervous system device**

   Z45.41 Encounter for adjustment and management of cerebrospinal fluid drainage device
Encounter for adjustment and management of cerebral ventricular (communicating) shunt

   Z45.42 Encounter for adjustment and management of neuropacemaker (brain) (peripheral nerve) (spinal cord)

   Z45.49 Encounter for adjustment and management of other implanted nervous system device
AHA: 2014, 3Q, 19

✓5ᵗʰ **Z45.8 Encounter for adjustment and management of other implanted devices**

   ✓6ᵗʰ **Z45.81 Encounter for adjustment or removal of breast implant**
Encounter for elective implant exchange (different material) (different size)
Encounter removal of tissue expander without synchronous insertion of permanent implant
> *EXCLUDES 1* *complications of breast implant (T85.4-)*
> *encounter for initial breast implant insertion for cosmetic breast augmentation (Z41.1)*
> *encounter for breast reconstruction following mastectomy (Z42.1)*

      Z45.811 Encounter for adjustment or removal of right breast implant

      Z45.812 Encounter for adjustment or removal of left breast implant

      Z45.819 Encounter for adjustment or removal of unspecified breast implant ▽

   Z45.82 Encounter for adjustment or removal of myringotomy device (stent) (tube)

   Z45.89 Encounter for adjustment and management of other implanted devices
AHA: 2014, 4Q, 26-28

Z45.9 Encounter for adjustment and management of unspecified implanted device ▽

✓4ᵗʰ **Z46 Encounter for fitting and adjustment of other devices**
> *INCLUDES* removal or replacement of other device
> *EXCLUDES 1* *malfunction or other complications of device—see Alphabetical Index*
> *EXCLUDES 2* *encounter for fitting and management of implanted devices (Z45.-)*
> *issue of repeat prescription only (Z76.Ø)*
> *presence of prosthetic and other devices (Z95-Z97)*

Z46.Ø Encounter for fitting and adjustment of spectacles and contact lenses

Z46.1 Encounter for fitting and adjustment of hearing aid
> *EXCLUDES 1* *encounter for adjustment and management of implanted hearing device (Z45.32-)*

Z46.2 Encounter for fitting and adjustment of other devices related to nervous system and special senses
> *EXCLUDES 2* *encounter for adjustment and management of implanted nervous system device (Z45.4-)*
> *encounter for adjustment and management of implanted visual substitution device (Z45.31)*

Z46.3 Encounter for fitting and adjustment of dental prosthetic device
Encounter for fitting and adjustment of dentures

Z46.4 Encounter for fitting and adjustment of orthodontic device

✓5ᵗʰ **Z46.5 Encounter for fitting and adjustment of other gastrointestinal appliance and device**
> *EXCLUDES 1* *encounter for attention to artificial openings of digestive tract (Z43.1-Z43.4)*

   Z46.51 Encounter for fitting and adjustment of gastric lap band

   Z46.59 Encounter for fitting and adjustment of other gastrointestinal appliance and device

Z46.6 Encounter for fitting and adjustment of urinary device
> *EXCLUDES 2* *attention to artificial openings of urinary tract (Z43.5, Z43.6)*

✓5ᵗʰ **Z46.8 Encounter for fitting and adjustment of other specified devices**

   Z46.81 Encounter for fitting and adjustment of insulin pump
Encounter for insulin pump instruction and training
Encounter for insulin pump titration

   Z46.82 Encounter for fitting and adjustment of non-vascular catheter

   Z46.89 Encounter for fitting and adjustment of other specified devices
Encounter for fitting and adjustment of wheelchair

Z46.9 Encounter for fitting and adjustment of unspecified device ▽

✓4ᵗʰ **Z47 Orthopedic aftercare**
> *EXCLUDES 1* *aftercare for healing fracture—code to fracture with 7th character D*

Z47.1 Aftercare following joint replacement surgery
Use additional code to identify the joint (Z96.6-)

Z47.2 Encounter for removal of internal fixation device
> *EXCLUDES 1* *encounter for adjustment of internal fixation device for fracture treatment—code to fracture with appropriate 7th character*
> *encounter for removal of external fixation device—code to fracture with 7th character D*
> *infection or inflammatory reaction to internal fixation device (T84.6-)*
> *mechanical complication of internal fixation device (T84.1-)*

✓5ᵗʰ **Z47.3 Aftercare following explantation of joint prosthesis**
Aftercare following explantation of joint prosthesis, staged procedure
Encounter for joint prosthesis insertion following prior explantation of joint prosthesis
AHA: 2015, 1Q, 16

   Z47.31 Aftercare following explantation of shoulder joint prosthesis
> *EXCLUDES 1* *acquired absence of shoulder joint following prior explantation of shoulder joint prosthesis (Z89.23-)*
> *shoulder joint prosthesis explantation status (Z89.23-)*

EXCLUDES 1 Not coded here   *EXCLUDES 2* Not included here   N Newborn Age: Ø   P Pediatric Age: Ø-17   M Maternity Age: 12-55   A Adult Age: 15-124   PDx Primary Dx

1190   ICD-10-CM 2018

Z47.32   **Aftercare following explantation of hip joint prosthesis**
     EXCLUDES 1   *acquired absence of hip joint following prior explantation of hip joint prosthesis (789.62-)*
       hip joint prosthesis explantation status (Z89.62-)

Z47.33   **Aftercare following explantation of knee joint prosthesis**
     EXCLUDES 1   *acquired absence of knee joint following prior explantation of knee prosthesis (Z89.52-)*
       knee joint prosthesis explantation status (Z89.52-)

√5th **Z47.8**   **Encounter for other orthopedic aftercare**

Z47.81   **Encounter for orthopedic aftercare following surgical amputation**
     Use additional code to identify the limb amputated (Z89.-)

Z47.82   **Encounter for orthopedic aftercare following scoliosis surgery**

Z47.89   **Encounter for other orthopedic aftercare**
     AHA: 2015, 1Q, 8

√4th **Z48**   **Encounter for other postprocedural aftercare**
     EXCLUDES 1   ▶*encounter for aftercare following injury – code to Injury, by site, with appropriate 7th character for subsequent encounter*◀
       encounter for follow-up examination after completed treatment (Z08-Z09)
     EXCLUDES 2   *encounter for attention to artificial openings (Z43.-)*
       encounter for fitting and adjustment of prosthetic and other devices (Z44-Z46)
     AHA: 2015, 4Q, 38; 2015, 1Q, 6-7

√5th **Z48.0**   **Encounter for attention to dressings, sutures and drains**
     EXCLUDES 1   *encounter for planned postprocedural wound closure (Z48.1)*

Z48.00   **Encounter for change or removal of nonsurgical wound dressing**
     Encounter for change or removal of wound dressing NOS

Z48.01   **Encounter for change or removal of surgical wound dressing**

Z48.02   **Encounter for removal of sutures**
     Encounter for removal of staples

Z48.03   **Encounter for change or removal of drains**

Z48.1   **Encounter for planned postprocedural wound closure**
     EXCLUDES 1   *encounter for attention to dressings and sutures (Z48.0-)*

√5th **Z48.2**   **Encounter for aftercare following organ transplant**

Z48.21   **Encounter for aftercare following heart transplant**   HCC

Z48.22   **Encounter for aftercare following kidney transplant**

Z48.23   **Encounter for aftercare following liver transplant**   HCC

Z48.24   **Encounter for aftercare following lung transplant**   HCC

√6th **Z48.28**   **Encounter for aftercare following multiple organ transplant**

     Z48.280   **Encounter for aftercare following heart-lung transplant**   HCC

     Z48.288   **Encounter for aftercare following multiple organ transplant**

√6th **Z48.29**   **Encounter for aftercare following other organ transplant**

     Z48.290   **Encounter for aftercare following bone marrow transplant**   HCC

     Z48.298   **Encounter for aftercare following other organ transplant**

Z48.3   **Aftercare following surgery for neoplasm**
     Use additional code to identify the neoplasm

√5th **Z48.8**   **Encounter for other specified postprocedural aftercare**

√6th **Z48.81**   **Encounter for surgical aftercare following surgery on specified body systems**
     NOTE   These codes identify the body system requiring aftercare. They are for use in conjunction with other aftercare codes to fully explain the aftercare encounter. The condition treated should also be coded if still present.
     EXCLUDES 1   *aftercare for injury—code the injury with 7th character D*
       aftercare following surgery for neoplasm (Z48.3)
     EXCLUDES 2   *aftercare following organ transplant (Z48.2-)*
       orthopedic aftercare (Z47.-)
     AHA: 2015, 4Q, 38

     Z48.810   **Encounter for surgical aftercare following surgery on the sense organs**

     Z48.811   **Encounter for surgical aftercare following surgery on the nervous system**
       EXCLUDES 2   *encounter for surgical aftercare following surgery on the sense organs (Z48.810)*

     Z48.812   **Encounter for surgical aftercare following surgery on the circulatory system**
       AHA: 2012, 4Q, 96

     Z48.813   **Encounter for surgical aftercare following surgery on the respiratory system**

     Z48.814   **Encounter for surgical aftercare following surgery on the teeth or oral cavity**

     Z48.815   **Encounter for surgical aftercare following surgery on the digestive system**

     Z48.816   **Encounter for surgical aftercare following surgery on the genitourinary system**
       EXCLUDES 1   *encounter for aftercare following sterilization reversal (Z31.42)*

     Z48.817   **Encounter for surgical aftercare following surgery on the skin and subcutaneous tissue**

     Z48.89   **Encounter for other specified surgical aftercare**

√4th **Z49**   **Encounter for care involving renal dialysis**
     Code also associated end stage renal disease (N18.6)

√5th **Z49.0**   **Preparatory care for renal dialysis**
     Encounter for dialysis instruction and training

Z49.01   **Encounter for fitting and adjustment of extracorporeal dialysis catheter**   HCC
     Removal or replacement of renal dialysis catheter
     Toilet or cleansing of renal dialysis catheter

Z49.02   **Encounter for fitting and adjustment of peritoneal dialysis catheter**   HCC

√5th **Z49.3**   **Encounter for adequacy testing for dialysis**

Z49.31   **Encounter for adequacy testing for hemodialysis**   HCC

Z49.32   **Encounter for adequacy testing for peritoneal dialysis**   HCC
     Encounter for peritoneal equilibration test

√4th **Z51**   **Encounter for other aftercare and medical care**
     Code also condition requiring care
     EXCLUDES 1   *follow-up examination after treatment (Z08-Z09)*

Z51.0   **Encounter for antineoplastic radiation therapy**   PDx

√5th **Z51.1**   **Encounter for antineoplastic chemotherapy and immunotherapy**
     EXCLUDES 2   *encounter for chemotherapy and immunotherapy for nonneoplastic condition—code to condition*

Z51.11   **Encounter for antineoplastic chemotherapy**   PDx
     AHA: 2015, 3Q, 19

Z51.12   **Encounter for antineoplastic immunotherapy**   PDx

Z51.5   **Encounter for palliative care**
     AHA: 2017, 1Q, 48

Z51.6   **Encounter for desensitization to allergens**

Chapter 21. Factors Influencing Health Status and Contact with Health Services

√5ᵗʰ **Z51.8 Encounter for other specified aftercare**
EXCLUDES 1 *holiday relief care (Z75.5)*

Z51.81 Encounter for therapeutic drug level monitoring
Code also any long-term (current) drug therapy (Z79.-)
EXCLUDES 1 *encounter for blood-drug test for administrative or medicolegal reasons (Z02.83)*
DEF: Drug monitoring: Measurement of the level of a specific drug in the body or measurement of a specific function to assess effectiveness of a drug.

Z51.89 Encounter for other specified aftercare
AHA: 2012, 4Q, 95-97

√4ᵗʰ **Z52 Donors of organs and tissues**
INCLUDES autologous and other living donors
EXCLUDES 1 *cadaveric donor—omit code examination of potential donor (Z00.5)*
AHA: 2012, 4Q, 99

√5ᵗʰ **Z52.0 Blood donor**
√6ᵗʰ **Z52.00 Unspecified blood donor**
Z52.000 Unspecified donor, whole blood PDx ▽
Z52.001 Unspecified donor, stem cells PDx ▽
Z52.008 Unspecified donor, other blood PDx ▽

√6ᵗʰ **Z52.01 Autologous blood donor**
Z52.010 Autologous donor, whole blood PDx
Z52.011 Autologous donor, stem cells PDx
Z52.018 Autologous donor, other blood PDx

√6ᵗʰ **Z52.09 Other blood donor**
Volunteer donor
Z52.090 Other blood donor, whole blood PDx
Z52.091 Other blood donor, stem cells PDx
Z52.098 Other blood donor, other blood PDx

√5ᵗʰ **Z52.1 Skin donor**
Z52.10 Skin donor, unspecified PDx ▽
Z52.11 Skin donor, autologous PDx
Z52.19 Skin donor, other PDx

√5ᵗʰ **Z52.2 Bone donor**
Z52.20 Bone donor, unspecified PDx ▽
Z52.21 Bone donor, autologous PDx
Z52.29 Bone donor, other PDx

Z52.3 Bone marrow donor PDx
Z52.4 Kidney donor PDx
Z52.5 Cornea donor PDx
Z52.6 Liver donor PDx

√5ᵗʰ **Z52.8 Donor of other specified organs or tissues**
√6ᵗʰ **Z52.81 Egg (Oocyte) donor**
Z52.810 Egg (Oocyte) donor under age 35, anonymous recipient PDx ♀
Egg donor under age 35 NOS
Z52.811 Egg (Oocyte) donor under age 35, designated recipient PDx ♀
Z52.812 Egg (Oocyte) donor age 35 and over, anonymous recipient PDx ♀
Egg donor age 35 and over NOS
Z52.813 Egg (Oocyte) donor age 35 and over, designated recipient PDx ♀
Z52.819 Egg (Oocyte) donor, unspecified PDx ♀ ▽
Z52.89 Donor of other specified organs or tissues PDx

Z52.9 Donor of unspecified organ or tissue ▽
Donor NOS

√4ᵗʰ **Z53 Persons encountering health services for specific procedures and treatment, not carried out**
√5ᵗʰ **Z53.0 Procedure and treatment not carried out because of contraindication**
Z53.01 Procedure and treatment not carried out due to patient smoking
Z53.09 Procedure and treatment not carried out because of other contraindication

Z53.1 Procedure and treatment not carried out because of patient's decision for reasons of belief and group pressure

√5ᵗʰ **Z53.2 Procedure and treatment not carried out because of patient's decision for other and unspecified reasons**
Z53.20 Procedure and treatment not carried out because of patient's decision for unspecified reasons ▽

Z53.21 Procedure and treatment not carried out due to patient leaving prior to being seen by health care provider
Z53.29 Procedure and treatment not carried out because of patient's decision for other reasons

√5ᵗʰ **Z53.3 Procedure converted to open procedure**
Z53.31 Laparoscopic surgical procedure converted to open procedure
Z53.32 Thoracoscopic surgical procedure converted to open procedure
Z53.33 Arthroscopic surgical procedure converted to open procedure
Z53.39 Other specified procedure converted to open procedure

Z53.8 Procedure and treatment not carried out for other reasons
Z53.9 Procedure and treatment not carried out, unspecified reason ▽

Persons with potential health hazards related to socioeconomic and psychosocial circumstances (Z55-Z65)

√4ᵗʰ **Z55 Problems related to education and literacy**
EXCLUDES 1 *disorders of psychological development (F80-F89)*
Z55.0 Illiteracy and low-level literacy
Z55.1 Schooling unavailable and unattainable
Z55.2 Failed school examinations
Z55.3 Underachievement in school
Z55.4 Educational maladjustment and discord with teachers and classmates
Z55.8 Other problems related to education and literacy
Problems related to inadequate teaching
Z55.9 Problems related to education and literacy, unspecified ▽
Academic problems NOS

√4ᵗʰ **Z56 Problems related to employment and unemployment**
EXCLUDES 2 *occupational exposure to risk factors (Z57.-)*
problems related to housing and economic circumstances (Z59.-)
Z56.0 Unemployment, unspecified ▽
Z56.1 Change of job A
Z56.2 Threat of job loss
Z56.3 Stressful work schedule
Z56.4 Discord with boss and workmates
Z56.5 Uncongenial work environment
Difficult conditions at work
Z56.6 Other physical and mental strain related to work
√5ᵗʰ **Z56.8 Other problems related to employment**
Z56.81 Sexual harassment on the job
Z56.82 Military deployment status
Individual (civilian or military) currently deployed in theater or in support of military war, peacekeeping and humanitarian operations
Z56.89 Other problems related to employment
Z56.9 Unspecified problems related to employment ▽
Occupational problems NOS

√4ᵗʰ **Z57 Occupational exposure to risk factors**
Z57.0 Occupational exposure to noise
Z57.1 Occupational exposure to radiation
Z57.2 Occupational exposure to dust
√5ᵗʰ **Z57.3 Occupational exposure to other air contaminants**
Z57.31 Occupational exposure to environmental tobacco smoke
EXCLUDES 2 *exposure to environmental tobacco smoke (Z77.22)*
Z57.39 Occupational exposure to other air contaminants
Z57.4 Occupational exposure to toxic agents in agriculture
Occupational exposure to solids, liquids, gases or vapors in agriculture
Z57.5 Occupational exposure to toxic agents in other industries
Occupational exposure to solids, liquids, gases or vapors in other industries
Z57.6 Occupational exposure to extreme temperature
Z57.7 Occupational exposure to vibration
Z57.8 Occupational exposure to other risk factors
Z57.9 Occupational exposure to unspecified risk factor ▽

EXCLUDES 1 Not coded here   EXCLUDES 2 Not included here   N Newborn Age: 0   P Pediatric Age: 0-17   M Maternity Age: 12-55   A Adult Age: 15-124   PDx Primary Dx

1192   ICD-10-CM 2018

✓4ᵗʰ **Z59 Problems related to housing and economic circumstances**
  EXCLUDES 2 *problems related to upbringing (Z62.-)*

  Z59.0 Homelessness

  Z59.1 Inadequate housing
    Lack of heating
    Restriction of space
    Technical defects in home preventing adequate care
    Unsatisfactory surroundings
    EXCLUDES 1 *problems related to the natural and physical environment (Z77.1-)*

  Z59.2 Discord with neighbors, lodgers and landlord

  Z59.3 Problems related to living in residential institution
    Boarding-school resident
    EXCLUDES 1 *institutional upbringing (Z62.2)*

  Z59.4 Lack of adequate food and safe drinking water
    Inadequate drinking water supply
    EXCLUDES 1 *effects of hunger (T73.0)*
       inappropriate diet or eating habits (Z72.4)
       malnutrition (E40-E46)

  Z59.5 Extreme poverty

  Z59.6 Low income

  Z59.7 Insufficient social insurance and welfare support

  Z59.8 Other problems related to housing and economic circumstances
    Foreclosure on loan
    Isolated dwelling
    Problems with creditors

  Z59.9 Problem related to housing and economic circumstances, unspecified ▽

✓4ᵗʰ **Z60 Problems related to social environment**

  Z60.0 Problems of adjustment to life-cycle transitions
    Empty nest syndrome
    Phase of life problem
    Problem with adjustment to retirement [pension]

  Z60.2 Problems related to living alone

  Z60.3 Acculturation difficulty
    Problem with migration
    Problem with social transplantation
    DEF: A problem in adapting to a different culture or environment not based on any coexisting mental disorder.

  Z60.4 Social exclusion and rejection
    Exclusion and rejection on the basis of personal characteristics, such as unusual physical appearance, illness or behavior.
    EXCLUDES 1 *target of adverse discrimination such as for racial or religious reasons (Z60.5)*

  Z60.5 Target of (perceived) adverse discrimination and persecution
    EXCLUDES 1 *social exclusion and rejection (Z60.4)*

  Z60.8 Other problems related to social environment

  Z60.9 Problem related to social environment, unspecified ▽

✓4ᵗʰ **Z62 Problems related to upbringing**
  INCLUDES current and past negative life events in childhood
    current and past problems of a child related to upbringing
  EXCLUDES 2 *maltreatment syndrome (T74.-)*
    problems related to housing and economic circumstances (Z59.-)

  Z62.0 Inadequate parental supervision and control

  Z62.1 Parental overprotection

  ✓5ᵗʰ **Z62.2 Upbringing away from parents**
    EXCLUDES 1 *problems with boarding school (Z59.3)*

    Z62.21 Child in welfare custody ℗
      Child in care of non-parental family member
      Child in foster care
      EXCLUDES 2 *problem for parent due to child in welfare custody (Z63.5)*

    Z62.22 Institutional upbringing
      Child living in orphanage or group home

    Z62.29 Other upbringing away from parents

  Z62.3 Hostility towards and scapegoating of child ℗

  Z62.6 Inappropriate (excessive) parental pressure

  ✓5ᵗʰ **Z62.8 Other specified problems related to upbringing**

    ✓6ᵗʰ **Z62.81 Personal history of abuse in childhood**
      Z62.810 Personal history of physical and sexual abuse in childhood
        EXCLUDES 1 *current child physical abuse (T74.12, T76.12)*
           current child sexual abuse (T74.22, T76.22)

    Z62.811 Personal history of psychological abuse in childhood
      EXCLUDES 1 *current child psychological abuse (T74.32, T76.32)*

    ~~**Z62.812 Personal history of neglect in childhood**~~
      EXCLUDES 1 *current child neglect (T74.02, T76.02)*

    Z62.819 Personal history of unspecified abuse in childhood ▽
      EXCLUDES 1 *current child abuse NOS (T74.92, T76.92)*

  ✓6ᵗʰ **Z62.82 Parent-child conflict**
    Z62.820 Parent-biological child conflict
      Parent-child problem NOS
    Z62.821 Parent-adopted child conflict
    Z62.822 Parent-foster child conflict

  ✓6ᵗʰ **Z62.89 Other specified problems related to upbringing**
    Z62.890 Parent-child estrangement NEC
    Z62.891 Sibling rivalry
    Z62.898 Other specified problems related to upbringing

  Z62.9 Problem related to upbringing, unspecified ▽

✓4ᵗʰ **Z63 Other problems related to primary support group, including family circumstances**
  EXCLUDES 2 *maltreatment syndrome (T74-, T76)*
    parent-child problems (Z62.-)
    problems related to negative life events in childhood (Z62.-)
    problems related to upbringing (Z62.-)

  Z63.0 Problems in relationship with spouse or partner
    ▶Relationship distress with spouse or intimate partner◀
    EXCLUDES 1 *counseling for spousal or partner abuse problems (Z69.1)*
       counseling related to sexual attitude, behavior, and orientation (Z70.-)

  Z63.1 Problems in relationship with in-laws

  ✓5ᵗʰ **Z63.3 Absence of family member**
    EXCLUDES 1 *absence of family member due to disappearance and death (Z63.4)*
       absence of family member due to separation and divorce (Z63.5)

    Z63.31 Absence of family member due to military deployment
      Individual or family affected by other family member being on military deployment
      EXCLUDES 1 *family disruption due to return of family member from military deployment (Z63.71)*

    Z63.32 Other absence of family member

  Z63.4 Disappearance and death of family member
    Assumed death of family member
    Bereavement
    AHA: 2014, 1Q, 25

  Z63.5 Disruption of family by separation and divorce
    Marital estrangement

  Z63.6 Dependent relative needing care at home

  ✓5ᵗʰ **Z63.7 Other stressful life events affecting family and household**

    Z63.71 Stress on family due to return of family member from military deployment
      Individual or family affected by family member having returned from military deployment (current or past conflict)

    Z63.72 Alcoholism and drug addiction in family

    Z63.79 Other stressful life events affecting family and household
      Anxiety (normal) about sick person in family
      Health problems within family
      Ill or disturbed family member
      Isolated family

  Z63.8 Other specified problems related to primary support group
    Family discord NOS
    Family estrangement NOS
    High expressed emotional level within family
    Inadequate family support NOS
    Inadequate or distorted communication within family

  Z63.9 Problem related to primary support group, unspecified ▽
    Relationship disorder NOS

☑ Additional Character Req   ✓×7ᵗʰ Placeholder Alert   Manifestation   HCC CMS-HCC Condition   ▽ Unspecified Code   ▶◀ Revised Text   ● New Code   ▲ Revised Code Title

ICD-10-CM 2018   1193

✓4ᵗʰ **Z64 Problems related to certain psychosocial circumstances**

    Z64.0 Problems related to unwanted pregnancy ♀

    Z64.1 Problems related to multiparity ♀

    Z64.4 Discord with counselors
        Discord with probation officer
        Discord with social worker

✓4ᵗʰ **Z65 Problems related to other psychosocial circumstances**

    Z65.0 Conviction in civil and criminal proceedings without imprisonment

    Z65.1 Imprisonment and other incarceration

    Z65.2 Problems related to release from prison

    Z65.3 Problems related to other legal circumstances
        Arrest
        Child custody or support proceedings
        Litigation
        Prosecution

    Z65.4 Victim of crime and terrorism
        Victim of torture

    Z65.5 Exposure to disaster, war and other hostilities
        EXCLUDES 1 *target of perceived discrimination or persecution (Z60.5)*

    Z65.8 Other specified problems related to psychosocial circumstances
        ▶Religious or spiritual problem◀

    Z65.9 Problem related to unspecified psychosocial circumstances ▽

Do not resuscitate status (Z66)

Z66 Do not resuscitate
    DNR status
    DEF: Medical order written by a physician that instructs others not to perform cardiopulmonary resuscitation (CPR), intubation, or advanced life support (ACLS); prevents unnecessary invasive treatment to prolong life should breathing stop or cardiac arrest occur.

Blood type (Z67)

✓4ᵗʰ **Z67 Blood type**
    AHA: 2015, 3Q, 40

    ✓5ᵗʰ **Z67.1 Type A blood**
        Z67.10 Type A blood, Rh positive
        Z67.11 Type A blood, Rh negative

    ✓5ᵗʰ **Z67.2 Type B blood**
        Z67.20 Type B blood, Rh positive
        Z67.21 Type B blood, Rh negative

    ✓5ᵗʰ **Z67.3 Type AB blood**
        Z67.30 Type AB blood, Rh positive
        Z67.31 Type AB blood, Rh negative

    ✓5ᵗʰ **Z67.4 Type O blood**
        Z67.40 Type O blood, Rh positive
        Z67.41 Type O blood, Rh negative

    ✓5ᵗʰ **Z67.9 Unspecified blood type**
        Z67.90 Unspecified blood type, Rh positive ▽
        Z67.91 Unspecified blood type, Rh negative ▽

Blood Types

Antigen A   Antigen B

Blood Type A   Blood Type B

Anti-B antibody   Anti-A antibody

Blood Type AB   NO ANTIBODIES   NO ANTIGENS

Antigen A   Antigen B   Blood Type O

Body mass index [BMI] (Z68)

✓4ᵗʰ **Z68 Body mass index [BMI]**
    Kilograms per meters squared
    NOTE BMI adult codes are for use for persons 21 years of age or older.
        BMI pediatric codes are for use for persons 2-20 years of age. These percentiles are based on the growth charts published by the Centers for Disease Control and Prevention (CDC).
    AHA: 2017, 1Q, 39
    DEF: Index used to help determine whether an individual is underweight, a healthy weight, overweight, or obese.

▲   **Z68.1 Body mass index [BMI] 19.9 or less, adult** Ⓐ

    ✓5ᵗʰ **Z68.2 Body mass index [BMI] 20-29, adult**
        Z68.20 Body mass index [BMI] 20.0-20.9, adult Ⓐ
        Z68.21 Body mass index [BMI] 21.0-21.9, adult Ⓐ
        Z68.22 Body mass index [BMI] 22.0-22.9, adult Ⓐ
        Z68.23 Body mass index [BMI] 23.0-23.9, adult Ⓐ
        Z68.24 Body mass index [BMI] 24.0-24.9, adult Ⓐ
        Z68.25 Body mass index [BMI] 25.0-25.9, adult Ⓐ
        Z68.26 Body mass index [BMI] 26.0-26.9, adult Ⓐ
        Z68.27 Body mass index [BMI] 27.0-27.9, adult Ⓐ
        Z68.28 Body mass index [BMI] 28.0-28.9, adult Ⓐ
        Z68.29 Body mass index [BMI] 29.0-29.9, adult Ⓐ

    ✓5ᵗʰ **Z68.3 Body mass index [BMI] 30-39, adult**
        Z68.30 Body mass index [BMI] 30.0-30.9, adult Ⓐ
        Z68.31 Body mass index [BMI] 31.0-31.9, adult Ⓐ
        Z68.32 Body mass index [BMI] 32.0-32.9, adult Ⓐ
        Z68.33 Body mass index [BMI] 33.0-33.9, adult Ⓐ
        Z68.34 Body mass index [BMI] 34.0-34.9, adult Ⓐ
        Z68.35 Body mass index [BMI] 35.0-35.9, adult Ⓐ
        Z68.36 Body mass index [BMI] 36.0-36.9, adult Ⓐ
        Z68.37 Body mass index [BMI] 37.0-37.9, adult Ⓐ
        Z68.38 Body mass index [BMI] 38.0-38.9, adult Ⓐ
        Z68.39 Body mass index [BMI] 39.0-39.9, adult Ⓐ

    ✓5ᵗʰ **Z68.4 Body mass index [BMI] 40 or greater, adult**
        Z68.41 Body mass index [BMI] 40.0-44.9, adult HCC Ⓐ
        Z68.42 Body mass index [BMI] 45.0-49.9, adult HCC Ⓐ
        Z68.43 Body mass index [BMI] 50-59.9, adult HCC Ⓐ
        Z68.44 Body mass index [BMI] 60.0-69.9, adult HCC Ⓐ
        Z68.45 Body mass index [BMI] 70 or greater, adult HCC Ⓐ

    ✓5ᵗʰ **Z68.5 Body mass index [BMI] pediatric**
        Z68.51 Body mass index [BMI] pediatric, less than 5th percentile for age
        Z68.52 Body mass index [BMI] pediatric, 5th percentile to less than 85th percentile for age
        Z68.53 Body mass index [BMI] pediatric, 85th percentile to less than 95th percentile for age
        Z68.54 Body mass index [BMI] pediatric, greater than or equal to 95th percentile for age

Persons encountering health services in other circumstances (Z69-Z76)

✓4ᵗʰ **Z69 Encounter for mental health services for victim and perpetrator of abuse**
    INCLUDES counseling for victims and perpetrators of abuse

    ✓5ᵗʰ **Z69.0 Encounter for mental health services for child abuse problems**

        ✓6ᵗʰ **Z69.01 Encounter for mental health services for parental child abuse**

            Z69.010 Encounter for mental health services for victim of parental child abuse Ⓟ
                ▶Encounter for mental health services for victim of child abuse by parent
                Encounter for mental health services for victim of child neglect by parent
                Encounter for mental health services for victim of child psychological abuse by parent
                Encounter for mental health services for victim of child sexual abuse by parent◀

EXCLUDES 1 Not coded here   **EXCLUDES 2** Not included here   N Newborn Age: 0   P Pediatric Age: 0-17   M Maternity Age: 12-55   Ⓐ Adult Age: 15-124   PDₓ Primary Dx

1194   ICD-10-CM 2018

Z69.011 **Encounter for mental health services for perpetrator of parental child abuse**
►Encounter for mental health services for perpetrator of parental child neglect
Encounter for mental health services for perpetrator of parental child psychological abuse
Encounter for mental health services for perpetrator of parental child sexual abuse◄
EXCLUDES 1   *encounter for mental health services for non-parental child abuse (Z69.02-)*

✓6ᵗʰ **Z69.02** **Encounter for mental health services for non-parental child abuse**

Z69.020 **Encounter for mental health services for victim of non-parental child abuse**   P
►Encounter for mental health services for victim of non-parental child neglect
Encounter for mental health services for victim of non-parental child psychological abuse
Encounter for mental health services for victim of non-parental child sexual abuse◄

Z69.021 **Encounter for mental health services for perpetrator of non-parental child abuse**
►Encounter for mental health services for perpetrator of non-parental child neglect
Encounter for mental health services for perpetrator of non-parental child psychological abuse
Encounter for mental health services for perpetrator of non-parental child sexual abuse◄

✓5ᵗʰ **Z69.1** **Encounter for mental health services for spousal or partner abuse problems**

Z69.11 **Encounter for mental health services for victim of spousal or partner abuse**
►Encounter for mental health services for victim of spouse or partner neglect
Encounter for mental health services for victim of spouse or partner psychological abuse
Encounter for mental health services for victim of spouse or partner violence, physical◄

Z69.12 **Encounter for mental health services for perpetrator of spousal or partner abuse**
►Encounter for mental health services for perpetrator of spouse or partner neglect
Encounter for mental health services for perpetrator of spouse or partner psychological abuse
Encounter for mental health services for perpetrator of spouse or partner violence, physical
Encounter for mental health services for perpetrator of spouse or partner violence, sexual◄

✓5ᵗʰ **Z69.8** **Encounter for mental health services for victim or perpetrator of other abuse**

Z69.81 **Encounter for mental health services for victim of other abuse**
►Encounter for mental health services for perpetrator of non-spousal adult abuse
Encounter for mental health services for victim of non-spousal adult abuse
Encounter for mental health services for victim of spouse or partner violence, sexual◄
Encounter for rape victim counseling

Z69.82 **Encounter for mental health services for perpetrator of other abuse**   ●

✓4ᵗʰ **Z70** **Counseling related to sexual attitude, behavior and orientation**
INCLUDES   encounter for mental health services for sexual attitude, behavior and orientation
EXCLUDES 2   *contraceptive or procreative counseling (Z30-Z31)*

Z70.0 **Counseling related to sexual attitude**

Z70.1 **Counseling related to patient's sexual behavior and orientation**
Patient concerned regarding impotence
Patient concerned regarding non-responsiveness
Patient concerned regarding promiscuity
Patient concerned regarding sexual orientation

Z70.2 **Counseling related to sexual behavior and orientation of third party**
Advice sought regarding sexual behavior and orientation of child
Advice sought regarding sexual behavior and orientation of partner
Advice sought regarding sexual behavior and orientation of spouse

Z70.3 **Counseling related to combined concerns regarding sexual attitude, behavior and orientation**

Z70.8 **Other sex counseling**
Encounter for sex education

Z70.9 **Sex counseling, unspecified**   ▽

✓4ᵗʰ **Z71** **Persons encountering health services for other counseling and medical advice, not elsewhere classified**
EXCLUDES 2   *contraceptive or procreation counseling (Z30-Z31)*
sex counseling (Z70.-)

Z71.0 **Person encountering health services to consult on behalf of another person**
Person encountering health services to seek advice or treatment for non-attending third party
EXCLUDES 2   *anxiety (normal) about sick person in family (Z63.7)*
expectant (adoptive) parent(s) pre-birth pediatrician visit (Z76.81)

Z71.1 **Person with feared health complaint in whom no diagnosis is made**
Person encountering health services with feared condition which was not demonstrated
Person encountering health services in which problem was normal state
"Worried well"
EXCLUDES 1   *medical observation for suspected diseases and conditions proven not to exist (Z03.-)*

Z71.2 **Person consulting for explanation of examination or test findings**

Z71.3 **Dietary counseling and surveillance**
Use additional code for any associated underlying medical condition
Use additional code to identify body mass index (BMI), if known (Z68.-)

✓5ᵗʰ **Z71.4** **Alcohol abuse counseling and surveillance**
Use additional code for alcohol abuse or dependence (F10.-)

Z71.41 **Alcohol abuse counseling and surveillance of alcoholic**

Z71.42 **Counseling for family member of alcoholic**
Counseling for significant other, partner, or friend of alcoholic

✓5ᵗʰ **Z71.5** **Drug abuse counseling and surveillance**
Use additional code for drug abuse or dependence (F11-F16, F18-F19)

Z71.51 **Drug abuse counseling and surveillance of drug abuser**

Z71.52 **Counseling for family member of drug abuser**
Counseling for significant other, partner, or friend of drug abuser

Z71.6 **Tobacco abuse counseling**
Use additional code for nicotine dependence (F17.-)

Z71.7 **Human immunodeficiency virus [HIV] counseling**

✓5ᵗʰ **Z71.8** **Other specified counseling**
EXCLUDES 2   *counseling for contraception (Z30.0-)*
~~*counseling for genetics (Z31.5)*~~
~~*counseling for procreative management (Z31.6-)*~~

Z71.81 **Spiritual or religious counseling**

Z71.82 **Exercise counseling**

Z71.83 **Encounter for nonprocreative genetic counseling**
EXCLUDES 1   *counseling for procreative genetics (Z31.5)*
counseling for procreative management (Z31.6)

Z71.89 **Other specified counseling**

Z71.9 **Counseling, unspecified**   ▽
Encounter for medical advice NOS

✓ Additional Character Req   ✓x7ᵗʰ Placeholder Alert   Manifestation   HCC CMS-HCC Condition   ▽ Unspecified Code   ►◄ Revised Text   ● New Code   ▲ Revised Code Title

√4ᵗʰ Z72   Problems related to lifestyle
> **EXCLUDES 2**   *problems related to life-management difficulty (Z73.-)*
> *problems related to socioeconomic and psychosocial circumstances (Z55-Z65)*

    Z72.0   Tobacco use
       Tobacco use NOS
> **EXCLUDES 1**   *history of tobacco dependence (Z87.891)*
> *nicotine dependence (F17.2-)*
> *tobacco dependence (F17.2-)*
> *tobacco use during pregnancy (O99.33-)*

    Z72.3   Lack of physical exercise

    Z72.4   Inappropriate diet and eating habits
> **EXCLUDES 1**   *behavioral eating disorders of infancy or childhood (F98.2- F98.3)*
> *eating disorders (F50.-)*
> *lack of adequate food (Z59.4)*
> *malnutrition and other nutritional deficiencies (E40-E64)*

    √5ᵗʰ Z72.5   High risk sexual behavior
       Promiscuity
> **EXCLUDES 1**   *paraphilias (F65)*

       Z72.51   High risk heterosexual behavior
       Z72.52   High risk homosexual behavior
       Z72.53   High risk bisexual behavior

    Z72.6   Gambling and betting
> **EXCLUDES 1**   *compulsive or pathological gambling (F63.0)*

    √5ᵗʰ Z72.8   Other problems related to lifestyle

       √6ᵗʰ Z72.81   Antisocial behavior
> **EXCLUDES 1**   *conduct disorders (F91.-)*

          Z72.810   Child and adolescent antisocial behavior   P
             Antisocial behavior (child) (adolescent) without manifest psychiatric disorder
             Delinquency NOS
             Group delinquency
             Offenses in the context of gang membership
             Stealing in company with others
             Truancy from school

          Z72.811   Adult antisocial behavior   A
             Adult antisocial behavior without manifest psychiatric disorder

       √6ᵗʰ Z72.82   Problems related to sleep
          Z72.820   Sleep deprivation
             Lack of adequate sleep
> **EXCLUDES 1**   *insomnia (G47.0-)*

          Z72.821   Inadequate sleep hygiene
             Bad sleep habits
             Irregular sleep habits
             Unhealthy sleep wake schedule
> **EXCLUDES 1**   *insomnia (F51.0-, G47.0-)*

       Z72.89   Other problems related to lifestyle
          Self-damaging behavior

    Z72.9   Problem related to lifestyle, unspecified   ▽

√4ᵗʰ Z73   Problems related to life management difficulty
> **EXCLUDES 2**   *problems related to socioeconomic and psychosocial circumstances (Z55-Z65)*

DEF: State of emotional, mental, and physical exhaustion; causing difficulties in managing personal, school, or work circumstances; usually due to prolonged stress; poor interpersonal relationship skills, or parenting skills.

    Z73.0   Burn-out
    Z73.1   Type A behavior pattern
    Z73.2   Lack of relaxation and leisure
    Z73.3   Stress, not elsewhere classified
       Physical and mental strain NOS
> **EXCLUDES 1**   *stress related to employment or unemployment (Z56.-)*

    Z73.4   Inadequate social skills, not elsewhere classified
    Z73.5   Social role conflict, not elsewhere classified
    Z73.6   Limitation of activities due to disability
> **EXCLUDES 1**   *care-provider dependency (Z74.-)*

    √5ᵗʰ Z73.8   Other problems related to life management difficulty
       √6ᵗʰ Z73.81   Behavioral insomnia of childhood
> **DEF:** Behaviors on the part of the child or caregivers that cause negative compliance with a child's sleep schedule; results in lack of adequate sleep.

          Z73.810   Behavioral insomnia of childhood, sleep-onset association type   P

          Z73.811   Behavioral insomnia of childhood, limit setting type   P
          Z73.812   Behavioral insomnia of childhood, combined type   P
          Z73.819   Behavioral insomnia of childhood, unspecified type   P ▽

       Z73.82   Dual sensory impairment
       Z73.89   Other problems related to life management difficulty

    Z73.9   Problem related to life management difficulty, unspecified   ▽

√4ᵗʰ Z74   Problems related to care provider dependency
> **EXCLUDES 2**   *dependence on enabling machines or devices NEC (Z99.-)*

    √5ᵗʰ Z74.0   Reduced mobility
       Z74.01   Bed confinement status
          Bedridden
       Z74.09   Other reduced mobility
          Chair ridden
          Reduced mobility NOS
> **EXCLUDES 2**   *wheelchair dependence (Z99.3)*

    Z74.1   Need for assistance with personal care
    Z74.2   Need for assistance at home and no other household member able to render care
    Z74.3   Need for continuous supervision
    Z74.8   Other problems related to care provider dependency
    Z74.9   Problem related to care provider dependency, unspecified   ▽

√4ᵗʰ Z75   Problems related to medical facilities and other health care
    Z75.0   Medical services not available in home
> **EXCLUDES 1**   *no other household member able to render care (Z74.2)*

    Z75.1   Person awaiting admission to adequate facility elsewhere
    Z75.2   Other waiting period for investigation and treatment
    Z75.3   Unavailability and inaccessibility of health-care facilities
> **EXCLUDES 1**   *bed unavailable (Z75.1)*

    Z75.4   Unavailability and inaccessibility of other helping agencies
    Z75.5   Holiday relief care
    Z75.8   Other problems related to medical facilities and other health care
    Z75.9   Unspecified problem related to medical facilities and other health care   ▽

√4ᵗʰ Z76   Persons encountering health services in other circumstances
    Z76.0   Encounter for issue of repeat prescription
       Encounter for issue of repeat prescription for appliance
       Encounter for issue of repeat prescription for medicaments
       Encounter for issue of repeat prescription for spectacles
> **EXCLUDES 2**   *issue of medical certificate (Z02.7)*
> *repeat prescription for contraceptive (Z30.4-)*

    Z76.1   Encounter for health supervision and care of foundling   PDx
    Z76.2   Encounter for health supervision and care of other healthy infant and child   PDx P
       Encounter for medical or nursing care or supervision of healthy infant under circumstances such as adverse socioeconomic conditions at home
       Encounter for medical or nursing care or supervision of healthy infant under circumstances such as awaiting foster or adoptive placement
       Encounter for medical or nursing care or supervision of healthy infant under circumstances such as maternal illness
       Encounter for medical or nursing care or supervision of healthy infant under circumstances such as number of children at home preventing or interfering with normal care

    Z76.3   Healthy person accompanying sick person
    Z76.4   Other boarder to healthcare facility
> **EXCLUDES 1**   *homelessness (Z59.0)*

    Z76.5   Malingerer [conscious simulation]
       Person feigning illness (with obvious motivation)
> **EXCLUDES 1**   *factitious disorder (F68.1-)*
> *peregrinating patient (F68.1-)*

> **DEF:** Act of intentionally exaggerating an illness or disability in order to receive personal gain; or to avoid punishment or responsibility.

    √5ᵗʰ Z76.8   Persons encountering health services in other specified circumstances
       Z76.81   Expectant parent(s) prebirth pediatrician visit
          Pre-adoption pediatrician visit for adoptive parent(s)
       Z76.82   Awaiting organ transplant status
          Patient waiting for organ availability

EXCLUDES 1 Not coded here   **EXCLUDES 2** Not included here   N Newborn Age: 0   P Pediatric Age: 0-17   M Maternity Age: 12-55   A Adult Age: 15-124   PDx Primary Dx

1196   ICD-10-CM 2018

Z76.89   **Persons encountering health services in other specified circumstances**
Persons encountering health services NOS
AHA: 2014, 2Q, 10

Persons with potential health hazards related to family and personal history and certain conditions influencing health status (Z77-Z99)

Code also any follow-up examination (Z08-Z09)

✓4ᵗʰ Z77   **Other contact with and (suspected) exposures hazardous to health**

    INCLUDES   contact with and (suspected) exposures to potential hazards to health

    EXCLUDES 2   contact with and (suspected) exposure to communicable diseases (Z20.-)
     exposure to (parental) (environmental) tobacco smoke in the perinatal period (P96.81)
     newborn affected by noxious substances transmitted via placenta or breast milk (P04.-)
     occupational exposure to risk factors (Z57.-)
     retained foreign body (Z18.-)
     retained foreign body fully removed (Z87.821)
     toxic effects of substances chiefly nonmedicinal as to source (T51-T65)

✓5ᵗʰ Z77.0   **Contact with and (suspected) exposure to hazardous, chiefly nonmedicinal, chemicals**

    ✓6ᵗʰ Z77.01   **Contact with and (suspected) exposure to hazardous metals**

      Z77.010   **Contact with and (suspected) exposure to arsenic**

      Z77.011   **Contact with and (suspected) exposure to lead**

      Z77.012   **Contact with and (suspected) exposure to uranium**
        EXCLUDES 1   retained depleted uranium fragments (Z18.01)

      Z77.018   **Contact with and (suspected) exposure to other hazardous metals**
        Contact with and (suspected) exposure to chromium compounds
        Contact with and (suspected) exposure to nickel dust

    ✓6ᵗʰ Z77.02   **Contact with and (suspected) exposure to hazardous aromatic compounds**

      Z77.020   **Contact with and (suspected) exposure to aromatic amines**

      Z77.021   **Contact with and (suspected) exposure to benzene**

      Z77.028   **Contact with and (suspected) exposure to other hazardous aromatic compounds**
        Aromatic dyes NOS
        Polycyclic aromatic hydrocarbons

    ✓6ᵗʰ Z77.09   **Contact with and (suspected) exposure to other hazardous, chiefly nonmedicinal, chemicals**

      Z77.090   **Contact with and (suspected) exposure to asbestos**

      Z77.098   **Contact with and (suspected) exposure to other hazardous, chiefly nonmedicinal, chemicals**
        Dyes NOS

✓5ᵗʰ Z77.1   **Contact with and (suspected) exposure to environmental pollution and hazards in the physical environment**

    ✓6ᵗʰ Z77.11   **Contact with and (suspected) exposure to environmental pollution**

      Z77.110   **Contact with and (suspected) exposure to air pollution**

      Z77.111   **Contact with and (suspected) exposure to water pollution**

      Z77.112   **Contact with and (suspected) exposure to soil pollution**

      Z77.118   **Contact with and (suspected) exposure to other environmental pollution**

    ✓6ᵗʰ Z77.12   **Contact with and (suspected) exposure to hazards in the physical environment**

      Z77.120   **Contact with and (suspected) exposure to mold (toxic)**

Z77.121   **Contact with and (suspected) exposure to harmful algae and algae toxins**
Contact with and (suspected) exposure to (harmful) algae bloom NOS
Contact with and (suspected) exposure to blue-green algae bloom
Contact with and (suspected) exposure to brown tide
Contact with and (suspected) exposure to cyanobacteria bloom
Contact with and (suspected) exposure to Florida red tide
Contact with and (suspected) exposure to pfiesteria piscicida
Contact with and (suspected) exposure to red tide

Z77.122   **Contact with and (suspected) exposure to noise**

Z77.123   **Contact with and (suspected) exposure to radon and other naturally occuring radiation**
    EXCLUDES 2   radiation exposure as the cause of a confirmed condition (W88-W90, X39.0-)
      radiation sickness NOS (T66)

Z77.128   **Contact with and (suspected) exposure to other hazards in the physical environment**

✓5ᵗʰ Z77.2   **Contact with and (suspected) exposure to other hazardous substances**

    Z77.21   **Contact with and (suspected) exposure to potentially hazardous body fluids**

    Z77.22   **Contact with and (suspected) exposure to environmental tobacco smoke (acute) (chronic)**
     Exposure to second hand tobacco smoke (acute) (chronic)
     Passive smoking (acute) (chronic)
     EXCLUDES 1   nicotine dependence (F17.-)
      tobacco use (Z72.0)
     EXCLUDES 2   occupational exposure to environmental tobacco smoke (Z57.31)

    Z77.29   **Contact with and (suspected) exposure to other hazardous substances**
     AHA: 2016, 2Q, 33

Z77.9   **Other contact with and (suspected) exposures hazardous to health**

✓4ᵗʰ Z78   **Other specified health status**

    EXCLUDES 2   asymptomatic human immunodeficiency virus [HIV] infection status (Z21)
     postprocedural status (Z93- Z99)
     sex reassignment status (Z87.890)

    Z78.0   **Asymptomatic menopausal state**   Ⓐ♀
Menopausal state NOS
Postmenopausal status NOS
    EXCLUDES 2   symptomatic menopausal state (N95.1)

    Z78.1   **Physical restraint status**
     EXCLUDES 1   physical restraint due to a procedure - omit code
     DEF: Application of mechanical restraining devices or manual restraints; used to limit physical mobility of a patient.

    Z78.9   **Other specified health status**

✓4ᵗʰ Z79   **Long term (current) drug therapy**

    INCLUDES   long term (current) drug use for prophylactic purposes

    Code also any therapeutic drug level monitoring (Z51.81)

    EXCLUDES 2   drug abuse and dependence (F11-F19)
     drug use complicating pregnancy, childbirth, and the puerperium (O99.32-)
     long term (current) use of oral antidiabetic drugs (Z79.84)
     long term (current) use of oral hypoglycemic drugs (Z79.84)

    ✓5ᵗʰ Z79.0   **Long term (current) use of anticoagulants and antithrombotics/antiplatelets**
     EXCLUDES 2   long term (current) use of aspirin (Z79.82)

     Z79.01   **Long term (current) use of anticoagulants**

     Z79.02   **Long term (current) use of antithrombotics/antiplatelets**

    Z79.1   **Long term (current) use of non-steroidal anti-inflammatories (NSAID)**
     EXCLUDES 2   long term (current) use of aspirin (Z79.82)

    Z79.2   **Long term (current) use of antibiotics**

    Z79.3   **Long term (current) use of hormonal contraceptives**
     Long term (current) use of birth control pill or patch

    Z79.4   **Long term (current) use of insulin**   **HCC**

✓ Additional Character Req   ✓7ᵗʰ Placeholder Alert   Manifestation   **HCC** CMS-HCC Condition   ▽ Unspecified Code   ►◄ Revised Text   ● New Code   ▲ Revised Code Title

ICD-10-CM 2018   **1197**

✓5ᵗʰ **Z79.5 Long term (current) use of steroids**

    Z79.51 Long term (current) use of inhaled steroids

    Z79.52 Long term (current) use of systemic steroids

✓5ᵗʰ **Z79.8 Other long term (current) drug therapy**

    ✓6ᵗʰ **Z79.81 Long term (current) use of agents affecting estrogen receptors and estrogen levels**

      Code first, if applicable:
      malignant neoplasm of breast (C50.-)
      malignant neoplasm of prostate (C61)
      Use additional code, if applicable, to identify:
      estrogen receptor positive status (Z17.0)
      family history of breast cancer (Z80.3)
      genetic susceptibility to malignant neoplasm (cancer) (Z15.0-)
      personal history of breast cancer (Z85.3)
      personal history of prostate cancer (Z85.46)
      postmenopausal status (Z78.0)
      EXCLUDES 1 ► hormone replacement therapy ◄ (Z79.890)

      Z79.810 Long term (current) use of selective estrogen receptor modulators (SERMs)
       Long term (current) use of raloxifene (Evista)
       Long term (current) use of tamoxifen (Nolvadex)
       Long term (current) use of toremifene (Fareston)

      Z79.811 Long term (current) use of aromatase inhibitors
       Long term (current) use of anastrozole (Arimidex)
       Long term (current) use of exemestane (Aromasin)
       Long term (current) use of letrozole (Femara)

      Z79.818 Long term (current) use of other agents affecting estrogen receptors and estrogen levels
       Long term (current) use of estrogen receptor downregulators
       Long term (current) use of fulvestrant (Faslodex)
       Long term (current) use of gonadotropin-releasing hormone (GnRH) agonist
       Long term (current) use of goserelin acetate (Zoladex)
       Long term (current) use of leuprolide acetate (leuprorelin) (Lupron)
       Long term (current) use of megestrol acetate (Megace)

    Z79.82 Long term (current) use of aspirin

    Z79.83 Long term (current) use of bisphosphonates

    Z79.84 Long term (current) use of oral hypoglycemic drugs
      Long term (current) use of oral antidiabetic drugs
      EXCLUDES 2 long term (current) use of insulin (Z79.4)

    ✓6ᵗʰ **Z79.89 Other long term (current) drug therapy**

      Z79.890 Hormone replacement therapy

      Z79.891 Long term (current) use of opiate analgesic
       Long term (current) use of methadone for pain management
       EXCLUDES 1 methadone use NOS (F11.9-)
       use of methodone for treatment of heroin addiction (F11.2-)

      Z79.899 Other long term (current) drug therapy
       AHA: 2015, 4Q, 34; 2015, 3Q, 21

✓4ᵗʰ **Z80 Family history of primary malignant neoplasm**

    Z80.0 Family history of malignant neoplasm of digestive organs
      Conditions classifiable to C15-C26

    Z80.1 Family history of malignant neoplasm of trachea, bronchus and lung
      Conditions classifiable to C33-C34

    Z80.2 Family history of malignant neoplasm of other respiratory and intrathoracic organs
      Conditions classifiable to C30-C32, C37-C39

    Z80.3 Family history of malignant neoplasm of breast
      Conditions classifiable to C50-

    ✓5ᵗʰ **Z80.4 Family history of malignant neoplasm of genital organs**
      Conditions classifiable to C51-C63

      Z80.41 Family history of malignant neoplasm of ovary

      Z80.42 Family history of malignant neoplasm of prostate

      Z80.43 Family history of malignant neoplasm of testis

      Z80.49 Family history of malignant neoplasm of other genital organs

    ✓5ᵗʰ **Z80.5 Family history of malignant neoplasm of urinary tract**
      Conditions classifiable to C64-C68

      Z80.51 Family history of malignant neoplasm of kidney

      Z80.52 Family history of malignant neoplasm of bladder

      Z80.59 Family history of malignant neoplasm of other urinary tract organ

    Z80.6 Family history of leukemia
      Conditions classifiable to C91-C95

    Z80.7 Family history of other malignant neoplasms of lymphoid, hematopoietic and related tissues
      Conditions classifiable to C81-C90, C96-

    Z80.8 Family history of malignant neoplasm of other organs or systems
      Conditions classifiable to C00-C14, C40-C49, C69-C79

    Z80.9 Family history of malignant neoplasm, unspecified
      Conditions classifiable to C80.1

✓4ᵗʰ **Z81 Family history of mental and behavioral disorders**

    Z81.0 Family history of intellectual disabilities
      Conditions classifiable to F70-F79

    Z81.1 Family history of alcohol abuse and dependence
      Conditions classifiable to F10-

    Z81.2 Family history of tobacco abuse and dependence
      Conditions classifiable to F17-

    Z81.3 Family history of other psychoactive substance abuse and dependence
      Conditions classifiable to F11-F16, F18-F19

    Z81.4 Family history of other substance abuse and dependence
      Conditions classifiable to F55

    Z81.8 Family history of other mental and behavioral disorders
      Conditions classifiable elsewhere in F01-F99

✓4ᵗʰ **Z82 Family history of certain disabilities and chronic diseases (leading to disablement)**

    Z82.0 Family history of epilepsy and other diseases of the nervous system
      Conditions classifiable to G00-G99

    Z82.1 Family history of blindness and visual loss
      Conditions classifiable to H54-

    Z82.2 Family history of deafness and hearing loss
      Conditions classifiable to H90-H91

    Z82.3 Family history of stroke
      Conditions classifiable to I60-I64

    ✓5ᵗʰ **Z82.4 Family history of ischemic heart disease and other diseases of the circulatory system**
      Conditions classifiable to I00-I52, I65-I99

      Z82.41 Family history of sudden cardiac death

      Z82.49 Family history of ischemic heart disease and other diseases of the circulatory system

    Z82.5 Family history of asthma and other chronic lower respiratory diseases
      Conditions classifiable to J40-J47
      EXCLUDES 2 family history of other diseases of the respiratory system (Z83.6)

    ✓5ᵗʰ **Z82.6 Family history of arthritis and other diseases of the musculoskeletal system and connective tissue**
      Conditions classifiable to M00-M99

      Z82.61 Family history of arthritis

      Z82.62 Family history of osteoporosis

      Z82.69 Family history of other diseases of the musculoskeletal system and connective tissue

    ✓5ᵗʰ **Z82.7 Family history of congenital malformations, deformations and chromosomal abnormalities**
      Conditions classifiable to Q00-Q99

      Z82.71 Family history of polycystic kidney

      Z82.79 Family history of other congenital malformations, deformations and chromosomal abnormalities

    Z82.8 Family history of other disabilities and chronic diseases leading to disablement, not elsewhere classified

EXCLUDES 1 Not coded here   *EXCLUDES 2* Not included here   N Newborn Age: 0   P Pediatric Age: 0-17   M Maternity Age: 12-55   A Adult Age: 15-124   PDx Primary Dx

1198   ICD-10-CM 2018

√4th **Z83 Family history of other specific disorders**

EXCLUDES 2 *contact with and (suspected) exposure to communicable disease in the family (Z20.-)*

Z83.0 Family history of human immunodeficiency virus [HIV] disease
Conditions classifiable to B20

Z83.1 Family history of other infectious and parasitic diseases
Conditions classifiable to A00-B19, B25-B94, B99

Z83.2 Family history of diseases of the blood and blood-forming organs and certain disorders involving the immune mechanism
Conditions classifiable to D50-D89

Z83.3 Family history of diabetes mellitus
Conditions classifiable to E08-E13

√5th **Z83.4 Family history of other endocrine, nutritional and metabolic diseases**
Conditions classifiable to E00-E07, E15-E88

Z83.41 Family history of multiple endocrine neoplasia [MEN] syndrome

Z83.42 Family history of familial hypercholesterolemia

Z83.49 Family history of other endocrine, nutritional and metabolic diseases

√5th **Z83.5 Family history of eye and ear disorders**

√6th **Z83.51 Family history of eye disorders**
Conditions classifiable to H00-H53, H55-H59
EXCLUDES 2 *family history of blindness and visual loss (Z82.1)*

Z83.511 Family history of glaucoma

Z83.518 Family history of other specified eye disorder

Z83.52 Family history of ear disorders
Conditions classifiable to H60-H83, H92-H95
EXCLUDES 2 *family history of deafness and hearing loss (Z82.2)*

Z83.6 Family history of other diseases of the respiratory system
Conditions classifiable to J00-J39, J60-J99
EXCLUDES 2 *family history of asthma and other chronic lower respiratory diseases (Z82.5)*

√5th **Z83.7 Family history of diseases of the digestive system**
Conditions classifiable to K00-K93

Z83.71 Family history of colonic polyps
EXCLUDES 1 ~~family history of malignant neoplasm of digestive organs (Z80.0)~~
EXCLUDES 2 ▶family history of malignant neoplasm of digestive organs (Z80.0)◀

Z83.79 Family history of other diseases of the digestive system

√4th **Z84 Family history of other conditions**

Z84.0 Family history of diseases of the skin and subcutaneous tissue
Conditions classifiable to L00-L99

Z84.1 Family history of disorders of kidney and ureter
Conditions classifiable to N00-N29

Z84.2 Family history of other diseases of the genitourinary system
Conditions classifiable to N30-N99

Z84.3 Family history of consanguinity

√5th **Z84.8 Family history of other specified conditions**

Z84.81 Family history of carrier of genetic disease

Z84.82 Family history of sudden infant death syndrome
Family history of SIDS

Z84.89 Family history of other specified conditions

√4th **Z85 Personal history of malignant neoplasm**
Code first any follow-up examination after treatment of malignant neoplasm (Z08)
Use additional code to identify:
alcohol use and dependence (F10.-)
exposure to environmental tobacco smoke (Z77.22)
history of tobacco dependence (Z87.891)
occupational exposure to environmental tobacco smoke (Z57.31)
tobacco dependence (F17.-)
tobacco use (Z72.0)
EXCLUDES 2 *personal history of benign neoplasm (Z86.01-)*
personal history of carcinoma-in-situ (Z86.00-)

√5th **Z85.0 Personal history of malignant neoplasm of digestive organs**
AHA: 2017, 1Q, 9

Z85.00 Personal history of malignant neoplasm of unspecified digestive organ   ▽

Z85.01 Personal history of malignant neoplasm of esophagus
Conditions classifiable to C15

√6th **Z85.02 Personal history of malignant neoplasm of stomach**

Z85.020 Personal history of malignant carcinoid tumor of stomach
Conditions classifiable to C7A.092

Z85.028 Personal history of other malignant neoplasm of stomach
Conditions classifiable to C16

√6th **Z85.03 Personal history of malignant neoplasm of large intestine**

Z85.030 Personal history of malignant carcinoid tumor of large intestine
Conditions classifiable to C7A.022-C7A.025, C7A.029

Z85.038 Personal history of other malignant neoplasm of large intestine
Conditions classifiable to C18

√6th **Z85.04 Personal history of malignant neoplasm of rectum, rectosigmoid junction, and anus**

Z85.040 Personal history of malignant carcinoid tumor of rectum
Conditions classifiable to C7A.026

Z85.048 Personal history of other malignant neoplasm of rectum, rectosigmoid junction, and anus
Conditions classifiable to C19-C21

Z85.05 Personal history of malignant neoplasm of liver
Conditions classifiable to C22

√6th **Z85.06 Personal history of malignant neoplasm of small intestine**

Z85.060 Personal history of malignant carcinoid tumor of small intestine
Conditions classifiable to C7A.01-

Z85.068 Personal history of other malignant neoplasm of small intestine
Conditions classifiable to C17

Z85.07 Personal history of malignant neoplasm of pancreas
Conditions classifiable to C25

Z85.09 Personal history of malignant neoplasm of other digestive organs

√5th **Z85.1 Personal history of malignant neoplasm of trachea, bronchus and lung**

√6th **Z85.11 Personal history of malignant neoplasm of bronchus and lung**

Z85.110 Personal history of malignant carcinoid tumor of bronchus and lung
Conditions classifiable to C7A.090

Z85.118 Personal history of other malignant neoplasm of bronchus and lung
Conditions classifiable to C34

Z85.12 Personal history of malignant neoplasm of trachea
Conditions classifiable to C33

√5th **Z85.2 Personal history of malignant neoplasm of other respiratory and intrathoracic organs**

Z85.20 Personal history of malignant neoplasm of unspecified respiratory organ   ▽

Z85.21 Personal history of malignant neoplasm of larynx
Conditions classifiable to C32

Z85.22 Personal history of malignant neoplasm of nasal cavities, middle ear, and accessory sinuses
Conditions classifiable to C30-C31

√ Additional Character Req   √x7th Placeholder Alert   Manifestation   HCC CMS-HCC Condition   ▽ Unspecified Code   ▶◀ Revised Text   ● New Code   ▲ Revised Code Title

Chapter 21. Factors Influencing Health Status and Contact with Health Services

✓6ᵗʰ **Z85.23 Personal history of malignant neoplasm of thymus**

    Z85.230 Personal history of malignant carcinoid tumor of thymus
        Conditions classifiable to C7A.091

    Z85.238 Personal history of other malignant neoplasm of thymus
        Conditions classifiable to C37

Z85.29 Personal history of malignant neoplasm of other respiratory and intrathoracic organs

Z85.3 Personal history of malignant neoplasm of breast
    Conditions classifiable to C50.-

✓5ᵗʰ **Z85.4 Personal history of malignant neoplasm of genital organs**
    Conditions classifiable to C51-C63

    Z85.40 Personal history of malignant neoplasm of unspecified female genital organ ♀▽

    Z85.41 Personal history of malignant neoplasm of cervix uteri ♀

    Z85.42 Personal history of malignant neoplasm of other parts of uterus ♀

    Z85.43 Personal history of malignant neoplasm of ovary ♀

    Z85.44 Personal history of malignant neoplasm of other female genital organs ♀

    Z85.45 Personal history of malignant neoplasm of unspecified male genital organ ♂▽

    Z85.46 Personal history of malignant neoplasm of prostate ♂

    Z85.47 Personal history of malignant neoplasm of testis ♂

    Z85.48 Personal history of malignant neoplasm of epididymis ♂

    Z85.49 Personal history of malignant neoplasm of other male genital organs ♂

✓5ᵗʰ **Z85.5 Personal history of malignant neoplasm of urinary tract**
    Conditions classifiable to C64-C68

    Z85.50 Personal history of malignant neoplasm of unspecified urinary tract organ ▽

    Z85.51 Personal history of malignant neoplasm of bladder

✓6ᵗʰ   **Z85.52 Personal history of malignant neoplasm of kidney**
        EXCLUDES 1 personal history of malignant neoplasm of renal pelvis (Z85.53)

        Z85.520 Personal history of malignant carcinoid tumor of kidney
            Conditions classifiable to C7A.093

        Z85.528 Personal history of other malignant neoplasm of kidney
            Conditions classifiable to C64

    Z85.53 Personal history of malignant neoplasm of renal pelvis

    Z85.54 Personal history of malignant neoplasm of ureter

    Z85.59 Personal history of malignant neoplasm of other urinary tract organ

Z85.6 Personal history of leukemia
    Conditions classifiable to C91-C95
    EXCLUDES 1 leukemia in remission C91.0-C95.9 with 5th character 1

✓5ᵗʰ **Z85.7 Personal history of other malignant neoplasms of lymphoid, hematopoietic and related tissues**

    Z85.71 Personal history of Hodgkin lymphoma
        Conditions classifiable to C81

    Z85.72 Personal history of non-Hodgkin lymphomas
        Conditions classifiable to C82-C85

    Z85.79 Personal history of other malignant neoplasms of lymphoid, hematopoietic and related tissues
        Conditions classifiable to C88-C90, C96
        EXCLUDES 1 multiple myeloma in remission (C90.01)
            plasma cell leukemia in remission (C90.11)
            plasmacytoma in remission (C90.21)

✓5ᵗʰ **Z85.8 Personal history of malignant neoplasms of other organs and systems**
    Conditions classifiable to C00-C14, C40-C49, C69-C75, C7A.098, C76-C79

✓6ᵗʰ   **Z85.81 Personal history of malignant neoplasm of lip, oral cavity, and pharynx**

        Z85.810 Personal history of malignant neoplasm of tongue

        Z85.818 Personal history of malignant neoplasm of other sites of lip, oral cavity, and pharynx

        Z85.819 Personal history of malignant neoplasm of unspecified site of lip, oral cavity, and pharynx ▽

✓6ᵗʰ **Z85.82 Personal history of malignant neoplasm of skin**

    Z85.820 Personal history of malignant melanoma of skin
        Conditions classifiable to C43

    Z85.821 Personal history of Merkel cell carcinoma
        Conditions classifiable to C4A

    Z85.828 Personal history of other malignant neoplasm of skin
        Conditions classifiable to C44

✓6ᵗʰ **Z85.83 Personal history of malignant neoplasm of bone and soft tissue**

    Z85.830 Personal history of malignant neoplasm of bone

    Z85.831 Personal history of malignant neoplasm of soft tissue
        EXCLUDES 2 personal history of malignant neoplasm of skin (Z85.82-)

✓6ᵗʰ **Z85.84 Personal history of malignant neoplasm of eye and nervous tissue**

    Z85.840 Personal history of malignant neoplasm of eye

    Z85.841 Personal history of malignant neoplasm of brain

    Z85.848 Personal history of malignant neoplasm of other parts of nervous tissue

✓6ᵗʰ **Z85.85 Personal history of malignant neoplasm of endocrine glands**

    Z85.850 Personal history of malignant neoplasm of thyroid

    Z85.858 Personal history of malignant neoplasm of other endocrine glands

Z85.89 Personal history of malignant neoplasm of other organs and systems

Z85.9 Personal history of malignant neoplasm, unspecified ▽
    Conditions classifiable to C7A.00, C80.1

✓4ᵗʰ **Z86 Personal history of certain other diseases**
    Code first any follow-up examination after treatment (Z09)

✓5ᵗʰ **Z86.0 Personal history of in-situ and benign neoplasms and neoplasms of uncertain behavior**
    EXCLUDES 2 personal history of malignant neoplasms (Z85.-)
    AHA: 2017, 1Q, 9

✓6ᵗʰ   **Z86.00 Personal history of in-situ neoplasm**
        Conditions classifiable to D00-D09

        Z86.000 Personal history of in-situ neoplasm of breast
            Personal history of cervical intraepithelial neoplasia III [CIN III]

        Z86.001 Personal history of in-situ neoplasm of cervix uteri ♀

        Z86.008 Personal history of in-situ neoplasm of other site
            Personal history of vaginal intraepithelial neoplasia III [VAIN III]
            Personal history of vulvar intraepithelial neoplasia III [VIN III]

✓6ᵗʰ   **Z86.01 Personal history of benign neoplasm**

        Z86.010 Personal history of colonic polyps
            AHA: 2017, 1Q, 14

        Z86.011 Personal history of benign neoplasm of the brain

        Z86.012 Personal history of benign carcinoid tumor

        Z86.018 Personal history of other benign neoplasm
            AHA: 2017, 1Q, 14

    Z86.03 Personal history of neoplasm of uncertain behavior

✓5ᵗʰ **Z86.1 Personal history of infectious and parasitic diseases**
    Conditions classifiable to A00-B89, B99
    EXCLUDES 1 personal history of infectious diseases specific to a body system
        sequelae of infectious and parasitic diseases (B90-B94)

    Z86.11 Personal history of tuberculosis

    Z86.12 Personal history of poliomyelitis

    Z86.13 Personal history of malaria

    Z86.14 Personal history of Methicillin resistant Staphylococcus aureus infection
        Personal history of MRSA infection

EXCLUDES 1 Not coded here   EXCLUDES 2 Not included here   N Newborn Age: 0   P Pediatric Age: 0-17   M Maternity Age: 12-55   A Adult Age: 15-124   PDx Primary Dx

1200   ICD-10-CM 2018

Z86.19   **Personal history of other infectious and parasitic diseases**

Z86.2   **Personal history of diseases of the blood and blood-forming organs and certain disorders involving the immune mechanism**
Conditions classifiable to D50-D89

✓5ᵗʰ **Z86.3**   **Personal history of endocrine, nutritional and metabolic diseases**
Conditions classifiable to E00-E88

Z86.31   **Personal history of diabetic foot ulcer**
EXCLUDES 2   *current diabetic foot ulcer (E08.621, E09.621, E10.621, E11.621, E13.621)*

Z86.32   **Personal history of gestational diabetes**   ♀
Personal history of conditions classifiable to O24.4-
EXCLUDES 1   *gestational diabetes mellitus in current pregnancy (O24.4-)*

Z86.39   **Personal history of other endocrine, nutritional and metabolic disease**

✓5ᵗʰ **Z86.5**   **Personal history of mental and behavioral disorders**
Conditions classifiable to F40-F59

Z86.51   **Personal history of combat and operational stress reaction**   A

Z86.59   **Personal history of other mental and behavioral disorders**

✓5ᵗʰ **Z86.6**   **Personal history of diseases of the nervous system and sense organs**
Conditions classifiable to G00-G99, H00-H95
EXCLUDES 2   *personal history of anaphylactic shock (Z87.892)*

Z86.61   **Personal history of infections of the central nervous system**
Personal history of encephalitis
Personal history of meningitis

Z86.69   **Personal history of other diseases of the nervous system and sense organs**

✓5ᵗʰ **Z86.7**   **Personal history of diseases of the circulatory system**
Conditions classifiable to I00-I99
EXCLUDES 2   *old myocardial infarction (I25.2)*
personal history of anaphylactic shock (Z87.892)
postmyocardial infarction syndrome (I24.1)

✓6ᵗʰ **Z86.71**   **Personal history of venous thrombosis and embolism**

Z86.711   **Personal history of pulmonary embolism**
Z86.718   **Personal history of other venous thrombosis and embolism**

Z86.72   **Personal history of thrombophlebitis**

Z86.73   **Personal history of transient ischemic attack (TIA), and cerebral infarction without residual deficits**
Personal history of prolonged reversible ischemic neurological deficit (PRIND)
Personal history of stroke NOS without residual deficits
EXCLUDES 1   *personal history of traumatic brain injury (Z87.820)*
sequelae of cerebrovascular disease (I69.-)
AHA: 2012, 4Q, 92

Z86.74   **Personal history of sudden cardiac arrest**
Personal history of sudden cardiac death successfully resuscitated

Z86.79   **Personal history of other diseases of the circulatory system**

✓4ᵗʰ **Z87**   **Personal history of other diseases and conditions**
Code first any follow-up examination after treatment (Z09)

✓5ᵗʰ **Z87.0**   **Personal history of diseases of the respiratory system**
Conditions classifiable to J00-J99

Z87.01   **Personal history of pneumonia (recurrent)**
Z87.09   **Personal history of other diseases of the respiratory system**

✓5ᵗʰ **Z87.1**   **Personal history of diseases of the digestive system**
Conditions classifiable to K00-K93

Z87.11   **Personal history of peptic ulcer disease**
Z87.19   **Personal history of other diseases of the digestive system**
AHA: 2017, 1Q, 14

Z87.2   **Personal history of diseases of the skin and subcutaneous tissue**
Conditions classifiable to L00-L99
EXCLUDES 2   *personal history of diabetic foot ulcer (Z86.31)*

✓5ᵗʰ **Z87.3**   **Personal history of diseases of the musculoskeletal system and connective tissue**
Conditions classifiable to M00-M99
EXCLUDES 2   *personal history of (healed) traumatic fracture (Z87.81)*

✓6ᵗʰ **Z87.31**   **Personal history of (healed) nontraumatic fracture**

Z87.310   **Personal history of (healed) osteoporosis fracture**
Personal history of (healed) fragility fracture
Personal history of (healed) collapsed vertebra due to osteoporosis

Z87.311   **Personal history of (healed) other pathological fracture**
Personal history of (healed) collapsed vertebra NOS
EXCLUDES 2   *personal history of osteoporosis fracture (Z87.310)*

Z87.312   **Personal history of (healed) stress fracture**
Personal history of (healed) fatigue fracture

Z87.39   **Personal history of other diseases of the musculoskeletal system and connective tissue**

✓5ᵗʰ **Z87.4**   **Personal history of diseases of genitourinary system**
Conditions classifiable to N00-N99

✓6ᵗʰ **Z87.41**   **Personal history of dysplasia of the female genital tract**
EXCLUDES 1   *personal history of intraepithelial neoplasia III of female genital tract* ▶*(Z86.001, Z86.008)*◀
personal history of malignant neoplasm of female genital tract (Z85.40-Z85.44)

Z87.410   **Personal history of cervical dysplasia**   ♀
Z87.411   **Personal history of vaginal dysplasia**   ♀
Z87.412   **Personal history of vulvar dysplasia**   ♀

Z87.42   **Personal history of other diseases of the female genital tract**   ♀

✓6ᵗʰ **Z87.43**   **Personal history of diseases of the male genital organs**

Z87.430   **Personal history of prostatic dysplasia**   ♂
EXCLUDES 1   *personal history of malignant neoplasm of prostate (Z85.46)*

Z87.438   **Personal history of other diseases of male genital organs**   ♂

✓6ᵗʰ **Z87.44**   **Personal history of diseases of the urinary system**
EXCLUDES 1   *personal history of malignant neoplasm of cervix uteri (Z85.41)*

Z87.440   **Personal history of urinary (tract) infections**
Z87.441   **Personal history of nephrotic syndrome**
Z87.442   **Personal history of urinary calculi**
Personal history of kidney stones
Z87.448   **Personal history of other diseases of urinary system**

✓5ᵗʰ **Z87.5**   **Personal history of complications of pregnancy, childbirth and the puerperium**
Conditions classifiable to O00-O9A
EXCLUDES 2   *recurrent pregnancy loss (N96)*

Z87.51   **Personal history of pre-term labor**   ♀
EXCLUDES 1   *current pregnancy with history of pre-term labor (O09.21-)*

Z87.59   **Personal history of other complications of pregnancy, childbirth and the puerperium**   ♀
Personal history of trophoblastic disease

✓ Additional Character Req   ✓x7ᵗʰ Placeholder Alert   Manifestation   HCC CMS-HCC Condition   ▽ Unspecified Code   ▶◀ Revised Text   ● New Code   ▲ Revised Code Title

✓5ᵗʰ **Z87.7 Personal history of (corrected) congenital malformations**
Conditions classifiable to Q00-Q89 that have been repaired or corrected

EXCLUDES 1   congenital malformations that have been partially corrected or repaired but which still require medical treatment—code to condition

EXCLUDES 2   other postprocedural states (Z98.-)
personal history of medical treatment (Z92.-)
presence of cardiac and vascular implants and grafts (Z95.-)
presence of other devices (Z97.-)
presence of other functional implants (Z96.-)
transplanted organ and tissue status (Z94.-)

✓6ᵗʰ **Z87.71 Personal history of (corrected) congenital malformations of** genitourinary system

Z87.710 Personal history of (corrected) hypospadias   ♂

Z87.718 Personal history of other specified (corrected) congenital malformations of genitourinary system

✓6ᵗʰ **Z87.72 Personal history of (corrected) congenital malformations of** nervous system and sense organs

Z87.720 Personal history of (corrected) congenital malformations of eye

Z87.721 Personal history of (corrected) congenital malformations of ear

Z87.728 Personal history of other specified (corrected) congenital malformations of nervous system and sense organs

✓6ᵗʰ **Z87.73 Personal history of (corrected) congenital malformations of** digestive system

Z87.730 Personal history of (corrected) cleft lip and palate

Z87.738 Personal history of other specified (corrected) congenital malformations of digestive system

Z87.74 Personal history of (corrected) congenital malformations of heart and circulatory system

Z87.75 Personal history of (corrected) congenital malformations of respiratory system

Z87.76 Personal history of (corrected) congenital malformations of integument, limbs and musculoskeletal system

✓6ᵗʰ **Z87.79 Personal history of other (corrected) congenital malformations**

Z87.790 Personal history of (corrected) congenital malformations of face and neck

Z87.798 Personal history of other (corrected) congenital malformations

✓5ᵗʰ **Z87.8 Personal history of other specified conditions**
EXCLUDES 2   personal history of self harm (Z91.5)

Z87.81 Personal history of (healed) traumatic fracture
EXCLUDES 2   personal history of (healed) nontraumatic fracture (Z87.31-)

✓6ᵗʰ **Z87.82 Personal history of other (healed)** physical injury and trauma
Conditions classifiable to S00-T88, except traumatic fractures

Z87.820 Personal history of traumatic brain injury
EXCLUDES 1   personal history of transient ischemic attack (TIA), and cerebral infarction without residual deficits (Z86.73)

Z87.821 Personal history of retained foreign body fully removed

Z87.828 Personal history of other (healed) physical injury and trauma

✓6ᵗʰ **Z87.89 Personal history of other specified conditions**

Z87.890 Personal history of sex reassignment

Z87.891 Personal history of nicotine dependence
EXCLUDES 1   current nicotine dependence (F17.2-)
AHA: 2017, 2Q, 27

Z87.892 Personal history of anaphylaxis
Code also allergy status such as:
allergy status to drugs, medicaments and biological substances (Z88.-)
allergy status, other than to drugs and biological substances (Z91.0-)

Z87.898 Personal history of other specified conditions
AHA: 2013, 1Q, 21

✓4ᵗʰ **Z88 Allergy status to drugs, medicaments and biological substances**
EXCLUDES 2   allergy status, other than to drugs and biological substances (Z91.0-)
AHA: 2015, 3Q, 23

Z88.0 Allergy status to penicillin

Z88.1 Allergy status to other antibiotic agents status

Z88.2 Allergy status to sulfonamides status

Z88.3 Allergy status to other anti-infective agents status

Z88.4 Allergy status to anesthetic agent status

Z88.5 Allergy status to narcotic agent status

Z88.6 Allergy status to analgesic agent status

Z88.7 Allergy status to serum and vaccine status

Z88.8 Allergy status to other drugs, medicaments and biological substances status

Z88.9 Allergy status to unspecified drugs, medicaments and biological substances status   ▽

✓4ᵗʰ **Z89 Acquired absence of limb**
INCLUDES   amputation status
postprocedural loss of limb
post-traumatic loss of limb
EXCLUDES 1   acquired deformities of limbs (M20-M21)
congenital absence of limbs (Q71-Q73)

✓5ᵗʰ **Z89.0 Acquired absence of** thumb and other finger(s)

✓6ᵗʰ **Z89.01 Acquired absence of** thumb

Z89.011 Acquired absence of right thumb

Z89.012 Acquired absence of left thumb

Z89.019 Acquired absence of unspecified thumb ▽

✓6ᵗʰ **Z89.02 Acquired absence of other** finger(s)
EXCLUDES 2   acquired absence of thumb (Z89.01-)

Z89.021 Acquired absence of right finger(s)

Z89.022 Acquired absence of left finger(s)

Z89.029 Acquired absence of unspecified finger(s)   ▽

✓5ᵗʰ **Z89.1 Acquired absence of** hand and wrist

✓6ᵗʰ **Z89.11 Acquired absence of** hand

Z89.111 Acquired absence of right hand

Z89.112 Acquired absence of left hand

Z89.119 Acquired absence of unspecified hand ▽

✓6ᵗʰ **Z89.12 Acquired absence of** wrist
Disarticulation at wrist

Z89.121 Acquired absence of right wrist

Z89.122 Acquired absence of left wrist

Z89.129 Acquired absence of unspecified wrist ▽

✓5ᵗʰ **Z89.2 Acquired absence of** upper limb above wrist

✓6ᵗʰ **Z89.20 Acquired absence of** upper limb, unspecified level

Z89.201 Acquired absence of right upper limb, unspecified level   ▽

Z89.202 Acquired absence of left upper limb, unspecified level

Z89.209 Acquired absence of unspecified upper limb, unspecified level   ▽
Acquired absence of arm NOS

✓6ᵗʰ **Z89.21 Acquired absence of** upper limb below elbow

Z89.211 Acquired absence of right upper limb below elbow

Z89.212 Acquired absence of left upper limb below elbow

Z89.219 Acquired absence of unspecified upper limb below elbow   ▽

✓6ᵗʰ **Z89.22 Acquired absence of** upper limb above elbow
Disarticulation at elbow

Z89.221 Acquired absence of right upper limb above elbow

Z89.222 Acquired absence of left upper limb above elbow

Z89.229 Acquired absence of unspecified upper limb above elbow   ▽

EXCLUDES 1 Not coded here   EXCLUDES 2 Not included here   N Newborn Age: 0   P Pediatric Age: 0-17   M Maternity Age: 12-55   A Adult Age: 15-124   PDx Primary Dx

1202   ICD-10-CM 2018

✓6th Z89.23 Acquired absence of shoulder
Acquired absence of shoulder joint following explantation of shoulder joint prosthesis, with or without presence of antibiotic-impregnated cement spacer

     Z89.231   Acquired absence of right shoulder
     Z89.232   Acquired absence of left shoulder
     Z89.239   Acquired absence of unspecified shoulder ▽

✓5th Z89.4 Acquired absence of toe(s), foot, and ankle

   ✓6th Z89.41 Acquired absence of great toe
     Z89.411   Acquired absence of right great toe   HCC
     Z89.412   Acquired absence of left great toe   HCC
     Z89.419   Acquired absence of unspecified great toe   HCC ▽

   ✓6th Z89.42 Acquired absence of other toe(s)
     EXCLUDES 2   acquired absence of great toe (Z89.41-)
     Z89.421   Acquired absence of other right toe(s)   HCC
     Z89.422   Acquired absence of other left toe(s)   HCC
     Z89.429   Acquired absence of other toe(s), unspecified side   HCC ▽

   ✓6th Z89.43 Acquired absence of foot
     Z89.431   Acquired absence of right foot   HCC
     Z89.432   Acquired absence of left foot   HCC
     Z89.439   Acquired absence of unspecified foot   HCC ▽

   ✓6th Z89.44 Acquired absence of ankle
     Disarticulation of ankle
     Z89.441   Acquired absence of right ankle   HCC
     Z89.442   Acquired absence of left ankle   HCC
     Z89.449   Acquired absence of unspecified ankle   HCC ▽

✓5th Z89.5 Acquired absence of leg below knee

   ✓6th Z89.51 Acquired absence of leg below knee
     Z89.511   Acquired absence of right leg below knee   HCC
     Z89.512   Acquired absence of left leg below knee   HCC
     Z89.519   Acquired absence of unspecified leg below knee   HCC ▽

   ✓6th Z89.52 Acquired absence of knee
     Acquired absence of knee joint following explantation of knee joint prosthesis, with or without presence of antibiotic-impregnated cement spacer
     Z89.521   Acquired absence of right knee
     Z89.522   Acquired absence of left knee
     Z89.529   Acquired absence of unspecified knee ▽

✓5th Z89.6 Acquired absence of leg above knee

   ✓6th Z89.61 Acquired absence of leg above knee
     Acquired absence of leg NOS
     Disarticulation at knee
     Z89.611   Acquired absence of right leg above knee   HCC
     Z89.612   Acquired absence of left leg above knee   HCC
     Z89.619   Acquired absence of unspecified leg above knee   HCC ▽

   ✓6th Z89.62 Acquired absence of hip
     Acquired absence of hip joint following explantation of hip joint prosthesis, with or without presence of antibiotic-impregnated cement spacer
     Disarticulation at hip
     Z89.621   Acquired absence of right hip joint
     Z89.622   Acquired absence of left hip joint
     Z89.629   Acquired absence of unspecified hip joint ▽

   Z89.9 Acquired absence of limb, unspecified ▽

✓4th Z90 Acquired absence of organs, not elsewhere classified
   INCLUDES   postprocedural or post-traumatic loss of body part NEC
   EXCLUDES 1   congenital absence—see Alphabetical Index
   EXCLUDES 2   postprocedural absence of endocrine glands (E89.-)

   ✓5th Z90.0 Acquired absence of part of head and neck
     Z90.01   Acquired absence of eye
     Z90.02   Acquired absence of larynx

     Z90.09   Acquired absence of other part of head and neck
       Acquired absence of nose
       EXCLUDES 2   teeth (K08.1)

   ✓5th Z90.1 Acquired absence of breast and nipple
     Z90.10   Acquired absence of unspecified breast and nipple ▽
     Z90.11   Acquired absence of right breast and nipple
     Z90.12   Acquired absence of left breast and nipple
     Z90.13   Acquired absence of bilateral breasts and nipples

   Z90.2 Acquired absence of lung [part of]
   Z90.3 Acquired absence of stomach [part of]

   ✓5th Z90.4 Acquired absence of other specified parts of digestive tract

     ✓6th Z90.41 Acquired absence of pancreas
       Code also exocrine pancreatic insufficiency (K86.81)
       Use additional code to identify any associated:
       insulin use (Z79.4)
       diabetes mellitus, postpancreatectomy (E13.-)
       Z90.410   Acquired total absence of pancreas
         Acquired absence of pancreas NOS
       Z90.411   Acquired partial absence of pancreas
     Z90.49   Acquired absence of other specified parts of digestive tract

   Z90.5 Acquired absence of kidney
   Z90.6 Acquired absence of other parts of urinary tract
     Acquired absence of bladder

   ✓5th Z90.7 Acquired absence of genital organ(s)
     EXCLUDES 1   personal history of sex reassignment (Z87.890)
     EXCLUDES 2   female genital mutilation status (N90.81-)

     ✓6th Z90.71 Acquired absence of cervix and uterus
       Z90.710   Acquired absence of both cervix and uterus ♀
         Acquired absence of uterus NOS
         Status post total hysterectomy
       Z90.711   Acquired absence of uterus with remaining cervical stump ♀
         Status post partial hysterectomy with remaining cervical stump
       Z90.712   Acquired absence of cervix with remaining uterus ♀

     ✓6th Z90.72 Acquired absence of ovaries
       Z90.721   Acquired absence of ovaries, unilateral ♀
       Z90.722   Acquired absence of ovaries, bilateral ♀
     Z90.79   Acquired absence of other genital organ(s)

   ✓5th Z90.8 Acquired absence of other organs
     Z90.81   Acquired absence of spleen
     Z90.89   Acquired absence of other organs

✓4th Z91 Personal risk factors, not elsewhere classified
   EXCLUDES 2   contact with and (suspected) exposures hazardous to health (Z77.-)
     exposure to pollution and other problems related to physical environment (Z77.1-)
     ▶female genital mutilation status (N90.81-)◀
     personal history of physical injury and trauma (Z87.81, Z87.82-)
     occupational exposure to risk factors (Z57.-)

   ✓5th Z91.0 Allergy status, other than to drugs and biological substances
     EXCLUDES 2   allergy status to drugs, medicaments, and biological substances (Z88.-)

     ✓6th Z91.01 Food allergy status
       EXCLUDES 2   food additives allergy status (Z91.02)
       Z91.010   Allergy to peanuts
       Z91.011   Allergy to milk products
         EXCLUDES 1   lactose intolerance (E73.-)
       Z91.012   Allergy to eggs
       Z91.013   Allergy to seafood
         Allergy to shellfish
         Allergy to octopus or squid ink
       Z91.018   Allergy to other foods
         Allergy to nuts other than peanuts
     Z91.02   Food additives allergy status

     ✓6th Z91.03 Insect allergy status
       Z91.030   Bee allergy status
       Z91.038   Other insect allergy status

✓ Additional Character Req   ✓x7th Placeholder Alert   Manifestation   HCC CMS-HCC Condition   ▽ Unspecified Code   ▶◀ Revised Text   ● New Code   ▲ Revised Code Title

ICD-10-CM 2018   Z89.23–Z91.038   1203

✓6ᵗʰ **Z91.04** **Nonmedicinal substance allergy status**

Z91.040 **Latex allergy status**
Latex sensitivity status

Z91.041 **Radiographic dye allergy status**
Allergy status to contrast media used for diagnostic X-ray procedure

Z91.048 **Other nonmedicinal substance allergy status**

Z91.09 **Other allergy status, other than to drugs and biological substances**

✓5ᵗʰ **Z91.1** **Patient's noncompliance with medical treatment and regimen**

Z91.11 **Patient's noncompliance with dietary regimen**

✓6ᵗʰ **Z91.12** **Patient's intentional underdosing of medication regimen**
Code first underdosing of medication (T36-T50) with fifth or sixth character 6
EXCLUDES 1　adverse effect of prescribed drug taken as directed—code to adverse effect poisoning (overdose)—code to poisoning

Z91.120 **Patient's intentional underdosing of medication regimen due to financial hardship**

Z91.128 **Patient's intentional underdosing of medication regimen for other reason**

✓6ᵗʰ **Z91.13** **Patient's unintentional underdosing of medication regimen**
Code first underdosing of medication (T36-T50) with fifth or sixth character 6
EXCLUDES 1　adverse effect of prescribed drug taken as directed—code to adverse effect poisoning (overdose)—code to poisoning

Z91.130 **Patient's unintentional underdosing of medication regimen due to age-related debility**

Z91.138 **Patient's unintentional underdosing of medication regimen for other reason**

Z91.14 **Patient's other noncompliance with medication regimen**
Patient's underdosing of medication NOS

Z91.15 **Patient's noncompliance with renal dialysis** HCC

Z91.19 **Patient's noncompliance with other medical treatment and regimen**
▶Nonadherence to medical treatment◀

✓5ᵗʰ **Z91.4** **Personal history of psychological trauma, not elsewhere classified**

✓6ᵗʰ **Z91.41** **Personal history of adult abuse**
EXCLUDES 2　personal history of abuse in childhood (Z62.81-)

Z91.410 **Personal history of adult physical and sexual abuse** Ⓐ
EXCLUDES 1　current adult physical abuse (T74.11, T76.11) current adult sexual abuse (T74.21, T76.11)

Z91.411 **Personal history of adult psychological abuse** Ⓐ

Z91.412 **Personal history of adult neglect** Ⓐ
EXCLUDES 1　current adult neglect (T74.01, T76.01)

Z91.419 **Personal history of unspecified adult abuse** Ⓐ▽

Z91.49 **Other personal history of psychological trauma, not elsewhere classified**

Z91.5 **Personal history of self-harm**
Personal history of parasuicide
Personal history of self-poisoning
Personal history of suicide attempt

✓5ᵗʰ **Z91.8** **Other specified personal risk factors, not elsewhere classified**

Z91.81 **History of falling**
At risk for falling

Z91.82 **Personal history of military deployment** Ⓐ
Individual (civilian or military) with past history of military war, peacekeeping and humanitarian deployment (current or past conflict)
Returned from military deployment

Z91.83 *Wandering in diseases classified elsewhere*
Code first underlying disorder such as:
Alzheimer's disease (G30.-)
autism or pervasive developmental disorder (F84.-)
intellectual disabilities (F70-F79)
unspecified dementia with behavioral disturbance (F03.9-)

✓6ᵗʰ **Z91.84** **Oral health risk factors**

Z91.841 **Risk for dental caries, low**

Z91.842 **Risk for dental caries, moderate**

Z91.843 **Risk for dental caries, high**

Z91.849 **Unspecified risk for dental caries** ▽

Z91.89 **Other specified personal risk factors, not elsewhere classified**
AHA: 2017, 1Q, 45

✓4ᵗʰ **Z92** **Personal history of medical treatment**
EXCLUDES 2　postprocedural states (Z98.-)

Z92.0 **Personal history of contraception**
EXCLUDES 1　counseling or management of current contraceptive practices (Z30.-)
long term (current) use of contraception (Z79.3)
presence of (intrauterine) contraceptive device (Z97.5)

✓5ᵗʰ **Z92.2** **Personal history of drug therapy**
EXCLUDES 2　long term (current) drug therapy (Z79.-)

Z92.21 **Personal history of antineoplastic chemotherapy**

Z92.22 **Personal history of monoclonal drug therapy**

Z92.23 **Personal history of estrogen therapy**

✓6ᵗʰ **Z92.24** **Personal history of steroid therapy**

Z92.240 **Personal history of inhaled steroid therapy**

Z92.241 **Personal history of systemic steroid therapy**
Personal history of steroid therapy NOS

Z92.25 **Personal history of immunosupression therapy**
EXCLUDES 2　personal history of steroid therapy (Z92.24)

Z92.29 **Personal history of other drug therapy**

Z92.3 **Personal history of irradiation**
Personal history of exposure to therapeutic radiation
EXCLUDES 1　exposure to radiation in the physical environment (Z77.12)
occupational exposure to radiation (Z57.1)

✓5ᵗʰ **Z92.8** **Personal history of other medical treatment**

Z92.81 **Personal history of extracorporeal membrane oxygenation (ECMO)**

Z92.82 **Status post administration of tPA (rtPA) in a different facility within the last 24 hours prior to admission to current facility**
Code first condition requiring tPA administration, such as:
acute cerebral infarction (I63.-)
acute myocardial infarction (I21-, I22-)
AHA: 2013, 4Q, 124

Z92.83 **Personal history of failed moderate sedation**
Personal history of failed conscious sedation
EXCLUDES 2　failed moderate sedation during procedure (T88.52)

Z92.84 **Personal history of unintended awareness under general anesthesia**
EXCLUDES 2　unintended awareness under general anesthesia during procedure (T88.53)

Z92.89 **Personal history of other medical treatment**

✓4ᵗʰ **Z93** **Artificial opening status**
EXCLUDES 1　artificial openings requiring attention or management (Z43.-)
complications of external stoma (J95.0-, K94.-, N99.5-)

Z93.0 **Tracheostomy status** HCC
AHA: 2013, 4Q, 129

Z93.1 **Gastrostomy status** HCC

Z93.2 **Ileostomy status** HCC

Z93.3 **Colostomy status** HCC

Z93.4 **Other artificial openings of gastrointestinal tract status** HCC

✓5ᵗʰ **Z93.5** **Cystostomy status**

Z93.50 **Unspecified cystostomy status** HCC ▽

Z93.51 **Cutaneous-vesicostomy status** HCC

Z93.52 **Appendico-vesicostomy status** HCC

Z93.59 **Other cystostomy status** HCC

Z93.6 Other artificial openings of urinary tract status   `HCC`
Nephrostomy status
Ureterostomy status
Urethrostomy status

~~**Z93.8 Other artificial opening status**~~   `HCC`

Z93.9 Artificial opening status, unspecified   `HCC` ▽

✓⁴ᵗʰ **Z94 Transplanted organ and tissue status**
   `INCLUDES` organ or tissue replaced by heterogenous or homogenous transplant
   `EXCLUDES 1` *complications of transplanted organ or tissue—see Alphabetical Index*
   `EXCLUDES 2` *presence of vascular grafts (Z95.-)*

Z94.0 Kidney transplant status

Z94.1 Heart transplant status   `HCC`
   `EXCLUDES 1` *artificial heart status (Z95.812)*
     heart-valve replacement status (Z95.2-Z95.4)

Z94.2 Lung transplant status   `HCC`

Z94.3 Heart and lungs transplant status   `HCC`

Z94.4 Liver transplant status   `HCC`

Z94.5 Skin transplant status
Autogenous skin transplant status

Z94.6 Bone transplant status

Z94.7 Corneal transplant status

✓⁵ᵗʰ **Z94.8 Other transplanted organ and tissue status**
   Z94.81 Bone marrow transplant status   `HCC`
   Z94.82 Intestine transplant status   `HCC`
   Z94.83 Pancreas transplant status   `HCC`
   Z94.84 Stem cells transplant status   `HCC`
   Z94.89 Other transplanted organ and tissue status

Z94.9 Transplanted organ and tissue status, unspecified ▽

✓⁴ᵗʰ **Z95 Presence of cardiac and vascular implants and grafts**
   `EXCLUDES 1` ~~*complications of cardiac and vascular devices, implants and grafts (T82.-)*~~
   `EXCLUDES 2` ▶*complications of cardiac and vascular devices, implants and grafts (T82.-)*◀

Z95.0 Presence of cardiac pacemaker
Presence of cardiac resynchronization therapy (CRT-P) pacemaker
   `EXCLUDES 1` *adjustment or management of cardiac device (Z45.0-)*
     adjustment or management of cardiac pacemaker (Z45.0)
     presence of automatic (implantable) cardiac defibrillator with synchronous cardiac pacemaker (Z95.810)

Z95.1 Presence of aortocoronary bypass graft
Presence of coronary artery bypass graft

Z95.2 Presence of prosthetic heart valve
Presence of heart valve NOS

Z95.3 Presence of xenogenic heart valve

Z95.4 Presence of other heart-valve replacement

Z95.5 Presence of coronary angioplasty implant and graft
   `EXCLUDES 1` *coronary angioplasty status without implant and graft (Z98.61)*

✓⁵ᵗʰ **Z95.8 Presence of other cardiac and vascular implants and grafts**
   ✓⁶ᵗʰ **Z95.81 Presence of other cardiac implants and grafts**
     Z95.810 Presence of automatic (implantable) cardiac defibrillator
Presence of automatic (implantable) cardiac defibrillator with synchronous cardiac pacemaker
Presence of cardiac resynchronization therapy defibrillator (CRT-D)
Presence of cardioverter-defibrillator (ICD)
     Z95.811 Presence of heart assist device   `HCC`
     Z95.812 Presence of fully implantable artificial heart   `HCC`
     Z95.818 Presence of other cardiac implants and grafts

✓⁶ᵗʰ **Z95.82 Presence of other vascular implants and grafts**
   Z95.820 Peripheral vascular angioplasty status with implants and grafts
     `EXCLUDES 1` *peripheral vascular angioplasty without implant and graft (Z98.62)*
   Z95.828 Presence of other vascular implants and grafts
Presence of intravascular prosthesis NEC

Z95.9 Presence of cardiac and vascular implant and graft, unspecified ▽

✓⁴ᵗʰ **Z96 Presence of other functional implants**
   `EXCLUDES 2` *complications of internal prosthetic devices, implants and grafts (T82-T85)*
     fitting and adjustment of prosthetic and other devices (Z44-Z46)

Z96.0 Presence of urogenital implants

Z96.1 Presence of intraocular lens
Presence of pseudophakia

✓⁵ᵗʰ **Z96.2 Presence of otological and audiological implants**
   Z96.20 Presence of otological and audiological implant, unspecified ▽
   Z96.21 Cochlear implant status
   Z96.22 Myringotomy tube(s) status
   Z96.29 Presence of other otological and audiological implants
Presence of bone-conduction hearing device
Presence of eustachian tube stent
Stapes replacement

Z96.3 Presence of artificial larynx

✓⁵ᵗʰ **Z96.4 Presence of endocrine implants**
   Z96.41 Presence of insulin pump (external) (internal)
   Z96.49 Presence of other endocrine implants

Z96.5 Presence of tooth-root and mandibular implants

✓⁵ᵗʰ **Z96.6 Presence of orthopedic joint implants**
   Z96.60 Presence of unspecified orthopedic joint implant ▽
   ✓⁶ᵗʰ **Z96.61 Presence of artificial shoulder joint**
     Z96.611 Presence of right artificial shoulder joint
     Z96.612 Presence of left artificial shoulder joint
     Z96.619 Presence of unspecified artificial shoulder joint ▽
   ✓⁶ᵗʰ **Z96.62 Presence of artificial elbow joint**
     Z96.621 Presence of right artificial elbow joint
     Z96.622 Presence of left artificial elbow joint
     Z96.629 Presence of unspecified artificial elbow joint ▽
   ✓⁶ᵗʰ **Z96.63 Presence of artificial wrist joint**
     Z96.631 Presence of right artificial wrist joint
     Z96.632 Presence of left artificial wrist joint
     Z96.639 Presence of unspecified artificial wrist joint ▽
   ✓⁶ᵗʰ **Z96.64 Presence of artificial hip joint**
Hip-joint replacement (partial) (total)
     Z96.641 Presence of right artificial hip joint
     Z96.642 Presence of left artificial hip joint
     Z96.643 Presence of artificial hip joint, bilateral
     Z96.649 Presence of unspecified artificial hip joint ▽
   ✓⁶ᵗʰ **Z96.65 Presence of artificial knee joint**
     Z96.651 Presence of right artificial knee joint
     Z96.652 Presence of left artificial knee joint
     Z96.653 Presence of artificial knee joint, bilateral
     Z96.659 Presence of unspecified artificial knee joint ▽
   ✓⁶ᵗʰ **Z96.66 Presence of artificial ankle joint**
     Z96.661 Presence of right artificial ankle joint
     Z96.662 Presence of left artificial ankle joint
     Z96.669 Presence of unspecified artificial ankle joint ▽
   ✓⁶ᵗʰ **Z96.69 Presence of other orthopedic joint implants**
     Z96.691 Finger-joint replacement of right hand
     Z96.692 Finger-joint replacement of left hand
     Z96.693 Finger-joint replacement, bilateral
     Z96.698 Presence of other orthopedic joint implants

☑ Additional Character Req   ✓ˣ⁷ᵗʰ Placeholder Alert   Manifestation   `HCC` CMS-HCC Condition   ▽ Unspecified Code   ▶◀ Revised Text   ● New Code   ▲ Revised Code Title

ICD-10-CM 2018   **1205**

Z96.7 Presence of other bone and tendon implants
Presence of skull plate

✓5ᵗʰ **Z96.8 Presence of other specified functional implants**

    Z96.81 Presence of artificial skin

    Z96.89 Presence of other specified functional implants

Z96.9 Presence of functional implant, unspecified   ▽

✓4ᵗʰ **Z97 Presence of other devices**

    EXCLUDES 1 *complications of internal prosthetic devices, implants and grafts (T82-T85)*
        fitting and adjustment of prosthetic and other devices (Z44-Z46)

    EXCLUDES 2 *presence of cerebrospinal fluid drainage device (Z98.2)*

Z97.0 Presence of artificial eye

✓5ᵗʰ **Z97.1 Presence of artificial limb (complete) (partial)**

    Z97.10 Presence of artificial limb (complete) (partial), unspecified   ▽

    Z97.11 Presence of artificial right arm (complete) (partial)

    Z97.12 Presence of artificial left arm (complete) (partial)

    Z97.13 Presence of artificial right leg (complete) (partial)

    Z97.14 Presence of artificial left leg (complete) (partial)

    Z97.15 Presence of artificial arms, bilateral (complete) (partial)

    Z97.16 Presence of artificial legs, bilateral (complete) (partial)

Z97.2 Presence of dental prosthetic device (complete) (partial)
Presence of dentures (complete) (partial)

Z97.3 Presence of spectacles and contact lenses

Z97.4 Presence of external hearing-aid

Z97.5 Presence of (intrauterine) contraceptive device   ♀

    EXCLUDES 1 *checking, reinsertion or removal of implantable subdermal contraceptive (Z30.46)*
        checking, reinsertion or removal of intrauterine contraceptive device (Z30.43-)

Z97.8 Presence of other specified devices

✓4ᵗʰ **Z98 Other postprocedural states**

    EXCLUDES 2 *aftercare (Z43-Z49, Z51)*
        follow-up medical care (Z08- Z09)
        postprocedural complication—see Alphabetical Index

Z98.0 Intestinal bypass and anastomosis status

    EXCLUDES 2 *bariatric surgery status (Z98.84)*
        gastric bypass status (Z98.84)
        obesity surgery status (Z98.84)

Z98.1 Arthrodesis status

Z98.2 Presence of cerebrospinal fluid drainage device
Presence of CSF shunt

Z98.3 Post therapeutic collapse of lung status
Code first underlying disease

✓5ᵗʰ **Z98.4 Cataract extraction status**
Use additional code to identify intraocular lens implant status (Z96.1)

    EXCLUDES 1 *aphakia (H27.0)*

    Z98.41 Cataract extraction status, right eye

    Z98.42 Cataract extraction status, left eye

    Z98.49 Cataract extraction status, unspecified eye   ▽

✓5ᵗʰ **Z98.5 Sterilization status**

    EXCLUDES 1 *female infertility (N97.-)*
        male infertility (N46.-)

    Z98.51 Tubal ligation status   ♀

    Z98.52 Vasectomy status   Ⓐ ♂

✓5ᵗʰ **Z98.6 Angioplasty status**

    Z98.61 Coronary angioplasty status

        EXCLUDES 1 *coronary angioplasty status with implant and graft (Z95.5)*

    Z98.62 Peripheral vascular angioplasty status

        EXCLUDES 1 *peripheral vascular angioplasty status with implant and graft (Z95.820)*

✓5ᵗʰ **Z98.8 Other specified postprocedural states**

✓6ᵗʰ **Z98.81 Dental procedure status**

    Z98.810 Dental sealant status

    Z98.811 Dental restoration status
        Dental crown status
        Dental fillings status

    Z98.818 Other dental procedure status

Z98.82 Breast implant status

    EXCLUDES 1 *breast implant removal status (Z98.86)*

Z98.83 Filtering (vitreous) bleb after glaucoma surgery status

    EXCLUDES 1 *inflammation (infection) of postprocedural bleb (H59.4-)*

Z98.84 Bariatric surgery status
Gastric banding status
Gastric bypass status for obesity
Obesity surgery status

    EXCLUDES 1 *bariatric surgery status complicating pregnancy, childbirth, or the puerperium (O99.84)*

    EXCLUDES 2 *intestinal bypass and anastomosis status (Z98.0)*

Z98.85 Transplanted organ removal status
Transplanted organ previously removed due to complication, failure, rejection or infection

    EXCLUDES 1 *encounter for removal of transplanted organ—code to complication of transplanted organ (T86.-)*

Z98.86 Personal history of breast implant removal

✓6ᵗʰ **Z98.87 Personal history of in utero procedure**

    Z98.870 Personal history of in utero procedure during pregnancy   ♀

        EXCLUDES 2 *complications from in utero procedure for current pregnancy (O35.7)*
                supervision of current pregnancy with history of in utero procedure during previous pregnancy (O09.82-)

    Z98.871 Personal history of in utero procedure while a fetus

✓6ᵗʰ **Z98.89 Other specified postprocedural states**

    Z98.890 Other specified postprocedural states
        Personal history of surgery, not elsewhere classified

    Z98.891 History of uterine scar from previous surgery

        EXCLUDES 1 *maternal care due to uterine scar from previous surgery (O34.2-)*

✓4ᵗʰ **Z99 Dependence on enabling machines and devices, not elsewhere classified**

    EXCLUDES 1 *cardiac pacemaker status (Z95.0)*

Z99.0 Dependence on aspirator

✓5ᵗʰ **Z99.1 Dependence on respirator**
Dependence on ventilator

    Z99.11 Dependence on respirator [ventilator] status   HCC
        AHA: 2015, 1Q, 21

    Z99.12 Encounter for respirator [ventilator] dependence during power failure   HCC PDx

        EXCLUDES 1 *mechanical complication of respirator [ventilator] (J95.850)*

Z99.2 Dependence on renal dialysis   HCC
Hemodialysis status
Peritoneal dialysis status
Presence of arteriovenous shunt for dialysis
Renal dialysis status NOS

    EXCLUDES 1 *encounter for fitting and adjustment of dialysis catheter (Z49.0-)*

    EXCLUDES 2 *noncompliance with renal dialysis (Z91.15)*

    AHA: 2016, 1Q, 12; 2013, 4Q, 125

Z99.3 Dependence on wheelchair
Wheelchair confinement status
Code first cause of dependence, such as:
    muscular dystrophy (G71.0)
    obesity (E66.-)

EXCLUDES 1 Not coded here   EXCLUDES 2 Not included here   Ⓝ Newborn Age: 0   Ⓟ Pediatric Age: 0-17   Ⓜ Maternity Age: 12-55   Ⓐ Adult Age: 15-124   PDx Primary Dx

1206   ICD-10-CM 2018

✓5ᵗʰ **Z99.8** **Dependence on other enabling machines and devices**

Z99.81 **Dependence on supplemental oxygen**
Dependence on long-term oxygen
AHA: 2013, 4Q, 129

Z99.89 **Dependence on other enabling machines and devices**
Dependence on machine or device NOS

Appendixes

Appendix A: 10 Steps to Correct Coding

Follow the 10 steps below to correctly code encounters for health care services.

Step 1: Identify the reason for the visit or encounter (i.e., a sign, symptom, diagnosis and/or condition).

The medical record documentation should accurately reflect the patient's condition, using terminology that includes specific diagnoses and symptoms or clearly states the reasons for the encounter.

Choosing the main term that best describes the reason chiefly responsible for the service provided is the most important step in coding. If symptoms are present and documented but a definitive diagnosis has not yet been determined, code the symptoms. **For outpatient cases, do not code conditions that are referred to as "rule out," "suspected," "probable," or "questionable."** Diagnoses often are not established at the time of the initial encounter/visit and may require two or more visits to be established. Code only what is documented in the available records and only to the highest degree of certainty known at the time of the patient's visit, unless it is an inpatient medical record, in which case uncertain diagnoses may be reported if documented at the time of discharge.

Step 2: After selecting the reason for the encounter, always consult the alphabetic index before verifying code selection in the tabular section.

The most critical rule is to begin code selection in the *alphabetic index.* Never turn first to the tabular list. The index provides cross-references, essential and nonessential modifiers, and inclusion terms not found in the tabular list. To prevent coding errors, always use both the alphabetic index (to identify a code) and the tabular list (to verify a code), as the index does not include the important instructional notes found in the tabular list. An added benefit of using the tabular list, which groups like things together, is that while looking at one code in the list, a coder might see a more specific one that would have been missed had the coder relied solely on the alphabetic index. Additionally, many of the codes require a fourth, fifth, sixth, or seventh, character to be valid, and many of these characters can be found only in the tabular list.

Step 3: Locate the main term entry.

The alphabetic index is a listing of conditions, which may be expressed as nouns or eponyms, with critical use of adjectives. Some conditions known by several names have multiple main entries. Reasons for encounters may be located under general terms such as admission, encounter, and examination. Other general terms such as history of, status post, or presence (of) are used to locate factors influencing health.

Step 4: Read cross-references listed with the main term or the subterm.

Cross-references such as *"see"* and *"see also"* are identified by italicized type and should always be checked to ensure that all alternative terms are researched.

Step 5: Review entries for modifiers.

Nonessential modifiers are the terms in parentheses following the main term entry. These parenthetical terms are supplementary words or explanatory information that may or may not appear in the diagnostic statement and do not affect code selection. The subterms listed under the main term are essential modifiers that do affect coding assignment. Each line of indent represents a more specific code entry. The nonessential modifiers apply to the subterms following a main term except when they are mutually exclusive, in which case the subterm takes precedence. For example, if "acute" is listed as a nonessential modifier but there is a subentry for "chronic," then the nonessential modifier of "acute" does not apply.

Step 6: Interpret abbreviations, cross-references, default codes, additional characters, and brackets.

The abbreviation NEC (not elsewhere classified) that follows some main terms or subterms indicates that there is no specific code for the condition even though the medical documentation may be very specific. The code next to the main term is called the default code. It represents the condition most commonly associated with the main term or the unspecified code for the main term. Additional characters may be required to construct the code; the tabular list must be referenced to determine what those specific characters should be. The alphabetic index uses brackets [ ] to enclose manifestation codes that can be

used only as secondary codes to the underlying condition code immediately preceding it. Both codes must be reported in this multiple-coding situation.

Step 7: Choose a potential code and locate it in the tabular list.

The coder must follow any Includes, Excludes 1 and Excludes 2 notes, and other instructional notes, such as "Code first" and "Use additional code," listed in the tabular list for the chapter, category, subcategory, and subclassification level of code selection that direct the coder to use a different or additional code. Any codes in the tabular range, A00.0- through T88.9-, may be used to identify the diagnostic reason for the encounter. The tabular list encompasses many codes describing disease and injury classifications (e.g., infectious and parasitic diseases, neoplasms, symptoms, nervous and circulatory system etc.).

Codes that describe symptoms and signs, as opposed to definitive diagnoses, should be used for reporting purposes when an established diagnosis has not been made (confirmed) by the physician. Chapter 18 of the ICD-10-CM code book, "Symptoms, Signs, and Abnormal Clinical and Laboratory Findings, Not Elsewhere Classified" (codes R00.--R99), contains many, but not all, codes for symptoms.

ICD-10-CM classifies encounters with health care providers for circumstances other than a disease or injury using codes in chapter 21, "Factors Influencing Health Status and Contact with Health Services" (codes Z00-Z99). Circumstances other than a disease or injury often are recorded as chiefly responsible for the encounter.

Step 8: Determine whether the code is at the highest level of specificity.

A code is invalid if it has not been coded to the full number of characters (greatest level of specificity) required. Codes in ICD-10-CM can contain from three up to seven alphanumeric characters. A three-character code is to be used only if the category is not further subdivided into four-, five-, six-, or seven-character codes. Placeholder character X is used both to allow for future expansion and as a placeholder for empty characters in a code that requires a seventh character but has no fourth, fifth, or sixth character. Certain categories require seventh characters that apply to all codes in that category. Always check the category level for applicable seventh characters for that category.

Step 9: Assign the code.

Having reviewed all relevant information concerning the possible code choices, assign the code that most completely describes the condition.

Repeat steps one through nine for all additional documented conditions that meet the following criteria:

- Conditions that currently exist at the time of the visit
- Conditions that require or affect patient care, treatment, or management

Step 10: Sequence codes correctly.

Sequencing is the order in which the codes are listed on the claim. List first the ICD-10-CM code for the diagnosis, condition, problem, or other reason for the encounter/visit, which is shown in the medical record to be chiefly responsible for the services provided. List additional codes that describe any coexisting conditions. Follow the official coding guidelines (see section II, "Selection of Principal Diagnosis"; section III, "Reporting Additional Diagnoses"; and section IV, "Diagnostic Coding and Reporting Guidelines for Outpatient Services") on proper sequencing of codes.

Coding Examples

Diagnosis: Anorexia

Step 1: The reason for the encounter was the condition, anorexia.

Step 2: Consult the alphabetic index.

Step 3: Locate the main term "Anorexia."

Step 4: There are no cross-references to check.

Step 5: Note that there are two possible subterms (essential modifiers), "hysterical" and "nervosa," neither of which is documented in this instance and therefore cannot be used in code selection. The code listed next to the main term is called the default code selection.

Step 6: There are no abbreviations, cross-references, additional character icons, or brackets.

Step 7: Turn to code R63.0 in the tabular list and read the instructional notes. In this case the Excludes 1 note indicates that anorexia nervosa and loss of appetite determined to be of nonorganic origin should be coded to a code from chapter 5. The diagnostic statement does not indicate nonorganic origin.

Step 8: There is no further division of the category past the fourth character subcategory. Therefore, the subcategory code level is the highest level of specificity.

Step 9: The default code, R63.0 Anorexia, is the correct code selection

Step 10: Since anorexia is listed as the chief reason for the health care encounter, the first-listed, or principal, diagnosis is R63.0. Note that this is a chapter 18 symptom code but can be assigned since the provider did not establish a more definitive diagnosis.

Diagnosis: Acute bronchitis

Step 1: The reason for the encounter was the condition, acute bronchitis.

Step 2: Consult the alphabetic index.

Step 3: Locate the main term "Bronchitis."

Step 4: There are cross-references to interpret.

Step 5: Review entries for modifiers. Since "acute" is not listed as a nonessential modifier, read past the "with" modifier until you find the subterm "acute or subacute" with a nonessential modifier of "with bronchospasm or obstruction," code J20.9.

Step 6: There are no abbreviations, cross-references, additional character icons, or brackets.

Step 7: Since there are no more appropriate subterms, turn to code J20.9 in the tabular list. The Includes note under category J20 does refer to other alternative terms for acute bronchitis. Note that the inclusion term list is not exhaustive but is only a representative selection of diagnoses that are included in the subcategory. The Excludes 1 note refers bronchitis and tracheobronchitis NOS to category J40. There are several Excludes 2 notes that, if applicable, can be coded in addition to this code.

Step 8: Note that the subcategories included in J20 represent acute bronchitis due to various infectious organisms that would be selected if identified in the documentation. In this case, the organism was not identified and there is no further division of the category past the fourth character subcategory. Therefore, the subcategory code level is the highest level of specificity.

Step 9: Assign code J20.9 Acute bronchitis, unspecified.

Step 10: Repeat steps 1-9 for any additional code assignments.

Diagnosis: Infectious diarrhea

Step 1: The reason for the encounter was the condition, infectious diarrhea.

Step 2: Consult the alphabetic index.

Step 3: Locate the main term "Diarrhea" in the alphabetic index.

Step 4: There are no cross-references to check.

Step 5: Review entries for modifiers. Note that the nonessential modifiers (in parentheses) after the main term do not include the term "infectious," which means that the coder should search the subterms for the term "infectious." The subterm "infectious" refers to code A09.

Step 6: There are no abbreviations, cross-references, additional character icons, or brackets.

Step 7: Locate code A09 in the tabular list, and read all instructional notes under the main category and subcategories. The Includes notes does not list the term "infectious diarrhea" under code A09; however, as instructed by the alphabetic index, you should code the condition to A09. The ICD-10-CM code book implies that infectious diarrhea is the same as infectious gastroenteritis, enteritis, and colitis.

Step 8: There is no further division of the category past the third-character category level. Therefore, the category code level is the highest level of specificity. The final code assignment would be A09.

Step 9: Assign code A09 Infectious gastroenteritis and colitis, unspecified.

Step 10: Since infectious diarrhea is listed as the chief reason for the health care encounter, the first-listed, or principal, diagnosis is A09.

Diagnosis: Decubitus ulcer of right elbow with skin loss and necrosis of subcutaneous tissue

Step 1: The reason for the encounter was the condition, decubitus ulcer.

Step 2: Consult the alphabetic index.

Step 3: Locate the main term "Ulcer" in the alphabetic index.

Step 4: There are no cross-references to check.

Step 5: This entry does not have any important nonessential modifiers; however, there are other terms such as ulcerated, ulcerating, etc., that are included as main terms. Locate the subterm "decubitus" and note that there is an italicized cross-reference to "see Ulcer, pressure, by site." Go to the subterm "pressure" and locate "elbow," which refers to code L89.0-.

Step 6: Note that the code L89.0 is followed by a dash and an additional character icon, which indicate that more characters are required. From here, the tabular list can be consulted at code L89.0-.

Step 7: Locate code L89.0 in the tabular list, and check the category level L89 for any instructional, Includes, and Excludes 1 and 2 notes. Note that "decubitus" is an Includes note under L89 Pressure ulcer. Excludes 2 notes indicate that if this were documented as a diabetic pressure ulcer, it would be necessary to use a code from chapter 4.

Step 8: Read through the subcategory codes under L89.0 and note that the fifth character describes laterality. Locate the right elbow at subcategory L89.01. See that an additional sixth character is now needed to complete the code. The sixth character specifies the stage of the ulcer, which can be determined either by the specific documentation of the stage (e.g., stage 1, stage 2) or in this case, a description that matches one of the Includes notes that follow each stage code. For example, the description in this case of "skin loss and necrosis of the subcutaneous tissue" matches the Includes notes under L89.013 Pressure ulcer of right elbow, stage 3.

Step 9: Assign code L89.013 Pressure ulcer of right elbow, stage 3

Step 10: Since the decubitus ulcer is listed as the chief reason for the health care encounter, the first-listed, or principal, diagnosis is L89.013. However, according to the Code first instructional note at the L89 category level, gangrene would be sequenced before the pressure ulcer if it were documented.

Diagnosis: First visit for bimalleolar fracture of the right ankle due to trauma

Step 1: The reason for the encounter was the condition, bimalleolar fracture of the right ankle.

Step 2: Consult the alphabetic index.

Step 3: Locate the main term "Fracture" in the alphabetic index.

Step 4: Note that the first main term for Fracture is pathological with cross-reference to "see also Fracture, traumatic." Locate the main term "Fracture, traumatic."

Step 5: Review entries for nonessential modifiers. Locate the subterms "ankle," "bimalleolar." Note that "displaced" is a nonessential modifier following "bimalleolar," indicating that S82.84- is the default code unless the fracture is specified as nondisplaced.

Step 6: Note that code S82.84- is followed by a dash and an additional character icon, both of which indicate that more characters are required. From here, the tabular list can be consulted at code S82.84.

Step 7: Locate code S82.84 Bimalleolar fracture of lower leg, in the tabular list and check the category level S82 for any instructional, Includes, and Excludes 1 and 2 notes. See the instructional notes indicating that fractures not specified as displaced or nondisplaced default to displaced, and fractures not designated as open or closed default to closed. See also the list of appropriate seventh characters to be added to all codes from category S82.

Step 8: Read through the subcategory codes under S82.84, and note that the sixth character specifies displaced or nondisplaced and laterality. Locate the displaced bimalleolar fracture of the right lower leg at code S82.841. See that an additional seventh character is still needed to complete the code. The seventh character specifies the type of encounter and whether the fracture is open or closed. Use character A listed in the box at the category level to describe initial encounter, closed fracture.

Step 9: Assign code S82.841A Displaced bimalleolar fracture of right lower leg, initial encounter for closed fracture.

Step 10: Since this is an injury code, code additionally any external cause, place of occurrence, and activity codes, with the injury (fracture) sequenced first.

Code	Description
A09	Infectious gastroenteritis and colitis, unspecified
A33	Tetanus neonatorum
A34	Obstetrical tetanus
A35	Other tetanus
A46	Erysipelas
A55	Chlamydial lymphogranuloma (venereum)
A57	Chancroid
A58	Granuloma inguinale
A64	Unspecified sexually transmitted disease
A65	Nonvenereal syphilis
A70	Chlamydia psittaci infections
A78	Q fever
A86	Unspecified viral encephalitis
A89	Unspecified viral infection of central nervous system
A90	Dengue fever [classical dengue]
A91	Dengue hemorrhagic fever
A94	Unspecified arthropod-borne viral fever
A99	Unspecified viral hemorrhagic fever
B03	Smallpox
B04	Monkeypox
B09	Unspecified viral infection characterized by skin and mucous membrane lesions
B20	Human immunodeficiency virus [HIV] disease
B49	Unspecified mycosis
B54	Unspecified malaria
B59	Pneumocystosis
B64	Unspecified protozoal disease
B72	Dracunculiasis
B75	Trichinellosis
B79	Trichuriasis
B80	Enterobiasis
B86	Scabies
B89	Unspecified parasitic disease
B91	Sequelae of poliomyelitis
B92	Sequelae of leprosy
C01	Malignant neoplasm of base of tongue
C07	Malignant neoplasm of parotid gland
C12	Malignant neoplasm of pyriform sinus
C19	Malignant neoplasm of rectosigmoid junction
C20	Malignant neoplasm of rectum
C23	Malignant neoplasm of gallbladder
C33	Malignant neoplasm of trachea
C37	Malignant neoplasm of thymus
C52	Malignant neoplasm of vagina
C55	Malignant neoplasm of uterus, part unspecified
C58	Malignant neoplasm of placenta
C61	Malignant neoplasm of prostate
C73	Malignant neoplasm of thyroid gland
D34	Benign neoplasm of thyroid gland
D45	Polycythemia vera
D62	Acute posthemorrhagic anemia
D65	Disseminated intravascular coagulation [defibrination syndrome]
D66	Hereditary factor VIII deficiency
D67	Hereditary factor IX deficiency
D71	Functional disorders of polymorphonuclear neutrophils
D77	Other disorders of blood and blood-forming organs in diseases classified elsewhere
E02	Subclinical iodine-deficiency hypothyroidism
E15	Nondiabetic hypoglycemic coma
E35	Disorders of endocrine glands in diseases classified elsewhere
E40	Kwashiorkor
E41	Nutritional marasmus
E42	Marasmic kwashiorkor
E43	Unspecified severe protein-calorie malnutrition
E45	Retarded development following protein-calorie malnutrition
E46	Unspecified protein-calorie malnutrition
E52	Niacin deficiency [pellagra]
E54	Ascorbic acid deficiency
E58	Dietary calcium deficiency
E59	Dietary selenium deficiency
E60	Dietary zinc deficiency
E65	Localized adiposity
E68	Sequelae of hyperalimentation
F04	Amnestic disorder due to known physiological condition
F05	Delirium due to known physiological condition
F09	Unspecified mental disorder due to known physiological condition
F21	Schizotypal disorder
F22	Delusional disorders
F23	Brief psychotic disorder
F24	Shared psychotic disorder
F28	Other psychotic disorder not due to a substance or known physiological condition
F29	Unspecified psychosis not due to a substance or known physiological condition
F39	Unspecified mood [affective] disorder
F53	Puerperal psychosis
F54	Psychological and behavioral factors associated with disorders or diseases classified elsewhere
F59	Unspecified behavioral syndromes associated with physiological disturbances and physical factors
F66	Other sexual disorders
F69	Unspecified disorder of adult personality and behavior
F70	Mild intellectual disabilities
F71	Moderate intellectual disabilities
F72	Severe intellectual disabilities
F73	Profound intellectual disabilities
F78	Other intellectual disabilities
F79	Unspecified intellectual disabilities
F82	Specific developmental disorder of motor function
F88	Other disorders of psychological development
F89	Unspecified disorder of psychological development
F99	Mental disorder, not otherwise specified
G01	Meningitis in bacterial diseases classified elsewhere
G02	Meningitis in other infectious and parasitic diseases classified elsewhere
G07	Intracranial and intraspinal abscess and granuloma in diseases classified elsewhere
G08	Intracranial and intraspinal phlebitis and thrombophlebitis
G09	Sequelae of inflammatory diseases of central nervous system
G10	Huntington's disease
G14	Postpolio syndrome
G20	Parkinson's disease
G26	Extrapyramidal and movement disorders in diseases classified elsewhere
G35	Multiple sclerosis
G53	Cranial nerve disorders in diseases classified elsewhere
G55	Nerve root and plexus compressions in diseases classified elsewhere
G59	Mononeuropathy in diseases classified elsewhere
G63	Polyneuropathy in diseases classified elsewhere
G64	Other disorders of peripheral nervous system
G92	Toxic encephalopathy
G94	Other disorders of brain in diseases classified elsewhere
H22	Disorders of iris and ciliary body in diseases classified elsewhere
H28	Cataract in diseases classified elsewhere
H32	Chorioretinal disorders in diseases classified elsewhere
H36	Retinal disorders in diseases classified elsewhere
H42	Glaucoma in diseases classified elsewhere
I00	Rheumatic fever without heart involvement
I10	Essential (primary) hypertension
I32	Pericarditis in diseases classified elsewhere
I38	Endocarditis, valve unspecified

I39	Endocarditis and heart valve disorders in diseases classified elsewhere
I41	Myocarditis in diseases classified elsewhere
I43	Cardiomyopathy in diseases classified elsewhere
I52	Other heart disorders in diseases classified elsewhere
I76	Septic arterial embolism
I81	Portal vein thrombosis
I96	Gangrene, not elsewhere classified
J00	Acute nasopharyngitis (common cold)
J13	Pneumonia due to Streptococcus pneumoniae
J14	Pneumonia due to Hemophilus influenzae
J17	Pneumonia in diseases classified elsewhere
J22	Unspecified acute lower respiratory infection
J36	Peritonsillar abscess
J40	Bronchitis, not specified as acute or chronic
J42	Unspecified chronic bronchitis
J60	Coalworker's pneumoconiosis
J61	Pneumoconiosis due to asbestos and other mineral fibers
J64	Unspecified pneumoconiosis
J65	Pneumoconiosis associated with tuberculosis
J80	Acute respiratory distress syndrome
J82	Pulmonary eosinophilia, not elsewhere classified
J90	Pleural effusion, not elsewhere classified
J99	Respiratory disorders in diseases classified elsewhere
K23	Disorders of esophagus in diseases classified elsewhere
K30	Functional dyspepsia
K36	Other appendicitis
K37	Unspecified appendicitis
K67	Disorders of peritoneum in infectious diseases classified elsewhere
K77	Liver disorders in diseases classified elsewhere
K87	Disorders of gallbladder, biliary tract and pancreas in diseases classified elsewhere
L00	Staphylococcal scalded skin syndrome
L14	Bullous disorders in diseases classified elsewhere
L22	Diaper dermatitis
L26	Exfoliative dermatitis
L42	Pityriasis rosea
L45	Papulosquamous disorders in diseases classified elsewhere
L52	Erythema nodosum
L54	Erythema in diseases classified elsewhere
L62	Nail disorders in diseases classified elsewhere
L80	Vitiligo
L83	Acanthosis nigricans
L84	Corns and callosities
L86	Keratoderma in diseases classified elsewhere
L88	Pyoderma gangrenosum
L99	Other disorders of skin and subcutaneous tissue in diseases classified elsewhere
N08	Glomerular disorders in diseases classified elsewhere
N10	Acute tubulo-interstitial nephritis
N12	Tubulo-interstitial nephritis, not specified as acute or chronic
N16	Renal tubulo-interstitial disorders in diseases classified elsewhere
N19	Unspecified kidney failure
N22	Calculus of urinary tract in diseases classified elsewhere
N23	Unspecified renal colic
N29	Other disorders of kidney and ureter in diseases classified elsewhere
N33	Bladder disorders in diseases classified elsewhere
N37	Urethral disorders in diseases classified elsewhere
N51	Disorders of male genital organs in diseases classified elsewhere
N62	Hypertrophy of breast
N72	Inflammatory disease of cervix uteri
N74	Female pelvic inflammatory disorders in diseases classified elsewhere
N86	Erosion and ectropion of cervix uteri
N96	Recurrent pregnancy loss
O68	Labor and delivery complicated by abnormality of fetal acid-base balance

O76	Abnormality in fetal heart rate and rhythm complicating labor and delivery
O80	Encounter for full-term uncomplicated delivery
O82	Encounter for cesarean delivery without indication
O85	Puerperal sepsis
O94	Sequelae of complication of pregnancy, childbirth, and the puerperium
P09	Abnormal findings on neonatal screening
P53	Hemorrhagic disease of newborn
P60	Disseminated intravascular coagulation of newborn
P84	Other problems with newborn
P90	Convulsions of newborn
P95	Stillbirth
Q02	Microcephaly
R05	Cough
R12	Heartburn
R17	Unspecified jaundice
R21	Rash and other nonspecific skin eruption
R32	Unspecified urinary incontinence
R34	Anuria and oliguria
R37	Sexual dysfunction, unspecified
R42	Dizziness and giddiness
R51	Headache
R52	Pain, unspecified
R54	Age-related physical debility
R55	Syncope and collapse
R58	Hemorrhage, not elsewhere classified
R61	Generalized hyperhidrosis
R64	Cachexia
R69	Illness, unspecified
R75	Inconclusive laboratory evidence of human immunodeficiency virus [HIV]
R81	Glycosuria
R99	Ill-defined and unknown cause of mortality
Y09	Assault by unspecified means
Y66	Nonadministration of surgical and medical care
Y69	Unspecified misadventure during surgical and medical care
Y95	Nosocomial condition
Z08	Encounter for follow-up examination after completed treatment for malignant neoplasm
Z09	Encounter for follow-up examination after completed treatment for conditions other than malignant neoplasm
Z21	Asymptomatic human immunodeficiency virus [HIV] infection status
Z23	Encounter for immunization
Z66	Do not resuscitate

Appendix C: Pharmacology List 2018

This section enables the coder to quickly review drugs, drug actions, and indications that are often associated with overlooked or undocumented diagnoses. The coder should review the patient's medication record and know what condition the physician is treating with the prescribed medication based on documentation in the medical record. When documentation is lacking, the coder can reference this section to locate the drug, determine the drug action, confirm drug indications, and when necessary query the physician.

Drug	Z Code	Drug Action	Indications
Abilify [aripiprazole]		Antipsychotic	Depression, bipolar disorder, schizophrenia, autism symptoms
Acarbose [acarbose]	Z79.84	Blood glucose regulator	Diabetes mellitus
Accupril [quinapril hydrochloride]		ACE inhibitor; antihypertensive	Congestive heart failure; essential hypertension
Acetaminophen with codeine [acetominophen/codeine phosphate]	Z79.891	Analgesic, general; analgesic-narcotic	Pain, moderate to severe
Actemra [tocilizumab]		Antirheumatic	Rheumatoid arthritis
Actimmune [interferon gamma-1b]	Z79.899	Antineoplastic interferons; antiviral interferons	Chronic granulomatous disease; malignant osteopetrosis
Activella [estradiol/norethindrone acetate]	Z79.890	Estrogen therapy	Menopause symptoms; vaginal and vulvar atrophy; osteoporosis prevention
Actonel [risedronate sodium]	Z79.83	Electrolytic and renal agent; bone resorption inhibitor	Decrease in bone loss in multiple myeloma patients; Paget's disease; hyperparathyroidism; osteoporosis
Actoplus Met [metformin hydrochloride/pioglitazone hydrochloride]	Z79.84	Blood glucose regulator	Diabetes mellitus
Actos [pioglitazone hydrochloride]	Z79.84	Blood glucose regulator	Diabetes mellitus
Adalat CC [nifedipine]		Calcium channel blocker	Vasospastic angina; chronic stable angina; essential hypertension
Advair [fluticasone propionate/salmeterol xinafoate]	Z79.51	Corticosteroids--inhaled; antiasthmatic	Prophylaxis and treatment of asthma and COPD
Advil [ibuprofen]	Z79.1	Nonsteroidal anti-inflammatory drug (NSAID)	Pain or fever relief
Aerospan [flunisolide]	Z79.51	Corticosteroids--inhaled; antiasthmatic	Prophylaxis and treatment of asthma
Afrezza [human insulin recombinant]	Z79.4	Blood glucose regulator	Diabetes mellitus
Aggrastat [tirofiban hydrochloride]	Z79.02	Antithrombotic platelet aggregation inhibitor	Unstable angina or heart attacks
Aggrenox [aspirin/dipyridamole]	Z79.02	Antithrombotic platelet aggregation inhibitor	Lessening of the chance of heart attack or stroke
Akne-Mycin [erythromycin]	Z79.2	Antibacterial	Severe acne treatment
Aldactone [spironolactone]		Cardiovascular agent; antihypertensive agent; diuretic; electrolytic and renal agent	Severe heart failure; ascites associated with cirrhosis; hypokalemia
Aleve [naproxen sodium]	Z79.1	Nonsteroidal anti-inflammatory drug (NSAID)	Reduction of temporary aches and pains
Allegra [fexofenadine hydrochloride]		Antihistamine	Seasonal allergic rhinitis
Allopurinol [allopurinol]		Antigout	Gouty arthritis, renal calculus, hyperuricemia, hyperuricemia secondary to leukemia, hyperuricemia secondary to lymphoma
Alora [estradiol]	Z79.890	Estrogen therapy	Menopause symptoms
Alphagan P [brimonidine tartrate]		Antiglaucoma agent (ophthalmic) antihypertensive, ocular	Open angle glaucoma or another condition in which pressure in the eye is too high (ocular hypertension)
Alprazolam [alprazolam]		Antianxiety; sedative/hypnotic	
Altabax [retapamulin]	Z79.2	Antibacterial	Skin infections
Altace [ramipril]		ACE inhibitor; antihypertensive	Congestive heart failure, essential hypertension
Altavera [ethinyl estradiol/levonorgestrel]	Z79.3	Contraceptive	Contraception
Alvesco [ciclesonide]	Z79.51	Corticosteroids--inhaled; antiasthmatic	Prophylaxis and treatment of asthma
Alyacen [ethinyl estradiol/norethindrone]	Z79.3	Contraceptive	Contraception
Amaryl [glimepiride]	Z79.84	Blood glucose regulator	Diabetes mellitus
Ambien [zolpidem tartrate]		Sedative/hypnotic	Insomnia
A-Methapred [methylprednisolone sodium succinate]	Z79.52	Corticosteroids	Severe inflammation
Amikacin [amikacin sulfate]		Aminoglycoside antibiotic	Active in treatment of gram-negative bacterial infections such as *Pseudomonas, Escherichia coli (E. coli), Proteus, Klebsiella-Enterobacter-Serratia*

Drug	Z Code	Drug Action	Indications
Aminophylline [aminophylline]		Bronchodilator, pulmonary vasodilator, smooth muscle relaxant	Relief and/or prevention of symptoms from asthma and reversible bronchospasms in bronchitis and emphysema
Amitriptyline hydrochloride [amitriptyline hydrochloride]		Anorexiant/CNS stimulant; antidepressant	Depression
Amoxicillin [amoxicillin]	Z79.2	Penicillin	Effective for infections with a broad spectrum of bactericidal activity against many gram-positive and gram-negative micro-organisms; otitis media, gonorrhea, skin, respiratory, gastrointestinal, and genitourinary infections
Ampicillin [ampicillin sodium]	Z79.2	Antibacterial	Bacterial infections
Amrix [cyclobenzaprine hydrochloride]		Muscle relaxant	Adjunct to rest and physical therapy for muscle spasms
Anaprox [naproxen sodium]	Z79.1	Nonsteroidal anti-inflammatory drug (NSAID)	Pain, inflammation, or fever relief
Anastrozole [anastrozole]	Z79.811	Aromatase inhibitor	Postmenopausal breast cancer
Ancef [cefazolin sodium]	Z79.2	Semisynthetic cephalosporin antibiotic	Respiratory tract infections due to *Streptococcus pneumoniae*, *Klebsiella species*, *Haemophilus influenzae (H. influenzae)*, *Staphylococcus aureus*, and group A betahemolytic streptococci; urinary tract infections due to *E. coli, Proteus mirabilis, Klebsiella* species and some strains of *Enterobacter* and enterococci; skin and skin structure infections, biliary tract infections, bone and joint infections, genital infections, septicemia, and endocarditis
Angeliq [drospirenone/estradiol]	Z79.890	Estrogen therapy	Menopause symptoms
Angiomax [bivalirudin]	Z79.02	Antithrombotic platelet aggregation inhibitor	Prevention of blood clots
Antabuse [disulfiram]		Alcohol treatment	Alcoholism
Antineoplastic/chemotherapy	Z79.899	Antineoplastic	Cancer
Anzemet [dolasetron mesylate]		Antiemetic/antinauseant	Management of nausea/vomiting following surgery or from effects of chemotherapy or cancer
Apidra [insulin glulisine recombinant]	Z79.4	Blood glucose regulator	Diabetes mellitus
Aranelle [ethinyl estradiol/norethindrone]	Z79.3	Contraceptive	Contraception; acne
Aranesp [darbepoetin alfa]		Erythropoiesis-stimulating agent (ESA)	Lower than normal blood cell count (anemia) from disorders such as CKD and neoplasms
Argatroban [argatroban]	Z79.02	Antithrombotic platelet aggregation inhibitor	Prophylaxis and treatment of venous thrombosis in thrombocytopenia patients
Aricept [donepezil hydrochloride]		Acetylcholine sterase inhibitor	Symptoms of mild to moderate Alzheimer's disease; can improve thinking ability in some patients
Arimidex [anastrozole]	Z79.811	Aromatase inhibitor	Postmenopausal breast cancer
Aristospan [triamcinolone hexacetonide]	Z79.52	Corticosteroids	Severe inflammation
Arixtra [fondaparinux sodium]	Z79.01	Anticoagulant	Venous thrombosis and pulmonary embolism
Arnuity Ellipta [fluticasone furoate]	Z79.51	Corticosteroids--inhaled; antiasthmatic	Prophylaxis and treatment of asthma
Aromasin [exemestane]	Z79.811	Aromatase inhibitor	Postmenopausal breast cancer
Arthrotec [diclofenac sodium/misoprostol]	Z79.1	Analgesic	Arthritis in patients who may develop stomach ulcers from taking nonsteroidal anti-inflammatory drugs (NSAIDs) alone; used to help relieve some symptoms of arthritis, such as inflammation, swelling, stiffness, and joint pain
Ashlyna [ethinyl estradiol/levonorgestrel]	Z79.3	Contraceptive	Contraception
Asmanex [mometasone furoate]	Z79.51	Corticosteroids--inhaled; antiasthmatic	Prophylaxis and treatment of asthma
Astagraf XL [tacrolimus]	Z79.899	Immunosuppressant	Prophylaxis of organ transplant rejection
Astramorph [morphine sulfate]	Z79.891	Narcotic analgesic	Pain
Atelvia [risedronate sodium]	Z79.83	Bisphosphonates	Prevention of thinning of the bones (osteoporosis)
Atenolol [atenolol]		Antianginal; antihypertensive; beta blocker	Chronic stable angina pectoris; essential hypertension; reduces cardiovascular mortality in those with definite or suspected acute myocardial infarction
Ativan [lorazepam]		Antianxiety; sedative/hypnotic	Anxiety disorder associated with depressive symptoms; controls tension, agitation, irritability, and insomnia
Atrovent [ipratropium bromide]		Antiasthmatic/bronchodilator	Chronic bronchitis, emphysema; bronchial asthma
Augmentin [amoxicillin/clavulanate potassium]	Z79.2	Antibacterial	Middle ear, lower respiratory, sinus, skin and skin structures, and urinary tract infections
Avandia [rosiglitazone maleate]	Z79.84	Blood glucose regulator	Diabetes mellitus

Drug	Z Code	Drug Action	Indications
Avapro [irbesartan]		Antihypertensive	Hypertension
Aviane [ethinyl estradiol/levonorgestrel]	Z79.3	Contraceptive	Contraception
Avonex [interferon beta-1a]	Z79.899	Antiviral interferon	Relapsing multiple sclerosis
Axid AR [nizatidine]		Histamine H2-receptor antagonist	Acid/peptic disorder; gastroesophageal reflux; duodenal, gastric, and peptic ulcers
Aygestin [norethindrone acetate]	Z79.3	Contraceptive	Contraception; menstrual disorders
Azactam [aztreonam]	Z79.2	Antibacterial	Severe or life-threatening bacterial infections
Azithromycin [azithromycin]	Z79.2	Antibacterial	Treatment of bacterial infections
Bactrim [sulfamethoxazole/trimethoprim]	Z79.2	Antibacterial	Urinary tract infections, acute otitis media, acute exacerbation of chronic bronchitis, shigellosis, and *Pneumocystis carinii*
Bactroban [mupirocin]	Z79.2	Dermatologic; topical anti-infective	Topical treatment of impetigo
Balziva [ethinyl estradiol/norethindrone]	Z79.3	Contraceptive	Contraception
Basaglar [insulin glargine]	Z79.4	Blood glucose regulator	Diabetes mellitus
Bayer [acetylsalicylic acid]	Z79.82	Aspirin	Prophylaxis and treatment of heart attacks, angina, or strokes; reduction of fever, pain, and inflammation
Beconase AQ [beclomethasone dipropionate monohydrate]		Corticosteroids; antiasthmatic	Bronchial asthma, prevention of nasal polyps, perennial allergies, seasonal allergies, and vasomotor rhinitis
Bekyree [desogestrel/ethinyl estradiol]	Z79.3	Contraceptive	Contraception
Betoptic [betaxolol hydrochloride]		Cardioselective beta-adrenergic receptor blocking agent	Lowering of intraocular pressure; also used for treatment of ocular hypertension and chronic open-angle glaucoma
Beyaz [drospirenone/ethinyl estradiol/levomefolate calcium]	Z79.3	Contraceptive	Contraception; acne
Biaxin [clarithromycin]		Macrolide	Acid/peptic disorder or ulcer, acute exacerbation chronic bronchitis, HIV, lower and upper respiratory tract infections, sinus infection, prophylaxis mycobacterium avium complex, pharyngitis, pneumonia, tonsillitis
Binosto [alendronate sodium]	Z79.83	Bisphosphonates	Prevention of thinning of the bones (osteoporosis)
Boniva [ibandronate sodium]	Z79.83	Bisphosphonates	Prevention of thinning of the bones (osteoporosis)
Brevicon [ethinyl estradiol/norethindrone]	Z79.3	Contraceptive	Contraception; acne
Briellyn [ethinyl estradiol/norethindrone]	Z79.3	Contraceptive	Contraception
Brilinta [ticagrelor]	Z79.02	Antithrombotic platelet aggregation inhibitor	Unstable angina or heart attacks and prevention of blood clots
Bufferin [acetylsalicylic acid]	Z79.82	Aspirin	Prophylaxis and treatment of heart attacks, angina or strokes; reduction of fever, pain, and inflammation
Buprenex [buprenorphine hydrochloride]	Z79.891	Narcotic analgesic	Moderate to severe pain
Buprenorphine HCl [buprenorphine hydrochloride]	Z79.891	Narcotic analgesic	Moderate to severe pain
Buspirone [buspirone hydrochloride]		Antianxiety agent	Generalized anxiety disorder
Butorphanol Tartrate [butorphanol tartrate]		Narcotic analgesic	Moderate to severe postsurgical pain
Butrans [buprenorphine]	Z79.891	Narcotic analgesic	Chronic pain
Calan [verapamil hydrochloride]		Antianginal; antiarrhythmic, antiarthritic, antihypertensive, calcium channel blocker	Angina pectoris at rest and chronic stable, arrhythmia, atrial fibrillation, atrial flutter, paroxysmal supraventricular tachycardia, ventricular arrhythmia, essential hypertension
Caldolor [ibuprofen]	Z79.1	Nonsteroidal anti-inflammatory drug (NSAID)	Pain or fever relief
Cambia [diclofenac potassium]	Z79.1	Nonsteroidal anti-inflammatory drug (NSAID)	Migraine headaches
Camila [norethindrone]	Z79.3	Contraceptive	Contraception; menstrual disorders
Cardizem CD [diltiazem hydrochloride]		Antianginal, antiarrhythmic, antihypertensive, channel blocker, coronary vasodilator	Chronic stable angina, atrial fibrillation, atrial flutter, essential hypertension, paroxysmal supraventricular tachycardia
Cardura [doxazosin mesylate]		Antihypertensive	Benign prostatic hyperplasia, essential hypertension
Catapres [clonidine hydrochloride]		Antihypertensive	Hypertension
Cefprozil [cefprozil]		Antibiotic: second generation cephalosporins	Acute exacerbation and chronic bronchitis, lower and upper respiratory tract infections, pharyngitis, tonsillitis

Appendix C: Pharmacology List 2018

Drug	Z Code	Drug Action	Indications
Ceftin [cefuroxime axetil]		Antibiotic: second generation cephalosporins	Acute exacerbation and chronic bronchitis, middle ear infection, sexually transmitted gonorrhea infection, upper respiratory tract infection, urinary tract infection, pharyngitis, tonsillitis
Ceftriaxone [ceftriaxone sodium]	Z79.2	Antibacterial	Bacterial infections
Celebrex [celecoxib]	Z79.1	Antirheumatic, nonsteroidal anti-inflammatory	Relief of some symptoms caused by arthritis, such as inflammation, swelling, stiffness, and joint pain
Celestone Soluspan [betamethasone acetate/ betamethasone sodium phosphate]	Z79.52	Corticosteroids; antiasthmatic	Asthma; severe inflammation
Celexa [citalopram hydrobromide]		Antidepressant	Depression
Cellcept [mycophenolate mofetil]	Z79.899	Immunosuppressant	Prophylaxis of organ transplant rejection
Centany [mupirocin]	Z79.2	Antibacterial	Topical treatment of skin infections
Cephalexin [cephalexin]	Z79.2	Antibacterial	Bacterial infections
Chantix [varenicline tartrate]		Smoking cessation aid	Nicotine addiction, smoking
Cipro [ciprofloxacin hydrochloride]	Z79.2	Anti-infective; quinolone	Cystitis, infectious diarrhea, gonorrhea, bone and joint infection, gastrointestinal tract infection, lower and upper respiratory tract infections, sinus infection, urinary tract infection, nosocomial pneumonia, chronic prostatitis
Ciprofloxacin [ciprofloxacin]	Z79.2	Antibacterial	Bacterial infections
Clarithromycin [clarithromycin]	Z79.2	Antibacterial	Skin and respiratory bacterial infections
Claritin [loratadine]		Antihistamine	Seasonal allergic rhinitis, chronic idiopathic urticaria
Cleocin [clindamycin phosphate]	Z79.2	Antibacterial	Bacterial infections
Climara [estradiol]	Z79.890	Estrogen therapy	Osteoporosis prevention and menopausal symptoms; vaginal and vulvar atrophy; hypoestrogenism; ovarian failure
Clindamycin [clindamycin phosphate]	Z79.2	Antibacterial	Bacterial infections
Clonazepam [clonazepam]		Anticonvulsant	Absence, akinetic, and myoclonic epilepsy, Lennox-Gastaut syndrome
Clonidine [clonidine hydrochloride]		Antihypertensive	Hypertension
Clopidogrel bisulfate [clopidogrel bisulfate]	Z79.02	Antithrombotic platelet aggregation inhibitor	Treatment of unstable angina or heart attacks and prevention of blood clots
Codeine [codeine sulfate]	Z79.891	Narcotic analgesic	Mild to moderate pain
Cogentin [benztropine mesylate]		Antiparkinsonism	Parkinson's disease
Colace [docusate sodium]		Gastrointestinal agent; laxative, stool softener	Constipation
Colocort [hydrocortisone]	Z79.52	Corticosteroids	Inflammation of the colon
CombiPatch [ethinyl estradiol/norethindrone acetate]	Z79.890	Estrogen therapy	Menopause symptoms; vaginal and vulvar atrophy; osteoporosis prevention
Combivent [ipratropium bromide/albuterol sulfate]		Antiasthmatic/bronchodilator	Chronic bronchitis, emphysema; bronchial asthma
Compro [prochlorperazine]		Antiemetic, antipsychotic	Nausea, vomiting, and manic phase of bipolar syndrome or schizophrenia
Cortef [hydrocortisone]	Z79.52	Corticosteroids	Severe inflammation
Cortenema [hydrocortisone]	Z79.52	Corticosteroids	Inflammation of the colon
Cortifoam [hydrocortisone acetate]	Z79.52	Corticosteroids	Colon and rectum inflammation
Cortisone acetate [cortisone acetate]	Z79.52	Corticosteroids	Inflammation
Cortisporin [hydrocortisone acetate/neomycin sulfate/polymyxin B sulfate]		Topical anti-infective, topical steroid	Dermatosis
Coumadin [warfarin sodium]	Z79.01	Anticoagulant	Prophylaxis and treatment of venous thrombosis, treatment of atrial fibrillation with embolization (pulmonary embolism), arrhythmias, myocardial infarction, and stroke prevention
Cozaar [losartan potassium]		Antihypertensive	Essential hypertension
Crestor [rosuvastatin calcium]		HMG-CoA reductase inhibitor (statin)	Hypercholesterolemia, hyperlipidemia, hyperproteinemia
Crixivan [indinavir sulfate]		HIV inhibitor	HIV, asymptomatic HIV
Cryselle [ethinyl estradiol/norgestrel]	Z79.3	Contraceptive	Contraception
Cyclafem [ethinyl estradiol/norethindrone]	Z79.3	Contraceptive	Contraception
Cyclessa [desogestrel/ethinyl estradiol]	Z79.3	Contraceptive	Contraception

Drug	Z Code	Drug Action	Indications
Cyclosporine [cyclosporine]	Z79.899	Immunosuppressant	Prophylaxis of organ transplant rejection
Cytomel [liothyronine sodium]		Thyroid hormone	Treatment of hypothyroidism or prevention of euthyroid goiters
Daptomycin [daptomycin]	Z79.2	Antibacterial	Skin and underlying tissue bacterial infections
Dasetta [ethinyl estradiol/norethindrone]	Z79.3	Contraceptive	Contraception
Daypro [oxaprozin]	Z79.1	Nonsteroidal anti-inflammatory drug (NSAID)	Osteoarthritis and rheumatoid arthritis
Daysee [ethinyl estradiol/levonorgestrel]	Z79.3	Contraceptive	Contraception
Delestrogen [estradiol valerate]	Z79.890	Estrogen therapy	Menopause symptoms
Demerol [meperidine hydrochloride]	Z79.891	Narcotic analgesic	Moderate to severe pain
Depakote [divalproex sodium]		Anticonvulsant	Bipolar affective disorder; complex absence, complex partial, and mixed pattern epilepsy; migraine headache
Depo-Medrol [methylprednisolone acetate]	Z79.52	Corticosteroids	Arthritis and joint disorders
Depo-Provera [medroxyprogesterone acetate]	Z79.3, Z79.890	Antineoplastic; contraceptive; progestin	Amenorrhea; carcinoma, endometrium, adjunct; carcinoma, renal; contraception; hemorrhage
Depo-SubQ Provera [medroxyprogesterone acetate]	Z79.3	Contraceptive	Contraception; menstrual disorder pain
Desogen [desogestrel/ethinyl estradiol]	Z79.3	Contraceptive; estrogen/progestin	Contraception
Detrol [tolterodine tartrate]		Muscarinic receptor antagonist	Overactive bladders in patients with urinary frequency, urgency, or urge incontinence
Dexamethasone Intensol [dexamethasone]	Z79.52	Corticosteroids	Arthritis; allergic disorders; breathing disorders; lupus
Didronel [etidronate disodium]	Z79.83	Bisphosphonates	Paget's disease and irregular bone growth
Dificid [fidaxomicin]	Z79.2	Antibacterial	*Clostridium difficile*
Diflucan [fluconazole]		Antifungal agent	Oropharyngeal and esophageal candidiasis and cryptococcal meningitis in AIDS patients
Digoxin [digoxin]		Cardiotonic glycoside	Heart failure, atrial flutter, atrial fibrillation, and supraventricular tachycardia
Dilantin [phenytoin sodium]		Anticonvulsant	Control of grand mal and psychomotor seizures
Dilaudid [hydromorphone hydrochloride]	Z79.891	Narcotic analgesic	Moderate to severe pain
Diovan [valsartan]		ACE inhibitor	Essential hypertension
Divigel [estradiol]	Z79.890	Estrogen therapy	Menopause symptoms
Dolophine HCl [methadone hydrochloride]	Z79.891	Narcotic analgesic	Pain; treatment of opioid addiction
Doxycycline [doxycycline]	Z79.2	Antibacterial	Treatment of bacterial infections; acne
Duavee [bazedoxifene acetate/conjugated estrogens]	Z79.890	Estrogen therapy	Treatment of menopause symptoms; osteoporosis prevention
Duetact [glimepiride/pioglitazone hydrochloride]	Z79.84	Blood glucose regulator	Diabetes mellitus
Duexis [famotidine/ibuprofen]	Z79.1	Nonsteroidal anti-inflammatory drug (NSAID)	Symptomatic treatment of osteoarthritis and rheumatoid arthritis; reduction of risk of ulcers
Dulera [formoterol fumarate/mometasone furoate]	Z79.51	Corticosteroids -inhaled; antiasthmatic	Prophylaxis and treatment of asthma
Duragesic [fentanyl]	Z79.891	Narcotic analgesic	Chronic pain
Duramorph [morphine sulfate]	Z79.891	Narcotic analgesic	Moderate to severe pain
Dyloject [diclofenac sodium]	Z79.1	Nonsteroidal anti-inflammatory drug (NSAID)	Pain relief
Dynacin [minocycline hydrochloride]	Z79.2	Antibacterial	Severe acne treatment
E.E.S. [erythromycin ethylsuccinate]	Z79.2	Antibacterial	Bacterial infections
Ecotrin [acetylsalicylic acid]	Z79.82	Aspirin	Prophylaxis and treatment of heart attacks, angina or strokes; reduction of fever, pain and inflammation
Effexor XR [venlafaxine hydrochloride]		Antidepressant	Depression
Effient [prasugrel hydrochloride]	Z79.02	Antithrombotic platelet aggregation inhibitor	Lessening of the chance of heart attack or stroke
Elestrin [estradiol]	Z79.890	Estrogen therapy	Menopause symptoms

Drug	Z Code	Drug Action	Indications
Eligard [leuprolide acetate]	Z79.818	Agents affecting estrogen receptors and estrogen levels	Endometriosis; uterine fibroids; symptoms of prostate cancer
Elinest [norgestrel/ethinyl estradiol]	Z79.3	Contraceptive	Contraception
Eliquis [apixaban]	Z79.01	Anticoagulant	Venous thrombosis
Embeda [morphine sulfate/naltrexone hydrochloride]	Z79.891	Narcotic analgesic	Moderate to severe pain
Emoquette [ethinyl estradiol/desogestrel]	Z79.3	Contraceptive	Contraception
Enjuvia [conjugated synthetic b estrogens]	Z79.890	Estrogen therapy	Osteoporosis prevention and to treat menopausal symptoms; vaginal and vulvar atrophy; hypoestrogenism; ovarian failure
Enpresse [ethinyl estradiol/levonorgestrel]	Z79.3	Contraceptive	Contraception
Enskyce [desogestrel/ethinyl estradiol]	Z79.3	Contraceptive	Contraception
Entocort EC [budesonide]	Z79.52	Corticosteroids	Crohn's disease; ulcerative colitis
Envarsus XR [tacrolimus]	Z79.899	Immunosuppressant	Prophylaxis of organ transplant rejection
Epinephrine [epinephrine]		Bronchodilator, cardiotonic	Most commonly, relief of respiratory distress due to bronchospasm and restoration of cardiac rhythm in cardiac arrest
Epivir, Epivir-HBV [lamivudine]		HIV and HBV inhibitor	HIV, hepatitis B (HBV), asymptomatic HIV
Errin [norethindrone]	Z79.3	Contraceptive	Contraception
Ertapenem [ertapenem sodium]	Z79.2	Antibacterial	Stomach, urinary tract, pelvis, skin and lung infections
ERYC [erythromycin]	Z79.2	Antibacterial	Lower respiratory tract infections
Erygel [erythromycin]	Z79.2	Antibacterial	Treatment of bacterial infections; rheumatic fever attacks
EryPed [erythromycin ethylsuccinate]	Z79.2	Antibacterial	Treatment of bacterial infections; rheumatic fever attacks
Ery-Tab [erythromycin]	Z79.2	Acne product; macrolide; ocular anti-infective; topical anti-infective	Acne vulgaris, intestinal amebiasis, infectious conjunctivitis, diphtheria, endocarditis, prevention, treatment of erythrasma infections: endocervical, gynecologic, lower and upper respiratory tract, ophthalmic, and rectal; skin and skin structures, and urethral; Legionnaires' disease, pelvic inflammatory disease, pertussis, pneumonia, rheumatic fever, prophylaxis, syphilis
Erythrocin [erythromycin lactobionate]	Z79.2	Antibacterial	Bacterial infections
Erythromycin [erythromycin]	Z79.2	Antibacterial	Respiratory tract infections
Estarylla [ethinyl estradiol/norgestimate]	Z79.3	Contraceptive	Contraception
Estrace [estradiol]	Z79.890	Estrogen therapy	Vaginal cream used to treat vaginal and vulvar atrophy
Estraderm [estradiol]	Z79.890	Estrogen therapy	Osteoporosis prevention and to treat menopausal symptoms, vaginal and vulvar atrophy, hypoestrogenism, ovarian failure
Estrasorb [estradiol hemihydrate]	Z79.890	Estrogen therapy	Menopause symptoms
EstroGel [estradiol]	Z79.890	Estrogen therapy	Menopause symptoms
Estrostep Fe [ethinyl estradiol/norethindrone acetate]	Z79.3	Contraceptive	Contraception
Evista [raloxifene hydrochloride]	Z79.810	Estrogen receptor modulator, selective osteoporosis prophylactic	Prevention of thinning of the bones (osteoporosis) only in postmenopausal women
Exalgo [hydromorphone hydrochloride]	Z79.891	Narcotic analgesic	Moderate to severe pain
Exemestane [exemestane]	Z79.811	Aromatase inhibitor	Postmenopausal breast cancer
Factive [gemifloxacin mesylate]	Z79.2	Antibacterial	Bacterial lung infections
Falmina [ethinyl estradiol/levonorgestrel]	Z79.3	Contraceptive	Contraception
Fareston [toremifene citrate]	Z79.810	Selective estrogen receptor modulator (SERM)	Metastatic breast cancer in postmenopausal women
Faslodex [fulvestrant]	Z79.818	Agents affecting estrogen receptors and estrogen levels	Metastatic breast cancer in postmenopausal women
Feldene [piroxicam]	Z79.1	Nonsteroidal anti-inflammatory drug (NSAID)	Treatment of pain and inflammation due to arthritis
Femara [letrozole]	Z79.811	Aromatase inhibitor	Postmenopausal breast cancer
Femcon Fe [ethinyl estradiol/norethindrone]	Z79.3	Contraceptive	Contraception; acne
Femhrt [ethinyl estradiol/norethindrone acetate]	Z79.3, Z79.890	Contraceptive; estrogen therapy	Contraception; menopause symptoms; osteoporosis prevention
Femring [estradiol acetate]	Z79.890	Estrogen therapy	Osteoporosis prevention and to treat menopausal symptoms; hypoestrogenism; ovarian failure

Drug	Z Code	Drug Action	Indications
Femtrace [estradiol acetate]	Z79.890	Estrogen therapy	Menopause symptoms
Fentanyl [fentanyl]	Z79.891	Narcotic analgesic	Postprocedural or chronic pain
Fentora [fentanyl citrate]	Z79.891	Narcotic analgesic	Breakthrough cancer pain
Fioricet with codeine [acetaminophen/butalbital/caffeine/codeine phosphate]	Z79.891	Narcotic analgesic	Tension headaches
Flagyl [metronidazole]	Z79.2	Antibacterial	Treatment of bacterial infections
Flavoxate hydrochloride [flavoxate hydrochloride]		Urinary tract spasmolytic	Relief of dysuria, urgency, nocturia, suprapubic pain, frequency, and incontinence associated with cystitis, prostatitis, urethritis, and urethrocystitis/urethrotrigonitis
Flomax [tamsulosin hydrochloride]		Alpha-adrenergic blocker, benign prostatic hypertrophy therapy agent	Signs and symptoms of benign enlargement of the prostate (benign prostatic hyperplasia, or BPH)
Flonase [fluticasone propionate]		Corticosteroid-inhalation/nasal; topical steroid	Corticosteroid-responsive dermatosis; perennial allergic and seasonal allergic rhinitis
Flovent HFA [fluticasone propionate]	Z79.51	Corticosteroid-inhaled/nasal; topical steroid	Corticosteroid-responsive dermatosis, perennial allergic and seasonal allergic rhinitis
Fortamet [metformin hydrochloride]	Z79.84	Blood glucose regulator	Diabetes mellitus
Fortaz [ceftazidime]	Z79.2	Antibacterial	Pneumonia and lower respiratory infections
Fosamax [alendronate sodium]	Z79.83	Calcium metabolism	Osteoporosis; Paget's disease
Fosinopril sodium [fosinopril sodium]		ACE inhibitor; antihypertensive	Essential hypertension
Fragmin [dalteparin sodium]	Z79.01	Anticoagulant	Prophylaxis and treatment of blood clots
Fulvestrant [fulvestrant]	Z79.818	Agents affecting estrogen receptors and estrogen levels	Treatment of metastatic breast cancer in postmenopausal women
Gengraf [cyclosporine]	Z79.899	Immunosuppressant	Prophylaxis of organ transplant rejection
Gentamicin sulfate [gentamicin sulfate]	Z79.2	Antibacterial	Severe bacterial infections
Gildagia [ethinyl estradiol/norethindrone]	Z79.3	Contraceptive	Contraception
Gildess [ethinyl estradiol/norethindrone acetate]	Z79.3	Contraceptive	Contraception
Glimepiride [glimepiride]	Z79.84	Blood glucose regulator	Diabetes mellitus
Glucophage [metformin hydrochloride]	Z79.84	Blood glucose regulator	Diabetes mellitus
Glucotrol [glipizide]	Z79.84	Oral blood-glucose-lowering agent	Diabetes mellitus
Glucovance [glyburide/metformin hydrochloride]	Z79.84	Blood glucose regulator	Diabetes mellitus
Glumetza [metformin hydrochloride]	Z79.84	Blood glucose regulator	Diabetes mellitus
Glyburide (micronized) [glyburide]	Z79.84	Blood glucose regulator	Diabetes mellitus
Heparin sodium [heparin sodium]	Z79.01	Anticoagulant	Prophylaxis and treatment of venous thrombosis, pulmonary embolism; prevention of cerebral thrombosis, and treatment of consumptive coagulopathies
Humalog [insulin lispro recombinant]	Z79.4	Blood glucose regulator	Diabetes mellitus
Humulin [insulin recombinant]	Z79.4	Blood glucose regulator	Diabetes mellitus
Hydrochlorothiazide [hydrochlorothiazide]		Diuretic, antihypertensive	Management of hypertension and in adjunctive therapy for edema associated with congestive heart failure, hepatic cirrhosis, corticosteroid, and estrogen therapy
Hydrocodone [acetaminophen/hydrocodone bitartrate]	Z79.891	Narcotic analgesic	Moderate to severe pain
Hydrocodone bitartrate and acetaminophen [acetaminophen/hydrocodone bitartrate]	Z79.891	Analgesic, general; analgesic-narcotic; antitussive/expectorant	Pain, moderate to severe
Hydrocortisone [hydrocortisone]	Z79.52	Corticosteroids	Addison's disease; arthritis; immune disorders; allergies; breathing problems
Hydromorphone HCl [hydromorphone hydrochloride]	Z79.891	Narcotic analgesic	Moderate to severe pain
Hyzaar [hydrochlorothiazide/ losartan potassium]		Antihypertensive	Hypertension
Ibuprofen [ibuprofen]	Z79.1	Nonsteroidal anti-inflammatory drug (NSAID)	Pain or fever relief
Imitrex [sumatriptan succinate]		Antimigraine	Migraine headache

Drug	Z Code	Drug Action	Indications
Imuran [azathioprine]	**Z79.899**	Immunosuppressant	Rheumatoid arthritis
Inderal [propranolol hydrochloride]		Beta-adrenergic blocking agent	Management of hypertension, long-term management of angina pectoris due to coronary atherosclerosis, cardiac arrhythmias
Indocin [indomethacin]	**Z79.1**	Nonsteroidal anti-inflammatory drug (NSAID)	Treatment of pain and inflammation
Integrilin [eptifibatide]	**Z79.02**	Antithrombotic platelet aggregation inhibitor	Treatment of unstable angina or heart attacks and prevention of blood clots
Intron [interferon alfa 2-b]	**Z79.899**	Antineoplastic interferons; antiviral interferons	Cancer; hepatitis
Introvale [levonorgestrel/ethinyl estradiol]	**Z79.3**	Contraceptive	Contraception
Invanz [ertapeneum sodium]	**Z79.2**	Antibacterial	Stomach, urinary tract, pelvis, skin and lung infections
Invokamet [canagliflozin/metformin hydrochloride]	**Z79.84**	Blood glucose regulator	Diabetes mellitus
Iprivask [desirudin recombinant]	**Z79.02**	Antithrombotic platelet aggregation inhibitor	Prophylaxis and treatment of venous thrombosis and pulmonary embolism
Isoniazid [isoniazid]	**Z79.2**	Antibacterial	Prophylaxis and treatment of tuberculosis
Isordil [isosorbide dinitrate]		Smooth muscle relaxant	Acute anginal attacks
Isuprel [isoproterenol hydrochloride]		Adrenergic agent	Bronchodilator for asthma, chronic pulmonary emphysema, bronchitis, and other conditions accompanied by bronchospasm; can be used in cardiogenic shock cases
Jantoven [warfarin sodium]	**Z79.01**	Anticoagulant	Prophylaxis and treatment of venous thrombosis, pulmonary embolism; prevention of cerebral thrombosis, and treatment of consumptive coagulopathies
Janumet [metformin hydrochloride/sitagliptin phosphate]	**Z79.84**	Blood glucose regulator	Diabetes mellitus
Januvia [sitagliptin phosphate]	**Z79.84**	Blood glucose regulator	Diabetes mellitus
Jencycla [norethindrone]	**Z79.3**	Contraceptive	Contraception
Jentadueto [linagliptin/metformin hydrochloride]]	**Z79.84**	Blood glucose regulator	Diabetes mellitus
Junel [ethinyl estradiol/norethindrone acetate]	**Z79.3**	Contraceptive	Contraception
Kadian [morphine sulfate]	**Z79.891**	Narcotic analgesic	Moderate to severe pain
Kariva [desogestrel/ethinyl estradiol]	**Z79.3**	Contraceptive	Contraception
Kazano [alogliptin benzoate/metformin hydrochloride]	**Z79.84**	Blood glucose regulator	Diabetes mellitus
Keflex [cephalexin]	**Z79.2**	Antibacterial	Bone, middle ear, skin and skin structures, upper respiratory tract and urinary tract infections; acute prostatitis
Kefzol [cefazolin sodium]	**Z79.2**	Antibacterial	Skin, ear, urinary tract, and upper respiratory bacterial infections
Kelnor [ethynodiol diacetate/ethinyl estradiol]	**Z79.3**	Contraceptive	Contraception
Kenalog [triamcinolone acetonide]	**Z79.52**	Corticosteroids	Eczema; allergic reactions; psoriasis
Kimidess [ethinyl estradiol/desogestrel]	**Z79.3**	Contraceptive	Contraception
Klaron [sulfacetamide sodium]	**Z79.2**	Antibacterial	Acne
Klonopin [clonazepam]		Anticonvulsant, anxiolytic - benzodiazepine	Epilepsy, seizures, panic disorder
Klor-Con [potassium chloride]		Replaces potassium and maintains potassium level	Hypokalemia
Kombiglyze [metformin hydrochloride/saxagliptin hydrochloride]	**Z79.84**	Blood glucose regulator	Diabetes mellitus
K-Tab [potassium chloride]		Replaces potassium and maintains potassium level	Hypokalemia
Kurvelo [ethinyl estradiol/levonorgestrel]	**Z79.3**	Contraceptive	Contraception; menstrual disorders
Lamisil [terbinafine hydrochloride]		Antifungal	*Tinea cruris* (jock itch), *T. pedis* (athlete's foot), *T. corporis* (ringworm)
Lanoxin [digoxin]		Cardiotonic glycoside	Congestive heart failure
Lantus [insulin glargine recombinant]	**Z79.4**	Blood glucose regulator	Diabetes mellitus
Larin [ethinyl estradiol/norethindrone acetate]	**Z79.3**	Contraceptive	Contraception

Drug	Z Code	Drug Action	Indications
Lasix [furosemide]		Antihypertensive; diuretic	Management of edema associated with congestive heart failure, renal disease, including nephrotic syndrome and hypertension
Lescol [fluvastatin sodium]		HMG-CoA reductase inhibitor (statin)	Hypercholesterolemia, hyperlipidemia, hyperlipoproteinemia
Lessina [ethinyl estradiol/levonorgestrel]	Z79.3	Contraceptive	Contraception
Letrozole [letrozole]	Z79.811	Aromatase inhibitor	Postmenopausal breast cancer
Levaquin [levofloxacin]	Z79.2	Fluoroquinolone antibacterial	Acute exacerbation chronic bronchitis; cellulitis; furuncle; impetigo; infections of the lower and upper respiratory tracts, sinus, skin and skin structures, and urinary tract; pneumonia, community-acquired; pyoderma
Levemir [insulin detemir recombinant]	Z79.4	Blood glucose regulator	Diabetes mellitus
Levonest [levonorgestrel/ethinyl estradiol]	Z79.3	Contraceptive	Contraception; menstrual disorders; acne
Levora [levonorgestrel/ethinyl estradiol]	Z79.3	Contraceptive	Contraception
Levothroid [levothyroxine sodium]		Thyroid hormone	Treatment of hypothyroidism
Levoxyl [levothyroxine sodium]		Synthetic thyroid hormone	Euthyroid goiter; hypothyroidism
Lexapro [escitalopram oxalate]		Antidepressant—selective serotonin reuptake inhibitor (SSRI)	Depression, anxiety
Librium [chlordiazepoxide hydrochloride]		Antianxiety agent	Acute withdrawal symptoms, especially from alcohol, or for other anxiety-producing conditions
Lidocaine hydrochloride [lidocaine hydrochloride]		Antiarrhythmic	Management of ventricular arrhythmias or during cardiac manipulation, such as cardiac surgery
Liletta [levonorgestrel]	Z79.3	Contraceptive	Intrauterine device for contraception
Lincocin [lincocin hydrochloride]	Z79.2	Antibacterial	Serious bacterial infections
Lipitor [atorvastatin calcium]		HMG-CoA reductase inhibitor (statin)	Hypercholesterolemia, hyperlipidemia, hyperproteinemia
Lithium [lithium carbonate]		Antimanic	Control of manic episodes in bipolar disorders
Lo Loestrin Fe [ethinyl estradiol/norethindrone acetate]	Z79.3	Contraceptive	Contraception
Lo Minastrin Fe [ethinyl estradiol/norethindrone acetate]	Z79.3	Contraceptive	Contraception
Loestrin [ethinyl estradiol/norethindrone acetate]	Z79.3	Contraceptive	Contraception
Lomotil [diphenoxylate hydrochloride/atropine sulfate]		Antidiarrheal	Treatment of symptoms of chronic and functional diarrhea
Lopid [gemfibrozil]		Lipid regulating agent	Hypercholesterolemia, hyperlipidemia, hyperlipoproteinemia, hypertriglyceridemia
Lopressor [metoprolol tartrate]		Antihypertensive, betablocker antianginal; antihypertensive; betablocker	Essential hypertension therapy, angina pectoris, and myocardial infarction
Lorazepam [lorazepam]		Antianxiety; sedative/hypnotic	Anxiety disorder associated with depressive symptoms; controls tension, agitation, irritability, and insomnia
Loryna [drospirenone/ethinyl estradiol]	Z79.3	Contraceptive	Contraception
LoSeasonique [ethinyl estradiol/levonorgestrel]	Z79.3	Contraceptive	Contraception
Lotensin [benazepril hydrochloride]		ACE inhibitor; antihypertensive	Essential hypertension
Lotrel [amlodipine besylate/benazepril hydrochloride]		Antihypertensive	Hypertension
Lotrisone [clotrimazole/ betamethasone dipropionate]		Antifungal-corticosteroid	Relief of redness, swelling, itching, and other discomfort of fungus infections
Lovastatin [lovastatin]		HMG-CoA reductase inhibitor (statin)	Hypercholesterolemia; hyperlipidemia, hyperlipoproteinemia
Lovenox [enoxaparin sodium]	Z79.01	Anticoagulant	Prophylaxis and treatment of venous thrombosis and pulmonary embolism
Low-Ogestrel [norgestrel/ethinyl estradiol]	Z79.3	Contraceptive	Contraception
Lupron [leuprolide acetate]	Z79.818	Agents affecting estrogen receptors and estrogen levels	Treatment of metastatic breast cancer in postmenopausal women; prostate cancer symptoms
Macrobid [nitrofuantoin]	Z79.2	Antibacterial	Bacterial urinary tract infections
Macrodantin [nitrofurantoin]		Antibacterial	Urinary tract infection; prophylaxis
Marlissa [ethinyl estradiol/levonorgestrel]	Z79.3	Contraceptive	Contraception
Maxipime [cefepime hydrochloride]	Z79.2	Antibacterial	Treatment of bacterial infections

Drug	Z Code	Drug Action	Indications
Meclizine hydrochloride [meclizine hydrochloride]		Antihistamine	Management of nausea and vomiting, and dizziness associated with motion sickness
Medrol [methylprednisolone]	Z79.52	Glucocorticoid; anti-inflammatory	Acute/chronic adrenal insufficiency, congenital adrenal hyperplasia, adrenal insufficiency secondary to pituitary insufficiency; nonendocrine disorders, including arthritis, rheumatic carditis, bronchial asthma, cerebral edema, and allergic, collagen, intestinal tract, liver, ocular, renal, and skin diseases
Mefoxin [cefoxitin sodium]	Z79.2	Antibacterial	Bacterial infections
Megace ES [megestrol acetate]	Z79.818	Agents affecting estrogen receptors and estrogen levels	Endometrial or advanced breast cancers; weight loss due to AIDS
Menest [esteriefied estrogens]	Z79.890	Estrogen therapy	Menopause symptoms; ovarian failure
Menostar [estradiol]	Z79.890	Estrogen therapy	Menopause symptoms; osteoporosis prevention
Mepron [atovaquone]	Z79.2	Antibacterial	Pneumonia
Merrem [meropenem]	Z79.2	Antibacterial	Bacterial infections of skin or stomach; bacterial meningitis
Metformin [metformin hydrochloride]	Z79.84	Blood glucose regulator	Diabetes mellitus
Methadone HCl [methadone hydrochloride]	Z79.891	Narcotic analgesic	Pain; treatment of opioid addiction
Methadose [methadone hydrochloride]	Z79.891	Narcotic analgesic	Acute and chronic pain
Methergine [methylergonovine maleate]		Oxytocic agent	Routine management of postpartum hemorrhage after delivery of placenta
Methylprednisolone [methylprednisolone]	Z79.52	Corticosteroids	Inflammatory disorders
Metro [metronidazole]	Z79.2	Antibacterial	Bacterial infections
Metronidazole [metronidazole]	Z79.2	Antibacterial	Bacterial infections
Miacalcin [calcitonin salmon]		Calcitonin; a peptide hormone	Hypercalcemia, osteoporosis, postmenopausal symptoms, Paget's disease
Microgestin [ethinyl estradiol/norethindrone acetate]	Z79.3	Contraceptive	Contraception
Micronor [norethindrone]	Z79.3	Contraceptive	Contraception
Minastrin [ethinyl estradiol/norethindrone acetate]	Z79.3	Contraceptive	Contraception
Minivelle [estradiol]	Z79.890	Estrogen therapy	Menopause symptoms; osteoporosis prevention
Minocin [minocycline hydrochloride]	Z79.2	Antibacterial	Bacterial infections; acne
Mirena [levonorgestrel]	Z79.3	Contraceptive	Intrauterine device for contraception; menstrual disorders
Mobic [meloxicam]	Z79.1	Nonsteroidal anti-inflammatory drug (NSAID)	Pain and inflammation due to osteoarthritis and rheumatoid arthritis
Modicon [ethinyl estradiol/norethindrone]	Z79.3	Contraceptive	Contraception
Monoclonal antibodies	Z79.899	Monoclonal antibodies	Cancer; prophylaxis of organ transplant rejection
Monodox [doxycycline]	Z79.2	Antibacterial	Bacterial infections; acne
Monoket [isosorbide mononitrate]		Antianginal; coronary vasodilator, nitrate	Angina pectoris
Mono-Linyah [norgestimate/ethinyl estradiol]	Z79.3	Contraceptive	Contraception; menstrual disorders; acne
Monurol [fosfomycin tromethamine]	Z79.2	Antibacterial	Bacterial bladder infections
Morphine [morphine sulfate]	Z79.891	Narcotic analgesic	Moderate to severe pain
Motrin [ibuprofen]	Z79.1	Analgesic, general; analgesic, non-narcotic; antiarthritic; antigout; antipyretic; NSAID	Osteoarthritis and rheumatoid arthritis, dysmenorrhea, fever; pain, mild to moderate
Moxatag [amoxicillin]	Z79.2	Antibacterial	Bacterial tonsillitis and pharyngitis
MS Contin [morphine sulfate]	Z79.891	Narcotic analgesic	Moderate to severe pain
Multaq [dronedarone hydrochloride]		Cardiac rhythm regulator	Treatment of patients with recent episodes of atrial fibrillation or atrial flutter
Mycobutin [rifabutin]	Z79.2	Antibacterial	Mycobacterium avium complex (MAC) prophylactic
Myzilra [ethinyl estradiol/levonorgestrel]	Z79.3	Contraceptive	Contraception
Nabumetone [nabumetone]	Z79.1	Non-steroidal anti-inflammatory drug (NSAID)	Osteoarthritis and rheumatoid arthritis
Nalfon [fenoprofen calcium]	Z79.1	Nonsteroidal anti-inflammatory drug (NSAID)	Pain or inflammation relief

Drug	Z Code	Drug Action	Indications
Naprelan [naproxen sodium]	Z79.1	Nonsteroidal anti-inflammatory drug (NSAID)	Pain or inflammation relief
Naprosyn [naproxen]	Z79.1	Anti-inflammatory analgesic, general; analgesic, non-narcotic; antiarthritic; antigout; NSAID	Rheumatoid, gouty arthritis and osteoarthritis; ankylosing spondylitis; bursitis; dysmenorrhea; pain, mild to moderate; tendonitis
Natazia [estradiol valerate/dienogest]	Z79.3	Contraceptive	Contraception; menstrual disorders
Nebupent [pentamidine isethionate]	Z79.2	Antibacterial	Serious bacterial lung infection in high-risk patients with HIV
Nefazodone hydrochloride [nefazodone hydrochloride]		Antidepressant	Depression
Nembutal sodium [pentobarbital sodium]		Sedative; hypnotic	Adjunct medication in diagnostic procedures or for emergency use with convulsive disorders
NeoProfen [ibuprofen lysine]	Z79.1	Nonsteroidal anti-inflammatory drug (NSAID)	Pain or fever relief
Neoral [cyclosporine]	Z79.899	Immunosuppressant	Prophylaxis of organ transplant rejection
Neurontin [gabapentin]		Anticonvulsant	Epilepsy, partial
Nexium [esomeprazole magnesium]		Proton pump inhibitor	Gastroesophageal reflux disease (GERD), erosive esophagitis
Nexplanon [etonogestrel]	Z79.3	Contraceptive	Implantable contraception
Nitrofurantoin [nitrofurantoin]	Z79.2	Antibacterial	Bacterial urinary tract infections
Nitropress [sodium nitroprusside]		Vasodilator	Potent, rapid action in reducing blood pressure in hypertensive crisis or for controlling bleeding during anesthesia by producing controlled hypotension
Nitrostat [nitroglycerin]		Muscle relaxant antianginal; antihypertensive; coronary vasodilator	Prophylaxis and treatment of angina pectoris; heart failure associated with myocardial infarction; hypertension, perioperative; surgery, adjunct
Norco [acetaminophen/hydrocodone bitartrate]	Z79.891	Narcotic analgesic	Moderate to severe pain
Norinyl [mestranol/norethisterone]	Z79.3	Contraceptive	Contraception
Norpace [disopyramide phosphate]		Antiarrhythmic	Coronary artery disease, for prevention, recurrence, and control of unifocal, multifocal, and paired PVCs
Nor-QD [norethindrone]	Z79.3	Contraceptive	Contraception
Nortrel [ethinyl estradiol/norethindrone]	Z79.3	Contraceptive	Contraception
Norvasc [amlodipine besylate]		Calcium channel blocker	Hypertension, chronic stable angina, and vasospastic angina
Novolin [insulin recombinant]	Z79.4	Blood glucose regulator	Diabetes mellitus
NovoLog [insulin recombinant]	Z79.4	Blood glucose regulator	Diabetes mellitus
Nucynta [tapentadol hydrochloride]	Z79.891	Narcotic analgesic	Moderate to severe pain
NuvaRing [etonogestrel/ethinyl estradiol]	Z79.3	Contraceptive	Vaginal ring for contraception
Ogestrel [norgestrel/ethinyl estradiol]	Z79.3	Contraceptive	Contraception
Onglyza [saxagliptin hydrochloride]	Z79.84	Blood glucose regulator	Diabetes mellitus
Opana [oxymorphone hydrochloride]	Z79.891	Narcotic analgesic	Moderate to severe pain
Oracea [doxycycline]	Z79.2	Antibacterial	Rosacea
Orapred ODT [prednisolone sodium phosphate]	Z79.52	Corticosteroids	Inflammatory disorders
Orbactiv [oritavancin diphosphate]	Z79.2	Antibacterial	Bacterial skin infections
Orphenadrine citrate [orphenadrine citrate]		Muscle relaxant	Acute spasms, tension, and post-trauma cases
Orsythia [ethinyl estradiol/levonorgestrel]	Z79.3	Contraceptive	Contraception
Ortho Cyclen [ethinyl estradiol/norgestimate]	Z79.3	Contraceptive	Contraception
Ortho-Novum [norethindrone/ethinyl estradiol]	Z79.3	Contraceptive	Contraception
Ortho-Tri-Cyclen [ethinyl estradiol/norgestimate]	Z79.3	Contraceptive	Contraception
Oseni [alogliptin benzoate/pioglitazone hydrochloride]	Z79.84	Blood glucose regulator	Diabetes mellitus
Osphena [ospemifene]	Z79.810, Z79.890	Selective estrogen receptor modulator (SERM)	Postmenopausal dyspareunia due to vaginal atrophy; osteoporosis prevention and treatment of menopause symptoms
Oxazepam [oxazepam]		Antianxiety agent	Anxiety, tension, and alcohol withdrawal

Drug	Z Code	Drug Action	Indications
Oxycodone HCl [oxycodone hydrochloride]	Z79.891	Narcotic analgesic	Moderate to severe pain
OxyContin [oxycodone hydrochloride]	Z79.891	Narcotic analgesic	Moderate to severe pain
Pavabid [papaverine hydrochloride]		Vasodilator	Relief of cerebral and peripheral ischemia
Paxil [paroxetine hydrochloride]		Antidepressant	Anxiety with panic disorder and depression; obsessive-compulsive disorder
PCE [erythromycin]	Z79.2	Antibacterial	Bacterial infections
PediaPred [prednisolone sodium phosphate]	Z79.52	Corticosteroids	Inflammatory disorders
Pegintron [peginterferon alfa-2b]	Z79.899	Antiviral interferon	Hepatitis C
Penicillin-VK [penicillin V potassium]	Z79.2	Natural penicillin	Chorea prevention; endocarditis prevention, secondary to tooth extraction; erysipelas; infections of the skin and skin structures, upper respiratory tract; rheumatic fever, prophylaxis; scarlet fever; Vincent's gingivitis; Vincent's pharyngitis
Pentam [pentamidine isethionate]	Z79.2	Antibacterial	Serious bacterial lung infections
Pepcid [famotidine]		Histamine H2-receptor inhibitor	Acid/peptic disorder; adenoma, secretory; gastroesophageal reflux; duodenal and gastric ulcer; Zollinger-Ellison syndrome
Percocet [oxycodone hydrochloride/acetaminophen]	Z79.891	Analgesic, general; analgesic-narcotic	Pain, moderate to severe
Persantine [dipyridamole]	Z79.02	Platelet inhibitor	Therapy for chronic angina pectoris, preventing clots post heart valve surgery
Pfizerpen [penicillin g potassium]	Z79.2	Antibacterial	Severe bacterial infections
Phenobarbital [phenobarbital sodium]		Barbiturate	Grand mal epilepsy
Philith [ethinyl estradiol/norethindrone]	Z79.3	Contraceptive	Contraception
Pimtrea [desogestrel/ethinyl estradiol]	Z79.3	Contraceptive	Contraception
Pirmella [ethinyl estradiol/norethindrone]	Z79.3	Contraceptive	Contraception
Pitocin [oxytocin]		Synthetic oxytocin	Induction or stimulation of labor at term
Plan B One-Step [levonorgestrel]	Z79.3	Contraceptive	Contraception
Plasmanate [plasma, plasma protein fraction]		Blood volume expander	Hypovolemic shock, burn patients, and hemorrhages when whole blood is unavailable
Plavix [clopidogrel bisulfate]	Z79.02	Antithrombotic platelet aggregation inhibitor	Lessening of the chance of heart attack or stroke
Ponstel [mefenamic acid]	Z79.1	Nonsteroidal anti-inflammatory drug (NSAID)	Pain
Portia [ethinyl estradiol/levonorgestrel]	Z79.3	Contraceptive	Contraception
Pradaxa [dabigatran etexilate mesylate]	Z79.01	Anticoagulant	Prophylaxis and treatment of blood clots in patients with atrial fibrillation
Prandimet [metformin hydrochloride/repaglinide]	Z79.84	Blood glucose regulator	Diabetes mellitus
Prandin [repaglinide]	Z79.84	Blood glucose regulator	Diabetes mellitus
Pravachol [pravastatin sodium]		HMG-CoA reductase inhibitor (statin)	Hypercholesterolemia, hyperlipidemia, hyperlipoproteinemia
Precose [acarbose]	Z79.84	Blood glucose regulator	Diabetes mellitus
Prednisolone [prednisolone]	Z79.52	Corticosteroids	Inflammatory disorders
Prednisone [prednisone]	Z79.52	Adrenocorticoid, corticosteroid	Used for its immunosuppressant effects and for relief of inflammations; used in arthritis, polymyositis and other systemic diseases
Pregnyl [chorionic gonadotropin]		Gonadotropic hormone	Prepubertal cryptorchidism, hypogonadism, corpus luteum insufficiency and infertility
Prelone [prednisolone]	Z79.52	Corticosteroids; antiasthmatic	Inflammatory disorders
Premarin [conjugated estrogens]	Z79.890	Antineoplastic; estrogen	Vasomotor symptoms associated with menopause; atrophic vaginitis; kraurosis vulvae, female hypogonadism; primary ovarian failure
Prempro [conjugated estrogens/medroxyprogesterone acetate]	Z79.890	Estrogen/progestin	Menopause, osteoporosis, atrophic vaginitis
Prevacid [lansoprazole]		Proton pump inhibitor (PPI)	Acid/peptic disorder, erosive esophagitis, duodenal ulcer, Zollinger-Ellison syndrome
Previfem [ethinyl estradiol/norgestimate]	Z79.3	Contraceptive	Contraception

Drug	Z Code	Drug Action	Indications
Priftin [rifapentine]	Z79.2	Antibacterial	Prophylaxis and treatment of tuberculosis
Prilosec [omeprazole magnesium]		Proton pump inhibitor	Acid/peptic disorder; endocrine adenoma; erosive esophagitis; systemic mastocytosis; gastroesophageal reflux; duodenal, peptic and gastric ulcer; Zollinger-Ellison syndrome
Primaxin [cilastatin sodium/imipenem]	Z79.2	Antibacterial	Skin, stomach, female reproductive organs or lower respiratory tract infections
Prinivil [lisinopril]		Synthetic peptide derivative, long-acting angiotensin converting enzyme inhibitor	Congestive heart failure, essential hypertension
Procardia [nifedipine]		Antianginal agent; calcium channel blocker	Management of vasospastic angina and chronic stable angina, essential hypertension
Prograf [tacrolimus]	Z79.899	Immunosuppressant	Prophylaxis of organ transplant rejection
Promethazine hydrochloride [promethazine hydrochloride]		Anesthesia, adjunct to; antiemetic; antihistamine; antitussive/expectorant; sedative/hypnotic; vertigo/motion sickness/vomiting	Anesthesia; adjunct; angioedema; conjunctivitis; dermographism; hypersensitivity, motion sickness; pain; perennial, seasonal, and allergic rhinitis; sedation, obstetrical; urticaria
Protonix [pantoprazole]		Proton pump inhibitor (PPI)	Short-term treatment and maintenance therapy of erosive esophagitis associated with gastroesophageal reflux disease (GERD)
Protopic [tacrolimus]	Z79.899	Immunosuppressant	Atomic dermatitis (eczema)
Proventil-HFA [albuterol sulfate]		Antiasthmatic/bronchodilator	Asthma
Provera [medroxyprogesterone acetate]	Z79.3, Z79.890	Antineoplastic; contraceptive; progestin	Amenorrhea; carcinoma, endometrium, adjunct; carcinoma, renal; contraception; hemorrhage
Prozac [fluoxetine hydrochloride]		Serotonin reuptake inhibitor	Bulimia nervosa; depression; obsessive-compulsive disorder
Pulmicort [budesonide]	Z79.51	Corticosteroids -inhaled; antiasthmatic	Prophylaxis and treatment of asthma
Qnasl [beclomethasone dipropionate]		Corticosteroid	Perennial allergies, seasonal allergies, and vasomotor rhinitis
Qtern [dapagliflozin propanediol/saxagliptin hydrochloride]	Z79.84	Blood glucose regulator	Diabetes mellitus
Quartette [levonorgestrel/ethinyl estradiol]	Z79.3	Contraceptive	Contraception
Quasense [ethinyl estradiol/levonorgestrel]	Z79.3	Contraceptive	Contraception
Quinidine gluconate [quinidine gluconate]		Antiarrhythmic	Management of cardiac arrhythmias
Qvar [beclomethasone dipropionate]	Z79.51	Corticosteroids -inhaled; antiasthmatic	Prevention and control of symptoms related to asthma
Raloxifene [raloxifene hydrochloride]	Z79.810	Selective estrogen receptor modulator (SERM)	Prevention of thinning of the bones (osteoporosis) only in postmenopausal women
Rapamune [sirolimus]	Z79.899	Immunosuppressant	Prophylaxis of organ transplant rejection
Rayos [prednisone]	Z79.52	Corticosteroids; antiasthmatic	Arthritis, blood disorders, allergies, asthma
Rebif [interferon beta-1a]	Z79.899	Antiviral interferon	Relapsing multiple sclerosis
Reclast [zoledronic acid]	Z79.83	Bisphosphonates	Prevention of thinning of the bones (osteoporosis); Paget's disease; bone cancer
Repaglinide [repaglinide]	Z79.84	Blood glucose regulator	Diabetes mellitus
Reprexain [hydrocodone bitartrate/ibuprofen]	Z79.891	Opioid analgesic/Nonsteroidal anti-inflammatory drug (NSAID)	Pain, inflammation, or fever relief
Restoril [temazepam]		Sedative/hypnotic	Insomnia
Retrovir [zidovudine]		Antiretroviral agent	Indicated in symptomatic HIV infection
Rifadin [rifampin]	Z79.2	Antibacterial	Prophylaxis and treatment of tuberculosis
Rimactane [rifampin]	Z79.2	Antibacterial	Prophylaxis and treatment of tuberculosis
Riomet [metformin hydrochloride]	Z79.84	Blood glucose regulator	Diabetes mellitus
Risperdal [risperidone]		Antipsychotic/antimanic	Schizophrenia; bipolar I disorder
Ritalin [methylphenidate hydrochloride]		Central nervous system (CNS) stimulant	Treatment of depression and hyperkinetic activity in children
Roxicet [oxycodone hydrochloride/acetaminophen]	Z79.891	Analgesic, general; analgesic-narcotic	Pain, moderate to severe
Roxicodone [oxycodone hydrochloride]	Z79.891	Narcotic analgesic	Pain relief
Ryzodeg [insulin aspart/insulin degludec]	Z79.4	Blood glucose regulator	Diabetes mellitus
Sabril [vigabatrin]		Anticonvulsant	Refractory complex partial seizures
Safyral [drospirenone/ethinyl estradiol/levomefolate calcium]	Z79.3	Contraceptive	Contraception

Drug	Z Code	Drug Action	Indications
Sandimmune [cyclosporine]	Z79.899	Immunosuppressant	Prophylaxis of organ transplant rejection
Savaysa [edoxaban tosylate]	Z79.01	Anticoagulant	Prophylaxis and treatment of venous thrombosis, pulmonary embolism; prevention of blood clots due to atrial fibrillation
Seasonale [levonorgestrel/ethinyl estradiol]	Z79.3	Contraceptive	Contraception
Seasonique [ethinyl estradiol/levonorgestrel]	Z79.3	Contraceptive	Contraception
Septra [sulfamethoxazole trimethoprim]	Z79.2	Antibacterial	Treatment of urinary tract infections, acute otitis media, acute exacerbations of chronic bronchitis, and shigellosis
Serevent [salmeterol xinafoate]		Bronchodilator	Asthma
Seromycin [cycloserine]	Z79.2	Antibacterial	Tuberculosis; urinary tract infections
Setlakin [ethinyl estradiol/levonorgestrel]	Z79.3	Contraceptive	Contraception
Simulect [basiliximab]	Z79.899	Immunosuppressant	Prophylaxis of organ transplant rejection
Sinemet [carbidopa/levodopa]		Antiparkinsonian	Parkinson's disease
Singulair [montelukast sodium]		Antiasthmatic, leukotriene receptor antagonist	Treatment of mild to moderate asthma to decrease the symptoms of asthma and the number of acute asthma attacks
Sirolimus [sirolimus]	Z79.899	Immunosuppressant	Prophylaxis of organ transplant rejection
Sitagliptin [sitagliptin/metformin hydrochloride]	Z79.84	Blood glucose regulator	Diabetes mellitus
Sivextro [tedizolid phosphate]	Z79.2	Antibacterial	Skin infections including MRSA
Skyla [levonorgestrel]	Z79.3	Contraceptive	Intrauterine device for contraception
Solodyn [minocycline hydrochloride]	Z79.2	Antibacterial	Bacterial infections
Soltamox [tamoxifen citrate]	Z79.810	Selective estrogen receptor modulator (SERM)	Breast cancer
Solu-Cortef [hydrocortisone sodium succinate]	Z79.52	Corticosteroids; antiasthmatic	Asthma; severe inflammation; allergic reactions
Solu-Medrol [methylprednisolone sodium succinate]	Z79.52	Adrenocorticosteroid	Anti-inflammatory and antiallergenic for shock and ulcerative colitis
Sprintec [norgestimate/ethinyl estradiol]	Z79.3	Contraceptive	Contraception
Streptomycin sulfate [streptomycin sulfate]	Z79.2	Antibacterial	Severe bacterial infections
Sublimaze [fentanyl citrate]	Z79.891	Narcotic analgesic	Pain relief
Supprelin LA [histrelin acetate]	Z79.818	Agents affecting estrogen receptors and estrogen levels	Precocious puberty; prostate cancer symptoms
Suprax [cefixime]	Z79.2	Antibacterial	Bacterial infections
Syeda [drospirenone/ethinyl estradiol]	Z79.3	Contraceptive	Contraception
Sylatron [peginterferon alfa-2b]	Z79.899	Antineoplastic interferons; antiviral interferons	Prevention of recurrent malignant melanoma
Symbicort [budesonide/formoterol fumarate dihydrate]	Z79.51	Corticosteroids -inhaled; antiasthmatic	Prophylaxis and treatment of asthma and COPD
Synarel [nafarelin acetate]	Z79.818	Agents affecting estrogen receptors and estrogen levels	Endometriosis symptoms; precocious puberty
Synercid [dalfopristin/quinupristin]	Z79.2	Antibacterial	Severe blood infections
Synjardy [empagliflozin/metformin hydrochloride]	Z79.84	Blood glucose regulator	Diabetes mellitus
Synthroid [levothyroxine sodium]		Thyroid hormone	Treatment of hypothyroidism
Tacrolimus [tacrolimus]	Z79.899	Immunosuppressant	Prophylaxis of organ transplant rejection
Tagamet HB [cimetidine]		Acid reducer	Treatment of active duodenal ulcer, short-term treatment of active, benign gastric ulcer, and treatment of pathological hypersecretory conditions
Tamoxifen [tamoxifen citrate]	Z79.810	Selective estrogen receptor modulator (SERM)	Metastatic breast cancer in postmenopausal women
Tazicef [ceftazidime]	Z79.2	Antibacterial	Confirmed or suspected bacterial infections
Teflaro [ceftaroline fosamil]	Z79.2	Antibacterial	Bacterial skin infections; pneumonia
Tegretol [carbamazepine]		Anticonvulsant; analgesic	Epilepsy, especially with complex symptomatology; specific analgesic for trigeminal neuralgia

Drug	Z Code	Drug Action	Indications
Tenormin [atenolol]		Antianginal; antihypertensive; beta blocker	Treatment of hypertension; lowering blood pressure lowers the risk of fatal and nonfatal cardiovascular events, primarily strokes and myocardial infarctions
Terazosin hydrochloride [terazosin hydrochloride]		Alpha-blocker; antihypertensive; diuretic	Benign prostatic hypertrophy; essential hypertension
Tetracycline HCl [tetracycline hydrochloride]	Z79.2	Antibacterial	Bacterial infections
Tiazac [diltiazem hydrochloride]		Antianginal, antiarrhythmic, antihypertensive, channel blocker, coronary vasodilator	Chronic stable angina, atrial fibrillation, atrial flutter, essential hypertension, paroxysmal supraventricular tachycardia
Tivorbex [indomethacin]	Z79.1	Nonsteroidal anti-inflammatory drug (NSAID)	Pain, inflammation and joint stiffness
Tobradex [tobramycin/dexamethasone]		Aminoglycoside ocular anti-infective; anti-inflammatory	Infectious conjunctivitis; dermatosis, corticosteroid-responsive with secondary infection; foreign body in eye; corneal inflammation; uveitis
Tobramycin [dexamethasone/tobramycin]	Z79.2	Antibacterial	Bacterial eye infections
Toprol-XL [metoprolol succinate]		Antianginal antihypertensive beta blocker	Angina pectoris, essential hypertension
Toremifene [toremifene citrate]	Z79.810	Selective estrogen receptor modulator (SERM)	Metastatic breast cancer in postmenopausal women
Torisel [temsirolimus]	Z79.899	Antineoplastic	Renal cell carcinoma
Toujeo Solostar [insulin glargine recombinant]	Z79.4	Blood glucose regulator	Diabetes mellitus
Trazodone hydrochloride [trazodone hydrochloride]		Antidepressant	Depression
Trelstar [triptorelin pamoate]	Z79.818	Agents affecting estrogen receptors and estrogen levels	Prophylaxis of chemo-induced menopause; prostate cancer symptoms
Tresiba [insulin degludec]	Z79.4	Blood glucose regulator	Diabetes mellitus
Triamterene and hydrochlorothiazide [triamterene/ hydrochlorothiazide]		Antihypertensive, diuretic	Edema; essential hypertension
Tri-Estarylla [ethinyl estradiol/norgestimate]	Z79.3	Contraceptive	Contraception; acne
Tri-Legest [ethinyl estradiol/norethindrone acetate]	Z79.3	Contraceptive	Contraception
Tri-Linyah [ethinyl estradiol/norgestimate]	Z79.3	Contraceptive	Contraception
Tri-Lo-Estarylla [ethinyl estradiol/norgestimate]	Z79.3	Contraceptive	Contraception
Tri-Lo-Sprintec [ethinyl estradiol/norgestimate]	Z79.3	Contraceptive	Contraception
Trimethoprim [trimethoprim]	Z79.2	Antibacterial	Acute exacerbation chronic bronchitis; travelers' diarrhea; infections of the middle and lower respiratory tracts, and urinary tract; pneumonia, pneumocystis; shigellosis
Tri-Norinyl [ethinyl estradiol/norethindrone]	Z79.3	Contraceptive	Contraception
Tri-Previfem [ethinyl estradiol/norgestimate]	Z79.3	Contraceptive	Contraception
Tri-Sprintec [ethinyl estradiol/norgestimate]	Z79.3	Contraceptive	Contraception; acne
Trivora [ethinyl estradiol/ levonorgestrel]	Z79.3	Contraceptive	Contraception
Tygacil [tigecycline]	Z79.2	Antibacterial	Bacterial skin or digestive system infections; pneumonia
Tylenol with codeine [acetaminophen/codeine phosphate]	Z79.891	Narcotic analgesic	Pain and cough
Ultram [tramadol hydrochloride]	Z79.891	Analgesic, non-narcotic (opiate, narcotic-like)	Pain, moderate to moderately severe
Unasyn [ampicillin sodium/sulbactam sodium]	Z79.2	Antibacterial	Bacterial infections
Vagifem [estradiol]	Z79.890	Estrogen therapy	Menopause symptoms
Valium [diazepam]		Antianxiety, muscle relaxant, anticonvulsant	Anxiety, tension, withdrawal from alcohol, muscle spasms and anticonvulsant therapy; epilepsy, generalized tonic-clonic; status epilepticus; stiff-man syndrome; tetanus

Drug	Z Code	Drug Action	Indications
Vancocin HCl [vancomycin hydrochloride]	Z79.2	Antibacterial	Serious bacterial infections
Vancomycin HCl [vancomycin hydrochloride]	Z79.2	Antibacterial	Serious bacterial infections
Vantas [histrelin acetate]	Z79.818	Agents affecting estrogen receptors and estrogen levels	Prostate cancer symptoms; breast cancer; endometriosis
Vasotec [enalaprilat maleate]		ACE inhibitor; antihypertensive	Congestive heart failure; essential hypertension
Velivet [desogestrel/ethinyl estradiol]	Z79.3	Contraceptive	Contraception
Ventolin HFA [albuterol sulfate]		Antiasthmatic/bronchodilator	Asthma
Verapamil HCL [verapamil hydrochloride]		Antianginal, antiarrhythmic, antiarthritic, antihypertensive, calcium channel blocker	Angina pectoris, chronic stable angina, atrial fibrillation, atrial flutter, paroxysmal supraventricular tachycardia, ventricular arrhythmia, essential hypertension
Viagra [sildenafil citrate]		Phosphodiesterase-5 (PDE5) inhibitor	Erectile dysfunction
Vibativ [telavancin hydrochloride]	Z79.2	Antibacterial	Pneumonia; severe bacterial skin infections
Vibramycin [doxycycline calcium]	Z79.2	Antibacterial	Bacterial infections
Vicoprofen [hydrocodone bitartrate/ibuprofen]	Z79.891	Opioid analgesic/ Nonsteroidal anti-inflammatory drug (NSAID)	Pain, inflammation, or fever relief
Victoza [liraglutide (rDNA) injection]		Glucagon-like peptide-1 (GLP-1) receptor agonist	Diabetes mellitus
Vienva [ethinyl estradiol/levonorgestrel]	Z79.3	Contraceptive	Contraception
Viorele [desogestrel/ethinyl estradiol]	Z79.3	Contraceptive	Contraception
Virazole [ribavirin]		Antiviral	Respiratory syncytial virus (RSV)
Vistaril [hydroxyzine pamoate]		Antianxiety agent, antiemetic	Treatment of nausea and vomiting, for reducing narcotic requirement in surgery and as tranquilizer for tension, anxiety, or agitation states
Vivelle [estradiol]	Z79.890	Estrogen therapy	Menopause symptoms; osteoporosis prevention
Voltaren [diclofenac sodium]	Z79.1	Nonsteroidal anti-inflammatory drug (NSAID)	Treatment of pain, inflammation, and joint stiffness due to arthritis
Warfarin [warfarin sodium]	Z79.01	Anticoagulant	Prophylaxis and treatment of venous thrombosis, treatment of atrial fibrillation with embolization (pulmonary embolism), arrhythmias, myocardial infarction, and stroke prevention
Wellbutrin SR, Wellbutrin XL [bupropion hydrochloride]		Antidepressant; CNS	Depression; smoking cessation
Wera [ethinyl estradiol/norethindrone]	Z79.3	Contraceptive	Contraception
Xalatan [latanoprost]		Prostaglandin F2α analogue	Glaucoma, open-angle; ocular hypertension
Xanax, Xanax XR [alprazolam]		Antianxiety; sedative/hypnotic	Anxiety disorders with panic disorder and depression
Xarelto [rivaraxaban]	Z79.01	Anticoagulant	Prophylaxis and treatment of venous thrombosis, pulmonary embolism; prevention of blood clots due to atrial fibrillation
Xifaxan [rifaximin]	Z79.2	Antibacterial	*E. coli* diarrhea
Xigduo [dapagliflozin propanediol/metformin hydrochloride]	Z79.84	Blood glucose regulator	Diabetes mellitus
Xigris [drotrecogin alfa]		Biologic response modifier	Severe sepsis
Yasmin [drospirenone/ethinyl estradiol]	Z79.3	Contraceptive	Contraception
Yaz [drospirenone/ethinyl estradiol]	Z79.3	Contraceptive	Contraception; menstrual disorders
Zantac [ranitidine hydrochloride]		Histamine H2-receptors inhibitor	Acid/peptic disorder, erosive esophagitis, gastrointestinal hypersecretion, mastocytosis, gastroesophageal reflux, peptic ulcer, Zollinger-Ellison syndrome
Zerbaxa [ceftolozane sulfate/tazobactam sodium]	Z79.2	Antibacterial	Complicated urinary tract and intra-abdominal infections
Zestoretic [lisinopril/hydrochlorothiazide]		ACE inhibitor; antihypertensive	Congestive heart failure; essential hypertension
Zestril [lisinopril]		ACE inhibitor; antihypertensive	Congestive heart failure; essential hypertension
Ziac [bisoprolol fumarate/ hydrochlorothiazide]		Antihypertensive	Essential hypertension
Zinacef [cefuroxime sodium]	Z79.2	Antibacterial	Bacterial infections
Zipsor [diclofenac potassium]	Z79.1	Nonsteroidal anti-inflammatory drug (NSAID)	Pain and inflammation relief

Drug	Z Code	Drug Action	Indications
Zithromax [azithromycin]	Z79.2	Macrolide	Infections of the cervix, lower respiratory tract, skin and skin structures, urethra, nongonococcal; mycobacterium avium complex; pharyngitis, streptococcal pneumonia; tonsillitis
Zmax [azithromycin]	Z79.2	Antibacterial	Pneumonia; sinusitis
Zocor [simvastatin]		HMG-CoA reductase inhibitor (statin)	Hypercholesterolemia, hyperlipidemia, hyperlipoproteinemia, hypertriglyceridemia
Zoladex [goserelin acetate]	Z79.818	Agents affecting estrogen receptors and estrogen levels	Prostate cancer symptoms and advanced breast cancer
Zoloft [sertraline hydrochloride]		Antidepressant	Anxiety with panic disorder and depression; obsessive-compulsive disorder
Zometa [zoledronic acid]	Z79.83	Bisphosphonates	Multiple myeloma; Paget's disease
Zorvolex [diclofenac]	Z79.1	Nonsteroidal anti-inflammatory drug (NSAID)	Pain, inflammation or fever relief
Zosyn [piperacillin sodium/tazobactam sodium]	Z79.2	Antibacterial	Bacterial infections
Zovia [ethynodiol diacetate/ethinyl estradiol]	Z79.3	Contraceptive	Contraception
Zovirax [acyclovir]		Antiviral	Genital herpes and herpes zoster infections
Zyloprim [allopurinol]		Antigout	Gouty arthritis, renal calculus, hyperuricemia, hyperuricemia secondary to leukemia, hyperuricemia secondary to lymphoma
Zyprexa [olanzapine]		Antipsychotic/antimanic	Psychotic disorders; schizophrenia
Zyrtec [cetirizine hydrochloride]		Antihistamine	Perennial allergic and seasonal allergic rhinitis; chronic urticaria
Zyvox [linezolid]	Z79.2	Antibacterial	Serious bacterial infections

Appendix D: Z Codes for Long-Term Drug Use with Associated Drugs

Z79.01 Long term (current) use of anticoagulants
- Arixtra
- Coumadin
- Eliquis
- Fragmin
- Heparin
- Jantoven
- Lovenox
- Pradaxa
- Savaysa
- Warfarin
- Xarelto

Z79.02 Long term (current) use of antithrombotics/antiplatelets
- Aggrastat
- Aggrenox
- Angiomax
- Argatroban
- Brilinta
- Clopidogrel bisulfate
- Effient
- Integrilin
- Iprivask
- Persantine
- Plavix

Z79.1 Long term (current) use of non-steroidal anti-inflammatories (NSAID)
- Advil
- Aleve
- Anaprox
- Arthrotec
- Caldolor
- Cambia
- Celebrex
- Daypro
- Duexis
- Dyloject
- Feldene
- Ibuprofen
- Indocin
- Mobic
- Motrin
- Nabumetone
- Nalfon
- Naprelan
- Naprosyn
- NeoProfen
- Ponstel
- Tivorbex
- Voltaren
- Zipsor
- Zorvolex

Z79.2 Long term (current) use of antibiotics
- Akne-Mycin
- Altabax
- Amoxicillin
- Ampicillin
- Ancef
- Augmentin
- Azactam
- Azithromycin
- Bactrim
- Bactroban
- Ceftriaxone
- Centany
- Cephalexin
- Cipro
- Ciprofloxacin
- Clarithromycin
- Cleocin
- Clindamycin
- Daptomycin
- Dificid
- Doxycycline
- Dynacin
- E.E.S.
- Ertapenem
- ERYC
- Erygel
- EryPed
- Ery-Tab
- Erythrocin
- Erythromycin
- Factive
- Flagyl
- Fortaz
- Gentamicin sulfate
- Invanz
- Isoniazid
- Keflex
- Kefzol
- Klaron
- Levaquin
- Lincocin
- Macrobid
- Maxipime
- Mefoxin
- Mepron
- Merrem
- Metro
- Metronidazole
- Minocin
- Monodox
- Monurol
- Moxatag
- Mycobutin
- Nebupent
- Nitrofurantoin
- Oracea
- Orbactiv
- PCE
- Penicillin-VK
- Pentam
- Pfizerpen
- Priftin
- Primaxin
- Rifadin
- Rimactane
- Septra
- Seromycin
- Sivextro
- Solodyn
- Streptomycin sulfate
- Suprax
- Synercid
- Tazicef
- Teflaro
- Tetracycline HCl
- Tobramycin
- Trimethoprim
- Tygacil
- Unasyn
- Vancocin HCl
- Vancomycin HCl
- Vibativ
- Vibramycin
- Xifaxan
- Zerbaxa
- Zinacef
- Zithromax
- Zmax
- Zosyn
- Zyvox

Z79.3 Long term (current) use of hormonal contraceptives
- Altavera
- Alyacen
- Aranelle
- Ashlyna
- Aviane
- Aygestin
- Balziva
- Bekyree
- Beyaz
- Brevicon
- Briellyn
- Camila
- Cryselle
- Cyclafem

Cyclessa
Dasetta
Daysee
Depo-Provera
Depo-SubQ Provera
Desogen
Elinest
Emoquette
Enpresse
Enskyce
Errin
Estarylla
Estrostep Fe
Falmina
Femcon Fe
Femhrt
Gildagia
Gildess
Introvale
Jencycla
Junel
Kariva
Kelnor
Kimidess
Kurvelo
Larin
Lessina
Levonest
Levora
Liletta
Lo Loestrin Fe
Lo Minastrin Fe
Loestrin
Loryna
LoSeasonique
Low-Ogestrel
Marlissa
Microgestin
Micronor
Minastrin
Mirena
Modicon
Mono-Linyah
Myzilra
Natazia
Nexplanon
Norinyl
Nor-QD
Nortrel
NuvaRing
Ogestrel
Orsythia
Ortho Cyclen
Ortho-Novum
Ortho-Tri-Cyclen
Philith

Pimtrea
Pirmella
Plan B One-Step
Portia
Previfem
Provera
Quartette
Quasense
Safyral
Seasonale
Seasonique
Setlakin
Skyla
Sprintec
Syeda
Tri-Estarylla
Tri-Legest
Tri-Linyah
Tri-Lo-Estarylla
Tri-Lo-Sprintec
Tri-Norinyl
Tri-Previfem
Tri-Sprintec
Trivora
Velivet
Vienva
Viorele
Wera
Yasmin
Yaz
Zovia

Z79.4   **Long term (current) use of insulin**
Afrezza
Apidra
Basaglar
Humalog
Humulin
Lantus
Levemir
Novolin
NovoLog
Ryzodeg
Toujeo Solostar
Tresiba

Z79.51   **Long term (current) use of inhaled steroids**
Advair
Aerospan
Alvesco
Arnuity Ellipta
Asmanex
Dulera
Flovent
Pulmicort
Qvar

Symbicort

Z79.52   **Long term (current) use of systemic steroids**
A-Methapred
Aristospan
Celestone Soluspan
Colocort
Cortef
Cortenema
Cortifoam
Cortisone acetate
Depo-Medrol
Dexamethasone Intensol
Entocort EC
Hydrocortisone
Kenalog
Medrol
Methylprednisolone
Orapred ODT
PediaPred
Prednisolone
Prednisone
Prelone
Rayos
Solu-Cortef
Solu-Medrol

Z79.810 **Long term (current) use of selective estrogen receptor modulators (SERMs)**
Evista
Fareston
Osphena
Raloxifene
Soltamox
Tamoxifen
Toremifene

Z79.811 **Long term (current) use of aromatase inhibitors**
Anastrozole
Arimidex
Aromasin
Exemestane
Femara
Letrozole

Z79.818 **Long term (current) use of other agents affecting estrogen receptors and estrogen levels**
Eligard
Faslodex
Fulvestrant
Lupron
Megace ES
Supprelin LA
Synarel

Trelstar
Vantas
Zoladex

Z79.82   Long term (current) use of aspirin
Bayer
Bufferin
Ecotrin

Z79.83   Long term (current) use of bisphosphonates
Actonel
Atelvia
Binosto
Boniva
Didronel
Fosamax
Reclast
Zometa

Z79.84   Long term (current) use of oral hypoglycemic drugs
Acarbose
Actoplus Met
Actos
Amaryl
Avandia
Duetact
Fortamet
Glimepiride
Glucophage
Glucotrol
Glucovance
Glumetza
Glyburide
Invokamet
Janumet
Januvia
Jentadueto
Kazano
Kombiglyze
Metformin
Onglyza
Oseni
PrandiMet
Prandin
Precose
Qtern
Repaglinide
Riomet
Sitagliptin
Synjardy
Xigduo

Z79.890 Hormone replacement therapy
Activella
Alora
Angeliq

Climara
CombiPatch
Delestrogen
Divigel
Duavee
Elestrin
Enjuvia
Estrace
Estraderm
Estrasorb
EstroGel
Femhrt
Femring
Femtrace
Menest
Menostar
Minivelle
Osphena
Premarin
Prempro
Provera
Vagifem
Vivelle

Z79.891 Long term (current) use of opiate analgesic
Acetaminophen with codeine
Astramorph
Buprenex
Buprenorphine HCl
Butrans
Codeine
Demerol
Dilaudid
Dolophine HCl
Duragesic
Duramorph
Embeda
Exalgo
Fentanyl
Fentora
Fioricet with codeine
Hydrocodone
Hydrocodone bitartrate and acetaminophen
Hydromorphone HCl
Kadian
Methadone HCl
Methadose
Morphine
MS Contin
Norco
Nucynta
Opana
Oxycodone HCl
OxyContin

Percocet
Reprexain
Roxicet
Roxicodone
Sublimaze
Tylenol with codeine
Ultram
Vicoprofen

Z79.899 Other long term (current) drug therapy
Actimmune
Antineoplastic/chemotherapy
Astagraf XL
Avonex
Cellcept
Cyclosporine
Envarsus XR
Gengraf
Imuran
Intron
Monoclonal antibodies
Neoral
Pegintron
Prograf
Protopic
Rapamune
Rebif
Sandimmune
Simulect
Sirolimus
Sylatron
Tacrolimus
Torisel

Appendix E: Z Codes Only as Principal/First-Listed Diagnosis

Z00.00	Z01.20	Z02.3	Z03.810	Z34.01	Z38.5	Z51.12	Z52.5
Z00.01	Z01.21	Z02.4	Z03.818	Z34.02	Z38.61	Z52.000	Z52.6
Z00.110	Z01.30	Z02.5	Z03.89	Z34.03	Z38.62	Z52.001	Z52.810
Z00.111	Z01.31	Z02.6	Z04.1	Z34.80	Z38.63	Z52.008	Z52.811
Z00.121	Z01.411	Z02.71	Z04.2	Z34.81	Z38.64	Z52.010	Z52.812
Z00.129	Z01.419	Z02.79	Z04.3	Z34.82	Z38.65	Z52.011	Z52.813
Z00.2	Z01.42	Z02.81	Z04.41	Z34.83	Z38.66	Z52.018	Z52.819
Z00.3	Z01.810	Z02.82	Z04.42	Z34.90	Z38.68	Z52.090	Z52.89
Z00.5	Z01.811	Z02.83	Z04.6	Z34.91	Z38.69	Z52.091	Z76.1
Z00.70	Z01.812	Z02.89	Z04.71	Z34.92	Z38.7	Z52.098	Z76.2
Z00.71	Z01.818	Z02.9	Z04.72	Z34.93	Z38.8	Z52.10	Z99.12
Z00.8	Z01.82	Z03.6	Z04.8	Z38.00	Z39.0	Z52.11	
Z01.00	Z01.83	Z03.71	Z04.9	Z38.01	Z39.1	Z52.19	
Z01.01	Z01.84	Z03.72	Z31.81	Z38.1	Z39.2	Z52.20	
Z01.10	Z01.89	Z03.73	Z31.83	Z38.2	Z42.1	Z52.21	
Z01.110	Z02.0	Z03.74	Z31.84	Z38.30	Z42.8	Z52.29	
Z01.118	Z02.1	Z03.75	Z33.2	Z38.31	Z51.0	Z52.3	
Z01.12	Z02.2	Z03.79	Z34.00	Z38.4	Z51.11	Z52.4	

Appendix F: Centers for Medicare & Medicaid Services Hierarchical Condition Categories (CMS-HCC)

In the 1970s, Medicare began demonstration projects that contracted with health maintenance organizations (HMO) to provide care for Medicare beneficiaries in exchange for prospective payments. In 1985, this project changed from demonstration status to a regular part of the Medicare program, Medicare Part C. The Balanced Budget Act (BBA) of 1997 named Medicare's Part C managed care program Medicare+Choice, and the Medicare Modernization Act (MMA) of 2003 again renamed it to Medicare Advantage (MA).

Medicare is one of the world's largest health insurance programs, and about one-fourth of the beneficiaries on Medicare are enrolled in a MA private health care plan. Due to the great variance in the health status of Medicare beneficiaries, risk adjustment provides a means of adequately compensating those plans with large numbers of seriously ill patients while not overburdening other plans that have healthier individuals. Medicare Advantage (MA) plans have been using the HCC/risk adjustment model since 2004.

The Risk Adjustment Model

The primary purpose of a risk adjustment model is to predict (on average) the future health care costs for specific consortiums enrolled in Medicare Advantage (MA) health plans. CMS is then able to provide capitation payments to these private health plans. Capitation payments are an incentive for health plans to enroll not only healthier individuals but those with chronic conditions or who are more seriously ill by removing some of the financial burden.

The MA risk adjustment model uses hierarchical condition categories (HCC) to assess the disease burden of its enrollees. HCC diagnostic groupings were created after examining claims data so that enrollees with similar disease processes, and consequently similar health care expenditures, could be pooled into a larger data set in which an average expenditure rate could be determined. The medical conditions included in HCC categories are those that were determined to most predictably affect the health status and health care costs of any individual. Several important principles to the risk adjustment model and the development of the HCC categories include but are not limited to:

1. The HCC diagnostic categories should be clinically meaningful.
   - Diagnostic categories are well-defined.
   - Clinically specific diseases or medical conditions are grouped to each category.
2. The HCC diagnostic categories should predict medical expenditures.
   - The diagnoses grouped to a specific category should have as close to the same cost burden not only in the current year but also in the future.
3. The HCC diagnostic categories should have adequate sample sizes and discretionary categories excluded to be as accurate and stable in their estimate of costs as possible.
   - A diagnostic category that groups extremely rare diseases or conditions would not be reliably effective in determining current or future costs.
   - Codes that are not credible as cost predictors or may be subject to coding variation should be excluded, when possible.
4. The HCC diagnostic categories should be both hierarchical and accumulative.
   - Hierarchical measurement is used within a specific disease process.
   - Disease processes that are unrelated to each other are measured accumulatively.
5. The diagnostic classification should encourage specificity and should not reward coding proliferation.
   - More diagnosis codes and vague diagnosis codes do not equal greater disease burden.

More than 9,000 ICD-10-CM diagnosis codes map to 79 HCCs in the current risk adjustment model. Diagnoses are excluded from mapping when they do not predict future cost or are vague or variable in diagnosis, coding, or treatment, such as symptoms or osteoarthritis. Also excluded are diagnosis codes from laboratories, radiology, and home health claims.

Risk Adjustment Factors

The CMS-HCC risk adjustment model uses "risk adjustment factors" to calculate a risk score for each member. This score summarizes that particular patient's expected cost of care relative to other members'. Each member's risk score is based on demographic and health status information and is calculated as the sum of these demographic and health factors weighted by their estimated marginal contributions to total risk. The model also takes into account where the patient resides (community or institutional), Medicaid eligibility (full or partial benefit), the patient's Medicare enrollment status (new or established), age, disability status, whether the patient is frail or has end-stage renal disease (ESRD), and even prescription drug use.

No procedure codes, ICD-10-PCS or CPT, are included in the MA risk adjustment model. The model relies solely on diagnostic and demographic data. Not all ICD-10-CM diagnoses map to an HCC, and there is no specific code sequencing involved. The CMS-HCC model is accumulative as well as hierarchical. The accumulative functionality allows a patient to have more than one HCC category assigned, providing a more complete clinical picture and prediction of resource consumption. The hierarchical aspect of the model provides a means of ranking diagnoses that are similar in disease process, by severity. The hierarchy of the condition categories ensures the patient's conditions are classified to the most severe condition within the related group. Less severe conditions within a particular hierarchy are superseded by more severe diagnoses within the same group. The hierarchy and accumulative relationship permits this model to characterize the person's illness level within each disease process, while still allowing the effects of unrelated disease processes to be counted in the patient's overall score.

Certain combinations of coexisting diagnoses for an individual can increase medical costs. The CMS-HCC model adjusts for these higher costs by the addition of "disease interaction" factors. For each patient, multiple HCCs assigned, along with demographic and disease interaction factors, are used to calculate a single, combined risk adjustment factor (RAF). The RAF score for an individual member represents all of the HCCs that have been submitted from all sources for that member to CMS during the course of an entire calendar year.

There are separate CMS-HCC models for new enrollees and continuing enrollees. The new enrollee model uses demographic factors only, such as age, sex, and disability status, and is used when the enrollee has less than 12 months of medical history. The community model accounts for age, sex, original reason for Medicare entitlement (age or disability), Medicaid eligibility, and clinical conditions as measured by HCCs. In the second step, expected costs are adjusted for outliers based on the member's risk score and whether the patient has ESRD.

Demographic data (age, sex, eligibility) as well as health status (diagnoses codes submitted on claims to CMS) of an MA population are used to determine the reimbursement to the health plan to care for their members.

RAF scores, which range from 0.118 to 2.4888, indicate patient health status. A RAF score of 1.0 or below is the benchmark CMS uses to indicate the average healthy patient with the same demographic and diagnostic factors. These patients are expected to use average or lower-than-average resources. When the RAF score is higher than 1.0, CMS considers the patient to be sicker than the average patient with the same criteria and expects greater-than-average resource utilization.

A low RAF score may accurately indicate a healthier patient, but it may also falsely indicate a healthier patient due to incomplete or inaccurate coding, incomplete or insufficient record documentation, or patients who fail to complete an annual assessment.

A high RAF score may accurately indicate a sicker patient, or it may be falsely inflated from overcoding due to diagnoses that are reported but not documented, or from copying and pasting from previous encounters or problem lists of resolved conditions.

Documentation Requirements

Payment is made per HCC category (not per diagnosis code). No matter how many times in the year the diagnosis codes are reported, a single payment is made to the MA plan each year. Each year the list of HCCs and the RAF for each patient is "reset." This means the annual health assessment is extremely important, and adequate documentation is critical. Accurate risk adjustment payment relies on complete medical record documentation and diagnosis coding. CMS requires that all applicable diagnosis codes be reported and that all diagnoses be reported to the highest level of specificity and that these be substantiated by the medical record.

CMS's Guiding Principle:

The risk adjustment diagnosis must be based on clinical medical record documentation from a face-to-face encounter, coded according to the *ICD-10-CM Guidelines for Coding and Reporting*; assigned based on dates of service within the data collection period, submitted to the MA organization from an appropriate risk adjustment provider type and an appropriate risk adjustment physician data source.

A "face-to-face" health service encounter between a patient and healthcare provider describes an encounter between the patient and the provider (MD, DO), including qualified nonphysician practitioners (NPP) (e.g. nurse practitioner or physician's assistant), which is face-to-face with the patient. CMS provides a current listing of acceptable physician specialty types for risk adjustment data submission within the 2012 Regional Technical Assistance Participant Guide. The only exception to the face-to-face encounter requirement is pathology services (professional component only). Currently, CMS does not provide a listing of all services that are considered face-to-face visits for risk adjustment data, but does provide guidance on what types of services are not acceptable for risk adjustment in the Participant Guide. For example, diagnostic radiology does not qualify because diagnostic radiologists typically do not document confirmed diagnoses. Other examples of services that are not acceptable include diagnostic reports that have not been interpreted, such as laboratory reports.

It is essential that the medical record documentation show evidence by provider authentication that the direct face-to-face service was personally furnished by the physician or qualified NPP. Examples of these services include office visits, hospital visits, preoperative anesthesia assessment, and surgical and invasive procedures.

Risk adjustment relies on annual health information. Each enrollee is assigned an individual risk score based on the health status information obtained from the diagnosis codes on the claims. The CMS-HCC model relies on ICD-10-CM coding specificity for accurate risk adjustment by using the most specific code available that is substantiated by the documentation in the medical record. Providers should fully document and accurately code the evaluation and management of all severe and chronic conditions to ensure a full, complete, and accurate clinical record of the patient's condition and reflect the work involved in caring for the patient, particularly those with complex and challenging health issues. All conditions affecting the treatment or management of the patient's health should be documented at least once a year, as applicable to care provided, to accurately describe the true complexity and severity of the patient's health. If the diagnosis coding on the claim is not accurate or complete, the claim may indicate that the provider did much less medical decision-making, evaluation, and management than was actually performed.

Documentation for a valid reportable diagnosis must clearly indicate evidence of M.E.A.T., for each diagnosis:

M	managed
E	evaluated
A	assessed
T	treated

It is recommended that providers use the Subjective and Objective observation, Assessment and Plan (S.O.A.P.) format for progress notes to document evidence of M.E.A.T. A problem list, active condition list, past medical history list, etc., are not suitable examples of documentation of M.E.A.T. Diagnoses and documentation may not be captured from past encounters that have been copied and pasted. Each encounter must be unique and reflect only that visit as it occurred. Chronic conditions require long-term attention and management, and should be reported when treated but are often inadequately documented due to familiarity with the patient. Insufficient documentation influences the assignment of diagnosis codes and directly affects the patient's risk score.

Documentation should be concise, include the reason for the face-to-face visit, and support the need for the patient to be monitored, evaluated, assessed, and/or treated for the conditions listed through clinical rationale and/or plan of care described in clear (legible) notes. Each page of progress notes should be properly authenticated and include the patient's name and the date.

Providers should document each clinical diagnosis to the highest degree of specificity per encounter, including all complications and/or manifestations, including clear links to causal conditions. Only confirmed conditions should be documented—no rule-out conditions or abnormal findings without clinical significance. All known conditions, including chronic conditions, that affect the care and treatment of the patient at least once per year should be noted.

Providers should specifically document the condition and test or report results, and document the status of any changes to the condition, using terminology such as decreased, increased, worsening, improving, or unchanged. Documentation should include supporting evidence of the results or plan of care.

Documentation Tips

- Document all cause-and-effect relationships.

- Report the most specific diagnosis code available that is supported by the documentation.

- Include all current diagnoses as part of the current medical decision-making, and document for every visit.

- Identify diagnoses that are current or chronic problems rather than a past medical history or previous resolved condition.

- Document history of heart attack, status codes, etc., that affect the patient's care as "history of" or "PMH" when they no longer exist or are not current conditions.

- Ensure each progress note has the date, signature, and credentials/specialty.

- Document the thought processes used to assess each condition.

- Know high revenue HCCs that are often undiagnosed or undercoded.

- Avoid "unspecified" codes.

- Ensure the codes reported are accurate.

- Ensure each encounter is billed.

- Review rejection reports, and audit reports to assess risks.

Audits

Because reimbursement is by patient, rather than based on an average of the entire population, and is based upon documentation, there is the potential for upcoding. Audits are conducted by the MA plan and CMS recovery auditors.

Initial Validation Audit (IVA)

CMS requires that the MA plan validate HCCs. This is usually performed by an independent auditor working with the plan or a contracted vendor to validate the MA plan's data submitted to CMS.

The MA plan submits the one best medical record that supports each HCC identified for the beneficiary.

Risk Adjustment Data Validation Audit

Risk adjustment data validation (RADV) audits were introduced in 2011 and updated for 2015. They are performed by CMS to validate the integrity and accuracy of risk-adjusted payments by verifying that the diagnosis codes the MA plans submit are supported by the medical record documentation for a member.

MA plans can be selected by CMS for RADV audits annually and if chosen are required to submit their members' medical records to CMS. Providers are required to assist the MA plan by providing the medical record documentation included in the audit. Even though each diagnosis needs to be reported only once in a calendar year, during a RADV audit up to five dates of service may be submitted to support any one HCC.

To be validated, medical record documentation must meet certain criteria and standards. Even if the diagnosis is documented and coded correctly, any deficiency in the documentation can make the encounter and the HCC invalid. Diagnoses that cannot be validated are considered payment errors. The results of the audit are communicated to the MA plan, which then communicates these results to the provider. Under- and overpayments are subject to payment adjustment. The results of RADV audits can be extrapolated over the MA plan population to calculate potential payment errors and overpayments/recoupments. Regulations include a RADV appeal process, a document dispute process, and a procedure for obtaining physician-signature attestations.

The following items are reviewed during the validation process:

- The record is for the correct enrollee.

- The record is from the correct calendar year for the payment year being audited.

- The record is legible.

- The date of service is present on the records and is for a face-to-face visit.

- The record is from a valid provider type.

- Valid credentials and/or a valid physician specialty are documented on the record.

- The record contains a signature from an acceptable type of physician.

- There is a diagnosis on the record.

- The diagnosis supports an HCC.

- The diagnosis supports the submitted HCC.

Mitigate audit risk by coding each reportable diagnosis each time it meets reporting guidelines. Audit regularly to assess areas of risk and in need of improvement and to capture conditions documented but not coded. Check for additional qualifying HCCs. Ensure claims are submitted and that corrected claims are submitted when indicated. There are three claims submission deadlines: January, March, and September. CMS adjusts each member's risk score twice a year, with the final reconciliation in August of the year after the plan year.

If providers emphasize correct coding and documentation and perform internal audits to determine where the risks are and prepare for audits, incorrect payment is less likely.

Illustrations

Chapter 3. Diseases of the Blood and Blood-forming Organs and Certain Disorders Involving the Immune Mechanism (D50–D89)

Red Blood Cells

White Blood Cell

Platelet

Coagulation

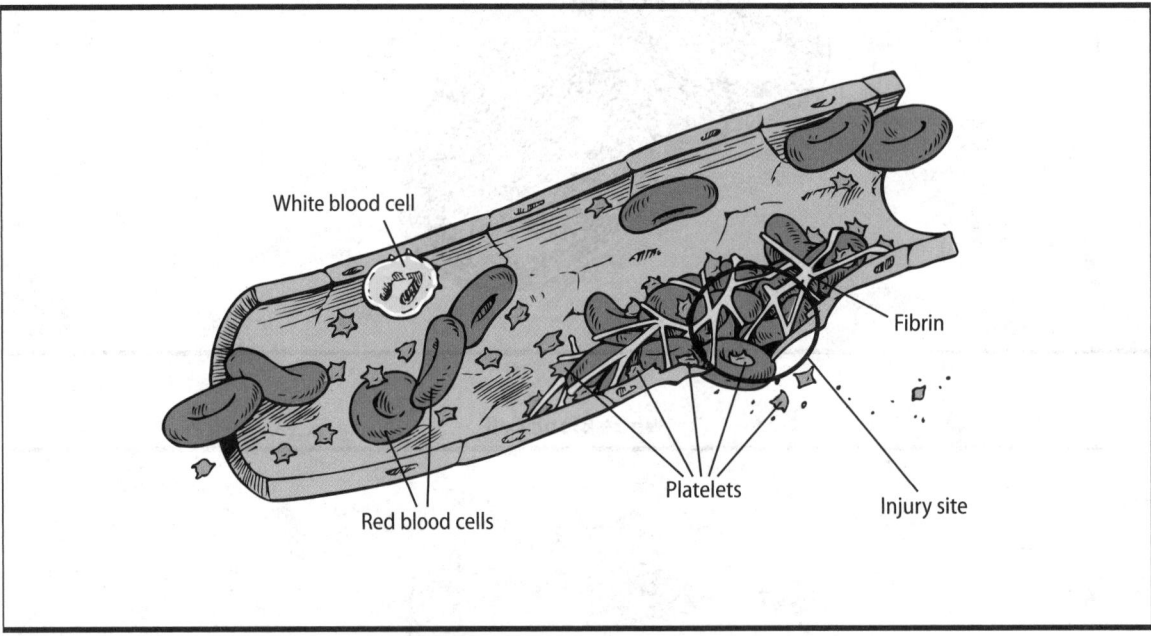

Spleen Anatomical Location and External Structures

Spleen Interior Structures

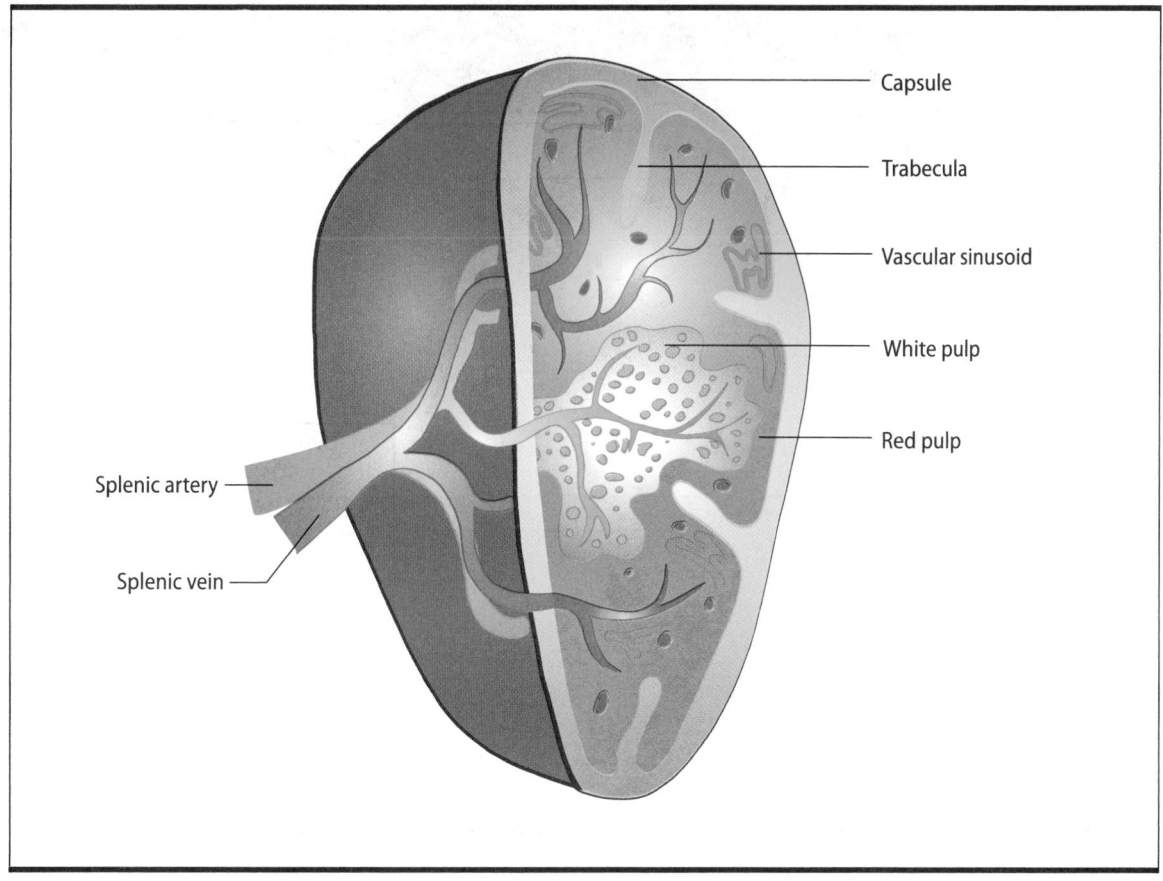

Chapter 4. Endocrine, Nutritional and Metabolic Diseases (E00–E89)

Endocrine System

Thyroid

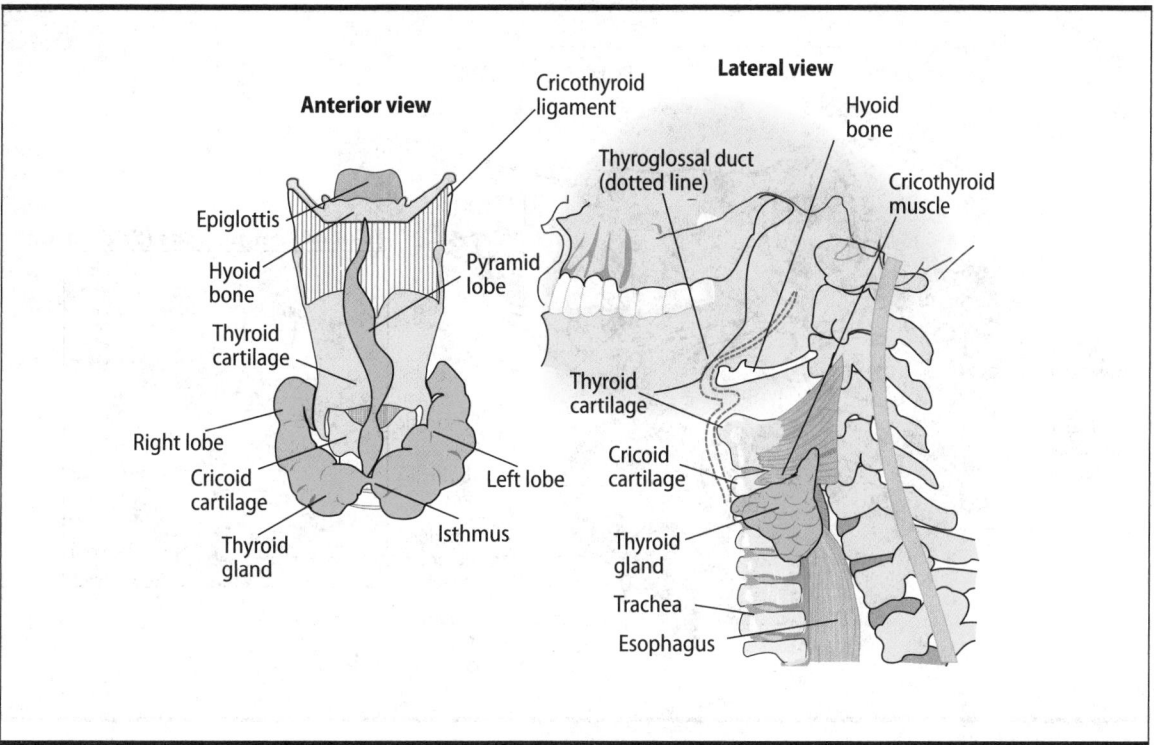

Anterior view

Cricothyroid ligament

Epiglottis

Hyoid bone

Thyroid cartilage

Right lobe

Cricoid cartilage

Thyroid gland

Pyramid lobe

Left lobe

Isthmus

Lateral view

Thyroglossal duct (dotted line)

Hyoid bone

Cricothyroid muscle

Thyroid cartilage

Cricoid cartilage

Thyroid gland

Trachea

Esophagus

Thyroid and Parathyroid Glands

Posterior view

Epiglottis

Pharynx

Thyroid gland

Parathyroid gland

Pancreas

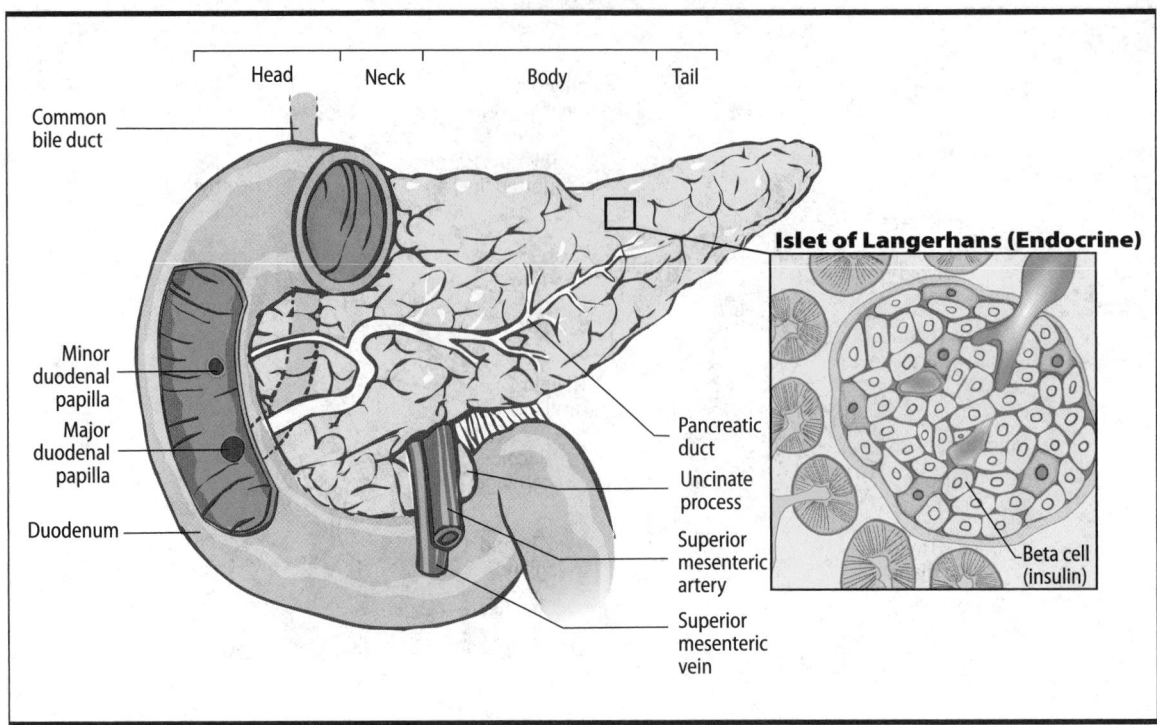

Head · Neck · Body · Tail

Common bile duct

Minor duodenal papilla

Major duodenal papilla

Duodenum

Pancreatic duct

Uncinate process

Superior mesenteric artery

Superior mesenteric vein

Islet of Langerhans (Endocrine)

Beta cell (insulin)

Anatomy of the Adrenal Gland

Adrenal glands

Kidney

Capsule

Cortex

Medulla

Structure of an Ovary

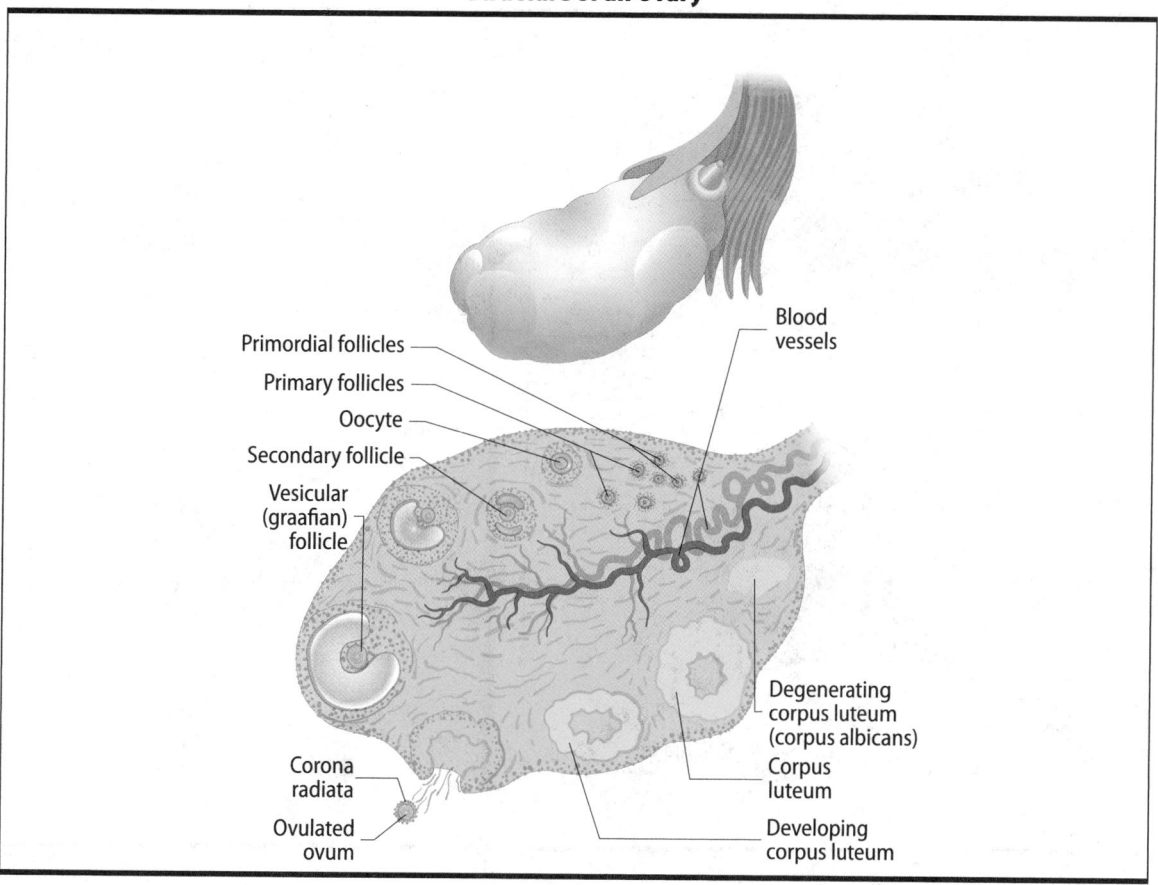

Testis and Associated Structures

Thymus

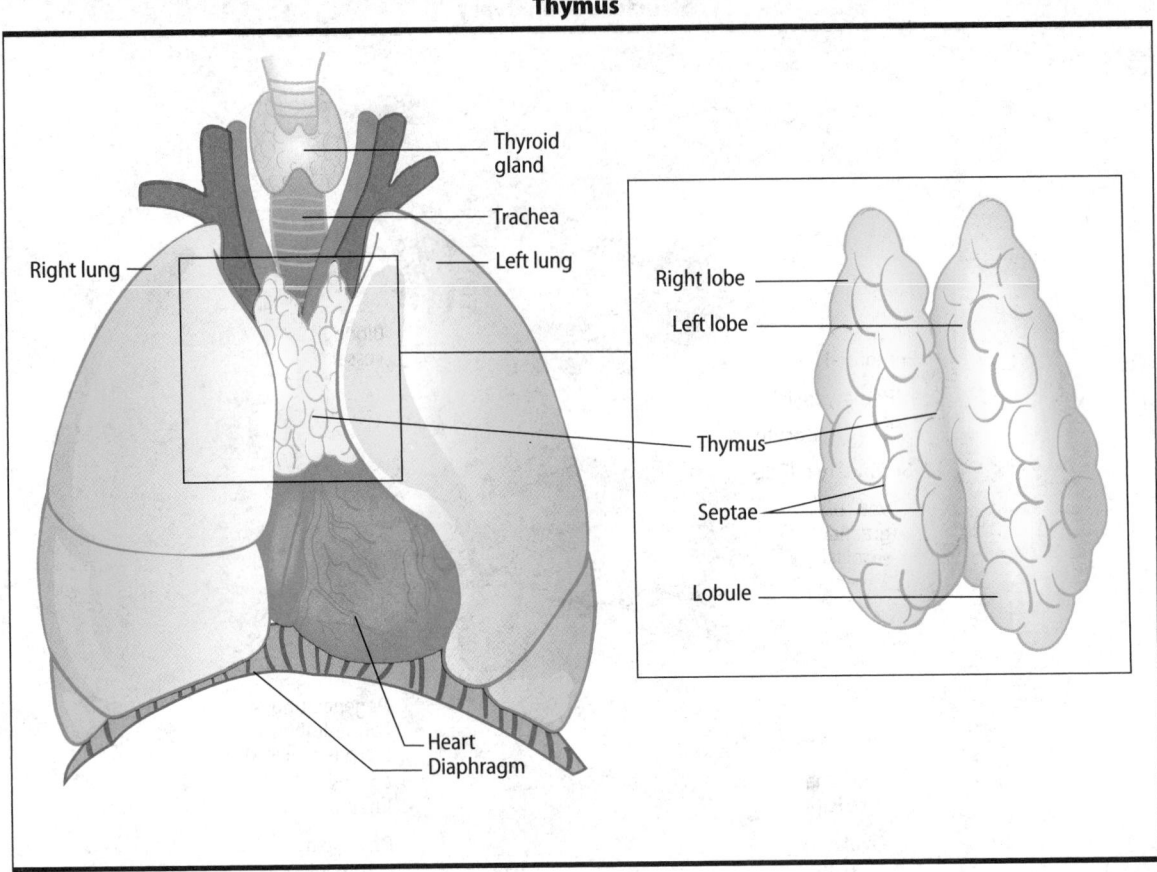

Chapter 6. Diseases of the Nervous System (GØØ–G99)

Brain

Cranial Nerves

Peripheral Nervous System

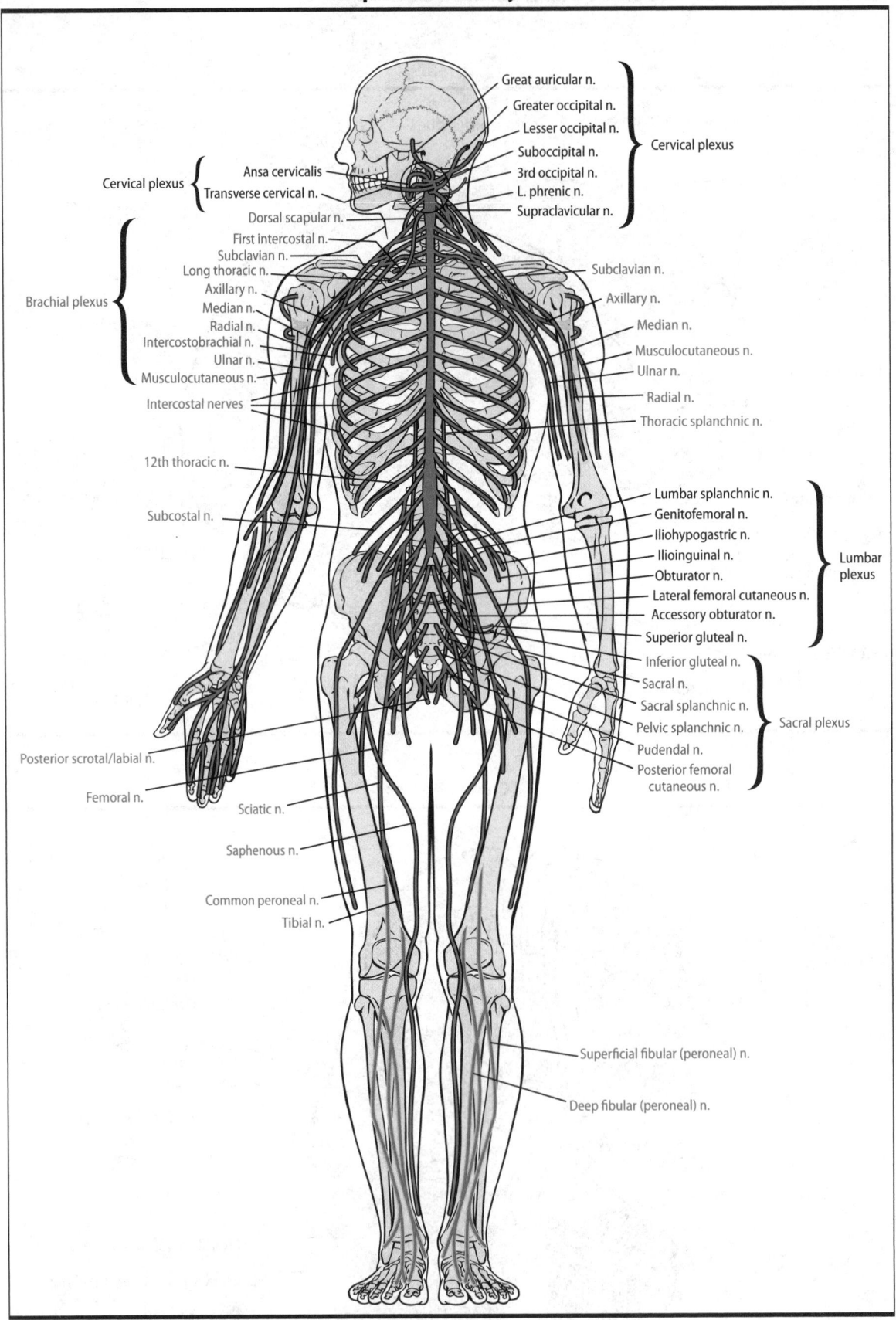

Spinal Cord and Spinal Nerves

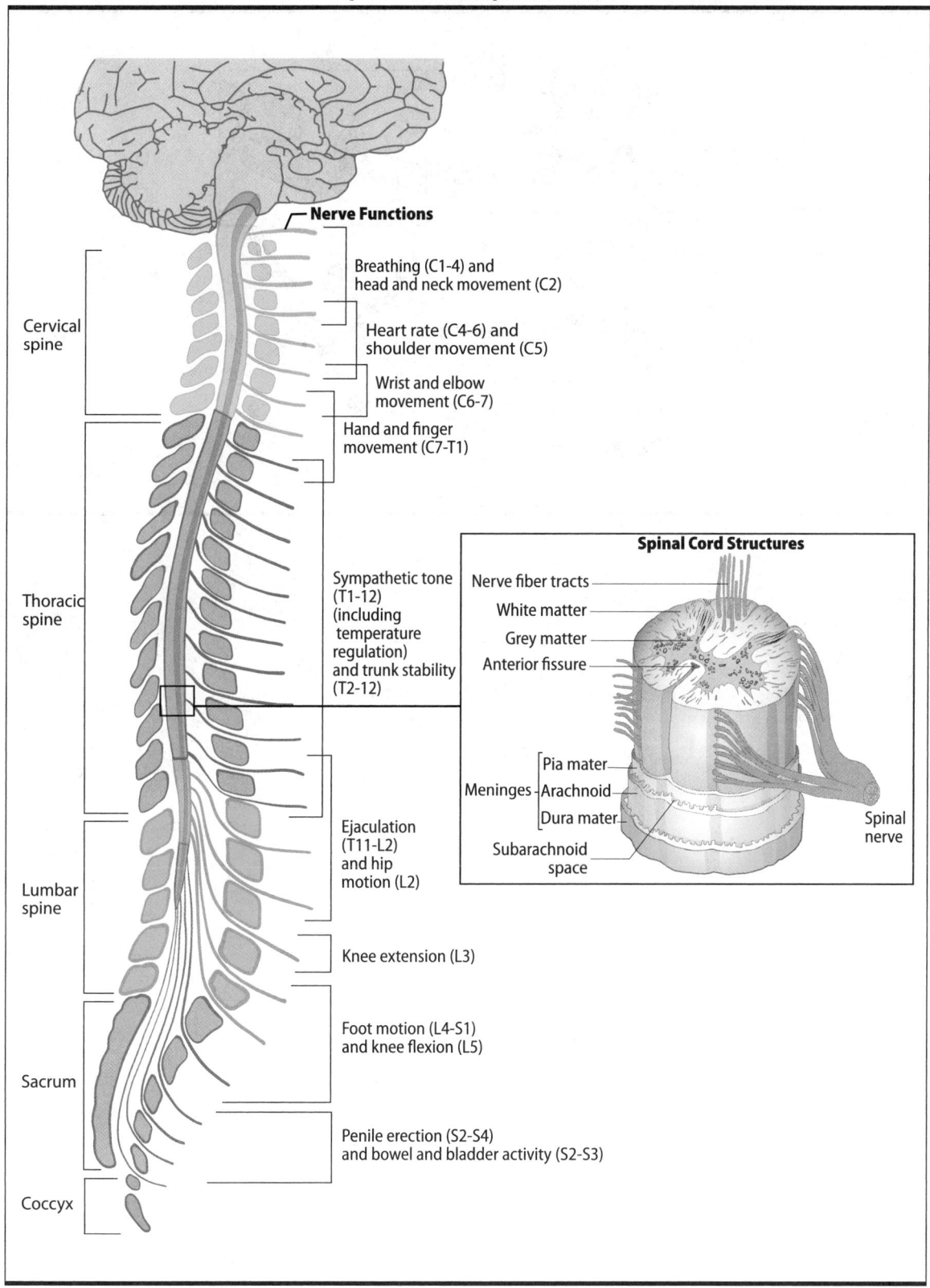

Nerve Functions

Breathing (C1-4) and head and neck movement (C2)

Heart rate (C4-6) and shoulder movement (C5)

Wrist and elbow movement (C6-7)

Hand and finger movement (C7-T1)

Cervical spine

Thoracic spine

Sympathetic tone (T1-12) (including temperature regulation) and trunk stability (T2-12)

Spinal Cord Structures

Nerve fiber tracts

White matter

Grey matter

Anterior fissure

Pia mater
Meninges — Arachnoid
Dura mater
Subarachnoid space

Spinal nerve

Ejaculation (T11-L2) and hip motion (L2)

Lumbar spine

Knee extension (L3)

Foot motion (L4-S1) and knee flexion (L5)

Sacrum

Penile erection (S2-S4) and bowel and bladder activity (S2-S3)

Coccyx

Nerve Cell

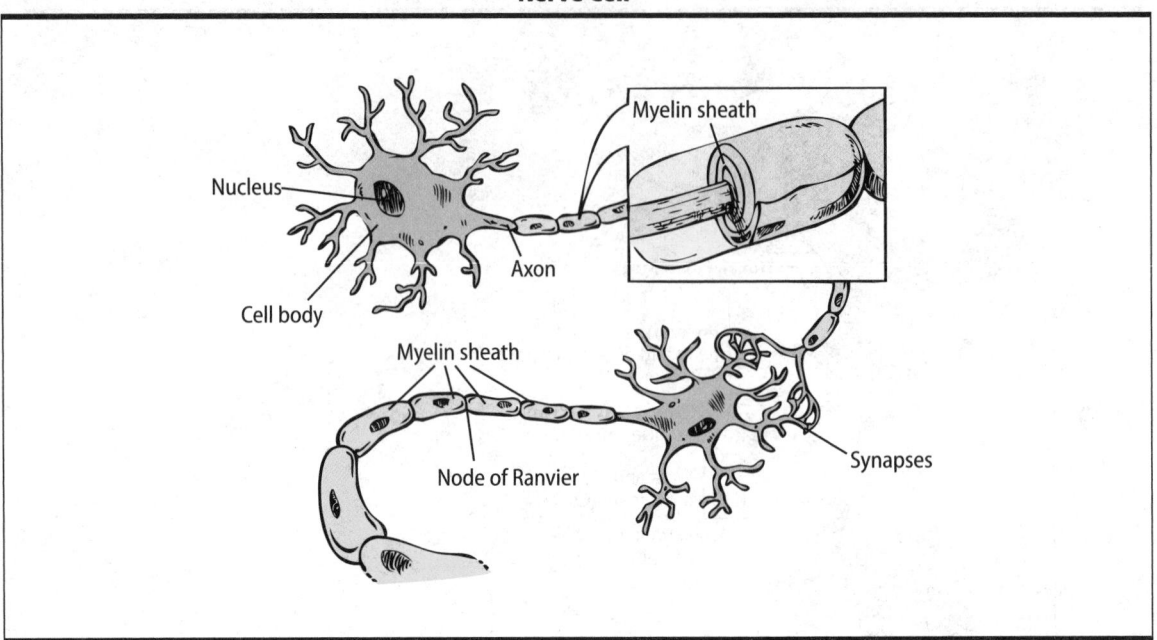

Chapter 7. Diseases of the Eye and Adnexa (H00–H59)

Eye

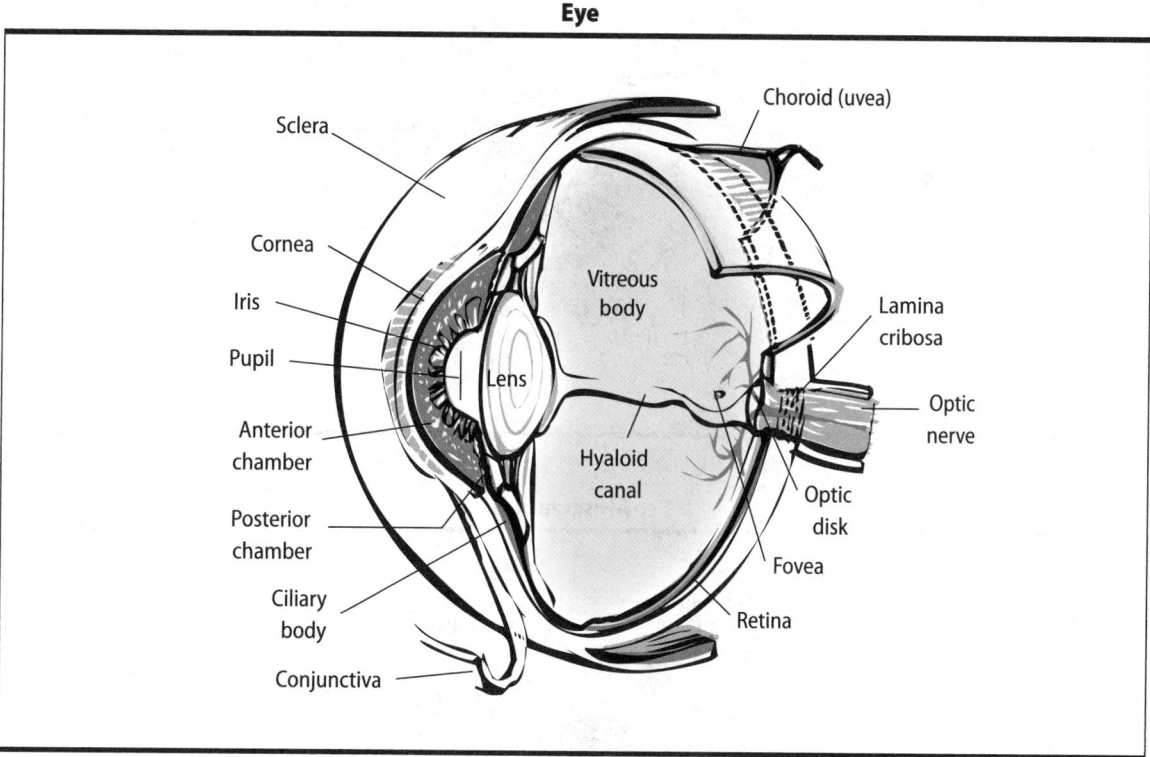

Posterior Pole of Globe/Flow of Aqueous Humor

Lacrimal System

Eye Musculature

Eyelid Structures

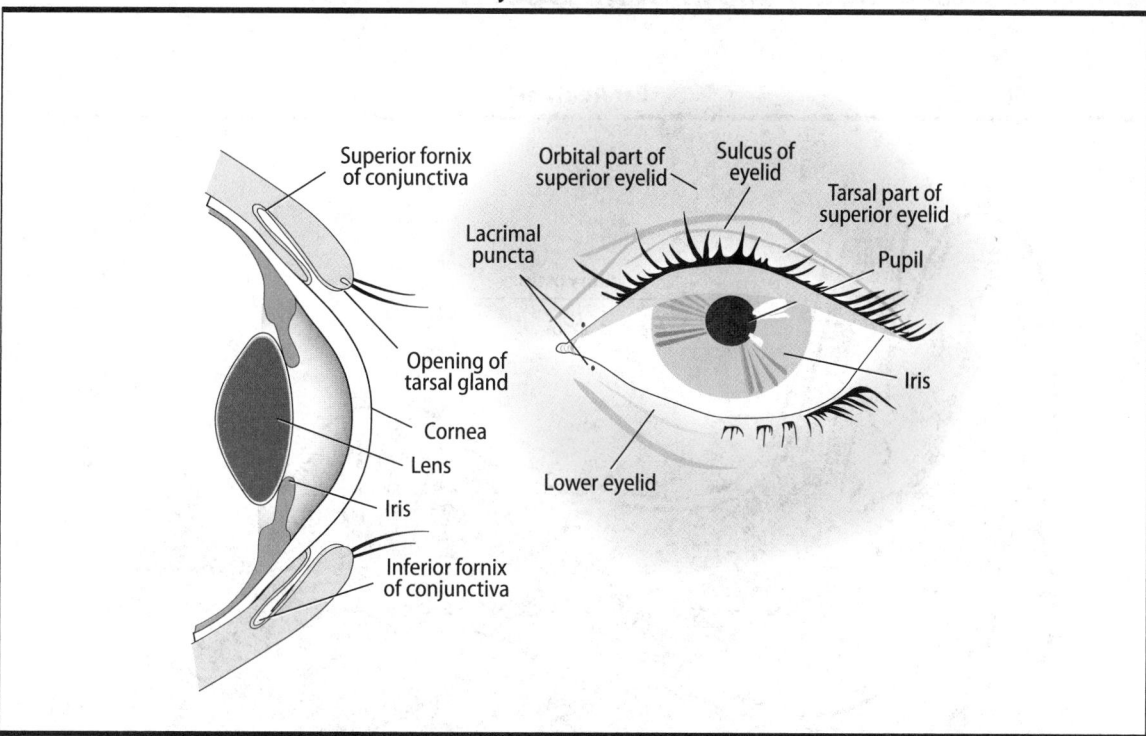

Chapter 8. Diseases of the Ear and Mastoid Process (H6Ø–H95)

Ear Anatomy

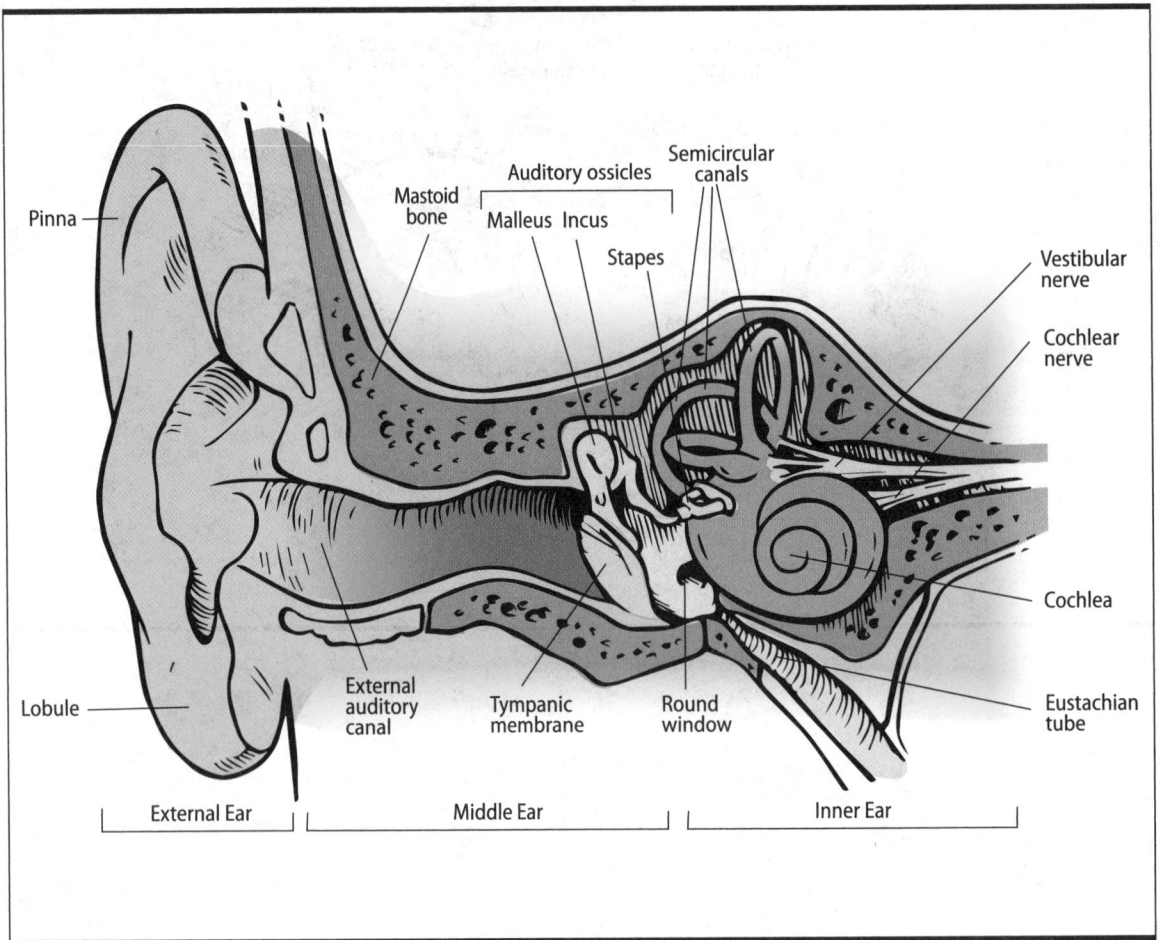

Chapter 9. Diseases of the Circulatory System (I00–I99)

Anatomy of the Heart

Superior vena cava

Aortic valve

Right atrium

Tricuspid valve

Right ventricle

Inferior vena cava

Aorta

Pulmonary artery

Pulmonary vein

Pulmonary valve

Left atrium

Mitral valve

Chorda tendinae

Left ventricle

Heart Cross Section

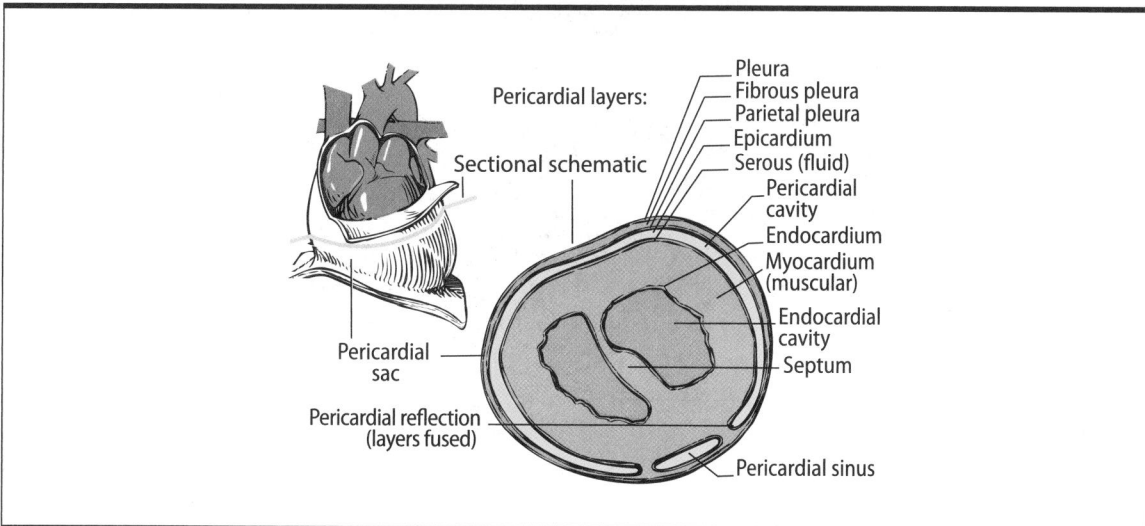

Pericardial layers:

Sectional schematic

Pleura
Fibrous pleura
Parietal pleura
Epicardium
Serous (fluid)
Pericardial cavity
Endocardium
Myocardium (muscular)
Endocardial cavity
Septum
Pericardial sinus

Pericardial sac

Pericardial reflection (layers fused)

Heart Valves

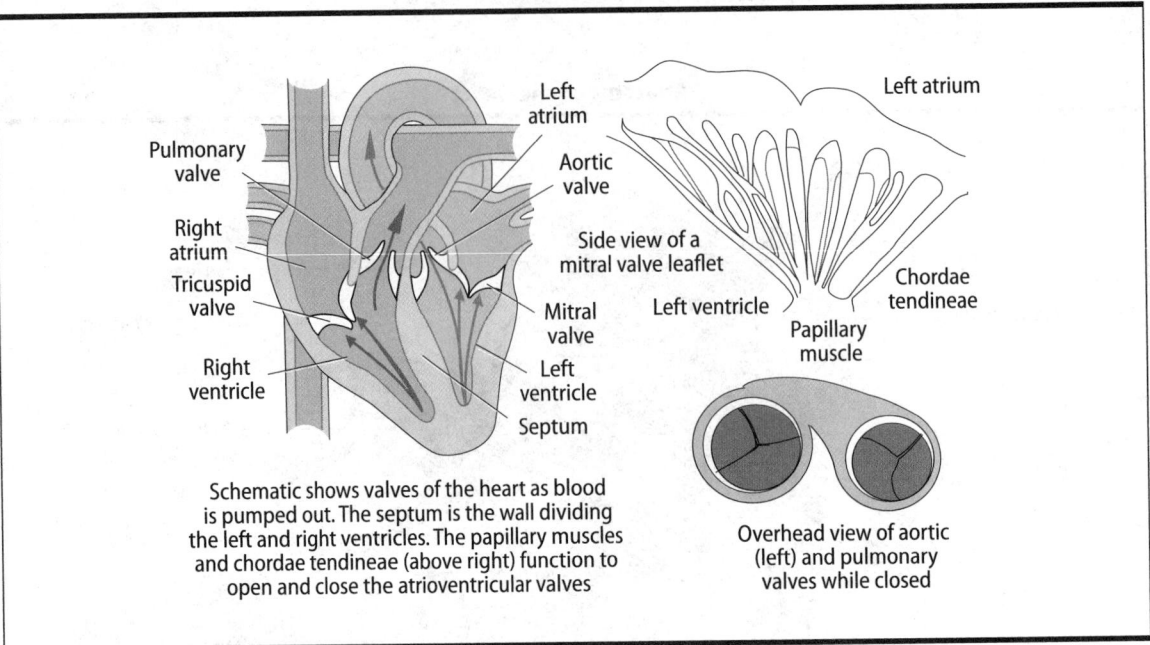

Schematic shows valves of the heart as blood is pumped out. The septum is the wall dividing the left and right ventricles. The papillary muscles and chordae tendineae (above right) function to open and close the atrioventricular valves

Overhead view of aortic (left) and pulmonary valves while closed

Heart Conduction System

Coronary Arteries

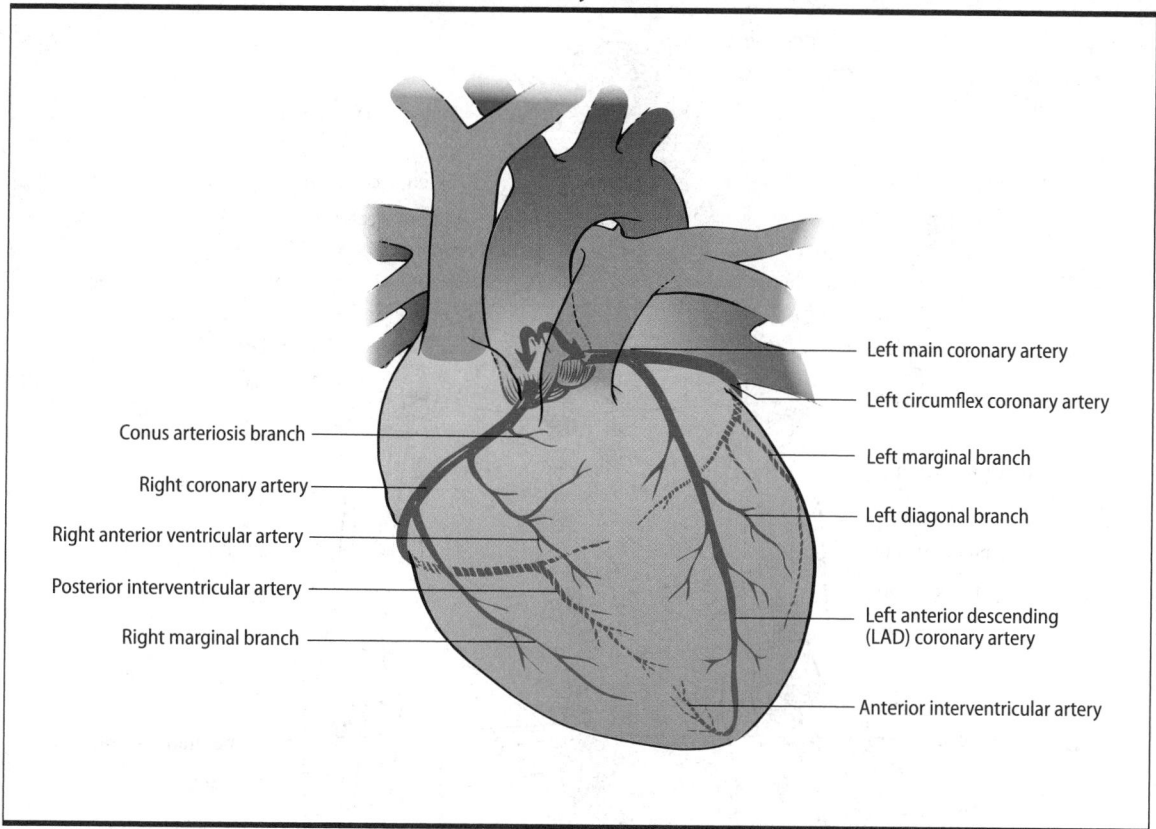

Conus arteriosis branch

Right coronary artery

Right anterior ventricular artery

Posterior interventricular artery

Right marginal branch

Left main coronary artery

Left circumflex coronary artery

Left marginal branch

Left diagonal branch

Left anterior descending (LAD) coronary artery

Anterior interventricular artery

Arteries

Veins

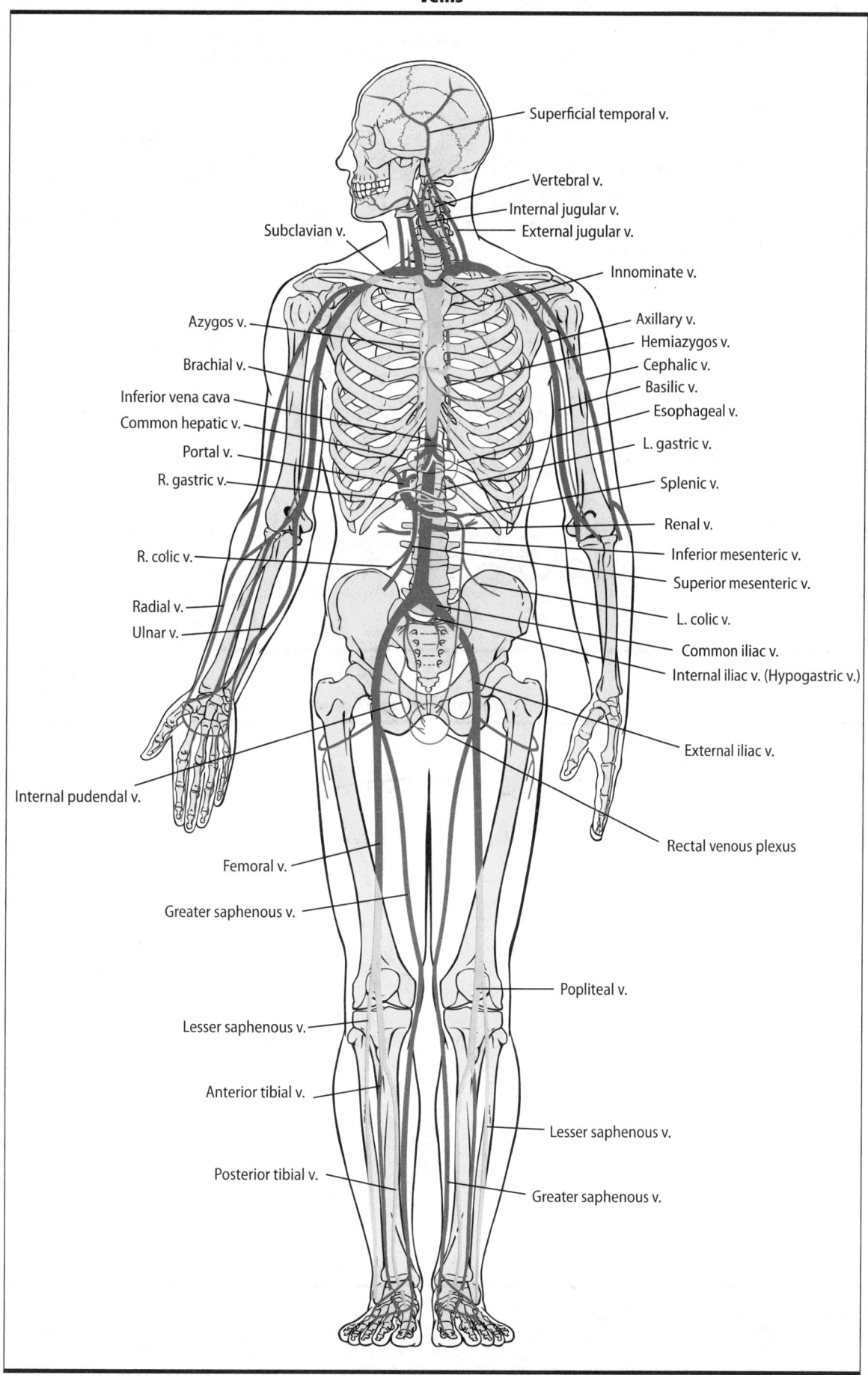

Internal Carotid and Vertebral Arteries and Branches

Side View

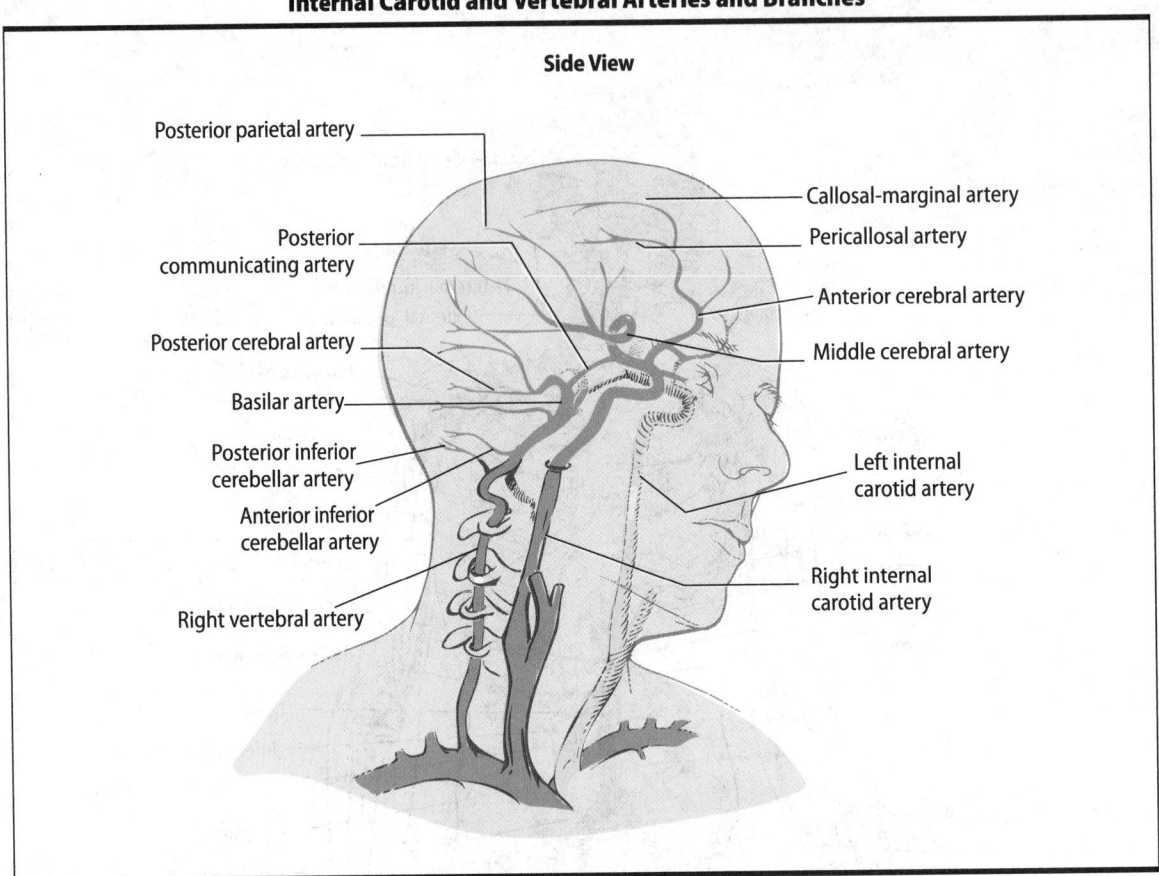

External Carotid Artery and Branches

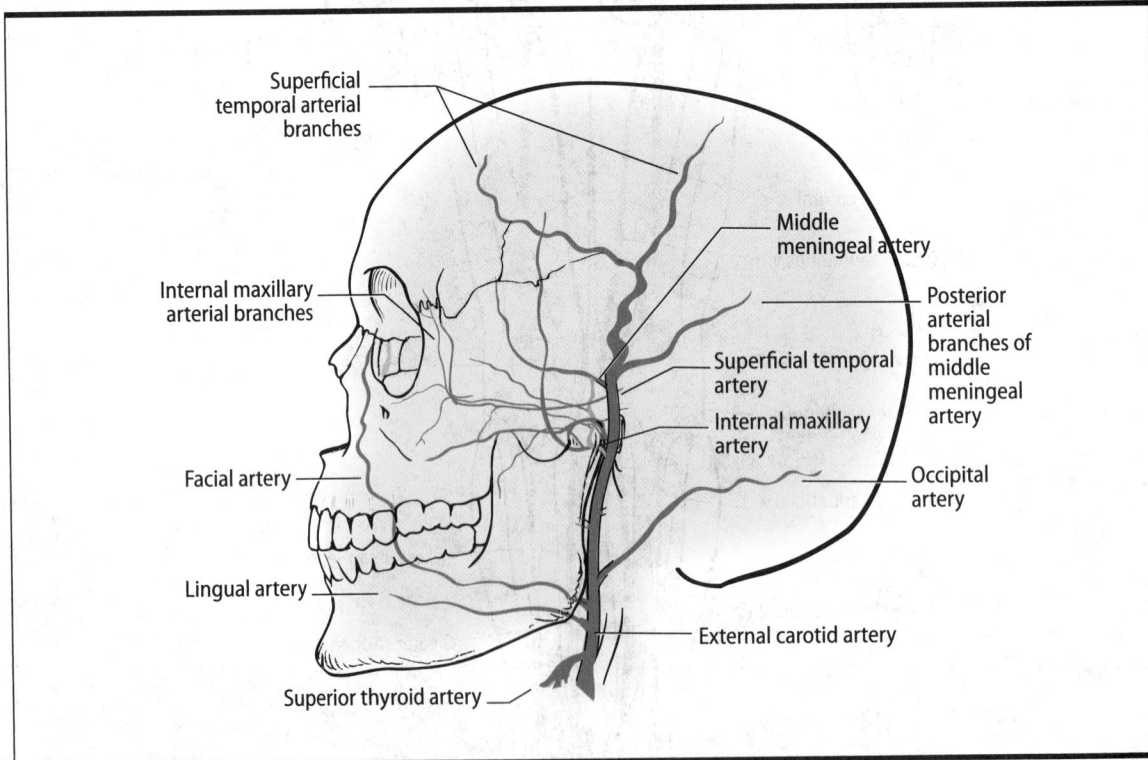

Branches of Abdominal Aorta

Portal Venous Circulation

Lymphatic System

Axillary Lymph Nodes

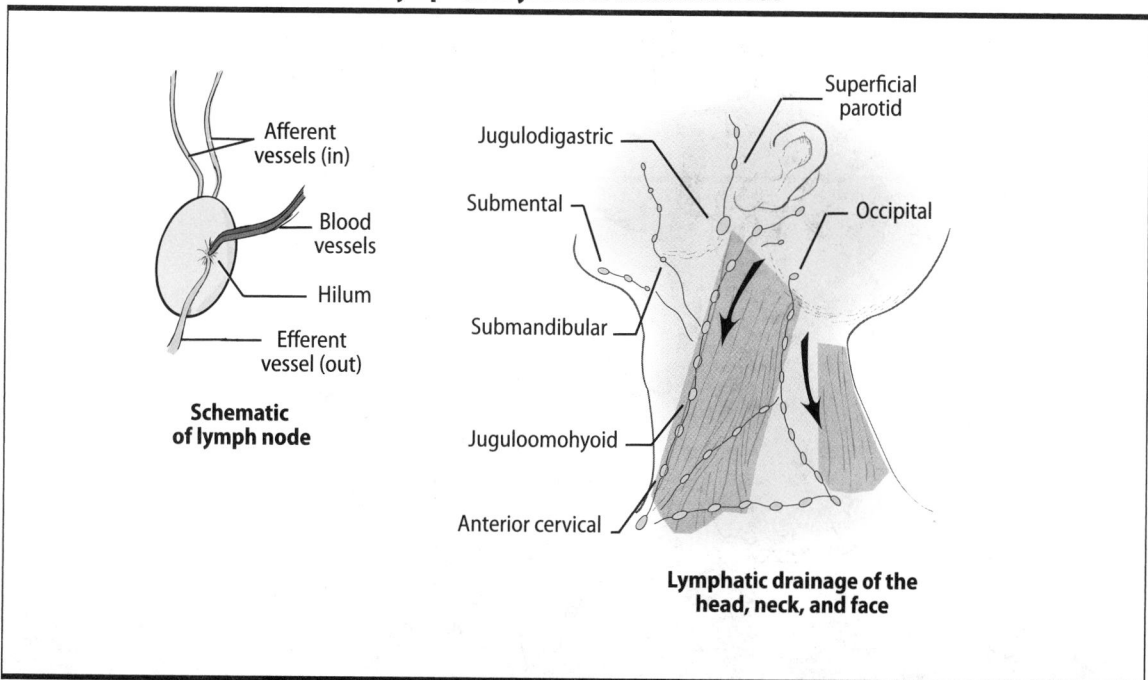

Parasternal nodes

Sternum

Clavicle

Deltoid muscle

Brachialis muscle

Lateral nodes

Subscapular nodes

Pectoral nodes

Axillary lymph nodes

Central nodes

Latissimus dorsi muscle

Rectus abdominis muscle

Lymphatic System of Head and Neck

Afferent vessels (in)

Blood vessels

Hilum

Efferent vessel (out)

Schematic of lymph node

Jugulodigastric

Submental

Submandibular

Juguloomohyoid

Anterior cervical

Superficial parotid

Occipital

Lymphatic drainage of the head, neck, and face

Lymphatic Capillaries

Schematic of lymphatic capillaries

Tissue cells

Valves

Endothelial cells

Fluids and particles can enter
the capillary through overlapping valves

Lymphatic Drainage

Lymphatic drainage of the colon follows blood supply

Middle colic nodes

Paracolic nodes

Left colic nodes

Ascending colon

Cecum

Rectum

Chapter 10. Diseases of the Respiratory System (J00–J99)

Respiratory System

Upper Respiratory System

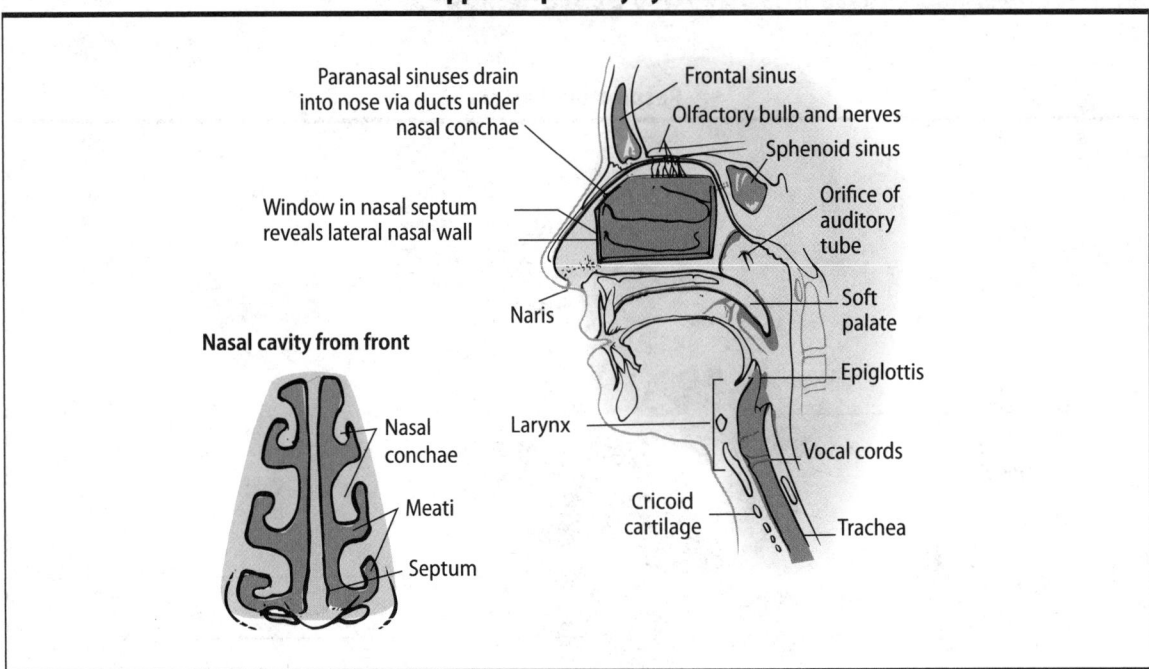

Paranasal sinuses drain into nose via ducts under nasal conchae

Frontal sinus

Olfactory bulb and nerves

Sphenoid sinus

Orifice of auditory tube

Window in nasal septum reveals lateral nasal wall

Nasal cavity from front

Naris

Soft palate

Epiglottis

Nasal conchae

Larynx

Vocal cords

Meati

Cricoid cartilage

Trachea

Septum

Lower Respiratory System

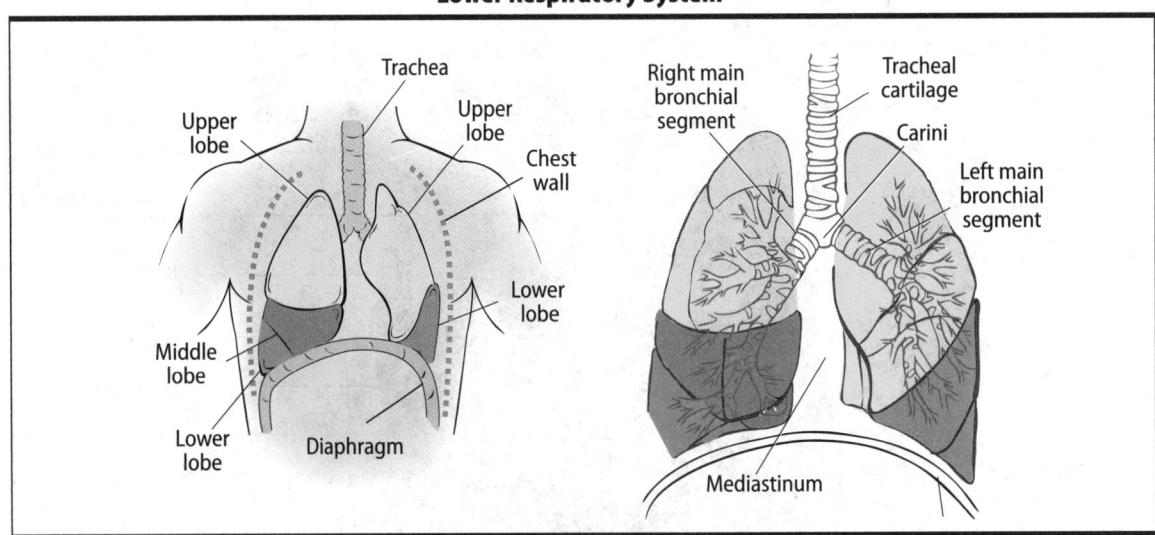

Trachea

Upper lobe

Upper lobe

Chest wall

Right main bronchial segment

Tracheal cartilage

Carini

Left main bronchial segment

Lower lobe

Middle lobe

Lower lobe

Diaphragm

Mediastinum

Paranasal Sinuses

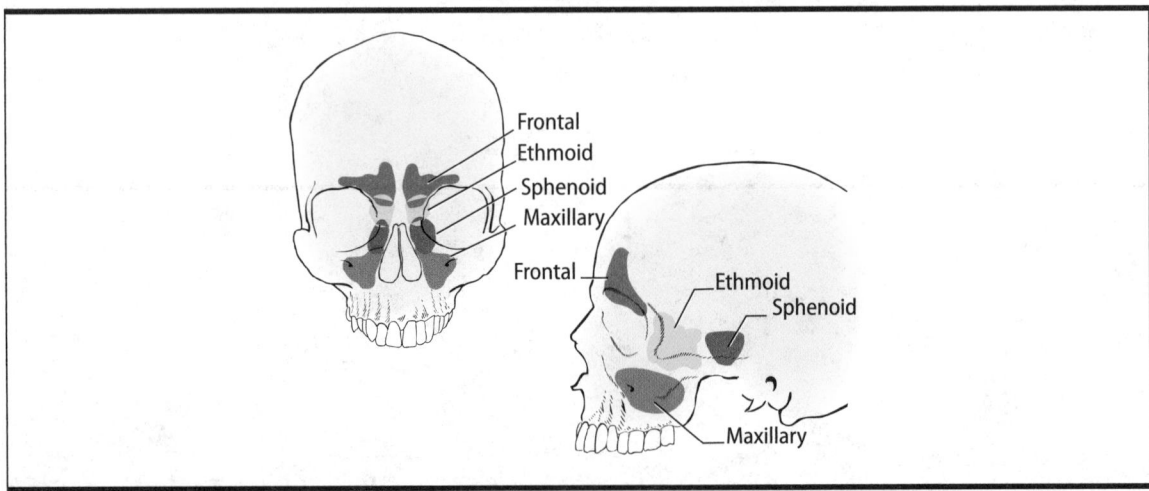

Frontal

Ethmoid

Sphenoid

Maxillary

Frontal

Ethmoid

Sphenoid

Maxillary

Lung Segments

Alveoli

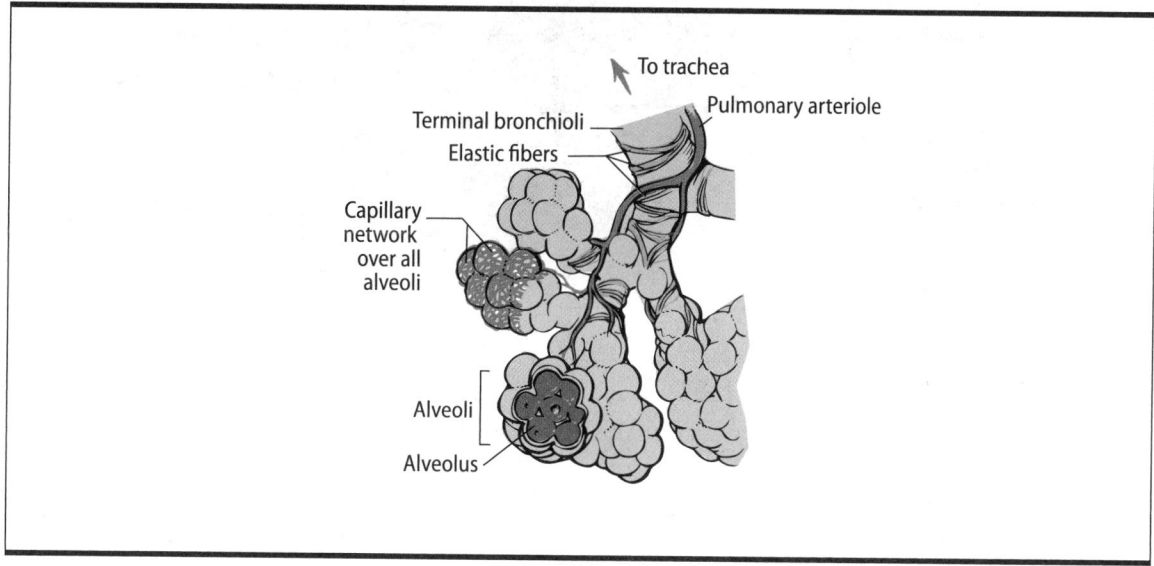

Chapter 11. Diseases of the Digestive System (KØØ–K95)

Digestive System

Omentum and Mesentery

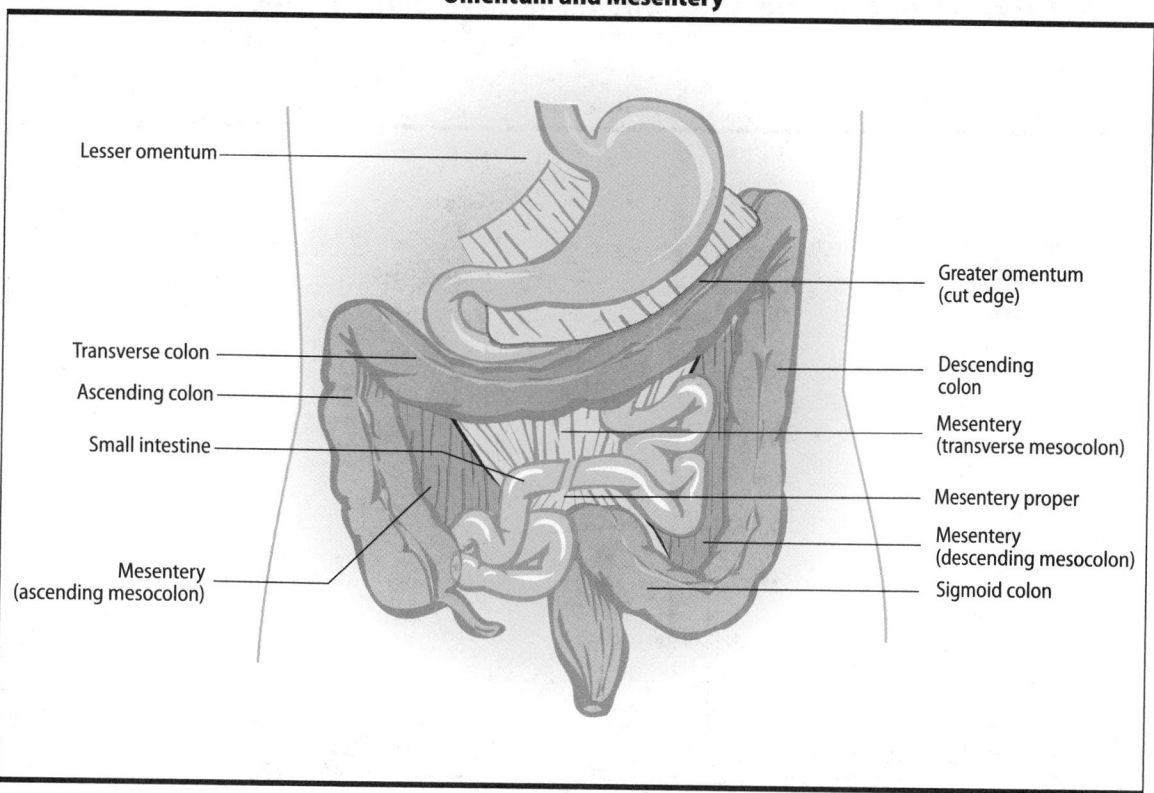

Lesser omentum

Greater omentum (cut edge)

Transverse colon

Descending colon

Ascending colon

Mesentery (transverse mesocolon)

Small intestine

Mesentery proper

Mesentery (descending mesocolon)

Mesentery (ascending mesocolon)

Sigmoid colon

Peritoneum and Retroperitoneum

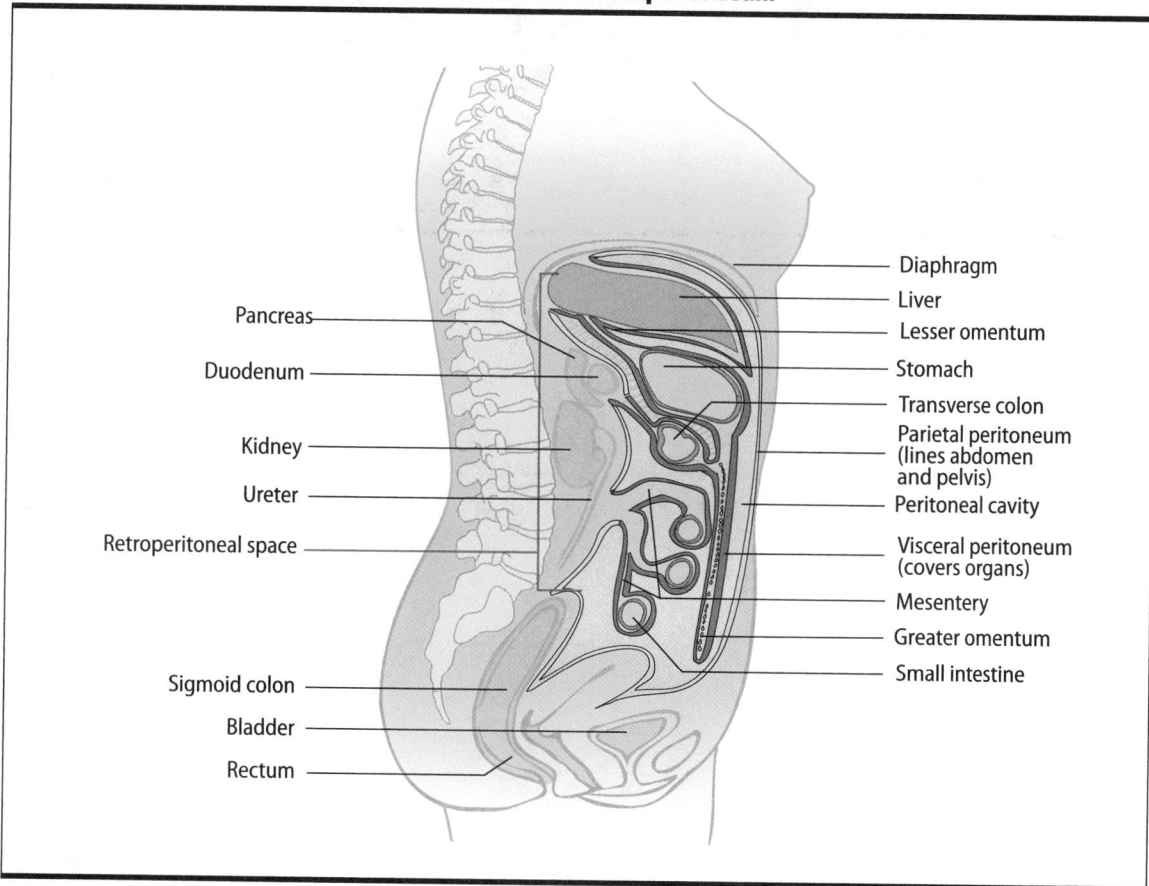

Pancreas

Diaphragm

Liver

Duodenum

Lesser omentum

Stomach

Kidney

Transverse colon

Parietal peritoneum (lines abdomen and pelvis)

Ureter

Peritoneal cavity

Retroperitoneal space

Visceral peritoneum (covers organs)

Mesentery

Greater omentum

Sigmoid colon

Small intestine

Bladder

Rectum

Chapter 12. Diseases of the Skin and Subcutaneous Tissue (L00–L99)

Nail Anatomy

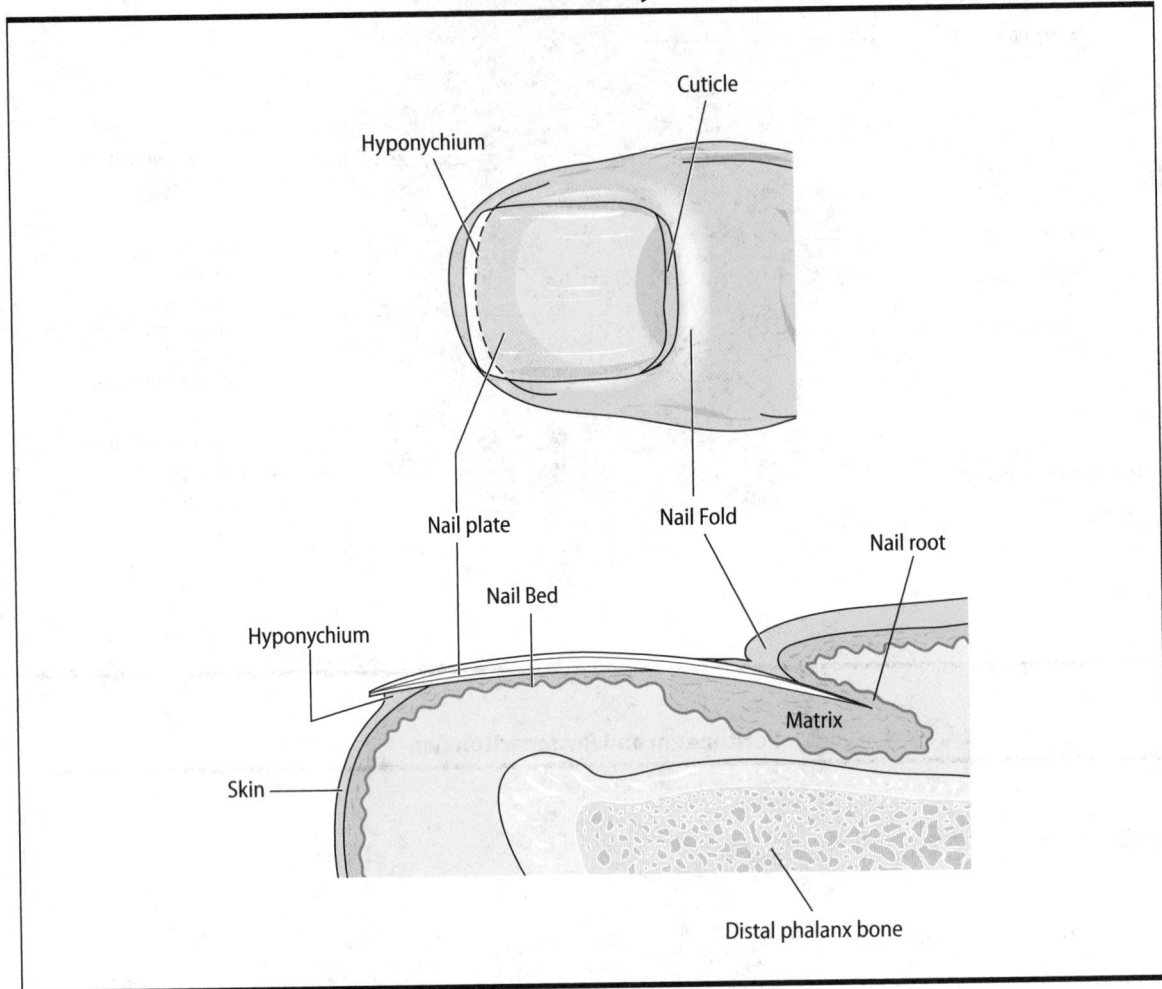

Skin and Subcutaneous Tissue

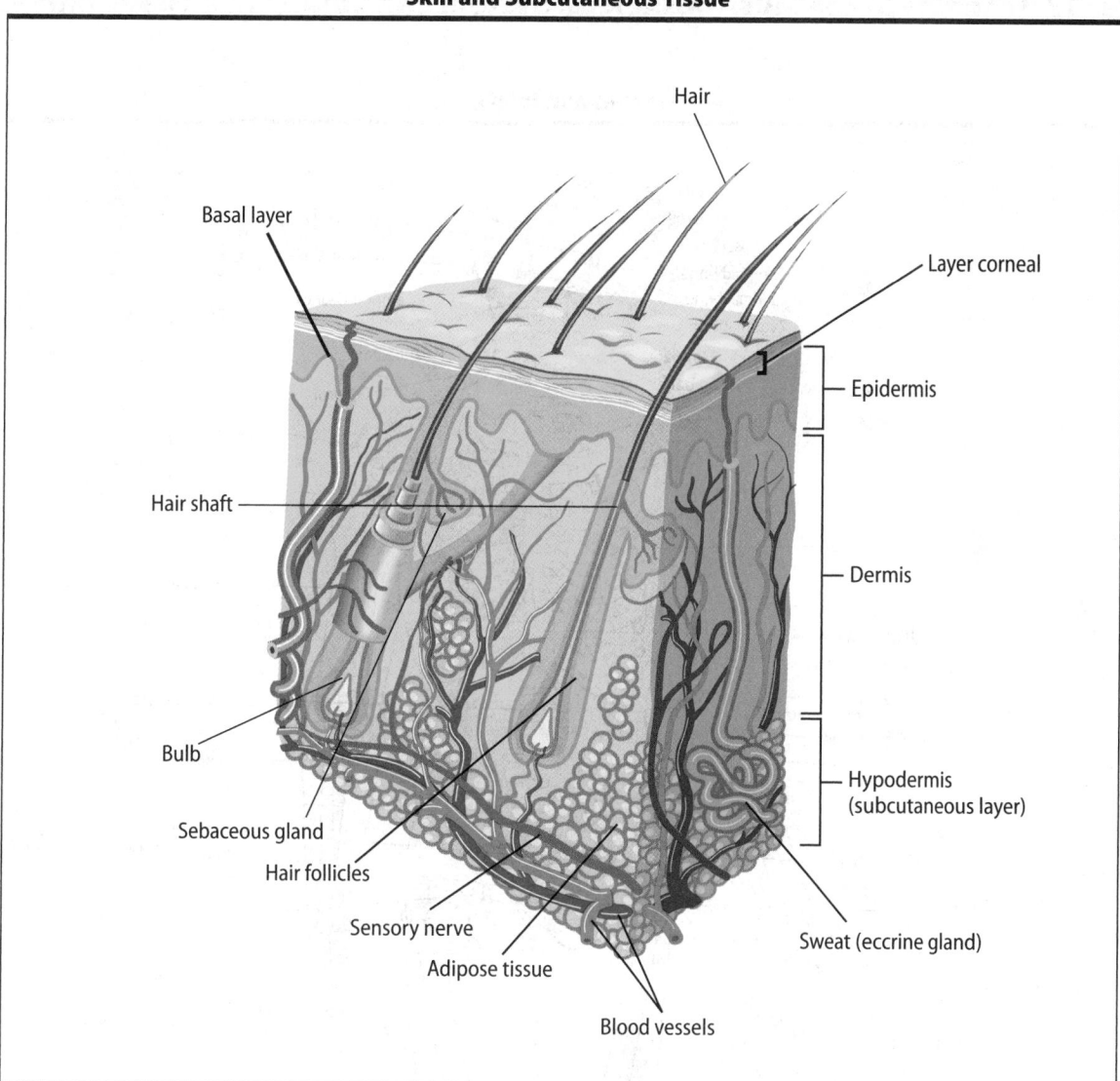

Chapter 13. Diseases of the Musculoskeletal System and Connective Tissue (MØØ–M99)

Bones and Joints

Shoulder Anterior View

Shoulder Posterior View

Elbow Anterior View

Elbow Posterior View

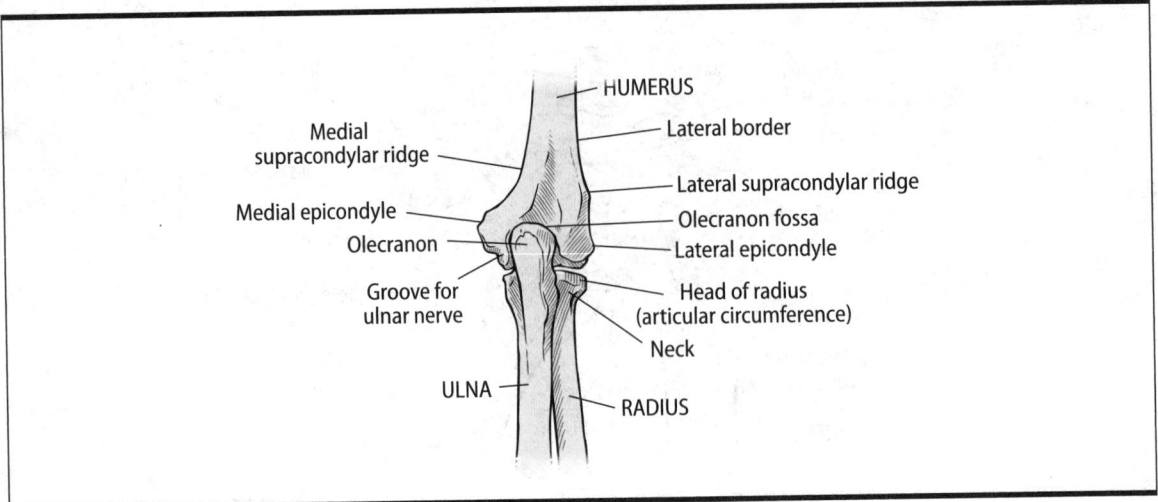

- HUMERUS
- Lateral border
- Medial supracondylar ridge
- Lateral supracondylar ridge
- Medial epicondyle
- Olecranon fossa
- Olecranon
- Lateral epicondyle
- Groove for ulnar nerve
- Head of radius (articular circumference)
- Neck
- ULNA
- RADIUS

Hand

- Phalanges (digits)
- Distal phalanx
- Middle phalanx
- Interphalangeal joints
- Proximal phalanx
- Metacarpophalangeal joint
- Distal phalanx (thumb)
- Metacarpals
- Proximal phalanx (thumb)
- 5   4   3   2   1
- Carpometacarpal joint
- Hamate
- Trapezium
- Pisiform
- Trapezoid
- Carpals
- Scaphoid
- Triquetral   Lunate   Cuboid

Hip Anterior View

Hip Posterior View

Knee Anterior View

Knee Posterior View

Foot

Muscles

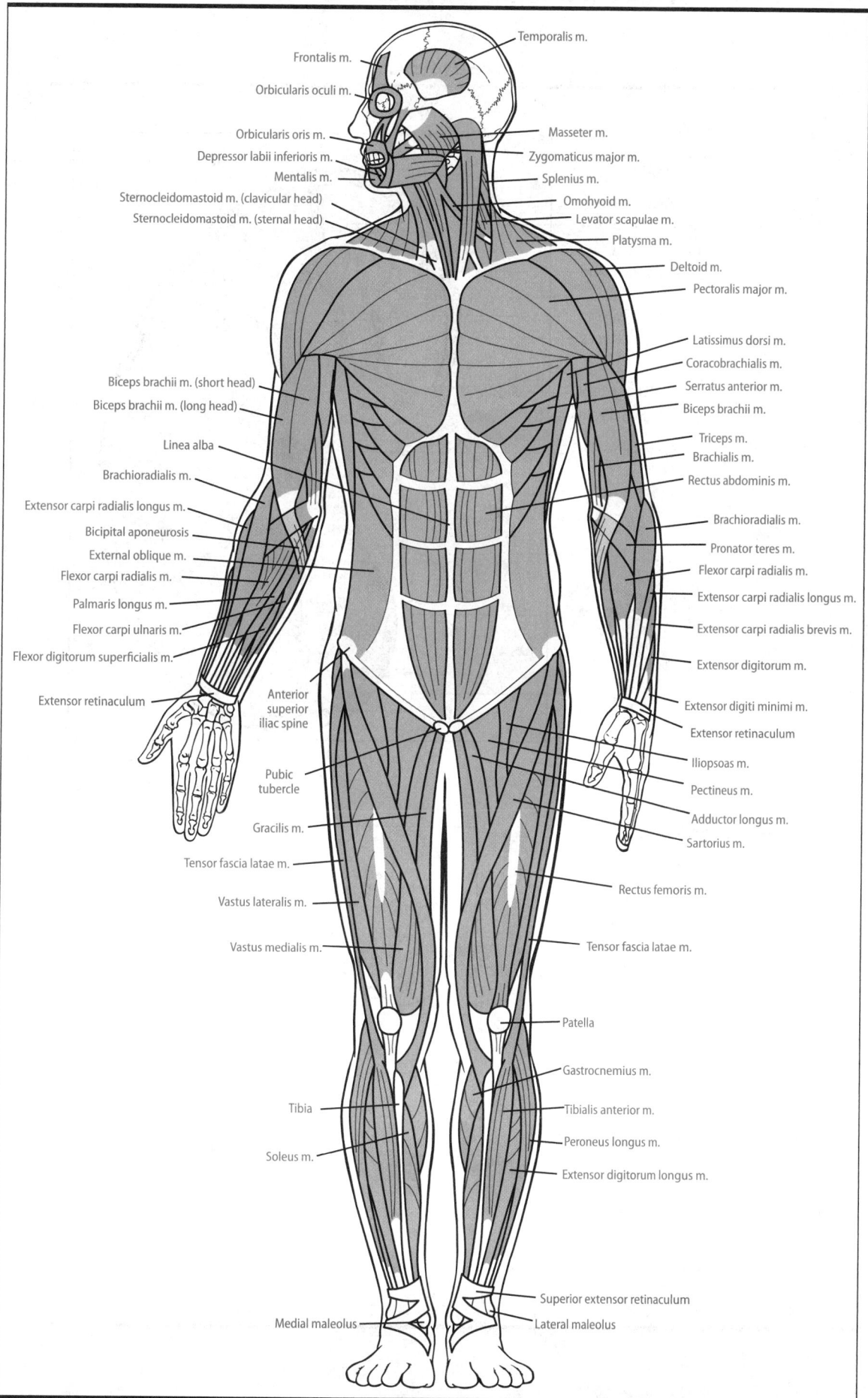

Temporalis m.
Frontalis m.
Orbicularis oculi m.
Orbicularis oris m.
Depressor labii inferioris m.
Mentalis m.
Masseter m.
Zygomaticus major m.
Splenius m.
Sternocleidomastoid m. (clavicular head)
Omohyoid m.
Sternocleidomastoid m. (sternal head)
Levator scapulae m.
Platysma m.
Deltoid m.
Pectoralis major m.
Latissimus dorsi m.
Coracobrachialis m.
Biceps brachii m. (short head)
Serratus anterior m.
Biceps brachii m. (long head)
Biceps brachii m.
Linea alba
Triceps m.
Brachialis m.
Brachioradialis m.
Rectus abdominis m.
Extensor carpi radialis longus m.
Brachioradialis m.
Bicipital aponeurosis
Pronator teres m.
External oblique m.
Flexor carpi radialis m.
Palmaris longus m.
Extensor carpi radialis longus m.
Flexor carpi ulnaris m.
Extensor carpi radialis brevis m.
Flexor digitorum superficialis m.
Extensor digitorum m.
Extensor retinaculum
Anterior superior iliac spine
Extensor digiti minimi m.
Extensor retinaculum
Iliopsoas m.
Pubic tubercle
Pectineus m.
Adductor longus m.
Gracilis m.
Sartorius m.
Tensor fascia latae m.
Rectus femoris m.
Vastus lateralis m.
Vastus medialis m.
Tensor fascia latae m.
Patella
Gastrocnemius m.
Tibialis anterior m.
Tibia
Peroneus longus m.
Soleus m.
Extensor digitorum longus m.
Superior extensor retinaculum
Medial maleolus
Lateral maleolus

Chapter 14. Diseases of the Genitourinary System (N00–N99)

Urinary System

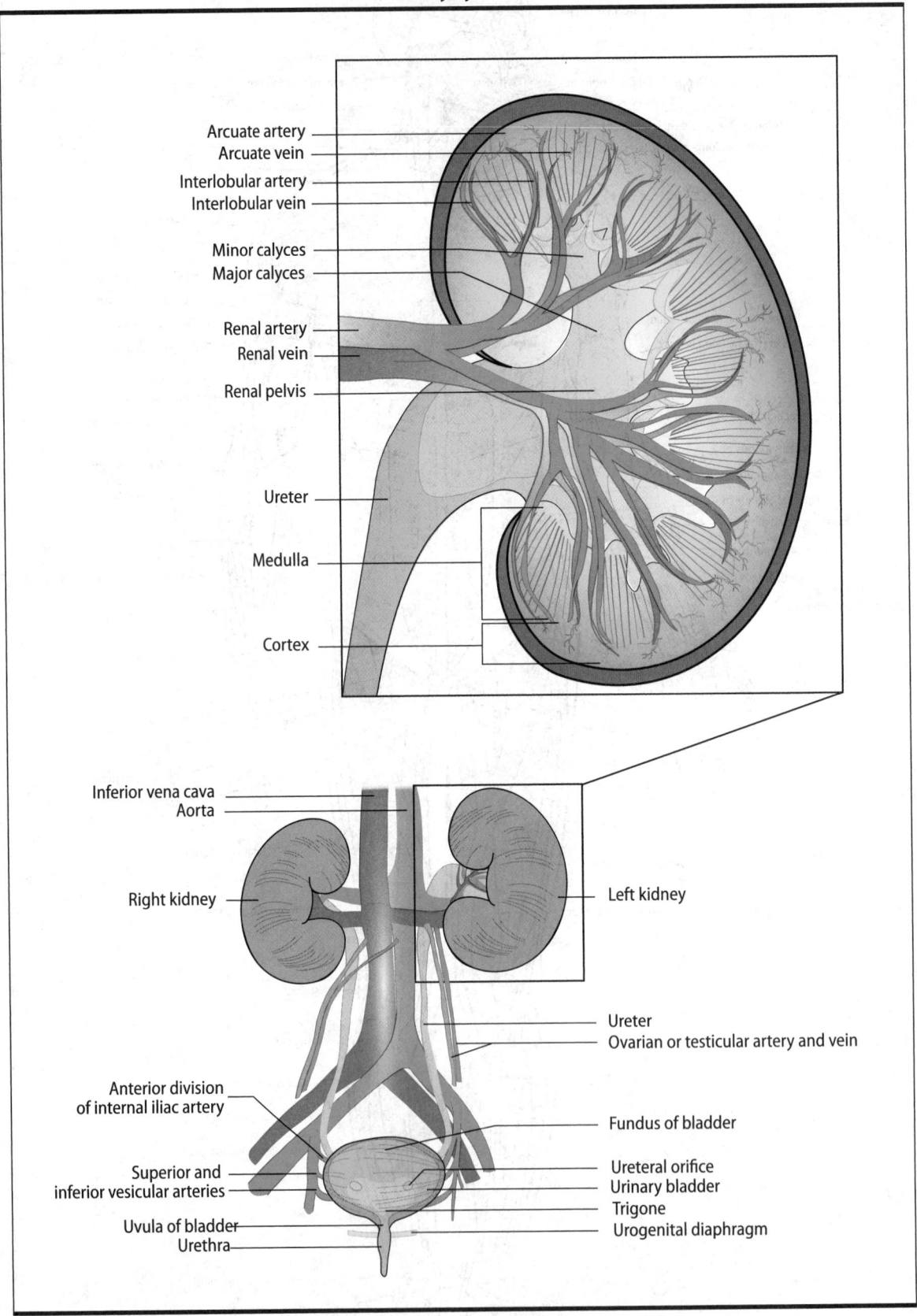

Arcuate artery
Arcuate vein
Interlobular artery
Interlobular vein

Minor calyces
Major calyces

Renal artery
Renal vein

Renal pelvis

Ureter

Medulla

Cortex

Inferior vena cava
Aorta

Right kidney

Left kidney

Ureter
Ovarian or testicular artery and vein

Anterior division
of internal iliac artery

Fundus of bladder

Superior and
inferior vesicular arteries

Ureteral orifice
Urinary bladder
Trigone

Uvula of bladder
Urethra

Urogenital diaphragm

Male Genitourinary System

Female Internal Genitalia

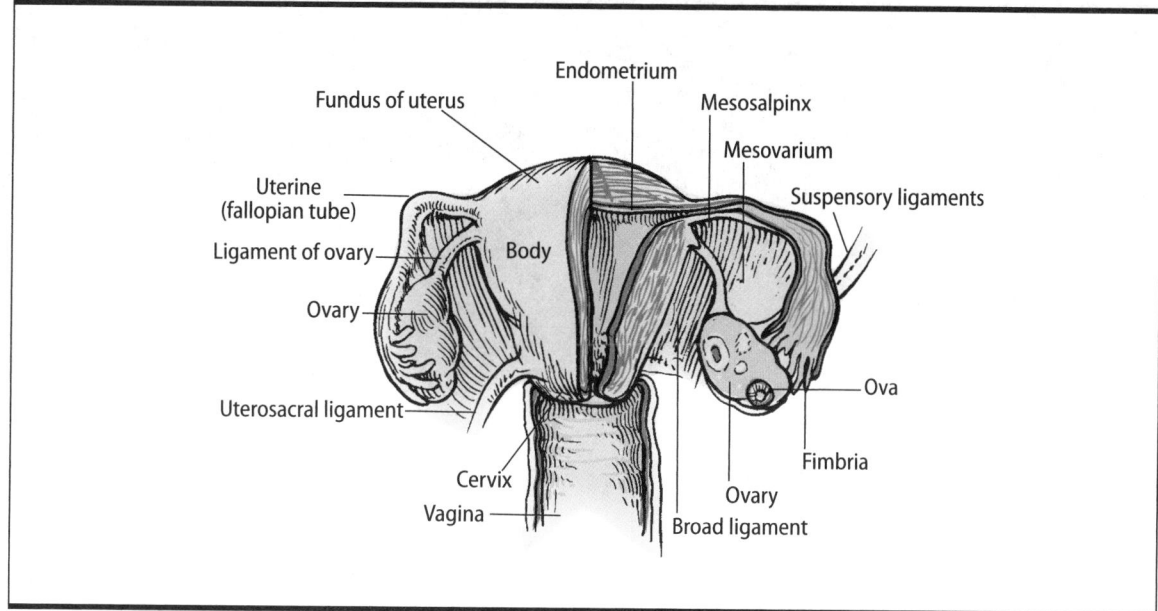

Female Genitourinary Tract Lateral View

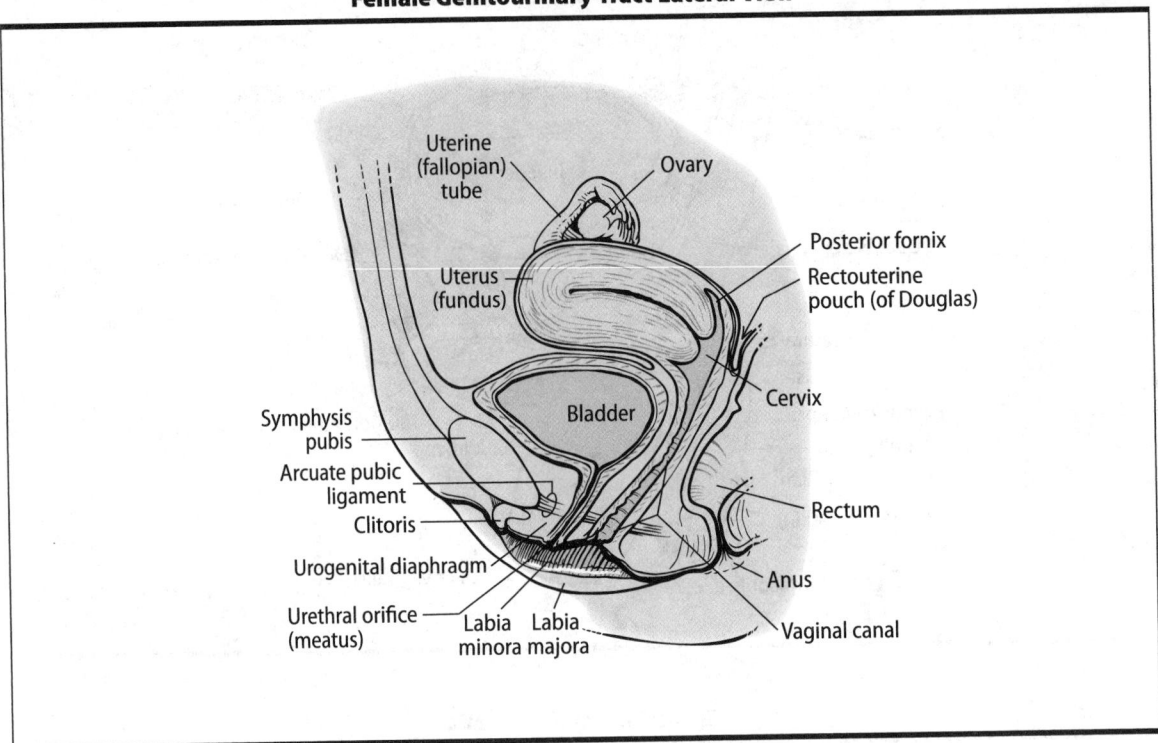

Chapter 15. Pregnancy, Childbirth and the Puerperium (O00–O9A)

Term Pregnancy – Single Gestation

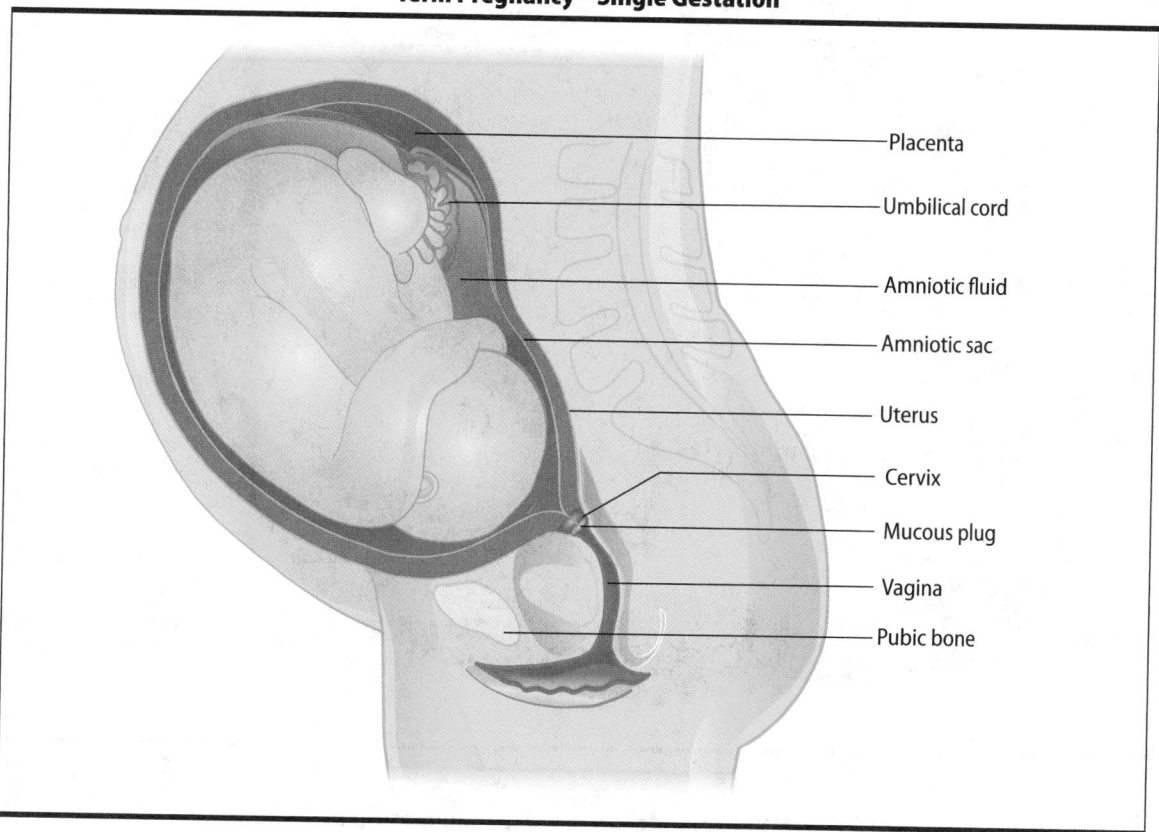

Placenta

Umbilical cord

Amniotic fluid

Amniotic sac

Uterus

Cervix

Mucous plug

Vagina

Pubic bone

Twin Gestation–Dichorionic–Diamniotic (DI-DI)

2 Chorionic sacs

2 Amniotic sacs

2 Fetuses

2 Umbilical cords

2 Placentas

Twin Gestation–Monochorionic–Diamniotic (MO-DI)

1 Chorionic sac

2 Amniotic sacs

2 Fetuses

2 Umbilical cords

1 Placenta

Twin Gestation–Monochorionic–Monoamniotic (MO-MO)

1 Chorionic sac

1 Amniotic sac

2 Fetuses

2 Umbilical cords

1 Placenta

Chapter 19. Injury, Poisoning and Certain Other Consequences of External Causes (SØØ–T88)

Types of Fractures

Normal	Transverse	Open/Compound	Oblique	Oblique displaced

Comminuted	Segmental	Avulsed	Spiral	Greenstick

Salter-Harris Fracture Types

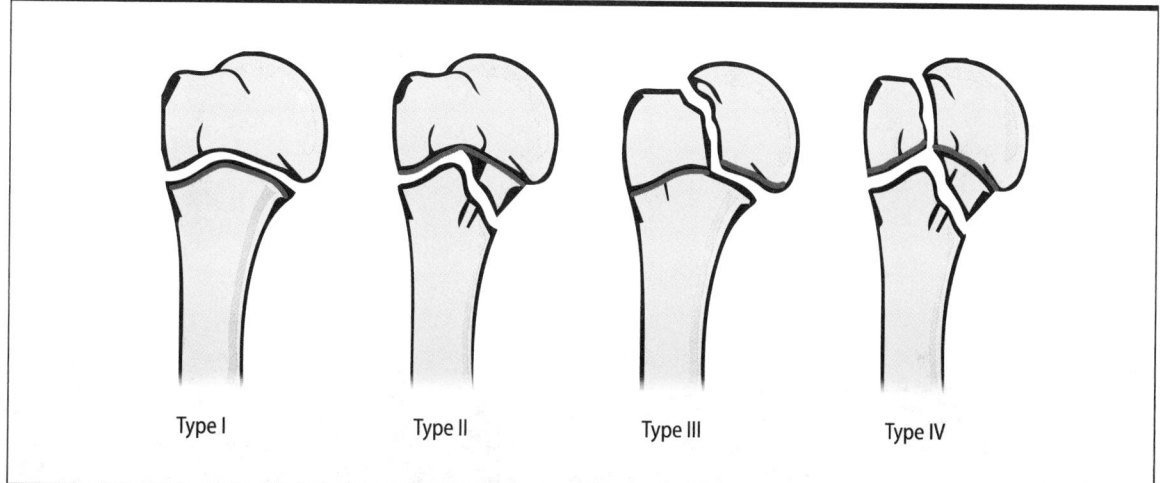

Type I	Type II	Type III	Type IV

Notes

Notes